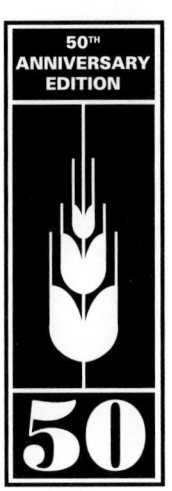

MODERN NUTRITION

IN HEALTH AND DISEASE

TENTH EDITION

SENIOR EDITOR

MAURICE E. SHILS, M.D., SC.D.

Professor Emeritus of Medicine
Cornell University Medical College
Attending Physician, Retired
Memorial Sloan-Kettering Cancer Center
New York, New York
Adjunct Professor (Nutrition), Retired
Department of Public Health Sciences
Wake Forest University, School of Medicine
Winston-Salem, North Carolina

ASSOCIATE EDITORS

MOSHE SHIKE, M.D.

Director of Clinical Nutrition
Memorial Sloan-Kettering Cancer Center
Professor of Medicine
Weill Medical College, Cornell University
New York, New York

A. CATHARINE ROSS, PH.D.

Dorothy Foehr Huck Professor of Nutrition
Department of Nutritional Science
The Pennsylvania State University
University Park, Pennsylvania

BENJAMIN CABALLERO, M.D., PH.D.

Director, Center for Human Nutrition
Professor of International Health and Pediatrics
Bloomberg School of Public Health and School of Medicine
Johns Hopkins University
Baltimore, Maryland

ROBERT J. COUSINS, PH.D.

Boston Family Professor of Nutrition
Center for Nutritional Sciences
University of Florida
Gainesville Florida

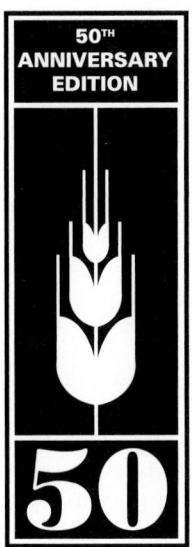

MODERN NUTRITION
IN HEALTH AND DISEASE
TENTH EDITION

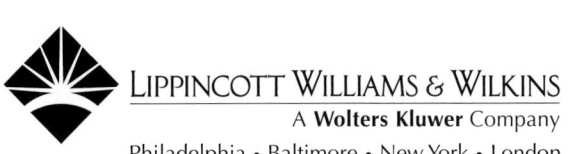

LIPPINCOTT WILLIAMS & WILKINS
A **Wolters Kluwer** Company

Philadelphia • Baltimore • New York • London
Buenos Aires • Hong Kong • Sydney • Tokyo

Acquisitions Editor: David B. Troy
Managing Editor: Matthew J. Hauber
Marketing Manager: Marisa A. O'Brien
Associate Production Manager: Kevin P. Johnson
Designer: Holly Reid McLaughlin
Cover and Interior Designer: Karen Klinedinst
Compositor: TechBooks
Printer: Quebecor World-Tuanton

The publisher is not responsible (as a matter of product liability, negligence, or otherwise) for any injury resulting from any material contained herein. This publication contains information relating to general principles of medical care that should not be construed as specific instructions for individual patients. Manufacturers' product information and package inserts should be reviewed for current information, including contraindications, dosages, and precautions.

Printed in the United States of America

Library of Congress Cataloging-in-Publication Data

Modern nutrition in health and disease / senior editor, Maurice E. Shils ; associate editors, Moshe Shike . . . [et al.].—10th ed.
   p. ; cm.
Includes bibliographical references and index.
ISBN 0-7817-4133-5 (alk. paper)
   1. Nutrition.   2. Diet therapy.   I. Shils, Maurice E. (Maurice Edward), 1914-   II. Shike, Moshe.
[DNLM: 1. Diet Therapy. 2. Nutrition. WB 400 M689 2006] QP141.M64 2006 613.2—dc22

                                                                                                    2005014447

The publishers have made every effort to trace the copyright holders for borrowed material. If they have inadvertently overlooked any, they will be pleased to make the necessary arrangements at the first opportunity.

To purchase additional copies of this book, call our customer service department at (800) 638-3030 or fax orders to (301) 824-7390. International customers should call (301) 714-2324.

Visit Lippincott Williams & Wilkins on the Internet: http://www.LWW.com. Lippincott Williams & Wilkins customer service representatives are available from 8:30 am to 6:00 pm, EST.

04 05 06 07 08
1 2 3 4 5 6 7 8 9 10

PREFACE

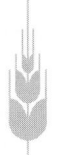

The first edition of *Modern Nutrition in Health and Disease* appeared 50 years ago. A brief history of the editions and publishers in all editions to date is presented on page ___.

This edition continues the goal of providing an updated, comprehensive, and authoritative text and reference source authored by experts in their fields. The close interconnection of nutrition with various chronic diseases has become even more obvious since the publication of the previous edition. Accordingly, we have included more chapters and more information related to these interconnections with emphasis on the need for different approaches in the understanding, evaluation, prevention, and management of these interrelated diseases.

This new edition combines the expertise of many repeat contributors with their updated chapters. We welcome new contributors in 63 chapters. A complete list of the names of all authors and their affiliations is presented just before the Table of Contents. We extend our appreciation to all for their informative contributions.

The organization is, except for changes in Part I, similar to recent past editions. That part now has three key nutrition history vignettes. The Appendices have been updated, particularly with the inclusion of the Dietary Reference Intakes of all nutrients by gender and age.

We invite comments and suggestions from our readers.

MAURICE E. SHILS, M.D., Sc.D.
Winston-Salem, NC

MOSHE SHIKE, M.D.
New York, NY

A. CATHARINE ROSS, Ph.D.
University Park, PA

BENJAMIN CABALLERO, M.D., Ph.D.
Baltimore, MD

ROBERT COUSINS, Ph.D.
Gainesville, FL

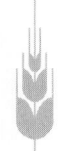

The new edition of *Modern Nutrition in Health and Disease* had the misfortune of losing through untimely deaths the expertise of James Allen Olson, Ph.D. and Roland Louis Weinsier, M.D., Dr.P.H. Dr. Olson had been a member of the Editorial Board of the eighth and ninth editions but died unexpectedly on September 22, 2000 in the early discussions of the tenth edition.

Dr. Weinsier, who had joined the Editorial Board for this edition, became seriously ill during the early period of author recruitment.

Nutritional science lost two eminent investigators and leaders in their areas of nutrition research and education. We honor our two colleagues with the following brief summaries in memoriam.

The Editors

JAMES ALLEN OLSON, Ph.D. (1925–2000)

James Allen Olson, Distinguished Professor of Liberal Arts and Sciences at Iowa State University, passed away suddenly on September 22, 2000, age 75. Dr. Olson served as an editor for the eighth and ninth editions of Modern Nutrition in Health and Disease.

Dr. Olson graduated from Gustavus Adolphus College in Minnesota and received his Ph.D. from Harvard University. During his predoctoral and postdoctoral training, he worked in the laboratories of Christian Anfinsen (Harvard), Sir Ernst Chain (Rome), and Konrad Bloch (Harvard). His career was nearly as varied and colorful as the carotenoids and retinoids he loved to study. He held an academic appointment in the Department of Biochemistry at the University of Florida College of Medicine. He took an extended leave to develop the biochemistry program at Mahidol University, Bangkok, Thailand, where he worked for 8 years with support from the Rockefeller Foundation. He established a graduate biochemistry program to train Thai scientists, but several American scientists also worked in his laboratory there. Mahidol University awarded Dr. Olson an honorary doctorate of science in 1999. In 1975, Dr. Olson returned to the United States and became the Chairman of the Department of Biochemistry and Biophysics, Iowa State University, until 1985. He was named Distinguished Professor of Liberal Arts and Sciences in 1985 and continued an active research program at Iowa State until his death. He continued his interests in international nutrition and in the health of all Asian peoples through his service on the US-Japan Malnutrition Panel, one of six panels of the US-Japan Cooperative Medical Science Program. Dr. Olson's expertise in nutritional assessment and knowledge of nutritional deficiencies prevalent in Asian countries

served this panel very well. A brief history of the formation and functions of this panel, which Dr. Olson chaired in the early 1990s (Olson JA, Proc Soc Exp Biol Med 1992; 200:147) provides insight into this continuing cooperative international health and nutrition activity.

Dr. Olson's abiding fascination for the biochemistry of carotenoids and vitamin A, and for using them to improve human health, was evidenced by more than 400 research publications and reviews, spanning from public health to basic biochemistry. Some highlights included the discovery and study of water-soluble retinoids and the application of stable isotopic compounds to assess the carotenoid and retinoid status of animals and humans. He is also well known for the development of the modified relative dose-response test, a tool to assess marginal vitamin A status, which has been used worldwide to assess vitamin A status.

He organized VARIG (Vitamin A Research Interaction Group) and later CARIG, a similar group for researchers on carotenoids, which began as informal meetings in his room at the Federation of American Societies for Experimental Biology (FASEB) meetings, grew to occupy the president's suite and, in the case of CARIG, to become a well-organized group that has sponsored regular workshops at experimental biology meetings. Dr. Olson cochaired the first Carotenoids Gordon Conference, in 1992, as well as the third FASEB Summer Conference on Vitamin A and Retinoids in the 1980s. He was president of the American Society of Nutritional Sciences from 1986 to 1989.

In his memory as a distinguished scientist and to celebrate his many contributions, Iowa State University convened a Symposium in 2001, "Functions and Actions of Retinoids and Carotenoids: Building on the Vision of James Allen Olson," the proceedings of which were published in the *Journal of Nutrition* (2004;134[Suppl 1]:220S–93S].

ROLAND LOUIS WEINSIER, M.D., Dr.P.H. (1942–2002)

Dr. Weinsier received his medical degree from the University of Florida in 1968 and completed his internship and residency in internal medicine at the University of Virginia. He followed with both masters and doctoral degrees in public health (nutrition) from Harvard University. In 1975, after serving as a major in the United States Air Force, he joined the Department of Medicine at the University of Alabama at Birmingham as Director of its Division of Clinical Nutrition. Roland devoted himself to clinical nutrition and instituted a nutrition support service, an outpatient clinic that eventually became four separate clinics, and a major first-year medical school course in nutrition. The last was increasingly recognized by medical students as the preferred course of the basic science curriculum.

He had a sustained interest in nutrition education in medical and dental schools, regionally and nationally, and helped to establish the American Society for Clinical Nutrition Award for Excellence in Medical/Dental Nutrition Education in 1991; he received the award in 1995.

His early clinical research was directed to studies of the nutritional status of hospitalized patients. In 1977, he became the Director of the Division of Clinical Nutrition in the newly formed Department of Nutrition Sciences. This department was administratively in the School of Health Related Professions with financial support from the Schools of Medicine and Dentistry. In 1979, that department was awarded the first Clinical Nutrition Research Unit grant supported by the National Cancer Institute. In 1983, Dr. Weinsier became Full Professor, and in 1988, he succeeded Charles E. Butterworth, Jr., M.D. as Department Chairman.

Based on his observations of the relationships among food intake, exercise, obesity, and diabetes, he established a research group focusing on obesity, energy metabolism, and body composition. His more recent findings noted inadequate physical activity as the principal cause for the rising prevalence of obesity and a difference between African-Americans and whites in body composition and muscle fiber efficiency that could explain their different propensities for obesity. These data led him to questioning the set-point theory for the etiology of obesity. In his 2001 American Society for Parenteral and Enteral Nutrition *Jonathan E. Rhoads Honorary Research Lecture,* Dr. Weinsier outlined the evidence for his view.

In 1999, he relinquished the chair of the Department of Nutrition Sciences, and in 2000, he was awarded a Clinical Nutrition Research Unit grant funded by the National Institute of Diabetes, Digestive and Kidney Diseases. As Director of this unit, he expanded his obesity investigations.

Roland was elected a member of the Editorial Board for the tenth edition of *Modern Nutrition in Health and Disease* in August, 2000 and participated actively in the initial planning meeting in January 2002. In the spring of 2002, he was diagnosed with cancer, and despite treatment, he died on November 27, 2002.

On November 22, 2002, a *Festschrift* was held in honor of Dr. Weinsier at the University of Alabama, Birmingham Medical Center. Many distinguished physicians and basic scientists who had worked with him were among the speakers and attendees.

A BRIEF HISTORY OF MODERN NUTRITION IN HEALTH AND DISEASE

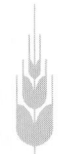

The title and objective of this work evolved from a book originally designated *Dietotherapy*. This was initiated by Michael G. Wohl, M.D., formerly Clinical Professor of Medicine at Temple University School of Medicine, Chairman of the Commission on Nutrition, Medical Society of Pennsylvania and also of the Committee on Nutrition, Philadelphia County Medical Society. With Robert S. Goodhart, M.D. as coeditor, the next edition had the title, *Modern Nutrition in Health and Disease,* subtitiled *Dietotherapy;* this was published in 1955. Dr. Goodhart, as a Fellow in Medicine in the 1930s, spent time in the laboratory of Dr. Severo Ochoa in England, doing research on the biochemical basis of thiamin; he later became an associate Dean at New York University School of Medicine, and, after World War II, the Scientific Director of the National Vitamin Foundation. From its onset, the book has taken a broad approach to nutritional science with a strong clinical view.

On the fiftieth anniversary of its appearance and the tenth edition with this title, a brief history of these editions seems appropriate because these editions have established themselves as a very major resource in this field, and as a whole, provide a half-century overview of the major nutritional advances in nutrition and related sciences, both basic and clinical.

The ninth edition is also on line through OVID as one of a collection of books in medical sciences sold to medical libraries. It also has been published in Spanish and Portuguese editions. Presumably, the tenth edition will follow suit.

Undoubtedly, new basic and clinical research affecting nutrition applications will continue to appear and will undoubtedly influence the Editors and Publisher to seek additional methods of providing updated information in this important field through more rapid methods of communication, although, one hopes that editions in book form will continue to be published.

The Editors

EDITION NO.[a]	PUBLICATION YEAR	EDITORS	PUBLISHER
1	1950	Drs. Michael Wohl, Robert Goodhart	Lea & Febiger
2	1955	Drs. Michael Wohl, Robert Goodhart	Lea & Febiger
3	1964	Drs. Michael Wohl, Robert Goodhart	Lea & Febiger
4	1968	Drs. Michael Wohl, Robert Goodhart	Lea & Febiger
5	1973	Drs. Robert Goodhart, Maurice E. Shils	Lea & Febiger
6	1980	Drs. Robert Goodhart, Maurice E. Shils	Lea & Febiger
7	1988	Drs. Maurice E. Shils, Vernon Young	Lea & Febiger
8	1994	Drs. Maurice E. Shils, James A. Olson, Moshe Shike	Lea & Febiger[b]
9	1998	Drs. Maurice E. Shils, James A. Olson, Moshe Shike, A. Catharine Ross	Lippincott Williams & Wilkins
10	2005	Drs. Maurice E. Shils, Moshe Shike, A. Catharine Ross, Benjamin Caballero, Robert J. Cousins	Lippincott Williams & Wilkins

[a]Year of the first printing

[b]Lea & Febiger, Philadelphia, was purchased shortly before the publication of the 8th edition by the Waverly Company, owner of Williams and Wilkins, Publishers, Baltimore. Shortly before publication of the 9th Edition, the Waverly Company was purchased by Wolters Kluwer Publishers and merged with Lippincott, the Medical Publisher in Philadelphia.

ACKNOWLEDGMENTS

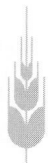

The preparation, editing, and production of this extensive work have succeeded because of the expertise, effort, and dedication of many individuals in addition to the numerous authors who are listed in the Contributors pages.

The Editors have worked personally with some of the staff of Lippincott Williams and Wilkins in Baltimore, while other members have been involved "behind the scenes" at the editorial, publication, distribution, and marketing stages.

During the period of planning and contract development, the Editors had the good fortune initially to work with Susan B. Katz, Vice-President and Publisher for Medical Education and Health Professions and with David Troy, the Senior Acquisitions Editor and his assistant, Elizabeth Connolly, and through them with various individuals in various specialty groups and in arranging the Editors' conference.

From the initiation of the editorial work to its completion, we have worked closely and cooperatively with Matthew J. Hauber, Manager, Product Development, in the many details of developing and preparing manuscripts for publication. We were also very fortunate in the publisher's selection of Holly Lukens as its chief copyeditor. We also express our appreciation to Chris Miller of Techbooks, Inc., who, with her staff, managed page proof production before the final printing.

We are also very indebted to those who worked closely and efficiently with us in preparing and distributing manuscripts and diskettes and in managing communications, and page proofs: Betty Shils, Nicole Goode, Virginia Mauldin, Beverly Satchell, and Madeline Stull. We express our appreciation to our respective spouses for their understanding and support.

The Editors

CONTRIBUTORS

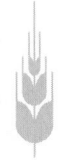

Phyllis B. Acosta, Dr.P.H., R.D., L.D.
Director, Metabolic Diseases
Ross Products Division, Abbott Laboratories
Columbus, Ohio

David H. Alpers, M.D.
Professor of Medicine
Associate Director, Center for Human Nutrition
Washington University School of Medicine
St. Louis, Missouri

James W. Anderson, M.D.
Professor of Medicine and Clinical Nutrition
Metabolic Research Group
University of Kentucky
Lexington, Kentucky

Aśok C. Antony, M.D.
Professor of Medicine
Division of Hematology-Oncology, Department
of Medicine
Indiana University School of Medicine
Chief, Hematology Oncology Section,
Medicine Service
Roudebush Veterans Affairs Hospital
Indianapolis, Indiana

Michelle Asp, B.A., M.S. student
School of Allied Medical Professions
Medical Dietetics Division
The Ohio State University
Columbus, Ohio

Joseph E. Baggott, Ph.D.
Assistant Professor of Nutrition Sciences
School of Health Related Professions and Medicine
Assistant Professor of Biochemistry and
Molecular Biology
Schools of Medicine and Dentistry
University of Alabama at Birmingham
Birmingham, Alabama

Connie Watkins Bales, Ph.D., R.D.
Associate Director
Geriatric Research Education and Clinical Center
Durham VA Medical Center and
Associate Research Professor
Department of Medicine
Duke University Medical Center
Durham, North Carolina

Stephen Barrett, M.D.
Consumer Advocate
Board Chairman, Quackwatch, Inc.
Allentown, Pennsylvania

Richard N. Baumgartner, Ph.D.
Professor, Division of Epidemiology
and Preventive Medicine
Department of Internal Medicine
University of New Mexico School of Medicine
Albuquerque, New Mexico

Wayne R. Bidlack, Ph.D.
Dean, College of Agriculture
Professor, Animal and Veterinary Science and Human
Nutrition and Food Science
California State Polytechnic University, Pomona
Pomona, California

Abby S. Bloch, Ph.D., R.D.
Formerly, Director of Clinical Nutrition
Support Kitchen
Memorial Sloan-Kettering Cancer Center
Adjunct Assistant Professor, Department of Nutrition
and Food Studies
New York University School of Education
New York, New York
Adjunct Assistant Professor, Department of Primary Care
School of Health Related Professions
University of Medicine and Dentistry of New Jersey
Newark, New Jersey

Christelle Bourgeois, Ph.D.
Senior Post-Doctoral Fellow
Pulmonary-Critical Care Medicine Branch
National Heart, Lung, and Blood Institute, National
Institutes of Health
Bethesda, Maryland

Irwin G. Brodsky, M.D., M.P.H.
Consultant, Maine Centers for Endocrinology
and Diabetes
Maine Medical Center
Portland, Maine

Patricia Brown, R.N., M.S., O.C.N.
Nurse Clinician, Clinical Nutrition Service
Memorial Sloan-Kettering Cancer Center
New York, New York

Rex O. Brown, Pharm.D., B.C.N.S.P.
Professor and Executive Vice Chair, Department of
Pharmacy
University of Tennessee Health Science Center
Memphis, Tennessee

Alan L. Buchman, M.D., M.S.P.H.
Associate Professor of Medicine
Division of Gastroenterology
Feinberg School of Medicine
Northwestern University
Chicago, Illinois

Raymond F. Burk, M.D.
Professor of Medicine and Pathology
Division of Gastroenterology
Department of Medicine
Vanderbilt University School of Medicine
Nashville, Tennessee

Nancy F. Butte, Ph.D.
Professor of Pediatrics
Children's Nutrition Research Center
Baylor College of Medicine
Houston, Texas

Roger F. Butterworth, Ph.D., D.Sc.
Professor of Medicine
University of Montreal
Director, Neuroscience Research Unit (CHUM)
Hôpital Saint-Luc
Montreal, Quebec
Canada

Kirstin J. Byrne, M.S.
Research Coordinator
Department of Psychiatry
University of Pennsylvania School of Medicine
Philadelphia, Pennsylvania

Benjamin Caballero, M.D., Ph.D.
Director, Center for Human Nutrition
Professor of International Health and Pediatrics
Bloomberg School of Public Health and School
of Medicine
Johns Hopkins University
Baltimore, Maryland

Joseph G. Cannon, Ph.D.
Professor of Medical Technology and Physiology
Medical College of Georgia
Augusta, Georgia

Ralph Carmel, M.D.
Director of Research, Department of Medicine
New York Methodist Hospital
Brooklyn, New York
Professor of Medicine
Weill Medical College, Cornell University
New York, New York

Kenneth J. Carpenter, Ph.D.
Professor Emeritus of Nutrition
University of California, Berkeley
Berkeley, California

Victoria A. Catenacci, M.D.
Clinical Fellow
Division of Endocrinology, Metabolism and Diabetes
University of Colorado at Denver and Health
Science Center
Denver, Colorado

Daniel Cervantes-Laurean, Ph.D.
Assistant Professor of Chemistry and Biochemistry
South Dakota State University
Brookings, South Dakota

Lingtak-Neander Chan, Pharm.D.
Associate Professor, School of Pharmacy
University of Washington
Seattle, Washington

Robert Chin, Jr., M.D.
Associate Professor of Medicine
Section on Pulmonary and Critical Care Medicine
Wake Forest University School of Medicine
Winston-Salem, North Carolina

Christopher R. Chitambar, M.D.
Professor of Medicine
Director, Hematology & Oncology Fellowship Program
Division of Neoplastic Diseases
Medical College of Wisconsin
Milwaukee, Wisconsin

Steven M. Cohn, M.D., Ph.D.
Associate Professor of Medicine
Associate Director, Digestive Health Research Center
University of Virgina School of Medicine
Charlottesville, Virginia

J. Joseph Connon, M.D.
Professor of Medicine
St Michael's Hospital and the University of Toronto
Toronto, Ontario, Canada

Arthur Cooper, M.D., M.S.
Associate Professor of Pediatric Surgery
College of Physicians & Surgeons, Columbia University
Chief, Pediatric Surgical Critical Care
Harlem Hospital Center
New York, New York

Janelle W. Coughlin, Ph.D.
Clinical Instructor of Psychiatry and Behavioral Sciences
Johns Hopkins University School of Medicine
Baltimore, Maryland

Robert J. Cousins, Ph.D.
Boston Family Professor of Nutrition
Center for Nutritional Sciences
University of Florida
Gainesville Florida

Alan D. Dangour, M.Sc., Ph.D.
Nutrition and Public Health Intervention Research Unit
London School of Hygiene and Tropical Medicine
University of London
London, United Kingdom

Steven R. Davis, Ph.D.
Assistant Professor of Nutritional Sciences
University of Connecticut
Storrs, Connecticut

Bess Dawson-Hughes, M.D.
Professor of Medicine, Senior Scientist
Human Nutrition Research Center, Tufts University
Boston, Massachusetts

Denise M. Deming, Ph.D.
Associate Scientific Leader
Department of Human Nutritional Products
DSM Nutritional Products, Inc.
Parsippany, New Jersey

Margo A. Denke, M.D.
Clinical Professor of Medicine
University of Texas Health Science Center
San Antonio, Texas

Dominick P. DePaola, D.D.S., Ph.D.
President and CEO
The Forsyth Institute
Boston, Massachusetts

William H. Dietz, M.D., Ph.D.
Director, Division of Nutrition and Physical Activity
Centers for Disease Control and Prevention
Atlanta, Georgia

John T. Dunn, M.D.*
Professor Emeritus of Medicine
University of Virginia
Executive Director, International Council for the Control of Iodine Deficiency Disorders
Charlottesville, Virginia

Erin E. Dweik, MEd., R.D., L.D.
Moreland Hills, Ohio

Raed A. Dweik, M.D.
Associate Professor of Medicine
Director, Pulmonary Vascular Program
Department of Pulmonary, Allergy, and Critical Care Medicine
The Cleveland Clinic Foundation
Cleveland, Ohio

Johanna T. Dwyer, D.Sc., R.D.
Professor of Medicine and Community Health
Friedman School of Nutrition Science and Policy and Medical School
Tufts University and Tufts-New England Medical Center Hospital
Boston, Massachusetts

Curtis D. Eckhert, Ph.D.
Professor and Chair, Department of Environmental Health Sciences
School of Public Health
University of California
Los Angeles, California

Louis J. Elsas, II, M.D.
Director, The Dr. John T. MacDonald Foundation
Center for Medical Genetics
University of Miami
Miami, Florida

Mary P. Faine, M.S., R.D.
Assistant Professor and Director, Nutrition Education
University of Washington School of Dentistry
Warren G. Magnuson Health Science Center
Seattle, Washington

Gabriel Fernandes, Ph.D.
Professor of Medicine
University of Texas Health Science Center at San Antonio
San Antonio, Texas

John W. Finley, Ph.D.
Chief Technology Officer
A.M. Todd
Montgomeryville, Pennsylvania

---

*Deceased.

Kenneth D. Fisher, Ph.D.
President
KD Consultants
Rockville, Maryland

Samuel J. Fomon, M.D.
Emeritus Professor of Pediatrics
College of Medicine
University of Iowa

Cutberto Garza, M.D., Ph.D.
Professor of Nutrition
Division of Nutritional Sciences
Cornell University
Ithaca, New York

Edward Giovannucci, M.D., Sc.D.
Professor of Nutrition and Epidemiology
Harvard School of Public Health
Boston, Massachusetts

Jesse F. Gregory, III, Ph.D.
Professor of Food Science and Human Nutrition
University of Florida
Gainesville, Florida

Ian J. Griffin, M.D.
Assistant Professor of Pediatrics
US Department of Agriculture/ Agricultural Research
Service Children's Nutrition Research Center
Baylor College of Medicine
Houston, Texas

Anne M. Griffiths, M.D.
Professor of Pediatrics
Faculty of Medicine, University of Toronto
Director of Inflammatory Bowel Diseases Program
The Hospital for Sick Children
Toronto, Ontario, Canada

Scott M. Grundy, M.D., Ph.D.
Professor of Clinical Nutrition and Internal Medicine
and the Center for Human Nutrition
University of Texas Southwestern Medical Center at Dallas
Dallas, Texas

Angela S. Guarda, M.D.
Assistant Professor of Psychiatry and Behavioral Sciences
Johns Hopkins University School of Medicine
Director of the Johns Hopkins Eating Disorders Program
Baltimore, Maryland

Alfred E. Harper, Ph.D.
Professor Emeritus of Biochemistry and of Nutritional
Sciences
University of Wisconsin, Madison
Madison, Wisconsin

Peter J. Havel, D.V.M., Ph.D.
Research Endocrinologist
Nutrition Department
University of California, Davis
Davis, California

Robert P. Heaney, M.D.
John A. Creighton University Professor
Creighton University
Omaha, Nebraska

Susan L. Hefle, Ph.D.
Associate Professor and Co-Director, Food Allergy
Research & Resource Program
University of Nebraska
Lincoln, Nebraska

Douglas C. Heimburger, M.D., M.S.
Professor of Nutrition Sciences and Medicine
University of Alabama at Birmingham
Birmingham, Alabama

William C. Heird, M.D.
Professor of Pediatrics
Children's Nutrition Research Center
Baylor College of Medicine
Houston, Texas

Eva Hertrampf, M.D.
Instituto de Nutrición y Tecnología de los
Alimentos (INTA)
University of Chile
Santiago, Chile

Steven R. Hertzler, Ph.D., R.D., L.D.
Assistant Professor of Human Nutrition
The Ohio State University
Columbus, Ohio

Steven B. Heymsfield, M.D.
Professor of Medicine
Obesity Research Center
St. Luke's/Roosevelt Hospital
College of Physicians & Surgeons, Columbia
University
New York, New York

James O. Hill, Ph.D.
Director, Clinical Research Unit
Center for Human Nutrition
University of Colorado Health Science Center
Denver, Colorado

L. John Hoffer, M.D., Ph.D.
Professor, Faculty of Medicine, McGill University
Senior Physician, Divisions of Endocrinology
and Internal Medicine
Lady Davis Institute for Medical Research
Sir Mortimer B. Davis Jewish General Hospital
Montreal, Quebec, Canada

Michael F. Holick, M.D., Ph.D.
Professor of Medicine, Physiology, and Biophysics
Boston University School of Medicine
Boston, Massachusetts

John R. Hoyle, M.D.
Assistant Professor of Medicine (Cardiology)
Section on Cardiology, Department of Medicine
Wake Forest University School of Medicine
Winston-Salem, North Carolina

Gary R. Hunter, Ph.D., C.S.C.S.
Professor of Human Studies and Nutrition Sciences
University of Alabama at Birmingham
Birmingham, Alabama

Khursheed N. Jeejeebhoy, M.B.B.S., Ph.D.
Professor of Medicine
University of Toronto
St. Michael's Hospital
Toronto, Ontario, Canada

Margaret M. Johnson, M.D.
Assistant Professor of Medicine
Mayo Graduate School of Medicine
Jacksonville, Florida

Patricia K. Johnston, M.S., Ph.D.
Professor Emeritus
Department of Nutrition
School of Public Health
Loma Linda University
Loma Linda, California

Christopher A. Jolly, Ph.D.
Assistant Professor
Department of Human Ecology
University of Texas at Austin
Austin, Texas

Peter J.H. Jones, Ph.D.
Professor
School of Dietetics and Human Nutrition
McGill University, Macdonald Campus
Ste-Anne de Bellevue
Quebec, Canada

Frederic R. Kahl, M.D.
Professor of Medicine (Cardiology)
Section on Cardiology, Department of Medicine
Wake Forest University School of Medicine
Winston-Salem, North Carolina

Robert Karp, M.D.
Professor of Pediatrics
Director, Social/Community Pediatrics Initiative
SUNY-Downstate Medical Center
Brooklyn, New York

Arie Katz, M.D.
Molecular and Clinical Nutrition Section
Digestive Diseases Branch
National Institute of Diabetes and Digestive
and Kidney Diseases
National Institutes of Health
Bethesda, Maryland

Richard Katz, M.D.
Associate Professor
Johns Hopkins University School of Medicine
and Mt. Washington Pediatric Hospital
Baltimore, Maryland

Nancy L. Keim, Ph.D.
Research Nutrition Scientist
Western Human Nutrition Research Center
University of California, Davis
Davis, California

Darlene G. Kelly, M.D., Ph.D.
Associate Professor, Mayo College of Medicine
Consultant, Division of Gastroenterology
and Hepatology
Department of Internal Medicine
Mayo Clinic
Rochester, Minnesota

Rubina Khan, MSc, Ph.D. student
The Ohio State University Interdisciplinary Ph.D.
Program in Nutrition
Department of Human Nutrition
Columbus, Ohio

Yeonsoo Kim, M.S., Ph.D. student
The Ohio State University Interdisciplinary Ph.D.
Program in Nutrition
Department of Human Nutrition
Columbus, Ohio

Janet C. King, Ph.D.
Professor of Internal Medicine and Nutrition
University of California Berkeley and Davis and
Children's Hospital Oakland Research Institute
Oakland, California

John M. Kinney M.D.
Professor of Surgery
College of Physicians & Surgeons, Columbia University
New York, New York
Visiting Professor, Rockefeller University
New York, New York

Samuel Klein, M.D.
William H. Danforth Professor of Medicine
and Nutritional Science
Director, Center for Human Nutrition
Washington University School of Medicine
St. Louis, Missouri

James P. Knochel, M.D.
Chair, Department of Internal Medicine
Clinical Professor Post
Presbyterian Hospital
Dallas, Texas

Joel D. Kopple, M.D.
Professor of Medicine and Public Health
David Geffen School of Medicine at UCLA and UCLA
School of Public Health
Chief, Division of Nephrology and Hypertension
Harbor-UCLA Medical Center
Los Angeles, California

Jane Morley Kotchen, M.D., M.P.H.
Professor of Epidemiology
Medical College of Wisconsin
Milwaukee, Wisconsin

Theodore A. Kotchen, M.D.
Professor of Medicine and Epidemiology
Associate Dean for Clinical Research
Medical College of Wisconsin
Milwaukee, Wisconsin

Stephanie Krauthamer-Ewing, M.P.H.
Research Coordinator
Department of Psychiatry
University of Pennsylvania School of Medicine
Philadelphia, Pennsylvania

David Kritchevsky, Ph.D.
Caspar Wistar Scholar
Wistar Institute
Philadelphia, Pennsylvania

Stanley Kubow, Ph.D.
Associate Professor
School of Dietetics and Human Nutrition
McGill University, Macdonald Campus
Ste-Anne de Bellevue
Quebec, Canada

Marie Fanelli Kuczmarski, Ph.D., R.D., L.D.
Professor of Health, Nutrition, and Exercise Sciences
University of Delaware
Newark, Delaware

Robert J. Kuczmarski, Dr.P.H., R.D., L.D.
Director, Obesity Prevention and Treatment Program
National Institutes of Diabetes and Digestive and
Kidney Diseases
National Institutes of Health
US Public Health Service
Bethesda, Maryland

Kenneth A. Kudsk, M.D.
Professor of Surgery, Vice Chair of Surgical Research
School of Medicine
University of Wisconsin—Madison
Madison, Wisconsin

Richard A. Lawrence, Ph.D.
Research Fellow
Department of Medicine
University of Texas Health Science Center
at San Antonio
San Antonio, Texas

Orville A. Levander, Ph.D.
Research Chemist
Nutrient Requirements and Functions Laboratory
Beltsville Human Nutrition Research Center
US Department of Agriculture, Agricultural Research
Service
Beltsville, Maryland

Roy J. Levin, Ph.D.
Reader in Physiology (Retired)
Department of Biomedical Science
University of Sheffield
Sheffield, Yorkshire
United Kingdom

Mark Levine M.D.
Chief, Molecular and Clinical Nutrition Section
Digestive Diseases Branch
National Institute of Diabetes and Digestive and Kidney
Diseases
National Institutes of Health
Bethesda, Maryland

Charles S. Lieber, M.D., M.A.C.P.
Professor of Medicine and Pathology
Mount Sinai School of Medicine
Chief, Section of Liver Disease and Nutrition
Director, Alcohol Research Center
Bronx Veterans Affairs Medical Center
New York, New York

Stephen F. Lowry, M.D.
Professor and Chair, Department of Surgery
Robert Wood Johnson Medical School
University of Medicine and Dentistry of New Jersey
New Brunswick, New Jersey

Joanne R. Lupton, Ph.D.
Regent's Professor, University Faculty Fellow and
William W. Allen Endowed Chair in Nutrition
Texas A&M University
College Station, Texas

Amy D. Mackey, Ph.D.
Research Scientist
Pediatric Research Department
Ross Products Division, Abbott Laboratories
Columbus, Ohio

Ramasamy Manikam, Ph.D.
Assistant Professor, Director, Behavior Psychology
Division of Pediatric
Gastroenterology and Nutrition
University of Maryland School of Medicine
and Mt. Washington Pediatric Hospital
Baltimore, Maryland

Richard D. Mattes, M.P.H., Ph.D.
Professor of Foods and Nutrition
Purdue University
West Lafayette, Indiana

Dwight E. Matthews, Ph.D.
Professor of Medicine
Professor and Chair, Department of Chemistry
University of Vermont
Burlington, Vermont

Donald B. McCormick, Ph.D.
Fuller E. Callaway Professor of Biochemistry,
Emeritus
Department of Biochemistry
Emory University
Atlanta, Georgia

Sharon S. McDonald, M.S.
Scientific Consultant Office of Dietary
Supplements
National Institutes of Health
Raleigh, North Carolina

Donald S. McLaren, M.D. Ph.D.
Formerly, Professor of Clinical Nutrition
School of Medicine
American University of Beirut, Lebanon
West Sussex, United Kingdom (Retired)

Gayle Minard, M.D.
Professor of Surgery
University of Tennessee Health Science Center
Memphis, Tennessee

Donald M. Mock, M.D., Ph.D.
Professor of Biochemistry and Molecular Biology and
Pediatrics
University of Arkansas for Medical Sciences
Little Rock, Arkansas

Sarah L. Morgan, M.D., R.D., M.S.
Professor of Nutrition Sciences
Director, Division of Clinical Nutrition and Dietetics
Department of Nutrition Sciences
School of Health Related Professions
Professor of Medicine
School of Medicine
University of Alabama at Birmingham
Birmingham, Alabama

John E. Morley, M.B., B.Ch.
Dammert Professor of Gerontology
Director, Division of Geriatric Medicine
Saint Louis University School of Medicine
Director, Geriatric Research, Education
and Clinical Center
Veterans' Administration Medical Center
St. Louis, Missouri

Joel Moss, M.D., Ph.D.
Chief, Pulmonary-Critical Care Medicine Branch
National Heart, Lung, and Blood Institute, National
Institutes of Health
Bethesda, Maryland

Mihai D. Niculescu, M.D., Ph.D.
Research Associate
Department of Nutrition
School of Public Health and School of Medicine
University of North Carolina at Chapel Hill
Chapel Hill, North Carolina

Man S. Oh, M.D.
Professor of Medicine
SUNY Health Science Center at Brooklyn
Brooklyn, New York

Sebastian J. Padayatty, Ph.D.
Staff Clinician
Molecular and Clinical Nutrition Section
Digestive Diseases Branch
National Institute of Diabetes and Digestive
and Kidney Diseases
National Institutes of Health
Bethesda, Maryland

J. Martin Perez, M.D.
Assistant Professor of Surgery
Robert Wood Johnson Medical School
University of Medicine and Dentistry
of New Jersey
New Brunswick, New Jersey

Mary Frances Picciano, Ph.D.
Senior Nutrition Research Scientist
Office of Dietary Supplements
National Institutes of Health
Bethesda, Maryland

Ronald L. Prior, Ph.D.
Research Chemist
US Department of Agriculture/Agriculture
Research Service
Arkansas Children's Nutrition Center
Little Rock, Arkansas

Sara A. Quandt, Ph.D.
Professor, Section on Epidemiology
Department of Public Health Sciences
Wake Forest University School of Medicine
Winston-Salem, North Carolina

Massimo Raimondo, M.D.
Assistant Professor of Medicine
Mayo Clinic
Jacksonville, Florida

Dana Rathkopf, M.D.
Medical Oncology Fellow
Department of Medicine
Memorial Sloan-Kettering Cancer Center
New York, New York

Gerald M. Reaven, M.D.
Professor of Medicine (Active Emeritus)
Falk Cardiovascular Research Center
Division of Cardiovascular Medicine
Stanford University School of Medicine
Stanford, California

Charles J. Rebouche, Ph.D.
Associate Professor of Pediatrics
University of Iowa
Iowa City, Iowa

Deborah L. Renaud, M.D.
Division of Child and Adolescent Neurology
Mayo Clinic
Rochester, Minnesota

Diane Rigassio-Radler, Ph.D., R.D.
Assistant Professor, Graduate Programs in
Clinical Nutrition, Department of Primary Care
School of Health Related Professions
Clinical Assistant Professor, Department of Diagnostic
Sciences
New Jersey Dental School
Newark, New Jersey

Christine Seel Ritchie M.D., M.S.P.H.
Associate Professor of Medicine
Birmingham-Atlanta Geriatric Research, Education, and
Clinical Center and the VA Deep South Center on
Effectiveness
Department of Medicine, Division of Geriatric
Medicine
University of Alabama at Birmingham
Birmingham VA Medical Center
Birmingham, Alabama

Gustavo C. Román M.D.
Professor of Medicine/Neurology
University of Texas Health Science Center at San
Antonio and Veterans Administration Hospital
San Antonio, Texas.

Alayne G. Ronnenberg, Sc.D.
Assistant Professor of Nutrition
School of Public Health and Health Sciences
University of Massachusetts
Amherst, Massachusetts

A. Catharine Ross, Ph.D.
Professor of Nutrition, Dorothy Foehr
Huck Chair
Department of Nutritional Sciences
The Pennsylvania State University
University Park, Pennsylvania

Robert K. Rude, M.D.
Professor of Medicine
Keck School of Medicine
University of Southern California
Los Angeles, California

Joan Sabaté, M.D.
Chair, Department of Nutrition
School of Public Health
Loma Linda University
Loma Linda, California

Gordon S. Sacks, Pharm.D.
Clinical Associate Professor
Schools of Pharmacy and Medicine
University of Wisconsin—Madison
Madison, Wisconsin

Dennis Savaiano, Ph.D.
Dean and Professor, School of Consumer and Family
Sciences
Purdue University
West Lafayette, Indiana

Mark Schattner, M.D.
Clinical Assistant Physician, Gastroenterology and
Nutrition Service
Department of Medicine
Memorial Sloan-Kettering Cancer Center
New York, New York

Linda Schuberth, M.S. O.T.R.
Senior Occupational Therapist
Feeding Disorders Program
Kennedy Krieger Institute
Baltimore, Maryland

Gary K. Schwartz, M.D.
Member and Attending Physician
Department of Medicine
Gastrointestinal Oncology Service
Memorial Sloan-Kettering Cancer Center
New York, New York

James S. Scolapio, M.D.
Associate Professor of Medicine
Mayo Clinic
Jacksonville, Florida

Richard D. Semba, M.D., M.P.H.
Associate Professor of Ophthalmology
Division of Ocular Immunology
Johns Hopkins University School of Medicine
Baltimore, Maryland

Moshe Shike, M.D.
Director, Clinical Nutrition and Attending Physician
Section on Gastroenterology and Nutrition
Memorial Sloan-Kettering Cancer Center
Professor of Medicine Weill Medical College,
Cornell University
New York, New York

Maurice E. Shils, M.D., Sc.D.
Professor Emeritus of Medicine, Cornell University
Medical College
Attending Physician, Retired, Memorial Sloan-Kettering
Cancer Center
New York, New York

Gerard P. Smith, M.D.
Professor Emeritus of Behavioral Neuroscience in
Psychiatry
Weill Medical College, Cornell University
New York-Presbyterian Hospital
White Plains, New York

Robert E. Smith, Ph.D.
President
R.E. Smith Consulting, Inc.
Newport, Vermont

Michael B. Sporn, M.D.
Professor of Pharmacology and Medicine
Dartmouth Medical School
Hanover, New Hampshire

Meir J. Stampfer, M.D., Dr.P.H.
Chair, Department of Epidemiology
Professor of Epidemiology and Nutrition
Harvard School of Public Health
Boston, Massachusetts

William F. Stenson, M.D.
Professor of Medicine and Gastroenterology
Washington University
St. Louis, Missouri

Martha H. Stipanuk, Ph.D.
Professor
Division of Nutritional Sciences
Cornell University
Ithaca, New York

Barbara J. Stoecker, Ph.D.
Professor of Nutritional Sciences
Oklahoma State University
Stillwater, Oklahoma

Patrick J. Stover, Ph.D.
Associate Professor of Nutritional Biochemistry
Division of Nutritional Sciences
Cornell University
Ithaca, New York

Bruce Suckling, M.D.
Senior Pulmonary Fellow
Section on Pulmonary and Critical Care Medicine
Wake Forest University School of Medicine
Winston-Salem, North Carolina

John W. Suttie, Ph.D.
Professor Emeritus of Biochemistry
University of Wisconsin-Madison
Madison, Wisconsin

Benjamin M. Chionglo Sy, M.D.
Senior Pulmonary Fellow
Department of Pulmonary, Allergy and Critical Care
Medicine
The Cleveland Clinic Foundation
Cleveland, Ohio

Christine L. Taylor, Ph.D.
Director, Office of Nutritional Products, Labeling and
Dietary Supplements
Center for Food Safety and Applied Nutrition
Food and Drug Administration
College Park, Maryland

Steve L. Taylor, Ph.D.
Professor and Co-Director, Food Allergy Research and
Resource Program
University of Nebraska
Lincoln, Nebraska

James A. Thomas, Ph.D.
Professor of Biochemistry and Biophysics
Department of Biochemistry, Biophysics, and Molecular
Biology
Iowa State University
Ames, Iowa

Benjamin Torún, M.D., Ph.D.
Director, Center for Research and Teaching in Latin
America (CIDAL)
Guatemala City, Guatemala
Investigator Emeritus
Institute of Nutrition of Central America and Panama
(INCAP)
Guatemala City, Guatemala

Riva Touger-Decker, Ph.D. R.D.
Associate Professor and Program Director
Graduate Programs in Clinical Nutrition, Department of
Primary Care
School of Health Related Professions
Director, Division of Nutrition, Department of
Diagnostic Sciences
New Jersey Dental School
Newark, New Jersey

Maret G. Traber, Ph.D.
Professor of Nutrition and Exercise Sciences
Linus Pauling Institute
Oregon State University
Corvallis, Oregon

Margarita S. Treuth, Ph.D.
Associate Professor, Center for Human Nutrition
Bloomberg School of Public Health
Johns Hopkins University
Baltimore, Maryland

Paula R. Trumbo, Ph.D.
Team Leader, Nutrition Science Evaluation
Office of Nutritional Products, Labeling and Dietary
Supplements
Center for Food Safety And Applied Nutrition
Food and Drug Administration
College Park, Maryland

R. Elaine Turner, Ph.D., RD
Associate Professor, Food Science and
Human Nutrition Department
University of Florida
Gainesville, Florida

Judith R. Turnlund, Ph.D., R.D.
Research Nutrition Scientist, US Department of
Agriculture, Agricultural Research Service
Western Human Nutrition Research Center
University of California, Davis
Davis, California

Ricardo Uauy, M.D., Ph.D.
Professor
Instituto de Nutrición y Tecnología de los Alimentos
(INTA)
University of Chile
Santiago, Chile
Nutrition and Public Health Intervention
Research Unit
London School of Hygiene and Tropical Medicine
University of London
London, United Kingdom

Jaime Uribarri, M.D.
Associate Professor of Medicine
Mount Sinai Medical School
New York, New York

Jerry Vockley, M.D., Ph.D.
Chief of Genetics
Children's Hospital of Pittsburgh
Professor of Pediatrics
University of Pittsburgh School of Medicine
Pittsburgh, Pennsylvania

Thomas A. Wadden, Ph.D.
Professor of Psychology
Department of Psychiatry
University of Pennsylvania School of Medicine
Philadelphia, Pennsylvania

Wei Wang, Ph.D.
Instructor, College of Agriculture
Department of Animal and Veterinary Sciences
California State Polytechnic University
Pomona, California

Connie M. Weaver, Ph.D.
Distinguished Professor and Head, Department
of Foods and Nutrition
Purdue University
West Lafayette, Indiana

Walter C. Willett, M.D., Dr.P.H.
Chair, Department of Nutrition
Fredrick John Stare Professor of Epidemiology and
Nutrition
Harvard School of Public Health
Channing Laboratory, Department of Medicine
Brigham & Women's Hospital, Harvard
Medical School
Boston, Massachusetts

Melvin H. Williams, Ph.D.
Eminent Scholar Emeritus
Department of Exercise Science
Old Dominion University
Norfolk, Virginia

Richard J. Wood, Ph.D.
Director, Mineral Bioavailability Laboratory
Jean Mayer USDA Human Nutrition Research Center
on Aging at Tufts University
Associate Professor, Dorothy J. and Gerald R. Friedman
School of Nutrition Science and Policy
Tufts University
Boston, Massachusetts

Holly R. Wyatt, M.D.
Assistant Professor of Medicine
Division of Endocrinology, Metabolism, and Diabetes
University of Colorado at Denvel and Health
Science Center
Denver, Colorado

Allison A. Yates, Ph.D., R.D.
Director of Nutritional Sciences
ENVIRON Health Sciences Institute
Arlington, Virginia

Elizabeth A. Yetley, Ph.D.
Senior Nutrition Research Scientist
Office of Dietary Supplements
National Institutes of Health
Bethesda, Maryland

Steven H. Zeisel, M.D., Ph.D.
Professor and Chair, Department of Nutrition
School of Public Health, Professor of Medicine School
of Medicine
University of North Carolina at Chapel Hill
Chapel Hill, North Carolina

CONTENTS

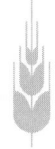

PART I. HISTORICAL LANDMARKS IN NUTRITION

1 alpha   Evolution of Knowledge of Essential Nutrients
KENNETH J. CARPENTER AND ALFRED E. HARPER / 3

1 beta   Human Energy Metabolism
JOHN M. KINNEY / 10

1 gamma   Management of Infantile Diarrhea and Dehydration
SAMUEL J. FOMON / 17

PART II. SPECIFIC DIETARY COMPONENTS

A. Major Dietary Constituents and Energy Needs

2.   Proteins and Amino Acids / 23
DWIGHT E. MATTHEWS

3.   Carbohydrates / 62
NANCY L. KEIM, ROY J. LEVIN, AND PETER J. HAVEL

4.   Dietary Fiber / 83
JOANNE R. LUPTON AND PAULA R. TRUMBO

5.   Lipids, Sterols, and Their Metabolites / 92
PETER J.H. JONES AND STANLEY KUBOW

6.   Cholesterol and Other Dietary Sterols / 123
DAVID KRITCHEVSKY

7.   Energy Needs: Assessment and Requirements / 136
NANCY F. BUTTE AND BENJAMIN CABALLERO

B. Minerals

8.   Electrolytes, Water, and Acid-Base Balance / 149
MAN S. OH AND JAIME URIBARRI

9.   Calcium / 194
CONNIE M. WEAVER AND ROBERT P. HEANEY

10.   Phosphorus / 211
JAMES P. KNOCHEL

11.   Magnesium / 223
ROBERT K. RUDE AND MAURICE E. SHILS

12.   Iron / 248
RICHARD J. WOOD AND ALAYNE G. RONNENBERG

13.   Zinc / 271
JANET C. KING AND ROBERT J. COUSINS

14.   Copper / 286
JUDITH R. TURNLUND

15.   Iodine / 300
JOHN T. DUNN

16.   Selenium / 312
RAYMOND F. BURK AND ORVILLE A. LEVANDER

17A.   Manganese / 326
ALAN L. BUCHMAN

17B.   Chromium / 332
BARBARA J. STOECKER

18.   Other Trace Elements / 338
CURTIS D. ECKHERT

C. Vitamins

19.   Vitamin A and Carotenoids / 351
A. CATHARINE ROSS

20.   Vitamin D / 376
MICHAEL F. HOLICK

21.   Vitamin E / 396
MARET G. TRABER

22.   Vitamin K / 412
JOHN W. SUTTIE

23.   Thiamin / 426
ROGER F. BUTTERWORTH

24.   Riboflavin / 434
DONALD B. McCORMICK

25.   Niacin / 442
CHRISTELLE BOURGEOIS, DANIEL CERVANTES-LAUREAN, AND JOEL MOSS

26.   Vitamin B_6 / 452
AMY D. MACKEY, STEVEN R. DAVIS, AND JESSE F. GREGORY III

27.   Pantothenic Acid / 462
PAULA R. TRUMBO

28.   Folic Acid / 470
RALPH CARMEL

29.   Cobalamin (Vitamin B_{12}) / 482
RALPH CARMEL

30.   Biotin / 498
DONALD M. MOCK

31.   Vitamin C / 507
MARK LEVINE, ARIE KATZ, AND SEBASTIAN J PADAYATTY

32.   Choline and Phosphatidylcholine / 525
STEVEN H. ZEISEL AND MIHAI D. NICULESCU

D. Other Compounds with Health Relevance

33.   Carnitine / 537
CHARLES J. REBOUCHE

34.   Homocysteine, Cysteine, and Taurine / 545
MARTHA H. STIPANUK

35.   Glutamine / 563
ALAN L. BUCHMAN

36.   Arginine and Nitric Oxide / 571
BENJAMIN M. CHIONGLO SY, ERIN E. DWEIK, AND RAED A. DWEIK

37.   Phytochemicals / 582
RONALD L. PRIOR

E. Signs of Clinical Deficiencies

38.   Clinical Manifestations of Nutrient Deficiencies and Toxicities: A Resume / 595
DOUGLAS C. HEIMBURGER, DONALD S. McLAREN, AND MAURICE E. SHILS

PART III. NUTRITION IN INTEGRATED BIOLOGIC SYSTEMS

A. Intercellular Regulation: Tutorials

39.   Nutritional Regulation of Gene Expression and Nutritional Genomics / 615
ROBERT J. COUSINS

40.   Polymorphisms: Effect on Nutrient Utilization and Metabolism / 627
PATRICK J. STOVER AND CUTBERTO GARZA

41.   Hormones and Growth Factors / 636
IRWIN G. BRODSKY

42.   Cytokines and Eicosanoids / 655
JOSEPH G. CANNON

43. Nutrition and the Immune System / 670
GABRIEL FERNANDES, CHRISTOPHER A. JOLLY, AND RICHARD A. LAWRENCE

44. Oxidant Defense in Oxidative and Nitrosative Stress / 685
JAMES A. THOMAS

B. Metabolic Regulation: Tutorials

45. Nutrition and the Chemical Senses / 695
RICHARD D. MATTES

46. Controls of Food Intake / 707
GERARD P. SMITH

47. Physical Activity, Fitness, and Health / 720
GARY R. HUNTER

48. Metabolic Consequences of Starvation / 730
L. JOHN HOFFER

PART IV. NUTRITION NEEDS AND ASSESSMENT DURING THE LIFE CYCLE

49. Body Composition and Anthropometry / 751
STEVEN B. HEYMSFIELD AND RICHARD W. BAUMGARTNER

50A. Nutrition During Pregnancy / 771
R. ELAINE TURNER

50B. Lactation / 784
MARY FRANCES PICCIANO AND SHARON S. MCDONALD

51. Infancy and Childhood / 797
WILLIAM C. HEIRD AND ARTHUR COOPER

52. Adolescence / 818
MARGARITA S. TREUTH AND IAN J. GRIFFIN

53. Adulthood / 830
DOUGLAS C. HEIMBURGER

54. The Elderly / 843
CONNIE WATKINS BALES AND CHRISTINE SEEL RITCHIE

PART V. PREVENTION AND MANAGEMENT OF DISEASE

A. Pediatric and Adolescent Disorders

55. Malnutrition among Children in the United States: The Impact of Poverty / 861
ROBERT KARP

56. Pediatric Feeding Problems / 875
RICHARD KATZ, RAMASAMY MANIKAM, AND LINDA SCHUBERTH

57. Protein-Energy Malnutrition / 881
BENJAMIN TORÚN

58. Inherited Metabolic Disease: Amino Acids, Organic Acids, and Galactose / 909
LOUIS J. ELSAS, II, AND PHYLLIS B. ACOSTA

59. Inherited Metabolic Diseases: Defects of β-Oxidation / 960
JERRY VOCKLEY AND DEBORAH L. RENAUD

60. Childhood Obesity / 979
WILLIAM H. DIETZ

61. Nutritional Management of Infants and Children with Specific Diseases or Other Conditions / 991
ARTHUR COOPER AND WILLIAM C. HEIRD

B. Disorders of Metabolism

62. Metabolic Syndrome: Definition, Relationship to Insulin Resistance, and Clinical Utility / 1004
GERALD M. REAVEN

63. Obesity: Etiology / 1013
JAMES O. HILL, VICTORIA A. CATENACCI, AND HOLLY R. WYATT

64. Obesity: Management / 1029
THOMAS A. WADDEN, KIRSTIN J. BYRNE, AND STEPHANIE KRAUTHAMER-EWING

65. Diabetes Mellitus: Medical Nutrition Therapy / 1043
JAMES W. ANDERSON

C. Prevention and Management of Cardiovascular Disease

66. Nutrient and Genetic Regulation of Lipoprotein Metabolism / 1067
MARGO A. DENKE

67. Nutrition in the Management of Disorders of Serum Lipids and Lipoproteins / 1076
SCOTT M. GRUNDY

68. Nutrition, Diet, and Hypertension / 1095
THEODORE A. KOTCHEN AND JANE MORLEY KOTCHEN

69. Congestive Heart Failure / 1108
JOHN R. HOYLE AND FREDERIC R. KAHL

D. Disorders of the Alimentary Tract

70. Alimentary Tract in Nutrition / 1115
SAMUEL KLEIN, STEVEN M. COHN, AND DAVID H. ALPERS

71. Assessment of Malabsorption / 1143
DARLENE G. KELLY

72. Nutrition and Dental Medicine / 1152
DOMINICK P. DePAOLA, RIVA TOUGER-DECKER, DIANE RIGASSIO-RADLER, AND MARY P. FAINE

73. The Esophagus and Stomach / 1179
WILLIAM F. STENSON

74. Intestinal Disaccharidase Depletions / 1189
STEVEN R. HERTZLER, YEONSOO KIM, RUBINA KHAN, MICHELLE ASP, AND DENNIS SAVAIANO

75. Short Bowel Syndrome / 1201
KHURSHEED N. JEEJEEBHOY

76. Inflammatory Bowel Disease / 1209
ANNE M. GRIFFITHS

77. Celiac Disease / 1219
J. JOSEPH CONNON

78. Nutrition in Pancreatic Disorders / 1227
MASSIMO RAIMONDO AND JAMES S. SCOLAPIO

79. Nutrition in Liver Disorders and the Role of Alcohol / 1235
CHARLES S. LIEBER

E. Prevention and Management of Cancer

80. Molecular Basis of Carcinogenesis / 1260
DANA RATHKOPF AND GARY K. SCHWARTZ

81. Epidemiology of Diet and Cancer Risk / 1267
WALTER C. WILLETT AND EDWARD GIOVANNUCCI

82. Chemoprevention of Cancer / 1280
MICHAEL B. SPORN

83. Nutrition Support of the Patient with Cancer / 1290
MARK SCHATTNER AND MOSHE SHIKE

F. Prevention and Management of Skeletal and Joint Disorders

84. Bone Biology in Health and Disease / 1314
ROBERT P. HEANEY

85. Nutrition and Diet in Rheumatic Diseases / 1326
SARAH L. MORGAN AND JOSEPH E. BAGGOTT

86. Osteoporosis / 1339
BESS DAWSON-HUGHES

G.   Psychiatric, Behaviorial, and Neurological Disorders

87.   Behavioral Disorders Affecting Food Intake: Eating Disorders and Other Psychiatric Conditions / 1353
JANELLE W. COUGHLIN AND ANGELA S. GUARDA

88.   Nutritional Disorders of the Nervous System / 1362
GUSTAVO C. ROMÁN

H.   Nutrition in Surgery, Infection, and Trauma

89.   The Hypercatabolic State / 1381
STEPHEN F. LOWRY AND J. MARTIN PEREZ

90.   Nutrition and Infection / 1401
RICHARD D. SEMBA

91.   Nutrition in the Care of the Patient with Surgery, Trauma, and Sepsis / 1414
KENNETH A. KUDSK AND GORDON S. SACKS

I.   Other Systemic Disorders

92.   Nutritional Aspects of Hematologic Diseases / 1436
CHRISTOPHER R. CHITAMBAR AND AŚOK C. ANTONY

93.   Nutrition, Respiratory Function, and Disease / 1462
BRUCE SUCKLING, MARGARET M. JOHNSON, AND ROBERT CHIN, JR.

94.   Nutrition, Diet, and the Kidney / 1475
JOEL D. KOPPLE

95.   Food Allergies and Intolerances / 1512
STEVE L. TAYLOR AND SUSAN L. HEFLE

96.   Nutrition in the Older Person / 1531
JOHN E. MORLEY

J.   Drug-Nutrient Interactions

97.   Drug-Nutrient Interactions / 1539
LINGTAK-NEANDER CHAN

K.   Systems of Nutritional Support

98.   Enteral Feeding / 1554
MOSHE SHIKE

99.   Parenteral Nutrition / 1567
REX O. BROWN AND GAYLE MINARD

100.   Chronic Disease Management: The Team Approach / 1598
MAURICE E. SHILS, ABBY S. BLOCH, AND PATRICIA BROWN

101.   Nutritional and Medical Ethics: The Interplay of Medical Decisions, Patients' Rights, and the Judicial System / 1608
MAURICE E. SHILS

PART VI.   DIET AND NUTRITION IN HEALTH OF POPULATIONS

102.   Foundations of a Healthy Diet / 1625
WALTER C. WILLETT AND MEIR J. STAMPFER

103.   Nutritional Implications of Vegetarian Diets / 1638
PATRICIA K. JOHNSTON AND JOAN SABATÉ

104.   Dietary Reference Intakes: Rationale and Applications / 1655
ALLISON A. YATES

105.   Dietary Guidelines: National Perspectives / 1673
JOHANNA T. DWYER

106.   Nutrition Monitoring in the United States / 1687
MARIE FANELLI KUCZMARSKI AND ROBERT J. KUCZMARSKI

107.   Food-Based Dietary Guidelines for Healthier Populations: International Considerations / 1701
RICARDO UAUY, EVA HERTRAMPF, AND ALAN D. DANGOUR

108.   The Nutrition Transition: Global Trends in Diet and Disease / 1717
BENJAMIN CABALLERO

109.   Sports Nutrition / 1723
MELVIN H. WILLIAMS

110.   Social and Cultural Influences on Food Consumption and Nutritional Status / 1741
SARA A. QUANDT

111.   Fads, Frauds, and Quackery / 1752
STEPHEN BARRETT

112.   Alternative Nutrition Therapies / 1762
STEPHEN BARRETT

PART VII.   ADEQUACY, SAFETY, AND OVERSIGHT OF THE FOOD SUPPLY

113.   Food Processing: Nutrition, Safety, and Quality / 1777
JOHN W. FINLEY, DENISE M. DEMING, AND ROBERT E. SMITH

114.   Designing Functional Foods / 1789
WAYNE R. BIDLACK AND WEI WANG

115.   Food Additives, Contaminants, and Natural Toxicants and Their Risk Assessment / 1809
STEVE L. TAYLOR

116.   Nutrition Labeling of Foods and Dietary Supplements / 1827
KENNETH D. FISHER, ELIZABETH A. YETLEY, AND CHRISTINE L. TAYLOR

PART VIII.   APPENDICES
ABBY S. BLOCH AND MAURICE E. SHILS

Table of Contents / 1840
Section I.   Conversion Factors, Weights and Measures, and Metabolic Water Formation / 1846
Section II.   National and International Recommended Dietary Reference Values / 1852
Section III.   Energy and Protein Needs and Anthropometric Data / 1901
Section IV.   Nutrients, Lipids, and Organic Compounds in Beverages and Selected Foods / 1964
Section V.   Therapeutic Diets / 1994
Section VI.   Web Sites of Interest to the Health Professional / 2024

Index / 2027

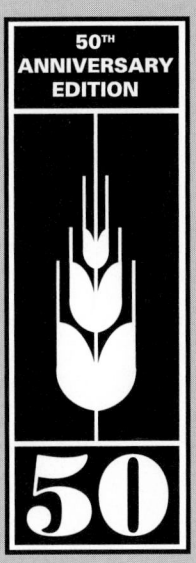

50TH
ANNIVERSARY
EDITION

50

PART I

HISTORICAL LANDMARKS
IN NUTRITION

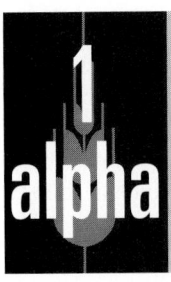

EVOLUTION OF KNOWLEDGE OF ESSENTIAL NUTRIENTS
KENNETH J. CARPENTER AND ALFRED E. HARPER

EARLY IDEAS 3
NITROGEN 3
PROTEIN 4
ENERGY 4
CALORIMETRY 4
INORGANIC ELEMENTS 4
AMINO ACIDS 5
DISCOVERY OF VITAMINS .6
VITAMIN NOMENCLATURE 7
FATTY ACIDS 7
NUTRITIONAL CLASSIFICATION OF DIET ESSENTIALS 7
CONDITIONAL ESSENTIALITY 8
MODIFICATIONS OF NUTRITIONAL NEEDS 8
    Premature Infants 8
    Genetic Defects 8
NUTRITIONAL AVAILABILITY 8

EARLY IDEAS

Early knowledge in nutritional science was acquired in several ways: initially, from practical experience in agriculture regarding what feeds gave improved growth and productivity of farm animals; subsequently, from efforts to discover the causes of diseases associated with consumption of certain diets; and also from intellectual curiosity.

Life is mysterious in all sorts of ways, and one that puzzled thinkers among our ancestors was that the wide variety of foods consumed could be turned into the tissues of the animal or human consuming them. Thus, a weaned calf eating nothing but grass continued to grow, but the blood, muscle, and skin being formed from it differed from grass in every obvious property. The ancient Greeks concluded that, despite this, the differences were superficial, and the food and the products formed from it were all made of the same single substance. Regarding why we continue to need food when we have stopped growing, it was assumed that our organs and tissues were continually wearing out and needing to be replaced (1).

In the seventeenth century, French botanists observed that one fairly constant difference between products from the plant and animal kingdoms was that plant materials left to decay would become acidic, whereas animal tissues that putrefied gave off an alkaline vapor. This does not sound like a very promising observation. However, in 1728, Jacopo Beccari (of the Academy at Bologna) announced that, by making a ball of dough from white wheaten flour and then washing out the "white floury particles" [starch], he was left with the insoluble gluten that had all properties of "animal glue" and gave an alkaline vapor on putrefaction. He concluded that it was this "animal" fraction that made wheat such a good food because "our bodies must be composed of the same substances as our nourishment" (2).

NITROGEN

In late-eighteenth century France, the main chemical elements were identified, and methods for their determination were established. In particular, the alkaline vapor from putrefying animal matter was identified as ammonia, which contained the element "nitrogen." In contrast, fats, sugars, and starches contained only carbon, hydrogen, and oxygen. If adults needed food only to replace animal tissues, how could materials that lacked nitrogen be truly nutritious?

François Magendie, a skeptical Parisian surgeon and physiologist in the early 1800s, wrote: "Although the subject of nutrition has been the subject of ingenious hypotheses, their only use has been to try to satisfy our imagination." He set out to obtain "some facts" by feeding dogs a series of palatable single foods that contained no nitrogen. On sucrose, dogs began to lose weight after 10 days, and they died in a month. Further trials with olive oil, gum, and then butter all gave the same results. Magendie concluded that dogs needed to obtain nitrogen from their food, rather than being able to use atmospheric nitrogen, and that: "diversity and multiplicity of aliments is an important rule of hygiene . . . indicated to us by our instincts" (3).

The French Academy of Sciences then invited Magendie to investigate whether gelatin, obtained relatively cheaply by boiling bones, could be used as a substitute for meat in hospitals. After another decade of research with dogs in which "unexpected results had contradicted every reasonable expectation" (or, in other words, the dogs fed gelatin as their major source of nitrogen failed to thrive), he urged that "chemists should investigate what the extractable parts of meat are that combine with gelatin or fibrin to make it a complete food; it could perhaps be iron or other salts, fatty material or lactic acid." We now know, of course, that gelatin lacks adequate quantities of several essential amino acids that are present in muscle meats.

One novelty of Magendie's work was his unstated assumption that information obtained with an animal would be relevant to human needs. This is taken for granted now, but he may have acquired the idea from French studies in comparative anatomy at that time that showed how physically similar we were to other animal species.

PROTEIN

In 1839, a Dutch physician, Gerrit Mulder, claimed that complex nitrogen compounds such as egg albumin, serum albumin, fibrin, and wheat gluten were all composed of a common radical (which he called "protein") together with small proportions of sulfur and phosphorus (4). Egg albumin was then designated as $Pr_{10}SP$ and serum albumin as $Pr_{10}S_2P$. After intense controversy over the constancy of the proportions of sulfur and phosphorus, the hypothesis was abandoned, and the term "protein" was adopted for any member of this class of complex compounds containing approximately 16% nitrogen.

ENERGY

Justus Liebig, the leading German organic chemist at this time, turned himself into an authority in physiologic chemistry. He asserted that protein was "the only true nutrient," and that as well as making up the working tissues of the body, it served as the source of energy for muscular contraction by an explosive breakdown that was followed by the synthesis and then excretion of urea. However, it had been known from the time of Lavoisier's work in the 1780s that expiration of carbon dioxide by humans increased with physical activity and that the oxidation of sugars and fats accounted, at least approximately, for the energy needed for animal heat production (5).

Then, Edward Smith in London found that prisoners engaged in "hard labor" (climbing a rotating drum treadmill) on alternate days excreted no more urea in the 24 hours that included their period of labor than on their days of rest. Smith concluded that the major factor affecting urea excretion was recent protein intake (6).

Adolf Fick and Johannes Wislicenus in Switzerland took the next step in establishing the sources of muscular energy as the result of a mountain climb (3). To minimize their protein metabolism, they ate only snacks that were almost protein free for 12 hours before and during the day of their easy 1956-m ascent by a path up a local mountain. That day, they excreted only 5.6 g of urinary nitrogen per head. This would require the degradation of no more than 35 g of protein. Other work at this time had determined the metabolizable energy of protein to be 4.37 kcal/g, so 35 g of protein would yield 153 kcal.

The energy needed to raise the temperature of 1 kg water by 1°C [i.e., 1 kcal] had been found equivalent to the work of raising 1 kg by 423 m against the force of gravity on the Earth's surface. Thus, the net work of one climber (average weight, 71 kg) was 1956 m × 71 kg = 139,000 kg · m, equivalent to 328 kcal, which was more than twice the amount of energy obtainable from 35 g protein (3). Fick and Wislicenus concluded that fats and carbohydrates in the diet could be, and usually were, the principal sources of muscular energy for the animal kingdom.

Liebig's school in Germany still claimed that a high-protein diet gave nervous energy and "a will to work," that German workmen instinctively selected diets containing more than 100 g protein/day, and that 118 g/day should remain the standard for such men. Wilbur Atwater, the pioneering nutritionist at the US Department of Agriculture at the end of the nineteenth century, accepted this conclusion. However, Russell Chittenden, working at Yale University in New Haven, Connecticut, early in the twentieth century, demonstrated that even 70 g of protein per day provided a margin of safety for a moderately active man of average weight (7) and that Liebig's proposed standard was excessive.

CALORIMETRY

In the second half of the nineteenth century, sophisticated calorimetry equipment was being developed in Germany, as well as by Atwater in Connecticut. These instruments were large enough for a subject to live in them for several days, with both heat output and respiratory exchange (oxygen consumption and carbon dioxide production) measured continuously. The findings from such studies in the period around 1900 confirmed that the body heat released, plus the mechanical work performed (as estimated from the respiratory exchange and urea excretion), corresponded to the amount of energy predicted to be expended from measurements made during combustion in vitro of the amounts of materials metabolized. Investigators also found that energy released from the metabolism of fats and carbohydrates could be used for mechanical work with approximately equal efficiency (8).

By about 1905, it appeared to many workers that nutrition was at last understood, and the only concerns in practice were to supply sufficient protein and energy (the latter as fat and carbohydrates) together with some minerals. However, after a period of self-satisfaction, the subject was turned upside down in the next 15 years. To quote from Gowland Hopkins' 1929 Nobel Prize lecture: "The quantitative character of the data obtained . . . induced a feeling that knowledge of these needs had become highly adequate and was approximating even to finality . . . [but it was] . . . leading to doctrinal teaching which contained inherent errors" (9).

INORGANIC ELEMENTS

Throughout the nineteenth century, investigators recognized that animal tissues contained minerals, but it was generally assumed (for no apparent reason) that these minerals would not, in practice, be deficient in the diet. The first suggested exception was for the relatively newly discovered element iodine. In parts of Europe, eating dried seaweed or burned sponges had been traditional folk treatments for the condition of goiter, a gross swelling of the thyroid gland in the neck. In 1820, Charles Coindet in Switzerland suggested that it was the iodine in these materials that was active. He found it to be effective, but later workers apparently overdosed, resulting in toxic effects, so the idea was abandoned (10). It was only in the 1920s, after the relationship between iodine intake and occurrence of goiter had been studied carefully, that iodine began to be used routinely to eradicate goiter in the central portions of the United States (11).

Rickets, characterized by deficient bone mineralization, was another serious problem among infants growing up in industrial cities in the nineteenth century. The minerals in bone are largely present as a form of calcium phosphate. However, the geographic distribution of rickets was correlated with the lack of sunshine, rather than with particularly low intakes of calcium and/or phosphate, as discussed later (12).

Blood had long been known to be relatively rich in iron, and in 1832 Pierre Blaud in France had demonstrated the value of giving ferrous sulfate to anemic patients. However, as the result in part of faulty analyses apparently showing that white bread was a good source of iron, it came to be thought that anemia was the consequence of intestinal disturbance and autointoxication, rather than deficiency; this erroneous concept was corrected only in the 1890s by Ralph Stockman in Edinburgh (13), who established clearly the relationship between iron intake and the incidence of chlorosis (anemia).

From 1920 onward, systematic investigation was undertaken to determine which of the mineral elements found in animal tissues in very small quantities (the so-called trace elements) were actually essential and required in the diet. The systematic work with young rats required the preparation of diets with an extremely low level of the mineral under investigation but adequate levels of all the others. In this way, both zinc and manganese were found to be nutritional essentials. However, one discovery occurred by chance. To compare the relative value of different iron salts in treating anemia, rats at the University of Wisconsin were made anemic by feeding them a milk diet. Surprisingly, none of the iron salts proved effective in reversing the condition, but the ash from certain foods was effective. Further investigation showed that it was the small quantity of copper salts in the ash that was required, in addition to iron, to produce a response (10).

In 1957, the element selenium, previously considered only toxic, was also found to be nutritionally essential, and it became clear that deficiency of this element was actually a practical problem among farm animals in several countries, as well as occurring at toxic levels in some areas (14). It was also discovered that selenium deficiency was the

TABLE 1.1. NUTRIENTS ESSENTIAL FOR HUMANS

Water	(Choline[a])
Amino acids (L isomers)	Energy sources
Histidine	Fatty acids
Isoleucine	Linoleic acid
Leucine	α-Linolenic acid
Lysine	Minerals
Methionine	Calcium
Phenylalanine	Phosphorus
Threonine	Magnesium
Tryptophan	Iron
Valine	Zinc
Vitamins	Copper
Ascorbic acid	Manganese
Vitamins A, D, E, K	Iodine
Thiamin	Selenium
Riboflavin	Molybdenum
Niacin	Chromium
Vitamin B_6 (pyridoxine)	Electrolytes
Pantothenic acid	Sodium
Folic acid	Potassium
Biotin	Chloride
Vitamin B_{12} (cobalamin)	Ultratrace elements[b]

[a] In experimental animals, choline is a conditional nutrient useful when methionine is not present in adequate amounts as a "methyl" donor, and this may also be true for humans.
[b] See Chapter 18. None have so far been proved by adequate studies to be essential for humans, but it remains possible that one or more may be found to be essential in exceedingly small amounts.

major cause of cardiomyopathy seen among the population of the Keshan area of China where the soil had a particularly low selenium content. It was then realized that cardiomyopathy occurring among patients who had been receiving total parenteral nutrition for prolonged periods could also result from lack of this element, and selenium is now routinely added to most total parenteral nutrition formulas (see Chapters 16 and 99).

It is understandable that farm animals should have been particularly susceptible to mineral element deficiencies, because they usually received only plant foods grown locally that reflected the characteristics of the local soils, including any possible mineral deficiencies, whereas humans (at least in industrialized countries) obtain a mix of foods produced in different areas. The elements that have been found to be required by humans are all listed in Table 1.1.

AMINO ACIDS

By 1900, investigators reluctantly accepted that, although most of the animal kingdom relied on plants as their source of protein, after the proteins were eaten they were broken down in the digestive tract to free amino acids that, after absorption, were used to rebuild proteins for the animal body (15).

In 1906, Hopkins, working at Cambridge University, obtained evidence that the amino acid tryptophan was essential in the diet for the survival of mice receiving zein as their sole protein source. A few years later, Thomas Osborne and Lafayette Mendel, working at Yale, added the further finding that tryptophan and lysine were needed for the growth of rats receiving zein, which lacked both these amino acids. Tryptophan was therefore the first organic compound to be identified as an essential nutrient for the animal kingdom (3).

By 1930, 19 individual amino acids were known to be present in proteins, but it was found that a mixture of them could not replace dietary protein in supporting the growth of young rats. Did this mean that a dietary requirement existed for some kind of "protein core"? William Rose and his research group at the University of Illinois studied this problem for many years. The original mixture of amino acids had not included methionine because it was thought at that time that only one sulfur-containing amino acid (i.e., cyst[e]ine) was needed. When growth and survival of rats were not improved by including methionine in the mixture but were improved by inclusion of a quantity of protein hydrolyzate, it became evident that protein hydrolyzates contained another as yet unidentified compound that was an essential nutrient. McCoy and Meyer (16) in Rose's laboratory conducted a classic isolation study with protein hydrolyzate as the starting material. They obtained a product that converted the inadequate amino acid mixture to one that supported the growth of rats without the need for inclusion of protein or protein hydrolyzate in the diet. The compound was identified as a new amino acid, 2-amino-3-hydroxybutanoic acid and was named threonine.

Subsequently, emphasis in the research in Rose's laboratory shifted to estimation of the quantitative requirements of rats for amino acids. After estimating the minimum amount of each amino acid required by the rat, Rose and his research group began to study the amino acid needs of human adults. These investigators demonstrated that humans could also be kept in nitrogen balance with a diet in which the protein component was replaced with free amino acids (17). They then studied the quantitative requirements of men for each of the amino acids. Ruth Leverton and her associates at the US Department of Agriculture studied the requirements of women, and the amino acids found to be nutritionally essential for humans are listed in Table 1.1.

DISCOVERY OF VITAMINS

In the 1880s, it was shown that beriberi, a disease rife among Japanese sailors and characterized by neuropathy, could be prevented by changes in the diet. In Indonesia (then the Dutch East Indies), investigators found that "something" in rice polishings (i.e., the byproduct from further milling of dehusked rice grains) could prevent the disease appearing among prisoners who were living mainly on white rice. This was observed after Christiaan Eijkman had produced a model of the disease (polyneuritis) in chickens, and the "something" was shown to be easily

destroyed (therefore not a mineral) and to be neither protein nor fat. Assays with chickens and other birds allowed fractionation of the active factor from the polishings. This factor, to be named thiamin, was isolated in 1926 and was found to cure chickens of the disease when only 2 ppm was added to their feed (18).

Scurvy had long been a problem, not just among sailors who had been at sea for long periods, but also on land, whenever access to fresh food was restricted, most recently during the siege of Paris in 1870. Unfortunately, by 1900, Pasteur's concept of diseases arising from microbial infection had taken such a hold that even scurvy was thought of as being caused by ptomaines present in infected meat. However, the accidental discovery of a model for the disease in guinea pigs fed a grain diet allowed the assay of materials for their antiscorbutic activity. This was followed in the 1930s by the isolation of ascorbic acid and then by its synthesis (19).

In 1912, Casimir Funk, a Polish biochemist working in London on the isolation of the antiberiberi factor, concluded that it must be an amine and suggested that pellagra, scurvy, and rickets were all the result of deficiencies of members of the same class of compounds, which he called "vital amines" and shortened to "vitamines" (14). This did not prove to be the case, but the term "vitamin" (with the 'e' omitted) was retained by international agreement for organic compounds required only in trace amounts.

In the United States, attention was attracted to the question of unknown nutrients by the results from a feeding trial with dairy cattle at the College of Agriculture of the University of Wisconsin, Madison. One group of heifers was fed for 3 years solely on wheat products (grain, hay, straw, gluten) and another only on corn products in proportions such that each mix had the same analysis for nitrogen, fiber, ash, and moisture. The second group did very well, but those receiving only wheat gave little milk, and their calves, if not born dead, were blind and weak (20).

E.V. McCollum, a young chemist recruited from Yale, was charged with discovering what was wrong with the wheat diet. He decided that he could make quicker progress using rats, which matured and reproduced so much faster than cattle. In a relatively short time, McCollum and Marguerite Davis discovered that young rats fed a basal diet made up of casein, lactose, mixed minerals, and olive oil would stop growing after 8 to 14 weeks but would start again if they were given butter as the fat source, or even the small, nonsaponifiable fraction of butterfat (21, 22). This finding was confirmed by Osborne and Mendel at Yale.

However, some other workers, using more highly purified lactose, found that rats would stop growing even when the animals were given McCollum's diet with added butterfat. It transpired that the lactose that McCollum had been using in his "purified" diet still contained at least one water-soluble growth factor. This finding was confirmed; the butterfat factor was called "vitamin A" and the water-soluble factor "vitamin B," with the latter assumed to be identical to the water-soluble factor in rice polishings that had been studied by Eijkman. However, when crude sources of "vitamin B" were replaced by more highly purified preparations, investigators soon realized that even this could not be the whole story, and the growth-promoting and antipolyneuritis activities of foods that were sources of "vitamin B" must come from more than one factor. Clarification of this problem took much more work (10).

VITAMIN NOMENCLATURE

After the designation of vitamins A and B, it was decided to call the antiscorbutic factor vitamin C. As more of the vitamins to be considered in later chapters were discovered, they were at first given further letters of the alphabet (D, E, and K), but some of the activities for which workers claimed the assignment of a letter (e.g., F, G, H, and M) were dropped after their chemical identity was established, because their existence was considered doubtful at best (as for vitamin H), or because it seemed clearer to use the chemical name, such as folic acid for the group of compounds with "vitamin M" activity.

As vitamin B was discovered to include many activities, the collective term vitamin B complex was used, and the individual members were identified as B_1, B_2, and so on. Then, some of these fractions became subdivided, and, as the factors were identified, they came to be known by their chemical names, such as thiamin and riboflavin, to minimize confusion. The only exceptions are the groups of compounds closely related to pyridoxal, which have the same biologic activity and are still commonly referred to as vitamin B_6, and those related to (and with the same activity as) cobalamin, which are still commonly described as vitamin B_{12}.

FATTY ACIDS

In the early 1800s, a French chemist demonstrated that ordinary animal fats and vegetable oils consisted of glycerol combined with a variety of fatty acids differing in their melting points. Investigators gradually came to know that the acids differed chemically in both the length of their carbon chains and the degree of unsaturation of those carbon chains with hydrogen atoms. In 1845, Boussingault confirmed, by means of a balance trial, that a pig could synthesize its body fat from dietary carbohydrate; from then on, it was generally assumed that fat, although a convenient and palatable source of energy in the diet, was not actually essential (23).

In 1929, however, George and Mildred Burr at the University of Minnesota found that rats consuming a diet with all traces of lipids scrupulously removed, except for the fat-soluble vitamins, failed to reach mature weight, lost fur, and had scaly tails. This condition was prevented by giving small amounts of the methyl ester of the doubly unsaturated linoleic acid, but not by giving either saturated fatty acids or the monounsaturated oleic acid (24).

In the 1960s, evidence accumulated that infants given formulas low in linoleic acid also grew more poorly on average than other infants receiving more of this substance and showed thicker skins. Then, in 1972, an infant who could be fed only parenterally and who was not receiving any lipid (except fat-soluble vitamins) was found to develop severe dermatosis of the feet; this cleared up quickly after oral administration of linoleic acid.

Investigators had already shown that fish needed a triunsaturated fatty acid such as linolenic acid (as well as a source of linoleic acid) in their diets. However, even in multigenerational studies with rats, no clear disadvantage was observed in those animals not receiving linolenic acid in addition to linoleic acid, even though a long-chain fatty acid derived from linolenic acid was retained in their eyes (see Chapter 5). Evidence for a human requirement for linolenic acid was obtained in 1982. A child who had been fed only parenterally for several years developed blurred vision that disappeared after the child was given linolenic acid specifically. Comparable results were subsequently obtained with monkeys (25).

Further advances in knowledge of the functions of the essential fatty acids are discussed at length in later chapters.

NUTRITIONAL CLASSIFICATION OF DIET ESSENTIALS

Further research between 1920 and 1948 revealed that other nutrients, specifically vitamins and trace minerals, were dietary essentials. In addition, doubtful claims were made, sometimes for commercial reasons, perhaps offering a special "vitamin X" that maintained the body's resistance to one or other diseases. Therefore, reason exists to have a list of nutrients with good evidence of dietary essentiality.

The list of essential nutrients varies among species, owing to differences in their ability to convert inactive precursors to the active compound. The obvious example is vitamin C, required in the diets of humans and guinea pigs; although cats and dogs, and most other animals, still need vitamin C in their tissues, they can make it for themselves. Table 1.1 lists the nutrients generally accepted as being essential for humans. The criteria for this essentiality is that absence of the nutrient from the diet results in characteristic signs of a deficiency disease and these signs are prevented only by the nutrient itself or a specific precursor of it.

In most cases a specific precursor and the nutrient itself differ from each other only by a single group that our bodies can either modify or exchange. Thus, vitamin B_6 can be supplied as pyridoxine, pyridoxal, or pyridoxamine. Niacin can be used as either nicotinic acid or nicotinamide. Tryptophan is a much further removed precursor for niacin. It can be metabolized, nonetheless, via an extensive series of reactions requiring a transformation of the indole ring it contains to a pyridine ring, to yield niacin. Because niacin can be synthesized in the body from tryptophan present in the diet in excess of the amount needed for protein synthesis, one could describe niacin as being only conditionally essential, the condition being a relative deficiency of tryptophan.

Again, vitamin D (cholecalciferol) can be produced from 7-dehydrocholesterol by ultraviolet irradiation. This occurs in human skin exposed to sunlight (that has not been filtered through cloud or smog), which is by far our most important natural source of the vitamin. Rickets could therefore be classified as a disease caused by a deficit of sunlight rather than a dietary deficiency, thus making the description of "D" as a vitamin a historical accident.

Vitamin A (retinol) is, under natural conditions, obtained by herbivores from carotenoids (mainly β-carotene) present in plants, that they can hydrolyze, although rather inefficiently, to obtain retinol. With regard to efficiency of utilization of vitamin precursors, great differences occur among species. Thus, the cat family, obligate carnivores, can obtain neither retinol from carotene nor niacin from tryptophan. The preceding paragraphs refer only to humans.

Most amino acids can still be used even if their amino group has been replaced by a keto or hydroxyl group. This is because of the transamination reactions that are occurring constantly in our bodies. Such compounds may not be of practical importance for humans, but the hydroxy analog of methionine was synthesized and used as a dietary supplement in poultry feed before methionine itself could be produced economically. The unnatural D isomer of a few amino acids can also be used, as a consequence of being first metabolized to the nonisomeric keto form and then reaminated to the active L form.

CONDITIONAL ESSENTIALITY

Cystine was the first nutrient shown to fall into this category. Workers in the 1920s found that young rats receiving 10 to 12% casein in their dry diets as a source of protein grew faster when 0.5% cystine (or its reduced form cysteine) was added to the diet, so that it was naturally considered to be an essential nutrient. However, after the discovery of methionine as a second sulfur-containing amino acid, investigators discovered that rats did not grow without it, and that, when enough was provided, there was no longer any need for the presence of cysteine/cystine in the diet. This finding was explained by the presence of a metabolic pathway for the catabolism of methionine, in excess of that needed for protein synthesis, into cysteine. Tyrosine and phenylalanine exhibit a similar relationship, with the latter being the only precursor of the former. Cyst(e)ine and tyrosine supplied in the diet do, of course, spare what would otherwise be higher requirements for methionine and phenylalanine, respectively.

Other amino acids that are essential components of proteins but can be synthesized from ammonium ions and

a variety of common carbon compounds in the body used to be called "nonessential," but this designation seemed possibly misleading, and the term "dispensable" is now preferred (26).

MODIFICATIONS OF NUTRITIONAL NEEDS

Premature Infants

Some enzymes of amino acid metabolism develop late during gestation, and investigators have found that premature infants can lack the ability of mature infants to synthesize cysteine and tyrosine, and so they need them as such in their diet (27). Investgators have also reported that these infants may lack the ability to elongate and desaturate linoleic acid and α-linolenic acid to the biologically important eicosanoids, so these substances may need to be supplied directly in some way (28). Indications also exist that such infants may not be able to synthesize taurine in the quantities they need and possibly carnitine also (29, 30).

Genetic Defects

Some individuals lack essential enzyme pathways. This means that throughout life, they may remain unable to synthesize substances that are biologically essential but not normally needed in the diet. Such compounds include carnitine and tetrahydrobiopterin (30). Three tests have been proposed to establish a condition of conditional essentiality: (a) an abnormally low plasma concentration of the nutrient in question; (b) appearance of some chemical, structural, or functional abnormalities; and (c) correction of both by a dietary supplement of the nutrient (31).

"Many mutations in a gene result in the corresponding enzyme having a decreased binding affinity for a coenzyme resulting in a lower rate of reaction. About 50 human genetic diseases due to defective enzymes can be remedied or ameliorated by the administration of high doses of the vitamin component of the corresponding coenzyme" (32). In the genetic disease acrodermatitis enteropathica, which impairs zinc absorption, the need for zinc is increased three- to fourfold (see Chapter 13).

NUTRITIONAL AVAILABILITY

Nutrients will not be able to correct a deficiency if they are supplied in a form that is not available. Digestion and absorption of nutrients can be influenced by a variety of factors; among these are solubility, release from substances with which they interact in foods, binding by another food constituent after release, and linking through bonds that are not readily broken by digestive enzymes. With regard to minerals in particular, iron, given in its elemental, metallic form, has been found to cure or prevent anemia resulting from deficiency of iron, but only if the iron is extremely finely divided to give a very high surface area so gastric acid can react with it to form a soluble salt in an adequate amount. Some metal compounds are also so inert and insoluble that they resist absorption from the digestive tract.

Again, requirements may be increased when the diet also contains another component that binds a nutrient and reduces its digestibility. Thus, phytic acid present in unleavened grains and oilseed products binds with multivalent cations. This situation has been responsible for serious problems of zinc deficiency in the Middle East even when the dietary zinc content has met the usual standards (33). High dietary levels of even ordinary essential nutrients can reduce the availability of other nutrients, in some cases through competition for absorption from the intestinal tract. Thus, excesses of iron and molybdenum increase the needs for manganese and copper, respectively (34).

The need for vitamin E is increased when the diet contains a high level of polyunsaturated fat, for example, as a result of taking a fish oil supplement. The extra vitamin is, in this case, required within the tissues to protect cellular structures against damage from reactive products of lipid peroxidation (35).

Many suggestions have been made that vitamins E and C and carotenoids, which all serve as antioxidants, could be of general value, at levels far higher than those needed to prevent deficiencies, in countering chronic and degenerative diseases that are major causes of death in affluent societies, but it has been difficult to define what the ideal levels would be or how to test for them.

REFERENCES

It is editorial policy to use modern articles or books in preference to early papers that may be difficult to access, but in this historical essay, those chosen include some primary references.

1. Guggenheim KY. Nutrition and Nutritional Diseases: The Evolution of Concepts. Lexington, MA: Collamore Press, 1981.
2. Bailey CH. Cereal Chem 1941;18:555–61.
3. Carpenter KJ. Protein and Energy: A Study of Changing Ideas in Nutrition. New York: Cambridge University Press, 1994.
4. Vickery HB. Yale J Biol Med 1950;22:387–93.
5. Holmes FL. Lavoisier and the Chemistry of Life. Madison, WI: University of Wisconsin Press, 1985:440–6.
6. Carpenter KJ. J Nutr 1991;121:1515–21.
7. Chittenden RH. Physiological Economy in Nutrition. New York: Stokes, 1904.
8. Lusk G. A history of metabolism. In: Barker LF, ed. Endocrinology and Metabolism, vol 3. New York: Appleton, 1922:3–78.
9. Hopkins FG. The earlier history of vitamin research. In: Nobel Lectures: Physiology or Medicine, 1922–1941. Amsterdam: Elsevier, 1965:211–22.
10. McCollum EV. A History of Nutrition. Cambridge, MA: Houghton Mifflin, 1957.
11. Marine D. Harvey Lect 1923–24;19:96–122.
12. De Luca HF. Historical overview. In: Feldman D, Glorieux FH, Pike JW, eds. Vitamin D. New York: Academic Press, 1997:3–11.
13. Carpenter KJ. J Nutr 1990;120:141–7.
14. Combs GF Jr, Levander OA, Spallholz JE et al, eds. Selenium in Biology and Medicine. 2 vols. New York: Avi, 1987.
15. Fruton JS. Molecules and Life. New York: Wiley, 1972.
16. McCoy RH, Meyer CE, Rose WC . J Biol Chem 1935;112: 283–302.
17. Rose WC. Fed Proc 1949;8:546–52.
18. Carpenter KJ. Beriberi, White Rice and Vitamin B. Berkeley, CA: University of California Press, 2000.
19. Carpenter KJ. The History of Scurvy and Vitamin C. New York: Cambridge University Press, 1986.
20. Harper AE. J Nutr 1997;127[Suppl]:1027S–8S.
21. Day HG. J Nutr 1997;127[Suppl]:1029S–31S.
22. McCollum EV. From Kansas Farm Boy to Scientist: The Autobiography of Elmer Verner McCollum. Lawrence, KS: University of Kansas Press, 1964.
23. Carpenter KJ. J Nutr 1998;128[Suppl]:423S–6S.
24. Burr GO, Burr MM. J Biol Chem 1930;86:587–621.
25. Neuringer F, Connor WE, Van Petten C et al. J Clin Invest 1984; 73:272–6.
26. Harper AE. J Nutr 1974;104:965–7.
27. Snyderman SE. Human amino acid metabolism. In: Velázquez A, Bourges H, eds. Genetic Factors in Nutrition. New York: Academic Press, 1984:269–78.
28. McCormick DB. The meaning of nutritional essentiality in today's context of health and disease. In: Roche AF, ed. Nutritional Essentiality: A Changing Paradigm. Report of the 12th Ross Conference on Medical Research. Columbus, OH: Ross Products Division, Abbott Laboratories, 1993:11–5.
29. Gaull GE. J Am Coll Nutr 1986;5:101–6.
30. Hoppel C. Carnitine: Conditionally essential? In: Roche AF, ed. Nutritional Essentiality: A Changing Paradigm. Report of the 12th Ross Conference on Medical Research. Columbus, OH: Ross Products Division, Abbott Laboratories, 1993:52–7.
31. Rudman D, Feller A. J Am Coll Nutr 1986;5:101–6.
32. Ames BN, Elson-Schwab I, Silver EA. Am J Clin Nutr 2002; 75:616–58.
33. Reinhold JG, Nasr K, Lahimgarzadeh A et al. Lancet 1973;i: 283–8.
34. Hill CH. Mineral interrelationships. In: Prasad AS, ed. Trace Elements in Human Health and Disease. New York: Academic Press, 1976:281–300.
35. DuPont J, Holub BJ, Knapp HR et al. Am J Clin Nutr 1996;63: 991S–3S.

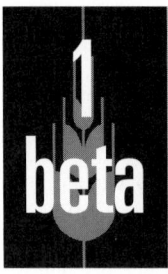

HUMAN ENERGY METABOLISM[1]

JOHN M. KINNEY

1050 TO 1600 VITALISM: THE ENERGY OF LIFE 10
THE 1600s: HARVEY AND THE OXFORD
   PHYSIOLOGISTS 11
THE 1700s: FOUR PIONEERS OF GAS EXCHANGE 11
    Joseph Black (1728–1799) 11
    Joseph Priestley (1733–1804) 11
    Carl Wilhelm Scheele (1742–1786) 11
    Antoine Laurent Lavoisier (1743–1794) 12
THE 1800s: HEAT, FOOD, AND CALORIMETRY 12
1890 TO 1920: CALORIMETRY SPREADS TO AMERICA ..13
1880 TO 1960: METABOLIC BODY SIZE 14
1900 TO 1950: MALNUTRITION AND CALORIMETRY ...14
1975 FORWARD: BEDSIDE GAS EXCHANGE 14
1982 FORWARD: DOUBLY LABELED WATER METHOD ..15

One of the most remarkable aspects of the human body is the relationship among food, work, and heat. In one sense, the human body is an engine that consumes fuel to perform work. The energy that does not appear as work is dissipated as heat. The human body may be considered a machine that does its own maintenance and powers a convective system that distributes fuel and oxygen to the local sites of utilization and removes the waste products as well as the heat. In addition to the internal maintenance of tissues and regulation of energy balance, the body may move and do work. The healthy body maintains relatively large stores of organic materials that can be used for reserve energy, whereas body heat reserves are comparatively limited in relation to the normal rate of heat production.

The human machine has an optimum range for body composition and also an optimum operating temperature, or body heat content. However, the range for the former can vary considerably, whereas the range for the latter is protected within narrow limits. The ability of physiologically normal humans to think, move, and work without delay or prior preparation illustrates a unique degree of independent energy utilization. This constant and ready availability of energy underlies animal life in general and human life in particular.

Normal life may be defined as the conversion of energy to perform meaningful work at an acceptable metabolic cost. Illness and injury may be defined as energy conversion, work requirements, or metabolic costs that have become excessive relative to the supply. Therefore, death may be defined as the irreversible loss of the ability to use energy to perform sufficient work in one or more vital organs.

The common measurements of nutritional status performed on hospitalized patients relate to concentrations, particularly in the blood or urine. Only a few clinical measurements are available that indicate the rate of a process rather than a concentration. This is particularly true of energy metabolism, in which conventional measurements of clinical care do not document the rate of energy expenditure, or heat production.

1050 TO 1600 VITALISM: THE ENERGY OF LIFE

The concept that life is associated with a "vital force" or vital heat dates back to the earliest cultures. Those who accepted in vitalism believed that life represented a new and foreign principle, or substance, imposed on materials that constituted the body. Hippocrates believed that the essence of life was an "ether," similar to the "pneuma" described in the works of Plato. To some, this pneuma had the attributes of a material substance comparable to oxygen, whereas to others it was an intangible material essential to all of life. Aristotle believed that the innate heat of the heart was the source of life and that all its powers were related to nutrition, sensation, movement, and thought. The heart was the source of life, and death would occur if the heart lost its heat. Galen believed that venous blood originating in the liver traveled to the right side of the heart, where a separation took place between the dead portion moving to the lungs to be refreshed under the influence of the life-giving pneuma. These concepts formed the strongest and longest-lived biologic doctrine that medicine has ever known. As late as the eighteenth century, vital heat was used in explanations by the foremost physicians and physiologists of the time.

The achievements of Copernicus, Galileo, and Newton did much to challenge vitalism in astronomy and the physical sciences during the 1500s. However, comparable changes in biology and medicine came approximately a century later.

---

[1]**Abbreviations: BMR,** basal metabolic rate; **DLW,** doubly labeled water; **H-B,** Harris-Benedict.

THE 1600s: HARVEY AND THE OXFORD PHYSIOLOGISTS

William Harvey stood at the threshold not only of modern medicine but also of a modern approach to science in general. Harvey's doctrine of the circulation of blood depended on the concept of innate heat for much of his theory. He considered the heart to be "the innate fire and the beginning of life." Not only was Harvey a pioneering investigator, but while at Oxford he also developed around him a remarkable group of early physiologists. Three of these men, Robert Boyle, Robert Hooke, and John Mayow, introduced a conceptual framework involving animal heat, respiration, and combustion. Boyle and Hooke experimented with a vacuum pump and showed that neither a flame nor a chick could survive in a vacuum. Further studies showed that atmospheric air contained a quality that allowed it to support both respiration and combustion, which would cease in its absence. The nature of physiologic ideas changed during the seventeenth century, and the concept of animal heat reflected these changes.

At the beginning of the century, innate heat was thought to arise in the heart, but at the end of the century not only was a causal explanation sought in heat production, but also that explanation resembled some aspects of the theory of combustion.

THE 1700s: FOUR PIONEERS OF GAS EXCHANGE

Ancient humans had probably recognized that where a fire would not burn, an animal could not live. Boyle and other investigators realized that a similar alteration in the volume of air was caused by combustion and respiration. The four following scientists played special roles in identifying the two gases central to energy metabolism: Priestley was a clergyman, Scheele a pharmacist, and Lavoisier a financier and reformer; Black was the only one with genuine academic credentials.

Joseph Black (1728–1799)

Joseph Black entered Glasgow University at the age of 16 to study medicine. In an effort to find an improved mixture for dissolving bladder stones, he discovered that the addition of acids liberated a gas that he called "fixed air" and that was later recognized as carbon dioxide. He showed that it was also present in expired air and was released during a fire.

Black's investigations aroused great interest and lead to a professorship in chemistry at the University of Edinburgh in 1766. Of particular interest to British scholars were new discoveries made by "those French chemists" and the attack on the "phlogiston" theory that was launched from Paris and disquieted many, including Priestley.

It is Joseph Priestley and Carl Wilhelm Scheele who share the credit for discovering oxygen, although they had only a hazy notion of the role the gas played in chemical processes of combustion and respiration. Both believed the phlogiston theory, in which all combustible materials contained the hypothetic substance phlogiston, which, on burning, was released into the air while the dephlogisticated ash remained behind.

Joseph Priestley (1733–1804)

Joseph Priestley was born of poor and pious parents in Yorkshire. After attending a clerical college, he became a separatist minister with variable success. While a language teacher at an academy, Priestley published several books on the history of electricity that won him membership in the Royal Society and the friendship of Benjamin Franklin. Priestley moved to Leeds, where he lived adjacent to a brewery. Immense quantities of carbon dioxide were seen to bubble up from the vats during fermentation. He then started to experiment with this "fixed air," leading to the invention of soda water, which he described in his first chemical publication. Priestley was hired by the Earl of Shelburne to raise the intellectual standards on his lands, a position that left Priestley free to pursue both his theologic studies and his scientific experiments. He isolated ten different gases, from nitrogen oxide to ammonia. He invariably tested each isolated gas to see whether a light would burn and a mouse would live in it. In 1774, he discovered oxygen. Sadly, he missed the significance of the oxygen he had discovered because of his steadfast belief in the phlogiston theory. He observed that ordinary air, in which a candle no longer would burn and a mouse no longer live, could regain its former properties when green plants were included in the sealed vessel.

Priestley accepted a post as minister of a Unitarian church in Birmingham whose congregation was proud to have so famous a scholar as their pastor. He entered eagerly into the controversial discussions on political and religious matters then taking place between the nonconformists and the Church of England. At the height of the feeling against the nonconformists, two churches were burned down, and Priestley's home and laboratory were destroyed. Shortly afterward, Priestley and his family sailed to America and settled in rural Pennsylvania. The Priestley home and laboratory are maintained as a historic landmark by the American Chemical Society; a US stamp was issued in his honor.

Carl Wilhelm Scheele (1742–1786)

Carl Wilhelm Scheele was born of German parents but grew up in Sweden, where he became an apothecary's apprentice. He spent his nights carrying out experiments that he had read about in his books. After serving for 10 years as a pharmacist, he became the owner of his own pharmacy. His chemical achievements had become highly esteemed, and this reputation allowed him to be established as a pharmacist without the usual formal education.

For the greater part of his life, Scheele was almost unknown in his own country, even after his chemical triumphs had made him known abroad.

As a chemist, Scheele was far ahead of his time. Using extremely primitive laboratory tools, he was able to characterize many more chemical substances than anyone before him. He discovered manganese, barium, chlorine, and oxygen. Scheele was led astray, like Priestley, in the belief that heat was generated by a combustion of phlogiston with oxygen.

Antoine Laurent Lavoisier (1743–1794)

Antoine Laurent Lavoisier was born in Paris of a middle class family in which every effort was made to provide for his upbringing and education. His early breadth of interest in research was evident when he won a special medal for an original plan to replace poor street lighting in the city while he was only 22 years of age. Cultivating chemistry as a side line was a usual practice at that time. Lavoisier was given more and more government assignments, including improving Parisian drinking water and reorganizing the prison system. He began to study methods of making niter, which could improve the notoriously poor French gunpowder. In a relatively short time, French gunpowder was of such fine quality that it was proven superior to that of other nations, particularly Britain.

Lavoisier found that diamonds lost weight and much of their brilliance when they were heated, yet this was not the case if they were heated in the absence of air. This finding started his interest in gases and in the growing evidence against the phlogiston theory. Lavoisier found that phosphorus and sulfur gained weight when burning in air. He believed that the increase in weight was the result of a gain in some constituent of air. Lavoisier used a large burning lens in 1772 to show that when lead oxide was roasted with charcoal, an enormous volume of "air" was liberated.

In 1774, Priestly paid a visit to Lavoisier and told of the recent discovery of a hitherto unknown gas that he had produced by heating mercuric oxide. The resultant gas was not fixed air and caused a candle to burn more brightly and a mouse to live longer. In subsequent studies, Lavoisier concluded that the "eminently respirable air" burned carbon to form the weak acid, carbon dioxide; hence Lavoisier called the new substance "oxygen," meaning "acid-former." In 1777, half of Lavoisier's chemical revolution was over. The second half was to be in respiration, based on the concept that oxygen burned the carbon in foodstuffs to form the carbon dioxide exhaled in the breath, whereas the heat released was the source of animal warmth. Lavoisier and Laplace demonstrated this theory quantitatively with a guinea pig in 1783. Respiration was seen to be clearly a slow form of combustion. The nonrespirable part of the air (later called nitrogen) was exhaled unaltered.

Lavoisier brought about a revolution in chemistry by ridding it of the phlogiston theory and by introducing oxidation and a new theory of chemical composition. He published a chemistry textbook in 1789 that became an international model for chemical instruction, thereby establishing Lavoisier's title as "father of modern chemistry."

THE 1800s: HEAT, FOOD, AND CALORIMETRY

The early part of the nineteenth century was characterized by many confrontations between physiologists and chemists. The rapid development of methods for identifying and analyzing organic compounds made it essential to investigate such vital phenomena as respiration, digestion, and nutrition in the light of the new chemical knowledge. Those who were trained as chemists sought to treat biologic problems by an extension of the methods they had found to be successful in their own discipline. This was strange to investigators accustomed to dealing with organisms by anatomic studies or vivisection. The chemical approach was defined most clearly in the efforts of Lavoisier and his followers, who sought to extend the theory of respiration that he had put forward at the end of the eighteenth century.

Some Parisian chemists in the early nineteenth century were engaged in experiments to determine whether the heat actually produced by an animal matched the heat theoretically caused by the chemical reactions of respiration. However, two well-known physiologists of the time, Francois Magendie of France and Johannes Muller of Germany, both doubted Lavoisier's theories. Many biologists at that time doubted whether a given chemical process could ever account for animal heat and even questioned any chemical explanation of related biologic phenomena. When Claude Bernard began his physiologic training, he was quickly exposed to both the prominence and the doubts concerning the chemical theories of respiration and animal heat production. He developed a growing conviction that chemical theories were useful only when they were coupled with direct animal experimentation.

During the 1840s, biochemical thought was being led by the brilliant German chemist, Justus Liebig, and his French counterpart, Jean-Baptist Dumas. An extended confrontation developed between them over the source of animal fat; Liebig contended that fat could arise from sugar, whereas Dumas maintained that there was "preformed fat" even in corn. Boussingault, a French colleague of Dumas, established metabolic balance studies in 1844 in a massive effort to use detailed analysis of food intake and carcass analysis of farm animals to define the source of animal fat. His experiments proved, in both the goose and the pig, that animals could form fat from other classes of food. Liebig copied this balance method to account for the rate of exchange of carbon compounds in animal metabolism, thus applying the advantages of the new organic chemistry that he himself was creating to basic problems in biology.

The word "energy" was used at the beginning of the 1800s to refer to mechanical energy and that heat was associated with motion. Joseph Black rejected the idea that heat was based on motion and instead chose to believe that heat was a fluid with particles that were self-repulsive. Many biologists believed that the nature of heat remained unsolved. The work of Hermann von Helmholtz, a towering scientific personality, influenced all branches of nineteenth-century science from theoretic mechanics to applied physiology. He believed that "vital forces" and especially vital heat could be thought of as mechanical forces. From 1840 to 1855, an English group with James Prescott Joule became preoccupied with problems of the conversion among various "mechanical powers." The efforts of Helmholtz and Mayer in Germany led to the formulation of the law of conservation of energy. At the beginning of the nineteenth century, the central concepts in physics were related to space, time, mass, and force; by the end of the century, however, the concepts of force had changed to those of energy.

Pioneering contributions to metabolism and nutrition came from Germany during the second half of the nineteenth century, particularly from the school established by Carl von Voit. He remains best known for the respiration apparatus designed with his teacher Max von Pettenkofer in Munich. They designed a respiration calorimeter able to measure carbon dioxide output, although they were unable to measure oxygen consumption. This made it possible to establish the daily carbon balance as well as nitrogen balance in a human subject. Max Rubner was trained in the laboratories of Carl von Voit in Munich. He refined the calorimeter and discovered that the heat produced or absorbed was the same irrespective of the pathway providing the end products. He proposed the standard respiratory quotients (carbon dioxide/oxygen) and caloric values for the major foods that are still in use today. He originated the concept that heat had to be lost through the surface of body and so body surface area should have a linear correlation with the energy metabolism of the body. He performed classic studies in the dog that showed that direct measurement of heat production agreed with the indirect calculations from gas exchange, consistent with the law of the conservation of energy.

1890 TO 1920: CALORIMETRY SPREADS TO AMERICA

Many investigators who had received their training in Germany set up their own laboratories elsewhere in Europe or in the United States with a continuing interest in calorimetry (1). W.O. Atwater, an American nutritionist who had studied with Voit, joined forces with the physicist E.B. Rosa to construct a large calorimeter at Wesleyan University in Connecticut that was capable of measuring the heat given off by a man confined in it for prolonged periods. This apparatus confirmed many of Rubner's

experiments and showed conclusively that the food metabolized during external work was equal to the heat produced. The physiologist F.G. Benedict extended Atwater's work by the construction of special facilities in the Carnegie Institution in Boston where simultaneous measurement of gas exchange and heat production could be made.

Calorimetry was developed at the Cornell University Medical College in New York under the direction of Graham Lusk (2) and at the Russell Sage Institute at Bellevue Hospital in New York under the direction of Eugene DuBois (3), both close friends of Rubner. DuBois (3) published extensive studies on the basal metabolic rate (BMR) in different kinds of fever and numerous medical conditions but remains best remembered for demonstrating the use of the BMR in the diagnosis and treatment of thyroid disorders. During the 1920s, there was a major shift away from energy metabolism and calorimetry. Biochemists were becoming interested in enzyme function, and nutritionists were busy searching for new vitamins. Interest in calorimetry was relegated to measuring the BMR as an indicator of thyroid function. This remained a standard hospital measurement until around 1950, when chemical methods for thyroid function caused hospitals to abandon the BMR measurement, thus terminating the last remaining quantitative measure of energy metabolism as part of conventional patient care.

From a thermodynamic standpoint, the human body does not expend energy, but merely converts it from one form to another. Heat cannot be used to perform work in the body. Thus, the body takes in energy in a highly organized form as food and returns an equivalent amount of energy to the environment as heat. The energy balance of the body represents two matched balances that must proceed simultaneously: a substrate balance that determines body composition and a thermal balance that determines body heat content (4).

The development of equipment to measure the production of heat in an animal directly dates back to Lavoisier and Laplace in 1780. Sporadic animal studies continued through the following century, although efforts in Voit's laboratory were unsuccessful in humans. Why were human studies considered important? It was to demonstrate that the law of conservation of energy applied to living persons. Adherents to vitalism still contended that life was special and God–given and was therefore not subject to the laws of energy transfer that applied to steam engines or laboratory chemicals. Atwater and Rosa in 1899 constructed a calorimeter in which they demonstrated that the first law of thermodynamics applied to the human body, a monumental contribution to both human biology and nutrition. After World War II, the study of human heat regulation required more elaborate instrumentation. One of the first of the new gradient layer calorimeters for human studies was built at the Naval Medical Research Institute in Bethesda, Maryland, by Benzinger and his group (5). This new approach was based on thermocouples that measured the passage of heat directly across the jacket of the inclosure, thus providing a rapid response with changes such as exercise. The interest in this new method led, by some accounts, to a broad revival of interest in the field of calorimetry.

1880 TO 1960: METABOLIC BODY SIZE

Rubner in 1883 studied the metabolic rate of fasting dogs of varying sizes and concluded that fasting homeotherms produce daily 1000 kcal of heat/m^2 of body surface. Lusk published a factor to correct for comparisons of animals of different shapes. DuBois and DuBois developed a formula in 1916 that allowed the calculation of surface area of stout and slim individuals more accurately than previous formulas. In attempting to avoid the assumptions involved in the surface law and ill-defined terms related to body surface area, Harris and Benedict (6) established predictions empirically for men and women involving only weight, height, and age. Many other equations have been proposed, but the Harris-Benedict (H-B) equations have been widely used for predicting daily caloric needs of hospitalized patients. Kleiber (7) observed that the basal rate of oxygen consumption within any species is roughly proportional to the body weight to the 0.67 power. This relationship, which has come to be known as the Kleiber law, states that the metabolic rate between species is proportional to the weight to the 0.75 power over a range of animals from mice to elephants.

Some investigators have reported that H-B equations provide values in close agreement with measured gas exchange, whereas others have found that H-B equations overestimate the measured values by 10 to 15% (8). Cunningham (9) examined the results of the H-B equation when compared with the prediction equation of Moore (10) for total body water and the estimated lean body mass. This estimated lean body mass was found to be the best single predictor of the BMR, whereas the influence of sex and age added little to the estimation. These findings suggested that estimations of BMR based on body surface area owed their usefulness to a hidden correlation to the lean body mass in each sex. The "active protoplasmic mass" referred to without measurement by various investigators over past decades appears similar to the "body cell mass" estimated by Moore and coworkers (10) from the isotope dilution measurement of total exchangeable potassium.

1900 TO 1950: MALNUTRITION AND CALORIMETRY

It is part of the common wisdom that the malnourished or partially starved individual will lose weight. However, the use of body weight as a form of nutritional assessment presents a series of questions and uncertainties. Numerous studies have shown that dietary restriction causes a reduction in energy expenditure. One of the most complete studies of human starvation was conducted by Benedict and associates in 1912 (11). A physiologically normal 40-year-old man was maintained continuously for 31 days while receiving only distilled water. He spent his nights sleeping in a bed calorimeter, and his days were occupied with respiration experiments and other tests. He experienced a 22% loss of body weight. Yet the most striking feature of the experiment was the reduction of basal metabolism. The average of direct and indirect measurements of calorimetry showed that, by the end of the third week, his heat production had decreased by 30% at a time when he had lost only 16.7% of his body weight. DuBois stated: "It is evident that the fall in energy metabolism was caused not only by the decreased body and protoplasmic mass, but also by some specific and unknown factor which tends to protect the organism from the evil results of starvation" (3).

A monumental study of partial starvation was conducted by Keys and coworkers (12) during World War II at the University of Minnesota. Young men were given approximately 1600 kcal/day with low-quality protein to simulate the food intake of those under the Nazi occupation. Over a period of 6 months, these men lost approximately 24% of their body weight while the basal energy expenditure decreased by an average of 39%. This finding and other evidence supported the idea that the metabolic rate is reduced more in starvation than would be expected from the reduction in body size. However, at the end of the study, the rate of decrease of the BMR approached zero. Certain of these subjects showed evidence of congestive heart failure during the early days of nutritional rehabilitation. This finding was interpreted as the result of increasing the energy expenditure of the body faster than the depleted myocardium could regain its pumping capacity.

1975 FORWARD: BEDSIDE GAS EXCHANGE

Portable instruments to measure gas exchange at the bedside became available during the 1980s (13). These appeared relatively easy to use but required careful calibration and standardized procedures for meaningful data. Measurements were often performed in patients who had no measurements of nitrogen excretion from which to calculate the proportion of protein in the energy expenditure. Weir (14) analyzed this problem and showed that an estimate of nitrogen excretion could be substituted for the actual measurement in calculating indirect calorimetry, and the usual error would be no more than 2% of the measured value. The gas exchange capabilities of these portable instruments were often designed so the devices could also be used for stress testing and in various aspects of sports medicine. A major stimulus to the use of beside calorimetry came from the introduction of nutritional support in the 1960s. This was particularly associated with the early enthusiasm for total parenteral nutrition that roughly coincided with the introduction of intensive care units for specialized care. Conditions associated with severe weight loss were thought to be the result of extreme resting hypermetabolism (i.e., estimates of two to three times normal were suggested for major burns). Such erroneous estimates probably contributed to the excessive nutrient intakes in the early days of total parenteral nutrition (particularly the high carbohydrate loads given during the early days of "hyperalimentation" in the United States).

The search for the proper clinical application of indirect calorimetry continues today. Some clinicians have concluded that H-B equations can substitute for actual measurements in routine hospital patients. However, some of the pitfalls and errors of reliance on H-B equations were reviewed by McClave and coworkers (15). Although the equations may be acceptable for estimating energy expenditure of groups of patients, the application to an individual patient becomes more uncertain. The general consensus appears to be that the more severe the illness or injury of a patient, the more actual calorimetry measurements are needed rather than reliance on predictive equations.

1982 FORWARD: DOUBLY LABELED WATER METHOD

The doubly labeled water (DLW) method was developed by Lifson and McClintock (16) during the 1960s, following an earlier observation that the oxygen in respired carbon dioxide was in rapid equilibrium with the oxygen in body water. It was concluded that isotopically labeled oxygen in body water would leave the body as water and carbon dioxide, whereas isotopically labeled hydrogen in body water would leave the body as water. Therefore, the turnover rates of isotopic hydrogen- and oxygen-labeled water would differ in an amount proportional to carbon dioxide production. Energy expenditure and other components of material balance, such as oxygen consumption, water intake, and metabolic water production, can be calculated along with the carbon dioxide production by the use of calorimetric equations and the respiratory quotient. This method was validated in animals of differing body composition and food intake and was shown to be readily acceptable in human subjects (17, 18). The equilibration time of up to a week or more provides a single average value for energy expenditure.

The greatest advantage is to allow studies in free-living subjects. The method soon demonstrated that obese subjects generally expend more energy than lean controls in proportion to the fat-free mass. Comparisons were conducted by Seale and coworkers (19) of DLW, direct and indirect calorimetry, and metabolizable energy intake. The daily energy expenditure over 13 days was 15% greater than by DLW when the 24-hour energy expenditure was measured with the calorimeter. Rosenbaum and cowork-

ers (20) also compared DLW with a weight-maintaining energy intake and 24-hour measurements of chamber calorimetry. Results were not significantly different between the DLW and caloric titration, whereas the chamber measurements were significantly lower, presumably because of limitations on physical activity in the chamber. Saltzman and Roberts (21) used the advantages of the DLW to demonstrate that energy expenditure is a critical factor contributing to successful energy regulation in normal individuals, as well as the dysregulation of energy balance that characterizes obesity.

The history of energy metabolism is a fascinating example of how progress depends alternately on new concepts and at other times on new technology that allows elements of the problem to be revealed and objectively measured.

REFERENCES

1. Webb P. Human Calorimeters. New York: Praeger Scientific, 1985.
2. Lusk G. The Elements of the Science of Nutrition. 4th ed. Philadelphia: WB Saunders, 1931:17–174.
3. DuBois EF. Basal Metabolism in Health and Disease. Philadelphia: Lea & Febiger, 1924:17–164.
4. Kinney JM. Energy metabolism: heat, fuel and life. In: Kinney JM, Jeejeebhoy KN, Hill GL et al., eds. Nutrition and Metabolism in Patient Care. Philadelphia: WB Saunders, 1988:3–34.
5. Benzinger TH, Huebscher RG, Minard D et al. J Appl Physiol 1958;12[Suppl 1]:1–24.
6. Harris J, Benedict FA. Biometric Study of Basal Metabolism in Man. Washington, DC: Carnegie Institution, 1919;279:40–4.
7. Kleiber M. The Fire of Life: An Introduction to Animal Energetics. Huntington, NY: Robert E. Kreiger, 1975.
8. Daly JM, Heymsfield SB, Head CA et al. Am Soc Clin Nutr 1980;42:1170–4.
9. Cunningham JJ. Am J Clin Nutr 1980;33:372–4 .
10. Moore FD, Oleson KH, McMurray JD et al. The Body Cell Mass and Its Supporting Environment. Philadelphia: WB Saunders, 1963.
11. Benedict FG. A Study of Prolonged Fasting. Publication 203. Washington, DC: Carnegie Institution, 1915.
12. Keys A, Brozek J, Henschel A et al. The Biology of Human Starvation, vol 1. Minneapolis, MN: University of Minnesota Press, 1950.
13. Kinney JM. JPEN J Parenter Enteral Nutr 1987;11:90S–4S.
14. Weir JB deV. J Physiol 1949;109:1–9.
15. McClave SA, Snider HL, Ireton-Jones C. Nutr Clin Pract 2002; 17:133–6.
16. Lifson N, McClintock RJ. Theoret Biol 1966;12:46–74.
17. Schoeller DA, van Santen E. J Appl Physiol 1982;53:955–9.
18. Schoeller D. J Nutr 1999;129:1765–8.
19. Seale JL, Rumpler WV, Conway JM et al. Am J Clin Nutr 1990; 52:66–71.
20. Rosenbaum M, Ravussin E, Matthews DE et al. Am J Physiol 1996;270:R496–504.
21. Salzman E, Roberts SB. Nutr Rev 1995;53:209–20.

SELECTED READINGS

Concepts of Heat
Elkana Y. The Discovery of the Conservation of Energy. Cambridge, MA: Harvard University Press, 1974.

McKie D, Heathcote NH, Andrade ENdaC. The Discovery of Specific and Latent Heats. London: Edward Arnold, 1935:11–53.

Mendelsohn E. Heat and Life: The Development of the Theory of Animal Heat. Cambridge, MA: Harvard University Press, 1964.

Singer C. A Short History of Anatomy and Physiology from the Greeks to Harvey. New York: Dover, 1957:46–184.

Gas Exchange and Metabolism

Blaxter K. Energy Metabolism in Animals and Man. Cambridge: Cambridge University Press, 1989.

Holmes FL. Claude Bernard and Animal Chemistry. Cambridge, MA: Harvard University Press, 1974:14–117.

Holmes FL. Lavoisier and The Chemistry of Life. Madison, WI: University of Wisconsin, 1985.

Robinson E, McKie D. Partners in Science: Letters of James Watt and Joseph Black. Cambridge, MA: Harvard University Press, 1970.

Uglow J. The Lunar Men: Five Friends whose Curiosity Changed the World. New York: Farrar, Straus and Giroux, 2002: 230–48.

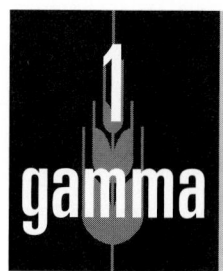

MANAGEMENT OF INFANTILE DIARRHEA AND DEHYDRATION[1]

SAMUEL J. FOMON

INFANTILE DIARRHEA 17
   Early Studies of Diarrhea 17
   Parenteral Administration of Potassium 18
HYPERNATREMIC DEHYDRATION 18
   Renal Function 18
   Insensible Water Loss 18
   Influence of Diet 19
   Epidemiologic Data 19
FINAL COMMENT 19

In pediatrics, as in medicine generally, the gradual accumulation of knowledge in seemingly disparate areas often serves as the basis for changes in patient management and in prevention of disease. In pediatrics, there were exciting early reports on development of an understanding of the role of vitamins, particularly ascorbic acid, and vitamins D and B_6. Among the minerals, the enormous decline in the prevalence of iron deficiency anemia has been a major success story. These events and many others are interwoven into the background of mode of infant feeding. From the 1920s until the early 1970s, the frequency of breast-feeding declined, and most infants were fed formulas, at first prepared in the home and later purchased from infant formula companies (1). Much was learned about infant nutrition from flaws in the design or manufacture of infant formulas (e.g., vitamin B_6 deficiency, chloride deficiency).

Beginning in the 1970s, parents and physicians gradually became convinced that breast-feeding promoted the well-being of infants more than did formula feeding, and most infants today are breast-fed, at least for the early months of life. The return to breast-feeding, although unquestionably desirable, has been associated with an increase in deficiency of iron and vitamin D—nutrients present in much greater concentrations in infant formulas than in human milk. A current educational challenge is dissemination of information about nutritional supplementation of breast-fed infants. Ranking high on the list of current pediatric problems is the management, including nutritional management, of the small preterm infant.

With so many areas to choose from, I have elected to review two areas of fluid and electrolyte balance—diarrhea and hypertonic (hypernatremic) dehydration. Until the 1950s, diarrhea was a prominent cause of infant mortality. Based on research in the 1940s and earlier, a rational and effective treatment of infantile diarrhea was developed, and, by the 1960s, diarrhea was no longer a major contributor to infant mortality. The problem of hypernatremic dehydration was gradually eliminated in the United States in the 1960s and 1970s and was eliminated more suddenly in the United Kingdom in the 1970s.

INFANTILE DIARRHEA

Early Studies of Diarrhea

In the 1920s and 1930s, most physicians believed that the composition of the cellular and extracellular water compartments of the body were resistant to change. Thus, potassium was largely restricted to cellular fluid, whereas chloride and, to a lesser extent, sodium, were predominantly extracellular electrolytes (2). However, as early as 1850, Schmidt, as cited by Darrow (2), demonstrated that in cholera and dysentery, potassium, in addition to water, sodium, and chloride, was lost from the body. This observation was confirmed in clinical studies by other German workers, who noted that the loss of potassium was greater than could be accounted for by the loss of nitrogen. Thus, the loss of potassium could not be entirely explained by cell death with excretion of nitrogen and potassium from the dead cells. In the United States, Holt, Courtney, and Fales (3) also reported that the loss of potassium in diarrheal fluid was greater than could be accounted for by loss of nitrogen, and this finding was later confirmed by Butler and colleagues (4).

Numerous studies relevant to shifts of water and electrolytes between extracellular and cellular compartments were carried out with experimental animals in the early and mid-1930s, but the plethora of studies in the late 1930s and early 1940s, as reviewed by Darrow (5), together with the clinical studies already mentioned, was compelling. Despite this evidence, Govan and Darrow (6) in 1946 wrote, "for all practical purposes no fundamental new principle in the treatment of diarrhea has been introduced in the last twenty years." The treatment of diarrhea in 1946 remained as

---

[1] **Abbreviation: PRSL,** potential renal solute load.

recommended in 1926 by Powers (7), except that repair solutions were more commonly delivered intravenously than intraperitoneally. The solutions contained sodium chloride, sodium bicarbonate (or sodium lactate), and glucose. Blood transfusions were frequently given to maintain the circulation. Food was not given until the diarrhea subsided.

Parenteral Administration of Potassium

The question of why attempts were not made to repair the deficit in potassium appears to be answered by the word *fear*. As stated by Butler and colleagues (4): "Since repair solutions must be placed in the vascular or interstitial compartment, they cannot contain with safety the intracellular components, such as potassium and phosphate, at concentrations above the small values prescribed for them in extracellular fluids."

In a landmark study in 1945 at the Harriet Lane Home in Baltimore, Maryland Govan and Darrow (6) determined mortality from diarrhea during the summer-fall epidemic of diarrhea. The epidemic was so severe that only the most seriously ill infants could be admitted. From the end of June through August, 17 of 53 patients died after receiving conventional treatment. From September through October, potassium was included in the treatment regimen, and only 3 of 50 patients died. The quantity of potassium administered in one infusion was calculated to raise the plasma potassium by 4 or 5 mmol/L under the conservative assumption that all the potassium would remain in extracellular fluid and thus, if the initial plasma potassium concentration was 5 mmol/L, would not reach a concentration high enough to cause heart block. The infusion solution was composed of sodium chloride, potassium chloride, and sodium lactate. After a near-death episode from potassium intoxication in an infant with low urine output, the regimen was altered so, on admission, a transfusion of blood was given to support the circulation, followed by an infusion of normal saline. When urine output was judged to be adequate, infusion of the solution of sodium chloride, potassium chloride, and sodium lactate was begun. The results were dramatic not only with respect to mortality but also because of the demonstration that potassium therapy could be used with relative safety.

In the light of current knowledge and practice, it may seem surprising that the results of Govan and Darrow (6) did not result in immediate and widespread use of potassium in treatment of diarrhea; however, fear of parenteral administration of potassium lingered. Presumably, to decrease this fear, Darrow modified the treatment regimen, giving potassium-containing solutions subcutaneously rather than intravenously. A study involving 153 patients with diarrhea was carried out collaboratively among three institutions in 1948 (8), and evidence of potassium toxicity was not observed. By the middle to late 1950s, potassium therapy became widespread in the treatment of severe diarrhea. In 1951, Darrow

received the Borden Award of the American Academy of Pediatrics for his contributions to the understanding and treatment of diarrhea.

HYPERNATREMIC DEHYDRATION

Hypernatremic dehydration develops when water loss from the body exceeds loss of electrolytes. It is a serious condition that may be associated with seizures and death (9–11). Diets that are quite high in potential renal solute load (PRSL)[1] are generally well tolerated by healthy infants, but such diets are hazardous when infants are ill. During illness, fluid intake is often decreased, and insensible water loss is often increased by fever. These circumstances, superimposed on the limited renal concentrating ability of the infant, predispose to development of hypernatremic dehydration.

Renal Function

When referenced to surface area, a number of researchers reported that glomerular filtration rate, urea clearance, and several other indices of renal function were lower in infants during the first week or first few weeks of life than in adults, as reviewed by McCance and Young (12). However, renal concentrating ability of the infant was little studied until considerably later. The systematic studies of the relation between age and urine concentration under conditions of water deprivation carried out by Winberg (13) (with the addition of an injection of pitressin) and by Poláček and colleagues (14) demonstrated that the ability to concentrate the urine increased from birth until at least 18 months of age and, perhaps more importantly, was variable from infant to infant. Whereas the older child and adult can usually achieve a urine concentration of 1400 mOsm/L, the concentrating ability of some infants is limited to less than 1000 mOsm/L.

Insensible Water Loss

Water loss from the body occurs through skin and lungs (insensible or evaporative loss) and in feces and urine. Loss of water from skin and lungs accounts for the greatest part of water requirement and has been the focus or much research (15–17). Under thermoneutral conditions in healthy term infants, insensible water loss generally ranges from 30 to 70 mL/kg/day and accounts for approximately 80% of total nonrenal water losses. When infants are exposed to elevated environmental temperatures, water losses from skin and lungs may increase greatly (17–19). During 3 days of exposure to an environmental temperature of 32.5 °C and humidity of 30 to 40%, evaporative water losses by seven infants were reported by Cooke and associates (17) to range from 42 to 145 mL/kg/day.

---

[1] PRSL consists of dietary solutes and metabolic products of protein digestion that would require renal excretion if none were cycled into synthesis of new tissue and none were lost through nonrenal routes.

Influence of Diet

In the belief that casein, the major protein of cow milk, was greatly inferior to the whey proteins of human milk, many infant formulas in the 1960s provided 13 to 15% of energy from protein (20). This quantity of protein, when supplied from cow milk, is associated with relatively high concentrations of sodium, potassium, chloride, and phosphorus, leading to high PRSL. Formulas with high PRSL that were commonly fed in the mid-1900s were demonstrated to be associated with development of hypernatremic dehydration (21, 22). Water requirements in relation to the PRSL of the diet were explored by several researchers (23–26). Based on these studies, Fomon and Ziegler (26) recommended that the PRSL of infant formulas be no more than 30 to 35 mOsm/L.

Epidemiologic Data

Epidemiologic data indicate that infants fed formulas providing PRSLs of 39 mOsm/100 kcal or more (e.g., from the evaporated milk formulas commonly fed in the 1940s and 1950s) are at much greater risk of developing hypernatremic dehydration during illness than are breast-fed infants (average PRSL of human milk is about 14 mOsm/L) or those fed currently marketed milk-based formulas (PRSL ~20 mOsm/100 kcal).

Strong circumstantial evidence for the role of dietary PRSL in the development of hypernatremia was provided by observations in the United Kingdom during the 1970s. In the early 1970s, most infants were fed formulas made from National Dried Milk (PRSL similar to that of evaporated milk–based formulas fed in the United States). The formulas fed to such infants presented high PRSLs, and the incidence of hypernatremic dehydration was high (27–29). In 1974, health authorities recommended use of feedings with a lower PRSL (30), and governmental acceptance of this recommendation in 1976 (31) led to discontinuation of feeding National Dried Milk and use of formulas with lower PRSL. Reports (31–34) documented the decrease in the incidence of hypernatremic dehydration in the following years. The close temporal relation between changes in feeding practices and the decline in incidence of hypernatremic dehydration strongly suggested that feedings providing a high PRSL were causally related to development of hypernatremic dehydration.

In the United States, the trend in feeding practices that led to use of formulas with a relatively modest PRSL occurred more gradually, and epidemiologic data comparable to those for the United Kingdom are not available. Nevertheless, once evaporated milk formulas were no longer widely fed, the incidence of hypernatremic dehydration certainly decreased. In hospitals in Bronx, New York, diarrhea and dehydration were reported (35) to account for about 12% of infant admissions from the 1960s through the 1980s. The dehydration was hypernatremic in 19.5% of these infants from 1963 to 1972, 9.3% from 1973 to 1980, and 4.5% in the 1980s.

FINAL COMMENT

Development of effective treatment for infantile diarrhea and prevention of hypernatremic dehydration were possible because pediatric and other researchers accumulated information that could be interpreted by clinicians and eventually put into practice. For the future, there are many challenges in other areas. Perhaps most obvious is the daunting task of providing adequate nutrition to the small preterm infant. Management of preterm infants with birth weights more than 1500 g has become reasonably successful, but management of those with birth weights less than 1000 g continues to present huge problems. As discussed by Heird in Chapter 51, much progress has been made in defining the nutritional requirements of preterm infants. It would be difficult to overestimate the enormity of the task of delivering the required nutrients when one considers the immaturity of the gastrointestinal tract, the need to maintain fluid and electrolyte balance, and the frequent life-and-death decisions that must be made regarding respiratory therapy and prevention and treatment of infections. Nutritional management of the small preterm infant is likely to rank for years among the most important frontiers in pediatrics.

REFERENCES

1. Fomon SJ. J Nutr 2001;131:409S–20S.
2. Darrow DC. J Pediatr 1946;28:515–40.
3. Holt LE, Courtney AM, Fales HL. Am J Dis Child 1915;9:213–24.
4. Butler AM, McKhann CF, Gamble JL. J Pediatr 1933;3:84–92.
5. Darrow DC. Annu Rev Physiol 1944;6:95–122.
6. Govan CD, Darrow DC. J Pediatr 1946;28:541–9.
7. Powers GF. Am J Dis Child 1926;32:232–57.
8. Flett J, Jr Pratt EL, Darrow DC. Pediatrics 1949;4:604–19.
9. Kerpel-Fronius E, Varga F, Kun K. Arch Dis Child 1950;25:156–8.
10. Finberg L. Pediatrics 1959;23:40–5.
11. Morris-Jones PH, Houston IB, Evans RC. Lancet 1967;2:1385–9.
12. McCance RA, Young WF. J Physiol 1941;99:265–82.
13. Winberg J. Acta Paediatr 1959;48:318–28.
14. Poláček E, Vocel J, Neugebauerová L et al. Arch Dis Child 1965;40:291–5.
15. Levine SZ, Wyatt TC. Am J Dis Child 1932;44:732–41.
16. Pratt EL, Bienvenu B, Whyte MM. Pediatrics 1948;1:181–7.
17. Cooke RE, Pratt EL, Darrow DC. Yale J Biol Med 1950;22:227–49.
18. Levine SZ, Wilson JR, Kelly M. Am J Dis Child 1929;37:791–806.
19. Darrow DC, Cooke RE, Segar WE. Pediatrics 1954;14:602–17.
20. Fomon SJ. Infant Nutrition. Philadelphia: WB Saunders, 1967:195–224.
21. Pratt EL, Snyderman SE. Pediatrics 1953;11:65–9.
22. Finberg L, Harrison HE. Pediatrics 1955;16:1–12.
23. Calcagno PL, Rubin MI. J Pediatr 1960;56:717–27.

24. Janovský M, Martínek J, Slechtová R. Physiol Bohemoslov 1968;17:143–51.
25. Bergmann KE, Ziegler EE, Fomon SJ. Water and renal solute load. In: Fomon SJ, Infant Nutrition. 2nd ed. Philadelphia: WB Saunders, 1974:245–66.
26. Fomon SJ, Ziegler EE. J Pediatr 1999;134:11–4.
27. Jacobs SI, Hotzel A, Wolman B et al. Arch Dis Child 1970;45:656–63.
28. Ironside AG, Tuxford AF, Heyworth B. BMJ 1970;3:20–4.
29. Taitz LS, Byers HD. Arch Dis Child 1972;47:257–60.
30. Working Party of the Panel on Malnutrition. Report on Health and Social Subjects 9. Department of Health and Social Security Working Party. London: Her Majesty's Stationary Office, 1974.
31. Arneil GC, Chin KC. Lancet 1979;2:840.
32. Davies DP, Ansari BM, Mandal BK. Am J Dis Child 1979;133: 148–50.
33. Sunderland R, Emery JL. BMJ 1979;2:575–6.
34. Manuel PD, Walker-Smith JA. Arch Dis Child 1980;55:124–7.
35. Finberg L. comment on Ziegler EE, Fomon SJ. J Pediatr 1989;78[Suppl A]:1788.

SELECTED READINGS

Fomon SJ, Ziegler EE. Renal solute load and *potential* renal solute load in infancy. J Pediatr 1999;134:11–4.
King CK, Duggan C. Acute diarrhea. In: Walker WA, Watkins JA, Duggan C, eds. Nutrition in Pediatrics: Basic Science and Clinical Applications. 3rd ed. Hamilton, Ontario, Canada: Decker, 2003:738–91.

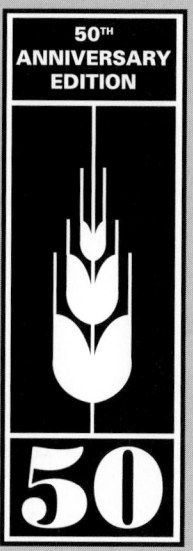

50TH ANNIVERSARY EDITION

PART II

SPECIFIC DIETARY COMPONENTS

A. Major Dietary Constituents and Energy Needs / 23

B. Minerals / 149

C. Vitamins / 351

D. Other Compounds with Health Relevance / 537

E. Signs of Clinical Deficiencies / 595

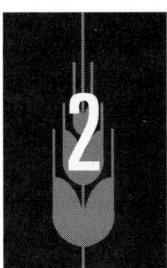

PROTEINS AND AMINO ACIDS[1]

DWIGHT E. MATTHEWS

AMINO ACIDS 24
   Basic Definitions 24
   Amino Acid Pools and Distribution 27
   Amino Acid Transport 28
PATHWAYS OF AMINO ACID SYNTHESIS
   AND DEGRADATION 29
   Amino Acid Degradation Pathways 29
   Synthesis of Dispensable Amino Acids 32
   Incorporation of Amino Acids into
      Other Compounds 33
   Purine and Pyrimidine Biosynthesis 34
TURNOVER OF PROTEINS IN THE BODY 35
METHODS OF MEASURING PROTEIN TURNOVER
   AND AMINO ACID KINETICS 35
   Nitrogen Balance 35
   Using Arteriovenous Differences to Define
      Organ Balances 38
   Tracer Methods Defining Amino Acid Kinetics 38
CONTRIBUTION OF SPECIFIC ORGANS TO PROTEIN
   METABOLISM 46
   Whole-Body Metabolism of Protein
      and Contributions of Individual Organs 46
   Role of Skeletal Muscle in Whole-Body Amino
      Acid Metabolism 48
   Whole-Body Adaptation to Fasting
      and Starvation 48
   The Fed State 48
   Gut and Liver as Metabolic Organs 49
PROTEIN AND AMINO ACID REQUIREMENTS 50
   Protein Requirements 51
   Amino Acid Requirements 53
   Assessment of Protein Quality 55
   Protein and Amino Acid Needs in Disease 57

Proteins are associated with all forms of life, and much of the effort to determine how life began has centered on how proteins were first produced. Amino acids joined together in long strings by peptide bonds form proteins that twist and fold in three-dimensional space producing centers to facilitate the biochemical reactions of life that either would run out of control or not run at all without them. Life could not have begun without these enzymes, thousands of different types of which are found in the body. Proteins are prepared and secreted to act as cell-cell signals in the form of hormones and cytokines. Plasma proteins produced and secreted by the liver stabilize the blood by forming a solution of the appropriate viscosity and osmolarity. These secreted proteins also transport a variety of compounds through the blood.

The largest source of protein in higher animals resides in muscle. Through complex interactions, entire sheets of proteins slide back and forth to form the basis of muscle contraction and all aspects of our mobility. Muscle contraction provides for pumping oxygen and nutrients throughout the body, for inhalation and exhalation of our lungs, and for movement. Many of the underlying causes of noninfectious diseases are the result of derangements in the sequence of proteins. The incredible advances in molecular biology have provided tremendous information about DNA and RNA and have introduced the field of genomics. This research is not driven to understand DNA per se, but rather to understand the purpose and function of the proteins that are translated from the genetic code. Now we have the emerging field of proteomics that does study the expression, modification, and regulation of proteins.

Three major classes of substrates are used for energy: carbohydrates, fat, and protein. Protein differs from the other two primary sources of dietary energy by inclusion of nitrogen (N). Protein on average is 16% by weight N. The component amino acids of proteins contain one N in the form of an amino group and additional N, depending on the amino acid. When amino acids are oxidized to carbon dioxide (CO_2) and water to produce energy, N is also produced as a waste product that must be eliminated via incorporation into urea. Conversely, N must be available when the body synthesizes amino acids de novo. The synthetic routes of other N-containing compounds in the body (e.g., nucleic acids for DNA and RNA synthesis) obtain their N during synthesis from donation of N from

[1]**Abbreviations: Apo-B,** apolipoprotein B; **ATP,** adenosine triphosphate; **AV,** arteriovenous; **BCAA,** branched-chain amino acid; **CO₂,** carbon dioxide; **CoA,** coenzyme A; **DAA,** dispensable amino acid; **DAAO,** direct amino acid oxidation; **EAR,** estimated average requirement; **IAA,** indispensable amino acid; **IAAO,** indicator amino acid oxidation; **KIC,** α-ketoisocaproate; **N,** nitrogen; **RDA,** recommended dietary allowance; **TCA,** tricarboxylic acid; **TML,** trimethyllysine; **VLDL,** very-low-density lipoprotein; **WHO/FAO/UNU,** World Health Organization/Food and Agriculture Organization/United Nations University.

TABLE 2.1. BODY COMPOSITION OF A NORMAL MAN IN TERMS OF ENERGY COMPONENTS

COMPONENT	MASS (kg)	ENERGY (kcal)	AVAILABILITY[a] (d)
Body water and minerals	49	0	0
Protein	6	24,000	13
Glycogen	0.2	800	0.4
Fat	15	140,000	78
Total:	70.2	164,800	91.4

[a] Availability is the duration for which the energy supply would last based on an 1800 kcal/day resting energy consumption.

Data from Cahill GF. N Engl J Med 1970;282:668–75.

amino acids. Therefore, when we think of amino acid metabolism in the body, we really mean N metabolism.

Protein and amino acids are also important in the energy metabolism of the body. As Cahill pointed out (1), protein is the second largest store of energy in the body after adipose tissue fat stores (Table 2.1). Carbohydrate is stored as glycogen, and although important for short-term energy needs, it is of very limited capacity for providing for energy needs beyond a few hours. Amino acids from protein are converted to glucose by the process called gluconeogenesis to provide a continuing supply of glucose after the glycogen is consumed during fasting. Yet, protein stores must be conserved for the numerous critical roles in which protein functions in the body. Loss of more than about 30% of body protein results in reductions in muscle strength for breathing, immune function, and organ function and, ultimately, in death. Hence, the body must adapt to fasting by conserving protein, as is seen by a dramatic decrease in N excretion within the first week of onset of starvation.

Body protein is made up of 20 different amino acids, each with different metabolic fates in the body, with different activities in different metabolic pathways in different organs, and with differing compositions in different proteins. When amino acids are liberated after absorption of dietary protein, the body makes a complex series of decisions concerning the fate of those amino acids: to oxidize them for energy, to incorporate them into proteins in the body, or to use them in the formation of a number of other N-containing compounds. The purpose of this chapter is to elucidate the complex pathways and roles amino acids play in the body, with a focus on nutrition.

AMINO ACIDS

Basic Definitions

The amino acids that we are familiar with and all those incorporated into mammalian protein are "α"-amino acids. By definition, they have a carboxyl-carbon group and an amino-N group attached to a central α-carbon

(Fig. 2.1). Amino acids differ in structure by the substitution of one of the two hydrogens on the α-carbon with another functional group. Amino acids can be characterized by their functional groups, which are often organized at neutral pH into the classes of (a) nonpolar, (b) uncharged but polar, (c) acidic (negatively charged), and (d) basic (positively charged) groups. Within any class are considerable differences in shape and physical properties. Thus, amino acids are often grouped into other functional subgroups. For example, amino acids with an aromatic group, phenylalanine, tyrosine, tryptophan, and histidine, are often associated together, although the tyrosine is clearly polar and histidine is also basic. Other common groupings are the aliphatic or neutral amino acids (glycine, alanine, isoleucine, leucine, valine, serine, threonine, and proline). Proline is different in that its functional group is also attached to the amino group, forming a five-membered ring. Because of the ring, proline is actually an *imino* acid, not an amino acid. Serine and threonine contain hydroxyl groups. There is also another important subgroup: the branched-chain amino acids ([BCAAs] isoleucine, leucine, and valine), which share common enzymes for the first two steps of their degradation. The acidic amino acids, aspartic acid and glutamic acid, are often referred to as their ionized, salt forms: *aspartate* and *glutamate*. These amino acids become *asparagine* and *glutamine* when an amino group is added in the form of an amide group to their carboxyl tails.

The sulfur-containing amino acids are methionine and cysteine. Cysteine is often found in the body as an amino acid dimer called *cystine* in which the thiol groups (the two sulfur atoms) are connected to form a disulfide bond. Particular attention should be paid when reading the literature to note the distinction between the names *cysteine* and *cystine*, because the former is a single amino acid, and the latter is a dimer with different properties. Other amino acids that contain sulfur, such as homocysteine, are not incorporated into protein.

All amino acids exist as charged particles in solution: in water, the carboxyl group rapidly loses a hydrogen to form a carboxyl anion (negatively charged), whereas the amino group gains a hydrogen to become positively charged. The amino acids, therefore, become "bipolar" (often called a *zwitterion*) in solution, but without a net charge (the positive and negatively charges cancel). However, the attached functional group may distort that balance. The acidic amino acids will lose the hydrogen on the second carboxyl group and become negatively charged in solution. In contrast, the basic group amino acids will in part accept a hydrogen on the second N and form a molecule with a net positive charge. Although the other amino acids do not specifically accept or donate additional hydrogens in neutral solution, their functional groups do influence the relative polarity and acid-base nature of the bipolar portion of the amino acids and give each amino acid different properties in solution.

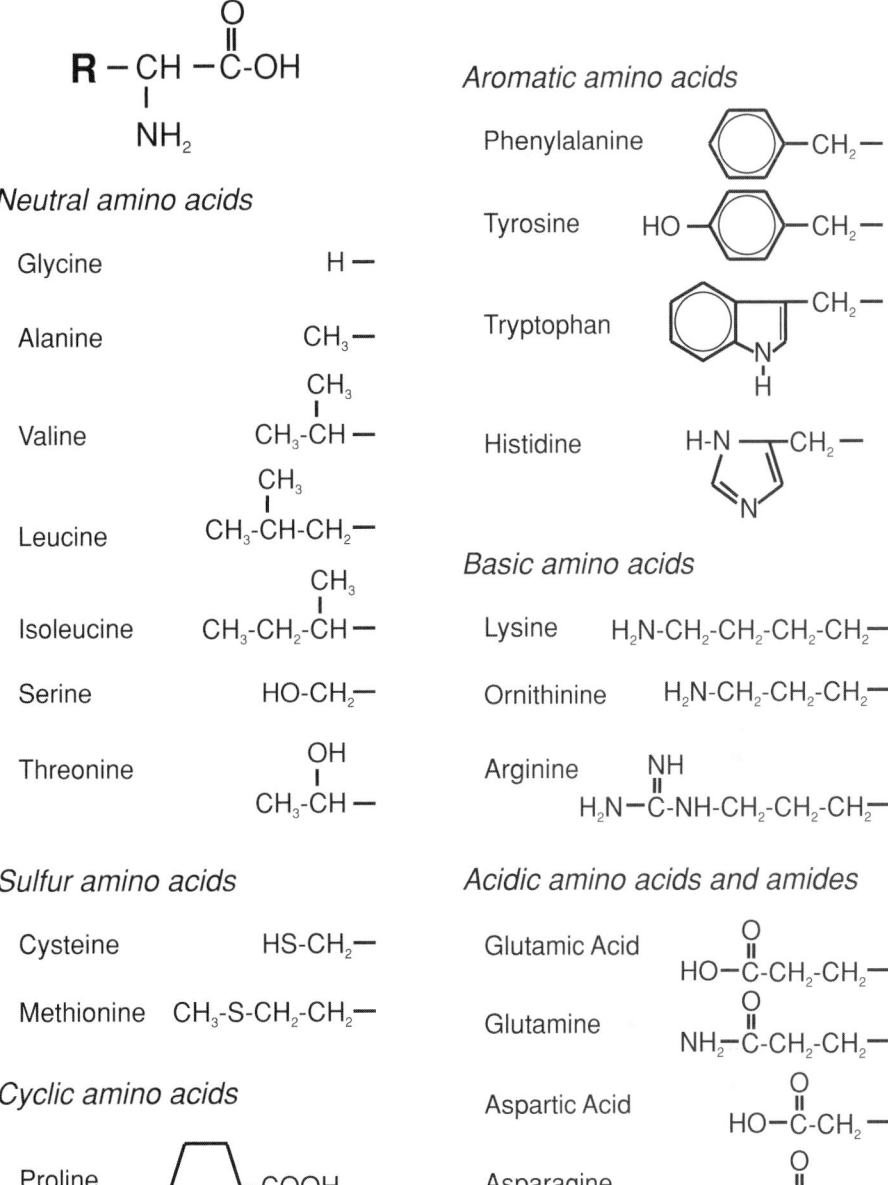

Figure 2.1. Structural formulas of the 21 common α-amino acids. The α-amino acids all have a carboxyl group, an amino group, and a differentiating functional group attached to the α-carbon. The generic structure of amino acids is shown in the **upper left corner** with the differentiating functional marked by an *R*. The functional group for each amino acid is shown below. Amino acids have been grouped by functional class. Proline is actually an imino acid because of its cyclic structure involving its nitrogen (N).

The functional groups of amino acids also vary by size. The molecular weights of the amino acids are shown in Table 2.2. Amino acids range from the smallest, glycine, to the largest, bulky molecule (e.g., tryptophan). Most amino acids crystallize as uncharged molecules when purified and dried. The molecular weights shown in Table 2.2 are reflective of their molecular weight as crystalline amino acids. However, the basic and acidic amino acids tend to form much more stable crystals as salts, rather than as free amino acids. Glutamic acid can be obtained as the free amino acid with a molecular weight of 147 and as its sodium salt, monosodium glutamate, which has a crystalline weight of 169. Lysine is typically found as a hydrogen chloride-containing salt. Therefore, when amino acids

are represented by weight, it is important to know whether the weight is based on the free amino acid or on its salt.

Another important property of amino acids is optical activity. Except for glycine, which has its functional group as a single hydrogen, all amino acids have at least one chiral center: the α-carbon. The term "chiral" comes from Greek for *hand* in that these molecules have a left ("*levo*" or "L") and right ("*dextro*" or "D") handedness to them around the α-carbon atom. Because of the tetrahedral structure of the carbon bonds, there are two possible arrangements of a carbon center with the same four different groups bonded to it that are not superimposable; the two configurations, called *stereoisomers*, are mirror images of each other. The body recognizes only the "L" form of amino acids for most

TABLE 2.2. COMMON AMINO ACIDS IN THE BODY

	STANDARD ABBREVIATION		
	3-LETTER	1-LETTER	MOLECULAR WEIGHT[a]
Indispensable (essential) amino acids			
Isoleucine	Ile	I	131
Leucine	Leu	L	131
Lysine	Lys	K	146
Methionine	Met	M	149
Phenylalanine	Phe	F	165
Threonine	Thr	T	119
Tryptophan	Trp	W	204
Valine	Val	V	117
Histidine[b]	His	H	155
Dispensable (nonessential) amino acids			
Alanine	Ala	A	89
Arginine	Arg	R	174
Aspartic acid	Asp	D	133
Asparagine	Asn	N	132
Glutamic acid	Glu	E	147
Glutamine	Gln	Q	146
Glycine	Gly	G	75
Proline	Pro	P	115
Serine	Ser	S	105
Conditionally dispensable amino acids			
Cysteine	Cys	C	121
Tyrosine	Tyr	Y	181
Some special amino acids			
Citrulline			175
Homocysteine	Hcy		135
Hydroxylysine	Hyl		162
Hydroxyproline	Hyp		131
3–Methylhistidine			169
Ornithine	Orn		132

[a] Molecular weight (daltons) is rounded to the nearest whole number and represents the number of grams per mole of amino acid. Because glutamine is degraded to glutamate when proteins are hydrolyzed, the sum of the glutamine and glutamate together is often abbreviated *Glx*. The same is true also for the sum of asparagine and aspartate: *Asx*. The one-letter abbreviations are often used to indicate protein sequences.
[b] The essentiality for histidine has only been shown for infants, but probably small amounts are needed for adults as well (4).

reactions in the body, although some enzymatic reactions operate with a lower efficiency when given the "D" form. Because we do encounter some "D" form amino acids in the foods that we eat, the body has some mechanisms for clearing these amino acids through renal filtration.

Any number of molecules could be designed that complete the basic definition of an amino acid: a molecule with a central carbon to which an amino group, a carboxyl group, and a functional group are attached. However, a relatively limited variety appears in nature; only 20 are incorporated directly into mammalian protein. Amino acids are selected for protein synthesis when coupled to transfer RNA (tRNA). To synthesize protein, strands of DNA are transcribed into messenger RNA (mRNA). tRNA binds to mRNA in three-base groups. Different combinations of three-consecutive RNA molecules in the mRNA code for different tRNA molecules. However, the three-base combinations of mRNA are recognized by only 20 different tRNA molecules, and 20 different amino acids are incorporated into protein during protein synthesis.

Of these 20 amino acids in proteins, some are synthesized de novo in the body either from other amino acids or from simpler precursors. These amino acids may be deleted from our diet without impairing health or blocking growth. These amino acids are *nonessential* and *dispensable* from the diet. However, no pathways exist for the synthesis of several other amino acids in humans, and hence these amino acids are *essential* or *indispensable* to the diet. The classification of amino acids as nondispensable/dispensable or essential/nonessential for humans is shown in Table 2.2. Both the standard three-letter abbreviation and the one-letter abbreviation used in representing amino acid sequences in proteins are also presented in Table 2.2 for each amino acid. Some dispensable amino acids may become *conditionally indispensable* under conditions when synthesis becomes limited or when adequate amounts of precursors are unavailable to meet the needs of the body (2–4). The history and rationale of the classification of amino acids in Table 2.2 are discussed in greater detail later.

Besides the 20 amino acids that are recognized by tRNA for incorporation into protein, other amino acids appear commonly in the body. These amino acids have important metabolic functions. Examples are ornithine and citrulline, which are linked to arginine through the urea cycle. Other amino acids appear as modifications of amino acids after they have been incorporated into proteins. Examples are hydroxyproline and hydroxylysine, which are produced when proline and lysine residues in collagen protein are hydroxylated, and 3-methylhistidine, which is produced by posttranslational methylation of select histidine residues of actin and myosin proteins. Because no tRNA exists to code for these amino acids, they cannot be reused when a protein containing them is broken down (hydrolyzed) to its individual amino acids.

Amino Acid Pools and Distribution

The distribution of amino acids is complex. Not only are 20 different amino acids incorporated into a variety of different proteins in many different organs in the body, but also amino acids are consumed in the diet from numerous protein sources. In addition, each amino acid is maintained in part as a free amino acid in solution in blood and inside cells. Overall, a wide range of concentrations is found among amino acids across the various protein and free pools that exist. We consume protein in food that is enzymatically hydrolyzed in the alimentary tract, thus releasing free individual amino acids that are then absorbed by the gut lumen and are transported into the portal blood. Amino acids then pass into the systemic circulation and are extracted by different tissues. Although the concentrations of individual amino acids vary among different free pools such as plasma and intracellular muscle, the abundance of individual amino acids is relatively constant in a variety of proteins throughout the body and in nature. Table 2.3

shows the composition of amino acids in egg protein and in muscle and liver proteins (5). The data are expressed as *moles* of amino acid. The historical expression of amino acids is on a weight basis (e.g., *grams* of amino acid). Comparing amino acids by weight skews the comparison toward the heaviest amino acids and makes them appear more abundant than they actually are. For example, tryptophan (molecular weight 204) appears almost three times as abundant as glycine (molecular weight 75) when quoted in terms of weight.

An even distribution of all 20 amino acids would be 5% per amino acid, and the median amino acid content centers around this value for the proteins shown in Table 2.3. Tryptophan is the least common amino acid in many proteins. Considering the effect that tryptophan's large size has on the conformation of proteins, it is not surprising to find less tryptophan in protein. Other amino acids of modest size and limited polarity, such as alanine, leucine, serine and valine, are relatively abundant in protein (8–10% per amino acid). Although the abundance of the indispensable amino acids is similar across the protein sources in Table 2.3, some vegetable proteins are deficient or low in some indispensable amino acids. In the body, certain proteins are particularly rich in specific amino acids to produce specific functions in the protein. For example, collagen is a fibrous protein abundant in connective tissues in tendons, bone, and muscle. Collagen fibrils are arranged in different ways, depending on the functional type of collagen. Glycine comprises about one third of collagen, and there is also considerable proline and hydroxyproline (proline converted after it has been incorporated into collagen). The glycine and proline residues allow the collagen protein chain to turn tightly and intertwine, and the hydroxyproline residues provide for hydrogen bond cross-linking. Generally, the alterations in amino acid concentrations do not vary dramatically among proteins as they do in collagen, but such examples demonstrate the diversity and functionality of the different amino acids in proteins.

The abundance of amino acids varies among amino acids over a far wider range in the free pools of extracellular and intracellular compartments. Typical values of free amino acid concentrations in plasma and in intracellular muscle are shown in Table 2.4. The primary points of Table 2.4 are as follows: (a) amino acid concentrations vary widely among amino acids, and (b) free amino acids are generally concentrated inside cells. Although a significant correlation exists between plasma and muscle free intracellular amino acid levels, the relationship is not linear (6). Concentrations of amino acids range from as low as approximately 20 μM for aspartic acid and methionine to a high of approximately 500 μM for glutamine. The median level for plasma amino acids is 100 μM. No defined relationship exists between the nature of amino acids (indispensable versus dispensable) and amino acid concentrations or type of amino acids (e.g., the three BCAAs plasma concentrations range, 50–250 μM). One notable point is that the concentration of the acidic amino

TABLE 2.3. AMINO ACID CONCENTRATIONS IN MUSCLE AND LIVER PROTEIN AND IN HIGH-QUALITY EGG PROTEIN

| | COMPOSITION (μmol/g PROTEIN) | | |
| | | MAMMALIAN | |
AMINO ACID	HEN EGG	MUSCLE	LIVER
Alanine	810	730	750
Arginine	360	380	328
Aspartate + asparagine	530	600	600
Cysteine	190	120	140
Glutamate + glutamine	810	990	800
Glycine	450	670	610
Histidine	150	180	170
Isoleucine	490	360	380
Leucine	650	610	690
Lysine	425	580	510
Methione	200	170	170
Phenylalanine	340	270	310
Proline	350	430	430
Serine	770	480	510
Threonine	410	390	390
Tryptophan	80	55	80
Tyrosine	220	170	200
Valine	600	470	520

Data from Block RJ, Weiss KW. Amino Acid Handbook: Methods and Results of Analysis. Springfield, IL: Charles C Thomas, 1956.

TABLE 2.4. TYPICAL CONCENTRATIONS OF FREE AMINO ACIDS IN THE BODY

AMINO ACID		PLASMA	CONCENTRATION (mM) INTRACELLULAR MUSCLE	GRADIENT INTRACELLULAR/ PLASMA
Aspartic acid	D	0.02		
Phenylalanine	I	0.05	0.07	1.4
Tyrosine	CI	0.05	0.10	2.0
Methionine	I	0.02	0.11	5.5
Isoleucine	I	0.06	0.11	1.8
Leucine	I	0.12	0.15	1.3
Cysteine	CI	0.11	0.18	1.6
Valine	I	0.22	0.26	1.2
Ornithine		0.06	0.30	5.0
Histidine	I	0.08	0.37	4.6
Asparagine	D	0.05	0.47	9.4
Arginine	D	0.08	0.51	6.4
Proline	D	0.17	0.83	4.9
Serine	D	0.12	0.98	8.2
Threonine	I	0.15	1.03	6.9
Lysine	I	0.18	1.15	6.4
Glycine	D	0.21	1.33	6.3
Alanine	D	0.33	2.34	7.1
Glutamic acid	D	0.06	4.38	73.0
Glutamine	D	0.57	19.45	34.1
Taurine[a]		0.07	15.44	221.0

CI, conditionally indispensable; D, dispensable; I, indispensable.
[a] Taurine is not an amino acid per se, but is highly concentrated in free form in muscle.

Data from Bergström J, Fürst P, Noree LO et al. J Appl Physiol 1974;36:693–7.

acids, aspartate and glutamate, is very low outside cells in plasma. In contrast, the concentration of glutamate is among the highest inside cells, such as muscle (see Table 2.4).

Important to bear in mind are the differences in the relative amounts of N contained in extracellular and intracellular amino acid pools and in protein itself. For a physiologically normal person, there are approximately 55 mg of amino acid N/L outside cells in extracellular space and approximately 800 mg of amino acid N/L inside cells; this means that free amino acids are approximately 15-fold more abundant inside cells than outside cells (6). The second point is that the total pool of free amino acid N is small compared with protein-bound amino acids. Multiplying the free pools by estimates of extracellular water (0.2 L/kg) and intracellular water (0.4 L/kg) provides a measure of the total amount of N present in free amino acids: 0.33 gN/kg body weight. In contrast, body composition studies have shown that the N content of the body is 24 g N/kg body weight (7, 8). Therefore, free amino acids make up only approximately 1% of the total amino N pool versus more than 99% of the amino acids that reside in proteins.

Amino Acid Transport

The gradient of amino acids within and outside cells is maintained by active transport. From a simple scan of

Table 2.4, it is clear that different transport mechanisms must exist for different amino acids to produce the range of concentration gradients observed. Many different transporters exist for different types and groups of amino acids (9–11). Amino acid transport is probably one of the more difficult areas of amino acid metabolism to quantify and characterize. The affinities of the transporters and their mechanisms of transport set the intracellular levels of the amino acids. Generally, the indispensable amino acids have lower intracellular/extracellular gradients than do the dispensable amino acids (see Table 2.4) and are transported by different carriers. The amino acid transporters are membrane-bound proteins that recognize different amino acid shapes and chemical properties (e.g., neutral, basic, or anionic). Transport occurs both into and out of cells. Transport may be thought of as a process that sets the intracellular/extracellular gradient, or the transporters may be thought of as processes that set the rates of amino acid influx into and efflux from cells, which then define the intracellular/extracellular gradients (9). Perhaps the more dynamic concept of transport defining flows of amino acids is more appropriate, but in real life it is the gradient (e.g., intracellular muscle amino acid levels) that is measurable, not the rates.

The transporters fall into two classes: sodium-independent and sodium-dependent carriers. The sodium-dependent carriers cotransport a sodium atom into the cell along with the amino acid. The high extracellular/intracellular sodium gradient (140 mEq outside and 10 mEq inside) facilitates the inward transport of amino acids by the sodium-dependent carriers. These transporters generally produce larger gradients and accumulations of amino acids inside cells than outside them. The sodium entering the cell may be transported out via the sodium-potassium pump that transports a potassium ion in for the removal of a sodium ion.

Few of the transporter proteins have been identified; most information concerning transport has been accrued through kinetic studies of membranes using amino acids and competitive inhibitors or amino acid analogs to define and characterize individual systems. Table 2.5 lists the different amino acid transporters characterized to date and the amino acids they transport. The neutral and bulky amino acids (the BCAAs, phenylalanine, methionine, histidine) are transported by system L. System L is sodium independent and operates with a high rate of exchange and produces small gradients. Other important transporters are systems ASC and A. These transporters use the energy available from the sodium-ion gradient as a driving force to maintain a steep gradient for the various amino acids transported (e.g., glycine, alanine, threonine, serine, and proline) (9, 10). The anionic transporter (X_{AG-}) also produces a steep gradient for the dicarboxylic amino acids, glutamate and aspartate. Other important carriers are system N and N^m for glutamine, asparagine, and histidine. System y^+ handles much of the transport of the basic

TABLE 2.5. AMINO ACID TRANSPORTERS

SYSTEM	AMINO ACID TRANSPORTED	TISSUE LOCATION	pH DEPENDENCE
Sodium dependent			
A	Most neutrals (Ala, Ser)	Ubiquitous	Yes
ASC	Most neutrals	Ubiquitous	No
B	Most neutrals	Intestinal brush border	Yes
N	Gln, Asn, His	Hepatocytes	Yes
N^m	Gln, Asn	Muscle	No
Gly	Gly, sarcosine	Ubiquitous	
X_{AG-}	Glu, Asp	Ubiquitous	
Sodium independent			
L	Leu, Ile, Val, Met, Phe, Tyr, Trp, His	Ubiquitous	Yes
T	Trp, Phe, Tyr	Red blood cells, hepatocytes	No
y^+	Arg, Lys, Orn	Ubiquitous	No
asc	Ala, Ser, Cys, Thr	Ubiquitous	Yes

Data from compilations in references 9 to 11.

amino acids. Some overall generalizations can be made in terms of the type of amino acid transported by a given carrier, but the system is not readily simplified because individual carrier systems transport several different amino acids, whereas individual amino acids are often transported by several different carriers with different efficiencies. Thus, amino acid gradients are formed and amino acids are transported into and out of cells via a complex system of overlapping carriers.

PATHWAYS OF AMINO ACID SYNTHESIS AND DEGRADATION

Several amino acids have their metabolic pathways linked to the metabolism of other amino acids. These codependencies that link the pathways of amino acids become important when nutrient intake is limited or when metabolic requirements are increased. Two aspects of metabolism are reviewed here: (a) synthesis of amino acids and (b) amino acid degradation. Degradation serves two useful purposes: (a) production of energy from the oxidation of individual amino acids ($\approx$4 kcal/g protein, almost the same energy production as for carbohydrate), and (b) conversion of amino acids into other products. The latter is also related to amino acid synthesis: the degradation pathway of one amino acid may be the synthetic pathway of another amino acid. The other important aspect of amino acid degradation is production of other nonamino acid, N-containing compounds in the body. The need for synthesis of these compounds may also drain the pools of their amino acid precursors, thus increasing the need for these amino acids in the diet. When amino acids are degraded for energy rather than converted to other compounds, the ultimate products become CO_2, water and urea. The CO_2 and water are produced through classic pathways of intermediary metabolism involving the tricarboxylic acid (TCA) cycle. The urea is produced because other forms of waste N, such as ammonia, are toxic if their levels rise in the blood and inside cells. For mammals, urea production

is a means of removal of waste N from the oxidation of amino acids in the form of a nontoxic, water-soluble compound.

More detailed descriptions of the amino acid pathways can be found in standard textbooks of biochemistry. Keep in mind when consulting such texts that pathways for non-mammalian systems (e.g., *Escherichia coli* and yeast) are often presented, and these pathways often have little importance to human biochemistry. When consulting reference material, the reader needs to be aware of the system of life from which the metabolic pathways and enzymes are being discussed. Discussion here is relevant to human biochemistry. Presented first is a discussion of the routes of degradation of each amino acid when the pathway is directed toward oxidation of the amino acid for energy. Next follows a discussion of the pathways of amino acid synthesis, and finally comes the use of amino acids for other important compounds in the body.

Amino Acid Degradation Pathways

Complete amino acid degradation ends up with the production of N, which is removed by incorporation into urea. Carbon skeletons are eventually oxidized as CO_2 via the TCA cycle (also known as the Krebs cycle or the citric acid cycle). The inputs to the cycle are acetyl coenzyme A (CoA) and oxaloacetate forming citrate, which is degraded to α-ketoglutarate and then to oxaloacetate. The carbon skeletons from amino acid may enter the Krebs cycle via acetate as acetyl CoA or via oxaloacetate/α-ketoglutarate. These latter two precursors are direct metabolites of the amino acids aspartate and glutamate. Alternative to the complete oxidation of the carbon skeletons to CO_2 is the use of these carbon skeletons for the formation of fat and carbohydrate. Fat is formed from elongation of acetyl units, and so amino acids whose carbon skeletons degrade to acetyl CoA and ketones may alternatively be used for synthesis of fatty acids. Glucose is split in glycolysis to pyruvate, and pyruvate is the immediate product of alanine. Pyruvate may be converted back to glucose by elongation to oxaloacetate. Amino acids whose degradation pathways go toward formation of pyruvate, oxaloacetate, or α-ketoglutarate may be used for synthesis of glucose. Therefore, the degradation pathways of many amino acids can be partitioned into two groups with respect to the disposal of their carbon: amino acids whose carbon skeleton may be used for synthesis of glucose (gluconeogenic amino acids) or those whose carbon skeletons degrade for potential use for fatty acid synthesis.

The amino acids that degrade directly to the primary gluconeogenic and TCA cycle precursors, pyruvate, oxaloacetate, and α-ketoglutarate, do so by rapid and reversible transamination reactions:

$$\text{L-glutamate} + \text{oxaloacetate} \leftrightarrow \alpha\text{-ketoglutarate} + \text{L-aspartate}$$

by the enzyme aspartate aminotransferase, which of course also can be:

$$\text{L-aspartate} + \alpha\text{-ketoglutarate} \leftrightarrow \text{oxaloacetate} + \text{L-glutamate}$$

and:

$$\text{L-alanine} + \alpha\text{-ketoglutarate} \leftrightarrow \text{pyruvate} + \text{L-glutamate}$$

by the enzyme alanine aminotransferase. What is quickly apparent is that the amino-N of these three amino acids may be rapidly exchanged and each amino acid rapidly converted to/from a primary compound of gluconeogenesis and the TCA cycle. As discussed later, compartmentation among different organ pools is the only limiting factor for complete and rapid exchange of the N of these amino acids.

The indispensable amino acids leucine, isoleucine, and valine are grouped together under the heading of the BCAAs because the first two steps in their degradation pathway are common to all three amino acids:

$$\left.\begin{array}{l}\text{Leucine} \\ \text{Isoleucine} \\ \text{Valine}\end{array}\right\} + \alpha\text{-ketoglutarate} \leftrightarrow \text{glutamate} + \left\{\begin{array}{l}\alpha\text{-ketoisocaproate} \\ \alpha\text{-keto-}\beta\text{-methylvalerate} \\ \alpha\text{-ketovalerate}\end{array}\right.$$

The reversible transamination to keto acids is followed by irreversible decarboxylation of the carboxyl group to liberate CO_2. The BCAAs are the only indispensable amino acids that undergo transamination and therefore are unique among indispensable amino acids.

Together, the BCAAs, alanine, aspartate, and glutamate make up the pool of amino-N that can move among amino acids via reversible transamination. As shown in Figure 2.2, glutamic acid is central to the transamination process. In addition, N can leave the transaminating pool via removal of the glutamate N via glutamate dehydrogenase, or it can enter by the reverse process. The amino acid glutamine is intimately tied to glutamate as well: all glutamine is made

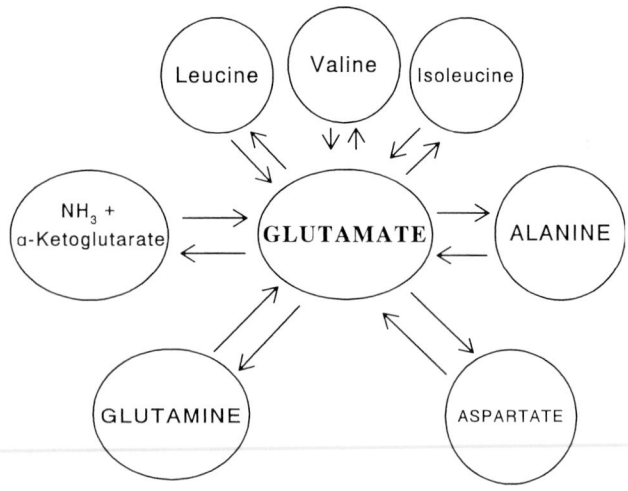

Figure 2.2. Movement of amino-nitrogen (N) around glutamic acid. Glutamate undergoes reversible transamination with several amino acids. Nitrogen is also removed from glutamate by glutamate dehydrogenase, thus producing an α-ketoglutarate and an ammonia. In contrast, the enzyme glutamine synthetase will add an ammonia to glutamate to produce glutamine. Glutamine is degraded back to glutamate by liberation of the amide-N to release an ammonia by a different enzymatic pathway (glutaminase).

from amidation of glutamate, and glutamine is degraded by removal of the amide-N to form ammonia and glutamate. A similar process occurs for formation and degradation of asparagine from aspartate. In terms of N metabolism, Figure 2.2 shows that the center of N flow in the body is through glutamate. This role becomes even clearer when we look at how urea is synthesized in the liver. The inputs into the urea cycle are a CO_2, adenosine triphosphate (ATP), and ammonia to form carbamoyl phosphate, which condenses with ornithine to form citrulline (Fig. 2.3). The second N enters via aspartate to form arginosuccinate, which is then cleaved into arginine and fumarate. The arginine is hydrolyzed by arginase to ornithine, liberating urea. The resulting ornithine can reenter the urea cycle. As mentioned briefly later, some amino acids may liberate ammonia directly (e.g., glutamine, asparagine, and glycine), but most transfer through glutamate first, which is then degraded to α-ketoglutarate and ammonia. The pool of aspartate is small in the body, and aspartate cannot be the primary transporter of the second N into urea synthesis. Rather, aspartate must act like arginine and ornithine: as a vehicle for the introduction of the second N. If so, the second N is delivered by transamination via glutamate, again placing glutamate at another integral point in the degradative disposal of amino acid N.

An outline of the degradative pathways of the various amino acids is presented in Table 2.6. Rather than show individual reaction steps, the major pathways for degradation, including the primary end products, are presented. The individual steps may be found in textbooks of biochemistry or in reviews on the subject, such as the very good chapter by Krebs (12). Because of the importance of

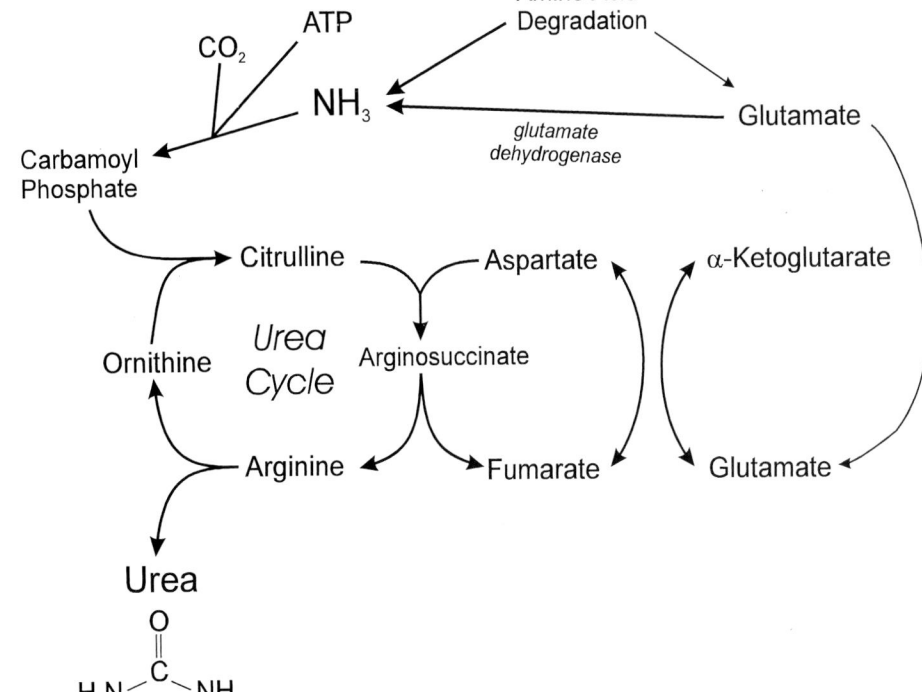

Figure 2.3. Urea cycle disposal of amino acid nitrogen (N). Urea synthesis incorporates one N from ammonia and another from aspartate. Ornithine, citrulline, and arginine sit in the middle of the cycle. Glutamate is the primary source for the aspartate N; glutamate is also an important source of the ammonia into the cycle. ATP, adenosine triphosphate.

TABLE 2.6. PATHWAYS OF AMINO ACID DEGRADATION

METABOLIC PATHWAY	IMPORTANT ENZYMES	NITROGEN END PRODUCTS	CARBON END PRODUCTS
Amino acids converted to other amino acids			
Asparagine	Asparaginase	Aspartate + NH_3	
Glutamine	Glutaminase	Glutamate + NH_3	
Arginine	Arginase	Ornithine + urea	
Phenylalanine	Phenylalanine hydroxylase	Tyrosine	
Proline		Glutamate	
Serine	Serine hydroxymethyltransferase	Glycine	
Cysteine		Taurine	
Amino acids transaminating to form glutamate			
Alanine		Glutamate	Pyruvate
Aspartate		Glutamate	Oxaloacetate
Cysteine		Glutamate	Pyruvate + SO_4^{-2}
Isoleucine		Glutamate	Succinate
Leucine		Glutamate	Ketones
Ornithine		Glutamate	α-Ketoglutarate
Serine		Glutamate	3-Phosphoglycerate
Valine		Glutamate	Succinate
Tyrosine		Glutamate	Ketone + fumarate
Other pathways			
Glycine		NH_3	Carbon dioxide
Histidine		NH_3	Urocanate
Methionine		NH_3	Ketobutryate
Serine	Serine dehydratase	NH_3	Pyruvate
Threonine	Serine dehydratase	NH_3	Ketobutyrate
Tryptophan		NH_3	Kynurenine
Lysine		2 Glutamates	Ketones

NH_3, ammonia.

transamination, the majority of the N from amino acid degradation appears via N transfer to α-ketoglutarate to form glutamate. In some cases, the aminotransferase catalyzes the transamination reaction with glutamate bidirectionally, as indicated in Figure 2.2, and these enzymes are distributed in multiple tissues. In other cases, the transamination reactions are liver specific, are compartmentalized, and act specifically to degrade, not reversibly exchange N. For example, when leucine labeled with the stable isotope tracer ^{15}N was infused into dogs for 9 hours, considerable amounts of the ^{15}N tracer were found in circulating glutamine + glutamate, alanine, the other two BCAAs, but not in tyrosine (13), a finding indicating that the transamination of tyrosine did not proceed backward.

Another reason why the entries in Table 2.6 do not show individual steps is that the specific pathways of the metabolism of all the amino acids are not clearly defined. For example, two pathways for cysteine are shown. Both are active, but how much cysteine is metabolized by which pathway is not as clear. Methionine is metabolized by conversion to homocysteine. The homocysteine is not directly converted to cysteine; rather, homocysteine condenses with a serine to form cystathionine, which is then broken apart to liberate cysteine, ammonia, and ketobutyrate. However, the original methionine molecule appears as ammonia and ketobutyrate. The cysteine carbon-skeleton comes from the serine. So the entry in Table 2.6 shows methionine degraded to ammonia, yet this degradation pathway is the major synthesis pathway for cysteine. Because of the importance of the sulfur-containing amino acids, a more extensive discussion of the metabolic pathways of these amino acids may be found in a later chapter.

Glycine is degraded by more than one possible pathway, depending on the text used for reference. However, the primary pathway appears to be the glycine cleavage enzyme system that breaks glycine into CO_2 and ammonia and transfers a methylene group to tetrahydrofolate (14). This pathway has been shown to be the prominent pathway in rat liver and in other vertebrate species (15). Although this reaction degrades glycine, its importance is the production of a methylene group that can be used in other metabolic reactions.

Synthesis of Dispensable Amino Acids

The indispensable amino acids are those amino acids that cannot be synthesized in sufficient amounts in the body and therefore must be in the diet in sufficient amounts to meets the body's needs. Therefore, discussion of amino acid synthesis applies only to the dispensable amino acids. Dispensable amino acid synthesis falls into two groups: (a) amino acids that are synthesized by transferring a N to a carbon skeleton precursor that has come from the TCA cycle or from glycolysis of glucose and (b) amino acids that are synthesized specifically from other amino acids. Because this latter group of amino acids depends on the

availability of other, specific amino acids, these amino acids are particularly vulnerable to becoming indispensable if the dietary supply of a precursor amino acid becomes limiting. In contrast, the former group is rarely rate limited in synthesis because of the ample precursor availability of carbon skeletons from the TCA cycle and from the labile amino-N pool of transaminating amino acids.

The pathways of dispensable amino acid synthesis are shown in Figure 2.4. As with amino acid degradation, glutamate is central to the synthesis of several amino acids by providing the N for synthesis. Glutamate, alanine, and aspartate may share amino-N transaminating back and forth among them (see Fig. 2.2). As Figure 2.4 is drawn, glutamate derives its N from ammonia with α-ketoglutarate, and that glutamate goes on to promote the synthesis of other amino acids. Kitagiri and Nakamura (16) argued that we have little capacity to form glutamate from ammonia and that the primary source of glutamate N comes from other amino acids via transamination. These amino acids ultimately result from dietary protein intake. Under circumstances of adequate dietary intake, the transaminating amino acids shown in Figure 2.2 supply more than adequate amino-N to glutamate. The transaminating amino acids act to provide a buffer pool of N that can absorb an

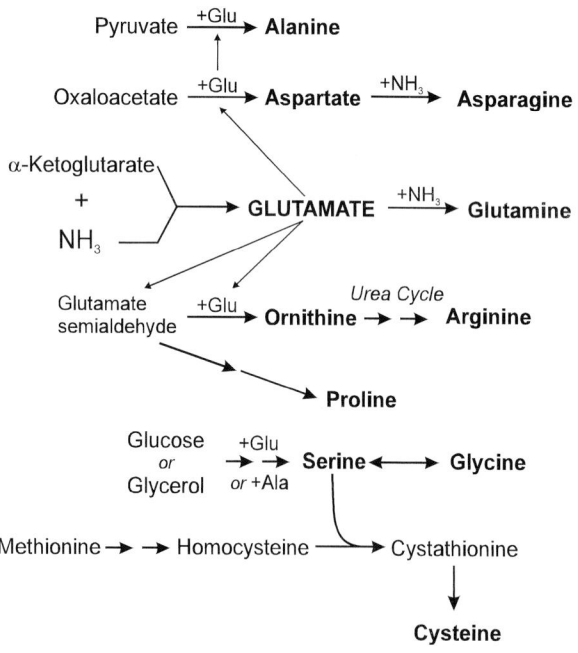

Figure 2.4. Pathways of the synthesis of dispensable amino acids. Glutamate is produced from ammonia and α-ketoglutarate. That glutamate becomes the nitrogen (N) source added to carbon precursors (pyruvate, oxaloacetate, glycolysis products of glucose, and glycerol) to form most of the other dispensable amino acids. Cysteine and tyrosine are different in that they require indispensable amino acid input for their production.

increase in N from increased degradation or supply N when there is a drain. From this pool, glutamate provides material to maintain synthesis of ornithine and proline, of which the latter is particularly important in protein synthesis of collagen and related proteins.

Serine is produced from 3-phosphoglycerate that comes from glycolysis of glucose. Serine may then be used to produce glycine through a process that transfers a methylene group to tetrahydrofolate. This pathway is listed in Table 2.6 as a degradative pathway for serine, but it is also a source of glycine and one-carbon unit generation (14, 15). In contrast, this pathway actively operates backward, forming serine from glycine in humans. When [^{15}N]glycine is given orally, the primary transfer of ^{15}N is to serine (17). Therefore, significant reverse synthesis of serine from glycine occurs. The other major place where ^{15}N appears was in glutamate and glutamine, a finding indicating that the ammonia released by glycine oxidation is immediately picked up and incorporated into glutamate and the transaminating N-pool via glutamate dehydrogenase.

All the amino acids shown in Figure 2.4 have *active* routes of synthesis in the body (12), in contrast to the indispensable amino acids, for which no routes of synthesis exist in humans. This statement should be a simple definition of "indispensable" versus "dispensable." However, we define in nutrition a "dispensable" amino acid as an amino acid that is *dispensable* from the diet (3). This definition is different from defining the presence or absence of enzymatic pathways for an amino acid's synthesis. For example, two of the dispensable amino acids depend on the degradation of indispensable amino acids for their production: cysteine and tyrosine. Although serine provides the carbon skeleton and amino group of cysteine, methionine provides the sulfur through condensation of homocysteine and serine to form cystathionine (18). From the foregoing discussion, neither the carbon skeleton nor the amino group of serine is likely to be in short supply, but provision of sulfur from methionine may become limiting. Therefore, cysteine synthesis depends heavily on the availability of the indispensable amino acid, methionine. The same is also true for tyrosine. Tyrosine is produced by the hydroxylation of phenylalanine, which is also *the* degradative pathway of phenylalanine. The availability of tyrosine is strictly dependent on the availability of phenylalanine and the liver's ability to perform the hydroxylation.

Incorporation of Amino Acids into Other Compounds

Table 2.7 lists some of the compounds that amino acids are converted directly into or are used as important parts of the synthesis of other compounds in the body. The list is not inclusive and is meant to highlight important compounds in the body that depend on amino acids for their synthesis. Other important uses of amino acids are for the synthesis of taurine (19, 20) that is the "amino acid–like"

TABLE 2.7. IMPORTANT PRODUCTS SYNTHESIZED FROM AMINO ACIDS

AMINO ACID	INCORPORATED INTO
Arginine	Creatine
	Nitric oxide
Aspartate	Purines and pyrimidines
Cysteine	Glutathione
	Taurine
Glutamate	Glutathione
	Neurotransmitters
Glutamine	Purines and pyrimidines
Glycine	Creatine
	Glutathione
	Porphyrins (hemoglobin and cytochromes)
	Purines
Histidine	Histamine
Lysine	Carnitine
Methionine	One-carbon methylation/transfer reactions
	Creatine
	Choline
Serine	One-carbon methylation/transfer reactions
	Ethanolamine and choline
Tyrosine	Catecholamines
	Thyroid hormone
Tryptophan	Serotonin
	Nicotinic acid

2-aminoethanesulfonate, found in far higher concentrations inside skeletal muscle than any amino acid (6). Another important, sulfur-containing compound is glutathione (21–23), a tripeptide composed of glycine, cysteine, and glutamate.

Carnitine (24) is important in the transport of long-chain fatty acids across the mitochondrial membrane before fatty acids can be oxidized. Carnitine is synthesized from ε-N,N,N-trimethyllysine (TML) (25). TML synthesis from free lysine has not been demonstrated in mammalian systems; rather, TML appears to arise from methylation of peptide-linked lysine. The TML is liberated when the proteins containing the TML are broken down (25). TML can also arise from hydrolysis of ingested meats. In contrast to 3-methylhistidine, TML can be found in proteins of both muscle and other organs such as liver (26). In rat muscle, TML is about one eighth as abundant as 3-methylhistidine. Using such comparisons of 3-methylhistidine to TML concentration in muscle protein and rates of 3-methylhistidine release in the rat (27), Rebouche estimated that the protein breakdown in a rat would release approximately 2 μmol TML/day that could be used for the estimated approximately 3 μmol/day of carnitine synthesized (25). These calculations suggest that carnitine requirements can be met from synthesis from TML from protein plus that carnitine that enters from dietary intake.

Amino acids are the precursors for a variety of neurotransmitters that contain N. Glutamate may be an exception in that it serves both as a precursor for neurotransmitter production and itself is a primary neurotransmitter (28).

Glutamate appears important in a variety of neurodegenerative diseases from amyotrophic lateral sclerosis to Alzheimer disease. (29). Tyrosine is the precursor for catecholamine synthesis. Tryptophan is the precursor for serotonin synthesis. Various studies have reported the importance of plasma concentrations of these and other amino acids on the synthesis of their neurotransmitter products. The most common putative relationship cited is the administration of tryptophan increasing brain serotonin levels.

Creatine and Creatinine

Most of the creatine in the body is found in muscle, where it exists primarily as creatine phosphate (30). When muscular work is performed, the creatine phosphate provides the energy through hydrolysis of its "high-energy" phosphate bond, thus forming creatine with transferal of the phosphate to form an ATP. The reaction is reversible and is mediated by the enzyme ATP-creatine transphosphorylase (also known as creatine phosphokinase).

The original pathway of creatine synthesis from amino acid precursors was defined by Bloch and Schoenheimer in an elegant series of experiments using ^{15}N-labeled compounds (31). Creatine is synthesized outside muscle in a two-step process (Fig. 2.5). The first step occurs in the kidney and involves the transfer of guanidino group of arginine onto the amino group of glycine to form ornithine and guanidinoacetate. Methylation of the guanidinoacetate occurs in the liver via S-adenosylmethionine to create creatine. Although glycine donates an N and carbon backbone to creatine, arginine must be available to provide the guanidino group, as well as methionine for donation of the methyl group. Creatine is then transferred to muscle, where creatine is phosphorylated. When creatine phosphate is hydrolyzed in muscle to form creatine, most of the creatine is recycled back to the phosphate form when ATP requirements are reduced to restore the creatine phosphate supply. However, a nonenzymatic process forming creatinine continually dehydrates some of the muscle creatine pool. Creatinine is not retained by muscle, but is released into body water, is then removed by the kidney from blood, and is excreted into urine (32).

The daily rate of creatinine formation is remarkably constant (≈1.7% of the total creatine pool/day) and dependent on the mass of the creatine/creatine-phosphate pool, which is proportional to muscle mass (33). Thus, daily urinary output of creatinine has been used as a measure of total muscle mass in the body. Urinary creatinine excretion increases within a couple days after a creatine load has been added to the diet, and several more days are required after removal of creatine from the diet before urinary creatinine excretion returns to baseline, a finding indicating that creatine in the diet per se affects creatinine production (34). Therefore, consumption of creatine and creatinine in meat-containing foods will increase urinary creatinine measurements. Although urinary creatinine

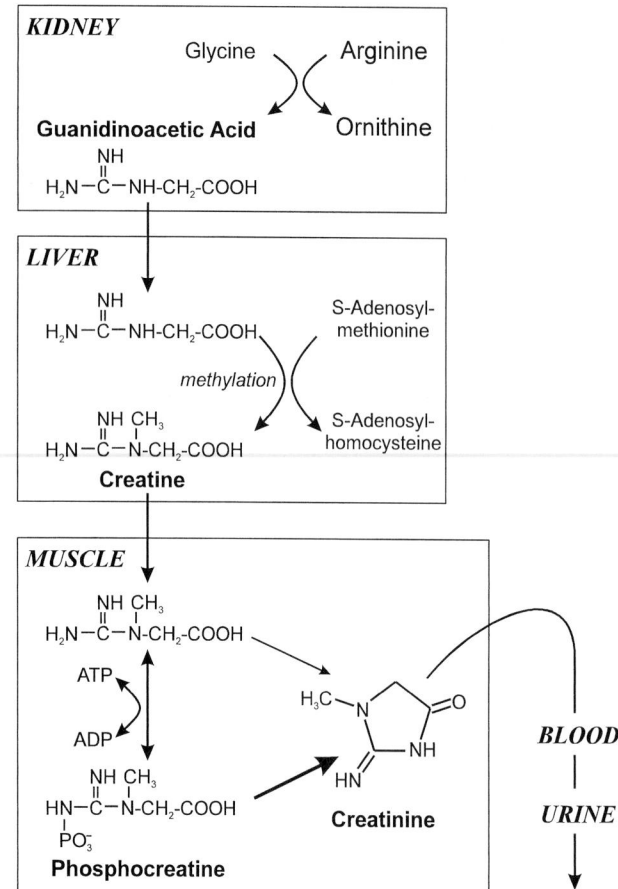

Figure 2.5. Synthesis of creatine and creatinine. Creatine is synthesized in the liver from guanidinoacetic acid that is synthesized in the kidney. Creatine taken up by muscle is primarily converted to phosphocreatine. Although there is some, limited direct dehydration of creatine directly to creatinine, the majority of the creatinine comes from dehydration of phosphocreatine. Creatinine is rapidly filtered by the kidney into urine. ADP, adenosine diphosphate; ATP, adenosine triphosphate.

measurements have been used primarily to estimate the adequacy of 24-hour urine collections, with adequate control of food composition and intake, creatinine excretion measurements are useful and accurate indices of body muscle mass (35, 36), especially when the alternatives are much more difficult and expensive radiometric approaches.

Purine and Pyrimidine Biosynthesis

The purines (adenine and guanine) and the pyrimidines (uracil and cytosine) are involved in many intracellular reactions when high-energy diphosphates and triphosphates have been added. These compounds also form the building blocks of DNA and RNA. Purines are heterocyclic double-ring compounds synthesized using phosphoribosylpyrophosphate sugar as a base to which the amide N of glutamine is added, followed by the attachment of a glycine molecule, a methylene group from tetrahydrofolate, and an amide N from another glutamine to form the imidazole ring. Then CO_2 is added, followed by the amino

N of aspartic acid and another carbon to form the final ring to produce inosine monophosphate, a purine attached to a ribose phosphate sugar. The other purines, adenine and guanine, are formed from inosine monophosphate by the addition of a glutamine amide-N or aspartate amino-N to make guanosine monophosphate or adenosine monophosphate, respectively. These compounds can be phosphorylated to make the high-energy diphosphate and triphosphate forms: adenosine diphosphate, ATP, guanosine diphosphate, and guanosine triphosphate.

In contrast to purines, pyrimidines are not synthesized after attachment to a ribose sugar. The amide-N of glutamine is condensed with a CO_2 to form carbamoyl phosphate, which is further condensed with aspartic acid to make orotic acid, the pyrimidine's heterocyclic 6-member ring. The enzyme forming carbamoyl phosphate is present in many tissues for pyrimidine synthesis, but it is not the same enzyme as found in the liver that makes urea (see Fig. 2.3). However, a block in the urea cycle causing a lack of adequate amounts of arginine to prime urea synthesis cycle in the liver will result in diversion of unused carbamoyl phosphate to orotic acid and pyrimidine synthesis (37). Uracil is synthesized as uridine monophosphate by forming orotidine monophosphate from orotic acid followed by decarboxylation. Cytosine is formed by adding the amide group of glutamine to uridine triphosphate to form cytidine triphosphate.

TURNOVER OF PROTEINS IN THE BODY

As indicated earlier, proteins in the body are not static. Just as every protein is synthesized, it is also degraded. The concept that proteins are continually made and degraded in the body at different rates was first described by Schoenheimer and Rittenberg, who first applied isotopically labeled tracers of amino acids to the study of amino acid metabolism and protein turnover in the 1930s. We now know that the rate of turnover of proteins in the body spans a broad range and that the rate of turnover of individual proteins tends to follow their function in the body; that is, those proteins whose concentrations need to be regulated (e.g., enzymes) or that act as signals (e.g., peptide hormones) have relatively high rates of synthesis and degradation as a means of regulating concentrations. Conversely, structural proteins such as collagen and myofibrillar proteins or secreted plasma proteins have relatively long lifetimes. However, there must overall be a balance between synthesis and breakdown of proteins. Balance in healthy adults who are neither gaining or losing weight will be that the amount of N consumed as protein in the diet will match the amount of N lost in urine, feces, and other routes. However, considerably more protein is mobilized in the body every day than is consumed (Fig. 2.6).

Although no definable entity such as "whole-body protein" exists, the term is very useful for understanding the amount of energy and resources spent by the body in producing and breaking down protein in the body. Several methods using isotopically labeled tracers have been defined to quantitate the whole-body turnover of proteins. An important point of Figure 2.6 is that the overall turnover of protein in the body is severalfold greater than the input of new dietary amino acids (38). A physiologically normal adult may consume 90 g of protein that is hydrolyzed and absorbed as free amino acids. Those amino acids mix with amino acids entering from protein breakdown from a variety of proteins. Approximately one third of the amino acids appear from the large, but slowly turning over, pool of muscle protein. In contrast, considerably more amino acids appear and disappear from proteins in the visceral and internal organs. These proteins make up a much smaller proportion of the total mass of protein in the body, but they have rapid synthesis and degradation rates. The overall result is that approximately 340 g of amino acids will enter the free pool daily, of which only 90 g will come from dietary amino acids. The question becomes the following: How do we assess the turnover of protein in the human body? As noted from Figure 2.6, the issue quickly becomes complex. Much effort has been spent in defining methods that can express in quantifiable and meaningful terms various aspects of human protein metabolism. The methods that have been developed and applied with success to date are listed in Table 2.8. These methods, which range from simple and noninvasive to expensive and complicated, are described in the following sections.

METHODS OF MEASURING PROTEIN TURNOVER AND AMINO ACID KINETICS

Nitrogen Balance

The oldest (and most widely used) method to follow changes in body N has been the N balance method. Because of its simplicity, the N balance technique has been the standard of reference for defining minimum levels of dietary protein and indispensable amino acid intakes in persons of all ages (39). Subjects are placed for several days on a specific level of amino acid and/or protein intake,

---

TABLE 2.8. METHODS OF MEASURING PROTEIN METABOLISM IN HUMANS

Nitrogen balance
Arterial-venous measurement of amino acids and/or tracer across a tissue bed
End-product method
Turnover of individual components:
   Indispensable amino acids (index of protein breakdown)
   Dispensable amino acids (de novo synthesis and gluconeogenesis)
   Urea (amino acid oxidation)
Tracer *into* a specific protein to measure protein synthesis
Tracer *out of* a specific protein to measure protein degradation

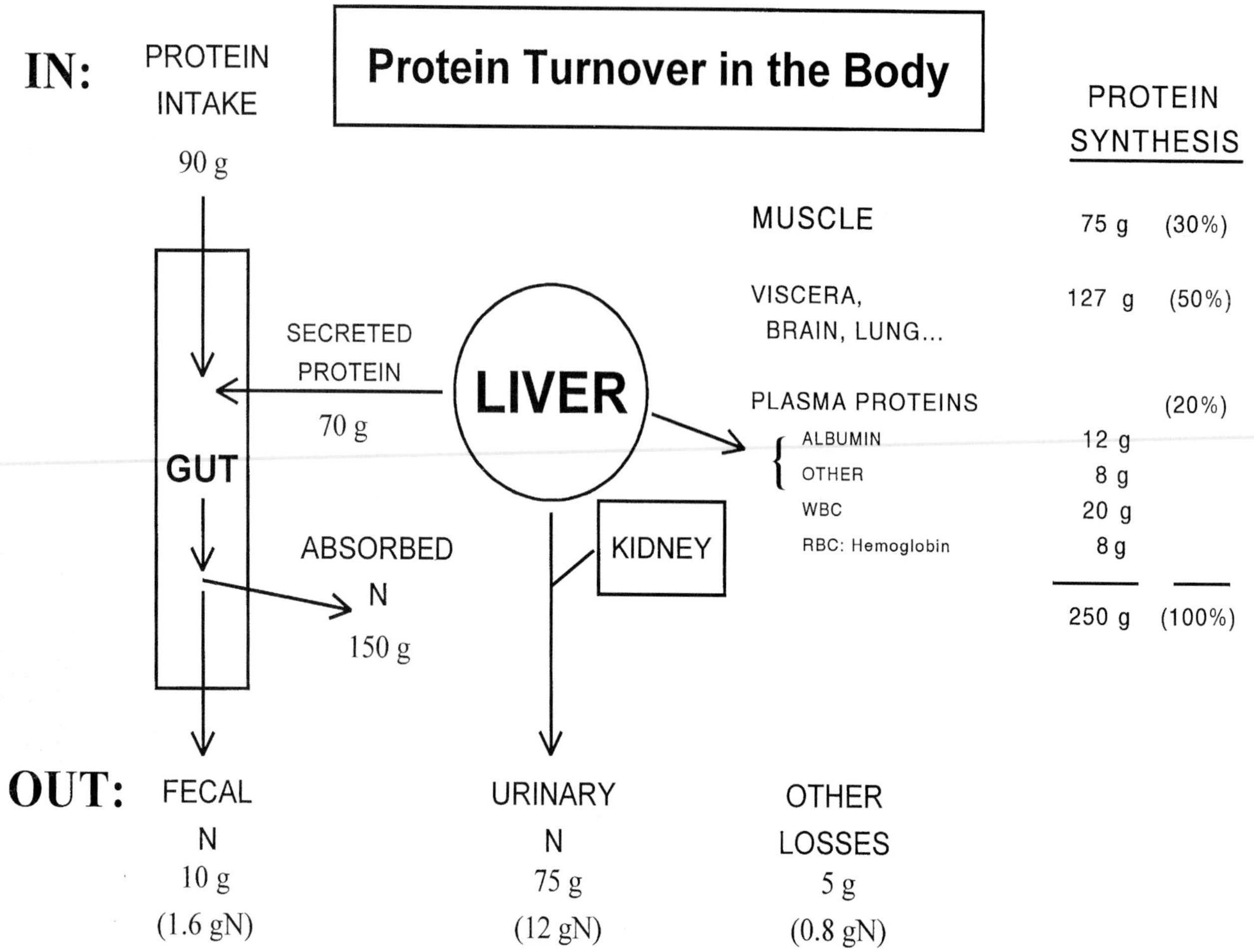

IN:

PROTEIN INTAKE

90 g

Protein Turnover in the Body

PROTEIN SYNTHESIS

MUSCLE	75 g	(30%)
VISCERA, BRAIN, LUNG...	127 g	(50%)
PLASMA PROTEINS		(20%)
ALBUMIN	12 g	
OTHER	8 g	
WBC	20 g	
RBC: Hemoglobin	8 g	
	250 g	(100%)

SECRETED PROTEIN
70 g

GUT

LIVER

ABSORBED
N
150 g

KIDNEY

OUT:

FECAL
N
10 g
(1.6 gN)

URINARY
N
75 g
(12 gN)

OTHER
LOSSES
5 g
(0.8 gN)

Figure 2.6. Relative rates of protein turnover and intake in a healthy 70-kg human. Under normal circumstances, dietary intake (IN = 90 g) will match nitrogen (N) losses (OUT = 90 g). Protein breakdown will then match synthesis. Protein intake is only 90/(90 + 250) ≈ (25% of total turnover of N in the body per day. (Redrawn from Hellerstein MK, Munro HN. In: Arias IM, Jakoby WB, Popper H et al., eds. The Liver: Biology and Pathobiology. 2nd ed. New York: Raven Press, 1988:965–83.)

and their urine and feces are collected over a 24-hour period to measure their N excretion. A week or more may be required before collection will reflect adaptation to a dietary changed. A dramatic example of adaptation is the

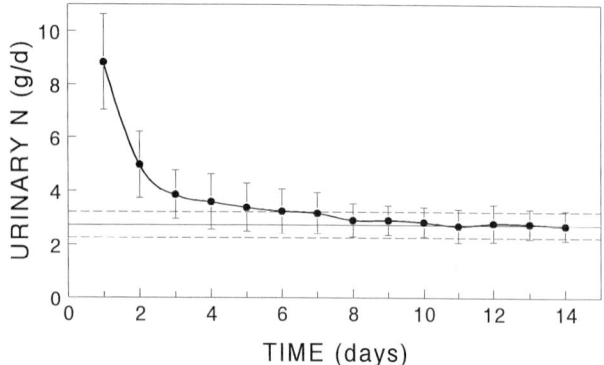

Figure 2.7. Time required for urinary nitrogen (N) excretion to stabilize after changing from an adequate to a deficient protein intake in young men. *Horizontal solid and broken lines* are mean ±1 standard deviation for N excretion at the end of the measurement period. (Data from Scrimshaw NS, Hussein MA, Murray E et al. J Nutr 1972;102: 1595–604.)

placement of healthy persons on a diet containing a minimal amount of protein. As shown in Figure 2.7, urinary N excretion drops dramatically in response to the protein-deficient diet over the first 3 days and stabilizes at a new lower level of N excretion by day 8 (40).

The N end products excreted in the urine are not only end products of amino acid oxidation (urea and ammonia), but also of other substances such as uric acid from nucleotide degradation and creatinine (Table 2.9). Fortunately, most of the nonurea, nonammonia N is relatively constant over a variety of situations and is a relatively small proportion of the total N in the urine. Most of the N is excreted as urea, but ammonia N excretion will increase significantly when subjects become acidotic, as is apparent in Table 2.9 when subjects fasted for 2 days (41). Table 2.9 also illustrates how urea production is related to N intake and how the body adapts its oxidation of amino acids to follow amino acid supply; that is, with ample supply, excess amino acids are oxidized and urea production is high, but with insufficient supply of dietary amino acids, amino acids are conserved and urea production is greatly decreased.

TABLE 2.9. COMPOSITION OF THE MAJOR NITROGEN-CONTAINING SPECIES IN URINE

N SPECIES	HIGH-PROTEIN DIET (g N/d)	LOW-PROTEIN DIET	FASTING (day 2)
Urea	14.7 (87%)	2.2 (61%)	6.6 (75%)
Ammonia	0.5 (3%)	0.4 (11%)	1.0 (12%)
Uric acid	0.2 (1%)	0.1 (3%)	0.2 (2%)
Creatinine	0.6 (4%)	0.6 (17%)	0.4 (5%)
Undetermined	0.8 (5%)	0.3 (8%)	0.5 (6%)
Total:	16.8 (100%)	3.6 (100%)	8.7 (100%)

Data from Folin (1905) and Cathcart (1907) cited in Allison JB, Bird JWC. Elimination of nitrogen from the body. In: Munro HN, Allison JB, eds. Mammalian Protein Metabolism. New York: Academic Press, 1964:483–512.

N appears in the feces because the gut does not completely absorb all dietary protein and reabsorb all N secreted into the gastrointestinal tract (see Fig. 2.6). In addition, N is lost from skin via sweat as well as via shedding of dead skin cells. Additional losses occur through hair, menstrual fluid, nasal secretions, and so forth. As N excretion in the urine decreases in the case of subjects on a minimal-protein diet (see Fig. 2.7), it becomes increasingly important to account for N losses through nonurine, nonfecal routes (42). The loss of N by these various routes is shown in Table 2.10. Most of the losses that are not readily measurable are minimal (<10% of total N loss under conditions of a protein-free diet in which adaptation has greatly reduced urinary N excretion) and can be discounted by use of a simple offset factor for nonurine, nonfecal N losses. The assessment of losses comes into play in the finer definition of where zero balance occurs as a function of dietary protein intake for the purpose of determining amino acid and protein requirements. As discussed later, small changes in N balance corrections make significant changes in the assessment of protein requirements using N balance.

Although the N balance technique is very useful and easy to apply, it provides no information about the inner workings of the system. An interesting analogy for the N balance technique is illustrated in Figure 2.8, in which the simple model of N balance is represented by a gumball machine. Balance is taken between "coins in" and "gumballs out." However, we should not come to the conclusion that the machine turns coins into gum, although that conclusion is easy to reach with the N balance method. What the N balance technique fails to provide is information about what occurs *within* the system (i.e., inside the gumball machine). Inside the system is where the changes in whole-body protein synthesis and breakdown actually occur (shown as the *smaller arrows* into and out of the *Body N Pool* in Fig. 2.8). A further illustration of this point is made at the bottom of Figure 2.8, in which a positive increase in N balance has been observed going from zero (case 0) to positive balance (cases A to D). A positive N balance could be obtained with identical increases in N balance by any of four different alterations

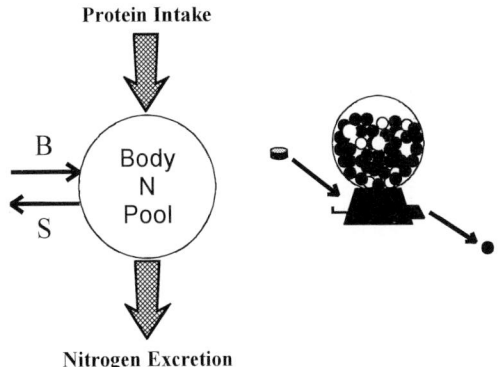

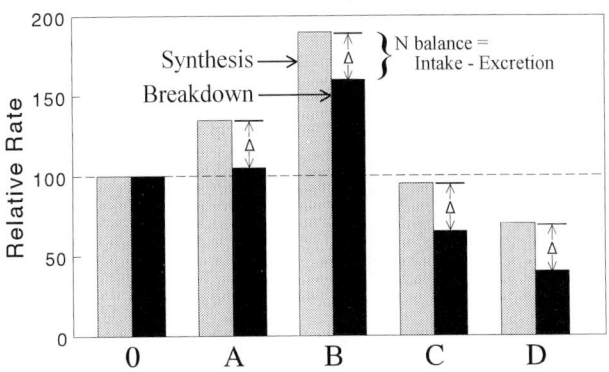

TABLE 2.10. OBLIGATORY NITROGEN LOSSES BY ADULT MEN ON A PROTEIN-FREE DIET

	DAILY NITROGEN LOSS	
	AS NITROGEN (mg N/kg/d)	AS PROTEIN EQUIVALENT (g PROTEIN/kg/d)
Urine	37	0.23
Feces	12	0.08
Cutaneous	3	0.02
Other	2	0.01
Total	54	0.34
Upper limit (+2 standard deviations)	70	0.44

Data from Munro HN. Amino acid requirements and metabolism and their relevance to parenteral nutrition. In: Wilkinson AW, ed. Parenteral Nutrition. London: Churchill Livingstone, 1972:34–67.

Figure 2.8. Illustration of the nitrogen (N) balance technique. N balance is simply the difference between input and output that is similar to the introduction of a coin into a gumball machine resulting in the release of a gumball. The perception of only the "in" and "out" observations is that the machine changed the coin directly into a gumball or that the dietary intake becomes directly the N excreted without consideration of amino acid entry from protein breakdown (B) or uptake for protein synthesis (S). This point is further illustrated with four different hypothetic responses to a change from a zero N balance (case 0) to a positive N balance (cases A to D). A positive N balance can obtained by increasing protein synthesis (A), by increasing synthesis more than breakdown (B), by decreasing breakdown (C), or by decreasing breakdown more than synthesis (D). The N balance method does not distinguish among the four possibilities.

in protein synthesis and breakdown: a simple increase in protein synthesis (case A), a decrease in protein breakdown (case C), an increase in both protein synthesis and breakdown (case B), or a decrease in both (case D). The effect is the same positive N balance for all four cases, but the energy implications are considerably different. Because protein synthesis costs energy, cases A and B are more expensive, whereas cases C and D require less energy than the starting case 0. To resolve these four cases, we have to look directly at rates of protein turnover (breakdown and synthesis) using a labeled tracer.

Using Arteriovenous Differences to Define Organ Balances

Just as the N balance technique can be applied across the whole body, so can the balance technique be applied across a whole organ or tissue bed. These measurements are made from the blood delivered to the tissue and from the blood emerging from the tissue via catheters placed in an artery to define arterial blood levels and the vein draining the tissue to measure venous blood levels. This latter catheter makes the procedure particularly invasive when applied to organs such as gut and liver, kidney, or brain (43–46). Less invasive are measures of muscle metabolism inferred from measurement of arteriovenous (AV) differences across the leg or the arm (45). Even measurements across fat depots have been performed (47). However, the AV difference provides no information about the mechanism within the tissue that causes the observed uptake or release. More information is gleaned from measurement of amino acids that are not metabolized within the tissue, such as the release of indispensable amino acids tyrosine or lysine that are not metabolized by muscle. Their AV differences across muscle should reflect the difference between net amino acid uptake for muscle protein synthesis and release from muscle protein breakdown. 3-Methylhistidine, an amino acid that is produced by posttranslational methylation of selected histidine residues in myofibrillar protein and that cannot be reused for protein synthesis when it is released from myofibrillar protein breakdown, is quantitatively released from muscle tissue when myofibrillar protein is degraded (27, 48). Its AV difference can used as a specific marker of myofibrillar protein breakdown (49–51).

The limited data set of simple balance values across an organ bed is greatly enhanced when a tracer is administered and its balance is also measured across an organ bed. This approach allows for a complete solution of the various pathways operating in the tissue for each amino acid tracer used. In some cases, the measurement of tracer can become very complicated, requiring measurement of multiple metabolites to provide a true metabolite balance across the organ bed (52). Another approach using a tracer of a nonmetabolized indispensable amino acid was

described by Barrett and colleagues (53). This method requires a limited set of measurements with simplified equations to define specifically rates of protein synthesis and breakdown in muscle tissue. The conceptual simplicity of this approach with a limited set of measurements required makes it extremely useful for defining muscle specific changes in response to a variety of perturbations, such as local infusion of insulin into the same muscle bed (54). This approach has been expanded by others (55–57).

Tracer Methods Defining Amino Acid Kinetics

To follow flows of *endogenous* metabolites in the body, isotopically labeled tracers are used. The labeled tracers are identical to the endogenous metabolites in terms of chemical structure by substitution of one or more atoms with isotopes different from those usually present. The substitution of isotopes is done to make the tracers distinguishable (measurable) from the normal metabolites. We usually think first of the radioactive isotopes (e.g., ^{3}H for hydrogen and ^{14}C for carbon) as tracers that can be measured by the particles they emit when they decay, but nonradioactive, stable isotopes can also be used. Because isotopes of the same atom differ only in the number of neutrons that are contained, they can be distinguished in a compound by mass spectrometry that determines the abundance of compounds by mass. Most of the lighter elements have one *abundant* stable isotope and one or two isotopes of higher mass of *minor abundance*. The major and minor isotopes are ^{1}H and ^{2}H for hydrogen, ^{14}N and ^{15}N for N, ^{12}C and ^{13}C for carbon, and ^{16}O, ^{17}O, and ^{18}O for oxygen. Except for some isotope effects that can be significant for both the radioactive (^{3}H) and nonradioactive (^{2}H) hydrogen isotopes, a compound that is isotopically labeled will be essentially indistinguishable from the corresponding unlabeled endogenous compound in the body. Because they do not exist in nature and so little of the radioactive material is administered, radioisotopes are considered "weightless" tracers that do not add material to the system. Radioactive tracer data are expressed as counts or disintegrations per minute per unit of compound. Because the stable isotopes are naturally occurring (e.g., $\approx$1% of all carbon in the body is ^{13}C), the stable isotope tracers are administered and measured as "the excess above the naturally occurring abundance" of the isotope in the body as either the *mole ratio* of the amount of tracer isotope divided by the amount of unlabeled material or the *mole fraction* (usually expressed as a percentage: *mole % excess* or *atom % excess*, the latter being an older and less appropriate term in the literature) (58).

The basis of most tracer measurements to determine amino acid kinetics is the simple concept of tracer dilution. This concept is illustrated in Figure 2.9 for the determination of the flow of water in a stream. If you infuse a dye of known concentration (enrichment) into the stream,

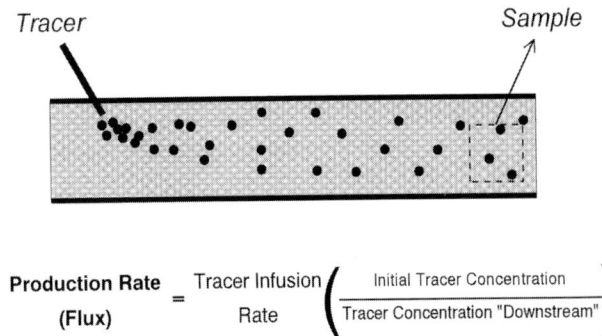

$$\text{Production Rate (Flux)} = \frac{\text{Tracer Infusion Rate}}{} \left(\frac{\text{Initial Tracer Concentration}}{\text{Tracer Concentration "Downstream"}} \right)$$

Figure 2.9. Basic principle of the "dye-dilution" method of determining tracer kinetics.

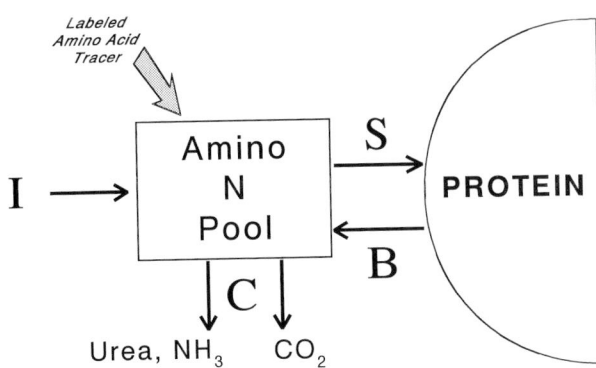

Figure 2.10. Single-pool model of whole-body protein metabolism measured using a labeled amino acid tracer. Amino acid enters the free pool from dietary intake (I) and amino acid released from protein breakdown (B) and leaves the free pool via amino acid oxidation (C) to urea, ammonia (NH_3), and carbon dioxide (CO_2) and via uptake for protein synthesis (S). N, nitrogen.

go downstream after the dye has mixed well with the stream water, and take a sample of the dye, then you can calculate from the measured dilution of the dye the rate at which water must be flowing in the stream to make that dilution. The necessary information required is infusion rate of dye (tracer infusion rate) and measured concentration of the dye (enrichment or specific activity of the tracer). The calculated value is the flow of water through the stream (flux of unlabeled metabolite) causing the dilution. This simple dye-dilution analogy is the basis for almost all kinetic calculations in a wide range of formats for a wide range of applications. A few of the more important approaches are discussed in the following sections.

Models for Whole-Body Amino Acid and Protein Metabolism

The limitations to using tracers to define amino acid and protein metabolism are largely driven by how the tracer is administered and where it is sampled. The simplest method of tracer administration is orally, but intravenous administration is preferred to deliver the tracer *systemically* (to the whole body) into the free pool of amino acids. The simplest site of sampling of the tracer dilution is also from the free pool of amino acids via blood. Therefore, most approaches to measuring amino acid and protein kinetics in the whole body using amino acid tracers have assumed a single, free pool of amino N, as shown in Figure 2.10. Amino acids enter the free pool from dietary amino acid intake (enteral or parenteral) and from amino acids released from protein breakdown. Amino acids leave the free pool by amino acid oxidation to end products (CO_2, urea, and ammonia) and from amino acid uptake for protein synthesis. The free amino acid pool can be viewed from the standpoint of all of the amino acids together (as discussed for the end-product method) or from the viewpoint of a single amino acid and its metabolism per se. The reason the model in Figure 2.10 is called a "single-pool model" is because protein is not viewed as a pool per se, but rather as a source of entry of unlabeled amino acids into the free pool and also as a route of amino acid removal for protein synthesis. Only a small portion of the

proteins in the body is assumed to turn over during the time course of the experiment. Obviously, these assumptions are not true: many proteins in the body are turning over rapidly (e.g., most enzymes). Those proteins that do turn over during the time course of the experiment will become labeled and appear as part of the free amino acid pool. However, these proteins make up only a fraction of the total protein; the remainder turns over slowly (e.g., muscle protein). Most amino acids entering via protein breakdown and leaving for new protein synthesis are coming from proteins that are turning over slowly. These flows are the "B" and "S" arrows of the traditional single-pool model of whole-body protein metabolism shown in Figure 2.10.

End-Product Approach

The earliest model of whole-body protein metabolism in humans was applied by San Pietro and Rittenberg in 1953 using [^{15}N]glycine (59). Glycine was used as the first tracer because glycine is the only amino acid without an optically active α-carbon center, and therefore it is easy to synthesize with a ^{15}N label. At that time, measurement of the tracer in plasma glycine was very difficult. Thus, San Pietro and Rittenberg proposed a model based on something that could be readily measured, urinary urea and ammonia. The assumption was that the urinary N end products reflected the average enrichment of ^{15}N of all the free amino acids oxidized. Although glycine ^{15}N was the tracer, the tracee was assumed to be *all* free amino acids (assumed to be a single pool). However, it quickly became obvious that the system was more complicated and that a more sophisticated model and solution were required. In essence, the method languished until 1969, when Picou and Taylor-Roberts (60) proposed a simpler method that also followed the glycine ^{15}N tracer into urinary N. Their method dealt only with the effect of the dilution of the ^{15}N tracer in the free amino acid pool as a whole, rather than invoking solution of tracer specific equations of a specific model. Their assumptions were

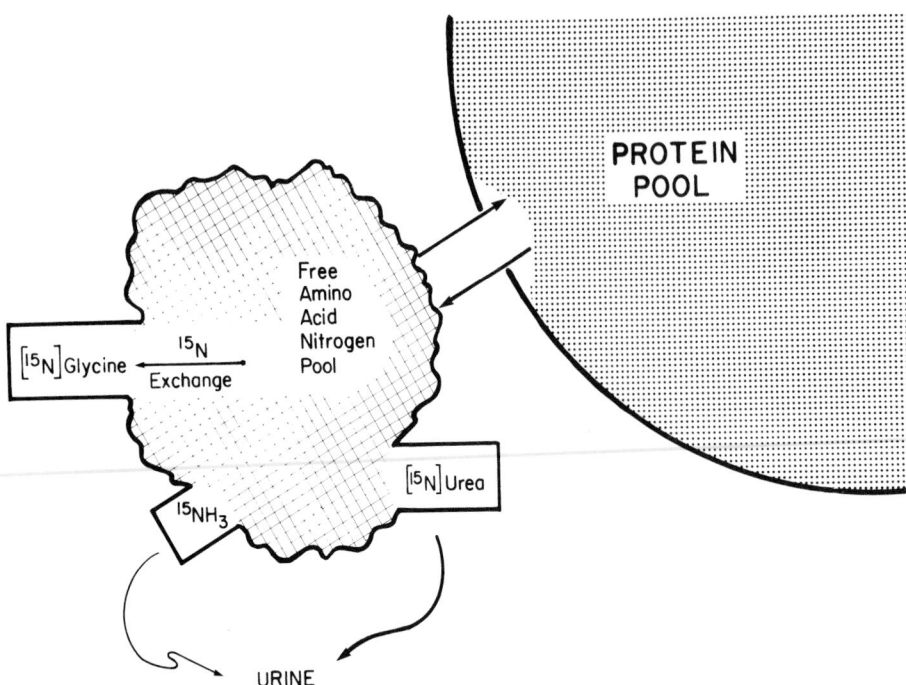

Figure 2.11. Model for measurement of protein turnover using [^{15}N]glycine as the tracer and measurement of the dilution of the ^{15}N tracer in urinary end products, urea and ammonia. (From Bier DM, Matthews DE. Fed Proc 1982;41: 2679–85, with permission.)

similar to the earlier Rittenberg approach in that they assumed that the ^{15}N tracer mixes (scatters) among the free amino acids in some distribution that is not required to be known, but is representative of amino acid metabolism per se. This distribution of ^{15}N tracer could be measured in the end products of amino acid metabolism, urea and ammonia. These assumptions allow the model to become "fuzzy" as shown in Figure 2.11, in that an explicit definition of the inner workings is not required. The [^{15}N]glycine tracer is administered (usually orally), and urine samples are obtained to measure the ^{15}N dilution in the free amino acid pool (61). The ^{15}N in the free amino acid pool is diluted with unlabeled amino acid entering from protein breakdown and from dietary intake. The turnover of the free pool (Q, typically expressed as mg N/kg/day) is calculated from the measured the dilution of ^{15}N in the end products via the same approach illustrated in Figure 2.9:

$$Q = i / E_{UN}$$

where i is the rate of [^{15}N]glycine infusion (mg ^{15}N/kg/day), and E_{UN} is the ^{15}N enrichment in atom % excess ^{15}N in urinary N (either urea and/or ammonia). The free pool is assumed to be in steady state (neither increasing or decreasing over time), and therefore, the turnover of amino acid will be equal to the rate of amino acids entering via whole-body protein breakdown (B) and dietary intake (I) and also equal to the rate of amino acids leaving via uptake for protein synthesis (S) and via amino acid oxidation to the end products urea and ammonia (C):

$$Q = I + B = C + S$$

Because dietary intake should be known and urinary N excretion is measured, the rate of whole-body protein

breakdown can be determined: B = Q − I, as well as the rate of whole-body synthesis: S = Q − C. In these calculations, the standard value of 6.25 g protein = 1 g N is used to interconvert protein and urinary N. Attention to the units (g of protein versus g of N) is important, because both units are often used concurrently in the same report.

Occasionally, the term "net protein balance" or "net protein gain" appears in the literature. Net protein balance is defined as the difference between the measured protein synthesis and breakdown rates (S-B) that can be determined from whole-body protein breakdown and synthesis measured as shown earlier. However, as can be seen by rearranging the balance equation for Q: S − B = I − C, which is simply the difference between intake and excretion, that is, N balance. The S-B term is a misnomer in that it is based solely on the N balance measurement, not on the administration of the ^{15}N tracer.

Without question, the end-product method of Picou and Taylor-Roberts is a cornerstone method for protein metabolic research in humans and is especially well suited for studies of infants and children because it is noninvasive, requiring only oral administration of tracer and collection only of urine. However, the end-product method is not without its problems, the most serious of which are mentioned in the following paragraphs.

When the [^{15}N]glycine tracer is given orally at short intervals (e.g., every 3 hours) the time required to reach a plateau in urinary urea ^{15}N is about 60 hours regardless of whether adults (17, 62), children, or infants (63, 64) are studied. The delay in attaining a plateau results from the time required for the ^{15}N tracer to equilibrate within the free glycine, serine, and urea pools (17, 61). An additional problem is plateau definition. Often, the urinary urea ^{15}N time course does not show by either visual inspection or curve-fitting regression the anticipated single exponential rise to plateau. To avoid this problem, Waterlow and colleagues (65) suggested measuring the ^{15}N in ammonia after a *single dose* of [^{15}N]glycine. The advantage is that the ^{15}N tracer passes through the body ammonia pool within 24 hours. Tracer administration and urine collection are greatly simplified, and the modification does not depend on defining a plateau in urinary urea ^{15}N. The caveat here is the dependence of the single-dose end-product method on *ammonia* metabolism. Urinary ammonia ^{15}N enrichment is also usually different from the urinary urea ^{15}N enrichment (66) because the amino-^{15}N precursor for ammonia synthesis is of renal origin, whereas the amino-^{15}N precursor for urea synthesis is of hepatic origin. Which enrichment should be used? Probably the urea ^{15}N, but it is difficult to prove either way.

The primary difficulty with the end-product method is highlighted by a report in which several different ^{15}N-labeled amino acid tracers, including ^{15}N-glycine and some ^{15}N-labeled proteins, were compared as tracers for the end-product method. Widely divergent results were determined for protein turnover (results ranging from 2.6–17.8 g/kg/day), depending on the ^{15}N label administered (67). The differences reflected differences in the metabolism and distribution of the ^{15}N label when placed into different amino acids and illustrated how dependent the end-product approach is on the metabolism of the amino acid tracer. Therefore, it is difficult to determine whether a change in end-product ^{15}N enrichment may be attributable either to a change in protein turnover *or* to a change in the distribution of ^{15}N resulting from changes in tracer metabolism *that may be independent* from changes in protein metabolism. To make these distinctions, measurement of the kinetics of the amino acid tracer in the body needs to be performed as well.

Measurement of the Kinetics of Individual Amino Acids

Alternative to measuring the turnover of the whole amino-N pool per se, the kinetics of an individual amino acid can be followed from the dilution of an infused tracer of that amino acid. The simplest models consider only indispensable amino acids that have no de novo synthesis components. The kinetics of indispensable amino acids mimics the kinetics of protein turnover, as shown in Figure 2.10. The same type of model can be constructed, but cast specifically in terms of a single indispensable amino acid, and the same steady-state balance equation can be defined:

$$Q_{aa} = I_{aa} + B_{aa} = C_{aa} + S_{aa}$$

where Q_{aa} is the turnover rate (or flux) of the indispensable amino acid, I_{aa} is the rate that the amino acid is entering the free pool from dietary intake, B_{aa} is the rate of amino acid entry from protein breakdown, C_{aa} is the rate of amino acid oxidation, and S_{aa} is the rate of amino acid uptake for protein synthesis. The most common method for defining amino acid kinetics has been a primed infusion of an amino acid tracer until isotopic steady state (constant dilution) is reached in blood. The flux for the amino acid is measured from the dilution of the tracer in the free pool. Knowing the tracer enrichment and infusion rate and measuring the tracer dilution in blood samples taken at plateau, the rate of unlabeled metabolite appearance is determined (58, 68, 69):

$$Q_{aa} = i_{aa} \bullet [E_i/E_p - 1]$$

where i_{aa} is the infusion rate of tracer with enrichment E_i (mole % excess) and E_p is the blood amino acid enrichment.

For a carbon-labeled tracer, the amino acid oxidation rate can be measured from the rate of $^{13}CO_2$ or $^{14}CO_2$ excretion (58, 68). The choice of a carbon label that is quantitatively oxidized is critical. For example, the ^{13}C of a L-[1-^{13}C]leucine tracer is quantitatively released at the first irreversible step of leucine catabolism. In contrast, a ^{13}C-label in the leucine tail will end up in acetoacetate or acetyl CoA, which may or may not be quantitatively oxidized (70). Other amino acids, such as lysine, have even more nebulous pathways of oxidation.

Before the oxidized carbon label is recovered in exhaled air, it must pass through the body bicarbonate pool. Therefore, information about body bicarbonate kinetics is required (71). To complete the oxidation rate calculation based on the measured recovery of the administered carbon label as CO_2, we must know what fraction of bicarbonate pool turnover is release of CO_2 into exhaled air versus retention for alternative fates in the body. In general, only approximately 80% of the bicarbonate produced is released immediately as expired CO_2, as determined from infusion of a labeled bicarbonate and measurement of the fraction infused that is recovered in exhaled CO_2 (72). The other approximately 20% is retained in bone and metabolic pathways that "fix" carbon. The amount of bicarbonate retained is somewhat variable (ranging from 0–40% of its production) and needs to be determined when different metabolic situations are investigated. When retention of bicarbonate in the body may change with metabolic perturbation, parallel studies measuring the recovery of an administered dose of ^{13}C- or ^{14}C-labeled bicarbonate are indispensable in interpretation of the oxidation results (73, 74).

The rates of amino acid release from protein breakdown and of uptake for protein synthesis are calculated by subtracting dietary intake and oxidation from the flux of an indispensable amino acid, just as is done with the end-product method. The primary distinction is that the measurements are specific to a single amino acid's kinetics (micromole of amino acid per unit of time), rather than directly in terms of N per se. Flux components can be extrapolated to whole-body protein kinetics by dividing the amino acid rates by the assumed concentration of the amino acid in body protein (as shown in Table 2.3).

The principal advantages in measuring the kinetics of an individual metabolite are as follows: (a) the results are specific to *that* metabolite, thus improving the confidence of the measurement; and (b) the measurements can be performed quickly because turnover time of the free pool is usually rapid (a tracer infusion study can be completed in less than 4 hours using a priming dose to reduce the time required to come to isotopic steady state). Drawbacks to the measurement of the kinetics of an individual amino acid are as follows: (a) an appropriately labeled tracer may not be available to follow the pathways of the amino acid studied, especially with regard to amino acid oxidation; and (b) metabolism of amino acids occurs within cells, but the tracers are typically administered into and sampled from the blood outside cells.

α-Ketoisocaproate as a Measure of Leucine Cellular Transport. Amino acids do not freely pass through cells; they are transported. For the neutral amino acids (leucine, isoleucine, and valine, phenylalanine, and tyrosine), transport in and out of cells may be rapid, and only a small concentration gradient between plasma and intracellular milieus exists (see Table 2.4). However, even that small gradient will limit exchange of intracellular and extracellular amino acids. For leucine, this phenomenon can be defined using α-ketoisocaproate (KIC), which is formed from leucine inside cells by transamination. Some of the KIC formed is then decarboxylated, but most of it is either reaminated to reform leucine (75) or released from cells into plasma. Thus, plasma KIC enrichment can be used as a marker of intracellular leucine enrichment from which it came (76).

Previous workers showed that, generally, plasma KIC enrichment is approximately 25% lower than plasma leucine enrichment (69, 76, 77). If plasma KIC enrichment is substituted for the plasma leucine tracer enrichment into the calculation of leucine kinetics, then the measured leucine flux and oxidation and, likewise, estimates of protein breakdown and synthesis are increased by approximately 25%. However, when protein metabolism is studied under two different conditions and the resulting leucine kinetics is compared, the same relative response will be obtained regardless of whether leucine or KIC enrichment is used for the calculation of kinetics (76). The prudent approach is to measure both species and to note occasions when the KIC-to-leucine enrichment ratio has changed, to signal a possible change in the partitioning of amino acids between intracellular and extracellular spaces (78).

Use of KIC to represent intracellular leucine is an application of a *concept* that adds definition to the model shown in Figure 2.12, but it does not require a more rigorous *model* to describe leucine kinetics. Because of confusion over what is a suitable model to describe leucine kinetics, experiments were performed to develop a true

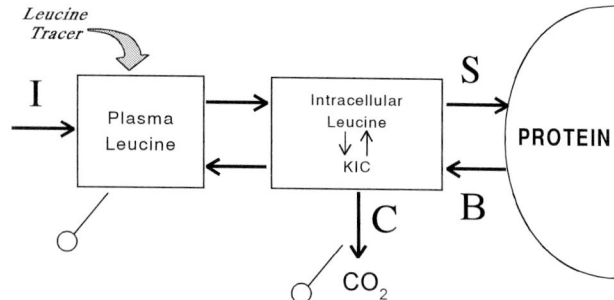

Figure 2.12. Two-pool model of leucine kinetics. The leucine tracer is administered to the plasma pool (*large arrow*) and is sampled either from plasma or from exhaled carbon dioxide (CO_2) (*circles with sticks*). Plasma leucine exchanges with intracellular leucine where metabolism occurs: uptake for protein synthesis (S) or conversion to α-ketoisocaproate (KIC). Oxidation (C) occurs from KIC. Unlabeled leucine enters into the free pool via dietary intake (I) or via protein breakdown (B) into intracellular pools.

multicompartmental model for the leucine-KIC system (79). A model consisting of four leucine and three KIC pools was required to account for leucine kinetics. Clearly, the kinetics of individual metabolites is far more complex than one- or two-compartment models. However, the conventional model using KIC as the precursor enrichment for calculating leucine kinetics as shown in Figure 2.12 agreed well with the multicompartmental model, a finding meaning that under many metabolic circumstances, the simpler approaches should follow accurately directional changes without requiring introduction of complicated compartmental models. These and intermediate models have been reviewed (69, 80), and the various assumptions, limitations, strengths, and weaknesses have been discussed. The leucine/KIC tracer system remains the single most commonly applied measure of whole-body amino acid kinetics to reflect changes in protein metabolism (78).

Most amino acids do not have a convenient metabolite that can be readily measured in plasma to define aspects of their intracellular metabolism, but an intracellular marker for leucine does not necessarily authenticate leucine as the tracer for defining whole-body protein metabolism. Various investigators measured the turnover rate of many of the amino acids, both indispensable and dispensable, in humans for purposes of defining aspects of the metabolism of these amino acids. The general trend of what the amino acid kinetic data from these studies represent was reviewed by Bier (69). The fluxes of indispensable amino acids should represent their release rates from whole-body protein breakdown for postabsorptive humans who have no dietary intake. Therefore, if the Waterlow model of Figure 2.10 is a reasonable representation of whole-body protein turnover, the individual rates of indispensable amino acid turnover should be proportional to each amino acid's content in body protein, and a linear relationship of amino acid flux and amino acid abundance in body protein should exist. That relationship is shown in Figure 2.13 for data

Figure 2.13. Fluxes of individual amino acids, measured in postabsorptive humans, plotted against amino acid concentration in protein. The *closed circles* are for dispensable amino acids, and the *open circles* represent indispensable amino acids. The *regression line* is for the flux of the indispensable amino acids versus their content in protein. *Error bars* represent the range of reported values that were taken from various reports in the literature of studies of amino acid kinetics in healthy persons eating adequate diets of nitrogen and energy intake studied in the postabsorptive state. The amino acid content of protein data are taken for muscle values from Table 2.3. The regression line slope of 4.1 g protein/kg/day is similar to other estimates of whole-body protein turnover. (Redrawn from DM Bier. Diabetes Metab Rev 1989;5:111–32, with additional data.)

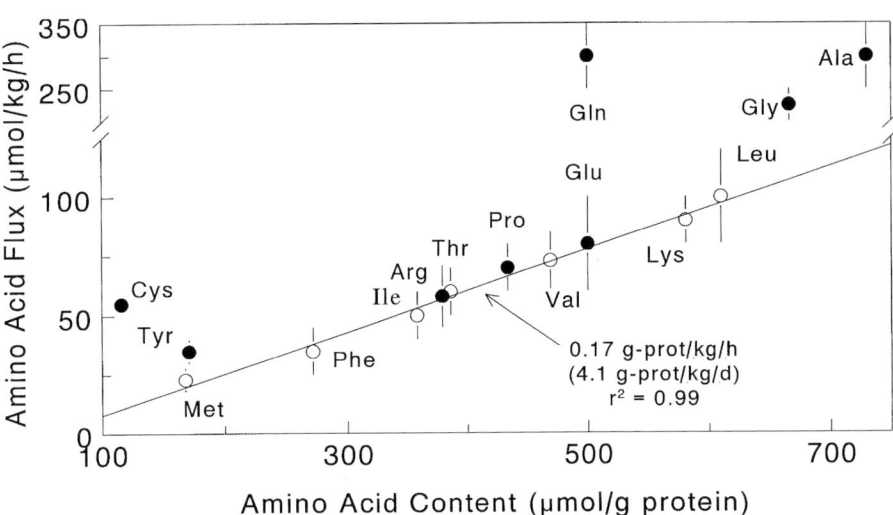

gleaned from a variety of studies in persons measured in the postabsorptive state (without dietary intake during the infusion studies) who previously consumed diets of adequate N and energy intake. A correlation of amino acid flux and amino acid composition in protein exists across a variety of amino acid tracers and studies. This correlation suggests that even if there are problems defining intracellular/extracellular concentration gradients of tracers to assess true intracellular events, changes in fluxes measured for the various indispensable amino acids are still reflective of changes in breakdown in general.

Because dispensable amino acids are synthesized in the body, their fluxes are expected to be higher than their expected flux based on the regression line in Figure 2.13 by the amount of de novo synthesis that occurs. Because de novo synthesis and disposal of the dispensable amino acids would be expected to be based on the metabolic pathways of individual amino acids, the degree to which individual dispensable amino acids lie above the line should also be variable. For example, tyrosine is a dispensable amino acid because it is made from the hydroxylation of phenylalanine, which is also the pathway of phenylalanine disposal. The rate of tyrosine de novo synthesis *is* the rate of phenylalanine disposal. In the postabsorptive state, 10 to 20% of an indispensable amino acid's turnover goes to oxidative disposal. For phenylalanine with a flux of approximately 40 μmol/kg/hour, phenylalanine disposal produces approximately 6 μmol/kg/hour of tyrosine. We would predict from the tyrosine content of body protein that tyrosine release from protein breakdown would be 21 μmol/kg/hour, and the flux of tyrosine (tyrosine release from protein breakdown plus tyrosine production from phenylalanine) would be 21 + 6 = 27 μmol/kg/hour. The measured tyrosine flux approximates this prediction (see Fig. 2.13) (81).

Compared with tyrosine, which has a de novo synthesis component limited by phenylalanine oxidation, most dispensable amino acids have very large de novo synthesis components because of their corresponding metabolic pathways. For example, arginine is at the center of the urea cycle (see Fig. 2.3). Normal synthesis for urea is 8 to 12 g/day N. That amount of urea production translates into an arginine de novo synthesis of approximately 250 μmol/kg/hour, which is four times the expected approximately 60 μmol/kg/hour of arginine released from protein breakdown. As can be seen in Figure 2.13, however, the *measured* arginine flux approximates the arginine release from protein breakdown (82). The large de novo synthesis component does not exist in the measured flux. The explanation for this low flux is that the arginine involved in urea synthesis is very highly compartmentalized in the liver, and this arginine does not exchange with the tracer arginine infused intravenously.

Similar disparities are seen between the measured fluxes of glutamine and glutamate determined with intravenously infused tracers and their anticipated fluxes from their expected de novo synthesis components. The predicted flux for glutamate should include transamination with the BCAAs, alanine and aspartate, as well as glutamate's contribution to the production and degradation of glutamine. However, the glutamate flux measured in postabsorptive adult subjects infused with [^{15}N]glutamate is 80 μmol/kg/hour, barely higher than the anticipated rate of glutamate release from protein breakdown (see Fig. 2.13). The size of free glutamate pool was also determined in this study from the tracer dilution. The tracer-determined pool of glutamate was very small and approximated only the pool size predicted for extracellular water. The much larger intracellular pool that exists in muscle (see Table 2.4) was not seen with the intravenously administered tracer. The flux measured for glutamine is considerably larger (350 μmol/kg/hour), a finding reflecting a large de novo synthesis component (see Fig. 2.13). However, the pool size determined with the $[^{15}N]$glutamine tracer also was a small pool, one not much larger than glutamine in extracellular water. The large intracellular muscle free pool of glutamine was not found (83). The results of this study showed that the glutamine and glutamate tracers, administered intravenously, define pools of glutamine and glutamate that reflect primarily extracellular free glutamine and glutamate. The large intracellular pools (especially those in muscle) are tightly compartmentalized and do not readily mix with extracellular glutamine and glutamate. The glutamate tracer does not detect intracellular events such as glutamate transamination. The same is true of the glutamine tracer. However, the prominent role of glutamine in the body *is interorgan transport*, that is, production by muscle and release for utilization by other tissues (84, 85), and that event is measured by the glutamine tracer (as is obvious from Figure 2.13, in which the tracer-determined glutamine flux shows the highest flux measured of any amino acid).

Splanchnic Bed Metabolism of Dietary Amino Acids. The model in Figure 2.10 does not consider the potential first-pass effect of the splanchnic bed (gut and liver) on regulating the delivery of nutrients from the oral route. Under normal circumstances, the amino acid tracer is infused intravenously to measure whole-body systemic kinetics. However, enterally delivered amino acids pass through the gut and liver before entering the systemic circulation. Any metabolism of these amino acids by gut or liver on the first pass during absorption will not be "seen" by an intravenously infused tracer in terms of systemic kinetics. Therefore, another pool with a second arrow showing the first-pass removal by gut and liver should precede the input arrow for "I" (Fig. 2.14) to indicate the role

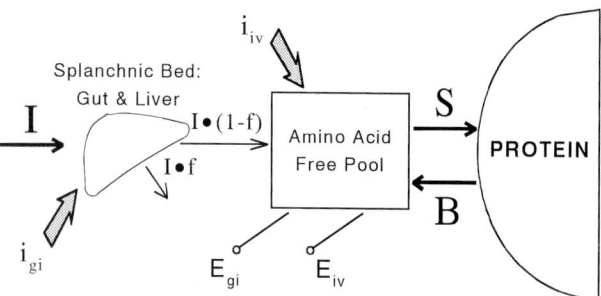

Figure 2.14. Model of whole–body protein metabolism for the fed state in which the first-pass uptake of dietary intake is considered. A labeled amino acid tracer is administered by the gastrointestinal route (i_{gi}) to follow dietary amino acid intake (I). The fraction of dietary amino acid sequestered on the first-pass by the splanchnic bed (f) can be determined by administering the tracer by both the gastrointestinal and the intravenous route (i_{iv}) and comparing the enrichments in blood for the two tracers (E_{gi} and E_{iv}, respectively).

of the splanchnic bed. A fraction "f" of the dietary intake ($I \bullet f$) is sequestered on the first pass, and only $I \bullet (1-f)$ enters systemic circulation.

Two approaches to addressing this problem are used. The first does not evaluate the fraction sequestered explicitly, but it builds the tracer administration scheme into the first-pass losses. Simply add the amino acid tracer to the dietary intake so the tracer administration *is* the oral route (I_{gi}) and enrichments in blood (E_{gi}) come after any first-pass metabolism by the splanchnic bed (86, 87). This approach is especially useful for studying the effect of varying levels of amino acid intake, but it does not evaluate per se the amount of material sequestered by the splanchnic bed.

The second approach applies the tracer both by the intravenous route and by the enteral route. The intravenous tracer infusion (I_{iv}) and plasma enrichment (E_{iv}) are used to determine systemic kinetics, and the enteral tracer infusion and its plasma enrichment determines systemic kinetics plus the effect of the first pass. By the difference, the fraction, f, is readily calculated (88). This approach can be applied even in the postabsorptive state to determine basal uptake of amino acid tracers by the splanchnic bed. Numerous indispensable and dispensable amino acids have been studied, and first-pass fractional uptake values for these different amino acids have been determined. In general, the splanchnic bed extracts between 20 and 50% of the indispensable amino acids leucine (88–91), phenylalanine (88, 92, 93), and lysine (94, 95). More than half of the dispensable amino acids are extracted by the splanchnic bed on the first pass, including alanine (96), arginine (90), and glutamine (93, 97–99), but splanchnic bed extracts almost all enteral glutamate (97, 100).

Synthesis of Specific Proteins

The foregoing methods deal with measurements at the whole-body level, but they do not address specific proteins and their rates of synthesis and degradation. To do so requires obtaining samples of the proteins that can be purified. Some proteins are readily sampled, such as proteins in blood such as the lipoproteins, albumin, fibrinogen, and other secreted proteins. Other proteins require tissue sampling, such as obtaining a muscle biopsy. If a protein or group of proteins can be sampled and purified, then its (their) synthetic rate can be determined directly from the rate of tracer incorporation into the proteins. Proteins that turn over slowly (e.g., muscle protein or albumin) incorporate only a small amount of tracer during a tracer infusion. Because the incorporation rate of tracer is approximately linear during this time, protein synthesis can be measured by obtaining only two samples. This technique has been especially useful for evaluating protein synthesis of myofibrillar protein with a limited number of muscle biopsies (101, 102). Once a tissue biopsy has been obtained, the sample may be fractionated into cellular components and the synthetic rate of proteins in organelles (e.g., mitochondria) or specific proteins of muscle (e.g., actin and myosin) determined (103, 104). For proteins that turn over at a faster rate, the tracer concentration rises exponentially in the protein toward a plateau value of enrichment that matches that of the precursor amino acids used for its synthesis, that is, the intracellular amino acid enrichment. The types of protein that have been measured under these conditions have been the lipoproteins, especially apolipoprotein B (Apo-B) in very-low-density lipoprotein (105–107).

The determination of the protein fractional synthetic rate is a "precursor-product" method that requires both knowledge of the rate of tracer incorporation into the protein being synthesized and knowledge of the enrichment of the amino acid precursor used for synthesis. For muscle, L-[1-^{13}C]leucine is often used as the tracer, and plasma KIC ^{13}C enrichment is used to approximate the intracellular muscle leucine enrichment (101). Various other schemes have been used to estimate intracellular liver amino acid tracer enrichment. Hippuric acid is excreted in urine after formation in the liver by conjugation of benzoic acid and glycine. Therefore, urinary hippuric acid can be used as an index of hepatic intracellular glycine ^{15}N enrichment (108). Although the evidence is not specific, suggestions have been made that the hippuric acid does not accurately reflect the glycine precursor pool from which the export proteins are synthesized. However, in the absence of better approach, using the hippuric acid ^{15}N enrichment is clearly better than using another tracer of which the hepatic intracellular enrichment is completely unknown. For proteins such as VLDL Apo-B that turnover quickly (typically 4–8 hours), tracer incorporation into the protein will approach a plateau within the period of tracer infusion. If the tracer enrichment in the protein does not reach a plateau during the time course of the tracer infusion, curve fitting can usually predict the plateau. When the standard precursor-product relationship holds (i.e., the product is made only from the precursor), the protein plateau amino acid enrichment will reflect the precursor enrichment, thus simplifying the kinetic calculation (107). Cryer and colleagues (105) were able to use the plateau in VLDL Apo-B to measure the precursor enrichment in normal subjects, but they still had to use urinary hippurate in hyperlipidemic subjects who had large, slow-turnover VLDL pools that did not approach plateau during the course of the 8-hour infusion.

Degradation of Specific Proteins

Measurement of protein degradation is much more limited in terms of the methods available. To measure protein degradation, the protein must be prelabeled. Three methods have been used: (a) removal of the protein from the body, followed by iodination with radioactive iodine, and reinjection back into the body to follow the disappearance of the labeled protein; (b) administration of a labeled amino acid to label proteins via incorporation of the tracer via protein synthesis, followed by measurement of labeled amino acid release from degradation of the protein; and (c) use of posttranslational amino acids such as 3-methylhistidine.

The use of iodination limits this methodology to readily removable and reinjectable proteins, that is, proteins in plasma. Therefore, the applications of this method are limited, but they have found use in lipoprotein metabolism (109–111). The method is not without problems: the proteins that are iodinated will not have the same structure after removal and iodination as they had before removal from the body, and the iodination process may cause untoward effects. However, properly applied, the method can be very specific for measuring the kinetics of select proteins.

Alternatively, proteins may be labeled by long infusions of amino acid tracer. After the tracer infusion is stopped, the tracer enrichment will disappear quickly from plasma. At that point, serial sampling of the protein and measurement of the decrease in tracer enrichment with time will give its degradation rate. However, another problem occurs: 80% or more of the amino acids released from protein breakdown will be reused for synthesis of new proteins. Therefore, recycling of amino acid tracer from protein degradation back into the new proteins occurs. Because there is generally not a large starting enrichment in the proteins measured, the recycling of low enrichments of tracer becomes an important and greatly complicating problem in the interpretation of the labeled protein data by this method.

3-Methylhistidine and Other Posttranslational Modified Amino Acids. In the body, certain enzymes can modify the structure of proteins after they have been synthesized. The posttranslational changes are generally modest, occur to specific amino acids, and are often the addition of a hydroxyl group (e.g., conversion of proline to hydroxyproline in collagen [112]) or methylation of N-moieties of amino acid residues such as histidine or lysine. Because tRNAs do not code for these hydroxylated or methylated amino acids, they are not reused for protein synthesis once the protein containing them is degraded, and their release and collection in urine can be used as a measure of the degradation rate of the proteins that contained them.

Because of the quantitative importance of muscle to whole-body protein metabolism, measurement of the release of 3-methylhistidine is an important tool for following myosin and actin breakdown, which are both primary proteins in skeletal muscle and the primary proteins containing 3-methylhistidine (27, 113). Analyses of rat carcasses demonstrated that muscle accounts for three fourths of the 3-methylhistidine pool in body proteins (27), and administered ^{14}C-3-methylhistidine has been shown to be quantitatively recovered in the urine of rats (114) and humans (115). There are caveats, however, to the use of 3-methylhistidine excretion for measurement of myofibrillar protein breakdown. Dietary meat will distort urinary 3-methylhistidine collection (116). As much as 5% of the 3-methylhistidine released in the urine may be acetylated in the liver first (a pathway that is much more predominant in the rat), and the urinary samples may have to by hydrolyzed before measurement of the 3-methylhistidine.

Myofibrillar protein and 3-methylhistidine are not specific to skeletal muscle (117, 118). Although skin and gut only contain a small pool of myofibrillar protein (compared with the large mass of myofibrillar protein found in skeletal muscle), skin and gut protein turn over rapidly and, therefore, can contribute a significant amount of 3-methylhistidine to the urine. Some work suggests that skin and gut contributions, although noticeable, can be accommodated in the calculation of human skeletal muscle turnover from urinary 3-methylhistidine excretion (113, 119, 120).

A more specific approach to 3-methylhistidine measurement of skeletal muscle myofibrillar protein breakdown is to measure the specific release of 3-methylhistidine from skeletal muscle via AV blood measurements across a muscle bed, such as leg or arm (121). This measurement of protein breakdown from the 3-methylhistidine AV difference can be combined with the AV difference measurement of an indispensable amino acid that is not metabolized in muscle, such as tyrosine. The AV difference of tyrosine across an arm or leg defines net protein balance, that is, the difference between protein breakdown and synthesis. If we subtract this protein balance measurement from the myofibrillar protein breakdown measurement from the AV difference of 3-methylhistidine, we obtain an estimate of muscle protein synthesis (50, 122). A final twist is to include coinfusion of an isotopically labeled 3-methylhistidine tracer and to measure the AV difference of the tracer in conjunction with the concentration of 3-methylhistidine. This approach provides the most complete and detailed kinetic picture of 3-methylhistidine movement and myofibrillar protein breakdown assessment (123, 124).

CONTRIBUTION OF SPECIFIC ORGANS TO PROTEIN METABOLISM

Whole-Body Metabolism of Protein and Contributions of Individual Organs

From the preceding discussion of tracers of amino acid and protein metabolism, it is clear that the body is not static, and all compounds are being made and degraded over time. A general balance of the processes occurring are shown in Figure 2.6 for an average adult. In diabetic patients treated with insulin, Nair and colleagues measured leucine and phenylalanine kinetics in the whole body as well as leucine and phenylalanine tracer balances across a leg and across the splanchnic bed (125). The results obtained from this work measure directly in humans what has been assumed from a composite of measurements shown in Figure 2.6. They also found that approximately 250 g of protein turns over in a day, based on the leucine and phenylalanine fluxes. Muscle protein turnover accounted for 65 g/day, and splanchnic protein turnover accounted for 62 g/day. If secreted proteins are synthesized at a rate of 48 g/day, then nonsplanchnic, nonmuscle organs account for another 75 g/day. The proportion of skeletal muscle mass in the body is consistent with skeletal muscle's contribution to whole-body protein turnover: skeletal muscle comprises about one third of the protein in the body (7) and accounts for about one fourth of the turnover.

If amino acids could be completely conserved, that is, if none were oxidized for energy or synthesized into other compounds, then all amino acids released from proteolysis could be completely reincorporated into new protein synthesis. Obviously, that is not the case, and when no dietary intake occurs, whole-body protein breakdown must be greater than protein synthesis by an amount equal to net disposal of amino acids by oxidative and other routes. Therefore, we need to consume enough amino acids during the day to make up for the losses that occur both during this period and during the nonfed period. This concept becomes the basis for methods defining amino acid and protein requirements discussed later.

As shown in Figure 2.6, if approximately 90 g of protein is eaten in a day, of which 10 g is lost to the feces, the net absorption will be 80 g. At the same time, considerably more protein is synthesized and degraded in the body. The total turnover of protein in the body, including both dietary intake and endogenous metabolism, is $90 + 250 = 340$ g/day, of which oxidation of dietary protein accounts for $(75 + 5)/340 = 24\%$ of the turnover of protein in the body per day. When dietary protein intake is restricted, adaptation occurs whereby the body reduces N losses (e.g., see Fig. 2.7) and protein intake/oxidation becomes a much smaller proportion of total protein turnover.

The preceding discussion defines turnover of protein in various parts of the body, but it does not integrate flows of material per se or highlight the relationship of amino acids to metabolites that are used for energy, such as glucose and fatty acids. Clearly, interorgan cooperation must occur to maintain protein homeostasis simply because some tissues such as muscle have large amino acid reservoirs, yet all tissues have amino acid needs. A regular feeding schedule means that part of the day is a fasting period when endogenous protein is used for energy and gluconeogenesis. The fed period then supplies amino acids from dietary protein to replenish these losses and to provide additional amino acids that can be used for energy during the feeding portion as well. Such a normal diurnal feeding and fasting pattern causes movement of amino acids among organs. Such movement takes on particular importance in situations of trauma and stress in which

TABLE 2.11. CONTRIBUTION OF DIFFERENT ORGANS AND TISSUES TO ENERGY EXPENDITURE

	WEIGHT		METABOLIC RATE	
ORGAN OR TISSUE	kg	(% OF TOTAL)	kcal/kg TISSUE/d	(% OF TOTAL)
Kidneys	0.3	(0.5)	440	(8)
Brain	1.4	(2.0)	240	(20)
Liver	1.8	(2.6)	200	(21)
Heart	0.3	(0.5)	440	(9)
Muscle	28.0	(40.0)	4	(22)
Adipose tissue	15.0	(40.0)	4	(4)
Other (e.g., skin, gut, bone)	23.2	(33.0)	12	(16)
Total	70.0	(100)		(100)

Data for a 70-kg man from Elia M. Organ and tissue contribution to metabolic rate. In: Kinney JM, Tucker HN, eds. Energy Metabolism: Determinants and Cellular Corollaries. New York: Raven Press, 1992:61–79.

adaptation, or rather lack of adaptation, of amino acid metabolism to physiologic insults or pathophysiologic states occurs.

As Cahill and Aoki have emphasized (1, 126), the primary consideration of the body is to maintain and distribute energy supplies (oxygen and oxidative substrates). The caloric needs of different tissues in the body are shown in Table 2.11. As can be seen from the table, the brain makes up only approximately 2% of body weight yet has 20% of the energy needs (127). The brain also lacks the ability to store energy (e.g., glycogen depots), so it depends continually on delivery of energy substrates via the blood from other organs (Fig. 2.15A). In the postabsorptive state, the primary energy substrate for the brain is glucose. In infancy and early childhood, in which the brain makes up a significantly greater proportion of body mass, glucose production and utilization rates are proportionately higher (128). The pioneering studies of Cahill, Felig, and Wahren

have provided us with a wealth of data concerning flows of amino acids and glucose from organ balance studies in humans studied over a range of nutritional states (44, 45, 129–131). Some basic concepts may be defined from these studies.

As shown in Figure 2.15A, in the postabsorptive state the body provides energy for the brain in the form of glucose primarily from hepatic glycogenolysis and secondarily from glucose synthesis (gluconeogenesis) from amino acids. Other substrates, such as glycerol released from triglyceride lipolysis, may also be used for gluconeogenesis, but amino acids provide the bulk of the gluconeogenic substrate. The pathways of conversion are discussed earlier for those amino acids whose carbon skeletons can be easily rearranged to form gluconeogenic precursors. The remaining amino acids released from protein breakdown and not used for gluconeogenesis may be oxidized. The amino acid N released by this process is removed from the

Figure 2.15. Interorgan flow of substrates in the body to maintain energy balance in the postabsorptive state (**A**) and after adaptation to starvation (**B**). The schematic diagrams are patterned after the work of Cahill. In all states, energy needs of the brain must be satisfied. In the postabsorptive state, glucose from liver glycogenolysis provides the majority of the glucose needed by the brain. After liver glycogen stores have been depleted (fasting state), gluconeogenesis from amino acids from muscle stores predominates as the glucose source. Eventually, the body adapts to starvation by production and utilization of ketone bodies instead of glucose, thereby sparing amino acid loss for gluconeogenesis. AA's, amino acids; Ala and Gln, alanine and glutamine, respectively; TG and FFA, triglycerides and free fatty acids, respectively. (Redrawn from GF Cahill Jr, Aoki TT. In: Kinney JM, ed. Report of the First Ross Conference on Medical Research. Columbus, OH: Ross Laboratories, 1980:129–34.)

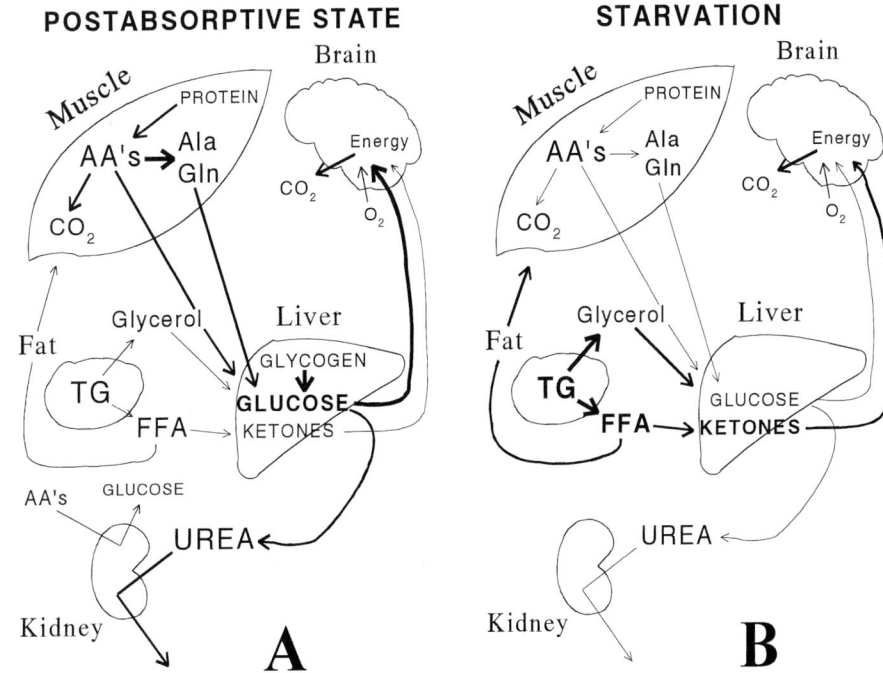

body by incorporation into urea via synthesis in the liver and excretion into urine via the kidney. Gluconeogenesis also occurs in the kidney, but the effect and magnitude are masked from AV measurements because the kidney is also a glucose consumer. With respect to amino acids, the net effects of the kidney are the uptake and utilization of amino acids for gluconeogenesis (132, 133).

Role of Skeletal Muscle in Whole-Body Amino Acid Metabolism

A very interesting observation made early in AV difference studies across the human leg or arm was that more than 50% of the amino acids released from skeletal muscle are in the form of alanine and glutamine (134), yet alanine and glutamine comprise less than 20% of amino acids in protein (see Table 2.3). To this day, the specific purpose of the alanine and glutamine release is not well defined. Several possible reasons exist. First, skeletal muscle oxidizes dispensable amino acids and the BCAAs in situ for energy. Because amino acid oxidation produces waste N and because ammonia is neurotoxic, release of waste N as ammonia needs to be avoided. Because both alanine and glutamine are readily synthesized from intermediates derived from glucose (alanine from transamination of pyruvate from glycolysis and glutamine from α-ketoglutarate), they are excellent vehicles to remove waste N from muscle while avoiding ammonia release. Alanine removes one and glutamine removes two Ns per amino acid. These observations have led to the proposal of a glucose-alanine cycle in which glucose made by the liver is taken up by muscle where glycolysis liberates pyruvate. The pyruvate is then transaminated to alanine and is released from muscle. That alanine is extracted by the liver and is transaminated to pyruvate, which is then used for glucose synthesis (134). This scheme has been expanded to explain the utilization of BCAAs by muscle for energy and disposal through alanine of their amino-N groups. Such a scheme resolves a problem related to the BCAAs. In contrast to the other indispensable amino acids that are metabolized only in liver, the BCAAs are readily oxidized in other tissues, especially muscle. Thus, if the BCAAs, which comprise approximately 20% of amino acids in muscle protein, are oxidized for energy by the muscle, then the glucose-alanine cycle could provide a means of removal of the N that is generated in the process.

Whole-Body Adaptation to Fasting and Starvation

As indicated in Figure 2.15A, lipolysis (breakdown of adipose triglyceride to free fatty acids and glycerol) plays a lesser role in postabsorptive energy supply, especially to the brain. However, glycogen stores are limited and will become depleted in less than 24 hours. That point in time when liver glycogen stores are exhausted is by definition the beginning of the *fasting* state. Now glucose needs of the brain must be met completely by gluconeogenesis,

which means sacrificing amino acids from protein. Because protein is critical to body function, from enzyme activity to muscle function related to breathing and circulation, unrestrained use of amino acids for glucose production would rapidly deplete protein and would cause death in a matter of days. Clearly, this result does not occur because people may survive without food, and obese persons may be fasted for weeks without protein intake (1). Adaptation occurs in starvation by the brain's switching from a glucose-based to a ketone-based fuel supply. Free fatty acids released from lipolysis are converted into ketone bodies in the liver that can then be used by the brain and other tissues for energy. That conversion begins in the fasting state and is complete under long periods of fasting (Fig. 2.15B). In starvation, tissues such as muscle may use free fatty acids directly for energy, and the brain uses ketone bodies. The body's dependence on glucose as a fuel has been greatly reduced, thereby conserving protein. This adaptation process is complete within a week of the onset of starvation (126).

The Fed State

Although the body can accommodate to starvation, it is not a normal occurrence in our lives. The adaptations that are seen in everyday life evolve around the postabsorptive period and the fed period. Basically, we go through our nights after completing absorption of the last meal using nutrient stores of glycogen and protein, as depicted in Figure 2.15A. During the fed portion of the day, three things occur to the dietary intake of amino acids and glucose: (a) they are used to replete protein and glycogen that were lost during the postabsorptive period; and intake in amounts above what is needed to replete nighttime losses are either (b) oxidized or (c) stored to increase protein, glycogen, or fat for growth or for storage of excess calories. Although muscle contains the bulk of body protein, all organs are expected to lose protein during the postabsorptive period and, therefore, need repletion during the fed period. What is poorly understood is how the individual amino acids that enter through the diet are distributed among the various tissues in the amounts they are needed for each tissue. Just as each amino acid has its own separate metabolic pathways, the rates and fates of absorption and utilization are expected to be different among amino acid. Thus, dietary protein requirements cannot be discussed without also considering the requirements of individual amino acids.

Digestion and Absorption of Protein

Two organs have particular potentially important regulatory roles during feeding: the gut and the liver. All dietary intake passes first through the gut and then through the liver via portal blood flow. Digestion of protein begins with pepsin secretion in gastric juice and with proteolytic enzymes secreted from pancreas and mucosa of the small intestine (135). These enzymes are secreted in their "pro" (or zymogen) form and become activated by cleavage of a small peptide portion. The pancreatic proenzymes become activated by intestinal enterokinase secreted into the intestinal juice to cleave trypsinogen to trypsin. The presence of dietary protein in the gut appears to signal the secretion of the enzymes. As trypsin becomes activated, it binds to proteins to initiate hydrolysis. An excess of trypsin occurs when either more trypsin is secreted than protein is present or when most of the dietary protein has been hydrolyzed. At this point, the presence of unbound trypsin appears to signal a feedback regulation system to the pancreatic acinar cells to inhibit synthesis and secretion of trypsinogen. Some plants, such as soybeans, contain protein inhibitors of proteolytic enzymes such as trypsin. These proteins may often be denatured by heating (i.e., by cooking). Feeding unheated soybean to rats results in hypertrophy of the pancreas, presumably resulting from hypersecretion because binding of the trypsin to the protein inhibitor removes the feedback signal of free trypsin on the pancreas (136).

The events of protein digestion and absorption as shown in Figure 2.16 are well established (135, 137–140). Proteins are successively broken down into smaller peptides on the basis of the amino acid residues targeted by the proteolytic enzymes. For example, pepsin has a relatively low specificity for neutral amino acids such as leucine or phenylalanine, whereas trypsin shows specificity for basic targets: lysine and arginine. In addition,

exopeptidases attack the free ends of the peptide chains at the carboxyl terminus for pancreatic carboxypeptidases and amino terminus for aminopeptidases secreted in intestinal juice.

The free amino acids are absorbed by active transport into the mucosa by transporters specific to different types of amino acids (138, 139). At the same time, peptides, in particular dipeptides and tripeptides, are also assimilated on the luminal side intact. Peptide hydrolases present in the brush border and cytosol of the mucosal cells complete the hydrolysis of these peptides before their release into the portal blood system. There are specific transport systems for peptide uptake into mucosal cells separate from the transporters for amino acids. It is thought that one fourth of dietary protein is absorbed as dipeptides and tripeptides (141). For example, patients with the rare genetic Hartnup disease with a defect in renal and gut transport of selected amino acids cannot transport free tryptophan into mucosal cells, but they do indeed absorb tryptophan when it is administered as a dipeptide (142, 143).

Figure 2.16 shows that, in addition to dietary protein, protein is added directly to the lumen in the form of secreted proteins and sloughed cells. Because the small intestine is continually being remodeled with cells formed in the crypts migrating toward the villus tips, epithelial and other cells are continuously being sloughed off the tips of the villi. Although the exact amounts of protein secreted and cells sloughed are unknown, a reasonable estimate is that, of the 70 g of protein added to the lumen, 20 g may come from secreted proteins and 50 g may come from sloughed cells (137). As indicated in Figure 2.16, the majority of this protein is very efficiently reabsorbed.

To a limited but important extent, some proteins and large peptides enter directly from the gut intact into the basolateral blood. Absorption of intact proteins or large portions of proteins is a tenable physiologic explanation for numerous diseases involving food allergies and idiosyncrasies. The gut is generally viewed as an impermeable barrier where nutrients cross by active transport or where a break in the barrier occurs through cell injury. Small amounts of some proteins may pass this barrier by several possible mechanisms, such as through "leaks" between epithelial cell junctions or possibly by transport through uptake into vesicles from the lumen to the submucosal side of the epithelial cells (144). Again, the amount of protein entering intact is small, but it may be important in situations of immune response to the proteins or in delivery of some peptide drugs.

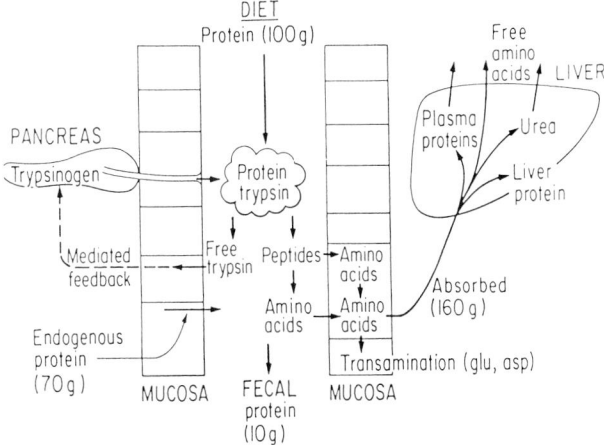

Figure 2.16. Digestion and absorption of dietary protein in the intestine. The secretion and feedback system of the pancreatic trypsinogen/trypsin is shown. In addition to the assumed dietary protein load of 100 g, an additional protein load of approximately 70 g occurs from secretion of protein and sloughing of mucosal cells. Under normal conditions, almost all the protein is recovered by hydrolysis and absorption. Amino acids are absorbed by active transport through the mucosal cells into the portal blood system. Some amino acids are immediately metabolized by gut and liver during absorption. (From Crim MC, Munro HN. In: Shils ME, ed. Defined Formula Diets for Medical Purposes. Chicago: American Medical Association, 1977;5–15, with permission.)

Gut and Liver as Metabolic Organs

The gut and liver facilitate absorption and delivery of dietary amino acids to the systemic blood and other tissues in the body. During this process, the gut and liver see all nutrients being absorbed and may sequester on the first pass during absorption any fraction of the dietary amino acids before these amino acid ever enter the systemic circulation. The liver has a natural role in this process because it is the organ that inactivates/modifies toxic substances in the blood. Therefore, the liver would be expected to regulate the flow of dietary amino acids into the systemic circulation following a meal. In addition, the liver is the only site in the body for metabolizing indispensable amino acids, except the BCAAs (which are metabolized by several tissues, most notably muscle). As mentioned earlier and discussed later in terms of determining amino acid requirements, amino acids consumed during feeding in excess of the body's current needs would be expected to be oxidized. Therefore, a potential role for the liver is removal of excess amino acids, especially indispensable amino acids that cannot be oxidized in other tissues, on the first pass during amino acid absorption. The role of the gut and liver as active metabolic organs that metabolize dietary amino acids was shown in catheterized dogs by Elwyn and associates in 1968 (145). They demonstrated the active metabolism of the key dispensable amino acids, alanine, glutamine, and glutamate and described how the BCAAs passed intact through the splanchnic bed. Several groups have shown similar results in humans using splanchnic bed and/or leg/arm AV catheterization with respect to passage of amino acids following meal feeding (45, 146–148). These studies have made several consistent observations.

As discussed earlier, the first observation was that most of the BCAAs in a meal pass through the splanchnic bed to be extracted and used by peripheral tissues. As shown in later studies using labeled amino acid tracers administered enterally and intravenously (see Fig. 2.14), the BCAA leucine has the lowest fractional extraction by the gut and liver on the first pass when delivered enterally. The amount of leucine oxidized by liver in the postabsorptive state is minimal (<2%) (88). Under conditions of feeding, the amount of enteral leucine extracted by the gut and liver on the first pass rises only slightly (89). However, the liver has been shown to be a significant producer of KIC from leucine and will convert enteral KIC to leucine, a finding indicating that the first step in BCAA metabolism is active, that is, transamination (88, 149). This step does not irreversibly remove leucine; rather, it forms only a ketoacid that can be reformed into leucine in a peripheral tissue such as muscle. Alternatively, the KIC produced by liver and released can be oxidized.

Of particular interest has been the observation that the gut extracts glutamate and glutamine and releases alanine and ammonia (145). Early experiments of enteral glutamate infusion in dogs suggested that the glutamate sequestered is converted directly to alanine on the basis of glutamate uptake with resulting alanine release (150). Unfortunately, any interpretation of such an observation without proof from isotopic tracer studies would fall under the gumball machine analogy of Figure 2.8. Nonetheless, the observation has been intriguing, especially when added to the consistent observation of a large AV gradient for glutamine across the gut, indicating uptake (151–154).

PROTEIN AND AMINO ACID REQUIREMENTS

The most fundamental question in nutrition concerning protein and amino acids is simply this: What amount of protein is required in the diets of humans to maintain health? This question has several subparts. First, we must evaluate the intake of both protein and the amounts of the individual amino acids in that protein. Second, this question needs to be evaluated in humans over (a) the complete range of life and development, (b) in sickness and in health, and (c) under different conditions of work and environment. These questions and the methods used to answer them are discussed later in terms of their individual components.

When we discuss the amino acid composition of a specific protein source, we generally focus on the amount of indispensable acids contained in it because these are the amino acids *indispensable* to our diet. Which amino acids are dispensable and which are indispensable were originally elucidated by testing whether a diet deficient in a particular amino acid would support growth in a rat. However, important species differences between rats and humans limit this comparison. Furthermore, the growth retardation model, which is effective with the rat, is not applicable to humans. An alternative for studying amino acid requirements in humans is the N balance technique. A diet that is adequate in total N, but deficient in an indispensable amino acid, cannot produce a positive N balance because protein can be synthesized only if each amino acid is present in adequate amounts. The dispensable amino acids can be synthesized if protein intake is adequate, but limited intake of an indispensable amino acid limits the amount of protein that can be synthesized. The body is then faced with a dietary excess of the other *non-limiting* indispensable and dispensable amino acids that it cannot put into protein. Therefore, these amino acids must be oxidized to urea, and a negative N balance results.

The classic studies of Rose and colleagues measured N balance in humans fed diets deficient in individual amino acids. They determined that eight amino acids produced a negative N balance when they were deficient in the diet of adult humans (155–157). Although the enzymatic pathways are missing for the synthesis of these indispensable amino acids, several of these amino acids (such as the BCAAs) have a catabolic pathway in which the first step in their catabolism is reversible, that is, transamination to form branched-chain keto acids (149). Using the rat growth model, investigators have shown that growth can be supported by supplying the keto acids of these indispensable amino acids. Various formulations have been proposed for supplying the carbon skeleton of several indispensable amino acids (e.g., the BCAAs) without adding N, which is detrimental in disease states such as renal disease (158).

Another related question to ask is this: Do dispensable amino acids ever become indispensable? If a dispensable amino acid is used in the body faster than it is made, it becomes indispensable for that *condition* (2). Tyrosine and cysteine are made from phenylalanine and methionine, respectively, but if insufficient phenylalanine or methionine is consumed, tyrosine and cysteine also become deficient and *indispensable*. This question must be evaluated across the range of life from infancy to the elderly as well as in sickness and health. For example, enzymes for amino acid metabolism mature at different rates in the growing fetus and newborn infant. Histidine is indispensable in infants, but not necessarily in healthy children or adults (159). Therefore, the classification of "indispensable" or "dispensable" is dependent on (a) species, (b) maturation (i.e. infant, growing child, or adult), (c) diet, (d) nutritional status, and (e) pathophysiologic condition. Also to be considered is whether a particular amino acid *given in excess of requirement* has properties that may ameliorate or improve a clinical condition. These considerations must somehow be evaluated for each population group in which they are important.

Protein Requirements

Determination of the requirement of protein must consider both the amount of amino acid N and its quality, that is, its ability to be digested and absorbed and its indispensable amino acid content. The simplest approach to the measurement of the nutritional quality of a protein is to measure the ability of that protein to promote growth in young, growing animals, such as rats. Their growth depends on synthesis of new protein, which depends on indispensable amino acid intake. Because alterations in rat growth can be measured in several days, the growing rat has been often used as the model to compare differences in quality (composition) of protein/amino acid diets. Because this approach cannot ethically be applied to humans, other approaches for assessing *human* requirements have been applied: the *factorial method* and the *balance method*.

Factorial Method

When a person is placed on a protein-free diet, rates of amino acid oxidation and urea production will decrease over a several day period as the body tries to conserve its resources, but amino acid oxidation and urea production do not drop to zero (see Fig. 2.7). There will always be some *obligatory* oxidation of amino acids and urea formation and miscellaneous losses of N (see Table 2.10). The factorial method assesses all routes of losses possible for adult humans on a N-free diet. The minimum daily requirement of protein is assumed to be that amount that matches the sum of the various obligatory N losses.

Whereas nonurinary nonfecal N losses are often ignored in N balance studies of adequate protein intake, they are of critical importance in the assessment of protein requirements by the factorial method. Various studies have been performed to assess these losses, and the results have been tabulated in a World Health Organization/Food and Agriculture Organization/ United Nations University (WHO/FAO/UNU) panel publication (160) and have been summarized again in a US Food and Nutrition Board report (161). The obligatory N losses include the following: (a) urinary N, estimated to be 38 mg/kg/day of N; (b) fecal losses of enzymes and desquamated intestinal cells that cannot be fully reabsorbed, estimated to be 12 mg/kg/day; and (c) loss of N through sweat, hair, skin; and nail turnover and growth, menstrual flow, seminal fluid, ammonia in breath, nasal secretions, and so forth, estimated to be 2 to 3 mg/kg/day on a protein-free diet and 5 to 8 mg/kg/day on a diet of normal protein intake (42). The summation of these directly measurable losses gives a total obligatory minimum daily loss of 54 mg/kg/day of N (range, 41–69 mg/kg/day), corresponding to a protein intake of 0.34 g/kg/day (where 1 g N = 6.25 g protein) (161).

This value of 54 mg/kg/day of N is an "average value" that must be raised if it is to indicate a requirement that will apply to most adults in the population. The 1973 WHO/FAO report (162) suggested a coefficient of variability among individuals of 15%. Adding twice this amount (+2 standard deviations) gives a protein requirement that will include 97.5% of the adult population. Thus, the 0.34 g/kg/day protein becomes 0.44 g/kg/day after roundoff (163). For adults, the *dietary protein requirement* is considered to be this amount *plus* an adjustment for the inefficiency of utilization of dietary protein and for the quality (amino acid composition and digestibility) of the source of protein consumed. For children and pregnant or lactating women, an additional (theoretically determined) amount of protein is added to this recommendation to account for growth and milk formation (161). Clearly, this approach is based on extrapolation of N losses from protein-starvation conditions and may reflect an adaptation to N deprivation, which may not be reflective of normal metabolism and N requirements of healthy persons near the actual requirement level. Rand and Young (164) also pointed out that the relationship between protein intake and N retention is curvilinear, thus making it troublesome to extrapolate obligatory N loss to a protein requirement. Hence, an alternative method is needed to produce an alternative assessment of protein requirements.

Balance Method

In the balance method, subjects are fed varying amounts of protein or amino acids, and the *balance* of a particular parameter, usually *N balance*, is measured. An adequate amount of dietary protein is that level of intake that will maintain a neutral or slightly positive N balance. The balance method can be used to titrate N intake in infants, children, and women during pregnancy in whom the end point is a balance positive enough to allow for appropriate accretion of new tissue. The balance method is also useful for testing the validity of the factorial method estimates. In general, N balance studies in which dietary protein intake is titrated give higher measures of protein requirements than predicted by the factorial method. Several reasons exist for this result.

The N balance method has important errors associated with it that are not minor (42, 162, 164, 165). Urine collections tend to underestimate N losses, and intake tends to be overestimated. Miscellaneous cutaneous and hair losses, which are "best guesses," may have small but substantial errors. However, these factors affect both methods. What has been noticed specifically with the balance method that "titrates" dietary intake to determine zero balance is that the response to increasing protein intake is nonlinear (164). As protein intake is increased from a grossly deficient toward an adequate status, the improvement in N balance is at first proportional to the amount of protein added to the diet. As the balance point is approached, however, the slope of the ratio of balance to protein intake progressively decreases; that is, more protein than predicted by linear extrapolation is required to achieve a zero N balance (162). This refractoriness in reaching N equilibrium has been estimated to add 30% to the amount of intake needed to equal output. As a result, the factorial method estimate of 0.44 g/kg/day is increased to a median estimated average requirement (EAR) of 0.66 g/kg/day (165).

Most studies of N balance have been performed at presumably adequate levels of energy intake. However, N balance is affected by energy intake. Decreasing energy intake to less than requirements causes the N balance measurement to go from zero to negative when the protein intake is near the requirement. Most recommendations are based, nonetheless, on the assumption that energy intake will be adequate (166). Other factors affecting N balance indirectly are the quality and the digestibility of the protein being consumed. Generally, it is assumed that protein of lesser quality and digestibility than egg white will be consumed. A correction factor that increases protein requirements by 25 to 30% is added to compensate for consumption of lesser-quality protein (160).

Recommended Dietary Allowances for Protein

In 1989, the Food and Nutrition Board subcommittee of the US Institute of Medicine, National Research Council updated their recommended dietary allowances (RDA) for protein and amino acids (161) that were largely based on the 1985 FAO/WHO/UNU committee report (160). In 2002, the Food and Nutrition Board released a new report on dietary reference intakes for a range of macronutrients, including protein and amino acids (167). The RDA values for protein shown in Table 2.12 are based on the 2002 report and reflect N balance data (rather than factorial

TABLE 2.12. RECOMMENDED INTAKES OF HIGH-QUALITY REFERENCE PROTEIN FOR NORMAL HUMANS

AGE (y)	WEIGHT (kg)		EAR[a] (g/kg/d)	RDA[b] (g/kg/d)
0–0.5	6			1.52[c]
0.5–1	9		1.1	1.5
1–3	13		0.88	1.10
4–8	20		0.76	0.95
9–13	36		0.76	0.95
	Male	Female		
14–18	61	54	0.72	0.85
>18	70	58	0.66	0.80

[a]EAR, estimated average requirement: the intake that meets the estimated nutrient needs of half of the individuals in a group.
[b]RDA, recommended dietary allowance: the intake that meets the nutrient need of almost all (97.5%) individuals in a group.
[c]Value for infants in the first half-year of life is the adequate intake estimate determined in that population that appears to sustain a defined nutritional status, including growth rate, normal circulating nutrient values, and other functional indicators of health. This value is not equivalent to an RDA.

Data from Food and Nutrition Board, Institute of Medicine. Proteins and amino acids. In: Dietary Reference Intakes for Energy, Carbohydrate, Fiber, Fat, Fatty Acids, Cholesterol, Protein, and Amino Acids (Macronutrients). Washington, DC: National Academy Press, 2002;10:1–143, with permission.

method data) from studies in which a high-quality, highly digestible source of protein was used. Data are presented for the EAR for protein. The EAR reflects that protein intake that produced zero N balance in half of the population. That value was then increased by two standard deviations to encompass 97.5% of the population to obtain the RDA for the reference protein. For example, from studies of young men, the EAR value of 0.66 g/kg/day was increased to 0.80 g/kg/day for the RDA (167).

Special cases occur in which growth and accretion of tissue must be accounted for in the RDAs: during pregnancy, during lactation, and in infants and children. In pregnancy, total protein deposited was estimated to be 925 g based on maternal weight gain and an average birth weight at term. The rates of protein accretion were then divided by trimesters with adjustments for variation in birth weight (+15%) and an assumed efficiency of conversion of dietary protein to fetal, placental, and maternal tissues (+70%) to produce increments in reference protein intake of +1.0, +6.3, and +10.6 g protein/day for the first, second, and third trimesters, respectively (167). The amount of additional protein needed to be added to the diet during the last two trimesters to compensate for uncertainties about rates of tissue deposition and maintenance of those increases is estimated to be an EAR of +21 g protein/day or an RDA of +25 g/day additional protein over prepregnancy needs (167).

Women who are lactating also require additional protein intake. Using the factorial method and data for the protein content of human milk, the volume of milk produced, and adjustment for the estimated 50% conversion efficiency of dietary protein into newly synthesized milk protein, an increase of +23.4 g protein/day needs to be added to the EAR of women in their first month of lactation. The EAR drops to +22 g/day in month 2 and to +18.3 g/day for months 4 to 6 of lactation (167). To compensate for variance among women, the EAR value is increased to an RDA of +25 g /day additional protein for women in their first month of lactation.

Amino Acid Requirements

The recommendations for the intake of individual amino acids are largely based on the pioneering work of W. C. Rose and his colleagues in the 1950s (155, 156). Irwin and Hegsted reviewed these and other studies of amino acid requirement levels published before 1971 (168). Rose's studies are all N balance studies in which young male subjects were placed on diets in which N intake consisted of a mixture of crystalline amino acids. The intake of a single amino acid could be altered and the N balance measured. Because of the expense of the amino acid diets and the great difficulty in performing serial N balance studies at different intakes, Rose and colleagues were able to study only a very limited number of subjects per amino acid. Problems with interpreting the N balance data for a limited number of subjects cloud the extrapolation of these data to populations (169–171); yet the data of Rose have been the primary basis for the amino acid recommendations in adults for years.

Direct Amino Acid Oxidation Method

An alternative approach has been taken by Young and colleagues (170, 172, 173). Their approach is based on the method of Harper and others to assess amino acid requirements in growing animals using amino acid oxidation as an index of dietary sufficiency. Animals fed an insufficient amount of a specific individual amino acid reduce their oxidation of the deficient amino acid to obligatory levels. The oxidation of the dietary deficient amino acid will remain at obligatory oxidation levels until the requirement level is met. As dietary amino acid intake rises to more than the requirement, the excess amino acid will be oxidized. Therefore, a two-line curve of amino acid oxidation should appear when plotted against amino acid intake: a flat line below requirement (indicating obligatory oxidation) and a rising curve above the requirement (indicating oxidation of excess amino acid intake). The requirement level for the amino acid should be the intersection of the two curves, that is, where oxidation of excess amino acid begins (174).

The direct amino acid oxidation (DAAO) method uses the breakpoint in amino acid oxidation as a function of the intake of the test amino acid to determine requirement. Amino acid oxidation is determined by administering a [13]C- or ^{14}C-labeled amino acid tracer of the test amino acid being manipulated in the diet. The tracer amino acid is administered at the end of each diet period. The DAAO

method has been used by Young and El-Khoury to estimate amino acid requirements for isoleucine, leucine, lysine, phenylalanine/tyrosine, and valine in healthy adults (172, 173). Their estimates are two to three times greater than the former RDAs for adults (161).

Indicator Amino Acid Oxidation Method

Zello and colleagues (175) took a different approach to the measurement of amino acid requirements. Rather than administer and measure the oxidation of a tracer of the same amino acid that is being manipulated in the diet, they used the oxidation of a tracer of another indispensable amino acid tracer as an *indicator* of N balance. N balance becomes negative when a single amino acid is deficient in the diet because of increased urea production resulting from oxidation of excess indispensable amino acids that cannot be incorporated into protein when the one test amino acid is deficient. As discussed earlier, measurement of the increase in urea production is fraught with problems, which is why the oxidation of the indicator amino acid is measured using an amino acid tracer. As the dietary intake of the test amino acid is decreased to less than requirement levels, the oxidation of the indicator amino acid will increase as excess amino acids are wasted. An example of this method is shown in Figure 2.17, in which [1-13C]phenylalanine is infused as the indicator amino acid in young men consuming different levels of dietary threonine intake (176). The intake of all other amino acids is held constant (including that of the indicator, phenylalanine). At threonine intakes greater than the requirement, phenylalanine oxidation is constant, but phenylalanine

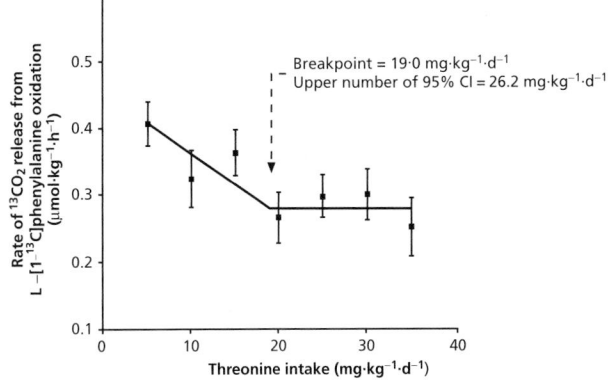

Figure 2.17. Oxidation of the indicator amino acid tracer [1-13C]phenylalanine to carbon-13 dioxide ([13]CO$_2$) in young men fed different dietary intakes of threonine. Phenylalanine oxidation is constant above the dietary requirement threonine, but it progressively increases as threonine intake drops below requirement because limitation of threonine intake limits the body's ability to synthesize protein causing the excess amino acids to be oxidized, including the indicator amino acid, phenylalanine. Thus, the breakpoint between the two lines indicates the threonine requirement in these subjects. CI, confidence interval. (From Wilson DC, Rafii M, Ball RO et al. Am J Clin Nutr 2000;71:757–64. Reproduced with permission by the *American Journal of Clinical Nutrition.* Copyright American Society for Clinical Nutrition.)

oxidation progressively increases as threonine intake is decreased to less than the threonine requirement. The breakpoint between the two curves in Figure 2.17 indicates the mean EAR for threonine intake. The RDA for threonine intake would be set two confidence intervals above the EAR.

The key to this method is the availability of an indicator amino acid tracer whose oxidation can be accurately and precisely measured that is different from the test amino acid being manipulated in the diet (175). Using this approach and [1-^{13}C]phenylalanine as the indicator amino acid, Zello and Kriengsinyos and their colleagues determined a requirement level for dietary lysine of 37 mg/kg/day (177, 178), which supports Young's higher estimate of lysine requirements by the DAAO method. However, the indicator amino acid oxidation (IAAO) method, as it has been applied, has raised some concerns. The first is the same as with the DAAO method: the tracer studies are performed only in the fed state. The second concern is that relatively short (e.g., 3-day) adaptation periods are used for the different dietary intakes tested. Classic N balance studies require 7 to 10 days for equilibration to occur in urinary N output, but this constraint is not required using the indicator tracer to measure oxidation directly. Thus, short adaptation periods can and are typically used with the IAAO method. The impact of these short adaptation periods has not been fully defined.

Twenty-Four-Hour Tracer Balance Method

A final twist has been added to the DAAO and IAAO methods to account for the fact that we oxidize amino acids 24 hours a day, not just during periods of feeding. El-Khoury and colleagues infused a [1-^{13}C]leucine tracer for 24 hours into subjects receiving different intakes of leucine to determine leucine requirements by the DAAO method (179, 180). Borgonha and colleagues infused

[1-^{13}C]leucine for 24 hours as an IAAO tracer into subjects receiving different intakes of threonine to determine threonine requirements (181). Similar studies such as these two from Young's group have been performed to redefine amino acid requirements in humans and have been used to put together recommendations for amino acid intakes (182) that are considerably greater for several indispensable amino acids than have been determined previously, largely by the N balance method (160–162).

When the Food and Nutrition Board prepared the most recent 2002 report on RDAs of indispensable amino acids, they considered the myriad of new data from recent stable isotope tracer studies in making their current recommendations (167). Their current recommendations are shown in Table 2.13 for infants, children, and adults. The RDAs for infants decreased with the 2002 report for most amino acids. The RDAs for children were reduced primarily for the BCAAs, but the RDAs for amino acids for which DAAO and IAAO method data were available increased significantly and now follow the pattern promoted by Young and Borgonha (182) (see Table 2.13).

Histidine

Although histidine has been shown to be indispensable to the diet of the rat, it has been difficult to define as indispensable to the diet of adult humans (168). In the 1973 FAO/WHO report, no requirement for histidine was given for adults (162), but in the 1985 WHO/FAO/UNU report (160), a requirement for histidine of 8 to 12 mg/kg/day was listed. This requirement in adults is based on extrapolation of data from infants (161). The limited studies of adults indicate that the requirement for histidine may be less than 2 mg/kg/day (183). However, this requirement has not been clearly documented in physiologically normal subjects (157). Proving histidine to be indispensable in adults has largely been restricted to studies of renal failure

TABLE 2.13. ESTIMATES OF RECOMMENDED DIETARY AMINO ACID ALLOWANCES (mg/kg/d) BY AGE GROUP

AMINO ACID	INFANTS 7–12 mo	CHILDREN 1–3 y	CHILDREN 4–13 y	ADULTS >19 y	PROPOSED BY YOUNG AND BORGONHA
Histidine[a]	32	21	16	14	—
Isoleucine	43	28	22	19	23
Leucine	96	62	48	42	40
Lysine	89	58	45	38	30
Methionine + cysteine	43	28	22	19	13
Phenylalanine + tyrosine	84	54	41	33	39
Threonine	49	32	24	20	15
Tryptophan	13	8	6	5	6
Valine	58	37	28	24	20

[a]Although no requirement for histidine has been quantified beyond infancy, histidine has been recommended for children and adults based on the histidine content of the recommended dietary allowance for protein of each of these age groups.

Data for the first four columns from Food and Nutrition Board, Institute of Medicine. Proteins and amino acids. In: Dietary Reference Intakes for Energy, Carbohydrate, Fiber, Fat, Fatty Acids, Cholesterol, Protein, and Amino Acids (Macronutrients). Washington, DC: National Academy Press, 2002;10:1–143; data in the last column from Young VR, Borgonha S. J Nutr 2000;130:1841S–9S, based on direct amino acid oxidation and indicator amino acid oxidation tracer studies.

(4). The currently RDA for histidine is 14 mg/kg/day (see Table 2.13), largely based on histidine content of protein and the RDA for protein.

Why is it so difficult to define whether histidine is indispensable in adults when there is little evidence that a metabolic pathway for histidine synthesis exists in humans (12)? The difficulties occur because the requirement for histidine is small and the stores of histidine in the body are large (4, 157). Histidine is particularly abundant in hemoglobin and carnosine (the dipeptide β-alanylhistidine, which is present in large quantities in muscle). Furthermore, gut flora synthesizes an unknown amount of histidine, which may be absorbed and used. Histidine must be removed from the diet for more than a month to observe effects, and those effects are indirect measures of histidine insufficiency (a fall in hemoglobin and rise in serum iron), rather than alteration in conventional indices (N balance). Pencharz' group placed four adults on a histidine-free diet for 48 days and periodically measured protein turnover using [1-^{13}C]phenylalanine (159). A small, significant fall in protein turnover was noted over time, but urinary excretion of N or 3-methylhistidine was unaffected. No direct effect of histidine requirement could be determined in adults in this study. Thus, even though little direct evidence for histidine synthesis in humans exists, our estimates for the necessity of dietary histidine intake in adults are still largely inferential.

Arginine

In contrast to histidine, arginine is synthesized in large amounts in the body for the production of urea. However, as with cysteine and tyrosine, the synthesis of arginine depends on the availability of precursors, ornithine and citrulline. Although adequate amounts of arginine, ornithine, and citrulline are normally present in the liver to operate the urea cycle, the synthesis of ornithine, from which arginine and citrulline are produced, may be limited (12). Because arginine is synthesized in the body from ornithine, it is *not* an indispensable amino acid, but it is *indispensable* for optimal growth in several species of young mammals (157).

Rose and colleagues observed an adequate N balance in adult subjects fed an arginine-free diet, and Snyderman and associates found no health problems or lack of weight gain in infants fed an arginine-free diet (reviewed in 4). Carey and colleagues (184) placed adult subjects on a diet devoid of arginine for 5 days. They measured indices of urea cycle activity: plasma ammonia concentration, daily urinary excretion of orotic acid, and urinary N excretion. They found no alterations caused by the arginine-free diet. These results would lead to the conclusion that arginine is dispensable to the diet of humans; yet, little evidence indicates that the body synthesizes ornithine from glutamate in substantial amounts (see Fig. 2.4).

Castillo and colleagues measured arginine, ornithine, and citrulline kinetics simultaneously using stable isotopically labeled tracers in healthy adults (82). These studies showed that the fluxes of all three amino acids are very low in blood and do not reflect the active urea cycle component, which appears to be highly compartmentalized in the liver. Ornithine and citrulline fluxes were comparable, but were only one third the rate of arginine turnover, and a relatively small fraction of the ornithine tracer appeared in plasma arginine or citrulline. The low flux of ornithine suggests that very little synthesis occurs, but direct measurements of ornithine synthesis are lacking. Inferential measurements do suggest ornithine synthesis. For example ^{15}N tracer is transferred from glycine into glutamate and into the metabolic products of glutamate, including ornithine and proline (17).

Assessment of Protein Quality

Quality of a protein is defined by its ability to support growth in animals. Higher-quality protein produces a faster growth rate. Such growth rate measurements evaluate the actual factors important in a protein: (a) pattern and abundance of indispensable amino acids, (b) relative amounts of dispensable versus indispensable amino acids in the mixture, (c) digestibility when eaten, and (d) presence of toxic materials such as trypsin inhibitors or allergenic stimuli. Methods to define the quality of a formula or protein source have fallen generally into two categories: empiric biologic assays and scoring systems.

Biologic Assays

It is assumed that the "highest-quality protein" is that protein that supports maximal growth in a young animal. Because rats grow quickly, have limited protein stores, and a high metabolic rate, it is easy to detect deficiencies and imbalances in amino acid patterns in young growing rats in a short period. The *protein efficiency ratio* has been defined as the weight gained (in grams) divided by the amount of test protein consumed (in grams) by a young growing rat over a several-day period. Obviously, duration of diet, age, starting body weight, and species of rat employed will be important variables. Typically, 21-day-old male rats fed 9 to 10% protein (by weight) for 10 days to 4 weeks have been used. In one series of tests, casein produced a protein efficiency ratio of 2.8, soy protein 2.4, and wheat gluten 0.4. Clearly, a casein diet produced much better growth compared with gluten. Such an approach has been useful in defining the relative efficacy of clinical formulas used in enteral and parenteral nutrition (185). The formula that provides the optimal mixture of indispensable and dispensable amino acids should induce the most rapid growth. However, this method's results will be skewed in application to humans depending on the extent that human requirements for individual amino acids do not mimic those of the rat. However, the method has been very useful in comparing a new protein source against reference proteins, such as egg protein, and it does evaluate other factors such as relative digestibility.

Scoring Systems

Rather than use growth in an animal species as an indicator of protein quality, various methods have been developed to assign a quantitative value to the pattern of amino acids in a nutritional formula or to a particular dietary protein source. Thus, assignment is based on the amounts and importance of the individual amino acids in a formula. These "scoring" methods can be applied to define protein quality in terms of amino acid content for any species. Block and Mitchell pointed out in 1946 that all amino acids have to be provided simultaneously at the sites of protein synthesis in the body in the same proportions that go into protein (186). Assuming that any dispensable amino acid would not be limiting, they proposed that the value of a protein could be determined from the indispensable amino acid most limiting in abundance relative to the optimum amount needed. From this idea of "most limiting amino acid" came the concept of chemical scoring, which has been incorporated into the important reports assessing dietary needs of humans (161, 162, 167, 182, 187). The key to the method is that the test protein is defined "against" a reference protein, deemed to be of the "highest quality" in terms of amino acid composition. Historically, proteins that support maximal growth in animals were considered the proteins of the "highest" quality. Those proteins from the most widely available sources for human consumption—eggs and cow's milk—were consequently used as reference proteins. In 1973, the FAO/WHO adopted using the amino acid requirement pattern recommended for various age groups (see Table 2.13) as the basis for calculating chemical score (162, 188). Some of the scoring patterns that have been used are shown in Table 2.14. Typically, data for the 2- to 5-year-old child are taken as being most representative.

The scoring system is easy to apply because no animal studies or clinical studies are required to compare different nutritional formulations. The *chemical score* of a protein is calculated in two steps. First a score is calculated for each indispensable amino acid (IAA in the following equation) in the protein against the reference protein:

$$\text{IAA score} = \frac{(\text{content of the IAA in the } test \text{ protein/mixture})}{(\text{content of the IAA in } reference \text{ protein/mixture})} \cdot 100$$

Next, the lowest score is selected; the amino acid with the lowest score is defined as the *limiting amino acid*. The chemical score of the limiting amino acid is the protein's score. Typically, the limiting amino acids in dietary proteins are lysine, the sulfur-containing amino acids, threonine, and/or tryptophan. The BCAAs and phenylalanine/tyrosine are not usually limiting. The scoring method points out the obvious: proteins not balanced among the indispensable amino acids are not as good as those that are. Schaafsma (189) raised the question whether the use of fecal digestibility is appropriate in calculating the amino acid score of dietary proteins because it may overestimate true digestibility as a result of colonic bacteria uptake, and perhaps ileal digestibility may be more appropriate (190).

Ratio of Indispensable to Dispensable Amino Acids in Protein

Protein requirements diminish from infancy onward (see Table 2.12) because rates of accretion of new protein diminish with maturity. However, when the change in requirements for indispensable amino acids in Table 2.13 are compared with the total protein requirements in Table 2.12 with age, a greater drop with age is seen in indispensable amino acid requirements than in protein requirements. Indispensable amino acids make up more than 30% of protein requirements in infancy and early childhood, drop to 20% in later childhood, and decrease further to 11% in adulthood. As indispensable amino acids become a decreasingly important part of the amino acid requirements with age, dispensable amino acid intake could increase and become an increasingly greater proportion of our intake. However, such substitution does not necessarily happen. Except for possibly changing the type of protein eaten (e.g., decreased intake of milk proteins), we continue to eat protein presumably at or above the RDA. If that protein is of high quality, such as egg protein,

TABLE 2.14. AMINO ACIDS REQUIREMENT PATTERNS OF HUMANS COMPARED WITH THE COMPOSITION OF EGG PROTEIN

AMINO ACID	INFANTS 1 y	CHILDREN 2–5 y	CHILDREN 10–12 y	ADULTS	HEN EGG PROTEIN
			(mg AMINO ACID/g PROTEIN)		
Histidine	16	19	19	11	22
Isoleucine	40	28	28	13	24
Leucine	93	66	44	19	54
Lysine	60	58	44	16	70
Methionine + cysteine	33	25	22	17	57
Phenylalanine + tyrosine	72	63	22	19	93
Threonine	50	34	28	9	47
Tryptophan	10	11	9	5	17
Valine	54	35	25	13	66

Data from FAO/WHO/UNU. Energy and Protein Requirements. Technical report series no. 724. Geneva: World Health Organization, 1985.

it provides almost half of its amino acids as indispensable amino acids. Therefore, consumption of high-quality protein by adults at levels appropriate to meet the RDA for protein provides a severalfold excess of individual indispensable amino acids beyond requirements. In general, it is not difficult for adults to meet the minimum for indispensable amino acid intake, as recommended or as proposed by Young and Borgonha (172, 182), when protein is consumed at or above requirement.

Amino Acid Availability from Dietary Protein Sources

The foregoing methods provide schemes for determining protein quality based on either animal growth or amino acid composition using scoring. A particular drawback concerning the scoring system is that it does not consider other factors inherent in the test protein or the effect of how the protein is prepared for consumption. How food is prepared may significantly affect the bioavailibility of individual amino acids. As discussed earlier, some plants contain protein inhibitors of proteolytic digestive enzymes. Although soy protein is limiting in terms of its methionine content (191), rats fed soy protein grow poorly because of trypsin inhibition (136). Heat processing of the soy protein inactivates these inhibitors and improves growth (191). However, heat processing itself may damage amino acids. For example, heat treatment of protein in the presence of reducing sugars can promote reactions altering the lysine amino groups in the protein. This reaction, called the Maillard or "browning" reaction, can be seen in milk processing in which lactose reacts with lysine at high temperatures. Oxidative or alkaline processing conditions may also alter other indispensable and dispensable amino acids, inducing loss of methionine or formation of amino acid products that have toxic properties. Likewise, storage conditions may affect the nutritional quality of the protein. Thus, processing or "cooking" of the protein source as well as storage conditions and other factors must be considered in evaluating the quality of the protein.

Protein and Amino Acid Needs in Disease

Most of the discussion up to this point has centered around amino acid and protein metabolism in physiologically normal individuals. Although the effect of disease on amino acid and protein requirements is beyond the limits of this chapter, a few important general points need to be made. The first is that energy and protein needs are tied together, as illustrated in Figure 2.15. When metabolic rate rises, body protein will be mobilized for use as a fuel (amino acid oxidation) and for supply of carbon for gluconeogenesis. Several disease states produce an increase in metabolic rate. The first is infection, in which the onset of fever is a hallmark of increased metabolic rate. The second is injury, be it trauma, burn injury, or surgery. Along with onset of a hypermetabolic state comes a characteristic

increase in the loss of protein measured by increased urea production. Sir David Cuthbertson reported in 1931 that a simple bone fracture causes significant loss of N in the urine (192). Since then, numerous studies of the hypermetabolic state of injury and infection have been performed.

For most people, the injuries we suffer are minimal and self-limiting; that is, the fever goes away in a couple of days or the injury heals. In physiologically normal, healthy people, the impact of the injury on overall protein metabolism is as minimal as would be a bout of fasting. However, in chronic, long-term illness or in patients otherwise weakened by age or other factors, the onset of a hypermetabolic state may produce a significant and dangerous loss of body N.

The second point is that although the diagnosis of a metabolic condition that needs correcting may be straightforward (e.g., finding an increased loss of N and wasting of body protein), correcting the problem by administration of nutritional support is not as simple. The underlying illness usually resists or complicates simple nutritional replacement of amino acids. Trauma and infection are classic problems for which prevention of N loss is very difficult. Supplying additional nutrients either enterally (by mouth or feeding tube) or parenterally (by intravenous administration) may blunt, but will not reverse, the N loss seen in injury (193, 194).

Simple tools have been used to identify the hypermetabolic state: indirect calorimetry to measure energy expenditure and N balance to follow protein loss. These measurement methods have shown that blunting the N loss in such patients is not as simple as supplying more calories, more amino acids, or different formulations of amino acids. What becomes clear is that, although a nutritional problem exists, nutritional replacement will not correct the problem; instead, the metabolic factors that cause the condition must be identified and corrected. Wilmore categorized the factors that produce the hypermetabolic state into three groups: stress hormones (cortisol, catecholamines, glucagon), cytokines (e.g., tumor necrosis factor, interleukins), and lipid mediators (e.g., prostaglandins, thromboxanes) (193). Strategies have been developed to address these various components. For example, insulin and growth hormone have been administered to provide anabolic hormonal stimuli to improve N balance. Alternatively, studies have been conducted in healthy persons in whom one or more of the potential mediators are administered to define the effect of the mediator on amino acid and protein metabolism (194, 195). For example, studies of the infusion of individual hormones while isotopically labeled amino acid tracers are also infused have given us some insight into the mechanisms of hormone action on the regulation of amino acid oxidation, protein breakdown, and synthesis in humans (195).

In some situations, administration of a specific amino acid may produce a pharmacologic effect in ameliorating the disease state. Examples are the administration of glutamine and arginine or the limiting of sulfur amino acid intake. Glutamine is the most highly concentrated amino acid inside muscle cells and in plasma (84). Glutamine is an important nutrient to many cells, especially the gut and white cells, in which the glutamine may be used as a source of energy and also for critical processes such as the synthesis of nucleotides (196). Glutamine is an essential nutrient for cell culture media. Because a hallmark of injury is a drop in the intracellular level of muscle glutamine, presumably as a result of increased utilization by other tissues, glutamine has been proposed as a nutrient that becomes conditionally indispensable in trauma and infection (193, 197).

Arginine is another dispensable amino acid with important properties for promoting immune system function. Arginine is the precursor for nitric oxide synthesis (198) and has been proposed as a nutrient for altering immune function and improving wound healing (199, 200). We believe that adequate ornithine is synthesized to maintain arginine supplies under normal conditions, but we do not know whether additional demands for arginine can be met endogenously or whether arginine becomes a conditionally indispensable nutrient. For example, Yu and colleagues (201) measured arginine kinetics using stable isotope tracers in pediatric patients with burn injury and determined little net de novo arginine synthesis, a finding suggesting that, under conditions of burn injury, insufficient arginine is made to meet the body's presumed increased need for arginine when the immune system is under challenge.

Elevated plasma homocysteine has been identified as an independent risk factor for vascular disease (202). Homocysteine is produced by the hydrolysis of S-adenosylhomocysteine, which is derived from S-adenosylmethionine, a major methyl group donor (e.g., in creatine synthesis in Fig. 2.5). Homocysteine may be "remethylated" to reform methionine or degraded via condensation with serine to form cystathionine, which then goes on to form cysteine (see Fig. 2.4). High concentrations of homocysteine will occur when either or both of the disposal pathways of homocysteine is impaired. Because these reactions of homocysteine metabolism are dependent on vitamin B_6 (pyridoxal 5'-phosphate) and folate, supplementation of the diet with vitamin B_6 and folate will often be effective in lowering plasma homocysteine levels (202). Alternatively, the dietary intake of sulfur amino acids may be reduced by ingesting relatively more of a sulfur amino acid–poor dietary protein, such as soy protein.

Although supplementation of specific amino acids or cofactors may produce beneficial responses, on some occasions supplementation may produce undesirable effects on the disease state. Supplementing glutamine in the diets of patients with cancer may be counterproductive because the glutamine (which is essential for fast-growing cell lines in culture) may promote accelerated tumor growth (203). Similarly, arginine supplementation may stimulate nitric oxide synthesis because of the increased availability of the precursor for its formation.

However, nitric oxide production produces both helpful and detrimental effects (198). In these and other applications of specific nutrients, the use of isotopically labeled tracers is particularly helpful because the metabolic fate of the administered nutrient may be followed (labeled nitrate production from nitric oxide synthesis from ^{15}N-labeled arginine), as well as measurement of the promotion or suppression of protein synthesis and proteolysis in specific tissues. Definition of amino acid and protein requirements in various diseases is quite difficult to assess and requires a multifactorial approach. These are the real challenges facing us in nutrition today and in the days ahead.

REFERENCES

1. Cahill GF. N Engl J Med 1970;282:668–75.
2. Chipponi JX, Bleier JC, Santi MT et al. Am J Clin Nutr 1982; 35:1112–6.
3. Harper AE. Dispensable and indispensable amino acid interrelationships. In: Blackburn GL, Grant JP, Young VR, eds. Amino Acids: Metabolism and Medical Applications. Boston: John Wright, 1983:105–21.
4. Laidlaw SA, Kopple JD. Am J Clin Nutr 1987;46:593–605.
5. Block RJ, Weiss KW. Amino Acid Handbook: Methods and Results of Analysis. Springfield, IL: Charles C Thomas, 1956.
6. Bergström J, Fürst P, Noree LO et al. J Appl Physiol 1974;36: 693–7.
7. Cohn SH, Vartsky D, Yasumura S et al. Am J Physiol 1980;239: E524–30.
8. Heymsfield SB, Waki M, Kehayias J et al. Am J Physiol 1991; 261:E190–8.
9. Christensen HN. Physiol Rev 1990;70:43–77.
10. Souba WW, Pacitti AJ. JPEN J Parenter Enteral Nutr 1992;16: 569–78.
11. Rennie MJ, Tadros L, Khogali S et al. J Nutr 1994;124 [Suppl]: 1503S–8S.
12. Krebs HA. The metabolic fate of amino acids. In: Munro HN, Allison JB, eds. Mammalian Protein Metabolism, vol 1. New York: Academic Press, 1964:125–76.
13. Ben Galim E, Hruska K, Bier DM et al. J Clin Invest 1980; 66:1295–304.
14. Yoshida T, Kikuchi G. Arch Biochem Biophys 1970;139:380–92.
15. Yoshida T, Kikuchi G. J Biochem (Tokyo) 1972;72:1503–16.
16. Katagiri M, Nakamura M. Biochem Biophys Res Commun 2003;312:205–8.
17. Matthews DE, Conway JM, Young VR et al. Metabolism 1981;30:886–93.
18. Stipanuk MH. Annu Rev Nutr 1986;6:179–209.
19. Jacobsen JG, Smith LH Jr. Physiol Rev 1968;48:424–511.
20. Hayes KC. Nutr Rev 1985;43:65–70.
21. Beutler E. Annu Rev Nutr 1989;9:287–302.
22. Griffith OW. Free Radic Biol Med 1999;27:922–35.
23. Wu G, Fang YZ, Yang S et al. J Nutr 2004;134:489–92.
24. Rebouche CJ, Seim H. Annu Rev Nutr 1998;18:39–61.
25. Rebouche CJ. Fed Proc 1982;41:2848–52.
26. Watkins CA, Morgan HE. J Biol Chem 1979;254:693–701.
27. Young VR, Munro HN. Fed Proc 1978;37:2291–300.
28. Meldrum BS. J Nutr 2000;130:1007S–15S.
29. Rothstein JD, Martin LJ, Kuncl RW. N Engl J Med 1992;326: 1464–8.
30. Wyss M, Kaddurah-Daouk R. Physiol Rev 2000;80:1107–213.

31. Bloch K, Schoenheimer R. J Biol Chem 1941;138:167–94.

32. Heymsfield SB, Arteaga C, McManus C et al. Am J Clin Nutr 1983;37:478–94.

33. Walser M. JPEN J Parenter Enteral Nutr 1987;11:73S–8S.

34. Crim MC, Calloway DH, Margen S. J Nutr 1975;105:428–38.

35. Welle S, Thornton C, Totterman S et al. Am J Clin Nutr 1996; 63:151–6.

36. Wang Z-M, Gallagher D, Nelson M et al. Am J Clin Nutr 1996; 63:863–9.

37. Milner JA, Visek WJ. Nature 1973;245:211–2.

38. Hellerstein MK, Munro HN. Interaction of liver and muscle in the regulation of metabolism in response to nutritional and other factors. In: Arias IM, Jakoby WB, Popper H, et al., eds. The Liver: Biology and Pathobiology. 2nd ed. New York: Raven Press, 1988:965–83.

39. Harper AE. Am J Clin Nutr 1985;41:140–8.

40. Scrimshaw NS, Hussein MA, Murray E et al. J Nutr 1972;102: 1595–604.

41. Allison JB, Bird JWC. Elimination of nitrogen from the body. In: Munro HN, Allison JB, eds. Mammalian Protein Metabolism. New York: Academic Press, 1964:483–512.

42. Munro HN. Amino acid requirements and metabolism and their relevance to parenteral nutrition. In: Wilkinson AW, ed. Parenteral Nutrition. London: Churchill Livingstone, 1972: 34–67.

43. Owen OE, Reichle FA, Mozzoli MA et al. J Clin Invest 1981;68: 240–52.

44. Owen OE, Morgan AP, Kemp HG et al. J Clin Invest 1967;46: 1589–95.

45. Wahren J, Felig P, Hagenfeldt L. J Clin Invest 1976;57:987–99.

46. Brundin T, Wahren J. Am J Physiol 1994;267:E648–55.

47. Frayn KN, Khan K, Coppack SW et al. Clin Sci 1991;80: 471–4.

48. Young VR, Haverberg LN, Bilmazes C et al. Metabolism 1973; 23:1429–36.

49. Pisters PWT, Pearlstone DB. Crit Rev Clin Lab Sci 1993;30: 223–72.

50. Möller-Loswick A-C, Zachrisson H, Hyltander A et al. Am J Physiol 1994;266:E645–52.

51. Louard RJ, Bhushan R, Gelfand RA et al. J Clin Endocrinol Metab 1994;79:278–84.

52. Cheng KN, Dworzak F, Ford GC et al. Eur J Clin Invest 1985; 15:349–54.

53. Barrett EJ, Revkin JH, Young LH et al. Biochem J 1987; 245: 223–8.

54. Gelfand RA, Barrett EJ. J Clin Invest 1987;80:1–6.

55. Biolo G, Chinkes D, Zhang XJ et al. JPEN J Parenter Enteral Nutr 1992;16:305–15.

56. Biolo G, Fleming RYD, Maggi SP et al. Am J Physiol 1995;268: E75–84.

57. Tessari P, Inchiostro S, Zanetti M et al. Am J Physiol 1995;269: E127–36.

58. Wolfe RR. Radioactive and Stable Isotope Tracers in Biomedicine: Principles and Practice of Kinetic Analysis. New York: Wiley-Liss, 1992.

59. San Pietro A, Rittenberg D. J Biol Chem 1953;201:457–73.

60. Picou D, Taylor-Roberts T. Clin Sci 1969;36:283–96.

61. Bier DM, Matthews DE. Fed Proc 1982;41:2679–85.

62. Steffee WP, Goldsmith RS, Pencharz PB et al. Metabolism 1976;25:281–97.

63. Duffy B, Gunn T, Collinge J et al. Pediatr Res 1981;15: 1040–4.

64. Yudkoff M, Nissim I, McNellis W et al. Pediatr Res 1987;21: 49–53.

65. Waterlow JC, Golden MHN, Garlick PJ. Am J Physiol 1978; 235:E165–74.

66. Fern EB, Garlick PJ, McNurlan MA et al. Clin Sci 1981;61: 217–28.

67. Fern EB, Garlick PJ, Waterlow JC. Clin Sci 1985;68:271–82.

68. Matthews DE, Motil KJ, Rohrbaugh DK et al. Am J Physiol 1980;238:E473–9.

69. Bier DM. Diabetes Metab Rev 1989;5:111–32.

70. Toth MJ, MacCoss MJ, Poehlman ET et al. Am J Physiol 2001;281:E233–41.

71. Saccomani MP, Bonadonna RC, Caveggion E et al. Am J Physiol 1995;269:E183–92.

72. Allsop JR, Wolfe RR, Burke JF. J Appl Physiol 1978;45:137–9.

73. El-Khoury AE, Sánchez M, Fukagawa NK et al. J Nutr 1994; 124:1615–27.

74. Leese GP, Nicoll AE, Varnier M et al. Eur J Clin Invest 1994; 24:818–23.

75. Matthews DE, Bier DM, Rennie MJ et al. Science 1981;214: 1129–31.

76. Matthews DE, Schwarz HP, Yang RD et al. Metabolism 1982; 31:1105–12.

77. Schwenk WF, Beaufrère B, Haymond MW. Am J Physiol 1985;249:E646–50.

78. Matthews DE. Ital J Gastroenterol 1993;25:72–8.

79. Cobelli C, Saccomani MP, Tessari P et al. Am J Physiol 1991; 261:E539–50.

80. Cobelli C, Saccomani MP. JPEN J Parenter Enteral Nutr 1991; 15:45S–50S.

81. Tessari P, Barazzoni R, Zanetti M et al. Am J Physiol 1996;271: E733–41.

82. Castillo L, Sánchez M, Vogt J et al. Am J Physiol 1995;268: E360–7.

83. Darmaun D, Matthews DE, Bier DM. Am J Physiol 1986;251: E117–26.

84. Souba WW, Herskowitz K, Austgen TR et al. JPEN J Parenter Enteral Nutr 1990;14:237S–43S.

85. Souba WW. Annu Rev Nutr 1991;11:285–308.

86. Cortiella J, Matthews DE, Hoerr RA et al. Am J Clin Nutr 1988;48:988–1009.

87. Tessari P, Pehling G, Nissen SL et al. Diabetes 1988;37:512–9.

88. Matthews DE, Marano MA, Campbell RG. Am J Physiol 1993;264:E109–18.

89. Hoerr RA, Matthews DE, Bier DM et al. Am J Physiol 1991; 260:E111–7.

90. Castillo L, Chapman TE, Yu YM et al. Am J Physiol 1993;265: E532–9.

91. Biolo G, Tessari P. Metabolism 1997;46:164–7.

92. Krempf M, Hoerr RA, Marks L et al. Metabolism 1990;39:560–2.

93. Haisch M, Fukagawa NK, Matthews DE. Am J Physiol 2000; 278:E593–602.

94. Hoerr RA, Matthews DE, Bier DM et al. Am J Physiol 1993; 264:E567–75.

95. Metges CC, El Khoury AE, Henneman L et al. Am J Physiol 1999;277:E597–607.

96. Battezzati A, Haisch M, Brillon DJ et al. Metabolism 1999; 48:915–21.

97. Matthews DE, Marano MA, Campbell RG. Am J Physiol 1993; 264:E848–54.

98. Hankard RG, Darmaun D, Sager BK et al. Am J Physiol 1995;269 :E663–70.

99. Boza JJ, Dangin M, Moennoz D et al. Am J Physiol 2001; 281: G267–74.

100. Battezzati A, Brillon DJ, Matthews DE. Am J Physiol 1995; 269: E269–76.

101. Nair KS, Halliday D, Griggs RC. Am J Physiol 1988;254: E208–13.

102. Welle S, Thornton C, Statt M et al. Am J Physiol 1994;267: E599–604.

103. Rooyackers OE, Adey DB, Ades PA et al. Proc Natl Acad Sci USA 1996;93:15364–9.

104. Rooyackers OE, Balagopal P, Nair KS. Muscle Nerve 1997; S93–6.

105. Cryer DR, Matsushima T, Marsh JB et al. J Lipid Res 1986;27: 508–16.

106. Lichtenstein AH, Hachey DL, Millar JS et al. J Lipid Res 1992; 33:907–14.

107. Reeds PJ, Hachey DL, Patterson BW et al. J Nutr 1992; 122: 457–66.

108. Arends J, Schäfer G, Schauder P et al. Metabolism 1995; 44: 1253–8.

109. Ikewaki K, Rader DJ, Schaefer JR et al. J Lipid Res 1993; 34: 2207–15.

110. Brinton EA, Eisenberg S, Breslow JL. Arterioscler Thromb 1994;14:707–20.

111. Ikewaki K, Zech LA, Brewer HB Jr et al. J Lab Clin Med 2002; 140:369–74.

112. Laurent GJ. Am J Physiol 1987;252:C1–9.

113. Long CL, Dillard DR, Bodzin JH et al. Metabolism 1988;37: 844–9.

114. Young VR, Alexis SD, Baliga BS et al. J Biol Chem 1972;247: 3592–600.

115. Long CL, Haverberg LN, Young VR et al. Metabolism 1975; 24:929–35.

116. Elia M, Carter A, Bacon S et al. Clin Sci 1980;59:509–11.

117. Millward DJ, Bates PC, Grimble GK et al. Biochem J 1980; 190:225–8.

118. Rennie MJ, Millward DJ. Clin Sci 1983;65:217–25.

119. Sjölin J, Stjernström H, Henneberg S et al. Metabolism 1989; 38:23–9.

120. Rathmacher JA, Flakoll PJ, Nissen SL. Am J Physiol 1995;269: E193–8.

121. Lundholm K, Bennegård K, Edén E et al. Cancer Res 1982;42: 4807–11.

122. Morrison WL, Gibson JNA, Rennie MJ. Eur J Clin Invest 1988; 18:648–54.

123. Vissers YL, Von Meyenfeldt MF, Braulio VB et al. Clin Sci 2003;104:585–90.

124. Vesali RF, Klaude M, Thunblad L et al. Metabolism 2004;53: 1076–80.

125. Nair KS, Ford GC, Ekberg K et al. J Clin Invest 1995;95: 2926–37.

126. Cahill GF Jr, Aoki TT. Partial and total starvation. In: Kinney JM, ed. Assessment of Energy Metabolism in Health and Disease. Report of the First Ross Conference on Medical Research. Columbus, OH: Ross Laboratories, 1980:129–34.

127. Elia M. Organ and tissue contribution to metabolic rate. In: Kinney JM, Tucker HN, eds. Energy Metabolism: Determinants and Cellular Corollaries. New York: Raven Press, 1992:61–79.

128. Bier DM, Leake RD, Haymond MW et al. Diabetes 1977;26: 1016–23.

129. Owen OE, Felig P, Morgan AP et al. J Clin Invest 1969;48: 574–83.

130. Pozefsky T, Felig P, Tobin JD et al. J Clin Invest 1969;48: 2273–82.

131. Felig P, Owen OE, Wahren J et al. J Clin Invest 1969;48:584–94.

132. Stumvoll M, Chintalapudi U, Perriello G et al. J Clin Invest 1995;96:2528–33.

133. Cersosimo E, Judd RL, Miles JM. J Clin Invest 1994;93: 2584–9.

134. Felig P. Annu Rev Biochem 1975;44:933–55.

135. Alpers DH. Digestion and absorption of carbohydrates and proteins. In: Johnson LR, Alpers DH, Christensen J, et al., eds. Physiology of the Gastrointestinal Tract. 3rd ed. New York: Raven Press, 1994:1723–49.

136. Green GM, Olds BA, Matthews G et al. Proc Soc Exp Biol Med 1973;142:1162–7.

137. Crim MC, Munro HN. Protein and amino acid requirements and metabolism in relation to defined formula diets. In: Shils ME, ed. Defined Formula Diets for Medical Purposes. Chicago: American Medical Association, 1977:5–15.

138. Matthews DM. Protein Absorption: Development and Present State of the Subject. New York: Wiley-Liss, 1991.

139. Ganapathy V, Brandsch M, Leibach FH. Intestinal transport of amino acids and peptides. In: Johnson LR, Alpers DH, Christensen J, et al., eds. Physiology of the Gastrointestinal Tract. 3rd ed. New York: Raven Press, 1994:1773–94.

140. Freeman HJ, Kim YS. Annu Rev Med 1978;29:99–116.

141. Alpers DH. Fed Proc 1986;45:2261–7.

142. Asatoor AM, Cheng B, Edwards KDG et al. Gut 1970;11: 380–7.

143. Jepsen JB. Hartnup disease. In: Stanbury JB, Wyngaarden JB, Fredrickson DS, eds. The Metabolic Basis of Inherited Disease. 4th ed. New York: McGraw-Hill, 1978:1563–77.

144. Gardner ML. Absorption of intact proteins and peptides. In: Johnson LR, Alpers DH, Christensen J, et al., eds. Physiology of the Gastrointestinal Tract. 3rd ed. New York: Raven Press, 1994:1795–820.

145. Elwyn DH, Parikh HC, Shoemaker WC. Am J Physiol 1968;215:1260–75.

146. Aoki TT, Brennan MF, Muller WA et al. Am J Clin Nutr 1976;29:340–50.

147. DeFronzo RA, Felig P. Am J Clin Nutr 1980;33:1378–86.

148. Elia M, Livesey G. Clin Sci 1983;64:517–26.

149. Matthews DE, Harkin R, Battezzati A et al. Metabolism 1999;48:1555–63.

150. Neame KD, Wiseman G. J Physiol (Lond) 1957;135:442–50.

151. Windmueller HG. Adv Enzymol 1982;53:201–37.

152. Windmueller HG. Metabolism of vascular and luminal glutamine by intestinal mucosa in vivo. In: Häussinger D, Sies H, eds. Glutamine Metabolism in Mammalian Tissues. Berlin: Springer–Verlag, 1984:61–77.

153. Cersosimo E, Williams PE, Radosevich PM et al. Am J Physiol 1986;250:E622–8.

154. Abumrad NN, Williams P, Frexes–Steed M et al. Diabetes Metab Rev 1989;5:213–26.

155. Rose WC, Wixom RL, Lockhart HB et al. J Biol Chem 1955; 217:987–95.

156. Rose WC. Nutr Abstr Rev 1957;27:631–47.

157. Visek WJ. Annu Rev Nutr 1984;4:137–55.

158. Walser M. Clin Sci 1984;66:1–15.

159. Kriengsinyos W, Rafii M, Wykes LJ et al. J Nutr 2002;132: 3340–8.

160. FAO/WHO/UNU. Energy and Protein Requirements. Technical report series no. 724. Geneva: World Health Organization, 1985.

161. Food and Nutrition Board, National Institute of Medicine. Recommended Dietary Allowances. 10th ed. Washington, DC: National Academy Press, 1989.

162. FAO/WHO. Energy and Protein Requirements. Echnical report series no. 522. Geneva: World Health Organization, 1973.

163. Munro HN. Historical perspective on protein requirements: objectives for the future. In: Blaxter K, Waterlow JC, eds. Nutritional Adaptation in Man. London: John Libbey, 1985:155–68.

164. Rand WM, Young VR. J Nutr 1999;129:1920–6.

165. Rand WM, Pellett PL, Young VR. Am J Clin Nutr 2003; 77:109–27.

166. Young VR, Yu YM, Fukagawa NK. Acta Paediatr Scand Suppl 1991;80:5–24.

167. Food and Nutrition Board, Institute of Medicine. Proteins and amino acids. In: Dietary Reference Intakes for Energy, Carbohydrate, Fiber, Fat, Fatty Acids, Cholesterol, Protein, and Amino Acids (Macronutrients). Washington, DC: National Academy Press, 2002;10:1–143.

168. Irwin MI, Hegsted DM. J Nutr 1971;101:539–66.

169. Millward DJ, Price GM, Pacy PJH et al. Proc Nutr Soc 1990;49:473–87.

170. Young VR, Bier DM, Pellett PL. Am J Clin Nutr 1989;50:80–92.

171. Young VR. Am J Clin Nutr 1987;46:709–25.

172. Young VR. J Nutr 1994;124[Suppl]:1517S–23S.

173. Young VR, El-Khoury AE. Proc Natl Acad Sci USA 1995;92:300–4.

174. Young VR, Moldawer LL, Hoerr R et al. Mechanisms of adaptation to protein malnutrition. In: Blaxter K, Waterlow JC, eds. Nutritional Adaptation in Man. London: John Libbey, 1985:189–217.

175. Zello GA, Wykes LJ, Ball RO et al. J Nutr 1995;125:2907–15.

176. Wilson DC, Rafii M, Ball RO et al. Am J Clin Nutr 2000;71:757–64.

177. Zello GA, Pencharz PB, Ball RO. Am J Physiol 1993;264:E677–85.

178. Kriengsinyos W, Wykes LJ, Ball RO et al. J Nutr 2002;132:2251–7.

179. El-Khoury AE, Fukagawa NK, Sánchez M et al. Am J Clin Nutr 1994;59:1000–11.

180. El-Khoury AE, Fukagawa NK, Sánchez M et al. Am J Clin Nutr 1994;59:1012–20.

181. Borgonha S, Regan MM, Oh SH et al. Am J Clin Nutr 2002;75:698–704.

182. Young VR, Borgonha S. J Nutr 2000;130:1841S–9S.

183. Kopple JD, Swendseid ME. J Nutr 1981;111:931–42.

184. Carey GP, Kime Z, Rogers QR et al. J Nutr 1987;117:1734–9.

185. Bjelton L, Sandberg G, Wennberg A et al. Assessment of biological quality of amino acid solutions for intravenous nutrition. In: Kinney JM, Borum PR, eds. Perspectives in Clinical Nutrition. Baltimore: Urban & Schwarzenberg, 1989:31–41.

186. Block RJ, Mitchell HH. Nutr Abstr Rev 1946;16:249–78.

187. Reeds PJ. Proc Nutr Soc 1990;49:489–97.

188. Pellett PL. Am J Clin Nutr 1990;51:723–37.

189. Schaafsma G. J Nutr 2000;130:1865S–7S.

190. Darragh AJ, Hodgkinson SM. J Nutr 2000;130:1850S–6S.

191. Young VR, Scrimshaw NS, Torun B et al. J Am Oil Chem Soc 1979;56:110–20.

192. Cuthbertson DP. Injury 1980;11:175–89.

193. Wilmore DW. N Engl J Med 1991;325:695–702.

194. Lowry SF. Proc Nutr Soc 1992;51:267–77.

195. Matthews DE, Battezzati A. Substrate kinetics and catabolic hormones. In: Kinney JM, Tucker HN, eds. Organ Metabolism and Nutrition: Ideas for Future Critical Care. New York: Raven Press, 1994:1–22.

196. Souba WW, Klimberg VS, Plumley DA et al. J Surg Res 1990;48:383–91.

197. Labow BI, Souba WW. World J Surg 2000;24:1503–13.

198. Griffith OW, Stuehr DJ. Annu Rev Physiol 1995;57:707–36.

199. Brittenden J, Heys SD, Ross J et al. Clin Sci 1994;86:123–32.

200. Ziegler TR, Gatzen C, Wilmore DW. Annu Rev Med 1994;45:459–80.

201. Yu YM, Sheridan RL, Burke JF et al. Am J Clin Nutr 1996;64:60–6.

202. Verhoef P, Stampfer MJ, Buring JE et al. Am J Epidemiol 1996;143:845–59.

203. Souba WW. Ann Surg 1993;218:715–28.

SELECTED READINGS

Food and Nutrition Board, Institute of Medicine. Recommended Dietary Allowances. 10th ed. Washington, DC: National Academy Press, 1989.

Food and Nutrition Board, Institute of Medicine. Dietary Reference Intakes for Energy, Carbohydrate, Fiber, Fat, Fatty Acids, Cholesterol, Protein, and Amino Acids (Macronutrients). Washington, DC: National Academy Press, 2002.

Munro HN, Allison JB. Mammalian Protein Metabolism, vol 1. New York: Academic Press, 1964.

Nissen S. Modern Methods in Protein Nutrition and Metabolism. San Diego: Academic Press, 1992.

Wolfe RR. Radioactive and Stable Isotope Tracers in Biomedicine: Principles and Practice of Kinetic Analysis. New York: Wiley-Liss, 1992.

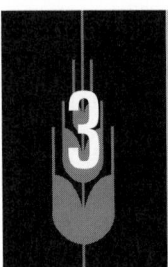

CARBOHYDRATES[1]

NANCY L. KEIM, ROY J. LEVIN, AND PETER J. HAVEL

HISTORICAL HIGHLIGHTS 62
DEFINITION 62
DIETARY CARBOHYDRATES 63
   Starch 63
     Starch Breakdown 63
     Resistant Starch 64
     Dietary Fiber 65
     Sugars: Functions and Properties 66
GETTING GLUCOSE INTO CELLS:
   THE TRANSPORTERS 66
   Human Facilitative-Diffusion Glucose
     Transporter Family 67
   Study of Glucose Transporters by Use
     of Transgenic and Knockout Mice 69
BLOOD GLUCOSE: METABOLIC
   AND HORMONAL REGULATION 69
   Metabolic Regulation 69
   Hormonal Regulation of Carbohydrate
     Metabolism 70
TRANSEPITHELIAL HEXOSE TRANSPORT:
   INTESTINE AND KIDNEY .72
   Sodium-Glucose Cotransporters 72
   Electrogenic Glucose-Linked Sodium Transfer 73
GLUCOSE STORAGE 76
   Glycogen 76
   Carbohydrates and Athletic Performance 77
DISORDERS OF CARBOHYDRATE DIGESTION,
   ABSORPTION, OR METABOLISM 77
   Carbohydrate Intolerance 77
   Diagnostic Tests to Evaluate Carbohydrate
     Digestion, Absorption, or Metabolism 78
DIETARY REFERENCE INTAKES
   FOR CARBOHYDRATE 79
CARBOHYDRATES AND CHRONIC DISEASE 79
   Sugar and Dental Caries .79
   Health Impact of Fructose Consumption 79

HISTORICAL HIGHLIGHTS

The initial history of simple carbohydrates is the story of sugar cane and the human passion for sweetness. Although there is some dissension, sugar cane's origin is thought to be Papua New Guinea. It was probably cultivated from wild plants (still in existence) about 10,000 years ago at the time of the global Neolithic agricultural revolution. The slow diffusion of migrants brought sugar cane to India, Southeast Asia, and China. Sugar was mentioned by an Indian author in 325 BCE. After the Arabs defeated the Romans, they brought the sugar cane from Persia to Europe and the Mediterranean, where it failed to thrive, apart from the Moroccan coast. The returning Crusaders brought sugar to the European courts, where it became an important and desirable luxury dietary constituent. Sugar cane was introduced to the Caribbean by Christopher Columbus on his second voyage, in 1493. The plants came from his father-in-law's plantation established in Madeira in 1492 (Canary Islands). These plants thrived and were dispersed to Central and South America and throughout the Caribbean. By the early seventeenth century, raw sugar was being handled by refineries in England and France. Beets (unlike sugar cane, which needed a tropical or semitropical climate) could be grown in temperate climates and were first recognized as a source of sugar by Marggraf in 1747. Napoleon used beets to bypass the British sugar blockade of the French Caribbean Islands. By 1813, sugar production was approximately 35,000,000 kg (35,000 tons). Sugar from beets represents about 40% of the world sugar market. Kirchoff, a Russian chemist, reported in 1812 that starch, the plant storage form of carbohydrate, when boiled with dilute acid, produced a free sugar known to be contained in grapes (glucose). Schmidt, in 1844, designated carbohydrates as compounds that contained carbon, hydrogen, and oxygen and showed that sugar was found in the blood. Liver glycogen, the animal storage form of carbohydrate, was discovered by the accomplished French physiologist Claude Bernard in 1856. Sugar is now produced in practically every country in the world and is consumed as a basic or staple food.

DEFINITION

What are carbohydrates? The formal definition is a class of substances having the formula $C_n(H_2O)_n$; that is, the molar

---

[1]**Abbreviations: AI,** adequate intake; **ATP,** adenosine triphosphate; **Ca^{2+},** calcium; **GLUT,** glucose transporter; **K^+,** potassium; **K_m,** Michaelis-Menten constant; **Na^+,** sodium; **RDA,** recommended dietary allowance; **RS,** resistant starch; **SGLT,** sodium-linked glucose transporter.

ratio of carbon to hydrogen to oxygen is 1:2:1. This definition, however, fails for oligosaccharides, polysaccharides, and the sugar alcohols (sorbitol, maltitol, mannitol, galactitol, and lactitol). Of the complex carbohydrate macromolecules known, the main member is plant starch (and the animal polymer glycogen), but the group includes pectins, cellulose, and gums. Simple carbohydrates include the hexose monosaccharides (glucose, galactose, and fructose) and the disaccharides maltose (glucose-glucose), sucrose (glucose-fructose), and lactose (glucose-galactose). Other carbohydrates include trioses (glycerose, $C_3H_6O_3$), tetroses (erythrose, $C_4H_8O_4$), and pentoses (ribose, $C_5H_{10}O_5$). The last are important constituents of nucleic acids. In general, oligosaccharides are defined as yielding three to ten monosaccharides on hydrolysis, whereas polysaccharides yield more than ten. The polysaccharides serve both energy storage and structural functions. Starch is the storage carbohydrate of plants, whereas animals store carbohydrate as glycogen (liver contains up to 6% and muscle about 1% glycogen by weight). Many different types of starch exist, depending on the plant source. Inulin, for example, is a starch found in the tubers and roots of dahlias, artichokes, and dandelions and, when hydrolyzed, yields only fructose; hence it is a fructosan. The oligosaccharide cellulose consists of glucose units linked by β (1-4) bonds to form long, straight chains strengthened by hydrogen bonding. It is the chief structural framework of plants and cannot be digested by humans because we do not secrete an intestinal carbohydrase that hydrolyzes the β (1-4) linkage. Thus, cellulose is considered to be a dietary fiber that provides bulk to plant-based foods. Bacterial enzymes, however, can break down cellulose. A small amount is hydrolyzed by this process in the human colon, but cellulose makes only a minor contribution to overall energy requirements.

DIETARY CARBOHYDRATES

Carbohydrates represent a large family of naturally occurring compounds and derivatives of these compounds (Fig. 3.1). However, only relatively small numbers of carbohydrates are produced commercially and used in the food industry or are of significant metabolic importance. Dietary carbohydrate is a major macronutrient for both humans and omnivorous animals. Human adults in the Western world obtain approximately half their daily caloric requirements from dietary carbohydrate; in developing countries, it has been the major source, at least until the recent introduction of Western foods to many such countries. Of ingested carbohydrate, approximately 60% is in the form of polysaccharides, mainly starch, but the disaccharides sucrose and lactose represent 30 and 10%, respectively (Table 3.1). Monosaccharides (glucose and fructose) are naturally present in fruits and also are found in manufactured foods and drinks, primarily in the form of high-fructose corn syrup. Some oligosaccharides, such as

raffinose and stachyose, are found in small amounts in various legumes. They cannot be broken down by the enzymes of the pancreas and small intestine (Table 3.2), but they are digested by bacterial enzymes, especially in the colon.

The important dietary polysaccharides have to be broken down into their constituent monosaccharides before they can be absorbed and metabolized. This breakdown is initially carried out by the carbohydrase α-amylase secreted by the salivary glands and the pancreas and completed by disaccharidases located in the brush-border membrane of the enterocytes in the small intestine (see Table 3.2 for the major intestinal glycosidases) (1).

Starch

Starch, by far the most important dietary polysaccharide, consists only of glucose units and is thus a homopolysaccharide and is designated a glucosan or glucan. It is actually composed of two such homopolymers (Fig. 3.2): amylose, which has linear (1-4) linked α-D-glucose, and amylopectin, a highly branched form containing both (1-4) and (1-6) linkages at the branch points. Plants have both forms as insoluble, semicrystalline granules and differing ratios of amylopectin and amylose, depending on the plant source (Table 3.3). The salivary and pancreatic amylases act on the interior (1-4) linkages but cannot break the outer glucose-glucose links. Thus, the final breakdown products formed by the amylases are α-(1-4)–linked disaccharides (maltose) and trisaccharides (maltotriose).

Starch Breakdown

The breakdown of starch begins in the mouth, with salivary amylase. It is often assumed that as this enzyme is swallowed into an acid stomach, the enzymic carbohydrate breakdown is stopped (although acid hydrolysis may still occur) because salivary amylase is inhibited by a pH lower than 4. However, starch and its end products and the proteins and amino acids present in a mixed meal all buffer the acid of the stomach and allow some amount of hydrolysis to continue. Thus, the quantitative involvement of salivary amylase in the breakdown of starch may be underestimated. Pancreatic α-amylase added to the emptying gastric contents (chyme) in the duodenum cannot hydrolyze the (1-6) branching links and has little specificity for the (1-4) links adjacent to the branching points. Amylase action produces large oligosaccharides (α-limit dextrins) containing on average about eight glucose units with one or more (1-6) links. These α-limit dextrins are split by the enzymatic action of glucoamylase (α-limit dextrinase), which sequentially removes a single glucose unit from the nonreducing end of a linear α-(1-4)-glucosyl oligosaccharide. Maltose and maltotriose are then broken down by secreted and brush-border disaccharidases, especially sucrase-isomaltase, into free glucose, which is then transported into and across the enterocytes by hexose transporters (Table 3.4).

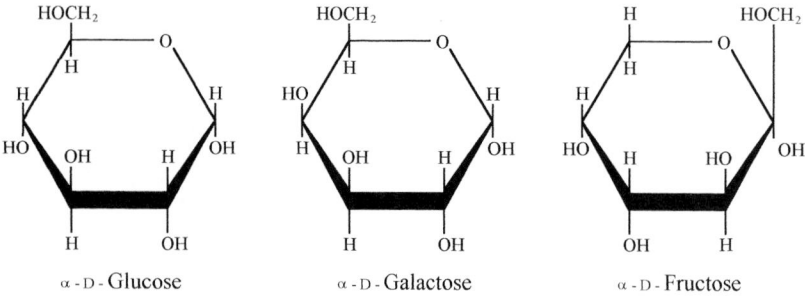

α-D-Glucose   α-D-Galactose   α-D-Fructose

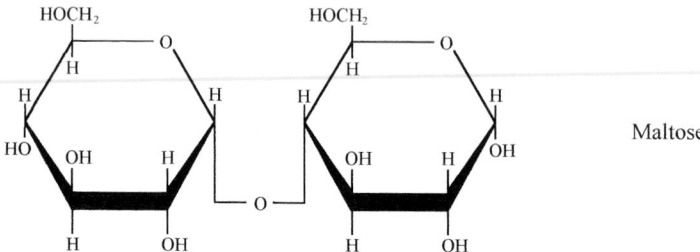

Maltose

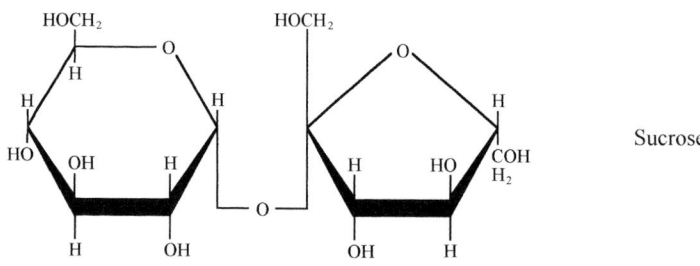

Sucrose

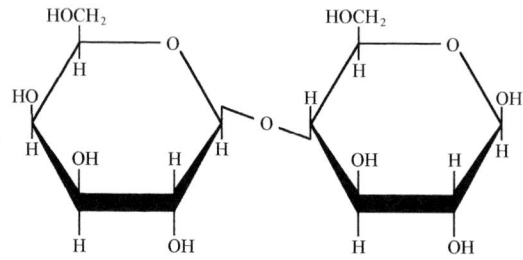

Lactose

Figure 3.1. Structures of the common dietary monosaccharides and disaccharides in perspective. Haworth representation.

The initial breakdown of starch into α-limit dextrins, the intraluminal or cavital digestion phase, occurs mainly in the bulk fluid phase of the intestinal contents. In humans, there appears to be little of the so-called contact or membrane digestion in which adsorption of amylase onto the brush-border surface of enterocytes facilitates its enzymatic activity (2).

Normally, α-amylase is not a limiting factor in the assimilation of starches in humans, but newborn babies, and especially premature ones, cannot assimilate starch because the pancreas secretes insufficient α-amylase to digest it. However, within a month, the secretion of α-amylase is usually sufficient for full digestion (3).

Resistant Starch

Starch is most frequently eaten after cooking. The heat of cooking gelatinizes the starch granules, thus increasing their susceptibility to enzymatic (α-amylase) digestion. However, a proportion of the starch, called resistant starch

TABLE 3.1. PRINCIPAL DIETARY CARBOHYDRATES

FOOD SOURCE	GRAINS	STARCHY VEGETABLES	LEGUMES	FRUITS	SUGARS AND SWEETENERS	MILK
	Rice	Yam	Soybeans	Apple	Cane sugar	
	Wheat	Potato	Dried peas	Orange	Beet sugar	
	Oats	Sweet corn	Lima beans	Grapes	Sorghum	
	Barley	Cassava		Peach	Honey	
	Rye			Pineapple	Corn syrup	
	Maize			Banana		
Polysaccharide	Starch	Starch	Starch			
Oligosaccharide			Raffinose, stachyose			
Disaccharide	Maltose			Sucrose	Sucrose	Lactose
Monosaccharide				Fructose	Fructose	
				Glucose	Glucose	

(RS), is undigestible even after prolonged incubation with the enzyme. In cereals, RS represents 0.4 to 2% of the dry matter; in potatoes, 1 to 3.5%; and in legumes, 3.5 to 5.7%. RS has been categorized as the sum of the starch and degradation products not absorbed in the small intestine of a healthy person (4). Three main categories are recognized: RS1, physically enclosed starch (partially milled grains and seeds); RS2, ungelatinized crystalline granules of the B-type x-ray pattern (as found in bananas and potatoes); and RS3, retrograded amylose (formed during the cooling of starch gelatinized by moist heating). RSs escape digestion in the small intestine, but then enter the colon, where they can be fermented by the local resident bacteria (>400 different types). In this respect, RS is somewhat similar to dietary fiber. Estimates of the RS and unabsorbed starch represent about 2 to 5% of the total starch ingested in the average Western diet, approximately 10 g/day (5). The end products of the fermentation of the RS in the colon are short-chain fatty acids (e.g., acetic, butyric, propionic), carbon dioxide, hydrogen, and methane (released as flatus).

Refractory starches stimulate bacterial growth in the colon. Although the short-chain fatty acids stimulate crypt cell mitosis in animals, it is not known whether they do the same in the human colon (6). However, if the human colon is removed from the mainstream of foodstuffs flowing down the lumen of the gastrointestinal tract, then the colonocytes lose their absorptive function, and ionic absorption is reduced. Luminal short-chain fatty acids from bacterial fermentation are used by colonocytes as metabolic substrates and appear to be required for normal colonic function (7).

Dietary Fiber

Dietary fiber was originally defined as "the remnants of plant cell walls not hydrolyzed by the alimentary enzymes of man," but the definition was subsequently modified to include "all plant polysaccharides and lignins which are resistant to hydrolysis by the digestive enzymes of man" (8). Soluble dietary fiber includes pectin and hydrocolloids, and insoluble fiber includes cellulose and hemicellulose. Grains, cereals, legumes, fruits, and vegetables are heterogeneous with respect to the mix of the various fiber types they contain, but the concentration of dietary fiber within a food group is generally similar. Pectins are found in greatest proportions in fruits and vegetables, hemicelluloses are the major fiber type in grains, and cellulose is the primary fiber type in legumes (9). Soluble and insoluble fibers are fermented by the luminal bacteria of the colon. High-fiber diets maintained for the long term reduce the incidence of colon cancer, but the mechanisms involved in the effects of fiber to prevent colon cancer are not well understood. Investigators have suggested that the bulk action of fiber speeds colonic transit and reduces the

TABLE 3.2. MAJOR GLYCOSIDASES OF THE MAMMALIAN ENTEROCYTE BRUSH BORDER

GLYCOSIDASE	ENZYME COMPLEX	ENZYME ACTIVITY
Maltase-sucrase	Sucrase-isomaltase	80% of maltase; some α-limit dextrinase; all of sucrose; most of isomaltase
Maltase-isomaltase		
Maltase-glucomylase (2)	Glucoamylase	All glucoamylase; most of α-limit dextrinase; 20% maltase; small % isomaltase
Trehalase		All trehalase
Lactase	β-glycosidase	All neutral lactase and cellobiose
Glycosyl-ceramidase (phlorizin hydrolase)		Most of aryl-β-glycosidase

Adapted from Dahlqvist A, Semenza G. J. Pediatr Gastroenterol 1988; 4:857–67, with permission.

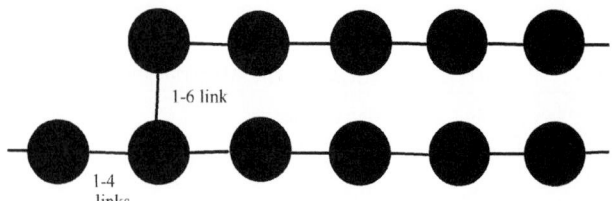

Figure 3.2. Starch is composed of amylose (15–20%) and amylopectin (80–85%). Amylose is a nonbranching helical chain structure of glucose residues, whereas amylopectin (a portion shown above) has branched chains of 24 to 30 glucose residues *(solid black)* joined by (1→4) glucosidic linkages with (1-6) linkages creating the branching points.

TABLE 3.3. AMYLOSE AND AMYLOPECTIN CONTENT OF VARIOUS PLANT STARCHES

PLANT	AMYLOSE (%)	AMYLOPECTIN (%)
Maize (standard)	24	76
Potato	20	80
Rice	18.5	81.5
Tapioca	16.7	83.3
Wheat	25	75

Sugars: Functions and Properties

Sugars, unlike starch, have an obvious impact on human taste because they are sweet. The classic view of taste recognizes four: sweet, sour, salty, and bitter, with all other taste sensations considered mixtures of these. A more modern concept is that sweetness is not a unitary quality, and individual variation exists in the ability to "taste" different sweetness qualities for different sweeteners. Human neonates recognize and like sweetness, a finding that is not surprising because the lactose in their major food, human milk, gives it a sweet taste. Estimates of relative sweetness of various carbohydrates by humans are usually made against the standard, sucrose (100%). On this scale, glucose (sweet with a bitter side taste) is 61 to 70, fructose (sweet, fruity) 130 to 180, maltose (sweet, syrupy) 43 to 50, and lactose 15 to 40. Investigators have speculated that during human evolution, the quest for foods containing maximal energy caused primitive humans to acquire a recognition that sweetness indicated safety and energy.

Today, sugars (primarily sucrose, glucose, and fructose) are used extensively in foods to provide sweetness, energy, texture, and bulk and also for appearance, preservation (by raising the osmotic pressure), and fermentation (in bread, alcoholic beverages). The palatability, appearance, and shelf life of a huge variety of foods and drinks are enhanced by adding sucrose; examples are as follows: breads, cakes, and biscuits; preserves and jellies; confectionery; dairy products; cured, dried, and preserved meats; breakfast cereals; and frozen and canned vegetables. As a result of the addition of sugars to so many food products, sugar consumption has increased since the 1970s. In certain Western countries, soft drinks, juice beverages, and the increased use of high-fructose corn syrup are the major sources of dietary sugar. This "hidden sugar" makes accurate assessment of dietary sugar intake difficult.

GETTING GLUCOSE INTO CELLS: THE TRANSPORTERS

A major source of metabolic energy for most, if not all, mammalian cells is the oxidation of D-glucose. The lipid-rich membranes of such cells, however, are relatively impermeable to hydrophilic polar molecules such as glucose. Specific transport processes have evolved to allow the cellular entry and exit of glucose. Carrier proteins located in the plasma membranes of cells can bind glucose and allow it to traverse the lipid membrane barrier, thus releasing the hexose into the cellular cytoplasm or body fluids.

TABLE 3.4. HUMAN FACILITATED-DIFFUSION GLUCOSE TRANSPORTER FAMILY (GLUT 1–5)

TYPE	AMINO ACIDS (N)	CHROMOSOME LOCATION	K_m (mmol/L) FOR HEXOSE UPTAKE[a]	MAJOR EXPRESSION SITES
GLUT 1 (red cell)	492	1	1–2 (red cells)	Placenta, brain, kidney, colon
GLUT 2 (liver)	524	3	15–20 (hepatocytes)	Liver, β-cell, kidney, small intestine
GLUT 3 (brain)	496	12	10 (*Xenopus* oocytes)	Brain, testis
GLUT 4 (muscle/fat)	509	17	5 (adipocytes)	Skeletal and heart muscle, brown and white fat
GLUT 5 (small intestine)	501	1	6–11* *(fructose) (*Xenopus* oocytes)	Small intestine, sperm

K_m, Michaelis-Menten constant; N, nitrogen.
[a]The approximate K_m values refer to the uptake of glucose (fructose in the case of GLUT 5) in the designated tissue or cells in parentheses and are shown to give an approximate index of the affinity of the transporter for glucose.

Two distinct classes have been described: (a) a family of facilitative glucose transporters (see Table 3.4) and (b) sodium (Na⁺)-glucose cotransporters (symporters). The former class consists of membrane integral proteins found on the surface of all cells. They transport D-glucose down its concentration gradient (from high to low), a process described as *facilitative diffusion*. The energy for the transfer comes from dissipation of the concentration difference of the glucose. Such glucose transporters allow glucose to enter cells readily, but they can also allow it to exit from cells according to the prevailing concentration difference. In contrast, the Na⁺-glucose cotransporters participate in the uphill movement of D-glucose against its concentration difference; that is, they perform *active transport*. They are especially expressed in the specialized brush borders of the enterocytes of the small intestine and the epithelial cells of the kidney (proximal) tubule. They occur at lower levels in the epithelial cells lining the lung and in the liver (10). Cooperation between the two classes of glucose transporters, together with the hormones involved in carbohydrate metabolism, allows a fine control of glucose concentration in the plasma, thus maintaining a continuous supply of the body's main source of cellular energy.

Human Facilitative-Diffusion Glucose Transporter Family

Several major hexose transporters have been identified and cloned since the characterization of the first, glucose transporter 1 (GLUT 1), by molecular cloning (11). They are numbered GLUT 1 to GLUT5 in the order of their discovery, and are all proteins with similar molecular structures containing between 492 and 524 amino acid residues. Mueckler and colleagues (11), using hydropathic and secondary structure predictions, proposed a two-dimensional orientation model of GLUT 1 in the plasma membrane (Fig. 3.3). The molecule has three major domains: (a) 12 α-spanning the membrane with the N and C termini of the protein on the cytoplasmic side of the cell membrane, (b) an intracellular domain of 65 hydrophilic amino acids (between membrane [M] regions 6 and M7 of Fig. 3.3), and (c) an extracellular 33-amino acid segment (between Ml and M2) containing the site for an asparagine-linked oligosaccharide at asparagine 45.

The prediction was that the polypeptide backbone of the molecule traverses or spans the plasma membrane 12 times. Both the amino- and carboxy-terminal ends of the molecule are on the cytoplasmic side of the membrane, whereas an N-glycosylation site is present on the first extracytoplasmic loop (Ml and M2). These basic topologic features have been confirmed by studies using proteolytic digestion and sequence-specific antibodies. GLUT 1, purified from human red cells and reconstituted in liposomes, appears to be predominantly in the α-helical form,

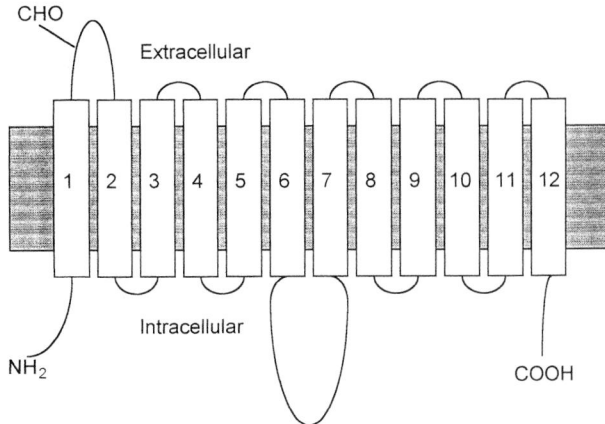

Figure 3.3. Highly schematic diagram illustrating the predicted secondary structure model of the glucose transporter molecule (GLUT 1) in the cell membrane *(shaded)*. The putative membrane-spanning α-helices are shown as rectangles numbered *1* to *12* connected by chains *(lines)* of linked amino acids. (Adapted from Mueckler M, Caruso C, Baldwin SA et al. Science 1985;229:941–5, with permission.)

and the transmembrane segments form α-helices at right angles to the plane of the lipid membrane (12). The molecular structure of GLUT 1, shown in Figure 3.3, is, of course, a two-dimensional model. Studies using radiation inactivation of the carrier in intact red cells have indicated that GLUT 1 probably exists as homotetramer (13). The structures, properties, expression sites, and roles of each of the five facilitative glucose transporter isoforms are briefly described here and are summarized in Table 3.4. Because of the recognized importance of these transporters in health and disease, numerous reviews have been published (14–18), and they should be consulted for greater detail.

GLUT 1 (Erythroid-Brain Carrier)

GLUT 1 is the glucose transporter in the human red cell. The first to be characterized by molecular cloning (11), it consists of 492 amino acid residues (see Table 3.4). The gene for its expression is located on chromosome 1. GLUT 1 is widely distributed in many tissues including heart, kidney, adipose cells, fibroblasts, placenta, retina, and brain, but little is expressed in muscle or liver. There is particularly high expression in the endothelial cells of the microvessels of the brain, where GLUT 1 forms part of the blood-brain barrier (19). The transport process for D-glucose in the red cell is asymmetric, because the affinity (Michaelis-Menten constant [K_m]) for D-glucose uptake is approximately 1 to 2 mmol/L, whereas the K_m for the exit of glucose is 20 to 30 mmol/L. This asymmetry appears to be allosterically regulated by the binding of intracellular metabolites and inhibited by adenosine triphosphate (ATP) (20). The asymmetry allows the transporter to be effective when the extracellular glucose is low and the intracellular demand high.

GLUT 2 (Liver Glucose Transporter)

Many biochemical studies indicated that the glucose transporter in liver cells was distinct from that of the red cells. Moreover, adult liver cells had only very low levels of GLUT 1 mRNA. Cloning of the second glucose carrier, GLUT 2, was accomplished by screening rat and human cDNA libraries with a cDNA probe for GLUT 1. GLUT 2 has 55% identity in amino acid sequence with GLUT 1, and it displays the same topologic organization in the cell membrane as predicted for GLUT 1. Human GLUT 2 contains 524 amino acids (see Table 3.4), compared with rat GLUT 1 of 522 residues, and they show 82% identity in amino acid sequences, an excellent example of conservation of structure among species. GLUT 2 is preferentially expressed in liver (sinusoidal membranes), kidney (tubule cells), small intestine (enterocytes), and the insulin-secreting β-cells of the pancreas.

In the liver cell, GLUT 2 has a low affinity for glucose ($K_m = 17$ mmol/L) and shows symmetric transport, that is, a similar K_m for influx and efflux. This high-capacity, low-affinity transporter is useful for rapid glucose efflux following gluconeogenesis. GLUT 2 can also transport galactose, mannose, and fructose (21). The ability to transport fructose is seen only with GLUT 2 and GLUT 5 (see later).

GLUT 3 (Brain Glucose Transporter)

GLUT 3 was originally cloned from a human fetal muscle cDNA library (22). It contains 496 amino acid residues (see Table 3.4) and shows 64% identity with GLUT 1 and 52% identity with GLUT 2. Its amino acid sequence again suggests that its membrane topology is similar to that of GLUT 1 (see Fig. 3.3). GLUT 3 mRNA appears to be present in all tissues, but its highest expression is in adult brain, kidney, and placenta. Adult muscle, however, shows only very low levels. In the brain, it is mainly expressed in neurons. GLUT 3 mRNA is found in fibroblasts and in smooth muscle. Because both these cell types are found in practically all tissues, the ubiquitous expression of GLUT 3 is understandable. Its affinity for glucose transport is relatively low ($K_m \approx 10$ mmol/L) but significantly higher than that of GLUT 1 (17 mmol/L). GLUT 3 is also found in spermatozoa. Such cells undertake glycolysis in the male genital tract and take up glucose from epididymal fluid.

GLUT 4 (Insulin-Responsive Glucose Transporter)

Glucose is transported across the cell membranes of adipocytes (fat cells), and its rate of transport can be speeded up 20- to 30-fold within 2 or 3 minutes by addition of insulin, without evidence of protein synthesis. Studies showed that this stimulation of glucose transport resulted in part from translocation of GLUT 1 from an intracellular pool into the membrane. Careful quantitative measurements showed, however, that this could account for only a 12- to 15-fold increase in glucose transport. It became obvious that another transporter would have to be involved to account for the much larger insulin-stimulated transport. This new transporter, GLUT 4, was first identified in rat adipocytes by use of a monoclonal antibody. Subsequently, it has been cloned from rat, mouse, and human DNA (21). It is a protein with 509 amino acid residues (see Table 3.4), with 65% identity with GLUT 1, 54% identity with GLUT 2, and 58% identity with GLUT 3. Rat and mouse GLUT 4s have 95 and 96% identity, respectively, with human GLUT 4. As with the previous GLUT transporters, the two-dimensional orientation of the structure in the cell membrane is similar to that proposed for GLUT 1 (see Fig. 3.3).

GLUT 4 is the major glucose transporter of the insulin-sensitive tissues, brown and white fat, and skeletal and cardiac muscle. It occurs primarily in intracellular vesicles in the cells of these tissues. Insulin stimulation causes a rapid increase in the number of glucose transporters on the membranes of these cells because the vesicles are translocated toward the membrane and then fuse with it, releasing the molecule. This process ensures a high density of glucose transporters and enhances the ability to move glucose from the surrounding cellular fluid into the interior of the cell, that is, increased maximal velocity for glucose uptake. Because of this mechanism, the position of GLUT 4 and its regulation are important components of glucose homeostasis, and its role in diabetes has been much studied.

GLUT 5 (Fructose Transporter?)

GLUT 5 was isolated from human (23), rat, and rabbit enterocyte cDNA libraries. It consists of 501 amino acid residues (see Table 3.4), and it has only 42, 40, 39, and 42% identity with GLUTs 1, 2, 3, and 4, respectively. It is said to be primarily expressed in the jejunum (both in the brush border and basolateral membrane), but its mRNA has been detected, albeit at low levels, in human kidney, skeletal muscle, and adipocytes, microglial cells, and the blood-brain barrier. GLUT 5 appears to transport glucose poorly and is really the transporter for fructose. It is found in high concentrations in mature human spermatozoa (24), which are known to use fructose as an energy source (human seminal fluid contains high concentrations of fructose, which is manufactured by the seminal vesicles). In oocytes injected with GLUT 5 mRNA to effect GLUT 5 expression, the K_m for fructose uptake was 6 to 11 mmol/L. With importance to the regulation of energy homeostasis, the expression of GLUT5 in pancreatic β-cells is very low (25), and consequently fructose has little if any effect to stimulate insulin secretion (26).

Other Transporters

The major glucose transporters in cells have been the identified and cloned (GLUT 1–5). There are reports, however, of many newer members of this family of sugar transport proteins including GLUT 6 to GLUT 12 (27, 28). Thus, the list of both Na^+-dependent and facilitative carbohydrate transport proteins identified continues to grow. Because these transporters exhibit a wide range of properties with variable combinations of these proteins distributed across different cell and tissue types (29, 30), the capacity exists for far greater complexity in sugar transport, storage, and metabolism than originally considered at the time the first transporters were initially identified.

Study of Glucose Transporters by Use of Transgenic and Knockout Mice

Although many metabolic inhibitors are available for use in examining metabolic pathways, the specificity of these agents is often questionable. With molecular techniques, however, metabolic pathways can be altered in quite specific ways, even in intact animals. A protein (e.g., enzyme/carrier) can be overexpressed, expressed in a tissue that normally does not contain it, or eliminated in a particular cell type. Site-directed mutations allow a molecule to be dissected and particular component groups removed or altered so their role in the molecule's functioning can be studied (see Chapter 39). Application of these techniques to the investigation of metabolic pathways is yielding interesting insights into the biologic roles of glucose transport proteins.

Transgenic mice were established that expressed high levels of human GLUT 1, properly located in the muscle sarcolemma. The increase in the GLUT 1 expression resulted in a three- to fourfold increase in glucose transport into specific muscles, a finding confirming that GLUT 1 plays a major role in controlling glucose entry into resting muscle. Strangely, insulin did not increase the entry of glucose into the transgenic mice muscles even though GLUT 4 levels in these mice were the same as those of control mice. Possibly, the GLUT 1 levels were elevated in the transgenic animals to a degree that glucose transport was not limited by transporter activity. Muscle glucose concentrations were four- to fivefold and glycogen tenfold higher in the transgenic mice, even though they showed 18% (fed) to 30% (fasted) decreases in plasma glucose concentration. Oral glucose loads did not increase plasma levels as much as in normal mice and glucose disposal was enhanced. Thus, increasing the number of GLUT 1 transporters affected not only muscle metabolism, but also whole-body glucose homeostasis.

Selective overexpression of GLUT 4 in muscle or adipose tissue protects against the development of diabetes in several rodent models (31). Mice with genetic ablation of GLUT 4 in all tissues exhibit impaired glucose tolerance despite postprandial hyperinsulinemia and decreased glucose lowering after insulin injection, a finding indicating that they are insulin resistant; however, these animals do not develop overt diabetes (32). Investigators had shown that glucose disposal in rodents, and mice in particular, has a large insulin-independent component that may protect against diabetes induced by ablation of GLUT 4. In addition, the background strain of the animals used for genetic manipulations can have major influence on the phenotypic outcome. For example, overt diabetes and glucose toxicity were observed in mice with a muscle-specific inactivation of GLUT 4 (33). Finally, adipose-specific GLUT 4 ablation not only markedly impairs glucose uptake in isolated adipocytes from these animals but also induces insulin resistance in skeletal muscle and liver, despite preservation of GLUT 4 expression in these tissues (34). These results suggest that some factors regulated by adipose glucose transport are involved in the control of insulin action in extra-adipose tissue and thus whole-body insulin sensitivity.

Because increased expression of the insulin-responsive transporter GLUT 4 occurs in human and rodent adipocytes and is associated with obesity, the question arises whether increasing the GLUT 4 levels in adipocytes plays a role in obesity. Transgenic mice were produced that expressed human GLUT 4 in their adipocytes. Basal-level glucose transport into adipocytes was increased approximately 20-fold compared with wild-type animals, but insulin only stimulated glucose uptake by a factor of 2.5, rather than the 15-fold increase of controls. Again, the possible explanation is that glucose transport is already so high in the adipocytes of transgenic animals that the number of transporters activated by insulin has a reduced relative contribution to the overall transport. Although the fat cell size was unchanged in the transgenic mice, the number of fat cells was more than doubled, and total body lipid nearly tripled, reflecting the increase in cell number. The results suggest that a specific increase in GLUT 4 in adipocytes can contribute to obesity.

One major limitation of using transgenic and "knockout" mice is that the induced genetic alterations occur early on in the developing animal. Thus, observed phenotypic outcomes in these animals may result from the presence or absence of the transgene at the time of the laboratory measurements, or, alternatively, the genetic alteration could initiate a plethora of events contributing to the observed phenotype. The development of conditional transgenic or knockout models in which transgenic manipulations allow temporal expression or inactivation of specific genes will help to overcome this limitation (35) (see Chapter 39).

BLOOD GLUCOSE: METABOLIC AND HORMONAL REGULATION

Metabolic Regulation

Glucose is one of the most highly regulated circulating substrates. The concentration of glucose in the blood after an overnight fast has a normal range of 3.9 to 5.8 mmol/L (70–105 mg/100 mL). When a carbohydrate meal is ingested, the level may temporarily rise to 6.5 to 7.2

mmol/L, and during prolonged fasting it can fall to 3.3 to 3.9 mmol/L. One of the major reasons that blood glucose levels are so closely regulated is that the brain normally depends on a continuous supply, although it can adapt to lower levels and use ketone bodies from fat breakdown (36) if adaptation occurs slowly during prolong fasting or starvation. The adaptation to use ketones becomes essential during starvation (see Chapter 48), because the adult human brain uses about 140 g/day of glucose (37), and only about 130 g/day of glucose can be obtained from non-carbohydrate sources. Injection of sufficient insulin to lower blood glucose levels acutely can rapidly lead to convulsions and even death if not promptly corrected.

Glucose enters the circulating pool from both exogenous (diet) and endogenous (hepatic production via glycogenolysis and gluconeogenesis) sources. In physiologically normal postabsorptive humans, the plasma appearance rate is 8 to 10 g/hour, the circulating pool being replaced every 2 hours. At normal blood glucose levels, the liver is a net producer of glucose. Dietary carbohydrates in a meal are hydrolyzed by amylases in the intestine and sucrase and lactase at the intestinal brush border. Starches yield glucose, sucrose yields one molecule of glucose and one of fructose, and lactose yields one molecule of glucose and one of galactose. After absorption, these monosaccharides are transported by the portal blood flow into the liver. The rising levels of glucose and insulin, as well as the indirect effect of insulin to inhibit lipolysis to reduce the portal delivery of free fatty acids to the liver, lead to a decrease of hepatic glucose production. As glucose entering the blood during a meal arrives at the liver and peripheral tissues, the first metabolic step is phosphorylation. Phosphorylation in nonhepatic tissues is catalyzed by hexokinase, an enzyme subject to feedback inhibition by its product, glucose-6-phosphate. The liver enzyme glucokinase is not so affected, has a lower affinity for glucose, and can increase its activity over the normal range of glucose found in the portal blood. Thus, hexokinase possesses the ideal characteristics required for the uptake of the large amounts of glucose arriving at the liver during a consumption of a high-carbohydrate meal. Fructose can be converted into glucose in the liver or metabolized to lactate and released. Thus, little fructose is found in the peripheral circulation even after a meal containing fructose, and more than 95% of all circulating hexose consists of glucose.

Cori Cycle

Glucose can be formed in the liver and kidney from two other groups of compounds that undergo gluconeogenesis. Those in the first group, such as some amino acids (especially alanine during starvation) and propionate, are converted into glucose without being recycled; those in the second group are formed from glucose during its partial metabolism in various tissues. Both muscle and red blood cells metabolize glucose to form lactate, which on entering the liver can be resynthesized into glucose. This newly formed glucose is then available for recirculation back to the tissue, a process known as the Cori, or lactic acid, cycle. The Cori cycle may account for approximately 40% of the normal plasma glucose turnover, particularly during exercise.

Hormonal Regulation of Carbohydrate Metabolism

The level of glucose in the blood is regulated by both hormonal and metabolic mechanisms. The major hormones controlling the glucose level are insulin, glucagon, and epinephrine (adrenaline), but other hormones including thyroid hormone, glucocorticoids, growth hormone, and adiponectin also play a role.

Insulin and Diabetes Mellitus (Type 1 and Type 2)

Insulin has a central role in regulating glucose metabolism. It is secreted by the β-cells in the islets of Langerhans in the pancreas; the daily output of insulin by the human pancreas is approximately 40 to 50 U, or 15 to 20% of pancreatic insulin stores. The glucose level in the blood is the major signal controlling insulin release; high blood glucose levels (hyperglycemia) stimulate the secretion of insulin, whereas low glucose levels (hypoglycemia) result in reduced insulin secretion. When the pancreas is unable to secrete insulin or secretes too little, the medical condition is known as diabetes mellitus (see also Chapter 65). This disease, the third most prevalent in the Western world, is normally classified as type 1, or insulin-dependent, diabetes mellitus or type 2, non–insulin-dependent, diabetes mellitus. Type 2 diabetes is strongly associated with obesity and accounts for approximately 90% of all diabetes. Type 1 diabetes is caused by autoimmune-mediated destruction of pancreatic β-cells resulting in an absolute inability to produce insulin and the need for daily injections of the hormone to prevent ketoacidosis and death. The onset of insulin-dependent diabetes mellitus occurs in children and younger adults predominantly and becomes manifest when greater than 80 to 90% of the β-cells are destroyed. Most cases of type 2 diabetes occur in mature adults, although the number of cases reported in children has increased dramatically since the mid-1990s in association with the increase of childhood obesity in Westernized countries. A form of type 2 diabetes occurs in pregnancy and is termed gestational diabetes. In type 2 diabetes, patients have reduced secretion of insulin accompanied by reduced metabolic responses to insulin in certain key insulin-sensitive tissues including liver and skeletal muscle (i.e., peripheral insulin resistance). The causes of this insulin resistance are yet to be identified; however, ectopic fat (triglyceride) deposition in liver and muscle is strongly associated with insulin resistance. Findings about the role of GLUT 4 in insulin insensitivity are conflicting. Some researchers have reported no changes in GLUT 4 mRNA expression or protein levels (38), but others have found a small (18%) decrease (39). The insulin resistance may be, in part, the result of a defect in translocation of GLUT 4 to the muscle membrane (21); however, defects at numerous control points in insulin receptor function, including impaired phosphorylation and the postreceptor signal transduction cascade, have been implicated in the etiology of insulin resistance. (For an in-depth discussion of insulin action and insulin resistance, see reference 40 and Chapters 62 and 65.)

Mechanism of Insulin Secretion

The mechanism of the regulation of insulin secretion by the external glucose level has been studied using patch clamp techniques to control the ionic channels in the β-cell membrane. The resting membrane potential of the β-cells is maintained by the Na^+-K^+/ATPase and ATP-sensitive K^+ channels (K_{ATP} channels). Normally, these channels are open, but they close in response to events triggered by the metabolism of glucose, when there is a concomitant increase in the ratio of ATP to adenosine diphosphate (41). This depolarizes the cell membrane and opens voltage-gated Ca^{2+} channels. The resulting increase in the intracellular free Ca^{2+} concentration activates secretion of insulin through exocytosis—the fusion of insulin-containing granules with the plasma membrane and the release of their contents (42). Certain drugs (sulfonylureas), such as tolbutamide and glibenclamide, cause insulin secretion by inhibiting the K_{ATP} channels of the β-cells and are used medically to treat type 2 diabetes. K_{ATP} channels are a heteromultimeric complex of the inward rectifier K^+ channel (K_{IR} 6.2) and a receptor for sulfonylureas, SUR1, a member of the ATP-binding cassette or traffic family of plasma membrane proteins (43).

In addition to glucose, other nutrients, including certain amino acids and fatty acids, can contribute to increased insulin secretion. Gastrointestinal hormones, including glucagon, secretin, and the known incretin hormones, glucagon-like peptide-1, and glucose-dependent insulinotropic polypeptide, augment meal-induced insulin secretion (44). The pancreatic islet is well innervated by the autonomic nervous system and the classic neurotransmitters, including acetylcholine and norepinephrine, as well as neuropeptides including galanin, vasoactive intestinal polypeptide, and pituitary adenylate cyclase–activating polypeptide modulate insulin secretion (45). Neural regulation by the parasympathetic nervous system augments insulin responses to meal ingestion and improves postprandial glucose tolerance (46, 47), whereas the sympathetic nervous system inhibits insulin secretion during periods of stress to increase glucose availability for the central nervous system (48). In pregnancy, the hormones placental lactogen, estrogens, and progestin all increase insulin secretion. For a detailed overview of the biology of insulin secretion, see Taborsky and Ahren (49).

Insulin lowers blood glucose levels by facilitating its entrance into insulin-sensitive tissues and uptake by the liver. It does this by increasing the level of transporters in tissues such as muscle. In the liver, however, insulin stimulates the storage of glucose as glycogen or enhances its metabolism via the glycolytic pathway. Surprisingly, glucose entry into liver cells is not mediated by changes in glucose transporter function, even though these transporters are present in hepatocyte membranes (50). There is a functional specialization in the liver in regard to the disposition of GLUT 1 and GLUT 2. GLUT 2 has higher expression in the periportal hepatocytes than in the perivenous hepatocytes. In the perivenous region, however, GLUT 1 is also present in the sinusoidal membranes of the hepatocytes, which form rows around the terminal hepatic venules. Periportal hepatocytes are more gluconeogenic than the more glycolytic perivenous cells (51). Why hepatocytes have GLUT 2 in their membranes is an enigma, because it is certainly not necessary for the entrance or release of glucose. Investigators have suggested that GLUT 2 may be involved in transporting fructose, because GLUT 5, the fructose transporter, is not expressed in the liver. However, GLUT 1 expression correlates well with the glycolytic activity of cells; in general, the higher the activity, the greater the concentration of GLUT 1. Thus, the presence of GLUT 1 in the perivenous liver cells may aid the efficient functioning of their glycolytic pathway.

Although insulin has a primary influence on glucose homeostasis, it also influences many other cellular functions (Table 3.5). Glucose has a profound effect on the secretion of insulin, and insulin strongly affects the normal storage of ingested fuels and cellular growth and differentiation (as exemplified in Table 3.5). Thus, indirectly, glucose also influences these cellular events, a finding that underscores the crucial role of glucose in influencing metabolism and catabolism, both directly and indirectly.

Glucagon

Glucagon is secreted by the α-cells of the islets of Langerhans in the pancreas. A major stimulus for its secretion is hypoglycemia (low blood glucose levels). Glucagon acts on the liver to cause glycogenolysis, the breakdown of glycogen, by activating the enzyme phosphorylase. It also

TABLE 3.5. INFLUENCE OF GLUCOSE VIA INSULIN

POSITIVE EFFECTS	NEGATIVE EFFECTS
Glucose uptake	Pyruvate→glucose
Amino acid uptake	Apoptosis
Acetyl-coenzyme A→fatty acid	Gene expression
Glucose→glycogen	
Protein synthesis	
DNA synthesis	
Sodium-potassium pump	
Gene expression	

enhances gluconeogenesis (formation of glucose) from amino acids and lactate. Thus, the major actions of glucagon oppose those of insulin. Pancreatic α- and β-cells in the islets have a close anatomic and functional relationship with intraislet regulation of glucagon by insulin and of insulin by glucagon (52). The suppression of glucagon secretion by glucose during hyperglycemia is mediated in part by the actions of increased intraislet insulin release (53).

Glucagon must bind its specific receptor in the plasma membrane to activate cellular responses. This specific glucagon receptor is a member of a superfamily of G-protein–coupled receptors, and it is also a member of a smaller subfamily of homologous receptors for peptides structurally related to glucagons: glucagon-like peptide-1, glucode-dependent insulinotropic polypeptide, vasoactive intestinal peptide, secretin, growth hormone–releasing factor, and pituitary adenylate cyclase–activating polypeptide. Using specific glucagon receptor mRNA expression in rat tissues, glucagon receptor mRNA was observed to be relatively abundant in liver, adipose tissue, and pancreatic islets, as expected, but also in heart, kidney, spleen, thymus, and stomach. Low levels were found in adrenal glands, small intestine, thyroid, and skeletal muscle. No expression was observed in testes, lung, large intestine, or brain (54). Importantly, glucagon acts as the first line of defense against low blood sugar levels (hypoglycemia). Activation of the autonomic nervous system (both parasympathetic and sympathoadrenal divisions) is an important mediator of increased glucagon secretion during hypoglycemia, and this mechanism appears to become impaired in people with diabetes and thus leaves these patients at increased risk of hypoglycemia during insulin treatment (55).

Other Counterregulatory Hormones

Epinephrine. Epinephrine is secreted by the chromaffin cells of the adrenal medulla. It is often called the "fight-or-flight" hormone because adrenal epinephrine release is triggered in response to many types of stress, such as fear, excitement, hypoglycemia, hypoxia, and blood loss (hypotension). Epinephrine acts on liver and muscle to increase glycogenolysis by stimulating phosphorylase, thus releasing glucose for use by muscle and the central nervous system.

Thyroid. In humans, fasting blood glucose levels are elevated in hyperthyroid patients and are lower than normal in hypothyroid patients. Thyroid hormones enhance the action of epinephrine in increasing glycolysis and gluconeogenesis and can potentiate the actions of insulin on glycogen synthesis and glucose utilization. Thyroid hormones have a biphasic action in animals; at low doses, they enhance glycogen synthesis in the presence of insulin, but at large doses, they increase glycogenolysis.

Glucocorticoids. Glucocorticoids (11-oxysteroids) are secreted by the adrenal cortex in response to adrenocorticotrophic hormone released from the anterior pituitary. They increase gluconeogenesis and inhibit the utilization of glucose in the extrahepatic tissues and thus are antagonistic to insulin's actions. The increased gluconeogenesis stimulated by the glucocorticoids is enhanced by increased protein catabolism, leading to increased availability of glucogenic amino acids to the liver and increased activity of transaminases and other enzymes involved with hepatic gluconeogenesis.

Growth Hormone. Growth hormone is secreted by the anterior pituitary. Its secretion is enhanced by hypoglycemia. It has direct and indirect effects on decreasing glucose uptake in specific tissues such as muscle. Part of this effect may be the result of the liberation of fatty acids from adipose tissue, which then inhibits glucose metabolism. If growth hormone is administered on a long-term basis or is released from a pituitary tumor, it results in a persistent modest elevation of circulating glucose levels. However, if the pancreatic β-cells' capacity to secrete insulin becomes exhausted, overt diabetes will ensue.

TRANSEPITHELIAL HEXOSE TRANSPORT: INTESTINE AND KIDNEY

Sodium-Glucose Cotransporters

The intestine and the kidney are two major organs that have epithelia with the specific function of vectorially transferring hexoses across their cells into the bloodstream. In the intestine, the transporters of the mature enterocytes capture the hexoses from the lumen after breakdown of dietary polysaccharides into simple hexoses, D-glucose, D-galactose, and D-fructose. In the kidney, the cells of the proximal tubule capture the glucose from the glomerular filtrate to return it to the blood. These glucose transporters, localized in the brush-border membranes of the epithelial cells, differ from the GLUT 1 to GLUT 5 types and share no sequence homology. They are thus members of quite a different protein family.

Moreover, they transport glucose across the cell membrane by having both hexose and Na$^+$ binding sites, hence the name Na$^+$-glucose cotransporters. They couple cellular glucose transfer to the inwardly directed electrochemical gradient of Na$^+$. The low intracellular concentration of Na$^+$ ions, maintained by Na$^+$-K$^+$/ATPase or the Na$^+$ pump at the basolateral borders of the cells, powers the uphill transfer of glucose through the agency of the cotransporter. The affinity of the sugar molecule for its cotransporter binding site is greater when the Na$^+$ ions are attached to the transporter than when they are removed. Thus, the external binding of Na$^+$ and its subsequent intracellular dissociation (because of the lower intracellular Na$^+$ ion concentration) causes the binding, then release, of glucose, allowing it to be transported uphill against its concentration gradient. It is then transported across the basolateral membranes of the cells of the small intestine and kidney, usually by GLUT 2, but in the S3 segments of straight kidney tubules GLUT 1 is found. In this part of the kidney,

GLUT 1 is probably involved both in the transepithelial transfer of glucose and in its uptake from the blood to provide energy for cellular glycolysis.

The low concentration of the cotransporters in cell membranes (0.05–0.7%), their hydrophobic nature, and their sensitivity to proteolysis and denaturation made them nearly impossible to prepare by normal biochemical extraction and purification techniques. The first to be cloned and sequenced, by the technique known as functional expression cloning, was sodium-linked glucose transporter-1 (SGLT-1), the form found in the rabbit small intestine (56). Amphibian eggs of the toad *Xenopus laevis* can express almost any RNA that is injected into them and make the corresponding protein. Poly(A)$^+$ mRNA isolated from the rabbit small intestinal mucosa and microinjected into *Xenopus* oocytes stimulated Na$^+$-dependent uptake of the hexose analogue α-methyl glucoside that could be blocked by the plant glycoside phlorizin, a high-affinity competitor for the sugar site of the transporter (17). Phlorizin has no effect on the GLUT 1–5 transporters; they are inhibited by the mold metabolite phloretin, which is the aglycone of phlorizin. Phloretin has no effect on the Na$^+$-glucose transporter but blocks the GLUT 1–5 transporters. The predicted topologic organization of SGLT-1 in the cell membranes was surmised from its amino acids and, like the glucose transporter family, it is a large polypeptide with 12 putative membrane-spanning α-helices (Fig. 3.4). The polypeptide is glycosylated at one site, but this has little effect on its function (57). Radiation inactivation analysis of SGLT-1 suggests that the functional form in the membrane is a tetramer. Human SGLT-1 cDNA encodes a transporter with 84% amino acid sequence identity to the rabbit SGLT-1. It is composed of 664 amino acids. The gene for human SGLT-1 is located on chromosome 22 at qll.2 → qter.

More recently, it has been shown that three different isoforms of the SGLT cotransporters exist, designated SGLT-1, SGLT-2 (672 amino acids), and SGLT-3

(18). The cotransporters SGLT-1 and SGLT-2 have different glucose-Na$^+$ coupling ratios; the former high-affinity cotransporter (Km ≈ 0.8 mmol glucose/L), primarily expressed in the small intestine, transports each glucose molecule with two Na$^+$ ions, whereas the latter, lower-affinity (Km ≈ 1.6 mmol glucose/L) cotransporter, expressed in the kidney tubules, transports glucose with one Na$^+$. SGLT-3, isolated from pig intestine, is a low-affinity cotransporter. It has approximately 60% homology in amino acid sequence to SGLT-2 (58).

Glucose-Galactose Malabsorption

The importance of human SGLT-1 for intestinal glucose absorption is exemplified in glucose-galactose malabsorption, a rare inborn error of glucose transport. This condition gives rise to severe watery diarrhea in neonates that is lethal unless glucose- and galactose-containing foods are removed from the diet. The diarrhea occurs because the unabsorbed hexoses enter the colon and are fermented into diarrheogenic compounds. The lack of hexose absorption in two sisters with the condition appears to result from a single base change at nucleotide position 92, where a guanine is replaced by adenine. The mutation changed amino acid 28 of their SGLT-1 from aspartate to asparagine, making the SGLT-1 cotransporter defective and inactive. A single amino acid alteration in the 664 that make up the molecule makes it unable to function as a cotransporter (59). Thus, in humans who lack a functional SGLT-1, it appears that absorption of glucose and galactose cannot proceed normally. Experimental studies measuring the absorption of glucose in human jejunum in vivo showed that more than 95% of glucose absorption occurred by a carrier-mediated process, a finding that agrees with the described pathophysiology of glucose-galactose malabsorption (60, 61).

Electrogenic Glucose-Linked Sodium Transfer

Because SGLT cotransporters carry both glucose and Na$^+$ ions across the cell membrane without counterions, movement of the charged Na$^+$ ions creates an electrical potential difference across the cell membrane and subsequently across the epithelium. The transfer of glucose (or galactose) across the intestine or kidney tubule is called electrogenic (potential generating) or rheogenic (current generating). This electrical activity has been of inestimable value in the assessment of the kinetics of active hexose transport in native tissues and injected *Xenopus* eggs. This linking of the electrogenic Na$^+$ ion transfer with the hexose also enhances the net absorption of fluid across the small intestine. It is so effective that it overcomes the terrible excessive fluid secretory consequences of cholera toxin action in the small bowel. The application of this principle—oral rehydration therapy—is a highly effective and cheap treatment to keep patients hydrated and alive. A simple solution of NaCl and glucose (or even rice water) has probably saved more lives than any drug! (See also Chapter 57.)

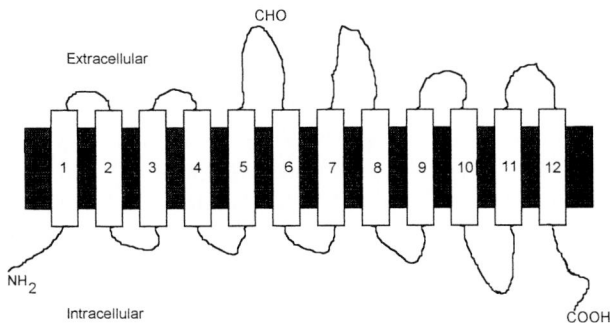

Figure 3.4 Highly schematic diagram illustrating the predicted secondary structure model of the sodium-glucose cotransporter (SGLT-1) molecule in the cell membrane *(solid)*. The putative membrane-spanning α-helices are shown as rectangles numbered *1* to *12* connected by linked amino acid chains *(lines)*. An outer glycosylation site is shown *(CHO)*. It has little effect on carrier function. (Adapted from Wright EM. Turk E, Zabel B et al. J Clin Invest 1991;88:1435–40, with permission.)

Galactose

Metabolism and Transport. Galactose is a hexose monosaccharide whose dietary intake is usually in the form of the disaccharide lactose (milk sugar). Lactose is split by the digestive enzyme lactase into its hexose moities, glucose and galactose. Galactose shares the same transport mechanisms as glucose in the enterocytes, namely, apical SGLT cotransporters and the basolateral GLUT 2. It enters the portal blood and is practically cleared in its passage through the liver, so little or no galactose above 1 mmol/L is seen in the systemic blood, even after ingesting as much as 100 g of lactose. Ingestion of galactose without glucose, however, induces higher plasma concentrations. Alcohol is said to depress galactose uptake and metabolism by the liver, thus leading to an increased level in the blood (galactosemia). In the liver cells, galactose is converted by the enzyme galactokinase into galactose-1-phosphate. This, in turn, is converted by a two-stage enzymic transformation into glucose-1-phosphate, which is converted into glycogen. Although in theory glucose-1-phosphate can enter the glycolytic pathway, it does not normally do so to any great extent. Most tissues have enzymes that can metabolize galactose. However, even in the complete absence of dietary galactose, glucose can be converted into galactose and supply cellular needs for galactose if required. Many structural elements of cells and tissues (glycoproteins and mucopolysaccharides) contain galactose.

Cataracts and Inborn Errors. Galactose levels in peripheral blood normally do not go higher than 1 mmol/L. If they do (galactosemia), then various tissues can remove galactose from the blood and convert it into galactitol (dulcitol) by the enzyme aldehyde reductase. Because it is nonmetabolized, galactitol builds up in the tissues and causes pathologic changes because of the high osmotic pressure created. In the lens of the eye, such a situation causes cataracts (62). Cataracts can also occur in two inborn errors of galactose metabolism caused by deficiencies of the enzymes galactose-1-phosphate uridyltransferase and galactokinase. The former enzyme deficiency creates classic galactosemia. Unless it is treated promptly in the neonate by withdrawing galactose from the diet (taken in from the lactose content of normal milk), either death or severe mental retardation can occur. Cataracts can also occur as a complication of diabetes mellitus, in which blood glucose is raised to high levels and is transported into the lens, where it is metabolized to sorbitol, thus causing the lens to swell and become opaque.

Fructose

Absorption. Fructose, a monosaccharide ketohexose, is present as the free hexose naturally occurring in honey and fruit or produced by isomerization of glucose from corn and added to soft drinks and many other sweetened beverages and foods as high-fructose corn syrup. Fructose is also produced from hydrolysis of the dietary disaccharide sucrose (yielding glucose and fructose). Although fructose is absorbed across the enterocytes of the small intestine, it is not a substrate for the SGLT cotransporters. The evidence for this is threefold: (a) fructose absorption is normal in those with glucose-galactose malabsorption, who have defective SGLT-1 cotransporters; (b) fructose absorption is not reduced by phlorizin, the classic inhibitor of SGLT 1 cotransporters; and (c) fructose absorption is neither Na^+-sensitive nor electrogenic like that of glucose or galactose. Studies on the expression of human GLUT 5 transporter in *Xenopus* oocytes showed that the transporter exhibited selectivity for high-affinity fructose transport that was not blocked by cytochalasin B, a potent inhibitor of facilitative glucose transport by glucose transporters (24). Because GLUT 5 is also expressed in high levels in the brush border of enterocytes in the small intestine (63), this isoform is likely to be the fructose transporter of the small intestine. Indirect evidence for the likelihood of fructose transporting by GLUT 5 is the finding that it is expressed in high concentration in human spermatids and spermatozoa (63), cells known to metabolize fructose. GLUT 2, localized to the basolateral membrane of enterocytes, although having a much lower affinity for fructose transport than GLUT 5, probably mediates the exit of the absorbed fructose from the enterocytes into the blood. Investigators have reported that GLUT 5 is also localized on the basolateral membrane in the human jejunum (64), so fructose could also exit from the enterocytes by this transporter. In humans, absorption of fructose from sucrose ingestion is more rapid than that from equimolar amounts of fructose ingestion. The numerous explanations for this phenomenon include differences in gastric emptying, enhanced fluid absorption initiated by the glucose entraining fructose, and cotransport of fructose and glucose by a disaccharidase-related transport system (65, 66).

Metabolism. Fructose absorbed and entering into the portal blood is almost totally cleared in a single passage through the liver, although a substantial amount of ingested fructose can be metabolized through glycolysis to lactate and released. Thus, essentially little measurable fructose is present in the blood after consumption of moderate mounts of fructose with meals. After a large oral dose of 1 g free fructose/kg body weight, the blood level will increase to 0.5 mmol/L in 30 minutes and then slowly decrease during the next 90 minutes. In the liver, fructose is phosphorylated by the abundant enzyme fructokinase into fructose-1-phosphate, which is cleaved by hepatic aldolase into glyceraldehyde and dihydroxyacetone phosphate. Dihydroxyacetone phosphate is an intermediary metabolite in both the glycolytic and gluconeogenic pathways. Glyceraldehyde, although not an intermediary in either pathway, can be converted by various liver enzymes into glycolytic intermediary metabolites available to be metabolized ultimately to produce glycogen. This glycogen can then be broken down into glucose by glycogenolysis. Thus, a relatively small but measurable amount of ingested fructose is converted to glucose by the liver. In addition, small "catalytic" amounts of fructose appear to enhance hepatic glucose uptake, perhaps by activation of glucokinase (67–69), and this finding suggests that including limited amounts of dietary fructose may be beneficial in the management of postprandial blood glucose excursion in patients with diabetes mellitus (70, 71). However, caution should be exercised in recommending fructose in the dietary management of diabetes because larger amounts could contribute to weight gain and could exacerbate hyperlipidemia or insulin resistance (see later) or induce protein fructosylation and/or oxidative damage (72–74) involved in the pathogenesis of diabetic complications.

When large amounts of fructose are ingested, such as occurs when a large serving of beverage sweetened with sucrose (50% fructose) or high-fructose corn syrup (55% fructose) is rapidly consumed, the glycolytic pathway becomes saturated with intermediates that can be used for the glycerol moiety of triglyceride synthesis or can enter the pathway of de novo lipogenesis to form fatty acids that are then esterified to triglycerides. This preferential increase of lipogenic precursors after fructose ingestion occurs in large part because, unlike glucose metabolism via phosphofructokinase, fructokinase is not subject to allosteric negative feedback inhibition by ATP and citrate (75) (Fig. 3.5). Thus, although only a small percentage (1–3%) of ingested glucose-containing carbohydrate enters de novo lipogenesis and is incorporated into triglyceride in physiologically normal individuals, a proportionally much greater amount of carbon from ingested fructose is metabolized to form triglycerides. This is thought to be a major reason that ingestion of fructose increases circulating triglyceride levels, particularly in the postprandial state (see later).

Inborn Errors of Fructose Metabolism. Six genetically determined abnormalities in the metabolism of fructose have been described in humans (76). These abnormalities are caused by deficiencies in fructokinase, aldolase A and B, fructose-1,6-diphosphatase, and glycerate kinase and by fructose malabsorption. Limiting dietary fructose produces a favorable result in each of these conditions except aldolase A deficiency. Fructokinase deficiency, manifest in the liver, causes fructosemia (high levels in blood) and fructosuria (excretion in urine). In contrast to the low levels of fructose observed in the blood of physiologically normal persons after ingestion of 1 g of free fructose/kg, the concentration in the fructokinase-deficient person approaches 3 mmol/L and is sustained for many hours. Despite the sustained high levels of fructose in the blood, cataracts do not develop, in sharp contrast to the cases of galactokinase deficiency and diabetes mellitus (see specific sections).

The three aldolases, A, B, and C, catalyze the reversible conversion of fructose-1,6-diphosphate into glyceraldehyde-3-phosphate and dihydroxyacetone phosphate. Each aldolase is coded for by a different gene: A is on chromosome 16, B on 9, and C on 17. Expression of the enzymes is regulated during development so A is produced in embryonic tissues and adult muscle, B in adult liver, kidney, and intestine, and C in adult nervous tissue. Deficiency of aldolase A produces a syndrome of

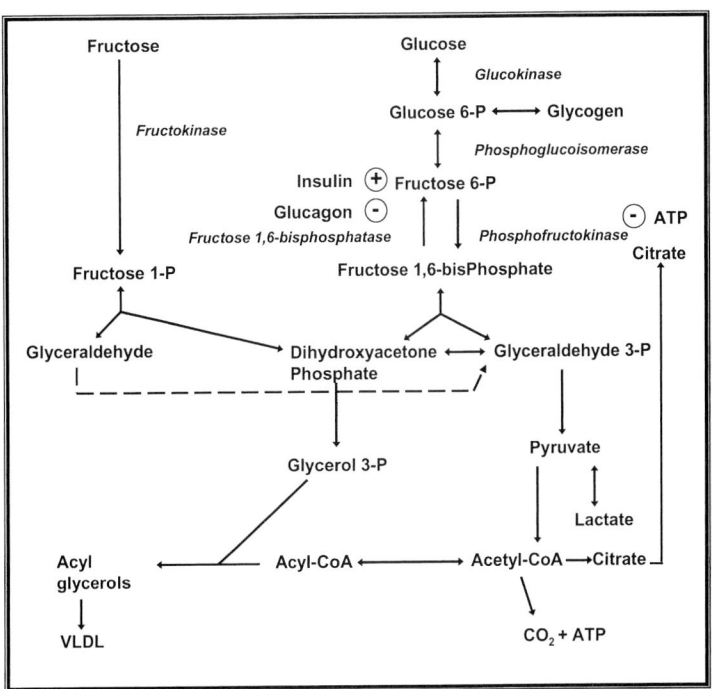

Figure 3.5. Fructose and glucose utilization in the liver. Hepatic fructose metabolism begins with phosphorylation by fructokinase. Fructose carbon enters the glycolytic pathway at the triose phosphate level (dihydroxyacetone phosphate to and glyceraldehyde-3-phosphate [P]). Thus, fructose bypasses the major control point by which glucose carbon enters glycolysis (phosphofructokinase) where glucose metabolism is limited by feedback inhibition by citrate and adenosine triphosphate (ATP). This allows fructose to serve as an unregulated source of both glycerol-3-phosphate and acetyl-coenzyme A (CoA) for hepatic lipogenesis. VLDL, very-low-density lipoprotein. (Adapted from Elliott SS, Keim NL, Stern JS et al. Am J Clin Nutr 2002;76: 911–22, with permission.)

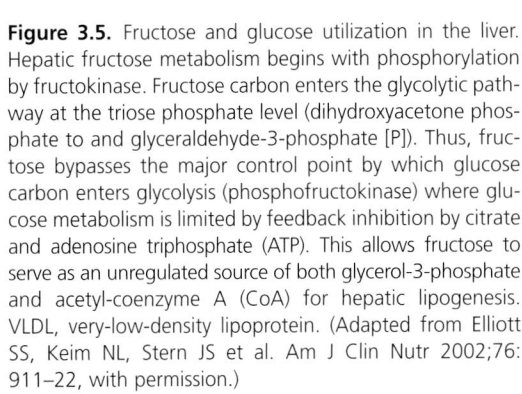

mental retardation, short stature, hemolytic anemia, and abnormal facial appearance. Deficiency of aldolase A probably results in these defects because it is normally involved in fetal glycolysis. No treatment exists for the condition. Deficiency of aldolase B (hereditary fructose intolerance), the most frequent of the three deficiencies, was first observed in 1956 (77). When fructose is ingested, vomiting, failure to thrive, and liver dysfunction occur.

Deficiency of fructose-1,6-diphosphatase was first described in 1970. Patients exhibit hypoglycemia, acidosis, ketonuria, and hyperventilation. Urinalysis shows many changes in organic acids, but excretion of glycerol is diagnostic. Treatment is to avoid dietary fructose. D-Glyceric aciduria is rare and is caused by D-glycerate kinase deficiency. The presentation of the disease is highly variable, from no clinical symptoms to severe metabolic acidosis and psychomotor retardation, findings that suggest that perhaps among the ten described cases, other, different enzyme deficiencies are present.

In fructose malabsorption, ingestion of the ketohexose in quantity creates abdominal bloating, flatulence, and diarrhea. Persons with this condition appear to have a defect in fructose absorption. No assessments of intestinal GLUT 5 or its controlling gene have yet been made in any of these patients. If either glucose or galactose is ingested with fructose, fructose absorption is enhanced, and often no symptoms of malabsorption occur (66, 76).

GLUCOSE STORAGE

Glycogen

Glucose is stored in the liver and muscles of animals and humans as the branched polymer glycogen; the equivalent polymer in plants is starch. Glycogen is more branched than amylopectin and has ten to 18 long chains of α-D-glucopyranose residues (in α(1→4) glucoside links) with branching by α(1→6) glucoside bonds (Fig. 3.6). Although it occurs in concentrations of up to 6% of liver mass but only 1% of muscle, muscle mass is so much greater that it represents three to four times as much glycogen as stored in the liver. Muscle glycogen is mainly used by the muscle, but liver glycogen is for storage, hydrolysis and export as glucose, and the maintenance of blood glucose. The liver has glycogen stores for only 12 to 18 hours of fasting before glycogen is depleted.

Formation and Breakdown of Glycogen

Glucose is first enzymatically phosphorylated and then reacts with uridine triphosphate to give uridine diphosphate glucose glucose). The enzyme glycogen synthetase adds this onto a preexisting glycogen chain (primer and/or protein backbone), splitting off the uridine diphosphate. The glucose residue added by 1→4 linkages is attached at the outer end of the molecule so the branches of the glycogen tree become elongated. After 11 glucose residues,

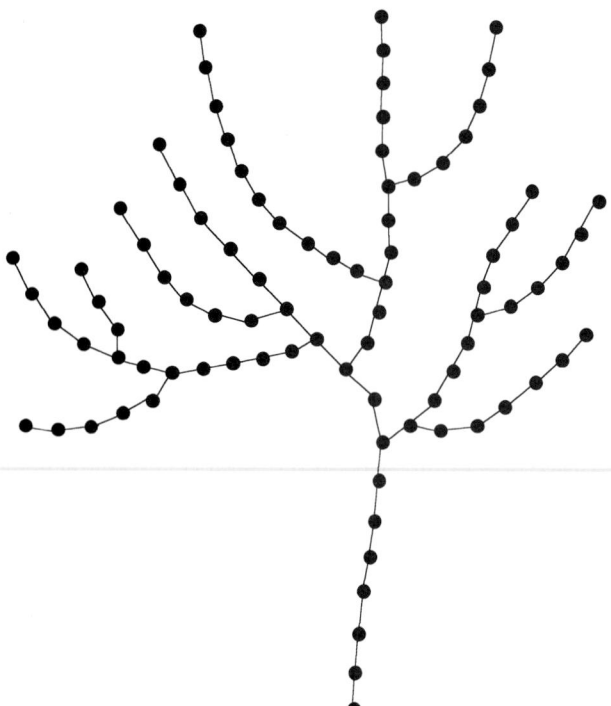

Figure 3.6. A highly schematic diagram of a portion of a glycogen molecule. Each *solid black circle* represents a glucose moiety joined by 1→4 and 1→6 links. The branching of the structure, caused by the 1→6 links, is more random than is shown.

another enzyme, called the "branching enzyme" (amylol (1→4)–(1→6) transglucosidase), transfers part of the 1→4 chain of glucose residues (>6) to a neighboring chain to form a 1→6 link and create a branch point. Glycogen grows by further 1→4 and 1→6 additions. As the number increases, the total number of reactive sites in the molecule also increases, which hastens both glycogenesis and glycogenolysis. Breakdown of glycogen is mediated by three enzymes: (a) phosphorylase acting at the 1→4 linkages; (b) α(1→4)–α(1→4) glucan transferase, which transfers a trisaccharide unit from one branch to another, exposing 1→6 branch points; and (c) the "debranching enzyme" (amylo(1→6)-glucosidase), which splits the linkage. Removal of the branch allows further action by the phosphorylase. In the liver and kidney (but not in muscle), a specific enzyme, glucose-6-phosphatase, dephosphorylates the glucose so it can diffuse from the cells into the bloodstream. The enzymes controlling glycogen metabolism are regulated by a complex series of phosphorylations and dephosphorylations and by allosteric mechanisms under hormonal influence (see the earlier discussions of insulin and glucagon).

Glycogen Storage Diseases

Glycogen storage diseases include more than ten genetic differences involving either enzymes or transporters. They are characterized as storing glycogen in abnormal quantity, location, or structure. Five types of glycogen storage disease have been described (76): type I (glucose-6-phosphatase deficiency), type II (acid α-glucoside deficiency), type III (amylo-1,6-glycosidase deficiency), type IV (branching enzyme deficiency), and type V (muscle phosphorylase deficiency). This classification was later expanded to at least seven types: type VI (liver phosphorylase or phosphorylase B kinase deficiency); and type VII (muscle fructokinase deficiency). For details, consult the review by Hers (78). In types I, III, and VI, the liver cannot convert glycogen into glucose, thus causing hepatomegaly (enlarged liver), hypoglycemia, hypoinsulinism, hyperglucagonemia, hyperlipidemia, and growth retardation. In types V and VII (but also in type II and a subgroup of type VI), the muscle is affected and cannot provide glycolytic fuel for contraction. Symptoms are often mild, however, and become apparent only when young adulthood is reached and strenuous exercise is taken. In a several of the glycogen storage diseases, liver transplantation is the only "curative" treatment.

Carbohydrates and Athletic Performance

Carbohydrate present in limited amounts in muscle (300 g glycogen), liver (90 g glycogen), and body fluids (30 g glucose) is a major fuel for physical performance. The ATP stored in muscle cells can only give high-power output for a few seconds. It can be resynthesized anaerobically for a further few seconds (5–8 seconds) by using the phosphate from creatinine phosphate. These short, intense bursts of muscular activity occur in sprints (100 m), track and field events, and sports such as tennis, hockey, football, gymnastics, and weightlifting. If the maximum effort lasts for 30 seconds or longer, then breakdown of muscle glycogen can supply the energy, with buildup of muscle lactic acid. Most physical activity, however, requires an energy source that can power muscles for longer periods. Both duration and intensity of exercise determine the mix of fuel used. At light to moderate activity levels, as duration of exercise lengthens, the contribution of fat to energy production increases. In contrast, as the intensity of activity increases from rest to light to moderate to intense, the contribution of carbohydrate to energy production increases. The change to using carbohydrate is not a linear response but accelerates with the intensity of the work. At higher exercise intensities, the versatility of carbohydrate as a fuel source is demonstrated, because it can produce energy under conditions of a limited oxygen supply. Endurance athletes use more fat and so conserve the carbohydrate stored in muscle and liver and maintain blood glucose concentrations for longer periods. Ultimately, the amount of carbohydrate stored sets the limits for continued performance, and fatigue arises when the glycogen stores becomes depleted. The store of carbohydrate usually suffices for just 1 to 3 hours of physical exertion, depending on the intensity of effort (see also Chapters 47 and 109).

Dietary Manipulation of Glycogen Stores: Carbohydrate Loading

Dietary manipulation can be used to increase the stores of glycogen in muscle and liver. Glycogen increases when more carbohydrate is eaten. The practice is called carbohydrate loading. The traditional protocol called for 3 days of exhausting physical exercise on a low-carbohydrate diet followed by 3 days of rest on a high-carbohydrate diet. In general, athletes dislike both phases; in the first, they feel exhausted both mentally and physically and are at increased risk of injury; and in the second, they feel bloated because the glycogen retains extra water. For these reasons, the traditional protocol has been modified to eliminate the initial carbohydrate depletion phase. Now the process relies solely on the tapering of exercise with a high-carbohydrate diet several days before the event to augment glycogen stores. For athletes in general, it makes sense to eat plenty of carbohydrate to maximize glycogen storage, because the usual training periods of several hours per day deplete it. Little doubt exists that a high-carbohydrate diet improves glycogen storage and athletic performance (see also Chapter 47). What to advise athletes to ingest just before an event is still debated. A meal or snack taken 3 to 4 hours before exercise should include about 200 to 300 g of carbohydrate, or about 1 hour before exercise, about 13 to 60 g of carbohydrate can be taken to maximize maintenance of blood glucose, but solid food is not advisable immediately before strenuous exercise. During endurance events, beverages containing simple carbohydrates (solutions of glucose, fructose, or sweetened fruit juices) can be provided to aid in the maintenance of blood glucose. Fructose ingestion is said to cause less increase in blood glucose and insulin levels and thus a slower loss of muscle glycogen (79). After glycogen-depleting exercise, carbohydrate intake of about 200 to 400 grams spaced over 4 to 6 hours after exercise will aid in the restoration of muscle glycogen.

DISORDERS OF CARBOHYDRATE DIGESTION, ABSORPTION, OR METABOLISM

Carbohydrate Intolerance

In certain clinical disorders, sugar digestion or absorption is disturbed and gives rise to sugar intolerance, creating symptoms by the undigested or unabsorbed sugar and causing water to enter the intestine, a process that activates peristalsis and induces passage of frequent fluid stools. The undigested carbohydrate can also enter the colon and become fermented into diarrheic agents. The disorders are usually classified as either congenital or secondary to some other disease, to impaired digestion of disaccharides, or to impaired absorption of the monosaccharides. The congenital deficiencies, although relatively rare, are life-threatening: examples are sucrase-maltase deficiency (watery diarrhea after ingesting sucrose-containing foods), alactasia (absence of lactase, diarrhea from ingestion of milk), glucose-galactose malabsorption (diarrhea from ingestion of glucose, galactose, or lactose), and the very rare trehalase deficiency (intolerance to trehalose in mushrooms). Sugar intolerance secondary to underlying gastrointestinal disease is the most common type, especially in pediatrics (see Chapter 51). Infections of the gastrointestinal tract, for example, often induce a temporary intolerance to lactose.

Lactose Intolerance

Adult mammals and most human groups after weaning keep only a fraction of the intestinal lactase activity of neonates (who need it to digest the lactose of breast milk). The persistence of lactase activity in Europeans has been regarded as the exception to the rule, because most human groups are hypolactasic and lactose malabsorbers (80). However, small amounts of dietary lactose, as in up to 250 mL of milk, can be tolerated by most adult lactose maldigesters. The decrease in lactase in adults is a developmentally programmed event, and feeding high-lactose diets does not prevent the decrease. The mechanisms of the decline in activity have been studied in rats. As the animal matures, more and more mRNA message for lactase is needed to maintain the decreasing lactase activity in the enterocytes, a finding suggesting that translational events may be of great importance in lactase gene expression (81) (see also Chapter 74).

Diagnostic Tests to Evaluate Carbohydrate Digestion, Absorption, or Metabolism

Breath Hydrogen Tests

Carbohydrates that have not been digested or absorbed reach the colon and become fermented by the resident bacteria. Hydrogen gas is produced and is excreted in the breath. Measuring breath hydrogen thus provides an estimate of whether malabsorption of a sugar or carbohydrate occurs. This test was first used to detect lactose intolerance and has since been used in numerous studies on carbohydrate intolerance (82). It has certain weaknesses; for example, it gives no indication of the amount of carbohydrate absorbed before the sugar reached the colon, and the hydrogen in the breath is only a fraction of that formed.

Sugar Tolerance Tests

Clinical quantitative assessment of the efficiency of the digestion and absorption of carbohydrates in humans rests mainly on relatively simple tests in which carbohydrate loads (≥50 g) are ingested and blood samples are taken to estimate the sugar levels attained at various time intervals after ingestion. The levels are then compared with those obtained in physiologically normal subjects. The most commonly used test is the oral glucose tolerance test.

Typically, nonpregnant adults take 75 g of glucose over 5 minutes, and the glucose is estimated in serum at 0, 30, 60, 90, and 120 minutes. A pregnant woman takes 100 g of glucose and has another estimate at 180 minutes. A child takes 1.75 g/kg up to the maximum of 75 g (83). Values greater than normal indicate some form of inadequate handling of the ingested glucose. This test is often used to evaluate glucose disposal and identify prediabetic and diabetic states. The reproducibility of the oral glucose tolerance test has been claimed to be poor, even when repeated in the same individual (84). An oral tolerance test also exists for galactose. Because the liver is a major site of galactose metabolism, the test has been used to assess liver function. Similar oral tolerance tests exist for fructose and the disaccharides lactose (lactase deficiency) and sucrose (sucrase deficiency).

Glycemic Index

Nutritionists use a form of oral tolerance test to assess the glycemic potential of different foods. For each food item under evaluation, a measured quantity containing 50 g of carbohydrate is ingested, and blood glucose concentrations are measured over a period of 2 hours. By calculating the incremental area under the 2-hour blood glucose curve, the incremental area in blood glucose is then compared with equivalent incremental area obtained by ingesting a reference food, usually a 50-g glucose load or a portion of white bread containing 50 g of carbohydrate. This normalized value, expressed as a percentage of the value obtained with the reference food, is designated the *glycemic index* of the food (85). The average glycemic index of a meal can be calculated by summing the products of the glycemic index for each food multiplied by the amount of carbohydrate in the food portion and dividing by the total amount of carbohydrate in the meal. Another concept, the *glycemic load*, combines the glycemic index with the total amount of carbohydrate to characterize the full glycemic potential of a mixed meal or diet plan. The glycemic load is determined by calculating the sum of the products of the glycemic index for each constituent food multiplied by the amount of carbohydrate in the each food. These classifications have been useful for the dietetic management of diabetes and hypoglycemia (see also Chapter 65). More recently, epidemiologic evidence has linked the glycemic index and the glycemic load with the risk of developing chronic diseases such as type 2 diabetes (86, 87), cardiovascular disease (88), and diet-related cancers of the colon and breast (89–91), thus raising the issue that restricting foods with a high glycemic index and the overall glycemic load may be potentially useful in disease prevention. However, before public health recommendations can be made, long-term clinical trials are needed to demonstrate that the glycemic property of a diet truly plays a role in preventing or delaying the onset of these chronic diseases. The value of the glycemic index remains controversial; there are arguments in support of (92) and opposed to (93) the use of the glycemic index in health and disease. In addition, foods are not consumed in isolation (as they are tested for their glycemic indices) but generally in the form of meals containing a mixture of macronutrients and carbohydrate types, including fiber. Thus, the glycemic effects of any particular food in the context of a mixed meal may be quite different than when a food is tested as the sole ingested food item. However, the glycemic index does illustrate that carbohydrate foods can differ widely in their effects on blood glucose and hormonal responses after a meal (see later). (The safety and value of low-carbohydrate diets are addressed in Chapters 64 and 111.)

DIETARY REFERENCE INTAKES FOR CARBOHYDRATE

The recommended dietary allowance (RDA) for carbohydrate is set at 130 g/day for adults and children ages 1 through 18 years (94). This value is based on the amount of available carbohydrate that can provide an adequate supply of glucose for brain and central nervous system cells without the need for glucose production from ingested proteins or triacylglycerols. It also assumes that energy intake is sufficient, and the central nervous system is not relying on a partial replacement of glucose fuel by ketoacids. For infants, an RDA value has not been established, but the adequate intake (AI) is set at 60 g/day for infants 0 to 6 months of age. This value is equal to the amount of carbohydrate consumed in human milk and is considered optimal for growth and development during the first 6 months of life. For infants ages 7 to 12 months, the AI is set at 95 g/day. This value is based on the amount of carbohydrate consumed from human milk and complementary foods in the diets of infants of this age group. No gender differences exist for carbohydrate RDA or AI values.

The amount of dietary carbohydrate that supports optimal health is not known, but an acceptable macronutrient distribution range has been set, with carbohydrate contributing between 45 to 65% of energy intake. The potential for adverse effects of overconsumption of carbohydrate was considered. Specifically, the effects of glycemic index, total sugar intake, and added sugar intake on increasing the risk for coronary heart disease, cancer, diabetes or obesity were examined. Currently, evidence available is insufficient to support an upper limit of carbohydrate intake related to the glycemic index of the diet or total or added sugar intake.

CARBOHYDRATES AND CHRONIC DISEASE

Sugar and Dental Caries

Dental caries is a disease created by bacterial plaque on the enamel of teeth. Gradual and progressive demineralization of the enamel, dentin, and cementum occurs. Many studies have suggested that carbohydrates, especially sugars and in particular sucrose, are important dietary components that promote dental caries. However, despite a huge amount of laboratory and clinical research, the relationship between sugar and caries is still poorly characterized. A major reason for this is the complexity of the problem because the formation of caries involves interactions such as nutrients and food components of diet, plaque bacteria, salivary flow and composition, minerals and fluoride status, genetics, age, and even race (see also Chapter 72). The most common organism in dental plaque associated with caries is *Streptococcus mutans*, but other bacteria also appear to contribute. Most studies have focused on the acids (lactic and acetic) generated from sugars (sucrose) by the bacteria, but the complex formation and accumulation of plaque from the insoluble dextran made from sucrose may also be important features (95, 96).

Health Impact of Fructose Consumption

The consumption of simple sugars comprises a significant portion of dietary energy intake and has increased significantly in the past 2 to 3 decades. The mean annual consumption of sucrose plus fructose in developed countries is approximately 25% of the caloric intake. The proceedings of a workshop on the health aspects of dietary sugars summarized this topic (97). Although precise data on total fructose intake are not available, mean per capita intake in the United States from the combined consumption of sucrose and high-fructose corn syrup is probably in the range of 25 to 35 kg/year/person. Fructose has been proposed to contribute to metabolic diseases including hyperlipidemia, insulin resistance, and obesity (75). The idea that fructose has these adverse metabolic effects is based on a substantial number of studies reporting that feeding high-sucrose/fructose diets to experimental animals induces weight gain, hyperliplidemia, insulin resistance, and hypertension, similar to data from a smaller number of human studies (75).

Because of the differences in the hepatic metabolism of fructose and glucose discussed earlier, fructose is more lipogenic than glucose and is therefore more readily converted in the liver to triglyceride, which can be exported and stored in adipose tissue. In addition, several studies have demonstrated that fructose increases circulating triglyceride levels in the postprandial period (98, 99), and evidence indicates that this effect is more pronounced in persons with existing hyperlipidemia or insulin resistance (100, 101). Thus, long-term consumption a diet high in fructose may increase the risk of atherosclerosis or other cardiovascular disease. In addition, recent data indicate that compared with glucose, consuming fructose with meals, which does not stimulate insulin secretion, results in a reduction of circulating leptin concentrations and an

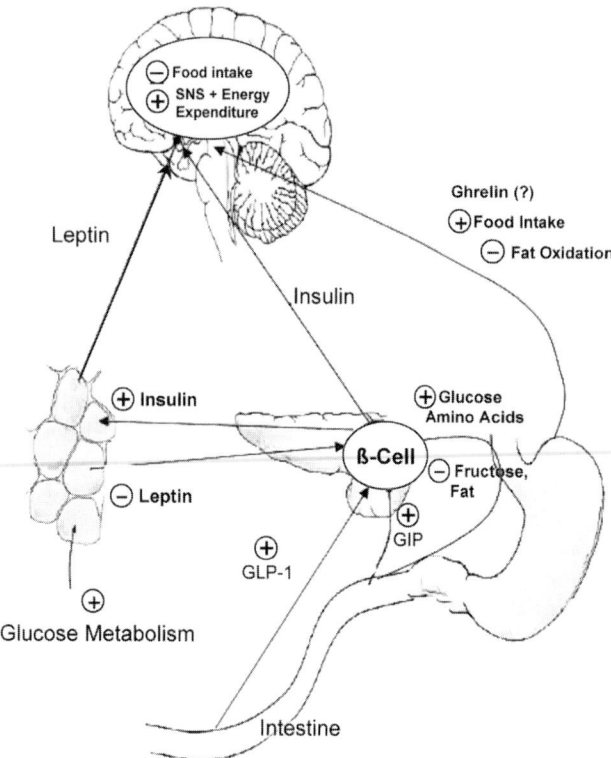

Figure 3.7. Long-term signals regulating food intake and energy homeostasis. Insulin and leptin are important long-term regulators of food intake and energy balance. Both insulin and leptin act in the central nervous system to inhibit food intake and to increase energy expenditure, most likely by activating the sympathetic nervous system (SNS). Insulin is secreted from the β-cells in the endocrine pancreas in response to circulating nutrients (glucose and amino acids) and to the incretin hormones, glucose-dependent insulinotropic polypeptide (GIP) and glucagon-like peptide-1 (GLP-1), which are released during meal ingestion and absorption. Insulin can also act indirectly by stimulating leptin production from adipose tissue via increased glucose metabolism. In contrast, dietary fat and fructose do not stimulate insulin secretion and therefore do not increase leptin production. Ghrelin, a hormone produced by endocrine cells in the stomach, increases food intake and decreases fat oxidation and appears to have an anabolic role in long-term regulation of energy balance. Ghrelin secretion is normally suppressed after meals, but it is not suppressed by fructose consumption. The long-term signals interact with the short-term signals in the regulation of energy homeostasis and appear to set sensitivity to the satiety-producing effects of short-term signals such as cholecystokinin. (Adapted from Havel PJ. Exp Biol Med (Maywood) 2001;226:963–77, with permission.)

attenuated postprandial suppression of ghrelin, a hormone produced by the stomach that stimulates hunger and increases food intake (99) (see Chapters 46 and 63). Thus, with respect to the hormones insulin, leptin, and ghrelin that are involved in the long-term endocrine regulation of food intake, energy balance, and body adiposity (102, 103), dietary fructose behaves more like dietary fat than do other types of carbohydrate that are composed of glucose (Fig. 3.7). The lack of effect of fructose on these hormones suggests that chronic consumption of a diet high in fructose could contribute, along with dietary fat and inactivity, to increased energy intake, weight gain, and obesity.

Acknowledgments

Dr. Havel acknowledges research funding from the International Life Science Institute, the American Diabetes Association, the United States Department of Agriculture, and the National Institutes of Health (DK-35747, DK-58108, HL-075675, and RR-019975).

REFERENCES

1. Dahlqvist A, Semenza G. J Pediatr Gastroenterol 1988;4:857–67.
2. Ugolev AM, Delaey P. Biochim Biophys Acta 1973;300:102–28.
3. Gray CM. J Nutr 1992;122:172–7.
4. Asp N-G, ed. Am J Clin Nutr 1994;59[Suppl]:679S–794S.
5. Wursch P. World Rev Nutr Diet 1989;60:99–256.
6. Wursch P. Dietary fibre and unabsorbed carbohydrates. In: Gracey M, Kretchmer N, Rossi E, eds. Sugars in Nutrition. Nestle Nutrition Workshop series. New York: Raven Press, 1991;25:153–68.
7. Roediger EEW. Dis Colon Rectum 1990;33:858–62.
8. Trowell H. Southgate DT, Wolever TMS et al. Lancet 1976;1:967.
9. Marlett JA. J Am Diet Assoc 1992;92:175–86.
10. Lee W-S, Kanal Y, Wells RG et al. J Biol Chem 1994;269:12032–9.
11. Mueckler M, Caruso C, Baldwin SA et al. Science 1985;229: 941–5.
12. Alvarez J, Lee DC, Baldwin SA et al. J Biol Chem 1987;262: 3502–9.
13. Cuppoletti J, Jung CY, Green FA. J Biol Chem 1981;256:1305–6.
14. Bell GI, Kayano T, Buse JB et al. Diabetes Care 1990;13: 198–208.
15. Silverman M. Annu Rev Biochem 1991;60:757–94.
16. Thorens B. Annu Rev Physiol 1993;55:591–608.
17. Hediger MA, Rhoads DB. Physiol Rev 1994;74:993–1026.
18. Hediger MA, Kanal Y, You G. J Physiol 1995;482[Suppl]: 7S–17S.
19. Maher F, Vanucci SJ, Simpson LA. FASEB J 1994;8:1003–11.
20. Diamond DL, Carruthers A. J Biol Chem 1993;284:6437–44.
21. Could GW, Holman GD. Biochem J 1993;295:329–41.
22. Kayano T, Kukumoto H, Eddy RL et al. J Biol Chem 1988;263: 15245–8.
23. Kayano T, Burant CF, Fukumoto H et al. J Biol Chem 1990;265: 13726–82.
24. Burant CF, Takeda J, Brot-Laroche E. J Biol Chem 1992;267: 14523–6.
25. Sato Y, Ito T, Udaka N et al. Tissue Cell 1996;28:637–43.
26. Curry DL. Pancreas 1989;4:2–9.
27. Joost HG, Thorens B. Mol Membr Biol 2001;18:247–56.
28. Joost HG, Bell GI, Best JD et al. Am J Physiol 2002; 282: E974–6.
29. Wood IS, Trayhurn, P. Br J Nutr 2003;89:3–9.
30. Uldry M, Thorens B. Pflugers Arch 2004;447:480–9.
31. Wallberg-Henriksson H, Zierath JR. Mol Membr Biol 2001;18: 205–11.
32. Katz EB, Stenbit AE, Hatton K. Nature 1995;377:151–6.
33. Kim JK, Zisman A, Fillmore JJ et al. J Clin Invest 2001;108: 153–60.
34. Abel ED, Peroni O, Kim JK et al. Nature 2001;409:729–33.
35. Misra RP, Duncan SA. Endocrine 2002;19:229–38.
36. Owen E, Morgan AP, Kemp HG et al. J Clin Invest 1967;46: 1589–95.
37. Cahill GF, Owen OE, Felig P. Physiologist 1968;11:97–102.
38. Pedersen O, Bak JF, Andersen P et al. Diabetes 1990:39: 865–70.
39. Dohm GL, Elton GW, Friedman E et al. Am J Physiol 1991;260: E459–63.

40. Olefsky G. Insulin resistance. In: Porte D Jr, Sherwin RS, Baron A, eds. Ellenberg and Rifkin's Diabetes Mellitus. 6ᵗʰ ed. New York: McGraw-Hill, 2003:367–400.

41. Ashcroft FM, Harr;son DE, Ashcroft SJH. Nature 1984;312: 446–8.

42. Dunne MJ, Petersen OH. Biochim Biophys Acta 1991;1071: 67–82.

43. Inagaki N, Gonoi T, Clement IV et al. Science 1995;270:1166–70.

44. Vahl T, D'Alessio D. Curr Opin Clin Nutr Metab Care 2003; 6:461–8.

45. Ahren B. Diabetologia 2000;43:393–410.

46. D'Alessio DA, Kieffer TJ, Taborsky GJ Jr et al. J Clin Endocrinol Metab 2001;86:1253–9.

47. Ahren B, Holst JJ. Diabetes 2001;50:1030–8.

48. Havel PJ, Taborsky GJ Jr. Stress-induced activation of the neuroendocrine system and its effects on carbohydrate metabolism. In: Porte D Jr, Sherwin RS, Baron A, eds. Ellenberg and Rifkin's Diabetes Mellitus. 6ᵗʰ ed. New York: McGraw-Hill, 2003:127–49.

49. Taborsky GJ Jr, Ahren B. β-cell function and insulin secretion. In: Porte D Jr, Sherwin RS, Baron A, eds. Ellenberg and Rifkin's Diabetes Mellitus. 6ᵗʰ ed. New York: McGraw-Hill, 2003:43–66.

50. Thorens B, Cheng Z-Q, Brown D et al. Am J Physiol 1990;259: C279–85.

51. Jungermann K, Katz N. Physiol Rev 1989;69:708–64.

52. Pipeleers D. Diabetologia 1987;30:277–91.

53. Greenbaum CJ, Havel PJ, Taborsky GJ Jr et al. J Clin Invest 1991;88:767–73.

54. Hansen LH, Abrahamsen N, Nishimura E. Peptides 1995;16: 1163–6.

55. Taborsky GJ Jr, Ahren B, Havel PJ. Diabetes 1998;47:995–1005.

56. Hediger MA, Coady MJ, Ikeda T et al. Nature 1987;330:379–81.

57. Wright EM, Turk E, Zabel B et al. J Clin Invest 1991;88:1435–40.

58. Mackenzie B, Panayotova-Heiermann M, Loo DDF et al. J Biol Chem 1994;269:22488–91.

59. Turk E, Zabel B. Mundlos S et al. Nature 1991;350:354–6.

60. Fine KD, Santa Ana CA, Porter JL et al. Gastroenterology 1993; 105:1117–25.

61. Levin RJ. Am J Clin Nutr Suppl 1994;59:690S–98S.

62. Van Heyningen R. Nature 1959;184:194–5.

63. Davidson NO, Hausman AML, Ifkovits CA. Am J Physiol 1992; 262:C795–800.

64. Blakemore SJ, Aledo JC, James J. et al. Biochem J 1995;309: 7–112.

65. Fujisawa T, Riby J, Kretchmer N. Gastroenterology 1991;101: 360–7.

66. Riby JE, Fujisawa T, Kretchmer N. Am J Clin Nutr 1993;58 [Suppl]:748S–3S.

67. Shiota M, Galassetti P, Monohan M et al. Diabetes 1998;47: 867–73.

68. Moore MC, Cherrington AD, Mann SL et al. J Clin Endocrinol Metab 2000;85:4515–9.

69. Petersen KF, Laurent D, Yu C et al. Diabetes 2001;50: 1263–8.

70. McGuinness OP, Cherrington AD. Curr Opin Clin Nutr Metab Care 2003;6:441–8.

71. Moore MC, Davis SN, Mann SL et al. Diabetes Care 2001;24: 1882–7.

72. Dills WL Jr. Am J Clin Nutr 1993;58[Suppl]:779S–87S.

73. Levi B, Werman MJ. J Nutr 1998;128:1442–9.

74. Bell RC, Carlson JC, Storr KC et al. Br J Nutr 2000;84:575–82.

75. Elliott SS, Keim NL, Stern JS et al. Am J Clin Nutr 2002;76: 911–22.

76. Hommes FA. Am J Clin Nutr 1993;58[Suppl]:788S–95S.

77. Cori GT. Harvey Lect 1954;48:148–71.

78. Hers H-G. Glycogen storage diseases. In: Gracey M, Kretchmer N, Rossi E, eds. Sugars in Nutrition. Nestle Nutrition Workshop series. New York: Raven Press, 1991:249–65.

79. Stanton R. Sugars in the diet of athletes. In: Gracey M, Kretchmer N, Rossi E, eds. Sugars in Nutrition. Nestle Nutrition Workshop series. New York: Raven Press, 1991:267–78.

80. Kretchmer N. Gastroenterology 1971;61:805–13.

81. Nudell DM, Santiago NA, Zhu J-S. Am J Physiol 1993;265: G1108–15.

82. Levitt MD, Donaldsen RM. J Lab Clin Med 1970;75: 937–45.

83. Potparic O, Gibson J, eds. A Dictionary of Clinical Tests. Lancashire, UK: Parthenon Publishing, 1993.

84. McDonald GW, Fisher GF, Burnham C. Diabetes 1965;14: 473–80.

85. Jenkins DJA, Wolever TMS, Taylor RH et al. Am J Clin Nutr 1981;34:362–6.

86. Salmeron J, Manson JE, Stampfer MJ et al. JAMA 1997;277: 472–7.

87. Salmeron J, Ascherio A, Rimm EB et al. Diabetes Care 1997; 20:545–50.

88. Liu S, Willet WC, Stampfer MJ et al. Am J Clin Nutr 2000;71: 1455–61.

89. Hu FB, Manson JE, Liu S et al. J Natl Cancer Inst 1999;91: 542–7.

90. Franceschi S, Dal Maso L, Augustin LS et al. Ann Oncol 2001; 12:173–8.

91. Augustin LS, Dal Maso L, La Vecchia C et al. Ann Oncol 2001;12:1533–8.

92. Jenkins DJA, Kendall CWC, Augustin LSA et al. Am J Clin Nutr 2002;76[Suppl]:266S–73S.

93. Pi-Sunyer FX. Am J Clin Nutr 2002;76[Suppl]:290S–8S.

94. Institute of Medicine, Food and Nutrition Board. Dietary Reference Intakes for Energy, Carbohydrate, Fiber, Fat, Fatty Acids, Cholesterol, Protein, and Amino Acids (Macronutrients). Washington, DC: National Academy Press, 2002; http://www.nap/edu.

95. Bowen W. Simple carbohydrates as microbiological substrates. In: Conning D, ed. Biological Functions of Carbohydrates. International symposium, 1993;64–7.

96. Navia JM. Am J Clin Nutr 1994;59[Suppl]:719S–27S.

97. Lineback DR, Jones JM. Am J Clin Nutr 2003;78[Suppl]: 893S–7S.

98. Bantle JP, Raatz SK, Thomas W et al. Am J Clin Nutr 2000;72: 1128–34.

99. Teff KL, Elliott SS, Tschop MR et al. J Clin Endocrinol Metab 2004;89:2963–72.

100. Abraha A, Humphreys SM, Clark ML et al. Br J Nutr 1998;80: 169–75.

101. Jeppesen J, Chen YI, Zhou MY et al. Am J Clin Nutr 1995;61: 787–91.

102. Havel PJ. Exp Biol Med (Maywood) 2001;226:963–77.

103. Havel PJ. Diabetes 2004;53[Suppl]:143S–51S.

SELECTED READINGS

American College of Sports Medicine, American Dietetic Association and Dietitians of Canada. Joint position statement: nutrition and athletic performance. Med Sci Sports Exerc 2000;32:2130–45; J Am Diet Assoc 2000;12:1543–56; Diet Canada 2000;61:176–92.

Elliott SS, Keim NL, Stern JS et al. Fructose, weight gain, and the insulin resistance syndrome. Am J Clin Nutr 2002;76:911–22.

Gould GW, Holman GD. The glucose transporter family: structure, function and tissue specific expression. Biochem J 1993;295:329–41.

Havel PJ. Peripheral signals conveying metabolic information to the brain: short-term and long-term regulation of food intake and energy homeostasis. Exp Biol Med 2001;226:963–77.

Joost HG, Thorens B. The extended GLUT-family of sugar/polyol transport facilitators: nomenclature, sequence characteristics, and potential function of its novel members. Mol Membr Biol 2001;18:247–56.

Lineback DR, Jones JM. Sugars and health workshop. Am J Clin Nutr 2003;78[Suppl]:814S–97S.

Wood IS, Trayhurn P. Glucose transporters (GLUT and SGLT): expanded families of sugar transport proteins. Br J Nutr 2003;89: 3–9.

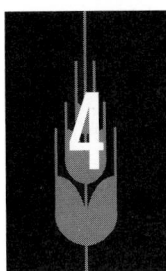

DIETARY FIBER[1]

JOANNE R. LUPTON AND PAULA R. TRUMBO

WHAT IS DIETARY FIBER? SCIENTIFIC RATIONALE
   BEHIND THE VARIOUS DIFFERENT DEFINITIONS 84
     Should the Definition Be Formal or Based
       on Analytic Procedures? 84
     Should Dietary Fiber Be Solely
       from Plant Sources? .84
     Should Low-Molecular-Weight Carbohydrates
       Be Considered Dietary Fiber? 84
     Should Resistant Starch Be Considered
       Dietary Fiber? 84
     Does Fiber Have to Be Intact from Food? 84
     Must Fiber Have Specific Health Benefits? 84
CHEMICAL NATURE OF DIETARY FIBER 85
     Analytic Methods to Determine Dietary Fiber 85
EFFECTS OF FIBER ON GASTROINTESTINAL
   PHYSIOLOGY AND ENERGY 86
     Effect of Fiber on the Stomach 86
     Effect of Fiber on the Small Intestine 86
     Effect of Fiber on the Large Intestine 86
     Contribution of Fiber to Energy 87
DIETARY FIBER AND DISEASE OR OTHER
   HEALTH-RELATED CONDITIONS 87
     Fiber, Satiety, and Obesity 87
     Fiber and Glucose Intolerance, Insulin
       Response, and Diabetes 87
     Fiber and Heart Disease 87
     Dietary Fiber and the Prevention of Colon,
       Breast, and Other Cancers 88
CONSEQUENCES OF OVERCONSUMPTION OF FIBER . . .88
     Gastrointestinal Distress 88
     Mineral Bioavailability 89
INTAKE OF FIBER IN THE UNITED STATES:
   AMOUNTS AND FOOD SOURCES 89
CURRENT RECOMMENDATIONS FOR FIBER INTAKE 89
     The New Adequate Intake for Total Fiber
       and the Science behind It 89

It would seem that the most fundamental prerequisite for a chapter on dietary fiber would be a consensus on its definition, yet no universally accepted definition of fiber exists. In fact, there is considerable ongoing debate as to whether fiber must be relatively intact in a plant source to earn the name "dietary fiber" or whether it can be synthesized in a laboratory. An equally contentious issue is whether dietary fiber sources must prove that they provide physiologic benefit to be called "dietary fiber" or whether the fact that they are not digested by mammalian enzymes and therefore pass relatively intact into the large intestine is sufficient justification. Key ways in which the definitions of dietary fiber differ from each other and the significance of these differences are explained at the onset of this chapter, together with the chemical structure of different fiber components and the major analytic procedures for measuring dietary fiber.

Dietary fiber has numerous important physiologic effects on the gastrointestinal tract, which may be attributed in large part to the physicochemical properties of the fiber sources. For example, in the upper gastrointestinal tract, an important attribute of fiber is its viscosity, which may lead to a delay in gastric emptying, interference with or prolonged absorption of other nutrients (e.g., cholesterol, glucose), and thus a lowering of blood cholesterol or an attenuation of the postprandial rise in blood glucose levels. In the large intestine, the fermentability of the fiber is its dominant attribute; the less fermentable fibers are good bulking agents and promote laxation, whereas some of the more fermentable fibers produce gases and short-chain fatty acids (one of which, butyrate, is the primary aerobic fuel for cells of the colon).

Fiber intake has been linked to risk reduction of a variety of different diseases, primarily diabetes, heart disease, and colon cancer, yet the data are not definitive in any of these areas, and the most recent reports from large-scale, well-conducted trials with fiber and adenomatous polyp recurrence (a surrogate marker for colon cancer) failed to show a protective effect of fiber against this disease. Nevertheless, taken collectively, the data support a health benefit from the consumption of fiber-containing foods. This benefit is reflected in the assignment of a daily dietary reference intake value for fiber of 14 g fiber/1000 calories. Because the current average intake of fiber is only approximately half this recommendation, it is likely that more fiber sources will be incorporated into foods in the future. Therefore, an understanding of fiber and the of strength of the evidence behind its purported physiologic effects and health benefits is important.

---

[1]**Abbreviations: AI,** adequate intake; **CHD,** coronary heart disease; **DRI,** dietary reference intake; **LDL,** low-density lipoprotein.

WHAT IS DIETARY FIBER? SCIENTIFIC RATIONALE BEHIND THE VARIOUS DIFFERENT DEFINITIONS

Hipsley, who defined dietary fiber as "unavailable carbohydrate from plant cell walls" (1), is generally attributed with the first definition of dietary fiber, although "unavailable carbohydrate" had been defined as early at 1929 by McCance and Lawrence (2). The original Hipsley definition has gone through important iterations resulting in an understanding of dietary fiber as "the plant polysaccharides and lignin which are resistant to hydrolysis by digestive enzymes of man" (3), a concept that forms the basis for many definitions today. However, no single "official" definition of dietary fiber exists today, and, in fact, current definitions may differ from each other in substantive ways. Examples of major ways in which definitions may differ are as follows: whether a formal definition is used or whether it is analytically based; whether fiber is solely from plants; whether low-molecular-weight substances such as oligosaccharides, disaccharides, monosaccharides, and sugar alcohols are included; whether resistant starch is considered dietary fiber; whether the fiber has to be relatively intact from food; and whether dietary fiber has to provide a physiologic benefit. The issues behind each of these differences in fiber definition are briefly discussed later. For a complete review of the various definitions of dietary fiber and how they differ from each other, see the *Dietary Reference Intakes Proposed Definition of Dietary Fiber* (4).

Should the Definition Be Formal or Based on Analytic Procedures?

The most basic way in which one definition can differ from another is whether the definition itself dictates the types of assays that need to be used to determine "dietary fiber" or whether the assays and their results determine the definition. A clear distinction between these two options is illustrated by the definitions of dietary fiber in the United States and Canada. In the United States, no formal definition of "dietary fiber" Exists. Instead, numerous accepted analytic procedures can be used to determine "dietary fiber" (5), so the amount of fiber in a product can be reported on the Nutrition Facts Panel on food labels. In Canada, however, a formal definition of dietary fiber does exist (6), and all procedures to analyze for dietary fiber must conform to the definition.

Should Dietary Fiber Be Solely from Plant Sources?

Although most definitions of dietary fiber are restricted to plant sources, the definitions that are based on analytic methods may include fiber from animal sources. Thus, compounds such as chitosan or glycosaminoglycans are often included in reported fiber values. Currently, these compounds do not constitute a large part of fiber intake. However, technically a food manufacturer could add these animal-derived substances to food and report them as dietary fiber.

Should Low-Molecular-Weight Carbohydrates Be Considered Dietary Fiber?

An alcohol precipitation step in most total fiber analyses excludes monosaccharides and disaccharides, oligosaccharides, and fructans, and thus these substances would not be considered dietary fiber if one of these analytic methods constituted the definition of fiber. Most would argue that it is appropriate for monosaccharides and disaccharides to be excluded because they are formally characterized as sugars rather than fiber, but some disagreement exists on oligosaccharides and fructans. In particular, the oligosaccharides in beans (raffinose, stachyose, and verbacose) do not precipitate in alcohol, nor do certain manufactured carbohydrates, such as methylcellulose and polydextrose.

Should Resistant Starch Be Considered Dietary Fiber?

Although resistant starch is characterized as dietary fiber by some organizations and countries (7), but not others (8), the properties of resistant starch mimic some of those of traditional dietary fiber. Resistant starch may occur naturally in the diet, it can be manufactured, and it can occur as a product of the processing of foods. Manufactured resistant starch is increasing in the US diet. Foods that contain significant amounts of resistant starch include legumes (9), green bananas (10), and potatoes that have been cooked and allowed to cool (11).

Does Fiber Have to Be Intact from Food?

Reasonable scientists disagree about whether dietary fiber has to be intact and in the food or whether fiber can be extracted or synthesized and still be called "dietary fiber." The primary reason for this ongoing debate is that although a very large database is available on the physiologic effects and potential health benefits of high-fiber foods, it is not clear that the same effects and benefits would accrue if the fiber were extracted from the food or synthesized in the laboratory. It is possible for an isolated fiber to be even more effective than its original food source, but it is also possible that an isolated fiber may lose its efficacy.

Must Fiber Have Specific Health Benefits?

Probably the most contentious issue among experts in the field of dietary fiber is whether a nonabsorbable substance has to have a proven beneficial physiologic effect to be called "dietary fiber." Some workers suggest that the fact that fiber is not digested and absorbed and therefore passes relatively intact into the colon is a beneficial effect per se. Others argue that to be beneficial, a fiber must result in some health benefit. For example, Health

Canada requires that "novel fibers," to be introduced into the food supply, must modulate blood glucose levels, lower low-density lipoprotein (LDL) cholesterol, or contribute to laxation (6). With new fiberlike substances coming on the market, this distinction of whether or not a fiber has to have a proven health benefit will assume increasing importance.

The National Academy of Sciences' Institute of Medicine, Food and Nutrition Board formed a committee to determine the definition of dietary fiber (4) and a second panel to determine the physiologic effects of dietary fiber and its relationship with health and disease (12). The definition determined by these panels is as follows: "*Dietary Fiber* consists of nondigestible carbohydrates and lignin that are intrinsic and intact in plants. *Functional Fiber* consists of isolated, nondigestible carbohydrates that have beneficial physiological effects in humans. *Total Fiber* is the sum of Dietary Fiber and Functional Fiber." Whether this definition will be adopted by the US Food and Drug Administration remains to be determined.

CHEMICAL NATURE OF DIETARY FIBER

As noted earlier, characterization of the chemical nature of different dietary fibers depends, in part, on what types of fibers are included in the definition. Most definitions of dietary fiber state that it includes nonstarch polysaccharides and lignin. However, some definitions do *not* include lignin, and others *do* include resistant starch. The major nonstarch polysaccharides that comprise dietary fiber are cellulose, β-glucans, hemicelluloses, pectins, and gums (13). Cellulose and β-glucans are polymers of glucose, but unlike starch, the bonds between glucose units are β1-4 linkages rather than α1-4 linkages, and because mammalian enzymes cannot break the β linkage, these polymers are not digested and absorbed. Hemicelluloses are a diverse groups of fibers containing xylans, galactans, or mannans as their backbone and various side chains such as arabinose and galactose. Pectins have galacturonic acid residues as their backbone that differ in their degree of methoxylation, which, in turn, affects their solubility and viscosity. Although not a carbohydrate, lignin (a phenylpropane polymer) is considered part of dietary fiber because it is usually tightly bound to polysaccharides in the plant (14). Gums include galactomannans or arabinogalactans and are found in the nonstructural components of plants along with mucilages. In contrast, pectins, hemicelluloses, cellulose, and lignin are part of the plant cell wall (15). For a more extensive description of the chemistry of different fibers, see the chapter by Southgate in *Handbook of Dietary Fiber in Human Nutrition* (15).

Analytic Methods to Determine Dietary Fiber

Historically, crude fiber analysis was developed to measure indigestible material in animal feed (16), and it was later used with a compensation factor to calculate dietary fiber.

The factor is no longer considered to be accurate because all soluble polysaccharides are lost in this procedure. Other methods have replaced crude fiber analysis. Similarly, as the importance of soluble fibers to human health has become recognized, the neutral detergent fiber and acid detergent fiber assays have also become inadequate because they do not estimate the content of soluble polysaccharides and thus underestimate the total fiber content of a food. It is not possible to use a simple conversion factor to account for the soluble fiber component because foods vary greatly in their soluble fiber content. Two other general categories of methods for measuring total dietary fiber are in use today: enzymatic/gravimetric methods and enzymatic/chemical methods. A complete discussion of analytic methodology for fiber analysis may be found in the *Dietary Reference Intakes Proposed Definition of Dietary Fiber* (4), together with a table listing which specific fractions are and are not recovered by the particular assay. In general, the enzymatic/gravimetric methods are simpler to perform and can be automated, but they lack the specific information on monosaccharide content that is provided in some of the enzymatic/chemical methods.

Briefly, the principal enzymatic/gravimetric procedure in use is the Prosky method, or a modification thereof, which measures both soluble and insoluble fiber (17). It has been adopted as an official method for dietary fiber analysis in the United States and many other countries. Several enzymatic/chemical methods are available, and each has modifications. For example, the Southgate procedure includes the colorimetric analysis of component monosaccharides (18). Some researchers consider the Southgate procedure to overestimate dietary fiber because starch is not completely solubilized in this assay procedure and would thus count as dietary fiber. The Englyst procedure, a variation of the Southgate method, replaces colorimetric detection of monosaccharides with their separation by gas chromatography (19). It also provides for more complete removal of starch. An advantage of this method is that it results in considerable information on the specific monosaccharides in fiber-containing foods. A disadvantage is that it is more complex and time consuming than the Prosky method. The Uppsala Method of Theander and colleagues (Association of Analytical Chemists 994.13) (20) measures neutral polysaccharides, uronic acids, and Klason lignin. A major difference between the Theander approach and that of Englyst is the inclusion of Klason lignin by Theander and its exclusion by Englyst.

In summary, the current methods to determine dietary fiber rely on either the weight or monosaccharide profile of the dietary fiber residue. The gravimetric procedures are simpler and faster. The Southgate method may lead to overestimation by including some starch. The Theander method and the enzymatic procedures include lignin, whereas the Englyst method only includes nonstarch polysaccharides. If the total amount of dietary fiber is of interest, methods based on those of Prosky should be satisfactory. However, if the exact characterization of the monosaccharides within the fiber source is or interest, methods based on those of Englyst or Theander are required.

EFFECTS OF FIBER ON GASTROINTESTINAL PHYSIOLOGY AND ENERGY

The effects of fiber on the gastrointestinal tract depend on specific properties of fiber, most importantly viscosity (for effects on the upper gastrointestinal tract) and fermentability for the colon. Until recently, the term "soluble fiber" was used to characterize those fibers that are viscous and are capable of attenuating blood glucose concentration and lowering LDL cholesterol levels (21, 22). However, not all soluble fibers are viscous. Insoluble fibers were thought to contribute to fecal bulk and thus improve laxation (23, 24). Again, not all insoluble fibers promote laxation, so a recommendation has been made to phase out the terms "soluble" and "insoluble" dietary fiber and to replace those terms with functional definitions that are physiologically meaningful such as "viscous" and "fermentable" (4).

Effect of Fiber on the Stomach

Because fiber is not digested by human enzymes, it remains intact in the stomach, as well as in the small intestine. The presence of viscous fibers in the stomach can delay the rate of emptying of ingested foods from the stomach into the duodenum by forming a viscous, gel-like consistency (25–27). Not all studies have shown a delayed gastric emptying effect (25, 28), and this inconsistency in findings may result from the presence of other food components and the amount or type of fiber consumed.

Effect of Fiber on the Small Intestine

The gel-like environment in the small intestine produced from viscous fiber has been shown to inhibit the activity of enzymes associated with fat, carbohydrate, and protein digestion (29–31). As a result, the intestinal absorption of fat, cholesterol, carbohydrate, and protein has been reported to be reduced with fiber consumption, as determined by increased fecal content of these macronutrients (32–36), resulting in decreased metabolizable energy (34). Delayed gastric emptying or a reduced rate of carbohydrate digestion, as a result of fiber consumption, has been reported to reduce the glycemic index of meals (37–39). Limited evidence suggests that dietary fiber may be beneficial in reducing the risk of and treatment for duodenal ulcers. A prospective study showed that high intakes of fiber reduced the risk of duodenal ulcers (40). Specifically, fiber from fruits and vegetables, but not cereal fiber, was associated with this risk reduction. It was speculated in the report of this study that because emptying of the liquid phase of a meal occurred more rapidly in persons with duodenal ulcers (41), the delayed gastric emptying of the liquid phase with fiber intake could explain this benefit.

Guar gum, a viscous fiber, was reported to help alleviate pain and to provide better tolerance for certain foods when it was given to patients with duodenal ulcers (42).

Effect of Fiber on the Large Intestine

Fermentation

The effect of fiber on the large intestine depends in large part on its fermentability, which, in turn, depends on both the physiochemical properties of the fiber and the colonic microflora. Fiber sources such as oat bran, pectin, and guar are highly fermented, whereas others such as cellulose and wheat bran may be poorly fermented (43–45). In general, fruits and vegetables (rich in hemicelluloses and pectins) contain more fermentable fiber than do cereals (rich in celluloses) (43–45). The degree of fermentability affects fecal bulking ability and, in general, the greater the fecal bulk, the greater the laxative effect. The poorly fermentable fibers contribute more to fecal bulk, and if they also attract water (e.g., wheat bran), they make a significant contribution to laxation. Conversely, when a fiber is fermented, hydrogen, carbon dioxide, methane, and other gases are formed, as are short-chain fatty acids, the principal anions in the colon. Although the highly fermentable fibers are not good bulking agents, they produce large amounts of short-chain fatty acids including butyrate, which is considered the primary energy source for the colon (46) and is hypothesized to be protective against colon cancer.

Short-Chain Fatty Acids and the Butyrate Paradox

The literature on the ability of butyrate (the four-carbon short-chain fatty acid produced from fiber fermentation) to decrease the growth of human colon cancer cell lines by decreasing cell proliferation and/or increasing cell death is substantial (47, 48). In contrast, many in vivo studies, providing butyrate in the diet (49), in drinking water (50), as a slow-release pellet (51), or as a fiber source that is fermented to butyrate in the colon (52) failed to find a chemoprotective effect of butyrate. This dichotomy between in vivo and in vitro studies has been termed the "butyrate paradox." Numerous explanations for this paradox are possible, including the finding that butyrate may have one effect on cancer cells (the subject of the in vitro studies) and a different effect on normal cells (the subject of the in vivo studies) because signal transduction processes are different in these two cell types. Cell culture conditions (e.g., a buffered pH) do not apply in vivo, and amounts of butyrate and the timing of an intervention may differ in these two types of studies. Whether or not butyrate is protective against colon cancer development remains the subject of active debate.

Laxation

Cummings (53) reviewed more than 100 studies of the effect of fiber intake on stool weight and calculated the increase in weight of the stool as a function of fiber intake. A wide range of the contribution of dietary fiber to fecal weight (e.g., an increase of 5.7 g fecal bulk/g of wheat bran fed compared with 1.3 g/g of pectin in the diet) was reported. In general, the greater the weight of the stool, the more rapid is the rate of passage through the colon (23, 54), thus the better the laxative effect. The same properties that result in increased laxation (water-holding capacity and bulking ability) are thought to reduce intracolonic pressure and to lower the risk for diverticular disease (55).

Contribution of Fiber to Energy

The amount of energy contributed by dietary fiber is the subject of considerable debate. Some fiber researchers say that the contribution is negligible because of some interference with the absorption of energy-containing macronutrients, coupled with a very small contribution to metabolizable energy through the production of absorbed fermentation products (i.e., primarily short-chain fatty acids). In other words, the combination of a decrease in energy from decreased absorption of macronutrients and a very small contribution of energy from microbial fermentation of fiber results in a zero net balance. Other fiber researchers supply higher values for dietary fiber in the range of 1.5 to 2.5 kcal/g (56, 57). In the United States, dietary fiber is currently assigned an energy value for food-labeling purposes of 0 kcal/g if it is insoluble and 4 kcal/g (the same as for carbohydrates and proteins) if it is soluble. Methods used to determine the energy value of dietary fiber were reviewed by Fahey and Grieshop (58).

DIETARY FIBER AND DISEASE OR OTHER HEALTH-RELATED CONDITIONS

Fiber, Satiety, and Obesity

Dietary fiber, particularly viscous fiber, has been reported to reduce hunger (59). Increased satiety with dietary fiber intake has been attributed, in part, to delayed emptying of the gastric contents (27, 60), and this, in turn, can cause an extended feeling of fullness (61). Some studies have not shown an effect on satiety with fiber intake, and this difference has been partially attributed to the level of fiber consumed (62). Based on a review of published studies, the consumption of an additional 14 g/day of fiber is associated with a 10% decrease in energy intake (59).

Several intervention studies demonstrated that consuming fiber as part of a weight-reducing diet assists in weight loss (63–65). Observational data showed that dietary fiber intake is positively associated with a lower incidence of obesity and a lower body mass index (66, 67). A large prospective cohort of female nurses showed that weight gain was inversely associated with consumption of high-fiber, whole-grain foods (68).

Fiber and Glucose Intolerance, Insulin Response, and Diabetes

Numerous intervention studies demonstrated a beneficial effect of dietary fiber, particularly viscous fibers, on plasma glucose and insulin response in patients with type 2 diabetes (69–73). When 10.8 g of beet fiber was added to the diet, the glucose plateau level and area under the curve were lower compared with their values when patients consumed diets without beet fiber (72). The ability of viscous fibers to lower the glycemic response of a meal has been attributed to delayed gastric emptying (71) and a slowed rate of digestion and absorption (74). Results of a large prospective cohort study concluded that the consumption of fiber-containing foods can reduce the risk of type 2 diabetes (75, 76). Whole-grain foods (e.g., bran, brown rice, whole-grain cereals, and dark bread) were associated with a lower risk of type 2 diabetes (75, 77). Cereal fiber intake was negatively associated with the risk of type 2 diabetes (76, 78).

Fiber and Heart Disease

Large prospective epidemiologic studies showed a protective effect of dietary fiber against coronary heart disease (CHD) and formed the basis for new recommendations from the Institute of Medicine for fiber intake (12). Mechanisms by which fibers may protect against CHD include lowering blood cholesterol, attenuating blood triglyceride levels, decreasing hypertension, and normalizing postprandial blood glucose levels. Data in support of each of these purported mechanisms are briefly described.

Decreasing Total and Low-Density Lipoprotein Cholesterol Levels

Numerous small-scale clinical intervention trials showed a cholesterol-lowering effect of ingesting different types of viscous fibers (e.g., pectin, guar, oat bran, psyllium), as reviewed by Fernandez (79). Studies continue to investigate in more detail the relationship of different types of fibers with a reduction in LDL and total cholesterol. However, the protective effect of fiber against CHD is not limited to soluble fibers. In fact, the epidemiologic studies support the relationship of all fiber-containing foods with a decreased risk of CHD, especially cereal fibers, as reviewed by Truswell (80).

Glycemic Response and Insulin Resistance

As noted earlier in the discussion of fiber and diabetes, fiber has been shown to ameliorate hyperglycemia in patients with diabetes, and patients with this disease have an elevated risk of cardiovascular disease. In addition, hyperglycemia is independently associated with the risk of cardiovascular disease in the general population (81). Purported mechanisms by which hyperglycemia may contribute to CHD include the induction of oxidative stress, which may increase blood pressure, accelerate blood clot formation, and reduce blood flow. Moreover, hyperglycemia may increase insulin levels, which could increase the risk for CHD through the insulin resistance syndrome (81).

Blood Triglycerides

One concern with low-fat, high-carbohydrate diets that are currently recommended to protect against the development of heart disease is that these diets may increase blood triglyceride levels (an independent risk factor for CHD) (82). Fiber intake may play a role in the reduction of blood triglycerides. A review of pertinent studies suggests that if the high-carbohydrate diet is also a high-fiber diet, one will see a small reduction in fasting triglyceride levels, rather than an increase, as usually seen with high-carbohydrate, low-fiber diets (83).

Lowering Blood Pressure

Many aspects of diet can affect blood pressure, particularly salt and protein intake, but a metaanalysis of fiber trials showed a small independent effect of dietary fiber on lowering blood pressure (84). In addition, the effects of combining a fiber intervention with other dietary changes may be additive. An additive effect was shown in a trial conducted in hypertensive patients in whom protein and fiber supplements in combination resulted in a decrease in systolic blood pressure of 5.9 mm Hg (85).

Dietary Fiber and the Prevention of Colon, Breast, and Other Cancers

Colon Cancer

For many years, it was thought that dietary fiber was protective against colorectal cancer. The data in support of such a protective effect were primarily the significant differences in rates of colorectal cancer among different countries with different fiber intakes (86), as well as the findings from migratory studies showing that persons take on the cancer risk factor rates of the population to which they move (87). However, more recently, three well-conducted large-scale clinical intervention trials were conducted, with colon polyp recurrence as the end point, and not one of the three trials showed a protective effect of fiber against colon cancer. One trial involved the addition of 13.5 g/day of wheat bran fiber versus 2 g/day of wheat bran fiber (88). No difference was reported between the control group and the intervention group in terms of polyp recurrence. A large-scale National Institutes of Health trial comprising eight clinical centers tested intervention with a diet that was low in fat, high in fiber, and high in fruits and vegetables. No difference between the intervention group and the control group was noted. In a large European trial, the intervention was 3.5 g/day psyllium (89). That trial actually showed a slightly promotive rather than protective effect of the psyllium intervention. Therefore, the clinical

intervention trials do not support the concept of a protective effect of fiber against colon cancer. However, whether fiber is protective against this disease is still an unresolved issue. Explanations for the reason that these large-scale clinical intervention trials failed to show a protective effect of fiber against polyp reoccurrence include the following: polyp recurrence may not be a good surrogate marker for colon cancer; the amount of fiber may not have been sufficient; the timing of the intervention may not have been optimal; the type of fiber may not have been correct; and confounding dietary factors may have been present.

Breast Cancer

Epidemiologic studies on the relationship between fiber intake and the incidence of breast cancer appear to show a negative association when fiber intakes are very different, as they are, for example, in England versus Wales (90), in Italy versus the United States (91), and in China versus the United States (92), but not in prospective cohort studies when the difference between the highest and lowest intake levels is not as marked, such as within New York State (93), within parts of the United States (94), and within the Netherlands (95). The mechanism by which fiber may protect against breast cancer that has received the most attention is through decreasing serum estrogen concentrations. Estrogens are excreted from the body by way of the gastrointestinal tract, but they may be reabsorbed if they are in their unconjugated form. Fiber can bind directly to unconjugated estrogens, thus interfering with their reabsorption (96–98), and fiber can also decrease the numbers of deconjugating bacteria (99).

Other Cancers

Most of the scientific research on fiber and cancer is directed to colon cancer and breast cancer. However, because of data showing a reduction of blood estrogen levels with high fiber intake (96–98), some researchers have hypothesized a protective effect against hormone-related cancers such as endometrial, ovarian, and prostate cancer. At this time, the data are equivocal on the relationship between fiber intake and endometrial cancer (100, 101). Studies have shown a decreased risk of ovarian cancer with a high intake of dietary fiber. No significant associations have been documented between dietary fiber intake and the risk of prostate cancer (102).

CONSEQUENCES OF OVERCONSUMPTION OF FIBER

Gastrointestinal Distress

Because viscous fibers are fermented in the large intestine, high intakes may result in gastrointestinal discomfort (e.g., flatulence, abdominal fullness). When 4 to 12 g/day of hydrolyzed guar gum were consumed, moderate to severe flatulence was reported (103). When as much as 32 g/day of resistant starch was consumed, 91% of persons studied reported bloated feelings (104). A metaanalysis of eight studies demonstrated that psyllium was well tolerated with no deleterious side effects (105).

Mineral Bioavailability

Because viscous fibers create a gel-like environment in the small intestine and because certain fiber-containing foods also contain phytate, numerous studies examined their effect on the absorption of micronutrients in humans. Most studies showed that viscous fiber (e.g., gums, pectin) consumption does not impair the intestinal absorption or balance of calcium (106, 107), magnesium (106–108), iron (109), or zinc (107, 109). In fact, some animal studies demonstrated that some viscous fibers may increase mineral absorption (110, 111). However, when 12 g/day of bran was added to a meal, iron absorption was reduced by 51 to 74%, and this reduction was not the result of the presence of phytate (112).

INTAKE OF FIBER IN THE UNITED STATES: AMOUNTS AND FOOD SOURCES

Information on total fiber consumption in the United States was obtained in the Continuing Survey of Food Intakes by Individuals during 1994 to 1996 and 1998. Usual intakes of dietary fiber ranged from 16.5 to 18 g/day for men and 12 to 14 g/day for women (12). This amount is primarily dietary fiber that exists naturally in foods, because very small amounts of isolated fibers are used as added ingredients. Information is also available on types of fibers consumed. Dietary fiber occurs naturally in most vegetables, fruits, and grains. Approximately one third of dietary fiber occurs as hemicellulose, and one fourth to one third as cellulose. Approximately 15 to 20% of dietary fiber is present as pectin. Some foods are good sources of certain types of dietary fiber. For example, most resistant starch is consumed from pasta and potatoes, and most inulin and oligofructose is consumed from wheat and onions. Isolated soluble fibers, such as inulin, carageenan, and guar gum, are added at low amounts to low-fat foods to create a creamy texture. Sources of soluble fiber (mostly viscous fibers) in different types of foods (e.g., cereals, beans, fruits) were described by Anderson and Bridges (113). Cellulose is ubiquitous and is found in all plants. β-Glucans are high in oats and barley. Fruits such as apples and oranges are good sources of pectin.

CURRENT RECOMMENDATIONS FOR FIBER INTAKE

The New Adequate Intake for Total Fiber and the Science behind It

For the first time, there is a dietary reference intake value for total fiber: 14 g fiber daily/1000 kcal (12). This adequate intake (AI) value is based on the strength of the relationship

TABLE 4.1. ADEQUATE INTAKE FOR TOTAL FIBER

AGE	ADEQUATE INTAKE (g/d)	
	MALES	FEMALES
0–6 mo	ND	ND
7–12 mo	ND	ND
1–3 y	19	19
4–8 y	25	25
9–13 y	31	26
14–18 y	38	26
19–50 y	38	25
>50 y	30	21
Pregnant women		28
Lactating women		29

ND, not determined.

between fiber intake and risk reduction for CHD as described earlier in the section on fiber and heart disease. The actual numbers (Table 4.1) were determined from three prospective cohort studies: the Health Professionals Follow-up Study (114), the Nurses' Health Study (115), and the Finnish Men's study (116), because these studies were adequately powered and provided intake data on both fiber and energy. This made it possible to calculate the number of grams of fiber/1000 kcal required to be in the most protected quintile for CHD (14 g of fiber/1000 kcal, as noted earlier). To convert g of fiber/1000 kcal to AI values, the average energy intake level for each sex and age group was used. Thus, for example, the AI for total fiber in foods is set at 38 and 25 g/day for young men and women, respectively. As persons age and energy intake diminishes, the AI for total fiber decreases proportionally. Because evidence on the adverse affects of long-term consumption of high levels of dietary fiber is limited, a tolerable upper intake level was not set (12). Unlike fibers that are consumed as they naturally occur in foods, those fibers that are extracted and concentrated or synthesized and added in high quantities to foods or supplements are more likely to cause adverse effects.

Appendix Table A-2-a through A-2-k summarize additional information on the basis and usage of the DRIs and actual nutritional data thus far published.

REFERENCES

1. Hipsley EH. BMJ 1953;2:420–2.
2. McCance RA, Lawrence RD. The Carbohydrate Content of Foods. London: His Majesty's Stationer's Office, 1929.
3. Trowell HC, Southgate DAT, Wolever TMS et al. Lancet 1976; 1:967.
4. Food and Nutrition Board, Institute of Medicine. Dietary Reference Intakes Proposed Definition of Dietary Fiber. Washington, DC: National Academy Press, 2001.
5. Food and Drug Administration. Fed Reg 1987;52:28590–691.
6. Health and Welfare Canada. Report of the Expert Advisory Committee on Dietary Fibre. Ottawa: Supply and Services Canada, 1985.
7. Life Sciences Research Office (LSRO). Physiological Effects and Health Consequences of Dietary Fiber. Bethesda, MD: LSRO, 1987.

8. Committee on Medical Aspects of Food and Nutrition Policy (COMA). Committee news. Food Safety Information Bulletin No. 97. Aberdeen, Scotland: Food Standards Agency, MAFF, Department of Health, 1998.

9. Marlett JA, Longacre MJ. Cereal Chem 1996;73;63–8.

10. Englyst HN, Cummings JH. Am J Clin Nutr 1986;44:42–50.

11. Englyst HN, Cummings JH. Am J Clin Nutr 1987;45:423–31.

12. Food and Nutrition Board, Institute of Medicine. Dietary, Functional, and Total Fiber. Dietary Reference Intakes for Energy, Carbohydrate, Fiber, Fat, Fatty Acids, Cholesterol, Protein, and Amino Acids. Washington, DC: National Academy Press, 2002.

13. Asp N-G. Am J Clin Nutr 1995;61:930S–7S.

14. Jung HG, Fahey GC. J Anim Sci 1983;57:206–19.

15. Southgate DAT. Dietary fiber parts of food plants and algae. In: Spiller GA, ed. CRC Handbook of Dietary Fiber in Human Nutrition. Boca Raton, FL: CRC Press, 1993:19–20.

16. Williams RD, Olmsted WH. J Biol Chem 1935;108:653–66.

17. Prosky L, Asp N-G, Furda I et al. J Assoc Off Anal Chem 1985; 68:677–9.

18. Southgate DAT. J Sci Food Agric 1969;20:331–5.

19. Englyst H, Cummings JH. J Assoc Off Anal Chem 1988;71: 808–14.

20. Theander O, Aman P, Westerlund E et al. The Uppsala method for rapid analysis of total dietary fiber. In: Furda I, Brine CJ, eds. New developments in dietary fiber. New York, New York: Plenum Press, 1990:273–81.

21. Anderson JW, Hanna TJ. J Nutr 1999;129:1457S–66S.

22. Jenkins DJA, Wolever TMS, Leeds AR et al. BMJ 1978;1: 1392–94.

23. Birkett AM, Jones GP, de Silva AM et al. Eur J Clin Nutr 1997; 51:625–32.

24. Cummings JH, Roberfroid MB, Andersson H et al. Eur J Clin Nutr 1997;51:417–23.

25. van Nieuwenhoven MA, Kovacs EMR, Brummer RJM et al. J Am Coll Nutr 2001;20;87–91.

26. Vincent R, Roberts A, Frier M et al. Gut 1995;37:216–9.

27. French SJ, Read NW. Am J Clin Nutr 1994;59:87–91.

28. Rigaud D, Paycha F, Meulemans A et al. Eur J Clin Nutr 1998; 52:239–45.

29. Leng-Peschlow E. Digestion 1989;44:200–10.

30. Hansen WE, Schulz G. Hepatogastroenterology 1982;29:157–60.

31. Isaksson G, Lundquist I, Ihse I. Gastroenterol 1982;82:918–24.

32. Baer DJ, Rumpler WV, Miles CW et al. J Nutr 1997;127: 579–86.

33. Barroso AJ, Contreras F, Bagachi D et al. J Med 2002;33: 209–25.

34. Miles CW. J Nutr 1992;122:306–11.

35. Kay RM, Truswell AS. Am J Clin Nutr 1977;30:171–5.

36. Savioli G, Lugli R, Pradelli JM. Dig Dis Sci 1985:301–7.

37. Wolever TMS, Vuksan V, Eshuis H et al. J Am Coll Nutr 1991; 10:364–71.

38. Lafrance L, Rabasa-Lhoret R, Poisson D et al. Diabet Med 1998;15:972–8.

39. Jenkins AL, Jenkins DJA, Zdravkovic U et al. Eur J Clin Nutr 2002;56:622–8.

40. Aldoori WH, Giovannucci EL, Stampfer MJ et al. Am J Epidemiol 1997;145:42–50.

41. Heading RC, Tothill P, Mclaoughlin GP et al. Gastroenterology 1976;71:45–50.

42. Harju EJ, Larmi TK. JPEN J Parenter Enteral Nutr 1985; 9:496–500.

43. Cummings JH. Proc Nutr Soc 1984;43:35–44.

44. Cummings JH, Englyst HN. Am J Clin Nutr 1987;45:1243–55.

45. McBurney MI, Thompson LU. Nutr Cancer 1990;13:271–80.

46. Roediger WE. Gastroenterology 1982;83:424–9.

47. Hague A, Manning AM, Hanlon KA et al. Int J Cancer 1993;55:498–505.

48. Heerdt BG, Houston MA, Augenlicht LH. Cancer Res 1994; 54:3288–94.

49. Deschner EE, Ruperto JF, Lupton JR. Cancer Lett 1990; 53:79–82.

50. Freeman HJ. Gastroenterology 1986;91:596–602.

51. Caderni G, Luceri C, De Filippo C et al. Carcinogenesis 2001; 22:525–7.

52. Zoran DL, Turner ND, Taddeo SS et al. J Nutr 1997;127: 2217–25.

53. Cummings JH. The effect of dietary fiber on fecal weight and composition. In: Spiller GA, ed. CRC Handbook of Dietary Fiber in Human Nutrition. Boca Raton, FL: CRC Press, 1993:263–349.

54. Burkitt DP, Walker ARP, Painter NS. Lancet 1972;2:1408–12.

55. Brodribb AJM, Humphreys DM. BMJ 1976;1:425–8.

56. Livesey G. Am J Clin Nutr 1990;51:617–37.

57. Smith T, Brown JC, Livesey G. Am J Clin Nutr 1998;68:802–19.

58. Fahey GC, Grieshop CM. Analysis of the net energy value of two soluble fibers. In: Life Sciences Research Office, Bethesda, MD: American Society of Nutritional Sciences, 2000:1–28.

59. Howarth NC, Saltzman E, Roberts SB. Nutr Rev 2001;59: 129–39.

60. DiLorenzo C, Willimans CM, Hajnal F et al. Gastroenterology 1988;95:1211–15.

61. Bergmann JF, Chassany O, Triki R et al. Gut 1992;33:1042–3.

62. Delargy HJ, Burley VJ, O'Sullivan KR et al. Eur J Clin Nutr 1995;49:754–66.

63. Birketvedt GS, Aseth J, Florholmen JR et al. Acta Med (Hradec Kralove) 2000;43:129–32.

64. Rigaud D, Ryttig KR, Angel AL et al. Int J Obes 1990;14:763–9.

65. Rossner S, von Zweigbergk DV, Ohlin A et al. Acta Med Scand 1987;222:83–8.

66. Miller WC, Niederpruem MG, Wallace JP et al. J Am Diet Assoc 1994;94:612–5.

67. Appleby PN, Thorogood M, Mann JI et al. Int J Obes Relat Metab Disord 1988;22:454–60.

68. Liu S, Willett WC, Manson JE et al. Am J Clin Nutr 2003;78: 920–7.

69. Tappy L, Gugolz E, Wursch P. Diabetes Care 1996;19:831–4.

70. Hanai H, Ikuma M, Sata Y et al. Biosci Biotechnol Biochem 1997;61:1358–61.

71. Leclere CJ, Champ M, Billot J et al. Am J Clin Nutr 1994;59: 914–21.

72. Hagander B, Asp NG, Efendic S et al. Diabetes Res 1986;3:91–6.

73. Groop PH, Aro A, Stenman S et al. Am J Clin Nutr 1993;58: 513–8.

74. Jenkins DJ, Ghafari H, Wolever TM et al. Diabetologia 1982; 22:450–5.

75. Liu S, Manson JE, Stampfer MJ et al. Am J Public Health 2000; 90:1409–15.

76. Hu FB, Manson JE, Stampfer MJ et al. N Engl J Med 2001; 345:790–7.

77. Montonen J, Knekt P, Jarvinen R et al. Am J Clin Nutr 2003; 77:622–9.

78. Salmeron J, Manson JE, Stampfer MJ et al. JAMA 1997;277: 472–7.

79. Fernandez ML. Curr Opin Lipidol 2001;12:35–40.

80. Truswell AS. Eur J Clin Nutr 2002;56:1–14.

81. Ludwig DDS. JAMA 2002;287:2414–23.

82. Parks EJ. Br J Nutr 2002;87:S247–53.

83. Anderson JW. Curr Atheroscler Rep 2000;2:536–41.

84. He J, Bazzano LA, Ogden LG et al. Circulation 2001;103:1366.

85. Burke V, Hodgson JM, Beilin LJ et al. Hypertension 2001;38: 821–6.

86. Boyle P, Zaridze DG, Smans M. Int J Cancer 1985;36:9–18.

87. Haenszel W, Kurihara M. J Natl Cancer Inst 1968;40:43–68.

88. Alberts D. N Engl J Med 2000;342:1156–62.

89. Bonithon-Kopp C, Kronborg O, Giacosa A et al. Lancet 2000; 356:1300–6.

90. Ingram DM. Nutr Cancer 1981;3:75–80.

91. Taioli E, Nicolosi A, Wynder EL. Nutr Cancer 1991;16:259–65.

92. Yu H, Harris RE, Gao YT. Int J Epidemiol 1991;20:76–81.

93. Graham S, Zielezny M, Marshall J et al. Am J Epidemiol 1992; 136:1327–37.

94. Willett WC, Hunter DJ, Stampfer MJ et al. JAMA 1992;268: 2037–44.

95. Verhoeven DTH, Assen N, Goldbohm RA et al. Br J Cancer 1997;75:149–55.

96. Shultz TD, Howie BJ. Nutr Cancer 1986;8:141–7.

97. Gorbach SL, Goldin BR. Prev Med 1987;16:525–9.

98. Goldin BR, Adlercreutz H, Gorbach SL. N Engl J Med 1982; 307:1542–7.

99. Rose DP. Nutr Cancer 1990;13:1–8.

100. Barbone E, Austin H, Partridge EE. Am J Epidemiol 1993;137: 393–403.

101. McCann S, Freudenhemi JL, Marshall JR et al. Cancer Causes Control 2000;11:965–74.

102. Andersson S, Wolk A, Bergstrom R et al. Int J Cancer 1996;68: 716–22.

103. Patrick PG, Gohman SM, Marx SC et al. J Am Diet Assoc 1998; 98:912–4.

104. Heijen M-L, van Amelsvoort JMM, Deurenberg P et al. Am J Clin Nutr 1998;67:322–31.

105. Anderson JW, Allgood LD, Lawrence A et al. Am J Clin Nutr 2000;71:472–9.

106. Sandberg AS, Ahderinne R, Andersson H et al. Hum Nutr Clin Nutr 1983;37:171–83.

107. Spencer H, Norris C, Derler J et al. J Nutr 1991;121: 1976–83.

108. Behall KM, Scholfield DJ, Lee K et al. Am J Clin Nutr 1987; 46:307–14.

109. Coudray C, Bellanger J, Castiglia-Delavaud C et al. Eur J Clin Nutr 1997;51:375–80.

110. Kim M, Atallah MT, Amarsiriwardena C et al. J Nutr 1996; 126:1883–90.

111. Schulz AGM, van Amelsvoort JMM, Beynen AC. J Nutr 1993; 123:1724–31.

112. Simpson KM, Morris ER, Cook JD. Am J Clin Nutr 1981; 34:1469–78.

113. Anderson JW, Bridges SR. Am J Clin Nutr 1988;47:440–7.

114. Rimm EB, Ascherio A, Giovannucci E et al. JAMA 1996;275: 447–51.

115. Wolk A, Manson JE, Stampfer MJ et al. JAMA 1999;281: 1998–2004.

116. Pietinen P, Rimm EB, Korhonen P et al. Circulation 1996;94: 2720–7.

SELECTED READINGS

Food and Nutrition Board, Institute of Medicine. Dietary Reference Intakes Proposed Definition of Dietary Fiber. Washington, DC: National Academy Press, 2001.

Food and Nutrition Board, Institute of Medicine. Dietary, Functional, and Total Fiber. Dietary Reference Intakes for Energy, Carbohydrate, Fiber, Fat, Fatty Acids, Cholesterol, Protein, and Amino Acids. Washington, DC: National Academy Press, 2002.

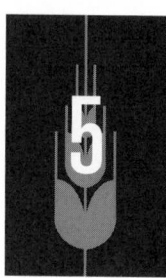

LIPIDS, STEROLS, AND THEIR METABOLITES[1]

PETER J.H. JONES AND STANLEY KUBOW

HISTORICAL INTRODUCTION 92
CHEMISTRY AND STRUCTURE 93
   Triglycerides and Fatty Acids 93
   Phospholipids 94
   Sterols 94
DIETARY CONSIDERATIONS 95
DIGESTION AND ABSORPTION 95
   Digestion in the Mouth and Esophagus 95
   Intestinal Digestion .95
   Absorption 98
   Digestion and Absorption of Phospholipids 98
   Digestion and Absorption of Sterols 98
TRANSPORT AND METABOLISM 99
   Solubility of Lipids 99
   Exogenous Transport System 99
   Endogenous Transport System 101
   Apoproteins, Lipid Transfer Proteins,
      and Lipoprotein Metabolism 101
   Dietary Factors Influencing Plasma Lipoproteins . .103
OXIDATION AND CONVERSION OF LIPIDS TO OTHER
   METABOLITES 103

Fatty Acid Oxidation 103
Peroxidative Modification of Lipids 104
INTRACELLULAR MOVEMENT AND BIOSYNTHESIS
   OF LIPIDS 107
   Fatty Acids 107
   Cholesterol 109
FUNCTIONS OF ESSENTIAL FATTY ACIDS 110
   Membrane Functions and Integrity 111
BIOSYNTHESIS AND FUNCTION OF EICOSANOIDS 111
ESSENTIAL FATTY ACID REQUIREMENTS 114
   n-6 Fatty Acid Requirements 114
   n-3 Fatty Acid Requirements 116

HISTORICAL INTRODUCTION

It was in 1918 that Aron first proposed that fat may be essential for normal growth and development of animals. Butter, apart from its caloric value, was deemed to have an important nutritional value because of the presence of certain lipid molecules. In 1927, Evans and Burr subsequently demonstrated that a deficiency of fat severely affected both growth and reproduction of experimental animals, despite the addition of the fat-soluble vitamins A, D, and E to the diet. These authors suggested that fat contained a new essential substance, termed vitamin F. The work of Evans and Burr in 1929 was the first to show the nutritional importance of specific lipids in fat. Weanling rats fed a fat-free diet showed impaired growth, scaly skin, tail necrosis, and increased mortality, conditions that were reversed by feeding linoleic acid (C18:2n-6). In further experiments, the same authors described impaired fertility and augmented water consumption as additional symptoms of a deficiency of either C18:2n-6 or α-linolenic acid (C18:3n-3). Hence the term *essential fatty acids* (EFAs) was coined by Burr and Burr for those fatty acids (FAs) not synthesized in mammals and for which deficiencies could be reversed by dietary addition.

Arachidonic acid (C20:4n-6) was determined to be an EFA in 1938. It was found to be approximately three times as effective as C18:2n-6 in relieving EFA deficiency (EFAD) symptoms. C18:2n-6 was subsequently found to undergo biotransformation to C20:4n-6, thus, C18:2n-6 was judged to be the primary unsaturated FA required by animals in

---

[1] **Abbreviations: ACAT,** acyl coenzyme A:cholesterol acyltransferase; **ADP,** adenosine diphosphate; **AI,** adequate intake; **ATP,** adenosine triphosphate; **BS,** bile salt; **BSSL,** bile salt–stimulated lipase; **CCK,** cholecystokinin; **CE,** cholesteryl ester; **CETP,** cholesterol ester transfer protein; **CH,** cholesterol; **CO,** cyclooxygenase; **CoA,** coenzyme A; **DAG,** diacylglycerol; **DG,** diglyceride; **DHA,** docosahexaenoic acid; **EAR,** estimated average requirement; **EFA,** essential fatty acid; **EFAD,** essential fatty acid deficiency; **EPA,** eicosapentaenoic acid; **FA,** fatty acid; **FABP,** fatty acid binding protein; **HDL,** high-density lipoprotein; **12-HETE,** 12-L-hydroxyeicosatetraenoic acid (12-HETE); **HMG,** hydroxymethylglutaryl; **12-HPETE,** 12-hydroperoxyeicosatetraenoic acid; **IDL,** intermediate-density lipoprotein; **IP,** inositol phosphate; **LCAT,** lecithin:cholesterol acyl transferase; **LCFA,** long-chain fatty acid; **LDL,** low-density lipoprotein; **LO,** lipoxygenase; **LT,** leukotriene; **MCFA,** medium-chain fatty acid; **MDA,** malondialdehyde; **MG,** monoglyceride; **MUFA,** monounsaturated fatty acid; **NAD,** nicotinamide adenine dinucleotide; **NIH,** National Institutes of Health; **PC,** phosphatidylcholine; **PE,** phosphatidylethanolamine; **PG,** prostaglandin; **PGHS,** prostaglandin H synthase; **PL,** phospholipid; **PP,** pyrophosphate; **PPAR,** peroxisome proliferator-activated receptor; **PUFA,** polyunsaturated fatty acid; **SAFA,** saturated fatty acid; **SCFA,** short-chain fatty acid; **TBARS,** thiobarbituric acid reactive substance; **TG,** triglyceride; **TRL,** triglyceride-rich lipoprotein; **TXA,** thromboxane; **VLCFA,** very-long-chain fatty acid; **VLDL,** very-low-density lipoprotein.

the diet. Although various researchers were able to generate EFAD in a variety of species via the feeding of EFA-deficient diets, EFAD was only first described in humans in 1958. Infants fed a milk-based formula diet lacking in EFA showed severe skin symptoms that were alleviated by the addition of C18:2n-6.

In human adults, EFAD was subsequently described as a consequence of parenteral nutrition in which fat-free solutions containing only glucose were continuously infused. The resulting skin rashes and low plasma concentrations of polyunsaturated FAs (PUFAs) were reversed by infusion of intravenous emulsions containing C18:2n-6. Holman and colleagues in 1982 reported the first example of deficiency symptoms attributed to C18:3n-3 deficiency in a 6-year-old girl maintained parenterally for 5 months on a safflower oil–based emulsion rich in C18:2n-6. Deficiency symptoms, including neuropathy and low serum concentrations of C18:3n-3, were corrected by changing the parenteral nutrition recipe to include a soybean oil emulsion rich in n-3 FA (1). Neuringer and associates in 1984 demonstrated C18:3n-3 deficiency in the offspring of rhesus monkeys who showed a loss in visual activity (2). C18:3n-3 deficiency was also described in nine patients who had received 0.02 to 0.09% of calories as n-3 FA via gastric tube feeding over a period of 2.5 to 12 years (3). The scaly dermatitis and depressed concentrations of n-3 FA in plasma and erythrocytes of the patients were eliminated with supplementation of C18:3n-3.

CHEMISTRY AND STRUCTURE

Fats and lipids are defined as a class of compounds soluble in organic solvents such as acetone, ether, and chloroform. Fats and lipids vary considerably in size and polarity, ranging from hydrophobic triglycerides (TGs) and sterol esters to more water-soluble phospholipids (PLs) and cardiolipins. Dietary lipids also include cholesterol (CH) and phytosterols. Unlike other macronutrients, the nonwater miscibility of lipids necessitates that these compounds undergo specialized processing during digestion, absorption, transport, storage, and utilization. This specialization in metabolic handling distinguishes dietary lipids and their metabolites from other dietary macronutrients.

Triglycerides and Fatty Acids

TGs, or triacylglycerols, make up by far the largest proportion of dietary lipids consumed by humans. A TG is composed of three FAs esterified to a glycerol molecule in one of three stereochemically distinct bonding positions, named sn-1, sn-2, and sn-3. Variation in the type of FAs and in their bonding pattern to glycerol further increases the heterogeneity of the TG composition. For most dietary oils, approximately 90% of the TG mass consists of FAs. These FAs are generally nonbranched hydrocarbon chains with an even number of carbons ranging from 4 to 26 carbon atoms. Smaller quantities of longer-chain FAs have also been identified in mammalian tissues and thus may exist in human diets (4). Very-long-chain fatty acids (VLCFAs) occur in brain and specialized tissues such as retina and spermatozoa (5). Adipose tissue contains FAs of varying lengths.

In addition to differences in chain length, FAs vary in the number and arrangement of double bonds along the hydrocarbon chain. Major FAs are given in Figure 5.1. Systems for identifying the position of double bonds along the hydrocarbon chain entail carbon counting from either end of the molecule. The less common "Δ" system of identification of double bonds counts from the carboxyl end of the fatty acyl chain. More commonly used is identification of the position of the first carbon of a double bond relative to the methyl terminus of the FA. Double bonds identified relative to the methyl end use the terms "n" or "ω" to indicate distance of the first bond along the carbon chain. For example, an FA described as "n-6" or "ω-6," indicates that the initial double bond is situated between the sixth and seventh carbon atoms from the methyl end. To contain a single double bond, a FA must be at least 12 carbon atoms in length. These monounsaturated fatty acids (MUFAs) typically possess a double bond at the n-9 or n-7 position. Addition of further double bonds produces a PUFA. Each subsequent double bond almost invariably occurs three carbon atoms further along the carbon chain from the bond preceding it. Therefore, the number of double bonds within a FA is restricted depending on its chain length. FAs of 18 carbon atoms or greater that possess more than a single double bond will contain the first bond of their series only at the n-9, n-6 or n-3 position. For a 16-carbon atom FA, the first double bond may be located at the n-7 position. A maximum of 6 double bonds occurs in dietary FA.

The essentiality of a FA depends on the position of the first double bond from the methyl terminus. During de novo FA formation, human biosynthetic enzymes are capable of inserting double bonds at the n-9 position or higher; however, these enzymes cannot insert double bonds at any position closer to the methyl end. For this reason, FAs with double bonds at the n-6 and n-3 positions are, as individual classes, considered essential. EFAs must therefore be obtained from plants or other organisms that possess the enzymatic pathways for their construction. Mammalian tissues contain four families of PUFAs (n-3, n-6, n-7, n-9) designated according to the number of carbon atoms from the terminal methyl group to the first carbon of the first double bond. Among all FAs, only those of n-6 and n-3 classes are essential to the diet. All other FAs can be synthesized by humans from an excess of dietary energy.

Double bonds in foods we consume most commonly occur as the *cis* configuration. Also present in foods are *trans* bonds which are a result of hydrogenation, the process used to increase the viscosity of oils, and the microbial

COMMON NAME	GENEVA NOMENCLATURE	CODE	FORMULA
butyric acid	butanoic acid	C4:0	$CH_3(CH_2)_2COOH$
caproic acid	hexanoic acid	C6:0	$CH_3(CH_2)_4COOH$
caprylic acid	octanoic acid	C8:0	$CH_3(CH_2)_6COOH$
capric acid	decanoic acid	C10:0	$CH_3(CH_2)_8COOH$
lauric acid	dodecanoic acid	C12:0	$CH_3(CH_2)_{10}COOH$
myristic acid	tetradecanoic acid	C14:0	$CH_3(CH_2)_{12}COOH$
palmitic acid	hexadecanoic acid	C16:0	$CH_3(CH_2)_{14}COOH$
stearic acid	octadecanoic acid	C18:0	$CH_3(CH_2)_{16}COOH$
palmitoleic acid	9-hexadecaenoic acid	C16:1, n-7 *cis*	$CH_3(CH_2)_5CH{=}CH(CH_2)_7COOH$
oleic acid	9-octadecaenoic acid	C18:1, n-9 *cis*	$CH_3(CH_2)_7CH{=}CH(CH_2)_7COOH$
elaidic acid	9-octadecaenoic acid	C18:1, n-9 *trans*	$CH_3(CH_2)_7CH{=}CH(CH_2)_7COOH$
linoleic acid	9, 12-octadecadienoic acid	C18:2, n-6,9 all *cis*	$CH_3(CH_2)_4CH{=}CHCH_2CH{=}$ $CH(CH_2)_7COOH$
α-linolenic acid	9, 12, 15-octadecatrienoic acid	C18:3, n-3,6,9 all *cis*	$CH_3CH_2CH{=}CHCH_2CH{=}CHCH_2CH{=}$ $CH(CH_2)_7COOH$
γ-linolenic acid	6,9,12-octadecatrienoic acid	C18:3, n-6,9,12 all *cis*	$CH_3(CH_2)_4CH{=}CHCH_2CH{=}HCH_2CH{=}$ $CH(CH_2)_4COOH$
columbinic acid	5,9,12-octatrienoic acid	C18:3, n-6 *cis*, 9 *cis*, 13 *trans*	$CH_3(CH_2)_4CH{=}CHCH_2CH{=}HCH_2CH{=}$ $CHCH_2CH_2CH{=}CH(CH_2)_3COOH$
arachidic acid	eicosanoic acid	C20:0	$CH_3(CH_2)_{18}COOH$
behenic acid	docosanoic acid	C22:0	$CH_3(CH_2)_{20}COOH$
eicosenoic acid	11-eicosenoic acid	C20:1, n-9 *cis*	$CH_3(CH_2)_7CH{=}CH(CH_2)_9COOH$
erucic acid	13-docosaenoic acid	C22:1, n-9 *cis*	$CH_3(CH_2)_7CH{=}CH(CH_2)_{11}COOH$
brassidic acid	13-docosaenoic acid	C22:1, n-9 *trans*	$CH_3(CH_2)_7CH{=}CH(CH_2)_{11}COOH$
nervonic acid	15-tetracosaenoic acid	C24:1, n-9 *cis*	$CH_3(CH_2)_7CH{=}CH(CH_2)_{13}COOH$
"Mead" acid	5,8,11-elcosatrienoic acid	C20:3, n-9,12,15 all *cis*	$CH_3(CH_2)_7CH{=}CHCH_2CH{=}CHCH_2CH{=}$ $CH(CH_2)_3COOH$
dihomo-γ-linolenic acid	8,11,14-eicosatetraenoic acid	C20:3, n-6,9,12 all *cis*	$CH_3(CH_2)_4CH{=}CHCH_2CH{=}HCH_2CH{=}$ $CH(CH_2)_6COOH$
arachidonic acid	5,8,11,14-eicosatetraenoic acid	C20:4, n-6,9,12,15 all *cis*	$CH_3(CH_2)_4CH{=}CHCH_2CH{=}HCH_2CH{=}$ $CHCH_2CH{=}CH(CH_2)_3COOH$
timnodonic acid	5,8,11,14,17-eicosapentaenoic acid	C20:5, n-3,6,9,12,15 all *cis*	$CH_3(CH_2CH{=}CH)_5(CH_2)_3COOH$
clupanodonic acid	7,10,13,16,19-docosapentaenoic acid	C22:5, n-3,6,9,12,15 all *cis*	$CH_3(CH_2CH{=}CH)_5(CH_2)_5COOH$
docosahexenoic acid	4,7,10,13,16,19-docosahexaenoic acid	C22:6, n-3,6,9,12,15,18 all *cis*	$CH_3(CH_2CH{=}CH)_6(CH_2)_2COOH$

Figure 5.1. Names, codes, and formulas of fatty acids mentioned in this chapter.

metabolism in ruminants. *Trans* bonds reduce internal rotational mobility of the fatty acyl chain and are less reactive to electrophilic addition such as halogenation, hydration, and hydrogenation (6, 7). Most dietary *trans* FAs are monoenes, 18 carbons in length. The major *trans* FA, elaidic acid (C18:1n-9 *trans*), has a melting point of 44°C, versus 13°C for oleic acid (C18:1n-9). *Trans* bonds are also found in FAs containing more than a single double bond. An example is conjugated linoleic acid, which contains both a *cis* and a *trans* double bond separated by only two, instead of three, carbons atoms.

Phospholipids

Some dietary lipids occur as PLs. PLs are distinct from TGs in that they contain polar head groups that confer amphipathic properties to the molecule. PLs are insoluble amphiphiles with a hydrophilic, often zwitterionic, head group, and hydrophobic tails composed of two longer-chain FAs. These head groups are attached to the primary glycerol moiety via phosphate linkages. The polar head group can vary in size and charge and can include inositol, choline, serine, ethanolamine, and glycerol.

Sterols

CH, an amphipathic molecule, is madeup of a steroid nucleus and branched hydrocarbon tail. It is found in the diet both in free form and esterified to FA, particularly C18:2n-6. CH is found only in foods of animal origin; plant oils are CH free. Although free of CH, plant materials do contain phytosterols, compounds that are chemically related to CH. Common dietary phytosterols are listed in Figure 5.2 (see also Chapter 6). Phytosterols differ in their chemical side-chain configuration and steroid ring-bonding pattern. The most common dietary phytosterols are β-sitosterol, campesterol, and stigmasterol. The Δ-5 hydrogenation of phytosterols forms saturated phytosterols, which include campestanol and sitostanol. These saturated phytosterols are found in very small amounts in normal diets, but they can be commercially produced. Plant sterols and stanols are often deliberately

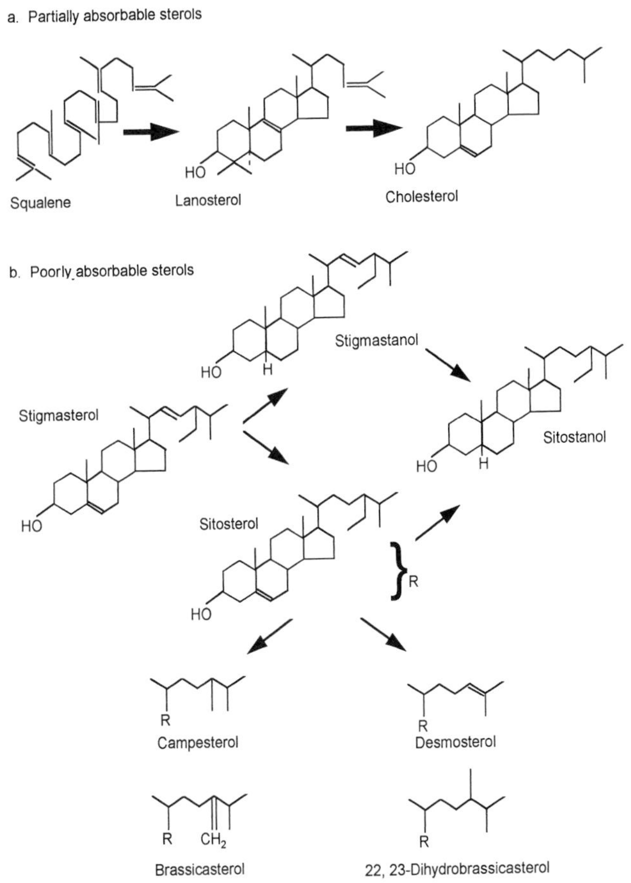

a. Partially absorbable sterols

Squalene   Lanosterol   Cholesterol

b. Poorly absorbable sterols

Stigmastanol

Stigmasterol

Sitosterol   Sitostanol

R

Campesterol   Desmosterol

R   CH₂   R

Brassicasterol   22, 23-Dihydrobrassicasterol

Figure 5.2. Molecular structure of the more important sterols in food (side chains only are shown for the bottom four structures).

esterified to FAs such as C18:2n-6 to improve their solubility in dietary oils.

DIETARY CONSIDERATIONS

Fat intake of average North Americans represents 35 to 40% of total calories consumed (8, 9). More than 95% of the total fat intake is constituted by TGs, with the remainder occurring in the form of PLs, free FAs, CH, and plant sterols. The total quantity of dietary TGs in the North American diet amounts to about 100 to 150 g/day. In addition to dietary intake, lipids enter the gastrointestinal tract both via release from mucosal cells and biliary expulsion into the lumen and by bacterial contributions.

In almost no other instance can food choice influence nutrient composition as much as in the case of fats. As dietary TGs vary widely in FA composition, so does FA consumption (Table 5.1). Large differences exist in the FA composition of oils from both plant and animal sources. Short-chain FAs (SCFAs) (four carbons) and medium-chain fatty acids (MCFAs) (six to 12 carbons) are found in vegetable oils and dairy fat, whereas fish oils and certain plants contain FAs of the n-3 family. n-3 long-chain FAs (LCFAs) can be found in a few terrestrial plants and range-fed,

nonruminant game animals. MUFAs are found in plant oils, although meat fats also contain moderate amounts. As a rule, n-6 PUFAs are found in vegetable fats and not in meat products, except in the case of C20:4n-6. Plant-derived oils vary widely in composition, largely because of genetic and environmental factors. In the case of animal fats, the composition of the feed also influences the final FA composition.

Intake of *trans* FAs in the North American diet has not been firmly established, but it appears to range from 2 to 7% of total energy intake (7, 10). Amounts of *trans* FAs in the diet have remained relatively constant over past decades, partly as the rise in vegetable fat consumption has been counterbalanced by a decline in the *trans* FA content of many foods made with vegetable fat (6). Methodologic limitations in measuring the various isomeric forms of dietary *trans* FA contribute to the imprecision of our knowledge of consumption levels.

The dietary contribution of CH varies significantly across foods. Typically, 250 to 700 mg of CH is consumed each day in the North American diet, with a larger proportion of this amount esterified to FA. Reduction of dietary CH levels can readily be achieved through exclusion of animal fats and eggs from the diet. North American diets typically contain about 250 mg/day of plant sterols, with vegetarian diets containing much larger amounts (11). Most plant sterols are found as β-sitosterol, campesterol, and stigmasterol.

DIGESTION AND ABSORPTION

Digestion in the Mouth and Esophagus

Digestion of dietary lipids and their metabolites evokes a series of specific processes enabling absorption through the water-soluble environment of the gut (Table 5.2). Digestion begins in the oral cavity with the process of salivation and mastication. Lingual lipase, released from the serous glands of the tongue with saliva, commences the process of hydrolysis of free FAs from TGs. The mechanical dispersing action of chewing enlarges the surface area on which lingual lipase can act. Lingual lipase cleaves at the sn-3 position, preferentially hydrolyzing shorter-chain FAs found in foods such as milk. Hydrolysis continues into the stomach, where gastric lipase promotes further lipid digestion and prefers TGs containing SCFAs. The composition of fat entering the upper duodenum is made up of 70% TGs with the remainder consisting of a mixture of partially digested hydrolysis products.

Intestinal Digestion

Intestinal digestion requires bile salts (BSs) and pancreatic lipase. BSs, PLs, and sterols are the three principal lipid components of bile, the emulsifying fluid produced by the liver. The BS molecule consists of a steroid nucleus and an aliphatic side chain conjugated by an amide bond with taurine or glycine. The number and orientation of the hydroxyl groups on the steroid nucleus vary. The hydroxyl and

TABLE 5.1. AVERAGE TRIGLYCERIDE FATTY ACID COMPOSITION OF IMPORTANT EDIBLE FATS[a]

| FOOD | AVERAGE FAT% | SATURATED | | | MONO- AND POLYUNSATURATED | | | |
		TOTAL[b]	16:0	18:0	18:1	18:2	18:3	20:4
Milk (cow)	3.5	65[b]	25	11	26	1–3	2	tr
Butter	80				Identical to milk			
Lard (pig)	100	42	20	13	46	6–8	2	2
Pork	36				Approx. as lard			
Tallow	100	53	29	20	42	2	tr	
Beef	25				Approx. as tallow			
Chicken	15	30	25	4	42	21		
Egg	11				Identical to chicken			
Turkey	20				Approx. or chicken			
Groundnut oil	100	19[c]	11	3	40–55[c]	20–43[c]		
Groundnut	50				Identical (variable, climate dependent)			
Sesame oil	100	15	9	5	39	40	1	
Soybean oil	100	15	11	4	23	51	7	
Corn oil	100	13	11	2	25	55	tr	
Sunflower seed oil	100	12	8	4	24	60–70	tr	
Olive oil	100	17	14	3	71	10	tr	
Cottonseed oil	100	30	25	3	18	51	tr	
Safflower seed oil	100	10	7	3	15[d]	75[d]	tr	
Palm oil	100	52	45	5	38	10		
Coconut oil	100	88[b]	8	3	6	2		
Palm kernel oil	100	80[b]	7	2	14	1		
Rapeseed oil	100	7	5	2	53	22	10[e]	
Cashew nut	68	24	14	10	30	35	tr	
Walnut	63	10	7	2	15	60	10	
Herring (menhaden)	16–25	30	19	4	13	1	1+[f]	
Mackerel[g]	26	25	17	5	18	1	[g]	

[a] The figures given are approximations, as climate, species, fodder composition, etc. cause great variations. The data given are compiled from refer 165,186.

[b] The balance of saturated fatty acids is formed by fatty acids with chain lengths <12 (butter 14%) and 12 and 14 (butter 16%, coconut and palm kernel 65–70%).

[c] Circa 4% of C20:0 and C22:0 groundnuts from Argentina and Virginia have relatively low C18:1 and high C18:2 concentrations.

[d] Also safflower seed oil with the reverse C18:1/18:2 composition is available.

[e] Contrary to new rapeseed varieties, such as Canbra and LEAR, old varieties of rapeseed oil and also mustard seed oil have 10% C20:1 n-9, and 30–50% C22:1 n–9.

[f] Menhaden herring oil has 11% C20:5 n-3, 9% C22:6 n-3, but Norwegian herring oil has 13% C20:1 n-9, 21% C22:1 n-11, 7% C20:5 n-3, and 7% C22:6 n-3.

[g] Dependent on fishing grounds, mackerel oil is similar to menhaden or to Norwegian/North Sea herring.

ionized sulfonate or carboxylate groups of the conjugate impart water solubility to BSs. Primary BSs, defined as those synthesized directly from hepatic CH, include the trihydroxy and dihydroxy BSs, cholate, and chenodeoxycholate, respectively. Secondary BSs, including deoxycholate and lithocholate, are produced from primary BSs via bacterial action on cholate and chenodeoxycholate in the gut. Further modifications of secondary BSs by hepatocytes or bacteria produce sulfate esters of lithocholate and ursodeoxycholate. Biliary phosphatidylcholine (PC), the main PL in bile, typically contains palmitic acid (C16:0) in the sn-1 position and an unsaturated 18- or 20-carbon FA in the sn-2 position.

Pancreatic lipase, the principal enzyme of TG digestion, acts to hydrolyse ester bonds at the sn-1 and sn-3 positions of the glycerol moiety (Fig. 5.3). BSs inhibit lipase activity through displacement of the enzyme from its substrate at the surface of the lipid droplet. Colipase,

TABLE 5.2. FACTORS INVOLVED IN THE DIGESTION OF FATS

SOURCE	FACTOR	LOCATION OF ACTION	FUNCTION
Food (breast milk)	Bile salt–stimulated lipase	Duodenum	Converts monoglycerides and free fatty acids to glycerol and free fatty acids
Oral cavity	Lingual lipase	Mouth; esophagus; stomach	Cleave triglycerdes at sn-3 position
Stomach	Gastric lipase	Stomach; duodenum	Cleave triglycerides at sn-3 position
Pancreas	Pancreatic lipase	Duodenum	Splitting of sn-1 and sn-3 positions
Liver	Bile salts	Duodenum	Emulsification of fats and reabsorption is small intestine and colon

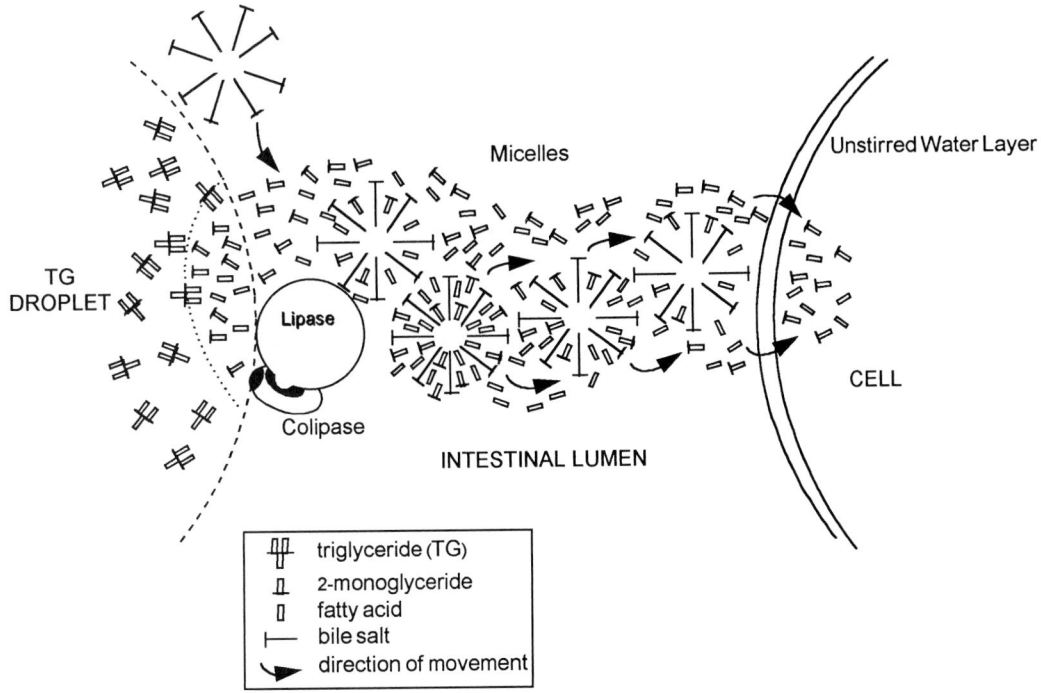

Figure 5.3. Transport hypothesis of fatty acids and 2-monoglycerides through lipase-mediated hydrolysis, micellar transfer, and cellular uptake stages.

also a pancreatic protein, reverses BS inhibition on pancreatic lipase by binding lipase and ensuring its adhesion to the droplet. Then, through its affinity to BSs, PLs, and CH, colipase facilitates shuttling of hydrolysis product monoglycerides (MGs) and free FAs from the lipid droplet into the BSs containing micelle. FAs linked at the sn-2 position of MGs, PLs, and cholesteryl ester (CE) are resistant to hydrolysis by lipase. Lipolysis by pancreatic lipase is extremely rapid; MGs and free FAs are produced faster than their subsequent incorporation into micelles (12). Synthesis of both lipase and colipase is stimulated by the hormone secretin and the presence of dietary TG in the small intestine. Release of BSs and pancreatic lipase is also regulated by hormonal actions. The presence of amino acids and fat digestion products in the digesta evokes release of cholecystokinin (CCK) and secretin into circulation. CCK stimulates production of exocrine pancreatic enzymes, whereas secretin enhances the output of pancreatic electrolytes. CCK also induces synthesis of hepatic bile and its release through contraction of the gallbladder.

In breast-fed infants, digestion of TGs is accomplished by concerted action of gastric lipase, colipase-dependent pancreatic lipase, and a BS-stimulated lipase (BSSL) present in breast milk. Whereas gastric lipase initiates digestion of the milk fat globule, BSSL nonselectively converts resulting MGs and free FAs to glycerol and free FAs, a process that increases absorptive efficiency.

Micellar solubilization of fat hydrolysis products occurs through the amphipathic actions of BSs and PLs, which are secreted at a ratio of approximately 1:3. CH is present in bile only in the unesterified form, which is the major sterol form (13). The polar termini of BSs orient themselves toward the water milieu of the chyme, whereas the nonpolar termini containing hydrocarbon groups face the center of the micelle. BSs and PLs naturally aggregate such that the nonpolar termini form a hydrophobic core. For micelles to form, a threshold concentration of BS must be reached, termed the critical micellar concentration. The typical biliary critical micellar concentration of BSs is 2 millimolar (mM). BS concentrations within the proximal duodenum generally remain well in excess of this threshold.

Incorporation of MG, hydrolysed from TGs into micelles, increases the ability of the particle to solubilize free FA and CH. BS micelles generally possess the highest affinity for MG and unsaturated free LCFAs (14). Both diglycerides (DGs) and TGs have limited incorporation into micelles. On formation, mixed micelles containing FAs, MGs, CH, PLs, and BSs migrate to the unstirred water layer adjacent to the brush border surface.

Fat digestion has been the focus of clinical attention in light of the increasing global prevalence of obesity. Creation of fat substitutes having properties similar to those of a naturally occurring fat, but that are resistant to the action of pancreatic lipase, has been actively pursued. Olestra, formed by chemical combination of sucrose with FAs, possesses mouth feel and texture properties similar to those of TGs. However, Olestra passes through the intestine undigested and unabsorbed (15). The molecule is heat stable and has been approved for use in certain foods. The efficacy of Olestra in long-term weight control has yet to be confirmed (16). Consumption of Olestra is not without the risk of side effects, which may include anal leakage and reduced absorption of fat-soluble vitamins.

Absorption

The process of lipid absorption appears to occur in large part through passive diffusion. Micelles containing fat digestion products exist in dynamic equilibrium with each other; the peristaltic, churning action of the intestine maintains a high frequency of intermicellar contact. This contact results in partitioning of constituents from more to lesser-populated micelles, with consequent equalization of the overall micellar concentration of digestion products. Thus, during digestion of a bolus of fat, micelles evenly accrue digestion products. The 2-MG and free FAs are released through the action of pancreatic lipase until saturation capacity of the micelles is achieved.

Penetration of micelles across the unstirred water layer bordering the intestinal mucosal cells represents the first stage of absorption. Micelles, but not lipid droplets, approach and enter this water layer for two reasons. First, micelles are much smaller (30–100 Å) particles than emulsified droplets of fat (25,000±20,000 Å). Second, the hydrophobic nature of the larger lipid droplet results in reduced solubilization at the site of the unstirred water layer.

Transport of micellar products across the unstirred water layer into the enterocyte occurs as described in Figure 5.3. Micelles closest to the plasma membrane of the brush border partition their digestion products across the water envelope in a concentration-dependent fashion. Digestion products continue to be shuttled between micelles across the unstirred water layer, thus creating a chain-reaction effect. This action hinges on the lower cellular concentration of digestion products at the enterocyte. Intestinal FA binding proteins (FABPs) assist in transmucosal shunting of digestion product FAs, and possibly MGs and BSs. Elevated FABP activity in the distal bowel has been shown to be associated with higher FA absorption (17).

The overall efficiency of fat absorption in human adults is about 95% and is more or less independent of the amount of fat consumed. However, the qualitative nature of the dietary fat influences overall efficiency. In general, efficiency increases with the degree of FA unsaturation (18). Evidence also suggests that as FA chain length increases, absorption efficiency decreases. Likewise, the positional distribution of FAs on dietary TGs is an important determinant of the eventual efficiency of absorption. Studies with structured lipids have shown that when octanoate, palmitate, or linoleate was substituted at different sn positions on a TG molecule, the positional distribution altered characteristics of digestion, absorption, and lymphatic transport of these FAs (19, 20). The natural tendency of C16:0 to locate at the sn-2 position in breast milk may therefore explain the high digestibility of this milk fat.

FAs with chain lengths less than 12 carbon atoms are also absorbed passively by the gastric mucosal boundary and are taken up by the portal vein (21).

Micellar BSs are not absorbed with fat digestion products, but rather are reabsorbed further along the gastrointestinal tract. Passive intestinal absorption of unconjugated BSs occurs throughout the small intestine and colon. Active transport components predominate in the ileum and include the brush border membrane receptor, cytosolic bile acid binding proteins, and basolateral anion exchange proteins. The enterohepatic recirculation of BSs is approximately 98% efficient (22). Although bile acid production and secretion are not normally rate limiting in lipid absorption, investigators have proposed that bile acid synthesis may be subnormal in infants. Dietary taurine supplementation has been shown to result in higher bile acid excretion and FA absorption in preterm and small for gestational age infants (23).

Digestion and Absorption of Phospholipids

Dietary PLs comprise only a small portion of ingested lipid; however, PLs are secreted in large quantities in bile. PLs assist in emulsification of TG droplets, as well as micellar solubilization of CH and other lipid-soluble components of diet. PLs, in particular PC, are also essential in the stabilization of the micelle within the unstirred water layer. PLs of both dietary and biliary origins are digested through cleavage by phospholipase A_2, a pancreatic enzyme secreted in bile. In contrast to pancreatic lipase, phospholipase A_2 cleaves FAs at the sn-2 position of PLs, thus yielding lysophosphoglycerides and free FAs. These products undergo absorption through a similar process as described earlier.

Digestion and Absorption of Sterols

CH within the intestine originates from both diet and bile. The amount of CH in the diet varies markedly depending on the degree of inclusion of foods from nonplant sources, whereas biliary CH secretion is more consistent. Dietary and biliary CH differ in several ways. Dietary CH is up to 65% esterified; while, biliary CH exists in free form, this is likely responsible for the different absorption efficiencies between dietary (34%) and biliary (46%) CH (24). Biliary CH is also absorbed at a more proximal site than diet-derived CH within the small intestine.

Being hydrophobic, CH requires a specialized system for digestion and absorption to occur within a water-soluble environment. Notably, absorption efficiency for CH is much less than that of TG. The major rate-limiting factor associated with the lower absorption of CH is its poor micellar solubility. Using various methodologies, investigators have demonstrated that 40 to 65% of CH is absorbed over the physiologic range of human CH intake (23).

The digestion of dietary CE involves release of the esterified FAs through the action of a BS-dependent CE hydrolase secreted by the pancreas. Removal of esterified FAs does not appear to be rate limiting; mixtures of free and esterified CH were absorbed with equal efficiency in rats (25). Free sterol then undergoes solubilization within mixed micelles in the upper small intestine. Water-soluble lipid exchange proteins of low molecular weight, located on the luminal side of the brush border membrane, may be involved in the transmembrane movement of CH and PLs (26). The concentration of sphingomyelin within the apical membrane of the intestinal cell may also exist as a factor regulating the rate of CH uptake from micelles.

The amount of CH in the circulatory lipoproteins appears to be marginally responsive to the amount of dietary CH within the normal, physiologic range. Likely, compensatory changes in CH absorption (27) and biosynthesis (28) serve to protect circulatory CH levels from shifting greatly in the presence of changes in dietary intake. In contrast to CH, plant sterol absorption is very limited and differs across dietary phytosterols. For the major plant sterol, β-sitosterol, typical absorption efficiency is 4 to 5%, about one tenth of that of CH (29). Absorption efficiency is higher for campesterol, about 10% (29), and is almost nonexistent for sitostanol (30). This structure-specific discrimination depends on both the number of carbon atoms at the C24 position of the sterol side chain and the degree of hydrogenation of the sterol nucleus double bond. Differences in absorption across phytosterols are reflected in their circulating concentrations. Plasma campesterol levels are usually higher than those of sitosterol, whereas circulating levels of highly saturated sitostanol are almost undetectable (11).

Reasons for the markedly reduced absorption of phytosterols are twofold. First, solubilization of phytosterols within micelles may be considerably less than that of CH. Second, inadequate esterification of phytosterols may occur within enterocyte membranes. Acyl coenzyme A:CH acyltransferase (ACAT)–dependent esterification of CH exceeds that of β-sitosterol by at least 60-fold (31).

Dietary phytosterols appear to compete with each other and with CH for absorption. Sitosterol consumption results in a reduction in absorption of CH, which in turn, lowers circulating CH levels. Addition of sitostanol to diets causes a depression in absorption of circulating levels of both CH and nonsaturated plants sterols (11), apparently through a reduction in intestinal absorption of both types of sterols (see also Chapter 6). Saturated and unsaturated plant sterols and their esters are useful in lowering serum total and low-density lipoprotein (LDL) CH levels (32).

TRANSPORT AND METABOLISM

Solubility of Lipids

Transport of largely hydrophobic lipids through the circulation is achieved in large part through use of aggregates of lipids and protein called lipoproteins. Principal lipid components of lipoproteins are TGs, CH, CE, and PLs. Protein constituents termed apolipoproteins, or apoproteins, serve to increase both particle solubility and recognition by enzymes and receptors located at the outer surface of lipoproteins. The major lipoprotein classes are listed in Table 5.3. Lipoproteins differ in composition; however, all types feature hydrophilic apoproteins, PL polar headgroups, and CH hydroxyl groups facing outward at the water interface with PL acyl tails and CH steroid nuclei oriented toward the interior of the aggregate. CEs and TG molecules form the core of the lipoprotein particle; in this manner, hydrophobic lipids can be internally solubilized and transported within a water medium. Although lipoproteins are characterized into subclasses, they represent a continuous spectrum of lipoprotein particles varying in size, density, composition, and function. Internal transport of lipids can be divided into exogenous and endogenous systems, reflecting lipids of dietary and internal origins, respectively.

Exogenous Transport System

The exogenous transport system transfers lipids of intestinal origin to peripheral and hepatic tissues (Fig. 5.4). Such lipids may originate from diet or secretions in the intestine. The exogenous system commences in the enterocyte with reorganization of absorbed FAs, 2-MG, lysoPLs, PLs, smaller amounts of glycerol, CH, and phytosterols into molecules more readily packaged within the primary

TABLE 5.3. PHYSICAL-CHEMICAL CHARACTERISTICS OF THE MAJOR LIPOPROTEIN CLASSES

LIPOPROTEIN	DENSITY (g/dL)	MOLECULAR MASS (DALTONS)	DIAMETER (nm)	LIPID (%)[a]		
				TRIGLYCERIDE	CHOLESTEROL	PHOSPHOLIPID
Chylomicrons	0.95	1400×10^6	75–1200	80–95	2–7	3–9
VLDL	0.95–1.006	10–80×10^6	30–80	55–80	5–15	10–20
IDL	1.006–1.019	5–10×10^6	25–35	20–50	20–40	15–25
LDL	1.019–1.063	2.3×10^6	18–25	5–15	40–50	20–25
HDL	1.063–1.21	1.7–3.6×10^5	5–12	5–10	15–25	20–30

HDL, high-density lipoprotein; IDL, intermediate-density lipoprotein; LDL, low density lipoprotein; VLDL, very-low-density lipoprotein.
[a] Percentage composition of lipids, apolipoproteins make up the rest.
From Ginsberg HN. Med Clin North Am 1994;78:1-20, with permission from WB Saunders.

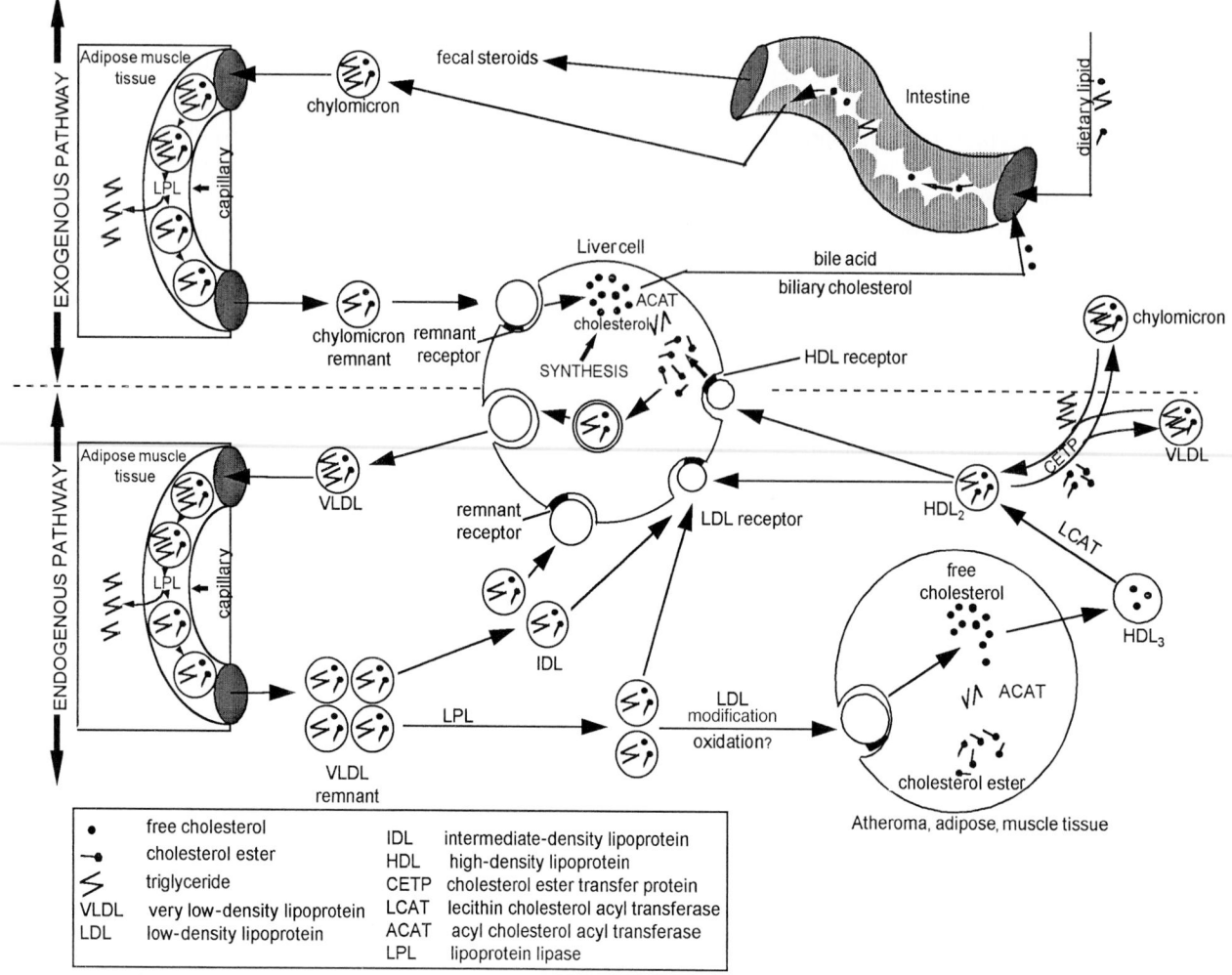

Figure 5.4. Exogenous and endogenous pathways of lipid transport.

secretory unit, the chylomicron. Chylomicrons are assembled in the enterocyte endoplasmic reticulum membrane in conjunction with the Golgi apparatus. Chylomicron TGs are reassembled predominantly using the monoacylglycerol pathway. Absorbed FAs are activated by microsomal FA-coenzyme A (CoA) synthase to yield acyl-CoA, then combined sequentially with 2-MG through the action of MG and DG-acyltransferases. In addition, about 20% of TG resynthesis occurs by the α-glycerophosphate pathway. α-Glycerophosphate, synthesized de novo within the enterocyte from absorbed free glycerol or triose phosphates, combines with two fatty acyl-CoA units to form phosphatidic acid. After dephosphorylation, the 1,2-DG is converted to TG by addition of a further fatty acyl-CoA. Phosphatidic acid is also converted to PL with addition of FA, as is the majority of lysoPL entering the enterocyte. The extent of the contribution of the phosphatidic acid pathway to TG synthesis is influenced by the PL requirement of the enterocyte for chylomicron structure and assembly. Absorbed free CH is in large part reesterified using fatty acyl-CoA by the microsomally located ACAT (33).

The process of synthesis of new lipid appears to be a driving force in assembly and secretion of lipoproteins. Uptake of dietary LCFAs, incorporation into TGs by the glycerol-3-phosphate pathway, and assembly of lipoproteins all require FABP (34).

Not all FAs requires chylomicron incorporation and transport. FAs of less than 14 carbons in length and those containing several double bonds undergo, to a variable degree, direct internal transport via the portal circulation. Direct portal transfer of fats occurs either as lipoprotein-bound TGs or as albumin-bound free (unesterified) FAs. Portal transfer results in more immediate delivery of FAs to the liver compared with chylomicron transit. The FA structure-dependent specificity in these studies has raised questions about whether all FAs can be regarded as equivalent in the context of energy and lipid metabolism. An accumulating body of evidence suggests that consumption of fats containing SCFAs and MCFAs is associated with portal transit to liver, resulting in higher rates of fat oxidation.

Chylomicrons released from mucosal cells circulate through the lymphatic system and reach the superior vena cava by way of the thoracic duct. Release into the circulation is followed by TG hydrolysis at the capillary surface of tissues by lipoprotein lipase. Hydrolysis of TG within the core of the chylomicron results in movement of FAs into tissues and subsequent production of TG-depleted chylomicron remnant particles. Chylomicron remnants then pick up CE from high-density lipoproteins (HDLs) and are rapidly taken up by the liver.

Endogenous Transport System

The endogenous shuttle for lipids and their metabolites consists of three interrelated components. The first, involving very-low-density lipoproteins (VLDLs), intermediate-density lipoproteins (IDLs), and LDLs, coordinates movement of lipids from liver to peripheral tissues. The second, involving HDLs, encompasses a series of events that returns lipids from peripheral tissues to the liver. The third component of the system, not involving lipoproteins, effects the free FA-mediated transfer of lipids from storage reservoirs to metabolizing organs.

Components of the endogenous lipoprotein system are illustrated in Figure 5.4. The system begins with assembly of VLDL particles, mostly in the liver. Assembly of nascent VLDL starts in the endoplasmic reticulum and depends on the presence of adequate core lipids, CE, and TGs. Investigators have estimated, using stable isotope tracers, that most TG FA within VLDL is preformed (35, 36). Some proportion of VLDL particles may also originate from intestinal tissue. Addition of surface lipids, mainly PLs and free CH, occurs in the Golgi apparatus before the particle is secreted.

Following secretion of VLDL particles into the circulation, certain interchanges with tissues and lipoproteins occur. A major event is deposition of lipids into peripheral tissues. Hydrolysis of VLDL TG occurs through the action of lipoprotein lipase, an enzyme located on the endothelial side of vessel tissue that mediates hydrolysis of chylomicron TG. Lipase-generated free FA can be used as energy sources, structural components for lipids including PLs, leukotrienes (LTs), and thromboxanes (TXAs), or converted back to TGs and stored. TGs and PLs from both chylomicron remnants and LDLs also undergo hydrolysis by the enzyme hepatic lipase. When hepatic lipase is absent, accumulation of large LDL particles and TG-rich lipoproteins occurs. Through TG depletion, the VLDL particle is converted to a denser, smaller, CH and TG-rich lipoprotein (TRL) remnant. High circulatory levels of TRL remnants are associated with progression of coronary artery disease. TRL remnants themselves can be cleared from plasma through hepatic lipoprotein receptors or converted to smaller LDL. LDL is the major CH-carrying lipoprotein. Although LDL levels are associated with heart disease risk in general, evidence suggests that a predominance of smaller, denser LDL particles in the circulation confers an elevated risk of coronary heart disease (37).

LDL receptors allows the liver to catabolize LDL. Modified or oxidized LDL can also be taken up by a scavenger receptor on macrophages in various tissues, including the arterial wall.

The second component of the endogenous transport system, perhaps nebulously termed "reverse CH transport," involves movement of CH from peripheral tissues to the liver. Since 1975, when Miller and Miller described the protective effect of HDLs on atherosclerosis, much work has been undertaken to better understand the structure and function of HDLs (38). HDL particles are highly heterogeneous, with subcomponents originating from both the intestinal tract and liver. Investigators have proposed that HDL particles participate in reverse CH transport by acquiring CH from tissues and other lipoproteins and transporting it to the liver for excretion. Membrane receptors of the adenosine triphosphate (ATP)–binding casette transporter family (ABCA1) mediate unidirectional efflux of cellular CH and PLs to lipid-poor HDLs, whereas receptors of the scavenger receptor family (SR-B1) mediate bidirectional lipid transfer (39). Circumstantial clinical evidence suggests that elevated HDL levels are associated with a reduced coronary risk, whereas the link between subnormal HDL levels and higher risk has been established (40).

The third component of the endogenous lipid transport system involves non–lipoprotein-associated movement of free FAs through the circulation. These FAs, derived largely as products of cellular TG hydrolysis, are secreted by adipose tissue into plasma, where they bind with albumin. Evidence suggests that SAFA and C18:1n-9 are more slowly mobilized than PUFAs, at a rate that is independent of their relative proportion in adipose tissue (41, 42). Albumin-bound FAs are removed in a concentration gradient–dependent manner by metabolically active tissues and used largely as energy sources.

Apoproteins, Lipid Transfer Proteins, and Lipoprotein Metabolism

The orchestration of inter-organ movement of exogenous and endogenous lipids within lipoproteins is not incidental, but coordinated by a series of apoproteins. Apoproteins confer greater water solubility, coordinate the movement and activities of lipoproteins by modulating enzyme activity, and mediate particle removal from the circulation by specific receptors. Indeed, rates of synthesis and catabolism of the major lipoproteins are regulated to a large extent by apoproteins residing on a particular surface recognized by specific cellular receptors. Much has been learned concerning the role of apoproteins through the study of genetic defects and their effects on modification of apoprotein structure and thus lipoprotein function (43).

Lipoproteins vary in apoprotein content. Apolipoprotein B (Apo-B) is the major protein contained in chylomicrons, VLDLs, IDLs, and LDL particles. A larger

Apo-B-100 is associated with VLDLs and LDLs of hepatic origin, whereas a lesser molecular weight Apo-B-48 species is found in chylomicrons and intestinally derived VLDLs. Apo-B-48 is thought to be generated from the same messenger RNA as is Apo-B-100. Within the intestine, only about one half of the B-100 protein is translated. During apoprotein assembly, hydrophobic Apo-B associates with PLs in the endoplasmic reticulum immediately after translation, and then it requires the presence of adequate core lipid CE and TGs. This process of assembly of Apo-B–containing lipoproteins may be influenced by FA composition.

Apo-E is synthesized in liver and is present on all forms of lipoproteins. Apo-E binds both heparin-like molecules present on all cells and the LDL receptor. Apo-E displays genetic polymorphism; at least three alleles of the Apo-E gene produce six or more possible genotypes that differ in their ability to bind the LDL receptor. Interactions between Apo-E genotype and CH absorption and synthesis have been suggested.

Most HDL particles contain apoproteins A-I, A-II, A-IV, and C. Apo-A-I and A-IV are believed to be activators of lecithin:CH acyl transferase (LCAT), an enzyme that esterifies CH in plasma. Apo-A-I also appears to be the crucial structural protein for HDL. Three C apoproteins exist, C-I, C-II, and C-III; each possesses distinct functions, and all are synthesized in the liver. Apo-C-II, present in chylomicrons, VLDLs, IDLs, and HDLs, is important in activation of the enzyme lipoprotein lipase, along with Apo-E. Apo-C-III, present on chylomicrons, IDLs, and HDLs, may inhibit PL action.

Apoproteins play a role in inter-organ lipid movement and distribution at several levels. For instance, VLDL undergoes modification through lipoprotein lipase action in peripheral tissues, with resulting formation of LDL particles. Apo-C-II, activating lipoprotein lipase, hydrolyses VLDL and chylomicron TG. It is believed that HDL exchanges Apo-E and Apo-C for Apo-A-I and Apo-A-IV on chylomicrons in the circulation. Apo-E is important in the hepatic clearance of TG-depleted chylomicron remnants.

Apoproteins are critical in the removal of particles from the circulation. LDL is taken up into tissues by two processes, mostly in liver cells, but also in adipocytes, smooth muscle cells, and fibroblasts. The first process is receptor dependent and involves the interaction of Apo-B-100 and LDL with specific LDL receptors on cell surfaces. Quantitatively, most LDL receptors exist in the liver (see Fig. 5.4). Postcontact events involve clustering of these receptors in coated pits and LDL internalization. The second process is receptor independent. In contrast to receptor-dependent LDL uptake, receptor-independent transport is nonsaturable and does not appear to be regulated. The rate of receptor-independent transfer is low; however, this form of transport increases as a direct function of plasma LDL levels, so uptake by this pathway can be substantial at high plasma LDL levels.

The LDL receptor is sensitive to both the total amount and unesterified fraction of CH within the cell. Receptor integrity, particularly for LDL, is implicated in the progression of atherosclerosis. Individuals with genetically inherited abnormalities in their LDL receptors have greatly elevated LDL levels as a result of faulty receptor-apoprotein interactions (43). Similarly, genetic problems with apoprotein structure can result in similar elevations of LDL. CH in LDL particles can undergo chemical modification by oxidation and glycation and can then be taken up by macrophage LDL scavenger receptors in an unregulated fashion, potentially resulting in foam cell production and atherogenesis. CH present at higher concentrations also favors formation of β-VLDLs, particles that float at a density of less than 1.006 but have β-electrophoretic mobility. β-VLDLs can arise from chylomicron remnants or can be formed by hepatocytes. These particles interact with LDL receptors on macrophages, depositing large amounts of CE into the macrophage. Substantial increases in CE content convert macrophages to foam cells. LDL receptors on macrophages do not appear to be suppressed as CE concentration increases, unlike those on fibroblasts or smooth muscle.

Formation of HDL also critically depends on apoproteins. Coalescence of PL-apoprotein complexes results in aggregation of Apo-A-I, Apo-A-II, Apo-A-IV, and possibly Apo-E, to form nascent HDL particles. These CH-poor, smaller Apo-A-I–containing forms of HDL are heterogeneous in size and can be classified overall as pre-β or discoidal HDLs. Subsequently, discoidal HDL undergoes changes in size and composition in plasma and extracellular spaces as a result of acquiring free CH from cell membranes of peripheral tissues. HDL binding proteins have been identified on plasma membranes of cells including macrophages, fibroblasts, hepatocytes, and adipocytes. Free CH taken up by HDL undergoes esterification by the enzyme LCAT and moves to the core of the HDL particle. LCAT transfers a sn-2-acyl group of PC or phosphatidylethanolamine (PE) to the free hydroxyl residue of CH. Esterification prevents reentry of CH into peripheral cells. An additional protein contributing to the compositional shifts in HDL is PL transfer protein, which provides PC to HDLs. As HDL becomes enriched with CE, Apo-C-II and C-III are picked up from other proteins to form three spheric categories of HDLs. In order of increasing size and lipid content, these are HDL$_3$, HDL$_{2a}$, and HDL$_{2b}$. Spheric HDLs are likely to go through repeated cycles of increase and decrease in size over their circulatory life span of 2 to 3 days.

Removal of spheric HDL from the circulation and metabolism can proceed via two routes. First, HDL$_2$ can transfer CE to either Apo-B–containing lipoproteins or directly to cells. Movement of CH from HDL$_2$ occurs through CE transfer protein (CETP), which mediates the transfer of CE from HDL$_2$ to VLDLs and chylomicrons in exchange for TGs. Apo-B–containing particles subsequently transport CE to liver. CETP is produced in liver and associates with HDL. As a result of CETP, HDL_2 reconverts to the HDL_3 form. Other apoproteins on HDL that play a role in reverse CH transport and can activate LCAT, include Apo-A-IV, Apo-C-1, and Apo-E. Second, entire particles of HDL_2 can be taken up by LDL receptors and possibly by a separate Apo-E receptor present on hepatocytes.

Actions of HDL other than reverse CH transport may include protection of lipoproteins from oxidative modification, direct removal of CH from atherosclerotic lesions, and a role in the metabolism of eicosanoids (40). Investigators have demonstrated that HDL can inhibit oxidative modification of LDL in vitro and may contribute to the antiatherogenic potential of HDL in vivo (44).

Plasma albumin may also be important in the process of reverse CH transport. Through passive diffusion, albumin picks up CH from peripheral cells and passes it to lipoproteins including HDLs and LDLs. A large proportion of CH efflux has been shown to persist in the absence of Apo-A-I, a finding suggesting mainly albumin-dependent shuttling (45).

Dietary Factors Influencing Plasma Lipoproteins

Dietary factors profoundly influence lipoprotein levels and metabolism, which, in turn, alter an individual's susceptibility to atherosclerosis. Several major dietary impactors have been identified including dietary fat, CH, fiber, protein, alcohol consumption, and energy balance. Classic clinical studies originally revealed that consumption of saturated fats produced an elevation in circulating total and LDL CH levels (46). Plasma CH-raising effects of SAFAs, particularly myristic (C14:0) and C16:0 acids, have been well established. Newer technologies that reduce saturated fat content in dairy products result in lower plasma CH levels when people consume these products (47). The CH-raising effect is believed to result from a shift of the regulatory pool of liver CH from CE to free CH under dietary conditions in which hepatocytes become enriched with C14:0 and C16:0 acids. Higher levels of free CH in the liver suppress LDL receptor activity and drive up circulatory levels. Postmeal accumulation of VLDLs is more prolonged in persons consuming diets rich in SAFAs versus diets containing n-6 PUFAs (48).

Conversely, metabolic studies showed that consumption of n-6 PUFA lowers circulatory CH values, although epidemiologic data failed to demonstrate any direct protective effect of dietary PUFAs on coronary heart disease risk. Consumption of n-3 PUFAs is more strongly inversely correlated with the incidence of heart disease. Whether this action results from lipid lowering or from changing eicosanoid-related thrombosis susceptibility has not been firmly established. n-3 PUFAs, which lower circulating TG levels, have only a minor impact on human lipoprotein CH levels. The role of n-3 FAs in reducing heart disease risk through their antiarrythmic action is becoming increasingly recognized (49).

Consumption of monounsaturated fats also results in lower CH levels, although to no greater extent than n-6 PUFA. Consumption of *trans* FAs has also been shown to raise LDL and lower HDL levels in a dose-dependent fashion. Investigators have suggested that dietary *trans* fat consumption may increase CETP activity, thus explaining the higher circulatory LDL levels associated with *trans* fat consumption (50). The role of dietary CH in hyperlipidemia has engendered considerable debate. Within the range of CH intakes normally consumed, changing dietary CH content seems to produce little alteration in circulating CH levels or subsequent metabolism (51). Certain persons demonstrate a hypersensitivity to dietary CH that may result in a misleading perception of the response to dietary CH within an overall population.

Dietary fiber is an additional factor influencing CH levels (see also Chapter 4). In general, insoluble fibers such as cellulose, hemicellulose, and lignin from grain and vegetables have limited effects on CH levels; whereas more soluble forms such as gums and pectins found in legumes and fruit possess greater CH-lowering properties. Fiber exhibits CH-lowering action by at least three mechanisms other than simple replacement of hypercholesterolemic dietary ingredients. First, fiber may act as a bile acid sequestering agent. Second, fiber likely reduces the rate of insulin rise by slowing carbohydrate absorption, thus slowing CH synthesis. Third, fiber may produce SCFAs, which are absorbed by the portal circulation and inhibit CH synthesis.

Qualitative protein intake is an additional factor that may influence circulating CH levels because consumption of animal versus plant protein increases circulating CH levels. Alcohol intake exists as another, albeit controversial, dietary factor associated with heart disease risk. The relationship between alcohol consumption and CH levels is "J" shaped. At lower levels of intake, wine and spirits, but not beer, produce a more favorable lipid profile, lowering LDL and raising HDL CH values. Further, consumption of excess calories resulting in obesity is associated with higher circulating CH levels. Studies have shown that both CH and TG levels fall during weight loss (52). The distribution of excess weight appears to have a stronger association with circulating lipid level than the amount of weight (53). In summary, these dietary factors suggest that substitution of energy-dense and saturated fat–rich, animal-based foods by those obtained from plant sources is warranted to maintain a desirable profile of circulating lipids.

OXIDATION AND CONVERSION OF LIPIDS TO OTHER METABOLITES

Fatty Acid Oxidation

In an individual of stable weight, the amount of fat consumed equals that quantity partitioned to meet energy needs. FAs represent the most efficient energy source compared with other macronutrients because of their high content in bonds between carbon and hydrogen. Such bonds are stronger, and therefore contain more oxidizable energy, compared with those between carbon and other atoms, as found in carbohydrates, protein, and alcohol. FAs used for energy go through stages including transport to oxidative tissues, transcellular uptake, mitochondrial transfer, and subsequent β-oxidation.

FA partitioned for oxidation undergoes activation to fatty acyl-CoA. Fatty acyl-CoA is then taken up by mitochondria to be oxidized. However, LCFAs and their CoA derivatives cannot cross the mitochondrial membrane without carnitine, synthesized in humans from lysine and methionine. Using transferase enzymes, activated FAs bind covalently to carnitine. After intramitochondrial transmission, FAs are reactivated with CoA, whereas carnitine recycles to the cytoplasmic surface.

Mitochondrial β-oxidation of FAs entails the consecutive release of two-carbon acetyl-CoA units from the carboxyl terminus of the acyl chain. Before release of each unit, the β-carbon atoms of the acyl chain undergo cyclic degradation through four stages: dehydrogenation (removal of hydrogen), hydration (addition of water), dehydrogenation (removal of hydrogens), and cleavage. Completion through these four reactions represents one cycle of β-oxidation. For unsaturated bonds within FAs, the initial dehydrogenation reaction is omitted. The entire cycle is repeated until the fatty acyl chain is completely degraded. Absence in cellular or subcellular compartments of chain-shortened n-6 or n-3 FAs indicates that once an FA commences cyclic degradation by β-oxidation, the process continues until the acyl chain is completely broken down. (See Chapter 59 for a review of inherited effects of β-oxidation on lipid metabolism.)

Peroxisomal FA β-oxidation is similar to mitochondrial oxidation, yet several differences exist between these two organelles. First, very long acyl-CoA synthetase, the enzyme responsible for the activation of VLCFAs, is present in peroxisomes and endoplasmic reticulum but not in mitochondria, a finding likely explaining why VLCFAs are oxidized predominantly in peroxisomes. Second, the initial reaction in peroxisomal β-oxidation (desaturation of acyl-CoA) is catalyzed by a flavin adenine dinucleotide–containing fatty acyl-CoA oxidase, presumed to be the rate-limiting enzyme, whereas an acyl-CoA dehydrogenase is the first enzyme in the mitochondrial pathway. Third, peroxisomal β-oxidation is not directly coupled to the electron transfer chain that conserves energy by means of oxidative phosphorylation. In peroxisomes, electrons generated in the first oxidation step are transferred directly to molecular oxygen yielding hydrogen peroxide that is disposed of by catalase, whereas energy produced in the second oxidation step (nicotinamide adenine dinucleotide [NAD^+] reduction) is conserved in the form of high-energy-level electrons of reduced NAD (NADH). Fourth, the second (hydration) and third (NAD^+-dependent dehydrogenation) steps are catalyzed by a multifunctional protein that also displays Δ^3, Δ^2-enoyl CoA isomerase activity required for oxidation of unsaturated FAs.

Dietary Modulation of Fatty Acid Oxidation

Considerable interest has surrounded structure-dependent induction of FA oxidation. Thus, food selection may influence the partitioning of dietary fat for oxidation versus retention for storage and structural use in humans. This issue is of health interest for at least two reasons. First, consumption of fats associated with greater retention may result in an increased tendency toward obesity. Second, the greater accumulation of less preferentially oxidized FAs in cells may confer structural or functional changes resulting from shifts in membrane PL FA patterns or in prostaglandin (PG)/ TXA ratios. The influence of tissue FA composition on functional ability such as insulin sensitivity is well recognized (54).

Discriminative oxidation of certain FAs has been well defined; for others, it has been suggested. Clinically, short- and medium-chain TG consumption is associated with increased energy production, possibly owing to direct portal transfer of SCFAs MCFAs from gut to liver. The lack of requirement for carnitine in mitochondrial membrane transit by SCFAs may also be responsible for their more rapid oxidation. For LCFAs, increasing evidence suggests that n-6 and n-3 PUFAs are more rapidly oxidized for energy compared with SAFAs. In animals, labeled PUFAs are more readily converted to carbon dioxide than SAFAs (55), whereas PUFA consumption exhibits greater thermogenic effect (56), oxygen consumption (57), and sympathetic nervous system stimulation (58). Whole-body FA balance data also support the concept that C18:2n-6 is more readily used for energy than are SAFAs (59). Although these findings have yet to be confirmed in humans, consumption of fats containing PUFAs appear to enhance the contribution of dietary fat to total energy production in healthy persons (60) and influence the utilization of other FAs for energy (61); however, mechanisms remain to be defined. Portal venous transfer rates, release rates of FAs from adipose tissue, hepatic FA oxidation enzyme activities, and mitochondrial entry rates of FAs generally increase with the degree of acyl chain unsaturation.

Peroxidative Modification of Lipids

Lipids are oxidized by reactive oxygen species produced as byproducts of normal metabolism. Reactive oxygen species include superoxide (O_2), hydroxyl radical ($\cdot OH$), hydrogen peroxide, singlet oxygen ($^1O_2$), and hypochlorous acid ($HOCl^-$). In healthy individuals, the generation of reactive oxygen species should be in balance with antioxidant defenses. Circumstances that enhance oxidant exposure, such as increased formation of reactive oxygen species caused by chemicals and drugs, or compromised antioxidant capability, such as decreased antioxidant vitamin levels via malnutrition, are referred to as oxidative stress. Possible free radical effects on cells include oxidative damage to proteins, carbohydrates, and DNA. Oxidative stress has also long been known to be capable of inducing lipid oxidation and, in the presence of oxygen, lipid peroxidation of cell membranes.

It is generally accepted that the process of lipid oxidation proceeds by way of a free radical mechanism called autoxidation, which includes initiation, propagation, and termination stages and predominantly occurs with PUFAs. Polyunsaturated acyl chains of membrane PLs are particularly sensitive to lipid peroxidation. Lipid oxidation is self-propagating in cellular membranes, catalyzed by both nonenzymatic and enzymatic mechanisms. The peroxidation of PUFAs is classically depicted as a series of three or four basic reactions; however, the process becomes more complex as both the degree of unsaturation and the severity of peroxidative conditions increase. The following initiation, propagation, and termination reactions characterize the general schema of autoxidation:

(1) Initiation: $X\cdot + LH \rightarrow L\cdot + XH$

(2) Propagation: $L\cdot + O_2 \rightarrow LOO\cdot$

(3) $LOO\cdot + LH \rightarrow L\cdot + LOOH$

(4) Termination: $LO\cdot + LO\cdot \rightarrow$ nonradical polymers

(5) $LOO\cdot + LOO\cdot \rightarrow$ nonradical polymers

(6) $L\cdot + L\cdot \rightarrow$ nonradical polymers

(7) $LOO\cdot + L\cdot \rightarrow$ nonradical polymers

The initiation of a peroxidation sequence in a membrane or PUFA results from the attack of any free radical that has sufficient reactivity to abstract a hydrogen atom from an allelic methylene group of an unsaturated FA, including the $HO\cdot$ and $HO_2\cdot$ radicals. The initiating free radical ($X\cdot$) abstracts a hydrogen atom from the carbon chain generating a lipid carbon-centered radical ($L\cdot$, reaction 1). This carbon-centered lipid radical tends to be stabilized by a molecular rearrangement to produce a conjugated diene, which then readily reacts with molecular oxygen to yield a hydroperoxyl radical ($LOO\cdot$, reaction 2). The peroxyl radical can propagate the oxidizing chain reaction by abstracting electrons from other susceptible PUFAs, forming another lipid free radical and a molecule of lipid hydroperoxide ($LOOH$) (reaction 3). The overall chain reaction has a pyramidal effect through which relatively few initiating radicals break down PUFAs. These reactions continue until the chain is terminated, either by the combination of two radicals to form a nonradical product (reactions 4–7) or by termination of the propagation reaction in the presence of a hydrogen or an electron donor. Termination may also occur as the result of hydrogen abstraction from vitamin E (α-tocopherol) or another lipid antioxidant to form hydroperoxides. Vitamin E is termed a chain-breaking antioxidant because it donates a hydrogen atom to lipid radicals, thereby terminating the propagative process

and lipid peroxidation. Lipid peroxidation can also be inhibited by a reduction of lipid hydroperoxides by selenoperoxidases, such as glutathione peroxidase, to their corresponding alcohols.

Lipid peroxides are rapidly decomposed in vivo by metal ions and their complexes. The alkoxyl or peroxyl radical byproducts of lipid hydroperoxide breakdown are capable of propagating the chain reaction of lipid peroxidation (62). Although lipid peroxides are highly toxic, they are poorly absorbed in vivo. The toxicity of peroxides has in part been attributed to their capability to oxidize the thiol groups of proteins, glutathione, and other sulfhydryl compounds and to form insoluble deposits called lipofuscin in the artery wall or neural tissue (62).

The end products of lipid peroxidation include aldehydes and hydrocarbon gases. Short-chain aldehydes can attack amino groups on protein molecules to form crosslinks between different protein molecules. The most commonly measured product is malondialdehyde (MDA), known to react with proteins and amino acids (Fig. 5.5). Several studies have shown a positive relationship between in vivo lipid peroxidation and urinary excretion of MDA. MDA adduct formation with proteins, PLs, and nucleic acids may be a cause of disease because the presence of MDA adducts with serine, lysine, ethanolamine, and guanidine has been detected in urine (63).

Isoprostanes are a family of eicosanoids produced nonenzymatically by random oxidation of PLs by oxygen free radicals. They are normally present in the plasma and urine, and human urinary concentrations are an order of magnitude higher than those of many enzymatically derived eicosanoids (64). $F_{(2)}$-isoprostanes are $PGF_{(2\alpha)}$ isomers

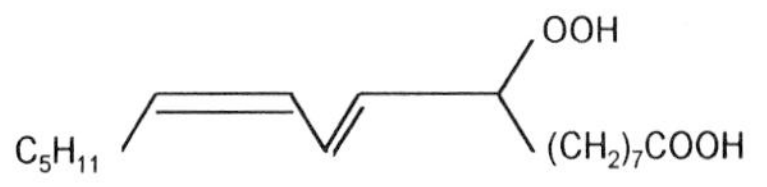

9-HYDROPEROXY-10-TRANS, 12-CIS-OCTADECADIENOIC ACID (LINOLEIC ACID-9-HYDROPEROXIDE)

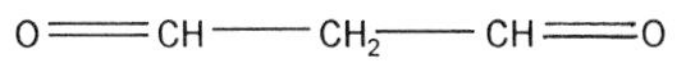

MALONDIALDEHYDE

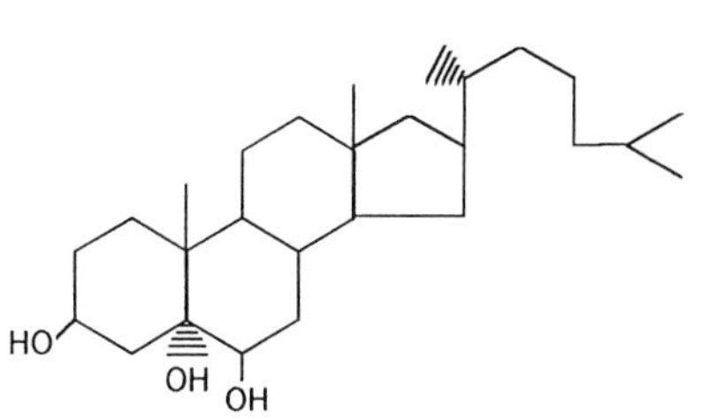

CHOLESTANE-3β, 5α, 6β-TRIOL (CHOLESTANETRIOL)

Figure 5.5. Three oxidation products associated with toxicity.

derived from arachidonic acid. These compounds have been demonstrated to have biologic activity including acting as potent pulmonary and renal vasoconstrictors (65). Levels of one of the isoprostanes, 8-isoprostane (8-iso PGF$_{2\alpha}$), are elevated with oxidative stress, and this has been suggested to act as a mediatory factor in a variety of disease states linked to oxidative stress (66). Isoprostanes may also appear as artifacts in tissue samples that have undergone oxidative degradation during prolonged or improper storage, and 8-isoprostane levels have been used to determine sample integrity for lipid-containing tissue samples.

Lipid peroxidation has been implicated in the pathogenesis of diseases including cancer and atherosclerosis. Although products of lipid peroxidation are readily measurable in blood, the significance and occurrence of lipid peroxidation are controversial. A major criticism has been that lipid peroxidation may not be initially involved in causing the underlying pathologic features because lipid peroxidation byproducts could be produced in excess as a consequence of the primary disease process. In addition, many methods of analysis produce some disruption of cell structure. Such disruption could produce misleading findings, because lipid peroxidation may accompany tissue damage; however, some studies have dissociated lipid peroxidation from in vitro cell death (67).

The PL components of cellular membranes are highly vulnerable to oxidative damage as a result of the susceptibility of their PUFA side chains to peroxidation. Membrane lipid peroxidation results in loss of PUFAs, decreased membrane fluidity, and increased permeability of the membrane to substances such as calcium ions. Lipid peroxidation can lead to loss of enzyme and receptor activity and can have deleterious effects on membrane secretory functions. Continued lipid peroxidation can lead to complete loss of membrane integrity, as can be observed from the hemolysis associated with lipid peroxidation of erythrocyte membranes.

Many different dietary components have been reported to influence membrane susceptibility to oxidative damage. Cellular lipid peroxidation strongly depends on PUFA intake, as well as on intake of vitamin E and other lipid antioxidants (see also Chapters 21 and 44). In isolated human erythrocytes, the production of lipid peroxidation products following hydrogen peroxide–induced oxidative stress has been measured as thiobarbituric acid reactive substances (TBARSs). Multivariate analysis has shown that the unsaturation index was the best predictor of erythrocyte-TBARS variability (68). A relatively stable C18:2n-6/vitamin E ratio in vegetable oils provides protection from risk of excessive lipid peroxidation and vitamin E deficiency at high PUFA intakes. Fish oils are an exception to the observation of a natural association between PUFA and vitamin E in edible fats and oils and the stability of PUFA to oxidation in the diet and body. The highly unsaturated n-3 pentaenoic and hexaenoic FAs, found in high concentrations in fish and marine oils with relatively low vitamin E

contents, markedly increase the in vivo susceptibility of these oils to peroxidation (69). TBARSs increased with higher concentrations of total n-3 PUFAs in isolated human erythocytes, whereas TBARSs decreased with higher concentrations of total MUFAs (68).

Numerous studies have suggested that oxidized lipids may exert atherogenic effects (70). Oxidized free FAs affect cell proliferation and survival, cell signaling, and chemotaxis, which have been indicated to be important mediators of atherogenesis. Oxidized PLs that contain oxidized FAs have also been shown to exert adverse effects on vascular cells (71). Cells are exposed regularly to oxidized FAs through endogenous metabolism via products produced by lipoxygenase and cyclooxygenase action as well as via absorption of end products of lipolysis of dietary oxidized lipids. Dietary oxidized lipids may contribute to the atherogenicity of lipoproteins by increasing oxidative stress and oxidized LDLs in the plasma and arterial walls (70). The typical Western diet contains large quantities of PUFAs that are exposed to heating or processing, thus generating oxidized FAs (71, 72). Oxidized FAs, such as 13-hydroxylinoleic acid, share structural similarities with the monohydroxy bile acid, lithocholic acid, which is required for intestinal absorption of CH. Such dietary oxidized FAs may thus act as BS enhancers to increase the solubilization and absorption of dietary CH, thereby leading to higher plasma CH concentrations (70).

The effects of oxygen free radicals on membrane CH may be as important as the effects observed on membrane PLs, because oxidized CH derivatives, the oxysterols or CH oxides, have been suggested to play a key role in the development of atherosclerosis (73). This concept has been fostered by increasing evidence of the role of oxidatively modified lipoproteins in atherogenesis. CH readily undergoes oxidation (74), and the metabolites derived display a wide variety of actions on cellular metabolism including angiotoxic, mutagenic, and carcinogenic effects (73). Common CH oxidation products include CH-5α, 6α-epoxide, CH-5β,6β-epoxide, and cholestane-3β,5α,6β triol (see Fig. 5.5). CH oxides disturb endothelial integrity by perturbing vascular permeability, whereas purified CH has no effect. CH oxidation products have been detected in human serum lipoproteins and human atheromatous plaques (75). Substantial amounts of oxidized CH are detected in a variety of foods of animal origin exposed to oxidizing conditions (74). These highly atherogenic oxysterols may also be ingested and absorbed from processed foods or generated by free radical oxidation of lipoproteins. To date, however, it is unclear whether CH oxides merely serve as markers for oxidatively modified lipoproteins or whether they contribute to the toxicity of oxidized lipoproteins. In addition, analysis of oxysterols is beset by difficulties that include artifact generation and decomposition of oxysterols during sample manipulation (74).

LDL oxidation has been implicated as a causal factor in the development of human atherosclerosis (76). Unsaturated lipids in LDL are subject to peroxidative degradation, and the susceptibility of LDL to oxidation has been correlated to the degree of coronary atherosclerosis (77). Autoantibodies exist in human serum, and oxidized LDL is present in atherosclerotic plaque, findings indicating that oxidized LDL exists in vivo (78). Possible sources of oxidation include endothelial cells, smooth muscle cells, monocytes and macrophages, and other inflammatory cells. In the presence of the promoter copper, peroxidation of LDL results in the formation of hydroxyalkenals and MDAs that modify Apo-B by reacting with its amino lysine groups. This modification of Apo-B could, in turn, impair its uptake by the LDL receptor. Oxidatively modified LDL may exert atherogenic effects via its cytotoxic and chemotactic properties and the promotion of LDL uptake via the scavenger receptors on macrophages, leading to the formation of lipid-enriched foam cells.

Nutritional and biochemical studies suggest that diet can modulate the susceptibility of plasma LDLs to oxidative degradation by altering the concentration of PUFAs and antioxidants in the lipoprotein particle. The first target of peroxidation in the oxidation of LDLs consists of PUFAs of PLs on the LDL surface. In studies of LDLs isolated from healthy persons and animals, a diet rich in C18:2n-6 increased the susceptibility of plasma LDL to copper-induced oxidation and to in vitro macrophage uptake, as compared with a diet high in C18:1n-9 (79). C18:1n-9 and other MUFAs do not contain the easily oxidized conjugated double bonds found in PUFAs. In addition, C18:1n-9 has a high affinity for transition metals, making them unavailable for LDL peroxidation. Studies have shown consistently that MUFA-rich diets induce an increased resistance of LDLs to oxidative modification (80). Depending on the dose used, subjects treated with n-3 PUFAs showed either an increase or no change in LDL oxidation (81).

Other studies have shown that increasing the amount of vitamin E in the LDL particle via oral supplementation will decrease LDL susceptibility to in vitro oxidative damage (82, 83). A difficulty with in vitro assays of plasma lipoprotein oxidation is that these assays are subject to influences by a variety of plasma substrates and conditions, making their relevance to physiologic situations uncertain. The lower incidence of cardiovascular disease associated with populations consuming more olive oil may be partly the result of an inhibition of LDL oxidation by the antioxidant action of olive oil, as well as by those antioxidants found in fruits and vegetables.

INTRACELLULAR MOVEMENT AND BIOSYNTHESIS OF LIPIDS

Fatty Acids

The biosynthesis of SAFAs occurs in the extramitochondrial compartment by a group of enzymes known as FA synthetases. Compared with many animal species, human FA synthesis occurs predominantly in the liver and is much less active in adipose tissue. The FA biosynthetic pathway is almost identical in all organisms examined to date. The starting point is acetyl-CoA. Acetyl-CoA and oxaloacetate are cleaved from citrate that is transported from the mitochondria. The first reaction in the FA biosynthetic pathway proper is the conversion of acetyl-CoA to malonyl-CoA. This reaction is catalyzed by acetyl-CoA carboxylase, which is rate limiting for FA synthesis. Acetyl-CoA then combines sequentially with a series of malonyl-CoA molecules as follows:

$$\text{Acetyl-CoA} + 7 \text{ malonyl-CoA} + 14 \text{ NADPH} + 14\text{H}+$$

$$\rightarrow \text{C16:0 (palmitic acid)} + 7 \text{ CO}_2 + 8 \text{ CoASH} + 14 \text{ NADP} + +6 \text{ H}_2\text{0}$$

In mammals, complete de novo synthesis results in C16:0. Other FAs can be formed from C16:0 by chain elongation via microsomal malonyl-CoA–dependent elongase. Mammals possess a series of desaturases and elongases to generate long-chain PUFAs from the metabolism of C16:0, C18:0, C18:2n-6, and C18:3n-3 (Fig. 5.6). These reactions take place predominantly in the endoplasmic reticulum membranes. Desaturase reactions are catalyzed by membrane-bound desaturases with broad chain-length specificity that includes Δ^9, Δ^6, Δ^5, and Δ^4 fatty acyl-CoA desaturases. These are involved in the desaturation of the C16:1n-7, C18:1n-9, C18:2n-6, and C18:3n-3 families. The Δ^4 desaturation required for the formation of C22:6n-3 from C22:5n-3, and C22:5n-6 from C22:4n-6, respectively, has been shown to involve three steps. These steps require an elongation reaction followed by membrane (microsomal) desaturation and shortening in peroxisomes (84). The desaturase enzymes are highly specific for the position of the double bond. The FA desaturase system involves three integral components, namely, the desaturase, NADH-cytochrome b_5 reductase, and cytochrome b_5, which are constituents of microsomal membranes. Desaturases require electrons supplied mostly by NADH-cytochrome b_5 reductase, in addition to the activated substrate in the form of acyl-CoA.

Precursors for the n-7 and n-9 families of PUFAs are MUFAs that are synthesized via microsomal Δ^9 oxidative desaturation of C16:0 and C18:0 to form C16:1n-7 and C18:1n-9, respectively (see Fig. 5.6). Additional double bonds can be further introduced into existing MUFAs C16:1n-7 and C18:1n-9 and also into C18:2n-6 via Δ^6 desaturase (see Fig. 5.6). Until recently, humans and other mammals were thought incapable of synthesizing long-chain n-3 (C18:3n-3) and n-6 (C18:2n-6) EFAs. More recent studies, however, suggest that C18:2n-6 and C18:3n-3 can be synthesized in humans and other mammals via elongation of the dietary precursors C16:2n-6 and C16:3n-3, respectively (85). Edible green plants can contain amounts of up to 14% of C16:2n-6 and C16:3n-3 (85). In a practical sense, a dietary supply of EFAs is still important because humans likely do not obtain sufficient quantities of 16-carbon precursors.

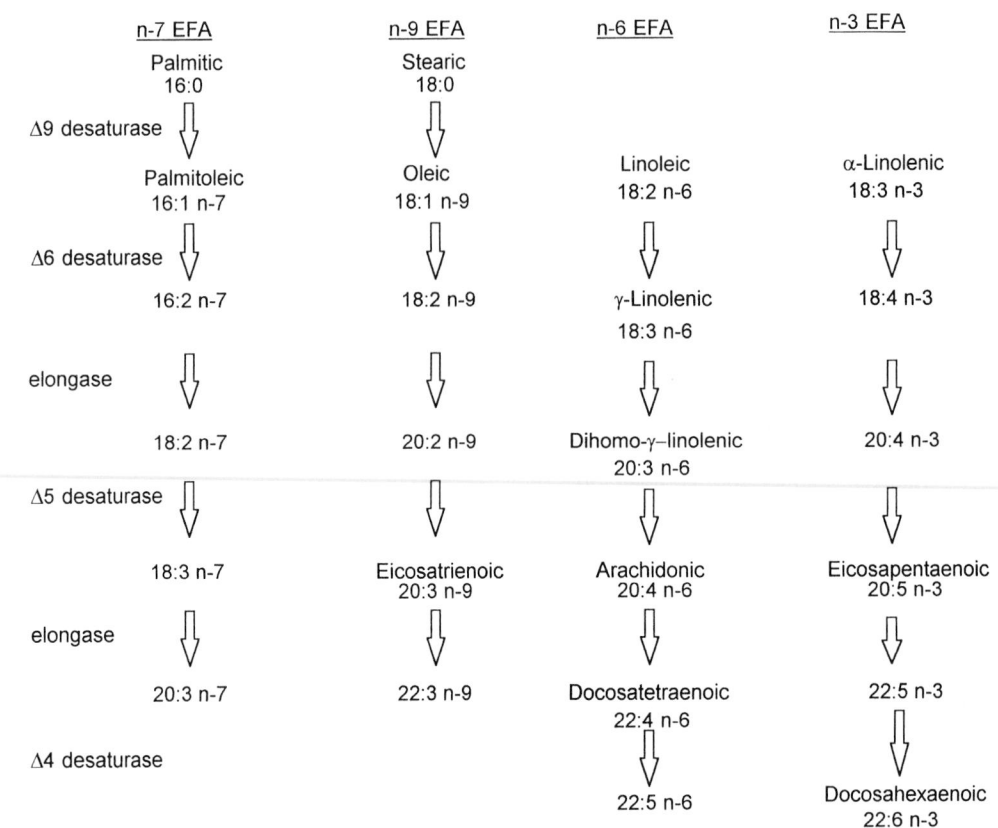

Figure 5.6. Effects of desaturase and elongase on essential fatty acids.

In the mammalian organism, the FAs from the n-3 and n-6 FAs cannot be interconverted because of a lack of Δ^{12} or Δ^{15} desaturase enzymes, although such interconversions can take place in plants. Δ^{6} Desaturase is the regulatory enzyme in these reactions and requires the presence of an n-9 *cis* double bond. Hence, *trans* FA such as C18:1n-9 *trans*, formed either by rumen bacteria or by chemical hydrogenation of FA with *cis* double bonds, cannot be desaturated by this enzyme. The n-3, n-6, and n-9 FA families compete with each other, especially at the rate-limiting Δ^{6} desaturase step. In general, the desaturase enzymes display the highest affinity for the utmost unsaturated substrate. The order of preference is: α-linolenic family (n-3) > linoleic family (n-6) > oleic acid family (n-9) > palmitoleic acid family (n-7) > elaidic acid family (n-9, *trans*). Competition also exists among the families of PUFAs for the elongase enzymes and for the acyl transferases involved in the formation of PLs.

Because of the competitive nature of FA desaturation and elongation, each class of EFA can interfere with the metabolism of the other. This competition has nutritional implications. An excess of n-6 EFA will reduce the metabolism of C18:3n-3, possibly leading to a deficit of its metabolites including eicosapentaenoic acid (EPA) (C20:5n-3). This is a matter of concern in relation to infant formulas, which may contain an excess of C18:2n-6 and no balancing of n-3 EFAs. Conversely, because long-chain n-3 EFAs

markedly decrease Δ^{6} desaturation of C18:2n-6, an excessive intake of fish oils could lead to an impairment of C18:2n-6 metabolism and a deficit of n-6 EFA derivatives. High doses of fish oil in humans can cause a large reduction in the levels of C20:3n-6 in plasma PLs with a smaller effect on C20:4n-6 content (86). Although C18:1n-9 can inhibit Δ^{6} desaturase activity, high dietary intakes are necessary. In the presence of C18:2n-6 or C18:3n-3, little desaturation of C18:1n-9 occurs. During EFAD, C20:3n-9 is synthesized from C18:1n-9 because of the nearly complete absence of competitive effects of n-3 and n-6 EFAs. The presence of C20:3n-9 in tissues instead of C20:4n-6, C20:5n-3, and C22:6n-3 is an indicator of EFAD, which reverses on EFA feeding (87). In the catalytic hydrogenation process of vegetable oils and fish oils for the production of some margarines and shortenings, various geometric and positional isomers of unsaturated FA are formed in varying amounts. After absorption, these isomers may compete with the EFAs and endogenously synthesized FAs for desaturation and chain elongation.

In a phenomenon called *retroversion*, very-long-chain C22 PUFAs, present in marine oils, may be shortened by two carbons with concomitant saturation of a double bond. For example, C22:6n-3 is converted to C22:5n-3 and to C20:5n-3 (88). This peroxisomal pathway is also active in converting C22:5n-6 to C20:4n-6 (89). As a result of competition among various PUFA families for desaturases, elongases, and acyl transferases, and owing to retroversion, a characteristic pattern of end products accumulates in tissue lipids for each family. Hence, the major PUFA product for the palmitoleate n-7 family is C20:3n-7, the oleate n-9 is C20:3n-9, linoleate is C20:4n-6 and some C20:3n-6. The most common products for the n-3 FA family are C20:5n-3 and C22:6n-3.

The efficiency of the multistage synthesis of human PUFAs is unclear. Stable isotope studies have indicated that in healthy subjects the conversion of dietary C18:3n-3 to C20:5n-3 appears to be limited, and the conversion to C22:6n-3 is minor (90, 91). Whole-body conversion of 18:3n-3 to 22:6n-3 in humans has generally been shown to be less than 5% and appears to depend on dietary concentration of n-6 FAs and long = chain PUFAs (91). Investigators have suggested that activities of the various required desaturase and elongase enzymes differ with developmental stage or pathologic state. The regulation of desaturase activity could be of biologic importance because the higher homologs of EFAs are physiologically important regulatory metabolites.

Dietary factors and hormonal status can influence desaturase activities. Fat-free diets result in an increase in Δ^5 and Δ^6 desaturation, which may reflect a homeostatic response to maintain membrane fluidity (92). Protein and EFAD increase dΔ^6 desaturase activity, whereas, conversely, low-protein diets and alcohol consumption decrease Δ^6 activity. Although glucose refeeding after a fast induces Δ^6 desaturase activity, a glucose-rich diet actually decreases enzymatic activity. Insulin stimulates Δ^6 desaturase activity, whereas activity is depressed by glucagon, epinephrine, glucocorticoids, and thyroxines. Diabetes is also known to depress Δ^6, Δ^5 desaturases, and Δ^4 desaturation activity, which are restored by insulin injection (93). Zinc may also play a role in the regulation of Δ^6 desaturase activity because the dermal and growth effects of both EFAD and zinc deficiency are similar (94). This concept is supported by observations that administration of C18:3n-6, which bypasses the Δ^6 desaturase step, corrects most of the symptoms of zinc deficiency, whereas administration of C18:2n-6 has no effect. Because the typical Western diet contains sufficient C20:4n-6, obtained from meat and dairy products, those with decreased desaturase activity could suffer from a deficiency of C20:3n-6, the precursor of the PG$_1$ series. Some authors have suggested that certain individuals may have an increased need for EFA derivatives as a result of a disease condition, aging, or a metabolic block in desaturase activity. Evening primrose, borage, and black current seed oils contain C18:3n-6 that bypasses the step requiring Δ^6 desaturase and have been used therapeutically for a variety of clinical conditions including psoriasis (95).

Cholesterol

Current evidence indicates that three distinct pathways modulate the intracellular trafficking of CH. Separate translocational systems exist for endogenously synthesized and LDL-derived exogenous CH. A third transport system also exists for CH destined for steroid synthesis.

CH biosynthesis represents a major vector in the total body CH supply in humans, with up to 60 to 80% being synthesized during consumption of the typical North American diet. Animal studies demonstrate that even though all organs incorporate acetate into sterol, the liver is the primary biosynthetic organ (96). Conversely, investigators have estimated that the net contribution of human liver biosynthesis does not exceed 10% of total CH biosynthesis. The role of extrahepatic organs in human cholesterogenesis remains undefined, but the level of production of CH by extrahepatic tissues is considered substantial.

Acetate can be converted into mevalonic acid by a sequence of reactions starting with acetate + CoA + ATP $\rightarrow$ acetyl-CoA + pyrophosphate (PP) + AMP. However, most of the acetyl-CoA used for sterol synthesis is not derived from this reaction, but rather is generated within the mitochondria by the β-oxidation of FAs or the oxidative decarboxylation of pyruvate. Pyruvate is converted into citrate, which diffuses into the cytosol and is hydrolyzed to acetyl-CoA and oxaloacetate by citrate-ATP lyase:

$$\text{Citrate} + \text{ATP} + \text{CoA} \rightarrow \text{acetyl-CoA} + \text{oxaloacetate} + \text{adenosine diphosphate (ADP)} + \text{H}_2\text{O}$$

Citrate participating in this reaction acts as a carrier to transport acetyl carbon across the mitochondrial membranes, which are impermeable to acetyl-CoA. Subsequently, in the cytosol, acetyl-CoA is converted into mevalonate:

$$2\ \text{acetyl-CoA} \rightarrow \text{acetoacetyl-CoA} + \text{CoA}$$

$$\text{Acetoacetyl-CoA} + \text{acetyl-CoA} + \text{H}_2\text{O} \rightarrow \text{hydroxymethylglutaryl (HMG)-CoA} + \text{CoA}$$

$$\text{HMG-CoA} + 2\ \text{NADPH} + 2\ \text{H}^+ \rightarrow \text{mevalonate} + 2\ \text{NADP}^+ + \text{CoA}$$

Mevalonic acid is phosphorylated, isomerized, and converted to geranyl- and farnesyl-pyrophosphate, which, in turn, forms squalene. Squalene is then oxidized and cyclized to a steroid ring, lanosterol. In the last steps, lanosterol is converted into CH by the loss of three methyl groups, saturation of the side chain, and a shift of the double bond from Δ^8 to Δ^5. During the later stages of CH biosynthesis, intermediates are bound to a sterol carrier protein.

CH biosynthesis in humans is sensitive to numerous dietary factors. Adding CH to the diet at physiologic levels results in modest increases in circulating CH levels, with a mild reciprocal inhibition of synthesis (28, 51) (see also Chapter 6). Dietary fat selection exhibits a more pronounced influence on human cholesterogenesis because consumption of polyunsaturated fats is associated with enhanced biosynthesis compared with other plant or animal fats. Both differences in FA composition and levels of plant sterol levels may be contributing factors (35). Higher meal frequency has been shown to reduce human biosynthesis rates, and this finding may explain the lower circulating CH synthesis rates seen with consumption of more numerous smaller meals (97). Insulin, which is associated with hepatic CH synthesis in animals, may be released in greater amounts when less frequent but larger meals are consumed. Circadian periodicity occurs, peaking at night, and is tied to the timing of meal consumption. In considering dietary factors capable of modifying CH synthesis, energy restriction exhibits the greatest effect. Persons who fast for 24 hours exhibit complete cessation of CH biosynthesis (18). Exactly how synthesis responds to more minor energy imbalance has not been examined.

An emerging view is that CH synthesis acts both passively and actively in relation to circulatory CH levels, depending on dietary perturbation. Passively, the liver responds to high CH levels through LDL receptor–mediated suppression of synthesis (43). The modest suppression in the presence of increasing dietary and circulating levels reflects the limited hepatic contribution to total body production of CH (28). Substitution of PUFAs in place of other fats results in a decrease in the ratio of hepatic intracellular free to esterified CH, which, in turn, upregulates both LDL receptor number and cholesterogenesis. In both ways, CH synthesis responds passively to external stimuli. In contrast, nonhepatic synthesis is less sensitive to dietary CH level and fat type, whereas hepatic synthesis is more responsive to synthesis pathway substrate availability (98). In this manner, several dietary factors actively modify CH synthesis and levels. Such differential sensitivity may explain the more pronounced decrement in CH synthesis and levels occurring after energy deficit in humans.

CH serves as a required precursor for other important steroid compounds including sex hormones, adrenocorticoid hormones, and vitamin D. Steroidal sex hormones, including estrogen, androgen, and progesterone, involve removal of the CH side chain at C-17 and rearrangement of the double bonds in the steroid nucleus. Corticosteroid hormone production involves similar rearrangements of the CH molecule. 7-Dehydrocholesterol is the precursor of cholecalciferol (vitamin D) formed at the skin surface through the action of ultraviolet irradiation (see Chapter 20). Steroid hormone metabolites are excreted principally through the urine. It is estimated that in humans, approximately 50 mg/day of CH is converted to steroid hormones.

Vertebrates are incapable of converting plant sterols to CH. However, insects and prawns have been shown capable of transforming phytosterols into steroid hormones or bile acids through a CH intermediate.

FUNCTIONS OF ESSENTIAL FATTY ACIDS

After ingestion, EFAs (C18:2n-6 and C18:3n-3) are distributed among adipose TGs, other tissue stores, and tissue structural lipids. A proportion of C18:2n-6 and C18:3n-3

contributes to provide energy, with these PUFAs apparently oxidized more rapidly than SAFAs or MUFAs. In contrast, long-chain PUFAs derived from EFAs (i.e., C20:3n-6, C20:4n-6, C20:5n-3, and C22:6n-3) are less readily oxidized. These acids, when present preformed in the diet, are incorporated into structural lipids about 20 times more efficiently than after synthesis from dietary C18:2n-6 and C18:3n-3. The liver is the site of most of the PUFA metabolism that transforms dietary 18-carbon EFAs into long-chain PUFAs with 20 or 22 carbons. Long-chain PUFAs are transported to extrahepatic tissues for incorporation into cell lipids, even though differential uptake and acylation of PUFAs occur among different tissues. The final tissue composition of long-chain PUFAs is an outcome of the foregoing complex processes along with the influence of dietary factors. The major elements in the diet that determine the final distribution of long-chain PUFAs in cell PLs include the relative proportions of n-3, n-6, and n-9 FA families and the preformed long-chain PUFAs versus their shorter-chain precursors (99).

Membrane structural PLs contain high concentrations of PUFAs and the 20- and 22-carbon PUFAs that predominate from the two families of EFAs. C20:4n-6 is the most important and abundant long-chain PUFA found in membrane PLs; and is the primary precursor of eicosanoids. The concentration of free C20:4n-6 is strictly regulated via phospholipases and acyltransferases. Most nonacylated C20:4n-6 is bound to cytosolic protein. In terms of EFAs from the n-3 PUFA series, C20:5n-3 and C22:6n-3 are most prevalent in membrane PLs. The long-chain PUFAs derived from EFAs are incorporated primarily in the 2-acyl position in bilayer PLs of mammalian plasma, mitochondrial, and nuclear membranes. The 20-carbon FAs, when released from their PLs, can be transformed into intracellular metabolites (i.e., inositol triphosphate, as well as diacylglycerol [DAG]) and extracellular metabolites (i.e., platelet activating factor and eicosanoids), which participate in many important cell-signaling responses. The relative proportions in tissue PL of C20:4n-6 and other long-chain PUFAs (C18:3n-6, C20:4n-6, and C20:5n-3) are important because these PUFAs can compete for or inhibit enzymes involved with the generation of intracellular and extracellular biologically active products. In addition, dietary C18:1n-9, C18:2n-6, C18:2n-6 *trans*, C18:3n-6, C18:3n-3, and long-chain n-3 PUFAs (C20:5n-3 and C22:6n-3) can compete with C20:4n-6 for the acyltransferases for esterification into PL pools and can thereby inhibit C20:4n-6-mediated membrane functions (see Fig. 5.6).

FAs and eicosanoids have been demonstrated to regulate gene transcription through peroxisome proliferator-activated receptors (PPARs), which are nuclear hormone receptors that play an important role in the genetic regulation of FA oxidation and lipogenesis. Chawla and associates (100, 101) reviewed the various families of nuclear receptors with important functions in lipid physiology, including the PPARs, which act as FA sensors. Four PPAR isotypes have been identified: α, β, γ, and, most recently, δ. PPARs are ligand-dependent transcription factors and act such that activation of target gene transcription depends on the binding of the ligand to the receptor. Certain ligands, such as PUFAs and oxidized Fas, are shared by all three isotypes. Several eicosanoids and FAs bind with high affinity to PPAR-α, including long C18:2n-6, conjugated linoleic acid, and eicosanoids such as LTB_4 (102). PPAR-α operates in the catabolism of FAs in the liver because it promotes FA oxidation under conditions of lipid catabolism such as fasting (103). Hepatic oxidation of FAs to acetyl-CoA and subsequent metabolism to ketone bodies are strongly stimulated by PPAR-α, whose expression is elevated with fasting. PPAR-β regulates the expression of acyl-CoA synthetase 2 in brain tissue (103). PPAR-γ promotes lipogenesis in adipose tissue under anabolic conditions, because PPAR-γ target genes in adipose tissue include FA transport protein, acyl-CoA synthase, lipoprotein lipase, and adipocyte FA binding protein (103). PPAR-γ could participate in the development of atherosclerosis by stimulating the cellular uptake of oxidized LDLs. Oxidized FAs entering cells via oxidized LDLs can activate PPAR-γ to stimulate cellular uptake of oxidized LDLs further (103). PPAR-δ has been characterized as a mediator of lipoprotein signaling in macrophages (101).

Membrane Functions and Integrity

Because fragile membranes in erythrocytes and mitochondria are typical of EFAD, an early function attributed to EFAs was their role as integral components of PLs required for plasma and intracellular membrane integrity. EFAD results in a progressive decrease of C20:4n-6 in membrane PLs, with a concomitant increase in C18:1n-9 and its product, C20:3n-9. The fluidity and other physical properties of membrane PLs are largely determined by the chain length and degree of unsaturation of their component FAs. These physical properties, in turn, affect the ability of PLs to perform structural functions such as the maintenance of normal activities of membrane-bound enzymes. Dietary SAFAs, MUFAs, and PUFAs, the major determinants of the composition of stored and structural lipids, have been shown to alter the activity and affinity of receptors, membrane permeability, and transport properties (104).

The heterogeneity and selectivity of PUFAs with respect to their tissue membrane distribution among different organs may be related to their structural and functional roles (104). For example, long-chain derivatives of n-3 PUFA are concentrated in biologic structures involved in fast movement as required in transport mechanisms in the brain and its synaptic junctions, as well as the retina (105). Approximately 50% of the PLs in the disc membrane of the retinal rod outer segment in which rhodopsin resides contains C22:6n-3 (106). The

C22:6n-3 is concentrated in the major PL classes (i.e., PC, PE, and phosphotidylsenine in the disc membrane), whereas C20:4n-6 is found in the minor PL components such as phosphatidylinositol. This observation has led to speculation that C22:6n-3 plays a structural role in these membranes, whereas C20:4n-6 may play more of a functional role (107).

In addition to their structural role and their movement across membranes, structural lipids can also modulate cell function by either acting as intracellular mediators of signal transduction or as modulators of cell-cell interactions. These actions are initiated by phospholipases. Phospholipase A_2 cleaves FAs, usually PUFAs, present at the 2 position of PLs. PUFAs released under action of phospholipase A_2 produce metabolites released extracellularly to act on other cells. These metabolites include platelet activating factor, a choline-containing PL with an acetate residue in the 2-position, and eicosanoids. Phospholipase C acts on phosphoinositides to break the bond between glycerol and phosphoric acid, thus releasing DAGs and inositol phosphates (IPs) intracellularly that are involved in signal transduction. After receptor stimulation, DAGs and IPs act intracellularly as second messengers to activate protein kinase C and to release intracellular stores of calcium, respectively (5). Activated protein kinase C mediates the transduction of a wide variety of extracellular stimuli such as hormones and growth factors, leading to regulation of cellular processes, including cell proliferation and differentiation. PL can act as a cofactor for some isoforms of protein kinase C by enhancing binding to DAG (108). In addition, unesterified PUFAs can activate protein kinase C with differing potencies (109). Because dietary PUFAs can modulate PUFA composition of structural lipids, the generation of intracellular and extracellular products can be greatly affected by dietary lipids. As an example, the formation of IP by thrombin-stimulated rabbit platelets is depressed in fish oil–fed rabbits relative to those fed either corn or olive oil (110).

BIOSYNTHESIS AND FUNCTION OF EICOSANOIDS

Some of the most potent effects of PUFAs are related to their enzymatic conversion into a series of oxygenated metabolites called eicosanoids, so-called because their precursors are PUFAs with chain lengths of 20 carbon units. Eicosanoids include PG, TXA, LT, hydroxy FAs, and lipoxins. PG and TXA are generated via cyclooxygenase (CO) enzymes, whereas LTs, hydroxy acids, and lipoxins are produced from lipoxygenase (LO) metabolism. Under stimulation, a rapid and transient synthesis of active eicosanoids activates specific receptors locally in the tissues in which they are formed. Eicosanoids modulate cardiovascular, pulmonary, immune, reproductive, and secretory functions in many cells. They are rapidly converted to their inactive forms via selective catabolic enzymes.

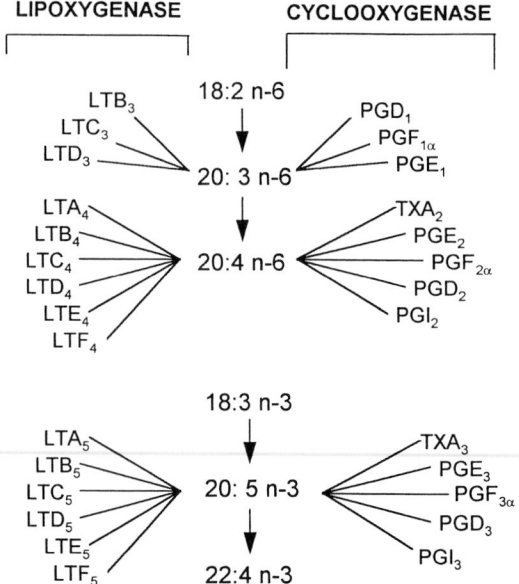

Figure 5.7. Formation of prostaglandin (PG), thromboxane (TXA), and leukotriene (LT) from dihomo-γ-linolenic acid (DHGA) (C20:3n-6), arachidonic acid (C20:4n-6), and eicosapentaenoic acid (C20:5n-3) via cyclooxygenase and lipoxygenase pathways.

Humans depend on the dietary presence of the n-3 and n-6 structural families of PUFAs for adequate biosynthesis of eicosanoids. Three direct precursor FAs have been identified from which eicosanoids are formed by the action of membrane-bound CO or specific LO enzyme systems. These are C20:3n-6, C20:4n-6, and C20:5n-3. Series of prostanoids and LTs, containing different biologic properties, are generated from each of these FAs (Fig. 5.7). The first irreversible, committed step in the synthesis of PGs and LTs is a hydroperoxide-activated FA oxygenase action exerted by either PGH synthase (PGHS) or LO enzymes on the nonesterified precursor PUFA (Fig. 5.8).

Stimulation of normal cells via specific physiologic or pathologic stimuli such as thrombin, ADP, or collagen initiates a calcium-mediated cascade. This cascade involves phospholipase A_2 activation that releases PUFAs on position 2 of the cell membrane. The greatest proportion of PUFAs available to phospholipase A_2 action contains C20:4n-6. Hydrolytic release from PL esters appears to occur indiscriminately with n-3 and n-6 types of PUFAs involving all major classes of PLs such as PC, PE, and phosphatidylinositol. These FAs serve as direct precursors for a generation of eicosanoid products via CO and LO enzymatic action (see Fig. 5.8). Enzymatic biotransformation of the PUFA precursors to PG is catalyzed via two PG synthase isozymes, designated PGH synthase-1 (PGHS-1) and PGH synthase-2 (PGHS-2) (111). PGHS-1 is located in the endoplasmic reticulum, and PGHS-2 is located in the nuclear envelope. Both forms are bifunctional enzymes that catalyze the oxygenation of C20:4n-6 to PGG_2 via CO reaction and the reduction of PGG_2, thus forming a transient hydroxyendoperoxide (PGH_2) via the peroxidase reaction (see Fig. 5.8). The PGH_2 intermediate is rapidly converted to PGI_2 by vascular endothelial cells, to TXA_2 by an isomerase in platelets, or to other prostanoids depending on the tissues involved. The PGHS-2 generates prostanoids associated with mitogenesis and inflammation and is inhibited by glucocorticoids. Conversely, PGHS-1 is expressed only after cell activation and is inhibited by nonsteroidal anti-inflammatory drugs such as aspirin but not by glucocorticoids.

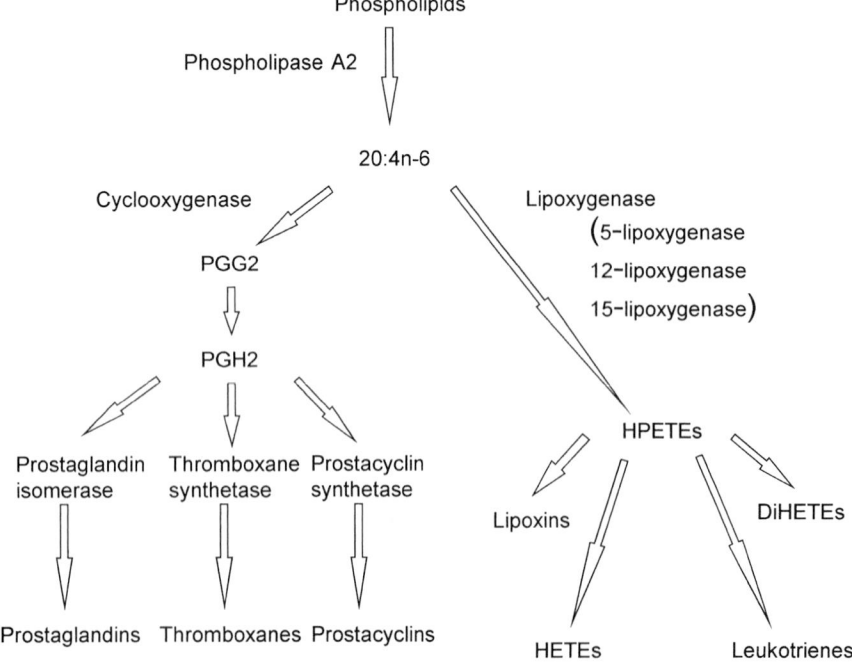

Figure 5.8. Major pathways of synthesis of eicosanoids from arachidonic acid. diHETE, dihydroxyeicosatetraenoic acid; HETE, hydroxyfatty acid; HPETE, hydroperoxyeicosatrienoic acid; PG, prostaglandin. (From Innis SM. Essential dietary lipids. In: Ziegler EE, Filer LJ, eds. Present Knowledge in Nutrition. 7th ed. Washington, DC: ILSI Press, 1996:58–66, with permission.)

C20:4n-6 can be oxygenated via the 5-, 12-, and 15-LO pathways (see Fig. 5.7). The 5-LO pathway generates mainly LTB$_4$, LTC$_4$, LTD$_4$ from C20:4n-6; these are implicated as important mediators in a variety of proliferative and synthetic immune responses. LTB$_4$ in particular has been indicated to be a key proinflammatory mediator in inflammatory and proliferative disorders (111). From C20:4n-6, the 12-LO pathway generates 12-L-hydroxyeicosatetraenoic acid (12-HETE) and 12-hydroperoxyeicosatetraenoic acid (12-HPETE). A proinflammatory response can be generated by 12-HETE in a variety of cell types. Products generated from C20:4n-6 metabolism by the 15-LO reaction include 15-hydroxyeicosatetraenoic acid (15-HETE), which has anti-inflammatory action and may inhibit 5-LO and 12-LO activities (112).

Because the major eicosanoids are synthesized from C20:4n-6, the availability of C20:4n-6 in PL pools of tissue may be a primary factor in regulating the quantities of eicosanoids synthesized by tissues in vivo. In addition, the intensity of the n-6 eicosanoid signal from the released PUFAs will be stronger as C20:4n-6 becomes proportionally greater in the PUFAs. The levels of C20:4n-6 in tissue PL pools are affected by the elongation and desaturation of dietary C18:2n-6 and by the intake of C20:4n-6 (170–220 mg/day in the Western diet) (113). Although dietary concentrations of C18:2n-6 up to 2 to 3% of calories increase tissue C20:4n-6 concentrations, intakes of C18:2n-6 greater than 3% of calories are poorly correlated with tissue C20:4n-6 content (114). Because C18:2n-6 constitutes approximately 6 to 8% of the North American diet, moderate dietary changes in C18:2n-6 would not be expected to modulate tissue C20:4n-6 levels. Intakes of C18:2n-6 greater than 12%, however, may actually decrease tissue C20:4n-6 as a result of inhibition of Δ^6 desaturase. In contrast, dietary C20:4n-6 is much more effective in enriching C20:4n-6 in tissue PLs (114), and, compared with C18:2n-6, relatively low dietary levels of C20:4n-6 may be physiologically significant in enhancing eicosanoid metabolism (113).

Feeding diets high in n-3 FAs results in substitution of C20:4n-6 by n-3 PUFAs in membrane PLs. This process can suppress the response of C20:4n-6–derived eicosanoids by decreasing availability of the C20:4n-6 precursor and by the competitive inhibition of C20:5n-3 for eicosanoid biosynthesis (115). Although less pronounced than the effect observed with C20:5n-3 and C22:6n-3 dietary supplementation, C18:3n-3–enriched diets suppressed PGE$_2$ production by peripheral blood mononuclear cells in monkeys (115). C18:3n-3 could competitively inhibit desaturation and elongation of C18:2n-6 for the conversion into C20:4n-6. The eicosanoids derived from n-3 are homologs of those derived from C20:4n-6 with which they compete (Fig. 5.9), and they are associated with less active responses than n-6 eicosanoids when bound to the specific receptors.

Diets rich in competing and moderating FAs (n-3 PUFA, C18:3n-6) may produce changes in the production of eicosanoids, which are more favorable with respect to

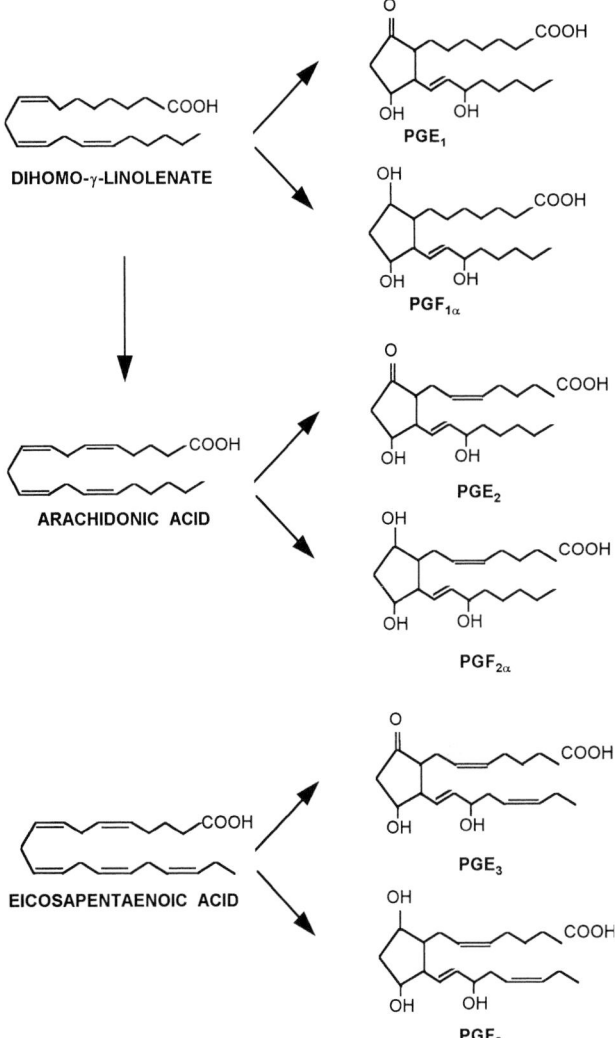

Figure 5.9. Prostaglandin formation.

inflammatory reactions. For instance, the PGE$_3$ formed from C20:5n-3 has less of an inflammatory effect than PGE$_2$ derived from C20:4n-6. The LTB$_5$ derived from C20:5n-3 is substantially less active in proinflammatory functions than the LTB$_4$ formed from C20:4n-6, including the aggregation and chemotaxis of neutrophils. Two 15-LO products, 15-HEPE and 17-hydroxydocosahexaenoic acid, are derived from C20:5n-3 and C22:6n-3, respectively (112). Both metabolites are potent inhibitors of LTB$_4$ formation.

Overproduction of C20:4n-6-derived eicosanoids has been implicated in many inflammatory and autoimmune disorders such as thrombosis, immune inflammatory disease (i.e., arthritis, lupus nephritis), cancer, and psoriatic skin lesions, among others. Because the typical US resident appears to maintain n-6 PUFA in PLs near the maximal capacity, some investigators have suggested that the n-6–rich diet in the United States may contribute to the incidence and severity of eicosanoid-mediated diseases such as thrombosis and arthritis (116). Platelet aggregation and activation are indicated to play a critical role in the progression toward vascular occlusion and myocardial infarction. Therefore, the counterbalancing roles of TXA_2 and PGI_2 in cardiovascular functions have been emphasized. C20:4n-6 is required for platelet function as a precursor of the proaggregatory TXA_2. Biosynthesis of TXA_2 is the rate-limiting step in the aggregation of platelets, a key event in the process of thrombosis. The effects of TXA_2 are counteracted by PGI_2, a potent anti-aggregatory agent that prevents adherence of platelets to blood vessel walls. Because of displacement of C20:4n-6 from membrane PL by C18:2n-6, C18:3n-6, and C20:3n-6, stepwise increases in dietary C18:2n-6 from 3 to 40% of calories actually decreased platelet aggregation, a finding indicating inhibition of eicosanoid synthesis by these n-6 PUFAs. However, the antithrombotic influence of C18:2n-6 is substantially less than that observed after high intakes of n-3 PUFA–rich fish oils (117). This has been related to the observations that PGI_3 generated from C20:5n-3 has antiaggregatory potency. Conversely, TXA_3 derived from C20:5n-3 has a very weak proaggregatory effect, whereas TXA_2 synthesis is reduced (118). Long-term ingestion of aspirin (119) and n-3 PUFAs reduces the intensity of TXA_2 biosynthesis, which could decrease rates of cardiovascular mortality. However, the epidemiologic studies on the effects of dietary n-3 FAs on cardiovascular disease have been inconsistent. One prospective study demonstrated no protective effect of fish consumption on cardiovascular disease mortality and morbidity (120), whereas another showed protective effects in elderly persons who ate only small amounts of fish (121). However, a more recent large clinical intervention trial involving fish oil supplementation showed a rapid onset of reduction in fatal arrhythmias and sudden cardiac death with no effect on recurrent nonfatal myocardial infarction (122). The early protective effect of n-3 PUFA intake on total mortality and sudden death could indicate that the major protective effect of n-3 PUFAs may be exerted by antiarrhythmic as opposed to antiatherothrombotic action (123).

Results of several studies suggest that C18:3n-6 and n-3 EFAs are involved in the regulation of cell-mediated immunity, and administration of these FAs may be beneficial in suppressing pathologic immune responses. For example, patients with rheumatoid arthritis who consume fish oils high in n-3 PUFAs have consistently obtained symptomatic benefit in double-blind randomized controlled trials (123). Although it appears that an inhibition of the proinflammatory eicosanoids LTB_4 and PGE_2 can account for a large part of the protective effects of n-3 PUFAs, decreased production of the cytokines interleukin-1β and tumor necrosis factor are also likely involved (124).

ESSENTIAL FATTY ACID REQUIREMENTS

n-6 Fatty Acid Requirements

In studies of EFAs, C18:2n-6 and C20:4n-6 have been emphasized because mammals have been found to have an absolute requirement for the n-6 family of FAs. The

EFAs are required for the stimulation of growth, maintenance of skin and hair growth, regulation of CH metabolism, lipotropic activity, and maintenance of reproductive performance, among other physiologic effects. On a molecular level, EFAs are components of specific lipids and maintain the integrity and optimal levels of unsaturation of tissue membranes. Since EFAs are necessary for the normal function of all tissues, the list of symptoms of EFAD is long (125). Detailed studies on the symptoms of EFAD have been done in young rats, in which EFAD was found to be avoided by providing 1 to 2% of calories as C18:2n-6 (126). In these rat studies, classic signs of EFAD included reduced growth rates, scaly dermatitis with increased loss of water by a change of skin permeability, male and female infertility, and depressed inflammatory responses. Also observed during EFAD are kidney abnormalities, abnormal liver mitochondria, decreased capillary resistance, increased fragility of erythrocytes, and reduced contraction of myocardial tissue (127).

Linoleic acid, C18:2n-6, is specifically required in the skin to maintain the integrity of the epidermal water barrier. In this regard, C18:2n-6 seems to be required as an integral component of the acylglucoceramides. Animals with EFAD lose considerable amounts of water through the skin, and this limits growth rates. Repletion of C18:2n-6 at 1% of calories corrects excessive transepidermal water loss, and growth is restored (128). Although transdermal water loss during EFAD may reflect the role of C18:2n-6 as a key component of skin acylglucoceramides, the major metabolic effects of C18:2n-6 derive from its further metabolism to C20:4n-6 and consequent conversion to eicosanoids. In EFAD, platelet adherence and aggregation are impaired because of limited TXA synthesis secondary to limiting supplies of C20:4n-6 and possible inhibition by accumulated eicosatrienoic acid C20:3n-9. The action of eicosanoids in modulating the release of hypothalamic and pituitary hormones has been indicated to be a major factor in the role of the n-3 and n-6 EFAs in supporting growth and development (128). Skin is subject to rapid infection, and surgical wounds heal very slowly in persons who have EFAD. This probably reflects the lack of C20:4n-6, which is required for eicosanoid-mediated protective inflammatory and immune cell functions and for tissue proliferation (116). Monocyte and macrophage function is defective in EFAD because of impaired production of eicosanoids. The scaliness of the skin in an EFA-deficient patient has been ascribed to insufficient synthesis of PG, and the efficacy of various EFAs of the n-6 type against the scaly dermatitis has been demonstrated at low dose levels.

Columbinic acid (C18:3n-6, 9, 13 *cis, cis, trans*), found in the seed oil of the columbine, *Aquilegia vulgaris*, and dihomocolumbinic acid (C20:3n-6, 9, 13 *cis, cis, trans*) have been used to differentiate between the roles of EFAs as structural components in biomembranes and their roles as eicosanoid precursors (129). Neither columbinic acid nor dihomocolumbinic acid can be converted to PG; however, columbinic acid can be incorporated into membrane PLs, in contrast to dihomocolumbinic acid. Because EFAD results in decreased tissue concentrations of C20:4n-6, EFAD symptoms are worsened further by the dietary addition of dihomocolumbinic acid. Columbinic acid, when given to EFA-deficient rats either orally or by topical skin application, efficiently restored their growth rate and normal skin function (118). However, when EFA-deficient rats treated with columbinic acid became pregnant, they died of inadequate labor during parturition because uterine labor depends on normal PG biosynthesis (130).

One of the most often used and sensitive diagnostic indicators of EFAD in all species tested including humans is the triene(n-9):tetraene (n-6) ratio (125), whereas C20:3n-9 (triene) is the major product derived from nonessential FAs. C20:4n-6 with four double bonds (tetraene) is the major metabolite of C18:2n-6. The triene:tetraene ratio in plasma remains less than 0.4 when dietary EFAs are adequate, and it increases to more than 0.4 in relation to EFAD. Dietary intake of adequate amounts of EFAs decreases the formation of triene as a consequence of competitive inhibition among families of PUFAs for desaturases and acyl transferases. If EFAs are not available, the biosynthesis of PUFAs with three double bonds derived from C18:1n-9 and C16:n-7 continues, leading to the accumulation of n-9 FA, specifically C20:3n-9, which in turn results in the increase of the plasma triene:tetraene ratio. Feeding diets with 0.1 to 0.5% of C18:2n-6 normalizes an abnormally high triene:tetraene ratio in a few days (131). The optimum dietary C18:2n-6 intake required to give a ratio of less than 0.4 and to prevent symptoms of EFAD is 1–3% of total calories. The triene:tetraene ratio, however, does not resolve whether the EFAD is caused by a lack of either n-3 or n-6 EFAs, because an adequate intake (AI) of either C18:2n-6 or C18:3n-3 will prevent synthesis of C20:3n-9 (132). A lower plasma threshold of 0.2 has been suggested for the triene:tetraene ratio because the average ratio was found to be 0.1 ± 0.08 (SD) in populations exhibiting normal n-6 PUFA status (133, 134).

The exact human requirement of EFA is not clearly defined but is apparently very low. The first study of EFAD in human adults maintained on a diet extremely low in fat for 6 months did not produce dramatic symptoms (135). Investigators have suggested that, because adults contain approximately a kilogram of C18:2n-6 in body stores, depletion of EFA stores to produce deficiency symptoms would require maintenance of more than 6 months on an EFAD diet. Most diets contain enough EFA or their metabolic products to meet daily EFA requirements; thus, EFAD is relatively rare in humans. When it does occur in humans, some of the symptoms characteristic in animals, such as abnormal skin conditions, increased susceptibility to infection, and an increase in triene:tetraene ratio, are observed. Data are lacking on the n-6 PUFA requirement in healthy persons because normal n-6 FA intake is higher than the levels needed to maintain

a triene:tetraene ratio of less than 0.2, and thus metabolic feeding studies to establish requirements have not been performed. As a result, an estimated average requirement EAR has not been set based on the correction of a deficiency (136).

An important role of C20:4n-6 in optimal fetal development has been suggested because C20:4n-6 exerts growth-promoting effects (137). Crawford and associates demonstrated lower intakes of C20:4n-6 by mothers of low-birth-weight infants relative to mothers with normal-birth-weight infants (138). However, lower C20:4n-6 concentrations in plasma and in plasma PC have been associated with depressed intrauterine and extrauterine growth despite adequate dietary C18:2n-6 levels (139). In a double-blind randomized control trial, depressed plasma PC C20:4n-6 concentrations induced by supplementation of formulas with C20:5n-3 rich marine oils were associated with slower growth rates in preterm infants (140). Supplementation of formula with a low C20:5n-3 concentration marine oil caused relatively minor decreases in plasma PC C20:4n-6 concentrations and in weight-to-length ratio in preterm infants (141).

Long-chain EFAs of 20- and 22-carbon chain length are incorporated about ten times more efficiently into the developing brain than the parent EFAs. Whether term or preterm infants have sufficient enzymatic activity to synthesize their own long-chain PUFAs from EFAs to meet their requirement for brain growth and development is controversial. Studies using stable isotopically labeled FAs, however, showed that the conversion of C18:2n-6 to C20:4n-6 can occur as early as 26 weeks of gestation (142). The studies also indicated that the rates of conversion of C18:2n-6 and C18:3n-3 to C20:4n-6 and C22:6n-3, respectively, decrease with increasing gestational age (142). Despite knowledge that the developing and mature brain can desaturate and elongate C18:2n-6 and C18:3n-3 to their respective long-chain PUFA products, and that brain and retina can incorporate C20:4n-6 and C22:6n-3 from plasma, the quantitative importance of these two pathways is uncertain. Lower levels of C20:4n-6 in the red blood cell PLs of formula-fed infants as compared with breast milk–fed infants has led to debate on whether C20:4n-6 is an essential nutrient for infants for optimal central nervous system development (143). The lower erythrocyte C20:4n-6 levels of formula versus breast-fed babies can be normalized by inclusion of C20:4n-6 in formula. Stable isotope studies have indicated in vivo C20:4n-6 synthesis in term infants; but, the activity of this synthesis is low, and only approximately 6% of total plasma C20:4n-6 is renewed in this manner (144). However, postmortem studies of brain FA composition have shown that brain C20:4n-6 is maintained in formula-fed infants (145).

The concept has emerged that n-3 and n-6 families compete for eicosanoid production because an optimal ratio of n-3 and n-6 FA is required in the diet to provide a proper balance among different eicosanoids. Various authorities have recommended that at least 3% of daily calories be provided as linoleate to prevent EFAD; however, equal amounts of C18:2n-6 and various SAFAs have been recommended to reduce serum CH for the prevention of atherosclerosis (131). The advocacy for the increased intake of vegetable oils rich in C18:2n-6 has resulted in the consumption of C18:2n-6 of approximately 6 to 7% of calories in the United States, leading to a ratio of consumption of n-6 to n-3 PUFAs of more than 10 (131). Although this amount of C18:2n-6 may be beneficial for the reduction of elevated plasma CH on a high-fat diet, investigators have argued that an n-6:n-3 PUFA ratio exceeding 10 is imbalanced as compared with n-6:n-3 ratios of 2 to 4 found in food lipids of hunter-gatherer societies (116, 131). Concern exists that a high intake of C18:2n-6 relative to n-3 PUFAs may lead to excessive or imbalanced eicosanoid production conducive to various pathophysiologic processes. The optimal ratio of n-6 to n-3 in the diet is not yet clear and may vary according to developmental stage, the presence of long-chain EFAs, and other factors. An unresolved issue is whether plant oils rich in C18:3n-3 have the same protective effect against cardiovascular disease as marine-derived longer-chain PUFAs, owing to the relatively limited conversion of C18:3n-3 to C20:5n-3 and C22:6n-3 (146). Some authorities have suggested that the ratio of n-6 to n-3 EFAs should be in the range of 4:1 to 10:1 (147), whereas other researchers believe that optimal n-6:n-3 ratios are 4:1 or lower (148, 149).

n-3 Fatty Acid Requirements

Requirements for n-3 FAs have been less definitive because it has been difficult to demonstrate their essentiality in animal studies; n-3 FA levels in mammalian tissues are generally much lower than those of n-6 FAs. Biochemical studies have indicated that differences in the metabolism and tissue distribution between the two series of EFAs exist. C20:4n-6 and C20:3n-6 tend to predominate in liver and platelets, whereas the main biologic activity of the long-chain n-3 EFA appears to reside in retina, testes, and central nervous system. C18:3n-3 is similar to C18:2n-6 with regard to growth rate, capillary resistance, erythrocyte fragility, and mitochondrial function. Dietary C18:3n-3 and C20:5n-3 are inferior to C18:2n-6 and the other n-6 PUFAs with respect to resolving skin lesions and preventing transepidermal water loss. Because of the inability of C18:3n-3 to normalize all physiologic functions during EFAD and because EFA activities attributed to C18:3n-3 were also expressed equally or more potently by C18:2n-6, n-3 FAs were until recently designated as nonessential or partially essential.

However, since the mid-1980s, studies have suggested that n-3 FAs may be essential in the development of neural tissue and visual function, beyond the requirement of n-6 FAs, for which they can partially substitute. Across mammalian species, the levels of C22:6 n-3 in brain and retinal PLs have been observed to be extremely stable despite wide variations in dietary composition (150). The strong affinity of brain lipids for C22:6n-3 suggested a requirement for n-3 EFAs, but this requirement is difficult to study because n-3 EFAD develops only under extreme dietary conditions (143, 150). In particular, C22:6n-3 is selectively retained by the brain, and depletion of C22:6n-3 is difficult after weaning. Multigenerational studies in rats have been needed to produce drastic reductions in brain C22:6n-3. For example, feeding rats fat-free diets from weaning reduced retinal C22:6n-3 concentrations in adults by only 10 to 20%. In the first generation, feeding diets containing 2.5% C18:2n-6 and free of n-3 PUFAs decreased C22:6n-3 concentrations by 60% and in the second generation by more than 87% (151).

An essential role for C22:6n-3 in brain and retinal PLs was described by Neuringer and Connor, who demonstrated C18:3n-3 deficiency in rhesus monkeys fed diets with safflower oil (n-6:n-3 ratio of 255:1) as the sole source of fat during gestation (152). Their offspring reared on the same diet developed abnormal electroretinograms when compared with the control group, consisting of offspring fed soybean oil (n-6:n-3 ratio of 7). Decreased concentrations of C18:3n-3 and long-chain n-3 PUFAs in plasma PLs were observed from those offspring who showed loss of visual activity. Learning capacity, as tested in a spatial reversal learning task, was not affected, possibly because of the observed compensatory increase of n-6 PUFAs, particularly C22:5n-6, in PLs. Retinal n-3 PUFA deficiency was reversed at the ages of 10 and 24 months by feeding a fish oil diet rich in C20:5n-3 and C22:6n-3 (152). Although such extremely high n-6:n-3 ratios rarely occur in human nutrition because of the wide availability of n-3 PUFAs in foods, these ratios have been induced by total parenteral nutrition. A 6-year-old child developed peripheral neuropathy and periods of blurred vision after receiving total parenteral nutrition, the sole source of lipid being a safflower oil emulsion (1). After 5 months, she experienced episodes of numbness, weakness, inability to walk, leg pain, and blurred vision. Very low serum concentrations of C18:3n-3 and other n-3 PUFAs were detected. Replacement of the lipid source by a soybean oil emulsion, containing C18:3n-3, caused all the symptoms of deficiency to disappear, and serum concentrations of n-3 PUFAs returned to normal (1). Reports on the neurologic symptoms in an infant associated with a parentally fed, C18:3n-3–poor formula, and the deficiency symptoms in adults that were corrected by C18:3n-3, support the essentiality of this FA in the diet (1, 153). In the foregoing cases, however, investigators argued that the C18:3n-3 deficiency symptoms could be accounted for by low levels of vitamin E or total EFAD (145). An EAR has not been set based on the correction of deficiency because of a lack of data on the n-3 FA requirement in healthy persons (136).

Because human brain gray matter and retinal membranes contain significant amounts of C22:6n-3, the requirement for n-3 EFAs may be more critical during the last trimester of gestation and the first months of life, when rapid accretion of these FAs occurs in the central nervous system (143, 150). The brain PL acquires only long-chain derivatives of EFAs, not their 18-carbon precursors, and C22:6n-3 is the predominant PUFA in PL in synaptosomal membranes and photoreceptors (150). C22:6n-3 also accounts for approximately 50 to 60% of FAs in the PL of the photoreceptor discs within which rhodopsin and the G-protein reside. Much of C22:6n-3 acquired by the brain is accrued during the suckling period, when the brain undergoes rapid development. Animal studies have demonstrated an impairment in the visual process, altered learning behavior, and low brain C22:6n-3 content resulting from a deficiency in C18:3n-3 and its metabolites C20:5n-3 and C22:6n-3 (143, 150). Permanent learning defects and alterations in synaptic function in the brain, observed in EFAD during pregnancy, can be prevented by feeding n-3 EFAs (152, 154). In addition, a correlation has been noted between dietary-induced changes in C22:6n-3 in the retina and a modification of electrical potentials induced in rod outer segments by light stimulation (155).

Although adequate dietary intakes of n-3 EFAs appear to be critical for central nervous system development, the optimum requirements for n-3 EFAs for infants are not known. Human milk provides C18:3n-3 and C22:6n-3, both often absent from infant formulas on the market. Formula-fed infants thus depend on endogenous synthesis of long-chain PUFAs. Infant formulas provide nutrition that results in growth rates equal or superior to those of breast milk–fed infants. The capability of term and preterm infants to convert C18:3n-3 to C22:6n-3 has been demonstrated via stable isotope studies with a greater capability for conversion observed in preterm infant tissues (142). A suggestion exists, however, that long-chain n-3 PUFAs may not be synthesized from their parent EFAs at optimal rates for brain development during the first few weeks after birth, particularly in preterm infants. Clandinin and colleagues indicated that an infant's requirement for neural accumulation of long-chain PUFAs could be met from the intake of long-chain PUFAs alone, without the need for endogenous synthesis (156). Using the FA composition of red blood cell PLs as an index of cerebral membrane composition, infants fed human milk were found to have a significantly better C22:6n-3 status than formula-fed infants (157). The extent to which diet-induced changes in red blood cell membranes reflects changes in brain PL is not clear. However, postmortem studies indicate a lower C22:6n-3 brain content in formula-fed infants versus infants receiving breast milk (158). In a randomized trial of n-3 PUFA supplementation of formulas fed to term infants, C22:6n-3–treated infants had better visual acuity than infants fed standard formula (159). Several other large randomized controlled trials, however, showed no consistent effect of long-chain PUFA formula supplementation of C22:6n-3 or C22:6n-3 plus

C20:4n-6 on visual, psychomotor, or mental development (160). A more recent randomized, prospective supplementation study that evaluated visual and cognitive development at 39 months of age showed no adverse effects or benefits of infant formula supplemented with C22:6n-3 or C22:6n-3 and C20:4n-6 on growth, visual development, and neurodevelopmental outcomes at 39 months (161).

Preterm infants may be especially susceptible to n-3 EFAD because of their relatively immature desaturase and elongase enzyme systems and their low fat stores. Intake of formula containing marine oil by preterm infants was demonstrated in two randomized clinical trials to normalize blood levels of C22:6n-3 and to improve certain aspects of visual function relative to breast-fed infants (162). In one of the randomized studies, however, marine oil supplementation was associated with decreases in linear growth, some measures of cognitive development, and blood C20:4n-6 content. These results are of concern in view of the important role of C20:4n-6 in growth and development (140). However, the use of a more physiologic formulation containing pure C22:6n-3 versus the mixture of C20:5n-3 and C22:6n-3 given over a shorter interval resulted in better cognitive and visual performance and a less detrimental effect on growth (141, 163). Large clinical trials (164, 165) have not shown reduced growth in infants provided with formulas containing C18:2n-6:C18:3n-3 ratios of 5:1 to 10:1 despite an earlier study indicating adverse effects on growth in infants fed formulas containing a ratio of 5:1 (166). Because of concerns regarding the impact of supplementation of long-chain n-3 FAs without C20:4n-6 on growth and development, neural development was not used to set an EAR for n-3 FAs in infancy (136). Recommendations for infant formulas for acceptable ranges of the ratio of total n-3:n-6 FAs or the C18:2n-6:C18:3n-3 ratio have ranged from 5:1 to 16:1 (167).

Pregnancy

The rapidly developing fetal organs such as the liver and brain incorporate large amounts of long-chain n-3 and n-6 EFAs into membrane PL (168). The accumulation of EFAs during human pregnancy has been approximated to be 620 g, which includes the demand for fetal, placental, mammary gland, and uterine growth, as well as the increased maternal blood volume. On the basis of this estimate of expected EFA acquisition by maternal tissues and the conceptus, investigators have suggested that the maternal EFA consumption during pregnancy be increased from 3 to 4.5% of calories (169). In circumstances of relatively low dietary intake of n-6 EFAs (i.e., 2–4% of calories), EFAD may be more likely to develop during periods of rapid cell division and growth. A National Institutes of Health (NIH) Working Group in 1999 proposed intakes of EPA and docosahexaenoic acid (DHA) of 650 mg/day or more and a minimum of 300 mg DHA/day during pregnancy and lactation (170). Because of insufficient evidence concerning C18:2n-6 and C18:3n-3 requirements during pregnancy, the AI of these FAs was based on their median intake in the United States, where no evidence of deficiencies of these FAs exists among the healthy population (136). During lactation, the AI for C18:2n-6 is set as 13 g/day, whereas the AI for C18:3n-3 is established as 1.4 g/day.

Lactation

In well-nourished mothers, approximately 4 to 5% of total calories in human milk is present as C18:2n-6 and C18:3n-3, and 1% further as long-chain PUFAs derived from these FAs, amounting to about 6% of total energy as EFA and its metabolites. The efficiency of conversion of dietary EFAs into milk FAs is not clear; however, an additional 1 to 2% of calories in the form of EFAs is recommended during the first 3 months of lactation. Another 2 to 4% of calories more than the basic requirement is recommended thereafter (169). Because of insufficient evidence concerning C18:2n-6 and C18:3n-3 requirements during lactation, the AI of these FAs was based on their median intake in the United States, where no evidence of deficiencies of these FAs exists in the healthy population (136). During pregnancy, the AI for C18:2n-6 is set as 13 g/day, whereas the AI for C18:3n-3 is established as 1.3 g/day.

Infancy and Childhood

The optimum requirements for EFAs of n-6 and n-3 families for infants are still not known, although normal growth of infants has been well demonstrated to depend on an adequate supply of EFAs. The apparent minimum requirements for C18:2n-6 for growing children are from 1 to 4.5% of total calories, to ensure an adequate supply of EFAs for tissue proliferation, membrane integrity, and eicosanoid formation (147, 171). From 0 to 6 months of age, an AI for C18:2n-6 was set as 4.4 g/day or approximately 8% of calories, as based on the average amount of n-6 FA provided by human milk. From 7 to 12 months, the AI for C18:2n-6 is 4.6 g/day or 6% of calories (136). The AI for C18:2n-6 in children and adolescents was set on the basis of the median intake of C18:2n-6 in the United States because no data are available concerning the amount needed to correct a deficiency, given that the deficiency is nonexistent in the free-living US population. The AI for C18:2n-6 was set as 7 to 10 g/day from 1 to 8 years of age. The AI for C18:2n-6 was set as 12 and 16 g/day for boys aged 9 to 13 and 14 to 18 years, respectively. The AI for C18:2n-6 was established as 10 and 11 g/day for girls aged 9 to 13 and 14 to 18 years, respectively. The need for n-3 EFAs has been indicated to be higher during growth and development. Estimates based on FA compositional data from autopsy tissue and breast milk n-3 EFA concentrations have ranged from 0.5 to 1.2% of calories (171). The Canadian Nutrition Recommendations suggest infant

dietary intakes of 1% C18:3n-3 of energy in the absence of intake of long-chain n-3 PUFAs as compared with 0.5% C18:3n-3 of energy when a supply of long-chain n-3 EFAs is available in the diet (147). However, the bioequivalency of C18:3n-3 versus its long-chain products, C20:5n-3 and C22:6n-3, has not yet been determined, although long-chain PUFAs clearly contribute to the C20:5n-3 and C22:6n-3 content of plasma and erythrocyte PL (150). Another question that needs to be addressed is whether long-chain PUFAs, especially C22:6n-3, are conditionally essential for the optimal visual and neural development of preterm and term infants. The AI for C18:3n-3 was established as 0.5 g/day or approximately 1% of calories as based on the average amount of n-3 FAs provided by human milk. For infants from 7 to 12 months of age, the AI for C18:3n-3 is 0.5 g/day (136). The AI for C18:3n-3 in children and adolescents was set on the basis of the median intake of C18:3n-3 in the United States, because deficiency is basically nonexistent in the free-living US population. The AI for C18:3n-3 was set as 0.7 to 0.9 g/day from 1 to 8 years of age. The AI for C18:3n-3 was set as 1.2 and 1.6 g/day for boys aged 9 to 13 and 14 to 18 years, respectively. The AI for C18:3n-3 was established as 1.0 and 1.1 g/day for girls aged 9 to 13 and 14 to 18 years, respectively.

Adulthood

For adults, appropriate minimum amounts of n-6 EFA are in the range of 1 to 4% of energy to prevent signs of EFAD (150). The C18:3n-3 requirements for adults have been suggested to range from 0.2 to 0.3% of energy to 1% of energy, although more studies are needed to clarify the amounts needed to meet the minimal requirements in humans (3, 172). The NIH Working Group recommended AIs of 2 to 3% of total calories for linoleic acid, 1% of total calories for α-linolenic acid, and 0.3% of total calories for EPA and DHA (170). There is insufficient information to set an EAR for C18:2n-6 and C18:3n-3 requirements for healthy adults. Thus, an AI for C18:2n-6 and C18:3n-3 was established on the basis of the highest median intakes of these FAs among different age groups of men and women in the United States, where no evidence of a C18:2n-6 or C18:3n-3 deficiency exists in the healthy population. Because C18:2n-6 is used readily for energy, the AI for men and women older than 50 years was lowered, given that their energy expenditure is lower than that of young adults. The AI for C18:2n-6 for men aged 19 to 50 years is 17 g/day, and it is 14 g/day for men more than 50 years of age. For women, the AI was set as 12 g/day between 19 and 50 years of age and 11 g/day for women of aged 51 years and older. The AI for C18:3n-3 is 1.6 g/day for men and 1.1 g/day for women. EPA and DHA can contribute toward reversing n-3 FA deficiency (3). Because these long-chain n-3 FAs can provide up to 10% of the total n-3 FA intake, this percentage can contribute toward the AI for C18:3n-3 (136).

Nutrient Interrelationships

Several dietary components are known to affect EFA requirements as a result of their interactions with EFA utilization or metabolism. Dietary SAFAs have been found to increase EFA requirements slightly as evaluated by growth and dermal symptoms of deficiency and the triene:tetraene ratio in plasma (173). This effect has been related to the action of SAFAs in raising plasma CH that forms esters with PUFAs, thereby depleting the availability of the EFA pool for PL. In addition, in several animal species an induction of serum CH via a high-CH diet can aggravate EFAD. *Cis*-MUFAs (mainly C18:1n-9 and its product C20:3n-9) can replace EFAs in the lipids of EFAD in animals and humans. High dietary levels of C18:1n-9 suppressed desaturation of EFAs such that when dietary concentrations of C18:1n-9 were ten times higher than those of C18:2n-6, triene:tetraene ratios indicative of an EFAD were observed (174). Partial hydrogenation of vegetable oils in the production of margarines and shortenings forms SAFAs and a variety of *trans* and positional isomers. The estimated average daily *trans* FA intake is 8 to 10 g or 6 to 8% of the total dietary FAs. *Trans*-MUFAs have been found to increase the EFA requirement in animals when fed at moderate levels and can influence the desaturase reactions critical to the metabolism of PUFAs (175). The *trans* FAs can also raise plasma levels of LDL and total CH, and this could further increase EFA utilization. *Trans* FAs can be transferred from the maternal diet via placental transfer to the fetus or through lactation. The *trans* isomers of C18:1n-9 and C18:2n-6 have been suggested to have potential adverse effects on fetal and infant growth and development through inhibition of the desaturation of C18:2n-6 and C18:3n-3 to C20:4n-6 and C22:6n-3, respectively (176). Plasma *trans* isomers have also been negatively correlated with infant birth weight and head circumference (177). Because animal and in vitro studies have used much higher amounts of *trans* FAs than typically seen in a normal human diet, it is controversial whether deleterious effects can occur with amounts consumed in a normal human diet containing sufficient amounts of C18:2n-6 (176).

High-Risk Clinical Situations

Although the development of human EFAD has traditionally been regarded as rare, use of the sensitive triene:tetraene ratio as a diagnostic index has served to indicate the existence of EFAD in certain high-risk clinical conditions. EFAD appears to be exacerbated by increased metabolic demands associated with either growth or the hypermetabolism seen following stress, injury, or sepsis (178).

The supply of C18:2n-6 is of concern in premature infants because of borderline stores of EFA and high caloric expenditure (178). Unless C18:2n-6 is supplied to premature infants in parenteral or enteral diets, early onset of EFAD may occur. Biochemical changes in the plasma and clinical signs indicative of EFAD can develop rapidly within 5 to 10 days of life in premature infants (178, 179).

In patients receiving long-term intake parenteral nutrition without lipids, the continuous glucose infusion results in high circulating levels of insulin that inhibit lipolysis and depress the release of EFA from adipose fat stores (150). Investigators have documented that the development of EFAD in infants, children, and adults maintained on continuous fat-free or minimal-fat parenteral nutrition was reversed by oral or intravenous administration of C18:2n-6 (178). Parenteral nutrition containing only amino acids and completely free of glucose does not produce evidence of EFAD (180). Clinical signs of EFAD include alopecia, scaly dermatitis, increased capillary fragility, poor wound healing, increased platelet aggregation, increased susceptibility to infection, fatty liver, and growth retardation in infants and children (180).

The development of EFAD has been described in several human diseases including cystic fibrosis (181), acrodermatitis enteropathica (174), peripheral vascular disease (182), and multiple sclerosis (183). Enteral supplementation of vegetable oils high in C18:2n-6 has been demonstrated to improve EFAD in patients with cystic fibrosis (181). Children with cystic fibrosis may require 7 to 10% of energy as C18:2n-6 to prevent reduced weight gain and growth, and infants with cystic fibrosis may require formula with a C18:2n-6 content greater than 12% of total calories (181, 184). Patients with anorexia nervosa may have EFAD exhibited by plasma PL profiles showing lowered n-6 and n-3 PUFA concentrations (185). Low total plasma PUFA concentrations, particularly those of 20- and 22-carbon n-3 PUFAs, have been noted in patients with acquired immunodeficiency syndrome (186). The development of EFAD as measured by the triene:tetraene ratio has been demonstrated in elderly patients with peripheral vascular disease (187), in patients with fat malabsorption after major intestinal resection, during low-fat, high-protein dietary supplementation for treatment of kwashiorkor (188), and after serious accidents and burns. Oral or intravenous feeding of C18:2n-6–containing TGs has been found to correct the biochemical and clinical abnormalities in these conditions.

Editor's note: Appendix Tables A-2-a through A-2-k summarize the basis and usage of the DRIs and the actual DRI data thus far published. Appendix Tables A-2-d-4, A-2-d-5 and A-2-d-6 contain the data for fat, linoleic and alpha linolenic acids mentioned in this chapter and in the author's reference 136.

Acknowledgments

We extend special thanks to Lily Lam, Catherine Vanstone, and Nick Osicka for their invaluable contribution to researching and writing this chapter. The graphic artwork of Helen Rimner is also gratefully acknowledged. Finally, appreciation is extended to the helpful students who offered suggestions on improving the quality and composition of the chapter.

REFERENCES

1. Holman RT, Johnson SB, Hatch TF. Am J Clin Nutr 1982;35:617-23.
2. Neuringer M, Connor WE, Van Petten C et al. J Clin Invest 1984;73:272.
3. Bjerve KS. J Intern Med 1989;225[Suppl]:171S–5S.
4. Poulos A, Beckman K, Johnson DW et al. Adv Exp Med Biol 1992;318:331–40.
5. Xi ZP, Want JY. J Nutr Sci Vitaminol 2003;49:210–3.
6. Muller H, Kirkhus B, Pedersen JI. Lipids 2001;36:83–91.
7. ASCN Task Force on Trans Fatty Acids. Am J Clin Nutr 1996;63:663–70.
8. Posner BM, Cupples LA, Franz MM et al. Int J Epidemiol 1993;22:1014–25.
9. Anonymous. MMWR Morb Mortal Wkly Rep 1994;43:116–7, 123–5.
10. Chen ZY, Ratnayake WM, Fortier L et al. Can J Physiol Pharmacol 1995;73:718–23.
11. Ling WH, Jones PJH. Life Sci 1995;57:195–206.
12. Vandermeers A, Vandermeers-Piret MC, Rathe J et al. Biochim Biophys Acta 1974;370:257–68.
13. Hay DW, Carey MC. Hepatology 1990;12[Suppl]:6S–14S.
14. Hofmann AF, Mekhijian HS. Bile acids and the intestinal absorption of fat and electrolytes in health and disease. In: Nair PP, Kritchevsky D, eds. The Bile Acids, vol 2. New York: Plenum Press, 1973.
15. Bergholz CM. Crit Rev Food Sci Nutr 1992;32:141–6.
16. Rolls BJ, Pirraglia PA, Jones MB et al. Am J Clin Nutr 1992;56:84–92.
17. Reinhart GA, Mahan DC, Lepine AJ et al. J Anim Sci 1993;71:2693–9.
18. Jones PJ, Scanu AM, Schoeller DA. J Lab Clin Med 1988;111:627–33.
19. Tso P, Karlstad MD, Bistrian BR et al. Am J Physiol 1995;268:G568–77.
20. de Fouw NJ, Kivits GA, Quinlan PT et al. Lipids 1994;29:765–70.
21. Bracco U. Am J Clin Nutr 1994;60[Suppl]:1002S–9S.
22. Grundy SM, Metzger AL, Adler RD. J Clin Invest 1972;51:3026–43.
23. Wasserhess P, Becker M, Staab D. Am J Clin Nutr 1993;58:349–53.
24. Samuel P, McNamara DJ. J Lipid Res 1983;24:265–76.
25. Mattson FH, Jandacek RJ, Webb MR. J Nutr 1976;106:747–52.
26. Lipka G, Schulthess G, Thurnhofer H et al. J Biol Chem 1995;270:5917–25.
27. Quintao EC, Sperotto G. Adv Lipid Res 1987;22:173–88.
28. Jones PJH, Pappu AS, Hatcher L et al. Atheroscler Thromb 1996;16:1222–8.
29. Miettinen TA, Tilvis RS, Kesaniemi YA. Am J Epidemiol 1990;131:20–31.
30. Vanhanen HT, Miettinen TA. Clin Chim Acta 1992;205:97–107.
31. Child P, Kuksis A. Biochem Cell Biol 1986;64:847–53.
32. Katan MB, Grundy SM, Jones P et al. Mayo Clin Proc 2003;78:965–78.
33. Sugiyama Y, Ishikawa E, Odaka H et al. Atherosclerosis 1995;113:71–8.
34. Levy E, Mehran M, Seidman E. FASEB J 1995;9:626–35.
35. Leitch CA, Jones PJ. J Lipid Res 1993;34:157–63.
36. Hellerstein MK, Christiansen M, Kaempfer S et al. J Clin Invest 1991;87:1841–52.
37. Austin MA, Hokanson JE, Brunzell JD. Curr Opin Lipidol 1994;5:395–403.
38. Miller GJ, Miller NE. Lancet 1975;1:16–9.
39. Yancey PG, Bortnick AE, Kellner-Weibel G et al. Arterioscler Thromb Vasc Biol 2003;23:712–9.
40. Barter PJ, Rye KA. Atherosclerosis 1996;121:1–12.
41. Raclot T, Groscolas R. J Lipid Res 1995;36:2164–73.
42. Connor WE, Lin DS, Colvis C. J Lipid Res 1996;37:290–8.
43. Brown MS, Goldstein JL. J Clin Invest 1983;72:743–7.
44. Mackness MI, Durrington PN. Atherosclerosis 1995;115:243–53.
45. Goldberg IJ. J Lipid Res 1996;37:693–707.
46. Hegsted DM, McGandy RB, Myers ML et al. Am J Clin Nutr 1965;17:281–95.
47. Noakes M, Nestel PJ, Clifton PM. Am J Clin Nutr 1996;63:42–6.
48. Bergeron N, Havel RJ. Arterioscler Thromb Vasc Biol 1996;16:497.
49. Jones PJH, Lau V. Nutr Rev 2003;132:329–32.
50. van Tol A, Zock PL, van Gent T et al. Atherosclerosis 1995;115:129–34.
51. Grundy SM, Barrett-Connor E, Rudel LL et al. Arteriosclerosis 1988;8:95–101.
52. Andersen RE, Wadden TA, Bartlett SJ et al. Am J Clin Nutr 1995;62:350–7.
53. Lemieux S, Prud'homme D, Moorjani S et al. Atherosclerosis 1995;118:155–64.
54. Clandinin MT, Cheema S, Field CJ et al. Ann NY Acad Sci 1993;683:151–63.
55. Leyton J, Drury PJ, Crawford MA. Br J Nutr 1987;57:383–93.
56. Takeuchi H, Matsuo T, Tokuyama K. J Nutr 1995;125:920–5.
57. Shimomura Y, Tamura T, Suzuki M. J Nutr 1990;120:1291–6.
58. Matsuo T, Shimomura Y, Saitoh S et al. Metab Clin Exp 1995;44:934–9.
59. Chen ZY, Menard CR, Cunnane SC. Am J Physiol 1995;268:R498–505.
60. Jones PJ, Schoeller DA. Metab Clin Exp 1988;37:145–51.
61. Clandinin MT, Wang LC, Rajotte RV et al. Am J Clin Nutr 1995;61:1052–7.
62. Kubow S. Free Radic Biol Med 1992;12:63–81.
63. Draper HH, Hadley M. Xenobiotica 1990;20:901–7.
64. Roberts LJ, Morrow JD. Free Radic Biol Med 2000;28:505–13.
65. Cracowski JL, Devillier P, Durand T et al. J Vasc Res. 2001;38:93–103.
66. Greco A, Minghetti L, Levi G. Neurochem Res 2000;25:1357–64.
67. Welsch CW, Welsch MA, Huelskamp LJ et al. Int J Oncol 1995;6:55–64.
68. Girelli D, Olivieri O, Stanzial AM et al. Clin Chim Acta 1994;227:45–57.
69. Draper HH. Adv Nutr Res 1990;8:119–45.
70. Penumetcha M, Khan N, Parthasarathy S. J. Lipid Res 2000;41:1473–80.
71. Loidl A, Sevcsik E, Riesenhuber G et al. J Biol Chem 2003;278:32921–8.
72. Dobarganes C. Marquez-Ruiz G. Curr Opin Clin Nutr Metab Care 2003;6:157–63.
73. Addis PB, Warner GJ. In: Aruoma OI, Halliwell B, eds. Free Radicals and Food Additives. London: Taylor and Francis, 1991:77–119.
74. Smith LL. Lipids 1996;31:453–87.
75. Peng SK, Philips GA, Xia GZ et al. Atherosclerosis 1987;64:1–6.
76. Holvoet P, Collen D. FASEB J 1994;8:1279–84.
77. Regnstrom J, Nilsson J, Tornvall P et al. Lancet 1992;339:1183–6.
78. Palinski W, Rosenfeld ME, Yla-Herttuala S et al. Proc Natl Acad Sci USA 1989;86:1372–6.
79. Louheranta AM, Porkkalasarataho EK, Nyyssönen MK et al. Am J Clin Nutr 1996;63:698–703.

80. Tsimikas S, Philis-Tsimikas A, Alexopoulos S et al. Arterioscler Thromb Vasc Biol 1999;19:122–30.

81. Bonanome A, Biasia F, Deluca M et al. Am J Clin Nutr 1996;63:261–6.

82. Jialal I, Fuller CJ, Huet BA. Arterioscler Thromb Vasc Biol 1995;15:190–8.

83. Upritchard JE, Schuurman C, Wiersma A et al. Am J Clin Nutr 2003;5:985–92.

84. Sprecher H. Curr Opin Clin Nutr Metab Care 1999;2:135–8.

85. Cunnane SC, Ryan MA, Craig KS et al. Lipids 1995;30:781–3.

86. Kinsella JE, Broughton KS, Whelan J. J Nutr Biochem 1990;1:123–41.

87. Holman RT. Biological activities of and requirement for polyunsaturated acids. In: Holman RT, ed. Progress in the Chemistry of Fats and Other Lipids, vol 9. New York: Pergamon Press, 1970:611–82.

88. Schlenk H, Sand DM, Gellerman JL. Biochim Biophys Acta 1969;187:201–7.

89. Hagve TA, Christophersen BO. Biochim Biophys Acta 1986;875:165–73.

90. Gerster H. Int J Vitam Nutr Res 1998;68:159–73.

91. Brenna JT. Curr Opin Clin Nutr Metab Care 2002;5:127–32.

92. Blond JP, Bezard J. Biochim Biophys Acta 1991;1084:255–60.

93. Mimouni V, Narce M, Huang YS et al. Prostaglandins Leukot Essent Fatty Acids 1994;50:43–7.

94. Cunnane SC. Prog Food Nutr Sci 1988;12:151–88.

95. Horrobin DF. Am J Clin Nutr 1993;57[Suppl]:732S–6S.

96. Dietschy JM. Klin Wochenschr 1984;62:338–45.

97. Jenkins DJ, Khan A, Jenkins AL et al. Metab Clin Exp 1995;44:549–55.

98. Wu-Pong S, Elias PM, Feingold KR. J Invest Dermatol 1994;102:799–802.

99. Galli C, Marangoni F, Galella G. Prostaglandins Leukot Essent Fatty Acids 1993;48:51–5.

100. Chawla A, Repa JJ, Evans RM et al. Science 2001;294:1866–70.

101. Chawla A, Lee CH, Barak Y et al. Proc Natl Acad Sci USA 2003;100:1268–73.

102. Desvergene B, Wahli W. Endocr Rev 1999;20:649–88.

103. Kersten S, Beatrice D, Wahli W. Nature 2000;405:421–4.

104. Murphy MG. J Nutr Biochem 1990;1:68–79.

105. Tinoco J. Prog Lipid Res 1982;21:1–45.

106. Stinson AM, Wiegand RD, Anderson RE. Exp Eye Res 1991;52:213–8.

107. Litman BJ, Mitchell DC. Lipids 1996;31[Suppl]:193S–7S.

108. Huang KP. Trends Neurosci 1989;12:425–32.

109. Nishizuka Y. Science 1992;258:607–14.

110. Medini L, Colli S, Mosconi C et al. Biochem Pharmacol 1990;39:129–33.

111. Goetzl EJ, An S, Smith WL. FASEB J 1995;9:1051–8.

112. Ziboh VA. Proc Soc Exp Biol Med 1994;205:1–11.

113. Li B, Birdwell C, Whelan J. J Lipid Res 1994;35:1869–77.

114. Whelan J, Surette ME, Hardardottir I et al. J Nutr 1993;123:2174–85.

115. Wu D, Meydani SN, Meydani M et al. Am J Clin Nutr 1996;63:273–80.

116. Lands WE. FASEB J 1992;6:2530–6.

117. Emken EA. Am J Clin Nutr 1992;56[Suppl]:798S.

118. von Schacky C, Fischer S, Weber PC. J Clin Invest 1985;76:1626–31.

119. Anonymous. Lancet 1988;2:349–60.

120. Morris MC, Manson JE, Rosner B et al. Am J Epidemiol 1995;142:166–75.

121. Kromhout D, Feskens EJ, Bowles CH. Int J Epidemiol 1995;24:340–5.

122. Marchioli R, Barzi F, Bomba E et al. Circulation 2002;105:1897–903.

123. Kremer JM. Lipids 1996;31[Suppl]:243S–7S.

124. Caughey GE, Mantzioris E, Gibson RA et al. Am J Clin Nutr 1996;63:116–22.

125. Holman RT. Essential fatty acid deficiency. In: Holman RT, ed. Progress in the Chemistry of Fats and Other Lipids, vol 9. New York: Pergamon Press, 1971:275–348.

126. Kinsella JE. Adv Food Nutr Res 1991;35:1–184.

127. Vergroesen AJ. Bibl Nutr Dieta 1976;23:19–26.

128. Hansen HS. Trends Biochem Sci 1986;11:263–5.

129. Houtsmuller UM. Prog Lipid Res 1981;20:889–96.

130. Paulsrud JR, Pensler L, Whitten CF et al. Am J Clin Nutr 1972;25:897–904.

131. Kinsella JE, Lokesh B, Stone RA. Am J Clin Nutr 1990;52:1–28.

132. Mohrhauer H, Holman RT. J Lipid Res 1963;4:151–9.

133. Mascioli EA, Lopes SM, Champagne C et al. Nutrition 1996;12:245–9.

134. Jeppesen PB, Hoy C-E, Mortensen PB. Am J Clin Nutr 1998;68:126–33.

135. Brown WR, Hansen AE, Burr GO et al. J Nutr 1938;16:511–24.

136. Food and Nutrition Board, Institute of Medicine. Dietary Reference Intakes for Energy, Carbohydrate, Fiber, Fat, Fatty Acids, Cholesterol, Protein, and Amino Acids (Macronutrients). Washington, DC: National Academy Press, 2002.

137. Carlson SE. J Nutr 1996;126:1092–8.

138. Crawford MA, Costeloe K, Doyle W et al. Essential fatty acids in early development. In: Bracco U, Deckelbaum RJ, eds. Polyunsaturated Fatty Acids in Human Nutrition. New York: Raven Press, 1992:93–110.

139. Koletzko B, Braun M. Ann Nutr Metab 1991;35:128–31.

140. Carlson SE, Cooke RJ, Werkman SH et al. Lipids 1992;27:901–7.

141. Carlson SE, Werkman SH, Tolley EA. Am J Clin Nutr 1996;63:687–97.

142. Uauy R, Mena P, Wegher B et al. 2000;Pediatr Res 47:127–35.

143. Innis SM. Can J Physiol Pharmacol 1994;72:1483–92.

144. Koletzko B, Decsi T, Demmelmair H. Lipids 1996;31:79–83.

145. Makrides M, Neumann MA, Gibson RA. Lipids 1996;31:115–9.

146. Sanderson P, Finnegan YE, Williams CM et al. Br J Nutr 2002;88:573–9.

147. Canada Health and Welfare, Health Protection Branch, Bureau of Nutritional Sciences. 1990 Nutrition Recommendations. Ottawa: Canada Health and Welfare, 1990.

148. Bezard J, Blond JP, Bernard A et al. Reprod Nutr Dev 1994;34:539–68.

149. Gibson RA, Makrides M, Neumann MA et al. J Pediatr 1994;125[Suppl]:48S–55S.

150. Innis SM. Prog Lipid Res 1991;30:39–103.

151. Anderson GJ. J Lipid Res 1994;35:105–11.

152. Neuringer M, Connor WE. Nutr Rev 1986;44:285–94.

153. Bjerve KS, Fischer S, Wammer F et al. Am J Clin Nutr 1989;49:290–300.

154. Galli C, Spagnuolo C, Bosisio E et al. Adv Prostaglandins Thromboxane Res 1978;4:181–9.

155. Wheeler TG, Benolken RM, Anderson RE. Science 1975;188:1312–4.

156. Clandinin MT, Chappell JE, Heim T. Prog Lipid Res 1981;20:901–4.

157. Carlson SE, Rhodes PG, Ferguson MG. Am J Clin Nutr 1986;44:798–804.

158. Farquharson J, Jamieson EC, Abbasi KA et al. Arch Dis Child 1995;72:198–203.

159. Makrides M, Neumann MA, Simmer K et al. Lancet 1995;345:1463–8.

160. Auestad N, Montalto MB, Wheeler RE et al. Pediatr Res 1995;37:302A.

161. Auestad N. Scott DT, Janowsky JS et al. Pediatrics 2003;112: E177–83.

162. Carlson SE, Werkman SH, Rhodes PG et al. Am J Clin Nutr 1993;58:35–42.

163. Werkman SH, Carlson SE. Lipids 1996;31:91–7.

164. Auestad N, Halter R, Hall RT et al. Pediatrics 2001;108: 372–81.

165. Makrides M, Neumann MA, Jeffrey B et al. Am J Clin Nutr 2000;71:120–9.

166. Jensen CL. Prager TC, Fraley JK et al. J Pediatr. 1997;131:200–9.

167. Life Science Research Office (LSRO). Fat. In: Raiten DJ, Talbot, JM, Waters JH, eds. Assessment of Nutrient Requirements for Infant Formulas. Bethesda, MD: LSRO, 1998:19–46.

168. Clandinin MT, Jumpsen J, Suh M. J Pediatr 1994;125[Suppl]: 25S–32S.

169. Food and Agriculture Organization (FAO)/World Health Organization Expert Consultation. The Role of Fats and Oils in Human Nutrition. FAO Food and Nutrition paper 3. Rome: FAO, 1978.

170. Simopoulos AP, Leaf A, Salem N. Workshop on the essentiality of and recommended dietary intakes for *n*-6 and *n*-3 fatty acids. Bethesda, MD: National Institutes of Health, 1999.

171. European Society of Paediatric Gastroenterology and Nutrition. Acta Paediatr Scand 1987;336:1–14.

172. Bjerve KS, Fischer S, Alme K. Am J Clin Nutr 1987;46:570–6.

173. Alfin-Slater RB, Morris RS, Hansen H et al. J Nutr 1965;87: 168–72.

174. Holman RT. Adv Exp Med Biol 1977;83:515–34.

175. Lands WE, Blank ML, Nutter LJ et al. Lipids 1966;1:224–9.

176. Larqué E, Zamora S,Gil A. Early Hum Dev 2001;65[Suppl]: S31–S41.

177. Craig-Schmidt MC. Lipids 2001;36:997–1006.

178. Sardesai VM. J Nutr Biochem 1992;3:154–67.

179. Farrell PM, Gutcher GR, Palta M et al. Am J Clin Nutr 1988; 48:220–9.

180. Stegink LD, Freeman JB, Wispe J et al. Am J Clin Nutr 1977; 30:388–93.

181. Mischler EH, Parrell SW, Farrell PM et al. Pediatr Res 1986; 20:36–41.

182. Kingsbury KJ, Brett C, Stovold R et al. Postgrad Med J 1974; 50:425–40.

183. Dworkin RH, Bates D, Millar JH et al. Neurology 1984; 34:1441–5.

184. van Egmond AW, Kosorok MR, Kosick R et al. Am J Clin Nutr 1996;63:746–52.

185. Holman RT, Adams CE, Nelson RA et al. J Nutr 1995;125: 901–7.

186. Begin ME, Manku MS, Horrobin DF. Prostaglandins Leukot Essent Fatty Acids 1989;37:135–7.

187. Friedman Z, Frolich JC. Pediatr Res 1979;13:932–6.

188. Naismith DJ. Br J Nutr 1973;30:567–76.

189. Linscheer WG, Vergroesen AJ, Lipids. In: *Modern Nutrition in Health and Disease*, 8th ed. Shils ME, Olson JA, Shike M, eds Lea and Febiger, Philadelphia, 1994.

SELECTED READINGS

Chawla A, Repa JJ, Evans RM et al. Nuclear receptors and lipid physiology: opening the X-files. Science 2001; 2941866–70.

Din JN, Newby DE, Flapan AD.Omega 3 fatty acids and cardiovascular disease: fishing for a natural treatment. BMJ 2004;328:30–5.

Grundy SM, Abate N, Chandalia M. Diet composition and the metabolic syndrome: what is the optimal fat intake? Am J Med 2002;113:25–9.

Innis SM. Essential dietary lipids. In: Ziegler EE, Filer LJ, eds. Present Knowledge in Nutrition. 7th ed. Washington, DC: ILSI Press, 1996: 58–66.

Jequier E, Bray GA. Low-fat diets are preferred. Am J Med 2002;113: 41–6.

Masson LF, McNeill G, Avenell A. Genetic variation and the lipid response to dietary intervention: a systematic review. Am J Clin Nutr 2003;77:1098–111.

6 CHOLESTEROL AND OTHER DIETARY STEROLS[1]

DAVID KRITCHEVSKY

CHOLESTEROL 123
    Atherosclerosis 124
    Influence of Fat Structure 127
    Influence of *Trans* Unsaturated Fat 127
    Influence of Protein 128
    Influence of Carbohydrate 129
    Influence of Fiber 129
PHYTOSTEROLS 130
    Effect on Cholesterolemia 130
    Toxicity Studies 131

CHOLESTEROL

Cholesterol is probably the physiologically important compound with which the general public is most acquainted. If one were to subject the "average person" to a word association test, the words associated with cholesterol would be bad, unhealthy, and dangerous. This negative image of cholesterol is the result of its relation to coronary disease. In fact, cholesterol is not only one of the most widely disseminated compounds present in the body but also one of the most important. Its relationship to coronary disease is, in many instances, statistical; its absolute necessity for maintenance of life is real. In 1903, an editorial in the *Journal of the American Medical Association* was devoted to cholesterol (then called cholesterin). The editorial stated that cholesterin was "one of the most inert of body constituents and it seems impossible that it plays any part in metabolic processes" (1). Accrual of our present knowledge of cholesterol has been stimulated by discovery of its presence in the arteries.

In 1815, Chevreul showed that cholesterol could be differentiated from other biologic waxes by virtue of its being unsaponifiable. Chevreul also gave the molecule its original name, cholesterine (Greek: *chole*, bile; *stereos*, solid). After the substance was shown to contain a hydroxyl group, its name was changed to the more descriptive cholesterol.

The pathway of cholesterol biosynthesis was elucidated through the brilliant work of Bloch, Lynen, Popjak, Cornforth, and their colleagues. The pattern of biosynthesis was beginning to appear at the time the first book on cholesterol was written in 1958 (2), and precise knowledge of the biosynthetic scheme was available by the time the best book on cholesterol appeared in 1981 (3). All 27 carbon atoms of cholesterol are derived from the two carbon atoms of acetate. Fifteen of cholesterol's carbons come from the methyl group and 12 from the carboxyl group. Fusion of three acetate residues produces β-hydroxy β-methylglutaryl (HMG) coenzyme A (CoA). HMG-CoA is reduced to give the six carbon acid, mevalonic acid. This conversion of HMG-CoA is a rate-limiting step in cholesterol biosynthesis. Mevalonate phosphate is converted to isopentenyl pyrophosphate, which is isomerized to 3,3-dimethallyl pyrophosphate. Isopentenyl pyrophosphate and 3,3-dimethallyl pyrophosphate combine to give to a ten carbon atom isoprenoid, geranyl pyrophosphate. Addition of another five carbon unit provides the 15 carbon atom farnesyl pyrophosphate. Fusion of two farnesyl units gives the 30 carbon atom hydrocarbon, squalene. Squalene is cyclyzed to give a 30 carbon atom steroid, lanosterol. This cyclization is another control point in cholesterol biosynthesis. Lanosterol is a hydroxysteroid, containing two double bonds. Three methyl groups are oxidized, one double bond is hydrogenated and one isomerized to yield the 3 β-hydroxy Δ^5steroid, cholesterol. The last unknown enzyme of mammalian cholesterol biosynthesis, 3-ketosteroid reductase, has only recently been identified (4). The level of effort that was expended to elucidate the cholesterol synthetic pathway in the 1940s is now being applied toward understanding the molecular biology of cholesterol synthesis and cellular transport. We now know that lipid synthesis is regulated by sterol regulatory element-binding proteins that activate the expression of more than 30 genes controlling cholesterol synthesis and uptake of fatty acids, triglycerides, and phospholipids.

Cholesterol is an integral component of the membrane of every cell. In addition, it is the precursor of the bile acids, pregnenolone, progesterone, corticosteroids, sex hormones, and vitamin D. Cholesterol represents about 0.2% of total body weight. The brain and central nervous

---

[1]**Abbreviations: ABC,** adenosine triphosphate-binding cassette; **ApoA,** apolipoprotein A; **ApoB,** apolipoprotein B; **ApoE,** apolipoprotein E; **CLA,** conjugated linoleic acid; **CoA,** coenzyme A; **HDL,** high-density lipoprotein; **HDL-C,** high density lipoprotein cholesterol; **HMG,** hydroxymethyl glutaric acid; **IDL,** intermediate-density lipoprotein; **LDL,** low-density lipoprotein; **LDL-C,** low-density lipoprotein cholesterol; **TC,** total cholesterol; **VLDL,** very-low-density lipoprotein.

system, connective tissue, muscle, and skin account for about 75% of the body cholesterol. Its function there is principally that of an insulator, but work on metabolism of brain cholesterol is beginning to appear. There is some evidence that 24-hydroxycholesterol (cerebrosterol) levels in the brain are correlated with Alzheimer disease (5). The cholesterol in muscle is largely inert. The cholesterol pool on which so much emotional and intellectual energy has been expended (blood and liver) represents a small fraction (~10%) of the body pool. Our conception of the role of cholesterol in the cell membrane is expanding. The cell membrane contains mainly cholesterol and phospholipids, and its role was initially thought to be structural, namely, in maintaining the rigidity of the fluid membrane.

Plasma membrane cholesterol is not evenly distributed, but rather localized in cholesterol-rich and cholesterol-poor domains. Cholesterol is involved in lipid raft assembly. Lipid rafts consist of cholesterol sandwiched between sphingomyelin and glycosylphosphatidyl inositol and appear in the exoplasmic leaflet of the membrane bilayer. Each raft can incorporate specific proteins and dictate the extent of their lateral diffusion to the cell surface as well as to other organelles. There is evidence that lipid rafts are involved in signaling cascades and in the immune response (6, 7). There is still much to learn concerning cholesterol movement in membranes and the physiologic consequences thereof.

Studies by Mueller, conducted in 1915 and 1916, suggested that dietary fat was necessary for absorption of dietary cholesterol (8, 9). However, the observation that crystalline cholesterol, when fed to rabbits, led to severe atherosclerosis (10) showed that fat was not essential for cholesterol absorption. Bile, however, is obligatory for cholesterol absorption (11). Cholesterol is absorbed via micelles (12), which also contain bile acids, phospholipid, monoglycerides, and free fatty acids. In the course of digestion, dietary triglycerides are partially hydrolyzed and absorbed as 2-monoglycerides (13). The micelle reaches the mucosal cell membrane, where it is disaggregated, and the cholesterol is taken up by the enterocyte. Initially, cholesterol appears in the blood as a component of chylomicrons, relatively large lipoprotein entities that are principally composed of triglycerides. Very-low-density lipoproteins (VLDLs), whose source is also the intestine,

contain triglycerides and free and esterified cholesterol. The VLDLs are metabolized to intermediate-density lipoprotein (IDL) and low-density lipoprotein (LDL). As the triglyceride levels diminish, the density of the particles increases. The high-density lipoproteins (HDLs) are derived primarily from the liver and intestine; HDL_2 contains about 33% protein, and HDL_3 contains 57% protein. Human serum also carries a small quantity of albumin-bound free fatty acids. The characteristics of the lipoproteins are summarized in Table 6.1.

The apolipoproteins have specific physiologic functions. The ratio of apolipoprotein A (ApoA) to ApoB is often measured as a risk factor for coronary heart disease. Polymorphism of ApoE appears to influence chances for successful treatment of hyperlipidemia. The ApoE alleles are designated E2, E3, and E4. The most common pattern is homozygosity for E3 (E3/E3 phenotype). There is evidence that subjects bearing the E4 allele have higher cholesterol levels than those with the E3/E3 pattern. The characteristics of the apolipoproteins are summarized in Table 6.2 (see also Chapter 66).

The mechanisms whereby cholesterol actually reaches the cell have been examined for several decades. The discovery of adenosine triphosphate–binding cassette (ABC) transporters, sterol transport molecules present in the surface cells of the intestine, may help to explain the mode of intracellular cholesterol movement. These transporters are members of a large family of membrane proteins that transport various substances across cell membranes. The cassette transporters associated principally with sterol movement are ABCA-1, 5, and 6. This area of research is proliferating. Wenzel and associates (14) reported cloning an additional subfamily of ABC transporters and described ABCA-10, an ABCA-6–like transporter. Cholesterol-binding proteins have been identified in the enterocyte brush border membrane (15). These proteins differ from the ABC family and suggest multiple regulated pathways of cholesterol transport.

Atherosclerosis

The observation that cholesterol is a constituent of the atherosclerotic plaque is more than 150 years old. Early

TABLE 6.1. CHARACTERISTICS OF MAJOR LIPOPROTEIN CLASSES

LIPOPROTEIN	DENSITY (g/dL)	MOL. WT. DALTON $\times 10^6$	DIAMETER (nm)	LIPID (%)		
				TG	CHOL	PL
CM	0.95	400	75–1200	80–95	2–7	3–9
VLDL	0.95–1.006	10–80	30–80	55–85	5–15	10–20
IDL	1.006–1.019	5–10	18–25	5–15	40–50	20–25
LDL	1.014–1.063	2.3	18–25	5–15	40–50	20–25
HDL	1.063–1.21	0.17–0.36	5–12	5–10	15–25	20–30

CHOL, cholesterol; CM, chylomicron; HDL, high-density lipoprotein; IDL, intermediate-density lipoprotein; LDL, low-density lipoprotein; PL, phospholipid; TG, triglyceride; VLDL, very-low-density lipoprotein.

TABLE 6.2. MAJOR APOLIPOPROTEINS AND THEIR FUNCTION

APOLIPROTEIN	MOLECULAR WEIGHT[a] (daltons)	RELATED LIPOPROTEIN	FUNCTION
ApoAI	28,000	CM, HDL	Structure; activate LCAT
ApoAII	17,000	CM, HDL	?
ApoAIV	46,500	CM, HDL	?
ApoB48	264,000	CM	Formation of chylomicrons
ApoB100	540,000	VLDL, IDL, LDL	Assembly and secretion of VLDL; structure of VLDL, IDL, LDL; ligand for LDL receptor
ApoCI	6,630	CM, VLDL, IDL, HDL	?
ApoCII	8,900	CM, VLDL, IDL, HDL	Activates lipoprotein lipase
ApoCIII	8,800	CM, VLDL, IDL, HDL	Inhibits lipoprotein lipases
ApoE	34,000	CM, VLDL, IDL, HDL	Ligand for binding to LDL receptors

Apo, apolipoprotein; CM, chylomicron; HDL, high-density lipoprotein; IDL, intermediate-density lipoprotein; LCAT, lecithin-cholesterol acyltransferase; LDL, low-density lipoprotein; VLDL, very-low-density lipoprotein.
[a] Approximate.

studies of the chemistry of normal aortas and atherosclerotic lesions from diseased aortas confirmed the presence of cholesterol.

Early attempts to induce atherosclerosis in rabbits combined diet and physical trauma. Using diet alone, early workers established aortic lesions by feeding cholesterol-rich fatty foods, but the use of pure cholesterol as the nutritional stimulus established it as the putative causative agent. Establishment of atherosclerosis in rats, dogs, monkeys, and chickens using cholesterol-rich diets with or without physiologic manipulation further established the idea that cholesterol was the initiator of atherosclerosis. Libby and colleagues (16) reviewed the role of cholesterol in atherogenesis.

Theories regarding the genesis of atherosclerotic lesions have paralleled the development of the field. It is accepted currently that atherosclerosis has its origins in inflammation (17). Atherosclerosis is characterized by aortic accumulation of lipids as well as other chemical entities. Oxidation products of LDL are readily taken up by macrophages to form the foam cells that characterize the atherosclerotic plaque (18). Oxidized LDL, rather than LDL per se, is now regarded as a prime inducer of the atherosclerotic process. The early view of simple lipid infiltration has given way to a complex series of reactions involving an array of adhesion molecules, growth factors, cytokines, and lipases, to name but a few. Lusis (19) reviewed the process based on current knowledge, and Blankenberg and associates (20) reviewed the various adhesion molecules and clarified the involvement of these molecules in the atherogenic process.

The relationship of cholesterol to the atherosclerotic process provided a springboard for studies of effects of blood and dietary cholesterol on progression of this disease. In animal studies, the effects of experimental procedures can be seen readily on necropsy, but in humans, progress is still measured externally, that is, through plasma lipids, lipoproteins, or other factors. The rapid advances being made in the area of noninvasive measurement of atherosclerosis should soon make it possible to follow treatment effects directly in vivo.

Assessment of serum lipid levels was originally used to follow treatment (dietary or pharmacologic effects). In 1950, Gofman and colleagues (21) demonstrated that blood lipids could be separated ultracentrifugally into a family of lipoprotein molecules depending on their hydrated density. This major lipoprotein classes are chylomicron, VLDL, IDL, LDL, and HDL (see Table 6.1). Elevated LDL is considered to be a major risk factor for coronary disease, and HDL, which is active in removal of cholesterol from cells, is a major protective factor in atherosclerosis. Assessment of risk may be done by measuring total cholesterol (TC) or LDL cholesterol (LDL-C) or the ratios TC/LDL-C, TC/HDL-C, or LDL-C/HDL-C. Molecular size dictates the ease with which lipoprotein molecules may enter the arterial wall (22). In human studies, small dense particles of LDL have been associated with a threefold increased risk of myocardial infarction (23).

Diagnosis of coronary risk depends on measurement of total serum or plasma cholesterol. Individual blood cholesterol levels vary seasonally over the course of the year (24), with elevations occurring during the winter months. Based on their observations in the Jerusalem Lipid Clinic, Harlap and associates (25) wrote: ". . . clinicians should take season into account when diagnosing hyperlipidemia and evaluating success or failure of its treatment." Gordon and colleagues (26) examined seasonal variations of plasma lipids and lipoproteins in the 1446 hypercholesterolemic men who comprised the placebo group in the Lipid Research Clinics Coronary Primary Prevention Trial. They found that total and LDL-C levels were significantly and inversely correlated with hours of daylight and that HDL-C levels varied significantly and positively with ambient temperature. These investigators concluded, "while the etiological mechanisms of seasonal plasma lipid and lipoprotein remain uncertain, there can no longer be any doubt that these cycles exist." These observations in no way reduce the importance of serum cholesterol as a risk factor and may possibly explain some apparently anomalous findings. Mustad and associates (27) reinvestigated this phenomenon and reported diet-independent seasonal variations in both young men who consumed a highly controlled experimental diet and in nonintervention controls.

Responses to dietary cholesterol vary broadly. Katan and colleagues (28) described hyporesponding and hyperresponding subjects. Hopkins (29) offered evidence that the range of human responsiveness may vary from zero to 100%. Sehayek and associates (30) described the U-shaped relationship between plasma lipoprotein levels and changes in dietary cholesterol absorption. Their findings emphasize the large interindividual variation in human dietary cholesterol absorption. These observations argue against the possibility of formulating a simple, all-inclusive guideline for the public.

Do elevated blood cholesterol levels represent a major risk factor throughout the life span? One view, based on the observation that 85% of deaths attributable to coronary heart disease occur in persons more than 65 years old (31), is that blood cholesterol levels should be monitored at all ages (32). In subjects older than 85 years, high TC has been associated with longevity (33). Schatz and colleagues (34) reported on cholesterol levels and all-cause mortality in elderly participants in the Honolulu Heart Program. They studied 3572 Japanese-American men aged 71 to 93 years, grouped by quartile of serum cholesterol level. There were roughly the same number of individuals in each quartile. The cholesterol levels per quartile were 149, 178, 199, and 232 mg/dL. The age-adjusted relative risk of coronary disease in the four quartiles was 1.0, 0.72, 0.60, and 0.65. These investigators advised a prudent approach to treatment in this age group.

The relationship between very low blood cholesterol levels and noncoronary deaths requires further investigation. A review (35) of a large number of trials, yielding 68,406 deaths, found that men whose blood cholesterol levels were less than 160 mg/dL (4.14 mmol/L) exhibited 20% more cancer deaths, 35% more deaths from injury, 40% more noncancer, noncardiovascular deaths, and 50% more deaths from digestive system disease. Risk of death surfaced during the course of the trials and not afterward, a finding suggesting metabolic problems that may have appeared during the course of therapy. The first large lipid-lowering trial that did not show an excess of noncoronary deaths was a large study using a statin drug (Simvastatin) (36). The problem seems to be related to cholesterol levels within a population because some populations normally exhibit cholesterol levels around 160 mg/dL, but no excess of cancer death.

The findings that risk of heart disease was associated with elevated blood cholesterol levels, coupled with the animal data, spurred interest in a connection between dietary and blood cholesterol and the risk of coronary disease. A reasonable assumption would be that high levels of dietary cholesterol inevitably lead to elevations in blood cholesterol. The data do not totally bear out this hypothesis. In 1950, Gertler and associates (37) segregated, from a large study, four groups of ten men each coming from the control group and from the group with coronary disease, respectively. The four groups represented the men with the highest or lowest serum cholesterol levels or the men who ate the most or least cholesterol. In every subgroup, the men with coronary disease exhibited significantly higher cholesterol levels than the controls, but in no group was there an apparent relationship between dietary and blood cholesterol. These data suggest that elevated serum cholesterol represents a risk factor but that level of cholesterol intake may not. Dawber and colleagues (38) found no correlation between cholesterol intake and serum cholesterol levels in the Framingham study, a finding confirming an earlier observation made in the course of that study. Gordon and colleagues (39) analyzed and compared the diets of men who did or did not exhibit overt coronary disease in three large prospective studies of heart disease: Framingham, Puerto Rico, and Honolulu. In all three venues, intake of cholesterol and the saturation level of dietary fat were the same in the groups with or without overt coronary disease. An exhaustive review of the effects of dietary cholesterol on human cholesterolemia and atherosclerosis found that a 100 mg/day change in dietary cholesterol resulted in an average change of 2.2 to 2.5 mg/dL in plasma TC level with a 1.9 mg/dL change in LDL-C and a 0.4 mg/dL change in HDL-C (40). A problem in discussions of cholesterol and heart disease is the interchanging reference to cholesterol in the diet and that in the blood. Whereas the cholesterol in the diet does not usually have a significant effect on blood cholesterol, the fat in the diet has profound effects on cholesterol levels in humans and on atherosclerosis in experimental animals.

In 1953, Keys (41) described atherosclerosis as a new public health problem and presented data in which the level of dietary fat in the diet was positively correlated with prevalence of heart disease in several populations. At that time, the emphasis was on amount, and not type of fat. Ahrens and associates (42) fed subjects a formula diet that contained 45% of energy as carbohydrate, 40% as fat, and 15% as protein. These investigators found that plasma cholesterol levels rose as fat saturation increased. McNamara and associates (43) fed normal subjects diets containing low (192–288 mg) or high (820–863 mg) levels of cholesterol and either saturated or unsaturated fat. The differences in plasma cholesterol levels in subjects fed polyunsaturated fat and low or high cholesterol was 2.8% and in those on saturated fat it was 2.1%. However, the differences in cholesterol levels between subjects fed low cholesterol and saturated or unsaturated fat was 11.5%, and on the high-cholesterol regimen it was 10.7%. Thus, the fat saturation influence was shown to be about four times stronger than the effect of dietary cholesterol.

In 1965, Keys (44) and Hegsted (45) and their colleagues devised formulas for predicting effects of changes in dietary fats on cholesterol levels. Generally, saturated fat had a positive coefficient and unsaturated fat a negative one. Stearic acid was regarded as neutral, and no effect was attributed to monounsaturated fat. Although many other such formulas have been published, those of Keys and Hegsted are still the ones referred to most often. Müller and colleagues (46) reviewed the many predicting equations and produced one of their own that, in addition to the usual array of fatty acid coefficients, contains coefficients for *trans* unsaturated fatty acids derived from hydrogenated vegetable or fish oils. These investigators concluded that myristic acid (14:0) is the most hypercholesterolemic fatty acid. They also showed that *trans* fatty acids are less hypercholesterolemic than either myristic (14:0) or palmitic (16:0) acids.

Hayes and Khosla (47) suggested that the two most important fatty acids relating to cholesterol levels are myristic acid, which is hypercholesterolemic at any concentration, and linoleic acid, which exerts an increasingly hypolipidemic effect until it reaches a dietary level of 6 to 7% of energy. After reviewing data from 420 dietary observations, Hegsted and colleagues (48) concluded that saturated fatty acids are the principal determinants of cholesterolemia. Thus, from the viewpoint of dietary fat, all other nutritional components being equal, saturated fat is regarded as the principal effector of cholesterolemia. Aside from putative effects on cholesterolemia, saturated fatty acids play important roles in other aspects of physiology. Thus, saturated fatty acids are necessary components of the physiologic economy, and their overall biologic role should be assessed accordingly.

Influence of Fat Structure

The structure of a fat may influence its atherogenicity without appreciably affecting cholesterolemia. Lard and tallow contain virtually the same amount of palmitic acid (24%), but in lard more than 90% of the palmitic acid is at the sn-2 position, whereas in tallow less then 15% of palmitic acid is at sn-2. When native lard or tallow is fed to rabbits as part of an atherogenic regimen, the diet containing lard is significantly more atherogenic. Randomization of lard and tallow provides two new fats each carrying about 8% of its palmitic acid complement at the sn-2 position. The two new fats are of equal atherogenicity (49). Randomization is a chemical process in which the fatty acids of a triglyceride are rearranged to provide a new fat in which every component fatty acid is present at each position of the glyceride to approximately one-third its total content. Cottonseed oil and palm oil carry most of their palmitic acid at the sn-1 and sn-3 positions. Randomization of either fat results in a new fat with a greater concentration of its palmitic acid at sn-2. Randomized cottonseed (50) or palm (51) oils are more atherogenic than

their native counterparts. A study using synthetic triglycerides has also shown the increased atherogenic potential of fats containing palmitic acid at the sn-2 position. There were no effects on serum lipids or on lipoprotein size (52).

Influence of *Trans* Unsaturated Fat

The double bonds in most naturally occurring unsaturated fats are in the *cis* configuration (see Chapter 5). However, *trans* double bonds do occur in certain plants, in milk, and in the body fat of ruminants. The principal source of dietary *trans* fatty acids in the developed world is as a component of the partially hydrogenated fats that are present in the processed fats in our diet. In the 1940s, it was discovered that hydrogenation of fats could be controlled to produce fats of varying physical properties that, in turn, would offer a variety of uses in commercial food preparation. The possible physiologic consequences of ingesting *trans* fat were a subject of concern as early as the 1940s. When fed as part of an adequate fat regimen, *trans* fats do not affect growth (53) or reproduction (54) in rats. When fed as sole source of fat, they exaggerate the symptoms of essential fat deficiency (55). *Trans* fat in a diet should be balanced with linoleic or another essential fatty acid. Hydrogenation of fat yields fatty acids with double bonds, *cis* and *trans*, at every fatty acid position from C4 to C16, so we are dealing with a heterogeneous material, and few data are available regarding effects of *cis* or *trans* double bonds at specific positions. Intake of *trans* fats of animal origin (usually 16:1t) has not been correlated with cardiovascular disease (56). Moreover, the deodorization process used in the manufacture of commercially available oils and fats yields a small amount of *trans* fat (57, 58).

Conjugated linoleic acid (CLA) is an all-inclusive term for a number of naturally occurring isomers of linoleic acid containing conjugated double bonds, both *cis* and *trans*. CLA occurs in the rumen of cows and other ruminants and in their milk and products thereof (e.g., cheese, yogurt). Dietary CLA reduces the incidence of chemically induced (59, 60) or transplanted (61) tumors in mice and rats and also reduces atherogenesis in rabbits (62, 63) and hamsters (64). Most naturally occurring CLA is in the form of the *cis*9,*trans*11 isomer, but the commercial product contains equal quantities (~45%) of the *cis*9,*trans*11, and *trans*10,*cis*12 isomers. The definition of what constitutes a health-threatening *trans* fat will have to be very precise.

Trans fats are transported in the body much like their *cis* counterparts. They are deposited in most body tissues, the level of deposition being proportional to the amount present in the diet, and they disappear from the tissues when the dietary *trans* fat stimulus is removed (65). Mitochondrial oxidation of *trans* fatty acids is slower than for the corresponding *cis* isomers (66) and desaturation and elongation proceed more slowly with *trans* fats (67). Cholesteryl esters of *trans* fatty acids are synthesized (68) and hydrolyzed (69) more slowly than with *cis* fatty acids. Deleterious effects of *trans* fatty acids on mitochondrial function in rats are negated if the diet contains sufficient linoleic acid (70).

Public health concerns over the possibly deleterious effects of *trans* fats in humans surfaced again in the 1980s and 1990s, and in both instances expert committees convened in the United States and Great Britain concluded that the levels then in current use posed no problems (71–74).

Numerous studies of the effects of *trans* fat on human cholesterolemia have been conducted, with varying results. Using published data, Emken (75) recalculated the findings relative to the levels of *trans* fat and linoleic acid in the diet and found that as the *trans* fat/linoleic acid ratio fell, so did cholesterolemia. Thus, when the *trans* fat/linoleic acid ratio was 2.45, plasma cholesterol levels rose by 21%; when the ratio was 0.35, the cholesterol levels only rose by 4%. In a graph that has become an icon, Ascherio and associates (76) showed that as the percentage of dietary *trans* fat increases, there is a significant linear upward trend in the ratio of LDL to HDL and hence an increase in risk. If one uses the same data and plots LDL-C/HDL-C against the percentage of dietary linoleic acid, a significant linear downward trend is seen.

Human data show that increase of dietary *trans* fat increases risk factors for coronary disease. Experimental data show that although *trans* fats significantly raise plasma cholesterol, they do not affect severity of atherosclerosis. This observation is true for rabbits fed atherogenic diets containing cholesterol (77) or free of cholesterol (78), as well as for monkeys fed cholesterol-free diets (79). Elson and colleagues (80) fed pigs seven different diets in which the fat content was 17%; the percentage of *trans* fat ranged from 0 to 48%. After 10 months, the average serum cholesterol of the control group, fed 17% saturated fat but no *trans* fat, was only 0 to 8% lower than cholesterol levels of the other six groups. Only five of 64 pigs (from three different groups) exhibited aortic sudanophilia covering more than 2% of the aortic surface.

The intake of *trans* fat in the United States was 7.70 g/person/day in 1970 and 7.55 g/person/day in 1980 (81). In that time span, age adjusted, all-cause mortality in the United States fell by 7% and heart disease deaths fell by 20% (82). These data do not bespeak an epidemic. A survey published in 1999 estimated the average per capita intake of *trans* fat in the United States population to be 5.3 g *trans* fatty acids per day, amounting to 2.6% of total energy intake (83). Innis and colleagues (84) pointed out that the wide variability in the *trans* fatty content of different foods may result in large errors in estimation of *trans* fatty acid intake.

Trans fats represent a small fraction of our fat intake and should not divert our attention from the broader aspects of fat and health. In an article published in 2003, Mensink and associates (85) asserted that although their findings relating to *trans* fat and other dietary effects on blood chemistry are consistent, they tell nothing about the actual individual effects of these findings on coronary disease, which must await human trials.

Influence of Protein

Dietary constituents other than fat also affect cholesterol metabolism. The first purely nutritional experimental atherosclerosis study was carried out by Ignatowski in 1908 (86). He hypothesized that animal protein per se was atherogenic. When he fed weanling rabbits milk and eggs, the animals were rendered atherosclerotic. His studies were carried out at the same time that Anitschkow and others were achieving experimental atherosclerosis by feeding cholesterol. Many concluded that the atherogenic ingredient in Ignatowski's diet was the cholesterol present in the eggs and milk, not the protein. Thus, the protein aspect was eclipsed, and it has not yet fully emerged from the shadow of cholesterol and fat.

Meeker and Kesten (87, 88) were the first to compare directly the effects of casein (animal) and soy (vegetable) protein on atherosclerosis in rabbits. The diet containing soy protein was significantly less atherogenic. Carroll and Hamilton (89) compared blood cholesterol levels in rabbits, fed semipurified diets containing 30% protein for 28 days. These investigators compared 12 proteins and found that the cholesterol levels in rabbits ranged from 235 mg/dL (6.08 mmol/L) (extracted whole egg) to 15 mg/dL (0.39 mmol/L) (soy protein isolate). Huff and associates (90) fed rabbits casein, an enzymatic hydrolysate of casein or a pure amino acid mixture approximating the amino acid composition of casein. After 28 days, the plasma cholesterol levels of the casein-and casein amino acid–fed groups were the same, whereas the cholesterol level of the hydrolyzate-fed rabbits was lower by 16%. In rabbits fed similar soy protein preparations, the hydrolyzate lowered plasma cholesterol by 41% (compared with intact soy protein), whereas the amino acid mixture raised cholesterol levels by 80%. Experiments with other amino acid mixtures led to the conclusion that the differences in cholesterolemia were the result of differences in digestion and absorption of the proteins. Kritchevsky (91) had speculated that the different effects on cholesterolemia of animal and vegetable protein were the result of the lysine/arginine ratio, which is higher in animal than in vegetable protein. Comparison was made of three animal proteins that had similar lysine content, but different arginine levels (92). The severity of atherosclerosis increased significantly as the lysine/arginine ratio rose. Because the lysine levels of the three proteins were similar, the result is caused by other amino acid variations.

Huff and Carroll (93) investigated the mechanisms underlying the protein effects and found that in rabbits, cholesterol was absorbed to a greater extent on a casein diet, but cholesterol oxidation and turnover were higher when soy protein was fed. Sugano and associates (94) reported that casein-rich diets lead to increases in serum insulin, but not glucagon, in rats. The glucagon level was increased proportionately with increasing levels of dietary arginine. These investigators concluded that insulin was associated with protein effects on serum lipids.

In 1957, Yerushalmy and Hilleboe (95), using the same data set from which Keys (41) had shown the strong relationship between dietary fat and atherosclerosis, pointed out an even stronger positive correlation between animal protein intake and the incidence of coronary heart disease.

Influence of Carbohydrate

In 1974, Grande (96) summarized the effects of sugars on serum lipids and cardiovascular disease. In normocholesterolemic individuals, substitution of complex carbohydrates for sucrose led to reduction of serum cholesterol levels. This could result from specific sugars or dietary fiber. Studies of carbohydrate effects in hyperlipidemic subjects have concentrated on triglyceride levels. In 1957, Yudkin hypothesized that sucrose consumption was a critical factor in the development of heart disease (97). Reviews by Walker (98) and Keys (99) pointed out that the theory was not supported by data. However, because so many aspects of diet and heart disease keep recycling, we should not be surprised if the sucrose-heart disease theory resurfaces. In general, the roles of carbohydrates in cholesterol metabolism and atherosclerosis have received less attention than have roles of other major nutrients.

Studies of carbohydrate effects on serum lipids have been concerned mainly with effects on triglycerides. In the early 1960s, serum triglyceride levels were proposed as risk factors for atherosclerosis (100, 101). Several investigators had observed that human subjects on a low-fat, high-carbohydrate diet showed little or no change in serum cholesterol, but very large increases in triglycerides. In 1985, Carlson and Böttiger (102) reported a 19-year follow-up of the Stockholm Prospective Study and still found serum triglyceride levels to be an independent risk factor for heart disease. Several more recent studies also showed elevated fasting triglyceride levels to be a strong risk factor for cardiovascular disease (103–105). The new interest in the role of triglyceride-rich lipoproteins in the development of coronary heart disease has been reviewed (106, 107). In 1988, Reaven (108) described syndrome X, which is characterized by insulin resistance, glucose intolerance, hypertension, hypertriglyceridemia, and upper body obesity. This group of symptoms is now referred to as the metabolic syndrome (109) (see also Chapter 62).

In rabbits fed cholesterol-free diets, sucrose and fructose were found to be more atherogenic than glucose or lactose (110, 111). Fructose feeding yielded the highest serum cholesterol levels and most severe atherosclerosis. In vervet monkeys fed a semipurified-cholesterol-free diet, fructose and sucrose were more cholesterolemic than

glucose. Fructose led to more severe aortic sudanophilia than either glucose or sucrose (112). Baboons fed the same diets (113) exhibited similar cholesterol levels in all groups but higher triglycerides in animals fed fructose or sucrose. When lactose was the dietary carbohydrate, neither lipemia nor aortic sudanophilia was affected in the absence of cholesterol. However, when cholesterol (0.1%) was added to the same high-carbohydrate diets, the lactose-fed baboons exhibited the highest serum cholesterol levels and significant levels of atherosclerosis (114). The levels of lactose fed in experimental studies are far greater than one finds in the human diet. However, a follow-up of the studies cited earlier could provide insights regarding carbohydrate effects on cholesterol metabolism.

Segall (115) reviewed the connection between lactose intake and atherosclerosis. He analyzed international statistical data relative to the intake of dairy products (butter, cheeses, milk) and ischemic heart disease and found the positive correlation greater for milk than for dairy fat. Segall pointed out that prevalence of lactose intolerance in a population correlated negatively with heart disease incidence. Segall is not the first investigator to suggest a causative role for milk in cardiovascular disease, but the first to target lactose specifically.

In humans, whole or skim milk and yogurt have been reported to exhibit hypocholesterolemic properties (116–118). African tribesmen such as the Masai ingest large quantities of milk and are not hypercholesterolemic. Ness and associates (119) provided evidence that milk consumption does not correlate with increased risk of coronary heart disease.

McLachlan (120) has proposed that β-casein A^1 is the milk component that leads to lipidemia and atherosclerosis. African cattle produce milk containing β-casein A^2 (121), which does not have the atherogenic potential of β-casein A^1–rich milks, and that may explain the lack of atherosclerosis in those African communities (Masai tribes, Samburu, Gambia) consuming large quantities of milk. The two casein variants differ in that β-casein A^1 carries a histidine residue at position 67, whereas β-casein A^2 has a proline at that position. β-Casein A^1 can be metabolized to release β-casomorphine, a heptapeptide (positions 60–66), whereas β-casein A^2 cannot, presumably because of the exchange of proline for histidine. Laugesen and Elliott (122), in a study of 20 affluent countries, correlated β-casein A^1 presence in milk with rates of ischemic heart disease and type 1 diabetes. No official guidelines are available relating to sugar intake as it may affect coronary disease (123, 124), but moderation in sugar intake is usually advised.

Influence of Fiber

What we refer to as dietary fiber has been discussed in the medical literature from the time of Hippocrates, and probably earlier. Most references were related to its laxative properties. In more recent times, fiber was called "roughage," and again laxation was the point of reference. The modern fiber era dates to the work of Surgeon Captain T.L. Cleave, whose article in the *Journal of the Royal Naval Med Services* in 1956 (125) defined the framework of the "fiber hypothesis." His work was popularized by the writings of Burkitt, Trowell, and Walker, which laid the groundwork for medical interest in fiber.

The basic definition of dietary fiber—material of plant origin indigestible by endogenous digestive systems—is still being debated as oligosaccharides and synthetic materials are shown to have fiber-like physiologic properties (see Chapter 4). The definition has expanded from major structural components of the cell wall (cellulose, noncellulose polysaccharides, pectic substances, and lignin) and now includes pectin, gums, mucilages, algal polysaccharides, and modified celluloses. There is still no total agreement whether the definition should be based on structure or function or origin or something in between. The first few chapters of Spiller's book on dietary fiber (126) are devoted to description of materials we call dietary fiber or other substances that exert fiber-like action. A satisfactory all-encompassing definition is not yet available.

Kritchevsky and Story (127) summarized the influences of dietary fiber on cholesterol metabolism in experimental animals. In most instances, 2.5 to 10% fiber was added to a semipurified diet. In rats, the soluble fibers—pectin, guar gum, locust bean gum, oat bran, and carrageenan—were hypocholesterolemic, but insoluble fibers such as cellulose, hemicellulose, and alfalfa were not. Soluble fibers are also hypocholesterolemic for guinea pigs and chickens.

Jenkins and colleagues (128) reviewed fiber effects on lipidemia in human subjects and found the viscous fibers such as pectin, guar, locust bean gum, and oat bran, as well as dried beans, lowered serum TC and LDL levels when these substances were fed to provide 12 to –30 g fiber daily. In discussing specific dietary fibers, these investigators cited data showing that lignin may have some hypolipidemic capacity, but cellulose has none. Pectin, regardless of origin (e.g., citrus pectin, apple pectin) is uniformly hypocholesterolemic, as is guar gum.

Several mechanisms by which fiber exerts a hypolipidemic effect have been suggested. These include altered site and rate of absorption, loss of bile acids resulting from their binding to fiber, and reduced postprandial glucose and insulin responses.

Because a requirement for dietary fiber has been generally accepted, research efforts in that area have waned. Most effort now is directed toward means of introducing fiber in the diet rather than investigations into mechanisms of action.

PHYTOSTEROLS

Plant sterols (phytosterols) are related structurally to cholesterol (Fig. 6.1) and probably perform in plants a function

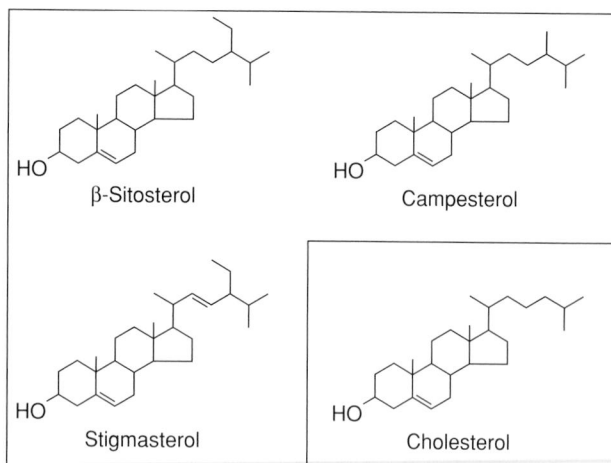

Figure 6.1. Structure of cholesterol and other sterols.

similar to one of cholesterol's roles in animals, namely, preserving cell structure. Phytosterols have a steroid nucleus with a hydroxyl group at the 3β position and a double bond between carbon atoms 5 and 6. The major phytosterols resemble cholesterol except for substitutions and/or double bonds in the side chain.

β-Sitosterol (24α-ethylcholesterol) comprises 45 to 95% of the total sterols of edible plants, campesterol (24α-methylcholesterol) accounts for up to 30% of the total sterol of seed oils, and stigmasterol (Δ^{22},24α-ethylcholesterol) is also a prominent component of seed oils. Sitosterol occurs in most plant oils, soybean oil being a particularly rich source. Tall oil (pine oil) is a major source of sitostanol. Ergosterol ($\Delta^{7,22}$,24α-methylcholesterol) is the principal sterol of yeast (96–100%) and is present in significant amounts in corn, cottonseed, peanut, and linseed oils. The unabsorbability of phytosterols was first observed in 1912.

Effect on Cholesterolemia

Peterson and associates (129) showed that addition of 1% phytosterols to the diet of chickens being fed 1% cholesterol brought their serum cholesterol levels into the normal range. They also showed (130) that addition of 1.3% soy sterol to a diet containing 1% cholesterol inhibited atherogenesis in chicks and that the lowering of serum cholesterol followed a dose-response relationship (131). Mattson and colleagues (132) reported that phytosterol esters inhibited cholesterol absorption as effectively as did free phytosterols. Phytosterols bearing methyl groups at the 4 position do not inhibit cholesterol absorption (133). It is generally accepted that the hypocholesterolemic action of phytosterols is the result of their interference with cholesterol absorption. In normal animals, phytosterols are absorbed to a slight extent. Studies of direct lymphatic absorption of β-sitosterol in rats indicate that it is absorbed to about 3 to 6% (134, 135). Vahouny and colleagues (136) found sitosterol, stigmasterol, and fucosterol

(24-ethylidene cholesterol) to be absorbed to the extents of 3.1, 4.3, and 3.1%, respectively.

In 1953, Pollak (137) demonstrated the serum cholesterol–lowering effect of plant sterols in human subjects. Feeding a cohort of 26 healthy men 5.7 to 10.0 g/day plant sterols for 13 days lowered their average cholesterol level by 17.7%. The next few years brought a virtual flood of articles describing studies in which subjects (average, 17±3) were fed varying levels of phytosterols (average, 13±1.1 g) for different lengths of time (average, 27±4 weeks) to achieve an average cholesterol lowering of 20±1.5%. These studies are discussed in detail in Pollak and Kritchevsky's *Sitosterol* (138).

Sugano and his co-workers were the first to investigate the hypocholesterolemic properties of sitostanol (139). They compared directly the effects of sitosterol and sitostanol in cholesterol-fed (0.5%) rats. They found that addition of 0.5% sitosterol lowered plasma and liver cholesterol levels by 17 and 82%, respectively. When sitostanol was fed, plasma cholesterol fell by 32% and liver cholesterol by 82% (140). Sitostanol has also been shown to be more hypocholesterolemic and antiatherogenic than sitosterol in rabbits (141). Heinemann and colleagues (142) showed that sitostanol (500 mg/day) was significantly hypolipidemic in human subjects.

The general problem faced in phytosterol-feeding studies has been their insolubility in almost all vehicles. Miettinen and associates (143) partially overcame the solubility problem by interesterifying sitostanol with rapeseed oil and incorporating the resulting ester mix into margarine. In a landmark study, they compared the effects of sitostanol containing margarine (1.8 or 2.6 g sitostanol daily) with a phytosterol-free margarine. Total serum cholesterol levels fell by 7.76% in subjects ingesting 1.8 g stanol/day and by 10.26% in those ingesting 2.6 g/day. In subjects ingesting 1.8 or 2.6 g sitostanol daily, LDL-C levels fell by 9.8 and 16.25%, respectively, and their LDL-C/HDL-C ratios fell by 11.19 and 16.56%. Weststrate and Meijer (144) demonstrated that a sitosterol ester–rich margarine was as effective as the stanol ester–rich margarine in effecting hypocholesterolemia. Both types of margarine have now been studied extensively and appear to have similar effects.

Hallikainen and Uusitupa (145) compared the hypolipidemic effects of wood (sitostanol) and vegetable (sitosterol) sterol esters in subjects prefed a high-fat diet for 4 weeks. Pine oil phytosterol esters were slightly more efficacious in lowering serum TC (18.6% versus 16.0%). In a similar study conducted in hyperlipidemic patients, the two preparations (wood versus vegetable) were shown to have equal hypocholesterolemic activity (146). Unesterified sterols and stanols lower LDL-C levels equivalently in hyperlipidemic subjects (147).

Reductions of total blood cholesterol are reflected in reductions in circulating LDL-C levels. Reduction in LDL levels implies lowering of levels of circulating carotenoids and vitamin E because they are transported in LDL. This issue has received considerable attention. Reductions in carotenoid and vitamin E levels are indeed observed often (148, 149), but when one corrects for reductions in LDL, there is no significant lowering of vitamin E levels, but β-carotene levels may be reduced by 8 to 19% (150). Not all studies show a reduction of circulating carotenoids (151–153). It has been shown that the problem can be averted by increasing the intake of carotenoid-rich foods (150).

Toxicity Studies

Almost a half century ago, the Eli Lilly Company introduced a cholesterol-lowering product that consisted of a suspension of phytosterols in a flavored, aqueous medium. Extensive safety tests were conducted using either β-sitosterol or mixed soy sterols (154). No detectable effects on growth, serum proteins, or blood urea nitrogen were observed. There were no abnormalities seen in any tissue or organ. The tests were carried out in rabbits (fed 4% phytosterol), rats (fed 5% phytosterol), or dogs (fed 0.5–1.0 g/kg/day phytosterols). The duration of the tests was 18 to 22 months.

With the expanded use of phytosterol-rich margarines and other foods there has been renewed interest in possible untoward effects. There is a new, extensive literature on safety testing of both sitosterol and sitostanol. After mixed phytosterol esters (0.1, 1.0, 2.0, 5.0%) were fed to male and female rats for 90 days, the authors performed a range of hematologic tests and examined total body and tissue weights. No significant effects were observed. A two-generation sitosterol feeding test in Wistar rats showed no untoward effects on fecundity, fertility, gestation time, live birth index, or sex ratio of pups. No evidence of estrogenic activity has been observed. Toxicity studies with phytostanol esters yielded results similar to those obtained with phytosterols. No adverse effects were seen when the esters were fed to Wistar rats at levels of 0.5 g/kg body weight/day. No estrogenic effects were observed, nor were there effects on reproduction or development. Neither phytosterol esters nor phytostanol esters were shown to be genotoxic in in vitro gene mutation assays using either bacterial or mammalian cells. These observations have been summarized (155).

Sitosterolemia

Sitosterolemia is a rare lipid storage disease that results in xanthomatosis and atherosclerosis (156, 157). In 1998, Berger and associates (158) estimated that there were 34 cases, world wide. The condition is precipitated by mutations in the adenosine triphosphate–binding cassette proteins ABCG5 and ABCG8 (159). The genetic basis of sitosterolemia was reviewed by Lee and colleagues (160) and more recently by Sehayek (161).

Serum Phytosterol Levels and Atherogenesis. Glueck and associates (162, 163) measured serum phytosterol levels in a large cohort of hypercholesterolemic subjects and found that high serum campesterol or stigmasterol levels were associated with a history (personal or familial) of coronary heart disease. These investigators also found high phytosterol levels to be closely correlated with high TC and LDL-C levels and suggested that increased absorption of phytosterols could be a heritable atherogenic trait different from the genetic disease. Sudhop and colleagues (164) studied subjects with or without a family history of coronary disease. The average cholesterol levels in 27 controls and 26 test subjects were 242±46 mg/dL (6.26±1.19 mmol/L) and 242±31 mg/dL (6.26±0.80 mmol/L), respectively. Serum campesterol levels in controls and probands were 0.38 and 0.50 mg/dL, respectively. Sitosterol levels in the two groups were 0.31 and 0.40 mg/dL, respectively. In both groups, the level of campesterol plus sitosterol was less than 1 mg/dL. The phytosterols in the control group represented 0.36% of cholesterol and in the probands they represented 0.37%. Elevated levels of serum phytosterols may indicate a defect in sterol absorption that is reflected in elevated cholesterol levels and hence risk. It appears unlikely that the observed levels of serum phytosterols would be atherogenic per se.

Lees and Lees (165) asserted that β-sitosterol came close to being the ideal drug for treatment of hypercholesterolemia. However, after finding relatively high levels of campesterol in the sera of some patients, these investigators suggested the possibility that plant sterols per se could be atherogenic (166). This thinking leads to the paradoxic situation in which the phytosterols, which lower blood cholesterol significantly and thus reduce risk of coronary heart disease, can themselves be atherogenic.

If phytosterols are atherogenic, one would expect to find them in atherosclerotic plaques, and to date nobody has. In 1943, Hardegger and colleagues (167) analyzed a large mass of human aortas and found only cholesterol and some oxidized cholesterol products. These investigators did not have the advantage of modern analytic techniques. Using modern chromatographic methodology, Brooks (168) and Hodis (169) and their co-workers recovered cholesterol and some of its oxidation products (7α-, 7β-, 24-, or 26-hydroxycholesterols) from human aortas. Vaya and associates (170) found the oxidation products reported by Brooks and Hodes as well as 7-keto- and β-epoxycholesterol. The presence of phytosterols was not noted by any of the investigators cited earlier.

Cook and associates (171) fed rabbits (two to three per group) 1% cholesterol, cholestanol, 7-dehydrocholesterol or lathosterol (Δ^7-cholesterol). Atherosclerotic plaques were observed in the rabbits fed cholesterol or cholestanol, whereas the other two sterols gave barely visible lesions. Triparanol is a compound that inhibits cholesterol synthesis late in the cycle with consequent accumulation of 24-dehydrocholesterol (desmosterol). When rabbits were fed normal or atherogenic diets with or without 0.2% triparanol,

desmosterol accumulated in both normal and atherosclerotic aortas (172).

To test whether phytosterols per se may be atherogenic, rabbits were fed a semipurified diet containing sitosterol or sitostanol esters for 60 days. Their aortas contained microgram quantities of cholesterol and nanogram amounts of sitosterol, campesterol, and sitosterol (173). Apparently, an unsubstituted side chain is required for incorporation of sterols into the arterial wall. Differences in absorption of cholesterol and phytosterols may depend, in part, on the configuration of the side chain. Campesterol (C24-methyl) may offer less of a barrier to absorption of sitosterol (C24-ethyl). A slight defect in the absorption mechanism may permit absorption of sitosterol and campesterol, with more of the latter being absorbed because the smaller side chain offers less resistance.

In a review of the pharmacologic effects of plant sterols, Moghadasian (174) pointed out that most adverse effects were observed in animals in which phytosterols were injected intraperitoneally or applied topically. In 1985, Pollak (175) reviewed the overall effects of plant sterols in humans and stated that the only undesirable side effect of a sitosterol regimen was occasional diarrhea. The accumulated data suggest that dietary phytosterols are a safe and effective way to lower blood cholesterol levels. Reviews dating from 1995 have arrived at the same conclusion (176–178). As with all dietary and pharmacologic treatments, continued monitoring is prudent.

Acknowledgments
This work is supported, in part, by a Research Career Award (HL00734) from the National Institutes of Health and the Commonwealth Universal Research Enhancement Program, Pennsylvania Department of Health.

REFERENCES

1. Editorial. JAMA 1903;41:1542–3.
2. Kritchevsky D. Cholesterol. New York: John Wiley & Sons, 1958.
3. Myant NB. The Biology of Cholesterol and Related Sterols. London: William Heinemann Medical Books, 1981.
4. Marijanovic Z, Laubner D, Möller G et al. Mol Endocrinol 2003;17:1715–25.
5. Locatelli S, Lütjohann D, Schmidt HHJ et al. Arch Neurol 2002; 59:213–6.
6. Danielsen EM, Hansen H. Biochim Biophys Acta. 2003;1617: 1–9.
7. Pizzo P, Viola A. Curr Opin Immunol. 2003:255–60.
8. Mueller JH. J Biol Chem 1915;22:1–9.
9. Mueller JH. J Biol Chem 1916;27:463–80.
10. Popjak G. Biochem J 1946;40:608–21.
11. Siperstein MD, Chaikoff IL, Reinhardt WO. J Biol Chem 1952; 198:111–4.
12. Biggs MW, Friedman M, Byers SD. Proc Soc Exp Biol Med 1951;78:641–3.
13. Kayden HJ, Senior JR, Mattson FA. J Clin Invest 1967;46: 1695–703.
14. Wenzel JJ, Kaminski WE, Prehler A et al. Biochem Biophys Res Commun 2003;306:1089–98.
15. Iqbal J, Anwar K, Hussain M. J Biol Chem 2003:278:31610–20.

16. Libby P, Aikawa M, Schönbeck U. Biochem Biophys Acta 2000; 340:115–26.
17. Ross R. N Engl J Med 1999;340:115–26.
18. Steinberg D. J Biol Chem 1997;272:20963–6.
19. Lusis AJ. Nature 2000;407:233–41.
20. Blankenberg S, Barbaux S, Tiret L. Atherosclerosis 2003; 59:213–6.
21. Gofman JW, Lindgren F, Elliott H et al. Science 1950;111: 166–71.
22. Stender S, Zilversmit DB. Arteriosclerosis 1981;1:38–49.
23. Austin MA, Breslow JL, Hennekens CH et al. JAMA 1988; 260:1917–21.
24. Kritchevsky D. Variation in Serum Cholesterol Levels. In: Weininger J, Briggs GM, eds. Nutrition Update, Vol. 2. New York: John Wiley & Sons, 1985:91–103.
25. Harlap S, Kark JD, Baras M et al. Isr J Med Sci 1982;18: 1158–65.
26. Gordon DJ, Hyde J, Trost DC et al. J Clin Epidemiol 1988;41: 679–89.
27. Mustad V, Derr J, Reddy CC et al. Arteriosclerosis 1996;126: 117–29.
28. Katan MB, Beynen AC, DeVries, JHM et al. Am J Epidemiol 1986;123:221–34.
29. Hopkins PN. Am J Clin Nutr 1992;55:1060–70.
30. Sehayek E, Nath C Heinemann T et al. J Lipid Res 1998;39: 2415–22.
31. Expert Panel on Detection, Evaluation and Treatment of High Blood Cholesterol in Adults. JAMA 2001;285:2486–97.
32. LaRosa JC. Am J Cardiol 2002;90:1330–2.
33. Weverling-Rijnsburger AWE, Blauw GJ, Lagaay AM et al. Lancet 1997;350:1119–23.
34. Schatz IJ, Masaki K, Yano K. Lancet 2001;358:351–5.
35. Muldoon M, Manuck S, Mathews K. BMJ 1990;301:309–14.
36. Scandinavian Simvastatin Survival Study Group. Lancet 1994; 304:1383–9.
37. Gertler MM, Garn SM, White PD. Circulation 1950;2: 696–702.
38. Dawber TR, Nickerson RJ, Brand FN et al. Am J Clin Nutr 1982;36:617–25.
39. Gordon T, Kagan A, Garcia-Palmieri M et al. Circulation 1981; 63:500–15.
40. McNamara DJ. Biochim Biophys Acta 2000;1529:310–20.
41. Keys A. J Mt Sinai Hosp 1953;20:118–39.
42. Ahrens EJ Jr, Insull W Jr, Blomstrand R et al. Lancet 1957;1: 943–53.
43. McNamara DJ, Kolb R, Parker TS et al. J Clin Invest 1987;79:1729–39.
44. Keys A, Anderson JT, Grande F. Metabolism 1965;14:776–87.
45. Hegsted DM, McGandy RB, Myers ML et al. Am J Clin Nutr 1965;17:281–95.
46. Muller H, Kirkus B, Pedersen JI. Lipids 2001;36:783–9.
47. Hayes KC, Khosla PR. FASEB J 1992;6:2600–7.
48. Hegsted DM, Ausman LM, Johnson JA et al. Am J Clin Nutr 1993;57:875–83.
49. Kritchevsky D, Tepper SA, Kuksis A et al. J Nutr Biochem 1998;9:582–5.
50. Kritchevsky D, Tepper SA, Wright S et al. Nutr Res 1998; 18:259–64.
51. Kritchevsky D, Tepper SA, Kuksis A et al. Nutr Res 2000; 20:887–92.
52. Kritchevsky D, Tepper SA, Chen SC et al. Lipids 2000;35: 621–5.
53. Alfin-Slater RB, Wells AF, Aftergood L et al. J Nutr 1957;63: 241–61.
54. Alfin-Slater RB, Wells P, Aftergood L et al. J Am Oil Chem Soc 1973;50:479–84.
55. Aaes-Jorgenson E, Funch JP, Dann H. Br J Nutr 1956;10: 317–24.
56. Willett WC, Stampfer MJ, Manson JE. Lancet 1993;341:581–5.
57. O'Keefe S, Gaskins-Wright S, Wiley V et al. J Food Lipids 1994; 1:165–76.
58. Exler J, Lemar L, Smith J. USDA Special Purpose Table 1. Washington, DC: US Department of Agriculture, 1994.
59. Ip C, Chin SF, Scimeca JA et al. Cancer Res 1990;51:6118–24.
60. Scimeca JA. Cancer Inhibition in Animals. In: Yurawecz MP, Mossaba MM, Kramer JKG et al, eds. Advances in Conjugated Linoleic Acid Research, Vol. 1. Champaign, IL: AOCS Press, 1999:420–33.
61. Visonneau S, Cesano A, Tepper, SA et al. Anticancer Res. 1977; 17:969–74.
62. Kritchevsky D. Conjugated Linoleic Acid in Experimental Atherosclerosis. In: Sebedio JL, Christie WW, Adolf R, eds. Advances in Conjugated Linoleic Acid Research, Vol. 2. Champaign, IL: AOCS Press, 2003:292–301.
63. Kritchevsky D, Tepper SA, Wright S et al. J Am Coll Nutr 2000; 19:472S–7S.
64. Wilson TA, Nicolosi RJ, Chrysam M et al. Nutr Res 2000;20: 1795–1805.
65. Moore CE, Alfin-Slater RB, Aftergood L. Am J Clin Nutr 1980; 33:2318–23.
66. Høy CE, Hølmer G. Lipids 1979;14:727–33.
67. Privett OS, Stearns EM Jr, Nickell EC. J Nutr 1967;92:303–10.
68. Kritchevsky D, Baldino AR. Artery 1978;4:480–6.
69. Sgoutas DS. Biochim Biophys Acta 1968;164:317–26.
70. Zevenbergen JL, Houtsmüller UMT, Gottenbos JJ. Lipids 1988;23:178–86.
71. Senti FR, ed. Health Aspects of Dietary Trans Fatty Acids. Bethesda, MD: FASEB, 1985.
72. British Nutrition Foundation Task Force Trans Fatty Acids. London: Br Nutr Foundation, 1987.
73. British Nutrition Foundation Task Force Trans Fatty Acids. London: British Nutrition Foundation, 1985.
74. Expert Panel on Trans Fatty Acids and Coronary Heart Disease. Am J Clin Nutr 1995;67:655S–708S.
75. Emken EA. Fat Nutr 1992;1:1–14.
76. Ascherio A, Katan MB, Zock PL et al. N Engl J Med 1999;340: 1994–8.
77. McMillan GC, Silver MD, Weigensberg BJ. Arch Pathol 1963; 76:106–12.
78. Ruttenberg H, Davidson LM, Little NA et al. J Nutr 1983; 113:835–44.
79. Kritchevsky D, Davidson LM, Weight M et al. Atherosclerosis 1984;51:123–33.
80. Elson CE, Benevenga NJ, Canty DJ et al. Atherosclerosis 1981;40:115–37.
81. Hunter JE, Applewhite TH. Am J Clin Nutr 1991;54:363–9.
82. National Center for Health Statistics. Health United States, 1994. Hyattsville, MD: DHHS Publ No (PHS-95-1232).
83. Allison DB, Egan K, Barraj LM et al. J Am Diet Assoc 1999; 99:166–74.
84. Innis SM, Green TJ, Halsey TK. J Am Coll Nutr 1999;18: 255–60.
85. Mensink RP, Zock PL, Kester ADM et al. Am J Clin Nutr 2003; 77:1146–55.
86. Ignatowski A. Virchow's Arch Pathol Anat Physiol Klin Med 1909;198:248–70.
87. Meeker DR, Kesten HD. Proc Soc Exp Biol Med 1940;45: 543–5.

88. Meeker DR, Kesten HD. Arch Pathol 1941;31:147–62.

89. Hamilton RMG, Carroll KK. Atherosclerosis 1976;24:47–62.

90. Huff MW, Hamilton RMG, Carroll KK. Atherosclerosis 1977; 28:187–95.

91. Kritchevsky D. J Am Oil Chem Soc 1979;56:135–46.

92. Kritchevsky D, Tepper SA, Czarnecki SK et al. Atherosclerosis 1982;41:429–31.

93. Huff MW, Carroll KK. J Lipid Res 1980;21:546–58.

94. Sugano M, Ishiwaki N, Negata Y et al. Br J Nutr 1982;48: 211–21.

95. Yerushalmy J, Hilleboe HE. NY State J Med 1957;57:2343–54.

96. Grande F. Sugars in Cardiovascular Disease. In: Sipple HL, McNutt KW, eds. Sugars in Nutrition. New York: Academic Press, 1974:401–37.

97. Yudkin J. Lancet 1957;2:155–62.

98. Walker ARP. Atherosclerosis 1971;14:137–52.

99. Keys A. Atherosclerosis 1971;14:193–202.

100. Albrink MJ, Man EB. Arch Intern Med 1959;103:4–8.

101. Carlson LA. Acta Med Scand 1960;167:399–413.

102. Carlson LA, Böttiger LE. Acta Med Scand 1985;218:207–11.

103. Austin MA. Arterioscler Thromb 1991;11:2–14.

104. Hokanson JE, Austin ME. J Cardiovasc Risk 1996;3:213–9.

105. Jeppesen J, Hein HO, Saudicani P et al. Circulation 1998;97: 1029–36.

106. Ginsberg HN. Circulation 2002;106:2137–42.

107. Durrington PN. Atherosclerosis 1998;141:S57–62.

108. Reaven GM. Diabetes 1998;37:1595–607.

109. Alberti KGMM, Zimmett PZ. Diabet Med 1998;15:539–53.

110. Kritchevsky D, Sallata P, Tepper SA. J Atheroscler Res 1968; 8:697–703.

111. Kritchevsky D, Tepper SA, Kitagawa M. Nutr Rep Int 1973; 7:193–202.

112. Kritchevsky D, Davidson LM, Kim HK et al. Exp Mol Pathol 1977;26:28–51.

113. Kritchevsky D, Davidson LM, Shapiro IL et al. Am J Clin Nutr 1974;27:29–50.

114. Kritchevsky D, Davidson LM, Kim HK et al. Am J Clin Nutr 1980;33:1869–87.

115. Segall JJ. Int J Cardiol 1994;46:197–207.

116. Mann GV. Am J Clin Nutr 1974;27:464–9.

117. Steinmetz KA, Childs MT, Stimson C et al. Am J Clin Nutr 1994;59:612–8.

118. Ashar MN, Prajapati JB. Folia Microbiol 2000;45:263–8.

119. Ness AR, Davey Smith G, Hart C. J Epidemiol Commun Health 2001;55:379–82.

120. McLachlan CNS. Med Hypotheses 2000;56:262–72.

121. Elliott RB, Harris DP, Hill JP et al. Diabetologia 1999;42:292–6.

122. Laugesen M, Elliott R. N Z Med J 2003;116:295–313.

123. Howard BV, Wylie-Rosett J. Circulation 2002;106:523–7.

124. Ruxton CHS. Br J Nutr 2003;90:245–7.

125. Cleave TL. J Royal Naval Med Serv 1956;42:55–83.

126. Spiller G, ed. CRC Handbook of Dietary Fiber in Human Nutrition. 2nd ed. Boca Raton, FL: CRC Press, 1993.

127. Kritchevsky D, Story JA. Influence of Dietary Fiber in Cholesterol Metabolism in Experimental Animals. In: Spiller GA, ed. CRC Handbook of Dietary Fiber in Human Nutrition. 2nd ed. Boca Raton, FL: CRC Press, 1993:163–78.

128. Jenkins DJA, Spadafora PJ, Jenkins AL et al. Fiber in the Treatment of Hyperlipidemia. In: Spiller GA, ed. Handbook of Dietary Fiber in Human Nutrition. 2nd ed. Boca Raton, FL: CRC Press, 1993:419–38.

129. Peterson DW. Proc Soc Exp Biol Med 1951;78:143–7.

130. Peterson DW, Nichols CW Jr, Shneour EA. J Nutr 1952; 47: 57–65.

131. Peterson DW, Shneour EA, Peek NF et al. J Nutr 1953; 191–201.

132. Mattson FH, Volpenhein RA, Erickson BA. J Nutr 1977; 107:1139–46.

133. Kritchevsky D, Tepper SA, Czarnecki SK et al. Nutr Res 1999; 19:1649–54.

134. Swell L, Trout EC Jr, Field H Jr et al. Proc Soc Exp Biol Med 1959;100:140–2.

135. Sylven C, Borgstrom B. J Lipid Res 1964;10:179–82.

136. Vahouny GV, Connor WG, Subramaniam S et al. Am J Clin Nutr 1983;37:805–9.

137. Pollak OJ. Circulation 1953;7:720–6.

138. Pollak OJ, Kritchevsky D. Sitosterol. Basel: Karger, 1981.

139. Sugano M, Kamo F, Ikeda I. Atherosclerosis 1976;24:301–9.

140. Sugano M, Morioka H, Ikeda I. J Nutr 1977;107:2011–9.

141. Ntanios FY, Jones PJH, Frohlich JJ. Atherosclerosis 1998; 138:101–10.

142. Heinemann T, Leiss O, von Bergmann K. Atherosclerosis 1986; 61:219–23.

143. Miettinen TA, Puska P, Gylling H et al. N Eng J Med 1995; 333:1308–12.

144. Weststrate JA, Meijer GW. Eur J Clin Nutr 1998;52:334–43.

145. Hallikainen MA, Uusitupa MJ. Am J Clin Nutr 1999;69:403–10.

146. Plat J, Mensink RP. Atherosclerosis 2000;148:101–12.

147. Vanstone CA, Raeini-Sarjaz M, Parsons WE et al. Am J Clin Nutr 2002;76:1272–8.

148. Judd JT, Baer DJ, Chen SC et al. Lipids 2002;37:33–42.

149. Amundsen AL, Ose L, Nenseter MS et al. Am J Clin Nutr 2002; 76:338–44.

150. Noakes M, Clifton P, Ntanios F et al. Am J Clin Nutr 2002; 75:79–86.

151. Maki KC, Davidson MH, Umporowicz DM et al. Am J Clin Nutr 2001;74:33–43.

152. Nestel P, Cehun M, Pomeroy S et al. Eur J Clin Nutr 2001;55: 1084–90.

153. Kwiterovich PO Jr, Chen SC, Virgel DG et al. J Lipid Res 2003;44:1143–55.

154. Shipley RE, Pfeiffer RR, Marsh MM et al. Circulation 1958; 6:373–82.

155. Kritchevsky D. Safety of Phytosterols and Phytosterol Esters as Functional Food Components. In: Dutta P, ed. Phytosterols as Functional Food Components and Neutraceuticals. New York: Marcel Dekker, 2003:347–63.

156. Bhattacharyya AK, Connor WE. J Clin Invest 1974;53:1033–43.

157. Salen G, Shore V, Tint GS et al. J Lipid Res 1989;30:1319–30.

158. Berger GMB, Pegoraro RJ, Patel SA et al. J Lipid Res 1998;39: 1046–54.

159. Berge KE, Tian H, Graf GA et al. Science 2000;290:1771–5.

160. Lee MH, Lu K, Patel SB. Curr Opin Lipidol 2001;11:141–9.

161. Sehayek E. J Lipid Res 2003;44:2030–8.

162. Glueck CJ, Speirs J, Tracy T et al. Metabolism 1991;40:842–8.

163. Glueck CJ, Streicher P, Illeg E. Clin Biochem 1992;25:331–4.

164. Sudhop T, Gottwald BM, von Bergmann K. Metabolism 2002;51:1519–21.

165. Lees RS, Lees AM. Effect of Sitosterol Therapy on Plasma Lipid and Lipoprotein Concentration. In: Greten H, ed. Lipoprotein Metabolism. Berlin: Springer-Verlag, 1976: 119–24.

166. Lees AM, Mok HYI, Lees RS et al. Atherosclerosis 1977;28: 325–38.

167. Hardegger E, Ruzicka L, Tagmann E. Helv Chem Acta 1943; 30:2205–21.

168. Brooks CJW, Steel G, Gilbert JD et al. Atherosclerosis 1971; 13:223–37.

169. Hodes HN, Crawford DW, Sevanian A. Atherosclerosis 1991; 89:117–26.
170. Vaya J, Aviram M, Mahmood S et al. Free Radic Res 2001;34: 485–97.
171. Cook RP, Kliman A, Fieser LF. Arch Biochem 1954;52: 439–50.
172. Kritchevsky D, Fumagalli R, Cattabeni F et al. Rev Farmacol Ter 1970;1:455–63.
173. Kritchevsky D, Tepper SA, Czarnecki SK et al. Lipids 2003; 38:1115–8.
174. Moghadasian M. Life Sci 2000;67:605–15.
175. Pollak OJ. Pharmacol Ther 1985;31:177–208.
176. Ling WH, Jones PJH. Life Sci 1995;57:195–206.
177. Jenkins DJA, Kendall CWC. J Am Coll Nutr 1999;18: 559–62.
178. Katan MB, Grundy SM, Jones P et al. Mayo Clin Proc 2003;78:965–78.

SELECTED READINGS

Ginsberg HN. Lipoprotein physiology. Endocrinol Metab Clin North Am 1998;27:503–19.

Kritchevsky D. Phytosterols in human health. In: Kotsonis FN, Mackey MA, eds. Nutritional Toxicology. 2nd ed. London: Taylor and Francis, 2002:173–89.

Lusis AJ. Atherosclerosis. Nature 2000;407:233–41.

Maxfield FR, Wüstner D. Intracellular cholesterol transport. J Clin Invest 2002;110:891–8.

Ross R. Atherosclerosis: an inflammatory disease. N Engl J Med 1999; 340:115–26.

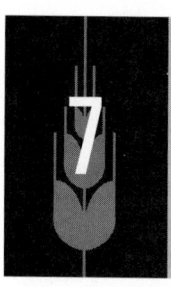

7 ENERGY NEEDS: ASSESSMENT AND REQUIREMENTS[1]

NANCY F. BUTTE AND BENJAMIN CABALLERO

ENERGETICS OF INTERMEDIATE METABOLISM 136
ENERGY BALANCE 138
MEASUREMENT OF ENERGY INTAKE AND ENERGY
  EXPENDITURE 139
HUMAN ENERGY REQUIREMENTS 141
  Basal Metabolism 141
  Thermogenesis 143
  Physical Activity 143
  Growth 144
  Pregnancy and Lactation 144
ASSESSMENT OF ENERGY REQUIREMENTS 144
DIETARY REFERENCE INTAKES: ESTIMATED ENERGY
  REQUIREMENT 145
  Infants and Children 145
  Adults 146
  Pregnancy and Lactation 146

ENERGETICS OF INTERMEDIATE METABOLISM

To sustain life, humans must eat. The chemical free energy of food is the only form of energy humans can use to maintain the structural and biochemical integrity of the body, to perform internal work of circulation, respiration, and muscle contraction, and to perform external work (1–3). Our ability to use the chemical free energy of food results from the development of the biochemical, structural, and physiologic apparatus that permits the transformation of chemical free energy into other energy forms essential for life. Part of the energy from food, on the order of 5%, is thermodynamically obligated for conversion to heat because the entropy of the metabolic end products is greater than the initial substances (Fig. 7.1). Conversion of food energy into high-energy biochemical

compounds is an inefficient process, with approximately 50% lost as heat. Through biochemical transformations, approximately 45% of the energy of food is available to the body primarily as adenosine triphosphate (ATP). Eventually, all the energy of food is lost from the body in the form of heat or external work.

Energy is provided in the diet by protein, carbohydrate, fat, and alcohol. The energy in foods is expressed as a unit of heat, the calorie. A calorie is defined as the amount of heat required to raise the temperature of 1 g of water by 1°C from 15°C to 16°C. The scientific international unit of energy is the joule (J), defined as the energy expended when 1 kg is moved 1 m by a force of 1 newton. In 1956, an international committee standardized the equivalency of these units as 1 cal = 4.1868 J, but the figure of 4.184 is more commonly used in nutrition studies. For practicality, a kilocalorie (kcal), which is 1000 times the energy of a calorie (cal), is commonly used in nutrition. Hence, 1 kcal = 4.184 kJ, and 1 kJ = 0.0239 kcal. Another less frequently used unit is the thermochemical calorie, which is the heat liberated by the combustion of 1 g of pure benzoic acid and is equivalent to 4.184 J (1).

The potential energy contribution of food is determined experimentally by measuring the heat evolved in a bomb calorimeter when foodstuffs are completely combusted to carbon dioxide (CO_2) and water (4). The actual amount of heat evolved per gram of foodstuff varies according to its chemical composition. Average values are 4.1 kcal/g of carbohydrate, 9.3 kcal/g of fat, and 5.4 kcal/g of protein. The body cannot oxidize nitrogen, and therefore energy resulting from the oxidation of the nitrogenous component of protein is unavailable to the body. Consequently, only 4.2 kcal/g protein is potentially available to the body. The physiologic fuel value is compromised further by the apparent digestibility of various foodstuffs that vary among food sources. These factors result in physiologic fuel values of 4 kcal/g for carbohydrate, 9 kcal/g for fat, and 4 kcal/g for protein, also known as the Atwater factors. The physiologic fuel value for alcohol is 7 kcal/g (Table 7.1).

Substrate oxidation rates are a function of dietary macronutrient intake and level of energy turnover (5). Protein oxidation is largely determined by protein intake, whereas the relative contributions of glucose or free fatty acids (FFAs) to the fuel mix are more variable. Glucose oxidation is adjusted to carbohydrate intake to maintain

---

[1]**Abbreviations: ATP,** adenosine triphosphate; **BEE,** basal energy expenditure; **BMR,** basal metabolic rate; **DLW,** doubly labeled water; **DRI,** dietary reference intake; **EE,** energy expenditure; **EER,** estimated energy requirement; **FFA,** free fatty acid; **FFM,** fat free mass; **FM,** fat mass; **HR,** heart rate; **NPRQ,** nonprotein respiratory quotient; **PAL,** physical activity level; **P:O ratio,** phosphorylation-to-oxidation ratio; **RMR,** resting metabolic rate; **RQ,** respiratory quotient; **SMR,** sleeping metabolic rate; **TEE,** total energy expenditure; **TEF,** thermic effect of food; **VCO₂,** carbon dioxide production; **VO₂,** oxygen consumption; **VO₂max,** maximal oxygen consumption.

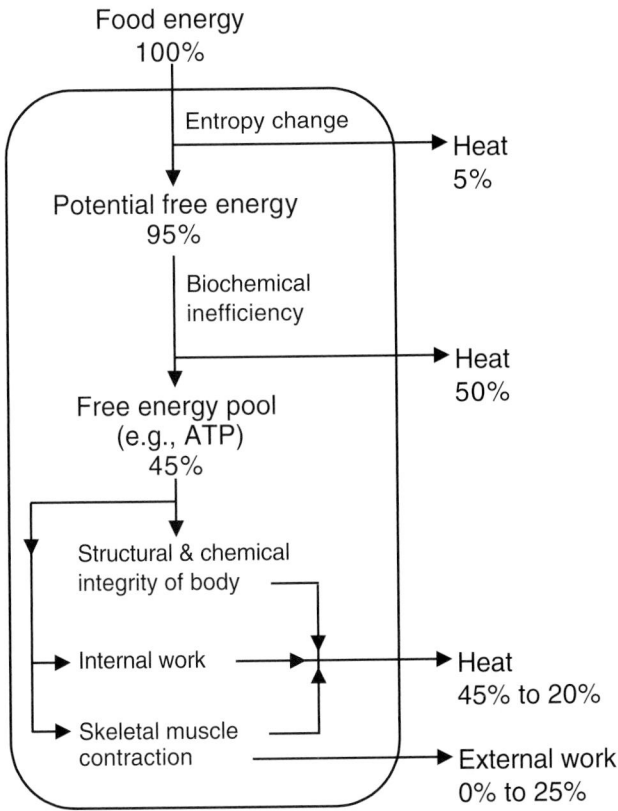

Figure 7.1. Energy utilization with the body. The distribution of food energy within the body and its transfer to the environment as heat or external work is illustrated (see text for further details). ATP, adenosine triphosphate. (From Brown AC. Energy metabolism. In: Ruch TC, Patton HD, eds. Physiology and Biophysics III: Digestion, Metabolism, Endocrine Function and Reproduction. Philadelphia: WB Saunders, 1973:85–104, with permission.)

stable glycogen stores. Fat intake, in contrast, does not promote its own oxidation, and under conditions of positive energy balance, some fat will be deposited. Most cells can use the metabolic intermediates of carbohydrates, fats, and proteins interchangeably to regenerate ATP, with a few exceptions. The brain preferentially uses glucose and is able to use ketone bodies after adaptation to starvation, but it does not use FFAs (6). Red blood cells also depend on glucose. At rest, the brain (20%), internal

organs (25–30%), and skeletal muscle (20%) account for the majority of energy turnover. During vigorous activity, skeletal muscle overwhelms the utilization of other tissues. In the postabsorptive state, FFAs are mainly oxidized by muscle, whereas during exertion, muscle's own glycogen reserve is used, with a subsequent shift toward use of FFAs mobilized from muscle fat stores and adipose tissue.

When alcohol is consumed, it promptly appears in the circulation and is oxidized at a rate determined largely by its concentration and by the activity of liver alcohol dehydrogenase. Oxidation of alcohol rapidly reduces the oxidation of the other substrates used for ATP regeneration. Ethanol oxidation proceeds in large part via conversion to acetate and oxidative phosphorylation. About 80% of the energy liberated by ethanol oxidation is used to drive ATP regeneration, and about 20% is released as heat (7). Alcoholic beverages can contribute to weight gain in healthy persons consuming an otherwise adequate diet (8), in contrast to the pharmacologic effect of excessive ethanol, which can inhibit normal eating and can cause emaciation in persons with alcoholism.

Flatt and Tremblay (5) computed the ATP yield from oxidation of macronutrients based on the phosphorylation-to-oxidation (P:O) ratio and the ATP required to initiate degradation, transport, activation, and handling of the metabolic fuels (Fig. 7.2). Assuming a P:O ratio of 3:1 for the reoxidation of mitochondrial reduced nicotinamide adenine dinucleotide, the oxidation of 1 mol of glucose produces 38 mol ATP, but 2 mol are used for activation; therefore, the net ATP yield is 95%. Allowing for the costs of recycling through the Cori cycle and glucose-alanine cycle and gluconeogenesis, the net postabsorptive ATP yield is about 82%. Accounting for the postprandial phase of digestion, absorption, and transport, the net ATP yield from dietary carbohydrate is 75%, such that the oxidation of 24 kcal of dietary carbohydrate is required to replace 1 mol of ATP. To calculate the ATP yield from dietary fat, the fatty acid oleate was used as an example. The oxidation of 1 mol of oleate yields 146 mol ATP, but expends 5.5 mol ATP in lipolysis/reesterification and activation to oleyl-CoA; therefore, the ATP yield for fat oxidation is about 96%. Accounting for the postprandial

TABLE 7.1. HEATS OF COMBUSTION, PHYSIOLOGIC ENERGY VALUES, HEAT EQUIVALENTS, AND CORRESPONDING VOLUMES OF OXYGEN AND CARBON DIOXIDE FOR CARBOHYDRATE, PROTEIN, FAT, AND ETHANOL OXIDATION

	ENERGY (kcal/g)			HEAT EQUIVALENTS			VOLUME	
FOOD	HEAT OF COMBUSTION	HUMAN OXIDATION	PHYSIOLOGIC VALUE	VO_2 (kcal/L)	VCO_2 (kcal/L)	RQ	Oxygen (L/g)	CO_2 (L/g)
Carbohydrate	4.1	4.1	4	5.05	5.05	1.00	0.81	0.81
Protein	5.4	4.2	4	4.46	5.57	0.80	0.94	0.75
Fat	9.3	9.3	9	4.74	6.67	0.71	1.96	1.39
Ethanol	7.1	7.1	7	4.86	7.25	0.67	1.46	0.98

RQ, respiratory quotient; VCO_2, carbon dioxide consumption; VO_2, oxygen consumption.

Data from Brown AC. Energy metabolism. In: Ruch TC, Patton HD, eds. Physiology and Biophysics III. Digestion, Metabolism, Endocrine Function and Reproduction. Philadelphia: WB Saunders, 1973:85–104.

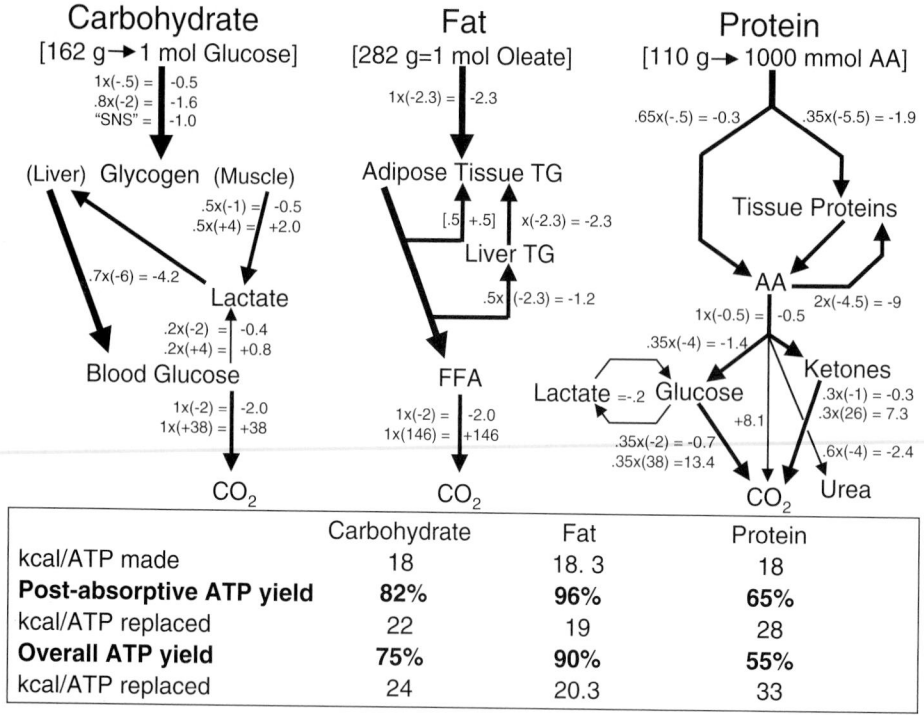

Figure 7.2. Adenosine triphosphate (ATP) yields from oxidation of carbohydrate, fat, and protein. Moles of substrate flowing through the metabolic pathways are in brackets, and the moles of ATP produced and expended per mole of substrate metabolized are in parenthesis, assuming a phosphorylation-to-oxidation (P:O) ratio of 3 for the reoxidation of mitochondrial reduced nicotinamide adenine dinucleotide. For example, 38 ATPs are produced during the oxidation of 1 mole of glucose, but because substrate handling, storage, and recycling costs, the postabsorptive ATP yield is approximately 82%, and the overall yield is 75%. AA, amino acid; FFA, free fatty acid; SNS, sympathetic nervous system; TG, triglyceride. (From Flatt JP, Tremblay A. Energy expenditure and substrate oxidation. In: Bray GA, Bouchard C, James WPT, eds. Handbook of Obesity. New York: Marcel Dekker, 1998, with permission.)

	Carbohydrate	Fat	Protein
kcal/ATP made	18	18.3	18
Post-absorptive ATP yield	**82%**	**96%**	**65%**
kcal/ATP replaced	22	19	28
Overall ATP yield	**75%**	**90%**	**55%**
kcal/ATP replaced	24	20.3	33

phase, the net ATP yield from dietary fat is approximately 90%. In the case of proteins, the oxidation of 1 mol of amino acids generates approximately 28.8 mol of ATP or 18 kcal/mol ATP. The costs of gluconeogenesis, ureagenesis, and protein resynthesis reduce the net postabsorptive ATP yield to 65%. Accounting for the postprandial phase, the overall ATP yield is 55%. Based on these estimates, the transport, storage, recycling, and activation dissipate about 10%, 25%, and 45% of the ATP produced in the oxidation of dietary fat, carbohydrate, and protein, respectively. Therefore, the corresponding net ATP yields are estimated to be 90%, 75%, and 55% with dietary fat, carbohydrate, and protein.

Lipogenesis from the conversion of dietary carbohydrate to fat is an inefficient process estimated at 25%. This pathway appears to be of minor importance in humans, because large amounts of dietary carbohydrate expand glycogen reserves, not body fat (9). Lipogenesis therefore does not account for the higher dissipation of dietary energy by carbohydrate compared with fat. Similarly, the energy dissipation by futile cycles or substrate cycles that dissipate ATP with no net change in the organism also appears to make only a minor contribution to overall energy economy. Futile cycles are thought to account for only a small percentage of total energy expenditure (TEE) (10).

ENERGY BALANCE

Energy balance is the accounting for the energy consumed in foods, losses in excreta, heat produced, and retention or secretion of organic compounds (4). Implicit in the delineation of energy balance is that energy is conserved. The energy balance may be expressed as follows:

$$E_{intake} - E_{feces} - E_{urine} - E_{combustible\ gas} - E_{expenditure} = E_{retention}\ or\ E_{secretion}$$

Digestible energy is the dietary energy absorbed by the gastrointestinal tract after accounting for loss in feces (11). Metabolizable energy is that energy available to the organism after accounting for losses in feces, urine, and combustible gases. Metabolizable energy is measured by meticulous energy balance techniques and was determined for human diets by Atwater in the early 1900s. The Atwater factors of 4, 9, and 4 kcal of metabolizable energy per gram of protein, fat, and carbohydrate, respectively, are widely used to express the energy content of foods in food composition tables, including those in the United States (12). The Atwater factors are applied to the protein estimated from its nitrogen content, fat determined by extraction, and carbohydrates determined by difference, after taking into account the water and ash in the food. In the United Kingdom, the metabolizable energy factors of 4, 9, and 3.75 kcal/g of protein, fat, and carbohydrate, respectively, are used in food composition tables (13). In this system, the metabolizable energy factor is applied to available carbohydrate, defined as the sum of free sugars, dextrins, starch, and glycogen, resulting in lower estimates of the caloric content of foods than in the Atwater system.

Humans can survive on foods with varying proportions of carbohydrates, fats, and proteins (14–18). The ability to shift from carbohydrate to fat as the main source of energy, coupled with substantial reserves of body fat, makes it possible to accommodate large fluctuations in energy intake and energy expenditure (EE). Energy balance is regulated by a complex set of neuroendocrine feedback mechanisms. Changes in energy intake or in EE trigger metabolic and behavioral responses aimed at restoring energy balance.

MEASUREMENT OF ENERGY INTAKE AND ENERGY EXPENDITURE

Several methods are used to assess dietary intake including weighed or observed diet records, dietary recalls and diaries, and food frequencies. It is now generally recognized that reported energy intakes tend to underestimate usual energy intake (19). Evidence of underreporting has been substantiated from measurements of TEE by the doubly labeled water (DLW) method (20, 21). Implausibly low energy intakes have been revealed when TEE was substantially greater than reported usual energy intakes in weight-stable individuals. Underreporting of food intake is pervasive, ranging from 10 to 45% depending on the age, gender, and body composition of the study subjects (22).

Methods for measuring EE include direct calorimetry, indirect calorimetry, and noncalorimetric methods (23). Direct calorimetry is the measurement of the heat emitted from the body over a given period (1, 24). A direct calorimeter chamber measures heat loss by radiation, convection, conduction, and latent heat arising from vaporization of water. Heat sink calorimeters capture the heat produced by liquid-cooled heat exchangers. Gradient layer calorimeters measure heat loss by a network of thermo-

couples in series surrounding the insulated chamber. Indirect calorimetry estimates heat production indirectly by measuring oxygen consumption (VO_2), CO_2 production (VCO_2), and the respiratory quotient (RQ), which is equal to the ratio of the VCO_2 to VO_2 (25). Indirect calorimetry arose from the observations of Lavoisier and Laplace that heat production of animals as measured by calorimetry was equal to that released when organic substances are burned and that the same quantities of oxygen were consumed by the two processes. The RQ reflects substrate utilization. The complete oxidation of glucose results in an RQ equal to 1.0. The complete oxidation of fat and protein results in an RQ averaging about 0.71 and 0.84, respectively, depending on chemical structure of the foodstuff. Specific RQs for FFAs range from 0.69 to 0.81. RQs of amino acids range from 0.56 to 1.00, with conventional food proteins ranging from 0.81 to 0.87. In mixed diets, the RQ is about 0.85. Lipogenesis, the conversion of carbohydrate to fat, can substantially increase the RQ. The conversion of fat to carbohydrate, in contrast, will lower the RQ to less than 0.70.

Substrate utilization can be determined from rates of VO_2, VCO_2, and urinary nitrogen (23, 25). First, gas exchange must be corrected for the incomplete oxidation of protein. One gram of urinary nitrogen represents the combustion of an amount of protein that would require 5.92 L of oxygen and produce 4.75 L of CO_2. The VO_2 and VCO_2 associated with the protein oxidized are subtracted from the total and are used to compute a nonprotein RQ. The amount of protein oxidized may be calculated directly from urinary nitrogen assuming that 1 g of nitrogen represents 6.25 g of

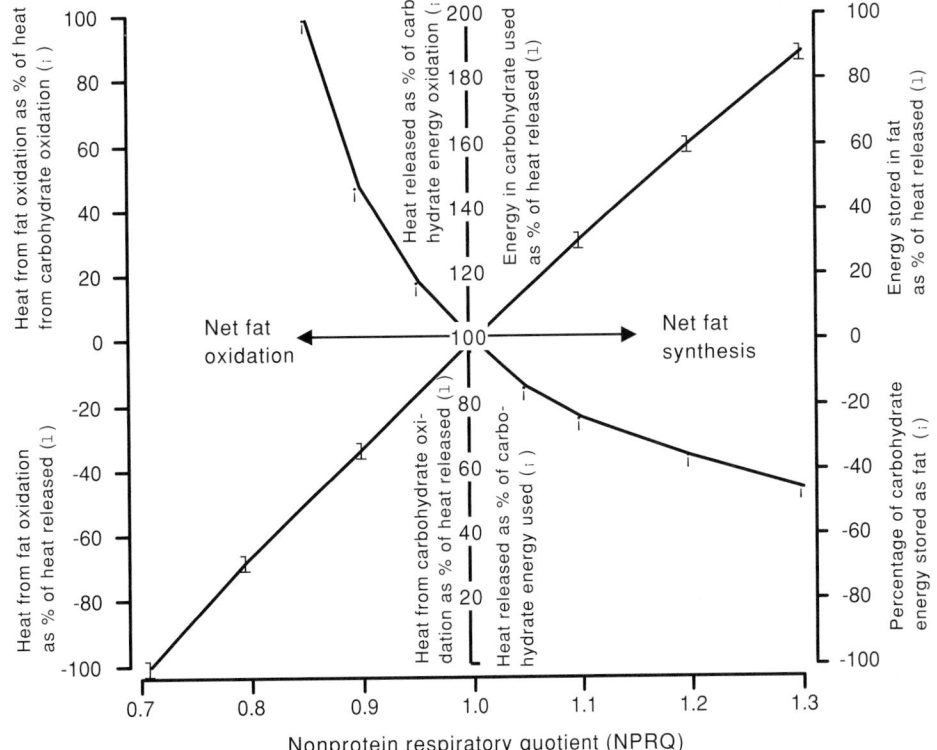

Figure 7.3. Carbohydrate and fat utilization as a function of nonprotein respiratory quotient (NPRQ). The two curves demonstrate carbohydrate utilization and fat oxidation and synthesis with the ordinate axes displaying heat from fat oxidation as a percentage of heat released (solid circles), heat from fat oxidation as a percentage of heat from carbohydrate oxidation (open circles), percentage of carbohydrate energy stored as fat (open circles), and energy stored in fat as a percentage of heat released (closed circles). (From Elia M, Livesey G. Theory and validity of indirect calorimetry during net lipid synthesis. Am J Clin Nutr 1988; 47:591–607, with permission. Copyright American Journal of Clinical Nutrition, American Society for Clinical Nutrition.)

TABLE 7.2. NONPROTEIN RESPIRATORY QUOTIENT AND THE RELATIVE QUANTITY OF CARBOHYDRATE AND FAT OXIDIZED AND ENERGY PER LITER OF OXYGEN

NONPROTEIN RESPIRATORY QUOTIENT	Carbohydrate (g/L O_2)	Fat (g/L O_2)	ENERGY (kcal/L O_2)
0.707	0.000	0.502	4.686
0.71	0.016	0.497	4.690
0.72	0.055	0.482	4.702
0.73	0.094	0.465	4.714
0.74	0.134	0.450	4.727
0.75	0.173	0.433	4.739
0.76	0.213	0.417	4.751
0.77	0.254	0.400	4.764
0.78	0.294	0.384	4.776
0.79	0.334	0.368	4.788
0.80	0.375	0.350	4.801
0.81	0.415	0.334	4.813
0.82	0.456	0.317	4.825
0.83	0.498	0.301	4.838
0.84	0.539	0.284	4.850
0.85	0.580	0.267	4.862
0.86	0.622	0.249	4.875
0.87	0.666	0.232	4.887
0.88	0.708	0.215	4.899
0.89	0.741	0.197	4.911
0.90	0.793	0.180	4.924
0.91	0.836	0.162	4.936
0.92	0.878	0.145	4.948
0.93	0.922	0.127	4.961
0.94	0.966	0.109	4.973
0.95	1.010	0.091	4.985
0.96	1.053	0.073	4.998
0.97	1.098	0.055	5.010
0.98	1.142	0.036	5.022
0.99	1.185	0.018	5.035
1.00	1.232	0.000	5.047

protein. The nonprotein RQ is then used to calculate the proportions of carbohydrate and fat oxidized when the nonprotein RQ (NPRQ) is less than 1.00 (Table 7.2). When the NPRQ is greater than 1.00, net fat synthesis occurs, as shown in Figure 7.3. When the NPRQ is greater than 1.00, carbohydrate is used both for storage of energy and for oxidation (25).

Weir demonstrated that the error in neglecting the effect of protein metabolism on the caloric equivalent of oxygen is 1% for each 12.3% of the total calories that arise from protein (26). The most widely used equation for the calculation of total heat output is by Weir:

$$EE \text{ (kcal)} = 3.941 \times VO_2 \text{ (L)} + 1.106 \text{ } VCO_2 \text{ (L)} - (2.17 \times UrN \text{ (g))} \text{ or}$$

$$EE \text{ (kcal)} = 3.941 \times VO_2 \text{ (L)} + 1 \text{ } VCO_2 \text{ (L)} / (1 + 0.082 \text{ p})$$

where UrN is urinary nitrogen and p is the fraction of calories resulting from protein. Under usual conditions, approximately 12.5% of total calories will arise from protein; therefore, the foregoing equation can be reduced to the following:

$$EE \text{ (kcal)} = 3.9 \times VO_2 \text{ (L)} + 1.1 \text{ } VCO_2 \text{ (L)}$$

Whole-body respiratory calorimeters are small rooms in which the subject may reside comfortably for longer periods unencumbered by respiratory gas collection devices. In these rooms, the concentrations of O_2 and CO_2 and airflow through the system are monitored continuously. Whole-body calorimeters provide a controlled experimental environment to measure TEE and its components. Portable indirect calorimetric systems also have been devised to measure EE in field, clinical, and laboratory settings (27–29). The Douglas bag method has been used historically for many measurements of basal and resting metabolism. In this method, all expired air is collected into a nonpermeable bag with a capacity up to 150 L. After a known period, the volume of expired air at standard temperature and pressure, dry, and the concentrations of O_2 and CO_2 are measured, from which VO_2 and VCO_2 and RQ are calculated. Commercial metabolic carts in laboratory and clinical settings have largely replaced the Douglas bag method. For field measurements, several portable respirometers have been designed with oxygen analyzers as well as gas flow meters and electronics to process and store data. These systems require airtight masks, breathing valves, and nose clips to measure respiratory gas exchange quantitatively. Hood devices and canopies have been designed for more comfort, but they restrict movement.

Other methods to assess EE applicable to field conditions include heart rate (HR) monitoring and DLW. The HR monitoring method is based on the linear relationship between HR and EE (30). Because of variations resulting from age, sex, body size fitness, and nutritional status, the relationship must be calibrated on an individual basis. Simultaneous measurements of EE and HR in subjects are performed across a range of activities to calibrate the individual. Other confounding factors such as ambient conditions, time of day, emotional state, hydration status, food and caffeine intake, and smoking may influence the EE:HR relationship. As a result, HR data on individuals are subject to error and may yield unreliable estimates of EE. When applied to groups of individuals, the HR monitoring method provides an acceptable estimate of TEE.

DLW is a stable (nonradioactive) isotope method that provides an estimate of TEE in free-living individuals. The DLW method was originally developed by Lifson for use in small animals (31, 32), and it was later adapted for humans (33, 34). Two stable isotopic forms of water ($H_2^{18}O$ and ^2H_2O) are administered to the individual, and their ^{18}O and ^2H disappearance rates from the body are monitored for 7 to 21 days, equivalent to one to three half-lives for these isotopes. The disappearance rate of ^2H_2O reflects water flux, whereas that of $H_2^{18}O$ reflects water flux plus VCO_2, because of the rapid equilibration of the body water and bicarbonate pools by carbonic anhydrase. The difference between the two disappearance rates is used to calculate VCO_2. Assuming a RQ, VO_2 and hence EE are calculated. When energy balance prevails, the average RQ may be estimated from the composition of the diet using the food quotient (35). If substantial gains or losses of body constituents are known to occur during the period of measurement, appropriate adjustments must be made in estimating the RQ. Under field conditions, this method is accurate within 5% or better. The advantage of this technique is the noninvasive, nonintrusive manner in which it measures TEE. In weight-stable individuals, the DLW method may be used to assess energy requirements. The disadvantages of the method are the high cost of ^{18}O and expensive, sophisticated mass spectrometric equipment and the expertise required to measure ^{18}O and ^2H.

HUMAN ENERGY REQUIREMENTS

Human energy requirements are composed of basal metabolism, thermogenesis, external work or physical activity, and energy costs of depositing new tissues during growth and pregnancy and secreting milk during lactation. The utilization of metabolizable energy is represented in terms of energy balance and thermal balance in Figure 7.4. Since the 1960s, a resurgence in whole-body energy metabolism has led to a reexamination of the major factors contributing to TEE (2). Additional history about human energetics is in chapter 1 beta.

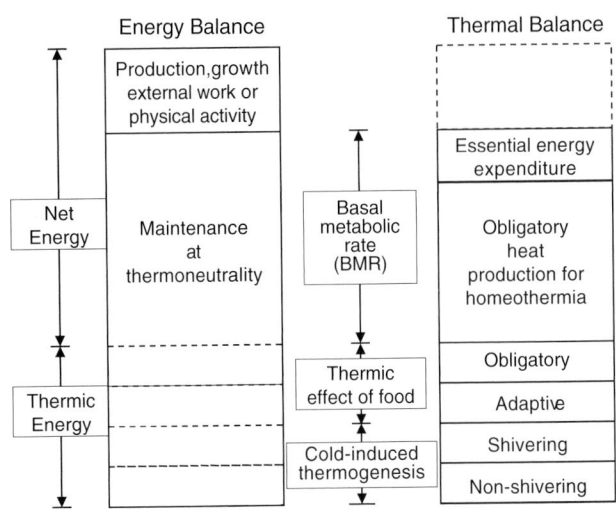

Figure 7.4. Utilization of metabolizable energy represented in terms of energy balance and thermal balance. (From Kinney JM. Energy metabolism: heat, fuel and life. In: Nutrition and Metabolism in Patient Care. Philadelphia: WB Saunders, 1988:3–34, with permission.)

Basal Metabolism

The basal metabolic rate (BMR) is defined as the rate of EE in the postabsorptive state after a 12-hour overnight fast. The BMR is measured while the subject is supine, awake, and motionless in a thermoneutral environment. The BMR represents the energy needed to sustain the metabolic activities of cells and tissues, plus the energy to maintain blood circulation and respiration in the awake state. The sleeping metabolic rate (SMR) is approximately 5 to 10% lower than the BMR (36). The BMR is affected by age, gender, body composition, and nutritional and health status. For practical considerations, the resting metabolic rate (RMR) is often measured instead of the BMR. By definition, the RMR is measured under the same experimental conditions as the BMR, except a 3- to 4-hour fasting period is required, and the time of day and prior physical activity are not controlled. The RMR is approximately 10 to 20% higher than the BMR. The BMR historically was normalized to body surface area, but it is now more appropriately normalized to body weight or fat free mass (FFM).

In 1932, Brody and Kleiber described the empiric relationship between BMR and body weight (1). The logarithm of metabolic rate was found to be a linear function of the logarithm of body weight, and therefore, metabolic rate could best be described as a power of body weight. When the BMR was measured across a wide range of species of varying sizes, it was estimated that

$$BMR = 70 \, WT^{3/4}$$

where WT, weight is in kg and BMR is in kcal/kg$^{3/4}$/day

However, the Brody-Kleiber relationship does not hold for all species or within a species. Within a species, the relationship between minimal metabolism and body weight varies with a power of weight less than the 0.75

TABLE 7.3. SCHOFIELD EQUATIONS FOR ESTIMATING BASAL METABOLIC RATE (kcal/d) FROM WEIGHT (kg)

		n	MULTIPLE CORRELATION	STANDARD ERROR
	Children: <3 y			
Males	BMR = 59.5 wt − 30.4	162	0.95	69.9
Females	BMR = 58.3 wt − 31.1	137	0.96	58.7
	3–10 y			
Males	BMR = 22.7 wt + 504.3	338	0.83	67.0
Females	BMR = 20.3 wt + 485.9	413	0.81	69.9
	10–18 y			
Males	BMR = 17.7 wt + 658.2	734	0.93	105.2
Females	BMR = 13.4 wt + 692.6	575	0.80	111.4
	Adults: 18–30 y			
Males	BMR = 15.0 wt + 692.1	2879	0.65	153.8
Females	BMR = 14.8 wt + 486.6	829	0.73	119.2
	30–60 y			
Males	BMR = 11.5 wt + 873.0	646	0.60	167.9
Females	BMR = 8.1 wt + 845.6	372	0.68	111.7
	>60 y			
Males	BMR = 11.7 wt + 587.7	50	0.71	164.8
Females	BMR = 9.1 wt + 658.4	38	0.68	108.3

BMR, basal metabolic rate; wt, weight.

From Schofield WN, Schofield C, James WPT. Hum Nutr Clin Nutr 1985;39C:1–96, with permission.

that relates to adults, because young individuals have higher metabolic rates per unit metabolic size.

In 1919, Harris and Benedict (37) published prediction equations for BMR based on sex, height, age, and weight:

$$\text{BMR}_{\text{women}} \text{ (kcal/day)} = 665 + (9.6 \times \text{Weight (kg)}) + (1.8 \times \text{Height (cm)}) - (4.7 \times \text{Age (years)})$$

$$\text{BMR}_{\text{men}} \text{ (kcal/day)} = 66 + (13.7 \times \text{Weight (kg)}) + (5 \times \text{Height (cm)}) - (6.8 \times \text{Age (years)})$$

Schofield and colleagues (38) compiled the most recent equations for predicting BMR using data on 7549 persons. The equations predicting BMR from weight and height or from weight alone are provided in Tables 7.3 and 7.4 for separate age-sex groups. Inclusion of height and weight was shown to be advantageous for the very young and the elderly; for older children and adults, weight-alone equations performed as well as the more complex equations. Although the Schofield equations predict the BMR reasonably in some populations, they seem to overestimate the BMR in tropical populations by 8 to 10% (39, 40). Other studies, however, did not collaborate these findings (41, 42). In addition, studies of well-nourished immigrants from tropic to temperate climates found similar BMR/kg body weight (43–45).

FFM contains the metabolically active compartments of the body and therefore is the major predictor of basal

TABLE 7.4. SCHOFIELD EQUATIONS FOR ESTIMATING BASAL METABOLIC RATE (kcal/d) FROM WEIGHT (kg) AND HEIGHT (m)

		n	MULTIPLE CORRELATION	STANDARD ERROR
	Children: <3 y			
Males	BMR = 1.67 wt + 1517 ht − 618	162	0.97	58.0
Females	BMR = 16.2 wt + 1023 ht − 413	137	0.97	51.6
	3–10 y			
Males	BMR = 19.6 wt + 130 ht + 415	338	0.83	66.8
Females	BMR = 17.0 wt + 162 ht + 371	413	0.81	69.4
	10–18 y			
Males	BMR = 16.2 wt + 137 ht + 516	734	0.93	105.0
Females	BMR = 8.4 wt + 466 ht + 200	575	0.82	108.1
	Adults: 18–30 y			
Males	BMR = 15.0 wt − 10.0 ht + 706	2879	0.65	153.2
Females	BMR = 13.6 wt + 283 ht + 98	829	0.73	117.7
	30–60 y			
Males	BMR = 11.5 wt − 2.6 ht + 877	646	0.60	167.3
Females	BMR = 8.1 wt + 1.4 ht + 844	372	0.68	111.4
	>60 y			
Males	BMR = 9.1 wt + 972 ht − 834	50	0.74	157.7
Females	BMR = 7.9 wt + 458 ht + 17.7	38	0.73	102.5

BMR, basal metabolic rate; ht, height; wt, weight.

From Schofield WN, Schofield C, James WPT. Hum Nutr Clin Nutr 1985;39C:1–96, with permission.

metabolism. The contribution of FFM and fat mass (FM) to the variability in RMR was examined in a meta-analysis of seven published studies (46). FFM was the single best predictor of RMR, accounting for 73% of the variability; FM accounted for only an additional 2%. Adjusted for FFM, the RMR did not differ between genders, but it did between lean and obese persons. In another meta-analysis, the relationship of the RMR to FFM was found to be nonlinear across a wide range of infants to adults (47). RMR/kg of weight or RMR/kg FFM falls as mass increases, because the relative contributions made by the most metabolically active tissues (brain, liver, and heart) decline as body size increases.

Basal metabolism declines with age at a rate of approximately 1 to 2% per decade in weight-constant persons (48). This decline is attributable to loss of FFM and gain of less metabolically active fat associated with aging. Endurance training may attenuate the decline in the BMR seen with aging (49). Gender differences in basal metabolism also are evident. Lower BMR in women is largely attributed to differences in body composition, although hormonal differences also may play a role. The BMR varies throughout the menstrual cycle (50, 51). The BMR is about 6 to 15% lower in the preovulatory (follicular) phase than the premenstrual (luteal) phase of the cycle. However, even when BMR data are adjusted for gender differences in FFM and FM, differences in BMR still exist, possibly because of variations in relative contributions of organs and tissues to FFM.

Ethnicity also may affect basal metabolism. Numerous studies documented lower BMR in African-American than white adults (52–55) and children (56–59). The BMR, expressed per kilogram of body weight or per kilogram of FFM, is on the order of 5 to 10% lower in African-Americans compared with whites. Differences in relative contributions of organs and tissues to FFM may explain the differences in BMR among ethnic groups.

Thermogenesis

Thermogenesis augments basal metabolism in response to stimuli unassociated with muscular activity. Stimuli include food ingestion and cold and heat exposure. Thermogenesis comprises two components, obligatory and facultative thermogenesis (23, 60). Obligatory thermogenesis depends on the energy cost of digesting, absorbing, and processing or storing nutrients. The magnitude of this component is determined by the metabolic fate of the ingested substrate. Obligatory thermogenesis also may be potentiated by exercise, a frequent meal pattern, and increased meal size. Facultative or regulatory thermogenesis represents the additional EE not accounted for by the known energy costs of obligatory thermogenesis. The sympathetic nervous system plays a role in modulating facultative thermogenesis.

The thermic effect of food (TEF) refers to the increase in EE elicited by food consumption (1). The increments in EE above BMR, divided by the energy content of the food consumed, vary from 5 to 10% for carbohydrate, 0 to 5% for fat, and 20 to 30% for protein. A mixed meal elicits an increase in EE equivalent to about 10% of the calories consumed.

Cold- and heat-induced thermogenesis refers to the increase in EE that is induced at ambient temperatures below or above the zone of thermoneutrality. Studies consistently suggest that low-normal temperatures of 20 to 22°C and high temperatures of 28 to 30°C are associated with an increase in sedentary EE of 2 to 5% compared with temperatures of 24 to 27°C. Because people usually adjust their clothing and environment to maintain comfort, the additional energy cost of thermoregulation has a minimal effect on TEE.

Other substances such as caffeine can increase the BMR by 10 to 30% for 1 to 3 hours (61). On a daily basis, normal caffeine consumption may cause a modest 3% increase in TEE (62). Drugs such as amphetamines, ephedrine, and some antidepressants stimulate the sympathetic nervous system and, in turn, increase metabolism, whereas propranalol, reserpine, or bethanidine may depress it. The effect of smoking on the BMR is unclear (63, 64), but one study showed a 10% increase in 24-hour EE in a room calorimeter associated with smoking 24 cigarettes (65).

Physical Activity

EE for physical activity represents the most variable component of TEE. Physical activity level (PAL) is defined as the ratio of daily TEE to BEE (TEE/BEE) and is commonly used to describe typical activity levels. PAL for sedentary individuals varied from 1.3 to 1.5, with an average value of 1.35 among nine studies (21). In whole-room calorimeter studies, the TEE/BEE ratio averaged 1.32 in groups with no exercise, 1.42 in those who did 30 to 75 minutes/day of exercise, and 1.60 in those who did 100 to 180 minutes/day (66). The value of 1.4 × BMR represents maintenance energy requirement and covers BMR, TEF, and minimal activity. In more active groups, the PAL ranges from 1.4 to 1.7, and from 2.0 to 2.8 in very active groups.

The energy costs of discrete physical activities have been made using indirect calorimetry (67, 68). Ainsworth and colleagues provided comprehensive tables to estimate the energy expended in discrete physical activities for adults (69).

The energetic efficiency for the conversion of dietary energy into physical work is remarkably constant in humans for non–weight-bearing activities (1, 3, 70a, 73, 102). The metabolic cost of performing specific physical activities is highly reproducible under standardized test conditions. Under optimal conditions, the net efficiency (external work/ internal energy conversion rate increase necessary to accomplish the work) of the body is about 25 to 27%, but under typical circumstances, the mechanical efficiency of the body is considerably less. However, this does not imply that the energy cost of activities is constant among individuals. Energy cost of activities among individuals varies because of differences in weight and skill. For weight-bearing physical activities, the cost is roughly proportional to body weight.

Excess postexercise oxygen consumption refers to the small increase in EE, which occurs for some time after the exercise has been completed. Excess postexercise oxygen consumption is estimated to be approximately 14% of the increment in expenditure that occurs during the exercise itself (70). A sustained increase in postexercise basal metabolism occurs only after intense and prolonged exercise (70–75% VO_2max for 80–90 minutes or longer), and even this increase is small relative to the energy expended in exercise. Moderate levels of exercise do not appear to increase markedly subsequent EE.

Substrate utilization during exercise depends mainly on relative intensity. Fat is the main energy source in muscle and at the whole-body level during rest and mild-intensity exercise (71). As exercise intensity increases, a shift from the predominant use of fat to carbohydrate occurs. Other factors such as exercise duration, gender, training status, and dietary history play secondary roles (72). Peak rate of fat oxidation is achieved at approximately 45% of VO_2max, and for exercises greater than 50% of VO_2max, the oxidation of FFAs declines in muscle, both as a percentage of total energy as well as on an absolute basis. The main carbohydrate energy source is muscle glycogen, supplemented by blood glucose and lactate. If exercise persists beyond 60 to 90 minutes, fat oxidation will rise as carbohydrate fuel sources become depleted. In this case, the intensity of exercise must drop because of depletion of muscle glycogen, decreased blood glucose, and fatigue (73).

Growth

In infants and children, the energy requirement includes the energy associated with the deposition of tissues. The energy requirement for growth relative to maintenance is low, except for the first months of life. As a percentage of total energy requirements, the energy cost of growth decreases from 35% at 1 month to 3% at 12 months of age, and it remains low until puberty, at which time it increases to 4% (102). During childhood, girls grow slightly more slowly than boys, and girls have slightly more body fat. During adolescence, the gender differences in body composition are accentuated (74–77). Adolescence in boys is characterized by rapid acquisition of FFM, a modest increase in FM in early puberty, followed by a decline. Adolescence in girls is characterized by a modest increase in FFM and a continual FM accumulation.

Pregnancy and Lactation

The additional energy requirements of pregnancy include increased basal metabolism and energy cost of physical activity and energy deposition in maternal and fetal tissues. The BMR increases as a result of the metabolic contribution of the uterus and fetus and the increased internal work

of the heart and lungs (78). In late pregnancy, the fetus accounts for about 50% of the increment in BMR. A 3-kg fetus uses approximately 8 mL O_2/kg/minute or 56 kcal/kg/day (79). The energy cost of weight-bearing activities was increased by 19% after 25 weeks of gestation (80). The gross energy cost of non–weight-bearing activities increased on the order of 10% and the net cost on the order of 6% in late pregnancy (80). The energy cost of tissue deposition can be calculated from the amount of protein and fat deposited in the fetus, placenta, amniotic fluid, uterus, breasts, blood, extracellular fluid, and adipose tissue. Hytten and Chamberlain (78) estimated that 925 g protein and 3.8 kg fat, equivalent to 41,500 kcal, were associated with a weight gain of 12.5 kg and a birth weight of 3.4 kg.

Consistent with the additional energy cost of milk synthesis, basal metabolism of lactating women increased on the order of 4 to 5% (81–84). Although TEE may be slightly lower in the first months postpartum, TEE does not appear to differ from nonpregnant, nonlactating values thereafter (81, 82, 85, 86). Energy cost of lactation is estimated from milk production rates and the energy density of human milk. Milk production rates averaged 0.78 L/day from 0 to 6 months postpartum (87–89) and 0.6 L/day from 6 to 12 months postpartum (90). Energy density measured by bomb calorimetry or proximate macronutrient analysis averaged from 0.67 (range, 0.64–0.74) kcal/g (91). Energy mobilized from maternal tissue stores can subsidize the energy cost of lactation. Gradual weight loss averaging –0.8 kg/month in the first 6 months postpartum is typical in well-nourished lactating women (81).

ASSESSMENT OF ENERGY REQUIREMENTS

Energy requirements are defined as the levels of metabolizable energy intake from food that will balance EE, plus cover the needs for growth, pregnancy, and lactation. Recommendations for the nutrient intakes of individuals are generally set to provide enough to meet or exceed the requirements of almost all healthy persons in a given gender-age group, as well as enough to allow reasonable fast recovery of losses that may have been incurred. For most nutrients, individual requirements correspond to the population average requirement plus two standard deviations as a safety factor to ensure that the requirements provide for the needs of nearly all (~95%) the healthy persons in the population. This is reasonable for nutrients for which modest excess intakes present no health risks. However, excess energy intake is eventually deposited in the form of body fat, which does provide a means to maintain metabolism during periods of limited food intake, although it can result in obesity.

Desirable levels of energy intake should be commensurate with EE, to achieve energy balance. However, energy balance was considered inadequate as a sole criterion for setting energy requirements in the 1985 *Technical Report* published by the Food and Agriculture Organization/World

Health Organization/United Nations University Expert Consultation on Energy and Protein Requirement (92). It stated:

> The energy requirement of an individual is a level of energy intake from food that will balance energy expenditure when the individual has a body size and composition, and level of physical activity, consistent with long-term good health; and that would allow for the maintenance of economically necessary and socially desirable physical activity. In children and pregnant or lactating women the energy requirement includes the energy needs associated with the deposition of tissues or the secretion of milk at rates consistent with good health.

This definition implies that desirable energy intakes should support healthy body weights and composition and adequate PALs. Although theoretically it is possible to maintain energy balance and to avoid excess weight gain by reducing dietary energy intake only, there are important advantages in optimizing both energy intake *and* output. First, some evidence suggests that the ability to control food intake may be reduced at very low PALs (93). Second, marked reductions in food intake may make it difficult to fulfill the requirements for essential nutrients such as vitamins and minerals. Implicit in this statement is that desirable energy intakes for obese persons are less than their EE, because weight loss and establishment of a lower body weight are desirable for them. For underweight persons, conversely, desirable energy intakes are greater than their EE to permit weight gain and maintenance of a higher body weight. Unlike other nutrients, body weight can be used to monitor the adequacy or inadequacy of habitual energy intake. Body weight provides a readily monitored indicator of the adequacy or inadequacy of habitual energy intake. Chronic energy deficiency or energy excess eventually will manifest as wasting or obesity. Weight-for-height indices and body mass index are used to assess the weight status of individual persons as well as population groups (94, 95).

The factorial method historically has been used to assess energy requirements (92, 96). In this approach, TEE is estimated from BEE (i.e., BMR extrapolated to 24 hours) and activity energy expenditure derived from the time devoted to different activities and the energy costs of each activity. Limitations of this approach include the accuracy of the BMR predictions, data availability of energy costs of all activities, and the difficulty in estimating random, spontaneous movement. Compared with the DLW method, the factorial method has been found to give significantly higher estimates of TEE (97, 98). Alternatively, the expansive DLW database of TEE measurements can be used to estimate energy requirements.

DIETARY REFERENCE INTAKES: ESTIMATED ENERGY REQUIREMENT

Dietary reference intakes (DRIs) are published by the Food and Nutrition Board of the Institute of Medicine and are intended for healthy persons in the United States and Canada (99). The estimated energy requirement (EER) is defined as the average dietary intake that is predicted to maintain energy balance in a healthy adult of a defined age, gender, weight, and height, and PAL consistent with health. In children and pregnant and lactating women, the EER is taken to include the needs associated with the deposition of tissues or the secretion of milk at rates consistent with health.

The EER was based on TEE measured by DLW method (99). A normative DLW database was compiled on TEE values of 407 adults and 525 normal-weight children. Four PALs were defined to reflect sedentary, low active, active, and very active levels of EE. The sedentary PAL category (PAL = $1.0 - 1.39$) reflects BEE, TEF, and activity energy expenditure. In addition to the activities that are required for independent living, the low PAL category (PAL = $1.4 - 1.59$) encompasses walking 2.5 miles/day or the equivalent EE in other activities; the active PAL category (PAL = $1.6 - 1.89$) includes walking 6 miles/day or its equivalent; and the very active PAL (PAL = $1.9 - 2.5$) reflects walking 12 miles/day or equivalent. Stepwise multiple linear regression was used to develop prediction equations of TEE from age, gender, weight, height, and PAL category. The general equation was as follows:

$$\text{TEE (kcal/day)} = A + B \times \text{Age (years)} + PC \times (D \times \text{Weight (kg)} + E \times \text{Height (m)})$$

where A is the constant term, B is the weight coefficient, PC is the physical activity coefficient for sedentary, low active, active, and very active PAL categories, D is the weight coefficient, and E is the height coefficient. EER was derived from TEE, plus an allowance for growth in the case of children. The equations for predicting EER of specific gender-age groupings are shown in Table 7.5. See Appendix Table A-2-a through A-2-h for more data om DRIs.

Infants and Children

The energy requirements of infants and young children should balance EE at PALs conducive to normal development and should allow for deposition of tissues at rates consistent with health. Because of the dominant contribution of the brain (60–70%), basal metabolism is highest during the first years of life (100). The BMR of term infants ranges from 43 to 60 kcal/kg/day or two to three times greater than in adults (101). The BMR and TEE are influenced by age (older greater than younger), gender (males greater than females), and feeding mode (breast-fed less than formula-fed infants) (102). The DRI for infants and young children was based on a single equation using weight alone to predict TEE, plus an allowance for growth.

Energy requirements of older children and adolescents are defined to promote normal growth and maturation and to support a desirable PAL consistent with health. Energy requirements of children and adolescents are highly variable as a result of differences in growth rate and

TABLE 7.5. EQUATIONS FOR ESTIMATED ENERGY REQUIREMENTS FOR GENDER-AGE GROUPINGS AND PHYSICAL ACTIVITY COEFFICIENTS FOR SEDENTARY, LOW ACTIVE, ACTIVE, AND VERY ACTIVE PHYSICAL ACTIVITY LEVELS

GENDER, AGE CATEGORY	EQUATIONS FOR ESTIMATED ENERGY REQUIREMENTS (kcal/d)	PA PAL = SEDENTARY	PA PAL = LOW ACTIVE	PA PAL = ACTIVE	PA PAL = VERY ACTIVE
Males, Females 0–3 mo	(89 × Weight [kg] − 100) + 175				
Males, Females 4–6 mo	(89 × Weight [kg] − 100) + 56				
Males, Females 7–12 mo	(89 × Weight [kg] − 100) + 22				
Males, Females 13–35 mo	(89 × Weight [kg] − 100) + 20				
Males, 3–8 y	88.5 − 61.9 × Age [y] + PA × (26.7 × Weight [kg] + 903 × Height [m]) + 20	1.00	1.13	1.26	1.42
Females, 3–8 y	135.3 − 30.8 × Age [y] + PA × (10.0 × Weight [kg] + 934 × Height [m]) + 20	1.00	1.16	1.31	1.56
Males, 9–18 y	88.5 − 61.9 × Age [y] + PA × (26.7 × Weight [kg] + 903 × Height [m]) + 25	1.00	1.13	1.26	1.42
Females, 9–18 y	135.3 − 30.8 × Age [y] + PA × (10.0 × Weight [kg] + 934 × Height [m]) + 25	1.00	1.16	1.31	1.56
Males, >19 y	662 − 9.53 × Age [y] + PA × (15.91 × Weight [kg] + 539.6 × Height [m]	1.00	1.11	1.25	1.48
Females, >19 y	354 − 6.91 × Age [y] + PA × (9.36 × Weight [kg] + 726 × Height [m])	1.00	1.12	1.27	1.45

PA, physical activity coefficient; PAL, physical activity level.

From Food and Nutrition Board, Institute of Medicine. Dietary Reference Intakes for Energy, Carbohydrate, Fiber, Fat, Fatty Acids, Cholesterol, Protein, and Amino Acids. 5th ed. Washington, DC: National Academy Press, 2002, with permission.

physical activity. Mean PALs estimated by DLW, HR monitoring, time-motion/diary, and time allocation records ranged from 1.3 to 1.5 for children less than 5 years of age, and 1.5 to 1.9 for children 6 to 18 years, living in urban, industrialized settings (103). Although absolute EE increases with age, weight-specific EE decreases across adolescence, primarily because of the decrease in BMR.

Haschke (104) estimated changes in body composition during adolescence from literature values of total body water, potassium, and calcium. FFM increases in boys, with peak deposition coinciding with peak rates of height gains. The percentage of FM increases during this period in girls, and it actually declines in boys.

The energy cost of growth is more accurately estimated from the individual costs of protein and fat deposition, because the composition of weight gain varies with age. Energy cost of growth ranges from 2.4 to 6.0 kcal/g (10 to 25 kJ/g), depending on the composition of the tissues deposited (105, 106). For the DRI, the energy cost of growth was estimated to be 175 kcal/day for the age interval 0 to 3 months, 60 kcal/day for 4 to 6 months, and 20 kcal/day for 7 to 35 months. Although the composition of newly synthesized tissues varies in childhood and adolescence, these variations have a minor impact on total energy requirements, because only approximately 20 to 25 kcal/day are required for growth.

Adults

In weight-stable adults, energy requirements are equal to their TEE. The DLW database was used to derive separate TEE predictive equations for men and women based on age, height, weight, and PAL category. The age-related decline in TEE was found to amount to approximately 10 and 7 kcal/year for men and women, respectively. Marked variation is apparent in PALs, which depend on the occupational and recreational lifestyles of adults.

Pregnancy and Lactation

Current DRIs are based on empiric longitudinal data of the changes in TEE and body composition of pregnant women. Total energy deposition during pregnancy as a result of 3.7 kg fat and 925 g protein is estimated at 39,862 kcal or 180 kcal/day. As pregnancy progresses, the increment in basal metabolism is offset partially by decreased physical activity. Longitudinal measurements of TEE throughout pregnancy indicate a median change in TEE of approximately 8 kcal/gestational week, with a range of −57 to 107 kcal/week. The DRI for the extra energy required during pregnancy (340 and 452 kcal/day during the second and third trimesters, respectively) was estimated from the sum of the median change in TEE plus the energy deposition during pregnancy. During the first trimester, no additional energy intake was recommended, because TEE changes little and weight gain is minor.

The EER during lactation is estimated from TEE, milk energy output, and energy mobilization from tissue stores. Based on milk production rates of 0.78 and 0.6 L/day from 0 to 6 months and 6 to 12 months postpartum, respectively, and an energy density of 0.67 kcal/g milk, the additional energy cost of lactation would be 523 kcal/day during the first 6 months and 402 kcal/day during the second 6 months of lactation. Based on the average weight loss (0.8 kg/month, equivalent to 170 kcal/day) of well-nourished women during 0 to 6 months postpartum, the net energy cost of lactation is 330 kcal/day from 0 to 6 months postpartum. No further weight loss is assumed; therefore, the full cost of lactation is 400 kcal/day for 6 to 12 months postpartum.

REFERENCES

1. Kleiber M. The Fire of Life: An Introduction to Animal Energetics. Huntington, NY: Robert E. Kreiger, 1975.
2. Kinney JM. Energy metabolism: heat, fuel, and life. In: Kinney JM, Jeejeebhoy KN, Hill GL et al., eds. Nutrition and Metabolism in Patient Care. Philadelphia: WB Saunders, 1988:3–34.
3. Brown AC. Energy metabolism. In: Ruch TC, Patton HD, eds. Physiology and Biophysics III. Digestion, Metabolism, Endocrine Function and Reproduction. Philadelphia: WB Saunders, 1973:85–104.
4. Blaxter K. Energy Metabolism in Animals and Man. Cambridge: Cambridge University Press, 1989:1–336.
5. Flatt JP, Tremblay A. Energy expenditure and substrate oxidation. In: Bray GA, Bouchard C, James WPT, eds. Handbook of Obesity. New York: Marcel Dekker, 1998.
6. Elia M. Fuels of the tissues. In: Garrow JS, James WPT, Ralph A, eds. Human Nutrition and Dietetics. Edinburgh: Churchill Livingstone, 2000:37–59.
7. Siler SQ, Neese RA, Hellerstein MK. Am J Clin Nutr 1999;70:928–36.
8. Suter PM, Schutz Y, Jequier E. N Engl J Med 1992;326:983–7.
9. Acheson KJ, Schutz Y, Bessard T et al. Endocrinol Metab 1984;9:E62–E70.
10. Wolfe RR. The role of triglyceride–fatty acid cycling and glucose cycling in thermogenesis and amplification of net substrate flux in human subjects. In: Muller MJ, Danforth E, Burger AG, eds. Hormones and Nutrition in Obesity and Cachexia. New York: Springer, 1990.
11. Consolazio CF, Johnson RE, Pecora LJ. The computation of metabolic balances. In: Physiological Measurements of Metabolic Functions in Man. New York: McGraw-Hill, 1963:313–25.
12. Watt BK, Merrill AL. Composition of Foods. ARS Handbook No. 8. Washington, DC: US Government Printing Office, 1963:160.
13. Paul AA, Southgate DAT. McCance & Widdowson's the Composition of Foods. 4th ed. London: Her Majesty's Stationery Office, 1978.
14. Flatt JP. Energetics of intermediary metabolism. In: Garrow JS, Halliday D, eds. Substrate and Energy Metabolism in Man. London: John Libbey, 1985:58–69.
15. Flatt JP. Rec Adv Obes Res 1978;2:211–28.
16. Flatt JP. Diabetes Metab Rev 1988;4:571–81.
17. Flatt JP. Am J Clin Nutr 1995;62:820–36.
18. Flatt JP. Am J Clin Nutr 1987;45:296–306.
19. Black AE, Prentice AM, Goldberg GR et al. J Am Diet Assoc 1993;33:572–9.
20. Schoeller D. Metabolism 1995;44:18–22.
21. Goldberg GR, Black AE, Jebb SA et al. Eur J Clin Nutr 1991;45:569–81.
22. Johnson RK, Soultanakis RP, Matthews DW. J Am Diet Assoc 1998;98:1136–40.
23. Jequier E, Acheson K, Schutz Y. Assessment of energy expenditure and fuel utilization in man. Annu Rev Nutr 1987;7:187–208.
24. Holmes FL. Lavoisier and the Chemistry of Life. Madison, WI: University of Wisconsin Press, 1985.
25. Livesey G, Elia M. Am J Clin Nutr 1988;47:608–28.
26. Weir JB. J Physiol 1949;109:1–9.
27. Webb P. Human Calorimeters. New York: Praeger, 1985.
28. McLean JA. Animal and Human Calorimetry. Cambridge: Cambridge University Press, 1987.
29. Murgatroyd PR, Shetty PS, Prentice AM. Int J Obes 1993;17:549–68.
30. Schutz Y, Weinsier RL, Hunter G. Obes Res 2001;9:368–79.
31. Lifson N, McClintock R. J Theoret Biol 1966;12:46–74.
32. Lifson N, Gordon GB, McClintock R. J Appl Physiol 1955;7:704–10.
33. Schoeller DA, Van Santen E. J Appl Physiol 1982;53:955–9.
34. Schoeller DA, Leitch CA, Brown C. Am J Physiol 1986;1:R1137–43.
35. Black AE, Prentice AM, Coward WA. Hum Nutr Clin Nutr 1986;40C:381–91.
36. Garby L, Kurzer MS, Lammert O et al. Hum Nutr Clin Nutr 1987;41:225–33.
37. Harris JA, Benedict FG. A Biometric Study of Basal Metabolism. Publication 279. Washington, DC: Carnegie Institution, 1919.
38. Schofield WN, Schofield C, James WPT. Hum Nutr Clin Nutr 1985;39C:1–96.
39. Henry CJK, Rees DG. Eur J Clin Nutr 1991;45:177–85.
40. Piers LS, Shetty PS. Eur J Clin Nutr 1993;47:586–91.
41. Henry CJK, Piggott SM, Emery B. Hum Nutr Clin Nutr 1987;41C:397–402.
42. Soares MJ, Francis DG, Shetty PS. Eur J Clin Nutr 1993;47:389–94.
43. Ulijaszek SJ, Strickland SS. Ann Hum Biol 1991;18:245–51.
44. Geissler CA, Aldouri MS. Ann Nutr Metab 1985;29:40–7.
45. Hayter JE, Henry CJK. Eur J Clin Nutr 1993;47:724–34.
46. Nelson KM, Weinsier RL, Long CL et al. Am J Clin Nutr 1992;56:848–56.
47. Weinsier RL, Schutz Y, Bracco D. Am J Clin Nutr 1992;55:790–4.
48. Keys A, Brozek J, Henschel A et al. The Biology of Human Starvation. Minneapolis, MN: University of Minneapolis Press, 1950.
49. Poehlman ET, Danforth E Jr. Am J Physiol 1991;261:E233–9.
50. Bisdee JT, James WP, Shaw MA. Br J Nutr 1989;61:187–99.
51. Solomon SJ, Kurzer MS, Calloway DH. Am J Clin Nutr 1982;36:611–6.
52. Albu J, Shur M, Curi M et al. Am J Clin Nutr 1997;66:531–8.
53. Carpenter WH, Fonong T, Toth MJ et al. Am J Physiol 1998;274:E98–101.
54. Foster GD, Wadden TA, Vogt RA. Obes Res 1997;5:1–8.
55. Jakicic JM, Wing RR. Int J Obes Relat Metab Disord 1998;22:236–42.
56. Kaplan AS, Zemel BS, Stallings VA. J Pediatr 1996;129:643–7.
57. Treuth MS, Butte NF, Wong WW. Am J Clin Nutr 2000;71:893–900.

58. Wong WW, Butte NF, Ellis KJ et al. J Clin Endocrinol Metab 1999;84:906–11.

59. Yanovski SZ, Renolds JC, Boyle AJ et al. Obes Res 1997;5: 321–5.

60. Jequier E. Clin Endocrinol Metab 1984;13:563–80.

61. Acheson KJ, Azhorska-Markiewicz B, Pittet P et al. Am J Clin Nutr 1980;33:989–97.

62. Garrow JS, Webster JD. Thermogenesis to small stimuli in human energy metabolism. In: van Es AJH, ed. Human Enery Metabolism. Wageningen, Netherlands: Agricultural University, 1985.

63. Warwick PM, Chapple RS, Thomson ES. Int J Obes 1987;11: 229–37.

64. Dallosso HM, James WPT. Int J Obes 1984;8:365–75.

65. Hofstetter A, Schutz Y, Jequier E et al. N Engl J Med 1986;314: 79–82.

66. Warwick PM. Predicting food energy requirements from estimates of energy expenditure. In: Truswell AS, Dreosti IE, English RM et al., Recommended Nutrient Intakes: Australian Papers. Sydney: Australian Professional Publications, 1990: 295–320.

67. Durnin JVGA, Passmore R. Energy, Work and Leisure. London: Heinemann Educational Books, 1967.

68. Passmore R, Durnin JVGA. Physiol Rev 1955;35:801–40.

69. Ainsworth BE, Haskell WL, Leon AS et al. Med Sci Sports Exerc 1993;25:71–80.

70. Bahr R, Ingnes I, Vaage O et al. J Appl Physiol 1987;62:485–90.

70a. Pahud P, Ravussin E, Jequier E. Appl Physiol 1980;48:770–5.

71. Brooks GA, Mercier J. J Appl Physiol 1994;76:2253–61.

72. Brooks GA, Fahey TD, White TP et al. Exercise Physiology: Human Bioenergetics and Its Applications. 3rd ed. Mountain View, CA: Mayfield Publishing, 2000.

73. Graham TE, Adamo KB. Can J Appl Physiol 1999;24:393–415.

74. Ellis KJ. Am J Clin Nutr 1997;66:1323–31.

75. Ellis KJ, Abrams SA, Wong WW. Am J Clin Nutr 1997;65: 724–731.

76. Forbes GB. Human Body Composition. Growth, Aging, Nutrition, and Activity. New York: Springer-Verlag, 1987:1–350.

77. Tanner JM. Growth at Adolescence. 2nd ed. Oxford: Blackwell Scientific Publications, 1962.

78. Hytten FE, Chamberlain G. Clinical Physiology in Obstetrics. 2nd ed. Oxford: Blackwell Scientific Publications, 1991.

79. Sparks JW. Biol Neonate 1980;38:113–9.

80. Prentice AM, Spaaij CJK, Goldberg GR et al. Eur J Clin Nutr 1996;50:S82–111.

81. Butte NF, Wong WW, Hopkinson JM. J Nutr 2001;131:53–8.

82. Forsum E, Kabir N, Sadurskis A et al. Am J Clin Nutr 1992;56:334–42.

83. Sadurskis A, Kabir N, Wager J et al. Am J Clin Nutr 1988;48: 44–9.

84. Spaaij CJK, van Raaij JMA, de Groot LCPGM et al. Am J Clin Nutr 1994;59:42–7.

85. Goldberg GR, Prentice AM, Coward WA et al. Am J Clin Nutr 1991;54:788–98.

86. Lovelady CA, Meredith CN, McCrory MA et al. Am J Clin Nutr 1993;57:512–8.

87. Allen JC, Keller RP, Archer P et al. Am J Clin Nutr 1991;54: 69–80.

88. Butte NF, Garza C, Stuff JE et al. Am J Clin Nutr 1984;39: 296–306.

89. Heinig MJ, Nommsen LA, Peerson JM et al. Am J Clin Nutr 1993;58:152–61.

90. Dewey KG, Finley DA, Lönnerdal B. J Pediatr Gastroenterol Nutr 1984;3:713–20.

91. Neville MC. Volume and caloric density of human milk. In: Jensen RG, ed. Handbook of Milk Composition. San Diego: Academic Press, 1995:99–113.

92. Food and Agriculture Organization/World Health Organization/United Nations University. Report of a Joint Consultation: Energy and Protein Requirements. Technical Report Series 724. Geneva: World Health Organization, 1985.

93. Stubbs RJ, Highes DA, Johnstone AM et al. Am J Clin Nutr 2004;79:62–9.

94. World Health Organization. Obesity: Preventing and Managing the Global Epidemic. Report of a World Health Organization Consultation on Obesity. Geneva: World Health Organization, 1998:1–276.

95. Kuczmarski RJ, Ogden CL, Grummer-Strawn LM et al. CDC Growth Charts: United States. Advance Data from Vital and Health Statistics. 314th ed. Hyattsville, MD: US Department of Health and Human Services, 2000:1–28.

96. National Research Council, Subcommittee on the Tenth Edition of the RDAs. Recommended Dietary Allowances. 10th ed. Washington, DC: National Academy Press, 1989.

97. Haggarty P, McNeill G, Abu Manneh MK et al. Br J Nutr 1994;72:799–813.

98. Jones PJ, Martin LJ, Su W et al. Can J Public Health 1997;88: 314–9.

99. Food and Nutrition Board, Institute of Medicine. Dietary Reference Intakes for Energy, Carbohydrate, Fiber, Fat, Fatty Acids, Cholesterol, Protein, and Amino Acids. 5th ed. Washington, DC: National Academy Press, 2002.

100. Holliday M, Potter D, Jarrah A et al. Pediatr Res 1967;1: 185–95.

101. Schofield WN, Schofield C, James WPT. Hum Nutr Clin Nutr 1985;39C:1–96.

102. Butte NF, Wong WW, Hopkinson JM et al. Am J Clin Nutr 2000;72:1558–69.

103. Torun B, Davies PSW, Livingstone MBE et al. Eur J Clin Nutr 1996;50:35S–81S.

104. Haschke F. Body Composition during Adolescence. In: Body Composition Measurements in Infants and Children. Columbus, OH: Ross Laboratories, 1989.

105. Butte NF, Wong WW, Garza C. Proc Nutr Soc 1989;48:303–12.

106. Roberts SB, Young VR. Am J Clin Nutr 1988;48:951–5.

107. Elia M, Livesey G. Am J Clin Nutr 1988;47:591–607.

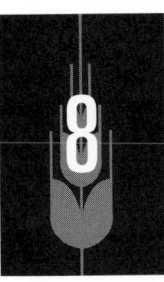

ELECTROLYTES, WATER, AND ACID-BASE BALANCE[1]

MAN S. OH AND JAIME URIBARRI

REGULATION OF INTRACELLULAR AND
  EXTRACELLULAR VOLUMES AND OSMOLALITY 149
  Volume of Body Fluids 150
  Composition of the Body Fluid 150
  Osmolar Relations and Regulations 151
  Types of Dehydration 158
  Principles of Fluid Therapy 159
POTASSIUM METABOLISM AND ITS DISORDERS 160
  Control of Transcellular Flux of Potassium 160
  Dietary Sources of Potassium 161
  Control of Renal Excretion of Potassium 161
  Plasma Renin Activity, Plasma Aldosterone
    Concentration, and Abnormalities in
    Potassium Metabolism 164
  Hypokalemia 164
  Hyperkalemia 166
PATHOPHYSIOLOGY OF WATER AND ANTIDIURETIC
  HORMONE METABOLISM 167
  Regulation of Thirst and Antidiuretic
    Hormone Release 167
  Polyuria 169
  Hyponatremia 171
  Hypernatremia 175
ACID-BASE DISORDERS 176
  Bicarbonate and Carbon Dioxide Buffer System ..176
  Terminology 176
  Whole-Body Acid-Base Balance 177
  Metabolic Acidosis 178
  Metabolic Alkalosis 183

Respiratory Acidosis 184
Respiratory Alkalosis 185
Mixed Acid-Base Disorders 185
CLINICAL PROBLEMS AND ANSWERS 186
  Regulation of Intracellular and Extracellular
    Volume and Osmolality 186
  Disorders of Potassium Metabolism 187
  Water and Antidiuretic Hormone Metabolism 188
  Acid-Base Disorders 189

REGULATION OF INTRACELLULAR AND EXTRACELLULAR VOLUMES AND OSMOLALITY

The body fluid is an aqueous solution containing many electrolytes and consists of intracellular and extracellular compartments. The intracellular fluid is not a single compartment, but each cell has its own separate environment, communicating with other cells only via interstitial fluid and plasma. Consequently, difference exists among cells in various tissues in their solute content and concentrations. Regardless of the nature of the solute and its electrical charge, however, osmotic equilibrium is maintained so each particle of solute throughout the body is surrounded by the same number of water molecules. Because cell membranes are permeable to water, osmolality is the same throughout the body fluids. Permeability of cell membranes to water depends on the ubiquitous presence of aquaporins (water channels), but in those cells lacking aquaporins, various ion channels probably provide sufficient water diffusion needed for osmotic equilibrium (1–3).

Operation of normal metabolic functions of the body requires maintenance of an optimal ionic strength of its environment, primarily the intracellular fluid, where most metabolic activities occur. The homeostatic mechanisms of the body are therefore constantly at work to provide such an environment. Because the extracellular fluid is not the site of major metabolic activity, substantial alteration in its ionic strength may occur without adverse effects on body function. The main function of the extracellular fluid is to serve as a conduit between cells and between organs. The plasma is a route of rapid transit, and the interstitial fluid serves as a slow supply zone, which, by flowing around the cell, permits the entire cell surface to be used as an area of exchange. The

---

[1]**Abbreviations: AA,** acetoacetic acid; **ADH,** antidiuretic hormone; **AG,** anion gap; **ATP,** adenosine triphosphate; **BB,** β-hydroxybutyric acid; **BUN,** blood urea nitrogen; **Ca²⁺,** calcium; **Cl⁻,** chloride; **DI,** diabetes insipidus; **ECG,** electrocardiogram, electrocardiographic; **EnaC,** epithelial sodium channel; **FFA,** free fatty acid; **GFR,** glomerular filtration rate; **H⁺,** hydrogen ion; **HCO₃⁻,** bicarbonate; **K⁺,** potassium; **LDH,** lactate dehydrogenase; **Mg²⁺,** magnesium; **Na⁺,** sodium; **NADH,** reduced nicotinamide adenine dincleotide; **NH₄⁺,** ammonium; **P,** phosphate; **PA,** plasma aldosterone; **Pco₂,** partial pressure of carbon dioxide; **PRA,** plasma renin activity; **ROMK,** renal outer medulla K channel; **RTA,** renal tubular acidosis; **SIADH,** syndrome of inappropriate antidiuretic hormone secretion; **TBW,** total-body water; **THAM,** tris-hydroxymethylaminomethane; **UA,** unmeasured anion; **UC,** unmeasured cation; **VRD,** volume regulatory decrease; **VRI,** volume regulatory increase.

ability of the extracellular fluid to function efficiently as a conduit requires maintenance of optimal extracellular volume, particularly of vascular volume. An additional important function of the extracellular fluid is regulation of the intracellular volume and its ionic strength. Because of the osmotic equilibrium between the cells and the extracellular fluid, any alteration in extracellular osmolality is followed by an identical change in intracellular osmolality, which is usually accompanied by a reciprocal change in cell volume (4).

Although cells and organs can be supplied with substrate and relieved of metabolic products with a much slower circulation, normal circulation is required to supply sufficient oxygen for the body's metabolic needs. Normal plasma volume is a prerequisite for maintenance of normal circulation. Because plasma is in equilibrium with the interstitial fluid, the maintenance of normal vascular volume requires normal extracellular volume. A low extracellular volume results in impaired organ perfusion, and an excessive extracellular volume leads to vascular congestion and pulmonary edema.

Volume of Body Fluids

Total-body water (TBW) can be determined by dilution of various substances including deuterium, tritium, and antipyrine. TBW measured with antipyrine in hospitalized adults without fluid and electrolyte disorders is about 54% of the body weight (5). The fractional water content is higher in infants and children, and it decreases progressively with aging. The water content also depends on the body content of fat; women and obese persons, because of their higher fat content, tend to have less water for a given weight. A useful short cut for the calculation of TBW, using the fact that 54% of body weight in kilograms is body water, and 1 kg is 2.2 lb, is as follows:

$$\text{TBW (L)} = \text{Body weight (lb)}/4$$

For an obese person, subtract 10% from the calculated body water, and for a lean person, add 10%. For a very obese person, subtract 20%. Women have about 10% less body water than men for the same body weight. Extracellular volume is measured directly, and intracellular volume is estimated as the difference between TBW and extracellular volume. The measurement of TBW is reliable, but the measurement of extracellular volume is not, because no ideal marker has been found. Markers such as sodium (Na^+), chloride (Cl^-), and bromide penetrate the cells to some extent, whereas other markers such as mannitol, inulin, and sucrose do not penetrate certain parts of the extracellular fluid. Thus, depending on the type of marker used, the extracellular fluid volume could vary from 27 to 53% of TBW (5).

Extracellular volume measured with Cl^- and expressed as a percentage of TBW varies from 42 to 53%, greater in older subjects and women. Extracellular volume measured with inulin or sulfate is smaller, about 30 to 33% of TBW (5). For discussion in this chapter, a value of 40% of TBW is

TABLE 8.1. VOLUMES OF BODY FLUID COMPARTMENTS[a]

Intracellular volume: 24 L (60%)
Extracellular volume: 16 L (40%)
   Interstitial volume: 11.2 L (28%)
   Plasma volume: 3.2 L (8%)
   Transcellular volume: 1.6 L (4%).

[a]A physiologically normal man weighing 73 kg (160 lb) with 40 L of total-body water is used as a model.

considered to represent extracellular volume. Extracellular volume is further divided into three fractions: interstitial (space between cells) volume (28% of TBW), plasma volume (8%), and transcellular water volume (4%) (Table 8.1). Transcellular water includes luminal fluid of the gastrointestinal (GI) tract, the fluids of the central nervous system, and fluid in the eye, as well as the lubricating fluids at serous surfaces.

Composition of the Body Fluid

Extracellular Composition

The concentrations of electrolytes in plasma are easily measured, and their values are well known. These concentrations increase by about 7% when expressed in plasma water, because about 7% of plasma is solids. Thus, plasma Na^+ is 140 mEq/L, but the concentration in plasma water is about 150 mEq/L. The concentrations of electrolytes in interstitial fluid are different from those in the plasma because of difference in protein concentrations between plasma and interstitial fluid. The differences in electrolyte concentrations between plasma and interstitial fluid can be predicted by the Donnan equilibrium (Table 8.2) (6). With normal plasma protein concentrations, the concentrations of diffusible cations are higher in plasma water than in interstitial water by about 4%, whereas the concentrations of diffusible anions are lower in the plasma than in the interstitial fluid by about 4%. The concentrations of calcium (Ca^{2+}) and magnesium (Mg^{2+}) in the interstitial fluid are lower than the values predicted by the Donnan equilibrium, because they are substantially protein bound.

Part of the interstitial space is occupied by a ground substance consisting of glycosaminoglycans, the most abundant of which is hyaluronan (hyaluronic acid), and this space excludes distribution of proteins. In the other part, proteins can distribute freely and communicate with lymphatics. The first part is a gel phase, and the second part is a free phase. Interspersed within the interstitial space is elastin, which provides the elastic property of the interstitial tissue; this property is necessary for generation of normal negative pressure of the interstitial space and positive pressure with the development of edema (7–9).

Intracellular Composition

Whereas Na^+, Cl^-, and bicarbonate (HCO_3^-) are the main solutes in the extracellular fluid, potassium (K^+), Mg^{2+},

TABLE 8.2. ELECTROLYTE CONCENTRATIONS IN EXTRACELLULAR AND INTRACELLULAR FLUIDS

	PLASMA		INTERSTITIAL FLUID		PLASMA WATER		CELL WATER (MUSCLE)	
	(mEq/L)	(mmol/L)	(mEq/L)	(mmol/L)	(mEq/L)	(mmol/L)	(mEq/L)	(mmol/L)
Na^+	140	140	145.3	145.3	149.8	149.8	13	13
K^+	4.5	4.5	4.7	4.7	4.8	4.8	140	140
Ca^{2+}	5.0	2.5	2.8	2.8	5.3	5.3	1×10^{-7}	0.5×10^{-7}
Mg^{2+}	1.7	0.85	1.0	0.5	1.8	0.9	7.0	3.5
Cl^-	104	104	114.7	114.7	111.4	111.4	3	3
HCO_3^-	24	24	26.5	26.5	25.7	25.7	10	10
SO_4^-	1	0.5	1.2	0.6	1.1	0.44	—	—
Phosphate	2.1	1.2[a]	2.3	1.3[a]	2.2	1.2[a]	107	57[b]
Protein	15	1	8	0.5	16	1	40	2.5[c]
Organic anions	5	5[d]	5.6	5.6[d]	5.3	5.3[d]	—	—

Ca^{2+}, calcium; Cl^-, chloride; HCO_3^-, bicarbonate; K^+, potassium; Mg^{2+}, magnesium; SO_4^-, sulfate.
[a] The calculation is based on the assumption that the pH of the extracellular fluid is 7.4 and the pK of $H_2PO_4^-$ is 6.8.
[b] The intracellular molal concentration of phosphate is calculated with the assumption that the pK of organic phosphates is 6.1 and the intracellular pH 7.0.
[c] The calculation is based on the assumption that each mmol of intracellular protein has on the average 15 mEq, but the nature of cell proteins is not clearly known.
[d] The assumption has been that all the organic anions are all univalent.

phosphate (P), and proteins are the dominant solutes in the cell. The intracellular concentrations of Na^+ and Cl^- cannot be measured with accuracy, and they are estimated by subtracting the amount that is extracellular from the total tissue value. Because concentrations of electrolytes in the extracellular fluid are high, a small error in extracellular water volume measurement will cause a large error in the measurement of intracellular concentration of these ions. The concentration of HCO_3^- is calculated from cell pH, and the HCO_3^- concentration shown in Table 8.2 is based on the assumption that average cell pH is 7.0.

The electrolyte composition of intracellular fluid is not identical throughout the tissues. For example, the concentration of Cl^- in muscle is very low, about 3 mEq/L, but it is about 75 mEq/L in erythrocytes. The concentration of K^+ in the muscle cell is about 140 mEq/L, but in platelets it is only about 118 mEq/L. The concentration of Na^+ in the muscle and red blood cell is about 13 mEq/L, but in the leukocytes it is about 34 mEq/L. The main P in the red blood cell is 2,3-diphosphoglycerate, but in the muscle they are adenosine triphosphate (ATP) and creatinine P. Because the muscle represents the bulk of the body cell mass, it is customary to use the electrolyte concentration of the muscle cells as representative of the intracellular electrolyte concentration. Because a substantial part of the anions inside the cell consists of polyvalent ions such as P and protein, the total ionic concentration in the cell in milliequivalents per liter is higher than that of the extracellular fluid, to maintain osmotic equilibrium with the extracellular fluid.

Osmolar Relations and Regulations

Measurement of Plasma Osmolality

When the osmolal concentration of the extracellular fluid increases by accumulation of solutes that are restricted to the extracellular fluid (effective osmols), such as glucose, mannitol, and Na^+, osmotic equilibrium is reestablished as water shifts from the cell to the extracellular fluid and thus increases intracellular osmolality to the same level as the extracellular osmolality (4, 6, 10). When the extracellular osmolality increases by accumulation of solutes that can enter the cell freely (ineffective osmols), such as urea and alcohol, the osmotic equilibrium is achieved by entry of those solutes into the cell. Because most of the solutes normally present in the extracellular fluid are effective osmols, loss of extracellular water (e.g., insensible losses) will increase effective osmolality and hence will cause a shift of water from the cells. Reduction in extracellular osmolality either by loss of normal extracellular solutes or by retention of water reduces effective osmolality for the same reasons and hence causes a shift of water into the cells.

The plasma osmolality can be measured with an osmometer or estimated as the sum of the concentration of all the solutes in the plasma. Because an osmometer does not distinguish between effective and ineffective osmols, effective osmolality can only be estimated. Urea is the only ineffective osmol that has substantial concentration in the plasma. Still, its normal concentration is only 5 mOsm/L. In the normal plasma, therefore, total osmolality is nearly equal to effective osmolality. Plasma osmolality is estimated as follows:

$$\text{Plasma osmolality} = \text{Plasma } Na^+ \text{ (mEq/L)} \times 2 + \text{Glucose (mg/dL)}/18 + \text{Urea (mg/dL)}/2.8$$

Many of the solutes that may accumulate abnormally in the body are anions of an acid, such as salicylate, glycolate, formate, lactate, and β-hydroxybutyrate. These substances should not be added in estimating plasma osmolality because they are largely balanced by Na^+ and therefore are already included in the value when plasma Na^+ is multiplied by 2. Nonelectrolyte solutes that accumulate abnormally in the serum, such as ethanol, ethylene glycol, methanol, and mannitol, will cause the measured osmolality to exceed the calculated osmolality, thus producing an osmolal gap (11, 12). This osmolal gap is a useful clinical clue to the presence of the toxic substances listed earlier. Accumulation of neutral and cationic amino acids can also cause a serum osmolal gap.

Effect of Hyperglycemia on Serum Sodium

The permeability of a membrane for a given solute varies with the cell type. For example, glucose does not accumulate in the muscle. It does not enter the muscle cell freely, and when it enters the cell with the help of insulin, it is quickly metabolized. Thus, glucose is an effective osmol for the muscle cell; for example, hyperglycemia will cause shift of water from the muscle cell. Conversely, glucose is an ineffective osmol for the red blood cells, liver, kidney cells, and some brain cells because it enters these cells freely. Glucose is generally categorized as an effective osmol mainly because the muscle cells represent the largest body cell mass. Accumulation of glucose or mannitol in the extracellular fluid is a well-known cause of hyponatremia. The relationship between change in serum Na^+ and change in glucose concentration in a physiologically normal adult is about 1.5 mEq/L of Na^+ for 100 mg/dL of glucose. This figure is valid, however, only when the volume of distribution of glucose is somewhere between 40 and 50% of TBW. As the volume of distribution of glucose in relation to TBW is increased, the effect of glucose on serum Na^+ decreases progressively. Decreased volume of distribution of glucose has an opposite effect. The change in serum Na^+ caused by hyperglycemia can be estimated with the following formula (6):

$$\Delta Na^+ \text{ (mEq/L)} = (5.6 - 5.6a)/2$$

where ΔNa^+ is a reduction in serum Na^+ in mEq/L for each 100 mg/dL increase in glucose, and "a" is the fraction of the volume of glucose distribution over TBW.

With marked expansion of extracellular volume, such as in congestive heart failure and other edema-forming states, the volume of distribution of glucose represents a much greater fraction of TBW, and hence a fall in serum Na^+ caused by hyperglycemia would be much less than usual. For example, when the volume of distribution of glucose is 80% of TBW (0.8), the decrease in serum Na^+ for 100 mg/dL rise in glucose would be only about 0.6 mEq/L; $(5.6 - 5.6 \times 0.8)/2 = 0.56$. When the glucose volume is 20% of TBW, ΔNa^+ would be 2.2 mEq/L for a 100 mg/dL increase in glucose.

Concept of Tonicity

In the strict sense, the tonicity of a solution is expressed only in reference to a physiologic system: A hypertonic solution is one that shrinks the cells, whereas a hypotonic solution is one that causes swelling of the cell. When the term tonicity is applied to a fluid in vitro, it is used almost interchangeably with total osmolality. Thus, a solution that contains a high concentration of urea is called hypertonic. Similarly, urine is said to be hypertonic if its osmolality is high, regardless of the nature of its solute (13).

Osmolality and Specific Gravity

Whereas osmolality of fluid depends on osmolal concentration of its solute, specific gravity is determined by the weight of the solute relative to the volume it occupies in solution. Plasma protein contributes little to osmolality because of its low molal concentration, but it is the major factor determining specific gravity of plasma. Urinary specific gravity and osmolality usually change in parallel, but discrepancy between the two occurs with heavy proteinuria and severe glycosuria (5).

Signs and Symptoms of Abnormal Cell Volume and Electrolyte Concentrations

Various signs and symptoms appear with increase or decrease in effective osmolality, which is accompanied by a reciprocal change in intracellular volume. Whether these manifestations are caused by abnormal cell volume or abnormal tonicity is not clearly known. Some of these clinical manifestations are probably caused by cell swelling and shrinkage. In contrast, some cerebral manifestations of hyperosmolality and hypoosmolality may persist even after the brain cell volume has been restored to normal. Because restoration of normal brain cell volume may not normalize electrolyte concentration, the persisting signs and symptoms may be attributed to abnormal electrolyte concentration of the brain cells rather than to the abnormal brain cell volume. The findings that some of the most serious cerebral manifestations of altered osmolality are related to brain cell volume and that brain cells have the capacity to regulate their volume with time explain why rapidity of alteration in osmolality is an important determinant of severity of symptoms (5).

Signs and Symptoms of Hypoosmolality. Whereas hyponatremia without hypoosmolality is possible, hypoosmolality without hyponatremia does not occur. A reduced concentration of Na^+ in the extracellular fluid, without low effective osmolality, causes no adverse effect, except that hyponatremia worsens manifestations of hyperkalemia. For example, when hyponatremia is caused by hyperglycemia or mannitol administration, the signs and symptoms are those of hyperosmolality and cell dehydration. When moderate hyponatremia is caused by salt depletion, some of the symptoms, such as easy fatigability and muscle cramps and spasms attributed to hyponatremia, are in part the result of reduced effective vascular volume. Most of the signs and symptoms of hyponatremia, such as nausea, vomiting, headache, papilledema, and mental confusion, are caused by brain swelling and increased intracranial pressure. Lethargy, weakness, hyperreflexia and hyporeflexia, delirium, coma, psychosis, focal weakness, ataxia, aphasia, generalized rigidity, and seizure are caused by increased cell volume and reduced electrolyte concentration of the brain cells. GI manifestations include abdominal cramps, temporary loss of sense of taste and flavor, decreased appetite, nausea, vomiting, salivation, and paralytic ileus. Cardiovascular effects of hypoosmolality are usually manifested as hypotension and other signs of low effective vascular volume. Hyponatremia can also be accompanied by muscle cramps, twitching, and rigidity (5, 14, 15).

Signs and Symptoms of Hyperosmolality. Increased effective osmolality need not be accompanied by hypernatremia. Accumulation of effective solutes other than Na^+ salts in the extracellular fluid can cause hyperosmolality and cell dehydration, but it may be accompanied by normal or low serum Na^+ concentration. However, hypernatremia is always accompanied by hyperosmolality and cell dehydration. Clinical signs and symptoms of hypernatremia are likely to be those of hyperosmolality and cell dehydration. Hence, clinical manifestations of hyperosmolality caused by glucose, mannitol, or glycerol mimic those of hypernatremia despite the low serum Na^+ concentration. As in the hypoosmolal states, the symptoms and signs of hyperosmolality depend on the rapidity of its development as well as the severity of hyperosmolality. A patient may be comatose when the serum Na^+ reaches 160 mEq/L rapidly, whereas the patient may remain conscious with a serum Na^+ concentration of 190 mEq/L if hypernatremia occurs gradually. Most of the symptoms and signs of hyperosmolality result from disturbed functions of the central nervous system. Acute hyperosmolality resulting from hypernatremia, both in human subjects and in animals, leads to subdural, cortical, and subarachnoid hemorrhages because sudden shrinkage of the brain cells creates negative pressure in the brain, given that the skull cannot collapse. Depression of mental state ranges from lethargy to coma. Generalized seizure may also be observed, although somewhat less commonly than in hypoosmolality. Muscular symptoms of hyperosmolality include muscular rigidity, tremor, myoclonus, hyperreflexia, spasticity, and rhabdomyolysis. In children, spasticity, chronic seizure disorder, and mental retardation may occur with chronic hyperosmolality (5).

Regulation of Intracellular Volume

When cells swell in response to extracellular hypoosmolality, the regulatory mechanism that works to reduce cellular solute content and thereby to reduce their volume is referred to as volume regulatory decrease (VRD). In shrunken cells, the volume regulatory mechanisms work to increase the solute content of the cells and thereby to increase their volume; this process is termed volume regulatory increase (VRI). Most cells are capable

of volume regulation with both VRD and VRI (16, 17). In contrast, the muscle cells do not have volume regulatory mechanisms. Red blood cells have a capacity to regulate the cell volume, but different species use different mechanisms for volume regulation. In general, VRD in blood cells is achieved by loss of electrolytes, namely, NaCl and KCl.

The initial defense against brain swelling in hyponatremia also seems to include osmotic inactivation as well as osmotic disequilibrium; the brain osmolality is significantly higher than that of serum in animals made acutely hyponatremic in 2 hours. As in the case of VRD, different species use different mechanisms to achieve VRI. VRI is accounted for by increases in Na^+, K^+, and Cl^- but also by accumulation of organic substances. The main organic solutes that accumulate in hyperosmolality are polyols (sorbitol and myoinositol), methylamines (betaine and glycerophosphodidylcholine), and amino acids (taurine, glutamine, glutamic acid, aspartic acid) (18).

Unlike the muscle cells, whose volume remain chronically altered as long as effective osmolality is abnormal, the brain cells have the ability to restore the volume to normal when effective osmolality remains chronically altered. In acute hyponatremia, the brain cell volume is initially increased. If the hypoosmolal state persists, the brain cell volume is normalized over a few days, as the cellular solute content decreases. Sudden normalization of osmolality from a chronic hypoosmolal state then causes extracellular shift of water and shrinkage of the brain to a subnormal level (Fig. 8.1). Similarly, in a chronic hyperosmolal state, brain volume is normalized by increasing total solute content of the brain, and a sudden reduction in osmolality from a chronic hyperosmolal state can therefore cause brain swelling (Fig. 8.2).

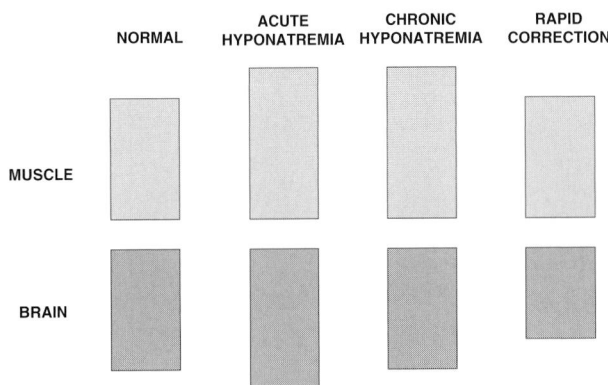

Figure 8.1. Volume changes of the brain and muscle in hyponatremia and after treatment. In acute hyponatremia, both the muscle and the brain swell in proportion to the degree of hyponatremia. As hyponatremia becomes chronic, the brain restores its volume to the original normal through the volume regulatory mechanisms, while the muscle remains swollen. As hyponatremia is rapidly corrected to normal serum sodium concentration, water shift from the cell normalizes the muscle volume, whereas the brain shrinks to a subnormal size.

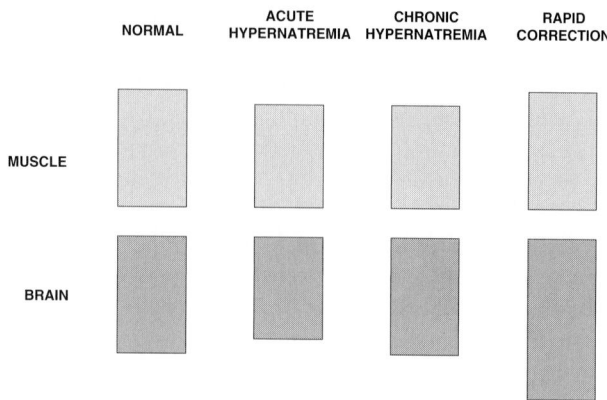

Figure 8.2. Volume changes of the brain and muscle in hypernatremia and after treatment. In acute hypernatremia, both the muscle and the brain shrink their volumes in proportion to the degree of hypernatremia. As hypernatremia becomes chronic, the brain restores its volume to the original normal through the volume regulatory mechanisms, while the muscle remains shrunken. As hypernatremia is rapidly corrected to normal serum sodium concentration, water shift into the cell normalizes the muscle volume, whereas the brain volume becomes abnormally increased.

Regulation of Extracellular Volume

Because the extracellular Na^+ concentration is maintained within a fairly narrow range through the regulation of antidiuretic hormone (ADH) release, the extracellular volume depends primarily on its Na^+ content. In most clinical situations, the extracellular volume correlates well with vascular volume, which, in turn, correlates positively with the effective vascular volume. Effective vascular volume is an imaginary volume that reflects cardiac output in relation to the tissue's demand for oxygen (6).

Hence, the main efferent mechanisms for the regulation of extracellular volume are designed to sense the changes in effective vascular volume, rather than the extracellular volume or vascular volume. This situation sometimes leads to a pathologic retention of salt. For example, salt is retained in congestive heart failure despite markedly expanded extracellular volume and vascular volume, because effective vascular volume is decreased.

Theoretically, the salt content of the body can be altered in two ways: by altering the intake of salt or by altering renal salt output. No well-developed mechanism influences salt intake in response to changes in effective vascular volume. Thus, alterations in salt content of the body are achieved primarily through changes in renal salt output. Changes in renal salt output can be achieved through physical and humoral factors. The physical factors for renal salt regulation work through changes in glomerular filtration rate (GFR) and in peritubular capillary oncotic and hydrostatic pressures. Humoral factors work primarily through their effects on renal tubular salt reabsorption, either by increasing or decreasing it, but they can also work through their effects on physical factors. Figure 8.3 shows the nomenclature of the nephron sites.

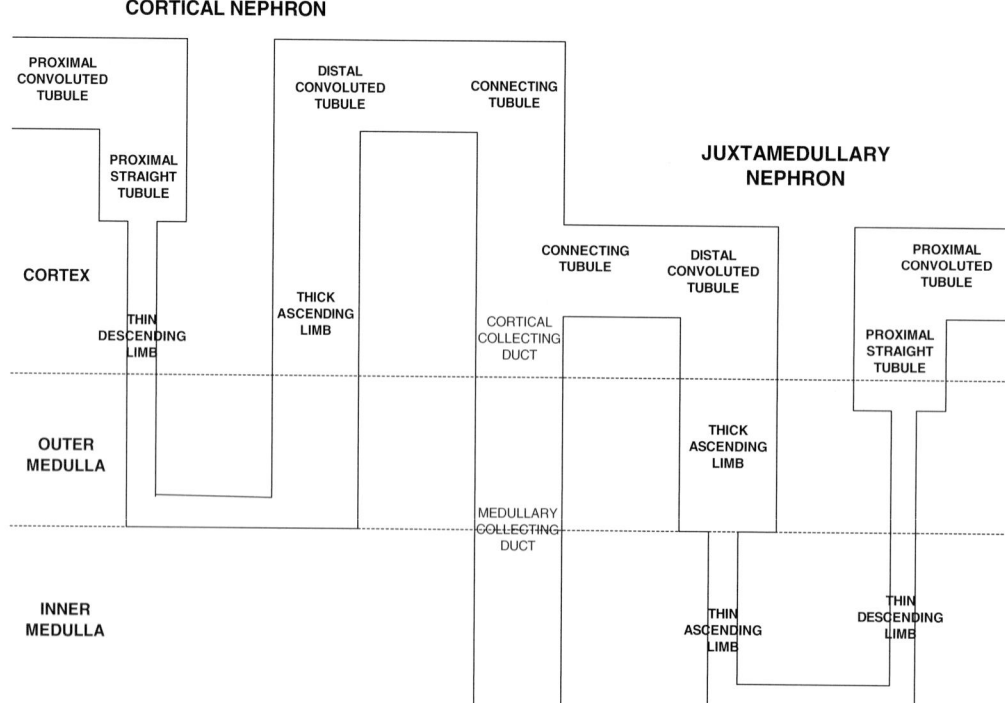

Figure 8.3. Distribution and subdivision of nephrons. The two major types of nephron are cortical and juxtamedullary. The loop of Henle of the cortical nephron does not enter the inner medulla and has no thin ascending limb. The juxtamedullary nephron has the thin ascending limb of Henle, which resides in the inner medulla. Both nephrons are further subdivided into eight or nine segments.

Figure 8.4. Mechanisms of sodium (Na^+) reabsorption at different nephron segments. The main source of energy for Na^+ reabsorption at all nephron segments is the basolateral Na^+-potassium-adenosine triphosphatase (Na^+-K^+-ATPase), which transports $3Na^+$ out of the cell in exchange for $2K^+$ into the cell, which creates a low intracellular Na^+ concentration and negative cellular potential. Both these conditions allow passive diffusion of Na^+ into the cell through the luminal membrane. In the proximal tubule, Na^+ entry is accompanied by exit of hydrogen ion (H^+) through the Na^+-H^+ exchanger type 3 (NHE-3). In the thick ascending limb of Henle, a Na^+ enters with a K^+ and 2 chlorides (Cl^-) through the Na^+- K^+- Cl^- cotransporter (NKCC). In the distal convoluted tubule, Na^+ enters with Cl^- through the NaCl cotransporter (NCCT), and in the cortical collecting duct, Na^+ enters through the epithelial Na^+ channel (ENaC).

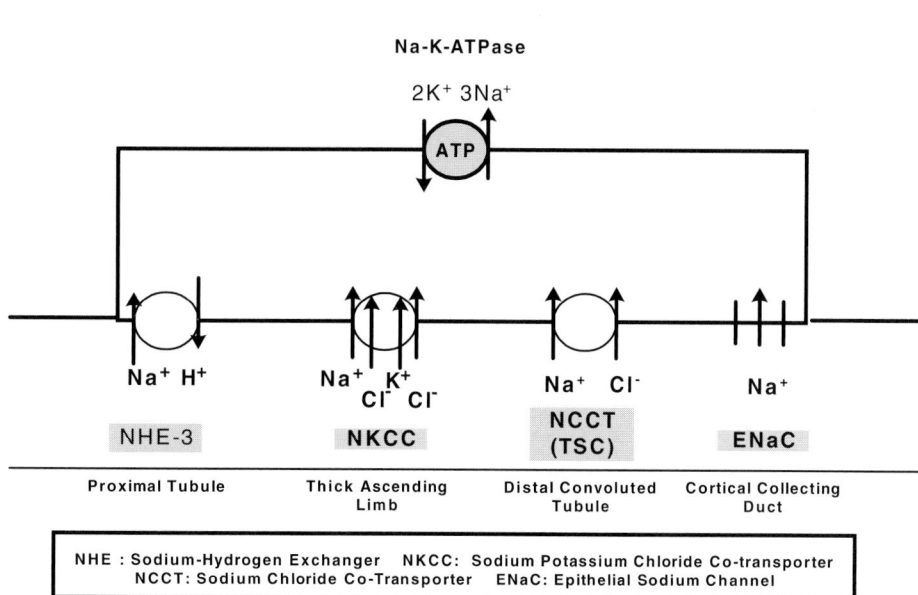

The ultimate source of energy for reabsorption of Na^+ at various nephron segments is Na^+-K^+-ATPase located on the basolateral membrane, which transports $3\ Na^+$ out of the cell in exchange for $2\ K^+$ into the cell. The resulting reduction in intracellular Na^+ concentration and the negative cellular electrical potential allow passive diffusion of Na^+ into the cell through the luminal membrane. Four major sites of Na^+ reabsorption in the nephron use four different mechanisms of Na^+ entry (Fig. 8.4). Numerous humoral factors have been proven or suggested as participating in the regulation of renal salt output. Those with well-proven physiologic effects are aldosterone, catecholamines, angiotensin II, and perhaps ADH and prostaglandins (6, 17).

Dietary Salt Intake and Blood Pressure. For most electrolytes, their total-body contents determine their concentrations in the extracellular fluid and hence those in the serum. Increased content of K^+ causes hyperkalemia, increased content of Mg^{2+} causes hypermagnesemia, and so on. Similarly, decreased K^+ and Mg^{2+} contents lead to hypokalemia and hypomagnesemia, respectively. This rule usually does not apply to Na^+ because serum Na^+ concentration, as the main determinant of the body fluid osmolality, is independently regulated by ADH. Consequently, a change in total-body Na^+ content is usually not accompanied by a change in serum Na^+ concentration. An increase in Na^+ content is accompanied by a nearly proportionate increase in water content, and serum Na^+ concentration remains about the same. Similarly, a decrease in Na^+ content does not usually result in hyponatremia as a proportionate amount of water is also lost. Only when Na^+ deficit is very great, hyponatremia occurs as volume

deficit-induced stimulation of ADH prevents renal excretion of water in an attempt to restore the effective vascular volume (19–22). Thus, total-body Na^+ content is reflected in the extracellular volume, which is the main determinant of effective vascular volume. Hence, a higher Na^+ content predicts increased effective vascular volume, and a lower Na^+ content predicts decreased effective vascular volume. This section briefly discusses the role of dietary intake of Na^+ as a determinant of body Na^+ content, effective vascular volume, and ultimately the latter's effect on the regulation of arterial blood pressure (6, 23–26).

Chronic increases in body Na^+ content occur either because of increased intake of Na^+ or decreased renal excretion of Na^+. Decreased renal excretion of Na^+, in turn, occurs either as a result of impaired function of salt-excreting mechanisms (primary renal Na^+ retention) or in response to reduced effective vascular volume (secondary renal Na^+ retention). Increased Na^+ content of the body that results from increased Na^+ intake or from primary renal Na^+ retention ultimately results in increased arterial blood pressure. The mechanism of increased blood pressure in these settings is mediated by increased effective vascular volume. Hypertension does not occur with secondary renal Na^+ retention as in congestive heart failure or ascites formation, because the cause of secondary renal Na^+ retention in those states is low effective vascular volume.

Effective vascular volume can be best assessed by volume of cardiac output in relation to tissue's requirement for perfusion. Hence, increased effective vascular volume indicates increased cardiac output beyond the tissue's requirement for perfusion. Chronic increase in cardiac output to a level beyond its requirement causes arteriolar constriction through the autoregulation mechanism. With chronic arteriolar constriction, cardiac output gradually returns to baseline, whereas peripheral vascular resistance remains increased; hypertension that results is caused mainly by increased peripheral vascular resistance with little contribution from increased cardiac output. The role of primary renal Na^+ retention as a cause of hypertension is clearly documented and is well accepted in various acute and chronic renal diseases, primary hyperaldosteronism, and many congenital disorders that are characterized by increased renal Na^+ reabsorption such as Liddle syndrome, Gordon syndrome, and apparent mineralocorticoid excess. In contrast to the well accepted role of primary renal Na^+ retention, the role of increased Na^+ intake as a cause of hypertension is still hotly debated, and raging controversy continues.

The pioneering rat studies by Dahl and colleagues first demonstrated the important role of dietary salt intake in the regulation of blood pressure (27). Furthermore, epidemiologic studies have shown that hypertension is rare in communities where salt intake is low, whereas the incidence of hypertension is high with high salt intake. For example, the Yanomamo Indians of Brazil, who eat little or no salt, have virtually no hypertension (28), whereas the northern Japanese, who eat 20 to 30 g/day salt, have the highest stroke rates. Many reports based on metaanalysis on effects of salt restriction on blood pressure concluded that salt restriction is beneficial in reducing blood pressure (29–33). Cutler, Elliot, and collaborators concluded that a 3- to 6-g reduction in daily salt consumption would drop blood pressure by 5/3 mm Hg (systolic/diastolic) in hypertensive persons and 2/1 mm Hg (systolic/diastolic) in normotensive persons (29).

Intersalt, led by Stamler and Rose, compared blood pressure and salt consumption, as measured by 24-hour urine samples, from 52 communities around the globe, from the highest to the lowest extremes of salt intake (32). One hundred male subjects and 100 female subjects from each decade of life between 20 and 60 years were chosen at random from each population group of 52 communities. The results did not confirm the existence of a linear relationship between salt intake and blood pressure. Of the 52 populations, four were primitive societies such as the Yanomamo with low blood pressure and daily salt intake lower than 3.5 g. Among the subjects in the remaining 48 communities, no clear relationship was found between Na^+ intake and blood pressure. However, an association appeared when all the subjects were treated as a single large population rather than 52 distinct populations, and the investigators concluded that reducing salt intake from 10 to 4 g/day would reduce blood pressure by 2.2/0.1 mm Hg. However, the more potent association was shown between salt intake and the rise in blood pressure with age: populations that ate less salt experienced a smaller rise with advancing age than did populations that ate more salt. Intersalt projected that reducing salt intake by 6 g/day would reduce

the average rise in blood pressure between the ages of 25 and 55 years by 9/4.5 mm Hg (32). The reinterpretation of the same Intersalt data by correcting regression dilution bias led to the conclusion that reducing daily salt intake by 6 g would drop blood pressure by 4.3/1.8 mm Hg, a benefit three times larger than originally estimated (33).

The Trials of Hypertension Prevention, Phase II (TOHP II), published in 1997, found that short-term Na^+ reduction and weight loss each lowered blood pressure in persons who were overweight and had slightly elevated blood pressures, but long-term implementation was judged to be difficult (34). In 1998, the Trial of Nonpharmacologic Interventions in the Elderly (TONE), a multicenter clinical trial involving 2400 people with "high normal" blood pressure, found that a 4-g reduction in daily salt intake correlated with a 2.9/1.6-mm Hg drop in blood pressure after 6 months (35).

Some reports based on metaanalysis of similar data concluded that the effect of salt restriction on blood pressure was negligible. Metaanalysis of 56 clinical trials by Midgley and associates concluded that benefit from salt reduction is small and does not support current dietary recommendations (36). The Scottish Heart Health Study, launched in 1984 by Tunstall-Pedoe and colleagues, on the basis of the data obtained by questionnaires, physical examinations, and 24-hour urine collections in 7300 Scottish men, concluded that increased K^+ intake but not reduced Na^+ intake seemed to have a beneficial effect on blood pressure (37). In 1997, Tunstall-Pedoe and associates published a 10-year follow-up and stated that Na^+ intake showed no relationship with either coronary heart disease or death (38).

Despite conflicting data and conflicting opinions, the National Heart, Lung, and Blood Institute is supporting the position of the National High Blood Pressure Education Program, which recommends that a high-salt diet is hazardous to health and that US residents should consume no more than 2400 mg/day Na^+ (6 g salt) (39).

Why such conflicting data? Two main reasons exist. First, too many variables affect blood pressure, and salt intake is intimately associated with many other dietary factors that influence blood pressure such as caloric intake, K^+ intake, Ca^{2+} and Mg^{2+} intake, and intake of fruits and vegetables. Consequently, isolating the influence of salt intake on blood pressure from these other variables is difficult. Second, increase in Na^+ content of the body does not result in immediate increase in blood pressure, but its effect could be delayed for years to decades. For example, children with genetic defects in renal Na^+ transport do not uniformly develop hypertension at early ages, and in some instances the development of hypertension may be delayed for decades (40). Yet most prospective studies that correlated Na^+ intake to hypertension were of short duration.

No one questions the antihypertensive effect of diuretics whose main effect is reducing Na^+ content of the body, notwithstanding certain claim that some diuretics may have direct vasodilatory effects. The question is then how much of a reduction in total-body Na^+ content can be achieved by reducing salt intake, for example. from 10 to 6 g/day. When salt intake is reduced, salt output eventually decreases to a level equal to intake, because prolonged imbalance between intake and output is theoretically impossible. Reduction in salt intake is initially not accompanied by reduction is renal salt output, so salt output exceeds salt intake temporarily. This imbalance creates a reduction in extracellular volume and hence effective vascular volume. The kidney, sensing reduced effective vascular volume, reduces salt output. As long as salt output exceeds salt intake, the body Na^+ content keeps decreasing. Only when salt output decreases sufficiently to equal the reduced salt intake, a new balance is struck, and the volume change stops. The question is how sensitive the kidney is in sensing a reduction in effective vascular volume. Those persons who have substantial salt loss before a new balance is achieved are likely to have a greater decrease in blood pressure than those who lose little salt before a new salt balance (23, 24). (See Chapter 68 for more on hypertension and diet.) In conclusion, dietary salt restriction is clearly beneficial, but its benefit may not be obvious in a short-term trial.

Sodium and Chloride Content of Food. Na^+ and Cl^-, being the major extracellular solutes, are contained in any food products that contain interstitial fluid, but the amounts contained in the interstitial fluid of food are quite small because the interstitial fluid represents a small fraction of total fluid content of foods. Intracellular content of both ions is quite low. For these reasons, high intake of Na^+ and Cl^- results invariably from salt added to food in prepared foods or during cooking. Therefore, the Na^+ content of food tends to parallel the Cl^- content. However, many natural foods contain more Cl^- than Na^+, and this explains why a usual 24-hour urinary excretion rate of Cl^- exceeds that of Na^+. For example, most nuts, vegetables, and fruits, and cereals contain more Cl^- than Na^+ (41). The exceptions to this rule are meat, fish, and eggs; these contain more Na^+ than Cl^- (Fig. 8.5).

Nonrenal Control of Water and Electrolyte Balance

Water is lost from the skin primarily as a means of eliminating heat. Water loss from the skin without sweat is called insensible perspiration. Sweat contains about 50 mEq/L of Na^+ and 5 mEq/L of K^+. Because the main purpose of water loss from the skin is elimination of heat, water loss from the skin depends mainly on the amount of heat generated in the body:

$$\text{Water loss from the skin} = 30 \text{ mL/100 cal}$$

The water content of inspired air is less than that of the expired air, and hence water is lost during normal ventilation. Because the ventilatory volume is determined by the amount of carbon dioxide (CO_2) production, which is, in turn, determined by the caloric expenditure, ventilatory

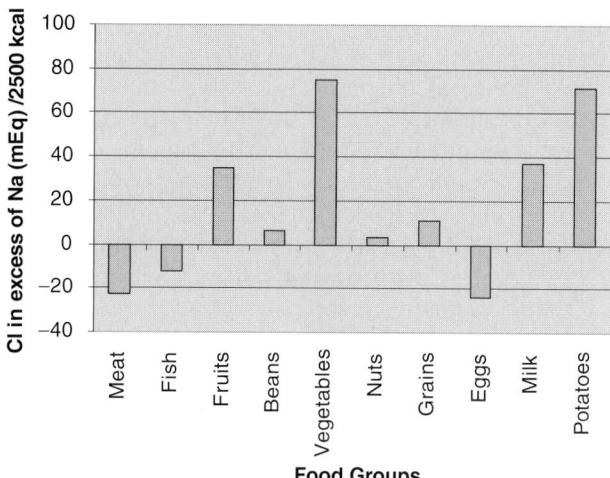

Figure 8.5. The chloride-sodium (Cl-Na) difference of major food groups. Sodium in food is mostly present as NaCl as salt is added during cooking or ingestion. In most natural foods without added salt, Cl content exceeds that of Na. Meat, fish, and eggs are exceptions and contain more Na than Cl.

water loss in normal environmental conditions depends also on caloric expenditure:

$$\text{Respiratory water loss} = 13 \text{ mL/100 cal at normal partial pressure of } CO_2 (P_{CO_2})$$

By coincidence, the quantity of water lost during normal respiration is about equal to the metabolic water production. Hence, in calculating water balance, respiratory water loss may be ignored in the measurement of insensible water loss, provided metabolic water gain is also ignored. Respiratory water loss increases with hyperventilation or fever disproportionately to metabolic water production (5).

The net activity of the GI tract to the level of the jejunum is secretion of water and electrolytes. The net activity from jejunum to colon is reabsorption. Most of the fluid entering the small intestine is absorbed in the small intestine, and the remainder by the colon, leaving only about 100 mL of water to be excreted daily in the feces. The contents of the GI tract are isotonic with plasma, and any fluid that enters the GI tract becomes isotonic. Thus, if water is ingested and vomited, solute is lost from the body.

Route of Fluid and Electrolyte Loss

Fluid and electrolytes may be lost from the GI tract for a variety of reasons such as diarrhea, vomiting or gastric drainage, and drainage or fistula from the bile ducts, pancreas, and intestine. Although diarrheal fluid is close to isotonic in terms of total electrolyte concentrations (Na^+, K^+, Cl^+, and HCO_3^-), diarrhea caused by nonabsorbable solutes, such as lactulose, mannitol, sorbitol, or disaccharide (e.g., in a patient with disaccharide malabsorption), causes much greater water loss than electrolyte loss. Because of the loss of HCO_3^- and K^+, diarrhea tends to cause metabolic acidosis and hypokalemia. Because vomitus contains HCl (100 mEq/L at pH 1.0), vomiting tends to produce metabolic alkalosis. The gastric fluid contains little Na^+ in relation to water; therefore, vomiting without fluid intake invariably causes hypernatremia (42–44).

Obstruction of the bowel may cause transfer of fluid from the extracellular space into the intestinal lumen. Because the composition of the sequestered fluid is similar to that of the extracellular fluid, effective arterial volume will be reduced without much alteration in composition. The patient may give evidence of extracellular volume depletion without weight loss.

The loss through skin increases with fever, increased metabolism, sweating, and burns. The fluid lost through the skin is markedly hypotonic.

Water is lost through the lung with ventilation, and the amount depends on the ventilatory volume. Fever and hyperventilation increase water loss through the lung.

The kidney may lose Na^+ excessively in certain situations, which include diuretic therapy, aldosterone deficiency or unresponsiveness to aldosterone, and relief of urinary obstruction. Other causes include drainage from the pleural and peritoneal cavity, seepage from burns and from transected lymphatics, and fluid loss during hemodialysis and peritoneal dialysis.

Types of Dehydration

Depending on the quantity of salt loss in relation to water loss, several types of dehydration are encountered. The net alteration in body composition is determined by the sum of that which has been lost and that which has been added. The net change in dehydration may be the following: (a) isotonic dehydration, in which net salt and water loss are equal; (b) hypertonic dehydration, characterized by loss of water alone or of water in excess of salt; or (c) hypotonic dehydration, characterized by salt loss in excess of water loss.

Isotonic Dehydration

Salt may be lost isotonically through the GI tract or directly from the extracellular fluid by aspiration of pleural effusion or ascites, among other causes. With GI fluid loss, salt is lost with equal or larger amount of water loss, and then the osmolality of the body fluids is subsequently adjusted to isotonicity by oral intake or urinary excretion of water. Isotonic fluid loss reduces only the extracellular fluid volume. Treatment calls for isotonic salt solution.

Hypertonic Dehydration

The primary aberration in hypertonic dehydration is water deficit. Two major mechanisms account for abnormal water deficit: inadequacy of water intake and excessive water loss. Dehydration resulting from excessive water loss usually develops more rapidly than dehydration caused by reduced water intake. Inadequacy of water intake is always caused by one of the following two mechanisms:

(a) defective thirst resulting from a defective thirst center or impaired consciousness; or (b) lack of available water or inability to drink water.

Water loss may occur excessively through the kidney (e.g., osmotic diuresis and diabetes insipidus [DI]) or through the nonrenal routes (e.g., sweating, osmotic diarrhea, vomiting of HCl). In terms of Na^+ balance, loss of HCl with water is almost equivalent to the loss of pure water because it leaves behind $NaHCO_3$ replacing $NaCl$ in the extracellular fluid. Even when excessive water loss is the cause of hypertonic dehydration, one of the conditions that limit water intake must be present to maintain hypertonicity. Otherwise, stimulation of thirst by increased osmolality will lead to increased water drinking and correction of hypernatremia. Salt content of the body in hypertonic dehydration may be normal, increased, or decreased, and the extent of extracellular volume depletion depends on the degree of salt retention. Conversely, intracellular volume depletion depends solely on the magnitude of hypertonicity. Salt administered or ingested in a state of water deficit is retained, resulting in increased salt content of the body. Water requirement to decrease serum Na^+ concentration to a desired level can be determined using the following formula:

$$\text{Water requirement} = (\text{Actual } Na^+/\text{Goal } Na^+ - 1) \times \text{TBW} = \Delta Na^+/\text{Goal } Na^+ \times \text{TBW}$$

where ΔNa^+ is difference between actual and normal Na^+ concentration.

Water requirement calculated using this formula is based on the assumption that water is lost without gain or loss of salt. If salt retention is part of the reason for hypernatremia, administration of the total amount calculated by the foregoing formula will cause overexpansion of volume. However, if the kidney is functioning normally, the excess salt and water will be excreted. Rapid correction of hypernatremia to normal levels offers no advantage and is potentially harmful because it may cause brain edema. It is advisable to reduce serum Na^+ at a rate no greater than 0.7 mEq/L/hour, or 10% of the original serum Na^+/day. In acute hypernatremia, the speed of correction can be faster.

Hypotonic Dehydration

Fluids lost from the body, especially GI tract losses, are almost always either hypotonic or isotonic in relation to extracellular Na^+ concentration, and loss of such fluid cannot cause hypotonicity of body fluid. Hypotonic dehydration occurs because the patient loses a salt solution and replaces it with water or with a solution containing less Na^+ and K^+ than the fluid that has been lost. In the presence of normal renal function, net loss of salt alone without net water loss is difficult to achieve because the resultant hyponatremia would suppress ADH, resulting in water loss. Decreased effective vascular volume then causes the release of ADH to prevent further depletion of the extracellular volume, and

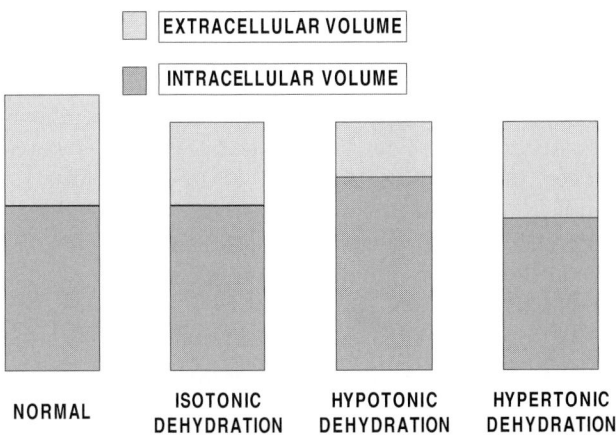

Figure 8.6. Three types of dehydration. Total-body water and extracellular volume are reduced in all three types, but intracellular volume is reduced in hypertonic dehydration, whereas it is expanded in hypotonic dehydration. For these reasons, for a given reduction in total-body water, extracellular volume depletion is most severe with hypotonic dehydration and is least severe with hypertonic dehydration.

hyponatremia develops. Hypoosmolality of the extracellular fluid causes a shift of water into the cells to achieve osmotic equilibrium. Hence cell volume is increased despite extracellular volume contraction. Patients with hypotonic dehydration therefore present with more evidence of compromised circulation, for a given degree of body water loss, than patients with isotonic or hypertonic dehydration (45) (Fig. 8.6). However, acute hyponatremia per se may also diminish vascular tone and cardiac output.

Hypotonic dehydration may be treated by estimating the amount of salt needed to restore the osmolality of the body fluids to normal, administering this amount of salt in the form of hypertonic saline, and administering normal saline to complete restoration of the extracellular volume. The Na^+ requirement to increase serum Na^+ concentration is calculated using the following equation:

$$Na^+ \text{ requirement} = \Delta Na^+ \times TBW$$

where ΔNa^+ is desired serum Na^+ minus actual serum Na^+.

Even though the administered Na^+ would be distributed mainly in the extracellular fluid, TBW is used for this calculation because increase in serum Na^+ is accompanied by an exactly proportionate increase in serum osmolality ($Na^+ \times 2 = $ osmolality). The estimation of the amount of solutes required to increase serum osmolality is always based on TBW, because increase in extracellular osmolality is not possible without increase in intracellular osmolality to the same extent (5).

As an alternative therapeutic approach, one can raise serum Na^+ with isotonic or hypotonic saline; as extracellular fluid volume increases, ADH will be suppressed; as free water is excreted, serum Na^+ will return to normal. This approach is recommended in patients who suffer more from hypovolemia than from hypotonicity. In patients with chronic hyponatremia, rapid correction of hyponatremia is dangerous because of the possible development of central pontine myelinolysis (osmotic demyelination syndrome), a demyelinating disease primarily affecting the central pons. The disorder causes a severe motor nerve dysfunction, such as quadriplegia, and it is more likely to occur with rapid treatment of chronic hyponatremia than of acute hyponatremia (46–49). Although the current recommendation is to increase serum Na^+ at a rate less than 0.5 mEq/L/hour (50, 51), this complication may be avoided by increasing serum Na^+ more slowly (no faster than 8 mEq/L/24 hours; about 0.35 mEq/L/hour) (52). Although hypertonic saline is the main culprit, administration of isotonic saline may also cause rapid correction of hyponatremia and central pontine myelinolysis (52, 53).

Principles of Fluid Therapy

Goals of Salt and Water Replacement

The goal of therapy is to restore the patient to a state of normal hemodynamics and normal body fluid osmolality. The program of water and electrolyte therapy has several components: (a) existing deficits must be identified and made up, (b) daily basal requirements for electrolytes and water must be supplied, and (c) ongoing losses must be quantified and provided for in the treatment plan (44, 54).

Basal Requirements

The basal requirement for water depends on sensible (urinary) and insensible losses of water. Fever increases respiratory water loss by increasing the vapor pressure of the expired air, and it increases loss of water from the skin by increasing the vapor pressure on the skin surface and the basal metabolic rate. Urinary loss of water depends on the total amount of solute excreted and urine osmolality. The solute excretion depends mainly on salt ingestion and protein intake, but severe glycosuria causes osmotic diuresis and increases the water requirement.

Daily Water Requirements

In the absence of fever and sweating, water loss through the skin is relatively fixed, but the urinary water excretion varies greatly and depends on the total amount of solute to be excreted and urine osmolality. For example, for a total solute excretion of 600 mOsm/day, the urine volume will be 500 mL if urine is concentrated to 1200 mOsm/L and 15 L if urine osmolality is 40 mOsm/L. For such a person, the minimum water requirement would be 1100 mL (500 mL for urinary water loss plus 600 mL for skin water loss at 2000 cal/day). Conversely, the maximal allowable water intake would be 15.6 L. If the concentration mechanism is impaired and the kidney can increase the urine osmolality to only 600 mOsm/L, the minimum water requirement would be 1.6 L. Similarly, if impairment in urine dilution results in a minimal urine osmolality of 300 mOsm/L, the maximal allowable water intake would be 2.6 (600/300 + 0.6) L. Clearly, in the absence of abnormality in urine concentration and dilution, a large range of water intake will cause neither dehydration nor overhydration. However, for various reasons, underestimation of water requirement is safer than overestimation. First, the excessive amount of water gain with impaired urine dilution tends to be greater than water deficit resulting from impaired urine concentration. Second, clinically impairment in urine dilution, such as syndrome of inappropriate ADH secretion (SIADH), is more common than impairment in urine concentration. Finally, in a conscious patient, thirst is an effective defense mechanism, whereas patients with severe hyponatremia often lapse into coma without warning (5).

POTASSIUM METABOLISM AND ITS DISORDERS

Total-body K^+ in hospitalized adults is about 43 mEq/kg body weight, and only about 2% of this is found in the extracellular fluid. The gradient of K^+ across the cell membrane determines the membrane potential (Em) according to the Nernst equation (55, 56):

Em (mV) = −61 Log (Intracellular K^+/Extracellular K^+)

The normal ratio of intracellular K^+ to extracellular K^+ is about 30, and therefore normal Em is −90 mV. The membrane potential tends to increase with hypokalemia and to decrease with hyperkalemia. In hypokalemia, both intracellular K^+ and extracellular K^+ tend to decrease, but the extracellular concentration tends to decrease proportionately more than the intracellular concentration. Hence, the ratio of intracellular K^+ to extracellular K^+ tends to increase. In hyperkalemia, the membrane potential tends to decrease because an increase in the extracellular K^+ is proportionately greater than that in the intracellular K^+.

Control of Transcellular Flux of Potassium

Transmembrane electrical gradients cause diffusion of cellular K^+ out of cells and Na^+ into cells. Because the Na^+-K^+ pump, which reverses this process, is stimulated by insulin and catecholamines (through β_2-adrenergic receptors), alterations in levels of these hormones can affect K^+ transport and its serum levels (57–60). Efflux of K^+ can also be stimulated by acidosis (Fig. 8.7). The effect of acidosis and alkalosis on transcellular K^+ flux depends not only on the pH but also on the type of anion that accumulates. In general, metabolic acidosis causes greater K^+ efflux than respiratory acidosis. Metabolic acidosis resulting from inorganic acids, such as sulfuric acid and hydrochloric acid, causes greater K^+ efflux than that resulting from organic acids, such as lactic acid and keto acids. Acidosis causes efflux of K^+ from the cell because of shift

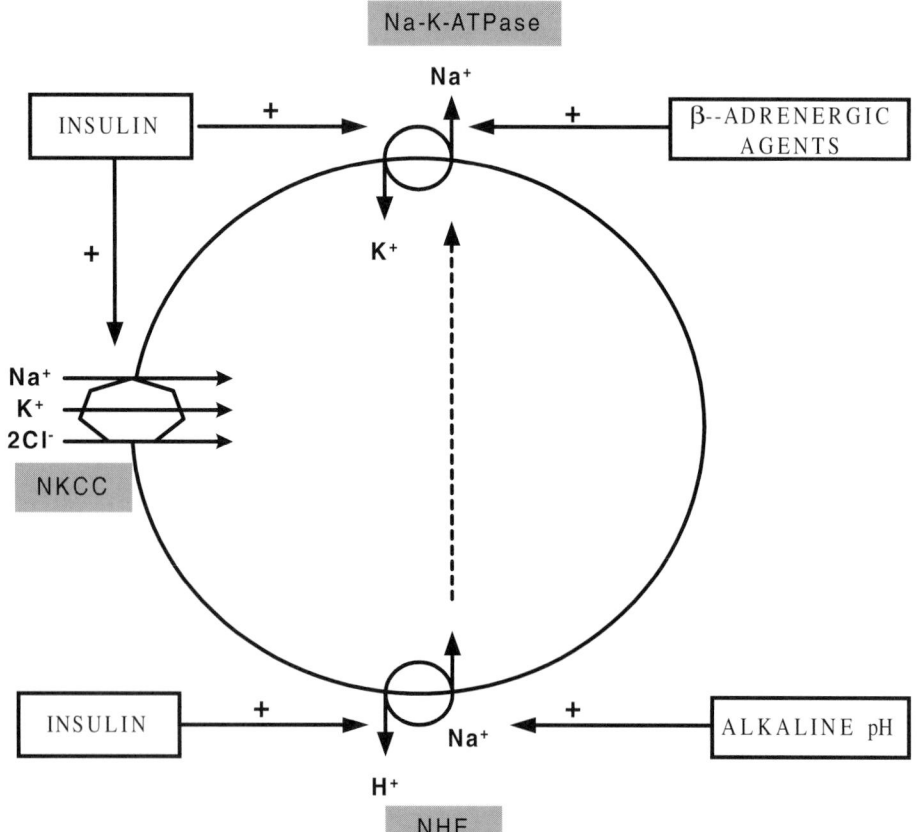

Figure 8.7. Control of transcellular movement of potassium (K^+). K^+ enters the cell through Na^+-K^+-ATPase (stimulated by β-adrenergic agents or insulin) or through the Na-K-Cl cotransporter (NKCC; stimulated by insulin). Stimulation of either transporters increases intracellular movement of K^+. Stimulation of the Na-H exchanger (NHE) by a high extracellular pH or insulin increases the intracellular Na^+ concentration, which, in turn, stimulates Na^+-K^+-ATPase.

of hydrogen ion (H^+) into the cell in exchange for K^+. A modifying factor appears to be the anion accumulation in the cells. In organic acidosis, much of H^+ entering the cell is balanced by organic anions, and therefore efflux of K^+ is prevented. In respiratory acidosis, the anion that accumulates in the cell to balance the incoming H^+ is HCO_3^- (61). Alkalosis tends to lower serum K^+. As with acidosis, K^+ influx varies with the type of alkalosis. In respiratory alkalosis, probably because of a drop in cellular HCO_3^- concentration, K^+ influx is not as much as in metabolic alkalosis. When pH is kept normal with proportionately increased concentration of HCO_3^- and P_{CO_2}, K^+ tends to move into the cells; accumulation of HCO_3^- in the cell must be accompanied by Na^+ and K^+. Similarly, when pH is kept normal with proportionately low HCO_3^- and low P_{CO_2}, K^+ tends to move out of the cells.

Dietary Sources of Potassium

K^+, being the major intracellular cation, is widely distributed in all foods, although the content varies greatly depending on the type of food (Fig. 8.8). In general, among food groups that are the main caloric sources of the modern diet, K^+ content is higher in meats and fishes than in nuts and cereals. Potatoes have particularly high K^+ content. However, the highest K^+ content is in fruits and vegetables; the K^+ content of vegetables is particularly high when it is expressed as the content per calorie (41, 62). Among the plant sources of food, K^+ contents of polished rice and light wheat flour are particularly low, whereas K^+ contents of potato, soy bean, and buckwheat are quite high (Fig. 8.9). Although citrus fruits and bananas are often cited by health professionals as particularly rich sources of K^+, many other foods contain K^+ at higher concentration. For example, tomatoes, apricots, and cantaloupes contain far more K^+ than oranges and bananas when expressed as milliequivalents of K^+ per calorie (Fig. 8.10) (41). See also Appendix Table A-22-a.

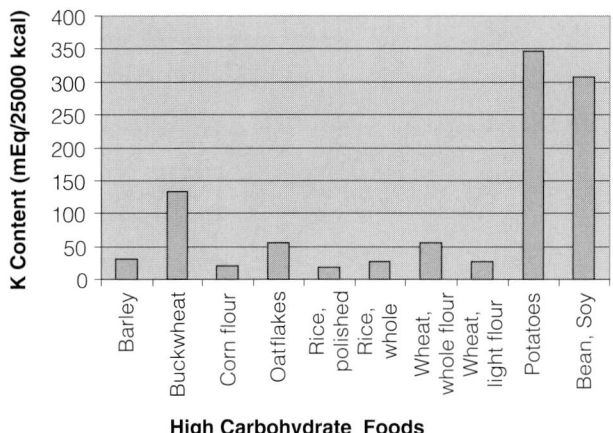

Figure 8.9. Potassium (K) contents of major carbohydrate containing foods. Grains, especially polished rice and light wheat flour, contain little potassium, whereas potatoes and soy beans contain large quantities of potassium.

Control of Renal Excretion of Potassium

About 90% of the daily K^+ intake (60–100 mEq) is excreted in the urine and 10% in the stool. K^+ filtered at the glomerulus is mostly (70–80%) reabsorbed by active and passive mechanisms in the proximal tubule. In the ascending limb of the loop of Henle, K^+ is reabsorbed together with Na^+ and Cl^-; the concentration of K^+ at the beginning of the distal convoluted tubule is about 1 mEq/L, with fluid volume of about 25 L. Thus, K^+ excreted in the urine is largely what has been secreted into the cortical collecting duct by mechanisms shown in Figure 8.11. Na^+-K^+-ATPase located on the basolateral side of the cortical collecting duct pumps K^+ into the cell while it pumps Na^+ out of the cell. The luminal Na^+ enters the cell through ENaC (epithelial Na channel), thus providing a continuous supply of Na^+. The negative

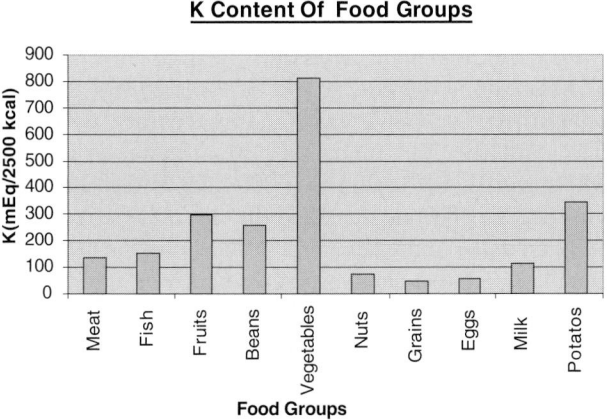

Figure 8.8. Potassium (K) contents of major food groups. When expressed by the caloric content of food, vegetables contain the highest amounts of potassium. The potassium content of grains is quite low.

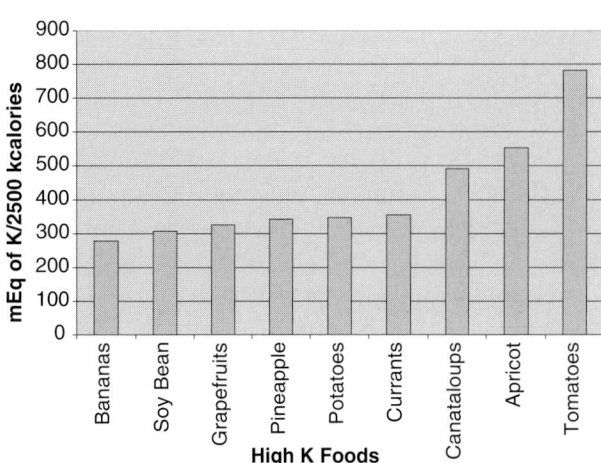

Figure 8.10. Potassium (K) contents of major fruits. Although oranges and bananas are most often cited as fruits of high potassium content, many other fruits contain far more potassium. For example, the potassium content of apricots is more than twice that of oranges.

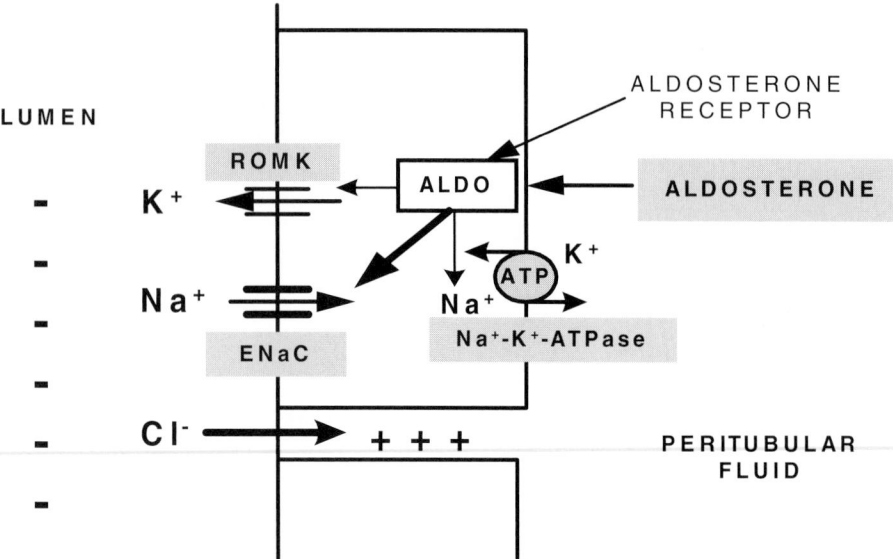

Figure 8.11. Control of potassium (K$^+$) secretion at the cortical collecting duct. Sodium (Na$^+$) enters from the luminal fluid into the cell through the epithelial Na$^+$ channel (EnaC) and is transported out of the cell through Na$^+$-K$^+$-adenosine triphosphatase (ATPase) on the basolateral membrane. These processes create the luminal electrical potential that is more negative than the electrical potential of the peritubular fluid. The electrical charge imbalance created by Na$^+$ reabsorption is partly matched by paracellular reabsorption of chloride and partly by entry of K$^+$ into the lumen through the renal outer medulla K$^+$ channel (ROMK), a K$^+$ channel. Aldo, aldosterone.

luminal potential that develops as a result of Na$^+$ reabsorption causes reabsorption of Cl$^-$ through the paracellular channels. Because Na$^+$ reabsorption is not followed one to one by Cl$^-$ reabsorption, the charge imbalance is corrected by secretion of K$^+$ through a specialized K$^+$ channel, the renal outer medulla K channel (ROMK). Aldosterone increases K$^+$ secretion by increasing passive entry of Na$^+$ from the lumen to the cell through increased expression of ENaC on the luminal membrane. The resulting increase in cellular concentration of Na$^+$ indirectly stimulates Na$^+$-K$^+$-ATPase, but aldosterone can also directly stimulate Na$^+$-K$^+$-ATPase and ROMK activities. The peritubular K$^+$ concentration and pH also influence K$^+$ secretion through their effects on Na$^+$-K$^+$-ATPase activity. High serum K$^+$ concentration and alkaline pH stimulate the enzyme activity, and low serum K$^+$ and acidic pH inhibit the activity.

When Na$^+$ is accompanied by anions that are less permeable than Cl$^-$, luminal negativity is increased, resulting in enhanced K$^+$ secretion. Examples of such anions include sulfate, HCO$_3^-$, and anionic antibiotics such as penicillin and carbenecillin. HCO$_3^-$ in the tubular fluid enhances K$^+$ secretion not only through its effect as a poorly reabsorbable anion but also by enhancing ROMK activity. An increase in renal K$^+$ excretion in patients who vomit may be explained by this mechanism. ADH also increases the luminal K$^+$ channel activity. K$^+$ secretion is increased by rapid urine flow by maintaining a low luminal K$^+$ concentration. Renal K$^+$ wasting during osmotic diuresis could be explained by this mechanism. The more Na$^+$ is presented to the distal nephron, the more can be absorbed, and more K$^+$ is secreted "in exchange." The increased Na$^+$ delivery to the collecting duct also increases renal K$^+$ excretion by its effect on urine flow (63–65).

Potassium Recycling and Its Role in Renal Potassium Excretion

Most of the mutations and evolutionary adaptations that have shaped the modern human physiology have occurred in paleolithic times and times beyond that. The dietary pattern of humans in preagriculture eras was vastly different from that of the modern era. The main difference appears to be extremely high K$^+$ intake, resulting from high intake of meat, fruits, and vegetables, and low Na$^+$ intake in the past. Most of the K$^+$ excreted in the urine is derived from secretion by the cortical collecting duct, and the absolute requirement for K$^+$ secretion is the amount of Na$^+$ delivery. The amount of Na$^+$ delivered to the collecting duct exceeds the amount of K$^+$ secreted. That is because K$^+$ secreted into the luminal fluid comes from what is transported into the principal cells by 3Na$^+$-2K$^+$-ATPase located on the basolateral membrane of the cell in exchange for Na$^+$ transport out of the cell; Na$^+$ transported out is what has entered from the luminal fluid into the cell through the ENaC. At the coupling ratio of 3:2 for Na$^+$ reabsorption to K$^+$ secretion, the maximal quantity of K$^+$ that can be secreted would be two thirds of the Na$^+$ reabsorbed. The delivery of Na$^+$ to the cortical collecting duct with the Na$^+$ intake of 150 mEq/day is a mere 450 mEq/day. Of these, about 300 mEq is reabsorbed in the cortical collecting duct, and the remaining 150 mEq is excreted in the urine. Under these situations, the maximum amount of K$^+$ that can be secreted would be 200 mEq. It is obvious that excretion of a large amount of K$^+$ requires an increased delivery of Na$^+$ to the cortical collecting duct (66, 67).

Because Na$^+$ delivery to the cortical collecting duct depends on Na$^+$ intake (through its influence on effective vascular volume and proximal reabsorption of Na$^+$), one would have predicted that the amount of Na$^+$ delivered to the cortical collecting duct was far less in prehistoric times than modern times, given that Na$^+$ intake in prehistoric times must have been far less than the modern values. Yet, in prehistoric times, a daily dietary load of K$^+$ probably exceeded 300 mEq/day. Hence, Na$^+$ delivery to the cortical collecting duct must have been much larger than the values predicted from the likely Na$^+$ intake. There must be a mechanism that allows delivery of a large quantity of Na$^+$ to the cortical collecting duct and thereby enables excretion of a large K$^+$ load in the presence of low Na$^+$ intake. That mechanism is K$^+$ recycling, discussed in the following paragraph.

Some of the K$^+$ leaving the cortical collecting duct is reabsorbed in the medullary collecting duct, and the remainder is excreted in the urine. The magnitude of K$^+$ reabsorbed in the medullary collecting duct is not known, but some of the reabsorbed K$^+$ is secreted into the proximal straight tubule and the thin descending limb and then is reabsorbed in the thick ascending limb. The countercurrent exchange mechanism of vasa recta helps to maintain a high concentration of K$^+$ in the medullary interstitium (Fig. 8.12). The K$^+$ concentration of the medullary interstitium rises progressively from the cortex toward the papillary tip, and the magnitude of rise in interstitial K$^+$ concentration of the medulla depends on the amount of K$^+$ excreted, which depends ultimately on K$^+$ intake. Thus, the greater the K$^+$ intake is, the greater the K$^+$ reabsorption and K$^+$ recycling will be. Yet, the main physiologic role of the K$^+$ recycling is increasing renal excretion of K$^+$. This may seem contradictory. However, the K$^+$ recycling allows an increased urinary excretion of K$^+$ because increased secretion of K$^+$ by the cortical collecting duct is greater in magnitude than the increase in K$^+$

reabsorption by the outer medullary collecting duct. An increased interstitial K$^+$ concentration induced by the K$^+$ recycling inhibits Na$^+$ reabsorption in the medullary thick ascending limb, with a resultant increase in the delivery of Na$^+$ to the cortical collecting duct. In other words, an increased K$^+$ recycling creates a situation that resembles the state following administration of a loop diuretic or in a person with Bartter syndrome. The main determinant of K$^+$ recycling is not serum K$^+$ concentration but the quantity of K$^+$ excreted in the urine, which ultimately depends on the K$^+$ intake.

The mechanism of inhibition of Na$^+$ reabsorption in the thick ascending limb by a high concentration of K$^+$ in the medullary interstitium is not understood. One plausible explanation is the depolarization of the epithelial cells of the medullary thick ascending limb, which inhibits Cl$^-$ reabsorption through the Cl$^-$ channel. Remember that the Cl$^-$ reabsorption across the basolateral membrane is against a concentration gradient and is powered by the favorable transmembrane voltage. The accumulation of chloride in the cell then secondarily would inhibit Cl$^-$ reabsorption through the Na$^+$-K$^+$-Cl$^-$ cotransporter (NKCC). Inhibition of renin secretion by a high K$^+$ intake can also be explained by the K$^+$ recycling; inhibition of NaCl reabsorption in the medullary thick ascending limb would increase the delivery of NaCl to the macula densa.

It is unlikely that hyperkalemia per se has much effect in the NaCl transport in the thick ascending limb. A marked increase in K$^+$ intake is accompanied by a modest increase in plasma K$^+$, and yet NaCl reabsorption by the thick ascending limb is greatly reduced. If plasma K$^+$ concentration were the signal that influences the Na$^+$ reabsorption in the thick ascending limb, impairment in Na$^+$

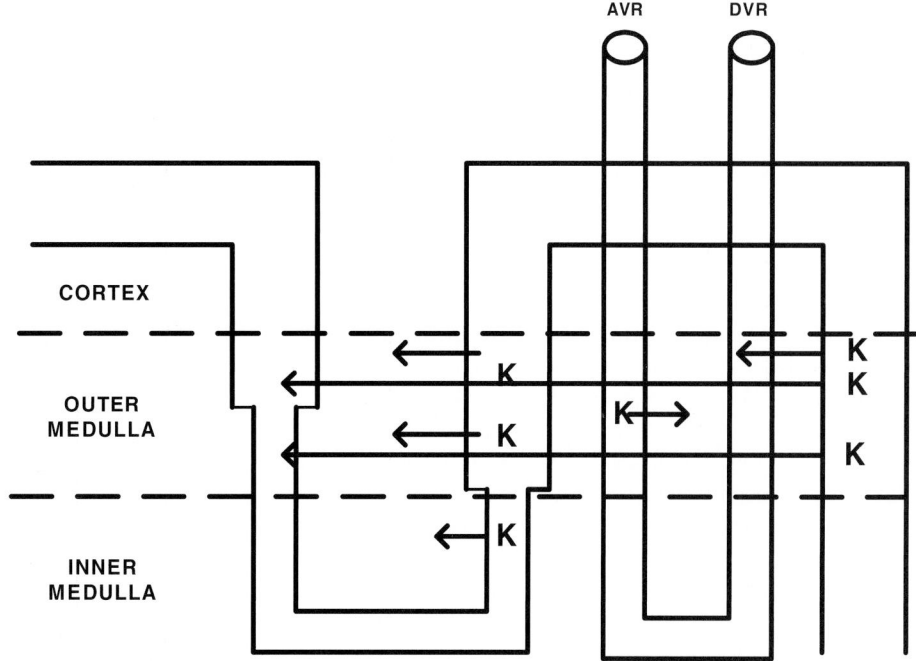

Figure 8.12. Renal recycling of potassium (K). The magnitude of recycling depends mainly on potassium intake, and the recycled potassium originates mainly from the medullary collecting duct. The main purpose of potassium recycling is to maintain a high concentration of potassium in the medullary interstitium, which inhibits sodium transport in the thick ascending limb of Henle. This results in increased delivery of sodium to the cortical collecting duct and enhances potassium secretion. AVR, ascending vasa recta, DVR, descending vasa recta.

reabsorption would be most severe in those disorders that result in impairment in K^+ excretion, such as hyporeninemic hypoaldosteronism. Yet no evidence exists for impaired salt reabsorption in the thick ascending limb of Henle in those conditions. Increased urinary excretion of K^+ with increased intake is mediated in part by a hyperkalemia-induced increase in aldosterone secretion. However, an increase in plasma K^+ with increased K^+ intake is quite modest and is unlikely to explain the marked increase in urinary K^+ excretion that occurs with increased K^+ intake.

Effect of Potassium Intake on Blood Pressure

Numerous studies have demonstrated that a high-K^+ diet lowers arterial blood pressure. Diets high in fruits and vegetables were shown to be beneficial in reducing blood pressure in the Dietary Approaches to Stop Hypertension study (68, 69). Because the diets used in the study diets had a high content of K^+, it is likely that some of the blood pressure–lowering effects of such diets may have come from their high K^+ content. A study of Scottish men showed that Na^+ content of the diet had no effect on blood pressure, whereas K^+ content had inverse correlation with blood pressure. Several other studies also demonstrated that an increase in K^+ by 40 mEq/day reduced blood pressure more than reduction in Na^+ intake of 60 to 80 mEq/day (68–71). The likely mechanism of a high-K^+ diet in reducing blood pressure is Na^+ diuresis that results from increased concentration of K^+ in the renal medulla owing to increased renal recycling of K^+, as discussed earlier. When a dietary approach is used to treat hypertension, increased K^+ intake is probably easier and more pleasant to implement than restriction of Na^+ intake.

Plasma Renin Activity, Plasma Aldosterone Concentration, and Abnormalities in Potassium Metabolism

Because abnormalities in plasma renin activity (PRA) and plasma aldosterone (PA) are frequently either responsible for or caused by abnormalities in K^+ metabolism, it is important to understand their relationships (72–75). The general principles are as follows. First, expansion of effective vascular volume caused by primary increase in aldosterone (primary aldosteronism) or by other mineralocorticoids will suppress PRA. When mineralocorticoids other than aldosterone are present in excess, they retain salt and water, and the resulting volume expansion leads to suppression of both PRA and PA. Second, an increase in PRA will always lead to increase in PA (secondary aldosteronism), unless the rise in PRA is caused by a primary defect in aldosterone secretion. PRA may be high because of (a) volume depletion secondary to renal or extrarenal salt loss, (b) abnormality in renin secretion (e.g., reninoma, hemangiopericytoma of afferent arteriole, malignant hypertension, renal artery stenosis), (c) increased renin substrate production (e.g., oral contraceptives), and (d) direct stimulation of the adrenal cortex by elevation in serum K^+ to release aldosterone. When renin is deficient primarily, aldosterone is always low, such as in hyporeninemic hypoaldosteronism.

Hypokalemia

Causes and Pathogenesis

Because the intracellular K^+ concentration greatly exceeds the extracellular concentration, K^+ shift into the cell can cause severe hypokalemia with little change in its intracellular concentration (76–84) (Table 8.3). Alkalosis, insulin, and β_2-agonists can cause hypokalemia by stimulating Na^+-K^+-ATPase activity (77, 78). Defective activity of dihydropyridine-responsive Ca^{2+} channels or voltage-dependent Na^+ channels has been documented in some patients, but the exact mechanism for hypokalemia is unknown. (82, 83). In barium poisoning, K^+ accumulates in the cell and hypokalemia develops, because of the inhibition of the K^+ channel by barium, resulting in inhibition of K^+ efflux from the cell, in the presence of continuous cellular uptake of K^+ through the action of Na^+-K^+-ATPase. K^+ accumulates in the cell along with anions as the cell mass increases during nutritional recovery, because K^+ is the main intracellular cation (84).

TABLE 8.3. CAUSES OF HYPOKALEMIA

Intracellular shift
 Alkalosis
 Periodic paralysis
 β_2-agonists
 Barium poisoning
 Insulin
 Nutritional recovery state
Poor intake
 Gastrointestinal loss
  Vomiting
  Diarrhea
  Intestinal drainage
  Laxative abuse
Excessive renal loss
 Primary aldosteronism (adrenal adenoma or hyperplasia); plasma renin activity is suppressed
 Secondary aldosteronism (the increase in aldosterone is secondary to increase in renin)
  Malignant hypertension, renal artery stenosis, reninoma
  Diuretics
  Bartter syndrome, Gitelman syndrome
 Excess mineralocorticoids other than aldosterone, e.g., Cushing syndrome, adrenocorticotropic hormone–producing tumor, licorice
 Chronic metabolic acidosis
 Delivery of poorly reabsorbed anions to the distal tubule, e.g., bicarbonate, ketone anions, carbenecillin
 Miscellaneous causes: magnesium deficiency, acute leukemia, Liddle syndrome

Poor intake of K^+ is rarely the sole cause of hypokalemia, because poor intake of K^+ is usually accompanied by poor caloric intake, which causes catabolism and release of K^+ from the tissues (84). Vomiting and diarrhea are common causes of hypokalemia (84). Diarrhea causes direct K^+ loss in the stool, but in vomiting hypokalemia is mainly the result of K^+ loss in the urine rather than in the vomitus. Vomiting causes metabolic alkalosis, and the subsequent renal excretion of HCO_3^- leads to renal K^+ wasting.

Renal loss of K^+ is the most common cause of hypokalemia. Renal K^+ wasting occurs when increased aldosterone concentration is accompanied by adequate distal delivery of Na^+ (85–100). In primary aldosteronism, distal delivery of Na^+ is increased because increased NaCl reabsorption in the cortical collecting duct by the action of aldosterone inhibits salt reabsorption in the proximal tubule and in the loop of Henle. In secondary aldosteronism, hypokalemia occurs only in conditions that are accompanied by increased distal Na^+ delivery. Examples include renal artery stenosis, diuretic therapy, and malignant hypertension. Heart failure does not lead to hypokalemia despite secondary aldosteronism unless distal delivery of Na^+ is increased by diuretic therapy. Bartter syndrome is caused by defective NaCl reabsorption in the thick ascending limb of Henle (92–96), whereas in Gitelman syndrome, the defect in NaCl reabsorption is in the distal convoluted tubule (97). Defective Na^+ reabsorption proximal to the aldosterone effective site results in adequate delivery of Na^+ to the cortical collecting duct and hence in hypokalemia.

In chronic metabolic acidosis, hypokalemia develops probably because reduced proximal reabsorption of NaCl allows increased delivery of NaCl to the distal nephron and also because metabolic acidosis directly stimulates aldosterone secretion. With licorice intake, renal K^+ wasting results from the sustained mineralocorticoid activity of cortisol because licorice inhibits the enzyme 11-β-hydroxysteroid dehydrogenase, which normally rapidly metabolizes cortisol in the kidney (98–100). Liddle syndrome is caused by increased Na^+ channel activity in the collecting duct; accumulation of Na^+ in the cell leads to stimulation of Na^+-K^+-ATPase activity, resulting in increased K^+ secretion (101). Figure 8.9 shows a schematic approach to the differential diagnosis of hypokalemia.

Clinical Manifestations

Low serum K^+ itself leads to characteristic electrocardiographic (ECG) changes, to alterations in cardiac rate, rhythm, and conduction, and to muscle weakness. Depletion of cell K^+ leads to numerous structural and functional alterations in various organs. These changes include skeletal muscle cell necrosis and acute rhabdomyolysis, nephrogenic DI, possibly owing to inhibition of ADH by excess prostaglandin, and cardiac cell necrosis. K^+ depletion is often associated with metabolic alkalosis, in part because

K^+ deficiency leads to increased renal production and retention of HCO_3^-. Reduced insulin secretion and reduced intestinal motility are other common disorders of hypokalemia. Hypokalemia produces abnormalities of rhythm and of rate of cardiac conduction through alteration in several physiologic states: Alteration in ventricular repolarization leads to depression of the ST segment, flattening and inversion of T waves, and appearance of U waves, the most common ECG abnormalities of hypokalemia. Combinations of altered states of polarization and conduction can produce arrhythmias, most commonly supraventricular and ventricular ectopic beats and tachycardia, atrioventricular conduction disturbances, and ventricular fibrillation. Rapidly developing hypokalemia is more likely to produce cardiac arrhythmias than more slowly developing hypokalemia. K^+ depletion intensifies digitalis toxicity through an unknown mechanism (5).

Treatment

Hypokalemia is usually treated either by K administration or by prevention of the renal loss of K^+. Renal loss of K^+ is prevented either by treating its cause (e.g., removal of aldosterone-producing adenoma or by discontinuation of diuretics) or by administering K-sparing diuretics (5, 102). The K-sparing diuretics in current use are aldosterone antagonists (e.g., spironolactone and eplerenone), triamterene, and amiloride. Aldosterone antagonists are effective in preventing renal K^+ loss only if an increased mineralocorticoid concentration is responsible for hypokalemia. In Liddle syndrome, spironolactone is ineffective because PA is reduced; triamterene and amiloride are effective regardless of the PA concentration. The daily dose of spironolactone ranges from 25 to 400 mg, and that of eplerenone is from 25 to 100 mg. The usual doses of triamterene range from 50 to 150 mg twice daily. Amiloride is administered at 5 mg/day, and it can be slowly increased up to 20 mg/day. Amiloride should be administered with food to avoid gastric irritation.

Because reduced delivery of Na^+ to the distal nephron always reduces K^+ secretion, a low-salt diet helps to reduce renal K^+ loss of any cause, independent of the PA concentration. In a nonemergency setting, K^+ should be given orally and in the form of KCl, KP, or the salt of organic acids. In the critical care setting, K^+ is usually given intravenously and primarily as KCl. The first goal in treating severe hypokalemia is elimination of cardiac arrhythmias. A decline in serum K^+ of 1 mEq/L generally indicates a loss of 150 to 200 mEq of K^+ and a decline of 2 mEq/L a loss in excess of 500 mEq, but the relationship is not rigidly fixed. For example in acidotic states, serum K^+ concentrations may be high in the presence of K^+ depletion.

To initiate rapid intravenous administration of K^+, it may be useful to estimate the number of liters of extracellular fluid as body weight in kilograms times 0.2. This value multiplied by desired increment in serum K^+/L represents the amount of K^+ that can be safely given in 20 to 30 minutes without danger of hyperkalemia. Although it is usually unnecessary to give K^+ at a rate greater than 10 to 20 mEq/hour, a rate in excess of 100 mEq/hour may be needed in certain life-threatening situations, such as in a patient with ketoacidosis, severe hypokalemia, and an ECG showing a dangerous arrhythmia. A glucose-containing solution should not be used as a vehicle for KCl when serum K^+ is to be increased rapidly; glucose will stimulate release of insulin, which will, in turn, drive K^+ into the cells. K^+ at concentrations exceeding 40 mEq/L may produce pain at the infusion site and may lead to sclerosis of smaller vessels. When a concentration in excess of 100 mEq/L is used, a femoral line is preferable. It is advisable to avoid central venous infusion of K^+ at high concentrations, lest depolarization of the conduction tissues may lead to cardiac arrest.

Hyperkalemia

Causes and Pathogenesis

Hyperkalemia may be caused by one of three mechanisms: (a) shift of K^+ from the cells to the extracellular fluid (103–111), (b) increased K intake, and (c) reduced renal K^+ excretion (Table 8.4). Hyperkalemic familial periodic paralysis, administration of succinylcholine in paralyzed patients (108–111), administration of cationic amino acids such as arginine and lysine, ε-aminocaproic acid (this probably becomes a cationic amino acid), rhabdomyolysis or hemolysis, and acute acidosis all cause hyperkalemia by extracellular K^+ shift. Rhabdomyolysis and hemolysis cause hyperkalemia only when they are

---

TABLE 8.4. CAUSES OF HYPERKALEMIA

Pseudohyperkalemia
  Thrombocytosis, severe leukocytosis, use of tourniquet with fist exercise, in vitro hemolysis
True hyperkalemia
  Extracellular shift
    Acute acidosis (especially inorganic acidosis)
    Catabolic states, periodic paralysis, succinylcholine
    Cationic amino acids
    Exercise while using a β-blocker
    Digitalis intoxication
  Excessive ingestion: rare if renal excretion of potassium is normal
  Decreased renal excretion
    Hypoaldosteronism: Addison disease; selective hypoaldosteronism (hyporeninemic hypoaldosteronism, heparin, congenital adrenal enzyme deficiencies, angiotensin-converting enzyme inhibitors)
    Tubular unresponsiveness to aldosterone (pseudohypoaldosteronism type I and II): congenital, salt-losing nephropathy
    Potassium-sparing diuretics
    Antirejection medications: cyclosporine, tacrolimus
    Severe dehydration

---

accompanied by renal failure. Although hyperkalemia is not as predictable with organic acidosis as with inorganic acidosis in experimental situations, hyperkalemia is common in diabetic ketoacidosis and phenformin-induced lactic acidosis. The more frequent occurrence of hyperkalemia in clinical organic acidosis may be explained by the longer duration of acidosis and the presence of other factors such as dehydration and renal failure and insulin deficiency in diabetic ketoacidosis (61).

Hyperkalemia can also occur in severe digitalis intoxication by extracellular shift of K^+ as digitalis inhibits the Na^+-K^+-ATPase pump. The kidney's ability to excrete K^+ is so great that hyperkalemia rarely occurs solely on the basis of increased intake of K. Thus, hyperkalemia is almost always the result of impaired renal excretion. The three major mechanisms of diminished renal K^+ excretion are reduced aldosterone or aldosterone responsiveness, renal failure, and reduced distal delivery of Na^+. Aldosterone deficiency may be part of a generalized deficiency of adrenal hormones (e.g., Addison disease), or it may represent a selective process (e.g., hyporeninemic hypoaldosteronism). Hyporeninemic hypoaldosteronism is the most common cause of all aldosterone deficiency states and by far the most common cause of chronic hyperkalemia among patients who are not undergoing dialysis (112, 113). Selective hypoaldosteronism can also occur with heparin therapy, which inhibits steroid production in the zona glomerulosa (114). In patients with reduced aldosterone secretion, any agent that limits the supply of renin or angiotensin II may provoke hyperkalemia, for example, angiotensin-converting enzyme inhibitors, nonsteroidal antiinflammatory agents, and β-blockers. The last category of drugs may compound the tendency to hyperkalemia by interfering with K^+ transport into cells. Renal tubular unresponsiveness to aldosterone (pseudohypoaldosteronism) may be congenital, but it is more often an acquired defect. This defect may involve only K^+ secretion (pseudohypoaldosteronism type II) or Na^+ reabsorption as well as K^+ secretion (pseudohypoaldosteronism type I) (115–119). Most cases of so-called "salt-losing nephritis" appear to represent the latter defect. Severe volume depletion may cause hyperkalemia despite secondary hyperaldosteronism because volume depletion causes a marked reduction in delivery of Na^+ to the cortical collecting duct.

Pseudohyperkalemia is defined as an increase in K^+ concentration only in the local blood vessel or in vitro, and it has no physiologic consequences (120–129). Prolonged use of a tourniquet with fist exercises can increase the serum K^+ level by as much as 1 mEq/L. Thrombocytosis and severe leukocytosis cause pseudohyperkalemia through K^+ release from the platelets and white blood cells, respectively, during blood clotting (see Table 8.4).

Clinical Manifestations

In severe hyperkalemia, paralysis of the skeletal muscle occurs. Rapidly ascending neuromuscular weakness or paralysis has been observed in very severe hyperkalemia. Hyperkalemia can also cause mental confusion and paresthesia. The main dangers of hyperkalemia are abnormalities of cardiac rhythm and of its rate of conduction. Increased velocity of repolarization results in tall, peaked T waves with shortened QT intervals. This is the earliest sign of hyperkalemia, and it begins to appear when K^+ concentration in serum rises to more than 5.5 mEq/L. However, as in hypokalemia, the rate of development of hyperkalemia is important in the development of cardiac abnormalities. Reduction in the resting potential of the cardiac conduction system and muscle by high extracellular K^+ concentration is associated with slowing of conduction. As hyperkalemia worsens, P waves flatten and QRS complexes widen progressively; then the P waves disappear entirely, and the QRS complexes merge with the T waves stimulating a sine wave. Other ECG findings include fascicular block and complete heart block (especially in digitalized patients), ventricular tachycardia, flutter and fibrillation, and cardiac arrest (5, 130, 131).

Treatment

Hyperkalemia may be treated by removal of K^+ from the body, by shifting extracellular K^+ into the cells, and by antagonizing K^+ action on the membrane of the cardiac conduction system (Table 8.5) (132–140). Removal of K^+ may be accomplished by several routes: through the GI tract with K^+ exchange resin given orally or by enema; through the kidney by diuretics, mineralocorticoids, and increased salt intake; and by hemodialysis or peritoneal dialysis. A K^+ exchange resin, Na polystyrene sulfonate (Kayexalate), is more effective when it is given with agents such as sorbitol or mannitol that cause osmotic diarrhea. One tablespoon of Kayexalate mixed with 100 mL of 10% sorbitol or mannitol can be given by mouth two to four times a day. When it is given as an enema, a larger quantity is given more frequently. However, sorbitol may cause intestinal necrosis (141–143), and other laxatives may be preferable (144, 145).

TABLE 8.5. TREATMENT OF HYPERKALEMIA

Reduction in body potassium content
  Reduction in intake
  Increased fecal excretion: potassium-exchange resin and
    sorbitol
  Increased renal excretion: mineralocorticoids, increased salt
    intake, diuretics
  Peritoneal or hemodialysis
Intracellular shift of potassium
  Glucose and insulin
  Administration of alkali
  β-Agonists: salbutamol, albuterol
Antagonism of the membrane effect of hyperkalemia
  Calcium salts
  Hypertonic sodium salts

Hemodialysis can rapidly remove K^+ from the body, but the disadvantage is that it takes time to set up the dialysis machine. Shift of K^+ into cells can be accomplished with glucose and insulin or by increasing the blood pH with $NaHCO_3^-$. HCO_3^- was not shown to be very effective against hyperkalemia in patients with renal failure. However, when given with insulin, HCO_3^- appears to have a synergistic effect (146). Specific $β_2$-agonists such as salbutamol and albuterol are effective in driving K^+ into cells by stimulating the Na^+-K^+–dependent ATPase (134).

Antagonism of the action of K^+ on the heart with intravenous Ca^{2+} salts has the fastest effect against hyperkalemia and is used in life-threatening hyperkalemia. CaCl and Ca gluconate are equally effective (137–139), but the latter is preferable because tissue damage is less when extravasation of the drug occurs during intravenous infusion.

Prolonged administration of diuretics and a high-salt diet comprise an effective treatment approach to hyporeninemic hypoaldosteronism. This regimen ensures the delivery of an adequate amount of Na^+ to the cortical collecting duct without causing further volume expansion. Mineralocorticoid may be required as an adjunct therapy for hyporeninemic hypoaldosteronism, and the agent most commonly used is a synthetic mineralocorticoid, fludrocortisone (Florinef). However, because renal salt retention may be an important mechanism in the pathogenesis of hyporeninemic hypoaldosteronism, mineralocorticoid replacement may lead to salt retention and worsening of hypertension (112). Reduced intake of K^+ is an additional measure to be added to any of the methods recommended earlier in the long-term management of hyperkalemia.

PATHOPHYSIOLOGY OF WATER AND ANTIDIURETIC HORMONE METABOLISM

Regulation of Thirst and Antidiuretic Hormone Release

A rise in effective osmolality shrinks the hypothalamic osmoreceptor cells, which then stimulate the thirst center in the cerebral cortex and stimulate ADH production in the supraoptic and paraventricular nuclei. Conversely, a decline in effective osmolality causes swelling of the osmoreceptor cells, resulting in inhibition of ADH production. ADH produced in the hypothalamus is carried through long axons and is secreted from the posterior pituitary (147–149). Stimulation and inhibition of osmoreceptor cells affect both production by the hypothalamus and secretion by the pituitary of ADH.

Regulation of ADH secretion by a change in effective osmolality is extremely sensitive. A rise in effective osmolality by only 2 to 3% stimulates ADH secretion sufficiently to result in a maximally concentrated urine, and decline in plasma osmolality of only 2 to 3% produces maximally dilute urine (<100 mOsm/L).

ADH release is also regulated by nonosmotic factors. Low effective vascular volume provokes thirst and ADH release, and high effective vascular volume has the reverse effects (150–152). These effects are mediated through baroreceptors and some humoral factors released in response to reduced blood flow. α Catecholamines suppress and β catecholamines enhance ADH output. Prostaglandins inhibit the effect of ADH on the kidney. Angiotensin II stimulates thirst and ADH release. Lack of glucocorticoid enhances ADH action on the kidney and also increases ADH release. Physical and emotional stress, such as major surgery, enhances ADH output, possibly in part through emetic stimuli. Many drugs affect ADH release or action; for example, ethanol inhibits the output of ADH. Lithium and demeclocycline inhibit the effect of ADH on the kidney. Chlorpropamide increases the action of ADH on the kidney. Some drugs may operate through the emetic stimulus, which is one of the most potent physiologic stimuli to ADH release. The urine may become osmotically concentrated in the absence of ADH if effective vascular volume is very low. The combination of reduced GFR and enhanced proximal reabsorption of filtrate reduces urine flow to the collecting duct so greatly that even the limited permeability of the membrane permits withdrawal of a sufficient amount of water to concentrate urine.

Three classes of ADH receptors are known: V1 receptors cause rise in vasomotor tone and certain metabolic effects, V2 receptors are associated with antidiuresis, and V3 receptors cause stimulation of ACTH secretion in the anterior pituitary (153–156). The antdiuretic effect of ADH is mediated by its effect on the collecting duct of the kidney to enhance permeability to water and on the outer medullary thick ascending limb of the loop of Henle to stimulate salt reabsorption. Vasopressinase, which normally breaks down ADH, may be increased in pregnancy and occasionally causes polyuria (157). Desmopressin (DDAVP), a synthetic analog of arginine vasopressin that resists vasopressinase and therefore has a prolonged effect, is useful in polyuria of pregnancy.

About 180 L of water are filtered daily; 120 L are reabsorbed in the proximal tubule and 35 L in the descending limb of Henle. About 25 L of dilute urine are delivered to the collecting duct. Even when ADH is totally absent, about 5 L of water are reabsorbed in the inner medullary collecting duct, and 20 L are excreted as the final urine. In the presence of maximal ADH, urine can be concentrated to as high as 1200 mOsm/L as water is reabsorbed in the cortical and medullary collecting duct, with urine volume as low as 0.5 L/day (Fig. 8.13).

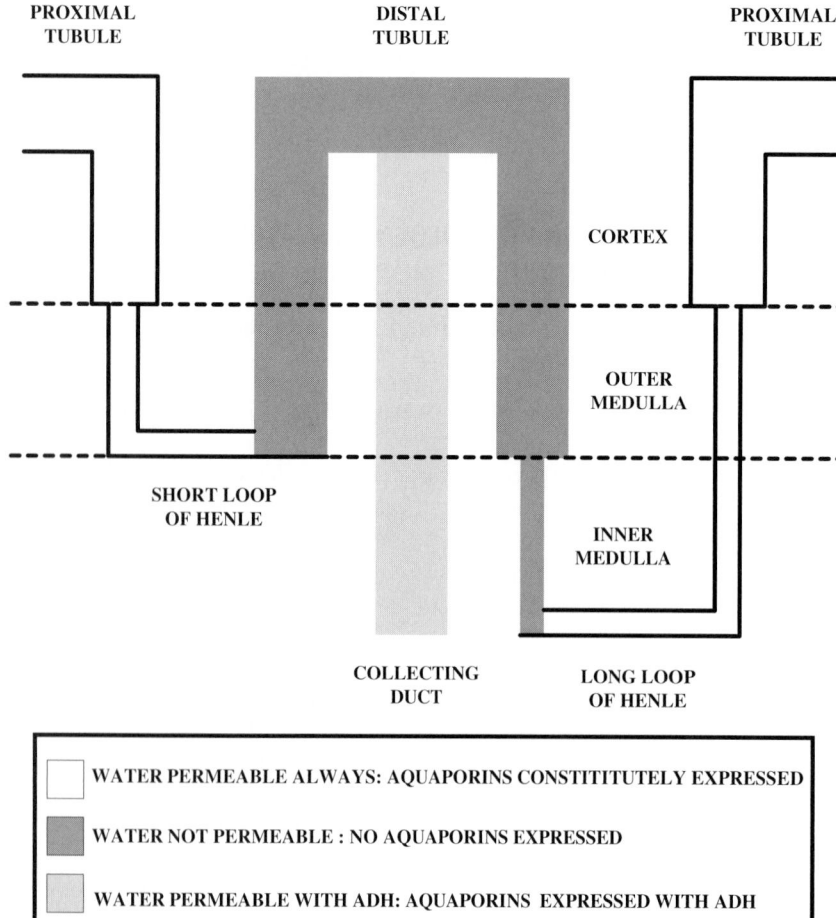

PROXIMAL TUBULE

DISTAL TUBULE

PROXIMAL TUBULE

CORTEX

OUTER MEDULLA

SHORT LOOP OF HENLE

INNER MEDULLA

COLLECTING DUCT

LONG LOOP OF HENLE

☐ WATER PERMEABLE ALWAYS: AQUAPORINS CONSTITITUTELY EXPRESSED

■ WATER NOT PERMEABLE : NO AQUAPORINS EXPRESSED

▨ WATER PERMEABLE WITH ADH: AQUAPORINS EXPRESSED WITH ADH

Figure 8.13. Transport of water at various nephron sites. The proximal tubule and the descending thin limb are always water permeable because aquaporins are constitutively expressed at these sites. The ascending thin limb and ascending thick limb of Henle, the distal convoluted tubule, and the connecting tubule have no aquaporins expressed and are always water impermeable. The collecting duct is water permeable with antidiuretic hormone (ADH) action.

In the proximal tubule, water reabsorption passively follows salt reabsorption, whereas in the descending thin limb, water reabsorption is unaccompanied by salt reabsorption, but is induced by the salt reabsorption that takes place in the ascending limb. Both thin and thick ascending limbs of Henle, distal convoluted tubules, and connecting tubules are water impermeable either in the presence or absence of ADH. The reabsorption of water in the collecting duct is regulated by ADH. Requirements for water conservation (and therefore for osmotic concentration of the urine) are medullary hypertonicity resulting from the action of countercurrent mechanism, sufficient ADH, and tubular membrane responsiveness to ADH (158–167).

Polyuria

Polyuria is arbitrarily defined as urine volume in excess of 2.5 L/day. The two types of polyuria are osmotic diuresis and water diuresis (5).

Osmotic Diuresis

Osmotic diuresis is defined as increased urine output resulting from an excessive rate of solute excretion; the commonly accepted level of solute excretion for osmotic diuresis is a rate in excess of 60 mOsm/hour or 1440 mOsm/day in the adult (5). Urine osmolality is usually greater than that of plasma, but it may be lower than plasma osmolality when it coexists with water diuresis. Solutes commonly responsible for osmotic diuresis include glucose, urea, mannitol, radiopaque media, and NaCl.

Water Diuresis

Water diuresis is characterized by excretion of a large volume of dilute urine. The polyuria is caused by reduced reabsorption of water in the collecting duct. Reasons for reduced water reabsorption in the collecting duct are lack of ADH (168–177) or unresponsiveness to ADH (nephrogenic DI). Nephrogenic DI can be either congenital or acquired. Congenital nephrogenic DI is caused by either a defective ADH receptor or an aquaporin defect (178–185).

The lack of ADH results from either primary deficiency (central DI) or physiologic suppression by low serum osmolality (primary polydipsia, dipsogenic DI) (168–170). The deficiency of ADH could be mild, moderate, or severe. When ADH deficiency is partial, urine osmolality may be fairly close to normal. ADH deficiency could be congenital or acquired (171–177). In a rare instance, ADH is made, but it cannot be released in response to a rise in body fluid osmolality because of a defect involving the osmoreceptor cells, such as in patients with hypothalamic lesions (174–176). In such instances, ADH may be released in response to hypovolemia or to drugs. During pregnancy, ADH deficiency may be caused by excessive production of vasopressinase (gestational DI) (154).

TABLE 8.6. CAUSES OF POLYURIA RESULTING FROM WATER DIURESIS

Lack of ADH
Central DI: congenital or acquired (idiopathic cell degeneration, tumors and granulomas, surgery, trauma, infarction, and infection of the pituitary or hypothalamus)
Dipsogenic DI (suppression by excessive water intake): psychogenic causes, organic brain disease, iatrogenic causes
Gestational DI: excess vasopressinase
Failure of the kidney to respond to ADH (nephrogenic DI)
Congenital nephrogenic DI: a defect in ADH receptor, a defect in aquaporin expression
Chronic renal failure
Acquired nephrogenic DI: lithium toxicity, demeclocycline toxicity, methoxyflurane toxicity, amyloidosis, light-chain nephropathy, hypercalcemia, hypokalemia, obstructive uropathy

ADH, antidiuretic hormone; DI, diabetes insipidus.

Causes of polyuria including central and nephrogenic DI are listed in Table 8.6.

Primary polydipsia is defined as increased water drinking that is not caused by physiologically stimulated thirst, that is, in the absence of hyperosmolality or volume depletion (168–170). Primary polydipsia is usually psychogenic in origin, hence the term psychogenic polydipsia. In contrast, polydipsia in patients with DI or diabetic patients with severe glycosuria is secondary polydipsia, which results from thirst stimulation in response to hyperosmolality. In primary polydipsia, increased urine output is caused by physiologic suppression of ADH secretion, and hence, serum Na$^+$ is usually at the low range of normal. In contrast, in central or nephrogenic DI serum Na$^+$ is in the high normal range. Occasionally, serum Na$^+$ is frankly low in severe primary polydipsia, a finding indicating that the capacity of the GI tract to absorb water exceeds the normal capacity of the kidney to excrete water.

Differential Diagnosis of Polyuria

The first step in the differential diagnosis should be the measurement of urine osmolality (186). Osmotic diuresis is ruled out or diagnosed solely on the basis of the rate of osmolal excretion: the excretion of osmols at a rate greater than 60 mOsm/hour or 1440 mOsm/day. For example, a urine output of 5 L/day at an osmolality of 400 mOsm/L equals an osmolal excretion rate of 2000 mOsm/day, and therefore it represents osmotic diuresis.

Conversely, excretion of 10 L of urine at 100 mOsm/L represents only 1000 mOsm/day, and this is water diuresis. For the differential diagnosis of water diuresis, the first step is to determine the serum Na$^+$ concentration. In DI, serum Na$^+$ tends to be high normal, and in primary polydipsia, it tends to be low normal. However, because of much overlap, the water deprivation test is needed to confirm the diagnosis. To perform this test, water is restricted overnight or until loss of 5% of the body weight. In primary polydipsia, maximum urine osmolality (>700 mOsm/L) can usually be achieved by water restriction. A submaximal response that improves significantly on administration of ADH indicates central DI; a submaximal response that fails to respond to ADH points to nephrogenic DI (Fig. 8.14).

Treatment

In osmotic diuresis, the cause of the increased solute excretion must be removed. Diabetes should be controlled to prevent osmotic diuresis resulting from glycosuria. Curtailing protein intake would reduce urea excretion.

Administration or stimulation of ADH secretion is helpful only for pituitary DI. Pitressin tannate in oil is no longer available. Desmopressin (DDAVP), a synthetic analog of ADH, is administered intranasally, subcutaneously, intravenously, or orally (187). Some patients may prefer oral agents, and the two that have been used extensively are chlorpropamide and thiazide diuretics. Chlorpropamide (100–250 mg/day) stimulates secretion of endogenous

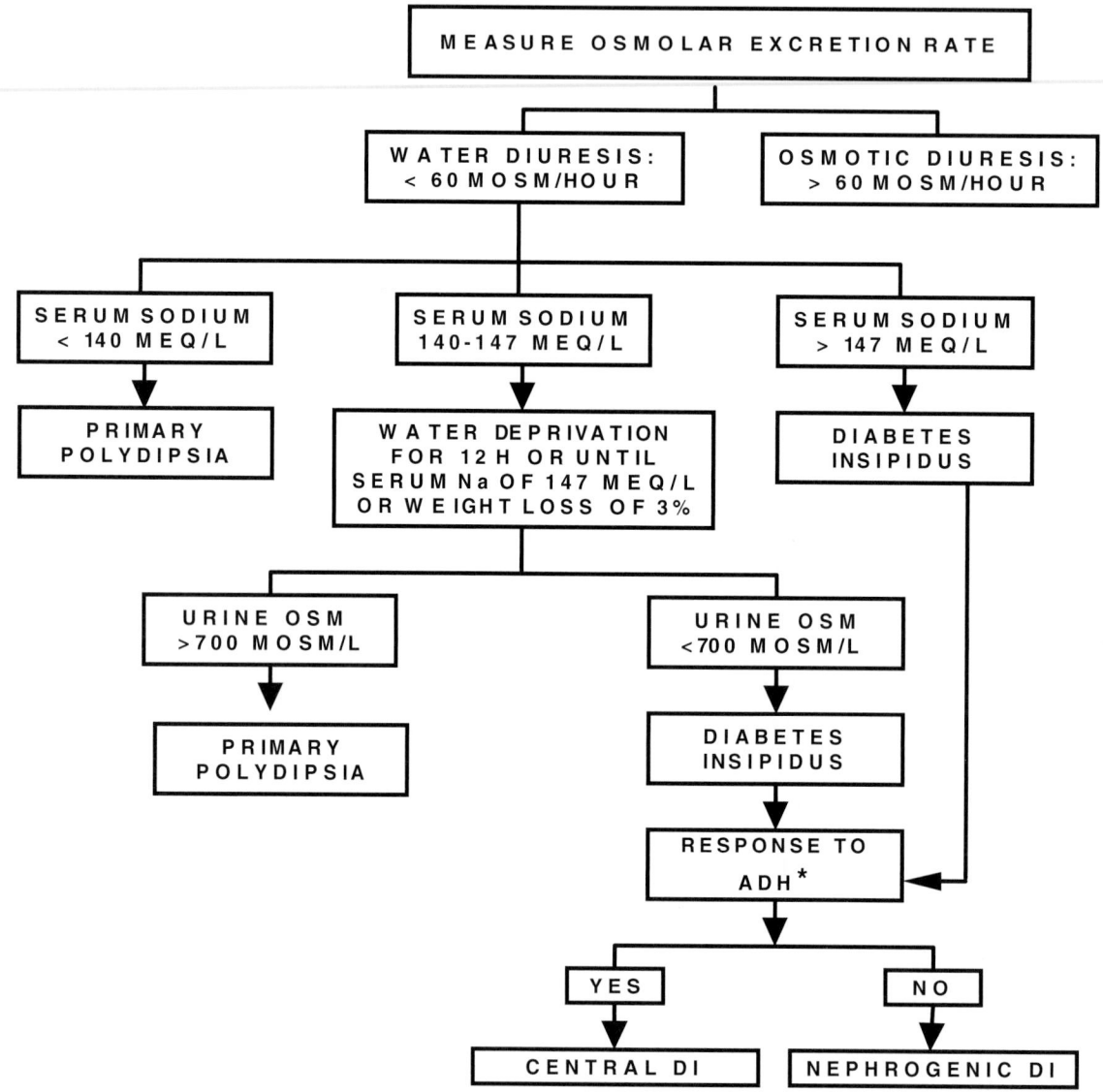

*RESPONSE TO ADH IS INCREASE IN URINE OSMOLALITY > 50% IF BASELINE URINE OSMOLALITY IS LESS THAN PLASMA OSMOLALITY, AND >20% IF THE BASELINE URINE OSMOLALITY IS GREATER THAN PLASMA OSMOLALITY.

Figure 8.14. Differential diagnosis of polyuria. By measuring osmolar excretion rate, osmotic diuresis is excluded. Among conditions that cause water diuresis, a high serum sodium concentration (>147 mEq/L) suggests diabetes insipidus (DI), and a low serum sodium concentration (<140 mEq/L) suggests primary polydipsia. When serum sodium is between these two values, a water deprivation test is done. The ability to concentrate urine normally (>700 mOsm/L) suggests primary polydipsia, and an inability to concentrate urine normally suggests DI. A good response to antidiuretic hormone (ADH) indicates central DI, and a poor response to ADH suggests nephrogenic DI.

TABLE 8.7. DRUG TREATMENT OF CENTRAL DIABETES INSIPIDUS

DDAVP (desmopressin), an analog of antidiuretic hormone, has a prolonged effect and few side effects and is easy to administer. Usual doses are as follows: parenteral, 2–4 μg BID; nasal, 10–40 μg BID–TID; oral, 100–800 μg TID–QID.

Lysine-vasopressin (lypressin) is used as a nasal spray QID.

Arginine vasopressin (Pitressin): Aqueous Pitressin is used by intravenous infusion in diagnostic tests.

Pitressin tannate in oil is no longer available.

Chlorpropamide may be used in partial central diabetes insipidus.

Thiazide diuretics and low-salt diet: Thiazide diuretics are used alone or in combination with a potassium-sparing diuretic to prevent hypokalemia.

ADH and may also enhance the effect of ADH (Table 8.7). Its use has been markedly curtailed since the advent of DDAVP. Thiazide diuretics produce vascular volume depletion and enhance reabsorption of fluid in the proximal tubule, thereby increasing urine concentration with reduction in the delivery of fluid to the distal diluting segment of the nephron. Addition of a thiazide diuretic to chlorpropamide may prevent the hypoglycemia that may occur if the latter is used alone.

Nephrogenic DI cannot be treated with ADH preparations or an agent that stimulates ADH release, but measures to reduce the distal delivery of salt and water (i.e., low-salt diet and thiazide diuretics) are effective (188, 189). A low-salt diet and a thiazide diuretic may also be used to treat central DI based on the same physiologic mechanisms.

Clozapine and propranolol have been successfully used to treat primary polydipsia in schizophrenic patients (190). Occasionally, patients with an upward reset of the osmostat for thirst may be managed with DDAVP. Drugs that interfere with urinary dilution, such as thiazide diuretics, should be avoided in primary polydipsia.

Hyponatremia

Hyponatremia, the most common electrolyte disorder, is defined as a reduced plasma Na^+ concentration to a value less than 135 mEq/L. Generally, clinical concern arises when the concentration is less than 130 mEq/L.

The term pseudohyponatremia is applied to a spurious reduction in serum Na^+ concentration resulting from a systematic error in the measurement. The most common, yet not widely known, cause of pseudohyponatremia is in vitro hemolysis, a well-known cause of pseudohyperkalemia (191). Because cell lysis does not change osmolality of the plasma, any rise in serum K^+ must be met by a reciprocal decrease in serum Na^+. However, the reduction in serum Na^+ from hemolysis is somewhat greater than the increase in serum K^+, by a factor of 1.3, because hemoglobin released from the red cells cause additional reduction in serum Na^+ as in hyperproteinemia; this additional error occurs only when samples are diluted before

measurement of serum Na^+. Other causes of pseudohyponatremia include hyperlipidemia, hyperproteinemia, and increased viscosity of the plasma (192, 193). The error in measurement in pseudohyponatremia results from the dilution of the sample. Measurements of serum Na^+ with a flame photometer can result in this type of error because the sample is always diluted. The same error also occurs even with an ion-specific electrode method, if the sample is diluted (indirect method). In pseudohyponatremia, plasma osmolality, which is customarily measured without dilution, is normal. However, a low plasma Na^+ concentration with a normal plasma osmolality need not indicate the presence of pseudohyponatremia; true hyponatremia may be accompanied by a normal plasma osmolality because of hyperglycemia, azotemia, or the presence of alcohol. In hypergammaglobulinemic states such as in multiple myeloma, serum Na^+ may be falsely low because of displacement of serum water by γ-globulins, but conversely, the Na^+ concentration is also truly low because cationic charges of γ-globulins displace Na^+ to maintain electrical neutrality (Table 8.8).

Hyponatremia induced by acute hyperglycemia is not pseudohyponatremia, because Na^+ concentration in the extracellular fluid is truly low; this occurs as a result of water shift from the cell caused by hyperglycemia. Serum Na^+ decreases by 1.5 mEq/L for every 100 mg/dL rise in serum glucose.

Causes and Pathogenesis

The immediate mechanisms responsible for a reduction in extracellular Na^+ concentration are shift of water from the cell caused by accumulation of extracellular solutes other than Na^+ salts (194–196), retention of excess water in the body, loss of Na^+ (197), and shift of Na^+ into the cells (Fig. 8.15). The appropriate physiologic response to hypotonicity is suppression of ADH release, which leads to rapid excretion of excess water and correction of hyponatremia. Persistence of hyponatremia therefore indicates the failure of this compensatory mechanism. In most instances, hyponatremia is maintained because the kidney fails to produce water diuresis, but sometimes ingestion of

TABLE 8.8. HYPONATREMIA WITH NORMAL EFFECTIVE OSMOLALITY

Accumulation of nonsodium cations
    Lithium intoxication
    Increased cationic γ-globulins (multiple myeloma)
    Severe hyperkalemia
    Severe hypermagnesemia
    Severe hypercalcemia
    Accumulation of cationic amino acids
Pseudohyponatremia
    In vitro hemolysis
    Pseudohyperkalemia of any cause
    Hyperlipidemia
    Hyperproteinemia

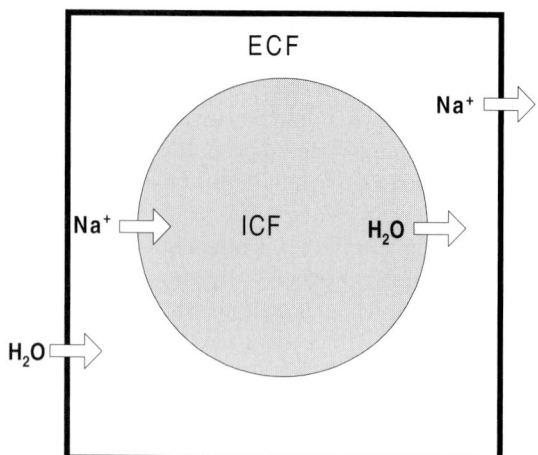

Figure 8.15. Pathogenetic mechanisms of hyponatremia. Reduction in extracellular sodium occurs by sodium (Na^+) loss from the extracellular fluid (ECF) either by loss into the outside or movement into the cell, or by gain of water in the ECF either from the outside or by shift out of the cell. ICF, intracellular fluid.

water in excess of the limits of normal renal compensation is responsible. The reasons for inability of the kidney to excrete water include renal failure, reduced delivery of glomerular filtrate to the distal nephron, and the presence of ADH.

The mechanism for impaired water excretion in renal failure is obvious and needs no further explanation. Reduced distal delivery of filtrate results from low GFR and enhanced proximal tubular reabsorption of salt and water, and these states are most commonly caused by volume depletion.

In most cases of hyponatremia, the main reason for the fall of serum Na^+ is abnormal retention of water, which is either ingested as such or administered as hypotonic fluids (197). However, in certain clinical settings, water retention can occur despite administration of isotonic fluid. The latter phenomenon occurs when urine is excreted containing Na^+ and K^+ at concentrations that exceed the sum of serum concentrations of the two ions. The physiologic requirement for the excretion of hypertonic urine is an increased amount of ADH in the presence of marked Na^+ diuresis. Clinical examples include (a) a patient who receives a large amount of isotonic fluid in the immediate postoperative period, (b) a patient with SIADH who is treated with isotonic fluid, and (c) a patient who receives a thiazide diuretic (198). The normal dilution of urine requires delivery of adequate amounts of fluid to the diluting segment and the reabsorption of solute without water at that segment. Increased body fluid tonicity causes release of ADH, which allows reabsorption of water in the collecting duct and helps to restore the body fluid tonicity. The response is considered appropriate when ADH is released in response to hypertonicity of the body fluid. However, release of ADH in the presence of hyponatremia is also considered appropriate if the effective

vascular volume is reduced. The term SIADH is therefore reserved for ADH secretion that occurs despite hyponatremia and despite a normal or increased effective vascular volume. Causes of SIADH include tumors, pulmonary diseases such as tuberculosis and pneumonia, central nervous system diseases, and drugs, among others (Table 8.9) (199–209). Hyponatremia in clinical states associated with reduced effective vascular volume such as congestive heart failure and cirrhosis of the liver is caused by a combination of reduced delivery of fluid to the distal nephron and increased secretion of ADH. Salt restriction and diuretics increase the severity of hyponatremia. ADH secretion may be present despite hyponatremia in myxedema (210) and glucocorticoid deficiency states. It is not clear, however, whether ADH secretion in these conditions is truly inappropriate or appropriate. Finally, mild hyponatremia may be caused by resetting of the osmostat at an osmolality lower than the usual level. In such cases, urine dilution occurs normally when the plasma osmolality is brought down below the reset level. Resetting of the

TABLE 8.9. CLASSIFICATION OF HYPONATREMIA BY PATHOGENESIS

Sodium loss
  Thiazide diuretics in the presence of ADH
  Saline infusion in the presence of ADH
Water retention
  Excessive water intake: primary polydipsia
  Advanced renal failure
  Appropriate ADH secretion: edema-forming states
    (congestive heart failure, nephritic syndrome, ascites), salt
    depletion states (gastrointestinal loss, diuretic
    therapy, aldosterone deficiency, hypothyroidism)
  Inappropriate ADH secretion
      Tumors: cancers of the lung, pancreas, duodenum,
        ureter, bladder, prostate, lymphoma, thymoma,
        mesothelioma, Ewing sarcoma
      Intrathoracic causes: bacterial and viral pneumonia,
        tuberculosis, lung abscess, aspergillosis, asthma,
        positive-pressure breathing, pneumothorax, cystic
        fibrosis
      Central nervous system abnormalities: encephalitis,
        meningitis, brain tumors and abscess, head trauma,
        subdural hematoma, cerebrovascular accidents,
        Guillain-Barré syndrome, acute intermittent porphyria,
        brain atrophy, schizophrenia, hydrocephalus, acute
        psychosis, multiple sclerosis, cavernous vein
        thrombosis, lupus cerebritis, Shy-Drager syndrome,
        Rocky Mountain spotted fever, delirium tremens,
        seizure disorder
      Drugs: arginine vasopressin and its analogs,
        sulfonylureas, tricyclic antidepressants, clofibrate,
        carbamazepine, vinca alkaloids, cylophosphamide,
        selective serotonin reuptake inhibitors, opiates,
        phenothiazines, haloperidol
  Surgical and emotional stress
  Emesis
  Endocrine causes: glucocorticoid deficiency and
    myxedema

ADH, antidiuretic hormone.

osmostat is a form of SIADH, because ADH secretion occurs inappropriately at hyponatremic levels without evidence of reduced effective vascular volume. Patients with chronic debilitating diseases such as pulmonary tuberculosis often manifest this phenomenon (211). Some authorities believe the existence of a cerebral salt-wasting syndrome, which is defined as renal loss of salt caused by humoral substances released in response to cerebral disorders such as acute subarachnoid hemorrhage. These patients are thought to manifest volume depletion that results in hyponatremia. However, a careful analysis of the existing data does not support existence of such entity, and those cases labeled as cerebral salt-wasting syndrome probably represent cases of SIADH (212).

Diagnosis

The presence of a low plasma Na^+ concentration and normal osmolality suggests pseudohyponatremia but does not confirm it. By coincidence, true hyponatremia may be accompanied by a high concentration of urea or alcohol, resulting in a normal osmolality. A more direct proof is the demonstration of a normal Na^+ concentration using a Na^+-specific electrode or demonstration of reduced water content of plasma. Pseudohyponatremia resulting from hyperlipidemia is caused by accumulation of chylomicrons, which consist mostly of triglyceride, and is obvious from the milky appearance of serum or plasma. Substantial hyponatremia resulting from hyperlipidemia requires accumulation of more than 5 to 6 g/dL of lipids, and such a degree of hyperlipidemia does not occur with hypercholesterolemia alone. Each gram per deciliter of lipid causes a false reduction in serum Na^+ by 1.7 mEq/L, and each gram per deciliter of protein causes a false reduction in serum Na^+ by 1.0 mEq/L. Pseudohyponatremia resulting from hyperproteinemia can be confirmed by measurement of plasma proteins (213, 214). Hyponatremia caused by mannitol or glucose is suspected from the history or by simultaneous measurements of plasma Na^+, osmolality, and glucose.

In evaluating hyponatremia associated with hypoosmolality, the main concern is distinguishing between SIADH and hyponatremia resulting from other causes, mainly volume depletion and edematous states. The major distinction between SIADH and other causes of hyponatremia lies in the status of effective vascular volume. Effective vascular volume is normal or increased in the former and reduced in the latter. However, no single diagnostic test measures effective vascular volume with certainty. Physical examination is notoriously inaccurate in determining mild to moderate volume depletion. A more reliable method for estimating effective vascular volume is the measurement of certain laboratory parameters, all of which depend on renal responses to changes in effective vascular volume. These parameters include urinary Na^+, serum urea nitrogen, serum creatinine, and serum uric

acid. Urinary Na^+ excretion of greater than 20 mEq/L, serum urea nitrogen less than 10 mg/dL, serum creatinine less than 1 mg/dL, and serum urate less than 4.0 mg/dL are all suggestive of normal or increased effective vascular volume. A bit more reliable than serum urea nitrogen in determining the status of effective vascular volume is fractional excretion of urea, because the former depends also on protein intake. Fractional excretion of urea of less than 35% is considered an indicator of low effective vascular volume (215).

Fractional excretion of Na^+ instead of actual Na^+ concentration has also been used, and a value less than 0.5% is thought to represent low effective vascular volume (216). In contrast, the measurement of urine osmolality has virtually no diagnostic value and often misleads physicians. Contrary to the common belief, urine osmolality in SIADH need not be greater than plasma osmolality. Furthermore, a high urine osmolality does not necessarily support the diagnosis of SIADH, because most other causes of hyponatremia are also accompanied by urine osmolality higher than plasma osmolality. The only situation in which urine osmolality may be appropriately low in the presence of hyponatremia is the hyponatremia caused by primary polydipsia, and this is usually apparent when a careful history reveals polyuria and polydipsia (Fig. 8.16). In all other causes of hyponatremia, urine osmolality is inappropriately increased (i.e., >100 mOsm/L) (213).

Treatment

Hyponatremia is treated either by the addition of Na^+ or by removal of water. Salt is given to patients with hyponatremia resulting from salt depletion. Water is removed in hyponatremic states with normal or increased body Na^+ content (217, 218). The speed of correction of hyponatremia should depend on the speed of development and on the patient's symptoms. Clearly, severe symptomatic hyponatremia is a life-threatening condition, but dangers are associated with treatment of hyponatremia. In the past, volume overload was thought to be the main danger associated with administration of a large quantity of salt-containing solution. Now, central pontine myelinolysis (also known as osmotic demyelinating disease) is considered a major danger associated with rapid correction of hyponatremia (50, 51). This demyelinating disease of the central pons and other areas of the brain is characterized by motor nerve dysfunction including quadriplegia. This complication tends to occur more often with chronic hyponatremia than with acute hyponatremia and is more frequently observed in malnourished and debilitated patients. The commonly accepted rate of correction of chronic hyponatremia is 0.5 mEq/L/hour or less. However, there are reported cases of central pontine myelinolysis with a rate of correction of hyponatremia less than 0.5 mEq/L. The more prudent rate of correction would be a speed less than 0.35 mEq/L/hour or less than 8 mEq/24

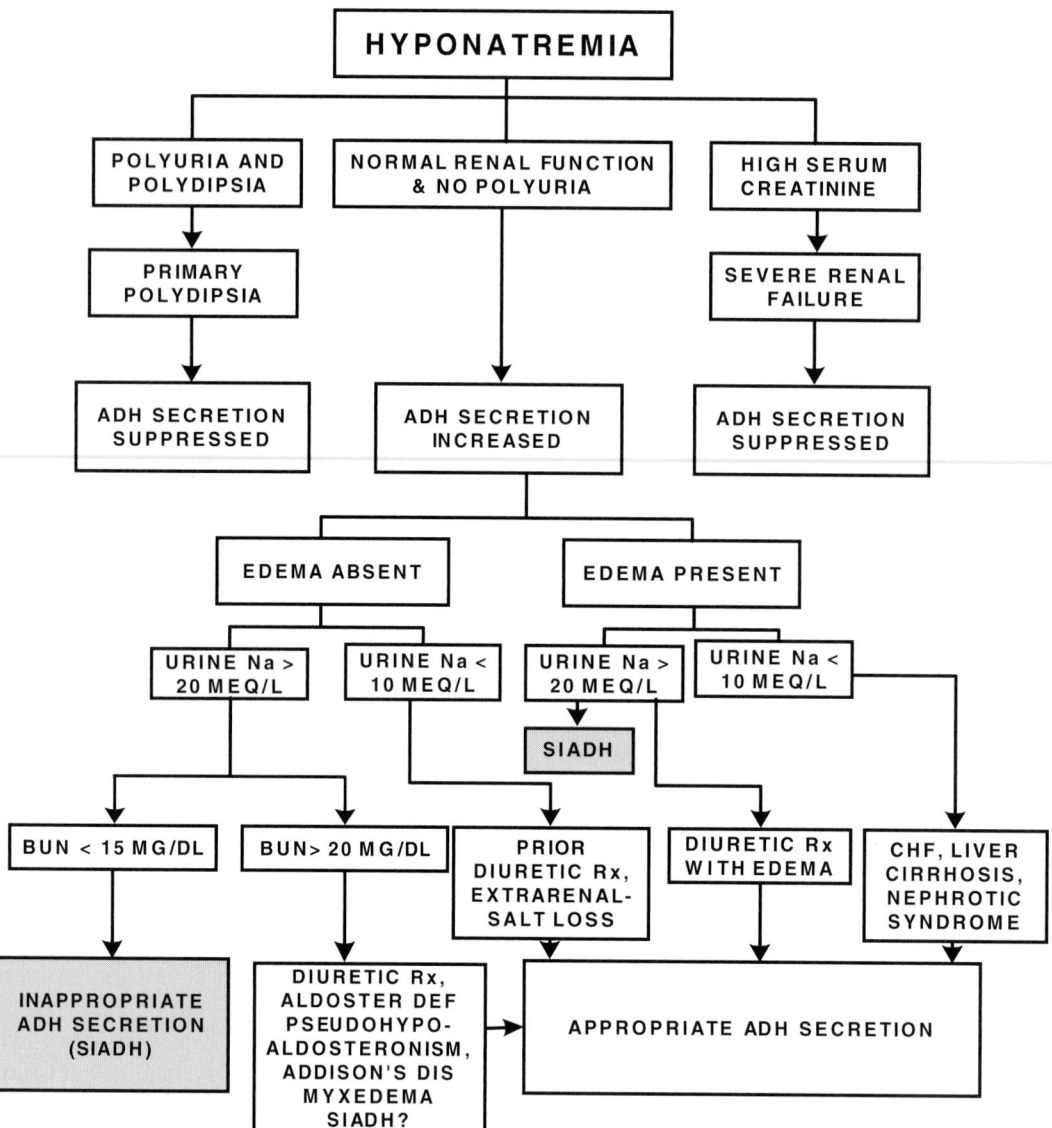

Figure 8.16. Differential diagnosis of hyponatremia. The main aim is to distinguish hyponatremia resulting from inappropriate antidiuretic hormone (ADH) secretion and that resulting from appropriate ADH secretion. This goal is best achieved by measurement of urine sodium (Na) and blood urea nitrogen (BUN). CHF, congestive heart failure; SIADH, syndrome of inappropriate ADH.

hours (52, 53). Because the danger of central pontine myelinolysis is limited mainly to those with asymptomatic chronic hyponatremia, rapid correction (at a rate of 1–2 mEq/L/hour) should be restricted to those with acute symptomatic hyponatremia. Even then, no advantage is conferred by a rapid increase of serum Na$^+$ to a level greater than 125 mEq/L (53). For patients admitted with hypotonic dehydration and chronic asymptomatic hyponatremia, the traditional recommendation has been administration of isotonic saline. As the volume expansion suppresses ADH release induced by low effective vascular volume, a rise in serum Na$^+$ follows rapid water excretion, provided the renal function is adequate. Sometimes, rapid excretion of water following isotonic saline administration in these patients may lead to the development of central pontine myelinolysis. Use of 0.45% alternating with 0.9%

NaCl solution may therefore be safer. If K$^+$ depletion coexists, the appropriate treatment is with 0.45% NaCl containing 40 mEq/L K$^+$.

Acute Treatment. For hyponatremia with Na$^+$ depletion and symptomatic hypoosmolality, intravenous administration of Na$^+$ as hypertonic saline will correct hypoosmolality effectively. The amount of Na$^+$ necessary to increase the Na$^+$ to a desired level is calculated as follows (53, 219):

$$\text{Na}^+ \text{ requirement (mEq)} = \text{TBW} \times \Delta\text{Na}$$

where ΔNa$^+$ is the desired serum Na$^+$ minus actual serum Na$^+$. Na$^+$ may be administered as a 3 or 5% NaCl solution.

When accumulation of excess water is primarily responsible for hyponatremia, as in SIADH, water may be rapidly removed by administration of intravenous osmotic diuretics such as mannitol or urea. More readily available is a loop diuretic, such as furosemide, to be given simultaneously with hypertonic saline. Furosemide causes loss of water and Na^+, but hypertonic saline replaces mainly the lost Na^+; the net result is removal of water. The response to furosemide cannot be predicted with precision, and frequent follow-up measurements of serum Na^+ level must be made. However, no theoretic advantage exists for replacing exactly the amount of Na^+ lost in urine with hypertonic saline. Administration of hypertonic saline alone usually causes salt and water diuresis, but addition of a loop diuretic makes the correction of hyponatremia more predictable by preventing excretion of concentrated urine. Another advantage of addition of a diuretic is prevention of fluid overload.

Chronic Treatment. Chronic hyponatremia may be treated by a reduction in water intake or by an increase in renal water excretion. Reduction of water intake is preferable but is not always feasible. If water restriction is difficult or unsuccessful, the latter approach may be used. Increased renal water excretion can be achieved by the use of pharmacologic agents that interfere with urine concentration. Lithium and demeclocycline increase urine output by interfering with the renal effects of ADH. Demeclocycline is more effective and has fewer side effects, but it may cause nephrotoxicity in patients with liver disease. Administration of a loop diuretic such as furosemide in conjunction with increased salt and K^+ intake is safer than the foregoing methods. The diuretic prevents high medullary interstitial osmolality by limiting the reabsorption of salt in the loop of Henle and hence prevents urine concentration. Increased salt and K^+ intake increases water output by increasing the rate of solute excretion. Finally, vasopressin antagonists, not yet commercially available, may become an important addition to the chronic as well as acute treatment of hyponatremia in the future (220). The daily ingestion of urea has been used successfully (221), but again it is not readily available and is not as practical as a loop diuretic plus Na^+ and K^+ supplements.

Hypernatremia

Hypernatremia is defined as an increased Na^+ concentration in plasma water. Whereas hyponatremia may not be accompanied by hypoosmolality, hypernatremia is always associated with an increased effective plasma osmolality and hence with a reduced cell volume. However, the extracellular volume in hypernatremia may be normal, decreased, or increased.

Causes and Pathogenesis

Hypernatremia is caused by loss of water, gain of Na^+, or both (Table 8.10). Loss of water could be the result of increased loss or reduced intake, and gain of Na^+ is the result either of increased intake or of reduced renal

TABLE 8.10. CAUSES OF HYPERNATREMIA

Reduced water intake
  Reduced water intake
  Defective thirst resulting from altered mental state or thirst center defect
  Inability to drink water
  Lack of access to water
Increased water loss (water intake must be impaired)
  Gastrointestinal loss: vomiting, osmotic diarrhea
  Cutaneous loss: sweating and fever
  Respiratory loss: hyperventilation and fever
  Renal loss: diabetes insipidus, osmotic diuresis
Increased sodium content of the body (water intake must be impaired)
  Increased intake
  Hypertonic saline or sodium bicarbonate infusion
  Ingestion of sea water
  Renal salt retention; usually in response to primary water deficit

excretion. Increased loss of water can occur through the kidney (e.g., in DI or osmotic diuresis), the GI tract (e.g., gastric suction or osmotic diarrhea), or the skin. Reduced water intake occurs most commonly in comatose patients or in those with a defective thirst mechanism. Less frequent causes of reduced water intake include continuous vomiting, lack of access to water, and mechanical obstruction resulting from a condition such as esophageal tumor. Gain of Na^+ in a person with normal perception of thirst, ability to drink water, and availability of water does not result in hypernatremia because a proportional amount of water is retained to maintain normal body fluid osmolality. Whereas the physiologic defense against hyponatremia is increased renal water excretion, the physiologic defense against hypernatremia is increased water drinking in response to thirst. Because thirst is such an effective and sensitive defense mechanism against hypernatremia, it is virtually impossible to increase serum Na^+ by more than a few milliequivalents per liter if the water drinking mechanism is intact. Therefore, a patient with hypernatremia will always have reasons for reduced water intake. These reasons include defective thirst mechanism, inability to drink water, and unavailability of water. The excess gain of Na^+ leading to hypernatremia is usually iatrogenic, such as from hypertonic saline infusion, accidental entry into maternal circulation during abortion with hypertonic saline, or administration of hypertonic $NaHCO_3^-$ during cardiopulmonary resuscitation or treatment of lactic acidosis. Reduced renal Na^+ excretion leading to Na^+ gain and hypernatremia is usually in response to dehydration caused by primary water deficit. Water depletion resulting from DI, osmotic diuresis, or insufficient water intake leads to secondary Na^+ retention in those who continue to ingest or are given Na^+. Consequently, in chronic hypernatremia, Na^+ retention plays a more important role than water loss (186).

Whether hypernatremia is caused by Na^+ retention or water loss can be determined by examination of the patient's volume status. For example, if a patient with a serum Na^+ concentration of 170 mEq/L does not have obvious evidence of dehydration, hypernatremia is not caused entirely by water loss. To increase the serum Na^+ to 170 mEq/L by water deficit alone, one would have to lose more than 20% of TBW.

Treatment

Acute Treatment. Hypernatremia is treated either by addition of water or by removal of Na^+. The choice depends on the status of the body Na^+ and water content. If water depletion is the mechanism of hypernatremia, water is added. If Na^+ excess is the main problem, Na^+ needs to be removed. When the water deficit is severe, isotonic (0.9%) NaCl or 0.45% NaCl may be given initially to stabilize circulatory dynamics, followed by administration of hypotonic solutions to normalize the tonicity. Administration of 5% dextrose solution would also correct the extracellular volume depletion, but a larger volume is needed to expand the extracellular volume, and the ensuing rapid reduction of the plasma osmolality may result in cerebral edema. In acute symptomatic hypernatremia, serum Na^+ may be reduced by 6 to 8 mEq/L in the first 3 to 4 hours, but thereafter the rate of decline should not exceed 1 mEq/L/hour. As with hyponatremia, chronic hypernatremia usually does not cause central nervous system symptoms and therefore does not require rapid correction. A safe rate of correction is 0.7 mEq/L/hour, or about 10% of the serum Na^+ concentration over 24 hours. The amount of water needed to correct hypernatremia can be estimated with the following equation (186, 187):

$$\text{Water deficit (L)} = \text{TBW} \times (\text{Actual } Na^+ - \text{Desired } Na^+)/$$
$$\text{Desired } Na^+ = \text{TBW} \times (\Delta Na^+/\text{Desired } Na^+)$$

where ΔNa^+ is the difference between the desired and actual serum Na^+.

In hypernatremia with excess Na^+, reduction in serum Na^+ with fluids usually initiates natriuresis, but if natriuresis does not occur promptly, Na^+ may be removed with diuretics. Furosemide plus 5% dextrose solution may be an appropriate regimen to treat hypernatremia associated with excess Na^+. If a hypernatremic patient with Na^+ excess has renal failure, salt can be removed by dialysis. The total water requirement must also include insensible water loss (~300–500 mL/24 hours) and urinary electrolyte-free water loss. Urinary electrolyte-free water loss represents the urine water loss in excess of the volume necessary to contain urinary Na^+ plus K^+ at the same concentration as serum Na^+. If the urine electrolyte-free water excretion is a positive number, urine output increases serum Na^+ further, and if it is a negative number, the effect is to decrease serum Na^+. Urinary electrolyte-free water excretion is calculated as follows:

$$\text{Electrolyte-free water excretion} = V - (U_{Na^+ + K^+})V/S_{Na^+}$$

where V is urine volume, $U_{(Na^+ + K^+)}$ is the sum of concentrations of urine Na^+ and K^+, and S_{Na} is serum Na^+ concentration.

Chronic Treatment. Hypernatremic disorders that require chronic preventive therapy include DI and primary hypodipsia. Although DI is often listed as a cause of hypernatremia, in the absence of thirst defect it does not cause hypernatremia. Treatment is therefore directed toward the curtailment of polydipsia and polyuria, which are the main complaints of the patients. Patients with primary hypodipsia should be educated to drink water on schedule. In some instances, stimulation of the thirst center with chlorpropamide has been effective (186).

ACID-BASE DISORDERS

Bicarbonate and Carbon Dioxide Buffer System

All body buffers are in equilibrium with protons (H^+) and therefore with pH as shown in the following equation (222):

$$pH = pK + \log A^-/HA$$

where A^- is a conjugate base of an acid HA.

Because HCO_3^- and CO_2 are the major buffers of the body, pH is typically expressed as a function of their ratio, as in the Henderson-Hasselbalch equation:

$$pH = 6.1 + \log HCO_3^-/P_{CO_2} \times 0.03,$$

where 6.1 is the pK of the HCO_3^- and CO_2 buffer system, and 0.03 is the solubility coefficient of CO_2.

The equation can be further simplified by combining the two constants, pK and solubility coefficient of CO_2:

$$\begin{aligned} pH &= 6.1 + \log HCO_3^-/P_{CO_2} \times 0.03 \\ &= 6.1 + \log 1/0.03 + \log HCO_3^-/P_{CO_2} \\ &= 7.62 + \log HCO_3^-/P_{CO_2} \ (5) \end{aligned}$$

Hence,

$$\begin{aligned} pH &= 7.62 - \log P_{CO_2}/HCO_3 \\ &= 7.62 + \log HCO_3^- - \log CO_2 \end{aligned}$$

When H^+ is expressed in nanomolars instead of a negative log value (pH), P_{CO_2} can be related to HCO_3^- in an equation:

$$H(nM) = 24 \times P_{CO_2} \ (mm\ Hg)/HCO_3^- \ (mM)$$

The Henderson-Hasselbalch equation indicates that pH depends on the ratio of HCO_3^-/P_{CO_2}. pH increases when the ratio increases (alkalosis), and pH decreases when the ratio decreases (acidosis). The ratio may be increased by an increase in HCO_3^- (metabolic alkalosis) or by a decrease in P_{CO_2} (respiratory alkalosis). The ratio may be decreased by a decrease in HCO_3^- (metabolic acidosis) or by an increase in P_{CO_2} (respiratory acidosis).

Terminology

The term acidosis or alkalosis refers to a pathologic process leading to acidic or alkaline pH, whereas acidemia and alkalemia refer to acidic and alkaline pH. Patients could have acidosis but actually have alkaline pH. For example, we may say that a patient has combined respiratory acidosis and metabolic alkalosis. Obviously, the patient cannot have acidic and alkaline pH at the same time, and those terms must refer to pathologic processes. However, clinicians often use the two terms interchangeably.

Whole-Body Acid-Base Balance

Net Acid Production

On a typical US diet, the daily production of nonvolatile acid is about 90 mEq/day. The main acids are sulfuric acid (~40 mEq/day), which originates from metabolism of sulfur-containing amino acids such as methionine and cystine, and incompletely metabolized organic acids (~50 mEq/day). The source of sulfuric acid is protein, but the sulfate content varies greatly with the types of protein that are ingested (223). In general, when sulfur content is expressed as mEq/100 g of proteins, proteins of animal sources (meat, fish, milk, and egg) contain higher amounts of sulfate for a given amount of protein than proteins of plant origin (cereal, beans, and nuts). The sulfur content per calorie is much greater in fruits, vegetables, and potatoes, but these food groups are not important sources of protein in the amounts usually eaten (Fig. 8.17). The total amount of acid or alkali content depends ont only on the sulfur content but also on alkali content of food, which is present mainly as salts of organic acids. When both factors are considered, milk has a net alkali value, whereas meat and fish have a net acid value. As a whole, fruits and vegetables contain a large amount of net alkali because they contain large amounts of organic anions (Fig. 8.18). The total amount of organic acids produced normally is much more than 50 mEq/day, but the bulk of organic acids produced in the body is metabolized; only a small amount is lost in the urine as organic anions that escape metabolism

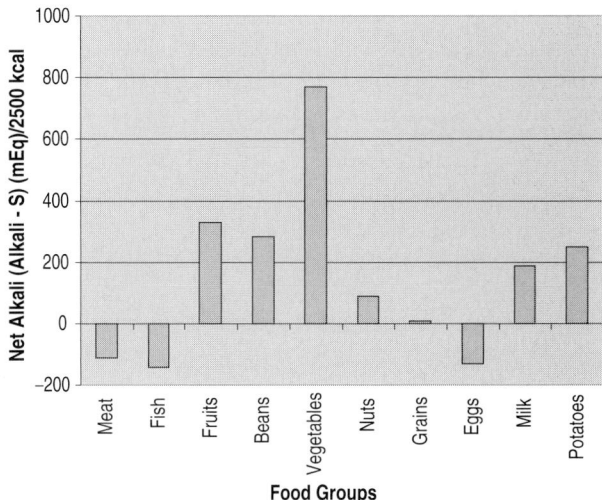

Figure 8.18. Net alkali content of food expressed as the alkali content of food minus sulfur (S) content. Only meat, fish, and eggs have negative alkali content. Vegetables have the highest alkali content when expressed by the caloric content.

(e.g., citrate) or as a metabolic end product (e.g., urate). On typical US diets, the amount of alkali absorbed from the GI tract is about 30 mEq/day (224–226). Thus, the net amount of acid produced daily can be estimated as follows:

$$Net\ acid\ production = (Urine\ sulfate + Urine\ organic$$
$$anions) - Net\ alkali\ absorbed\ from\ the\ GI\ tract$$

Determination of the net alkali (or acid) content of diet is based on the metabolic fates of the chemicals in diet after absorption into the body rather than its in vitro states. For example, citric acid in the food is considered neutral, because it would be metabolized to CO_2 and water in the body, whereas K^+ citrate is an alkali because it would be converted to K^+ HCO_3^- after metabolism. Similarly, arginine Cl^- is an acid, because metabolism of arginine in the body would result in the formation of HCl (223). Thus, net alkali value of diet is best determined by the total amount of noncombustible cations (Na^+, K^+, Ca^{2+}, and Mg^{2+}) relative to the total amount of noncombustible anions (Cl^- and P):

$$Net\ alkali\ content$$
$$= (Na^+ + K^+ + Ca^{2+} + Mg^{2+}) - (Cl^- + 1.8\ P)$$

All units are expressed as milliequivalents per day, except P, which is expressed as millimoles per day multiplied by 1.8, because P valence depends on pH, and at pH 7.4 the average valence of P is 1.8 . Only the foregoing six ions are considered in the equation because other noncombustible ions are present in negligible amounts in the normal food. Sulfate is not included here because sulfate is formed in the body only after metabolism of sulfur-containing amino acids. The amount of alkali absorbed from the food is not equal to the amount present in the food, because the absorption of divalent noncombustible ions, Ca^{2+}, Mg^{2+}, and P, is incomplete. Hence, traditionally the

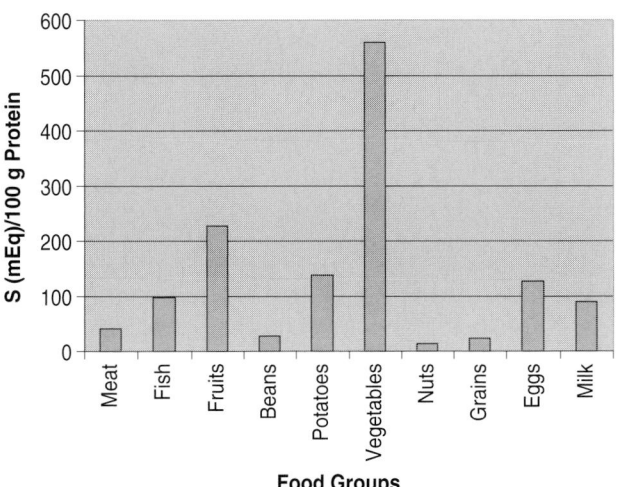

Figure 8.17. Sulfur (S) content of food groups.

measurement of the net GI alkali absorption required analysis of the food as well as the stool, which necessitated prolonged collection of stool (227). Thus, the net GI alkali absorption is expressed as follows:

$$\text{Net GI alkali absorbed} = \text{Net alkali of food} - \text{Net alkali of stool}$$

The analysis of the food for the measurement of net alkali content is cumbersome, and the analysis of the stool is even more cumbersome. Such analyses typically require admitting the patients to a special metabolic unit.

A newer method has been developed to measure net GI alkali absorption. In this method, urine electrolytes, instead of diet and stool electrolytes, are measured. The method is based on the principle that noncombustible ions absorbed from the GI tract would eventually be excreted in the urine, and therefore the individual amounts of these electrolytes excreted in the urine would equal those absorbed from the GI tract. Hence,

$$\text{Net GI alkali absorption} = \text{Urine} (Na^+ + K^+ + Ca^{2+} + Mg^{2+}) - \text{Urine} (Cl^- + 1.8\ P)$$

Twenty-four hour urine can be collected in outpatient settings, while the patients are eating their usual diets. The amount of net alkali absorbed on a typical US diet stated earlier, 30 mEq/day, was measured by the analysis of urine electrolytes using the foregoing formula (224–228).

Net Acid Excretion

The most important function of the kidney in acid-base homeostasis is excretion of acid, which is tantamount to generation of alkali. Acid is excreted in the form of ammonium (NH_4^+) and titratable acid. Another important function of the kidney is excretion of HCO_3^-. Usually, the main function of renal excretion of HCO_3^- is prevention of metabolic alkalosis, but a small amount of HCO_3^- is normally excreted in the urine ($\sim$10 mEq/d). Thus, net acid excretion, which is equivalent to net renal production of alkali, can be determined by subtracting HCO_3^- excretion from acid excretion.

$$\text{Net acid excretion} = \text{Acid excretion} - HCO_3^- \text{ excretion}$$
$$= NH_4^+ + \text{Titratable acid} - HCO_3^-$$

Normally, about two thirds of acid excretion occurs in the form of NH_4^+, but in acidosis NH_4^+ excretion may increase as much as tenfold. Excretion of titratable acid is usually modest because of the limited amount of buffer that produces titratable acid (i.e., P, creatinine, and urate), but it may be increased markedly in disease states (e.g., β-hydroxybutyrate in diabetic ketoacidosis). Maintenance of acid-base balance requires that net acid production equals net acid excretion (Fig. 8.19). Metabolic acidosis develops when net acid production exceeds net acid excretion, and metabolic alkalosis develops when net acid excretion exceeds net acid production.

Metabolic Acidosis

Classification By Net Acid Excretion

All metabolic acidoses result from reduction in HCO_3^- content of the body, with two minor and clinically unimportant exceptions: acidosis resulting from dilution of the body fluid by administration of a large amount of saline solution (dilution acidosis) and acidosis that results from shift of H^+ from the cell. Reduction in HCO_3^- content may be caused by a primary increase in acid production (extrarenal acidosis) or by a primary reduction in net acid

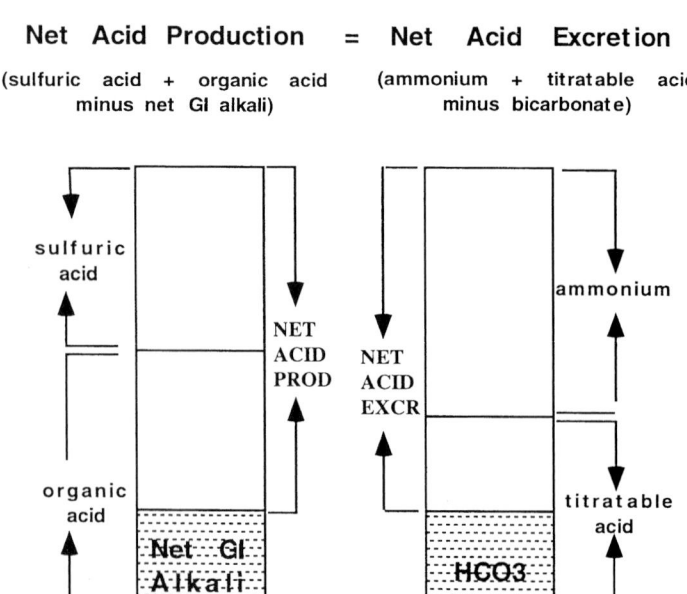

Net Acid Production = Net Acid Excretion

(sulfuric acid + organic acid minus net GI alkali)   (ammonium + titratable acid minus bicarbonate)

Figure 8.19. Net acid production and net acid excretion. In states of acid-base balance, net acid production equals net acid excretion. GI, gastrointestinal; HCO_3^-, bicarbonate.

TABLE 8.11. CAUSES OF METABOLIC ACIDOSIS ACCORDING TO NET ACID EXCRETION

Renal acidosis: absolute or relative reduction in net acid excretion
   Uremic acidosis
   Renal tubular acidosis
      Distal renal tubular acidosis (type I)
      Proximal renal tubular acidosis (type II)
      Aldosterone deficiency or unresponsiveness (type IV)
Extrarenal acidosis: increase in net acid excretion
   Gastrointestinal loss of bicarbonate
   Ingestion of acids or acid precursors: ammonium chloride, sulfur
   Acid precursors or toxins: salicylate, ethylene glycol, methanol, toluene, acetaminophen, paraldehyde
   Organic acidosis
      L-lactic acidosis
      D-lactic acidosis
      Ketoacidosis

excretion (renal acidosis) (Table 8.11). In this classification, nonrenal loss of HCO_3^- or an alkali precursor is considered as part of increased acid production. In extrarenal acidosis, net acid excretion is markedly increased as the kidney compensates to overcome acidosis. Conversely, net acid excretion may be restored to normal in chronic renal acidosis as acidosis stimulates renal H^+ excretion. Normal net acid excretion in the presence of acidic pH suggests a defect in renal acid excretion and therefore renal acidosis. If the renal acid excretion capacity is normal, net acid excretion should be supernormal in the presence of acidic pH. (Fig. 8.20).

Renal Acidosis

Renal acidosis is further classified into two types: uremic acidosis and renal tubular acidosis (RTA). In uremic acidosis, reduced net acid excretion results from reduced

nephron mass (i.e., renal failure), whereas in renal tubular acidosis reduction in net acid excretion results from a specific tubular dysfunction. Because development of renal acidosis depends on the rate of net acid excretion as well as the rate of net acid production, which varies greatly according to the diet, the level of renal failure at which uremic acidosis develops depends on the dietary intake of acid. On a usual diet, uremic acidosis may develop when GFR falls to less than 20% of normal (229).

Three types of RTA are known. Type I RTA, also called classic RTA or distal RTA, is characterized by inability to reduce urine pH to less than 5.5. Because acidification of urine to a very low urine pH occurs at the collecting duct, the likely site of defect is the collecting duct, which is a part of the distal nephron, hence the term distal RTA. Because H^+ secretion in the collecting duct is somewhat impaired also in type IV RTA, some authors consider both type I and type IV RTA a form of distal RTA. Still, most authorities use the terms type I RTA and distal RTA synonymously. In type I RTA, net acid excretion usually remains persistently less than daily net acid production, and therefore the patients develop progressively severe metabolic acidosis. Type I RTA can develop as a primary disorder or secondary to drug toxicity, tubulointerstitial renal diseases, or other renal diseases (230).

Type II RTA, also called proximal RTA, causes defective proximal HCO_3^- reabsorption characterized by reduced renal HCO_3^- threshold. Urine can be made free of HCO_3^- and acidified normally when serum HCO_3^- decreases to a low level. Most patients with proximal RTA have evidence of generalized proximal tubular dysfunction (i.e., Fanconi syndrome), which is manifested by bicarbonaturia, aminoaciduria, glycosuria, phosphaturia, and uricosuria. Of these conditions, renal glycosuria (glycosuria in the presence normal blood glucose) is most useful in diagnosing Fanconi syndrome. Type II RTA may be a primary disorder or secondary to genetic or acquired renal

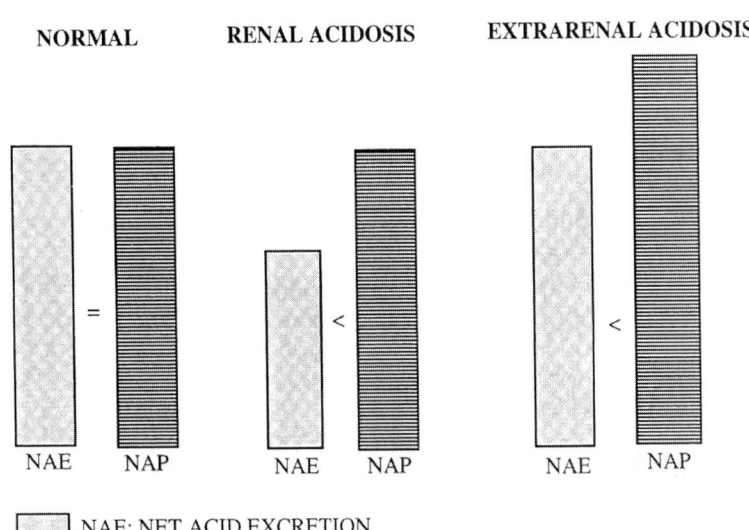

Figure 8.20. Genesis of renal and extrarenal acidosis. Normally, net acid excretion (NAE) equals net acid production (NAP). Acidosis occurs when net acid production is more than net acid excretion. In renal acidosis, the imbalance is caused by a primary decrease in net acid excretion, and in extrarenal acidosis, the imbalance is caused by a primary increase in net acid production.

dysfunction. Hypokalemia is a characteristic finding of both type I and type II RTA, but it tends to be more severe in type I than in type II. Type III RTA, a term to describe a hybrid form of types I and II RTA, is no longer in use.

Type IV RTA is caused by aldosterone deficiency or tubular unresponsiveness to aldosterone, resulting in impaired renal tubular K^+ secretion and hence hyperkalemia. Although reduced H^+ secretion in the collecting duct plays a role, the major mechanism of acidosis in type IV RTA is hyperkalemia-induced impairment in ammonia production in the proximal tubule. Type IV RTA is far more common than either type I or type II RTA, and the most common cause of type IV RTA is hyporeninemic hypoaldosteronism.

Organic Acidosis

Extrarenal acidosis may result from administration or ingestion of acid, overproduction of endogenous acid, or loss of HCO_3^-. Among these, overproduction of endogenous acid, especially that of lactic acid and ketoacids, is the most important mechanism. Only a marked overproduction of acid leads to acidosis because of the enormous capacity to metabolize organic acids. For example, a physiologically normal person produces approximately 1300 mEq of lactic acid daily, without resulting in acidosis. Organic acids are titrated immediately by the body's alkaline buffers. When they react with HCO_3^-, organic anions and CO_2 are formed. When the anions are retained in the body fluid, the result is metabolic acidosis with increased anion gap (AG). When the anions are excreted in the urine, the AG returns to normal, and acidosis becomes hyperchloremic. Retention of these anions per se is not responsible for acidosis. Their presence merely provides a clue to the mechanism of a reduced HCO_3^- concentration. Their removal from the body fluid, by dialysis or by renal excretion, would not improve the pH. The retained organic anions are potential HCO_3^-; when they are metabolized, HCO_3^- is regenerated. Thus, loss of organic anions in the urine is tantamount to loss of HCO_3^-. If an organic anion produced is entirely retained, subsequent metabolism will result in the complete recovery of the lost alkali. Characteristically, organic acidosis is rapid in onset and in recovery.

Lactic Acidosis. Lactic acid is produced from pyruvic acid by the action of the enzyme lactate dehydrogenase (LDH) and the cofactor reduced nicotinamide adenine dincleotide (NADH). Metabolism of lactic acid requires its conversion back to pyruvic acid, using the same enzyme and NAD^+ as a cofactor. For this reason, both production and metabolism of lactic acid are reciprocally influenced by the same factors; an increased concentration of pyruvic acid and an increased $NADH/NAD^+$ ratio increase lactic acid production and at the same time reduce its metabolism. Consequently, in most cases of lactic acidosis, lactic acid production is increased, and at the same time its

metabolism is reduced. By far the most common cause of lactic acidosis is tissue hypoxia, which results from circulatory shock, severe anemia, severe heart failure, acute pulmonary edema, cardiac arrest, carbon monoxide poisoning, seizures, and vigorous muscular exercise, among other causes (231, 232). Normally, lactic acid is produced by the extrahepatic tissues and is metabolized by the liver, but every organ in the body, except red blood cells, is capable of producing and metabolizing lactic acid. Red blood cells can produce lactic acid but cannot metabolize it. Lactic acidosis in acute alcoholism and severe liver disease is caused by impaired lactic acid utilization (Table 8.12).

Lactic acidosis, unless specified, refers to the acidosis caused by L-lactic acid, which is the isomer normally produced in the human body because the enzyme LDH, responsible for production of lactic acid, is an L-isomer. D-Lactic acidosis is caused by the accumulation of D-lactic acid and is characterized by severe acidosis and neurologic manifestations. Affected patients behave as if they are intoxicated with alcohol despite normal blood ethanol levels. The mechanism of D-lactic acidosis is the colonic overproduction of D-lactic acid by bacteria. Necessary requirements for overproduction of D-lactic acid in the colon are delivery of a large amount of substrate to the colon (i.e., malabsorption syndrome) and proliferation of D-LDH–forming bacteria in the colon (233, 234). Treatment of D-lactic acidosis is oral administration of antibiotics.

Ketoacidosis. Ketoacids, acetoacetic acid (AA) and β-hydroxybutyric acid (BB), are produced in the liver from free fatty acids (FFAs) and are metabolized by the extrahepatic tissues. Increased production of keto acids is the main mechanism for keto acid accumulation, although decreased utilization of keto acids by the brain with the patient in a coma may accelerate keto acid accumulation. Increased production requires a high concentration of FFAs and its conversion to ketoacids in the liver. Insulin deficiency is responsible for increased mobilization of FFAs from the adipose tissue, and glucagon excess and insulin deficiency stimulate conversion of FFAs to ketoacids in the liver. The initial step in ketoacid production from FFAs is the entry of FFAs into the mitochondria,

TABLE 8.12. CAUSES OF L-LACTIC ACIDOSIS

Type A lactic acidosis: resulting from tissue hypoxia
　　Circulatory shock
　　Severe hypoxemia
　　Heart failure
　　Severe anemia
　　Grand mal seizure
Type B lactic acidosis: no tissue hypoxia
　　Acute alcoholism
　　Drugs and toxins, (e.g., phenformin, antiretroviral drugs)
　　Diabetes mellitus
　　Leukemia
　　Deficiency of thiamin or riboflavin
　　Idiopathic

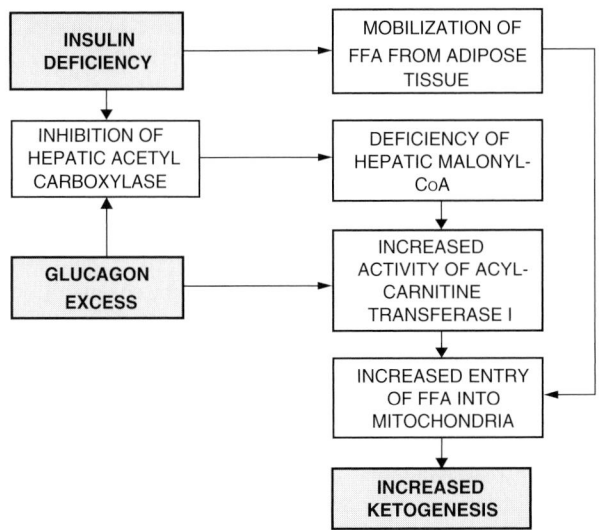

Figure 8.21. Mechanism of ketoacidosis. Mainly insulin deficiency and partly glucagon excess are responsible for ketoacidosis. Insulin deficiency causes mobilization of fatty acid from the adipose tissue. Activation of acyl-carnitine transferase is required for fatty acid to enter the mitochondria to become ketoacids, and this occurs as a result of deficiency of malonyl coenzyme A (CoA), which, in turn, is caused by insulin deficiency and glucagon excess. FFA, free fatty acid.

which requires acyl-carnitine transferase. This step is stimulated by glucagons excess. The next step is metabolism of FFAs to acetyl-coenzyme A, and then finally to ketoacids. Diversion of acetyl-coenzyme A to fatty acid resynthesis requires the enzyme acetyl-coenzyme A carboxylase, and inhibition of this enzyme by insulin deficiency, glucagon excess, and excess of stress-induced hormones further contributes to increased ketoacid synthesis (Fig. 8.21).

Two major ketoacids in the body are AA and BB. BB is produced from AA with the enzyme BB dehydrogenase and the cofactor NADH. The same enzyme and NAD$^+$ are required to convert BB to AA. Consequently, the ratio of NADH to NAD$^+$ is the sole determinant of the BB/AA ratio. The clinical diagnosis of ketoacidosis is usually made with Acetest, which detects AA but not BB. Although BB is the predominant acid in typical ketoacidosis (the usual BB/AA ratio is ~2.5–3.0), the reaction to Acetest represents a fair estimate of the total concentration of ketoacids as long as the ratio remains within a usual range. When the BB/AA ratio is greatly increased, Acetest may be negative or only slightly positive despite retention of a large amount of total ketones in the form of BB. Such condition is called β-hydroxybutyric acidosis and is commonly seen in alcoholic ketoacidosis (235, 236).

Serum Anion Gap

Serum AG is estimated as follows:

$$Na^+ - (Cl^- + HCO_3^-) \text{ or } (Na^+ + K^+) - (Cl^- + HCO_3^-)$$

Because normal serum K$^+$ concentration is quantitatively a minor component of serum electrolytes, the fluctuation in

its concentration does not greatly affect the overall result, and hence the first of the two equations is more commonly used to estimate the AG. The normal value is about l2 mEq/L (8–l6 mEq/L). Some authors subtract the normal AG from the observed AG as we have defined it; calculated this way, the normal AG should be zero. The term AG implies a gap between cation and anion concentrations, which obviously is not true; the concentration of total cations in the serum must be exactly equal to the concentration of total anions. Although the total concentration of unmeasured anions (UAs, i.e., all anions other than Cl$^-$ and HCO$_3^-$) is about 23 mEq/L, the AG, Na$^+$ − (Cl$^-$ + HCO$_3^-$), is only l2 mEq/L because there are about 11 mEq/L of unmeasured cations (UCs, i.e., all cations other than Na$^+$). Let us assume that total serum cations = Na$^+$ + UCs and that total serum anions = Cl$^-$ + HCO$_3^-$ + UAs. Because total serum cations = total serum anions, Na$^+$ + UC = (Cl$^-$ + HCO$_3^-$) + UA. Hence, Na$^+$ − (Cl$^-$ + HCO$_3^-$) = UA − UC. Because the AG = Na$^+$ − (Cl$^-$ + HCO$_3^-$), the AG = UA − UC (Fig. 8.22) (237).

The AG is estimated from the concentrations of Na$^+$, Cl$^-$, and HCO$_3^-$, but alterations in the AG can be predicted more readily from changes in UAs or UCs than from changes in Na$^+$, Cl$^-$, or HCO$_3^-$. Figure 8.16 shows this relationship graphically. It is apparent that a change in the AG must involve changes in UAs or UCs, or a laboratory error involving the measurement of Na$^+$, Cl$^-$, or HCO$_3^-$. The AG can be increased by increased UAs or decreased UCs or by a laboratory error resulting in a false increase in serum Na$^+$ or a false decrease in serum Cl$^-$ or HCO$_3^-$. AG can be decreased by decreased UAs or increased UAs or by a laboratory error resulting in a false decrease in serum Na$^+$ or a false increase in serum Cl$^-$ or HCO$_3^-$. The equation also predicts that a change in UA may not change AG if UC is also changed by the same extent in the same direction. For example, hypermagnesemia resulting from Mg sulfate intoxication does not

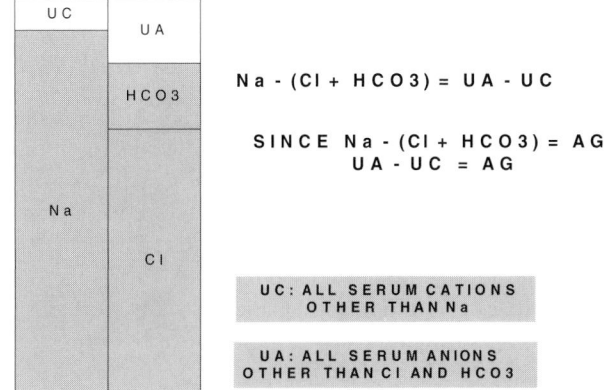

Figure 8.22. The anatomy of anion gap. When unmeasured cation (UC) is defined as all serum cations other than sodium (Na), and unmeasured anion (UA) as all serum anions other than chloride (Cl) or bicarbonate (HCO3), the serum anion gap (AG) can be stated as UA minus UC.

reduce the AG, although high serum Mg^{2+} increases UC. That is because the sulfate accumulation also causes an increase in UA.

Decreased AG is most commonly the result of a reduction in serum albumin concentration, whereas increased AG is most often caused by accumulation of anions of acids, such as sulfate, lactate, ketone anions. Because bromide is a UA, bromide intoxication should lead to increased AG. However, bromide intoxication is accompanied by low serum AG because bromide causes a false increase in serum Cl^-. A change in serum Na^+ usually does not alter AG because serum Cl^- usually changes in the same direction. For the same reason, HCO3⁻ concentrations cannot be used to predict a change in AG. For example, when serum HCO_3^- concentration increases in metabolic alkalosis, Cl^- concentration almost invariably decreases reciprocally to maintain electrical neutrality, so the AG is unchanged. When HCO_3^- concentration decreases, Cl concentration may remain unchanged or be increased. If HCO_3^- is replaced by another anion, Cl^- concentration remains unchanged, hence normochloremic acidosis with increased AG. Examples are organic acidosis and uremic acidosis. When HCO_3^- concentration decreases without another anion replacing it, electrical neutrality is maintained by a higher Cl^- concentration, hence hyperchloremic acidosis with a normal AG. Proper interpretation of a serum AG requires the knowledge of the existence of conditions that influence the AG even though they may have no direct effect on metabolic acidosis. For example, if a person with hypoalbuminemia develops lactic acidosis, the AG could be normal because the low albumin concentration and the lactate accumulation have opposite effects on the AG. Not knowing the effect of serum albumin on AG, one could have overlooked the existence of lactic acidosis on the basis of a normal AG.

Diagnosis

One approach to the differential diagnosis of metabolic acidosis is to calculate the serum AG. If the AG is increased, the likely conditions include organic acidosis, uremic acidosis, and acidosis resulting from certain toxins (Table 8.13). If the AG is normal, the likely conditions include RTA and acidosis resulting from diarrheal loss of HCO_3^-. Contrary to the common misconception, most cases of uremic acidosis are accompanied by a normal AG; only in advanced chronic and acute renal failure is the AG increased. Furthermore, most patients with ketoacidosis pass through a phase of hyperchloremic acidosis (normal AG) during the recovery phase.

Another approach to the differential diagnosis of metabolic acidosis is to classify the acidosis into renal and extrarenal. Two major causes of extrarenal acidosis are organic acidosis and diarrheal loss of HCO_3^-. The presence of organic acidosis is usually obvious from clinical

TABLE 8.13. CLASSIFICATION OF METABOLIC ACIDOSIS BY ANION GAP

Metabolic acidosis with increased anion gap (normochloremic acidosis)
  Ketoacidosis
  L-Lactic acidosis
  D-lactic acidosis
  β-Hydroxybutyric acidosis
  Uremic acidosis
  Ingestion of toxins: salicylate, methanol, ethylene glycol, toluene, acetaminophen
Metabolic acidosis with normal anion gap (hyperchloremic acidosis)
  Renal tubular acidosis
  Uremic acidosis (early)
  Acidosis following respiratory alkalosis
  Intestinal loss of bicarbonate
  Administration of chloride-containing acid: HCl, NH_4Cl
  Ketoacidosis during recovery phase

findings, such as evidence of tissue hypoxia in lactic acidosis, or hyperglycemia and ketonemia in ketoacidosis. Diarrhea as the cause of metabolic acidosis is first suspected from the patient's history, but the history is often misleading because the severity of diarrhea cannot be easily determined. The measurement of the urine AG is useful in determining the severity of diarrhea. The urine AG, which is measured as Urine $(Na^+ + K^+) -$ Urine Cl^-, is reduced or negative when diarrhea is severe. Diarrheal loss of HCO_3^- leads to metabolic acidosis, which, in turn, causes increased urinary excretion of NH_4^+ as a part of renal compensatory mechanisms. Vomiting causes metabolic alkalosis and hence urinary excretion of HCO_3^-, leading to an increased urine AG.

Once extrarenal acidosis is excluded, renal acidosis is the only alternative diagnosis. Of the two types of renal acidosis, uremic acidosis can be readily diagnosed by the measurement of serum creatinine and blood urea nitrogen (BUN). If renal acidosis is confirmed but uremic acidosis is ruled out, the diagnosis must be RTA. Among the three types of RTA, type IV RTA will be suspected by the presence of hyperkalemia. Hypokalemia suggests either type I or type II RTA. If spontaneous urine pH is less than 5.5, type I RTA is ruled out. If urine pH is higher than 5.5, urine pH should be measured after oral administration of 40 mg of furosemide or 10 mg of torsemide. The latter drug has higher sensitivity and specificity. If the urine pH remains at greater than 5.5, the likely diagnosis is type I RTA. The evidence of Fanconi syndrome (the best evidence is renal glycosuria) suggests type II RTA.

Treatment

Restoration of normal blood pH and HCO_3^- concentration is the ultimate aim of therapy for metabolic acidosis (235). Rapid restoration of normal pH is usually unnecessary and may be undesirable for several reasons. When the pH is increased acutely, restoration of a normal concentration of the red blood cell 2,3-diphosphoglycerate lags behind. In addition, a sudden increase in extracellular pH can cause paradoxic acidosis of the cerebrospinal fluid. Rapid restoration of a normal serum HCO_3^- level in metabolic acidosis would also be undesirable because persistent hyperventilation would produce a very high blood pH. The initial aim in the treatment of severe metabolic acidosis should be to increase the blood pH to a level at which adverse cardiovascular effects of severe acidemia can be avoided. Although the risk of acidosis varies with the age and the cardiovascular status of patients, it is considered prudent, at least in older subjects, to keep the blood pH gerater than 7.2. The blood pH may be increased by the administration of alkali (see later) or in the case of organic acidosis by allowing alkali to be generated by metabolism of retained organic anions (OA^-):

$$OA^- + H_2CO_3 \rightarrow OAH + HCO_3^-$$
$$\uparrow$$
$$CO_2 + H_2O$$

Successful treatment of the cause of organic acidosis increases the serum HCO_3^- concentration by the foregoing mechanism. When ketoacidosis is treated with insulin and fluid, the outcome is usually predictable: a substantial increase in the plasma HCO_3^- concentration. Thus, exogenous alkali is seldom necessary in ketoacidosis. In contrast, response to treatment in lactic acidosis is usually poor. In type A lactic acidosis (resulting from hypoxia), the prognosis depends on the cause of hypoxia. In most cases of circulatory shock, the prognosis is extremely poor. The prognosis of lactic acidosis caused by acute alcohol intoxication is fairly good. With seizure-induced lactic acidosis, recovery is usually complete within hours after the control of the seizure. Type B lactic acidosis can be treated with the administration of alkali in the hope of spontaneous recovery, but administration of HCO_3^- tends to be self-defeating because it results in further production of lactic acid. Rising cell pH stimulates glycolysis and therefore increases production of lactic acid. Discouraged by the poor results of HCO_3^- therapy and offering theoretic arguments against alkali therapy, some authors have recommended against the use of HCO_3^- in the treatment of all types of lactic acidosis, but the judicious use of HCO_3^- is beneficial in severe metabolic acidosis.

Three types of alkali can be used for the treatment of metabolic acidosis: HCO_3^-, salts of organic acids, and THAM (tris-hydroxymethylaminomethane; tromethamine) (238–242). Organic salts used as a HCO_3^- substitute include lactate, acetate, gluconate, and citrate. Each milliequivalent of the organic salts produces 1 mEq of HCO_3^-. However, the increase in HCO_3^- concentration is delayed because these salts require metabolism. Furthermore, when metabolism is impaired (e.g., in lactic acidosis) certain organic salts may have no effect. The amount and speed of administration of HCO_3^- and organic salts vary widely

depending on the severity of acidosis. THAM causes increase in pH by production of HCO_3^- by reacting with H_2CO_3 in the following reaction:

$$THAM + H_2CO_3 \rightarrow THAM\text{-}H^+ + HCO_3^-$$
$$\uparrow$$
$$CO_2 + H_2O$$

Because formation of HCO_3^- by THAM occurs at the expense of carbonic acid, rapid infusion of THAM results in a marked reduction in P_{CO_2}; the rate should not exceed 2 mmol/minute. Administration of THAM probably has no advantage in treatment of metabolic acidosis in most situations, but it should be more advantageous than HCO_3^- in treating metabolic acidosis complicated by respiratory acidosis.

For a given quantity of administered HCO_3^-, the rise in serum HCO_3^- is less in severe than in mild metabolic acidosis (i.e., the apparent volume of distribution of HCO_3^- is greater in severe than mild metabolic acidosis). However, the absolute increase in pH for a given dose of HCO_3^- administered is greater in more severe metabolic acidosis than in mild acidosis because the increase in serum HCO_3^- is proportionately greater, although less in absolute magnitude, with severe acidosis than with mild acidosis. In practice, however, no need exists to estimate HCO_3^- requirements accurately to achieve a certain specific level. Because changes in P_{CO_2} following acute increase in serum HCO_3^- cannot be accurately predicted, it is difficult to predict the pH for a given increase in HCO_3^-. The best approach is to administer two to three ampules of $NaHCO_3^-$ (44.5 or 50 mEq/ampule) by intravenous injection, and then to repeat a blood gas measurement 20 or 30 minutes after HCO_3^- injection to determine the need for further therapy. For treatment of chronic acidosis, citrate, available as Shohl solution, is more palatable than HCO_3^-. If the patient also requires K^+ supplementation, as in a patient with distal RTA, K^+ citrate can be used. The amount of alkali needed to correct acidosis must be determined by trial and error. For treatment of uremic acidosis in patients undergoing dialysis, $NaHCO_3^-$ is the most commonly used alkali in hemodialysis fluids and Na lactate in peritoneal dialysis fluids (5).

Metabolic Alkalosis

Causes and Pathogenesis

At normal serum HCO_3^- concentration, HCO_3^- filtered at the glomerulus is virtually completely reabsorbed. As serum HCO_3^- concentration rises to more than the normal level, HCO_3^- reabsorption is incomplete, and bicarbonaturia begins. A slight increase in serum HCO_3^- to more than 24 mEq/L causes marked bicarbonaturia. Hence, when renal tubular HCO_3^- handling and GFR are normal, it is very difficult to maintain a high plasma HCO_3^- concentration unless an enormous amount of HCO_3^- is given. Therefore, maintenance of metabolic

TABLE 8.14. MECHANISMS AND CAUSES TO MAINTAIN HIGH EXTRACELLULAR BICARBONATE CONCENTRATION

Reduced effective vascular volume, e.g., diuretic therapy, vomiting, edema formation
Potassium deficiency
Chloride deficiency (?) when accompanied by volume depletion, e.g., vomiting
High partial pressure of carbon dioxide
Secondary hypoparathyroidism, e.g., milk-alkali syndrome, hypercalcemia of malignancy resulting from an osteolytic mechanism
Advanced renal failure

TABLE 8.15. MECHANISMS AND CAUSES TO INCREASE EXTRACELLULAR BICARBONATE CONCENTRATION

Loss of hydrochloric acid from the stomach, e.g., gastric suction, vomiting
Administration of bicarbonate or bicarbonate precursors, e.g., sodium lactate, sodium acetate, sodium citrate
Shift of hydrogen ion into the cell, e.g., potassium depletion
Rapid contraction of extracellular volume without loss of bicarbonate, e.g., contraction alkalosis by the use of loop diuretics
Increased renal excretion of acid, e.g., diuretic therapy, high aldosterone state, potassium depletion, high partial pressure of carbon dioxide, secondary hypoparathyroidism

alkalosis requires two conditions: a mechanism to increase plasma HCO_3^- and a mechanism to maintain the increased concentration. HCO_3^- concentration may be increased by administration of alkali, gastric loss of HCl through vomiting or nasogastric suction, or renal generation of HCO_3^-. Plasma HCO_3^- concentration can be maintained at a high level, if HCO_3^- is not filtered at the glomerulus because of advanced renal failure or if filtered HCO_3^- is reabsorbed avidly because of increased renal threshold for HCO_3^- (243). The two most common causes of increased renal HCO_3^- threshold are volume depletion and K^+ depletion (Table 8.14).

The renal threshold for HCO_3^- is increased in K^+ depletion because of enhanced tubular reabsorption of HCO_3^- and a decrease in GFR, which could reduce the filtered load of HCO_3^-. When metabolic alkalosis is caused by volume depletion of nonrenal causes, urinary excretion of Cl^- is reduced. Measurement of urinary Na^+ is an unreliable index of volume depletion in metabolic alkalosis because excretion of HCO_3^- causes obligatory loss of Na^+ despite volume depletion. Metabolic alkalosis accompanied by low urinary Cl^- can be corrected by administration of Cl^--containing fluid, such as NaCl or KCl solution, hence the term Cl^--responsive metabolic alkalosis (e.g., vomiting-induced alkalosis). Patients with Cl^--responsive metabolic alkalosis are volume depleted (244). However, when volume depletion is caused by primary renal Na^+ loss, urinary loss of Cl^- is not reduced despite volume depletion. Metabolic alkalosis accompanied by normal excretion of Cl^- in urine is called Cl^--resistant metabolic alkalosis (e.g., hypokalemia-induced alkalosis); administration of Cl^- does not correct alkalosis in such condition. In edema-forming conditions, administration of Cl^- may not improve metabolic alkalosis even though the pattern of urinary excretion of Cl^- would suggest Cl^--responsive metabolic alkalosis because fluid administration usually does not restore the effective vascular volume to normal. Common clinical conditions that increase serum HCO_3^- are shown in Table 8.15.

Treatment

When increased renal HCO_3^- threshold in metabolic alkalosis is caused by reduced effective vascular volume and

hypokalemia, correction of these abnormalities leads to rapid restoration of serum HCO_3^- concentration in most patients. Correction of low effective vascular volume is accomplished by administration of normal saline or half-normal saline. Sometimes, discontinuation of an offending agent (e.g., a diuretic) and restoration of normal salt intake are sufficient. If volume depletion is to be corrected, Cl^- must be given to replace the excreted HCO_3^-, either as NaCl or KCl (237, 245). In certain clinical situations such as edema-forming states, treatment of reduced effective vascular volume with salt solution is not effective. In such situations, acetazolamide (Diamox), a carbonic anhydrase inhibitor, will treat metabolic alkalosis as well as edema. Acetazolamide administration usually reduces the renal HCO_3^- threshold to a subnormal level, but HCO_3^- threshold may remain supernormal despite the drug in severe volume depletion. Correction of metabolic alkalosis by renal excretion of HCO_3^- requires adequate renal function. In renal failure, metabolic alkalosis can be treated by administration of dilute HCl or acidifying salts or by dialysis. Acidifying salts include NH_4^+Cl, arginine Cl, and lysine Cl. Metabolism of these salts results in release of HCl, which then titrates HCO_3^-. Direct administration of HCl into large veins has also been used. If continuous acid loss from the stomach is the cause of metabolic alkalosis, an inhibitor of acid secretion such histamine (H_2)-blockers or proton pump inhibitors may be used.

Respiratory Acidosis

Causes and Pathogenesis

The causes are usually quite apparent. They include diseases of the lung (most common), respiratory muscle, respiratory nerve, thoracic cage, and airways and suppression of the respiratory center by stroke, drugs such as phenobarbital, or severe hypothyroidism (Table 8.16).

Treatment

All cases of respiratory acidosis are caused by alveolar hypoventilation, but in severe respiratory acidosis, efforts should be made to normalize ventilation. When restoration

TABLE 8.16. CAUSES OF RESPIRATORY ACIDOSIS

TABLE 8.16. CAUSES OF RESPIRATORY ACIDOSIS

Lung diseases: chronic obstructive lung disease, advanced interstitial lung disease, acute asthma
Thoracic deformity or airway obstruction
Diseases of respiratory muscle and nerve: myasthenia gravis, hypokalemia paralysis, botulism, amyotrophic lateral sclerosis, Guillain-Barré syndrome
Depression of the respiratory center: barbiturate intoxication, stroke

of effective ventilation is delayed and the patient is comatose or has cardiac arrhythmias, acidosis can be treated temporarily with the administration of alkali. However, administration of HCO_3^- is not very effective in correcting the brain pH because of the slow penetration of HCO_3^- into the central nervous system.

Administration of non-HCO_3^- buffer has a theoretic advantage in superacute respiratory acidosis because it reduces PCO_2 as it increases the HCO_3^- concentration by the following reaction (238–242):

$$Buff^- + H_2CO_3 \rightarrow HBuff + HCO_3^-$$
$$\uparrow$$
$$CO_2 + H_2O$$

Non-HCO_3^- buffers ($Buff^-$) used in these settings are as follows: THAM (tris buffer, tromethamine), which is an amine buffer; Carbicarb, which is an equal combination of HCO_3^- and CO_3^-; and Tribonat, which is a mixture of THAM, Na acetate, HCO_3^-, and P.

In experimental animal studies, administration of a sufficient amount of these agents can keep PCO_2 at a lower level and can maintain a higher intracellular pH than a comparable amount of HCO_3^-. However, evidence is lacking that these agents actually improve survival during cardiopulmonary resuscitation. When used in pigs during resuscitation of electrically induced cardiac arrest, THAM showed an unexpected vasodilatory effect causing reduction in perfusion pressure. This effect has not been reported in human studies. In chronic respiratory acidosis, hypoxia poses a greater problem than acidosis. Acidosis is reasonably well controlled with renal compensation. When ventilation cannot be improved, hypoxemia can be treated with nasal oxygen supplement, but removal of the hypoxic drive with oxygen supplementation in patients with chronic hypercapnia may result in severe respiratory depression (CO_2 narcosis).

Various drugs have been tried in an attempt to stimulate respiration in acute and chronic respiratory acidosis. Apnea of prematurity has been treated with respiratory stimulants such as doxapram and the methylxanthines caffeine citrate and theophylline. Caffeine citrate is the consensus drug of choice for premature babies with respiratory depression. In chronic obstructive pulmonary disease, theophylline, doxapram, and progesterone derivatives including progesterone, medroxyprogesterone, and chlormadinone have been tried (246, 247).

Respiratory Alkalosis

Causes and Pathogenesis

With the exception of respirator-induced alkalosis and voluntary hyperventilation, respiratory alkalosis is always the result of stimulation of the respiratory center. The two most common causes of respiratory alkalosis are hypoxic stimulation of the respiratory center and stimulation through the pulmonary receptors caused by various lung lesions, such as pneumonia, pulmonary congestion, and pulmonary embolism. Certain drugs, such as salicylate and progesterone, stimulate the respiratory center directly (248–250). Respiratory alkalosis is common in gram-negative sepsis through an unknown mechanism. Blood pH tends to be extremely high when respiratory alkalosis is caused by psychogenic stimulation of the respiratory center because the condition is usually superacute, and therefore no time exists for compensation (Table 8.17).

Treatment

In chronic respiratory alkalosis, treatment is usually not needed because of the excellent compensation restores the blood pH to either normal or nearly normal values. In acute respiratory alkalosis resulting from psychogenic hyperventilation, the patient should be sedated to depress the respiratory center. PCO_2 can also be increased by the use of a rebreathing bag.

Mixed Acid-Base Disorders

The term mixed acid-base disorder refers to a clinical condition in which two or more primary acid-base disorders coexist. They generally present with one obvious disturbance with what appears to be an inappropriate (excessive or inadequate) compensation. The "inappropriateness" of the compensatory process is the result of a separate primary disorder. The appropriate degrees of compensation for primary acid-base disorders have been determined by analysis of data from a large number of patients and are expressed in the form of equations in Table 8.18. When the two disorders influence the blood pH in opposite directions, the blood pH will be determined by the dominant disorder. If the disorders cancel out each other's effects, blood pH can be normal. When any degree of compensation for acid-base disorders exists, both PCO_2 and HCO_3^- change in the same direction (i.e., both are

TABLE 8.17. CAUSES OF RESPIRATORY ALKALOSIS

Diseases of the lung: any intrapulmonary disorder such as pneumonia, pulmonary fibrosis, pulmonary congestion, pulmonary embolism
Hypoxemia
Central nervous system lesions
Gram-negative sepsis
Drugs: salicylate, progesterone

TABLE 8.18. FORMULAS FOR PREDICTING NORMAL ACID-BASE COMPENSATION

Metabolic acidosis: $\Delta Pco_2 = \Delta HCO_3^- \times 1.2 \pm 2$
Metabolic alkalosis[a]: $\Delta Pco_2 = \Delta HCO_3^- \times 0.7 \pm 5$
Acute respiratory acidosis: $\Delta HCO_3^- = \Delta Pco_2 \times 0.07 \pm 1.5$
Chronic respiratory acidosis: $\Delta HCO_3^- = \Delta Pco_2 \times 0.4 \pm 3$
Acute respiratory alkalosis: $\Delta HCO_3^- = \Delta Pco_2 \times 0.2 \pm 2.5$
Chronic respiratory alkalosis: $\Delta HCO_3^- = \Delta Pco_2 \times 0.5 \pm 2.5$
ΔHCO_3^- and ΔPco_2 represent the difference between normal and actual values.

HCO_3^-, bicarbonate; Pco_2, partial pressure of carbon dioxide.
[a] No matter how high the serum HCO_3^- rises, Pco_2 rarely rises above 60 mm Hg in metabolic alkalosis.

high or both are low). If Pco_2 and HCO_3^- have changed in opposite directions (e.g., Pco_2 is high and HCO_3^- is low, or Pco_2 is low and HCO_3^- is high), the presence of a mixed acid-base disorder is certain. Appropriateness of compensation can be determined by consulting Table 8.18. Compensation could be excessive, insufficient, or appropriate. One can also have an approximate idea about the appropriateness of compensation from the degree of pH deviation without consulting the formula for normal compensation.

In general, compensation is most effective in respiratory alkalosis (pH is often normalized); the next best is respiratory acidosis (pH may become normal), and the third best is metabolic acidosis. Compensation is least effective in metabolic alkalosis, probably because hypoxemia, an inevitable consequence of hypoventilation, stimulates ventilation. If a patient has low Pco_2 and low HCO_3^- with normal pH, the likely diagnosis is compensated respiratory alkalosis rather than compensated metabolic acidosis (5).

CLINICAL PROBLEMS AND ANSWERS

Regulation of Intracellular and Extracellular Volume and Osmolality

Problems

1. A 45-year-old patient with chronic alcoholism was brought in a coma to the emergency room. The patient had the following laboratory values: serum Na^+, 115 mEq/L; serum osmolality, 400 mOsm/L; serum glucose, 1000 mg/dL; BUN, 42 mg/dL; and total serum osmolality, 400 mOsm/L.
   a. Is the patient's intracellular volume increased, decreased, or normal?
   b. When serum glucose is normalized by metabolism, will serum Na^+ increase, decrease, or remain the same?
   c. When glucose is normalized by metabolism, will extracellular osmolality increase, decrease, or remain the same?
2. Which of the following patients has an increased intracellular volume?
   a. A diabetic patient with serum Na^+ of 110 mEq/L and serum glucose of 2000 mg/dL?

   b. An alcoholic patient with serum Na^+ of 125 mEq/L and serum alcohol of 500 mg/dL?
   c. A uremic patient with serum Na^+ of 150 mEq/L and serum urea nitrogen of 140 mg/dL?
   d. A patient with serum Na^+ of 150 mEq/L with anasarca?
   e. A patient who developed hyponatremia after receiving 200 g of mannitol?
3. A patient, weighing 120 lb has serum Na^+ of 110 mEq/L. How much Na^+ is needed to increase serum Na^+ to 120 mEq/L? Assume that TBW volume is kept constant.
4. A patient has TBW of 40 L and serum Na^+ concentration of 180 mEq/L. What is the amount of water required to reduce serum Na^+ to 163 mEq/L?
5. Match lettered conditions with numbered laboratory data:
   a. Vomiting
   b. Diarrhea
   c. Ciuretic therapy
      i. Low serum K^+, low serum HCO_3^-, urine Cl^- more than the sum of urine Na^+ and K^+
      ii. Low serum K^+, high serum HCO_3^- normal urine Cl^-
      iii. Low serum K^+, high serum HCO_3^-, low urine Cl^-
6. Three patients with identical size, weight, and body composition are admitted to the hospital after acute weight loss of 2.2 lb overnight, but with different serum Na^+ concentrations. Patient A has serum Na^+ of 120 mEq/L, patient B serum Na^+ 140 mEq/L, and patient C serum Na^+ 160 mEq/L. Which patient has the smallest extracellular volume?

Answers

1. a. The intracellular volume is normal because effective serum osmolality is normal, even though total serum osmolality is increased. Alcohol is not an effective osmol. The effective osmolality in this patient is: $(115 \times 2) + (1000/18) = 285$ mOsm/L
   b. Metabolism of glucose will cause loss of osmols from the extracellular fluid and hence a shift of water into cells. Serum Na^+ therefore will increase.
   c. The extracellular osmolality decreases as glucose enters the cell and is metabolized.
2. Answer is b. Only this patient has reduced effective osmolality. The laboratory data do not show an actual value of osmolality, but effective osmolality is expected to be low with low serum Na^+ because ethanol is an ineffective osmol. In choice e, serum osmolality is also not given, but mannitol accumulation in the extracellular fluid is expected to increase the effective osmolality causing shift of water from the cell.
3. Na^+ requirement = Δserum $Na^+ \times$ TBW = $10 \times 30 = 300$ mEq, where Δserum Na^+ is actual serum Na^+ minus the goal serum Na, and TBW is calculated as body weight (lb)/4. Although the administered Na^+

would remain mostly in the extracellular fluid, TBW is used to calculate the Na^+ requirement because an increase in serum Na^+ causes an increase in serum osmolality that is exactly twice the value of the increase in serum Na^+. One important principle to understand is that one must use TBW rather than extracellular volume to calculate the required amount of solute to increase the serum osmolality. An increase in extracellular osmolality is impossible without the increase in intracellular osmolality by the same extent; otherwise, water will continue to come out of the cell. The use of TBW to calculate the amount required to correct a deficit of an extracellular solute applies only to Na^+ and not to other solutes. Even for Na^+, the formula is applicable only when serum Na^+ is half of serum osmolality. For example, in severe hyperglycemia, serum Na^+ in mEq/L is not half of serum osmolality in mOsm/L, and the formula cannot be used.

4. The formula to calculate the amount of water removal to reduce serum Na^+ is: (Δserum Na^+/ goal serum Na^+) $\times$ TBW. Hence, the answer is: $(17/163) \times 40 = 4.17$ L.

5. a-iii, b-i, c-ii. Diarrhea causes loss of HCO_3^- and K^+ in the stool and thus hypokalemia and metabolic acidosis. Because the loss of HCO_3^- in diarrhea is accompanied by the loss of K^+ and Na^+, urinary excretion of Na^+ and K^+ tends to be less than that of Cl^-. The higher concentration of Cl^- in urine is accompanied by increased excretion of NH_4^+, which occurs in response to metabolic acidosis. Both vomiting and diuretic therapy cause hypokalemia and metabolic alkalosis, but the former is accompanied by low urine Cl^- because Cl^- is lost in the vomitus.

6. Patient A has the smallest extracellular volume because A has the largest intracellular volume. Because they all started with the same total body weight and lost the same amount of water (2.2 lb = 1 L), the current TBW must be the same for all three patients. Remember that acute weight loss is considered to be entirely water loss. For the same TBW, the one with the largest intracellular volume must have the smallest extracellular volume.

Disorders of Potassium Metabolism

Problems

1. A 64-year-old man is admitted to the hospital with severe pneumonia, fever, and bacteremia. White blood cell count is 28,500, and platelet count is 700,000. As part of his general evaluation, a blood sample is sent for serum electrolyte concentrations. Serum K^+ is reported at 5.7 mEq/L. A rapid evaluation of the ECG shows no abnormalities. The patient is not acidotic, and renal function is nearly normal. What is the likely cause of this patient's hyperkalemia?

2. A 60-year-old woman with diabetes mellitus since age 48 is admitted to the hospital because of shortness of breath. Blood pressure is 160/107 mm Hg. She has slight edema. Serum Na^+ is 140 mEq/L, Cl^- is 114,

HCO_3^- is 15, and K^+ is 6.5 mEq/L. Blood glucose concentration is 170 mg/dL. She is treated with diuretics and with Kayexalate and sorbitol. Serum K^+ the next day is 4.0 mEq/L. What is the likely cause of this patient's hyperkalemia?

3. A 45-year-old woman complains of severe weakness and is afraid of falling when she does her regular aerobic exercise. The only remarkable physical findings: a transient drop in blood pressure on standing up, sluggish tendon reflexes, and muscle weakness. Blood test shows serum K^+ of 2.6 mEq/L. ECG shows ST depression and sagging T waves. An additional complaint is moderate polyuria. Urinary K^+ excretion is 9 mEq in 24 hours. Blood pH is normal. What is the likely cause of this patient's hypokalemia?

4. A patient with chronic hypokalemia (serum K^+ of 2.8 mEq/L) and recently diagnosed hypertension has presented to you. You are suspecting primary hyperaldosteronism as the likely diagnosis and have ordered a 24-hour urinary K^+ measurement. Which of the following is most likely to be found if your suspicion was correct?

   a. Higher than usual average amount
   b. Usual average amount
   c. Lower than usual average amount

Answers

1. The likely cause is pseudohyperkalemia resulting from thrombocytosis. Leukocytosis can also cause pseudohyperkalemia, but only when white cell counts are extremely high. However, the absence of ECG abnormality should not be taken as evidence for pseudohyperkalemia because chronic hypokalemia, even when it is quite severe, is often accompanied by normal ECG.

2. The most likely cause is hyporeninemic hypoaldosteronism, mainly because it is the most common cause of chronic hyperkalemia. Furthermore, diabetic nephropathy is the most common disorder associated with hyporeninemic hypoaldosteronism. The presence of hypertension further suggests hyporeninemic hypoaldosteronism rather than Addison disease. Lacking both glucocorticoids and mineralocorticoids, Addison disease is expected to cause hypotension. One could predict hypotension in patients with hyporeninemic hypoaldosteronism because they are lacking in both renin and aldosterone. However, they are usually hypertensive, a finding suggesting that the effective vascular volume is increased in these patients. In fact, the most widely accepted pathogenetic mechanism of the hyporeninemia is the primary volume expansion resulting from renal salt retention. Low serum HCO_3^- is probably the result of type IV RTA, a common complication of hyporeninemic hypoaldosteronism.

3. Nonrenal loss of K^+, such as laxative abuse or diarrhea, is the likely cause of her hypokalemia. The clue is the

low excretion of urine K^+. A diuretic therapy or primary hyperaldosteronism would be accompanied by normal rate of K^+ excretion. Vomiting is also a common cause of hypokalemia, but the main route of K^+ loss in vomiting is the kidney rather than the stomach, because the increased urine HCO_3^- causes renal K^+ wasting.

4. b is correct. Although renal K^+ loss is the cause of hypokalemia in primary hyperaldosteronism, a prolonged imbalance between K^+ intake and output in chronic K^+ wasting states is impossible. Because hypokalemia is antikaliuretic, renal K^+ excretion ultimately returns to normal.

Water and Antidiuretic Hormone Metabolism

Problems

1. A 63-year-old man, weighing 120 lb, with alcoholic cirrhosis of the liver was admitted to the hospital for complaints of progressive weakness and vomiting for several days, but without neurologic abnormality. On examination, he had poor skin turgor and no subcutaneous fat. Serum Na^+ was 108 mEq/L, Cl^- 78 was mEq/L, K^+ 2.3 was mEq/L, and HCO_3^- was 29 mEq/L. Urine osmolality was 650 mOsm/L, BUN was 15 mg/dL, serum creatinine was 1.1 mg/dL, uric acid was 5.5 mg/dL, urine Na^+ was 45 mEq/L, and urine pH was 7.5. The patient was treated with 1 L of normal saline (154 mEq/L of Na^+), with addition of 40 mEq/L of K^+ every 6 hours for the first 24 hours. In 16 hours, the serum Na^+ had risen to 121 mEq/L, and in 24 hours it was 128 mEq/L. Three days later, the patient was unable to speak or swallow. Computed tomography scan and magnetic resonance imaging of the brain showed a hypodense area in the central pons.
   a. Why was hyponatremia corrected so fast with normal saline? Did K^+ administration play a role?
   b. How do you explain the neurologic abnormality?
   c. Does urine osmolality on admission suggest SIADH? If the value were 200 mOsm/L, would you have ruled out SIADH?
   d. Does urine Na^+ on admission suggest SIADH or a volume depletion state?

2. A 65-year-old woman, weighing 150 lb, was admitted to the hospital because her family believed that she was weak and "not quite herself." She had no specific complaints and was able to answer questions. Physical examination suggested moderate dehydration, and the resident estimated her fluid loss at about 4 L. She had a 10-cm curved scar over the area of the frontal lobe of the brain. BUN was 45 mg/dL, creatinine was 1.3, serum Na^+ was 182 mEq/L, urine osmolality was 550 mOsm/L, and urinary Na^+ was 75 mEq/L. After 2 μg of DDAVP was administered, the urine osmolality rose to 750 mOsm/L.

True or False:

   a. The patient's hypernatremia is entirely the result of water loss.
   b. Computed tomography scan of the head would show marked brain shrinkage consistent with severe hyperosmolality.
   c. The patient has central DI.
   d. The patient has a thirst defect as well as a defect in water conservation.
   e. The patient should immediately receive an infusion of DDAVP and water sufficient to lower her serum Na^+ to 140 mEq/L within the next 12 to 16 hours.
   f. From the information given, can you prove that the patient does not have osmotic diuresis?

3. A 72-year-old healthy man ingests a diet that allows him to excrete a total of 800 mOsm/day of solute and 2 L of water.
   a. What will be his average urine osmolality on the diet indicated?
   b. What will be his average urine osmolality if he increases salt intake and excretes 1000 mOsm of solute and drinks less water to decrease urine output to 1 L/day?
   c. What will be his average urine osmolality if he reduces his food intake and excretes only 320 mOsm of solute and drinks enough water to increase urine output to 4 L/day?
   d. What would his fluid balance be if the patient developed lung cancer and had a high blood level of ADH that prevented urine osmolality from falling to less than 400 mOsm/L while ingesting the original diet and drinking the original volume of water?

Answers

1. a. As volume depletion was corrected, water diuresis occurred. Administration of K^+ has almost the same effect as that of Na^+ for the following reasons. K^+ is retained mostly in the cell, and therefore its replacement requires a shift of K^+ into the cells in exchange for extracellular shift of Na^+. Thus, K^+ replacement has the same effect on extracellular Na^+ concentration as Na^+ replacement. Alternatively, if the administered K^+ is excreted in the urine, it will be accompanied by water. The loss of water causes a rise in serum Na^+.
   b. A rapid increase in serum Na^+ in a patient with chronic hyponatremia can cause central pontine myelinolysis, and the patient has characteristic clinical findings of this disorder.
   c. Urine osmolality is rarely useful in differential diagnosis of hyponatremia because virtually every patient with hyponatremia has inappropriately concentrated urine (i.e., urine osmolality in excess of 100 mOsm/L in the presence of hyponatremia). The only exception is hyponatremia caused by primary polydipsia, in which urine osmolality is expected to

be less than 100 mOsm/L. However, the polyuria and polydipsia of primary polydipsia make the diagnosis obvious. Urine osmolality values of 650 and 200 mOsm/L are both consistent with SIADH, but they are also consistent with most other causes of hyponatremia.

d. Urine Na^+ concentration on admission argues against dehydration. Conversely, a high urine pH (7.5) indicates an increased excretion of HCO_3^-, which can cause Na^+ diuresis despite dehydration. When urine pH is high, urine Cl^- concentration is a more reliable indicator of the volume status.

2. a. False. If water deficit were the sole cause of hypernatremia, serum Na^+ concentration of 182 mEq/L would require a loss of 9.2 L of water for a person with TBW of 40 L. The amount of water deficit needed to raise serum Na^+ to 182 mEq/L is calculated as follows: $(\Delta Na^+ \times TBW)/goal\ Na^+ = (42 \times 40)182 = 9.2$ L. The patient was judged to be only moderately dehydrated by the resident, who estimated the loss of water at 4 L. Obviously, a big part of hypernatremia was caused by the retention of Na^+.

b. False. Because the hypernatremia was chronic as shown by the lack of severe neurologic abnormalities, the brain volume would be nearly normal.

c. True. Urine osmolality of 550 mOsm/L is inappropriately low for the patient's severe hypernatremia, and therefore the patient has DI. The subsequent response to exogenous ADH indicates that it was central DI.

d. True, the patient has deficiency of ADH and a thirst defect. In fact, if ADH deficiency were the only defect the patient had, the patient would have been polydipsic and polyuric but not hypernatremic.

e. False. Because the patient has chronic hypernatremia with a near-normal brain volume, rapid correction of hyponatremia can cause brain edema and therefore should be avoided.

f. To rule out osmotic diuresis, one must know the rate of solute excretion, which requires urine osmolality and urine volume. Because only urine osmolality is known, osmotic diuresis cannot be ruled out in this case.

3. a. 800 mosm/2 L = 400 mOsm/L

b. (1000 mOsm/L)/1 = 1,000 mOsm/L

c. (320 mOsm/L)/4 = 80 mOsm/L

d. The patient will retain water and develop hyponatremia.

Acid-Base Disorders

Problems

1. A 46-year-old alcoholic man with type 1 diabetes mellitus is brought to the hospital after he was discovered unconscious. In the ambulance, his vital signs were as follows: blood pressure, 80/40 mm Hg; pulse, 120/minute; and respiration rate, 40/minute. The examinations of the chest and abdomen were normal, except for a surgical scar in the middle line of the upper abdomen. The emergency room physician subsequently learned that a day before the patient became ill, he drank whiskey and skipped his usual insulin dose. He gave no history of malabsorption syndrome. The inital laboratory tests: urinalysis: 4+ glucose, 4+ ketones, 1+ protein, no red blood cells; serum Na^+, 144 mEq/L; Cl^-, 109 mEq/L; K^+, 5.5 mEq/L; CO_2, 14 mmol/L; glucose, 920 mg/dL; creatinine, 2.1 mg/dL; BUN, 90 mg/dL; serum ketone, 2+; serum lactate, 2.5 mEq/L; and measured serum osmolality, 360 mOsm/L. Arterial blood gases: pH, 7.32; Pco_2, 28 mm Hg; and Po_2, 105 mm Hg on room air.

a. Does the patient have ketoacidosis?

b. Is the respiratory compensation appropriate?

c. If net acid excretion were 70 mEq/day (usual normal value, 40–100 mEq/day) in this patient at the time of admission, would this have ruled out renal acidosis?

2. The serum AG can be best predicted from this formula: $AG = UA - UC$, where UAs are defined as any anions other than Cl^- and HCO_3^-, and UCs are any cations other than Na^+.

a. Bromide is a UA according to the foregoing definition. However, bromide intoxication lowers the AG. Why?

b. Why is serum the AG usually normal in hypermagnesemia as a result of Mg sulfate?

c. What is the effect of high serum Na^+ or Cl^- on the serum AG?

3. The HCO_3^-/Pco_2 ratio determines pH. Normal blood pH is 7.4 with normal HCO_3^- of 24 mm Hg and normal Pco_2 of 40 mm Hg; the normal ratio is 24/40. If Pco_2 is 20 mm Hg and HCO_3^- 14 mM, will pH be higher or lower than 7.4?

4. A patient has the following data: serum Na^+, 138; K^+, 4.2 mEq/L; Cl^-, 114; and HCO_3^-, 12 mEq/L. Within seconds, you know the diagnosis: hyperchloremic metabolic acidosis and suspect two conditions, diarrhea and RTA, as the likely cause.

a. What serum electrolyte value argues against RTA in this patient?

b. What is the most common cause of type IV RTA?

c. What test would you need to diagnose diarrhea as the cause?

d. Do you think your diagnosis, hyperchloremic acidosis, is premature? What test is essential before such a conclusion ?

e. If blood pH were 7.4, what would be Pco_2? What would be your diagnosis?

f. If a drug were responsible for this type of acid-base disorder, what would it be?

5. Why are there two phases of compensation (acute and chronic) for respiratory acidosis and respiratory alkalosis, but only one phase of compensation for metabolic acidosis and metabolic alkalosis?

6. Predict changes in serum AG in the following conditions as increased (I), decreased (D), or unchanged (U).
   a. Low serum Na^+
   b. Low serum Cl^-
   c. Lithium intoxication
   d. Hypoalbuminemia
   e. Lactic acidosis
   f. Bromide intoxication
   g. Diarrhea-induced metabolic acidosis
   h. Hypermagnesemia resulting from Mg sulfate overdose

Answers

1. a. The increased serum AG suggests organic acidosis or advanced uremic acidosis. The serum creatinine of 2.1 mg/dL rules out advanced uremic acidosis. Among the organic acidoses, lactic acidosis is ruled out by serum lactate level of only 2.5 mEq/L (the value must be at least 6 mEq/L). Usual ketoacidosis requires a stronger Acetest reaction. However, β-hydroxybutyric acidosis, a subtype of ketoacidosis, can occur with a modest elevation in AA, with which Acetest primarily reacts.
   b. Yes. Using the formula for normal compensation in Table 8.18, you will realize that Pco_2 of 28 mm Hg is an appropriate compensation for HCO_3^- of 14 mEq/L.
   c. If net acid excretion were only 70 mEq/day, you would have to suspect renal acidosis. In extrarenal acidosis, net acid excretion is markedly increased.

2. a. Bromide is measured as Cl^- in most hospital laboratories. This results in pseudohyperchloremia and hence a low serum AG.
   b. Because both UA (sulfate) and UC (Mg^{2+}) are increased.
   c. The effects of high serum Na^+ or Cl^- on the serum AG cannot be predicted without knowing how other ions are altered.

3. The pH would be higher than 7.4, because Pco_2 is exactly a half of the normal value, but HCO_3^- is slightly higher than the normal value. Thus, the ratio of HCO_3^-/Pco_2 is slightly increased.

4. a. In type I and II RTA, serum K^+ is low, and in type IV RTA serum K^+ is high. Therefore, a normal serum K^+ concentration in this patient argues against RTA.
   b. Hyporeninemic hypoaldosteronism.
   c. The urine AG should be measured, and it is expected to be reduced or negative. The low urine AG in diarrhea results from increased renal excretion of NH_4^+.
   d. Chronic respiratory alkalosis can also be accompanied by low serum HCO_3^- and high serum Cl^-. The blood pH will decide between chronic respiratory alkalosis and hyperchloremic metabolic acidosis. In the former, the blood pH would be slightly high or high normal, and in the latter, the blood pH would be low.
   e. The normal blood pH suggests chronic respiratory alkalosis more than chronic metabolic acidosis. In chronic respiratory alkalosis, compensation often results in normal pH. Salicylate and progesterone are two drugs that can produce chronic respiratory alkalosis.

5. Compensation in respiratory acid-base disorders has two distinct stages. The first stage, which is completed within a second, is the result of tissue buffering. The second stage is the result of renal compensation, which requires several days to complete. Thus, no matter how acute respiratory acid-base disorder may be, the acute phase of compensation is always completed. In contrast, metabolic acid-base disorders have only one stage of compensation, the ventilatory adjustment, which requires 12 to 24 hours to complete.

6. a: U; b: U; c: D; d: D; e: I; f: D; g: U; h: U

REFERENCES

1. Agre P, King LS, Yasui M et al. J Physiol 2002;542:3–16.
2. Nielsen S, Frokiaer J, Marples D et al. Physiol Rev 2002;82:205–44.
3. Goodman BE. Adv Physiol Educ 2002;26:146–57.
4. Hill LL. Pediatr Clin North Am 1990;37:241–56.
5. Carroll HJ, Oh MS. Water, Electrolyte, and Acid-Base Metabolism. Philadelphia: JB Lippincott, 1989.
6. Oh MS, Carroll HJ. In: Arieff AI, DePronzo RA, eds. Fluid, Electrolyte, and Acid-Base Disorders. 2nd ed. New York: Churchill Livingstone, 1995.
7. Reed RK, Laurent UB. Am Rev Respir Dis 1992;146:37S–9S.
8. Aukland K, Reed RK. Physiol Rev 1993;73:1–78.
9. Burton RF. Comp Biochem Physiol A 1988;90:11–6.
10. Weisberg HF. Ann Clin Lab Sci 1978;8:155–64.
11. Gennari FJ. N Engl J Med 1984;310:102–5.
12. Kruse JA, Cadnapaphornchai P. Crit Care 1994;9:185–97.
13. Pradella M, Dorizzi RM, Rigolin F. Crit Rev Clin Lab Sci 1988;26:195–242.
14. Arieff AI, Llack F, Massry SG. Medicine (Baltimore) 1976;55:121–9.
15. Fishman RA, Brain EDE. N Engl J Med 1975;293:706–11.
16. Gullans SR, Verbalis JG. Annu Rev Med 1993;44:289–301.
17. Hill LL. Pediatr Clin North Am 1990;37:241–56.
18. Videen JS, Micaelis T, Pinto P et al. J Clin Invest 1995;95:788–793.
19. Potts PD, Ludbrook J, Gillman-Gaspari TA et al. Neuroscience 2000;95:499–511.
20. Schreihofer AM, Anderson BK, Schiltz JC et al. Am J Physiol 1999;276:R251–8.
21. Kuramochi G, Kobayashi I. Am J Nephrol 2000;20:42–7.
22. Osborn JL. Hypertension 1991;17[Suppl]:I91–6.
23. Oh MS, Carroll HJ. In: Seldin DW, GiebischG, eds. The Kidney. 3rd ed. Philadelphia: Lippincott Williams & Wilkins, 2000:33–59.
24. Guyton AC, Coleman TG, Cowley AV Jr et al. Am J Med 1972;52:584–94.
25. Walser M. Kidney Int 1985;217:837–41.
26. Hollenberg NK. Kidney Int 1980;17:423–429.
27. Dahl LK, Leitl G, Heine M. Exp Med 1972;136:318–30.
28. Oliver WJ, Cohen EL, Neel JV. Circulation 1975;52:146–51.
29. Cutler JA, Follmann D, Allender PS. Am J Clin Nutr 1997;65[Suppl]:643S–51S.
30. He FJ, MacGregor GA. J Hum Hypertens 2002;16:761–70.
31. Alam S, Johnson AG. J Hum Hypertens 1999;13:367–74.

32. Stamler J, Rose G, Elliott P et al. Hypertension 1991;17 [Suppl]:I9–15.
33. Elliott P, Stamler J, Nichols R et al. BMJ 1996;312:1249–53.
34. Trials of Hypertension Prevention, Phase II. Arch Intern Med 1997;157:657–67.
35. Whelton PK, Appel LJ, Espeland MA et al. JAMA 1998;279:839–46.
36. Midgley JP, Matthew AG, Greenwood CM et al. JAMA 1996;275:1590–7.
37. Bolton-Smith C, Woodward M, Tunstall-Pedoe H. Eur J Clin Nutr 1992;46:75–84.
38. Tunstall-Pedoe H, Woodward M, Tavendale R et al. BMJ 1997;315:722–9.
39. Whelton PK, He J, Appel LJ et al. JAMA 2002;288:1882–8.
40. Watson B Jr. Curr Hypertens Rep 2003;5:273–6.
41. Lentner C. Geigy Scientific Tables, vol 1: Units of Measurement, Body Fluids, Composition of the Body, Nutrition. Basel: Ciba-Geigy, 1986:243–60.
42. Walker JEC, Wells RE Jr, Merrill EW. Am J Med 1961;30:259.
43. Kinney JM Moore FD. In: Bland JH, ed. Clinical Metabolism of Body Water and Electrolytes. Philadelphia: WB Saunders, 1963:337.
44. Arieff AI. In: Maxwell MH, Kleeman CR, eds. Clinical Disorders of Fluid and Electrolyte Metabolism. 2nd ed. New York: McGraw-Hill, 1972:567.
45. Winkler AW, Danowski TS. J Clin Invest 1947;26:1002.
46. Tomlinson BE, Pierides AM, Bradley WG. Q J Med 1976;45:373–86.
47. Laureno R. Ann Neurol 1983;13:232–42.
48. Sterns RH, Thomas DJ, Herndon RM. Kidney Int 1989;35:69–75.
49. Verbalis JG, Martinez AJ. Kidney Int 1991;39:1274–82.
50. Sterns RH. Semin Nephrol 1990;10:503–14.
51. Sterns RH. Crit Care Med 1992;20:534–9.
52. Oh MS, Kim HJ, Carroll HJ. Nephron 1995;70:143–50.
53. Oh MS, Carroll HJ. Crit Care Med 1992;20:94–103.
54. Shoemaker WC, Walker WF. Year Book of Surgery. Chicago: Year Book Medical Publishers, 1970.
55. Veech RL, Kashiwaya Y, King MT. Integr Physiol Behav Sci 1995;30:283–307.
56. Goldman DE. J Gen Phyiol 1943;27:37–60.
57. Meister B, Aperia A. Semin Nephrol 1993;13:41–9.
58. Feraille E, Carranza ML, Gonin S et al. Mol Biol Cell 1999;10:2847–59.
59. Sweeney G, Klip A. Mol Cell Biochem 1998;182:121–33.
60. Goguen JM, Halperin ML. Diabetologia 1993;36:813–6.
61. Perez GO, Oster JR, Vaamonde CA. Nephron 1981;27:233–43.
62. Frassetto L, Morris RC Jr, Sellmeyer DE et al. Eur J Nutr 2001;40:200–13.
63. Giebisch GH. Kidney Int 2002;62:1498–512.
64. Halperin ML, Kamel KS. Lancet 1998;352:135–40.
65. Giebisch G. Am J Physiol 1998;274:F817–33.
66. Stokes JB. J Clin Invest 1982;70:219–29.
67. Jamison RL. Kidney Int 1987;31:695–703.
68. Sacks FM, Willett WC, Smith A et al. Hypertension 1998;31:131.
69. Moore TJ, Vollmer WM, Appel LJ et al. Hypertension 1999;34:472–7.
70. Geleijnse JM, Kok FJ, Grobbee DE. J Hum Hypertens 2003;17:471–80.
71. Espeland MA, Kumanyika S, Yunis C et al. J Ann Epidemiol 2002;12:587–95.
72. Bock HA, Hermle M, Brunner FP et al. Kidney Int 1992;41:275–80.
73. Hollenberg NK. Hypertension 2000;35:150–4.
74. Laragh JH. J Hum Hypertens 1995;9:385–90.
75. Hall JE. Compr Ther 1991;17:8–17.
76. Clemessy JL, Favier C, Borron SW et al. Lancet 1995;346:877–80.
77. Matsumura M, Nakashima A, Tofuku Y. Intern Med 2000;39:55–7.
78. Rakhmanina NY, Kearns GL, Farrar HC 3rd. Pediatr Emerg Care 1998;14:145–7.
79. Jordan P, Brookes JG, Nikolic G et al. J Toxicol Clin Toxicol 1999;37:861–4.
80. Ogawa T, Kamikubo K. Am J Med Sci 1999;318:69–75.
81. Cannon SC. Neuromuscul Disord 2002;12:533–43.
82. Jurkat-Rott K, Mitrovic N, Hang C et al. Proc Natl Acad Sci USA 2000;97:9549–54.
83. Bradberry SM, Vale JA. J Toxicol Clin Toxicol 1995;33:295–310.
84. Steen B. Acta Med Scand Suppl 1981;647:61–6.
85. Torpy DJ, Gordon RD, Lin JP et al. J Clin Endocrinol Metab 1998;83:3214–8.
86. Stowasser M, Bachmann AW, Jonsson JR et al. Clin Exp Pharmacol Physiol 1995;22:444–6.
87. Stowasser M, Bachmann AW, Jonsson JR et al. J Hypertens 1995;13:1610–3 .
88. Abdelhamid S, Lewicka S, Vecsei P et al. J Clin Endocrinol Metab 1995;80:737–44.
89. Litchfield WR, New MI, Coolidge C et al. J Clin Endocrinol Metab 1997;82:3570–3.
90. Litchfield WR, Coolidge C, Silva P et al. J Clin Endocrinol Metab 1997;82:1507–10.
91. Vargas-Poussou R, Huang C, Hulin P et al. J Am Soc Nephrol 2002;13:2259–66.
92. Sakakida M, Araki E. J Clin Endocrinol Metab 2003;88:781–6.
93. Finer G, Shalev H, Birk OS et al. J Pediatr 2003;142:318–23.
94. Kunchaparty S, Palceo M, Berkman J et al. Am J Physiol 1999;277:F643–9.
95. Seyberth HW, Rascher W, Schweer H et al. J Pediatr 1985;107:694–701.
96. Zelikovic I, Szargel R, Hawash A. Kidney Int 2003;63:24–32.
97. Schulthesis PJ, Lorenz JN, Menton P et al. J Biol Chem 1998;273:29150–5.
98. Krozowski Z, Li KX, Koyama K et al. J Steroid Biochem Mol Biol 1999;69:391–401.
99. Heilmann P, Heide J, Hundertmark S et al. Exp Clin Endocrinol Diabetes 1999;107:370–8.
100. Song D, Lorenzo B, Reidenberg MM. J Lab Clin Med 1992;120:792–7.
101. Warnock DG. Contrib Nephrol 2001;136:1–10.
102. Cohn JN, Kowey PR, Whelton PK et al. Arch Intern Med 2000;160:2429–36.
103. Wasserman K, Stringer WW, Casaburi R et al. J Appl Physiol 1997;83:631–43.
104. Perazella MA, Biswas P. Am J Kidney Dis 1999;33:782–5.
105. McIvor ME, Cummings CC. Toxicol Lett 1987;38:169–76.
106. McIvor ME, Cummings CC, Mower MM et al. Toxicology 1985;37:233–9.
107. Emser W. Arch Neurol 1982;39:727–30.
108. Delphin E, Jackson D, Rothstein P et al. Anesth Analg 1987;66:1190–1192.
109. Cooperman LH. JAMA 1970;213:1867–71.
110. Gronert GA, Theye RA. Anesthesiology 1975;43:89–99.
111. Larach MG, Rosenberg H, Gronert GA et al. Clin Pediatr 1997;36:9–16.
112. Phelps KR, Lieberman RL, Oh MS et al. Metabolism 1980;29:186–99.

113. Oh MS, Carroll HJ, Clemmons JE et al. Metabolism 1974;23: 1157–66.
114. Phelps KR, Oh MS, Carroll HJ. Nephron 1980;25:254–8.
115. Wilson FH, Kahle KT, Sabath E et al. Proc Natl Acad Sci USA 2003;100;680–4.
116. Kahle KT, Wilson FH, Leng Q et al. Nat Genet 2003;35: 372–6.
117. Wilson FH, Disse-Nicodeme S, Choate KA et al. Science 2001; 293:1107–12.
118. Sebastian A, Rector FC Jr, Schambelan M. Kidney Int 1981; 19:716–27.
119. Brautbar N, Levi J, Rosler A et al. Arch Intern Med 1978;138: 607–10.
120. Stewart GW, Ellory JC. Clin Sci 1985;69:309–19.
121. Stewart GW, Corrall RJ, Fyffe JA et al. Lancet 1979;2:175–7.
122. Kim HJ, Chung CH, Moon CO et al. Korean J Intern Med 1990;5:97–100.
123. Zaltzman M, Bezwoda WR. S Afr Med J 1982;61:209–10.
124. Bellevue R, Dosik H, Spergel G et al. J Lab Clin Med 1975; 85:660–4.
125. Iolascon A, Stewart GW, Ajetunmobi JF et al. Blood 1999;93: 3120–3.
126. Hayward LJ, Sandoval GM, Cannon SC. Neurology 1999;52: 1447–53.
127. Iolascon A, Stewart GW, Ajetunmobi JF et al. Blood 1999;93: 3120–3.
128. Delaunay J, Stewart G, Iolascon A. Curr Opin Hematol 1999; 6:110–4.
129. Don BR, Sebastian A, Cheitlin M et al. N Engl J Med 1990; 322:1290–2.
130. Campistol JM, Almirall J, Montoliu J et al. Nephrol Dial Transplant 1989;4:233–5.
131. Clark BA, Brown RS. Endocrinol Metab Clin North Am 1995;24:573–91.
132. Greenberg A. Semin Nephrol 1998;18:46–57.
133. Mandelberg A, Krupnik Z, Houri S et al. Chest 1999;115: 617–22.
134. Wong SL, Maltz HC. Ann Pharmacother 1999;33:103–6.
135. Ngugi NN, McLigeyo SO, Kayima JK. East Afr Med J 1997; 74:503–9.
136. Allon M, Shanklin N. Am J Kidney Dis 1996;28:508–14.
137. Martin TJ, Kang Y, Robertson KM et al. Anesthesiology 1990;73:62–5.
138. Edwards BD, Chalmers RJ, O'Driscoll JB et al. Anesthesiology 1990;73:62–5.
139. Broner CW, Stidham GL, Westenkirchner DF et al. J Pediatr 1990;117:986–9.
140. Heining MP, Band DM, Linton RA. Anaesthesia 1984;39: 1079–82.
141. Lillemoe KD, Romolo JL, Hamilton SR et al. Surgery 1987; 101:267–72.
142. Gerstman BB, Kirkman R, Platt R. Am J Kidney Dis 1992;20: 159–61.
143. Rogers FB, Li SC. J Trauma 2001;51:395–7.
144. Emmett M, Hootkins RE, Fine KD et al. Gastroenterology 1995;108:752–60.
145. Gruy-Kapral C, Emmett M, Santa Ana CA et al. Am Soc Nephrol 1998;9:1924–30.
146. Kim HJ, Han SW. Nephron 2002;92[Suppl 1]:33–40.
147. McKinley MJ, Allen AM, Burns P et al. Clin Exp Pharmacol Physiol Suppl 1998;25:61S–7S.
148. Ibata Y, Okamura H, Tanaka M et al. Front Neuroendocrinol 1999;20:241–68.
149. Wells T. Mol Cell Endocrinol 1998;136:103–7.
150. Bourque CW, Oliet SH. Annu Rev Physiol 1997;59:601–19.
151. Olsson K. Acta Paediatr Scand Suppl 1983;305:36–9.
152. Schrier RW, Berl T, Anderson RJ. Am J Physiol 1979;236: F321–32.
153. Aguilera G, Rabadan-Diehl C. Exp Physiol 2000;85:19S–26S.
154. Nielsen S, Frokiaer J, Marples D et al. Physiol Rev 2002;82: 205–44.
155. Ma XM, Aguilera G. Endocrinology 1999;140:5642–50.
156. Mouri T, Itoi K, Takahashi K, et al. Neuroendocrinology 1993; 57:34–9.
157. Molitch ME. Semin Perinatol 1998;22:457–70.
158. Pallone TL, Turner MR, Edwards A et al. Am J Physiol 2003; 284:R1153–75.
159. Hogg RJ, Kokko JP. In: Brenner BM, Rector FC, eds. The Kidney. Philadelphia: WB Saunders, 1986:251–79.
160. de Rouffignac C, Jamison RL. Kidney Int 1987;31:501–672.
161. Oh MS, Halperin ML. Nephron 1997;75:3.
162. Sands JM, Kokko JP. Kidney Int Suppl 1996;57:93S–9S.
163. Burg MB. Am J Physiol 1995;268:F983–9.
164. Schmidt-Nielson B. Fed Proc 1977;36:2493.
165. Knepper MA. Am J Physiol 1983;245:F634.
166. Hogg RJ, Kokko JP. Kidney Int 1978;14:428.
167. Gregger R, Schlatter E, Lang F. Pflugers Arch 1983;396: 308–14.
168. Rendell M, McGrane D, Cuesta M. JAMA 1978;240:2557–9.
169. Hariprassad MK, Eisinger RP, Nadler IM et al. Arch Intern Med 1980;140:1639–42.
170. Levine S, McManus BM, Blackbourne BD et al. Am J Med 1987;82:153–155.
171. Vokes TJ, Gaskill MB, Robertson GL. Ann Intern Med 1988;108:190–5.
172. Arai K, Akimoto H, Inokami T et al. Nippon Jinzo Gakkai Shi 1999;41:804–12.
173. Leggett DA, Hill PT, Anderson RJ. Australas Radiol 1999;43: 104–7.
174. Siggaard C, Rittig S, Corydon TJ et al. J Clin Endocrinol Metab 1999;84:2933–4.
175. Rutishauser J, Kopp P, Gaskill MB et al. Mol Genet Metab 1999;67:89–92.
176. Ito M, Jameson JL, Ito M. J Clin Invest 1997;99:1897–905.
177. Shibata S, Mori K, Teramoto S. No Shinkei Geka 1978;6: 795–801.
178. Weir B. Neurosurgery 1992;30:585–91.
179. Lam GS, Asplin JR, Halperin ML. Clin Sci (Colch) 2000;98: 313–9.
180. Nielsen S, Frokiaer J, Marples D et al. Physiol Rev 2002;82: 205–44.
181. Spruce BA, Baylis PH, Kerr DN et al. Postgrad Med J 1984;60: 493–4.
182. Li C, Wang W, Kwon TH et al. Am J Physiol 2001;281: F163–71.
183. Canada TW, Weavind LM, Augustin KM. Ann Pharmacother 2003;37:70–3.
184. Marples D, Christensen S, Christensen EI et al. J Clin Invest 1995;95:1838–45.
185. Wang W, Kwon TH, Li C et al. Am J Physiol 2002;282:F34–44.
186. Oyama H, Kida Y, Tanaka T et al. Neurol Med Chir (Tokyo) 1995;35:380–4.
187. Oh MS, Carroll HJ. Crit Care Med 1992;20:94–103.
188. Fukuda I, Hizuka N, Takano K. Endocr J 2003;50:437–43.
189. Magaldi AJ. Nephrol Dial Transplant 2000;15:1903–5.
190. Kirchlechner V, Koller DY, Seidl R et al. Arch Dis Child 1999; 80:548–52.
191. Leadbetter RA, Shutty MS Jr. J Clin Psychiatry 1994;55 [Suppl B]:110–3.

192. Oh MS, Dawood M, Carroll HJ. Proceedings of the American Society of of Nephrology, Boston, 1993.
193. Weisberg LS. Am J Med 1989;86:315–8.
194. Milionis HJ, Liamis GL, Elisaf MS. Can Med Assoc J 2002; 166:1056–62.
195. Agraharkar M, Agraharkar A. Am J Kidney Dis 1997;30:717–9.
196. Akan H, Sargin S, Turkseven F et al. Br J Urol 1996;78:224–7.
197. Agarwal R, Emmett M. Am J Kidney Dis 1994;24:108–11.
198. Gowrishankar M, Lin SH, Mallie JP et al. Clin Nephrol 1998; 50:352–60.
199. Sonnenblick M, Friedlander Y, Rosin AJ. Chest 1993;103: 601–60.
200. Bartter FC, Schwartz WB. Am J Med 1967;42:790–99.
201. Ajaelo I, Koenig K, Snoey E. Acad Emerg Med 1998;5:839–40.
202. Fallon JK, Kicman AT, Hutt AJ et al. Lancet 1998;351:1784.
203. Gold PW, Robertson GL, Ballenger JC et al. J Clin Endocrinol Metab 1983;57:952–7.
204. Hensen J, Haenelt M, Gross P. Eur J Endocrinol 1995;132: 459–64.
205. North WG. Exp Physiol 2000;85:27S–40S.
206. Arlt W, Dahia PL, Callies F et al. Clin Endocrinol (Oxf) 1997;47:623–7.
207. Johnson BE, Chute JP, Rushin J et al. Am J Respir Crit Care Med 1997;156:1669–78.
208. Argani P, Erlandson RA, Rosai J. Am J Clin Pathol 1997; 108:537–43.
209. Ferlito A, Rinaldo A, Devaney KO. Ann Otol Rhinol Laryngol 1997;106:878–83.
210. Friedmann AS, Memoli VA, North WG. Cancer Lett 1993;75:79–85.
211. Koide Y, Oda K, Shimizu K et al. Endocrinol Jpn 1982;29: 363–8.
212. Hill AR, Uribarri J, Mann J et al. Am J Med 1990;88:357–64.
213. Oh MS, Carroll HJ. Nephron 1999;82:110–4.
214. Oh MS. Nephron 2002;92[Suppl 1]:2–8.
215. Carvounis CP, Nisar S, Guro-Razuman S. Kidney Int 2002;62: 2223–9.
216. Musch W, Thimpont J, Vandervelde D et al. Am J Med 1999: 348–55.
217. Halperin ML, Bichet DG, Oh MS. Clin Nephrol 2001;56: 339–45.
218. Sterns RH. Am J Med 1990;88:557–60.
219. Sterns RH. Ann Intern Med 1987;107:656–64.
220. Oh MS, Kim IIJ. Nephron 2002;92[Suppl 1]:56–9.
221. Verbalis JG. J Mol Endocrinol 2002;29:1–9.
222. Soupart A, Silver S, Schrooeder B et al. J Am Soc Nephrol 2002;13:1433–41.
223. Ramsay AG. Appl Ther 1965;7:730–6.
224. Lemann J Jr, Relman AS. J Clin Invest 1959;38:2215–23.
225. Oh MS. Nephron 1991;59:7–10.
226. Oh MS. Kidney Int 1989;36:915–7.
227. Oh MS, Carroll HJ. Contrib Nephrol 1992;100:89–104.
228. Lennon EJ, Lemann J Jr, Litzow JR. J Clin Invest 1966;45: 1601–7.
229. Relman AS, Lennon, EJ, And Lemann, J. Jr. J Clin Invest 1961; 40:1621–1630.
230. Bommer J, Keller C, Gehlen F et al. Clin Nephrol 1996;46: 280–5.
231. Rodriguez Soriano J. J Am Soc Nephrol 2002;13:2160–70.
232. Luft FC. J Am Soc Nephrol 2001;12[Suppl 17]:15S–9S.
233. Arenas-Pinto A, Grant AD, Edwards S et al. Sex Transm Infect 2003;79:340–3.
234. Uribarri J, Oh MS, Carroll HJ. Medicine (Baltimore) 1998;77: 73–82.
235. Oh MS, Phelps KR, Traube M et al. N Engl J Med 1979;301: 249–52.
236. Delaney MF, Zisman A, Kettyle WM. Endocrinol Metab Clin North Am 2000;29:683–705.
237. Umpierrez GE, Khajavi M, Kitabchi AE. Am J Med Sci 1996; 311:225–33.
238. Oh MS, Carroll HJ. N Engl J Med 1977;297:814–7.
239. McLaughlin ML, Kassirer JP. Drugs 1990;39:841–55.
240. Schneiderman R, Rosenkrantz TS, Knox I et al. Biol Neonate 1993;64:287–94.
241. von Planta M, Gudipati C, Weil MH et al . J Clin Pharmacol 1988;28:594–9.
242. Dybvik T, Strand T, Steen PA. Resuscitation 1995;29:89–95.
243. Kamel KS. Clin Nephrol 1996;46:112–6.
244. Blecic S, De Backer D, Deleuze M et al. Ann Emerg Med 1991;20:235–8.
245. Palmer BF, Alpern RJ. J Am Soc Nephrol 1997;8:1462–9.
246. Oh MS, Carroll HJ. Nephron 2002;91:379–82.
247. Martin WJ, Matzke GR. Clin Pharm 1982;1:42–8.
248. Saaresranta T, Polo-Kantola P, Irjala K et al. Chest 1999;115: 1581–7.
249. Bayliss DA, Millhorn DE. J Appl Physiol 1992;73:393–404.
250. Gabow PA, Anderson RJ, Potts DE et al. Arch Intern Med 1978;138:1481–4.

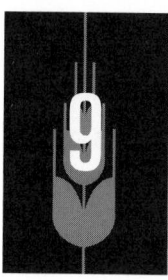

CALCIUM[1]

CONNIE M. WEAVER AND ROBERT P. HEANEY

BIOLOGIC ROLES OF CALCIUM 194
   Calcium and the Cell 194
OCCURRENCE AND DISTRIBUTION IN NATURE 195
METABOLISM 195
   Homeostatic Regulation 195
   Absorption 196
   Physiologic Factors Affecting Absorption 198
   Excretion 199
DIETARY CONSIDERATIONS .200
   Food Sources and Bioavailability 200
   Nutrient-Nutrient Interactions 201
FUNCTIONS 202
   Intracellular Messenger 202
   Cofactor for Extracellular Enzymes and Proteins . .204
   Bones and Teeth 204
ASSESSMENT OF CALCIUM STATUS 204
DEFICIENCY 204
REQUIREMENTS AND RECOMMENDED INTAKES 205
   Infancy 206
   Childhood and Adolescence 206
   Peak Bone Mass 206
   Adults 206
   Pregnancy 207
   Lactation 207
ADEQUACY OF CALCIUM INTAKE 207
TOXICITY 208
CLINICAL DISORDERS INVOLVING CALCIUM 208

BIOLOGIC ROLES OF CALCIUM

In higher mammals, the most obvious role of calcium is structural or mechanical and is expressed in the mass, hardness, and strength of the bones and teeth. However, calcium has another fundamental function: shaping key biologic proteins to activate their catalytic and mechanical properties. A significant portion of the regulatory apparatus

of the body is concerned with the protection of this second function (e.g., all the activities and roles of parathyroid hormone [PTH], calcitonin [CT], and vitamin D). The structural role is discussed in greater detail in Chapter 84, whereas the cell metabolic, regulatory, and nutritional aspects of this critical element are discussed in this chapter.

Calcium and the Cell

The calcium ion (Ca^{2+}) has an ionic radius of 0.99 Å and is able to form coordination bonds with up to 12 oxygen atoms (1). The combination of these two features makes calcium nearly unique among all cations in its ability to fit neatly into the folds of the peptide chain. By binding with the oxygen atoms of glutamic and aspartic acid residues projecting from the peptide backbone, calcium stiffens the protein molecule and fixes its tertiary structure. Magnesium and strontium, which are chemically similar to calcium in the test tube, have different ionic radii and do not bond so well with protein. Lead and cadmium ions, by contrast, substitute quite well for calcium, and, in fact, lead binds to various calcium-binding proteins with greater avidity than does calcium itself. (Fortunately, neither element is present in significant quantity in the milieu in which living organisms thrive. Nevertheless, the ability of lead to bind to the calcium-binding proteins is a part of the basis for lead toxicity.)

Binding of calcium to a large number of cell proteins (see Table 9.1 for some examples) results in the activation of their unique functions (2). These proteins range from those involved with cell movement and muscle contraction to nerve transmission, glandular secretion, and even cell division. In most of these situations, calcium acts both as a signal transmitter from the outside of the cell to the inside and an activator or stabilizer of the functional proteins involved. In fact, ionized calcium is the most common signal transmitter in all of biology. It operates from bacterial cells all the way up to cells of highly specialized tissues in higher mammals.

When a cell is activated (e.g., a muscle fiber receives a nerve stimulus to contract), the first thing that happens is that calcium channels in the plasma membrane open up to admit a few Ca^{2+} ions into the cytosol. These bind immediately to a wide array of intracellular activator proteins, which, in turn, release a flood of calcium from the intracellular storage vesicles (the sarcoplasmic reticulum,

[1]Abbreviations: Ca^{2+}, calcium ion; CaR, calcium-sensing receptor; CT, calcitonin; DG, diacylglycerol; DRI, dietary reference intake; EAR, estimated average requirement; ECF, extracellular fluid; InsP$_3$, inositol-1,4,5-triphosphate; Na$^+$, sodium ion; PIP$_2$, phosphatidylinositol-4,5-bisphosphate; PTH, parathyroid hormone; RDA, recommended dietary allowance.

TABLE 9.1. EXAMPLES OF CELL PROTEINS BINDING OR ACTIVATED BY CALCIUM

PROTEIN	FUNCTION
Calmodulin	Modulator/regulator of several protein kinases
Troponin C	Modulator of muscle contraction
Calretinin, retinin	Activator of guanyl cyclase
Calneurin B	Phosphatase
Protein kinase C	Widely distributed protein kinase
Phospholipase A_2	Synthesis of arachidonic acid
Caldesmon	Regulator of muscle contraction
Parvalbumin	Calcium storage
Calbindin	Calcium storage
Calsequestrin	Calcium storage

in the case of muscle). This second step very quickly raises cytosol calcium concentration and leads to activation of the contraction complex. Two of the many reactions involving calcium-binding proteins are of particular interest here: (a) troponin c, after it has bound calcium, initiates a series of steps that lead to the actual muscle contraction; and (b) calmodulin, a second and widely distributed calcium-binding protein, activates the enzymes that break down glycogen to release energy for contraction. In this way, Ca^{2+} both triggers the contraction and fuels the process. When the cell has completed its assigned task, the various pumps quickly lower the cytosol calcium concentration, and the cell returns to a resting state. These processes are described in more detail later in this chapter.

If all the functional proteins of a cell were fully activated by calcium at the same time, the cell would rapidly self-destruct. For that reason, cells must keep free Ca^{2+} concentrations in the cytosol at extremely low levels, typically on the order of 0.1 μmol. This is 10,000-fold lower than the concentration of Ca^{2+} in the extracellular water outside the cell. Cells maintain this concentration gradient by a combination of mechanisms: (a) a cell membrane with limited calcium permeability; (b) ion pumps that move calcium rapidly out of the cytosol, either to the outside of the cell or into storage vesicles within the cell; and (c) a series of specialized proteins in the storage vesicles that have no catalytic function in their own right, but that serve only to bind (and hence sequester) large quantities of calcium. Low cytosolic $[Ca^{2+}]$ ensures that the various functional proteins remain dormant until the cell activates certain of them, and it does this simply by letting $[Ca^{2+}]$ rise in critical cytosolic compartments. In contrast to proteins, which are activated by rising cystolic $[Ca^{2+}]$, certain enzymes, such as several proteases and dehydrogenase, are activated or stabilized by bound calcium independent of changes in intracellular $[Ca^{2+}]$.

OCCURRENCE AND DISTRIBUTION IN NATURE

Calcium is the fifth most abundant element in the biosphere (after iron, aluminum, silicon, and oxygen). It is the stuff of limestone and marble, coral and pearls, sea shells and egg shells, and antlers and bones. Because calcium salts exhibit intermediate solubility, calcium is found both in solid form (rocks) and in solution. It was probably present in abundance in the watery environment in which life first appeared. Today, seawater contains approximately 10 mmol/L of calcium (approximately eight times higher than the calcium concentration in the extracellular water of higher vertebrates), and even fresh waters, if they support an abundant biota, will typically contain calcium at concentrations of 1 to 2 mmol. In most soils, calcium exists as an exchangeable cation in the soil colloids. It is taken up by plants, whose parts typically contain from 0.1% to as much as 8% calcium. Generally, calcium concentrations are highest in the leaves, are lower in the stems and roots, and are lowest in the seeds.

In land-living mammals, calcium accounts for 2 to 4% of gross body weight. A 60-kg adult human woman typically contains about 1000 to 1200 g (25–30 mol) of calcium in her body. More than 99% of that total is in the bones and teeth. About 1 g is in the plasma and extracellular fluid (ECF) bathing the cells, and 6 to 8 g are in the tissues themselves (mostly sequestered in calcium storage vesicles inside of cells; see earlier).

In the circulating blood, the calcium concentration is typically 2.25 to 2.5 mmol. About 40 to 45% of this quantity is bound to plasma proteins, about 8 to 10% is complexed with ions such as citrate, and 45 to 50% is dissociated as free ions. In the ECF outside the blood vessels, total calcium is on the order of 1.25 mmol, which differs from the plasma concentration because of the absence of most plasma proteins from the ECF. It is the calcium concentration in the ECF that the cells see and that is tightly regulated by the parathyroid, CT, and vitamin D hormonal control systems.

With advancing age, humans commonly accumulate calcium deposits in various damaged tissues, such as atherosclerotic plaques in arteries, healed granulomas, and other scars left by disease or injury, and often in the rib cartilages as well. These deposits are called dystrophic calcification and rarely amount to more than a few grams of calcium. These deposits are not caused by dietary calcium but by local injury, coupled with the widespread tendency of proteins to bind calcium. Calcification in tissues other than bones and teeth is generally a sign of tissue damage and cell death. This process is greatly exaggerated in conditions such as end-stage kidney disease, when the calcium × phosphorus product by ECF exceeds 2.5 to 3.0 $mmol^2$.

METABOLISM

Homeostatic Regulation

Plasma calcium, which is in exchange with ECF calcium, is tightly regulated at approximately 2.5 mM (9–10 mg/dL). If serum calcium is more than 10% away from the population mean, there is reason to suspect disease. The regulation of serum calcium concentration involves a system of controlling factors and feedback mechanisms (Fig. 9.1).

Plasma calcium concentrations are detected by surface Ca^{2+}-sensing receptors (CaRs) found in parathyroid and the clear cells of thyroid glands, kidney, intestine, bone marrow, and other tissues. When plasma calcium concentrations are elevated, PTH release is inhibited and CT release is stimulated.

When plasma calcium concentration falls, the parathyroid gland is stimulated to release PTH. PTH increases renal phosphate clearance and renal tubular reabsorption of calcium; it activates bone resorption loci, it augments osteoclast activity at existing resorption loci, and it activates vitamin D to enhance intestinal calcium absorption. Activation of vitamin D occurs in two steps. An initial hydroxylation is catalyzed by vitamin D-25-hydroxylase (CYP27), a microsomal cytochrome P450 enzyme system in the liver. The second hydroxylation by 25-OH-D-1-α- hydroxylase

(CYP1α) in the proximal convoluted tubule cells of the kidney converts the vitamin to its active potent form, 1,25-dihydroxy vitamin D or calcitriol (see Chapter 20 for additional details). This latter step is stimulated by PTH and is augmented by a fall in serum phosphate. PTH and $1,25(OH)_2D$ act synergistically to enhance renal tubular reabsorption of calcium and to mobilize calcium stores from bone. PTH acts in a classic negative feedback loop to raise the ECF $[Ca^{2+}]$, thereby closing the loop and reducing PTH release. Although this sophisticated regulatory mechanism allows a rapid response that corrects transient hypocalcemia, in the presence of a chronically calcium-deficient diet, it maintains ECF $[Ca^{2+}]$ at the cost of depleting the skeleton. The three tissues supporting serum calcium levels (i.e., gut, kidney, and bone) operate independently of one another, and altered responsiveness of any of these can increase bone fragility. For example, low fractional calcium absorption capacity was associated with increased hip fracture risk in elderly women (3).

When plasma calcium concentration rises in response to increased calcium absorption or increased bone resorption, extracellular Ca^{2+} binds to CaRs on the surface of parathyroid cells, and this stimulates a conformational change in the receptors leading to an inhibition of PTH secretion from the parathyroid (4). With increased tubular reabsorption, the renal excretory threshold is exceeded, and extra calcium is excreted in the urine.

In infants and children, a principal defense against hypercalcemia is release of CT by the C cells of the thyroid gland. CT is a peptide hormone with binding sites in the kidney, bone, and central nervous system. Absorption of calcium from an 8-oz feeding in a 6-month-old infant dumps 150 to 220 mg calcium into the ECF. This is enough, given the small size of the ECF compartment at that age (1.5–2 L), to produce fatal hypercalcemia if other adjustments are not made. What happens is that CT is released, in part in response to the rise in serum calcium, but even before that, in response to gut hormones signaling coming absorption. This burst of CT slows or halts osteoclastic resorption, thus stopping bony release of calcium. Then, later, when absorption stops, CT levels fall also, and osteoclastic resorption resumes. By contrast, CT has little significance in adults because absorption is lower to begin with, and the ECF is vastly larger. As a result, absorptive calcemia from a high-calcium diet raises ECF $[Ca^{2+}]$ by only a few percentage points, and thyroid ablation has little impact on calcium homeostasis.

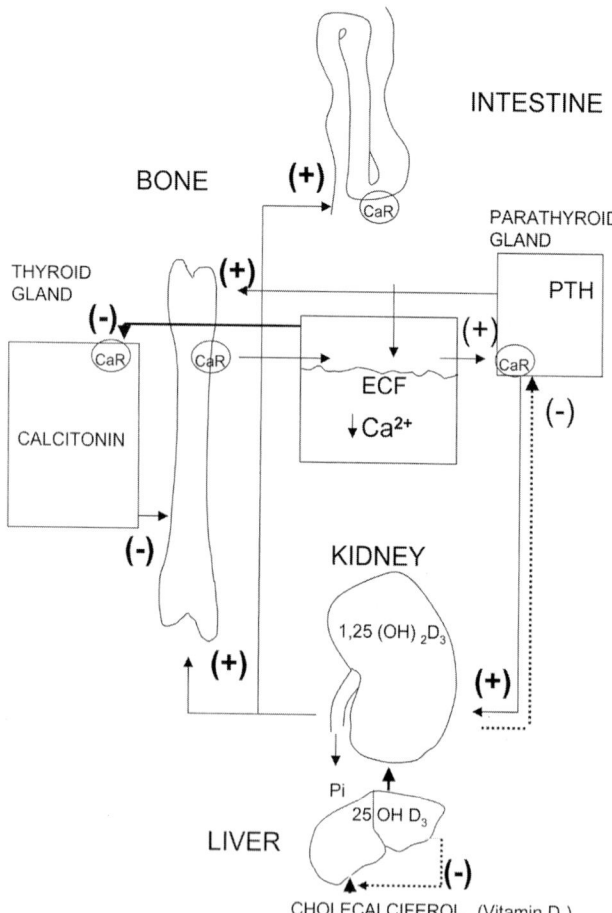

Figure 9.1. Homeostatic regulation of serum calcium depicting the positive and negative controls in effect when plasma calcium (Ca^{2+}) falls to less than 2.5 mM. The calcium-sensing receptor, CaR, has been localized in each of the cells depicted, but its direct role in calcium homeostasis at the intestine has not been demonstrated. ECF, extracellular fluid, PTH, parathyroid hormone.

Absorption

Calcium usually is freed from complexes in the diet during digestion and is released in a soluble and probably ionized form for absorption. However, small-molecular-weight complexes such as calcium oxalate and calcium carbonate can be absorbed intact (5).

Fractional calcium absorption (absorptive efficiency) generally varies approximately inversely with intake, but the absolute quantity of calcium absorbed increases with intake (6,7). However, only 20% of the variation in calcium absorption can be accounted for by usual calcium intake (8). Rather, individuals seem to have preset absorptive efficiencies; approximately 60% of the variance in calcium absorption among individuals can be accounted for by their individual fractional calcium absorption (9).

Mechanisms of Absorption

Calcium absorption occurs by two pathways (Fig. 9.2): (a) transcellular: saturable (active) transfer, which involves a calcium binding protein, calbindin; and (b) paracellular: a nonsaturable (diffusional) transfer that is a linear function of calcium content of the chyme.

The relationship between calcium intake and absorbed calcium is shown in Figure 9.3. At lower calcium intakes, the active component contributes to absorbed calcium. As calcium intakes increase and the active component becomes saturated, an increasing proportion of calcium is absorbed by passive diffusion. Figure 9.3 illustrates that the adaptive component, (i.e., the change in active transport produced by intakes that differ from the group mean) is rather small. This demonstrates our inefficiency to compensate for a fall in calcium intake.

Active absorption is most efficient in the duodenum and next in the jejurnum, but total calcium absorbed is greatest in the ileum, where residence time is greatest. In one rat study, net calcium absorption was distributed as 62% in the ileum, 23% in the jejunum, and 15% in the duodenum (10). Absorption from the colon accounts for about 5 to 23% (or about 1% of ingested calcium) of the

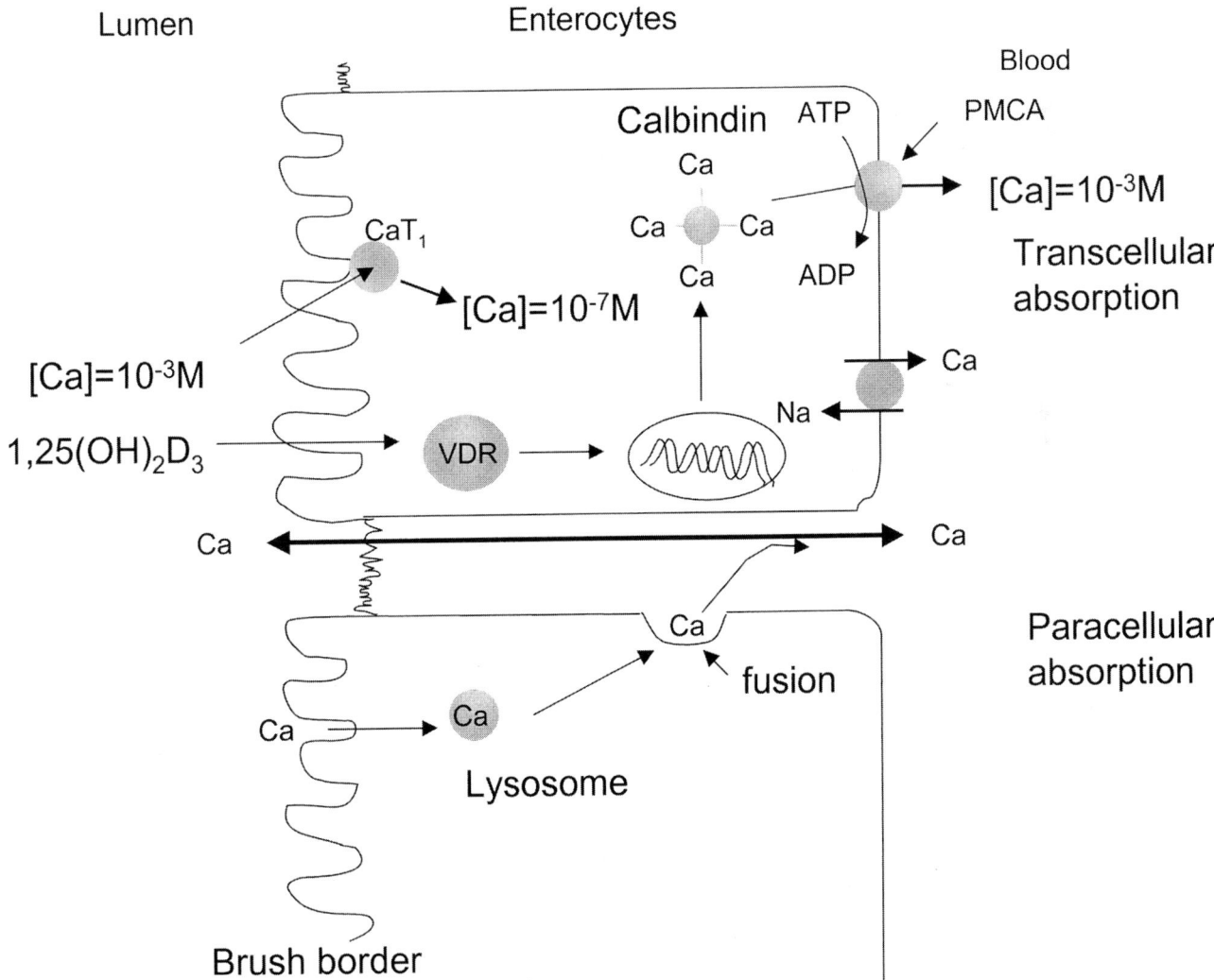

Figure 9.2. Calcium (Ca) absorption showing active, transcellular absorption and passive, paracellular absorption. Paracellular absorption is bidirectional; transcellular absorption is unidirectional. Calcium enters the cytosol down a concentration gradient. Calcium enters the cell via CaT_1 and is transported across the enterocyte against an uphill gradient with the aid of vitamin D–induced calbindin, probably at least partially via endosomes and lysosomes. Finally, it is extruded at the basolateral membrane primarily via the plasma membrane calcium ATPase pump (PMCA) and secondarily via the Na^+/Ca^{2+} exchanger or by exocytosis. ADP, adenosine diphosphate; ATP, adenosine triphosphate; VDR, vitamin D receptor.

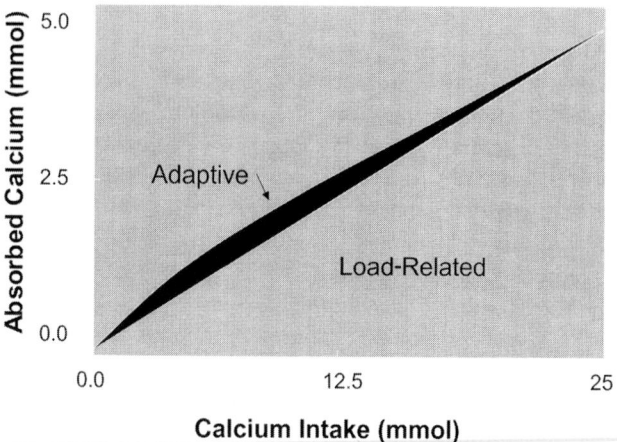

Figure 9.3. Relationship between calcium intake and absorbed calcium in women tested on their usual calcium intakes (adaptive) and in women tested with no prior exposure to the test load (load-related, a physiochemical effect).

total absorption in physiologically normal individuals, but it may be important in patients with small bowel resections and when colonic bacteria break down dietary complexes.

Transcellular Calcium Transport. Calcium entry into the epithelial cells occurs through a calcium channel, CaT_1 (11) although it is not a rate-limiting step (12). Calcium transfer occurs down a steep electrochemical gradient and does not require energy. The main regulator of transport across the epithelial cell against the energy gradient is $1,25(OH)_2$ vitamin D. As illustrated in Figure 9.3, $1,25(OH)_2D$, which is responsive to serum calcium levels, regulates the synthesis of calbindin by binding with vitamin D receptor (VDR) in the cytoplasm and translocating to the nucleus, where it binds to response elements to initiate transcription of calbindin mRNA. Intestinal calbindin, a 9-kDa protein in mammals and a 28-kDa protein in birds, is capable of binding 2 Ca^{2+} per molecule. Calbindin operates by binding Ca^{2+} on the surface of the cell, then internalizing the ions via endocytic vesicles, which probably fuse with lysosomes. After release of the bound calcium in the acidic lysosomal interior, the calbindin returns to the cell surface, and the Ca^{2+} ions exit the cell via the basolateral membrane (13). Calbindin serves both as a Ca^{2+} translocator and a cytosolic Ca^{2+} buffer to resist toxicity (14). Using ion microscopic imaging of injected $^{44}Ca^{2+}$, calcium entry into the villus was observed in vitamin D–deficient chicks, but the rapid transfer of Ca^{2+} through the cytoplasm to the basolateral pole did not occur in the absence of the ability to synthesize calbindin (15).

Vitamin D–induced calcium transport also involves activation of a calcium-dependent adenosine triphosphate (ATP) pump (PMCAlb) to effect extrusion of calcium against an electrochemical gradient into the ECF (16). Relative Ca^{2+} binding capacities across the enterocyte are

brush border, 1; calbindin, 4; and the ATP-dependent Ca^{2+} pump, 10; this gradient ensures unidirectional transfer of Ca^{2+} (17). About 20% of calcium extrusion occurs through the Na^+/Ca^{2+} exchanger (18).

Paracellular Calcium Transport. In the paracellular pathway, calcium transfer occurs between the cells. Theoretically, this can be in both directions, but normally the predominant direction is from lumen into blood because much of the transfer is by solute drag, which is predominantly from lumen into ECF. Rate of transfer depends on ingested calcium load and tightness of the junctions. Calcitriol also enhances flux of ions including Ca^{2+} (19). Water probably carries calcium through the junctions by solvent drag (20). Some compounds are thought to enhance calcium transfer through the tight junctions.

Physiologic Factors Affecting Absorption

Various host factors affect fractional calcium absorption (Table 9.2). Vitamin D status, intestinal transit time, and mucosal mass are the best established (21). Phosphorus deficiency, as may occur through prolonged use of aluminum-containing antacids, can cause hypophosphatemia, increased circulating levels of $1,25(OH)_2D$, and elevated calcium absorption.

Stage of life also influences calcium absorption. In infancy, absorption is dominated by diffusion. Therefore, the vitamin D status of the mother does not affect fractional calcium absorption of young breast-fed infants. Both active calcium transport and passive calcium transport are increased during pregnancy and lactation. Calbindin and plasma $1,25(OH)_2$ and PTH levels increase during pregnancy. From midlife onward, absorption efficiency declines by about 0.2 absorption percentage points per year, and at menopause, there is an additional 2% decrease (22). Decreased calcium absorption efficiency with age is related to increased intestinal resistance to $1,25(OH)_2 D$, as illustrated by a steeper slope in the relationship between fractional calcium absorption and serum $1,25(OH)_2D_3$ in elderly postmenopausal women than in young premenopausal women (23). The age-related decrease in calcium absorption from intestinal resistance to $1,25(OH)_2D_3$ has been associated with decreased VDR levels (24), as well as reduced estrogen levels (23).

TABLE 9.2. PHYSIOLOGIC FACTORS AFFECTING CALCIUM ABSORPTION

INCREASED ABSORPTION	DECREASED ABSORPTION
Vitamin D adequacy	Vitamin D deficiency
Increased mucosal mass	Decreased mucosal mass
Calcium deficiency	Menopause
Pregnancy	Decreased stomach acid (without a meal)
Postweaning status	Rapid intestinal transit time
Mucosal permeability	Estrogen deficiency

Decreased stomach acid, as occurs in achlorhydria, reduces the solubility of insoluble calcium salts (e.g., carbonate, phosphate), which could, in theory, reduce absorption of calcium unless fed with a meal (25). Absorption of calcium supplements improves when they are taken with food irrespective of gastric acid status, perhaps by slowing gastric emptying, and thereby extending the time in which the calcium-containing chyme is in contact with the absorptive surface.

VDR polymorphisms have been studied for their relationship to calcium absorption efficiency. One study showed a significant association between the VDR Fok1 polymorphism and calcium absorption in children (26).

Excretion

Loss of calcium from the body occurs in urine, feces, and sweat. Differences in losses between adult women and adolescent girls on equal and adequate calcium intakes are given in Figure 9.4 (27–29). This figure demonstrates the conservation of calcium at the kidney for building bone during the rapid period of skeletal growth during puberty. African-American girls absorb more calcium and excrete less calcium than white girls, and this results in greater net bone deposition (28). African-American women average 10% higher bone mineral content than white women (30).

Turnover of the miscible calcium pool in healthy adults is about 16%/day, and the rapidly exchanging component (of which the ECF is a part) is about 40%/day. The filtered load of the kidney is determined by the glomerular filtration rate and the plasma concentration of ultrafilterable cacium (ionized plus that bound to small molecular weight anions). In adults, this is about 175 to 250 mmol/day (7–10 g/day). More than 98% of this calcium is reabsorbed by the renal tubule as the filtrate passes through the nephron, but 2.5 to 5 mmol (100–200 mg) is excreted in the urine daily. Endogenous fecal excretory loss is similar to the amount excreted in the urine. Loss in the sweat is typically 0.4 to 0.6 mmol (16–24 mg)/day (29), and there are additional diurnal losses from shed skin, hair, and nails, bringing the total to as much as 1.5 mmol (60 mg)/day. Dermal losses from children average 1.3 mmol (52 mg)/day (31). Higher losses can occur under conditions of exertion (32).

Endogenous Fecal Calcium

Fecal calcium includes calcium that is unabsorbed from the diet plus calcium that enters the gut from endogenous sources, including shed mucosal cells and digestive secretions. Endogenous fecal calcium losses are approximately 2.5 to 3.0 mmol (100–120 mg)/day. These losses are inversely proportional to absorption efficiency and are directly related to gut mass (and hence to food intake).

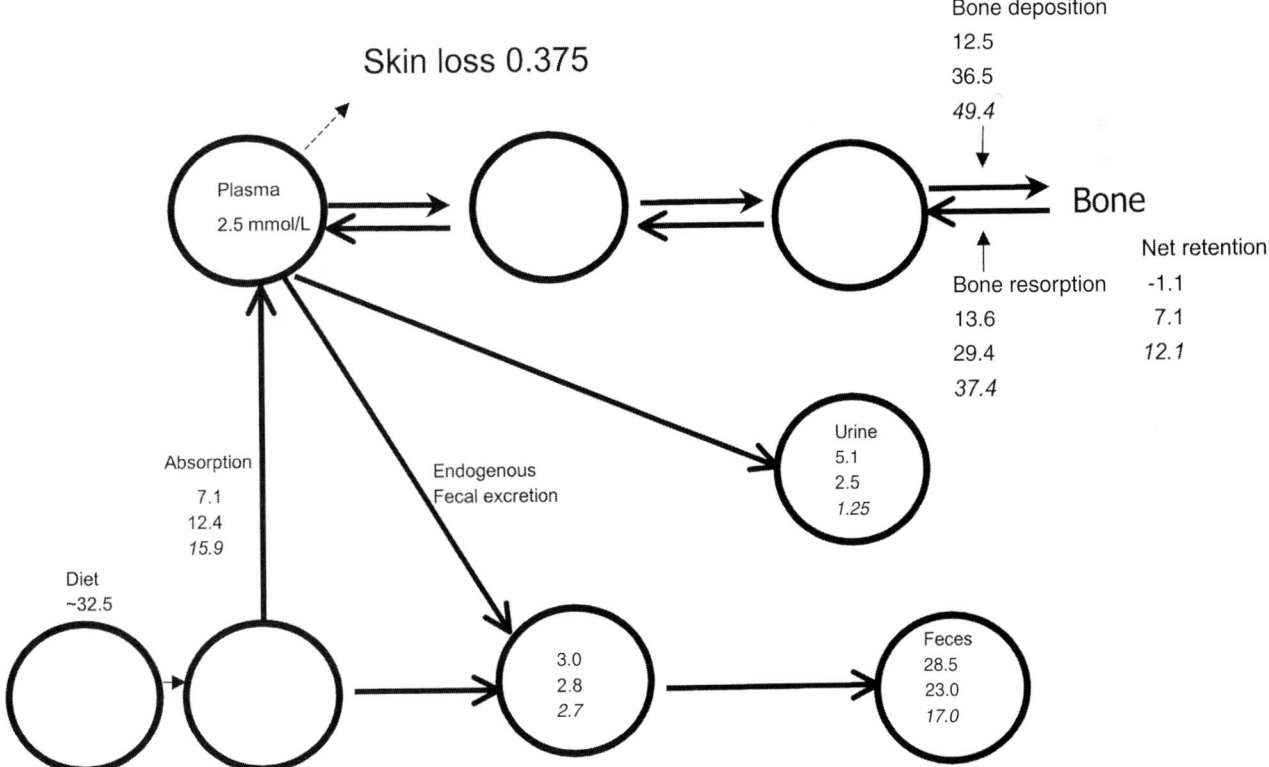

Figure 9.4. Calcium metabolism. Daily mass transfer (mmol) in white adult women (*upper values*) adolescent girls (*middle values*), and African-American girls (*italicized, lower values*). Data were taken from references 27 and 28, except skin loss in adults was taken from reference 29. *Circles* represent compartments determined from kinetic modeling and do not necessarily represent discrete physiologic entities.

Urinary calcium increases during childhood up to adolescence. Endogenous fecal calcium values in adolescent girls do not differ significantly from those of young women (see Fig. 9.4).

Urinary Excretion

In the kidney, an increase in ECF Ca^{2+} concentration decreases the glomerular filtration rate, has a diuretic action in the proximal tubule, and inhibits the actions of antidiuretic hormone (33). Machinery for calcium transport described earlier for the intestinal epithelial cells is also present in the nephron. Paracellular transport dominates in the proximal tubule as reabsorption occurs across a concentration gradient, and it also occurs in the thick ascending limb of the loop of Henle, the distal nephron, and the collecting ducts.

Both active transport and passive transport are calcium load dependent, are detected through CaRs, are stimulated by PTH and $1,25(OH)_2D$, and have a microvillar myosin I–calmodulin complex that could serve as a calcium transporter (34). PTH acts on proximal tubular cells to upregulate CYP1α expression. Calcium enters renal epithelial cells via a calcium channel, ECaC or CaT_2 (35). Active transport occurs in the distal convoluted tubule against a concentration gradient. In the mammalian kidney, vitamin D regulation works through calbindin-$D_{28}k$, which binds 4 Ca^{2+} per molecule and shares no sequence homology with calbindin-D_9k of the intestine. This calcium-binding protein has been cloned and is regulated by both transcriptional and posttranscriptional mechanisms. Administration of $1,25(OH)_2D$ to rats induces calbindin-$D_{28}k$ mRNA and VDR mRNA in vitamin D–sufficient animals (36). However, in the absence of vitamin D, hypercalciuria is not observed, as would be predicted if mechanisms were similar to those in the gut. A fall in filtered load is associated with slight reductions in urine calcium. Even so, renal calcium clearance is reduced in vitamin D deficiency and is increased in PTH deficiency, a finding indicating that the major effect on conservation of calcium is exerted by PTH.

During the rapid growth of adolescence, urinary calcium is little influenced by load. Absorbed calcium is diverted to bone growth at calcium intakes typically ingested, except for obligatory losses of urine, skin, and endogenous secretions (37). Sodium intake is a principal determinant of obligatory urine loss and in adolescent girls is more strongly correlated with urine calcium than is dietary calcium (37). Tubular reabsorption decreases in postmenopausal women.

DIETARY CONSIDERATIONS

Dietary sources and calcium intakes have altered considerably during human evolution. Early humans derived calcium from roots, tubers, nuts, and beans in quantities believed to exceed 37.5 mmol (1500 g)/day (38) and perhaps up to twice this when consuming food to meet the caloric demands of a hunter-gatherer of contemporary body size. After domestication of grains, calcium intakes decreased substantially because the staple foods became grains (fruits), the plant parts that accumulate the least calcium. Pre–iron age milling practices were based on limestone and hence added appreciable calcium as calcium carbonate to the otherwise low-calcium flour. Consequently, the modern human on average consumes insufficient calcium to optimize bone density. The food group that supplies the bulk of the calcium in the Western diet is now the dairy food group.

Food Sources and Bioavailability

For adults, dairy products supply 78% of the calcium in the US diet, grain products about 11%, and vegetables and fruits about 6% (39). Although corn tortillas processed with lime and dried beans provide the bulk of dietary calcium for some ethnic groups, it is difficult for most persons to ingest sufficient quantities of calcium from foods available in a cereal-based economy without liberal consumption of dairy products. Thus, food manufacturers have developed calcium-fortified products. Many persons have turned to dietary supplements in order to meet their calcium needs. However, calcium is not the only nutrient important to health that is supplied by dairy products (Table 9.3). Users of milk in the United States, compared with nonusers, get 35% more vitamin A, 38% more folate, 56% more riboflavin, 22% more magnesium, and 24% more potassium, in addition to 80% more calcium (40).

TABLE 9.3. CONTRIBUTION OF MILK TO NUTRIENTS CONSUMED BY INDIVIDUALS IN THE UNITED STATES AND RANK ORDER RELATIVE TO CONTRIBUTION FROM OTHER FOODS (USING US DEPARTMENT OF AGRICULTURE'S 1994 TO 1996 CONTINUING SURVEY OF FOOD INTAKES BY INDIVIDUALS)

NUTRIENT	PERCENTAGE OF TOTAL (%)	RANK ORDER OF MILK
Calcium	28.3	1
Riboflavin	14.9	1
Phosphorus	14.0	1
Vitamin B_{12}	12.6	3
Potassium	10.2	1
Vitamin A	9.0	2
Magnesium	8.3	1
Protein	7.5	3
Zinc	6.1	3
Fat	4.2	8
Energy	4.2	5
Vitamin B_6	4.0	6
Carbohydrate	3.3	9

[1] From Cotton PA, Subar AF, Friday JE et al. Dietary sources of nutrients among US adults, 1994 to 1996. J Am Diet Assoc 2004;104:921–30.

Aside from gross calcium content, potential calcium sources vary importantly in bioavailability. Fractional calcium absorption from various dairy products is similar, at approximately 30% (41). The calcium from most supplements is absorbed as well as from milk, because solubility of the salts at neutral pH has little impact on calcium absorption (42). A few calcium salts, including calcium citrate malate and calcium ascorbate, have superior absorbability. However, adjuvants added to supplements or food matrices can substantially alter bioavailability.

Several plant constituents form indigestible salts with calcium, thereby decreasing absorption of their calcium. The most potent inhibitor of calcium absorption is oxalic acid, found in high concentration in spinach, rhubarb, and, to a lesser extent, sweet potatoes and dried beans (43). Calcium absorption from spinach is only 5% compared with 27% from milk ingested at a similar load (44). When these two foods of dissimilar bioavailability are coingested during the same meal, calcium fractional absorption from milk is depressed 30% of the difference between milk and spinach fed alone by the presence of spinach, and calcium fraction absorption from spinach is enhanced by 37% of the difference between milk and spinach by the presence of milk (45). The absence of complete exchange and the failure to find equal absorption from the two foods intermediate between the values for the foods fed singly suggest that calcium does not completely form a common dietary pool, as has been reported for iron and zinc.

Phytic acid, the storage form of phosphorus in seeds, is a modest inhibitor of calcium absorption. The phytic acid content of seeds, which depends on the phosphorus content of the soil where the plants are grown, influences calcium absorption (46). Fermentation, such as occurs during bread making, reduces phytic acid content by virtue of the phytase present in yeast. This results in increased calcium absorption (47). Since the early balance studies of McCance and Widdowson, who reported negative calcium balance with consumption of whole wheat products (48), it has been assumed that fiber negatively affects calcium balance through physical entrapment or through cationic binding with uronic acid residue (49). However, it is more likely that the phytic acid associated with fiber-rich foods is the component that affects balance because purified fibers do not negatively affect calcium absorption (50). Only concentrated sources of phytate such as wheat bran ingested as extruded cereal (47) or dried beans (51) substantially reduce calcium absorption. For other plants rich in calcium (primarily the *Brassica* genus, which includes broccoli, kale, bok choy, cabbage, and mustard and turnip greens), calcium bioavailability is as good as that from milk (52). The *Brassicas* are an anomaly in the plant kingdom in that they do not accumulate oxalate as a mechanism to detoxify excess calcium to protect against cell death.

Several foods and the number of servings required to equal the amount of absorbable calcium in one serving of milk are given in Table 9.4.

True enhancers of calcium absorption have not been well characterized. Lactose appears to enhance calcium absorption in infants. However, in adults, calcium absorption from various dairy products is equivalent regardless of the lactose content, chemical form of calcium, or presence of flavorings (53). Some nondigestible oligossacharides and milk proteins appear to have weak calcium absorption enhancing capacity, but not in all circumstances (54).

Nutrient-Nutrient Interactions

Several nutrients and food constituents affect aspects of calcium homeostasis by means other than through a simple effect on digestibility, as described earlier. Several dietary components influence urinary calcium excretion. A major determinant of urinary calcium is urinary sodium, which reflects dietary sodium (55, 56). Sodium and calcium share some of the same transport systems in the proximal tubule, so each 100 mmol (2.3-g) increment of sodium excreted by

TABLE 9.4. FOOD SOURCES OF BIOAVAILABLE CALCIUM[a]

FOOD	SERVING SIZE (g)	CALCIUM CONTENT (mg)	FRACTIONAL[b] ABSORPTION (%)	ESTIMATED[c] ABSORBABLE CALCIUM/SERVING (mg)	SERVINGS NEEDED TO EQUAL 1 c MILK
Milk (or 1 c yogurt or 1½ oz. cheddar cheese)	260	300	32.1	96.3	1.0
Beans, dried	177	50	15.6	7.8	12.3
Broccoli	71	35	61.3	21.5	4.5
Bok choy	85	79	52.7	41.6	2.3
Kale	65	47	58.8	27.6	3.5
Spinach	90	122	5.1	6.2	15.5
Tofu, calcium set	126	258	31.0	80.0	1.2

[a] Adapted from reference 51.
[b] Adjusted for load; for milk, this is fractional absorption (Fx abs) = 0.889-0.0964. In load; for low-oxalate vegetables, after adjusting by the ratio of Fx abs determined for kale relative to milk at the same load, the equation becomes Fx abs = 0.959-0.0964 In load.
[c] *Calcium* content (mg) × Fx abs.

the kidney pulls out approximately 0.6 to 1.0 mmol (24–40 mg) accompanying calcium (57). Because urinary calcium losses account for 50% of the variability in calcium retention, dietary sodium has a tremendous potential to influence bone loss at preliminary calcium intakes in women; each extra gram of sodium per day is projected to produce an additional rate of bone loss of 1% per year if the calcium loss in the urine comes from the skeleton (58). A longitudinal study of postmenopausal women showed a negative correlation between urinary sodium excretion and bone density of the hip (55). The authors concluded, from the range of values available to them, that bone loss could have been prevented by either a daily dietary calcium increase of 891 mg or halving the daily sodium intake.

Another dietary component that influences urinary calcium excretion is protein. Each gram of protein metabolized increases urinary calcium by about 1 mg; thus, doubling purified dietary proteins or amino acids in the diet increases urinary calcium by about 50% (59). The acid load of the sulfate produced in the metabolism of sulfur-containing amino acids is mainly responsible for this increase. However, protein-rich foods typically also contain phosphorus, which has a hypocalciuric effect, thereby offsetting the hypercalciuric effect of the protein. Although urinary calcium loss is unchanged by the inclusion of protein and phosphorus-rich foods such as meat, cereal, beans, and dairy products, the phosphorus increases the calcium content of the digestive secretions, and therefore, increases endogenous calcium losses in the feces. In a controlled feeding study, whole-body tracer calcium retention was similar on low-meat and high-meat diets, a finding suggesting no practical detrimental impact of meat protein consumption on bone (60). At the other extreme, inadequate protein intakes compromise bone health and contribute to osteoporosis in elderly persons (61).

Although widely varying intakes of dietary phosphorus and calcium have produced no changes in calcium balance (62) (presumably because of the offset of increased endogenous secretion of calcium by the decrease in urinary calcium), some investigators have been concerned about the popular trend toward high phosphate consumption in soft drinks. Elevated PTH levels, if sustained, could lead to bone resorption, but this effect has been reported in diets that have both elevated phosphorus and low calcium levels (63). Other investigators (64) reported the same elevated PTH levels with lower calcium intakes without elevated phosphorus intakes. Thus, low calcium level alone accounts for the observed elevation in PTH.

Although caffeine in high amounts acutely increase urinary calcium (65), 24-hour urinary calcium was not altered in a double-blind, placebo-controlled trial (66). Daily consumption of caffeine equivalent to 2 to 3 cups of coffee accelerated bone loss from the spine and total body in postmenopausal women who consumed less than 744 mg calcium/day (67). The relationship between caffeine intake and bone loss in this observational study may be the result of a small decrease in calcium absorption (68) or a confounding factor such as a probable inverse association between milk intake and caffeine intake.

Fat intake has a negative impact on calcium balance only during steatorrhea. In this condition, calcium forms insoluble soaps with fatty acids in the gut.

Increased use of calcium supplements and fortified foods has raised concern about high calcium intakes on producing relative deficiencies of several minerals. High calcium intakes have produced relative magnesium deficiencies in rats (69). However, calcium intake does not affect magnesium retention in humans (70). Similarly, except for a single report in postmenopausal women (71), decreased zinc retention has not been associated with high calcium intakes. The nature of this interaction is unclear and requires further study. Iron absorption from nonheme sources is decreased by half from radiolabeled test meals in the presence of calcium intakes up to 300 mg calcium/day, after which there is no further reduction. Thus, practically speaking, it is prudent to set iron requirements assuming that persons are going to ingest the amount of calcium in at least one glass of milk with each meal (72). The inhibition of iron absorption by calcium does not appear to be a gut effect and may involve competition with the transport of iron in the intestinal mucosa (73), possibly at the level of mobilferrin (see Chapter 12). Supplementation of calcium for up to 12 weeks does not produce changes in iron status (74), probably because of compensating upregulation of iron absorption, nor does long-term supplementation reduce total body iron mass accumulation in adolescent girls (75). Single-meal iron absorption studies quite possibly exaggerate inhibitory effects that disappear in the context of the whole diet.

FUNCTIONS

Intracellular Messenger

Ionized calcium is the most common signal transduction element in cells because of its ability to bind to proteins reversibly. To effect a regulatory change, an internal or external stimulus (physical, electrical, or chemical) causes a change in $[Ca^{2+}]$ at a specific site in the cell by releasing a store of Ca^{2+} from within or by causing Ca^{2+} to enter the cell from the outside (Fig. 9.5). $[Ca^{2+}]$ is maintained at about 0.1 μM in the cytosol via many binding and specialized extrusion proteins. This is necessary because Ca^{2+} is not metabolized like other second-messenger molecules. A released Ca^{2+} ion probably migrates less than 0.1 to 0.5 μm, existing as a free ion only about 50 microseconds before encountering a binding protein. The endoplasmic reticulum (sarcoplasmic reticulum in muscles) with its Ca^{2+}-ATP pumps is the major intracellular calcium sink housing Ca^{2+} binding proteins. Accumulation of Ca^{2+} in the cytosol would lead to cell death as it would precipitate phosphate (vital in energy transfer).

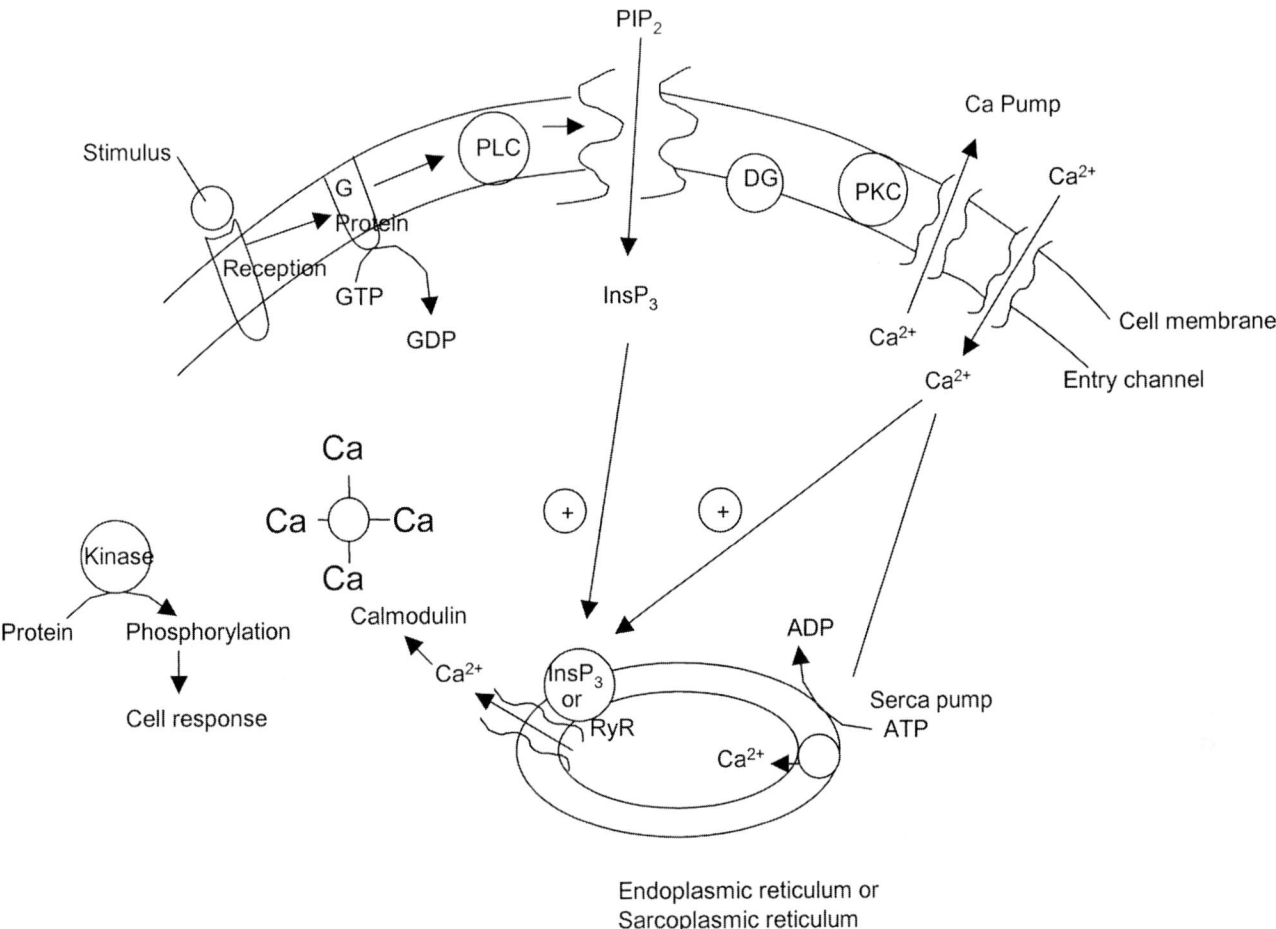

Figure 9.5. Intracellular calcium signaling. Ca pump, plasma membrane Ca^{2+} ATPase pump; DG, diacylglycerol; GDP, guanosine diphosphate; GTP, guanosine triphosphate; $InsP_3$, inositol-(1,4,5)-triphosphate; $InsP_3R$, $InsP_3$ receptor; PIP_2, phosphatidylinositol-4,5-bisphosphate; PKC, protein kinase C; PLC, phospholipase C; RYR, ryanodine receptor; SERCA, smooth endoplasmic reticulum Ca^{2+} ATPase pump. (Adapted from Clapham DE. Cell 1995;80:259–68, with permission.)

The $[Ca^{2+}]$ is perceived by the body through the CaR. Thus, Ca^{2+} itself is one stimulus represented in Figure 9.5 detected by the G-protein–coupled receptor, CaR. In this way, calcium is an important expracellular "first" messenger as well as a key intracellular second messenger. The plasma membrane is important in maintaining calcium homeostasis because the resting membrane is only slightly permeable to entering Ca^{2+}, and a Ca^{2+}-Mg^{2+}-ATPase pump pumps Ca^{2+} out of the cell cytosol back to the ECF space. The pump is activated by calmodulin, an intracellular Ca^{2+} receptor protein that lowers the K_m (Michaelis-Menten constant) of Ca^{2+} from a level of 0.4 to 0.8 μM to 0.2 μM and increases the total capacity of the pump. Thus, a momentary increase of cytosolic $[Ca^{2+}]$ caused by an influx of Ca^{2+} is quickly returned to preexcitation levels. Other less important pathways of Ca^{2+} flux across the plasma membrane include influx pathways, potential-operated (voltage-dependent) channels, receptor-operated channels, and Na^+ channels, and efflux pathway, a Na^+/Ca^{2+} exchange pathway maintained by the Na^+ pump. Calcium messenger systems include trigger proteins in excitable cells and sustained responses in nonexcitable and excitable cells (1).

Sustained Responses

When an external or internal stimulus such as a hormone or neurotransmitter binds to a receptor in the plasma membrane, a series of responses occurs, as depicted in Figure 9.5. Receptors can be G protein–coupled receptors, as shown in the figure, or receptor tyrosine kinases. Phospholipase C is activated, which breaks down phosphatidylinositol-4,5-bisphosphate (PIP_2) in the cell membrane into inositol-1,4,5-triphosphate ($InsP_3$) and diacylglycerol (DG). Released into the cytosol, $InsP_3$ binds to receptors in the endoplasmic reticular (or sarcoplasmic reticular in muscles) membrane, and this induces liberation of Ca^{2+} from internal stores. Ca^{2+} can also enter the cytosol via plasma membrane Ca^2-selective voltage-independent channels. Cystolic Ca^{2+} concentrations can change from 0.1 to 10 μM. The increased cytosolic Ca^{2+} binds to calmodulin, which, in turn, activates kinases to phosphorylate specific proteins. This system accounts for the secretion of aldosterone from adrenal cells in response to angiotension II, insulin secretion from β cells, and contraction of smooth muscles.

Meanwhile the lipid portion of PIP_2, DG, remains in the membrane and activates another membrane-attached enzyme, protein kinase C, which stimulates activity of the calcium pump. Thus, waves of Ca^{2+} are initiated by extra Ca^{2+} cycling in and out of cells (76). As Ca^{2+} concentration returns to resting levels following action of Ca^{2+} pumps, recovery occurs in about 1 second, setting the stage for another Ca^{2+} spike. With the cloning of CaR, signal transduction pathways influenced by CaR are rapidly being discovered. CaR activates phospholipases and mitogen-activated protein kinase and inhibits adenylate cyclase (77).

Trigger Proteins

Calcium receptor protein pathways are almost universal and are present in both excitable and nonexcitable cells. They are important for fast switch processes where Ca^{2+} acts as an on-off switch. Examples of excitable cells are skeletal muscle and neurons. Excitable cells contain voltage-dependent Ca^{2+} channels in the plasma membrane in addition to the system described above for nonexcitable cells which allow dramatic increases in intracellular Ca^{2+}. Entering Ca^{2+} activates ryanodine receptors to release Ca^{2+} from internal stores. We have much yet to learn about how one diffusible ion can regulate such diverse cellular processes as proliferation, differentiation, neuronal adaptation, and movement.

Cofactor for Extracellular Enzymes and Proteins

Calcium is necessary to stabilize or allow maximal activity for a number of proteases and blood clotting enzymes. These functions are not significantly affected by changes in extracellular Ca^{2+} concentration. Those that do not seem to be calmodulin activated by the system described earlier include glyceraldehyde phosphate dehydrogenase, pyruvate dehydrogenase, and α-ketoglutarate dehydrogenase.

Bone and Teeth

The role of calcium in bones and teeth is described more fully in Chapter 84. Calcium exists primarily as the insoluble hydroxyapatite with the general formula $Ca_{10}(PO_4)_6(OH)_2$. Calcium comprises 39.9% of the weight of bone mineral.

Aside from the obvious structural role, the skeleton is an important reservoir of calcium to maintain plasma calcium concentrations. Mobilization of calcium from bone may involve as yet unidentified calcium-binding sites (78).

The bone calcium pool in adults turns over every 8 to12 years on average, but turnover does not occur in the teeth. Remodeling of bone continues throughout life. Bone resorbing osteoclasts begin this process by attaching to a bone surface and then extruding packets of citric and lactic acids (to dissolve bone mineral) and proteolytic enzymes (to digest organic matrix). Later, bone-forming osteoblasts synthesize new bone to replace resorbed bone. Usually, these processes are coupled. Bone formation exceeds resorption during growth. Bone resorption exceeds formation during development of osteoporosis. Osteoblasts have receptors for PTH, $1,25(OH)_2$ vitamin D, estrogen, and prostaglandin E_2. Osteoclasts have receptors for CT and a variety of cytokines. Bone resorption is enhanced by PTH and is inhibited by CT.

ASSESSMENT OF CALCIUM STATUS

Assessment of calcium nutrient status presents challenges unique among the nutrients. The skeleton, as noted in Chapter 84, functions as a very large calcium reserve both for the maintenance of ECF calcium concentrations and for the critical cellular functions of calcium. This reserve is so large that deficiency of calcium at a cell or tissue level is essentially never encountered, at least for nutritional reasons. However, because the mechanical function of the skeleton is directly proportional to skeletal mass (i.e., to the size of the calcium reserve), it follows that any reduction whatsoever in the reserve will result in a decrease in bone strength. In this sense, calcium is the only nutrient for which the reserve has a major function in its own right. Assessment of the size of that reserve can be done by total-body bone mineral estimation using dual energy X-ray absorptiometry (see Chapter 86). A problem arises in the interpretation of the results: the reserve can be low not only for nutritional causes, but for other reasons as well, such as lack of adequate physical activity, weight loss, gonadal hormone deficiency, and various medical diseases and their treatments.

In a research setting, calcium balance (intake minus excretion) can be used to determine whether losses of calcium from the body are being met by the intake of the controlled diet. If someone is in negative balance, calcium is being lost from bone. However, calcium status of a free-living population on self-selected calcium intakes cannot be readily assessed.

The other aspect of calcium metabolism, the concentration of $[Ca^{2+}]$ in blood and ECF, can, however, readily be measured. Low serum $[Ca^{2+}]$ usually means some abnormality of parathyroid function; serum $[Ca^{2+}]$ is rarely ever low because of dietary calcium deficiency. This is basically because (as noted earlier) the skeleton serves as a very large calcium reserve and protects the ECF $[Ca^{2+}]$ essentially without limit. As described elsewhere in this chapter, it is the function of the parathyroid glands to draw down calcium from these reserves for the maintenance of ECF $[Ca^{2+}]$.

DEFICIENCY

Overt, uncomplicated, calcium metabolic deficiencies are almost nonexistent given the large skeletal reserves as discussed earlier. One possible exception is the report in children aged 7 to12 year with daily calcium intakes of 3.1 mol (125 mg) (79). Abnormal biochemistry results were observed, including hypocalcemia and elevated alkaline phosphatase levels.

Adequate calcium intakes have been definitively established as protective against osteoporosis. The primary strategies for reducing the risk of osteoporosis are to maximize development of peak bone mass during growth and to reduce bone loss later in life. Achieving optimal calcium intakes is a goal for both of these aims. Further details on the role of calcium in preventing this debilitating disease may be found in Chapter 86.

The intracellular messenger function of calcium, described earlier, is not affected by variations in calcium intake in the range usually encountered in the populations of industrialized nations. However, it nevertheless plays a role in calcium deficiency indirectly. Some of the consequences of low calcium intake involve systems not directly related to the calcium economy. It has been known for several years that tissues uninvolved in calcium homeostasis possess receptors for $1,25(OH)_2$ vitamin D, but their function was not understood. It has been shown that high circulating levels of $1,25(OH)_2D$, such as would occur in response to low calcium intake (see earlier), open calcium channels in the membrane of certain cells (e.g., smooth muscle and adipocytes) thereby elevating cytosolic $[Ca^{2+}]$, with all the consequences described earlier (i.e., activation of various tissue-specific responses, such as contraction in arteriolar smooth muscle and upregulation of fat synthesis and downregulation of lipolysis in adipocytes). In this way, low calcium intakes contribute to the development or severity of disorders such as obesity and hypertension (80).

The effect of dietary calcium in reducing the risk for colonic tumors has been suggested in numerous studies. Dietary calcium may protect against abnormal epithelial growth. One proposed mechanism is that Ca^{2+} precipates bile acids and fatty acids that can otherwise stimulate colon cell proliferation. Intakes of 1800 mg/day for men and 1500 mg/day for women have been recommended to reduce the incidence of colon cancer (81). However, two prospective studies showed that the occurrence of colorectal adenoma was related neither to calcium intake nor to milk consumption (82). Rectal mucosal proliferation was not decreased with calcium supplementation in patients with large bowel proliferation (83), but recurrence of adenomas was (84). The evidence for a protective effect of calcium on colon cancer in animal studies is strong, but the role of calcium in colon cancer of humans requires further study.

High calcium intakes decrease the risk of kidney stones (see the discussion of toxicity later in this chapter) (85). Unabsorbed calcium in the gut forms a highly insoluble oxalate salt, thereby reducing absorption of oxalate from the diet. Large calcium supplements are the accepted therapy for the kidney stone problem of intestinal hyperoxalosis.

An emerging set of etiologies accompanying the increase in the population that is overweight has a dietary component. Consumption of dairy products (which may be partially or wholly related to calcium consumption) is associated with a lower risk of developing insulin resistance syndrome and its components, such as obesity, hyperinsulinemia, and insulin resistance (86). Low-fat dairy products are also part of the Dietary Approaches to Stop Hypertension (DASH) diet recommended for managing hypertension by the Joint National Committee on Prevention, Detection, Evaluation, and Treatment of High Blood Pressure (87).

REQUIREMENTS AND RECOMMENDED INTAKES

The calcium requirement is the amount of dietary calcium required to replace losses in the urine, feces, and sweat, plus the calcium needed for bone accretion during periods of skeletal growth. Once the body's calcium retention capacity is saturated, further increases in dietary calcium intake will result in increases in excretion. The intake level at which this saturation occurs (i.e. the intake for maximal calcium retention) was the primary basis to define the recommended intakes in the 1997 dietary reference intakes (DRIs). Recommendations across the life span for optimal calcium intakes by the National Academy of Science Food and Nutrition Board are given in Table 9.5. Because the approach of using intakes for maximal retention to set calcium requirements was new, the DRI committee decided to use an adequate intake for calcium instead of an estimated average requirement (EAR)/recommended dietary allowance (RDA). With more experience in deriving an EAR/RDA from the relationship of calcium intake and maximal calcium retention, it should be possible to set an EAR/RDA for calcium in the next revision of the DRIs. The basic definitions and uses of the DRIs are summarized in Appendix Tables A-2-a to A-2-k. Calcium requirements from bone health throughout life are not uniform

TABLE 9.5. CALCIUM RECOMMENDATIONS DURING THE LIFE SPAN

GROUP	ADEQUATE INTAKE (mg/d)
Infants	
Birth–6 mo	210
6 mo–1 y	270
Children	
1–5 y	500
4–8 y	800
Adolescents 8–18 y	1,300
Adults	
19–50 y	1,000
>50 y	1,200
Pregnant and lactating adolescents and women	
14–18 y	1,300
>19 y	1,000

From Food and Nutrition Board, Institute of Medicine. Dietary Reference Intakes Calcium, Phosphorus, Magnesium, Vitamin D, and Fluoride. Washington, DC: National Academy Press, 1997.

because of changes in skeletal growth and age-related changes in absorption and excretion. The many studies of the relationship of calcium or dairy product intake and skeletal health for all ages were reviewed (88). In all but two of 52 randomized, controlled intervention trials, increasing calcium intake increased calcium balance, increased bone gain during growth, reduced bone loss in later years, or reduced fracture incidence. Furthermore, about three fourths of the 86 observational studies showed a positive relationship of calcium intake and bone health.

Infancy

A term human infant contains approximately 0.65 to 0.75 mol (26–30 g) calcium. By the end of the first year of life, total body calcium increases to approximately 2 mol (80 g). The rate of calcium deposition in relation to body size is higher than at any other period during life. Required intakes of calcium are based on adequate intakes determined from the mean intake of human milk for infants fed primarily human milk during the first 6 months and milk plus solids during the second 6 months.

Childhood and Adolescence

Calcium accretion continues throughout childhood. Rate of growth slows between the ages of 2 and 8 years. Between the ages of 9 and 17 years, approximately 45% of the adult skeleton is acquired, but the rate is not uniform. Maximal accretion occurs during the pubertal growth spurt, which occurs for most girls between the ages of 12 and 14 years and for boys between 14 and 16 years (89). Likely regulators of the pubertal growth spurt and skeletal maturation include insulinlike growth factor 1 and sex steroid hormones (90). The intake required for mean maximal calcium retention in adolescent girls is 1300 mg/day (91). Calcium intake greater than this level, compared with lower levels, increases bone calcium accretion through increased absorbed calcium and suppressed bone resorption (92). However, there is some debate whether calcium intakes lower than recommended in Table 9.5 will lead to suboptimal adult bone mass. Animal studies show that adequate calcium intakes following calcium deficiency during pubertal growth fail to recover adult tibia bone volume (93). However, the differential gain in bone mass in randomized, controlled trials in humans wanes after cessation of calcium supplementation (94), similar to other nutrients, although it sometimes remains statistically significant on follow-up (95).

Peak Bone Mass

After adult height is achieved, calcium accretion continues to occur during the phase of bone consolidation. At the end of consolidation, when the maximum amount of bone has been accumulated, the adult is said to have achieved his or her peak bone mass. In girls and women, 90% of total body bone mineral content is achieved by age 16.9 years, 95% by 19.8 years, and 99% by age 22.1 years (96). However, the timing of peak bone mass varies with the skeletal site. The hip achieves peak bone mass first at approximately age 16.7 years for the trochanter, 17.2 years for the femoral neck, and 18.5 years for the Ward triangle, whereas the spine can add mass throughout most of the third decade of life in women (97). The skull accumulates bone throughout life, as does the femur shaft (98).

Approximately 60 to 80% of peak bone mass is genetically predetermined. These include diverse genes controlling all aspects of calcium utilization from those influencing skin pigmentation, which affects vitamin D synthesis, thereby influencing active calcium absorption efficiency, to those controlling renal tubule reabsorption efficiency, to those controlling body size. Additionally, certain environmental factors affect bone mass (99). The main determinant of bone density in adolescent girls is calcium intake (100). During this period, urinary calcium is relatively unaffected by calcium intake (91). Aside from calcium intake, other lifestyle choices that affect peak bone mass include physical activity, intake of other nutrients that affect calcium balance (covered elsewhere in this chapter), anorexia, and substance abuse. Beyond the timing of peak bone mass, lifestyle choices can affect the rate of bone loss, but the window of opportunity to build bone has passed.

Adults

The mature woman has 23 to 25 mol (920-1000 g) body calcium, and the mature man has appoximately 30 mol (1200 g) total body calcium. The population coefficient of variation around these means is about 15%. Total body bone mass remains relatively constant over the reproductive years, as decreases in the proximal femur and other sites after age 18 are offset by continued growth of the forearm, total spine, and head. Then, age-related bone loss occurs, which varies with the individual, but is most rapid during the first 3 years after menopause in women. The average adult loses bone at a rate of approximately 1%/year. Age-related decreases in calcium absorption and increases in urinary calcium contribute to this loss. These physiologic changes are more abrupt at the menopause in women. The explanation for bone loss during aging includes a variety of causes such as declining calcium intakes (discussed later), decreased efficiency of calcium conservation, declining physical activity, decreased levels of gonadal hormones, decreased circulating levels of $1,25(OH)_2D$, and intestinal resistance to $1,25(OH)_2D$. The calcium intake required by older adults to achieve mean maximal retention or minimal loss was determined to be 1200 mg/day by the Panel on Calcium and Related Nutrients (see Table 9.5) using the balance data of Spencer and associates (101).

Calcium intakes required to prevent bone loss are also sufficient to protect against the risk of hypertension. The calcium intake threshold for reducing the risk of high blood pressure is likely to be 12.5 to 15 mmol/day

(500–600 mg/day). Optimal calcium intakes to reduce the risk of other diseases are not known.

Pregnancy

Fetal skeletal calcium accretion is not great until the third trimester. During the third trimester, approximately 5 mmol/day (200 mg/day) of calcium is required for fetal growth. The mother's calcium absorption increases beginning by the second trimester to meet fetal demands and to store calcium for the subsequent lactational drain (102). From prepregnant status to the third trimester, fractional calcium absorption increases 60 to 70% (103) At low calcium intakes, the mother's skeleton is compromised to meet the calcium demands of the fetus, and the fetal skeleton is protected except at exceptionally low calcium intakes (104). In one study, calcium supplementation increased bone density of neonates of malnourished women in India (105). There is no evidence to date that multiple births are harmful to women even with low calcium intakes. During pregnancy, biologically active PTH falls, CT increases during early pregnancy, and prolactin increases ten- to 20-fold.

Lactation

Calcium transfer to breast milk varies mainly with changes in volume; calcium concentration is relatively constant at 7±0.65 mmol/L (280±26 mg/L) and is independent of the calcium content of the mother's diet. Wide variability in the amount of calcium transferred to milk daily has not generally been associated with bone mineral growth or status in infancy (106). However, low dairy consumption by pregnant African-American adolescents was associated with decreased fetal femur length (107). Daily calcium transfer from maternal serum to breast milk increases from 4.2 mmol/day (168 mg/day) at 3 months following parturition to 7 mmol/day (280 mg/day) at 6 months following parturition. The increase in intestinal calcium absorption at the end of pregnancy gradually disappears after childbirth and during the lactation period. To meet the need of milk production, some renal conservation occurs, but more importantly, the maternal skeleton is depleted at a rate of about 1% per month; this loss is not prevented with calcium and vitamin D supplementation (108). Increased bone turnover during lactation may be under the control of PTH-related peptide produced by the lactating mammary gland (109). A postlactation anabolic phase allows recovery of bone density to prelactation levels. Whether this recovery is complete in all individuals, such as older lactating women, is not known. Epidemiologic studies have found no association between pregnancy and lactation and the risk of osteoporotic fractures (109).

ADEQUACY OF CALCIUM INTAKE

The median calcium intakes by age, for both sexes in the United States, collected by the US Department of Agriculture's 1994 continuing Survey of Food Intakes by

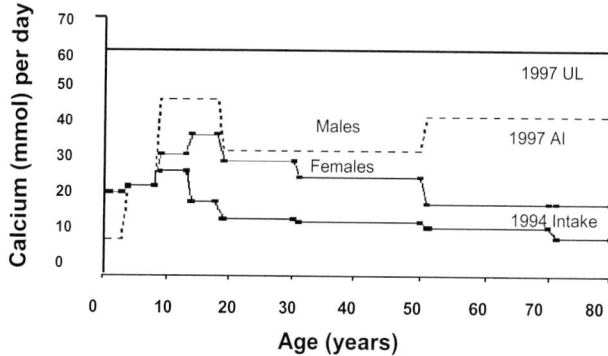

Figure 9.6. Mean calcium intakes by age for US men and women assessed by 24-hour dietary recall adjusted for day-to-day variation (110) compared with 1997 adequate intakes (AI) and upper levels (UL) for calcium, 40 mg calcium = 1 mmol.

Individuals (CSFII) and adjusted for day-to-day variation, are shown in Figure 9.6 (110), compared with the adequate intakes and upper levels for calcium set by the DRI Committee. It is obvious that men typically consume more calcium at all stages of life than do women. Calcium intakes are highest in boys during their adolescent growth spurt. In contrast, just as girls enter their period of most rapid skeletal growth, intakes decline. Mean calcium intakes of girls older than 9 years were less than the DRI. Milk intake drops more than 25% from early childhood to late adolescence, and this explains the drop in calcium intake (111). Low calcium intakes are also associated with low intakes of other nutrients including vitamin B_6, vitamin B_{12}, thiamin, riboflavin, and magnesium (112).

Assessment of calcium intakes of populations is important for determining nutritional status and for drawing conclusions about the relationship between diet and health and disease. However, assessing a person's usual calcium intake is fraught with errors. Calcium intake can be assessed with food frequency questionnaires, diet recalls, diet records, or by duplicate plate analysis. The last approach eliminates many of the errors associated with other methods but is not practical for assessing large groups. Food frequency questionnaires assess calcium better than some other nutrients because dairy foods are the major source of calcium, and persons recall dairy product consumption reasonably well. However, hidden calcium taken in as food additives (e.g., anticaking agents), water, fortified foods, and components of pharmaceuticals can be easily overlooked. When calcium intakes from fortified foods were considered in assessing diets of Asian, Hispanic, and white 10- to 18-year-old children, higher calcium intakes were observed than previously reported in national surveys, but most subgroups still fell below the recommended intakes for that age (113). The gap between calcium intakes and recommended intakes is greatest for African-Americans (114). Diet recall and diet records suffer from errors in estimating portion size, from variability in food composition, and from inadequacies of existing food composition tables. Multiple diet records can improve the estimate of a person's average calcium intake. However, the generally large variability in calcium intake from day to day precludes confidence in estimates of usual calcium intake of an individual person (115,116).

TOXICITY

Nutritional toxicity of calcium means an elevation of blood calcium levels (hypercalcemia) by reason of overconsumption of calcium or an elevation of urine calcium excretion to the point that either the kidneys calcify or renal stones develop. Hypercalcemia, particularly if severe, results in lax muscle tone, constipation, large urine volumes, nausea, and ultimately confusion, coma, and death. It essentially never occurs from ingestion of natural food sources. A good illustration of the safety of food calcium sources is provided by nomadic, pastoral peoples, such as the Masai (117). Because their diets consist mostly of the milk of their herds and flocks, they have calcium intakes greater than 5000 mg/day (and often higher), roughly five to ten times what people of industrialized nations ingest. Such pastoral peoples are not known to have any unusual incidence of hypercalcemia or kidney stones.

Hypercalcemia is reported only with ingestion of large quantities of calcium in the form of supplements, usually taken with absorbable alkali (which raises the pH of the urine and predisposes to calcium deposits in the kidneys). In the past, this outcome sometimes occurred in the treatment of peptic ulcer with large quantities of milk, calcium carbonate, and sodium bicarbonate and was termed the milk alkali syndrome. Even so, this complication was unusual, and most persons can consume large quantities of calcium supplements for years without difficulty. Upper levels were set at 2.5 g/day for all ages to protect against hypercalcemia.

Kidney stones are not usually caused by dietary calcium. More often, patients with kidney stones have high urine calcium levels because they have a renal leak of calcium. Accordingly, they often have some degree of reduction of their skeletal calcium reserves. Lowering calcium intake in such individuals rarely affects their kidney stone problem, but it always leads to further reduction in bone mass. Although high calcium intakes may contribute to kidney stone formation in certain susceptible persons, in general, the stone problem is actually helped by *increasing* calcium intakes (85), unless calcium is taken as a supplement without food (118). This is because urinary oxalate excretion is a more important risk factor for stones than is urinary calcium excretion. A high-calcium diet binds oxalate of dietary origin in the gut and prevents its absorption, thereby reducing urinary oxalate load.

CLINICAL DISORDERS INVOLVING CALCIUM

As noted earlier, low calcium intakes, coupled with low calcium absorption efficiency and high obligatory calcium losses from the body, deplete skeletal calcium reserves. In other words, low intakes cause subnormal bone mass (and strength). This is one of the contributing causes of the disorder called osteoporosis, which is covered in Chapter 86. Medical science recognizes no clear disorder of intracellular calcium regulation. However, cell injury, damage, or serious dysfunction is always associated with a rise in cytosolic calcium concentration, probably reflecting impaired ability of the cell to maintain the normal 10,000-fold gradient between the interior and exterior of the cell. Moreover, it is likely that the rise in cytosolic calcium worsens the cell damage and hastens cell death (119).

The most common disorders of calcium metabolism (other than osteoporosis, which is multifactorial in etiology), involve regulation of ECF [Ca^{2+}]. Usually, these conditions are the result of disorders of parathyroid gland function and are not nutritional. As noted elsewhere in this chapter, the skeletal calcium reserves are so vast, relative to the size of the ECF [Ca^{2+}] compartment, that simple dietary deficiency of calcium essentially never compromises ECF [Ca^{2+}] regulation. There are, however, a few rare exceptions that are worth noting because they illustrate how the system operates.

During growth, when the demands of skeletal mineralization are highest, extremely low-calcium diets may lead to hypocalcemia, despite maximal secretory output of the parathyroid glands. One consequence of the hypersecretion of PTH is a lowering of serum phosphate levels. The combination of low calcium and low phosphorus levels in the ECF results both in undermineralization of newly deposited bone matrix and in osteoblast dysfunction. The result is rickets. Usually, rickets would be produced by vitamin D deficiency, by hypophosphatemia from other causes, or by osteoblast toxicity. However, as this example shows, it can sometimes be caused by calcium deficiency alone (116).

Another example of nutritional hypocalcemia occurs as a result of magnesium deficiency, most often noted in severe alcoholism or as a result of intestinal fistulas or malabsorption causing excessive magnesium loss from the body. Magnesium, of course, is an essential cation for many cell metabolic processes (see Chapter 11), and with severe magnesium depletion, many organs and systems function abnormally. The system regulating ECF [Ca^{2+}] is an example. Both PTH release from the parathyroid glands and bony response to PTH are dependent on magnesium, and both are defective in magnesium deficiency (117). Evidence that both steps are impaired is provided by the finding that PTH levels in magnesium-deficient patients fail to rise adequately in response to the hypocalcemia, and exogenous PTH fails to elevate their bone remodeling, as it should. Magnesium repletion corrects both problems.

Acknowledgments
This work was supported in part by US Public Health Service grants AR40553, RR00750, and AR39221.

REFERENCES

1. Clapham DE. Cell 1995;80:259-68.
2. Carafoli E, Penniston JT. Sci Am 1985;253:70–8.
3. Ensrud KE, Duong T, Cauley JA et al. Ann Intern Med 2000;132:345–53.
4. Chattopadhyay N, Brown EM. Cell Signal 2000;12:361–6.
5. Hanes D, Weaver CM, Wastney ME. FASEB J 1995;9:A283(abst 1642).
6. Heaney RP, Saville PD, Recker RR. J Lab Clin Med 1975;85:881–90.
7. Heaney RP, Weaver CM, Fitzsimmons ML. J Bone Miner Res 1990;5:1135–8.
8. Heaney RP. Am J Clin Nutr 1991;54:242S–57S.
9. Heaney RP, Weaver CM, Fitzsimmons ML et al. J Bone Miner Res 1990;5:1139–42.
10. Marcus CS, Lengermann FW. J Nutr 1962;77:155–60.
11. Peng JB, Cheng XZ, Berger UV et al. J Biol Chem 1999;274:22739–46.
12. Song Y, Kato S, Fleet JC. J Nutr 2003;133:374–80.
13. Nemere I, Leathers V, Norman AW. J Biol Chem 1986;261:16106–14.
14. Nemer I. J Nutr 1992;122:657–61.
15. Fulmer CA. J Nutr 1992;122:644–50.
16. Wasserman RH, Fullmer CS. J Nutr 1995;125:1971S–9S.
17. Wassermann RH, Chandler JS, Meyer SA et al. J Nutr 1992;122:662–71.
18. Ghijsen WE, DeJong MD, Van Os CHM. Biochim Biophys Acta 1983;730:85–94.
19. Chirayath MV, Gajdzik L, Hulla W et al. Am J Physiol 1998;274:G389–96.
20. Korback U. J Nutr 1992;122:672–7.
21. Barger-Lux MJ, Heaney RP, Lanspa SJ et al. J Clin Endocrinol Metab 1995;80:406–11.
22. Heaney RP, Recker RR, Steagman MR et al. J Bone Miner Res 1989;4:469–75.
23. Pattanaungkul S, Riggs BL, Yergey AL et al. J Clin Endocrinol Metab 2000;85:4023–27.
24. Ebeling PR, Sandgren ME, Dimagno EP et al. J Clin Endocrinol Metab 1992;75:176–82.
25. Recker RR. N Engl J Med 1985;43:133–7.
26. Ames SK, Ellis KJ, Gunn SK et al. J Bone Miner Res 1999;14:740–6.
27. Wastney ME, Ng J, Smith D et al. Am J Physiol 1996;271:R208–16.
28. Bryant RJ, Wastney ME, Martin BR et al. J Endocrinol Metab 2003;88:1043–7.
29. Charles P, Jenson FT, Mosekilde L et al. Clin Sci 1983;65:415–22.
30. Looker AC, Wahner HW, Dunn WL et al. Osteoporos Int 1998;8:468–89.
31. Palacios C, Wigertz K, Martin B et al. Nutr Res 2003;23:401–11.
32. Klesges RC, Ward KD, Shelton ML et al. JAMA 1996;276:226–30.
33. Humes HD, Ichikawa I, Troy JL et al. J Clin Invest 1978;61:32–40.
34. Coluccio LM. Eur J Cell Biol 1991;56:286–94.
35. Hoenderop JGJ, van der Kemp AWCM, Hartog A et al. J Biol Chem 1999;274:8375–8.
36. Christakos S, Gill R, Lee S et al. J Nutr 1992;122:678–82.
37. Matkovic V, Heaney RP. Am J Clin Nutr 1992;55:992–6.
38. Eaton SB, Konner M. N Engl J Med 1985;312:283–9.
39. Gerrior S, Bente L. Nutrient Content of the U.S. Food Supply, 1909–94. Home Economics Research Report No 53. Washington, DC: US Department of Agriculture, Center for Nutrition Policy and Promotion, 1997.
40. Fleming KH, Heimback JT. J Nutr 1994;124:1426S–30S.
41. Nickel KP, Martin BR, Smith DL et al. J Nutr 1996;126:1406–11.
42. Heaney RP, Recker RR, Weaver CM. Calcif Tissue Int 1990;46:300–4.
43. Heaney RP, Weaver CM. Am J Clin Nutr 1989;50:830–2.
44. Heaney RP, Weaver CM, Recker RR. Am J Clin Nutr 1988;47:707–9.
45. Weaver CM, Heaney RP. Calcif Tissue Int 1991;56:436–42.
46. Heaney RP, Weaver CM, Fitzsimmons ML. Am J Clin Nutr 1991;53:745–7.
47. Weaver CM, Heaney RP, Martin BR et al. J Nutr 1991;121:1769–75.
48. McCance RA, Widdowson EM. J Physiol 1942;101:44–85.
49. James WPT, Branch WJ, Southgate DAT. Lancet 1978;1:638–9.
50. Heaney RP, Weaver CM. J Am Geriatr Soc 1995;43:1–3.
51. Weaver CM, Proulx WR, Heaney RP. Am J Clin Nutr 1999;70:543S–8S.
52. Heaney RP, Weaver CM, Hinders SM et al. J Food Sci 1993;58:1378–80.
53. Recker RR, Bammi A, Barger-Lux MG et al. Am J Clin Nutr 1988;47:93–5.
54. Cashman KD. Br J Nutr 2002;87:S169–S77.
55. Devine A, Criddle RA, Dick IM et al. Am J Clin Nutr 1995;62:740–5.
56. Matkovic V, Ilich JZ, Andon WB et al. Am J Clin Nutr 1995;62:417–25.
57. Itoh R, Suyama Y. Am J Clin Nutr 1996;63:735–40.
58. Shortt C, Madden A, Fllynn A. et al. Eur J Clin Nutr 1988;42:595–603.
59. Heaney RP. J Am Diet Assoc 1993;93:1259–60.
60. Roughead ZK, Johnson LK, Lykken GI et al. J Nutr 2003;133:1020–6.
61. Dawson-Hughes B. J Nutr 2003;82S–4S.
62. Spencer H, Kramer L, Osis D et al. J Nutr 1978;108:447–57.
63. Calvo MS, Kumar R, Heath H. J Clin Endocrinol Metab 1990;70:1334–40.
64. Barger-Lux MJ, Heaney RP. J Clin Endocrinol Metab 1993;76:103–7.
65. Hasling C, Sondergraad K, Charles P et al. J Nutr 1992;122:1119–26.
66. Barger-Lux MJ, Heaney RP, Stegman MR. Am J Clin Nutr 1990;52:722–5.
67. Harris SS, Dawson-Hughes B. Am J Clin Nutr 1994;60:573–8.
68. Barger-Lux MJ, Heaney RP. Osteoporos Int 1995;5:97–102.
69. Evans GE, Weaver CM, Harrington DD et al. J Hypertens 1990;8:327–37.
70. Andon, MB, Ilich JZ, Tzagournio MA et al. Am J Clin Nutr 1996;63:950–3.
71. Wood RJ, Zheng JJ. Am J Clin Nutr 1997;65:1803–9.
72. Gleerup A, Rossander-Hulten L, Gramatkovski E et al. Am J Clin Nutr 1995;61:97–104.
73. Halberg L, Rossander-Hulten L, Brune M et al. Eur J Clin Nutr 1992;46:317–27.
74. Whiting SJ. Nutr Rev 1995;53:77–80.

75. Ilich-Ernst JZ, McKenna AA, Badenhop NE et al. Am J Clin Nutr 1998;68:880–7.
76. Berridge MJ. Nature 1993;361:315–25.
77. Brown EM. Annu Rev Nutr 2000;20:501–33.
78. Bronner F, Stein WD. J Nutr 1995;125:1987S–95S.
79. Pettifore JM. Am J Clin Nutr 1979;32:2477–83.
80. Barger-Lux MJ, Heaney RP. J Nutr 1994;124:1406S–11S.
81. Garland CF, Garland FC, Gorham ED. Am J Clin Nutr 1991;54:193S–201S.
82. Kampman E, Giovannucci E, vant Veer P et al. Am J Epidemiol 1994;139:16–29.
83. Baron JA, Tosteson TD, Wargovich MJ et al. J Natl Cancer Inst 1995;87:1307–7.
84. Baron JA, Beach M, Mandel JS et al. N Engl J Med 1999;340:101–7.
85. Curhan GC, Willett WC, Renion EB et al. N Engl J Med 1993;328:833–8.
86. Pereira MA, Jacobs DR, Van Horn L et al. JAMA 2002;287:2081–9.
87. Chobanian AV, Bakris GL, Black HR et al. JAMA 2003:289:2560–72.
88. Heaney RP. J Am Coll Nutr 2000;19:83S–99S.
89. Bailey DA, McKay HA, Mirald RL et al. J Bone Miner Res 1999;14:1672–9.
90. Weaver CM. Endocrinology 2002;17:43–48.
91. Jackman LA, Millane SS, Martin BR et al. Am J Clin Nutr 1997;66:327–33.
92. Wastney ME. J Clin Endocrinol Metab 2000;85;4470–5.
93. Peterson CA. J Bone Miner Res 1995;10:81–95.
94. Lee WTK, Leung SSF, Leung DMY et al. Am J Clin Nutr 1996;64;71–7.
95. Bonjour JP. Lancet 2001;358:1208–13.
96. Teegarden D, Proulx WR, Martin BR et al. J Bone Miner Res 1995;10:711–5.
97. Matkovic V, Jelic T, Wardlaw GM et al. J Clin Invest 1994;93:799–808.
98. Heaney RP, Barger-Lux MJ, Davis KM et al. Osteoporos Int 1997;7:426–30.
99. Heaney RP, Abrams S, Dawson-Hughes B et al. Osteoporos Int 2000;11:985–1009.
100. Matkovic V, Fortana D, Tominac C et al. Am J Clin Nutr 1990;52:878–88.
101. Spencer K, Kramer L, Lesniak M et al. Clin Orthop 1984;184:270–80.
102. Heaney RP, Skillman TG. J Clin Endocrinol Metab 1971;331:661–70.
103. Ritchie LD, Fung EB, Holloran BP et al. Am J Clin Nutr 1998;67:693–701.
104. Naylor KE, Igbal,P, Fledeluis C et al. J Bone Miner Res 2000;15:129–37.
105. Wargovich MJ. J Am Coll Nutr 1988;7:295–300.
106. Prentice A, Laskey A, Jarjou LMA. Lactation and bone development: implications for the calcium requirements of infants and lactating mothers. In: Bonjour JP, Tsang RC, eds. Nutrition and Bone Development, vol 41. Philadelphia: Lippincott-Raven, 1999:127–45.
107. Chang SC, O'Brien KO, Nathanson MS et al. Am J Clin Nutr 2003;77:1248–54.
108. Kalkwarf HJ, Specker BC, Henbi JE et al. Am J Clin Nutr 1996;63:526–31.
109. Kalkwarf HJ, Specker BL. Endocrine 2002;17:49–53.
110. Nusser SM, Carriquiry AL, Dodd KW et al. J Am Stat Assoc 1996;14404–9.
111. Rampersaud GD, Bailey LB, Kauwell GP. J Am Diet Assoc 2003;103:97–100.
112. Barger-Lux MJ, Heaney RP, Packard PT et al. Clin Appl Nutr 1992;2:39–44.
113. Novotny R, Peck L, Auld G et al. J Am Coll Nutr 2003;224:64–70.
114. Dietary Intake of Macronutrients, Micronutrients, and Other Dietary Constituents: United States, 1998–1994. *http://www.cdc.gov/nchs/data/series/sr11/sr11 s45.pdf*
115. Weaver CM, Martin BR, Peacock M. In: Burckhardt P, Heaney RP, eds. Nutritional Aspects of Osteoporosis, vol 7. New York: Raven Press, 1995:123–8.
116. Barger-Lux MJ, Heaney RP. In: Burckhardt P, Heaney RP, eds. Nutritional Aspects of Osteoporosis New York: Raven Press 1995;7:243–251.
117. Jackson RT, Latham MC. Am J Clin Nutr 1979;32:779–82.
118. Curhan GC, Willett WC, Speizer FE. Ann Intern Med 1997;126:494–504.
119. Rasmussen H, Palmieri GMA. Altered cell calcium metabolism and human diseases. In: Rubin RP, Weiss GB, Putnsy JW Jr, eds. Calcium in Biological Systems. New York: Plenum, 1985:551–60.

SELECTED READINGS

Weaver CM. Calcium. In: Bowman BA, Russell, RM, eds. Present Knowledge in Nutrition. 8th ed. Washington, DC: ILSI Press, 2001:273–80.

Brown EM, MacLeod RJ. Physiol Rev 2001;81:239–97.

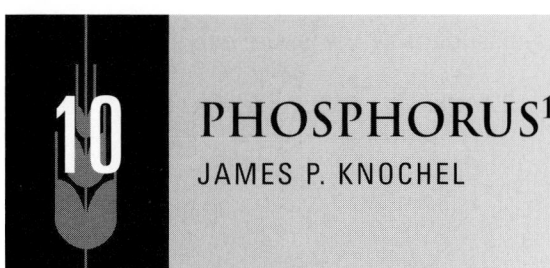

10 PHOSPHORUS[1]

JAMES P. KNOCHEL

CHEMISTRY AND PROPERTIES 211
METABOLISM 212
    Dietary Sources 212
    Absorption 212
    Total Body Content 212
    Renal Handling 212
    Functions 213
HYPOPHOSPHATEMIA 213
    Hypophosphatemia without Phosphorus
        Deficiency 213
    Hypophosphatemia with Phosphorus Deficiency . .214
    Effects of Phosphorus Deficiency and
        Hypophosphatemia .215
    Treatment 220
HYPERPHOSPHATEMIA 220
    Treatment 221

Hypophosphatemia and phosphorus deficiency are common among seriously ill, hospitalized patients. Although both conditions have many causes, they are most commonly seen during treatment of diabetic ketoacidosis, in alcoholic withdrawal, and while administering nutrients (without adequate phosphorus) to a starved or wasted patient.

Refeeding a starved person or administering nutrients to an undernourished sick patient may result in a predictable derangement of blood composition, a variety of specific organ dysfunctions, and sudden death secondary to arrhythmias. This condition has been termed the refeeding syndrome. Old historical records describe epidemics of death when starving persons gained access to food, engorged themselves, then become sick and died. One report describes the deaths of Jews who had been entrapped and starved by the Romans. Some of the captives escaped, stuffed themselves with food, and died. Flavius Josephus pointed out very clearly that death occurred in those who overindulged themselves but not in those who were skillful enough to restrain their appetites (1). Similar descriptions of death during refeeding were related by physicians observing liberated prisoners during World War II. Although the appearance of anasarca suggested beriberi precipitated by feeding carbohydrates, incorporation of brewer's yeast did not prevent the disease. As foretold from biblical descriptions (1), it was finally realized that refeeding with small amounts of food or milk would prevent this disaster. Because laboratory measurements were not available then, it was never clearly appreciated that overaggressive refeeding could cause serious derangements of plasma chemistry. However, more recent studies of patients with anorexia nervosa treated with parenteral nutrition or overzealously with a normal diet showed that hypophosphatemia and phosphorus deficiency play major roles in the metabolic complications of these patients.

CHEMISTRY AND PROPERTIES

At normal blood pH, phosphate ions exist as four parts of HPO_4^{-2} and one part of $H_2PO_4^{-1}$. Thus, $(4 \times 2^-) + (1 \times 1^-) \div (4 + 1) = 1.8$, which is the average valence of phosphate in arterial plasma. In most laboratories, phosphorus is reported as inorganic P, and its normal range is 3.0 to 4.5 mg/dL, or because the molecular weight of phosphorus is 30 daltons, 1.0 to 1.5 mM/L. About 5 to 10% of phosphorus is bound to protein; thus, most of the element is freely filtered by the glomerulus.

Children have higher values for plasma phosphorus concentration, perhaps the result of growth hormone and insulinlike growth factor activities (2). Plasma phosphorus concentration regulates erythrocyte synthesis and stores of 2,3-diphosphoglycerate (2,3-DPG), which is bound to hemoglobin (3). This substance plays an important role in hemoglobin affinity for oxygen. When 2,3-DPG is elevated, as it is in children, hemoglobin releases its oxygen more easily, and as a result, blood hemoglobin concentration and hematocrit are set at lower values. Nevertheless, oxygen delivery to tissues is normal. This phenomenon is also seen in patients with end-stage renal disease. If phosphate-binding antacids are administered to cause hypophosphatemia, 2,3-DPG in erythrocytes falls, and blood hemoglobin levels rise to complement the reduction of oxygen delivery that would occur otherwise (2).

[1]Abbreviations: **ADP**, adenosine diphosphate; **AMP**, adenosine monophosphate; **ATP**, adenosine triphosphate; **CPK**, creatine phosphokinase; **2,3-DPG**, 2,3-diphosphoglycerate; **FGF-23**, fibroblast growth factor-23; **FRP-4**, frizzled related protein-4; **PTH**, parathyroid hormone; **TPN**, total parenteral nutrition; **XLH**, X-linked hypophosphatemic rickets.

TABLE 10.1. CRITERIA AND DIETARY REFERENCE INTAKE VALUES FOR PHOSPHORUS BY LIFE-STAGE GROUP

LIFE-STAGE GROUP[a]	CRITERION	EAR (mg/d)[b]	RDA (mg/d)[c]	AI (mg/d)[d]
0–6 mo	Human milk content	—	—	100
6–12 mo	Human milk and solid food	—	—	275
1–3 y	Factorial approach	380	460	—
4–8 y	Factorial approach	405	500	—
9–13 y	Factorial approach	1,055	1,250	—
14–18 y	Factorial approach	1,055	1,250	—
19–30 y	Serum P_i[e]	580	700	—
31–50 y	Serum P_i	580	700	—
51–70 y	Extrapolation of serum P_i from 19–50 y	580	700	—
>70 y	Extrapolation of serum P_i from 19–50 y	580	700	—
Pregnancy				
≤18 y	Factorial approach	1,055	1,250	—
19–50 y	Serum P_i	580	700	—
Lactation				
≤18 y	Factorial approach	1,055	1,250	—
19–50 y	Serum P_i	580	700	—

[a] All groups except pregnancy and lactation are males and females.
[b] EAR, estimated average requirement: the intake that meets the estimated nutrient needs of 50% of the individuals in a group.
[c] RDA, recommended dietary allowance: the intake that meets the nutrient needs of almost all (97–98%) of individuals in a group.
[d] AI, adequate intake: the observed average or experimentally set intake by a defined population or subgroup that appears to sustain a defined nutritional status, such as growth rate, normal circulating nutrient values, or other functional indicators of health. AI is used if sufficient evidence is not available to derive an EAR. For healthy breast-fed infants, AI is the mean intake. The AI is not equivalent to an RDA.
[e] P_i, inorganic phosphate concentration.
From Food and Nutrition Board, Institute of Medicine. Dietary Reference Intakes for Calcium, Phosphorus, Magnesium, Vitamin D, and Fluoride. Washington, DC: National Academy Press, 1997 (prepublication copy; Table S-2 in original).

METABOLISM

Dietary Sources

The current recommendations for daily dietary phosphorus intake by the Food and Nutrition Board of the Institute of Medicine are shown in Table 10.1 as follows: (a) 0 to 6 months, 100 mg (provided by human milk); 6 to 12 months, 275 mg (provided by milk plus food); (b) 1 through 8 years, 460 to 500 mg; (c) 9 to 18 years, 1250 mg; (d) 19 to 70 years, 700 mg; and during pregnancy or lactation, 1250 mg.

Protein-rich foods and cereal grains are rich sources of phosphorus. In the United States, about one-half of phosphorus in the diet comes from milk, meat, poultry, and fish. Cereals provide 12%. Processed meats and cheese contain more phosphorus than natural products.

Absorption

Phosphorus from soluble products such as meat is more readily available than from other sources. Milk casein contains a phosphopeptide resistant to enzymatic hydrolysis; human milk, being lower in casein, may have more phosphorus available for absorption than cow's milk. Phytic acid in cereal grains reduces bioavailability. A low phytase content of corn and oats reduces phosphorus bioavailability, and accordingly, these grains may be rachitogenic (4).

Absorption of phosphorus occurs throughout the length of the small intestine and is under control of vitamin D and specific phosphate transporters. Absorption is reduced by numerous phosphate-binding antacids.

Total Body Content

A physiologically normal 70-kg man contains about 700 g (23 mol) of phosphorus. Eighty percent is contained in bone and 9% in skeletal muscle. Most intracellular phosphorus exists as organic compounds, such as creatine phosphate, adenosine monophosphates, and triphosphates. As potassium is the most concentrated cation in the cell, phosphate is the most abundant anion. Total tissue phosphorus and nitrogen contents exist in a molar ratio of 0.03 in health.

Renal Handling

In health, the kidneys retain about 80% of phosphorus filtered by the glomerulus. The major regulators of phosphate balance by the kidney are glomerular filtration, tubular reabsorption, and parathyroid hormone (PTH). Phosphorus is reabsorbed mainly in the proximal tubule paired with sodium via type II sodium/inorganic phosphorus cotransporters (5). PTH reduces phosphorus reabsorption by the proximal tubular cells. The fractional clearance rises with hyperphosphatemia and falls with hypophosphatemia. Expansion of extracellular volume independently raises phosphate clearance (2). Vitamin D plays a small role in renal phosphate balance. Nevertheless, serum phosphorus levels play a major role in renal conversion of 25-hydroxyvitamin D_3 to 1, 25-dihydroxyvitamin D_3 (see Chapter 20).

Functions

Phosphorus is a critically important element in every cell of the body. It is a major component of bone, in which it exists as hydroxyapatite. Plasma membranes require phosphorus as a component of phospholipids. All energy production and storage in the body depend on adequate sources of phosphorus including adenosine triphosphate, creatine phosphate, and other phosphorylated compounds. Phosphorus is a critical component of virtually all enzymes, cellular messengers such as the G-proteins, and carbohydrate fuels. Certain hormones depend upon phosphorylation for their activation. Phosphorus is of vital importance for acid-base regulation; it serves not only as one of the most important buffers at the bone surface but also in renal regulation of proton balance.

HYPOPHOSPHATEMIA

Hypophosphatemia without Phosphorus Deficiency

Hypophosphatemia, defined as a plasma concentration lower than 2.5 mg/dL (0.83 mM), is especially common in hospitalized patients who are seriously ill. It often occurs in the absence of a total body phosphorus deficit (Table 10.2). For example, hyperventilation and respiratory alkalosis can reduce plasma phosphorus to values as low as 0.3 mg/dL (0.1 mM) in physiologically normal persons (6). By reducing plasma carbon dioxide tension, cytosolic carbon dioxide tension falls, intracellular pH rises, and phosphofructokinase activity increases, resulting in phosphorylation of glucose. As a result, cytosolic phosphate falls, plasma phosphate enters the cell, and hypophosphatemia follows. Hyperventilation, respiratory alkalosis,

TABLE 10.2. CAUSES OF HYPOPHOSPHATEMIA

HYPOPHOSPHATEMIA WITHOUT PHOSPHORUS DEFICIENCY	HYPOPHOSPHATEMIA WITH PHOSPHORUS DEFICIENCY
Pseudohypophosphatemia	Decreased dietary intake
Mannitol ingestion	Decreased intestinal absorption
High bilirubin	Vitamin D deficiency
Acute leukemia	Malabsorption
Shift from serum into cells	Steatorrhea
Respiratory alkalosis	Secretory diarrhea
Sepsis	Vomiting
Heat stroke	Phosphate-binding antacids
Neuroleptic malignant syndrome	Increased excretion into the urine
Hepatic coma	Hyperparathyroidism
Salicylate poisoning	Renal tubule defects
Gout	Fanconi syndrome
Panic attacks	X-linked hypophosphatemic rickets
Psychiatric depression	Hereditary hypophosphatemic rickets with hypercalciuria
Hormonal effects	Polyostotic fibrous dysplasia
Insulin	Panostotic fibrous dysplasia
Glucagon	Neurofibromatosis
Epinephrine	Kidney transplantation
Androgens	Oncogenic osteomalacia
Cortisol	Aldosteronism
Anovulatory hormones	Licorice ingestion
Nutrient effects	Volume expansion
Glucose	Inappropriate secretion of antidiuretic hormone
Fructose	Mineralocorticoid administration
Glycerol	Corticosteroid therapy
Lactate	Diuretics
Amino acids	Aminophylline therapy
Xylitol	
Cellular uptake syndromes	
Recovery from hypothermia	
Burkitt lymphoma	
Histiocytic lymphoma	
Acute myelomonocytic leukemia	
Acute myelogenous leukemia	
Chronic myelogenous leukemia in blast crisis	
Treatment of pernicious anemia	
Erythropoietin therapy	
Erythrodermic psoriasis	
Hungry bone syndrome	
After parathyroidectomy	
Acute leukemia	

and hypophosphatemia in the absence of phosphorus deficiency can occur in hepatic coma, (7), in acute psychiatric disorders, in hypothermia, in the systemic inflammatory response syndrome (SIRS), with severe pain, during recovery from exercise, and in fever from either heat stroke or the neuroleptic malignant syndrome. Administration of glucose or amino acids stimulates release of insulin, and administration of insulin per se causes cellular uptake of phosphorus and hypophosphatemia (2, 3).

Administration of intravenous fructose, a dangerous procedure that can cause severe liver injury in physiologically normal persons, induces only modest hypophosphatemia but, more importantly, causes a severe depression of free phosphate ions in the cell as a result of phosphate trapping (2, 8). In this process, fructose is phosphorylated in the liver to fructose-1-phosphate without feedback inhibition of continued fructose uptake. For example, when glucose is transported into a hepatocyte, the glucose-6-phosphate formed inhibits glucokinase, thereby downregulating the process of glucose uptake. In the case of fructose, fructose-1-phosphate does not inhibit fructokinase, and accordingly, the unregulated uptake of fructose continues, resulting in hypophosphatemia and the near disappearance of phosphate ions in the cytoplasm, thus the term phosphate trapping. The cytosolic phosphate trapping causes a sharp elevation of the phosphorylation potential: adenosine triphosphate(ATP)/[adenosine diphosphate (ADP) $\times$ inorganic phosphate]. Because the phosphorylation potential regulates ATP production, a decreased cytosolic phosphorus increases this ratio, which, in turn, diminishes mitochondrial ATP stores and energy production. When ATP stores fall below a critical level, cellular injury follows. Cytosolic hypophosphatemia also activates adenosine monophosphate (AMP) deaminase, and the resulting inosine monophosphate is irreversibly converted to uric acid. This explains the hyperuricemia and uricosuria that occur as a result of intravenous fructose infusion. Injury resulting from intravenous (not oral) fructose is seen only in those tissues capable of metabolizing fructose, including the liver, the proximal tubules of the kidney, and probably the small intestinal epithelium.

Hypophosphatemia with Phosphorus Deficiency

Hypophosphatemia in association with phosphorus deficiency (see Table 10.2) is most commonly seen in patients with chronic alcoholism during withdrawal and in patients recovering from diabetic ketoacidosis. Long-term ingestion of ethanol in large quantities causes depletion of body phosphorus stores both in humans and in experimental animals (2). Indeed, phosphorus deficiency in this setting may play an important role in alcoholic myopathy and acute rhabdomyolysis (2, 9).

Hypophosphatemia occurs in as many as 50% of hospitalized patients with alcoholism (2). Most patients with

chronic alcoholism who are not acutely ill show either a normal or a slightly depressed serum phosphorus concentration (10). It is commonly observed that hospitalized patients with alcoholism have been unable to eat for a period of days before admission to the hospital because of alcoholic ketoacidosis or, alternatively, alcohol withdrawal. Two important factors generally explain hypophosphatemia in such patients. First, administration of intravenous fluids containing nutrients (e.g., glucose) without phosphorus is commonly responsible. Second, the usual hyperventilation and respiratory alkalosis that prevail in patients in alcohol withdrawal may result in hypophosphatemia that may be severe. Studying patients with alcoholism on the first day of hospitalization, before the decline of serum phosphorus, urinary phosphorus excretion rates may equal 1 g or more (11). This is a large quantity of phosphorus excretion for a person who has virtually no phosphorus intake. Phosphaturia in such instances has been ascribed to the associated ketoacidosis (12), lactic acidosis, or proximal tubular injury (11). Nevertheless, consequent to administration of nutrients, correction of volume depletion, reversal of ketoacidosis, and the development of respiratory alkalosis, serum phosphorus virtually disappears from the urine. Thus, the development of hypophosphatemia is caused by a shift of phosphorus out of extracellular fluid into the intracellular compartment. Hypokalemia and hypomagnesemia occur less commonly in these patients.

Measurement of muscle composition in patients with severe chronic alcoholism discloses a complex derangement in which total phosphorus and magnesium are abnormally low and sodium, chloride, and calcium contents are abnormally elevated (10, 13, 14). In some patients, potassium content of skeletal muscle is also low. Although the average value for total phosphorus content in patients with alcoholism is 20.4 mMol/dg of dried fat free muscle, some patients demonstrate values as low as 12 mMol/dg. If one assumes that all muscle tissue is uniformly affected, and that skeletal muscle occupies 40% of the body mass, the total deficiency of phosphorus in skeletal muscle alone extrapolates to a value of 1800 mMol in those patients with the lower values.

The causes of phosphorus deficiency in patients with chronic alcoholism are multifactorial. Long-term administration of intoxicating quantities of ethanol to dogs for 2 months causes equally severe phosphorus deficiency in skeletal muscle despite a generous intake of all essential nutrients, including phosphorus (13, 14). Our observations suggest that alcohol exerts toxicity on the muscle cell and is responsible for disorganization of muscle composition, despite a nutritious diet (15). The precise cause whereby these effects occur is unknown. Because ethanol interferes with sodium transport in a variety of tissues, including skeletal muscle (14, 15), and because phosphate transport in nearly all tissues examined depends on normal sodium transport, perhaps deranged sodium transport is somehow responsible for loss of phosphate from muscle. It has been proposed that cytosolic production of the anion acetaldehyde during metabolism of ethanol may electrically dislocate phosphate from the cell (16).

Alcohol may also damage the renal proximal tubule epithelium. It has been reported that urinary γ-glutamyltranspeptidase, a tubular brush border membrane enzyme, and the fractional clearance of lysome, a marker of proximal tubular function, are elevated in 61% of patients with chronic alcoholism (17). Reduced capacity for phosphate reabsorption is seen in 82% of hypophosphatemic patients with alcoholism but in none who were normophosphatemic. Other investigatorss have described a renal phosphorus leak causing hypophosphatemia that resolves on abstinence from alcohol (11). PTH is inhibited by acute alcoholic intoxication and therefore is unlikely to be responsible for these abnormalities (18). Poor phosphorus intake, use of phosphate-binding antacids, impairment in vitamin D metabolism, magnesium deficiency, vomiting, or diarrhea may also cause such a deficit of phosphorus.

Simple dietary deficiency as a cause of phosphorus deficiency and hypophosphatemia is very rare because of the abundance of phosphorus in all foods and the capacity to retain phosphorus avidly. However, if phosphorus is deprived in the diet while a person ingests a phosphate-binding drug, for example, aluminum hydroxide gel, severe and potentially fatal phosphorus deficiency may occur. In fact, refeeding a diet containing inadequate phosphorus to a starving person may allow tissue to be resynthesized without adequate phosphorus. This refeeding or nutritional recovery syndrome is heralded by hypophosphatemia with or without hypokalemia, progressively severe weakness, and a multitude of tissue and organ dysfunctions that are described subsequently in more detail.

Hyperparathyroidism causes only mild hypophosphatemia in most instances. Malabsorption of fat causes modest hypophosphatemia, mainly by losses into the urine. Thus, steatorrhea causes the sequence of reduced absorption of vitamin D, vitamin D deficiency, malabsorption of calcium, hypocalcemia, increased production of PTH, phosphaturia, and hypophosphatemia.

Primary impairment of phosphorus absorption by the renal tubule is seen in several conditions. Dietary vitamin D deficiency and acquired Fanconi syndrome are well-recognized examples.

Patients with hypophosphatemic disorders including X-linked hypophosphatemic rickets (XLH), autosomal dominant hypophosphatemic rickets, and oncogenic osteomalacia have substances in their circulation that inhibit phosphate reabsorption in the kidney and also inhibit formation of 1α-25-$(OH)_2$ D synthesis. Thus, both renal phosphate wasting and intestinal absorption of phosphorus occur. These substances include fibroblast growth factor-23 (FGF-23) and secreted frizzled related protein-4 (FRP-4), which are known as phosphatonins. In XLH,

there is a defect in a phosphate-regulating gene with homology to endopeptidases located on the X chromosomes (PHEX). This enzyme normally degrades FGF-23 and FRP-4, but in this defect, large quantitites of these phosphatonins accumulate in the blood. In patients with oncogenic osteomalacia, the tumor produces a substance that prevents degradation of FGF-23 and FRP-4. XLH and autosomal dominant hypophosphatemic rickets may become targets for gene therapy. Successful removal of responsible tumors may cure oncogenic osteomalacia. Discovery of these phosphaturic substances has greatly expanded our knowledge of phosphate regulation (19–23).

Extracellular volume-expanded states including the syndrome of inappropriate secretion of antidiuretic hormone and primary aldosteronism also reduce phosphorus absorption (2). Acute infusion of sodium chloride solutions causes phosphaturia and hypophosphatemia by two mechanisms. First, the resulting volume expansion per se appears to reduce tubular reabsorption of phosphorus, and, in addition, acute reduction of serum calcium by hemodilution causes release of PTH and phosphaturia.

Two important conditions causing excessive loss of phosphorus into the urine are chronic respiratory acidosis and diabetic ketoacidosis. A reduction of intracellular pH causes degradation of organic phosphates that allows phosphorus to enter plasma. Both conditions, untreated, are usually associated with a normal or even elevated serum phosphorus concentration. Because of this, phosphorus is lost into the urine, and depletion occurs. The associated osmotic diuresis in diabetic ketoacidosis abets phosphorus losses. Effective treatment of either condition unveils the phosphorus deficiency. Thus, relief from hypercarbia allows cell pH to rise; glucose phosphorylation increases, and phosphorus in serum falls to potentially very low levels. Treatment of diabetic ketoacidosis with insulin, fluids, and electrolytes results in rapid appearance of hypophosphatemia as phosphorus is taken up by cells. Therefore, phosphorus needs to be provided during therapy of diabetic ketoacidosis.

Effect of Phosphorus Deficiency and Hypophosphatemia

Phosphorus deficiency impairs growth. This is seen especially in the various forms of vitamin D deficiency in humans, such as celiac sprue and in those diseases causing renal tubular loss of phosphorus. Numerous experimental studies have documented the role of phosphorus in growth. Early phosphorus deficiency is often associated with losses of potassium, magnesium, and nitrogen. Reductions of major cell components are almost invariably associated with abnormalities of cellular ion transport, eventually resulting in accumulation of sodium, chloride, calcium, and water.

Osteomalacia, defined as a defect in bone mineralization, often occurs in long-standing phosphorus deficiency.

Experimental phosphorus deprivation in conjunction with phosphate-binding antacid ingestion in human volunteers (24) resulted in profound muscle weakness and bone pain.

Distinct from osteomalacia, dietary phosphorus deprivation acutely results in skeletal demineralization, even before the serum phosphorus concentration falls (2). Although the substance responsible for this phenomenon is unknown, it appears to be either a hormone or a cytokine, but not PTH. In physiologically normal adults, phosphorus deprivation causes release of calcium from the skeleton and hypercalcuria. However, hypercalemia does not occur. In contrast, in growing children, or in adults with various diseases affecting bone such as Paget disease, hyperparathyroidism, or metastatic malignancy involving bone, the skeletal response to phosphorus deprivation is more brisk, and hypercalcemia may occur. In experimental animals, dissolution of hydroxyapatite from the skeleton with phosphorus deprivation is prevented by colchicine (25).

Myopathy and Rhabdomyolysis

Chronic phosphorus deficiency in humans causes proximal myopathy (26). Proximal muscle atrophy and weakness may be striking. Osteomalacia usually accompanies this disorder. Laboratory findings characteristically show normal values for creatine phosphokinase (CPK) and aldolase activities; phosphorus in serum is modestly depressed, calcium may be low or normal, and alkaline phosphatase activity is usually sharply elevated.

Selective phosphorus deficiency causes a reversible injury to muscle cells of the dog (27). These changes include a depressed resting muscle transmembrane electrical potential, increased cellular content of sodium, chloride, and water, and a decreased content of phosphorus. Serum CPK activity is normal. Chronic phosphorus deficiency apparently does not cause acute rhabdomyolysis. However, acute hypophosphatemia may precipitate rhabdomyolysis if it is superimposed on chronic phosphorus depletion (28, 29). Most cases have occurred either during acute alcohol withdrawal or in patients with severe, chronic alcoholism who are treated with nutrients devoid of phosphorus (13). In patients with alcoholism, rhabdomyolysis usually appears within the first few days in the hospital and is marked by a sudden elevation of CPK activity. The clinical manifestations include severe muscle pain, profound weakness, muscle tenderness, stiffness, swelling, and rarely muscular paralysis and diaphragm failure. Some patients are relatively asymptomatic and show very few abnormal muscle findings despite severe elevations of serum creatine kinase or aldolase activities. In either situation, muscle creatine kinase activity in serum is consistently elevated, sometimes exceeding 100,000 IU/L. Other classic laboratory findings may be seen, such as myoglobinuria, hyperkalemia, hypocalcemia, hyperuricemia, and hypoalbuminemia (30). Hypophosphatemia and phosphorus deficiency may be obscured by release of

residual phosphate from necrotic skeletal muscle and correction of the hypophosphatemia (29, 31).

Rhabdomyolysis during the course of total parenteral nutrition (TPN) is very rare. It has not been observed when important intracellular element deficiencies are prevented. It appears that rhabdomyolysis does not occur with acute hypophosphatemia in the absence of preexisting damage to muscle cells (32). When chronically phosphorus-depleted dogs with hypophosphatemic myopathy were given TPN without phosphorus, serum phosphorus rapidly declined to values lower than 1.0 mg/dL, and they became very ill, displaying marked weakness, inability to swallow their secretions, muscle fasciculations, and, in some, convulsions. These dogs also showed a pronounced elevation of CPK activity in serum. Histologic examination of skeletal muscle showed frank rhabdomyolysis. However, when phosphorus-deficient dogs were given TPN with phosphorus, serum phosphorus did not fall, CPK activity did not increase, and muscle histology remained normal (28).

The apparent prerequisite that muscle injury must exist before hypophosphatemia can cause acute, florid rhabdomyolysis expresses itself both positively and negatively in several clinical settings. Patients with chronic alcoholic myopathy develop frank rhabdomyolysis if they became acutely hypophosphatemic (31, 32), and patients with the neuroleptic malignant syndrome (33) develop florid rhabdomyolysis that appears to correlate inversely with the degree of hypophosphatemia. Negative expressions of this relationship are exemplified by the rarity of rhabdomyolysis in the patient who becomes hypophosphatemic during treatment of diabetic ketoacidosis or in the patient with simple starvation who becomes hypophosphatemic during TPN therapy (34). In either of the latter instances, usually no evidence indicates preexisting skeletal muscle damage.

Physiologically normal dogs deprived of calories but otherwise fed a diet replete with all other nutrients developed acute hypophosphatemia when they were given TPN. They showed no evidence of rhabdomyolysis (28). Organs were sampled to determine their total phosphorus, sodium, potassium, chloride, magnesium, and calcium content. Although hypophosphatemia appeared quickly and usually attained levels lower than 1 mg/dL by the second or third day of hyperalimentation, CPK levels did not become abnormally high. Total phosphorus content fell substantially in skeletal muscle, liver, and bone. In contrast, total phosphorus content of cerebral cortex, left ventricle, adrenal gland, pancreas, renal cortex, renal medulla, thyroid, and spleen remained within normal limits. Despite sharp reductions in total muscle phosphorus and inorganic phosphorus concentration in serum, ATP, ADP, and inorganic phosphorus content of muscle tissue remained normal in dogs with acute hypophosphatemia that were not already phosphorus deficient. Thus, the phosphorylation potential, which was 855 mmol/L in control animals, remained essentially unchanged at a value of 863 mmol/L in the hypophosphatemic animals (32).

In contrast to the acute hypophosphatemic model, chronic phosphorus deficiency caused a pronounced change in muscle content of high-energy components. ATP, ADP, and inorganic phosphate each fell by approximately 50%, thus seriously reducing the total adenine nucleotide pool. In addition, the increased value for the phosphorylation potential indicates a reduced rate of mitochondrial respiration, hence a reduced rate of ATP synthesis (32).

Our studies also suggest that not only bone but also skeletal muscle is apparently an endogenous reservoir for phosphorus. Thus, in the event of acute phosphorus depletion causing hypophosphatemia, muscle phosphorus is rapidly mobilized to provide phosphorus for vital organs. A low value for ATP, such as that observed in dogs with chronic phosphorus deficiency, implies that the cell is in jeopardy. Thus, in the event of a superimposed insult, such as more pronounced hypophosphatemia or perhaps anorexia from a variety of influences in the phosphorus-deficient state, ATP levels must necessarily fall further. A large amount of evidence suggests that when ATP levels decline to critically low values, cellular death may supervene. Additional evidence indicates that if sodium transport is sufficiently impaired that sodium ions accumulate in muscle cytoplasm, activity of sodium-calcium exchange is decreased (35), so calcium may accumulate in the cell in sufficient quantities to activate lysosomal enzymes and lead to destruction of the cell.

An important species difference appears to exist among rats, dogs, and humans in terms of the effect of phosphorus depletion and hypophosphatemia on skeletal muscle (36). Humans and dogs respond to phosphorus depletion in a virtually identical manner. In contrast, rats fed a phosphorus-deficient diet without added phosphate-binding antacids showed no changes of sodium, adenine nucleotides, resting transmembrane potential difference, potassium, or water contents of skeletal muscle, although serum phosphorus declined from 8.3 to 2.8 mg/dL (37). Similarly, only a very slight change in phosphate content of muscle and no change in calcium content or transport occurred. It appears that in experimental phosphate depletion, dogs are the ideal model if one wishes to replicate human disease.

Hypophosphatemic Cardiomyopathy and Arrhythmias

Calculated stroke work increases after phosphorus administration in seriously ill patients with hypophosphatemia. These improvements occur independently of Starling effects and probably represent an improvement in myocardial contractility (2, 38, 39).

In phosphorus-deficient dogs (40), left ventricular end-diastolic pressure increased and stroke work decreased. Myocardial stroke work fell independently of the Frank-Starling effect. Left ventricular ejection velocity and ventricular contractility are both reduced by phosphorus

deficiency (41). Isoproterenol, which usually increases stroke work of the left ventricle, fails to do so in the presence of phosphorus deficiency. The phosphorylation potential of left ventricular muscle became substantially elevated in dogs with chronic phosphorus deficiency. This occurred because of 30% reduction of cytosolic inorganic phosphate concentration. The resulting alteration of the phosphorylation potential infers that the capacity for mitochondrial energy production is reduced. All abnormalities return to normal with phosphorus repletion.

Phosphorus-depleted rats show reductions of myocardial inorganic phosphorus and of glycogen, glucose-6-phosphate, cytidine triphosphate, phosphatidylcholine, phosphatidylethanolamine, total phospholipid phosphorus (42), and impaired fatty acid oxidation. Such abnormalities of lipid metabolism suggest defective phospholipid biosynthesis and may explain cellular membrane injury. Others have shown that feeding growing pigs aluminum hydroxide gel to induce phosphorus deficiency causes low levels of ATP and glucose-6-phosphate in the myocardium (43).

Approximately 20% of hypophosphatemic patients showed cardiac arrhythmias, even though they have no underlying heart disease, hypokalemia, hypomagnesemia, hyperlactatemia, or hypoxia (44). After repletion of the anion, the severity of arrhythmias decreases. Arrhythmias have been described in patients with anorexia nervosa who become hypophosphatemic (45) and in those with sepsis (46). Hypophosphatemia in patients with acute myocardial infarction increases the risk for ventricular tachycardia (47).

In vivo metabolism of inorganic phosphorus and its compounds can be studied using ^{31}P nuclear magnetic resonance spectroscopy. Using this technique, the concentration of phosphocreatine and ATP in the normal human heart has been estimated to be 11.0 ± 2.7 (SD) mmol/g and 6.9 ± 1.6 mmol/g wet weight, respectively (48). This technique should be a useful tool to study disorders of the heart associated with phosphorus deficiency and hypophosphatemia. Reversible myocardial dysfunction has been described after correction of hypophosphatemia (49).

Respiratory Insufficiency

Several clinical reports have described patients treated with TPN who have developed respiratory failure (2, 50). These patients became seriously ill because of respiratory acidosis and hypoxia. Most were in intensive care unit settings and were desperately ill, receiving glucose or amino acids intravenously. Some demonstrated abnormalities of central nervous system function or peripheral neuropathy. Although profound weakness or muscle paralysis in some of the patients suggested the Guillain-Barré syndrome, usually the cerebrospinal fluid was normal. Some patients could not be weaned from the ventilators at the anticipated time.

Most patients who have developed acute respiratory failure from hypophosphatemia induced by TPN had serious preexisting conditions. These include chronic intestinal fistulas, malabsorption syndrome, Crohn disease, ulcerative colitis, small bowel resection, exocrine pancreatic insufficiency, chronic alcoholism associated with malnutrition, and gastrointestinal cancer. Others have suffered from chronic respiratory acidosis or cor pulmonale. Serum phosphorus concentrations have been less than 1.0 mg/dL when respiratory failure occurred. In some cases, the patients were also hypokalemic. However, respiratory failure persisted despite correction of hypokalemia, and patients responded to subsequent administration of phosphate salts and correction of hypophosphatemia (51). Phosphorus-deficient dogs also showed diminished diaphragm function as a result of muscular weakness (52).

One important study was conducted on eight such patients with a mean serum phosphorus level of 1.65±0.54 mg/dL, to characterize contractility of the diaphragm during electrical phrenic nerve stimulation (53). Correction of hypophosphatemia resulted in a twofold increase in transdiaphragmatic pressure generated by phrenic nerve stimulation. Infusions of fructose 1, α-diphosphate in hypophosphatemic patients with respiratory failure has also been reported to improve pulmonary function (54).

Oddly enough, frank clinically evident rhabdomyolysis rarely occurs in patients who have developed respiratory failure. As pointed out in the earlier discussion of rhabdomyolysis, this condition apparently does not appear to occur as a consequence of acute hypophosphatemia per se unless significant muscle cell injury preexists. Thus, almost all cases of hypophosphatemic rhabdomyolysis occur in patients with alcoholism, who probably all have preexistent muscle cell damage. This relationship may also explain the observation that the respiratory insufficiency syndrome and the hypophosphatemic neurologic syndromes are hardly ever seen in patients with alcoholism after admission to the hospital because rhabdomyolysis usually corrects their hypophosphatemia spontaneously. It seems that chronic alcoholism protects against hypophosphatemic respiratory failure. Most patients who develop hypophosphatemic respiratory insufficiency have slowly become hypophosphatemic during administration of nutrients following correction of respiratory acidosis. In these patients, muscle cells have presumably not been damaged sufficiently that hypophosphatemic rhabdomyolysis could occur.

Erythrocyte Dysfunction

Phosphorus deficiency impairs oxygen release from hemoglobin (55) and rarely causes hemolysis (56–59). The red cell is the only tissue in the body that produces 2,3-DPG (55). 2,3-DPG is bound to hemoglobin and serves to enhance dissociation of oxygen from the hemoglobin molecule. The interaction of 2,3-DPG with oxyhemoglobin has been well characterized. Deficiency of erythrocyte 2,3-DPG impairs release of oxygen from oxyhemoglobin

and thus causes hypoxia (55). Coexistent acidosis reverses this effect by the Bohr effect (60). Reduced 2,3-DPG in erythrocytes may play an important role in neurologic disturbances that occur in hypophosphatemia (55, 61).

As pointed out earlier, most patients with diabetic ketoacidosis become hypophosphatemic during treatment. However, in most such patients, there has not been adequate time to permit development of severe phosphorus deficiency. Because they usually recover rapidly with appropriate treatment, serum phosphorus recovers spontaneously on resumption of food intake, and 2,3-DPG levels ordinarily do not fall (2). Conversely, patients with newly discovered diabetes that has been out of control for prolonged periods have more opportunity to develop serious phosphorus depletion (2).

Hemolysis in hypophosphatemia is rare. Superimposed events such as alcoholic ketoacidosis or coincidental aspirin poisoning requiring hemodialysis have also been present (2). Serum phosphorus concentration was less than 0.5 mg/dL. Severe acidosis, quite independently of hypophosphatemia, may inhibit phosphofructokinase and, in turn, inhibit synthesis of 2,3-DPG and ATP (60). If ATP falls to levels less than 15% of normal, hemolysis may supervene (62). That most patients with diabetic ketoacidosis are not severely phosphorus deficient probably explains why frank hemolysis has never been reported in such patients. Simple improvement of acidosis in most patients with diabetic ketoacidosis leads to correction of the metabolic abnormalities despite hypophosphatemia.

Leukocyte Dysfunction

One of the most important side effects of TPN therapy is infection by bacterial and fungal organisms. Patients receiving hyperalimentation usually have serious diseases complicated by malnutrition and as such are compromised hosts. The cannula, a foreign body in the circulation, is commonly colonized. Plasma hypertonicity may inhibit phagocytic activity (63). Patients with malnutrition tend to be glucose intolerant and thus prone to hyperglycemia. Moreover, it is customary to administer hypertonic solutions for parenteral hyperalimentation.

Hypophosphatemia and phosphorus deficiency cause a 50% reduction of chemotactic, phagocytic, and bactericidal activity of granulocytes. Leukocyte ATP falls (63). All abnormalities are corrected by phosphate repletion or in vitro by incubation of the leukocytes with adenosine and phosphate. These effects are seen only when hypophosphatemia is severe.

The mechanism by which hypophosphatemia impairs granulocytic function is probably related to impairment of ATP synthesis. Microtubule contractions regulate the mechanical properties of leukocytes and thus pseudopod and vacuole formation. Microfilaments require ATP as their source of energy (2, 64). Actin and myosin are found in the cytoplasm of granulocytes. Phosphorus deficiency is also associated with a rise in intracellular calcium that may independently impair phagocytosis (65). Hypophosphatemia not only limits mechanical functions of the granulocyte but may also impair the requirement for the increased rate of synthesis of phosphoinositides and other organic phosphate compounds that are necessary for bactericidal activity during phagocytosis (66).

Platelet Disorders

Malnourished dogs treated with parenteral nutrition become hypophosphatemic and show seven abnormalities of platelet function and structure (67). These include the following: (a) thrombocytopenia; (b) an increase in platelet diameter suggesting increased platelet production; (c) megakaryocytosis of the marrow; (d) a five- to tenfold acceleration of the rate of labeled platelet disappearance from blood; (e) impairment of clot retraction; (f) a 50% reduction in platelet ATP content; and (g) hemorrhage into the gut and skin. None of these abnormalities is seen if phosphorus supplements are provided. Despite these abnormalities, there appears to be little evidence that hypophosphatemia is a primary cause of hemorrhage in humans.

Metabolic Acidosis

Three mechanisms permit urinary excretion of hydrogen ions. First, disodium hydrogen phosphate is converted to monosodium dihydrogen phosphate by exchange of luminal sodium ions for cellular hydrogen ions, and the hydrogen ions thus excreted are measurable as titratable acidity. Second, ammonia produced in the tubular cell diffuses into the tubular lumen and combines with hydrogen ion to become ammonium ion. Third, a small quantity of hydrogen is excreted as free hydrogen ion, thus accounting for the acid pH. The acid pH facilitates formation of ammonium ion in the tubular lumen. Because the ammonium ion is essentially not reabsorbable, ammonium excretion is enhanced in proportion to urinary acidification.

Severe metabolic acidosis may occur in the presence of phosphate deficiency and severe hypophosphatemia (68). Removal of phosphorus from the diet and simultaneous administration of phosphate-binding antacids lead to prompt mobilization of bone mineral and hypercalciuria (69). As hypophosphatemia becomes more severe, phosphate ions virtually disappear from the urine, thereby eliminating the capacity to excrete hydrogen ions as titratable acid.

Ordinarily, metabolic acidosis would be expected to augment renal production of ammonia. However in phosphate deficiency, ammonia formation decreases, presumably as a result of an increase of intracellular pH (70), and reduces urinary acidification by formation of ammonium ion (71). Thereby, the decrease in ammonia production and the unavailability of buffer phosphate in the urine substantially reduce excretion of metabolic acids.

One would predict that metabolic acidosis would regularly develop when excretion of titratable acid or ammonium into the urine is severely limited. However, metabolic acidosis in phosphorus deficiency is rare. The explanation is that during mobilization of bone mineral, mobilization of carbonate also occurs, and carbonate is an important component of bone apatite. During osteolysis associated with phosphorus deprivation, sufficient carbonate is mobilized from bone to titrate all metabolic acid retained in the body. However, should something prevent mobilization of bone mineral, then severe metabolic acidosis may occur. This has been described in experimental vitamin D deficiency and in children with severe lactase deficiency and protein-calorie malnutrition during refeeding without providing adequate phosphate in the diet (68). Addition of phosphate to their diet increased excretion of titratable acid into the urine and corrected metabolic acidosis. In experimental phosphorus deficiency, administration of diphosphonate or colchicine to impede calcium mobilization from bone caused metabolic acidosis (25).

Nervous System Dysfunction

Nervous system dysfunction is a well-recognized complication of severe hypophosphatemia. Malnourished dogs receiving parenteral nutrition became hypophosphatemic and developed ataxia, convulsions, and death (28, 72). Experimental human phosphorus deficiency caused weakness, apathy, a bedridden state, and intention tremors (24).

Many different clinical manifestations have been reported involving almost all levels of the nervous system from higher cortical function, brainstem, to peripheral nerves and muscle (73). The most florid examples of hypophosphatemia-induced nervous system dysfunction have been reported during the course of nutritional recovery syndrome. In such patients, hypophosphatemia usually occurs after approximately 1 week or more of parenteral nutrition with solutions of glucose and/or amino acids not containing enough phosphorus to prevent hypophosphatemia. The sequence of abnormalities consists of irritability, apprehension, muscular weakness, numbness, paresthesias, dysarthria, confusion, obtundation, convulsive seizures, coma, and death (74, 75). Such a clinical state could be confused with that of delirium tremens in the patient with alcoholism, because even lucid visual and auditory hallucinations may occur (76, 77). One report (55) described paresthesias about the mouth and the limbs, mental obtundation, and hyperventilation in three of eight patients who became hypophosphatemic during parenteral nutrition. At the same time, these patients displayed a sharp drop in red cell 2,3-DPG content that correlated with slowing of the electroencephalogram. Both abnormalities disappeared and the patients recovered symptomatically as hypophosphatemia was corrected. Most notably, such symptoms do not occur when adequate phosphorus is provided to prevent hypophosphatemia during parenteral nutrition. Emphasis has been placed on the importance of central nervous system complications in patients who slowly develop severe hypophosphatemia during the course of TPN (2, 55, 72–75).

Symptoms of brainstem dysfunction such as ptosis, dysphagia, dysphonia, impairment in the ability to swallow secretions, respiratory weakness, and hypercarbia in a setting of profound muscle weakness have been reported. Distortions of color perception and even amblyopia may occur. Some patients with slowly developing hypophosphatemia develop all clinical features of the Guillain-Barré syndrome with ascending paralysis, areflexia, and respiratory muscle paralysis (2). Other cases closely resemble Wernicke encephalopathy in which dramatic improvement has been observed following correction of hypophosphatemia. However, when hypophosphatemia is prolonged, recovery after correction may be delayed. Asterixis has also been described. Peripheral neuropathy documented by nerve conduction studies has also been reported. Psychiatric manifestations may include paranoid delusions, extreme anxiety, and visual and auditory hallucinations. A syndrome resembling encephalitis has been described in children with malnutrition who became ill after 1 week of refeeding. Although phosphorus levels were not measured, the possibility of hypophosphatemia seems likely. These children developed coarse tremors, resembling parkinsonism, mainly involving the upper extremities, but also the legs, neck, and tongue. They remained alert. Hypotonia has also been described in infants undergoing treatment for protein-calorie malnutrition (78). A positive correlation appeared to exist between hypophosphatemia and death during treatment. Obviously, all levels of nervous system dysfunction may be seen. As one may suspect, smooth muscle function is also apparently affected by severe hypophosphatemia, as evinced by ileus.

It is worth reemphasizing that in patients who develop syndromes of central or peripheral nervous system dysfunction, and also in those who develop respiratory failure as a result of hypophosphatemia, rhabdomyolysis is virtually nonexistent. Presumably, the apparent requirement for preexistent skeletal muscle injury is missing. The failure to develop rhabdomyolysis results in inexorable and progressive hypophosphatemia and thus permits full expression of nervous system failure.

Treatment

Milk is an excellent source of phosphorus, containing 33 mmol/L (100 mg/dL). Phosphate salts are also available for oral use. They are less likely to cause diarrhea in phosphorus-deficient patients than in physiologically normal persons. Phosphorus salts cannot be given by intramuscular or subcutaneous injection, but sodium phosphate and potassium phosphate are available for intravenous use. The potassium salt should be given when hypokalemia and

hypophosphatemia coexist. Two prospective studies of hypophosphatemic patients in acute intensive care unit situations showed that a 15-mmol dose of either sodium or potassium phosphate may be given in 100 mL of 0.9% sodium chloride intravenously over a period of 2 hours (79). A second study showed that, depending on the severity of hypophosphatemia, doses ranging from 0.16 to 0.64 mmol/kg may be given over a period of 1 or 2 hours as a single dose on a daily basis (80). Serum phosphorus should be measured within several hours of the infusion and at least daily under such conditions. Oral administration of phosphate salts or milk should be resumed as quickly as possible (2). A safe dosage regimen for treatment of patients with alcoholism who are hypophosphatemic, phosphorus deficient, hypokalemic, and hypomagnesemic is the infusion each 8 to 12 hours of 1 L of 0.5 normal sodium chloride in 5% glucose containing 9 mmol of potassium phosphate and 4.2 mmol of magnesium sulfate (2.0 mL of 50% magnesium sulfate solution).

Intravenous administration of phosphate salts either too rapidly or in excess of recommended doses may cause hyperphosphatemia. This should be avoided because it can cause metastatic calcification in the eyes and blood vessels of the kidneys, heart, and lungs.

Acute hypophosphatemia not associated with phosphorus deficiency, typified by that observed in patients with acute respiratory alkalosis as a result of sepsis, may not require treatment because it will resolve on correction of the alkalosis.

HYPERPHOSPHATEMIA

The complications of hyperphosphatemia may be acute or chronic. Those seen acutely include hypocalcemia with tetany, acute nephrocalcinosis with renal failure, acute pulmonary calcification with diffusion block, ocular band keratopathy, and acute calcification of the coronary arteries, the aorta, and its major branches. Calcium and phosphorus crystal depositions are more likely to occur in the presence of metabolic or respiratory alkalosis. The long-term effects of hyperphosphatemia primarily involve the kidneys, coronary arteries, skeleton, and parathyroid glands.

Hyperphosphatemia in adults is defined as an elevation of serum phosphorus higher than 5 mg/dL (1.67 mmol/L). Hyperphosphatemia is a common finding with many causes. Spurious hyperphosphatemia may occur in patients with thrombocytosis when blood is allowed to clot to obtain serum. Undelayed collection of plasma from heparinized samples will show lower values. Certain autoanalyzers cause spurious hyperphosphatemia because of chemical interference. Abnormal positively charged serum proteins, as in plasma cell dyscrasias, may bind phosphorus and cause marked elevations exceeding 13 mg/dL (4.3 mM).

Decreased renal excretion of phosphorus is the most common cause of hyperphosphatemia. Because PTH is phosphaturic, hyperphosphatemia is a cardinal feature of hypoparathyroidism, either as a primary disorder or in patients whose renal cyclic AMP response to PTH is abnormal (pseudohypoparathyroidism type I) or those whose phosphaturic response to PTH is suppressed (pseudohypoparathyroidism type II) (2).

Severe hypomagnesemia causes marked suppression of PTH in plasma despite hypocalcemia but does not usually cause hyperphosphatemia (81, 82). Hyperphosphatemia occurs in tumoral calcinosis, pseudoxanthoma elasticum, infantile hypophosphatasia, and hyperostosis because of decreased renal excretion. Untreated severe hyperthyroidism apparently increases cellular catabolism sufficiently to elevate serum phosphorus despite increased phosphorus loss in the urine. Acromegaly or administration of growth hormone causes hyperphosphatemia. Presumably, the higher phosphorus levels in children partly reflect growth hormone activity (83) or insulinlike growth factor I activity (84). Hyperphosphatemia occurs in untreated adrenal insufficiency because of volume contraction, metabolic acidosis, and possibly reduced glomerular permeability. Mild hyperphosphatemia may occur with biphosphonate therapy because of increased tubular reabsorption of phosphorus.

Hyperphosphatemia, sometimes with levels up to 46 mg/dL, has occurred secondary to increased absorption from the gut following administration of excess phosphate salts by mouth or from the colon as a result of enemas that contain phosphorus. Overmedication with vitamin D and production of vitamin D by granulomatous tissue such as in sarcoidosis and tuberculosis can cause hyperphosphatemia (2). Both acute metabolic acidosis and acute respiratory acidosis may decompose cellular organic phosphates, reduce phosphorylation, and result in diffusion of phosphorus from the cell and hyperphosphatemia. Lactic acidosis is especially important as a cause of hyperphosphatemia. Reduced insulin levels secondary to clonidine administration also can cause hyperphosphatemia. Cellular release of phosphorus may cause hyperphosphatemia, particularly in rhabdomyolysis, infarction of other tissues, or hemolysis. The tumor lysis syndrome, usually seen in patients whose tumor responds briskly to chemotherapy, consists of hyperphosphatemia, hypocalcemia, hyperkalemia, metabolic acidosis, hyperuricemia, and, in many cases, acute renal failure. Severe hyperphosphatemia after intravenous infusion of phosphate salts is a particular danger in patients who are acidotic or oliguric. Finally, infusion of compounds containing phospholipids for parenteral nutrition has caused hyperphosphatemia.

Treatment

Hyperphosphatemia is potentially serious because of potential metastatic calcification. Before initiating treatment for hyperphsosphatemia, its cause should be identified and corrected whenever possible. Although only an approximate guide, a calcium-phosphorus product (serum calcium/mg/dL × serum phosphorus mg/dL) greater than 70 indicates a potential threat of calcification. Calcification is more likely to occur in the presence of an elevated blood pH or elevated level of PTH.

In the absence of renal insufficiency, hydration or volume expansion by infusing hypotonic saline increases fractional clearance of phosphorus by the kidney. Aluminumbased antacids bind phosphorus in the gut and prevent absorption. Although long-term use of these compounds may result in aluminum toxicity, their use for a short time in acute hyperphosphatemia is safe and may be very helpful. Hyperphosphatemia in the presence of renal insufficiency often requires either peritoneal dialysis or hemodialysis.

REFERENCES

1. Josephus F. Complete Works of Flavius Josephus. Grand Rapids, MI: Kreger Publications, 1960:56.
2. Knochel J, Agarwal R. Hypophosphatemia and hyperphosphatemia. In: Brenner B, ed. The Kidney. 5th ed. Philadelphia: WB Saunders, 1996:1086–1133.
3. Guest GM, Rapoport S. Am J Dis Child 1939;58:1072–89.
4. Simons PCM, Versteegh HAJ, Jongbloed AW et al. J Nutr 1990; 64:525–40.
5. Murer H, Hernando N, Forester I et al. Physiol Rev 2000;80: 1373–1409.
6. Paleologas M, Stone E, Braute S. Clin Sci (Lond) 2000;98: 619–25.
7. Chung PY, Sitrin MD, Te HS. Liver Transplant 2003;9:248–53.
8. Bode JC, Zelder O, Rumpelt HJ et al. Eur J Clin Invest 1973;3: 436–41.
9. Kumar D, McAlister FA. Can J Gastroenterol 1999;13:165–7.
10. Anderson R, Cohen M, Haller R et al. Mineral Electrolyte Metab 1980;4:106–12.
11. DeMarchi S, Cecchin E, Basile A et al. N Engl J Med 1993;329: 1927–34.
12. Elisaf M, Merkouropoulos M, Tsianos EV et al. Miner Electrol Metab 1994;20:274–81.
13. Blachley JD, Ferguson ER, Carter NW et al. Trans Assoc Am Phys 1980;93:110–22.
14. Ferguson ER, Blachley JD, Carter NW et al. Am J Physiol 1984; 246:F700–9.
15. Blachley JD, Johnson JH, Knochel JP. Am J Med Sci 1985;289: 22–6.
16. Veech RL, Gates DN, Crutchfield C et al. Clin Exp Res 1994;18: 1040–56.
17. Angeli P, Gatta A, Caregaro L et al. Gastroenterology 1991;100: 502–12.
18. Peng T, Cooper CW, Munson PL. Endocrinology 1972;91: 586–93.
19. Drezner MK. Kidney Int 2000;57:9–18.
20. White KE, Carn G, Lorenz-Depiereux B et al. Kidney Int 2001; 60:2079–86.
21. Fukumoto S, Yamashita T. Curr Opin Nephrol Hypertens 2002; 11:385–9.
22. Schiavi SC, Kumar R. Kidney Int 2003;65:1–14.
23. Jonsson KB, Zahradnik R, Larson T et al. N Engl J Med 2003; 348:1705–8.
24. Lotz M, Zisman E, Bartter FC. N Engl J Med 1968;278:409–15.

25. Emmet M, Goldfarb S, Agus ZS et al. J Clin Invest 1977;59:291–8.
26. Ravid M, Robson M. JAMA 1976;236:1380.
27. Fuller TJ, Carter NC, Barcenas C et al. J Clin Invest 1976;57:1019–24.
28. Knochel JP, Barcenas C, Cotton JR et al. J Clin Invest 1978;62:1240–6.
29. Knochel JP, Bilbrey GL, Fuller TJ et al. Ann NY Acad Sci 1975;252:274–86.
30. Knochel JP. Am J Med 1982;72:521–35.
31. Knochel JP. Am J Med 1992;92:455–7.
32. Knochel JP, Haller R, Ferguson E. Adv Exp Med Biol 1980;128:323–34.
33. Harsch H. J Clin Psychiatry 1987;48:328–33.
34. Wada S, Nagase T, Koike Y et al. Intern Med 1992;31:478–82.
35. Welsh DG, Lindinger MI. J Appl Physiol 1996;80:1263–9.
36. Knochel JP. Adv Exp Biol Med 1982;151:191–8.
37. Kretz J, Sommer G, Boland R et al. Klin Wochenschr 1980;58:833–7.
38. Zazzo JF, Troche G, Ruel P et al. Intensive Care Med 1995;21:826–31.
39. Bollaert PE, Lev, B, Nace L et al. Chest 1995;107:1698–1701.
40. Fuller TJ, Nichols WW, Brenner BJ et al. J Clin Invest 1978;62:1194.
41. Fuller TJ, Nichols WW, Brenner BJ et al. Adv Exp Biol Med 1977;103:395–400.
42. Brautbar N, Baczynski R, Carpenter C et al. Am J Physiol 1982;242:F699–704.
43. Haglin L, Essen-Gustavsson B, Lindholm A. Acta Vet Scand 1994;35:263–71.
44. Venditti FJ, Marotta C, Panezai FR et al. Miner Electrol Metab 1987;13:19–25.
45. Beumont PJ, Large M. Med J Aust 1991;155:519–22.
46. Schwartz A, Gurman G, Cohen G et al. Eur J Intern Med 2002;13:434.
47. Ognibene A, Ciniglio R, Greifenstein A et al. South Med J 1994;87:65–9.
48. Bottomley PA, Hardy CJ, Roemer PB. Magn Reson Med 1990;14:425–34.
49. Machiels JP, Dive A, Donckier J et al. Am J Emerg Med 1998;16:371–3.
50. Fiaccadori E, Coffsini E, Fracchia C et al. Chest 1994;105:1392–8.
51. Newman JH, Neff TA, Ziporin P. N Engl J Med 1977;296:1101–3.
52. Planas RF, McBrayer RH, Koen PA. Adv Exp Med Biol 1982;151:283–90.
53. Aubier M, Murciano D, Lecogguic Y et al. N Engl J Med 1985;313:420–4.
54. Marchezani F, Valerio G, Dardes N et al. Respiration 2000;67:177–82.
55. Travis SF, Sugerman HJ, Ruberg RL et al. N Engl J Med 1971;285:763–8.
56. Lichtman MA, Miller DR, Cohen J et al. Ann Intern Med 1971;74:562–8.
57. Jacob HS, Amsden P. N Engl J Med 1971;285:1446.
58. Kaiser U, Barth N. Acta Haematol 2001;106:133–5.
59. Melvin JD, Watts RG. Am J Hematol 2002;69:223–4.
60. Astrup P. Adv Exp Med Biol 1970;6:67.
61. Funabiki Y, Tatsukawa H, Ashida K et al. Intern Med 1998;37:911–2.
62. Nakoa K, Wada T, Kamiyana T. Nature 1962;194:877–8.
63. Craddock PR, Yawata Y, Van Santen L et al. N Engl J Med 1974;290:1403.
64. Stossel T.P. Phagocytosis. N Engl J Med 1974;290:717–23.
65. Kiersztejn M, Chervu I, Smogorzewski M et al. J Am Soc Nephrol 1992;2:1484–9.
66. Lichtman MA. N Engl J Med 1974;290:1432–3.
67. Yawata Y, Hebbel RP, Silvis S et al. J Lab Clin Med 1974;84:643–53.
68. Kohaut EC, Klish WJ, Beachler CW et al. Am J Clin Nutr 1977;30:861.
69. Pronove P, Bell NH, Bartter FC. Metabolism 1961;10:364–71.
70. Gold LW, Massry SG, Arieff AI et al. J Clin Invest 1973;52:2556–62.
71. Arruda JAL, Julka NK, Rubinstein H et al. Metabolism 1980;29:826–36.
72. Yawata Y, Craddock P, Hebbel R et al. Clin Res 1973;31:729.
73. Knochel JP. Neurological manifestations of hypophosphatemia and phosphorus depletion. In: Murer H, Knochel JP, Prilipko L et al., eds. Phosphate Metabolic in Neurological Disorders: Proceedings of the WHO Meeting. Geneva: World Health Organization, 1998:43–52.
74. Silvis SE, DiBartolomeo AG, Aaker HM. Am J Gastroenterol 1980;73:215–22.
75. Silvis SE, Paragas PD. J Lab Clin Med 1972;62:513–20.
76. Treloar A, Crook M, Parker L et al. Lancet 1991;338:1467–8.
77. Zurkirchen MA, Misteli M, Conen D. Schweiz Med Wochenschr 1994;124:1807–12.
78. Freiman I, Pettifor JM, Moodley GM. J Pediatr Gastroenterol Nutr 1982;1:547–50.
79. Rosen GH, Boullata JI, O'Rangas EA et al. Crit Care Med 1995;23:1204–10.
80. Clark CL, Sacks GS, Dickerson RN et al. Crit Care Med 1995;23:1504–11.
81. Shils ME. Medicine (Baltimore) 1969;48:61–85.
82. Shils ME. Magnesium. In: Shils ME, Shike M, Olson J, eds. Modern Nutrition in Health and Disease. 8th ed. Philadelphia: Lea & Febiger, 1994:164–84.
83. Haramati A, Mulroney SE, Lumpkin MD. Pediatr Nephrol 1990;4:387–91.
84. Suzuki K, Nonaka K, Ichihara K et al. Bone Miner 1986;1:51–8.

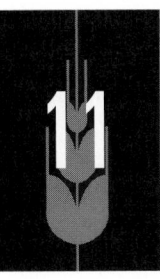

MAGNESIUM[1]

ROBERT K. RUDE AND MAURICE E. SHILS

BIOCHEMISTRY AND PHYSIOLOGY 223
    Enzyme Interactions 223
    Structural Modification of Nucleic Acids and
        Membranes 224
    Ion Channels 224
BODY COMPOSITION AND HOMEOSTASIS 225
    Composition 225
    Cellular Magnesium Homeostasis 225
    Body Homeostasis 227
ASSESSING MAGNESIUM REQUIREMENTS 229
    Assessment of Magnesium Need 229
    Assessment of Dietary Magnesium Intake 230
ASSESSING MAGNESIUM STATUS 231
    Analytic Procedures for Magnesium 231
    Biologic Indicators 231
RISK FACTORS AND CAUSES OF MAGNESIUM
    DEFICIENCY 233
    Prevalence 233
    Key Disorders 233
CLINICAL PRESENTATIONS OF MAGNESIUM
    DEFICIENCY 234
    Laboratory Animals 234
    Humans 234
MANAGEMENT OF MAGNESIUM DEPLETION 239
    Adolescents and Adults .240
    Infants and Young Children 240
MAGNESIUM EXCESS 240
    Causes of Hypermagnesemia 240
    Clinical Presentations of Magnesium Excess 241
    Management of Hypermagnesemia 242

Magnesium (Mg) plays an essential role in a wide range of fundamental biologic reactions. Hence, it is not surprising that Mg deficiency may lead to serious clinical symptoms.

[1]**Abbreviations: AAS,** atomic absorption spectrophotometry; **ADP,** adenosine diphosphate; **AMI,** acute myocardial infarction; **ATP,** adenosine triphosphate; **cAMP,** cyclic adenosine monophosphate; **DRI,** dietary reference intake; **IP₃,** inositol triphosphate; **ISE,** ion-selective electrode; **Mg,** magnesium; **Na,** sodium; **NHANES,** National Health and Nutrition Examination Survey III; **NMR,** nuclear magnetic resonance; **PGI₂,** prostacylin; **PTH,** parathyroid hormone; **RDA,** recommended dietary allowance; **UL,** upper intake level; **USDA,** United States Department of Agriculture.

Kruse and associates made the first systematic observations of Mg deficiency in rats and dogs in the early 1930s (1). The first description of clinical depletion in humans, published in 1934, involved a small number of patients with various underlying diseases (2). In the early 1950s, Flink initiated studies documenting depletion of this ion in patients with alcoholism and in patients receiving Mg-free intravenous solutions (3). Although the diets ordinarily consumed by healthy Americans fall below the recommended dietary allowance (RDA) (4), they do not appear to lead to symptomatic Mg depletion. Some clinical disorders, however, as discussed in this chapter, have been associated with a low-Mg diet.

BIOCHEMISTRY AND PHYSIOLOGY

Mg is widely distributed in nature and is the eighth most abundant element on earth and the second most abundant cation in sea water (5, 6). It has therefore been incorporated widely in biology and is the fourth most abundant cation in the body and the second most prevalent intracellular cation (5, 6). The chemistry of Mg dictates its role in biologic processes (5, 6). Its ionic radius is small; however, the hydrated radius is large. It exists as a hexacoordinate in a rigid octahedron structure. It exchanges water slowly and thus is quite stable. Because of its positive charge, Mg binds to negatively charged molecules. Most intracellular Mg ($[Mg^{2+}]_i$) binds to ribosomes, membranes, and other macromolecules in the cytosol and nucleus. Mg provides specific structure and catalytic activity for enzymes, as discussed in the following section.

Enzyme Interactions

Mg is involved in more than 300 essential metabolic reactions (7). Mg ion (Mg^{2+}) forms complexes with a variety of organic molecules having biologic activities. The relatively high—in comparison with other electrolytes—extracellular and intracellular concentrations of Mg^{2+} tend to favor binding to such molecules. The binding of functional groups is, in descending order: phosphates > carboxylates > hydroxyls, in terms of both relative importance and binding affinities (5, 8, 9). Mg^{2+} is essential for many enzymatic reactions and has two general interactions: (a) Mg^{2+} binds to the substrate, thereby forming a complex with which the enzyme interacts, as in the reaction of kinases with Mg adenosine triphosphate (MgATP); and (b) Mg^{2+} binds directly to the enzyme and alters its structure and/or serves a catalytic role (e.g, exonuclease, topoisomerase, and RNA- and DNA polymerases) (8, 9). Other divalent metal ions (especially manganese) activate many of the same enzymes but usually have less specificity and/or are present in much smaller quantities. Overall, the predominant action of Mg is related to ATP utilization. ATP has a strategic position in "free-energy" currency for virtually all cellular processes by providing high-energy phosphate. It exists in all cells primarily as $MgATP^{2-}$.

Some examples of the numerous enzymes in both classes mentioned earlier emphasize the important role of Mg (5, 6, 10, 11). They include hexokinase, which phosphorylates glucose by way of MgATP and other enzymes necessary for the glycolytic cycle. Mg is required in steps of the citric acid cycle; three of the four key enzymes in the gluconeogenesis pathway from noncarbohydrate sources require Mg. It is required in lipid metabolism, amino acid activation via RNA and DNA polymerases, the transketolase reaction involving thiamin, and the transfer of carbon dioxide to biotin in carboxylation reactions. Glutathione, a key intracellular antioxidant, has an Mg^{2+} requirement for its synthesis. The ubiquitin-proteosome pathway of protein degradation also requires Mg^{2+} and ATP. Protein kinases, enzymes that catalyze the transfer of the α-phosphate from MgATP (e.g. in intracellular signaling), number more than 100 (11).

Mg plays a critical role in the second messenger systems. Cyclic adenosine monophosphate (cAMP) is formed from MgATP and in addition this enzyme, adenylate cyclase, is activated by Mg^{2+} through two binding sites (11–13). Mg^{2+} is also an important physiologic regulator of the phospholipase C second messenger system. First, an Mg^{2+}-dependent guanine nucleotide regulating protein is involved in activation of phospholipase C (14, 15). Mg^{2+} has also been shown to be a noncompetitive inhibitor of inositol triphosphate (IP_3)-induced calcium (Ca^{2+}) release (16). It is clear that the effect of Mg depletion on cellular function in terms of the second messenger systems is most complex, involving substrate availability, G-protein activity, release and sensitivity to intracellular Ca^{2+}, and phospholipid metabolism.

Structural Modification of Nucleic Acids and Membranes

Another important role of Mg is its ability to form complexes with nucleic acids. The negatively charged ribose phosphate structure of nucleic acids has a high affinity for Mg^{2+}; the resulting stabilization of numerous ribonucleotides and deoxyribonucleotides induces important physicochemical changes that affect DNA maintenance, duplication, and transcription (7–9, 17–19). In addition, the binding of hydrated Mg^{2+} by transfer RNA (tRNA) and modified tRNA and its DNA analogs results in structures that cannot be duplicated by the binding of other metals (7–9, 17, 19).

Mg, Ca^{2+}, and some other cations react with hydrophilic polyanionic carboxylates and phosphates of the various membrane components to stabilize the membrane and thereby affect fluidity and permeability. This process influences ion channels, transporters, and signal transducers (6).

Ion Channels

Ion channels constitute a class of proteins across the cell membrane that allow passage of ions into or out of cells when the channels are open. Ion channels are classified according to the type of ion they allow to pass such as sodium (Na^+), potassium (K^+), or Ca^{2+} (20, 21). Mg^{2+} plays an important role in the function of a number of ion channels.

A deficit of Mg results in cellular K^+ depletion. Several mechanisms may contribute to the K^+ loss. Mg^{2+} is necessary for the active transport of K^+ out of cells by Na^+, K^+ ATPase. Mg-depleted animals and humans have been found to have a reduced concentration of Na^+/K^+-ATPase pumps in skeletal muscle, and this may contribute to the decrease in cellular K^+ (22). ATPase is also dependent on Mg^{2+}, and therefore Na^+ and K^+ transport may be impaired during Mg deficiency (23). Another mechanism for the K^+ loss is an increased efflux of K^+ from cells via other Mg^{2+}-sensitive K^+ channels, as has been seen in skeletal muscle (22) and in heart muscle (24, 25). These K^+ channels normally allow K^+ to pass more readily inward than outward. Mg appears to regulate the outward movement of K^+ so in the absence of Mg^{2+}, K^+ is transported equally well in both directions. Therefore, a deficiency in Mg^{2+} may lead to a reduced amount of intracellular K^+. Because the resting membrane potential of heart muscle cells is determined in part by the intracellular K^+ concentration, a decreased intracellular K^+ concentration will result in a less negative resting membrane potential. The arrhythmogenic effect of Mg deficiency, as discussed later, may therefore be related to its effect on maintenance of intracellular K^+.

Mg has been called nature's physiologic Ca^{2+} channel blocker (26). During Mg depletion, intracellular Ca^{2+} rises. This may be caused by both an increase from extracellular Ca^{2+} and release from intracellular Ca^{2+} stores. Mg^{2+} has been demonstrated to decrease the inward Ca^{2+} flux through slow Ca^{2+} channels (21, 25). In addition, Mg^{2+} will decrease the transport of Ca^{2+} out of the sarcoplasmic reticulum into the cell cytosol. As stated earlier, the inverse ability of IP_3 to release Ca^{2+} from intracellular stores in response to changes in Mg^{2+} concentrations would also allow a greater rise in intracellular Ca^{2+} during a fall in Mg^{2+}.

BODY COMPOSITION AND HOMEOSTASIS

Composition

The distribution of Mg in various body compartments of apparently healthy adults is summarized in Table 11.1. Approximately 60% of Mg is in the skeleton, of which two thirds of it is within the hydration shell and one third on the crystal surface (27), and it may serve as a reservoir for maintaining extracellular Mg and $[Mg^{2+}]_i$. Only 1% of Mg is in the extracellular fluid, and the rest is intracellular.

Reference values for Mg in serum and blood cells and in adults, infants, and children have been published (28–30). Mg is the most abundant divalent mineral cation in cells and is second only in electrolyte quantity to monovalent K.

TABLE 11.1. DISTRIBUTION AND CONCENTRATIONS OF MAGNESIUM (Mg) IN A HEALTHY ADULT (TOTAL BODY: 833–1170 MMOL[a], or 20–28 g)

SITE	PERCENTAGE OF TOTAL-BODY Mg	CONCENTRATION/ CONTENT
Bone	53	0.5% of bone ash
Muscle	27	9 mmol/kg wet weight
Soft tissue	19	9 mmol/kg wet weight
Adipose tissue	0.012	0.8 mmol/kg wet weight[b]
Erythrocytes	0.5	1.65–2.73 mmol/L[c]
Serum	0.3	0.88 ± 0.06 mml/L[d]
% Total		
Free	65	0.56 ± 0.05 m/mol/L[e]
Complexed	8	
Bound	27	
Mononuclear		2.91 ± 0.6 fmol/cell[g]
Blood cells[f]		2.79 ± 0.6 fmol/cell[h]
		3.00 ± 0.4 fmol/cell[i]
Platelets		2.26 ± 0.29 mmol/L[j]
$[Mg^{2+}]_i$[k]		0.5–1.0 mmol/L
Cerebrospinal fluid		1.25 mmol/L
Free 55%		
Complexed 45%		
Secretions		
Saliva, gastric, bile		0.3–0.7 mmolL
Sweat		0.3 mmol/L (38°C)[l]
		0.09 mmol/h[m]

[a] 1 mmol = 2 mEq = 24.3 mg.
[b] From Snyder et al. Report of the Task Group on Reference Man. Elmsford, NY: Pergamon Press, 1975:306.
[c] Mg falls slowly with aging.
[d] Similar at various ages.
[e] From Huijgen HJ, Van Ingen HE, Kok WT et al. Clin Biochem 1996;29:261–6.
[f] Monocytes and lymphocytes in venous blood.
[g] From Elin RJ, Hosseini JM. Clin Chem 1985;31:377–80. 1 fmol = 24.3 fg.
[h] From Reinhart RA, Marx JJ Jr, Haas RG et al. Clin Clim Acta 1987;167:187–95.
[i] From Yang et al. J Am Coll Nutr 1990;9:328.
[j] From Niemala JE et al. Clin Chem 1996;42:S280.
[k] Intracellular free Mg concentration.
[l] From Consolazio CF, Matoush LO, Nelson RA et al. J Nutr 1963;79:407.
[m] From Wenk C, Kohut M, Kunz G et al. Z Ernahrungswiss 1993;32:301–7.

Cellular Magnesium Homeostasis

As stated earlier, Mg is compartmentalized within the cell, and most of it is bound to proteins and negatively charged molecules. Significant amounts of Mg are found in the nucleus, mitochondria, the endoplasmic and sarcoplasmic reticulum, and the cytoplasm (5, 6, 31, 32). Total cell Mg concentration has been reported to range between 5 and 20 mM (31, 32). Ninety to 95% of that in the cytosol is bound to ligands such as ATP, adenosine diphosphate (ADP), citrate, proteins, and nucleic acids. The remainder is free Mg^{2+}, constituting 1 to 5% of the total cellular Mg (33–35). The process that maintains or modifies the relationships between total and ionized internal and external Mg is incompletely understood. (5, 6, 31, 32, 36).

The concentration of free ionized Mg^{2+} that has been measured in the cytoplasm of mammalian cells has ranged from 0.2 to 1.0 mM, depending on cell type and means of measurement (6, 37–40). The Mg^{2+} concentration in the cell cytoplasm is maintained relatively constant even when the Mg^{2+} concentration in the extracellular fluid is experimentally varied to either high or low nonphysiologic levels (41–43). The relative constancy of the Mg^{2+} in the intracellular milieu is attributed to the limited permeability of the plasma membrane to Mg and to the operation of specific Mg transport systems that regulate the rates at which Mg is taken up or extruded from cells (5, 6, 32). Although the concentration differential between the cytoplasm and the extracellular fluid for Mg^{2+} is minimal, Mg^{2+} enters cells down an electrochemical gradient because of the relative electronegativity of the cell interior. Maintenance of the normal intracellular concentrations of Mg^{2+} requires that Mg be actively transported out of the cell. Mg transport into or out of cells appears to require the presence of carrier-mediated transport systems, possibly regulated by the concentration of Mg^{2+} within the cell (32, 44, 45). The efflux of Mg from the cell appears to be coupled to Na transport and requires energy (5, 6, 32, 46). Maintenance of this process would require the subsequent extrusion of Na by Na^+/K^+-ATPase. Evidence also indicates an Na-independent efflux of Mg, however (45, 46). Mg influx appears to be linked to Na transport but by a different mechanism than efflux (45, 47). The molecular characteristics of the Mg transport proteins have not been described. Studies in prokaryotes, however, have identified four separate transport proteins for Mg (48, 49).

Studies have demonstrated that tissues vary with respect to the rates at which Mg exchange occurs and the percentage of total Mg, which is readily exchangeable (6, 36). The rate of Mg exchange in heart, liver, and kidney exceeded that in skeletal muscle, lymphocytes, red blood cells, brain, and testis. These studies do show that, albeit slow in some tissues, a continuous equilibration of Mg between cells and the extracellular fluid occurs. Increased cellular Mg content has been reported for rapidly proliferating cells, a finding indicating a relationship between the metabolic state of a cell and the relative rates of Mg transport (50).

Mg transport in mammalian cells is influenced by hormonal and pharmacologic factors. Mg^{2+} efflux was stimulated after short-term exposure of isolated perfused rat heart and liver (32, 51–54) or thymocytes (55) to α- and β-agonists and permeant cAMP. Because $[Mg^{2+}]_i$ did not change, a redistribution from the mitchondria was suggested, given that cAMP can induce Mg^{2+} release from this compartment (56). Current data suggest that two adrenergic signaling pathways mobilize Mg^{2+} from two distinct cellular pools (57). In contrast, Mg^{2+} influx was stimulated by β-agonists after a more prolonged exposure in hepatocytes, as well as in adipocytes and vascular smooth muscle, presumably mediated by protein kinase A (32, 45, 58). However, the rate of Mg^{2+} uptake by the mouse lymphoma S49 cell line is inhibited by β-adrenergic agents (59). Activation of protein kinase C by diacylglycerol or by phorbol esters also stimulates Mg^{2+} influx and does not alter efflux (32, 60, 61).

Growth factors may also influence Mg^{2+} uptake by cells. Epidermal growth factor has been shown to increase Mg^{2+} transport into a vascular smooth muscle cell line (62). Insulin and dextrose were found to increase ^{28}Mg uptake by certain tissues, including skeletal and cardiac muscle, in which total cellular Mg content increased as well (5, 6, 63). Increased amounts of total $[Mg^{2+}]_i$ following treatment with insulin in vitro have been reported in uterine smooth muscle and chicken embryo fibroblasts (64, 65). The mechanism of insulin-induced Mg transport is likely the result of an effect on protein kinase C (5, 6). Insulin-induced transport of Mg into cells could be one factor responsible for the fall in the serum Mg concentration observed during insulin therapy of diabetic ketoacidosis (66). The effect of insulin on total cellular Mg may differ from its effects on intracellular free Mg^{2+}. Measurements of the intracellular free Mg^{2+} in frog skeletal muscle failed to show an effect of insulin; however, other studies demonstrated that insulin increases Mg^{2+} in human red blood cells, platelets, and lymphocytes (67–69).

Despite these changes in cellular Mg, the ionized fraction does not change, a finding suggesting that these changes affect shifts in Mg binding within the cell (6). Investigators have hypothesized that this hormonally regulated Mg uptake system controls $[Mg^{2+}]_i$ concentration in cellular subcytoplasmic compartments. The Mg^{2+} concentration in these compartments would then serve to regulate the activity of Mg-sensitive enzymes. An overall schema of cellular Mg homeostasis is shown in Figure 11.1.

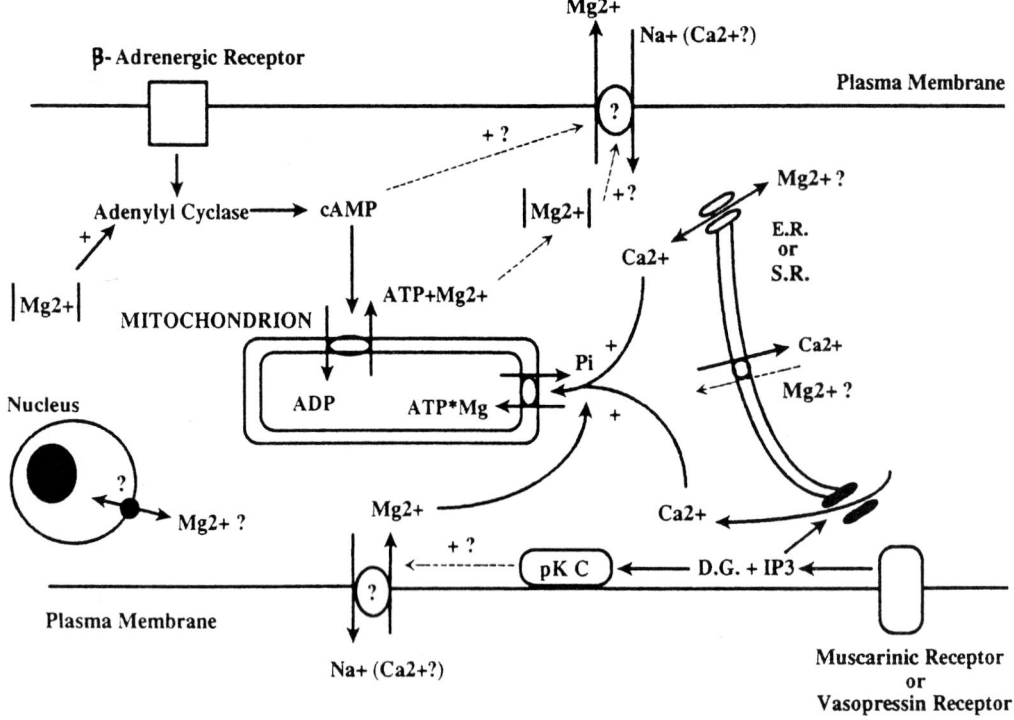

Figure 11.1. Schema of regulation of cellular magnesium (Mg^{2+}) homeostasis in the mammalian cell. The pathways are indicated for cellular Mg^{2+} release **(upper section)** and for its uptake **(lower section)**. Stimulated by β-adrenergic agonists, cyclic adenosine monophosphate (cAMP) is increased in the cytosol, which modulates mitochondrial adenine nucleotide translocase and increases the efflux of Mg^{2+} from the mitochondrion by means of an exchange of one Mg-adenosine triphosphate (ATP) for adenosine diphosphate (ADP). Activation of muscarinic receptors (in cardiac cells) or vasopressin receptors (in the liver) may stimulate an Mg^{2+} influx mechanism either by decreasing cAMP or by enhancing protein kinase C (pK C) activity by diacylglycerol (D.G.). Vasopressin receptor activation is coupled with production of inositol triphosphate (IP₃) from phosphatidylinositol bisphosphate, which induces release of calcium ion (Ca^{2+}) from the endoplasmic reticulum (E.R.) or the sarcoplasmic reticulum (S.R.). Ca^{2+} release may be associated with either Mg^{2+} influx or Mg redistribution in the nucleus or endoplasmic reticulum. (From Romani A, Marfella C, Scarpa A. Miner Electrolyte Metab 1993;19:282–9, with permission.)

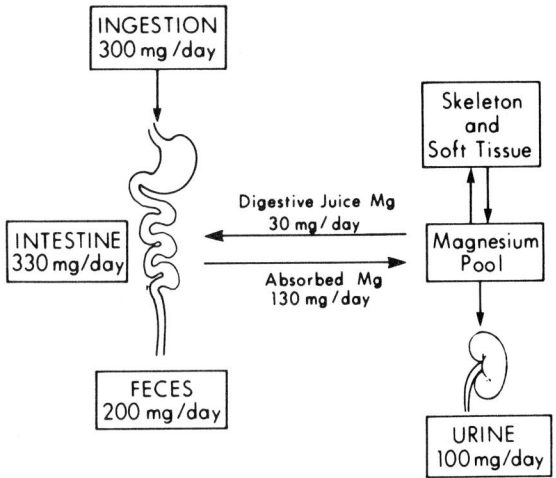

Figure 11.2. Magnesium homeostasis in humans. A schematic representation of its metabolic economy indicating (*a*) its absorption from the alimentary tract, (*b*) its distribution into tissue pools with major distribution into bone, and (*c*) its dependence on the kidney for excretion. Homeostasis depends on the integrity of intestinal and renal absorptive processes. (From Slatapolsky E. In: Klahr S, ed. Pathophysiology of Calcium, Magnesium and Phosphorus Metabolism in the Kidney and Body Fluids. New York: Plenum Publishing, 1984, with permission.)

Body Homeostasis

Homeostasis of the individual with respect to a mineral depends on the amounts ingested, the efficiency of intestinal and renal absorption and excretion, and all other relevant factors. A schema for Mg balance is given in Figure 11.2.

Dietary Intake

Mg is widely distributed in plant and animal sources but in differing concentrations (see Appendix Table A-22-a). The major food sources of the element beyond childhood to ages 60 to 65 years in the United States as percentages of the daily intake have been listed (70). Vegetables, fruits, grains, and animal products accounted for approximately 16% each; dairy product contributions fell from about 20% in adolescents to about 10% for those beyond the third decade; beverages of various types yielded percentages of about 4% among adolescents and increased to 15% in older age groups.

The 1994, the United States Department of Agriculture (USDA) Continuing Survey of Food Intakes by Individuals indicated that the mean daily Mg intake was 323 mg in males and 228 mg in females (4), findings similar to those of the National Health and Nutrition Examination Survey III (NHANES III) (71). These values fall below the current RDA recommendation of approximately 420 mg for males and 320 mg for females (4). Indeed, it has been suggested that 75% of persons in the United States have dietary Mg intake that falls below the recommended intake (72, 73) (see the later discussion of Mg requirements).

When calculating individual intake from food composition tables, caution is advised because "there is less than 75% analytical data for important sources of this food component" (74). An example is the analyzed versus calculated values (using the USDA database) for the 234 foods in the US Food and Drug Administration Total Dietary Study for eight age-sex groups, representing the core items of the US food supply. The analyzed figures were 115 to 124% greater than the calculated values (unadjusted for missing values in the database) among the age groups reported (70, 75). Inadequate or few data exist for this ion in some products (76).

Intestinal Absorption

In humans, the primary sites of intestinal Mg absorption are the jejunum and the ileum, although absorption can occur at other sites including the colon (77–79). Under a normal dietary Mg intake, 30 to 40% of is absorbed. Based on the time of appearance of ^{28}Mg in the blood following its oral ingestion, absorption begins within 1 hour, stabilizes at the rate of 4 to 6%/hour from the second to the eighth hour, then decreases rapidly, and ceases at the tenth hour (80). Both a passive paracellular mechanism and an active transport process for Mg absorption exist (Fig. 11.3). The paracellullar mechanism depends on a transcellular potential difference generated by Na transport and accounts for about 90% of intestinal Mg absorption (78, 79). An Mg-specific transport protein/channel that is not yet well defined accounts for the remainder of Mg absorption. Absorption of Mg as a function of intake is curvilinear (see Fig. 11.3) and reflects this active saturable

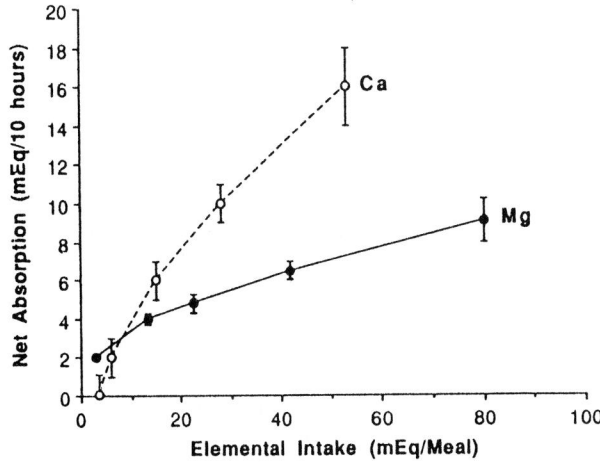

Figure 11.3. Net magnesium (Mg) and calcium (Ca) absorption in healthy humans. The data were obtained under conditions described in reference 80 and in the text. Mean values S.E. are indicated by *vertical bars*. The absorption data for magnesium represent a curved function compatible with a saturable process (at about 10 mEq/meal in this study) and a linear function reflecting passive diffusion at higher intakes. (From Fine KD, Santa Ana CA, Porter JL et al. J Clin Invest 1991;88:396–402, with permission.)

process and passive diffusion. Net Mg absorption increases with further Mg intake; however, fractional Mg absorption falls. When small amounts of Mg were fed in the form of a standard meal supplemented by varying amounts of Mg (81) or when Mg was given as ^{28}Mg (82), fractional absorption fell progressively from approximately 65 to 70% with intake of 7 to 36 mg (0.3–1.5 mmol) down to 11 to 14% with intake of 960 to 1000 mg (40 mmol).

Data on absorption fractions from balance studies using differing diets have been quite variable, ranging from 35 to 70% (83). When free-living adults eating self-selected diets were evaluated periodically over the course of a year, the mean absorptive fraction averaged 21% with an average intake of 323 mg (13.4 mmol) by men and 27% with an average intake of 234 mg (9.75 mmol) by women (84).

Bioavailability: Influence of Other Dietary Factors

The fractional absorption of ingested Mg by healthy persons is influenced by its dietary concentration, as discussed earlier, as well as by the presence of dietary components inhibiting or promoting Mg absorption. Long-term balance studies in healthy persons, for the most part, indicated that increasing oral Ca intake does not significantly affect Mg absorption or retention (85–87). Increased amounts of Mg in the diet have been associated with either decreased Ca absorption (88) or no effect (81, 89). Although increased Mg intake may not affect intestinal Ca absorption, renal tubular mechanisms may increase Ca excretion (81) as discussed later.

Some reports indicated decreased Mg absorption at high levels of dietary phosphate, whereas others found no consistent effect (90–92). Increased amounts of absorbable oral Mg have been noted to decrease phosphate absorption, perhaps secondary to formation of insoluble Mg phosphate (81). Decreased absorption of Mg associated with high phosphate intake did not change Mg balance because of associated decreased urinary excretion of Mg (81).

A major increase in zinc intake (from 12 to 142 mg/day) decreased Mg absorption and balance very significantly (93). Vitamin B_6 depletion induced in young women was associated with negative Mg balance because of increased urinary excretion (94). The presence of excessive amounts of free fatty acids and oxalate may also impair Mg absorption (95).

Increased intakes of dietary fiber have been reported to decrease Mg utilization in humans, presumably by decreasing absorption. However, the introduction of uncontrolled variables, including multiple differences among dietary components in addition to fiber contents, complicates interpretation of the data (92, 96, 97). When isolated fiber was added to a basal diet, the effects of fiber per se were negative for dephytinized barley fiber (98) and positive for cellulose (99).

Absorbability of Magnesium Salts in Humans

Multiple salts of Mg are available as dietary supplements including oxide, hydroxide, citrate, chloride, gluconate,

lactate, and aspartate. The fractional absorption of a salt depends on its solubility in intestinal fluids and the amounts ingested; for example, 5 mmol (120 mg) of the acetate in gelatin capsules has been found to be an optimal dose in terms of net absorption (81). Absorption of enteric-coated Mg chloride is 67% less than that of the acetate in gelatin capsules (81). In one study, Mg citrate was found to have high solubility, even in water, whereas Mg oxide was poorly soluble even in acid solution; better absorption of the citrate salt was demonstrated in humans (100). Little difference in absorption has been demonstrated among other salts, however (101–103). Mg oxide and various salts in large doses act as an osmotic laxative, with resultant diarrhea; the physician faced with a patient with diarrhea of uncertain origin should consider measuring fecal Mg levels (89).

Regulation of Magnesium Absorption

No hormone or factor has been described that regulates Mg metabolism. The effect of vitamin D on Mg absorption is unclear. Vitamin D and its active metabolites have been shown to increase intestinal Mg absorption in some studies (78, 79). The active metabolite of vitamin D, $1,25(OH)_2$-vitamin D, increases intestinal absorption in physiologically normal human subjects (104) and in patients with chronic renal failure (105, 106). Similar data are available in animal models (78). In balance studies, vitamin D and its metabolites increased intestinal Mg absorption but much less than Ca (107, 108). Mean Mg balance was not affected. In patients with impaired Ca absorption who were given vitamin D or its active form, those with both osteomalacia and osteoporosis had equivocal improvement in Mg absorption (108). Patients with osteomalacia or hypoparathyroidism or hyperparathyroidism had only small increases in Mg absorption compared with Ca (108, 109). Mg was absorbed by persons with no detectable plasma $1,25(OH)_2$-vitamin D, and, in contrast to Ca absorption, no significant correlation exists between plasma $1,25(OH)_2$-vitamin D and Mg absorption (109). Persons with absorptive hypercalciuria resulting from increased intestinal Ca absorption have normal Mg absorption (110, 111).

Renal Regulation

Filtration and Tubular Absorption. The kidney is the critical organ regulating Mg homeostasis. Mg handling is a filtration/reabsorption process. The kidney plays a critical role in excreting the Mg that is not retained for tissue growth or turnover replacement (112–114). About 10% (~100 mmol or 2400 mg) of the total body Mg is normally filtered daily through the glomeruli in the healthy adult; of this, only about 5% is excreted in the urine. Approximately 75% of the serum Mg is ultrafilterable at the glomeruli. The fractional absorption of the filtered load in the various segments of the nephron is summarized in Figure 11.4. Approximately 15 to 20% of filtered Mg is reabsorbed in

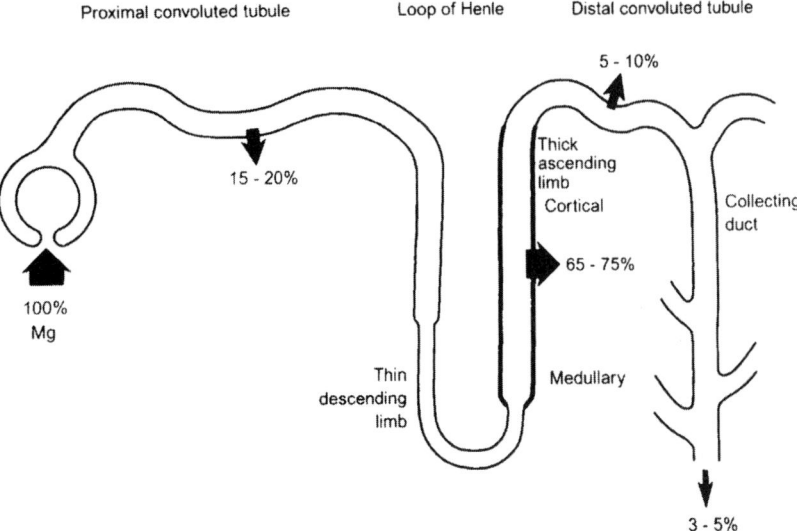

Figure 11.4. Fractional segmental reabsorption of filtered magnesium (Mg^{2+}) in the nephron. The percentage absorption of filtered Mg^{2+} has been determined by micropuncture techniques in various laboratory animals as the Mg^{2+} proceeds through the nephron. Approximately 15 to 20% of the Mg^{2+} is reabsorbed in the proximal convoluted tubule. The major site for Mg^{2+} reabsorption is the thick ascending limb of the loop of Henle, primarily in its cortical portion. Here, 65 to 75% of Mg^{2+} leaves the lumen. In the distal convoluted tubule, 5 to 10% of Mg^{2+} is reabsorbed. (From Cole DE, Quamme GA. J Am Soc Nephol 2000;11:1937-7, with permission).

the proximal convoluted tubule, presumably by a paracellular mechanism. The majority, 65 to 75%, is reclaimed in the cortical thick ascending limb of Henle. The mechanism also appears to be paracellular transport. A gene, paracellin-1, has been shown to encode for a protein thought to mediate Mg transport at this site. The distal convoluted tubule reabsorbs 5 to 10% of filtered Mg via an active transcellular pathway (112–114).

Hormonal and Other Regulator Influences on Absorption. Micropuncture studies in rodents showed that arginine vasopressin, glucagon, calcitonin, parathyroid hormone (PTH), and (to a lesser degree) an adrenergic agonist and insulin, when added individually to the bath of mouse segments of the cortical thick ascending limb of loop of Henle and/or the distal convoluted tubule, significantly increased Mg absorption (112, 114, 115). The physiologic significance of these observations, however, is unclear. Proof that Mg balance is normally regulated hormonally would require that certain changes in serum Mg levels liberate one or more of these hormones into the blood and act on the tubule (115).

Although the regulatory mechanisms are unclear, certain conditions affect absorption, principally in the ascending thick limb. Inhibition occurs with hypermagnesemia and hypercalcemia (112–114). This is thought to occur because these cations bind to a Ca-sensitive receptor on the basolateral aspect of these tubular cells, decrease transepithelial voltage, and thereby decrease the paracellular absorption of both Mg and Ca. Decreased Mg intake in experimental animals and humans rapidly decreases Mg excretion, even before serum/plasma Mg levels fall below the normal range, a finding suggesting an adaption of the kidney to Mg insufficiency (112–114).

The close relationship between Mg and K is clearly demonstrated in renal function. In the rat and in humans, Mg depletion results in K loss. In the Mg-deficient rat, K^+ entry into the tubule lumen occurs at the distal convoluted tubule and is associated with a rise in plasma aldosterone levels (116).

Tissue Sources

Extracellular Mg and $[Mg^{2+}]_i$ and that in bone compartments fall during Mg depletion. Bone may serve as an important reservoir for Mg. Human iliac crest changes indicate a broad range of loss during depletion with a weighted average of 18%, or 1.2 mmol/kg body weight (117). In young Mg-deficient rats and mice, the major body loss was from bone (~30% of that in bone), with much less from muscle; however, age and duration of study affected the amounts lost (117–119). During starvation in a study of human obesity associated with acidosis, significant amounts of Mg were lost from lean body mass and bone (120). In an experimental human study of about 3 weeks' duration with resulting asymptomatic hypomagnesemia, no significant decrease in muscle Mg was noted; presumably, bone and other soft tissues were the sources of loss (121).

Sweat Losses

The amount of Mg lost in sweat is very small in comparison with other cations. For example, in a 10-km run in 40.5 minutes with an average body weight (fluid) loss of 1.45 kg, the actual ion losses per kg of weight loss were as follows: Na, 800 mg; K, 200 mg; Ca, 20 mg; and Mg, 5 mg (122).

ASSESSING MAGNESIUM REQUIREMENTS

Assessment of Magnesium Need

The Food and Nutrition Board of the Institute of Medicine has periodically published standards of adequacy. Table 11.2 compares the 1989 RDAs with those of the 1997 dietary reference intakes (DRIs) by age and gender.

TABLE 11.2. COMPARISON OF 1989 AND 1997 RECOMMENDATIONS FOR DAILY INTAKES OF MAGNESIUM

	1989[a]			1997[b]			
AGE (y)	MALE (mg)	FEMALE (mg)	AGE (y)	MALE	FEMALE		
0–0.5	40	40	0–0.5	30[c]	30[c]	AI	
0.5–1.0	60	60	0.5–1.0	74[d]	75[d]	AI	
1–3	80	80	1–3	80	80		
4–6	120	120	4–8	130	130		
7–10	170	170	9–13	240	240		
11–14	270	280	14–18	410	360		
15–18	400	300	19–30	400	310		
19–24	350	280	31–50	420	320		
25–50	350	280	51–70	420	320		
51+	350	280	>70	420	320		
Pregnant	320	<18			400		
		19–30			350		
		31–50			360		
Lactating							
First 6 months		<18			400		
Second 6 months		19–30			350		
		31–50			320		

AI, adequate intake.

[a] Food and Nutrition Board, National Research Council. Recommended Dietary Allowances. 10th ed. Washington, DC: National Academy Press, 1989.
[b] Food and Nutrition Board, Institute of Medicine. Dietary Reference Intakes for Calcium, Phosphorus, Magnesium, Vitamin D, and Fluoride. Washington, DC: National Academy Press, 1997.
[c] Intake from human milk by healthy breast-fed infants.
[d] Human milk plus solid food.

The latter are uniformly higher for children 4 years or more and for adults.

Because excessive Mg intake from nonfood sources causes adverse effects, the DRIs (4) established tolerable upper intake levels (UL) for such sources. The UL for adolescents and adults is 350 mg (14.6 mmol)/day. This is based on the lowest observed adverse effect level of 360 mg (15 mmol)/day.

According to DRI Table S-3 (4), infant levels are based on estimates of Mg content of adequate human intake, whereas most other ages have data based on balance studies. We previously discussed the difficulties in performing balance studies with specific reference to the difficulties in achieving zero balance (i.e., equilibrium) and uncertainties presented by variability in subject energy expenditure and body build (123). Tables 6-1, 6-4, and 6-5 in reference 4 have data on balance and supplementation studies used in developing the RDAs. It is apparent from these tables that the numbers of persons studied are quite limited and their age variations are quite large; only one study (by Spencer and colleagues) had long adaptation and balance periods, and few of the subjects in the various studies were in Mg equilibrium. Suffice it to say, until we have both adequate knowledge and useful methodology in estimating changes in the various body pools of Mg with the varying and controlled intakes of Mg over appropriate periods, we will rely on rather crude methods of estimating the needs of significant numbers of healthy persons. Appendix Tables A-2-a through A-2-k provide information on the DRIs, definitions, and use of all DRI data published to date. Appendix

Tables A-3-b-1 and A-3-b-2 represent the 1989 and 1990 US and Canadian RDAs for comparison.

Assessment of Dietary Magnesium Intake

Estimates of Mg intakes in NHANES III (1988–1991) indicated that children 2 to 11 years old grouped by gender, age, and race/ethnicity had median intakes well above their RDAs. Those ages 1 to 5 years in the lower fifth percentile took in about 90% of the RDA, which includes a safety factor (74–76). Conversely, boys and men and girls and women from 12 to more than 60 years old, grouped by race and ethnicity, with the exception of non-Hispanic white boys and men, had low median intakes in terms of the RDA (76).

The basis for the claims that many adolescents and adults in the United States are at risk of Mg depletion rests on the accuracy of two indices: the dietary intake data summarized in NHANES and the RDA. If either or both of these are seriously inaccurate, the extent of potential depletion will be either higher or lower. The *Third Report on Nutrition Monitoring in the United States* (1995) analyzed intake in relation to the RDA for age and gender; it concluded that Mg presents a potential public health issue requiring further study (76). One reason given was that the medium intakes of Mg from food were lower than the RDAs in various population groups.

Assessment of Mg status of large numbers of healthy persons at various dietary Mg intakes has not been performed. It is therefore impossible to estimate what level of intake would place one at risk for a problem associated with Mg deficiency. Serum Mg was determined by atomic absorption spectrometry in 15,820 healthy persons in the NHANES I (1971–1974) survey; 95% of adults ages 18 to 74 years had serum levels in the range of 0.75 to 0.96 mmol/L (1.50–1.92 mEq/L), with a mean of 0.85 mmol/L. The levels of the fifth percentile were at or above the lower levels of normal (i.e., 0.70–0.73 mmol/L) (124, 125). Although serum Mg concentration correlated with blood pressure, this parameter may not reflect true body Mg status.

ASSESSING MAGNESIUM STATUS

Because Mg is mostly within cells or in bone, assessment of Mg status is most difficult. Certain laboratory techniques are used in clinical and research investigations.

Analytic Procedures for Magnesium

Various methods have been developed to measure Mg in foods, excreta, blood, cells, and cell compartments.

Atomic Absorption Spectrophotometry

Atomic absorption spectrophotometry (AAS) has been widely used to determine total Mg in many sources and still remains the reference method because it provides greater accuracy and precision than other methods (126, 127). Numerous metallochromic indicators and dyes change color when they are bound to Mg, and clinical laboratories now almost exclusively use one of the these chromophores in automated instruments with varying precision compared with AAS. With experience and proper calibration, these methods are acceptable (127). Inductively coupled plasma emission spectroscopy is useful for determination of certain minerals including Mg in serum, urine, and, after wet washing, stool or foods (128).

Ionized Magnesium and Ion-Selective Electrodes

Electrodes have been developed that can measure ionized Mg in serum, plasma, and whole blood (33–35, 129). Ca^{2+} and lipophilic cations (e.g., acetylcholine and cation substitutes) may interfere. In determination of ionized Mg, free Ca is simultaneously determined, and a correction factor is applied. The current clinical chemistry literature indicates that ion-selective electrodes (ISEs) from various manufacturers differ in accuracy from each other and from AAS and may give misleading results in sera with low Mg concentrations (34, 35, 130). Several reports have reviewed the combination of methods that allows measurement of all known serum Mg parameters (34, 35, 129). ISEs for Mg have also been developed and applied for study of $[Mg^{2+}]_i$ homeostasis (34, 35).

Nuclear Magnetic Resonance Spectroscopy

Certain intracellular metabolites exist in equilibrium between uncomplexed and complexed Mg^{2+}. Because the resonances of such molecules may shift on Mg^{2+} complexation, nuclear magnetic resonance (NMR) spectra can provide information on $[[Mg^{2+}]_i$. ATP is the most useful endogenous indicator because of the ^{31}P nuclei and its high concentration and broad distribution in cells. The observed shift difference between α- and β-phosphate resonances was originally used as the parameter of choice; however, the α/β peak height ratio of ATP provides a more sensitive measure of $[Mg^{2+}]$ (33, 34, 131, 132). This method is used to measure $[Mg^{2+}]_i$ noninvasively in many tissues and cells. Technical issues in methodology have been discussed (33, 133). Exogenous magnetic resonance spectroscopy indicators have been developed to measure cytosolic Mg^{2+}; such indicators gain sensitivity and selectivity, for example, by using fluoridated compounds, because essentially no fluoride background resonance normally exists in cells. Biologic and technical issues with these indicators have been reviewed (33). These methods are reserved as research tools.

Fluorescent Indicators

Several fluorescent indicators undergo a change in fluorescence on binding to Mg^{2+}. FURAPTRA possesses properties that allow it to function as an intracellular indicator for free Mg^{2+}. The measurable shift in the excitation spectrum allows determination by a ratio method of the ion concentration in cell suspensions and in individual cells. Calibration and a relatively high affinity for Ca^{2+} must be considered in using this method (33, 34, 133). As with NMR, this is a research tool.

Magnesium Isotopes

Isotopes have been used as biologic tracers to follow the absorption, distribution, and excretion of the Mg ion. The radioisotope ^{28}Mg has been used in human studies (5, 134). Its value is limited by its radioactivity, its short half-life of 21.3 hours, and its short supply. The percentage of distribution of stable Mg in nature is 78.99% ^{24}Mg, 10.0% ^{25}Mg, and 11.01 ^{26}Mg. The last has been used for tracer studies (135), including absorption studies in humans (136). The $^{25}Mg:^{26}Mg$ ratio has been used to measure intestinal absorption (137).

Energy-Dispersive X-Ray Analysis

Energy-dispersive x-ray analysis has been used to measure $[Mg^{2+}]_i$ in sublingual epithelial cells and atrial biopsy specimens in various conditions (138).

Biologic Indicators

Total Serum Magnesium

In otherwise healthy laboratory animals and humans, instituting a Mg-restricted diet results in a fairly early and progressive decline in total serum Mg. In contrast, some reports have noted normal serum and plasma levels associated with a variety of illnesses but with low values in various blood cells and other organs (see later). Consequently, total serum and plasma Mg values in such situations may be considered unreliable indicators of depletion. Despite this, total serum Mg is the only test available to clinicians to assess Mg status rapidly and therefore is the most widely used method. Its lack of accuracy, however, has stimulated the search for more reliable laboratory markers for Mg status.

Ionized Serum Magnesium

Mg bound to protein and other serum and plasma ligands varies with changes in the concentrations of such ligands and in acid-base conditions; acidosis decreases binding, and alkalosis increases it. The level of ionized Mg may be more relevant under certain circumstances than that of total Mg (33–35, 129). Improved ISEs for determining ionized Mg in whole blood, serum, and plasma greatly simplify this determination; they are available commercially but require calibration (33–35). As discussed earlier, intermethod differences for ionized Mg exist and therefore reference ranges must exist for each analyzer and may not be comparable to those of a different manufacturer (139).

Erythrocytes

In experimental human Mg deficiency, the Mg content of red cells measured following hemolysis decreases more slowly and to a lesser extent than does total serum Mg (140). Mg ion concentrations measured by ^{31}P magnetic resonance spectroscopy in erythrocytes of healthy volunteers on a Mg-deficient diet for 3 weeks and in erythrocytes of other hypomagnesemic patients were significantly lower than those in the baseline period of normal magnesemic groups; in all subjects, $[Mg^{2+}]_i$ correlated with serum levels (141). Technical issues, however, appear to limit the use of this method in assessing Mg status in any given person (33, 34, 141).

Blood Mononuclear Cells

Some reports indicate that Mg concentrations in human mononuclear cells are a better guide to Mg nutriture than is the serum level (142, 143), but other reports are contradictory (144–146).

Urine Magnesium Excretion

In someone with normal renal function, 24-hour Mg excretion that is more than 10 to 15% of the amount ingested from an adequate diet suggests good nutriture. When a major reduction in the amounts ingested and/or absorbed is noted, there is a fairly rapid and progressive reduction in urinary excretion of this ion by the normal kidney; in early stages of such depletion, total serum Mg

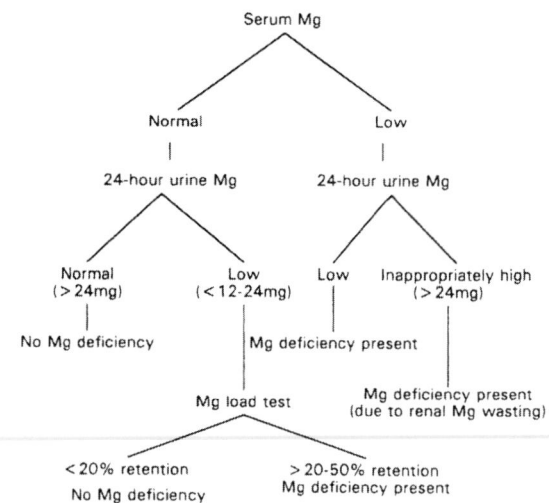

Figure 11.5. Algorithm of a diagnostic approach to suspected magnesium (Mg) deficiency, in which urine Mg levels are emphasized to distinguish the key factors leading to Mg depletion. (From Al Ghamdi SMG, Cameron EC, Sutton RAL. Am J Kidney Dis 1994;24:737–52, with permission.)

may still be within normal limits, but urine levels may be significantly reduced (147, 148). In situations in which renal Mg wasting occurs (see Tables 11.3 & 11.4), the resulting hypomagnesemia is associated with urinary Mg excretion of more than 1 mmol/day (149–151) (Fig. 11.5). Such a relationship suggests renal tubular dysfunction if the cause of the hypomagnesemia is otherwise uncertain.

Magnesium Load/Retention Test

The intravenous load or retention test provides an estimate of the proportion of infused Mg that is retained over a given period (143, 151, 152). Persons retaining more than the percentage retained by Mg-replete persons (e.g., 20–25%) are considered to have some body depletion. The test was initially validated in weanling rats and then in mature rats given differing amounts of Mg while Mg was measured in plasma, urine, and bone (152). A suggested clinical protocol that has been tested in relatively large numbers of hypomagnesemic patients, patients with chronic alcoholism, and animal controls has been published (143, 150). It is an invasive, time-consuming, nonstandardized, and expensive test, requiring hospitalization or other close supervision for the partial or full 24 hours after infusion, with careful urine collection for laboratory analysis. This type of test again raises the important question of how much depletion must occur in various body pools before Mg deficiency becomes biochemically and clinically significant.

Combined Laboratory Testing

An algorithm combining serum Mg level with renal excretion and the load test is presented in Figure 11.5. Although blood and urine levels together with history usually suffice to make the diagnosis, the load test may be included when semiqualitative data on the severity of pool depletion are desired or when the urinary data are equivocal (151).

RISK FACTORS AND CAUSES OF MAGNESIUM DEFICIENCY

Prevalence

The many risk factors for Mg depletion (Table 11.3) suggest that this condition is not rare in acutely or chronically ill patients. Of 2300 patients surveyed in a Veterans Administration hospital, 6.9% were hypomagnesemic; 11% of patients having routine Mg determinations were hypomagnesemic (153). When patients were hypokalemic, hypomagnesemia occurred in 42%; 29% of those with hypophosphatemia were hypomagnesemic, as were 27% of those with hyponatremia and 22% of those with hypocalcemia (153). The true prevalence of Mg depletion is not known, because this ion is not included in routine electrolyte testing in many clinics or hospitals (154). Similar high rates of depletion have been reported in studies of patients in intensive care units (155–157).

TABLE 11.3. CAUSES OF MAGNESIUM DEFICIENCY

Gastrointestinal disorders
  Prolonged nasogastric suction/vomiting
  Acute and chronic diarrhea
  Intestinal and biliary fistulas
  Malabsorption syndromes
  Extensive bowel resection or bypass
  Acute hemorrhagic pancreatitis
  Protein-calorie malnutrition
  Primary intestinal hypomagnesemia (neonatal)
Renal loss
  Long-term parenteral fluid therapy
  Osmotic diuresis (glucose, urea, manitol)
  Hypercalcemia
  Alcohol
  Diuretics (furosemide, ethacrynic acid)
  Aminoglycosides
  Cisplatin
  Cyclosporine
  Amphotericin B
  Pentamidine
  Tacrolimus
  Metabolic acidosis
  Renal disorders with magnesium wasting
  Primary renal hypomagnesemia
Endocrine and metabolic disorders
  Diabetes mellitus (glycosuria)
  Phosphate depletion
  Primary hyperparathyroidism (hypercalcemia)
  Hypoparathyroidism (hypercalciuria, hypercalcemia
    from overtreatment with vitamin D)
Primary aldosteronism
Hungry bone syndrome
Chronic renal disease
Excessive lactation

Key Disorders

Gastrointestinal Disorders

Gastrointestinal disorders (see Table 11.3) may lead to Mg depletion in various ways. The Mg content of upper intestinal tract fluids is approximately 1 mEq/L. Vomiting and nasogastric suction therefore may contribute to Mg depletion. The Mg content of diarrheal fluids and fistulous drainage is much higher (≤ 15 mEq/L), and consequently Mg depletion is common in acute and chronic diarrhea, regional enteritis, ulcerative colitis, and intestinal and biliary fistulas (158–160). Malabsorption syndromes caused by nontropical sprue, radiation injury resulting from therapy for disorders such as carcinoma of the cervix, and intestinal lymphangiectasia may also produce Mg deficiency (161–163). Steatorrhea and resection or bypass of the small bowel, particularly the ileum, often result in intestinal Mg loss or malabsorption (164, 165). Finally, acute severe pancreatitis is associated with hypomagnesemia that may result from the clinical problem causing the pancreatitis, such as alcoholism, or from saponification of Mg in necrotic parapancreatic fat (166, 167). A primary defect in intestinal Mg absorption, which presents early in life with hypomagnesemia, hypocalcemia, and seizures, has been described as an autosomal recessive disorder linked to chromosome 9q22 (168). This disorder appears to be caused by mutations in *TRPM6*, which expresses a protein involved with active intestinal Mg transport.

Renal Disorders

Excessive excretion of Mg into the urine may be the basis of Mg depletion (see Table 11.3). Renal Mg reabsorption is proportional to tubular fluid flow as well as to Na and Ca excretion. Therefore, long-term parenteral fluid therapy, particularly with saline, volume expansion states such as primary aldosteronism, and hypercalciuric states may result in Mg depletion (169–171). Hypercalcemia have been shown to decrease renal Mg reabsorption, probably mediated by Ca binding to the Ca-sensing receptor in the thick ascending limb of Henle and decreasing transepithelial voltage, and this is the likely cause of renal Mg wasting and hypomagnesemia observed in many hypercalcemic states (172, 173). Osmotic diuresis from glucosuria will result in urinary Mg wasting (171).

Many pharmaceutical drugs may cause renal Mg wasting and depletion. The major site of renal Mg reabsorption is at the loop of Henle; therefore, diuretics such as furosemide and ethacrynic acid have been shown to result in marked Mg wasting (174). Aminoglycosides cause a reversible renal lesion that results in hypermagnesuria and hypomagnesemia (175, 176). Similarly, amphotericin B therapy has been reported to result in renal Mg wasting. Other renal Mg-wasting agents include cisplatin, cyclosporine, tacrolimus, and pentamidine (177–179). A rising blood alcohol level has been associated with hypermagnesuria and is one factor contributing to Mg depletion in chronic alcoholism. Metabolic acidosis caused by diabetic ketoacidosis, starvation, or alcoholism may also result in renal Mg wasting (180, 181).

Several renal Mg wasting disorders have been described that may be genetic or sporadic (182). One form, which is autosomal recessive, results from mutations in the paracellin-1 gene on chromosome 3 (183). This disorder is characterized by low serum Mg as well as by hypercalciuria and nephrocalcinosis (184). Another autosomal dominant form of isolated renal Mg wasting and hypomagnesemia has been linked to chromosome 11q23 and is identified as a mutation on the Na^+/K^+-ATPase γ-subunit of gene *FXYD2* (185). Gitelman syndrome (familial hypokalemia-hypomagnesemia syndrome) is an autosomal recessive disorder caused by a genetic defect of the thiazide-sensitive Na chloride cotransporter gene on chromosome 16 (186). Other undefined genetic defects also exist (187).

Hypomagnesemia may accompany numerous other disorders, as reviewed in the literature (188). Phosphate depletion has been shown experimentally to result in urinary Mg wasting and hypomagnesemia. Hypomagnesemia may also accompany the "hungry bone" syndrome, a phase of rapid bone mineral accretion in subjects with hyperparathyroidism or hyperthyroidism following surgical treatment. Finally, chronic renal tubular, glomerular, or interstitial diseases may be associated with renal Mg wasting. Rarely, excessive lactation may result in hypomagnesemia.

Diabetes Mellitus

Special consideration must be given to diabetes mellitus. It is the most common disorder associated with Mg deficiency (171, 189, 190). The mechanism for Mg depletion in patients with diabetes is generally thought to result from renal Mg wasting secondary to osmotic diuresis generated by hyperglycosuria. Mg deficiency has been reported to result in impaired insulin secretion as well as insulin resistance (189, 190). The mechanism is unclear but it may be caused by abnormal glucose metabolism because Mg is a cofactor in several enzymes in this cycle. In addition, Mg depletion may decrease tyrosine kinase activity at the insulin receptor, and Mg may influence insulin secretion by the β cell. Diabetic patients given Mg therapy appear to have improved control of the disease. Two studies reported that the incidence of type 2 diabetes is significantly greater in people on a lower-Mg diet (189, 190). Mg status should therefore be assessed in patients with diabetes mellitus because a vicious cycle may occur, with diabetes out of control leading to Mg loss and the subsequent Mg deficiency resulting in impaired insulin secretion and action and worsening diabetes control.

CLINICAL PRESENTATIONS OF MAGNESIUM DEFICIENCY

Many different laboratory and domestic animals, subhuman primates, and human subjects have been studied in the course of Mg deficiency induced by diets low in this element (191). These observations, along with those in persons who have Mg deficiency from secondary causes, have identified the manifestations of this deficit.

Laboratory Animals

Manifestations of Mg depletion vary among species. Although most studied, the rat is strikingly different from other species in certain of its acute deficiency signs, including hyperemia of ears and feet induced by histamine release from basophils, hyperirritability associated with characteristic and usually fatal tonic-clonic convulsions, and high levels of serum Ca. Mice on the same diet did not have hyperemia and often died with a single abrupt and massive convulsion (192). Although early studies suggested that the Mg-deficient mouse became hypocalcemic, more current study observed hypercalcemia similar to that seen in the rat (193). Mg-deficient dogs and monkeys developed spasticity, weakness, tremors, and occasionally nonfatal convulsions with hypocalcemia; increasing Ca intake did not increase serum calcium or prevent the neuromuscular changes (194).

Other changes in Mg-deficient young rats include reduced growth rate, alopecia, and skin lesions. Chronic deficiency in the rat leads to edema, hypertrophic gums, leukocytosis, and splenomegaly. Various thymic abnormalities have also been noted (195). Crystalluria in the kidney with calcification and degenerative changes in various organs, especially the kidney, muscle, heart, and aorta, are prominent in deficient rats (196, 197), guinea pigs (198), dogs (196), and certain other species maintained on low-Mg diets, particularly when the Ca content is high compared with that of human diets (194, 198).

Humans

Clinical evaluation includes a history and physical examination taken by a health practitioner sensitive to the causes, signs, and symptoms associated with Mg depletion. This usually provides enough information to decide whether the patient is at no risk, is already at risk, or is symptomatically depleted. Risk factors are listed earlier in Table 11.3. Symptoms and signs of deficiency are given in Table 11.4. Symptomatic human deficiency has been induced experimentally by dietary restriction. Deficiency also occurs in certain predisposing and complicating disease states (see Table 11.4). The clinical presentation of Mg deficiency in disease states may coexist or may be masked by the signs and symptoms of the primary disorder.

TABLE 11.4. MANIFESTATIONS OF MAGNESIUM DEPLETION

Bone and mineral metabolism
  Hypocalcemia
    Impaired parathyroid hormone secretion
    Renal and skeletal resistance to parathyroid hormone
    Resistance to vitamin D
  Osteoporosis (putative)
Neuromuscular manifestations
  Positive Chvostek and Trousseau signs
  Spontaneous carpal-pedal spasm
  Seizures
  Vertigo, ataxia, nystagmus, athetoid and chorioform movements
  Muscular weakness, tremor, fasciculation, and wasting
  Psychiatric: depression, psychosis
Potassium homeostasis
  Hypokalemia
    Renal potassium wasting
    Decreased intracellular potassium
Cardiovascular manifestations
  Cardiac arrhythmia
    Electrocardiographic: prolonged PR and QT intervals, U waves
    Atrial tachycardia, premature contractions, and fibrillation
    Junctional arrhythmias
    Ventricular premature contractions, tachycardia, fibrillation
    Sensitivity to digitalis intoxication
    Torsade de pointes
  Myocardial ischemia/infarction (putative)
  Hypertension (putative)
  Atherosclerotic vascular disease (putative)
Preeclampsia

Moderate to Severe Magnesium Deficiency

When Mg deficiency is recognized in the clinical setting, it is usually moderate to severe. Biochemical, neuromuscular, and cardiac complications are the most prevalent findings in the Mg-deficient patient.

Hypocalcemia. Ca is the major regulator of PTH secretion. Mg, however, modulates PTH secretion in a manner similar to that of Ca. Studies have demonstrated that acute elevations of Mg inhibit PTH secretion, whereas an acute reduction stimulates PTH secretion (200–202). Extracellular Ca^{2+} and Mg^{2+} do not act directly but rather modulate a cell-surface, extracellular, Ca^{2+}-sensing receptor; the resulting inward current mobilizes intracellular Ca^{2+} stores, presumably by activating phosphoinositide-specific phospholipase C on a pathway to inhibition of PTH secretion (203). These results support the in vitro and in vivo findings that extracellular $[Mg^{2+}]$ has an appreciably smaller effect than $[Ca^{2+}]$ in suppressing PTH secretion (204). Acute changes in the serum Mg concentration may therefore modulate PTH secretion and should be considered in the evaluation of the determination of serum PTH concentrations.

Although acute changes in the extracellular Mg concentrations influence PTH secretion qualitatively similar to changes in Ca, it is clear that Mg deficiency markedly perturbs mineral homeostasis (202, 205). Hypocalcemia is a prominent manifestation of Mg deficiency in humans (202, 205), as well as in most other species (206, 207). In human patients, Mg deficiency must become moderate to severe before symptomatic hypocalcemia develops. Mg therapy alone restores serum Ca concentrations to normal in these patients within days (205). Ca and/or vitamin D therapy will not correct the hypocalcemia (202, 205). Even mild degrees of Mg depletion, however, may result in a significant fall in the serum Ca concentration, as demonstrated in experimental human Mg depletion (206, 208).

One major factor resulting in the fall in the serum Ca is impaired parathyroid gland function. Determination of serum PTH concentrations in hypocalcemic hypomagnesemic patients has shown that most patients have low or normal serum PTH levels (205, 209, 210). Normal serum PTH concentrations are thought to be inappropriately low in the presence of hypocalcemia. The administration of Mg will result in an immediate rise in the serum PTH concentration (205, 210, 211). The serum PTH concentration will gradually fall to normal within several days of therapy with return of the serum Ca concentration to normal (205, 208, 210). The impairment in PTH secretion appears to occur early in Mg depletion. Experimental human experimental Mg deficiency shows similar, but not as marked, changes in the serum PTH concentrations (208). Heterogenous serum PTH values may be explained by the severity of Mg depletion. As the serum Mg concentration falls, the parathyroid gland will react normally with an increase in PTH secretion. As $[Mg^{2+}]_i$ depletion develops, however, the ability of the parathyroid to secrete PTH is impaired, resulting in a fall in the serum PTH levels with a resultant fall in the serum Ca concentration.

The presence of normal or elevated serum concentrations of PTH in the presence of hypocalcemia (205, 210) suggests that there may also be end-organ resistance to PTH action. Clinical studies have reported skeletal resistance to exogenous PTH in hypocalcemic Mg-deficient patients as assessed by a rise in serum Ca and increase in urinary hydroxyproline excretion (205, 212, 213). PTH has also been shown to have a reduced calcemic effect in Mg-deficient animals (213-216).

The renal response to PTH in Mg deficiency has been assessed by determining urinary excretion of cAMP and/or phosphate. In studies of severely Mg-depleted patients, an impaired response to PTH has been observed (205, 212, 217). A decrease in urinary cAMP excretion in response to PTH has also been described in the Mg-deficient dog and rat (215, 216).

The mechanism for impaired PTH secretion and action in Mg deficiency remains unclear. Investigators have suggested a possible defect in the second messenger systems in Mg depletion. PTH is thought to exert its biologic effects through the intermediary action of cAMP (218, 219). Adenylate cyclase has been universally found to require Mg for cAMP generation both as a component of the substrate (MgATP) and as an obligatory activator of enzyme activity (220). It is clear that some patients and animal models with severe Mg deficiency have reduced urinary excretion of cAMP in response to exogenously administered PTH (205).

Although cAMP is an important mediator of PTH action, current studies do not suggest an important role in mediating Ca^{2+}-regulated PTH secretion (221, 222). PTH has also been shown to activate the phospholipase C second messenger system (222), leading to an acute transient rise in cytosolic Ca^{2+} with subsequent activation of calmodulin-dependent protein kinases. Mg depletion could perturb this system via several mechanisms because an Mg^{2+}-dependent guanine nucleotide regulating protein is involved in activation of phospholipase C (223, 224), and Mg^{2+} has also been shown to be a noncompetitive inhibitor of IP_3-induced Ca^{2+} release (225). The effect of Mg depletion on cellular function in terms of the second messenger systems is most complex, potentially involving substrate availability, G-protein activity, release and sensitivity to intracellular Ca^{2+}, and phospholipid metabolism.

Mg is also important in vitamin D metabolism and/or action. Patients with hypoparathyroidism, malabsorption syndromes, and rickets have been reported to be resistant to therapeutic doses of vitamin D until Mg was simultaneously administered, as reviewed in the literature (202). Patients with hypocalcemia and Mg deficiency have also been reported to be resistant to pharmacologic doses of vitamin D (217, 226), 1α-hydroxy vitamin D (227) and 1,25-dihydroxy-vitamin D (228). Similarly, an impaired calcemic response to vitamin D has been found in Mg-deficient rats (229), lambs (230), and calves (231).

The exact nature of altered vitamin D metabolism and/or action in Mg deficiency is unclear. Patients with Mg deficiency and hypocalcemia frequently have low serum concentrations of 25-hydroxy-vitamin D (232, 233), and therefore nutritional vitamin D deficiency may be one factor. Therapy with vitamin D, however, results in high serum levels of 25-hydroxy-vitamin D without correction of the hypocalcemia (220), a finding suggesting that the vitamin D nutrition is not the major reason. Serum concentrations of 1,25-dihydroxy-vitamin D have also been found to be low or low normal in most hypocalcemic Mg-deficient patients (232–234). Because PTH is a major trophic for 1,25-dihydroxy vitamin D formation, the low serum PTH concentrations could explain the low 1,25-dihydroxy vitamin D levels, suggesting that human Mg deficiency impairs the ability of the kidney to synthesize 1,25-dihydroxy vitamin D. This suggestion is supported by the observation that the ability of exogenous administration of 1-34 human PTH to physiologically normal subjects after 3 weeks of experimental Mg depletion resulted in a significantly lower rise in serum 1,25-dihydroxy-vitamin D concentrations than before institution of the diet (208). Mg is known to support the 25-hydroxy-1α-hydroxylase in vitro (235).

Hypokalemia. A common feature of Mg depletion is hypokalemia (236). Experimental human Mg deficiency demonstrated a negative K balance resulting from increased urinary loss (206). During Mg depletion, patients have a loss of K from the cell with intracellular K depletion, which is enhanced by the inability of the kidney to conserve K. Attempts to replete the K deficit with K therapy alone are not successful without simultaneous Mg therapy. The reason for this disrupted K metabolism may be related to Mg dependence of Na^+/K^+-ATPase (237). This enzyme uses the energy derived from ATP hydrolysis to pump Na and K actively across the plasma membrane against their respective concentration gradients to maintain the physiologically normal intracellular concentrations of these cations. Cyclic binding and release of Mg occur between the enzyme complex and the intracellular space during the Na and K exchange (238). During Mg depletion, intracellular Na and Ca rise, and Mg and K fall (239). Mg also appears to be important in regulation of K channels in cardiac cells that are characterized by inward rectification (240). This biochemical feature may be a contributing cause of the electrocardiographic findings and cardiac dysrhythmias discussed later.

Neuromuscular Manifestations. Neuromuscular hyperexcitability is a common presenting complaint of a patient with Mg deficiency (241). Latent tetany, as elicited by a positive Chvostek and Trousseau sign, or spontaneous carpal-pedal spasm may be present. Generalized seizures may also occur. Although hypocalcemia may contribute to the neurologic signs, Mg deficiency without hypocalcemia has been reported to result in neuromuscular hyperexcitability (242). Other signs occasionally seen include vertigo, ataxia, nystagmus, and athetoid and choreiform movements. Muscular tremor, fasciculation, wasting, and weakness may be present. Reversible psychiatric aberrations also have been reported (241, 243).

Several mechanisms may exist by which Mg deficiency results in these neuromuscular problems. Mg has been shown to stabilize the nerve axon. Lowering the serum Mg concentration decreases the threshold of axonal stimulation and increases nerve conduction velocity (244). Mg also has been shown to influence the release of neurotransmitters, such as glutamate, at the neuromuscular junction by competitively inhibiting the entry of Ca into the presynaptic nerve terminal (245, 246). It is likely that a decrease of extracellular Mg would allow a greater influx of Ca into the presynaptic nerves and the subsequent release of a greater quantity of neurotransmitters, resulting in hyperresponsive neuromuscular activity (247).

Cardiac Dysrhythmias. Cardiac dysrhythmias are an important consequence of Mg deficiency. Experimental Mg deficiency in animals results in electrocardiographic alterations as well as changes in conduction velocity and automaticity (239, 248, 249). Mg depletion also renders the heart more susceptible to the dysrhythmogenic effects of isoproterenol and cardiac glycosides (250, 251). Electrocardiographic abnormalities in human Mg deficiency include prolonged PR and QT intervals. Intracellular K depletion and hypokalemia are complicating features of Mg deficiency and may contribute to these electrocardiographic abnormalities. Mg-deficient patients with cardiac dysrhythmias have been treated successfully by Mg administration (252–255). Supraventricular dysrhythmias including premature atrial complexes, atrial tachycardia, atrial fibrillation, and junctional arrhythmias have been described (250, 255–257). Ventricular premature complexes, ventricular tachycardia, and ventricular fibrillation are more serious complications (252, 255, 258–260). Such dysrhythmias may be resistant to usual therapy (253, 261). Because $[Mg^{2+}]_i$ depletion may be present despite a normal serum Mg concentration, Mg deficiency always must be considered as a potential factor in cardiac dysrhythmias.

Acute Myocardial Infarction. Acute myocardial infarction (AMI), the leading cause of death in the United States, accounts for more than 300,000 deaths per year. Mg may be a risk factor because it has been shown to play a role in systemic and coronary vascular tone (see later) and cardiac dysrhythmias (see earlier) and by inhibiting platelet aggregation (262, 263). In the 1980s, debate arose over the clinical utility of adjunctive Mg therapy for AMI (264). Three major trials define our understanding to date regarding Mg therapy in AMI: the Second Leicester Intravenous Magnesium Intervention Trial (LIMIT-2), the Fourth International Study of Infarct Survival (ISIS-4), and the Magnesium in Coronaries (MAGIC) trial (265–267).

Before 1992, several small controlled trials suggested that adjunctive Mg therapy reduced mortality from AMI by 50% (268). LIMIT-2 was the first study involving large numbers of participants (265). Over a 6-year period, 2316 participants with suspected AMI were randomized to receive adjunctive Mg therapy or placebo. At 28 days, the Mg-treated group showed an approximately 25% lower mortality rate (7.8% versus 10.3%; $p < .04$). Until the release of ISIS-4, many considered adjunctive therapy with Mg part of standard therapy for acute coronary syndromes.

The ISIS-4 trial randomized more than 58,000 participants over a 3-year period to examine the effects of captopril, nitrates, and Mg on AMI (266). The strength of the study was the large number of participants enlisted. The primary end point was mortality at 35 days. Unlike in LIMIT-2, the mortality rate in the Mg-treated group was not significantly different from the control group (7.64% versus 7.24%). The conclusion was that Mg therapy was not indicated in suspected AMI.

Despite the null result, some investigators suggested that the ISIS-4 design masked the benefits of Mg therapy (268). Two major criticisms involved the timing of the Mg therapy and the severity of illness. ISIS-4 randomized participants up to 24 hours after presentation, although most

were randomized within 8 hours. The leading theory regarding the role of Mg therapy in AMI involves the prevention of ischemia-reperfusion injury (267).

The MAGIC trial was designed to address the issues regarding ISIS-4 study design; namely, early intervention in higher-risk patients would more likely show the benefit of Mg therapy (267). Over a 3-year period, 6213 participants were randomized to three treatment arms or strata. Patients in the treatment strata received the first dose of Mg therapy within 6 hours of the onset of symptoms. The first stratum included patients who were 64 years or older and eligible for reperfusion therapy, and the second stratum included patients of any age who were not eligible for reperfusion therapy. Both strata were considered high-risk groups. The third stratum received placebo. The Mg-treated group mortality at 30 days was not significantly different from the placebo group mortality (15.3% versus15.2%). After adjustment for factors shown to affect mortality risk, no benefit of Mg was observed. Thus, early intervention with Mg therapy in higher-risk patients did not offer a survival advantage in the MAGIC trial.

The overall evidence from clinical trials does not support the routine application of adjunctive Mg therapy in patients with AMI. Prior studies may have shown benefit, but they were smaller and possibly more prone to type 1 statistical errors of chance (268). Both the ISIS-4 and MAGIC trials were large, and both found no benefit of adjunctive Mg therapy.

Chronic Latent Magnesium Deficiency

Investigators have suggested that mild degrees of Mg deficiency present over time may contribute to disease states such as hypertension, coronary artery disease, preeclampsia, and osteoporosis.

Hypertension. Epidemiologic and clinical evidence suggests that Mg influences vascular tone and may play an important role in regulating blood pressure (269). Numerous studies have demonstrated an inverse relationship between populations with a low dietary intake of Mg and blood pressure (270–272). Hypomagnesemia and reduction of $[Mg^{2+}]_i$ have also been inversely correlated with blood pressure. One study of hypertensive patients revealed low serum Mg concentrations (273), but another study did not (274). Patients with essential hypertension were found to have reduced free Mg^{2+} concentrations in red blood cells (275, 276). The Mg^{2+} levels were inversely related to both systolic and diastolic blood pressures. The possible relationship between hypertension and Mg deficiency is an important consideration because the two often coexist in high proportions in populations such as patients with diabetes and those with alcoholism (277).

Intervention studies with Mg therapy in hypertension have led to conflicting results, however. Several studies have shown a positive blood-pressure lowering effect of Mg supplements (278–280), whereas others have not

(281, 282). Other dietary factors may also play a role. A diet of fruits and vegetables, which increased Mg intake from 176 to 423 mg/day (along with an increase in K), significantly lowered blood pressure (283). The addition of nonfat dairy products increased Ca intake as well as lowered blood pressure further.

The mechanism by which Mg may affect blood pressure is not clear. Mg administration increases the production of the vasodilatory prostaglandin, prostacyclin (PGI_2) (284). In addition, Mg depletion heightens the vasoconstrictive effect of angiotensin II and norepinephrine in vitro and in vivo (285, 286). In contrast, increasing the Mg concentration reduces the pressor responses to these agents (285, 286). Mg deficiency is also associated with an increase in platelet aggregation and release of the potent vasoconstrictor, thromboxane A_2 (287). This effect may be reversed with Mg supplementation (288). These events may be affected by the influence of Mg on Ca channel activity. A rise in intracellular Ca^{2+} in response to angiotensin II and in platelets is crucial for smooth muscle contraction and platelet aggregation. Mg causes a reduction in intracellular Ca^{2+} in vascular smooth muscle and in platelets (289). Therefore, hypomagnesemia is likely to cause increased intracellular Ca^{2+}, increased smooth muscle contraction, and platelet aggregation.

Atherosclerotic Vascular Disease. Another potential cardiovascular complication of Mg deficiency is the development of atheromatous disease (290). Mg deficiency in rats has been associated with increased serum and plasma phospholipid and triglyceride levels, variable total cholesterol levels, low free cholesterol levels, increased levels of oleic and linoleic acids, decreased stearic and arachidonic acid levels, and modifications of lipoprotein concentrations (291, 292). Plasma prostanoid (PGE_2, prostaglandin F_2 [PGF_2], 6-keto-PGF_α, and thromboxane A_2) levels were significantly higher in both plasma and tissues of Mg-deficient rats than in controls (293). In contrast to pair-fed controls, the hyperlipidemia in Mg-depleted young rats was associated with increased oxidation of very low-density and low-density lipoproteins. Increased lipid oxidation occurred in liver, heart, and muscle of the Mg-deficient rats (294). Mg depletion, by inhibiting adenylate cyclase activity and thereby lowering cAMP levels, may permit increased cyclooxygenase activity and stimulation of prostanoid synthesis (292). Because certain biochemical and pathologic changes differ in the Mg-deficient rat and in other species, experimental comparison with other species is necessary before generalizing the lipid and prostanoid changes noted earlier.

Lipid alterations have been reported in hypomagnesemic human subjects (290); however, they are often complicated by factors related to underlying lipoprotein abnormalities occurring in diabetes, coronary artery disease, myocardial infarction, and other diseases. Epidemiologic studies have related water hardness (Ca and Mg content) inversely to cardiovascular death rates (280, 295).

Platelet hyperactivity is a recognized risk factor in the development of cardiovascular diseases. Mg has been shown to inhibit platelet aggregation against numerous aggregation agents (287). Patients with diabetes who have Mg depletion have been shown to have increased platelet aggregations (288). Mg therapy in these patients returned the response toward normal. The antiplatelet effect of Mg may be related to the finding that Mg inhibits the synthesis of thromboxane A_2 and 12-hydroxyeicosatetraenoic acid, eicosanoids thought to be involved in platelet aggregation (287, 288). Mg also inhibits the thrombin-induced Ca influx in platelets as well as stimulates synthesis of PGI_2, the potent antiaggregatory eicosanoid (284, 287).

Preeclampsia. Preeclampsia complicates one in 2000 pregnancies in developed countries and consists of hypertension, proteinuria, edema, and multiple-organ failure (296). In developing countries, the incidence is as high as one in 100 (297, 298) and is responsible for more than 50,000 maternal deaths a year. The principal treatment for both conditions is delivery of the fetus. In addition, Mg therapy has been used for decades in both preeclampsia and eclampsia and contributes to the very low mortality rate in developed countries (299). Despite decades of use, no large randomized trial examining the efficacy of Mg therapy had been performed until the Magnesium Sulphate for Prevention of Eclampsia (MAGPIE) trial in 2002. Endothelial dysfunction is the central feature in the pathophysiology of preeclampsia (300). Multiple causes of endothelial dysfunction have been implicated, such as ischemia, oxidative stress, abnormal maternal immune response, and genetic factors (300). Three main features of endothelial dysfunction are vasoconstriction, platelet activity, and leukocyte activity, all of which are affected by Mg therapy (301–303). Moreover, the neuronal effects of Mg, as previously described, may also contribute to its therapeutic efficacy. A trial comparing women with preeclampsia treated with Mg sulfate ($MgSO_4$) with nimodipine, a specific cerebral arterial vasodilator, showed a lower risk (0.8% versus 2.6%) of eclampsia in the Mg-therapy group (304). The results of the trial suggest that the mechanism of Mg therapy involves more than cerebral arterial vasodilation and is likely multifactorial.

As in other critical illnesses, the Mg status of women with preeclampsia has been difficult to establish. No difference was found in the plasma Mg levels of women with preeclampsia and in healthy pregnant women; however, women with preeclampsia had a decreased red blood cell Mg level (305). In a comparison between women with preeclampsia and women with preterm labor, no differences were found before Mg therapy in ionized or serum Mg levels (306). Although subtle deficits in total-body Mg may contribute to hypertension during pregnancy, the role of Mg may relate more to its stabilizing neuronal and vascular effects, rather than to correction of an electrolyte deficit.

The MAGPIE trial was the largest trial to date examining hypertensive disease in preeclamptic women (307).

More than 10,000 women with preeclampsia were randomized to receive Mg therapy or placebo. The Mg-therapy group experienced eclampsia significantly less often than the placebo group (0.8% versus 1.9%; relative risk [RR], 0.42; 95% confidence interval [CI], 0.29–.60). Moreover, the relative risk of death in the Mg-therapy group was lower (RR, 0.55; 95% CI, 0.26–1.14). Interestingly, neither benefit nor harm was shown for the fetus with Mg therapy. Mg therapy is clearly indicated for women with preeclampsia. It has been shown to decrease the incidence of eclampsia and likely decreases overall mortality.

Osteoporosis. The effect of dietary Mg depletion on bone and mineral homeostasis in animals has been studied since the 1940s. Most studies have been performed in the rat. Dietary restriction has usually been severe, ranging from 0.2 to 8 mg/100 g chow (normal = 50–70 mg/100 g). A universal observation has been a decrease in growth of both the whole body and the skeleton (308–314). The epiphyseal and diaphyseal growth plate is characterized by thinning and decrease in the number and organization of chrondrocytes (310). Reduced osteoblastic bone formation has been observed by quantitative histomorphometry (311, 314, 315). Serum and bone alkaline phosphatase (31, 310, 316), serum and bone osteocalcin (311, 312, 317), and bone osteocalcin mRNA (311, 312) have been reduced, suggesting decreased osteoblastic function. An increase in the number and activity of osteoclasts in the Mg-deficient rat and mouse has been reported (315, 318). Bone from Mg-deficient rat has been described as brittle and fragile (309, 319). Biomechanical testing has directly demonstrated skeletal fragility in both rat and pig (311, 312, 320–322).

In humans, epidemiologic studies have demonstrated a correlation between bone mass and dietary Mg intake in appendicular (radius, ulna, and heel) skeleton (323–325). Longitudinal observation over 4 years demonstrated that loss of bone mass was inversely related to Mg intake in premenopausal women ($p < .05$), with a similar trend in the postmenopausal group ($p < .085$). In other studies of bone mineral density of the axial skeleton (lumbar spine and hip), a significant relationship between dietary Mg intake and bone mineral density has been observed (326–330). These epidemiologic studies link dietary Mg intake to bone mass. Exceptions appear to include women in the early postmenopausal period, in whom the effect of acute sex steroid deficiency may mask the effect of dietary factors such as Mg. Therefore, further investigations are needed to provide a firm relationship of dietary Mg inadequacy with osteoporosis.

Few studies have been conducted assessing Mg status in patients with osteoporosis (331–334). Low serum and red blood cell Mg concentrations as well as high retention of parenterally administered Mg have suggested an Mg deficit; however, these results are not consistent from one study to another. Similarly, whereas low skeletal Mg content has been observed in some studies, others have found normal or even high Mg content.

The effect of dietary Mg supplementation on bone mass in patients with osteoporosis has not been extensively studied (335–338). The effect of Mg supplements on bone mass has generally led to an increase in bone mineral density, although study design limits useful information. Larger, long-term, plabeco-controlled, double-blind investigations are required.

Osteoporosis appears to occur with greater than usual frequency in certain populations in which Mg depletion is also common. These include patients with diabetes mellitus (339–344), chronic alcoholism (345–347), and malabsorption syndromes (348, 349).

Several potential mechanisms may account for a decrease in bone mass in Mg deficiency. Mg is mitogenic for bone cell growth, and this may directly result in a decrease in bone formation (350). Mg also affects crystal formation; a lack of Mg results in a larger, more perfect crystals that may affect bone strength (331).

Mg deficiency can perturb Ca homeostasis and can result in a fall in both serum PTH and $1,25(OH)_2D$, as discussed earlier (205, 208). Because $1,25(OH)_2D$ stimulates osteoblast activity (351) and the synthesis of osteocalcin and procollagen (352), decreased formation of $1,25(OH)_2D$ may be a major cause of decreased bone formation such as that observed in experimental Mg deficiency (313, 321, 353). Similarly, PTH has been demonstrated to be trophic for bone (354), and therefore impaired PTH secretion or PTH skeletal resistance may result in osteoporosis.

Acute Mg depletion in the rat and mouse has demonstrated an immediate rise in substance P followed by a rise in inflammatory cytokines (tumor necrosis factor-α and interleukins-1β, 6, 11) (355). These cytokines could contribute to an increase in osteoclastic bone resorption and could explain the uncoupling of bone formation and bone resorption observed in the rat and mouse (315, 318). Whether these possibilities are valid for suboptimal chronic dietary Mg deficit in human osteoporosis is unknown. Further studies are needed to explore these possibilities.

MANAGEMENT OF MAGNESIUM DEPLETION

The physician should consider all predisposing factors in patients at risk, should anticipate hypomagnesemia, and should institute early treatments to *prevent* its occurrence or minimize its severity. These measures include instituting control of underlying disease, minimizing therapeutic insult, and initiating medical and dietary changes designed to maximize Mg retention by the intestine and kidney. When Mg depletion is evident, its cause must be determined. Before treatment is initiated, Mg, Ca, K, and Na levels in the blood and urine and the acid-base balance in blood must be determined. The amount, route, and duration of

Mg administration depend on the severity of Mg depletion and its causes.

Adolescents and Adults

Seizures, acute arrhythmias, and severe generalized spasticity require immediate intravenous infusion with one of several protocols, depending on the state of renal function. One to 2 g MgSO$_4$ · 7H$_2$O (8.2–16.4 mEq Mg^{2+}) is usually infused over 5 to 10 minutes, followed by continuous infusion of 6 g over 24 hours or until the condition is controlled (143). Infusion of Ca gluconate may accompany the Mg if blood levels are low. Alternatively, 2 g of the sulfate is given over 1 minute, followed by 1.0 mEq/kg (0.5 mmol) during the first 24 hours, followed by 0.5 mEq/kg for the next 3 days (356). Other protocols (357, 358) have been used to suppress the ventricular arrhythmia torsade de pointes. In all instances, correction of electrolyte (especially K) and acid-base imbalances should accompany the Mg therapy. Additionally, levels of serum Mg and other electrolytes should be determined at least twice daily in such patients.

Less severe manifestations (e.g., paresthesias with latent or active tetany associated with persisting intestinal or renal losses) are likewise best treated by the intravenous route, again in conjunction with appropriate therapy for the underlying condition and with correction of other electrolyte and acid-base abnormalities. When renal function is good, 6 g (48 mEq) of MgSO$_4$ may be given intravenously over 24 hours in saline or dextrose solutions, with other nutrients as required (143). This may be continued for 3 to 5 days until the signs and symptoms and/or electrolytes abnormalities are corrected. When the intravenous route cannot be used, equivalent periodic intramuscular injections can be given, although these are painful and may lead to fibrotic reactions. This regimen is continued for 2 or more days, and the situation is then reassessed. The dosages given must always exceed the daily losses as indicated by serum levels and urinary excretion.

The return to the normal or slightly higher range of serum Mg levels with any of these schedules is relatively rapid. However, repletion of Mg lost from bone and other tissues requires more prolonged Mg therapy at lower and/or less frequent doses, preferably by mouth. This regimen is continued until—or, if necessary, beyond—the time necessary to attain a persisting, relatively normal serum Mg concentration and a urine output of 20% or more of the oral intake in the case of intestinal malabsorption. When intestinal absorption is normal and renal Mg wasting is present, supplements should be added to the usual diet to tolerance (onset of diarrhea) to maintain normal serum levels; this supplement should be 20% or more above the amount of Mg lost in fecal water plus urine, as measured when only the diet is given. In some instances, oral Mg may not be sufficient, and intramuscular and/or intravenous may be required. Patients with continuing severe Mg and K losses in the urine (as in cisplatin nephrotoxicity) may require long-term supplements by intravenous infusion via an indwelling central catheter for home administration.

When depletion is modest and persistent, initial efforts should be directed to increased intake of Mg-rich foods. When necessary and feasible, supplementary oral Mg may be taken as small gelatin capsules packed with the sulfate, chloride, acetate, citrate, or other salts with good solubility in enteric fluids. Three hundred to 600 mg may be given in divided doses three to six times per day, with a full glass of water to prevent or minimize Mg-related diarrhea (83) and to ensure solubilization. For the patient receiving enteral feeding, one of these salts may be dissolved in the formula. Improvement of existing steatorrhea by dietary or other medical means will decrease fecal Mg losses. Again, treatment of underlying disease and replacement of K deficits are essential.

Infants and Young Children

Symptomatic Mg depletion in infants responds well to relatively small amounts of intravenous or intramuscular Mg. When renal function is normal, parenteral administration is recommended: 3.6 to 6.0 mg (0.15–0.25 mmol or 0.3 to 0.5 mEq)/kg body weight as 50% MgSO$_4$ over the first several hours, followed by an equal amount, either intramuscularly or intravenously, over the remainder of the day (359). Ca may also be infused initially, together with K and other electrolytes as indicated. When convulsions or arrhythmias are present in patients beyond infancy, treatment may be initiated with an oral bolus of the 50% MgSO$_4$ at a dose of 20 to 100 mg (1.65–8.25 mEq/kg) over 1 minute; this is followed by 1.0 mEq/kg given continuously thereafter (360).

In patients with chronic malabsorption (e.g., primary hypomagnesemia), 12 to 18 mg/kg (0.5–0.75 mmol) in multiple, divided oral doses is suggested; this dosage schedule raises serum levels to near normal without inducing diarrhea (359).

MAGNESIUM EXCESS

Mg excess or intoxication is not a common clinical problem, however mild to moderate elevation in the serum Mg have been observed in up to 12% of admissions in acute care hospitals (361). Mg intoxication is usually due to excessive administration of Mg salts, usually in the presence of impaired renal function.

Causes of Hypermagnesemia

Preeclampsia and Eclampsia

Excessive Mg administration is observed in preeclampsia and eclampsia. As discussed earlier, preeclampsia and eclampsia are the most important causes of maternal death in the United States and in many other countries (257, 258, 362). High-dose parenteral MgSO$_4$ is the drug of choice in North America for preventing eclamptic convulsions that may occur in association with severe hypertension and other problems in late pregnancy or during labor (307, 363). A loading dose and then maintenance doses are given to maintain a high serum level of approximately 2 to 3 mmol/L (4–6 mEq/L) (363) or slightly higher (364). Patients with normally functioning kidneys can excrete 40 to 60 g of MgSO$_4$ · 7H$_2$O per day when Mg is given constantly by infusion. The high doses used are rarely associated with serious side effects, because patients are closely monitored, with modification of dosage as indicated.

In one study, fetuses delivered from mothers receiving high-dosage Mg had hypermagnesemia of the umbilical vein and artery blood at about the elevated levels of the mother. However, serum levels fell progressively to normal levels in neonates by 48 hours (365).

Magnesium Overdose

Mg-containing cathartics have been given orally with activated charcoal in single or multiple doses (each of 30 g MgSO$_4$. 7H$_2$0 [245 mEq Mg^{2+}]) in an effort to decrease blood levels of drugs, as part of the treatment of patients with suspected drug overdose. In one study, despite initially normal serum creatinine concentrations (366), nine of 14 patients were hypermagnesemic by the third dose at 8 hours, including four with Mg levels of 3.0 mEq/L and one of 5.0. The presence of drugs that decreased gut motility (e.g., anticholinergics or opioids) appeared related to the higher levels (367).

Renal Failure

In addition to the planned therapeutic hypermagnesemia noted earlier, elevated serum levels occur when Mg-containing drugs, usually antacids or cathartics, are ingested on a long-term basis and in relatively large amounts by patients with advanced renal insufficiency. Because 20% or more of Mg^{2+} from various salts may be absorbed, impaired renal clearance can induce significant hypermagnesemia. The common association of age- or disease-related impairment of glomerular filtration, which may be exacerbated by ingestion of potentially nephrotoxic medications (e.g., steroidal antiinflammatory drugs for arthritic pain), and the long-term use of Mg-containing antacids and/or laxatives contribute to the danger of significant hypermagnesemia in such patients.

Hypermagnesemia may occur at symptomatic levels in patients with gastrointestinal disorders such as obstipation, severe constipation, ulceration, obstruction, or perforation when Mg-containing cathartics or antacids are taken, even in moderate dosages, and renal insufficiency is mild or moderate (368).

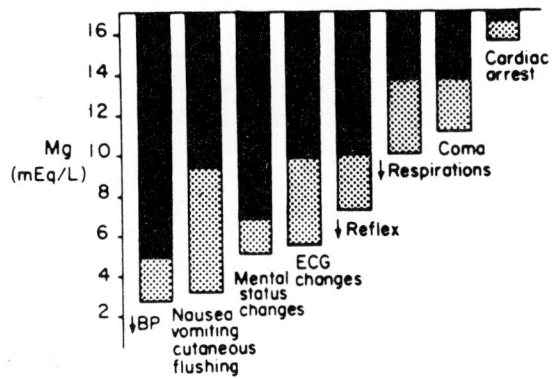

Figure 11.6. The progression in toxic effects as hypermagnesemia becomes more severe. An early sign is a lowering of blood pressure (BP). Nausea, vomiting, and hypotension may occur in the range of 3 to 9 mEq/L; bradycardia and urinary retention also occur in this range. Electrocardiogram (ECG) changes, hyporeflexia, and secondary central nervous system depression may appear in the range of 5 to 10 mEq/L, followed at higher concentrations by life-threatening respiratory depression, coma, and asystolic cardiac arrest. Mg, magnesium. (From Mordes JP, Wacker EC. Pharmacol Rev 1978;29:274–300, with permission.)

Clinical Presentations of Magnesium Excess

The many potentially toxic and even lethal effects of Mg excess are summarized in Figure 11.6 (369). One of the earliest effects is a fall in blood pressure, progressing with increasing hypermagnesemia; this appears to result from inhibition of Ca^{2+} flux and the vasoconstrictive action of norepinephine and angiotensin II (370). Mg at levels higher than normal relax vascular smooth muscle in vitro and reduce pressor responses (371). In humans, when serum Mg levels were roughly twice normal, systolic and diastolic blood pressures fell by an average of 10 and 8 mm Hg, respectively; renal blood flow increased significantly; and the pressor effect of angiotensin II was blunted (370). Urinary excretion of 6-keto-PGF$_{1\alpha}$ increased markedly. Cyclooxygenase inhibition with indomethacin or ibuprofen completely blocked the Mg-induced fall in blood pressure, the rise in urinary 6-keto-PGF$_{1\alpha}$, and the rise in renal blood flow. The Ca channel blocker nifedipine also prevented the Mg-induced rise in 6-keto-PGF$_{1\alpha}$ and fall in blood pressure. These findings indicate that the effect of Mg was mediated by PGI$_2$ release and increased Ca^{2+} flux.

With increased serum Mg levels, circulating PTH levels may drop, with associated hypocalcemia (372, 373). With maternal hypocalcemia in treatment of eclampsia, the fetus at delivery may have normal (374) or low (375) serum Ca value.

Some of the effects of very high serum Mg levels, such as lethargy, confusion, and deterioration in renal function, may be related to the hypotension (376). Electrocardiographic changes, such as prolongation of the PR and QT intervals, occur at 5 mEq/L (2.5 mmol). Tachycardia (probably secondary to hypotension) or bradycardia may occur. At 6 mEq/L and greater, muscle weakness and hyporeflexia may occur, presumably resulting from decreased release of acetylcholine and impaired transmission at the neuromuscular junction; hypocalcemia may contribute to the progressive muscle weakness and respiratory difficulty. Complete heart block and cardiac arrest may occur at about 15 mEq/L (369).

Management of Hypermagnesemia

Prevention or treatment of mild– to moderate hypermagnesemia (≥1.5 mmol) requires reducing Mg intake when absorption from all sources exceeds the renal excretory capability. At higher levels, when hemodynamic instability and muscle weakness are apparent, all Mg intake should be stopped, and an acute infusion of 5 to 10 mEq of Ca over 5 to 10 minutes should be given; Ca antagonizes the toxic effects (376). Continued saline and Ca infusion will increase Mg excretion. Peritoneal dialysis or hemodialysis will remove Mg readily in the patient with poor renal function (376).

REFERENCES

1. Kruse HD, Orent ER, McCollum EV. J Biol Chem 1932;96:519–36.
2. Hirschfelder AD, Haury VG. JAMA 1934;102:1138–41.
3. Flink EB. J Am Coll Nutr 1985;4:17–31.
4. Food and Nutrition Board, Institute of Medicine. Dietary Reference Intakes for Calcium, Phosphorus, Magnesium, Vitamin D, and Fluoride. Washington, DC: National Academy Press, 1997.
5. Maguire ME, Cowan JA. Biometals 2002;15:203–10.
6. Wolf FI, Cittadini A. Mol Aspects Med 2003;24:3–9.
7. Cowan JA. Biometals 2002;15:225–35.
8. Cowan JA. Introduction to the biological chemistry of magnesium. In: Cowan JA, ed. The Biological Chemistry of Magnesium. New York: VCH Publishers, 1995:1–24.
9. Black CB, Cowan JA. Magnesium dependent enzymes in nucleic acid biochemistry; and Magnesium dependent enzymes in general metabolism. In: Cowan JA, ed. The Biological Chemistry of Magnesium. New York: VCH Publishers, 1995:137–58.
10. Vernon WB. Magnesium 1988;7:234–48.
11. Garfinkel D, Garfinkel L. Magnesium 1988;7:249–61.
12. Knighton DR, Zheng J, Ten Eyck LF et al. Science 1991;253:407–14.
13. Maguire ME. Trends Pharmacol Sci 1984;5:73–7.
14. Babich M, King KL, Nissenson RA. J Bone Miner Res 1989;4:549–56.
15. Litosch I. J Biol Chem 1991;266:4764–71.
16. Volpe P, Alderson-Lang BH, Nickols GA. Am J Physiol 1990;258:C1077–85.
17. Smith D. Magnesium as the catalytic center of RNA enzymes. In: Cowan JA, ed. The Biological Chemistry of Magnesium. New York: VCH Publishers, 1995:111–36.
18. Agris PF. Vitam Horm 1996;52:81–126.
19. Sreedhara A, Cowan JA. Biometals 2002;15:211–23.
20. Ackerman MJ, Clapham DE. N Engl J Med 1997;336:1575–86.
21. O'Rourke B. Biochem Pharmacol 1993;46:1103–12.
22. Dorup, I. Acta Physiol Scand 1994;150:7–46.
23. Ryan MF. Ann Clin Biochem 1991;28:19–26.
24. Matsuda, H. Annu Rev Physiol 1991;53:289–98.
25. White, R.E, Hartzell H.C. Biochem Pharmacol 1989;38:859–67.
26. Iseri LT, French JH. Am Heart J 1984;108:188–93.
27. Wallach S. Magnes Trace Elem 1990;9:1–14.
28. Endres DB, Rude RK. In: Bustis CA, Ashwood ET, eds. Tietz Textbook of Clinical Chemistry. Philadelphia: WB Saunders, 1999:1395–457.
29. Gevens WB, Monnens LAH, Willems JL. Miner Electrolyte Metab 1993;19:308–13.
30. Cook LA, Mimouni FB. J Am Coll Nutr 1997;16:161–3.
31. Gunther T. Magnesium 1986;5:53–9.
32. Romani A, Marfella C, Scarpa A. Miner Electrolyte Metab 1993;19:282–9.
33. Grubbs RD. Biometals 2002;15:251–9.
34. Saris N, Mervaala E, Karppanen H et al. Clin Chim Acta 2000;294:1–26.
35. Gunzel D, Schlue W. Biometals 2002;15:237–49.
36. Murphy E. Circ Res 2000;86:245–8.
37. Grubbs RD, Maguire ME. Magnesium 1987;6:113–27.
38. Raju B, Murphy E, Levy LA et al. Am J Physiol 1989;256:C540–8.
39. Murphy E, Freudenrich CC, Levy LA et al. Proc Natl Acad Sci USA 1989;86:2981–4.
40. London RE. Annu Rev Physiol 1991;53:241–58.
41. Long-Jun D, Quamme GA. J Clin Invest 1991;88:1255–64.
42. London RE. Annu Rev Physiol 1991;53:241–58.
43. Quamme GA, Dai L, Rabkin SW. Am J Physiol 1993; 265:H281–8.
44. Erdos JJ, Maguire ME. J Physiol (Lond) 1983;337:351–71.
45. Gunther T. Miner Electrolyte Metab 1993;19:259–65.
46. Gunther T, Vormann J. FEBS Lett 1990;271:149–51.
47. Gunther T, Hollriegl V. Biochim Biophys Acta 1993;1149:49–54.
48. Smith DL, Maguire ME. Miner Electrolyte Metab 1993;19:266–76.
49. Kehres DG, Mguire ME. Biometals 2002;15:261–70.
50. Cameron IL, Smith NKR, Pool TB et al. Cancer Res 1980;40:1493–500.
51. Jakob A, Becker J, Schottle G et al. FEBS Lett 1989;246:127–30.
52. Romani A, Scarpa A. FEBS Lett 1990;269:37–40.
53. Gunther T, Vormann J, Hollriegl V. Magnes Bull 1991;13:122–4.
54. Romani A, Scarpa A. Nature 1990;346:841–4.
55. Gunther T, Vormann J. Magnes Trace Elem 1990;9:279–82.
56. Romani A, Scarpa A. Arch Biochem Biophy 1992;298:1–12.
57. Fagan TE, Scarpa A. Arch Biochem Biophy 2002;401:277–82.
58. Ziegler A, Somlyo AV, Somlyo AP. Cell Calcium 1992;13:593–602.
59. Maguire ME. Trends Pharmacol Sci 1984;5:73–7.
60. Grubbs RD, Maguire ME. J Biol Chem 1986;261:12550–4.
61. Romani A, Marfella C, Scarpa A. FEBS Lett 1992;296:135–40.
62. Grubbs RD. Am J Physiol 1991;260:C1158–64.
63. Lostroh AJ, Krahl ME. Biochim Biophys Acta 1973;291:260–8.
64. Aikawa JK. Proc Soc Exp Biol Med 1960;103:363–6.
65. Sanui H, Rubin AH. J Cell Physiol 1978;96:265–78.
66. Hua H, Gonzales J, Rude RK. Magnes Res 1995;8:359–66.
67. Kumar D, Leonard E, Rude RK. Arch Intern Med 1978;138:660.
68. Barbagallo M, Gupta RK, Resnick LM. Diabetologia 1993;36:146–9.
69. Hwang DL, Yen CF, Nadler JL. J Clin Endocrinol Metab 1993;76:549–53.
70. Pennington JAT, Young B. J Am Diet Assoc 1991;91:179–83.
71. Alaimo K, McDowell MA, Briefel RR et al. Advance Data from Vital and Health Statistics. No. 258. Hyattsville, MD: US

Department of Health and Human Services, National Center for Health Statistics, 1994.

72. Marier JR. Magnesium 1986;5:1–8.

73. Ford ES, Mokdad AH. J Nutr 2003;133:2879–82.

74. US Department of Health and Human Services (DHHS), Department of Agriculture. Nutrition Monitoring in the United States: An Update Report on Nutrition Monitoring. DHHS publication no. 89–1255. Washington, DC: US Government Printing Office, 1989.

75. Pennington JAT, Wilson DB. J Am Diet Assoc 1990;90:375–81.

76. American Society for Experimental Biology, Life Sciences Research Office, Interagency Board for Nutrition Monitoring and Related Research. Third Report on Nutrition Monitoring in the United States. Washington, DC: US Government Printing Office, 1995.

77. Rude RK. Magnesium homeostasis. In: Bilezikian JB, Raisz L, Rodan G, eds. Principles of Bone Biology. 2nd ed. San Diego: Academic Press, 2001:339–58.

78. Kerstan D, Quamme GA. Physiology and pathophysiology of intestinal absorption of magnesium. In: Massry SG, Morii H, Nishizawa Y, eds. Calcium in Internal Medicine. London: Springer-Verlag, 2002:171–83.

79. Schweigel M, Martens H. Front Biosci 2000;5:666–77.

80. Graham LA, Ceasar JJ, Burgen ASU. Metab Clin Exp 1960; 9:646–59.

81. Fine KD, Santa Ana CA, Porter JL et al. J Clin Invest 1991; 88:396–402.

82. Roth P, Werner E. Int J Appl Radiat Isot 1979;30:523–6.

83. Spencer H, Lesniak M, Gatza LA et al. Gastroenterology 1980; 79:26–34.

84. Lakshmann FL, Rao RB, Kim WW. Am J Clin Nutr 1984; 40[Suppl 6[:1380–9.

85. Spencer H, Osis D. Magnesium 1988;7:271–80.

86. Andon MB, Illich JZ, Tzagournis MA et al. Am J Clin Nutr 1996;63:950–3.

87. Lewis NM, Marcus MSK, Behling AR et al. Am J Clin Nutr 1989;49:527–33.

88. Spencer H, Osis D. Magnesium 1988;7:271–80.

89. Fine KD, Santa Ana CA, Fordtran JS. N Engl J Med 1991; 324: 1012–7.

90. Hardwick LL, Jones MR, Brautbar N et al. J Nutr 1991; 121:13–23.

91. Greger JS, Smith SA, Snedeker SM. Nutr Res 1981;1: 315–25.

92. Vormann J. Mol Aspects Med 2003;24:27–37.

93. Spencer H, Norris C, Williams D. J Am Coll Nutr 1994; 13: 479–84.

94. Turnlund JR, Betschart AA, Liebman M et al. Am J Clin Nutr 1992;56:905–10.

95. Franz KB. In: Itokawa Y, Durlach J, eds. Magnesium in Health and Disease. London: John Libbey and Co, 1989:71–8.

96. Kelsey JL, Behall KM, Prather ES. Am J Clin Nutr 1979; 32:1876–80.

97. Siener R, Hesse A. Br J Nutr 1995;73:783–90.

98. Wisker E, Nagel R, Tanudjaja TK et al. Am J Clin Nutr 1991; 54:553–9.

99. Slavin JL, Marlett JA. Am J Clin Nutr 1980;33:1932–9.

100. Lindberg JS, Zobitz MM, Poindexter JR et al. J Am Coll Nutr 1990;9:48–55.

101. Bohmer T, Roseth A, Holm H et al. Magnes Trace Elem 1990; 9:272–8.

102. White J, Massey L, Gales SK et al. Clin Ther 1992;14:678–96.

103. Kuhn I, Jost V, Wieckhorst G et al. Methods Find Exp Clin Pharmacol 1992;14:269–72.

104. Krejs GJ, Nicar MJ, Zerwekh JE et al. Am J Med 1983; 75:973–6.

105. Schmulen AC, Lerman M, Pak CYC et al. Am J Physiol 1980; 238:G349–52.

106. Kerstan , Quamme GA. In: Massry SG, Morii H, Nishizawa Y, eds. Calcium in Internal Medicine. London: Springer-Verlag, 2002:171–183.

107. Hodgkinson A, Marshall DH, Nordin BEC. Clin Sci 1979; 57:121–3.

108. Heaton FW, Hodgkinson A, Rose GA. Clin Sci 1964;27:31–40.

109. Wiltz DR, Gary RW, Dominquez JH et al. Am J Clin Nutr 1979;32:2052–60.

110. Brannan PG, Vergne-Marini P, Pak YC et al. J Clin Invest 1976;57:1412–8.

111. Norman DA, Fordtran JS, Brinkley LJ et al. J Clin Invest 1981;67:1599–603.

112. Quamme GA. Kidney Int 1997;52:1180–95.

113. Quamme GA, de Rouffignac C. Front Biosci 2000;5:694–711.

114. Satoh J, Romero MF. Biometals 2002;15:285–95.

115. de Rouffignac C, Mandon B, Wittner M et al. Miner Electrolyte Metab 1993;19:226–31.

116. Francisco LL, Sawin LL, DiBona GF. Proc Soc Exp Biol Med 1981;168:382–8.

117. Wallach S. Magnesium 1988;7:262–70.

118. Rude RK, Kirchen ME, Gruber HE et al. Magnes Res 1999; 4:257–67.

119. Rude RK, Gruber HE, Wei LY et al. Cacif Tissue Int 2003; 72:32–41.

120. Drenick EG, Hung JF, Swendseid ME. J Clin Endocrinol l969;29:1341–8.

121. Dunn MJ, Walser M. Metabolism 1966;15:884–95.

122. Wenk C, Kohut M, Kunz G et al. Z Ernahrungswiss 1993;32:301–7.

123. Shils ME, Rude RK. J Nutr 1996;126:2398S–403S.

124. Wood RJ, Suter PM, Russell RM. Am J Clin Nutr 1995; 62:493–505.

125. Lowenstein FW, Stanton MF. J Am Coll Nutr 1986;5:399–414.

126. Elin RJ. Magnes Trace Elem 1991–92;10:60–6.

127. Toffaletti J, Alvarus B, Bird C et al. Magnesium 1988;7:84–90.

128. Nixon DE, Moyer TP, Johnson P et al. Clin Chem 1986;32: 1660–5.

129. Huijgen HJ, Van Ingen HE, Kok WT et al. Clin Biochem 1996; 29:261–6.

130. Csako G, Rehak N, Elin RJ. Clin Chem 1996;42:S279(abst 763).

131. Hoffenberg EF, Kozlowski P, Salerno TA et al. J Surg Res 1996; 62:135–43.

132. Golding EM, Dobson GP, Golding RM. Magn Reson Med 1996;35:174–85.

133. London RE. Annu Rev Physiol 1991;53:241–58.

134. Aikawa JK, Gordon GS, Rhoades EL. J Appl Physiol 1960; 15:503–7.

135. Haigney MC, Silver B, Tanglao E et al. Circulation 1995;92.

136. Schwartz R. Fed Proc 1982;41:2709–13.

137. Schuette SA, Ziegler EE, Nelson SE et al. Pediatr Res 1990;27: 36–40.

138. Haigney MC, Silver B, Tanglao E. et al. Circulation 1995;92: 2190–7.

139. Cecco SA, Hristova MEN, Rehak NN. Clin Chem 1997;108: 564–9.

140. Shils ME. Medicine (Baltimore) 1969;48:61–85.

141. Rude RK, Stephen A, Nadler J. Magnes Trace Elem 1991–92; 10:117–21.

142. Elin RJ, Hosseini JM. Clin Chem 1985;31:377–80.

143. Ryzen E. Magnesium 1989;8:201–12.

144. Ryan MF, Ryan MP. Ir J Med Sci 1979;148:108–9.

145. Ralston MA, Murname MR, Kelley RE et al. Circulation 1989;
80:573–80.

146. Elin RJ, Hosseini JM, Gill JR Jr. J Am Coll Nutr 1994;13:463–6.

147. Quamme GA, Rabkin SW. Biochem Biophys Res Commun
1990;167:1406–12.

148. Fleming CR, George L, Stoner GL et al. Mayo Clin Proc
1996;71:21–4.

149. Sutton RAL, Domrongkitchaiporn S. Miner Electrolyte Metab
1993;19:232–40.

150. Rude RK. Magnesium Disorders. In: Kokko JP, Tannen RL,
eds. Fluids and Electrolytes. 3rd ed. Philadelphia: WB Saunders, 1996.

151. Al Ghamdi SMG, Cameron EC, Sutton RAL. Am J Kidney Dis
1994;24:737–52.

152. Cadell JL, Reed GF. Magnesium 1989;8:65–70.

153. Whang R, Oei T, Aikawa JK et al. Arch Intern Med
1984;144:1794–6.

154. Whang R, Hampton EM, Whang DD. Ann Pharmacother
1994;28:220–6.

155. Ryzen E, Wagers PW, Singer FR. et al. Crit Care Med 1985;
13:19–21.

156. Chernow B, Bamberger S, Stoiko M et al. Chest 1987;
955:391–7.

157. Fiaccadori E, del Canale S, Coffrini E et al. Crit Care Med
1988;16:751–60.

158. Thoren L. Acta Chir Scand 1963;306[Suppl]:5–60.

159. LaSala MA, Lifshitz F, Silverber M et al. J Pediatr Gastroenterol Nutr 1985;4:75–81.

160. Nyhlin H, Dyckner T, Ek B, Wester PO. J Am Coll Nutr 1985;
4:531–8.

161. Heaton FW, Fourman P. Lancet 1965;2:50–2.

162. Booth CC, Hanna S, Babouris N et al. BMJ 1963;2:141–4.

163. Goldman AS, Van Fossan DD, Baird EE. Pediatrics 1962;29:
948–52.

164. Dyckner T, Hallberg D, Hultman E et al. J Am Coll Nutr
1982;1:239–46.

165. Van Gaal L, Delvigne C, Vandewoude M et al. J Am Coll Nutr
1987;6:397–400.

166. Weir GC, Lesser PB, Drop LJ et al. Ann Intern Med 1975;
83:185–9.

167. Ryzen E, Rude RK. West J Med 1990;152:145–8.

168. Schlingmann KP, Weber S, Peters M et al. Nat Genet 2002:
31:166–70.

169. Massry SG, Coburn JW, Chapman LW et al. Am J Physiol 1967;
213:218–24.

170. Coburn JW, Massry SG, Kleeman CR. Nephron 1970;7:131–43.

171. McNair P, Christensen MS, Christiansen C et al. Eur J Clin
Invest 1982;12:81–5.

172. Quamme GA. Am J Physiol 1989;256:F197–210.

173. Quamme GA. Kidney Int 1997;52:1180–95.

174. Quamme GA. Am J Physiol 1981;241:F340–7.

175. Zaloga GP, Chernow B, Pock A et al. Surg Gynecol Obstet
1984;158:561–5.

176. Kes P, Reiner Z. Magnes Trace Elem 1990;9:54–60.

177. Meyer KB, Madias NE. Miner Electrolyte Metab 1994;20:
201–13.

178. Lam M, Adelstein BJ. Am J Kidney Dis 1986;8:164–9.

179. Allen RD, Hunnisett AG, Morris PJ. Lancet 1985;6:1283–4.

180. Mendelson JH, Ogata M, Mello NK. Ann NY Acad Sci
1969;169:918–33.

181. Lau K, Nichols FR, Tannen RL. J Lab Clin Med 1987;109:
27–33.

182. Kondrad M, Weber S. J Am Soc Nephrol 2003;14:249–60.

183. Simon DB, Lu Y, Choate KA et al. Science 1999;285:103–6.

184. Praga M, Vara J, Gonzalez-Parra E et al. Kidney Int 1995;
47:1419–25.

185. Meij IC, Saar K, van den Heuvel LPWJ et al. Am J Hum Genet
1999;64:180–8.

186. Simon DB, Nelson-Williams C, Bia MJ et al. Nat Genet 1996;
12:24–30.

187. Kantorovich V, Adams JS, Gaines JE et al. J Clin Endocrinol
Metab 2002;87:612–7.

188. Rude RK. Magnesium disorders. In: Kokko JP, Tannen RL, eds.
Fluids and Electrolytes. 3rd ed. Philadelphia: WB Saunders,
1996:421–45.

189. Song Y, Buring JE, Manson JE et al. Diabetes Care 2004;
27:59–65.

190. Lopez-Ridaura R, Stampfer MJ, Willett WC et al. Diabetes
Care 2004;27:134–40.

191. Shils ME: Magnesium. In: O'Dell BL, Sunde RA, eds. Handbook of Nutritionally Essential Mineral Elements. New York:
Marcel Dekker, 1997:117–52.

192. Alcock NW, Shils ME. Proc Soc Exp Biol Med 1974; 146:
137–41.

193. Rude RK, Gruber HE, Wei LY et al. Calcif Tissue Int
2003;72:32–41.

194. Shils ME. Magnesium deficiency and calcium and parathyroid
hormone interrelations. In: Prasad A, ed. Trace Elements in
Human Health and Disease, vol 2. New York: Academic Press,
1976:23–46.

195. Alcock NW, Shils ME, Lieberman PH et al. Cancer Res
1973;33:2196–204.

196. Whang R, Oliver J, Welt LG et al. Ann NY Acad Sci 1969;
162:766–74.

197. Heggtveit HA. Ann NY Acad Sci 1969;162:758–65.

198. Morris ER, O'Dell BL. J Nutr 1963;81:175–81.

199. Bunce GE, Chiemchaisri V, Phillips PH. J Nutr 1962;76:
23–9.

200. Sherwood LM, Herrman I, Bassett CA. Nature 1970;225:
1056–7.

201. Ferment O, Garnier PE, Touitou Y. J Endocrinol 1987;113:
117–22.

202. Rude RK. In: Bilezikian JP, ed. The Parathyroids. New York:
Raven Press, 1994:829–42.

203. Brown EM, Gamba G, Riccardi D et al. Nature 1993;366:
575–80.

204. Hebert SC. Kidney Int 1996;50:2129–39.

205. Rude RK, Oldham SB, Singer FR. Clin Endocrinol 1976;5:
209–24.

206. Shils ME. Ann NY Acad Sci 1980;355:165–80.

207. Anast CS, Forte LF. Endocrinology 1983;113:184–9.

208. Fatemi S, Ryzen E, Flores J et al. J Clin Endocrinol Metab
1991;73:1067–72.

209. Suh SM, Tashjian AH, Matsuo N et al. J Clin Invest
1973;52:153–60.

210. Rude RK, Oldham SB, Sharp CF Jr et al. J Clin Endocrinol
Metab 1978;47:800–6.

211. Anast CS, Mohs JM, Kaplan SL et al. Science 1972;177:606–8.

212. Estep H, Shaw WA, Watlington C et al. J Clin Endocrinol
1969;29:842–8.

213. Woodard JC, Webster PD, Carr AA. Digest Dis 1972;17:612–8.

214. Mac Manus J, Heaton FW, Lucas PW. J Endocrinol 1971;49:
253–8.

215. Levi J, Massry SG, Coburn JW et al. Metabolism 1974;23:
323–35.

216. Forbes RM, Parker HM. J Nutr 1980;110:1610–7.

217. Medalle R, Waterhouse C, Hahn TJ. Am J Clin Nutr 1976;29: 854–8.
218. Bitensky MW, Keirns JJ, Freeman J. Am J Med Sci 1973; 266: 320–47.
219. Neer E. J Cell 1995;80:249–57.
220. Northup JK, Smigel MD, Gilman AG. J Biol Chem 1982;257: 11416–23.
221. Brown EM. Physiol Rev 1991;71:371–411.
222. Dunlay R, Hruska K. Am J Physiol 1990;258:F223–31.
223. Babich M, King KL, Nissenson RA. J Bone Miner Res 1989;4: 549–56.
224. Litosch I. J Biol Chem 1991;266:4764–71.
225. Volpe P, Alderson-Lang BH, Nickols GA. Am J Physiol 1990; 25:C1077–85.
226. Leicht E, Biro G, Keck E et al. Klin Wochenschr 1990; 68:678–84.
227. Selby PL, Peacock M, Bambach CP. Br J Surg 1984;71:334–7.
228. Graber ML, Schulman G. Ann Intern Med 1986;104:804–6.
229. Lifshitz F, Harrison HC, Harrison HE. Proc Soc Exp Biol Med 1967;125:472–6.
230. McAleese DM, Forbes RM. Nature 1959;184:2025–6.
231. Smith RH. Biochim J 1958;70;201–5.
232. Rude RK, Adams JS, Ryzen E et al. J Clin Endocrinol Metab 1985;61:933–40.
233. Fuss M, Bergmann P, Bergans A et al. J Clin Endocrinol Metab 1989;31:31–8.
234. Leicht E, Schmidt-Gayk N, Langer HJ et al. Magnes Res 1992; 5:33–6.
235. Fisco F, Traba ML. Magnes Res 1992;5:5–14.
236. Whang R, Hampton EM, Whang DD. Ann Pharmacother 1994;28:220–6.
237. Hexum T, Samson FE Jr, Himes RH. Biochim Biophys Acta 1970;212:322–31.
238. Beauge L, Campos MA. J Physiol (Lond) 1986;375:1–25.
239. Chang C, Bloom S. J Am Coll Nutr 1985;4:173–85.
240. Zhang S, Sawanobori T, Adaniya H et al. Am J Physiol 1995; 268:H2321–8.
241. Rude RK and Oldham S. In: Cohen RD, Lewis B, Albert KGMM et al, eds. The Metabolic and Molecular Basis of Acquired Disease. London: Bailliere Tindall, 1990:1124–48.
242. Wacker WE, Moore FD, Ulmer DD et al. JAMA 1962;180: 161–3.
243. Cole DE, Quamme GA. J Am Soc Nephrol 2000;11:1937–47.
244. Mordes JP, Wacker WE. Pharmacol Rev 1978;29:273–300.
245. Del Castillo J, Engbaek L. J Physiol (Lond) 1954;124:370–84.
246. Jenkinson DH. J Physiol (Lond) 1957;138:434–44.
247. Augustine GJ, Charlton MP, Smith SJ. Annu Rev Neurosci 1987;10:633–93.
248. Carpentier RG, Posner P, Bloom S. J Cardiovasc Pharmacol 1985;7:919–23.
249. Laban E, Charbon GA. J Am Coll Nutr 1986;5:521–32.
250. Guideri G, Lehr D, Horowitz S. J Am Coll Nutr 1985;4:139–55.
251. Seller RH, Cangiano J, Kim KE et al. Am Heart J 1970; 79:57–68.
252. Zehender M, Meinertz T, Faber T et al. J Am Coll Cardiol 1997;29:1028–34.
253. Kasaoka S, Tsuruta R, Nakashima K et al. Japan Circ J 1996; 60:871–5.
254. Moran JL, Gallagher J, Peake SL et al. Crit Care Med 1995; 23:1816–24.
255. Delva P. Mol Aspects Med 2003;24:53–62.
256. Iseri LT, Freed J, Bures AR. Am J Med 1975;58:837–46.
257. Iseri LT, Fairshter RD, Hardemann JL et al. Am Heart J 1985; 110:789–94.
258. Shechter M, Hod H, Chouraqui P et al. Am J Cardiol 1995; 75:321–3.
259. Tsuji H, Venditti FJ Jr, Evans JC et al. Am J Cardiol 1994; 74:232–5.
260. Kafka H, Langevin L, Armstrong P. Arch Intern Med 1987; 147:465–9.
261. Chadda KD, Lichstein E, Gupta P. Am J Cardiol 1973;31: 98–100.
262. Shechter M, Merz CN, Rude RK et al. Am Heart J 2000;140: 212–8.
263. Leclerc JR. Crit Care Med 2002;30:S332–40.
264. Delva P. Mol Aspects Med 2003;24:63–78.
265. Woods KL, Fletcher S, Roffe C et al. Lancet 1992;330:1553–8.
266. Collins R, Peto R, Flather M et al. Lancet 1995;345:669–85.
267. Antman E, Cooper H, Domanski M et al. Lancet 2002; 360:1189–96.
268. Woods KL, Abrams K. Prog Cardiovasc Dis 2002;44:267–74.
269. Touyz RM. Mol Aspects Med 2003;24:107–36.
270. Joffres MR, Reed DM, Yano K. Am J Clin Nutr 1987;45: 469–75.
271. Ma J, Folsom AR, Melnick SL et al. J Clin Epidemiol 1995; 48:927–40.
272. Witteman JCM, Willett WC, Stampfer MJ et al. Circulation 1989;80:1320–7.
273. Albert DB, Morita Y, Iseri LT. Circulation 1958;17:761–4.
274. Gadallah M, Massry SG, Bigazzi R et al. Am J Hypertens 1991;4:404–9.
275. Resnick LM, Gupta RK, Laragh JH. Proc Nat Acad Sci USA 1984;81:6511–5.
276. Touzy RM. Mol Aspects Med 2003;24:107–36.
277. Resnick L, Gupta R, Bhargara K. Hypertension 1991;17: 951–7.
278. Dyckner T, Wester PO. BMJ 1983;286:1847–9.
279. Geleijhnse JM, Witteman JC, Bak AA et al. BMJ 1994; 309: 436–40.
280. Witteman JC, Grobbee DE, Derkx FH et al. Am J Clin Nutr 1994;60:129–35.
281. Sachs FM, Brown LE, Appel L et al. Hypertension 1995;26: 950–6.
282. Yamamoto ME, Applegate WB, Klag MJ et al. Ann Epidemiol 1995;5:96–107.
283. Appel LJ, Moore TJ, Obarzanek E et al. N Engl J Med 1997;336:1117–24.
284. Nadler JL, Goodson S, Rude R. Hypertension 1987;9:379–83.
285. Altura BM, Altura BT. Magnes Bull 1986;8:338–50.
286. Rude R, Manoogian C, Ehrlich L et al. Magnesium 1989; 8:266–73.
287. Hwang D, Yen C, Nadler J. Am J Hypertens 1992;5:700–6.
288. Nadler J, Malayan S, Luong H et al. Diabetes Care 1992; 15:835–41.
289. Gilbert DAE, Singer H, Rembold C. J Clin Invest 1992;89: 1988–94.
290. Maier JAM. Mol Aspects Med 2003;24:137–46.
291. Cunnane SC, Soma M, McAdoo KR et al. J Nutr 1985;115: 1498–503.
292. Geuex E, Mazur A, Cardot P et al. J Nutr 1991;121:1222–7.
293. Nigam S, Averdunk R, Gunther T. Prostaglandins Leukot Med 1986;23:1–10.
294. Rayssiguier Y, Geuex E, Bussiere L et al. J Am Coll Nutr 1993; 12:133–7.
295. Sachs FM, Brown LE, Appel L et al. Hypertension 1995; 26:950–6.
296. Douglas K, Redman C. BMJ 1994;309:1395–400.
297. Crowther CA. S Afr Med J 1985;68:927–9.

298. Bergstrom S, Povey G, Songane F et al. J Perinat Med 1992;20:153–8.

299. Greene MF. N Engl J Med 2003;348:275–6.

300. Isler CM, Martin JN Jr. Semin Nephrol 2002;22:54–64.

301. Johnson JS, Hand WL, King-Thompson NL. Cell Immunol 1980;53:236–45.

302. Laurant P, Touyz RM. J Hypertens 2000;18:1177–91.

303. Rukshin V, Shah PK, Cercek B et al. Circulation 2002; 105: 1970–5.

304. Belfort MA, Anthony J, Saade GR et al. N Engl J Med 2003; 348:302–11.

305. Kisters K, Barenbrock M, Louwen F et al. Am J Hypertens 2000;13:765–9.

306. Taber EB, Tan L, Chao CR et al. Am J Obstet Gynecol 2002;186:1017–21.

307. Duley L, Farrell B, Spark P et al. Lancet 2002;359:1877–90.

308. Lai CC, Singer L, Armstrong WD. J Bone Joint Surg 1975;57: 516–22.

309. McCoy H, Kenny MA, Gillham B. Nutr Rep Int 1979;19: 233–40.

310. Mirra JM, Alcock NW, Shils ME et al. Magnesium 1982; 1:16–33.

311. Carpenter TO, Mackowiak SJ, Troiano N et al. Am J Physiol 1992;263:E107–14.

312. Boskey AL, Rimnac CM, Bansal M et al. J Orthop Res 1992;10: 774–83.

313. Kenney MA, McCoy H, Williams L. Calcif Tissue Int 1994;54: 44–9.

314. Gruber HE, Massry SG, Brautbar N. Miner Electrolyte Metab 1994;20:282–6.

315. Rude RK, Kirchen ME, Gruber HE et al. Magnes Res 1999;12: 257–67.

316. Loveless BW, Heaton FW. Br J Nutr 1976;36:487–95.

317. Creedon A, Flynn A, Cashman K. Br J Nutr 1999;82:63–71.

318. Rude RK, Gruber HE, Wei LY et al. Calcif Tiss Int 2003; 72:32–41.

319. Duckworth J, Godden W, Warnock GM. Biochem J 1940; 34:97–108.

320. Miller ER, Ullrey DE, Zutaut CL et al. J Nutr 1965;85: 13–20.

321. Heroux O, Peter D, Tanner A. Can J Physiol Pharmacol 1975;53:304–10.

322. Smith BS, Nisbet DI. J Comp Pathol 1968;78:149–59.

323. Yano K, Heilbrun LK, Wasnich RD et al. Am J Clin Nutr 1985; 42:877–88.

324. Angus RM, Sambrook PN, Pocock NA et al. Bone Miner 1988; 4:265–77.

325. Tranquilli AL, Lucino E, Garzetti GG et al. Gynecol Endocrinol 1994;8:55–8.

326. Houtkooper LB, Ritenbaugh C, Aickin M et al. J Nutr 1995; 125:1229–37.

327. New SA, Bolton-Smith C, Grubb DA et al. Am J Clin Nutr 1997;65:1831–9.

328. New SA, Robins SP, Campbell MK et al. Am J Clin Nutr 2000;71:142–51.

329. Tucker KL, Hannan MT, Chen H et al. Am J Clin Nutr 1999;69:727–36.

330. Wang MC, Moore EC, Crawford PB et al. Osteoporos Int 1999;9:532–5.

331. Cohen L, Kitzes AL. Magnesium 1983;2:70–5.

332. Cohen L, Laor A, Kitzes R. Magnesium 1983;2:139–43.

333. Reginster JY, Maertens de Noordhout B, Albert A et al. Magnesium 1985;4:208.

334. Reginster JY, Strause L, Deroisy R et al. Magnesium 1989;8: 106–9.

335. Abraham GE. J Nutr Med 1991;2:165–78.

336. Eisinger J, Clairet D. Magnes Res 1993;6:247–9.

337. Stendig-Lindberg G, Tepper R, Leichter I. Magnes Res 1993;6: 155–63.

338. Rude RK, Olerich M. Osteoporosis Int 1996;6:453–61.

339. Levin ME, Boisseau VC, Avioli LV. N Engl J Med 1976; 294:241–5.

340. McNair P, Christiansen C, Christensen MS et al. Eur J Clin Invest 1981;11:55–9.

341. McNair P, Madsbad S, Christensen MS et al. Acta Endocrinol 1979;90:463–72.

342. Hui SL, Epstein S, Johnston CC Jr. J Clin Endocrinol Metab 1985;60:74–80.

343. Saggese G, Bertelloni S, Baroncelli GI et al. Helv Paediatr Acta 1988;43:405–14.

344. Krakauer JC, McKenna MJ, Buderer, NF. et al. Diabetes 1995;44:775–82.

345. Bikle DD, Genant HK, Cann C et al. Ann Intern Med 1985;103:42–8.

346. Lindholm J, Steiniche T, Rasmussen E et al. J Clin Endocrinol Metab 1991;73:118–24.

347. Peris P, Pares A, Guanabens N et al. J. Alcohol Alcohol 1992; 27:619–25.

348. Molteni N, Caraceni MP, Bardella MT et al. Am J Gastroenterol 1990;85:51–3.

349. Mora S, Weber G, Barera G et al. Am J Clin Nutr 1993;57:224–8.

350. Liu CC, Yeh JK, Aloia JF. J Bone Miner Res 1988;3:S104.

351. Azria M. Calcif Tissue Int 1989;45:7–11.

352. Franceschi RT, Romano PR, Park K-H et al. In: Norman AW, Schaefer K, Grigoleit HG et al, eds. Vitamin D Molecular Cellular and Clinical Endocrinology. Berlin: W de Gruyter, 1988: 624–625.

353. Jones JE, Schwartz R, Krook L. Calcif Tissue Int 1980;31: 231–8.

354. Marcus R. In: Bilezikian JP, ed. The Parathyroids. New York: Raven Press, 2001:853–63.

355. Weglicki WB, Dickens BF, Wagner TL et al. Magnes Res 1996;9:3–11.

356. Flink E. Acta Med Scand Suppl 1981;647:125–37.

357. Ramee SR, White CJ, Savarinth JT. et al. Am Heart J 1985;109:164–6.

358. Tzivoni D, Keren A. Am J Cardiol 1990;65:1397–9.

359. Stromme JH, Steen-Johnson J, Harnaes K et al. Pediatr Res 1981;15:1134–9.

360. Allen DB, Greer FR. Calcium and magnesium deficiency beyond infancy. In: Tsang RC, ed. Calcium and Magnesium Metabolism in Early Life. Boca Raton, FL: CRC Press, 1995.

361. Wong ET, Rude RK, Singer FR et al. Am Soc Clin Pathol 1983;79:348–52.

362. Roberts JM, Redman CWG. Lancet 1993;341:1447–51.

363. Cunningham FG, Lindheimer MD. N Engl J Med 1992;326: 927–32.

364. Cholst IN, Steinberg SF, Tropper PJ et al. N Engl J Med 1984;310:1221–5.

365. McGuinness GA, Weinstein MM, Cruikshank DP et al. Obstet Gynecol 1980;56:595–600.

366. Smilkstein MJ, Steedle D, Kulig KW et al. Clin Toxicol 1988;26:51–65.

367. Nelson KB. Editorial. JAMA 1996;276:1843–33.

368. Kattan M. Editorial. J Pediatr 1996;129:783–5.

369. Mordes JP, Wacker EC. Pharmacol Rev 1978;29:274–300.

370. Rude RK, Mamoogian C, Ehrich P et al. Magnesium 1989; 8:266–73.

371. Altura BM, Altura BT. Magnes Bull 1986;8:338–50.

372. Cholst IN, Steinberg SF, Tropper PJ et al. N Engl J Med 1984;310:1221–5.

373. Eisunbud E, LoBoe CL. Arch Intern Med 1976;136: 688–91.

374. McGuinness GA, Weinstein MM, Cruikshank DP et al. Obstet Gynecol 1980;56:595–600.

375. Donovan EF, Tsang RC, Steichen JJ et al. J Pediatr 1980;96:305–10.

376. Clark BA, Brown RS. Am J Nephrol 1992;12:336–43.

IRON[1]

RICHARD J. WOOD AND ALAYNE G. RONNENBERG

HISTORICAL BACKGROUND 248
IRON BIOCHEMISTRY 248
   Iron Is a Limited Biologic Resource 248
   Iron Is a Generator of Free Radicals 249
   Biologic Importance of Iron-Containing Proteins . .249
IRON PHYSIOLOGY 249
   Iron Partitioning in the Body 249
   Overview of Iron Kinetics 249
   Iron Loss 251
IRON CELL BIOLOGY 251
   Mechanisms of Cellular Iron Uptake and Storage . .251
   Iron Regulatory Protein–Dependent Control
      of Intracellular Iron Homeostasis 252
   Mitochondrial Iron Metabolism 254
   Iron Metabolism in Specialized Cell Types 255
IRON IN MEDICINE 258
   Genetic Disorders Affecting Iron Metabolism 258
   Clinical Disorders Affecting Iron Metabolism 261
IRON NUTRITION 262
   Dietary Iron Intake 262
   Dietary Iron Bioavailability 263
   Dietary Reference Intakes 264
   Assessment of Iron Status 266
   Anemia and Iron Deficiency 267
   Health Consequences of Elevated Iron Stores 268

HISTORICAL BACKGROUND

The history of iron in medicine and nutrition has been reviewed in the literature (1, 2). Iron had early medicinal uses. The ancient Egyptians used rust (iron oxide) as a

treatment for baldness, whereas the ancient Greeks used a mixture of wine and iron in attempts to restore male potency. During the seventeenth century, iron was used to treat chlorosis ("green disease"), a disease subsequently shown to be the result of iron deficiency. However, it would not be until 1932 that the importance of iron in chlorosis was finally settled. An early study of iron nutrition published in 1895 described the diets of patients with chlorosis as containing only 1 to 3 mg/day iron compared with a usual dietary content in healthy, physiologically normal persons of 8 to 11 mg/day.

IRON BIOCHEMISTRY

Iron Is a Limited Biologic Resource

Iron is a metal that is found in abundance on Earth and is a biologically essential element involved in the metabolism of all living organisms. However, despite its geologic abundance, iron is a limiting biologic important metal in the environment. This apparent paradox is because almost all the Earth's iron is found in insoluble iron oxide complexes or metallic iron and is not readily available for biologic needs. This fact of geochemistry has led to the evolution of various cellular mechanisms to capture iron from the environment in a biologically useful form. For example, one common environmental iron retrieval mechanism found in microbes involves iron-regulated secretion of iron chelator molecules, called siderophores, into the local microbial environment (3). Chelation is the process wherein metal ions are attached to organic molecules through the formation of coordination bonds. The iron-laden siderophore is captured by the microbe via siderophore receptors on the cell surface, and the iron is internalized. Under low iron conditions, iron-regulated gene expression can result in the coordinated upregulation of both iron siderophores and siderophore receptors. Additional microbial iron transport adaptations include ways of using iron-containing proteins found in blood of higher organisms and the ability to reduce ferric (Fe^{+3}) iron to ferrous (Fe^{+2}) iron. Simple eukaryotic organisms, such as yeast, have developed complicated metabolic systems to regulate iron nutrition (4). Many of these iron utilization mechanisms in lower organisms have analogous counterparts in higher organisms, including humans.

[1]**Abbreviations: ACD,** anemia of chronic disease; **ALAS2,** erythroid isoform of 5-aminolevulinate synthase; **ATP,** adenosine triphosphate; **Dcytb,** duodenal cytochrome b; **DMT1,** divalent metal transporter 1; **DRI,** dietary reference intake; **EAR,** estimated average requirement; **FPN1,** ferroportin 1; **HLA,** human leukocyte antigen; **IRE,** iron-responsive element; **IRP,** iron regulatory protein; **NHANES,** National Health and Nutrition Examination Survey; **NRAMP,** natural resistance-associated macrophage protein; **RBC,** red blood cell; **RDA,** recommended dietary allowance; **RES,** reticuloendothelial system; **SNP,** single nucleotide polymorphism; **TfR,** transferrin receptor; **UL,** tolerable upper intake level; **USDA,** United States Department of Agriculture; **UTR,** untranslated region.

Iron Is a Generator of Free Radicals

In an aqueous environment, iron can be found in two principal oxidation states as either ferrous (Fe^{+2}) or ferric (Fe^{+3}) iron. Conversion between these two iron states is accomplished relatively easily. At the oxygen concentration found under physiologic conditions, iron is mostly found in the more stable oxidized ferric form. Conversely, important biologic processes such as transmembrane transport, deposition of iron into ferritin, and the synthesis of heme all require that iron be in its reduced ferrous state. This leads to a critical role of ferrireductases in iron metabolism. The redox capabilities of iron can also be the basis of potential toxicity resulting from the Haber-Weiss-Fenton sequence (shown later) that leads to the generation of hydroxyl radical (OH •) subsequent to the formation of superoxide (O_2^-•) following the one-electron reduction of dioxygen (O_2) by ferrous iron. The hydroxyl radical can attack proteins, nucleic acids and carbohydrates and initiate chain-propagating lipid peroxidation (5).

Haber-Weiss-Fenton reactions:

$$Fe^{+2} + O_2 \rightarrow Fe^{+3} + O_2^- \bullet$$

$$2\,O_2^- \bullet + 2H^+ \rightarrow H_2O_2 + O_2$$

$$Fe^{+2} + H_2O_2 \rightarrow OH\bullet + OH^- + Fe^{+3}$$

Biologic Importance of Iron-Containing Proteins

Two biologically important iron-containing chemical moieties are iron-sulfur complexes or clusters and heme. Both these chemical forms of iron lie at the very base of the chemistry of life as we know it. For example, plant iron-sulfur clusters found in ferredoxin are needed in the early steps of photosynthesis. In certain nitrogen-fixing bacteria, an iron-sulfur cluster is a constituent of the enzyme nitrogenase needed for converting atmospheric nitrogen into ammonia. In animals, the iron-sulfur cluster in the enzyme aconitase links the iron content of the cell with the activity of the tricarboxylic acid cycle, a series of linked enzymatic steps important for cellular energy production via oxidative phosphorylation reactions involving carbohydrate and lipids. Mitochondrial aconitase catalyzes the conversion of citrate to isocitrate in the tricarboxylic acid cycle. Heme is composed of a porphyrin ring structure with a central iron atom. The primary function of heme iron is as the oxygen-carrying constituent of the proteins hemoglobin in erythrocytes and myoglobin in muscle tissue. Peroxidase enzymes also contain heme and are important in protecting the cell from oxidative injury by reducing peroxides to water. Myeloperoxidase is a heme-containing peroxidase enzyme unique to neutrophils and monocytes that binds superoxide anion radicals or hydrogen peroxide and is able to form a wide variety of oxidant products. Heme iron also functions as the active site of cytochromes, enzymes needed in the electron transport chain.

In addition to proteins containing heme or iron-sulfur clusters are numerous important iron metalloenzymes. For example, aromatic amino acid hydroxylases are iron-containing monooxygenases. Monooxygenases add one oxygen atom to the substrate that is hydroxylated. These metalloenzymes require tetrahydrobiopterin as a cofactor and are involved in the synthesis of the following: tyrosine (phenylalanine hydroxylase); DOPA (tyrosine hydroxylase), a precursor of dopamine; and 5-hydroxy-tryptophan (tryptophan hydroxylase), a precursor of serotonin. Other iron metalloenzymes include dioxygenases that add both oxygen atoms to a single substrate. For example, 5-lipoxygenase is a dioxygenases that plays an essential role in the biosynthesis of proinflammatory leukotrienes.

IRON PHYSIOLOGY

Iron Partitioning in the Body

The average person's body contains approximately 3 to 4 g of iron. Most (~2 g) of body iron is found in the blood as hemoglobin iron. Storage iron (ferritin and hemosiderin) is found mostly in the liver. Under normal circumstances, storage iron content is approximately 300 to 1000 mg in girls and women and 500 to 1500 mg in boys and men. In iron overload disorders, however, body iron can reach 40,000 to 50,000 mg (6). In iron overload disorders, excess body iron is deposited primarily in the liver, spleen, and bone marrow. The third largest iron compartment is found in the myoglobin (130 mg) in muscle tissue. Only a very small amount of the body's total iron content is contained in iron metalloenzymes (8 mg). Likewise, the iron bound to transferrin in the plasma represents only about 3 mg. However, as much as ten times this amount of iron must cycle through the transferrin iron compartment daily to meet the ongoing needs of erythropoiesis.

Overview of Iron Kinetics

Absorption: Exogenous Iron Supply

An overview of the movement of iron in the body is shown in Figure 12.1. Dietary iron is composed of heme iron derived exclusively from animal (meat) foods, or nonheme iron found in both animal and plant-based foods. The usual Western-style diet contains about 10% of its iron as heme iron. Dietary iron is absorbed in the upper small intestine. From a typical daily dietary iron intake of 10 to 15 mg, only about 1 to 2 mg is absorbed. Heme iron bioavailability is usually much greater than nonheme iron. In iron deficiency, the absorption efficiency of nonheme iron is greatly increased. Additional amounts of iron can be absorbed in iron-deficient subjects if they consume high-dose iron supplements. In nursing infants, another source of dietary iron is from lactoferrin found in mother's milk. Regardless of its dietary source, iron absorbed from the intestine joins the small, but rapidly turning over,

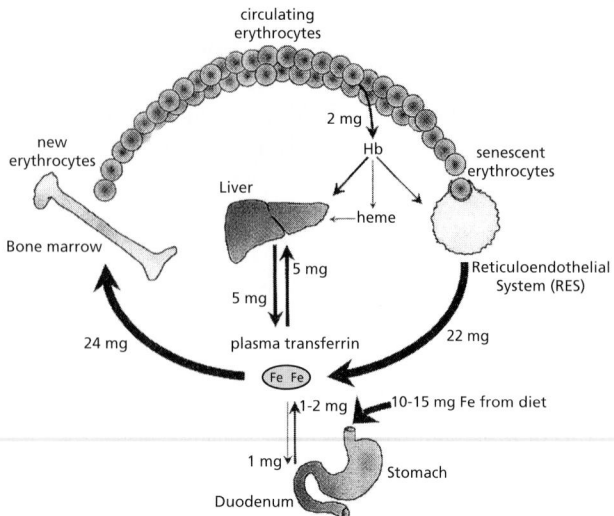

Figure 12.1. Overview of iron flux in the body. Only a relatively small amount of dietary iron intake is absorbed. Absorbed iron is contributed to the circulating pool of plasma iron carried on the protein transferrin. At any point in time, only a small fraction of total body iron is bound to transferrin, but the daily flux of iron through this compartment is considerable. Plasma transferrin needs to deliver about 24 mg of iron daily to the bone marrow because of the need of erythrocyte precursors for hemoglobin synthesis in the ongoing process of replacement of worn-out red blood cells. Most of this iron need is supplied by the reticuloendothelial system (RES) that is responsible for destruction of erythrocytes and reclamation of iron. About 10% of red blood cell destruction occurs intravascularly. The released hemoglobin and any heme generated from hemoglobin degradation are delivered to the RES or liver, and the iron is reclaimed. The liver acts as the main site of iron storage in the body. (From Knutson M, Wessling-Resnick M. Iron metabolism in the reticuloendothelial system. Crit Rev Biochem Mol Biol 2003;38:61–88, with permission of CRC Press LLC.)

circulating pool of protein-bound plasma iron carried on transferrin. Under normal circumstances, the efficiency of iron absorption is closely linked to body iron needs and iron stores. Iron absorption is known to be increased in iron deficiency anemia, the latter stages of pregnancy during rapid fetal growth, when erythropoiesis is stimulated, and in hereditary hemochromatosis. In contrast, iron absorption is decreased in certain chronic inflammatory diseases, such as rheumatoid arthritis, or whenever erythropoiesis is decreased.

The Transferrin Iron Pool: Iron Delivery

Iron absorbed from the intestine, or released from macrophages during red blood cell (RBC) breakdown, is carried in plasma as ferric iron (Fe^{+3}) by transferrin, an 80-kDa glycoprotein consisting of a single polypeptide chain and two N-linked complex-type glycan chains (7). The protein contains two iron-binding sites. Essentially all the iron in plasma is bound to transferrin. One milligram of diferric transferrin contains 1.4 μg iron. Normally, only about one third of the iron-binding capacity of transferrin is saturated. The plasma half-life of transferrin is 8.5 to

10 days. In contrast, the plasma clearance of transferrin-bound iron is much faster (half-life, 60–90 min). Transferrin is responsible for delivering significant quantities of iron (~24 mg/day) to the bone marrow to supply the daily needs of erythrocyte precursors for hemoglobin synthesis. Thus, most (70–90%) of the iron on transferrin is delivered to the bone marrow for hemoglobin synthesis in RBC precursors. The remainder of the iron is used by other tissues for synthesis of iron-containing compounds, such as myoglobin, cytochromes, and iron-containing enzymes. During pregnancy, a substantial need exists for transferrin-mediated iron delivery to the placenta to meet the iron need for fetal growth. The large size of transferrin hinders its glomerular filtration at the kidney. Thus, the amount of iron in the renal ultrafiltrate is very low and is the reason that very little iron is lost in the urine under normal circumstances.

Reticuloendothelial System: Iron Reclamation

Most of the iron used for hemoglobin synthesis is supplied to the plasma transferrin pool by the macrophages of the reticuloendothelial system (RES), which is responsible for the reclamation of iron from worn-out RBCs. Within 12 hours of RBC breakdown, 60% of the iron is recycled into new hemoglobin. The remainder enters the ferritin storage pool. In cases of increased or ineffective erythropoiesis, release of stored iron is increased to meet the demands of hemoglobin synthesis. In contrast, in infectious, inflammatory, or neoplastic diseases, a cytokine-mediated anemia of chronic disease (ACD) develops that is associated with decreased iron reutilization and accumulation of reticuloendothelial iron stores. Normally, in adults, only about 20 to 25 mg iron/day is needed to sustain hemoglobin synthesize in the ongoing process of replacing worn-out erythrocytes, which have a usual life span of 120 days. Normal bone marrow can increase RBC production up to sixfold, however, if needed. Under these conditions of maximal hemoglobin synthesis, as much as 100 to 125 mg iron/day can be needed for hemoglobin synthesis.

To illustrate the large daily iron needs for hemoglobin synthesis, consider that a person with a blood volume of 5 L and a hemoglobin concentration of 150 g/L will have 750 g hemoglobin in circulation. Because hemoglobin has an iron content of 0.34%, this represents 2.55 g iron (750 × 0.0034) that will be needed every 4 months (or ~21 mg iron/day) to replace worn-out erythrocytes.

Some circulating erythrocytes (~10%) are broken down intravascularly, and hemoglobin is released directly into the plasma. This free hemoglobin is bound by a special protein (haptoglobin) and is delivered to the liver and RES. Any heme that is released into the bloodstream from degraded hemoglobin during the intravascular destruction of erythrocytes will be bound by another protein, hemopexin, and delivered to the liver and RES.

Liver: Iron Storage Depot and Possible Control Point for Iron Regulation

Liver is the primary site of iron storage in the body, and it likely serves as the central control point of whole-body iron regulation. Within the cell, iron is sequestered in the cytosol inside the ferritin macromolecule, but it can be released as iron is needed. A recent serendipitous observation in knockout mice (8) implicated the liver-derived peptide hepcidin (HAMP) as a candidate central regulatory molecule that could explain both iron-dependent and inflammation-dependent changes in iron absorption (9, 10). Iron absorption efficiency and circulating hepcidin are inversely correlated. High circulating hepcidin is associated with low iron absorption. In hereditary hemochromatosis, hepcidin concentrations are inappropriately low, a finding suggesting a possible role of this peptide in the hyperabsorption of iron in this genetic disorder. This notion is further supported by the observation that the phenotypic expression of iron overload in persons with the C282Y HFE mutation may be modulated by concomitant mutations in hepcidin (11). Likewise, overexpression of hepcidin can prevent iron overload normally seen in HFE knockout mice (12). Investigators have suggested that some regulatory signal, which could be hepcidin, somehow programs intestinal crypt cells (13) that will then mature into absorptive enterocytes with innate iron transport characteristics reflecting iron status or needs of the host. However, alternative models of intestinal iron regulation based on more direct effects on mature enterocytes (14–16) are also possible.

Iron Loss

Endogenous losses of iron in male subjects estimated from ferrokinetic studies are about 1 mg/day (0.013 mg/kg body weight) (17). About one half of daily endogenous iron losses occur through the intestine, most of that accounted for by occult blood loss (0.35 mg/day) and the remainder from ferritin iron in sloughed enterocytes (0.10 mg/day) and iron in biliary secretions (0.10 mg/day). Iron loss in the shedding of skin cells is about 0.2 mg/day, and a small amount (0.08 mg/day) is lost in the urine. In iron overload, as much as 4 mg iron/day can be lost through the gastrointestinal tract. Vigorous exercise can also result in increased gastrointestinal blood loss. In one study using radioactively labeled RBCs to measure gastrointestinal blood loss, baseline blood loss of less than 1.5 mL/day increased to 4.9 to 6.6 mL/day during intensive training periods (18). Important determinants of iron loss in women include periodic bleeding associated with menstruation and pregnancy-associated blood loss and fetal iron needs. In addition, body iron is lost in men and women from miscellaneous blood loss (e.g., hemorrhage, blood donation). The iron content of whole blood is about 0.5 mg/mL at a blood hemoglobin concentration of 150 g/L. The importance of menstruation on iron loss in women can then be appreciated if one considers that the periodic monthly menstrual blood loss is about 1.5 ounces (43 mL), which would be equivalent to about 0.7 mg iron/day (43 × 0.5/30). Moreover, the upper limit of normal blood loss is about twice that amount. Additional factors, such as the use of oral or mechanical (intrauterine device) contraceptive methods or the onset of menopause, alter menstrual blood loss and affect iron loss in women. Because of their increased iron requirements resulting from periodic blood loss, women of reproductive age are at relatively high risk of developing iron deficiency and anemia. Body iron stores are also further markedly affected by net iron losses associated with each pregnancy. Lactation is not an important source of net iron loss in women. The iron content of human milk is 0.35 mg/L. Thus, typical milk volumes of 0.78 L/day produced during lactation are associated with an additional 0.27 mg/day iron loss. However, the cessation of menstruation associated with lactation serves to offset this additional iron loss in women who are breast-feeding.

IRON CELL BIOLOGY

Mechanisms of Cellular Iron Uptake and Storage

Some important proteins involved in cellular iron metabolism are listed in Table 12.1. Iron uptake by cells is controlled by the number of transferrin receptors (TfRs) expressed on the plasma membrane. Especially high numbers of TfRs are associated with erythrocyte precursors as a result of the significant cellular iron needs for hemoglobin synthesis. The expression of TfR in these cells is regulated by an Ets-1 transcription factor–mediated transcriptional mechanism (19), which differs from the post-transcriptional mode of regulation found in other cell types. TfR numbers diminish with further maturation of the normoblast as hemoglobin synthesis declines and are absent in the mature reticulocyte (20). Circulating transferrin-bound iron is taken up into cells by a cell-surface TfR (TfR-1). The TfR complex functions as a dimer of two identical 90-kDa transferrin receptors. TfRs are class II membrane receptors and are internalized in response to binding of the diferric transferrin ligand to their extracellular domains. This internalization process involves uptake of the entire TfR-diferric transferrin complex into an endocytic vesicle (Fig. 12.2). Once formed, the vesicle is acidified by the action of a membrane proton pump. The slightly acidic environment in the endosome facilitates the release of Fe^{+3} from transferrin, which is then reduced to Fe^{+2}. The Fe^{+2} is transported out of the endosome by divalent metal transporter 1 (DMT1), the plasma membrane proton-coupled iron transporter. The transferrin cycle is completed when the endosome containing the TfR and iron-free apotransferrin recycles back to the plasma membrane where the neutral pH environment facilitates the dissociation of apotransferrin from the TfR. The apotransferrin released into the plasma is then free to be reloaded with ferric iron. Cellular iron uptake via the TfR

TABLE 12.1. SOME IMPORTANT PROTEINS INVOLVED IN IRON METABOLISM

PROTEIN	STRUCTURE AND FUNCTION
PROTEINS INVOLVED IN IRON TRANSPORT	
Duodenal cytochrome b (Dcytb)	Membrane ferric reductase
Divalent metal transporter 1 (DMT1)	Single-chain membrane-spanning glycoprotein acts as membrane iron transporter
Hephaestin (HEPH)	Transmembrane-bound ceruloplasmin-like ferroxidase
Ferroportin 1 (FPN1)	Membrane iron exporter
Transferrin	Plasma and extracellular fluid iron-binding transport protein
Transferrin receptor 1	Membrane receptor dimer composed of two 90-kDa units involved in receptor-mediated endocytosis of ferric transferrin
Transferrin receptor 2	Membrane receptor involved in receptor-mediated endocytosis of ferric transferrin in liver and intestinal crypt cell
Lactoferrin	Iron-binding protein secreted into milk and found in neutrophils with possible antibactericidal activity
PROTEINS INVOLVED IN IRON STORAGE	
Ferritin	Spheric intracellular iron storage protein composed of 24 L- and H-ferritin subunits; binds up to 4500 iron atoms
Hemosiderin	Partially degraded form of ferritin found in greater abundance in tissues with iron overload
PROTEINS INVOLVED IN IRON REGULATION	
HFE	Hemochromatosis gene product that interacts with transferrin receptor to regulate transferrin receptor affinity and recycling rate
Iron regulatory protein (IRP)	Cytosolic RNA-binding proteins (IRP-1 and IRP-2) that coordinate translational regulation of transferrin receptor, ferritin, and other iron responsive element (IRE)–containing mRNAs
Ceruloplasmin (CP)	Plasma copper-dependent ferroxidase
Hepcidin (HAMP)	Liver-produced peptide involved in regulation of iron absorption
PROTEINS INVOLVED IN MITOCHONDRIAL IRON METABOLISM	
Frataxin (FRDA)	Mitochondrial iron homeostasis
ATP-binding cassette 7 transporter (ABC7)	Transporter involved in mitochondrial iron homeostasis and maturation of iron-sulfur cluster-containing proteins
Ferrochelatase	Enzyme responsible for iron incorporation into heme

can be modulated by HFE, the protein defective in hereditary hemochromatosis, which can influence the rate of the TfR cycle (13).

In addition to transferrin-mediated iron uptake into cells, some tissues, such as the liver, also have a non–transferrin-bound iron uptake capacity. Evidence for this pathway includes the observation that iron accumulates in the liver and some other tissues in patients with the genetic disorder atransferrinemia. TfR expression is regulated in most cell types in response to cellular iron status through an iron regulatory protein (IRP)–dependent posttranscriptional mechanism that involves stabilization of the TfR mRNA. In contrast, a second form of TfR (TfR-2) (21), which has been recently identified in liver, is not regulated by iron. TfR-2 is clearly important, however, because mutations in this gene result in iron overload (HFE3) disease in humans (22) and mice (23).

The storage of excess iron in cells is accomplished by its sequestration within the ferritin molecule. A small amount of ferritin is also found in plasma and has been shown to be a good measure of iron stores. Serum ferritin concentrations up to and including 12 µg/L are found in the absence of stainable iron in bone marrow and indicate depleted

iron stores. Ferritin protein is a large, spheric molecule composed of 24 L-ferritin and H-ferritin monomers. Pores are evident on the surface of the ferritin molecule and may allow iron to be transferred into the center core region, where iron is deposited as inorganic ferric oxyhydroxide (24). The capacity of each ferritin shell is 4300 iron atoms, but most have about 2000 iron atoms. Iron can be removed from the ferritin core, but the details of this process are poorly understood. A second storage form of iron is in the less well-characterized molecule hemosiderin that is believed to be an aggregated ferritin partially stripped of protein. Under conditions of excess iron, more of the metal is stored as hemosiderin than ferritin.

Iron Regulatory Protein–Dependent Control of Intracellular Iron Homeostasis

Iron is essential for cellular function. Excess cellular iron can be dangerous to the cell because of increased oxidation of DNA, proteins, and cell membranes resulting from the generation of free radicals by iron-driven Fenton reactions (25). It is necessary, therefore, to maintain tight control on the availability of iron. Cellular iron balance is regulated by

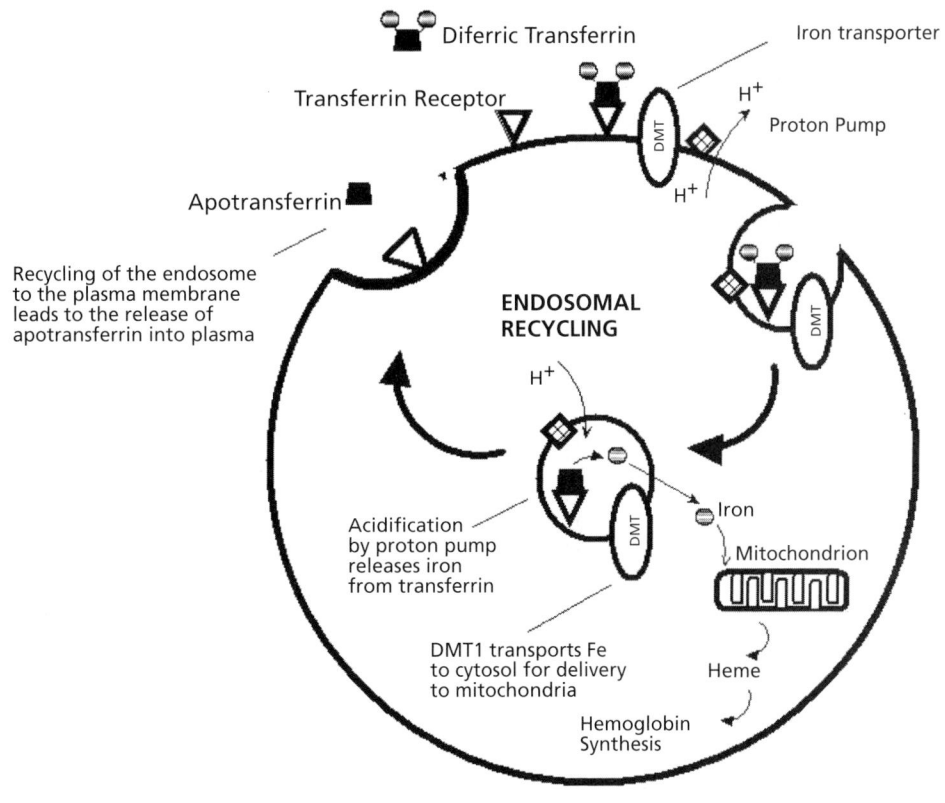

ERYTHROID PRECURSOR

Figure 12.2. Transferrin receptor cycle. Apotransferrin in the plasma can bind two atoms of iron as ferric (Fe^{+3}) iron. Diferric transferrin has increased binding affinity for transferrin receptors found on the surface of cells. Transferrin receptors transport iron into cells by a process that involves the formation of endosomes wherein the plasma membrane invaginates and forms an endosomal vesicle. Both the transferrin receptor and diferric transferrin are taken up into the cell, along with some other cell membrane proteins including divalent metal transporter 1 (DMT1), a proton-dependent transporter of the reduced ferrous (Fe^{+2}) form of iron. During its cycling through the cell, the internal compartment of the endosome is acidified by the action of a proton pump. The acidic environment facilitates the release of ferric iron from transferrin. The iron is presumably reduced by a ferrireductase (not shown) to ferrous iron that is transported out of the endosome by DMT1. The recycling of the transferrin-transferrin receptor complex is completed when the endosome fuses with the plasma membrane leading to the exposure of apotransferrin to the more neutral environment of the extracellular fluid, which facilitates its release from the transferrin receptor. The apotransferrin is then free to bind additional ferric iron atoms, and the transferrin receptor is available once again to capture additional iron for the cell and repeat the cycle. The iron delivered to the cell is primarily used by mitochondria for incorporation into heme, especially in erythrocyte precursor cells, or into iron-sulfur clusters.

an elegant posttranscriptional mechanism involving IRP-1 and IRP-2. IRP is an approximately 90-kDa molecular weight protein that can bind in an iron-dependent manner "stem-loop" secondary structure formed in mRNA by a nucleotide sequence called the iron-responsive element (IRE).

The coordinated control of ferritin and TfR protein concentrations by the IRP-IRE regulatory system is illustrated in Figure 12.3. When the chelatable iron pool in the cytosol is low, the physiologic responses of the cell to restore iron balance are to increase the expression of TfR to allow for greater uptake of iron from the plasma and to decrease the synthesis of the iron storage protein ferritin. In this low-iron situation, the 4Fe-4S iron-sulfur cluster in the IRP is converted to 3Fe-4S. In this 3Fe-4S configuration, the IRP has high affinity for binding to the IRE (26) found in the ferritin and TfR mRNAs. The IRE is found as a single IRE in the 5′

untranslated region (UTR) of ferritin mRNAs and as multiple IREs in the 3′ UTR of the TfR mRNA. This differential positioning of the IRE-found ferritin and TfR mRNA results in different effects when the IRP binds. In the ferritin example, IRP binding to the 5′ UTR IRE inhibits the translation of the mRNA into protein because of an inability to recruit the 43S preinitiation complex (27), whereas in the TfR example, the binding of IRPs to the IREs in the 3′ UTR of the TfR mRNA stabilizes the mRNA and leads to an increase in the mRNA pool and increased translation of TfR protein. Thus, the balance of iron in each cell can be coordinately controlled by the rate of synthesis of ferritin and TfR that is controlled by the iron-sulfur cluster switch in IRP that acts as a biologic sensor of cellular iron status (28).

Conversely, when cellular iron levels rise sufficiently to restore the 4Fe-4S cluster configuration in IRP, the RNA-

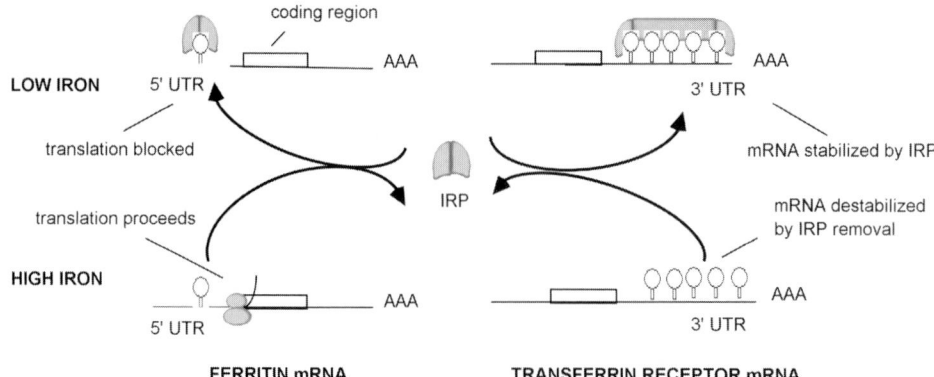

Figure 12.3. Iron regulatory protein (IRP)–dependent control of intracellular iron homeostasis. The iron-responsive element (IRE) is found in either the 5′- or 3′-untranslated region (UTR) of certain mRNAs and allows for the IRP-dependent regulation of protein translation, as in the case of ferritin, or stabilization of the mRNA pool, as seen with the transferrin receptor mRNA. The binding affinity of IRP-1 for the IRE is dependent on cellular iron status. Under low-iron conditions in the cell, homeostasis is achieved by reducing the synthesis of ferritin, an iron storage protein, and increasing the expression of transferrin receptor protein, which is responsible for bringing iron into the cell. When cellular iron conditions are low, IRP-1 binds to the IRE stem-loop structure in the 5′- UTR of the ferritin mRNA. IRP binding at the 5′-UTR position blocks recruitment of the preinitiation complex and prevents ferritin translation. At the same time, binding of IRP under these low-iron conditions to the multiple IREs found in the 3′-UTR of transferrin receptor mRNAs stabilizes the mRNA and leads to a rise in the concentration of transferrin receptor mRNA and an increased production of transferrin receptor protein, which can be directed to the cell surface and is then available to increase cellular iron uptake. Under high-iron conditions, the opposite effect occurs, wherein removal of the IRP protein from IRE allows ferritin synthesis to proceed (providing additional cellular iron-binding capacity), and the transferrin receptor mRNA pool declines because of an increase in its degradation rate. Thus, less transferrin receptor protein is produced, and cellular iron uptake decreases. The iron-related change in IRP-1 mRNA binding depends on the ability to switch the 4Fe-4S cluster in IRP-1 to 3Fe-4S. The IRE binding of a second IRP protein (IRP-2) that does not contain an iron-sulfur cluster is not iron dependent, but cellular iron status controls the rate of IRP-2 degradation leading to a similar type of iron-dependent control.

binding affinity of IRP is decreased and the 3′ UTR translational block on ferritin synthesis is removed, leading to increased ferritin and a greater intracellular iron sequestering capacity. At the same time, IRP can no longer bind to the 3′ UTR of TfR mRNA. The removal of IRP from the IRE in the TfR mRNA exposes a "rapid turnover determinant" in the 3′ UTR that contains a site for endonucleolytic cleavage of the mRNA (29, 30). This reduces the half-life of TfR mRNA from 3 hours to 30 minutes, thus reducing mRNA availability.

In addition to the IRE found in ferritin mRNA and TfR mRNA, IRE or IRE-like motifs have also been recognized in several other mRNAs coding for proteins involved in iron metabolism. These other potential IRP target mRNAs are as follows: the erythroid isoform of 5-aminolevulinate synthase (ALAS2) that is involved in heme synthesis; DMT1, which is responsible for nonheme iron uptake; ferroportin 1 (FPN1/IREG-1), a transporter needed for cellular iron export; and mitochondrial aconitase, an enzyme involved in mitochondrial citrate efflux (30). With the exception of DMT1, all the IREs in these target mRNAs are found in the 5′ UTR, a finding suggesting that the synthesis of these proteins will be blocked under low-iron conditions.

Mitochondrial Iron Metabolism

Much of the iron taken up by cells is first used by mitochondria. For example, a large part of the daily cellular iron flux is related to use by erythroblast mitochondrial

ferrochelatase, which inserts iron into protoporphyrin IX to form heme, which is needed for hemoglobin synthesis. Mitochondria also require iron for synthesis of various iron-sulfur proteins. Iron-sulfur clusters are synthesized in mitochondria and are incorporated into proteins. Disruption of mitochondrial iron metabolism can have important disease implications. For example, Friedreich ataxia is one of the most common autosomal recessive forms of ataxia and is characterized by mitochondrial iron overload and degeneration of the central and peripheral nervous system, cardiomyopathy, skeletal abnormalities, and increased risk of diabetes. The genetic mutation in this abnormality is in a nuclear-encoded gene for the mitochondrial iron-binding protein frataxin (FRDA). A GAA-repeat expansion in the *FRDA* gene interferes with gene transcription and leads to frataxin deficiency, which ultimately disrupts mitochondrial iron handling. The specific function of frataxin is under active investigation, but recent evidence suggests that it is primarily important for its role in the maturation of cellular iron-sulfur cluster proteins (31). In yeast, the export of iron-sulfur proteins from mitochondria is mediated by the inner mitochondrial membrane transporter ATM1p (32), a yeast ortholog of ABC7, a member of the adenosine triphosphate (ATP)-binding cassette (ABC) transporter family. Missense mutations in ABC7 are associated with mitochondrial iron accumulation and cause the genetic disorder known as X-linked sideroblastic anemia with cerebellar ataxia. Iron accumulation in mitochondria involves two mitochondrial solute carriers, MRS3 (*mitochondrial RNA splicing protein*) and MRS4 (33), although other systems of mitochondrial iron acquisition probably also exist (34). A nuclear-coded mitochondrial H-type ferritin has also been described and may play an important role in mitochondrial iron metabolism (35).

Iron Metabolism in Specialized Cell Types

Enterocyte

A current view of iron transport across the enterocyte is shown in Figure 12.4. The main barriers of cellular iron transport in the intestine include transport across the apical membrane of the enterocyte, iron movement across the cytosol, transport across the basolateral membrane, and passage through the interstitial space and capillary wall (36). Nonheme iron in the intestinal lumen is first presented to the brush border membrane, found on the apical aspect of the absorptive enterocyte, where it encounters at least two important membrane proteins: duodenal cytochrome b (Dcytb) (37) and DMT1 (also known as NRAMP2 (natural resistance-associated macrophage protein 2) and DCT1) (38, 39). The uptake of heme iron by the enterocyte is via a separate pathway than nonheme iron. Heme is absorbed intact, by a putative apical membrane heme receptor (40). Once in the cytosol, heme is split by heme oxygenase, and iron is released to enter a common intracellular iron pool with absorbed nonheme iron.

Dcytb is a membrane-bound ferric reductase that converts oxidized ferric (Fe^{+3}) iron to reduced ferrous (Fe^{+2}) iron. Dcytb also has a putative binding site for ascorbic acid, a potential electron donor (41). Ferrous iron is transported across the apical membrane by DMT1, a membrane iron transporter that can also transport other divalent ions (38). Both Dcytb (42) and DMT1 (38) expression are increased in iron deficiency. The potential adverse oxidative reactivity of free iron and emerging information about the important trafficking role of metal "chaperone" proteins (43) suggest that iron will always be protected in some bound state with intracellular proteins. However, these putative iron transport proteins have not been adequately characterized to date in higher organisms. Exit of ferrous iron across the basolateral membrane of the enterocyte is mediated by FPN1 (44), also known as IREG-1 (iron-regulated protein 1) (45) or MTP-1 (metal protein transporter-1) (46). FPN1 expression increases in iron deficiency (47). The export of iron depends on a second basolateral membrane protein called hephaestin, a ceruloplasmin-like, membrane-bound protein that has copper-dependent ferroxidase activity (48). The Fe^{+3} resulting

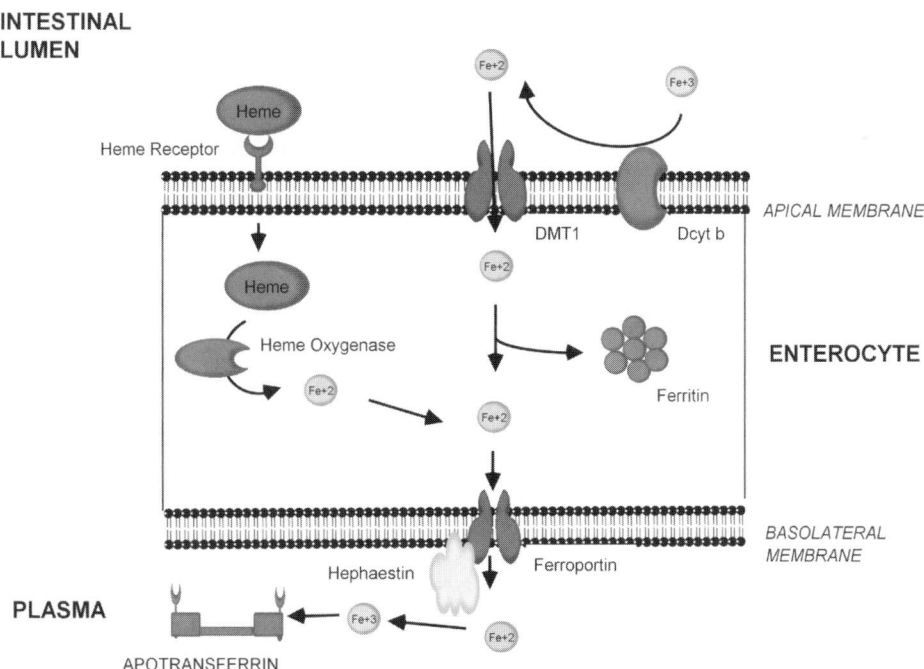

Figure 12.4. Molecular mechanism of enterocyte iron transport. Dietary ferric iron (Fe^{+3}) in the intestinal lumen is reduced by a cell-surface ferrireductase (duodenal cytochomes b [Dcyt b]) to ferrous (Fe^{+2}) iron. Ferrous iron is transported into the enterocyte by divalent metal transporter 1 (DMT1). Iron entering the enterocyte can be sequestered into ferritin, an iron storage protein, or transported across the basolateral membrane. The export of iron from the enterocyte is accomplished by ferroportin. However, iron export from the enterocyte is dependent on another protein called hephaestin, which is a ceruloplasmin-like molecule that has copper-dependent ferroxidase activity. In the absence of functional hephaestin, iron accumulates in the enterocyte. Hephaestin presumably functions by converting ferrous iron to ferric iron that is then available to bind to plasma apotransferrin. Iron may also be found in meat as heme iron. The enterocyte has a putative heme receptor that can bind heme and deliver it into the enterocyte. Once in the cytosol, the ferrous iron in heme is released by the action of heme oxygenase. The released iron then enters a common pool with any absorbed nonheme iron and is available for export out of the cell by ferroportin.

from the oxidation of Fe^{+2} by hephaestin could then bind to circulating apotransferrin. In *sla* (sex-linked anemic) mice, a genetic mutation leads to hephaestin deficiency, and the transfer of iron out of the enterocyte is blocked, leading to iron deficiency anemia (48). However, it is still unclear whether the ferroxidase activity of hephaestin is critical for iron release because recent studies in rats (49) and Caco-2 cells, a human intestinal cell line (50), found that copper deficiency leads to increased, not decreased, iron absorption. Iron depletion in rats does not appear to affect hephaestin levels markedly (51). Another important protein that plays a role in the regulation of iron absorption and metabolism is HFE, the protein mutated in hereditary hemochromatosis. In the intestine, HFE is expressed exclusively in the intestinal crypt cell, where it associates with TfR-2 and programs the iron absorption of the maturing enterocyte. HFE is also found in the macrophage and hepatocyte, two other cell types important in iron metabolism. In this genetic disorder, inappropriately high rates of iron absorption occur despite chronic body iron loading. The absorption defect is caused by a disruption in the functioning of the HFE protein. In hemochromatosis, it is likely that altered HFE function leads to the development of a low iron content in the enterocyte because of a reduced TfR recycling rate (13) and concomitant upregulation of the iron transporter protein DMT1 leading to inappropriately high iron absorption in the presence of accumulating body iron burdens.

Erythroblast

The erythroblast refers to all nucleated RBCs that are precursors of erythrocytes. In the adult, erythroblasts are produced within the bone marrow of the vertebra, sternum, and ribs. The least mature recognizable cell type in the erythroblast lineage in the marrow is the proerythroblast. Each proerythroblast will eventually develop into eight to 32 mature RBCs. Cells of subsequent stages of maturation are known as erythroblasts (or normoblasts). Ferritin has been shown by electron microscopy in the cytoplasm of normoblasts as either isolated molecules or within membrane enclosed structures referred to as sidersomes, but little hemoglobin is as yet present (52). Further maturation of the normoblast is associated with increased amounts of hemoglobin. Ferrochelatase is an important mitochondrial enzyme involved in the last step of heme biosynthesis wherein iron is incorporated into protoporphyrin IX. Ferrochelatase interacts with a mitochondrial ATP-binding cassette (ABC) transporter protein called ABC7, which is needed for heme transport (53). Achievement of a critical hemoglobin concentration leads to nuclear damage, cessation of cell division, and the eventual extrusion of the degenerated nucleus from the cell. In iron deficiency, hemoglobin synthesis is reduced, and this allows additional cell division to occur, leading to the development of smaller (microcytic) erythrocytes (52).

The denucleated cell is known as a reticulocyte. Reticulocytes leave the bone marrow and enter into circulation. Normally, only about 1% of circulating RBCs are reticulocytes; however, under some circumstances, this percentage can increase significantly when the bone marrow produces reticulocytes at a very rapid rate. As the reticulocyte matures into the erythrocyte in the peripheral blood, additional intracellular organelles continue to be lost, including eventually the ribosomes. Because mature RBCs lack ribosomes, hemoglobin synthesis no longer occurs. Hemoglobin accounts for 90% of the dry weight of the erythrocyte and is primarily responsible for oxygen transport by the blood.

Macrophage

The RES is composed of circulating monocytes and tissue macrophages and plays an important role in iron metabolism (54). Monocytes are released from bone marrow into the blood. After migrating to tissues, the monocytes differentiate into macrophages. The predominant tissue location of macrophages is the liver, intestine, bone marrow, spleen, and kidney. Macrophages in the spleen, liver, and bone marrow are mainly responsible for recycling iron from senescent RBCs. Macrophages can acquire iron by erythrophagocytosis, by receptor-mediated uptake of hemoglobin, and possibly by receptor-mediated uptake of transferrin (Fig. 12.5). Phagocytosis of senescent erythrocytes is the main source of macrophage iron. The erythrocyte is broken down by hydrolytic enzymes in the phagosome. Hemoglobin is degraded by proteolytic digestion releasing heme that then crosses the phagosomal membrane to be broken down by heme oxygenase in the endoplasmic reticulum. About 10 to 20% of erythrocyte breakdown occurs intravascularly. Hemoglobin released intravascularly is bound by haptoglobin and is cleared from circulation by hepatic parenchymal cells. Some hemoglobin may also be removed from plasma by the CD163 hemoglobin scavenger receptor on monocytes and macrophages. Under conditions such as hemolytic anemia, some free hemoglobin may be found in the plasma and can be broken down, releasing heme. The heme is bound by hemopexin, a plasma glycoprotein, and is delivered to the liver. Specific hepatic hemopexin receptors remove the heme-hemopexin complex from circulation. Some heme may also be taken up by the RES. In culture, macrophages express high levels of TfRs; however, the extent to which iron uptake by macrophages occurs by this mechanism in vivo is unknown. Macrophages do express IRP1 and IRP2, findings suggesting that the IRE-IRP iron regulatory system operates in this cell type. Cellular iron transport in macrophages is accomplished by two proteins (Nramp1 and Nramp2) of the NRAMP family. Nramp1 is expressed exclusively in monocytes and macrophages and is involved in the transport of iron in the phagosomes, although it is unclear whether it transports iron in or out of this

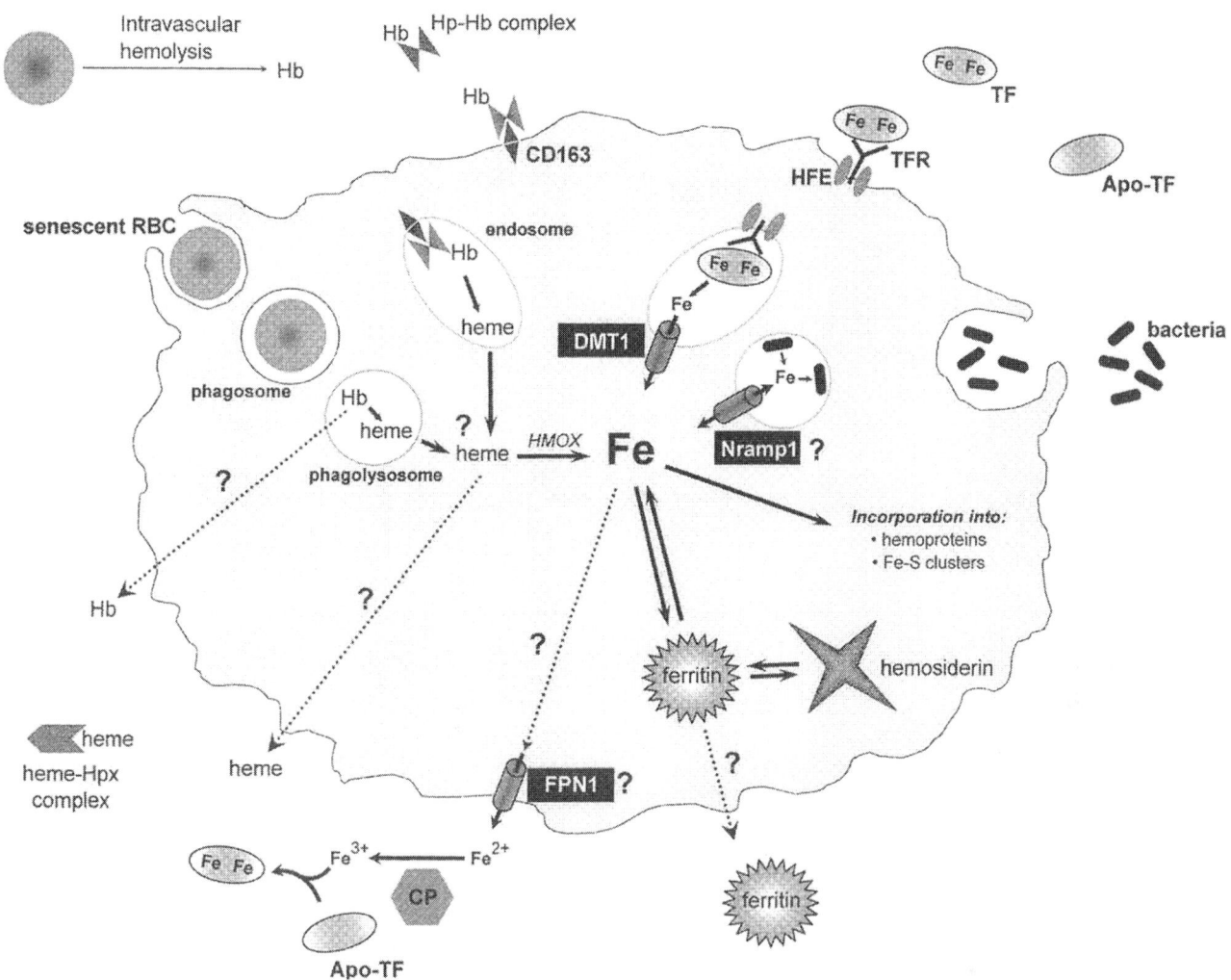

Figure 12.5. Macrophage iron metabolism. Macrophages play an important role in iron recycling and supply the majority of iron used by erythrocyte precursors in the bone marrow in the synthesis of hemoglobin. Senescent red blood cells are taken up by macrophages into phagosomes and are broken down. Heme recovered from degraded hemoglobin in the phagosome is released into the cytosol, where it is catabolized by heme oxygenase (HMOX), releasing iron that may then be sequestered by ferritin, the iron storage protein, or incorporated into hemoproteins or Fe-S clusters. Macrophages also take up transferrin-bound iron via transferrin receptors (TFRs) located on the plasma membrane. The iron released from transferrin is transported from endosomal vesicles by divalent metal transporter 1 (DMT1). A similar iron transporter (Nramp1) is found in macrophages and plays a role in the inactivation of phagocytosed bacteria. HFE, the protein mutated in hereditary hemochromatosis, is found in association with the transferrin receptor and can modulate transferrin receptor function. Ferrous iron in the cytosol may exit the macrophage via ferroportin (FPN1). Ferrous iron exported from the macrophage is oxidized by ceruloplasmin (CP; a copper-dependent plasma ferroxidase) and can then be bound as ferric iron by apotransferrin. Other sources of iron taken up by macrophages likely include free plasma hemoglobin (Hb) resulting from any intravascular breakdown of red blood cells (RBCs). In addition, any hemoglobin complexed with haptoglobin (Hp) in plasma is recognized by the macrophage CD163 receptor. This complex is endocytosed, and the heme is released to the cytosol where the iron can be reclaimed by the action of HMOX. Some heme, hemoglobin, and ferritin may be released directly into the plasma from macrophages. In plasma, heme is bound by hemopexin (Hpx). (From Knutson M, Wessling-Resnick M. Iron metabolism in the reticuloendothelial system. Crit Rev Biochem Mol Biol 2003;38:61–88, with permission of CRC Press LLC.)

organelle (54). Nramp1 shares 64% amino acid identity with Nramp2, also known as DMT1. DMT1 is ubiquitously expressed and has been more fully characterized as an iron transporter than Nramp1. DMT1 is responsible for transporting iron released from diferric transferrin out of the endosome into the cytosol in other cell types and likely functions in the same way in the RES. In macrophage cell lines, DMT1 is not regulated by iron. Following phagocytosis and breakdown of the RBC in

macrophages, released iron that is not used for other functions can be sequestered in the cytosol by ferritin. The reticuloendothelial cells of the bone marrow contain similar amounts of iron as the liver, approximately 100 to 300 mg. In addition to ferritin, the macrophage also stores excess iron in hemosiderin, an insoluble, aggregated form of partially digested ferritin. The highest concentrations of hemosiderin are found in the RES (55). Iron is released from macrophages, mostly in a low-molecular-weight form that can bind to plasma transferrin. However, transferrin does not appear to be critical for iron release from macrophages. Conversely, ceruloplasmin, a copper-dependent plasma ferroxidase, is needed for iron release. Most (80%) of circulating iron in plasma is en route between the RES and bone marrow. At present, the molecular mechanism of iron release from the macrophage is uncertain (54). These cells express FPN1, which has been shown to be important for iron export from the enterocyte. However, FPN1 may also play a role in the transit of iron intracellularly following heme breakdown. The molecular factors involved in regulating the release of iron from the RES and the specific role of ferroportin require clarification.

IRON IN MEDICINE

Genetic Disorders Affecting Iron Metabolism

Hereditary Hemochromatosis

Genetic disorders affecting proteins involved in iron metabolism are shown in Table 12.2. Hereditary hemochromatosis is an inherited disorder characterized by iron overload. Hemochromatosis was recognized as a clinical entity in the nineteenth century (56). Hereditary hemochromatosis is a human leukocyte antigen (HLA)–linked autosomal recessive disorder that is now appreciated to be caused in the majority of cases by a single nucleotide polymorphism (SNP) (Fig. 12.6) in the *HFE* gene (57). The SNP in the *HFE* gene causes a cysteine-to-tyrosine residue substitution at position 282 in the HFE protein (C282Y HFE), a major histocompatibility complex class I–like protein (57) expressed on the plasma membrane. The prevalence of the C282Y HFE mutation is five of 1000 in white people (58). Approximately 10% of the non-Hispanic white population in the United States is estimated to be heterozygous for the C282Y HFE mutation compared with 2% of non-Hispanic blacks

and 3% of Mexican-Americans (59). A second SNP in *HFE* that results in a histidine-to-aspartic acid residue substitution in the HFE protein (H63D) may also play some role in hereditary hemochromatosis. The prevalence estimates in the US population are 5.4% for the C282Y HFE mutation and 13.5% for the H63D HFE mutation (59).

The primary cause of iron overload in hereditary hemochromatosis is inappropriately elevated intestinal iron absorption. Persons with hereditary hemochromatosis may chronically absorb 2 mg/day iron irrespective of high body iron burdens. Following phlebotomy, iron absorption may rise to 10 mg/day. Our understanding of the likely molecular mechanism of this intestinal defect in iron homeostasis was greatly enhanced by the discovery in 1996 of the HFE mutation associated with hereditary hemochromatosis (57). The amino acid substitution in C282Y HFE caused by the mutation disrupts the normal association of the HFE protein with β_2-microglobulin (60) and leads to premature degradation of HFE and reduced cell-surface HFE expression. Based on findings generated in transfected Chinese hamster ovary cells overexpressing both HFE and β_2-microglobulin, a hypothetic model of the possible cellular defect in the enterocyte in hereditary hemochromatosis that leads to excess iron absorption has been presented (13). The loss of normal HFE protein expression on the cell membrane of the enterocyte leads to a reduced recycling rate of the TfR and causes lower enterocyte uptake of iron from diferric transferrin and consequently low cellular iron content. The low enterocyte iron content continues to drive high expression of intestinal DMT1 and ferroportin iron transporters and to cause inappropriately high iron absorption in the presence of accumulating body iron stores. Because the body cannot homeostatically rid itself of iron, the excess absorbed iron leads to increased body iron burdens that can eventually cause pathologic tissue and organ damage.

TABLE 12.2. GENETIC DISORDERS AFFECTING PROTEINS INVOLVED IN IRON METABOLISM

GENETIC DISORDER	DEFECTIVE GENE	PHYSIOLOGIC AND CLINICAL MANIFESTATIONS
Hereditary (HLA-linked) hemochromatosis	*HFE*	Increased intestinal iron absorption and iron overload; liver and heart disease, diabetes, gonadal failure, arthritis, skin pigmentation
Juvenile hemochromatosis	Unknown	Similar to hereditary hemochromatosis, but earlier clinical onset and less prominent liver involvement
African dietary iron overload	Unknown	Iron overload; liver disease, diabetes, ascorbate deficiency, osteoporosis
Atransferrinemia	Transferrin gene	Transfusion-dependent iron deficiency anemia, growth retardation, poor survival
Aceruloplasminemia	Ceruloplasmin	Iron overload from inability to release iron from tissues; progressive neurodegeneration of the retina and basal ganglia; diabetes
Hyperferritinemia and autosomal dominant congenital cataracts	IRE of the L-ferritin gene	Increased serum ferritin levels with bilateral nuclear cataracts
Friedreich ataxia	Frataxin	Mitochondrial damage; spinocerebellar ataxia with cardiomyopathy
X-linked sideroblastic anemia with ataxia	ABC7	Spinocerebellar ataxia with mild anemia

IRE, iron-responsive element; HLA, human leukocyte antigen; ABC7, ATP-binding cassette 7 transporter.

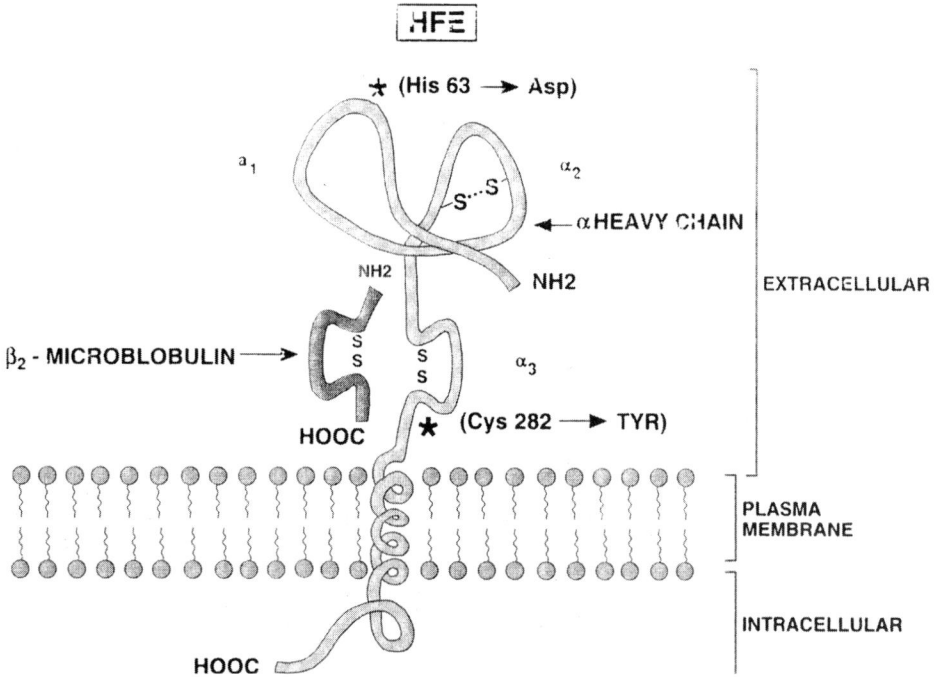

Figure 12.6. Mutations in the HFE, a major histocompatibility complex (MHC) class I–like protein, are responsible for the majority of cases of hereditary hemochromatosis. HFE is composed of three main structural domains (α_1, α_2, and α_3 loops) in the extracellular portion of the protein. Common mutations in HFE associated with hereditary hemochromatosis occur in the α_3 loop (resulting in a tyrosine-for-cysteine shift at amino acid position 282; C282Y HFE) and the α_1 loop (resulting in a aspartate-for-histidine amino acid shift at amino acid position 63; H63D HFE). The C282Y HFE mutation is the most common cause of hereditary hemochromatosis (85%) and has been shown to disrupt the association of HFE protein with β_2-microglobulin. This disrupted interaction prevents proper posttranslational maturation of HFE protein and leads to premature HFE degradation preventing normal cell-surface expression. HFE may function to influence the rate of transferrin receptor recycling. Defective HFE functioning leads to low intracellular iron levels in the enterocyte triggering increased absorption of dietary iron, which increases the risk of iron overload and organ damage and can lead to the development of clinical symptoms of hemochromatosis. (From Testa U. Proteins of Iron Metabolism. Boca Raton, FL: CRC Press, 2002, with permission.)

Adverse health consequences of significant iron overload in hereditary hemochromatosis include increased risk of mortality from liver cancer and cardiopathy. If the propensity of iron overload is recognized early enough in patients with hereditary hemochromatosis, organ failure can be prevented by periodic phlebotomy with favorable clinical outcomes. Historically, clinically evident hemochromatosis was considered a rare disease (2). The clinical definition of hemochromatosis required the presence of iron overload (determined by liver biopsy) associated with organ injury, such as skin pigmentation, hepatomegaly, arthropathy, diabetes mellitus, heart failure, and hypogonadism (58). With the development of biochemical measures of iron status, a shift in the definition of hemochromatosis from a clinical entity to a disease characterized by elevated transferrin saturation gained in prominence, leading to the suggestion that hemochromatosis was much more prevalent than previously recognized. This trend was further reinforced by the discovery in 1996 of the C282Y HFE mutation causing hereditary hemochromatosis (57) and the findings of large-scale population screening efforts (59) confirming the high prevalence of the occurrence of the C282Y HFE mutation in certain populations. Hereditary hemochromatosis could now be defined as the presence of two

hemochromatosis alleles with or without organ injury and with or without the presence of iron overload (58). The development of serious pathologic findings in patients with iron overload, the availability of high-throughput methods to identify persons carrying the genetic mutation associated with hereditary hemochromatosis, and the ability to prevent iron overload with periodic phlebotomy create a potentially compelling argument for universal screening for hereditary hemochromatosis. However, at present this course of action has not been recommended as a public health measure, in large part because of the apparent low penetrance of the clinical phenotype in persons with the C282Y HFE mutation (61). In a large study in the United States, 41,038 persons attending a health appraisal clinic were screened for the C282Y and H63D HFE mutations, and data on signs and symptoms of clinically evident hemochromatosis were obtained by questionnaire. Although 152 homozygotes for hereditary hemochromatosis were identified, only one subject had signs and symptoms suggestive of clinical manifestations of hemochromatosis, a finding suggesting that fewer than 1% of homozygotes develop frank clinical hemochromatosis. However, the clinical consequences of being an HFE homozygote remain controversial (62).

Other less common forms of hereditary hemochromatosis have been described. Hemochromatosis type 2 (HFE2 or "juvenile hemochromatosis") is autosomal recessive and recently has been identified to be caused in most cases by a glycine-to-valine (G320V) amino acid substitution in the *HFE2* gene found on chromosome 1q, whose protein product has been called hemojuvelin (63). The *HFE2* gene is expressed in liver, heart, and skeletal muscle. In addition, a second form of juvenile hemochromatosis (HFE2B) has been mapped to 19q13 and is caused by a defect in the gene encoding hepcidin antimicrobial peptide (HAMP). Hemochromatosis type 3 (HFE3) is autosomal recessive and results from a polymorphism in the gene encoding TfR-2 *(TFR-2)*. Hemochromatosis type 4 (HFE4) is an autosomal dominant disorder and is caused by mutation in the *SLC11A3* gene, which encodes FPN1, an iron exporter protein.

African Hemochromatosis

African hemochromatosis was first recognized in people of Bantu linguistic stock and is sometimes referred to as Bantu siderosis (2). This disease, found in sub-Saharan Africa, has a suspected non–HLA-linked genetic basis (64) and is associated with the consumption of traditional beers containing significant levels of iron contamination from the brewing process in nongalvanized metal pots. Iron intake from beer brewed in this context may exceed 100 mg/day. Clinical evidence of iron overload becomes evident in late adolescence, with a marked manifestation between ages 40 and 60 years, especially in men who typically have greater levels of alcohol consumption. Urban African populations with diets containing normal amounts of iron also can develop iron overload (65). This non-HFE dependent form of iron overload may be common in populations with African ancestry (6).

Hereditary Sideroblastic Anemia

In X-linked hereditary sideroblastic anemia, patients have excessive mitochondrial iron accumulation leading to the development of ringed sideroblasts in which nucleated RBCs are seen with a full or partial ring of Prussian blue–positive stained granules surrounding the nucleus (66). The unique characteristic of amorphous iron deposits in erythroblast mitochondria is found in the heterogeneous group of disorders known as sideroblastic anemias. The basis for mitochondrial iron accumulation in sideroblastic anemia stems from low heme generation resulting from impaired iron utilization in heme synthesis caused by a defect in ALAS2. Iron continues to be transported into the erythroid cell despite reduced heme synthesis, and iron is transported to the mitochondria, where it accumulates. The progeny of the ringed sideroblasts are hypochromic and microcytic erythrocytes reflecting impaired hemoglobin synthesis. The presence of siderotic mitochondria retained in some circulating erythrocytes (Pappenheimer bodies) evident in Wright-stained blood smears is nearly pathognomonic for sideroblastic anemias (66). Sideroblastic anemias can result from both hereditary and nonhereditary causes and lead to an increase in total body iron. Serum iron levels are elevated often to the point of complete saturation of transferrin, and iron absorption is increased because of ineffective erythropoiesis. Elevated serum ferritin reflects body iron stores in this condition of erythropoietic hemochromatosis, which is similar in clinical and pathologic features to hereditary hemochromatosis. Acquired sideroblastic anemias resulting from idiopathic or myelodysplastic or myeloproliferative disorders are more common than inherited forms of this disorder. Reversible sideroblastic anemia has been associated with alcoholism, certain drugs (isoniazid, chloramphenicol), copper deficiency, and hypothermia. Isoniazid used in the treatment of tuberculosis interferes with vitamin B_6 metabolism and leads to a decrease in heme production.

Congenital Atransferrinemia

Congenital atransferrinemia is a very rare (eight described cases) autosomal recessive disorder characterized by extremely low or absent plasma transferrin. Serum iron and total iron-binding capacity are near zero. Despite the lack of transferrin, dietary iron is readily absorbed and circulates loosely bound to albumin and other plasma constituents (6). Because of the lack of transferrin, this iron cannot be used by the erythrocyte, and severe microcytic hypochromic anemia develops. Absorbed iron is deposited by a transferrin-independent mechanism in liver, pancreas, heart, thyroid, and kidneys. Patients die in the absence of transferrin infusion or blood transfusions and are at risk of iron overload.

Congenital Aceruloplasminemia

Congenital aceruloplasminemia is another rare autosomal recessive disorder of iron metabolism resulting from mutation in the ceruloplasmin gene and is characterized by a deficiency of ceruloplasmin ferroxidase activity (6). Patients with aceruloplasminemia present with diabetes mellitus and progressive neurodegeneration of the retina and basal ganglia in middle age. No abnormal copper deposits develop in tissue in patients with this disease. Marked iron accumulation appears in the liver, pancreas, brain, and some accumulation of iron occurs in spleen, heart, kidney, thyroid, and retina. Serum iron is low, serum iron-binding capacity is normal, and serum ferritin is moderately elevated. The unique central nervous system involvement noted in aceruloplasminemia sets apart this form of iron overload from hereditary hemochromatosis, African dietary iron overload, or iron overload as a consequence of transfusion or iron-loading anemias (6).

Hyperferritinemia with Autosomal Dominant Congenital Cataract

Hyperferritinemia with autosomal dominant congenital cataract is a genetic disorder characterized by early-onset, bilateral nuclear cataracts and elevated (1000–2500 μg/L) plasma ferritin. The genetic defect is caused by point mutations in the iron response element (IRE) of the L-ferritin mRNA that disrupts high-affinity binding with the IRP that controls ferritin synthesis.

Hereditary Ataxias

Friedreich ataxia is one of the most common forms of autosomal recessive ataxia. In this genetic disorder, the spinocerebellar tracts, dorsal columns, and pyramidal tracts are primarily involved. The disorder is usually manifest before adolescence and is generally characterized by incoordination of limb movements, dysarthria, nystagmus, diminished or absent tendon reflexes, Babinski sign, impairment of position and vibratory senses, scoliosis, pes cavus (claw foot), and hammer toe. Friedreich ataxia is caused by a deficiency of the mitochondrial protein frataxin, which is required for mitochondrial iron efflux. The absence of this protein leads to oxidative stress and respiratory deficiency, eventually producing cellular damage.

X-linked sideroblastic anemia with ataxia is a rare form of hereditary sideroblastic (characterized by stainable iron in erythrocyte precursors) anemia. In this genetic disease, patients have nonprogressive cerebellar ataxia in infancy or early childhood. The causative mutation is in the *ABC7* (ATP-binding cassette) transporter gene, which is highly homologous to the yeast *ATM1* gene that encodes an inner mitochondrial protein involved in heme transport.

Clinical Disorders Affecting Iron Metabolism

Anemia of Chronic Disease

Anemia, usually of mild to moderate severity, can be frequently encountered in the clinical setting in patients with infectious, inflammatory, or neoplastic diseases that persist for more than 1 or 2 months and is referred to as the anemia of chronic disorders or ACD (67). In most cases, the anemia is mild, and therapy should focus on correction of the underlying disease process. ACD is frequently encountered in geriatric populations. ACD is characterized specifically by hypoferremia in the presence of ample iron stores in the RES and therefore does not include all anemias that may develop in patients with chronic disorders. In ACD, the anemia usually develops during the first 2 months of the disease and then generally does not progress further. The pathogenesis of ACD involves raised cytokine levels, shortened erythrocyte survival, and impaired bone marrow response, which is related to impaired erythropoietin response to anemia and poor response of erythrocyte precursors in the bone marrow to available erythropoietin, and probable abnormalities in iron metabolism. In ACD, serum iron, iron-binding capacity, and transferrin saturation are typically reduced, and free protoporphyrin in erythrocytes is increased, mimicking the signs of iron deficiency anemia. Interpretation of serum ferritin as an indicator of iron stores in persons with ACD is complicated. Serum ferritin is increased by inflammatory-related cytokine-driven processes in ACD. Normally, serum ferritin of 12 μg/L or less is indicative of depleted iron stores. However, serum ferritin concentrations may be as high as 160 μg/L despite the absence of stainable marrow iron in persons with ACD (68). Thus, the identification of iron deficiency in patients who also have ACD is problematic. Investigators have suggested that a patient with ACD and a serum ferritin lower than 30 μg/L probably definitely has iron deficiency, whereas a serum ferritin greater than 200 μg/L would preclude a diagnosis of iron deficiency. However, intermediate serum ferritin values would require an examination of a Prussian blue–stained marrow specimen to make the diagnosis of iron deficiency (67). If available, an indication of an elevated serum TfR concentration would be useful to help define iron deficiency in the patient with ACD.

Alcoholic Cirrhosis and Iron Overload

A close association exists between excessive alcohol consumption and the clinical expression of hemochromatosis (69). Among 206 patients with classic HFE-associated hemochromatosis, liver cirrhosis was nine times more likely to occur (66 versus 7%) in persons who consumed more than 60 g/day alcohol compared with those who drank less than that amount (70), a finding suggesting that alcohol consumption in the presence of a propensity for iron loading may be detrimental. This position is supported by the observations in an experimental animal model in which dietary iron loading exacerbated the development of alcohol-induced liver cirrhosis (71).

Shunt Hemochromatosis

Establishment of a shunt between the portal and venous circulation, often to relieve pressure in esophageal varices, is associated with the development of shunt hemochromatosis (2). Hepatic iron concentrations have been measured in patients with nonalcoholic cirrhosis who had previously undergone portacaval shunting and then liver transplantation. Mean hepatic iron concentration was significantly increased in shunt-treated patients compared with a control group (20 nmol/g versus 9 nmol/g). Mean hepatic iron index (hepatic iron/age) was higher in the shunt group than controls (0.5 versus 0.19). In a group of patients who received serial biopsies, the mean annual rate of hepatic iron accumulation was significantly greater in the shunt group (4.75 nmol/g/year versus 0.93 nmol/g/year in controls). However, it was concluded that the extent of iron loading in shunt-treated patients was unlikely to result in tissue damage (72).

Prolonged Oral Iron Therapy

The intestine has a remarkable ability to block iron absorption. This protective effect of the intestine is important given the normal avid retention of absorbed iron and the tendency toward chronic iron accumulation, as seen in persons with hereditary hemochromatosis who absorb inappropriately high amounts of dietary iron. Consumption of high doses of supplemental iron in menstruating women will not result in the development of iron overload (2). However, the wide use of dietary supplements in the United States, many of which contain iron, deserves attention in persons who are homozygotes for hereditary hemochromatosis in particular and those other persons who are not bleeding and are not iron deficient. A study of elderly men and women in the United States found that taking iron supplements increased the risk of high iron stores, defined as a serum ferritin concentration greater than 300 ng/mL in men and 200 ng/mL in women, by fourfold (73). Although the adverse health effects of moderately elevated body iron stores have not been well supported, it would seem prudent for the elderly to avoid iron supplements in the absence of documented iron deficiency.

Severe Chronic Anemia and Transfusional Hemochromatosis

Excessive iron absorption is likely to occur in patients with ineffective erythropoiesis, including those patients with sideroblastic anemia and thalassemia major (2), and it can lead to death from cardiac and hepatic complications of hemochromatosis. Iron overload is likely to occur whenever chronic anemia is treated by numerous blood transfusions over many years. These patients often require long-term treatment with iron chelating agents.

Porphyria Cutanea Tarda

Porphyria cutanea tarda is an autosomal dominant disorder characterized by light-sensitive dermatitis and associated with the excretion of large amounts of uroporphyrin in urine. The onset of light-sensitive dermatitis in later adult life, associated with the excretion of large amounts of uroporphyrin in urine, characterizes this form of porphyria. The onset is often associated with alcoholism. Iron overload is frequently present, and it may be associated, coincidentally or causally, with varying degrees of liver damage or fibrosis.

IRON NUTRITION

Dietary Iron Intake

Dietary iron concentration is usually about 5 to 7 mg/1000 kcal. When consuming an average American or European-type diet, 10 to 20 mg iron/day can be expected to be consumed at typical adult energy intakes. By analogy, consumption of energy-restricted diets for any reason is likely to provide inadequate amounts of iron unless special effort is made to include iron-rich foods or iron supplements. Likewise, extensive use of calorie-dense fast foods in the diet that are relatively poor sources of iron per kilocalorie of energy should be especially avoided in population groups at risk of iron deficiency. For example, potato is an important vegetable in the diets of children in the United States, and its consumption has increased markedly over the past few decades. According to US Department of Agriculture (USDA) surveys (74), in 1965 white potatoes accounted for one third of all vegetable intake in children, whereas by 1996 potatoes accounted for half of all vegetable consumption. Comparisons of iron content per 1000 kcal energy for four types of potato preparation are shown in Table 12.3.

Comparison of trends in dietary intake in adolescent children in the United States between 1965 and 1996 (74) shows that total iron intake increased from 14 mg/day in 1965 to 17 mg/day in 1996. However, still only about 40% of girls met the recommended dietary intakes for iron. During this same period, grain consumption increased and meat consumption declined, a finding suggesting a shift of dietary iron to rely more on less bioavailable fortification iron. Elemental iron used in many iron-fortified cereal products has relatively low bioavailability (75).

Figure 12.7 shows the findings of the National Health and Nutrition Examination Survey (NHANES) III concerning estimates of iron intake in the United States by age and gender group in comparison with the current recommended dietary intake for iron of each group.

Table 12.4 lists some high-iron food sources in the US diet. For further information, the reader is directed to the USDA Internet site (www.nal.usda.gov/fnic/cgi-bin/nut_search.pl), which provides convenient capabilities for identification of the iron content of most foods. Iron-fortified formulas make an important contribution to dietary iron intake of infants. The consumption of iron-fortified foods, especially ready-to-eat breakfast cereal products, can supply significant quantities of dietary iron. However, the bioavailability of iron from fortified breakfast cereals is not well documented.

TABLE 12.3. EFFECT OF FOOD PREPARATION ON IRON DENSITY OF POTATO

FOOD ITEM	IRON (mg/100 g)	ENERGY (kcal/100 g)	IRON DENSITY (mg/1000 kcal)
Baked potato	0.35	93	3.8
Potato chips	1.63	536	3.0
French fried potatoes	0.78	342	2.3
Hash brown potatoes	0.55	265	2.1

From US Department of Agriculture National Nutrient Data Base (www.nal.usda.gov/fnic/cgi-bin/nut_search.pl).

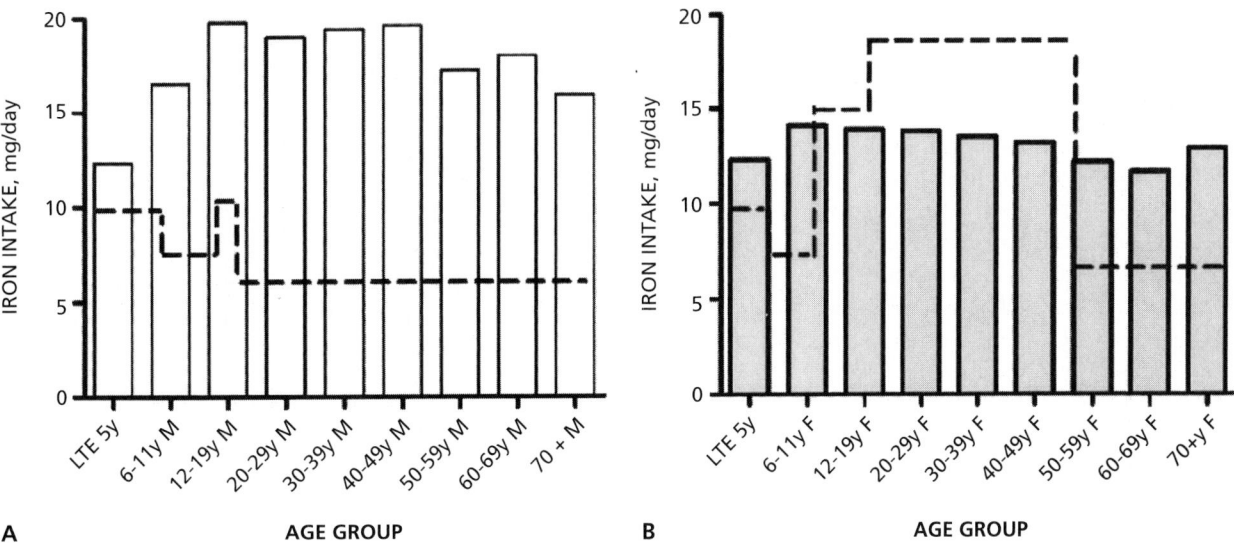

Figure 12.7. Average dietary iron intake in the United States (1999–2000) compared with the current recommended dietary allowance (RDA) for iron. Bar graphs depict the average daily iron intake of various age groups in the United States. The graph on the **left** with *clear bars* is for boys and men. The graph on the **right** with *shaded bars* is for girls and women. The *dotted line* represents the iron RDA for that particular age group and gender. As is evident, boys and men have higher iron intakes than girls and women and on average exceed the current RDA in all age categories. In contrast, iron intakes in girls and in premenopausal women are less than adequate. (Data from United States Department of Agriculture (USDA). USDA Continuing Survey of Food Intakes by Individuals. Washington, DC: USDA, 1996.)

Iron Intakes in Developing Countries

In many developing countries, iron intake is inadequate, and the bioavailability of iron in these diets is low because of high concentrations of inhibitors, such as phytate, in the staple grain food sources. A study of dietary mineral content of representative diets in nine Asian countries, which represented more than 50% of the world's population,

TABLE 12.4. SOME HIGH-IRON FOOD SOURCES

FOOD	SERVING SIZE	IRON (mg/SERVING)
Clams, canned	3 oz	23.8
Ready-to-eat cereal, Total Raisin Bran	1 cup	18.0
Soybeans, boiled	1 cup	8.8
Beans, baked, canned, with pork and tomato sauce	1 cup	8.3
Rice, white, enriched, dry	1 cup	8.0
Lentils, boiled	1 cup	6.6
Spinach, boiled	1 cup	6.4
Fast food hamburger, large, double patty	1 sandwich	5.9
Beef liver	3 oz	5.2
Fast food, chicken fillet sandwich	1 sandwich	4.9
Infant formula, ready-to-feed, iron-fortified	100 g	1.2

From US Department of Agriculture (http://www.nal.usda.gov/fnic/foodcomp/Data/SR16/wtrank/sr16w303.pdf).

found a fourfold country-to-country variation in iron intake (76). In Africa, the use of nongalvanized steel drums to ferment homemade beverages in some populations can lead to excess iron intake. A study of homemade Zimbabwean beer (77) found a median iron content of 52 mg/L in traditional "7-day" beer (*doro rematanda*). Conversely, these homemade brews could have an important impact on iron status in women at risk of iron deficiency anemia. In a study of rural African women (78), a group of women who drank traditional high-iron beer had no evidence of iron deficiency anemia compared with a 13% prevalence of anemia in a group who did not consume beer. A safer low-tech alternative to boost iron intake could be an increased use of iron cooking pots (79).

Dietary Iron Bioavailability

The absorbability of iron from food is dependent on gastrointestinal conditions in the host and on intrinsic food-based factors. In the host, gastric acidity is an important factor determining iron bioavailability from food because an acidic environment in the stomach can solubilize food iron and can thus allow the opportunity for chelation of iron to soluble low-molecular-weight compounds, such as ascorbic acid and other organic acids, thereby preventing the formation of alternative insoluble iron complexes. Ionic iron can exist in two different valence states: reduced ferrous iron (Fe^{+2}) or oxidized ferric (Fe^{+3}) iron. Ferrous iron is more soluble than ferric iron, particularly in neutral environment found in the more distal small intestine, and this is one explanation of the generally higher bioavailability of ferrous iron-containing dietary supplements.

A naturally occurring chelated form of food iron is heme iron, found in high amounts in red or dark meats. Heme iron has an important nutritional benefit because the bioavailability of this form of dietary iron is high and generally is not affected by important iron absorption inhibitors in the diet, such as polyphenols and phytate, although heme iron has been reported to be inhibited by calcium (80). Breast milk iron bioavailability is higher than from infant formula, and this could be related to the lactoferrin content of breast milk. However, the role of lactoferrin in milk iron bioavailability remains uncertain.

Measurement of Food Iron Bioavailability

Studies have been done comparing the fractional absorption of iron isotopes added either extrinsically by mixing with the test food or intrinsically by incorporating the isotope directly into food during growth. These comparison studies demonstrated that ingested nonheme food iron enters an apparent "common pool" in the gut lumen from which intestinal iron absorption takes place (81). The development of the "extrinsic tag method" for estimating iron bioavailability from individual foods simplified estimation of food iron absorption and spurred a large number of human studies determining iron bioavailability of individual foods, the interaction of various combinations of foods consumed together in meals, as well as the effect of specific enhancing and inhibiting substances in food (82). Important enhancers and inhibitors of nonheme iron absorption are shown in Table 12.5. These human studies demonstrated that nonheme iron bioavailability among various foods can be markedly different. Algorithms have been developed, based on experimental measures of iron absorption from a large number of human iron absorption studies, to predict iron absorption and bioavailability of dietary iron based on knowing the subjects iron status (serum ferritin) and the content of enhancers and inhibitory substances in the meal (83). The prevention of the formation of insoluble iron complexes in the intestinal lumen is important for the bioavailability of food iron because free iron (or low-molecular-weight iron complexes) must interact with molecular iron-binding sites on iron transport proteins, such as DMT1, on the apical (brush border) surface of the absorptive enterocyte.

TABLE 12.5. ENHANCERS AND INHIBITORS OF NONHEME IRON BIOAVAILABILITY

ENHANCERS	INHIBITORS
Ascorbic acid	Polyphenols (especially galloyl groups)
Meat	Phytate
Alcohol	Calcium
	Myricetin
	Chlorogenic acid (coffee)

Dietary Reference Intakes

Recommended Dietary Allowance

The Food and Nutrition Board of the Institute of Medicine is responsible for setting dietary intake guidelines (dietary reference intakes [DRI]) for the United States and Canada. The various DRIs are presented in text and tables in the Appendix, Section II, Tables A-2-a to A-2-h and represent optimal dietary nutrient intake levels and guidelines for upper safe limits of nutrient intakes. To derive a recommended dietary allowance (RDA) for iron, an estimated average requirement (EAR) was made on the basis of available scientific data, along with additional considerations of population variation (84 and http://books.nap.edu/books/0309072794/html/290.html#pagetop). The EARs and RDAs for iron for various groups are shown in Table 12.6.

Ideally, a functional indicator of iron deficiency, such as reduced work capacity, delayed psychomotor development in infants, impaired cognitive function, or adverse effects on mother or fetus, could provide the basis for

TABLE 12.6. ESTIMATED AVERAGE REQUIREMENT AND RECOMMENDED DIETARY ALLOWANCE FOR IRON

	EAR[a] (mg/d)		RDA[b] (mg/d)	
GROUP	MALE	FEMALE	MALE	FEMALE
0–6 mo			0.27[c]	0.27[c]
7–12 mo	6.9	6.3	11	11
1–3 y	3	3	7	7
4–8 y	4.1	4.1	10	10
9–13 y	5.9	5.7	8	8
14–18 y	7.7	7.9	11	15
19–30 y	6	8.1	8	18
31–50 y	6	8.1	8	18
51–70 y	6	5	8	8
>70 y	6	5	8	8
Pregnancy				
≤18 y		23[d]		27
18–50 y		22		27
Lactation				
≤18 y		7		10
18–50 y		6.5		9

[a] Estimated average requirement (EAR) is defined as the intake that meets the estimated iron needs of half of the individuals in the group.
[b] Recommended dietary allowance (RDA) is defined as the intake that meets the needs of almost all individuals in the group.
[c] For breast-fed infants 0 to 6 months old, an adequate intake (AI) estimate is used instead of an RDA. The AI is the observed average intake by the target population that appears to sustain a defined condition. The AI is used if there is not sufficient scientific evidence to derive an EAR.
[d] The iron cost of pregnancy is based on basal losses (250 mg), fetal and placental deposition (320 mg), and increased hemoglobin mass (500 mg). The total iron need for pregnancy is 1070 mg. However, about 250 to 350 mg of iron is not lost with the placenta or from blood loss, resulting in a net iron need during pregnancy of 700 to 800 mg.

From Food and Nutrition Board, Institute of Medicine. Dietary Reference Intakes for Vitamin A, Vitamin K, Arsenic, Boron, Chromium, Copper, Iodine, Iron, Manganese, Molybdenum, Nickel, Silicon, Vanadium, and Zinc. Washington, DC: National Academy Press, 2001, with permission.

establishing an iron requirement (84). However, this has not been possible because of complications related to the development of anemia. A series of biochemical indicators of iron depletion and deficiency can be employed to assess iron status and to indicate the early stages of anemia and serve as surrogates of functional iron deficiency. However, these measures were not chosen as the basis of establishing an iron requirement because of a lack of sufficient sensitivity in these measures to provide an adequate margin of safety in calculating iron requirements (84). The calculation of the EAR for iron was based on the need to maintain a normal, functional iron concentration and a minimal store of body iron, set at a serum ferritin concentration of 15 µg/L.

Factorial Modeling Method for Estimating the Physiologic Requirement for Absorbed Iron. The factorial modeling method was used by the DRI committee to derive an estimate of the need for absorbed iron and is based on calculating the individual components of an iron requirement, which include basal iron losses, menstrual losses, and accretion. A summation of such losses and accretions would estimate the amount of iron that needs to be absorbed from the diet. In the case of iron, some of the components have a skewed distribution necessitating the use of sophisticated mathematic approaches to arrive at accurate descriptions of the population distribution and estimates of the population median to arrive at an average requirement for absorbed iron and to derive the RDA for iron.

Basal iron losses, estimated from radiolabeled iron studies in 41 men from South Africa, the United States, and Venezuela (17), are 14 µg/kg body weight (0.9–1.0 mg/day). Median menstrual blood losses, estimated in women of reproductive age in three large studies in Egypt (85), England (86), and Sweden (87), are 20 to 30 mL, and fewer than 10% of women have blood losses exceeding 80 mL per period. Accretion of iron in pregnancy and for growth of children can be estimated from changes in blood volume, fetal and placental iron concentration, and the increase in total body erythrocyte mass.

The absorption of dietary iron is affected by both the size of the iron stores and components of the diet that influence iron bioavailability. For the purposes of estimating the dietary iron requirement in adults living in the United States and Canada, iron absorption was estimated as 18%. This level of absorption was based on the assumption that 90% of dietary iron was from nonheme iron absorbed at 16.8% efficiency and 10% of dietary iron is heme iron absorbed at 25% efficiency.

Additional Considerations in Estimating Iron Requirements and Dietary Iron Needs. Special considerations concerning the iron requirements of certain subpopulations (Table 12.7) have been recognized and should be taken into account when considering dietary iron needs. Women using oral contraceptives have about a 60% reduction in blood loss during menstruation that lowers their RDA to about 11 mg/day. In contrast, the use of hormone replacement therapy in postmenopausal women can be associated with uterine bleeding that would increase their iron needs in comparison with postmenopausal women not using hormone replacement therapy. It is well known that the iron bioavailability of plant-based diets is generally lower than mixed Western-type diets that contain meat. Therefore, an adjustment of the underlying assumption of dietary iron bioavailability from 18% for mixed diets to 10% for vegetarian diets would increase the iron requirement by 1.8 times for vegetarians. Moreover, it is also recognized that vegetarian diets with limited variety of foodstuffs, as may often be found in developing countries, may approach 5% bioavailability, thereby greatly increasing the risk of iron deficiency anemia by long-term consumption of inadequate amounts of bioavailable iron. This situation may be further worsened by the presence of intestinal parasites in some populations. These common infections have been estimated to affect 1 billion people in the world and, in some cases, such as hookworm infestation, can cause significant blood loss. Thus, successful anemia intervention programs in areas of endemic intestinal parasite infection need to consider not only iron supplementation but also treatment of this underlying cause of blood loss. Additional situations of increased iron needs are in persons who donate blood and in endurance athletes. A donation of 0.5 L of blood represents a loss of about 200 to 250 mg iron. Frequent blood donation can be

TABLE 12.7. GROUPS NEEDING SPECIAL CONSIDERATION IN ESTIMATING DIETARY IRON REQUIREMENTS

GROUP	COMMENT
Women using oral contraceptives	60% reduction in menstrual blood loss; lowers RDA to 11 mg/d
Postmenopausal women using HRT	Associated with uterine bleeding; increases RDA compared with women not using HRT
Vegetarian diets	Lower iron bioavailability increases dietary iron requirement by 1.8 times; situation worsened when limited variety of foods available, may increase dietary iron requirement by 3 to 4 times greater than mixed Western diet
Intestinal parasites (e.g., hookworm)	Increased blood loss raises risk of iron depletion
Persons who donate blood on a regular basis	Increased iron needs
Endurance athletes	Increased iron needs by 30 to 70%

HRT, hormone replacement therapy; RDA, recommended dietary allowance.

problematic, especially in women who usually have lower iron stores than men. Lower iron status has been noted in persons who exercise frequently. Part of this difference in iron status may reflect differences in dietary intake patterns, but there also appears to be a physiologic component reflecting increased blood loss. Investigators have suggested that intense physical exercise increases gastrointestinal blood loss and hemoglobinuria stemming from erythrocyte rupture within the foot during running. Thus, the estimated average requirement for iron is about 30 to 70% higher for those who engage in regular intense exercise (84).

Tolerable Upper Levels of Iron Intake

From a medical perspective, acute accidental iron poisoning is recognized as the most common cause of poisoning deaths in children under the age of 6 years in the United States. Symptoms of acute iron poisoning can occur with iron doses between 20 to 60 mg/kg. Gastrointestinal irritation alone usually occurs at the lower range of iron dose with increasing risk of systemic poisoning at the higher doses.

The establishment of DRIs by the Food and Nutrition Board of the Institute of Medicine includes both RDAs and estimates of tolerable upper intake levels (ULs). The UL is defined as the highest level of daily nutrient intake that is likely to have no adverse health effects for almost all persons (84). From this perspective, episodes of acute iron poisoning were not considered in the derivation of the UL for iron. However, high-dose iron supplementation is associated with the development of gastrointestinal side effects (constipation, diarrhea, nausea, vomiting) and was used as the criterion to establish the iron UL. These untoward gastrointestinal effects of iron supplementation have been reported at iron supplement doses of 50 mg/day. The UL for iron for all persons 14 years old and older, including pregnant and lactating women, is 45 mg/day and is slightly lower (40 mg/day) for everyone younger, including infants. The primary data used in the derivation of the UL were from an iron supplementation trial in men and women from Sweden (88). In that double-blind, placebo-controlled trial, adverse gastrointestinal effects were observed in subjects taking 60 mg/day nonheme iron as ferrous fumarate. The iron UL of 45 mg/day was approximated by adding the usual dietary iron intake to the intake from the nonheme iron supplement to estimate a lowest-observed-adverse-effect level and dividing by an uncertainty factor of 1.5. Individuals with a genetic predisposition to iron overload represent a distinct iron-sensitive population that is not considered in deriving the UL for dietary iron.

Assessment of Iron Status

Iron depletion and the development of iron deficiency and eventually anemia occur in stages and can be assessed by

TABLE 12.8. NORMAL SERUM CLINICAL CHEMISTRY VALUES FOR MEASURES OF IRON STATUS

IRON MEASURE	NORMAL RANGE[a]
Hemoglobin (whole blood)	120–160 g/L (female) (7.4–9.9 mmol/L) 130–180 g/L (male) (8.1–11.2 mmol/L)
Iron	50–150 μg/dL (9–27 μmol/L)
Iron-binding capacity	250–370 μg/dL (45–66 μmol/L)
Ferritin	10–200 μg/L (female) 15–400 μg/L (male)
Transferrin saturation	20–45 % (0.2–0.45)
Transferrin	2.3–3.9 g/L
Erythrocyte protoporphyrin	<70 μg/dL red blood cells
Mean cell volume	>80 fl (adult)
Soluble transferrin receptor	≤9 mg/L[b]

[a]Values are given in common units, and, where applicable, SI units are shown below within parentheses.
[b]Values depend on the specific assay used.

Data from http://harrisons.accessmedicine.com/server-java/Arknoid/amed/harrisons/co_appendices/appa_p01.html; and Sauberlich H. Laboratory Tests for the Assessment of Nutritional Status. 2nd ed. Boca Raton, FL: CRC Press, 1999:486.

measuring various biochemical indices. Normal values for these iron status biochemical measures are shown in Table 12.8. Iron enzyme activity can be affected by iron deficiency (89), although not all enzymes are equally sensitive to iron depletion. For example, catalase is relatively resistant to iron deficiency, whereas aconitase and cytochrome c are readily depleted. However, the measurement of the activity of iron-dependent enzymes has not been successfully used as a routine measure of iron status.

Laboratory measurements are essential for a proper diagnosis of iron deficiency. A battery of such measures is available, and these tests are most informative when multiple measures of iron status are examined in the context of the patient's nutritional and medical history. Early stages of iron depletion are characterized by a reduced plasma iron and elevated plasma transferrin concentration, measured by the plasma total iron-binding capacity. These changes result in a decreased transferrin saturation, which is defined as plasma iron divided by total iron-binding capacity times 100. However, marked biologic variation can occur in these values as a result of diurnal variation, the presence of infection or inflammatory conditions, and recent dietary iron intake. Blood erythrocyte protoporphyrin is a sensitive early indicator of iron deficiency and can be used for screening iron status. Erythrocyte protoporphyrin is elevated when the iron supply is limited; however, it is also affected when hemoglobin synthesis is blunted by other factors, such as lead poisoning or inflammation, and it can also be increased in hemolytic anemia. Serum ferritin is a good indicator of body iron stores under most circumstances. On the basis of quantitative phlebotomy studies, 1 μg/L serum ferritin represents about 8 to 10 mg stored iron (90). However, ferritin is an acute-phase reactant protein, and plasma concentrations can be elevated irrespective of a change in iron stores by infection and inflammation. Plasma-soluble TfR concentrations reflect tissue iron deficiency and are not affected by inflammation. The concentration of plasma TfR increases progressively with increased tissue iron deficiency. Anemia, the end stage of iron deficiency, is reflected by a decrease in blood hemoglobin concentration and hematocrit. However, anemia is not exclusive to iron deficiency and can be caused by other nutritional deficiciencies, as well as nonnutritional causes, such as chronic inflammatory conditions (ACD). Erythrocyte indices, such as mean cell volume, are helpful in screening for microcytic anemia resulting from iron deficiency and can also be used to distinguish the mild anemia resulting from thalassemic traits (90).

Anemia and Iron Deficiency

Anemia

Anemia is a hematologic condition defined as an abnormally low concentration of blood hemoglobin. Estimates suggest that at least 1 billion persons in the world are anemic. The most common cause of anemia is iron deficiency, but other micronutrient deficiencies, such as folic acid and vitamin B_{12} deficiency, as well as other causes (chronic infection and inflammation, and hereditary hemoglobinopathies) can also result in anemia. Moreover, these conditions can coexist and contribute to the severity of the observed anemia. Hematologic characteristics in anemia vary depending on the cause and are described in detail in Chapter 92.

Iron Deficiency

Iron deficiency is defined as a functional tissue deficit of iron resulting from depleted iron stores and is characterized by changes in iron metabolism and iron-related biochemical indices. Iron deficiency occurs when iron absorption cannot keep pace over an extended period with the metabolic demands for iron or the rate of iron loss, which is primarily related to blood loss. Anemia is often encountered in pregnant women and is caused by several factors, including the need for additional iron for maternal tissue accumulation in early gestation, expansion and dilution of blood volume, and the need to transfer considerable quantities of iron (3–4 mg/day) to the fetus during the last trimester of gestation.

Iron deficiency can exist with or without anemia. Some subtle functional changes may occur in the absence of anemia, but the strongest evidence to date suggests that most functional deficits occur with the development of anemia. However, even mild and moderate forms of iron deficiency anemia can be associated with functional impairments affecting cognitive function (91), immunity (92), work capacity (93), and the ability to regulate body temperature properly (94). Numerous studies have reported a relation between maternal anemia during pregnancy, particularly iron deficiency anemia, and shortened gestation, preterm birth (95, 96), and lower infant birth weight (97, 98). Maternal anemia during pregnancy increases the risk of low birth weight by about threefold (99).

The primary causes of iron deficiency are as follows: low intake of bioavailable iron; high iron requirement as a result of rapid growth, pregnancy, or menstruation; and excess blood loss caused by pathologic infestations, such as hookworm causing gastrointestinal blood loss or shistosomiasis causing urinary blood loss. When iron stores are depleted and insufficient iron is available for erythropoiesis, hemoglobin synthesis in erythrocyte precursors becomes impaired, and the hematologic signs of iron deficiency anemia appear. In very severe cases, iron deficiency anemia can be life-threatening, particularly at the time of parturition, when significant maternal hemorrhage can occur.

Prevalence of Iron Deficiency and Iron Deficiency Anemia. Global estimates of iron deficiency and iron deficiency anemia are only rough estimates, based on available prevalence estimates of anemia to which various assumptions are then applied, and they may be grossly overinflated (100). These global prevalence estimates assume that a given fraction of anemic persons is anemic because of iron deficiency. Estimates of the number of iron-deficient persons in the world are, in turn, based on a multiple of the number of persons with iron deficiency anemia found in studies done in the United States. The validity of these underlying assumptions is open to challenge, particularly in any populations in which anemia caused by other factors is common (101). With these caveats in mind, it has been estimated that 2 to 5 billion persons in the world are iron deficient, and many of these have iron deficiency anemia. Conversely, surveys in the United States indicate that iron deficiency anemia is relatively uncommon, although iron deficiency still persists, particularly in infants 1 to 2 years old and in women of reproductive age. The overall prevalence of iron deficiency, based on abnormalities of at least two of three biochemical measures of iron status (serum ferritin, transferrin saturation, erythrocyte protoporphyrin), range from 2% in boys and men 16 to 69 years old to 16% in girls and women 16 to 19 years old, whereas the prevalence of iron deficiency anemia (iron deficiency plus low hemoglobin) ranges from less than 1% in men to 4% in women 20 to 49 years old in the United States, based on NHANES surveys (102). Current estimates suggest that the prevalence of iron deficiency is about twice as high among non-Hispanic black and Mexican-American women (19–22%) compared with non-Hispanic white women (10%). The latter estimate is similar to the prevalence estimates of depleted iron stores (defined as a serum ferritin <16 μg/L) in premenopausal Danish women surveyed in 1984 and 1994 (103).

Conditions Associated with Iron Deficiency

Helicobacter pylori. Infection with the bacteria *Helicobacter pylori* is common and has been estimated to be present in half the world's population (104). In general, *H. pylori* infections are more commonly found in populations living in the developing rather than the developed world. A possible link between *H. pylori* infection and anemia was first suggested in 1993 (105). Accumulating evidence supports the suggestion that *H. pylori* infection is associated with an increased risk of anemia and lower iron stores (106–108), and it can play a role in iron deficiency anemia that is refractory to iron supplementation (109). The physiopathologic mechanism through which *H. pylori* infection increases the risk of anemia is uncertain at present, although raised intragastric pH and lower ascorbic acid concentrations found in patients with *H. pylori* gastritis may be important factors (110).

Lead Poisoning. Iron deficiency can be a risk factor for heavy metal contamination (111). For example, higher blood lead levels are found in children with iron deficiency (112, 113). A possible mechanism for this iron-lead association is an increase in intestinal lead absorption (114), which may result from an increase in the intestinal divalent metal transporter DMT1 in response to iron deficiency. DMT1 has an affinity for several divalent metals, including lead (38). Blood lead levels are higher in iron-deficient children with each increasing level of environmental exposure (112). Moreover, a strong biologic basis for a causal relation between human iron deficiency and lead contamination is the finding of a prospective longitudinal study of children followed in an urban primary care clinic that showed children with iron deficiency were at increased risk of *subsequent* lead poisoning (115). These findings suggest that nutritional supplementation may have a role along with environmental remediation in preventing lead poisoning.

Health Consequences of Elevated Iron Stores

Dietary Iron Excess

Although current evidence is insufficient to support the notion that high iron intakes alone generally lead to secondary iron overload, excessive dietary iron intake can clearly be detrimental under certain circumstances. For example, a high prevalence of iron overload has been noted in South African and Zimbabwean blacks and has been associated with consumption of traditional beer made from fermented maize that has a high iron (80 mg/L) content (116) as a result of high levels of iron contamination from iron-containing brewing vessels. Moreover, several dietary factors, including heme (meat) iron and iron supplementation, have been associated with an increased risk of moderately elevated iron stores (based on serum ferritin >300 μg/L in men and 200 μg/L in women) in elderly white persons in the United States (73). The role of moderately elevated iron stores in the development of chronic disease remains an area of scientific controversy.

Elevated Serum Ferritin as a Risk Factor for Chronic Disease

Excess body iron is a possible source of oxidant stress because of its ability to participate in the generation of free radicals. In 1981, the hypothesis was put forth that increased body iron in men compared with women was instrumental in explaining the gender difference in cardiovascular disease risk (117). Interest in the potential role of iron in cardiovascular disease was rekindled about a decade later by epidemiologic support of the iron-heart disease hypothesis from studies in Finland (118). In the Finnish study, iron stores were estimated on the basis of serum ferritin concentrations. Men with a serum ferritin concentration greater than 200 μg/L had a 2.2-fold increase in risk of acute myocardial infarction. Many studies of the iron-heart disease hypothesis followed with mixed findings. Based on a systematic review of many prospective studies of iron status and cardiovascular disease (119), there does not appear to be strong and consistent support of an association between iron status and coronary heart disease. A potential role for high iron stores (high serum ferritin) in other chronic diseases, including cancer and type 2 diabetes, has been suggested but remains inconclusive. The interpretation of epidemiologic studies in which serum ferritin is used as a biomarker of iron stores must be done with caution because these studies can be confounded (120). Serum ferritin is a useful measure of elevated iron stores under most circumstances. However, it is also an acute-phase protein, and serum ferritin concentrations are artificially raised in the presence of chronic inflammation, which has become increasingly appreciated as an important independent risk factor for many chronic diseases. Despite associations in some studies of high serum ferritin with heart disease, type 2 diabetes, and colon cancer, adverse health effects of moderately elevated iron stores in the general population remain controversial.

Acknowledgment

This work was supported in part by funds provided by the USDA Agricultural Research Service under Cooperative Agreement No. 58-1950-001 and National Institutes of Health grant number DK064327. The contents of this publication do not necessarily reflect the views or policies of the USDA, nor does mention of trade names, commercial products, or organizations imply endorsement by the US government.

REFERENCES

1. Beutler E. Blood Cells Mol Dis 2002;29:297–308.
2. Fairbanks V. Iron in medicine and nutrition. In: Shils M, Olson J, Shike M, eds. Modern Nutrition in Health and Disease. 8th ed. Philadelphia: Lea & Febiger, 1994:185–213.
3. Guerinot ML. Annu Rev Microbiol 1994;48:743–72.
4. Askwith C, Kaplan J. Trends Biochem Sci 1998;23:135–8.
5. Aisen P, Enns C, Wessling-Resnick M. Int J Biochem Cell Biol 2001;33:940–59.
6. Sheth S, Brittenham GM. Annu Rev Med 2000;51:443–64.
7. Testa U. Proteins of Iron Metabolism. Boca Raton, FL: CRC Press, 2002:559.

8. Nicolas G, Bennoun M, Devaux I et al. Proc Natl Acad Sci USA 2001;98:8780–5.
9. Weinstein DA, Roy CN, Fleming MD et al. Blood 2002;100:3776–81.
10. Nicolas G, Bennoun M, Porteu A et al. Proc Natl Acad Sci USA 2002;99:4596–601.
11. Merryweather-Clarke AT, Cadet E, Bomford A et al. Hum Mol Genet 2003;12:2241–7.
12. Nicolas G, Viatte L, Lou DQ et al. Nat Genet 2003;34:97–101.
13. Waheed A, Grubb JH, Zhou XY et al. Proc Natl Acad Sci USA 2002;99:3117–22.
14. Frazer DM, Wilkins SJ, Becker EM et al. Gut 2003;52:340–6.
15. Martini LA, Tchack L, Wood RJ. J Nutr 2002;132:693–6.
16. Frazer DM, Anderson GJ. Blood Cells Mol Dis 2003;30:288–97.
17. Green R, Charlton R, Seftel H et al. Am J Med 1968;45:336–53.
18. Nachtigall D, Nielsen P, Fischer R et al. Int J Sports Med 1996;17:473–9.
19. Marziali G, Perrotti E, Ilari R et al. Oncogene 2002;21:7933–44.
20. Geminard C, Nault F, Johnstone RM et al. J Biol Chem 2001;276:9910–6.
21. Kawabata H, Yang R, Hirama T et al. J Biol Chem 1999;274:20826–32.
22. Roetto A, Daraio F, Alberti F et al. Blood Cells Mol Dis 2002;29:465–70.
23. Fleming RE, Ahmann JR, Migas MC et al. Proc Natl Acad Sci USA 2002;99:10653–8.
24. Theil EC. J Nutr 2003;133:1549S–53S.
25. Halliwell B, Gutteridge JM. FEBS Lett 1992;307:108–12.
26. Rouault TA, Tang CK, Kaptain S et al. Proc Natl Acad Sci USA 1990;87:7958–62.
27. Muckenthaler M, Gray NK, Hentze MW. Mol Cell 1998;2:383–8.
28. Eisenstein RS. Annu Rev Nutr 2000;20:627–62.
29. Casey JL, Koeller DM, Ramin VC et al. EMBO J 1989;8:3693–9.
30. Eisenstein RS, Ross KL. J Nutr 2003;133:1510S–6S.
31. Muhlenhoff U, Richhardt N, Ristow M et al. Hum Mol Genet 2002;11:2025–36.
32. Kispal G, Csere P, Guiard B et al. FEBS Lett 1997;418:346–50.
33. Foury F, Roganti T. J Biol Chem 2002;277:24475–83.
34. Muhlenhoff U, Stadler JA, Richhardt N et al. J Biol Chem 2003;278(42):40612–20.
35. Drysdale J, Arosio P, Invernizzi R et al. Blood Cells Mol Dis 2002;29:376–83.
36. Morgan EH, Oates PS. Blood Cells Mol Dis 2002;29:384–99.
37. McKie AT, Latunde-Dada GO, Miret S et al. Biochem Soc Trans 2002;30:722–4.
38. Gunshin H, Mackenzie B, Berger UV et al. Nature 1997;388:482–8.
39. Fleming MD, Trenor CC 3rd, Su MA et al. Nat Genet 1997;16:383–6.
40. Grasbeck R, Majuri R, Kouvonen I et al. Biochim Biophys Acta 1982;700:137–42.
41. Chung J, Wessling-Resnick M. Crit Rev Clin Lab Sci 2003;40:151–82.
42. McKie AT, Barrow D, Latunde-Dada GO et al. Science 2001;291:1755–9.
43. O'Halloran TV, Culotta VC. J Biol Chem 2000;275:25057–60.
44. Donovan A, Brownlie A, Zhou Y et al. Nature 2000;403:776–81.
45. McKie AT, Marciani P, Rolfs A et al. Mol Cell 2000;5:299–309.
46. Abboud S, Haile DJ. J Biol Chem 2000;275:19906–12.
47. Chen H, Su T, Attieh ZK et al. Blood 2003;102:1893–9.
48. Vulpe CD, Kuo YM, Murphy TL et al. Nat Genet 1999;21:195–9.
49. Thomas C, Oates PS. Am J Physiol 2003;285:G789–95.
50. Linder MC, Zerounian NR, Moriya M et al. Biometals 2003;16:145–60.
51. Frazer DM, Vulpe CD, McKie AT et al. Am J Physiol 2001;281:G931–9.
52. Dessypris E. Erythropoiesis. In: Lee R, Foerster J, Lukens J et al, eds. Wintrobe's Clinical Hematology. 10th ed. Philadelphia: Lippincott Williams & Wilkins, 1999:169–92.
53. Taketani S, Kakimoto K, Ueta H et al. Blood 2003;101:3274–80.
54. Knutson M, Wessling-Resnick M. Crit Rev Biochem Mol Biol 2003;38:61–88.
55. Bothwell T, Charlton R, Cook J et al. Iron Metabolism in Man. Oxford: Blackwell Scientific, 1979.
56. Trousseau A. Clin Med Hotel-Dieu Paris 1865;2:663–98.
57. Feder JN, Gnirke A, Thomas W et al. Nat Genet 1996;13:399–408.
58. Edwards C. Hemochromatosis. In: Lee G, Foester J, Lukens J et al, eds. Wintrobe's Clinical Hematology. 10th ed. Baltimore: Lippincott Williams & Wilkins, 1999:1056–70.
59. Steinberg KK, Cogswell ME, Chang JC et al. JAMA 2001;285:2216–22.
60. Waheed A, Parkkila S, Zhou XY et al. Proc Natl Acad Sci USA 1997;94:12384–9.
61. Beutler E, Felitti VJ, Koziol JA et al. Lancet 2002;359:211–8.
62. Ajioka RS, Kushner JP. Blood 2003;101:3351–3.
63. Papanikolaou G, Samuels ME, Ludwig EH et al. Nat Genet 2003;36:77–82.
64. Gordeuk V, Mukiibi J, Hasstedt SJ et al. N Engl J Med 1992;326:95–100.
65. Gangaidzo IT, Moyo VM, Saungweme T et al. Gut 1999;45:278–83.
66. Bottomley S. Sideroblastic anemias. In: Lee G, Foerster J, Lukens J et al, eds. Wintrobe's Clinical Hematology. 10th ed. Philadelphia: Lippincott Williams & Wilkins, 1998:1022–45.
67. Means Jr R. The anemia of chronic disorders. In: Lee G, Foerster J, Lukens J et al, eds. Wintrobe's Clinical Hematology. 10th ed. Philadelphia: Lippincott Williams & Wilkins, 1998:1011–21.
68. Coenen JL, van Dieijen-Visser MP, van Pelt J et al. Clin Chem 1991;37:560–3.
69. Fletcher LM, Powell LW. Alcohol 2003;30:131–6.
70. Fletcher LM, Dixon JL, Purdie DM et al. Gastroenterology 2002;122:281–9.
71. Tsukamoto H, Horne W, Kamimura S et al. J Clin Invest 1995;96:620–30.
72. Adams PC, Bradley C, Frei JV. Hepatology 1994;19:101–5.
73. Fleming DJ, Tucker KL, Jacques PF et al. Am J Clin Nutr 2002;76:1375–84.
74. Cavadini C, Siega-Riz AM, Popkin BM. West J Med 2000;173:378–83.
75. Hurrell R, Bothwell T, Cook JD et al. Nutr Rev 2002;60:391–406.
76. Iyengar GV, Kawamura H, Parr RM et al. Food Nutr Bull 2002;23:124–8.
77. Saungweme T, Khumalo H, Mvundura E et al. Cent Afr J Med 1999;45:136–40.
78. Mandishona EM, Moyo VM, Gordeuk VR et al. Eur J Clin Nutr 1999;53:722–5.
79. Adish AA, Esrey SA, Gyorkos TW et al. Lancet 1999;353:712–6.
80. Hallberg L, Brune M, Erlandsson M et al. Am J Clin Nutr 1991;53:112–9.

81. Hallberg L. Proc Nutr Soc 1974;33:285–91.

82. Hallberg L. Annu Rev Nutr 1981;1:123–47.

83. Hallberg L, Hulthen L. Am J Clin Nutr 2000;71:1147–60.

84. Food and Nutrition Board, Institute of Medicine. Dietary Reference Intakes for Vitamin A, Vitamin K, Arsenic, Boron, Chromium, Copper, Iodine, Iron, Manganese, Molybdenum, Nickel, Silicon, Vanadium, and Zinc. Washington, DC: National Academy Press, 2001.

85. Hefnawi F, el-Zayat AF, Yacout MM. Int J Gynaecol Obstet 1980;17:348–52.

86. Cole SK, Billewicz WZ, Thomson AM. J Obstet Gynaecol Br Commonw 1971;78:933–9.

87. Hallberg L, Hogdahl AM, Nilsson L et al. Acta Obstet Gynecol Scand 1966;45:320–51.

88. Frykman E, Bystrom M, Jansson U et al. J Lab Clin Med 1994; 123:561–4.

89. Dallman PR. Annu Rev Nutr 1986;6:13–40.

90. Yip R. Iron. In: Bowman B, Russell R, eds. Present Knowledge in Nutrition. 8th ed. Washington, DC: ILSI Press, 2001: 311–28.

91. Beard JL, Connor JR. Annu Rev Nutr 2003;23:41–58.

92. Failla ML. J Nutr 2003;133:1443S–7S.

93. Viteri FE, Torun B. Clinics Haematol 1974;3:609–26.

94. Beard J, Green W, Miller L et al. Am J Physiol 1984;247: R114–9.

95. Klebanoff MA, Shiono PH, Selby JV et al. Am J Obstet Gynecol 1991;164:59–63.

96. Scholl TO, Hediger ML. Am J Clin Nutr 1994;59:492S–500S.

97. Singla PN, Tyagi M, Kumar A et al. J Trop Pediatr 1997;43: 89–92.

98. Agarwal KN, Agarwal DK, Mishra KP. Indian J Med Res 1991;94:277–80.

99. Rasmussen K. J Nutr 2001;131:590S–601S.

100. Stoltzfus R. J Nutr 2001;131:565S–7S.

101. Ronnenberg AG, Goldman MB, Aitken IW et al. J Nutr 2000; 130:2703–10.

102. Anonymous. MMWR Morb Mortal Wkly Rep 2002;51:897–9.

103. Milman N, Byg KE, Ovesen L et al. Eur J Haematol 2003;71: 51–61.

104. Go MF. Aliment Pharmacol Ther 2002;16[Suppl 1]:3–15.

105. Dufour C, Brisigotti M, Fabretti G et al. J Pediatr Gastroenterol Nutr 1993;17:225–7.

106. Seo JK, Ko JS, Choi KD. J Gastroenterol Hepatol 2002;17:754–7.

107. Peach HG, Bath NE, Farish SJ. Med J Aust 1998;169:188–90.

108. Milman N, Rosenstock S, Andersen L et al. Gastroenterology 1998;115:268–74.

109. Barabino A. Helicobacter 2002;7:71–5.

110. Annibale B, Capurso G, Lahner E et al. Gut 2003;52:496–501.

111. Goyer R. Annu Rev Nutr 1997;17:37–50.

112. Bradman A, Eskenazi B, Sutton P et al. Environ Health Perspect 2001;109:1079–84.

113. Willows ND, Gray-Donald K. Sci Total Environ 2002;289: 255–60.

114. Crowe A, Morgan EH. Biol Trace Elem Res 1996;52:249–61.

115. Wright RO, Tsaih SW, Schwartz J et al. J Pediatr 2003;142: 9–14.

116. Bothwell T, Seftel H, Jacobs P et al. Am J Clin Nutr 1964;14: 47–51.

117. Sullivan JL. Lancet 1981;1:1293–4.

118. Salonen JT, Nyyssonen K, Korpela H et al. Circulation 1992; 86:803–11.

119. Danesh J, Appleby P. Circulation 1999;99:852–4.

120. Fleming DJ, Jacques PF, Massaro JM et al. Am J Clin Nutr 2001;74:219–26.

SELECTED READINGS

Aisen P, Enns C, Wessling-Resnick M. Chemistry and biology of eukaryotic iron metabolism. Int J Biochem Cell Biol 2001;33:940–59.

Eisenstein RS. Iron regulatory proteins and the molecular control of mammalian iron metabolism. Annu Rev Nutr 2000;20:627–62.

Heath AL, Fairweather-Tait SJ. Health implications of iron overload: the role of diet and genotype. Nutr Rev 2003;61:45–62.

Miret S, Simpson RJ, McKie AT. Physiology and molecular biology of dietary iron absorption. Annu Rev Nutr 2003;23:283–301.

Sauberlich H. Laboratory Tests for the Assessment of Nutritional Status. 2nd ed. Boca Raton, FL: CRC Press, 1999:486.

Sheth S, Brittenham GM. Genetic disorders affecting proteins of iron metabolism: clinical implications. Annu Rev Med 2000;51:443–64.

13 ZINC[1]

JANET C. KING AND ROBERT J. COUSINS

HISTORY 271
CHEMISTRY 271
BIOCHEMICAL AND PHYSIOLOGIC FUNCTIONS 272
    Catalytic Functions 272
    Structural Functions 272
    Regulatory Functions 272
BIOAVAILABILITY 273
    Factors Affecting Bioavailability 273
    Nutrient Interactions 273
    Food Sources 274
METABOLISM 274
    Body Zinc 274
    Zinc Transporters 275
    Absorption 275
    Zinc Turnover and Transport 276
    Dietary and Physiologic Adaptation Mechanisms ..277
    Storage, Recycling, and Conservation 277
    Excretion and Losses 277
ZINC DEFICIENCY: ANIMALS AND HUMANS 278
CAUSES AND EFFECTS OF DEFICIENCY 279
    Malabsorption Disorders 279
    Alcoholism 280
    Diabetes 280
    Infections 280
    Other Diseases 280
DIETARY CONSIDERATIONS AND REQUIREMENTS 280
    Absorption versus Endogenous Losses 280
    Estimated Average Requirement 281
    World Health Organization Standards 281
EVALUATION OF ZINC STATUS 281
    Individuals 281
    Populations 282
ZINC TOXICITY AND UPPER LIMITS OF INTAKE 282

---

[1]**Abbreviations: AIDS,** acquired immunodeficiency syndrome; **AMD,** age-related macular degeneration; **Cu,** copper; **DRI,** dietary reference intake; **EAR,** estimated average requirement; **Fe,** iron; **HIV,** human immunodeficiency virus; **IGF,** insulinlike growth factor; **K_d,** dissociation constant; **LOAEL,** lowest observed adverse effect level; **MTF1,** metal-response element (MRE)–binding transcription factor; **NO,** nitric oxide; **RDA,** recommended dietary allowance; **UL,** tolerable upper intake level; **Zn,** zinc.

HISTORY

Zinc (Zn) essentiality in plants was established in 1869, in experimental animals in 1934, and in humans in 1961. The biochemical basis for essentiality is traced to the discovery of Zn as a requirement for activity of carbonic anhydrase in 1940 and Zn finger protein domains in 1985. Detailed reviews are available (1–4). A syndrome of anemia, hypogonadism, and dwarfism was reported in a 21-year-old Iranian farmer in 1961 who was subsisting on a diet of unrefined flat bread, potatoes, and milk. Shortly thereafter, a similar syndrome was observed in 45 adolescent boys in Egypt who were also subsisting on a diet of flat bread and a few vegetables. Administration of a hospital diet containing flesh foods improved growth and corrected the hypogonadism. Subsequent studies showed that the syndrome was primarily the result of a lack of Zn in the diet. Since discovery of Zn deficiency in humans, interest in the biochemical and clinical aspects of Zn nutrition has increased markedly.

CHEMISTRY

Zn^{2+} is a stronger Lewis acid (electron acceptor) than iron (Fe^{3+}), but weaker than copper (Cu^{2+}). This characteristic favors strong binding to thiolate and amine electron donors (5). Zn exhibits fast ligand exchange, which is believed important for some biochemical functions. Zn does not exhibit redox chemistry directly, but Zn^{2+} release from a Zn-thiolate cluster by an oxidant produces disulfide bonds. Zn-S thiolate bonds, therefore, are sensitive to cellular redox (6).

Analytic procedures focus on atomic absorption spectrophotometry and inductively coupled plasma emission. Both have working ranges suitable for biologic samples and have generated much of the literature quoted in this chapter. Zn reference standards are available from the National Institute of Standards and Technology. Of the Zn radioisotopes, only ^{65}Zn (half-life, 245 days) has been widely used in research. Stable isotopes of Zn and corresponding natural abundances are as follows: ^{64}Zn, 49%; ^{66}Zn, 29%; ^{67}Zn, 4%; ^{68}Zn, 19%; and ^{70}Zn, 1%. These have been effectively used in experiments with humans. Highly specific fluorescent probes for Zn are increasingly available and are being applied to understand Zn metabolism at the cellular and molecular level (7).

BIOCHEMICAL AND PHYSIOLOGIC FUNCTIONS

Zn-dependent biochemical mechanisms that determine physiologic functions have received extensive study, but clear relationships have not been fully defined. Zn has a ubiquitous subcellular distribution, which hampers this situation. Consequently, Zn contrasts with Fe, which exists in defined cellular components and has defined physiologic roles. Three general functional classes—catalytic, structural, and regulatory—define Zn's role in biology (7).

Catalytic Functions

Zn serves a catalytic role in enzymes from all six classes of enzymes (8). More than 300 Zn metalloenzymes have been identified, but when the same enzyme identified in different species is counted only once, the number is much lower. How Zn is donated to apometalloenzymes, or any metalloprotein, is not known (7). Zn binding is a posttranslational protein modification, which likely requires a metal donor molecule and/or pH appropriate for Zn solubility, perhaps coordinated by events in the endoplasmic reticulum or a vesicular compartment. An enzyme is considered a Zn metalloenzyme if Zn removal causes loss of activity without irreversibly altering the protein and selective reconstitution with Zn restores activity. Examples are the nucleotide polymerases (RNA polymerases I, II, and III), alkaline phosphatase, and the carbonic anhydrases.

Unequivocal evidence of a direct link between signs of Zn deficiency or toxicity and a specific metalloenzyme has not been shown in complex organisms. It is generally believed that an overt physiologic defect would occur only if the Zn-requiring enzyme were rate limiting in a critical biochemical pathway. Older literature has examples of Zn-enzyme-disease relationships, such as alcohol dehydrogenase with liver disease and RNA polymerases with growth retardation. Such enzyme changes are not considered to represent a critical function for Zn. Of continued interest is fructose 1,6-bisphosphatase, which is allosterically regulated by Zn (9) and could influence gluconeogenesis. Reports documenting Zn-responsive control of enzymes for intermediary metabolism, perhaps operating through hormonal effects on intracellular Zn concentrations (10), have been advanced.

Structural Functions

The structural function for Zn had its origin in 1985 with identification of frog *(Xenopus)* oocyte transcription factor TFIIIA as having coordinating Zn motifs (11). These motifs ("Zn fingers") use cysteine and histidine to form a tetrahedral Zn^{2+} coordination complex. These have the general structure -C-X_2-C-X_n-C-X_2-C-, where C designates cysteine or histidine and X designates other amino acids. Zn fingers have two to four cysteines and up to two histidines. Removal of Zn from Zn finger proteins alters folding and results in loss of function and probably

degradation. The fate of apo-Zn finger proteins has not been widely studied. Classic examples of Zn finger transcription factors are the retinoic acid and calcitriol receptors. The human transcriptome has 2500 Zn finger protein genes (12). This represents approximately 8% of the genome, a finding suggesting that a significant portion of the Zn requirement is allocated to maintain occupancy of Zn finger proteins. The mouse transcriptome has a comparable number of Zn finger genes (13). Binding affinity (apparent stability constants) of the fingers varies widely (dissociation constant $[K_d] = 10^8 – 10^{11} M^{-1}$). By comparison, metallothionein binds Zn strongly ($K_d = 10^{12} M^{-1}$). Ability to activate apo-Zn finger proteins has led to the concept that metallothionein acts as a Zn donor/acceptor protein for Zn binding motifs (14). Although this may be correct, metallothionein knockout mice apparently produce Zn finger proteins in amounts sufficient for health, so other mechanisms must play a role in Zn donation to Zn finger motifs. Because Zn binding by fingers exhibits a spectrum of affinities (14), some sites may be particularly facile. This has led to speculation that more facile sites are potentially influenced by the dietary Zn supply (15).

Originally viewed as a DNA-binding domain of transcription factors, Zn finger proteins were subsequently shown to have a broad cell distribution and also to bind RNA molecules and other proteins for protein-protein interactions. This finding broadens their biologic role to include transcriptional and translational control, modulation of those processes, and signal transduction. Interest in Zn finger motifs is considerable because of their potential as targets for therapeutic interventions, including gene therapy (16, 17). Overall, Zn fingers contribute to the body's need for Zn and provide a rationale for the tight homeostatic control of Zn metabolism; their basic function may explain some of the nonspecificity that characterizes a Zn deficiency state.

Zn/sulfur clusters, such as those in metallothionein, may act as redox units (6). The low redox potential of these thiol clusters, when oxidized by cellular oxidants, results in Zn release. The glutathione/oxidized glutathione redox couple and some selenium compounds influence Zn release, which potentially integrates metallothionein into cellular redox mechanisms. Nitric oxide (NO) may also mobilize Zn from this protein's thiolate clusters (18). Increased oxidative stress (19) that accompanies Zn deficiency may be explained by induction of NO synthase (20).

Regulatory Functions

Regulation of specific genes is a biochemical role of Zn. Originally identified as an active component of the metalloregulatory mechanism for *metallothionein* gene regulation (21), the metal-response element (MRE)–binding transcription factor (MTF1) now is believed to provide Zn responsiveness to many genes (22). Null mutation of the *MTF1* gene produces embryonic lethality (23), whereas a null mutation of the *metallothionein* gene yields viable mice (24). MTF1 has six Zn finger domains of dissimilar Zn-binding affinity which, on Zn occupancy, lead to nuclear translocation and stabilization of MTF1-chromatin binding through MREs of the gene promoter (25). Polymorphisms in the Zn finger domain of the human *MTF1* gene (26) suggest the possibility of genetic variation in the response of MTF1-regulated genes to dietary Zn intakes. cDNA arrays have recently shown that Zn-deficient human monocyte/macrophages have gene clusters that are either positively or negatively responsive to Zn (27). This includes genes associated with apoptosis and receptor-mediated immune regulation. Reciprocal expression of Zn-responsive genes, including Zn transporters, that maintain Zn homeostasis may be regulated by transcription factors that provide opposite responses to Zn status (27).

Regulatory roles of Zn may include receptor-mediated signal transduction. Antigen-dependent T-cell activation occurs when the cysteine-rich motif of the T-cell receptor's (CD4) cytoplasmic tail forms a Zn coordination site with a comparable motif of cytoplasmic protein-tyrosine kinase (p56^{lck}) (28). A defect in such a process may relate to immune dysfunctions associated with poor Zn nutrition (29). The *lck* gene upregulates in Zn-deficient mice (30, 31). Similarly, involvement of Zn in regulating insulinlike growth factor (IGF) binding to soluble and cell-surface IGF receptors has been shown (32). Extracellular Zn may activate phospholipase C and calcium ion release from the endoplasmic reticulum and, hence, cellular signaling through a Zn-sensing membrane receptor (33) or through regulation of protein tyrosine kinases and phosphatases (34). Such mechanisms suggest that the hypozincemia of stress and infection may have a signaling role via a Zn-sensing receptor.

Zn is abundant in the central nervous system, particularly in presynaptic vesicles of excitatory neurons. Zn is released with synaptic activity or membrane depolarization, presumably for endogenous signaling purposes (35). Trafficking of Zn in neuronal tissues is governed in part through the unique tissue-specific expression of *metallothionein-3* and *ZnT3* genes (35, 36). Zn and glutamate colocalize, a finding suggesting that Zn has a regulatory role in functioning of the glutamatergic synapses (35).

BIOAVAILABILITY

The bioavailability of Zn refers to the fraction of Zn intake that is retained and used for physiologic functions. Zn bioavailability in healthy individuals is determined by three factors: the individual's Zn status, the total Zn content of the diet, and the availability of soluble Zn from the diet's food components (37). If the individual's Zn status is discounted, Zn absorption is largely determined by its solubility in the intestinal lumen, which, in turn, is affected by the chemical form of Zn and the presence of specific inhibitors and enhancers of Zn absorption.

Factors Affecting Bioavailability

In general, Zn is absorbed more efficiently from aqueous sources in the absence of food and from animal products. Phytate (myoinositol hexaphosphate), which is present in plant products, especially cereals and legumes, irreversibly binds Zn in the intestinal lumen and accounts for the lower efficiency of absorption from plant foods. The negative effect on absorption is exerted by the inositol hexaphosphates and pentaphosphates. Phytates with less phosphate have little to no affect on Zn absorption (38). When plant staple foods are fermented (as occurs with leavened breads and porridges prepared from fermented cereals), the fermenting organisms produce phytases that break down phytate and increase the amount of absorbable Zn (39). Because phytate is a major inhibitor of Zn absorption, the phytate-Zn molar ratio is used to estimate the likely absorption of Zn from a mixed diet. It can be calculated as follows: (phytate content of foods/660)/(Zn content of foods/65.4), where 660 and 65.4 represent the molecular or atomic weights of phytate and Zn, respectively (40). It is generally considered that phytate-Zn molar ratios greater than 15 have relatively poor Zn bioavailability, those between 5 and 15 have medium bioavailability, and those less than 5 have good bioavailability. Because calcium has the propensity to form complexes with phytate and Zn that are insoluble, it has been proposed that the phytate-Zn molar ratio should be multiplied by the dietary calcium concentration to improve the prediction of Zn bioavailability (41). The interaction with calcium is complex, however, and not all studies show that calcium further modulates the impact of phytate on Zn absorption (37). Fiber is often implied as having a negative effect on Zn absorption, but the reason is usually that most high-fiber foods are also high-phytate foods (37).

The amount and source of protein in a meal influence Zn absorption. Fractional Zn absorption tends to increase linearly with increased protein intakes (42). In addition, animal protein (e.g., beef, eggs, and cheese) improves the bioavailability of Zn from plant food sources possibly because amino acids released from the animal protein keep Zn in solution (37). The binding of Zn to low-molecular-weight ligands or chelators that can be absorbed also has a positive effect on Zn absorption because the solubility of Zn is increased. Certain chelators (e.g., ethylenediamine tetraacetic acid), amino acids (histidine or methionine), and organic acids (citrate) have been used to enhance Zn absorption. These have been shown to have mixed benefit. Recently, plant breeding or genetic engineering strategies that either reduce the content of inhibitors (e.g., phytate) or increase the expression of compounds that enhance Zn absorption (e.g., amino acids) have been considered to improve the bioavailability of Zn from plant foods (43).

Nutrient Interactions

Interactions with other divalent cations in the intestinal lumen may also influence Zn bioavailability. High doses of

TABLE 13.1. ZINC AND PHYTATE CONTENT OF DIFFERENT FOODS AND ESTIMATED AMOUNT OF ABSORBABLE ZINC[a]

FOOD TYPE	ZINC CONTENT (mg/100 g)	PHYTATE CONTENT (mg/100 g)	PHYTATE-ZINC MOLAR RATIO	ESTIMATED ABSORBABLE ZINC[a] (mg/100 g)
Liver, kidney	4.2–6.1	0	0	2.1–3.1
Meat (beef, pork)	2.9–4.7	0	0	1.4–2.4
Poultry (chicken, duck)	1.8–3.0	0	0	0.9–1.5
Seafood (without oysters)	0.5–5.2	0	0	0.2–2.6
Dairy products	0.4–3.1	0	0	0.2–1.6
Eggs (chicken, duck)	1.1–1.4	0	0	0.6–0.7
Seeds and nuts	2.9–7.8	1,760–4,710	22–88	0.3–0.8
Bread (made with white flour and yeast)	0.9	30	3	0.4
Whole-grain cereal	0.5–3.2	211–618	22–53	0.1–0.3
Beans, lentils	1.0–2.0	110–617	19–56	0.1–0.2
Refined cereal grains (e.g., white flour, white rice)	0.4–0.8	30–439	16–54	0.1
Vegetables	0.1–0.8	0–116	0–42	<0.1–0.4
Fruits	0–0.2	0–63	0–31	<0.1–0.2
Tubers	0.3–0.5	93–131	26–31	<0.1–0.2

[a] Amount of absorbable zinc estimated as 45–55% if phytate/zinc molar ratio is <5, as 30–35% if phytate-zinc molar ratio = 5 to 15, and as 10–15% if phytate/zinc molar ratio is >15.

From Brown KH, Wuehler SE, eds. Zinc and Human Health: Results of Recent Trials and Implications for Program Interventions and Research. Ottawa: Micronutrient Initiative, 2000.

Fe (25, 50, or 75 mg) in a water solution inhibited the absorption of Zn from a 25-mg Zn dose (44), but the interaction is less pronounced when intakes are closer to "physiologic levels" (37). Nevertheless, reports exist of Fe supplementation reducing Zn absorption in persons with increased Fe and Zn needs (e.g., pregnant and lactating women, patients with ileostomies) (45–47). The interaction between calcium intake at high supplementation levels and Zn absorption have not been resolved (48, 49). Modest increases in Cu intake do not interfere with Zn absorption (50). High levels of tin and cadmium inhibit Zn absorption, but the extent to which lower, physiologic levels affect absorption in humans is unknown.

Food Sources

The quality of dietary Zn sources is determined by the amount and bioavailability of Zn from the foods. Organ and flesh of mammals, fowl, fish, and crustaceans are the richest food sources of Zn, and because these foods do not contain phytate, they are particularly good sources of absorbable Zn (Table 13.1). Eggs and dairy foods also are free of phytate, but they have slightly lower Zn contents than organ and flesh foods. Cereals and legumes contain a modest amount of Zn, but their high phytate content reduces the amount absorbed. Many breakfast cereals are fortified with Zn. Fruits and vegetables are low in Zn.

METABOLISM

Body Zinc

Total-body Zn in human adults is between 1.5 g (women) and 2.5 g (men), making it slightly less abundant than Fe. The tissue distribution of Zn, however, is ubiquitous, with some tissues, such as the prostate, having a curiously high overall concentration. Zn concentrations of some tissues in a physiologically normal man are shown in Table 13.2.

TABLE 13.2. APPROXIMATE ZINC CONTENT OF MAJOR ORGANS AND TISSUES IN A NORMAL ADULT MAN

TISSUE	APPROXIMATE ZINC CONCENTRATION		TOTAL ZINC CONTENT	
	WET WEIGHT (μM/g)	(μg/g)	mM	(g)
Skeletal muscle	0.78	(51)	24	(1.53)
Bone	1.54	(100)	12	(0.77)
Skin	0.49	(32)	2	(0.16)
Liver	0.89	(58)	2	(0.13)
Brain	0.17	(11)	0.6	(0.04)
Kidneys	0.85	(55)	0.3	(0.02)
Heart	0.35	(23)	0.15	(0.01)
Hair	2.30	(150)	<0.15	(<0.01)
Blood plasma	0.02	(1)	<0.15	(<0.01)

Modified from Mills CF, ed. Zinc in Human Biology. London: Springer-Verlag, 1989.

Eighty-six percent of the total-body Zn is in skeletal muscle and bone. Within organs, regional differences in Zn abundance can be striking, such as hippocampus of the cerebral hemispheres and β cells of the pancreas and kidney cortex. These foci of Zn concentration are believed to be functionally relevant. About 95% of body Zn is intracellular, with the majority of Zn found in the cytosol. A variable amount of cytosolic Zn may reside in vesicles. The finite amount of "free" Zn^{2+} in cells is a subject of some debate, but it is agreed to be very low (35, 51). The high binding affinities of nucleic acids, protein thiols, and nitrogen ligands account for this low concentration, which may be as low as a few atoms per cell (52).

Zinc Transporters

It has become clear in the few years following discovery of Zn transporters that all aspects of Zn metabolism in human cells must be viewed within the context of transporter gene regulation by diet and hormones/cytokines, their tissue specificity of expression and interactions, as well as mutations and polymorphisms in these genes, and their phenotypic consequences.

Two families of Zn transporter proteins have been defined. The ZnT family (solute carrier; Slc30) and the ZIP family (Slc39) have numerous members (53, 54). ZnTs are believed to facilitate Zn efflux across the cell membrane or into intracellular vesicles. At least nine mammalian ZnTs (ZnT1–ZnT9) are recognized. In contrast, ZIPs facilitate Zn influx into cells or from vesicles. At least 15 mammalian ZIP transporters are known. Genes from both families exhibit tissue-specific expression. Subcellular localization does not appear uniform; rather, localization may be a function of physiologic conditions and body Zn status (55, 56). Some metal-metal interactions could be explained by specific transporters exhibiting multiple ion specificity (57). Evidence from GenBank suggests that some transporter genes exhibit single nucleotide polymorphisms, which may have physiologic significance. Evidence exists that human ZnT and ZIP genes exhibit either upregulation or downregulation in response to Zn (27) and may contribute to the tight homeostatic control of Zn.

Absorption

Understanding on the molecular level of how Zn is absorbed by the gastrointestinal tract has recently advanced significantly and has merged well with past concepts of absorption kinetics and homeostatic regulation. Evidence from model systems suggest that Zn is transported as free solute (Zn^{2+}) and/or as a complex which can liberate Zn^{2+} before or after membrane transport. Nevertheless, how Zn is liberated from complexes in the neutral pH of the intestinal lumen for transport as a free solute is not known.

Absorption is from the entire intestinal tract (58, 59). Perfusion studies suggest that the human jejunum exhibits the highest rate of absorption (60). Other studies in humans and animals suggest that the duodenum is quantitatively most important to the overall mass of Zn absorbed because the duodenal lumen has the highest initial Zn concentration after a meal (61). Endogenous secretions, including those from the pancreas, contribute to this luminal Zn abundance. As described later, the estimated average requirement (EAR) and recommended dietary allowance (RDA) are now based on endogenous Zn excretion, of which intestinal secretion is the major contributor. Overall, the extent of absorption is a function of the collective solubility of ingested Zn. Apparent absorption averages 33% and is a factor used to compute the RDA (62).

The nature of absorbed Zn is not clear. As the Zn-binding macromolecules of food are liberated and degraded to smaller Zn-binding molecules during digestion, bioavailability is generally improved. As mentioned in the previous section, no specific complex appears to have a preferential role in promoting Zn absorption. Systemic factors that influence endogenous intestinal Zn secretion or result in poor hydrolysis of luminal constituents (e.g., pancreatic insufficiency, inflammatory bowel diseases) affect intestinal Zn absorption and retention.

Cellular Uptake/Transport

Zn absorption is down a concentration gradient from a relatively high luminal concentration (micromolar range) after a meal. Kinetic measurements with different systems place the K_m (affinity) for Zn uptake in the range of 30 to 100 μM (63–65). Of note is the increase in maximum velocity during Zn-deficient conditions, a finding suggesting upregulation of Zn transport when dietary Zn consumption is less than physiologic needs (64, 66, 67). Apical uptake of Zn^{2+}, a divalent cation, requires adjustment for positive charge gain through counter cation loss or anion gain.

Zn uptake kinetics by the small intestine show mediated (saturable or active transport) and nonmediated (or passive transport) components (63, 64, 68). The saturable component may represent the sum of Zn transporter activity of enterocytes and/or vesicular compartmentalization. Of particular note is the apically localized transporter ZIP4 (SLC39A4). Transfection of the *ZIP4* gene into cells increases saturable Zn uptake, and ZIP4 mRNA and protein expression upregulate in murine Zn deficiency (56). Both features are consistent with the homeostatic increase in the saturable component of Zn absorption during Zn deficiency conditions. A mutation of the human *ZIP4* gene is responsible for the Zn malabsorption disorder, acrodermatitis enteropathica (69, 70). Defective ZIP4 in this disorder leads to Zn-responsive immune dysfunction and cognitive abnormalities (71) and suggests ZIP4 has a quantitatively important role in human Zn uptake. Numerous other Zn transporter genes are expressed in the intestine of rodents, a finding suggesting that multiple transporters participate in compartmentalization and/or release of Zn by enterocytes. At higher luminal Zn concentrations, such as after a Zn supplement, the nonmediated (nonsaturable) component of Zn absorption makes a higher quantitative contribution to absorption (63, 64). This mode of luminal-to-vascular Zn transport could represent a linear phase of transcellular movement or paracellular diffusion. Some Zn chelates may be absorbed by the paracellular route.

Expression of the *metallothionein* gene in the intestine is responsive to dietary Zn (72). Some, but not all, metabolic and gene knockout/overexpression studies show that this Zn-binding protein influences the transcellular phase of Zn absorption (72, 73), acts as an inducible Zn buffer that exhibits rapid ligand exchange, and may influence the Zn transfer process. Because many Zn transporter genes expressed in enterocytes exhibit responsiveness to dietary Zn supply, a complex regulatory process for Zn absorption is envisioned.

Albumin appears to be the major portal carrier for Zn after transfer across the basolateral surface of enterocytes (74). Changes in the systemic levels of albumin or other blood components may alter Zn release from intestinal cells.

Homeostatic Regulation

Absorption efficiency is the primary mode of maintaining control of total-body Zn. Fecal Zn output is directly related to the dietary Zn content. This output is the sum of control over absorption efficiency and regulation of secretion into the gastrointestinal tract. When dietary Zn intake decreases, reduced intracellular concentration increases the rate of absorption, resulting in higher fractional absorption (75, 76). Concomitantly, there is a reduction in Zn secretion into the intestinal lumen via pancreatic secretions and from the intestine via transepithelial flux in the serosal to mucosal direction. The relationship between endogenous Zn loss and absorbed Zn (Fig. 13.1) is the basis around which the new EAR for Zn was formulated (62). Normally, in humans, absorption amounts to 3 to 4 mg (45–60 μmol) Zn/day. In severe Zn restriction, the endogenous fecal losses can be reduced to less than 1 mg/day (77). Absorption adapts to physiologic need such that it increases during lactation and decreases with aging. Some conditions of stress, such as infectious disease, may alter absorption efficiency (7).

Zinc Turnover and Transport

Plasma Zn comprises only 0.1% of total-body Zn and, depending on species, represents 20 to 30% of the Zn in whole blood. Plasma concentrations are normally maintained within strict limits (~10 μg/dL; 15 μM), with serum concentrations slightly higher in nonhemolyzed samples. Reduction of Zn status in humans produces some decrease in these levels, but results are not consistent (78). Acute Zn depletion markedly reduces these levels (79). Acute disease can decrease plasma Zn as a result of the acute-phase response (80), but acute starvation increases

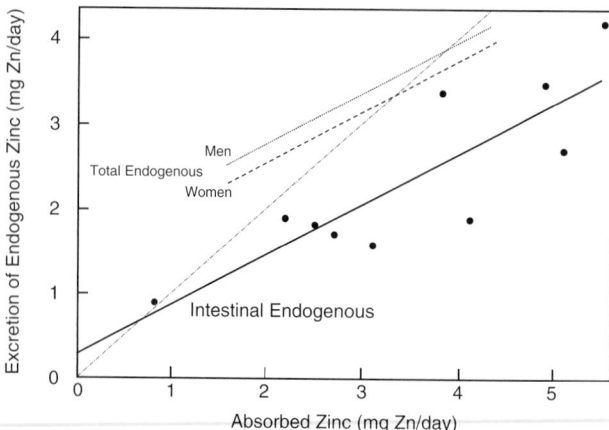

Figure 13.1. The relationship between zinc losses and absorbed zinc in adult humans. The line starting at the origin (*dotted and dashed line*) represents a hypothetical, perfect agreement between endogenous loss and absorbed zinc. The *heavy solid line* represents the linear regression of actual intestinal excretion of endogenous zinc versus absorbed zinc based on data from ten metabolic studies with isotopes. Other losses, added to intestinal endogenous losses, were used to obtain lines (*dotted lines* and *dashed lines*) for total endogenous losses for men and women. The intersect of the line of perfect agreement with that for total endogenous losses represents the amount of zinc that must be absorbed to compensate for those losses. (From Food and Nutrition Board, Institute of Medicine. Zinc. In: Dietary Reference Intakes for Vitamin A, Vitamin K, Arsenic, Boron, Chromium, Copper, Iodine, Iron, Manganese, Molybdenum, Nickel, Silicon, Vanadium, and Zinc. Washington, DC: National Academy Press, 2001:442–501.)

the levels above normal as a result of tissue Zn release in association with catabolism (81). Transient postprandial reductions in plasma Zn are about 15% and may reflect hormonally regulated Zn redistribution (82). A transient increase in plasma Zn occurs when consumption is greater than the RDA (83, 84). In rodents, the dietary Zn intake markedly influences the plasma Zn concentration (2, 7).

Plasma Zn is distributed among many proteins. Albumin, which represents up to 70% of the total Zn in plasma is metabolically influenced (7). At its normal plasma concentration of 600 μM, albumin has a molar ratio with Zn of 40:1. Zn is easily exchanged from albumin (K_d = 7.5 M). Recent evidence suggests an interaction of the albumin Zn binding site with fatty acids (85). α_2-Macroglobulin, a protease inhibitor and carrier of growth factors, binds Zn tightly and represents most of the remaining protein-bound Zn in plasma (2, 7). The ultrafilterable plasma Zn is about 0.2 nM (0.01%), primarily as cysteine and histidine complexes (86). Alterations in this non–protein-bound component of the plasma Zn pool could influence urinary Zn loss and other metabolic and functional parameters. Zn chemistry is such that virtually none circulates in a free ionized form. The flux of Zn through the plasma compartment is approximately 130 times/day (87).

Blood Zn is 70 to 80% cellular, with the concentration of leukocytes (6 mg Zn/10^6 cells) greater than that of erythrocytes (1 mg Zn/10^6 cells) (88). Erythrocyte Zn is found mostly with carbonic anhydrase (>85%), Cu-Zn superoxide dismutase, and various other proteins including metallothionein (89). Leukocytes actively synthesize proteins, and cDNA array analyses have shown that leukocyte genes are very sensitive to Zn (27). Genes expressed in circulating leukocytes may respond to plasma Zn levels.

Kinetic data with both radioactive and stable isotopes have provided important information on Zn pool turnover in humans. Two metabolic pools (rapid [≈ 12.5 days] and slow [≈ 300 days]) have been identified (90, 91). Kinetically active tissues are first liver and then pancreas, kidney, and spleen. Slow turnover is found in muscle and red blood cells, followed by bone and the nervous system. A comparable metabolic model with rats identified the thymus, skin, spleen, intestine, and, especially, the bone marrow as important organs for Zn metabolism (92). An exchangeable Zn pool whose size is influenced by Zn intake has been defined in human subjects (93). It is decreased after severe dietary Zn restriction and may reflect the pool of Zn available to tissues and provide a measure of Zn status. The exchangeable Zn pool encompasses all the Zn in the plasma compartment and some in the hepatic compartment. General features of Zn metabolism are shown in Figure 13.2.

Dietary and Physiologic Adaptation Mechanisms

Hormonal regulation of Zn metabolism has been identified through transient fluctuations in plasma Zn. Persons experience a reproducible reduction in this level postprandially, perhaps related to meal-induced changes in insulin and other hormones (82). Plasma Zn increases during acute fasting (81) are likely caused by hormonally influenced muscle catabolism, with concomitant Zn release. Plasma Zn is transiently reduced following acute stresses (infection, trauma, surgery) (94, 95). Biologic significance of hypozincemia associated with stress has not been identified, but some underlying mechanisms are partially established. Metallothionein, the Zn-binding/exchange protein, is inducible by many mediators that decrease plasma Zn. Cytokines, primarily interleukin-6, which initiate the hepatic acute phase response, are major regulators of metallothionein expression (96, 97). Similarly responsive Zn transporter genes will complement this metabolic adaptation. These may be modified through Zn transporter gene polymorphisms.

Storage, Recycling, and Conservation

Zn does not have a specific "storage site." Conservation mechanisms are such that tissue Zn levels are maintained during Zn restriction, however. Supplemental Zn, at levels higher than the requirement, may provide some reserve in animals during a deficiency (98). Occurrence of a comparable reserve in humans has not been investigated. Retention of body Zn is accomplished through powerful retention mechanisms and recycling.

Recycling of Zn through the erythron is analogous to that for Fe. Red blood cells contain between 20 to 40 μg Zn/g hemoglobin (88, 99), and the average circulating hemoglobin content is 750 g in adults. This represents a red blood cell Zn pool of 15 to 30 mg. The average life span of a red blood cell is 120 days; therefore, turnover for this Zn pool is between 0.12 and 0.25 mg/day (15 or 30 mg/120 days). This finding shows that a meaningful amount of Zn needs to be supplied to the erythrocyte pool daily.

Excretion and Losses

Secretion into the gastrointestinal tract is the major route of Zn excretion. This is the combined contribution from the pancreatic secretions (enterohepatic circulation), sloughing of mucosal cells into the intestinal lumen, and transepithelial flux of intestinal Zn in the serosal to mucosal direction (2, 7). Zn lost via pancreatic secretions comprises an ill-defined mixture, but it certainly includes Zn metalloenzymes. Pancreatic Zn secretion is therefore stimulated by meals. Quantitatively, this may constitute the major route of fecal elimination. Gastrointestinal excretion is directly related to dietary Zn intake (Fig. 13.3). Estimates are as low as less than 1 mg/day in severe dietary Zn restriction (0.3 mg/day) (77). At realistic intakes of 7 to 15 mg/day, excretion is 3.0 to 4.6 mg/day (4, 62), and it increases proportionately at higher intakes.

Urinary Zn output is low (<1 mg/day), and it is refractory to change over a wide intake range (4–25 mg/day) (77, 100). Starvation or trauma and other conditions that increase muscle protein catabolism will increase urinary Zn as the load of amino acids filtered by the kidney increases. Some supplements that bind Zn tenaciously (e.g., Zn picolinate) may promote Zn loss in the urine (101). Glucagon

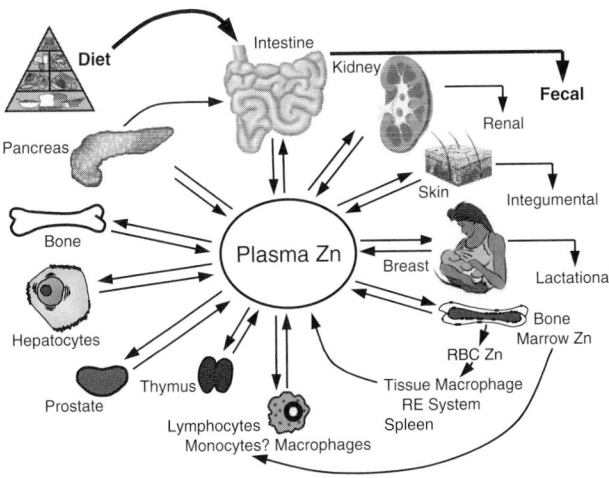

Figure 13.2. Diagrammatic representation of mammalian zinc (Zn) metabolism. Tissues of high metabolic activity and/or particular functional significance are shown as deriving zinc from the plasma pool (*double arrows*). Systems contributing to absorption, recycling, and loss of zinc are shown as *unidirectional arrows*. RBC, red blood cell; RE, reticuloendothelial.

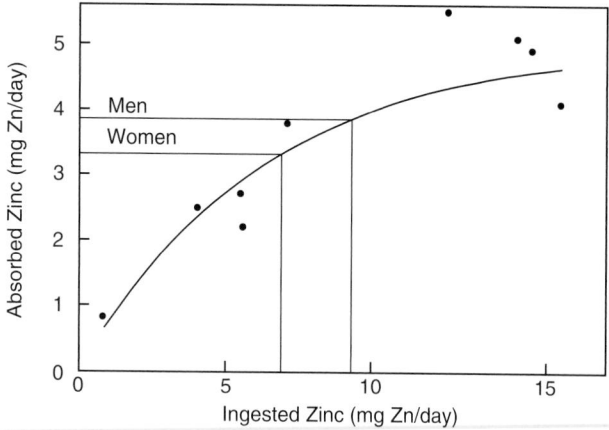

Figure 13.3. Relationship of absorbed zinc to ingested zinc in human subjects losses. (From Food and Nutrition Board, Institute of Medicine. Zinc. In: Dietary Reference Intakes for Vitamin A, Vitamin K, Arsenic, Boron, Chromium, Copper, Iodine, Iron, Manganese, Molybdenum, Nickel, Silicon, Vanadium, and Zinc. Washington, DC: National Academy Press, 2001:442–501.)

has been shown to regulate Zn reabsorption by the renal tubular system (102). Certain Zn transporters are expressed in the kidney. Investigators have proposed that ZnT1, an efflux transporter, is oriented such that it contributes to Zn reabsorption (103). Although not well explored, it is generally held that Zn transporter expression responding to dietary Zn intake regulates endogenous Zn secretion into the intestine and Zn conservation by the renal supply.

Other losses of Zn include integument (1 mg/day), semen (1 mg/ejaculate), menstruation (0.1–0.5 mg total), and parturition (100 mg/fetus, 100 mg/placenta). Lactation produces losses of 2.2 mg/day at 4 weeks and 0.9 mg/day at 35 weeks (62) (see Fig. 13.2). Some women do not produce milk with normal amounts of Zn, but altered expression of the transporter ZnT4 in mammary gland does not explain the defect (104).

ZINC DEFICIENCY: ANIMALS AND HUMANS

Tissue damage (including peroxidation, cytotoxicity/cytoprotection, apoptosis, decreased cell proliferation, stress intolerance, immune deficiency including cytokine imbalances, developmental changes) has been reported in Zn-deficient animals and humans (2, 29, 105–108). However, the biochemical functions of Zn, described in the previous section, are so basic to cellular growth, development, and activity that there is little wonder the exact factors responsible for these effects of Zn deficiency have yet to be defined. Outcomes of Zn functions in integrative systems can be placed in four general categories: (a) redox, peroxidation, and tissue damage; (b) apoptosis regulation; (c) cell proliferation and growth; and (d) immune regulation. These provide a framework to help understand the complexities of Zn deficiency.

Zn, as described, does not undergo redox directly, yet tissue peroxidation and oxidative injury are occasionally observed in Zn-deficient animals. Fe accumulation leading to reactive oxygen or nitrogen radical generation could be a factor (109). NO causes oxidative Zn release from sulfhydryl binding sites and leads to dysfunction (18). Upregulation of inducible NO synthetase in Zn deficiency may exacerbate NO-induced Zn release and cell injury (110). Animal-based evidence suggests that Zn protects against xenobiotic radical damage. Similarly, Zn may be a factor in regulating apoptosis (programmed cell death) through influences at various steps in the signaling cascades involved. Cells with characteristically high turnover rates, such as immune and epithelial cells, could be most vulnerable. Consequently, immune dysfunction and skin and intestinal disorders associated with Zn deficiency could be outcomes of altered apoptosis (51, 106, 111). Reduced growth and cell proliferation observed in Zn deficiency could also be related to abnormal apoptosis. Further, direct effects on hormones that influence cell division or food intake (e.g., IGF or leptin), or the genes that produce these hormones or their receptor or alter their signal transduction pathways could also explain the decreased growth as an outcome of Zn deficiency (31, 32, 112, 113). Finally, immune dysfunction and the susceptibility to infection in Zn deficiency could involve atypical regulation of cytokine genes that, in turn, would disrupt the balance of cell-mediated versus humoral immunity (106–108). Alternatively, failure of Zn-dependent structural factors needed for antigen presentation or microbial killing could be an outcome that leads to parasitic and microbial infections secondary to Zn deficiency.

Essentiality of Zn in animals was first identified in rats (1934) and subsequently in pigs (1955). Most prominent signs of deficiency include skin lesions, a reduction in growth, and a reduction in food intake (1, 2). Essentiality in humans was not shown until 1961 (114). Human Zn deficiency is characterized by skin lesions, reductions in growth, delayed puberty, hypogonadism, host defense defects including infections of the epithelium, and poor appetite (Table 13.3). The response to nutrient deficiencies has been classified as either type I or type II. In a type I deficiency, growth continues, body stores are consumed, and then there is a reduction in the specific bodily functions that depend on the deficient nutrient. Fe fits this category. Type II nutrient deficiencies cause growth to stop; the body nutrient is avidly conserved, and, if necessary, weight is lost to make the nutrient internally available and thus maintain the concentration of the nutrient in the tissues. Zn deficiency is characterized as a type II nutrient deficiency (2). As such, reduced growth occurs without a concomitant reduction in Zn levels of tissues, coupled with nonspecific signs, particularly in the most metabolically active tissues. In human adults, depletion of Zn is a slow process because of adaptive mechanisms that involve homeostatic control of absorption and endogenous losses.

TABLE 13.3. CLINICAL MANIFESTATIONS OF MARGINAL TO SEVERE HUMAN ZINC DEFICIENCY[a]

Growth retardation
Delayed sexual maturation and impotence
Hypogonadism and hypospermia
Diarrhea and intestinal inflammation
Alopecia
Acroorificial skin lesions
Other epithelial lesions: glossitis, alopecia, nail dystrophy
Immune deficiencies: lymphopenia, thymic defects, reduced
    phagocytosis, depressed T-cell function, impaired cytokine
    production
Behavioral disturbances, including impaired hedonic tone
Impaired taste (hypogeusia)
Delayed healing of wounds, burns, and decubitus ulcers
Impaired appetite and food intake
Eye lesions, including photophobia and lack of dark adaptation
    and photic injury

[a] Some signs have been observed in severe deficiency or are reversed
by zinc supplementation.

Repletion of a Zn deficiency appears to be rapid. Evidence from experimental animal studies suggests that some biochemical markers of Zn deficiency are normalized in a period of 24 hours. The clinical spectrum of severe Zn deficiency contrasts with what is expected with the far more prevalent condition of moderate Zn deficiency (4). Other possible signs of marginal Zn deficiency include dysfunctions in taste (hypogeusia) and smell (hyposmia). These observations have not been rigorously tested, but recent evidence suggests that olfactory receptors are Zn metalloproteins (115). Zn-related oxidative injury to retinal pigment epithelium, which is rich in Zn, has been advanced as a factor in age-related macular degeneration (AMD). A beneficial effect of Zn in treatment of that disease was shown only when Zn was provided in a supplement containing a variety of antioxidants (116).

Our current understanding of human Zn deficiency, much of which is marginal Zn deficiency, is based on responses to Zn supplementation. General agreement exists, from studies done in many parts of the world, that physical growth of children in some population groups benefits from Zn supplementation. In numerous studies, cognitive performance and other measures of neuropsychologic performance have concomitantly improved on Zn supplementation. In other studies, impressive reductions in childhood morbidity and mortality have been produced through Zn supplementation. Most of this relates to a reduction in secretory diarrhea and upper respiratory infections, including pneumonia (117, 118).

CAUSES AND EFFECTS OF DEFICIENCY

Zn deficiency can be attributed to five general causes occurring either in isolation or in combination (58). These are inadequate intake, increased requirements, malabsorption, increased losses, and impaired utilization. Primary, or diet-induced, Zn deficiency occurs when intake of absorbable Zn is inadequate. Dietary surveys show widespread, worldwide prevalence of inadequate Zn intakes. Using data from the Food and Agriculture Organization's food balance sheets, Brown and Wuehler determined the mean daily per capita intake of Zn in the food supply of 178 countries and estimated the prevalence of the population at risk for low Zn intakes (i.e., less than the weighed mean normative requirement suggested by the World Health Organization [WHO]) (119). Overall, nearly half of the world's population was at risk. The risk was considerably lower in European and North American populations (1–13%) than in Asian, African, and Eastern Mediterranean regions (68–95%). Data from national surveys show that the median Zn intakes of men and women in the United States are 13 and 9 mg/day, respectively (62).

Low intakes of absorbable Zn are exacerbated by physiologic or pathologic conditions that increase Zn requirements. Increased Zn needs for growth place infants, children, adolescents, and pregnant and lactating women at increased risk of Zn depletion. Pathologic conditions such as preterm birth, low birth weight, and diarrheal disorders reduce Zn absorption because of immaturity of the gastrointestinal tract, or they increase intestinal losses and further increase the risk of Zn deficiency among infants and children (118).

Severe Zn deficiency is characterized by erythematous, visiculobullous, and pustular rashes primarily adjacent to the body orifices and at the extremities (see Table 13.3). After the onset of dermatitis, the hair may change and become hypopigmented and acquire a reddish hue. Patchy loss of hair is a common feature.

Malabsorption Disorders

Malabsorptive syndromes and inflammatory bowel diseases that alter the integrity of the mucosal cell can reduce Zn absorption and precipitate secondary Zn deficiency states, particularly if Zn intakes are also marginal. Crohn disease, celiac sprue, short bowel syndrome, and jejunoileal bypass predispose to Zn deficiency. Crohn disease, or regional enteritis, is a type of inflammatory bowel disease. Low serum Zn concentrations and depressed urinary Zn excretion have been reported in patients with Crohn disease (120). Zn depletion in Crohn disease may result from impaired absorption, increased excretion, hypoalbuminemia, or an internal redistribution of Zn (121). Supplementation with 25 mg elemental Zn/day for 8 weeks reduced the permeability of the small intestine in patients with Crohn disease (122).

Decreased plasma Zn levels have also been reported in patients with celiac sprue (see Chapter 77) (123). Zn absorption may be impaired, and the activity of the disaccharidase enzymes may be reduced (124). Patients with short bowel syndrome (see Chapter 75) are at risk of Zn depletion because the absorptive surface of the bowel is reduced, transit time is increased, and intestinal reabsorption of Zn from the pancreatic juice is impaired if much of the distal bowel is removed.

Low levels of plasma Zn have been reported in patients with intestinal bypass surgery. Although the dietary Zn intakes of these patients seems adequate, absorption, as measured by an oral Zn tolerance test, suggests that Zn uptake is impaired (125). A poor Zn status may contribute to the frequent occurrence of infections following jejunoileal bypass surgery.

Alcoholism

Patients with alcoholic cirrhosis often have hyperzincuria, hypozincemia, and low liver Zn concentrations (126). The hyperzincuria is attributed to a shifting of Zn in the plasma to ligands that are easily excreted and that inhibit tubular Zn reabsorption. Long-term alcohol feeding in monkeys, rats, and pigs lowered hepatic Zn and plasma Zn concentrations. Poor dark adaptation in patients with alcoholism has been linked to Zn deficiency–induced reduction in retinol alcohol dehydrogenase activity in the retina (127).

Diabetes

Rats with genetic or chemically induced diabetes accumulate Zn in the liver and kidney and have hyperzincuria (128). Patients with type 1 or type 2 diabetes may exhibit hyperzincuria, which tends to increase with the severity of the disease (129). The mechanisms underlying the altered Zn metabolism in diabetic patients have not been identified. Atypical Zn responsiveness of metallothionein and specific Zn transporter genes in rodent pancreas suggests that this organ is very sensitive to Zn status. Zn supplementation has improved the immune function of patients with diabetes (130).

Infections

Because Zn is required for the synthesis of immune regulatory proteins and for maintaining normal immune function, poor Zn status may increase the susceptibility to infectious diseases such as diarrheal disorders or viral infections. At the same time, chronic, long-term infections may lower plasma Zn concentrations as a result of an acute-phase response and sequestration of zinc in the liver and other tissues. Zn lozenges taken within 24 hours of the onset of cold symptoms and continued every 2 to 3 hours while awake have been used for reducing the duration of the common cold (131). A meta-analysis of the effectiveness of Zn lozenges in reducing the duration of the common cold failed to find a significant effect (131). Intranasal Zn treatment also had no effect on the incidence and severity of the common cold (132). Taking Zn lozenges every 2 to 3 hours while awake results in a total Zn intake that exceeds the recommended tolerable upper intake level (UL) for Zn of 40 mg/day. Some persons have reported gastrointestinal disturbances and mouth irritation while using Zn lozenges (133).

Zn metabolism is also altered in the late stages of the acquired immunodeficiency syndrome (AIDS); excessive losses of Zn from diarrhea increase the requirement for Zn. Furthermore, plasma Zn concentrations may be low as a result of cytokine-directed redistribution of the element in the liver and other tissues. In a randomized controlled trial of Zn supplementation (45 mg Zn/day for 1 month) in patients with AIDS, opportunistic infections were reduced in comparison with a placebo (134). However, the human immunodeficiency virus (HIV) requires Zn, and Zn supplementation may also enhance disease progression. Until further information is available on optimal Zn intakes for HIV-infected persons, the amount of supplemental Zn taken by patients with AIDS should not exceed the UL.

Other Diseases

Drugs that chelate Zn, such as penicillamine (used to treat Wilson disease) and diethylenetriamine pentaacetate, make it less available for tissue utilization and cause Zn deficiency (135). These drugs, used to treat Fe overload in patients with thalassemia, have caused Zn deficiency. Prepubertal children with sickle cell disease may have Zn deficiency and may benefit from Zn supplementation to improve linear growth and weight gain. Children with sickle cell disease who were supplemented with 10 mg/day of Zn had significantly greater increases in height (0.66± 0.29 cm/year), sitting height (0.97±0.40 cm/year), knee height (3.8±1.2 mm/year), and arm circumference z scores (0.27±0.12 cm/year) (136).

Zn is found in high concentrations in the retina and is hypothesized to reduce the risk of AMD. In two large randomized controlled trials, moderate Zn intake from food or in supplements was not associated with a reduction in AMD in long-term studies of 8 or 10 years (137). Other ongoing studies are under way to determine the effects of higher Zn intakes on AMD.

DIETARY CONSIDERATIONS AND REQUIREMENTS

Absorption versus Endogenous Losses

Dietary Zn requirements are derived from the amount of absorbed Zn needed to replace endogenous losses or by the factorial approach (40, 62). Previously, factorial estimates of Zn requirements were derived from merely summing all losses and approximating the dietary requirement by dividing those losses by an average fractional absorption value for the typical diet consumed by the population. In the recent publication of the dietary reference intakes (DRIs) for Zn (Table 13.4), the factorial approach was improved by incorporating the influence of variations in absorbed Zn and dietary Zn with the estimates of endogenous losses and fractional Zn absorption. Although the nonintestinal losses (i.e., renal and integumental, along

TABLE 13.4. RECOMMENDED ZINC INTAKES (mg/d)

	AGE (y)	MALES RDA[a]	FEMALES RDA[a]	AGE (y)	MALES WHO HIGH[c]	MALES WHO MODERATE[c]	FEMALES WHO HIGH[c]	FEMALES WHO MODERATE[c]
Infants	0–0.5	2.0[b]	2.0[b]	—	—	—	—	—
	0.5–1	3.0	3.0	0.5–1	3.3	5.6	3.3	5.6
Children or Adolescents	1–3	3.0	3.0	1–3	3.3	5.5	3.3	5.5
	4–8	5.0	5.0	3–6	3.9	6.5	3.9	6.5
	9–13	8.0	8.0	6–10	4.5	7.5	4.5	7.5
	11–18	11.0	9.0	10–12	5.6	9.3	5.0	8.4
	—	—	—	12–15	7.3	12.1	6.1	10.3
	—	—	—	15–18	7.8	13.1	6.2	10.2
Adults	19–	11.0	8.0	18–	5.6	9.4	4.0	6.5
	71+			60+				
Pregnancy	>19	—	11.0	—	—	—	8.0[d]	13.3[d]
Lactation	>19	—	12.0	—	—	—	7.6[e]	12.7[e]

WHO, World Health Organization.

[a] Data from Institute of Medicine, ed. Zinc. In: Dietary Reference Intakes for Vitamin A, Vitamin K, Arsenic, Boron, Chromium, Copper, Iodine, Iron, Manganese, Molybdenum, Nickel, Silicon, Vanadium, and Zinc. Washington, DC: National Academy Press, 2001:442–501.
[b] Adequate intake that reflects the observed mean zinc intakes of infants principally fed human milk.
[c] Dietary zinc bioavailability based on estimates of fractional absorption from test meals.
[d] Third trimester.
[e] 0–3 months' lactation.

with smaller quantities of seminal and menstrual losses) are constant over the usual range of Zn intakes, intestinal endogenous losses are positively correlated with the quantity of Zn absorbed. The total need for absorbed Zn, therefore, was determined by adding the nonintestinal to the intestinal losses and regressing the total losses to absorbed Zn. The intercept of the line of equality (i.e., where absorbed Zn equals endogenous Zn) with the regression line predicts the amount of absorbed Zn needed to replace total endogenous losses (see Figs. 13.1 and 13.3).

Estimated Average Requirement

The relationship between ingested and absorbed Zn is asymptotic (i.e., the fractional absorption declines slightly with increasing intakes). This relationship is then used to determine the average Zn intake required to absorb enough Zn to replace total endogenous losses (see Fig. 13.3). This is the EAR or the daily Zn intake that meets the requirements of half of the healthy persons in a life stage and gender group for replacing total endogenous Zn losses. An RDA, which meets the needs for 97 to 98% of persons, is estimated based on the assumption that the coefficient of variation for Zn requirements is 10%. A UL was also established (see later). The various DRIs are presented in text and tables in Appendix Section II, Table A-2-a through A-2-h.

World Health Organization Standards

Standards for Zn intake established by the WHO (40) are based on sums of total endogenous Zn losses (without considering the influence of variations in absorbed Zn). However, because the bioavailability of Zn varies widely worldwide, the WHO set standards for high-, moderate-, and low-availability diets in which about 50, 30, and 15% of the dietary Zn is absorbable, respectively. Because the estimated fractional absorption of Zn used for the DRI recommendations was 0.41 for men and 0.48 for women, the RDAs are comparable to the high- and moderate-availability WHO estimates in Table 13.4.

EVALUATION OF ZINC STATUS

Individuals

The efficient regulation of Zn homeostasis complicates the diagnosis of Zn deficiency, and no accepted, reliable indicators of individual Zn status exist. Only when Zn deficiency is very severe is it possible to make a definitive diagnosis of Zn deficiency (see Table 13.3.), but the possibility of Zn deficiency in an individual person can be evaluated from low dietary intakes, poor bioavailability, and suggestive clinical signs (e.g., growth retardation, delayed sexual maturation, dermatitis, or defects in immune function). Measuring a functional response to supplemental Zn confirms Zn deficiency, but this approach is limited by cost of the assessment and the need for several months to document the functional response, such as growth, with confidence.

Zn does not have a well-established index that can be used in the clinical laboratory to evaluate status. The relative ease of plasma Zn measurements, using blood in which lithium heparin is used to prevent Zn contamination from the anticoagulant, is attractive. However, Zn homeostatic control is efficient, so plasma Zn levels are maintained within narrow limits over a wide range of intake levels (62). The normal plasma Zn concentration range is 12 to 18 μM (8–12 μg/dL). Acute dietary Zn restriction under experimental conditions in human subjects will reduce plasma Zn significantly (79). Postprandial effects on plasma Zn levels (82) and those associated with acute and chronic disease (2, 7) are factors that limit this parameter as an indicator. Extensive numbers of intervention studies have used plasma or serum Zn despite the limited responsiveness of this index (1, 78, 95). Hair, saliva, leukocyte, and erythrocyte Zn concentrations give mixed results as status indicators. A Zn tolerance test, based on the plasma Zn increase after an oral Zn dose of 25 to 50 mg, has not attained widespread use (138). Similarly, many Zn metalloenzymes, including plasma alkaline phosphatase, erythrocyte Cu-Zn superoxide dismutase, and lymphocyte 5'-nucleotidase, have not proved reliable (62). Specific hormones, immune mediators, and circulating hepatic proteins lack specificity as indicators.

Expression of some genes associated with Zn metabolism is Zn responsive, and this has been suggested as an approach to evaluate Zn status (139). Erythrocyte metallothionein protein decreases and increases in a Zn-responsive fashion, but it has been evaluated only under controlled conditions (83, 89, 140–142). Mononuclear cell metallothionein mRNA levels respond to Zn deficiency (143) and supplementation (83, 142) in human subjects, but these levels have not been evaluated as clinical indicators. Combinations of indicators may prove of value (78).

Populations

The risk of poor Zn status in a population can be estimated from measurements of the intake of absorbable Zn, the prevalence of a pathologic state associated with poor Zn nutriture (i.e., stunting or increased infections), and serum Zn concentrations. Although several physiologic factors (e.g., low serum albumin, pregnancy, use of oral contraceptives) affect serum Zn levels, serum Zn concentrations can be used to estimate the risk of Zn deficiency in populations. Cutoff levels, based on National Health and Nutrition Examination Survey II data that control for time of day or fasting status, gender, and physiologic state, have been established for use in population surveys (144). The suggested cutoff for the 2.5th percentile is 74 μg/dL (11.3 μmol/L) in fasting men and 70 μg/dL (10.7 μmol/L) in fasting women.

ZINC TOXICITY AND UPPER LIMITS OF INTAKE

Dietary aspects of Zn toxicity have been well reviewed (2, 62, 145). Acute Zn toxicity causes gastric distress, dizziness, and nausea. Zn has an emetic effect at doses as low as 50 mg. This can be a problem in supplementation trials. Acetate and gluconate Zn salts are better tolerated than Zn sulfate. Liquefied preparations are used in some intervention trials with children. Poisoning by consumption of US pennies (those made after 1982 are mostly Zn with Cu veneer) has been reported. Toxicity and fatalities have occurred with large total parenteral nutrition doses (146).

Gastric problems are observed in chronic toxicity. Other effects include reduction in immune function (lymphocyte stimulation by phytohemagglutinin) and decreased high-density cholesterol (145); these occur at a Zn intake of 100 to 300 mg/day intake for 6 weeks. At lower levels of supplemental Zn, these effects may not be relevant (83, 147). At an intake of 60 mg/day for 10 weeks, erythrocyte superoxide dismutase activity was reduced (62). In animals (dogs and chicks), the pancreas is a target of Zn toxicity (2, 148). This toxicologic effect has not been studied in humans. Hypocupremia was observed in Zn-treated (150 mg Zn/day) patients with sickle cell anemia (149). The phenomenon may relate to reduced Cu absorption, possibly through Zn induction of intestinal metallothionein, which preferentially binds Cu over Zn, thus rendering Cu unavailable for release from enterocytes (150). Clinically, this Zn-Cu interaction has been used to treat Wilson disease, a Cu accumulation disorder, with supplemental Zn. Sideroblastic anemia was observed secondary to Cu deficiency induced by high Zn intake (151).

Zn has been implicated in the pathogenesis of Alzheimer disease. Zn may bind to the normal glycoprotein, β-amyloid protein (Aβ), alter its secondary structure, and cause its aggregation and accumulation as amyloid plaque, a hallmark of this disease (152). A direct link between Alzheimer disease and Zn consumption has been implied, but not clearly defined. Again, not directly linked to Zn consumption but potentially relevant in clinical situations is the toxic effect of Zn ions to cortical neurons (153). After transient forebrain ischemia, Zn accumulates and may contribute to neurodegeneration and neuronal death. Overexpression of ZnT1 reduces this neuronal damage, likely through a Zn efflux process (154).

Metallothionein induction by supplemental Zn has potential clinical and toxicologic ramifications. Expression is induced in human red blood cells and mononuclear cells with a Zn supplement of 15 mg/day (83). Because the physiologic role of the protein is not known, this could be either a physiologic or toxicologic response. This protein has cytoprotective properties against certain chemotherapeutic drugs (155), and induction may alter their effectiveness (156).

A UL for Zn has been calculated (57). After considering adverse effects, including those mentioned earlier, a lowest observed adverse effect level (LOAEL) was derived based on the observation that erythrocyte superoxide dismutase activity was lower at an intake of 50 mg/day. Assuming that dietary Zn intake was 10 mg/day, the LOAEL was calculated to be 60 mg Zn/day (50 mg+10 mg). An uncertainty factor for the LOAEL estimate of 1.5 was applied, and the UL was estimated at 40 mg Zn/day (60/1.5) for adults 19 years of age and older. Dietary intake data of non–breast-fed preschool children in the United States show that, in children less than 1 year of age, 86% or more exceed the UL for Zn (157).

REFERENCES

1. Hambidge KM, Casey CE, Krebs NF. Zinc in trace elements. In: Mertz W, ed. Trace Elements in Human and Animal Nutrition. 5th ed. Orlando, FL: Academic Press, 1986:1–137.
2. Mills CF, ed. Zinc in Human Biology. New York: Springer-Verlag, 1989:371–81.
3. Prasad AS, ed. Biochemistry of Zinc. New York: Plenum, 1993:1–303.
4. Hambidge M. J Nutr 2000;130[Suppl]:1344S–9S.
5. da Silva JJR, Williams RJP, eds. The Biological Chemistry of the Elements: The Inorganic Chemistry of Life. Oxford: Clarendon Press, 1991:1–561.
6. Maret W. J Nutr 2000;130[Suppl]:1455S–8S.
7. Cousins RJ. Zinc. In: Filer LJ and Ziegler EE, eds. Present Knowledge in Nutrition. 7th ed. Washington, DC: International Life Science Institute–Nutrition Foundation, 1996:293–306.
8. McCall KA, Huang C, Fierke CA. J Nutr 2000;130[Suppl]:1437S–46S.
9. Pedrosa FO, Pontremoli S, Horecker BL. Proc Natl Acad Sci USA 1977;74:2742–5.
10. Brand IA, Kleineke J. J Biol Chem 1996;271:1941–9.
11. Klug A, Schwabe JWR. FASEB J 1995;9:597–60.
12. Blasie CA, Berg JM. Biochemistry 2002;41:15068–73.
13. Ravasi T, Huber T, Zavolan M et al. Genome Res 2003;13:1430–42.
14. Roesijadi G, Bogumil R, Vasak M et al. J Biol Chem 1998;273:17425–32.
15. Cousins RJ. Integrative aspects of zinc metabolism and function: Underwood Memorial Lecture. In: Roussel AM, Anderson RA, Favier AE, eds. Trace Elements in Man and Animals 10. New York: Plenum, 2000:1–7.
16. Kang JS, Kim JS. J Biol Chem 2000;275:8742–8.
17. Roberts JP. Drug Discov Today 2003;8:726–7.
18. Pearce LL, Wasserloos K, St Croix CM et al. J Nutr 2000;130[Suppl]:1467S–70S.
19. Powell SR. J Nutr 2000;130[Suppl]:1447S–54S.
20. Cui L, Blanchard RK, Cousins RJ. J Nutr 2003;133:51–6.
21. Cousins RJ. Annu Rev Nutr 1994;14:449–69.
22. Lichtlen P, Wang Y, Belser T et al. Nucl Acids Res 2001;29:1514–23.
23. Günes C, Heuchel R, Georgiev O et al. EMBO J 1998;17:2846–54.
24. Dalton TP, Fu K, Palmiter RD et al. J Nutr 1996;126:825–33.
25. Jiang H, Daniels PJ, Andrews GK. J Biol Chem 2003;278:30394–402.
26. Otsuka F, Okugaito I, Ohsawa M et al. Biochim Biophys Acta 2000;1492:330–40.
27. Cousins RJ, Blanchard RK, Popp MP et al. Proc Natl Acad Sci USA 2003;100:6952–7.
28. Huse M, Eck MJ, Harrison SC. J Biol Chem 1998;273:18729–33.
29. Fraker PJ, King LE, Laakko T et al. J Nutr 2000;130[Suppl]:1399S–406S.
30. Lepage LM, Giesbrecht JC, Taylor CG. J Nutr 1999;129:620–27.
31. Moore JB, Blanchard RK, Cousins RJ. Proc Natl Acad Sci USA 2003;100:3883–8.
32. McCusker RH, Novakofski J. J Endocrinol 2004;180:227–46.
33. Hershfinkel M, Moran A, Grossman N et al. Proc Natl Acad Sci USA 2001;98:11749–54.
34. Maret W. Proc Natl Acad Sci USA 2001;98:12325–7.
35. Frederickson CJ, Suh SW, Silva D et al. J Nutr 2000;130[Suppl]:1471S–83S.
36. Palmiter RD, Cole TB, Quaife CF et al. Proc Natl Acad Sci USA 1996;93:14934–9.
37. Lonnerdal B. J Nutr 2000;130[Suppl]:1378S–83S.
38. Han O, Failla ML, Hill AD et al. J Nutr 1994;124:580–7.
39. Hotz C, Gibson RS, Temple L. Int J Food Sci Nutr 2001;52:133–42.
40. World Health Organization. Trace Elements in Human Nutrition and Health. Geneva: World Health Organization, 1996:1–361.
41. Fordyce EJ, Forbes RM, Robbins KR et al. J Food Sci 1987;52:440–4.
42. Sandstrom B. Proc Nutr Soc 1992;51:211–8.
43. Lonnerdal B. J Nutr 2003;133[Suppl]:1490S–3S.
44. Solomons NW, Jacob RA. Am J Clin Nutr 1981;34:475–82.
45. O'Brien KO, Zavaleta N, Caulfield LE et al. J Nutr 2000;130:2251–5.
46. Chung CS, Nagey DA, Veillon C et al. J Nutr 2002;132:1903–5.
47. Troost FJ, Brummer RM, Dainty JR et al. Am J Clin Nutr 2003;78:1018–23.
48. McKenna AA, Ilich JZ, Andon MB et al. Am J Clin Nutr 1997;65:1460–4.
49. Wood RJ, Zheng JJ. Am J Clin Nutr 1997;65:1803–9.
50. August D, Janghorbani M, Young VR. Am J Clin Nutr 1989;50:1457–63.
51. Truong-Tran AQ, Ho LH, Chai F et al. J Nutr 2000;130[Suppl]:1459S–66S.
52. Outten CE, O'Halloran TV. Science 2001;292:2488–92.
53. Eide DJ. Pflugers Arch Eur J Physiol 2004;447:796–800.
54. Palmiter RD, Huang L. Pflugers Archiv Eur J Physiol 2004;447:744–51.
55. Liuzzi JP, Bobo JA, Cui L et al. J Nutr 2003;133:342–51.
56. Dufner-Beattie J, Wang F, Kuo YM et al. J Biol Chem 2003;278:33474–81.
57. McMahon RJ, Cousins RJ. J Nutr 1998;128:667–70.
58. Solomons NW, Cousins RJ. Zinc. In: Solomons NW, Rosenberg IH, eds. Absorption and Malabsorption of Mineral Nutrients. New York: Alan R Liss, 1984:125–97.
59. Cousins RJ. Theoretical and practical aspects of zinc uptake and absorption. In: Laszlo JA, Dintzis FR, eds. Mineral Absorption in the Monogastric GI Tract: Chemical, Nutritional and Physiological Aspects. New York: Plenum, 1989:3–12.
60. Lee HH, Prasad AS, Brewer GJ et al. Am J Physiol 1989;256:G87–G91.
61. Matseshe JW, Phillips SF, Malagelada J-R et al. Am J Clin Nutr 1980;33:1946–53.
62. Food and Nutrition Board, Institute of Medicine, ed. Zinc. In: Dietary Reference Intakes for Vitamin A, Vitamin K, Arsenic, Boron, Chromium, Copper, Iodine, Iron, Manganese, Molybdenum, Nickel, Silicon, Vanadium, and Zinc. Washington, DC: National Academy Press, 2001:442–501.
63. Steel L, Cousins RJ. Am J Physiol 1985;248:G46–G53.
64. Hoadley JE, Leinart AS, Cousins RJ. Am J Physiol 1987;252:G825–G31.
65. Menard MP, Cousins RJ. J Nutr 1983;113:1434–42.
66. Ziegler EE, Serfass RE, Nelson SE et al. J Nutr 1989;119:1647–53.
67. Lee DY, Prasad AS, Hydrick-Adair C et al. J Lab Clin Med 1993;122:549–56.
68. Raffaniello RD, Lee SY, Teichberg S et al. J Cell Physiol 1992;152:356–61.
69. Wang K, Zhou B, Kuo YM et al. Am J Hum Genet 2002;71:66–73.
70. Kury S, Dreno B, Bezieau S et al. Nat Genet 2002;31:239–40.
71. Oleske JM, Westphal ML, Shore S et al. Am J Dis Child 1979;133:915–8.

72. Davis SR, McMahon RJ, Cousins RJ. J Nutr 1998;128:825–31.
73. Coyle P, Philcox JC, Rofe AM. J Nutr 1999;129:372–9.
74. Smith KT, Failla ML, Cousins RJ. Biochem J 1979;184:627–33.
75. Fung EB, Ritchie LD, Woodhouse LR et al. Am J Clin Nutr 1997;66:80–8.
76. Morgan PN, Costa FM, King JC et al. FASEB J 1990;4:A648.
77. Baer MT, King JC. Am J Clin Nutr 1984;39:556–70.
78. King JC. J Nutr 120:1474–9.
79. Gordon PR, Woodruff CW, Anderson HL et al. Am J Clin Nutr 1982;35:113–9.
80. Falchuk KH. N Engl J Med 1977;296:1129–34.
81. Fell GS, Fleck A, Cuthbertson DP et al. Lancet 1973;2:280–2.
82. King JC, Hambidge KM, Westcott JL et al. J Nutr 1994;124:508–16.
83. Cao J, Cousins RJ. J Nutr 2000;130:2180–7.
84. Jackson MJ. J Clin Pathol 1977;30:284–7.
85. Stewart AJ, Blindauer CA, Berezenko S et al. Proc Natl Acad Sci USA 2003;100:3701–6.
86. Magneson GR, Puvathingal JM, Roy WJ. J Biol Chem 1987;262:11140–5.
87. Lowe NM, Shames DM, Woodhouse LR et al. Am J Clin Nutr 1997;65:1810–9.
88. Milne DB, Ralston NVC, Wallwork JC. Clin Chem 1985;31:65–9.
89. Grider A, Bailey LB, Cousins RJ. Proc Natl Acad Sci USA 1990;87:1259–62.
90. Foster DM, Aamodt RL, Henkin RI et al. Am J Physiol 1979;237:R340–9.
91. Wastney ME, Aamodt RL, Rumble WF et al. Am J Physiol 1986;251:R398–R408.
92. Dunn MA, Cousins RJ. Am J Physiol 1989;256:E420–30.
93. Miller LV, Hambidge KM, Naake VL et al. J Nutr 1994;124:268–76.
94. Henkin RI, Foster DM, Aamodt RL et al. Metabolism 1984;33:491–501.
95. Cousins RJ. Systemic transport of zinc. In: Mills CF, ed. Zinc in Human Biology. New York: Springer-Verlag, 1989;79–93.
96. Cousins RJ, Leinart AS. FASEB J 1988;2:2884–90.
97. Huber KL, Cousins RJ. J Nutr 1993;123:642–8.
98. Emmert JL, Baker DH. Poult Sci 1995;74:1011–21.
99. Diaz-Gomez NM, Domenech E, Barroso F et al. Pediatrics 2003;111:1002–9.
100. Jackson MJ, Jones FA, Edwards RHT et al. Br J Nutr 1984;51:199–208.
101. Seal CJ, Heaton FW. J Nutr 1985;115:986–93.
102. Victery W, Levenson R, Vander AJ. Am J Physiol 1981;240:F299–F305.
103. Cousins RJ, McMahon RJ. J Nutr 2000;130[Suppl]:1384S–7S.
104. Michalczyk A, Varigos G, Catto-Smith A et al. Hum Genet 2003;113:202–10.
105. Kondoh M, Tasaki E, Araragi S et al. Eur J Biochem 2002;269:6204–11.
106. Rink L, Kirchner H. J Nutr 2000;130[Suppl]:1407S–11S.
107. Shankar AH, Prasad AS. Am J Clin Nutr 1998;68:447S–63S.
108. Koski KG, Scott ME. Annu Rev Nutr 2001;21:297–321.
109. Mackenzie GG, Keen CL, Oteiza PI. Dev Neurosci 2002;24:125–33.
110. Blanchard RK, Cousins, RJ. Modulation of gene expression by dietary zinc. In: Packer L, Rimbach G, eds. Nutrigenomics: Role of Antioxidants in Gene Expression. New York: Marcel Dekker, 2004.
111. Ibs KH, Rink L. J Nutr 2003;133[Suppl]:1452S–6S.
112. MacDonald RS. J Nutr 2000;130[Suppl]:1500S–8S.
113. Shay NF, Mangian HF. J Nutr 2000;130[Suppl]:1493S–9S.
114. Prasad AS. BMJ 2003;326:409–10.
115. Wang J, Luthey-Schulten ZA, Suslick KS. Proc Natl Acad Sci USA 2003;100:3035–9.
116. Age-Related Eye Disease Study Research Group. J Nutr 2000;130[Suppl]:1516S–9S.
117. Black MM. J Nutr 2003;133[Suppl]:1473S–6S.
118. Black RE. J Nutr 2003;133[Suppl]:1485S–9S.
119. Brown KH, Wuehler SE. Zinc and Human Health: The Results of Recent Trials and Implications for Program Interventions and Research. Ottawa: Micronutrient Initiative, 2000:1–68.
120. McClain CJ. J Am Coll Nutr 1985;4:49–64.
121. Matsui T. J Gastroenterol 1998;33:924–5
122. Sturniolo GC, Di Leo V, Ferronato A et al. Inflamm Bowel Dis 2001;7:94–8.
123. Elmes M, Golden MK, Love AHS. Q J Mol Med 1978;55:293–306.
124. Jones PE, Peters TJ. Gut 1981;22:194–8.
125. Andersson KE, Bratt L, Dencker H et al. Eur J Clin Pharmacol 1976;9:423–8.
126. Halsted CH, Keen CL. Eur J Gastroenterol Hepatol 1990;2:399–405.
127. McClain CJ, Su LC. Alcohol Clin Exp Res 1983;7:5–10.
128. Uriu-Hare JY, Stern JS, Keen CL. Diabetes 1989;38:1282–90.
129. Walter RM Jr, Uriu-Hare JY, Olin KL et al. Diabetes Care 1991;14:1050–6.
130. Niewoehner CB, Allen JI, Boosalis M et al. Am J Med 1986;81:63–8.
131. Jackson JL, Peterson C, Lesho E. Arch Intern Med 1997;157:2373–6.
132. Turner RB. Clin Infect Dis 2001;33:1865–70.
133. Garland ML, Hagmeyer KO. Ann Pharmacother 1998;32:63–9.
134. Kupka R, Fawzi W. Nutr Rev 2002;60:69–79.
135. Weismann K. Dan Med Bull 1986;33:208–11.
136. Zemel BS, Kawchak DA, Fung EB et al. Am J Clin Nutr 2002;75:300–7.
137. Cho E, Stampfer MJ, Seddon JM et al. Ann Epidemiol 2001;11:328–36.
138. Sullivan JF, Jetton MM, Burch RE. J Lab Clin Med 1979;93:485–92.
139. Cousins RJ, Blanchard RK, Moore JB et al. J Nutr 2003;133[Suppl]:1521S–6S.
140. Thomas EA, Bailey LB, Kauwell GA et al. J Nutr 1992;122:2408–14.
141. Kauwell GP, Bailey LB, Gregory JF III et al. J Nutr 1995;125:66–72.
142. Sullivan VK, Burnett FR, Cousins RJ. J Nutr 1998;128:707–13.
143. Allan AK, Hawksworth GM, Woodhouse LR et al. Br J Nutr 2000;84:747–56.
144. Hotz C, Peerson JM, Brown KH. Am J Clin Nutr 2003;78:756–64.
145. Fosmire G. Am J Clin Nutr 1990;51:225–7.
146. Brocks A, Reid H, Glazer G et al. BMJ 1977;1:1390–1.
147. Bonham M, O'Connor JM, McAnena LB. Biol Trace Elem Res 2003;93:75–86.
148. Lü J, Combs GF. J Nutr 1988;118:681–9.
149. Prasad AS, Brewer GJ, Shoomaker EB et al. JAMA 1978;240:2166–8.
150. Yuzbasiyan-Gurkan V, Grider A, Nostrant T et al. J Lab Clin Med 1992;120:380–6.
151. Fiske DN, McCoy HE, Kitchens CS. Am J Hematol 1994;46:147–50.
152. Huang X, Cuajungco MP, Atwood CS et al. J Nutr 2000;130[Suppl]:1488S–92S.
153. Choi DW, Koh JY. Zinc and brain injury. Annu Rev Neurosci 1998;21:347–75.
154. Kim AH, Sheline CT, Tian M et al. Brain Res 2000;886:99–107.

155. Kelley SL, Basu A, Teicher BA et al. Science 1988;241:1813–5.
156. Doz F, Berens ME, Deschepper CF et al. Cancer Chemother Pharmacol 1992;29:219–26.
157. Arsenault JE, Borwn KH. Am J Clin Nutr 2003;78:1011–7.

SELECTED READINGS

Food and Nutrition Board, Institute of Medicine, ed. Zinc. In: Dietary Reference Intakes for Vitamin A, Vitamin K, Arsenic, Boron, Chromium, Copper, Iodine, Iron, Manganese, Molybdenum, Nickel, Silicon, Vanadium, and Zinc. Washington, DC: National Academy Press, 2001:442–501.

Hambidge M, Cousins RJ, Costello RB, eds. Zinc and health: Current status and future directions. J Nutr 2000;130[Suppl]:1341S–520S.

King JC, ed. 11th International Symposium on Trace Elements in Man and Animals. J Nutr 2003;133[Suppl]:1429S–587S.

Liuzzi JP, Cousins RJ. Mammalian zinc transporters. Annu Rev Nutr 2004;24:151–72.

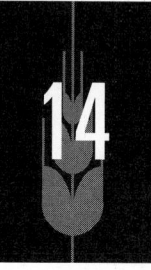

14 COPPER[1]

JUDITH R. TURNLUND

HISTORICAL HIGHLIGHTS 286
CHEMISTRY, BIOCHEMISTRY, AND FUNCTIONS 286
    Chemistry 286
    Biochemistry 287
    Physiologic Functions 288
ANALYTIC METHODS 289
METABOLISM 290
    Genetic Regulation 290
    Absorption and Bioavailability 291
    Transport and Transfer 291
    Excretion 291
    Storage 291
    Homeostatic Mechanisms 291
DIETARY CONSIDERATIONS AND REQUIREMENTS 292
    Evaluation of Copper Status 292
    Dietary Requirements and Recommendations 292
    Food Sources 293
    Dietary Intake 293
    Interactions 294
CAUSES AND EFFECTS OF DEFICIENCY 295
    Copper Deficiency in Animals 295
    Copper Deficiency in Humans 295
CAUSES AND EFFECTS OF TOXICITY 295
    Copper Toxicity in Animals 295
    Copper Toxicity in Humans 296
IMPACTS OF STRESS AND DISEASE 296
    Clinical Conditions with Increased Risk of
        Copper Depletion .296
    Clinical Conditions Accompanied by
        Copper Accumulation 296
    Conditions with Increased Serum Copper 296
    Genetic Defects in Copper Metabolism 297

HISTORICAL HIGHLIGHTS

Copper has been used therapeutically since at least 400 BC, when Hippocrates prescribed copper compounds for pulmonary and other diseases (1). The use of copper compounds in the treatment of diseases reached its peak in the nineteenth century and subsequently declined when the treatments were not successful.

Copper was identified as a normal constituent of blood, and its toxicity was described in the late nineteenth century. By 1900, anemia that could not be prevented by iron supplements had been observed in animals kept on a whole-milk diet. In 1928, Hart reported that this anemia in rats was responsive to iron only when copper supplements were also given (2). Experiments in several animal species produced similar results and suggested that copper deficiency anemia occurs in all species. Detailed reviews of the early history of copper have been published (1, 3).

Human disease was first linked to copper metabolism shortly after Wilson disease was described in 1912 and long before the condition was recognized as an inborn error of metabolism in 1953 (1). As early as 1930, a relationship between anemia in humans and copper deficiency was suspected, but copper supplements improved only hemoglobin synthesis in some instances, so the hypothesis was not well accepted. Since about 1950, increasing numbers of diseases that are not specifically disorders of copper metabolism have been associated with altered, usually increased, levels of copper in blood or other tissues. Menkes disease, another genetic disorder, was described in 1962 and was recognized as a disorder of copper absorption in 1972. Conclusive evidence of copper deficiency in humans was not reported until 1964 (4), and a dietary recommendation was first introduced in 1980 (5).

CHEMISTRY, BIOCHEMISTRY, AND FUNCTIONS

Chemistry

Copper, a transition metal with an atomic mass of 63.54 daltons, has two stable isotopes, ^{63}Cu and ^{65}Cu, with natural abundances of 69.2 and 30.8%, respectively. There are seven radioisotopes of copper, most with a half-life of seconds or minutes. The two with the longest half-life, ^{67}Cu (61.9 hours) and ^{64}Cu (12.9 hours), and either the stable isotope ^{65}Cu or ^{63}Cu, are used as tracers of copper metabolism.

Copper has two oxidation states, Cu^+ and Cu^{2+}, and it may shift back and forth between the two during enzyme action. It may occur rarely as Cu^{3+} (6). Only minute

---

[1]**Abbreviations: AA,** atomic absorption spectroscopy; **ATP,** adenosine triphosphate; **GFAA,** graphite furnace atomic absorption spectrometry; **ICP,** inductively coupled plasma; **MS,** mass spectrometry; **MT,** metallothionein; **PAM,** peptidylglycine-α-amidating monooxygenase; **SOD,** superoxide dismutase; **TIMS,** thermal ionization mass spectrometry; **TPN,** total parenteral nutrition; **UL,** tolerable upper intake level.

quantities of Cu^+ ions can exist in solution; thus Cu^+ compounds are highly insoluble and are strongly complexed (7). Copper is most often found in biologic systems as Cu^{2+}. At least three types of bound Cu^{2+}, each with distinctly different physicochemical properties, are found in copper-containing enzymes. Type 1 is a deep blue protein seen in many copper-containing oxidases. Type 2, characteristic of many multicopper oxidases, is not blue but is detectable by electron paramagnetic resonance. Type 3, neither blue nor detectable by electron paramagnetic resonance, is also found in certain enzymes. A single protein may contain one or more types of copper (6, 8).

Biochemistry

Copper functions in vivo as a part of numerous proteins, including many important enzymes. Detailed descriptions of these proteins and their functions have been published (6, 8, 9). The copper proteins known to be present in humans are listed in Table 14.1 and are described briefly in the following paragraphs. Many other copper-containing proteins are found in plants, lower organisms, and some animal species. Some of the better known of these include ascorbate oxidase, carboxypeptidase A, hemocianin, laccase, and uricase.

Copper-Containing Enzymes Found in Humans

Amine Oxidases. Several important amine oxidases are cuproproteins. Relatively small amounts of these enzymes

---

TABLE 14.1. COPPER-CONTAINING PROTEINS IN HUMANS

Copper-containing enzymes
  Amine oxidases
    Amine oxidase[a] (flavin-containing) [monoamine oxidase, tyramine oxidase]
    Amine oxidase (copper-containing) [diamine oxidase, histaminase]
    Lysyl oxidase
    Peptidlyglycine-α-amidating monooxygenase (PAM)
  Ferroxidases
    Ferroxidase I [ceruloplasmin]
    Ferroxidase II
  Cytochrome c oxidase [cytochrome oxidase]
  Dopamine β-monooxygenase [dopamine β-hydroxylase]
  Superoxide dismutase [hemocuprin, erythrocupin]
    Extracellular superoxide dismutase
    Copper/zinc superoxide dismutase
  Monophenol monooxygenase [tyrosinase]
  Prion protein
Copper-binding proteins
  Metallothionein
  Albumin
  Transcuprein
  Blood clotting factors V and VIII
Low-molecular-weight ligands
  Amino acids
  Peptides

[a] The recommended names of enzymes are followed by other common names in brackets.

---

are found circulating in blood plasma, where they inactivate and catabolize physiologically active amines such as histidine, tyramine, and polyamines. They are found in tissues throughout the body. Their activity is elevated in conditions in which connective tissue activation and deposition take place, including liver fibrosis, congestive heart failure, hyperthyroidism, childhood, and senescence (9).

Monoamine Oxidase. Monoamine oxidase is involved in inactivation of catecholamines. It reacts with substances such as serotonin, norepinephrine, tyramine, and dopamine. The enzyme is inhibited by tricyclic antidepressant drugs.

Diamine Oxidase. Numerous copper-dependent diamine oxidase enzymes are found in cells throughout the body. Diamine oxidase inactivates histamine, by acting in the small intestine, where histamine stimulates acid secretion, and in allergic reactions throughout the body, where histamine is released in response to exposure to antigens. It also inactivates polyamines involved in cell proliferation, a finding suggesting that diamine oxidase may play a role in limiting excessive growth. Diamine oxidase activity is highest in the small intestine. Activity is also high in the kidney, where diamine oxidase inactivates diamines filtered from the blood, and in maternal placenta, where it may inactivate amines produced by the fetus.

Lysyl Oxidase. Lysyl oxidase, a unique amine oxidase, acts on lysine and hydroxylysine side chains of collagen and elastin. It deaminates the lysine of newly formed, immature elastin and collagen, after which cross-links are formed. The enzyme functions in the formation of connective tissue, including bone, blood vessels, vasculature, skin, lungs, and teeth. The concentrations are highest during development. Long-term estrogen treatment increases the activity of lysyl oxidase, and malignant transformation decreases activity.

Peptidylglycine-α-amidating monooxygenase (PAM). The cuproenzyme peptidylglycine-α-amidating monooxygenase (PAM), which is also ascorbate dependent, was identified more recently than most of the enzymes discussed here. It is involved with the synthesis of many bioactive peptides and may be influenced by copper deficiency (10). PAM is found in many tissues, including the adrenal medulla, pituitary, pancreas, and cardiac atria (11).

Ferroxidases

Ceruloplasmin. Ceruloplasmin, also called ferroxidase I, is an α_2-glycoprotein with a molecular weight of about 150,000 daltons. It contains six (possibly seven) atoms of copper per molecule, including Cu^{2+} atoms of all three types described earlier in the discussion of chemistry. Four copper atoms appear to be involved in the oxidation/reduction reactions the enzyme catalyzes. The role of the other atoms is not yet understood. This enzyme catalyzes the oxidation of ferrous iron and plays a role in the transfer of iron from storage to sites of hemoglobin synthesis. Ceruloplasmin also oxidizes aromatic amines and phenols.

Most of the copper in blood plasma is bound to ceruloplasmin. Estimates of the ceruloplasmin fraction range from 60 to 95% (12). The fraction of plasma copper associated with ceruloplasmin appears to be relatively constant within an individual, but it varies considerably among individuals (13).

Ferroxidase II. Ferroxidase II is another enzyme that catalyzes the oxidation of ferrous iron (11). It accounts for only about 5% of the ferroxidase activity in human plasma, but it plays a more important role in some animal species.

Cytochrome *c* Oxidase. This enzyme, present in the mitochondria of cells throughout the body, is the terminal link in the electron transport chain. It reduces oxygen to form water, and permits the formation of adenosine triphosphate (ATP) in mitochondrial energy production. Cytochrome *c* oxidase is considered a crucial enzyme in the mammalian cell, because it is rate limiting in electron transport (14). It contains two or three copper atoms per molecule. The activity of this enzyme is highest in the heart and high in brain, liver, and kidney tissues.

Dopamine β-Hydroxylase. This enzyme catalyzes the conversion of dopamine to the neurotransmitter norepinephrine in the brain. Estimates of the copper content of dopamine β-hydroxylase range from two to eight atoms per molecule, with the most recent estimates being the higher amount (15). Dopamine β-hydroxylase concentration is two to three times higher in gray matter of the brain than in white matter, and it is present in the adrenal gland, where it is required for epinephrine production.

Superoxide Dismutase

Extracellular Superoxide Dismutase. Extracellular superoxide dismutase (SOD), a copper-containing enzyme, is present in high amounts in the lungs, thyroid, and uterus and in small amounts in blood plasma. It functions as a scavenger of superoxide radicals and protects against oxidative damage.

Copper/Zinc Superoxide Dismutase. This enzyme, which contains two copper atoms per molecule, is present within most cells of the body, primarily within the cytosol. It protects intracellular components from oxidative damage, converting the superoxide ion to hydrogen peroxide. It requires both zinc and copper for catalytic function (16). High concentrations are found in brain, thyroid, liver, pituitary, erythrocytes, and kidney of humans. Erythrocyte levels of SOD are high in patients with alcoholism and persons with Down syndrome.

Tyrosinase. Tyrosinase catalyzes the conversion of tyrosine to dopamine and the oxidation of dopamine to dopaquinone, steps that take place in the synthesis of melanin. It is present in the melanocytes of the eye and skin and is responsible for the color in hair, skin, and eyes. Deficiency of tyrosinase in skin leads to albinism.

Prion Protein. Prion protein has been found to be a copper-dependent antioxidant enzyme. It is important for maintaining a healthy central nervous system and is abnormal in bovine spongiform encephalopathy (mad cow disease)

(9). Defects in normal prion protein metabolism impair the ability of neurons to respond to oxidative stress.

Copper-Binding Proteins

Metallothionein. Metallothioneins (MTs) are small, nonenzymatic 61 amino acid proteins, rich in cysteine, which is responsible for binding copper (9). Each molecule can bind 11 or 12 copper atoms, as well as zinc and cadmium. MT appears to play a role in metal storage and sequesters excess metal ions, thus preventing toxicity. The concentration is highest in the liver, where metals accumulate in MT fractions. MT is found in many other human tissues, including small amounts in the blood plasma. The presence in blood plasma has prompted the suggestion that MT also plays a role in copper transport, but if so, the role would be minor.

Albumin. Albumin, a protein with a molecular weight of 68,000 daltons, has one high-affinity site for copper and is the most prevalent protein in blood plasma and interstitial fluids. Albumin binds and transports copper and may also play a role in binding excess copper that would otherwise be toxic. Estimates of the fraction of the copper in blood plasma that is bound to albumin range from 10 to 12% (9, 11).

Transcuprein. Transcuprein, a plasma protein with a molecular weight of about 270,000 daltons, binds copper and is found in human plasma. It has not yet been completely characterized, and its functions are not clear, but it may play a role in copper transport. A considerably smaller fraction of serum copper is bound to transcuprein than to albumin (9).

Blood Clotting Factors V and VIII. Each of these nonenzymatic components of the blood clotting process contains one atom of copper per molecule (11, 17). Although this suggests that copper is required for blood clotting, impaired blood clotting is not among the reported manifestations of copper deficiency.

Low-Molecular-Weight Ligands

Amino acids and small peptides also carry a small fraction of the copper in the blood plasma. Estimates range from less than 1 to 4% (18). Histidine, glutamine, threonine, and cystine are examples of amino acids that bind copper in the plasma, and at least one copper peptide complex, glycyl-histidine-lysine, has been isolated from human plasma. The role of these complexes is not known, but the copper carried by low-molecular-weight ligands is thought to exchange with nonceruloplasmin copper in the blood. The ligands may carry copper to cells (19).

Physiologic Functions

Many of the physiologic functions of copper can be deduced from reactions the cuproenzymes catalyze. Others are based on symptoms of copper deficiency. Detailed reviews of the physiologic functions of copper have been published (1, 3).

Connective Tissue Formation

Copper, through the enzyme lysyl oxidase, is essential for cross-linking of collagen and elastin, which are required for the formation of strong, flexible connective tissue. Thus, it plays a role in bone formation, skeletal mineralization, and the integrity of the connective tissue in the heart and vascular system. Lysyl oxidase activity declines during severe copper deficiency in weanling rats, and the resulting defects in connective tissue formation may be responsible for the multiple effects of copper deficiency on cardiac system integrity and bone formation (20). Copper depletion in humans also results in modest changes in lysyl oxidase activity in the skin (21), but the degree of change does not compromise function, because a large excess is present.

Iron Metabolism

Several mechanisms have been proposed for the role of copper in iron metabolism and erythropoiesis (22). Ceruloplasmin and ferroxidase II oxidize ferrous iron, so it can be transported from the intestinal lumen and storage sites to sites of erythropoiesis. This may explain why anemia develops with copper deficiency, yet iron accumulates in the intestinal lumen and liver. Copper may also be required for the formation of normal bone marrow cells, necessary for the production of red blood cells.

Central Nervous System

Copper plays multiple roles in the central nervous system. It is required for the formation and maintenance of myelin, a protective layer composed primarily of phospholipids covering neurons. Phospholipid synthesis depends on cytochrome c oxidase activity, and this may explain why copper deficiency leads to poor myelination, necrosis of nerve tissue, and neonatal ataxia in copper-deficient animals. The role of cuproenzymes in catecholamine metabolism (the conversion of dopamine to norepinephrine by dopamine β-hydroxylase and the degradation of serotonin, norepinephrine, tyramine, and dopamine by monoamine oxidase) implies a function in normal neurotransmission (10).

Melanin Pigment Formation

The role of copper in the pigmentation of skin, hair, and eyes is related to the requirement for tyrosinase in melanin synthesis. Depigmentation of hair and skin is observed with copper deficiency in several animal species and in Menke disease in humans.

Cardiac Function and Cholesterol Metabolism

The role of copper in cardiac function has been explored in numerous laboratory animals (23). Cardiac myopathy and various other conditions appear when weanling, but not older, rats, are deprived of copper. Cardiac symptoms have not been reported in the few cases of frankly copper-deficient human patients, although links to human heart irregularities have been suggested (24). The roles of copper in cardiovasular disease have been reviewed (25). Blood cholesterol increases in animals fed copper-deficient diets, but results of studies on the effects of low-copper diets on human blood cholesterol are not consistent. Levels increased in some and declined in others, and copper supplementation increased low-density lipoprotein in a study in men (26).

Immune Function

Evidence suggests a role for copper in immune function. Both low and high copper intakes influence immune function in laboratory animals (27). Humoral and cellular factors of the immune system are suppressed by copper deficiency (11). With severe copper deficiency, laboratory animals show numerous changes in the immune system, including changes in T lymphocytes and T-helper cells, B cells and monocytes, and interleukin-2 (28, 29). Some indices of immune function declined with copper depletion in young men, but they were not reversed by a higher copper intake (30).

Other Functions

Other physiologic functions suggested for copper are not as well understood as those described earlier. These include roles for copper in thermal regulation and glucose metabolism. A role in blood clotting through factors V and VIII is known but has not yet been clearly associated with clinical manifestations of copper deficiency. Copper is known to be both prooxidant and antioxidant. Two key antioxidant enzymes, ceruloplasmin and SOD, decrease in copper deficiency and may result in impaired antioxidant status (31). The effect of dietary copper on these functions warrants further investigation.

ANALYTIC METHODS

Atomic spectroscopy is the method of choice for determining the copper content of foods and biologic tissues. Samples can be analyzed directly in liquids with low organic content, but destruction of organic material is necessary for solid samples or those with high organic content. A review of the different atomic spectroscopy approaches describes the principles and advantages of each (32). Atomic absorption spectroscopy (AA) and inductively coupled plasma (ICP) emission spectroscopy are used most often. Samples are atomized for AA either with an air-acetylene flame (flame AA) or with a graphite furnace (GFAA) for electrothermal ionization. Flame AA is the fastest and easiest of the two approaches, but GFAA has the advantage of much lower detection limits; detection limits for copper are about

1.5 μg/mL by flame AA and 0.014 μg/mL by GFAA. AA is usually the method of choice when copper is the only mineral be analyzed. Flame AA is preferred, but GFAA is used when sample concentrations are too low for flame AA. The primary advantage of ICP is that several elements can be determined simultaneously. It is more sensitive than flame AA and less sensitive than GFAA. Detection limits for copper by ICP are about 0.4 μg/mL and depend on the type of nebulizer used. With highly efficient nebulization, greater sensitivity can be obtained.

Stable isotopes of copper are employed as tracers of its metabolic fate (33). They are used to determine copper absorption, utilization, excretion, and kinetics. When they are combined with computer modeling (34), pool sizes and turnover can be determined. Mass spectrometry (MS) is used most often to measure the copper isotope ratios. The two preferred MS methods for the purpose are ICP-MS and thermal ionization mass spectrometry (TIMS) (35). Of the two, ICP-MS is usually the method of choice. It is faster, is easier to learn and use than TIMS, and has lower detection limits. However, TIMS can achieve the greatest precision, so it is preferred when isotopic enrichment is very low.

METABOLISM

Mammalian copper metabolism is depicted schematically in Figure 14-1. Some copper in the diet is absorbed into the body through the intestinal mucosa, transported via the portal blood to the liver, and incorporated into ceruloplasmin. Ceruloplasmin is released into the blood and delivers copper to tissues throughout the body. Albumin-bound copper exchanges with tissue copper, and numerous low-molecular-weight moieties also supply copper to the tissues (19). Most endogenous copper is secreted into the gastrointestinal tract, where it combines with unabsorbed dietary copper and is eliminated from the body. A small amount of copper is eliminated through other excretory routes.

Genetic Regulation

Certain genes have been identified that influence copper metabolism (36). Copper ions can regulate the genetic expression of proteins responsible for copper storage, electron transport, and catalytic activity (11). The discovery of genes encoding for copper transporters and chaperones, thereby regulating copper uptake and distribution, has resulted in major advances in the understanding of the

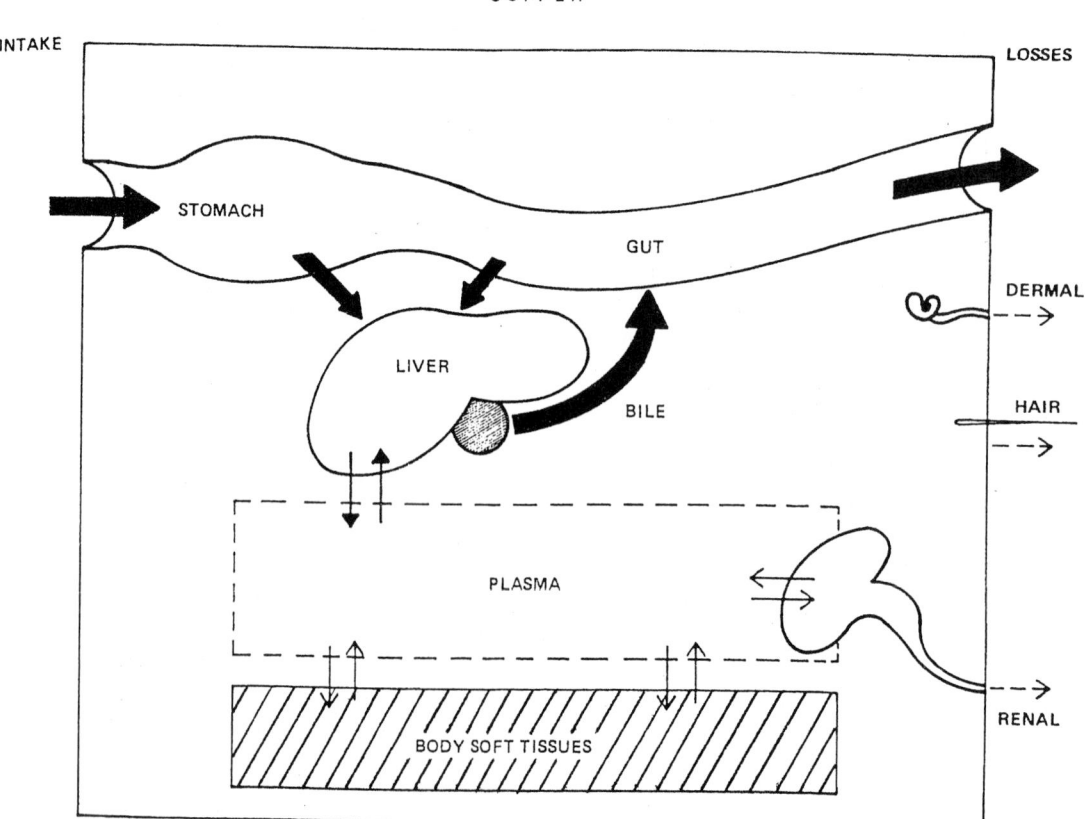

Figure 14.1. Schematic representation of the metabolism of copper in mammals. (From Solomons NW. Zinc and copper. In: Shils ME, Young VR, eds. Modern Nutrition in Health and Disease. 8th ed. Philadelphia: Lea & Febiger, 1988.)

copper metabolism (37). Copper transporters and chaperones are discussed in more detail later, under transport and transfer. Defects in two specific genes, both encoding for copper ATPases, are responsible for Menkes and Wilson diseases.

Absorption and Bioavailability

Estimates of the bioavailability of dietary copper to humans are usually based on absorption (38). The amount of copper in the diet appears to influence bioavailability more than the composition of the diet or specific dietary components unless the levels are extremely high or low or the diet composition is unusual.

Studies conducted with laboratory animals have begun to provide some basic information on the mechanism of copper absorption (3, 9). Copper is absorbed primarily in the small intestine, with a small amount absorbed in the stomach. Absorption is probably by a saturable, active transport process at lower levels of dietary copper; at high levels of dietary copper, passive diffusion plays a role. Absorption may be regulated by the need for copper, with MT in intestinal cells and the copper transporter Ctr1 involved in regulation.

By using a stable isotope of copper as a tracer, the ability to determine copper absorption has become much more reliable (38). Early estimates of copper absorption in humans ranged from 15 to 97% (1). Estimates of copper absorption varied widely in part because of inadequate methods and because the level of dietary copper was not known or controlled. A series of stable isotope studies of copper absorption since demonstrated that the level of copper in the diet strongly influences absorption (38, 39). As dietary copper increases, the fraction absorbed declines and the amount absorbed increases. Absorption declined from 75% at 0.4 mg (6 µmol) copper/day to 12% at 7.5 mg (120 µmol) copper/day. The amount absorbed increased from 0.3 to 0.9 mg (5–15 µmol), or only tripled with 20 times the amount of dietary copper. This demonstrates that copper homeostasis is maintained in part by regulation of absorption.

Transport and Transfer

Following absorption, copper is transported bound primarily to albumin and to transcuprein and low-molecular-weight ligands (9, 14). The newly absorbed copper disappears rapidly from the plasma. Most is taken up by the liver, and some is taken up by the kidney. Once in the liver, copper is incorporated into ceruloplasmin within hours. Some is incorporated into MT in the liver of animals, particularly when copper intake is high; a role for MT in cellular detoxification has been proposed (40). A role for copper in the kidney is not known, but copper is probably filtered by the glomerulus and reabsorbed in the tubules (41).

Copper bound to ceruloplasmin is released from the liver into the blood and is delivered to cells with specific ceruloplasmin receptors on their surface. Ceruloplasmin binds to these receptors; the copper is reduced, dissociates from ceruloplasmin, and is released into the cells (42).

One suggested sequence leading to excretion of copper in bile is that ceruloplasmin with part of the copper removed may return to the liver, where it is partially degraded (9). Copper-containing ceruloplasmin fragments are then transferred to the bile and are excreted into the gastrointestinal tract. In addition to this sequence, glutathione (not a cuproenzyme) may play a role in the rapid transfer of excessive copper to the bile (43).

Much has been learned in the last few years about transporter proteins and chaperones responsible for copper transport, cellular uptake and release, and the distribution of copper (9, 11, 37). Among those identified to date are two copper transporters, Ctr1 and Dmt1, that appear to be responsible for transfer of copper into cells. The newly discovered copper chaperone proteins carry copper to specific intracellular sites and enzymes. Two that have be identified are Atox/HAH1 and Ccs. Atox/HAH1 delivers copper to ATPases, and Ccs delivers copper to SOD.

Excretion

The primary route of copper excretion is via bile into the gastrointestinal tract. Little of this copper is reabsorbed. It combines with a small amount of copper from intestinal cells and from pancreatic and intestinal fluids and unabsorbed dietary copper and is then eliminated in the feces. Other routes of excretion contribute little to total copper losses. Healthy humans excrete only 10 to 30 µg (0.2–0.5 µmol) of copper in the urine (13, 44), but urinary losses can increase markedly in some conditions, such as renal tubular defects (41). Sweat and integumentary losses are usually less than 50 µg (0.8 µmol)/day (13).

Storage

The adult human body contains only about 50 to 120 mg (0.79 to 1.9 mmol) of copper (3), very little compared with other trace elements such as iron and zinc. Animal data suggest that copper is stored in the liver bound to MT-like proteins. Ruminants and a few other animal species can store much more copper in the liver than can humans or most other animal species. Copper may also be held, at least temporarily, bound to intestinal MT.

Homeostatic Mechanisms

Absorption of ingested copper is regulated, and absorption is much more efficient when dietary copper is low. The importance of an individual's copper status in absorption is not understood. When a low-copper diet is consumed, the efficiency of absorption increases within days, and it remains about the same over time when a low-copper diet is continued (39). This finding suggests the dietary content is more important than copper status in regulation of absorption. A newly discovered point of regulation is retention of copper in the cells of the intestinal mucosa (45). When dietary copper is high, excess copper is sequestered by the intestinal mucosa and does not enter the systemic circulation. These cells turn over rapidly, and exfoliated cells are eliminated in the stools. Another point of homeostatic control of total body copper is the excretion of copper into the bile and from there into the gastrointestinal tract. Animals and humans increase endogenous copper excretion when the diet is high in copper and excrete little during copper deficiency or when dietary copper is low (39, 46, 47). When a stable isotope of copper was administered to rats, tissue copper was conserved in copper-restricted rats. Intravenous doses of a stable isotope of copper were administered to human subjects. When dietary copper was 2.5 mg/day (39 μmol/day), 20% of the dose was excreted and eliminated in the stools in 6 days, whereas only 7% of the dose was eliminated when the diet contained 0.4 mg/day (6 μmol/day). The homeostatic regulation of copper absorption and excretion protects against copper deficiency and toxicity over a broad range of dietary intakes.

DIETARY CONSIDERATIONS AND REQUIREMENTS

Evaluation of Copper Status

Biochemical Indices

Currently used indices of copper status easily detect severe copper deficiency. Serum copper and ceruloplasmin concentrations fall to levels far below the normal range and respond quickly to copper supplementation (41). Ceruloplasmin has generally been considered the most reliable index of copper status (48), but some consider red cell SOD equally or more sensitive (49). SOD values have not yet been reported in cases of severe copper deficiency in humans, and a level that would indicate copper deficiency has not been established. The normal ranges of these indices vary among laboratories, but they are approximately as follows: 10.0 to 24.6 μmol/L (64–156 μg/dL) for serum copper; 180 to 400 mg/L (18–40 mg/dL) for ceruloplasmin; and 0.47 ± 0.067 mg/g for erythrocyte SOD (48).

Although serum copper and ceruloplasmin clearly reflect severe deficiency, they may not be sensitive to marginal copper status. In addition, ceruloplasmin is an acute-phase reactant, and, as a result, serum copper and ceruloplasmin are elevated in various conditions. Serum copper and ceruloplasmin could be within the normal range or even elevated, masking copper deficiency when one of these conditions occurs at the same time.

The search for a reliable index of marginal copper status has been unsuccessful, although numerous possibilities have been suggested (41). Copper levels in the hair, nails, or saliva do not appear to reflect copper status. Urinary copper varies greatly among individuals and declines only when dietary copper is very low (39). Cytochrome oxidase in red cells, or possibly in platelets or white cells (24), may be sensitive to copper status, but more data are needed. A single index is not sufficient to assess copper nutriture. Other indices have the potential to provide information on copper status, such as leukocyte copper (44) and changes in lysyl oxidase activity (21).

Functional Tests

Most functional tests that could be of value in assessing copper status, such as assessment of immune function or antioxidant status, lack the necessary specificity to diagnose copper deficiency. However, in conjunction with the more established indices of copper status, these tests may be valuable. Stable isotope measurements of total body copper, the exchangeable copper pool size, or copper turnover may prove useful in evaluating copper status, but research in this area has just begun (50). Compartmental models of copper metabolism should aid in evaluating copper status (34).

Dietary Requirements and Recommendations

Laboratory Animals

The copper requirements of laboratory animals are influenced by other components of the diet, including those discussed later under interactions. They differ among species as well. Approximately 6 μg copper/g diet appears to be adequate for young animals of most species (3), including pigs, rats, and guinea pigs. This amount can be lower under optimal conditions and higher with confounding factors or for specific functions.

Humans

Copper depletion/repletion studies, to establish the minimum requirements of healthy humans, were not done until recently with a copper intake low enough to produce systematic depletion of copper status. Studies conducted under highly controlled and closely monitored conditions have now been conducted. Relatively few cases of frank copper deficiency have been reported, and these were accompanied by confounding factors such as malnutrition, malabsorption, and excessive gastrointestinal losses, which limited their value in establishing a minimum requirement for healthy individuals.

The most relevant example of a long-term diet containing less than the minimum copper requirement may be the following: An enteral diet containing 15 μg copper/100 kcal (0.56 pmol/J) produced copper deficiency in six of six severely handicapped patients between the ages of 4 and 24 years after they had consumed the diet for 12 to 66 months. Serum copper values of 1.8 to 7.2 μmol/L (11.7 to 45.7 μg/dL) and ceruloplasmin values of 30 to 125 mg/L (3 to 12.5 mg/dL) were found, accompanied by other manifestations of copper deficiency. These values increased to within the normal range after 3 months of copper supplementation (51). By extrapolation, although it may not be valid to extrapolate from these growing, severely handicapped individuals to healthy adults, copper deficiency could be expected to develop, eventually if the diet contained 15 μg copper/100 kcal, or 0.44 mg copper/2900 kcal for men and 0.29 mg copper/1900 kcal for women (0.56 pmol/J). The foregoing example, combined with one study in which healthy young men maintained copper balance and status at 0.79 mg/day (12 μmol/day) (38) and another in which young men did not maintain status at 0.37 mg/day (6 μmol/day) (39), suggests that the minimum copper requirement of men is somewhere between 0.4 and 0.8 mg/day (6 and 12 μmol/day).

The newly established dietary reference intakes (DRIs) for copper (52) for all age groups and during pregnancy and lactation are shown in Table 14-2 and Appendix Table A-2-g. The DRIs include the following: an estimated average requirement (EAR), the intake that meets the needs of half of the individuals in a group; recommended dietary allowance (RDA), the intake that meets the nutrient needs of almost all (98–98%) the individuals in a group; adequate intake (AI) for infants, the mean intake of healthy infants receiving human milk, and a tolerable upper intake level, the highest level that is likely to pose no risk of adverse effects to almost all individuals. See Appendix

Tables A-2-a, A-2-b, A-2-g, and A-2-h for further definitions of the DRIs and for summary tables. For adults, the EAR for copper is 0.7 mg/day, the RDA is 0.9 mg/day, and the tolerable upper intake level (UL) is 10 mg/day. Additional increments are added for pregnancy and lactation, as shown in Table 14-2. The World Health Organization estimated the adult basal copper requirement to be 0.6 mg/day (9 μmol/day) for women and 0.7 mg/day (11 μmol/day) for men. (53). Their requirement for individuals, which includes a factor of safety to include additional increment for almost all dietary conditions, is 0.7 mg/day (11 μmol/day) for women and 0.8 mg/day (12.5 μmol/day) for men.

Food Sources

The richest sources of dietary copper contain from 0.3 to more than 2 mg/100 g (50–>300 nmol/g). These include shellfish, nuts, seeds (including cocoa powder), legumes, and the bran and germ portions of grains, liver, and organ meats. Most grain products, most products containing chocolate, fruits and vegetables such as dried fruits, mushrooms, tomatoes, bananas, grapes, and potatoes, and most meats have intermediate amounts of copper, from 0.1 to 0.3 mg/100 g (20–50 nmol/g). Other fruits and vegetables, chicken, many fish, and dairy products contain relatively low concentrations (<0.1 mg/100 g [20 nmol/g]) of copper (54). Cow's milk is particularly low in copper. The major sources of copper in the US diet are meat, nuts, beans or peas, and main dishes (55). (See Appendix Table A-22-b for a detailed list.)

Because information on the copper content of foods is incomplete and databases often contain missing values, copper intake is underestimated unless missing values are replaced with imputed values (56). A table of the copper content of foods compiled when much of the available data were from the 1930s and 1940s reported consistently higher copper concentrations (57) than tables that exclude pre-1960 data, a finding suggesting that early values were too high. However, a critical evaluation of the reliability of post-1960 published values for the copper content of foods demonstrated that improvement is still needed (54). The copper content of foods can vary because of a combination of factors, including analytic method, sampling procedure, recipe, cooking method, and the part of the country from which samples are collected. Careful analysis of the copper content of high-copper foods from the US Food and Drug Administration's total-diet study varied by an average of 24%, which is in the middle of average variation of other minerals in the same foods (55, 56).

Dietary Intake

Estimates of dietary intake of Americans before 1970 were considerably higher than current estimates. This reflects marked improvements in analytic techniques for measuring copper and awareness of the importance of

TABLE 14.2. DIETARY REFERENCE INTAKE VALUES FOR COPPER[a]

AGE	EAR (μg/d)[b]	RDA (μg/d)[c]	AI (μg/d)[d]	UL (μg/d)[e]
0–6 mo			200	ND[f]
7–12 mo			220	ND
1–3 y	260	340		1,000
4–8 y	340	440		3,000
9–13 y	540	700		5,000
14–18 y	685	890		8,000
19–50 y	700	900		10,000
>51 y	700	900		10,000
Pregnancy				
14–18 y	785	1,000		8,000
19–50 y	800	1,000		10,000
Lactation				
14–18 y	985	1,300		8,000
19–50 y	1,000	1,300		10,000

[a] 1 μg copper = 0.0157 μmol

[b] Estimated average requirement. The intake that meets the estimated nutrient needs of half of the individuals in a group.

[c] Recommended dietary allowance. The intake that meets the nutrient needs of almost all (97–98%) of individuals in a group.

[d] Adequate intake. The mean intake of healthy infants receiving human milk.

[e] Tolerable upper intake levels. The highest level that is likely to pose no risk of adverse health effects to almost all individuals.

[f] Not determinable. The source of intake should be from food only.

avoiding copper contamination of analytic samples. The usual diet was thought to contain 2 to 5 mg (30–80 μmol) of copper, but studies, including one study of 132 diet composites, now show that few diets contain more than 2 mg (30 μmol)/day (53, 56). As with all nutrients, copper intake can vary widely, depending on food choices. Diets in countries where more whole-grain products, legumes, and organ meats are eaten contain more copper.

The median intake in the United States, based on the Third National Health and Nutrition Examination Survey and the Continuing Survey of Food Intake by Individuals is approximately 1.0 to 1.1 mg/day for women and 1.2 to 1.6 mg/day for men (52). About 15% of adults consume supplements including copper, and when supplement intake was included, mean intake increased to 1.3 to 2.2 mg/day. These mean intakes are higher than the current RDA and suggest that healthy individuals consuming a reasonably well-balanced diet should meet their dietary copper requirement.

Interactions

Interactions with Other Nutrients

Nutrients known to affect the bioavailability of copper when included in the diet of humans or animals in extreme amounts are iron, zinc, molybdenum, ascorbic acid, and carbohydrates. In addition, high or low levels of dietary copper may affect metabolism of some of these nutrients. Interactions between dietary copper and other nutrients or dietary components have been reviewed (48).

Iron. Copper and iron may interact in numerous ways. As discussed later, copper deficiency alters iron metabolism. Anemia, often accompanied by accumulation of iron in the liver, has been reported in all species studied, including humans. An excess of copper produced anemia in the pig. Excessive iron in the form of inorganic iron salts decreased copper status and, in time, resulted in clinical signs of copper deficiency in several animal species (58).

Zinc. When the diet contains excessive zinc over a sufficient period, the copper status of animals and humans has been impaired; the effect is reversed by copper supplements. One explanation for this interaction is that high dietary zinc induces intestinal MT. Copper does not play an important role in the induction of MT, but it has a stronger affinity for MT than zinc. Copper displaces zinc in intestinal MT and is trapped (3, 59). Copper depletion was observed in human study subjects when supplements of 50 mg (280 μmol) or more of zinc were given for extended periods. The UL for zinc, 40 mg/day for adults, was based on the effect of excess zinc on copper status (60). High doses of copper have in some cases reduced the effects of zinc deficiency in animals, but these effects were inconsistent (61). In one

study, a high-copper diet reduced zinc absorption slightly and increased the excretion of zinc in young men, but it did not impair zinc status (62).

Molybdenum. Interactions between copper and molybdenum have been observed frequently in ruminants (3). Slight excesses of molybdenum in the presence of sulfide produce molybdenum toxicity and secondary copper deficiency. A similar response in rats requires much more molybdenum and is independent of sulfur. A single report of a high-molybdenum diet in humans increasing urinary copper excretion suggested that a similar interaction could occur in humans, but results were not confirmed in other studies. The toxicity of molybdenum in ruminants is ameliorated when dietary copper is increased.

Ascorbic Acid. Ascorbic acid supplements have produced copper deficiency in laboratory animals and may affect the copper status of humans. Plasma ascorbic acid concentrations in premature infants were negatively correlated with plasma ceruloplasmin concentrations and plasma antioxidant activity (63). Daily ascorbic acid supplements of 1500 mg (8.5 mmol) given to young men caused ceruloplasmin activity to decline. Copper absorption was not impaired by 600 mg (3.4 mmol) of ascorbic acid, but ceruloplasmin declined, and the results suggested that the oxidase activity of ceruloplasmin may be impaired by excessive ascorbic acid (48).

Carbohydrates. The type of carbohydrate in the diet affects the rate and severity of copper depletion in rats. These animals are more resistant to copper deficiency when the carbohydrate source is cornstarch than when it is sucrose or fructose. The interaction between carbohydrate source and copper in humans is not clear. Erythrocyte SOD levels of humans in one study were lower with a high-fructose diet compared with a high-cornstarch diet, but copper retention increased (64). In addition, research in young pigs, whose cardiovascular and gastrointestinal systems are similar to those in humans, suggests that the interaction observed in rats may not apply to humans (65, 66).

Interactions with Nonnutrient Components of the Diet and Drugs

Fiber and phytate in the diet influence the bioavailability of several minerals, but their effect on copper absorption and metabolism is not clear. Rat studies demonstrated both inhibition and enhancement of copper absorption by phytate (48). Copper utilization may be influenced by both phytate and fiber in the diets of humans.

Relatively little is known about interactions of copper with drugs. Penicillamine is used to chelate endogenous copper in the treatment of Wilson disease. Its use results in the excretion of up to 5 mg/day (79 μmol/day) of copper in the urine (67). Antacids may interfere with copper absorption (48) when they are used in very high amounts.

CAUSES AND EFFECTS OF DEFICIENCY

Copper Deficiency in Animals

Copper deficiency has been produced experimentally and observed in areas with copper-deficient soil in rats, mice, guinea pigs, rabbits, chicks, pigs, dogs, cattle, goats, and sheep. Detailed descriptions of deficiency symptoms and comparisons among species have been published (1, 3, 68). Animal studies have provided definitive information on the manifestations of copper deficiency. However, the deficiencies produced in animals were more severe than those reported in humans, and species differences make extrapolation to humans difficult.

Anemia, neutropenia, and osteoporosis are observed with copper deficiency in all species. Other well-established manifestations of copper deficiency observed in animal species are as follows: skeletal abnormalities, fractures, and spinal deformities; neonatal ataxia; depigmentation of hair and wool; impaired keratinization of hair, fur, and wool; reproductive failure, including low fertility, fetal death, and resorption; cardiovascular disorders including degeneration of myocardium, cardiac hypertrophy and failure, rupture of blood vessels, and electrocardiographic changes; and impaired immune function. Changes in lipid and cholesterol metabolism, increased lipid peroxidation, and impaired glucose metabolism have been observed in some studies. Hypercholesterolemia may be linked to glutathione metabolism (43). Some of the manifestations of copper deficiency are considered controversial because they have only been observed in one or two species or under specific dietary conditions such as unusually high levels of fructose or zinc (3).

Copper Deficiency in Humans

For years following the discovery of copper deficiency in laboratory animals, it was considered unlikely that copper deficiency could occur in humans. Although copper deficiency in humans is relatively rare, it has been reported several times since 1964 under special circumstances. Reviews of copper deficiency in humans have been published (22, 41).

Copper deficiency has been clearly documented in infants recovering from malnutrition, in premature and low-birth-weight infants fed milk diets, and in patients receiving prolonged total parenteral nutrition (TPN) solutions without added copper. In established cases, blood was sampled for determination of serum copper and ceruloplasmin before administration of copper supplements, and manifestations of copper deficiency were reversed following copper supplementation.

Frank copper deficiency is accompanied by hypocupremia and low ceruloplasmin levels. Levels fall to 30% of normal and lower. Serum copper values as low as 0.5 μmol/L (3 μg/dL) and ceruloplasmin values as low as 35 mg/L (3.5 mg/dL) have been reported (68). Usual features of copper deficiency are anemia, leukopenia, and

neutropenia. The anemia is most often described as normocytic and hypochromic, but it is sometimes normochromic and sometimes microcytic. Osteoporosis is often observed when bones are still growing and may be accompanied by flaring of the metaphyses and fractures at the margins of the metaphyses.

The possibility of mild copper deficiency resulting from marginal copper intake over a long period has been suggested. Possible manifestations, in addition to the features of severe deficiency, are conditions such as arthritis, arterial disease, loss of pigmentation, myocardial disease, and neurologic effects (41). Glucose intolerance, increased serum cholesterol, and cardiac arrythmias have been linked to marginal copper intake (3). These conditions were not accompanied by the low ceruloplasmin or serum copper levels or other features of severe deficiency, but serum copper levels declined in one person with these symptoms. Dietary copper intake in these studies was within the range of intakes consumed by a large segment of the population, 0.8 to 1 mg (13–16 μmol)/day, and these effects were not produced in other studies at this level of dietary copper (13). Further research is required to establish whether these conditions are related to copper status, but this is complicated by ethical considerations related to feeding very low copper intakes, the possibility that some persons may have a higher copper requirement than others, and possible nutrient interactions.

CAUSES AND EFFECTS OF TOXICITY

Copper toxicity can occur in all animal species. It has been observed in sheep, cattle, pigs, rats, and poultry, as well as in humans. The effects of copper poisoning and the levels required for deleterious effects to develop have been reviewed (3).

Copper Toxicity in Animals

Tolerance to high levels of copper differs greatly from one species to another, with sheep being the most susceptible to copper poisoning and rats having high tolerance to excessive copper. Because of species differences and the effects of the levels of zinc, iron, and molybdenum in the diet, the minimum toxic copper level varies. Deleterious effects were observed in pigs at 250 μg copper/g (4 μmol/g) diet, but these effects could be avoided by increasing the amount of iron and zinc in the diet. Poultry exhibit slowed growth and egg production at 500 μg/g (8 μmol/g), and fatality can occur at 1200 μg/g (19 μmol/g). Sheep have developed copper toxicosis from diets containing 12 μg/g (0.19 μmol/g), and some breeds of sheep are more susceptible to excess copper than others. Copper chloride is more toxic than copper sulfate; lower levels of copper are toxic when the molybdenum content of the diet is low. Single doses of 20 to 100 mg (0.31–1.8 mmol) copper/kg body weight have been toxic. Cattle are susceptible to toxicity when diets contain

3 to 12 times the required level of copper. Ruminants can store more copper in their livers than other animals, and symptoms of toxicity appear when the capacity of the liver to sequester copper has been exceeded. Manifestations of copper toxicity include weakness, tremors, anorexia, and jaundice. Tissue copper levels increase, producing liver, kidney, and brain damage, and hemolytic crisis may follow. The immune function of mice was impaired following supplements of 100 ppm copper in the drinking water (69).

Copper Toxicity in Humans

Acute copper poisoning has been observed to occur in the following ways: accidental consumption by children, ingestion of several grams in suicide attempts, application of copper salts to burned skin, drinking of water from contaminated water supplies, or consumption of acidic food or beverages that had been stored in copper containers. Excessive copper produces epigastric pain, nausea, vomiting, and diarrhea, which usually prevents the more serious manifestations of copper toxicity. Serious manifestations include coma, oliguria, hepatic necrosis, vascular collapse, and death. Chronic copper toxicosis has been observed in dialysis recipients following months of hemodialysis when copper tubing was used and in vineyard workers using copper compounds as pesticides. The amount of oral copper required to produce toxic effects is not well established, but liver damage in two infants may have been related to consuming water with 2 to 3 mg copper/L (31–47 μmol copper/L) in early infancy (70). An extremely wide range of oral copper, beginning at 0.07 mg/kg (1.1 μmol/kg)/day, has been associated with gastrointestinal effects. An increased incidence of nausea and other gastrointestinal effects has been reported at copper levels higher than 3 mg/L (71). The new DRIs for copper include a UL, defined as the highest level of intake that is likely to pose no risk of adverse effects. The UL for copper was set at 10 mg/day for adults. This was based on observations that levels much higher than this amount resulted in liver failure after 2 years of consumption (52). The World Health Organization recommends intakes lower than 10 mg/day for women and 12 mg/day for men (53).

Subtle deleterious effects of high dietary copper have been observed. Low-density lipoprotein cholesterol increased when copper supplements were given to men (26). Copper has a critical role in neurologic diseases, and there is speculation that copper-induced production of hydroxy radicals may contribute to the neurodegeneration in Alzheimer disease (72).

IMPACTS OF STRESS AND DISEASE

Clinical Conditions with Increased Risk of Copper Depletion

Copper deficiency has been documented during TPN, in premature infants fed milk formulas, in infants recovering from malnutrition (usually associated with chronic diarrhea),

in infants undergoing chronic peritoneal dialysis, and in severely handicapped patients (73). Two cases of copper deficiency were observed in full-term infants fed only cow's milk. Increased gastrointestinal losses resulting from diarrhea or fistulas increase copper losses and the risk of copper depletion. Diseases of malabsorption such as celiac disease and nontropical sprue increase the risk of copper depletion because of both malabsorption and increased losses, and it appears that the copper status of patients with cystic fibrosis may be compromised (74). Prolonged use of antacids and long-term therapy with very high doses of zinc in treatment of sickle cell anemia have resulted in hypocupremia and some manifestations of copper deficiency.

Parenteral Nutrition

The realization that trace element deficiencies sometimes follow prolonged parenteral nutrition prompted recommendations that several trace elements, including copper, be added to the solutions. Guidelines for their preparation and addition were established in 1979, and these elements are now added routinely. Copper deficiency usually develops after months of parenteral nutrition without added copper; the risk of deficiency is increased substantially in persons with excessive gastrointestinal losses (75). Free amino acid solutions increase urinary copper losses, adding to the risk. Adults receiving TPN who did not have excessive gastrointestinal fluid losses could maintain balance and normal serum and ceruloplasmin levels on only 0.25 mg (3.9 μmol) copper/day. These values did not increase after supplementation with copper. In contrast, serum copper and ceruloplasmin values declined steadily in others receiving a TPN solution in which copper was not detectable, and these indices increased when oral feeding was resumed. Stable adult patients receiving TPN need about 0.3 mg (4.7 μmol) copper/day to maintain balance. The requirements are increased to 0.4 to 0.5 mg (6–8 μmol)/day with excessive gastrointestinal losses and should be reduced in patients with cholestasis and impaired biliary excretion (76) (see Chapter 99 for more information).

Clinical Conditions Accompanied by Copper Accumulation

Copper can accumulate in the liver in any disease that causes impaired biliary excretion, even without excessive intake. Two such diseases, Wilson disease and Indian childhood cirrhosis, are discussed later. Liver copper levels are also very high in primary biliary cirrhosis and biliary atresia. Copper chelation rather than dietary copper restriction is recommended to reduce the liver copper stores in these diseases (77).

Conditions with Increased Serum Copper

Serum copper and ceruloplasmin levels rise progressively during pregnancy, usually reaching twice-normal levels by term. This is partly the result of redistribution of copper, and the change is accompanied by increased total body copper (78). Serum copper and ceruloplasmin levels rise, often to two to three times normal values, in inflammatory conditions, infectious diseases, hematologic diseases, diabetes, coronary and cardiovascular diseases, uremia, and malignant diseases, and following surgery (1, 3). Smoking and some drugs will also increase serum copper concentrations. Ceruloplasmin is an acute-phase reactant, and the rise in ceruloplasmin is probably responsible for the increase in serum copper in the foregoing conditions. The mechanism for the increase or the role for ceruloplasmin is not well understood, but it is under investigation in several laboratories (9).

Genetic Defects in Copper Metabolism

The two best-known defects in copper metabolism in humans are Menkes disease and Wilson disease. Several defects in production of cuproenzymes have been identified, including overproduction of SOD in Down syndrome, absence of tyrosinase in albinism, changes in lysyl oxidase in cutis laxa (Ehlers-Danlos syndrome), and myopathy resulting from a reduction in cytochrome c oxidase. Genetic defects in copper metabolism have also been observed in mice and dogs. The reader is referred to reviews of genetic diseases of copper metabolism (67, 79).

Menkes Disease

Menkes disease is a fatal X-linked disorder characterized by mental retardation, abnormal hair, and maldistribution of copper (79). It occurs in one in 50,000 to 100,000 live births and is usually fatal by the age of 3 years. A defect in the gene (*MNK* gene) encoding for the MNK protein, ATP7A, appears to be responsible for the condition (36, 37). ATP7A plays an important role in copper efflux from cells. When ATP7A is defective, copper is trapped in the intestinal mucosa and others cells and is not available for transport to peripheral organs and tissues. Serum copper and ceruloplasmin levels are low, as are levels in liver and brain, but copper accumulates in intestinal mucosa, muscle, spleen, and kidney. Synthesis of ceruloplasmin, SOD, and cytochrome oxidase is impaired. Abnormalities in connective tissue cross-linking caused by dysfunction of lysyl oxidase result in defective arteries in the brain and elsewhere and in osteoporosis. Progressive nerve degeneration in the brain results in intellectual deterioration, hypotonia, and seizures. Hypothermia is common. Skin and hair are poorly pigmented, and hair is characteristically "kinky." The anemia and neutropenia common to nutritional copper deficiency are not found in Menkes disease, a difference that cannot be explained. Administration of parenteral copper increases serum copper and ceruloplasmin, but it does not improve brain function or slow the progressive deterioration.

Wilson Disease

Wilson disease is an autosomal recessive disease of copper storage. The prevalence of the defect is uncertain, but it has been estimated at approximately one in 200,000 in the United States. The gene *(Wilson gene)* encoding for the Wilson protein, ATP7B, is defective (37). ATP7B, expressed primarily in the liver and neuronal tissue, is needed for copper efflux from tissues. Copper accumulates in the liver, the brain, and the cornea of the eye (Kayser-Fleisher rings). Urinary copper excretion is abnormally high, but ceruloplasmin values are usually low. If the disease goes untreated, copper accumulation in the liver and brain results in neurologic damage and cirrhosis. Acute hepatitis, hemolytic crisis, and hepatic failure may ensue. Early diagnosis and treatment can prevent the severe consequences of the disease. Dietary copper restriction was advocated for Wilson disease at one time, but chelation therapy, usually using D-penicillamine, is much more effective in reducing copper stores (77). Avoidance of large quantities of foods rich in copper may also be recommended, but diets very low in copper are not necessary. D-penicillamine is an antimetabolite of pyridoxine, so daily pyridoxine supplements of 12.5 to 25 mg (75–150 nmol) are recommended. The treatment induces removal of excess copper and prevents reaccumulation through excretion of 1 to 5 mg (16–79 μmol) copper/day in the urine. As an alternative to penicillamine, tetrathiomolybdate, 20 mg six times/day, followed by oral zinc supplements, is sometimes used to eliminate excess copper accumulation (67).

Childhood Cirrhosis. Indian childhood cirrhosis, a heredity disease accompanied by rapid copper accumulation in the liver, was once fatal, but now it can be treated with chelators, with improved chances of recovery. A genetic defect is present, but high copper intake is required for symptoms to appear. The incidence of Indian childhood cirrhosis in India has decreased markedly in recent years, but diseases mimicking it have appeared in other parts of the world (70).

REFERENCES

1. Mason KE. J Nutr 1979;109:1979–2066.
2. Hart EB, Steenbock J, Waddell J et al. J Biol Chem 1928;77: 797–812.
3. Davis GK, Mertz W. Copper. In: Mertz W, ed. Trace Elements in Human and Animal Nutrition, vol 1, 5th ed. San Diego: Academic Press, 1987:301–64.
4. Cordano A, Baerti JM, Graham GG. Pediatrics 1964;34:324–36.
5. National Research Council. Recommended Dietary Allowances. Washington D.C.: National Academy of Sciences, 1980.
6. Owen CA Jr. Biochemical Aspects of Copper: Copper Proteins, Ceruloplasmin, and Copper Protein Binding. Park Ridge, NJ: Noyes Publications, 1982.
7. Dyer FF, Leddicotte GW. The Radiochemistry of Copper. Washington, DC: National Academy of Sciences, National Research Council, 1961.

8. Weser U, Schubotz LM, Younes M. Chemistry of copper proteins and enzymes. In: Nriugu JO, ed. Copper and the Environment. Part II: Health Effects. New York: J. Wiley & Sons, 1979: 197–239.

9. Linder MC. Biochemistry and molecular biology of copper in mammals. In: Massaro EJ, ed. Handbook of Copper Pharmacology and Toxicology. Totowa, NJ: Humana Press, 2003: 3–32.

10. Prohaska JR. J Nutr Biochem 1990;1:452–61.

11. Harris ED. Copper. In: O'Dell BL, Sunde RA, eds. Clinical Nutrition in Health and Disease: Handbook of Nutritionally Essential Mineral Elements, vol 2. New York: Marcel Dekker, 1997:231–73.

12. Wirth PL, Linder MC. J Natl Cancer Inst 1985;75:277–84.

13. Turnlund JR, Keen CL, Smith RG. Am J Clin Nutr 1990;51: 658–64.

14. Frieden E. Clin Physiol Biochem 1986;4:11–9.

15. McCracken J, Desai PR, Papadopoulos NJ et al. Biochem 1988; 27:4133–7.

16. Harris ED. J Nutr 1992;122:636–40.

17. Mann KG, Lawler CM, Vehar GA et al. J Biol Chem 1984; 259:12949–51.

18. Linder MC. The Biochemistry of Copper. New York: Plenum Press, 1991.

19. Cousins RJ. Physiol Rev 1985;65:238–309.

20. Werman MJ, Barat E, Bhathena SJ. J Nutr 1995;125:857–63.

21. Werman MJ, Bhathena SJ, Turnlund JR. J Nutr Biochem 1997; 9:201–4.

22. Williams DM. Semin Hematol 1983;20:118–27.

23. Medeiros DM, Davidson J, Jenkins JE. Proc Soc Exp Biol Med 1993;203:262–73.

24. Milne DB. Clin Chem 1994;40:1479–84.

25. Strain JJ. Proc Nutr Soc 1994;53:583–98.

26. Medeiros DM, Milton A, Brunett E et al. Biol Trace Element Res 1991;30:19–35.

27. Prohaska JR, Failla ML. Copper and immunity. In: Klurfeld DM, ed. Human Nutrition: A Comprehensive Treatise. New York: Plenum Press, 1993:309–32.

28. Bonham M, O'Conner JM, Hannigan BM et al. Br J Nutr 2002; 87:393–403.

29. Failla ML, Hopkins RG. Nutr Rev 1998;56:S59–S64.

30. Kelley DS, Daudu PA, Taylor PC et al. Am J Clin Nutr 1995; 62:412–6.

31. Johnson MA, Fisher JG. Crit Rev Food Sci Nutr 1992; 32:1–31.

32. An overview of atomic spectroscopy. In: Guide to Atomic Spectroscopy Techniques and Applications: AA, GFAA, ICP, ICP-MS. Norwalk, CT: PerkinElmer, 2000:3–10.

33. Patterson KY, Veillon C. Exp Biol Med 2001;226:271–82.

34. Scott KC, Turnlund JR. J Nutr Biochem 1994;5:342–50.

35. Crews HM, Ducros V, Eagles J et al. Analyst 1994;119: 2491–514.

36. Harris ED, Qian Y, Reddy MCM. Mol Cell Biochem 1998; 188:57–62.

37. Puig S, Thiele DJ. Curr Opin Chem Biol 2002;6:171–80.

38. Turnlund JR, Keyes WR, Anderson HL et al. Am J Clin Nutr 1989;49:870–8.

39. Turnlund JR, Keyes WR, Peiffer GL et al. Am J Clin Nutr 1998; 67:1219–25.

40. Bremner I. J Nutr 1987;117:19–29.

41. Danks DM. Ann Rev Nutr 1988;8:235–57.

42. Harris ED, Percival SS. Copper transport: insights into a ceruloplasmin-based delivery system. In: Kies C, ed. Copper Bioavailability and Metabolism. New York: Plenum Press, 1990: 95–102.

43. Bunce GE. Nutr Rev 1993;51:305–7.

44. Turnlund JR, Scott KC, Peiffer GL et al. Am J Clin Nutr 1997; 65:72–8.

45. Turnlund JR, Domek JM, Nair PP et al. J Trace Elem Exp Med 2003;16:105–8.

46. Levenson CW, Janghorbani M. Anal Biochem 1994;221: 243–9.

47. Harvey LJ, Majask-Newman G, Dainty JR et al. Br J Nutr 2003;90:161–8.

48. Turnlund JR. J Am Diet Assoc 1988;88:303–10.

49. Uauy R, Castillo-Duran C, Fisberg M et al. J Nutr 1985; 115:1650–5.

50. Turnlund JR. J Nutr 1989;119:7–14.

51. Higuchi S, Higashi A, Nakamura T et al. J Pediatr Gastroenterol Nutr 1988;7:583–7.

52. Institute of Medicine. Copper. In: Food and Nutrition Board, ed. Dietary Reference Intakes: Vitamin A, Vitamin K, Arsenic, Boron, Chromium, Copper, Iodine, Iron, Manganese, Molybdenum, Nickel, Silicon, Vanadium, and Zinc. Washington, DC: National Academy Press, 2002:224–57.

53. Copper. In: World Health Organization, ed. Trace elements in human nutrition and health. Geneva: World Health Organization, 1996:123–43.

54. Lurie DG, Holden JM, Schubert A et al. J Food Comp Anal 1989;2:298–316.

55. Pennington JAT, Schoen SA, Salmon GD et al. J Food Comp Anal 1995;8:171–217.

56. Pennington JAT, Wilson DB. J Am Diet Assoc 1990;90:375–81.

57. Pennington JT, Calloway DH. J Am Diet Assoc 1973;63: 143–53.

58. Gawthorne JM. Copper interactions. In: Howell JM, Gawthorne JM, eds. Copper in Animals and Man, vol 1. Boca Raton, FL: CRC Press, 1987:79–100.

59. Luza SC, Speisky HC. Am J Clin Nutr 1996;63:812S–20S.

60. Institute of Medicine. Zinc. In: Food and Nutrition Board, ed. Dietary Reference Intakes for Vitamin A, Vitamin K, Arsenic, Boron, Chromium, Copper, Iodine, Iron, Manganese, Molybdenum, Nickel, Silicon, Vanadium, and Zinc. Washington, DC: National Academy Press, 2002:442–501.

61. Kirchgessner M. Interactions of copper with other trace elements. In: Nriugu JO, ed. Copper and the Environment. Part II: Health Effects. New York: J. Wiley & Sons, 1979:433–72.

62. Turnlund JR, Keyes WR, Anderson HL. High dietary copper decreases zinc absorption, as determined with the stable isotope ^{67}Zn. In: Momcilovic B, ed. Trace Elements in Man and Animals. 7th ed. Zagreb, Yugoslavia: Institute for Medical Research and Occupational Health, University of Zagreb, 1991:5/ 13–5/15.

63. Powers HJ, Loban A, Silvers K et al. Free Radic Res 1995;22: 57–65.

64. Reiser S, Smith JC, Mertz W et al. Am J Clin Nutr 1985;42: 242–51.

65. Schoenemann HM, Failla ML, Steele NC. Am J Clin Nutr 1990; 52:147–54.

66. O'Dell BL. Nutr Rev 1990;48:425–34.

67. Brewer GJ, Yuzbasiyan-Gurkan V. Medicine (Baltimore) 1992; 71:139–64.

68. Fujita M, Itakura T, Takagi Y et al. JPEN J Parenter Enteral Nutr 1989;13:421–5.

69. Pocino M, Baute L, Malave I. Fund Appl Toxicol 1991;16: 249–56.

70. Muller-Hocker J, Meyer U, Wiebecke B et al. Path Res Pract 1988;183:39–45.

71. Pizzaro F, Olivares M, Uauy R et al. Environ Health Perspect 1999;107:117–21.

72. Multhaup G, Schlicksupp L, Hesse L et al. Science 1996;271: 1406–9.

73. Shaw JCL. Copper deficiency in term and preterm infants. In: Fomon SJ, Zlotkin S, eds. Nutritional Anemias. New York: Raven Press, 1992:105–17.

74. Percival SS, Bowser E, Wagner M. Am J Clin Nutr 1995; 62: 633–8.

75. Spiegel JE, Willenbucher RF. JPEN J Parenter Enteral Nutr 1999;23:169–72.

76. Fleming CR. Am J Clin Nutr 1989;49:573–9.

77. Smithgall JM. J Am Diet Assoc 1985;85:609–11.

78. McArdle HJ. Food Chem 1995;54:79–84.

79. Bankier A. J Med Genet 1995;32:213–5.

SELECTED READINGS

Davis GK, Mertz W. Copper. In: Mertz W, ed. Trace Elements in Human and Animal Nutrition, vol 1. San Diego: Academic Press, 1987: 301–64.

Harris ED. Copper. In: O'Dell BL, Sunde RA, eds. Handbook of Nutritionally Essential Elements. New York: Marcel Dekker, 1997: 231–73.

Institute of Medicine Food and Nutrition Board, ed. Dietary Reference Intakes: Vitamin A, Vitamin K, Arsenic, Boron, Chromium, Copper, Iodine, Iron, Manganese, Molybdenum, Nickel, Silicon, Vanadium, and Zinc. Washington, DC: National Academy Press, 2002:224–57.

Linder MC. Biochemistry and molecular biology of copper. In: Massaro EJ, ed. Handbook of Copper Pharmacology and Toxicology. Totowa, NJ: Humana Press, 2003:3–32.

Mason KE. A conspectus of research on copper metabolism and requirements of man. J Nutr 1979;109:1979–2066.

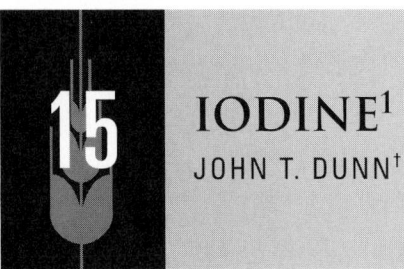

IODINE[1]

JOHN T. DUNN[†]

OVERVIEW 300
HISTORICAL HIGHLIGHTS 300
CHEMISTRY 301
    Properties 301
    Distribution 301
METABOLISM 301
ACTIONS OF THYROID HORMONES 302
ASSESSMENT OF IODINE NUTRITION 302
    Iodine Balance 302
    Urinary Excretion of Iodine 302
    Radioiodine Studies .302
    Serum Thyroid-Stimulating Hormone 302
    Serum Thyroglobulin and Hormones 303
    Thyroid Size 303
RECOMMENDED INTAKES 303
DIETARY SOURCES 304
CONSEQUENCES OF DEFICIENCY 304
    Fetal and Infant Mortality 304
    Neurologic Deficits .304
    Reproductive Damage 305
    Hypothyroidism 305
    Goiter 305
    Iodine-Induced Hyperthyroidism 306
    Socioeconomic Damage 306
    Complicating Factors 306
CONSEQUENCES OF EXCESS 306
    Hypothyroidism 306
    Autoimmune Thyroid Disease 306
    Thyroid Cancer 307
SUPPLEMENTATION 307
    Iodized Salt 307
    Iodized Water 307
    Iodized Oil 308
    Iodine Tablets, Solutions, and Other Vehicles 308

NATIONAL IODINE NUTRITION PROGRAMS 308
    Iodine Nutrition 308
    Iodized Salt Oversight 308
    Education and Advocacy 308
GLOBAL IODINE NUTRITION STATUS 309
ACHIEVING AND SUSTAINING OPTIMAL IODINE
    NUTRITION 309
SUMMARY 310

OVERVIEW

The nutritional importance of iodine stems from its role as an essential component of thyroid hormones (the word *iodine* refers both generally to the element in any form and specifically to I_2, also called molecular iodine). Iodine deficiency is widespread globally. Its worst consequences are for the developing fetus and child, leading to death, complications of pregnancy, and irreversible mental retardation. Good means exist for its correction, especially with iodized salt, and their implementation is a major public health objective at present.

This chapter describes the chemistry and physiology of iodine and its role in the thyroid, nutritional requirements, the consequences of deficiency and excess, supplementation measures, the current status of its global nutrition, and the campaign to provide optimal iodine nutrition for all. Several reviews and reference sources offer more details (1–6).

HISTORICAL HIGHLIGHTS

Bernard Courtois is credited with discovering iodine in 1811, when he saw violet vapors condense into crystals during the manufacture of saltpeter, a process involving burned seaweed extract (7). Shortly afterward, iodine was identified as a chemical element, and given its name, from the Greek word for violet. It could be detected by the sensitive reaction of free iodine with starch, and many substances such as marine sponges and peat were found to contain it. In 1825, Boussingault detected iodine in brines in the Andes and pioneered its use for goiter prophylaxis.

Knowledge of endemic goiter, now known to result from iodine deficiency, goes back many centuries. Although writings and sculptures suggest the presence of goiter at least

[1]**Abbreviations: DIT,** diiodotyrosine; **FNB,** Food and Nutrition Board; **ICCIDD,** International Council for the Control of Iodine Deficiency Disorders; **IQ,** intelligence quotient; **KI,** potassium iodide; **KIO₃,** potassium iodate; **MIT,** iodotyrosine; **RDA,** recommended dietary allowance; **T₃,** 3,5,3′-triiodothyronine; **T₄,** thyroxine; **Tg,** thyroglobulin; **TPO,** thyroperoxidase; **TRH,** thyrotropin-releasing hormone; **TSH,** thyrotropin (thyroid-stimulating hormone); **UNICEF,** United Nations Children's Fund; **WHO,** World Health Organization.

[†]Deceased.

2000 years ago, true thyroid enlargement was frequently confused with other abnormalities in neck anatomy and was not identified definitively. Beginning in the eleventh, the School of Salerno in present-day Italy studied goiter, developed surgical procedures for it, and prescribed medication that included iodine-containing marine sponges. In subsequent centuries, goiter was ascribed to various causes, and its relationship with the thyroid and iodine was not clearly recognized until the beginnings of modern physiology in the late nineteenth century.

Similarly, the history of endemic cretinism is clouded by diagnostic vagary in separating it from other causes of dwarfism and retardation. Its association with endemic goiter was recognized in the seventeenth century, but its relation to the thyroid gland took 2 more centuries to establish.

The late nineteenth and early twentieth centuries saw dramatic increases in knowledge about iodine and the thyroid. The iodine-containing hormone thyroxine (T_4) was isolated in 1914. Pioneering studies by Marine in the United States and others in Switzerland established that iodine administration could prevent endemic goiter, and prophylactic salt iodization was introduced in the early 1920s. Many advances in knowledge of thyroid physiology and iodine utilization have since occurred, but the fundamental facts about iodine nutrition remain: the thyroid needs adequate iodine for production of its hormone; iodine deficiency causes cretinism, mental retardation, and goiter; and these consequences can be eliminated by the use of iodized salt and other prophylactic measures.

CHEMISTRY

Properties

Iodine is an element with atomic number 53 and an atomic weight of 126.9. The densest of the common halogens, it consists of solid blue-black crystals with a melting point of 113.6°C. It is a mild oxidizing agent at acid pH, with oxidation states of -1, $+1$, $+3$, $+5$, and $+7$. It is readily soluble in many organic solvents, but only sparingly in water.

Distribution

Iodine is sixty-first among the first 96 elements, making it one of the least common, a trace element (8, 9). It is usually found as an inorganic salt, in rocks, soil, plants, animals, and water. The largest amount is in sea water, but at a very low concentration, less than 0.05 ppm. Usable sources are sodium nitrate deposits, underground brines, and sea life. The two major production sites are northern Chile and Japan, with small amounts in the United States, central Asia, and Indonesia. Iodide and iodate are the common commercial forms. The estimated distribution of iodine's industrial usage is radiocontrast media (23%),

iodophors and biocides (17%), chemicals (17%), pharmaceuticals (8%), human nutrition (8%), nylon (6%), animal feed (5%), and herbicides (4%).

METABOLISM

Iodine enters the human body in a variety of forms, but most is broken down to iodide in the gut and is quickly absorbed into the circulation (10, 11). From there, its main fates are concentration by the thyroid and excretion by the kidney. Small amounts are also concentrated by the salivary glands, choroid plexus, and mammary glandt. The metabolism of molecular iodine (I_2) may differ somewhat from that of iodide ($I-$), with less uptake by the thyroid and more to fatty tissues, including the mammary gland.

The sodium/iodide symporter, a 65-kDa protein spanning the thyroid's basal membrane, complexes with sodium and iodide to transport iodide actively from the circulation into the thyroid cell. The iodide then migrates to the cell's apical membrane. There it is oxidized in a complex series of reactions to iodinate tyrosyl residues within the peptide chains of thyroglobulin (Tg), a 660-kDa glycoprotein synthesized on the endoplasmic reticulum and glycosylated in the Golgi. Key components in this process include the following: thyroperoxidase (TPO), an approximately 107-kDa hemoglycoprotein located at the apical membrane; and hydrogen peroxide, whose generation requires calcium, reduced nicotinamide adenine dinucleotide phosphate (NADPH), and an NADPH oxidase.

The initial iodination produces iodotyrosine (MIT) and diiodotyrosine (DIT), still within the peptide structure of Tg. Further action of TPO forms T_4, by coupling two molecules of DIT, and 3,5,3'-triiodothyronine (T_3), by coupling a molecule each of MIT and DIT; T_4 and T_3 are the active thyroid hormones. Tg, still containing hormones, is stored in the follicular lumen until needed, and then it is processed by micropinocytosis, formation of endocytic vesicles, and digestion by endosomal and lysosomal proteases, finally to release the free hormones into the circulation. There they attach to binding proteins made in the liver and are carried to target tissues for action in cells. The iodine remaining as DIT and MIT in Tg is recycled within the thyroid, a valuable mechanism for its conservation.

Several factors modulate hormone synthesis and release. The most important is thyrotropin (thyroid-stimulating hormone [TSH]), a hormone produced by the pituitary and responsive to circulating levels of T_4; it stimulates all the major steps above–iodine concentration, synthesis of Tg and TPO, Tg iodination, T_4 formation within Tg, and Tg proteolysis. It also promotes peripheral conversion of T_4 to T_3, the active form of the hormone. TSH secretion is controlled by thyrotropin-releasing hormone (TRH), secreted by the hypothalamus and responsive both to thyroid hormone and to TSH feedback.

The amount of available iodine is another important influence. When iodine is scarce, the fraction concentrated by the thyroid from the circulation increases, and relatively more T_3 (which contains less iodine than T_4) is synthesized; iodine excess produces the opposite effects and can inhibit hormone formation. Other factors are the molecular chaperones that monitor cell machinery and genetic variability in the several proteins involved.

ACTIONS OF THYROID HORMONES

Key target tissues are liver, kidney, muscle, and developing brain. About 98% of circulating thyroid hormone is T_4, but its metabolic action is through its conversion to T_3 in tissues, a process catalyzed by selenium-containing 5′-deiodinases. Two forms of these enzymes exist, one for pituitary, the central nervous system, and brown adipose fat and the other for liver, kidney, and muscle. At the cell nucleus, T_3 acts with receptors similar to those for steroids and retinoic acid. At the gene level, these receptors bind to hormone response elements and modify their translation, expressed in the cytoplasm by modulation of protein synthesis. The affected proteins vary among tissues; examples include growth hormone, liver enzymes controlling lipogenesis, myosin, and various brain enzymes. In a general way, thyroid hormones promote synthesis of enzymes and other proteins to increase metabolic activity in tissues. Thus, hyperthyroidism is characterized by increases in nervous activity, temperature, energy consumption, and heart rate, whereas hypothyroidism involves an overall slowing of metabolism, including lower body temperature and mental and physical sluggishness.

The action of T_4 at the pituitary level is especially critical. Low circulating levels of T_4 cause the pituitary to increase its release of TSH, thus stimulating the thyroid to produce more hormone, a compensatory reaction. Goiter (thyroid enlargement) is a product of this stimulation. When circulating levels of T_4 are high, the reverse reaction occurs, and TSH secretion is suppressed. Clinicians use the circulating TSH concentration as the most sensitive indicator of thyroid function.

ASSESSMENT OF IODINE NUTRITION

Iodine Balance

Studies carried out a generation ago uncovered many difficulties with this approach (12). Iodine intake was difficult to control, and variability in baseline conditions limited the extrapolation of results. The thyroid adapts quite efficiently to iodine availability, thus presenting a changing compartment that complicated interpretation of excretion data. The measurement techniques at that time were tedious and did not include modern determinations for serum TSH and thyroid hormones. Balance took a long time (months) to achieve, even on metabolic units, and would be logistically impractical to repeat now. Conclusions from these studies place the iodine requirement for adults somewhere in the range of 100 to 200 µg/day.

Urinary Excretion of Iodine

Urinary iodine excretion is currently the most useful tool for assessing iodine status. More than 90% of iodine intake eventually appears in urine, casual samples are easy to collect, and good analytic techniques are available. For field studies of populations, it is usually satisfactory to obtain casual specimens and to report direct concentrations, rather than relating it to urinary creatinine or obtaining 24-hour collections (13). Although the degree of hydration and other factors will affect the concentration in individuals, these variations are minimized by the use of population medians. International organizations recommend the median urinary iodine concentration as the yardstick for assessing iodine nutrition in communities (Table 15.1) (12, 14).

Radioiodine Studies

Another approach to assessing iodine requirements is by investigating thyroid performance, because iodine is an essential component of the hormones. The thyroidal accumulation of administered radioiodine was about 90 to 100 µg in adults in one study (15), and another reported iodine uptake of 21 to 97 µg/day in four subjects (16); application of these results is limited by the techniques and the uncertain baseline iodine status.

Serum Thyroid-Stimulating Hormone

The most useful marker of thyroid function in *individuals* is the serum TSH, and its sensitivity can be enhanced by measuring its response to TRH. However, the distribution of TSH values among physiologically normal persons is

TABLE 15.1. RECOMMENDATION ON DIETARY INTAKES OF IODINE

	RDA[a] (µg/d)	AI[b] (µg/d)	UL[c] (µg/d)
Women	150		1,100
Men	150		1,100
Pregnancy	220		1,100
Lactation	290		1,100
Infants			
0–6 mo		110	
7–12 mo		130	
Children			
1–3 y	90		200
4–8 y	90		300
9–13 y	120		600
14–18 y	150		900

[a] RDA, recommended dietary allowance.
[b] AI, adequate intake; estimated from intakes in healthy populations.
[c] UL, tolerable upper limit; infants not included, because of insufficient data.

From Food and Nutrition Board, Institute of Medicine. Dietary Reference Intakes for Vitamin A, Vitamin K, Arsenic, Boron, Chromium, Copper, Iodine, Iron, Manganese, Molybdenum, Nickel, Silicon, Vanadium, and Zinc. Washington, DC: National Academy Press, 2001:258–89, with permission.

skewed and fairly wide, and defining normal thyroid function is not easy. For population studies, the median serum TSH is slightly elevated in iodine deficiency, but not sufficiently so to be higher than the cutoffs for normal unless the deficiency is severe.

An important exception is the TSH in newborns. Most industrialized countries employ routine screening of newborns with bloodspot TSH to detect congenital hypothyroidism, a condition occurring in about one of every 4000 births in iodine-sufficient communities; the usual cause is failure of the thyroid to develop properly. If detected and treated immediately, the neurologic damage from the fetal hypothyroidism can be minimal. In iodine deficiency, the incidence of elevated TSH levels in newborns increases, in rough proportion to its severity, so-called *transient neonatal hypothyroidism*. For example, one of every 112 newborns had elevated TSH levels in iodine-deficient Freiburg, Germany, compared with one of every 1428 in iodine-sufficient Stockholm (17). Depending on the degree of iodine deficiency, this transient hypothyroidism usually resolves spontaneously, but it emphasizes that iodine deficiency poses a threat to the developing brain.

Serum Thyroglobulin and Hormones

Some Tg is normally secreted by the thyroid and can be measured in the serum. Levels increase nonspecifically with thyroid hyperplasia, as in iodine deficiency, and correlate fairly well with goiter. The serum T_4 and T_3 concentrations increase and decrease, respectively, in iodine deficiency, but not enough to be clinically useful.

Thyroid Size

Thyroid size is another good marker of iodine nutrition. Although it is not the worst consequence of iodine deficiency, goiter is one of the earliest and most visible. It can be estimated crudely by palpation and visual observation, but much more reliably by ultrasonography. This technique is not difficult to learn and can be performed in the field; global normative values for iodine-sufficient children are available for comparison (18, 19).

RECOMMENDED INTAKES

The Food and Nutrition Board (FNB) of the US Institute of Medicine, National Academy of Sciences, recommends 150 µg/day for nonpregnant nonlactating adults, with lower amounts for children and more during pregnancy and lactation (see Table 15.1) (12). Children require more iodine per kilogram of weight than adults, because of their more active metabolism and turnover. These recommendations are fairly close to those of World Health Organization (WHO)/ International Council for the Control of Iodine Deficiency Disorders (ICCIDD)/United Nations Children's Fund (UNICEF) and of several national regulatory bodies (20). Some factors in their derivation have been the

amounts of iodine that prevent goiter and provide the lowest serum TSH, calculations from the amount of replacement T_4 (and therefore T_4's iodine) necessary to achieve euthyroidism in athyreotic subjects, and disposal rates of administered T_4. When possible, the FNB used its estimated average requirement methodology to estimate Recommended Dietary Allowances (RDAs); when data were insufficient, it offered an adequate intake.

Children 8 to 10 years old have been used to assess the iodine nutrition in communities, because they are conveniently surveyed in schools and show the effects of fairly recent iodine intake, especially on thyroid size. The recommended dietary intakes have been keyed to urinary iodine excretion in these children to classify the community iodine nutrition (Table 15.2). A urinary iodine concentration of 100 µg/L is considered the lower cutoff for iodine sufficiency.

Pregnancy and lactation are conditions that require special attention (21). The pregnant woman needs more iodine because the condition of pregnancy increases her metabolism and requires more thyroid hormone; in addition, she must provide adequate iodine for the fetal thyroid as well as her own, and her renal threshold for iodine may be lowered. Current guidelines are scant in setting optimal urinary iodine levels for pregnancy. From the RDA of 220 µg for pregnancy, and estimating a daily urine output of about 1.5 L, the urinary iodine in pregnancy should be at least 150 µg/L, probably higher. Similarly, to meet the RDA of 290 µg in lactation, the urinary iodine concentration should be close to 200 µg/L. Ways to meet these requirements are discussed later, in the discussion on achieving optimal iodine nutrition.

Iodine excess is more difficult to define. Many people regularly ingest large amounts of iodine without apparent harm. Several investigating teams gave graded increments of iodine to healthy iodine-sufficient persons and established the amount of iodine required to increase the serum TSH, or the TSH response to TRH. The FNB used these data to derive a tolerable upper limit of 1.1 mg/day of iodine for adults (12). The WHO/ICCIDD/UNICEF

TABLE 15.2. MEDIAN URINARY IODINE CONCENTRATION AS AN INDEX OF COMMUNITY IODINE NUTRITION

MEDIAN URINARY IODINE CONCENTRATION (µg/L)	IODINE NUTRITION
<20	Severe deficiency
20–49	Moderate deficiency
50–99	Mild deficiency
100–199	Optimal nutrition
200–299	More than adequate nutrition
>299	Possible excess

From International Council for the Control of Iodine Deficiency Disorders, United National Children's Fund (UNICEF), World Health Organization (WHO). Assessment of the Iodine Deficiency Disorders and Monitoring Their Elimination. Geneva: WHO Publication WHO/NHD/01.1, 2001:1–107 (also available at www.iccidd.org), with permission.

recommendations were similar, 1.0 mg/day. Although these are useful signposts, their application needs to be adjusted to the characteristics of different populations, discussed more fully later. The issue of excess is important because iodine exposure can come from many sources that are usually unrecognized and uncontrolled.

DIETARY SOURCES

These sources vary with country and population sector. In the United States, dairy products are the most important source. One article reported 116 μg iodine in an 8-oz glass of milk in the Boston area (22). Seafood has a moderate amount of iodine. Meat and some grains are additional sources. Bread formerly contained considerable iodine because iodate was used in the baking process, a practice largely discontinued, but one survey found several brands with more than 300 μg per slice (22). Iodized salt contributes only slightly, because most US residents obtain their salt from processed food, which does not usually contain iodized salt. The food colorant erythrosine has large amounts of iodine, but most is not bioavailable. Moreover, in the United States, significant iodine exposure comes from various iodine-containing medicines, radiocontrast dyes, topical antiseptics, and vitamin and mineral preparations. Except for iodized salt, all these sources contain iodine for commercial reasons without attention to their effects on nutrition. The National Health and Nutrition Examination Survey studies of the Centers for Disease Control and Prevention showed a pronounced drop in median urinary iodine between the 1970s and 1990s, from 321 to145 μg/L, perhaps related to withdrawal of iodate from breadmaking (23).

In Japan, the frequent ingestion of iodine-rich seaweed produces one of the world's highest iodine intakes. Europeans generally ingest less iodine than do US residents, but the major sources are similar. In contrast, people in developing countries obtain most of their food locally, without external sources of iodine unless they use iodized salt.

CONSEQUENCES OF DEFICIENCY

Increased fetal and infant mortality, irreversible mental and neurologic retardation, other reproductive complications, hypothyroidism, goiter, and late hyperthyroidism are the worst consequences of iodine deficiency, in approximate order of importance (1, 2, 11). These conditions are referred to as the iodine deficiency disorders. For the community, they impose wasted reproductive effort, increased child mortality, poor educability, impaired economic productivity, and increased health costs. Until about 40 years ago, it was commonly assumed that iodine-deficient populations would include a few unfortunates who were obvious cretins, and the remainder would have goiter ("only a cosmetic issue") but were otherwise normal. Now we recognize these consequences as part of a continuum from severe to subtle manifestations, and *everyone* in the community is at potential risk, roughly correlated with the degree of iodine deficiency.

Fetal and Infant Mortality

Studies on this topic are necessarily observational, but several clearly demonstrate an association between iodine deficiency and decreased fetal and infant survival (21). Treatment of women during pregnancy (mean 28 weeks) resulted in higher birth weights and fewer newborn deaths in a severely deficient area of the Congo (24). Newborn mortality was halved by administration of iodized oil in an Indonesian study (25). Addition of potassium iodate (KIO_3) to irrigation in western China reduced infant mortality to about half its previous level (26). In Papua New Guinea, iodized oil treatment during fetal life correlated with a higher survival rate at age 15 years (27). Increased abortions and developmental abnormalities are well known in domestic and experimental animals exposed to iodine deficiency.

Neurologic Deficits

Thyroid hormone is essential for proper maturation of the central nervous system. It modulates key synthetic processes in the brain and is especially crucial for myelination (28). This dependence is present throughout the fetal period and in the first several years of life. Iodine deficiency any time during this period risks causing irreversible brain damage. Severely deficient communities show a spectrum stretching from obvious gross retardation to mild intellectual blunting recognized only on careful examination. In such places, *most* people may have some impairment.

The extreme result of hypothyroidism (and of iodine deficiency) during development is *cretinism*. Its cardinal manifestation is mental retardation. Other common features include hearing and speech loss, short stature, and spasticity. Cretinism can occur sporadically, in the absence of iodine deficiency, from other causes of hypothyroidism during development, such as toxic exposure and genetic abnormalities in thyroid hormone production or utilization. When cretinism occurs in communities with endemic goiter, iodine deficiency is the presumed cause. Both sporadic and endemic cretins share mental retardation, but aspects of the pathogenesis can differ between the two subtypes. The fetal thyroid is not active until around 12 weeks of gestation, so maternal T_4 is provided transplacentally during that period; the mother of the sporadic cretin can usually do this satisfactorily because her own thyroid and iodine supply are normal. However, the fetus of the iodine-deficient mother is at risk for inadequate hormone exposure throughout the 9 months of pregnancy.

The clinical description of endemic cretinism is divided into neurologic and myxedematous types. Typically, the former include persons who are mentally retarded, often deaf mutes, but frequently of normal height and strength, and who may have goiters. Detailed examinations have described proximal extrapyramidal signs, dystonia, gait abnormalities, primitive reflexes, squint (29), and subtypes including severe hypotonicity, ataxia, autism, and severe thalamic signs (30). The myxedematous cretins, most extensively described in Africa, are mentally retarded and are also short and hypothyroid. Much literature in the past puzzled over these two types, and numerous examples of overlap appeared. Coexistent selenium deficiency has been proposed as a contributing factor in the myxedematous type of cretinism, by impairing the actions of selenium-containing thyroidal enzymes that prevent hydrogen peroxide buildup and tissue damage (31).

One of the worst results of iodine deficiency is intellectual impairment. This is often overlooked in field observations, especially when it is mild and not tested. However, many investigations using a range of instruments provide convincing data that iodine-deficient children are not as bright as iodine-sufficient peers, even when all apparent confounding variables are controlled. A careful metaanalysis of 18 studies from four continents using several different tests concluded that iodine deficiency had cost individuals an average of 12.5 intelligence quotient (IQ) points (32) Similarly, an analysis of data from 37 studies of 12,291 Chinese children found higher IQs in those from iodine-sufficient areas and in those whose community iodine deficiency had been corrected before their conception; the loss from iodine deficiency was estimated at 12.45 IQ points (33). Such estimates have generated considerable international interest among political leaders and emphasize the damage that continuing iodine deficiency brings to a country's intellectual health and productivity.

Deafness is a frequent feature of severe iodine deficiency, usually accompanied by intellectual impairment. Most neurologic cretins have some hearing loss. The defect is usually neural, but auditory and mixed types have also been found. Radiologic studies have shown arrested cochlear development and petrous bone abnormalities, findings implying damage occurring in the second trimester of gestation (34). The hearing deficits can be prevented by correction of iodine deficiency before conception. Audiometry has shown subtle hearing impairment even when the iodine deficiency is mild, a finding that provides another reason to urge the correction of iodine deficiency of any degree.

Reproductive Damage

The most severe reproductive consequences of iodine deficiency are on the fetus, as detailed earlier, but they involve the mother as well (21). Hypothyroidism can cause anovulation, first trimester abortions, gestational hypertension, and abnormal fetal presentations. Any pregnancy, whether successful or not, makes increased demands on the maternal thyroid, and the thyroid may not be able to meet these demands because of insufficient iodine. Iodine stores may continue depleted as the woman faces another pregnancy, thereby increasing the chances of further damage to her and to the pregnancy. Thyroid enlargement may not regress between pregnancies, and the gland may eventually become nodular, leading to possible neck compression, thyroid autonomy, and even late hyperthyroidism.

Hypothyroidism

Depending on its severity and the success of the thyroid's compensatory mechanisms, iodine deficiency carries the risk of inadequate hormone production. Features of adult hypothyroidism include lethargy, sleepiness, slowed mentation, sluggish physical movement, cold intolerance, and increased susceptibility to cardiovascular and infectious diseases; many of these are correctable with adequate treatment, but some complications, such as those involving the cardiovascular system, may remain. Hypothyroidism in fetal and early postnatal life causes additional damage to the developing brain, described earlier, and is largely irreversible.

Goiter

Goiter is the most obvious manifestation of iodine deficiency, but not the most dangerous. Although other causes of goiter exist, a prevalence of more than 5% in a community suggests iodine deficiency as the etiologic agent. The thyroid volumes taken as normal in countries with mild iodine deficiency, such as much of western Europe, are much larger than those considered acceptable in the United States. Initially, the enlargement is diffuse, and it can be regarded as an adaptation to the threat of hypothyroidism, through the compensatory action of increased TSH secretion by the pituitary. Still, its presence warns that the thyroid is working under pressure. During periods in life when the thyroid is more active, such as adolescence and pregnancy, women may develop goiters even though iodine deficiency is not otherwise evident in them or in their communities. Once someone has been iodine deficient for several years, the thyroid may never return entirely to a normal size, even after adequate iodine supplementation. Glands that are initially hyperplastic eventually develop nodules (lumps), that can be inert ("colloid" nodules), cystic, autonomous (capable of secreting excess hormone), and occasionally malignant (usually follicular carcinoma).

Although dwarfed by the effects of iodine deficiency on the brain, goiters still have clinical importance. They may enlarge enough to compress neighboring structures in the neck, especially the trachea and esophagus, and may require surgical intervention. The presence of nodules from iodine deficiency can raise the specter of thyroid cancer, which usually presents as a nodule, requiring various diagnostic maneuvers and perhaps eventual surgery.

Iodine-Induced Hyperthyroidism

Autonomous nodules are adenomas (benign tumors) that secrete thyroid hormone at their own rate, uncontrolled by TSH and other regulatory mechanisms. When these nodules are exposed to an increase in iodine supply, they may increase their manufacture of thyroid hormones and make more than a person needs, so he or she becomes hyperthyroid. This situation occurs more frequently in older persons who have had enough time to develop such nodules, but the young are not immune. Iodine-induced hyperthyroidism is properly regarded as an iodine deficiency disorder because it results from a goiter that developed in response to insufficient iodine. It may occur in some members of a population whose iodine deficiency has recently been corrected. It can be treated satisfactorily by measures used for hyperthyroidism from other causes. It is important that medical personnel be aware of this possibility and treat it promptly. The increased incidence after introduction of iodine sufficiency usually subsides within a year or two (35).

Socioeconomic Damage

Iodine deficiency affects the community as well as individual community members. Hypothyroidism makes people less energetic and inefficient, thus hindering productive work. School performance is poorer; children drop out earlier and repeat grades more often. Domestic animals share the area's iodine deficiency; the results are more stillbirths, lower weights, and impaired production of milk, eggs, meat, and wool. Health costs rise, to cover the various complications of goiter, abnormal thyroid function, reproductive problems, and care of the ill and retarded. Such costs are difficult to quantitate, but for Germany, they were estimated at about 1 billion dollars annually, from effects on the thyroid alone (36). Correction of severe iodine deficiency in one Chinese village was associated with a reduction in goiter prevalence (from 80 to 4.5%), an absence of new cretins (from a previous 11% prevalence), improvement in district school performance ranking (from fourteenth [last] to third), decline in school failure rate (from >50 to 2%), and approximately tenfold increases in farm production and per capita income (37).

Complicating Factors

Other deficiencies can worsen the effects of iodine lack, and these frequently coexist in the same populations. Laboratory and clinical investigations have shown that iodine treatment in iodine-deficient children is significantly more effective if coexisting iron deficiency anemia is corrected (38). Similar studies have concluded that treatment of iodine deficiency is more effective if vitamin A deficiency is also corrected. As noted earlier, selenium deficiency may be a factor in the development of myxedematous cretinism.

Certain toxic substances (termed *goitrogens*) complicate iodine deficiency (39). Thiocyanate, an inhibitor of thyroidal iodine concentration, is a derivative of cassava, a widely used food staple in many of the developing countries with iodine deficiency. Depending on the method of cassava preparation, its thiocyanate can worsen the iodine-starved thyroid's ability to make hormone. Thiocyanate also occurs in tobacco smoke, and it further compromises the thyroid in iodine-deficient smokers (40). Some forms of millet, another food staple in much of the world, also have potent thyroid-inhibitory properties that contribute to the effects of iodine deficiency. Many other goitrogens have been described, in polluted water, humic substances, edible plants, and elsewhere. Most are not major problems, except in persons with coexisting iodine deficiency.

CONSEQUENCES OF EXCESS

Too much iodine does far less damage than too little. Generally, humans can tolerate fairly large amounts without serious harm (41). Issues of concern are hypothyroidism, autoimmune thyroid disease, and papillary thyroid cancer. Iodine-induced hyperthyroidism, which has its roots in iodine deficiency, is discussed earlier.

Hypothyroidism

Large amounts of iodine can reduce thyroid hormone output (41). Most persons can adapt to an iodine load by decreasing iodine transport into the thyroid. If not, they become hypothyroid. Iodine can saturate the TPO receptors in the thyroid and can prevent coupling of MITs in Tg to make hormone. It can also block release of hormone from the gland. Some common medical sources of excess iodine are radiocontrast media, sterilizing agents, and drugs (e.g., amiodarone). Large doses of iodine are frequently used clinically to control hyperthyroidism from various causes.

Autoimmune Thyroid Disease

This term includes several clinical entities involving autoantibodies directed at thyroid antigens, including Tg, TPO, and the TSH receptor (42). These can variously cause hyperthyroidism (Graves disease), goiter, hypothyroidism, and thyroiditis (Hashimoto disease). They are quite common in the iodine-sufficient United States, causing an estimated 15 to 20% of women eventually to become hypothyroid. Graves disease is the most frequent cause of hyperthyroidism in the United States, in contrast to iodine-deficient countries, where nodular goiter prevails. Studies have shown that increased iodine in the diet is associated with a higher incidence of autoimmune thyroid disease, including both hyperthyroidism and hypothyroidism. In experimental animals, the immunogenicity of injected Tg is proportional to its degree of iodination. A high-iodine diet induced autoimmune changes in the human thyroid, examined histologically and immunologically, and these changes subsided on stopping the diet (43). These and other examples led to the conclusion that iodine contributes in the pathogenesis of these disorders.

Thyroid Cancer

Three broad histologic types of thyroid cancer exist: papillary, follicular, and anaplastic. The first two, especially papillary, generally have an excellent prognosis with standard surgical treatment, occasionally with additional radioiodine. Careful pathologic examination of thyroid glands from routine autopsies in iodine-sufficient countries revealed a high incidence of microscopic papillary cancers, up to 30 to 40%. Many of these were only several millimeters in size and clearly do not cause damage. Correction of iodine deficiency is associated with a shift in the ratio of follicular to papillary cancers. Some studies also showed that the incidence of papillary cancer increases with population iodine intake, but many of these cancers were the small incidental ones, so the importance of this increase is not clear; the subject needs further study. For the present, it is prudent to be aware of this possibility, and it adds another reason to avoid prolonged iodine excess.

SUPPLEMENTATION

Iodine is the obvious treatment for iodine deficiency. Several acceptable approaches are available. For public health purposes, the most practical is iodization of salt, and this continues to be the mainstay of national prophylactic programs. Sometimes, other measures are needed, for both individual persons and communities. These include iodized water, iodized vegetable oil, iodine tablets, and occasionally other vehicles. The success of any iodization effort depends on quality control of the product and on regular monitoring of iodine nutrition in the target, usually by surveying representative urine samples for iodine concentration.

Iodized Salt

Salt has several appeals as a fortification vehicle. It is a necessary nutrient, so everyone must have it, regardless of age, gender, geography, or socioeconomic condition. Salt deposits are situated unevenly on land, and frequently salt is one of the very few commodities that remote communities cannot provide for themselves. The iodization technology is straightforward and can be adapted to a wide range of salt production methods. At its simplest, a measured amount of salt enriched with KIO_3 or potassium iodide (KI) is mixed manually with a larger reservoir of salt to achieve the desired iodization level. In more sophisticated designs, a solution of KIO_3 or KI is added by spray or drip to salt moving on a conveyor belt. Portable iodization instruments, consisting of a rotating drum or other mixing chamber and a means of adding iodine either by

dry mixing or spray, have been widely used at small-scale salt production sites. Large producers can easily add an iodization step to their assembly.

The two major iodine fortificants are KIO_3 and KI. The latter is less expensive, has a higher iodine content (76%), and is more soluble. KIO_3, with an iodine content of 59%, is more stable. KIO_3 is preferred when the salt is fairly crude with various impurities and high humidity, in hot climates, with porous packaging, and adverse storage conditions; it is the form most widely used, especially in the developing world. In temperate countries with high-quality crystalline salt, like the United States and much of northern Europe, KI is satisfactory and is generally used.

Salt iodization is usually in the range of 15 to 50 µg iodine/g salt (15–50 ppm). It is important to specify the *iodine* content, not that of the KIO_3 or KI; some national regulations and recommendations confuse this point. Factors in choosing a level include the daily average per capita salt consumption of the population (this can vary from 2 to 20 g, with most in the 5- to 10-g range), the availability of iodine from other sources, whether iodized salt will be used in commercial food processing as well as at home, and whether iodine is lost from salt between production and consumption. Most countries have chosen levels of 20 to 40 ppm. Because salt moves across national borders, the harmonization of iodization levels within regions is desirable.

The issue of including iodized salt in commercial food processing is important. In industrialized countries such as the United States and Canada, most dietary salt intake comes from processed food, and its salt is not usually iodized, so the discretionary salt added in the kitchen or at table is only about 15% of the total intake. In Europe, some countries require or encourage iodized salt usage in the food industry, whereas others do not. Developing countries depend less on processed food for their salt and more on that added at home, but this may change, and the issue should be addressed.

Another variation among national laws is whether salt for domestic animals must be iodized. Animals, like humans, need iodine, and progressive farming practice routinely provides iodine in some form; this is why dairy products are the most important source of dietary iodine in the United States and in many Western countries. Another reason for iodizing animal salt is that many people in developing countries use the same salt for themselves and their animals; the availability of inexpensive crude uniodized salt for animals is powerful competition for iodized salt in the market.

Iodized Water

Water, like salt, is a human necessity, so its iodization treats iodine deficiency in all whom it reaches (44). In the 1920s, bags of iodine salts were thrown into the reservoir inlet in Rochester, New York, and tap water in homes contained iodine. More recently, several other approaches have been used. In the simplest, a small amount of a concentrated solution of KIO_3 or KI is added to standing drinking water for the school or home. Slightly more complicated systems divert a small amount of flowing water and slowly release a concentrated iodine solution into it before returning it to the main outflow. Iodine salts can also be added at the outflow from closed reservoirs. All these methods require minimal instrumentation or expense, but they do need competent oversight to ensure continuing availability of the right amount of iodine. Another system slowly releases KI from porous polyethylene baskets that can be placed in wells. DeLong and colleagues (26) periodically dripped KIO_3 into irrigation ditches in western China, so iodine reached both humans and animals; these investigators found this approach highly effective in correcting iodine deficiency, at very low cost.

Iodine (I_2, or molecular iodine), but not KIO_3 or KI, is antibacterial and is frequently used for water purification, both for communities and for individual persons, such as campers. Many iodine-deficient communities also have polluted water, so this effect of iodine can be useful in a prophylactic program. Water purification schemes based on iodine may greatly augment the community's iodine intake, and iodine excess should be avoided.

Iodized Oil

Many radiocontrast dyes used medically are iodinated vegetable oils. A typical agent, lipiodol, contains 480 mg/mL iodine. Beginning in the late 1950s, iodized oil has been widely used to correct iodine deficiency in many countries (45). A single oral administration of 200 to 400 mg can provide adequate iodine for up to a year; intramuscular injection prolongs coverage for 3 years or more. The iodine is stored in the thyroid and in fat tissue and also at the site of injection when that route is used. Release after oral administration is high in the first week, then much slower, so the amount provided is uneven, in contrast to daily supplements of iodized salt or water. Iodized oil is also more expensive and requires direct contact with each targeted person. However, its use can be implemented quickly without the delays inherent in introducing iodization into salt commerce. Its greatest application has been for especially vulnerable targets, women and children in moderate or severely deficient areas, who are unlikely to benefit from salt iodization in the near future.

Iodine Tablets, Solutions, and Other Vehicles

Alternatives to iodized salt are occasionally needed, as additional iodine for vulnerable groups or as primary supplementation while awaiting successful implementation of salt. Daily addition of 150 μg or more of iodine as KI can help to cover the increased needs during pregnancy and lactation; this is most conveniently done in industrialized countries by including KI in routine vitamin and mineral mixtures. Often, health personnel in remote villages

need simpler ways to correct iodine deficiency. Their medicine chest probably contains Lugol iodine or a similar preparation as an antiseptic; these preparations can be diluted to provide appropriate iodine supplementation, or solutions of KI can be prepared and distributed easily and cheaply (46).

Various other vehicles have been occasionally used for iodine delivery, such as bread, sugar, candy, tea, dried bananas, and fish sauce. These may be appropriate for specific populations and food habits, but in general, first consideration should be given to iodized salt. Any approach should focus on the most vulnerable groups, women and young children in poor, remote areas.

NATIONAL IODINE NUTRITION PROGRAMS

Iodine nutrition is a public health issue and therefore a concern of the government. Most countries delegate responsibility to some governmental agency, usually a division of nutrition within a ministry of health. The most successful programs have a designated chief, an assigned budget, and high visibility. The principal activities are monitoring and assessment of iodine nutrition, oversight of iodized salt or other supplementation measures, and education and advocacy.

Iodine Nutrition

Surveys should be carried out regularly in representative portions of the population, usually by measuring urinary iodine concentrations. The results should be analyzed and made public promptly, to initiate any necessary corrective action.

Iodized Salt Oversight

The program must work effectively with salt producers to ensure that properly iodized salt is available to consumers at a reasonable price. In addition to the producers' own quality control, independent governmental monitoring of iodine in the salt should be carried out regularly at both production and consumption levels, with corrective action or penalties for deviations from prescribed standards.

Education and Advocacy

All relevant parties—governmental decision makers, the health sector, salt producers, citizens groups, and the general public—must understand the consequences of iodine deficiency and the importance of its correction. The message should be pitched to a level appropriate for the audience and should emphasize iodine deficiency's irreversible damage to the developing brain. Success requires some adjustments, especially by salt producers and consumers, and the educational campaign must make them appreciate and accept—and ultimately demand—the benefits of iodized salt.

GLOBAL IODINE NUTRITION STATUS

Iodine is distributed unevenly over the earth. Low amounts are typically associated with young mountains (Himalayas, Andes, Alps), frequent flooding (India, Bangladesh), or areas remote from the sea (Central Asia, Central Africa), but deficiency occurs in many other geographic areas as well, including the seaside. Virtually every country in the world has had some iodine-deficient areas.

The last two decades have seen a strong international effort against iodine deficiency. The World Summit for Children in 1990 pledged the elimination of this deficiency by 2000, a goal recently pushed back to 2005. National governments and international organizations have aggressively pursued universal salt iodization, especially for developing countries. The success has been considerable, although much more needs to be done.

ICCIDD reports that about half of the world's countries, containing about half of its population, still have a significant iodine deficiency in at least part of their territory, enough to need corrective measures (Table 15.3) (47, 48). Coverage with adequately iodized salt now reaches about 70% of the people in previously iodine-deficient countries. Most of these countries have legislation and programs for iodized salt, but they are much less advanced in monitoring of iodine nutrition and in plans for sustaining iodine sufficiency once achieved. Environmental iodine deficiency is a chronic situation unlikely to change, so complacency after a successful iodization program invites regression; good examples of this have been documented in Guatemala and elsewhere (49).

Iodine excess occurs in Japan (high seaweed consumption) and Chile (high environmental iodine, wide use of iodine for water purification, and iodization of salt at excessive levels in the recent past). Several other countries showed signs of iodine excess when salt iodization was inappropriately high, but iodine levels returned to normal on lowering the amount of iodine in salt.

TABLE 15.3. GLOBAL IODINE NUTRITION

	MILLIONS (%)
By population	
Deficient	3,034 (50)
Sufficient	2,839 (47)
Excessive	210 (3)
Unknown	6 (0)
By number of countries[a]	
Deficient	84 (53)
Sufficient	72 (45)
Excessive	3 (2)

[a] Of 159 largest countries.

From International Council for the Control of Iodine Deficiency Disorders, 2002; www.iccidd.org, with permission.

ACHIEVING AND SUSTAINING OPTIMAL IODINE NUTRITION

An international consultation proposed criteria for charting progress against iodine deficiency (14). These criteria were principally that the median iodine concentration in urine samples representative of the population was greater than 100 μg/L, and at least 90% of households received adequately iodized salt, if that was the designated vehicle. In addition, the consultation required programmatic indicators to ensure that progress could be sustained. The latter can be grouped as monitoring of iodine nutrition and of salt, education, national coalitions, designated responsibility, and data collection and reporting. Most of these have already been presented in preceding sections of this chapter, but national coalitions deserve further discussion here.

A national coalition for optimal iodine nutrition should represent all relevant sectors that will actively promote and sustain the effort. The structure and composition of such coalitions will vary with the unique circumstances in each country. Generally, all sectors associated with iodine deficiency or its solution should be included. Examples are governmental institutions (health, nutrition, commerce, education, agriculture, law, standards), health workers, the salt industry, educators, consumers, mothers, civic organizations, the media, and affected communities. In one model, the ministry of health is in charge of the coalition; it assembles the members and chairs meetings. In another model, the coalition is independent of the government, although advisory to it and supportive of its programs. The government must clearly be involved, because it has ultimate responsibility for this public health issue. However, day-to-day running of the coalition is often best left in nongovernmental hands, given that iodine nutrition is only one of many issues governments face, and personnel and organizational structure in governmental programs change frequently, thus endangering continuity. The most successful coalitions have been led by prominent citizens, often health professionals, who are determined to eliminate iodine deficiency and who invest their energy and skill toward this goal over a long period, working in close harmony with the government. Macedonia and Croatia are good examples, and promising initiatives have started in South Africa, Russia, India, Peru, and Thailand (5, 6).

Many pitfalls face an initially successful iodization program. Some are changes in governmental knowledge and interest (with decentralization and replacement of regimes and personnel), natural or civil disasters that disrupt the salt trade, overlooking of the economic consequences of iodized salt for consumer and producer, continued dependence on international donors, failure to make all levels of the population aware of the consequences of iodine deficiency and the ease of its correction, absence of regular monitoring of iodine nutrition and its public reporting, and complacency at all levels. Examples of these and other problems are available and remind us that iodine deficiency is a geologic reality that will return if programs against it are not maintained (49).

SUMMARY

Iodine is a necessary component of the thyroid hormones, which are required for life and health. Iodine is distributed unevenly over the earth, and about half of the world's population lives in countries with significant deficiency. The worst consequences of deficiency occur during pregnancy and include fetal and infant death, irreversible brain damage, and maternal complications. Additional problems for the rest of the community are hypothyroidism, goiter, and socioeconomic stagnation. Iodization of salt is the best and most practical of several good means for correcting iodine deficiency. Excess iodine intake occasionally occurs but can be avoided; its consequences are minor compared with those of deficiency. A massive global effort to eliminate iodine deficiency is under way. Results so far have been impressive, but much more remains to be done. Once iodine sufficiency is achieved, a great danger is that the effort will lapse and deficiency will recur. This can best be prevented by constant monitoring of iodine nutrition and prompt corrective action when needed.

Acknowledgments
I am grateful to many colleagues in ICCIDD and others who have taught me and stimulated my interest in iodine over several decades, especially Drs. Ann Dunn, John Stanbury, Francois Delange, Basil Hetzel, Eduardo Pretell, and Lewis Braverman.

REFERENCES

1. Dunn JT. Iodine deficiency and its elimination by iodine supplementation. In: Braverman LE, ed. Diseases of the Thyroid. 2nd ed. Totowa, NJ: Humana Press, 2003:329–45.
2. Delange F. Iodine deficiency. In: Braverman LE, Utiger RD, eds. Werner & Ingbar's The Thyroid: A Fundamental and Clinical Text. 8th ed. Philadelphia: Lippincott Williams & Wilkins, 2000:295–316.
3. Dunn JT, Pretell EA, Daza CH et al, eds. Towards the Eradication of Endemic Goiter, Cretinism, and Iodine Deficiency. Washington, DC: Pan American Health Organization, 1986:1–419.
4. Hetzel BS, Dunn JT, Stanbury JB, eds. The Prevention and Control of Iodine Deficiency Disorders. Amsterdam: Elsevier, 1987: 1–354.
5. International Council for the Control of Iodine Deficiency Disorders. IDD Newslett 1992–present, www.iccidd.org.
6. International Council for the Control of Iodine Deficiency Disorders. Country information: CIDDS Database, www.iccidd.org.
7. Merke F. History and Iconography of Endemic Goitre and Cretinism. Lancaster, UK: MTP Press, 1984:1–339.
8. Lauterbach A, Ober G, Rios S et al, eds. Iodine: High Performance Chemistry. Santiago, Chile: SQM, 2001:1–85.
9. Anonymous. IDD Newslett 2001;17:62–3.
10. Dunn JT, Dunn AD. Thyroglobulin: chemistry, biosynthesis, and proteolysis. In: Braverman LE, Utiger RD, eds. Werner & Ingbar's The Thyroid: A Fundamental and Clinical Text. 8th ed. Philadelphia: Lippincott Williams & Wilkins, 2000:91–104.
11. Dunn JT, Dunn AD. Thyroid physiology. In: Besser GM, Thorner MO, eds. Comprehensive Clinical Endocrinology. 3rd ed. St Louis: Mosby, 2002:131–8.
12. Food and Nutrition Board, Institute of Medicine. Dietary Reference Intakes for Vitamin A, Vitamin K, Arsenic, Boron, Chromium, Copper, Iodine, Iron, Manganese, Molybdenum, Nickel, Silicon, Vanadium, and Zinc. Washington, DC: National Academy Press, 2001:258–89.
13. Dunn JT, Crutchfield HE, Gutekunst R et al. Methods for Measuring Iodine in Urine. Wageningen, Netherlands: International Council for Control of Iodine Deficiency Disorders, 1993:1–71.
14. International Council for the Control of Iodine Deficiency Disorders, United National Children's Fund (UNICEF), World Health Organization (WHO). Assessment of the Iodine Deficiency Disorders and Monitoring Their Elimination. Geneva: WHO Publication WHO/NHD/01.1, 2001:1–107 (also available at www.iccidd.org).
15. Oddie TH, Fisher DA, Long JM. J Clin Endocrinol 1964;24: 924–33.
16. DeGroot LJ. J Clin Endocrinol Metab 1966;26:149–73.
17. Delange F, Heidemann P, Bourdoux P et al. Biol Neonat 1986; 49:322–30.
18. Vitti P, Martino E, Aghini-Lombardi F et al. J Clin Endocrinol Metab 1994;79:600–3.
19. Zimmermann MB, Hess SY, Molinari L et al. IDD Newslett 2003;19:62–3.
20. Thomson CD. IDD Newslett 2002;18:38–42.
21. Dunn JT, Delange F. J Clin Endocrinol Metab 2001;86:2360–3.
22. Pearce EN, Pino S, He X et al. J Clin Endocrinol Metab (in press).
23. Hollowell JG, Staehling NW, Hannon WH et al. J Clin Endocrinol Metab 1998;83:3401–8.
24. Thilly C, Lagasse R, Roger G et al. Impaired fetal and postnatal development and high perinatal death rate in a severe iodine deficient area. In: Stockigt JR, Nagataki S, eds. Thyroid Research VIII. Proceedings of the Eighth International Thyroid Congress. Canberra: Australian Academy of Science, 1980:20–3.
25. Cobra C, Muhilal Rusmil K, Rustama D et al. J Nutr 1997;127: 574–8.
26. DeLong GR, Leslie PW, Wang S-H et al. Lancet 1997;350: 771–3.
27. Pharoah POD, Connolly KJ. Int J Epidemiol 1987;16:68–73.
28. Stanbury JB, ed. The Damaged Brain of Iodine Deficiency. New York: Cognizant Communication Corp, 1994:1–335.
29. Halpern J-P. The neuromotor deficit in endemic cretinism and its implications for the pathogenesis of the disorder. In: Stanbury JB. ed. The Damaged Brain of Iodine Deficiency. New York: Cognizant Communication Corp, 1994:15–24.
30. DeLong R, Tai M, Xue-Yi C et al. The neuromotor deficit in endemic cretinism. In: Stanbury JB, ed. The Damaged Brain of Iodine Deficiency. New York: Cognizant Communication Corp, 1994:9–13.
31. Delange F. Endemic cretinism: In: Braverman LE, Utiger RD, eds. Werner & Ingbar's The Thyroid: A Fundamental and Clinical Text. 8th ed. Philadelphia: Lippincott Williams & Wilkins, 2000:743–54.
32. Bleichrodt N, Born MO. A metaanalysis of research on iodine and its relationship to cognitive development. In: Stanbury JB, ed. The Damaged Brain of Iodine Deficiency. New York: Cognizant Communication Corp, 1994:195–200.
33. Quian M, Wang D, Watkins WE et al. 7th Asia and Oceania Thyroid Association Congress Abstract Book, 2003:34.
34. Boyages SC. The neuromuscular system and brain in hypothyroidism. In: Braverman LE, Utiger RD, eds. Werner & Ingbar's

The Thyroid. A Fundamental and Clinical Text. 8ᵗʰ ed. Philadelphia: Lippincott Williams & Wilkins, 2000:803–10.

35. Stanbury JB, Ermans AE, Bourdoux P et al. Thyroid 1998;8:83–100.
36. Pfannenstiel P. IDD Newslett 1998;14:11–2.
37. Li J, Wang X. IDD Newslett 1987;3:4–5.
38. Zimmermann MB. IDD Newslett 2003;19:52–54.
39. Engel A, Lamm SH. Goitrogens in the environment. In: Braverman LE, ed. Diseases of the Thyroid. 2ⁿᵈ ed. Totowa, NJ: Humana Press, 2003:307–328.
40. Knudsen N, Bulow I, Laurberg P et al. Arch Intern Med 2002;162:439–43.
41. Roti E, Vagenakis AG. Effects of excess iodide: clinical aspects. In: Braverman LE, Utiger RD, eds. Werner & Ingbar's The Thyroid. A Fundamental and Clinical Text. 8ᵗʰ ed. Philadelphia: Lippincott Williams & Wilkins, 2000:316–29.
42. Davies TF. Graves' disease. In: Braverman LE, Utiger RD, eds. Werner & Ingbar's The Thyroid. A Fundamental and Clinical Text. 8ᵗʰ ed. Philadelphia: Lippincott Williams & Wilkins, 2000: 518–31.
43. Kahaly GJ, Dienes HP, Beyer J et al. Eur J Endocrinol 1998;139:290–7.
44. International Council for the Control of Iodine Deficiency Disorders. IDD Newslett 1997;13:33–9.
45. Dunn JT. Iodized oil in the treatment and prophylaxis of IDD. In: Hetzel BS, Dunn JT, Stanbury JB, eds. The Prevention and Control of Iodine Deficiency Disorders. Amsterdam: Elsevier, 1987:135–8.
46. Todd CH, Dunn JT. Am J Clin Nutr 1998;67:1279–83.
47. International Council for the Control of Iodine Deficiency Disorders. IDD Newslett 2003;19:24–5.
48. Delange F, Burgi H, Chen ZP et al. Thyroid 2002;12:915–24.
49. Dunn JT. Thyroid 2000;19:681–583.

16   SELENIUM[1]

RAYMOND F. BURK AND ORVILLE A. LEVANDER

CHEMICAL FORMS 312
DIETARY CONSIDERATIONS .313
   Food Sources 313
   Bioavailability 314
   Nutrient-Nutrient Interrelationships 314
METABOLISM 314
   Absorption 315
   Transport 315
   Incorporation into Protein 315
   Excretion 316
BIOCHEMICAL FUNCTIONS .316
   Glutathione Peroxidases .316
   Iodothyronine Deiodinases 316
   Thioredoxin Reductases .316
   Selenoprotein P 317
   Selenoprotein W 317
   Selenophosphate Synthetase 317
BIOLOGIC ACTIVITY 317
DEFICIENCY IN HUMANS AND ANIMALS 317
EVALUATION OF NUTRIENT STATUS 319
   Analytic Evaluation 319
   Biochemical Evaluation .320
REQUIREMENTS AND RECOMMENDED INTAKES 320
TOXICITY IN HUMANS AND ANIMALS 322
HIGH-RISK CLINICAL SITUATIONS 323

Selenium first attracted biologic interest in the 1930s when it was found to cause poisoning of livestock that grazed in areas with high-selenium soils (1). In 1957, Schwarz and Foltz reported that small amounts of selenium prevented liver necrosis in vitamin E–deficient rats, a finding indicating that selenium was an essential nutrient and not only a toxin (2). Soon thereafter, deficiencies of selenium and vitamin E were shown to be involved in several economically important nutritional diseases of cattle, sheep, swine, and poultry (3). The first demonstration of a biochemical function for

selenium in animals came in 1973 when the element was discovered to be a constituent of the enzyme glutathione peroxidase (GSHPx) (4).

The importance of selenium in human nutrition was documented in 1979 when Chinese scientists reported that selenium supplementation prevented the development of a cardiomyopathy known as Keshan disease in children living in low-selenium areas (5), and New Zealand workers reported a clinical response to selenium in a selenium-depleted patient (6). Information about the role of selenium in human nutrition increased rapidly in the 1980s, and a recommended dietary allowance (RDA) for selenium was established in 1989 (7) and revised in 2000 (8). Dietary recommendations from the World Health Organization (WHO) were issued in 1996 (9). Since the late 1980s, research has provided extensive new information on selenoproteins and the molecular biology of selenium.

CHEMICAL FORMS

Most selenium in biologic systems is present in proteins as a constituent of amino acids. Reflecting the similarity of selenium chemistry to that of sulfur, those amino acids are usually selenocysteine and selenomethionine. Selenocysteine (Fig. 16.1) contains selenium in an exposed position, a selenol, and is therefore chemically highly reactive. It almost always performs catalytic functions in proteins. Selenomethionine, conversely, contains selenium bound covalently to two carbon atoms and is therefore considerably less reactive than selenocysteine. It is not known to have a biochemical function distinct from that of methionine.

A selenoprotein contains stoichiometric amounts of selenium. Selenocysteine is the form of the element in the primary structure of all the animal selenoproteins identified so far and in nearly all the bacterial selenoproteins. The presence of selenium in an unidentified form (not selenocysteine) that is coordinated with molybdenum in nicotinic acid hydroxylase from *Clostridium barkeri* (10) indicates that selenoproteins containing forms of the element other than selenocysteine exist in nature.

Numerous proteins contain selenium in nonstoichiometric amounts and are referred to as selenium-containing proteins. This designation has low utility because virtually

---

[1] **Abbreviations: AI,** adequate intake; **DRI,** dietary reference intake; **EAR,** estimated average requirement; **GSH,** glutathione; **GSHPx,** glutathione peroxidase; **NOAEL,** no-observed-adverse-effect level; **RDA,** recommended dietary allowance; **SECIS,** selenocysteine insertion sequence; **UL,** tolerable upper intake level; **WHO,** World Health Organization.

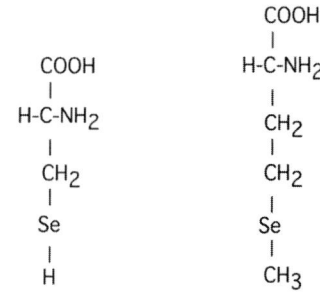

Figure 16.1. Selenium-containing amino acids found in animals. Selenocysteine is the biologically active form of the element found in selenoproteins. Its selenol is largely ionized at physiologic pH and is a stronger nucleophile than the thiol of cysteine. These chemical properties contribute to its catalytic function in selenoenzymes. Selenomethionine contains selenium covalently bound to two carbon atoms. Thus, its selenium is shielded and is not as chemically active as the selenium in selenocysteine. Selenomethionine appears to be distributed nonspecifically in the methionine pool.

all proteins that contain methionine contain selenomethionine in proportion to the relative abundance of these two amino acids in the organism (see later).

Selenium enters the food chain through plants that incorporate it into compounds that usually contain sulfur. The result is that plant selenium is in the form of selenomethionine and, to a lesser extent, selenocysteine and other analogs of sulfur amino acids. No evidence has been presented that plants require selenium for incorporation into a specific molecule that is necessary for their existence.

Some plants express an enzyme that methylates free selenocysteine, producing Se-methylselenocysteine (11). This is a detoxification product, and it cannot be incorporated into protein. It accumulates to high concentrations and can be responsible for selenium poisoning in animals that eat the plants.

Selenophosphate is an important intermediate compound in selenium metabolism. It is produced by selenophosphate synthetase and serves as the selenium donor for the production of selenium-containing transfer RNAs as well as for selenocysteine destined for incorporation into selenoproteins (12).

Methylated forms of selenium are produced as excretory metabolites and rapidly appear in the urine and breath (13, 14). Small molecule forms of the element have been detected in blood plasma, but their identities have not been established (15).

DIETARY CONSIDERATIONS

Food Sources

Although SI units (Système International d'Unités, or International System of Units) are increasingly used to express concentrations of nutrients in body fluids and tissues, food composition tables primarily express values in micrograms per gram (μg/g). In this regard, 1 μg of selenium equals 0.0127 μmol of selenium. The richest food sources of selenium are organ meats and seafoods (0.4–1.5 μg/g fresh weight), followed by muscle meats (0.1–0.4), cereals and grains (<0.1–>0.8), dairy products (<0.1–0.3), and fruits and vegetables (<0.1) (16). The reason for the wide variation in the selenium content of cereals and grains is that plants do not appear to require selenium and thus contain variable amounts, depending on how much soil selenium is available for uptake (phytoavailability). For example, one study showed that the selenium content of corn collected in the People's Republic of China ranged from 0.005 to 8.1 μg/g, depending on whether the samples came from areas with soils that were poor or rich in phytoavailable selenium (17). The importance of geographic origin as a determinant of the selenium content of grains was also indicated by the reported decline in the selenium content of the British diet from 65 to 31 μg/day after Britain switched its source of wheat from North America to Europe (18). Foods from animal sources vary somewhat in selenium content, but the degree of variation is less than in plants because of the homeostatic control of selenium in animals under different conditions of exposure. The US Department of Agriculture National Nutrient Database for Standard Reference, Release 16 provides analytic or inferred values for the selenium content of hundreds of food items expressed as microgams of selenium per common measure, such as cups, teaspoons, and slices (19). The selenium content of a large number of foods is given in Appendix Table A-22-b. Drinking water generally contributes negligible selenium to the overall intake, except in some localized highly seleniferous areas (20).

The Total Diet Study conducted by the US Food and Drug Administration showed that a typical diet in the United States provided an average daily selenium intake of 100 and 70 μg for men and women, respectively, between 1982 and 1986 (21). Lower daily selenium intakes, 30 μg or less, have been reported in countries with selenium-poor soils, such as New Zealand (22). Because of the increasing evidence that good selenium status may confer human health benefits, the government of Finland started adding selenium to the fertilizers used in that low-selenium country in 1984 as a way of improving the selenium status of the general population. Daily dietary selenium intakes increased from 39 μg in 1984 to 120 μg in 1990, resulting in an increase in serum selenium concentrations from 0.95 to 1.5 μmol/L in 1990 (23).

During 1991 to 1998, the amount added to fertilizers was decreased, and the serum selenium concentration gradually declined to 1.10 μmol/L. Then, in 1998, the selenium in fertilizer was increased again, and a trend of increasing serum selenium values was noted. Despite more than 15 years of elevated serum selenium concentrations as a result of their fertilizer intervention, the Finns were unable to ". . . find any change in the declining trend [in coronary heart disease] that could be attributed to Se supplementation. . . . Neither do the data on cancer incidence in Finland suggest any specific effects due to increased dietary Se intake . . ." (24). Extremely low dietary selenium intakes have been reported in Keshan disease–affected areas of China, from 3 to 22 μg/dayday (17). Conversely, very high dietary intakes (≤6690 μg/day) have been observed in a region of China with endemic human selenosis (17). The food in this area had been grown on soil contaminated with selenium leached from a highly seleniferous coal fly ash.

Bioavailability

Only a few investigations have been carried out to determine the nutritional bioavailability of selenium in foods consumed by humans. A commonly used experimental procedure to estimate selenium availability has been to follow increases in hepatic GSHPx activity after feeding various food sources of selenium to rodents previously depleted of selenium (25). On this basis, selenium fed as mushrooms, tuna, and wheat was 5, 57, and 83% as available to rats, respectively, as sodium selenite (25, 26). A human bioavailability trial performed in Finland with men of moderately low selenium status showed significant differences among various forms of selenium tested (e.g., selenate, wheat, yeast) depending on the criterion of availability used (increase in platelet GSHPx activity, elevation of plasma or red blood cell selenium content, retention of selenium) (27). This study pointed out the need to consider several variables in such trials including short-term increases in GSHPx activity, long-term tissue retention of selenium, and metabolic conversion of retained selenium to biologically active forms.

Nutrient-Nutrient Interrelationships

Because of its role in the GSHPxs and thioredoxin reductases, selenium probably interacts with any nutrient that affects the antioxidant-prooxidant balance of the cell. For example, the selenium requirement of chicks is inversely proportional to the dietary vitamin E intake (28). Selenium also protects against the toxicity of mercury, cadmium, and silver (29, 30), and a physiologic role for selenium in counteracting heavy metal pollutants has been proposed (31). The low bioavailability of the selenium in tuna may result from complexation with mercury, but this issue needs further investigation (26).

METABOLISM

Selenium enters the body in several forms (Fig. 16.2). The two major ones are selenomethionine, derived ultimately from plants, and selenocysteine, mainly from animal selenoproteins. Selenomethionine does not appear to be specifically recognized as a selenium compound and is

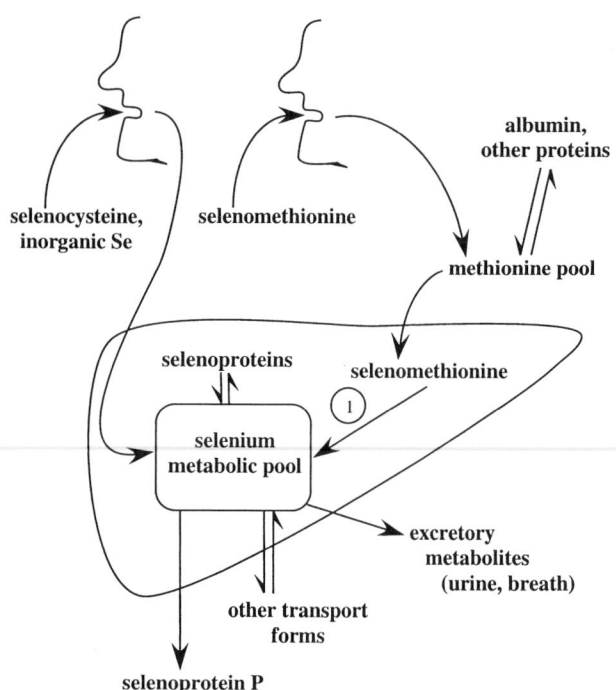

Figure 16.2. Relationship of dietary form of selenium with tissue forms of the element. Ingested selenocysteine and inorganic selenium forms selenite and selenate enter the selenium metabolic pool (more detail in Fig. 16.3) directly. Selenomethionine enters the methionine pool and is incorporated into methionine-containing proteins throughout the body. When selenomethionine is metabolized to selenocysteine by the transsulfuration pathway (1) in the liver or kidney, it enters the selenium metabolic pool. In liver, the selenium metabolic pool produces selenoprotein P for export and hepatic selenoproteins. Homeostasis of selenium is maintained by the production of excretory metabolites and transport forms of selenium that have not been identified.

metabolized in the methionine pool. It is measured as tissue selenium because it is present in methionine-containing proteins in blood and tissues. The selenium in selenomethionine is made available for specific use when the amino acid is catabolized by the transsulfuration pathway (see also Chapter 34) in liver or kidney (see Fig. 16.2). The selenium then enters regulated selenium metabolism and can be incorporated into selenoproteins, transported to other organs, or excreted.

Figure 16.3 is an outline of selenium metabolism in a typical nonliver or kidney cell. The selenium in selenomethionine cannot be used by peripheral cells until it has been liberated by the transsulfuration pathway in liver or kidney. Free selenocysteine, whether derived from catabolism of intracellular or extracellular selenoproteins, is degraded by selenocysteine β-lyase (32). The resulting selenide can enter the anabolic pathway by conversion to selenophosphate or be modified for transport out of the cell in an unknown form. The further metabolism of selenide is the likely point of homeostatic regulation of selenium in the cell. The mechanism by which this form of selenium is directed into the anabolic pathway or into the transport pathway has not been determined.

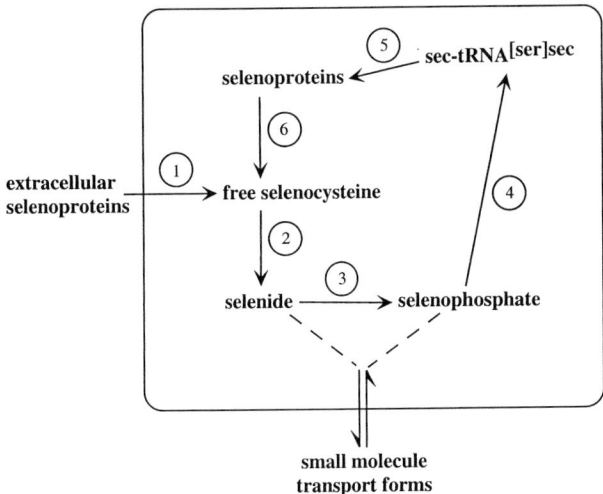

Figure 16.3. Selenium metabolic pool in a typical nonliver or kidney cell. Selenium enters the cell as selenocysteine from extracellular selenoproteins (probably mainly selenoprotein P) (127) or from unidentified small molecule forms. Free selenocysteine is produced by catabolism of (6) cellular selenoproteins or (1) extracellular selenoproteins. Free selenocysteine does not accumulate because it is metabolized by (2) selenocysteine β–lyase (128). The resulting selenide is transformed into selenophosphate by (3) selenophosphate synthetase, using the cosubstrate adenosine triphosphate. It appears likely that an interorgan transport form of selenium enters and/or leaves this part of the pathway. Selenophosphate is a substrate for (4) selenocysteine synthase, which forms sec-tRNA[ser]sec (see Fig. 16.4A). sec-tRNA[ser]sec is used in the synthesis of selenoproteins (5) (see Fig. 16.4C).

Absorption

Absorption appears to play no role in the homeostatic regulation of selenium. Virtually complete absorption occurs when the element is supplied as selenomethionine (33) and, presumably, as selenocysteine. Absorption of selenite and selenate is greater than 50%, but it varies significantly, influenced by luminal factors (34). Thus, selenium absorption is usually in the range of 50 to 100% and is not affected by selenium nutritional status.

Transport

Knowledge of the extracellular transport of selenium is incomplete. Two selenoproteins, selenoprotein P and extracellular GSHPx (GSHPx-3), have been identified in plasma, and both contain the element as selenocysteine in their primary structures. Work using mice with targeted deletion of the selenoprotein P gene has shown that this protein is involved in supplying selenium to the brain and to the testis (35, 36). However, raising selenium intake compensates for deletion of selenoprotein P, a finding indicating that other forms of selenium can be taken up by the brain (35). Low-molecular-weight forms of the element have been recognized as minor components of the plasma selenium (15), and they may serve transport functions. Chemical identification of these forms has not yet been made.

Incorporation into Protein

The animal selenoproteins characterized so far contain selenocysteine in their primary structures. The mechanism by which selenocysteine, the twenty-first amino acid, is synthesized and then incorporated into selenoproteins is complex.

Figure 16.4A shows how selenium is attached to its tRNA as selenocysteine. tRNA[ser]sec, a unique tRNA with the anticodon for UGA, is charged with serine by seryl tRNA ligase. The serine in the resulting ser-tRNA[ser]sec is then converted to selenocysteine by a process requiring selenophosphate synthesized by selenophosphate synthetase. Two isoforms of selenophosphate synthetase have been identified (37, 38), one of which is itself a selenoprotein. In prokaryotes, a pyridoxal phosphate enzyme catalyzes the selenophosphate-dependent conversion of serine to selenocysteine (39). The corresponding enzyme in animals has not yet been characterized.

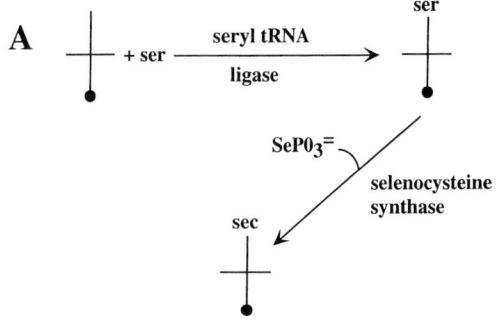

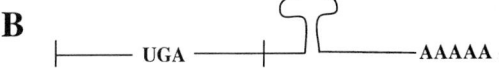

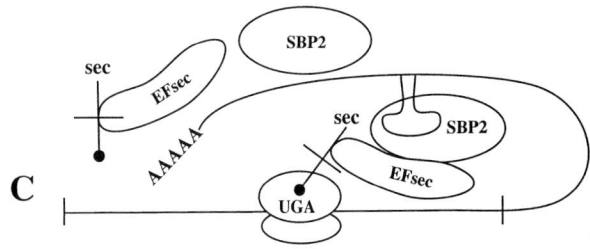

Figure 16.4. Selenoprotein synthesis. **A.** A unique tRNA with the anticodon for UGA, tRNA[ser]sec, is charged with serine. Then, using selenophosphate as a substrate, selenocysteine synthase (not yet identified in animals) converts the serine to selenocysteine, thus producing sec-tRNA[ser]sec. **B.** The mRNA of a selenoprotein has a UGA in the open-reading frame where the selenocysteine is incorporated and a specialized stem-loop structure, known as a selenocysteine insertion sequence (SECIS) element, in the 3' untranslated region. **C.** Two trans-acting proteins, SBP2 (SECIS-binding protein 2) and EFsec (elongation factor for selenocysteine), facilitate the recognition of the sec-tRNA[ser]sec by the UGA. SBP2 binds to the SECIS element and interacts with EFsec that has the sec-tRNA[ser]sec attached. This complex delivers the sec-tRNA[ser]sec to the ribosome for incorporation into the growing polypeptide chain.

Figure 16.4*B* represents a typical selenoprotein mRNA. UGA in the open reading frame codes for insertion of selenocysteine. A stem-loop structure with several conserved features is present in the 3′ untranslated region. This stem-loop structure is known as a selenocysteine insertion sequence (SECIS) element. Absence of the SECIS element or modification of its essential features results in the UGA in the open-reading frame functioning as a termination codon instead of designating selenocysteine insertion (40). The stem loop in prokaryotes is adjacent to the UGA codon (39). It binds a complex consisting of a unique elongation factor and sec-tRNA[ser]sec and approximates them to the UGA codon, thus facilitating selenocysteine insertion into the protein at that point.

Figure 16.4*C* shows that, in eukaryotes, two protein factors facilitate delivery of the sec-tRNA[ser]sec to the ribosome for incorporation into the growing polypeptide chain. One factor, SBP2, binds to the SECIS element (41). The other, EF_{sec}, binds to the sec-tRNA[ser]sec (42, 43). These two proteins presumably bind to each other to form a complex that delivers the sec-tRNA[ser]sec to the ribosome. Although this overall mechanism appears to account for insertion of selenocysteine, important details, such as how SBP2 and EF_{sec} interact with the ribosome, remain to be discovered, and it is also possible that additional protein factors will be found.

Excretion

Homeostasis of selenium in the body is achieved through regulation of its excretion. As dietary intake increases from the deficient range into the adequate range, urinary excretion of the element increases and accounts for maintenance of homeostasis (44). At very high intakes, volatile forms of selenium are exhaled, and the breath becomes a significant route of excretion. No evidence indicates that fecal selenium is regulated. Thus, under physiologic conditions, urinary excretion is the primary means whereby body selenium is regulated.

Most excretory metabolites of selenium appear to be methylated forms produced in the liver or kidneys. One study indicated that a large fraction of urinary selenium is a methylated selenosugar (14). A smaller percentage is trimethylselenonium ion (13). Selenium in the breath is largely dimethylselenide (13). The biochemical mechanism by which formation of these metabolites is regulated is not known.

BIOCHEMICAL FUNCTIONS

Twenty-five selenoprotein genes have been identified in the human genome by bioinformatics methods (45). The selenoproteins that result from expression of these genes are responsible for the biochemical function of selenium. However, most of the proteins have not been characterized well enough to identify their activities. Some of the better-known selenoproteins are discussed briefly to show the breadth of selenium biochemical function. New information on selenium function can be expected as the newly recognized selenoproteins are characterized.

Glutathione Peroxidases

The GSHPxs use reducing equivalents from glutathione (GSH) to catabolize hydroperoxides. Five selenium-containing GSHPxs, all separate gene products, have been identified in the human genome, as reviewed in the literature (45, 46). The cellular GSHPx, GSHPx-1, is the most abundant member of the group and is present in all cells. GSHPx-2, originally designated GSHPx-GI, is also a cellular enzyme but is found predominantly in tissues of the gastrointestinal tract (47). GSHPx-3 is present in plasma and milk (48). Phospholipid hydroperoxide GSHPx, GSHPx-4, is present inside cells and differs in several respects from other members of the group. It can catalyze reduction of fatty acid hydroperoxides that are esterified in phospholipids (49), and alternative processing can produce a form with a signal that localizes the protein to the mitochondrion (50). This enzyme has two special functions in the spermatozoan. It is a constituent of the mitochondrial capsule (51), and it is involved in chromatin packing in the sperm head (52). GSHPx-6 is present in the olfactory apparatus (45). It is a selenoprotein in humans, but the selenocysteine is replaced by cysteine in the mouse. Its function is not known.

Selenium deficiency decreases GSHPx activity. However, the effect varies according to tissue and enzyme. Brain GSHPx is relatively well preserved in selenium deficiency, as is GSHPx-4 in all tissues. GSHPx activities in plasma and liver are very sensitive to selenium supply and are used as indices of selenium nutritional status (see the later discussion of evaluation of nutrient status).

The GSHPxs catabolize hydrogen peroxide and fatty acid–derived hydroperoxides. They have generally been considered to protect cells from these oxidant molecules. However, many oxidant molecules have functions in metabolism and in signaling pathways. Thus, the GSHPxs have regulatory roles in the cell because they affect the concentrations of oxidant molecules. Moreover, the GSHPxs have different localizations and different substrate specificities that could be part of a regulatory strategy.

Iodothyronine Deiodinases

The iodothyronine deiodinases, types I to III, have all been shown to be selenoproteins (40, 53, 54). These enzymes catalyze the deiodination of thyroxine, triiodothyronine, and reverse triiodothyronine and thereby regulate the concentration of the active hormone triiodothyronine. Several thiols can serve as the reducing substrate for these enzymes, but GSH is likely to be the physiologic substrate (40).

Thioredoxin Reductases

Thioredoxin reductase is a flavin-containing selenoprotein, dependent on reduced nicotinamide-adenine dinucleotide phosphate, that reduces the internal disulfide of thioredoxin (55). Three isoforms have been identified. One is present in the cytosol and another in the mitochondrion (56). The third is expressed in the testis. These reductases provide reducing equivalents to a variety of enzymes. Many of them are oxidant defense enzymes, but others function in DNA synthesis and cell signaling. The hepatic activity of the enzyme declines in selenium deficiency (57).

Selenoprotein P

This selenoprotein was identified in plasma in 1977 but resisted purification and characterization for many years (58). It has now been purified (59) as well as characterized at the nucleic acid level (60). Selenoprotein P is an extracellular glycoprotein found in plasma and also associated with endothelial cells (61). Its cDNA indicates that it has a typical signal peptide for secretion from the cell and that its open-reading frame contains ten to 17 UGAs that designate selenocysteine incorporation (60, 62). Four isoforms of the protein have been identified in rat plasma. One function of selenoprotein P is to supply selenium to the brain to maintain normal neurologic function and to the testis for spermatogenesis (35, 36).

Selenoprotein P contains a large fraction of the plasma selenium, about 45% in a typical North American (63). The concentration of selenoprotein P declines in selenium deficiency and can be used as an indicator of selenium status (64).

Selenoprotein P has been associated with the oxidant defense properties of selenium. Selenium-deficient rats are susceptible to diquat-induced lipid peroxidation and liver necrosis; protection by selenium correlates with selenoprotein P concentration in plasma (65). Investigators have speculated that its endothelial cell location indicates that it protects those cells from oxidant molecules generated by inflammation or by xenobiotic metabolism.

Selenoprotein W

This selenoprotein was originally identified in muscle and was postulated to play a role in the development of white muscle disease, a selenium deficiency condition in sheep. It has now been identified in many other tissues and shown to exist in several forms (66). One form has GSH bound to it, a finding suggesting that selenoprotein W undergoes redox changes. Some evidence indicates that it can protect against oxidative injury. Selenoprotein W concentration decreases in selenium deficiency (67).

Selenophosphate Synthetase

Two selenophosphate synthetases have been identified in animals. One contains a selenocysteine residue in its primary structure, and the other contains a cysteine residue at the same position (37, 38). Because regulation of selenium homeostasis appears to reside at the level of this activity,

work on the function of these enzymes could reveal the mechanism of selenium regulation.

BIOLOGIC ACTIVITY

Deficiency of selenium leads to marked changes in many biochemical systems. Certain drug-metabolizing enzymes, including the cytochrome P450 system, are affected, some with activities increased and others with activities decreased (68). GSH S-transferase activities in rat liver, kidney, and lung rise in selenium deficiency. The underlying causes of these changes have not been established, but they are presumably related to decreases in selenoprotein levels. GSH metabolism is affected by selenium deficiency. In the rat, plasma GSH concentration is increased two to three times above the concentration in selenium-replete animals (69). This has been traced to increased synthesis of GSH by the liver and release of it into the plasma (69).

Changes in thyroid hormone metabolism were characterized many years ago in selenium-deficient animals (70) and are now explained by the discovery that the iodothyronine deiodinases are selenoenzymes. Other metabolic effects, such as changes in glucose metabolism, have not yet been traced to a selenoprotein (71).

Selenium deficiency in itself does not usually cause clinical illness in free-living humans or animals. Only when laboratory animals are raised through several generations on a selenium-deficient regimen do they exhibit pathologic changes from selenium deficiency alone. However, first-generation selenium-deficient animals exhibit heightened sensitivity to certain stresses; these are the basis of most naturally occurring conditions of selenium deficiency. One of those stresses is vitamin E deficiency. Simultaneous selenium and vitamin E deficiencies lead to numerous pathologic conditions in animals (3). Selenium-deficient animals are more susceptible to injury by certain chemicals such as the redox cyclers paraquat, diquat, and nitrofurantoin. These injuries are generally oxidative and may be related to decreased levels of the selenoenzymes that defend against oxidative injury.

Selenium can influence the outcome of infections. The increased virulence of Coxsackievirus B3 in selenium-deficient mice is described later. Additionally, potential selenocysteine-incorporation codons have been described in certain viral genomes, including that of human immunodeficency virus (72). This points to a viral strategy of appropriating the selenium of the cell and of disrupting selenium-dependent functions in it.

DEFICIENCY IN HUMANS AND ANIMALS

Combined deficiency of selenium and vitamin E causes liver necrosis in rats and swine, exudative diathesis in chickens, and white muscle disease in sheep and cattle (3). In animals fed a selenium-deficient diet containing adequate levels of vitamin E, signs attributable to selenium deficiency included hair loss and growth retardation, as well as reproductive failure in rats fed a deficient diet for two generations (73) and pancreatic degeneration in chicks fed amino acid–based diets severely deficient in selenium (74). This pancreatic atrophy in the chick, however, can be prevented by feeding high levels of vitamin E or other antioxidants (75). Pancreatic atrophy can be induced in chicks fed practical rations from a selenium-deficient zone of China, but this disorder is less severe than that seen with the amino acid diet, a finding suggesting the presence of partially protective factors in the practical diet (76). In one study, adult squirrel monkeys fed a low-selenium diet for 9 months lost weight and developed alopecia, myopathy, nephrosis, and hepatic degeneration (77). However, in another study, consistent signs of selenium deficiency proved to be more difficult to produce in rhesus monkeys, even in offspring born to mothers fed a selenium-deficient diet (78). Investigators hypothesized that elevated GSH transferase activity in the tissues of rhesus monkeys may account for their relative resistance to selenium deficiency.

Several lines of evidence indicate that selenium is a nutritionally essential trace element for humans. First of all, selenoproteins are present in the human being (45, 79). Second, favorable responses have been obtained after selenium supplementation of depleted patients undergoing long-term total parenteral nutrition. Finally, selenium deficiency has been found to play a role in Keshan disease.

In 1979, Chinese scientists first described in English the relationship of selenium to Keshan disease, an endemic cardiomyopathy affecting children and young women that occurs in a long belt running from northeastern to southwestern China (5). The acute form is characterized by sudden onset of insufficient heart function, whereas patients with chronic disease exhibit moderate to severe heart enlargement with varying degrees of heart insufficiency (80). The histopathologic features include multifocal necrosis and fibrosis of the myocardium. Keshan disease is related to a low dietary selenium intake and low blood and hair selenium levels (81). A series of intervention trials encompassing more than a million subjects has demonstrated the protective effects of selenium supplements (82). However, selenium cannot reverse the cardiac failure once it occurs. Marginal to deficient vitamin E status has also been observed in persons residing in endemic areas (83), and other complicating nutritional deficiencies (e.g., protein) may exacerbate the condition. Nonetheless, selenium deficiency appears to be the fundamental underlying condition predisposing persons to the development of Keshan disease. With improved economic and living conditions in China, the disease has disappeared.

Because certain features of the disease could not be explained solely on the basis of selenium status (e.g., seasonal variation), investigators suggested that a cardiotoxic agent, such as a virus, may also be necessary for the disease to occur (84). Scientists in Beijing provided evidence for a nutrition-infection interaction in the etiology of Keshan disease because a Coxsackievirus B4 isolate from a patient with Keshan disease caused more severe cardiopathology when it was inoculated into selenium-deficient mice than when it was inoculated into normal mice (85). Beck and colleagues (86) also found that a myocarditic strain of Coxsackievirus B3 (CVB3/20) produced more heart damage in selenium-deficient mice than in physiologically normal mice. Likewise, normal mice infected with a benign (amyocarditic) strain of Coxsackievirus B3 (CVB3/0) suffered no heart damage, whereas a moderate degree of heart damage was observed in infected, selenium-deficient mice (87). Virus isolated from the selenium-deficient mice infected with originally benign CVB3/0 retained its cardiotoxicity when it was subsequently inoculated into physiologically normal mice, a finding indicating that the avirulent virus had converted to a virulent strain by a genotypic change. Sequence analysis of the genome of this newly virulent virus revealed that six of the seven virulence-determining sites had been altered (88). To our knowledge, this was the first report of an effect of host nutritional status on the genetic composition of a pathogen. More recent research revealed a similar phenomenon with the influenza virus (89); that is, passage of a mild strain of influenza A through a selenium-deficient mouse resulted in a more virulent strain. The newly virulent influenza strain had 29 point mutations in its gene for the M1 matrix protein. These results with the CVB3/0 and influenza A viruses suggest that diet-driven mutations may be a general feature of RNA viruses.

Kashin-Beck disease is a preadolescent or adolescent osteoarthritis endemic in China that has been associated with poor selenium status (90). Necrotic degeneration of the chondrocytes is the most striking pathologic feature of this disease. Dwarfism and joint deformation result from these cartilage abnormalities. Aside from selenium deficiency, numerous other etiologic factors have been suggested for this condition (e.g., mycotoxins in grain, mineral imbalance, organic contaminants in drinking water) (91). Attempts to improve the clinical condition of subjects with Kashin-Beck disease by administering selenium have not been successful (92). However, it is still possible that selenium deficiency permits the development of the illness.

A major unresolved issue in selenium biology is whether the element has a beneficial cancer preventive effect in humans. The epidemiologic evidence linking low-selenium status and an increased incidence of cancer is conflicting (93, 94) and is often based on small differences in plasma selenium levels between controls and subjects who later developed cancer (95). Some animal experiments show that high levels of dietary selenium can protect against certain chemically or virally induced cancers (94), but examples exist in which selenium itself can stimulate tumorigenesis in rodent models (96).

Human nutritional intervention studies suggest that selenium supplements may have some beneficial effects against cancer. For example, a study of about 30,000 poorly nourished rural Chinese persons found that overall cancer mortality could be reduced 13% by giving a supplement containing selenium, vitamin E, and β-carotene (97). However, these results may not be directly applicable to Western populations of better nutritional status. In the United States, Clark and associates (98) reported the effect of selenium supplementation on development of basal or squamous cell carcinoma of the skin in persons with a history of this disease. A total of 1,312 patients, representing a follow-up of 8,271 person-years, was enrolled in this multicenter, double-blind, randomized, placebo-controlled cancer prevention trial. The intervention consisted of oral administration of 200 μg/day of selenium as selenized yeast or placebo. Although no effect of the selenium was seen on the primary end points of the trial (incidence of basal and squamous cell carcinoma of the skin), significant reductions were observed in several secondary end points, including a 37% reduction in total cancer incidence; 63, 58, and 46% declines in the incidence of prostate, colorectal, and lung cancers, respectively; and a 50% decrease in total cancer mortality.

The original report by Clark and colleagues was subjected to several reanalyses, prompted by a follow-up study showing that baseline plasma selenium concentration could predict the effect of subsequent selenium supplementation on prostate cancer (99). Only the persons in the lower two tertiles of plasma selenium concentration had a statistically significantly lower incidence of prostate cancer resulting from selenium supplementation.

The first of these reevaluations showed that the effect of selenium supplementation on overall cancer incidence also was strongly influenced by the participants' baseline plasma selenium concentrations (100). Persons in the lowest two tertiles (<1.56 μmol/L) experienced reductions in total cancer incidence with selenium supplementation, whereas those in the highest tertile showed a statistically nonsignificant 20% elevation in total cancer incidence. If the lowest and highest tertiles were compared directly, those in the highest tertile experienced an almost twofold, and statistically significant, elevation of cancer incidence compared with participants in the lowest tertile. The authors concluded that "these results provide little support for the use of 200 micrograms selenium/day to protect against cancer among average-risk individuals with plasma concentrations at or above the United States estimated average of 123 ng/mL [1.56 μmol/L]."

The second reexamination of the study by Clark and associates found that selenium supplementation caused a nonsignificant 26% decrease in the overall incidence of lung cancer (versus a significant 44% decrease in the original study) based on the original data set plus 25 additional months of follow-up (101). Subgroup analysis revealed a significant (*p* = .04) decline of 58% in lung cancer incidence among persons with baseline plasma selenium in the lowest tertile (<1.34 μmol/L). Those in the highest tertile (>1.56 μmol/L), however, had an apparent, but nonsignificant, increase in lung cancer incidence of 20%. The authors concluded that "selenium supplementation for chemoprevention of lung cancer should be targeted at populations with low plasma selenium concentrations."

The third reexamination of the study by Clark and colleagues found that selenium supplementation continued to reduce the overall incidence of prostate cancer significantly (102). However, the only men to benefit from selenium treatment were those in the lower two tertiles of baseline plasma selenium concentration (<1.56 μmol/L). The authors compared their results with those from the Physicians' Health Study, which showed that β-carotene reduced the incidence of prostate cancer only among those persons who had low baseline plasma β-carotene concentrations initially.

The fourth reexamination of the study by Clark and colleagues using the expanded data set continued to show a nonsignificant association between selenium supplementation and time to multiple basal cell carcinoma (103). However, statistically significant positive associations were observed between selenium supplementation and squamous cell carcinoma and nonmelanoma skin cancer. The deleterious effect of selenium on squamous cell carcinoma was most pronounced in younger participants, those who had never smoked, and those with baseline plasma selenium concentrations in the highest tertile (>1.56 μmol/L) resulting in 52, 53, and 55% increases, respectively.

Given the uncertainty generated by the expanded data set derived from the Nutritional Prevention of Cancer Trial (98), the advice from 1996 of Colditz (104) that it would be "premature to change individual behavior, to market specific selenium supplements, or to modify public health recommendations based on the results of this one randomized trial" would seem to be as germane now as it was then. Additional studies of selenium as a cancer chemopreventive agent are needed, and some are under way.

EVALUATION OF NUTRIENT STATUS

Selenium status can be evaluated by dietary and biochemical means. No known physical examination signs are associated with selenium deficiency.

Analytic Evaluation

Random urine samples are of little use in assessing selenium status because these samples are affected by dilution and by the selenium content of the previous meal (105). Blood selenium levels, which vary widely in different countries (16), are thought to reflect dietary intakes and selenium nutriture when they are evaluated under steady-state conditions. However, a direct correlation of dietary selenium with muscle levels or total body selenium has yet to be established (105). Average blood selenium levels reported in different areas of the United States range between 2.03 and 3.29 μmol/L (106), whereas extreme values of 0.10 and 95.0 μmol/L have been reported in areas of China affected by Keshan disease and endemic selenosis, respectively (17).

Plasma (or serum) selenium levels, which respond to selenium supplementation more rapidly than whole blood levels, are the most commonly used index of selenium status. Average plasma selenium levels observed in areas of the United States with marginally adequate (Maryland) or low (Ohio) levels of soil selenium were 1.70 and 1.51 μmol/L, respectively (107, 108). Levels less than 0.63 μmol/L are often seen in healthy residents of the south island of New Zealand (22). Serum selenium concentrations fall soon after birth and then gradually increase to adult values (105). Response to selenium supplementation was observed in a patient from New Zealand who was receiving total parenteral nutrition and who had a plasma level of 0.11 μmol/L (6). Measurement of plasma, serum, and whole blood selenium concentrations has become much easier with the introduction of graphite furnace atomic absorption spectrometry with Zeeman background correction (109). This procedure lends itself to large-scale epidemiologic surveys because no pretreatment of the samples is required other than dilution (i.e., no wet ashing is needed). This method was used to measure serum selenium concentrations of 18,597 persons in the Third National Health and Nutrition Examination Survey (1988–1994) as a way of helping to establish normal selenium ranges in the US population. The mean value of all subjects was 1.58 μmol/L, with fifth and ninety-fifth percentiles of 1.27 and 1.95 μmol/L, respectively (110).

Determination of total selenium in blood or blood fractions provides no information about the speciation of selenium in blood. The compartmentalization of selenium can influence the interpretation of blood selenium levels (Fig. 16.5). Intake of diets rich in selenomethionine can raise blood selenium concentrations markedly, because this form of selenium is not subject to homeostatic regulation. Moreover, serum selenium does not reflect the buildup of selenium in the skeletal muscle of animals when high levels of selenomethionine are fed (111). Hair selenium was used in China to evaluate selenium status (82), but this approach may not be valid in Western countries where shampoos containing selenium are used. Toenail selenium has been suggested as a convenient noninvasive index of selenium status (112). However, hair and nail selenium levels, at least in rats, are influenced by the form of selenium fed and the methionine content of the diet (111).

Assessment of selenium status by calculating the dietary intake from food composition tables is a risky procedure because of the wide variation in the selenium content of foods. Unless one is certain that the database used is applicable to the diet in question, the safest approach is

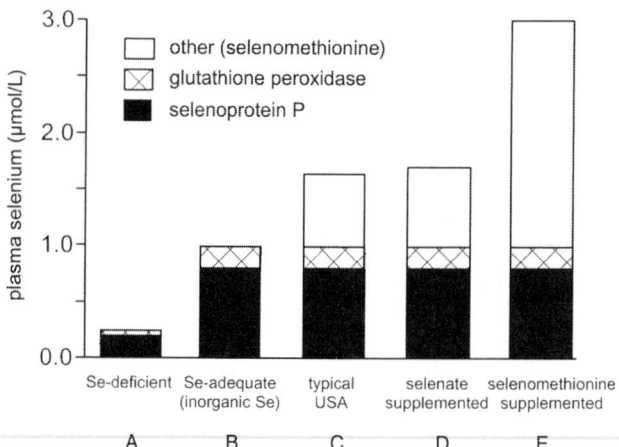

Figure 16.5. Pools of selenium in plasma proteins. The two selenoproteins in plasma are glutathione peroxidase (GSHPx-3) and selenoprotein P. Selenomethionine is distributed in the methionine pool and is present as such in most proteins. These three pools make up more than 95% of plasma selenium. The bar labeled *A* represents plasma from a Keshan disease–affected area in China (64). Bar *B* represents plasma from a selenium-adequate person who had consumed only inorganic selenium and therefore did not have any selenium in the form of selenomethionine (64). Bar *C* represents plasma from someone consuming more than the recommended dietary allowance of selenium, with much of it in the form of selenomethionine (63). Bar *D* represents plasma from the person in bar *C* after a month of supplementation with 400 μg/day selenium as selenate (63). Bar *E* represents plasma from the person in bar *C* after a month of supplementation with 400 μg/day selenium as selenomethionine (63). The selenium-deficient person has subnormal selenoproteins and selenium. All selenium adequate samples have the same selenoprotein contents. Plasma selenium concentration in selenium-adequate persons depends on selenomethionine intake.

direct chemical analysis of the diet. Nonetheless, it is possible to obtain reasonable agreement between calculated and analyzed selenium intakes if the appropriate database is available (113).

Biochemical Evaluation

Measurement of selenoproteins, such as plasma selenoprotein P and GSHPx, is useful in assessing selenium nutriture. However, neither value rises after the selenium requirement has been met. Beyond that point, values plateau and can only be used to indicate that selenium nutriture is adequate. Plasma selenium will continue to rise if increasing amounts of selenium are fed as selenomethionine (see Fig. 16.5). Thus, adequate selenium nutriture can be assumed if plasma GSHPx activity and selenoprotein P concentration are normal, or if plasma selenium concentration is 1 μmol/L or greater. Higher plasma selenium concentrations usually parallel selenomethionine intake.

REQUIREMENTS AND RECOMMENDED INTAKES

In 1980, the National Research Council established an estimated safe and adequate daily dietary selenium intake for adults of 50 to 200 μg (114). This recommendation was the first dietary standard for selenium and was based primarily on extrapolation from animal experiments because few human data were available at that time. A nutritionally generous level of selenium for most animals appears to be about 0.1 μg/g of dry diet. If it is assumed that humans consume 500 g of diet (dry basis) daily then, based on the animal results, humans would need 50 μg/day of selenium. Because of uncertainties about the bioavailability of selenium from different diets and possible individual variations in requirements, the dietary recommendation was given as a range.

Since the mid-1980s, numerous human studies have been carried out that have greatly increased our understanding of human selenium requirements. Some of the first attempts to delineate human selenium requirements more precisely involved balance studies, but comparison of international balance data revealed that people could maintain selenium balance over a broad range of intake (95). Therefore, the balance method proved not especially useful in clarifying human selenium requirements. Another approach was to conduct dietary surveys in areas with and without human selenium deficiency; that is, with and without Keshan disease. Such surveys showed that Keshan disease was not present in areas where the selenium intake was at least 19 and 13 μg/day for men and women, respectively (84). These values can be considered minimum dietary requirements for selenium.

Human selenium requirements have also been estimated by determining the dietary selenium intake needed to maximize the activity of the selenoenzyme GSHPx. In these studies, the diets of Chinese men of very low selenium status (residents of an area where Keshan disease is endemic) were supplemented with graded doses of selenomethionine (115). Plasma GSHPx activity tended to be greatest in those persons who received 30 μg/day or more of supplemental selenium over several months. That intake plus their habitual dietary intake (11 μg/day) yielded 41 μg/day as the lowest amount tested that caused a plateau of enzyme activity.

Maximization of plasma GSHPx activity was accepted by the US National Research Council as the basis for its RDA for selenium in 1989 (7). The Chinese value of 41 μg/day was multiplied by body weight and safety factors to come up with recommendations of 70 and 55 μg/day for men and women, respectively. Recommendations for children were extrapolated from the adult values on the basis of body weight.

Although North Americans should easily achieve the selenium RDA through consumption of a typical mixed US diet, persons living in countries with selenium-poor soils would have difficulty in attaining such intakes (see earlier section on dietary considerations). For that reason, an expert consultation group of the WHO produced dietary selenium standards that were considerably lower than the RDAs produced in the United States (9). Moreover, the WHO advisory group presented the values in

their report in the form of safe ranges of population mean intakes; this meant that their recommendations were applicable only to large groups of people and not to individuals. The purpose was to make the WHO document more relevant from the public health point of view (diet planning for large groups and/or diagnostic assessment of dietary intakes of populations). In addition, the WHO stipulated a two-tiered system of population mean intake based on two distinct levels of requirement: basal and normative. The basal requirement referred to the "intake needed to prevent pathologically relevant and clinically detectable signs of impaired function attributable to inadequacy of the element," whereas the normative requirement referred to the "intake that serves to maintain a level of tissue storage or other reserve that is judged . . . to be desirable."

The population minimum mean intake of selenium likely to meet basal requirements was given as 21 and 16 μg/day for men and women, respectively, with lower values for children and infants extrapolated on the basis of basal metabolic rate. These figures were calculated from Chinese epidemiologic dietary survey data, which showed the amount of selenium that would need to be consumed to protect against Keshan disease. The population mean intake of selenium that would meet the normative requirements was given as 40 and 30 μg/day for men and women, respectively. Again, lower values for children and infants were extrapolated on the basis of basal metabolic rate. These figures were calculated from Chinese experimental data, which showed the amount of ingested selenium that was needed to achieve two thirds of the maximum attainable activity of plasma GSHPx. This is in contrast to the RDA approach in the United States, which favored the dietary intake needed to achieve full activity of the enzyme. The decision to use two thirds of maximal GSHPx activity was based on the observation that "abnormalities in the ability of blood cells to metabolize hydrogen peroxide became apparent only when the GSHPx activity in these cells declines to one-quarter or less of normal." (9).

In the year 2000, the US Institute of Medicine published its *Dietary Reference Intakes*, a set of dietary standards consisting not only of the RDAs but also the adequate intake (AI), the tolerable upper intake level (UL; described in the section on toxicity), and the estimated average requirement (EAR) (8). These terms and their derivations are discussed in Chapter 104. Two intervention trials, one in China and the other in New Zealand, provided selenium EARs of 52 and 38 μg/day, respectively, based on the amount of dietary selenium needed to maximize plasma GSHPx activity. The 2000 Committee (8) took the average of the two EARs, 45 μg/day, and multiplied by 1.2 to account for individual variation to yield an RDA of 55 μg/day (Table 16.1). Because women of childbearing age are prone to Keshan disease, their RDA was kept at 55 μg/day despite their smaller size. No data were available to derive an EAR for children or adolescents, so

TABLE 16.1. CRITERIA AND DIETARY REFERENCE INTAKE VALUES FOR SELENIUM BY LIFE STAGE GROUP

LIFE STAGE GROUP	CRITERION	EAR (μg/d)	RDA (μg/d)	AI (μg/d)
0–6 mo	Human milk content			15
7–12 mo	Human milk + solid food			20
1–3 y	Extrapolation from adult	17	20	
4–8 y	Extrapolation from adult	23	30	
9–13 y	Extrapolation from adult	35	40	
14–18 y	Extrapolation from adult	45	55	
>18 y	Maximizing plasma glutathione peroxidase activity	45	55	
Pregnancy				
14–18 y	Accretion of selenium by fetus + age-specific requirement	49	60	
19–50 y	Accretion of selenium by fetus + age-specific requirement	49	60	
Lactation				
14–18 y	Loss of selenium in milk + age-specific requirement	59	70	
19–50 y	Loss of selenium in milk + age-specific requirement	59	70	

AI, adequate intake; EAR, estimated average requirement; RDA, recommended dietary allowance.

From Food and Nutrition Board, Institute of Medicine. Dietary Reference Intakes for Vitamin C, Vitamin E, Selenium, and Carotenoids. Washington, DC: National Academy Press, 2000. All groups except Pregnancy and Lactation are males and females.

their RDAs were extrapolated downward from young adult values using an adjustment for metabolic body size and growth. The criteria and DRIs for selenium by life stage groups are given in Table 16.1. Older and younger adults seem to have similar selenium requirements, and the aging process seems to have little effect on selenium absorption or utilization. Therefore, the RDA for elderly persons was kept the same as that for young adults. For infants, it was not possible to establish an RDA because "no functional criteria of selenium status have been demonstrated that reflect response to dietary intake." Rather, the "recommended intakes of selenium are based on an AI that reflects the observed mean selenium intake of infants fed principally with human milk." Thus, the AI for selenium is 15 and 20 μg/day for the first and second 6 months of life, respectively. The selenium RDA during pregnancy and lactation can be calculated by adding the amount of selenium acquired by the fetus or the amount of selenium lost in the breast milk, respectively, to the EAR for the nonpregnant, nonlactating woman. In pregnancy, it was calculated that the fetal demand is about 4 μg/day, thereby leading to an RDA of 60 μg/day. For lactation, the amount of selenium lost in the breast milk is 14 μg/day, giving rise to an RDA of 70 μg/day.

TOXICITY IN HUMANS AND ANIMALS

The level of dietary selenium needed to cause chronic selenium toxicity in animals is 4 to 5 μg/g (3). In livestock, chronic selenosis (alkali disease) is characterized by cirrhosis, lameness, hoof malformations, hair loss, and emaciation (3). Laboratory rats poisoned with selenium on a long-term basis exhibit growth depression and cirrhosis. The mechanism of selenium toxicity is not known, and the toxic effects of selenium may be modified by adaptation and certain dietary factors (16). No sensitive and specific biochemical test is currently available to indicate overexposure to

selenium (116). However, the plasma selenium level serves as an index of selenium intake when the form ingested is selenomethionine (see Fig. 16.5).

Public health surveys carried out in seleniferous areas of the United States failed to establish any symptom specific for selenium poisoning (117–119). Field studies conducted in Venezuela showed that the incidence of dermatitis, loose hair, and diseased nails was greater in children from a seleniferous area than in those from Caracas (120), a nonseleniferous area, but no differences were seen in the various biochemical tests performed. A report from China described an outbreak of endemic selenium poisoning in humans (17). The most common sign of intoxication was loss of hair and nails. In high-incidence areas, lesions of the skin, nervous system, and teeth were observed. Biochemical analyses showed a change in the ratio of plasma selenium to erythrocyte selenium at selenium intakes greater than 750 μg/day (121). Signs of selenosis (nail changes) were seen in susceptible patients at intakes of 910 μg/day or more, corresponding to a blood selenium level of 13.3 μmol/L or higher. No signs or symptoms of selenium overexposure were observed among residents of seleniferous ranches in South Dakota or Wyoming whose dietary intake was as high as 724 μg/day (119). However, an episode of human selenium poisoning was reported in the United States in 1984 involving 13 persons who consumed a "health food" supplement that exceeded the label declaration for selenium by 182 times because of a manufacturing error (122, 123). The total amount of selenium consumed by these persons was thought to have been between 27 and 2387 mg. Signs and symptoms of poisoning included nausea, diarrhea, irritability, fatigue, peripheral neuropathy, hair loss, and nail changes.

As part of its DRIs, the Institute of Medicine established a UL, defined as "the highest level of daily nutrient intake that is likely to pose no risk of adverse health effects in almost all individuals." For selenium, the adult UL was based on hair and nail brittleness and loss as the critical toxicologic end points. To calculate the UL, the committee used a data set provided by five Chinese persons who had recovered in 1992 from an earlier episode of selenium poisoning in 1986 (124). During the selenosis phase, these persons were consuming 913 to 1907 µg/day of selenium (calculated from corresponding blood selenium concentrations). Six years later during the recovery phase, the mean selenium intake of the same persons was 800 µg/day. The Chinese investigators suggested that the latter intake represented a no-observed-adverse-effect level (NOAEL), and, in fact, 800 µg/day was used to calculate the UL according to the following formula:

$$UL = NOAEL/UF$$

where UF is an uncertainty factor that encompasses all relevant uncertainties associated with extrapolating from the observed data set to the general population. To protect sensitive persons, a UF of 2 was used to calculate the UL:

$$UL = 800/2 = 400 \ \mu g/day$$

An intake of 400 µg/day was also suggested as a maximum safe dietary selenium intake by Chinese investigators familiar with selenotic episodes in their country (125). Moreover, the WHO proposed 400 µg/day as the upper limit of its safe range of adult population mean intake of selenium (9).

The Institute of Medicine committee also calculated ULs for infants, children, and adolescents. A NOAEL of 7 µg/kg was identified based on the lack of adverse effects in infants consuming breast milk containing 60 µg/L. Consuming 0.78 L/day of such milk would provide an average of 47 µg/day to a 7-kg infant or 7 µg/kg/day. The 7 µg/kg/day was then used to calculate ULs for all age groups through adolescence adjusted according to body weight. Because no reports of teratogenicity or selenosis in infants born to mothers with high but not toxic intakes of selenium have been published, the ULs for pregnant and lactating women were kept the same as for nonpregnant and nonlactating women.

HIGH-RISK CLINICAL SITUATIONS

Although selenium-deficient animals are clearly at risk to develop injury from oxidative stresses of various kinds (see earlier), it is not certain that people with low selenium status share those risks. The reason is that the deficiency that occurs in free-living human beings is not as severe as the one produced in laboratory animals. Plasma GSHPx activity is around 1% of control in selenium-deficient rodents, but it is 10 to 20% of control in selenium-deficient Chinese persons (83).

Nevertheless, Keshan disease occurs in selenium-deficient Chinese children, and the precipitating cause is not known. Chinese researchers have postulated that the selenium-deficient state makes the children susceptible to another stress, perhaps a viral infection. Thus, selenium deficiency of the degree seen in some parts of China can be considered to put the children at risk of Keshan disease.

No population in North America or in Europe has been reported to have selenium deficiency as severe as that seen in the persons in China. Tibet and Africa have low-selenium areas where people are selenium deficient, and conditions associated with thyroid abnormalities have been attributed to selenium deficiency in those populations (92, 126).

With the investigation of selenoproteins, the possibility exists that genetic causes of selenium deficiency will be found that could be treated by feeding supranutritional amounts of selenium (35). The tools for these investigations in human beings are available now.

Acknowledgment

The authors are grateful to Mrs. Kristina J. Allen for manuscript preparation.

REFERENCES

1. Moxon AL, Rhian MA. Physiol Rev 1943;23:305–37.
2. Schwarz K, Foltz CM. J Am Chem Soc 1957;79:3292–93.
3. National Research Council. Selenium in Nutrition, rev. Washington, DC: National Academy of Sciences, 1983.
4. Rotruck JT, Pope AL, Ganther HE et al. Science 1973;179: 588–90.
5. Keshan Disease Research Group. Chin Med J 1979;92:471–6.
6. Van Rij AM, Thomson CD, McKenzie JM et al. Am J Clin Nutr 1979;32:2076–85.
7. National Research Council. Recommended Dietary Allowances, 10th ed. Washington, DC: National Academy of Sciences, 1989.
8. Food and Nutrition Board, Institute of Medicine. Dietary Reference Intakes for Vitamin C, Vitamin E, Selenium, and Carotenoids. Washington, DC: National Academy Press, 2000.
9. World Health Organization (WHO). Trace Elements in Human Nutrition and Health. Geneva: WHO, 1996.
10. Gladyshev VN, Khangulov SV, Stadtman TC. Proc Natl Acad Sci USA 1994;91:232–6.
11. Neuhierl B, Böck A. Methods Enzymol 2002;247:203–7.
12. Stadtman TC. Annu Rev Biochem 1996;65:83–100.
13. Bopp BA, Sonders RC, Kesterson JW. Drug Metab Rev 1982; 13:271–318.
14. Kobayashi Y, Ogra Y, Ishiwata K et al. Proc Natl Acad Sci USA 2002;99:15932–6.
15. Kato T, Read R, Rozga J et al. Am J Physiol 1992;262:G854–8.
16. International Programme on Chemical Safety. Environmental Health Criteria 58: Selenium. Geneva: World Health Organization, 1987.
17. Yang GQ, Wang S, Zhou R et al. Am J Clin Nutr 1983;37:872–81.
18. Rayman MP. BMJ 1997;314:387–8.
19. United States Department of Agriculture (USDA), Agricultural Research Service. USDA National Nutrient Database for Standard Reference, release 16. Nutrient Data Laboratory Home Page, http://www.nal.usda.gov/fnic/foodcomp, 2003.
20. National Research Council. The contribution of drinking water to mineral nutrition in humans. In: Drinking Water and Health, vol 3. Washington, DC: National Academy of Sciences, 1980.
21. Pennington JAT, Young BE, Wilson DB. J Am Diet Assoc 1989; 89:659–64.

22. Robinson MF. Nutr Rev 1989;47:99–107.

23. Varo P, Alfthan G, Huttunen JK, Aro A. Nationwide selenium supplementation in Finland: effects on diet, blood and tissue levels, and health. In: Burk RF, ed. Selenium in Biology and Medicine. New York: Springer-Verlag, 1994:197–215.

24. Eurola M, Alftan G, Aro A et al. Results of the Finnish selenium monitoring program 2000–2001. Agrifood research reports 36. FIN-31600 Jokioinen, Finland: MTT Agrifood Research Finland, 2003.

25. Levander OA. Fed Proc 1983;42:1721–5.

26. Chansler MW, Mutanen M, Morris VC et al. Nutr Res 1986;6: 1419–28.

27. Levander OA, Alfthan G, Arvilommi H et al. Am J Clin Nutr 1983;37:887–97.

28. Thompson JN, Scott ML. J Nutr 1969;97:335–42.

29. Levander OA, Cheng L. Ann NY Acad Sci 1980;355:227–39.

30. Suzuki KT, Sasakura C, Yoneda S. Biochim Biophys Acta 1998; 1429:102–12.

31. Parizek J, Ostadalova I, Kalouskova A et al. The detoxifying effects of selenium: interrelations between compounds of selenium and certain metals. In: Mertz W, Cornatzer WE, eds. Newer Trace Elements in Nutrition. New York: Marcel Dekker, 1971:85–122.

32. Esaki N, Nakamura T, Tanaka H et al. J Biol Chem 1982;257: 4386–91.

33. Swanson CA, Patterson BH, Levander OA et al. Am J Clin Nutr 1991;54:917–26.

34. Van Dael P, Davidsson L, Ziegler EE et al. Pediatr Res 2002; 51:74–5.

35. Hill KE, Zhou J, McMahan WJ et al. J Biol Chem 2003;278: 13640–6.

36. Schomburg L, Schweizer U, Holtmann B et al. Biochem J 2003;370:397–402.

37. Low SC, Harney JW, Berry MJ. J Biol Chem 1995;270: 21659–64.

38. Guimaraes MJ, Peterson D, Vicari A et al. Proc Natl Acad Sci USA 1996;93:15086–91.

39. Böck A. Incorporation of selenium into bacterial selenoproteins. In: Burk RF, ed. Selenium in Biology and Human Health. New York: Springer-Verlag, 1994:9–24.

40. Berry MJ, Larsen PR. Endocr Rev 1992;13:207–19.

41. Driscoll DM, Copeland PR. Annu Rev Nutr 2003;23:17–40.

42. Tujebajeva RM, Copeland PR, Xu XM et al. EMBO Rep 2000;1:158–63.

43. Fagegaltier D, Hubert N, Yamada K et al. EMBO J 2000;19: 4796–805.

44. Burk RF, Brown DG, Seely RJ et al. J Nutr 1972;102:1049–55.

45. Kryokov GV, Castellano S, Novoselov SV et al. Science 2003; 300:1439–43.

46. Arthur JR. Cell Mol Life Sci 2000;1825–35.

47. Chu FF, Doroshow JH, Esworthy RS. J Biol Chem 1993;268: 2571–6.

48. Avissar N, Slemmon JR, Palmer IS, Cohen HJ. J Nutr 1991; 121:1243–9.

49. Ursini F, Maiorino M, Brigelius-Flohe R et al. Methods Enzymol 1995;252B:38–53.

50. Pushpa-Rekha TR, Burdsall AL, Oleksa LM et al. J Biol Chem 1995;270:26993–9.

51. Ursini F, Heim S, Kiess M et al. Science 1999;285:1393–6.

52. Pfeifer H, Conrad M, Roethlein D et al. FASEB J 2001;15: 1236–8.

53. Salvatore D, Bartha T, Harney JW et al. Endocrinol 1996;137: 3308–15.

54. Croteau W, Whittemore SL, Schneider MJ et al. J Biol Chem 1995;270:16569–75.

55. Holmgren A, Björnstedt M. Methods Enzymol 1995;252: 199–208.

56. Sun QA, Zappacosta F, Factor VM et al. J Biol Chem 2001;276: 3106–14.

57. Hill KE, McCollum GW, Boeglin ME et al. Biochem Biophys Res Commun 1997;234:293–5.

58. Herrman JL. Biochim Biophys Acta 1977;500:61–70.

59. Yang JG, Morrison-Plummer J, Burk RF. J Biol Chem 1987; 262:13372–5.

60. Hill KE, Lloyd RS, Yang JG et al. J Biol Chem 1991;266: 10050–3.

61. Burk RF, Hill KE, Boeglin ME et al. Histochem Cell Biol 1997; 108:11–5.

62. Saijoh K, Saito N, Lee MJ et al. Mol Brain Res 1995;30:301–11.

63. Burk RF, Hill KE, Motley AK. Biofactors 2001;14:107–14.

64. Hill KE, Xia Y, Åkesson B et al. J Nutr 1996;126:138–45.

65. Burk RF, Hill KE, Awad JA et al. Hepatology 1995;21:561–9.

66. Vendeland SC, Beilstein MA, Chen CL et al. J Biol Chem 1993; 268:17103–7.

67. Yeh JY, Gu QP, Beilstein MA et al. J Nutr 1997;127:394–402.

68. Reiter R, Wendel A. Biochem Pharmacol 1983;32:3063–7.

69. Hill KE, Burk RF, Lane JM. J Nutr 1987;117:99–104.

70. Beckett GJ, MacDougall DA, Nicol F et al. Biochem J 1989;259:887–92.

71. Fischer WC, Whanger PD. J Nutr 1977;107:1493–501.

72. Taylor EW, Ramanathan CS, Jalluri RK et al. J Med Chem 1994;37:2637–54.

73. McCoy KEM, Weswig PH. J Nutr 1969;98:383–9.

74. Thompson JN, Scott ML. J Nutr 1970;100:797–809.

75. Whitacre ME, Combs GF Jr, Combs SB et al. J Nutr 1987;117:460–7.

76. Combs GF Jr, Liu CH, Lu ZH et al. J Nutr 1984;114:964–76.

77. Muth OH, Weswig PH, Whanger PD et al. Am J Vet Res 1971; 32:1603–5.

78. Butler JA, Whanger PD, Patton NM. J Am Coll Nutr 1988;7: 43–56.

79. Awasthi YC, Beutler E, Srivastava SK. J Biol Chem 1975;250: 5144–9.

80. Ge K, Xue A, Bai J et al. Virchows Arch [A] 1983;401:1–15.

81. Keshan Disease Research Group. Chin Med J 1979;92:477–82.

82. Yang G, Chen J, Wen Z et al. Adv Nutr Res 1984;6:203–31.

83. Xia Y, Hill KE, Burk RF. J Nutr 1989;119:1318–26.

84. Yang G, Ge K, Chen J et al. World Rev Nutr Diet 1988;55: 98–152.

85. Ge KY, Bai J, Deng XJ et al. The protective effect of selenium against viral myocarditis in mice. In: Combs GF Jr, Spallholz JE, Levander OA et al, eds. Selenium in Biology and Medicine, part B. New York: Van Nostrand Reinhold, 1987:761–8.

86. Beck MA, Kolbeck PC, Rohr LH et al. J Infect Dis 1994;170: 351–7.

87. Beck MA, Kolbeck PC, Rohr LH et al. J Med Virol 1994; 43:166–70.

88. Beck MA, Shi Q, Morris VC et al. Nat Med 1995;1:433–6.

89. Nelson HK, Shi Q, Van Dael P et al. FASEB J 2001;15:1846–8.

90. Allander E. Scand J Rheum 1994;23:1–6.

91. World Health Organization. Kashin Beck Disease and Noncommunicable Diseases. Beijing: Chinese Academy of Preventive Medicine, 1990.

92. Moreno-Reyes R, Mathieu F, Boelaert M et al. Am J Clin Nutr 2003;78:137–44.

93. Willett WC, Stampfer MJ. BMJ 1988;297:573–4.

94. Ip C. J Nutr 1998;128:1845–54.

95. Levander OA. Annu Rev Nutr 1987;7:227–50.

96. Birt DF, Pour PM, Pelling JC. The influence of dietary selenium on colon, pancreas and skin tumorigenesis. Wendel A, ed.

Selenium in Biology and Medicine. Berlin, Springer-Verlag, 1989:297–304.

97. Blot WJ, Li JY, Taylor PR et al. J Natl Cancer Inst 1993;85:1483–92.

98. Clark LC, Combs GF, Turnbull BW et al. JAMA 1996;276:1957–63.

99. Clark LC, Dalkin B, Krongrad A et al. Br J Urol 1998;81:730–4.

100. Duffield-Lillico AJ, Reid ME, Turnbull BW et al. Cancer Epidemiol Biomarkers Prev 2002;11:630–9.

101. Reid ME, Duffield-Lillico AJ, Garland L et al. Cancer Epidemiol Biomarkers Prev 2002;11:1285–91.

102. Duffield-Lillico AJ, Dalkin BL, Reid ME et al. BJU Int 2003;91:608–12.

103. Duffield-Lillico AJ, Slate EH, Reid ME et al. J Natl Cancer Inst 2003;95:1477–81.

104. Colditz GA. JAMA 1996;276:1984–5.

105. Thomson CD, Robinson MF. Am J Clin Nutr 1980;33:303–23.

106. Allaway WH, Kubota J, Losee F et al. Arch Environ Health 1968;16:342–8.

107. Levander OA, Morris VC. Am J Clin Nutr 1984;39:809–15.

108. Snook JT, Palmquist DL, Moxon AL et al. Am J Clin Nutr 1983;38:620–30.

109. McMaster D, Bell N, Anderson P et al. Clin Chem 1990;36:211–6.

110. Niskar AS, Paschal DC, Kieszak SM et al. Biol Trace Elem Res 2003;91:1–10.

111. Salbe AD, Levander OA. J Nutr 1990;120:200–6.

112. Morris JS, Stampfer MJ, Willett WC. Biol Trace Elem Res 1983;5:529–37.

113. Welsh SO, Holden JM, Wolf WR et al. J Am Diet Assoc 1981;79:277–85.

114. National Research Council. Recommended Dietary Allowances, 9th ed. Washington, DC: National Academy of Sciences, 1980.

115. Yang GQ, Qian PC, Zhu LZ et al. Human selenium requirements in China. In: Combs GF Jr, Spallholz JE, Levander OA et al, eds. Selenium in Biology and Medicine. New York: Van Nostrand Reinhold, 1987:589–607.

116. Levander OA. Selenium: Biochemical actions, interactions and some human health implications. In: Prasad AS, ed. Clinical, Biochemical and Nutritional Aspects of Trace Elements. New York: Alan R. Liss, 1982:345–68.

117. Smith MI, Franke KW, Westfall BB. U.S. Public Health Rep 1936;51:1496–505.

118. Smith MI, Westfall BB. US Public Health Rep 1937;52: 1375–84.

119. Longnecker MP, Taylor PR, Levander OA et al. Am J Clin Nutr 1991;53:1288–94.

120. Jaffe WG. Effect of selenium intake in humans and in rats. In: Proceedings of the Symposium on Selenium-Tellurium in the Environment. Pittsburgh, PA: Industrial Health Foundation, 1976:188–93.

121. Yang G, Yin S, Zhou R et al. J Trace Elem Electrolytes Health Dis 1989;3:123–30.

122. Jensen R, Clossen W, Rothenberg R. MMWR Morbid Mortal Wkly Rep 1984;33:157–8.

123. Helzlsouer K, Jacobs R, Morris S. Fed Proc 1985;44:1670.

124. Yang GQ, Zhou RH. J Trace Elem Electrolytes Health Dis 1994;8:159–65.

125. Yang GQ, Xia YM. Biomed Environ Sci 1995;8:187–201.

126. Ngo DB, Dikassa L, Okitolonda W et al. Trop Med Int Health 1997;2:572–81.

127. Saito Y, Takahashi K. Eur J Biochem 2002;269:5746–51.

128. Esaki N, Nakamura T, Tanaka H et al. Biochemistry 1981;20:4492–6.

SELECTED READINGS

Hatfield DL ed. Selenium: Its Molecular Biology and Role In Human Health. Boston: Kluwer Academic Publishers, 2001.

Selenium. In: Food and Nutrition Board, Institute of Medicine. Dietary Reference Intakes for Vitamin C, Vitamin E, Selenium, and Carotenoids. Washington, DC: National Academy Press, 2000:284–324.

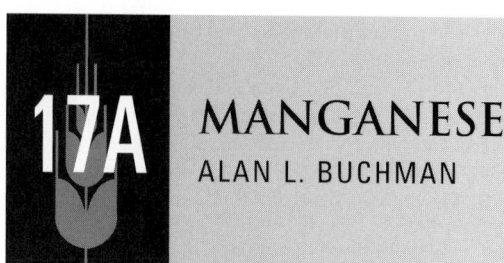

17A MANGANESE
ALAN L. BUCHMAN

HISTORY, CHEMISTRY, AND BIOCHEMISTRY 326
     Associated Enzymes 326
DIETARY CONSIDERATIONS .326
     Parenteral Nutrition 327
     Nutrient-Nutrient Interactions 327
ABSORPTION, TRANSPORT, AND EXCRETION 328
ANALYTIC METHODS 328
DEFICIENCY 329
     Human Deficiency 329
     Experimental Animal 329
TOXICITY 329
     Tolerable Upper Intake Levels 330

HISTORY, CHEMISTRY, AND BIOCHEMISTRY

Manganese (Mn) was first isolated as a free metal in 1774 following the reduction of its dioxide with carbon. It was first found as a constituent of animal tissues in 1913, although a state of deficiency (in animals) was not described until 1931 (1–3). Mn is a hard, brittle metal. Its oxidation state ranges between −3 and +7, although the most stable valence is +2 and the most abundant is 4+. Mn^{2+}, the only form absorbed by humans, is oxidized to Mn^{3+}, the oxidative state, over time in plasma. The human body contains approximately 10 to 20 mg of Mn, with 5 to 8 mg turned over on a daily basis. Its biologic half-life ranges from approximately 12 to 40 days (4).

Associated Enzymes

Mn is essential as a cofactor for the metalloenzymes superoxide dismutase (SOD), xanthine oxidase, arginase, galactosyl transferase, and pyruvate carboxylase (5). It functions as a constituent of these metalloenzymes and/or as an enzyme activator. SOD activity is depressed in Mn-deficient animals (6). SOD protects the cell against antioxidant processes, including radiation, chemical and ultraviolet light–associated injury. Mn binding to arginase has significant importance in nitrogen metabolism via the ornithine cycle (7). It hydrolyzes L-arginine to urea and

L-ornithine. Decreased arginase results in increased plasma ammonia in rats (8). Pyruvate carboxylase is involved in gluconeogenesis, but its activity appears minimally affected by Mn deficiency except in newborns (6, 9). Mn also activates numerous enzymes including various decarboxylases, glutamine synthetase, hydrolases, kinases, and transferases such as glycosyl transferases, the latter of which are involved in polysaccharide biosynthesis (10). Depressed galactosyl transferase activity may account for connective tissue defects observed in Mn-deficient animals (11). Activation of these enzymes by Mn probably involves Mn binding to the protein that induces a conformational change or binding to a substrate such as ATP. Mn is not essential to most of these enzyme systems, which can also be activated by other metals, except for glycosyltransferases. Therefore, at least in nonprimate animals, Mn deficiency can result in defective cartilage formation in animals.

DIETARY CONSIDERATIONS

Dietary Mn is found primarily in whole-grain cereals, legumes, nuts, and tea. Appendix Table A-22-b provides specific data on the Mn content of many foods. A 1982 study of 10,000 French households found that the average daily Mn intake was 2 mg/day, based on purchases of food designed to total 2000 kcal /day (8360 kJ/day) (12). Other dietary surveys in the United States, Canada, and New Zealand have shown intake to range between 2.0 and 4.7 mg/day, with vegetarians having significantly greater intake (13). Daily food intake ranges between 2 and 6 mg and up to 11 mg/day in vegetarian diets (13).

Orally consumed adult nutritional formulas have a range of Mn content from 0.7 to 1.2 mg per 237-mL (14, 15). The actual concentration may differ from that shown in the label (16). In a study of 116 milk samples from 24 lactating women in Champaign-Urbana, Illinois, the concentration of Mn was found to range between 1.9 and 27.5 µg/L (0.03 and 0.50 µmol/L) with a mean value of 4.9±3.9 µg/L (0.09±0.07 µmol/L), with infants consuming approximately 0.4 µg/kg/day (17). Bovine-based infant formula contains 30 to 75 µg/L (0.54–1.35 µmol/L) and soy-based formula contains approximately 100 to 300 µg/L of Mn (18) (1.8–5.4 µmol/L). Cow's milk has significantly more Mn than human milk (19). For adults, most

Abbreviations: AI, adequate intake; **Mn,** manganese; **MRI** magnetic resonance imaging; **SOD,** superoxide dismutase; **TPN,** total parenteral nutrition.

TABLE 17A.1. CRITERIA AND DIETARY REFERENCE INTAKE VALUES FOR MANGANESE BY LIFE-STAGE GROUP

		AI (mg/d)[a]	
LIFE-STAGE GROUP	CRITERION	MALE	FEMALE
0–6 mo	Average manganese intake from human milk	0.003	0.003
7–12 mo	Extrapolation from adult AI	0.6	0.6
1–3 y	Median manganese intake from Food and Drug Administration (FDA) Total Diet Study	1.2	1.2
4–8 y	Median manganese intake from FDA Total Diet Study	1.5	1.5
9–13 y	Median manganese intake from FDA Total Diet Study	1.9	1.6
14–18 y	Median manganese intake from FDA Total Diet Study	2.2	1.6
≥19 y	Median manganese intake from FDA Total Diet Study	2.3	1.8
Pregnancy			
14–18 y	Extrapolation of adolescent female AI based on body weight		2.0
19–50 y	Extrapolation of adult female AI based on body weight		2.0
Lactation			
14–18 y	Median manganese intake from FDA Total Diet Study		2.6
19–50 y	Median manganese intake from FDA Total Diet Study		2.6

[a] AI, adequate intake. The observed average or experimentally determined intake by a defined population or subgroup that appears to sustain a defined nutritional status, such as growth rate, normal circulating nutrient values, or other functional indicators of health. The AI is used if sufficient scientific evidence is not available to derive an estimated average requirement (EAR). For healthy infants receiving human milk, the AI is the mean intake. **The AI is not equivalent to a recommended dietary allowance.**
From Food and Nutrition Board, Institute of Medicine. Dietary Reference Intakes for Vitamin A, Vitamin K, Arsenic, Boron, Chromium, Copper, Iodine, Iron, Manganese, Molybdenum, Nickel, Silicon, Vanadium, and Zinc. Washington, DC: National Academy Press, 2001.

studies have shown that an intake of 2 to 5 mg/day is sufficient to remain in positive Mn balance, although there is significant individual variation. For example, men absorb less Mn, but they retain it longer than do women (20).

The dietary reference intakes of the Food and Nutrition Board, Institute of Medicine for Mn are given in Table 17A.1. From the criteria list, it is apparent that none of the data are based on quantitative biochemical data. Insufficient data were available for a recomended dietary allowance to be formulated; hence, the adequate intake (AI) value of Mn is indicated. For infants, the AI reflects the mean intake of Mn from breast milk. For adults, the AI was set based on median intakes reported in the US Food and Drug Administration Total Diet Study. Although there is no documented need for dietary Mn supplementation, absorption of Mn supplements is substantially greater in the fasting state (15). The tolerable upper intake levels for children and adults are given in Appendix Table A-2-h.

Parenteral Nutrition

For patients who require parenteral nutrition, the American Society for Parenteral and Enteral Nutrition has recommended 0.06 to 0.1 mg/day in adults and 0.001 to 0.15 mg/kg for children, depending on age (21). Contamination in total parenteral nutrition (TPN) components is low (~3 to 20 µg/day), with nearly all Mn in TPN therefore derived from the addition of a multitrace metal complex (16, 22). However, at the low end of probable requirements, such contamination could supply up to one third of the daily need. Data on various concentrations of

Mn in patients who received long-term TPN indicated that blood concentrations could be maintained at adequate levels at 60 to 120 µg/day (1.5–3.0 µg/kg) (23). However, human deficiency, even in the absence of Mn supplementation, has not clearly been described in the patient receiving TPN, and as such, supplementation may not be required. Mn supplementation should cease in the presence of biliary obstruction or cholestasis jaundice, because of decreased Mn excretion with subsequent accumulation in tissues (see the later discussion of toxicity).

Nutrient-Nutrient Interactions

The addition of large doses of Mn (four to eight times the AI) leads to a decrease in iron absorption by about one third (24). Mn supplementation leads to decreased iron absorption in iron-deficient animals, although this has not been demonstrated in humans (25). It has also been suggested that Mn absorption is enhanced in iron sufficiency and is decreased in iron deficiency (26). It is therefore possible that Mn is recognized by the intestinal iron transport mechanism, and factors that regulate iron absorption may also then regulate Mn absorption. In no other known situations does Mn ingestion has any affect on other nutrient, metal, or medication absorption. Adding calcium to human milk and increasing dietary phytate have been shown to reduce Mn absorption (27, 28).

Because of biliary excretion (29), balance studies are not particularly useful in the determination of daily requirements. Therefore, most estimates of absorption are based on whole-body retention after 10 to 30 days using ^{54}Mn.

ABSORPTION, TRANSPORT, AND EXCRETION

Dietary Mn is absorbed in the divalent and tetravalent state via both diffusion and what appears to be an active transport mechanism that is rapidly saturable (30, 31). Approximately 6 to 16% of dietary Mn is absorbed (mean, 9%), with a retention half-life of 8 to 33 days (16, 32, 33). Mena found that retention was 15.4% in premature infants at 10 days, but only 8% in term newborns and 1 to 3% in adults (34). The better absorption from human milk than from bovine milk or soy-based formula may be related to the decreased concentration of Mn in human milk or the increased binding of Mn in human milk to lactoferrin, the increased calcium content of bovine milk, and, for soy-based formula, the relatively large amounts of phytic acid (35, 36). No other dietary factors are known to affect Mn absorption, including ascorbic acid. Homeostatic mechanisms control intestinal absorption; lower amounts are absorbed during periods of significant exposure (37). However, the cellular mechanisms that govern absorption and the mechanism that controls absorption are unknown. Absorption is increased in patients with hemochromatosis (32), as well as in patients with iron deficiency (34). Mn absorption is decreased in the presence of a large calcium load (38). Mn sulfate is the most soluble salt and is therefore the form found in most nutritional supplements (39). After absorption into the portal circulation, Mn may remain either free or bound preferably to transferrin (40), but also to α_2-macroglobulin (41, 42), and albumin (43) to a lesser extent, all three of which are rapidly taken up by the liver.

In serum, Mn appears to be bound primarily to transferrin (42), and an α_2-macroglobulin (44), although binding to transferrin at least, does not appear to be essential for Mn uptake by extrahepatic tissues (45). The divalent form of Mn is firmly bound within the erythrocyte. The mechanism by which Mn is transported to and taken up by extrahepatic tissues has not yet been clearly elucidated, but it appears to involve internalization within endosomal vesicles as well as voltage-regulated calcium channels (46). Mn crosses the blood-brain barrier via carrier-mediated transport, although the specific carrier has not been elucidated (47, 48). Over time, Mn^{2+} is oxidized to Mn^{3+} in plasma (49, 50), possibly by ceruloplasmin (44), which is also bound to transferrin (44). The latter may be the moiety that accumulates in tissues (50). When Mn is oxidized, it becomes more tightly bound to transferrin (44).

The trivalent form of Mn is transported and is bound to transferrin, albumin, and the β-globulin transmanganin (51). It is taken up by the liver, pancreas, and kidney, although it is not clear that Mn^{3+} is stored in tissues except for bone, where 25% of the estimated 10 to 20 mg of total-body Mn can be found (52). Metabolically active tissues with high numbers of mitochondria as well as pigmented structures appear to have greater Mn concentrations (6). Animal studies have indicated Mn is then secreted into bile against a concentration gradient (53).

Excretion occurs primarily via the bile, and, as such, nearly all is excreted in the feces (29). Studies in the rat have indicated that approximately 11% of intravenously infused Mn that is excreted into the biliary system is reabsorbed in the intestine, although some variation may exist among species. However, as little as 1% of an intravenously administered dose of ^{54}Mn was present in the blood 10 minutes after injection (54). This finding indicates enterohepatic circulation of Mn and shows that all is not eliminated necessarily via the biliary tract (55). Very little Mn is excreted in the urine, and urinary excretion does not correlate with dietary intake (56).

ANALYTIC METHODS

Flame atomic absorption spectrophotometry is the accepted method for quantitation of Mn in biologic samples, although in the presence of low Mn concentration, graphite furnace atomic absorption is preferable (29). Inductively coupled plasma source mass spectrometry may also be used, although this technique is much more expensive (16). Whole blood concentration reflects current exposure, rather than chronic toxicity or deficiency (57). Normal whole blood concentration is 4 to 15 µg/L (73–274 nmol/L) when measured by atomic absorption, and it is increased in cirrhosis (58). Serum concentration of Mn is not generally useful, given that elevated intracerebral concentration may occur in the presence of normal serum concentration. In addition, serum concentrations are subject to error as the concentration may approach the limits of detection. Finally, even slight sample hemolysis may increase either plasma or serum Mn concentration dramatically.

Red blood cell Mn may also be measured because erythrocytes account for 60 to 80% of the Mn in whole blood and are a good indicator of tissue stores (59). When blood is obtained for analysis, the potential for contamination from Mn-containing disposable steel syringe needles must be considered; the error value may be as great as 80% (60). It is therefore appropriate to discard the initial sample obtained by syringe before obtaining blood for analysis. Ethylenediamine tetraacetic acid is the preferred anticoagulant because heparin may also be contaminated with Mn. Because the concentration of Mn in erythrocytes is some 25 times greater than in serum, contamination has a less significant effect on the measurement of erythrocyte Mn as compared with serum Mn. Care must also be taken to avoid Mn-contaminated water used for dilutions during analysis (61). A three-step purification procedure including deionization, double distillation, and re-deionization is advised to achieve true blanks. In addition, because of significant contamination potential from dust, the analytic apparatus should be covered.

DEFICIENCY

Human Deficiency

Human deficiency has not been well documented. One patient who was studied in a metabolic ward while he received 0.34 mg/day of Mn accidently for 17 weeks developed delayed blood clotting, hypocholesterolemia, weight loss, slowed nail and hair growth, and reddening of his beard (62). This was a patient who had been placed on an experimental vitamin K–free diet in an attempt to induce vitamin K deficiency. The Mn level in food was determined from food tables created before 1970, when analytic methods were not as accurate as more recent methods, and additional Mn from contamination was not considered. Unfortunately, neither blood Mn nor Mn loss was measured. Prothrombin time failed to respond to a 0.5-mg dose of vitamin K, and it responded incompletely to a 10-mg dose injected intramuscularly. In addition, the fall in cholesterol was only 20 mg/dL. It is not reported whether these findings, other than the prothrombin time, improved following resumption of a normal diet. Finally, only one patient in the study developed these characteristics and failed to respond to vitamin K supplementation despite identical experimental diets. Improvement in clotting ability occurred when a standard diet was provided without any additional Mn supplementation. Another case of proported Mn deficiency, reported in abstract form only, described a TPN-dependent neonate who developed irregularities in bone calcification as well as bone demineralization in the presence of very low serum Mn concentration (63). These abnormalities corrected reportedly following an unspecified amount of Mn supplementation over a 4-month period. Finally, Friedman and associates described clinical and laboratory findings in a group of seven male college students who were placed on a purported Mn-deficient diet in a research setting for 39 days (64). The serum cholesterol concentration decreased, although the subjects had been place on a low-cholesterol diet 3 weeks before baseline evaluation, for unclear reasons. The cholesterol concentration continued to decline, however, following Mn supplementation during the repletion phase of the study. *Miliaria crystallina* dermatitis developed in five of the seven subjects during the Mn depletion period and resolved following Mn supplementation. Plasma, serum, and whole blood Mn concentration did not change during the study. Based on measured Mn losses and calculated retention (difficult to determine accurately because of Mn's enterohepatic circulation), the investigators calculated the minimum Mn requirement to be 98.5 to 1037 μ g/day (mean, 743 μ g/day).

Experimental Animal

In various nonprimate animal species, Mn deficiency has been associated with skeletal abnormalities (10, 65), ataxia (66), decreased fertility (67), cornea degeneration (68),

and abnormalities in carbohydrate and lipid metabolism, including impaired insulin production (69) and decreased serum high-density lipoprotein concentration (70–73).

TOXICITY

Toxicity affects primarily the central nervous system and was first described in 1837 in Chilean Mn miners who were exposed to Mn-containing dust and developed *locura manganica* (Mn madness) (74). Workers with significant occupational exposure to Mn have been observed to exhibit a manic stage initially, with insomnia, depression, and delusions, followed by anorexia, apathy, arthralgias, asthenia, headaches, irritability, lethargy, and lower extremity weakness early. Eventually, progressive alterations in gait and balance as well as tremor and Parkinson's-like symptoms develop (including tremor and rigidity), consistent with Mn deposition in the basal ganglia. Symptoms may improve, but not completely resolve, and they may even continue to progress despite withdrawal from Mn exposure and improvement of magnetic resonance imaging (MRI) findings (75–77). More recently, the potential for airborne Mn toxicity has been suggested when Mn^{2+} is released in the exhaust fumes from methylcyclopentadienyl Mn tricarbonyl, a lead-replacement additive in gasoline used to increase octane. It is in use in parts of Europe and Canada (78).

Mn deposits primarily in the globus pallidus and subthalamic area, but also in the internal capsule and white matter, resulting in an increased signal observed on T1-weighted images of a brain MRI scan. However, these lesions may also be seen in other diseases including cirrhosis and neurofibromatosis type 1, as well as in patients with basal ganglia calcification. Mn appears to alter dopaminergic neurotransmission by some unknown mechanism. It has been postulated that Mn binding to dopaminergic receptors leads to autooxidation of dopamine with subsequent dopamine depletion and the formation of free radicals (79).

Several cases of possible Mn toxicity have been reported in patients receiving TPN at home, although not all patients were symptomatic (80–83). Whole blood concentration correlates with both MRI intensity of the globus pallidus and T1 value (84). Brain Mn deposition may occur even with a daily Mn dose of 0.1 mg (22). In some patients, the increased signal intensity in the globus pallidus dissipates following removal of supplemented Mn (although not Mn present through contamination) from the TPN solutions, although the Parkinson's-like symptoms often fail to improve in the absence of medical therapy (80, 81). Tremor has improved in other patients following withdrawal of Mn and decrease in whole blood Mn concentration (85, 86). The homeostatic mechanism that controls Mn absorption becomes irrelevant when Mn is intravenously infused. Despite the lack of well-demonstrated evidence that Mn deficiency occurs in patients who require long-term TPN, supplementation of the parenteral solutions has been advised (87). This supplementation is in addition to that contained in the various TPN components as a contaminant (88). It is currently unknown, however, whether Mn accumulation and brain deposition of Mn are direct results of Mn toxicity or are caused by a decrease in biliary excretion mediated by TPN and TPN-associated liver disease (89). Significantly elevated whole blood Mn concentrations have been described in patients with cholestatic jaundice (81–83). It has been postulated that TPN-associated liver disease may, in part, be related to Mn toxicity. However, given that Mn excretion is decreased in liver disease, especially cholestasis, and bile flow is decreased during TPN (90), it is likely the elevated Mn concentrations and brain deposition in these patients are sequelae of the liver disease, rather than its cause. Mn toxicity is discussed further in Chapter 99, on parenteral nutrition.

Toxicity from increased dietary intake of Mn has not been well described in healthy humans. No adverse effects have been observed in persons ingesting an estimated 13 to 20 mg/day of Mn (56, 91, 92), although blood levels may increase significantly in association with lymphocyte Mn-dependent SOD activity (56).

Tolerable Upper Intake Levels

The Food and Nutrition Board chose reasonable no-observed-adverse-effect levels of total Mn from food, water, and supplements: 2, 3, and 6 mg/day for children at ages 1 to 3 years, 4 to 8 years, and 9 to 13 years, respectively; 9 mg/day for ages 14 to 18 years and during pregnancy and lactation for adolescents; and 11 mg/day for adults more than 19 years old and for adults during pregnancy and lactation. Based on the Food and Drug Administration Total Diet Study, the highest daily dietary intake at the ninety-fifth percentile was 6.3 mg (by men aged 31 to 50 years) (12) (see Appendix Table A-2-h).

REFERENCES

1. Kemmerer AR, Elvehjem CA, Hart EB. J Biol Chem 1931;92: 623–30.
2. Orent ER, McCollum EV. Science 1931;73:501–6.
3. Orent ER, McCollum EV. J Biol Chem 1931;92:651–78.
4. Mahoney JP, Small WJ. J Clin Invest 1968;47:643–53.
5. Schroder HA, Balassa JJ, Tipton IH. J Chronic Dis 1966;19: 545–71.
6. Keen CL, Ensunsa JL, Clegg MS. Metal Ions Biol Systems 2000; 37:89–121.
7. Kuhn NJ, Ward S, Piponski M et al. Arch Biochem Biophys 1995; 320:24–34.
8. Brock AA, Chapman SA, Ulman EA et al. J Nutr 1994;124: 340–4.
9. Baly DL, Keen CL, Hurley LS. J Nutr 1985;115:872.
10. Staley GP, Van der Lugt JJ, Axsel G et al. J S Afr Vet Assoc 1994.
11. Baly DL, Keen CL, Hurley LS. J Nutr 1985;115:872–9.
12. Food and Nutrition Board, Institute of Medicine. Dietary Reference Intakes for Vitamin A, Vitamin K, Arsenic, Boron, Chromium, Copper, Iodine, Iron, Manganese, Molybdenum, Nickel, Silicon, Vanadium, and Zinc. Washington, DC: National Academy Press, 2001.
13. Couzy F, Aubree E, Magnolia C et al. J Trace Elem Electrolytes Health Dis 1988;2:79–83.
14. Gibson RS. Am J Clin Nutr 1994;59:1223S–32S.
15. Sandstrom B, Davidsson L, Eriksson R et al. J Trace Elem Electrolytes Health Dis 1987;1:33–8.
16. Stobbaerts RFJ, Ieven M, Deelstra H et al. Z Emahrungswiss 1992;31:138–46.
17. Krachler M, Rossipal E. Ann Nutr Metab 2000;44:68–74.
18. Stastny D, Vogel RS, Picciano MF. Am J Clin Nutr 1984; 39:872–78.
19. Lonnerdal B. Physiol Rev 1997;77:643–649.
20. Finley JW, Johnson PE, Johnson LK. Am J Clin Nutr 1994; 60:949–55.
21. National Advisory Group on Standards and Practice Guidelines for Parenteral Nutrition. JPEN J Parenter Enteral Nutr 1998;22:49–66.
22. Bertinet DB, Tinivella M, Balzola FA et al. JPEN J Parenter Enteral Nutr 2000;24:223–7.
23. Shike M, Ritchie ME, Shils ME. Clin Nutr 1986;34:804A.
24. Rossander-Hulten L, Brune M, Sandstrom B et al. Am J Clin Nutr 1991;54:152–6.
25. Thompson ABR, Olatunbosun P, Valberg LS. J Lab Clin Med 1971;78:642–55.
26. Finley JW. Am J Clin Nutr 1999;70:37–43.
27. Davidsson L, Cedarblad A, Lonnerdal B et al. Am J Clin Nutr 1991;54:1065–70.
28. Davidsson L, Almgren A, Jullerat MA et al. Am J Clin Nutr 1995; 62:984–87.
29. Ishihara N, Matsushiro T. Arch Environ Health 1986;41:324–30.
30. Garcia-Aranda JA, Wapnir RA, Lifshitz F. J Nutr 1983; 113:2601–7.
31. Bell JG, Keen CL, Lonnerdal B. J Toxicol Environ Health Res 1989;26:387–98.
32. MacDonald NS, Figueroa WG. UCLA Rep (US Atomic Energy Com) 1969;June 30:51–33.
33. Davidsson L, Cederblad A, Hagebo E et al. J Nutr 1988; 118:1517–21.
34. Mena I. In: Bronner FL, Coburn JW, eds. Disorders of Mineral Metabolism. New York: Academic Press. 1981 233–70.
35. Ekmekcioglu C. Nahrung 2000;44:390–7.
36. Davidson L, Almgren A, Juillerat MA et al. Am J Clin Nutr 1995;62:984–7.
37. Mena I, Horiuchi K, Burke K et al. Neurology 1969;19:1000–6.
38. Freeland-Graves JH, Lin PH. J Am Coll Nutr 1991;10:38–43.
39. Wong-Valle J, Henry PR, Ammerman CB et al. J Anim Sci 1989;67:2409–14.
40. Rabin O, Hegedus L, Bourre JM et al. J Neurochem 1993; 61:509–17.
41. Davis CD, Wolf TL, Greger JL. J Nutr 1992;122:1300–8.
42. Davidsson L, Lonnerdal B, Sandstrom B et al. J Nutr 1989; 119:1461–4.
43. Davis CD, Zech L, Greger JL. Proc Soc Exp Biol Med 1993; 202:103–8.
44. Harris WR, Chan Y. J Inorg Chem 1994;54:1–19.
45. Davidsson L, Lonnerdal B, Sandstrom B et al. J Nutr 1989; 119:1461–4.
46. Ruth JA, Garrick MD. Biochem Pharmacol 2003;66:1–13.
47. Ascher M, Ascher JL. Neurosci Biobehav Rev 1991:15:333–40.
48. Rabin O, Hegedus L, Bourren JM et al. J Neurochem 1993; 61:509–17.
49. Aisen P, Aesa R, Redfield AG. J Biol Chem 1969;244:4628–33.

50. Gibbons RA, Dixon SN, Hallis K et al. Biochem Biophys Acta 1976;444:1–10.
51. Cotzias GC, Bertinchamps AJ. J Clin Invest 1960;39:979.
52. Sumino K, Hayakawa K, Shibata T et al. Arch Environ Health 1975;30:487–94.
53. Klassen C. Toxicol Appl Pharmacol 1974;29:458–68.
54. Cotzias GC, Horiuchi K, Fuenzalida S et al. Neurology 1968;18:376–82.
55. Cikrt M. Arch Toxikol 1973;31:51–9.
56. David CD, Greger JL. Am J Clin Nutr 1992;55:747–52.
57. Tsalev DL, Langmyhr FJ, Gunderson N. Bull Environ Contam Toxicol 1977;17:660–6.
58. Hauser RA, Zesiewica TA, Martinez C et al. Can J Neurol Sci 1996;23:95–8.
59. Milne DB, Sims RL, Ralston NVC. Clin Chem 1990;36:450–2.
60. Versieck J. Crit Rev Clin Lab Sci 1985;22:97–184.
61. Neve J, Leclercq N. Clin Chem 1991;37:723–8.
62. Doisy EA Jr. Trace Sub Environ Health 1972;6:193–9.
63. Norose N, Terai M, Norose K. J Trace Elem Exp Med 1992;5:100–1.
64. Friedman BJ, Freeland-Graves JH, Bales CW et al. J Nutr 1987;117:133–43.
65. Smart ME. Vet Clin North Am Food Anim Pract 1985;1:13–23.
66. Erway L, Hurley LS, Fraser AS. J Nutr 1970;100:643–54.
67. Hidiroglou M. J Diary Sci 1979;62:1195–206.
68. Gong H, Amemiya T. Cornea 1999;18:472–82.
69. Baly DL, Curry DL, Keen CL et al. J Nutr 1984;114:1438–46.
70. Leach RM Jr, Lilburn MS. World Rev Nutr Diet 1978;32:123–34.
71. Everson GJ, Shrader RE. J Nutr 1968;94:89–94.
72. Amdur MO, Norris LC, Heuser GF. J Biol Chem 1946; 164:783–4.
73. Kawano J, Ney DM, Keen CL et al. J Nutr 1987;117:902–6.
74. Couper J. Br Ann Med Pharm Vital Statis Gen Sci 1837;1:41–2.
75. Rodier J. Br J Ind Med 1955;12:21–35.
76. Huang CC, Lu CS, Chu NS et al. Neurology 1993;43:1479–83.
77. Huang CC, Chu NS, Lu CS et al. Neurology 1998;50:698–700.
78. Kaiser J. Science 2003;300:926–8.
79. Mergler D. Can J Neurol Sci 1996;23:93–4.
80. Mirowitz SA, Westrich TJ. Radiology 1992;18:535–6.
81. Ejima A, Imamura T, Nakamura S et al. Lancet 1992;339:426.
82. Taylor S, Manara AR. Anaethesia 1994;49:1013.
83. Azaz A, Thomas A, Miller V et al. Arch Dis Child 1995;73:89.
84. Takagi Y, Okada A, Sando K et al. Am J Clin Nutr 2002;75:112–8.
85. Komaki H, Maisawa SI, Sugai K et al. Brain Dev 1999;21:122–4.
86. Nagatomo S, Umehara F, Hanada K et al. J Neurol Sci 1999; 162:102–5.
87. American Society for Parenteral and Enteral Nutrition (ASPEN) Board of Directors. JPEN J Parenter Enteral Nutr 1998;22:49–66.
88. Buchman AL, Neely M, Grossie VB Jr et al. Nutrition 2001; 17:600–6.
89. Alves G, Thiebot J, Tracqui A et al. JPEN J Parenteral Enteral Nutr 1997;21:41–5.
90. Messing B, Bories C, Kunstlinger F et al. Gastroenterology 1983;84:1012–9.
91. Greger JL. Neurotoxicology 1999;20:205–12.
92. Schroeder HA, Balassa JJ, Tipton IH. J Chronic Dis 1966; 19:545–71.

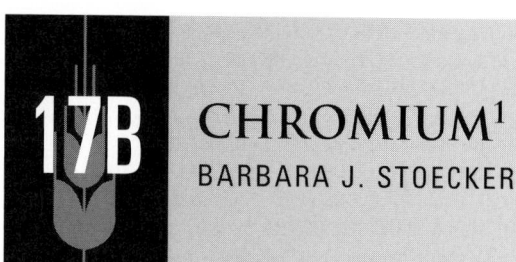

17B CHROMIUM[1]
BARBARA J. STOECKER

HISTORICAL INTRODUCTION .332
CHEMISTRY AND NOMENCLATURE 332
BIOLOGIC ACTIVITY 332
DIETARY CONSIDERATIONS .332
   Food Sources 332
   Bioavailability 333
   Nutrient-Nutrient Interrelationships 333
   Nutrient-Drug Interrelationships 333
   Adequacy of Intakes 333
METABOLISM 334
   Digestion 334
   Absorption 334
   Transport 334
   Storage 334
   Homeostatic Regulation 334
   Excretion 334
FUNCTIONS 334
KEY CAUSES OF DEFICIENCY
   AND THEIR MANIFESTATIONS 335
EVALUATION OF NUTRIENT STATUS 335
REQUIREMENTS AND RECOMMENDED INTAKES 335
   Humans 335
   Experimental Animals .336
TOXICOLOGY 336

HISTORICAL INTRODUCTION

In 1959, chromium was identified as an element that potentiates insulin action and restores normal glucose tolerance in rats (1). Subsequently, infants recovering from malnutrition responded to an oral supplement of 250 μg (4.8 μmol) chromium as chromium chloride with improved glucose removal rates. In a patient receiving total parenteral nutrition (TPN), Jeejeebhoy and colleagues demonstrated that infusing 250 μg (4.8 μmol) chromium as chromium chloride markedly reduced exogenous insulin requirements as well as lowering circulating glucose and free fatty acid levels (2). Other investigators confirmed the benefits of supplementation with chromium chloride in two additional patients receiving TPN. For citations to additional references concerning chromium, the reader is referred to several reviews (3–8).

CHEMISTRY AND NOMENCLATURE

Chromium (MW, 52 g/mol) occurs in multiple valence states, and marked differences based on valence characterize absorption, tissue distribution, and potential toxicity of chromium (9, 10). Most chromium in the food supply is in the trivalent state (9). Any chromium (VI) in food or water as a contaminant should be reduced to chromium (III) by the acidic environment of the stomach (11). Chromium (III) can bind with ligands such as acetate, picolinate, and niacin to form complexes.

Chromium (VI), which usually occurs as chromate or dichromate, is a strong oxidizing agent. Because of their oxidative ability, chromium (VI) compounds are irritating and are potential health hazards (7).

BIOLOGIC ACTIVITY

Chromium salts differ substantially in solubility (9), and these solubility differences are important in determining the absorption and use of chromium. In addition, the different ligands with which chromium (III) can be complexed may enhance or hinder both its absorption and tissue retention.

A "glucose tolerance factor" form of chromium was hypothesized originally by Mertz (9) to contain chromium bound to nicotinic acid and the amino acids glycine, cysteine, and glutamic acid. The complex enhanced glucose tolerance and was a low-molecular-weight, dialyzable compound. Vincent and colleagues characterized a low-molecular-weight, carboxyl-rich chromium-binding oligopeptide, which they named chromodulin. This compound contains glycine, cysteine, aspartic acid, and glutamic acid (8).

DIETARY CONSIDERATIONS
Food Sources

Chromium is widely distributed, albeit in small quantities, throughout the food supply. Whole grains and cereals contain higher concentrations of chromium than fruits or vegetables (12). Chromium may be added or removed during food processing (13). Refined sugars and flour usually are

---

[1]**Abbreviations: AI,** adequate intake; **EAR,** estimated average requirement; **TPN,** total parenteral nutrition.

lower in chromium than less refined products (12); however, acidic foods take up chromium from contact with stainless steel (13). Processed meats are quite high in chromium (12).

Bioavailability

Because of the very low chromium concentrations in biologic tissues, its bioavailability is difficult to assess in humans. However, the solubility of chromium salts varies, and chromium absorption is sensitive to physiochemical reactions within the gastrointestinal tract (9, 11). Several studies in rats have examined the tissue distribution of chromium-51 (^{51}Cr) that was chelated to different ligands. Anderson and colleagues (14) reported that chromium concentrations in kidney were significantly higher after feeding a complex containing chromium dinicotinic acid, diglycine, cysteine, and glutamic acid for 3 weeks than after feeding eight other chromium compounds. However, the identified complex did not produce such clear concentration differences in liver, spleen, muscle, lung, and heart (14).

High-fiber intakes raise concerns about the bioavailability of dietary trace minerals. One study in rats indicated that phytate impaired, and oxalate enhanced, absorption of ^{51}Cr. Two other studies in rats found no reduction in ^{51}Cr absorption with lower concentrations of phytate in the diet (3–8).

Nutrient-Nutrient Interrelationships

Chromium uptake is enhanced by simultaneous administration with ascorbate in both human beings and experimental animals. Offenbacher (15) administered 1 mg (19.2 μmol) chromium as chromium chloride with and without 100 mg (0.56 mmol) ascorbate and monitored plasma chromium concentrations for 8 hours. The plasma chromium concentration was consistently enhanced by the presence of ascorbate. In rats dosed with ^{51}CrCl$_3$, oral supplementation with ascorbate increased [^{51}Cr] in urine without reducing tissue concentrations, a finding that also suggests that ascorbate enhanced ^{51}Cr absorption (16).

Absorption of ^{51}Cr from ^{51}CrCl$_3$ was enhanced in zinc-deficient rats, and oral administration of zinc decreased ^{51}Cr absorption in zinc-deficient rats. Chromium absorption also was higher in iron-deficient mice than in iron-replete mice, as reviewed in the literature (4). These observations raise the issue of mineral-mineral competition for absorption.

Tissue chromium concentrations generally were higher in mice fed starch as a carbohydrate source than in those fed sucrose, fructose, or glucose (17). Nineteen men and 18 women consumed a diet containing either 35% of total calories from complex carbohydrates and 15% from simple sugars (reference diet) or a diet containing 35% of total calories from simple sugars and 15% from complex carbohydrates (high-sugar diet); the high-sugar diet enhanced urinary chromium losses in most, for a significantly increased mean excretion (18).

Nutrient-Drug Interrelationships

Some commonly used medications affect absorption of ^{51}Cr from ^{51}CrCl$_3$ in rats. Administration by gavage of large doses of antacids composed of calcium carbonate or magnesium hydroxide significantly reduced [^{51}Cr] in blood, tissues, and urine 6 to 12 hours after oral dosing with ^{51}CrCl$_3$ (16, 19). Aspirin and indomethacin, which block the synthesis of prostaglandins, increased ^{51}Cr absorption (19, 20), whereas oral dosing with 16,16-dimethyl prostaglandin E$_2$ decreased ^{51}Cr absorption (20). Total chromium administration was low (<180 ng [<3.5 nmol]) per rat) in these studies but was consistent with the low intakes required to demonstrate signs of chromium depletion in rodents.

Adequacy of Intakes

Lack of an appropriate indicator of status makes assessment of adequacy of chromium intakes problematic. Chromium balance was monitored for 12 days in a metabolic unit in two normal male subjects consuming a mean of 36.9 and 36.7 μg (0.71 μmol) chromium/day from the diet. Apparent net retention was 0.6 and 0.2 μg (12 and 4 nmol)/day, respectively, a finding indicating that the subjects were in equilibrium (21). Bunker and colleagues (22) conducted a 5-day balance study with 22 apparently healthy elderly people between 69 and 86 years of age. Mean daily intake was 24.5 μg (471 nmol), with a mean retention of 0.2 μg (4 nmol), again indicating apparent adequacy of less than 25 μg (<480 nmol) chromium intake/day. In another study, subjects with serum glucose concentrations lower than 100 mg/dL (<5.6 mmol/L) 90 minutes after an oral glucose load were fed diets containing less than 20 μg/day chromium for a total of 9 weeks without apparent change in their glucose tolerance (23). Their glucose, insulin, and glucagon values also did not change in response to 4 weeks of chromium supplementation. Conversely, on feeding the same diet to subjects who initially presented with glucose values between 100 and 200 mg/dL (5.57–11.1 mmol/L) 90 minutes after a glucose load, glucose, insulin, and glucagon sums (over a glucose tolerance test) showed significant reductions after 4 weeks of supplementation with 200 μg chromium as chromium chloride.

Studies with low dietary intakes (<5–15 μg/1000 kcal) are needed to determine an estimated average requirement (EAR). Additionally, studies in which diets are supplemented with doses such as 25 or 50 μg (0.48–0.96 umol) chromium, which would double or triple usual dietary intakes (~15 μg/1000 kcal) are needed to allow fine-tuning of dietary recommendations (7).

One well-conducted analysis of breast milk found the chromium concentration to be approximately 0.18 ng/mL (3.43 nmol/L) (24). Thus, exclusively breast-fed infants would receive approximately 130 ng/day (2.5 nmol) chromium (24). Based on this study, the adequate intake (AI) for infants 0 to 6 months old has been set at 29 ng/kg/day. The

AI for infants 7–12 months old is 611 ng/kg/day. No studies of the bioavailability of chromium from breast milk have been conducted in human infants.

METABOLISM

Digestion

Solubility of any mineral in food is affected by reduction potential, pH, and processing techniques, as well as by complex formation. Transition-series minerals, including chromium, can form hydrates that may become hydroxides as gastrointestinal pH is increased. The hydroxides may precipitate or form large aggregates with reduced solubility (9).

Absorption

Dowling and colleagues, as reviewed in the literature (4), used an in situ double-perfusion technique in which both the intestinal vasculature and the intestinal lumen were perfused to investigate absorption mechanisms. Amino acids in the test meal and the presence of either albumin or transferrin in the vascular perfusate enhanced chromium absorption.

Chromium-depleted guinea pigs dosed with less than 200 ng (<3.8 nmol) ^{51}Cr as ^{51}CrCl$_3$ absorbed a higher percentage of ^{51}Cr than did controls fed adequate chromium diets (25). In humans, Anderson and Kozlovsky (26) similarly reported that a higher percentage of dietary chromium intake was absorbed when dietary intakes were low, a finding that also indicates some homeostatic control of absorption.

Transport

Chromium is transported primarily by transferrin (27). Incubation of serum with iron reduced the amount of ^{51}Cr bound by transferrin (27).

Storage

Chromium is a bone-seeking element (28), and its uptake in bone appears to be rapid. Several investigators have noted that chromium accumulates in bone, spleen, liver, and kidney. O'Flaherty emphasized the need for physiologically based kinetic modeling to understand the behavior of bone-seeking minerals (28). Early modeling work using rats indicated three pools for chromium with half-lives of less than 1 day, approximately 1 week, and 7 to 12 weeks. A model in humans suggested four compartments, with different half-lives for diabetic and physiologically normal subjects in at least some of the compartments (29). The half-life of chromium in the compartment that turned over most slowly was 346 days; this compartment presumably is related to long-term tissue deposition.

Homeostatic Regulation

Studies in guinea pigs (25) and humans (26) indicate that chromium absorption is higher when chromium intakes are low. Specifically, in humans, Anderson and Kozlovsky (26) noted that when dietary chromium intakes reached 40 μg (0.77 μmol)/day, apparent absorption (measured by urinary excretion) dropped to 0.5% per day.

Excretion

Most ingested chromium is excreted in the feces. In balance studies, Offenbacher and associates recovered a mean of 98.1% of the dietary chromium in stools (21). At physiologic levels, excretion via the bile does not appear to be a major contributor to fecal chromium (5). Urinary excretion increased fourfold following a supplemental dose of 200 μg (3.8 μmol) chromium as CrCl$_3$ (30). In addition, tannery workers who were occupationally exposed to trivalent chromium had significantly higher urinary chromium excretion than controls, and their urinary chromium declined significantly during a weekend without exposure to chromium (31).

Increased chromium excretion induced by stress may be an important factor exacerbating chromium deficiency (32). Ascorbate-depleted guinea pigs had high circulating cortisol concentrations (33), and they excreted more ^{51}Cr from an oral dose of ^{51}CrCl$_3$ than did controls (33). Patients who had experienced physical trauma excreted more chromium than normal in urine (34). Furthermore, the urinary chromium excretion of distance runners was approximately doubled on the day of a 6-mile run, compared with a rest day (35).

FUNCTIONS

Chromium potentiates the action of insulin in vitro and in vivo. Vincent (8) proposed that a chromium-containing oligopeptide, called "chromodulin," binds to an activated insulin receptor stimulating its kinase activity. Mertz (36) summarized the results of 15 controlled studies in which subjects with impaired glucose tolerance were supplemented with defined chromium (III) compounds. In 12 of these studies, chromium supplementation improved the efficiency of insulin or had beneficial effects on the blood lipid profiles. The reasons for lack of response to chromium in the remaining 3 studies are uncertain; however, chromium depletion is not the only cause of impaired glucose tolerance. Furthermore, chromium status of subjects in supplementation trials still cannot be adequately assessed; a nonpharmacologic response to chromium supplementation would be expected only if the subjects were chromium depleted.

More recently, Althuis and colleagues (37) conducted a metaanalysis of randomized clinical trials assessing the effects of chromium on glucose, insulin, or glycated hemoglobin. These investigators found no association between chromium and glucose or insulin in nondiabetic subjects. Data from a large study with diabetic patients in China showed that chromium reduced glucose, insulin, and glycated hemoglobin (38, 39), whereas data from three small studies did not show significant improvement with chromium supplementation (39). Scientists from several countries have continued to report positive effects of chromium supplements on glucose control in diabetic patients (40, 41), but none have measured chromium intake or status.

Intense public interest has emerged in using chromium as an ergogenic (muscle-building) aid. This enthusiasm is surprising, given the equivocal effects on body composition seen to date in human studies (42, 43). Two studies used very sensitive techniques to estimate body composition. Lukaski and associates (44) supplemented 36 young men with placebo, chromium chloride, or chromium picolinate as these subjects participated in an 8-week weight-training program. Fat-free mass, mineral-free mass, and body fat were estimated by dual x-ray absorptiometry. Although resistive exercise increased lean body mass, no effect of chromium supplementation on either fat-free mass or body fat was found. Hallmark and colleagues (45) likewise supplemented 16 untrained healthy men undergoing a 12-week resistive-exercise program with 200 μg (3.8 μmol)/day chromium as picolinate or with placebo. Based on food records, these men were consuming approximately 36 μg (0.7 μmol) chromium/day from their diets. The authors assessed body composition with hydrodensitometry and found no significant differences in lean body mass, percentage body fat, or strength measurements as a result of chromium supplementation.

Chromium supplementation trials have also been conducted in rapidly growing food animals. Barrows were fed a fortified, corn-soybean meal basal diet supplemented with 0 or 200 μg (3.8 μmol)/kg diet of chromium as chromium picolinate. In this study, addition of chromium picolinate to the diet increased the accretion of muscle tissue and decreased the total gain of fat (46). In a study using gilts of a similar size, basal diets were supplemented with 300 μg (5.8 μmol) chromium/kg diet as chromium picolinate, and recombinant porcine somatotropin was administered to half of the pigs in a 2 × 2 factorial design. All gilts treated with recombinant porcine somatotropin demonstrated better growth than controls. Diets supplemented with chromium picolinate, however, produced no differences in growth performance (47).

Effects of chromium on morbidity in livestock stressed by shipping or disease exposure have received attention among producers. Chromium significantly decreased serum cortisol (48, 49) and increased serum immunoglobulin M and total immunoglobulins in stressed and growing calves (49). Supplemental chromium also lowered serum cortisol after a disease challenge (48, 49).

KEY CAUSES OF DEFICIENCY AND THEIR MANIFESTATIONS

Chromium deficiency was reported in two patients who did not receive supplemental chromium in their TPN solutions. The first, a female patient who had received

TPN for more than 3.5 years, developed unexplained weight loss and peripheral neuropathy. Glucose removal from the plasma was impaired, and her respiratory quotient was low, findings indicating preferential use of fat for fuel. Addition of 250 μg (4.8 μmol) chromium to the daily TPN infusate for 2 weeks restored the glucose removal rate and increased her respiratory quotient (2). The second patient developed severe hyperglycemia and rapid weight loss after 5 months of TPN therapy without added chro-mium. Several other cases have also been discussed (3–8). Some TPN solutions contain a fairly high basal level of chromium (34, 50), and some patients who receive TPN may be exposed to excessive amounts of trivalent chromium, primarily as a contaminant from amino acids in the solutions. Chromium absorption from oral doses is so low, that only 0.5–2.0%, an intravenous dose of 20 μg can be considered equivalent to 1000–4000 μg of oral intake; this suggests the need for restraint in adding chromium to TPN solutions.

Nielsen (32) hypothesized that alterations in metabolism secondary to malnutrition, disease, injury, or stress may be responsible for deficiencies of the ultratrace elements. Some studies in animals and humans lend support to his hypothesis. Trauma patients excreted more urinary chromium than physiologically normal controls (34). Strenuous exercise causes "dumping" of chromium in the urine (35). Guinea pigs excreted more ^{51}Cr from $^{51}CrCl_3$ when they were stressed by ascorbate depletion (25). Many of the studies in farm animals that report beneficial effects of chromium supplementation also involved some type of stress: shipping, exposure to infectious agents, crowding, or high temperatures.

Finally, some commonly used medications may interfere with chromium absorption. The long-term effects of these medications have not been investigated in relation to chromium; however, studies have indicated negative effects of antacids on iron and copper status.

EVALUATION OF NUTRIENT STATUS

Currently, no reliable indicator of chromium status exists. Chromium in blood is very difficult to measure because the extremely low concentrations approach the detection limits of even sensitive instruments. Furthermore, serum or plasma chromium levels may not be in equilibrium with other body pools. No enzyme has been identified for which chromium is specific. Thus, both nutritional measures and clinical assessments are difficult. In the absence of reliable indicators of chromium status, considerable diversity no doubt exists in the chromium status of patients in supplementation trials.

REQUIREMENTS AND RECOMMENDED INTAKES

Humans

Data were insufficient to set an EAR or recommended dietary allowance for chromium. Therefore, an AI was established based on estimated mean intakes (7).

Anderson and Kozlovsky (26) determined the chromium content of self-selected diets of 10 male and 22 female subjects for 7 consecutive days. The 7-day average intake for male subjects was 33 μg (0.63 μmol)/day (range, 22–48 μg), and for female subjects it was 25 μg (0.48 μmol)/day, (range, 13–36 μg). These investigators observed that when dietary chromium intake was 10 μg (0.19 μmol), urinary excretion (representing absorption) was approximately 2%. With increasing intake to 40 μg (0.77 μmol), however, chromium absorption decreased to 0.5% (26). For healthy adults, the average urinary chromium excretion is approximately 0.2 μg/day (3–8).

A mean chromium intake of 13.4 μg/1000 kcal was used as a basis for deriving AI estimates for chromium for adults ages 19 through 50 years, resulting in an AI of 35 μg/day for men and 25 μg/day for women (7). Based on median energy intakes for men and women 50 through 70 years of age of 2100 and 1500 kcal/day, respectively (51), the AI for chromium for adults ages 51 and older was set at 30 μg/day for men and 20 μg/day for women (7). (See Appendix Tables A-2-a through—h for more DRI data.)

Experimental Animals

In experimental animals, dietary concentrations lower than 50 μg (0.96 μmol) chromium/kg diet are necessary to produce symptoms associated with chromium deficiency. The American Institute of Nutrition-93 diet includes addition of chromium at the level of 1 mg (19.2 μmol) chromium/kg diet as chromium potassium sulfate and defines it as a "potentially beneficial mineral element" (52). Many experimental animals obtain enough chromium in their unsupplemented feed, however, to prevent well-recognized symptoms of deficiency.

TOXICOLOGY

Risk assessment for chromium is affected by its oxidation state. Trivalent chromium, which is the predominant form in the food supply, has low oral toxicity, at least partially because it is very poorly absorbed (7, 9).

A report by Stearns and colleagues (53) generated some controversy about the safety of chromium (III) supplements. Relatively high concentrations of chromium picolinate, chromium chloride, or chromium nicotinate were added to Chinese hamster ovary cells in culture. Chromium picolinate and picolinic acid tested positive in an assay used to predict mutagenicity, whereas chromium nicotinate and chromium chloride did not (53). Many supplementation trials have been conducted in human subjects with chromium chloride and with chelated chromium compounds without reports of toxicity; however, some groups recently suggested that chromium (III) picolinate produces significantly more oxidative stress and potential DNA damage than other chromium supplements (42, 54). The Panel on Micronutrients of the Food and Nutrition Board found insufficient toxicity data to establish an upper level recommendation for soluble chromium III salts (7). However, because of the current widespread use of chromium supplements, more research would be appropriate to evaluate the risk and cost-to-benefit ratios of trivalent chromium supplements.

In contrast, chromium (VI), a product of manufacturing, is included in health risk assessments at Environmental Protection Agency superfund sites. Fortunately, certain foods and substances in our gastrointestinal tract have substantial capacity for reduction of chromium (VI) to chromium (III) (6, 10, 11). For example, Kuykendall and associates (55) gave volunteers 5 mg (96 μmol) of chromium (VI), alone or fully reduced to chromium (III) with orange juice (before ingestion). These investigators demonstrated no DNA-protein cross-links in leukocytes resulting from acute ingestion of either chromium (III) or (VI) and suggested that all the chromium (VI) was reduced to chromium (III) intragastrically before absorption (55). Data from such human trials have been used to formulate a physiologically based human kinetic model for ingestion of chromium (III) and chromium (VI) (10).

To evaluate the in vivo genotoxicity of chromium (VI) further, Mirsalis and colleagues (56) administered chromium (VI) to mice at concentrations of 1, 5, or 20 mg (19.2, 96, or 384 μmol)/L in drinking water. These levels represent the range from a relevant human exposure level to the upper limit of palatability in rodents. These investigators concluded that either the animals had sufficient reductive capacity in their gastrointestinal tracts to prevent uptake of chromium (VI) or even these high doses were insufficient to exert a genotoxic effect via oral administration (56).

Route of exposure has an impact on toxicity. Chromium (VI) is known to be a human pulmonary carcinogen. Stainless steel welding may be the most common source of occupational exposure to chromium. Various research groups have suggested that products formed during intracellular reduction of chromium (VI) to chromium (III) may be responsible for the DNA damage ascribed to chromium (VI) (54, 57).

REFERENCES

1. Schwarz K, Mertz W. Arch Biochem Biophys 1959;85:292–5.
2. Jeejeebhoy KN, Chu RC, Marliss EB et al. Am J Clin Nutr 1977; 30:531–8.
3. Anderson RA. Chromium. In: Mertz W, ed. Trace Elements in Human and Animal Nutrition. New York: Academic Press, 1987: 225–44.
4. Offenbacher EG, Pi-Sunyer FX, Stoecker BJ. Chromium. In: O'Dell BL, Sunde RA, eds. Handbook of Nutritionally Essential Mineral Elements. New York: Marcel Dekker, 1997:389–411.
5. Stoecker BJ. Chromium. In: Bowman BA, Russell RM, eds. Present Knowledge in Nutrition. Washington, DC: International Life Sciences Institute, 2001:366–72.
6. Stoecker BJ. Chromium. In: Merian E, Anke M, Ihnat M et al., eds. Elements and Their Compounds in the Environment. Weinheim: Wiley-VCH Verlag, 2004:709–29.
7. Panel on Micronutrients, Food and Nutrition Board, Institute of Medicine. Chromium. In: Dietary Reference Intakes for Vitamin A,

Vitamin K, Arsenic, Boron, Chromium, Copper, Iodine, Iron, Manganese, Molybdenum, Nickel, Silicon, Vanadium, and Zinc. Washington, DC: National Academy Press, 2001:197–223.

8. Vincent JB. Proc Nutr Soc 2004;63:41–7.

9. Mertz W. Physiol Rev 1969;49:163–239.

10. O'Flaherty EJ, Kerger BD, Hays SM et al. Toxicol Sci 2001;60:196–213.

11. De Flora S, Camoirano A, Bagnasco M et al. Carcinogenesis 1997;18:531–7.

12. Anderson RA, Bryden NA, Polansky MM. Biol Trace Elem Res 1992;32:117–21.

13. Offenbacher EG, Pi-Sunyer FX. J Agric Food Chem 1983;31:89–92.

14. Anderson RA, Bryden NA, Polansky MM et al. J Trace Elem Exp Med 1996;9:11–25.

15. Offenbacher EG. Trace Elem Elect 1994;11:178–81.

16. Seaborn CD, Stoecker BJ. Nutr Res 1990;10:1401–7.

17. Seaborn CD, Stoecker BJ. J Nutr 1989;119:1444–51.

18. Kozlovsky AS, Moser PB, Reiser S et al. Metabolism 1986;35:515–8.

19. Davis ML, Seaborn CD, Stoecker BJ. Nutr Res 1995;15:201–10.

20. Kamath SM, Stoecker BJ, Davis-Whitenack ML et al. J Nutr 1997;127:478–82.

21. Offenbacher EG, Spencer H, Dowling HJ et al. Am J Clin Nutr 1986;44:77–82.

22. Bunker VW, Lawson MS, Delves HT et al. Am J Clin Nutr 1984;39:797–802.

23. Anderson RA, Polansky MM, Bryden NA et al. Am J Clin Nutr 1991;54:909–16.

24. Anderson RA, Bryden NA, Patterson KY et al. Am J Clin Nutr 1993;57:519–23.

25. Seaborn CD, Stoecker BJ. Nutr Res 1992;12:1229–34.

26. Anderson RA, Kozlovsky AS. Am J Clin Nutr 1985;41:1177–83.

27. Hopkins LL Jr, Schwarz K. Biochim Biophys Acta 1964;90:484–91.

28. O'Flaherty EJ. Toxicol Lett 1995;82-83:367–72.

29. Do Canto OM, Sargent T III, Liehn JC. Chromium (III) metabolism in diabetic patients. In: Sive Subrananian KN, Wastney ME, eds. Kinetic Models of Trace Element and Mineral Metabolism. Boca Raton, FL: CRC Press, 1995:416.

30. Anderson RA, Polansky MM, Bryden NA et al. Am J Clin Nutr 1982;36:1184–93.

31. Randall JA, Gibson RS. Proc Soc Exp Biol Med 1987;185:16–23.

32. Nielsen FH. Nutr Rev 1988;46:337–41.

33. Seaborn CD, Cheng NZ, Adeleye B et al. Biol Trace Elem Res 1994;41:279–94.

34. Borel JS, Majerus TC, Polansky MM et al. Biol Trace Elem Res 1984;6:317–26.

35. Anderson RA, Polansky MM, Bryden NA. Biol Trace Elem Res 1984;6:327–36.

36. Mertz W. J Nutr 1993;123:626–33.

37. Althuis MD, Jordan NE, Ludington EA et al. Am J Clin Nutr 2002;76:148–55.

38. Anderson RA, Cheng NZ, Bryden NA et al. Diabetes 1997;46:1786–91.

39. Cheng NZ, Zhu XX, Shi HL et al. J Trace Elem Exp Med 1999;12:55–60.

40. Ghosh D, Bhattacharya B, Mukherjee B et al. J Nutr Biochem 2002;13:690–7.

41. Bahijri SMA, Mufti AMB. Biol Trace Elem Res 2002;85:97–109.

42. Vincent JB. Sports Med 2003;33:213–30.

43. Lukaski HC. Annu Rev Nutr 1999;19:279–302.

44. Lukaski HC, Bolonchuk WW, Siders WA et al. Am J Clin Nutr 1996;63:954–65.

45. Hallmark MA, Reynolds TH, DeSouza CA et al. Med Sci Sports Exerc 1996;28:139–44.

46. Mooney KW, Cromwell GL. J Anim Sci 1995;73:3351–7.

47. Myers MJ, Farrell DE, Evock-Clover CM et al. Pathobiology 1995;63:283–7.

48. Kegley EB, Spears JW, Brown TT Jr. J Dairy Sci 1996;79:1278–83.

49. Chang X, Mowat DN. J Anim Sci 1992;70:559–65.

50. Leung FY, Galbraith LV. Biol Trace Elem Res 1995;50:221–8.

51. Briefel RR. Am J Clin Nutr 1994;59[Suppl]:164S–7S.

52. Reeves PG, Nielsen FH, Fahey GC Jr. J Nutr 1993;123:1939–51.

53. Stearns DM, Wise JP, Sr., Patierno SR et al. FASEB J 1995;9:1643–9.

54. Bagchi D, Stohs SJ, Downs BW et al. Toxicology 2002;180:5–22.

55. Kuykendall JR, Kerger BD, Jarvi EJ et al. Carcinogenesis 1996;17:1971–7.

56. Mirsalis JC, Hamilton CM, O'Laughlin KG et al. Environ Mol Mutagen 1996;28:60–3.

57. Stearns DM, Kennedy LJ, Courtney KD et al. Biochemistry 1995;34:910–9.

18 OTHER TRACE ELEMENTS[1]
CURTIS D. ECKHERT

ULTRATRACE ELEMENTS: OVERVIEW 339
ARSENIC 339
   Historical Overview 339
   Chemistry 339
   Suitable Analytic Methods 339
   Absorption and Bioavailability 339
   Transport, Distribution, Metabolism,
      and Excretion 340
   Modes and Mechanisms of Action 340
   Dietary Considerations .340
   Health Effects 340
BORON 341
   Historical Overview 341
   Chemistry 341
   Suitable Analytic Methods 342
   Absorption and Bioavailability 342
   Transport, Distribution, and Excretion 342
   Modes and Mechanisms of Action 342
   Dietary Considerations .343
   Health Effects 343
MOLYBDENUM 343
   Historical Overview 343
   Chemistry 343
   Suitable Analytic Methods 344
   Absorption and Bioavailability 344
   Transport, Distribution, and Excretion 344
   Modes and Mechanisms of Action 344
   Dietary Considerations .344
   Health Effects 345
NICKEL 345
   Historical Overview 345
   Chemistry 345
   Suitable Analytic Methods 345
   Absorption and Bioavailability 345
   Transport, Distribution, and Excretion 345

Modes and Mechanisms of Action 346
   Dietary Considerations .346
   Health Effects 346
SILICON 346
   Historical Overview 346
   Chemistry 346
   Suitable Analytic Methods 346
   Absorption and Bioavailability 346
   Transport, Distribution, and Excretion 346
   Modes and Mechanisms of Action 346
   Dietary Considerations .347
   Health Effects 347
VANADIUM 347
   Historical Overview 347
   Chemistry 347
   Suitable Analytic Methods 347
   Absorption and Bioavailability 347
   Transport, Distribution, and Excretion 347
   Modes and Mechanisms of Action 348
   Dietary Considerations .348
   Health Effects 348

Elements ingested through food and water in milligrams or less per day are called trace elements (1). The term reflects concentrations recorded as "trace" in feed and food. Trace signified that the levels of an element were measurable in some samples but were less than the detectable limits of analytic instrumentation in others. The practice was dropped because of the statistical difficulties of combining numbers and words. The importance of trace elements in human health is tied to their participation in biologic processes and their fate and transport through the environment. Trace elements are present in soil, water, and atmospheric particles as weathered products of rock and volcanic eruptions. Humans contribute to the transport of these elements into the living environment through agriculture and the release of industrial pollutants.

Two concepts are important to keep in mind when considering the value of trace elements to human health. The first is that metals and metalloids have been adapted by biologic systems because of their versatility in performing catalytic, structural, and signaling functions. In metal-poor environments such as the ocean, organisms survive because

---

[1] **Abbreviations: ADP,** adenosine diphosphate; **AI-2,** autoinducer 2; **As,** arsenic; **ATP,** adenosine triphosphate; **B,** boron; **cADPR,** cyclic adenosine diphosphate ribose; **DARP,** dissimilatory arsenate-reducing prokaryote; **DRI,** dietary reference intake; **ICP,** inductively coupled plasma; **Mo,** molybdenum; **MS,** mass spectrometry; **NAD$^+$,** oxidized nicotinamide adenine dinucleotide; **Ni,** nickel; **Si,** silicon; **UL,** tolerable upper intake level; **V,** vanadium.

the function of metalloproteins can be maintained using different metals with similar ionic radii and electronic structure. The term *essential* applies more to the biologic function than to the element. The second concept is chemical reactivity. In living systems, reactive metal atoms are not "free," but they are stabilized by coordinate bonds either to functional groups of amino acids in energetically strained (entatic) catalytic sites of proteins or to ligands such as nucleobases, nucleotides, and tetrapyrroles (2). In metalloenzymes, the strained state of metal coordination geometry stores most of the energy needed to reach the critical high-energy transition state of the enzyme-substrate complex, so only small geometric changes are required to produce the activation energy needed to initiate enzymatic catalysis. One of the coordination sites on the metal atom is open for substrate binding and in the relaxed state binds an easily replaced ligand such as water. The reactivity of a metal confined in this manner performs an essential biologic function. However, at concentrations that exceed the capacity to coordinate or bind metal atoms, the same reactivity can damage neighboring molecules. In short, at low levels of intake, the benefit of a trace element may be relative to the availability of other elements, but at high intakes, the probability of toxicity approaches certainty.

ULTRATRACE ELEMENTS: OVERVIEW

This chapter addresses several of the ultratrace elements: arsenic (As), boron (B), molybdenum (Mo), nickel (Ni), silicon (Si), and vanadium (V). Ultratrace elements have estimated dietary requirements less than 1 mg/kg diet and are present in tissues at concentrations in the range of micrograms per kilogram. The elements Mo, Ni, and V are metals, whereas As, B, and Si are metalloids, elements that have properties of both metals and nonmetals. Only Mo has been shown to be essential for human health. Evidence suggests the other elements are beneficial to human health, but the underlying chemical and physiologic mechanisms remain obscure. The importance of As also rests on its presence in drinking water at concentrations that induce toxicity to millions of people around the world. All the elements covered in this section are known to undergo biologic processing in some species. However, the dietary reference intake (DRI) process did not, with the exception of Mo, make specific dietary recommendations for the ultratrace elements covered in this chapter.

ARSENIC

Historical Overview

As has been used as a poison for thousands of years. The value of inorganic salts of As as agricultural pesticides was recognized by the ancient Syrians, and its use continues to this day (3). Organic arsenicals such as roxarsone (4-hydroxy-3-nitrophenyl As acid) are used in swine production to prevent coccidiosis and in poultry to improve

growth. As trioxide is such a powerful human poison that it was called "inheritance powder" in the Middle Ages (4). As played a paradoxic role in the origin of the green environmental movement in Europe (5). One of the movement's founders, William Morris (1834–1896), was born into a family that controlled the largest As mine of the 1800s. Pollution from the mine both harmed the ecology of Devon, England, and caused As pock skin lesions and lung disease in its population. Morris did not want to be associated with the harm caused by the mine and sold his family interest to start an interior design business. The new company produced wallpaper patterned with the Scheele green dye, a pigment produced from copper arsenite. Fungi grew in the damp wallpaper paste and converted the As salt into toxic trimethyl arsine that was slowly released into wallpapered rooms. The most famous victim of As wallpaper poisoning was the exiled Napoleon Bonaparte (5a).

Chemistry

As is a metalloid widely distributed in nature and associated with the ores of metals such as copper, lead, and gold (4, 6). It exists in four oxidation states: As(−III), As(0), As(III), and As(V). The predominant form of inorganic As in aqueous and aerobic environments is arsenate [As(V) as $H_2AsO_4^-$ and $HAsO_4^{2-}$]. In anoxic environments, arsenite [As(III) as $H_3AsO_3^0$ and $H_2AsO_3^-$] predominates. Adsorption of arsenate to the surface of minerals such as ferrihydrite and alumina constrains its hydrologic mobility. Arsenite is less strongly adsorbed to minerals, so its oxyanion is more mobile in environmental water (7). Tissue accumulation is influenced by methyltransferases. Isomers and polymorphisms of these enzymes have been proposed to explain risk differences in As toxicity that occur both within and among populations (8).

Suitable Analytic Methods

Atomic absorption spectrophotometry, inductively coupled plasma (ICP) atomic emission spectrometry, and ICP-mass spectrometry (ICP-MS) are the most common methods used to quantitate As (9). Measurements of total As are obtained by digesting tissue by wet ashing with nitric, sulfuric, and/or perchloric acids. The As is then reduced to arsine (AsH3), a gas that is trapped and measured by AAS. The determination of organoarsenicals and specific inorganic species requires prior separation using a procedure such as high-performance liquid chromatography or gel chromatography.

Absorption and Bioavailability

Soluble forms of ingested As are readily absorbed from water (90%) and food (60–70%) by the human gastrointestinal tract (10, 11). Less soluble arsenosugars that occur in plant products such as seaweed are poorly absorbed (12). The proportion of inhaled As absorbed ranges from

30 to 34% (13). As bound to the skin is slowly released into the circulation (14).

Transport, Distribution, Metabolism, and Excretion

As accumulates in the liver, kidney, muscles, heart, spleen, pancreas, lungs, and brain (15). Tissue clearance is rapid, and 2 weeks after ingestion, the majority is confined to keratin-rich tissues such as skin, hair, and nails, and, to a lesser extent, bones and teeth. Arsenicals are methylated by As methyltransferase to methylarsonic acid and dimethylarsinic acid (8). The liver is the major site of methylation using S-adenosylmethione as the methyl donor. Arsenicals containing As(III) are the preferred substrates for enzymatically catalyzed methylation. Inorganic and organic As(V) is first reduced to As(III) by glutathione or other thiols, then methylated and cycled between the As(V) and As(III) oxidation states to form dimethylated products:

$$As^VO_4^{3-} + 2e \rightarrow As^{III}O_3^{3-} + CH_3^+ \rightarrow CH_3As^VO_3^{2-} + 2e \rightarrow$$
$$CH_3As^{III}O_2^{2-} + CH_3^+(CH_3)_2As^VO_2^- + 2e \rightarrow$$
$$(CH_3)_2As^{III}O^- + CH_3^+$$

The mammalian enzyme responsible for catalyzing transfer of the methyl group from S-adenosyl-L-methionine to trivalent and dimethylated arsenicals is S-adenosyl-L-methionine:As(III) methyltransferase (8). Methylated metabolites are still cytotoxic, but they are rapidly excreted (16). The relative proportions of urinary As metabolites are 40 to 60% dimethylarsinic acid, 20 to 25% inorganic As, and 15 to 25% methylarsinic acid (17).

Methylation efficiency in humans decreases when concentrations are high (18). When concentrations of inorganic As exceed the methylating capacity of the liver, the substance accumulates in soft tissues. Pretreatment of cells with small amounts of As over prolonged periods increases the methylating efficiency and thereby decreases the risk of toxicity.

As is excreted primarily through the kidneys, with small amounts of inorganic As eliminated in feces, sweat, skin desquamation, hair, and nails. Following a low-level exposure to inorganic As, most urinary As is present in the form of methylated metabolites. A single intravenous injection of radiolabeled trivalent inorganic As(III) in human volunteers showed that most of the As is removed by urinary excretion within 2 days, with a small amount of excretion continuing during the subsequent 2 weeks. The biologic half-life of As from fish is estimated to be less than 20 hours, and total clearance occurs over 48 hours. Blood concentrations may appear normal while levels in the urine remain elevated.

Modes and Mechanisms of Action

Reduced As(III) reacts strongly with sulfhydryl groups in proteins leading to the inactivation of enzymes (19). Mitochrondria are the primary cellular targets of As(III) where it accumulates, uncouples oxidative phosphorylation, and reduces the synthesis of adenosine triphosphate (ATP). As is a cocarcinogen with ultraviolet radiation (20). This probably results from the ability of arsenites to inhibit the DNA repair following ultraviolet damage (20). Methylation of As also competes for S-adenosylmethionine and thus leads to hypomethylation of DNA and potential damage (21, 22).

A group of bacteria called dissimilatory arsenate-reducing prokaryotes (DARPs) uses As(V) as a nutrient (6). These bacteria are found in anoxic environments, in the gastrointestinal tracts of animals, and in the subsurface aquifer sediments of Bangladesh (2, 6). DARPs use As in respiration by linking the oxidation of lactate to the reduction of As(V) to As(III).

Dietary Considerations

The total dietary intake of As from food is about 50 µg/day, of which 10 µg is inorganic. Less than 4 µg/day is derived from drinking water (23). Saltwater fish contain the highest concentration of As (1662 ng/g), in which it occurs as arsenobetaine, a nontoxic organic form. Cereals and bakery products provide about 23.5 ng/g and fats and oils 19 ng/g (24). The major contributors of inorganic As are rice, flour, spinach, and grape juice (25). As intakes ranged from 0.5 to 0.81 µg/kg/day, with a median intake of 2.0 to 2.9 and 1.7 to 2.1 µg/day for men and women, respectively (26). The concentration in human milk ranges from 0.2 to 6 µg/kg wet weight. Drinking water is the primary source of inorganic As(III) and As(V). The Food and Nutrition Board of the Institute of Medicine did not set a DRI for As (27).

Health Effects

Deficiency Symptoms

Signs of As deficiency have been observed in goats, miniature pigs, and rats (28). Myocardial damage was observed in lactating goats, with evidence of mitochrondrial membrane damage. Other manifestations include reduced growth, impaired fertility, and increased perinatal mortality. Deficiency symptoms depend on available methylating capacity (28).

Toxic Effects

Acute As poisoning causes an acute paralytic syndrome, characterized by cardiovascular collapse and loss of brain function resulting from necrosis of white and gray matter secondary to vasodilation (29, 30). The symptoms of As toxicity are dose dependent and include encephalopathy, gastrointestinal symptoms, skin pigmentation and dermatitis, peripheral vascular disease and neuropathy, genotoxicity, and cancer. Acute ingestion of 1 mg/kg/day inorganic As causes anemia and hepatotoxicity. Ingestion of 10 mg/kg/day or higher leads to encephalopathy and gastrointestinal disturbances. Long-term ingestion of 10 μg/kg/day in drinking water can produce arsenicism. This is an occlusive peripheral vascular disease commonly referred to as black foot disease because, in extreme cases, feet turn black and develop gangrene.

Long-term ingestion of low levels of inorganic As occurs over an extensive region of Southern Asia and increases the risk of cancers of the skin, bladder, and lung (31). As poisoning is a problem in Bangladesh and West Bengal, India on a scale never before encountered for a natural or synthetic toxic substance (32, 33). The problem arose from the high water demands needed by the large populations and intensive agriculture. In the 1970s, the United Nations Children's Fund (UNICEF) and other relief international agencies drilled 6 to 10 million shallow drinking-water wells to bypass sewage-tainted surface waters that were causing outbreaks of cholera. The sediments in the area contained As bound in minerals to iron oxides. By 1998, 61% of the shallow wells were contaminated with As; millions of people were exposed to high levels, with reports of more than 200,000 cases of arsenicosis. The release of As from the minerals may have been initiated by the reduction of iron oxides that coated grains of sand in the sediment by DARPs, inorganic carbon from peat, and methane (33).

The Food and Nutrition Board did not establish a DRI or tolerable upper intake level (UL) for dietary As. The US Environmental Protection Agency's maximum contaminant level for drinking water As is 10 μg/L (16).

BORON

Historical Overview

B was formed along with hydrogen, carbon, nitrogen, and oxygen during the nucleosynthesis of low-weight elements following the Big Bang (34). With the exception of B, these elements are presumed to be critical for the formation of life. Primitive conditions of Earth supported the chemical synthesis of amino acids, nucleic acid bases, and simple carbohydrates, such as diglyceroaldehyde, a precursor in the formation of pentose sugars such as ribose. In the prebiotic environment, diglyceroaldehyde would have been unstable and degraded in a "browning" reaction. This fact made it difficult to understand how the RNA world could have emerged from the prebiotic chemical environment. However, Scientists at the University of Florida and the University of Southern California found the answer to this puzzle. They demonstrated that borate can stabilize glyceroaldehyde, thus allowing it to combine with enediolate and to stabilize ribose in the interstellar environment (35). This postulated role, in the transition between interstellar chemistry and the RNA world, places B at center stage in the history of life. This section addresses the following question: "Does Boron have a role in the DNA world"?

Borates have been used as a medicines and preservatives for 4000 years (36). Early humans filled bags with borax ($Na_2B_4O_7.10H_2O$) at the Tibetan lakes and hauled them by sheep over the Himalayas to India. Borates in soils are high in the Fertile Cresent stretching from the Mediterranean to Kazakhstan, as well as in parts of Southern California. Between the mid-1800s and 1900, borates were used for the treatment of epilepsy, with noted side effects of indigestion, dermatitis, alopecia, and anorexia at doses greater than 5 mg B/kg/day (37). In the 1870s, borax and boric acid were used to preserve fish, meat, cream, and butter. However, a report in 1904 showed that borax reduced appetite and caused indigestion, and so it was banned as a general preservative (29).

B deficiencies are a major reason for crop failure throughout the world. Warrington identified B as an essential plant nutrient in 1923 (38). Despite much effort, it took 73 years to discover that the essentiality of B was based on its role in stabilizing the cytoskeletal system during growth (39). Roles for B in bacterial defense and interspecies communication have also been discovered during the last few years and are discussed in the section on Modes and Mechanisms of Action.

The evidence that B is essential for vertebrates is less convincing, because a molecular role for the element has not been identified in animals. Hunt and Nielsen conducted a series of studies in chickens and suggested that B was beneficial under conditions of calcium, vitamin D, or magnesium deficiency (40). The first evidence of a specific vertebrate requirement for B was a dose-dependent increase in growth of embryonic rainbow trout embryos (*Oncorhynchus mykiss*) (41). Further investigation showed that B was essential for the formation of viable blastula in zebrafish (42) and for the survivability and normal morphogenesis of frog (*Xenopus*) embryos (43). Retinal degeneration was also observed in B-deprived zebrafish adults (44). A biochemical role has not been proven in humans, but B has been shown to modulate several important biologic processes in animals deprived of other nutrients.

Chemistry

B is the fifth element in the Periodic Table and is assigned to group IIIA. It has an atomic weight of 10.81 and exists as a mixture of stable isotopes ^{10}B and ^{11}B with respective abundances of 19.8 and 80.2% in the natural environment. B is a metalloid with an electronic structure of $1s^22s^2p$ and an oxidation state of +3. Three (trigonal) covalent bonds with oxygen form boric acid and four (tetrahedral) borates. B also has a strong tendency to form a fourth bond to complete the octet of valence electrons in molecules such as halides.

The chemistry of B in nature is dominated by its affinity for oxygen. Soluble forms of B include boric acid $B(OH)_3$ and the monovalent anion $B(OH)_4^-$, with the predominant form depending on the pH of the solvent. Boric acid is a weak Lewis acid with a negative logarithm of the constant for the ionization equilibrium (pK_a) of 9.2. The structures of borate minerals contain trigonal BO_3, or tetrahedral BO_4 units forming large B-oxygen anions. The principal geologic forms of borate include the following: tincal (borax), $Na_2B_4O_7.10H_2O$; kernite (borax pentahydrate), $Na_2[B_4O_5(OH)_4].2H_2O$; colemanite, $Ca[B_3O_4(OH)_3].H_2O$; and ulexite, $NaCa[B_5O_6(OH)_6].5H_2O$ (44). Elemental B does not occur naturally. Boric acid is the major form of B in physiologic fluids, and much remains to be learned about its interaction with other biomolecules in mammalian cells. Boric acid and borate form complexes with nucleotides by binding to the *cis*-diol groups of ribose (45).

Suitable Analytic Methods

The primary means of analysis are ICP-atomic emission spectropmetry and ICP-MS (46). Mammalian samples are problematic because they are near the level of detection for most instruments. Samples are digested with nitric acid in Teflon vessels before analysis and require the use of an internal standard for accurate analysis.

Absorption and Bioavailability

Boric acid and borates are rapidly absorbed from the gastrointestinal tract with more than 90% efficiency (27). They are not absorbed across skin, but occupational and consumer product exposures from inhaled dust can contribute a small amount to the overall total exposure.

Transport, Distribution, and Excretion

The major chemical form of B in blood and other body fluids is boric acid. Boric acid is not metabolized and is distributed throughout all tissues. More than 90% is eliminated in the urine of humans and rats following first-order kinetics. The half-life of renal clearance is about 21 hours, with renal resorption occurring if the ratio of B to creatinine is less than 1 (47). This finding suggests that B is under homeostatic regulation.

Locksley and Sweet conducted a dose-response mouse study using intraperitoneal injections of borax (48). Tissue B concentrations increased proportionally over a range of 1.8 to 71 mg B/kg. Ku and colleagues (49) evaluated the tissue concentrations of male rats fed 1575 mg B/kg diet that provided 93 to 96 mg B/kg/day for 7 days. B tissue concentrations are given in Table 18.1. After treatment, the highest concentration and percentage of increase occurred in bone, a finding providing evidence that bone is the major depository for B. The seminal vesicles had the next highest concentration and are known to be a target of toxic exposure levels in rats.

Modes and Mechanisms of Action

Chemical roles have been identified for B in three different biologic processes. It is a structural component of plants, a structural component of antibiotics, and a structural component of a pheromone released by bacterial populations that coordinates colony-wide gene expression.

In vascular plants, polysaccharide chains of the most complex carbohydrate known, rhamnoglacturonan II, provide scaffolding to maintain the architecture of cells when they elongate hundreds of times their length during growth. Borate esters link dimers of rhamnoglacturonan II together to stabilize cells as they expand under tremendous turgid pressure (39). A transporter has also been identified in plants that moves borate anions from the roots to the shoots. It is not known whether B anion transporters are present in animals, but homology studies using the plant transporter suggest that one may exist in the human kidney (50, 51).

TABLE 18.1. TISSUE BORON LEVELS IN RATS FOLLOWING 7 DAYS' EXPOSURE TO A 1575 mg/kg BORON DIET[a]

TISSUE	CONTROL (μg B/g)	DAY 7 (μg B/g)	FOLD INCREASE
Bone	1.17±0.19	47.40±1.14	40
Seminal vesicles	1.64±0.23	23.70±6.56	14
Adrenals	7.99	21.90	3
Kidney	1.55±0.03	19.80±1.65	13
Seminal vesicle fluid	2.05	19.20	9
Epididymis	0.81±0.15	16.81±3.7	21
Plasma	1.94±0.17	16.00±0.71	8
Testis	0.97±0.10	16.00±1.19	16
Large intestine	3.08±0.17	14.90±0.7	5
Prostate	1.20	14.80	12
Hypothalamus	0.91	14.30	16
Muscle	3.69±0.54	14.23±0.19	4
Brain	0.76±0.02	13.50±0.86	18
Liver	0.66±0.10	13.13±0.54	20
Adipose	1.71±0.17	3.78±0.13	2

B, boron.
[a] Values are mean ± SEM, n = 3 samples pooled from two animals or if given without SEM, 1 sample pooled from six animals.

Data from Ku WW, Chapin RE, Moseman RF et al. Toxicol Appl Pharmacol 1991;111:145–51.

Myxobacteria synthesize ion carrier antibiotics containing a single negatively charged B atom. The antibacterial compounds are boromycin, aplasmomycin, borophycin, and tartrolon B (52–54). Gram-positive and gram-negative bacteria also synthesize a bacterial signaling molecule, autoinducer 2 (AI-2), which contains a single B atom in its structure (55). AI-2 coordinates gene expression between different species of bacteria through a process called quorum sensing that enables bacteria to sense and respond to cell density. Quorum sensing is involved in the formation of biofilms on water surfaces and important in the etiology of dental plaque and spreading infections of gram-negative and gram-positive bacteria.

A mechanism for B action in mammals has yet to be discovered, but this is not because of a shortage of hypotheses. Hunt proposed that B acts by altering energy substrate utilization, mineral metabolism, and vitamin metabolism, by altering the activity of enzymes, by binding to polyhydroxy compounds, by perturbing the immune system, and more (56–59). Many of the phenomenologic observations may be explained by the affinity of B for oxidized nicotinamide adenine dinucleotide (NAD^+) (60). Extracellular NAD^+ binds to a plasma membrane receptor, CD38. The CD38 receptor is a adenosine diphosphate (ADP)–ribosyl cyclase that converts NAD^+ to cyclic ADP ribose (cADPR) and releases it intracellularly where cADPR binds to the ryanodine receptor and releases calcium ion from the endoplasmic reticulum. MS has shown that boric acid binds NAD^+ and cADPR (45, 61), and physiologic studies have shown that it inhibits the ability of NAD^+ to release calcium ion stores in human prostate cells (61). CD38/ADP-ribosyl cyclase activity is involved in nearly all the processes in which B has been shown to have an effect, including fertilization and early cleavage, insulin release, osteoblast metabolism, immune cell responses, and nerve physiology.

Dietary Considerations

Plant foods and their byproducts contain B because it is an essential structural component of plant cells. Foods that are particularly rich in B include avocados, dates, prunes, nuts, honey, and wine (62). Geographic variability in dietary B intake is considerable (62, 63). A comparison of dietary intakes in the United States, Germany, Kenya, and Mexico showed that residents of the United States consumed the lowest amounts of B and residents of Mexico the highest (63). The major contributors to total (100%) boron dietary intake in the United States were coffee (6.7%), milk (5.1%), apples (5.1%), beans (4.8%), and potatoes (4.8%) (64).

Health Effects

Beneficial Effects

Three human clinical trials were performed to deplete body B levels. Depleted subjects showed changes in neuropsychologic function, steroid metabolism, and blood cell indicators (65, 66). Epidemiologic screening identified an inverse relationship between dietary B intake and the risk of prostate cancer (67). Boric acid inhibits prostate-specific antigen, a serine protease, and inhibits the growth of prostate tumors in mice (68) and human cancer cell lines (69).

B was shown in numerous studies to alter bone in chicks (39), pigs (70), and rats (71, 72). In pigs, supplementation levels of 5 mg B/kg diet increased bone bending moment in males, but not in females. In male rats, B supplementation did not change tibia or femur resistance to bending, but dietary levels of 200 mg/kg diet did increase vertebral resistance to crush force (71). In contrast, supplementation of ovariectomized female rats did not provide protection against osteopenia or improve vertebrae strength (72).

Toxicity

Animal studies identified reproductive and developmental toxicity as the most sensitive adverse effect of excess B. The primary reproductive effect is the degeneration of the spermatogenic epithelium of the testes leading to impaired spermatogenesis, reduced fertility, and sterility (73). The toxic mechanism for the reproductive effects remains unknown. The primary developmental toxicologic effects are fetal rib malformations and decreased fetal weight at birth (74). Boric acid and borates are not considered carcinogens. The Food and Nutrition Board has not established a DRI for B, but it has set the following ULs for different age groups: 3 mg B/day, 1 to 3 years; 6 mg B/day, 4 to 8 years; 11 mg B/day, 9 to 13 years, 17 mg B/day, 14 to 18 years; and 20 mg/day, pregnant and lactating women more than 19 years old, and all adults (27).

MOLYBDENUM

Historical Overview

Mo has an essential role in the nitrogen cycle through molybdoenzymes involved in nitrogen fixation and the conversion of nitrate to ammonia by nitrate reductase. Mo was recognized as essential for the activity of human xanthine oxidase in 1953 and sulfite oxidase in 1971 (75, 76). Human essentiality is based on observations of genetic defects that cause a deficiency in the Mo cofactor resulting in seizures and death of newborns within days of birth (77).

Chemistry

The earth's crust contains about 1 mg/kg Mo (78). It is an essential element for plants and occurs at concentrations ranging from less than 0.5 to more than 100 mg/kg in plant dry matter (79). The stable hexavalent form, molybdate(VI), MoO_4^{2-}, is very soluble at pH 7 and resembles the sulfur-transporting ion, SO_4^{2-}. Molybdate aggregates into clusters at oxidation states below +VI, but this is suppressed in biologic systems by coordination of the Mo atom to dithiolene sulfurs on molybdopterin to form the molybdopterin cofactor. The molybdopterin cofactor is identical in all species and serves as the coenzyme in molybdoenzymes.

Physiologically relevant oxidations states for Mo are between +IV and +VI with redox potentials of −0.3 V (80). At these oxidation states, Mo has an affinity toward negatively charged O and S ligands such as oxide, sulfide, thiolates, or hydroxide and nitrogen ligands. The most important biologic function in mammalian systems is the transfer of oxygen to a two-electron substrate using one-electron transferring compounds such as flavin adenine dinucleotide. Coupling electron transfer and oxide exchange leads to the transfer of an oxygen atom from the metal center to the substrate.

$$LMo^{VI}O_2 + X \leftrightarrow LMo^{IV}O + XO$$

Three mammalian hydroxylases are molybdenoenzymes. They include the mitochondrial enzyme sulfite oxidase, which catalyzes the oxidation of sulfite to sulfate in the metabolism of sulfur from methionine and cysteine, and two enzymes that hydroxylate heterocyclic substrates including purines and pyridines, xanthine oxidase, and aldehyde oxidase. Xanthine oxidase catalyzes the conversion of xanthine and its derivatives such as caffeine to uric acid and uric acid derivatives. Aldehyde oxidase is a metalloflavoprotein composed of flavin adenine dinucleotide, Mo, and iron in a 1:1:4 ratio. It is involved in the formation of cotinine, a major metabolite of nicotine that occurs in the urine of cigarette smokers.

Suitable Analytic Methods

The most widely used method of Mo analysis relies on its ability to bind dithiol reagents. Biologic samples are wet ashed in sulfuric acid followed by extraction with toluene-3,4-dithiol. The Mo-mercaptide complex is extracted in organic solvent and is measured at 680 nm. For the analysis of lower concentrations, electrothermal atomic absorption spectroscopy and ICP emission spectroscopy are used (81).

Absorption and Bioavailability

In its most stable hexavalent form as molybdate(VI) (MoO_4^{2-}), Mo is water soluble and is absorbed over a wide range of intakes. The extrinsic addition of stable isotopes of Mo to diets has been used to measure absorption, retention, and excretion (82). Mo is rapidly absorbed and excreted from the kidney, with retention regulated primarily by urinary excretion. Absorption averaged 89% when daily Mo intake ranged from 25 to 122 μg/day and 93% when average intakes ranged from 466 to 1488 μg/day. The finding that sulfate anions are competitive inhibitors of absorption in rats and sheep suggests that they share a common transport mechanism (83).

Transport, Distribution, and Excretion

Mo blood concentrations range widely in the literature (84). Isotope dilution studies reported plasma values of 5 nmol/L in subjects with an intake of 22 μg/day, 20 μmol/L at an intake of 467 μg/day, and 44 μmol/L at an intake of 1490 μg/day (85). Mo accumulates as the molybdopterin cofactor in the liver, kidney, adrenal gland, and bone at concentrations that range from 0.1 to 1 mg/g wet weight (86). A pool of enzyme free metal-pterin complex, the Mo cofactor, occurs in the mitochrondrial outer membrane. The molybdoenzyme, sulfite oxidase, occurs in the mitochrondrial intermembrane space, and xanthine dehydrogenase and aldehyde oxidase are cytosolic enzymes (87).

The excretion of intrinsically labeled food was determined by incorporating ^{97}Mo into soybeans and kale grown in hydroponic systems (88, 89). Purées of extrinsically and intrinsically and labeled soybean and kale were fed to 12 women. The mean 8-day absorption of Mo was 87% from extrinsic sources, 86.1% from kale, and 56.7% from soybean. The mean urinary excretion was 60.8% of absorbed dose for extrinsic Mo and 56.6% from kale and 63.9% from soy.

Modes and Mechanisms of Action

Evidence for Mo essentiality rests on clinical observations (90). The first was a case of sulfite oxidase deficiency in a child resulting from an inborn error in metabolism. The symptoms included seizures, mental retardation, and dislocated ocular lenses, with the appearance of the unusual amino acid S-sulfocysteine in the plasma and urine, and high urinary levels of sulfite, thiosulfate and taurine. A postmortem examination confirmed sulfite oxidase deficiency. Since then, nearly 50 additional cases of sulfite oxidase deficiency have been identified (90). The second observation was loss of sulfite oxidase activity in a patient with Crohn disease who was supported on total parenteral nutrition for 18 months (91). Symptoms developed after 1 year and included tachycardia, tachypnea, night blindness, and coma. Biochemical evaluation showed an elevation in plasma methionine, low serum uric acid, and reduced urinary levels of sulfate, thiosulfate, and uric acid. All symptoms were eliminated by addition of 300 μg/day of ammonium molybdate to the total parenteral nutrition solution.

Dietary Considerations

Mo absorption is inhibited by high intakes of sulfate, possibly because they compete for the same transport proteins (92). Mo produced a copper deficiency in ruminants and nonruminants left grazing on a pasture contaminated with high concentrations of Mo from industrial and mining waste (93). Tungsten, the element immediately below Mo in group 6B in the Periodic Table, has a similar ionic radius and electronic structure and forms a complex with molybdopterin

TABLE 18.2. RECOMMENDED DIETARY ALLOWANCES FOR MOLYBDENUM

AGE (y) AND BOTH SEXES	RDA (μg/d)
Children 1–3	17
Children 4–8	22
Children 9–13	34
Children 14–18	43
Adults 19–>70	45
Pregnancy and lactation	50

RDA, recommended dietary allowance.

Adapted from Food and Nutrition Board, Institute of Medicine. Dietary Reference Intakes for Vitamin A, Vitamin K, Arsenic, Boron, Chromium, Copper, Iodine, Iron, Manganese, Molybdenum, Nickel, Silicon, Vanadium, and Zinc. Washington, DC: National Academy Press, 2001.

that activates molybdoenzymes. Tungsten can induce Mo deficiency as measured by a decrease in molybdoenzymes activity, but it is not considered to be significant to livestock or humans because it is rarely found in the environment. Data from the Total Diet Study indicated that the average Mo intake in the United States is 76 μg/day for women and 109 μg/d for men (94). Rich sources include legumes, grains, and nuts (27). The recommended dietary allowances are given in Table 18.2. The recommended adequate intake for term infants is 0.3 μg/(kg/day) (27), but concern has been expressed that the value should be between 4 and 6 μg/(kg/day) for premature infants (95).

Health Effects

Beneficial Effects

Human Mo deficiency has not been observed, and no beneficial effects from taking supplements of the element have been documented. Observations of Mo deficiency have been limited to genetic defects that interfere with the Mo cofactor's ability to activate molybdoenzymes.

Toxicity

Mo toxicity has been induced in rats; it causes renal insufficiency at levels of 80 mg/kg/day, but not at 40 mg/kg/day (96). In rabbits, a dose of 5 mg/kg/day induced weight loss and histopathologic changes in the kidney and liver (97). The Food and Nutrition Board used a lowest-observed adverse effect level of 0.9 mg/kg/day and an uncertainty factor of 30 to determine the UL (27). The ULs for different age groups are as follows: 300 μg Mo/day, 1 to 3 years; 600 μg Mo/day, 4 to 8 years; 1100 μg Mo/day, 9 to 13 years, 1700 μg Mo/day, 14 to 18 years; and 2000 μg Mo/day, pregnant and lactating women oilder than 19 years (27).

NICKEL

Historical Overview

Ni was first shown to promote the growth of bacteria in 1965 (98). The biologic importance of Ni was subsequently shown in both bacteria and plants, based on its catalytic role in four enzymes, urease, hydrogenases, carbon monoxide dehydrogenase, and methyl-coenzyme M reductase. Between 1975 and 1978, diets were used to induce deficiency symptoms in rats (99, 100), chicks (101), pigs (102), and goats (103). The nutritional importance of Ni in humans is unknown and remains largely unstudied.

Chemistry

Ni is in the first transition series of the Periodic Table with oxidation states of –I, 0, II, III, and IV. State II is the most important in biologic systems. Ni coordinates with the amino acids histidine, glutamic acid, and aspartate in metal centers of proteins (2) and binds to histidine and cysteine on albumin and a macroglobulin called nickeloplasmin (104). Tissue concentrations decrease with age and are lower in 90-year-old adults than 1-year-old children (105).

Suitable Analytic Methods

Analysis of biologic Ni samples usually uses atomic absorption spectrophotometry. Samples are prepared using wet or dry ashing and are transferred to a graphite tube furnace for electrothermal volatilization. Liquid samples can also be analyzed using ICP-MS.

Absorption and Bioavailability

Dietary Ni is poorly absorbed, with reported values from 1 to 5% (105–108). A stable isotope study using ^{62}Ni reported that 29 to 40% of the metal was absorbed (109). The highest concentrations in the blood occurred 2 to 3 hours after oral intake of Ni sulfate (107, 109). Absorption is increased under conditions of low Ni and iron availability. Entry into brush border epithelial cells is saturable. Movement of Ni from epithelial cells into blood is not regulated, and Ni ions move in both directions (107).

Transport, Distribution, and Excretion

The majority of Ni occurs in human serum bound to albumin (110), and about 26% is bound to nickeloplasmin, an α-macroblobulin that contains 0.9 g/mol of Ni (104). In human serum, 40% of Ni occurs in the ultrafiltrable fraction bound to amino acids such as histidine, cysteine, and aspartic acid, as well as other low molecular mass ligands. In cells, Ni is bound to low-molecular-mass ligands, proteins, and DNA (107). Ni occurs in all tissues with concentrations dependent on age, sex, and dietary intake. Reported human tissue (wet) concentrations include the following: pubic hair, 700 ng/g; lymph node, 810 ng/g; testis, 549 ng/g; lung, 230–160 ng/g; bone, 230 ng/g; muscle, 100 ng/g; skin, 100 ng/g; and liver, 80 ng/g (104). More than 90% of ingested Ni is excreted in the feces. Of the Ni that is absorbed, 51 to 82% is excreted in the urine (109), but some is also lost through sweat (111). Renal reabsorption of Ni occurs in humans, a finding suggesting some homeostatic regulation (111).

Modes and Mechanisms of Action

Ni has not been shown to be essential for any human biochemical processes. Ni is an essential component of ureases in jackbeans, ruminal bacteria, and several other plants, algae, and fungi. Ureases catalyze the degradation of urea to carbon dioxide and ammonia. It is also essential for hydrogenases in methanogenic bacteria that catalyze the conversion of hydrogen and carbon dioxide to methane. Methanogenic and acetogenic bacteria also require Ni in carbon monoxide dehydrogenase, an enzyme that converts carbon monoxide to carbon dioxide. Finally, methanogens use Ni in methyl-coenzyme M reductase in the last step in the formation and liberation of methane (107, 112).

Dietary Considerations

The Food and Drug Administration's Total Diet Study of 1984 showed that the mean Ni consumption of infants and children was 69 to 90 μg/day, and the median values for adolescents, adults, and the elderly were 71 to 97 μg/day, 74 to 100 μg/day, and 80 to 97 μg/day, respectively (94). The major contributors to the diet are mixed dishes and soups (19–30%), grains and grain products (12–30%), vegetables (10–24%), legumes (3–16%), and desserts (4–18%) (94).

Health Effects

Beneficial Effects

No beneficial human health effects from consuming dietary Ni are known. Nielsen reviewed the health effects of dietary Ni restriction in animals (105). The major observations in Ni-deprived pigs and rats were delayed sexual maturity, perinatal mortality, rough coat, and disorganization of the rough endoplasmic reticulum of the liver.

Toxicity

The Food and Nutrition Board used a no observed adverse effect level of 5 mg/kg/day based on decreased weight gain in rats. An uncertainty factor of 300 was derived by multiplying uncertainties of 10 for extrapolation from rat to human, human variation, and safety for potential toxic reproductive effects. The ULs for children aged 1 to 3, 4 to 8, and 9 to 13 years were 0.2, 0.3, and 0.6 mg/day of soluble Ni salts, respectively. The UL for adolescents and all adults was 1.0 mg/day (27).

SILICON

Historical Overview

The accumulation of Si in bone of chickens and rats was first reported in the 1970s and 1980s, but an essential chemical role remains to be discovered in animals (113–116). The best evidence for biologic essentiality is in plants and diatoms. A gene family of Si transport proteins was identified in diatoms in 1997 (117).

Chemistry

Si is the second most abundant element in the earth's crust. The chemistry of Si in the natural world is dominated by its affinity for oxygen, to which it is tetrahedrally coordinated in minerals (118). In aqueous solution at neutral pH ($2 < $ pH $ < 9$) and [Si] less than 100 mg/L, it takes the form of monosilicic acid, $Si(OH)_4$ (119). It also forms stable complexes with mannitol and other polyhydroxy aliphatic hexose sugars containing two hydroxyls in the *theo* position. This results in the formation of stable polyolate complexes containing five and six coordinated Si atoms. The ease of formation and the stability of these polysilicate anions are most likely the basis for its absorption and accumulation in tissue (119).

Suitable Analytic Methods

Atomic absorption spectrophotometry is used for the analysis of biologic samples. Samples are prepared using wet or dry ashing and are transferred to a graphite tube furnace for electrothermal volatilization. Liquid samples can also be analyzed using ICP-MS.

Absorption and Bioavailability

The mean uptake of Si in men and women from the Total Diet Study was 40 and 19 mg/day, respectively (94). Humans readily absorb silicic acid, and absorption is increased by dietary fiber (120).

Transport, Distribution, and Excretion

Si is freely transported in the blood, possibly in a polymeric form (121). It is freely diffusible into tissue from plasma and readily excreted. The excretion of Si in humans is increased as dietary Si intake is increased (122).

Modes and Mechanisms of Action

Carlisle used an electron microprobe to determine that Si localizes to the active growth areas of bone of growing mice and rats (123). The localized concentration reaches a maximum during the final stages of calcification and then dissipates. In rats, Si appears to promote bone mineralization. Carlisle suggested that Si is involved with phosphorus in events leading to calcification. Chemical mechanisms were never elucidated to explain this effect.

Observations in diatoms suggested to me that the basis of Si's effect on bone could lie in proton buffering (124). Diatoms are the primary oceanic consumers of atmospheric carbon dioxide and are responsible for a quarter of the total global production of fixed carbon. Carbon dioxide concentrations at the atmospheric ocean interface are lower than levels needed to saturate the carbon fixating enzyme, ribulose-1,5-bisphosphate carboxylase-oxygenase. Si has an important role in concentrating carbon dioxide substrate levels for the enzyme. Specific transporters remove Si from the ocean and transport it to vesicles where it is polymerized and is then transported the exterior surface of the cell. The polymerized silica serves as the proton donor for an extracellular carbonic anhydrase because proton exchange from water is too slow.

It is reasonable to assume that if diatom carbonic anhydrase prefers protons from polymerized silica over water, then mammalian enzymes could do the same. Indeed, this is the case. An examination of mammalian (bovine) carbonic anhydrase demonstrated that polymerized silica is a better proton donor than water (124). This begs the question whether carbonic anhydrase is involved in bone metabolism. The answer is yes, genetic deficiencies of carbonic anhydrase II in humans are associated with osteoclast dysfunction and osteopetrosis (125). Given this information, it may be that the meticulous use of Si free amino acid diets by Carlisle and her colleagues produced localized proton deficits that were responsible for some of the adverse effects on bone growth and maturation.

Dietary Considerations

The mean intake of Si in men and women from the Total Diet Study was 40 and 19 mg/day, respectively (94). The magnitude of difference between intakes on low-fiber diets and high-fiber diets is approximately 21 versus 46 mg/day (120).

Health Effects

Beneficial Effects

No beneficial effects of dietary Si have been confirmed in humans. In rats and mice, dietary Si has been shown to be important for the maturation of bone and for protection against aluminum-induced neurotoxicity (120).

Toxicity

Si causes urolithiasis, a deposition of calculi or uroliths containing monosilicic acid in the kidney, bladder, and urethra of grazing animals (123). In humans, adverse effects are primarily limited to silicosis, a lung disease resulting from the inhalation of silica particles. No dose-response data are available with which to establish a UL for Si.

VANADIUM

Historical Overview

V was reported to improve the growth of chickens, rats, and goats by several laboratories in the 1970s (126). However, experimental results from different laboratories were inconsistent, and Nielsen suggested that the effects were probably caused by poorly controlled experimental diets that provided V at levels 10 to 100 times that found in normal diets (127). In 1986 and 1989, Anke compared V-supplemented goats (2 μg/g diet) with V-deprived goats (10 ng/g diet) using better-formulated diets (126). V-deficient goats exhibited higher rates of spontaneous abortion and offspring that developed convulsions and succumbed to death at a rate of 41% during the first 3 months of life (126). Serum creatinine and β-lipoprotein concentrations were elevated, and serum glucose concentrations were depressed in V-deprived goats. Rats studies showed that thyroid weights were increased in animals deprived of V (128). No evidence indicates that dietary V is beneficial for humans, although pharmacologic levels promote the action of insulin and reduce blood glucose levels (129, 130).

Chemistry

V is a transition metal with six oxidations, of which three are biologically relevant: +III, +IV, and +V (131). Common compounds include V pentoxide (V_5O_5), sodium metavanadate ($NaVO_3$), sodium orthovanadate (Na_3VO_4), vanadyl sulfate ($VOSO_4$), and ammonium vanadate (NH_4VO_3). Vanadate (V) ions compete with phosphate ions and inhibit sodium ion ATPase. The *ortho*-vanadate ion, VO_4^{3-} resembles the *ortho*-phosphate ion, PO_4^{3-}. Unlike the phosphate ion, V is easily reduced to IV and III with biologic reductants such as glutathione (132, 133). V-dependent enzymes include nitrogenase in bacteria, iodoperoxidase, and bromoperoxidase in algae and lichens (131).

Suitable Analytic Methods

Atomic absorption spectrophotometry is used for the analysis of biologic samples. Samples are prepared using wet or dry ashing and are transferred to a graphite tube furnace for electrothermal volatilization. Liquid samples can also be analyzed using ICP-MS.

Absorption and Bioavailability

Less than 5% of ingested V is absorbed (134, 135). Most V is in the form of the vanadyl ion VO^{2+} (IV) in the stomach. Absorption occurs in the duodenum and upper gastrointestinal tract (136). The vanadate anion (V) is absorbed three to five times more readily than the vanadyl ion (IV). The vanadate anion (V) enters cells through nonspecific anionic channels and is reduced by glutathione (137, 138).

Transport, Distribution, and Excretion

V is rapidly cleared from plasma and accumulates in kidney, liver, testes, bone, and spleen. The vanadate anion (V) binds to the iron binding proteins, lactoferrin, transferrin, and ferritin. Tissue levels are markedly increased in rats fed V-supplemented diets (136). V is excreted primarily through the kidney, with a small amount through the bile. Tissues with the highest concentrations include lung, teeth, thyroid, and bone (136).

Modes and Mechanisms of Action

Vanadate (V) anions inhibit phosphate-dependent enzymes and sodium/potassium–ATPase hydrolysis. The V atom has a larger ionic radius than phosphorus and forms a stable five-coordinate intermediate or transition state, thereby inhibiting catalysis (131, 139). Vanadyl (IV) complexes potentiate the effect of insulin (128).

Dietary Considerations

Dietary intake of V ranges from 6 to 18 μg/day (140). Grains and grain products contribute 13 to 30% of dietary V. Marine organisms, such as tunicates and brown algae, lichen and mushrooms are rich sources of V (141).

Health Effects

Beneficial Effects

No cases of human V deficiency have been reported. V deficiency in goats leads to an increase in abortion, convulsions, bone malformations, and early death. V is used in pharmacologic quantities to potentate the effect of insulin.

Toxicity

V causes abdominal cramps, diarrhea, hemolysis, increased blood pressure, and fatigue. The primary toxic effect in humans occurs from the inhalation of vanadate dust in industrial settings. The Food and Nutrition Board did not determine a UL for dietary V, but the Environmental Protection Agency's oral reference dose is 0.009 mg/kg/day (27).

REFERENCES

1. O'Dell BL, Sunde RA, eds. Handbook of Nutritionally Essential Mineral Elements. New York: Marcel Dekker, 1997:1–11.
2. Kaim W, Schwederski B, eds. Some general principles. In: Bioinorganic Chemistry: Inorganic Elements in the Chemistry of Life. West Sussex, UK: John Wiley & Sons, 1994:6–38.
3. Czarnecki DL, Baker GH. Poultry Sci 1982;61:516.
4. Nriagu JO. Arsenic poisoning through the ages. In: Frankenberger WT Jr, ed. Environmental Chemistry of Arsenic. New York: Marcel Dekker, 2002:1–26.
5. Megard A. Nature 2003;423:688.
5a. Jones DE, Ledingham KW. Nature 1982;299:626–7.
6. Oremland RS, Stolz JF. Science 2003;300:939–43.
7. Smedley PL, Kinniburgh DG. Appl Geochem 2002;17:517.
8. Lin S, Shi Q, Nix FB et al. J Biol Chem 2002;277:10795–803.
9. US Department of Health and Human Services, Agency for Toxic Substances and Disease Registry, Division of Toxicology/Toxicology Information Branch. Toxicological Profile for Arsenic. Atlanta, GA: US Department of Health and Human Services, Agency for Toxic Substances and Disease Registry, 2000: 301–6.
10. Vahter M. Metabolism of arsenic. In: Fowler BA, ed. Biological and Environmental Effects of Arsenic. Amsterdam: Elsevier, 1983:171–98.
11. Hopenhayn-Rich C, Biggs ML, Fuchs A et al. Epidemiology 1996;7:117–24.
12. Yamauchi H, Kaise T, Yamamura Y. Bull Environ Contam 1986; 36:350–5.
13. Holland RH, McCall MS, Lanz HC. Cancer Res 1959;19: 1154–6.
14. Wester RC, Maibach HI Sedik L. Fundam Appl Toxicol 1993; 20:336–40.
15. Benramdane L, Accominotti M, Fanton L. Clin Chem 1999; 45:301–6.
16. Abernathy CO, Thomas DJ, Calderon RL. J Nutr 2003;133: 1536S–8S.
17. Marafante E, Vahter M, Norin H et al. J Appl Toxicol 1987;7: 111–7.
18. Marcus WL, Rispin AS. Threshold carcinogenicity using arsenic as an example. In: Cothern CR, Mehlman MA, Marcus WL, eds. Advances in Modern Environmental Toxicology, vol 15: Risk Assessment and Risk Management of Industrial and Environmental Chemicals. Princeton, NJ: Princeton Scientific Publishing, 1988:133–58.
19. Abernathy Co, Liu YP, Longfellow D et al. Environ Health Perspect 1999;107:593–597.
20. Rossman TG, Uddin AN, Burns FJ et al. Toxicol Appl Pharmacol 2001;176:64–71.
21. Costa M. Am J Clin Nutr 1995;61[Suppl 3]:666S–9S.
22. Oremland RS, Newman DK, Wail BW et al. In: Frankenberger Jr, ed. Environmental Chemistry of Arsenic. New York: Marcel Dekker, 2002:273–96.
23. Borum DR, Abernathy CO. Human oral exposure to inorganic arsenic. In: Chappell WR, Abernathy CO, Cothern CR, eds. Arsenic: Exposure and Health Effects. Science and Technology Letters. Northwood, UK: Elsevier, 1994:21–9.
24. Bagla P, Kaiser J. Science 1996;274:174–5.
25. Dabeka RW. Sci Total Environ 1989;89:279–89.
26. Schoof RA, Yost LJ, Eickhoff J et al. Food Chem Toxicol 1999; 37:839–46.
27. Food and Nutrition Board, Institute of Medicine. Dietary Reference Intakes for Vitamin A, Vitamin K, Arsenic, Boron, Chromium, Copper, Iodine, Iron, Manganese, Molybdenum, Nickel, Silicon, Vanadium, and Zinc. Washington, DC: National Academy Press, 2001.
28. Gunderson EL. AOAC Int 1995;78:1352–63.
29. Nielsen FH. Ultratrace minerals. In: Shils ME, Olson JA, Shike M et al, eds. Modern Nutrition in Health and Disease. 9th ed. Baltimore: Williams & Wilkins, 1999:283–303.
30. Civantos DP, Lopez Rodriguez A, Aguado-Borruey JM et al. Chest 1995;108:1774–5.
31. Brouwer OF, Okenhout W, Edelbroek PM et al. Clin Neurol Neurosurg 1992;94:307–10.
32. National Research Council. Arsenic in Drinking Water. Washington, DC: National Academy Press.
33. Stokstad E. Science 2002;298:1535–36.
34. Copi CJ, Schramm DN, Turner ST. Science 1995;267:192–8.
35. Ricardo A, Carrigan MA, Olcott AN et al. Science 2004;303: 196.
36. Woods WG. Environ Health Perspect 1994;102[Suppl 7]:5–11.
37. Culver BD, Hubbard SA. J Trace Elem Exp Med 1996;9: 175–84.
38. Warrington K. Ann Bot 1923;37:629–72.
39. O'Neill MA, Eberhard S, Albersheim P et al. Science 2001; 294:846–9.
40. Hunt C, Nielsen F. Interaction between boron and cholecalciferol in the chick. In: Gawthorne J, White C, eds. Trace Element Metabolism in Man and Animals. 1981;4:567–600.
41. Eckhert CD. J Nutr 1998;128:2488–93.
42. Rowe RI, Eckhert CD. J Exp Biol 1999;37:1649–54.

43. Fort, DJ, Propst TL, Stover EL et al. Biol Trace Elem Res 1998;66:237–59.
44. Eckhert CD, Rowe RI. J Trace Elem Exp Med 1999;12:213–9.
45. Kim DH, Marbois BN, Faull KF et al. J Mass Spectrom 2003;38:632–40.
46. Downing RG, Strong PL. Biol Trace Elem Res 1998;66:23–37.
47. Pahl MV, Culver BD, Strong PL et al. Toxicol Sci 2001;60: 252–6.
48. Locksley HB, Sweet WH. Proc Soc Exp Biol Med 1954;86: 56–63.
49. Ku WW, Chapin RE, Moseman RF et al. Toxicol Appl Pharmacol 1991;111:145–51.
50. Takano J, Noguchi K, Yasumori M et al. Nature 2002;420: 337–40.
51. Frommer WB, von Wirén N. Nature 2002;410:282–3.
52. Dunitz JD, Hawley DM, Mikloš D et al. Helv Chim Acta 1971;54:1709–13.
53. Chen TSS, Ching-Jer C, Floss HG. J Am Chem Soc 1979;101: 5826–7.
54. Schummer D, Irschik H, Reichenbach H et al. Liebigs Ann Chem 1994;283–9.
55. Chen X, Schauder S, Potier N et al. Nature 2002;415:545–9.
56. Hunt CD. J Trace Elem Exp Med 1996;9:185–213.
57. Hunt C. Environ Health Perspect 1994;102[Suppl 7];35–43.
58. Hunt CD. Biol Trace Elem Res 1998;66:205–25.
59. Hunt CD. J Trace Elem Exp Med 2003;216:291–306.
60. Kim DH, Faull KF, Norris AJ et al. J Mass Spectrom 2004;39: 743–51.
61. Barranco W, Eckhert CD. FASEB J 2004;18:A491 (351.2).
62. Naghii MR, Wall L, Samman S. J Am Coll Nutr 1996;15:614–9.
63. Rainey CJ, Nyquist LA, Christensen RE et al. J Am Diet Assoc 1999;99:335–40.
64. Rainey C, Nyquist L. Biol Trace Elem Res 1998;66:79–86.
65. Penland JG. Environ Health Perspect 1994;102[Suppl 7];65–72.
66. Nielsen FH. Environ Health Perspect 1994;102[Suppl 7]: 59–63.
67. Cui Y, Winton MI, Zhang et al. Oncol Rep 2004;11:887–92.
68. Gallardo-Williams MT, Maronpot RR, Wine RN et al. Prostate 2003;54:44–9.
69. Barranco WT, Eckhert CD. Cancer Lett 2004(in press).
70. Armstrong TA, Spears JW, Grenshaw TD et al. J Nutr 2000;139: 2575–81.
71. Chapin RE, Ku WW, Kenney MA et el. Fundam Appl Toxicol 1997;35:205–15.
72. Gallardo-Williams MT, Maronpot RR, Turner CH et al. Biol Trace Elem Res 2003;93:155–70.
73. Fail PA, Chapin RE, Price CJ et al. Reprod Toxicol 1998; 12:1–18.
74. Ku WW, Chapin RE. Environ Health Perspect 1998;102[Suppl 7]:99–105.
75. Richert DA, Westerfield WW. J Biol Chem 1953;203:915–23.
76. Cohen HJ, Fridovich I, Rajagopalan KV. J Biol Chem 1971;246: 374–82.
77. Johnson JL. Molybdenum. In: O'Dell BL, Sunde RA, eds. Handbook of Nutritionally Essential Mineral Elements. New York: Marcel Dekker, 1997:413–38.
78. Davis GK, Jorden R, Kubota H et al. In: Geochemistry and the Environment, vol 1. Washington, DC: National Academy of Sciences, 1974:68–79.
79. Stone LR, Erdman JA, Fedder GL et al. J Range Manage 1983;36:280–5.
80. Kaim W, Schwederski B, eds. Biological functions of the "early" transition metals: molybdenum, tungsten, vanadium and chromium. In: Bioinorganic Chemistry: Inorganic Elements in

the Chemistry of Life. West Sussex, UK: John Wiley & Sons, 1994:215–41.
81. Mills CF, Davis GK. Molybdenum. In: Mertz W, ed. Trace Elements in Human and Animal Nutrition. 5th ed. San Diego: Academic Press, 1986:429–63.
82. Turnlund JR, Keyes WR, Anderson HL et al. Am J Clin Nutr 1989;49:870–8.
83. Cardin CJ, Mason J. Biochim Biophys Acta 1975;455:937.
84. Allaway WH, Kubota J, Losee F et al. Arch Environ Health 1968;16:342–8.
85. Turnlund JR, Keyes WR. J Nutr Biochem 2004;25:90–5.
86. Schroeder HA, Balassa JJ, Tipton IH. J Chronic Dis 1970;23: 481–99.
87. Johnson JL, Jones HP, Rajogopalan KV. J Biol Chem 1977;252: 4994–5003.
88. Turnlund JR, Keyes WR, Peiffer GL. Am J Clin Nutr 1995;61: 1102–9.
89. Turnlund JR, Keyes WR, Peiffer GL. Am J Clin Nutr 1995;61: 790–6.
90. Johnson JL, Wadman SK. Molybdenum cofactor deficiency and isolated sulfite oxidase deficiency. In: Scriver CR, Beaudet AL, Sly WS et al, eds. The Metabolic and Molecular Bases of Inherited Disease. 7th ed. New York: McGraw-Hill, 1995:2271–83.
91. Abumrad N, Schnieder AJ, Steel D et al. Am J Clin Nutr 1981: 34:2551.
92. Mills CF, Bremner I. Nutritional aspects of molybdenum in animals. In: Coughlan MP, ed. Molybdenum and Molybdenum–Containing Enzymes. Oxford: Pergamon Press, 1980: 517–42.
93. Ladefoged O, Sturup S. Vet Hum Toxicol 1995;37:63–5.
94. Pennington JAT, Jones JW. J Am Diet Assoc 1987;87:1644–50.
95. Sievers E. J Nutr 2003;133:236–7.
96. Bompart G, Pecher C, Prevot D et al. Toxicol Lett 1990;52: 293–300.
97. Asmangulyan TA. Gig Sanit 1965;30:6–11.
98. Bartha R, Ordal EJ. J Bacteriol 1965;89:1015–9.
99. Schnegg A Kirchgessner M. Z Tierphysiol Tierernahr Futtermittelkd 1975;36:63–74.
100. Nielsen FH, Myron DR, Givand SH et al. J Nutr 1975;105: 1620–30.
101. Anke M, Grün M, Dittrich D et al. Low nickel rations for growth and reproduction in pigs. In: Hoekstra WG, Sutte JW, Ganther HE et al, eds. Trace Element Metabolism in Animals, vol 2. Baltimore: University Park Press 1974:715–8.
102. Anke M, Hennig A. Grün et al. Arch Tierernahr 1977;27:25–38.
103. Spears JW. J Anim Sci 1984;59:823–35.
104. Sunderman FW Jr. Ann Clin Lab Sci 1977;7:377–98.
105. Nielsen FH. Nickel. In: Mertz W, ed. Trace Elements in Human and Animal Nutrition, vol 1, 5th ed. San Diego: Academic Press, 1987:245–73.
106. Zimmerli B, Candrian U, Schlatter C. Mitt Gegiete Lebensm Hyg 1987;78:344–96.
107. Eder K, Kirchgessner M. Nickel. In: O'Dell BL, Sunde RA, eds. Handbook of Nutritionally Essential Mineral Elements. New York: Marcel Dekker, 1997:439–541.
108. Solomons NW, Viteri F, Shyler TR et al. J Nutr 1982;112:39–50.
109. Patriarca M, Lyon TD, Fell GS. Am J Clin Nutr 1997;66: 616–21.
110. Tabata M, Sarkar B. J Inorg Biochem 1992;45:93–104.
111. Nieboer E, Rickey TT, Sanford WE. Nickel metabolism in man and animals. In: Sigel H, ed. Nickel and Its Role in Biology. New York: Marcel Dekker, 1988:91–121.
112. Kaim W, Schwederski B, eds. Nickel-containing enzymes: the remarkable career of a long overlooked biometal. In: Bioinorganic

Chemistry: Inorganic Elements in the Chemistry of Life. West Sussex, UK: John Wiley & Sons 1994:172–86.

113. Schwarz K, Milne BD. Nature 1972;239:333–4.
114. Carlisle EM. J Nutr 1980;110:352–9.
115. Carlisle J. Nutr 1980;110:1046–55.
116. Carlisle EM. Calcif Tissue Int 1981;33:27–34.
117. Hildebrand, Volcani BE, Gallmann W et al. Nature 1997;385:688–9.
118. Coradin T, Lopez PJ. Chem Biochem 2003;3:1–9.
119. Kinrad SD, Del Nin JW, Schach AS et al. Science 1999;285:1542–45.
120. Kelsay JL, Behall KM Prather ES. Am J Clin Nutr 1979;32:1876–80.
121. Policard A, Collet A, Moussard DH et al. J Biophys Biochem Cytol 1961;9:236.
122. Holt PF. Br J Ind Med 1950;7:12.
123. Carlisle EM. Silicon. In. Mertz W, ed. Trace Element Metabolism in Human and Animal Nutrition, vol 2. Orlando, FL: Academic Press, 1986:373–90.
124. Milligan AJ, Morel FMM. Science 2002;297:1848–50.
125. Kocher MS, Kasser JR. Am J Orthop 2003;32:222–8.
126. Anke M. The essentiality of ultra trace elements for reproduction and pre- and postnatal development. In: Chandra RK, ed. Trace Elements in Nutrition of Children II. Nestle Nutrition Workshop Series, vol 23. New York: Raven Press, 1991:119–44.
127. Nielsen FH. J Nutr 1985;115:1239–47.
128. Uthus EO, Nielsen FH. Magnes Trace Elem 1990;9:219–26.
129. Shechter Y. Diabetes 1990;39:1.
130. Fantus IG, Kadota S. Deragon G et al. Biochemistry 1989;28:8864–71.
131. Kaim W, Schwederski B, eds. Unequally distributed electrolytes: function and transport of alkali and alkaline earth metal cations. In: Bioinorganic Chemistry: Inorganic Elements in the Chemistry of Life. West Sussex, UK: John Wiley & Sons 1994:265.
132. Degani H, Gochin M, Karlish SJD et al. Biochemistry 1981;20:5795–9.
133. Liochev SI, Fridovich I. Arch Biochem Biophys 1990;279:1–7.
134. Byrne RR, Kosta L. Sci Total Environ 1978;10:17–30.
135. Myron DR, Kimmerman TJ, Shuler TR et al. Am J Clin Nutr 1978;31:527–31.
136. Nielsen FH. Vanadium. In: O'Dell BL, Sunde RA, eds. Handbook of Nutritionally Essential Mineral Elements. New York: Marcel Dekker, 1997:619–30.
137. Boyd DW, Kustin K. Adv Inorg Biochem 1984;6:311–65.
138. Nechay BR. Annu Rev Pharmacol Toxicol 1984;4:501–24.
139. Tracy AS, Jaswal, Greser MJ et al. Inorg Chem 1990;29:4283.
140. Pennington JAT, Jones JW. J Am Diet Assoc 1987;87:1644–50.
141. Wever R, Kustin K. Adv Inorg Chem 1990;53:81.

SELECTED READINGS

Food and Nutrition Board, National Institute of Medicine. Dietary Reference Intakes for Vitamin A, Vitamin K, Arsenic, Boron, Chromium, Copper, Iodine, Iron, Manganese, Molybdenum, Nickel, Silicon, Vanadium, and Zinc. Washington, DC: National Academy Press, 2001.

Kaim W, Schwederski B, eds. Bioinorganic Chemistry: Inorganic Elements in the Chemistry of Life. West Sussex, UK: John Wiley & Sons, 1994.

Mertz W, ed. Trace Elements in Human and Animal Nutrition, vols 1 and 2, 5th ed. San Diego: Academic Press, 1987.

Nielsen FH. Ultratrace Minerals. In: Shils ME, Olson JA, Shike M, et al, eds. Modern Nutrition in Health and Disease. 9th ed. Baltimore: Williams & Wilkins, 1999:283–303.

O'Dell BL, Sunde RA, eds. Handbook of Nutritionally Essential Mineral Elements. New York: Marcel Dekker, 1997.

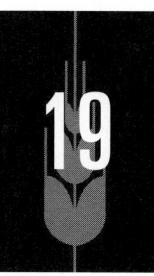

19   VITAMIN A AND CAROTENOIDS[1]

A. CATHARINE ROSS

HISTORICAL OVERVIEW 351
TERMINOLOGY, CHEMISTRY, AND PROPERTIES 352
    Retinoids 352
    Provitamin A 352
    Methods of Analysis 353
NUTRITIONAL SOURCES, UNITS, AND
    RECOMMENDED DIETARY ALLOWANCES 353
    Units 353
PHYSIOLOGIC PROCESSING OF VITAMIN A 355
    Retinoid-Binding Proteins and Receptors 355
    Absorption and Hepatic Metabolism 356
    Plasma Retinol 359
FUNCTIONS 362
    Vision and Ocular Retinoid Metabolism 362
    Cellular Differentiation 363
    Uses of Retinoids 366
DEFICIENCY AND TOXICITY 367
    Vitamin A Deficiency 367
    Hypervitaminosis A, Adverse Effects, and
        the Upper Level 367
    Assessment of Vitamin A Status 369
SUMMARY 371

HISTORICAL OVERVIEW

Ancient medical writings of Egyptian and Greek physicians revealed that the liver of ox was recommended as a cure for night blindness in early times (1). Strangely, the writings are

[1]**Abbreviations: APL,** acute promyelocytic leukemia; **ARAT,** acyl-coenzyme A:retinol acyltransferase; **BMD,** bone mineral density; **CRABP,** cellular retinoic acid-binding protein; **CRALBP,** cellular retinal-binding protein; **CRBP,** cellular retinol-binding protein; **DR,** direct repeat; **EAR,** estimated average requirement; **HIV,** human immunodeficiency virus; **IOM,** Institute of Medicine; **IRBP,** interstitial retinoid-binding protein; **IU,** international unit; $\mathbf{K_m}$, Michaelis-Menten constant; **LRAT,** lecithin:retinol acyltransferase; **MRDR,** modified dose response test; **NHANES,** National Health and Nutrition Examination Survey; **RA,** retinoic acid; **RAE,** retinol activity equivalent; **RALDH,** retinal dehydrogenase; **RAR,** retinoic acid receptor; **RARE,** retinoic acid receptor-response element; **RBP,** retinol-binding protein; **RDA,** recommended dietary allowance; **RDH,** retinol dehydrogenase; **RDR,** relative dose response; **RE,** retinol equivalent; **REH,** retinyl ester hydrolase; **RPE,** retinal pigment epithelium; **RXR,** retinoid X receptor; **TTR,** transthyretin; **UL,** tolerable upper intake level; **WHO,** World Health Organization.

interpreted to indicate that the liver was applied on the eyes, although perhaps some of it was also eaten. The modern era of vitamin A research began in 1913 with the independent discoveries by Osborne and Mendel at Yale University and McCollum and Davis at the University of Wisconsin of what was then known as "fat-soluble A." McCollum and Davis described the ability of certain "lipins," which they extracted from butter, eggs, or cod liver oil, to promote the survival and growth of young rats fed diets containing lard or olive oil as the only fat. Soon thereafter, Steenbock recognized that a yellow lipid fraction extracted from yellow-orange vegetables had a similar biologic activity. It was inferred that the yellow substance of vegetable origin, later identified as β-carotene, was a precursor of the nearly colorless "lipin," later identified as the lipid alcohol retinol.

In every decade since the 1910s, important new discoveries about vitamin A have been made. During the 1920s to 1950s, vitamin A deficiency was linked to xerophthalmia, abnormal tissue differentiation, and impaired immune functions (2). Retinol was synthesized de novo by Karrer and others. Arens and van Dorp (3) synthesized the acid form of vitamin A, retinoic acid (RA), and showed its ability to restore growth, but not vision, in vitamin A–deficient rats. Wald, Hubbard, and others clarified the role of vitamin A in vision by showing that "retinene" (retinal) is the essential chromophore of the visual pigment rhodopsin (4).

During the 1960s to 1980s, several proteins that are crucial for the transport and metabolism of retinol or other forms of vitamin A were isolated and purified. The purification of retinol-binding protein (RBP) and several forms of cellular retinoid-binding proteins (CRBP and CRABP) in the 1960s to 1980s greatly improved the understanding of the plasma transport of retinol and its intracellular metabolism. In 1987, the laboratories of Chambon and Evans independently reported the cloning of the first nuclear retinoid receptor, RARα, which they showed to be a new member the steroid/thyroid hormone receptor superfamily. The retinoid receptor family is now known to include six types: three RA receptors, RARα, β, and γ, and three retinoid X receptors, RXRα, β, and γ. These receptors mediate the ability of RA to activate or inhibit the transcription of responsive genes (5). In the 1980s, research originally designed to understand the prevalence of xerophthalmia led to the surprising discovery that mortality rates were higher in children classified as having only "mild" subclinical vitamin A deficiency. These unanticipated results served as the impetus for a series of randomized controlled trials to test the ability of vitamin A supplementation to reduce young child mortality in at-risk populations (6, 7).

The term carotenoids was coined in 1831 by Wackenroder to describe the orange-yellow pigments he discovered in carrots (8). Nearly a century later, Karrer and colleagues determined the structure of β-carotene. The work of several investigators showed certain carotenoids to be a physiologic precursor of vitamin A (retinol). However, of the 600 or so carotenoids that have been isolated from natural sources, only a very few, mainly β-carotene, α-carotene, and β-cryptoxanthin, possess vitamin A activity.

Currently, vitamin A research continues to span a very wide range of interests, from public health programs designed to eliminate vitamin A deficiency to basic research to help one better to understand the mechanisms of retinoid actions. Retinoids, including numerous synthetic analogs related to vitamin A, have gained wide clinical use in dermatology and for the treatment of acute promyelocytic leukemia (APL). Retinoids continue to hold promise as cancer chemopreventive agents because of their ability to inhibit cell proliferation and to promote cell differentiation.

TERMINOLOGY, CHEMISTRY, AND PROPERTIES

Vitamin A is a nutritional term for a family of essential fat-soluble dietary compounds that are structurally related to the lipid alcohol retinol. Vitamin A includes the provitamin A carotenoids, discussed later. The term *retinoids* refers to retinol, its endogenous metabolites, and a large number of synthetic analogs. Most of these compounds possess limited activity as compared with the broad spectrum of biologic activities of vitamin A.

Retinoids

Certain structural features are shared by all the natural retinoids and provitamin A carotenoids. They all have at least one β-ionone ring linked to a side chain composed of conjugated carbon-carbon (C) double bonds. The double bonds may exist in *cis* or *trans* conformation. All-*trans*-retinol (Fig. 19.1A) contains a β-ionone ring, five conjugated C-C double bonds, and a primary hydroxyl group at C-15 (molecular weight 286.44). Most tissues contain retinol esterified with a fatty acid (retinyl palmitate or stearate), whereas most pharmaceutical preparations contain synthetically produced retinyl palmitate or acetate. All these forms generate retinol and are nutritionally equivalent. In vivo, retinol is oxidized and isomerized to 11-*cis*-retinal (Fig. 19.1B) and subsequently to all-*trans*- and 9-*cis*-RA (Fig. 19.1C and D). Many other natural retinoids are known (9); some of them have an additional keto, hydroxyl, or epoxide substituent that renders them more polar, although they are still lipid soluble. Conjugation with a molecule such as glucuronic acid imparts aqueous solubility. A prominent example is retinoyl-β-glucuronide (Fig. 19.1E). Some synthetic retinoids (e.g., Acitretin; Fig. 19.1F) have few structural features in common with natural retinoids, and yet they may share significant biologic activities with natural compounds. It seems that for some functions, the overall shape of the molecule may be more important than its precise chemical features.

Provitamin A

Provitamin A carotenoids are produced only by plants and a few lower organisms (e.g., algae) (10). In plants, carotenoids are present in association with chlorophyll and other photosynthetic pigments in chloroplasts. Although more than 600 carotenoids are known (10), only a few of them—α-carotene, β-carotene and β-cryptoxanthin—are important sources of vitamin A. All provitamin A carotenoids have one or two β-ionone rings. β-Carotene (Fig. 19.2A), a 40-carbon molecule that is symmetric around its central 15,15′ C-C double bond, is synthesized by the tail-to-tail condensation of two 20-carbon molecules of geranylgeranyl diphosphate to form lycopene, which lacks a closed ring structure (Fig. 19.2B) (10); lycopene is then converted to β-carotene (molecular weight 536.88) by the enzyme lycopene-β-cyclase. Oxygen may be added to the ionone ring to produce xanthophylls such as lutein (Fig. 19.2C) and

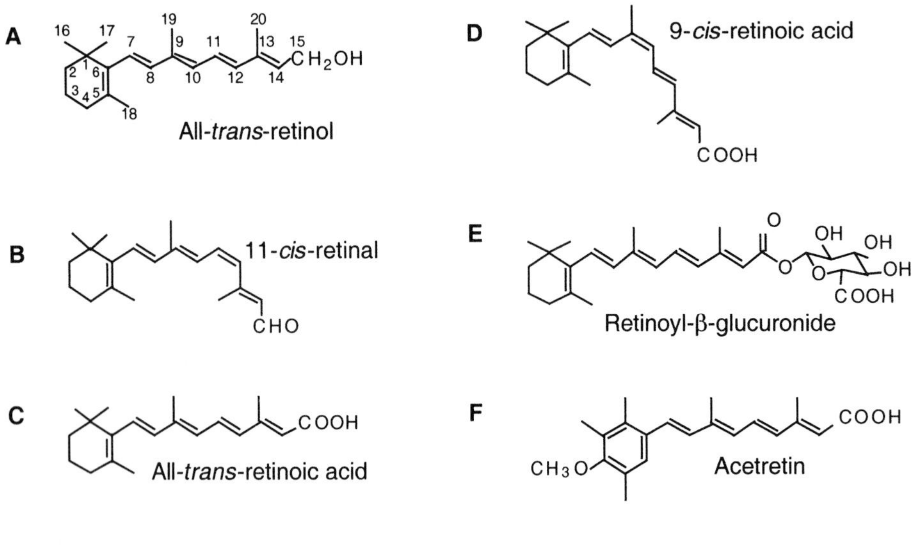

Figure 19.1. Structures of common naturally occurring retinoids (**A–E**), and a representative synthetic retinoid, Acitretin (**F**).

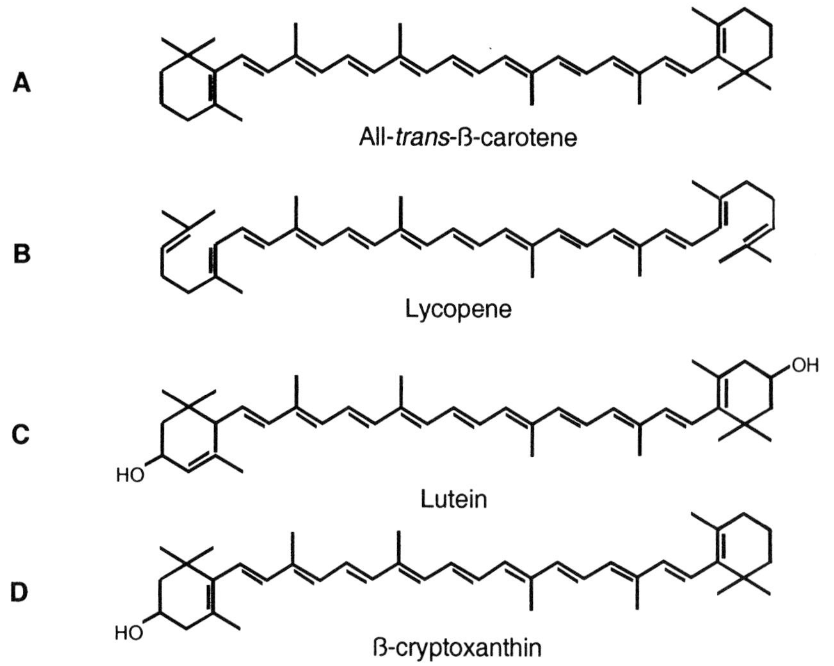

Figure 19.2. Common carotenes and carotenoids in the diet and human plasma: β (β,β')-carotene (**A**), lycopene (**B**), lutein (**C**), and β-cryptoxanthin (**D**).

zeaxanthin, which differs from lutein only in the position of the double bond in one of the β-ionone rings (10). Dietary β-carotene is present at relatively high levels in carrots and yellow and green leafy vegetables; α-carotene is present in carrots and red palm oil; and β-cryptoxanthin (Fig. 19.2D) is found in sweet red pepper, oranges, and papaya, according to the US Department of Agriculture Nutrition Coordinating Center Carotenoids Database (11). In general, the all-*trans* form of each carotenoid is more abundant and has greater stability as compared with carotenoids containing one or more *cis* bonds.

Methods of Analysis

Modern methods of retinoid and carotenoid analysis are based on solvent extraction of samples followed by chromatographic separation of molecular species, most often by high-performance liquid chromatography, with detection by ultraviolet absorption at single or multiple wavelengths (12). Some metabolic and biochemical studies in animals and humans have been conducted using deuterium- or carbon-13–labeled compounds. Isotopically enriched forms of vitamin A and isotope dilution methods have proved useful for determining the mass of retinol stored in body pools (see the later section on indicators and tests), whereas labeled carotenoids have been used to determine the bioavailability and tissue distribution of carotenoids (see the later section on plasma carotenoids).

NUTRITIONAL SOURCES, UNITS, AND RECOMMENDED DIETARY ALLOWANCES

The nutritional need for vitamin A can be met by sufficient amounts, from any source, of preformed vitamin A (retinol and its esters), provitamin A carotenoids, or various combinations of both. The highest concentrations of vitamin A are found in liver and fish liver oils. Yellow and green leafy vegetables, eggs, and whole-milk products provide most of the vitamin A consumed in developed countries (13). Carotenoid-containing vegetables and fruits such as mangoes are the major source of vitamin A in most of the developing world.

Units

Because preformed vitamin A and provitamin A differ in their bioavailability, which affects their biologic activity, it has been necessary to use equivalency factors (units) to compare the amounts contained in foods. One of the earliest established units, the international unit (IU), does not take into account the poor absorption of carotenoids by the human digestive system. By definition, 1 IU = 0.30 µg all-*trans*-retinol or 0.6 µg of all-*trans* β-carotene. The IU was replaced in 1967 by the retinol equivalent (RE) (14), which takes into account the lower nutritional value of provitamin A carotenoids compared with β-carotene. In this system, 1 RE equals 1 µg retinol, 6 µg β-carotene, or 12 µg other provitamin A carotenoids (all in their all-*trans* configurations). After it was shown that the bioactivity of carotenoids in foods is less than had previously been thought, another unit, the retinol activity equivalent (RAE), was adopted in 2001 (13). In RAE units, 1 µg RAE is equal to 1 µg of pure all-*trans*-retinol, 2 µg of all-*trans*-β-carotene in oil (a highly absorbable form), 12 µg of food-based all-*trans*-β-carotene, or 24 µg of other, food-based, all-*trans* provitamin A carotenoids (13) (see Appendix Table A-1-b for conversion factors).

The recommended dietary allowances (RDAs) for vitamin A that were established in 2001 are expressed in micrograms RAE/day (13). Current US and Canadian RDAs for vitamin A are given in Table 19.1, which includes estimated average requirements (EARs), RDAs, and the criteria used to establish them. The adequate intake for infants is based on estimates of the vitamin A content of human breast milk and the volume of breast milk consumed by 0- to 6-month-old and 7- to 12-month-old nursing infants (13). The EAR for adult men and women was determined using a factorial method that takes into consideration the proportion of vitamin A stores lost per day (0.5%), minimum acceptable liver vitamin A reserves (20 μg/g) (15), and the efficiency of storage of ingested vitamin A (13). Because data to calculate an EAR were not available for adolescents and children, the values for these age groups are based on adult EAR values scaled down on the basis of metabolic weight (see Table 19.1). The EAR for pregnancy includes the woman's vitamin A requirement and an additional amount to cover the vitamin A that is transferred to her growing fetus. Similarly, the EAR for lactating women includes an additional amount to cover the secretion of vitamin A in breast milk (13). For all age and sex groups, the RDAs were calculated from the EARs, assuming a coefficient of variation of 20%. The rationale for the tolerable upper intake levels (ULs) for vitamin A is discussed later in this chapter.

No dietary reference intake values were set specifically for carotenoids because no specific requirement could be identified for carotenoids, except as provitamin A (13). The RDA for vitamin A may be obtained by consuming any mixture of Provitamin A preformed vitamin A that provides an adequate intake in micrograms RAE. When the new conversion factors and RAE are used, a larger consumption of provitamin A–containing foods is needed to meet the RDA values. Sample menus were developed for the 2001 Institute of Medicine (IOM) report to illustrate that it is feasible to meet the RDA for vitamin A from purely vegetarian diets (13). Still, the recognition that carotenoid bioavailability is very low from some foods, especially fibrous vegetables, has led to concern that people in some parts of the world may have difficulty meeting their vitamin A requirement from locally available foods (16).

Appendix Table A-23-a lists the vitamin A content of a large number of foods. The Appendices also contain the 1989 to 1990 US and Canadian RDA tables (Appendix Table A-3a and b) and current nutrient recommendations issued by the United Kingdom, Japan, Korea, and the World Health Organization (WHO) (Appendix Tables A-4 through A-8). Appendix Tables A-2b through A-2k have additional DRI data.

TABLE 19.1. CRITERIA AND DIETARY REFERENCE INTAKE VALUES FOR VITAMIN A BY LIFE-STAGE GROUP

| LIFE-STAGE GROUP | CRITERION | EAR (μg RAE/d)[a] | | RDA (μg RAE/d)[b] | | AI[c] (μg/d) |
		MALE	FEMALE	MALE	FEMALE	
0–6 mo	Average vitamin A intake from human milk					400
7–12 mo	Extrapolation from 0–6 mo AI					500
1–3 y	Extrapolation from adult EAR	210	210	300	300	
4–8 y	Extrapolation from adult EAR	275	275	400	400	
9–13 y	Extrapolation from adult EAR	445	420	600	600	
14–18 y	Extrapolation from adult EAR	630	485	900	700	
>18 y	Adequate liver vitamin A stores	625	500	900	700	
Pregnancy						
14–18 y	Adolescent female EAR plus estimated daily accumulation by fetus		530		750	
19–50 y	Adult female EAR plus estimated daily accumulation by fetus		550		770	
Lactation						
14–18 y	Adolescent female EAR plus average amount of vitamin A secreted in human milk		885		1,200	
19–50 y	Adult female EAR plus average amount of vitamin A secreted in human milk		900		1,300	

a, From reference 13.

[a] EAR, estimated average requirement, the intake that meets the estimated nutrient needs of half of the individuals in a group, as retinol activity equivalents (RAEs).

[b] RDA, recommended dietary allowance, the intake that meets the nutrient need of almost all (97–98%) of individuals in a group.

[c] AI, adequate intake, the observed average or experimentally determined intake by a defined population or subgroup that appears to sustain a defined nutritional status, such as growth rate, normal circulating nutrient values, or other functional indicators of health. The AI is used if sufficient scientific evidence is not available to derive an EAR. For healthy infants receiving human milk, the AI is the mean intake. The AI is not equivalent to an RDA.

From Food and Nutrition Board, Institute of Medicine. Dietary Reference Intakes for Vitamin A, Vitamin K, Arsenic, Boron, Chromium, Copper, Iodine, Iron, Manganese, Molybdenum, Nickel, Silicon, Vanadium, and Zinc. Washington, DC: National Academy Press, 2001.

PHYSIOLOGIC PROCESSING OF VITAMIN A

Numerous retinoids are formed during metabolism. Most of them exist at one of three oxidation levels: alcohol (retinol and its esters), aldehyde (retinal in various isomeric forms), and carboxylic acid (RA in its various isomeric forms). More highly oxidized metabolites are formed by oxidation of the ionone ring, and water-soluble retinoids may be formed by the addition of a hydrophilic adduct such as glucuronic acid. A schematic of the main reactions of retinoid metabolism is shown in Figure 19.3.

Retinoid-Binding Proteins and Receptors

Several retinoid-binding proteins are crucial to vitamin A metabolism. These proteins (a) confer aqueous solubility to lipophilic retinoids, (b) serve as chaperones that guide the transport and metabolism of specific retinoids, and (c) mediate certain retinoid functions. The principal groups of retinoid-binding proteins are as follows: the plasma transport protein, RBP together with its cotransport protein transthyretin (TTR); cytosolic (cellular) retinoid-binding proteins found in the soluble fraction of many cells; and nuclear retinoid receptors (RAR and RXR; see later), which mediate the functions of RA in gene expression.

By contrast to the retinoids, the carotenoids are transported by various plasma lipoproteins. No specific cytosolic binding proteins or nuclear receptors have yet been found for carotenoids.

Retinol-Binding Protein and Transthyretin

Nearly all (90–95%) plasma vitamin A is in the form of retinol, bound through hydrophobic interactions to a 21-kDa protein, RBP. RBP is a member of the lipocalin family of hydrophobic ligand-binding proteins. Its tertiary structure, which has been described as a "β-barrel," includes an interior cavity into which one molecule of retinol can fit, thus forming holo-RBP. The hydroxyl group of retinol is oriented toward RBP's outer surface (17-19). In plasma, RBP circulates bound noncovalently with TTR (previously known as thyroxin-binding globulin and as prealbumin), and this complex further stabilizes the binding

of retinol to RBP (17, 19, 20). TTR is a tetrameric protein (~56 kDa) having two identical thyroxine-binding sites. TTR and RBP interact in plasma to form a complex of approximately 75 kDa, but the concentration of TTR exceeds that of RBP, and therefore most of the TTR in plasma circulates independently from RBP. TTR is also present at high concentration in cerebrospinal fluid (20). Numerous inherited variants of TTR have been described, some of which affect thyroxine and/or RBP binding; however, most are associated with familial amyloidotic polyneuropathy (20).

The gene for RBP is located on human chromosome 10q23–24, spanning 10 kb of genomic DNA. The cDNA of approximately 1000 bp encodes a 199-amino acid proprotein, including a 16-amino acid signal peptide that is removed cotranslationally to produce the mature 183-amino acid RBP. The mRNA for RBP is most abundant in the liver, a finding implying the liver is a primary site of RBP synthesis. However, that RBP mRNA is also present at lower levels in the kidney and several other organs (21) suggests that these organs may also secrete RBP (see the later section on in vivo kinetics of retinol).

Cellular Retinoid-Binding Proteins

The cellular retinoid-binding protein family is composed of several proteins of similar size (~14.6 kDa) and shape (17). Whereas these cellular retinoid-binding proteins are found in nearly all cells, they differ in tissue distributions (17), and therefore investigators have suggested that these proteins are involved with different requirements for retinol and RA in different tissues (22). All the cellular retinoid-binding proteins bind one molecule of ligand. The cellular retinoid-binding proteins CRBP-I, CRBP-II, CRBP-III, and CRBP-IV bind all-*trans*-retinol; however, some of them, such as CRBP-II, also bind retinal, whereas CRBP-III also binds *cis*-retinols with nearly equal affinity. CRBP-I is expressed nearly ubiquitously and is most abundant in the liver, kidneys, and the male reproductive tract. CRBP-II is most abundant in small intestine villous-associated enterocytes (23); CRBP-III is relatively abundant in the heart, skeletal muscle, kidney, and liver (24, 25), and CRBP-IV is most abundant in the kidney, heart, and transverse colon (26). Two cellular RA-binding proteins, CRABP-I and CRABP-II, preferentially bind all-*trans*-RA (23). Most adult tissues express CRABP-I, generally at lower levels than the CRBPs, whereas CRABP-II is mainly restricted to the skin, reproductive organs, and choroid plexus. Both CRABP-I and CRABP-II are expressed in embryos but usually not together in the same cells.

Besides the cellular retinoid-binding proteins mentioned earlier, two other proteins are restricted to ocular tissues (see the later section on vision and ocular retinoid metabolism). Cellular retinal-binding protein (CRALBP) is a 45-kDa protein located in the retina that is involved in the visual cycle (17, 27). A larger protein, referred to as

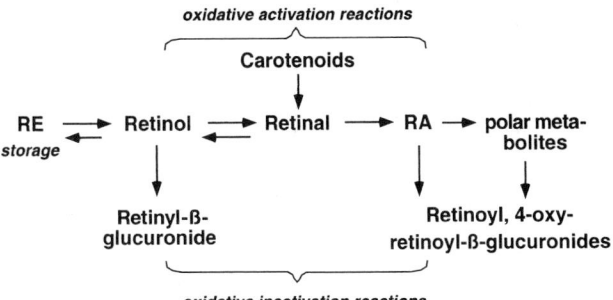

Figure 19.3. Schematic overview of retinoid metabolism. RA, retinoic acid; RE, retinyl ester.

interstitial retinoid-binding protein (IRBP), is synthesized by photoreceptor cells (and by the pineal gland) and is secreted into the interphotoreceptor space, where it appears to function as a retinoid chaperone during the transport of retinoids between the retina and retinal pigment epithelium (RPE) (17, 27).

Nuclear Retinoid Receptors

The retinoid receptor gene family is part of the larger superfamily of steroid/thyroid hormone receptors. The retinoid receptor family comprises six genes: RARα, β, and γ, and RXRα, β, and γ. Although similar in structure, these receptors differ in spatial and temporal expression, both in adult and in embryonic tissues.

The RAR and RXR proteins share a similar protein organization that includes a DNA-binding domain, a hinge region, a ligand-binding domain, and a C-terminal domain that functions in receptor dimerization and ligand-dependent receptor activation (5, 28–30). The principal ligand of the RAR is all-*trans*-RA. The binding of ligand induces a change in the receptor protein's conformation that facilitates its interaction with other receptors (e.g., RXR) and with a multiprotein complex that may contain coactivator or repressor molecules along with the basal transcription factors required for gene transcription (5, 30). The level of RAR expressed by cells is regulated by transcription, posttranscriptional modification (e.g., phosphorylation), and active proteolysis (31, 32).

The RXR are homologous to yet distinct from the RAR. The principal RXR ligand is believed to be 9-*cis*-RA (33, 34); however, alternative ligands such as unsaturated fatty acids have been proposed (35, 36). The RXRs (α, β, or γ) interact with the RARs to form a functional heterodimer that is capable of binding to specific DNA sequences in retinoid-responsive genes, as discussed later in this section. However, the RXRs also form heterodimers with several other proteins in the steroid/thyroid hormone gene family including the vitamin D receptor, thyroid hormone receptor, peroxisome proliferator-activated receptors, and drug/xenobiotic binding receptors (29). Thus, the RXRs function in a wide range of hormone-responsive pathways. Retinoid analogs termed "rexinoids" have been synthesized that are able to activate the RXRs selectively (34).

Most retinoid receptor functions are believed to require ligand binding; however, the RARs and RXRs may also function in a ligand-independent manner. An active repressive complex capable of inhibiting gene transcription has been proposed to be ligand independent (37, 38).

DNA nucleotide sequences to which RAR-RXR heterodimers bind are referred to as RA receptor-response elements (RAREs). The typical RARE consensus sequence is a hexanucleotide of $A(orG),GGTCA$, which occurs twice in a direct repeat (DR) with either five or two intervening nucleotides (DR-5 or DR-2, respectively). RAREs are most often located in the 5′ regulatory region of retinoid-responsive genes. Some of the genes that encode retinoid-binding proteins and receptors contain an RARE in their own promoter, thus providing a means for RA to induce some of the proteins that mediate RA's own metabolism and functions.

Absorption and Hepatic Metabolism

The small intestine, liver, and peripheral tissues play crucial roles in vitamin A metabolism (Fig. 19.4), with extensive interorgan recycling of retinoids occurring among them.

Intestinal Metabolism

Vitamin A, whether ingested as preformed vitamin A (retinyl esters) or as provitamin A carotenoids, requires

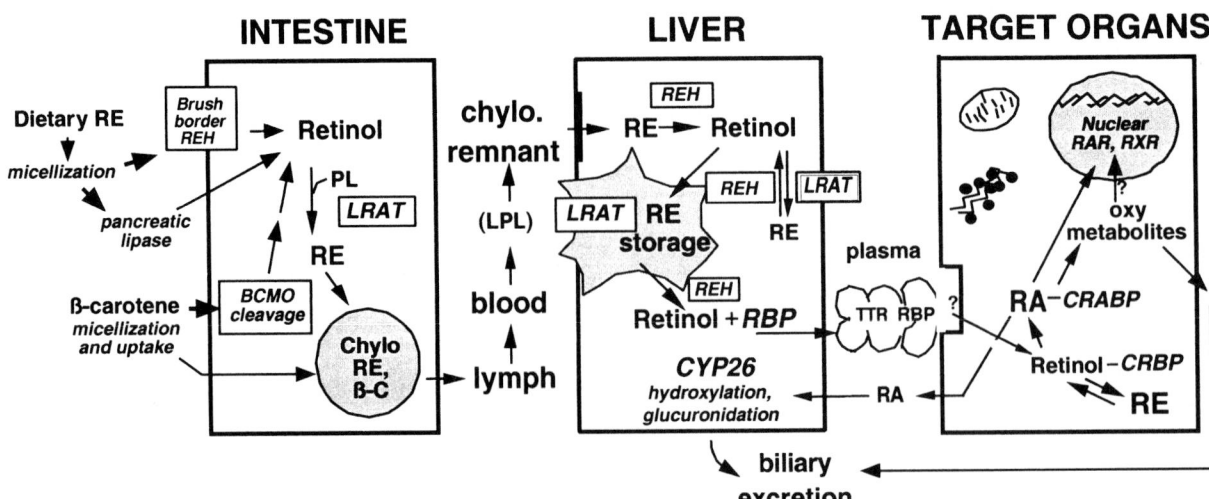

Figure 19.4. Schematic overview of intraorgan transport and physiologic processing of vitamin A. BCMO, β-carotene monooxygenase; chylo, chylomicron; β-C, β-carotene; CRABP, cellular retinoic acid-binding protein; CRBP, cellular retinol-binding protein; CYP26, cytochrome P450 26; LPL, lipoprotein lipase; LRAT, lecithin:retinol acyltransferase; PL, phospholipid; RA, retinoic acid; RAR, retinoic acid receptor; RBP, retinol-binding protein; RE, retinyl esters; REH retinyl ester hydrolase; RXR, retinoid X receptor; TTR, transthyretin.

processing in the intestine to release the nutrient in an absorbable form. The vitamin A-containing fat must first be emulsified, and micelles must be formed. In the case of retinyl esters, the ester bond must be hydrolyzed. Most nonhuman species metabolize nearly all the β-carotene they absorb into retinol and retinyl esters. However, humans, bovines, and some other species absorb a portion of ingested carotenoids directly and incorporate the unmetabolized carotenoids into chylomicrons, thus accounting for the presence of β-carotene and other carotenoids in the plasma and milk of these species. Any condition that interferes with luminal emulsification or lipolysis, such as a relative lack of bile salts or dietary fat ($<\sim5\%$), is likely to reduce the intestinal absorption of retinol (13). Several retinyl ester hydrolases (REHs) have been characterized (39). The predominant intestinal REH is thought to be colipase-dependent pancreatic lipase (40), which also hydrolyzes luminal triglycerides (see Chapter 5). Other REHs located on the enterocyte microvillus membrane may also hydrolyze dietary retinyl esters (41). Once dietary vitamin A is emulsified and retinyl esters are hydrolyzed, most of the retinol is passively absorbed by the enterocytes. The efficiency of absorption of preformed vitamin A ingested in physiologic amounts is relatively high (70–90%). When intake increases, absorption remains high (60–80%), and therefore relatively large quantities of retinol can be absorbed (13). The relatively unlimited absorption of retinol is beneficial from the perspective of allowing for the rapid restoration of vitamin A in depleted individuals, but it is also part of the etiology of hypervitaminosis A (see later).

Similar to preformed vitamin A, carotenoids must be emulsified and solubilized into micelles before they are absorbed into the mucosa by passive diffusion. The efficiency of absorption of a moderate dose of β-carotene in oil is about 9 to 22%. As intake increases, absorption efficiency drops (13). In most animals and humans, the majority of β-carotene is cleaved within the small intestinal mucosa and is absorbed as retinol. In humans and a few animal species, some β-carotene is absorbed intact. In a study of two patients fed radiolabeled β-carotene, the ratio of labeled retinyl esters to intact β-carotene in lymph was about 2:1 (42).

The conversion of provitamin A carotenoids to vitamin A is catalyzed by carotene cleavage enzymes. Retinal, the first reaction product, is then either reduced to retinol or is oxidized to RA (see Fig. 19.3). Carotene cleavage enzymes have been cloned from several species (43). Whereas carotene cleavage was previously described as resulting from β-carotene dioxygenase activity, the mechanism of the expressed enzyme activity has been characterized as β-carotene monooxygenase (44), and the intestinal activity is now referred to by this name. The mRNA for carotene monooxygenase is most abundant in the jejunum, but it is also present in liver, lung, kidneys, and retina (44, 45). The cleavage of β-carotene at the central

15,15′ double bond can in theory yield two molecules of retinal. In some studies, experimental yields close to the theoretic yield of two molecules have been obtained (46). In other studies, however, the experimental yield has been lower. Based on a lower yield and the finding that β-apocarotenals (cleavage products with more or fewer than 15 carbons) may be produced during β-carotene cleavage, an alternative pathway of off-center (excentric) cleavage was proposed. β-Apocarotenals with more than 15 carbons could be shortened to produce retinal; however, this process would yield at most one molecule of retinal per molecule of β-carotene. A gene encoding an asymmetric carotene cleavage enzyme was cloned (47), providing a mechanism for the excentric cleavage pathway (48). However, central cleavage is believed to be the predominant pathway of intestinal β-carotene metabolism.

Besides provitamin A carotenoids, some carotenoids that lack vitamin A activity, such as lycopene, lutein and zeaxanthin, are also absorbed by the human intestine and are present at variable levels in plasma and tissues (46). Evidence suggests that such carotenoids may also undergo intestinal metabolism. Lycopene was cleaved in vitro to acycloretinal, acyclo-RA, and apolycopenals in a nonenzymatic manner (48).

Carotenoids, like retinoids, can exist in multiple isomeric forms. In foods, most β-carotene is the all-*trans*-β form, but certain foods contain *cis* isomers of β-carotene. Pott and colleagues (49) analyzed the β-carotene content of mangoes, a significant source of provitamin A carotenoids in parts of the developing world, and reported finding 9-*cis* and 13-*cis*-β-carotene as 19 to 64% of the total β-carotene, depending on the cultivar tested. For dried mangoes, the proportions of each isomer also depended on the method of drying (conventional versus solar). 9-*cis*-β-Carotene can be absorbed by the human intestine, although in studies using an intestinal epithelial cell line, CaCo-2, 9-*cis*-β-carotene was taken up and transported less efficiently than all-*trans*-β-carotene (50). The fate of various *cis* carotene isomers in vivo is not well known, but it may include isomerization to all-*trans*-carotenoids, either in the intestine (51) or after absorption, and cleavage to form *cis* products such as all-*trans*- and 9-*cis*- or 13-*cis*-retinal (46).

Most of the retinal produced in the intestine from carotene cleavage is reduced to retinol, is esterified with a long-chain fatty acid, and then is absorbed through the lymphatic system just as for preformed vitamin A. In chick intestine, the abilities to cleave β-carotene, to reduce retinal, and to esterify retinol were shown to develop coordinately along the villus-to-crypt axis of the duodenal villi (52, 53). A small portion of retinal produced from the cleavage of β-carotene is oxidized to RA, bound to albumin, and absorbed through the portal venous system (54).

Carotenoid Bioavailability. The bioavailability of carotenoids depends on the type of food consumed, the individual consuming it, and the physical state of the carotenoids (whether free in oily solution or bound within the food matrix), all factors in carotenoid absorption (55–58). Food processing can affect the bioavailability of carotenoids (59). On average, the plasma response after ingestion of 2 μg of β-carotene in an oily solution is similar to the response after ingestion of 1 μg of retinol (60). Factors that are known to reduce the bioavailability of provitamin A carotenoids include following: the presence of dietary fiber, particularly pectins, inadequate dietary fat; the use of nondigestible fat substitutes; interference by other nonprovitamin A carotenoids; and various clinical conditions including inadequate bile flow; lipid malabsorption; and reduced gastric acidity (61). Several studies have shown that the bioavailability of carotenoids present in foods is lower and more variable than it was previously believed to be. These studies led to the introduction of new conversion factors used to compute the nutritional equivalency of carotenoids and preformed vitamin A in foods in RAE units (13), as discussed earlier in the section on units.

Among individual persons, the plasma response to oral dosing with β-carotene, both as a supplement and in foods, can vary widely (62, 63). The average absorption of a large (~20-mg) single dose of β-carotene was 6.1% in a small study of healthy women (63) and 2.2% in a similar study of healthy men (64). However, the absorption efficiency was much higher, 57 and 52%, in two subjects given a much smaller dose of β-carotene (65). Moreover, some subjects showed no detectable response to β-carotene (62, 63, 66). This wide interindividual variation in absorption and plasma response could result from differences in the efficiency of uptake into the mucosa, intracellular cleavage, and/or postabsorptive clearance from plasma (46, 63, 67). After β-carotene has been absorbed from the intestine, its postabsorption conversion may occur over an extended period, up to 53 days after feeding in one study (67).

Retinol Esterification and Chylomicron Transport. Most intestinal retinol is esterified and transported in chylomicrons through the intestinal lymphatic system to the systemic circulation (68, 69) (Fig. 19.5). CRBP-II, which is abundant in enterocytes (68), is involved in the reduction of retinal (produced from β-carotene cleavage) to retinol and in the esterification of retinol to form retinyl esters.

Two enzymes, acyl-coenzyme A:retinol acyltransferase (ARAT) and lecithin:retinol acyltransferase (LRAT), have been implicated in intestinal retinol esterification. Under in vitro assay conditions, ARAT esterifies dispersed retinol using an acyl group derived from fatty acyl-coenzyme A (70); however, ARAT does not esterify retinol bound to CRBP-II. This characteristic and the relatively high Michaelis-Menten constant (K_m) (>20 μmol/L) of ARAT for retinol suggest that it may be most active when the level of retinol is high. Another microsomal enzyme, LRAT, esterifies retinol bound to CRBP-II and has a much lower K_m (<5 μmol/L) for retinol. The acyl donor

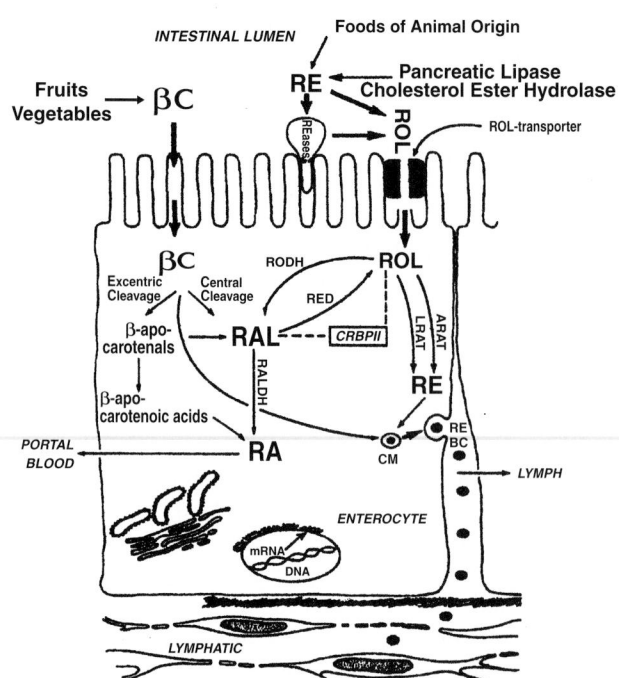

Figure 19.5. Aspects of the metabolism of natural retinoids and β-carotene in the intestinal epithelium. ARAT, acyl-CoA:retinol acyltransferase; βC, β-carotene; CM, chylomicron; CRBPII, cellular retinol-binding protein type II; LRAT, lecithin:retinol acyltransferase; RA, retinoic acid; RAL, retinal; RALDH, retinal dehydrogenase; RE, retinyl ester; REases, brush border retinyl ester hydrolases; RED, retinal reductase; RODH, retinol dehydrogenase; ROL, retinol. (From Silveira ER, Moreno FS. J Nutr Biochem 1998;9:446–56, with permission of *The Journal of Nutritional Biochemistry* [Elsevier]).

for LRAT is the sn-1 fatty acid of phosphatidyl choline in the microsomal membrane. Because LRAT can bind CRBP-I and CRBP-II, has a K_m in the physiologic range, and forms mainly retinyl palmitate and stearate, the main retinyl esters found in vivo, LRAT is likely to be the predominant means of retinyl ester formation in most tissues (71). In the intestine, the retinyl esters produced by LRAT mix with other neutral lipids during assembly of the lipid core of nascent chylomicrons (39). The amount of retinyl ester per chylomicron is directly proportional to the amount of vitamin A being absorbed and esterified during chylomicron assembly (71, 72). In the vitamin A–deficient state, retinyl esters are not detectable in chylomicrons; however, after ingestion of high doses of retinol, the concentration of chylomicron retinyl esters rises dramatically, and retinyl esters can be detected in this lipoprotein fraction of plasma (73). As noted later, the transport of retinyl esters by chylomicrons has implications for the delivery of vitamin A to tissues that metabolize these triglyceride-rich lipoproteins, such as the lactating mammary gland.

The concentration of vitamin A in lymph and plasma reaches a peak about 2 to 6 hours after its ingestion. Chylomicron triglycerides are rapidly hydrolyzed, and chylomicron remnants are rapidly cleared (see Chapter 5). Therefore, the half-life of chylomicron vitamin A in plasma is short, less than 20 minutes in physiologically normal subjects (74).

Hepatic Metabolism

Newly absorbed vitamin A is rapidly and efficiently (85–90%) taken up into liver when chylomicron remnants are cleared into hepatocytes by receptor-mediated endocytosis (71). If the circulation of remnants is prolonged, a proportion of chylomicron retinyl esters may transfer to low- and high-density lipoproteins and then enter cells by lipoprotein receptor-mediated pathways (75). Studies in rats first showed that chylomicron retinyl esters are hydrolyzed soon after their uptake (76, 77). In vitamin A–adequate rats given retinyl ester-labeled chylomicrons, the labeled retinol was transferred within several hours from hepatocytes, the site of initial uptake, into hepatic stellate cells (vitamin A–storing cells, Ito cells) (77), which contain the most concentrated, largest pool of vitamin A in liver. Vitamin A is believed to be transferred as retinol, followed by its reesterification in stellate cells that contain both LRAT activity and CRBP (78). In animals with adequate vitamin A status, about 50 to 85% of total body retinol is stored in the liver, more than 90% as retinyl esters (enriched in retinyl palmitate) (71) located in cytoplasmic lipid droplets in stellate cells (79). In contrast to the reesterification of retinol and storage in stellate cells in vitamin A–adequate rats (77), retinol was rapidly secreted from hepatocytes into plasma bound to RBP in vitamin A–deficient rats (80). These data imply that retinol molecules in hepatocytes can be channeled into either a secretory pathway or a storage pathway, depending on the animal's vitamin A status.

The liver plays a central role in whole-body retinoid homeostasis. First, the expression of LRAT mRNA and activity in the liver are closely regulated by vitamin A status (72), and both fall progressively as vitamin A deficiency develops. A reduction in hepatic LRAT activity as vitamin A deficiency develops may spare what little retinol remains in the liver for other processes, such as the secretion of retinol into plasma or the production of RA. As vitamin A status falls, apo-CRBP increases. Apo-CRBP stimulates the hydrolysis of retinyl esters by microsomal REH (81). Physiologic studies have shown that nearly all the vitamin A in the liver of experimental animals can be mobilized during long-term vitamin A deficiency (82). It is likely that the same is true for humans, because very low values have been observed in some autopsy specimens. Additionally, the liver's role in the secretion of holo-RBP is closely regulated by retinol, and RBP secretion falls off as vitamin A stores fall, as described further later. When vitamin A is administered to vitamin A–depleted animals, holo-RBP is rapidly secreted, LRAT mRNA and activity are rapidly induced (83–85), and retinyl esters are once again stored in liver and other tissues.

Several aspects of hepatic vitamin A metabolism are altered by inflammation. Stellate cells become activated and are induced to mobilize their vitamin A reserves (86, 87) while undergoing a transformation to a myofibroblastic phenotype (88, 89); these activated stellate cells are producers of collagen and are thought to contribute to the etiology of hepatic fibrosis (86). The synthesis of RBP and TTR by the liver is reduced during inflammation (90, 91). In one study, patients having inflammation had low levels of plasma RBP, retinol, all-*trans*- and 13-*cis*-RA concentrations, which were negatively correlated to the concentration of C-reactive protein used as a marker of inflammation (92). Based on this finding, Fex and colleagues (92) speculated that "the decrease in serum retinol and retinoic acid concentration, which occurs in inflammation may create an 'acute vitamin A deficiency,' which may be a factor contributing to the excess mortality associated with measles in children with marginal vitamin A deficiency and in patients with AIDS." (See the later section on vitamin A deficiency.)

Plasma Retinol

Plasma (or serum) vitamin A may be expressed as *total* (saponified) retinol or as *unesterified* retinol. The difference between total and unesterified retinol provides an estimate of *esterified retinol*. In the fasting plasma of healthy humans and many animals, more than 95% of total retinol is in its unesterified form. Plasma retinyl esters are elevated in the postprandial state because of the presence of retinyl esters in chylomicrons or their remnants. Plasma retinyl esters are also typically elevated in hypervitaminosis A (see later). However, in dogs and several other carnivores, high levels of plasma retinyl esters are the norm (93).

In healthy humans, plasma retinol concentrations are quite constant (ranging from ~1.5–3 μmol/L, i.e., 43–86 μg/dL). The molar concentration of RBP is slightly higher such that the molar ratio of retinol to RBP is about 0.9. In several National Health and Nutrition Examination Survey (NHANES) studies, retinol concentrations were lowest in young children, increased during adolescence, and were higher in men than in premenopausal women (30–60 years), then equal in men and women from age 70 years (94, 95). Retinol concentrations were elevated 15 to 35% in oral contraceptive users compared with nonusers (9, 96). Levels were lower in neonates than older children and lower in premature infants (<36 weeks' gestation) than in full-term infants (97). Indicator values of less than 0.35, less than 0.70, less than 1.05, and greater than 1.05 μmol retinol/L are often used to categorize severe deficiency, marginal deficiency, subclinical low plasma vitamin A, and vitamin A adequacy, respectively. Because normal plasma retinol levels differ with age, age should also be considered in interpreting these retinol levels (96).

Liver diseases usually result in lower levels of plasma retinol and RBP, in proportion to the severity of disease (98–100). Patients with both primary biliary cirrhosis and primary sclerosing cholangitis had significantly reduced levels of retinol and carotenoids compared with healthy controls in one study (101).

Relationship between Plasma Vitamin A and Liver Vitamin A Storage. Plasma retinol levels are not linearly related to liver vitamin A levels. In fact, plasma retinol concentrations nearly always remain within a narrow range and fall significantly only when nearly all liver vitamin A is depleted (<20–30 μg retinol/g) (15). When liver retinol levels rise to more than approximately 300 μg total retinol/g liver, plasma *total* retinol levels are also likely to increase, but the rise results from retinyl esters in lipoproteins (15), rather than from an elevation in holo-RBP. Retinyl esters are elevated in fasting plasma when chylomicron clearance is impaired and during hypervitaminosis A (see later); thus, further testing is needed to distinguish between these possibilities.

In Vivo Kinetics (Retinol). An important feature of retinol physiology is the recycling of retinol from the plasma to tissues and back to plasma. Computer-based kinetic modeling has shown that each molecule of retinol recycles an average of nine to 11 times between the liver, plasma, kidneys, and other tissues of rats before being irreversibly degraded (102, 103). In one study, the number of cycles per retinol molecule remained fairly constant even though the total-body vitamin A pool size of individuals varied 40-fold (102). Model-based compartmental analysis of plasma retinol in one healthy young man who had consumed 105 μmol of retinyl palmitate indicated that 50 μmol of retinol passed through his plasma each day, whereas only 4 μmol/day was degraded (103). Unlike retinol, RBP does not appear to be reused (104). It therefore appears that RBP must be synthesized *de novo* for retinol to recycle among organs. Overall, the body's capacity for vitamin A storage is high, whereas its ability to rapidly dispose of excess vitamin A is quite limited. The lack of efficient disposal mechanisms may help to explain why vitamin A can accumulate to toxic levels when intake greatly exceeds requirements.

Retinoids themselves can alter (usually reduce) plasma retinol levels and liver retinoid storage (105, 106). Numerous hepatotoxicants, such as 2,3,7,8-tetrachlorodibenzo-*p*-dioxin and carbon tetrachloride, reduce retinol storage and/or alter retinoid metabolism (107–110).

Plasma Carotenoids. Six species of carotenoids comprise about 60- to 70% of the total carotenoid pool in human plasma (111, 112). The median concentrations (μmol/L) of carotenoids measured in NHANES III for nonsmoking men (M) and women (F) were as follows: lycopene, 0.47 (M) and 0.41 (F); lutein plus zeaxanthin, 0.35 (M and F); β-cryptoxanthin, 0.13 (M and F); β-carotene, 0.22 (M) and 0.28 (F); and α-carotene, 0.065 (M) and 0.081 (F) (46). Smokers have lower mean values than nonsmokers (113). Plasma carotenoid levels tend to be more variable, both within and between subjects, than retinol levels (114). Different carotenoids turn over at different rates, as shown in studies of healthy nonsmokers fed

low-carotenoid diets in which the half-life of plasma carotenoids ranged from less than 12 days for β-carotene, α-carotene, and cryptoxanthin, to 12 to 33 days for lycopene, and to 33 to 61 days for zeaxanthin plus lutein (115, 116). Based on a multicompartmental model of the metabolism of a low physiologic dose (0.3 mg) of orally administered deuterated β-[^{14}C]carotene in one man (117), a minimum of 62% of the absorbed β-carotene was cleaved to produce vitamin A, and the turnover time for β-carotene in plasma was approximately 58 days (117).

Plasma Retinol Transport Proteins

Although several tissues express the RBP gene, the liver and, specifically, the hepatocytes are likely to produce most of it. RBP is translated as a 24-kDa preprotein that is cleaved cotranslationally to the mature 21-kDa protein. The newly synthesized protein then progresses through the secretory pathway to the Golgi apparatus (118), where some portion of it combines with retinol. In studies of cultured hepatocytes, only a portion of the newly synthesized RBP was secreted, whereas the remainder was subject to intracellular degradation (119). In the liver of vitamin A–deficient rats, RBP synthesis continues, but the secretion of holo-RBP is impaired by the lack of retinol, and apo-RBP accumulates in the parenchymal cells (120). Within minutes after the administration of retinol to vitamin A–deficient rats, the plasma concentrations of both retinol and RBP rose very rapidly, exceeded a normal concentration for an hour or so, and then subsided and stabilized at normal values (118, 120). The insight gained from these finding in rats led Underwood and coworkers to develop the relative dose response (RDR) test as a useful clinical indicator of the adequacy of vitamin A reserves in human liver (see the later section on assessment of vitamin A status).

The plasma concentrations of RBP and TTR, also produced by hepatocytes (20), are sensitive to changes nutritional and physiologic conditions because their half-lives are relatively short (~0.5 and 2–3 days, respectively [104]), and, therefore, a high rate of protein synthesis is necessary to maintain their normal levels. RBP and TTR concentrations are significantly reduced in protein-energy malnutrition (121, 122), during infection and inflammation, and after trauma (90, 91, 123, 124). The levels of RBP and TTR are considered useful clinical indicators of visceral protein status and the response to nutritional support (125–127).

Mice with a genetic lack of RBP have been useful for studying the effects of low or absent levels of RBP. Weanling RBP-deficient mice had low plasma retinol levels and impaired vision, but they recovered visual function when they were fed a diet with adequate vitamin A (128). Visual function also was improved when RBP-deficient mice were engineered to carry a human RBP transgene and therefore had human RBP in their circulation (129). Very low plasma retinol levels and impaired vision were also reported in two teenage sisters shown to have a mutation in their RBP gene that resulted in a single amino acid substitution in RBP protein (130). Despite very low plasma retinol, both siblings showed normal growth and development. Interestingly, plasma RA levels were not abnormal. It is likely that their diet, which was adequate in vitamin A, provided enough vitamin A from chylomicrons to compensate for the lack of holo-RBP (131). Because the retina was affected in these patients, and in mice lacking RBP, it appears that the retina is more dependent on holo-RBP than are most other organs.

Transport Kinetics and Tissue Uptake. Apo-RBP is readily filtered in the kidneys. The plasma half-life of apo-RBP is even shorter than that of holo-RBP, only approximately 4 hours (104). The formation of the complex of holo-RBP and TTR (20, 118) serves to prevent the rapid loss of RBP in the kidneys. Retinol is taken up from holo-RBP by many tissues, but the mechanism of its uptake is not well understood. Investigators have sought a receptor for RBP, but biochemical evidence is still scant. One promising mechanism has been described for kidney proximal tubule cells. Megalin, a multiligand receptor linked to transcytosis (132), was shown to bind RBP (133, 134) and TTR (135) and to facilitate the reuptake of retinol after renal filtration (see the later section on retinoid excretion). Retinyl esters associated with plasma lipoproteins may gain entry to cells by cell-surface apolipoprotein or scavenger receptors (75), whereas relatively polar retinoids such as RA and glucuronide adducts most likely enter cells by diffusion.

Retinoic Acid in Plasma and Tissues. In contrast to retinol, RA is bound to serum albumin (136). Plasma contains low (nanomolar) concentrations of several isomers of RA, including all-*trans*-RA, 13-*cis*-RA and 9-*cis*-RA, and metabolites such as 13-*cis*-4-oxo-RA (137, 138). Both dietary vitamin A and ingestion of supplements can produce rapid changes in RA and its metabolites in vivo. The levels of 13-*cis*-RA and 13-*cis*-4-oxo-RA in plasma increased two- to fourfold after healthy human subjects had ingested retinyl palmitate at levels that were well in excess of normal dietary levels (139) and after the consumption of a serving of turkey liver that provided the subjects with about 1 mg of total retinol/kg body weight (138). After administration of a high dose of RA to cynomolgus monkeys, retinoyl-β-glucuronide was a major metabolite (140), and it was rapidly cleared from plasma (141).

The rapid turnover of RA has been demonstrated in a variety of studies. When rats were given ^{14}C-all-*trans*-RA orally, less than 10% of the label remained in the body, mostly in the liver, kidney, and intestine after 8 days (136). A large intravenous dose of all-*trans*-RA was cleared rapidly in rhesus monkeys, initially by first-order kinetics with a half-life of 19 minutes (142), followed by a dose-dependent plateau suggesting that clearance was saturated. Cell, animal, and human studies have shown that all-*trans*-RA can induce its own catabolism. In healthy men, the area under the curve of all-*trans*-RA decreased following repeated oral administration of all-*trans*-RA (143), a finding indicating the induction of RA metabolism by RA itself. In monkeys, all-*trans*-RA was rapidly converted to 9-*cis*- or 13-*cis*-RA (140). In a graded-dose pharmacokinetic study in healthy men, orally administered 9-*cis*-RA was metabolized with a half-life of less than 2.4 hours, mainly to 4-oxo-9-*cis*-RA (144), but at the same time, some was isomerized into all-*trans*- and 13-*cis*-RA.

The concentration of RA in tissues is usually higher than the concentration of RA in plasma (145, 146). The contributions to tissue RA of plasma-derived RA and in situ-produced RA varied substantially among different rat organs; for example, more than 80% of the RA in liver was derived from plasma, but most of RA in the testis was produced locally, presumably from the oxidation of retinol (146).

RA concentrations are regulated both by biosynthesis (147, 148) and oxidation (149). Some tissues derive most of their RA by local metabolism (150) and others by uptake from plasma (146), consistent with RA's functioning as an autocrine or paracrine as well as an endocrine hormone. Multiple enzymes have been shown to be capable of producing and degrading RA, and the mechanisms of RA homeostasis may differ with tissues and/or cell type. The oxidation of retinol to RA is a tightly controlled process in which retinol is first oxidized to retinal. Several retinol dehydrogenases (RDHs) that are members of the short-chain dehydrogenase/reductase superfamily) have been isolated. RDHs tend to have broad substrate specificity for steroids as well retinoids. In assays of retinoid metabolism in vitro, some RDHs preferentially oxidized all-*trans*-retinol and others *cis* isomers of retinol (151). Some RDHs have been shown to interact with CRBP, and this may facilitate the metabolism of CRBP-bound retinol by particular enzymes (147, 152). Some members of the alcohol dehydrogenase gene family can oxidize retinol (147, 148, 153). In all, numerous enzymes involved in the oxidation reduction of retinol and retinal have been described, but their relative importance in vivo is still uncertain.

The second oxidation reaction in which retinal is converted to RA is irreversible. Again, multiple enzymes have been implicated, including members of the retinal dehydrogenase (RALDH) gene family (147, 154, 155), some of which interact with CRBP (17, 147), and some members of the cytochrome P450 gene family (156, 157).

How 9-*cis*- and 13-*cis*-RA are formed is not yet clear. Dietary 9-*cis*-β-carotene is likely to be metabolized to 9-*cis*-retinol, and isolated cells have been shown to oxidize 9-*cis*-retinol to 9-*cis*-RA and other products (158–160). In human serum, the levels of retinol, all-*trans*-RA, and 13-*cis*-RA were significantly and positively correlated with each other, findings suggesting that their metabolism may be coordinated (92). The cellular retinoid-binding protein, CRABP, by virtue of preferentially binding all-*trans*-RA, could indirectly affect the intracellular concentrations and the proportions of various isomers of RA in cells (17).

CRABP is also thought to facilitate the oxidation of RA to more polar products (17, 147). Microsomal cytochrome P450 enzymes have been described that can hydroxylate RA and catalyze its glucuronidation (161–163). One subfamily of cytochrome P450 enzymes, CYP26, is of special interest because its expression is inducible by RA. CYP26A1 has been cloned from several vertebrate species; in adults, it is most abundant in liver, intestine, and reproductive organs. The CYP26A1 gene promoter contains a nearly canonical RARE (164), and the expression of CYP26A1 mRNA in liver and several other tissues (165) is responsive to vitamin A and RA (165, 166). Besides CYP26A1, the CYP26 gene family includes CYP26B1, which is relatively highly enriched in cephalic tissue (167, 168), and CYP26C1, which is expressed in embryonic hindbrain structures (169) and seems to be the only form of CYP26 capable of oxidizing *cis* as well as *trans* isomers of RA (170).

Retinoid Excretion. The kidneys are the principal organ of catabolism and loss of RBP. The renal clearance of RBP is equivalent to approximately 7/8 L of plasma per day in a 70-kg person (104). Plasma holo-RBP is partially filtered through the glomerulus (19). As noted earlier, both TTR and RBP can bind to megalin (gp330), a multiligand receptor present on the apical surface of renal proximal tubule cells (132, 135) and perhaps other cell types. A portion of the RBP that is taken up is degraded intracellularly, whereas a portion undergoes transcytosis across the tubule cells; the latter process is believed to result in the recycling of retinol back to plasma (132). Mice lacking megalin failed to take up RBP into renal proximal tubules, and retinol and RBP excretion in urine was increased (133).

Chronic renal diseases affecting filtration are typically associated with higher levels of plasma retinol, RBP (104, 171), and TTR (126). In nephrectomized rats, serum retinol increased up to 70% within just 2 hours (106, 172). RBP also increased in the extracellular fluid space of rats with acute renal failure (106). Plasma apo-RBP, which normally is rapidly filtered in the glomerulus, may provide a feedback signal to the liver to stimulate the output of holo-RBP to maintain homeostasis (173). In severe infections causing significant proteinuria (174), and in diarrhea (175), urinary retinol excretion was detected.

FUNCTIONS

Vision and Ocular Retinoid Metabolism

Vitamin A plays two distinct roles in different parts of the eye: (a) in the retina, 11-*cis*-retinal functions directly in vision by undergoing photoisomerization; this process initiates a signal transduction cascade that relays information to the brain's visual cortex; and (b) in the conjunctival membranes and the cornea, RA acts as a differentiating agent to maintain the normal morphology and functions of the various cells in these tissues.

The retina includes two types of photoreceptor cells: the rods, which are specialized for the detection of motion and for visual acuity in dim light; and the cones, which are specialized for red, green, or blue color vision, which occurs at a higher level of light. 11-*cis*-Retinal is the specific photoreceptor; in rods, it is bound as a Schiff base to opsin forming rhodopsin. As noted by Saari concerning the role of opsin (176), "opsin is tailor-made to shift the absorption spectrum of the retinoid into the visible range, increase its quantum efficiency of photoisomerization, and trigger further biochemical responses." As illustrated in Figure 19.6, the absorption of a photon of light triggers the photoisomerization of 11-*cis*-retinal to all-*trans*-retinal. The photoisomerization process triggers a G-protein signal transduction cascade leading to a reduction in sodium conductance across the photoreceptor cell plasma membrane, which initiates signaling to neuronal cells (27). In actuality, simultaneous signals from millions of molecules of rhodopsin in thousands of rod cells are integrated into a signal that is transmitted by the optic nerve to the brain's visual cortex.

During photoisomerization, all-*trans*-retinal is released from opsin. For vision to continue, 11-*cis*-retinal must be regenerated. Rhodopsin is regenerated very quickly, within

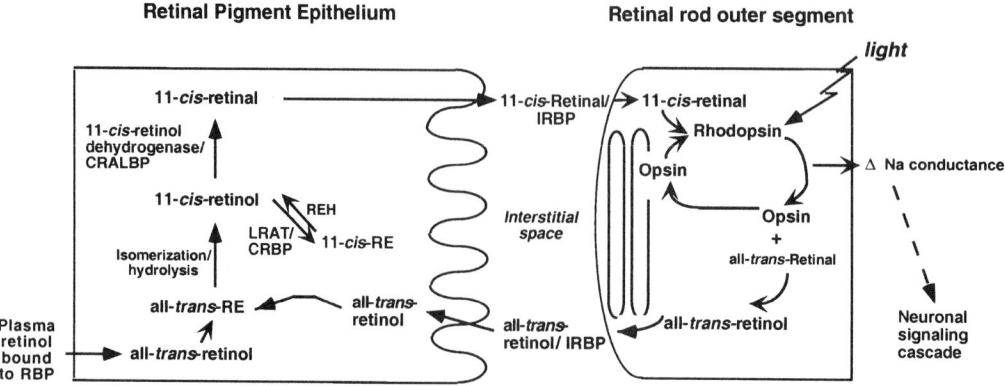

Figure 19.6. Retinoid metabolism in vision. CRALBP, cellular retinal-binding protein; CRBP, cellular retinol-binding protein; IRBP, interstitial retinoid-binding protein; LRAT, lecithin:retinol acyltransferase; RBP, retinol-binding protein; REH retinyl ester hydrolase.

minutes, when vitamin A is adequate (176). The regeneration process occurs in a series of so-called "dark reactions," most of which take place in the RPE (177), a layer of epithelial cells separated from the photoreceptor cells by the interphotoreceptor space. All-*trans*-retinal is first reduced to all-*trans*-retinol enzymatically (178) in the photoreceptor cell outer segments, and then it is transported, presumably by IRBP, to the RPE (27). Within the RPE cells, all-*trans*-retinol is then esterified by LRAT to form a local pool of stored retinyl esters. This small pool of retinyl esters provides a highly concentrated supply of vitamin A for the immediate replenishment of 11-*cis*-retinal after photobleaching. When this retinyl ester pool is depleted (e.g., in vitamin A deficiency), the regeneration of rhodopsin is delayed, and night blindness (poor dark adaptation after exposure to bright light) results (6). When vitamin A is adequate, retinyl esters in the RPE are rapidly hydrolyzed to produce all-*trans*-retinol and subsequently 11-*cis*-retinol. 11-*cis*-Retinol is then oxidized to regenerate 11-*cis*-retinal in a reaction facilitated by CRALBP (27), and 11-*cis*-retinal then is transported, probably by IRBP, to the rod cells for combination with opsin. In a conveyor-like fashion, 11-*cis*-retinal is bleached and regenerated several times before it is degraded (27).

Although the visual cycle has been most extensively studied in rods, a similar cycle occurs for the color-sensitive cone cells. In cones, retinal is bound to a red-, green-, or blue-specific cone opsin protein. A novel cone visual cycle has been deduced that involves the regeneration of retinal released from cone opsin in a pathway that involves both cones and nearby Müller cells (179). The cone visual cycle regenerates cone opsins 20 times more rapidly than rhodopsin is regenerated in the rod visual cycle (180).

In addition to night blindness resulting from vitamin A deficiency (6), which is readily reversible by vitamin A, night blindness also occurs in Sorsby fundus dystrophy, an autosomal dominant retinal degeneration. This condition improved within a week after provision of 50,000 IU (~15,000 μg) of vitamin A to patients at the early stages of disease (181, 182), a finding suggesting that their defect may involve impaired storage of vitamin A in the RPE.

Another light-sensitive protein, melanopsin, also contains retinal as its light-sensitive prosthetic group. Melanopsin is located in ganglion cells and has been implicated in the regulation of circadian rhythm (183).

Several mutations and deletions of vitamin A–metabolizing proteins affecting visual function have been described. Mutations in LRAT, RDHs, the retinyl ester-binding RPE-specific protein 65 (RPE65) (177, 184), and others, affect the regeneration of visual pigments and are associated with retinal dystrophy (RPE65, LRAT), fundus albipunctatis (RDH5), and other abnormalities (177, 185–187).

The cornea, an avascular tissue, depends on vitamin A delivered in tear fluid to maintain cell differentiation and structural integrity. The lacrimal gland synthesizes and secretes RBP, which apparently solubilizes the retinol in tears (188). As shown for liver, the synthesis of RBP in the lacrimal gland continues at a normal level during vitamin A deficiency (189). However, mucus production by the goblet cells of the conjunctival membranes is reduced, and the cornea becomes dry (xerosis) as vitamin A deficiency progresses (6). Bitôt spots (cellular debris) may develop, usually at the outer quadrant of the eyes. Although these changes are reversible if vitamin A is administered at this time, a continued lack of vitamin A results in extensive, irreparable damage to the cornea (keratomalacia and ulceration) (see Chapter 38).

Cellular Differentiation

Vitamin A deficiency has long been associated with abnormal epithelial morphology. In the mid-1920s, Wolbach and Howe first established the marked change in epithelial morphology in tissues of vitamin A–deficient rats (190). The epithelial lining of many tissues became flattened (squamous), dry, and keratinized. This research provided the first clue to the functions of vitamin A in cell differentiation, now known to be the result of RA's action as a regulator of gene transcription (191). In rapidly dividing cells, retinoids efficiently inhibit progression through the cell cycle and induce cell differentiation (192). Although nearly all studies of retinoid mechanisms have been conducted using isolated cells, good congruence exists between their actions in cells and their effects in intact animals and humans. For example, the expression of cell cycle–related gene cyclin proteins and proliferation-related proteins AP-1 were shown to be regulated in intact rats by vitamin A deficiency and supplementation (193), whereas myeloid cell differentiation is rapidly induced by all-*trans*-RA in patients with APL and in cells in vitro (194, 195) (see the later section on cancer chemoprevention and treatment).

Development

Embryonic development requires a closely timed sequence of gene expression, cell proliferation, and apoptosis. Research conducted in the 1940s and 1950s clearly demonstrated that experimental vitamin A deficiency causes birth defects and fetal mortality (196). Abnormalities observed in vitamin A–deficient rats included microphthalmia, craniofacial abnormalities, and abnormalities of the thymus, liver, vascular system, and heart (197, 198). Similar developmental abnormalities are often observed in vitamin A deficiency (199), in hypervitaminosis A (200), and after exposure to high doses of acidic retinoids during critical gestational periods (201).

Vertebrate embryogenesis does not appear to require RA prior to gastrulation; however, RA is clearly involved in the induction of morphogenesis in the postgastrulation period. The induction of retinoid signaling is thought to depend on RA produced by the embryo from maternally derived retinol. Various retinoid-binding proteins and retinoid biosynthetic enzymes (203, 204) are expressed early in embryonic development in temporally and spacially specific patterns (205), including the genes for nuclear retinoid receptors (206), cellular retinoid-binding proteins, and biosynthetic enzymes, such as RDH-1 (207) and RALDH-2 (203, 208, 209), as well as oxidative enzymes, such as cytochrome P450s (167, 205, 210–212). It may be inferred from the patterns of gene expression that RA production is first turned on and then suppressed in wavelike patterns. A concept central to embryology is that a biochemical gradient of diffusable morphogens serves to guide and control the development of the body's anterior-posterior and dorsal-ventral axes as well as the formation of the limbs and other structures. The production and catabolism of retinoids in temporally and spacially regulated patterns are believed to control the expression of other genes, including members of the home-obox-containing *Hox* gene family (213) and the *hedgehog* gene family (214). Some of these genes contain a functional RARE (202, 215) and therefore are direct targets of RA. Numerous studies have shown that retinoids are involved in the regulating the development of the limbs, central nervous system, cardiovascular system, ears and eyes, and skeletal system (213, 216).

Given the critical actions of RA in embryonic development, it was surprising to observe that knockout mice lacking a single form of RAR or RXR, and even double knockouts lacking both CRABP-I and CRABP-II, appear relatively normal (28). The absence of a severe phenotype in these mice could be the result of compensation by other proteins within the same gene family. Mice with compound receptor deletions (e.g., mice lacking both RARα and RARγ) did show a more severe phenotype. Indeed, their defects closely resembled those seen in genetically normal embryos of vitamin A–deficient mothers (197, 217).

Besides the well-demonstrated requirement for RA in early development, retinol may be a specific requirement later in gestation. In one study, pregnant rats required retinol for normal fetal development beyond gestational day 15 (218).

Retinoids and related proteins are also regulated in developmentally specific patterns in the perinatal periods. RBP is first detectable in rat liver at about gestational day 16. Organ-specific patterns have been described for the expression of retinoid-binding proteins and nuclear receptors and for the deposition of retinyl esters in liver, lungs, small intestine, and other tissues (219–222).

Immunity

Effective immunity requires a complex interplay of cell types. Depending on the infectious agent, the host response may involve primarily the innate or the adaptive arm of the immune system, or both. Cells of the T helper (CD4), cytotoxic (CD8), natural killer, and antigen-presenting cell sets (see Chapter 43) are often affected in experimental models of vitamin A deficiency, although B-cell responses may also be abnormal (223). In animals, vitamin A deficiency is generally associated with a dysregulated immune response characterized by an excess production of type 1 (or Th1) cytokines and in some cases a reduction type 2 (or Th2) activity (223). The innate arm of the immune system responsible for the first line of defense against pathogens is also dysregulated, as evidenced by impairments in neutrophil microbicidal activity, macrophage-mediated phagocytosis, and natural killer cell-mediated cytotoxicity (224). In the deficient state, an excess of proinflammatory (type 1) cytokine expression is often observed (225), and epithelial integrity may be altered (226). Vitamin A deficiency is known to impair epithelial barriers, as illustrated by increased bacterial translocation across the intestinal mucosa of vitamin A–deficient rats (227), a process that further induces inflammation. As noted earlier, inflammatory stimuli reduce the levels of plasma holo-RBP. Together, these results of impaired epithelial barrier functions and increased inflammatory may synergize in a vicious cycle. Marginal vitamin A deficiency and accompanying hyporetinemia may be exacerbated by inflammation (228), further impairing the delivery of vitamin A to tissues that require it for cell differentiation, repair, and recovery from infectious disease.

Poor resistance to infection was one of the earliest recognized pathologic features of vitamin A deficiency. Many studies have shown that vitamin A–deficient animals and persons are more susceptible to natural infections and respond poorly to many immune challenges. However, the effect of vitamin A deficiency, and vitamin A intervention, depends in part on the nature of the infectious agent and the type of immune response it elicits, as shown in a variety of experimental models (223, 224, 229, 230). Similarly, in clinical studies, the outcome of vitamin A treatment has varied with the type of infectious disease monitored. In children, vitamin A has proved effective in reducing the severity of measles (231), yet similar studies monitoring diarrhea have produced mixed results (232, 233), and vitamin A has had little if any benefit on respiratory tract infections and pneumonia (233). Neither vitamin A nor β-carotene supplementation reduced mortality or human immunodeficiency virus (HIV) transmission in two studies, whereas, contrary to expectations, vertical HIV transmission was increased in one study (234), even though RA markedly suppressed the rate of virus replication in vitro (235). Thus, the effects of vitamin A on specific infectious diseases have been uneven, despite the overwhelming evidence that vitamin A reduces all-cause mortality.

The potential for carotenoids to modulate immune responses has been demonstrated in vivo and in cell models (236). It is, however, often difficult to separate the actions of provitamin A carotenoids from those of the vitamin A generated from them. Nonetheless, several non-provitamin A carotenoids have been proposed to have an immunoregulatory role. Although the mechanisms of their effects are not clear, investigators have proposed that carotenoids alter gap junction proteins such as connexin, thus affecting cell-cell communications (237). Relatively nonspecific effects of carotenoids on membrane structure and signal transduction pathways could also affect immune outcomes, as could antioxidant mechanisms involving reactive oxidant species (236), as have been proposed for many other tissues (see next section).

Antioxidant Properties of Carotenoids

Carotenoids possess the ability to quench singlet oxygen. The interaction of carotenoids with singlet oxygen, which is more reactive than the triplet oxygen present in the air, yields triplet oxygen and an excited triplet carotenoid, which releases its energy into the surrounding solution (46). Carotenoids form both radical cations and radical anions, under suitable conditions and depending on prevailing conditions, may act as antioxidants or prooxidants (238). Carotenoid radicals can interact with other free radicals to quench them to nonradical products, or they can interact with other molecules to restore the carotenoid to the ground state, while producing a new free radical (10). Many inflammatory reactions generate oxidant molecules such as nitric oxide, peroxide, and peroxynitrite (see Chapter 44), and thus carotenoids could plausibly play a role in the control of inflammation and the regulation of immune responses, through their antioxidant properties.

Oxidation has been proposed as a factor in the etiology of age-related macular degeneration, the leading cause of irreversible vision loss in the developed world (177). The nonprovitamin A carotenoids lutein and zeaxanthin are the only carotenoids of dietary origin deposited in the macular region (239). Several case-control and randomized controlled intervention studies of lutein supplementation have provided both null and positive results on different biomarkers of oxidative stress (240). Lutein supplementation appears effective in increasing macular pigment concentration and may improve visual function in some, but not all, subjects with retinal disorders (240, 241).

Large numbers of epidemiologic studies have explored a possible association between carotenoid intake and reduced risk of cancer and cardiovascular disease (46, 242). Diets high in fruits and vegetables have been consistently associated with reduced disease risk. However, the data for specific nutrients such as carotenoids are less persuasive. The methods of diet assessment have varied among studies, and specific nutrient intakes have often been inferred from food frequency questionnaires. The statistical methods used to control for covarying nutrients and confounding factors, such as smoking, may not be adequate (243). Thus, it may not be surprising that although a diet high in fruits and vegetables has been repeatedly shown to reduce the risk of cancer, cardiovascular disease, and other diseases, the effects of individual nutrients have often been weaker or inconsistent (244).

To test whether β-carotene was specifically able to reduce cancer incidence, several large-scale randomized intervention studies were carried out in the United States and Finland in the 1990s. The three β-carotene intervention trials—the β-Carotene and Retinol Efficacy Trial (United States), the ∝-Tocopherol, β-Carotene Cancer Prevention Study (Finland), and the Physician's Health Study (United States)—all pointed to a lack of effect of synthetic β-carotene in decreasing cardiovascular disease or cancer risk in well-nourished populations (245, 246)]. In fact, lung cancer incidence was actually elevated in carotene-supplemented smokers in the Finnish study (relative risk 1.18), and in smokers and asbestos workers in the the β-Carotene and Retinol Efficacy Trial (relative risk 1.28), findings leading to the termination of the trial in advance of its completion date. These unexpected results were reviewed extensively (245, 247, 248), and numerous possible explanations were proposed. One hypothesis is that a large dose of β-carotene, such as was used in these trials, is metabolized differently than a smaller dietary dose, resulting in adverse effects. This idea was tested experimentally in a model of smoke-exposed, β-carotene–treated ferrets. In the lungs of these animals, retinoid oxidative enzymes were elevated and retinoid levels were reduced (249). Other possible explanations for the negative results of the human β-carotene intervention trials are that the positive effects of β-carotene shown in case-control studies were instead the result of other nutrients that covary with carotenoids, and carotenoids are only one of several factors in fruits and vegetables that must be consumed together to be effective. Carotenoids could also be surrogate markers of a generally healthy lifestyle that includes a diet low in fat and high in fruits and vegetables (250).

In contrast to the negative results for β-carotene discussed earlier, β-carotene (180 mg/day) has been used successfully for years, with minimal side effects, in the treatment of the photosensitivity disorder erythropoietic porphyria and similar diseases (251). β-Carotene, vitamin A, and retinoids have shown some benefit in remission of oral leukoplakia, although the lesions returned after cessation of treatment (252). High intakes of carotenoids, in contrast to retinoids, are considered nontoxic, although undesirable cosmetic effects (carotenodermia) may occur (253).

Lycopene, an acyclic nonprovitamin A carotene that is relatively abundant in tomatoes and tomato-based products, has received considerable attention for its possible role in cancer prevention, especially prostate cancer (254, 255). About half of the carotenoids found in plasma, including lycopene, are derived from consumption of tomatoes and tomato products (256). Higher intakes of tomato products, a characteristic of diets high in fruits and vegetables and the Mediterranean diet, in particular, have been associated with reduced prostate cancer risk in several, but not all, epidemiologic studies, as reviewed by Giovannucci (256). In a large prospective study in male health professionals the consumption of two to four servings/week of tomato sauce was associated with a 35 to 50% reduction in prostate cancer risk (256). However, several case-control studies did not show this association, and some investigators have reported results that differed for different tomato products. The lycopene contents of tomato and vegetable crops is variable and depends on the cultivars grown and the growing conditions. The assessment of lycopene intake varies with the method used to collect dietary data and the food composition database used to estimate nutrient contents. Thus, estimates of lycopene intake are currently imprecise and may compromise the ability to test the lycopene-prostate cancer hypothesis (256). At present, the idea that lycopene may reduce cancer risk is interesting, but it is based on imprecise and circumstantial evidence. It is reminiscent of earlier notions about β-carotene and cancer prevention. Several trials now under way may provide more convincing evidence regarding whether tomato products or purified lycopene can reduce the risk of diseases such as prostate cancer and macular degeneration.

Uses of Retinoids

Treatment and Prophylaxis of Vitamin A Deficiency

Even now, millions of children and pregnant women worldwide do not receive enough vitamin A in their diets. When vitamin A deficiency is clinically evident, it should be treated immediately with retinol (257). The use of vitamin A as prophylaxis to prevent vitamin A deficiency in vulnerable populations is now widely accepted as beneficial (257) (see also Chapter 90). Although the optimal dose and frequency of treatment are unknown, a periodic high dose (30–60 mg of retinol at 3–6-month intervals [6]) and a weekly dose at an RDA-based level of vitamin A (258) were both effective in reducing child mortality (257). A large dose provided infrequently is practical in places where health care services are limited. This strategy is effective because of the intestine's ability to absorb retinol efficiently and the liver's capacity to store retinyl esters and gradually release retinol as holo-RBP into plasma, thus ensuring normal plasma levels for several months after dosing.

Dermatology

All-*trans*-RA (tretinoin), 13-*cis*-RA (etretinate, Accutane), and numerous synthetic retinoids have formed the basis of effective treatments for severe forms of cystic acne and psoriasis since the mid-1980s. Both systemic and topical treatments were developed. Subsequently, topically applied retinoids were used to reverse the clinical and histologic features of photodamaged skin (259–262). Retinoids influence the physiology of the skin by several mechanisms, including by reducing cell proliferation, by promoting epidermal differentiation, by modulating dermal growth factors and their receptors (260), by inhibiting sebaceous gland activity (263), and by suppressing androgen formation (151).

These actions may account for the comedolytic and anti-comedogenic activity of systemic and topically applied retinoids (264).

The use of oral retinoids in dermatology is not without adverse effects. The risk of teratogenic effects early in pregnancy and of resultant birth defects has received the greatest attention, but depression and other psychiatric effects have also been claimed as adverse effects (265). The profile of adverse effects is dose dependent and is closely related to hypervitaminosis A (see later). The use of topical retinoids results in far less systemic exposure. A pharmacokinetic model used to assess the internal exposure to all-*trans*-RA when applied topically to skin indicated an internal exposure some four to six orders of magnitude below that of a minimally teratogenic oral dose (266).

Cancer Chemoprevention and Treatment

Many epidemiologic studies have suggested that a lower intake of vitamin A is associated with a higher risk of certain cancers, especially those of epithelial origin (243). Experimentally, vitamin A deficiency is associated with higher tumor incidence and with increased susceptibility to chemical carcinogens (267). In human cancers, several retinoid-binding proteins and nuclear retinoid receptors, most notably RARβ and CRBP-I, have been reported to be expressed at reduced levels in various types of cancer, including premalignant lesions (267, 268). Investigators have hypothesized that aberrant changes in tissue retinoid metabolism and retinoid signaling via nuclear receptors may contribute to tumor growth and cancer progression (267).

Some retinoids have proven to be effective in preventing or delaying cancer recurrence (269, 270). An outstanding example is APL, a form of leukemia characterized by a specific chromosomal translocation between the long arms of chromosomes 15 and 17 (t15,17). The most common breakpoint in chromosome 17 interrupts a copy of the gene for RARα, which is located at 17q21. Physicians in China were the first to report that all-*trans*-RA was effective in inducing a high rate of remission in APL patients. This result was then confirmed in several clinical trials in Europe and the United States. These studies led to the wide use of all-*trans*-RA for the differentiation therapy of APL (194, 195). Treatment appears to induce the expression of the remaining normal RARα allele rapidly, apparently allowing cells to differentiate sufficiently to attain a normal phenotype. Other chemotherapeutic agents are required either with or after treatment with RA to eliminate the remaining aberrant cells (195).

The use of RA in patients with APL revealed a new high-risk syndrome, referred to as the RA syndrome (195), a combination of fever, respiratory distress, hypotension, and renal failure, which was fatal in a significant percentage of patients. Treatment plans have since been modified to shorten the length of treatment with high-dose RA, followed by the use of conventional chemotherapy to eliminate the leukemogenic clone. Investigators have observed repeatedly that patients treated with all-*trans*-RA gradually become refractory to its differentiating activity, and those who have a disease relapse after withdrawal of chemotherapy are often resistant to further treatment with all-*trans*-RA (195). Resistance to RA appears to be related at least in part to an increase in the rate of RA-induced retinoid catabolism.

Other Uses

Clinical data and animal studies suggest that vitamin A may be useful in other situations requiring cell differentiation and tissue repair. The lungs normally undergo extensive postnatal development, and vitamin A has been implicated in accelerating lung maturation (alveolization). A Cochrane database review of very-low-birth-weight infants concluded that supplementing infants of less than 1500 g with vitamin A (5000 IU, or 1.5 mg three times weekly) is associated with a reduction in infant death or a lessening of the requirement for oxygen at 1 month of age (271).

Retinoids may be beneficial in the treatment of other lung conditions, including emphysema, as suggested by clinical data and animal studies (272). These findings are consistent with previous work suggesting a critical role of RA in lung alveolar development and repair (273). In a rat model of partial small bowel resection, vitamin A deficiency inhibited intestinal adaptation by reducing crypt cell proliferation, enhancing apoptosis, and reducing extracellular matrix synthesis and enterocyte migration rates (274). These preclinical results in animal models of lung and intestinal injury suggest that vitamin A could be important clinically to promote the healing of tissues and the recovery of function after tissue injury.

DEFICIENCY AND TOXICITY

Vitamin A Deficiency

Surveys made in the mid-1990s indicated that more than 3 million children, most living in developing countries, develop xerophthalmia each year, and between 250,000 and 500,000 of them become blind (2, 6). By WHO criteria, vitamin A deficiency is considered a public health problem based on the regional prevalence of traditional eye signs of severe deficiency (e.g., corneal xerosis, Bitôt spots), as well as population-based cutoff levels for subclinical indicators (e.g., low serum retinol, low breast milk retinol levels [275, 276]). Although estimates made in 2002 suggest that the number of affected children is declining, the prevalence of vitamin A deficiency, characterized by a low serum retinol level (<0.7 µmol/L) or xerophthalmia, still is unacceptably high (275), and international health programs to eliminate vitamin A deficiency remain a high priority (277). Vitamin A deficiency may worsen iron status, resulting in "vitamin A deficiency anemia" (278).

The prevalence of vitamin A deficiency in young children increases just after weaning (279). This increase is most likely a reflection of a combination of factors: (a) limited transfer of vitamin A from mother to fetus in utero, as has been shown in animal studies; (b) an inadequate amount of vitamin A in the mother's diet during lactation, resulting in a low breast milk vitamin A levels; and (c) an inadequate quantity of vitamin A in the child's postweaning diet (2). Animal studies have shown that increasing the amount of vitamin A in the mother's diet results in higher milk vitamin A concentrations and in higher vitamin A concentrations in the liver of the suckling young (280, 281). The uptake of chylomicron vitamin A into the mammary gland of lactating rats was directly proportional to the contents of chylomicron retinyl ester delivered to the mammary gland (73). Consistent with this finding, the vitamin A contents of the mother's milk increased as her vitamin A intake increased (281). Vitamin A supplementation increased the amount of vitamin A in mother's milk and in neonatal liver without having any effect on maternal plasma retinol concentration (280, 281). These results imply that the uptake of chylomicron vitamin A, which varies with diet, plays an important role in determining the concentration of vitamin A in breast milk (73).

The efficacy of vitamin A supplementation has been tested in numerous clinical trials in vulnerable populations. A metaanalysis of trials conducted in young children, most from regions of Southeast Asia and India with a high rate of xerophthalmia, showed conclusively that vitamin A reduces child mortality by 23 to 34% (6,7). Similarly, supplementation with a weekly low dose of vitamin A or β-carotene reduced pregnancy-related mortality in pregnant women in Nepal (282). Vitamin A supplementation in Indonesian women early in lactation increased their breast milk vitamin A concentration (276, 283) while reducing the frequency of low serum retinol levels in their infants (276). Because of the potential teratogenicity of high-dose vitamin A in early gestation, it is thought unwise to supplement women of reproductive age with vitamin A after the first 6 weeks postpartum, when they could once again become pregnant (257, 258). A study of supplementation in neonates showed reduced mortality at 6 months in infants who received vitamin A during the first 2 days of life (284).

Hypervitaminosis A, Adverse Effects, and the Upper Level

Hypervitaminosis A is inducible by either an acute or a chronic excess of vitamin A. Hypervitaminosis A is most often the result of excessive use of vitamin A–containing supplements (285). Some cases have resulted from food faddism, such as an excessive consumption of liver (286), or self-medication with vitamin A preparations. The severity of adverse effects is dosage dependent, and these effects may include severe headache, nausea, skin irritation, pain in bones and joints, coma, and death. Prescription retinoids can also produce side effects similar to those of hypervitaminosis A, although this condition is better referred to as retinoid toxicity. Retinoid toxicity is dosage dependent, and it varies with the structure of the retinoid (287, 288).

The 2001 IOM committee on micronutrients (13) focused on three potential critical adverse effects of hypervitaminosis A: (a) increased risk of birth defects in women of reproductive age, (b) liver abnormalities, and (c) reduced bone mineral density (BMD) that may result in osteoporosis.

Birth Defects (Teratogenesis)

Retinoid-induced birth defects are well documented in several animal models (289). After 13-*cis*-RA was introduced as a treatment for skin diseases, a high incidence (>20%) of spontaneous abortions and birth defects was observed in the fetuses of women who ingested therapeutic doses of 13-*cis*-RA during the first trimester of pregnancy. Because 13-*cis*-RA (isotretinoin, Accutane) and etretinate (Tegison, Tigason) are known teratogens in humans, these drugs are marketed in the United States with the contraindication for use during pregnancy. In 2004, a federal advisory committee recommended that the Food and Drug Administration mandate a registry of all users of Accutane, or its generic equivalent, in part to monitor appropriate contraceptive use by women taking the drug (290). The risk of teratogenesis may, however, persist for many months after discontinuation of the drug (289). The period of fetal organogenesis (first trimester) is of greatest concern. The teratogenicity of retinoids depends on the following: their structure, with molecules having a free carboxyl group being more potent; dosage of the retinoid; rate of its metabolism; and extent of placental transfer from mother to the fetus. Although pregnant women and nonhuman primates are generally more sensitive to retinoids than are rodents, the resulting fetal malformations (exencephaly, craniofacial malformations, eye defects, and cardiac abnormalities) are quite similar across species (291).

Rothman and colleagues (292) investigated the relationship of dietary vitamin A intake with birth defects by reviewing the birth records and dietary interviews for more than 22,000 pregnant women in the United States. Of 339 babies with birth defects, 121 were in sites that originated from the embryonic cranial neural crest. From a logistic-regression analysis, the authors concluded that the risk of birth defects was significantly higher in women who consumed more than 10,000 IU/day of vitamin A from supplements (1.4% of the group studied) during the periconceptual period. Other investigators believe that an intake of less than 30,000 IU/day should not be considered teratogenic (293). Concerns have been raised about the frequent consumption by pregnant or potentially pregnant women of foods very high in vitamin A such as liver (>100,000 IU [~33,000 μg retinol]/100 g [138]).

Liver Abnormalities

The IOM committee reviewed case reports of liver abnormalities associated with elevated, long-term, intakes of vitamin A. Human data are potentially confounded by other factors related to liver damage such as alcohol intake, hepatitis A, B, and C, hepatotoxic medication, or preexisting liver disease. In establishing the ULs, data were considered only if they showed the following: grossly elevated liver vitamin A levels or hypertrophy of stellate (Ito) cells; no alcoholism, because alcoholic liver disease is known to be associated with loss of cellular vitamin A and low plasma retinol (294–296); no concomitant liver hepatitis; and no hepatotoxic drug use. Consistency and specificity were found for the following liver abnormalities associated with prolonged high intakes of vitamin A: evidence of excessive vitamin A in perisinusoidal (stellate) cells, perisinusoidal fibrosis, hyperplasia, and hypertrophy of stellate cells. The level of intake reported for these cases ranged from 1500 to greater than 14,000 μg/day over periods of 1 to 30 years' duration.

Bone Mineral Loss

Animal, human, and laboratory research all support an association between a high intake of vitamin A and a loss of BMD, a risk factor for osteoporosis (see Chapter 86). In rats fed high levels of vitamin A (297), bone rarification preceded actual fractures. Vitamin A reduced the amount of total bone ash, increased epiphyseal plate width, and caused bone resorption both in the presence or absence of vitamin D_3 (298) and at various levels of calcium and phosphorus intake (299).

Reduced BMD, at least in elderly persons, may occur with retinol intakes not greatly in excess of RDA amounts. Melhus and colleagues (300) compared the intake of retinol determined from diet records with BMD in Swedish women with a first hip fracture and reported that retinol intake greater than 1500 μg/day, compared with less than 500 μg/day, was associated with lower BMD and a twofold increase in risk of hip fracture (300). A longitudinal study of Swedish men showed a significant dose-dependent increase in bone fractures in the highest versus middle quintile of serum retinol (301). A small, short-term metabolic study of healthy Swedish persons showed that consuming a dose of vitamin A similar in amount to a serving of liver can significantly blunt the plasma calcium response induced by 1,25-dihydroxy vitamin D (302). For more than 72,000 postmenopausal women enrolled in the Nurses' Health Study, the risk of hip fracture was higher for those whose intake of retinol was greater than 3000 μg/day, compared with women who consumed less than 1250 μg/day (303). In elderly persons in the United States, retinol-containing supplements are widely used. Fifty percent of women and 39% of men in a community study of older Americans reported using supplemental retinol, and, among female supplement users, BMD change was inversely associated with retinol intake (304).

Overall, the emerging results from human studies suggest that a chronically high intake of vitamin A, on the order of 3000 μg/day (approximately four times the RDA), may increase the risk of osteoporotic bone disease and fracture, at least in older men and women. Additional studies to evaluate the interactions of dietary vitamin A, vitamin D, and calcium on BMD and fracture risk are needed.

Upper Level

The Dietary Reference Intake Committee selected birth defects as the critical adverse effect to set the UL for vitamin A for women of reproductive age and liver abnormalities as the indicator for men and for women more than 50 years old (13). Although reduced BMD was recognized as an important potential adverse effect, it was not used as an indicator to set the UL because of a lack of sufficient dose-response data (13). The UL for vitamin A applies only to *preformed vitamin A* because no evidence indicates that β-carotene intake is associated with increased risk. The UL is 3000 μg/day of retinol for both women and men. The UL

established by the IOM is consistent with the American Teratology Society's recommendation that the daily intake of vitamin A be lower than 3000 μg in pregnant women.

Assessment of Vitamin A Status

Vitamin A status comprises a continuum from clinically evident deficiency to overt toxicity (296) (Table 19.2). In between these extremes, vitamin A status may, for convenience, be categorized as marginal, adequate, and excessive. These "in-between" categories span a wide range of body vitamin A reserves over which plasma retinol levels remain relatively constant, and clinical abnormalities are not observed. Thus, investigators have sought other indicators of vitamin A status, which may be useful for detecting subclinical changes in vitamin A status.

Indicators and Tests

Biochemical Indicators. Low vitamin A or RBP levels in plasma, breast milk, or tear fluid may indicate vitamin A

TABLE 19.2. TYPICAL FINDINGS ASSOCIATED WITH RANGES OF VITAMIN A STATUS

RANGE	PLASMA RETINOL	PLASMA RETINYL ESTERS IN THE FASTING STATE	LIVER STORES	CLINICAL SIGNS	VULNERABLE GROUPS AND MOST COMMON SITUATIONS
Deficient	<0.35 μmol/L[a]	Little, if any (<5 μg/g)	Severely depleted	Night blindness; other ocular manifestations; skin dryness	Preschool-age children and pregnant or lactating women with low vitamin A intakes; patients with chronic alcoholism; patients with chronic liver diseases
Marginal	0.35–0.7[b] μmol/L	Low (<2%) (5–20 μg/g)	Severely depleted	None (positive plasma response to vitamin A)[c]	Children, pregnant women in vulnerable populations, often with high rates of infection[d]
Adequate	>1.05–3 μmol/L	2–20%[b]	~20–300 μg/g	None	Typical of a well-nourished general population[b]
Excessive	Upper normal to >3 μmol/L[e]	Significantly present in fasting state in lipoproteins	High (>300 μg/g)	Not apparent or very mild; elevated liver enzymes in plasma	Long-term supplement use; frequent intake of foods (e.g., liver) high in preformed vitamin A
Toxic	Usually in normal concentration range	May be higher than retinol; lipoprotein associated	Very high in liver and increased in peripheral tissues	Headache; bone/joint pain; elevated liver enzymes and clinical signs of liver disease	Food faddists and users of high-dose vitamin A supplements; patients treated with retinoids[f]

[a] Very rarely, plasma retinol may be low because of hereditary familial low retinol-binding protein (see text); 0.35 μmol/L = 10 μg retinol/dL.

[b] The range 1.05 to 0.7 μmol/L is sometimes used to indicate marginal status and <0.7 μmol/L to indicate vitamin A deficiency. These ranges may be more appropriate for adults, in whom median plasma retinol levels are higher than those in children.

[c] Positive relative dose response (RDR) or modified RDR test.

[d] Low plasma retinol in inflammation may indicate an acute-phase response associated with reduced retinol-binding protein (RBP) production rather than deficient vitamin A storage (see text).

[e] Retinol and RBP are normal, whereas total retinol is elevated because of retinyl esters, and liver total retinol exceeds approximately 300 μg/g (reference 15).

[f] Retinoid administration typically reduces, not increases, plasma retinol levels.

deficiency. As discussed earlier, however, plasma retinol is of limited value in assessing marginal vitamin A reserves because plasma retinol levels are maintained until liver vitamin A reserves are nearly exhausted. Plasma RBP concentration is a good surrogate for serum retinol in vitamin A deficiency (305), but it is also likely to be low during protein-energy deficiency and in conditions of inflammation.

Liver vitamin A concentrations are considered a "gold standard," but they are seldom obtainable in human studies. Based on the analysis of plasma retinol and liver vitamin A in human liver specimens collected at autopsy or surgery and from animal studies, Olson concluded that liver concentrations of less than 5 µg total retinol/g are associated with very low plasma retinol, and liver concentrations of 5 to 20 µg/g are indicative of marginal vitamin A status (306). Indirect assays of liver vitamin A reserves have been developed, based on the rapid output of holo-RBP from the liver of vitamin A–deficient animals treated with vitamin A. In the RDR test (306), a small dose of retinol (1.6–3.5 µmol [450–1000 µg]) is given orally in oil. Plasma is sampled at baseline and again approximately 5 hours later, the peak of the plasma retinol response. An increase in excess of 20% of the predosing baseline value is generally interpreted as indicating that hepatic vitamin A reserves are not adequate to maintain the secretion of holo-RBP at its maximum level (307)]. The modified RDR (MRDR) test is similar in principle but uses vitamin A_2 (3,4-didehydroretinol), taking advantage of the normally low level of vitamin A_2 in plasma that rises substantially when 3,4-didehydroretinol-RBP is released from liver in response to the test dose (307–309). The RDR and MRDR have proved useful as indicators of low vitamin A reserves in clinical research settings and have been adapted for use in population-based studies.

Tracer methodologies using stable isotopes of retinol have been used as research tools to quantify total body retinol. Using a deuterated retinol dilution technique in rats, the calculated and experimentally measured values of total body vitamin A reserves were within 7% of each other, and the relationship was linear (r = 0.98) (310). In a study of human volunteers supplemented with vitamin A, the deuterated retinol dilution method detected changes in total body stores of vitamin A similar to those that were predicted (311). A similar retinol dilution method was applied in a field situation to the determination of retinol reserves of Peruvian children (312).

A low molar ratio of plasma RBP to TTR has been proposed as an indicator of marginal vitamin A deficiency (313, 314), with the advantage that it may be valid even during inflammation (313). It may, however, be no more sensitive and specific than serum retinol concentration or the MRDR test (315). An analysis of NHANES data showed that low plasma retinol is inversely related to the level of the C-reactive protein, a positive acute-phase protein and frequently measured marker of inflammation, a finding suggesting that persons with adequate vitamin A status and inflammation could be misclassified as having low (inadequate) vitamin A based on their lower serum retinol values (95). Several acute-phase plasma proteins are inversely correlated with plasma retinol (314, 316), but it remains to be determined whether the levels of acute-phase proteins can be used to "correct" low plasma retinol for the effects of inflammation (223).

Eye Signs. Conjunctival xerosis with Bitôt spots in young children (WHO classification X1B) is strongly associated with vitamin A deficiency (6). A prevalence of greater than 0.5% X1B in young children is one of the criteria used by the WHO to identify vitamin A deficiency as a public health problem (2). Tests of night blindness have been developed to be suitable for field use in young children (317). Night blindness is also significant in pregnant women in regions of low vitamin A intake (275). The histologic evaluation of the conjunctiva (conjunctival impression cytology) has also been proposed as a field-operative test (317). Low vitamin A status is detected as a relative lack of goblet cells and the presence of enlarged epithelial cells in the conjunctiva (317). See Color insert in Chapter 38.

Dietary Assessment. Dietary data are of greatest value in assessing the food habits of populations at risk of vitamin A deficiency (277). Vitamin A is concentrated in relatively few foods, which may be consumed infrequently. Comparisons of dietary histories and food frequency questionnaire methods were conducted in studies of Australian adults (318) and Indonesian children (319). For Australian men and women, the food frequency questionnaire overestimated β-carotene intake (149%) while underestimating retinol (63%), as compared with intake determined by four 1-week dietary records (318). In a study of Indonesian children at high risk of xerophthalmia, the vitamin A intake based on a 24-hour history corresponded to the population's vitamin A status as assessed by serum retinol, whereas the food frequency questionnaire seems to overestimate vitamin A intake (319). These comparisons suggest that, at least in populations, a diet history may provide a more accurate estimate of vitamin A intake, compared with a food frequency questionnaire.

Public Health Assessment Tools. Although serum retinol is not a sensitive indicator of the vitamin A status of individual persons, low serum retinol values in populations have greater significance. In 1994, the WHO updated its criteria for identifying countries in which vitamin A deficiency is considered a public health problem in children 6 to 71 months old by using a combination of ocular, biochemical, and nutritional indicators (320). Even when xerophthalmia is not prevalent, the presence of other indicators—low serum retinol, low breast milk retinol, and abnormal conjunctival cytology—still are warnings that mild, moderate, or severe vitamin A deficiency may be present (see Table 19.2). A child mortality rate greater than 70/1000 for children less than 5 years old is considered a surrogate indicator for vitamin A deficiency when other indicators are not available (321). A significant impetus for better public health assessment is the heightened awareness by health professionals and policy makers that marginal vitamin A deficiency significantly increases the severity of infectious diseases, and decreases survival, in young children (see Chapter 90).

SUMMARY

The fundamental roles of vitamin A in the form of retinal in vision and of RA in the regulation of gene transcription are now well defined. However, much remains to be learned concerning the physiologic and pharmacologic situations in which specific genes are regulated by RA or similar retinoids in vivo. The ability of vitamin A supplementation to reduce child mortality has served as a powerful reminder that micronutrient intake is still inadequate in much of the developing world. The confluence of new molecular data and important public health advances almost certainly ensures that vitamin A research will continue to be exciting and rewarding well into the twenty-first century.

Acknowledgments

I am indebted to the late James Allen Olson, co-editor of the ninth edition of Modern Nutrition in Health and Disease, *for his guidance and insights over the years, and I wish to acknowledge the use of some of his materials on carotenoids in this chapter. Support from National Institutes for Health grants DK-41479 and CA-90214 and Dorothy Foehr Huck chair is gratefully acknowledged.*

REFERENCES

1. Wolf G. FASEB J 1996;10:1102–7.
2. McLaren DS, ed. The Control of Xerophthalmia: A Century of Contributions and Lessons. Basel: Task Force Sight and Life, 2004.
3. Arens JF, van Dorp DA. Nature 1946;157:190–1.
4. Wald G. Science 1968;162:230–9.
5. Altucci L, Gronemeyer H. Trends Endocrinol Metab 2001; 12:460–8.
6. Sommer A, West KP Jr. Vitamin A Deficiency: Health, Survival, and Vision. New York: Oxford University Press, 1996.
7. Beaton GH, Martorell R, Aronson KA et al. Food Nutr Bull 1994;15:282–9.
8. Olson JA, Krinsky NI. FASEB J 1995;9:1547–50.
9. Vahlquist A. Dermatology 1999;199[Suppl]:3–11.
10. Britton G. FASEB J 1995;9:1551–8.
11. Holden JM, Eldridge AL, Beecher GR et al. J Food Comp Anal 1999;12:169–96.
12. Furr HC. J Nutr 2004;134[Suppl]:281S–5S.
13. Food and Nutrition Board, Institute of Medicine. Dietary Reference Intakes for Vitamin A, Vitamin K, Arsenic, Boron, Chromium, Copper, Iodine, Iron, Manganese, Molybdenum, Nickel, Silicon, Vanadium, and Zinc. Washington, DC: National Academy Press, 2001.
14. World Health Organization (WHO/FAO). Requirements of Vitamin A, Thiamine, Riboflavin, and Niacin. Report of a Joint Food and Agriculture Organization/World Health Organization Expert Committee. FAO nutrition meetings report series no. 41. WHO technical report series no. 362. Geneva: World Health Organization, 1967.
15. Olson JA. J Natl Cancer Inst 1984;73:1439–44.
16. West CE, Eilander A, van Lieshout M. J Nutr 2002;132[Suppl]: 2920S–6S.
17. Noy N. Biochem J 2000;348:481–95.
18. Newcomer ME, Ong DE. Biochim Biophys Acta 2000;1482: 57–64.
19. Monaco HL. Biochim Biophys Acta 2000;1482:65–72.
20. Robbins J. Clin Chem Lab Med 2002;40:1183–90.
21. Soprano DR, Blaner WS. Plasma retinol-binding protein. In: Sporn MB, Roberts AB, Goodman DS, eds. The Retinoids: Biology, Chemistry and Medicine. 2nd ed. New York: Raven Press, 1994:257–81.
22. Dong D, Ruuska SE, Levinthal DJ et al. J Biol Chem 1999; 274:23695–8.
23. Ong DE, Newcomer ME, Chytil F. Cellular retinoid-binding proteins. In: Sporn MB, Roberts AB, Goodman DS, eds. The Retinoids: Biology, Chemistry and Medicine. 2nd ed. New York: Raven Press, 1994:283–317.
24. Folli C, Calderone V, Ottonello S et al. Proc Natl Acad Sci USA 2001;98:3710–5.
25. Vogel S, Mendelsohn CL, Mertz JR et al. J Biol Chem 2001; 276:1353–60.
26. Folli C, Calderone V, Ramazzina I et al. J Biol Chem 2002; 277:41970–7.
27. Saari JC. Invest Ophthalmol Vis Sci 2000;41:337–48.
28. Chambon P. FASEB J 1996;10:940–54.
29. Mangelsdorf DJ, Thummel C, Beato M et al. Cell 1995;83: 835–9.
30. Wei LN. Annu Rev Pharmacol Toxicol 2003;43:47–72.
31. Boudjelal M, Voorhees JJ, Fisher GJ. Exp Cell Res 2002; 274:130-7.
32. Adachi S, Okuno M, Matsushima-Nishiwaki R et al. Hepatology 2002;35:332–40.
33. Levin AA, Sturzenbecker LJ, Kazmer S et al. Nature 1992; 355:359–61.
34. Dawson MI, Zhang XK. Curr Med Chem 2002;9:623–37.
35. De Urquiza AM, Liu SY, Sjöberg M et al. Science 2000;290: 2140–4.
36. Goldstein JT, Dobrzyn A, Clagett-Dame M et al. Arch Biochem Biophys 2003;420:185–93.
37. Hauksdottir H, Farboud B, Privalsky ML. Mol Endocrinol 2003;17:373–85.
38. Weston AD, Blumberg B, Underhill TM. J Cell Biol 2003;161: 223–8.
39. Harrison EH, Hussain MM. J Nutr 2001;131:1405–8.
40. van Bennekum AM, Fisher EA, Blaner WS et al. Biochemistry 2000;39:4900–6.
41. Rigtrup KM, McEwen LR, Said HM et al. Am J Clin Nutr 1994;60:111–6.
42. Goodman DS, Blomstrand R, Werner B et al. J Clin Invest 1966;45:1615–23.
43. von Lintig J, Wyss A. Arch Biochem Biophys 2001;385: 47–52.
44. Bhatti RA, Yu S, Boulanger A et al. Invest Ophthalmol Vis Sci 2003;44:44–9.
45. Wyss A, Wirtz GM, Woggon WD et al. Biochem J 2001;354: 521–9.
46. Olson JA. Carotenoids. In: Shils ME, Olson JA, Shike M et al, eds. Modern Nutrition in Health and Disease. 9th ed. Baltimore: Williams & Wilkins, 1999:525–41.
47. Kiefer C, Hessel S, Lampert JM et al. J Biol Chem 2001;276: 14110–6.
48. Nagao A. J Nutr 2004;134:237S–40S.
49. Pott I, Marx M, Neidhart S et al. J Agric Food Chem 2003;51: 4527–31.

50. During A, Hussain MM, Morel DW et al. J Lipid Res 2002;43:1086–95.

51. You CS, Parker RS, Goodman KJ et al. Am J Clin Nutr 1996;64:177–83.

52. Tajima S, Goda T, Takase S. Comp Biochem Physiol B Biochem Mol Biol 2001;128:425–34.

53. Tajima S, Goda T, Takase S. Life Sci 1999;65:841–8.

54. Wang XD, Krinsky NI. Subcell Biochem 1998;30:159–80.

55. Parker RS, Swanson JE, You CS et al. Proc Nutr Soc 1999;58:155–62.

56. Castenmiller JJ, West CE, Linssen JP et al. J Nutr 1999;129:349–55.

57. van het Hof KH, Gartner C, Wiersma A et al. J Agric Food Chem 1999;47:1582–6.

58. van Lieshout M, West CE, van Breemen RB. Am J Clin Nutr 2003;77:12–28.

59. Edwards AJ, Nguyen CH, You CS et al. J Nutr 2002;132:159–67.

60. van Lieshout M, West CE, Muhilal et al. Am J Clin Nutr 2001;73:949–58.

61. Tanumihardjo SA. Int J Vitam Nutr Res 2002;72:40–5.

62. Hickenbottom SJ, Lemke SL, Dueker SR et al. Eur J Nutr 2002;41:141–7.

63. Lin Y, Dueker SR, Burri BJ et al. Am J Clin Nutr 2000;71:1545–54.

64. Hickenbottom SJ, Follett JR, Lin Y et al. Am J Clin Nutr 2002;75:900–7.

65. Lemke SL, Dueker SR, Follett JR et al. J Lipid Res 2003;44:1591–600.

66. Wieringa FT, Dijkhuizen MA, West CE et al. Am J Clin Nutr 2003;77:651–7.

67. Tang G, Qin J, Dolnikowski GG et al. Am J Clin Nutr 2003;78:259–66.

68. Li E, Tso P. Curr Opin Lipidol 2003;14:241–7.

69. Silveira ER, Moreno FS. J Nutr Biochem 1998;9:446–56.

70. Helgerud P, Petersen LB, Norum KR. J Clin Invest 1983;71:747–53.

71. Ross AC. Hepatic metabolism of vitamin A. In: Zakim D, Boyer TD, eds. Hepatology: A Textbook of Liver Disease. 4th ed. Philadelphia: WB Saunders, 2002:149–68.

72. Ross AC, Zolfaghari R. J Nutr 2004;134.

73. Ross AC, Pasatiempo AM, Green MH. Exp Biol Med (Maywood) 2004;229:46–55.

74. Berr F. J Lipid Res 1992;33:915–30.

75. Blomhoff R, Skrede B, Norum KR. J Intern Med 1990;228:207–10.

76. Harrison EH, Gad MZ, Ross AC. J Lipid Res 1995;36:1498–506.

77. Blomhoff R, Green MH, Norum KR. Annu Rev Nutr 1992;12:37–57.

78. Matsuura T, Gad MZ, Harrison ER et al. J Nutr 1997;127:218–24.

79. Sato M, Suzuki S, Senoo H. Cell Struct Funct 2003;28:105–12.

80. Dixon JL, Goodman DS. J Cell Physiol 1987;130:14–20.

81. Boerman MHEM, Napoli JL. J Biol Chem 1991;266:22273–8.

82. Green MH, Green JB, Berg T et al. J Nutr 1988;118:1331–5.

83. Matsuura T, Ross AC. Arch Biochem Biophys 1993;301:221–7.

84. Zolfaghari R, Ross AC. J Lipid Res 2000;41:2024–34.

85. Ross AC. J Nutr 2003;133:291S–6S.

86. Safadi R, Friedman SL. Med Gen Med 2002;4:27.

87. Hendriks HF, Bosma A, Brouwer A. Semin Liver Dis 1993;13:72–80.

88. Pinzani M, Gentilini P, Abboud HE. J Hepatol 1992;14:211–20.

89. Blomhoff R, Wake K. FASEB J 1991;5:271–7.

90. Rosales FJ, Ritter SJ, Zolfaghari R et al. J Lipid Res 1996;37:962–71.

91. Ross AC, Stephensen CB. FASEB J 1996;10:979–85.

92. Fex GA, Larsson K, Nilsson-Ehle I. J Nutr Biochem 1996;7:162–5.

93. Schweigert FJ, Thomann E, Zucker H. Int J Vitam Nutr Res 1991;61:110–3.

94. Sowell A, Briefel R, Huff D et al. FASEB J 1996;10:A813.

95. Stephensen CB, Gildengorin G. Am J Clin Nutr 2000;72:1170–8.

96. Life Science Research Office. Assessment of the Vitamin A Nutritional Status of the U.S. Population Based on Data Collected in the Health and Nutrition Examination Surveys. Bethesda, MD: Federation of American Societies for Experimental Biology, 1985.

97. Shenai JP, Rush MG, Stahlman MT et al. J Pediatr 1990;116:607–14.

98. Bell H, Nilsson A, Norum KR et al. J Hepatol 1989;8:26–31.

99. Bankson DD, Rifai N, Silverman LM. Ann Clin Biochem 1988;25:246–9.

100. Janczewska I, Ericzon BG, Ericksson LS. Scand J Gastroenterol 1995;30:68–71.

101. Floreani A, Baragiotta A, Martines D et al. Aliment Pharmacol Ther 2000;14:353–8.

102. Green MH, Green JB. J Nutr 1994;124:2477–85.

103. Von Reinersdorff D, Green MH, Green JB. Adv Exp Med Biol 1998;445:207–23.

104. Goodman DS. Plasma retinol-binding protein. In: Sporn MB, Roberts AB, Goodman DS, eds. The Retinoids, vol 2. Orlando, FL: Academic Press, 1984:42–88.

105. Berni R, Clerici M, Malpeli G et al. FASEB J 1993;7:1179–84.

106. Ritter SJ, Green MH, Adams WR et al. J Nutr Biochem 1995;6:689–96.

107. Kelley SK, Nilsson CB, Green MH et al. Toxicol Sci 2000;55:478–84.

108. Schmidt CK, Hoegberg P, Fletcher N et al. Arch Toxicol 2003;77:371–83.

109. Nanni G, Majorani F, Maloberti G et al. Life Sci 2000;67:2293–304.

110. Rosengren RJ, Sauer J-M, Hooser SB et al. Fundam Appl Toxicol 1995;25:281–92.

111. Barua AB, Kostic D, Olson JA. J Chromatogr 1993;617:257–64.

112. Khachik F, Beecher GR, Goli MB et al. Anal Chem 1992;64:2111–22.

113. Dietrich M, Block G, Norkus EP et al. Am J Clin Nutr 2003;77:160–6.

114. Peng YM, Peng YS, Lin Y et al. Nutr Cancer 1995;23:233–46.

115. Rock CL, Swendseid ME, Jacob RA et al. J Nutr 1992;122:96–100.

116. Burri BJ, Neidlinger TR, Clifford AJ. J Nutr 2001;131:2096–100.

117. Dueker SR, Lin Y, Buchholz BA et al. J Lipid Res 2000;41:1790–800.

118. Gaetani S, Bellovino D, Apreda M et al. Clin Chem Lab Med 2002;40:1211–20.

119. Tosetti F, Ferrari N, Brigati C et al. Exp Cell Res 1992;200:467–72.

120. Smith JE, DeMoor LM, Handler CE et al. Biochim Biophys Acta 1998;1380:10–20.

121. Smith FR, Goodman DS, Arroyave G et al. Am J Clin Nutr 1973;26:982–7.

122. Smith FR, Goodman DS, Zaklama MS et al. Am J Clin Nutr 1973;26:973–81.

123. Aldred AR, Schreiber G. The negative acute phase proteins. In: Mackiewicz A, Kushner I, Bauman H, eds. Acute Phase Proteins

Molecular Biology, Biochemistry, and Clinical Applications. Boca Raton, FL: CRC Press, 1993:21–37.

124. Felding P, Fex G. Acta Physiol Scand 1985;123:477–83.
125. Raguso CA, Dupertuis YM, Pichard C. Curr Opin Clin Nutr Metab Care 2003;6:211–6.
126. Cano NJ. Clin Chem Lab Med 2002;40:1313–9.
127. Bernstein LH, Ingenbleek Y. Clin Chem Lab Med 2002;40:1344–8.
128. Vogel S, Piantedosi R, O'Byrne SM et al. Biochemistry 2002;41:15360–8.
129. Quadro L, Blaner WS, Hamberger L et al. J Biol Chem 2002;277:30191–7.
130. Biesalski HK, Frank J, Beck SC et al. Am J Clin Nutr 1999;69:931–6.
131. Ross AC. Am J Clin Nutr 1999;69:829–30.
132. Marino M, Andrews D, Brown D et al. J Am Soc Nephrol 2001;12:637–48.
133. Christensen EI, Moskaug JO, Vorum H et al. J Am Soc Nephrol 1999;10:685–95.
134. Leheste JR, Rolinski B, Vorum H et al. Am J Pathol 1999;155:1361–70.
135. Sousa MM, Norden AG, Jacobsen C et al. J Biol Chem 2000;275:38176–81.
136. Smith JE, Milch PO, Muto Y et al. Biochem J 1973;132:821–7.
137. Blaner WS, Olson JA. Retinol and retinoic acid metabolism. In: Sporn MB, Roberts AB, Goodman DS, eds. The Retinoids: Biology, Chemistry and Medicine. 2nd ed. New York: Raven Press, 1994:229–55.
138. Arnhold T, Tzimas G, Wittfoht W et al. Life Sci 1996;59:PL169–PL77.
139. Chen C, Mistry G, Jensen B et al. J Clin Pharmacol 1996;36:799–808.
140. Tzimas G, Nau H, Hendrickx AG et al. Teratology 1996;54:255–65.
141. Romans DA, Barua AB, Olson JA. Int J Vitam Nutr Res 2003;73:251–7.
142. Adamson PC, Balis FM, Smith MA et al. J Natl Cancer Inst 1992;84:1332–5.
143. Ozpolat B, Lopez–Berestein G, Adamson P et al. J Pharm Pharm Sci 2003;6:292–301.
144. Weber C, Dumont E. J Clin Pharmacol 1997;37:566–74.
145. Napoli JL, Posch KP, Fiorella PD et al. Biomed Pharmacother 1991;45:131–43.
146. Kurlandsky SB, Gamble MV, Ramakrishnan R et al. J Biol Chem 1995;270:17850–7.
147. Napoli JL. Enzymology and biogenesis of retinoic acid. In: Livrea MA, ed. Vitamin A and Retinoids: An Update of Biological Aspects and Clinical Applications. Basel: Birkhèuser Verlag, 2000:17–27.
148. Duester G. Chem Biol Interact 2001;130–132:469–80.
149. Luu L, Ramshaw H, Tahayato A et al. Adv Enzyme Regul 2001;41:159–75.
150. Duester G. Biochemistry 1996;35:12221–7.
151. Karlsson T, Vahlquist A, Kedishvili N et al. Biochem Biophys Res Commun 2003;303:273–8.
152. Lapshina EA, Belyaeva OV, Chumakova OV et al. Biochemistry 2003;42:776–84.
153. Ross AC, Zolfaghari R, Weisz J. Curr Opin Gastroenterol 2001;17:184–92.
154. Duester G, Mic FA, Molotkov A. Chem Biol Interact 2003;143:201–10.
155. Lin M, Napoli JL. J Biol Chem 2000;275:40106–12.
156. Chen H, Howald WN, Juchau MR. Drug Metab Dispos 2000;28:315–22.
157. Zhang QY, Raner G, Ding X et al. Arch Biochem Biophys 1998;353:257–64.
158. Paik J, Vogel S, Piantedosi R et al. Biochemistry 2000;39:8073–84.
159. Gamble MV, Shang E, Zott RP et al. J Lipid Res 1999;40:2279–92.
160. Shang E, Lai K, Packer AI et al. J Lipid Res 2002;43:590–7.
161. Sass JO, Forster A, Bock KW et al. Biochem Pharmacol 1994;47:485–92.
162. Samokyszyn VM, Gall WE, Zawada G et al. J Biol Chem 2000;275:6908–14.
163. McSorley LC, Daly AK. Biochem Pharmacol 2000;60:517–26.
164. Loudig O, Babichuk C, White J et al. Mol Endocrinol 2000;14:1483–97.
165. Wang Y, Zolfaghari R, Ross AC. Arch Biochem Biophys 2002;401:235–43.
166. Yamamoto Y, Zolfaghari R, Ross AC. FASEB J 2000;14:2119–27.
167. MacLean G, Abu-Abed S, Dolle P et al. Mech Dev 2001;107:195–201.
168. Trofimova-Griffin ME, Juchau MR. Dev Brain Res 2002;136:175–8.
169. Tahayato A, Dolle P, Petkovich M. Gene Expr Patterns 2003;3:449–54.
170. Taimi M, Helvig C, Wisniewski J et al. J Biol Chem 2004;279:77–85.
171. Smith FR, Goodman DS. J Clin Invest 1971;50:2426–36.
172. Gerlach TH, Zile MH. J Lipid Res 1991;32:515–20.
173. Gerlach TH, Zile MH. FASEB J 1991;5:86–92.
174. Stephensen CB, Alvarez JO, Kohatsu J et al. Am J Clin Nutr 1994;60:388–92.
175. Alvarez JO, Salazar-Lindo E, Kohatsu J et al. Am J Clin Nutr 1995;61:1273–6.
176. Saari JC. Retinoids in photosensitive systems. In: Sporn MB, Roberts AB, Goodman DS, eds. The Retinoids: Biology, Chemistry, and Medicine. 2nd ed. New York: Raven Press, 1994:351–85.
177. Thompson DA, Gal A. Prog Retin Eye Res 2003;22:683–703.
178. Haeseleer F, Huang J, Lebioda L et al. J Biol Chem 1998;273:21790–9.
179. Mata NL, Radu RA, Clemmons RS et al. Neuron 2002;36:69–80.
180. Arshavsky V. Neuron 2002;36:1–3.
181. Jacobson SG, Cideciyan AV, Regunath G et al. Nat Genet 1995;11:27–32.
182. Cideciyan AV, Haeseleer F, Fariss RN et al. Vis Neurosci 2000;17:667–78.
183. Wolf G. Nutr Rev 2002;60:257–60.
184. Gollapalli DR, Maiti P, Rando RR. Biochemistry 2003;42:11824–30.
185. Saari JC, Nawrot M, Kennedy BN et al. Neuron 2001;29:739–48.
186. Saari JC, Nawrot M, Garwin GG et al. Invest Ophthalmol Vis Sci 2002;43:1730–5.
187. Golovleva I, Bhattacharya S, Wu ZP et al. J Biol Chem 2003;278:12397–402.
188. Lee S-Y, Ubels JL, Soprano DR. Exp Eye Res 1992;55:163–71.
189. Ubels JL, Harkema JR. Invest Ophthalmol Vis Sci 1994;35:1249–53.
190. Wolbach SB, Howe PR. J Exp Med 1925;42:753–77.
191. Balmer JE, Blomhoff R. J Lipid Res 2002;43:1773–808.
192. Chen Q, Ross AC. Exp Cell Res 2004;297:68–81.
193. Borras E, Zaragoza R, Morante M et al. Eur J Biochem 2003;270:1493–501.

194. Pitha-Rowe I, Petty WJ, Kitareewan S et al. Leukemia 2003;17: 1723–30.

195. Parmar S, Tallman MS. Expert Opin Pharmacother 2003;4: 1379–92.

196. Wilson JG, Roth CB, Warkany J. Am J Anat 1953;92:189–217.

197. Clagett-Dame M, DeLuca HF. Annu Rev Nutr 2002;22: 347–81.

198. Gottesman ME, Quadro L, Blaner WS. Bioessays 2001;23: 409–19.

199. White JC, Highland M, Kaiser M et al. Dev Biol 2000;220: 263–84.

200. Perrotta S, Nobili B, Rossi F et al. Vitam Horm 2003;66: 457–591.

201. McCaffery PJ, Adams J, Maden M et al. Eur J Neurosci 2003;18:457–72.

202. Conlon RA. Trends Genet 1995;11:314–9.

203. Ulven SM, Gundersen TE, Weedon MS et al. Dev Biol 2000;220:379–91.

204. Martinez-Ceballos E, Burdsal CA. J Exp Zool 2001;290: 136–47.

205. Perlmann T. Nat Genet 2002;31:7–8.

206. Cui J, Michaille JJ, Jiang W et al. Dev Biol 2003;260:496–511.

207. Zhang M, Thomas BC, Napoli JL. Gene 2003;305:121–31.

208. Oosterveen T, Niederreither K, Dolle P et al. EMBO J 2003;22:262–9.

209. Niederreither K, Vermot J, Fraulob V et al. Proc Natl Acad Sci USA 2002;99:16111–6.

210. Sakai Y, Meno C, Fujii H et al. Genes Dev 2001;15:213–25.

211. Niederreither K, Abu-Abed S, Schuhbaur B et al. Nat Genet 2002;31:84–8.

212. Otto DM, Henderson CJ, Carrie D et al. Mol Cell Biol 2003;23:6103–16.

213. Morriss-Kay GM, Sokolova N. FASEB J 1996;10:961–8.

214. Helms JA, Kim CH, Hu D et al. Dev Biol 1997;187:25–35.

215. Niederreither K, Vermot J, Le Roux I et al. Development 2003;130:2525–34.

216. Underhill TM, Sampaio AV, Weston AD. Retinoid Signalling and Skeletal Development: The Molecular Basis of Skeletogenesis Novartis Foundation Symposium. Chichester, UK: Wiley, 2001:171–88.

217. Maden M. Nature Rev Neurosci 2002;3:843–53.

218. Wellik DM, Norback DH, DeLuca HF. Am J Physiol 1997;272:E25–9.

219. Levin MS, Li E, Ong DE et al. J Biol Chem 1987;262:7118–24.

220. E X, Zhang L, Lu J et al. J Biol Chem 2002;277:36617–23.

221. Biesalski HK, Nohr D. Mol Aspects Med 2003;24:431–40.

222. Zachman RD, Grummer MA. Retinoids and lung development. In: Zachman RD, Grummer MA, eds. Contemporary Endocrinology: Endocrinology of the Lung: Development and Surfactant Synthesis. Totowa, NJ: Humana Press, 2000:161–79.

223. Stephensen CB. Annu Rev Nutr 2001;21:167–92.

224. Ross AC. Clin Immunol Immunopathol 1996;80:S36–S72.

225. DeCicco KL, Zolfaghari R, Li N-Q et al. J Infect Dis 2000;182: S29–S36.

226. Reifen R. Proc Nutr Soc 2002;61:397–400.

227. Kozakova H, Hanson LA, Stepankova R et al. Microbes Infect 2003;5:405–11.

228. Rosales FJ, Ross AC. J Nutr 1998;128:960–6.

229. Ross AC, Hämmerling UG. Retinoids and the immune system. In: Sporn MB, Roberts AB, Goodman DS, eds. The Retinoids: Biology, Chemistry and Medicine. 2nd ed. New York: Raven Press, 1994:521–44.

230. Smith SM, Hayes CE. Proc Natl Acad Sci USA 1987;84: 5878–82.

231. D'Souza RM, D'Souza R. J Trop Pediatr 2002;48:323–7.

232. Walker-Smith JA. Curr Opin Infect Dis 2001;14:567–71.

233. Grotto I, Mimouni M, Gdalevich M et al. J Pediatr 2003;142: 297–304.

234. Stephensen CB. Nutr Rev 2003;61:280–4.

235. Hanley TM, Kiefer HL, Schnitzler AC et al. J Virol 2004;78: 2819–30.

236. Chew BP, Park JS. J Nutr 2004;134:257S–61S.

237. Bertram JS. Nutr Rev 1999;57:182–91.

238. Sies H, Stahl W. Am J Clin Nutr 1995;62:1315S–21S.

239. Curran Celentano J, Burke JD, Hammond BR Jr. J Nutr 2002; 132:535S–9S.

240. Granado F, Olmedilla B, Blanco I. Br J Nutr 2003;90:487–502.

241. Bartlett H, Eperjesi F. Ophthalmic Physiol Opt 2003;23: 383–99.

242. Mayne ST. FASEB J 1996;10:690–701.

243. Ross AC. Vitamin A and cancer. In: Carroll KK, Kritchevsky D, eds. Nutrition and Disease Update: Cancer. Champaign, IL: AOCS Press, 1994:27–109.

244. Riboli E, Norat T. Am J Clin Nutr 2003;78:559S–69S.

245. Patrick L. Altern Med Rev 2000;5:530–45.

246. Kritharides L, Stocker R. Atherosclerosis 2002;164:211–9.

247. Christen WG, Buring JE, Manson JE et al. Curr Opin Lipidol 1999;10:29–33.

248. Goodman GE. Curr Opin Oncol 1998;10:122–6.

249. Liu C, Russell RM, Wang XD. J Nutr 2003;133:173–9.

250. Mayne ST. J Nutr 2003;133[Suppl]:933S–40S.

251. Badminton MN, Elder GH. Int J Clin Pract 2002;56:272–8.

252. Lodi G, Sardella A, Bez C et al. Cochrane Database Syst Rev 2001:CD001829.

253. Mathews-Roth MM. Am J Clin Nutr 1990;52:500–1.

254. Khachik F, Carvalho L, Bernstein PS et al. Exp Biol Med (Maywood) 2002;227:845–51.

255. Hadley CW, Miller EC, Schwartz SJ et al. Exp Biol Med (Maywood) 2002;227:869–80.

256. Giovannucci E. Exp Biol Med (Maywood) 2002;227:852–9.

257. Sommer A. Curr Iss Public Health 1996;2:161–4.

258. Underwood BA. Prevention of vitamin A deficiency. In: Howson CP, Kennedy ET, Horwitz A, eds. Prevention of Micronutrient Deficiencies: Tools for Policymakers and Public Health Workers. Bethesda, MD: Institute of Medicine, 1998:103–64.

259. Ellis CN, Krach KJ. J Am Acad Dermatol 2001;45:S150–7.

260. Orfanos CE, Zouboulis CC, Almond-Roesler B et al. Drugs 1997;53:358–88.

261. Kang S, Fisher GJ, Voorhees JJ. Clin Geriatr Med 2001;17: 643–59, v–vi.

262. Millikan LE. Am J Clin Dermatol 2003;4:75–80.

263. Orfanos CE, Zouboulis CC. Dermatology 1998;196:140–7.

264. Krautheim A, Gollnick H. Clin Pharmacokinet 2003;42: 1287–304.

265. O'Donnell J. Am J Ther 2003;10:148–59.

266. Clewell HJ 3rd, Andersen ME, Wills RJ et al. J Am Acad Dermatol 1997;36:S77–85.

267. Sun SY, Lotan R. Crit Rev Oncol Hematol 2002;41:41–55.

268. Schmitt-Graff A, Ertelt V, Allgaier HP et al. Hepatology 2003; 38:470–80.

269. Lippman SC, Lotan R. J Nutr 2000;130 [Suppl]:479S–82S.

270. Camacho LH. J Biol Regul Homeost Agents 2003;17:98–114.

271. Darlow BA, Graham PJ. Cochrane Database Syst Rev 2002: CD000501.

272. Massaro D, Massaro GD. Am J Respir Cell Mol Biol 2003;28: 271–4.

273. McGowan SE. Chest 2002;121:206S–8S.

274. Swartz-Basile DA, Wang LH, Tang YZ et al. Am J Physiol 2003;285:G424–32.

275. West KP Jr. J Nutr 2002;132:2857S–66S.

276. Stoltzfus RJ, Humphrey JH. Adv Exp Med Biol 2002;503:39–47.

277. Underwood BA, Smitasiri S. Annu Rev Nutr 1999;19:303–24.

278. Semba RD, Bloem MW. Eur J Clin Nutr 2002;56:271–81.

279. Stephens D, Jackson PL, Gutierrez Y. Pediatr Nurs 1996;22:377–89.

280. Davila ME, Norris L, Cleary MP et al. J Nutr 1985;115:1033–41.

281. Green MH, Green JB, Akohoue SA et al. J Nutr 2001;131:1279–82.

282. West KP Jr, Katz J, Khatry SK et al. BMJ 1999;318:570–5.

283. Tanumihardjo SA, Muherdiyantiningsih, Permaesih D et al. Am J Clin Nutr 1996;63:32–5.

284. Rahmathullah L, Tielsch JM, Thulasiraj RD et al. BMJ 2003;327:254–7.

285. Office of Dietary Supplements, National Institutes of Health. http://odsodnihgov/factsheets/vitahtml, 2003.

286. Mahoney CP, Margolis T, Knauss TA et al. Pediatrics 1980;65:893–6.

287. Collins MD, Mao GE. Annu Rev Pharmacol Toxicol 1999;39:399–430.

288. Tzimas G, Nau H. Curr Pharm Des 2001;7:803–31.

289. Nau H. J Am Acad Dermatol 2001;45:S183–7.

290. Food and Drug Administration. http://www.fda.gov/ohrms/dockets/ac/04/briefing/4017b1.htm, 2004.

291. Biesalski HK. Toxicology 1989;57:117–61.

292. Rothman KJ, Moore LL, Singer MR et al. N Engl J Med 1995;333:1369–73.

293. Wiegand UW, Hartmann S, Hummler H. Int J Vitam Nutr Res 1998;68:411–6.

294. Friedman SL. Alcohol Clin Exp Res 1999;23:904–10.

295. Leo MA, Lieber CS. Am J Clin Nutr 1999;69:1071–85.

296. Russell RM. Am J Clin Nutr 2000;71:878–84.

297. Johansson S, Lind PM, Hakansson H et al. Bone 2002;31:685–9.

298. Rohde CM, Manatt M, Clagett–Dame M et al. J Nutr 1999;129: 2246–50.

299. Rohde CM, DeLuca H. J Nutr 2003;133:777–83.

300. Melhus H, Michaëlsson K, Kindmark A et al. Ann Intern Med 1998;129:770–8.

301. Michaelsson K, Lithell H, Vessby B et al. N Engl J Med 2003;348:287–94.

302. Johansson S, Melhus H. J Bone Miner Res 2001;16:1899–905.

303. Feskanich D, Singh V, Willett WC et al. JAMA 2002;287:47–54.

304. Promislow JH, Goodman-Gruen D, Slymen DJ et al. J Bone Miner Res 2002;17:1349–58.

305. de Pee S, Dary O. J Nutr 2002;132[Suppl]:2895S–901S.

306. Olson JA. Vitamin A, retinoids and carotenoids. In: Shils ME, Olson JA, Shike M, eds. Modern Nutrition in Health and Disease. 8th ed. Philadelphia: Lea & Febiger, 1994:287–307.

307. Makdani D, Sowell AL, Nelson JD et al. J Am Coll Nutr 1996;15:439–49.

308. Tanumihardjo SA, Cheng JC, Permaesih D et al. Am J Clin Nutr 1996;64:966–71.

309. Apgar J, Makdani D, Sowell AL et al. J Am Coll Nutr 1996;15:450–7.

310. Tanumihardjo SA. J Nutr 2000;130:2844–9.

311. Haskell MJ, Mazumder RN, Peerson JM et al. Am J Clin Nutr 1999;70:874–80.

312. Haskell MJ, Lembcke JL, Salazar M et al. Am J Clin Nutr 2003;77:681–6.

313. Rosales FJ, Ross AC. J Nutr 1998;128:1681–7.

314. Rosales FJ, Topping JD, Smith JE et al. Am J Clin Nutr 2000;71:1582–8.

315. Filteau SM, Willumsen JF, Sullivan K et al. Br J Nutr 2000;83:513–20.

316. Paracha PI, Jamil A, Northrop-Clewes CA et al. Am J Clin Nutr 2000;72:1164–9.

317. Congdon NG, West KP Jr. J Nutr 2002;132[Suppl]:2889S–94S.

318. Ambrosini GL, de Klerk NH, Musk AW et al. Public Health Nutr 2001;4:255–64.

319. Humphrey J, Friedman D, Natadisastra G et al. J Am Diet Assoc 2000;100:1501–10.

320. Underwood BA, Arthur P. FASEB J 1996;10:1040–8.

321. Schultink W. J Nutr 2002;132[Suppl]:2881S–3S.

SELECTED READINGS

McLaren DS, ed. The Control of Xerophthalmia: A Century of Contributions and Lessons. Basel: Task Force Sight and Life, 2004.

Ross AC, Zolfaghari R, Weisz J. Vitamin A: recent advances in the biotransformation, transport, and metabolism of retinoids. Curr Opin Gastroenterol 2001;17:184–92.

Russell RM. The vitamin A spectrum: from deficiency to toxicity. Am J Clin Nutr 2000;71:878–84.

Stoltzfus RJ, Humphrey JH. Vitamin A and the nursing mother-infant dyad: evidence for intervention. Adv Exp Med Biol 2002;503:39–47.

Khachik F, Carvalho L, Bernstein PS et al. Chemistry, distribution, and metabolism of tomato carotenoids and their impact on human health. Exp Biol Med (Maywood). 2002;227:845–51.

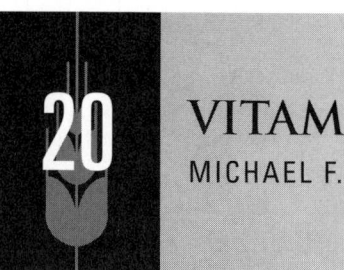

20 VITAMIN D[1]

MICHAEL F. HOLICK

HISTORY OF RICKETS 377
THE ANTIRACHITIC FACTOR: VITAMIN D 378
PHOTOBIOLOGY 378
  History 378
  Photosynthesis of Previtamin D_3 in Human Skin . .378
  Regulation of Previtamin D_3 Synthesis in
    Human Skin 379
  Effect of Age 380
  Sunscreens 381
  Season, Latitude, and Time of Day 381
INTESTINAL ABSORPTION .382
METABOLISM 383
  Vitamin D to 25-Hydroxyvitamin D 383
  25-Hydroxyvitamin D to
    1,25-Dihydroxyvitamin D 384
  Alternative Metabolism of 25-Hydroxyvitamin D . .384
  Regulation of Vitamin D Metabolism:
    Photochemical Regulation 385
BIOLOGIC FUNCTIONS 385
  Role in Calcium and Phosphorus Metabolism 385
  Other Biologic Actions of
    1,25-Dihydroxyvitamin D 386
  Extrarenal Production of 1,25-Dihydroxyvitamin
    D and Its Role in Cancer Prevention 387
USE AND INTERPRETATION OF ASSAYS FOR
  VITAMIN D AND ITS METABOLITES 387
  Vitamin D and 25-Hydroxyvitamin D Assays 387
  1,25-Dihydroxyvitamin D Assays 387
  Vitamin D Deficiency Epidemic 388
RECOMMENDATIONS 389
  Exposure to Sunlight 389
VITAMIN D SUPPLEMENTS 390
  Recommended Dietary Allowance of Vitamin D
    for Humans 390
  Vitamin D Intoxication .392
SUMMARY 392

[1]**Abbreviations: AI,** adequate intake; 1,25(OH)$_2$D, 1,25-dihydroxyvitamin D; 25(OH)D, 25-hydroxyvitamin D; **DRI,** dietary reference intake; **EAR,** estimated average requirement; **EST,** Eastern Standard Time; **RANK,** receptor activator of NFκB (**RANKL,** RANK ligand); **RDA,** recommended dietary allowance; **UL,** tolerable upper intake level; **UV,** ultraviolet.

Vitamin D has existed on Earth for at least 500 million years. It was first produced in ocean dwelling phytoplankton while they were exposed to sunlight for photosynthesis. Although the physiologic function of vitamin D in these lower life forms is unknown, vitamin D and its precursors may have acted either as a natural sunscreen to absorb high-energy ultraviolet (UV) radiation, thus protecting UV-sensitive organelles and macromolecules, or as a photochemical signal (1). For reasons that are not understood, terrestrial vertebrates during evolution became dependent on vitamin D for the development and maintenance of their ossified skeletons. The principal physiologic function of vitamin D in all vertebrates including humans is to maintain serum calcium and phosphorus concentrations in a range that supports cellular processes, neuromuscular function, and bone ossification. Vitamin D accomplishes this goal by enhancing the efficiency of the small intestine to absorb dietary calcium and phosphorus and by mobilizing calcium and phosphorus stores from bone.

Vitamin D is inherently biologically inactive and requires successive hydroxylations in the liver and kidney to form 1,25-dihydroxyvitamin D (1,25(OH)$_2$D; calcitriol), the biologically active form of vitamin D (2–4). 1,25(OH)$_2$D interacts with a specific nuclear receptor in its target tissues that results in a biologic response. Recent evidence suggests that 1,25(OH)$_2$D may also have rapid actions on intracellular calcium, phosphatidylinositol metabolism, and cyclic guanosine triphosphate metabolism (2–4).

The identification of vitamin D metabolites led to the development of assays for them. These assays have become valuable diagnostic tools for evaluating patients with hypocalcemic, hypercalcemic, and metabolic bone disorders.

The major target tissues for 1,25(OH)$_2$D are the intestine and bone; however, nuclear receptors for 1,25(OH)$_2$D have been identified in several other tissues and in cultured tumor cells. 1,25(OH)$_2$D inhibits the proliferation and induces terminal differentiation of many tumor and normal cultured cells that possess its receptor (2–4). These observations have been the impetus for a reevaluation of the physiologic and pharmacologic actions of 1,25(OH)$_2$D.

HISTORY OF RICKETS

Although historians state that rickets occurred in humans as early as the second century, the disease was not considered a significant health problem until the industrialization of northern Europe. In the seventeenth century, Whistler, DeBoot, and Glissen independently recognized that many of the children who lived in the crowded and polluted cities in northern Europe developed a severe bone-deforming disease that was characterized by enlargement of the epiphyses of the long bones and rib cage, bowing of the legs, bending of the spine, and weak and toneless muscles (Fig. 20.1) (5). The incidence of this debilitating bone disease increased dramatically in northern Europe and North America during the industrial revolution, and by the latter part of the nineteenth century, autopsy studies done

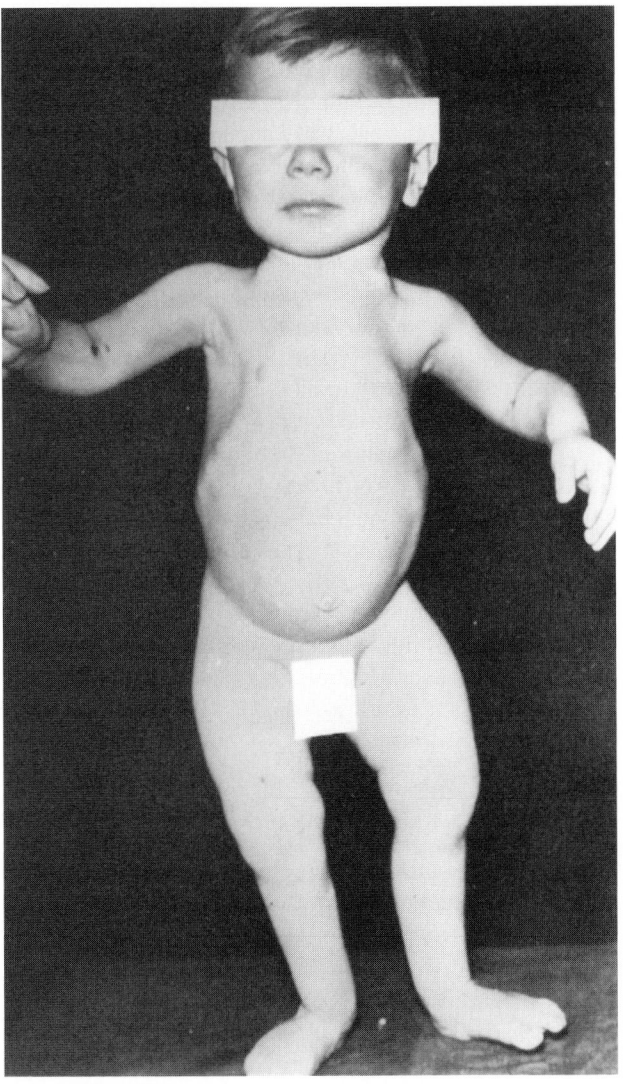

Figure 20.1. Child with rickets showing rachitic rosary of the rib cage, bowed legs, deformity of the long bones, and muscle weakness. (From Fraser D, Scriver CR. Hereditary disorders associated with vitamin-D resistance or defective phosphate metabolism. In: DeGroot L, ed. Endocrinology, vol 2. New York: Grune and Stratton, 1979, with permission.)

in Leiden, the Netherlands showed evidence that about 90% of the children had rickets (6). This disease was especially devastating for young women of childbearing age, who often had a deformed pelvis, resulting in a high incidence of infant and maternal morbidity and mortality. This high incidence led to the development and widespread use of cesarean sections in Great Britain.

From the earliest recognition of rickets in 1650, scientists and physicians throughout Europe began what would be a 270-year search for the cause and cure of this unfortunate childhood malady. In 1822, Sniadecki observed that children living in Warsaw had a high incidence of rickets, whereas children living in rural areas outside of Warsaw did not (7). Based on this observation, he advocated the use of exposure to sunlight as a means of curing this disease. Little attention was focused, however, on the environment as the cause of this disorder. In 1889, the British Medical Society conducted an epidemiologic survey and confirmed previous observations that the incidence of rickets was extremely high in the industrialized cities in Great Britain and was less known in rural districts of the British Highlands (8). This finding was much different from the incidence of rheumatism and malignant disease that was common in all districts in the British Isles (9). Unfortunately, these investigators were unable to relate the lack of exposure to sunlight with their observations. One year later, however, Palm published an extensive epidemiologic survey and came to the same conclusion as Sniadecki (10). He collected observations numerous physicians throughout the British Empire and the Orient. His information revealed that rickets was rare in children living in impoverished cities in China, Japan, and India, where people received poor nutrition and lived in squalor, whereas the children of middle class and poor residents of industrialized cities in the British Isles had a high incidence of rickets. Based on this survey, Palm urged the systematic use of sunbathing as a preventive and therapeutic measure in rickets and other diseases. He also advocated the education of the public to the appreciation of sunshine as a means of health.

Unfortunately, little attention was paid to the insightful observations of Sniadecki and Palm, and another 30 years passed before Huldschinsky demonstrated that exposure of rachitic children to radiation from a mercury vapor arc lamp was effective in curing this bone disease (11). When he exposed one arm of a rachitic child to the UV radiation, he demonstrated that rickets in the other arm was cured to the same degree as the exposed arm. He concluded that the phototherapy was not a local effect and speculated that something was made in the skin and could be transported to distal sites to carry out its antirachitic activity. Two years later, Hess and Unger exposed seven rachitic children on a roof of New York City hospital to varying periods of sunshine and reported that radiographic examinations showed improvement of rickets in each child as evidenced by calcification of the epiphyses (12).

THE ANTIRACHITIC FACTOR: VITAMIN D

During the eighteenth and nineteenth centuries, cod liver oil was used as a common folklore medicine for the prevention and cure of rickets. As early as 1827, Bretonneau treated acute rickets in a 15-month-old child with cod liver oil and noted the incredible speed with which the patient was cured. His student Trousseau advocated the use of oils from fish and sea mammals accompanied by exposure to sunlight for a rapid cure of rickets (13). This knowledge prompted an intense investigation to determine what nutritional factor was present in cod liver oil that was responsible for preventing rickets. In 1918, Mellanby reported that he could produce rickets in dogs by feeding them oatmeal and could cure the disease by adding cod liver oil to their diet (14). Two years later, McCollum and colleagues examined whether the antirachitic factor in cod liver oil was identical to or distinct from vitamin A (15). Cod liver oil was heated and oxidized in a manner that destroyed all vitamin A activity. When the oil was administered to rachitic rats, it maintained its antirachitic properties. Thus, the antirachitic factor present in cod liver oil clearly was not vitamin A but a new fat-soluble vitamin that was called vitamin D.

Powers and associates showed that exposure to radiation from a mercury arc lamp had the same antirachitic potency as cod liver oil (16). At the same time, Hess and Weinstock (17) and Steenbock and Black (18) found that exposure of food and a variety of other substances such as rat liver, human serum, cotton, olive and linseed oils, lettuce, growing wheat, and rat chow to UV radiation resulted in their having antirachitic properties. This concept led Steenbock to patent use of the addition of provitamin D to foods followed by UV irradiation to impart antirachitic activity. The addition of provitamin D_2 to milk followed by UV irradiation became widely practiced in the United States and Europe in the 1930s. This vitamin D fortification process eradicated rickets as a significant health problem in countries that used this practice. Today, the fortification of milk and infant formula with 400 IU (10 µg) of vitamin D_2 or vitamin D_3 has eliminated rickets as a health problem in the United States and Canada. In Europe, vitamin D fortification of milk is prohibited because of severe vitamin D intoxication that resulted from the indiscriminate addition of excessive amounts of vitamin D to infant formulas in the 1940s and 1950s. However, some foods, including cereals and margarine, are fortified with vitamin D in many European countries.

PHOTOBIOLOGY

History

The first vitamin D that was isolated was a photoproduct from the irradiation of the fungal sterol ergosterol. This was known as vitamin D (1), until it was realized that it

was a combination of substances. As a result, further purification of the irradiation mixture yielded a single compound, which was called ergocalciferol or vitamin D_2 (19) (Fig. 20.2). At the time of its identification, it was assumed that the vitamin D made in human skin during exposure to sunlight was vitamin D_2 (20). In the 1930s, however, it was reported that vitamin D obtained from the irradiation of ergosterol had little antirachitic activity in chicken, whereas the vitamin D that was isolated from the irradiation of cholesterol-like sterol yielded a potent antirachitic substance (21–24). The confusion about whether vitamin D_2 was identical to the substance produced in human skin was resolved when Windaus and Bock reported the synthesis of a new provitamin D analog that was similar to ergosterol, except the side chain was that of cholesterol (see Fig. 20.2) (25). This provitamin D was called provitamin D_3 or 7-dehydrocholesterol, and on irradiation, it gave rise to vitamin D_3 (cholecalciferol) (see Fig. 20.2). Vitamin D_3, unlike vitamin D_2, had equal antirachitic activity in chicks and rats and was identical to the vitamin D found in fish liver oils and mammalian skin. Therefore, it was concluded that 7-dehydrocholesterol, rather than ergosterol, was the parent compound in the skin, and its resulting photoproduct was vitamin D_3.

Because of the availability of large quantities of ergosterol, vitamin D_2 was the one used for fortification of milk in the United States and Canada and for pharmaceutical preparations. During the past 2 decades, vitamin D_3 has also been used to fortify milk and other food substances worldwide.

Originally, it was believed that during exposure to sunlight, provitamin D_3 was directly converted to vitamin D_3. This concept was then challenged by Velluz and colleagues, who reported that exposure of provitamin D_3 in an organic solvent to UV radiation at 0°C did not yield any vitamin D_3 (26). They reported the isolation of a new photoproduct, which they called previtamin D_3 (27), that was a thermally labile substance and underwent rearrangement of its double bonds to form vitamin D_3 by a temperature-dependent process.

Photosynthesis of Previtamin D₃ in Human Skin

The sun emits a broad spectrum of electromagnetic radiation. The high-energy photons that are most damaging to life on Earth (<290 nm) are absorbed by the thin layer of ozone that envelops the planet. The small band of radiation between 290 and 315 nm (UVB radiation) is responsible for the photolysis of provitamin D_3 in the epidermis and dermis. During exposure to sunlight, the 5,7-diene of provitamin D_3 absorbs radiation with energies between 290 and 315 nm (28), causing the cleavage of ring B between carbons 9 and 10 (see Fig. 20.2) and the formation of a 6,7-cis-conjugated triene to form a 9,10-seco (seco from the Greek term split) sterol known as previtamin D_3 (Fig. 20.3). In adult skin,

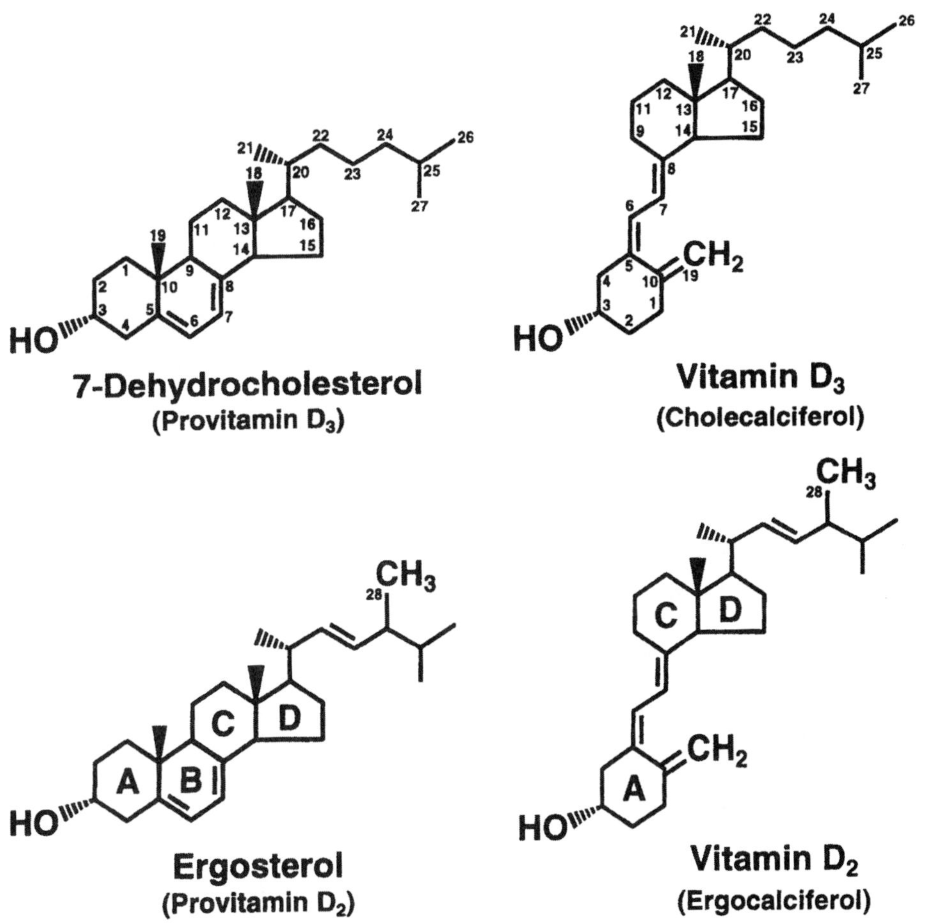

7-Dehydrocholesterol
(Provitamin D₃)

Vitamin D₃
(Cholecalciferol)

Ergosterol
(Provitamin D₂)

Vitamin D₂
(Ergocalciferol)

Figure 20.2. Structure of vitamins D₃ and D₂ and their respective precursors, 7-dehydrocholesterol and ergosterol. The only structural difference between vitamins D₂ and D₃ is their side chains; the side chain for vitamin D₂ contains a double bond among C22, C23, and a C24 methyl group. (From MacLaughlin JA, Holick MF. Mediation of cutaneous vitamin D₃ synthesis by UV radiation. In: Goldsmith LA, ed. Biochemistry and Physiology of the Skin. New York: Oxford University Press, 1983, with permission.)

approximately 60% of the cutaneous stores of provitamin D₃ are found in the epidermis, whereas the other 40% of these stores reside in the dermis (29). When white and black adults are exposed to sunlight, approximately 70 to 80% and 95 to 98% of the UVB photons are absorbed by the epidermis, respectively (30). Therefore, approximately 80 to 90% of the previtamin D₃ that is formed in the skin occurs in the actively growing layers of the epidermis, including the stratum basale and stratum spinosum, and less than 20% occurs in the dermis (31). In neonates, approximately 50% of the provitamin D₃ stores are found in both the epidermis and dermis. Because the thin neonatal epidermis transmits more UVB photons into the dermis, the dermis is also a major site for previtamin D₃ synthesis.

Once previtamin D₃ is made in the skin, it immediately begins to equilibrate thermally to vitamin D₃ (see Fig. 20.3). This thermal equilibration takes approximately 4 to 8 hours to reach completion at body temperature (37°C) in humans. This is because the previtamin D₃ is made in the plasma membrane of the skin cell. It is trapped in an *s-cis,s-cis* conformation. Once it isomerizes to vitamin D₃, its conformation is altered, causing the vitamin D₃ to be jettisoned from the plasma membrane into the extracellular space. The vitamin D binding protein in the circulation, in turn, attracts the vitamin D₃ into the dermal capillary bed (32).

Regulation of Previtamin D₃ Synthesis in Human Skin: Photochemical Regulation

Loomis speculated that melanin pigmentation evolved in persons who lived near the Equator as a mechanism to prevent sunlight-induced vitamin D intoxication (33). Although melanin is an excellent natural sunscreen that competes with provitamin D₃ for UVB photons, thereby limiting the cutaneous production of previtamin D₃ (29, 34), firm evidence exists that sunlight itself is responsible for regulating the total production of vitamin D₃ in human skin (29). Loomis based his theory on the concept that exposure to prolonged intense sunlight would result in an increase in the production of vitamin D₃ in the skin. Once previtamin D₃ is photosynthesized in the skin, however, it can either thermally isomerize to vitamin D₃ or, during exposure to sunlight, absorb UV radiation and isomerize to biologically inert isomers lumisterol and tachysterol (see Fig. 20.3). Thus, if a white person is exposed to sunlight at the Equator, provitamin D₃ is rapidly converted to previtamin D₃ during the initial few minutes of exposure. Prolonged exposure to sunlight, however, does not increase previtamin D₃ production, but rather previtamin D₃ is photodegraded to biologically inert isomers (see Fig. 20.3) (29, 35).

Vitamin D₃ is exquisitely sensitive to photodegradation when exposed to sunlight (see Fig. 20.3). The principal

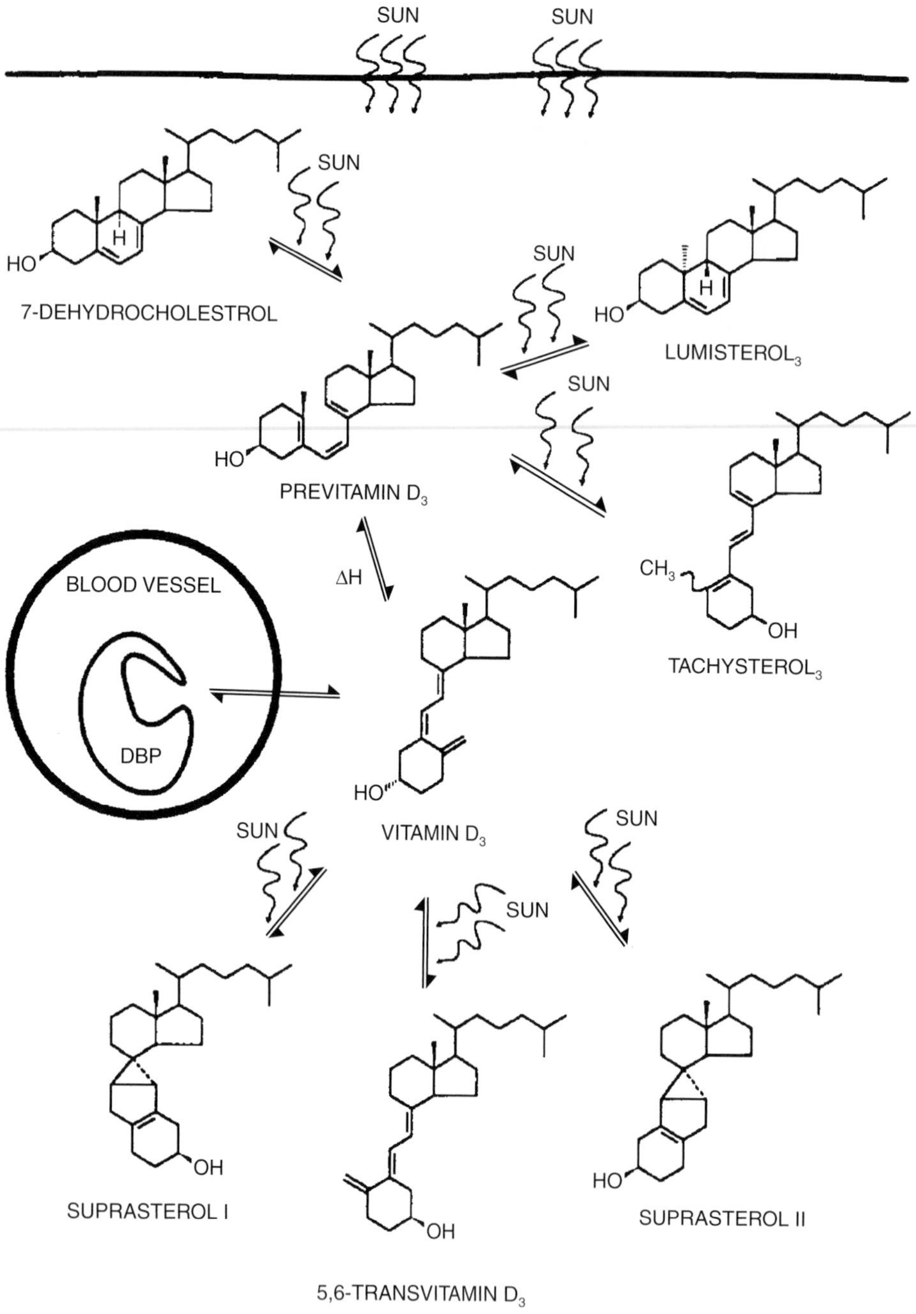

Figure 20.3. Photochemical events that lead to the production and regulation of cholecalciferol (vitamin D_3) in the skin. DBP, vitamin D–binding protein. (From Holick MF. McCollum Award lecture 1994: vitamin D—new horizons for the 21st century. Am J Clin Nutr 1994; 60:619–30, with permission.)

photoisomers that are formed are 5,6-*trans*-vitamin D_3 and supersterols I and II (see Fig. 20.3). Thus, once vitamin D_3 is made from previtamin D_3, it must exit the epidermis into the dermal capillary bed; otherwise, it will rapidly be photodegraded during exposure to sunlight (35, 36).

Effect of Age

The photoproduction of previtamin D_3 in any layer of skin depends on the concentration of provitamin D_3, the presence of chromophors that compete with provitamin D_3 for UVB photons, and the quantum of UVB photons that are able to penetrate the skin and are absorbed by provitamin D_3. The average concentration of provitamin D_3 in 1 cm² of young adult skin is approximately 0.8 μg/g for the epidermis and 0.15 to 0.5 mg/g for the dermis (31). An inverse relation exists between the concentrations of provitamin D_3 in the epidermis with age (Fig. 20.4) (37). The net effect of this age-related decrease is demonstrated in Figure 20.5. The circulating concentrations of vitamin D were measured in healthy young and elderly subjects who were exposed to the same quantity of whole-body UV radiation. The peak circulating concentrations of vitamin D in the elderly subjects were about 30% of that in young adults (38).

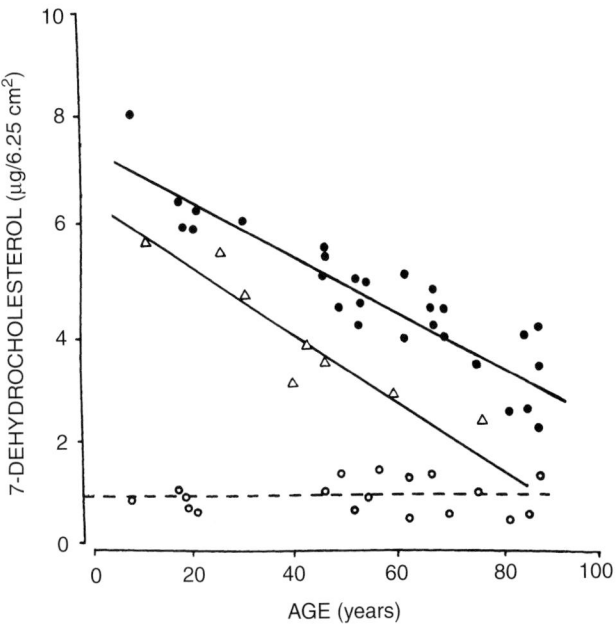

Figure 20.4. Effect of aging on 7-dehydrocholesterol concentrations in human epidermis and dermis. Concentrations of 7-dehydrocholesterol (provitamin D_3) per unit area of human epidermis (*closed circles*), stratum basal (*open triangles*), and dermis (*open circles*) were obtained from surgical specimens from donors of various ages. Linear regression analysis gave slopes of −0.05, −0.06, and −0.0005 for epidermis (r = −.89), stratum basal (r = −.92), and dermis (r = −.04), respectively. The slopes of epidermis and stratum basal are significantly different from the slope of dermis ($p < .001$). (From MacLaughlin JA, Holick MF. Aging decreases the capacity of human skin to produce vitamin D_3. J Clin Invest 1985;76:1536–38, with permission.)

Sunscreens

The awareness that the alarming increase in the incidence of skin cancer is related to chronic exposure to sunlight has led to the recommendation that people should wear sunscreen before going outdoors (39). The solar radiation that is responsible for causing wrinkles and skin cancer, however, is the same radiation that is responsible for producing previtamin D_3 in the skin. Thus, the application of a sunscreen with a sun protection factor of only 8 can markedly reduce the cutaneous production of previtamin D_3 (Fig. 20.6) (40). The use of sunscreens by children and young adults will affect their vitamin D status and will increase their risk of vitamin D deficiency (35). Elderly persons, being more conscious of their health, often apply a sunscreen on their skin before going outdoors. Long-term use of sunscreens can decrease circulating concentrations of 25-hydroxyvitamin D (25(OH)D), a hallmark for determining vitamin D deficiency. In one study, almost one half the persons who lived in Springfield, Illinois who always wore a sunscreen before going outdoors had overt vitamin D deficiency as determined by low circulating concentrations of 25(OH)D (41).

Season, Latitude, and Time of Day

At the turn of the twentieth century, a seasonal incidence of rickets was recognized in the industrialized cities of the United States and Europe. Rickets was seen less frequently in children at the end of the summer and more frequently at the end of the winter and early spring (9). As winter approaches, the solar zenith angle of the sun becomes more oblique. This configuration causes the UVB photons to be absorbed more efficiently by the stratospheric ozone layer, thereby decreasing the total number of photons that reach the Earth's surface. As a result, the cutaneous synthesis of previtamin D_3 is affected by time of day, season of the year, and latitude. As shown

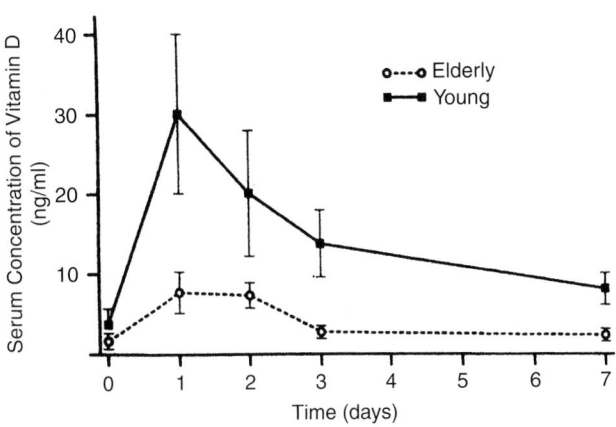

Figure 20.5. Circulating concentrations of vitamin D in healthy young and elderly volunteers exposed to ultraviolet radiation. To convert nanograms per milliliter to nanomoles per liter, multiply by 2.60. (From Holick MF, Matsuoka LY, Wortsman J. Age, vitamin D, and solar ultraviolet. Lancet 1989;2:1104–5, with permission.)

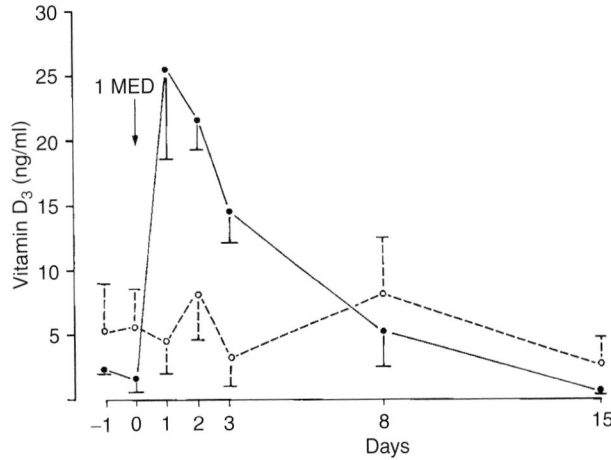

Figure 20.6. Mean (± SEM) serum vitamin D_3 concentrations in eight physiologically normal subjects. Four subjects (*open circles*) applied *p*-aminobenzoic acid with sun protection factor 8, and four applied vehicle (*closed circles*) to the entire skin before exposure to ultraviolet B (UVB). On day 0, all subjects underwent total-body exposure to 1 minimal erythema dose of UV radiation. To convert nanograms of vitamin D per milliliter to nanomoles per liter, multiply by 2.60. (From Matsuoka LY, Ide L, Wortsman J et al. Sunscreens suppress cutaneous vitamin D_3 synthesis. J Clin Endocrinol Metab 1987;64:1165–8, with permission.)

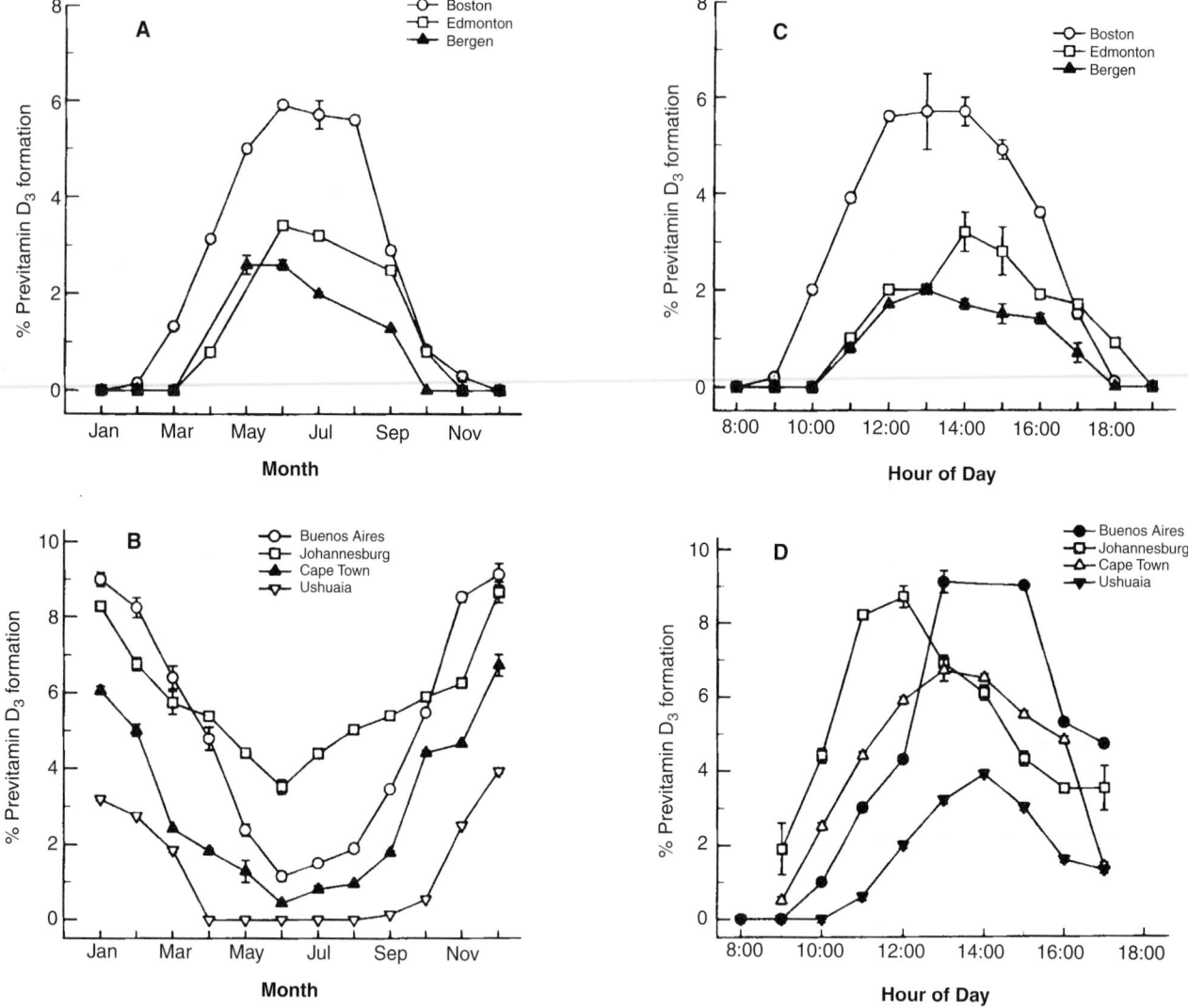

Figure 20.7. Influence of season, time of day, and latitude on the synthesis of previtamin D_3 in northern (**A** and **C**) and southern (**B** and **D**) hemispheres. The hour indicated in **C** and **D** is the end of the 1-hour exposure time. (From Chen TC. Photobiology of vitamin D. In: Holick MF, ed. Vitamin D: Physiology, Molecular Biology, and Clinical Applications. Totowa, NJ: Humana Press, 1999:17–37, with permission.)

in Figure 20.7, exposure to sunlight in Boston (42°N) promoted the cutaneous photosynthesis of previtamin D_3 in human skin from March through October. By November, however, the number of 290- to 315-nm photons that penetrated the stratospheric layer into Boston was insufficient to cause significant conversion of provitamin D_3 to previtamin D_3. Just 10° north in Edmonton (Alberta), Canada, this period was extended between mid-October and mid-March. Further south in Los Angeles (34°N) and Puerto Rico (18°N), the production of previtamin D_3 occurred throughout the year (42).

In Boston in the summer, exposure to sunlight beginning at 5:30 Eastern Standard Time (EST) to 18:30 EST resulted in the cutaneous production of previtamin D_3. By October, however, most of the UVB photons were absorbed by the ozone layer, and, as a result, exposure to sunlight before 10:00 EST and after 15:00 EST was ineffective in producing previtamin D_3 in the skin (see Fig. 20.7)

(43). These observations are beginning to provide guidelines for recommendations regarding the use of sunlight as a means of providing people with their vitamin D requirement. For example, it is reasonable to advise people, especially elderly persons, that exposure to morning or late afternoon sunlight in the summer is a good source for their vitamin D requirement. At these times, sunlight exposure is less damaging to the skin.

INTESTINAL ABSORPTION

In nature, only a few foods contain vitamin D: fish liver oils, fatty fish, and egg yolks. Several countries practice the fortification of some foods with vitamin D. In the United States, milk is the principal dietary component that is subject to fortification with either vitamin D_2 or vitamin D_3. However, the amount of vitamin D can vary. Studies have shown that up to 80% of milk samples tested did not contain 80 to 120% of the vitamin D, and about 14% had no detectable vitamin D (44–46). In other countries, some cereals, margarine, and breads have small quantities of vitamin D added to them.

When vitamin D is ingested, this fat-soluble compound is incorporated into the chylomicron fraction, and about 80% is absorbed into the lymphatic system (4). After the ingestion of a single dose of 50,000 IU of vitamin D_2, the circulating concentrations of vitamin D begin to increase within hours, peak at 12 hours, and gradually decline to near baseline by 72 hours (Fig. 20.8) (47). This provocative vitamin D absorption test has been useful in determining whether a patient with an intestinal malabsorption syndrome is capable of absorbing this fat-soluble vitamin. A blood sample is drawn just before and 12 or 24 hours after a single oral administration of 50,000 IU of vitamin D_2 (see Fig. 20.8). If no elevation in the circulating concentration of vitamin D is observed, complete malabsorption of vitamin D should be suspected; however, any increase in the circulating concentration of vitamin D reflects vitamin D absorption. The dose of vitamin D can therefore be tailored accordingly (4).

Patients who suffer from chronic intestinal malabsorption syndromes caused by chronic liver disease, cystic fibrosis, Crohn disease, Whipple disease, and sprue are more likely to develop vitamin D deficiency because the small intestine is unable to absorb this fat-soluble vitamin. Diseases that affect the more distal small intestine and large intestine, such as in ileocolitis caused by Crohn disease and ulcerative colitis, have little effect on absorption of vitamin D (see Fig. 20.8).

METABOLISM

Vitamin D to 25-Hydroxyvitamin D

Once vitamin D (the term vitamin D without a subscript relates to either or both vitamin D_2 or vitamin D_3 and its metabolites) enters the circulation, it is bound to the group-specific protein commonly known as the vitamin D–binding protein. Vitamin D is transported to the liver, where it undergoes its first hydroxylation on carbon 25, resulting in the formation of the major circulating form of vitamin D, (25(OH)D) (Fig. 20.9) (2–4, 21, 48). The

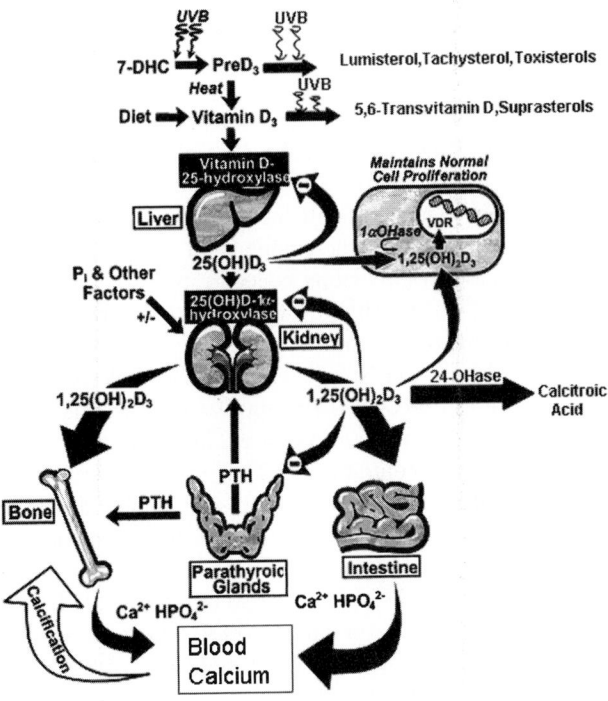

Figure 20.9. Schematic representation for cutaneous production of vitamin D and its metabolism and regulation for calcium homeostasis and cellular growth. During exposure to sunlight, 7-dehydrocholesterol (7-DHC) in the skin absorbs solar ultraviolet (UVB) radiation and is converted to previtamin D_3 (preD$_3$). Once formed, previtamin D_3 undergoes thermally induced transformation to vitamin D_3. Further exposure to sunlight converts preD$_3$ and vitamin D_3 to biologically inert photoproducts. Vitamin D coming from the diet or from the skin enters the circulation and is metabolized in the liver by the vitamin D-25-hydroxylase (25-OHase) to 25-hydroxyvitamin D_3 [25(OH)D$_3$]. 25(OH)D$_3$ reenters the circulation and is converted in the kidney by the 25–hydroxyvitamin D_3-1α-hydroxylase (1-OHase) to 1,25-dihydroxyvitamin D_3 [1,25(OH)$_2$D$_3$]. Various factors, including serum phosphorus (P$_i$) and parathyroid hormone (PTH), regulate the renal production of 1,25(OH)$_2$D. 1,25(OH)$_2$D regulates calcium metabolism through its interaction with its major target tissues, the bone and the intestine. 1,25(OH)$_2$D$_3$ also induces its own destruction by enhancing the expression of the 25-hydroxyvitamin D-24-hydroxylase (24-OHase). 25(OH)D is metabolized in other tissues for the purpose of regulation of cellular growth. (Copyright Michael F. Holick, 2003.)

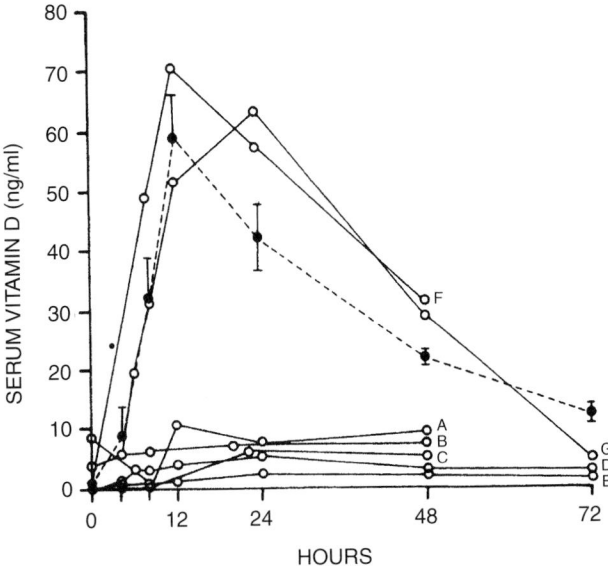

Figure 20.8. Serum vitamin D concentrations in seven patients (patients A to G) with intestinal fat malabsorption syndromes after a single oral dose of 50,000 IU (1.25 mg) of vitamin D_2. For comparison, the means and standard errors of vitamin D concentrations measured in seven physiologically normal control subjects after a similar dose are indicated by the *closed circles* and *dotted lines*. Two patients, one with Crohn ileocolitis (patient F) and one with ulcerative colitis (patient G), had essentially normal absorption curves. Five patients, however, showed a dramatic lack of response, with no values greater than 25.2 nmol/L (10 ng/mL). (From Lo CW, Paris PW, clemens TL et al. Vitamin D absorption in healthy subjects and in patients with intestinal malabsorption syndromes. Am J Clin Nutr 1985;42:644–9, with permission.)

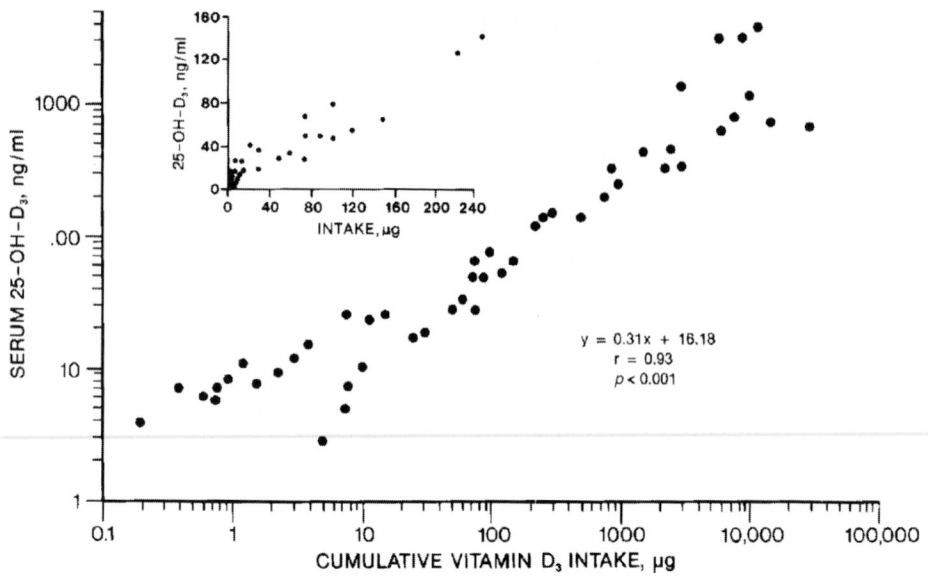

Figure 20.10. Serum levels of 25(OH)D₃, observed in response to various oral doses of vitamin D₃ given to vitamin D–deficient rats. A clear linear correlation extends well into the pharmacologic range for both parameters. To convert nanograms per milliliter to nanomoles per liter, multiply by 2.50. (From Holick MF. Vitamin D: Relevance for Clinical Medicine. Los Angeles: Nichols Institute, 1981, with permission.)

production of 25(OH)D by the liver is regulated by a negative feedback mechanism that is controlled by vitamin D, 25(OH)D, and 1,25(OH)₂D (49). This negative feedback control is not regulated tightly in as much as an increase in exposure to sunlight or dietary intake of vitamin D results in an increase in circulating concentrations of 25(OH)D (Fig. 20.10) (50, 51). Although the liver is the major site for 25(OH)D production, some extrahepatic sites are capable of this hydroxylation. It is likely that the cholesterol-25-hydroxylase can recognize vitamin D and hydroxylase the side chain on carbon 25 to produce 25(OH)D (4).

Circulating concentrations of 25(OH)D often are low in patients with severe parenchymal and cholestatic liver disease (52), in part because of the associated intestinal malabsorption of vitamin D as well as the decrease in the reservoir of the vitamin D-25-hydroxylase in the liver. Although low circulating concentrations of 25(OH)D can cause vitamin D deficiency bone disease, it is unlikely that these low levels are responsible for the debilitating osteoporosis-like bone disease associated with severe liver failure. Little correlation exists between the severity of osteopenia and fractures with circulating levels of 25(OH)D in patients with primary biliary cirrhosis and other chronic liver disorders. Furthermore, treatment of these patients with 25(OH)D or its metabolites has not provided any significant benefit (53). Because these patients are more prone to developing vitamin D deficiency as a result of associated fat malabsorption, however, it is prudent to increase their vitamin D intake (e.g., 50,000 IU vitamin D once or twice a month) and monitor circulating concentrations of 25(OH)D.

25-Hydroxyvitamin D to 1,25-Dihydroxyvitamin D

Although 25(OH)D is the major circulating form of vitamin D, it is biologically inert at physiologic concentrations. In order for it to become active, it must be hydroxylated on carbon 1 by a specific 25(OH)D-1α-hydroxylase (1-OHase)

that is present in the kidney (see Fig. 20.9) (1–4, 21). Although the kidney is the principal site for the production of 1,25(OH)₂D under most circumstances, the placenta also appears to play a role in producing 1,25(OH)₂D at a time of increased requirement for calcium by the fetus (54–56). In various reports, authors cite that extrarenal sites exist for the production of 1,25(OH)₂D. The 1-OHase is expressed in a wide variety of cultured cells, such as placental cells, human bone cells, keratinocytes, and stimulated monocytes, as well as many tissues including lung, colon, prostate, and breast, also produce 1,25(OH)₂D₃ (3, 4, 35, 57–59). 1,25(OH)₂D may be produced locally in cells to act in an autocrine or paracrine manner to regulate cell growth (35). In patients who have had bilateral nephrectomy or have chronic renal failure, the concentrations of 1,25(OH)₂D in the circulation usually are low or undetectable. Thus, the kidney is the principal organ responsible for activating vitamin D for the regulation of calcium metabolism. The extrarenally produced 1,25(OH)₂D carries out its biologic functions locally and then induces its catabolism so it never enters the circulation (35).

Alternative Metabolism of 25-Hydroxyvitamin D

25(OH)D as well as its biologically active metabolite 1,25(OH)₂D can act as substrates for a variety of hydroxylases. The principal site of metabolism is the side chain, where carbons 23, 24, and 26 undergo hydroxylation and oxidation to yield a plethora of metabolites of 25(OH)D and 1,25(OH)₂D (2–4, 21). Although the metabolic importance of these side-chain modifications is uncertain, most likely they are related to the deactivation and rapid clearance of 1,25(OH)₂D. This is particularly true for the C-23 and C-24 oxidations, which ultimately yield a biologically inactive, water-soluble metabolite, 1α-OH-24, 25, 26, 27-tetranor-23-COOH-vitamin D₃ (calcitroic acid) (2, 50). In addition to the multiple hydroxylations in the side chain,

$25(OH)D_3$ can have its A ring oxidized whereby the C-19 is replaced with a keto group. This reaction occurs in vivo in ruminants and in vitro in chick kidney homogenates, resulting in the conversion of $25(OH)D_3$ to the *cis*- and *trans*-isomers of 10-keto-19-nor-25-hydroxyvitamin D_3 (2, 4, 60). Although this keto metabolite is biologically inactive, it is of interest because it comigrates on many chromatographic systems with $1,25(OH)_2D_3$ and can be mistaken for $1,25(OH)_2D_3$. Additional chromatography using methylene chloride as one of the solvents separates these metabolites (4, 61). To date, more than 60 metabolites of vitamin D have been structurally identified (62). All these metabolites are biologically less active on a weight basis when compared with $1,25(OH)_2D$. At present, many investigators believe that most of the side-chain and A-ring metabolites exist only in intoxicated states and are not relevant to the physiologic actions of vitamin D.

Regulation of Vitamin D Metabolism

The synthesis of vitamin D in the skin and its metabolism to $1,25(OH)_2D_3$ is regulated tightly by the body. Sunlight regulates the total production of previtamin D_3 and vitamin D_3 in the skin. Once vitamin D enters the circulation, it can be stored in the fat for later use or metabolized in the liver to $25(OH)D$. This hydroxylation step is feedback regulated. The most critical step in the vitamin D metabolism pathway is the production of $1,25(OH)_2D$ by the kidney. During periods of calcium deprivation, circulating ionized calcium concentrations decline. The parathyroid glands immediately detect this decrease and increase the production and secretion of parathyroid hormone (63). The principal role of parathyroid hormone on calcium metabolism is to increase the tubular reabsorption of calcium from the renal tubular ultrafiltrate and by increasing the renal production of $1,25(OH)_2D$. $1,25(OH)_2D$ travels to the small intestine where it increases the efficiency of intestinal calcium absorption. $1,25(OH)_2D$ and parathyroid hormone act indirectly to induce monocytic stem cells to become mature functioning osteoclasts by stimulating the expression of RANK (receptor activator of $NF\kappa B$) ligand in (RANKL) osteoblasts (35). The mature osteoclasts mobilize calcium from bone (see Fig. 20.9).

It is generally believed that parathyroid hormone does not directly regulate the renal $25(OH)D$-1α-hydroxylase. Evidence suggests that the hypophosphatemic effect of parathyroid hormone is ultimately responsible for enhancing the renal 1α-hydroxylase activity (64). In healthy men, phosphorus restriction caused an increase in circulating concentrations of $1,25(OH)_2D$ to 80% above control values; this increase was related to an increase in the production rate without any change in the metabolic clearance of this hormone. With phosphorus supplementation, serum concentrations of $1,25(OH)_2D$ decreased abruptly, reaching a nadir within 2 to 4 days. After 10 days of supplementation, the mean concentration of $1,25(OH)_2D$ was 29% lower than the value measured when phosphorus intake was normal.

Under certain physiologic circumstances, factors other than calcium, phosphorus, and parathyroid hormone may also modulate the activity of $25(OH)D$-1-hydroxylase (4). The efficiency of intestinal calcium transport is enhanced when calcium demands by the body are increased during pregnancy, lactation, and skeletal growth. Because $1,25(OH)_2D$ is the principal hormone responsible for the regulation of calcium absorption in the small intestine, it is not surprising that growth hormone, estrogen, and prolactin can directly or indirectly enhance the renal production of $1,25(OH)_2D$ in various in vitro and in vivo animal models (65–69). Although estrogen appears to play a significant role in regulating the production of $1,25(OH)_2D$ in the laying hen, estrogen and progesterone likely do not play a significant role in the renal production of $1,25(OH)_2D$ (70–73). This statement is based on the observation that circulating free concentrations of $1,25(OH)_2D$ do not change in women before, during, and after menopause. Furthermore, circulating concentrations of $1,25(OH)_2D$ were not altered in young women with estrogen deficiency caused by anorexia nervosa (71). A few authors have suggested that circulating concentrations of $1,25(OH)_2D$ are slightly lower in osteoporotic women compared with age-matched control subjects. Estrogen replacement in postmenopausal women increased circulating concentrations of $1,25(OH)_2D$ (71).

The responsiveness of the renal $25(OH)D$-1α-hydroxylase to parathyroid hormone may be affected by either age or osteoporosis (74–76). When osteoporotic women were infused with a synthetic fragment of parathyroid hormone, circulating concentrations of $1,25(OH)_2D$ increased twofold within 24 hours in healthy young control subjects, whereas no significant increase was observed in older osteoporotic patients. Whether the moment-to-moment regulation of renal $25(OH)D$-1α-hydroxylase in response to parathyroid hormone is altered with aging or osteoporosis and its role in the disease process remain to be determined. One study suggested that the number of vitamin D receptors in the small intestine decreases in the elderly (77). This may help to explain why the efficiency of intestinal calcium absorption is decreased in elderly persons.

BIOLOGIC FUNCTIONS

Role in Calcium and Phosphorus Metabolism

The principal physiologic function of vitamin D in vertebrates, including humans, is to maintain intracellular and extracellular calcium concentrations within a physiologically acceptable range. Vitamin D accomplishes this goal through the action of $1,25(OH)_2D$ on regulating calcium and phosphorus metabolism in the intestine and bone. $1,25(OH)_2D$ interacts with a specific high affinity receptor in its respective target tissue (2–4). This rare intracellular protein has been cloned and belongs to the superfamily of the steroid hormone zinc-finger receptors (78). It selectively binds $1,25(OH)_2D_3$ to retinoic acid X receptor (RXR) to form a heterodimeric complex that interacts with specific DNA sequences known as vitamin D–responsive elements (62, 76, 79).

This nuclear binding activity results in the transcription of hormone-specific mRNA, which in turn govern the translation of several proteins including the epithelial calcium channel and the calcium-binding protein (calbindin 9k) (80). These proteins are thought to be important in the transcellular transport of calcium in the intestine. The net result is an increase in the absorption of calcium from intestinal contents into the circulation (see Fig. 20.9). $1,25(OH)_2D$ also enhances dietary phosphorus absorption in the jejunum and ileum by unknown mechanisms.

$1,25(OH)_2D$ has various effects on bone cells. In keeping with its principal physiologic function in maintaining serum calcium levels within an acceptable physiologic range for cellular activity, it enhances the mobilization of calcium and phosphorus from bone at times of calcium deprivation. $1,25(OH)_2D$ indirectly induces stem cell monocytes to become mature osteoclasts (35, 76, 81).

Osteoblasts have nuclear receptors for $1,25(OH)_2D$ (35, 76, 81, 82). $1,25(OH)_2D$ enhances the expression on the osteoblasts cell surface. The receptor for RANKL known as RANK is present on the cell surface of immature monocytic osteoclast precursor cells. The intimate coupling of the osteoblast's RANKL with the monocyte RANK results in signaling the monocyte to become a mature osteoclast (76–81). The mature osteoclasts release hydrochloric acid and hydrolytic enzymes that dissolve the mineral and matrix to release calcium and phosphorus into the extracellular space. In vitro studies have also shown that $1,25(OH)_2D$ increases alkaline phosphatase activity and the gene expression for osteocalcin and osteopontin in osteoblasts (76, 83, 84). Although vitamin D is regarded as essential for the development and maintenance of a healthy skeleton, little evidence suggests an active role of $1,25(OH)_2D$ in bone mineralization. Two studies in vitamin D–deficient rats either maintained on a high-calcium, high-phosphorus, vitamin D–deficient diet or infused with calcium and phosphorus to maintain serum calcium and phosphorus concentrations within the normal range showed that these animals were capable of mineralizing their bones in a similar fashion to groups of rats maintained on a normal-calcium, normal-phosphorus, vitamin D–sufficient diet (85, 86). These data suggest that vitamin D and its metabolites are not absolutely required for the bone ossification process. Instead, vitamin D is responsible for maintaining extracellular calcium and phosphorus concentrations in a supersaturated state that results in the mineralization of bone (87).

Other Biologic Actions of 1,25-Dihydroxyvitamin D

Much effort has been directed toward identifying actions of $1,25(OH)_2D$ that are not directly related to maintenance of calcium and phosphorus homeostasis. The impetus for this search resulted from the observation that various tissues that were not related to calcium metabolism possessed nuclear receptors for $1,25(OH)_2D$ (2, 35, 76, 80, 88). Since these initial observations, careful analysis has shown that these tissues, as well as activated B and T lymphocytes (89, 90) and several cultured normal and tumor cell lines, possess high-affinity, low-capacity $1,25(OH)_2D$ receptorlike proteins that are quantitatively similar to the intestinal receptor (2, 35, 76, 80).

The first insight into a noncalcemic action of $1,25(OH)_2D_3$ came when promyeloid leukemic cells (line M-1) that had nuclear receptors for $1,25(OH)_2D_3$ responded to this hormone by differentiating into macrophages (91). $1,25(OH)_2D_3$ induced time- and dose-dependent phagocytic activity and expression of cell-surface antigens including Fc and C3 receptors and lysozyme activity. Similar studies were done in a human promyelocytic leukemic cell line (HL-60). Cell growth was inhibited by as little as 10^{-9} M of $1,25(OH)_2D_3$ in a dose-dependent manner (92). $1,25(OH)_2D_3$ was also found to be an effective antiproliferative agent for cultured tumor cells, such as tumor breast, colon, lung, prostate, and melanoma cells, that possessed its nuclear receptor (35, 76, 80, 93).

The effect of $1,25(OH)_2D_3$ on leukemia cells is reversible. When clones of HL-60 cells that possessed less than 10% of nuclear binding activity for $1,25(OH)_2D_3$ were incubated with $1,25(OH)_2D_3$, little difference in their proliferative activity was noted (94). The effect of pharmacologic doses of $1,25(OH)_2D_3$ on the immune system has been dramatically demonstrated in animal models for autoimmune diseases. $1,25(OH)_2D_3$ markedly decreased the incidence of type 1 diabetes in NOD mice (35, 76, 95, 96). This calciotropic hormone also reduced development of thyroiditis and encephalomyelitis and prolonged the survival of transplanted skin allografts in mice (35, 76, 97–99). Of interest was that human epidermal cells have nuclear receptors for $1,25(OH)_2D_3$. $1,25(OH)_2D_3$ inhibited the proliferation and induced terminal differentiation of cultured murine and human keratinocytes in a dose-dependent manner (100, 101). These laboratory observations have been put to practical use by the development of $1,25(OH)_2D_3$ and its analogs as a safe and effective treatment for the hyperproliferative epidermal disorder psoriasis (102–107).

Investigators have recognized since 1979 that people who live at higher latitudes are at a higher risk of developing hypertension (108). It was also observed that hypertensive adults exposed to a tanning bed with UVB radiation had an increase in their 25(OH)D levels by more than 100% and complete resolution of their hypertension (109). When similar adults were exposed to UVA radiation under the same conditions, no increase in circulating concentration of 25(OH)D and no resolution of their hypertension were noted (109). It is now recognized that $1,25(OH)_2D$ modulates the renal production of the blood pressure hormone renin in a negative fashion, and this may, in part, explanain the role of vitamin D sufficiency in the prevention of hypertension (110).

Extrarenal Production of 1,25-Dihydroxyvitamin D and Its Role in Cancer Prevention

Since the late 1980s, investigators have recognized that the risk of developing and dying of breast, colon, prostate, ovarian, and many other cancers (35, 76, 111–116) is increased in relation to living at higher latitudes and being more prone to developing vitamin D deficiency. However, it was difficult to understand this relationship because it was also well recognized that increase in sun exposure resulting in an increase in the production of vitamin D_3 in the skin or an increase in the intake of dietary vitamin D did not raise the blood levels of the antiproliferative hormone $1,25(OH)_2D$ in the circulation (35, 76). The reason is that the production of $1,25(OH)_2D$ is tightly regulated in the kidneys by serum calcium, phosphorus, and parathyroid hormone (35, 76, 80).

Investigators had observed that activated macrophages and skin cells had the capacity to produce $1,25(OH)_2D$ because both cell types expressed the 1-OHase (35, 59). In 1998, it was found that normal and malignant prostate cells had 1-OHase activity (117). Investigators suggested that the reason that vitamin D deficiency was associated with an increased risk of dying of prostate cancer was that the prostate cells were not receiving an adequate amount of 25(OH)D to satisfy their production of the antiproliferative hormone $1,25(OH)_2D$. This concept was supported by the observation that prostate cancer cells that lacked the 1-OHase were unresponsive to $25(OH)D_3$ (118). However, when the same prostate cancer cells were transfected with the 1-OHase gene, the cellular growth of these cells was inhibited by the addition of $25(OH)D_3$ to the cells (118). Thus, it appears that by increasing 25(OH)D in the circulation increases tissue levels of 25(OH)D that can then be metabolized to $1,25(OH)_2D$. The local production of $1,25(OH)_2D$ may be critically important in regulating cell growth and therefore in decreasing risk of many common cancers including prostate, breast, colon, and esophagus. All these tissues have now been shown to express the 1-OHase (35, 76, 117–121).

USE AND INTERPRETATION OF ASSAYS FOR VITAMIN D AND ITS METABOLITES

Vitamin D and 25-Hydroxyvitamin D Assays

The first assays for vitamin D were chick and rat bioassays (122, 123). The rat bioassay, commonly known as the line test, was used widely to determine the concentration of vitamin D in fortified foods such as milk (123). The development of specific assays for vitamin D and its biologically important metabolites made these bioassays obsolete.

A specific assay to measure circulating concentrations of vitamin D_2 and vitamin D_3 has been developed (124, 125). This assay has been of great value in evaluating circulating concentrations of vitamin D after exposure to quantitative doses of UVB radiation (50). It has also been useful as a provocative test for determining which patients with intestinal malabsorption syndromes are at risk for developing vitamin D deficiency (47). Using this assay, the half-life of circulating vitamin D is approximately 24 hours. The serum concentration of vitamin D at any time depends on the most recent ingestion of vitamin D as well as the last exposure to sunlight. The normal range of serum vitamin D is 0 to 310 nmol/L (0 to 120 ng/mL). Consequently, serum vitamin D_2 and vitamin D_3 concentrations are of little value in determining the vitamin D status of a patient.

Circulating concentrations of 25(OH)D are measured by a specific competitive protein-binding assay using the vitamin D–binding protein (126–129). Because the half-life of circulating 25(OH)D is approximately 3 weeks, the steady-state concentration of 25(OH)D in the circulation represents the concentrations of vitamin D derived from both diet and from photoproduction over several weeks to several months (35, 76, 122). $25(OH)D_2$ and $25(OH)D_3$ can be measured separately (129, 130). Originally, it was thought that $25(OH)D_2$ was reflective of the dietary component of vitamin D and $25(OH)D_3$ was reflective of exposure to sunlight. Because milk and multivitamin preparations are now fortified with both forms of the vitamin, however, the separate measurement of these metabolites is of little value (122).

Measurement of the circulating concentration of 25(OH)D is most valuable for determining the vitamin D status of an individual. The normal circulating concentration of 25(OH)D is usually reported to be between 20 and 150 nmol/L (9 and 60 ng/mL). However, most experts recommend that a serum value lower than 50 nmol/L (20 ng/mL) is considered to indicate vitamin D deficiency (131–133). Although most diagnostic laboratories report the upper limit of the normal range for 25(OH)D to be 150 nmol/L (60 ng/mL), a circulating concentration of 250 nmol/L (100 ng/mL) in lifeguards after a full summer of exposure to sunlight is not surprising and is considered normal. Vitamin D intoxication is usually associated with 25(OH)D concentrations greater than 375 nmol/L (150 ng/mL) with attendant hypercalcemia and hyperphosphatemia (63, 76, 134).

The assay for serum 25(OH)D has clinical utility for determining vitamin D deficiency in patients with intestinal malabsorption syndromes, severe hepatic failure, and the nephrotic syndrome. It is the hallmark assay for determining vitamin D deficiency in very young and elderly persons (35, 76).

1,25-Dihydroxyvitamin D Assays

$1,25(OH)_2D$ levels in serum and plasma can be specifically measured with a competitive receptor-binding assay using a nuclear/cytosolic receptor for 1,25(OH)$_2$D or an anti-body assay (122, 129, 135–137). A bioassay has also been developed using cultured calvaria (138). This assay, which is tedious to conduct, directly measures the biologic activity of 1,25(OH)$_2$D in serum.

The half-life of circulating 1,25(OH)$_2$D has been estimated to be between 4 and 6 hours. The normal range of serum values is between 38 and 144 pmol/L (16 and 60 pg/mL). As vitamin D deficiency develops, the body responds by increasing the production and secretion of parathyroid hormone (see Fig. 20.9). Parathyroid hormone, in turn, enhances the 1-hydroxylation of 25(OH)D. Thus, secondary hyperparathyroidism associated with vitamin D deficiency accelerates the conversion of 25(OH)D to 1,25(OH)$_2$D. Because the circulating concentration of 25(OH)D is about three orders of magnitude higher than that of 1,25(OH)$_2$D, even low levels of 25(OH)D in the blood can provide enough substrate for the formation of 1,25(OH)$_2$D. Thus, a patient who is becoming vitamin D deficient will still have enough 25(OH)D substrate for the renal 25(OH)D-1-OHase. As a result, a patient who has low stores of vitamin D and is becoming vitamin D deficient can have low, normal, or even high circulating concentrations of 1,25(OH)$_2$D (35, 63, 76). When a patient who is vitamin D deficient enters a hospital and obtains vitamin D either from the short exposure to sunlight while on the way to the hospital or from dietary sources in the hospital, the vitamin D is rapidly metabolized to 25(OH)D and then to 1,25(OH)$_2$D.

When circulating concentrations of 25(OH)D dip to less than 50 nmol/L (20 ng/mL), the body is unable to satisfy its vitamin D requirement and, as a result, increases the production of parathyroid hormone. The finding that 1,25(OH)$_2$D levels are normal or increased as circulating concentrations of 25(OH)D drop to less than 50 nmol/L is consistent with the fact that the body's requirement at the target tissue level (i.e., intestine and bone) is not satisfied. The blood level of 1,25(OH)$_2$D does not provide any insight about the vitamin D status, and even though 1,25(OH)$_2$D can be normal or even elevated, the patient still is by definition vitamin D deficient because he or she has secondary hyperparathyroidism. As a result, circulating levels of 1,25(OH)$_2$D can be elevated to twice normal levels for several months (35, 50, 76). Thus, serum 1,25(OH)$_2$D concentrations are of little value in evaluating vitamin D deficiency. Needless to say, in an absolute vitamin D deficiency state, circulating concentrations of 1,25(OH)$_2$D are undetectable.

The measurement of circulating concentrations of 1,25(OH)$_2$D has been of great value to clinicians for evaluating patients with inherited and acquired disorders of 25(OH)D metabolism. Patients with chronic renal failure, hyperphosphatemia, hypoparathyroidism, pseudohypoparathyroidism, tumor-induced osteomalacia, hypercalcemia of malignancy (in most cases), or vitamin D–dependent rickets type I, which is an inborn error

reducing the conversion of 25(OH)D to 1,25(OH)$_2$D, often have low circulating concentrations of 1,25(OH)$_2$D (2–4, 35, 63, 70, 76, 122). Serum concentrations of 1,25(OH)$_2$D are greater than normal in some patients with the following: primary hyperparathyroidism; vitamin D–dependent rickets type II, which is an inborn error in which the recognition of 1,25(OH)$_2$D by target tissue receptors is defective; chronic granulomatous disorders such as sarcoidosis, tuberculosis, and silicosis; and lymphoma. Investigators now recognize that chronic granulomatous disorders and some lymphomas that activate macrophages and lymphoma cells, respectively, can 1α-hydroxylate 25(OH)D, a process that is inhibited by glucocorticoids (2–4, 63, 76, 108).

Vitamin D Deficiency Epidemic

By the turn of the twentieth century, more than of 90% of children in northeastern United States and in the industrialized cities in Europe suffered from the devastating consequences of rickets. The recognition that some sun exposure was essential for producing vitamin D$_3$ in the skin and the fortification of foods with vitamin D eradicated rickets as a significant health problem by the 1940s. Indeed, by the 1940s not only milk, but also a wide variety of foods and beverages including Bond bread, hot dogs, peanut butter, soda, and even Schlitz beer, were fortified with vitamin D (139). However, very few foods naturally contain or are now fortified with vitamin D (35, 76, 140). Until 2003, only milk, some cereals and some breads were fortified with vitamin D. However, in 2003 the US Food and Drug Administration gave approval for the fortification of juice products including orange juice with vitamin D (133). There is now 100 IU of vitamin D in 8 oz of orange juice and other fortified juice products, similar to what is found in milk.

Infants and young children, especially of those color as well as white children who always wear sun protection or avoid sunlight, are at risk for vitamin D deficiency (141, 142). Rickets is now being seen more frequently in urban hospitals, especially in young children of color who receive their nutrition solely from breast-feeding (143). There is little vitamin D in human milk and even less in the milk from women of color because they are often vitamin D deficient themselves. We recently observed that 76% of women of color at the time of the birth of their children were vitamin D deficient, and 81% of their infants also were vitamin D deficient (Lee J, Phillip B, Holick MF unpublished results). Young children who are always indoors playing with computers and watching television and who have minimum outdoor activities as well as young children and adolescents of color are at high risk of vitamin D deficiency (141, 142). At the end of winter, 48% of white girls aged 9 to 11 years who were living in Maine were found to be vitamin D deficient. Seventeen percent remained vitamin D deficient at the end of summer (141).

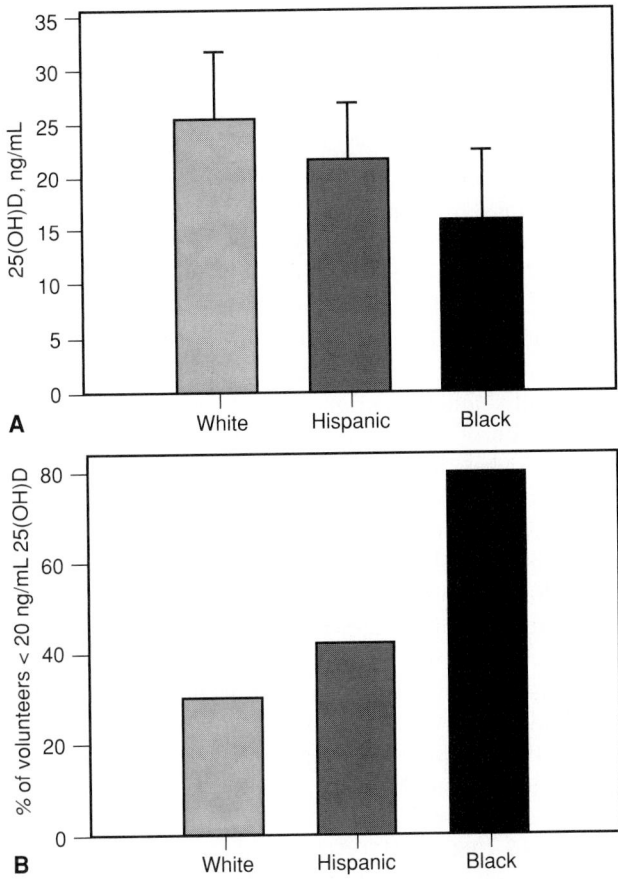

Figure 20.11 A. Serum 25(OH)D levels collected from free-living senior citizens in August in Boston. Mean + SEM. **B.** Percentage of free-living senior citizens who were vitamin D insufficient in August in Boston. (From Holick MF. Vitamin D- the underappreciated D-lightful hormone that is important for skeletal and cellular health. Opin Endocrinol Diabetes 2002;9:87–98, with permission.)

Even young adults are at risk of vitamin D deficiency. Forty-two percent of African-American women aged 15 to 49 years were found to be vitamin D deficient as part of the National Health and Nutrition Examination Survey III (144). Thirty-two percent of white young men and women aged 18 to 29 years were found to be vitamin D deficient at the end of winter in Boston (145).

On average, it is estimated that more than 50% of adults in the United States and Europe who are more than 50 years old are at risk of vitamin D deficiency. This is especially true for elderly persons, who are often infirm and seldom have an opportunity to be outdoors (146–150). In Boston at the end of summer in free-living elderly persons, vitamin D deficiency was found in 30% of whites, 42% Hispanics, and 84% of African-Americans (Fig. 20.11) (111).

RECOMMENDATIONS

Exposure to Sunlight

It is not often appreciated that casual exposure to sunlight during everyday activities provides most persons with their vitamin D requirement (35, 76, 140, 145). With the increased awareness from scientific and lay press about the causal relationship between long-term exposure to sunlight with skin cancer and skin wrinkling, sunscreen use is more prevalent (10). For children and young active adults, being outdoors for short periods of time (5–15 minutes) at least two or three times per week without sun protection will provide them with their vitamin D requirement. Elderly persons, in contrast, have a decreased capacity to produce vitamin D in their skin. In addition, they are likely to heed the warnings about the damaging effects of sunlight and use a sunscreen and wear more clothing, thus preventing the cutaneous synthesis of vitamin D_3. Because many elderly persons do not drink milk because of a lactase deficiency or because of their misconception that they no longer need to drink milk ("it is only for growing children"), their only source of vitamin D is either a multivitamin pill containing vitamin D or exposure to sunlight. If elderly persons do not take advantage of the beneficial effect of sunlight, they can develop vitamin D deficiency, which can result in secondary hyperparathyroidism.

This condition accelerates osteoporosis and can cause a mineralization defect in bones, resulting in adult rickets or osteomalacia. The net effect of this process on bone is likely to weaken bones and increase the risk of fracture (146–154). Results of several studies indicate that vitamin D deficiency does put elderly persons at risk of developing hip fractures. An epidemiologic survey in a controlled nursing home environment revealed that both free-living and institutionalized elderly persons who took a vitamin supplement or drank two to three glasses of milk per day were vitamin D sufficient. Of those persons who did not take a vitamin D supplement or drink milk, approximately 80% were overtly to borderline vitamin D deficient by the end of winter (150). Thus, especially for elderly people, exposure to sunlight in the morning or late afternoon in spring, summer, and fall (depending on skin sensitivity to sunlight) will provide the recommended vitamin D requirement and will permit them to store any excess vitamin D in fat for use during the winter months. Elderly persons need not be exposed to prolonged periods of sunlight, because the amount that they can produce in this period should satisfy their body's requirement.

Therefore, I recommend for the elderly population in Boston 5 to 15 minutes of exposure (depending on their sensitivity to sunlight) to a suberythemal amount of sunlight of arms and legs or face, hands, and arms three times a week. This recommendation is based on our observation that if you take a healthy person and expose the whole body to one minimal erythemal dose of simulated sunlight, the circulating vitamin D concentrations are comparable to the ingestion of 10,000 IU of vitamin D (111). After elderly persons are exposed to sunlight for a short period, they should apply a sunscreen, with a sun protection factor of at least 8, which will protect them from the chronic damaging effects of excessive exposure to sunlight (10).

VITAMIN D SUPPLEMENTS

Various pharmaceutical preparations are available by prescription. These include a capsule that contains 50,000 IU of vitamin D_2 and an oil preparation that contains 100,000 IU/mL. Pharmaceutical preparations containing 50,000 IU of vitamin D_2 have been of value in treating vitamin D deficiency in elderly patients and in patients with intestinal malabsorption syndromes, hepatic failure, and nephrotic syndrome. The dose is generally 50,000 IU once per week for 8 weeks. Circulating concentrations of 25(OH)D usually increase into the midnormal range approximately 100 nmol/L (40 ng/mL) (131). For persons unable to ingest a capsule containing vitamin D, an alternative source is an oil-based preparation. I usually recommend that patients take 1000 IU each day until circulating concentrations of 25(OH)D are in the midnormal range (Fig. 20.12). Once these concentrations have returned to normal, I recommend an over-the-counter multivitamin containing 400 IU of vitamin D and an additional vitamin D supplement of either 400 or 1000 IU vitamin D. This amount is usually sufficient to maintain adequate circulating concentrations of 25(OH)D.

Recommended Dietary Allowance of Vitamin D for Humans

Beginning in the 1930s, milk was fortified with 400 IU (10 μg) of vitamin D_2 per quart. This fortification process

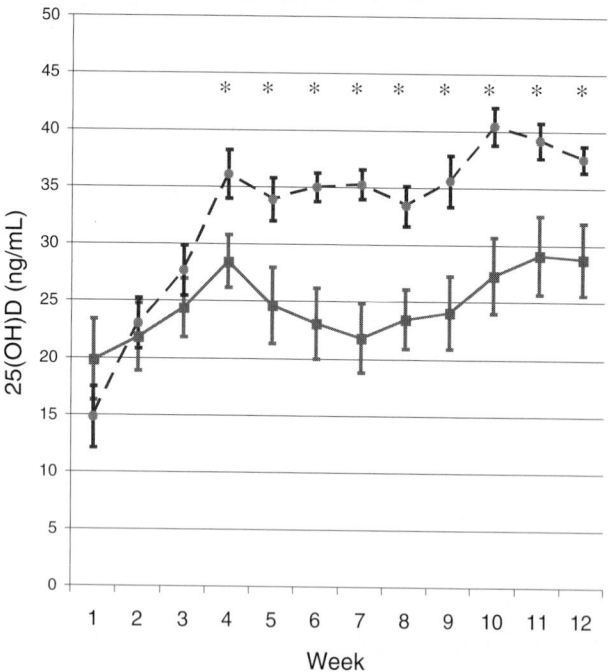

Figure 20.12. Weekly 25-hydroxyvitamin D (25(OH)D) levels in healthy adults ingesting vitamin D–fortified (1000 IU/8 oz/day) (*bars with circles*) and unfortified orange juice (*bars with squares*). Error bars represent standard error of the means (*p ≤ .01). (From Tangpricha V, Koutkia P, Rieke SM et al. Fortification of orange juice with vitamin D: a novel approach for enhancing vitamin D nutritional health. Am J Clin Nutr 2003;77:1478–83, with permission.)

eliminated rickets as a significant health problem in the United States and other countries that used this practice. In Britain during World War II, milk was supplemented with up to 2000 IU of vitamin D to compensate for wartime nutritional deprivation in children. Manufacturers often put 1.5 to two times as much vitamin D in the food preparations to compensate for anticipated vitamin D breakdown during shelf storage. As a result, an epidemic of hypercalcemia in neonates appeared in the 1940s and 1950s (155). This led to laws in Europe that prevented the fortification of milk and infant formulas with vitamin D.

In the United States, infant formula is fortified with 400 IU of vitamin D per quart. It has been estimated that a minimum of 100 IU of vitamin D daily is required to prevent rickets in infants. To provide a margin of safety, the recommended dietary allowance (RDA) was set at 300 IU for infants from birth to 3 months of age, which is approximately the amount consumed by formula-fed physiologically normal infants. Because human milk contains little vitamin D activity, it has been recommended that breast-fed infants receive exposure to sunlight or ingest formula supplemented with vitamin D. The RDA for children older than 3 months has been set at 400 IU to satisfy their requirement during rapid periods of bone growth and mineralization.

In the mid-1960s, studies in infants fed 300 IU, 350 to 550 IU, or 1380 to 2170 IU/day demonstrated no differences in growth in length or weight or in serum calcium concentrations. Earlier studies, however, suggested that daily ingestion of 2000 to 5000 IU of vitamin D in the diet caused hypercalcemia and all its clinical features (155). Vitamin D deficiency osteomalacia is associated with intakes of less than 100 IU/day of vitamin D. The RDA of 200 IU (5 μg) for adults is reasonable as long as sun exposure is adequate. Otherwise, 400 to 800 IU/day may be needed to prevent vitamin D deficiency (35).

Aging does not alter vitamin D absorption. Most studies evaluating the vitamin D requirement have been conducted in healthy persons who received some exposure to sunlight. Thus, the combination of exposure to sunlight with 200 IU of vitamin D is adequate for satisfying the body's requirement for this essential vitamin/prohormone. The amount of vitamin D that is required by adults who are not exposed to sunlight has been studied. Young adult submariners who received a vitamin D supplement that contained 600 IU of vitamin D_2 for their 3-month mission showed that circulating concentrations of 25(OH)D were maintained, whereas the submariners who did not receive the supplement had a significant decline in serum 25(OH)D levels (35). Tangpricha and colleagues found that adults who consumed 1000 IU/day of vitamin D_3 were able to maintain circulating concentrations of 25(OH)D in the range of 30 to 40 ng/mg (see Fig. 20.12) (133).

In the mid-1990s the Food and Nutrition Board of the Institute of Medicine was given the task of updating the reference values for dietary nutrient intakes for the healthy population in the United States and Canada (156). The committee recommended that the dietary reference intakes (DRIs) be reference values that can be used for planning and assessing diets for healthy populations and for many other purposes. The DRIs replaced the periodic revisions of the RDAs that have been published since 1941 by the National Academy of Sciences. The DRIs encompass the estimated average requirement (EAR), the RDA, the adequate intake (AI), and the tolerable upper intake level (UL). By definition, the RDA is the average daily dietary intake level that is sufficient to meet the nutrient requirements of nearly all (97–98%) individuals in a life stage and gender group. The RDA applies to individuals, not to groups. The EAR was defined as the nutrient intake value that is estimated to meet the requirement defined by a specific indicator of adequacy in 50% of individuals in a life stage and gender group. Thus, the RDA was set at 2 SDs above the EAR. It was suggested that if there were not adequate scientific data for specific life stage group to set an EAR, then no RDA could be set. As a result, the AI was developed based on the data available. The AI was set instead of the RDA if sufficient scientific evidence was not available to calculate the EAR. The AI was based on observed or experimentally determined estimates of average nutrient intake by group (or groups) of healthy people. The main intended use for the AI was for nutrient intake for an individual rather than group. The UL is the highest level of daily nutrient intake that is likely to pose no risk of adverse health effects to almost all individuals in the general population. Thus, because the EAR could not be determined for vitamin D, the Food and Nutrition Board reported AIs for vitamin D for age groups and gender. The no-observed-adverse-effect level was defined as the highest intake (or experimental dose) of a nutrient at which no adverse effects have been observed.

The UL was derived by dividing that level (or the lowest-observed-adverse-effect level) by all the relevant uncertainty factors. The size of the uncertainty factor varied depending on the confidence in the data and the nature of the adverse effect.

The committee noted that because most persons of all ages, all races, and both sexes obtain most of their vitamin D requirement from exposure to sunlight, it was difficult to determine an accurate value for the EAR, and therefore no RDA was proposed. The AI was determined based on a level of vitamin D intake that adequately sustained circulating concentrations of 25(OH)D for individuals in population groups who had limited, but uncertain sun exposure and stores increased by a safety factor of 100% for those unable to obtain sunlight. It was considered that when consumed by an individual person, the AI was sufficient to minimize the risk of low serum 25(OH)D, but the committee admitted that this value may actually represent an overestimate of the true biologic need. The committee concluded that the recommended AI assumes that no vitamin D is available from sun-mediated cutaneous synthesis. The AI and UL for different age groups and gender are outlined in Table 20.1. However, with recent new information, it is now clear that the data before 1997 that were reviewed by the committee did not provide a full appreciation for the dietary requirement of vitamin D to sustain healthy circulating concentrations of 25(OH)D. It is now recognized that 1000 IU/day of vitamin D is required in the absence of sun exposure to maintain circulating concentrations of 25(OH)D in a vitamin D sufficient range, that is, a 25(OH)D level of greater than 50 nmol/L.

The Institute of Medicine recommends the AI (see Table 20.1 and also Appendix Table A-2-c) for vitamin D to be 200 IU, 400 IU, and 600 IU for 1 to 50 years, 51 to 70 years, and 71 years and older, respectively (156); most

TABLE 20.1. CRITERIA AND DIETARY REFERENCE INTAKE VALUES AND TOLERABLE UPPER INTAKE LEVELS FOR VITAMIN D BY LIFE STAGE GROUP

		VITAMIN D	
LIFE STAGE GROUP	CRITERION	AI (μg/DAY)*	UL (μg/DAY)
0–6 mo	Serium 25(OH)D	5	25
7–12 y	Serium 25(OH)D	5	25
1–3 y	Serium 25(OH)D	5	50
4–8 y	Serium 25(OH)D	5	50
9–13 y	Serium 25(OH)D	5	50
14–18 y	Serium 25(OH)D	5	50
19–30 y	Serium 25(OH)D	5	50
31–50 y	Serium 25(OH)D	5	50
51–70 y	Serium 25(OH)D	10	50
>70 y	Serium 25(OH)D	15	50
Pregnancy			
≤18 y	Serium 25(OH)D	5	50
19–50 y	Serium 25(OH)D	5	50
Lactation			
≤18 y	Serium 25(OH)D	5	50
19–50 y	Serium 25(OH)D	5	50

*1 μg vitamin D is equivalent to 40 IU.

experts recommend 1000 IU/day (see Fig. 20.12) (35, 157). The UL, as outlined in Table 20.1, is also outdated. The UL of 2000 IU of vitamin D for children less than 1 year of age and the UL of 4000 IU for everyone older than 1 year of age is probably more reasonable (i.e., double that in Table 20.1).

Vitamin D Intoxication

Although vitamin D intoxication is of great concern for physicians, in fact it is extremely difficult to become intoxicated with vitamin D. Although the safe upper limit (UL) for vitamin D intake for children and adults was recommended to be 2000 IU/day by the Food and Nutrition Board, mounting evidence indicates that levels greater than 10,000 IU/day of vitamin D are more likely to cause vitamin D intoxication. By definition, vitamin D intoxication means a markedly elevated level of 25(OH)D in conjunction with hypercalcemia and high normal or elevated serum phosphorus levels. The consequence of vitamin D intoxication is similar to the consequences of hypercalcemia. Patients with hypercalcemia often complain of constipation, confusion, lethargy, polyuria, and polydypsia. In addition, vitamin D intoxication and hypercalcemia are associated with an increased risk of nephrocalcinosis, kidney stones, and soft tissue calcifications. Although the upper limit of normal for most commercial 25(OH)D assays is between 55 and 60 ng/mL, it is recognized that sun worshippers and lifeguards can often achieve a blood level of up to 125 ng/mL with no untoward consequences. Thus, typically patients who are vitamin D intoxicated have blood levels of 25(OH)D levels of greater than 150 ng/mL. To achieve these levels, a person needs to ingest more than 10,000 IU/day of vitamin D for prolonged periods. Recent examples that cause vitamin D intoxication include inad-

vertent ingestion of hundreds of thousands to a million units of vitamin D a day (134). These individuals achieved blood levels of 25(OH)D greater than 400 to 500 ng/mL.

The best treatment for vitamin D intoxication is to tell the patient to avoid any direct sun exposure without sun protection and to eliminate all vitamin D from diet and supplements. Correction of the hypercalcemia with hydration and diuresis often is adequate. Although glucocorticoids are often suggested as a means of managing vitamin D intoxication, frequently this is not necessary. More important, high-dose steroid therapy can have more serious consequences. Koutia and associates (134) followed a patient who was severely vitamin D intoxicated with a 25(OH)D level that was higher than 450 ng/mL for 3 years. This patient was conservatively treated and did not receive glucocorticoids. The 25(OH)D level gradually came down and after 3 years was still higher than 100 ng/mL. The patient, however, remained normocalcemic with no untoward consequences.

SUMMARY

Investigators have recognized that living at higher latitudes and thus being prone to vitamin D deficiency increases the risk of dying of many common cancers, of developing several autoimmune disorders including type 1 diabetes and multiple sclerosis, and of developing hypertension and cardiovascular heart disease (35, 157). Evidence also indicates that simply taking a multivitamin containing 400 IU/day of vitamin D can reduce the risk of developing multiple sclerosis and rheumatoid arthritis by 40 to 50%. The observations that children receiving 2000 IU/day of vitamin D from 1 year of age on reducing risk of type 1 diabetes by more than 80% and that children who

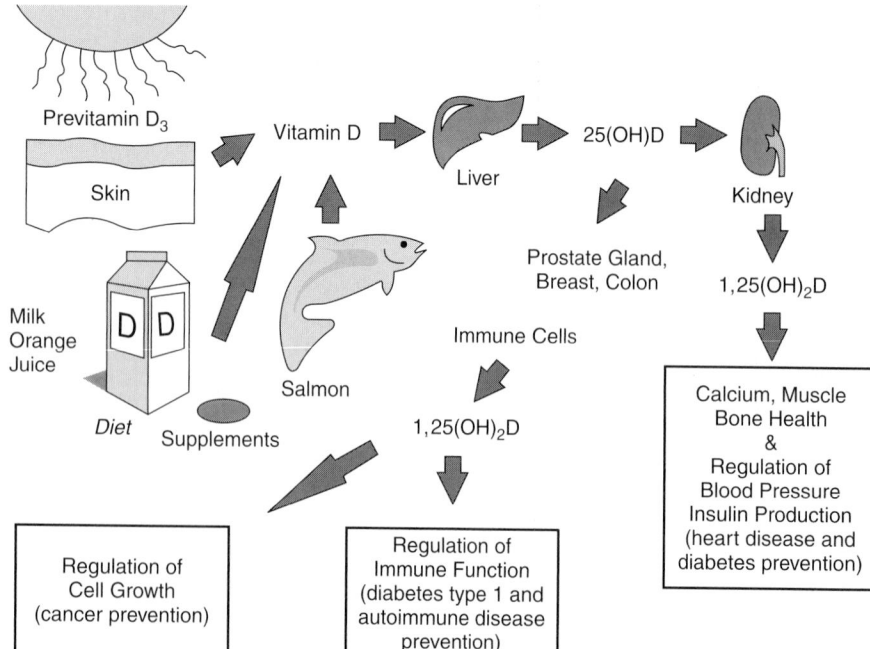

Figure 20.13. Schematic representation of the multitude of other potential physiologic actions of vitamin D for cardiovascular health, cancer prevention, regulation of immune function, and decreased risk of autoimmune diseases. (Copyright Michael F. Holick, 2003, with permission.)

were vitamin D deficient at 1 year of age onward and whose course was followed had a fourfold increased risk of developing type 1 diabetes make it clear that maintaining vitamin D sufficiency, especially during the formative childhood and adolescent years, is critically important not only for bone health, but also for the prevention of many serious chronic diseases, including cancer, cardiovascular heart disease, and autoimmune diseases. Indeed, it has been suggested that vitamin D deficiency during infancy and childhood may imprint an increased risk of these chronic diseases for the rest of one's life.

Compelling clinical research supports the recommendation that a 25(OH)D level of less than 20 ng/mL should be considered to be vitamin D deficient (131, 132). However, to maximize the effect of vitamin D on intestinal calcium absorption truly, Heaney and colleagues (158) reported that a 25(OH)D level higher than 30 ng/mL maximized intestinal calcium absorption.

Sensible exposure to sunlight during the spring, summer, and fall can satisfy most of our vitamin D requirement. In the absence of sun exposure, 1000 IU/day of vitamin D is effective in maintaining 25(OH)D levels in what is considered to be the healthy range of 30 to 40 ng/mL (133). Vigilance in maintaining a normal vitamin D status not only is important for bone health throughout our lives, but may also be important for the prevention of many chronic diseases (Fig. 20.13).

Acknowledgments

This work was supported in part by the following National Institutes of Health grants: AR36963 and M01RR0053327.

REFERENCES

1. Holick MF. Phylogenetic and evolutionary aspects of vitamin D from phytoplankton to humans. In: Pang PKT, Schreibman MP, eds. Vertebrate Endocrinology: Fundamentals and Biomedical Implications, vol 3. Orlando, FL: Academic Press, 1989:7–43.
2. DeLuca H. FASEB J 1988;2:224–36.
3. Reichel H, Koeffler HP, Norman AW. N Engl J Med 1989;320:981–91.
4. Holick MF. Vitamin D: photobiology, metabolism, and clinical applications. In: DeGroot LJ, ed. Endocrinology. Philadelphia: WB Saunders, 1995:990–1013.
5. Fraser D, Scriver CR. Hereditary disorders associated with vitamin–D resistance or defective phosphate metabolism. In: DeGroot LJ, ed. Endocrinology, vol 2. New York: Grune and Stratton, 1979.
6. Schmorl G. Med U Kinderh 1909;4:403.
7. Sniadecki J. 1840. Cited by Mozolowski W. Nature 1939;143:121.
8. Owen I. BMJ 1889;1:113–6.
9. Holick MF. Vitamin D₃: synthesis and biologic functions in skin. In: Mukhtar H, ed. Pharmacology of the Skin. Boca Raton, FL: CRC Press, 1991:183–202.
10. Palm TA. Practitioner 1890;45:270–9, 321–42.
11. Huldschinsky K. Dtsch Med Wochenschr 1919;45:712–3.
12. Hess AF, Unger LF. JAMA 1921;77:39.
13. Mayer J. Nutr Rev 1957;15:321–3.
14. Mellanby T. J Physiol (Lond) 1918;52:11–4.
15. McCollum EF, Simmonds N, Becker JE et al. J Biol Chem 1922;53:293–312.
16. Powers GF, Park EA, Shipley PG et al. Proc Soc Exp Biol Med 1921;19:120–1.
17. Hess AF, Weinstock M. J Biol Chem 1924;62:301–13.
18. Steenbock H, Black A. J Biol Chem 1924;61:408–22.
19. Holick MF, MacLaughlin JA, Parrish JA et al. The photochemistry and photobiology of vitamin D₃. In: Regan JD, Parrish JA, eds. The Science of Photomedicine. New York: Plenum Press, 1982.
20. Fieser LD, Fieser M. Vitamin D. In: Steroids. New York: Reinhold, 1959:90–168.
21. Holick MF. Vitamin D and the skin: photobiology, physiology and therapeutic efficacy for psoriasis. In: Heersche J, Kanis J, eds. Bone and Mineral Research. 7ᵗʰ ed. Amsterdam: Elsevier Science, 1990.
22. Massengale ON, Nussmeier M. J Biol Chem 1930;87:423–5.
23. Steenbock H, Kletzien SWF. J Biol Chem 1932;97:249–64.
24. Waddell J. J Biol Chem 1934;105:711–39.
25. Windaus A, Bock F. Hoppe-Seylers Z Physiol Chem 1937;245:168.
26. Velluz L, Petit A, Amiard G. Bull Soc Chim Fr 1948;15:1115–20.
27. Velluz L, Amiard G, Petit A. Bull Soc Chim Fr 1949;16:501–8.
28. MacLaughlin JA, Holick MF. Mediation of cutaneous vitamin D₃ synthesis by UV radiation. In: Goldsmith LA, ed. Biochemistry and Physiology of the Skin. Oxford: Oxford University Press, 1983.
29. Holick MF, MacLaughlin JA, Doppelt SH. Science 1981;211:590–3.
30. Anderson RR, Parrish JA. Optical properties of human skin. In: Regan JD, Parrish JA, eds. The Science of Photomedicine. New York: Plenum Press, 1982.
31. Holick M, MacLaughlin J, Clark M et al. Science 1980;210:203–5.
32. Holick MF, Tian XQ, Allen M. Proc Natl Acad Sci USA 1995;92:3124–6.
33. Loomis F. Science 1967;157:501–6.
34. Clemens TL, Henderson SL, Adams JS et al. Lancet 1982;1:74–6.
35. Holick MF. J Cell Biochem 2003;88:296–307.
36. Webb AR, DeCosta BR, Holick MF. J Clin Endocrinol Metab 1989;68:882–7.
37. MacLaughlin JA, Holick MF. J Clin Invest 1985;76:1536–8.
38. Holick MF, Matsuoka LY, Wortsman J. Lancet 1989;2:1104–5.
39. Montagna W, Carlisle MS. J Invest Dermatol 1979;73:47–53.
40. Matsuoka LY, Ide L, Wortsman J et al. J Clin Endocrinol Metab 1987;64:1165–8.
41. Matsuoka LY, Wortsman J, Hanifan N et al. Arch Dermatol 1988;124:1802–4.
42. Webb AR, Kline L, Holick MF. J Clin Endocrinol Metab 1988;67:373–8.
43. Lu Z, Chen T, Holick MF. Influences of season and time of day on the synthesis of vitamin D₃. In: Holick MF, Kligman A, eds. Proceedings: Biologic Effects of Light Symposium. Berlin: Walter De Gruyter, 1992:53–6.
44. Tanner JT, Smith J, Defibaugh P et al. J Assoc Off Analyt Chem 1988;71:607–10.
45. Holick MF, Shao Q, Liu WW et al. N Engl J Med 1992;326:1178–81.
46. Chen TC, Heath H III, Holick MF. N Engl J Med 1993;329:1507.
47. Lo CW, Paris PW, Clemens TL et al. Am. J Clin Nutr 1985;42:644–9.

48. Holick MF. Kidney Int 1987;32:912–29.
49. Bell NH. J Clin Invest 1985;76:1–6.
50. Adams JA, Clemens TL, Parrish JA et al. N Engl J Med 1981; 306:722–5.
51. Holick MF, Clark MB. Fed Proc 1978;37:2567–74.
52. Long RG, Skinner RK, Meinhard E et al. Gut 1976;17: 824–7.
53. Kaplan MM, Goldberg MJ, Matloff DS et al. Gastroenterology 1981;81:681–5.
54. Gray TK, Lester GE, Lorenc RS. Science 1979;204:1311–3.
55. Weisman Y, Vargas A, Duckett G et al. Endocrinology 1978; 103:1992–6.
56. Tanaka Y, Halloran B, Schnoes HK et al. Proc Natl Acad Sci USA 1979;76:5033–5.
57. Mason RS. Extra-renal production of 1,25(OH)$_2$D$_3$, the metabolism of vitamin D by non-traditional tissues. In: Norman AW, ed. Vitamin D: A Chemical, Biochemical and Clinical Update. Berlin: Walter de Gruyter, 1985.
58. Howard GA, Turner RT, Sherrard DJ et al. J Biol Chem 1981; 256:7738–40.
59. Bikle DD, Nemanic MD, Whitney JO et al. Biochemistry 1986; 25:1545–8.
60. Napoli J, Horst R. Vitamin D metabolism. In: Kumar R, ed. Vitamin D: Basic and Clinical Aspects. Boston: Martinus Nijhoff, 1984.
61. Gray TK, Millington DS, Maltby DA et al. Proc Natl Acad Sci USA 1985;82:8218–21.
62. Bouillon R, Okamura WH, Norman AW. Endocr Rev 1995;16: 200–57.
63. Holick MF, Potts JR Jr, Krane SM. Calcium, phosphorus and bone metabolism. In: Isselbacher KJ, Braunwald E, Wilson JD et al, eds. Harrison's Principles of Internal Medicine, 13th ed. New York: McGraw-Hill, 1990:2137–51.
64. Portale AA, Halloran BP, Murphy MM et al. J Clin Invest 1986; 77:7–12.
65. Fraser D. Physiol Rev 1980;60:551–663.
66. Adams ND, Garthwite TL, Gray RW et al. J Clin Endocrinol Metab 1979;49:628–30.
67. Kumar R, Abboud CF, Riggs BL. Mayo Clin Proc 1980;55:51–3.
68. Kumar R, Merimee TJ, Silva P et al. The effect of chronic growth hormone excess or deficiency on plasma 1,25-dihydroxy vitamin D levels in man. In: Norman AW, Schaeffer K, Herrath DV et al, eds. Vitamin D, Basic Research and Its Clinical Application. Berlin: Walter de Gruyter, 1979.
69. Turner RT. 1,25-Dihydroxyvitamin D-1-hydroxylase, measurements and regulation. In: Kumar R, ed. Vitamin D: Basic and Clinical Aspects. Boston: Martinus Nijhoff, 1984.
70. Krabbe S, Hummer L, Christiansen C. J Clin Endocrinol Metab 1986;62:503–7.
71. Rigotti NA, Nussbaum SR, Herzog DB et al. N Engl J Med 1984;311:1601–6.
72. Sowers MF, Wallace RB, Hollis BW. Bone Miner 1990;10: 139–48.
73. Hartwell D, Riis BJ, Christiansen C J Clin Endocrinol Metab 1990;71:127–32.
74. Riggs BL, Gallagher JC, DeLuca HF et al. Mayo Clin Proc 1978;53:701–6.
75. Slovik DM, Adams JS, Neer RM et al. N Engl J Med 1981;305: 372–4.
76. Holick MF. Vitamin D: photobiology, metabolism, mechanism of action, and clinical application. In: Favus MJ, ed. Primer on the Metabolic Bone Diseases and Disorders of Mineral Metabolism. 5th ed. Washington, DC: American Society for Bone and Mineral Research, 2003:129–37.
77. Ebeling PR, Sandgren ME, DiMagno EP et al. J Clin Endocrinol Metab 1992;75:176–82.
78. Pike JW. Nutr Rev 1985;43:161–8.
79. Darwish H, DeLuca HF. Crit Rev Eukaryot Gene Expr 1993;3: 89–116.
80. Bouillon R. Vitamin D: from photosynthesis, metabolism, and action to clinical applications. In: DeGroot LJ, Jameson JL, eds. Endocrinolgy. Philadelphia: WB Saunders, 2001:1009–28.
81. Khosla S. Endocrinology 2001;142:5050–5.
82. Merke J, Klaus G, Hugel U et al. J Clin Invest 1986;77:312–4.
83. Haussler MR, Donaldson CA, Kelly MA et al. Functions and mechanism of action of the 1,25-dihydroxyvitamin D$_3$ receptor. In: Norman AW, ed. Vitamin D: A Chemical, Biochemical and Clinical Update. Berlin: Walter de Gruyter, 1985.
84. Demay MB, Roth DA, Kronenberg HM. J Biol Chem 1989; 264:2279–82.
85. Underwood B, DeLuca HF. Am J Physiol 1984;246:E493–8.
86. Holtrop ME, Cox KA, Carnes DL. Am J Physiol 1986;251:E20.
87. Holick MF. J Nutr 1996;126:11595–645.
88. Stumpf WE, Sar M, Reid FA et al. Science 1979;206:1188–90.
89. Bhalla AK, Clemens T, Amento E et al. J Clin Endocrinol Metab 1983;57:1308–10.
90. Provvedine DM, Tsoukaas CD, Deftos LJ et al. Science 1983; 221:1181.
91. Abe E, Miyaura C, Sakagami H et al. Proc Natl Acad Sci USA 1981;78:4990–4.
92. Tanaka H, Abe E, Miyaura C et al. Biochem J 1982;204:713–9.
93. Eisman JA. 1,25-Dihydroxyvitamin D$_3$ receptor and role of 1,25-dihydroxyvitamin D$_3$ in human cancer cells in vitamin D. In: Kumar R, ed. Vitamin D: Basic and Clinical Aspects. Boston: Martinus Nijhoff, 1984.
94. Bar-Shavit Z, Kahn AJ, Stone KR et al. Endocrinology 1986;118:679–86.
95. Mathieu C, Waer M, Laureys J et al. Endocrinology 1994;136: 866–72.
96. Cantorna MT, Hayes CE, DeLuca HF. Proc Natl Acad Sci USA 1996;93:7861–4.
97. Fournier C, Gepner P, Sadouk MB et al. J Immunol Immunopathol 1990;54:53–63.
98. Holick MF. Photobiology and noncalcemic actions of vitamin D. In: Bilezikian JP, Raisz LG, Rodan GA, eds. Principles of Bone Biology. San Diego: Academic Press, 2002:587–601.
99. Binderup L. Biochem Pharmacol 1992;43:1885–92.
100. Hosomi J, Hosoi J, Abe E et al. Endocrinology 1983;113: 1950–7.
101. Smith EL, Walworth ND, Holick MF. J Invest Dermatol 1986; 86:709–14.
102. Smith EL, Pincus SH, Donovan L et al. J Am Acad Dermatol 1988;19:516–28.
103. Holick MF. Arch Dermatol 1989;125:1692–7.
104. Morimoto S, Kumahara Y. Med J Osaka Univ 1985;35:51.
105. Kragballe K. Arch Dermatol 1989;125:1642–52.
106. Kato T, Rokugo M, Terui T et al. Br J Dermatol 1986;115: 431–3.
107. Perez A, Chen C, Turner A et al. Br J Dermatol 1996;134: 238–46.
108. Rostand SG. Hypertension 1979;30:150–6.
109. Krause R, Buhring M, Hopfenmuller W et al. Lancet 1998;352: 709–10.
110. Li YC, Kong J, Wei M et al. J Clin Invest 2002;110: 229–38.
111. Holick MF. Opin Endocrinol Diabetes 2002;9:87–98.
112. Garland CF, Garland FC, Shaw EK et al. Lancet 1989;2:1176–8.
113. Garland CF, Garland FC, Gorham ED et al. Sunlight, vitamin D, and mortality from breast and colorectal cancer in Italy. In:

Biologic Effects of Light. New York: Walter de Gruyter, 1992: 39–43.

114. Hanchette CL, Schwartz GG. Cancer 1992;70:2861–9.

115. Grant WB. Cancer 2003;164:371–7.

116. Grant WB. Cancer 2002;94:1867–75.

117. Schwartz GG, Whitlatch LW, Chen TC et al. Cancer Epidemiol Biomarkers Prev 1998;7:391–5.

118. Whitlatch LW, Young MV, Schwartz GG. et al. J Steroid Biochem Mol Biol 2002;81:135–40.

119. Mawer EB, Hayes ME, Heys SE et al. J Clin Endocrinol Metab 1994;79:554–60.

120. Tangpricha V, Flanagan JN, Whitlatch LW et al. Lancet 2001; 357:1673–4.

121. Cross HS, Bareis P, Hofer H et al. Steroids 2001;66:287–92.

122. Holick MF. J Nutr 1990;120:1464–9.

123. Steenbock H, Black A. J Biol Chem 1924;61:408–22.

124. Clemens TL, Adams JS, Holick MF. Clin Chim Acta 1982;121: 301–8.

125. Chen T, Turner A, Holick MF. J Nutr Biochem 1990;1:272–6.

126. Haddad JG, Chu, KJ. J Clin Endocrinol Metab 1971;33:992–5.

127. Belsey R, Clark MB, Bernat M et al. Am J Med 1974;57:50–6.

128. Hollis BW, Burton JH, Draper HH. Steroids 1977;30:285–93.

129. Chen TC, Turner AK, Holick MF. J Nutr Biochem 1990;1: 315–9.

130. Jones G. Clin Chem 1978;24:287–98.

131. Malabanan A, Veronikis IE, Holick MF. Lancet 1998;351: 805–6.

132. Chapuy MC, Prezoisi P, Maamer M. Osteoporos Int 1997;7: 439–43.

133. Tangpricha V, Koutkia P, Rieke SM et al. Am J Clin Nutr 2003; 77:1478–83.

134. Koutkia P, Chen TC, Holick MF. N Engl J Med 2001;345: 66–7.

135. Hollis BW. Clin Chem 1986;32:2060–3.

136. Horst R. Recent advances in the quantitation of vitamin D and vitamin D metabolites. In: Kumar R, ed. Vitamin D: Basic and Clinical Aspects. Boston: Martinus Nijhoff, 1984.

137. Chen TC, Turner AK, Holick MF. J Nutr Biochem 1990;1: 320–7.

138. Stern PH, Hamstra AJ, DeLuca HF et al. J Clin Endocrinol Metab 1978;46:891–6.

139. Holick MF. Vitamin D: Importance for bone health, cellular health and cancer prevention. In: Holick MF, ed. Proceedings: Biologic Effects of Light Symposium 2001. Boston: Kluwer Academic Publishing, 2002:155–73.

140. Holick MF. Osteoporos Int 1998;8:24S–9S.

141. Sullivan SS, Rosen CJ, Chen TC et al. J Bone Miner Res 2003; S407(abst).

142. Gordon CM, DePeter KC, Grace E et al. Proceedings: Endocrine Society. Chevy Chase, MD: Endocrine Society Press, 2003:87(abst OR21-2).

143. Kreiter SR, Schwartz RP, Kirkman HN et al. J Pediatr 2000; 137:153–7.

144. Nesby-O'Dell S, Scanlon KS, Cogswell ME, et al. Am J Clin Nutr 2002;76:187–92.

145. Tangpricha V, Pearce EN, Chen TC et al. Am J Med 2002;112:659–62.

146. Harris SS, Soteriades E, Stina S et al. J Clin Endocrinol Metab 2001;85:4125–30.

147. Gloth FM, Tobin JD, Sherman SS et al. J Am Geriatr Soc 1991; 39:137–41.

148. Lips P, Duong T, Oleksik A et al. J Clin Endocrinol Metab 2001;86:1212–21.

149. Chel VGM, Ooms ME, Popp-Snijders C et al. J Bone Miner Res 1998;13:1238–42.

150. Webb AR, Pilbeam C, Hanafin N et al. J Clin Nutr 1990;51: 1075–81.

151. Chalmers J, Conacher DH, Gardner DL et al. J Bone Joint Surg 1967;49:403–23.

152. Doppelt SH, Neer RM, Daly M et al. Orthop Trans 1983;7: 512–3.

153. Sokoloff L. Am J Surg Pathol 1978;2:21–30.

154. Kavookjian H, Whitelaw G, Lin S et al. Orthop Trans 1990;14: 580.

155. Chesney RW. J Clin Nutr 1990;119:1825cc8.

156. Food and Nutrition Board, Institute of Medicine. Dietary Reference Intakes for Calcium, Phosphorus, Magnesium, Vitamin D, and Fluoride. Washington, DC: National Academy Press, 1997:S1–S13.

157. Holick MF. Am J Clin Nutr 2004;79:362–71.

158. Heaney RP, Dowell MS, Hale CA et al. J Am Coll Nutr 2003; 22:142–6.

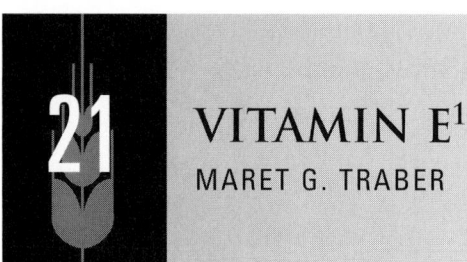

21 VITAMIN E¹

MARET G. TRABER

HISTORICAL HIGHLIGHTS 397
STRUCTURES, NOMENCLATURE, AND CHEMISTRY 397
    Units 398
    Antioxidant Activity 398
    Vitamin E Interactions: The Antioxidant
       Network 399
    Structure-Function Relationships of
       Vitamin E Forms 399
DIGESTION AND INTESTINAL ABSORPTION 399
    Vitamin E Absorption Requires Bile and
       Pancreatic Secretions 399
    Vitamin E Absorption Requires Chylomicron
       Synthesis and Secretion 400
PLASMA TRANSPORT 400
    Distribution of Vitamin E to Tissues during
       Triglyceride-Rich Lipoprotein Lipolysis 400
    Requirement for Very-Low-Density Lipoprotein
       Synthesis in The Preferential Secretion of
       α-Tocopherol from the Liver 400
    Plasma Vitamin E Kinetics 401
HEPATIC α-TOCOPHEROL TRANSFER PROTEIN 401
    Other Tocopherol Binding Proteins 401
DISTRIBUTION TO TISSUES 402
    Vitamin E Delivery to Tissues 402

Tissues with Slow Versus Fast Turning over
    Vitamin E Pools 402
    Storage Sites 403
METABOLISM AND EXCRETION 403
    Hepatic Metabolism .403
    Routes of Excretion .403
    Oxidation Products 403
CAUSES OF DEFICIENCY 404
    Genetic Defects in the α-Tocopherol
       Transfer Protein 404
    Genetic Defects in Lipoprotein Synthesis 405
    Fat Malabsorption Syndromes 405
    Total Parenteral Nutrition 405
PATHOLOGY OF HUMAN α-TOCOPHEROL
    DEFICIENCY 406
DIETARY CONSIDERATIONS, REQUIREMENTS,
    AND RECOMMENDED INTAKES 406
DIETARY REFERENCE INTAKES 406
    Adequacy of α-Tocopherol Intakes in Normal
       Populations in the United States 407
    Assessment of α-Tocopherol Status in
       Patients at Risk for Deficiency 407
    Controversial Topics .408
CONCLUSIONS 409

Vitamin E is unique in human nutrition because for decades it was "a vitamin looking for a disease" (1). Most water-soluble vitamins are enzyme cofactors; fat-soluble

---

¹**Abbreviations: ABC**, adenosine triphosphate binding cassette; **α-CEHC**, 2,5,7,8-tetramethyl-2-(2'-carboxyethyl)-6-hydroxychroman; **apo**, apolipoprotein; **α-TTP**, α-tocopherol transfer protein; **AVED**, ataxia and vitamin E deficiency; **DRI**, dietary reference intake; **EAR**, estimated average requirement; **γ-CEHC**, 2,7,8-trimethyl-2-(2'carboxyethyl)-6-hydroxychroman; **CYP**, cytochrome P450; **FNB**, Food and Nutrition Board; **HDL**, high-density lipoprotein; **IU**, international unit; **LDL**, low-density lipoprotein; **LPL**, lipoprotein lipase; **LRP**, low-density lipoprotein receptor–related protein; **MDR2**, P-glycoprotein; **NGT**, 2,7,8-trimethyl-2-(4,8,12-trimethyldecyl)-5-nitro-6-chromanol; **PKC**, protein kinase C; **PLTP**, phospholipid transfer protein; **PUFA**, polyunsaturated fatty acid; **RDA**, recommended dietary allowance; **ROO•**, peroxyl radical; **SPF**, supernatant protein factor; **SR**, scavenger receptor; **TAP**, tocopherol-associated protein; **TPGS**, d-α-tocopheryl polyethylene glycol-1000 succinate; **TPN**, total parenteral nutrition; **UL**, tolerable upper intake level; **VLDL**, very-low-density lipoprotein.

vitamins, such as vitamins A, D, and K, have specific roles in vision, bone formation, and blood clotting, respectively. Thus, it was anticipated that vitamin E would have a specific role in some metabolic function. However, in more than 80 years of investigation, this has not proven to be the case. The literature is replete with studies describing a variety of vitamin E deficiency symptoms in various species leading to confusion about the vitamin's function in humans. This range of symptoms is not surprising, however, given that the major function of vitamin E is that of an antioxidant. Consequently, vitamin E deficiency symptoms in target tissues depend not only on α-tocopherol content, uptake, and turnover, but also on the degree of oxidative stress and polyunsaturated fatty acid (PUFA) content. Furthermore, vitamin E activity dependes on an "antioxidant network" involving a wide variety of antioxidants and antioxidant enzymes that functions to maintain α-tocopherol in its unoxidized state, ready to intercept and scavenge radicals (2). In addition, vitamin E is fat-soluble and is transported in plasma lipoproteins and partitions into membranes and fat-storage sites, where it has the unique role of protecting PUFA from oxidation.

The biologic function of α-tocopherol cannot be fulfilled by just any antioxidant. Plasma α-tocopherol is regulated by the liver α-tocopherol transfer protein (α-TTP) (3–6), and in humans, a genetic defect in α-TTP results in severe vitamin E deficiency (7). α-TTP is necessary for facilitated hepatic α-tocopherol transfer to plasma.

This chapter describes the structure-function relationships of vitamin E, its antioxidant properties, its lipoprotein transport and delivery to tissues, and, finally, the role of vitamin E in human health and disease.

HISTORICAL HIGHLIGHTS

The first two decades of vitamin E history were reviewed by Mason (8), a pioneer in studies of vitamin E. Vitamin E deficiency was first described in 1922 by Evans and Bishop (9) at the University of California in Berkeley during their investigations of infertility in rancid lard–fed rats. In 1936, Evans and associates (10) isolated a factor from wheat germ with the biologic activity of vitamin E. They named this factor α-tocopherol, a name derived from the Greek *tokos* ("offspring") and *pherein* ("to bear") with an "ol" to indicate that it was an alcohol. Two other tocopherols, β and γ, were isolated from vegetable oils in the subsequent year, and it was noted that these had lower biologic activities than α-tocopherol (11). This was the first description that different naturally occurring forms of vitamin E exist and that α-tocopherol is the most effective form in preventing the symptoms of vitamin E deficiency.

These early observations formed the basis for determining the biologic activity of vitamin E. As defined by Machlin (12), the biologic activity of vitamin E is based on its ability to prevent or reverse specific symptoms of vitamin E deficiency (e.g., fetal resorption, muscular dystrophy, and encephalomalacia). The most often used, although most tedious and time-consuming, assay for the biologic activity of vitamin E is the fetal resorption assay (12). In this study, vitamin E–depleted virgin female rats are mated with normal male rats. After successful mating of these animals, various levels of single vitamin E forms are fed in several divided doses to the females, which are killed 20 to-21 days after mating. The numbers of living, dead, and resorbed fetuses are counted, and the percentage of live young is determined. Thus, the vitamin E biologic activity depends on the amount necessary to maintain the maximum number of live fetuses. Studies have demonstrated that α-TTP is present in pregnant mouse uterus and human placenta (13, 14), findings suggesting that α-tocopherol is especially important during pregnancy.

Vitamin E deficiency symptoms in various animal species were described by Machlin (12) in his comprehensive chapter on vitamin E. Necrotizing myopathy has been observed in vitamin E–deficient monkeys, pigs, rats, dogs, rabbits, goats, guinea pigs, horses, cows and calves, sheep and lambs, mink, chicken, ducks, turkeys, salmon, catfish, antelope, and elephants. Fetal death and resorption are reported symptoms of vitamin E deficiency in rats, mice, guinea pigs, cows, pigs, sheep, and chickens. Anemia has been observed in rats, pigs, monkeys, salmon, catfish, and chickens. Lipofuscin (a fluorescent pigment of "aging") frequently accumulates in tissues of vitamin E–deficient animals. Based on the symptoms observed in animals, investigators attempted to treat human patients with muscular dystrophy or with anemia by supplementation with vitamin E. Except for a few cases associated with oxidative stress, such as anemia of prematurity (15), infants fed formulas high in PUFA and iron (16), or children with anemia associated with protein-calorie malnutrition (17), these vitamin E trials were largely unsuccessful. These negative findings gave credence to the viewpoint, which we now know is incorrect, that vitamin E deficiency does not occur in humans.

Horwitt and colleagues (18, 19) attempted to induce vitamin E deficiency in men by feeding a diet low in vitamin E for 6 years to volunteers at the Elgin State Hospital in Illinois. After about 2 years, these patients' serum vitamin E levels decreased into the deficient range. Although their erythrocytes were more sensitive to peroxide-induced hemolysis, overt anemia did not develop. The data from the study by Horwitt and associates was used in 2000 to set the recommended dietary allowance (RDA) for vitamin E (20). These latest RDAs (also see Appendix tables) are discussed further later in this chapter.

It was not until the mid-1960s that vitamin E deficiency was described in children with fat malabsorption syndromes, principally abetalipoproteinemia and cholestatic liver disease, as reviewed by Sokol (21). By the mid-1980s, it was clear that the major human symptom of vitamin E deficiency was peripheral neuropathy characterized by the degeneration of the large caliber axons in the sensory neurons (21). Subsequently, patients with peripheral neuropathies without fat malabsorption, who were vitamin E-deficient, were described (22). Studies in such patients opened new avenues in vitamin E investigations because these patients were found to have a genetic defect in the hepatic α-TTP (7, 23).

STRUCTURES, NOMENCLATURE, AND CHEMISTRY

Vitamin E is the collective name for molecules that exhibit the antioxidant activity of α-tocopherol, including all tocol and tocotrienol derivatives, as reviewed by Sheppard and colleagues (24). The Food and Nutrition Board (FNB) of the Institute of Medicine (20) defined vitamin E for human requirements as only α-tocopherol. However, the antioxidant forms include four tocopherols and four tocotrienols, which have similar chromanol structures:

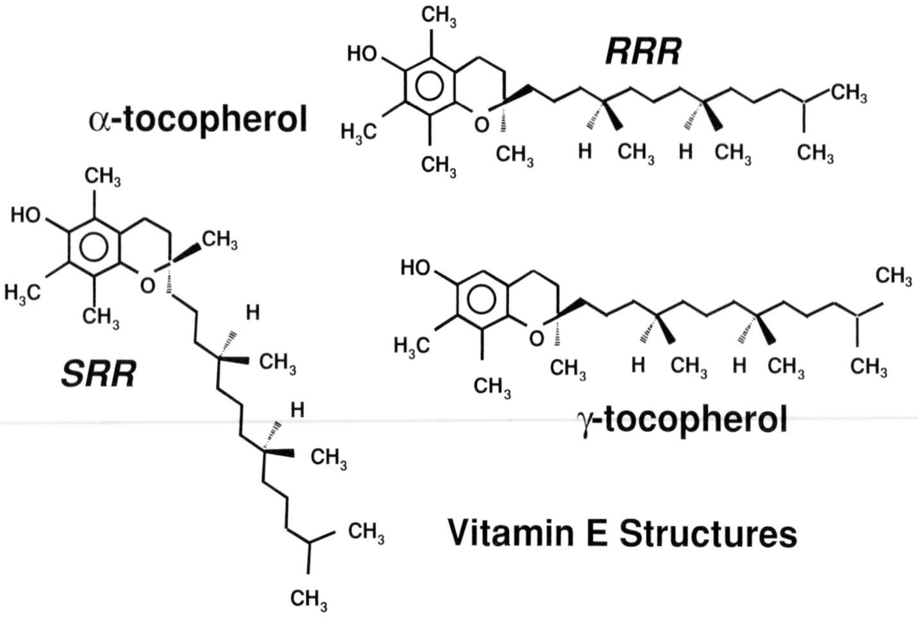

Figure 21.1. Structures of α- and γ-tocopherols. There are eight naturally occurring forms of vitamin E. Shown is *RRR*-α-tocopherol with naturally occurring stereochemistry; the three chiral centers can give rise to eight different stereoisomers in synthetic vitamin E (*all-rac*-α-tocopherol). These are *RRR*-, *RRS*-, *RSR*-, *RSS*-, *SRR*-, *SSR*-, *SRS*-, *SSS*-. Shown is *SRR*-α-tocopherol; its dramatic structural difference is readily apparent and explains why only 2*R*-α-tocopherols meet the human vitamin E requirement. Also shown is *RRR*-γ-tocopherol.

trimethyl (α-), dimethyl (β- or γ-), and monomethyl (δ-). Tocotrienols differ from tocopherols in that they have an unsaturated side chain. In this chapter, the term "vitamin E" includes all antioxidants with a chromanol head group. Functions of α-tocopherol, or other forms, are specifically indicated.

Unlike most other vitamins, chemically synthesized α-tocopherol is not identical to the naturally occurring form. α-Tocopherol synthesized by condensation of trimethyl hydroquinone with racemic isophytol (25) contains eight stereoisomers, arising from the three chiral centers: 2, 4', and 8'), and is designated *all-rac*-α-tocopherol (incorrectly called *d,l*-α-tocopherol) (Fig. 21.1). The naturally occurring and most biologically active form, *RRR*-α-tocopherol (formerly called *d*-α-tocopherol) constitutes only one of the eight stereoisomers present in *all-rac*-α-tocopherol. The FNB (20) further defined vitamin E for human requirements as only 2*R*-α-tocopherol; thus, only half of the stereoisomers in *all-rac*-α-tocopherol meet the vitamin E requirement. Previously, γ-tocopherol and other vitamin E forms were included as sources of vitamin E; these forms no longer are included because of a lack of evidence that they have health benefits in humans.

Units

This new vitamin E definition has lead to confusion about vitamin E units. The definition of the unit used on vitamin E supplement labels derives from units set by the US Pharmacopoeia (26). The now outdated vitamin E international unit (IU) was defined previously as 1 IU = 1 mg *all-rac*-α-tocopheryl acetate or 0.67 mg *RRR*-α-tocopherol or 0.74 mg *RRR*-α-tocopheryl acetate. However, the FNB (see Table 6.1 in reference (20) defined the vitamin E requirement in mg 2*R*-α-tocopherol and

provided conversion factors, such that *all-rac* is equal to 1/2 *RRR*-α-tocopherol.

Vitamin E as defined by FNB:

$$\text{IU } all\text{-}rac\text{-α-tocopherol or its esters}$$
$$= 0.45 \text{ mg } 2R\text{-α-tocopherol}$$

$$\text{IU } RRR\text{-α-tocopherol or its esters}$$
$$= 0.67 \text{ mg } 2R\text{-α-tocopherol}$$

Vitamin E supplements often contain esters of α-tocopherol, such as α-tocopheryl acetate, succinate, or nicotinate. The ester form prevents the oxidation of vitamin E and prolongs its shelf life. Except for persons with malabsorption syndromes, these esters are readily hydrolyzed in the gut and are absorbed in the unesterified form (27).

Antioxidant Activity

Vitamin E functions in vivo as a chain-breaking antioxidant that prevents the propagation of free radical damage in biologic membranes (28). Vitamin E is a potent peroxyl radical scavenger and especially protects PUFA within phospholipids of biologic membranes and in plasma lipoproteins. When lipid hydroperoxides are oxidized to peroxyl radicals (ROO•), these react 1000 times faster with vitamin E (Vit E-OH) than with PUFA (RH). The phenolic hydroxyl group of tocopherol reacts with an organic peroxyl radical to form the corresponding organic hydroperoxide and the tocopheroxyl radical (Vit E-O•):

In the presence of vitamin E: ROO• + Vit E-OH → ROOH + Vit E-O•

In the absence of vitamin E: ROO• + RH → ROOH + R•

R• + O$_2$ → ROO•

In this way, vitamin E acts as a chain breaking antioxidant and thus prevents the further auto-oxidation of lipids. Further information concerning the reactions of tocopherols and tocotrienols in vivo and in vitro can be found in the extensive review by Kamal-Eldin and Appelqvist (29).

Vitamin E Interactions: The Antioxidant Network

The tocopheroxyl radical (Vit E-O•) formed in membranes emerges from the lipid bilayer into the aqueous domain. It is here that the tocopheroxyl radical reacts with vitamin C (or other reductants serving as hydrogen donors, AH), thereby oxidizing the latter and returning vitamin E to its reduced state.

$$\text{Vit E-O•} + \text{AH} \rightarrow \text{Vit E-OH} + \text{A•}$$

Biologically important hydrogen donors, which have been demonstrated in vitro to regenerate tocopherol from the tocopheroxyl radical, include ascorbate (vitamin C) and thiols, especially glutathione. Subsequently, the vitamin C and thiyl radicals can be reduced via metabolic processes. This phenomenon has led to the idea of vitamin E recycling, in which the antioxidant function of oxidized vitamin E is continuously restored by other antioxidants. This antioxidant network depends on the supply of aqueous antioxidants and the metabolic activity of cells.

Structure-Function Relationships of Vitamin E Forms

Historically, the biologic activities of the various vitamin E forms were determined using the classical fetal resorption assay in rats (30). Overall, the highest biologic activity was found in molecules with three methyl groups and a free hydroxyl group on the chromanol ring with the phytyl tail meeting the ring in the *R*-orientation (see Fig. 21.1). This specific requirement for biologic, but not antioxidant, activity can best be rationalized by the preferential interactions of *RRR*-α-tocopherol with some stereospecific ligands in cells. One such ligand clearly is the hepatic protein, α-TTP. Hosomi and associates (3) demonstrated that α-TTP relative affinities of various forms of vitamin E (calculated from the degree of competition with *RRR*-α-tocopherol) were as follows: *RRR*-α-tocopherol, 100%; β-tocopherol, 38%; γ-tocopherol, 9%; δ-tocopherol, 2%; α-tocopherol acetate, 2%; α-tocopherol quinone, 2%; *SRR*-α-tocopherol, 11%; α-tocotrienol, 12%; trolox, 9%. These investigators concluded that the affinity of α-TTP for vitamin E analogs is one of the critical determinants for plasma concentrations and, thus, vitamin E biologic activity. These findings are emphasized in α-TTP knockout mice in which plasma and tissue α-tocopherol concentrations are 2 to 20% of control mice (4, 6).

In addition to its antioxidant function, structure-specific effects of α-tocopherol have been described. The most convincing work in this respect is on the regulation of vascular smooth muscle cell proliferation and protein kinase C

(PKC) activity (31–33) and on the suppression of arachidonic acid metabolism via phospholipase A_2 inhibition (34). Clement and associates (35) reported that α-tocopherol, but not β-tocopherol, prevents the phosphorylation of PKCα and thus decreases its activity. Tocopherols and tocotrienols have been reported to bind to various nuclear receptors (36); the physiologic significance of these findings is currently under intense investigation.

In vitro studies have shown that γ-, β-, or δ-tocopherols, unlike α-tocopherol, can be nitrated (37–39). Hoglen and associates (40) demonstrated that 5-nitro-γ-tocopherol (2,7,8-trimethyl-2-(4,8,12-trimethyldecyl)-5-nitro-6-chromanol [NGT]) is the major reactive product between peroxynitrite and γ-tocopherol. Thus, NGT, like 3-nitro-tyrosine, may serve as a useful in vivo biomarker for peroxynitrite interactions. NGT has been reported in the plasma of zymosan-treated rats (41), in the plasma from patients with coronary artery disease (42) and from cigarette smokers (43), and in brains collected post mortem from patients with Alzheimer disease (44).

DIGESTION AND INTESTINAL ABSORPTION

Vitamin E Absorption Requires Bile and Pancreatic Secretions

The absorption of vitamin E from the intestinal lumen depends on processes necessary for fat digestion and uptake into enterocytes (28). Pancreatic esterases are required for release of free fatty acids from dietary triglycerides. Bile acids, monoglycerides, and free fatty acids are important components of mixed micelles.

Esterases are also required for the hydrolytic cleavage of tocopheryl esters, a common form of vitamin E in dietary supplements. Generally, these esterases are quite effective; the apparent absorption of deuterated *RRR*-α-tocopherol was similar whether it was administered as α-tocopherol, α-tocopheryl acetate, or α-tocopheryl succinate (27).

Bile acids are needed for the formation of mixed micelles and are essential for vitamin E absorption. In the absence of either pancreatic or biliary secretions, vitamin E absorption and secretion into the lymphatic system are poor. In the absence of both, only negligible amounts of vitamin E are absorbed. Thus, vitamin E deficiency occurs as a result of malabsorption in patients with biliary obstruction, cholestatic liver disease, pancreatitis, or cystic fibrosis (28).

The bioavailability of vitamin E appears also to depend on the fat content of the food. Hayes and colleagues (45) reported that plasma α-tocopherol concentrations doubled when α-tocopheryl acetate (100–200 mg/day) was provided as a microdispersion in milk compared with providing the same dose in orange juice. Leonard and associates demonstrated that cereal fortified with *all-rac*-α-tocopheryl acetate (30 or 400 IU per serving) was more bioavailable than 400 IU taken in a capsule with fat-free milk (46). Again, this finding emphasizes that the physical properties of how vitamin E is presented to the intestinal absorptive surfaces have great bearing on its bioavailability.

Vitamin E Absorption Requires Chylomicron Synthesis and Secretion

The movement of vitamin E through the absorptive cells is not well understood; no intestinal tocopherol transfer proteins have been described (28). In the intestinal mucosa, chylomicrons containing triglycerides, free and esterified cholesterol, phospholipids, and apolipoproteins (apos), especially apoB48, are synthesized. In addition, fat-soluble vitamins, carotenoids, and other fat-soluble dietary components are incorporated into chylomicrons. Subsequently, chylomicrons containing these fats are secreted by the intestine into the lymph. Even in healthy persons, the efficiency of vitamin E absorption is low (<50%).

The critical role of bile acids for vitamin E absorption also suggests that the key step in vitamin E absorption is entry into the enterocyte, followed by packaging into chylomicrons (28). Borel and colleagues (47) showed that vitamin E absorption and secretion into chylomicrons occurred between 3 to 5 hours after dosing with an emulsion containing 57% fat, with no difference in absorption with small or large particle sizes. However, it appeared that vitamin E and triglyceride absorption were temporally separated (47). Thus, secretion in chylomicrons can be accomplished if vitamin E is absorbed into the enterocyte.

Often, differences in plasma concentrations of various forms of vitamin E are assumed to result from differences in the degree of intestinal absorption, but this is not the case, as reviewed in the literature (28). Discrimination between forms of vitamin E does not occur during their absorption by the intestine and their secretion in chylomicrons. Thus, all dietary forms of vitamin E are absorbed and secreted into chylomicrons.

PLASMA TRANSPORT

Distribution of Vitamin E to Tissues during Triglyceride-Rich Lipoprotein Lipolysis

During chylomicron catabolism in the circulation, some of the newly absorbed vitamin E is transferred to circulating lipoproteins and some remains with the chylomicron remnants (Fig. 21.2) (28). The process of chylomicron catabolism is quite rapid. During chylomicron delipidation by lipoprotein lipase, the size of the triglyceride core is reduced and excess surface is created. This excess surface is transferred to high-density lipoproteins (HDLs). Similarly, vitamin E is also transferred to HDLs. Because HDLs readily transfer vitamin E to other lipoproteins, vitamin E is distributed to all the circulating lipoproteins (see Fig. 21.2). Kostner and associates (48) demonstrated that the phospholipid transfer protein (PLTP) catalyzed

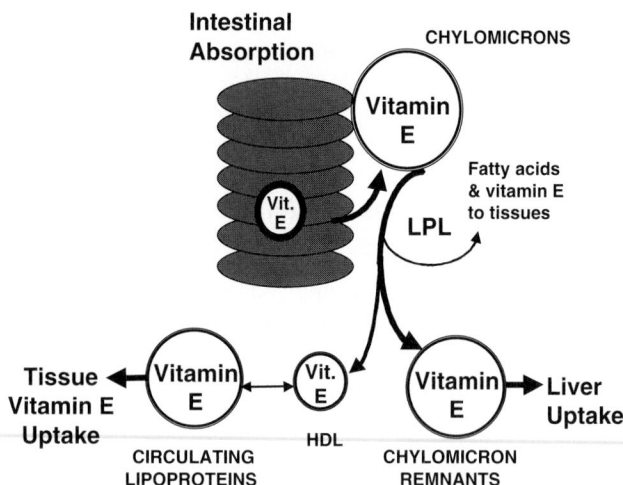

Figure 21.2. Pathways for absorption of vitamin E and its delivery to tissues during chylomicron catabolism. Vitamin E absorption requires bile acids (secreted from the liver) and fatty acids and monoglycerides (released from dietary fat by pancreatic enzymes) for micelle formation. Following uptake into enterocytes of the intestine, all forms of dietary vitamin E are incorporated into chylomicrons (28). These triglyceride-rich lipoproteins are secreted into the circulation, where lipolysis by lipoprotein lipase (LPL) bound to the endothelial lining of capillary walls takes place. The resultant chylomicron remnants are mainly taken up by the liver. During lipolysis, various forms of vitamin E can be transferred to tissues or to high-density lipoproteins (HDLs). Vitamin E can exchange between HDLs and other circulating lipoproteins, which can also deliver vitamin E to peripheral tissues.

vitamin E exchange between lipoproteins. The transfer activity was 2.45 ± 0.88 nmol/mL/hour, a rate that represents transfer of approximately 10% of the plasma vitamin E per hour.

Requirement for Very-Low-Density Lipoprotein Synthesis in the Preferential Secretion of α-tocopherol from the Liver

Following partial delipidation of chylomicrons by lipoprotein lipase and acquisition of apo E, the liver removes these remnants from the plasma. The mechanisms for chylomicron remnant uptake include both low-density lipoprotein (LDL) receptor–related protein (LRP) and the LDL receptor (49, 50). The remnants taken up by the liver likely contain a major portion of absorbed vitamin E.

Once chylomicron remnants reach the liver, the dietary fats are repackaged and secreted into the plasma in very-low-density lipoproteins (VLDLs) (28). Like chylomicrons, VLDLs have a triglyceride-rich core, but they have apoB 100 as a major apo instead of apoB 48. In the circulation, VLDLs are delipidated to form LDLs, which retain apoB 100. LDLs then interact with LDL receptors (apoB/E receptors) in peripheral tissues, as well as in the liver. During VLDL delipidation, similarly to that described earlier for chylomicron catabolism, vitamin E is transferred to HDLs, which can transfer vitamin E to all of the circulating lipoproteins.

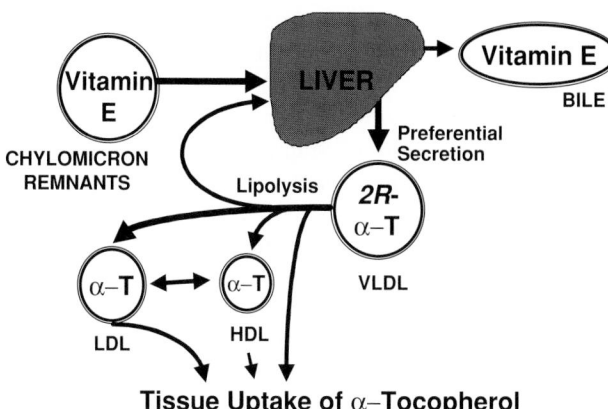

Tissue Uptake of α–Tocopherol

Figure 21.3. Pathways for the preferential delivery of α-tocopherol (α-T) to peripheral tissues. Chylomicron remnants containing various forms of vitamin E are taken up by the liver. In the liver, the α-tocopherol transfer protein seems preferentially to incorporate α-tocopherol into nascent very-low-density lipoproteins (VLDL) (28). Following VLDL secretion into plasma, lipolysis of VLDL by lipoprotein lipase and hepatic triglyceride lipase results in the preferential enrichment of circulating lipoproteins with *RRR*-α-tocopherol. The metabolism of these lipoproteins results in the delivery of *RRR*-α-tocopherol to peripheral tissues.

Unlike other fat-soluble vitamins, which have specific plasma transport proteins, vitamin E is transported nonspecifically in lipoproteins in the plasma. However, plasma vitamin E concentrations do depend on secretion of vitamin E from the liver (28). Remarkably, only one form of vitamin E, *RRR*-α-tocopherol, is preferentially secreted by the liver, as illustrated in Figure 21.3. Additionally, the newly absorbed α-tocopherol compared with circulating α-tocopherol appears to be preferentially secreted into the plasma from the liver (51). Thus, the liver, not the small intestine, discriminates among tocopherols.

Plasma Vitamin E Kinetics

A kinetic model of vitamin E transport in plasma has been developed using data from studies with deuterium-labeled stereoisomers of α-tocopherol (*RRR-* and *SRR-*) (52). In three patients with both ataxia and vitamin E deficiency (abbreviated AVED), who had genetically defective α-TTP, the fractional disappearance rates of deuterium-labeled *RRR-* and *SRR*-α-tocopherols in plasma were similar for the two stereoisomers, with a half-life of approximately 13 hours for both α-tocopherols. In control subjects, the fractional disappearance rates of deuterium-labeled *RRR*-α-tocopherol (0.4 ± 0.1 pools/day) were significantly ($p < .01$) slower than for *SRR-* (1.2 ± 0.6). The apparent half-life of *RRR*-α-tocopherol in physiologically normal subjects was approximately 48 hours, consistent with the "slow" disappearance of *RRR*-α-tocopherol from the plasma (52). Because *RRR*-α-tocopherol is returned to the plasma, its apparent turnover is slow. This hepatic recirculation of *RRR*-α-tocopherol

results in the daily replacement of nearly all the circulating *RRR*-α-tocopherol.

HEPATIC α-TOCOPHEROL TRANSFER PROTEIN

α-TTP (30–35 kDa) has been isolated from rat, human, mouse, and dog liver, and its cDNA sequences have been reported. The human protein has 94% homology to the rat protein and some homology both to the cellular retinaldehyde binding protein (CRALBP) in the retina (see Chapter 19) and to sec14, a PLTP (53). The gene has been localized to the 8q13.1-13.3 region of human chromosome 8 (53, 54).

Expression of α-TTP was first reported to be limited to hepatocytes (55). However, α-TTP mRNA has also been detected in rat brain, spleen, lung, and kidney (56), as well as α-TTP protein in human brain (57). Furthermore, α-TTP is present in pregnant mouse uterus and human placenta (13, 14), a finding suggesting that it functions to ensure adequate α-tocopherol concentrations during pregnancy.

α-TTP preferentially transfers α-tocopherol, compared with other dietary vitamin E forms, between liposomes and microsomes (58). Hypothetically, this ability to transfer tocopherol is necessary for the observed in vivo α-TTP action because nascent VLDLs secreted from the liver are preferentially enriched in *RRR*-α-tocopherol (59). However, when this hypothesis was tested in an α-TTP-expressing hepatic cell line (McARH7777 cells), α-TTP–mediated α-tocopherol secretion was not associated with VLDL secretion (60). Thus, the mechanism by which α-TTP facilitates α-tocopherol secretion into plasma is unknown. Progress in this area is highlighted by studies demonstrating the ability of the purified protein in vitro to fold properly, to bind, and to transfer vitamin E (61). The crystal structure has also been described (62, 63).

Other Tocopherol Binding Proteins

The search for proteins that regulate tissue α-tocopherol concentrations led to the identification of the tocopherol-associated protein (TAP), a 46-kDa cytosolic protein in bovine liver (64); the human homolog, hTAP, has been cloned (65). The highest amounts of hTAP mRNA are found in liver, brain, and prostate (65). TAP is controversial because its sequence is identical to that of supernatant protein factor (SPF). SPF stimulates squalene conversion to lanosterol and thus enhances cholesterol biosynthesis (66). The crystal structure of human SPF has been reported; the ligand binding cavity has a peculiar horseshoe shape (67). Provocatively, human TAP/SPF complexes with *RRR*-α-tocopheryl quinone, the oxidation product of α-tocopherol (68). The actual function of TAP/SPF remains under intense investigation.

Both α-TTP and TAP belong to a family of hydrophobic ligand binding proteins that have a *cis*-retinal binding motif sequence (CRAL_TRIO). This motif is also shared with CRALBP and yeast phosphatidylinositol transfer protein (Sec14p). Panagabko and associates (69) showed that all the CRAL_TRIO members bind α-tocopherol to some extent, but only α-TTP appears to have high enough affinity to serve as a physiologic α-tocopherol mediator (see the later section on genetic defects in α-TTP).

Dutta-Roy and colleagues (70, 71) reported that both the liver and the heart contain an α-tocopherol binding protein with a mass of 14.2 kDa. This protein is present in the liver in addition to α-TTP. The 14.2-kDa protein also transfers α-tocopherol in preference to γ- or δ-tocopherol. These investigators suggested that the 14.2-kDa tocopherol binding protein may regulate cellular α-tocopherol concentrations. Nalecz and associates (72) also reported the existence of various α-tocopherol binding proteins in cultured smooth muscle cells. No function has yet been proposed for these proteins.

DISTRIBUTION TO TISSUES

Vitamin E is transported in plasma lipoproteins in a nonspecific manner (28). No plasma specific vitamin E transport proteins have been described, but rather mechanisms of lipoprotein metabolism determine the delivery of vitamin E to tissues. Tissues likely acquire vitamin E by at least three major routes: (a) via lipoprotein lipase mediated lipoprotein catabolism, (b) via the LDL receptor, and (c) mediated by HDL. In addition, vitamin E rapidly exchanges among lipoproteins and between lipoproteins and membranes and may enrich membranes with vitamin E.

Vitamin E Delivery to Tissues

During chylomicron catabolism, peripheral tissues can acquire vitamin E from lipoproteins, which contain all the forms of vitamin E that were consumed (28). Following hepatic secretion of VLDL enriched with α-tocopherol, peripheral tissues take up primarily α-tocopherol. Delivery of vitamin E from both chylomicrons and VLDLs is likely mediated by lipoprotein lipase. This mechanism may be particularly important for tissues that express lipoprotein lipase, such as adipose tissue, muscle, and brain. Sattler and associates (73) tested this hypothesis directly by overexpressing lipoprotein lipase in mouse muscle and found increased delivery of α-tocopherol to muscle.

Another important mechanism for the delivery of tocopherols to tissues is via the LDL receptor (28). However, LDL receptor–dependent pathways are not the only receptors involved in tissue uptake of tocopherols.

HDL acquires vitamin E during chylomicron or VLDL catabolism, by exchange with other lipoproteins, or by removal of excess vitamin E from tissues. HDL, via the scavenger receptor-BI (SR-BI), are major α-tocopherol transporters to lung (74–77), brain (78, 79), and liver (80). SR-BI mediates selective cholesteryl ester uptake from HDL; that is, the lipids are transferred from HDL and the protein is released back into the circulation (81). Apparently,

SR-BI similarly delivers vitamin E to cells. Both LDL and HDL are SR-BI ligands, and thus LDL vitamin E may also be delivered by the SR-BI mechanism.

Vitamin E delivery by HDL to the liver appears analogous to reverse cholesterol transport (82) in that HDL via SR-BI delivers vitamin E for excretion into bile. Mardones and associates (83) reported in SR-BI–knockout mice, relative to wild-type mice, that plasma α-tocopherol concentrations were increased, whereas there was a 65 to 80% decrease in biliary α-tocopherol but no change in liver α-tocopherol. These investigators concluded that SR-BI–mediated hepatic α-tocopherol uptake was coupled to biliary excretion. Vitamin E–deficient rats have increased liver SR-BI protein, a finding suggesting that SR-BI is regulated by α-tocopherol (80). Increased SR-BI would serve to increase vitamin E delivery to the liver.

ABCA1 is an adenosine triphosphate binding cassette (ABC) transporter that transports cellular cholesterol and phospholipids to lipid-poor HDL. Oram and associates (84) have identified that ABCA1 is also responsible for the cellular secretion of α-tocopherol in association with HDL particles. Mice lacking ABCA1 have a severe deficiency of fat-soluble vitamins, including α-tocopherol (85). Clearly, ABCA1 is important in α-tocopherol trafficking, and its physiologic role appears to involve cellular tocopherol efflux, but further investigations into its role in regulating tissue vitamin E concentrations are warranted.

Circulating blood cells likely obtain their vitamin E by transfer of tocopherols from lipoproteins, especially HDLs (28). Patients with abetalipoproteinemia, who have HDLs, but not chylomicrons, VLDLs, LDLs, and other lipoproteins containing apoB, have plasma vitamin E concentrations approximately one tenth of normal, whereas their erythrocytes contain about two thirds of the vitamin E found in controls. Thus, HDLs have an important role in delivering vitamin E to circulating cells.

Tissues with Slow Versus Fast Turning over Vitamin E Pools

Deuterated α-tocopherol has been used to assess the kinetics and distribution of α-tocopherol into various tissues in rats (86), guinea pigs (87), and humans (88). From these studies, it is apparent that a group of tissues is in rapid equilibrium with the plasma α-tocopherol pool. Tissues such as erythrocytes, liver, and spleen quickly replace "old" with "new" α-tocopherol (89). Other tissues such as heart, muscle, and spinal cord have slower α-tocopherol turnover times. By far, the brain shows the slowest α-tocopherol turnover time. Remarkably, human brain α-tocopherol can be increased with vitamin E supplementation (88).

In general, the α-tocopherol content of the nervous system is spared during α-tocopherol depletion (90–92). Studies in adult beagle dogs demonstrated that the peripheral nerves are the most responsive of the nervous system to low dietary α-tocopherol concentrations (93).

Thus, it is not surprising that, in humans, the peripheral nerves (22) are the most susceptible clinically to α-tocopherol deficiency (94). In contrast, the brain retains α-tocopherol, perhaps because it expresses α-TTP (56, 57).

Storage Sites

The mechanisms for the release of tocopherols from tissues are unknown—no organ functions as a storage organ for α-tocopherol and releases it on demand (28). The bulk of vitamin E in the human body is localized in the adipose tissue. More than 90% of the human body pool of α-tocopherol is located in the adipose tissue, and more than 90% of adipose tissue α-tocopherol is in fat droplets, not membranes. Handelman and associates (95) estimated that more than 2 years are required for adipose tissue α-/γ-tocopherol ratios to reach new steady-state levels in response to changes in dietary intake. Thus, the analysis of adipose tissue α-tocopherol content provides a useful estimate of long-term vitamin E intakes. El-Sohemy and colleagues (96) reported in nearly 500 Costa Rican subjects that adipose tissue γ-tocopherol concentrations were related to dietary intakes, but adipose tissue α-tocopherol concentrations were not. Nonetheless, adipose tissue α-tocopherol concentrations were higher than γ-tocopherol concentrations, a finding suggesting that additional mechanisms, such as plasma α-tocopherol regulation by α-TTP, are important for determining adipose tissue α-tocopherol concentrations.

The availability of human adipose tissue α-tocopherol as a source of vitamin E during times of increased need remains controversial. During weight reduction in obese persons, triglyceride, but not α-tocopherol or cholesterol, was released from adipose tissue (97). However, in α-tocopherol–deficient persons, adipose tissue α-tocopherol content is lower than in physiologically normal subjects, but it is not clear whether this is caused by decreased delivery or increased export or utilization (98).

METABOLISM AND EXCRETION

Hepatic Metabolism

Unlike other fat-soluble vitamins, vitamin E is not accumulated in the liver to toxic levels, a finding suggesting that excretion and metabolism are important in preventing adverse vitamin E effects. The vitamin E metabolites, α-CEHC (2,5,7,8-tetramethyl-2-[2'-carboxyethyl]-6-hydroxychroman) and γ-CEHC (2,7,8-trimethyl-2-[2'carboxyethyl]-6-hydroxychroman), are derived from α-tocopherols and α-tocotrienols and from γ-tocopherols and γ-tocotrienols, respectively (99, 100). Based on studies in hepatocytes (100, 101), it is likely that liver can synthesize CEHCs, but the site of metabolism remains unresolved.

Vitamin E forms appear to be metabolized, similar to xenobiotics, by ω-oxidation by cytochrome P450s (CYPs), then conjugated and excreted in urine (102) or bile (103). Hepatic CYP4F2 is involved in ω-oxidation of α- and γ-tocopherols (104), but CYP3A may also be involved (100, 105–107). Like other xenobiotics, CEHCs are sulfated or glucuronidated (108–110). Xenobiotic transporters are likely candidates for mediating hepatic CEHC excretion because CEHCs are found in plasma, urine, and bile. These pathways may all be under the regulation of orphan nuclear receptors (36).

High α-tocopherol intakes, such as from most vitamin E supplements, lead to increases of plasma α-tocopherol, decreases of γ-tocopherol (111), and increases in both α-CEHC (112) and γ-CEHC excretion (99, 113). γ-CEHC excretion increases because γ-tocopherol is more actively metabolized to CEHCs than is α-tocopherol (99, 108, 114). Additionally, studies in patients with end-stage renal disease demonstrated that vitamin E supplementation was accompanied by a concomitant decrease (~1 μM) in circulating γ-tocopherol and an approximately 1-μM increase in γ-CEHC (113). Thus, metabolism appears to be a regulator of plasma γ-tocopherol concentrations.

Routes of Excretion

Most ingested vitamin E is eliminated by the fecal route because of its low intestinal absorption. Excretion of excess hepatic vitamin E into the bile has been demonstrated to be mediated by the ABC transporter, P-glycoprotein (MDR2) (115), a transporter that also facilitates biliary phospholipid excretion into bile.

The skin may be an important route for vitamin E excretion (28). Skin sebaceous glands secrete vitamin E to provide antioxidants to protect cutaneous lipids (116). Moreover, dietary α-tocopherol was secreted in human sebaceous gland lipids approximately 7 days after ingestion of vitamin E (117).

Oxidation Products

Because the tocopheroxyl radical can be reduced back to tocopherol by ascorbate or other reducing agents, the flux through the cyclic radical pathway may be much larger than the flux through the pathway of further metabolism of oxidized vitamin E. Liebler, Burr, and co-workers (118, 119) suggested that biologically relevant oxidation products formed from α-tocopherol include 4a,5-epoxy- and 7,8-epoxy-8a(hydroperoxy) tocopherones and their respective hydrolysis products, 2,3-epoxy-tocopherol quinone and 5,6-epoxy-α-tocopherol quinone. However, these products are formed during in vitro oxidation; their importance in vivo is unknown.

The primary oxidation product of α-tocopherol is α-tocopheryl quinone, which can be conjugated to yield the glucuronate after prior reduction to the hydroquinone. The glucuronate can be excreted into bile or further degraded in the kidneys to α-tocopheronic acid, which is excreted in the urine (120). Further oxidation products, including dimers and trimers, as well as other adducts have also been described (29).

CAUSES OF DEFICIENCY

α-Tocopherol deficiency occurs only rarely in humans and virtually never as a result of dietary deficiencies because of the nearly ubiquitous distribution of tocopherols in foods, especially oils and fats (28). α-Tocopherol deficiency does occur as a result of genetic abnormalities in α-TTP and as a result of various fat malabsorption syndromes, as shown in Table 21.1.

Genetic Defects in the α-Tocopherol Transfer Protein

Genetic defects in α-TTP are associated with a characteristic syndrome, AVED, previously called familial isolated vitamin E (FIVE) deficiency. Patients with AVED have neurologic abnormalities similar to those of Friedreich ataxia (28). The symptoms are characterized by progressive peripheral neuropathy with a specific "dying back" of the large caliber axons of the sensory neurons, with resulting ataxia.

These patients are responsive to oral α-tocopherol supplements. A dose of 800 to 1200 mg/day is usually sufficient to prevent further deterioration of neurologic function, and in some cases improvements have been noted, as reviewed by Sokol (22). Untreated patients have extraordinarily low plasma α-tocopherol concentrations (as low as 1/100 of normal), but if they are given α-tocopherol supplements, then plasma concentrations reach normal levels within hours! However, if α-tocopherol supplementation is halted, then plasma α-tocopherol concentrations fall within days to deficient levels.

TABLE 21.1. DISORDERS REQUIRING ADMINISTRATION OF α-TOCOPHEROL TO PREVENT DEFICIENCY

Genetic abnormalities
  α-Tocopherol transfer protein (ataxia with vitamin E deficiency)
  Apolipoprotein B (homozygous hypobetalipoproteinemia)
  Microsomal triglyceride transfer protein (abetalipoproteinemia)
Fat malabsorption syndromes
  Chronic cholestasis in children and adults
    Idiopathic neonatal hepatitis
    Familial cholestatic syndrome
    Alagille syndrome
    Paucity of interlobular bile ducts
    Extrahepatic biliary atresia
    Primary biliary cirrhosis
  Cystic fibrosis and pancreatic insufficiency
  Short bowel syndromes
    Crohn disease
    Mesenteric vascular thrombosis
    Intestinal pseudoobstruction
  Chronic steatorrhea
    Blind loop syndrome
    Intestinal lymphangiectasia
    Celiac disease
    Chronic pancreatitis
Total parenteral nutrition

Patients with AVED can be segregated into two groups. In one study, some patients could not discriminate between forms of vitamin E and some patients could discriminate, but all patients had difficulty maintaining plasma α-tocopherol concentrations (7). Ouahchi and associates(23) mapped their genetic defect to chromosome 8q13.1-13.3, the same chromosomal location as α-TTP (53, 54). Most of the patients described (23) were found to have a truncation of the C-terminal portion of α-TTP. The genetic defect in α-TTP has now been identified in some of the same patients through the use of deuterium-labeled tocopherols. A truncation of the terminal portion of α-TTP (23, 121) causes an inability to discriminate between *RRR-* and *SRR-*α-tocopherols (122). However, patients who are heterozygous for the α-TTP truncation mutation (23, 121) can discriminate between stereoisomers (23, 121). In addition to truncation mutations, defective transfer function of α-TTP has also been described. A patient who experienced neurologic difficulties only after reaching approximately 50 years of age (123) preferentially incorporated *RRR-*α-tocopherol into lipoproteins, but at a reduced rate (124). This patient was found to be homozygous for a thymine-to-guanine (T-to-G) transversion in the α-TTP gene that causes the histidine at position 101 to be replaced with glutamine (125). Gotoda and associates (125) screened 801 inhabitants near the patient's home on an isolated Japanese island, where 21 heterozygotes were found with this mutation. These heterozygotes had significantly lower serum vitamin E concentrations than a control population. The mutated gene, when expressed in COS-7 cells, produced a functionally defective α-TTP with approximately 11% of the activity of the wild-type α-TTP (125). Thus, the region around histidine 101 must be important for transfer activity. This region has a high degree of homology both with retinal CRALBP present and yeast sec14 protein (53). Because these latter two proteins are also lipid binding/transfer proteins, this region of all three proteins may be important for their lipid transfer roles.

Retinitis pigmentosa commonly accompanies human vitamin E deficiency (28). Importantly, α-tocopherol supplementation stops or slows the progression of retinitis pigmentosa caused by vitamin E deficiency (126). Mutations in proteins with the CRAL_TRIO motif, such as CRALBP (127) and α-TTP (128), are associated with retinitis pigmentosa. Moreover, the results from a trial of vitamin E and A supplements in patients with many common forms of retinitis pigmentosa without vitamin E deficiency showed a beneficial effect of 15,000 IU/day of vitamin A and a possible adverse effect of 400 IU vitamin E (129). Therefore, plasma vitamin E concentrations should be measured in patients with retinitis pigmentosa to evaluate their vitamin E status before supplementation is prescribed. Only those patients with retinitis pigmentosa who have vitamin E deficiency should be supplemented with α-tocopherol.

Genetic Defects in Lipoprotein Synthesis

Studies of patients with hypobetalipoproteinemia or abetalipoproteinemia (low to nondetectable circulating chylomicrons, VLDLs, or LDLs) have demonstrated that lipoproteins containing apoB are necessary for effective absorption and plasma transport of lipids, especially vitamin E (28). These patients have steatorrhea from birth because of the impaired ability to absorb dietary fat, which also contributes to their poor vitamin E status. Other clinical features include retarded growth, acanthocytosis, retinitis pigmentosa, and a chronic progressive neurologic disorder with ataxia.

Although the two groups of patients similarly lack apoB-containing lipoproteins, their underlying genetic defects are different. Homozygous hypobetalipoproteinemia patients have a defect in the apoB gene, and thus any apoB-containing lipoproteins that are secreted into the circulation turnover rapidly. Abetalipoproteinemic patients have genetic defects in microsomal triglyceride transfer protein, which prevents normal lipidation of apoB. Thus, the secretion of apoB-containing lipoproteins is virtually nonexistent. Clinically, both groups of subjects become vitamin E deficient and develop a characteristic neurologic syndrome—progressive peripheral neuropathy—if they are not given large vitamin E supplements. Daily doses of 100 to 200 mg/kg, or about 5 to 7 g, of RRR-α-tocopherol are recommended (22). Although plasma concentrations of α-tocopherol never reach normal levels, adipose tissue α-tocopherol concentrations do reach normal levels.

Fat Malabsorption Syndromes

Vitamin E deficiency occurs secondary to fat malabsorption because vitamin E absorption requires biliary and pancreatic secretions (see earlier). Failure of micellar solubilization and malabsorption of dietary lipids leads to vitamin E deficiency in children with chronic cholestatic hepatobiliary disorders, including disease of the liver and anomalies of intrahepatic and extrahepatic bile ducts. Children with cholestatic liver disease, who have impaired secretion of bile into the small intestine, have severe fat malabsorption. Neurologic abnormalities appear as early as the second year of life and become irreversible if the vitamin E deficiency is uncorrected.

Children with cystic fibrosis can also become vitamin E deficient because the impaired secretion of pancreatic digestive enzymes causes steatorrhea and vitamin E malabsorption, even when pancreatic enzyme supplements are administered orally. More severe vitamin E deficiency occurs if bile secretion is impaired.

Any disorder that causes fat malabsorption can lead to vitamin E deficiency. The list of disorders associated with acquired vitamin E deficiency, assembled by Sokol (22), includes chronic dysfunction or resection of the small bowel, Crohn disease, mesenteric vascular thrombosis or intestinal pseudoobstruction, blind loop syndrome, intestinal lymphangiectasia, celiac disease, and chronic pancreatitis. However, the development of neurologic symptoms of vitamin E deficiency in adults who acquire these disorders takes decades. Serum vitamin E levels may fall within 1 to 2 years of acquired lipid malabsorption in adolescents and adults; however, a 10- to 20-year interval between the identification of biochemical vitamin E deficiency and the onset of neurologic symptoms is generally observed in adults (22). The prolonged time for onset of symptoms results from the prior accumulation of vitamin E in most tissues and its relatively slow release from nervous tissues.

Vitamin E supplementation in patients with fat malabsorption syndromes is very difficult to achieve because these patients also malabsorb vitamin E. Sokol (22) suggested treatment with RRR-α-tocopherol (not the ester) at 25 to 50 mg/kg/day, advancing by 50 mg/kg/day up to 150 to 200 mg/kg/day if the ratio of serum α-tocopherol to total lipids does not become normal (>0.8 mg/g). The dose should be given with a meal before administration of any medication that may interfere with vitamin E absorption (e.g., cholestyramine, large doses of vitamin A or ferrous sulfate). In cases of severe cholestasis, intraluminal bile acid concentrations are much lower than the critical micellar concentration, with resulting failure of vitamin E absorption. Here intramuscular injections of vitamin E, such as Viprimol (DSM Nutritional Products, Parsippany, NJ) can be used to provide 1 to 2 mg/kg/day (22). A water-soluble ester of vitamin E, such as d-α-tocopheryl polyethylene glycol-1000 succinate (TPGS, Eastman Chemical Company, Kingsport, TN) is absorbed when it is administered orally, appears to be nontoxic, and reverses or prevents neurologic dysfunction (22). However, products such as TPGS should not be used if the patient suffers from renal failure or dehydration because the excretion of absorbed polyethylene glycol may be impaired (130).

Total Parenteral Nutrition

Patients receiving total parenteral nutrition (TPN) ideally are provided with all their required nutrients—vitamin E (10 mg/day) is given as part of a vitamin mix and as a component of a lipid emulsion, which also provides essential fatty acids and calories (28). Most intravenous preparations of lipid emulsions are made with soybean oil to provide PUFAs. However, the soybean oil emulsions contain high levels of γ-tocopherol, but not α-tocopherol. Evaluation of the vitamin E status of patients receiving TPN with lipid emulsions suggests that these patients may be receiving inadequate amounts of α-tocopherol. They have elevated levels of exhaled pentane and ethane, which are markers of lipid peroxidation in vivo (131), and adipose tissue α-tocopherol concentrations that are half normal values, findings suggesting depletion of tissue stores of vitamin E (98) (see Chapter 99 concerning vitamin E dosages in parenteral nutrition).

PATHOLOGY OF HUMAN α-TOCOPHEROL DEFICIENCY

The primary manifestations of human α-tocopherol deficiency include spinocerebellar ataxia, skeletal myopathy, and pigmented retinopathy (28). The progression of neurologic symptoms resulting from α-tocopherol deficiency in humans follows a distinct pattern. Hyporeflexia or areflexia is the earliest symptom observed. By the end of the first decade of life, untreated patients with chronic cholestatic hepatobiliary disease have a combination of spinocerebellar ataxia, neuropathy, and ophthalmoplegia. The progression of neurologic symptoms appears to depend on the level of oxidative stress accompanying the α-tocopherol deficiency.

Deficiency in children and adults results in progressive peripheral neuropathy with a dying back of the large-caliber axons in the sensory neurons, as reviewed in the literature (132). The large-caliber, myelinated axons of peripheral sensory nerves are the predominant target in human α-tocopherol deficiency. Diminished amplitudes of sensory nerve action potential are common, whereas delayed conduction velocity, an indicator of demyelination, is unusual. Thus, axonal degeneration rather than demyelination is the primary sensory nerve abnormality; that is, the axons degenerate first, then demyelination occurs.

Axonal dystrophy has been observed in the posterior columns of the spinal cord and the dorsal and ventral spinocerebellar tracts (132). Specifically, swollen, dystrophic axons (spheroids) have been observed in the gracile and cuneate nuclei of the brainstem. Lipofuscin accumulation has been observed in dorsal sensory neurons and peripheral Schwann cell cytoplasm. Electromyographic studies show denervation injury of muscles in patients with advanced α-tocopherol deficiency. Somatosensory-evoked potential testing has shown a central delay in sensory conduction, correlating with degeneration of the posterior columns of the spinal cord.

DIETARY CONSIDERATIONS, REQUIREMENTS, AND RECOMMENDED INTAKES

Only plants synthesize vitamin E. The richest food sources of vitamin E are edible vegetable oils (24). These oils contain all four homologs: α-, β-, γ-, and δ-tocopherols in varying proportions. RRR-α-tocopherol is especially high in wheat germ oil, safflower oil, and sunflower oil. Soybean and corn oils contain predominantly γ-tocopherol, as well as some tocotrienols. Cottonseed oil and palm oil contain both α- and α-tocopherols in equal proportion. In addition, palm oil contains large amounts of α- and γ-tocotrienols (133).

Previously, it was assumed for the purpose of calculating vitamin E intakes that γ-tocopherol could substitute for α-tocopherol with an efficiency of 10%, β-tocopherol of 50%, and α-tocotrienol of 30%. However, these forms of vitamin E are not equivalent to α-tocopherol, and the FNB recommended that specific forms of dietary vitamin E be reported and only 2R-α-tocopherol be counted to meet the requirement.

Probably, the most important source of α-tocopherol in the diet in the United States is the supplement pill. Supplemental vitamin E is sold as esters (e.g., acetate, succinate, nicotinate). Pills containing vitamin E with natural stereochemistry (RRR-α-tocopherol) are labeled "d-α-tocopherol." Pills containing synthetic vitamin E (all-rac-α-tocopherol) contain eight different stereoisomers and are labeled "dl." For each vitamin E IU, manufacturers are required to include 0.91 mg all-rac-α-tocopherol, but only 0.67 mg RRR-α-tocopherol. The FNB (20) stated that only 2R-α-tocopherol meets human requirements for vitamin E and redefined the equivalence such that 2 mg all-rac-α-tocopherol is needed to provide 1 mg 2R-α-tocopherol. Thus, a 400-IU pill of d-α-tocopherol contains 268 mg 2R-α-tocopherol (400 IU times 0.67 mg/IU), whereas a 400-IU pill of dl-α-tocopherol contains 180 mg 2R-α-tocopherol (400 IU times 0.91 mg/IU divided by 2). As of this writing, the IU has not been redefined in accordance with FNB recommendations.

DIETARY REFERENCE INTAKES

The dietary reference intakes (DRIs) for vitamin C, vitamin E, selenium, and carotenoids were published in 2000 by the Panel on Dietary Antioxidants and Related Compounds, FNB (20). The basis, definitions, and use of the DRIs and the data published to date are summarized in Appendix Tables A-2-a through A-2-b. The FNB changed the criteria for establishing DRIs from prevention of deficiency diseases to evaluation of the potential of a given nutrient for prevention of chronic diseases (134). Nevertheless, the "health benefits" of the antioxidant nutrients as described in the revised 2000 DRIs were primarily those related to the prevention of deficiency symptoms, because of a lack of evidence that increased antioxidants prevented chronic diseases (20). The DRIs distinguish between RRR- and all-rac-α-tocopherol because these structures are physically different and have different fates with respect to transport and metabolism.

The estimated average requirement (EAR) was based on the amount of 2R-α-tocopherol intake that reversed erythrocyte hemolysis in men who were vitamin E deficient as a result of consuming a vitamin E–deficient diet for 5 years, as reviewed in the literature (20). The criteria and DRI values for α-tocopherol by life stage are given in Table 21.2. The EAR of 12 mg 2R-α-tocopherol was chosen because intakes at this level and higher resulted in plasma α-tocopherol concentrations that prevented in vitro hydrogen peroxide–induced erythrocyte hemolysis. The assumption was made that men and women would have similar requirements because

TABLE 21.2. CRITERIA AND DIETARY REFERENCE INTAKE VALUES FOR VITAMIN E BY LIFE STAGE GROUP[a]

LIFE STAGE GROUP	CRITERION	EAR[b] (mg/d)	RDA[c] (mg/d)	AI[d] (mg/d)
0–6 mo	Average vitamin E intake from human milk			4
7–12 mo	Extrapolation from 0–6 mo AI			5
1–3 y	Extrapolation from adult EAR	5	6	
4–8 y	Extrapolation from adult EAR	6	7	
9–13 y	Extrapolation from adult EAR	9	11	
14 through 18 y	Extrapolation from adult EAR	12	15	
>18 y	Intakes sufficient to prevent hydrogen peroxide–induced erythrocyte hemolysis in vivo	12	15	
Pregnancy				
≤18 y	Adolescent EAR	12	15	
19–50 y	Adult EAR	12	15	
Lactation				
≤18 y	Adolescent EAR plus average amount of vitamin E secreted in human milk	16	19	
19–50 y	Adult EAR plus average amount of vitamin E secreted in human milk	16	19	

[a] In units of milligrams of 2R-α-tocopherol.

[b] EAR, estimated average requirement. The intake that meets the estimated nutrient needs of half the individuals in a group.

[c] RDA, recommended dietary allowance. The intake that meets the nutrient needs of almost all (97–98%) of individuals in a group.

[d] AI , adequate intake. The observed average or experimentally determined intake by a defined population or subgroup that appears to sustain a defined nutritional status, such as growth rate, normal circulating nutrient values, or other functional indicators of health. The AI is used if sufficient scientific evidence is not available to derive an EAR. For healthy infants receiving human milk, the AI is the mean intake. The AI is not equivalent to an RDA.

From Food and Nutrition Board, Institute of Medicine. Dietary Reference Intakes for Vitamin C, Vitamin E, Selenium, and Carotenoids: Washington, DC: National Academy Press, 2000.

women, despite their lower body weight, have a larger percentage of body fat needing antioxidant protection. The 2000 RDA for adults (both men and women >19 years) for vitamin E defined as 2R-α-tocopherol is 15 mg/day. The 1989 RDA for men and women, respectively, was 10 and 8 mg/day α-tocopherol equivalents (also included γ-tocopherol and other forms based on their biologic activities).

The tolerable upper intake level (UL) was set at 1000 mg/day for vitamin E (any form of supplemental α-tocopherol). This was one of the few ULs that was set using data in rats because sufficient and appropriate quantitative data assessing long-term adverse effects of vitamin E supplements in humans were not available. A meta-analysis of antioxidant-intervention trials in humans suggests that the doses of vitamin E supplements (400 or 800 IU) given in many clinical trials are not associated with adverse effects (135).

Adequacy of α-Tocopherol Intakes in Normal Populations in the United States

The amount of α-tocopherol consumed by most US adults is sufficient to prevent overt symptoms of deficiency, such as peripheral neuropathy (28). However, the actual quantities consumed by adults in the United States are closer to 8 mg, as assessed by various surveys (136–138). These low intakes may be real, or they may result from underreporting of fat intakes. Nevertheless, it is quite possible that

many people do not consume a diet that contains 15 mg α-tocopherol.

The major source of α-tocopherol in the American diet is desserts (136). Thus, it is not surprising that decreasing fat intake will decrease vitamin E intakes. In one study, as fat was reduced from 30 to 11% of energy intake, α-tocopherol intakes decreased from 9 to 4 mg daily in subjects' diets (139). In persons who have changed their diets to lower serum cholesterol by decreasing intake of saturated fats and increasing intake of PUFA-containing fats, usually corn oil or soybean oil, which contain high γ-tocopherol concentrations (24), the intake of oxidizable lipids is increased, whereas intake of α-tocopherol is decreased. To avoid excessive intakes of PUFAs, the ingestion of monounsaturated fats, such as olive or canola oils that are rich in α-tocopherol, is recommended (140).

Assessment of α-Tocopherol Status in Patients at Risk for Deficiency

The FNB determined that a plasma concentration of less than 12 μmol α-tocopherol/L was associated with increased evidence of α-tocopherol inadequacy; plasma concentrations in physiologically normal persons are approximately 20 μmol/L. Several parameters can be measured in patients who may be α-tocopherol deficient (Table 21.3). Although low serum or plasma α-tocopherol concentrations are indicative of vitamin E deficiency, measurement of plasma levels is insufficient for patients

---

TABLE 21.3. TECHNIQUES FOR ASSESSMENT OF α-TOCOPHEROL STATUS

Measurements of plasma vitamin E concentrations
   Normal values are >12 μmol α-tocopherol/L (μM) or 5 μg/mL
   Normal values are >0.8 mg α-tocopherol/g total lipid
      (cholesterol plus triglycerides) or 2.8 mg/g cholesterol
Measurements of adipose tissue vitamin E concentrations
   >100 μg α-tocopherol/mg triglyceride
Functional signs of vitamin E deficiency
   Increased red cell hemolysis
   Increased lipid peroxidation (e.g., F_2-isoprostanes)
   Increased expired ethane or pentane
Clinical signs of vitamin E deficiency
   Neurologic testing: abnormal sensory nerve function
   Histopathology of peripheral nerves
   Electrophysiologic measurements
Gene testing
   Genetic defects in α-tocopherol transfer protein
   Genetic defects on chromosome 8

TABLE 21.4. DISORDERS IN WHICH SUPPLEMENTAL α-TOCOPHEROL MAY BE BENEFICIAL

Premature infants: retinopathy of prematurity (147)
   Protection from retrolental fibroplasia
   Possible protection of intraventricular hemorrhage
   Increased risk of necrotizing enterocolitis or sepsis
Anemia of prematurity (165)
   Protection from vitamin E deficiency caused by inappropriate
      formulas
   May be beneficial in physiologic jaundice or anemia of the
      newborn
Cardiovascular disorders
   Decreased risk of coronary heart disease (144, 145, 152, 153,
      166)
   Decreased in vitro low-density lipoprotein oxidation (167,
      168)
   Decreased in vitro platelet aggregation (169)
Ischemia-reperfusion injury (160)
Immune response
   Improved responses in elderly patients (170)
Cataract (147)
Tardive dyskinesia (171, 172)
Alzheimer disease (143)

---

with various forms of lipid malabsorption. Calculation of effective plasma α-tocopherol concentrations needs to take into account plasma lipid levels. These are calculated by dividing the plasma α-tocopherol by the sum of plasma cholesterol and triglycerides (141).

Patients with elevated cholesterol or triglyceride concentrations may have α-tocopherol levels in the "normal" range, but these may not be sufficient to protect tissues. For example, Sokol and associates (142) showed that plasma α-tocopherol concentrations were in the normal range in patients with α-tocopherol deficiency as a result of cholestatic liver disease, a disorder that is also characterized by extraordinarily high serum lipid levels.

Patients with peripheral neuropathies or retinitis pigmentosa of unknown cause should be evaluated to assess whether they are α-tocopherol deficient. The ataxia of Friedreich ataxia is so remarkably similar to that of AVED that plasma concentrations of α-tocopherol in all patients with ataxia should be measured.

Controversial Topics

Epidemiologic studies and some intervention trials indicate a beneficial role of supplemental α-tocopherol in decreasing disease risk (Table 21.4). The risk of degenerative diseases, such as Alzheimer disease (143), cardiovascular disease and atherosclerosis (144, 145), cancer (146), cataract formation (147), and aging (148) have been the focus of numerous population studies evaluating α-tocopherol intakes. It is not clear whether such chronic diseases are a hallmark of long-term suboptimal vitamin E intakes. Studies that have examined vitamin E function at the molecular level have demonstrated that α-tocopherol modulates pathways important in heart disease (149, 150). Additionally, studies in animal models demonstrate that α-tocopherol can decrease atherosclerotic lesion formation (4, 151). However, the studies in humans given vitamin E

supplements to study α-tocopherol effects on heart attack risk have resulted in conflicting outcomes: beneficial effects (152–154), limited effects (155), no benefit (156), and possible harm (157–159). Boaz and associates (153) suggested that in the clinical trials in which vitamin E has had benefit, the subjects consuming the placebo had higher incidences of cardiovascular disease and perhaps greater oxidative stress; examples include patients with end-stage renal disease and heart transplants. Thus, higher intakes of α-tocopherol may be beneficial if chronic diseases, such as heart disease, stroke, cancer, diabetes, and Alzheimer disease, result, at least in part, from suboptimal protection by antioxidants. Importantly, the amounts of vitamin E that exerted beneficial effects in intervention studies are not achievable by dietary means.

The benefit arising from vitamin E supplementation in heart disease may result from the ability of vitamin E to interfere with clot formation. This is an important function in the prevention of thrombosis, which can lead to heart attacks or stroke. However, this effect also brings up the potential risks. Supplemental α-tocopherol may increase bleeding tendencies. Additionally, vitamin E may potentiate the effects of aspirin with respect to blood clotting (160). Certainly, the UL set by the FNB of 1000 mg α-tocopherol (1100 IU *dl*- or 1500 IU *d*-) should not be exceeded by supplement users (20).

Health benefits of γ-tocopherol have been touted because, unlike α-tocopherol, γ-tocopherol can be nitrated and thus may protect against peroxynitrite injury and because γ-CEHC, the γ-tocopherol metabolite, has potent cell signaling effects in vitro (161, 162). Moreover, Ohrvall and associates (163) reported low circulating γ-tocopherol levels in patients with coronary heart disease, a finding suggesting that higher γ-tocopherol levels could be protective. However, serum γ-tocopherol may be a marker of a healthier diet containing vegetable oil that is lower in saturated fat and higher in unsaturated fat—not necessarily that a higher circulating γ-tocopherol itself decreases the risk of coronary heart disease. Nonetheless, great interest exists in studying the human health benefits of γ-tocopherol (164).

CONCLUSIONS

More than 8 decades after its discovery, vitamin E remains an elusive nutrient. Its potential for decreasing the risks of acquiring chronic disease has spurred the interests of scientists and clinicians world wide. The description of vitamin E deficiency in patients with genetic abnormalities in α-TTP has opened new avenues of investigation of α-tocopherol transfer and binding proteins in various tissues. We are again brought back to the questions, "What is the function of vitamin E?" and "Why do we need a specific protein that recognizes only α-tocopherol if all the naturally occurring forms of vitamin E have nearly similar antioxidant functions?"

Acknowledgments

I gratefully acknowledge Jane Higdon, Ph.D., and Scott Leonard, M.S., of the Linus Pauling Institute, Oregon State University for critiquing this chapter. I was supported in part by National Institutes of Health grant number DK59576.

REFERENCES

1. Mason KE. Fed Proc 1977;36:1906–10.
2. Packer L. Sci Am Sci Med 1994;1:54–63.
3. Hosomi A, Arita M, Sato Y et al. FEBS Lett 1997;409:105–08.
4. Terasawa Y, Ladha Z, Leonard SW et al. Proc Natl Acad Sci USA 2000;97:13830–34.
5. Yokota T, Igarashi K, Uchihara T et al. Proc Natl Acad Sci USA 2001;98:15185–90.
6. Leonard SW, Terasawa Y, Farese RV Jr et al. Am J Clin Nutr 2002;75:555–60.
7. Cavalier L, Ouahchi K, Kayden HJ et al. Am J Hum Genet 1998;62:301–10.
8. Mason KE. The first two decades of vitamin E history. In: Machlin LJ, ed. Vitamin E: A Comprehensive Treatise. New York: Marcel Dekker, 1980:1–6.
9. Evans HM, Bishop KS. Science 1922;56:650–51.
10. Evans HM, Emerson OH, Emerson GA. J Biol Chem 1936;113:319–32.
11. Emerson OH, Emerson GA, Mohammed A et al. J Biol Chem 1937;122:99–107.
12. Machlin LJ, Vitamin E. In: Machlin LJ, ed. Handbook of Vitamins. 2nd ed. New York: Marcel Dekker, 1991 99–144.
13. Kaempf-Rotzoll DE, Horiguchi M, Hashiguchi K et al. Placenta 2003;24:439–44.
14. Kaempf-Rotzoll DE, Igarashi K, Aoki J et al. Biol Reprod 2002;67:599–604.
15. Oski FA, Barness LA. J Pediatr 1967;70:211–20.
16. Williams ML, Shoot RJ, O'Neal PL et al. N Engl J Med 1975;292:887–90.
17. Whitaker JA, Fort EG, Vimokesant S et al. Am J Clin Nutr 1967;20:783–89.
18. Horwitt MK, Harvey CC, Duncan GD et al. Am J Clin Nutr 1956;4:408–19.
19. Horwitt MK. Am J Clin Nutr 1960;8:451–61.
20. Food and Nutrition Board, Institute of Medicine. Dietary Reference Intakes for Vitamin C, Vitamin E, Selenium, and Carotenoids. Washington, DC: National Academy Press, 2000.
21. Sokol RJ. Annu Rev Nutr 1988;8:351–73.
22. Sokol RJ, Vitamin E deficiency and neurological disorders. In: Packer L, Fuchs J, eds. Vitamin E in Health and Disease. New York: Marcel Dekker, 1993:815–49.
23. Ouahchi K, Arita M, Kayden H et al. Nat Genet 1995;9:141–45.
24. Sheppard AJ, Pennington JAT, Weihrauch JL. Analysis and distribution of vitamin E in vegetable oils and foods. In: Packer L, Fuchs J, eds. Vitamin E in Health and Disease. New York: Marcel Dekker, 1993:9–31.
25. Kasparek S. Chemistry of tocopherols and tocotrienols. In: Machlin LJ, ed. Vitamin E: A Comprehensive Treatise. New York: Marcel Dekker, 1980:7–65.
26. United States Pharmacopeia. Vitamin E: The United States Pharmacopeia. Rockville, MD: United States Pharmacopeia Convention, 1980:846–48.
27. Cheeseman KH, Holley AE, Kelly FJ et al. Free Radic Biol Med 1995;19:591–8.
28. Traber MG. Vitamin E. In: Shils ME, Olson JA, Shike M et al, eds. Modern Nutrition in Health and Disease. 9th ed. Baltimore: Williams & Wilkins, 1999:347–62.
29. Kamal-Eldin A, Appelqvist LA. Lipids 1996;31:671–701.
30. Bunyan J, McHale D, Green J et al. Br J Nutr 1961;15:253–57.
31. Boscoboinik D, Szewczyk A, Hensey C et al. J Biol Chem 1991;266:6188–94.
32. Stauble B, Boscoboinik D, Tasinato A et al. Eur J Biochem 1994;226:393–402.
33. Tasinato A, Boscoboinik D, Bartoli G et al. Proc Natl Acad Sci USA 1995;92:12190–94.
34. Pentland AP, Morrison AR, Jacobs SC et al. J Biol Chem 1992;267:15578–84.
35. Clement S, Tasinato A, Boscoboinik D et al. Euro J Biochem 1997;246:745–49.
36. Traber MG. Arch Biochem Biophys 2004;423:6–11.
37. Green J, McHale D, Marcinkiewicz S et al. J Chem Soc 1959;3362–73.
38. Cooney RW, France AA, Harwood PJ et al. Proc Natl Acad Sci USA 1993;90:1771–75.
39. Christen S, Woodall AA, Shigenaga MK et al. Proc Natl Acad Sci USA 1997;94:3217–22.
40. Hoglen NC, Waller SC, Sipes IG et al. Chem Res Toxicol 1997;10:401–7.
41. Christen S, Jiang Q, Shigenaga MK et al. J Lipid Res 2002;43:1978–85.
42. Morton LW, Ward NC, Croft KD et al. Biochem J 2002;364:625–8.
43. Leonard SW, Bruno RS, Paterson E et al. Free Radic Biol Med 2003;38:813–9.
44. Williamson KS, Gabbita SP, Mou S et al. Nitric Oxide 2002;6:221–7.
45. Hayes KC, Pronczuk A, Perlman D. Am J Clin Nutr 2001;74:211–8.
46. Leonard SW, Good CK, Gugger ET et al. Am J Clin Nutr 2004;79:86–92.
47. Borel P, Pasquier B, Armand M et al. Am J Physiol 2001;280:G95–G103.
48. Kostner GM, Oettl K, Jauhiainen M et al. Biochem J 1995;305:659–67.

49. Herz J, Qiu SQ, Oesterle A et al. Proc Natl Acad Sci USA 1995; 92:4611–5.

50. Strickland DK, Kounnas MZ, Argraves WS. FASEB J 1995;9: 890–98.

51. Traber MG, Rader D, Acuff R et al. Am J Clin Nutr 1998;68: 847–53.

52. Traber MG, Ramakrishnan R, Kayden HJ. Proc Natl Acad Sci USA 1994;91:10005–08.

53. Arita M, Sato Y, Miyata A et al. Biochem J 1995;306:437–43.

54. Doerflinger N, Linder C, Ouahchi K et al. Am J Hum Genet 1995;56:1116–24.

55. Yoshida H, Yusin M, Ren I et al. J Lipid Res 1992;33: 343–50.

56. Hosomi A, Goto K, Kondo H et al. Neurosci Lett 1998;256: 159–62.

57. Copp RP, Wisniewski T, Hentati F et al. Brain Res 1999;822: 80–7.

58. Sato Y, Hagiwara K, Arai H et al. FEBS Lett 1991;288:41–5.

59. Traber MG, Rudel LL, Burton GW et al. J Lipid Res 1990;31: 687–94.

60. Arita M, Nomura K, Arai H et al. Proc Natl Acad Sci USA 1997; 94:12437–41.

61. Panagabko C, Morley S, Neely S et al. Protein Express Purif 2002;24:395–403.

62. Meier R, Tomizaki T, Schulze-Briese C et al. J Mol Biol 2003; 331:725–34.

63. Min KC, Kovall RA, Hendrickson WA. Proc Natl Acad Sci USA 2003;100:14713–18.

64. Stocker A, Zimmer S, Spycher SE et al. IUBMB Life 1999;48: 49–55.

65. Zimmer S, Stocker A, Sarbolouki MN et al. J Biol Chem 2000; 275:25672–80.

66. Shibata N, Arita M, Misaki Y et al. Proc Natl Acad Sci USA 2001;98:2244–49.

67. Stocker A, Tomizaki T, Schulze-Briese C et al. Structure 2002; 10:1533–40.

68. Stocker A, Baumann U. J Mol Biol 2003;332:759–65.

69. Panagabko C, Morley S, Hernandez M et al. Biochemistry 2003;42:6467–74.

70. Dutta-Roy A, Gordon M, Leishman D et al. Mol Cell Biochem 1993;123:139–44.

71. Dutta-Roy AK, Leishman DJ, Gordon MJ et al. Biochem Biophys Res Comm 1993;196:1108–12.

72. Nalecz K, Nalecz M, Azzi A. Eur J Biochem 1992;209:37–42.

73. Sattler W, Levak-Frank S, Radner H et al. Biochem J 1996; 15–9.

74. Guthmann F, Harrach-Ruprecht B, Looman AC et al. Eur J Cell Biol 1997;74:197–207.

75. Kolleck I, Witt W, Wissel H et al. Lung 2000;178:191–200.

76. Kolleck I, Sinha P, Rustow B. Am J Respir Crit Care Med 2002; 166:S62–6.

77. Rustow B, Haupt R, Stevens PA et al. Am J Physiol 1993;265: L133–9.

78. Goti D, Hrzenjak A, Levak-Frank S et al. J Neurochem 2001; 76:498–508.

79. Goti D, Hammer A, Galla HJ et al. J Neurochem 2000;74: 1374–83.

80. Witt W, Kolleck I, Fechner H et al. J Lipid Res 2000;41: 2009–16.

81. Trigatti BL, Krieger M, Rigotti A. Arterioscler Thromb Vasc Biol 2003;23:1732–8.

82. Oram JF, Lawn RM. J Lipid Res 2001;42:1173–9.

83. Mardones P, Strobel P, Miranda S et al. J Nutr 2002;132:443–9.

84. Oram JF, Vaughan AM, Stocker R. J Biol Chem 2001;276: 39898–902.

85. Orso E, Broccardo C, Kaminski WE et al. Nat Genet 2000;24: 192–6.

86. Ingold KU, Burton GW, Foster DO et al. Lipids 1987;22: 163–72.

87. Burton GW, Wronska U, Stone L et al. Lipids 1990;25:199–210.

88. Burton GW, Traber MG, Acuff RV et al. Am J Clin Nutr 1998; 67:669–84.

89. Burton GW, Traber MG. Annu Rev Nutr 1990;10:357–82.

90. Bourre J, Clement M. J Nutr 1991;121:1204–07.

91. Vatassery GT. Lipids 1978;13:828–31.

92. Meydani M, Macauley JB, Blumberg JB. Lipids 1986;21: 786–91.

93. Pillai SR, Traber MG, Steiss JE et al. Lipids 1993;28:1101–05.

94. Traber MG, Sokol RJ, Ringel SP et al. N Engl J Med 1987; 317: 262–65.

95. Handelman GJ, Epstein WL, Peerson J et al. Am J Clin Nutr 1994;59:1025–32.

96. El-Sohemy A, Baylin A, Ascherio A et al. Am J Clin Nutr 2001; 74:356–63.

97. Schaefer EJ, Woo R, Kibata M et al. Am J Clin Nutr 1983;37: 749–54.

98. Steephen AC, Traber MG, Ito Y et al. JPEN J Parenter Enteral Nutr 1991;15:647–52.

99. Lodge JK, Riddlington J, Vaule H et al. Lipids 2001;36:43–8.

100. Birringer M, Pfluger P, Kluth D et al. J Nutr 2002;132: 3113–8.

101. Parker RS, Swanson JE. Biochem Biophys Res Commun 2000;269:580–3.

102. Brigelius-Flohé R, Traber MG. FASEB J 1999;13:1145–55.

103. Kiyose C, Saito H, Kaneko K et al. Lipids 2001;36:467–72.

104. Sontag TJ, Parker RS. J Biol Chem 2002;277:25290–6.

105. Birringer M, Drogan D, Brigelius-Flohe R. Free Radic Biol Med 2001;31:226–32.

106. Parker RS, Sontag TJ, Swanson JE. Biochem Biophys Res Commun 2000;277:531–4.

107. Ikeda S, Tohyama T, Yamashita K. J Nutr 2002;132:961–6.

108. Swanson JE, Ben RN, Burton GW et al. J Lipid Res 1999;40: 665–71.

109. Stahl W, Graf P, Brigelius-Flohe R et al. Anal Biochem 1999; 275:254–9.

110. Pope SA, Burtin GE, Clayton PT et al. Free Radic Biol Med 2002;33:807–17.

111. Handelman GJ, Machlin LJ, Fitch K et al. J Nutr 1985;115: 807–13.

112. Schultz M, Leist M, Elsner A et al. Methods Enzymol 1997; 282:297–310.

113. Smith KS, Lee C-L, Ridlington JW et al. Lipids 2003;38:813–19.

114. Traber MG, Elsner A, Brigelius-Flohe R. FEBS Lett 1998;437: 145–8.

115. Mustacich DJ, Shields J, Horton RA et al. Arch Biochem Biophys 1998;350:183–92.

116. Thiele JJ, Weber SU, Packer L. J Invest Dermatol 1999;113: 1006–10.

117. Vaule H, Leonard SW, Traber MG. Free Radic Biol Med 2004; 36:456–63.

118. Liebler DC, Burr JA. Lipids 1995;30:789–93.

119. Liebler DC, Burr JA, Philips L et al. Anal Biochem 1996;236: 27–34.

120. Drevon CA. Free Radic Res Comm 1991;14:229–46.

121. Hentati A, Deng H-X, Hung W-Y et al. Ann Neurol 1996;39: 295–300.

122. Traber MG. Regulation of human plasma vitamin E. In: Sies H, ed. Antioxidants in Disease Mechanisms and Therapeutic Strategies, vol 38. San Diego, CA: Academic Press 1996:49–63.

123. Yokota T, Wada Y, Furukawa T et al. Ann Neurol 1987;22:84–87.
124. Traber MG, Sokol RJ, Kohlschütter A et al. J Lipid Res 1993;34:201–10.
125. Gotoda T, Arita M, Arai H et al. N Engl J Med 1995;333:1313–18.
126. Yokota T, Shiojiri T, Gotoda T et al. N Engl J Med 1996;335:1769–70.
127. van Soest S, Westerveld A, de Jong PT et al. Surv Ophthalmol 1999;43:321–34.
128. Yokota T, Shiojiri T, Gotoda T et al. Ann Neurol 1997;41:826–32.
129. Berson EL, Rosner B, Sandberg MA et al. Archiv Ophthalmol 1993;111:761–72.
130. Sokol RJ, Butler-Simon N, Conner C et al. Gastroenterology 1993;104:1727–35.
131. Lemoyne M, Van Gossum A, Kurian R et al. Am J Clin Nutr 1988;48:1310–15.
132. Sokol RJ, Kayden HJ, Bettis DB et al. J Lab Clin Med 1988;111:548–59.
133. Dial S, Eitenmiller RR. Tocopherols and tocotrienols in key foods in the U.S. diet. In: Ong ASH, Niki E, Packer L, eds. Nutrition, Lipids, Health, and Disease. Champaign, IL: AOCS Press 1995:327–42.
134. Yates AA, Schlicker SA, Suitor CW. J Am Diet Assoc 1998;699–706.
135. Vivekananthan DP, Penn MS, Sapp SK et al. Lancet 2003;361:2017–23.
136. Ma J, Hampl JS, Betts NM. Am J Clin Nutr 2000;71:774–80.
137. Ford ES, Sowell A. Am J Epidemiol 1999;150:290–300.
138. Kushi LH, Fee RM, Sellers TA et al. Am J Epidemiol 1996;144:165–74.
139. Mueller-Cunningham WM, Quintana R, Kasim-Karakas SE. J Am Diet Assoc 2003;103:1600–6.
140. Reaven P, Parthasarathy S, Grasse BJ et al. Am J Clin Nutr 1991;54:701–06.
141. Traber MG, Jialal I. Lancet 2000;355:2013–4.
142. Sokol RJ, Heubi JE, Iannaccone ST et al. N Engl J Med 1984;310:1209–12.
143. Sano M, Ernesto C, Thomas RG et al. N Engl J Med 1997;336:1216–22.
144. Rimm EB, Stampfer MJ, Ascherio A et al. N Engl J Med 1993;328:1450–56.
145. Stampfer MJ, Hennekens C, Manson JE et al. N Engl J Med 1993;328:1444–49.
146. Blot WJ, Li J-Y, Taylor PR et al. J Natl Cancer Inst 1993;85:1483–92.
147. Trevithick JR, Robertson JM, Mitton KP. Vitamin E and the eye. In: Packer L, Fuchs J, eds. Vitamin E in Health and Disease. New York: Marcel Dekker, 1993:873–926.
148. Packer L, Vitamin E. Biological activity and health benefits: overview. In: Packer L, Fuchs J, eds. Vitamin E in Health and Disease. New York: Marcel Dekker, 1993:977–82.
149. Davi G, Alessandrini P, Mezzetti A et al. Arterioscler Thromb Vasc Biol 1997;17:3230–5.
150. Jialal I, Devaraj S. Circulation 2003;107:926–8.
151. Pratico D, Tangirala RK, Rader DJ et al. Nat Med 1998;4:1189–92.
152. Stephens NG, Parsons A, Schofield PM et al. Lancet 1996;347:781–6.
153. Boaz M, Smetana S, Weinstein T et al. Lancet 2000;356:1213–18.
154. Salonen RM, Nyyssonen K, Kaikkonen J et al. Circulation 2003;107:947–53.
155. Gruppo Italiano per lo Studio della Streptochinasi nell'Infarcto Miocardico. Lancet 1999;354:447–55.
156. Yusuf S, Dagenais G, Pogue J et al. N Engl J Med 2000;342:154–60.
157. Cheung MC, Zhao XQ, Chait A et al. Arterioscler Thromb Vasc Biol 2001;21:1320–6.
158. Brown BG, Zhao XQ, Chait A et al. N Engl J Med 2001;345:1583–92.
159. Waters DD, Alderman EL, Hsia J et al. JAMA 2002;288:2432–40.
160. Steiner M, Glantz M, Lekos A. Am J Clin Nutr 1995;62:1381S–84S.
161. Jiang Q, Ames BN. FASEB J 2003;17:816–22.
162. Jiang Q, Christen S, Shigenaga MK et al. Am J Clin Nutr 2001;74:714–22.
163. Ohrvall M, Sundlof G, Vessby B. J Intern Med 1996;239:111–7.
164. Hensley K, Benaksas EJ, Bolli R et al. Free Radic Biol Med 2004;36:1–15.
165. Sinha S, Chiswick M. Vitamin E in the newborn. In: Packer L, Fuchs J, eds. Vitamin E in Health and Disease. New York: Marcel Dekker, 1993:861–70.
166. Fang JC, Kinlay S, Beltrame J et al. Lancet 2002;359:1108–13.
167. Jialal I, Grundy SM. J Lipid Res 1992;33:899–906.
168. Jialal I, Fuller CJ, Huet BA. Arterioscler Thromb Vasc Biol 1995;15:190–98.
169. Richardson PD, Steiner M. Adhesion of human platelets inhibited by vitamin E. In: Packer L, Fuchs J, eds. Vitamin E in Health and Disease. New York: Marcel Dekker, 1993:297–311.
170. Meydani SN, Hayek M, Coleman L. Ann NY Acad Sci 1992;669:125–39.
171. Dabiri LM, Pasta D, Darby JK et al. Am J Psychiatry 1994;151:925–26.
172. Lohr JB, Caligiuri MP. J Clin Psychiatry 1996;57:167–73.

SELECTED READINGS

Cavalier L, Ouahchi K, Kayden HJ et al. Ataxia with isolated vitamin E deficiency: heterogeneity of mutations and phenotypic variability in a large number of families. Am J Hum Genet 1998;62:301–10.

Food and Nutrition Board, Institute of Medicine. Dietary Reference Intakes for Vitamin C, Vitamin E, Selenium, and Carotenoids. Washington, DC: National Academy Press, 2000.

Hensley K, Benaksas EJ, Bolli R et al. New perspectives on vitamin E: gamma-tocopherol and carboxyethylhydroxychroman metabolites in biology and medicine. Free Radic Biol Med 2004;36:1–15.

Kaempf-Rotzoli DE, Traber MG, Arai H. Vitamin E and transfer proteins. Curr Opin Lipidol 2003;14:249–54.

Traber MG. Vitamin E, nuclear receptors and xenobiotic metabolism. Arch Biochem Biophys 2004;423:6–11.

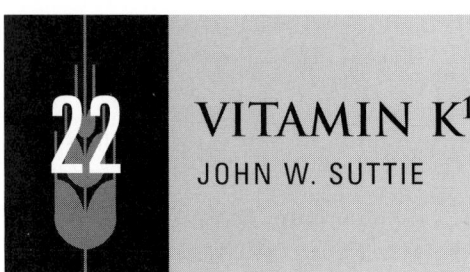

22   VITAMIN K[1]

JOHN W. SUTTIE

CHEMICAL STRUCTURE AND NOMENCLATURE 413
SOURCES AND UTILIZATION OF VITAMIN K 413
   Analysis, Food Content, and Bioavailability 413
   Absorption, Transport, and Metabolism
     of Vitamin K 414
   Utilization of Menaquinones from the
     Large Bowel 415
VITAMIN K–DEPENDENT PROTEINS 415
   Plasma Proteins Involved in Hemostasis 415
   Proteins Found in Calcified Tissue 416
   Other Proteins 416
BIOCHEMICAL ROLE OF VITAMIN K 417
   Vitamin K–Dependent Carboxylase 417
   Vitamin K–Epoxide Reductase 419
   Possible Metabolic Role for Menaquinone-4 420
CONSEQUENCES OF VITAMIN K DEFICIENCY 420
   Anticoagulant Therapy 420
   Hemorrhagic Disease of the Newborn 421
   Adult Deficiencies 421
ROLE IN SKELETAL HEALTH 422
OTHER POSSIBLE ROLES 423
DIETARY REQUIREMENTS 423

Vitamin K was discovered as investigators attempted to explain observations of hemorrhagic episodes in experimental animals fed diets with altered lipid content. In 1929, Henrik Dam (1) working in Copenhagen noted that chicks ingesting diets that had been extracted with nonpolar solvents to remove cholesterol developed subdural or muscular hemorrhages and that blood taken from these animals clotted slowly. These observations were not unique. A similar response was subsequently observed by other investigators in experiments designed to assess the nutritive value of different protein sources in purified chick diets (2) and in chicks fed fish meal or yeast as a

protein source (3). This hemorrhagic disease could not be cured by supplementation with any other known dietary factor, and Dam (4) proposed the existence of a new fat-soluble factor, vitamin K. A series of studies by Dam and his co-workers and independent studies by Almquist and Stokstad (5) at the University of California in Berkeley established that the factor was present both in the lipid extracts of green plants and in preparations of fish meal that had been subjected to bacterial action.

During the late 1930s it was established that menadione, 2-Me-1,4-naphthoquinone, had vitamin K activity, and Dam's collaboration with Karrer of the University of Zurich resulted in the isolation of the vitamin from alfalfa as a yellow oil. This form, vitamin K_1, was characterized as 2-methyl-3-phytyl-1,4-naphthoquinone (6) and was synthesized by Doisy's group at St. Louis University. The Doisy group also isolated a form of the vitamin from putrified fish meal which, in contrast to the oil isolated from alfalfa, was a crystalline product. Subsequent studies demonstrated that this compound, called vitamin K_2, contained an unsaturated polyprenyl side chain at the 3-position of the naphthoquinone ring. Early investigators recognized that the vitamin K activity of some sources of the vitamin, such as putrified fish meal, resulted from bacterial synthesis, and numerous different vitamers of the K_2 series had differing chain length polyprenyl groups at the 3-position.

At the time that vitamin K was isolated and characterized, the only plasma proteins known to be involved in blood coagulation were prothrombin and fibrinogen. Dam (7) isolated a crude prothrombin fraction from chick plasma and demonstrated that its activity was decreased when it was obtained from a vitamin K–deficient chick. The hemorrhagic condition resulting from obstructive jaundice or biliary problems was also shown to result from poor utilization of vitamin K, and these bleeding episodes were initially specifically attributed to a lack of prothrombin. A real understanding of thrombus formation and of the various soluble and cellular factors involved in regulating the generation of thrombin from prothrombin did not begin until the mid-1950s. As factors VII, IX, and X were discovered through the study of patients with clotting disorders, they were shown to be dependent on vitamin K for synthesis; for a considerable time, these three factors and prothrombin were the only proteins known to require vitamin K for their synthesis.

---

[1]**Abbreviations: AI,** adequate intake; **apo,** apolipoprotein; **DRI,** dietary reference intake; **EAR,** estimated average requirement; **Gla,** γ-carboxyglutamic acid; **Glu,** glutamic acid; **INR,** international normalized ratio; K_m, Michaelis-Menten constant; **MGP,** matrix Gla protein; **MK,** menaquinone; **OC,** osteocalcin; **PT,** prothrombin time; **RDA,** recommended dietary allowance; **ucOC,** under-γ-carboxylated osteocalcin; **VKDB,** vitamin K deficiency bleeding.

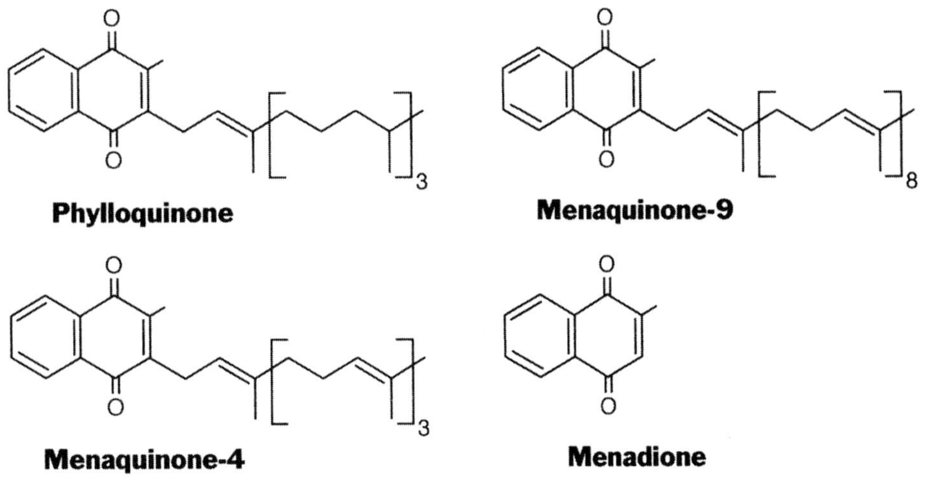

Figure 22.1. Structures of vitamin K active compounds. Phylloquinone (vitamin K_1) synthesized in plants is the main dietary form of vitamin K. Menaquinone-9 is a prominent member of a series of menaquinones (vitamin K_2) produced by intestinal bacteria, and menadione, (vitamin K_3), is a synthetic compound that can be converted to menaquinone-4 by animal tissues.

Phylloquinone

Menaquinone-9

Menaquinone-4

Menadione

CHEMICAL STRUCTURE AND NOMENCLATURE

The term vitamin K is used as a generic descriptor of 2-methyl-1,4-naphthoquinone (menadione or vitamin K_3) and all derivatives of this compound that exhibit an antihemorrhagic activity in animals fed a vitamin K–deficient diet (Fig. 22.1). The major dietary source of vitamin K, the form found in green plants, is generally called vitamin K_1, but it is preferably called phylloquinone (USP phytonadione). The compound 2-methyl-3-farnesylgeranylgeranyl-1,4-naphthoquinone, first isolated from putrified fish meal, is one of a series of vitamin K compounds with unsaturated side chains called multiprenylmenaquinones that are produced by a limited number of anaerobic bacteria and are present in large quantities in the lower bowel. This particular menaquinone (MK) has seven isoprenoid units, or 35 carbons in the side chain; it was once called vitamin K_2, but that term is currently used to describe any of the vitamers with an unsaturated side chain, and this compound would be identified as MK-7. Vitamins of the MK series with up to 13 prenyl groups have been identified, as well as several partially saturated members of this series, but the predominant forms found in the gut are MK-7 through MK-9. MK-4 (2-methyl-3-geranylgeranyl-1,4-naphthoquione) can be formed in animal tissues by alkylation of menadione (8) and is the biologically active tissue form of the vitamin used when menadione is used as the dietary form of vitamin K.

SOURCES AND UTILIZATION OF VITAMIN K

Analysis, Food Content, and Bioavailability

Until the development of high-performance liquid chromatography assays for vitamin K and methodology for the extraction of the vitamin from foods, reported values were based on biologic assays using vitamin K–deficient chicks and some measure of plasma procoagulant activity. Although widely quoted in older reviews of the nutritional aspects of vitamin K, these assays are of no current value.

Standardized procedures suitable for the assay of the vitamin K content of foods are now available (9), and sufficient values have been obtained (10) to provide a reasonable estimate of dietary intake of the vitamin (Table 22.1).

In general, foods with higher phylloquinone content are green leafy vegetables. Those providing substantial

TABLE 22.1. PHYLLOQUINONE CONCENTRATION OF COMMON FOODS[a]

FOOD ITEM	μg/100 g	FOOD ITEM	μg/100 g
Vegetables		**Fats and oils**	
Collards	440	Soybean oil	193
Spinach	380	Canola oil	127
Salad greens	315	Cottonseed oil	60
Broccoli	180	Olive oil	55
Brussels sprouts	177	Margarine	42
Cabbage	145	Butter	7
Bib lettuce	122	Corn oil	3
Asparagus	60		
Okra	40	**Prepared foods**	
Iceberg lettuce	35	Salad dressings	100
Green beans	33	Coleslaw	80
Green peas	24	Mayonnaise	41
Cucumbers	20	Beef chow mein	31
Cauliflower	20	Muffins	25
Carrots	10	Doughnuts	10
Tomatoes	6	Potato chips	15
Potatoes	1	Apple pie	11
		French fries	5
Protein sources		Macaroni/cheese	5
Dry soybeans	47	Lasagna	5
Dry lentils	22	Pizza	4
Liver	5	Hamburger/bun	4
Eggs	2	Hot dog/bun	3
Fresh meats	<1	Baked beans	3
Fresh fish	<1	Bread	3
Whole milk	<1		

[a] Median values.
Modified from Food and Nutrition Board, Institute of Medicine. Dietary Reference Intakes: Vitamin A, Vitamin K, Arsenic, Boron, Chromium, Copper, Iodine, Iron, Manganese, Molybdenum, Nickel, Silicon, Vanadium, and Zinc. Washington DC: National Academy Press, 2001.

amounts of the vitamin to the majority of the population are spinach (380 μg/100 g), broccoli (180 μg/100 g), and iceberg lettuce (35 μg/100 g). Less obvious until more recently was the major contribution of fats and oils to the daily vitamin K intake of many persons (11). The phylloquinone content of oils varies considerably, with soybean oil (190 μg/100 g) and canola oil (130 μg/100 g) quite high and corn oil (3 μg/100 g) a very poor source. Of course, the source of fat or oil has a major influence on the vitamin K content of margarine and prepared foods with a high fat content. The process of hydrogenation to convert plant oils to solid margarines or shortening converts some of the phylloquinone to 2′,3′-dihydrophylloquinone with a completely saturated side chain. The biologic activity of this form of the vitamin has not been accurately determined, and it has been found that the intake of this form of the vitamin by the US population is 20 to 25% that of phylloquinone (12).

Only limited information on the relative bioavailability of phylloquinone from various foods in human subjects is available. Phylloquinone (1000 μg) in the form of cooked spinach was found (13) to be only 4% as bioavailable, based on area under an absorption curve, as the same amount from a phylloquinone supplement. Three times as much phylloquinone was absorbed when butter was consumed with the spinach. In another study (14), investigators observed that when persons consumed 500 μg of phylloquinone as part of a meal containing 27% of energy from fat, the relative absorption of phylloquinone from a tablet was between five and six times higher than from spinach. In this study, phylloquinone absorption from fresh spinach, broccoli, or romaine lettuce did not differ but was highly variable among a limited number of study subjects. It is apparent from these limited studies that the bioavailability of phylloquinone from various vegetable sources should not be considered more than 15 to 20% as available as phylloquinone consumed as a supplement. The availability of phylloquinone from vegetable oil may presumably be higher, and in one study (15), phylloquinone added to corn oil was about twice as available as that in broccoli. A few foods, mainly cheeses, do contain a significant (50–70 μg/100 g) amount of long-chain MKs, mainly MK-8 and MK-9, and a fermented soybean product, natto, consumed mainly in the Japanese market contains nearly 100 μg/100 g of MK-7. A few data (16) indicate that the absorption of long-chain MKs from these products is substantially higher than the absorption of phylloquinone from green vegetables.

Absorption, Transport, and Metabolism of Vitamin K

Phylloquinone, the predominant dietary form of the vitamin, is absorbed from the intestine via the lymphatic system (17), and absorption is decreased in biliary insufficiency or various malabsorption syndromes. Phylloquinone in plasma is predominantly carried by the triglyceride-rich lipoprotein fraction containing very-low-density lipoproteins and chylomicrons, although significant amounts are located in the low-density-lipoprotein fraction (18, 19). In a comparative study (20), significant amounts of MK-4 were found in the high-density lipoprotein fraction, and the half-life of MK-9 was found to be substantially greater than either phylloquinone or MK-4. Plasma phylloquinone concentrations in a physiologically normal population (21) have been shown to have a mean of about 1.0 nmol/L (= 0.45 ng/mL) but values range widely, from 0.3 to 2.6 nmol/L. As expected from this route of transport, plasma phylloquinone concentrations are strongly correlated with plasma lipid levels (22, 23). The major route of entry of phylloquinone into tissues appears to be via clearance of chylomicron remnants by apolipoprotein E (apoE) receptors. The polymorphism of apoE has been found to influence the fasting plasma phylloquinone concentrations in patients undergoing hemodialysis therapy (23), and plasma phylloquinone concentrations were shown to decrease according to apoE genotype: apoE2 > apoE3 > apoE4. This response is correlated to the hepatic clearance of chylomicron remnants from the circulation, with apoE2 having the slowest rate of removal. Removal of circulating phylloquinone by osteoblasts has also been shown (24) to be modulated by apoE genotype. Details of the secretion of phylloquinone from liver and the movement of the vitamin between organs are not available.

The total human body pool of phylloquionone is very small, and early studies (17) using pharmacologic doses of radioactive phylloquinone indicated that the turnover is rapid. Limited data based on disappearance of small amounts of infused ^{3}H-phylloquinone from human subjects (25) are consistent with a body pool turnover of about 1.5 days and a body pool size of about 100 μg. Data based on liver biopsies of patients fed diets very low in vitamin K before surgery (26) indicated that about two thirds of hepatic phylloquinone was lost in 3 days, and these findings are consistent with a small pool size of phylloquinone that turns over very rapidly.

The major route of phylloquinone metabolite excretion is via the feces, and very little unmetabolized vitamin is excreted (27). Many details of the metabolic transformation of the vitamin are currently lacking. Investigators showed that the side chains of phylloquinone and MK-4 were shortened by the rat to seven carbon atoms, yielding a carboxylic acid group at the end that cyclized to form a γ-lactone (28). This lactone was excreted in the urine, presumably as a glucuronic acid conjugate. The metabolism of radioactive phylloquinone was also studied in humans (17), and investigators showed that about 20% of an injected dose of either 1 mg or 45 μg of phylloquinone was excreted in the urine in 3 days, and 40 to 50% was excreted in the feces via the bile. Two different aglycones of phylloquinone were tentatively identified as the five- and seven-carbon side-chain carboxylic acid derivatives, respectively. The investigators concluded that the γ-lactone previously identified was an artifact formed by the acidic extraction conditions used in previous studies. Evidence indicates that numerous unidentified metabolites exist (29), and treatment of patients with the oral anticoagulant warfarin, which results in a substantial conversion of the body pool of phylloquinone to phylloquinone-2,3-epoxide, also leads to the generation of new metabolites (30).

Utilization of Menaquinones from the Large Bowel

The human gut has long been known to contain substantial amounts of vitamin K in the form of long-chain MKs. Relatively few of the bacteria that comprise the normal intestinal flora are major producers of menaquiones, but obligate anaerobes of the *Bacteroides fragilis*, *Eubacterium*, *Propionibacterium*, and *Arachnia* groups are, as are facultatively anaerobic organisms such as *Escherichia coli*. The amount of vitamin K in the gut can be quite large, and the amounts found in total intestinal tract contents from five patients undergoing colonoscopy ranged from 0.3 to 5.1 mg (31), with MK-9 and MK-10 the major contributors. This amount is considerably larger than the daily dietary requirement for the vitamin. MKs, mainly MK-7, MK-8, and MK-9, have also been reported by some investigators to be present in plasma, usually at concentrations much lower than phylloquinone. Long-chain MKs, mainly MK-6, MK-7, MK-10, and MK-11, have, however, been found in human liver at levels that greatly exceed the phylloquinone concentration, which represents only about 10% of the total (32). Some evidence (33) indicates that the hepatic turnover of long-chain MKs is slower than that of phylloquinone, a finding that would account for the increased concentration observed, but a major question remaining is how these very lipophylic compounds that are present as constituents of bacterial membranes are absorbed from the lower bowel. Little evidence of the route of absorption and transport of these vitamins to the liver is available.

Vitamin K deficiency in the human adult that is characterized by vitamin K–responsive hypoprothrobinemia is a very rare condition, and numerous case reports of antibiotic-induced hypoprothrombinemia are often cited as evidence of the importance of bacterial MKs. A review of the available data (34) indicated that these cases of hypoprothrombinemia are not limited to the use of a single antibiotic. Penicillin, semisynthetic penicillins, and cephalosporins commonly have been involved, but aminoglycosides, trimethorprim, chloramphenicol, amphotericin B, erythromycin, and clindamycin have also been implicated. These antibiotic-induced hypoprothronemias have historically been assumed to result from a decrease in the synthesis of MKs by gut organisms, with the underlying assumption that MKs are important in satisfying at least a portion of the normal human requirement for vitamin K. However, in nearly all these case reports, evidence of decreased MK synthesis in the presence of antibiotic treatment is lacking, and the drugs themselves may have influenced hemostatic control. The difficulty in producing a clinically significant (increased prothrombin time [PT]) deficiency in human subjects by dietary restriction and the known rapid turnover of the body phylloquinone pool strongly suggest that MKs do contribute to maintaining adequate vitamin K status (32), but the magnitude of the contribution cannot be determined with the available data.

VITAMIN K–DEPENDENT PROTEINS

Plasma Proteins Involved in Hemostasis

Prothrombin (clotting factor II) is the circulating zymogen of the procoagulant thrombin, and it was the first protein shown to be dependent on vitamin K for its synthesis and also the first protein demonstrated to contain γ-carboxyglutamic acid (Gla) residues. Plasma clotting factors VII, IX, and X were all initially identified because their activity was decreased in the plasma of a patient with a hereditary bleeding disorder (35), and they were subsequently shown to depend on vitamin K for their synthesis. Until the mid 1970s, these four "vitamin K–dependent clotting factors" were the only proteins known to require this vitamin for their synthesis.

The blood coagulation process is essential for hemostasis and involves a complex series of events (Fig. 22.2) that lead to the generation of thrombin by proteolytic activation of protease zymogens (36, 37). The vitamin K–dependent clotting factors are involved in these activation and propagation events through membrane-associated complexes with each other and with accessory proteins (38). The amino terminal, Gla domain, of the four vitamin K–dependent procoagulants is very homologous, and the 10 to 13 Gla residues in each are in essentially the same position as in prothrombin. Following the discovery of Gla residues in vitamin K–dependent proteins, three more Gla-containing plasma proteins with similar homology were discovered. Protein C and protein S are involved in a thrombin-initiated inactivation of factor V, and therefore they play an anticoagulant rather than a procoagulant role in normal hemostasis (39). In addition to the approximately 40 residues of the Gla domain, the vitamin K–dependent proteins have other common features. The Gla domain of prothrombin is followed by two kringle domains, which are also found in plasminogen, and a serine protease domain. Factors VII, IX, and X and protein C contain two epidermal growth factor domains and a serine protease domain, whereas protein S contains four epidermal growth factor domains, but it is not a serine protease. The function of the seventh Gla-containing plasma protein (protein Z), which is not a protease zymogen, was not known for some time, but it has more recently been shown (40) to have an anticoagulant function under some conditions. Because these proteins play a critical role in hemostasis, they have been extensively studied, the cDNA and genomic organization of each of them are well documented (41), and many

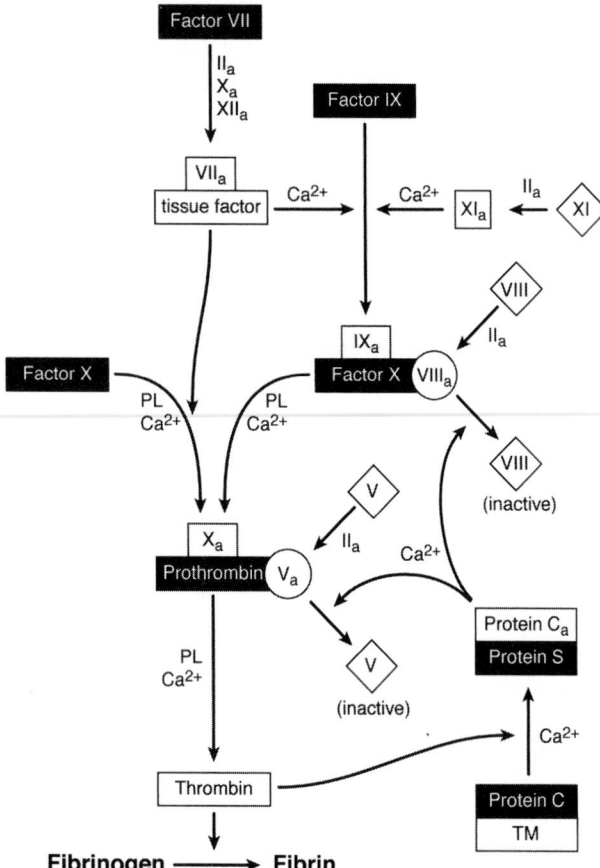

Figure 22.2. Vitamin K–dependent clotting factors involved in blood coagulation. The vitamin K–dependent procoagulants (prothrombin, factors VII, IX, X) circulate as zymogens of serine proteases until they are converted to their active (subscript a) forms. Initiation of this process occurs when vascular injury exposes tissue factor to blood (extrinsic pathway). The product of the activation of one factor can activate a second zymogen, and this cascade effect results in the rapid activation of prothrombin to thrombin and the subsequent conversion of soluble fibrinogen to the insoluble fibrin clot. Some of the steps in this activation involve an active protease, a second vitamin K–dependent protein substrate, and an additional plasma protein cofactor (*circles*) to form a calcium (Ca^{2+})-mediated association with a phospholipid (PL) surface. The formation of activated factor X can also occur through thrombin activation of factor XI and subsequently factor IX (intrinsic pathway). The other two vitamin K–dependent proteins participate in hemostatic control as anticoagulants, not procoagulants. Protein C is activated by thrombin (II_a) in the presence of an endothelial cell protein called thrombomodulin (TM). Activated protein C functions in a complex with protein S to inactivate V_a and VIII_a and to limit clot formation.

genetic variants of these proteins have been identified as risk factors in coagulation disorders (42).

Proteins Found in Calcified Tissue

The discovery of Gla residues in the plasma vitamin K–dependent proteins led to a search for other proteins with this modification, and the first vitamin K–dependent protein discovered that was not located in plasma was isolated from bone (43, 44). This 49-residue protein contained three Gla residues, was called osteocalcin (OC) or

bone Gla protein, and had little structural homology to the vitamin K–dependent plasma proteins. Although it is the second most abundant protein in bone, its function is not clearly defined. OC production by bone cells was blocked (45) when rats were maintained on a protocol of anticoagulant treatment and vitamin K administration to prevent bleeding problems. No defects in bone were seen (45) when bone OC was decreased to about 2% of normal after 2 months of this protocol. When the protocol was continued for 8 months (46), fusion of the proximal tibia growth plate was observed. OC appears to be involved in some manner in the control of tissue mineralization or skeletal turnover, but OC gene knockout mice were shown (47) to produce more dense bone rather than a defect in bone formation. Some of the OC produced in bone does appear in plasma at concentrations that are high in young children and approach adult levels at puberty. OC concentrations are increased in Paget disease and other conditions of rapid bone turnover, and OC is often measured (48, 49) as a diagnostic tool (see also Chapter 84).

A second low-molecular-weight (79-residue) protein with five Gla residues was also first isolated from bone (50) and was called matrix Gla protein (MGP). This protein has a structural relationship with OC but is also present in other tissues and is synthesized in cartilage and many other soft tissues (51). The protein has been difficult to study because of its hydrophobic nature, relative insolubility, and tendency to aggregate. As with OC, details of its physiologic role are unclear, but in studies with MGP knockout mice, death ensued from spontaneous calcification of arteries and cartilage (52). Arterial calcification was also demonstrated in a warfarin-treated rat model (53), and high MK intake was reported (54) to decrease the progression of atherosclerotic plaques in a hypercholesterolemic rabbit model. The significance of these observations is not yet established. Although evidence to support a specific function in calcified tissues is lacking, the plasma protein, protein S, which is produced in the liver, is also synthesized by bone cells.

Other Proteins

Limited numbers of other mammalian proteins have been found to contain Gla residues and therefore depend on vitamin K for their synthesis. One is Gas 6, a ligand for the tyrosine kinase Axl (55), which appears to be a growth factor for mesangial and epithelial cells. Two proline-rich Gla proteins (PRGP-1, PRGP-2) were discovered (56) as integral membrane proteins with an extracellular amino terminal domain that is rich in Gla residues. Subsequently, two other members of this transmembrane Gla protein family (TMG-3 and TMG-4) were cloned (57). The specifics of the role of these cell-surface receptors are not yet known. Vitamin K deficiency has been reported to alter brain sphingolipid synthesis (58,59), but the mechanism of the response has not been clearly identified. Other peptide-bound

Gla residues have been reported in mammalian tissue, but no specific proteins have been identified.

Vitamin K–dependent proteins are not confined to vertebrates, and many toxic venom peptides secreted by marine *Conus* snails are rich in Gla residues (60). Vitamin K–dependent proteins have also been found in snake venom (61), and the carboxylase has been cloned from numerous vertebrates, from the *Conus* snail, a tunicate, and from *Drosophila* (62–65). The strong sequence homology of the enzyme from these phyllogenetic systems suggests that this posttranslational modification of glutamic acid is of ancient evolutionary origin, and numerous vitamin K–dependent proteins are yet to be discovered.

BIOCHEMICAL ROLE OF VITAMIN K

Approximately 40 years elapsed between the discovery of vitamin K and the determination of its metabolic role. Beginning in the early 1960s, studies of prothrombin production in humans and experimental animals eventually led to an understanding of the metabolic role of vitamin K (66). Early theories that vitamin K controlled the production of specific proteins at a transcriptional level could not be proven. Abnormalities of clotting times in anticoagulated patients suggested a circulating inactive form of prothrombin, and an immunochemically similar, but biologically inactive, form of prothrombin was demonstrated to be present in increased concentrations in the plasma of patients treated with oral anticoagulants. More direct evidence of a posttranslational modification of a liver precursor protein was obtained when investigators demonstrated that the prothrombin produced when hypoprothrombinemic rats were given vitamin K and a protein synthesis inhibitor was not radiolabeled if radioactive amino acids were administered at the same time as the vitamin (67). These observations were consistent with the presence of a significant amount of a hepatic precursor protein pool in the hypoprothrombinemic rat that could be converted to prothrombin by a posttranslational modification.

Characterization of the abnormal prothrombin isolated from the plasma of cows fed the anticoagulant dicumarol led directly to an understanding of the metabolic role of vitamin K. This protein lacked the specific calcium-binding sites present in normal prothrombin and did not demonstrate the calcium-dependent association with negatively charged phospholipid surfaces that was known to be essential for prothrombin activation. Acidic peptides were obtained by proteolytic enzyme digestion of prothrombin, and they were subsequently shown (68, 69) to contain Gla, a previously unrecognized acidic amino acid. Peptides containing Gla residues could not be obtained by proteolysis of the abnormal prothrombin. All ten of the glutamic acid residues in the first 42 residues of bovine prothrombin were subsequently shown to be posttranslationally γ-carboxylated to form these effective calcium-binding groups.

Vitamin K–Dependent Carboxylase

The discovery of Gla residues in prothrombin led to the demonstration (70) that crude rat liver microsomal preparations contained an enzymatic activity (the vitamin K–dependent carboxylase) that promoted a vitamin K–dependent incorporation of ^{14}C bicarbonate into endogenous precursors of vitamin K–dependent proteins present in these preparations. Subsequent studies established that the fixed [14]carbon dioxide ($^{14}CO_2$) was present in Gla residues and that detergent-solubilized microsomal preparations retained this activity. In this preparation, small peptides containing adjacent glutamic acid (Glu)-Glu sequences such as Phe-Leu-Glu-Glu-Val were substrates for the enzyme, and they were used to study the properties of this unique carboxylase. The rough microsomal fraction of liver is highly enriched in carboxylase activity, and lower but significant activity is found in smooth microsomes. Initial studies were consistent with the hypothesis that the carboxylation event occurs on the luminal side of the rough endoplasmic reticulum.

A general understanding of the properties of this unique enzyme was gained from studies using this crude enzyme preparation, and these data have been adequately reviewed (66, 71). The vitamin K–dependent carboxylation reaction does not require adenosine triphosphate, and the energy to drive this carboxylation reaction is derived from the oxidation of the reduced, hydronaphthoquinone, form of vitamin K (vitamin KH_2) by oxygen to form vitamin K-2,3-epoxide (Fig. 22.3). The lack of a requirement for biotin and studies of the CO_2/bicarbonate requirement indicate that CO_2, rather than bicarbonate, is the active species in the carboxylation reaction. Studies of substrate specificity at the vitamin K binding site of the enzyme have shown that active substrates are 2-methyl-1,4-naphthoquinones substituted at the 3-position with a rather hydrophobic group. Although some differences in biologic activity can be measured, phylloquinone, MK-4, and the predominant intestinal forms of the vitamin, MK-6 and MK-8, are all effective substrates. The 2-ethyl and desmethyl analogs of the vitamin have little activity, and methyl substitution of the benzenoid ring has little effect or decreases substrate binding (72). Synthesis and assay of a large number of rather high Michaelis-Menten constant (K_m) low-molecular-weight peptide substrates of the enzyme have failed to reveal any unique sequences surrounding the Glu residue that are needed as a signal for carboxylation.

Only a few of the proteins secreted by the liver to the plasma are vitamin K dependent, so an efficient mechanism for recognizing the precursors of the vitamin K–dependent proteins is an essential prerequisite for efficient carboxylation. Cloning of the vitamin K–dependent proteins revealed that their primary gene products contain a very homologous domain between the amino terminus of the mature protein and the signal sequence that targets

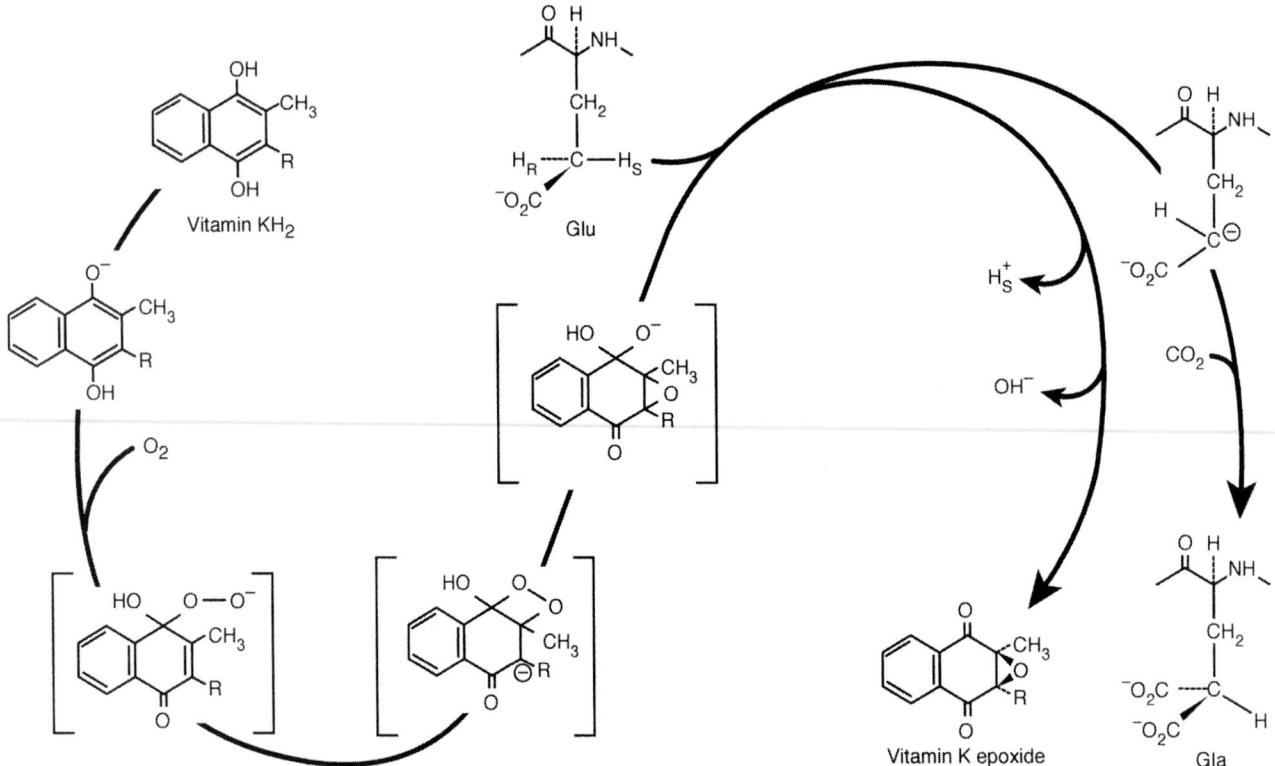

Figure 22.3. The vitamin K–dependent γ-glutamyl carboxylase. The available data support an interaction of oxygen with vitamin KH₂, the reduced (hydronaphthoquinone) form of vitamin K, to form an oxygenated intermediate that is sufficiently basic to abstract the γ-hydrogen of the glutamyl residue. The products of this reaction are vitamin K-2,3-epoxide and a glutamyl carbanion. Attack of carbon dioxide on the carbanion leads to the formation of a γ-carboxyglutamyl residue (Gla). The bracketed peroxy, dioxetane, and alkoxide intermediates have not been identified in the enzyme catalyzed reaction but are postulated based on model organic reactions, and the available data are consistent with their presence.

the polypeptide for the secretory pathway. This propeptide region appears to be both a "docking" or "recognition" site for the enzyme (41, 73) and a modulator of the activity of the enzyme by decreasing the apparent K_m of the Glu site substrate (74). All vitamin K–dependent proteins contain this approximately 18-residue sequence, which is cleaved before secretion of the protein. The propeptide sequence of these proteins exhibits significant homology, and some of the more highly conserved residues are essentially required for efficient binding to the enzyme. Although the carboxylase binding affinities of the propeptides for different proteins differ significantly (75), propeptides are required for efficient carboxylation, and glutamate-containing peptides with no homology to vitamin K–dependent proteins are good substrates for the carboxylase if a propeptide is attached (76, 77).

The role of vitamin K in the overall reaction catalyzed by the enzyme is to abstract the hydrogen on the γ-carbon of the glutamyl residue to allow attack of CO_2 at this position. Some studies that used substrates tritiated at the γ-carbon of each Glu residue defined the action and the stoichiometry (78). The association among epoxide formation, Gla formation, and γ-C-H bond cleavage was studied, and the reaction efficiency, defined as the ratio of Gla residues formed to γ-C-H bonds cleaved, was shown to be

independent of Glu substrate concentrations and approached unity at high CO_2 concentrations (79). Identification of an intermediate chemical form of vitamin K that could be sufficiently basic to abstract the γ-hydrogen of the glutamyl residue has been a challenge. A possible candidate is that first proposed by Dowd and colleagues (80), who suggested that an initial attack of oxygen at the naphthoquinone carbonyl carbon adjacent to the methyl group results in the formation of a dioxetane ring that generates an alkoxide intermediate. This intermediate is hypothesized to be the strong base that abstracts the γ-methylene hydrogen and leaves a carbanion that can interact with CO_2. This pathway leads to the possibility that a second atom of molecular oxygen can be incorporated into the carbonyl group of the epoxide product as well as the epoxide oxygen, and this partial dioxygenase activity was verified by Dowd and other investigators (81, 82). Although the general scheme (83) shown in Figure 22.3 is consistent with all the available data, the mechanism remains a hypothesis at this time.

Although a general understanding of the mechanism of the vitamin K–dependent carboxyase was gained through studies of very impure preparations, progress in purifying the enzyme was slow. Utililzation of bound propeptide as an affinity column allowed a 500- to 1000-fold increase in specific activity (84, 85), and the enzyme was eventually purified to near homogeneity (86) and was cloned (87). The carboxylase is a unique 758-amino acid residue protein with a sequence suggestive of an integral membrane protein with numerous membrane spanning domains in the N-terminus, and a C-terminal domain located in the lumen of the endoplasmic reticulum. Investigators have demonstrated (88) that the multiple Glu sites on the substrate for this enzyme are carboxylated processively as they are bound to the enzyme via their propeptide, while the Gla domain undergoes intramolecular movement to reposition each Glu for catalysis, and release of the carboxylated substrate is the rate-limiting step in the reaction (89). Further details of the morphology of the enzyme within the membrane and the location and identification of key active site residues are available in the literature (73, 75, 90–92).

Vitamin K–Epoxide Reductase

As vitamin K–dependent proteins are turned over, the Gla residues are not metabolized but are excreted in the urine (93). The amount of Gla excreted by a human adult is in the range of 50 μmol/day, so a similar amount must be formed each day. The dietary requirement of vitamin K is only about 0.2 μmol/day, and tissue stores are very low. Because

a mole of vitamin is oxidized for each mole of Gla formed, the vitamin K-2,3-epoxide generated by the carboxylase must be actively recycled by an enzyme called the vitamin K-epoxide reductase. The epoxide was shown (94) to be a major liver metabolite of vitamin K before it was known to be the second product of the vitamin K–dependent carboxylase. Investigators also demonstrated that the hepatic ratio of the epoxide relative to that of the vitamin was increased in animals administered the 4-hydroxycoumarin anticoagulant warfarin (95), and the general theory that warfarin inhibition of vitamin K action was indirect through an inhibition of the 2,3-epoxide reductase was developed (96). Blocking of this enzyme prevents the reduction of the epoxide to the quinone form of the vitamin and eventually to the carboxylase substrate, vitamin KH_2. Widespread use of warfarin as an anticoagulant rodenticide led to the appearance of strains of warfarin-resistant rats (97, 98), and the study of epoxide reductase activity in the livers of these animals was a key to an understanding (99–101) of the details of the vitamin K cycle (Fig. 22.4). Three forms of vitamin K can feed into this liver vitamin K cycle: the quinone (K), the hydronaphthoquinone (KH_2), and the 2,3-epoxide (KO). In normal liver, the ratio of vitamin K-2,3-epoxide to the less oxidized forms of the vitamin is about 1:10 but can increase to a majority of epoxide in an anticoagulated animal. In addition to the epoxide reductase,

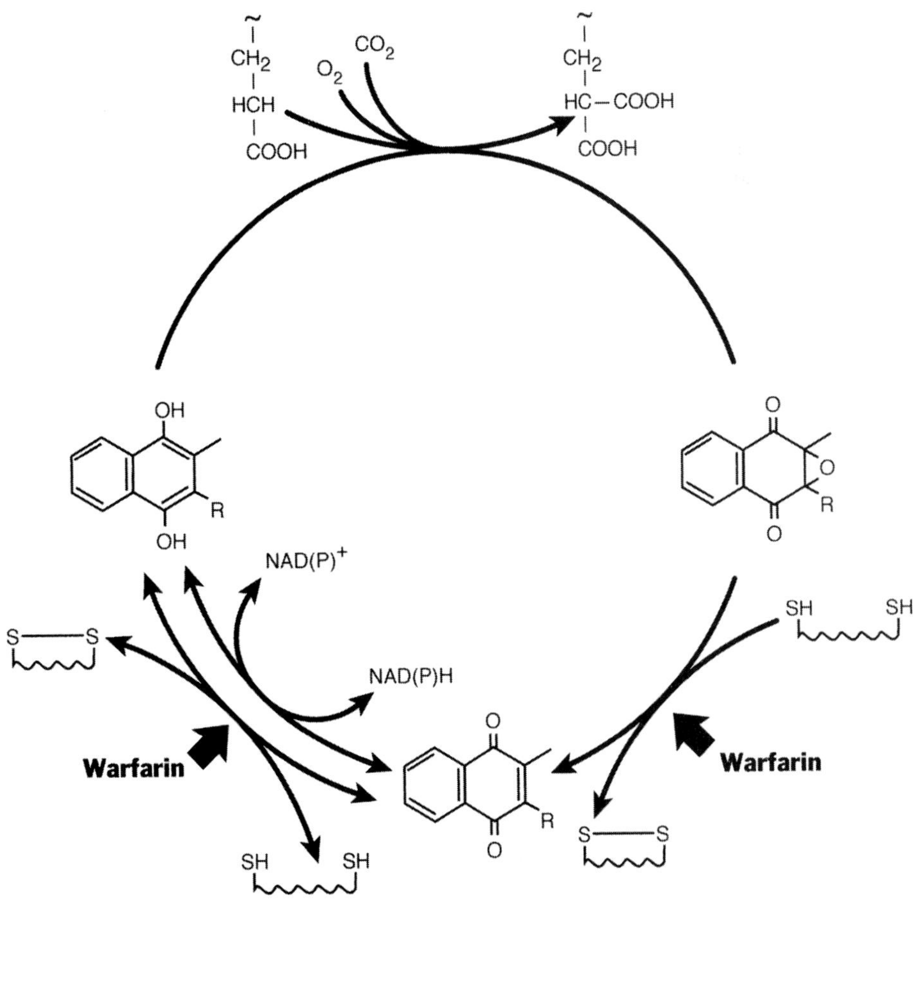

Figure 22.4. Tissue metabolism of vitamin K. Vitamin K epoxide formed in the carboxylation reaction is reduced to the quinone form of the vitamin by a warfarin-sensitive pathway, vitamin K–epoxide reductase, that is driven by a reduced dithiol. The naphthoquinone form of the vitamin can be reduced to the hydronaphthoquinone form either by the same warfarin-sensitive dithiol-driven reductase or by one or more of the hepatic reduced nicotinamide adenine dinucleotide (NADH) or NADH phosphate (NADPH)–linked quinone reductases, which are less sensitive to warfarin.

the quinone and hydronaphthoquinone forms of the vitamin can also be interconverted by reductases linked to reduced nicotinamide adenine dinucleotide phosphate. The epoxide reductase uses a sulfhydryl compound as a reductant in vitro, but the physiologic reductant has not been identified. Efforts to purify and characterize this enzyme have proceeded slowly, but the identification of the gene for this protein (102, 103) should lead to a rapid increase in an understanding of the details of this important step in vitamin K metabolism.

Possible Metabolic Role for Menaquinone-4

The ability of certain organisms found in the lower bowel to synthesize a range of long-chain MKs was recognized in the early 1930s, and human liver contains a mixture of long-chain MKs (mainly MK-7 to MK-11) that exceed the concentration of the major dietary source, phylloquinone (32). MK-4 is, however, not a major product of this bacterial synthesis of vitamin K. Investigators have known for some time that animals have the ability to convert menadione to MK-4 (8), and menadione is the form of vitamin K that is extensively used in poultry and swine rations. MK-4, rather than phylloquinone, is also the form of vitamin K routinely used in Japan and other Asian countries to prevent hemorrhagic disease of the newborn.

Observations of vitamin K metabolism in poultry in the early 1990s (104) demonstrated that the liver of chicks fed phylloquinone, rather than menadione, as a source of vitamin K also contained large amounts of MK-4. Subsequent studies demonstrated that high liver MK-4 concentrations were apparently limited to chicks, but certain extrahepatic tissues such as brain, salivary gland, and pancreas of rats and humans fed phylloquinone contained a much higher concentration of MK-4 than of phylloquinone (105, 106). Observations of the apparent conversion of phylloquinone to MK-4 in rats and pigeons in the early 1960s (107) were explained by a postulated bacterial cleavage of the phytol side chain of phylloquinone and the subsequent absorption of the released menadione and tissue alkylation to form MK-4. Tissue formation of MK-4 from phylloquinone fed to gnotobiotic rats (108, 109) and the demonstration that cultured kidney cells (109) can convert phylloquinone to MK-4 showed that bacterial action is not involved in the conversion.

Details of the mechanism of this conversion are lacking, but it seems unlikely that a metabolic pathway leading to MK-4 has evolved unless this vitamer has some specific role. This role is unlikely to involve the vitamin K–dependent carboxylase, because phylloquinone and MK-4 have similar activity as a substrate for this enzymatic activity. The shorter-chain MKs (MK-3 through MK-4) have been shown to induce apoptosis in leukemia and other malignant cell lines (110), and MK-4 has been identified as a ligand for the steroid xenobiotic receptor in bone cells (111), where it has a marked influence on the expression of proteins produced

by these cells to favor the expression of osteoblastic markers. These data suggest that MK-4 may be a control element for numerous cellular functions not yet identified, and that a role for vitamin K completely different from its essentiality for Gla protein synthesis does exist.

CONSEQUENCES OF VITAMIN K DEFICIENCY

Anticoagulant Therapy

The most common vitamin K deficiency is that acquired by treatment with oral anticoagulants. A naturally occurring antagonist of vitamin K was isolated at about the same time the vitamin was discovered. A hemorrhagic disease of cattle consuming improperly cured sweet clover hay was prevalent in the upper midwestern United States and in western Canada in the 1920s. By the early 1930s, investigators established that the cause of the prolonged clotting times was a decrease in the prothrombin activity of blood, and some investigators attempted to isolate the compound from spoiled sweet clover. It was first isolated, characterized as 3-3'-methylenebis-4-(hydroxycoumarin) by Link's group at the University of Wisconsin (112) and was called dicumarol (Fig. 22.5). Many analogs of dicumarol were synthesized and tested for their anticoagulant activity, and the compound first used as both a rodenticide and as therapy for thrombotic disease was warfarin. Several other coumarin derivatives have been developed for clinical use as oral anticoagulants. Although warfarin has a very favorable pharmacologic profile and is essentially the only coumarin derivative prescribed in North America, acenocoumarol, phenprocoumon, and ticlomarol are widely used in Europe. The pharmacology and clinical uses of these drugs are similar to those of warfarin.

The action of warfarin as an inhibitor of the vitamin K epoxide reductase results in an acquired deficiency of vitamin K at the tissue level and causes the secretion to the

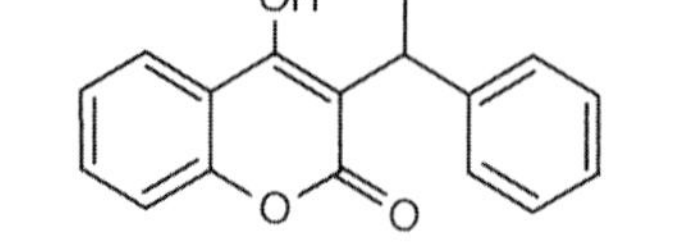

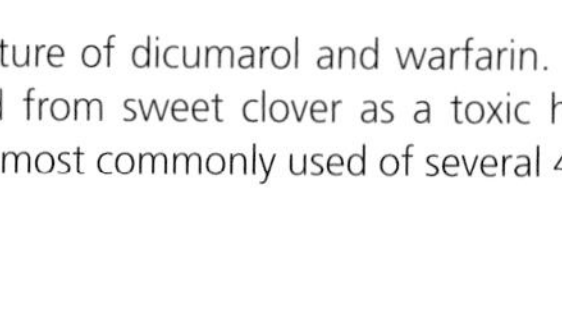

Figure 22.5. Structure of dicumarol and warfarin. Dicumarol was the compound isolated from sweet clover as a toxic hemorrhagic factor, and warfarin is the most commonly used of several 4–hydroxycoumarin anticoagulants.

plasma of vitamin K–dependent proteins lacking all or a portion of the normal number of Gla residues. The relationship between the concentration of various partially γ-carboxylated proteins and alterations in the assays used to monitor warfarin therapy is not yet clear. Although the activities of all the vitamin K–dependent clotting factors are altered by warfarin treatment, the available evidence suggests that efficacy of treatment is best correlated with prothrombin activity. The magnitude of the anticoagulant effect produced by a given dose of warfarin varies by as much as 20-fold among individuals and may vary by severalfold in an individual patient over time. Drug interactions have been found to be responsible for some of this variation, and drugs have been shown to alter displacement of warfarin from its plasma albumin carrier, induce the hepatic cytochrome P450 that metabolizes warfarin, interfere with warfarin clearance, or bind to warfarin in the gut. Alterations of vitamin K intake or absorption can also alter warfarin efficacy, and genetic variability is undoubtedly important. In extreme cases, a genetic alteration of the warfarin sensitivity of the epoxide reductase has been shown to result in an enzyme that is very difficult to inhibit to a desired therapeutic level (113).

The anticoagulant effect of warfarin therapy is monitored by measurement of the PT, which is really a measure of combined procoagulant status rather than a true measure of prothrombin activity. The PT is the clotting time of a mixture of citrate-anticoagulated plasma, calcium, and thromboplastin, a mixture of phospholipid and tissue factor or a tissue factor–containing tissue extract. Because thromboplastin reagents vary widely in their composition and functional characteristics, some reagents are much more sensitive than others to the effects of depressed levels of various clotting factors. Plasma from a warfarin-treated patient may therefore yield very different PTs when tested with different thromboplastins. To overcome this problem, the international normalized ratio (INR) is used as a standardized method for reporting PT results. The INR allows interconversion of PT ratios (patient PT/mean normal PT) by use of an international sensitivity index that corrects for differences in thromboplastin sensitivities. The goal of anticoagulant therapy is a steady-state level of vitamin K–dependent procoagulants in the range of 20 to 30% of normal (INR of 2–3) (114). The most common complication of anticoagulant therapy, bleeding, is directly related to the INR, with few episodes of bleeding at a stable INR of less than 4.0 and a relatively high incidence with INRs of more than 7.0. Overanticoagulation can be brought back to the desired level by lowering the warfarin dose or, if it is severely out of range, by subcutaneous or even slow intravenous infusion of phylloquinone.

Hemorrhagic Disease of the Newborn

The classic example of human vitamin K deficiency is that of hemorrhagic disease of the newborn or early vitamin K deficiency bleeding (VKDB) occurring during the first week of life in healthy-appearing neonates (115). Low placental transfer of phylloquinone, low clotting factor levels, a sterile gut, and the low vitamin K content of breast milk all contribute to the disease. Although the incidence is low, the mortality rate from intracranial bleeding is high, and prevention by oral or parenteral administration of vitamin K immediately following birth is the standard management approach. Late VKDB is a syndrome occurring between 2 and 12 weeks of age predominantly in exclusively breastfed infants (116, 117) or in infants with severe intestinal malabsorption problems. Although oral administration of vitamin appears to be as effective as parenteral administration to prevent early VKDB, it may not be as effective for preventing late VKDB. A report in the early 1990s (118) suggested that intramuscular injection of vitamin K to infants was associated with an increased incidence of certain childhood cancers. This led to a switch to oral administration of vitamin K in some countries and an increase in the incidence of late VKDB. Subsequent studies failed to show a correlation between the use of intramuscular vitamin K and the incidence of childhood leukemia or other cancers (119, 120). The current recommendations of the American Academy of Pediatrics (121) advise that "vitamin K (phylloquinone) should be given to all newborns as a single, intramuscular dose of 0.5 to 1 mg."

Adult Deficiencies

Reports of uncomplicated adult deficiencies of vitamin K are extremely rare, and most diets contain an adequate amount of vitamin K. The historical indication of vitamin K deficiency, hypoprothrombinemia that responded to vitamin K administration, depended on the relatively insensitive PTs to assess adequacy of the vitamin K–dependent clotting factors. Vitamin K deficiency has been reported in patients subjected to long-term total parenteral nutrition, and supplementation of the vitamin is advised under these circumstances. Although vitamin K has been included in pediatric intravenous multivitamin formulation for many years, it has only recently been a required component of adult formulations (see Chapter 99). Low lipid intake or the impaired lipid absorption resulting from the lack of bile salts also adversely affects vitamin K absorption. Depression of the vitamin K–dependent coagulation factors has frequently been reported in malabsorption syndromes and in other gastrointestinal disorders (e.g., cystic fibrosis, sprue, celiac disease, ulcerative colitis, regional ileitis, ascaris infection, and short bowel syndrome). These reports and numerous cases of the most commonly reported cause of vitamin K deficiency, a vitamin K–responsive hemorrhagic event in patients receiving antibiotics, have been extensively reviewed (34). These episodes have usually been assumed to result from decreased MK utilization by these patients, but it is possible that many cases may represent low dietary intake alone and that the presumed effect on gut bacteria was not related to the hypoprothrombinemia. The second- and third-generation cephalosporins have been implicated in many hypothrombinemic eposides (122), and it is likely that they are exerting a weak carboxylase inhibition (123) or a coumarinlike response (124, 125) that could be more important than an influence on the gut bacterial population.

Experimentally induced vitamin K deficiencies that are sufficiently severe to prolong PT measurements are rare. An often-cited study (126) investigated the vitamin K requirement of starved, intravenously fed debilitated patients given antibiotics to decrease intestinal vitamin K synthesis. A significant degree of vitamin K–responsive hypoprothrombinemia was clearly established in these subjects. More recently, controlled studies using diets containing approximately 10 μg/day or less of phylloquinone (127–129) demonstrated alterations using more sensitive markers of vitamin K status, but a clinically significant increase in PTs was not seen.

ROLE IN SKELETAL HEALTH

Three vitamin K–dependent proteins, OC, MGP, and protein S, are known to be synthesized in bone. The chondrodysplasia punctata, characterized by a hypoplasia of the nasal bridge and punctata calcification of the growth plate of rapidly growing bone, that is the characteristic feature of fetal warfarin syndrome resulting from oral anticoagulant treatment (130) during the first trimester of pregnancy, has focused attention on a possible role of vitamin K in skeletal tissue metabolism. Because of its relatively high concentration in bone, attention has been directed toward OC as a possible factor in bone health. Small amounts of this protein circulate in plasma, and concentrations are four- to fivefold higher in young children than in adults and reach the adult levels at puberty.

Investigators have shown significant interest in the observation that a fraction of the circulating OC in physiologically normal persons is not completely γ-carboxylated and can be influenced by vitamin K status (128–133). Although an immunochemical assay for the des-γ-carboxylated form of OC has been developed, most reports have defined under-γ-carboxylated OC (ucOC) as the fraction that does not adsorb to hydroxyapatite under standard conditions. Depending on assay conditions and the specific epitopes detected by the assay kits used, the fraction of ucOC reported in physiologically normal populations has ranged from 30 to 40 to less than 10%. It is clear that the normal dietary intake of vitamin K is not sufficient to γ-carboxylate OC maximally, and one study (134) established that supplementation with 1 mg phylloquinone/day is required to achieve maximal γ-carboxylation; this is about ten times the adequate intake (AI) of 120 μg/day for men and 90 μg/day for women that defines the current dietary reference intake (DRI) for vitamin K. Attempts to link this apparent marker of vitamin K insufficiency with bone health have included epidemiologic observations that low

vitamin K intake is associated with increased hip fracture risk (135, 136) and reports that ucOC is correlated with low bone mass (137, 138). These associations do not necessarily imply causation, and they may simply be surrogate markers of general nutrient deficiencies. Patients receiving oral anticoagulant therapy have very high ucOC levels, and numerous attempts to correlate this treatment with alterations in bone mineral density have not yielded consistent outcomes (139).

No evidence supports a link between increased ucOC and decreased mineralization. Rats maintained on a protocol in which a high intake of warfarin was accompanied by administration of large amounts of phylloquinone maintained adequate levels of plasma clotting factors, but γ-carboxylation of OC was effectively blocked. Using this protocol (46), investigators observed a mineralization disorder characterized by complete fusion of proximal tibia growth plate and cessation of longitudinal growth. These data suggest that a skeletal vitamin K–dependent protein, probably OC, is involved in regulating the deposition of bone mineral, but the outcome is not decreased mineralization. More recent studies using transgenic mice lacking the OC gene (47) complicated interpretation of many of the data by demonstrating an increase in bone mineralization, rather than a decrease.

Although near-maximal carboxylation of OC does not appear to be needed for bone mineralization, vitamin K supplementation is a common therapy for osteoporosis in Japan and other Asian countries. The standard amount supplemented is 45 mg of MK-4/day, a pharmacologic rather than nutritional approach. Positive responses in bone mineral density at specific sites or reduction in fracture rates of postmenopausal osteoporotic women have been noted (140, 141), and MK-4 has been reported (142, 143) to increase markers of bone formation or to increase bone mineral density in experimental animals or human subjects. The response to a similar amount of phylloquinone has not been studied, although supplementation of 1 mg phylloquinone/day to postmenopausal women between 50 and 60 years of age for 3 years was reported (144) to reduce ($p < .05$) the decrease in bone mineral density of the femoral neck. The decrease in mineral loss from the lumbar spine was not altered. Studies of the efficacy of 45 mg of MK-4 in maintaining the skeletal health of women in North America or Western Europe have not yet been reported.

MK-4 does have effects on cultured bone cells that are not seen with phylloquinone (145), and it has apoptotic effects on malignant cell lines (110) that are seen by other medium-chain MKs, but not by phylloquinone. Although most cells appear to obtain MK-4 by synthesis (108, 109), it is possible that high doses do have an effect on bone cells that would explain the responses reported. Efforts to reproduce the ability of MK-4 to decrease bone loss were studied in rat models, with success in some studies (146, 147), but not in others (148). A clear understanding of the influence of vitamin K status on bone health will likely require substantially more study.

OTHER POSSIBLE ROLES

Studies of the matrix Gla protein knockout mouse indicated that these animals died of massive calcifications of the large arteries within 8 weeks of birth (52), and rapid calcification of the elastic lamellae of arteries and heart valves was seen in a rat model in which matrix Gla protein carboxylation was blocked (53). Calcification of vascular smooth muscle cells appears to be associated with chondrocyte differentiation and cartilage formation (149), and investigators reported that the ability of γ-carboxylated MGP to prevent soft tissue calcification is mediated through an interaction with bone morphogenic protein-2 (150, 151). Reports of an association between low vitamin K intake and aortic calcification have been published (152), as well as reports of an inverse correlation between MK intake and aortic calcification, myocardial infarction, and sudden cardiovascular death (153). High intake of MK-4 was also reported to decrease atherosclerotic plaques in a rabbit model (54). Whether persons with a low vitamin K status are at risk of cardiovascular disease is not yet clear, and many additional data would be needed to classify low vitamin K intake as a risk factor for cardiovascular disease.

DIETARY REQUIREMENTS

Reference values for vitamin K intake have been established as part of the Dietary Reference Intakes Project of the Food and Nutrition Board, Institute of Medicine and have been published (10). Ample data are available to establish that essentially all persons do not consume sufficient vitamin K to γ-carboxylate their circulating OC maximally and that supplementation with about 1 mg/day of phylloquinone is needed to achieve this response. Because the clinical significance of this apparent deficiency has not been established, these indices of adequacy were not used to set a reference value.

The only indicator of vitamin K status with clinical significance is PT, and alterations in the PT by changes in dietary intake alone are uncommon to nonexistent. Because circulating phylloquionone concentration is very dependent on the previous day's intake, it is also not a satisfactory indicator of an AI. Intakes of vitamin K that are in the range of 10% of normal under controlled conditions have been demonstrated to result in decreases in urinary Gla excretion and increases in under-γ-carboxylated prothrombin, which can be measured by a commercially available immunoassay. However, no studies using a range of intakes that would allow the calculation of an estimated average requirement (EAR) are available. If available data allow the determination of an EAR, the recommended dietary allowance (RDA), the historical term that is used

TABLE 22.2. ADEQUATE INTAKES OF VITAMIN K[a]

POPULATION	VITAMIN K (μg/d)
0–6-mo-old infants	2.0
7–12-mo-old infants	2.5
1–3-y-old children	30
4–8-y-old children	55
9–13-y-old boys and girls	60
14–18-y-old boys and girls[b]	75
19–>70-y-old men	120
19–>70-y-old women[b]	90

[a] Dietary reference intakes.
[b] No alteration of intake for pregnancy or lactation.
From Food and Nutrition Board, Institute of Medicine. Dietary Reference Intakes: Vitamin A, Vitamin K, Arsenic, Boron, Chromium, Copper, Iodine, Iron, Manganese, Molybdenum, Nickel, Silicon, Vanadium, and Zinc. Washington DC: National Academy Press, 2001.

to indicate requirements and is defined as the intake sufficient for nearly all (97–98%) persons, can be calculated. Because insufficient data are available to determine an EAR, the value used was the AI. The value is defined as "the recommended average daily intake level based on observed or experimentally determined approximations or estimates of nutrient intake by a group (or groups) of apparently healthy people that are assumed to be adequate." AIs (Table 22.2) of infants are based on the phylloquinone content of human milk and assume that infants also receive prophylactic vitamin K at birth. AIs for children, adolescents, and adults are based on the highest median intake for each age group reported by the Third National Health and Nutrition Examination Survey. Based on those data, the intakes of pregnant or lactating women do not differ from those of the general population. Because indications of toxicity following the ingestion of large amounts of vitamin K are not available, the DRI process was unable to define an upper tolerable intake level for vitamin K. Appendix Tables A-2-a through A-2-k include a summary of the basic definitions and usage of the new DRIs as well as all the DRIs published to date. The 1989 RDAs for vitamin K are given in Appendix Table A-3-a. It is apparent that the RDAs are less for all ages beyond infancy than the AIs of the new DRIs.

REFERENCES

1. Dam H. Biochem Z 1929;215:475–92.
2. McFarlane WD, Graham WR, Richardson F. Biochem J 1931;25:358–66.
3. Holst WF, Halbrook ER. Science 1933;77:354.
4. Dam H. Nature 1935;135:652–3.
5. Almquist HJ, Stokstad ELR. J Biol Chem 1935;111:105–13.
6. MacCorquodale DW, Cheney LC, Binkley SB et al. J Biol Chem 1939;131:357–70.
7. Dam H, Schonheyder F, Tage-Hansen E. Biochem J 1936;30:1075–9.
8. Dialameh GH, Yekundi KG, Olson RE. Biochim Biophys Acta 1970;223:332–8.
9. Booth SL, Sadowski JA. Methods Enzymol 1997;282:446–56.

10. Food and Nutrition Board, Institute of Medicine. Dietary Reference Intakes: Vitamin A, Vitamin K, Arsenic, Boron, Chromium, Copper, Iodine, Iron, Manganese, Molybdenum, Nickel, Silicon, Vanadium, and Zinc. Washington DC: National Academy Press, 2001.

11. Peterson JW, Muzzey KL, Haytowitz D et al. J Am Oil Chem Soc 2002;79:641–6.

12. Booth SL, Webb DR, Peters JC. J Am Diet Assoc 1999;99: 1072–6.

13. Gijsbers BLMG, Jie K–S, Vermeer C. Br J Nutr 1996;76:223–9.

14. Garber AK, Binkley NC, Krueger DC et al. J Nutr 1999;129: 1201–3.

15. Booth SL, Lichtenstein AH, Dallal GE. J Nutr 2002;132: 2609–12.

16. Schurgers LJ, Vermeer C. Haemostasis 2000;30:298–307.

17. Shearer MJ, McBurney A, Barkhan P. Vitam Horm 1974;32: 513–42.

18. Kohlmeier M, Salomon A, Saupe J et al. J Nutr 1996;126: 1192S–6S.

19. Lamon–Fava S, Sadowski JA, Davidson KW et al. Am J Clin Nutr 1998;67:1226–31.

20. Schurgers LJ, Vermeer C. Biochim Biophys Acta 2002;1570: 27–32.

21. Sadowski JA, Hood SJ, Dallal GE et al. Am J Clin Nutr 1989; 50:100–8.

22. Saupe J, Shearer MJ, Kohlmeier M. Am J Clin Nutr 1993; 58: 204–8.

23. Kohlmeier M, Saupe J, Drossel HJ et al. Thromb Haemost 1995;74:1252–4.

24. Newman P, Bonello F, Wierzbicki AS et al. J Bone Miner Res 2002;17:426–33.

25. Olson RE, Chao J, Graham D et al. Br J Nutr 2002;88:543–53.

26. Usui Y, Tanimura H, Nishimura N et al. Am J Clin Nutr 1990; 51:846–52.

27. Taylor JD, Millar GJ, Jaques LB et al. Can J Biochem Physiol 1956;34:1143–52.

28. Wiss O, Gloor H. Vitam Horm 1966;24:575–86.

29. Matschiner JT. Occurrence and biopotency of various forms of vitamin K. In: DeLuca HF, Suttie JW, eds. The Fat-Soluble Vitamins. Madison, WI: University of Wisconsin Press, 1970:377–97.

30. Shearer MJ, McBurney A, Barkhan P. Br J Haematol 1973;24: 471–9.

31. Conly JM, Stein K. Am J Gastroenterol 1992;87:311–6.

32. Suttie JW. Annu Rev Nutr 1995;15:399–417.

33. Will BH, Suttie JW. J Nutr 1992;122:953–8.

34. Savage D, Lindenbaum J. Clinical and experimental human vitamin K deficiency. In: Lindenbaum J, ed. Nutrition in Hematology. New York: Churchill Livingstone, 1983:271–320.

35. Giangrande PLF. Br J Haematol 2003;121:703–12.

36. Dahlback B. Lancet 2000;355:1627–32.

37. Mann KG. Chest 2003;124:4S–10S.

38. Huang M, Rigby AC, Morelli X et al. Nature Struct Biol 2003; 10:751–6.

39. Esmon CT. Chest 2003;124:26S–32S.

40. Broze GJ Jr. Thromb Haemost 2001;86:8–13.

41. Ichinose A, Davie EW. The blood coagulation factors: their cDNAs, genes, and expression. In: Colman RW, Hirsh J, Marder VJ et al, eds. Hemostasis and Thrombosis. 3rd ed. Philadelphia: JB Lippincott; 1994:19–54.

42. Endler G, Mannhalter C. Clin Chim Acta 2003;330:31–55.

43. Hauschka PV, Lian JB, Gallop, PM. Proc Natl Acad Sci USA 1975;72:3925–9.

44. Price PA, Otsuka AS, Poser, JW et al. Proc Natl Acad Sci 1976; 73:1447–1451.

45. Price PA, Williamson MK. J Biol Chem 1981;256:12754–9.

46. Price PA, Williamson MK, Haba T et al. Proc Natl Acad Sci USA 1982;79:7734–8.

47. Ducy P, Desbois C, Boyce B et al. Nature 1996;382:448–52.

48. Price PA, Parthemore JG, Deftos LJ. J Clin Invest 1980;66: 878–83.

49. Delmas PD, Malaval L, Arlot ME et al. Bone 1985;6:339–41.

50. Price PA, Williamson MK. J Biol Chem 1985;260:14971–5.

51. Fraser JD, Price PA. J Biol Chem 1988;263:11033–6.

52. Luo G, Ducy P, McKee MD et al. Nature 1997;386:78–81.

53. Price PA, Faus SA, Williamson MK. Arterioscler Thromb Vasc Biol 1998;18:1400–7.

54. Kawashima H, Nakajima Y, Matubara Y et al. Jpn J Pharmacol 1997;75:135–43.

55. Manfioletti G, Brancolini C, Avanzi G et al. Mol Cell Biol 1993; 13:4976–85.

56. Kulman JD, Harris JE, Haldeman BA et al. Proc Natl Acad Sci USA 1997;94:9058–62.

57. Kulman JD, Harris JE, Xie L et al. Proc Natl Acad Sci USA 2001;98:1370–5.

58. Sundaram KS, Lev M. Arch Biochem Biophys 1990;277: 109–13.

59. Sundaram KS, Engelke JA, Foley AL et al. J Nutr 1996;126: 2746–51.

60. McIntosh JM, Olivera BM, Cruz LJ et al. J Biol Chem 1984; 259:14343–6.

61. Brown MA, Hambe B, Furie B et al. Toxicon 2002;40:447–53.

62. Wang C-P, Yagi K, Lin PJ et al. J Thromb Haemost 2002;1: 118–23.

63. Bandyopadhyay PK, Garret JE, Shetty RP et al. Proc Natl Acad Sci USA 2002;99:1264–9.

64. Li T, Yang CT, Jin D et al. J Biol Chem 2000;275:18291–6.

65. Walker CS, Shetty RP, Clark K. J Biol Chem 2001;276:7769–74.

66. Suttie JW. Annu Rev Biochem 1985;54:459–77.

67. Shah DV, Suttie JW. Proc Natl Acad Sci USA 1971;68:1653–7.

68. Stenflo J, Fernlund P, Egan W et al. Proc Natl Acad Sci USA 1974;71:2730–3.

69. Nelsestuen GL, Zytkovicz TH, Howard JB. J Biol Chem 1974; 249:6347–50.

70. Esmon CT, Sadowski JA, Suttie JW. J Biol Chem 1975; 250:4744–8.

71. Olson RE. Annu Rev Nutr 1984;4:281–337.

72. Cheung AY, Wood GM, Funakawa S et al. Vitamin K–dependent carboxylase: substrates, products, and inhibitors. In: Suttie JW, ed. Current Advances in Vitamin K Research. New York: Elsevier, 1988:3–16.

73. Furie B, Furie BC. N Engl J Med 1992;326:800–6.

74. Knobloch JE, Suttie JW. J Biol Chem 1987;262:15334–7.

75. Presnell SR, Stafford DW. Thromb Haemost 2002;87:937–46.

76. Furie BC, Ratcliffe JV, Tward J et al. J Biol Chem 1997;272: 28258–62.

77. Stanley TB, Wu S-M, Houben RJTJ. Biochemistry 1998;37: 13262–8.

78. Suttie JW. Vitamin K. In:Rucker RB, Suttie JW, McCormick DB et al, eds. Handbook of Vitamins. New York: Marcel Dekker, 2001:115–64.

79. Wood GM, Suttie JW. J Biol Chem 1988;263:3234–9.

80. Dowd P, Ham SW, Geib SJ. J Am Chem Soc 1991;113:7734–43.

81. Dowd P, Ham SW, Hershline R. J Am Chem Soc 1992;114: 7613–7.

82. Kuliopulos A, Hubbard BR, Lam Z et al. Biochemistry 1992;31: 7722–8.

83. Dowd P, Ham SW, Naganathan S et al. Annu Rev Nutr 1995;15: 419–40.

84. Harbeck MC, Cheung AY, Suttie JW. Thromb Res 1989;56: 317–23.

85. Hubbard BR, Ulrich MMW, Jacobs M et al. Proc Natl Acad Sci USA 1989;86:6893–7.

86. Wu S-M, Morris DP, Stafford DW. Proc Natl Acad Sci USA 1991;88:2236–40.

87. Wu S-M, Cheung W-F, Frazier D et al. Science 1991;254: 1634–6.

88. Stenina O, Pudota BN, McNally BA et al. Biochemistry 2001; 40:10301–9.

89. Hallgren KW, Hommema EL, McNally BA et al. Biochemistry 2002;41:15045–55.

90. Furie BC Furie B. Thromb Haemost 1997;78:595–8.

91. Furie B, Bouchard BA, Furie BC. Blood 1999;93:1798–808.

92. Berkner KL. J Nutr 2000;130:1877–80.

93. Shah DV, Tews JK, Harper AE et al. Biochim Biophys Acta 1978;539:209–17.

94. Matschiner JT, Bell RG, Amelotti JM et al. Biochim Biophys Acta 1970;201:309–15.

95. Bell RG, Matschiner, JT. Nature 1972;237:32–3.

96. Sadowski JA, Suttie, JW. Biochemistry 1974;13:3696–9.

97. Boyle CM. Nature 1960;188:517.

98. Lund M. Nature 1964;203:778.

99. Zimmermann A, Matschiner JT. Biochem Pharmacol 1974;23: 1033–40.

100. Fasco MJ, Hildebrandt EF, Suttie JW. J Biol Chem 1982;257: 11210–2.

101. Hildebrandt EF, Suttie JW. Biochemistry 1982;21:2406–11.

102. Rost S, Fregin A, Ivaskevicius V et al. Nature 2004;427:537–41.

103. Li T, Chang CY, Jim DY et al. Nature 2004;427:541–4.

104. Will BH, Usui Y, Suttie JW. J Nutr 1992;122:2354–60.

105. Thijssen HHW, Drittij-Reijnders MJ. Br J Nutr 1994;72: 415–25.

106. Thijssen HHW, Drittij-Reijnders MJ. Br J Nutr 1996;75: 121–7.

107. Billeter M, Martius C. Biochem Z 1960;333:430–9.

108. Ronden JE, Drittij-Reijnders M-J, Vermeer C et al. Biochim Biophys Acta 1998;1379:69–75.

109. Davidson RT, Foley AL, Engelke JA et al. J Nutr 1998;128: 220–3.

110. Yoshida T, Miyazawa K, Kasuga I. Int J Oncol 2003;23:627–32.

111. Tabb MM, Sun A, Zhou C. J Biol Chem 2003;278:43919–27.

112. Link KP. Circulation 1959;19:97–107.

113. O'Reilly RA, Aggeler PM. Fed Proc 1965;24:1266–73.

114. Williams EC, Suttie JW. Vitamin K antagonists. In: Verstraete M, Fuster V, Topol EJ, eds. Cardiovascular Thrombosis: Thrombocardiology and Thromboneurology. Philadelphia: Lippincott–Raven, 1988;285–300.

115. Lane PA, Hathaway WE. J Pediatr 1985;106:351–9.

116. Greer FR. Nutr Res 1995;15:289–310.

117. Von Kries R, Shearer M, McCarthy PT et al. Pediatr Res 1987;22:513–7.

118. Golding J, Greenwood R, Birmingham K et al. BMJ 1992;305: 341–6.

119. Roman E, Fear NT, Ansell P et al. Br J Cancer 2002;86:63–9.

120. Fear NT, Roman E, Ansell P et al. Br J Cancer 2003;89: 1228–31.

121. American Academy of Pediatrics Committee on Fetus and Newborn. Pediatrics 2003;112:191–2.

122. Weitekamp MR, Aber RC. JAMA 1983;249:69–71.

123. Lipsky JJ. Proc Natl Acad Sci USA 1984;81:2893–7.

124. Suttie JW, Engelke JA, McTigue J. Biochem Pharmacol 1986; 35:2429–33.

125. Creedon KA, Suttie JW. Thromb Res 1986;44:147–53.

126. Frick PG, Riedler G, Brogli H. J Appl Physiol 1967;23:387–9.

127. Allison PM, Mummah-Schendel LL, Kindberg CG et al. J Lab Clin Med 1987;110:180–8.

128. Booth SL, O'Brien-Morse ME, Dallal GE et al. Am J Clin Nutr 1999;70:368–77.

129. Sokoll IJ, Booth SL, O'Brien ME et al. Am J Clin Nutr 1997;65: 779–84.

130. Shaul WL, Emery H, Hall JG. Am J Dis Child 1975;129:360–2.

131. Sokoll, IJ, Sadowski JA. Am J Clin Nutr 1996;63:566–73.

132. Binkley NC, Krueger DC, Engelke JA et al. Am J Clin Nutr 2000;72:1523–8.

133. Knapen MHJ, Hamulyak K, Vermeer C. Ann Intern Med 1989; 111:1001–5.

134. Binkley NC, Krueger DC, Kawahara TN et al. Am J Clin Nutr 2002;76:1055–60.

135. Feskanich D, Weber P, Willett WC et al. Am J Clin Nutr 1999; 69:74–9.

136. Booth SL, Tucker KI, Chen H et al. Am J Clin Nutr 2000; 71: 1201–8.

137. Vergnaud P, Garnero P, Meunier PJ et al. J Clin Endocrinol Metab 1997;82:719–24.

138. Szulc P, Arlot M, Chapuy MC et al. J Bone Miner Res 1994; 9:1591–5.

139. Caraballo PJ, Gabriel SE, Castro MR et al. Osteoporos Int 1999;9:441–8.

140. Orimo H, Shiraki M, Tomita A et al. J Bone Miner Metab 1998;16:106–12.

141. Shiraki M, Shiraki Y, Aoki C et al. J Bone Miner Res 2000; 15:515–21.

142. Iwamoto I, Kosha S, Fujino T et al. Gynecol Obstet Invest 2002;53:144–8.

143. Ozuru R, Sugimoto T, Yamaguchi T et al. Endocrine J 2002; 49:363–70.

144. Braam LA, Knapen MH, Geusens P et al. Calcif Tissue Int 2003;73:21–6.

145. Binkley NC, Suttie JW. J Nutr 1995;125:1812–21.

146. Akiyama Y, Hara K, Kobayashi M et al. Jpn J Pharmacol 1999; 80:67–74.

147. Hara K, Akiyama Y, Ohkawa I et al. Bone 1993;14:813–8.

148. Binkley N, Krueger D, Engelke J et al. Bone 2002;30:897–900.

149. El–Maadawy S, Kaartinen MT, Schinke T et al. Connect Tiss Res 2003;44[Suppl]:272–8.

150. Sweatt A, Sane DC, Hutson SM et al. J Thromb Haemost 2002; 1:178–85.

151. Zebboudj AF, Imura M, Bostrom K. J Biol Chem 2002;277: 4388–94.

152. Jie KS, Bots ML, Vermeer C et al. Atherosclerosis 1995;116: 117–23.

153. Geleijnse JM, Vermeer C, Schurgers LJ et al. Thromb Haemost 2001;[Suppl ISTH XVIII]:473.

23

THIAMIN[1]
ROGER F. BUTTERWORTH

HISTORICAL LANDMARKS 426
CHEMISTRY AND BIOCHEMISTRY 426
DIETARY SOURCES AND REQUIREMENTS 426
THIAMINASES AND ANTITHIAMIN COMPOUNDS
    IN FOODS 427
ABSORPTION AND EXCRETION 428
ROLE OF THIAMIN IN CELL FUNCTION 428
    Enzyme Cofactor 428
    Component of Neuronal Membranes 429
SELECTIVE NEURONAL CELL DEATH RESULTING
    FROM THIAMIN DEFICIENCY 429
    Cellular Energy Failure 429
    Oxidative Stress 429
MEASUREMENT OF THIAMIN STATUS 430
    Erythrocyte Transketolase Activation Assay 430
    High-Performance Liquid Chromotography 430
HUMAN THIAMIN DEFICIENCY DISORDERS 430
    Beriberi 430
    Wernicke Encephalopathy (Wernicke-Korsakoff
        Syndrome) 431
    Thiamin Diphosphate–Dependent Enzymes
        in Brain in Neurodegenerative Diseases 431
    Other Thiamin-Related Disorders 432
    Clinical Response to Thiamin Administration 432

HISTORICAL LANDMARKS

Chinese medical texts referred to beriberi as early as 2700 BC, but it was not until AD 1884 that Takaki, a surgeon general in the Japanese navy, showed that the disease was the consequence of dietary inadequacy. Some years later, Eijkman, a military doctor in the Dutch Indies, discovered that fowl fed on a diet of cooked, polished rice developed paralysis that he attributed to a nerve poison in the endosperm of rice. An associate, Grijns, later correctly interpreted the connection between excessive consumption of polished rice and beriberi; he concluded that rice

contained an essential nutrient in the outer layers of the grain that was removed in polishing (1). In 1911, Funk isolated an antineuritic substance from rice bran that he called a "vitamine" on account of its containing an amino group. Dutch chemists, again working in Java, went on to isolate and crystallize the active agent whose structure (Fig. 23.1) was later determined by Williams, a US chemist, in 1934. Thiamin was finally synthesized in 1936.

CHEMISTRY AND BIOCHEMISTRY

Chemically, thiamin (also known as vitamin B or aneurin) is 3-(4-amino-2-methylpyrimid-5-ylmethyl)-5-(2-hydroxyethyl)-4-methylthiazonium (see Fig. 23.1) and has a molecular weight (as the hydrochloride salt) of 337.3 (2). Thiamin is a water-soluble vitamin. Aqueous solutions of thiamin are stable at acid pH but are unstable in alkaline solutions or when exposed to ultraviolet light. Both the pyrimidine and thiazole moities (see Fig. 23.1) are necessary for biologic activity(3). Thiamin is readily cleaved at the methylene bridge by sulfite treatment of pH 6.0.

DIETARY SOURCES AND REQUIREMENTS

Thiamin concentrations are highest in yeast and in the pericarp and germ of cereals (3, 4). Major dietary sources of thiamin are shown in Table 23.1. An extensive list of food sources and contents of this vitamin is given in Appendix Table A-23.

Most cereals and breads are nowadays fortified with thiamin. Conversely, milk and dairy products, seafood, and most fruits are poor sources of thiamin, and thiamin is absent from refined sugars. Thiamin is sensitive to high temperatures, and prolonged cooking of foods may result in a loss of thiamin content. Baking of bread, for example, leads to a 20 to 30% reduction in thiamin, and pasteurization of milk may also result in thiamin losses of up to 20%. In contrast, freezing of foods does not result in significant reductions of thiamin content. Because thiamin is a water-soluble vitamin, significant amounts are lost in discarded cooking water. Thiamin is also destroyed by x-rays and by ultraviolet irradiation of food stuffs (3, 4). Dietary reference intake values for thiamin by life stage group (4) are shown in Table 23.2.

Thiamin deficiency may result from inadequate dietary intake of the vitamin as well as from decreased absorption,

---

[1]**Abbreviations: HIV-AIDS,** human immunodeficiency virus–acquired immunodeficiency syndrome; **HPLC,** high-performance liquid chromatography; **αKGDH,** α-ketoglutarate dehydrogenase; **KP,** Korsakoff psychosis; **TDP,** thiamin diphosphate; **TTP,** thiamin triphosphate; **WE,** Wernicke encephalopathy.

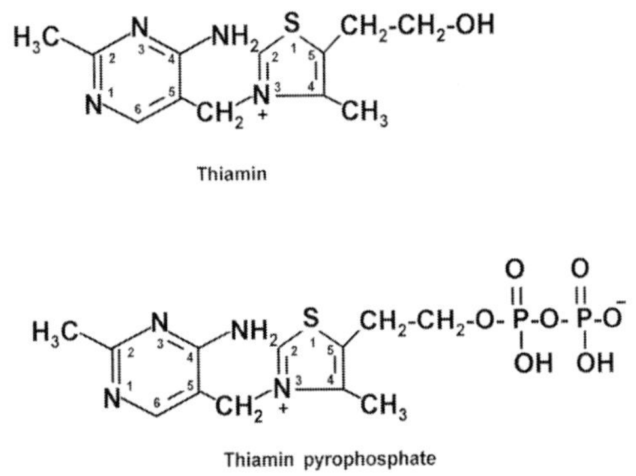

Figure 23.1. The thiamin molecule consists of a pyrimidine ring and a thiazole moiety, which are linked by a methylene (CH_2) bridge. Thiamin is a water-soluble white crystalline solid.

TABLE 23.1. THIAMIN CONTENT OF COMMON FOODS

FOOD TYPE	THIAMIN CONTENT (mg/100 g)
Wheat flour (wholemeal)	0.4–0.5
Rice	
Whole rice	0.5
Polished rice	0.03
Rice bran	2.3
Vegetables	
Peas	0.36
Other legumes	0.4–0.6
Potatoes	0.1
Cow's milk	0.04
Meats	
Beef	0.3
Lamb	0.2
Pork	≤1.0
Poultry	0.1
Refined sugars	Nil

defective transport, increased requirements (as discussed earlier), and enhanced losses (4). Populations at particularly high risk for the development of thiamin deficiency include patients with alcoholism, human immunodeficiency virus–acquired immunodeficiency syndrome (HIV-AIDS) (5), gastrointestinal and liver diseases, and persistent vomiting (hyperemesis gravidarum) (6), as well as those receiving parenteral nutrition (7) when thiamin is omitted from the formula in error or when the thiamin is destroyed by prolonged contact with the amino acid solution. Certain drugs such as the antihyperglycemic agent tolazamide may also cause thiamin deficiency (8). Thiamin deficiency is also seen in hunger strikers and in patients with anorexia nervosa.

THIAMINASES AND ANTITHIAMIN COMPOUNDS IN FOODS

Certain foods contain thiaminases, which rapidly degrade thiamin (3). Thiaminase I is also encountered in some raw fish, shellfish, and ferns, as well as in microorganisms such as *Clostridium thiaminolyticus*. Thiaminase II, which has an action distinct from that of thiaminase I, is found in other organisms such as *Candida aneurinolytica*. Thiaminases act during food storage or during passage through the gastrointestinal tract. Consequently, regular consumption of raw fish (with or without fermentation), raw shellfish, and ferns

TABLE 23.2. CRITERIA AND DIETARY REFERENCE INTAKE VALUES FOR THIAMIN BY LIFE STAGE GROUP

LIFE STAGE GROUP	CRITERION	EAR (mg/d)[a] Male	EAR (mg/d)[a] Female	RDA (mg/d)[b] Male	RDA (mg/d)[b] Female	AI[c] (mg/d)
0–6 mo	Average thiamin intake from human milk					0.2
7–12 mo	Extrapolation from adult requirements					0.3
1–3 y	Extrapolation from adult EAR	0.4	0.4	0.5	0.5	
4–8 y	Extrapolation from adult EAR	0.5	0.5	0.6	0.6	
9–13 y	Extrapolation from adult EAR	0.7	0.7	0.9	0.9	
14–18 y	Extrapolation from adult EAR	1.0	0.9	1.2	1.0	
18–>70 y	Depletion/repletion studies; erthrocyte transketolase activity	1.0	0.8	1.2	1.1	
Pregnancy 14–50 y	Adult female EAR plus estimated daily thiamin accumulation by fetus	1.2		1.4		
Lactation 14–50 y	Adolescent female EAR plus average amount of thiamin secreted in human milk	1.2		1.4		

[a] EAR, estimated average requirement, the intake that meets the estimated nutrient needs of half of the individuals in a group.

[b] RDA, recommended dietary allowance, the intake that meets the nutrient need of almost all (97–98%) of individuals in a group.

[c] AI, adequate intake, the observed average of experimentally determined intake by a defined population or subgroup that appears to sustain a defined nutritional status, such as growth rate, normal circulating nutrient values, or other functional indicators of health. The AI is used if sufficient scientific evidence is not available to derive an EAR. For healthy infants receiving human milk, the AI is the mean intake. The AI is not equivalent to an RDA.

From Food and Nutrition Board, Institute of Medicine. Dietary Reference Intakes for Thiamin, Riboflavin, Niacin, Vitamin B_6, Folate, Vitamin B_{12}, Biotin, and Choline. Washington, DC: National Academy Press, 1998:58–86, with permission.

are risk factors for the development of thiamin deficiency. Thiaminases are thermolabile.

Antithiamin compounds, conversely, are thermostable and have been identified in some ferns, teas, and betel nut, in which the toxic agents were found to be analogs of polyphenolic compounds such as tannic acid (tannin).

ABSORPTION AND EXCRETION

Thiamin is absorbed by the small intestine by two distinct mechanisms, namely, active transport (at concentrations <2 μmol/L) and passive diffusion (at higher concentrations) (3). Active thiamin transport is greatest in jejunum and ileum. Intestinal transport of thiamin is rate limiting in humans. Following uptake from the gastrointestinal tract, thiamin is transported by the portal blood to the liver.

Total thiamin concentrations in the normal adult human body have been estimated to be of the order of 25 to 30 mg. Relatively high concentrations are found in skeletal muscle, heart, liver, kidney, and brain. Thiamin turnover rates in brain are region dependent (Table 23.3), with highest turnover rates evident in more caudal brain structures and cerebellum compared with rostrally situated structures such as striatum and cerebral cortex (9). Given these relatively fast turnover rates and because thiamin is not stored to any large extent in any tissue, a continuous dietary supply is necessary. Thiamin and its acid metabolites (2-methyl-4-amino-5-pyrimidine carboxylic acid, 4-methyl-thiazole-5-acetic acid and thiamin acetic acid) are excreted principally in the urine (3).

ROLE OF THIAMIN IN CELL FUNCTION

Enzyme Cofactor

Following uptake into the cell, thiamin is rapidly phosphorylated to its diphosphate ester (thiamin diphosphate [TDP]), previously referred to as thiamin pyrophospate.

TABLE 23.3. THIAMIN TURNOVER RATES IN PERIPHERAL NERVE, SPINAL CORD, AND BRAIN REGIONS

THIAMIN TURNOVER RATE (μg/g tissue/h)	
Peripheral nerve	0.58
Spinal cord	0.39
Brain	
Cerebellum	0.55
Medulla oblongata	0.54
Pons	0.45
Hypothalamus	0.36
Midbrain	0.29
Striatum	0.27
Cerebral cortex	0.16

Adapted from Rindi G, Patrini C, Comincioli V et al. Thiamine content and turnover rates of some rat nervous regions, using labeled thiamine as a tracer. Brain Res 1980;181:369–80, with permission.

TDP is an essential cofactor for important enzymes involved in glucose and amino acid metabolism by the cell (10–12). Such enzymes include transketolase, a key enzyme component of the pentose shunt pathway, pyruvate dehydrogenase complex, an enzyme complex situated at the point of entry of pyruvate carbon into the tricarboxylic acid cycle, α-ketoglutarate dehydrogenase (αKGDH), a rate-limiting enzyme and constituent of the tricarboxylic acid cycle, and branched-chain keto acid dehydrogenases. The first three of these TDP-dependent enzymes are implicated in glucose and energy metabolism by the cell, as shown in simplified schematic form in Figure 23.2.

Not surprisingly, given the mitochondrial localization of the dehydrogenase and the importance of the pentose shunt pathway in cellular glucose metabolism, thiamin deficiency results in a plethora of metabolic consequences including the accumulation of lactate (13) and alanine (12), a reduction of tricarboxylic acid cycle intermediates, and reduced synthesis of high-energy phosphates (14). In the brain, where the tricarboxylic acid cycle is essential for

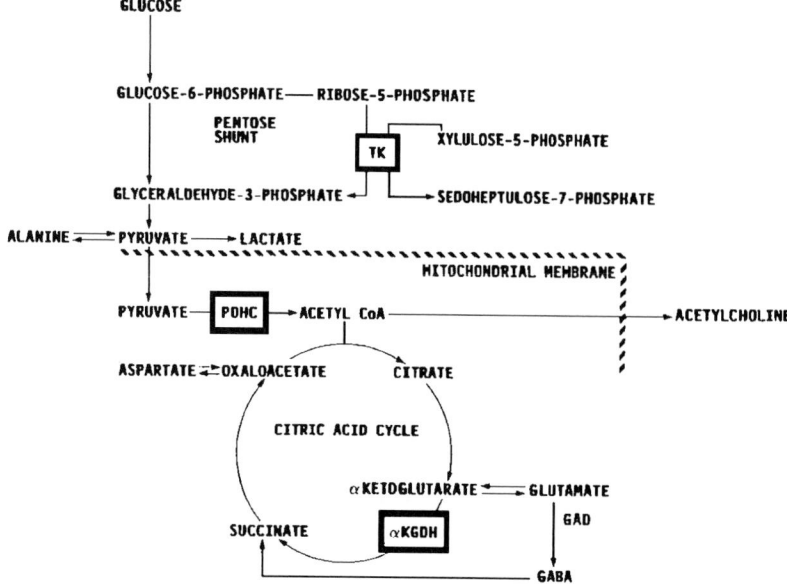

Figure 23.2. Thiamin diphosphate–dependent enzymes. αKGDH, α-ketoglutarate dehydrogenase; PDHC, pyruvate dehydrogenase complex; TK, transketolase.

the synthesis of neurotransmitters such as acetylcholine and γ-aminobutyric acid, thiamin deficiency also results in decreases in their synthesis (7, 11, 12) (see Fig. 23.2). Addition of thiamin to thiamin-deprived cellular preparations in vitro (15) or to intact thiamin-deficient animals (12) results in a rapid normalization in activities of TDP-dependent enzymes and their associated metabolites and neurotransmitters (12). This reversible metabolic phenomenon has been referred to as "the biochemical lesion" in thiamin deficiency.

Component of Neuronal Membranes

Electrical stimulation of nerve preparations results in the release of thiamin, a finding that led to the proposal that thiamin has a cellular function distinct from its role in the form of TDP as enzyme cofactor (discussed earlier). TDP may be further phosphorylated to thiamin triphosphate (TTP) by the enzyme TDP phosphoryltransferase, which is expressed in brain, liver, kidney, and heart. The precise role of TTP has yet to be determined, but investigators have suggested that it activates high-conductance chloride channels (16). TTP also has regulatory properties on certain proteins involved in the clustering of acetycholine receptors suggestive of a direct role in the regulation of cholinergic neurotransmission (17).

TTP is rapidly hydrolyzed to TDP (by the action of TTPase) then to thiamin monophosphate by the action of TDPase and finally to free thiamin by the action of thiamin monophosphatase). Recent studies suggest that thiamin phosphorylation-dephosphorylation reactions represent a compartmentalized series of processes in brain involving both neurons and surrounding glial cells (18). Genes coding for the enzymes involved in thiamin phosphorylation and dephosphorylation are currently being cloned and characterized, and this information is expected to assist greatly in our understanding of the role of these processes in cellular function.

SELECTIVE NEURONAL CELL DEATH RESULTING FROM THIAMIN DEFICIENCY

Investigators have proposed that thiamin deficiency leads to two distinct types of neuropathologic lesions. The first type comprises neuronal disintegration, mild endothelial swelling, and sparing of the neuropil, generally confined to the thalamus and inferior olives. Conversely, destruction of the neuropil, endothelial swelling, and neuronal sparing occur in mammillary bodies and periventricular brainstem nuclei (19). Several mechanisms have been proposed to explain the phenomenon of selective neuronal cell damage and death resulting from thiamin deficiency.

Cellular Energy Failure

As discussed earlier, thiamin deficiency is characterized by decreases in brain concentrations of TDP and a reduction in activities of TDP-dependent enzymes (12). Attention has been focused particularly on the role of decreased αKGDH in the pathogenesis of neuronal cell death resulting from thiamin deficiency because it is well established that αKGDH is a rate-limiting enzyme in the tricarboxylic acid cycle responsible for cellular energy production.

Prolonged reductions in activity of αKGDH resulting from thiamin deficiency lead to decreased glucose (pyruvate) oxidation and increased brain concentrations of alanine and lactate. Studies of oxidative metabolism in mitochondria isolated from the brains of thiamin-deficient animals reveal decreased respiration using α-ketoglutarate as substrate but no such changes in respiration using succinate (20), a finding consistent with decreased activities of αKGDH (see Fig. 23.2). Measurement of high-energy phosphates in brain in thiamin deficiency reveals decreased levels of adenosine triphosphate in brainstem (14). Decreased activity of αKGDH resulting from thiamin deficiency also results in decreased synthesis of amino acid neurotransmitters such as glutamate and γ-aminobutyric acid (12). Focal accumulation of lactate leading to reduced pH has also been described (13), and disintegration of mitochondria has also been reported in degenerating diencephalic neurons of thiamin-deficient animals (11).

Oxidative Stress

Increased production of reactive oxygen species has been reported in brain in thiamin deficiency (21). Other markers of oxidative stress in experimental thiamin deficiency include microglial activation (22) and increased expression and activity of inducible nitric oxide synthase leading to increased nitrotyrosine immunoreactivity in vulnerable regions of the brain (23). Vascular factors also contribute to oxidative damage to neurons in thiamin deficiency. Such factors include increased endothelial nitric oxide synthase, and targeted disruption (knockout) of the endothelial nitric oxide synthase (eNOS) gene has been shown to attenuate the neuronal cell death resulting from thiamin deficiency significantly (11). Antioxidants are neuroprotective in experimental thiamin deficiency (24).

The nature of the neuropathologic damage resulting from thiamin deficiency is similar to some degree to that encountered in excitotoxic brain injury (i.e., brain injury resulting from excessive stimulation of N-methyl-D-aspartate receptors by glutamate, a process known as excitotoxicity and shown to result in excessive accumulation of intracellular calcium leading to the activation of cell death mechanisms). Evidence consistent with a role for excitotoxicity in relation to neuronal cell loss resulting from thiamin deficiency includes the finding of increased extracellular concentrations of glutamate in vulnerable brain regions (25), and pretreatment of thiamin-deficient animals with the competitive N-methyl-D-aspartate receptor antagonist MK801 leads to significant neuroprotection (26). One explanation for the increases of extracellular brain glutamate in thiamin deficiency may relate to the finding of a selective downregulation of astrocytic glutamate transporters in brain structures vulnerable to thiamin deficiency (27).

MEASUREMENT OF THIAMIN STATUS

Measurements of blood thiamin levels and urinary thiamin excretion are not reliable indices of thiamin status. Consequently, these measurements have been replaced by indirect assays of thiamin status based on measurement and activation of the TDP-dependent enzyme transketolase in red blood cell hemolysates (28) or direct measurement of TDP in these hemolysates using high-performance liquid chromatography (HPLC) (29).

Erythrocyte Transketolase Activation Assay

This widely used assay is based on measurement of transketolase activity in hemolysates of red blood cells in the absence of (and in the presence of) added excess cofactor (TDP). The enzymatic reaction catalyzed by transketolase is as follows:

$$\text{Xylulose-5-phosphate} + \text{ribose-5-phosphate} \rightleftarrows$$
$$\text{sedoheptulose-7-phosphate} + \text{glyceraldehyde-3-phosphate}$$

Samples of hemolyzed whole blood are incubated with the enzyme substrate (ribose-5-phosphate) in a buffer at pH 7.4, 37°C with or without added TDP (10 mM). The product, sedoheptulose-7-phosphate produced per milliliter of blood per hour, is a measure of transketolase activity. The difference in enzymatic activity between the sample to which excess TDP has been added compared with that without added excess cofactor is then defined as the TDP effect.

In physiologically normal human volunteers, hemolysate transketolase activities are in the range of 90 to 160 μg sedoheptulose formed/mL/hour, and the TDP effect values range from 0 to 15% depending on the levels of circulating TDP in physiologically normal subjects. Patients with marginal thiamin deficiency manifest TDP effect values in the 15 to 25% range, and those with values in excess of 25% are generally considered to be thiamin deficient. Following parenteral thiamin administration to deficient persons, TDP effect values generally return to within normal ranges within 24 hours (28).

High-Performance Liquid Chromotography

The advent of HPLC led to the publication of several procedures to measure thiamin and its phosphate esters in blood directly. One of the most reliable of these methods makes use of HPLC and precolumn derivatization. Blood samples are hemolyzed and deproteinized with perchloric acid, and supernatants are then oxidized to their thiochrome derivatives following the addition of potassium ferricyanide and sodium hydroxide and subsequent neutralization. Analysis times are short using this technique, and recovery is excellent. Reference values for TDP in healthy volunteers are 120±17.5 nmol/L (20).

HUMAN THIAMIN DEFICIENCY DISORDERS

Human disorders resulting directly from thiamin deficiency include several forms of beriberi and Wernicke encephalopathy (WE; Wernicke-Korsakoff syndrome). In addition, abnormalities of TDP-dependent enzymes have been reported in a wide range of neurodegenerative and inherited metabolic diseases.

Beriberi

Clinical manifestations of beriberi vary with age. The three major forms of the disorder are dry beriberi, wet beriberi, and infantile beriberi (3). Dry beriberi is characterized principally by peripheral neuropathy consisting of symmetric impairment of sensory, motor, and reflex functions affecting distal more than proximal limb segments and causing calf muscle tenderness. Wet beriberi is associated with edema, tachycardia, cardiomegaly, and congestive heart failure in addition to peripheral neuropathy. Hemodynamic changes in wet beriberi include high cardiac output and low peripheral resistance. Rarely, patients manifest fulminant or "shoshin" beriberi, the major features of which are tachycardia and circulatory collapse.

Developing brain is more sensitive than adult brain to the deleterious effects of thiamin deficiency (30, 31); for example, it is well established that infantile beriberi occurs in infants breast-fed by mothers who themselves may be asymptomatic. Reports from many world populations continue to describe a high prevalence of thiamin deficiency and its complications in pregnant and lactating women, a population known to have increased thiamin requirements. Populations at particular high risk for the development of maternal thiamin deficiency include victims of trade embargoes as well as displaced persons in refugee camps (32).

Increased thiamin requirements during the third semester of pregnancy are thought to result from increased sequestration by the fetus and placenta. Thiamin concentrations are higher in umbilical cord blood compared with maternal blood, a finding consistent with preferential delivery of thiamin to the developing infant.

The major cause of maternal thiamin deficiency in many parts of the world continues to be the eating of a staple diet of polished rice together with ingestion of foods containing thiaminases or antithiamine compounds. Other causes of maternal thiamin deficiency include alcohol abuse, gastrointestinal disease, hyperemesis gravidarum, and HIV-AIDS. Investigators have shown that maternal thiamin deficiency contributes to intrauterine growth retardation (30), a condition that results in delayed myelination of the brain caused by reduced activity of TDP-dependent enzymes. Maternal thiamin deficiency may also contribute to the pathogenesis of the fetal alcohol syndrome.

Infantile beriberi commonly presents between the ages of 2 and 6 months. Infants may manifest cardiac, aphonic, or pseudomeningitic forms of the disorder. Infants with cardiac beriberi frequently exhibit a loud piercing cry, vomiting, and tachycardia (3). Convulsions are not uncommon, and death may ensue if thiamin is not administered promptly.

Wernicke Encephalopathy (Wernicke-Korsakoff Syndrome)

WE is a common neuropsychiatric complication of chronic alcoholism (10). It is also encountered in patients with severe gastrointestinal disease, those with HIV-AIDS (5), and with the injudicious administration of parenteral glucose or hyperalimentation without adequate B-vitamin supplementation (5). Activities of all three TDP-dependent enzymes are reduced in brain tissue obtained at autopsy from patients with WE (33).

In patients with alcoholism, thiamin deficiency results from inadequate dietary intake of the vitamin, reduced absorption from gastrointestinal disease, and reduced liver thiamin stores caused by hepatic steatosis or fibrosis (10). In addition, ethanol per se inhibits thiamin transport in the gastrointestinal system and blocks phosphorylation of thiamin to its cofactor form (TDP) (34).

The diagnosis of WE is based generally on the acute appearance of ocular palsies, nystagmus, and ataxia of gait, as well as disorders of mentation (1). In addition, more than 80% of patients with WE show signs of peripheral neuropathy. However, these diagnostic criteria are nonspecific, and the diagnosis of WE is missed in a large percentage of both patients with alcoholism (35) and those with HIV-AIDS (5). The reason for the high degree of underdiagnosis rests with the overzealous use of the classic triad of symptoms (ophthalmoplegia, ataxia, confusion) espoused by many textbooks. In practice, many cases of WE confirmed at autopsy do not manifest this triad of symptoms, and patients may show only psychomotor slowing or apathy (5). A rewriting of this textbook definition of WE is long overdue. In the meantime, thiamin deficiency should be suspected in all patients with grossly impaired nutritional status associated with chronic diseases, with particular attention being paid to patients with alcoholism, gastrointestinal diseases, HIV-AIDS, and persistent vomiting. Thiamin should be administered parenterally in a timely manner. It is essential to administer thiamin to all such patients before infusions of glucose or parenteral nutrition are given.

Korsakoff psychosis (KP) is generally considered to occur with deterioration of brain function in patients initially diagnosed with WE (1). However, KP may be present at the time of diagnosis of WE or even, in a small number of cases, present without WE symptoms. KP is an amnestic-confabulatory syndrome characterized by retrograde and anterograde amnesia, impairment of conceptual functions, and decreased spontaneity and initiative.

Neuropathology

In the acute stages of WE, hemorrhagic lesions of mammillary bodies and periventricular regions of the thalamus are observed (36). Multiple acute insults eventually give rise to a chronic lesion, characterized by loosening of the neuropil and cell loss, that manifests as mammillary body atrophy and ventricular dilatation. One also sees a significant loss of neurons in the superior cerebellar vermis in WE, a phenomenon also referred to as alcoholic cerebellar degeneration.

Magnetic resonance imaging permits the diagnosis and assessment of the extent of brain lesions. Mammillary body atrophy and loss of thalamic tissue leading to ventricular enlargement as well as cerebellar atrophy are clearly discernible (37).

Genetics

Although thiamin deficiency is very common in patients with alcoholism, only relatively small numbers (10–12%) go on to develop WE, an observation that led to the proposal of a genetic predisposition to the disorder. A great deal of attention in this regard has been paid to the TDP-dependent enzyme transketolase. Initially, investigators proposed that a reduction in affinity of transketolase for its cofactor (TDP) could represent one such genetic abnormality. Reports of both biochemical and chromatographic variants of transketolase in cells from patients with WE have appeared in the literature (38, 39). However, more recently the coding sequences of the transketolase gene were compared between cells from physiologically normal individuals and from patients with WE, and no significant differences were observed (40), a finding suggesting that, if alterations of transketolase do exist in these patients, these alterations are posttranslational. Further studies are required to clarify this issue.

Thiamin Diphosphate–Dependent Enzymes in Brain in Neurodegenerative Diseases

Brain tissue obtained at autopsy from patients with Alzheimer disease contains reduced activities of TDP-dependent enzymes (41, 42). Activities of αKGDH in particular are significantly reduced in both genetic and sporadic forms of Alzheimer disease. Decreased activities of αKGDH have also been described in the brains of patients with other neurodegenerative diseases including Parkinson disease and progressive subnuclear palsy (11). The most plausible explanation for the selective loss of αKGDH activity in these diseases may relate to the deleterious effects of oxidative stress resulting from the cell death cascade mechanisms in these disorders (11).

Other Thiamin-Related Disorders

Other disorders in which a putative role for thiamin has been implicated include subacute necrotizing encephalomyelopathy, opsoclonic cerebellopathy (a paraneoplastic syndrome), and Nigerian seasonal ataxia. In addition, several inherited disorders of TDP-dependent enzymes have been reported (43). Some of these latter disorders may respond to thiamin treatment.

Clinical Response to Thiamin Administration

Parenteral thiamin should be administered promptly to patients suspected of having beriberi or WE. Doses in the 50- to 100-mg range are initially administered intravenously or intramuscularly to replenish cellular thiamin stores (particularly liver) (3). Parenteral rather than oral thiamin administration is particularly important in patients with gastrointestinal disease and/or alcoholism, in whom thiamin absorption is likely to be impaired.

In wet beriberi, rapid improvement consisting of reduction in heart rate, respiratory rate, and clearing of pulmonary congestion occurs generally within 24 hours (3). Rapid improvements are also seen in infants with dry beriberi; recovery of impaired sensation and motor weakness, in contrast, may take several weeks or months.

Response to thiamin administration in patients with WE is variable, depending on the symptoms and the degree of neuronal cell loss. Ophthalmoplegia (nystagmus, ptosis) generally improves rapidly (within 24 hours), a finding suggesting that these symptoms are the result of biochemical (metabolic) lesions in ocular-motor and vestibular nuclei. Gait ataxia, convsersely, responds more sluggishly to thiamin administration because, in most cases, loss of cerebellar neurons has occurred (44). Similarly, the amnestic deficit that is generally thought to result from lesions in the medial-dorsal nucleus of the thalamus shows variable response to thiamin administration; most patients show some residual memory deficit. Improvements of peripheral neuropathy in both beriberi and WE syndrome may require several months of thiamin treatment (44).

REFERENCES

1. McCollum EV. A History of Nutrition. Cambridge, MA: Riverside Press, Houghton Mifflin, 1957.
2. International Union of Nutritional Sciences Committee on Nomenclature. J Nutr 1990;120:7–14.
3. Tanphaichitr V. Thiamin. In: Shils ME, Olsen JA, Shike M et al., eds Modern Nutrition in Health and Disease. 9th ed. Baltimore: Lippincott Williams & Wilkins, 1999.
4. Food and Nutrition Board, Institute of Medicine. Dietary Reference Intakes for Thiamin, Riboflavin, Niacin, Vitamin B$_6$, Folate, Vitamin B$_{12}$, Biotin, and Choline. Washington, DC: National Academy Press, 1998:58–86.
5. Butterworth RF, Gaudreau C, Vincelette J et al. Metab Brain Dis 1991;6:207–12.
6. Nightingale S, Bates D, Heath PD. Postgrad Med J 1982;58: 558–9.
7. Harper CG. Aust NZ J Med 1980;10:230–5.
8. Kwee IL, Nakada T. Med Intell 1983;309:599–600.
9. Rindi G, Patrini C, Comincioli V et al. Brain Res 1980;181: 369–80.
10. Butterworth RF. Drug Alcohol Rev 1993;12:315–22.
11. Gibson GE, Zhang H. Neurochem Int 2002;40:493–504.
12. Butterworth RF, Héroux M. J Neurochem 1989;52:1079–84.
13. Hakim AM. Ann Neurol 1984;16:673–9.
14. Aikawa H, Watanabe IS, Furuse T et al. J Neuropathol Exp Neurol 1984;43:276–87.
15. Pannunzio P, Hazell AS, Pannunzio M et al. J Neurosci Res 2000;62:286–92.
16. Cooper JR, Pincus JH. Neurochem Res 1979;4:233–9.
17. Bettendorff L. Metab Brain Dis 1994;9:183–209.
18. Butterworth RF. Nutr Res Rev 2004;16:277–83.
19. Trovik A. Science 1985;11:179–90.
20. Parker WD Jr, Haas R, Stumpf DA et al. Neurology 1984;34: 1477–81.
21. Langlais PJ, Anderson G, Guo SX et al. Metab Brain Dis 1997;12:137–43.
22. Todd KG, Butterworth RF. Glia 1999;25:190–8.
23. Calingasan NY, Park LCH, Calo LL et al. Am J Pathol 1998;153: 599–610.
24. Pannunzio P, Hazell AS, Pannunzio M et al. J Neurosci Res 2000;62:286–92.
25. Hazell AS, Butterworth RF, Hakim AM. J Neurochem 1993;61: 1155–8.
26. Langlais PJ and Mair MG. J Neurosci 1990;10:1664–74.
27. Hazell AS, Rama Rao KV, Danbolt NC et al. J Neurochem 2001;78:560–8.
28. Dreyfus PM. N Engl J Med 1962;267:596–8.
29. Brunnekreeft JWI, Eidhof H, Gerrits J. J Chromatogr 1989;491: 89–96.
30. Butterworth RF. Am J Clin Nutr 2001;74:712–3.
31. Fournier H, Butterworth RF. Metab Brain Dis 1990;5:77–84.
32. McGready R, Simpson JA, Cho T et al. Am J Clin Nutr 2001;74:808–13.
33. Butterworth RF, Kril JJ, Harper CG. Alcohol Clin Exp Res 1993; 17:1084–8.
34. Rindi G, Imarisio L, Patrini C. Biochem Pharmacol 1986;35: 3903–8.
35. Harper C. J Neurol Neurosurg Psychiatry 1979;42:226–31.
36. Kril JJ. Metab Brain Dis 1996;11:9–17.
37. Charness ME, DeLaPaz RL. Ann Neurol 1987;22:595–600.
38. Blass JP, Gibson GE. N Engl J Med 1977;297:1367–70.
39. Mekherjee AB, Svoronos S, Ghzanfari A et al. J Clin Invest 1987; 79:1039–43.
40. McCool BA, Plonk SG, Martin PR et al. J Biol Chem 1993;268: 1397–404.
41. Gibson GE, Sheu KF, Blass JP et al. Arch Neurol 1988;45: 836–40.
42. Butterworth RF, Besnard AM. Metab Brain Dis 1990;5:179–84.
43. Blass JP. Inborn errors of pyruvate metabolism. In: Stanbury JB, Wyngaarden JB, Frederckson DS et al., eds. Metabolic Basis of Inherited Disease. 5th ed. New York, McGraw-Hill, 1983: 193–203.
44. Maurice V, Adams RD, Collins GH. The Wernicke-Korsakoff Syndrome and Related Neurologic Disorders Due to Alcoholism and Malnutrition. 2nd ed. Philadelphia: FA Davis, 1989.

SELECTED READINGS

Butterworth RF. Thiamin deficiency and brain disorders. Nutr Res Rev 2004;16:277–83.

Food and Nutrition Board, Institute of Medicine. Dietary Reference Intakes for Thiamin, Riboflavin, Niacin, Vitamin B_6, Folate, Vitamin B_{12}, Biotin, and Choline. Washington, DC: National Academy Press, 1998:58–86.

Jordan F, Patel MS. Thiamin. In: Jordan F, Patel MS, eds. Catalytic Mechanisms in Normal and Disease States. New York: Marcel Dekker, 2004.

Maurice V, Adams RD, Collins GH. The Wernicke-Korsakoff Syndrome and Related Neurologic Disorders Due to Alcoholism and Malnutrition. 2nd ed. Philadelphia: FA Davis, 1989.

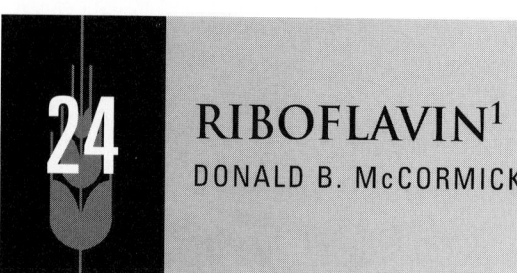

24 RIBOFLAVIN[1]
DONALD B. McCORMICK

HISTORY AND NATURAL FLAVINS 434
CHEMISTRY AND BIOCHEMISTRY 434
METHODS FOR ASSAY AND STATUS DETERMINATION .435
    Urinary Excretion 435
    Erythrocyte Assays 436
DIGESTION AND ABSORPTION 436
TRANSPORT AND METABOLISM 436
    Metabolic Interconversions 437
EXCRETION AND SECRETION 437
    Secretion in Milk 437
DEFICIENCY AND EXCESS 438
    Deficiency 438
    Excess 438
DIETARY CONSIDERATIONS .439

HISTORY AND NATURAL FLAVINS

A water-soluble, yellow fluorescent compound was known in the latter part of the nineteenth century (1) to occur in such natural materials as whey. Association of the pigment with vitaminic properties was not firmly established until its isolation in 1933 by several groups (2–4) following purification from the B$_2$ fraction of the "water-soluble" growth factors. By 1932, Warburg and Christian had isolated a yellow respiratory ferment (now called "old yellow enzyme") from yeast (5). This flavoprotein was dissociated into a protein apoenzyme and a yellow prosthetic coenzyme that was clearly similar to the yellow vitamin (6). In 1934, Stern and Holiday found that the coenzyme was an alloxazine derivative (7), and Theorell demonstrated that it was a phosphate ester (8). By 1935, the groups of Kuhn at Heidelberg (9, 10) and Karrer in Zurich (11, 12) had synthesized riboflavin, the name ultimately adopted to signify the vitamin that contains a riboselike side chain and is yellow (Latin, *flavus*). Theorell in 1937 secured the structure of the simpler coenzyme as riboflavin 5′-phosphate (flavin mononucleotide [FMN]) (13). By 1938, Warburg and Christian had isolated and characterized the more abundant and more complex prosthetic group, flavin adenine

dinucleotide (FAD) and showed its participation as the coenzyme of D-amino acid oxidase (14–17).

Intermediates and enzymes involved in the biosynthesis of riboflavin from guanosine triphosphate and ribulose-5-phosphate by some prokaryotes are now known (18, 19). In addition, diverse natural flavins have been found that have alterations in the side chain or ring system of the basic flavin structures (20). Some of these are the 8-dimethyl-amino group of roseoflavin produced by *Streptomyces davawensis* (21, 22), the side-chain aldehyde and acid products (schizoflavins [23]) resulting from oxidation of the 5′-hydroxymethyl of riboflavin by a fungal enzyme narrowly specific for the vitamin (24–26), and 5′-glycosides of riboflavin, which can be formed by plant and animal species (27, 28). No fewer than four 8α-modified forms of FAD occur covalently attached to important flavoproteins in the mammal: N^3-histidyl-linked succinate and sarcosine dehydrogenases of the inner mitochondrial membrane, S-cysteinyl-linked monoamine oxidase of the outer mitochondrial membrane, and the N^1-histidyl-linked L-gulonolactone oxidase of the liver microsomal fraction.

CHEMISTRY AND BIOCHEMISTRY

Riboflavin (vitamin B$_2$) was chemically specified as 6,7-dimethyl-9-(1′-D-ribityl)isoalloxazine, but with evolution of systematic nomenclature is now correctly given as 7,8-dimethyl-10-(1′-D-ribityl)isoalloxazine. The free vitamin is a weak base isolated or synthesized as a yellowish-orange amorphous solid. The 5′-hydroxymethyl terminus of the ribityl side chain in the vitamin is phosphorylated to become the simpler coenzyme, FMN, which can be further converted to the more complex and frequently encountered FAD with a pyrophosphate-bridged adenylate moiety (Fig. 24.1). The molecular weight of riboflavin is 376.4; thus, 1 mg equals 2.66 μmol. Chemical syntheses of riboflavin and similar isoalloxazines have been accomplished by several routes (29), most of which were adapted from the earlier procedures of Kuhn, Karrer, and Tishler and their associates, although more recent modifications continue to be introduced (30).

Riboflavin is only modestly soluble in aqueous solutions, although flavinium salts of strong acids formed at low pH (<1) and flavin anion formed at alkaline pH (>10) are considerably more soluble. Neutral and slightly

[1]**Abbreviations: FAD,** flavin adenine dinucleotide; **FMN,** flavin adenine mononucleotide; **MTHFR,** 5-methylenetetrahydrofolate reductase; **RDA,** recommended dietary allowance.

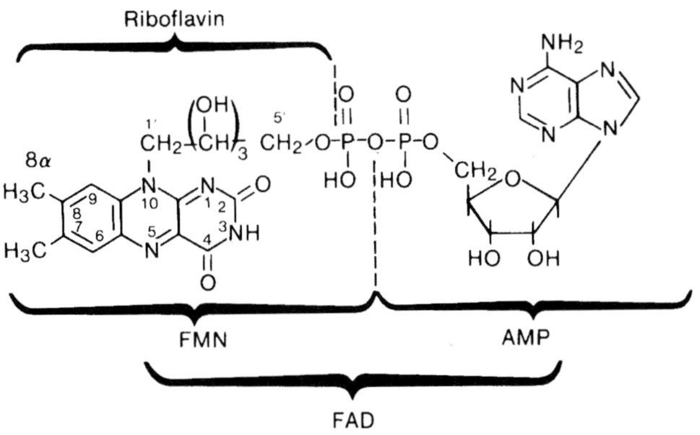

Figure 24.1. Riboflavin and flavin mononucleotide (FMN) as components of flavin–adenine dinucleotide (FAD). AMP, adenosine monophosphate.

alkaline solutions are yellow with a long-wavelength absorption maximum near 450 nm. Strongly acidic flavin solutions are paler, because their primary absorbance shifts with intensification to about 385 nm. Solutions of the neutral oxidized (quinoid) form of the vitamin are strongly fluorescent, with an emission wavelength at 525 nm. Riboflavin also has phosphorescent character reflecting triplet state reactivity following light excitation. The photoreactivity of light-excited riboflavin finds medical application in the photosensitized oxidation of bilirubin during phototherapy of neonatal jaundice (31–34) and in the photooxidation of nucleic acids of pathogens in blood products (35, 36). One consequence of flavin photochemistry is the photolability of the side chain. Riboflavin is photodegraded ultimately to yield vitaminically inactive lumiflavin (7,8,10-trimethyl-isoalloxazine) under alkaline conditions and lumichrome (7,8-dimethyl-alloxazine) at all pH values, especially in neutral to acidic solutions. Flavins are chemically and biologically reduced, often through the radical (semiquinone) forms, to the nearly colorless, nonfluorescent 1,5-dihydro forms that rapidly reoxidize on exposure to air (oxygen).

Chemical syntheses of flavocoenzymes involve phosphorylation of riboflavin (37), commonly with chlorophosphoric acid, to form crude FMN, which is purified chromatographically. Conversion of FMN to FAD usually involves condensation of activated adenosine monophosphate, such as adenosine-5'-phosphoromorpholidate, with an FMN salt (38, 39). Extension of these techniques has been useful in forming coenzyme analogs (40).

Stability of FMN is greater than FAD in acidic aqueous solutions because of the greater lability of the pyrophosphate linkage in the latter coenzyme. FAD is somewhat more stable in light because its adenine moiety quenches the excited isoalloxazine portion.

In bound coenzymic form, riboflavin participates in oxidation-reduction reactions in numerous metabolic pathways and in energy production via the respiratory chain

(41, 42). Various chemical reactions are catalyzed by flavoproteins (22, 42), and periodic symposia are held on the subject (43). The functions of flavocoenzymes (42, 44) include one-electron transfers, during which the biologically encountered, neutral, oxidized quinone level of flavin is half reduced to the radical semiquinone, which can exist in natural pH ranges as a neutral or anionic species. Further electron transfer can lead to a fully reduced hydroquinone. Additionally, a single-step, two-electron transfer from substrate to flavin can occur with hydride ion transfer, as from reduced pyridine nucleotide, or by base abstraction of a substrate proton together with carbanion addition.

Flavoprotein-catalyzed dehydrogenations occur that are both pyridine nucleotide dependent and independent reactions with sulfur-containing compounds, hydroxylations, oxidative decarboxylations, dioxygenations, and reduction of oxygen to hydrogen peroxide. The intrinsic abilities of flavins to be varyingly potentiated as redox carriers on differential binding to proteins, to participate in both one- and two-electron transfers, and in reduced (1,5-dihydro) form to react rapidly with oxygen permit wide scope in their operation. Investigators have even found a vitamin B2–based blue-light photoreceptor (cryptochrome) in the mammalian retinohypothalamic tract that is involved in setting the circadian clock (45). Mammalian cryptochromes 1 and 2 use both methylene tetrahydrofolate and FAD as prosthetic groups (46).

METHODS FOR ASSAY AND STATUS DETERMINATION

Numerous biochemical methods are aimed at the separation and quantification of the diverse natural flavins (47–50). High-performance liquid chromatography and fluorometry are useful procedures. Among the most sensitive methods are those that invoke specific binding to a riboflavin-binding apoprotein (51), such as riboflavin with egg white riboflavin-binding protein, FMN with apoflavodoxin, and FAD with apoproteins for D-amino acid oxidase or glucose oxidase. However, nutritional status is commonly assessed by measuring urinary excretion of the vitamin in fasting, random, or 24-hour specimens or by riboflavin load return tests, or by measurement of erythrocyte riboflavin concentration, or determination of the erythrocyte glutathione reductase activity coefficient (52, 53).

Urinary Excretion

Under conditions of adequate intake, the amount of urinary riboflavin excreted per day is more than 0.32 μmol (120 μg) or at least 0.21 μmol (80 μg)/g of creatinine. The rate of excretion expressed as milligrams of riboflavin/gram of creatinine is greater for children than adults, who can fall to less than 27 μg/g when deficient. Conditions causing negative nitrogen balance increase urinary riboflavin as a consequence of tissue depletion, whereas the administration of antibiotics and certain psychotropic drugs (phenothiazine) increase riboflavin loss by displacement. Load return tests may be used to gauge the degree to which the body is saturated with riboflavin for a given case; the result generally agrees with tests using other indicators. Only chromatography of suitable extracts followed by specific identification of each flavin can distinguish the vitamin itself from other urinary flavins (54).

Erythrocyte Assays

Because changes in erythrocyte riboflavin are rather small, some problem with sensitivity and interpretation of results exists. Nevertheless, values lower than 27 nmol (10 μg)/dL cells should be considered to reflect a deficient status. Again, high-performance liquid chromatography has been used to monitor the riboflavin composition and content of human blood more exactly (55, 56).

Currently, riboflavin status is most commonly assessed by the glutathione reductase activity in freshly lysed red cells, as detailed for routine clinical use (57) from the procedure described by Sauberlich and colleagues (58). Activities of holo and apo forms of the reductase in erythrocyte hemolysates are measured before and after addition of FAD and are expressed in terms of "activity coefficients" that represent the degree of stimulation of apoenzyme resulting from addition of FAD in vitro. Guidelines suggested for such coefficients are as follows: less than 1.2, acceptable; 1.2 to 1.4, low; greater than 1.4, deficient. Some drawbacks (52) are that the test cannot be used in persons with glucose-6-phosphate dehydrogenase deficiency, which occurs in about 10% of African-Americans, because of an increased avidity in the glutathione reductase for FAD in this disease. Moreover, in vitro treatment of blood with inosine and adenine elevates activity coefficients (59). In a study of piglets, the erythrocyte glutathione reductase activity coefficient was not significantly correlated with either total vitamin B_2 metabolites in the circulation or liver, a finding leading the authors to conclude that the erythrocyte glutathione reductase activity coefficient is not indicative of riboflavin status in the pig (60). However, the erythrocyte glutathione reductase activity coefficient increased and liver flavins concomitantly decreased during induction of riboflavin deficiency in a rat model (61).

DIGESTION AND ABSORPTION

The processes by which riboflavin and its natural derivatives are released by digestion of complexes with food proteins and then assimilated have been reviewed fairly comprehensively (20). Salient features are that coenzyme forms of the vitamin (mainly FAD and less FMN) are released from noncovalent attachment to proteins as a consequence of gastric acidification. Nonspecific action of pyrophosphatase and phosphatase on the coenzymes occurs in the upper gut. Several percent of 8α-(amino acid)riboflavins originally in covalent attachment to certain enzymes, such as mitochondrial succinate dehydrogenase and monoamine oxidase, and traces of other ring and side-chain substituted flavins are also released by these actions following proteolysis. The vitamin is primarily absorbed in the human in the proximal small intestine by a saturable transport system that is rapid and proportional to dose before leveling off at 66.5 μmol (25 mg) of riboflavin. Bile salts appear to facilitate uptake, and a modest amount of the vitamin circulates via the enterohepatic system. Active transport at lower levels of intake may be sodium dependent and involve phosphorylation. Recent studies indicate that a carrier-mediated transport in the colon is probably similar to that in the small intestine (62–65).

TRANSPORT AND METABOLISM

Some of the riboflavin circulating in human blood plasma is loosely associated with albumin, although significant amounts complex with other proteins. A subfraction of immunoglobulin G binds avidly to a small portion of the total free flavin in blood (66), and several immunoglobulins contribute significantly to the circulatory transport of the vitamin (67). As found earlier in other mammals such as the cow (68), pregnancy increases the level of a riboflavin carrier protein in humans as well (69, 70), and differential rates of uptake for the vitamin occur at the fetal and maternal surfaces of the placenta (71). A riboflavin transporter on the microvillus membrane of the human trophoblast-derived choriocarcinoma cell line BeWo appears to be modulated by cellular nucleotide levels and calmodulin (72). Entry of riboflavin into mammalian cells is carrier mediated (facilitated) at physiologic concentrations, but diffusion contributes to entry at higher levels (65, 73, 74). Uptake exhibits relative specificity, and a riboflavin-binding protein has been found in the plasma membrane of rat liver cells (75). The parenchymal hepatocyte does not depend on sodium for riboflavin import (76) as does the renal tubular cell (77). In both the human liver HepG2 cells (78) and renal HK-2 cells (79), the carrier-mediated system seems to be regulated by an intracellular calcium/calmodulin-mediated pathway. (65). Besides the saturable active component that dominates at near-physiologic riboflavin concentrations and a passive component evident at higher concentrations, a receptor-mediated endocytic component has also been implicated in riboflavin absorption (80). In all cases, metabolic trapping dependent on cytosolic flavokinase follows passage of the vitamin through the plasma membrane, which also contains nonspecific alkaline phosphatase that can catalyze release of vitamin from its internal phosphate ester (73).

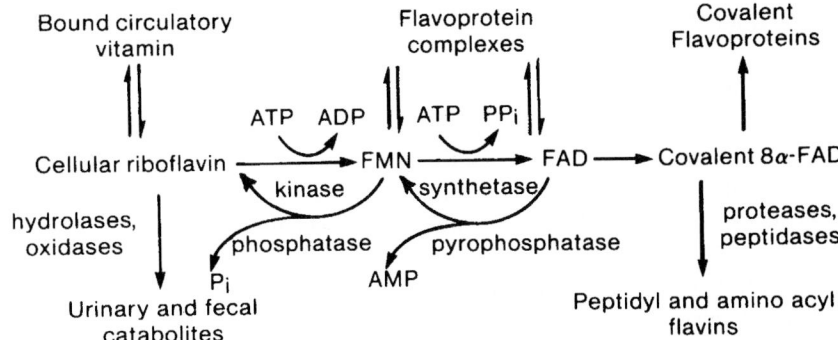

Figure 24.2. Cellular interconversions of flavins. ADP, adenine diphosphate; ATP, adenine triphosphate; FAD, flavin adenine dinucleotide; FMN, flavin mononucleotide; PPi, inorganic pyrophosphate.

Metabolic Interconversions

Metabolic interconversions of flavins at the cellular level are outlined in Figure 24.2. Conversion of riboflavin to coenzymes occurs mainly within the cytoplasm of most tissues, particularly in the small intestine, liver, heart, and kidney (20, 72, 81), but the mitochondria also exhibit a riboflavin/FAD cycle (82). The obligatory first step is the adenosine triphosphate–dependent phosphorylation of the vitamin catalyzed by flavokinase. The FMN product can be complexed with specific apoproteins to form several functional flavoproteins, but most FMN is further converted to FAD in a second adenosine triphosphate–dependent reaction catalyzed by FAD synthetase. It seems likely that the biosynthesis of flavocoenzymes is tightly regulated and dependent on riboflavin status (83). Thyroxine and triiodothyronine stimulate FMN and FAD synthesis in mammalian systems (84); this seems to involve a hormone-mediated increase in an active form of flavokinase (85). As a product of the synthetase, FAD is also an effective inhibitor at this step and may regulate its own formation (86). FAD is the predominant flavocoenzyme in tissues, where it is mainly complexed with numerous flavoprotein dehydrogenases and oxidases. Interaction between coenzyme and apoenzyme usually involves a characteristic dinucleotide-binding fold with the amino acid fingerprint of GXGXXG (87). Analysis of the structure-function relationships in 32 families of FAD-binding proteins revealed four different FAD-family folds, which among them differed in the shape of the binding pocket, the orientation of the FAD molecule, and its conformation (28). Less than 10% of the FAD can also become covalently attached via 8α-linkage to specific amino acid residues of a few important apoenzymes. Although flavination may be autocatalytic for some cases, a protein factor in the mitochondrial matrix has been reported to stimulate flavination of dimethylglycine dehydrogenase (88). Turnover of covalently attached flavocoenzymes requires intracellular proteolysis, and further degradation of the 8α-substituted coenzymes involves nonspecific pyrophosphatase cleavage of the 8α-FAD residue to adenosine monophosphate and the FMN derivative and action by nonspecific phosphatases on the 8α-FMN. A 5′-nucleotidase purified from human placenta possesses specific FAD pyrophosphatase activity when stimulated with cobalt ion (89).

EXCRETION AND SECRETION

Because little riboflavin is stored as such, the urinary excretion reflects dietary intake and catabolic and photodegradative events (20, 53). For physiologically normal adults who eat varied diets, riboflavin accounts for 60 to 70% of urinary flavin. Both 7- and 8-hydroxymethylflavins appear in urine from the human and rat and are the result of microsomal mixed-function oxidases (90, 91). 7-Hydroxymethylriboflavin (7α-hydroxyriboflavin) also appears as the only significant catabolite of the vitamin in human plasma (92). Smaller amounts of side-chain degradation products such as lumichrome, 10-formylmethylflavin, and 10-(2′-hydroxyethyl)flavin are also excreted and may result largely from production by colonic microorganisms (53, 93). Traces of 8α-flavin peptides and catabolites are found in urine and feces (54, 94). The α-D-glucoside attached to the side-chain 5′-position of riboflavin has been detected in liver (27) and urine (95), even though it is easily taken in and hydrolyzed by hepatocytes to liberate the free vitamin (96). A 5′-riboflavinyl peptide ester also occurs in human urine (97).

Secretion in Milk

Secretion of flavin into milk depends on dietary intake and reflects maternal status of riboflavin (98, 99). In milk from both cows (100) and humans (101), the flavin in highest concentration other than the free vitamin is FAD, which can account for more than one third of total flavin. Much of this is hydrolyzed to riboflavin during pasteurization. Fairly significant quantities of the 10-(2′-hydroxyethyl)flavin are notable, because this catabolite has antivitaminic activities as reflected in competitive inhibition of both cellular uptake (76) and subsequent flavokinase-catalyzed phosphorylation of riboflavin (102). Hence, this catabolite subtracts modestly from the biologic activity of the food. Several percent of both 7- and 8-hydroxymethylriboflavins are also present, with more of the former. Smaller amounts of other catabolites, including the 10-formylmethylflavin and lumichrome, account for most of the rest (100).

DEFICIENCY AND EXCESS

Deficiency

Although riboflavin is widely distributed in foodstuffs (see later), many people live for long periods on low intakes; consequently, minor signs of deficiency are common in many parts of the world (103). The incidence of biochemical riboflavin deficiency may be especially high in women and children in developing countries (104). Moreover, the deficiency encountered almost invariably occurs in combination with deficiency of other water-soluble vitamins (57). Clinical deficiency of riboflavin has been induced by feeding a riboflavin-deficient diet, by administration of an antagonist such as galactoflavin, or both. The deficiency syndrome is characterized by sore throat, hyperemia, and edema of the pharyngeal and oral mucus membranes, cheilosis, angular stomatitis (see Fig. 38.1D in Chapter 38), glossitis (magenta tongue; see Fig. 38.1E), seborrheic dermatitis, and normochromic, normocytic anemia associated with pure red cell cytoplasia of the bone marrow (57). However, some of these symptoms, such as glossitis and dermatitis, when encountered in the field may have resulted from other complicating deficiencies. Severe riboflavin deficiency can affect the conversion of vitamin B_6 to its coenzyme and may even curtail conversion of tryptophan to niacin (73).

Inadequate dietary intake, most commonly related to limited availability of food but sometimes exacerbated by poor storage or processing, remains the major cause of deficiency (105). Anorectic persons rarely ingest adequate amounts of riboflavin and other nutrients. Active persons who restrict their energy intake, who make poor dietary choices, or who have preexisting marginal vitamin intakes are at greatest risk of poor status of riboflavin and other B vitamins (106).

Metabolic Causes

Decreased assimilation results from abnormal digestion, absorption, or both. Lactose intolerance as a result of lactase insufficiency, mostly encountered among nonwhite populations, may result in low or negligible consumption of unaltered milk, which is a good source of the vitamin. Malabsorption can result from tropical sprue, celiac disease, malignancy and resection of the small bowel, and gastrointestinal and biliary obstruction. Poor absorption also results from disorders that increase motility and decrease gastrointestinal passage time, such as diarrhea, infectious enteritis, and irritable bowel syndrome, and excessive consumption of alcohol.

Rarely encountered, but usually significantly improved by therapeutic treatment with riboflavin, are certain inborn errors in which the genetic defect affects formation of a normal flavoprotein (84). This category includes defective FAD-dependent fatty acyl-coenzyme A dehydrogenases and poor formation of flavocoenzymes.

Although concern was expressed that plasma total homocysteine is a risk factor for cardiovascular disease, riboflavin did not prove to be an effective lowering agent in a general population (107); however, an effect is noted in a small segment of the population who have both low folate status and are homozygotes for the FAD-dependent 5-methylenetetrahydrofolate reductase (MTHFR) (108) (see Chapter 28). This enzyme supplies folate for the metabolism of homocysteine (see Chapter 34). Investigators have questioned whether the inefficient thermolabile genotype of this enzyme, associated with elevated homocysteine levels, may be sensitive to low riboflavin status. Plasma homocysteine was elevated in subjects with this thermolabile isoform of MTHFR when their riboflavin status was poor, but not when it was sufficient, a finding implying that the functioning of thermolabile MTHFR depends on maintaining adequate riboflavin status (109). The finding that phenobarbital induces microsomal oxidation of the 7-methyl function of the vitamin (90) lends credence to the belief that long-term use of barbiturates may jeopardize flavin status.

Increased Catabolism

Enhanced excretion of riboflavin occurs in catabolic patients undergoing nitrogen loss. The relationship of the vitamin with protein status has long been recognized. Certain antibiotics and phenothiazine drugs also increase excretion of riboflavin (110, 111).

Increased requirements can, of course, result from one or more of the factors mentioned earlier. For example, protein-calorie malnutrition commonly is accompanied by diminution in both intake and absorption of riboflavin.

Systemic infections even without gastrointestinal involvement sometimes lead to increased requirements that can result from decreased intake, defective absorption, poor utilization, and increased excretion. In mice infected with gram-positive or gram-negative bacteria, purified riboflavin-5-phosphate was reported to improve survival (112).

Excess

Toxicity from ingestion of excess riboflavin by experimental animals or humans is doubtful. The human gastrointestinal tract may be able to absorb less than 30 mg of riboflavin from a single dose orally administered (55). Pharmacokinetic analysis of riboflavin dynamics in healthy humans reflects the expected saturability of plasma levels, with excretion enhanced by renal tubular secretion (55). The limited solubility and absorptivity of this vitamin as encountered in multivitamin preparations and in natural foodstuffs and its ready excretion (which is typical of water-soluble vitamins) normally preclude a health risk. One report described a 15-year-old boy who suffered anaphylaxis after consuming riboflavin in either a pill or a soft drink (113).

TABLE 24.1. CRITERIA AND DIETARY REFERENCE INTAKE VALUES FOR RIBOFLAVIN BY LIFE STAGE GROUP

LIFE-STAGE GROUP	CRITERION	EAR (mg/d)[a] MALE	EAR (mg/d)[a] FEMALE	RDA (mg /d)[b] MALE	RDA (mg /d)[b] FEMALE	AI[c] (mg/d)
0–6 mo	Average riboflavin intake obtained from human milk					0.3
7–12 mo	Extrapolation from 0–6 mo AI					0.4
1–3 y	EARs and RDAs for riboflavin for	0.4	0.4	0.5	0.5	
4–8 y	children ages 1–18 y have been	0.5	0.5	0.6	0.6	
9–13 y	extrapolated from adult values using	0.8	0.8	0.9	0.9	
14–18 y	a metabolic body weight ratio multiplied	1.1	0.9	1.3	1.0	
	by a growth factor[a]	1.1	0.9	1.3	1.1	
>18–70 y	Normalization of erythrocyte	1.1	0.9	1.3	1.1	
>70 y	glutathione reductase activity coefficient					
Pregnancy, 14–50 y	Female EAR plus allowance for increased growth in maternal and fetal compartments and a small increase in energy utilization	1.2		1.4		
Lactation, 14–50 y	Female EAR plus replacement of riboflavin transferred in milk[d]	1.3		1.6		

[a] EAR, estimated average requirement. This is the intake that meets the estimated nutrient needs of half of the individuals in a group.

[b] RDA, recommended dietary allowance. The RDA for riboflavin is set by assuming a coefficient of variation (CV) of 10%. The RDA is defined as equal to the EAR plus twice the CV to cover the needs of 97 to 98% of the individuals in the group (therefore, for riboflavin the RDA is approximately 120% of the EAR).

[c] AI, adequate intake. The AI is used if sufficient scientific evidence is not available to derive an EAR. For healthy infants receiving human milk, the AI is the mean intake.

[d] It is assumed that 0.3 mg of riboflavin is transferred in their milk each day when milk production is 0.78 L/d (during the first 6 months of lactation), and that efficiency of use of dietary riboflavin for milk production is 70%; therefore, values are adjusted upward to 0.4 mg/day for the amount of the vitamin that should be replaced.

From Food and Nutrition Board, Institute of Medicine. Dietary Reference Intakes. Thiamin, Riboflavin, Niacin, Vitamin B_6, folate, Vitamin B_{12}, Pantothenic Acid, Biotin, and Choline. Washington, DC: National Academy Press, 1998, with permission.

DIETARY CONSIDERATIONS

Small amounts of riboflavin, occurring largely as digestible coenzymes, are present in most plant and animal tissues. Especially good sources are eggs, lean meats, milk, broccoli, and enriched breads and cereals. Such losses as occur during cooking are largely the result of leaching of the heat-stable but light-sensitive flavins into water. (See Appendix Table A-23-a for the riboflavin content of selected common foods.)

The requirement for riboflavin, in contrast to that for thiamin, does not increase when energy use is increased (114). Because of the interdependence of protein, energy intake, and metabolic body size, however, recommended dietary allowances (RDAs) calculated on theses bases do not differ significantly. Because the RDA values for riboflavin (see Appendix Table A-2-c-1), are given in milligrams/day, this mass unit has been used here. For conversion, 1 μmol riboflavin equals 0.376 mg, or inversely, 1 mg riboflavin equals 2.66 μmol. Clinical signs of deficiency in adults can be prevented with intakes of riboflavin greater than 0.4 mg/1000 kcal, but more than 0.5 mg/1000 kcal may be required to maintain tissue reserves in adults and children, as reflected in urinary excretion, red cell riboflavin, and erythrocyte glutathione reductase.

An adequate intake for infants, based on content in human milk (0.35 mg/L) and the volume that is consumed (0.78 L), is now suggested as 0.3 mg/day for the 0- to 6-month period and 0.4 mg/day for 7 to 12 months (Table 24.1). The RDAs for riboflavin (114) for children progress on the basis of age and body weight from 0.5 to 1.3 mg/day for the age ranges of 1 to 3 years up to 18 years, respectively, with slightly greater amounts recommended for boys than for girls. The RDA for women of 19 to more than 70 years is 1.1 mg/day, and for men it is 1.3 mg/day. Because pregnancy imposes extra demands, an additional 0.3 mg/day over the normal is recommended. During lactation, an additional 0.5 mg/day is deemed appropriate. When supplementation or therapy with riboflavin is warranted, oral administration of five to ten times the RDA usually is satisfactory. See Appendix Tables A-2-a through A-2-h for more data on DRIs.

REFERENCES

1. Blyth AW. J Chem Soc 1879;35:530–9.
2. Kuhn R, Gyorgy P, Wagner-Jayregg T. Ber Dtsch Chem Ges 1933;66B:317, 576–80, 1034–8.
3. Ellinger P, Koschara W. Ber Dtsch Chem Ges 1933;66B:315–7.
4. Booher LE. J Biol Chem 1933;102:39–46.
5. Warburg O, Christian W. Biochem Z 1932;254:438–58.
6. Warburg O, Christian W. Biochem Z 1933;266:377–411.
7. Stern KG, Holiday ER. Ber Dtsch Chem Ges 1934;67:1104–6.
8. Theorell H. Biochem Z 1934;272:155–6.
9. Kuhn R, Reinemund K, Kaltschmitt H et al. Naturwissenschaften 1935;23:260.

10. Kuhn R, Reinemund K, Weygand F et al. Chem Ber 1935;68: 1765–74.
11. Karrer P, Schöpp K, Benz F. Helv Chim Acta 1935;18:426–9.
12. Karrer P, Salomon H, Schöpp K et al. Helv Chim Acta 1935;18: 1143–6.
13. Theorell H. Biochem Z 1937;290:293–303.
14. Warburg O, Christian W. Biochem Z 1938;295:261.
15. Warburg O, Christian W. Biochem Z 1938;296:294.
16. Warburg O, Christian W, Griese A. Biochem Z 1938;297:417.
17. Warburg O, Christian W. Biochem Z 1938;298:150–68.
18. Bacher A, Eberhardt S, Fischer M et al. Annu Rev Nutr 2000; 20:153–67.
19. Bacher A, Eberhardt S, Eisenreich W et al. Vitam Horm 2001; 61:1–49.
20. Merrill AH Jr, Lambeth JD, Edmondson DE et al. Annu Rev Nutr 1981;1:281–317.
21. Otani S, Takatsu M, Nakano M et al. J Antibiot 1974;27:88–9.
22. Otani S. Studies on roseoflavin: isolation, physical, chemical, and biological properties. In: Singer TP, ed. Flavins and Flavoproteins. Amsterdam: Elsevier, 1976:323–7.
23. Tachibana S, Murakami T. Methods Enzymol 1980;66:333–8.
24. Kekelidze T, Edmondson DE, McCormick DB. Arch Biochem Biophys 1994;315:1000–3.
25. Chen H, McCormick DB. J Biol Chem 1997;272:20077–81.
26. Chen H, McCormick DB. Biochim Biophys Acta 1997;1342: 116–8.
27. Whitby LG. Methods Enzymol 1971;18:404–13.
28. Dym O, Eisenberg D. Protein Sci 2001;10:1712–28.
29. Lambooy JP. The alloxazines and isoalloxazines. In: Elderfield RC, ed. Heterocyclic Compounds, vol 9. New York: John Wiley & Sons, 1967:118–223.
30. Murthy YVSN, Massey V. Methods Enzymol 1997;280:436–60.
31. Rublatelli FF, Allegri G, Costa C et al. J Pediatr 1974;85:865–7.
32. Gromisch DS, Lopez R, Cole HS et al. J Pediatr 1977;90: 118–22.
33. Knobloch E, Mandys F, Hodr R. J Chromatogr 1988;428: 255–63.
34. Knobloch E, Hodr R. Czech Med 1989;12:134–44.
35. Goodrich RP. Vox Sang 2000;78[Suppl 2]:211–5.
36. Schuyler R. Trans Apheresis Sci 2001;25:189–90.
37. Flexer LA, Farkas WG. Cited in Merck Index. 11th ed. Rahway, NJ: Merck, 1989.
38. Moffatt JG, Khorana HG. J Am Chem Soc 1958;80:3756–61.
39. Moffatt JG, Khorana HG. J Am Chem Soc 1961;83:649–58.
40. Föry W, McCormick DB. Methods Enzymol 1971;18:458–64.
41. McCormick DB. Oxidation-reduction reactions. In: Encyclopedia of Life Sciences. London: Nature Publishing Group, 1999 (www.els.net).
42. Massey V. Biochem Soc Trans 2000;28:283–96.
43. Chapman S, Perham R, Scrutton N, eds. 14th International Symposium on Flavins and Flavoproteins. Berlin: Dr. Rudolf Weber, Agency for Scientific Publications, 2002.
44. McCormick DB. Coenzymes, biochemistry of. In: Meyers RA, ed. Encyclopedia of Molecular Biology and Molecular Medicine. New York: Weinheim, 1996:396–406.
45. Miyamoto Y, Sancar A. Proc Natl Acad Sci USA 1998; 95:6097–102.
46. Wolf G. Nutr Rev 2002;60:257–60.
47. McCormick DB, Wright LD. Methods Enzymol 1971;18: 132–598.
48. McCormick DB, Wright LD. Methods Enzymol 1980;66: 217–425.
49. Chytil F, McCormick DB. Methods Enzymol 1986;122: 185–248.
50. McCormick DB, Suttie JW, Wagner C. Methods Enzymol 1997;280:343–460.
51. Kodentsova VM, Vrzhensinskaya OA, Spirachev VB. Ann Nutr Metab 1995;39:455–60.
52. Nicholalds GE. Clin Lab Med 1981;1:685–98.
53. Briggs M, ed. Vitamins in Human Biology and Medicine. Boca Raton, FL: CRC Press, 1981.
54. Chastain JL, McCormick DB. Am J Clin Nutr 1987;46:830–4.
55. Zempleni J, Galloway JR, McCormick DB. Am J Clin Nutr 1996;63:54–66.
56. Ishida T, Horiike K. Nippon Rinsho 1989;48:589–91.
57. McCormick DB, Greene HL. Vitamins. In: Burtis CA, Ashwood ER, eds. Tietz Textbook of Clinical Chemistry. Philadelphia: WB Saunders, 1999:999–1028.
58. Sauberlich HE, Judd JH Jr, Nicholalds GE et al. Am J Clin Nutr 1972;25:756–62.
59. Trout GE. Proc Soc Exp Biol Med 1989;191:12–7.
60. Giguere A, Girad CL, Matte JG. Int J. Vitam Nutr Res 2002; 72:383–7.
61. Yates CA, Evans GS, Powers HJ. Br J Nutr 2001;86:593–9.
62. Yuasa H, Hirobe M, Tomei S et al. Biopharm Drug Dispos 2000;21:77–82.
63. Tomei S, Yuasa H, Inoue K et al. Drug Del 2001;8:119–24.
64. Said HM, Ortiz A, Moyer MP et al. Am J Physiol 2000;278: C270–6.
65. Said HM. Annu Rev Physiol 2004;419–46.
66. Merrill AH Jr, Froehlich JA, McCormick DB. Biochem Med 1981;25:198–206.
67. Innis WSA, McCormick DB, Merrill AH Jr. Biochem Med 1985;34:151–65.
68. Merrill AH Jr, Froehlich JA, McCormick DB. J Biol Chem 1979;254:9362–4.
69. Natraj U, George S, Kadam P. J Reprod Immunol 1988;13: 1–16.
70. Subramanian S, Adiga PR. Biochem Biophys Res Commun 1999;262:539–44.
71. Dancis J, Lehanka J, Levitz M. Am J Obstet Gynecol 1988;158: 204–10.
72. Huang SN, Swaan PW. J Pharmacol Exp Ther 2001;298:264–71.
73. McCormick DB. Physiol Rev 1989;69:1170–98.
74. Bowman BB, McCormick DB, Rosenberg IH. Annu Rev Nutr 1989;9:187–99.
75. Nokubo M, Ohta M, Kitani K. Biochim Biophys Acta 1989;981: 303–8.
76. Aw T-Y, Jones DP, McCormick DB. J Nutr 1983;113:1249–54.
77. Bowers-Komro DM, McCormick DB. Riboflavin uptake by rat kidney cells. In: Edmondson DE, McCormick DB, eds. Flavins and Flavoproteins. New York: Walter de Gruyter, 1988:449–53.
78. Said HM, Ortiz A, Ma TY et al. J Cell Physiol 1998;176:588–94.
79. Kumar CK, Yanagawa N, Ortiz A et al. Am J Physiol 1998;274: F104–10.
80. Foraker AB, Khantwal CM, Swaan PW. Adv Drug Del Res 2003;5:1467–83.
81. McCormick DB. Riboflavin. In: Brown ML, ed. Present Knowledge in Nutrition. 6th ed. Washington, DC: International Life Sciences Institute Press, 1990;146–54.
82. Barile M, Brizio C, Valenti D et al. Eur J Biochem 2000;267: 4888–9000.
83. Lee SS, McCormick DB. J Nutr 1983;113:2274–9.
84. Rivlin RS. Riboflavin. In: Bowman BA, Russell RM, eds. Present Knowledge in Nutrition. 8th ed. Washington, DC: International Life Sciences Institute Press, 2001;191–8.
85. Lee SS, McCormick DB. Arch Biochem Biophys 1985;237: 197–201.

86. Yamada Y, Merrill AH Jr, McCormick DB. Arch Biochem Biophys 1990;278:125–30.

87. Wierenga RK, De Maeyer MCH, Hol WGJ. Biochemistry 1985;24:1346–57.

88. Brizio C, Otto A, Brandsch R et al. Eur J Biochem 2000;267:4346–54.

89. Lee RS, Ford HC. J Biol Chem 1988;263:14878–83.

90. Ohkawa H, Ohishi N, Yagi K. J Biol Chem 1983;258:5623–8.

91. McCormick DB. Riboflavin. In: Modern Nutrition in Health and Disease. 9th ed. Shils ME, Shike M, Olson JA et al., eds. Baltimore: Williams & Wilkins, 1999:391–9.

92. Zempleni J, Galloway JR, McCormick DB. Int J Vitam Nutr Res 1996;66:151–7.

93. Chastain JL, McCormick DB. J Nutr 1987;117:468–75.

94. Chia CP, Addison R, McCormick DB. J Nutr 1978;108:373–81.

95. Ohkawa H, Ohishi N, Yagi K. J Nutr Sci Vitaminol 1983;29:515–22.

96. Joseph T, McCormick DB. J Nutr 1995;125:2194–8.

97. Chastain JL, McCormick DB. Biochim Biophys Acta 1988;967:131–4.

98. Ortega RM, Quintas ME, Martinez RM et al. J Am Coll Nutr 1999;18:324–9.

99. Allen LH. J Nutr 2003;133[Suppl]:3000S–7S.

100. Roughead Z, McCormick DB. J Nutr 1990;120:382–8.

101. Roughead Z, McCormick DB. Am J Clin Nutr 1990;52:854–7.

102. McCormick DB. J Biol Chem 1962;237:959–62.

103. Bates CJ. World Rev Nutr Diet 1987;50:215–67.

104. Lakshmi AV. Indian J Med Res 1998;108:182–90.

105. Blanck HM, Bowman BA, Serdula MK et al. Am J Clin Nutr 2002;76:430–5.

106. Manore MM. Am J Clin Nutr 2000;72[Suppl]:598S–606S.

107. McKinley MC, McNulty H, McPartlin J et al. Eur J Clin Nutr 2002;56:850–6.

108. Jacques PF, Kalmbach R, Bagley PJ et al. J Nutr 2002;132:283–8.

109. McNulty H, McKinley MC, Wilson B et al. Am J Clin Nutr 2002;76:436–41.

110. Goldsmith GA. Prog Food Nutr Sci 1975;1:559–609.

111. Pinto J, Huang YP, Rivlin RS. Clin Res 1979;27:444A.

112. Toyosawa T, Suzuki M, Kodman K et al. Infect Immun 2004;72:1820–3.

113. Ou LS, Kuo ML, Huang JL. Ann Allergy Asthma Immunol 2001;87:430–3.

114. Food and Nutrition Board, Institute of Medicine. Dietary Reference Intakes. Thiamin, Riboflavin, Niacin, Vitamin B_6, folate, Vitamin B_{12}, Pantothenic Acid, Biotin, and Choline. Washington, DC: National Academy Press, 1998.

SELECTED READINGS

Chapman S, Perham R, Scrutton N, eds. Flavins and Flavoproteins. 14th ed. Berlin: Rudolf Weber Agency for Scientific Publications , 2002.

Massey V. The chemical and biological versatility of riboflavin. Biochem Soc Trans 2000;28:283–96.

Rivlin RS, Pinto JT. Riboflavin (Vitamin B_2). In: Rucker RB, Suttie JW, McCormick DB et al., eds. Handbook of Vitamins. 3rd ed. New York: Marcel Dekker, 2001:255–73.

Said HM. Recent advances in carrier-mediated intestinal absorption of water-soluble vitamins. Annu Rev Physiol 2004;66:419–66.

Zempleni J, Galloway JR, McCormick DB. Pharmacokinetics of orally and intravenously administered riboflavin in healthy humans. Am J Clin Nutr 1996;63:54–66.

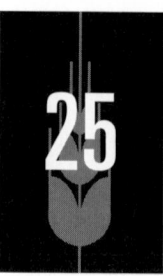

NIACIN[1]

CHRISTELLE BOURGEOIS, DANIEL CERVANTES-LAUREAN, AND JOEL MOSS

HISTORICAL BACKGROUND 442
CHEMISTRY AND NOMENCLATURE 442
DIETARY CONSIDERATIONS AND RECOMMENDED
    INTAKE 443
METABOLISM: ABSORPTION, DISTRIBUTION,
    AND EXCRETION 445
FUNCTIONS 446
    Pyridine Nucleotide Synthesis 446
    Oxidation-Reduction Reactions 446
    Nicotinamide Adenine Dinucleotide–Consuming
        Enzymes 446
DEFICIENCY AND MANIFESTATIONS 448
EVALUATION OF NUTRIENT STATUS 449
NIACIN AS A PHARMACOLOGIC AGENT 449
    Antihyperlipidemic Effects of Niacin 449
    Prevention of Oxidant-Induced Cell Injury
        in Pathophysiologic Conditions 449
AVAILABLE FORMULATIONS OF NIACIN 449
TOXICOLOGY 450

HISTORICAL BACKGROUND

Niacin (nicotinic acid), a member of the B group of vitamins, was initially studied because of its association with pellagra. Symptoms of this nutritional deficiency disease include dermatitis, diarrhea, and dementia, with death as the eventual outcome (1). Early in the last century, it was associated with poor nutrition, inadequate meat and milk intake, and use of corn as the principal constituent of the diet. By suggesting that pellagra was an amino acid deficiency in 1922, Goldberger and Tanner opened the way to the identification of niacin

and tryptophan as cures for pellagra and to the later elucidation of the biochemical pathway for conversion of tryptophan to nicotinic acid mononucleotide (NaMN) (Fig. 25.1).

CHEMISTRY AND NOMENCLATURE

The structures of niacin, also known as nicotinic acid, and nicotinamide, also termed niacinamide, are shown in Figure 25.2. The positively charged nitrogen in nicotinamide adenine dinucleotide (NAD) and NAD phosphate (NADP) confers unique chemical properties (Fig. 25.3A). In oxidation-reduction reactions catalyzed by dehydrogenases, addition of a hydride derived from a reduced substrate, at position 4 of the pyridine ring, yields reduced NAD (NADH) and an oxidized substrate (2) (Fig. 25.3B). Nucleophilic attack on the glycosylic bond that links the ribose to nicotinamide (see Fig. 25.3A) leads to nicotinamide release and substitution on the electrophilic ribose 1″ carbon. In the enzyme-catalyzed reaction, the nicotinamide of NAD is replaced with a nucleophilic acceptor molecule. Acceptors of the adenosine diphosphate (ADP)-ribose moiety can be amino acids in specific target proteins, as in reactions catalyzed by mono-ADP-ribosyltransferases (ARTs) (3). When the acceptor is the nitrogen at position 1 of the adenine moiety of NAD, cyclic ADP-ribose (Fig. 25.4A) is formed in a reaction catalyzed by ADP-ribose cyclase (4, 5). For the members of the poly(ADP-ribose) polymerase (PARP) family, the acceptor may be a carboxylate group of a protein, or the hydroxyl group in the 2′ position of an ADP-ribose monomer (forming 1″ to 2′ glycosidic linkages) already attached to a protein. Sequential additions of ADP-ribose molecules produce a polymer with branches, on average, every 40 to 50 residues (Fig. 25.4B). Members of the Sir2-like family of NAD-dependent deacetylases catalyze the transfer of an acetyl group from lysine in a protein, to the ADP-ribose moiety, releasing 2′-O-acetyl-ADP-ribose and nicotinamide. The former, by an intramolecular transesterification, readily isomerizes to 3′-O-acetyl-ADP-ribose (6, 7) (Fig. 25.5). Finally, the acceptor nucleophile may be water, a reaction catalyzed by NAD glycohydrolases (NADases) (8), yielding free ADP-ribose and nicotinamide.

---

[1]**Abbreviations: ADP,** adenosine diphosphate; **ApoA1,** apolipoprotein A1; **ART,** mono-adenosine diphosphate–ribosyltransferase; **ATP,** adenosine triphosphate; **ENDIT,** European Nicotinamide Diabetes Intervention Trial; **HDL,** high-density lipoprotein; **LDL,** low-density lipoprotein; **NAADP,** nicotinic acid adenosine diphosphate–ribose; **NAD,** nicotinamide adenine dinucleotide; **NADH,** reduced nicotinamide adenine dinucleotide; **NADP,** nicotinamide adenine dinucleotide phosphate; **NaMN,** nicotinic acid mononucleotide; **NMNAT,** nicotinamide/nicotinic acid mononucleotide adenylyltransferase; **PARP,** poly(adenosine diphosphate–ribose) polymerase.

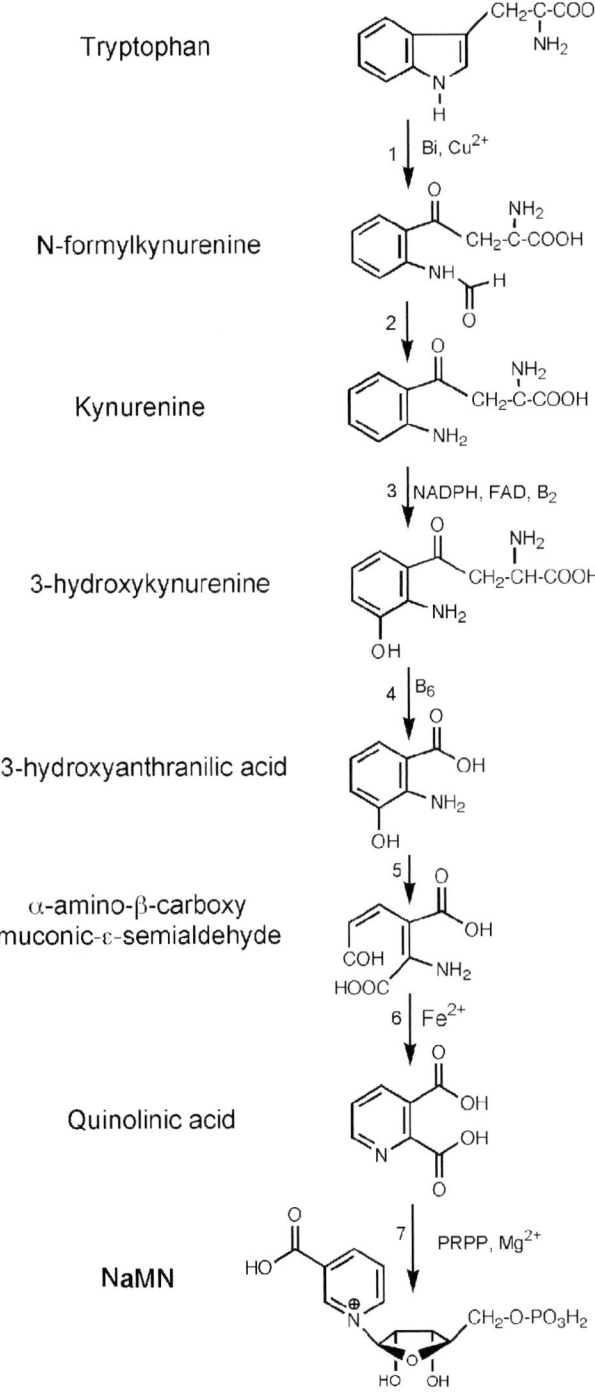

Figure 25.1. Metabolic conversion of tryptophan to nicotinic acid mononucleotide. *1*, tryptophan pyrrolase; *2*, kynurenine formamidease; *3*, kynurenine 3-monoxygenase; *4*, kynureninase; *5*, 3-hydroxyanthranilic acid oxygenase; *6*, nonenzymatic; *7*, quinolinic acid phosphoribosyltransferase. NaMN, nicotinic acid mononucleotide. (Adapted from Rongvaux A, Andris F, Van Gool F et al. Bioessays 2003;25:683–90.)

DIETARY CONSIDERATIONS AND RECOMMENDED INTAKE

The main sources of dietary niacin are meat, fish, and nuts (9). Although milk and eggs contain small amounts of preformed niacin, their content of tryptophan, a precursor of

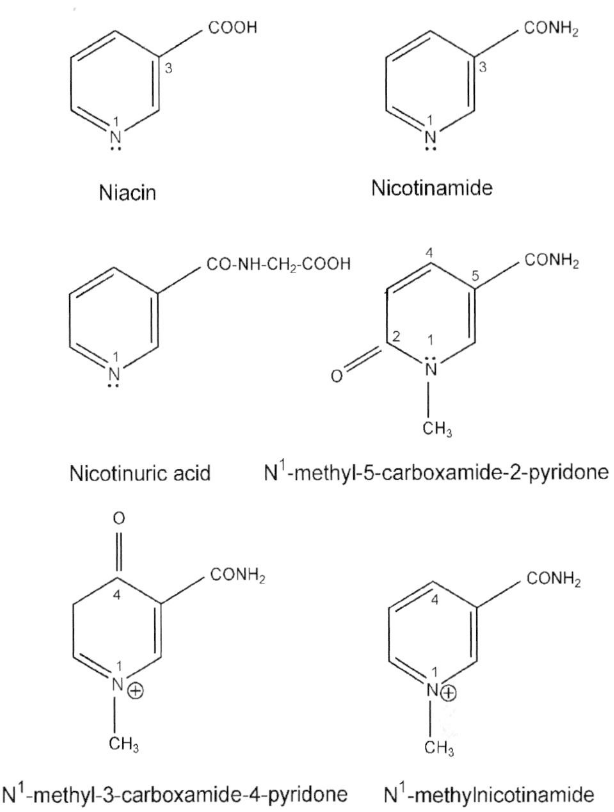

Figure 25.2. Chemical structures of niacin and nicotinamide and their metabolites. A unique metabolite of niacin is nicotinuric acid (glycine conjugate of niacin). The main metabolites of nicotinamide are N′-methylnicotinamide and its 2- and 4-pyridone analogs.

the "de novo" NAD synthesis pathway (see Fig. 25.1), provides significant amounts of niacin equivalents (NEs). It is estimated that 60 g of the amino acid is converted to 1 g of the vitamin, with a variation of about 30% (SD) among individuals. The efficiency of tryptophan conversion to niacin depends on nutritional history and hormonal factors (10). Quantitatively, tryptophan is primarily used for protein biosynthesis, even in conditions of niacin deficiency. Bioavailability of NEs should be taken into account when estimating the content of dietary niacin in food. Of niacin in maize, 70% is in a biologically unavailable form (11). Niacin availability may be improved, however, by specific processes such as the alkali treatment of corn used in the preparation of tortillas (10).

The recommended dietary allowance, as defined in the report of the Food and Nutrition Board's Standing Committee on the Scientific Evaluation of Dietary Reference Intakes and its 1998 Panel on Folate, Other B Vitamins, and Choline (11), is summarized in Table 25.1. These values were established according to the doses required to prevent pellagra (11.3–13.3 mg of NE/day). No data are available concerning relevant niacin requirements in pregnancy and lactation. Thus, niacin requirements were estimated based on an average increase in energy expenditure of 300 kcal/day during pregnancy and an average daily secretion of 1.4 mg of NE during lactation (11). In the United States, women 19 to 50 years old consume, on average, 17 mg of

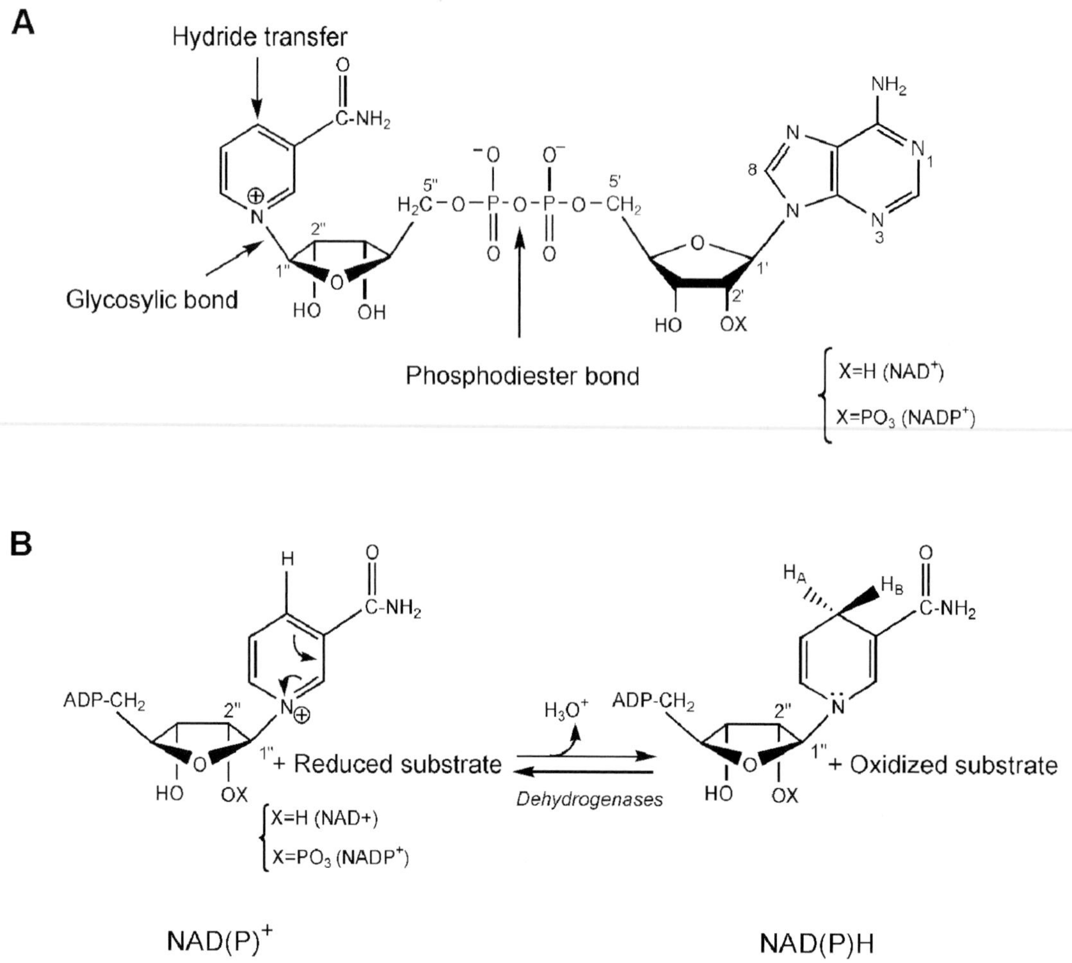

A

Figure elements labeled: Hydride transfer, Glycosylic bond, Phosphodiester bond, X=H (NAD⁺), X=PO₃ (NADP⁺)

B

ADP-CH₂ ... + Reduced substrate ⇌ (Dehydrogenases) ADP-CH₂ ... + Oxidized substrate, H₃O⁺

X=H (NAD+)
X=PO₃ (NADP⁺)

NAD(P)⁺   NAD(P)H

Figure 25.3. A. Structure of nicotinamide adenine dinucleotide (NAD). **B.** General reaction of oxidation-reduction of NAD(P) by dehydrogenases.

NE, daily, whereas men, in the same age range, consume 21 mg of NE (11). According to preliminary experimental data linking niacin status and genomic stability, these doses would not be sufficient to promote genomic stability (12).

The various dietary reference intakes are presented in Tables 25.1 and 25.2. Appendix TableA-2-a through A-2-k summarize additional information on the basis and usage of the DRIs and actual nutritional data thus for published.

TABLE 25.1. RECOMMENDED DAILY DIETARY ALLOWANCES FOR NIACIN (mg OF NE)[a]

	AGE (y)	MALES	FEMALES
Infants	0.0–0.5	2[b]	2[b]
	0.5–1.0	4[b]	4[b]
Children	1–3	6[c]	6[c]
	4–8	8[c]	8[c]
Adolescents	9–13	12[c]	12[c]
	14–18	16[c]	14[c]
Adults	>19	16	14
Pregnancy	14–50		18
Lactation	14–50		17

[a] 1 mg niacin = 60 mg tryptophan = 1 mg of niacin equivalent (NE).
[b] For infants, values correspond to the adequate intake level, which is based on the observed mean intake of preformed niacin by infants fed with human milk.
[c] No data are available for these age ranges; recommended dietary allowances were estimated by extrapolation from adult values.

Data from Food and Nutrition Board, Institute of Medicine. Dietary Reference Intakes for Thiamin, Riboflavin, Niacin, Vitamin B₁₂, Folate, Vitamin B₁₂, Pantothenic Acid, Biotin, and Choline. Washington, DC: National Academy Press, 1998:123–49.

TABLE 25.2. DAILY TOLERABLE UPPER INTAKE LEVEL FOR NIACIN (mg OF NE)[a]

	AGE (y)	UL
Infants	0.0–1.0	[b]
Children	1–3	10[c]
	4–8	15[c]
Adolescents	9–13	20[c]
	14–18	30[c]
Adults	>19	35
Pregnancy and	14–18	30
lactation	>19	35

UL, tolerable upper intake level.
[a] 1 mg niacin = 60 mg tryptophan = 1 mg of niacin equivalent (NE).
[b] Because of a lack of data on adverse effects of niacin for infants, UL could not be determined.
[c] No data are available for these age ranges; recommended dietary allowances were estimated by extrapolation from adult values.

Data from Food and Nutrition Board, Institute of Medicine. Dietary Reference Intakes for Thiamin, Riboflavin, Niacin, Vitamin B₆, Folate, Vitamin B₁₂, Pantothenic Acid, Biotin, and Choline. Washington, DC: National Academy Press, 1998:123–49.

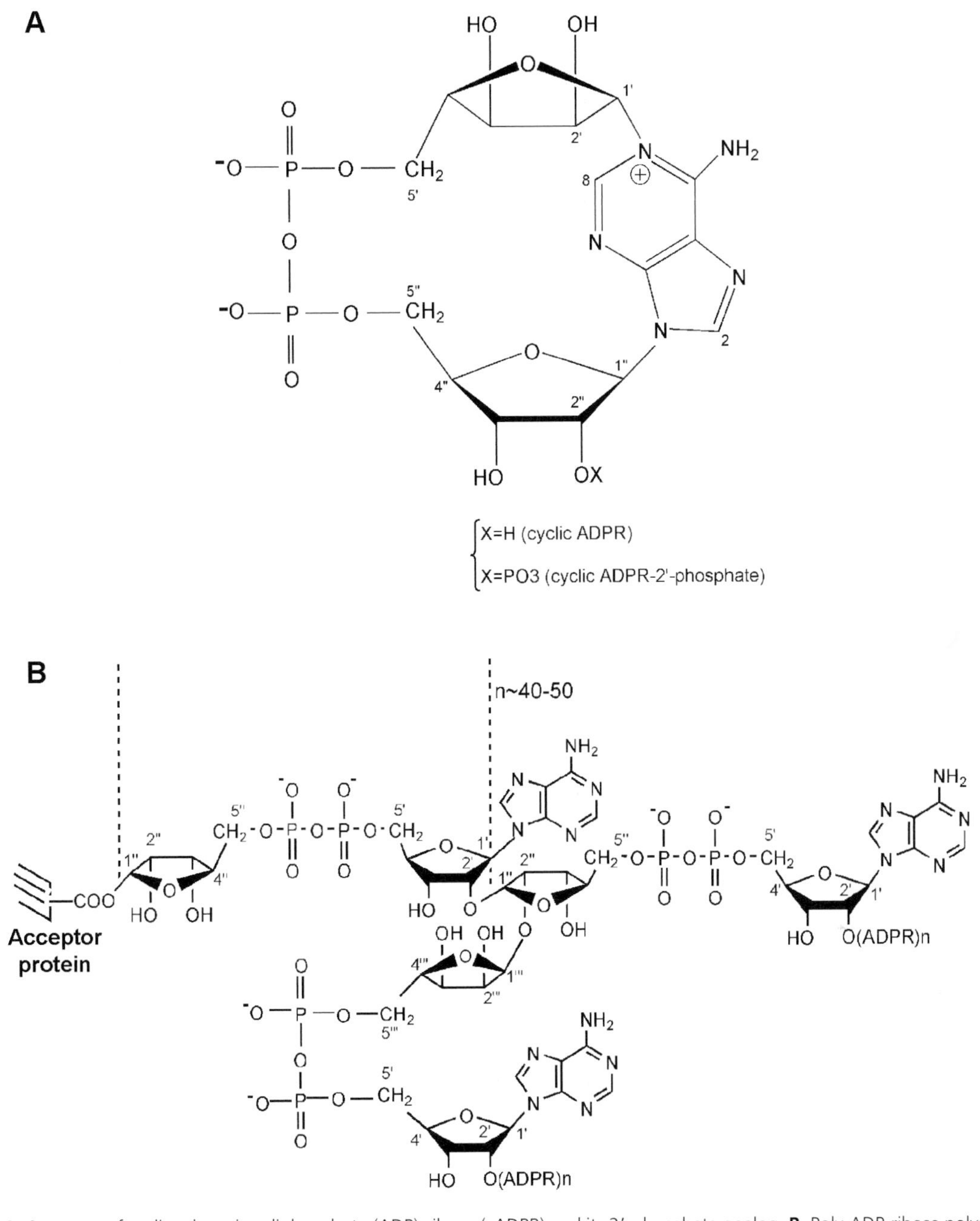

A

X=H (cyclic ADPR)

X=PO3 (cyclic ADPR-2'-phosphate)

B

Figure 25.4. A. Structure of cyclic adenosine diphosphate (ADP)-ribose (cADPR) and its 2'-phosphate analog. **B.** Poly-ADP-ribose polymer. The first monomer unit of ADP-ribose is linked to an acceptor protein through an α-glycosidic linkage on a carboxylate group. The linear polymer is formed with ADP-ribose units linked via α-1″-2″-glycosidic linkages and branches occurring, on average, every 40 to 50 residues via α-1″-2″-glycosidic linkages. Chemically, the glycosidic linkages attaching ADP-ribose units correspond to acetal bonds, which are acid sensitive. (Data from Kim H, Jacobson EL, Jacobson MK. Biochem Biophys Res Commun 1993;194:1143–7.)

METABOLISM: ABSORPTION, DISTRIBUTION, AND EXCRETION

Niacin and its amide are absorbed through the intestinal mucosa by simple diffusion. Fifteen to 30% of niacin is bound to protein, and the vitamin-protein complex, as well as free niacin, is then taken up by tissues. Adipose tissue is responsible for the rapid clearance of niacin after an intravenous dose. Metabolic trapping, in which niacin and nicotinamide are converted to NAD, accounts for reten-

tion of these vitamins (10). Neutral niacin as a zwitterionic species with a carboxylic anion and quaternary nitrogen cation may partition as a lipid-soluble molecule. In contrast, nicotinamide is lipid-soluble only in the neutral form (i.e., with an uncharged nitrogen in the pyridine ring). Receptor-mediated uptake of nicotinamide has, however, been reported (10). Niacin and nicotinamide are metabolized via different pathways. In liver, the major product of pharmacologic doses of niacin is the glycine conjugate, nicotinuric acid (see Fig. 25.2), whereas the main metabolites of

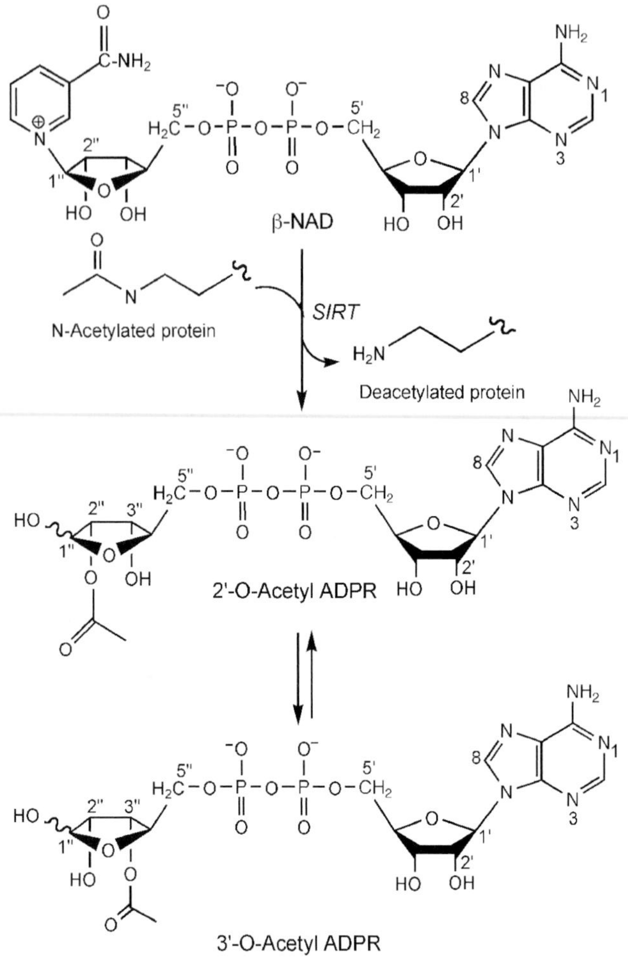

Figure 25.5. Sir2-like deacetylases catalyze the release of the acetyl group from N-acetyl-modified histones. Adenosine diphosphate ribose (ADPR) from oxidized nicotinamide adenine dinucleotide (NAD⁺) is used as an acceptor of the acetyl group, forming 2′-O-acetyl-ADP-ribose, which, in turn, forms 3′-O-acetyl-ADP-ribose via a nonenzymatic transesterification reaction.

nicotinamide are N^1-methylnicotinamide and its oxidized products, 2- and 4-pyridones (13) (see Fig. 25.2). Niacin and nicotinamide metabolites formed in the liver are excreted in urine. Quantification of excretion of nicotinuric acid and N^1-methylnicotinamide and its pyridones is useful in evaluating niacin nutriture.

FUNCTIONS

Pyridine Nucleotide Synthesis

Nicotinic acid, nicotinamide, and tryptophan are precursors of NAD and NADP. These nucleotides can be synthesized "de novo," using tryptophan from the diet to generate nicotinic acid mononucleotide (see Fig. 25.1), or through the "salvage pathway" (Fig. 25.6), using niacin and nicotinamide absorbed from nutrients or nicotinamide recycled from signaling reactions that involve NAD catabolism (14). Tryptophan metabolism, initiated

by tryptophan 2,3-dioxygenase, a tryptophan-inducible enzyme, occurs primarily in liver. Because quinolinic acid phosphoribosyltransferase activity has been detected only in liver and kidney in mammals, other tissues rely mostly on an exogenous supply of nicotinic acid/nicotinamide for NAD biosynthesis, hence the role of niacin and niacinamine as essential nutrients. The last step of NAD synthesis is catalyzed by nicotinamide/nicotinic acid mononucleotide adenylyltransferases (NMNAT1-3, in humans) (15–17), which use both NMN and NaMN as targets for the adenylyl-transfer reaction. These substances exhibit specific patterns of tissue expression and cell localization; hNMNAT1 is in the nucleus, hNMNAT2 in the cytoplasm, and NMNAT3 in both mitochondria and cytoplasm, findings suggesting the existence of several different sites of NAD synthesis, and therefore NAD pools, in the cell. In yeast, genes of the "de novo" synthesis pathway are silenced by an NAD-dependent histone deacetylase that functions as a sensor of nuclear NAD pool levels (18). NADP is formed directly from NAD by phosphorylation catalyzed by a specific kinase expressed in most tissues except skeletal muscle (19). A phosphatase has also been described that converts NADP to NAD (2). Nicotinamidase activity has been detected in lower eukaryotes (14).

Oxidation-Reduction Reactions

In oxidation-reduction reactions, dehydrogenases use NAD/P(H) as coenzymes to oxidize or reduce a substrate (see Fig. 25.3B). NADP dehydrogenases are preferentially involved in anabolic reactions (e.g., synthesis of fatty acids and cholesterol) (20). In contrast, NAD is used in catabolic reactions to transfer the potential free energy stored in macronutrients such as carbohydrates, lipids, and proteins to NADH, which is then used to form adenosine triphosphate (ATP), the primary energy currency of the cell.

Nicotinamide Adenine Dinucleotide–Consuming Enzymes

Unlike oxidation-reduction reactions, which change only the redox status of the pyridine nucleotide pool and do not alter its size, hydrolysis of NAD is required for the function of some enzymes that thereby link nutritional and metabolic status of the cell to the regulation of essential cell functions, such as gene silencing, maintenance of genome integrity, and innate immunity. Many of them yield nicotinamide in addition to other molecules, thus fueling the NAD salvage pathway for NAD resynthesis (see Fig. 25.6).

Adenosine Diphosphate–Ribose Cyclases

Cyclic ADP-ribose, generated by ADP-ribose cyclases, is an endogenous modulator of the calcium ion–releasing channel ryanodine receptors. The cyclases also catalyze

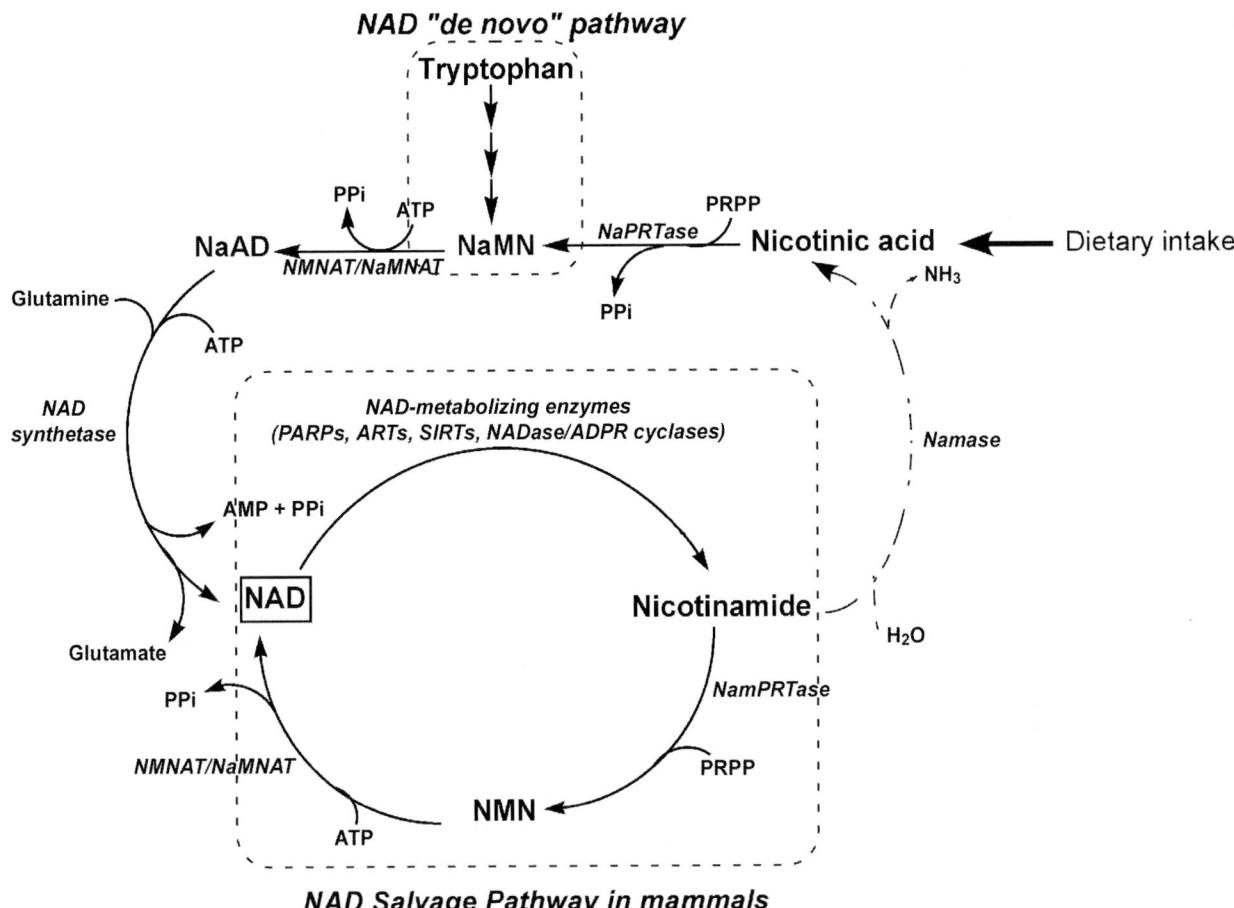

Figure 25.6. Biochemical pathways of niacin and nicotinamide metabolism. Salvage pathways differ among species. In lower eukaryotes and in procaryotes, Namase converts nicotinamide to nicotinic acid, whereas in mammals the nicotinamide to NMN conversion seems to predominate. ADP, adenosine diphosphate; ADPR cyclase, ADP-ribosyl cyclase; ARTs, mono-ADP-ribosyltransferases; ATP, adenosine triphosphate; NaAD, nicotinic acid adenine dinucleotide; NAD, nicotinamide adenine dinucleotide; NADase, NAD glycohydrolase; Namase, nicotinamidase; NaMN, nicotinic acid mononucleotide; NamPRTase, nicotinamide-5'-phosphoribosyltransferase; NaPRTase, nicotinic acid phosphoribosyltransferase; NMN, nicotinamide mononucleotide; NMNAT, nicotinamide-5'-mononucleotide adenosine-5'-triphosphate adenylyltransferase; PARPs, poly(ADP-ribosyl)polymerases; PPi, pyrophosphate; SIRTs, Sir2-like NAD-dependent deacetylases. (Data from Rongvaux A, Andris F, Van Gool F et al. Bioessays 2003;25:683–90.)

cyclic ADP-ribose hydrolysis, NAD+ hydrolysis, and a base-exchange reaction between NADP+ and nicotinic acid, which produces nicotinic acid ADP-ribose (NAADP), another regulator of intracellular calcium stores. The mammalian ADP-ribose cyclase family comprises the well-characterized ectoenzymes CD38 and CD157, and newly described intracellular cyclases, whose activities are under the control of G-protein–coupled receptors (21, 22). CD38 knockout mice have a defect in T-cell–dependent antibody response and an impaired innate immune response to bacterial pathogens, whereas inactivation of the CD157 gene perturbs the regulation of the humoral T-cell–independent immune response and mucosal thymus-dependent responses (23, 24). CD157 expression is upregulated in some patients with rheumatoid arthritis and may participate to the development of this autoimmune disease (25). CD38 has been proposed as a mediator of glucose-induced insulin secretion from pancreatic β cells via

the increase of intracellular calcium ion concentration (25), and it may be involved in the pathogenesis of autoimmune diabetes (26, 27).

Mono-Adenosine Diphosphate–Ribosyltransferases

These enzymes catalyze the transfer of ADP-ribose to specific amino acid acceptors (e.g., arginine, cysteine, asparagines, or histidine) in target proteins, altering the biologic properties of the protein (3). The family of ecto-ADP-ribosyltransferases (ecto-ART1-7) comprises glycosylphosphatidylinositol-linked or secreted enzymes. ART activity has been associated with myocyte differentiation (28, 29), modulation of neutrophil recruitment and chemotaxis (30–32), and inhibition of T cell cytotoxicity (33). Although intracellular mono-ADP-ribosyltransferases have yet to be identified, the existence of an intracellular ADP-ribosyl cycle is inferred from the demonstrated presence of

ADP-ribosylprotein hydrolases that can reverse the ADP-ribosylation of intracellular proteins. Intracellular ARTs have been implicated in the regulation of G-protein cell signaling, the control of the molecular chaperone protein GRP78/BiP pool in response to nutritional stress, the inhibition of protein translation, and the regulation of the structure and function of the Golgi complex and the cytoskeleton (3).

Poly(Adenosine Diphosphate–Ribose) Polymerases

The highly negatively charged ADP-ribose polymers synthesized by PARPs dramatically affect the function of target proteins. These polymers are rapidly metabolized by two enzymes, poly(ADP-ribose) glycohydrolase and lyase, making the target protein readily available for remodification (34). As many as 18 genes encoding nuclear or cytoplasmic proteins that carry the PARP signature, a highly conserved sequence in the PARP catalytic domain, have been reported (35). PARP1 and PARP2 are nuclear enzymes activated by DNA breaks and are important in the base-excision repair pathway. Tankyrase 1, a telomere-associated PARP, is also involved in the maintenance of genome integrity, by contributing to the control of telomere homeostasis. PARP1 participates in the regulation of many physiologic nuclear processes, such as transcription, chromatin structure, DNA replication, cell differentiation, protein degradation, and cell death (36, 37). PARP1 activation is now believed to play the role of an "apoptosis to necrosis switch," determining cell fate depending on the extent of DNA damage (38). According to this model, activation of PARP by limited DNA breakage promotes DNA repair, and cells survive without the risk of transmitting genetic mutations. When DNA damage is more severe, the apoptotic cascade induces caspases, which cleave and inactivate PARP1, promoting the death of cells with irreparable DNA damage. Extensive DNA breakage may trigger overactivation of PARP1, leading to depletion of cellular stores of NAD and ATP. Under these conditions, the ATP-dependent apoptosis pathway cannot proceed, and cells undergo necrosis, a process much more damaging to the surrounding cells.

Sir2-like Protein Deacetylases

Sir-2 like proteins (or sirtuins) were first identified as class III histone deacetylases, related to the yeast silent information regulator (Sir2), an enzyme that promotes the formation of euchromatin, and thereby gene silencing, in an NAD-dependent fashion. In yeast and worm, Sir2 is required for life span expansion in conditions of nutrient scarcity (39). In humans, the sirtuin family comprises seven members (hSIRT1-7) that can reverse acetylation of lysine in proteins, using NAD as the acetyl group acceptor (40–42). The nuclear SIRT1, the most closely related to yeast Sir2, deacetylates p53, thereby inhibiting apoptosis in response to DNA damage (43, 44). In mice, absence of SIRT1 leads to

p53 hyperacetylation, impaired development, a shorter life span, and sterility (45). Thus, in several species, SIRT1 and homologs appear to regulate diverse pathways that have one common feature: their impact on aging (39). SIRT2, mainly found in the cytoplasm, has α-tubulin as a substrate (40), and hSIRT3 deacetylase is a mitochondrial protein (46). The metabolite 2'-O-acetyl-ADP-ribose, by-product of SIRT activity (see Fig. 25.5), has been proposed as a possible second messenger, regulating other enzymatic processes (47). Nicotinamide, but not nicotinic acid, is a potent inhibitor of sirtuin activity; it has been proposed to serve as a physiologic regulator (48), the level of which would be controlled by the rate of its conversion to nicotinic acid through the NAD^+ salvage pathway, and /or to N-methyl nicotinamide, by the excretion pathway (49). Whether a decrease in nicotinamide or an increase in NAD levels is responsible for the increased activity of Sir2 during caloric restriction, is still debated (49, 50).

DEFICIENCY AND MANIFESTATIONS

Niacin deficiency causes pellagra. The classic symptoms of this disease in the late stages are dermatitis, diarrhea, and dementia, with symptoms including anxiety, insomnia, and, in advanced stages, disorientation, hallucinations, and delirium (51). Advanced stages of pellagra can be cured with nicotinamide in intramuscular doses of 50 to 100 mg three times a day for 3 to 4 days, followed by similar quantities orally, supplemented with 100 g of proteins daily. Because the biotransformation of tryptophan to nicotinic acid requires several vitamins and minerals (e.g., vitamin B_6, vitamin B_2, iron, copper) (see Fig. 25.1), diets deficient in these nutrients can predispose to pellagra. Similarly, isoniazid therapy of tuberculosis, which causes depletion of vitamin B_6, may trigger niacin deficiency. An excess of neutral amino acids in the diet (e.g., leucine) that can compete with tryptophan for uptake may also be a factor predisposing to niacin deficiency by impairing its synthesis from tryptophan (10).

Because numerous NAD-dependent enzymes (e.g., PARPs, sirtuins) can influence genomic stability, insufficient nicotinic acid intake is also likely to increase the risk of cancer and other diseases attributable to increased DNA damage (52–54). Investigators have suggested that maintenance of adequate NAD levels would prevent or retard, in the long term, the multistage process of carcinogenesis and age-related diseases (55). Several lines of evidence support this hypothesis in yeast and in rodents (56, 57). Furthermore, studies in rats suggest that niacin supplementation could decrease the risk of patients with cancer and compromised nutritional status to develop chemotherapy-related malignancies (57, 58).

Hartnup syndrome is an autosomal recessive disorder characterized by impaired synthesis of niacin from tryptophan, which results in pellagra-like symptoms (59). The disease results from defective transport of tryptophan and other neutral amino acids in the intestine and/kidney (60). Treatment with nicotinamide in large doses (40–250 mg/day) or tryptophan methyl ester (61) markedly improves the dermatitis and neurologic symptoms.

EVALUATION OF NUTRIENT STATUS

Niacin nutriture has been assessed in several ways by a variety of methods (62). Dowex-1 formate chromatography is used to separate pyridine nucleotides and N^1-methylnicotinamide. Measurement of N^1-methylnicotinamide and of its 2-pyridone derivative in urine (63) is most commonly used. Excretion of N^1-methylnicotinamide of less than 0.8 mg/day indicates niacin deficiency (62). A ratio of N^1-methyl-5-carboxamide-2-pyridone to N^1-methylnicotinamide of 1.3 to 2.0 is considered normal; in niacin deficiency, it is less than 1.0. Niacin status can also be assessed by measuring its physiologically active forms, NAD(H)/NADP(H), accurate determination of which depends on the method of extraction, because acid destroys NADH and NADPH, and alkali degrades NAD and NADP. A method devised by Lowry and associates in 1961, modified by Slater and Sawyer in 1962, and Nisselbaum and Green in 1969 (cited in [10]) uses appropriate dehydrogenases specific for either NAD or NADP and thiazolyl blue, which, when reduced by NADH and NADPH, forms a purple compound, formazan, in an amount proportional to the concentration of the coenzymes (oxidized and reduced). This assay is used to measure these pyridine nucleotides in tissue and blood. Assays of NAD/NADP in erythrocytes and cultured cells suggest that the intracellular NAD level may reflect niacin status, whereas NADP levels do not. Measurement of NAD/NADP content and tryptophan level in erythrocytes has been proposed to evaluate niacin deficiency (10).

NIACIN AS A PHARMACOLOGIC AGENT

Beyond its vitamin and nutrition-related roles, niacin in large doses (1–3 g/day), but not niacinamide (nicotinamide), is antihyperlipidemic. Nicotinamide is being investigated as preventive therapy for oxidant-induced cell injury in pathologic conditions and is used currently to treat Hartnup syndrome.

Antihyperlipidemic Effects of Niacin

In pharmacologic doses (2–6 g/day), nicotinic acid exerts wide-spectrum, antilipidemic effects with reduction of the ratio of low-density lipoprotein (LDL) to high-density lipoprotein (HDL) and thereby significant reduction in atherosclerotic cardiovascular disease and mortality (64). Current knowledge (65) suggests that nicotinic acid prevents the formation of LDL and VLDL (very low density lipoprotein) by inhibiting lipolysis of triglyceride in adipose tissue and triglyceride synthesis in liver. In adipose tissue, the antilipolytic effect of niacin is mediated by a recently

characterized Gi/o-protein–coupled receptor with high affinity for niacin, the activation of which inhibited cyclic adenosine monophosphate-stimulated lipolysis (66–69). These receptors are also expressed in spleen and macrophages (70). In vitro studies suggest that niacin promotes an increase in HDL by preventing uptake, by the liver, of apolipoprotein A1 (ApoA1), a major protein component of HDL, but not of cholesterol esters from HDL. According to a present model of reverse cholesterol transport, by increasing the amount of ApoA1 available for HDL synthesis, niacin would promote the removal of excess cholesterol from peripheral tissues and thereby lower the risk of atherosclerotic cardiovascular disease. Low-affinity receptors for niacin have also been characterized. Their patterns of expression are distinct and their signaling properties unknown (67, 68). When therapy with niacin alone fails to lower blood cholesterol levels sufficiently, niacin may be used with other lipid-lowering drugs that act through different mechanisms (e.g., bile acid–binding resins, statins) (71).

Prevention of Oxidant-Induced Cell Injury in Pathophysiologic Conditions

At high doses (≤3.5 g/day), nicotinamide is protective against cell death and inhibits the production of inflammatory mediators in animal and in vitro models. In addition to these properties that are consistent with PARP1 inhibition, nicotinamide also exhibits PARP1-independent pharmacologic effects (72) that may be attributable to its inhibitory effects on other signaling pathways (e.g., sirtuins) and its function as a precursor of pyridine nucleotides (73). Nicotinamide has been proposed as a possible means of increasing the survival of pancreatic β cells after diagnosis of type 1 diabetes (insulin-dependent diabetes mellitus) or of preventing the onset of the disease in high-risk persons (38). This notion was not confirmed, however, by the recently published European Nicotinamide Diabetes Intervention Trial (ENDIT), a large-scale evaluation of nicotinamide benefits in first-degree relatives of patients with type 1 diabetes (74). The present state of knowledge suggests that specific inhibitors of PARP1 would be needed for effective preventive action (75).

AVAILABLE FORMULATIONS OF NIACIN

The large doses of niacin used to treat hyperlipidemia are available in three different formulations: immediate-release niacin, sustained-release, and a more recent formulation, extended-release (76). Recommended doses of niacin are 1.5 to 2 g/day for sustained-release and up to 3 g/day of immediate-release niacin. The advantage claimed for sustained-release niacin over immediate-release niacin is absence of the flushing that occurs in some patients after ingestion of large doses of the latter, but evidence indicates that this formulation is more likely to be associated with gastrointestinal symptoms and hepatotoxicity. The newer, extended-release formulation achieves the efficacy of the immediate-release form and a reduced incidence of flushing without the hepatic problems caused by sustained-release niacin (77). To circumvent the hepatic effects of oral intake of niacin, proniacin formulations (e.g., esters of niacin) have been developed for topical application (78, 79). Following conversion of the esterified form by skin α-naphtylacetate-esterase activity, slower systemic delivery through the skin is accomplished, with lower concentrations of drug and sustained benefits of niacin (77).

TOXICOLOGY

Prostaglandin-induced flushing is the major specific side effect experienced by users of nicotinic acid in the initial days of treatment with pharmacologic doses of niacin. Because it occurs at lower doses than other effects (e.g., hepatotoxicity), it was chosen as a critical adverse effect for determining the tolerable upper intake level for all forms of niacin taken as a vitamin supplement or as a pharmacologic agent (see Table 25.2). These tolerable upper intake levels apply to the general population and may not be protective enough for persons with conditions that render them more susceptible to the adverse effects of excess niacin intake (e.g., hepatic dysfunction, cardiac arrhythmias, gout). In most patients, tolerance to nicotinic acid develops with continued use, and premedication with aspirin can be used to counteract flushing events. Symptoms can also be reduced by ingestion of the drug with food and/or by increasing the dose gradually. A lower incidence of flushing has been documented in patients using timed-release or extended-release forms of niacin (71). Because of potential hepatic toxicity, liver enzymes (aminotransferases and or alkaline phosphatase) should be monitored before the initiation of therapy, 6 weeks after initiation and/or any change of dose, and two or three times a year thereafter. If liver enzyme levels exceed three times the upper limit of normal, treatment should be discontinued. To avoid liver toxicity, a starting dose not exceeding 250 to 300 mg/day is recommended, with monthly increments not greater than 250 to 300 mg/day until a maximum of 3 g/day is reached.

Niacin may cause insulin resistance, which requires compensatory insulin secretion and, in patients with dysfunctional pancreatic β cells, may trigger hyperglycemia. Patients with diabetes mellitus therefore require special monitoring during niacin treatment. No adverse effects of the pharmacologic doses of nicotinamide used during the ENDIT study were reported (74). Investigators have been concerned, however, that saturation of the nicotinamide excretion pathway may divert methylation equivalents required for anabolic pathways to nicotinamide methylation and may lead to growth retardation in children (80). Furthermore, as a strong inhibitor of sirtuins, nicotinamide may interfere with cell survival (49). Thus, more data are needed on the long-term effects of therapeutic doses of nicotinamide.

Acknowledgments

We thank Dr. Martha Vaughan and Dr. Vincent Manganiello for useful discussions and critical review of the manuscript.

REFERENCES

1. Weiner M, Van Eys J. The discovery of nicotinic acid as a nutrient. In: Weiner M, ed. Nicotinic Acid: Nutrient-Cofactor-Drug. New York: Marcel Dekker, 1983:3–16.
2. Weiner M, Van Eys J. Assessment of the adequacy of niacin nutriture. In: Wiener M, ed. Nicotinic Acid: Nutrient-Cofactor-Drug. New York: Marcel Dekker, 1983:51–71.
3. Corda D, Di Girolamo M. EMBO J 2003;22:1953–8.
4. Kim H, Jacobson EL, Jacobson MK. Biochem Biophys Res Commun 1993;194:1143–7.
5. Lee HC, Aarhus R. Cell Regul 1991;2:203–9.
6. Jackson MD, Denu JM. J Biol Chem 2002;277:18535–44.
7. Sauve AA, Celic I, Avalos J et al. Biochemistry 2001;40:15456–63.
8. Kaplan NO. The pyridine coenzymes. In: Boyer PD, Lardy H, Myrback K, eds. The Enzymes. New York: Academic Press, 1960:105–69.
9. Bates CJ. Niacin: physiology, dietary sources and requirement. In: Sadler MJ, Strain JJ, Caballero B, eds. Encyclopedia of Human Nutrition. San Diego: Academic Press, 1999:1290–97; http://apress .gvpi.net/cgi-bin/om_isapi.dll?clientID= 498755058&infobase= apress_nutrition&softpage=nut_doc_frame_pg.
10. Cervantes-Laurean D, McElvaney G, Moss J. Niacin. In: Shils ME, Olson JA, Shike M et al, eds. Modern Nutrition in Health and Disease. 9th ed. Philadelphia: Williams & Wilkins, 1999:401–11.
11. Food and Nutrition Board, Institute of Medicine. Dietary Reference Intakes for Thiamin, Riboflavin, Niacin, Vitamin B₆, Folate, Vitamin B₁₂, Pantothenic Acid, Biotin, and Choline. Washington, DC: National Academy Press, 1998:123–49.
12. Fenech M. Food Chem Toxicol 2002;40:1113–7.
13. Shibata K. J Nutr 1989;119:892–5.
14. Rongvaux A, Andris F, Van Gool F et al. Bioessays 2003;25: 683–90.
15. Zhang X, Kurnasov OV, Karthikeyan S et al. J Biol Chem 2003;278:13503–11.
16. Emanuelli M, Carnevali F, Saccucci F et al. J Biol Chem 2001; 276:406–12.
17. Raffaelli N, Sorci L, Amici A et al. Biochem Biophys Res Commun 2002;297:835–40.
18. Bedalov A, Hirao M, Posakony J et al. Mol Cell Biol 2003;23: 7044–54.
19. Lerner F, Niere M, Ludwig A et al. Biochem Biophys Res Commun 2001;288:69–74.
20. Nelson DL, Cox MM. Principles of bioenergetics. In: Lehninger Principles of Biochemistry. 3rd ed. New York: Worth Publishers, 2000:490–526.
21. Sternfeld L, Krause E, Guse AH et al. J Biol Chem 2003;278: 33629–36.
22. Ceni C, Muller-Steffner H, Lund F et al. J Biol Chem 2003;278: 40670–8.
23. Partida-Sanchez S, Randall TD, Lund FE. Microbes Infect 2003;5:49–58.
24. Itoh M, Ishihara K, Hiroi T et al. J Immunol 1998;161:3974–83.
25. Ortolan E, Vacca P, Capobianco A et al. Cell Biochem Funct 2002;20:309–22.
26. Antonelli A, Baj G, Marchetti P et al. Diabetes 2001;50:985–91.

27. Marchetti P, Antonelli A, Lupi R et al. Diabetes 2002;51: 474S–7S.

28. Kharadia SV, Huiatt TW, Huang HY et al. Exp Cell Res 1992; 201:33–42.

29. Zolkiewska A, Moss J. J Biol Chem 1993;268:25273–6.

30. Paone G, Wada A, Stevens LA et al. Proc Natl Acad Sci USA 2002;99:8231–5.

31. Kefalas P, Saxty B, Yadollahi-Farsani M et al. Eur J Biochem 1999;259:866–71.

32. Terashima M, Hara N, Badruzzaman M et al. FEBS Lett 1997; 412:227–32.

33. Ohlrogge W, Haag F, Lohler J et al. Mol Cell Biol 2002;22:7535–42.

34. Davidovic L, Vodenicharov M, Affar EB et al. Exp Cell Res 2001;268:7–13.

35. Menissier de Murcia J, Ricoul M, Tartier L et al. EMBO J 2003; 22:2255–63.

36. Kraus WL, Lis JT. Cell 2003;113:677–83.

37. Tong WM, Cortes U, Wang ZQ. Biochim Biophys Acta 2001; 1552:27–37.

38. Virag L, Szabo C. Pharmacol Rev 2002;54:375–429.

39. Hekimi S, Guarente L. Science 2003;299:1351–4.

40. North BJ, Marshall BL, Borra MT et al. Mol Cell 2003;11: 437–44.

41. Frye RA. Biochem Biophys Res Commun 2000;273:793–8.

42. Frye RA. Biochem Biophys Res Commun 1999;260: 273–9.

43. Cheng HL, Mostoslavsky R, Saito S et al. Proc Natl Acad Sci USA 2003;100:10794–9.

44. Luo J, Nikolaev AY, Imai S et al. Cell 2001;107:137–48.

45. McBurney MW, Yang X, Jardine K et al. Mol Cell Biol 2003; 23:38–54.

46. Onyango P, Celic I, McCaffery JM et al. Proc Natl Acad Sci USA 2002;99:13653–8.

47. Borra MT, O'Neill FJ, Jackson MD et al. J Biol Chem 2002; 277:12632–41.

48. Bitterman KJ, Anderson RM, Cohen HY et al. J Biol Chem 2002;277:45099–107.

49. Anderson RM, Bitterman KJ, Wood JG et al. Nature 2003; 423:181–5.

50. Lin SJ, Guarente L. Curr Opin Cell Biol 2003;15:241–6.

51. Karthikeyan K, Thappa DM. Int J Dermatol 2002;41:476–81.

52. Ames BN. Mutat Res 2001;475:7–20.

53. Hageman GJ, Stierum RH. Mutat Res 2001;475:45–56.

54. Kirkland JB. Nutr Cancer 2003;46:110–8.

55. Lin SJ, Defossez PA, Guarente L. Science 2000;289:2126–8.

56. Anderson RM, Bitterman KJ, Wood JG et al. J Biol Chem 2002; 277:18881–90.

57. Spronck JC, Kirkland JB. Mutat Res 2002;508:83–97.

58. Boyonoski AC, Spronck JC, Gallacher LM et al. J Nutr 2002;132: 108–14.

59. Baron DN, Dent CE, Harris H et al. Lancet 1956;271:421–8.

60. Levy HL. Hartnup disorder. In: Scriver CR, Beudet AL, Sly WS et al, eds. The Metabolic and Molecular Basis of Inherited Diseases. New York: McGraw-Hill, 2003; http://genetics.accessmedicine. com/index.html.

61. Jonas AJ, Butler IJ. J Clin Invest 1989;84:200–4.

62. Sauberlich HE. Niacin. In: Laboratory Tests for the Assessment of Nutritional Status. 2nd ed. Boca Raton, FL: CRC Press, 1999: 161–74.

63. Lee YC, Gholson RK, Raica N. J Biol Chem 1969;244:3277–82.

64. Tavintharan S, Kashyap ML. Curr Atheroscler Rep 2001;3: 74–82.

65. Ganji SH, Kamanna VS, Kashyap ML. J Nutr Biochem 2003; 14:298–305.

66. Tunaru S, Kero J, Schaub A et al. Nat Med 2003;9:352–5.

67. Wise A, Foord SM, Fraser NJ et al. J Biol Chem 2003;278: 9869–74.

68. Soga T, Kamohara M, Takasaki J et al. Biochem Biophys Res Commun 2003;303:364–9.

69. Lorenzen A, Stannek C, Lang H et al. Mol Pharmacol 2001; 59:349–57.

70. Lorenzen A, Stannek C, Burmeister A et al. Biochem Pharmacol 2002;64:645–8.

71. Miller M. Mayo Clin Proc 2003;78:735–42.

72. Yang J, Klaidman LK, Adams JD. Mini Rev Med Chem 2002;2: 125–34.

73. Klaidman L, Morales M, Kem S et al. Pharmacology 2003;69: 150–7.

74. Gale EA. Diabetologia 2003;46:339–46.

75. Szabo C. Intensive Care Med 2003;29:863–6.

76. Kreisberg RA. Am J Med 1994;97:313–6.

77. Van den Berg H. Eur J Clin Nutr 1997;51[Suppl 1]:64S–5S.

78. Sugibayashi K, Hayashi T, Hatanaka T et al. Pharm Res 1996;13: 855–60.

79. Realdon N, Ragazzi E, Dal Zotto M. Pharmazie 1995;50: 603–6.

80. Petley A, Macklin B, Renwick AG et al. Diabetes 1995;44: 152–5.

81. Kim H, Jacobson EL, Jacobson MK. Science 1993;261:1330–3.

82. Vu CQ, Lu PJ, Chen CS et al. J Biol Chem 1996;271:4747–54.

83. Panzeter PL, Zweifel B, Althaus FR. Biochem Biophys Res Commun 1992;184:544–8.

SELECTED READINGS

Bays H, Stein EA. Pharmacotherapy for dyslipidaemia: current therapies and future agents. Expert Opin Pharmacother 2003;4:1901–38.

Kraut AM. Goldberger's War: The Life and Work of a Public Health Crusader. New York: Farrar-Strauss and Giroux, 2003.

Rucker RB, Suttie JW, McCormick DB et al, eds. Handbook of Vitamins. 3rd ed. New York: Marcel Dekker, 2001.

Sadler MJ, Strain JJ, Caballero B, eds. Encyclopedia of Human Nutrition. San Diego: Academic Press, 1999; http://apress.gvpi.net/cgi-bin/om_ isapi.dll?clientID=498755058&infobase=apress_nutrition&softpage= nut_doc_frame_pg.

Weiner M, Van Eys J. Nicotinic Acid: Nutrient-Cofactor-Drug. New York: Marcel Dekker, 1983.

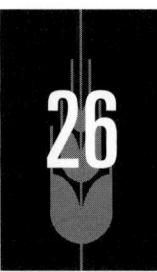

26   VITAMIN B$_6$[1]

AMY D. MACKEY, STEVEN R. DAVIS, AND JESSE F. GREGORY III

HISTORY 452
CHEMISTRY AND NOMENCLATURE 452
ABSORPTION AND BIOAVAILABILITY 453
    Absorption 453
    Bioavailability 453
TRANSPORT AND METABOLISM 454
FUNCTIONS 454
    Amino Acids 454
    One-Carbon Units 454
    Lipids 455
    Glycogenolysis and Gluconeogenesis 455
    Heme Biosynthesis 455
    Immune Function 455
    Interactions with Other Nutrients 455
VITAMIN B$_6$ IN FOODS AND SUPPLEMENTS 456
ASSESSMENT OF NUTRITIONAL STATUS 456
REQUIREMENTS 457
VITAMIN B$_6$ IN HEALTH AND DISEASE 457
    Pyridoxine-Responsive Inherited Disorders 457
    Vitamin B$_6$ Status in Relation to Disease
        States and Aging .458
PHARMACOLOGIC PYRIDOXINE THERAPY
    AND PYRIDOXINE TOXICITY 459
VITAMIN B$_6$–DRUG INTERACTIONS 459

Since vitamin B$_6$ was first reported in the 1930s, our understanding of its properties, metabolic function, and role in maintaining health has expanded enormously. In spite of these advances, areas of uncertainty still exist, including the optimal intake of the vitamin, the consequences of inadequacy, how best to assess nutritional status, and the effects of supplementation on health. Since the previous edition of this book (1), important advances have occurred regarding the role of vitamin B$_6$ nutritional status and incidence of chronic disease, and this aspect is given special consideration.

---

[1]**Abbreviations: ALAS**, δ-aminolevulinate synthase; **HPLC**, high-performance liquid chromatography; **4-PA**, 4-pyridoxic acid; **PL**, pyridoxal; **PLP**, pyridoxal 5′-phosphate; **PM**, pyridoxamine; **PMP**, pyridoxamine 5′-phosphate; **PN**, pyridoxine; **PNG**, pyridoxine 5′-β-D-glucoside; **PNP**, pyridoxine 5′-phosphate; **RDA**, recommended dietary allowance; **VD**, vascular disease.

HISTORY

Evidence of a water-soluble nutritional factor later identified as vitamin B$_6$ was first reported in 1934 (2, 3). Five laboratories reported the independent isolation and crystallization of pyridoxine (PN) in 1938 (4–9), and the proposed structure was confirmed through successful synthesis the following year. Studies of the nutritional requirements of lactic acid bacteria led to the recognition of pyridoxal (PL) and pyridoxamine (PM) (9–12). The coenzyme form of vitamin B$_6$ was demonstrated to be a phosphorylated derivative (13), and eventually was identified as the 5′-phosphate. The reader is referred to several excellent reviews for more detailed information on the interesting history of vitamin B$_6$ (14–16).

CHEMISTRY AND NOMENCLATURE

The term vitamin B$_6$ is the preferred generic descriptor (17) for the family of 2-methyl, 3-hydroxy, 5-hydroxymethyl-pyridine derivatives that exhibit the nutritional activity of PN. Pyridoxine has been used as a generic term especially in clinical contexts; however, it is strongly recommended that the consistent use of the generic vitamin B$_6$ rather than pyridoxine be adopted to reduce confusion in vitamin B$_6$ nomenclature.

Vitamin B$_6$ exists as three main derivatives of a 2-methyl, 3-hydroxy, 5-hydroxymethyl-pyridine nucleus that differ with respect to their substituent at the 4 position of the pyridine ring (Fig. 26.1). For the C-4 substituent, PN has a hydroxymethyl group, PL is an aldehyde, whereas PM has an aminomethyl group. Because PN is an alcohol, PN has been termed "pyridoxol" intermittently; this designator is obsolete, and its use should be discontinued. PN, PL, and PM all can exist with a phosphate group esterified at the C-5′ position (i.e., pyridoxine 5′-phosphate [PNP], pyridoxal 5′-phosphate [PLP], and pyridoxamine 5′-phosphate [PMP]). PLP and PMP are the coenzyme forms of vitamin B$_6$ and are interconverted as they function in the actions of the aminotransferase family of enzymes. Although PNP is not a coenzyme, it is an important intermediate in the metabolic pathway by which PLP is formed from dietary PN (Fig. 26.2). 4-Pyridoxic acid (4-PA), which is the major metabolically inactive catabolic

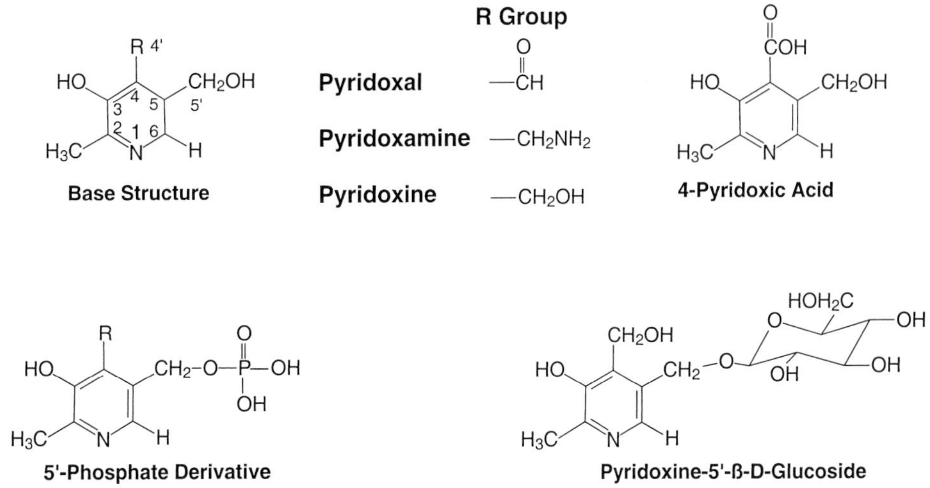

R Group

Pyridoxal   —CH (O)

Pyridoxamine —CH₂NH₂

Pyridoxine   —CH₂OH

Base Structure

4-Pyridoxic Acid

Figure 26.1. Chemical structures of vitamin B₆ forms.

5'-Phosphate Derivative

Pyridoxine-5'-ß-D-Glucoside

ABSORBTION AND BIOAVAILABILITY

Absorption

Intestinal absorption of vitamin B₆ is thought to take place in the jejunum by nonsaturable, passive diffusion of the nonphosphorylated forms (16). However, evidence from in vitro studies using eukaryotic cells suggests that vitamin B₆ absorption is pH dependent and exhibits both saturable and nonsaturable components (18). The in vitro model of absorption appears to occur via a carrier-mediated pathway that involves proton exchange (18, 19). Dietary PLP, PMP, and PNP are enzymatically dephosphorylated at the brush border membrane by alkaline phosphatase before absorption (1). Once absorbed, dietary PN, PL, and PM are phosphorylated by PL kinase for the purpose of metabolic trapping. Addition of the phosphate group at the 5' position of the pyridine ring creates a negative charge on the molecule that prevents the vitamers from leaking through the membrane in intestinal mucosal cells and in other tissues. To cross the basolateral membrane and enter into portal circulation, PN, PL, and PM are converted back to a nonphosphorylated form.

Bioavailability

The bioavailability of nutrients in foods and supplements is an important issue in evaluation the adequacy of diets and the efficacy of supplements in meeting nutritional requirements and in resolving inadequate status. The bioavailability of vitamin B₆ in humans consuming a mixed diet is approximately 75% (20), and data from pigs indicate that the digestibility of vitamin B₆ from animal sources is approximately 10% greater than from plant sources (21). As reviewed elsewhere (22), vitamin B₆ bioavailability is likely to be a function of the degree of entrapment in the food matrix (i.e., nondigestible residue) and the extent of utilization of glycosylated forms of vitamin B₆. PNG, the major glycosylated form of vitamin B₆ in the human diet, provides an average of approximately 15%

product of vitamin B₆ metabolism, has a carboxyl group at C-4 and is nutritionally and metabolically inactive. Also shown in Figure 26.1 is pyridoxine 5'-ß-D-glucoside (PNG), a glycosylated form of vitamin B₆ commonly found in foods of plant origin.

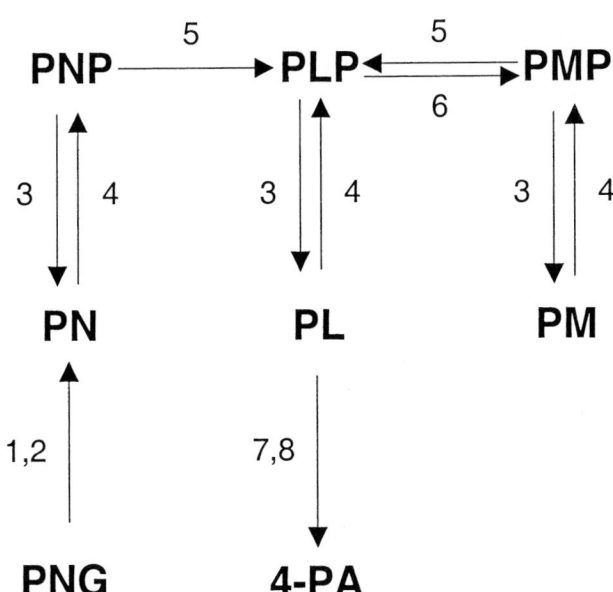

1: Lactase-phlorizin hydrolase
2: Pyridoxine-5'-ß-D-glucoside hydrolase
3: Phosphatases
4: Pyridoxal kinase
5: Pyridoxine (pyridoxamine) phosphate oxidase
6: Aminotransferase
7: Aldehyde oxidase
8: Aldehyde dehydrogenase

Figure 26.2. Overview of vitamin B₆ metabolism. 4-PA, 4-pyridoxic acid; PL, pyridoxal; PLP, pyridoxal-5'-phosphate; PM, pyridoxamine; PMP, pyridoxamine-5'-phosphate; PN, pyridoxine; PNG, pyridoxine-5'-ß-D-glucoside; PNP, pyridoxine-5'-phosphate.

of total daily vitamin B_6 intake (23), although this percentage could be much higher depending on food selection. The bioavailability of purified PNG was only approximately 30% in rats (24, 25) and approximately 50% in humans when compared with free PN (26, 27). Rat (24) and human (26, 27) studies using isotopically labeled PNG found that PNG was effectively absorbed, but it was not completely hydrolyzed in the small intestine to glucose and PN. Intestinal hydrolysis of PNG is catalyzed by two β-glucosidases: a novel, cytosolic enzyme designated PNG hydrolase (28); and the brush border membrane enzyme lactase-phlorizin hydrolase (29–31). PNG also can be absorbed intact, potentially hydrolyzed by glucosidase activity in the kidney, or it can be excreted unchanged in the urine (26, 27).

TRANSPORT AND METABOLISM

Vitamin B_6, mostly as PL, enters into portal circulation and is bound to albumin in the plasma and hemoglobin in erythrocytes for transport (32). Although PL and PLP constitute 75 to 80% of the circulating forms of vitamin B_6 (33), PN also is detected in the circulation bound to erythrocytes (34). Whereas the mechanism of uptake of PN and other forms by erythrocytes is not known, their retention is favored by rapid phosphorylation and binding to hemoglobin (33, 35, 36). Erythrocytes may serve as a component of vitamin B_6 transport between tissues (36).

The liver is the primary site of vitamin B_6 metabolism through which PLP is generated for hepatic use and export to extrahepatic tissues. Nonphosphorylated forms of vitamin B_6 are phosphorylated in the liver by PL kinase, which uses adenosine triphosphate-zinc as a cosubstrate and catalyzes the phosphorylation of PN, PL, and PM to yield PNP, PLP, and PMP, respectively (37). Conversion of PNP and PMP to PLP is catalyzed by the flavin-mononucleotide–dependent pyridoxamine (pyridoxine) 5′-phosphate oxidase in the liver (37). This reaction is critical to the metabolism of dietary vitamin B_6 because most extrahepatic tissues have comparatively little oxidase activity. Pyridoxamine (pyridoxine) 5′-phosphate oxidase is subject to strong product inhibition, which serves to avoid the production of excessive amounts of PLP (38). Dephosphorylation of PLP and PMP in the liver and other tissues is catalyzed by tissue nonspecific phosphatase (39), as well as a vitamin B_6–specific form of erythrocyte alkaline phosphatase (40). Two hepatic enzymes, riboflavin (flavin adenine dinucleotide)–dependent aldehyde oxidase and nicotinamide adenine dinucleotide–dependent aldehyde dehydrogenase, oxidize excess dephosphorylated PL in tissues to 4-PA, the major catabolic product of vitamin B_6 (39).

As stated earlier, PLP and PL are the predominant circulating forms of vitamin B_6. The turnover of vitamin B_6, as PLP, has been described using a compartmental model that includes five body pools: muscle, liver, plasma, erythrocytes, and one to combine all other pools (41). Total

body concentrations of vitamin B_6 are estimated to be 15 nmol/g, corresponding to approximately 1000 μmol in an adult human (42). PLP in the muscle pool represents 75 to 80% of total body vitamin B_6 largely as a coenzyme for glycogen phosphorylase (42).

Tissue uptake of vitamin B_6 from circulation requires dephosphorylation. After enzymatic removal of the 5′-phosphate group by plasma membrane tissue nonspecific phosphatase, vitamin B_6 can cross cellular membranes by a carrier-mediated transport system (43, 44). Vitamin B_6 in tissues is retained by phosphorylation and is concentrated to the mitochondria and cytosol.

FUNCTIONS

Vitamin B_6 functions as a coenzyme in a variety of enzymatic reactions in the metabolism of amino acids, one-carbon units, lipids, and the pathways of gluconeogenesis, heme, and neurotransmitter biosynthesis. PLP is the most common vitamin B_6 coenzyme. The structures of PLP and PMP accommodate the formation of Schiff base linkages with other amines and aldehydes (see Fig. 26.1). These structures make them well suited to serve as coenzymes for more than 100 different enzymes. PLP may affect steroid hormone function through modulation of steroid hormone receptor-mediated gene transcription, although the physiologic implications of this interaction are uncertain (45, 46).

Amino Acids

Nearly all amino acids require at least one PLP-dependent enzyme in their metabolism. PLP is a coenzyme for aminotransaminases that catalyze reversible conversions of amino acids to their corresponding α-keto acids with simultaneous transfer of the amino group to yield PMP. Amino acids also can be modified by PLP-dependent decarboxylation, dehydration, and desulfuration reactions. Metabolism of several amino acids involved in one-carbon metabolism is catalyzed by PLP-dependent reactions, as described later. PLP-dependent decarboxylation reactions are important in the biosynthesis of neurotransmitters (γ-aminobutyric acid, dopamine, and norepinephrine), including the conversion of L-aromatic amino acids to active neurotransmitters by dopa decarboxylase (e.g., 5-hydroxytryptophan conversion to serotonin) (47).

One-Carbon Units

PLP is a coenzyme for four enzymes in one-carbon metabolism and transsulfuration. Serine hydroxymethyltransferase and glycine decarboxylase transfer one-carbon units to tetrahydrofolate from serine and glycine, respectively (Fig. 26.3, reactions 1 and 2). Combined, these enzymatic reactions provide the majority of one-carbon groups used for purine and thymidine synthesis as well as methyl groups for remethylation of homocysteine

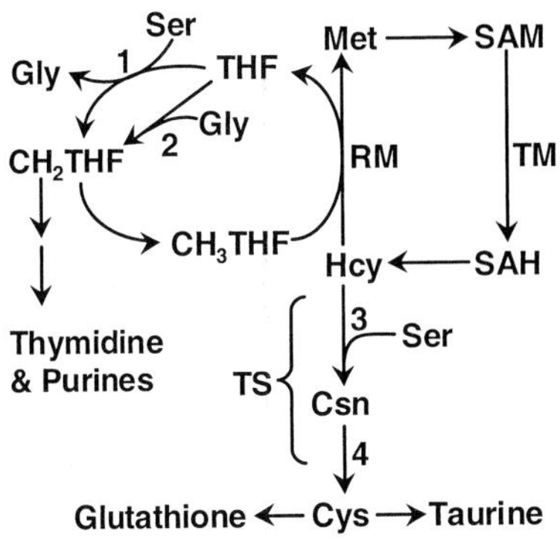

Figure 26.3. Pyridoxal 5'-phosphate (PLP) dependence of homocysteine (Hcy) and other one-carbon cycle reactions: (1) serine (Ser) hydroxymethyltransferase; (2) glycine (Gly) decarboxylase of the glycine cleavage system; (3) cystathionine (Csn) β-synthase; (4) cystathionine γ-lyase. CH$_2$THF, 5,10-methylenetetrahydrofolate; CH$_3$THF, 5-methyltetrahydrofolate; Cys, cysteine; Met, methionine; RM, remethylation; SAH, S-adenosylhomocysteine; SAM, S-adenosylmethionine; TM, transmethylation; TS, transsulfuration.

to methionine. Once incorporated into methionine, these methyl groups may be used for S-adenosylmethionine–dependent transmethylation reactions involved in the metabolism of creatine, DNA, RNA, lipids, proteins, and other molecules. The transsulfuration pathway, composed of the PLP-dependent enzymes cystathionine β-synthase and cystathionine γ-lyase (see Fig. 26.3, reactions 3 and 4), catabolizes homocysteine through condensation with serine to produce cystathione, followed by cleavage of that molecule to produce cysteine and α-ketobutyrate. One-carbon unit generation and transsulfuration are impaired in severely vitamin B$_6$–deficient rats (48, 49).

Lipids

The role of vitamin B$_6$ in lipid metabolism is not clearly defined. The arachadonic acid (50, 51) and docosohexaenoic acid (52) content of hepatic phospholipids and the arachadonic acid content of plasma (53) phospholipids were reduced in vitamin B$_6$–deficient rats. The biochemical mechanisms involved are uncertain; however, these observations may be explained by aberrations in the PLP-dependent enzymatic pathways involved in the transfer of one-carbon units, which could yield lower concentrations of methylated phospholipids. The biosynthetic pathway of carnitine, which is essential for intramitochondrial transport of long-chain fatty acids, requires the activity of PLP-dependent 3-hydroxytrimethyl-lysine aldolase. Vitamin B$_6$ deficiency was shown to reduce plasma carnitine concentrations in rats (54), but not in humans (1).

Glycogenolysis and Gluconeogenesis

Vitamin B$_6$, as PLP, plays a dual role in the synthesis of glucose. Glycogen phosphorylase relies on PLP as a coenzyme in the enzymatic cleavage of glycogen that sequentially releases glucose-1-phosphate units. The 5'-phosphate group of PLP, rather than the 4'-aldehyde group (as in the aminotransferase reactions), is required for general acid catalysis in glycogenolysis. PLP-dependent transaminases convert gluconeogenic amino acids to α-keto acids to create substrates for the production of glucose.

Heme Biosynthesis

Heme biosynthesis relies on the activity of PLP-dependent δ-aminolevulinate synthase (ALAS). This enzyme catalyzes the condensation of succinyl coenzyme A and glycine to form δ-aminolevulinate, which is the precursor for the porphyrin ring. Chronic vitamin B$_6$ deficiency can precipitate microcytic, hypochromic anemia in which the hemoglobin concentration of erythrocytes is reduced. Sideroblastic anemia is an inherited form of an ALAS deficiency. This anemia often can be successfully treated with PN supplementation; however, some mutations alter the PLP binding sites on the ALAS enzyme (55, 56) and thus diminish the efficacy of PN supplementation.

Immune Function

The importance of adequate vitamin B$_6$ status for proper immune function in animals, particularly cell-mediated and to a lesser degree humoral immunity, has been known since the 1950s, as reviewed by Chandra and Sudhakaran (57). Lymphocytes isolated from vitamin B$_6$–deficient persons display reduced proliferation, reduced interleukin-2 production in response to mitogens (58, 59), and reduced antibody production in response to immunization (57). Depressed lymphocyte proliferation may stem from impaired DNA synthesis as a result of reduced activity of serine hydroxymethyltransferase (see Fig. 26.3, reaction 1). Vitamin B$_6$ depletion-repletion studies in young and old subjects suggest that intake of vitamin B$_6$ equal to the current recommended ietary allowance (RDA) may be insufficient to maximize immunocompetence (58, 59), but the relevance of this observation to infectious disease susceptibility is uncertain.

Interactions with Other Nutrients

The interconversion and metabolism of vitamin B$_6$ depend on riboflavin, niacin, and zinc (see Fig. 26.2). Both PN (PM) phosphate and aldehyde oxidases require riboflavin in the forms of flavin mononucleotide and flavin adenine dinucleotide, respectively. Niacin, as nicotinamide adenine dinucleotide, serves as coenzyme for aldehyde dehydrogenase. The phosphorylation of vitamin B$_6$ is catalyzed by PL kinase, which requires zinc as cofactor. An insufficient dietary intake of these nutrients may adversely affect the metabolic utilization of vitamin B$_6$.

Niacin, folate, and carnitine require vitamin B$_6$ for their biosynthesis and metabolism. Biosynthesis of niacin from tryptophan requires PLP-dependent kynureninase. As discussed earlier, PLP-dependent serine hydroxymethyl-transferase and glycine decarboxylase are essential for normal folate metabolism (see Fig. 26.3, reactions 1 and 2).

VITAMIN B₆ IN FOODS AND SUPPLEMENTS

Vitamin B_6 traditionally has been measured in foods and biologic materials by microbiologic assays using the yeast *Saccharomyces uvarum* (60). Both microbiologic and high-performance liquid chromatography (HPLC) methods are now widely used (60–62). Microbiologic assays can be well suited to the measurement of total vitamin B_6, whereas properly configured HPLC methods allow the determination of the various forms of vitamin B_6, including the glycosylated forms.

Vitamin B_6 is widely distributed throughout the food supply. Appendix Table A-23-a lists the vitamin B_6 content of many foods, including cooked foods. Foods of animal origin such as meat, fish, eggs, and dairy products are rich in vitamin B_6, mostly as PL and PM and their phosphorylated forms. Many vegetables and whole-grain cereal products are good sources of the vitamin. The predominant forms of vitamin B_6 in foods of plant origin are PN and glycosylated PN (16). Plant tissues may contain up to 75% of their vitamin B_6 as PNG (63), which is presumed to be a storage form of the vitamin. According to the 1995 Continuing Survey of Food Intakes by Individuals (63a), the adult US population obtains most of its dietary vitamin B_6 from ready-to-eat fortified cereals, meat, fish, poultry, starchy vegetables, and noncitrus fruits.

Relatively little loss of vitamin B_6 occurs during food storage and handling, aside from losses occurring during the milling of grain, but losses of PL, PLP, PM, and PMP during cooking and thermal processing of foods can be significant (64). The nutritional impact of vitamin B_6 loss was acutely observed in the 1950s when infants were fed formula for which a change in thermal processing conditions led to excessive destruction of vitamin B_6 in the unfortified formula (65). Certain infants consuming this formula developed convulsive seizures that were alleviated by PN supplementation. This situation prompted the routine fortification of formulas with PN. Because of its greater stability than the other B_6 vitamers, PN hydrochloride is used in all types of food fortification and in most nutritional supplements. PN α-ketoglutarate also has been used as a vitamin B_6 supplement to enhance exercise performance; however, the evidence supporting this benefit is equivocal (66).

ASSESSMENT OF NUTRITIONAL STATUS

Vitamin B_6 nutritional status can be evaluated using direct measurement of B_6 vitamers in blood and/or urine or by indicators based on the biochemical function of vitamin B_6 (1, 16, 67, 68). The various indicators of vitamin B_6 status and their generally accepted cutoff values for adequacy are summarized in Table 26.1.

TABLE 26.1. INDICES FOR ASSESSMENT OF VITAMIN B₆ STATUS AND SUGGESTED MINIMAL VALUES FOR ADEQUATE STATUS

INDEX	ADEQUATE STATUS
Direct	
Plasma pyridoxal phosphate	>30 nmol/L[a]
Plasma total vitamin B_6	>40 nmol/L
Urinary 4-pyridoxic acid	>3 μmol/d
Urinary total vitamin B_6	>0.5 μmol/d
Indirect	
Erythrocyte alanine aminotransferase coenzyme stimulation index[b]	<1.25
Erythrocyte aspartate aminotransferase coenzyme stimulation index[b]	<1.80
2-g L-Tryptophan load, urinary xanthurenic acid	<65 μmol/d
3-g L-Methionine load, urinary cystathionine	<350 μmol/d
Dietary intake	
Vitamin B_6 intake, weekly average	>1.25–1.5 mg/d
Vitamin B_6/protein ratio	>0.016 mg/g

[a] Plasma PLP <20 nmol/L is considered indicative of deficiency; 1 mg PN = 5.92 μmol.

[b] Coenzyme stimulation index is the ratio of enzyme activity values measured with and without preincubation of the erythrocyte hemolysate with added pyridoxal phosphate. This index is proportional to the fraction of enzyme in apoenzyme form.

Adapted from Leklem J. J Nutr 1990;120[Suppl]:1503S–7S, with permission from the American Society for Nutritional Sciences.

The most commonly used direct measure of vitamin B_6 status is the concentration of PLP in plasma, which can be readily measured by HPLC or enzymatic methods. Plasma PLP concentration has been shown to correlate with tissue PLP concentration in rats (69) and with vitamin B_6 intake in controlled human dietary studies (16, 68). A plasma PLP concentration of more than 30 nmol/L traditionally has been considered to indicate adequate status in human adults (16, 68), whereas a concentration greater than 20 nmol/L has been used as a more conservative cutoff value (67). If the 20 nmol/L cutoff is used, we recommend that values in the range of 20 to 30 nmol/L be interpreted as indicative of marginal status. Certain genetic and physiologic conditions influence plasma PLP values (1); thus, conclusions regarding vitamin B_6 status based on plasma PLP should be considered presumptive until they are confirmed by an alternate method of status assessment. Even though plasma total vitamin B_6 has been used as an indicator of status, neither total B_6 concentrations nor the individual concentrations of other vitamers (e.g., PL, 4-PA) are as useful as PLP because of the lack of criteria for interpretation. Similarly, erythrocyte PLP is a potential indicator of vitamin B_6 status for which a consensus is lacking regarding its diagnostic utility. The diagnostic use of erythrocyte PLP also is limited because of unresolved methodologic issues. Urinary 4-PA excretion (>3 μmol/day) is indicative of vitamin B_6 adequacy (16, 68). Whereas urinary 4-PA is easily determined by HPLC, it must be considered a secondary status indicator because a complete 24-hour urine collection is usually required and 4-PA excretion is strongly affected by recent vitamin B$_6$ intake.

Functional indicators of vitamin B$_6$ status are based on measures of PLP-dependent processes either in vivo or in blood cells. Urinary excretion of xanthurenic acid, either basal or following a tryptophan load, was the first functional indicator. The tryptophan load test has not been widely used since an incident of toxicity occurred in the 1980s resulting from the presence of a toxic impurity in a batch of tryptophan. The methionine load test, as most widely used currently, involves the measurement of the rise in plasma homocysteine following an oral methionine load (70). Vitamin B$_6$ deficiency has little effect on fasting plasma homocysteine concentration (unlike folate deficiency) but yields a higher postmethionine load homocysteine concentration as a result of the impairment of the transsulfuration pathway. The many variations in the protocol of methionine load tests (i.e., doses and blood sampling times) complicate interpretation and comparison of published findings. Finally, the in vitro measurement of erythrocyte aspartate aminotransferase or alanine aminotransferase in the presence and absence of added PLP allows calculation of an activation coefficient, which is an indirect measure of the degree of deficiency through assessment of the proportion of the enzyme in apoenzyme form.

REQUIREMENTS

The Food and Nutrition Board (67) revised the requirements for vitamin B$_6$ in 1998 (Table 26.2). An estimated average requirement of 1.1 mg/day and an RDA of 1.3 mg/day for men and women (19–50 years) were established as a result of this reassessment. The RDAs were reduced from previous recommendations set in 1989 (1) (see also Appendix Table A-3-b-1.). To determine the requirement, plasma PLP concentration ($\geq$20 nmol/L) was used as the major vitamin B$_6$ status indicator because it best represents tissue stores (67). As reviewed in the report (67), vitamin B$_6$ requirements were based on data from controlled investigations examining dietary vitamin B$_6$ intake in combination with synthetic PN. Average vitamin B$_6$ intake, as estimated by nationally representative nutrient intake surveys in the United States, is approximately 1.5 mg/day for women and 2 mg/day for men. Although indicators of vitamin B$_6$ status have been shown to decline with increasing protein consumption in numerous studies, this effect has not been consistently observed (42). Thus, the current RDA is not expressed as a function of protein intake (42). Some controversy exists regarding the RDA for vitamin B$_6$ especially in light of findings results suggesting that an optimal intake is greater than the current RDA of 1.3 mg/day (58, 71). Further research is required to answer this question.

Limited data exist regarding the requirements of infants and children for vitamin B$_6$. The adequate intake established for infants up to 11 months of age was primarily derived from the vitamin B$_6$ content of human milk (0.13–0.24 mg/L) and milk intake from healthy, exclusively breast-fed infants (67, 72). The background, basis, definitions, and other dietary reference intakes are summarized in Appendix Tables A-2-h through A-2-k. Although insufficient dietary intake and, consequently, nutritional status of vitamin B$_6$ are not prevalent in the general population, significant portions of the population are at risk of suboptimal vitamin B$_6$ intake and status, including pregnant and lactating women (23, 73) and elderly persons (74).

VITAMIN B$_6$ IN HEALTH AND DISEASE

Pyridoxine-Responsive Inherited Disorders

Homocystinuria, which is an autosomal recessive disorder of genetic heterogeneity occurring at a frequency of one in 344,000, is primarily caused by deficient activity of the PLP-dependent enzyme cystathionine β-synthase (75). The result is disruption of homocysteine catabolism manifested as hyperhomocysteinemia, hypermethioninemia, and hypocystinemia. Clinical outcomes include dislocation of the optic lens, long bone malformation and osteoporosis, mental retardation, and thromboembolism; the last condition is the most frequent cause of death. Treatment includes a low-methionine diet designed to minimize homocysteine accumulation. In a subgroup (~1/2) of patients in one study, pharmacologic doses of PN (250–500 mg/day) partly ameliorated the biochemical and clinical consequences of the enzyme deficiency (76). The mechanism of responsiveness is likely related to overcoming reduced

TABLE 26.2. RECOMMENDED VITAMIN B$_6$ INTAKES BY AGE AND GENDER^a

	AGE (y)	MALES (mg/d)	FEMALES (mg/d)
Infant	0–0.5	0.1^b	0.1^b
	0.5–1	0.3^b	0.3^b
Children	1–3	0.5	0.5
	4–8	0.6	0.6
Adolescents	9–13	1.0	1.0
	14–18	1.3	1.2
Adults	19–30	1.3	1.3
	31–50	1.3	1.3
	51–70	1.7	1.5
	>70	1.7	1.5
Pregnancy			1.9
Lactation			2.0

^{a}1 mg of PN = 5.92 μmol.
^{b}Adequate intakes; all other values are presented as recommended dietary allowances.

From Food and Nutrition Board, Institute of Medicine. Vitamin B$_6$. In: Dietary Reference Intakes for Thiamin, Riboflavin, Niacin, Vitamin B$_6$, Folate, Vitamin B$_{12}$, Pantothenic Acid, Biotin, and Choline. Washington, DC: National Academy Press, 1998, with permission of the National Academy of Sciences (US), Washington, DC.

affinity of PLP for the mutant enzyme, and not correction of a preexisting vitamin B_6 deficiency.

PN-dependent seizure is a rare (~1 in 500,000) inherited condition of unknown genetic origin that is characterized by seizures that begin before or within days of birth, sometimes accompanied by abnormal behavior and vomiting (77, 78). Although PLP concentrations in plasma and blood cells are normal in these infants, seizures cease immediately on intravenous PN administration (100–500 mg), and the condition is controllable through daily PN supplementation (~0.2–3 mg/kg body weight). Reduced glutamate decarboxylase activity is presumed to cause the seizures, but this mechanism has been challenged (77).

Vitamin B_6 Status in Relation to Disease States and Aging

Patients affected by many disease states have lower vitamin B_6 status than otherwise healthy populations as indicated by low plasma PLP, elevated postmethionine load plasma homocysteine, or elevated urinary tryptophan catabolites. Plasma PLP concentrations are low in patients with malabsorption syndromes such as acute celiac disease (79), Crohn disease, and ulcerative colitis (80). The mechanism has not been investigated exhaustively, but reduced PN absorption occurs in celiac disease (79), and the inflammatory response may affect plasma PLP concentration in inflammatory bowel diseases (80).

Vitamin B_6 deficiency causes vascular damage in monkeys (81) and pigs (82), but not in all species studied. Plasma PLP concentrations characteristic of deficiency in one study were found in 5% of patients with vascular disease (VD), twice the incidence in controls (83). Many other cross-sectional and retrospective studies found associations of low human vitamin B_6 status with elevated risk of coronary artery disease, cerebrovascular disease, and peripheral VD, as reviewed by McKinley (84). Although most studies focused on the connection between vitamin B_6 status and homocysteine metabolism in VD, many found the association between vitamin B_6 and VD to be independent of fasting plasma total homocysteine concentration (83, 84). These associations are strongest in studies involving populations already diagnosed with VD, a finding suggesting that this relationship reflects negative effects of VD progression on vitamin B_6 status. The results of prospective studies of vitamin B_6 status and VD are equivocal (84). Most clinical trials of vitamin B_6 supplementation for VD risk reduction conducted thus far involve concurrent folate and vitamin B_{12} supplementation, and this protocol complicates assessment of the effects of vitamin B_6 alone. The results of two ongoing, large-scale, randomized trials of the effect of high dose PN therapy (40 mg/day) on VD may clarify the role of vitamin B_6 in these conditions (85).

Potential but unproven mechanisms whereby vitamin B_6 deficiency may affect VD include effects on lipid metabolism (86), endothelial function (87), thrombogenesis (86), and inflammation (88). Although vitamin B_6 deficiency can affect multiple pathways of homocysteine metabolism, the association between vitamin B_6 status and VD is independent of fasting total homocysteine (83, 84). The inhibitory role proposed for vitamin B_6 in platelet aggregation in vivo is unlikely (89).

Altered vitamin B_6 metabolism as observed in patients with breast cancer and within tumors suggests an association between vitamin B_6 and cancer (90). Data from epidemiologic studies suggest that low vitamin B_6 status is associated with a greater risk of certain cancers (91). For example, an increased risk of breast cancer was noted between extreme quintiles of plasma PLP concentration (<28.5 versus >48.2 nmol/L; odds ratio, 0.7 [92]) and extreme tertiles of vitamin B_6 intake (1.4 versus 2.6 mg/day, odds ratio, 0.54 [93]). An inverse association exists between vitamin B_6 exposure and cell proliferation in experimental cancer models, as reviewed in Komatsu and associates (94). Other potential protective effects of vitamin B_6 include modulation of steroid hormone action (45), maintenance of one-carbon metabolism, and maintenance of immune function (90). Few clinical trial data are available to assess causality for low vitamin B_6 status in cancer.

The nervous system relies on certain PLP-dependent enzymes for neurotransmitter synthesis, as explained earlier. Serotonin and γ-amino butyric acid are particularly sensitive to vitamin B_6 status in rats and may account for altered thyroid hormone levels and seizure activity observed in vitamin B_6–deficient animals (47). Moreover, these studies suggest a strong role for vitamin B_6 in cognitive development. Some evidence indicates a modest positive relationship between vitamin B_6 status in elderly persons and memory, but not mood (95, 96). As discussed earlier, seizures also occurred in infants consuming infant formula deficient in vitamin B_6 (97). Abnormal brain wave activity was observed in these infants, as well in some adults examined in vitamin B_6 deficiency studies (98). Vitamin B_6 status was reported to be lower than normal in patients with some psychiatric conditions, such as Alzheimer disease (99), but it is uncertain to what extent this reflects poor dietary intake after the onset of disease. Attempts to correct suspected neurotransmitter abnormalities with PN treatment in conditions such as headache, chronic pain, behavioral disorders, depression, autism, Down syndrome, schizophrenia, and various neuropathies have met with limited success (100).

Multiple links exist between vitamin B_6 status and diabetes, as reviewed by Leklem (46). The roles of vitamin B_6 in gluconeogenesis and glycogenolysis are described in the earlier section on vitamin B_6 functions. Low concentrations of plasma B_6 vitamers observed in patients with type 1 or type 2 diabetes may be related to increased plasma alkaline phosphatase activity or the acute suppressive effect of an oral glucose load on plasma PLP concentration (46). Moreover, supraphysiologic concentrations of

PLP inhibit protein glycation reactions in model systems, but such effects presumably result from the action of PLP as a competing aldehyde in such nonphysiologic in vitro conditions. The use of pharmacologic intakes of PN in treatment of specific symptoms of diabetes remains controversial (101).

Biochemical and functional indices indicate that declining vitamin B_6 status occurs with aging in both animals (102) and humans (74, 102). The cause of these observations is uncertain, but reduced dietary intake, impaired renal function, and effects of inflammation and the acute-phase response on vitamin B_6 metabolism are possible contributors (74). These indices, as well as immune function, are improved by PN supplementation (103, 104). In controlled nutritional studies, vitamin B_6 intakes needed to restore biochemical, functional, and immunologic indices of B_6 status in elderly persons to levels considered normal for younger populations were greater than the current RDA for this age group (59, 105).

Impaired renal function, including end-stage renal disease and chronic renal insufficiency, is associated with perturbed vitamin B_6 status, as indicated by low PLP and PL in plasma and red blood cells, elevated 4-PA, and elevated postmethionine load plasma homocysteine (106, 107). Elevated postmethionine load homocysteine concentrations in renal transplant recipients (108) and peripheral neuropathy symptoms associated with hemodialysis have been ameliorated with supplemental PN (250 mg/day) (109), although this dose raises concerns of potential toxicity. Low vitamin B_6 status in patients with renal disease may contribute to their elevated risk of VD.

Rheumatoid arthritis is associated with poor vitamin B_6 nutritional status, as evaluated by both plasma PLP and functional indices (110, 111). The inverse association of vitamin B_6 status and indicators of arthritis severity, combined with related data connecting low vitamin B_6 status and other conditions characterized by elevated markers of inflammation (e.g., VDs, inflammatory bowel disease, renal disease, and aging), suggests that inflammation impairs vitamin B_6 status by a currently unknown mechanism (110).

PHARMACOLOGIC PYRIDOXINE THERAPY AND PYRIDOXINE TOXICITY

In addition to the uses of supplemental PN mentioned earlier, PN treatment also improves hematopoeisis in patients with specific forms of sideroblastic anemia (112). Pharmacologic doses of vitamin B_6 also have been used, with little proof of efficacy, to alleviate the symptoms of dysmenorrhea, morning sickness, asthma, carpal tunnel syndrome, and hyperoxaluria, among others (101, 113). Those studies that show benefits of supplemental PN often are small and poorly controlled. Trials of PN therapy for premenstrual syndrome, the treatment that may represent the most frequent use of large PN doses, have

yielded equivocal results (114). Although efficacy is questionable in many cases, PN treatment at pharmacologic doses continues to be used, either prescribed or self-medicated, as stand-alone or adjunct therapy for many of the conditions mentioned earlier. Its persistent use is the result, in part, of low perceived toxicity of PN treatment compared with traditional medical approaches. However, long-term treatment with pharmacologic doses of PN (>500 mg/day) is associated with risk of neuropathies that are reversed largely on withdrawal from PN supplements, as reviewed elsewhere (67). To reduce this risk, the Food and Nutrition Board of the Institute of Medicine established a tolerable upper intake level of vitamin B_6 at 100 mg/day for adults (67). This quantity of vitamin B_6 intake is not approachable by dietary means other than supplementation.

VITAMIN B₆–DRUG INTERACTIONS

Numerous drugs, including cycloserine, hydralazine, phenelzine, gentamicin, penicillamine, isoniazid, and L-dopa, antagonize vitamin B_6 status by covalently binding to the carbonyl group of PLP or PL, which reduces the availability of the PLP coenzyme (115). The asthma drug theophylline interferes with PLP production by inhibition of PL kinase (116). Vitamin B_6 status usually is recovered through PN supplementation without reducing drug efficacy (115). PN supplementation was once contraindicated in L-dopa treatment for Parkinson disease because it enhances peripheral metabolism of the drug (113). However, concurrent treatment with a peripheral decarboxylase inhibitor preserves the effectiveness of L-dopa treatment during PN supplementation. Alcohol intake antagonizes vitamin B_6 status through production of acetaldehyde, which competes with PLP for binding sites of PLP-dependent enzymes (117). Because chronic alcoholism likely increases vitamin B_6 catabolism through this mechanism, PN supplementation may be advisable in treatment of this disease.

REFERENCES

1. Leklem JE. Vitamin B₆. In: Shils ME, Olson JA, Shike M et al, eds. Modern Nutrition in Health and Disease, 9th ed. Baltimore: Williams & Wilkins, 1999:413–21.
2. Birch T, Gyorgy P. Biochem J 1936;30:304–7.
3. Gyorgy P. Nature 1934;133:448–9.
4. Lepkovsky S. Science 1938;87:169–70.
5. Keresztesy J, Stevens J. Proc Soc Exp Biol Med 1938;38:64–5.
6. Gyorgy P. J Am Chem Soc 1938;60:983–4.
7. Kuhn R, Wendt G. Ber Deut Chem Ges 1938;71B:780–2.
8. Ichiba A, Michi K. Sci Papers Inst Phys Chem Res (Tokyo) 1938;34:623–6.
9. Snell E, Guirard B, Williams R. J Biol Chem 1942;143:519–30.
10. Snell E. J Am Chem Soc 1944;2082–8.
11. Snell E. J Biol Chem 1944;154:313–4.
12. Harris S, Heyl D, Folkers K. J Biol Chem 1944;154:315–6.
13. Gunsalus I, Bellamy W, Umbreit W. J Biol Chem 1944;155:685–6.

14. Snell E. Vitamin B_6 analysis: some historical aspects. In: Leklem JE,.Reynolds RD eds. Methods in Vitamin B_6 Nutrition. Analysis and Status Assessment. New York: Plenum Press, 1981:1–18.

15. Snell E. Annu Rev Nutr 1989;9:1–19.

16. Leklem JE. Vitamin B_6. In: Machlin LJ, ed. Handbook of Vitamins. New York: Marcel Dekker, 1991:341–92.

17. American Institute of Nutrition. J Nutr 1990;120:12–9.

18. Said HM, Oritz A, Ma TY. Am J Physiol 2003;285:C1219–25.

19. Stolz J, Vielreicher M. J Biol Chem 2003;278:18990–6.

20. Tarr JB, Tamura T, Stokstad ELR. Am J Clin Nutr 1981;34:1328–37.

21. Roth-Maier DA, Kettler SI, Kirchgessner M. Int J Food Sci Nutr 2002;53:171–9.

22. Gregory JF. Eur J Clin Nutr 1997;51[Suppl 1]:43S–8S.

23. Andon MB, Reynolds RD, Moser-Veillon PB et al. Am J Clin Nutr 1989;50:1050–8.

24. Ink SL, Gregory JF, Sartain DB. J Agric Food Chem 1986;34:857–62.

25. Trumbo PR, Gregory JF, Sartain DB. J Nutr 1988;118:170–5.

26. Gregory JF, Trumbo PR, Bailey LB et al. J Nutr 1991;121:177–86.

27. Nakano H, McMahon LG, Gregory JF. J Nutr 1997;127:1508–13.

28. McMahon LG, Nakano H, Levy MD et al. J Biol Chem 1997;272:32025–33.

29. Armada LJ, Mackey AD, Gregory JF. J Nutr 2002;132:2695–9.

30. Mackey AD, Henderson GN, Gregory JF. J Biol Chem 2002;277:26858–64.

31. Mackey AD, Lieu SO, Carman C et al. J Nutr 2003;133:1362–7.

32. Ink SL, Mehansho H, Henderson LM. J Biol Chem 1982;257:4753–7.

33. Coburn SP, Mahuren JD, Kennedy MS et al. Biofactors 1988;1:307–12.

34. Mehansho H, Henderson LM. J Biol Chem 1980;255:11901–7.

35. Fonda ML, Harker C. Am J Clin Nutr 1982;35:1391–9.

36. Anderson B, Perry G, Clements J et al. Am J Clin Nutr 1989;50:1059–63.

37. McCormick DB, Chen H. J Nutr 1999;129:325–7.

38. Merrill AH, Henderson JM. Ann NY Acad Sci 1990;585:110–7.

39. Van Hoof VO, De Broe ME. Crit Rev Clin Lab Sci 1994;31:197–293.

40. Fonda ML. J Biol Chem 1992;267:15978–83.

41. Coburn SP. Ann NY Acad Sci 1990;585:76–85.

42. Coburn SP, Lewis DL, Fink WJ et al. Am J Clin Nutr 1988;48:291–4.

43. Said HM, Oritz A, Vaziri ND. Am J Physiol 2002;282:F465–71.

44. Zhang Z, Gregory JF, McCormick DB. J Nutr 1993;123:85–9.

45. Allgood A, Cidlowski J. J Biol Chem 1992;267:3819–24.

46. Leklem J. Ann NY Acad Sci 1992;669:34–43.

47. Dakshinamurti K, Paulose C, Viswanathan M et al. Ann NY Acad Sci 1990;585:128–44.

48. Martinez M, Cuskelly G, Williamson J et al. J Nutr 2000;130:1115–23.

49. Sturman J, Cohen P, Gaull G. Biochem Med 1969;3:244–51.

50. Cunnane SC, Manku MS, Horrobin DF. J Nutr 1984;114:1754–61.

51. Delorme CB, Lupien PJ. J Nutr 1976;106:169–80.

52. Tsuge H, Hotta N, Hayakawa T. J Nutr 2000;130:333S–4S.

53. Bergami R, Maranesi M, Marchetti M et al. Int J Vitam Nutr Res 1999;69:315–21.

54. Cho YO, Leklem JE. J Nutr 1990;120:258–65.

55. Furuyama K, Fujita H, Nagai T. Blood 1997;90:822–30.

56. Hurford MT, Marshall-Taylor C, Vicki SL et al. Clin Chim Acta 2002;321:49–53.

57. Chandra R, Sudhakaran L. Ann NY Acad Sci 1990;585:404–23.

58. Kwak H-K, Hansen C, Leklem J et al. J Nutr 2002;132:3308–13.

59. Meydani S, Ribaya-Mercado J, Russel R et al. Am J Clin Nutr 1991;53:1275–80.

60. Gregory J. J Food Comp Anal 1988;1:105–23.

61. Gregory J, Sartain D. J Agric Food Chem 1991;39:899–905.

62. Toukairin-Oda T, Sakamoto E, Hirose N et al. J Nutr Sci Vitaminol (Tokyo) 1989;35:171–80.

63. Kabir H, Leklem JE, Miller LT. J Food Sci 1983;48:1422–5.

63a. US Department of Agriculture. CSFII/DHKS 1994–1996 Data Set and Documentation: The 1994 Continuing Survey of Food Intakes by Individuals and the 1994–1996 Diet and Health Knowledge Survey. On: CSFII/DHKS 1994–96 CD ROM. Riverdale, MD: Agricultural Research Service, 1996.

64. Gregory J. Vitamins. In: Fennema O, ed. Food Chemistry. New York: Marcel Dekker, 1996:531–616.

65. Coursin D. JAMA 1954;154:406–8.

66. Gregory JF. Vitamin B_6 Deficiency. In: Carmel R, Jacobsen DW, eds. Homocysteine in Health and Disease. New York: Cambridge University Press, 2001:307–20.

67. Food and Nutrition Board, Institute of Medicine. Vitamin B_6. In: Dietary Reference Intakes for Thiamin, Riboflavin, Niacin, Vitamin B_6, Folate, Vitamin B_{12}, Pantothenic Acid, Biotin, and Choline. Washington, DC: National Academy Press, 1998:150–95.

68. Leklem J. J Nutr 1990;120[Suppl]:1503S–7S.

69. Lumeng L, Ryan M, Li T. J Nutr 1978;108:545–53.

70. Ubbink J, van der Merwe A, Delport R et al. J Clin Invest 1996;98:177–84.

71. Hansen C, Shultz TD, Kwak H–K et al. J Nutr 2001;131:1777–86.

72. West KD, Kirksey A. Am J Clin Nutr 1976;29:961–9.

73. Reynolds RD, Polansky M, Moser PB. J Am Diet Assoc 1984;84:1339–44.

74. Bates C, Pentieva K, Prentice A et al. Br J Nutr 1999;81:191–201.

75. Mudd S, Levy H, Skovby F. Disorders of transsulfuration. In: Stanbury J, Wyngaarden J, Frederickson D, eds. The Metabolic and Molecular Bases of Inherited Disease. New York: McGraw–Hill, 2004:1279–327.

76. Barber G, Spaeth G. J Pediatr 1969;75:463–78.

77. Baxter P. Biochim Biophys Acta 2003;1647:36–41.

78. Gupta V, Mishra D, Mathur I et al. J Paediatr Child Health 2001;37:592–6.

79. Reinken L, Zieglauer H. J Nutr 1978;108:1562–5.

80. Saibeni S, Cattaneo M, Vecchi M et al. Am J Gastroenterol 2003;98:112–7.

81. Rhinehart J, Greenberg L. Am J Pathol 1949;25:481–91.

82. Smolin L, Crenshaw T, Kurtycz D et al. J Nutr 1983;113:2122–33.

83. Robinson K, Arheart K, Refsum H et al. Circulation 1998;97:437–43.

84. McKinley M. Proc Nutr Soc 2000;59:221–37.

85. Clarke R, Armitage J. Semin Thromb Hemost 2000;26:341–8.

86. Brattström L, Stavenow L, Galvard H. Scand J Clin Lab Invest 1990;50:873–7.

87. Miner S, Cole D, Evrovski J et al. J Heart Lung Transplant 2001;20:964–9.

88. Friso S, Jacques P, Wilson P et al. Circulation 2001;103:2788–91.

89. Schoene N, Chanmugam P, Reynolds R. Am J Clin Nutr 1986;43:825–30.

90. Brown R. Possible role for vitamin B-6 in cancer prevention and treatment. In: Leklem J, Reynolds RD, eds. Clinical and

Physiological Applications of Vitamin B-6. New York: Arlan R. Liss, 1987:279–301.

91. Ames B, Wakimoto P. Nat Rev Cancer 2002;2:694–704.

92. Zhang S, Willet W, Selhub J et al. J Natl Cancer Inst 2003;95: 373–80.

93. Levi F, Pasche C, Lucchini F et al. Int J Cancer 2001;91:260–3.

94. Komatsu S, Yanaka N, Matsubara K et al. Biochim Biophys Acta 2003;1647:127–30.

95. Bryan J, Calvaresi E, Hughes D. J Nutr 2002;132:1345–56.

96. Selhub J, Bagley L, Miller J et al. Am J Clin Nutr 2000;71S:614S–20S.

97. Coursin DB. JAMA 1954;154:406–8.

98. Kretsch M, Sauberlich H, Newburn E. Am J Clin Nutr 1991; 53:1266–74.

99. Miller J, Green R, Mungas D et al. Neurology 2002;58:1471–5.

100. Pfeiffer S, Norton J, Nelson L et al. J Autism Dev Disord 1995; 25:481–93.

101. Bender D. Br J Nutr 1999;81:7–20.

102. van den Berg H, Bode W, Mocking J et al. Ann NY Acad Sci 1990;585:96–104.

103. Schrijver J, Westermarck T, Tolonen M. Vitamin B-6 status and the effect of supplementation in Finnish and Dutch elderly. In: Leklem J, Reynolds RD, eds. Clinical and Physiological Applications of Vitamin B-6. New York: Arlan R. Liss, 1988: 127–32.

104. Talbott M, Miller L, Kerkvliet N. Am J Clin Nutr 1987;46: 659–64.

105. Ribaya-Mercado J, Russel R, Sahyoun N et al. J Nutr 1991;121:1062–71.

106. Lindner A, Bankson D, Stehman-Breen C et al. Am J Kidney Dis 2002;39:134–45.

107. Robinson K, Gupta A, Dennis V et al. Circulation 1996;94: 2743–8.

108. Bostom A, Gohh R, Beaulieu A et al. Ann Intern Med 1997;127:1089–92.

109. Okada H, Moriwaki K, Kanno Y et al. Nephrol Dial Transplant 2000;15:1410–3.

110. Chiang E, Bagley P, Selhub J et al. Am J Med 2003;114:283–7.

111. Chiang E, Bagley P, Roubenoff R et al. J Nutr 2003;133:1056–9.

112. Mason D, Emerson P. BMJ 1973;1:389–90.

113. Bernstein A. Ann NY Acad Sci 1990;585:250–60.

114. Wyatt K, Dimmock P, Jones P et al. BMJ 1999;318:1375–81.

115. Bhagavan B. Curr Concepts Nutr 1983;12:1–12.

116. Ubbink J, Delport R, Becker P et al. J Lab Clin Med 1989;113: 15–22.

117. Lumeng L. J Clin Invest 1978;62:286–93.

SELECTED READINGS

Food and Nutrition Board, Institute of Medicine. Vitamin B$_6$. Dietary Reference Intakes for Thiamin, Riboflavin, Niacin, Vitamin B$_6$, Folate, Vitamin B$_{12}$, Pantothenic Acid, Biotin, and Choline. Washington, DC: National Academy Press, 1998:150–95.

Gregory JF. Vitamin B$_6$ deficiency. In: Carmel R, Jacobsen DW, eds. Homocysteine in Health and Disease. New York: Cambridge University Press, 2001:307–20.

Leklem JE. Vitamin B$_6$. In: Rucker RB, Suttie JW, McCormick DB et al eds. Handbook of Vitamins. 3rd ed. New York: Marcel Dekker, 2001:339–96.

McCormick DB. Vitamin B-6. In: Bowman BA, Russell RM, eds. Present Knowledge in Nutrition. 8th ed. Washington, DC: ILSI Press, 2002: 207–13.

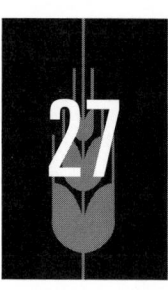

27 PANTOTHENIC ACID[1]
PAULA R. TRUMBO

HISTORICAL HIGHLIGHTS 462
CHEMISTRY AND BIOCHEMISTRY 462
PHYSIOLOGIC ASPECTS 462
   Digestion, Absorption, and Excretion 462
   Bioavailability 464
   Metabolism of Pantothenic Acid and Coenzyme A .464
ANALYTIC METHODS 465
DIETARY COMPONENTS AFFECTING PANTOTHENIC
   ACID STATUS 465
   Fat 465
   Protein 465
   Ascorbic Acid 465
DIETARY CONSIDERATIONS AND REQUIREMENTS ...465
   Food and Supplement Sources 465
   Dietary Intake 466
   Recommended Intakes 466
BIOCHEMICAL ASSESSMENT 466
   Blood Concentrations 466
   Urinary Excretion 466
CAUSES AND SYMPTOMS OF DEFICIENCY 467
   Alcoholism 467
   Diabetes Mellitus 467
CLINICAL BENEFITS 467
GENETIC MUTATIONS 467
ADVERSE EFFECTS OF OVERCONSUMPTION 467

HISTORICAL HIGHLIGHTS

Pantothenic acid belongs to the group of B vitamins. The name is a Greek derivation meaning "from everywhere." Earlier names used for pantothenic acid include vitamin B_5, chick antidermatitis factor, antidermatosis vitamin, and chick antipellagra factor. The vitamin was isolated by R.J. Williams and colleagues in 1931 (1), and this isolate was shown to be a single acidic substance essential for the growth of yeast in 1933 (2). The structure of pantothenic acid was later determined in 1939 (3). In 1940, Williams and colleagues successfully synthesized pantothenic acid (4), showed its relationship to inositol, thiamin, biotin, and

vitamin B_6 as to the growth of yeast (5), and developed assays for its isolation and measurement (6). In 1947, Lipmann and coworkers identified pantothenic acid as one of the components of coenzyme A (CoA). The accepted biochemical structure of CoA was published in 1953 (7). It was not until 1954 that Bean and Hodges (8) reported that pantothenic acid is essential in human nutrition. Pantothenic acid–containing CoA has since been shown to be essential to the respiratory tricarboxylic acid (TCA) cycle, fatty acid synthesis and degradation, and many other metabolic and regulatory processes.

CHEMISTRY AND BIOCHEMISTRY

Pantothenic acid is water soluble, and it exists as a yellow viscous oil and is unstable to acids, bases, and heat. Pantothenic acid, d(+)-α-(-dihydroxy-β,β-dimethylbutyryl-β-alanine), is synthesized by microorganisms via an amide linkage of β-alanine and pantoic acid (Fig. 27.1). Pantetheine consists of a β-mercaptoethylamine group added to pantothenate in humans. CoA is composed of 4′-phosphopantetheine linked by an anhydride bond to adenososine 5′-monophosphate, modified by a 3′-hydroxyl phosphate.

Besides serving as a component of CoA, 4′-phosphopantetheine is linked to certain proteins. 4′-Phosphopantetheine has been shown to be an essential cofactor in the biosynthesis of fatty acids (e.g., fatty acid synthetase), peptides (e.g., antibiotics), and polyketides (9).

Pantothenate, in the form of CoA, performs multiple roles in cellular metabolism. CoA facilitates the transfer of acetyl or acyl groups. β-Oxidation of fatty acids and the oxidative degradation of amino acids depend on CoA, by making the catabolic products available to the TCA cycle. Furthermore, acetyl CoA provides acetyl groups to oxaloacetic acid for the formation of citrate in the TCA cycle. The condensation of three acetyl CoA molecules yields hydroxyl-3-methylglutaryl-CoA, an intermediate in cholesterol synthesis.

PHYSIOLOGIC ASPECTS

Digestion, Absorption, and Excretion

Dietary CoA is hydrolyzed in the intestinal lumen to dephospho-CoA, pantetheine, and phosphopantetheine. Pantetheine is further hydrolyzed to pantothenic acid. Although

---

[1]**Abbreviations: AI,** adequate intake; **ATP,** adenosine triphosphate; **CoA,** coenzyme A; **PANK2,** pantothenate kinase 2; **TCA,** tricarboxylic acid.

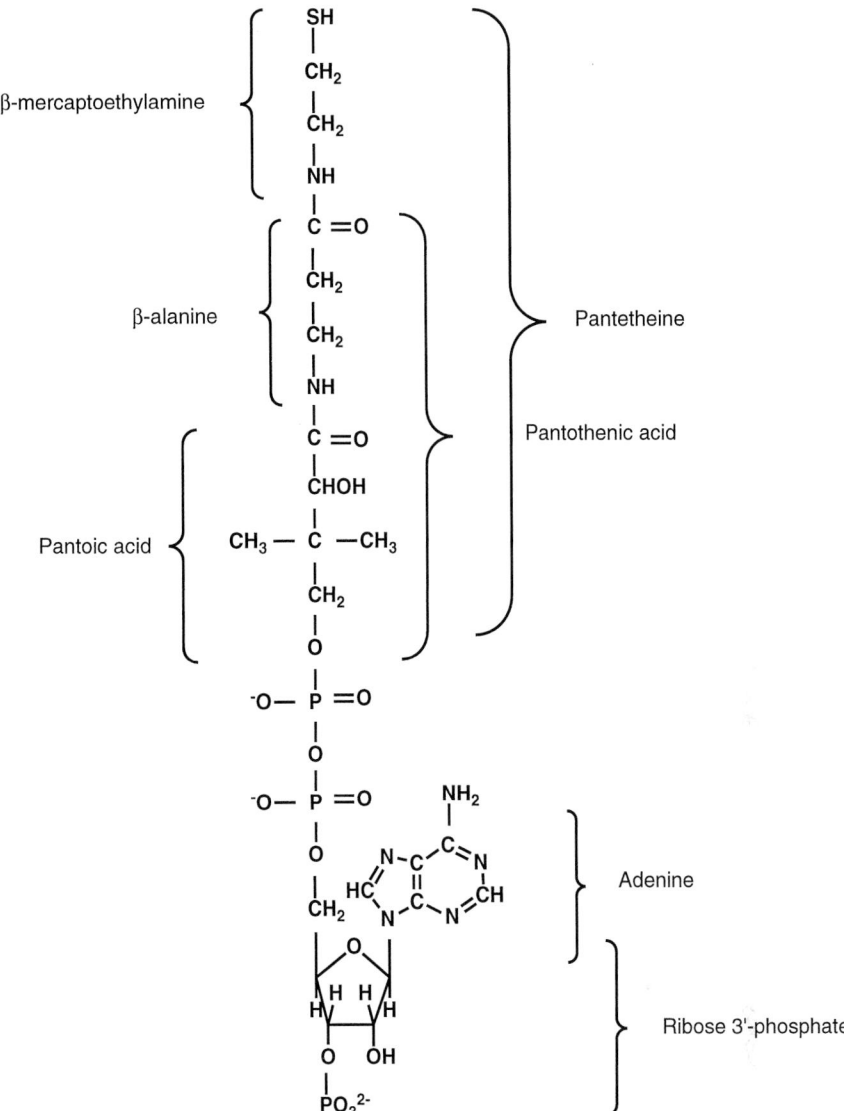

Figure 27.1. Coenzyme A and intermediates.

pantothenic acid may be absorbed by passive diffusion, it is absorbed into the bloodstream of animals by a saturable, sodium-dependent active transport mechanism (10). Studies in mice indicate that the kinetics for this active transport system is not affected by different dietary intake levels of the vitamin (11). Although animal studies have demonstrated that intestinal microflora synthesize pantothenic acid (11), the contribution to absorbed pantothenic acid in humans is unknown.

Absorbed pantothenic acid is transported via the red blood cells throughout the body (12). The vitamin also is transported in the free acid form in the plasma at a concentration of approximately 1 μg/mL[a] (13). Concentrations in red blood cells are higher than in plasma. Maximum pantothenate concentrations occurred 3 minutes following intravenous injection and subsequently decreased, a finding

suggesting that the vitamin is rapidly taken up by red blood cells and other tissues (14). A large increase in red blood cell pantothenate concentrations was observed in men following the injection of a multivitamin mixture that included 45 mg D-panthenol (15).

Animal studies have shown that, following the intraluminal administration of radiolabeled pantothenate or CoA, approximately 40% is located in muscle, 10% in the liver, and 10% in the intestine (16). Because pantothenic acid is an essential component for the biosynthesis of CoA, most tissues transport the vitamin via an active sodium cotransport mechanism (17, 18). Most of the pantothenic acid in tissues is present as CoA, with lesser amounts present as acyl carrier protein and free pantothenic acid.

Before urinary excretion, CoA is hydrolyzed to pantothenate in a multistep reaction. Pantothenic acid is excreted in urine and is typically measured by microbiologic assay. When subjects were given 100 mg/day of pantothenic acid, urinary excretion was only 60 mg/day, a

---

[a]Molecular weight of pantothenic acid = 219.24 g/mol; 1 mg = 4.56 μmol; 1 μg/mL = 4.56 μmolar (μM).

finding suggesting that the vitamin can be stored when intake levels are high or when the fractional bioavailability is relatively low.

Bioavailability

Data on the bioavailability of dietary pantothenic acid are limited. One study reported that dietary pantothenic acid was on average 50% (40–61%) bioavailable compared with the pure form of the vitamin (calcium pantothenate) given in a formula diet (19). Approximately 60% of ingested pantothenic acid was excreted in urine when subjects were fed three different experimental diets (20). Adults who consumed 5 to 7 mg/day of pantothenic acid excreted 2 to 7 mg/day in urine and 1 to 2 mg/day in the feces (21).

Metabolism of Pantothenic Acid and Coenzyme A

Synthesis

The first step in the synthesis of CoA is phosphorylation of pantothenic acid, which is catalyzed by pantothenate kinase. Following this is an adenosine triphosphate (ATP)-dependent condensation of 4'-phosphopantothenic acid with cysteine, yielding 4'-phosphopantothenoylcysteine which is decarboxylated to 4'-phosphopentatheine (22). CoA is formed via a series of transfers of adenosine monophosphate and phosphate from ATP to 4'-phopshopantetheine. Approximately 95% of CoA is located in the mitochondria. Because CoA does not cross the mitochondria membrane, it is thought that the final site of CoA synthesis occurs within the mitochondria (23).

Cellular Metabolism

Pantothenate, usually in the form of CoA, performs multiple roles in cellular metabolism (24). Acetyl-CoA is central to the energy-yielding oxidation of glycolytic products and other metabolites through the mitochondrial TCA cycle. The first step of the TCA cycle involves the condensation of acetyl-CoA with oxalacetate to yield citrate, and subsequently succinyl-CoA, which provides energy for guanosine diphosphate phosphorylation. The β-oxidation of fatty acids and the oxidative degradation of amino acids are also CoA-dependent processes; the catabolic products of these processes become available to the respiratory TCA cycle for further degradation and energy production.

Pantothenic acid is also required for the synthesis, by biosynthetically competent species, of numerous essential molecules including sphingolipids, leucine, arginine, and methinonine. CoA is also required for the synthesis of isoprenoid derivatives such as farnesol, cholesterol, steroid hormones, vitamin A, vitamin D, and heme A. Some of the isoprenoids are further bound to certain proteins such as viral Ras proteins. Succinyl-CoA is required for the synthesis of δ-aminolevulinic acid, which is the precursor of the porphyrin rings in hemoglobin and the cytochromes and the corrin ring

of vitamin B_{12}. CoA provides the essential acetyl group to the neurotransmitter acetylcholine and to serotonin in its conversion to melatonin and to the acetylated sugars present in glycoproteins and glycolipids (N-acetylgluocsamine, N-acetylgalactosamine, and N-acetylneuramic acid).

Protein Acetylation

Most soluble proteins are N-terminally acetylated by CoA. N-Acetylation appears to alter the structure of certain proteins, thereby altering the function or metabolism of the protein. Peptide hormones are acetylated, and this alters their hormone activity. For example, acetylation results in the activation of α-melanocyte-stimulating hormone and the inactivation of β-endorphin. Acetylation of histones alters the conformation of chromatin and changes its sensitivity to nucleases. Two classes of proteins are internally acetylated: histones and α-tubulin. Acetylation of histones neutralizes the charge of acetylated lysine residues, thereby weakening the interactions between the nucleosomes that depend on histone N-terminal tails. Histones that are highly acetylated tend to be associated with newly synthesized DNA or DNA that is transcriptionally active. Acetylated chromatin has a more unfolded conformation, as indicated by its increased sensitivity to nucleases (25). Hyperacetylation of histones H3 and H4 decreased the supercoiling within the nucleosome (26).

Acetylation and deacetylation regulate the assembly and disassembly of microtubules. Microtubules, which are essential components of the cellular cytoskeleton, are assembled from α- and β-tubulin dimers that polymerize and depolymerize continuously. Acetylation of α-tubulin occurs in the assembled microtubule and appears to stabilize microtubules (27). Deacetylation appears to be associated with depolymerization of microtubules (28).

Protein Acylation

Many different cellular proteins are covalently modified with long-chain fatty acids donated by fatty acyl CoA. The fatty acids, myristic acid and palmitic acid, are commonly added to proteins via acylation. This modification affects the location and activity of many proteins, including those involved with signal transduction. Myristolated proteins are located in the cytoplasm, plasma membrane, endoplasmic reticulum, and nuclear membrane. Myristolation of proteins is irreversible and often combines with other protein modifications for regulation of the protein's activity or localization. Because of the reversibility of palmitoylation, this process has a regulatory function. Guanosine triphosphate–binding proteins, Src and Src-related tyrosine kinases, and most viral and cellular Ras proteins comprise an extensive group of proteins that become modified by addition of myristate and/or palmitate. Palmitoylation is required for oncogenic viral Ras proteins to bind to the plasma membrane and transform cells and for vesicular transport through the Golgi stacks (29). Transmembrane receptors that are palmitolyated include the insulin receptor and the iron-transferrin receptor. Palmitate is acylated to numerous membrane proteins involved with the cytoskeleton including fibronectin and gap junction proteins (30). Several neuronal proteins are modified with palmitate. Acetylcholinesterase, which degrades the neurotransmitter acetylcholine, is bound to the cell membrane by palmitoylation (31). The reversible palmitoylation of proteins is involved with neural development by influencing neural motility and outgrowth in the developing brain (32).

ANALYTIC METHODS

Blood, urine, and tissue pantothenic acid concentrations are often measured by microbiologic growth assays, animal bioassay, or radioimmunoassay. Microbiologic assays for measuring pantothenic acid are highly sensitive and specific, but they are slow and tedious to perform. Results from radioimmunoassay compare favorably with those obtained by microbiologic methods. Samples containing bound vitamin (biologic sources excluding urine) must be hydrolyzed with enzymes or chemicals to release the pantothenate component of CoA before being assayed. Enzymes used to release pantothenic acid include papain, mylase-P, diastase, and clarase. Chemical methods are faster but less sensitive. High-performance liquid chromatography has been used for measuring pantothenic acid in foods (33). Radioimmunoassay has also been used to measure the pantothenic acid content in a wide variety of foods (34). Quantification of pantothenic acid in foods and biologic samples has been developed using stable isotope dilution assay (35), liquid chromatography tandem mass spectrometry (36) and enzyme-linked immunosorbent assay (37).

DIETARY COMPONENTS AFFECTING PANTOTHENIC ACID STATUS

No dietary factors are known to affect pantothenate absorption in humans. However, some animal studies have shown that dietary fat, protein, and ascorbic acid may have an effect.

Fat

When fed a diet deficient in pantothenic acid and high in fat, pigs exhibited a lower feed efficiency ratio. The onset of symptoms of pantothenic acid deficiency occurred more quickly when the fat content of the diet was increased (38). Feeding a high-fat diet has been shown to lower liver CoA concentration markedly (39). Liver total fat and cholesterol concentrations have been reported to be higher in animals fed a diet deficient in pantothenic acid (40).

Protein

Several studies have reported that diets with low intake of protein have a sparing action on pantothenic acid. When

deficient in pantothenic acid and fed a high-protein diet, rats excreted more pantothenic acid than rats fed a diet high in protein (41). Urinary pantothenic acid increased with increased protein intake of rats (42). It has been suggested that this effect may be caused, in part, by a more efficient conversion of pantothenic acid to CoA as a result of increased methionine intake because CoA concentrations were lowered in rats deficient in both pantothenic acid and methionine (43).

Ascorbic Acid

The consumption of high amounts of ascorbic acid has been show to delay the onset of pantothenic acid deficiency. When rats were fed a diet deficient in pantothenic acid and supplemented with either pantothenic acid or ascorbic acid, the severity of the deficiency was lessened (44). Weight gains were improved when rats deficient in pantothenic acid were supplemented with ascorbic acid (45).

DIETARY CONSIDERATIONS AND REQUIREMENTS

Food and Supplement Sources

Free and conjugated pantothenic acid is found in various plants and animals foods. Approximately 85% of dietary pantothenic acid exists as CoA or phosphopantetheine (46). Major sources of pantothenic acid include beef, chicken, liver, eggs, tomato products, broccoli, potatoes, and whole grains (34, 47) (Table 27.1). Pantothenic acid is added to a variety of foods, such as breakfast cereals and beverages and baby foods. Fruit products and corn-based and presweetened cereals are among the poorest sources of pantothenic acid.

A review of studies in North America and the United Kingdom reported that the average pantothenic acid concentration in mature breast milk ranges from 2.2 to 2.5 mg/L (48). The pantothenic acid concentration in human milk has been reported to be 6.7 mg/L, with no change occurring from 1 to 6 months postpartum (49).

TABLE 27.1. PANTOTHENIC ACID CONTENT OF FOODS

FOOD	PANTOTHENIC ACID (mg/100 g EDIBLE PORTION)
Beef, ground, cooked	0.33
Bran, 100%	1.73
Broccoli, raw	0.53
Cashew nuts	1.22
Chicken, fried	1.00
Eggs, hard-boiled	1.4
Liver, fried	5.92
Milk, canned	0.76
Mushrooms, cooked	2.16
Potato, baked	0.86
Rice, white	1.13
Tomato products	0.75

The pantothenic acid content in human milk correlates with maternal intake of the vitamin (50). In one study, within 4 days after parturition, the concentration of pantothenic acid in breast milk increased from 0.48 to 2.45 mg/L (51).

Pantothenic acid is relatively stable at neutral pH. However, cooking can destroy 15 to 50% of the vitamin (52). Processing of vegetables caused losses of up to 74% (13). Pasteurization of milk does not appear to destroy pantothenic acid (33).

Pure pantothenic acid exists as a viscous hygroscopic oil. Therefore, the vitamin occurs in supplements as either the calcium salt or the alcohol form, panthenol. Both forms are water soluble and are rapidly converted to pantothenic acid in the body. Because of its stability, panthenol is the form of choice in monopreparations, which are available in a variety of pharmaceutical forms (e.g., tablets, ointments, and creams). The common dose of pantothenic acid in multiple supplements is 10 mg; however, doses as high as 1000 mg are available as a monosupplement.

Dietary Intake

Nutrition surveys in the United States do not estimate intakes of pantothenic acid. The mean pantothenic acid intake of men and women of different ages in Quebec in 1990 fell from approximately 6 mg/day to approximately 3 mg/day with advancing age (53). Usual intakes of approximately 4 to 7 mg/day have been reported for adolescents and adults of various ages (53). The average dietary intake estimated for pregnant and lactating women was 2.75 mg/1000 kcal (54). The mean pantothenic acid intake of lactating women was 7.6 mg/day (49). The average dietary intake of pantothenic acid of elderly persons was estimated to be 5.9 mg/day (55).

Recommended Intakes

In 1989, an Estimated Safe and Adequate Daily intake of 4 to 7 mg/day of pantothenic acid was set because subjects were shown to excrete this level via the urine and feces (56). Based on a scientific review of the data for setting dietary reference intakes, it was determined that information for setting an estimated average requirement was insufficient, and therefore a recommended dietary allowance could not be set. However, an adequate intake (AI) was set for pantothenic acid for all life-stage and gender groups in 1998 (Table 27.2) (53). The AI for infants 0 to 6 months old represents the average daily intake of pantothenic acid for infants exclusively fed human milk. The AI for men and for nonpregnant and pregnant women is based on usual pantothenic acid intakes by adults in the United States. The AI for children 1 to 18 years old were set by extrapolating from the adult AI, based on body weight and growth factors. The AI during lactation is

TABLE 27.2. ADEQUATE INTAKE FOR PANTOTHENIC ACID

AGE (MALES AND FEMALES)	ADEQUATE INTAKE (mg/d)[a]
0–6 mo[b]	1.7
7–12 mo	1.8
1–3 y	2
4–8 y	3
9–13 y	4
14–18 y	5
≥19 y	5
Pregnant women	6
Lactating women	7

[a] Based on usual intakes for groups 1 year and older (see text).
[b] Based on the average contents of pantothenic acid in human milk consumed by infants (see text).

7 mg/day beacuse approximately 2 mg of pantothenic acid is secreted in human milk daily (53).

BIOCHEMICAL ASSESSMENT

Blood Concentrations

Blood levels of pantothenic acid blood lower than 100 μg/dL have been suggested to be indicative of inadequate intake (57). Whole blood pantothenic acid concentrations were reported to be significantly correlated with intake (58). Whole blood concentrations fell from 8.9 to 6.4 μmol/L when men were fed a diet devoid of pantothenic acid for up to 9 weeks (59). When men were supplemented with 10 mg/day of pantothenic acid for 9 weeks, no difference in whole blood concentrations was noted compared with baseline. Dietary pantothenic acid intake did not correlate with blood concentrations in a group of elderly persons; however, when a supplement containing pantothenic acid was taken, blood concentrations increased markedly (60).

Pantothenic acid intake and serum concentrations were reported to correlate in adolescents, whereas no correlation was observed in adults (61). Plasma concentrations were not reflective of changes in intake or status of pantothenic acid (15). The correlation between dietary and erythrocyte pantothenic acid values in a group of well-nourished adolescents was 0.4, and average erythrocyte concentrations were 1.5 μmol/L (334 ng/L) (58). At parturition, the pantothenic acid concentration was five times lower in the mother's serum compared with the infant's (51).

Urinary Excretion

A dose-response relationship exists between dietary intake and urinary excretion of pantothenic acid in women (21). This correlation was also confirmed in adolescents (58). Urinary pantothenic acid levels in women fed a diet low in pantothenic acid (2.8 mg/day) exceeded the intake level, a finding indicating that body stores were being lost or synthesis was occurring (21). The body has been shown to conserve pantothenic acid (62).

CAUSES AND SYMPTOMS OF DEFICIENCY

Because pantothenic acid is present to some extent in all foods, a deficiency in humans is rare, except in severe malnutrition, and it most likely occurs in conjunction with other nutrient deficiencies. During World War II, prisoners of war in Japan, the Philippines, and Burma experienced numbness in their toes and painful burning sensations in their feet. These symptoms were relieved with pantothenic acid supplementation, but not when other B-complex vitamins were given (63). When given a diet completely devoid of pantothenic acid (58) or when given an antagonist of pantothenic acid metabolism (64, 65), subjects experienced irritability, restlessness, sleep disturbances, numbness, and gastrointestinal disturbances.

Administration of pantothenate analogs to humans has occurred unintentionally, with deleterious side effects. Hopantenate is an analog of pantothenic acid, in which γ-aminobutyric acid replaces β-alanine. Hopantenate was used in Japan to stimulate retarded persons cerebrally and to alleviate tardive dyskinesia symptoms induced by tranquilizers. As a result, the patients exhibited severe side effects including lactic acidosis, hypoglycemia, hyperammonemia, and eventually acute encephalopathy (67). These effects were also demonstrated in dogs and were shown to result from a pantothenic acid deficiency. Dogs given an equivalent amount of pantothenic acid and calcium hopantenate did not develop the disorder (68).

Effects of a pantothenate-restricted diet have been studied in many animals (66). Rats developed hypertrophy of the adrenal cortex, followed by hemorrhage and necrosis. Furthermore, monkeys showed depressed heme synthesis and became anemic. Chickens developed dermatitis and poor feathering, and they also displayed axon and myelin degeneration within the spinal cord.

Alcoholism

Because alcohol consumption interferes with the metabolism of pantothenic acid, the requirement for pantothenic acid may be increased in heavy drinkers. Ethanol causes a decrease in the concentration of pantothenic acid in tissues, and the result is increased serum concentrations of the vitamin (69). Pantothenic acid excretion in patients with alcoholism was increased following the administration of pantothenic acid by mouth or by injection (70). CoA activity in the liver was shown to decrease markedly in rats provided 5 to 15% ethanol for 8 months (71).

Diabetes Mellitus

Humans deficient in pantothenic acid have been shown to have lower blood glucose concentrations and an increased sensitivity to insulin (72). Patients with diabetes mellitus have a higher urinary excretion of pantothenic acid than healthy persons (73). Alloxan-diabetic rats were reported to have decreased concentration of pantothenic acid in muscles and increased concentrations in kidneys, brain, heart, and pancreas (74).

CLINICAL BENEFITS

Pantothenic acid has been shown to be beneficial while not being associated with a deficiency of the vitamin. Pantothenic acid was shown to protect against peroxidation and carbon tetrachloride–induced liver damage in rats (75). Furthermore, pantothenic acid was reported to increase skeletal muscle energy metabolism in the murine model of muscular dystrophy (76). Pantothenic acid has been suggested to aid in wound healing (77, 78), by increasing the number of migrating dermal fibroblasts (79). Low blood concentrations of pantothenic acid have been reported in patients with rheumatoid arthritis (80). One randomized, double-blind study showed that daily supplementation with 1 g calcium pantothenate resulted in a significant reduction in pain symptoms in patients with rheumatoid arthritis (81) (see also Chapter 85).

GENETIC MUTATIONS

Many patients afflicted with the Hallevorden-Spatz syndrome, characterized by dystonia, parkinsonism, and iron accumulation in the brain, have been found to have pantothenate kinase 2 (PANK2)-associated neurodegeneration (82). PANK2 is one of four known pantothenate kinases. Hayflick and associates noted that this neurodegeneration is one of three known extrapyramidal disorders associated with increased brain iron concentration for which the molecular basis has been defined; the other disorders have mutations in the ferritin light-chain gene (83) and in the gene encoding ceruloplasmin (84). Acanthocytosis and a defect in plasma lipoproteins have also been noted in association with the PANK2 mutations (85). Hayflick and colleagues speculated that "supplemental pantothenate . . . could compensate for partial enzymatic deficiency in these patients, possibly altering ameliorating or retarding the symptoms" (82).

ADVERSE EFFECTS OF OVERCONSUMPTION

No adverse effects of overconsumption of pantothenic acid have been reported in humans. For this reason, the Institute of Medicine did not set a tolerable upper intake level for pantothenic acid (53). When patients were treated with up to 15 g/day pantothenic acid, symptoms of lupus erythematosus, nausea, and gastrointestinal distress were reported (86, 87). The toxic oral dose for mice (LD_{50}) was determined to be 10 g/kg, and this led to death by respiratory failure (50).

REFERENCES

1. Williams RJ, Bradway EM. J Am Chem Soc 1931;53:783.
2. Williams RJ, Lyman CM, Goodyear GH et al. J Am Chem Soc 1933;55:2912–27.

3. Williams RJ, Weinstock HH, Rohrmann E et al. J Am Chem Soc 1939;89:199–206.

4. Williams RJ, Mitchell HK, Weinstock HH et al. J Am Chem Soc 1940;62:1784–5.

5. Williams RJ, Eakin RE, Snell EE. J Am Chem Soc 1940;62:1204–7.

6. Pennington D, Snell EE, Williams RJ. J Biol Chem 1940;135:213–22.

7. Baddiley J, Thain EM, Novelli GD et al. Nature 1953;171:76–9.

8. Bean WB, Hodges RE. Proc Soc Exp Biol Med 1954;86:693–9.

9. Plesofsky-Vig N, Brambl R. Annu Rev Nutr 1988;8:461–82.

10. Fenstermacher DK, Rose DC. Am J Physiol 1986;250:G155–60.

11. Stein ED, Diamond JM. J Nutr 1989;119:1973–83.

12. Eissenstat BR, Wyse BW, Hansen RG. Am J Clin Nutr 1986;44:931–37.

13. Fox HM. Pantothenic acid. In: Machlin LJ, ed. Handbook of Vitamins. New York: Marcel Dekker, 1984:437.

14. Tahiliani AB, Beinlich CH. Vitam Horm 1991;46:165–8.

15. Baker H, Frank O, Thomson AD et al. Am J Clin Nutr 1969;22:1469–75.

16. Shibata K, Gross CJ, Henderson LM. J Nutr 1983;113:2107–15.

17. Barbarat B, Podevin RA. J Biol Chem 1986;14455–60.

18. Prasad PD, Ramamoorthy S, Leibach FH et al. Placenta. 1997;18:527–33.

19. Tarr JB, Tamura T, Stocksatd EL. Am J Clin Nutr 1981;34:1328–37.

20. Yu BH, Kies C. Plant Foods Hum Nutr 1993;43:87–95.

21. Fox HM, Linkswiler H. J Nutr 1961;75:451–4.

22. Brown G. J Biol Chem 1959;234:370–8.

23. Robishaw JD, Berkick D, Neely JR. J Biol Chem 1982;257:10967–72.

24. Combs GF. The Vitamins: Fundamental Aspects in Nutrition and Health. New York: Academic Press, 1992:352.

25. Ridsdale JA, Hendzel MJ, Delcuve GP et al. J Biol Chem 1990;265:5150–6.

26. Norton VG, Marvin KW, Yau P et al. J Biol Chem 1990;265:19848–52.

27. Plesofsky-Vig N, Brambl R. Annu Rev Nutr 1988;8:461–82.

28. Lim SS, Sammak PJ, Borisy GG. J Cell Biol 1989;109:253–63.

29. Pfanner N, Orci L, Glick BS et al. Cell 1989;59:95–102.

30. Maneti S, Dunia I, Benedetti EL. FEBS Lett 1990;262:356–8.

31. Randall WR. J Biol Chem 1994;269:12367–74.

32. Hess DT, Petterson Sim Smith DS et al. Nature 1993;366:562–5.

33. Romera JM, Ramirez M, Gil A. J Dairy Sci 1996;79:523–6.

34. Walsh JH, Wyse BW, Hansen RG. J Am Diet Assoc 1981;78:140–4.

35. Rychlik M. Analyst 2003;128:832–7.

36. Rychlik M. J Agr Food Chem 2000;48:1175–81.

37. Gonthier A, Boullanger P, Fayol V et al. J Immunoassay 1998;19:167–94.

38. Sewell RF, Price DG, Thomas MC. Fed Proc 1962;21:468–73.

39. Williams MA, Chu LC, McIntosh DJ et al. J Nutr 1968;94:377–82.

40. Guehring RR, Hurley LS, Morgan AF. J Biol Chem. 1952;11:138–41.

41. Nelson MM, Evans HM. Proc Soc Exp Biol Med 1945;60:319–23.

42. Tao HG, Fox HM. Nutr Rep Int 1980;22:239–43.

43. Dinning JS, Neatrour R, Day PL. J Nutr 1955;56:431–6.

44. Everson G, Northrop L, Chung NY et al. J Nutr 1954;54:305–9.

45. Barboriak JJ, Krehl WA. J Nutr 1957;63:601–9.

46. Bender DA, Bender AE, eds. Nutrition: A Reference Handbook. Oxford: Oxford University Press, 1997.

47. US Department of Agriculture (USDA), Agricultural Research Service. USDA National Nutrient Database for Standard Reference, Release 16, 2003. Nutrient Data Laboratory Home Page: http://www.nal.usda.gov/fnic/foodcomp

48. Picciano MF. Water-soluble Vitamins in Milk. In: Jensen RG, ed. Handbook of Milk Composition. San Diego: Academic Press, 1995.

49. Johnston L, Vaughan L, Fox HM. Am J Clin Nutr 1981;34:2205–9.

50. Song WO, Chan GM, Wyse BW et al. Am J Clin Nutr 1984;40:317–24.

51. Robinson AF, Folkers K, eds. Vitamins and Coenzymes. New York: John Wiley & Sons, 1964.

52. Schroeder HA. Am J Clin Nutr 1971;24:562–73.

53. Institute of Medicine. Dietary Reference Intakes for Thiamin, Riboflavin, Niacin, Vitamin B₆, Folate, Pantothenic Acid, Biotin, and Choline. Washington, DC: National Academy Press, 1998;357–73.

54. Song WO, Wyse BW, Hansen RG. J Am Diet Assoc 1985;85:192–8.

55. Srinivasan V, Christensen N, Wyse BW et al. Am J Clin Nutr 1981;34:1736–42.

56. National Research Council. Recommended Dietary Allowances. Washington, DC: National Academy Press. 1989:169–73.

57. Sauberlich HE, Skala, JH. Laboratory Tests for the Assessment of Nutritional Status. Cleveland, OH: CRC Press. 1974:88.

58. Eissenstat BR, Wyse BW, Hansen RG. Am J Clin Nutr 1986;44:931–7.

59. Fry PC, Fox HM, Tao HG. J Nutr Sci Vitaminol (Tokyo) 1976;22:399–446.

60. Wyse BW, Hansen RG. Fed Proc 1977;36:1169.

61. Kathman JV, Kies C. Nutr Res 1984;4:245–50.

62. Karnitz LM, Gross CJ, Henderson LM. Biochim Biophys Acta 1984;769:486–92.

63. Glusman M. Am J Med 1947;3:211–23.

64. Hodges RE, Ohlson MA, Bean WB. J Clin Invest 1958;37:1642–57.

65. Hodges RE, Bean WB, Ohlson MA et al. Clin Invest 1959;38:1421–5.

66. Robinson FA. The Vitamin C-factors of Enzyme Systems. Oxford: Pergamon Press, 1966:406–86.

67. Otsuka M, Akiba T, Okita Y et al. Jpn J Med 1990;29:324–8.

68. Noda S, Haratake J, Sasaki A et al. Liver 1991;11:134–42.

69. Leevy CM, Baker H. Arch Environ Health 1963;7:453–8.

70. Moiseenhok AG, Sheibak WM, Gurinovich VA. Int J Vitam Nutr Res 1987;57:71–4.

71. Maisyayunak AH, Tsverbaum AA, Rybalko MA. Vyest Akad Navuk BSSR Syer Biyal Navuk 1980;0:68–70.

72. Bean WB, Hodges RE, Daum K. J Clin Invest 1955;84:1973–6.

73. Hatano M, Hodges RE, Evans RC et al. Am J Clin Nutr 1967;20:960–7.

74. Martsinchyk AP, Amal'anchykp SN, Maisyaenak AG. Vyest Akad Novuk BSSR Biyal Navuk 1982;3:80–4.

75. Nagiel-Ostaszewski I, Lau-Cam CA. Res Commun Chem Pathol Pharmacol 1990;67:289–92.

76. Even PC, Decrouy A, Chinet A. Biochem J 1994;30:649–54.

77. Aprahamian M, Dentiger A, Stock-Damage C et al. Am J Clin Nutr 1985;41:578–89.

78. Lacroix B, Didier E, Grenier JF. Int J Vitam Nutr Res 1988;58:407–13.

79. Weimann BI, Hermann D. Int J Vitam Nutr Res 1999;69: 113–9.
80. Barton-Wright EC, Elliot WA. Lancet 1963;26:862–3.
81. Einstein P, Scheiner SA, eds. Overcoming the Pain of Inflammatory Arthritis: The Pain-Free Promise of Pantothenic Acid. Garden City, NY: Avery Publishing. 1999.
82. Hayflick SJ, Westaway SK, Levinson B et al. N Engl J Med 2003;348:33–40.
83. Curtis AR, Fey C, Morris CM et al. Nat Genet 2001;28: 350–4.
84. Gitlin JD. Pediatr Res 1998;44:271–6.
85. Ching KHL, Westaway SK, Levinson B et al. Neurology 2002; 58:1673–4.
86. Welsh AL. Arch Dermatol 1952;65:137–48.
87. Welsh AL. Arch Dermatol 1954;70:181–98.

SELECTED READINGS

Expert Group on Vitamins and Minerals. Review of Pantothenic Acid. London: Food Standards Agency, 2002.

Hayflick SJ, Westaway SK, Levinson B et al. Genetic, clinical, and radiographic delineation of Hallervorden-Spatz syndrome. N Engl J Med 2003;348:33–40.

US Department of Agriculture Nutrient Database for Pantothenic Acid, Release 16: http://www.nal.usda.gov/fnic/foodcomp/Data/SR16/wtrank/sr16a410.pdf

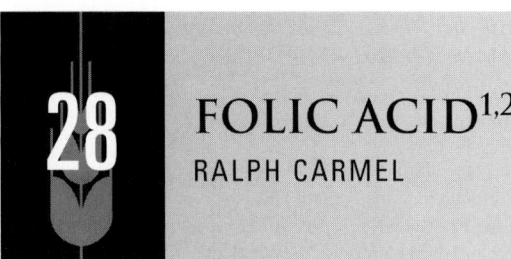

FOLIC ACID[1,2]

RALPH CARMEL

HISTORICAL BACKGROUND 470
BIOCHEMISTRY 470
ANALYTIC METHODS 471
    Assay of Folate 471
    Red Blood Cell Folate .472
    Homocysteine 473
NUTRITION AND BIOAVAILABILITY 473
    Food Fortification and Supplement Use 473
    Bioavailability 474
ABSORPTION 474
TRANSPORT, METABOLISM, AND EXCRETION 474
    Transport 474
    Cellular Uptake and Metabolism 474
DIETARY CONSIDERATIONS AND REQUIREMENTS . . .475
DEFICIENCY STATE 475
    Clinical Features 476
    Subclinical Features and Predispositions 476
    Responsiveness to Folate in Nondeficiency States .477
    Causes 478
    Treatment 479
INTERACTIONS 479
    Cobalamin 479
    Homocysteine 479
    Iron 479

HISTORICAL BACKGROUND

The history of folic acid and its deficiency is intertwined with that of cobalamin in many ways. The two vitamins share a critical biochemical interaction, the remethylation of methionine, and thus its metabolic consequences. As a result, they also share a dramatically disordered hematologic expression of deficiency, megaloblastic anemia, and a web of clinical, diagnostic, and therapeutic interrelationships, some of which pose challenges to optimal management.

Probable reports of folate deficiency go back nearly two centuries. Long before its cause was understood, megaloblastic anemia was characterized by Hayem's description of giant red blood cells (RBCs with macrocytosis) in 1877 (1) and by Ehrlich's description of the disordered nuclear appearance in the bone marrow in 1880 (2). More than 40 years later, the hematologic picture was completed with the description of the typical white blood cell changes.

In 1931, Wills (3) described responsiveness of "pernicious anemia of pregnancy," now a misnomer (see Chapter 29), and "tropical anemia" to a component of a yeast preparation, Marmite. Day and colleagues (4) identified a response of a macrocytic anemia in monkeys to "vitamin M." Other preparations were identified by properties such as support for growth of microorganisms, and the observation of such activity in spinach led to the name folic acid (5). Nutritional megaloblastic anemia was reversed by a component of liver unrelated to that curing cobalamin deficiency (6). The active component in all these preparations was proved to be folate, once folic acid was purified and characterized (7).

A separate line of investigation, stimulated by suggestions of acceleration of leukemia by folate therapy, led to the synthesis and use of antifolate drugs (8), which helped to usher in the modern era of cancer chemotherapy. The salutary effect of folic acid in folate deficiency also led to a wave of its inappropriate use in patients who actually suffered from deficiency of cobalamin (9–12); these events helped to focus attention on the interactions between the two vitamins. The demonstration that pure folate deficiency could arise on a nutritional basis alone and the sequence of events leading to its megaloblastic anemia were provided by a notable self-experiment by Herbert in 1962 (13). Technical and scientific developments related to homocysteine have fostered major advances in the understanding of the metabolic and clinical interactions between folate and homocysteine. As folate deficiency has become less common in the United States since 1998, interest has shifted to the possibility that even mild folate insufficiency, perhaps combined with genetic and acquired predispositions, may contribute as a risk factor to an array of chronic sequelae.

BIOCHEMISTRY

Folic acid (pteroylmonoglutamic acid), the stable, fully oxidized folate, consists of pteridine, *p*-aminobenzoic acid, and glutamic acid. Metabolic activity requires folate that is

---

[1] **Abbreviations: DFE,** dietary folate equivalent; **MCV,** mean corpuscular volume; **MTHFR,** N5,10-methylenetetrahydrofolate reductase; **NTD,** neural tube defect; **RBC,** red blood cell; **tHcy,** total homocysteine; **THF,** tetrahydrofolate.

[2] Système Internationale units: 1 μg folic acid = 2.266 nmol.

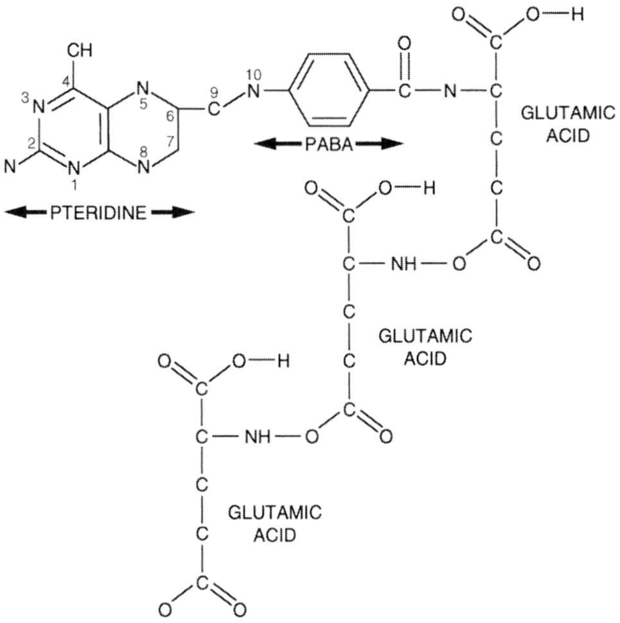

Figure 28.1. The biochemical structure of folate, shown as pteroyl triglutamate. The constituents, shown, from **left** to **right**, are pteridine and p-aminobenzoic acid (PABA), which together make up the pteroyl moiety, and one or more glutamate residues attached by γ-carboxyl linkage. Reduction at positions 5, 6, 7, and 8 to tetrahydrofolate confers metabolic activity. Various one-carbon moieties are attached to the nitrogen at positions 5 (e.g., N5-methyl, N5-formyl, N5-formimino) or 10 (e.g., N10-formyl), or bridging the two positions (e.g., N5,10-methylene, N5,10-methenyl). Each folate form takes part in specific reactions by donating, accepting, or transforming its one-carbon moiety. (From Carmel R. Megaloblastic anemias: disorders of impaired DNA synthesis. In: Greer JP, Foerster J, Lukens JL et al, eds. Wintrobe's Clinical Hematology. 11th ed. Philadelphia: Lippincott Williams & Wilkins, 2004, with permission.)

reduced at positions 5, 6, 7, and 8 in the pteridine ring to produce tetrahydrofolate (THF). The monoglutamate side chain of folates can be extended by folylpolyglutamate synthetase to form γ-carboxyl-linked polyglutamates of up to 11, but most often three to seven, glutamate residues (Fig. 28.1). The polyglutamated folates have greater metabolic activity and are also retained better by cells, whereas monoglutamated folates traverse cell membranes more readily (14).

Folate functions as a coenzyme or cosubstrate by accepting, transferring, or modifying one-carbon moieties that are attached to the N5 or N10 position of folate or bridge those two positions (15). Different folate forms are involved in these one-carbon transactions, which are important for the synthesis of thymidine for DNA and purines for RNA, the interconversion of key amino acids, and the generation of formates (Fig. 28.2). MethylTHF is the predominant folate in human plasma and tissues, but folate metabolism in the different compartments is complex (16). A particularly important reaction requires methylTHF for the cobalamin-dependent remethylation of homocysteine to methionine (reaction 4, Fig. 28.2).

Methionine is subsequently converted to S-adenosylmethionine (reaction 12, Fig. 28.2), which participates as the methyl donor in many important biologic methylation reactions (reaction 13) of proteins, nucleoproteins (e.g., the methylation of DNA cytosine), histones, neurotransmitters, and phospholipids (17). Another important folate-dependent reaction is the methylation of deoxyuridylate to thymidylate mediated by methyleneTHF (reaction 2, Fig. 28.2). This reaction's impairment initiates the process leading to megaloblastic anemia. The excess uracil that accumulates as a result and often replaces the diminished thymine in nucleoprotein synthesis requires excision repair. When the scale of misincorporation is so great that many opposing nucleotides are coincidentally excised, double-strand breaks occur, and chromosomal damage results (18, 19).

ANALYTIC METHODS

Assay of Folate

Folate can be measured in serum or cells, each of which reflects a person's folate status and stores in varying and sometimes indirect ways (20, 21). The earliest methods relied on the proportionate growth achieved by folate-requiring microorganisms on exposure to the folate in the test sample; the organisms often responded differently to various forms of folate (20). The microbiologic assays, although still regarded by some as the most reliable methods, were supplanted several decades ago by simpler radioisotopic assays usually based on binding of the sample's extracted folate, in competition with radiolabeled methylTHF, by an added protein capable of binding folate. Since the 1990s, clinical laboratories have embraced highly automated immunologic methods employing chemiluminescence or other nonisotopic detection. Folate results can vary so much by method and laboratory that comparisons of values obtained by different assays or from different laboratories are best viewed as only approximations (22).

Methodologic concerns include the following: (a) the nonequivalent recognition of diverse folate forms with some assays, a problem partially obviated by the predominance of methylTHF in serum but requiring conversions of all folates to methylTHF in other materials; (b) the suboptimal extraction of folates, especially from cells, tissues, and foods; and (c) inadequate validation and standardization of assay methods, a problem magnified in recent years because laboratories often carry out limited validation of individual assays that are sold as a part of a commercially packaged system of assays of a host of unrelated analytes and because automation and frequent rotation of personnel have diminished staff familiarity with individual assays.

The instability of folates can be an analytic obstacle. Whereas folic acid is relatively stable in solution, reduced folates, which predominate in blood, tissues, and food, tend to be oxidized readily (20). Adding ascorbic acid to

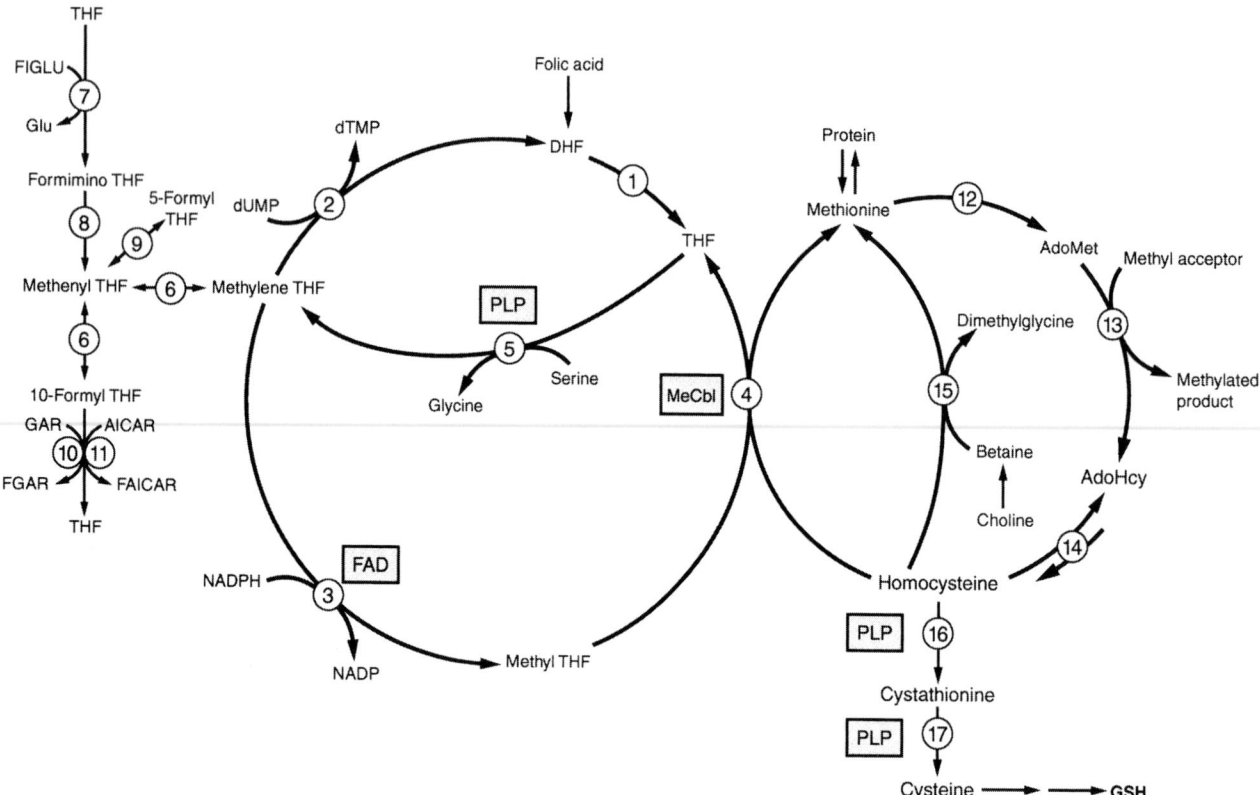

Figure 28.2. Folate metabolism and its linkage with cobalamin and with homocysteine-methionine metabolism. Vitamin cofactors are *highlighted within boxes*. Not all bidirectional reactions are shown as such. The enzymes for the listed reactions are as follows: (1) dihydrofolate reductase (this reaction is inhibited by antifols such as methotrexate); (2) thymidylate synthase (inadequacy of this pyrimidine metabolic step is important to the genesis of megaloblastic anemia); (3) methylene tetrahydrofolate (THF) reductase (the unidirectional nature of this reaction helps to seal the methylTHF "trap"); (4) methionine synthase (a reductive system mediated by methionine synthase reductase is critical to this enzyme's activity); (5) serine hydroxymethylase; (6) the two reactions, mediated by a protein with two enzymatic activities, methyleneTHF dehydrogenase and methenylTHF cyclohydrolase; (7) glutamate (Glu) formiminotransferase; (8) formiminoTHF cyclodeaminase; (9) methenylTHF synthase; (10) and (11) two reactions important in purine metabolism, mediated by glycinamide ribonucleotide (GAR) transformylase and aminoimidazolecarboxamide ribonucleotide (AICAR) transformylase, respectively. The following reactions comprise homocysteine-methionine metabolism: (12) methionine adenosyltransferase; (13) various *S*-adenosylmethionine (AdoMet)–dependent methyltransferases (mediating scores of important biologic methylations); (14) *S*-adenosylhomocysteine (AdoHcy) hydrolase (the kinetics of the reaction usually favor synthesis of AdoHcy); (15) betaine:homocysteine methyltransferase (this is an alternative pathway of homocysteine remethylation to reaction 4 in some tissues); (16) cystathionine β-synthase (the first step in homocysteine transsulfuration, the major catabolic pathway for homocysteine, which also influences redox activity); (17) cystathionine γ-lyase. AICAR, aminoimidazolecarboxamide ribonucleotide; DHF, dihydrofolate; dTMP, deoxythymidine monophosphate; dUMP, deoxyuridine monophosphate; FAD, flavine adenine dinucleotide (riboflavin); FAICAR, formyl AICAR; FGAR, formyl glycinamide ribonucleotide; FIGLU, formiminoglutamic acid; GAR, glycinamide ribonucleotide; GSH, glutathione; MeCbl, methylcobalamin; NADP, nicotinamide adenine dinucleotide phosphate (NADPH is the reduced form); PLP, pyridoxal 5'-phosphate. (From Carmel R. Megaloblastic anemias: disorders of impaired DNA synthesis. In: Greer JP, Foerster J, Lukens JL et al, eds. Wintrobe's Clinical Hematology. 11th ed. Philadelphia: Lippincott Williams & Wilkins, 2004, with permission.)

the sample stabilizes folate activity. However, few, if any, clinical laboratories add ascorbate to serum samples awaiting assay, and variable, sometimes substantial folate loss can occur within a few days of storage or with thawing and refreezing (23).

Traditionally, clinical signs of folate deficiency, primarily megaloblastic anemia, have been used to help define subnormal folate levels. Such signs of deficiency commonly have been associated with serum folate levels lower than 2.5 μg/L (also expressed as 5.7 nmol/L; 1 μg = 2.266 nmol), hence the common use of 2.5 μg/L as the cutpoint defining folate deficiency. However, metabolic studies have shown that plasma total homocysteine (tHcy) levels

tend to be slightly elevated and respond to folate supplementation in persons with folate levels as high as 4.5 or 5.0 μg/L (10.2 or 11.3 nmol/L) (24). The latter finding led to suggestions that serum folate levels between 2.5 and 5.0 μg/L be regarded as suspicious for borderline or mildly compromised folate status.

Red Blood Cell Folate

RBC folate, 60% of which is methylTHF (25), is a stable index of folate status because RBC folate content fluctuates very little throughout the cell's long life span and is not affected by transient events. In contrast, serum folate, which is largely a product of absorbed dietary folate and reabsorbed enterohepatic folate pools, fluctuates daily and need not correlate with tissue stores (20, 26). Only 14% of patients with low serum folate also have low RBC folate (20). RBC folate correlates with hepatic content (27), although weakly, and declines weeks to months later than serum folate, which often falls within 2 to 3 weeks after folate intake and/or absorption decrease (28). Unfortunately, RBC folate levels are also affected by phenomena unrelated to folate. Thus, blood transfusions or the presence of many very young RBC (reticulocytes), which have higher folate content than mature RBCs, alter RBC folate levels. The most important source of diagnostic confusion is that RBC folate content also falls in 63% of patients with cobalamin deficiency (29). In contrast, RBC folate is increased in iron deficiency (30).

RBC folate assay has more troublesome performance issues, and its results vary more among methods and laboratories than does serum folate assay (21, 22). Cutpoints ranging from 140 to 180 µg/L (317 to 408 nmol/L) have been used to define folate deficiency. The many methodologic and interpretive concerns led some investigators to downgrade the usefulness of RBC folate determination in clinical practice (31), but others believe that its usefulness outweighs the disadvantages (21).

Homocysteine

Plasma tHcy, which consists of reduced homocysteine and its oxidized forms, has become a common research tool for assessing folate status and, despite its indirect relationship to folate, is also used increasingly for clinical purposes. tHcy provides a fairly sensitive index of folate metabolic status because of the impaired conversion of homocysteine to methionine in folate deficiency (reaction 4, Fig. 28.2); plasma tHcy levels were elevated in 86% of patients with clinically expressed folate deficiency (32). Surveys also suggest that folate status is a major determinant of tHcy levels in healthy people (33–36).

However, tHcy abnormality lacks specificity: the tHcy level is also elevated in deficiencies of other vitamins (cobalamin, sometimes vitamin B_6, and perhaps riboflavin), renal insufficiency, inborn errors of metabolism and common genetic polymorphisms of various enzymes, severe alcohol abuse, and many other situations (37–39). Analysis of national survey data identified nine personal characteristics and laboratory findings other than folate status as significant predictors of tHcy levels (40). Blood sampling and processing conditions also affect tHcy levels because cells release homocysteine into serum and, to a lesser extent, plasma in vitro (41). The reference interval for tHcy has varied widely among laboratories and investigators (cutpoints as diverse as 11.7 and 16 µmol/L have been recommended), and men have higher levels than women (42).

The Institute of Medicine, in its assessment of the literature on folate, concluded that the diagnosis of folate deficiency cannot rely on tHcy data alone (34). However, tHcy may be the best biochemical tool for monitoring response to therapy; its level falls to normal within a few days after appropriate folate therapy but will not respond to inappropriate cobalamin therapy (43), whereas a vitamin level invariably rises whether the vitamin was used appropriately or not.

NUTRITION AND BIOAVAILABILITY

Folate, although named for leafy vegetables, is found in virtually all foods: dairy products, poultry and meat (liver and kidney are especially rich in folate), seafood, fruits and fruit juices, nuts, grain and cereal products, and, of course, vegetables (see Appendix Table A-23-a for the folate content of a number of foods). The highest concentrations of folate exist in yeast, spinach, liver, peanuts, lima and kidney beans, Brussels sprouts, and broccoli (20). The broad distribution helps explain why folate deficiency usually follows from a generally poor diet rather than from poor intake of any single food group.

The major forms of folate in food are methylTHF and formylTHF; the proportions of the folate forms vary with the food source (20). Studies and databases of the folate content of food are extensive but suffer from methodologic problems that have produced broad underestimates (34, 44). The major methodologic shortcomings include inadequate extraction of the folate and incomplete hydrolysis of the polyglutamated forms. New, more reliable databases must be developed.

Food Fortification and Supplement Use

Fortification of cereal and grain products with folic acid (140 µg/100 g) has been mandated in the United States since 1998 (and begun even earlier by some manufacturers), in the effort to prevent neural tube defects (NTDs) in newborns (45). Other countries have adopted similar programs using different amounts of folate (46, 47). In fact, the fortification target is often exceeded in the United States, reaching concentrations of 190 µg/100 g (48), and the daily intake of folate now may greatly exceed predictions (49). Further augmentation of fortification has been debated, but concern exists about still unknown but potential adverse effects, especially in persons with unrecognized cobalamin deficiency (47, 50). Indeed, cogent arguments exist for more nuanced and focused approaches in the future that take subgroup variations, genetic influences, and individualized considerations into account (51).

Following the introduction of fortification, serum folate levels increased significantly both in the general population and in patients seen by physicians (52). Clinically apparent folate deficiency with megaloblastic anemia has become very uncommon, although milder, usually subclinical folate insufficiency still exists, especially within some subsets of the general population. The effects of fortification have been augmented by the growing use of vitamin supplements in Western countries (34, 53). An incidental byproduct of these changes is that all US data on folate nutrition and folate status obtained before 1998 have only limited applicability today. Care must be taken to differentiate between pre-1998 and post-1998 data.

Bioavailability

Because the proportions of ingested folate that are assimilated vary with the ingested form, its protein binding, and its absorbability, a formula based on availability from several types of sources has been applied (34). Unreduced folic acid taken as a supplement exists as a monoglutamate and has an availability approaching 100% of the content of usual doses (54). Folate in food, usually reduced, often methylated, typically polyglutamated, and perhaps protein-bound, has a variable availability estimated to be not more than 50% (34, 55). Folic acid taken with food or used to fortify food has an intermediate availability, estimated at 85% or more of the content (56, 57). These estimates have been used to create the dietary folate equivalent (DFE), based on assigning an availability value in relation to the 100% availability of free folic acid (34). The recommended intake levels expressed in DFEs can be applied if the folate sources comprising the person's total intake are known.

No important interactions of folates with any other nutrients have been identified. Fiber appears not to modify folate availability substantially (34), and folate's effect on zinc absorption and status is controversial and, at best, minimal (34, 58).

ABSORPTION

Folate is absorbed by both saturable and unsaturable mechanisms. The saturable processes are specific and tend to occur in the upper small intestine. These processes mediate the absorption of a variety of folates, usually after the polyglutamated forms have been hydrolyzed to monoglutamates by glutamate carboxypeptidase, an enzyme found in the jejunal cells' brush borders. The major mediator of specific absorption is the reduced folate carrier, which has a high affinity for reduced folates and is located in the cellular brush border membranes (59, 60). After entering the intestinal cell, folates are usually converted to methylTHF, and a carrier-mediated mechanism exports them into the bloodstream. The entire process of specific absorption takes approximately an hour from the time of ingestion.

Nonspecific, unsaturable absorption predominates in the ileum and allows nearly all folate reaching that site to be absorbed in linear proportion to the amount presented (61). This mechanism assumes importance whenever ingested folate exceeds the limited capacity of specific jejunal absorption (~200 µg). The process can deliver large amounts of unreduced folic acid from supplements into the bloodstream without modification. This nearly

limitless capacity probably accounts for the 100% availability of folic acid supplements as well as the frequent effectiveness of oral folic acid even in patients who have intestinal diseases that impair absorption of food folates.

TRANSPORT, METABOLISM, AND EXCRETION

Transport

Once absorbed, folate is quickly cleared from the bloodstream (62) and enters various compartments for metabolism, storage, or enterohepatic recirculation (16). The rapid clearance helps to explain why serum folate levels fall within a few weeks or sometimes even days when intake diminishes (13, 20, 28). Most folate circulates in the blood attached nonspecifically to albumin and other proteins, although about one third circulates unattached. Only a tiny fraction of serum folate is bound by specific folate-binding proteins, several of which appear to be derived from folate receptors of cell membranes (59, 60). The roles of both the specific and nonspecific binding proteins are not well understood, and none seems to play a major role in cellular uptake. The specific binding proteins are also present in secretions such as breast milk, in which a role in protecting folate from bacterial uptake has been postulated.

Perhaps as much as 100 µg of folate undergoes enterohepatic recycling daily, with biliary excretion followed by reabsorption (62, 63). Most of the estimated 200 µg of folate that is excreted fecally every day is composed of unabsorbed food folate, bacterial folate, and folate from sloughed intestinal cells (64). Some folate is filtered by the glomerulus but is largely reabsorbed, and only a few micrograms of intact folate are lost in the urine daily (55).

Cellular Uptake and Metabolism

The reduced folate carrier, discussed earlier in the section on absorption, also participates in cellular uptake of reduced folates (and of the antifolate drug, methotrexate) in liver, brain, and other tissues. Folate receptor-α, which has a particularly high affinity for methylTHF monoglutamate (65), and folate receptor-β are found in other cells, including hematopoietic precursors, renal tubule cells, and placenta (59, 60), but their roles are unclear. The latter receptors also take up methotrexate, and they may facilitate intracellular entry of some viruses (66). Cellular folate uptake also occurs nonspecifically by passive diffusion. Once internalized, folate rapidly undergoes polyglutamation that enhances both its attachment to enzymes and its cellular retention. Most folate metabolism takes place in the liver, but several folate pools exist (16), with varying turnover rates of up to 100 days (64).

Folate metabolism, discussed earlier in this chapter, is summarized in Figure 28.2, along with its linkage to homocysteine-methionine metabolism. The contributory roles of several other vitamins, most importantly cobalamin, are also highlighted in Figure 28.2; for details of the metabolic interaction with cobalamin, involving the methylTHF trap hypothesis, see Chapter 29. Intracellular folate catabolism occurs largely by cleavage at the C9-N10 bond, and the acetylated product is excreted by the kidneys.

DIETARY CONSIDERATIONS AND REQUIREMENTS

The reduced folates found in food are labile and thus are subject to ready loss under certain food storage, preparation, and cooking conditions (20, 67) (see also Chapter 113). Some processes, such as boiling, especially if the water is then discarded, can lead to the loss of most of the folate content.

The main repository of folate is the liver, which has been variably estimated to contain about 4 to 15 mg of folate (68, 69). The total body content that can be approximated from these values averages 10 to 20 mg. Thus, daily losses of folate may approach 1 to 2% of body stores. This is compatible with a report that normal folate stores can be depleted enough to produce hematologic manifestations within 2 to 3 months (13) and more rapidly when stores are low or other adverse influences such as alcohol abuse coexist (27).

In the past, estimates of the daily requirements for folate were based on the amount needed to prevent clinical manifestations of folate deficiency, especially megaloblastic anemia, and/or to maintain normal levels of folate in serum or, more often, in RBCs. The application of sensitive and accurate metabolic tests showed that many healthy people with folate levels viewed as normal have mildly compromised folate metabolic status, as judged by mildly elevated tHcy levels that improve after folate supplementation. Furthermore, studies in healthy populations have shown a significant, inverse relationship of tHcy levels not only with serum folate levels but also with intake of folate (33). Given the intimate relation between folate intake and metabolic status that derives from both the low ratio of body stores to daily requirement and the infrequency of folate malabsorption, the exquisite influence of dietary intake is not surprising. Although tHcy elevation is often minimal and need not always represent folate deficiency, improving the metabolic status of at least some subgroups of seemingly healthy people may prove beneficial; this is discussed further in the section on deficiency.

Certain subpopulations are at increased risk of various degrees of folate insufficiency, such as infants (especially premature babies), adolescents, and some ethnic groups such as blacks, Hispanic-Americans, and South Asians (35, 53, 70); elderly persons, however, do not appear to be at increased risk unless other factors supervene (35, 36, 71). Folate deficiency is rare at birth. Newborns' folate levels exceed those of their mothers because the fetus obtains maternal folate efficiently (72, 73). However, infants' folate levels decline subsequently, especially in the presence of

TABLE 28.1. ADEQUATE INTAKE (AI) OR RECOMMENDED DIETARY ALLOWANCE (RDA) OF FOLATE PROPOSED BY THE FOOD AND NUTRITION BOARD, INSTITUTE OF MEDICINE

SUBGROUP	DFE[a]
Infants[b]	
0–6 mo old	9.4 μg/kg/d (AI)[b]
7–12 mo old	8.8 μg/kg/d (AI)[b]
1–3 y old[c]	150 μg/d (RDA)
4–8 y old[c]	200 μg/d (RDA)
9–13 y old[c]	300 μg/d (RDA)
14–18 y old[c]	400 μg/d (RDA)
Women of reproductive age[d]	400 μg/d (RDA) (plus 400 as folic acid supplement or fortification)[e]
All other adults[d]	400 μg/d (RDA)
Pregnant women[f]	600 μg/d (RDA)
Lactating women[g]	500 μg/d (RDA)

[a] The data are expressed in dietary folate equivalents (DFE). 1 μg DFE = 1 μg of food folate = 0.6 μg of synthetic folic acid fortifying food = 0.5 μg of synthetic folic acid supplement; 1 μg folic acid = 2.266 nmol.
[b] The Institute of Medicine panel estimated an adequate intake (AI) goal for infants, based on the maintenance of blood folate levels in infants fed human milk exclusively or, at later ages, either human milk or formula.
[c] Based on extrapolation from adult data (boys and girls).
[d] Based on the maintenance of some combination of normal blood folate and/or homocysteine values.
[e] This additional supplement was recommended solely to reduce the risk of neural tube defects in children.
[f] Based on the maintenance of normal blood folate values.
[g] Based on the replacement of daily folate secretion in milk plus maintenance of adequate maternal folate status.

Modified from Carmel R. Folate deficiency. In: Carmel R, Jacobsen DW, eds. Homocysteine in Health and Disease. Cambridge University Press, 2001, with permission. (Data from Food and Nutrition Board, Institute of Medicine. Folate. In: Dietary Reference Intakes: Thiamin, Riboflavin, Niacin, Vitamin B₆, Folate, Vitamin B₁₂, Pantothenic Acid, Biotin, and Choline. Washington, DC: National Academy Press, 1998.)

very high growth demands such as occur in premature infants (74).

The dietary recommendations summarized in Table 28.1 and expressed in DFEs to provide guidance related to bioavailability take into account both the variations in requirements in some of these groups and the liberalized definitions of folate insufficiency or folate responsiveness that are made possible by metabolic testing and to the goal of reducing the risk of NTDs. (See Appendix Tables A-2-a through A-2-k for more information on DRIs.)

DEFICIENCY STATE

Folate deficiency has sometimes dramatic clinical manifestations but can pose diagnostic challenges for several reasons. The main clinical expression, megaloblastic anemia, is indistinguishable from that seen in cobalamin deficiency, a finding that is not surprising in view of the important biochemical interaction between the two vitamins (see Fig. 28.2). Folate deficiency also rarely exists in a pure state because of its strong associations with poor diet, alcoholism, and sometimes malabsorption, all of which also affect other nutrients; indeed, even the rigorously planned experimental induction of folate deficiency was, in the end, marred by superimposed deficiencies of iron and potassium (13). For that reason, attribution of any unusual manifestions to folate deficiency always requires high standards of proof.

Clinical Features

The chief clinical expression of folate deficiency is megaloblastic anemia, which despite the term "anemia" affects other blood cells besides RBCs. Indeed, megaloblastic changes involve all dividing cells, such as epithelial cells in the gut and elsewhere (20), although the clinical consequences predominate in the blood system. The twin cellular hallmarks of megaloblastic anemia are macrocytosis and an abnormal nuclear maturation that is dissonant with the cells' apparently normal cytoplasmic maturation. The mechanisms are reviewed elsewhere (19).

Macrocytosis is most easily detected in RBCs, in which a quantitative measure, the erythroid mean corpuscular volume (MCV), is readily available as part of electronic cell sizing in routine blood counts. In adults, the MCV is normally between 83 and 97 fl. As newly minted macrocytes replace older normal RBCs, the MCV gradually rises to more than 97 fl before anemia is apparent; the MCV continues to rise, sometimes to levels exceeding 120 fl, as anemia develops and progressively worsens. However, macrocytosis also has many causes unrelated to folate deficiency. The most common causes are as follows: a direct alcohol effect on RBCs; liver disease; use of chemotherapeutic, immunosuppressive, or antiviral drugs; hypothyroidism; and maturational hematopoietic disorders such as the myelodysplastic syndrome (20, 38, 75). Indeed, most macrocytic anemias are nonmegaloblastic in origin and have nothing to do with folate (or cobalamin) deficiency. To complicate diagnostic matters further, common hematologic disorders that cause microcytosis (iron deficiency and thalassemia) can blunt or eliminate the expected macrocytosis if they coexist with the megaloblastic anemia (76, 77) (see also Chapter 92).

The megaloblastic changes produce large nuclei with dispersed chromatin that impart an immature appearance to the hematopoietic cells despite normal cytoplasmic maturation (Fig. 28.3). The granulocytes exhibit an additional, distinctive nuclear change not apparent in other cells. The segmented nuclei of mature neutrophilic granulocytes, normally having two to four lobes, become hypersegmented; this feature can be diagnosed when more than 3 or 4% of neutrophils have five-lobed nuclei or when any neutrophil with six or more lobes is recognized (see Fig. 28.3). The hypersegmentation in neutrophils is the earliest recognizable expression of megaloblastic anemia (13, 78), although the time interval by which it preceded macrocytosis in a landmark study (13) was overestimated as a result of the failure of the MCV to rise because iron deficiency

supervened. Hypersegmentation is also a more specific finding than macrocytosis, but it nevertheless occurs in some conditions unrelated to megaloblastic anemia (38).

The megaloblastic change induces ineffective hematopoiesis, in which blood cell precursors are generated in abundance in the bone marrow but do not survive to enter the bloodstream (19, 20). Biochemical markers of the massive, premature cell death become prominent once the anemia is florid; serum bilirubin and lactate dehydrogenase levels are typically elevated in advanced cases. The hematologic abnormality progresses from barely symptomatic, mild macrocytic anemia to severe pancytopenia, as granulocyte and platelet counts fall along with the worsened anemia that at this stage can also feature congestive heart failure and other signs of impaired oxygen delivery. Clinical expression can be worsened by other factors such as coexisting complications, or it can be ameliorated by highly efficient compensatory changes in oxygen delivery from RBC.

Occasionally, epithelial changes of the tongue and oral mucosa may produce soreness or shallow ulcerations (20). Epithelial changes in the gut sometimes also impair absorption of nutrients, including folate itself (79). A wellknown setting in which this may have clinical consequences is tropical sprue, in which the malabsorption itself can be improved by folate therapy, although not as effectively as when antibiotics are given (80, 81). The explanation for the occasional changes in skin, hair, or fingernail pigmentation that folate deficiency produces in nonwhites is unknown (82).

Controversy has surrounded the existence of neurologic consequences in folate deficiency (83). Opinion long had contrasted the rarity of neurologic dysfunction in folate deficiency with the high frequency of myeloneuropathy and mental changes in cobalamin deficiency. However, the volunteer with self-induced folate deficiency developed irritability and forgetfulness (13), mild neuropathy has been reported in folate-deficient patients (84–86), and an association with depression has been hypothesized (87), although results have been mixed concerning associations between folate deficiency and psychiatric disorders (88). Moreover, severe neurologic dysfunction characterizes many inborn errors of folate metabolism in children (89). In adults with acquired folate deficiency, however, neurologic consequences are infrequent and, if present, usually mild. Because acquired folate deficiency rarely exists alone, attribution of neurologic or mental changes directly to the lack of folate requires careful exclusion of all other possible explanations.

Subclinical Features and Predispositions

Metabolic folate insufficiency can be identified in asymptomatic persons (83). As mentioned earlier in the section on homocysteine, this diagnosis is made frequently now, most often by demonstrating an elevated plasma tHcy that

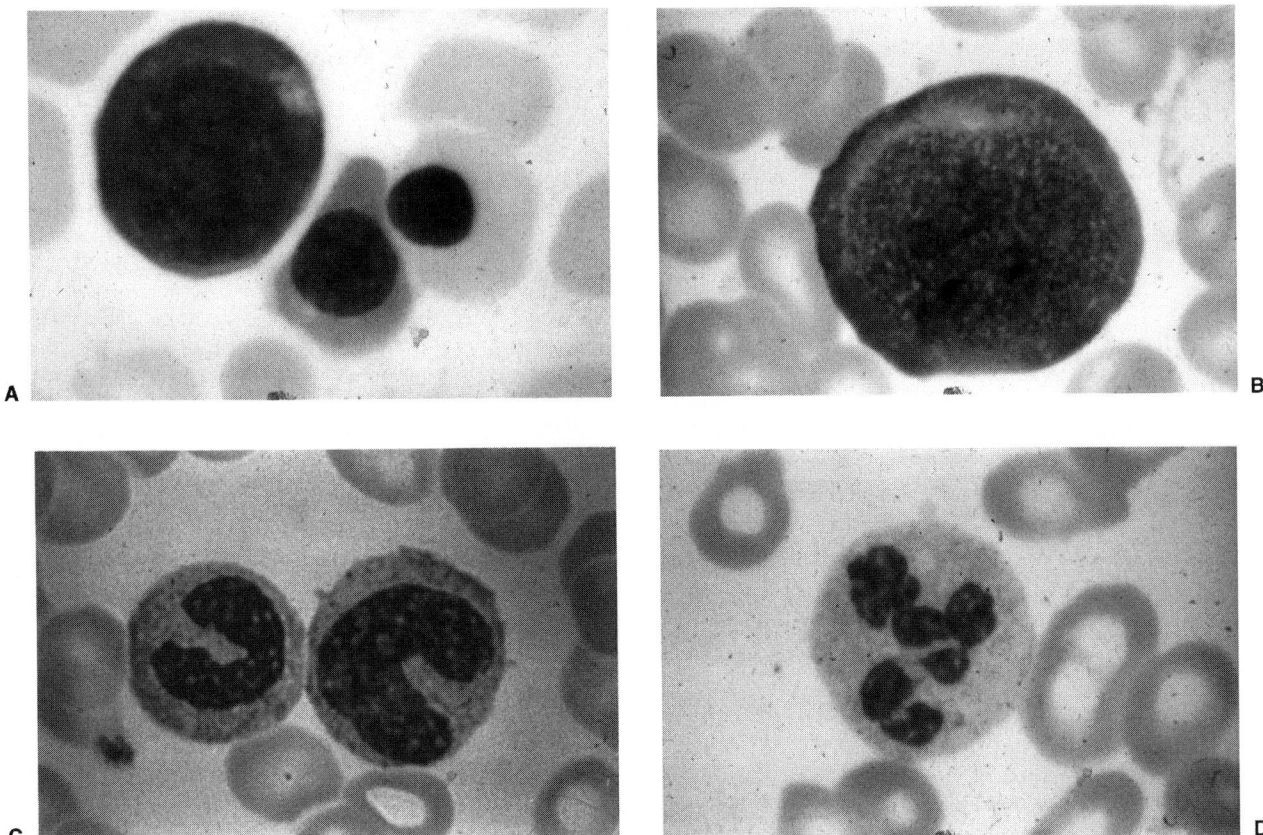

Figure 28.3. Megaloblastic changes in hematopoietic precursors in the bone marrow and their progeny in the peripheral blood, compared with normal cells. **A.** Normal erythroid precursor cells in bone marrow. Three nucleated precursors of increasing maturation are shown from **left** to **right**, with progressively smaller cell size and greater nuclear compactness; the cell on the **right** is ready to extrude its nucleus before becoming a mature erythrocyte and exiting into the bloodstream. **B.** Megaloblastic erythroid precursor cell at a maturation stage comparable to that of the normal large precursor cell on the **left** in A. Note the abnormal appearance of the nuclear chromatin in the megaloblastic cell, compared with its normal equivalent. **C.** Peripheral blood containing a megaloblastic "giant" band cell (a nearly mature neutrophilic granulocyte) that can be contrasted with the normal band cell to its left; note the larger size of both the megaloblastic cell and its nucleus and the slightly more dispersed nuclear chromatin. **D.** Megaloblastic peripheral blood smear showing a hypersegmented neutrophilic granulocyte; the nucleus has more than six lobes, whereas normal neutrophils typically have four nuclear lobes or fewer. In addition, the mature red blood cells (no nuclei) tend to be unusually large, some approaching the neutrophil in size; also note the abnormal shape of many red blood cells, many of which are oval instead of round and others of which have irregular shapes; these findings are typical of but not exclusive to megaloblastic anemia. (From Carmel R. Folate deficiency. In: Carmel R, Jacobsen DW, eds. Homocysteine in Health and Disease. Cambridge University Press, 2001, with permission.)

improves after folate therapy. However, such tHcy-based diagnosis requires caution. Even when it is folate responsive, hyperhomocysteinemia can reflect origins other than folate deficiency, including a mild genetic polymorphism and, in its seeming response to folate, coincidence or regression to the mean. Nevertheless, subclinical deficiency of folate appears to be common and, in still unknown ways, may contribute to or be a risk factor for vascular disease, presumably by its effect on homocysteine metabolism (37), and NTDs. Low dietary folate intake has been associated with increased coronary disease in prospective studies (90) and a 6-month study of 205 subjects suggested that taking folate and other vitamins reduced restenosis after coronary angioplasty (91), but the role of folate in relation to vascular disease still remains uncertain. The evidence linking compromised folate status with a host of other postulated associations, such as non-NTD birth defects, complications of pregnancy, and some cancers, especially colorectal cancer, is also unsettled (34, 36, 92–94). Folic acid supplementation clearly prevents some NTDs, but the benefits of folic acid in preventing vascular disease and cancer remain unproven, and its use for the latter two conditions is therefore not recommended at this time (34). Indeed, moderate reduction of homocysteine levels with folate, cobalamin, and vitamin B_6 had no effect on vascular outcomes in patients with stroke in a 2-year follow-up (95).

Responsiveness to Folate in Nondeficiency States

The example best illustrating the promise and ambiguities of the just-mentioned associations is provided by the NTD story. NTDs, occurring in approximately one in 1000 births in the United States but varying widely among ethnic groups and geographic locations, are the most common neurologic birth defects and can be disabling or lethal (96). Because neurulation begins at day 21 after conception, a time when most women are still unaware that they are pregnant, effective prevention cannot await the recognition of pregnancy. Giving 400 μg folic acid daily to women of reproductive age and 4 mg to those with known risk factors for NTD, such as having previous children with NTD or use of valproic acid, has unquestionably reduced the incidence of newborns with NTD (34, 97). The incidence has decreased by 20% since the introduction of folate fortification in the United States (98). Nevertheless, NTDs are rarely directly attributable to maternal folate deficiency but appear to be associated with a variety of still unidentified genetic and environmental risk factors. The risk factors may not even all be directly traceable to folate-related abnormality, although antibody to folate receptor was reported to be more common in women with previous NTD-affected pregnancies than in control subjects (99).

Causes

Poor dietary intake is the most common cause of folate deficiency by far (Table 28.2). Several weeks or a few months of poor general nutrition can induce deficiency because the ratio of body stores to daily requirements is only about 100:1. Restricted diets, such as those used to manage phenylketonuria, have also been associated with folate deficiency.

The likelihood of deficiency is also enhanced when marginal intake combines with other conditions that compromise folate status (28). The most common such condition is alcohol abuse (100), which affects the enterohepatic recycling of cobalamin, interferes with folate metabolism, forms aldehyde adducts with folates, and accelerates folate breakdown (101–104). Alcohol abuse is often associated with poor diet, especially when hard liquor is the alcohol of choice (beer contains folate). Any of the causes of folate deficiency shown in Table 28.2 can become aggravated by suboptimal intake. This applies even to conditions that are normally clinically inconsequential themselves, such as an increased requirement for folate or common but mild polymorphisms (e.g., the 677C→T mutation of the N5,10-methylenetetrahydrofolate reductase (*MTHFR*) gene), and metabolic or occasionally clinical insufficiency can result (105). Increased requirements for folate have been documented in pregnancy, lactation, adolescence, prematurity, and chronic hemolytic anemias such as sickle cell anemia (74, 106, 107). Routine folate supplementation is commonly given to patients undergoing hemodialysis, to pregnant women, and to patients with chronic hemolytic anemia. The advisability of routine folate supplementation for chronic hemolytic anemia has been questioned for several reasons (108–110), and the frequent hyperhomocysteinemia in adults with sickle cell disease seems unrelated to

TABLE 28.2. CAUSES OF AND CONTRIBUTING FACTORS TO FOLATE DEFICIENCY

Poor dietary intake
Sometimes combined with other causes of folate deficiency
Malabsorption
Diseases of small intestine (e.g., tropical sprue, celiac disease, Whipple disease, dermatitis herpetiformis)
Gastric diseases (e.g., atrophic gastritis, giant hypertrophic gastritis, partial gastric resection)[a]
Drugs and toxins (e.g., alcohol, sulfasalazine, p-aminosalicylic acid, gastric acid–suppressive drugs, pancreatic extracts for pancreatic insufficiency)[a]
Genetic (hereditary folate malabsorption)
Metabolic blocks
Acquired
  Drugs and toxins
    Dihydrofolate reductase inhibitors with potent activity in humans (e.g., methotrexate)
    Dihydrofolate reductase inhibitors with weak activity in humans (e.g., trimethoprim-sulfamethoxazole, pyrimethamine, triamterene)[a]
    Alcohol
    Sulfasalazine[a]
    Valproic acid[a]
Genetic
  Methylenetetrahydrofolate reductase deficiency
  Glutamate formiminotransferase deficiency
  Polymorphisms of the methylenetetrahydrofolate reductase gene[a]
Increased Requirements and Increased Losses
Hemodialysis for renal disease
Premature infants
Pregnancy
Lactation[a]
Chronic hemolytic anemia[a]
?Hyperthyroidism[a]
Unknown Mechanisms
Drugs (e.g., hydantoins, ?oral contraceptives)[a]

[a] These conditions rarely cause folate deficiency by themselves but can predispose to it when other complications, such as poor dietary intake, supervene.

folate status (111). All agree, however, that care must be taken that all persons with increased requirements have diets containing adequate folate.

Other causes of folate deficiency are malabsorptive disorders, which can be caused by diseases of the small bowel such as tropical sprue (80, 81), celiac disease (112), and, less often, inflammatory bowel disease (113). Limitations of folate absorption can also occur because of diminished gastric acid secretion (114–116), such as in atrophic gastritis, gastric surgery, use of acid-suppressive therapy, or acid neutralization by treatment of pancreatic insufficiency. A rare hereditary disorder causes folate malabsorption as well as diminished folate transport into the central nervous system, with severe neurologic consequences (117).

Various drugs interfere with folate metabolism (118), including folate antagonists such as the dihydrofolate reductase inhibitor, methotrexate, which is used to treat neoplastic disorders, rheumatoid arthritis, psoriasis, and inflammatory bowel disease (119). Other drugs, such as sulfasalazine, may act in multiple ways. Anticonvulsants are associated with folate deficiency, but the proposed mechanisms, such as an impairment of absorption attributed to hydantoins, are controversial. Increased folate breakdown and loss have also been proposed for anticonvulsants and other drugs (104). Reported associations between oral contraceptives and folate deficiency now appear doubtful.

Inborn errors of folate metabolism are rare but can be catastrophic. The most common of these disorders is MTHFR deficiency, which causes severe neurologic dysfunction, including myelopathy, seizures, and developmental disturbances, but does not cause anemia (89). The explanation for that paradoxic clinical phenotype is that methyleneTHF is preserved, and this allows adequate conversion of deoxyuridylate to thymidylate (reaction 2, Fig. 28.2), thereby avoiding anemia. The common 677C→T polymorphism of the *MTHFR* gene, which, unlike the severe disorder of MTHFR deficiency, causes only mild reduction of MTHFR activity, produces no obvious clinical disability but sometimes causes mild hyperhomocysteinemia and may be associated with an increased risk of NTDs (105, 120).

Treatment

Most folate deficiency states, which usually arise entirely or partially from dietary inadequacy, respond readily to dietary modification. However, folic acid supplements are usually given and are cheap and effective. Folic acid is not commonly available in doses greater than 400 µg in over-the-counter supplements; higher doses, rarely exceeding 1 mg, generally require a physician's prescription because of concerns about masking cobalamin deficiency. Even patients with malabsorptive diseases that limit the absorption of food folate usually respond to oral folic acid, which is readily absorbed by nonspecific mechanisms, although doses up to 5 mg may be needed sometimes. Folic acid can be given by injection, but this is needed only in special cases. Reduced folates, such as folinic acid (N5-formylTHF), need to be used only when folate metabolism is impaired by drugs such as methotrexate or by some inborn errors of metabolism. Toxicity of folic acid, even when given in high doses, is rare in humans (34, 121); given in very high doses intravenously, folic acid has sometimes exacerbated seizures in epileptic children taking anticonvulsants. By far the most serious potential toxicity occurs if folate is given to someone with unrecognized cobalamin deficiency, as discussed in the next section.

Because folate deficiency is usually accompanied by broad dietary inadequacy or malabsorption, and often by alcohol abuse, attention to these non–folate-related problems is also important in most cases. A special requirement is always to rule out the coexistence of cobalamin deficiency before instituting folate therapy.

INTERACTIONS

Cobalamin

The interaction with cobalamin is intimate. The metabolic and hematologic connections are described earlier in this chapter. The clinical interaction extends to issues of diagnosis and therapy as well (20, 21, 38, 122). Diagnostic confusion can easily develop because serum cobalamin levels regularly fall in folate deficiency, often to subnormal levels; the cobalamin levels rise after folate is repleted. In contrast, serum folate levels often rise with cobalamin deficiency, whereas RBC folate falls; both the folate changes reverse with cobalamin therapy.

Therapeutic confusion, with potentially serious neurologic consequences, can arise whenever folic acid is given instead of cobalamin, either inadvertently or intentionally, to patients who have cobalamin deficiency (20, 34, 123). The error is unfortunately common (124), and it may become further aggravated by fortification of the diet with folic acid and the increased use of supplements. Folic acid bypasses the methylTHF trap of cobalamin deficiency and thereby reverses the megaloblastic anemia of cobalamin deficiency. Although the hematologic improvement is often only partial and is never permanent (9, 123, 125), diagnostic delay and a failure to institute cobalamin treatment often result. The cobalamin deficiency can progress, with the potential risk that any neurologic deterioration that may occur (but is not inevitable) can become irreversible; occasionally, the progression may be at an accelerated pace. Unchecked progression can be catastrophic, but old reports have shown that sometimes the mistaken folate therapy can induce temporary and partial improvement of neurologic dysfunction, too (9, 125); these variations and paradoxes remain enigmatic. Most reports of neurologic deterioration have been in patients receiving more than 5 mg folic acid daily (10, 34, 126), but the problem can also occur at lower doses (34, 110). Although the Institute of Medicine endorsed a 1-mg folic acid intake from fortified food and supplements as the upper limit of safety for adults (34), no folic acid dose can be considered truly safe in the presence of untreated cobalamin deficiency.

Homocysteine

Together with cobalamin, vitamin B$_6$, and, to a lesser extent, riboflavin, folate plays an important role in homocysteine-methionine metabolism (see Fig. 28.2 and Chapter 34). Folate status is a major regulator of plasma tHcy levels (33, 34, 36). However, plasma methionine levels are surprisingly often normal in folate deficiency (127, 128), although even normal methionine levels tend to rise after folate therapy (129).

Iron

Iron has no known biochemical interaction with folate, but folate (and cobalamin) interacts in many physiologic, clinical, and diagnostic ways with iron. Like any anemia, megaloblastic anemia induces increased iron absorption in the gut. In addition, the huge cellular turnover that marks the ineffective erythropoiesis of megaloblastic anemia markedly raises tissue iron stores, serum ferritin and iron levels, and serum transferrin receptor levels. All these iron-related serum and tissue values revert to normal within 24 to 48 hours of folate therapy as the ineffective erythropoiesis reverses, and, before equilibrium is restored, the values sometimes become spuriously low as iron is rapidly mobilized by newly effective erythropoiesis (20). Occasionally, the high pretreatment iron-related findings mask a coexisting iron deficiency, which can remain undiagnosable until the megaloblastic process is reversed.

Although not directly related to each other, the coexistence of megaloblastic anemia and iron deficiency anemia is not unusual (20). Depending on the circumstances, the combination can produce dimorphic anemia with predominant macrocytosis (high MCV) caused by the folate deficiency, predominant microcytosis (low MCV) resulting from the iron deficiency, or normocytosis (normal MCV) because of the mixture (76). Sometimes, too, the iron deficiency anemia can actually blunt the megaloblastic changes themselves, both morphologically and, as demonstrated by the deoxyuridine suppression test, biochemically (76, 130).

REFERENCES

1. Hayem G. Bull Mem Soc Med Hop Paris 1877;14:155–66.
2. Ehrlich P. Berlin Klin Wochenschr 1880;17:405.
3. Wills L. BMJ 1931;1:1059–64.
4. Day PL, Langton WC, Shukers CF. J Nutr 1935;9:637–44.
5. Mitchell HK, Snell EE, Williams RJ. J Am Chem Soc 1941;63:2284.
6. Hoffbrand AV, Weir DG. Br J Haematol 2001;113:579–89.
7. Jukes TH, Stokstad TLR. Physiol Rev 1948;28:51–106.
8. Farber S, Diamond LK, Mercer RD et al. N Engl J Med 1948;238:787–93.
9. Hall BE, Watkins CH. J Lab Clin Med 1947;32:622–34.
10. Wagley P. N Engl J Med 1948;238:11–5.
11. Ross JF, Belding H, Paegel BL. Blood 1948;3:68–90.
12. Schwartz SO, Kaplan SR, Armstrong BE. J Lab Clin Med 1950;35:894–8.
13. Herbert V. Trans Assoc Am Phys 1962;75:307–20.
14. Moran RG. Semin Oncol 1999;26[Suppl 6]:24–32.
15. Shane B. Folate chemistry and metabolism. In: Bailey LB, ed. Folate in Health and Disease. New York: Marcel Dekker, 1995:1–22.
16. Cook RJ. Folate metabolism. In: Carmel R, Jacobsen DW, eds. Homocysteine in Health and Disease. Cambridge: Cambridge University Press, 2001:113–34.
17. Clarke S, Banfield K. S-Adenosylmethionine–dependent methyltransferases. In: Carmel R, Jacobsen DW, eds. Homocysteine in Health and Disease. New York: Cambridge University Press, 2001:65–80.
18. Blount BC, Mack MM, Wehr CM et al. Proc Natl Acad Sci USA 1997;94:3290–5.
19. Wickramasinghe SN. Semin Hematol 1999;36:3–18.
20. Chanarin I. The Megaloblastic Anaemias. 2nd ed. Oxford: Blackwell Scientific, 1979.
21. Zittoun J, Zittoun R. Semin Hematol 1999;36:35–46.
22. Gunter EW, Bowman BA, Caudill SP et al. 1996;42:1689–94.
23. O'Broin JD, Temperley IJ, Scott JM. Clin Chem 1980;26:522–4.
24. Brouwer DAJ, Welten HTME, Reijngoud D-J et al. Clin Chem 1998;44:1545–50.
25. Lucock M, Yates Z. Lancet 2002;360:1021–2.
26. Eichner ER, Hillman RS. J Clin Invest 1973;52:584–91.
27. Wu A, Chanarin I, Slavin G et al. Br J Haematol 1975;29:469–78.
28. Eichner ER, Pierce HI, Hillman RS. N Engl J Med 1971;284:933–8.
29. Hoffbrand AV, Newcombe BFA, Mollin DL. J Clin Pathol 1966;19:17–28.
30. Omer A, Finlayson NDC, Shearman DJC et al. Blood 1970;35:821–8.
31. Jaffe JP, Schilling RF. Am J Hematol 1991;36:116–21.
32. Savage DG, Lindenbaum J, Stabler SP et al. Am J Med 1994;96:239–46.
33. Selhub J, Jacques PF, Wilson PWF et al. JAMA 1993;270:2693–8.
34. Food and Nutrition Board, Institute of Medicine. Folate. In: Dietary Reference Intakes: Thiamin, Riboflavin, Niacin, Vitamin B_6, Folate, Vitamin B_{12}, Pantothenic Acid, Biotin, and Choline. Washington, DC: National Academy Press, 1998:196–305.
35. Selhub J, Jacques PF, Rosenberg IH et al. Ann Intern Med 1999;131:331–9.
36. Carmel R. Folate deficiency. In: Carmel R, Jacobsen DW, eds. Homocysteine in Health and Disease. Cambridge: Cambridge University Press, 2001:271–88.
37. Carmel R, Jacobsen DW, eds. Homocysteine in Health and Disease. Cambridge: Cambridge University Press, 2001.
38. Carmel R. Megaloblastic anemias: disorders of impaired DNA synthesis. In: Greer JP, Foerster J, Lukens JN et al, eds. Wintrobe's Clinical Hematology. 11th ed. Philadelphia: Lippincott Williams & Wilkins, 2004:1367–95.
39. Refsum H, Smith AD, Ueland PM et al. Clin Chem 2004;50:3–32.
40. Ganji V, Kafai MR. Am J Clin Nutr 2003;77:826–33.
41. Andersson A, Isaksson A, Hultberg B. Clin Chem 1992;38:1311–5.
42. Rasmussen K, Moller J, Lyngbak M et al. Clin Chem 1996;42:630–6.
43. Stabler SP, Marcell PD, Podell ER et al. J Clin Invest 1988;81:466–74.
44. Rader JI, Weaver CM, Angyal G. Food Chem 2000;70:275–89.
45. Food and Drug Administration. Fed Reg 1996;61:8781–97.
46. Health Canada. Can Gazette Part I 1997;131:3702–5.
47. Hirsch S, de la Maza P, Barrera G et al. J Nutr 2002;132:289–91.
48. Choumenkovitch SF, Selhub J, Wilson PWF et al. J Nutr 2002;132:2792–8.
49. Quinlivan EP, Gregory JF III. Am J Clin Nutr 2003;77:221–5.
50. Mills JL. N Engl J Med 2000;342:1442–5.
51. Stover PJ, Garza C. J Nutr 2002;132:2476S–80S.
52. Lawrence JM, Petitti DB, Watkins M et al. Lancet 1999;354:915–6.
53. Ford ES, Bowman BA. Am J Clin Nutr 1999;69:476–81.
54. Gregory JF III, Eur J Clin Nutr 1997;51:54S–9S.
55. Sauberlich HE, Kretsch MJ, Skala JH et al. Am J Clin Nutr 1987;46:1016–28.
56. Cuskelly GJ, McNulty H, Scott JM. Lancet 1996;347:657–9.
57. Pfeiffer CM, Rogers LM, Bailey LB et al. Am J Clin Nutr 1997;66:1388–97.

58. Butterworth CE, Tamura T. Am J Clin Nutr 1989;50:353–8.

59. Antony AC. Annu Rev Nutr 1996;16:501–21.

60. Sirotnak FM, Tolner B. Annu Rev Nutr 1999;19:91–122.

61. Rosenberg IH, Selhub J. Intestinal absorption of folates. In: Blakley R, Whitehead V, eds. Folates and Pterins, vol 3. New York: John Wiley & Sons, 1986;147–76.

62. Steinberg SE, Campbell CL, Hillman RS. J Clin Invest 1979; 64:83–8.

63. Whitehead VM. Pharmacokinetics and physiological disposition of folate and its derivatives. In: Blakley RL, Whitehead VM, eds. Folates and Pterins, vol 3. New York: John Wiley & Sons, 1986;177–205.

64. Stites TE, Bailey LB, Scott KC et al. Am J Clin Nutr 1997;65: 53–60.

65. Wang X, Shen F, Freisheim JH et al. Biochem Pharmacol 1992; 44:1898–901.

66. Chan SY, Empig CJ, Welte FJ et al. Cell 2001;106:117–26.

67. McKillop DJ, Pentieva K, Daly D et al. Br J Nutr 2002;88: 681–8.

68. Whitehead VM. Lancet 1973;1:743–5.

69. Hoppner K, Lampi B. Am J Clin Nutr 1980;33:862–4.

70. Michie CA, Chambers J, Abramsky I et al. Lancet 1998;351: 1105.

71. Rosenberg IH, Bowman BB, Cooper BA et al. Am J Clin Nutr 1982;36[Suppl]:1060–6.

72. Landon MJ, Oxley A. Arch Dis Child 1971;46:810–4.

73. Ek J. J Pediatr 1980;97:288–92.

74. Worthington-White DA, Behnke M, Gross S. Am J Clin Nutr 1994;60:930–5.

75. Savage DG, Ogundipe A, Allen RH et al. Am J Med Sci 2000; 319:343–52.

76. Spivak J. Arch Intern Med 1982;142:2111–4.

77. Green R, Kuhl W, Jacobson R et al. N Engl J Med 1982;307: 1322–5.

78. Lindenbaum J, Nath BJ. Br J Haematol 1980;44:511–3.

79. Elsborg L. Acta Haematol 1976;55:140–7.

80. Baker SJ. Crit Rev Trop Med 1982;1:197–245.

81. Haghighi P, Wolf PL. Crit Rev Clin Lab Sci 1997;34:313–41.

82. Gough KR, Read AE, McCarthy CF et al. Q J Med 1963;32: 243–57.

83. Green R, Miller JW. Semin Hematol 1999;36:47–64.

84. Reynolds EH, Rothfeld P, Pincus J. BMJ 1973; 2:398–400.

85. Manzoor M, Runcie J. BMJ 1976;1:1176–8.

86. Botez ML, Reynolds EH. Folic Acid in Neurology, Psychiatry, and Internal Medicine. New York; Raven Press, 1979.

87. Shorvon SD, Carney MWP, Chanarin I et al. BMJ 1980;281: 1036–8.

88. Hutto BR. Comp Psychiatry 1997;38:305–34.

89. Rosenblatt D, Fenton W. Inherited disorders of folate and cobalamin metabolism. In: Scriver C, Beaudet A, Sly W et al, eds. The Metabolic and Molecular Bases of Inherited Disease. 8th ed. New York: McGraw-Hill, 2001;3897–933.

90. Voutilainen S, Rissanen TH, Virtanen J et al. Circulation 2001; 103:2674–80.

91. Schnyder G, Roffi M, Pin R et al. N Engl J Med 2001;345: 1593–600.

92. Mason JB, Levesque T. Oncology 1996;10:1727–36.

93. Ray JG, Laskin CA. Placenta 1999;20:519–29.

94. Kim YI. J Nutr Biochem 1999;10:66–88.

95. Toole JF, Malinow MR, Chambless LE et al. JAMA 2004;291: 565–75.

96. Volpe JJ. Neurology of the Newborn. 3rd ed. Philadelphia: WB Saunders, 1995.

97. Berry RJ, Li Z, Erickson JD et al. N Engl J Med 1999;341: 1485–90.

98. Honein MA, Paulozzi LJ, Mathews TJ et al. JAMA 2001;285: 2981–6.

99. Rothenberg SP, da Costa MP, Sequeira JM et al. N Engl J Med 2004;350:134–42.

100. Lindenbaum J, Roman MJ. Am J Clin Nutr 1980;33:2727–35.

101. Steinberg S, Campbell C, Hillman R. Clin Toxicol 1980;17: 407–11.

102. Halsted CH. Am J Clin Nutr 1980;33:2736–40.

103. Shaw S, Jayatilleke E, Herbert V et al. Biochem J 1989;257: 277–80.

104. Suh JR, Herbig AK, Stover PJ. Annu Rev Nutr 2001;21:255–82.

105. deBree A, Verschuren WMM, Bjorke-Monsen AL et al. Am J Clin Nutr 2003;77:687–93.

106. Lindenbaum J. Folic acid requirement in situations of increased need. In: Food and Nutrition Board, National Research Council, ed. Folic Acid: Biochemistry and Physiology in Relation to the Human Nutrition Requirement. Washington, DC: National Academy Press, 1977:256–76.

107. Mackey AD, Picciano MF. Am J Clin Nutr 1999;69:285–92.

108. Rabb L, Grandison Y, Mason K et al. Br J Haematol 1983;54: 589–94.

109. Wang WC. J Pediatr Hematol Oncol 1999;21:176–8.

110. Dhar M, Bellevue R, Carmel R. N Engl J Med 2003;348: 2204–7.

111. Dhar M, Bellevue R, Brar S et al. Am J Hematol 2004;76: 114–20.

112. Hallert C, Tobiasson P, Walan A. Scand J Gastroenterol 1981; 16:263–7.

113. Elsborg L, Larsen L. Scand J Gastroenterol 1979;14:1019–24.

114. Russell RM, Krasinski SD, Samloff IM et al. Gastroenterol 1986;91:1476–82.

115. Elsborg L. Scand J Gastroenterol 1974;9:271–4.

116. Russell RM, Golner BB, Krasinski SD et al. J Lab Clin Med 1988;112:458–63.

117. Zittoun J. Baillieres Clin Haematol 1995;8:603–16.

118. Lambie D, Johnson R. Drugs 1985;30:145–55.

119. Morgan SL, Baggott JE. Folate antagonists in nonneoplastic disease: proposed mechanisms of efficacy and toxicity. In: Bailey LB, ed. Folate in Health and Disease. New York: Marcel Dekker, 1995:405–33.

120. Rozen R. Polymorphisms of folate and cobalamin metabolism. In: Carmel R, Jacobsen DW, eds. Homocysteine in Health and Disease. Cambridge: Cambridge University Press, 2001: 259–69.

121. Butterworth CE Jr, Tamura T. Am J Clin Nutr 1989;50:353–8.

122. Rothenberg SP. Semin Hematol 1999;36:65–74.

123. Carmel R. Cobalamin deficiency. In: Carmel R, Jacobsen DW, eds. Homocysteine in Health and Disease. Cambridge: Cambridge University Press, 2001:289–305.

124. Carmel R, Karnaze DS. Arch Intern Med 1986;146:1161–5.

125. Schwartz SO, Kaplan SR, Armstrong BE. J Lab Clin Med 1950;35:894–8.

126. Dickinson CJ. Q J Med 1995;88:357–64.

127. Maree KA, van der Westhuyzen J, Metz J. Int J Vitam Nutr Res 1989;59:136–41.

128. Stabler SP, Lindenbaum J, Savage DG et al. Blood 1993;81: 3404–13.

129. Guttormsen AB, Schneede J, Ueland PM et al. Am J Clin Nutr 1996;63:194–202.

130. van der Weyden M, Rother M, Firkin B. Br J Haematol 1972;22:299–307.

29 COBALAMIN (VITAMIN B$_{12}$)[1,2]

RALPH CARMEL

HISTORICAL BACKGROUND 482
BIOCHEMISTRY 483
ANALYTIC METHODS 484
    Serum Cobalamin 484
    Cellular Cobalamin 485
    Methylmalonic Acid 485
    Homocysteine 485
    Holotranscobalamin II 485
NUTRITION AND BIOAVAILABILITY 486
ABSORPTION 486
TRANSPORT, METABOLISM, AND EXCRETION 488
    Transcobalamin II 488
    Cellular Metabolism 488
    Transcobalamin I; Haptocorrin 488
DIETARY CONSIDERATIONS AND REQUIREMENTS 488
    Adults 488
    Children 489
DEFICIENCY STATE 489
    Hematologic Features 489
    Neurologic Features 489
    Other Clinical Manifestations 490
    Metabolic Explanations for the Clinical
        Manifestations 490
    Subclinical Cobalamin Deficiency 490
CAUSES OF DEFICIENCY 491
    Dietary Causes 491
    Pernicious Anemia and Other Causes
        of Malabsorption of Free Cobalamin 491
    Malabsorption of Food Cobalamin 492
    Drugs 492
    Metabolic Disorders 492
    Cobalamin-Related Disorders that Do Not
        Cause Cobalamin Deficiency 493
    Diagnostic Tests for Causes of Cobalamin
        Deficiency 493
TREATMENT OF DEFICIENCY 493

    Vegetarians and Other Patients with
        Normal Absorption 493
    Patients Who Cannot Absorb Free Cobalamin 493
    Patients with Malabsorption Limited
        to Food Cobalamin .494
    Patients with Inborn Errors of Metabolism 494
    Monitoring and Response to Cobalamin
        Therapy 494
    Characteristics of Cobalamin Preparations 494
INTERACTIONS 494
    Folate 494
    Iron 495
    Homocysteine 495
    Miscellaneous 495

HISTORICAL BACKGROUND

The history of cobalamin is inextricably bound to the disease that provides the most common setting for its clinical deficiency, even though cobalamin deficiency can arise from many other causes. The reader is referred to excellent reviews of the dramatic scientific and clinical story (1, 2). In 1849, Addison (3) reported several patients with a "remarkable form of anemia" that was accompanied by languor and restlessness, among other signs and symptoms. Although Addison mistakenly attributed the anemia to adrenal disease, his report is considered to be the first of the disease whose often fatal course later led Biermer (4) to name it "pernicious anemia" (PA). The dramatic name, then very apt, is misleading now because the easily treated disease is no longer pernicious and because anemia may be a minor or even absent feature. Indeed, the striking megaloblastic anemia is not specific to this disease or, for that matter, to cobalamin deficiency (Table 29.1). The history of the identification and elucidation of the megaloblastic anemia characteristic of both cobalamin deficiency and folate deficiency is discussed in Chapter 28.

The critical experiments that transformed the lethal course of PA were done by Minot and Murphy (5), who fed affected patients large amounts of liver and documented the hematologic improvement. For this, they shared a Nobel Prize. The second important contribution was Castle's discovery that patients with PA responded effectively to

---

[1]**Abbreviations: CoA,** coenzyme A; **IF,** intrinsic factor; **MCV,** mean corpuscular volume; **MMA,** methylmalonic acid; **PA,** pernicious anemia; **tHcy,** plasma total homocysteine; **TC,** transcobalamin; **THF,** tetrahydrofolic acid.

[2]Système Internationale units: 1 ng cobalamin = 0.738 pmol.

TABLE 29.1. BRIEF GLOSSARY OF POTENTIALLY CONFUSING TERMINOLOGY

Megaloblastic anemia: A form of anemia whose cellular and nuclear features are characteristic of but are not entirely specific to deficiency of cobalamin or folate. (The term anemia should not obscure the fact that leukocytes and platelets are also affected and are often decreased in number.)

Macrocytic anemia: Anemia with larger than normal red blood cells. Not all macrocytic anemias are megaloblastic and therefore cannot be automatically assumed to arise from cobalamin or folate deficiency or be taken as evidence of such deficiency. Indeed, most macrocytic anemias are unrelated to either cobalamin or folate deficiency.

Pernicious anemia: This name is reserved specifically for the gastric disorder in which cobalamin malabsorption occurs because of the lack of gastric intrinsic factor. The disorder's definition is therefore gastroenterologic, not hematologic. The presence or absence of anemia is irrelevant; indeed, many patients with pernicious anemia have little or no anemia. It may be useful to note common misuses of the name: pernicious anemia is not synonymous with megaloblastic anemia or with cobalamin deficiency, either of which can have many causes other than pernicious anemia.

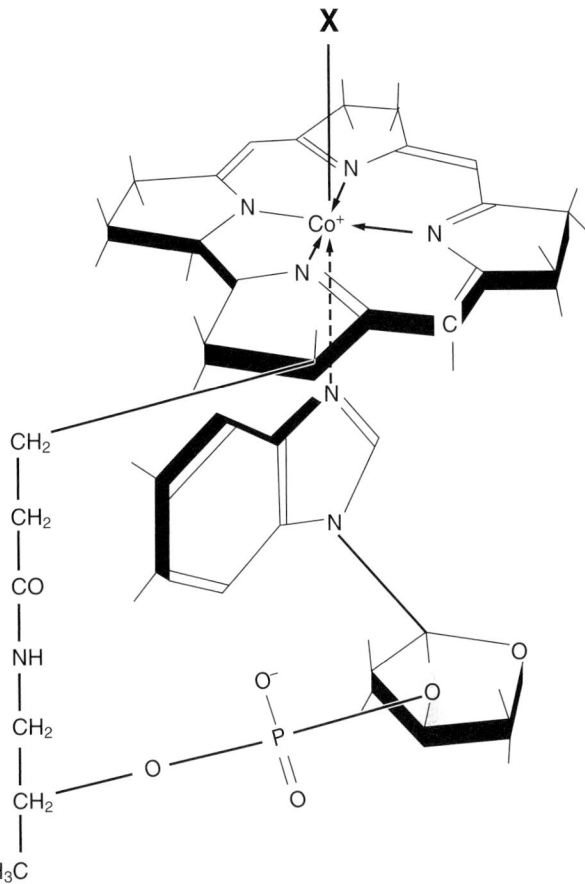

Figure 29.1. The structure of cobalamin. Attached to the central cobalt atom of the corrin tetrapyrrole and to one of the pyrrole rings is the α-ligand, the 5,6-dimethylbenzimidazole nucleotide, extending below the corrin plane. The β-ligand (marked as *X* in the figure) above the plane can be any of several moieties, such as methyl, 5′-deoxyadenosyl, hydroxyl, or cyanide. (From Carmel R. Megaloblastic anemias: disorders of impaired DNA synthesis. In: Greer JP, Foerster J, Lukens JL et al., eds. Wintrobe's Clinical Hematology. 11th ed. Philadelphia: Lippincott Williams & Wilkins, 2004, with permission.)

an "extrinsic factor" in the ingested liver or meat when it was combined with an "intrinsic factor" (IF) in gastric juice (6). This demonstration sealed the long-suspected connection of PA with achylia gastrica. The third critical achievement was the identification of cobalamin as the extrinsic factor. The purification of cobalamin (7, 8) was accompanied by elucidation of its structure by Hodgkin (9), who was also awarded a Nobel Prize for her crystallographic work.

With the availability of vitamin B₁₂ (cyanocobalamin), PA became easy to treat. Indeed, vitamin B₁₂ became one of the most frequently given injections in the United States and ultimately acquired the dubious status of a frequently misused placebo. Having lost its grim implications, cobalamin deficiency began to be viewed with complacency by some health professionals, at times to their patients' disadvantage.

The past decades have been marked by steady methodologic advances in the development of accurate and sensitive metabolic assays, which have led to identification of cobalamin deficiency at ever earlier stages of development. As a result, subclinical cobalamin deficiency is now understood to be far more common than the relatively rare state of clinical deficiency (10). Developments in molecular biology have also led to advances in understanding both the physiology of cobalamin transport and metabolism and the varied disorders that affect them. The vista is also opening for clearer insights into how genetic influences interact with the environment and with acquired disorders.

BIOCHEMISTRY

Cobalamin contains a planar tetrapyrrole (corrin), at whose center sits a cobalt atom that fluctuates among monovalent, divalent, and trivalent states (Fig. 29.1).

The reduced, monovalent cob(I)alamin is the active form. Linked to cobalt in the α position below the corrin plane is the 5,6-dimethylbenzimidazole nucleotide. Also linked to the cobalt atom but extending above the plane (β position) is any one of several interchangeable prosthetic moieties that lend their names to the cobalamin. The most important cobalamins are methylcobalamin, in which methyl is the prosthetic moiety, and deoxyadenosylcobalamin, in which 5′-deoxyadenosine is the β-linked moiety. Methylcobalamin predominates in cytoplasm and serves as the intermediate cofactor in the transfer of methyl from methyltetrahydrofolic acid (methylTHF) to methionine in the methionine synthase reaction (see Fig. 28.2 in Chapter 28). Deoxyadenosylcobalamin predominates in mitochondria, where it attaches as a cofactor to methylmalonyl-coenzyme A (CoA) mutase for the intramolecular rearrangement of methylmalonyl-CoA to succinyl-CoA in propionate metabolism. The two reactions just mentioned are the only known roles for cobalamin in human metabolism.

Other cobalamins that are found in plasma and cells include hydroxocobalamin, which is very stable and occurs widely, aquocobalamin, and sulfitocobalamin. Cyanocobalamin exists largely as a stable synthetic pharmaceutical that must be converted to other cobalamins to become metabolically active; the term vitamin B_{12} refers specifically to cyanocobalamin (7) but is often used as a broad name for cobalamins as a whole. Altered corrinoids with structural deletions also exist that are nonfunctional in humans but can find their way into tissues (11), perhaps because they can be bound to transcobalamin (TC) I as functional cobalamins are (12, 13).

ANALYTIC METHODS

Serum Cobalamin

Cobalamin in serum is more stable on long-term storage than other analytes such as folate and can be assayed by a variety of techniques. The earliest methods employed microorganisms, such as *Euglena gracilis*, whose growth was proportional to the cobalamin content of the unknown sample (14). The assays proved reliable and are considered the standard by some. However, their cumbersomeness led to their replacement by radioisotopic dilution methods that rely on competitive binding of the sample's cobalamin by IF as the added cobalamin-binding protein. After correction of problems caused by using binding proteins that contained non-IF binder, which bound nonfunctional as well as functional cobalamin and gave falsely high results, radioisotopic assay use became widespread (15). As clinical laboratories became more automated and because of a desire to avoid radioactive materials, immunologic techniques employing chemiluminescence detection replaced isotopic methods in the past decade. These immunologic assays are typically purchased as part of a fixed package of assays for diverse analytes.

The new methods are closely guarded commercial secrets, and confirmation of their reliability has been skimpy, unlike the extensive, diverse, and open testing that was done for the earlier microbiologic and isotopic techniques. Moreover, independent monitoring of performance is rarely done or published. Concerns have been raised about cobalamin assay performance (16).

The cutoff point between subnormal and normal serum cobalamin values varies from method to method and from laboratory to laboratory. Most laboratories use traditional cutpoints between 200 and 250 ng/L (alternately expressed as 148 and 185 pmol/L; 1 ng = 0.738 pmol) to define normality. Ethnic differences may exist; for example, blacks have higher cobalamin levels than whites at all ages (17).

The question of sensitivity of low serum cobalamin levels for cobalamin deficiency does not have a simple answer, and almost all the data derive from isotopic assays whose use has declined. The sensitivity was 97 to 100% in

patients selected because they had obvious clinical manifestations of deficiency, such as megaloblastic anemia or neurologic abnormalities (18), or because their physicians suspected deficiency (19). The lower the cobalamin level, too, the greater is the likelihood of clinically severe deficiency (14, 20, 21), although many exceptions exist (22). Despite its high sensitivity, the positive predictive value of a low cobalamin level was only 22% because cobalamin deficiency is relatively uncommon (19).

In contrast to symptomatic patients, sensitivity is only 58 to 78% in studies of clinically unselected persons, often elderly, who have only metabolic abnormalities without clinical manifestations, that is, those with subclinical deficiency (23, 24). Moreover, many asymptomatic elderly persons have metabolic signs suggestive of cobalamin deficiency despite normal serum cobalamin levels (25, 26). One result of these observations was a suggestion to raise the cutpoint for deficiency from the traditional 200 or 250 ng/L to 350 ng/L or higher (25). The reasoning was that a higher cutpoint would ensure that no case of cobalamin deficiency would be missed. The many disadvantages to doing so are reviewed elsewhere (27, 28).

Briefly, the arguments against such a revision of the normal range are as follows: (a) large numbers of persons with possible deficiency will remain undetected despite the revision because about 15% of elderly persons with cobalamin levels well above the new cutpoint (i.e., >350 ng/L) have metabolic deficiency by the same criteria (23, 24); (b) about two thirds of the persons redefined as cobalamin deficient by the cutpoint revision will, in fact, be metabolically normal and thus will not be deficient at all (24, 26); (c) of the 32 to 35% of persons with low-normal cobalamin levels who do turn out to have metabolic cobalamin deficiency, the vast majority will have only subclinical deficiency without clinical manifestations; and (d) because the proper management of subclinical deficiency remains controversial, it is not clear what clinical benefit derives from their aggressive identification, especially when it comes at the cost of mislabeling as deficient a much larger number of unquestionably nondeficient persons (28). These issues and their ramifications require further study before introducing wholesale changes of this magnitude.

As already noted, the specificity of low serum cobalamin levels may be more limited than their sensitivity. Table 29.2 lists the conditions that have been associated with low levels. The clinically notable causes of falsely low cobalamin levels include pregnancy, folate deficiency, and TC I deficiency (14, 15, 31, 32).

In clinical practice, spuriously elevated cobalamin levels are seen most often in patients with renal failure or for unknown reasons (33). Cobalamin therapy also elevates levels. Less common but often dramatic elevations regularly accompany the very high plasma TC I levels in patients with chronic myelogenous leukemia and acute promyelocytic leukemia and occasionally in some patients with metastatic cancer (34).

TABLE 29.2. CONDITIONS FREQUENTLY ASSOCIATED WITH LOW SERUM COBALAMIN LEVELS

Cobalamin deficiency
    Clinically expressed deficiency (can be severe or very mild)
    Subclinical deficiency (biochemical abnormalities only)
Normal cobalamin status
    Pregnancy
    Transcobalamin I deficiency (severe or mild)
    Human immunodeficiency virus infection; acquired
        immunodeficiency syndrome[a]
    Folate deficiency
    Multiple myeloma[a]
    Aplastic anemia; myelodysplastic syndrome
    Multiple sclerosis

[a] Most patients have no evidence of cobalamin deficiency or malabsorption, but some may have coexisting deficiency and/or malabsorption, as described in some patients with acquired immunodeficiency syndrome (29, 30), or coexisting pernicious anemia, as described in some patients with multiple myeloma.

Despite all its limitations, cobalamin assay at present remains the first test of choice in the patient with suspected cobalamin deficiency (28, 35). Additional tests available for patients in whom the diagnosis is in doubt are discussed next.

Cellular Cobalamin

Red blood cell cobalamin content is influenced by many factors other than cobalamin status and is rarely assayed for clinical purposes.

Methylmalonic Acid

Methylmalonic acid (MMA) is a byproduct of methylmalonyl-CoA, which accumulates when cobalamin deficiency limits the activity of methylmalonyl-CoA mutase. MMA can be measured with exquisite sensitivity by gas chromatography-mass spectrometry in serum and urine. Reference intervals have varied widely (36), although many laboratories now describe values higher than 280 nmol/L as abnormal. Serum MMA is elevated in 98% of patients with PA who have clinically expressed cobalamin deficiency, often to levels exceeding 1000 nmol/L (37). The levels respond within several days to cobalamin therapy and become normal after a week (18). MMA levels are usually only mildly elevated in asymptomatic patients with subclinical cobalamin deficiency, and the sensitivity of MMA in this setting is probably lower than in clinical deficiency (23, 24, 38).

Specificity of elevated MMA is superior to that of plasma total homocysteine (tHcy) (28, 35). A particularly important advantage is that MMA levels, unlike tHcy levels, remain normal in folate deficiency (18, 37). Nevertheless, specificity is limited, and MMA levels are often elevated in patients with renal insufficiency. Some authors have also attributed unexplained MMA elevations, especially in elderly patients, to plasma volume contraction, but did not

provide evidence. Homozygotes for methylmalonyl-CoA mutase deficiency, a rare inborn error, have greatly elevated MMA levels, but heterozygotes seem to have normal levels (39). Very elevated MMA levels are also seen in some asymptomatic babies; these elevations often remit spontaneously after the first year of life and appear to be benign, perhaps as manifestations of hepatic enzyme immaturity (40).

Were it not for the assay's technical demands and high costs, MMA measurement could be the metabolic test of choice for diagnosing cobalamin deficiency. Normal levels provide strong evidence against deficiency. However, it is uncertain what to make of the many elderly persons who have mild, unexplained MMA elevations without any other evidence to support cobalamin deficiency. The isolated MMA elevations often improve after cobalamin is given; this suggests that these values represent mild deficiency in many cases (24–26), but an assumption of deficiency cannot otherwise be made automatically. It is not clear whether the mild, transient elevations of MMA common in children during the first year of life (41) represent part of the spectrum of benign massive methylmalonic aciduria or bear some relation to unrecognized cobalamin deficiency. MMA levels sometimes decline after antibiotic therapy in people without apparent cobalamin deficiency (18); the explanation is unknown but thought to reflect propionate metabolism by intestinal bacteria.

Homocysteine

Measurement of tHcy and its many implications are discussed in Chapter 28. As noted there, diagnostic specificity is limited because many conditions affect tHcy levels. Surveys of healthy populations have shown that cobalamin status influences tHcy levels less than does folate status or renal status (26, 27). The impact of cobalamin status rises in elderly persons, however. Despite the 95% sensitivity of elevated tHcy for clinically expressed cobalamin deficiency and the finding that elevation is often striking in such cases (18, 37), the poor specificity limits the diagnostic usefulness of tHcy measurement. Like MMA, tHcy values fall after cobalamin deficiency is treated with cobalamin but not if folate is given (18).

Holotranscobalamin II

Because cobalamin levels can be falsely low or falsely normal, it was suggested that diagnostic specificity and sensitivity may be enhanced by measuring only the cobalamin that is attached to TC II (42). The cobalamin-TC II complex (holo-TC II) is thought to be the metabolically active fraction of circulating cobalamin because TC II is the critical carrier on which cobalamin depends for entry into cells (43). Only 30% or less of plasma cobalamin circulates as holo-TC II; the remainder is carried by TC I, which does not promote specific cellular uptake (34). Among the proposed diagnostic roles for holo-TC II, its potential as an early marker for cobalamin deficiency has been particularly enticing. The latter claim is under study now that an accurate holo-TC II assay has become available (44), but its practical value appears limited to date (45). Indeed, absorption status appears to have a slight, independent effect on holo-TC II levels (45a), which may complicate its diagnostic utility.

NUTRITION AND BIOAVAILABILITY

Cobalamin is synthesized by bacteria, as are corrinoids that are nonfunctional in humans. Animals ingest the microorganisms and incorporate the cobalamin into their flesh, organs, eggs, and milk in varying proportions of different cobalamin forms, which are eaten by humans (14, 46). Plants are very meager sources of cobalamin. Milk and cobalamin-fortified cereals are particularly efficient sources in the US diet, exceeding meat in their cobalamin bioavailability (47).

Because of the great disparities in efficiency between active and passive absorption, cobalamin availability depends very much on cobalamin release from food by pepsin and other gastric enzymes, the viability of the IF-mediated absorption system, and the amount of cobalamin ingested at any given time. The IF mechanism is particularly crucial because it affects absorption of both food-bound cobalamin and free cobalamin. If the IF system, including IF receptors, is intact, more than 50% of the cobalamin in a typical meal will be absorbed actively, but IF cannot accommodate much more than 2 μg cobalamin at a time (14) (Table 29.3). Larger cobalamin doses, such as are often found in supplements, exceed the binding capacity of available IF. When that happens, the excess

cobalamin becomes dependent on passive, nonspecific absorption, which is much less efficient (1–2% of the dose is absorbed) even though it is to a large extent nonsaturable and linearly related to the amount of cobalamin presented. It is not known whether the absorption characteristics of free cobalamin in supplements become altered when taken together with food.

ABSORPTION

Active, highly specific absorption of cobalamin predominates in the ileum and depends on IF and its receptor (43). This efficient process, designed to secure and concentrate the micronutrient maximally, is illustrated in Figure 29.2.

After ingestion, the cobalamin in food is released by gastric pepsin, whose activity becomes optimal at the acid pH of the normal stomach and degrades the food proteins to which cobalamin is attached (48) (see Fig. 29.2, panel 1). The parietal cell that provides the acid also synthesizes and secretes IF, a 48-kDa glycoprotein that binds cobalamin specifically. However, rather than binding immediately to IF, the released cobalamin is preferentially bound in the stomach by a glycoprotein secreted by salivary gland and other exocrine gland epithelial cells, called haptocorrin (also called R binder and, in plasma, TC I).

Pancreatic proteases, such as trypsin, degrade haptocorrin once haptocorrin leaves the stomach and is exposed to pancreatic alkalinization, which potentiates trypsin activity (49). The newly rereleased cobalamin within the duodenum and jejunum is now bound by the accompanying IF, as presumably is biliary cobalamin that is secreted and exposed to proteases there (13) (see Fig. 29.2, panel 2). The IF binds only intact, functional cobalamin and, unlike

TABLE 29.3. COBALAMIN ABSORPTION FROM A SINGLE ORAL DOSE GIVEN TO PERSONS WITH (A) NORMAL ABSORPTION AND (B) ABNORMAL ABSORPTION WITHOUT INTRINSIC FACTOR (PERNICIOUS ANEMIA)[a]

ORAL DOSE	(A) AMOUNT (AND %) ABSORBED BY BOTH INTRINSIC FACTOR–MEDIATED AND PASSIVE PROCESSES[b]		(B) AMOUNT (AND %) ABSORBED BY PASSIVE PROCESS ONLY[c]	
0.25 μg	0.19 μg	(75%)	—	
1 μg	0.56 μg	(56%)	≈0.02 μg	(≈2%)
2 μg	0.92 μg	(46%)	—	
3 μg	—		≈0.08 μg	(≈3%)
5 μg	1.4 μg	(28%)	—	
10 μg	1.6 μg	(16%)	≈0.2 μg	(≈2%)
50 μg	1.5 μg	(3%)	≈0.5 μg	(≈1%)
100 μg	—		≈1.8 μg	(≈1.8%)
500 μg	—		≈6 μg	(≈1.2%)

[a] Data are not available for the partially compromised absorption in patients with food-cobalamin malabsorption, whose absorption efficiency is unknown but is presumed to be intermediate between (A) normal and (B) severely impaired absorption.

[b] In normal subjects; as evident from comparing columns A and B, intrinsic factor–mediated absorption in normal subjects greatly exceeds passive diffusion until doses exceed 5 μg.

[c] Intrinsic factor activity is lost in patients with pernicious anemia, so absorption is by passive diffusion only. The numbers in this column were obtained in a different study than those for normal subjects in the left-hand column. Comparability may be limited, therefore, but the striking patterns illustrate the essential points.

Data from Chanarin I. The Megaloblastic Anaemias. 2nd ed. Oxford: Blackwell Scientific, 1979:94; and Berlin H, Berlin R, Brante G. Acta Med Scand 1968;184:247–58.

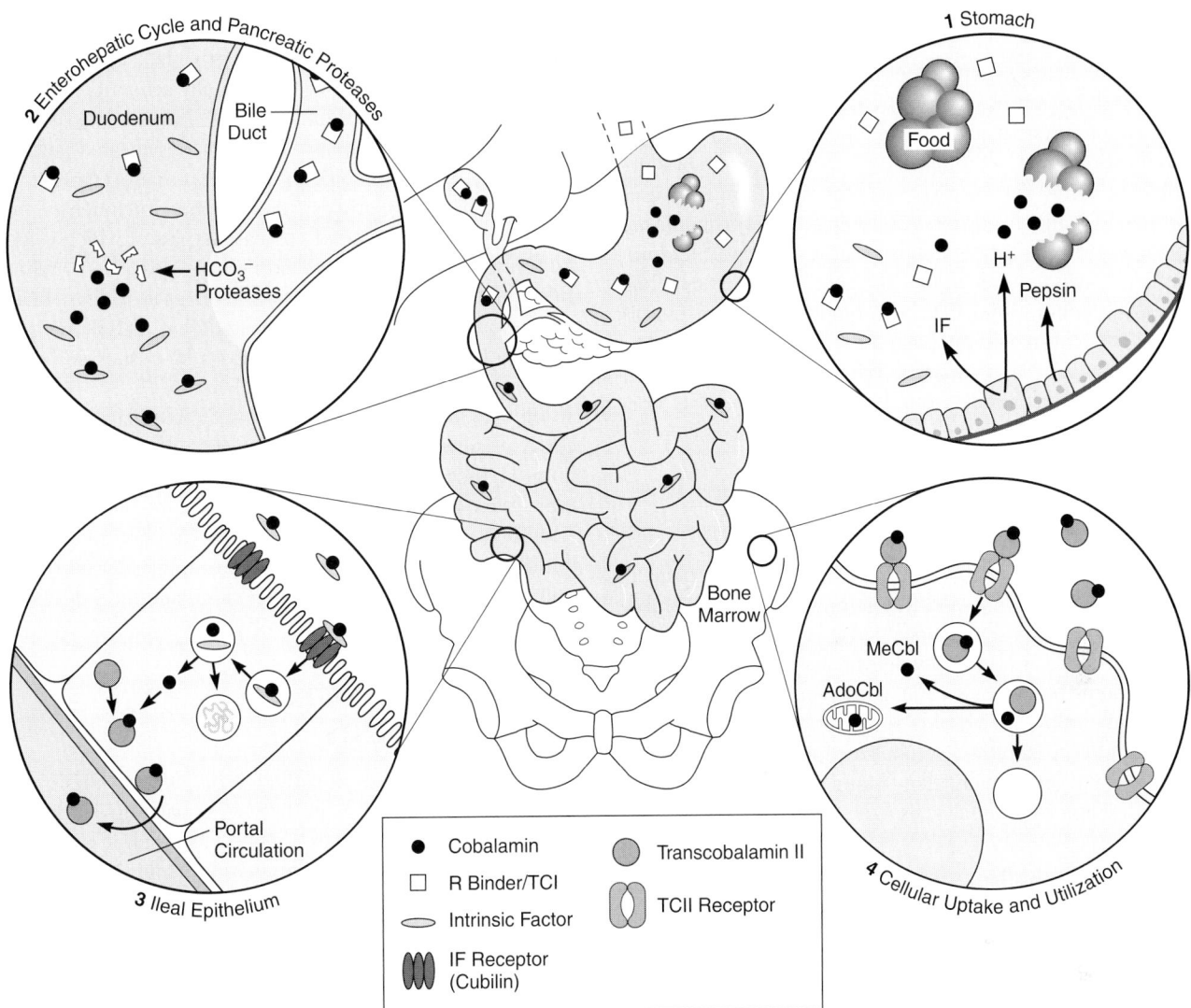

Figure 29.2. Absorption and cellular uptake cycle of cobalamin in humans: *1,* secretion of gastric intrinsic factor (IF), acid, and pepsin and release of cobalamin from food and binding to R binder (haptocorrin); *2,* biliary and pancreatic secretion and degradation of haptocorrin by pancreatic enzymes; *3,* ileal cell uptake of IF-cobalamin, lysosomal processing, and transfer of transcobalamin (TC) II–cobalamin to the portal circulation; *4,* cellular uptake (e.g., in bone marrow) of TC II–cobalamin, lysosomal processing, and release of cobalamin for attachment to enzymes. AdoCbl, adenosylcobalamin; MeCbl, methylcobabamin. (From Carmel R, Rosenblatt, DS. Disorders of cobalamin and folate metabolism. In: Handin RI, Lux SE, Stossel TP, eds. Blood: Principles and Practice of Hematology. 2nd ed. Philadelphia: Lippincott Williams & Wilkins, 2003. Originally adapted from Carmel R. Cobalamin deficiency. In: Carmel R, Jacobsen DW, eds. Homocysteine in Health and Disease. Cambridge: Cambridge University Press, 2001, with permission.)

haptocorrin, does not bind corrins that are inactive in humans (12).

The IF-cobalamin complex then travels to the distal small bowel (see Fig. 29-2, panel 3), where it is taken up by the IF receptor, cubilin, a nontransmembrane glycoprotein on gut epithelial cells, which is also found in kidney tubules and yolk sac (50); the function of cubilin is supported by the protein amnionless (51). After internalization, the cubilin-IF-cobalamin complex is split in the ileal cell endosomes (43). The cobalamin eventually reaches the abluminal surface of the ileal cell, where it is bound by TC II and exits into the bloodstream as holo-TC II (52). The time from oral ingestion to entry into the bloodstream takes up to 4 hours (14).

IF-mediated absorption of ingested cobalamin and, presumably, reabsorption of much of biliary cobalamin are efficient but, as mentioned, saturable. In addition, nonspecific absorption of cobalamin occurs by passive diffusion, without any mediation by proteins. This inefficient process, whereby 1 to 2% of the presented amount is absorbed (53), assumes importance only when the IF mechanism is damaged, as in patients with PA, or is overwhelmed by doses of free cobalamin greater than a few micrograms (see Table 29.3); it can also operate at all mucosal sites throughout the gut and elsewhere, such as the sublingual or nasal epithelium. The quantitative characteristics of active and passive absorption are compared in Table 29.3.

TRANSPORT, METABOLISM, AND EXCRETION

Cobalamin crosses membranes poorly and depends on several binding proteins for its transport. The IF-mediated absorption process just described is limited to the gastrointestinal tract, although IF fragments have been identified in urine (54) and IF receptors are found in renal tubular cell brush borders (50). Once the cobalamin has been absorbed into the bloodstream, its transport and utilization become dependent on another specific cobalamin-binding protein, TC II (sometimes called simply TC). TC I also binds cobalamin in the blood and elsewhere, but its role is uncertain. There is a sizeable hepatic clearance of cobalamin from TC I into bile, estimated at 1.4 μg daily, approximately 70% of which is normally reabsorbed while the remainder is lost in feces (13).

Transcobalamin II

TC II is synthesized by many cells, including especially endothelial cells (55, 65). Its gene shares considerable homology with IF but is located on a different chromosome (56–58). TC II rapidly delivers its cobalamin to cells throughout the body (see Fig. 29.2, panel 4). The half-life of plasma holo-TC II is only 90 minutes (59). Its first and major delivery is to the liver, but receptors specific for TC II are found on virtually all cells and internalize the holo-TC II complex by pinocytosis (43).

Cellular Metabolism

After uptake, cobalamin is released within endosomes and enters the cytoplasm, where it exists primarily as methylcobalamin or is taken up by mitochondria (see Fig. 29.2, panel 4). The methylcobalmin is bound to methionine synthase and helps to mediate homocysteine remethylation. Mitochondrial deoxyadenosylcobalamin is bound to methylmalonyl-CoA mutase and takes part in propionate metabolism. No other intracellular binding proteins have been identified for cobalamin, nor have any other metabolic roles.

The kidney is also rich in TC II receptors (60), and this feature may play an important role in minimizing urinary loss of cobalamin. The kidney is, along with the liver, the richest repository of cobalamin in the body.

Transcobalamin I; Haptocorrin

TC I in the plasma is immunologically and, except for variable differences in glycosylation, structurally identical to all haptocorrins in the body (34), as discussed in the section on absorption. Its gene has modest homology with IF and, like the gene for IF, is located on chromosome 11 (58). Plasma TC I appears to be derived from late granulocytic precursors, in whose specific granules it is synthesized (61). The concentration of TC I in the plasma is nearly equal to that of TC II (34). However, because TC I appears to have no specific cellular receptors, the TC I-cobalamin complex (holo-TC I) continues to circulate with a half-life of 9 to 10 days (59). Therefore, holo-TC I usually accounts for 70% or more of plasma cobalamin (62, 63). Animal data suggest that holo-TC I eventually becomes desialylated and is cleared by the nonspecific asialoglycoprotein receptors in the liver (64). This process may account for much of the enterohepatic clearance of cobalamin, part of which is lost in feces while most is reabsorbed, as described earlier. Because TC I binds nonfunctional corrins as well as cobalamin, some authors have suggested that TC I prevents uptake of potentially harmful analogs by tissues and promotes their excretion by hepatic clearance.

Besides the granulocyte-derived TC I in plasma, haptocorrin is also synthesized by exocrine glandular epithelium. Haptocorrin is therefore also found in saliva, breast milk, tears, and other secretions, usually in concentrations tenfold greater than in plasma (34). It has been speculated that haptocorrin prevents cobalamin uptake by intestinal microorganisms and may serve an antibacterial role there and in other secretions.

DIETARY CONSIDERATIONS AND REQUIREMENTS

Dietary considerations are affected by age and other characteristics. Nevertheless, in the end, cobalamin status and its clinical ramifications are dictated as much if not more by the ability to absorb cobalamin as by its intake. This fact is especially important in elderly persons, who constitute the population segment at greatest risk for cobalamin deficiency (65–67). The increased risk largely arises from their greater propensity for impaired cobalamin absorption, either by PA or food-cobalamin malabsorption (23, 65, 68, 69), and not their cobalamin intake, which appears to be adequate (23, 70, 71).

Adults

The estimated daily losses of 1 μg cobalamin are minute when compared with the total body stores of approximately 2500 μg (72). The recommended dietary allowance was revised slightly upward to 2.4 μg, with a recommendation of a 2.8 μg intake during pregnancy and lactation (46). The average US diet contains 4.0 to 6.2 μg cobalamin (73).

Evaluations of intake adequacy have usually been based on maintenance of normal serum cobalamin levels and avoidance of hematologic manifestations. These are not ideal assessment criteria today, the more so given the long time interval before inadequate cobalamin intake can even begin to affect those end points. It may be preferable to base recommendations on metabolic criteria, such as maintaining normal MMA levels. Data based on amounts of cobalamin needed to prevent relapse in patients with PA have also been used; although these data have some value, they reflect amounts given by injection to patients with malabsorption, which bear only a somewhat limited relationship to the normal setting and normal requirements.

The daily cobalamin requirement of only 0.1% of body stores accounts for the very important clinical facts that depletion of body stores takes years and that clinically apparent cobalamin deficiency only infrequently arises because of poor dietary intake (14). It is particularly instructive to compare the requirements-to-stores ratio with that for folate, which is approximately ten times higher (see Chapter 28). This difference in impact of diet was illustrated in the Framingham study: serum folate and cobalamin levels were significantly associated inversely with high tHcy levels, but cobalamin intake did not significantly affect tHcy, whereas folate intake did (70).

The use of cobalamin supplements, usually as part of a multivitamin preparation, is increasing, especially among elderly persons (46). This use of supplements may turn out to be valuable for them because of their greater risk of food-cobalamin malabsorption (68), but it provides no benefit to persons who have PA and absorb supplements poorly.

The cobabamin content of a variety of foods is given in Appendix Table A-23-a. The specific dietary reference intakes for children and adults are given in Appendix Table A-2-e.

Children

Maternal cobalamin transfer favors the fetus and seems unaffected by the frequent fall in maternal serum cobalamin levels that occurs in the last trimester of pregnancy (14). Adequate cobalamin intakes in children have been estimated in comparisons based on the effectiveness of human milk of known cobalamin content (46), but much depends on the criteria used to define deficiency in infants. Intakes of 0.4 to 0.5 μg are considered adequate in the first year of life (46). The first year of life is typically marked by slightly elevated serum MMA (41). However, the elevations may reflect hepatic enzyme immaturity rather than inadequate cobalamin status, and MMA levels decrease by the end of the year without intervention. The recommended cobalamin intake rises through childhood to 1.2 μg by the age of 4 to 8 years, 1.8 μg in preadolescence, and adult values in teenage years (46).

DEFICIENCY STATE

The clinical consequences of cobalamin deficiency closely resemble those of folate deficiency (see Chapter 28), the major exception being their dissimilar neurologic complications. Because of the great disparity in the time it takes to deplete the body stores of the two vitamins, clinical signs also take much longer to appear and progress more slowly in cobalamin deficiency. Even the early biochemical changes that precede clinical symptoms do not appear until many months or, more often, several years after the process that causes the deficiency (e.g., malabsorption) begins, whereas the changes appear within weeks in folate

deficiency. Patients with complete loss of IF require 3 to 5 years to become overtly cobalamin deficient (14). The process is even more protracted in vegans because their intact absorption permits normal reabsorption of biliary cobalamin. The slower development of cobalamin deficiency in patients with food-cobalamin malabsorption, (in which IF should be adequate for reabsorption of biliary cobalamin, than in patients with PA) may be similarly explained.

Hematologic Features

The hematologic picture is identical to that described for folate in Chapter 28, other than the time course difference just discussed. The erythroid mean corpuscular volume (MCV) rises long before anemia develops, so many patients display nonanemic macrocytosis for months (74). Moreover, some patients express only mild or no hematologic manifestations even with severe deficiency; 19 to 28% of patients with PA are not anemic at the time of diagnosis (10, 22, 37).

Neurologic Features

The much greater risk and severity of neurologic and psychiatric manifestations in cobalamin deficiency are the major clinical differences between it and folate deficiency. The frequency of neurologic abnormalities has never been established, but most agree that more than half of patients with PA display neurologic findings (75). The latter can be the earliest and, in 28% of cases, even the sole clinical expression of cobalamin deficiency (22, 75, 76). For unknown reasons, the severity of hematologic and neurologic manifestations tends to be inversely related to each other in the individual patient (75). Moreover, some patients seem predisposed to repeat the same form of expression on relapse (75, 77, 78).

Myelopathy and neuropathy are typical and can be severe. Histologically, the myelopathy is characterized by myelin loss followed by axonal degeneration and gliosis, and the larger, more myelinated fibers are preferentially affected (77). The myelopathy affects the posterior and lateral columns, which gives rise to the classic "subacute combined degeneration" of the spinal cord. Symptoms tend to be symmetric and to begin in the feet (14, 75). The early manifestations are diminished vibratory and position sense in the toes, later ascending to affect the legs and hands. Ataxia, spasticity, and often incontinence and other disabling manifestations can supervene as myelopathy progresses. Motor function is largely spared, although gait disturbances occur and patients can become wheelchair or bed bound because of the spasticity. Cerebral changes may range from diminished memory or mild personality changes to psychosis and occasionally delirium (14, 75, 76). Rare neurologic manifestations include optic neuritis, visual changes, and autonomic dysfunction.

Surprisingly large patches of demyelination may be seen with magnetic resonance imaging throughout the brain, in addition to the typical posterior and lateral column changes in the upper spinal cord. Electroencephalographic and other electrophysiologic abnormalities are common (79, 80) and may occur even in asymptomatic patients (81–84).

Not only are the neurologic and mental findings sometimes disabling, they can become permanently debilitating if not treated promptly. Unlike the anemia, partial or complete irreversibility may result. The failure of neurologic abnormalities to reverse is sometimes unpredictable but is often tied to the extent of the involvement and to therapeutic delay (14, 85, 86). High folate intake and folate therapy have also been suspected contributing factors, both because neurologically affected patients tend to have higher folate levels than unaffected patients (87, 88) and because folate therapy can delay recognition of cobalamin deficiency (14) and may rarely accelerate neurologic worsening (89). The interactions with folate are complex and poorly understood.

Alzheimer disease is often accompanied by unexplained low cobalamin levels (90, 91). However, unlike the milder cognitive dysfunction sometimes seen in cobalamin deficiency, the symptoms of Alzheimer disease do not respond to cobalamin therapy (83), and a causal connection has not been found. An even stronger association of Alzheimer disease with homocysteine and folate status has been suggested (92, 93) but is similarly murky. It has been aptly pointed out that attribution of neurologic problems to cobalamin deficiency requires more than just finding low serum cobalamin levels (94).

Other Clinical Manifestations

Abnormalities that reverse with cobalamin therapy include the following: occasional glossitis, sometimes so severe as to be the principal symptom in the patient (14); weight loss (95); transient intestinal malabsorption (96, 97); skin darkening, reddish hair, and nail pigment changes, especially in darker-skinned patients (98, 99); and biochemical evidence of impaired bone formation, such as decreased bone alkaline phosphatase and osteocalcin levels in the blood (100), although suggestions of an increased risk of osteoporosis and fractures are controversial.

Metabolic Explanations for the Clinical Manifestations

The limitation of cobalamin's role in human metabolism to two reactions, neither of which affect nucleoprotein metabolism directly, has puzzled those trying to explain the symptoms of cobalamin deficiency and the indistinguishability of the megaloblastic anemia in cobalamin and folate deficiencies. The "methylTHF trap" hypothesis (101, 102) provides a compelling explanation. The methylation of homocysteine to methionine by methionine synthase depends on its cofactors, methylTHF and cobalamin (reaction 4, Fig. 28.3 in Chapter 28). When cobalamin is lacking, this irreversible reaction is impaired, and methylTHF, the most abundant folate but one unable to flow through the folate cycle via any other reaction, is "trapped" and accumulates. The resultant decrease in reaction 12 of Figure 28.3 diminishes S-adenosylmethionine generation, which stimulates conversion of methyleneTHF to methylTHF (reaction 3) in an attempt to generate more S-adenosylmethionine. However, the compensatory effort only succeeds in accentuating the trapping of folate as methylTHF and depleting methyleneTHF availability for thymidylate synthesis (reaction 2). It is not clear what contribution, if any, poor methylation of DNA (reaction 13) makes to the megaloblastic anemia. An alternative or supplement to the methylTHF trap hypothesis is the suggestion that poor methionine synthesis ultimately depletes formates and the folates that use them (103).

The mechanism for the neurologic changes in cobalamin deficiency is unknown. Proposed hypotheses have included abnormal fatty acid synthesis and myelinization resulting from impaired propionic acid metabolism caused by deoxyadenosylcobalamin deficiency, the accumulation of nonfunctional cobalamin analogs, and possible effects of cytokines. However, a broad variety of observations now strongly favors the unavailability of methylcobalamin for methionine synthesis as the linchpin, although the metabolic details are elusive (104). S-adenosylmethionine depletion has been proposed as the cause of neurologic dysfunction in cobalamin deficiency and other states. However, patients with PA who have only neurologic abnormalities appear to have higher plasma S-adenosylmethionine levels, as well as cysteine and folate levels, than patients with anemia alone (88).

Subclinical Cobalamin Deficiency

Once thought to be rare, subclinical cobalamin deficiency (81, 90, 105) is the most common form of cobalamin deficiency and is at least ten times more common than deficiency accompanied by clinical signs and symptoms (10, 24). Subclinical deficiency is characterized by the following: (a) biochemical abnormalities such as a low cobalamin level, elevated MMA and tHcy levels, and/or abnormal deoxyuridine suppression test results; (b) responsiveness of the latter biochemical findings to cobalamin therapy; and (c) the absence of all clinical signs such as macrocytosis or megaloblastic anemia or symptoms of neurologic dysfunction. Most of the data for subclinical deficiency have been derived from studies in elderly persons, in whom the condition is particularly common (65–67). Low cobalamin levels occur in 10 to 15% of elderly persons (especially white men), almost all of whom seem healthy, absorb free cobalamin adequately as shown with the Schilling test, and appear to have adequate cobalamin intake (10, 65). Metabolic abnormalities suggestive of cobalamin deficiency have been found in 60 to 70% of people with low cobalamin levels (24, 25, 106). When tested, some persons also have had subtle neurologic and electrophysiologic test findings of still uncertain importance that reverse with cobalamin therapy (82–84).

Much remains unknown about subclinical deficiency. A few of the affected persons simply have very early PA (107) and therefore can be expected to progress inexorably to a symptomatic state because of their irreversible malabsorption. However, those without early PA have often remained asymptomatic for at least a decade (108). Still to be resolved are issues that include the clinical impact of subclinical deficiency, which seems by definition to be small, its course, which appears static in most observations, and whether it can regress spontaneously. The causes of subclinical deficiency are also not well understood in many cases. Malabsorption of free cobalamin, such as PA, is found in fewer than 5% of cases (107), whereas food-cobalamin malabsorption may account for 30 to 40% of cases (65, 68). No cause has been found in most patients, however. For all these reasons, and because millions of people fall into this category, it is important to answer the outstanding questions and to reach a consensus on what to do about subclinical deficiency (28, 65).

CAUSES OF DEFICIENCY

Identifying what caused the patient's cobalamin deficiency is an important task for the clinician. It affects how the deficiency is best managed, what its course and prognosis are likely to be, and what complications must be considered. The causes are grouped in Table 29.4 by categories of

TABLE 29.4. CAUSES OF COBALAMIN DEFICIENCY

Inadequate dietary intake
  Veganism
  Infants of vegan mothers (especially if also breast-fed by them)
  Long-term, highly restricted diets (e.g., phenylketonuria diet)
Gastrointestinal malabsorption
  Malabsorption of free cobalamin
    Pernicious anemia: acquired or hereditary
    Total gastrectomy
    Partial gastrectomy (~30% of cases)
    Ileal disease or damage (e.g., tropical sprue, ileal surgery)
    Hereditary cobalamin malabsorption (Imerslund-Gräsbeck syndrome)
    Bacterial overgrowth of the small bowel
    Parasitic infestation (e.g., *Diphyllobothrium latum*)
  Malabsorption limited to food-bound cobalamin
    Atrophic gastritis
    Partial gastrectomy (>50% of cases)
    Other gastric surgery (e.g., gastric stapling, vagotomy)
    Inhibitors of gastric acid secretion (e.g., omeprazole)
Metabolic disorders
  Acquired
    Nitrous oxide toxicity
  Hereditary
    Transcobalamin II deficiency
    cbl mutations

mechanisms that roughly adhere to the sequential steps from cobalamin intake through cellular utilization that are illustrated in Figure 29.2.

Dietary Causes

For reasons already discussed, adult vegans and strict vegetarians take many years to develop cobalamin deficiency. The consequences also tend to be mild (e.g., barely noticeable elevation of red cell MCV without anemia) or, more often, subclinical with biochemical changes only (109–111). Clinical consequences are more likely when poor intake begins in childhood, perhaps because of smaller body stores, the requirements of growth, and the greater vulnerability of the developing brain. Cognitive problems have been described in children, and metabolic abnormalities sometimes persist despite dietary correction (112, 113).

An instructive, often catastrophic illustration is the consequence to infants born to vegan mothers with subnormal breast milk cobalamin content who continue to rely heavily on breast-feeding their babies (97, 114–117). These children often develop severe neurologic complications, with seizures and developmental problems, whereas the mothers typically have only asymptomatic, subclinical cobalamin deficiency.

Although particularly common among Hindus and other lifelong vegetarians, dietary insufficiency may be common in other, unsuspected parts of the world also (118). However, the limited investigations done in most developing countries have not excluded the possibility that other undiagnosed disorders, such as tropical sprue, may contribute.

Pernicious Anemia and Other Causes of Malabsorption of Free Cobalamin

Malabsorption of free cobalamin, which is diagnosable with the Schilling test, is the most common setting in which clinically expressed deficiency arises. Chief among this group of disorders is PA, in which the loss of IF secretion leads to malabsorption of free cobalamin and hence also of food-bound cobalamin.

In the evolution of classic acquired (addisonian) PA, atrophic gastritis, typically autoimmune and usually confined to the gastric fundus while sparing the antrum, begins in late middle age. PA supervenes if the damage to parietal cells progresses beyond causing achlorhydria and to the eventual loss of IF (14, 119). It is important to remember, however, that this transformation is uncommon; gastritis with achlorhydria, which is widespread in middle-aged and older person and often causes food-cobalamin malabsorption, only infrequently progresses to PA. If IF secretion is lost, cobalamin depletion begins or accelerates, and deficiency appears several years later, usually after the age of 60 years. However, PA can also develop in young adults and even in adolescents (14), especially among black women but also, to a lesser degree, among Latin Americans (120, 121). The immune features of PA include two autoantibodies; the more prevalent one is directed against the hydrogen, potassium-adenosine triphosphatase pump of parietal cells, and the other, more diagnostically specific one is directed against IF. In addition, other autoimmune disorders frequently coexist. The most common are immune endocrine disorders, especially of the thyroid gland, which affect 5 to 10% of patients (122); other immune disorders include vitiligo, myasthenia gravis, immune cytopenias, and agammaglobulinemia (14). Iron deficiency coexists in half of cases (123). The most worrisome complication in PA is the increased risk of gastric cancer and carcinoid tumors (14, 119, 124, 125).

A much less common form of PA features the isolated loss of IF secretion resulting from mutations in the IF gene (126). Gastric status is otherwise normal in this congenital PA (or inherited IF deficiency), and neither immune phenomena nor risks of malignancy are seen (39, 127). Clinical cobalamin deficiency usually appears in the first few years of life.

Partial gastric resection sometimes causes malabsorption of free cobalamin, implying loss of IF or significant parasitization of cobalamin by upper small bowel bacteria and leading to cobalamin deficiency in 15 to 30% of patients (128, 129). More often, however, the partial resection causes only food-cobalamin malabsorption (130).

Overgrowth of the small bowel by bacteria resulting from blind loops, motility disorders, or giant diverticuli can divert ingested cobalamin to the microorganisms and can produce a malabsorptive picture and deficiency. The fish tapeworm, *Diphyllobothrium latum*, can do the same but is infrequently seen today.

More common causes of intestinal malabsorption of free cobalamin are disorders of the ileum, the major site for IF-mediated absorption (131). These include tropical sprue, damage to the ileum by surgical bypass, resection, or radiation, and ileal bladder reserve pouches. Other nutrients are often malabsorbed as well. Hereditary malabsorption of cobalamin (Imerslund-Gräsbeck syndrome or megaloblastic anemia-1) causes isolated cobalamin malabsorption early in life (39). Two different genetic mechanisms have been identified, one affecting the cubilin IF receptor gene (132, 133) and another the gene for amnionless, a protein important to the function of cubilin (51). Most of the affected children also have minor proteinuria, a finding reflecting defective cubilin function in the kidney.

Malabsorption of Food Cobalamin

A mild form of malabsorption limited to inadequate release of cobalamin from food was discovered in 1973 in cobalamin-deficient patients with normal Schilling test results (130). This food-cobalamin malabsorption was associated with atrophic gastritis, usually with diminished acid and pepsin secretion but always with intact IF secretion (68). It is associated with an increased rate of *Helicobacter pylori* infection (69, 134). Improvement of malabsorption has followed antibiotic therapy, but the offending organism has not been identified conclusively (134, 135). The postgastrectomy state and omeprazole therapy are regularly associated with food-cobalamin malabsorption (68), as are various gastric procedures to promote weight loss (136–138).

Long-standing food-cobalamin malabsorption accompanies 30 to 40% of cases of subclinical cobalamin deficiency (68, 81). More severe, clinically expressed deficiency usually develops only in the occasional patients whose gastric lesion transforms into PA (68).

Drugs

Many drugs such as colchicine or omeprazole and toxins such as alcohol can produce cobalamin malabsorption. However, only those drugs that continue to be used regularly for many years have any likelihood of leading to cobalamin deficiency in the patient. Drug-induced cobalamin deficiency is therefore rare.

Metabolic Disorders

Clinical cobalamin deficiency supervenes more quickly in metabolic disorders than in malabsorptive conditions because cobalamin uptake or metabolism is blocked directly at the cellular level. Serum cobalamin levels usually remain normal. The most common acquired metabolic disorder is long-term recurrent exposure to nitrous oxide, which oxidatively destroys cobalamin and the methionine synthase to which it is attached intracellularly (139). Inhalant abuse of nitrous oxide is particularly widespread among young people (140) and can produce severe neurologic or mental changes. Although nitrous oxide exposure during routine anesthesia is too transient to produce clinical problems, postoperative neurologic dysfunction can occur in patients with preoperatively unrecognized and untreated cobalamin deficiency (141, 142). Nitrous oxide anesthesia may also have contributed to the postoperative death of a child with a severe inborn error of folate metabolism (143).

Hereditary metabolic disorders are rare but can be severe and sometimes fatal. They include TC II deficiency, a variety of *cbl* mutations that affect methionine synthase or methionine synthase reductase, and other cobalamin-related metabolic defects. The reader is referred to an excellent review of this complex subject (39). TC II deficiency causes a failure of cellular uptake of cobalamin, with resulting megaloblastic anemia and, occasionally, neurologic complications and immune dysfunction. Developmental, neurologic, and hematologic manifestations often characterize the various *cbl* mutations, which can range from mild to lethal.

Cobalamin-Related Disorders that Do Not Cause Cobalamin Deficiency

Chronic pancreatic insufficiency produces abnormal Schilling test results in about half of affected patients because they lack pancreatic secretions to degrade haptocorrin and release its cobalamin to IF in the gut (see Fig. 29.2); cobalamin deficiency is rare, however. An increased cobalamin requirement has been reported in patients with hyperthyroidism or malignant diseases, but its clinical relevance appears negligible.

Serum cobalamin levels are low in patients with hereditary deficiency of TC I, which carries most of the cobalamin in plasma. Cobalamin deficiency does not occur because TC II continues delivering its cobalamin to cells normally, and the function of TC I is unknown (144). One family had a coexisting deficiency of lactoferrin, which has the same cellular sources as TC I (145). Patients with mild TC I deficiency, many of them presumptive heterozygotes for hereditary TC I deficiency, may account for 15% of all unexplained low cobalamin levels (32).

Diagnostic Tests for Causes of Cobalamin Deficiency

Serum cobalamin and metabolite assays identify cobalamin deficiency but not its cause. For the latter, tests related to malabsorption are a mainstay because cobalamin deficiency is so often malabsorptive in origin. The classic Schilling test relies on 24-hour urinary excretion to measure the absorption of oral, radioisotopically labeled, free cyanocobalamin (14). Subnormal excretion indicates malabsorption, as long as renal function is normal and urine collection is complete. If abnormal, the test can be repeated with an oral dose of IF to help localize the absorptive defect. Modified versions using food-bound or protein-bound, radiolabeled cyanocobalamin have been devised to assess absorption of food cobalamin (68, 130). Because these tests are limited to research laboratories only and the Schilling test's once wide availability has shrunk in the past few years, clinicans have been left to rely increasingly on surrogate tests of limited value to assess absorption.

Because PA is the most common cause of clinically symptomatic cobalamin deficiency, a major surrogate test is the assay for serum antibody to IF (146, 147). The antibody is highly specific for PA but, being present in only 50 to 70% of cases, has limited sensitivity; it also has no diagnostic value in other malabsorptive disorders. Serum gastrin levels are elevated and pespinogen I levels are decreased in 80 to 90% of patients with PA, but specificity of both tests is poor (148). The diagnostic approach to inborn errors of cobalamin metabolism is discussed elsewhere (39).

TREATMENT OF DEFICIENCY

Approximately 1 μg of cobalamin given by injection suffices to reverse the megaloblastic anemia of cobalamin deficiency. The goals of treatment are not just to reverse the signs and symptoms of deficiency but also to replete stores insofar as possible and to prevent relapses. Good management also requires ascertainment of the cause of the deficiency and monitoring of the response to therapy.

Vegetarians and Other Patients with Normal Absorption

When cobalamin absorption is completely normal, small doses of oral supplements can be used. Doses greater than 3 to 5 μg exceed the binding capacity of IF, and only a tiny fraction of the excess amount can be assimilated (see Table 29.3).

Patients Who Cannot Absorb Free Cobalamin

This category includes patients with PA and intestinal diseases and, indeed, affects most patients who have clinical signs and symptoms of cobalamin deficiency. The optimal goal of parenteral regimens is to replete cobalamin stores while minimizing the frequency of injections. Larger doses permit greater retention, despite proportionately greater excretory losses when the injected cobalamin exceeds the capacity of binding proteins and cell uptake (14). Common injection regimens use 100 or 1000 μg of cyanocobalamin, from which approximately 55 and 100 μg, respectively, is retained (Table 29.5). Such doses permit spacing

TABLE 29.5. RETENTION OF INTRAMUSCULAR INJECTION DOSES OF COBALAMIN: COMPARISON OF CYANOCOBALAMIN AND HYDROXOCOBALAMIN[a]

INTRAMUSCULAR INJECTION DOSE	CYANOCOBALAMIN		HYDROXOCOBALAMIN	
	AMOUNT RETAINED	% RETAINED	AMOUNT RETAINED	% RETAINED
10 μg	9.7 μg	(97%)	—	—
100 μg	55 μg	(55%)	92 μg	(92%)
500 μg	150 μg	(30%)	375 μg	(75%)
1,000 μg	150 μg	(15%)	710 μg	(71%)

[a]The amounts retained may be overestimated because they are based on losses by urinary excretion only. For example, it is conceivable that losses by other routes (e.g., biliary) may differ between the two forms of cobalamin.

Data from Chanarin I. The Megaloblastic Anaemias. 2ⁿᵈ ed. Oxford: Blackwell Scientific, 1979:311.

of the injections at monthly intervals. For unknown reasons, occasional patients seem to require more frequent injections. It is common practice to help replete stores with a short course of daily or weekly injections before embarking on monthly maintenance therapy.

It has long been known that even patients with PA can respond to oral cobalamin if the dose is large enough so that the approximately 1% nonspecific diffusion rate provides enough absorbed vitamin. The oral dose, usually of 1000 μg, must be given daily. This practice has been championed by some authors as a way of avoiding the discomfort, inconvenience, and cost of monthly injections. The hematologic and metabolic responses have been good (149), although the documentation involved many inappropriate patients who did not have cobalamin malabsorption. Oral therapy in patients with PA still requires caution. Suboptimal clinical responses have been described in some cases (150), more rapid relapse may follow discontinuance of oral than parenteral therapy (151), and an equivalent therapeutic efficacy of oral and parenteral cobalamin in patients with severe neurologic symptoms is not completely proven. It also remains to be seen whether compliance with the daily oral regimen in quotidian practice will match that seen in research studies.

Noncompliance is the major problem in all modes of treating cobalamin deficiency in general (78) and can be traced to both the patients' poor understanding of their medical problem and their physicians' sometimes complacent attitudes to cobalamin therapy. Relapse is a common outcome.

Patients with Malabsorption Limited to Food Cobalamin

Patients with food-cobalamin malabsorption absorb free, unbound cobalamin normally and theoretically should absorb cobalamin from supplements normally. However, that may not always be the case. Some patients seem to respond inadequately to oral doses as high as 50 μg (136–138), and limited responses to doses higher than that have been described as well (152–154). Reliable data on the oral doses needed for patients with food-cobalamin malabsorption, a particularly common problem in elderly persons but not exclusive to them, are not available.

Patients with Inborn Errors of Metabolism

Most such patients require parenteral therapy and sometimes auxiliary measures as well. The reader is referred to other sources for the details of this complex subject (39).

Monitoring and Response to Cobalamin Therapy

Monitoring the response to therapy has many virtues, chief of which is ultimate confirmation that the right diagnosis was made and the patient has benefited. Reticulocyte counts begin to rise within 2 to 3 days after cobalamin

is given and reach a peak at 7 to 10 days (14). The red blood cell count also begins to rise by the end of the week, followed by a decline in the MCV, and both become completely normal by 8 weeks. If they fail to do so, then either the diagnosis was incorrect or a second cause of anemia coexists. Neurologic response begins within the first few weeks, too, but its course and rate vary from patient to patient, some of whom may respond incompletely or not at all. Progression of symptoms despite therapy suggests that a process other than cobalamin deficiency is operative.

Biochemical improvement also begins within a few days. MMA and tHcy levels begin to fall, reaching normal levels after a week (155, 156). Either test provides a sensitive and specific means of monitoring; neither level will improve if folic acid is given instead. Retesting cobalamin levels after therapy serves little purpose, however; cobalamin levels rise after injection regardless of the injection's utility. Maintenance cobalamin therapy must be continued for as long as the underlying process causing the deficiency persists.

Characteristics of Cobalamin Preparations

Alternative routes of administering cobalamin (e.g., nasal or sublingual) have been developed, but their advantages have not been proven. Hydroxocobalamin is a suitable alternative to cyanocobalamin (see Table 29.5); it is used frequently in Europe because of its superior retention, which allows many patients to space out their injections to every second or third month (157). Methylcobalamin has been recommended for some purposes, but documentation of its benefits is still limited.

Cobalamin has little toxicity even at massive doses. Allergic reactions can occur, most often resulting from preservatives or other components of the preparation. Development of autoantibody to TC II was reported with depot preparations of cobalamin (158); serum cobalamin levels reached very high levels as a result, but no harmful effects were noted. Regarding tolerable upper intake levels, no adverse effects have been associated with excess cobalamin intake from food or supplements in healthy individuals; similarly, no adverse effects have occurred with periodic parenteral doses of 1000 to 5000 μg of vitamin B_{12} to patients with PA (46).

INTERACTIONS

Folate

The close metabolic, clinical, and therapeutic connections between cobalamin and folate are considered in this chapter and in Chapter 28. Table 29.6 reemphasizes and summarizes the key principles that underlie the differences in the characteristic expressions of the two vitamin deficiencies. Because of its narrow dietary sources and specific but vulnerable, IF-mediated absorption processes, cobalamin deficiency tends to be a relatively

TABLE 29.6. CHARACTERISTIC FEATURES OF COBALAMIN AND FOLATE PATHOPHYSIOLOGY THAT DIFFERENTIATE THEIR DEFICIENCY STATES

FEATURE	COBALAMIN	FOLATE
Ratio of stores to daily requirements	1,000:1	50–100:1

Clinical consequence: Cobalamin deficiency develops slowly; folate deficiency develops rapidly

Distribution of dietary sources	Narrow	Very broad

Clinical consequence: Dietary cobalamin deficiency involves narrow dietary restriction; dietary folate deficiency requires broad dietary restriction

Absorption	Relies on specific protein (intrinsic factor); limited capacity	Nonspecific processes predominate; high capacity

Clinical consequence: Malabsorption is a very common cause of cobalamin deficiency and is often limited to cobalamin; malabsorption is a less common cause of folate deficiency and is often part of a broad set of deficiencies

Time to onset of signs of deficiency	Several years	Weeks to months

Clinical consequence: Cobalamin deficiency requires a long, persistent causative process, whose onset may be historically remote from onset of symptoms; folate deficiency quickly follows a relatively brief causative process

pure, isolated deficiency, whereas folate deficiency, given the multiple dietary sources and nonspecific absorption processes of folate, is often part of a broader insufficiency of several nutrients.

Cobalamin deficiency, particularly its anemia, often responds to folate therapy. The response is typically incomplete and is usually transient, however. The possibility that the sharply increasing folate intake in the United States may compromise the early hematologic diagnosis of cobalamin deficiency and/or worsen its neurologic complications remains under scrutiny. A recent analysis of anemia rates in elderly patients with low cobalamin levels concluded that anemia rates have not diminished despite the fortification of the diet with folic acid (159). However, better data that focus only on macrocytic anemias are needed to answer the question more reliably. A report of progressive neurologic deterioration in a young black woman with sickle cell anemia and unrecognized PA who was taking folic acid illustrates the continuing dilemmas of routine folate supplementation (160).

Iron

More than half of patients with PA have iron deficiency at some time (123). Although blood loss cannot be identified in most cases, clinical prudence dictates a search for occult gastrointestinal blood loss, especially because of the increased risk of gastric cancer in patients with PA. It is likely that the atrophic gastritis underlying PA compromises absorption of iron as well, especially food iron, and that this fosters iron deficiency in PA. When iron and cobalamin deficiencies coexist, the expected hematologic characteristics of either entity may be blurred by the other, as discussed for combined folate and iron deficiency in Chapter 28. The mixed anemia may fail to respond if only one of the required hematinics is given alone.

Homocysteine

Cobalamin status affects tHcy levels not just with the striking elevations caused by florid cobalamin deficiency but also in mild tHcy elevations when cobalamin deficiency is mild or even subclinical. Serum cobalamin is an independent predictor of tHcy levels in surveys of healthy populations, second only to serum folate and, in elderly populations, nearly equal to folate (27).

Miscellaneous

A proposed deleterious effect of high doses of ascorbic acid on cobalamin status has not been confirmed.

REFERENCES

1. Kass L. Pernicious Anemia. Philadelphia: WB Saunders, 1976.
2. Wintrobe MM. Blood, Pure and Eloquent: A Story of Discovery, of People, and of Ideas. New York: McGraw-Hill, 1980.
3. Addison T. London Med Gaz 1849;43:517–8.
4. Biermer A. Schweiz Arzte 1872;2:15.
5. Minot GR, Murphy WP. JAMA 1926;87:470–6.
6. Castle WB. Am J Med Sci 1929;178:748–64.
7. Rickes EL, Brink NG, Koniuszy FR et al. Science 1948;107:396–7.

8. Smith EL, Parker LFJ. Biochem J 1948;43:viii–ix.

9. Hodgkin DC, Kamper J, Mackay M et al. Nature 1956;178: 64–6.

10. Carmel R. Annu Rev Med 2000;51:357–75.

11. Kondo H, Kolhouse JF, Allen RH. Proc Natl Acad Sci USA 1980; 77:817–21.

12. Kolhouse JF, Kondo H, Allen NC et al. N Engl J Med 1978;299: 785–92.

13. el Kholty S, Guéant JL, Bressler L et al. Gastroenterology 1991; 101:1399–408.

14. Chanarin I. The Megaloblastic Anaemias. 2nd ed. Oxford: Blackwell Scientific, 1979.

15. Zittoun J, Zittoun R. Semin Hematol 1999;36:35–46.

16. Carmel R, Brar S, Agrawal A et al. Clin Chem 2000;46:2017–8.

17. Carmel R. Semin Hematol 1999;36:88–100.

18. Lindenbaum J, Savage DG, Stabler SP et al. Am J Hematol 1990;34:99–107.

19. Matchar DB, McCrory DC, Millington DS et al. Am J Med Sci 1994;308:276–83.

20. Adams J, Boddy K, Douglas A. Br J Haematol 1972;23: 297–305.

21. Mollin DL, Anderson BB, Burman JF. Clin Haematol 1976;5: 521–46.

22. Carmel R. Arch Intern Med 1988;148:1712–4.

23. van Asselt DZB, de Groot LCPGM, van Staveren WA et al. Am J Clin Nutr 1998;68:328–34.

24. Carmel R, Green R, Jacobsen DW et al. Am J Clin Nutr 1999;70:904–10.

25. Pennypacker LC, Allen RH, Kelly JP et al. J Am Geriatr Soc 1992;40:1197–204.

26. Lindenbaum J, Rosenberg IH, Wilson PWF et al. Am J Clin Nutr 1994;60:2–11.

27. Carmel R. Cobalamin deficiency. In: Carmel R, Jacobsen DW, eds. Homocysteine in Health and Disease. Cambridge: Cambridge University Press, 2001:289–305.

28. Carmel R, Green R, Rosenblatt DS, Watkins D. Update on cobalamin, folate, and homocysteine. In: Broudy VC, Prchal JT, Tricot GJ, eds. Hematology 2003. Washington, DC: American Society of Hematology, 2003:62–81.

29. Remacha AF, Cadafalch J. Semin Hematol 1999;36:75–87.

30. Remacha AF, Cadafalch J, Sardà P et al. Am J Clin Nutr 2003;77:420–4.

31. Koebnick C, Heins UA, Dagnelie PC et al. Clin Chem 2002;48: 928–33.

32. Carmel R. Clin Chem 2003;49:1367–74.

33. Carmel R, Vasireddy H, Aurangzeb I et al. Clin Lab Haematol 2001;23:365–71.

34. Carmel R. Cobalamin–binding proteins in man. In: Silber R, Gordon AS, LoBue J et al., eds. Contemporary Hematology-Oncology, vol 2. New York: Plenum, 1981:79–129.

35. Bolann BJ, Soll JD, Schneede J et al. Clin Chem 2000;46: 1744–50.

36. Rasmussen K, Moller J, Lyngbak M et al. Clin Chem 1996;42: 630–6.

37. Savage DG, Lindenbaum J, Stabler SP et al. Am J Med 1994;96: 239–46.

38. Carmel R, Rasmussen K, Jacobsen DW et al. Br J Haematol 1996;93:311–8.

39. Rosenblatt D, Fenton W. Inherited disorders of folate and cobalamin metabolism. In: Scriver C, Beaudet A, Sly W et al., eds. The Metabolic and Molecular Bases of Inherited Disease. 8th ed. New York: McGraw-Hill, 2001:3897–933.

40. Sniderman LC, Lambert M, Giguère R et al. J Pediatr 1999; 134: 675–80.

41. Monsen ALB, Refsum H, Markestad T, Ueland PM. Clin Chem 2003;49:2067–75.

42. Lindemans J, Schoester M, van Kapel J. Clin Chim Acta 1983;132:53–61.

43. Seetharam B. Annu Rev Nutr 1999;19:173–95.

44. Ulleland M, Eilertsen I, Quadros EV et al. Clin Chem 2002;48: 526–32.

45. Carmel R. Clin Chem 2002;48:407–9.

45a. Chen X, Remacha AF, Sardà MP et al. Am J Clin Nutr 2005;81(Jan).

46. Food and Nutrition Board, Institute of Medicine. Dietary Reference Intakes: Thiamin, Riboflavin, Niacin, Vitamin B6, Folate, Vitamin B12, Pantothenic Acid, Biotin, and Choline. Washington, DC: National Academy Press, 1998:306–56.

47. Tucker KL, Rich S, Rosenberg I et al. Am J Clin Nutr 2000; 71:514–22.

48. del Corral A, Carmel R. Gastroenterology 1990;98:1460–6.

49. Allen RH, Seetharam B, Podell E et al. J Clin Invest 1978; 61:47–54.

50. Moestrup SK, Verroust PJ. Annu Rev Nutr 2001;21:407–28.

51. Fyfe JC, Madsen M, Hojrup P et al. Blood 2004;103:1573–9.

52. Quadros EV, Regec AL, Khan KMF et al. Am J Physiol 1999;277:G161–6.

53. Berlin H, Berlin R, Brante G. Acta Med Scand 1968;184: 247–58.

54. Waters HM, Dawson DW. Clin Lab Haematol 1999;21:169–72.

55. Carmel R, Neely SM, Francis RB, Jr. Blood 1990;75:251–4.

56. Eiberg H, Moller N, Mohr J et al. Clin Genet 1986;29:354–9.

57. Hewitt JE, Gordon MM, Taggart RT et al. Genomics 1991;10: 432–40.

58. Platica O, Janeczko R, Quadros EV et al. J Biol Chem 1991;266: 7860–3.

59. Hom BL. Scand J Haematol 1967;4:321–32.

60. Birn H, Willnow TE, Nielsen R et al. Am J Physiol 2002;282: F408–16.

61. Cowland JB, Borregaard N. J Leukoc Biol 1999;66:989–95.

62. Hall CA. Clin Sci Mol Med 1977;53:453–7.

63. Carmel R. Am J Clin Nutr 1985;41:713–9.

64. Burger RL, Schneider RJ, Mehlman CS et al. J Biol Chem 1975;250:7707–13.

65. Carmel R. Am J Clin Nutr 1997;66:750–9.

66. Nilsson-Ehle H. Drugs Aging 1998;12:277–92.

67. Baik HW, Russell RM. Annu Rev Nutr 1999;19:357–77.

68. Carmel R. Baillieres Clin Haematol 1995;8:639–55.

69. Carmel R, Aurangzeb I, Qian D. Am J Gastroenterol 2001;96: 63–70.

70. Selhub J, Jacques PF, Wilson PWF et al. JAMA 1993;270: 2693–8.

71. Howard JM, Azen C, Jacobsen DW et al. Eur J Clin Nutr 1998; 52:582–7.

72. Adams JF, Tankel HI, MacEwan F. Clin Sci 1970;39:107–13.

73. Life Sciences Research Office. Third Report on Nutrition Monitoring in the United States, vol. 2. Washington DC: US Government Printing Office, 1996.

74. Carmel R. Arch Intern Med 1979;139:47–50.

75. Healton EB, Savage DG, Brust JC et al. Medicine (Baltimore) 1991;70:229–45.

76. Lindenbaum J, Healton EB, Savage DG et al. N Engl J Med 1988;318:1720–8.

77. Pant SS, Asbury AK, Richardson EP Jr. Acta Neurol Scand Suppl 1968;44:1–36.

78. Savage D, Lindenbaum J. Am J Med 1983;74:765–72.

79. Fine EJ, Soria E, Paroski MW et al. Muscle Nerve 1990;13:158–64.

80. Hemmer B, Glocker FX, Schumacher M et al. J Neurol Neurosurg Psychiatry 1998;65:822–7.

81. Carmel R, Sinow RM, Karnaze DS. J Lab Clin Med 1987;109:454–63.

82. Karnaze DS, Carmel R. Arch Neurol 1990;47:1008–12.

83. Carmel R, Gott PS, Waters CH et al. Eur J Haematol 1995;54: 245–53.

84. van Asselt DZ, Pasman JW, van Lier HJ et al. J Gerontol 2001; 56A:M775–9.

85. Rundles RW. Blood 1946;1:209–19.

86. Ungley CC. Brain 1949;72:382–427.

87. Magnus EM. Eur J Haematol 1987;39:39–43.

88. Carmel R, Melnyk S, James SJ. Blood 2003;101:3302–8.

89. Ross JF, Belding H, Paegel BL. Blood 1948;3:68–90.

90. Karnaze DS, Carmel R. Arch Intern Med 1987;147:429–31.

91. Levitt AJ, Karlinsky H. Acta Psychiatr Scand 1992;86:301–5.

92. Clarke R, Smith AD, Jobst KA et al. Arch Neurol 1998;55: 1449–55.

93. Quadri P, Fragiacomo C, Pezzati R et al. Am J Clin Nutr 2004;80:114–22.

94. Moelby L, Nielsen G, Rasmussen K et al. Scand J Clin Lab Invest 1997;57:209–16.

95. Seaton DA, Goldberg A. Lancet 1960;1:1002–4.

96. Carmel R, Herbert V. Ann Intern Med 1967;67:1201–7.

97. Lindenbaum J, Pezzimenti J, Shea N. Ann Intern Med 1974; 80:326–31.

98. Jadhav M, Webb JKG, Vaishnava S et al. Lancet 1962;2;903–7.

99. Carmel R. Arch Intern Med 1985;145:484–5.

100. Carmel R, Lau KHW, Baylink DJ et al. N Engl J Med 1988;319: 70–5.

101. Noronha JM, Silverman M. On folic acid, vitamin B$_{12}$, methionine and formiminoglutamic acid metabolism. In: Heinrich HC, ed. Vitamin B$_{12}$ und Intrinsic Factor 2. Europäisches Symposion. Stuttgart: Enke, 1962:728–36.

102. Herbert V, Zalusky R. J Clin Invest 1962;41:1263–76.

103. Chanarin I, Deacon R, Lumb M et al. J Clin Pathol 1992;45:277–83.

104. Metz J. Annu Rev Nutr 1992;12:59–79.

105. Carmel R, Karnaze DS. JAMA 1985;253:1284–7.

106. Metz J, Bell AH, Flicker L et al. J Am Geriatr Soc 1996;44: 1355–61.

107. Carmel R. Arch Intern Med 1996;156:1097–100.

108. Waters WE, Withey JL, Kilpatrick GS et al. Br J Haematol 1971;20:521–6.

109. Refsum H, Yajnik CS, Gadkari M et al. Am J Clin Nutr 2001; 74:233–41.

110. Carmel R, Mallidi PV, Vinarskiy S et al. Am J Hematol 2002;70: 107–14.

111. Obeid R, Geisel J, Schorr H et al. Eur J Haematol 2002;69: 275–9.

112. van Dusseldorp M, Schneede J, Refsum H et al. Am J Clin Nutr 1999;69:664–71.

113. Louwman MWJ, van Dusseldorp M, van den Vijver FJR et al. Am J Clin Nutr 2000;72:762–9.

114. Higginbottom MC, Sweetman L, Nyhan WL. N Engl J Med 1978;299:317–23.

115. Graham SM, Arvela OM, Wise GA. J Pediatr 1992;121:710–4.

116. Monagle PT, Tauro GP. Clin Lab Haematol 1997;19:23–5.

117. Grattan-Smith PJ, Wilcken B, Procopis PG et al. Mov Disord 1997;12:39–46.

118. Stabler SP, Allen RH. Annu Rev Nutr 2004;24:299–326.

119. Carmel R. Pernicious anemia: definitions, expressions, and the long-term consequences of atrophic gastritis. In: Holt PR, Russell RM. eds. Chronic Gastritis and Hypochlorhydria in the Elderly. Boca Raton, FL: CRC Press, 1993:99–114.

120. Carmel R, Johnson CS. N Engl J Med 1978;298:647–50.

121. Carmel R, Johnson CS, Weiner JM. Arch Intern Med 1987;147:1995–6.

122. Carmel R, Spencer CA. Arch Intern Med 1982;142:1465–9.

123. Carmel R, Weiner JM, Johnson CS. JAMA 1987;257:1081–3.

124. Borch K. Scand J Gastroenterol 1986;21:21–30.

125. Sjoblom SM, Sipponen P, Miettinen M et al. Endoscopy 1988;20:52–6.

126. Yassin F, Rothenberg SP, Rao S et al. Blood 2004;103:1515–7.

127. Carmel R. Am J Hum Genet 1983;35:67–77.

128. Rygvold O. Scand J Gastroenterol Suppl 1974;9:57–64.

129. Sumner AE, Chin MM, Abraham JL et al. Ann Intern Med 1996;124:469–76.

130. Doscherholmen A, Swaim WR. Gastroenterology 1973;64: 913–9.

131. Fausa O. Scand J Gastroenterol Suppl 1974;9:75–9.

132. Aminoff M, Carter JE, Chadwick RB et al. Nature Genet 1999;21:309–13.

133. Kristiansen M, Aminoff M, Jacobsen C et al. Blood 2000;96:405–9.

134. Cohen H, Weinstein WM, Carmel R. Gut 2000;47:638–45.

135. Suter PM, Golner BB, Goldin BR et al. Gastroenterology 1991;101:1039–45.

136. Schilling RF, Gohdes PN, Hardie GH. Ann Intern Med 1984;101:501–2.

137. Provenzale D, Reinhold RB, Golner B et al. J Am Coll Nutr 1992;11:29–35.

138. Rhode BM, Arseneau P, Cooper BA et al. Am J Clin Nutr 1996;63:103–9.

139. Guttormsen AB, Refsum H, Ueland PM. Acta Anaesthesiol Scand 1994;38:753–6.

140. Ng J, Frith R. Lancet 2002;360:384.

141. Schilling RF. JAMA 1986;255:1605–6.

142. Kinsella LJ, Green R. Neurology 1995;45:1608–10.

143. Selzer RR, Rosenblatt DS, Laxova R et al. N Engl J Med 2003;349:45–50.

144. Carmel R. JAMA 1983;250:1886–90.

145. Lin JC, Borregaard N, Liebman HA et al. Am J Med Genet 2001;100:145–51.

146. Carmel R. Clin Exp Immunol 1992;89:74–7.

147. Waters HM, Dawson DW, Howarth JE et al. J Clin Pathol 1993;46:45–7.

148. Carmel R. Am J Clin Pathol 1988;90:442–6.

149. Kuzminski AM, Del Giacco EJ, Allen RH et al. Blood 1998;92: 1191–8.

150. Kondo H. Acta Haematol 1998;99:200–5.

151. Magnus EM. Scand J Haematol 1986;36:457–65.

152. Seal EC, Metz J, Flicker L et al. J Am Geriatr Soc 2002;50: 146–51.

153. Garcia A, Paris-Pombo A, Evans L et al. J Am Geriatr Soc 2002; 50:1401–4.

154. Rajan S, Wallace JI, Brodkin KI et al. J Am Geriatr Soc 2002;50:1789–95.

155. Stabler SP, Marcell PD, Podell ER et al. J Clin Invest 1986;77: 1606–12.

156. Stabler SP, Marcell PD, Podell ER et al. J Clin Invest 1988;81: 466–74.

157. Skouby AP. Acta Med Scand 1987;221:399–402.

158. Skouby A, Hippe E, Olesen H. Blood 1971;38:769–74.

159. Mills JL, Von Kohorn I, Conley MR et al. Am J Clin Nutr 2003;77:1474–7.

160. Dhar M, Bellevue R, Carmel R. N Engl J Med 2003;348: 2204–7.

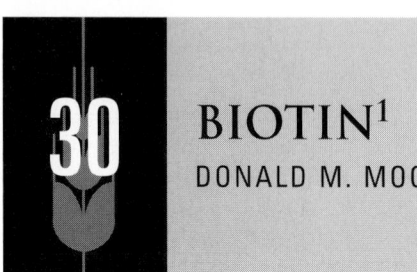

BIOTIN[1]
DONALD M. MOCK

HISTORY OF DISCOVERY .498
STRUCTURE, CHEMISTRY, AND BIOCHEMISTRY 498
   Structure 498
   Regulation 498
   Chemistry 499
   Biotin-Dependent Carboxylases 499
   Metabolism 500
   Measurement of Biotin and Metabolites 500
ABSORPTION 501
   Digestion of Protein-Bound Biotin 501
   Intestinal Absorption, Renal Reabsorption, and
      Uptake by Somatic Cells 501
   Intestinal Uptake 501
   Uptake by the Liver .501
   Renal Handling 502
   Transport in Blood 502
   Transport into the Central Nervous System 502
   Placental Transport .502
   Transport into Human Milk 502
BIOTIN DEFICIENCY 503
   Circumstances Leading to Deficiency 503
   Clinical Findings of Frank Deficiency 503
   Laboratory Findings .504
   Biochemical Pathogenesis 504
   Diagnosis 505
REQUIREMENTS AND ALLOWANCES 505
DIETARY SOURCES 505
TOXICITY 505

HISTORY OF DISCOVERY

Although a growth requirement for the "bios" fraction had been demonstrated in yeast, Boas first demonstrated the mammalian requirement for a factor, biotin, in rats fed egg-white protein. The severe dermatitis, hair loss, and neuromuscular dysfunction were termed "egg-white injury" and were cured by a factor present in liver. The critical event in this egg-white injury of both humans and rats is the highly specific and very tight binding (dissociation constant = 10^{-15}M) of biotin by avidin, a glycoprotein found in egg white. From an evolutionary standpoint, avidin probably serves as a bacteriostat in egg white; consistent with this hypothesis is the observation that avidin is resistant to a broad range of bacterial proteases in both the free and biotin-bound forms. Avidin is also resistant to pancreatic proteases; dietary avidin binds dietary biotin and microbial biotin and thus prevents absorption. Biotin is synthesized by many intestinal microbes; however, the contribution of microbial biotin to absorbed biotin remains unknown. Cooking denatures avidin and renders this protein susceptible to digestion and unable to interfere with absorption of biotin.

STRUCTURE, CHEMISTRY, AND BIOCHEMISTRY

Structure

The structure of biotin (Fig. 30.1) was elucidated independently by Kogl and by du Vigneaud in the early the 1940s (1). Eight stereoisomers exist, but only one (designated d-(+)-biotin or, simply, biotin) is found in nature and is enzymatically active. Biocytin (ε-N-biotinyl-L-lysine) is about as active as biotin on a molar basis in mammalian growth studies. Biotin is a bicyclic compound. One ring contains a ureido group (-N-CO-N-). The other contains sulfur and has a valeric acid side chain.

Regulation

In mammals, biotin serves as an essential cofactor for five carboxylases, each of which catalyzes a critical step in intermediary metabolism. Biotin exists in free and bound pools within the cells that are responsive to changes in biotin status (2). The pool size is likely determined by a balance among cellular uptake, cellular release, incorporation into apocarboxylases and histones, release from these biotinylated proteins during turnover, and catabolism to inactive metabolites.

Attachment of biotin to the apocarboxylase (see Fig. 30.1) is a condensation reaction catalyzed by holocarboxylase synthetase. An amide bond is formed between the carboxyl group of the valeric acid side chain of biotin and the ε-amino group of a specific lysyl residue in the apocarboxylase; these apocarboxylase regions contain sequences

---

[1] **Abbreviations: ACC,** acetyl-coenzyme A carboxylase; **CoA,** coenzyme A; **MCC,** methylcrotonyl-CoA carboxylase; **PC,** pyruvate carboxylase; **PCC,** propionyl-CoA carboxylase; **SMVT,** sodium-dependent multivitamin transporter.

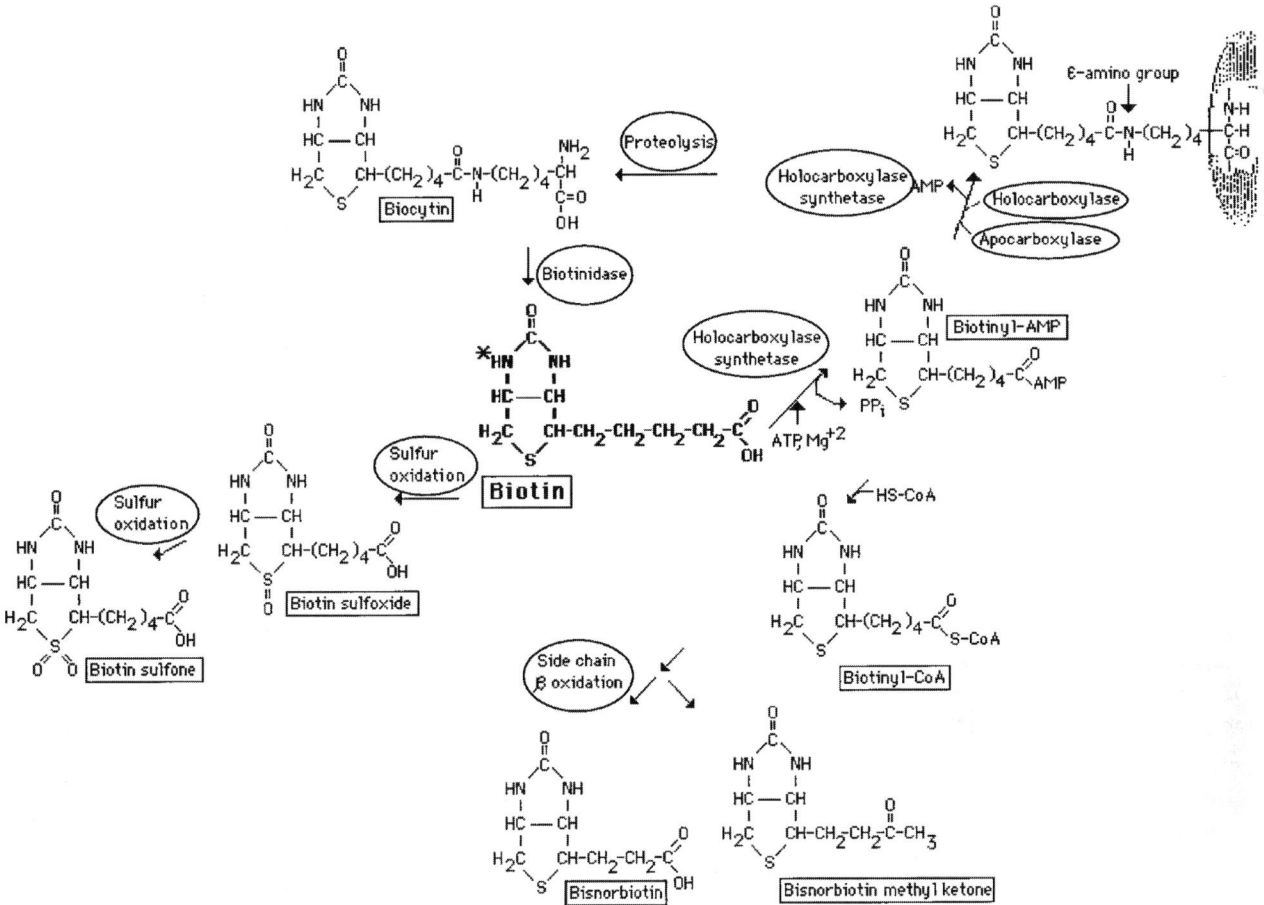

Figure 30.1. Biotin metabolism and degradation. *Ovals* denote enzymes or enzyme systems; *rectangles* denote biotin, intermediates, and metabolites. AMP, adenosine monophosphate; ATP, adenosine triphosphate; CoA, coenzyme A; Pp$_i$, pyrophosphate; *asterisk,* site of attachment of carboxyl moiety.

of amino acids that tend to be highly conserved within and among species for the individual carboxylases.

Regulation of intracellular mammalian carboxylase activity by biotin remains to be elucidated. In the normal turnover of cellular proteins, holocarboxylases are degraded to biocytin or biotin linked to an oligopeptide containing, at most, a few amino acid residues (see Fig. 30.1). Biotinidase (biotin amide hydrolase, EC 3.5.1.12) releases biotin for recycling.

The clinical manifestations of biotinidase deficiency appear to result largely from a secondary biotin deficiency. The genes for holocarboxylase synthetase and human biotinidase have been cloned, sequenced, and characterized (3).

Chemistry

All five of the mammalian carboxylases catalyze the incorporation of bicarbonate as a carboxyl group into a substrate and employ a similar catalytic mechanism. In the carboxylase reaction, the carboxyl moiety is first attached to biotin at the ureido nitrogen opposite the side chain; then the carboxyl group is transferred to the substrate. The reaction is driven

by the hydrolysis of adenosine triphosphate to adenosine diphosphate and inorganic phosphate. Subsequent reactions in the pathways of the five mammalian carboxylases release carbon dioxide from the product of the carboxylase reaction. Thus, these reaction sequences rearrange the substrates into more useful intermediates but do not violate the classic observation that mammalian metabolism does not result in the *net* fixation of carbon dioxide (4).

Biotin-Dependent Carboxylases

The five biotin-dependent mammalian carboxylases are acetyl-coenzyme A (CoA) carboxylase (ACC; EC 6.4.1.2) isoforms I and II (also known as α ACC and β ACC), pyruvate carboxylase (PC; EC 6.4.1.1), methylcrotonyl-CoA carboxylase (MCC; EC 6.4.1.4), and propionyl-CoA carboxylase (PCC; EC 6.4.1.3).

ACC catalyzes the incorporation of bicarbonate into acetyl CoA to form malonyl CoA (Fig. 30.2). Two isoforms of ACC are known: (a) isoform I of ACC is located in the cytosol and produces malonyl CoA, which is rate limiting in fatty acid synthesis (elongation); and (b) isoform II of ACC is located on the outer mitochondrial membrane and

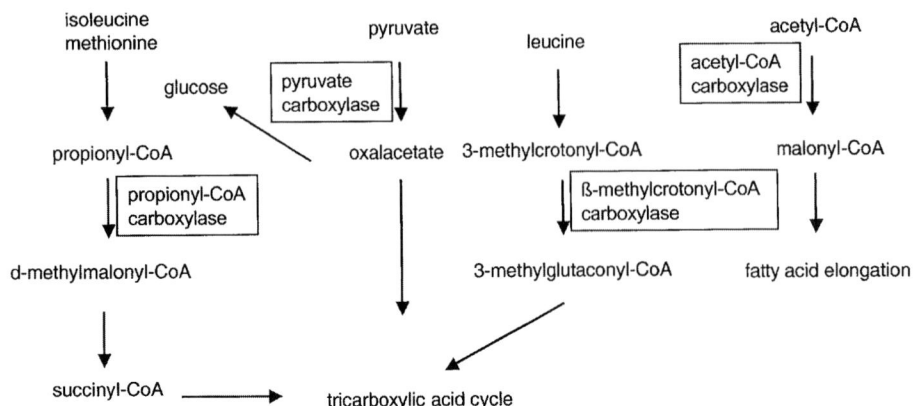

Figure 30.2. Interrelationship of pathways catalyzed by biotin-dependent enzymes (shown in *boxes*). CoA, coenzyme A.

controls fatty acid oxidation in mitochondria through the inhibitory effect of malonyl CoA on fatty acid transport into mitochondria. An inactive mitochondrial form of ACC may serve as storage for biotin (5).

The three remaining carboxylases are mitochondrial. PC catalyzes the incorporation of bicarbonate into pyruvate to form oxaloacetate, an intermediate in the Krebs tricarboxylic acid cycle (see Fig. 30.2). Thus, PC catalyzes an anaplerotic reaction. In gluconeogenic tissues (i.e., liver and kidney), the oxaloacetate can be converted to glucose. Deficiency of PC is probably the cause of the lactic acidemia, central nervous system lactic acidosis, and abnormalities in glucose regulation observed in biotin deficiency and biotinidase deficiency (see later). MCC catalyzes an essential step in the degradation of the branched-chain amino acid leucine (see Fig. 30.2). Deficient activity of MCC leads to metabolism of 3-methylcrotonyl CoA to 3-hydroxyisovaleric acid and 3-methylcrotonylglycine by an alternate pathway (1). Thus, increased urinary excretion of these abnormal metabolites reflects deficient activity of MCC (1).

PCC catalyzes the incorporation of bicarbonate into propionyl CoA to form methylmalonyl CoA; methylmalonyl CoA undergoes isomerization to succinyl CoA and enters the tricarboxylic acid cycle (see Fig. 30.2). In a fashion analogous to MCC deficiency, deficiency of PCC leads to increased urinary excretion of 3-hydroxypropionic acid and 3-methylcitric acid.

Metabolism

An alternate fate to being incorporated into carboxylases or excretion unchanged is catabolism to an inactive metabolite before excretion in urine (4). About half of biotin undergoes metabolism before excretion. Two principal pathways of biotin catabolism have been identified in mammals. In the first pathway, the valeric acid side chain of biotin is degraded by β-oxidation. β-Oxidation of biotin leads to the formation of bisnorbiotin, tetranorbiotin, and related intermediates that are known to result from β-oxidation of fatty acids. The cellular site of this β-oxidation of biotin is uncertain. Nonenzymatic decarboxylation of the unstable β-keto-biotin and β-keto-bisnorbiotin leads to formation of bisnor-

biotin methyl ketone and tetranorbiotin methyl ketone, which appear in urine. In the second pathway, the sulfur in the thiophane ring of biotin is oxidized leading to the formation of biotin L-sulfoxide, biotin D-sulfoxide, and biotin sulfone. Combined oxidation of the ring sulfur and β-oxidation of the side chain lead to metabolites such as bisnorbiotin sulfone. In mammals, degradation of the biotin ring to release carbon dioxide and urea is quantitatively minor.

On a molar basis, biotin accounts for approximately half of the total avidin-binding substances in human serum and urine (Table 30.1). Biocytin, bisnorbiotin, bisnorbiotin methyl ketone, biotin D,L-sulfoxide, and biotin sulfone account for most of the balance. Biotin metabolism is accelerated in some persons by anticonvulsants and during pregnancy, thereby increasing the ratio of biotin metabolites to biotin in urine.

Measurement of Biotin and Metabolites

For measuring biotin at physiologic concentrations (i.e., 100 pmol/L to 100 nmol/L), various assays have been proposed, and a few have been used to study biotin nutriture. For a more detailed review, see *Biotin* (6). All published studies of biotin nutriture have used one of three basic types of biotin assays: bioassays, avidin-binding assays, or fluorescent derivative assays.

TABLE 30.1. NORMAL RANGE FOR BIOTIN AND METABOLITES IN HUMAN SERUM AND URINE[a]

COMPOUND	SERUM (pmol/L)	URINE (nmol/24 h)
Biotin	133–329	18–127
Bisnorbiotin	21–563	6–39
Biotin D,L–sulfoxide	0–120	5–19
Bisnorbiotin methylketone	0–120[b]	2–13
Biotin sulfone	ND	1–8
Biocytin	0–26	1–13
Total biotinyl compounds	294–1021[b]	46–128

ND, not determined.
[a] Normal Ranges (minimum–maximum) are reported (n = 15 for serum; n = 16 for urine, except biocytin, n = 10).
[b] Including unidentified biotin metabolites.

Bioassays generally have adequate sensitivity to measure biotin in blood and urine, especially with recent modifications using injected agar plates or metabolic radiometry. However, the bacterial bioassays (and perhaps the eukaryotic bioassays as well) suffer interference from unrelated substances and variable growth response to biotin analogs. Bioassays give conflicting results if biotin is bound to protein (6).

Avidin-binding assays generally measure the ability of biotin to compete with radiolabeled biotin for binding to avidin (isotope dilution assays), to bind to avidin coupled to a reporter and thus prevent the avidin from binding to a biotin linked to solid phase, or to prevent inhibition of a biotinylated enzyme by avidin. Various novel reporter systems have been described (1, 7). Avidin-binding assays generally detect all avidin-binding substances, although the relative detectabilities of biotin and analogs vary among analogs and among assays (7). Chromatographic separation of biotin analogs with subsequent avidin-binding assay of the chromatographic fractions appears to be both sensitive and chemically specific. Values for the concentration of biotin in human plasma vary among the various bioassays and avidin-binding assays; reported mean values range from approximately 500 pmol/L to more than 10,000 pmol/L.

ABSORPTION

Digestion of Protein-Bound Biotin

The content of free biotin and protein-bound biotin in foods is variable, but most biotin in meats and cereals appears to be protein bound via an amide bond between biotin and lysine. Neither the mechanisms of intestinal hydrolysis of protein-bound biotin nor the determinants of bioavailability have been clearly delineated. Wolf and colleagues (8) have postulated that biotinidase plays a critical role in the release of biotin from covalent binding to protein. In patients with biotinidase deficiency, doses of free biotin that do not greatly exceed the estimated dietary intake (e.g., 50–150 μg per day) appear adequate to prevent the symptoms of biotinidase deficiency, a finding suggesting that biotinidase deficiency causes biotin deficiency, at least in part, through impaired intestinal digestion of protein-bound biotin.

Intestinal Absorption, Renal Reabsorption, and Uptake by Somatic Cells

At physiologic pH, the carboxylate group of biotin is negatively charged. Thus, biotin is at least modestly water soluble and requires a transporter to cross cell membranes such as enterocytes for intestinal absorption, somatic cells for utilization, and renal tubule cells for reclamation from the glomerular filtrate.

Intestinal Uptake

An excellent in-depth review of intestinal uptake of biotin has been published (9). In intact intestinal preparations such as loops and everted gut sacks, biotin transport exhibits two components (6). One component is saturable at a Michaelis-Menten constant of approximately 10 μM biotin transporter; the other is not saturable even at very large concentrations of biotin; this observation is consistent with passive diffusion. Absorption of biocytin, the biotinyl-lysine product of intraluminal protein digestion, is inefficient relative to biotin (10), consistent with biotinidase release of biotin from dietary protein (11). The transporter is present in the intestinal brush border membrane (9). Transport is highly structurally specific, temperature dependent, sodium coupled, and electroneutral; in the presence of a sodium ion gradient, biotin transport occurs against a concentration gradient (9).

In rats, biotin transport is upregulated with maturation and by biotin deficiency (9). Although carrier-mediated transport of biotin is most active in the proximal small bowel of the rat, the absorption of biotin from the proximal colon is still significant, a finding supporting the potential nutritional significance of biotin synthesized and released by enteric flora (9). Clinical studies have provided some evidence that biotin is absorbed from the human colon (6), but studies in swine indicated that absorption of biotin from the hindgut is much less efficient than from the upper intestine; further, biotin synthesized by enteric flora is probably not present at a location or in a form in which bacterial biotin contributes importantly to absorbed biotin. Exit of biotin from the enterocyte (i.e., transport across the basolateral membrane) is also carrier mediated (9). However, basolateral transport is independent of sodium ion, is electrogenic, and does not accumulate biotin against a concentration gradient.

Based on a study in which biotin was administered orally in pharmacologic amounts, bioavailability of biotin is approximately 100%. Thus, the pharmacologic doses of biotin given to treat biotin-dependent inborn errors of metabolism are likely to be well absorbed. Moreover, the finding of high bioavailability of biotin at pharmacologic doses provides at least some basis for predicting that bioavailability will also be high at the physiologic doses at which the biotin transporter mediates uptake.

Uptake by the Liver

Studies in various hepatic cell lines indicate that uptake of free biotin is similar to intestinal uptake (12, 13). Transport is mediated by a specialized carrier system that is sodium dependent, electroneutral, and structurally specific for a free carboxyl group. At large concentrations, transport is mediated by diffusion. Metabolic trapping, such as biotin bound covalently to intracellular proteins, is also important. After entering the hepatocyte, biotin diffuses into the mitochondria via a pH-dependent process.

Two biotin transporters have been described: (a) a multivitamin transporter present in many tissues and (b) a biotin transporter identified in human lymphocytes. In 1997, Prasad and co-workers discovered a sodium-coupled,

saturable, structurally specific transporter present in human placental choriocarcinoma cells that can transport pantothenic acid, lipoic acid, and biotin (14). This sodium-dependent multivitamin transporter has been named SMVT and is widely expressed in human tissues (15). Studies by Said and co-workers using RNAi specific for SMVT provided strong evidence that biotin uptake by Caco-2 and HepG2 cells occurs via SMVT (9); thus, intestinal absorption and hepatic uptake are likely mediated by SMVT.

The biotin transporter identified in lymphocytes is also sodium coupled, saturable, and structurally specific (16). Studies by Daberkow and co-workers provided evidence in favor of monocarboxylate transporter 1 as the lymphocyte biotin transporter (17).

A child with biotin dependence resulting from a defect in the lymphocyte biotin transporter was reported. SMVT gene sequence was normal (18). The investigators speculated that lymphocyte biotin transporter is expressed in other tissues and mediates some critical aspect of biotin homeostasis.

Ozand and collaborators described several patients in Saudi Arabia with biotin-responsive basal ganglia disease (19). Symptoms included confusion, lethargy, vomiting, seizures, dystonia, dysarthria, dysphagia, seventh nerve paralysis, quadriparesis, ataxia, hypertension, chorea, and coma. A defect in the biotin transporter system across the blood-brain barrier was postulated.

The relationship of these putative biotin transporters with each other and their relative roles in intestinal absorption, transport into various organs, and renal reclamation remain to be elucidated.

Renal Handling

Specific systems for the reabsorption of water-soluble vitamins from the glomerular filtrate may contribute importantly to conservation of the water-soluble vitamins (20). Animal studies using brush border membrane vesicles from human kidney cortex indicated that biotin is reclaimed from the glomerular filtrate against a concentration gradient by a saturable, sodium-dependent, structurally specific system (21). Subsequent egress of biotin from the tubular cells occurs via a basolateral membrane transport system that is not dependent on sodium. Biocytin does not inhibit tubular reabsorption of biotin (21). Studies in patients with biotinidase deficiency suggest a role for biotinidase in the renal handling of biotin (22, 23).

Transport in Blood

Biotin is transported in blood from the site of absorption in the intestine to the peripheral tissues and the liver (1). Wolf and co-workers (24) originally hypothesized that biotinidase could serve as a biotin-binding protein in plasma or perhaps even as a carrier protein for the transport of biotin into the cell. Based on protein precipitation and by equilibrium dialysis using ^{3}H-biotin, Chauhan and Dakshinamurti (25) concluded that biotinidase is the only protein in human serum that specifically binds biotin. However, using ^{3}H-biotin, centrifugal ultrafiltration, and dialysis to assess reversible binding in plasma from the rabbit, pig, and human, Lankford and I (26) found that less than 10% of the total pool of free plus reversibly bound biotin is reversibly bound to plasma protein; the biotin binding observed could be explained by binding to human serum albumin. Using acid hydrolysis and ^{3}H-biotinyl-albumin, Malik and I (27) found additional biotin covalently bound to plasma protein. The percentages of free to reversibly bound to covalently bound biotin in human serum are approximately 81 to 7 to 12%. The role of plasma proteins in the transport of biotin remains to be definitively established. Biotin concentrations in erythrocytes are equal to the concentrations in plasma (unpublished observation), but transport of biotin into erythrocytes is very slow, consistent with passive diffusion (18).

Transport into the Central Nervous System

Various animal and human studies suggest that biotin is transported across the blood-brain barrier (1, 28, 29). The transporter is saturable and is structurally specific for the free carboxylate group on the valeric acid side chain. Transport into the neuron also appears to involve a specific transport system, as well as subsequent trapping of biotin by covalent binding to brain proteins, presumably carboxylase.

Placental Transport

Biotin concentrations are three- to 17-fold greater in plasma from second-trimester human fetuses compared with their mothers, a finding consistent with active placental transport. (30). Specific systems for transport of biotin from the mother to the fetus have been reported (15, 31–33). The microvillus membrane of the placenta contains a saturable transport system for biotin that is sodium dependent and actively accumulates biotin within the placenta, consistent with SMVT (15, 31–33).

Transport into Human Milk

More than 95% of the biotin is free in the skim fraction of human milk (34). The concentration of biotin in human milk varies substantially in some women (35), and it exceeds the concentration in serum by one to two orders of magnitude, a finding suggesting a transport system into milk. Bisnorbiotin accounts for approximately 50% and biotin sulfoxide about 10% of the total biotin plus metabolites in early and transitional human milk (36). With postpartum maturation, the biotin concentration increases, but the bisnorbiotin and biotin sulfoxide concentrations still account for 25 and 8% at 5 weeks post partum. Current studies provide no evidence for a predominant

trapping mechanism or for a soluble biotin-binding protein.

BIOTIN DEFICIENCY

Circumstances Leading to Deficiency

The finding that physiologically normal persons have a requirement for biotin has been clearly documented in two situations: prolonged consumption of raw egg white and parenteral nutrition without biotin supplementation in patients with short gut syndrome and other causes of malabsorption (1). Biotin deficiency also has been clearly demonstrated in biotinidase deficiency. The mechanism by which biotinidase deficiency leads to biotin deficiency probably involves several processes: (a) gastrointestinal absorption of biotin may be decreased because deficiency of biotinidase in pancreatic secretions leads to inadequate release of protein-bound biotin; (b) salvage of biotin at the cellular level may be impaired during normal turnover of proteins to which biotin is linked covalently; and (c) renal loss of biocytin and biotin is probably abnormally increased.

The clinical findings and biochemical abnormalities caused by biotinidase deficiency are quite similar to those of biotin deficiency; common findings include periorificial dermatitis, conjunctivitis, alopecia, ataxia, and developmental delay (1). These clinical similarities suggest that the pathogenesis of biotinidase deficiency involves a secondary biotin deficiency. However, the reported signs and symptoms of biotin deficiency and biotinidase deficiency are not identical. Seizures, irreversible neurosensory hearing loss, and optic atrophy have been observed in biotinidase deficiency but have not been reported in human biotin deficiency.

Based on lymphocyte carboxylase activity and plasma biotin levels, Velazquez and co-workers reported that biotin deficiency occurs in children with severe protein-energy malnutrition (37). These investigators speculated that the effects of biotin deficiency may be responsible for part of the clinical syndrome of protein-energy malnutrition.

Accumulating data provide evidence that long-term anticonvulsant therapy in adults can lead to biotin depletion and that the depletion at the tissue level can be severe enough to interfere with amino acid metabolism (38–40). The mechanism may involve both accelerated biotin breakdown (40–42) and impairment of biotin absorption caused by the anticonvulsants (43, 44).

Concerns about the teratogenic effects of biotin deficiency have led to studies of biotin status during human gestation (45). Studies of biotin status during pregnancy (46, 47) and of biotin supplementation during pregnancy (48) provided evidence that a marginal degree of biotin deficiency develops in at least one third of women during normal pregnancy. Although the degree of biotin deficiency is not severe enough to produce overt manifestations of biotin deficiency, the deficiency is severe enough to produce metabolic derangements. A similar marginal degree of biotin deficiency causes high rates of fetal malformations in some mammals (49–51). Moreover, data from a multivitamin supplementation study provided significant, albeit indirect, evidence that the marginal degree of biotin deficiency that occurs spontaneously in normal human gestation is teratogenic (45).

Biotin deficiency has also been reported or inferred in several other circumstances:

1. Leiner's disease is a severe form of seborrheic dermatitis that occurs in infancy. Although some studies reported prompt resolution of the rash with biotin therapy (52, 53), biotin was ineffective in the only double-blind therapeutic trial reported (54).

2. Sudden infant death syndrome: Biotin deficiency in the chick produces a fatal hypoglycemia dubbed fatty liver-kidney syndrome; impaired gluconeogenesis from deficient activity of PC is the cause of the hypoglycemia. Hood, Johnson, Heard, and Emery (55, 56) proposed that biotin deficiency may cause sudden infant death syndrome by an analogous pathogenic mechanism. They supported their hypothesis by demonstrating that hepatic biotin was significantly lower at autopsy in infants with sudden infant death syndrome than in infants who died of other causes. Additional studies (e.g., levels of hepatic PC, urinary organic acids, and blood glucose) are needed to confirm or refute this hypothesis.

3. Dialysis: Patients undergoing long-term hemodialysis have been reported to have reduced (57) or increased plasma concentrations of biotin (58). Yatzidis and colleagues (59) reported nine patients undergoing long-term hemodialysis who developed either encephalopathy (four patients) or peripheral neuropathy (five patients); all responded to biotin therapy. The etiologic role of biotin deficiency in uremic neurologic disorders remains to be determined (59–61).

4. Gastrointestinal diseases or alcoholism: Reduced blood or liver concentrations of biotin or urinary excretion of biotin have been reported in alcoholism, gastric disease, and inflammatory bowel disease (1).

5. Brittle nails: Colombo and co-workers treated women with brittle fingernails with 2.5 mg/day biotin orally (62) and observed a 25% increase in nail thickness and improved morphology by electron microscopy.

Clinical Findings of Frank Deficiency

Whether caused by egg-white feeding or omission of biotin from total parenteral nutrition, the clinical findings of frank biotin deficiency in adults, older children, and infants are similar. Typically, the findings appear gradually after weeks to several years of egg-white feeding or parenteral nutrition. Thinning of hair and progression to loss of all hair including eyebrows and lashes are reported. A scaly (seborrheic), red (eczematous) skin rash is present in most patients; the rash may be distributed around the eyes, nose, mouth, and perineal orifices. The appearance of the rash is similar to that of cutaneous candidiasis; typically, *Candida* can be cultured from the lesions. These cutaneous manifestations, in conjunction with an unusual distribution of facial fat, have been dubbed biotin deficiency facies. Depression, lethargy, hallucinations, and paresthesias of the extremities are prominent neurologic symptoms in most adults. The most striking neurologic findings in infants are hypotonia, lethargy, and developmental delay.

Laboratory Findings

Although commonly used to assess biotin status in various clinical populations, the putative indices of human biotin status were previously studied during progressive biotin deficiency only twice: Mock and co-workers (63–66) induced progressive biotin deficiency in humans by feeding egg white to physiologically normal persons in a clinical research center for 3 weeks in one study and for 4 weeks in a second study. In both studies, the urinary excretion of biotin declined dramatically with time on the egg-white diet, and the urinary excretion of 3-hydroxyisovaleric acid excretion increased steadily, thus providing evidence that biotin depletion decreased the activity of MCC and altered leucine metabolism earlier in biotin deficiency than previously appreciated. However, the urinary excretion of 3-methylcrotonylglycine, 3-hydroxypropionic acid, and 3-methylcitric acid did not change as drastically and proved not to be as sensitive indicators of biotin deficiency as 3-hydroxyisovaleric acid excretion. Based on a study of only five subjects, 3-hydroxyisovaleric acid excretion in response to a leucine challenge may be even more sensitive than 3-hydroxyisovaleric acid excretion. In contrast, plasma concentrations of free biotin decreased to abnormal values in only half of the subjects These investigators concluded that plasma biotin is not an early or sensitive indicator of impaired biotin status.

In the second study, lymphocyte PCC activity decreased to abnormal values in all subjects by the twenty-eighth day of egg-white feeding and returned to normal in about 75% within 3 weeks of resuming a general diet with or without biotin supplement. The investigators concluded that lymphocyte PCC activity is an early and sensitive indicator of marginal biotin deficiency.

Odd-chain fatty acid accumulation is also a marker of biotin deficiency. The accumulation of odd-chain fatty acid is thought to result from PCC deficiency (see Fig. 30.2). Presumably, the accumulation of propionyl CoA leads to the substitution of propionyl CoA moiety for acetyl CoA in the ACC reaction and to the incorporation of a three- (rather than two-) carbon moiety during fatty acid elongation. These abnormalities develop more slowly and resolve more slowly than the abnormalities in organic acid excretion and lymphocyte PCC activity.

Biochemical Pathogenesis

The mechanisms by which biotin deficiency produces specific signs and symptoms remain to be completely delineated. However, several studies have given new insights into the biochemical pathogenesis of biotin deficiency. The tacit assumption of most of these studies is that the clinical findings of biotin deficiency result directly or indirectly from deficient activities of the five biotin-dependent carboxylases. On the basis of human studies in biotinidase deficiency and isolated PC deficiency as well as biotin deficiency in animals, the central nervous system effects of biotin deficiency (hypotonia, seizures, ataxia, and delayed development) are mediated through deficiency of brain PC and the attendant central nervous system lactic acidosis, rather than by disturbances in brain fatty acid composition (67–69). Abnormalities in metabolism of fatty acids are likely important in the pathogenesis of the skin rash and hair loss. My co-workers and I (70) reported that supplementation with ω-6 fatty acids strikingly delays the onset of the cutaneous manifestations of biotin deficiency. We concluded that an abnormality in ω-6 polyunsaturated fatty acid metabolism does play a pathogenic role in the cutaneous manifestations of biotin deficiency and that the effect of the ω-6 polyunsaturated fatty acid cannot be attributed to biotin sparing.

Exciting work has provided evidence for a potential role for biotin in gene expression; these findings likely will provide new insights into the pathogenesis of biotin deficiency. In 1995, Hymes and Wolf discovered that biotinidase can act as a biotinyl-transferase; biocytin serves as the source of biotin, and histones are specifically biotinylated (3). Approximately 25% of total cellular biotinidase activity is located in the nucleus. Zempleni and co-workers demonstrated that the abundance of biotinylated histones varies with the cell cycle, that biotinylated histones are increased approximately twofold compared with quiescent lymphocytes, and that histones are debiotinylated enzymatically in a process that is at least partially catalyzed by biotinidase (71–73). These observations suggest that biotin plays a role in regulating DNA transcription and regulation.

Although the mechanisms remain to be elucidated, biotin status has been shown to affect gene expression. Cell culture studies suggest that cell proliferation generates an increased demand for biotin, perhaps mediated by increased synthesis of biotin-dependent carboxylases (72). Rodriguez-Melendez and Velazquez and co-workers reported that biotin deficiency in rats reduces messenger RNA levels of holocarboxylase synthetase, but it has differential effects on the amount of mRNA and enzyme protein for the various carboxylases (74, 75).

Studies conducted in diabetic patients and rats support an effect of biotin status on carbohydrate metabolism.

Genes studied include glucokinase, phosphoenolpyruvate carboxykinase *(PEPCK)*, and expression of the asialoglycoprotein receptor on the surface of hepatocytes (76–78). The effect of biotin status on *PEPCK* expression was particularly striking when diabetic rats were compared with nondiabetic rats. However, most studies were performed in rats in which metabolic pathways were perturbed before administration of biotin. Thus, the role of biotin in regulation of these genes during normal biotin status remains unclear.

Diagnosis

Biotin deficiency can be diagnosed by demonstrating reduced urinary excretion of biotin, increased urinary excretion of the 3-hydroxyisovaleric acid, and resolution of the clinical and laboratory abnormalities with biotin supplementation. The clinical response to administration of biotin has been dramatic in all well-documented cases of biotin deficiency. Healing of the rash is striking within a few weeks, and growth of healthy hair is generally present by 1 to 2 months. Hypotonia, lethargy, and depression generally resolve within 1 to 2 weeks, followed by accelerated mental and motor development in infants. Pharmacologic doses of biotin (e.g., 1–10 mg) have been used to treat most patients.

REQUIREMENTS AND ALLOWANCES

Data providing an accurate estimate of the dietary and parenteral biotin requirements for infants, children, and adults are lacking (79). However, recommendations for biotin supplementation have been formulated for oral intake in infants through adults, for oral and parenteral intake of biotin for preterm infants, and for parenteral intake in infants through adults (80). The more recent recommendations for oral intake developed by the Food and Nutrition Board of the Institute of Medicine are listed in Table 30.2 and Appendix Tables A-2-a through A-2-h.

DIETARY SOURCES

No published evidence indicates that biotin can be synthesized by mammals; thus, higher animals must derive biotin from other sources. The ultimate source of biotin appears to be de novo synthesis by bacteria, primitive eukaryotic organisms such as yeast, molds, and algae, and some plant species.

Most measurements of biotin content of foods have used bioassays. (81, 82). Although one publication provides evidence that the values likely contain substantial errors (83), some worthwhile generalizations can be made. Biotin is widely distributed in natural foodstuffs, but the absolute content of even the richest sources is low when compared with the content of most other water-soluble vitamins. Foods relatively rich in biotin include egg yolk, liver, and some vegetables. Based on the data of Hardinge (81), the average dietary biotin intake has been estimated to be approximately 70 μg/day (300 nmol/day) for the Swiss population. This result is in reasonable agreement with the estimated dietary intake in Canada of 60 μg/day (84) and in Britain of 35 μg/day (85, 86).

TOXICITY

Daily doses up to 200 mg orally and up to 20 mg intravenously have been given to treat biotin-responsive inborn errors of metabolism and acquired biotin deficiency. Toxicity has not been reported.

Acknowledgments
Nell Matthews Mock and Shawna L. Stratton provided assistance in the preparation of this chapter.

REFERENCES

1. Mock DM. Biotin. In: Ziegler EE, Filer J, eds. Present Knowledge in Nutrition. 7th ed. Washington, DC: International Life Sciences Institutes, Nutrition Foundation, 1996:220–35.
2. Lewis B, Rathman S, McMahon R. J Nutr 2001;131:2310–5.
3. Wolf B. Disorders of biotin metabolism. In: Scriver CR, Beaudet AL, Sly WS et al, eds. The Metabolic and Molecular Basis of Inherited Disease. 8th ed. New York: McGraw-Hill, 2001: 3151–77.
4. Mock DM. Biotin. In: Shils ME, Olson JA, Shike M et al, eds. Modern Nutrition in Health and Disease. 9th ed. Baltimore: Williams & Wilkins, 1999:459–66.
5. Shriver BJ, Roman-Shriver C, Allred JB. J Nutr 1993;123:1140–9.
6. Mock DM. Biotin. In: Brown M, ed. Present Knowledge in Nutrition. 6th ed. Blacksburg, VA: International Life Sciences Institute, Nutrition Foundation, 1990:189–207.
7. Mock DM, Nyalala JO, Raguseo RM. J Nutr 2001;131:2208–14.
8. Wolf B, Heard G, McVoy JRS et al. J Inherit Metab Dis 1984;7:121–2.
9. Said H.M. Biotin In: Recent advances in carrier-mediated intestinal absorption of water-soluble vitamins (*arjournals.annualreviews.org/doi/abs/10.1146/annurev.physiol. 66.032102. 144611*). Accessed 12/17/2003.
10. Said HM, Redha R. Am J Physiol 1987;252:G52–5.
11. McMahon RJ. Annu Rev Nutr 2002;22:221–39.
12. Bowers-Komro DM, McCormick DB. Biotin uptake by isolated rat liver hepatocytes. In: Dakshinamurti K, Bhagavan HN, eds. Biotin. New York: New York Academy of Sciences, 1985:350–8.
13. Said HM, Ma TY, Kamanna VS. J Cell Physiol 1994;161:483–9.
14. Prasad PD, Ramamoorthy S, Leibach FH et al. Placenta 1997; 18:527–33.

TABLE 30.2. ADEQUATE INTAKE OF BIOTIN (μg/d)[a]

LIFE-STAGE GROUP	AGE	ADEQUATE INTAKE
Infants	0–6 mo	5
	7–12 mo	6
Children	1–3 y	8
	4–8 y	12
Males and females	9–13 y	20
	14–18 y	25
	≥19 y	30
Pregnancy		30
Lactation		35

[a] 1 μg biotin = 4 nmol.

15. Prasad PD, Wang H, Kekuda R et al. J Biol Chem 1998;273: 7501–6.
16. Zempleni J, Mock DM. Am J Physiol 1998;275:C382–8.
17. Daberkow RL, White BR, Cederberg RA et al. J Nutr 2003;133: 2703–6.
18. Mardach R, Zempleni J, Wolf B et al. J Clin Invest 2002;109: 1617–23.
19. Ozand PT, Gascon GG, Alessa M et al. Brain 1999;121:1267–79.
20. Bowman BB, McCormick DB, Rosenberg IH. Annu Rev Nutr 1989;9:187–99.
21. Baur B, Baumgartner ER. Pflugers Archiv 1993;422:499–505.
22. Baumgartner ER, Suormala T, Wick H. J Inherit Metab Dis 1985;8:59–64.
23. Baumgartner ER, Suormala T, Wick H. J Inherit Metab Dis 1985;7:123–5.
24. Wolf B, Grier RE, McVoy JRS et al. J Inherit Metab Dis 1985; 8:53–8.
25. Chauhan J, Dakshinamurti K. Biochem J 1988;256:265–70.
26. Mock DM, Lankford G. J Nutr 1990;120:375–81.
27. Mock DM, Malik MI. Am J Clin Nutr 1992;56:427–32.
28. Spector R, Mock DM. J Neurochem 1987;48:400–4.
29. Spector R, Mock DM. Neurochem Res 1988;13:213–9.
30. Mantagos S, Malamitsi-Puchner A, Antsaklis A et al. Biol Neonate 1998;74:72–4.
31. Karl PI, Fisher SE. Am J Physiol 1992;262:C302–8.
32. Schenker S, Hu Z, Johnson RF et al. Alcohol Clin Exp Res 1993; 17:566–75.
33. Hu Z-Q, Henderson GI, Mock DM et al. Proc Soc Biol Exp Med 1994;206:404–8.
34. Mock DM, Mock NI, Langbehn SE. J Nutr 1992;122:535–45.
35. Mock DM, Mock NI, Dankle JA. J Nutr 1992;122:546–52.
36. Mock DM, Stratton SL, Mock NI. J Pediatr 1997;131:456–8.
37. Velazquez A, Martin del Campo C, Baez A et al. Eur J Clin Nutr 1988;43:169–73.
38. Krause K–H, Berlit P, Bonjour J-P. Ann Neurol 1982;12:485–6.
39. Krause K–H, Berlit P, Bonjour J-P. Int J Vitam Nutr Res 1982;52:375–85.
40. Mock DM, Dyken ME. Neurology 1997;49:1444–7.
41. Wang K-S, Mock NI, Mock DM. J Nutr 1997;127:2212–6.
42. Mock DM, Mock NI, Lombard KA et al. J Pediatr Gastroenterol Nutr 1998;26:245–50.
43. Said HM, Redha R, Nylander W. Am J Clin Nutr 1989;49: 127–31.
44. Said HM, Redha R, Nylander W. Am J Clin Nutr 1989;49: 127–31.
45. Zempleni J, Mock DM. Proc Soc Exp Biol Med 2000;223:14–21.
46. Mock DM, Stadler D, Stratton S et al. J Nutr 1997;127:710–6.
47. Mock DM, Stadler DD. J Am Coll Nutr 1997;16:252–7.
48. Mock DM, Quirk JG, Mock NI. Am J Clin Nutr 2002;75: 295–9.
49. Mock DM, Mock NI, Stewart CW et al. J Nutr 2003;133: 2519–25.
50. Watanabe T, Endo A. Teratology 1990;42:295–300.
51. Watanabe T, Endo A. J Nutr 1991;121:101–4.
52. Nisenson A. J Pediatr 1957;51:537–48.
53. Nisenson A. Pediatrics 1969;44:1014–5.
54. Erlichman M, Goldstein R, Levi E et al. Arch Dis Child 1981; 567:560–2.
55. Johnson AR, Hood RL, Emery JL. Nature 1980;285:159–60.
56. Heard GS, Hood RL, Johnson AR. Med J Aust 1983;2:305–6.
57. Livaniou E, Evangelatos GP, Ithakissios DS et al. Nephron 1987; 46:331–2.
58. DeBari V, O. Frank, H. Baker et al. Am J Clin Nutr 1984; 39:410–5.
59. Yatzidis H, Koutisicos D, Agroyannis B et al. Nephron 1984; 36:183–6.
60. Koutsikos D, Fourtounas C, Kapetanaki A et al. Ren Fail 1996; 18:131–7.
61. Descombes E, Hanck AB, Fellay G. Kidney Int 1993; 43:1319–28.
62. Colombo VE, Gerber F, Bronhofer M et al. J Am Acad Dermatol 1990;23:1127–32.
63. Mock NI, Malik MI, Stumbo PJ et al. Am J Clin Nutr 1997;65 :951–8.
64. Mock DM, Henrich-Shell CL, Carnell N et al. J Nutr 2004;134: 317–20.
65. Mock DM, Henrich CL, Carnell N et al. Am J Clin Nutr 2002; 76:1061–8.
66. Mock DM, Henrich CL, Carnell N et al. J Nutr Biochem 2002;13:462–70.
67. Sander JE, Packman S, Townsend JJ. Neurology 1982; 32: 878–80.
68. Suchy SF, Rizzo WB, Wolf B. Am J Clin Nutr 1986;44:475–80.
69. Suchy SF, Wolf B. Am J Clin Nutr 1986;43:831–8.
70. Mock DM. J Pediatr Gastroenterol Nutr 1990;10:222–9.
71. Zempleni J, Mock DM. Arch Biochem Biophys 1999;371:83–8.
72. Zempleni J, Mock DM. Biomol Eng 2000;16:181.
73. Stanley JS, Griffin JB, Zempleni J. Eur J Biochem 2001;268: 5424–9.
74. Rodriguez-Melendez R, Perez-Andrade ME, Diaz A et al. Mol Genet Metab 1999;66:16–23.
75. Rodriguez-Melendez R, Cano S, Mendez ST et al. J Nutr 2001; 131:1909–13.
76. Chauhan J, Dakshinamurti K. J Biol Chem 1991;266:10035–8.
77. Dakshinamurti K, Desjardins PR. Can J Biochem 1968;46: 1261–7.
78. Collins JC, Paietta E, Green R et al. J Biol Chem 1988;263: 11280–3.
79. Mock DM, Said H. Biotin. American Society for Nutritional Sciences Web Site (*n.utrition.org/nutinfo*). Accessed 5/2001.
80. Greene HL, Hambridge KM, Schanler R et al. Am J Clin Nutr 1988;48:1324–42.
81. Hardinge MG, Crooks H. J Am Diet Assoc 1961;38:240–5.
82. Guilarte TR. Nutr Rep Int 1985;32:837–45.
83. Staggs CG, Sealey WM, McCabe BJ et al. J Food Composit Anal 2004 (in press).
84. Hoppner K, Lampi B, Smith DC. Can Inst Food Sci Technol J 1978;11:71–4.
85. Bull NL, Buss DH. Hum Nutr: Appl Nutr 1982;36A:125–9.
86. Lewis J, Buss DH. Br J Nutr 1988;60:413–24.

VITAMIN C[1]

MARK LEVINE, ARIE KATZ, AND SEBASTIAN J. PADAYATTY

HISTORY 507
CHEMICAL PROPERTIES, FORMATION,
    OXIDATION-REDUCTION, AND DEGRADATION 508
BIOCHEMISTRY 509
    General Principles of Vitamin C as
        an Electron Donor 509
    Reductive Functions 510
    Measurement 512
PHYSIOLOGY 512
    General Physiology and Tissue Distribution 512
    Transport and Accumulation 513
    Function In Vivo 514
PHARMACOKINETICS: DEPLETION-REPLETION STUDIES .514
    Plasma Concentrations Are Tightly Controlled
        as a Function of Dose 514
    Mechanisms of Tight Control 514
FUNCTIONAL CONSEQUENCES IN HUMANS 518
    Benefits of Vitamin C Consumption from Foods . .518
    Outcome Studies 518
    Effects in the Gastrointestinal Tract 520
    Genetics 520
    Pharmacologic Doses 520
    Summary: Functions in Relation to Concentration . .520
DEFICIENCY 520
    Scurvy 520
    Treatment and Prevention 521
ADVERSE EFFECTS 521
    Gastrointestinal Tract 521
    Blood 521
    Kidney 521
    Miscellaneous 521
DIETARY REFERENCE INTAKES 521
    Strategies for Deriving Recommendations 521
    Dietary Reference Intake Values for Vitamin C . . .521
    Use in Pregnancy 521
    Use in Disease 522
    Upper Limit 522

---

[1]**Abbreviations: DRI,** dietary reference intake; **EAR,** estimated average requirement; **HPLC,** high-performance liquid chromatography; **K_m,** Michaelis-Menten constant; **LDL,** low-density lipoprotein; **NHANES,** National Health and Nutrition Examination Survey; **NIH,** National Institutes of Health; **RDA,** recommended dietary allowance; **SVCT,** sodium-dependent vitamin C transporter.

Vitamin C (L-ascorbic acid, ascorbate) is a water-soluble micronutrient essential for human health. Vitamin C is synthesized by plants and most animals. Humans and other primates cannot synthesize vitamin C because of the lack of L-gulonolactone oxidase, the terminal enzyme in the biosynthetic pathway of vitamin C from glucose. The gene encoding this enzyme has undergone extensive mutations, and it is estimated to have become nonfunctional millions of years ago in a common primate ancestor (1). As a consequence, humans must obtain vitamin C exogenously, usually from foods. Vitamin C deficiency causes scurvy, a disease with an insidious onset but a fatal outcome unless vitamin C is administered (2, 3). The vitamin C knowledge base has undergone explosive growth since the mid-1990s. This chapter describes vitamin C history, chemistry, and biochemistry and advances in molecular biology, clinical pharmacokinetics, functional consequences, and dietary recommendations.

HISTORY

The earliest descriptions of what probably is scurvy appear in Egyptian hieroglyphs circa 3000 BC, and Hippocrates described the disease in 500 BC (4). Scurvy occurred whenever bodies of men depended on stored rations and had no access to vitamin C–containing foods, such as during military campaigns, ocean voyages, or scientific expeditions. Sixteenth and seventeenth century sailor-explorers described scurvy, its fatal outcome, and its cure with fruits, lime juice, or plant products. Scurvy was common until the nineteenth century, especially in northern latitudes whenever fruits and vegetables were scarce. The disease was endemic in many parts of Europe, and during sea voyages it was so widespread that it was the dread of sailors.

In 1753, James Lind published his *Treatise of the Scurvy*, showing clearly that scurvy was easily treated (2). In clinical experiments at sea, Lind divided 12 patients with severe scurvy into six groups. Each received different treatment, including cider, vinegar, seawater, or citrus fruit. The results unequivocally demonstrated that citrus fruit cured scurvy.

Despite Lind's findings, scurvy deaths continued at sea because the disease was still thought to be caused by additional environmental factors such as cold climate, dampness, lack of fresh air, and foggy weather. Only in 1795, largely through the efforts of the Scottish physician Sir Gilbert Blane, the British Royal Navy made it mandatory to issue an ounce of citrus juice (lemon, and later lime) daily to every sailor after 2 weeks at sea. This provision resulted in the nickname "limey" to denote a British sailor, but it was not enforced until 1804. Sailors in merchant navies continued to develop scurvy until citrus fruit provision became mandatory following the Merchant Shipping Act of 1854.

Unfortunately, scurvy remained widespread during the American Civil War and World War I, and in 1912 it was responsible for the dramatic and tragic end to Robert Scott's expedition to the South Pole. After World War I, research intensified to identify the antiscorbutic principle. Using ox adrenals, oranges, and cabbages, Albert Szent-Gyorgyi in 1928 isolated a six-carbon reducing substance. From 1928 to 1932, the laboratories of Szent-Gyorgyi and C.C. King independently confirmed that this substance was the antiscorbutic principle (5, 6). Albert Szent-Gyorgyi named it ascorbic acid and was awarded the Nobel Prize in 1937.

CHEMICAL PROPERTIES, FORMATION, OXIDATION-REDUCTION, AND DEGRADATION

Vitamin C (L-ascorbic acid, ascorbate) is a six-carbon α-ketolactone weak acid with a pK of 4.2 and a molecular weight of 176 (Fig. 31.1). Plants synthesize vitamin C from glucose and fructose. Vitamin C is abundant in plant leaves and in chloroplasts, and it may have a role in photosynthesis, stress resistance, plant growth, and development (7). Most mammals synthesize vitamin C from glucose in liver, whereas birds, reptiles, and amphibians usually synthesize the vitamin in kidney (1). Vitamin C cannot be synthesized by humans, nonhuman primates, guinea pigs, capybaras, Indian fruit bats, bulbuls, swallows, trout, salmon, and locusts (8). Because these species must ingest ascorbic acid to survive, for them it is a vitamin by definition. Species unable to synthesize vitamin C usually obtain sufficient amounts from plant diets, but they can develop scurvy in captivity when they are fed processed diets that are not adequately supplemented (9).

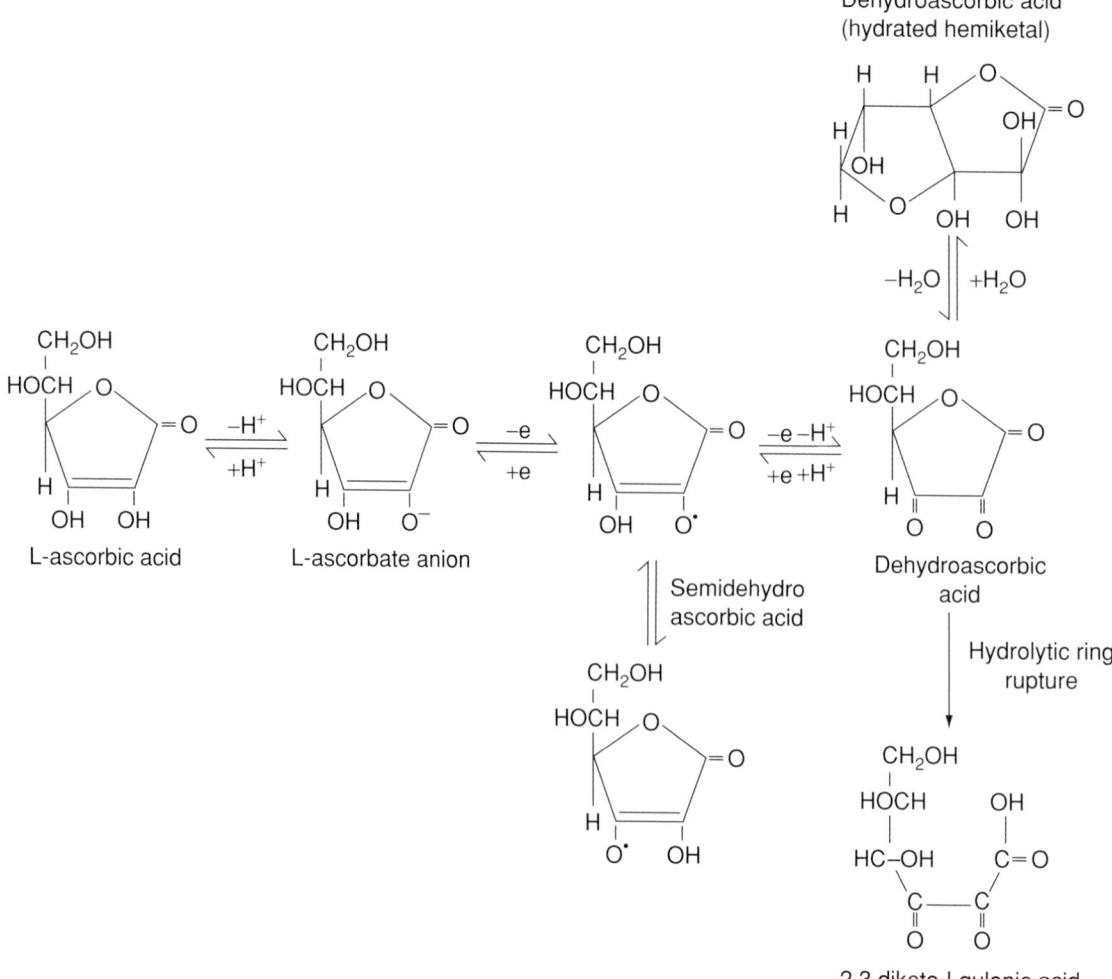

Figure 31.1. Ascorbic acid metabolism. (From Washko PW, Welch RW, Dhariwal KR et al. Ascorbic acid and dehydroascorbic acid analyses in biological samples. Anal Biochem 1992;204:1–14. Reproduced with permission of *Analytical Biochemistry*.)

Vitamin C is an electron donor, or reducing agent (see Fig. 31.1), and its functions are attributable to this action. Vitamin C sequentially donates two electrons from the double bond between carbons two and three. When these electrons are lost, vitamin C is oxidized and another compound is reduced, forestalling oxidation of the reduced compound. Thus, vitamin C is commonly known as an antioxidant.

With loss of the first electron, vitamin C is oxidized to the free radical ascorbyl radical (semidehydroascorbic acid). In comparison with other free radicals, ascorbyl radical is relatively stable and unreactive. Reactive, and therefore possibly harmful, free radicals can be reduced by vitamin C, and the less reactive ascorbyl radical is formed in their place. For these reasons, vitamin C is characterized as a good free radical scavenger, or antioxidant (10). Because of short half-lives, most free radicals cannot be measured directly, and instead they are measured indirectly by using other agents that form radical species with longer half-lives. However, the half-life of ascorbyl radical is long enough to be measurable directly by electron paramagnetic resonance. Ascorbyl radical half-life is dependent on concentration, presence of trace metals, and oxygen, and it can vary from milliseconds to minutes.

Ascorbyl radical is either reversibly reduced to vitamin C or, with loss of the second electron, is oxidized to form the more stable product dehydroascorbic acid (10). Dehydroascorbic acid stability depends on its concentration, temperature, and pH, but it often lasts only minutes (11, 12). Dehydroascorbic acid may exist in one of several different structural forms (13) (see Fig. 31.1). Its dominant form in vivo is uncertain, but it is possible that it is the hydrated hemiketal. Because dehydroascorbic acid is probably not an acid in vivo, the designation "dehydroascorbate" is incorrect. Formation of both ascorbyl radical and dehydroascorbic acid from vitamin C in biologic systems is mediated by oxidants such as molecular oxygen with or without trace metals (iron and copper), superoxide, hydroxyl radical, hypochlorous acid, and reactive nitrogen species.

In biologic systems, dehydroascorbic acid has two fates. One is hydrolysis, with irreversible rupture of the ring to yield 2,3-diketogulonic acid. Although 2,3-diketogulonic acid metabolism is not well characterized, its metabolic products are believed to include oxalate, threonate, xylose, xylonic acid, and lynxonic acid (11). Carbons from vitamin C were reported to be expired as carbon dioxide in animals, but this probably does not occur in humans (14). Of vitamin C metabolites formed by dehydroascorbic acid hydrolysis, oxalate is an end product with clinical significance. Excess oxalate excretion in urine, or hyperoxaluria, can result in oxalate kidney stones in some people. Whether gram doses of vitamin C contribute to hyperoxaluria remains a matter of debate (15, 16).

The second fate of dehydroascorbic acid is reduction, either to ascorbyl radical by one electron or directly to vitamin C by two electrons. Dehydroascorbic acid reduction in biologic tissues can be mediated chemically or by protein-dependent pathways (17, 18). Chemical reduction of dehydroascorbic acid is mediated in vivo by glutathione, with formation of glutathione disulfide. Enzymatic reduction of dehydroascorbic acid is mediated in vivo by an expanding list of proteins acting with another electron donor. At least some proteins mediate reduction substantially faster compared with chemical reduction alone. Regenerating enzymes dependent on reduced nicotinamide adenine dinucleotide phosphate include 3-α-hydroxysteroid dehydrogenase and thioredoxin reductase. Glutathione-dependent regenerating enzymes include glutaredoxin (thioltransferase), protein disulfide isomerase, and dehydroascorbate (sic) reductase, with Michaelis-Menten constants (K_ms) for dehydroascorbic acid ranging from approximately 250 μM to several millimolar. Protein-mediated reduction can result in ascorbate formation without ascorbyl radical as an intermediate, as described for glutaredoxin.

Ascorbyl radical can also be reduced to vitamin C. Although they have not been purified, several reducing activities have been reported in membranes of mitochondria, microsomes, and erthyrocytes. The cytosolic enzyme thioredoxin reductase also reduces ascorbyl radical (19).

In humans, reduction efficiency is only partial for both ascorbyl radical and dehydroascorbic acid. If reduction efficiency were complete, people would not develop scurvy. When vitamin C is removed from diets of healthy persons, they become vitamin C deficient by 30 days, even if they were initially vitamin C saturated (20, 21). Reduction efficiencies in vivo are uncertain, because these clinical data represent a summed measure of both oxidation and reduction rates. Nevertheless, some proportion of formed ascorbyl radical must disproportionate to dehydroascorbic acid, and some dehydroascorbic acid must undergo irreversible hydrolysis. It is possible that reduction efficiency can be regulated in vivo, but such processes are not characterized. For dehydroascorbic acid, the contribution of chemical versus protein-mediated reduction in vivo is also unresolved. In part, this is because of the relatively high K_m of most of the reducing proteins for dehydroascorbic acid, when compared with expected in vivo concentrations of dehydroascorbic acid.

BIOCHEMISTRY

General Principles of Vitamin C as an Electron Donor

Vitamin C is often called an outstanding antioxidant because of its reduction potential (redox potential) as an electron donor, taking into account anticipated concentrations in vivo. Under standard chemical conditions, the reduction potential of the couple dehydroascorbic acid/vitamin C is approximately +0.06 volt (11). Reduction potentials are based on the Nernst equation (22):

$$E = E° + \frac{R\,T}{n\,F} \quad \ln \frac{[\text{electron acceptor}]}{[\text{electron donor}]}$$

Because vitamin C loses electrons sequentially, with ascorbyl radical as an intermediate, the reduction potential for the dehydroascorbic acid/ascorbic acid couple is the sum of the dehydroascorbic acid/ascorbyl radical and ascorbyl radical/ascorbic acid couples. Under standard conditions, the redox potential of the couple ascorbyl radical/ascorbic acid is approximately +0.3 volt (10, 11). Based only on these redox potentials, ascorbic acid would not appear to be a good reducing agent. However, standard reduction potentials are measured assuming that each member of the redox pair is at 1 molar concentration, pH 7, at 25°C. Varying concentrations of each species are taken into account by the Nernst equation for calculating reduction potentials, and these can change when concentrations of electron donor and acceptor are different. Under physiologic concentrations, predicted concentrations are ascorbic acid >> dehydroascorbic acid >> ascorbyl radical. Using such estimates, the ascorbyl radical/ascorbic acid and the dehydroascorbic acid/ascorbyl radical redox potentials become favorable for reduction of many oxidizing compounds (10, 11).

In addition to its redox potential, other properties of ascorbic acid make it an excellent biochemical electron donor. After one electron loss, the product ascorbyl radical is relatively harmless under physiologic conditions because it is relatively nonreactive and reacts poorly with oxygen, producing little if any superoxide (10). Some of the fully oxidized product dehydroascorbic acid is reduced by cells back to ascorbic acid, as described earlier, which then becomes available for reuse (12).

Reductive Functions

Enzymatic Functions

Vitamin C is an electron donor for 11 enzymes (23, 24), three of which are in fungi and are involved in reutilization pathways for pyrimidines or the deoxyribose moiety of deoxynucleosides. In mammals, vitamin C is a cofactor for eight different enzymes that are either monooxygenases or dioxygenases (Table 31.1). The monooxygenases dopamine β-monooxygenase and peptidyl glycine α-monooxygenase incorporate a single oxygen molecule into a substrate, either dopamine for norepinephrine synthesis or a peptide with a terminal glycine for peptide amidation. The remaining enzymes are dioxygenases, which incorporate molecular oxygen (O_2), but with each oxygen atom incorporated in a different way (23, 24). Three different dioxygenase enzymes add hydroxyl groups to the amino acids proline or lysine in the collagen molecule, to stabilize its triple helix structure (25). Two different dioxygenase enzymes require

vitamin C in the biosynthetic pathway of carnitine, necessary for fatty acid transport into mitochondria for adenosine triphosphate synthesis (26). The remaining dioxygenase participates in tyrosine metabolism. Scurvy in part is perhaps the result of impaired function of these enzymes, with some scurvy signs attributed to impaired collagen synthesis (27).

Nonenzymatic Functions

Vitamin C as an Antioxidant In Vitro. Vitamin C may have nonenzymatic functions resulting from its redox potential and/or free radical intermediate. In vitro evidence suggests that vitamin C has a role as a chemical reducing agent both intracellularly and extracellularly (see Table 31.1) (28–40). Because in many tissues vitamin C achieves millimolar concentrations, it may prevent intracellular protein oxidation (35). Such protection could be relevant in tissues with high oxidant production and/or oxygen concentration, such as neutrophils, monocytes, macrophages, lung, and tissues of the eye exposed to light (41).

Extracellular vitamin C may protect against oxidants and oxidant-mediated damage. In vitro studies suggest that vitamin C may be the primary antioxidant in plasma for quenching aqueous peroxyl radicals as well as lipid peroxidation products (36, 42). In vitro, vitamin C is preferentially oxidized before other plasma antioxidants such as uric acid, tocopherols, and bilirubin. Vitamin C is a potent water-soluble antioxidant in biologic systems and may be advantageous because of the relative stability of the intermediate ascorbyl radical under physiologic conditions.

In vitro, extracellular vitamin C affects several pathways involved in atherogenesis. Vitamin C as an antioxidant can decrease lipid peroxidation and protect extracellular low-density lipoprotein (LDL) from metal catalyzed oxidation (36, 42, 43). Oxidized LDL has been postulated to be an initiating factor in atherogenesis, as described in the oxidative modification hypothesis (44). Vitamin C concentrations greater than 40 μM inhibit metal catalyzed LDL oxidation in vitro (42, 43). Vitamin C as a water-soluble antioxidant can regenerate oxidized α-tocopherol (vitamin E) as a lipid-soluble antioxidant added to liposomes in vitro (45). Because tocopherol also prevents LDL oxidation in vitro, (43) recycling of oxidized tocopherol by vitamin C was hypothesized to play a central role in prevention of atherosclerosis. Unfortunately, animal and clinical evidence to date has not supported a role for tocopherol recycling in vivo (46, 47).

Extracellular vitamin C could have other effects as an antioxidant. Vitamin C decreases adhesion of monocytes to endothelium and aggregation of platelets and leukocytes (48). Extracellular vitamin C may quench oxidants that leak from activated neutrophils (12) or macrophages that, in turn, may damage supporting tissues such as collagen or surrounding fibroblasts (49). As

TABLE 31.1. FUNCTION OF VITAMIN C[a]

		COFACTOR FOR ENZYMES
KNOWN ROLES	ENZYME	FUNCTION OF ENZYME (REFERENCE)
	Mammalian	
	Dopamine β–monooxygenase	Norepinephrine biosynthesis (28)
	Peptidyl-glycine α–amidating monooxygenase	Amidation of peptide hormones (29)
	Prolyl 4-hydroxylase	Collagen hydroxylation (25)
	Prolyl 3-hydroxylase	
	Lysyl hydroxylase	
	Trimethyllysine hydroxylase	Carnitine biosynthesis (26)
	γ-Butyrobetaine hydroxylase	
	4-hydroxyphenylpyruvate dioxygenase	Tyrosine metabolism (30)
	Fungi	
	Deoxyuridine 1'-hydroxylase	Reutilization pathways for pyrimidines or
	Thymine 7-hydroxylase	the deoxyribose moiety of deoxynucleosides (31)
	Pyridine deoxyribonucleoside 2' hydroxylase	
		REDUCING AGENT
	SITE	ACTION
	Small intestine	Promote iron absorption (32)
		ANTIOXIDANT
POSTULATED ROLES	SITE	ACTION
	Cells	Regulate gene expression and mRNA translation, prevent oxidant damage to intracellular proteins (33–35)
	Plasma	Quench aqueous peroxyl radicals and lipid peroxidation products (36)
	Stomach	Prevent formation of N-nitroso compounds (37)
		PROOXIDANT
	TARGET	EFFECT
	DNA	DNA damage (38)
	Lipid hydroperoxidase	Decomposition of lipid peroxidase leading to DNA damage (39)
	Ascorbyl radical targets	Cell damage (40)

[a] Known (enzymatic) and postulated (nonenzymatic) functions of vitamin C. The basis of the postulated functions is that vitamin C is a reducing agent, but under certain conditions it may be a prooxidant. Postulated functions have been demonstrated in vitro, but supporting in vivo data are sparse.

Adapted from Padayatty SJ, Daruwala R, Wang Y et al. Vitamin C: molecular actions to optimum intake. In: Cadenas E, Packer L, eds. Handbook of Antioxidants. 2nd ed. New York: Marcel Dekker, 2002:117–145, with permission of Marcel Dekker Inc, New York.

discussed later, extracellular vitamin C in the intestinal lumen may keep iron reduced, may facilitate iron absorption, and may quench reactive oxidants in stomach and duodenum.

Caution is necessary in extrapolating extracellular reducing reactions in vitro involving vitamin C to animals and humans (41). Reactions in vitro may not specifically require vitamin C as an antioxidant in vivo, and the type or concentration of the oxidant selected for use in vitro may not be relevant in vivo. Iron or copper can be added exogenously to produce oxidation in vitro, and these may also be present as contaminants in trace amounts in cell culture media and thereby initiate oxidation. In vivo, copper and iron are tightly bound to proteins and may not be available to oxidize vitamin C. Moreover, in vivo conditions are quite different from the conditions necessary for metal-catalyzed LDL oxidation in vitro, which requires free copper or iron and relatively long lag periods for oxidation induction.

Other Cell Functions. In cell systems in vitro, vitamin C has other intracellular functions that are not known to be enzymatically mediated. Vitamin C has been reported to regulate gene transcription or mRNA stabilization for the following genes: collagen types I and III, elastin, acetylcholine receptor, fra-1, AP-1, some forms of cytochrome P450, tyrosine hydroxlase, collagen integrins, and some ubiquitins (18). The mechanism of these effects is controversial. For example, the effect on collagen gene transcription may be an artifact resulting from vitamin C–mediated generation of lipid hydroperoxides in cell culture media (50). Vitamin C may regulate mRNA translation (51) and may also stabilize intracellular tetrahydrobiopterin, thereby enhancing endothelial nitric oxide synthesis (52).

Potential Functions as a Prooxidant. Other than its action with enzymes as a required electron donor, vitamin C action to lose electrons may not be specific. Vitamin C has been shown to have prooxidant actions in vitro, either by decomposition of lipid hydroperoxides or by increasing 8-oxo-adenine in DNA (38, 39). The relevance of these systems to in vivo physiology is unclear, because the vitamin C concentrations in these studies were not truly physiologic, the in vitro conditions were not representative of in vivo physiology, or experimental artifact may have complicated interpretation of the measurements. In vivo data do not support a prooxidant effect of physiologic concentrations of vitamin C (21). At pharmacologic concentrations, vitamin C is a prooxidant in vitro, but it is unclear whether this is an experimental artifact or has clinical relevance via ascorbyl radical (40, 53).

Measurement

Before 1980, ascorbic acid was measured by reacting it to form derivatives that were quantitated using colorimetric or spectrophotometric techniques. Ascorbic acid, dehydroascorbic acid, and 2,3-diketogulonic acid were detected by these methods. Their advantages are that they do not require sophisticated instruments, they can be set up relatively easily, and they do not require specialized operator training. For ascorbic acid, the disadvantages are interference from many compounds, nonspecificity for other reductants, relatively limited sensitivity especially at low concentrations, and sample instability. With these techniques, dehydroascorbic acid and 2,3-diketogulonic acid measurements have similar limitations and also are especially vulnerable to overestimation artifact. Spectrophotometric and colorimetric assays for ascorbic acid and dehydroascorbic acid have been widely used since the 1940s. Because these assays are still used, their limitations must be remembered (54, 55).

Since 1980, more sophisticated separation and detection methods have been applied to ascorbic acid measurement. One of the most useful assay techniques blends high-performance liquid chromatography (HPLC), for separation, to one of several detection systems. Common detectors are based on flow-by electrochemistry (amperometry), flow-through electrochemistry (coulometry), ultraviolet detection, and fluorescence detection. These methods must still solve the problems of sensitivity, specificity, interferences, and sample instability. The method class that solves these problems best, and is probably the most powerful, is HPLC with electrochemical detection. Disadvantages of this method are high equipment cost and the need for a trained operator. Other techniques for ascorbic acid measurement include enzymatic assay, capillary electrophoresis, and microdialysis (54, 55).

Unlike ascorbic acid, dehydroascorbic acid measurements remain problematic. Dehydroascorbic acid cannot be directly and sensitively detected using electrochemistry or spectrophotometry. Derivatization assays continue to be tried, sometimes by coupling HPLC (for separation) and a detection system. Unfortunately, these assays are frequently compromised by the derivatization procedures themselves, unknown sample stability, potential for high values owing to alteration of equilibrium between ascorbic acid and dehydroascorbic acid, and insufficient sensitivity. In addition, the availability and use of pure standards, which are best prepared fresh from ascorbate, are inconsistent. Dehydroascorbic acid is currently detected indirectly, by ascorbate sample measurements before and after reduction. Dehydroascorbic acid is calculated as the difference between reduced and unreduced samples. Because dehydroascorbic acid seems to be present, if at all, in many biologic samples as a small percentage of ascorbate, a large number is usually subtracted from a large number (56). As a consequence, indirect reduction assays have an increased chance of artifact error and are of limited value. An ideal dehydroascorbic acid has remained elusive, and new assays are needed (54, 55).

PHYSIOLOGY

General Physiology and Tissue Distribution

Absorbed vitamin C reaches the liver through the hepatic portal venous system. It is unknown what percentage of portal venous vitamin C passes directly through the liver sinusoidal system and what percentage is transported into hepatocytes and resecreted into the hepatic vein. Beyond the hepatic vein, vitamin C appears in the general circulation not bound to any proteins. As discussed further later, in blood ascorbic acid is either the dominant or only chemical species (56). If the oxidized form dehydroascorbic acid is present in blood, it is only in trace amounts. In the kidney, vitamin C is freely filtered through glomeruli and is reabsorbed in the proximal collecting tubule. When reabsorptive mechanisms are saturated, the remaining vitamin C is excreted as such in urine.

From blood, vitamin C is presumed to distribute freely in the extracellular space as a water-soluble micronutrient and is thereby available for cell transport. The vitamin is accumulated by many human tissues (Table 31.2) (57, 58). As an approximate conversion, 1 g of tissue can be considered equal to 1 mL internal volume. Using this conversion, the data in Table 31.2 show that vitamin C is accumulated by almost all tissues against a concentration gradient. Concentration gradients range from a minimum of approximately two- to fivefold to a maximum of approximately 100-fold for pituitary and adrenal. A notable exception is red blood cells, one of the few cell types in which the internal concentration is less than the plasma concentration. Because many of these measurements were performed before advent of HPLC assays, there may be some absolute quantitative inaccuracies compared with more recent measurements. Many samples were postmortem specimens, likely resulting in underestimated absolute

TABLE 31.2. VITAMIN C CONTENT OF HUMAN TISSUES[a]

ORGAN/TISSUE	VITAMIN C CONCENTRATION	ORGAN/TISSUE	VITAMIN C CONCENTRATION
Pituitary gland	40–50	Lungs	7
Adrenal gland	30–40	Skeletal muscle	3–4
Eye lens	25–31	Testes	3
Liver	10–16	Thyroid	2
Brain	13–15	Cerebrospinal fluid	3.8
Pancreas	10–15	Plasma	0.4–1
Spleen	10–15	Saliva	9.07–0.09
Kidneys	5–15		

[a] Ascorbic acid content of human tissues (mg/100 g of wet tissue, mg/100 mL for fluids) (57, 58). Values given are approximate and may vary with ascorbic acid intake, age, and possibly disease state.

Adapted from Hornig D. Ann NY Acad Sci 1975;258:103–18, with permission of the New York Academy of Sciences, New York.

values. Nevertheless, the data can be compared relatively, and they show that vitamin C is widely accumulated.

It is uncertain why almost all cells, tissues, and organs accumulate vitamin C in millimolar concentrations. For some cells and tissues, the potential role of the vitamin seems reasonably clear, as a specific enzyme cofactor. In the adrenal medulla, vitamin C appears to be a cofactor for norepinephrine biosynthesis from dopamine. Especially in pituitary and perhaps in pancreas, the main function of vitamin C may be as a cofactor for amidation of peptide hormones. In fibroblasts, osteoblasts, and chondrocytes, vitamin C may function as a cofactor for proline and lysine hydroxylation, and it may perhaps regulate collagen or elastin gene transcription. In other cells and tissues, vitamin C has postulated roles that have been incompletely characterized, often involving antioxidant action as an electron donor. Such cells and tissues include neutrophils, monocytes, lens, retina, cornea, peripheral and central neurons, liver, pancreas, skeletal muscle, and endothelial cells. In others cells and tissues, including lymphocytes, platelets, adrenal cortex, testis, and ovary, the purpose of accumulated vitamin C is unknown.

Transport and Accumulation

Ascorbic acid is accumulated intracellularly by two distinct pathways: transport as ascorbate and ascorbate recycling. In the former, ascorbic acid itself is transported by one of two known sodium dependent transporters, termed SVCT1 and 2 (sodium-dependent vitamin C transporter) (59, 60). These two transporters are in the nucleobase transporter superfamily and are dissimilar to other sodium-dependent transporters. SVCT1 is found in intestine, liver, and kidney and is an epithelial cell transporter. It has a K_m of approximately 100 to 200 μM and an apparent maximum velocity of approximately 1 mM, consistent with expected vitamin C concentrations from foods in the intestinal lumen. These kinetics properties are also consistent with the concentrations expected in the portal venous system and in the proximal renal tubule, although direct measurements of these concentrations are not available. SVCT2 is the tissue transporter and is widely distributed.

It has an apparent K_m of approximately 5 to 10 μM and an apparent maximum velocity of approximately 60 to 100 μM. These values are within the range observed in humans, as described later. Both transporters are sodium and energy dependent and do not transport dehydroascorbic acid.

The second mechanism for ascorbate accumulation in cells is ascorbate recycling. In this pathway, external ascorbic acid is oxidized to dehydroascorbic acid, which is then transported by facilitated glucose transporters and immediately reduced to ascorbic acid intracellularly (12). Glucose transporters 1 to 4 have been reported to transport dehydroascorbic acid, and the affinity of dehydroascorbic acid is equal to or more than that for glucose. Dehydroascorbic acid reduction may be mediated by glutathione and/or reducing proteins, as described earlier.

The dominant mechanism that drives vitamin C accumulation in vivo is still unresolved. Data from SVCT2 knockout mice show that sodium-dependent transport is the dominant mechanism of ascorbate accumulation in these animals (61). Other investigators propose that ascorbate recycling, the process of dehydroascorbic acid transport with intracellular reduction, may be the dominant pathway (62). A reasonable interpretation of the evidence is that ascorbate recycling is dependent on substrate availability, meaning dehydroascorbic acid availability. Although not completely certain given assay variability, it is likely that little or no dehydroascorbic acid is present in blood and plasma (56). Dehydroascorbic acid would have to form locally for ascorbate recycling to occur. This mechanism may be relevant for cells such as neutrophils that generate diffusible oxidants, so that extracellular ascorbic acid will be oxidized to dehydroascorbic acid. To determine the dominant mechanism of vitamin C accumulation in vivo, compounds are needed that are accumulated by one, but not both, mechanisms.

It is probable that other vitamin C transporters exist that have not been isolated or identified as vitamin C transporters. Such transporters are expected to mediate vitamin C efflux from cells. After vitamin C is transported, it must exit intestinal cells for transit to the mesenteric vein and renal tubule cells for reabsorption into the circulation. In addition, vitamin C has been reported to be released by the adrenal, ovary, testes, stomach, and brain (63–67). Because vitamin C is a charged molecule at physiologic pH and is not diffusible, transmembrane transport should be protein mediated. The relevant proteins remain to be identified.

Function in Vivo

Vitamin C function in vivo, other than to prevent gross deficiency, remains something of a puzzle. Nearly all tissues concentrate vitamin C, including many that lack enzymes known to require it, a finding implying that vitamin C must have other uncharacterized functions. Our knowledge of the eight vitamin C–dependent enzymes in vivo and the other nonenzymatic functions discussed earlier is still rudimentary. For example, some vitamin C functions are described simply with or without added vitamin C in vitro, but with no further characterization. It is attractive to think of vitamin C as a critical antioxidant or electron donor in vivo, but conclusive evidence is lacking. Because vitamin C is essential for life, a minimum amount must always be present. What are missing are experiments that characterize vitamin C concentration-dependent function in living cells. Such experiments may be thought of as kinetics in situ for vitamin C–dependent functions, whether enzymatic or nonenzymatic. Such kinetics were proposed to be one basis of recommended nutrient intake (9, 28). As part of determining dietary reference intakes, vitamin concentration function relationships are now sought for vitamin C and other vitamins, by the National Academy of Sciences (16). Although difficult to obtain, such data are essential for ideal intake recommendations.

PHARMACOKINETICS: DEPLETION-REPLETION STUDIES

Plasma Concentrations Are Tightly Controlled as a Function of Dose

To determine how vitamin C doses affect vitamin C concentrations, human depletion-repletion studies have been the study design of choice. Plasma vitamin C has been measured because samples are readily available, measurements should reflect extracellular concentrations, the vitamin is not protein bound, and dehydroascorbic acid is either not present or is at levels lower than detection limits (56).

Depletion-repletion studies have been conducted using either outpatient or inpatient designs. We will not review outpatient studies because true vitamin C consumption was uncertain, and this variable can be controlled in inpatients. In inpatient studies in prisoners, physical signs of scurvy were prevented by 10 mg/day of vitamin C, and body stores prevented scurvy for less than 6 weeks (3, 68, 69). Although for many years these data were the basis of vitamin C recommended dietary allowances (RDAs), the data were limited by an imprecise vitamin C assay, a diet that probably was deficient in other nutrients, a small number of subjects, and a narrow dose range.

Two inpatient depletion-repletion studies that addressed these concerns were conducted at the National Institutes of Health (NIH) using healthy men and women (20, 21). These studies are described in detail because they provide comprehensive dose-concentration data using modern assays, and some results were used to calculate vitamin C dietary reference intakes (DRIs). Seven men and 15 women were studied as inpatients for 5 to 7 months. Their diet had less than 5 mg/day of vitamin C, and it was supplemented to prevent other nutrient deficiencies. The diet caused depletion to a plasma concentration of 7 to 8 μM in 4 weeks in all subjects. Repletion followed and was designed to determine fasting steady-state plasma concentrations for daily oral vitamin C doses of 30, 60, 100, 200, 400, 1000, and 2500 mg. During repletion, subjects were given one dose until steady state was reached for that dose, and only then was the dose increased in sequence. Fasting steady-state plasma vitamin C was defined as five or more consecutive measurements in which plasma vitamin C concentrations in samples were obtained over at least 7 days with an SD of less than 10%. At steady state for each dose, bioavailability studies were performed as described later, samples were obtained for vitamin C measurements and isolation of neutrophils, other white blood cells were harvested by means of apheresis, and 24-hour urine samples were collected for vitamin C and metabolites. Subjects were then given the next higher dose of vitamin C, and the sampling sequence was repeated for each of the vitamin C doses. Pure vitamin C was administered in water in the fasting state.

The depletion-repletion design and plasma values from 15 women are shown in Figure 31.2. Every fasting steady-state calculation for every subject can be displayed as a function of dose for men and women (Fig. 31.3). At doses less than or equal to 100 mg/day, a steep sigmoidal relationship existed between dose and plasma concentration, and small dose changes produced large plasma concentration changes. At doses less than or equal to 100 mg/day, women achieved a higher fasting steady-state plasma concentration than men, for uncertain reasons. At doses greater than or equal to 400 mg/day, fasting steady-state plasma concentrations were 70 to 80 μM, and they increased little with higher doses. These data show that vitamin C plasma concentrations are tightly controlled as a function of oral dose in both sexes. Underlying mechanisms include intake, intestinal absorption, tissue distribution, utilization, and renal reabsorption and excretion, and these mechanisms are discussed next.

Mechanisms of Tight Control

Intake

Food Sources of Vitamin C. Fruits and seeds act as sink organs for plant ascorbate (7) (Table 31.3). Vitamin C is labile, and its content in plant foods may vary depending on season, transportation, shelf time, storage, and

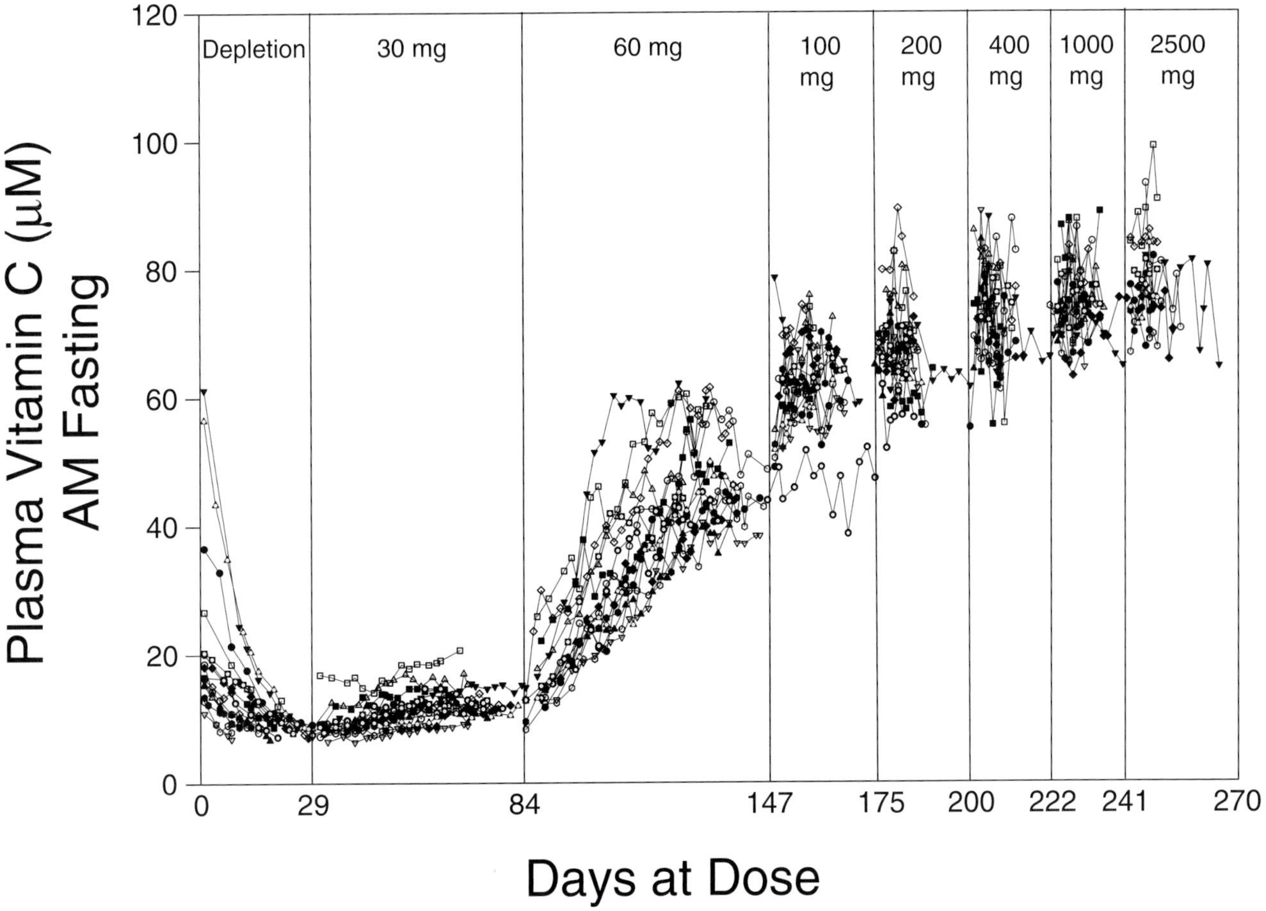

Figure 31.2. Fasting plasma vitamin C concentrations as a function of dose for 15 healthy women. Subjects consumed a vitamin C–deficient diet, resulting in plasma and tissue vitamin C depletion. Vitamin C in solution was then administered by mouth at the doses shown until steady state was reached for each dose. (From Levine M, Wang Y, Padayatty SJ et al. A new recommended dietary allowance of vitamin C for healthy young women. Proc Natl Acad Sci USA 2001;98:9842–6, with permission of the National Academy of Sciences, Washington DC.)

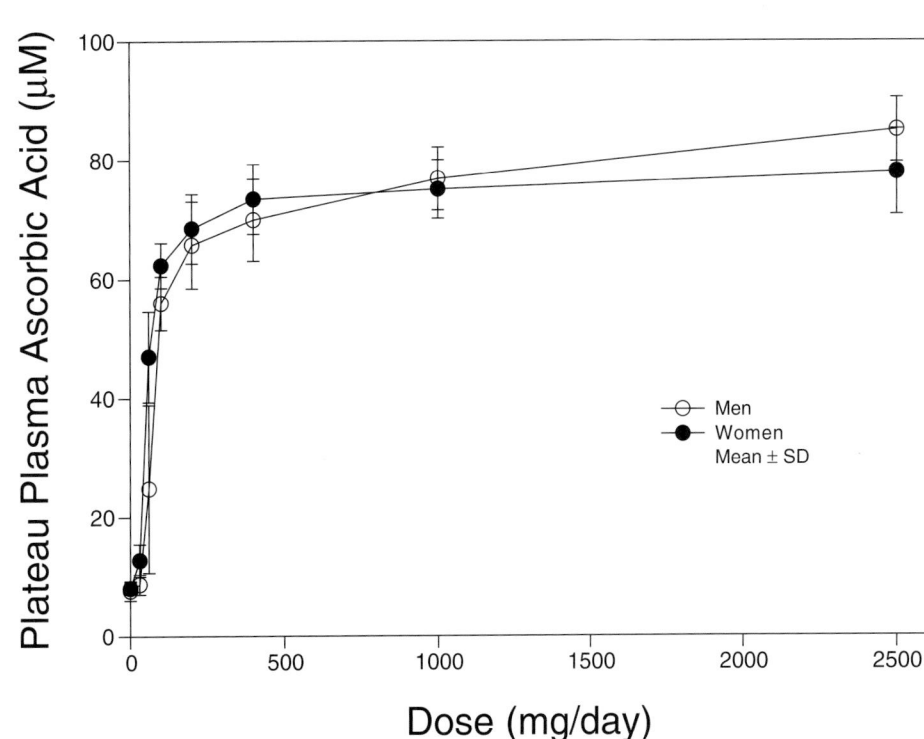

Figure 31.3. The relationship between oral doses of vitamin C and the mean fasting steady-state plasma ascorbic acid concentration in seven healthy men (20) and 15 healthy women (21). The daily doses of vitamin C were 30, 60, 100, 200, 400, 1000, and 2500 mg. The dose concentration curve is sigmoidal, with its steep portion between 30 and 100 mg of vitamin C daily. (Data from Levine M, Conry–Cantilena C, Wang Y et al. Vitamin C pharmacokinetics in healthy volunteers: evidence for a recommended dietary allowance. Proc Natl Acad Sci USA 1996;93:3704–9; and Levine M, Wang Y, Padayatty SJ et al. A new recommended dietary allowance of vitamin C for healthy young women. Proc Natl Acad Sci USA 2001;98:9842–6.)

TABLE 31.3. FOOD SOURCES OF VITAMIN C

SOURCE (PORTION SIZE)	VITAMIN C (mg)	SOURCE (PORTION SIZE)	VITAMIN C (mg)
Fruit		Vegetables	
Cantaloupe (1/4 medium)	60	Asparagus, cooked (1/2 cup)	10
Fresh grapefruit (1/2 fruit)	40	Broccoli, cooked (1/2 cup)	60
Honeydew melon (1/8 medium)	40	Brussels sprouts, cooked (1/2 cup)	50
Kiwi (1 medium)	75	Cabbage	
Mango (1 cup, sliced)	45	Red, raw, chopped (1/2 cup)	20
Orange (1 medium)	70	Red, cooked (1/2 cup)	25
Papaya (1 cup, cubes)	85	Raw, chopped (1/2 cup)	10
Strawberries (1 cup, sliced)	95	Cooked (1/2 cup)	15
Tangerines or tangelos (1 medium)	25	Cauliflower, raw or cooked (1/2 cup)	25
Watermelon (1 cup)	15	Kale, cooked (1/2 cup)	55
		Mustard greens, cooked (1 cup)	35
Juice		Pepper, red or green	
		Raw (1/2 cup)	65
Grapefruit (1/2 cup)	35	Cooked (1/2 cup)	50
Orange (1/2 cup)	50	Plantain, sliced, cooked (1/2 cup)	15
		Potato, baked (1 medium)	25
Fortified juice		Snow peas	
		Fresh, cooked (1/2 cup)	40
Apple (1/2 cup)	50	Frozen, cooked (1/2/ cup)	20
Cranberry juice cocktail (1/2 cup)	45	Sweet potato	
Grape (1/2 cup)	120	Baked (1 medium)	30
		Vacuum can (1 cup)	50
		Canned, syrup-pack (1 cup)	20
		Tomato	
		Raw (1/2 cup)	15
		Canned (1/2 cup)	35
		Juice (6 fluid oz)	35

From Levine M, Rumsey SC, Daruwala R et al. Criteria and recommendations for vitamin C intake. JAMA 1999;281:1415–23, with permission of the American Medical Association.

cooking practices. The US Department of Agriculture and the NIH's National Cancer Institute recommend five servings of fruits and vegetables per day (70), and a wide variety of these should be consumed. This will provide vitamin C intake in the range of 200 to 300 mg/day. Fruit and vegetable consumption restricted to a narrow selection may provide less vitamin C (71). Vitamin C is available as supplement in tablet and powder form, alone or in combination with other vitamins (41).

Intake in the United States. From the third National Health and Nutrition Examination Survey (NHANES III), part 1, from 1988 to 1991, median intake of vitamin C from diet in all men 20 to 59 years old was 85 mg/day and in all women 20 to 59 years old was 67 mg/day, with some variation as a function of race and ethnicity (72). As opposed to median intake, mean intake of vitamin C was somewhat higher, perhaps because of skewing by large-dose supplement users (16). Approximately 37% of men and 24% of women consumed less than 2.5 servings of fruits and vegetables per day (72). Five or more servings were eaten by approximately one fourth of women and less than one fifth of men. Estimated vitamin C intake was lower among some subgroups (15, 72). Some intake data did not take into account vitamin C consumption from supplements, estimated to be used by half of the US population, but it is unclear whether supplements change total vitamin C consumption substantially (73). Data from NHANES III

indicate a small increase in vitamin C ingestion in the United States compared with data from the earlier nutritional survey NHANES II. Nevertheless, 10 to 25% of the US population had mean vitamin C intakes at or below DRI values (16, 41). To summarize, vitamin C is in found in fruits and vegetables, but only a small fraction of the population eats recommended amounts of these vitamin C–rich foods. A more detailed list of foods and their vitamin C content is in Appendix Table A-23-a.

Intestinal Absorption

Bioavailability studies assess intestinal absorption. For vitamin C, most studies determined relative bioavailability, in which bioavailability of two forms of vitamin C was compared. Relative bioavailability data described vitamin C bioavailability from supplements. Supplement bioavailability was dependent on the preparation selected and was affected by binders and dissolution time in the gastrointestinal tract (74).

More valuable, but more difficult to perform, are absolute bioavailability measurements. No data are available to describe absolute bioavailability of vitamin C from foods. Absolute bioavailability of pure vitamin C was determined in the NIH study of healthy men for subjects at steady state. Bioavailability was calculated using either standard area under curve pharmacokinetic analyses or a

TABLE 31.4. BIOAVAILABILITY OF VITAMIN C[a]

DOSE (mg)	METHOD USING AREA UNDER CURVE ANALYSES MEAN (%) (SD)	METHOD USING MULTICOMPARTMENT MATHEMATIC MODEL MEDIAN (%)
15	—	89
30	—	87.3
50	—	58
100	—	80
200	112 (25)	72
500	73 (27)	63
1250	49 (25)	46

[a]Bioavailability of vitamin C in healthy men at steady state for each dose. Vitamin C bioavailability for three doses was calculated using area under curve analyses (20). This method could not be used for doses lower than 200 mg, when vitamin C did not have a constant volume of distribution or a constant rate of clearance (75).

Data from Levine M, Conry-Cantilena C, Wang Y et al. Proc Natl Acad Sci USA 1996;93:3704–9; and Graumlich JF, Ludden TM, Conry-Cantilena C et al. Pharm Res 1997;14:1133–9.

more complex three-compartment model (20, 75). According to convention, bioavailability was expressed as a percentage, with 100% indicating complete absorption. Vitamin C bioavailability was nearly complete at low doses, and it decreased to less than 50% for 1250 mg (Table 31.4). These data show that intestinal absorption contributes to tight control of vitamin C concentrations.

Tissue Distribution

Tight control of plasma vitamin C concentrations could be caused in part by concentration-dependent cell and tissue distribution. Vitamin C tissue transporter SVCT2 is widely distributed and has kinetic properties similar to the range of plasma concentrations in healthy persons (see Fig. 31.3). In healthy persons, only limited samples can be obtained and include the following: neutrophils, monocytes, lymphocytes, and platelets, all of which are blood components; semen and seminal fluid from men; and urine (76, 77).

We describe data from NIH depletion-repletion studies because a wide dose range was used, and vitamin C was measured in neutrophils, monocytes, and lymphocytes in men (20) and additionally in platelets in women (21) (Fig. 31.4). Intracellular vitamin C concentrations increased two- to threefold at doses increased from 30 to 100 mg/day. Cells achieved plateau concentrations before plasma (see Fig. 31.4), consistent with SVCT2 transporter kinetics. Other than the circulating cell data, reliable information on general in vivo tissue distribution with depletion is unavailable. For now, data in circulating cells may be regarded as proxy for concentrations in other tissues.

Utilization

Vitamin C concentrations may be affected by its rate of utilization. In theory, utilization rates may be affected by differences in transporter activity, recycling, enzyme efficiency, and presence or absence of conditions that could accelerate utilization, such as oxidative stress. Accelerated utilization is presumed to account for lower than expected vitamin C concentrations in smokers (78). In healthy persons, utilization rates differ (see Fig. 31.2) (9, 21, 69). They also may increase in disease, based on unexpectedly

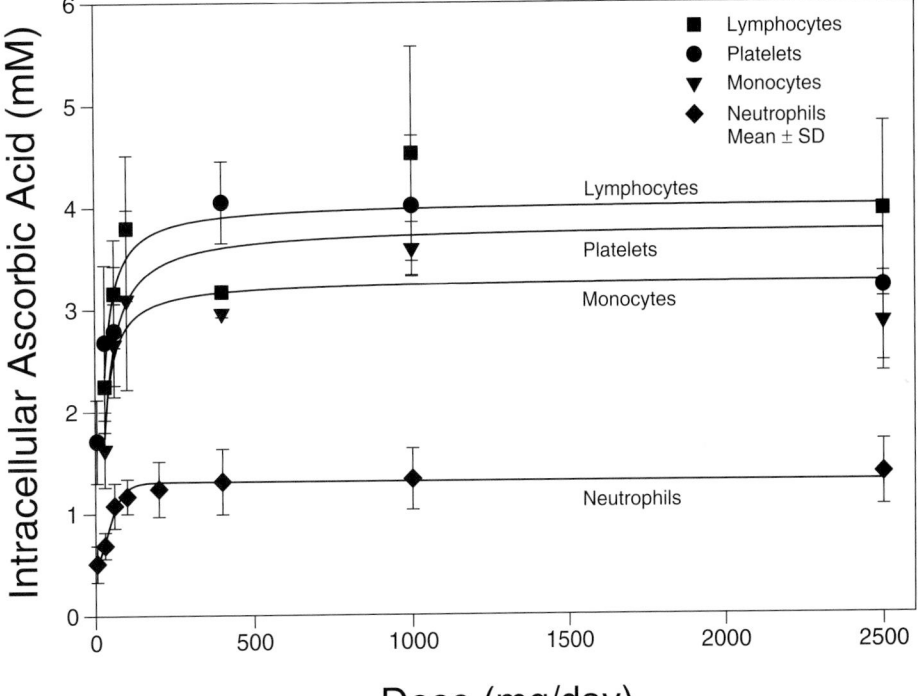

Figure 31.4. Intracellular vitamin C concentrations in circulating cells as a function of dose in healthy women. Cells were isolated when steady-state was achieved for each dose. (From Levine M, Wang Y, Padayatty SJ et al. A new recommended dietary allowance of vitamin C for healthy young women. Proc Natl Acad Sci USA 2001;98:9842–6, with permission of the National Academy of Sciences, Washington DC.)

low plasma vitamin C concentrations in patients with sepsis, critical illness, acute myocardial infarction, diabetes, and pancreatitis (79–82). Although these conditions may be associated with increased oxidants that could oxidize vitamin C, other explanations exist for observed low vitamin C concentrations (83). More research is indicated, because if vitamin C utilization changes in disease, there are clear implications for disease treatment and vitamin C replacement.

Renal Reabsorption and Excretion

In healthy persons, the normal kidney completely reabsorbs some substances (e.g., glucose, amino acids) from the glomerular filtrate. Individual nephrons have limited abilities to absorb specific substances. The upper limit of this ability is the tubular maximum. For substances such as phosphate in which the tubular maximum is within the range of plasma concentrations (84), the kidney has a central role in homeostasis. In the kidney, vitamin C undergoes glomerular filtration and tubular reabsorption. It is presumably freely filtered in the glomerulus and reabsorbed in proximal tubules (85). If a tubular maximum for ascorbic acid could be determined accurately, it would be valuable for intake recommendations.

Specific characteristics and mechanisms of vitamin C reabsorption remain open to interpretation and further investigation. Early experiments revealed that vitamin C reabsorption was never complete. Vitamin C clearance was constant and independent of plasma concentrations less than approximately 65 μM, and a low but steady amount of vitamin C appeared in urine, even at low plasma concentrations (86). Similar findings were reported in an outpatient study (87), but not in other inpatient studies (68, 69). In the NIH studies, no ascorbic acid in urine was detected at steady state for doses less than 100 mg in men and 60 mg in women. Exact threshold data have not been published from the NIH studies. However, the data imply that a true plasma threshold for ascorbic acid excretion exists, that below this threshold no vitamin C is present in urine, and that vitamin C plasma concentrations in humans could straddle a tubular maximum.

Even without a conclusive threshold, we can conclude that the kidney mediates tight control of vitamin C plasma and cell concentrations. In the NIH studies, no vitamin C was excreted at low doses. At higher doses, all the vitamin C administered intravenously or that was absorbed orally was excreted (Fig. 31.5). For example, when 1250 mg of vitamin C was given orally, approximately 600 mg was absorbed and subsequently excreted in the urine. With intravenous administration, which bypasses the confounding effects of intestinal absorption, virtually the entire administered dose was excreted at 500 and 1250 mg. It is unknown whether additional mechanisms, such as active secretion, participate in vitamin C excretion by the kidney.

In patients with end-stage renal disease, vitamin C cannot be excreted because no glomerular filtration occurs, and doses higher than 200 mg can accumulate to produce hyperoxalemia. Conversely, vitamin C is freely dialyzable and is lost during dialysis. Because of concerns of over-replacement, patients with end-stage renal disease who undergo dialysis often have chronically low plasma vitamin C concentrations (15).

FUNCTIONAL CONSEQUENCES IN HUMANS

Benefits of Vitamin C Consumption from Foods

Higher fruit and vegetable consumption and plasma vitamin C concentrations were inversely related to risk of ischemic heart disease, angina pectoris, acute myocardial infarction, stroke, diabetic complications, blood pressure in hypertensive patients, and overall mortality (88–93). Diets with at least 200 mg of vitamin C from fruits and vegetables were associated with lower risk of cancers, especially those of the oral cavity, esophagus, stomach, colon, and lung (94, 95). Based on extensive evidence, recommendations from the US Department of Agriculture and the National Cancer Institute are to consume at least five fruit and vegetable servings daily (70). It is unknown whether benefits of fruit and vegetable intake are the result of vitamin C itself, vitamin C plus other components of fruits and vegetables, or fruit and vegetable components independent of vitamin C (23, 88, 96). Vitamin C may be simply a surrogate marker for fruit and vegetable consumption or, perhaps, for other healthy lifestyle practices. Nevertheless, fruit and vegetable intake should be encouraged to maintain health.

Outcome Studies

Vitamin C from foods plus supplements was investigated for prevention of cancer, cardiovascular disease, stroke, and age-related eye diseases, with conflicting and often disappointing results (41, 97–100). In some observational studies, vitamin C consumption from both food and supplements correlated with reduced mortality (101) and with a lower risk for ischemic heart disease, (97) particularly when subjects had low vitamin C intake (98). In an interventional study, vitamins C plus E supplementation slowed progression of carotid atherosclerosis (102), but a protective effect for atherosclerosis was not observed by many others (41). In large-scale interventional studies, vitamin C was partially obtained from foods but was also consumed in combination with other antioxidant vitamins. Under these conditions, vitamin C did not provide the health benefits seen with fruit and vegetable consumption to prevent cancer or reduce vascular disease (103, 104). Observational data indicated that vitamin C supplementation may prevent cataract, (99) but a large prospective study showed no effect when vitamin C supplements were combined with vitamin E and β-carotene

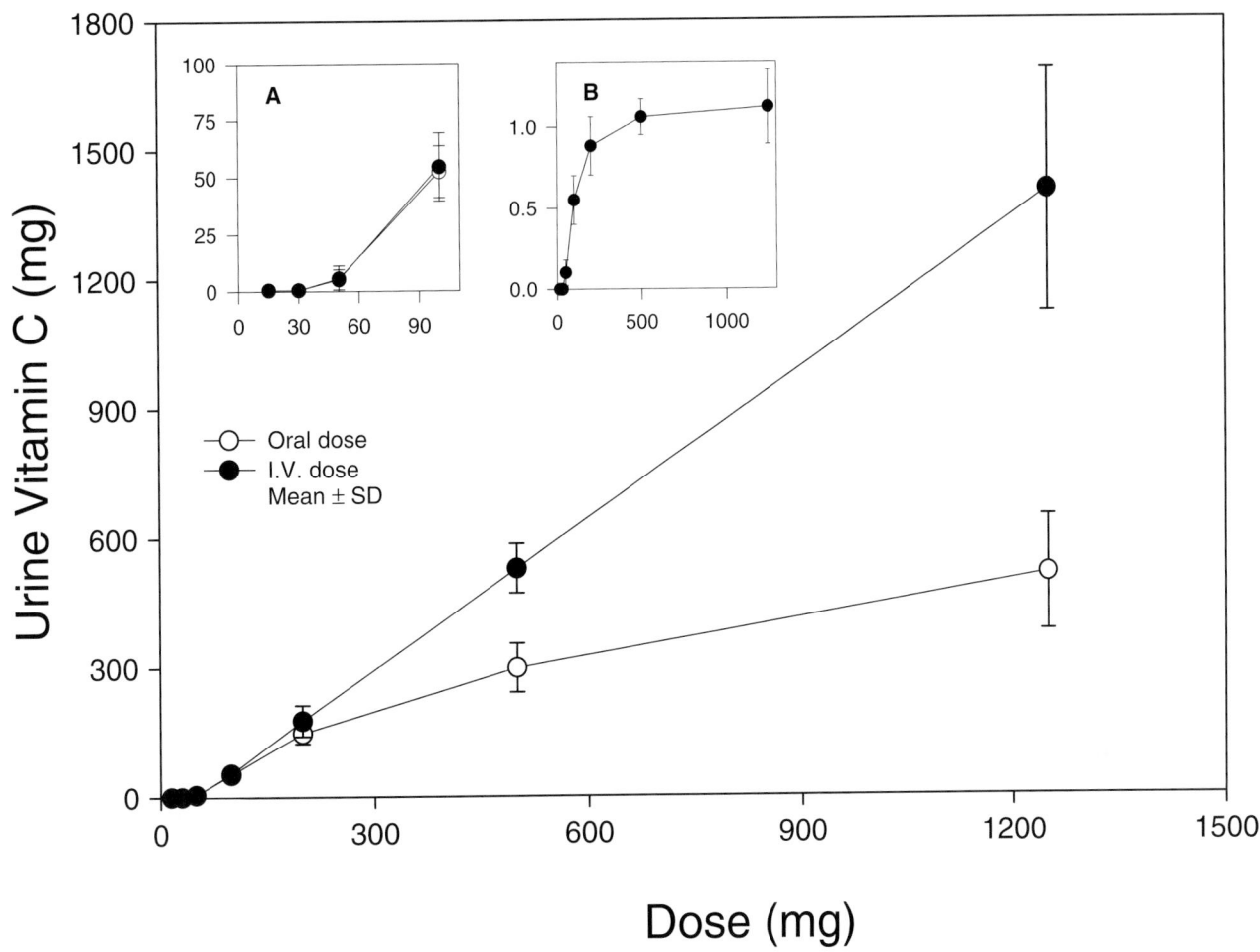

Figure 31.5. Urinary vitamin C excretion as a function of single vitamin C doses at steady state. Vitamin C excretion over 24 hours was determined after administration of single doses given either orally or intravenously. **Inset A.** Vitamin C excretion for single oral or intravenous doses of 15 to 100 mg. X–axis indicates dose, Y-axis indicates amount (milligrams) excreted in urine. **Inset B.** Fractional excretion (the fraction of the dose excreted) after intravenous administration of single doses of vitamin C. X-axis indicates dose, Y-axis indicates fractional excretion (vitamin C excreted in urine in milligrams divided by the vitamin C dose in milligrams). (From Levine M, Wang Y, Padayatty SJ et al. A new recommended dietary allowance of vitamin C for healthy young women. Proc Natl Acad Sci USA 2001;98:9842–6, with permission of the National Academy of Sciences, Washington DC.)

(105). In a large placebo-controlled study, combined supplements of vitamin C, vitamin E, β-carotene and zinc reduced the odds of developing advanced age-related macular degeneration (106). No large-scale interventional studies of disease prevention have been reported in which vitamin C was administered as the sole supplement.

Vitamin C as a supplement was also tested for potential effects on outcome for hypertension, endothelial dysfunction, and respiratory diseases. Vitamin C supplements had a modest effect on lowering blood pressure in some, but not all, subjects (107–109), and no large-scale studies are available. Vitamin C did not alter blood flow in healthy subjects and did not reverse endothelial dysfunction in patients with hypertension (110). Many studies show that vitamin C diminishes endothelial vasomotor dysfunction and induces vasodilatation when it is administered arterially, but intraarterial concentrations are far higher than

those achievable orally. Vitamin C supplements for 3 days potentiate nitroglycerin-induced vasodilatation, but it is unknown whether this effect persists in the long term (111). Vitamin C supplements probably do not prevent acute respiratory infections, except, perhaps, in some people who are vitamin C deficient (112). Vitamin C supplementation added no clinical benefit to care of patients with asthma (113).

Ascorbic acid supplements in a small study were effective in treating pressure sores, (114) although this finding has not been confirmed (115). The original findings may have simply indicated that the control subjects were deficient in vitamin C, and supplementation corrected deficiency. Even though data are scant, vitamin C supplements are used clinically in elderly patients for healing pressure sores, because of low risk, the possibility that the treatment population is deficient in vitamin C, and the difficulty in treating the condition.

Effects in the Gastrointestinal Tract

Vitamin C concentrations in gastric juice are three times higher than those in plasma (116). Vitamin C content is low in gastric juice of patients with atrophic gastritis and *Helicobacter pylori*, and eradication of the bacterium increases gastric vitamin C secretion (117).Vitamin C can potentially quench reactive oxygen metabolites in the stomach and duodenum and can prevent the formation of mutagenic N-nitroso compounds. Whether this has any clinical benefit is not known (37). Although high vitamin C dietary intake correlates with reduced risk of gastric cancer (95), it is unknown whether vitamin C itself or other substances found in vitamin C–rich plant-derived food are responsible for reduced cancer risk. In a population at high risk for gastric cancer, vitamin C supplementation, with and without anti-*Helicobacter pylori* treatment, was associated with regression of precancerous lesions (118). However, a large epidemiologic study showed no association between vitamin C supplementation and reduced mortality from stomach cancer (119).

In the small intestine, vitamin C promotes absorption of iron by keeping it reduced (Fe^{2+}). Vitamin C increased soluble nonorganic iron absorption by 1.5- to tenfold, depending on iron status, the dose of vitamin C, and the type of test meal. Vitamin C amounts of 20 to 60 mg, found in vitamin C–rich foods, enhanced small intestinal iron absorption (32). Iron absorption was usually increased by vitamin C supplementation (32), but its effect on raising hemoglobin concentration was modest (120). Clinically, vitamin C is administered with iron to increase its absorption, especially in pregnancy.

Genetics

It is possible that vitamin C transporters and/or reducing proteins have genetic variations, such as polymorphisms or splice variants, which alter function. Little information has been published to date (121), but insights from the Human Genome Project may facilitate such studies.

Pharmacologic Doses

In young adults, oral single doses of 1.25 g vitamin C produced transient peaks of about 140 μM (20, 21, 40) that returned to baseline within 12 hours. The highest tolerated oral doses ingested every few hours will produce plasma concentrations lower than 220 μM (40). Intravenous administration of vitamin C bypasses the absorptive barrier of the gastrointestinal tract and produces much higher plasma and urine vitamin C concentrations (40, 122). As examples, 1.25 g of intravenous vitamin C produced a peak plasma concentration of 885 μM, and predicted peak plasma concentration after intravenous administration of 10 g is 5580 μM (40). Whether such high plasma concentrations have therapeutic use remains to be established (40, 123).

Summary: Functions in Relation to Concentration

Fruit and vegetable intake is clearly beneficial and should be encouraged to promote health and prevent disease, but it is unknown whether the benefit is the result of vitamin C. When fruit and vegetable intake is excluded, no definitive data indicate that a daily intake of vitamin C itself or a particular vitamin C concentration attained in plasma or tissues results in a clinically beneficial outcome, other than to prevent scurvy (41). Ingestion of five to nine servings of fruits and vegetables will provide 200 to 400 mg of vitamin C, resulting in steady-state fasting plasma concentrations of 70 to 80 μM. It is unclear whether such vitamin C concentrations in vivo enhance a biochemical function or are responsible for changing clinical outcome. The relationships among intake, plasma concentrations, and outcome may be different in health and disease. It is possible that vitamin C utilization (79, 81) or renal loss (124) is increased in disease, and a higher intake may be needed to offset this effect.

DEFICIENCY

Scurvy

The earliest symptoms of scurvy are weakness and lassitude (2). Physical signs include the following: petechial hemorrhage; perifollicular hyperkeratosis; erythema and purpura; bleeding into the skin, subcutaneous tissues, muscles, and joints; coiled hairs; breakdown of wounds; arthralgias and joint effusions; swollen and friable gums; hypochondriasis and depression; Sjögren syndrome; fever; shortness of breath; and confusion (3, 125). Severe scurvy results in loss of teeth, bone damage, internal hemorrhage, and infection. Diagnosis is based on clinical findings and can be confirmed by low plasma vitamin C concentrations. Untreated, scurvy is fatal, and treatment should not be delayed for laboratory confirmation.

Frank scurvy is now rare in industrialized countries, and it occurs primarily in malnourished populations, including those with cancer cachexia and malabsorption, persons with alcoholism, poor and elderly persons whose diet is inadequate, institutionalized persons, drug addicts, and occasionally some persons on idiosyncratic diets (126). Subclinical vitamin C deficiency may be more common, but symptoms are nonspecific and are not easily attributed to lack of vitamin C. Infantile scurvy, or Barlow disease, affects infants and children 6 to 24 months old and is now rare, although it has recently been reported in infants fed an enteral formula (127). Manifestations include irritability, loss of appetite, leg tenderness that may present as pseudoparalysis, hemorrhages, low-grade fever, leg swelling, joint swelling, and gum swelling and discoloration. Scurvy may be confused with rickets because both can present with impaired bone growth (127, 128). Typical roentgenographic changes in the bones, along with clinical findings and a history of inadequate vitamin C intake, establish the diagnosis, confirmed by low plasma vitamin C concentrations.

Treatment and Prevention

Treatment should be initiated with vitamin C 100 mg three times daily. An initial intravenous dose of 100 mg of vitamin C may be given. Children may be given 100 to 200 mg/day either orally or parenterally. If diagnosis and treatment are prompt, permanent damage from scurvy can be prevented. Steady-state plasma concentrations achieved by a vitamin C dose of 60 mg/day will prevent deficiency for 10 to 14 days, and that achieved by 100 mg/day will probably prevent deficiency for approximately 1 month (20, 23).

ADVERSE EFFECTS

Gastrointestinal Tract

Vitamin C is generally safe and well tolerated, with few dose-related side effects (23). Because ingestion of 3 g or more at once can cause diarrhea and bloating, the tolerable upper intake level has been set at 2 g/day (see later). Vitamin C enhances iron absorption from the small intestine. Long-term vitamin C use could increase the risk of iron overload in susceptible patients, such as those with hemochromatosis, thalassemia major, sickle cell disease, sideroblastic anemia, and those who need multiple, frequent red blood cell transfusions (129). Such patients should avoid large doses of vitamin C, but not fruits and vegetables (130). In healthy persons, vitamin C in doses as high as 2 g over 18 months did not induce iron overabsorption (131).

Blood

Glucose-6-phosphate dehydrogenase deficiency is an X-linked inherited disease that may cause hemolytic crises, most often on exposure to oxidant stress. In people with this deficiency, hemolysis was precipitated by vitamin C given intravenously and by single oral doses of at least 6 g (132).

Kidney

Vitamin C doses of 3 g may cause transient hyperuricosuria, but this does not occur at doses lower than 1 g/day. Doses higher than 1 g/day may increase oxalate excretion in those with known or occult hyperoxaluria and may precipitate oxalate kidney stone formation (23). In large-scale studies of healthy people who had no prior history of kidney stones, increased vitamin C consumption from food and supplements did not increase kidney stone formation (133). In patients with renal failure who were undergoing chronic hemodialysis, hyperoxalemia was induced by repeated intravenous vitamin C doses greater than 500 mg. To prevent oxalosis, vitamin C intake in these patients should probably not exceed 200 mg/day (23).

Miscellaneous

Vitamin C, at doses of 250 mg and higher, may cause false-negative results for stool occult blood with guaiac-based tests. Vitamin C intake should be reduced to less than 250 mg for several days before such testing. Several harmful effects have been erroneously attributed to vitamin C, including hypoglycemia, rebound scurvy, infertility, mutagenesis, and destruction of vitamin B_{12} (23).

DIETARY REFERENCE INTAKES

Strategies for Deriving Recommendations

Recommendations for optimum intake of vitamin C ideally should be based on doses that produce good health, and clinical outcome should be shown for different intakes of vitamin C as a component of food. Without such data, other measures may reasonably be expected to reflect outcome. These include dietary availability, steady-state concentrations in plasma in relation to dose, steady-state concentrations in tissue in relation to dose, bioavailability, urinary excretion, adverse effects, biochemical and molecular function in relation to concentration, beneficial effects in relation to dose (direct effects and epidemiologic observations), and prevention of deficiency (23). Recent studies provided data on some of these aspects (20, 21). However, clinical outcome studies are needed to determine the optimal intake of vitamin C in health and disease (134).

Dietary Reference Intake Values for Vitamin C

DRI values for vitamin C were published by the Food and Nutrition Board, Institute of Medicine, US National Academy of Sciences (16). Estimated average requirement (EAR) calculations were based on neutrophil vitamin C concentrations in men, (20) putative vitamin C antioxidant action in neutrophils (135), and urinary vitamin C excretion in men (20), an approach reviewed elsewhere (134). The EAR for men 19 years and older was established as 75 mg/day. Based on body weight differences between genders, requirements for women were extrapolated, and the EAR for women 19 years and older was set at 60 mg/day. RDAs for vitamin C in the United States were calculated from these EAR values, and they were increased from 60 to 90 mg/day for men and to 75 mg/day for women (Table 31.5). Actual rather than extrapolated data for women were available only a year after the release of DRI values (21) and have not been incorporated into these guidelines. (Ed note. The original DRI table did not include data on smokers. The original DRIs are in Appendix Tables A-2-e & A-2-f.)

Use in Pregnancy

Plasma vitamin C concentrations decrease during pregnancy, perhaps secondary to hemodilution, active transfer to the fetus, or increased renal loss. Vitamin C deficiency during pregnancy is associated with increased risk of infection, premature rupture of membranes, premature delivery, and eclampsia. It is unknown whether vitamin C deficiency contributes to these conditions or simply indicates poor nutrition. An increased in intake from 75 mg/day in

TABLE 31.5. DIETARY INTAKE VALUES FOR VITAMIN C[a]

LIFE STAGE	GENDER	AGE (y)	EAR	RDA	AI	UL
Infants (months)		0–6			40	[b]
		7–12			50	
Children	Boys and girls	1–3	13	15		400
		4–8	22	25		650
	Boys	9–13	39	45		1,200
		14–18	63	75		1,800
	Girls	9–13	39	45		1,200
		14–18	56	65		1,800
Adults	Men	19–30	75	90		2,000
		31–0	75	90		
		51–70	75	90		
		>70	75	90		
	Women	19–30	60	75		
		31–50	60	75		
		51–70	60	75		
		>70	60	75		
Pregnancy		14–18	66	80		1,800
		19–30	70	85		2,000
		31–50	70	85		
Lactation		14–18	96	115		1,800
		19–30	100	120		2,000
		31–50	100	120		
Smokers	Men	>19	110	130[c]		
	Women	>19	95	115[c]		

AI, adequate intake; EAR, estimated average requirement; RDA, recommended dietary allowance; UL, tolerable upper intake level.

[a] Dietary reference intake values for vitamin C in milligrams, by life stage and gender.

[b] It is not possible to establish ULs for infants and children, for whom the source of vitamin C intake should be infant formula and food only.

[c] Whereas EARs were stated for smokers, RDAs for smokers were not explicitly documented. We calculated RDAs for smokers based on stated EAR × 1.2.

Modified from Food and Nutrition Board, Institute of Medicine. Dietary Reference Intakes for Vitamin C, Vitamin E, Selenium, and Carotenoids. Washington, DC: National Academy Press, 2000, in Levine M, Padayatty SJ, Katz A et al. Dietary allowances for vitamin C: recommended dietary allowances and optimal nutrient ingestion. In: Asard H, May JM, Smirnoff N, eds. Vitamin C Function and Biochemistry in Animals and Plants. London: BIOS Scientific Publishers, 2004:291–316, with permission of BIOS Scientific Publishers, London.

nonpregnant women to 85 mg/day during pregnancy was recommended based on data that 7 mg/day of vitamin C prevents scurvy in infants (16).

Use in Disease

The Food and Nutrition Board believed that data were insufficient to recommend additional vitamin C other than in pregnant women, lactating women, and smokers.

Upper Limit

The Food and Nutrition Board set the tolerable upper intake level for vitamin C at 2 g/day based on gastrointestinal adverse effects at higher doses (16).

Acknowledgments

We thank Dr. Y. Wang for his help in preparing this manuscript.

REFERENCES

1. Nishikimi M, Yagi K. Subcell Biochem 1996;25:17–39.
2. Lind J. Lind's treatise on scurvy. In: Stewart CP, Guthrie D, eds. Bicentenary Volume. Edinburgh: Edinburgh University Press, 1953.
3. Hodges RE, Hood J, Canham JE et al. Am J Clin Nutr 1971;24:432–43.
4. Clemeston CAB. Classical scurvy: a historical review. In: Vitamin C, vol 1. Boca Raton, FL: CRC Press, 1989:1–10.
5. Svirbely J, Szent-Gyorgyi A. Biochem J 1932;26:865–70.
6. King CG, Waugh WA. Science 1932;75:357.
7. Smirnoff N, Conklin PL, Loewus FA. Annu Rev Plant Physiol Plant Mol Biol 2001;52:437–67.
8. Cueto GR, Allekotte R, Kravetz FO. J Wildl Dis 2000;36:97–101.
9. Levine M. N Engl J Med 1986;314:892–902.
10. Buettner GR. Arch Biochem Biophys 1993;300:535–43.
11. Lewin S. Vitamin C: Its Molecular Biology and Medical Potential. London: Academic Press, 1976:5–39.
12. Wang Y, Russo TA, Kwon O et al. Proc Natl Acad Sci USA 1997;94:13816–9.
13. Tolbert BM, Ward JB. Dehydroascorbic acid. In: Seib PA, Tolbert BM, eds. Ascorbic Acid: Chemistry, Metabolism, and Uses. Washington, DC: American Chemical Society, 1982:101–23.
14. Baker EM, Halver JE, Johnsen DO et al. Ann NY Acad Sci 1975;258:72–80.
15. Levine M, Rumsey SC, Daruwala R et al. JAMA 1999;281:1415–23.
16. Food and Nutrition Board, Institute of Medicine. Dietary Reference Intakes for Vitamin C, Vitamin E, Selenium, and Carotenoids. Washington, DC: National Academy Press, 2000:95–184;420–1.
17. Winkler BS, Orselli SM, Rex TS. Free Radic Biol Med 1994;17:333–49.

18. Arrigoni O, De Tullio MC. Biochim Biophys Acta 2002;1569: 1–9.

19. May JM, Qu Z, Cobb CE. Free Radic Biol Med 2001;31: 117–24.

20. Levine M, Conry-Cantilena C, Wang Y et al. Proc Natl Acad Sci USA 1996;93:3704–9.

21. Levine M, Wang Y, Padayatty SJ et al. Proc Natl Acad Sci USA 2001;98:9842–6.

22. Nelson DL, Cox MM. Lehninger Principles of Biochemistry New York: Worth Publishers; 2000:515.

23. Levine M, Rumsey SC, Daruwala R et al. JAMA 1999;281: 1415–23.

24. Levine M, Rumsey SC, Wang Y et al. Vitamin C. In: Stipanuk MH, ed. Biochemical and Physiological Aspects of Human Nutrition. Philadelphia: WB Saunders, 2000:541–67.

25. Prockop DJ, Kivirikko KI. Annu Rev Biochem 1995;64:403–34.

26. Rebouche CJ. Am J Clin Nutr 1991;54:1147S–52S.

27. Gosiewska A, Wilson S, Kwon D et al. Endocrinology 1994;134: 1329–39.

28. Levine M, Dhariwal KR, Washko PW et al. Am J Clin Nutr 1991;54:1157S–62S.

29. Eipper BA, Milgram SL, Husten EJ et al. Protein Sci 1993;2: 489–97.

30. Lindblad B, Lindstedt G, Lindstedt S. J Am Chem Soc 1970;92: 7446–9.

31. Stubbe J. J Biol Chem 1985;260:9972–5.

32. Hallberg L, Brune M, Rossander-Hulthen L. Ann NY Acad Sci 1987;498:324–32.

33. Hitomi K, Tsukagoshi N. Subcell Biochem 1996;25:41–56.

34. Toth I, Rogers JT, McPhee JA et al. J Biol Chem 1995;270: 2846–52.

35. Stadtman ER, Berlett BS. Chem Res Toxicol 1997;10:485–94.

36. Polidori MC, Mecocci P, Levine M et al. Arch Biochem Biophys 2004;423:109–15.

37. Helser MA, Hotchkiss JH, Roe DA. Carcinogenesis 1992;13: 2277–80.

38. Podmore ID, Griffiths HR, Herbert KE et al. Nature 1998;392:559.

39. Lee SH, Oe T, Blair IA. Science 2001;292:2083–6.

40. Padayatty SJ, Sun H, Wang Y et al. Ann Intern Med 2004;140: 533–7.

41. Padayatty SJ, Katz A, Wang Y et al. J Am Coll Nutr 2003;22: 18–35.

42. Carr AC, Frei B. Am J Clin Nutr 1999;69:1086–107.

43. Jialal I, Fuller CJ. Can J Cardiol 1995;11:97G–103G.

44. Steinberg D. Nat Med 2002;8:1211–7.

45. Niki E. Ann NY Acad Sci 1987;498:186–99.

46. Burton GW, Wronska U, Stone L et al. Lipids 1990;25:199–210.

47. Jacob RA, Kutnink MA, Csallany AS et al. J Nutr 1996;126: 2268–77.

48. Lehr HA, Weyrich AS, Saetzler RK et al. J Clin Invest 1997;99: 2358–64.

49. Nualart FJ, Rivas CI, Montecinos VP et al. J Biol Chem 2003; 278:10128–33.

50. Houglum KP, Brenner DA, Chojkier M. Am J Clin Nutr 1991; 54:1141S–3S.

51. Toth I, Bridges KR. J Biol Chem 1995;270:19540–4.

52. Heller R, Unbehaun A, Schellenberg B et al. J Biol Chem 2001;276:40–7.

53. Clement MV, Ramalingam J, Long LH et al. Antioxid Redox Signal 2001;3:157–63.

54. Levine M, Wang Y, Rumsey SC. Methods Enzymol 1999;299: 65–76.

55. Rumsey SC, Wang Y, Levine M. Ascorbic acid and dehydroascorbic acid analyses in biological samples. In: Song WO,

56. Beecher GR, Eitenmiller RR, eds. Modern Analytical Methodologies on Fat and Water Soluble Vitamins, vol 154. New York: John Wiley and Sons, 2000:411–55.

56. Dhariwal KR, Hartzell WO, Levine M. Am J Clin Nutr 1991; 54:712–6.

57. Hornig D. Ann NY Acad Sci 1975;258:103–18.

58. Voigt K, Kontush A, Stuerenburg HJ et al. Free Radic Res 2002;36:735–9.

59. Daruwala R, Song J, Koh WS et al. FEBS Lett 1999;460:480–4.

60. Tsukaguchi H, Tokui T, Mackenzie B et al. Nature 1999;399: 70–5.

61. Sotiriou S, Gispert S, Cheng J et al. Nat Med 2002;8:514–7.

62. Huang J, Agus DB, Winfree CJ et al. Proc Natl Acad Sci USA 2001;98:11720–4.

63. Lipscomb HS, Nelson DH. Endocrinology 1960;66:144–6.

64. Koba H, Kawao K, Yamashita K. Tohoku J Exp Med 1971;104: 65–71.

65. Musicki B, Kodaman PH, Aten RF et al. Biol Reprod 1996;54: 399–406.

66. Rebec GV, Wang Z. J Neurosci 2001;21:668–75.

67. Schorah CJ, Sobala GM, Sanderson M et al. Am J Clin Nutr 1991;53:287S– 93S.

68. Baker EM, Hodges RE, Hood J et al. Am J Clin Nutr 1969;22: 549–58.

69. Baker EM, Hodges RE, Hood J et al. Am J Clin Nutr 1971;24: 444–54.

70. Lachance P, Langseth L. Nutr Rev 1994;52:266–70.

71. Johnston CS. JAMA 1999;282:2118.

72. Life Sciences Research Office, Federation of American Societies for Experimental Biology, Interagency Board for Nutrition Monitoring and Related Research. Third Report on Nutrition Monitoring in the United States. Report No. 2: VA53 and VA102. Washington, DC: US Government Printing Office, 1995.

73. Block G, Sinha R, Gridley G. Am J Clin Nutr 1994;59:232S–9S.

74. Mayersohn M. J Nutr Sci Vitaminol (Tokyo) 1992;Spec:446–9.

75. Graumlich JF, Ludden TM, Conry-Cantilena C et al. Pharm Res 1997;14:1133–9.

76. Fraga CG, Motchnik PA, Shigenaga MK et al. Proc Natl Acad Sci USA 1991;88:11003–6.

77. Jacob RA, Kelley DS, Pianalto FS et al. Am J Clin Nutr 1991;54:1302S–9S.

78. Alberg A. Toxicology 2002;180:121–37.

79. Bonham MJ, Abu-Zidan FM, Simovic MO et al. Br J Surg 1999;86:1296–301.

80. Riemersma RA, Carruthers KF, Elton RA et al. Am J Clin Nutr 2000;71:1181–6.

81. Long CL, Maull KI, Krishnan RS et al. J Surg Res 2003;109: 144–8.

82. Price KD, Price CS, Reynolds RD. Atherosclerosis 2001;158: 1–12.

83. Padayatty SJ, Levine M. Am J Clin Nutr 2000;71:1027–8.

84. Brenner BM, Rector FC. Brenner & Rector's The Kidney. 7th ed. Philadelphia: WB Saunders, 2004:553–5.

85. Martin M, Ferrier B, Roch-Ramel F. Am J Physiol 1983;244: F335–41.

86. Friedman GJ, Sherry S, Ralli EP. J Clin Invest 1940;19:685–9.

87. Kallner A, Hartmann D, Hornig D. Am J Clin Nutr 1979;32: 530–9.

88. Khaw KT, Bingham S, Welch A et al. Lancet 2001;357:657–63.

89. Gale CR, Ashurst HE, Powers HJ et al. Am J Clin Nutr 2001; 74:402–8.

90. Joshipura KJ, Hu FB, Manson JE et al. Ann Intern Med 2001; 134:1106–14.

91. Voko Z, Hollander M, Hofman A et al. Neurology 2003;61: 1273–5.
92. Sahyoun NR, Jacques PF, Russell RM. Am J Epidemiol 1996; 144:501–11.
93. Baynes J, Thorpe S. Diabetes 1999;48:1–9.
94. Ames B, Gold L, Willett W. Proc Natl Acad Sci USA 1995;92: 5258–65.
95. Byers T, Guerrero N. Am J Clin Nutr 1995;62:1385S–92S.
96. Joshipura KJ, Ascherio A, Manson JE et al. JAMA 1999;282: 1233–9.
97. Osganian SK, Stampfer MJ, Rimm E et al. J Am Coll Cardiol 2003;42:246–52.
98. Nyyssonen K, Parviainen MT, Salonen R et al. BMJ 1997;314:634–8.
99. Jacques PF, Chylack LT, Jr., Hankinson SE et al. Arch Ophthalmol 2001;119:1009–19.
100. Jacobs EJ, Henion AK, Briggs PJ et al. Am J Epidemiol 2002; 156:1002–10.
101. Enstrom JE, Kanim LE, Klein MA. Epidemiology 1992;3: 194–202.
102. Salonen RM, Nyyssonen K, Kaikkonen J et al. Circulation 2003; 107:947–53.
103. Blot WJ, Li JY, Taylor PR et al. Am J Clin Nutr 1995;62: 1424S–6S.
104. Heart Protection Study Collaborative Group. Lancet 2002;360: 23–33.
105. Age Related Eye Disease Study. Arch Ophthalmol 2001;119: 1439–52.
106. Age Related Eye Disease Study. Arch Ophthalmol 2001;119: 1417–36.
107. Duffy SJ, Gokce N, Holbrook M et al. Lancet 1999;354:2048–9.
108. Mullan BA, Young IS, Fee H et al. Hypertension 2002;40: 804–9.
109. Kim MK, Sasaki S, Sasazuki S et al. Hypertension 2002;40: 797–803.
110. Duffy SJ, Gokce N, Holbrook M et al. Am J Physiol 2001;280: H528–34.
111. Bassenge E, Fink N, Skatchkov M et al. J Clin Invest 1998;102: 67–71.
112. Hemila H, Douglas RM. Int J Tuberc Lung Dis 1999;3:756–61.
113. Fogarty A, Lewis SA, Scrivener SL et al. Clin Exp Allergy 2003; 33:1355–9.
114. Taylor TV, Rimmer S, Day B et al. Lancet 1974;2:544–6.
115. ter Riet G, Kessels AG, Knipschild PG. J Clin Epidemiol 1995; 48:1453–60.
116. Rathbone BJ, Johnson AW, Wyatt JI et al. Clin Sci 1989;76: 237–41.
117. Sobala GM, Schorah CJ, Shires S et al. Gut 1993;34:1038–41.
118. Correa P, Fontham ET, Bravo JC et al. J Natl Cancer Inst 2000;92:1881–8.
119. Jacobs EJ, Connell CJ, McCullough ML et al. Cancer Epidemiol Biomarkers Prev 2002;11:35–41.
120. Cook JD, Reddy MB. Am J Clin Nutr 2001;73:93–8.
121. Erichsen HC, Eck P, Levine M et al. J Nutr 2001;131: 2623–7.
122. Padayatty SJ, Levine M. Can Med Assoc J 2001;164:353–5.
123. Du WD, Yuan ZR, Sun J et al. World J Gastroenterol 2003; 9:2565–9.
124. Hirsch IB, Atchley DH, Tsai E et al. J Diabetes Complications 1998;12:259–63.
125. Hood J, Burns CA, Hodges RE. N Engl J Med 1970;282: 1120–4.
126. Anonymous. N Engl J Med 1995;333:1695–702.
127. Gorman SR, Armstrong G, Allen KR et al. J Pediatr Gastroenterol Nutr 2002;35:93–5.
128. Rajakumar K. Pediatrics 2001;108:E76.
129. Nienhuis AW. N Engl J Med 1981;304:170–1.
130. Barton JC, McDonnell SM, Adams PC et al. Ann Intern Med 1998;129:932–9.
131. Cook JD, Watson SS, Simpson KM et al. Blood 1984;64:721–6.
132. Rees DC, Kelsey H, Richards JD. BMJ 1993;306:841–2.
133. Gerster H. Ann Nutr Metab 1997;41:269–82.
134. Levine M, Padayatty SJ, Katz A et al. Dietary allowances for vitamin C: recommended dietary allowances and optimal nutrient ingestion. In: Asard H, May JM, Smirnoff N, eds. Vitamin C: Function and Biochemistry in Animals and Plants. London: BIOS Scientific Publishers, 2004:291–316.
135. Anderson R, Lukey PT. Ann NY Acad Sci 1987;498:229–47.

SELECTED READINGS

Asard H, May JM, Smirnoff N, eds. Vitamin C Function and Biochemistry in Animals and Plants. London: BIOS Scientific Publishers, 2004.

Carr AC, Frei B. Toward a new recommended dietary allowance for vitamin C based on antioxidant and health effects in humans. Am J Clin Nutr 1999;69:1086–107.

Food and Nutrition Board, Institute of Medicine. Dietary reference intakes for vitamin C, Vitamin E, Selenium, and Carotenoids. Washington, DC: National Academy Press, 2000.

Levine M, Rumsey SC, Daruwala R et al. Criteria and recommendations for vitamin C intake. JAMA 1999; 281:1415–23.

Padayatty SJ, Katz A, Wang Y et al. Vitamin C as an antioxidant: evaluation of its role in disease prevention. J Am Coll Nutr 2003; 22:18–35.

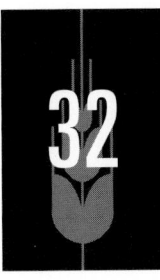

32   CHOLINE AND PHOSPHATIDYLCHOLINE[1]

STEVEN H. ZEISEL AND MIHAI D. NICULESCU

DIETARY SOURCES OF CHOLINE 526
METABOLISM 526
   Intestinal Absorption 526
   Increased Availability of Choline to Tissues
     during the Perinatal Period 528
   Uptake of Choline by Tissues 528
   Tissue Distribution and Transformation 528
   Methyl Group Transfer .528
   Phosphatidylcholine Biosynthesis 530
BIOCHEMICAL AND PHYSIOLOGIC CONSEQUENCES
   OF CHOLINE DEFICIENCY 531
CHOLINE AND THE DEVELOPING BRAIN 531
CHOLINE AND NEURONAL FUNCTION IN ADULTS 532
CARCINOGENESIS 533
CHOLINE AND EPIGENETIC CHANGES
   IN GENE EXPRESSION 533
HUMAN CHOLINE DEFICIENCY 533
SUMMARY 533

Choline is a quaternary amine that is widely distributed in foods. It is a dietary component essential for normal function of all cells. Choline ensures the structural integrity and signaling functions of cell membranes; it is the major source of methyl groups in the diet; it directly affects cholinergic neurotransmission; and it is required for lipid transport and metabolism (1). Most choline in the body is found in phospholipids such as phosphatidylcholine and sphingomyelin. Phosphatidylcholine (lecithin) is the predominant phospholipid (>50%) in most mammalian membranes. Although representing a smaller proportion of the total choline pool, important metabolites of choline include platelet-activating factor, acetylcholine, choline plasmalogens, lysophosphatidylcholine, phosphocholine, glycerophosphocholine, and betaine.

First discovered by Strecker in 1862, choline was chemically synthesized in 1866 (2). It was known to be a component of phospholipids, but the pathway for its biosynthesis was first described in 1941 by du Vigneaud (3). The route for its incorporation into phosphatidylcholine was not elucidated until 1956 (4). The importance of choline as a nutrient was first appreciated during the pioneering work on insulin (5). Depancreatized dogs, maintained on insulin, developed fatty infiltration of the liver and died. Administration of raw pancreas prevented hepatic damage; the active component was the choline moiety of pancreatic phosphatidylcholine. In 1935, the association between a low-choline diet and fatty infiltration of the liver in rats was recognized (6). The term "lipotropic" was coined to describe choline and other substances that prevented deposition of fat in the liver. Subsequently, researchers suggested that the liver disease associated with alcoholism could respond to choline therapy. However, few data supported this hypothesis until Lieber and colleagues showed that phosphatidylcholine supplementation prevented fibrosis and fatty liver caused by ethanol ingestion in baboons (7).

In 1975, several laboratories reported that administration of choline accelerated the synthesis and release of the acetylcholine by neurons (8). A revival of interest in choline ensued, resulting in a plethora of publications characterizing the metabolism, physiologic effects, and pharmacology of choline.

Breakdown products of choline phospholipids are molecules that can amplify external signals or that can terminate the signaling process by generating inhibitory second messengers (9, 10). These signals are a matter of life and death for cells. Since the mid-1990s and using both in vivo and in vitro models, we found that choline deficiency activates internal programs for cell suicide called apoptosis (11–14). Apoptosis is involved in normal cell turnover, embryogenesis, and elimination of cancer cells.

Although initially choline was not considered an essential nutrient for humans because an endogenous pathway exists for the de novo biosynthesis of choline (15), today it is accepted that the presence of a pathway for endogenous synthesis does not make it a dispensable nutrient for most animals or humans. Beginning in 1989, several investigators identified choline deficiency syndromes in humans (16–20). In 1998, the US Institute of Medicine's Food and Nutrition Board established an adequate intake (AI) and tolerable upper intake limit (UL) for choline (Table 32.1) (21). The UL for choline (see Table 32.1) was derived

---

[1]**Abbreviations: AI,** adequate intake; **CDP,** cytidine diphosphocholine; **CoA,** coenzyme A; **DRI,** dietary reference intake; **LTP,** long-term potentiation; **SRE,** sterol-responsive element; **TPN,** total parenteral nutrition; **UL,** tolerable upper intake limit; **VLDL,** very-low-density lipoprotein.

TABLE 32.1. DIETARY REFERENCE INTAKE VALUES FOR CHOLINE

POPULATION	AGE	AI	UL
Infants	0–6 mo	125 mg/d, 18 mg/kg	Not possible to
	6–12 mo	150 mg/d	establish[a]
Children	1–3 y	200 mg/dy	1,000 mg/d
	4–8 y	250 mg/d	1,000 mg/d
	9–13 y	375 mg/d	2,000 mg/d
Males	14–18 y	550 mg/d	3,000 mg/d
	≥19 y	550 mg/d	3,500 mg/d
Females	14–18 y	400 mg/d	3,000 mg/d
	≥19 y	425 mg/d	3,500 mg/d
Pregnancy	All ages	450 mg/d	Age-appropriate UL
Lactation	All ages	550 mg/d	Age-appropriate UL

AI, adequate intake; UL, tolerable upper intake limit.
[a] Source of intake should be food and formula only.

From Food and Nutrition Board, Institute of Medicine. Dietary Feference Intakes for Folate, Thiamin, Riboflavin, Niacin, Vitamin B$_{12}$, Panthothenic Acid, Biotin, and Choline, vol 1. Washington, DC: National Academy Press, 1998.

from the lowest observed adverse effect level (hypotension) in humans (21). Information on the definitions and purposes of the dietary reference intakes (DRIs) and DRI data are presented in Appendix Tables A-2-a to A-2-h. At present, clinical studies are under way to refine estimates of human choline requirements.

In this review, we discuss the expected biochemical and physiologic uses for choline and the expected effects of choline deficiency.

DIETARY SOURCES OF CHOLINE

Many of the foods we eat contain significant amounts of choline and esters of choline (22) (Table 32.2). Some of this choline is added during food processing, especially when preparing infant formula (23). In one study, when persons were switched from a diet of normal foods to a defined diet containing little choline, plasma choline and phosphatidylcholine concentrations decreased in most subjects (20). We estimate that persons consuming a free diet ingest approximately 1 g/day of choline in all forms (24). Foods also contain the choline metabolite betaine (22) (see Table 32.2), which cannot be converted to choline but can be used as a methyl donor, thereby sparing choline requirements. Human milk is rich in choline compounds (23), and bioavailability may differ from that in infant formulas (23, 25), which contain different choline compounds. Human milk has a significantly higher phosphocholine concentration, the same or lower glycerophosphocholine concentration, and similar phosphatidylcholine and sphingomyelin concentrations compared with either bovine milk or bovine-derived infant formulas; soy-derived infant formulas have lower glycerophosphocholine and sphingomyelin concentrations and higher phosphatidylcholine concentrations than do either human milk or bovine milk-derived formulas (23) (Fig. 32.1). Where does all this choline in human milk come from? Mammary epithelial cells are capable of concentrative uptake of choline from maternal blood (26). Two uptake processes occur: one is saturable

and obeys Michaelis-Menten kinetics; the other is nonsaturable and linear. Mammary epithelial cells can synthesize choline de novo (27) via phosphatidylethanolamine N-methyltransferase activity; this is the only pathway for synthesis of the choline moiety.

Rat pups denied access to milk have lower serum choline concentrations than do their milk-fed littermates (28). Thus, dietary intake of choline contributes to the maintenance of high serum choline concentrations in the neonate. In lactating women who have a low-choline diet, milk choline content is lower than in women with a more adequate diet (29). Dietary variation causes a fourfold change (comparing the choline-deficient and choline-supplemented diets) in milk phosphocholine content (23, 30). The free choline content of human milk is very high at the start of lactation and diminishes to quantities similar to those in commercial formulas by 30 days post partum (30).

METABOLISM

Intestinal Absorption

The extent to which dietary choline is bioavailable depends on the efficiency of its absorption from the intestine. In adults, some ingested choline is metabolized before it can be absorbed from the gut. Gut bacteria degrade it to form betaine and to make methylamines (31). The free choline surviving these fates is absorbed by the intestine by carrier-mediated transport (1, 32). At this time, no other component of the diet has been identified as competing with choline for transport by intestinal carriers. Both pancreatic secretions and intestinal mucosal cells contain enzymes (phospholipases A$_1$, A$_2$, and B) capable of hydrolyzing phosphatidylcholine in the diet. The free choline that is formed enters the portal circulation of the liver (33).

Infants have differences in the bioavailability of the water-soluble, choline-derived compounds (choline, phosphocholine, and glycerophosphocholine) and the lipid-soluble compounds (phosphatidylcholine and sphingomyelin)

TABLE 32.2. CHOLINE CONTENT OF SOME COMMON FOODS[a,b]

FOOD	CHOLINE	GPCho	PCho	PtdCho	SM	TOTAL CHOLINE	BETAINE
Dairy and Eggs							
Cheese	1.6	2.3	0.6	7.4	4.6	16.5	0.7
Eggs	0.6	0.6	0.6	238.4	10.7	251.0	0.6
Whole milk	3.7	7.5	1.8	0.6	0.6	14.3	0.6
Skim milk	2.8	9.7	1.7	0.7	0.7	15.6	1.9
Meat							
Beef	3.6	3.9	0.5	62.4	7.8	78.2	11.4
Chicken	5.3	1.2	3.4	44.4	11.5	65.8	5.6
Bacon	12.1	14.5	2.7	85.6	10.0	124.9	3.5
Pork	2.2	22.5	1.2	70.5	6.4	102.8	1.6
Atlantic cod	17.7	30.0	1.6	32.9	1.4	83.6	9.6
Salmon	8.6	5.9	1.1	48.0	1.8	65.5	2.1
Cereals and grains							
Wheat germ, toasted	69.2	33.8	4.2	44.9	ND	152.1	1395.0
Wheat bran	50.2	4.4	2.1	17.8	ND	74.4	1505.6
Wheat bread	18.0	4.9	0.3	3.3	ND	26.5	226.5
White bread	6.0	3.3	0.2	2.6	ND	12.2	104.8
Oat Bran	4.4	33.2	0.7	20.2	ND	58.6	35.7
Oats	1.2	1.6	ND	4.5	ND	7.4	3.1
Rice	0.7	0.9	ND	0.4	ND	2.1	0.3
Fruits and fruit products							
Apples	0.3	ND	ND	3.1	ND	3.4	0.1
Bananas	3.2	5.6	0.5	0.4	ND	9.8	0.1
Grapefruit	3.6	1.2	0.3	2.5	ND	7.5	0.1
Grapes	4.8	ND	0.6	0.2	ND	5.6	0.1
Oranges	4.7	1.1	0.5	2.1	ND	8.4	0.1
Vegetables							
Broccoli	8.5	1.3	9.3	21.0	ND	40.1	0.1
Carrots	6.8	0.0	1.1	0.8	ND	8.8	0.4
Cucumber	4.0	0.5	0.9	0.6	ND	6.0	0.1
Peppers	3.6	ND	1.2	0.7	ND	5.5	0.1
Spinach	1.7	ND	1.1	22.0	ND	24.8	725.4
Tomatoes	4.4	ND	1.8	0.5	ND	6.7	0.1
Yellow corn	8.9	0.6	1.7	10.7	ND	22.0	0.2
Peas	2.2	0.8	0.7	23.9	ND	27.5	0.1
Beverages							
White wine	3.6	1.6	ND	ND	ND	5.1	0.1
Brewed tea	0.4	ND	ND	ND	ND	0.4	1.0
Coffee	1.9	0.7	ND	0.0	0.0	2.6	0.1
Legumes and legume products							
Peanuts	17.6	1.3	1.8	31.8	ND	52.5	0.6
Peanut butter	25.0	1.3	1.6	35.1	ND	63.0	0.8
Beans, navy	14.0	0.8	0.6	11.6	ND	26.9	0.1
Soybean	47.3	2.9	1.1	64.6	ND	115.9	2.1
Fast food							
Cheese pizza	6.7	1.4	0.8	4.2	0.9	14.0	25.9
French fries	12.1	3.9	0.8	5.2	0.0	22.1	0.7
Fast food hamburger	5.7	4.5	0.9	20.3	2.8	34.2	33.3
Hot dog and bun	4.5	1.9	0.8	20.7	2.1	30.1	44.3

ND, not detected.

[a] Foods were stored in a glass container at −20°C overnight and then stored at −80°C until analyzed using liquid chromatography-electrospray ionization-isotope dilution mass spectrometry.

[b] Data (mean of duplicate determinations) are presented for choline compounds (mg choline moiety/100 g food). Total choline is the sum of choline, phosphocholine (PCho), glycerophosphocholine (GPCho), phosphatidylcholine (PtdCho), and sphingomyelin (SM) in the food.

From http://www.nal.usda.gov/fnic/foodcomp/Data/Choline/Choline.html (accessed 8-23-04).

present in milk (25) (see Fig. 32.1). Liver tissue metabolizes the glycerophosphocholine ingested in milk differently than it does either choline or phosphocholine. In addition, phosphatidylcholine-derived label is metabolized very differently from other choline esters, with most remaining as phosphatidylcholine in liver and probably incorporated into liver membranes. The various dietary sources of choline available in milk are therefore used differently by liver in the rat pup. Although the data obtained from the rat pup model cannot be directly extrapolated to

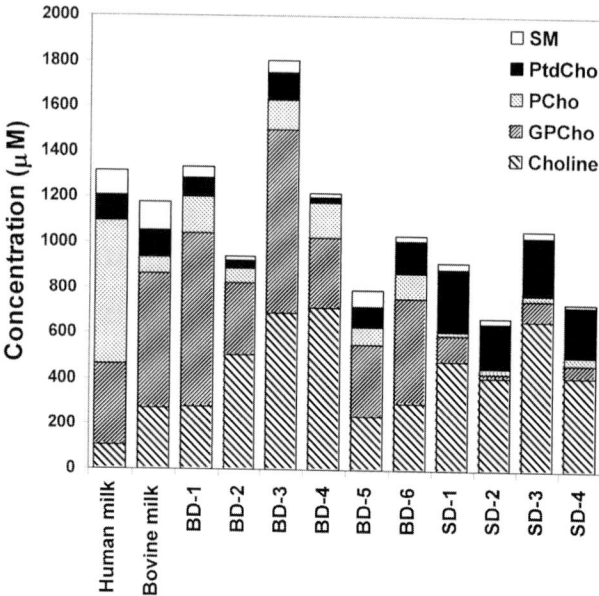

Figure 32.1. Choline in milk and infant formulas. Human milk contains different amounts of choline-containing compounds than do many infant formulas. BD, bovine-derived formula; GPCho, glycerophosphocholine; PtdCho, phosphatidylcholine; PCho, phosphocholine; SD, soy-derived formula (each brand identified with a different number); SM, sphingomyelin;. (Adapted from Holmes-McNary M, Cheng WL, Mar MH et al. Choline and choline esters in human and rat milk and in infant formulas. Am J Clin Nutr 1996;64:572–6, with permission.)

the human infant, these variations in the bioavailability and utilization should be considered when milk substitutes are developed. Human milk serves as a useful model for the safe and effective provision of choline to the neonate from a milk substitutes.

Increased Availability of Choline to Tissues during the Perinatal Period

Large amounts of choline are delivered to the fetus across the placenta, where choline transport systems pump it against a concentration gradient (34). The placenta is one of the few nonnervous tissues to store large amounts of choline as acetylcholine (35). Perhaps this is a special reserve storage pool that ensures delivery of choline to the fetus. In utero, the fetus is exposed to very high choline concentrations, with a progressive decline in blood choline concentration thereafter until adult levels are achieved after the first weeks of life (36). In fact, plasma or serum choline concentrations are six- to sevenfold higher in the fetus and newborn than they are in the adult (28, 37). High levels of choline circulating in the neonate presumably ensure enhanced availability of choline to tissues. Neonatal rat brain efficiently extracts choline from blood (38), and increased serum choline in the neonatal rat is associated with twofold higher choline concentration in neonatal brain than is present later in life. Supplementing choline during the perinatal period further increases choline metabolite concentrations in blood and brain (39).

Uptake of Choline by Tissues

All tissues accumulate choline by diffusion and mediated transport, but uptake by liver, kidney, mammary gland, placenta, and brain is of especial importance (1, 40). A specific carrier mechanism transports free choline across the blood-brain barrier at a rate that is proportional to serum choline concentration, and, in the neonate, this choline transporter has especially high capacity (38, 41). Hepatectomy increases the half-life of choline and results in an increase in blood choline concentration. The rate at which liver takes up choline is sufficient to explain the rapid disappearance of choline injected systemically. The kidney also accumulates choline (42). Some of this choline appears in the urine unchanged, but most is oxidized within the kidney to form betaine (43–46) and glycerophosphocholine (47). Both are important intracellular osmoprotectants within kidney. Mean free choline concentrations in the plasma of azotemic patients are several times greater than in physiologically normal controls (48). Hemodialysis rapidly removes choline from the plasma (49, 50). Clinical renal transplantation lowers plasma choline from 30 μM in the azotemic patient to 15 μM within 1 day (51).

Tissue Distribution and Transformation

Only a small fraction of dietary choline is acetylated (Fig. 32.2), catalyzed by the activity of choline acetyltransferase (8). This enzyme is highly concentrated in the terminals of cholinergic neurons, but it is also present in such nonnervous tissues as the placenta. The availability of choline and acetyl-coenzyme A (CoA) influences choline acetyltransferase activity. In brain, it is unlikely that choline acetyltransferase is saturated with either of its substrates, so choline (and possibly acetyl-CoA) availability determines the rate of acetylcholine synthesis (8). Increased brain acetylcholine synthesis is associated with an augmented release into the synapse of this neurotransmitter (52–54). Choline taken up by brain may first enter a storage pool (perhaps the phosphatidylcholine in membranes) before being converted to acetylcholine (55). The choline phospholipids in cholinergic neurons comprise a large precursor pool of choline available for use in acetylcholine synthesis (56). This may be especially important in neurons with increased demands for choline to sustain acetylcholine release (e.g., when particular cholinergic neurons fire frequently, or when the supply of choline from the extracellular fluid is inadequate).

Methyl Group Transfer

The methyl groups of choline can be made available from one-carbon metabolism, on conversion to betaine (57) (see Fig. 32.2). Formation of betaine involves oxidation to betaine aldehyde in the inner mitochondrial membrane (58) and then the oxidation of betaine aldehyde (catalyzed by betaine aldehyde dehydrogenase or by a nonspecific aldehyde dehydrogenase in the mitochondria and in the

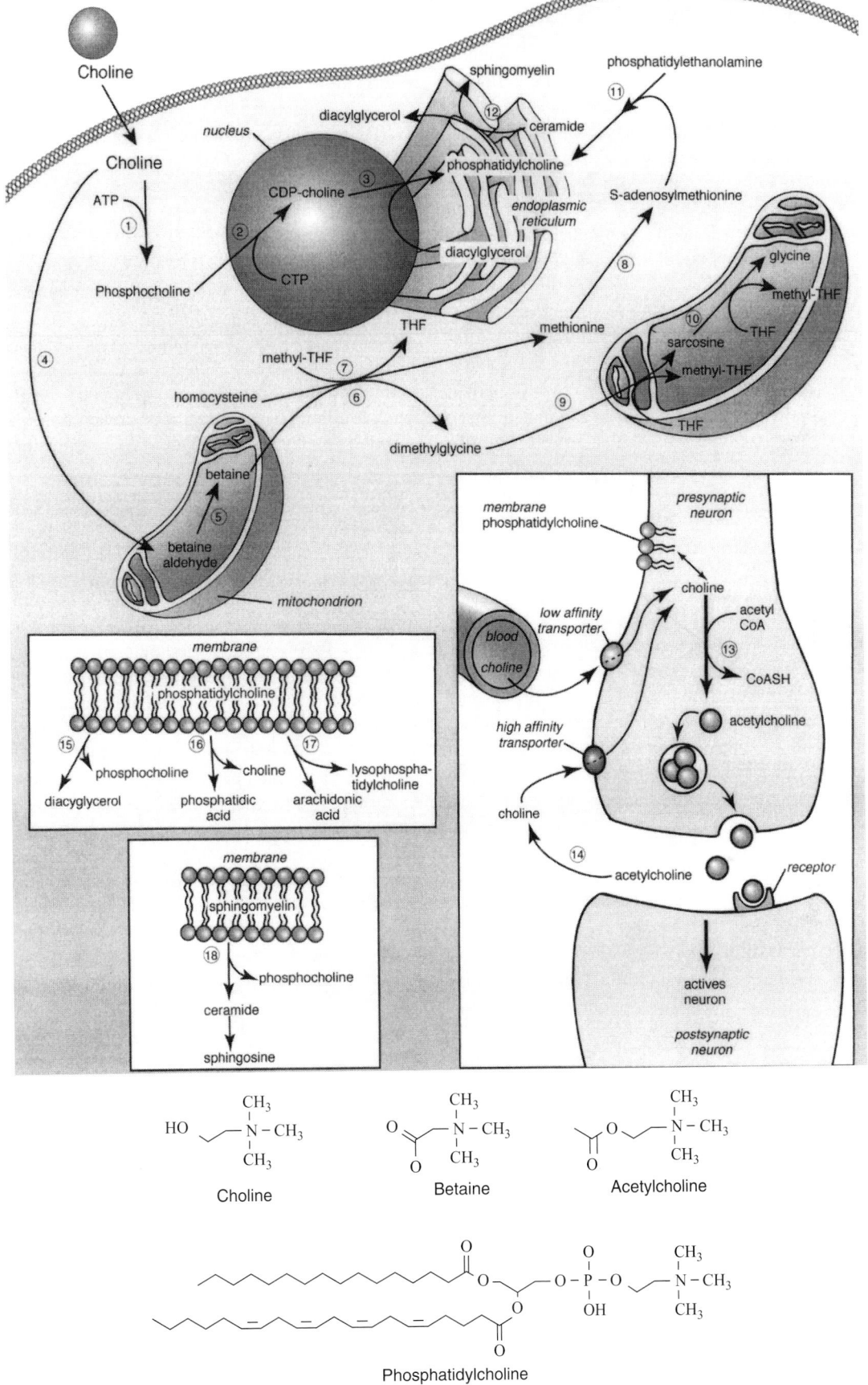

Figure 32.2. Metabolism of choline. The three major metabolic uses for choline are as a precursor for phosphatidylcholine biosynthesis, as a methyl donor, and as a precursor for acetylcholine biosynthesis. ATP, adenosine triphosphate; CDP-choline, cytidine diphosphocholine; CoA, coenzyme A; CoASH, coenzyme A acetylcholine synthesis; CTP, cytidine triphosphate; THF, tetrahydrofolate.

cytosol) to form betaine. Liver and kidney are the major sites for choline oxidation. Betaine cannot be reduced back to choline. Thus, the oxidation pathway acts to diminish the availability of choline to tissues while at the same time scavenging some methyl groups.

The demand for choline as a methyl-group donor is probably the major factor that determines how rapidly a diet deficient in choline will induce pathologic processes. The metabolism of choline, methionine, and methyl-folate is closely interrelated (see Fig. 32.2). The pathways intersect at the formation of methionine from homocysteine. Betaine:homocysteine methyltransferase catalyzes the methylation of homocysteine using the choline metabolite betaine as the methyl donor (59, 60). In an alternative pathway, 5-methyltetrahydrofolate:homocysteine methyltransferase regenerates methionine using a methyl group derived de novo from the one-carbon pool (61). Perturbing the metabolism of one of the methyl donors results in compensatory changes in the other methyl donors as a result of the intermingling of these metabolic pathways (62–66). Rats ingesting a choline-deficient diet showed diminished tissue concentrations of methionine and S-adenosylmethionine (66) and of total folate (63). Methotrexate, which is widely used in the treatment of cancer, psoriasis, and rheumatoid arthritis, limits the availability of methyl groups by competitively inhibiting dihydrofolate reductase, a key enzyme in intracellular folate metabolism. Rats treated with methotrexate have diminished pools of all choline metabolites in liver (67). Choline supplementation reverses the fatty liver caused by methotrexate administration (68–71). Genetically modified mice with defective methylene tetrahydrofolate reductase activity become choline deficient (72), an important observation because many persons have genetic polymorphisms that alter the activity of this enzyme (73, 74). The interrelationship between choline and folate is especially interesting because multiple clinical studies have demonstrated that persons with diminished folate status are much more likely to have babies with neural tube defects (21, 75). A large case control study recently reported that women in the highest quartile for dietary choline and betaine intake, as compared to the lowest quartile), had 25% of the risk for having a baby with neural tube defects (75a). In mice, depletion of choline was associated with development of neural tube defects (76, 77). In addition, the intermingling of choline and homocysteine metabolism is important because increased plasma homocysteine concentration is an independent risk factor for cardiovascular disease (78).

Phosphatidylcholine Biosynthesis

Elegant regulatory mechanisms control phosphatidylcholine biosynthesis and hydrolysis (79, 80). Synthesis occurs by two pathways (see Fig. 32.2). In the first, choline is phosphorylated and is then converted to cytidine diphosphocholine (CDP-choline). This high-energy intermediate, in combination with diacylglycerol, forms phosphatidylcholine and cytidine monophosphate. In the alternative pathway, phosphatidylethanolamine is sequentially methylated to form phosphatidylcholine, using S-adenosylmethionine as the methyl donor.

Choline kinase, the first enzyme in the CDP-choline pathway, has been purified, and its properties are reviewed elsewhere (81). It is a cytosolic enzyme that also catalyzes the phosphorylation of ethanolamine. The next step in the pathway, catalyzed by CTP:phosphocholine cytidylyltransferase, is the rate-limiting and regulated step in phosphatidylcholine biosynthesis (82, 83). A deficient activity of this enzyme in the lungs of prematurely born human infants contributes to the respiratory distress syndrome (84). Cytidylyltransferase is present in the cytosol and in the nucleus (85) as an inactive dimer of two 42-kDa subunits, and in the endoplasmic reticulum, Golgi apparatus, and nuclear envelope as an active membrane-bound form (79). Expression of the CTP:phosphocholine cytidylyltransferase$_\alpha$ gene is inhibited by a sterol-responsive element (SRE) in the promoter activated by cholesterol, 25-hydroxycholesterol, SREBP$_{1a}$, or SREBP$_2$ (86, 87). The state of phosphorylation of cytidylyltransferase and the membrane phosphatidylcholine and diacylglycerol content regulate the reversible translocation of the enzyme between cytosol and membranes (79). Cyclic adenosine monophosphate-dependent protein kinase phosphorylates the enzyme, which then translocates from membranes into the cytosol and becomes inactivated. This process reverses when the enzyme is dephosphorylated by protein phosphatase (88). The phosphatidylcholine content of the membrane also regulates the binding of the enzyme to membranes. Cytidylyltransferases bind to membranes more avidly when their phosphatidylcholine content decreases, whereas the reverse occurs when membrane phosphatidylcholine content increases (89, 90). This may explain why cytidylyltransferase activity increases in choline-deficient hepatocytes (91). Diacylglycerol is also a regulator of cytidylyltransferase. Treatments that increase intracellular diacylglycerol activate cytidylyltransferase (92).

The third enzyme in the CDP-choline pathway (CDP-choline:1,2-diacylglycerol choline-phosphotransferase) is present in the membranes of the endoplasmic reticulum. Its properties are reviewed elsewhere (93). Because it is not the rate-limiting enzyme in the pathway, CDP-choline does not accumulate in significant concentrations within cells. The efficacy of CDP-choline as a treatment for ischemia and memory disorders is currently being tested in clinical trials (94, 95).

The alternative pathway for phosphatidylcholine biosynthesis (through the methylation of phosphatidylethanolamine by phosphatidylethanolamine N-methyltransferase) is most active in liver, but it has also been identified in many other tissues, including brain and the mammary gland

(27, 96, 97). This is the major (perhaps only) pathway for de novo synthesis of the choline moiety in adult mammals. However, plants (98) and perhaps embryonic neurons (from chicken or rat) (99, 100) are capable of methylating phosphoethanolamine to form phosphocholine. Phosphatidylethanolamine-N-methyltransferase is membrane bound, and at least two isoforms exist (101). In adult liver, the availability of phosphatidylethanolamine, the S-adenosylmethionine/S-adenosylhomocysteine concentration ratio, and the composition of the boundary lipids that surround phosphatidylethanolamine-N-methyltransferase regulate its activity. S-adenosylhomocysteine, a product of the reactions, inhibits the methyltransferase. The availability of S-adenosylmethionine in the liver of choline-deficient animals limits the activity of this pathway. The *PEMT* gene is highly polymorphic; 98 single nucleotide polymorphisms were identified in the Japanese population (102), a finding suggesting the possibility of a wide range of variation in the protein structure and perhaps activity. This would have important consequences for human dietary requirements of phosphatidylcholine and choline. Phosphatidylethanolamine-N-methyltransferase (-/-) mice become choline deficient on normal diets, and choline supplementation can restore choline status (103, 104).

BIOCHEMICAL AND PHYSIOLOGIC CONSEQUENCES OF CHOLINE DEFICIENCY

Long-term ingestion of a diet deficient in choline has major consequences that include hepatic, renal, pancreatic, memory, and growth disorders (105). In most animals (except ruminants), choline deficiency results in liver dysfunction. Large amounts of lipid (mainly triglycerides) can accumulate in liver, eventually filling the entire hepatocyte. Fatty infiltration of the liver starts in the central area of the lobule and spreads peripherally. This process is different from that occurring in kwashiorkor or essential amino acid deficiency, in which fatty infiltration usually begins in the portal area of the lobule. Lipid accumulation within hepatocytes begins within hours after rats are started on a choline-deficient diet, peaks within the first 6 months (at >2000 mg/liver; in control rats it was 28 mg/liver) (106), and then diminishes as liver becomes fibrotic. Fatty liver occurs because triacylglycerol must be packaged as very-low-density lipoprotein (VLDL) to be exported from liver, and phosphatidylcholine is required for VLDL formation (107–109). Activation of peroxisome proliferator-activated receptor α (PPARα) receptors decreased the severity of choline deficiency–induced steatosis (110). Choline-deficient persons have diminished plasma low-density lipoprotein cholesterol (derived from VLDL) concentrations (20). This observation is consistent with the hypothesis that in humans, as in other species, choline is required for VLDL secretion.

Renal function is also compromised by choline deficiency (1), with abnormal concentrating ability, free water reab-sorption, sodium excretion, glomerular filtration rate, renal plasma flow, and gross renal hemorrhage. Infertility, growth impairment, bony abnormalities, decreased hematopoiesis, and hypertension have also been reported to be associated with diets low in choline content (1). Pancreatic function can also be compromised in animals fed diets deficient in methyl donor (111).

Females are less sensitive to choline deficiency than are males because estrogen enhances females' capacity to form the choline moiety de novo (112, 113). Pregnancy increases demands for choline significantly, and pregnant rats are as vulnerable to choline deficiency as are males (114). The need for choline is likely to be increased during lactation because so much must be secreted into milk, and the recommended human AI is appropriately increased to 550 mg/day (see Table 32.1).

Choline appears to be needed for normal carnitine transport into tissues (115–118). Choline deficiency is associated with decreased serum and urinary carnitine concentrations (119, 120).

CHOLINE AND THE DEVELOPING BRAIN

Nature has developed mechanisms to ensure that a developing animal receives adequate amounts of choline. As discussed earlier, in mammals the placenta regulates the transport of choline to the fetus. In this regard, choline concentration in amniotic fluid is tenfold greater than that present in maternal blood (Zeisel, unpublished observations). The capacity of brain to extract choline from blood is greatest during the neonatal period. A novel phosphatidylethanolamine-N-methyltransferase in neonatal rat brain is extremely active (97); this enzyme is not present in adult brain. Furthermore, in the brains of newborn rats, S-adenosylmethionine concentrations are 40 to 50 nmol/g of tissue (121), levels probably sufficient to enable the neonatal form of phosphatidylethanolamine-N-methyltransferase to maintain high rates of activity. As previously mentioned, human milk and rat milk provide large amounts of choline to the neonate. The existence of these multiple mechanisms, which ensure the availability of choline to the fetus and neonate, accords with the view that the choline supply must be crucial during this period.

Choline is needed for normal neural tube closure in early pregnancy (76, 77), and maternal dietary choline supplementation and choline deficiency during late pregnancy were associated with significant and irreversible changes in hippocampal function in the adult animal, including altered long-term potentiation (LTP) (122–124) and altered memory (125–130). More choline (about four times dietary levels) during days 11 to 17 of gestation in the rodent increased hippocampal progenitor cell proliferation (131, 132), decreased apoptosis in these cells (131, 132), enhanced LTP in the offspring when they were adult animals (122–124), and enhanced visuospatial and auditory memory by as much as 30% in the adult animals throughout their lifetimes

(125–127, 129, 130, 133, 134). Indeed, adult rodents have decrements in memory as they age, and offspring exposed to extra choline in utero do not show this "senility" (127, 133). Mother rodents fed choline-deficient diets during late pregnancy have offspring with diminished progenitor cell proliferation and increased apoptosis in fetal hippocampus (131, 132), insensitivity to LTP when they were adult animals (124), and decrements in visuospatial and auditory memory (130). The effects of perinatal choline supplementation on memory were initially found using radial-arm maze tasks and the Sprague-Dawley rat strain. However, other laboratories found similar results by using other spatial memory tasks, such as the Morris water maze (135, 136) and by using other strains of rats such as Long-Evans (137–139), and mice (140 and Williams, personal communication). Thus, choline deficiency during a critical period in pregnancy causes lifelong deficits in memory.

The mechanism whereby a choline supplement supplied to the dam results in a permanent change in memory of its offspring has not been elucidated. Although the initial hypothesis was that the effect of neonatal choline supplementation on memory is mediated by increased brain choline with subsequent increased acetylcholine release, the amounts of choline that accumulate in fetal brain after treatment of the pregnant dam are not of sufficient magnitude to enhance acetylcholine release (39). Rather, supplementing choline to dams results in significantly greater accumulation of phosphocholine and betaine in fetal brain than in fetuses of controls (39). Evidence indicates that these effects may occur via epigenetic mechanisms (see later).

Whether these findings in rodents apply as well to humans is not known. Of course, human and rat brains mature at different rates, with rat brain comparatively more mature at birth than the human brain. The architecture of the human hippocampus continues to develop after birth, and by 4 years of age it closely resembles adult structure (141). This area of brain is one of the few which nerve cells continue to multiply slowly throughout life (142, 143). Are we varying the availability of choline when we feed infant formulas instead of milk? Do the form and amount of choline ingested contribute to variations in memory observed among different persons? All are good questions that are worthy of additional research.

CHOLINE AND NEURONAL FUNCTION IN ADULTS

As discussed earlier, choline accelerates the synthesis and release of acetylcholine in nerve cells (8, 52, 53, 144–146). A specific carrier mechanism transports free choline across the blood-brain barrier at a rate that is proportional to serum choline concentration (41, 147). Phosphatidylcholine may be carried into neurons as part of an apolipoprotein E lipoprotein (148, 149). Choline derived from phosphatidylcholine may be especially important when extracellular choline is in short supply, as could be expected to occur in advanced age because of decreased brain choline uptake in older adults (150). Abnormal phospholipid metabolism in Alzheimer disease (151) results in reduced levels in brain (at autopsy) of phosphatidylcholine, phosphatidylethanolamine, choline, and ethanolamine and in increased levels of glycerophosphocholine and glycerophosphoethanolamine. For these reasons, choline and phosphatidylcholine have been used to treat neurologic disorders.

Mice and rats exhibit an age-related loss of memory function. In adult animals, long-term low dietary intake of choline exacerbated this memory loss, whereas choline-enriched diets diminished memory loss (152). Young choline-deficient mice performed as poorly as much older mice, whereas choline-supplemented older mice performed as well as young 3-month-old mice. Supplemented mice did have changes in the shape (more dendritic spines) of their neurons in the hippocampus (153). In a replicate experiment by these investigators, more modest effects were noted when 2.7 times normal dietary choline was added to drinking water of mice for 4 months starting at age 8.5 months. These treatments occurred after the memory centers of brain underwent most of their growth and development. No equivalent human studies have been reported. Studies have been performed on the effects of short-term administration of choline or lecithin on the memory of physiologically normal persons, and the results reported vary. In a double-blind study using physiologically normal college students, 25 g of phosphatidylcholine caused significant improvement in explicit memory, as measured by a serial learning task; this improvement could have resulted from the improved responses of slow learners (154). A single oral 10-g dose of choline chloride given to physiologically normal volunteers significantly decreased the number of trials needed to master a serial-learning word test (155). The precursor for formation of phosphatidylcholine, CDP-choline, also has been tested for its memory-enhancing effects. In a randomized, double-blind, placebo-controlled study, volunteers were treated with CDP-choline, 1000 mg/day, or placebo for 3 months. CDP-choline improved immediate and delayed logical memory (156). In a second study, oral administration of CDP-choline (500–1000 mg/day) for 4 weeks in elderly persons with memory deficits but without dementia resulted in improved memory in free recall tasks, but not in recognition tests (157). In a double-blind study, patients with early Alzheimer-type dementia were treated with 25 g/day phosphatidylcholine for 6 months. Modest improvements were observed compared with placebo in several memory tests (158, 159). Studies were also conducted in which choline's effect on memory was not observed in physiologically normal persons (160–162) or in patients with dementia (163–165).

CARCINOGENESIS

Choline is the only single nutrient for which dietary deficiency causes development of hepatocarcinomas in the absence of any known carcinogen (166). Choline-deficient rats not only have a higher incidence of spontaneous hepatocarcinoma, but also they are markedly sensitized to the effects of administered carcinogens (166). Choline deficiency is therefore considered to have both cancer-initiating and cancer-promoting activities.

Several mechanisms are suggested for the cancer-promoting effect of a choline-devoid diet. A progressive increase in cell proliferation that is related to regeneration after parenchymal cell death occurs in the choline-deficient liver (167, 168). Cell proliferation and its associated increased rate of DNA synthesis could be the cause of the heightened sensitivity to chemical carcinogens. Methylation of DNA is essential to the regulation of expression of genetic information, and the undermethylation of DNA observed during choline deficiency (despite adequate dietary methionine) may be responsible for carcinogenesis (169–172). Choline-deficient rats experience increased lipid peroxidation in liver (173, 174). Lipid peroxides in the nucleus are a possible source of free radicals that could modify DNA and cause carcinogenesis. Choline deficiency activates protein kinase C signaling (106, 175), usually involved in growth factor signaling in hepatocytes. Finally, a defect in cell suicide (apoptosis) mechanisms may contribute to the carcinogenesis of choline deficiency (176).

CHOLINE AND EPIGENETIC CHANGES IN GENE EXPRESSION

The disparate effects of choline in the diet may be mediated by changes in the expression of genes. Dietary choline deficiency not only depletes choline and choline metabolites in rats, but also decreases S-adenosylmethionine concentrations (66, 177), with resulting hypomethylation of DNA (178, 179). DNA methylation occurs at cytosine bases that are followed by a guanosine (CpG sites) (180), and it influences many cellular events, including gene transcription, genomic imprinting, and genomic stability (181–183). In mammals, about 60 to 90% of 5'-CpG-3' sites are methylated (184). When this modification occurs in promoter regions, gene expression is altered (185); increased methylation is associated with gene silencing or reduced gene expression (184). In choline-deficient cells in culture, methylation of the *CDKN3* gene promoter was decreased, resulting in overexpression of this gene (186). In choline-deficient liver, hypomethylation of specific CCGG sites occurred within several genes for which mRNA levels were increased, including c-*myc*, c-*fos* and c-Ha-*ras* (170). Hypomethylation of CpG sites and c-*myc* gene overexpression occurred in hepatocellular carcinomas induced by a choline-deficient diet in rats (179). It is also reasonable that maternal diet during pregnancy could alter the methylation

status of fetus. Feeding pregnant Pseudoagouti Avy/a mouse dams a choline methyl-supplemented diet altered epigenetic regulation of agouti expression in their offspring, as indicated by increased agouti/black mottling of their coats (187, 188). This change in the phenotype is the result of the metastability of a specific transposable element (when methylated), which is the cause of this epigenetic variation, rather than the direct influence of methylation on *agouti* gene expression (189). Whatever the exact mechanism, it becomes clear that the dietary manipulation of methyl donors (either deficiency or supplementation) can have a profound impact on gene expression and, by consequence, on the homeostatic mechanisms that ensure the normal function of physiologic processes.

HUMAN CHOLINE DEFICIENCY

We require dietary choline, and the AI is approximately 550 mg/day in men; the UL is 3 g/day (21) (see Table 32.1). As discussed earlier, normal diets likely deliver sufficient choline. Healthy men with normal folate and vitamin B_{12} status who have a choline-deficient diet have diminished plasma choline and phosphatidylcholine concentrations, and they develop liver damage, evidenced by elevated plasma alanine aminotransferase (20); they may also have muscle damage, as shown by elevated creatine phosphokinase (190). Studies of choline requirements in women, children, or infants have not been conducted. Thus, we do not know whether choline is needed in the diet of these groups. Women may need less dietary choline because of enhanced endogenous biosynthesis (113), but pregnancy and lactation require large amounts of choline, and likely increase the requirement for this nutrient (114).

Hepatic complications associated with total parenteral nutrition (TPN), which include fatty infiltration of the liver and hepatocellular damage, have been reported by many clinical groups. Frequently, TPN must be terminated because of the severity of the associated liver disease. Amino acid–glucose solutions used in human TPN contain no choline. The lipid emulsions used to deliver extra calories and essential fatty acids during TPN contain choline in the form of phosphatidylcholine (20% emulsion contains 13.2 mmol/L). Some of the liver disease associated with TPN is related to choline deficiency and is prevented with supplemental choline or phosphatidylcholine (18, 19, 191–193). Thus, choline seems to be an essential nutrient during long-term TPN.

SUMMARY

Choline is crucial for sustaining life. It modulates the basic signaling processes within cells, is a structural element in membranes, and is vital during critical periods in brain development. Choline metabolism is closely interrelated with the metabolism of methionine and folate. Although the normal human diet provides sufficient choline to sustain healthy organ function, populations vulnerable to choline deficiency exist, including the growing infant, the pregnant or lactating woman, and the patient fed by TPN. Studies of choline requirements in these groups need to be pursued vigorously.

Acknowledgments

Some of the work described in this chapter was supported by grants from the National Institutes of Health (DK55865, AG09525, ES012997, DK56350, RR00046).

REFERENCES

1. Zeisel SH, Blusztajn JK. Annu Rev Nutr 1994;14:269–6.
2. Strecker A. Ann Chem Pharm 1862;123:353–60.
3. du Vigneaud V, Cohn M, Chandler JP et al. J Biol Chem 1941; 140:625–41.
4. Kennedy EP, Weiss SB. J Biol Chem 1956;222:193–214.
5. Best CH, Huntsman ME. J Physiol 1932;75:405–12.
6. Best CH, Huntsman ME. J Physiol 1935;83:255–74.
7. Lieber CS, Robins SJ, Li J et al. Gastroenterology 1994;106: 152–9.
8. Blusztajn JK, Wurtman RJ. Science 1983;221:614–20.
9. Exton JH. Biochim Biophys Acta 1994;1212:26–42.
10. Merrill AH Jr, Liotta DC, Riley RE. Handbk Lipid Res 1995; 8:205–37.
11. Albright CD, Lui R, Bethea TC et al. FASEB J 1996;10:510–6.
12. Albright CD, Zeisel SH. Pathobiology 1997;65:264–70.
13. Holmes-McNary M, Baldwin J, Zeisel SH. J Biol Chem 2001; 276:41197–41204.
14. Shin OH, Mar MH, Albright CD et al. J Cell Biochem 1997;64: 196–208.
15. Bremer J, Greenberg D. Biochim Biophys Acta 1961;46:205–16.
16. Chawla RK, Wolf DC, Kutner MH et al. Gastroenterology 1989;97:1514–20.
17. Tayek JA, Bistrian B, Sheard NF et al. J Am Coll Nutr 1990; 9:76–83.
18. Buchman AL, Moukarzel A, Jenden DJ et al. Clin Nutr 1993; 12:33–7.
19. Buchman AL, Ament ME, Sohel M et al. JPEN J Parenter Enteral Nutr 2001;25:260–8.
20. Zeisel SH, daCosta K-A, Franklin PD et al. FASEB J 1991; 5:2093–8.
21. Food and Nutrition Board, Institute of Medicine. Dietary Reference Intakes for Folate, Thiamin, Riboflavin, Niacin, Vitamin B$_{12}$, Panthothenic Acid, Biotin, and Choline, vol 1. Washington, DC: National Academy Press, 1998.
22. Zeisel SH, Mar MH, Howe JC et al. J Nutr 2003;133:1302–7.
23. Holmes-McNary M, Cheng WL, Mar MH et al. Am J Clin Nutr 1996;64:572–6.
24. Zeisel SH, Growdon JH, Wurtman RJ et al. Neurology 1980; 30:1226–9.
25. Cheng W-L, Holmes-McNary MQ, Mar M-H et al. J Nutr Biochem 1996;7:457–64.
26. Chao CK, Pomfret EA, Zeisel SH. Biochem J 1988;254:33–8.
27. Yang EK, Blusztajn JK, Pomfret EA et al. Biochem J 1988; 256:821–8.
28. Zeisel SH, Wurtman RJ. Biochem J 1981;198:565–70.
29. Zeisel SH, Stanbury JB, Wurtman RJ et al. N Engl J Med 1982;306:175–6.
30. Zeisel SH, Char D, Sheard NF. J Nutr 1986;116:50–8.
31. Zeisel SH, Wishnok JS, Blusztajn JK. J Pharmacol Exp Ther 1983;225:320–4.
32. Kamath A, Darling I, Morris M. J Nutr 2003;133:2607–11.
33. Lekim D, Betzing H, Hoppe Seylers Z. Physiol Chem 1976; 357:1321–31.
34. Sweiry JH, Page KR, Dacke CG et al. J Dev Physiol 1986; 8:435–45.
35. Leventer SM, Rowell PP. Placenta 1984;5:261–70.
36. McMahon KE, Farrell PM. Clin Chim Acta 1985;149:1–12.
37. Ozarda IY, Uncu G, Ulus IH. Arch Physiol Biochem 2002; 110:393–9.
38. Cornford EM, Cornford ME. Fed Proc 1986;45:2065–72.
39. Garner SC, Mar M-H, Zeisel SH. J Nutr 1995;125:2851–8.
40. Lockman PR, Allen DD. Drug Dev Ind Pharm 2002; 28:249–71.
41. Cornford EM, Braun LD, Oldendorf WH. J Neurochem 1978;30:299–308.
42. Acara M, Rennick B. Am J Physiol 1973;225:1123–8.
43. Rennick B, Acara M, Glor M. Am J Physiol 1977;232:F443–7.
44. Guder WG, Beck FX, Schmolke M. Klin Wochenschr 1990;68: 1091–5.
45. Handler J, Kwon H. Kidney Int 1996;49:1682–3.
46. Garcia-Perez A, Burg MB. J Membrane Biol 1991;119:1–13.
47. Nakanishi T, Burg MB. Am J Physiol 1989;251:C795–801.
48. Ilcol YO, Donmez O, Yavuz M et al. Clin Biochem 2002;35: 307–13.
49. Ilcol YO, Gurun MS, Taga Y et al. Horm Metab Res 2002; 34:341–7.
50. Rennick B, Acara M, Hysert P et al. Kidney Int 1976; 10:329–35.
51. Acara M, Rennick B, LaGraff S et al. Nephron 1983;35:241–3.
52. Cohen EL, Wurtman RJ. Life Sci 1975;16:1095–1102.
53. Ulus IH, Wurtman RJ, Mauron C et al. Brain Res 1989;484: 217–27.
54. Wecker L. J Neurochem 1991;57:1119–27.
55. Blusztajn JK, Holbrook PG, Lakher M et al. Psychopharmacol Bull 1986;22:781–6.
56. Blusztajn JK, Liscovitch M, Richardson UI. Proc Natl Acad Sci USA 1987;84:5474–7.
57. Niculescu MD, Zeisel SH. J Nutr 2002;132:2333S–5S.
58. Lin CS, Wu RD. J Prot Chem 1986;5:193–200.
59. Sunden S, Renduchintala M, Park E et al. Arch Biochem Biophys 1997;345:171–4.
60. Millian NS, Garrow TA. Arch Biochem Biophys 1998;356:93–98.
61. Bailey LB, Gregory JF 3rd. J Nutr 1999;129:779–782.
62. Kim Y-I, Miller JW, da Costa K-A et al. J Nutr 1995;124: 2197–2203.
63. Selhub J, Seyoum E, Pomfret EA et al. Cancer Res 1991; 51:16–21.
64. Varela-Moreiras G, Selhub J, da Costa K et al. J Nutr Biochem 1992;3:519–22.
65. Pomfret EA, daCosta K, Schurman LL et al. Anal Biochem 1989;180:85–90.
66. Zeisel SH, Zola T, daCosta K et al. Biochem J 1989;259:725–9.
67. Pomfret EA, da Costa K, Zeisel SH. J Nutr Biochem 1990;1:533–41.
68. Freeman–Narrod M, Narrod SA, Yarbro JW. Med Pediatr Oncol 1977;3:9–14.
69. Custer RP, Freeman–Narrod M, Narrod SJ. J Natl Cancer Inst 1977;58:1011–15.
70. Aarsaether N, Berge RK, Aarsland A et al. Biochim Biophys Acta 1988;958:70–80.
71. Svardal AM, Ueland PM, Berge RK et al. Cancer Chemother Pharmacol 1988;21:313–8.
72. Schwahn BC, Chen Z, Laryea MD et al. FASEB J 2003;17: 512–4.

73. Rozen R. Clin Invest Med 1996;19:171–8.
74. Wilcken D, Wang X, Sim A et al. Arterioscler Thromb Vasc Biol 1996;16:878–82.
75. Centers for Disease Control. MMWR Morbid Mortal Wkly Rep 1992;41:1–7.
75a. Shaw GM, Carmichael SL, Yang W et al. Am J Epidemiol 2004;160:102–9.
76. Fisher MC, Zeisel SH, Mar MH et al. Teratology 2001;64:114–22.
77. Fisher MC, Zeisel SH, Mar MH et al. FASEB J 2002;16:619–21.
78. Boushey C, Beresford S, Omenn G et al. JAMA 1995;274:1049–57.
79. Vance DE. Biochem Cell Biol 1990;68:1151–65.
80. Kent C. Prog Lipid Res 1990;29:87–105.
81. Ishidate K, Nakazawa Y. Methods Enzymol 1992;209:121–34.
82. Kent C. Biochimica et Biophys Acta 1997;1348:79–90.
83. Pelech SL, Cook HW, Paddon HB et al. Biochim Biophys Acta 1984;795:433–40.
84. Farrell PM, Epstein MF, Fleischman AR et al. Biol Neonate 1976;29:238–46.
85. Wang Y, MacDonald JI, Kent C. J Biol Chem 1995;270:354–60.
86. Kast HR, Nguyen CM, Anisfeld AM et al. J Lipid Res 2001;42:1266–72.
87. Ridgway ND, Lagace TA. Biochem J 2003;372:811–9.
88. Wang Y, MacDonald JI, Kent C. J Biol Chem 1993;268:5512–8.
89. Watkins JD, Wang YL, Kent C. Arch Biochem Biophys 1992;292:360–7.
90. Jamil H, Hatch GM, Vance DE. Biochem J 1993;291:419–27.
91. Yao ZM, Jamil H, Vance DE. J Biol Chem 1990;265:4326–31.
92. Hatch GM, Jamil H, Utal AK et al. J Biol Chem 1992;267:15751–8.
93. Cornell R. Cholinephosphotransferase. In: Vance DE, ed. Phosphatidylcholine Metabolism. Boca Raton, FL: CRC Press, 1989:47–65.
94. Mosharrof AH, Petkov VD. Acta Physiol Pharmacol Bulg 1990;16:25–31.
95. Bonavita E, Chioma V, Dall'Oca P et al. Minerva Psichiatr 1983;24:53–62.
96. Vance DE, Walkey CJ, Cui Z. Biochim Biophys Acta 1997;1348:142–50.
97. Blusztajn JK, Zeisel SH, Wurtman RJ. Biochem J 1985;232:505–11.
98. Mudd SH, Datko AH. Plant Physiol 1989;90:306–10.
99. Andriamampandry C, Freysz L, Kanfer JN et al. J Neurochem 1991;56:1845–50.
100. Andriamampandry C, Freysz L, Kanfer JN et al. Biochem J 1989;264:555–62.
101. Cui Z, Vance JE, Chen MH et al. J Biol Chem 1993;268:16655–63.
102. Saito S, Iida A, Sekine A et al. J Hum Genet 2001;46:529–37.
103. Waite KA, Cabilio NR, Vance DE. J Nutr 2002;132:68–71.
104. Zhu X, Song J, Mar MH et al. Biochem J 2003;370:987–93.
105. Zeisel SH. Nutrition 2000;16:669–71.
106. da Costa K-A, Garner SC, Chang J et al. Carcinogenesis 1995;16:327–34.
107. Yao ZM, Vance DE. J Biol Chem 1988;263:2998–3004.
108. Yao ZM, Vance DE. J Biol Chem 1989;264:11373–80.
109. Yao ZM, Vance DE. Biochem Cell Biol 1990;68:552–8.
110. Rao MS, Papreddy K, Musunuri S et al. In Vivo 2002;16:145–52.
111. Longnecker DS. J Nutr 2002;132:2373S–6S.
112. Drouva SV, LaPlante E, Leblanc P et al. Endocrinology 1986;119:2611–22.
113. Drouva SV, Rerat E, Leblanc P et al. Endocrinology 1987;121:569–74.
114. Zeisel SH, Mar M-H, Zhou Z-W et al. J Nutr 1995;125:3049–54.
115. Daily Jr, Sachan D. J Nutr 1995;125:1938–44.
116. Dodson W, Sachan D. Am J Clin Nutr 1996;63:904–10.
117. Buchman A. Am J Clin Nutr 1997;65:574–5.
118. Carter AL, Frenkel R. J Nutr 1978;108:1748–54.
119. Hongu N, Sachan DS. J Nutr 2003;133:84–9.
120. Corredor C, Mansbach C, Bressler R. Biochim Biophys Acta 1967;144:366–74.
121. Hoffman DR, Cornatzer WE, Duerre JA. Can J Biochem 1979;57:56–65.
122. Pyapali G, Turner D, Williams C et al. J Neurophysiol 1998;79:1790–96.
123. Montoya DA, White AM, Williams CL et al. Brain Res Dev Brain Res 2000;123:25–32.
124. Jones JP, Meck W, Williams CL et al. Brain Res Dev Brain Res 1999;118:159–67.
125. Meck W, Williams C. Neuroreport 1997;8:3053–9.
126. Meck W, Williams C. Neuroreport 1997;8:2831–5.
127. Meck W, Williams C. Neuroreport 1997;8:3045–51.
128. Meck WH, Smith RA, Williams CL. Behav Neurosci 1989;103:1234–41.
129. Meck WH, Smith RA, Williams CL. Dev Psychobiol 1988;21:339–53.
130. Meck WH, Williams CL. Brain Res Dev Brain Res 1999;118:51–9.
131. Albright CD, Friedrich CB, Brown EC et al. Brain Res Dev Brain Res 1999;115:123–9.
132. Albright CD, Tsai AY, Friedrich CB et al. Brain Res Dev Brain Res 1999;113:13–20.
133. Meck WH, Williams CL. Neurosci Biobehav Rev 2003;27:385–99.
134. Williams CL, Meck WH, Heyer DD et al. Brain Res 1998;794:225–38.
135. Schenk F, Brandner C. Psychobiology 1995;23:302–13.
136. Brandner C. Brain Res 2002;928:85–95.
137. Tees RC. Behav Brain Res 1999;105:173–88.
138. Tees RC. Dev Psychobiol 1999;35:328–42.
139. Tees RC, Mohammadi E, Adam TJ. Soc Neurosci Abstr 1999;17:1401.
140. Ricceri L, Berger-Sweeney J. Behav Neurosci 1998;112:1387–92.
141. Dani S, Hori A, Walter G, eds. Principles of Neural Aging. Amsterdam: Elsevier, 1997.
142. van Praag H, Kempermann G, Gage FH. Nat Neurosci 1999;2:266–70.
143. Markakis EA, Gage FH. J Comp Neurol 1999;406:449–60.
144. Cohen EL, Wurtman RJ. Science 1976;191:561–2.
145. Haubrich DR, Wang PF, Clody DE et al. Life Sci 1975;17:975–80.
146. Trommer BA, Schmidt DE, Wecker L. J Neurochem 1982;39:1704–9.
147. Pardridge WM. Fed Proc 1986;45:2047–9.
148. Poirier J. Trends Neurosci 1994;17:525–30.
149. Weisgraber KH, Mahley RW. FASEB J 1996;10:1485–94.
150. Cohen BM, Renshaw PF, Stoll AL et al. JAMA 1995;274:902–7.
151. Nitsch RM, Blusztajn JK, Pittas AG et al. Proc Natl Acad Sci USA 1992;89:1671–5.
152. Bartus RT, Dean RL, Goas JA et al. Science 1980;209:301–3.
153. Mervis RF. J Neuropathol Exp Neurol 1982;41:363.
154. Ladd SL, Sommer SA, LaBerge S et al. Clin Neuropharmacol 1993;16:540–9.

155. Sitaram N, Weingartner H, Caine ED et al. Life Sci 1978;22:1555–60.

156. Spiers P, Myers D, Hochanadel G et al. Arch Neurol 1996;53:441–8.

157. Alvarez XA, Laredo M, Corzo D et al. Methods Find Exp Clin Pharmacol 1997;19:201–10.

158. Levy R. Lancet 1982;2:671–2.

159. Little A, Levy R, Chuaqui-Kidd P et al. J Neurol Neurosurg Psychiatry 1985;48:736–42.

160. Mohs RC, Davis KL. Psychiatry Res 1980;2:149–56.

161. Drachman DA, Glosser G, Fleming P et al. Neurology 1982;32:944–50.

162. Harris CM, Dysken MW, Fovall P et al. Am J Psychiatry 1983;140:1010–2.

163. Weinstein HC, Teunisse S, van Gool WA. J Neurol 1991;238:34–8.

164. Fitten LJ, Perryman KM, Gross PL et al. Am J Psychiatry 1990;147:239–42.

165. Brinkman SD, Smith RC, Meyer JS et al. J Gerontol 1982;3 7:4–9.

166. Newberne PM, Rogers AE. Annu Rev Nutr 1986;6:407–32.

167. Abanobi SE, Lombardi B, Shinozuka H. Cancer Res 1982;42:412–5.

168. Chandar N, Lombardi B. Carcinogenesis 1988;9:259–63.

169. Andry CD, Kupchik HZ, Rogers AE. Toxicol Pathol 1990; 18:10–7.

170. Christman JK, Sheikhnejad G, Dizik M et al. Carcinogenesis 1993;14:551–7.

171. Shivapurkar N, Wilson MJ, Hoover KL et al. J Natl Cancer Inst 1986;77:213–7.

172. Pogribny IP, Basnakian AG, Miller BJ et al. Cancer Res 1995;55:1894–901.

173. Banni S, Corongiu FP, Dessi MA et al. Free Radic Res Commun 1989;7:233–40.

174. Rushmore T, Lim Y, Farber E et al. Cancer Lett 1984; 24:251–5.

175. da Costa K, Cochary EF, Blusztajn JK et al. J Biol Chem 1993;268:2100–5.

176. Zeisel SH, Albright CD, Shin O-K et al. Carcinogenesis 1997;18:731–8.

177. Shivapurkar N, Poirier LA. Carcinogenesis 1983;4:1051–7.

178. Locker J, Reddy TV, Lombardi B. Carcinogenesis 1986;7:1309–12.

179. Tsujiuchi T, Tsutsumi M, Sasaki Y et al. Jpn J Cancer Res 1999;90:909–13.

180. Holliday R, Grigg GW. Mutat Res 1993;285:61–7.

181. Jaenisch R. Trends Genet 1997;13:323–9.

182. Jones PA, Gonzalgo ML. Proc Natl Acad Sci USA 1997;94:2103–5.

183. Robertson KD, Wolffe AP. Nat Rev Genet 2000;1:11–9.

184. Jeltsch A. Chembiochemistry 2002;3:382.

185. Bird AP. Nature 1986;321:209–13.

186. Niculescu MD, Yamamuro Y, Zeisel SH. J Neurochem 2004;89:1252–9.

187. Wolff GL, Kodell RL, Moore SR et al. FASEB J 1998;12:949–57.

188. Cooney CA, Dave AA, Wolff GL. J Nutr 2002;132:2393S–2400S.

189. Waterland RA, Jirtle RL. Mol Cell Biol 2003;23:5293–5300.

190. da Costa KA, Badea M, Fischer LM et al. Am J Clin Nutr 2004;80:163–70.

191. Buchman A, Dubin M, Moukarzel A et al. Hepatology 1995;22:1399–1403.

192. Buchman AL, Dubin M, Jenden D et al. Gastroenterology 1992;102:1363–70.

193. Misra S, Ahn C, Ament ME et al. JPEN J Parenter Enteral Nutr 1999;23:305–8.

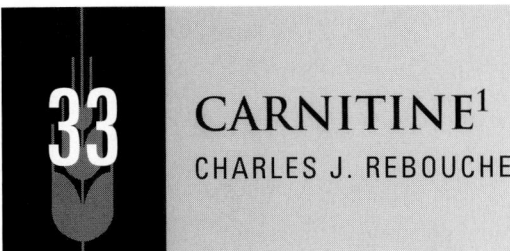

CARNITINE[1]

CHARLES J. REBOUCHE

HISTORICAL INTRODUCTION 537
CHEMISTRY, NOMENCLATURE, AND ANALYSIS 537
BIOCHEMICAL FUNCTIONS .538
    Mitochondrial Long-Chain Fatty
       Acid Oxidation 538
    Modulation of Acyl-Coenzyme
       A/Coenzyme A Ratio 538
    Proteins Associated with Carnitine Function 539
HOMEOSTATIC MECHANISMS 540
    Biosynthesis 540
    Dietary Sources, Absorption, and
       Bioavailability 540
    Transport and Excretion 541
CAUSES AND EFFECTS OF DEFICIENCY
    AND DEPLETION 542
NUTRIENT AND DRUG INTERACTIONS 542
EVALUATION OF STATUS 543
REQUIREMENTS AND RECOMMENDED
    INTAKES 543

HISTORICAL INTRODUCTION

Carnitine was first discovered in muscle extracts independently by Gulewitsch and Krimberg and by Kutscher in 1905, and the correct structure was assigned in 1927 by Tomita and Sendju (1). Between 1948 and 1952, Fraenkel and colleagues demonstrated the essential nature of this compound for the mealworm, *Tenebrio molitor*, and assigned the term "vitamin B_T" to carnitine (1). The role of carnitine in fatty acid oxidation was first discovered independently by Bremer and by Fritz and Yue between 1962 and 1963 (2). The origin of the methyl groups of carnitine was identified by Wolf and Berger and by Bremer in 1961 (2), and the origin of the carbon chain of carnitine from the essential amino acid lysine was first reported by Tanphaichitr, Horne, and Broquist in 1971 (3). Clinical syndromes associated with carnitine deficiency were first reported by Engel and colleagues in 1973 (4) and 1975 (5),

and carnitine deficiency associated specifically with a defect in carnitine transport was identified by Treem and colleagues in 1988 (6).

CHEMISTRY, NOMENCLATURE, AND ANALYSIS

L-Carnitine [R(-)-β-hydroxy-γ-(N,N,N-trimethylammonio)butyrate] is a zwitterionic quaternary amino acid (Fig. 33.1) with a molecular weight of 161.2 g/mol (inner salt). Only the L isomer is biologically active. L-Carnitine is present in biologic systems in both nonesterified and esterified forms. Short-chain (C_2–C_5) organic acids or medium (C_6–C_{12})– or long (C_{14}–C_{24})–chain fatty acids are transferred to and from coenzyme A (CoA) and the hydroxyl group of carnitine (see Fig. 33.1). These reversible reactions are catalyzed by a group of enzymes appropriately named carnitine acyltransferases.

Analysis of carnitine concentrations in biologic fluids and tissues has most commonly used the reaction of acetyl-CoA, either radiolabeled (7) or nonlabeled (8), with carnitine, catalyzed by commercially available carnitine acetyltransferase (CAT) (EC 2.3.1.7). Quantification was achieved by measurement of radiolabeled acetyl-L-carnitine formed in the enzymatic reaction or spectrophotometrically by reaction of CoA (released in the enzymatic reaction) with 5,5'-dithio-*bis*-2-nitrobenzoic acid. The spectrophotometric method has been adapted for use with automated analyzers. Different sample preparation procedures permit direct measurement of free (nonesterified) carnitine, total acid-soluble (free plus short- and medium-chain acyl-) carnitine, long-chain acylcarnitine esters, and total carnitine (free plus all acylcarnitine esters) but not individual species of the various esters present in biologic materials. Accurate quantification of carnitine and its esters by these methods depends on control of factors present in specimens to be analyzed and in reaction mixtures (e.g., salt concentration) that inhibit enzyme activity or alter the equilibrium of the reversible reaction catalyzed by CAT.

More recently, nonenzymatic methods to measure carnitine and individual species of acylcarnitine esters have been introduced. These include, after derivatization, separation by reversed-phase, high-performance liquid chromatography with on-line quantification by spectrophotometry (9) and electrospray tandem mass

---

[1] **Abbreviations: CACT,** carnitine-acylcarnitine translocase; **CAT,** carnitine acetyltransferase; **CoA,** coenzyme A; **COT,** carnitine octanoyltransferase; **CPT,** carnitine palmitoyltransferase; **K_t,** ligand concentration at which binding is half-maximal; **Na⁺,** sodium ion.

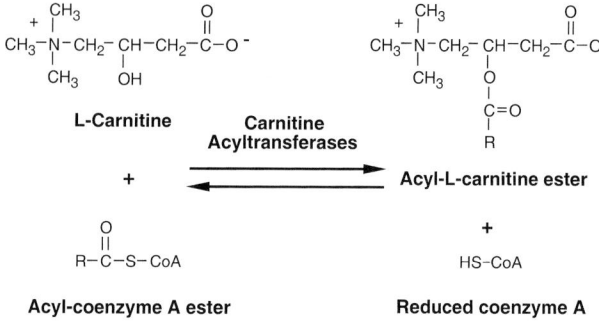

Figure 33.1. Carnitine structure and metabolic interconversions. CoA, coenzyme A.

spectrometry (10). The tandem mass spectrometry procedure has been applied to large-scale screening of neonates. Results of plasma free and total carnitine assays using this procedure compared favorably with results using the spectrophotometric assay (10).

BIOCHEMICAL FUNCTIONS

Mitochondrial Long-Chain Fatty Acid Oxidation

Long-chain fatty acids enter mitochondria only as acylcarnitine esters (Fig. 33.2). Carnitine palmitoyltransferase I (CPT I) (EC 2.3.1.21), located in the outer mitochondrial membrane, catalyzes transesterification of cytosolic long-chain fatty acids from CoA to carnitine. The acylcarnitine esters traverse the inner mitochondrial membrane via a carnitine-acylcarnitine translocase (CACT), and the acyl moieties are transesterified to intramitochondrial CoA by the action of CPT II, located on the matrix surface of the inner mitochondrial membrane. Thus, carnitine is essential for mitochondrial utilization of long-chain fatty acids for energy production.

Modulation of Acyl-Coenzyme A/Coenzyme A Ratio

CoA is a required cofactor in many cellular reactions. If nonesterified CoA is not available in a cellular compartment (e.g., cytosol, mitochondria, peroxisomes) because it is completely esterified, the flux through pathways that require this cofactor will diminish. Carnitine is a reservoir for excess acyl residues, generated, for example, by high rates of β-oxidation in mitochondria, in which the acyl residue is transesterified from CoA to carnitine, thus freeing CoA to participate in other cellular reactions (see Fig. 33.2). The acylcarnitine ester formed in this process may remain in the organelle or cell of origin, for use when needed, or it may be exported out of the cell for use by other cells or tissues or for excretion. Unlike CoA and its esters, carnitine and its esters readily exchange across most membranes, facilitated by specific carriers and transporters.

This function has important implications for cellular energy metabolism. For example, carnitine facilitates oxidation of glucose in working hearts by relieving inhibition of pyruvate dehydrogenase by fatty acids (11). The mechanism involves removal of acetyl groups generated from fatty acid β-oxidation by transesterification from acetyl-CoA to carnitine, thus freeing CoA to participate in the pyruvate dehydrogenase reaction sequence. Carnitine may also increase the rate of glucose production and oxidation secondarily by facilitating utilization of long-chain acyl-CoA in the hypothalamus. Inhibition of CPT I and the consequent increase in long-chain acyl-CoA concentration in the hypothalamus have been shown to promote anorexia and decreased hepatic glucose production (12).

Carnitine and extramitochondrial CPT are important in long-chain fatty acid utilization for phospholipid remodeling and biosynthesis. Carnitine acts as a reservoir for long-chain fatty acids destined for incorporation into phospholipids, as, for example, in erythrocytes during repair after oxidative insult (13), and in lung alveolar cells in synthesis

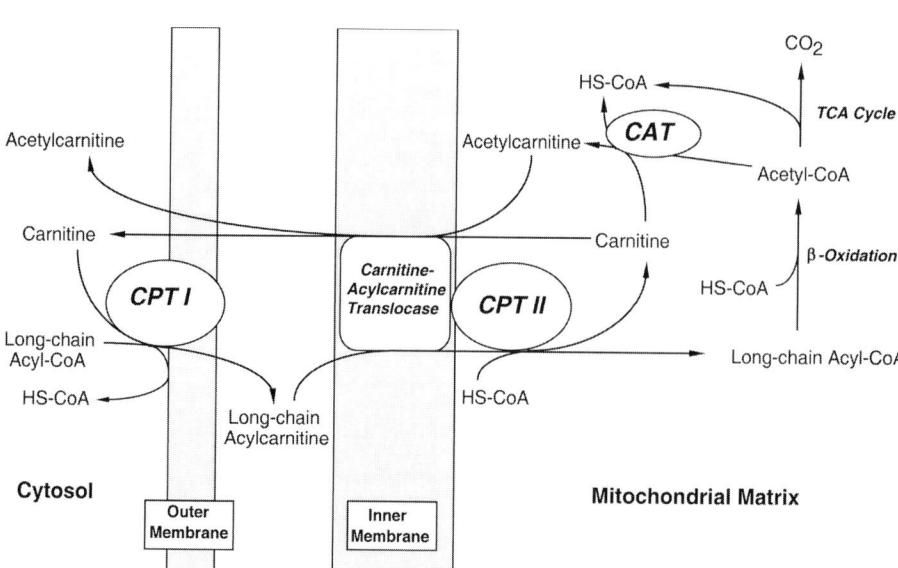

Figure 33.2. Carnitine function: facilitation of mitochondrial long-chain fatty acid oxidation and modulation of intramitochondrial acyl-coenzyme A (CoA)/CoA ratio. CAT, carnitine acyltransferase; CPT, carnitine palmitoyltransferase.

of dipalmitoylphosphatidylcholine, the major component of surfactant (14).

The ability of carnitine to act as a reservoir for activated acyl residues is important in abnormal cellular metabolism, in particular, in genetic diseases associated with defects in organic and fatty acid metabolism. For example, in propionyl-CoA carboxylase deficiency, propionyl-CoA is an end product that, if not cleared, would starve the cellular energy-producing machinery of nonesterified CoA. In patients with this disease, large amounts of propionylcarnitine are excreted, a finding indicating that cells and tissues adapt to the demand for nonesterified CoA by transesterification of excess propionyl residues to carnitine (15). Pharmacologic amounts of carnitine often are prescribed for treatment of this disease.

Proteins Associated with Carnitine Function

Carnitine Palmitoyltransferase

Two major forms of CPT have been identified: CPT I and CPT II. CPT I and CPT II are structurally distinct and products of different genes. CPT I is an integral protein of the mitochondrial outer membrane, consisting of two transmembrane segments. CPT I is potently inhibited by malonyl-CoA. This reversible inhibition is a primary metabolic regulator that partitions fatty acids to mitochondrial oxidation or to triglyceride formation. CPT I catalyzes the rate-limiting step in transfer of long-chain fatty acids into mitochondria. Two isoforms of CPT I are recognized: a "liver" isoform (L-CPT I) of molecular weight approximately 88 kDa and a "muscle" isoform (M-CPT I) of molecular weight approximately 82 kDa (16). These isoforms are encoded by different genes, *CPT1A* and *CPT1B* (17), and they differ in their affinity for carnitine and malonyl-CoA. L-CPT I is present throughout the mitochondrial outer membrane, but it is especially concentrated within the contact sites that occur between the outer and inner membranes (18). The different membrane environments in the outer membranes and contact sites result in different conformations of L-CPT I that specifically affect the long-chain acyl-CoA binding site. These conformational differences result in a lower Michaelis-Menten dissociation constant (K_m) for palmitoyl-CoA at the contact sites. Malonyl-CoA inhibition is noncompetitive generally in outer membranes, but competitive at contact sites. As a result of these changes, the concentration that inhibits 50% (IC_{50}) for malonyl-CoA is fivefold higher for L-CPT I in the contact sites relative to the rest of the membrane. These differences provide a potent additional mechanism for regulation of L-CPT I activity at contact sites (18).

CPT II is found on the matrix surface of the mitochondrial inner membrane. It is synthesized as a proenzyme of molecular weight 74 kDa. The N-terminal 25 residues are cleaved following import into mitochondria, and the result is a mature protein of 70 kDa (17). It is not inhibited by malonyl-CoA.

CPT activity is found extramitochondrially, in peroxisomes and endoplasmic reticulum. The activity present in peroxisomes generally is attributed to carnitine octanoyltransferase (COT; see later) present in this organelle. CPT activity in endoplasmic reticulum has been observed, as for example, in erythrocytes (13), but this activity has not been well characterized.

Carnitine Acetyltransferase

This enzyme catalyzes reversible transesterification of short-chain organic acids (two to eight carbons, with maximal activity directed to acetyl and propionyl residues) between CoA and carnitine. CAT is found in soluble form in mitochondria and peroxisomes and in membrane-associated form in endoplasmic reticulum (19). The enzyme has been purified from different tissues of various species. Molecular weights reported range from 51 to 75 kDa. Investigators generally accept that, based on enzyme kinetics and specificity, CAT in the various subcellular compartments provides for efficient synthesis, utilization, and/or disposal of short-chain organic acids generated by mitochondrial or peroxisomal metabolism of both physiologic and xenobiotic compounds.

Carnitine Octanoyltransferase

COT is a broad-specificity enzyme with highest affinity for medium-chain fatty acids (highest activity with hexanoyl-CoA as substrate). It is found mostly in peroxisomes, and its activity in liver is increased by peroxisomal proliferating agents. Peroxisomes generally oxidize very-long-chain fatty acids that are not metabolized in mitochondria. Chain-shortened products, primarily medium-chain esters of CoA, are transesterified to carnitine and are subsequently oxidized in mitochondria. Peroxisomal COT has a molecular weight of approximately 62 kDa and is immunologically distinct from CPT I, CPT II, and CAT (20). Like mitochondrial CPT I, it is inhibited by malonyl-CoA. COT accounts for the CPT activity observed in peroxisomal preparations.

COT activity also is found in rough and smooth endoplasmic reticulum. This 53-kDa protein is immunologically distinct from peroxisomal COT (21). Like mitochondrial CPT I, crude (membrane-bound) microsomal COT is inhibited by malonyl-CoA, but after solubilization with detergents, inhibition by malonyl-CoA is lost. Microsomal COT probably accounts for the CPT activity in endoplasmic reticulum. As with peroxisomal CAT and COT, reversible reaction kinetics of this enzyme favors formation of acylcarnitine esters at normal intracellular concentrations of its substrates (21).

Carnitine-Acylcarnitine Translocase

Entry of long-chain acylcarnitine esters into mitochondria occurs by rapid exchange diffusion (22), facilitated by a 32.5-kDa CACT in the inner mitochondrial membrane. The cDNA (23) and gene (24) coding for human CACT have been cloned. CACT is a member of the mitochondrial carrier family. The protein has been purified and functionally reconstituted into liposomes (25). It is inhibited by sulfhydryl-reactive reagents and some analogs of carnitine (e.g., sulfobetaines). The translocase has several other important functions in addition to its role in facilitating entry of long-chain acylcarnitine esters into mitochondria. It facilitates entry into mitochondria of short- and medium-chain acylcarnitine esters formed in peroxisomes from oxidation of very-long-chain fatty acids. CACT also facilitates removal of short-chain acylcarnitine esters from mitochondria, thus freeing CoA to recycle through the various pathways in the mitochondrial matrix.

HOMEOSTATIC MECHANISMS

Carnitine homeostasis in humans is maintained by the dynamic interactions of endogenous synthesis, acquisition from dietary sources, maintenance of concentration gradients across cell membranes, and regulation of renal reabsorption and excretion of carnitine.

Biosynthesis

Humans are able to synthesize carnitine from the essential amino acids lysine and methionine. Lysine provides the carbon chain and nitrogen atom, and three methionine molecules provide the methyl groups for one molecule of carnitine (26). Methylation of the epsilon amino group of lysine is catalyzed by one or more protein:lysine methyltransferases. Lysine residues destined for carnitine synthesis must be peptide linked; no evidence indicates that free lysine is enzymatically methylated in mammals. ε-N-Trimethyllysine is released for carnitine synthesis via normal mechanisms of protein hydrolysis.

ε-N-Trimethyllysine undergoes four sequential enzymatic reactions (26): hydroxylation at position two of the carbon chain, catalyzed by ε-N-trimethyllysine hydroxylase (EC 1.14.11.8); aldol cleavage between carbons two and three of the carbon chain, catalyzed by serine hydroxymethyltransferase (EC 2.1.2.1); oxidation of the resulting aldehyde by any of several oxidized nicotinamide adenine dinucleotide (NAD$^+$)–requiring aldehyde dehydrogenases, including one with high specificity for γ-N,N,N-trimethylaminobutyraldehyde (27); and a second hydroxylation, catalyzed by γ-butyrobetaine hydroxylase (EC 1.14.11.1). cDNAs coding for each of these four enzymes have been cloned and sequenced (27).

All enzymes in the pathway except γ-butyrobetaine hydroxylase are ubiquitous in mammalian tissues. The last enzyme in the pathway is not found in cardiac and skeletal muscle (26). γ-Butyrobetaine hydroxylase activity is highest in liver and testes, and in some species, including humans, it is abundant in kidney.

The normal rate of carnitine synthesis in humans is approximately 1.2 μmol/kg body weight/day (28). This estimate is obtained from normal rates of urinary carnitine excretion by strict vegetarians, who acquire very little carnitine (~0.1 μmol/kg body weight/day) from dietary sources. Direct measurement of the rate of carnitine synthesis by, for example, isotope incorporation from labeled precursors, technically is not feasible (28).

The rate of carnitine synthesis in mammals is regulated by the availability of ε-N-trimethyllysine, which, in turn, is determined by the extent of peptide-linked lysine methylation and by the rate of protein turnover (28). ε-N-Trimethyllysine destined for carnitine synthesis probably is derived from the general protein pool, and not from any single or small group of proteins. Provision of excess lysine in the diet may increase carnitine synthesis modestly (29), but the evidence is indirect, and the mechanism (e.g., increased flux through protein synthesis, methylation, and turnover or stimulation of a putative vestigial capability to methylate free lysine) has not been identified. The rate of carnitine biosynthesis does not appear to be affected by the magnitude of dietary carnitine intake, or by changes in renal handling of carnitine.

Dietary Sources, Absorption, and Bioavailability

Carnitine generally is abundant in food products of animal origin (Table 33.1). Fruits, vegetables, grains, and other plant-derived foods contain relatively little carnitine (28). Thus, a normal omnivorous diet provides approximately two to 12 μmol/kg body weight/day of carnitine, whereas a strict vegetarian diet contains about 0.1 μmol/kg body weight/day (28). Carnitine is available commercially as a diet supplement. Carnitine consumed orally in large quantities (~5 g/day by an adult) may cause diarrhea or "fish odor syndrome." No other toxic properties have been identified.

TABLE 33.1. CARNITINE CONTENT OF SELECTED FOODS

FOOD ITEM	CARNITINE CONTENT[a]
Meat products (cooked)	
Beef steak	592±260
Ground beef	582±32
Pork	172±32
Canadian bacon	146±52
Bacon	145±24
Fish	34.6±11.7
Chicken (breast)	24.3±8.0
Dairy products	
Whole milk	20.4
American cheese	23.2
Ice cream	23.0
Butter	3.07
Cottage cheese	6.96

[a] Units are μmol/100 g (solid foods) or μmol/100 mL (liquids). Values for meat products are based on precooked weight. All values are total (nonesterified plus esterified) carnitine.
Data from Rebouche CJ, Engel AG. J Clin Invest 1984;73:57–67.

Approximately 63 to 75% of carnitine is absorbed from the normal omnivorous diet (30). The remainder is almost entirely degraded by bacteria in the large intestine. The percentage of carnitine absorbed from supplements may be much lower. For example, from a 2-g supplement daily, approximately 20% is absorbed (31). Primary organic degradation products of carnitine are trimethylamine (excreted in urine as trimethylamine oxide) and γ-butyrobetaine (excreted primarily in feces). Carnitine is not degraded by enzymes of animal origin (32).

Absorption of carnitine likely involves a combination of active transport and passive diffusion across the intestinal mucosal barrier. Evidence has accumulated from in vivo and in vitro studies using several experimental preparations, to demonstrate that active transport of carnitine occurs across the apical brush border membrane of enterocytes, but not across the basal membrane (33). Paradoxically, in one study active, sodium ion (Na^+)–dependent carnitine transport into mouse intestinal basolateral membrane vesicles was observed (34). In the same study, the rate of Na^+-dependent carnitine transport into brush border membrane vesicles was much slower than for transport into basolateral membrane vesicles. Thus, absorption of carnitine may occur by active transport from the lumen into the enterocyte, by active transport or passive diffusion across the serosal surface, or by paracellular diffusion. A passive component, at least at the serosal surface, is strongly suggested by experimental studies in rats (35, 36) and Caco-2 cells (37) that demonstrated relatively rapid entry of carnitine into enterocytes from the luminal medium, but very slow appearance in the serosal perfusate or medium.

Transport and Excretion

Carnitine is concentrated in most tissues of the body. In humans, the intracellular concentrations of carnitine in skeletal muscle and liver are approximately 76 and 50 times higher, respectively, than that in extracellular fluid (~50 μmol/L). Approximately 97% of all carnitine in the body is in skeletal muscle. Four carnitine transporters have been identified: OCTN1, OCTN2, OCTN3, and $ATB^{0,+}$. OCTN1 is expressed in many tissues (but not human adult liver) (38), but it has relatively low affinity (ligand at which binding is half-maximal $[K_t] = 412$ μM) and specificity for carnitine (39). This pH-dependent, 63-kDa transporter may be responsible for secretion of carnitine and its short-chain esters across the renal epithelial brush border membrane (40, 41). Carnitine is transported into most tissues by a high-affinity ($K_t = 3-5$ μM), Na^+gradient–dependent organic cation transporter, OCTN2 (17, 42). This 63-kDa transporter is highly expressed in heart, placenta, skeletal muscle, kidney, pancreas, testis, and epididymis (39, 43) and is weakly expressed in brain, lung, and liver (43). OCTN2 binds carnitine, acetylcarnitine, and propionylcarnitine with comparable affinity (44). It is likely to be quantitatively the

most important carnitine transporter in all tissues except liver and testis.

OCTN3 is expressed primarily and at a high level in testis, and it has higher specificity for carnitine than OCTN1 or OCTN2 (39). Unlike with OCTN2, carnitine transport via OCTN3 is not driven by an inwardly directed Na^+ gradient. A murine Octn3-green fluorescent protein construct was expressed in HepG2 cells, where it localized in peroxisomes (45). The $ATB^{0,+}$ amino acid transporter cloned from mouse colon also transports carnitine (46). This transporter is expressed primarily in the lung, mammary gland, and intestine. Carnitine binds with low affinity ($K_t = 1-2$ mM) and low specificity, but the capacity of carnitine transport is high owing to energization by transmembrane gradients of Na^+ and chloride and by membrane potential (46). This transporter may have a role in absorption of carnitine (46). Its tissue distribution and function as a carnitine transporter in humans have not been examined.

The transporter responsible for entry of carnitine into human liver has not been determined. OCTN2 is expressed at a low level in human adult liver, but OCTN1 and $ATB^{0,+}$ are not expressed. γ-Butyrobetaine enters hepatocytes via a high-affinity ($K_t = 5$ μM), Na^+- and chloride-coupled transporter, but this transporter does not bind or transport carnitine (47). Experiments with perfused rat liver suggest protein-mediated release of carnitine (17). Regulated release of carnitine from liver would have significant implications for whole-body carnitine homeostasis, because liver is a primary site for carnitine biosynthesis in humans.

Carnitine and short-chain esters of carnitine are excreted by the kidney. At normal plasma carnitine concentrations, the rate of carnitine excretion is very low, but it increases rapidly as the plasma carnitine concentration is increased (Fig. 33.3), by increased oral consumption of carnitine or by intravenous infusion of carnitine (33). A "threshold" effect is observed at near-normal plasma carnitine concentrations, above which the rate of carnitine excretion soon parallels the increase of filtered load.

Efficient reabsorption has a major role in maintenance of carnitine homeostasis. Approximately 95% of filtered carnitine is reabsorbed in physiologically normal persons. The efficiency of carnitine reabsorption decreases as dietary intake of carnitine increases, independent of glomerular filtration rate and filtered load (48). This adaptive response serves to maintain circulating carnitine concentration in the presence of decreased input from dietary intake.

Carnitine transport across the renal brush border membrane is mediated by OCTN2. γ-Butyrobetaine and short-chain acylcarnitine esters also are efficiently reabsorbed, probably by the same transporter. The mechanism by which intracellular carnitine is transferred across the serosal membrane of the renal epithelial cell is not completely understood. Mouse renal basolateral membranes transport carnitine by a high-affinity, Na^+-dependent

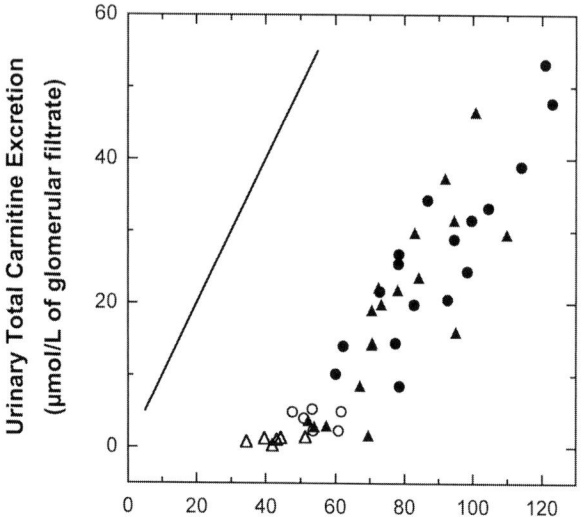

Figure 33.3. Total carnitine excretion as a function of plasma carnitine concentration in humans. Data are composite for 12 subjects (six omnivores *[circles]*, six strict vegetarians *[triangles]*) with *(filled symbols)* or without *(open symbols)* intravenous carnitine infusion. The *solid line* indicates filtered load of carnitine. (Experimental data reported in Rebouche CJ, Lombard KA, Chenard CA. Am J Clin Nutr 1993;58:660–5.)

process similar to renal brush border membrane vesicles, but whereas Western blot analysis revealed OCTN2 in the brush border membrane vesicles, it was not observed in basolateral membrane vesicles (34). Carnitine, short-chain acylcarnitine esters, and γ-butyrobetaine are secreted from renal epithelial cells into the tubular lumen (33). The brush border membrane carrier responsible for this process has not been identified.

CAUSES AND EFFECTS OF DEFICIENCY AND DEPLETION

Carnitine is not required in the normal human diet. No clinically recognizable condition of nutritional carnitine deficiency exists. Population groups that would be most vulnerable to nutritional carnitine deficiency are newborn infants and strict vegetarians. Infants, particularly premature infants, are born with relatively low stores of carnitine, and rapid growth places a demand for carnitine accretion. In the past, but not currently, commercial soy protein–based infant formulas did not contain carnitine. Infants consuming these formulas grew at a normal rate and displayed no evidence of clinically relevant carnitine deficiency, although some biochemical parameters relating to lipid metabolism (e.g., plasma free fatty acid concentration, rate of excretion of medium-chain dicarboxylic acids) were different compared with infants consuming the same formulas but supplemented with carnitine (28). Strict vegetarians (both adults and children) acquire very little carnitine in their diets. They have somewhat lower

plasma carnitine concentrations compared with omnivores, but no indication of clinically relevant carnitine deficiency (33).

Primary systemic carnitine deficiency of genetic origin occurs as a result of mutations in the carnitine transporter OCTN2. It is an autosomal recessive disorder characterized by progressive cardiomyopathy, skeletal myopathy, hypoglycemia, and hyperammonemia (49). The disease usually presents within the first 5 years of life, and it is fatal if untreated. No primary carnitine deficiency resulting from a defect in carnitine biosynthesis has been identified.

Carnitine deficiency or depletion occurs secondary to many genetic and acquired disorders and conditions (50) (see also Chapter 59). At least two basic mechanisms are responsible for these effects on carnitine status. In some disorders, the efficiency of carnitine reabsorption is impaired (e.g., medium-chain acyl-CoA dehydrogenase deficiency). In others, abnormal amounts of short-chain organic acids are produced and are removed from the body by urinary excretion as acylcarnitine esters (e.g., propionylcarnitine in propionyl-CoA carboxylase deficiency). In these disorders, the rate of excretion of carnitine as short-chain acylcarnitine esters exceeds the combined rates of endogenous synthesis and dietary carnitine intake, thus leading to a state of carnitine depletion.

NUTRIENT AND DRUG INTERACTIONS

Carnitine status and metabolism are affected by several nutrients and drugs. For example, rates of carnitine excretion by persons supplemented with choline are lower than corresponding rates of unsupplemented persons (51). Experimental vitamin C deficiency in guinea pigs is associated with decreased plasma carnitine concentration and increased rate of urinary carnitine excretion (52).

Valproic acid and pivalic acid–containing prodrugs (antibiotics) negatively affect human carnitine status (53). Valproic acid administration lowers circulating carnitine concentrations in some patients. The mechanism for this effect has not been identified. Pivalic acid is conjugated to some antibiotics to improve their rates of absorption. In the intestinal mucosa, pivalic acid is cleaved by nonspecific esterases. Pivalic acid is conjugated to carnitine and is quantitatively excreted in urine as pivaloylcarnitine. Prolonged treatment with these antibiotics leads to depletion of the circulating carnitine pool and, presumably, tissue carnitine pools as well.

Short-term treatment with the chemotherapeutic agents cisplatin (54) and ifosfamide (55) increase the rate of total carnitine excretion by approximately ten- and 30-fold, respectively, during the period of treatment. Plasma carnitine concentrations were modestly elevated with cisplatin treatment, suggesting loss of carnitine from tissues as well as diminished capacity to reabsorb carnitine contributed to the increased rate of carnitine excretion. On the other hand, metabolism of ifosfamide produces chloroacetaldehyde, which, after oxidation, is esterified to carnitine and excreted in urine. Both nonesterified carnitine and acylcarnitine esters excretion were elevated with ifosfamide treatment, a finding suggesting two mechanisms for increased urinary loss of carnitine: excretion and/or secretion of the abnormal acylcarnitine ester chloroacetyl-L-carnitine and diminished capacity to reabsorb carnitine.

EVALUATION OF STATUS

Carnitine status most often is reported as a function of circulating carnitine concentration, and the ratio of esterified to nonesterified carnitine. In general, plasma free carnitine concentration of 20 μmol/L or less, or total carnitine concentration of 30 μmol/L or less, is considered abnormally low. However, these values only demarcate the lower range of normal plasma carnitine concentrations; they do not reflect points at which functional carnitine deficiency is observed. A ratio of esterified to free carnitine of 0.4 or greater in plasma or serum (but not urine) is considered indicative of abnormal carnitine metabolism. This ratio is elevated primarily when mitochondrial energy metabolism is impaired, resulting in increased load of short-chain organic acids esterified to CoA, which are transesterified to carnitine for export from tissues into the circulation. Thus, in genetic disorders of fatty acid and organic acid oxidation (see Chapter 59), the ratio of esterified to free carnitine in the circulation often is elevated. This elevated ratio is associated with carnitine depletion resulting either from hyperexcretion of acylcarnitine esters or from decreased ability of the kidneys to reabsorb carnitine and its esters. Rates of carnitine excretion in urine do not provide a particularly useful measure of carnitine status, because these rates vary considerably with dietary carnitine intake and other physiologic parameters. No validated tests or measures of functional carnitine deficiency are available to assess carnitine status in humans.

REQUIREMENTS AND RECOMMENDED INTAKES

Carnitine is not a required nutrient for children and adults. Supplementation of formulas for infants (particularly premature infants) is recommended at a level normally found in human milk (28–95 μmol/L). These recommendations are based on observations of very low plasma and tissue carnitine concentrations and other biochemical differences observed in infants not fed exogenous carnitine (28). Exogenous carnitine is recommended for treatment of some genetic and acquired disorders (e.g., primary and secondary carnitine deficiency of genetic origin, end-stage renal disease requiring hemodialysis, and anticonvulsant polytherapy that includes valproic acid in children), but for these purposes, use of exogenous carnitine is pharmacologic rather than nutritional.

REFERENCES

1. Fraenkel G, Friedman S. Vitam Horm 1957;15:73–118.
2. Bremer J. Physiol Rev 1983;63:1420–80.
3. Tanphaichitr V, Horne DW, Broquist HP. J Biol Chem 1971; 246:6364–6.
4. Engel AG, Angelini C. Science 1973;173:899–902.
5. Karpati G, Carpenter S, Engel AG et al. Neurology 1975;25: 16–24.
6. Treem WR, Stanley CA, Finegold DN et al. N Engl J Med 1988; 319:1331–6.
7. Cederblad G, Lindstedt S. Clin Chim Acta 1972;37:235–43.
8. Marquis NR, Fritz IB. J Lipid Res 1964;5:184–7.
9. van Kempen ATG, Odle J. J Chromatogr 1992;584:157–65.
10. Stevens RD, Hillman SL, Worthy S et al. Clin Chim Acta 2000; 46:727–9.
11. Broderick TL, Quinney HA, Lopaschuk GD. J Biol Chem 1992; 267:3758–63.
12. Obici S, Feng Z, Arduini A et al. Nat Med 2003;9:756–61.
13. Ramsay RR, Arduini A. Arch Biochem Biophys 1993;302:307–14.
14. Arduini A, Zibellini G, Ferrari L et al. Mol Cell Biochem 2001; 218:81–6.
15. Roe CR, Millington DS, Maltby DA et al. J Clin Invest 1984; 73:1785–8.
16. McGarry JD. Biochem Soc Trans 1995;23:321–4.
17. Ramsay RR, Gandour RD, van der Leij FR. Biochim Biophys Acta 2001;1546:21–43.
18. Fraser F, Padovese R, Zammit VA. J Biol Chem 2001;276:20182–5.
19. Colucci WJ, Gandour RD. Bioorg Chem 1988;16:307–34.
20. Farrell SO, Fiol CJ, Reddy JK et al. J Biol Chem 1984;259: 13089–95.
21. Chung CD, Bieber LL. J Biol Chem 1993;268:4519–24.
22. Pande SV, Murthy MSR. Biochim Biophys Acta 1994;1226: 269–76.
23. Huizing M, Iocobazzi V, Ijlst L et al. Am J Hum Genet 1997;61: 1239–45.
24. Iacobazzi V, Naglieri MA, Stanley CA et al. Biochem Biophys Res Commun 1998;252:770–4.
25. Indiveri C, Tonazzi A, Palmieri F. Biochim Biophys Acta 1990; 1020:81–6.
26. Rebouche CJ. Am J Clin Nutr 1991;54[Suppl]:1147S–52S.
27. Vaz FM, Wanders RJC. Biochem J 2002;361:417–29.
28. Rebouche CJ. FASEB J 1992;6:3379–86.
29. Rebouche CJ, Bosch EP, Chenard CA et al. J Nutr 1989;119: 1907–3.
30. Rebouche CJ, Chenard CA. J Nutr 1991;121:539–46.
31. Rebouche CJ. Metabolism 1991;40:1305–10.
32. Rebouche CJ, Mack DL, Edmonson PF. Biochemistry 1984;23: 6422–6.
33. Rebouche CJ, Seim H. Annu Rev Nutr 1998;18:39–61.
34. Lahjouji K, Malo C, Mitchell GA et al. Biochim Biophys Acta 2002;1558:82–93.
35. Gross CJ, Henderson LM. Biochim Biophys Acta 1984;772: 209–19.
36. Gudjonsson H, Li BUK, Shug AL et al. Gastroenterology 1985; 88:1880–7.
37. Rebouche CJ. J Nutr Biochem 1998;9:228–35.
38. Tamai I, Yabuuchi H, Nezu J et al. FEBS Lett 1997;419:107–11.
39. Xuan W, Lamhonwah AM, Librach C et al. Biochem Biophys Res Commun 2003;306:121–8.
40. Yabuuchi H, Tamai I, Nezu J et al. J Pharmacol Exp Ther 1999; 289:768–73.
41. Tein I. J Inherit Metab Dis 2003;26:147–69.
42. Tamai I, Ohashi R, Nezu J et al. J Biol Chem 1998;273:20378–82.

43. Wu X, Prasad PD, Leibach FH et al. Biochem Biophys Res Commun 1998;246:589–95.

44. Wu X, Huang W, Prasad PD et al. J Pharmacol Exp Ther 1999;290:1482–92.

45. Lamhonwah AM, Skaug J, Scherer SW et al. Biochem Biophys Res Commun 2003;301:98–101.

46. Nakanishi T, Hatanaka T, Huang W et al. J Physiol (Lond) 2001; 532:297–304.

47. Berardi S, Stieger B, Wachter S et al. Hepatology 1998;28:521–5.

48. Rebouche CJ, Lombard KA, Chenard CA. Am J Clin Nutr 1993; 58:660–5.

49. Nezu J, Tamai I, Oku A et al. Nat Genet 1999;21:91–4.

50. Famularo C, Matricardi F, Nucera E et al. Carnitine deficiency: primary and secondary syndromes. In: De Simone C, Famularo C, eds. Carnitine Today. Austin, TX: RG Landes, 1997:119–61.

51. Daily JW III, Sachan DS. J Nutr 1995;125:1938–44.

52. Rebouche CJ. Metabolism 1995;44:1639–43.

53. Melegh B, Pap, M, Bock I et al. Pediatr Res 1993;34:460–4.

54. Heuberger W, Berardi S, Jacky E et al. Eur J Clin Pharmacol 1998;54:503–8.

55. Marthaler NP, Visarius T, Küpfer A et al. Cancer Chemother Pharmacol 1999;44:170–2.

SELECTED READINGS

Kerner J, Hoppel C. Genetic disorders of carnitine metabolism and their nutritional management. Annu Rev Nutr 1998;18:179–206.

Ramsay RR, Gandour RD, van der Leij FR. Molecular enzymology of carnitine transfer and transport. Biochim Biophys Acta 2001:1546: 21–43.

Rebouche CJ, Seim H. Carnitine metabolism and its regulation in microorganisms and mammals. Annu Rev Nutr 1998;18:39–61.

Tein I. Carnitine transport: pathophysiology and metabolism of known molecular defects. J Inherit Metab Dis 2003;26:147–169.

Vaz FM, Wanders RJC. Carnitine biosynthesis in mammals. Biochem J 2002;361:417–29.

34 HOMOCYSTEINE, CYSTEINE, AND TAURINE[1,2]

MARTHA H. STIPANUK

HISTORICAL INTRODUCTION 545
CHEMISTRY, NOMENCLATURE, AND CELLULAR/
    EXTRACELLULAR FORMS 546
    Plasma Levels 546
DIETARY CONSIDERATIONS, TYPICAL INTAKES,
    AND RECOMMENDED INTAKES 547
    Methionine and Cyst(e)ine 547
    Taurine 548
ABSORPTION, TRANSPORT, AND EXCRETION 549
    Transporters and Transport Defects 549
    Excretion 550
METHIONINE/HOMOCYSTEINE METABOLISM AND
    CYSTEINE FORMATION 550
    Metabolic Pathways 550
    Regulation of Remethylation Versus
        Transsulfuration 551
    Homocystinuria and Hyperhomocysteinemia 553
METABOLISM OF CYSTEINE 554
    Pathways of Cysteine Metabolism 554
    Cysteine Oxidation and Taurine Synthesis
        in Humans 555
ESSENTIAL FUNCTIONS OF CYSTEINE AND
    ITS METABOLITES 556
    Synthesis of Protein and Glutathione 556
    Functions of Inorganic Sulfur 556
    Functions of Taurine 557
POSSIBLE CAUSES OF DEFICIENCY OF CYSTEINE
    OR TAURINE 557
    Immaturity 557
    Hepatic Dysfunction 558
    Total Parenteral or Enteral Nutrition 558
    Drug Metabolism 558
MEASURES OF TAURINE STATUS AND OF CYSTEINE
    AND/OR SULFUR AMINO ACID STATUS 559
TOXICITY 559

HISTORICAL INTRODUCTION

The importance of sulfur amino acids for growth or protein synthesis has been recognized since 1915, when Osborne and Mendel (1) demonstrated that addition of cystine to a low-casein diet resulted in restoration of rapid growth of rats. The amino acid methionine was identified almost two decades after most of the amino acids in protein had been discovered (2) and was subsequently shown to also be an effective supplement to low-casein diets (3). Womack and associates (4) demonstrated that cyst(e)ine (Cys or CySH) was not essential for rats when dietary methionine was adequate and that the effect of Cys resulted from its ability to replace part, but not all, of the methionine in the diet. Rose and Wixom (5) demonstrated the same relation of methionine and Cys requirements in their studies of the amino acid requirements of men. Thus, only methionine is considered an essential amino acid, but in practice the methionine or total sulfur amino acid requirement is usually met by a combination of methionine and Cys. N-Acetylcysteine, which is readily deacetylated to Cys or CySH, is used clinically in the treatment of acetaminophen overdose and for prevention of radiocontrast-induced nephropathy.

More recently, the nutritional importance of taurine, a metabolite of Cys, and the clinical significance of homocysteine (Hcy or HcySH), a metabolite of methionine, have been recognized. Hcy was discovered by du Vigneaud in 1932 (6) as the product of methionine demethylation. The role of Hcy in the conversion of methionine sulfur to Cys (the transsulfuration pathway) was studied in the years to follow, and it was shown that Hcy could support the growth of animals fed diets deficient in Cys, methionine, or choline. Homocystinuria, an inborn error of metabolism, was identified in 1962 when mentally retarded persons were screened for abnormal urinary amino acid patterns (7). In the 1990s,

---

[1]**Abbreviations: Ca^{2+},** calcium; **Cys,** cysteine (any form), with thiol and disulfide forms indicated as **CySH, CySSCy,** and **CySSR;** cyst(e)ine, cysteine, and/or cystine; **EAR,** estimated average requirement; **Glu,** glutamate; **Gly,** glycine; **GSH,** glutathione; **Hcy,** homocysteine (any form), with thiol and disulfide forms indicated as **HcySH, HcySSHcy,** and **HcySSR; H$_2$S,** hydrogen sulfide; **K$_m$,** Michaelis constant; **Na$^+$,** sodium; **NADH,** reduced nicotinamide-adenine dinucleotide; **NHANES,** National Health and Nutrition Examination Survey; **pK$_a$,** negative log

of association constant of acid; **PLP,** pyridoxal 5′-phosphate; **RDA,** recommended dietary allowance; **SCMC,** S-carboxymethylcysteine; **tCys,** sum of all forms of Cys including that present as thiol, half-disulfide, mixed disulfide, and protein-bound disulfide; **tHcy,** sum of all forms of **Hcy;** homocyst(e)ine, homocysteine, and/or homocystine **THF,** tetrahydrofolate; **TPN,** total parenteral nutrition.

[2]List of Compounds: cysteine, 121.2 g/mol; glutathione (reduced form), 307.3 g/mol; homocysteine, 135.2 g/mol; methionine, 149.2 g/mol; taurine, 125.1 g/mol.

investigators recognized that small increases in plasma Hcy concentrations are associated with an increased risk of vascular disease and neural tube defects in the general population (8–11).

Taurine is an end product of Cys catabolism. It was first isolated from the bile of the ox (*Box taurus*) in 1827 (12). Interest in taurine surged following the discovery in 1975 that cats fed diets containing little or no taurine suffered retinal degeneration accompanied by low retinal and plasma taurine concentrations (13). This finding was soon followed by the observation that infants fed purified formulas lacking taurine had lower plasma and urine taurine levels than did infants fed pooled human milk (14, 15). As a consequence of increasing evidence of a possible role of taurine in development, taurine has been added to most human infant formulas since the mid-1980s. Numerous therapeutic applications of taurine have been suggested, including treatment of patients with hypertension, cardiovascular disease, diabetes, hepatic disorders, chronic renal failure, sepsis, and inflammatory disorders.

CHEMISTRY, NOMENCLATURE, AND CELLULAR/EXTRACELLULAR FORMS

The structures of CySH, HcySH, and taurine and their relations with precursor amino acids (methionine and serine) are shown in Figure 34.1. Like other amino acids with an asymmetric carbon atom, the L-isomers of methionine, Hcy, and Cys are the biologically active forms. Both HcySH and CySH have a free sulfhydryl group. The carbon skeleton of HcySH, which is derived from methionine, has one more carbon than does the carbon chain of CySH, which is derived from serine. Taurine, 2-aminoethane sulfonate, is formed from CySH by removal of the carboxyl group and oxidation of the sulfur to form a sulfonic acid group. The carboxyl (negative log of association constant of acid [pK_a] ~1.7), sulfonic (pK_a ~1.5), sulfhydryl (pK_a ~8.3),

and amino (pK_a ~9–11) groups all undergo ionization; the zwitterionic forms shown in Figure 34.1 are the dominant species at physiologic pH.

Technically, the terms Cys and Hcy refer to the thiol or reduced form (RSH) of these amino acids. However, Cys and Hcy, like other aminothiols, also exist in free oxidized forms, including the disulfide (RSSR) and mixed disulfides (RSSR′), and in the protein-bound oxidized form (via formation of disulfides with cysteinyl residues of proteins; PSSR) (16, 17). The thiol form of Cys (CySH) dominates intracellularly, whereas disulfide forms of Cys (protein-bound Cys, PSSCy, and cystine, CySSCy) dominate in the more oxidized extracellular environment. Intracellularly, low concentrations of Hcy are present in free (HcySH) and protein-bound (PSSHcy) forms. Extracellularly, Hcy is present predominantly as mixed disulfides of Hcy with protein (PSSHcy) or Cys (HcySSCy). High levels of the disulfide of Hcy (homocystine, HcySSHcy) are excreted by persons with the inborn error of metabolism known as homocystinuria.

Plasma Levels

The distribution of Cys and Hcy in plasma of healthy adults is shown in Figure 34.2. Cys is the major plasma thiol, with total Hcy (tHcy) present at 10% or less of the concentration for total Cys (tCys). Both Cys and Hcy are predominantly present as protein-bound disulfides, with intermediate concentrations of disulfides (predominantly CySSCy and HcySSCy) and with very low concentrations of free thiols. The Cys-containing peptides, cysteinylglycine (CysGly), γ-glutamylcysteine (γGluCys), and glutathione (GSH or γGluCysGly), are also present in plasma and tissues.

The protein binding and redox status of different plasma aminothiols are interactive as a result of presumed ongoing redox cycling and disulfide exchange reactions. For example, Hcy will displace protein-bound Cys or CysGly (18). After ingestion of a methionine load or of a protein-containing meal, protein-bound Cys tends to decrease, probably because of displacement of protein-bound Cys by Hcy (16, 19).

Measures of tHcy or tCys are useful in clinical studies because these measurements are not affected in vitro by disulfide exchange reactions and redistribution between forms. Mean fasting plasma tHcy was 11.9 μmol/L (median, 11.6), with a range of 3.5 to 66.8 μmol/L in 1160 subjects aged 67 to 95 years (20); mean plasma tHcy is slightly less for younger than for older adults and for women than for men (21–23). Results from clinical treatment of homocystinuria caused by cystathionine β-synthase deficiency in 25 patients in Ireland between 1971 and 1996 indicated that maintenance of a median plasma free Hcy less than 11 μmol/L was associated with the absence of any homocystinuria-related complications (24). Mean fasting plasma tCys concentrations in healthy adults range from about 220 to 320 μmol/L (16–19).

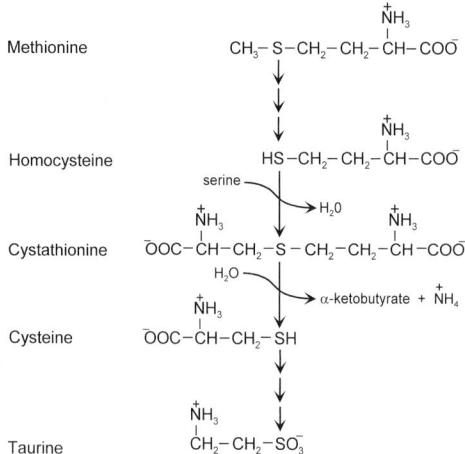

Figure 34.1. Structures and metabolic relations of sulfur amino acids.

	Reduced		Oxidized			Total	Reduced/Total Ratio
	Free			Protein-Bound			
Cysteine	CySH	14	RSSCy	88	PSSCy	196	250	0.056
Cysteinylglycine	HSCyGly	4	RSSCyGly	5	PSSCyGly	18	29	0.14
Homocysteine	HcySH	0.05	RSSHcy	1	PSSHcy	10	11	0.0045
Glutathione	GSH	4	RSSG	1.5	PSSG	1.6	6	0.67
γ-Glutamylcysteine	γ-GluCySH	0.6	RSSCyGlu	2	PSCyGlu	1	3	0.20

Figure 34.2. Concentrations (μmol/L) of various forms of the major aminothiols in human plasma. PS, sulfhydryl group of cysteinyl residue in protein; RS, unspecified thiol, usually CySH in plasma. The designation RSH is used to represent the reduced thiol form, RSSR or RSSR' to represent the disulfide of the thiol with itself or another thiol, and PSSR to represent protein-bound disulfides. Mean fasting values for plasma aminothiols are based on the data of Manssor and associates (16, 18) and Andersson and colleagues (17).

A wide range of plasma taurine concentrations has been reported for human subjects. Trautwein and Hayes (25) reviewed values reported in the literature and found that the reported mean plasma concentration of taurine in human subjects ranged from 39 to 116 μmol/L. Whole blood taurine ranged between 160 and 320 μmol/L with a mean of 225 μmol/L in a small sample of adults (25). Plasma taurine concentrations change more rapidly in response to changes in taurine intake than do whole blood concentrations, and whole blood taurine concentrations are not correlated with plasma taurine concentrations, except during periods of depletion or excess intake. Plasma taurine concentrations are somewhat lower in vegans than in omnivores and are somewhat lower in girls and women than in boys and men (26, 27).

Careful handling of blood samples is essential for measurement of plasma concentrations of aminothiols and taurine. Plasma tHcy concentrations may increase with storage of blood as a result of transsulfuration in blood cells unless the blood is rapidly cooled and processed (28). Hemolysis or contamination of the plasma fraction with platelets or white cells will interfere with analysis of plasma taurine, but not with measures of whole blood taurine (25).

DIETARY CONSIDERATIONS, TYPICAL INTAKES, AND RECOMMENDED INTAKES

Methionine and Cyst(e)ine

The sulfur amino acids, methionine and Cys (Table 34.1), are normally consumed as components of dietary proteins. Normal Western diets provide approximately 2 to 4 g/day of sulfur amino acids for adults (29). Based on the Third National Health and Nutrition Examination Survey (NHANES III;1988–1994), the mean methionine intake of 31- to 50-year-old men and women was 2.3±0.04 and 1.6±0.2 (SE) g/day, or 15.4 and 10.7 mmol/day, respectively.

TABLE 34.1. METHIONINE AND CYSTEINE CONTENT OF SELECTED FOODS

	AMOUNT		PATTERN	
	METHIONINE	CYSTEINE	METHIONINE	CYSTEINE
FOOD	(mg/100 g EDIBLE PORTION)		(mg/g PROTEIN)	
Cheese, cheddar	652	125	26	5
Milk, whole	83	30	25	9
Egg, whole, chicken	392	289	32	24
Chicken, flesh only, cooked roasted	800	370	28	13
Beef, round, separable lean only	557	224	26	11
Wheat flour, whole meal	186	278	14	21
Corn grits, regular, dry	196	237	22	22
Oats, regular, dry	266	398	17	25
Peanut butter	292	365	10	13
Soybean, green cooked	150	113	12	9
Brown rice, dry	142	152	19	21

Values taken or calculated from values in US Department of Agriculture. Agricultural Handbook No. 8. Washington, DC: Agriculture Research Service, US Department of Agriculture, 1976–1986.

Mean Cys intake for the same age group was 1.3±0.02 and 0.89±0.01 g/day, or 10.7 and 7.4 mmol/day, respectively. Thus, mean total sulfur amino acid intake was 26.1 and 18.1 mmol/day, respectively, for men and women. Sulfur amino acids tend to be more abundant in animal and cereal proteins than in legume proteins, and the ratio of methionine to Cys tends to be higher in animal proteins than in plant proteins (30).

For adults, the current estimated average requirement (EAR) for methionine and Cys intake is $15 \text{ mg} \cdot \text{kg}^{-1} \cdot \text{day}^{-1}$, and the recommended dietary allowance (RDA) is $19 \text{ mg} \cdot \text{kg}^{-1} \cdot \text{day}^{-1}$ (29). Considering that about one third of the sulfur amino acid requirement is taken in as Cys rather than methionine, the current RDA is consistent with the estimated safe intake of methionine ($21 \text{ mg} \cdot \text{kg}^{-1} \cdot \text{day}^{-1}$) reported by Di Buono and colleagues (24) but is less than the estimated safe intake ($25 \text{ mg} \cdot \text{kg}^{-1} \cdot \text{day}^{-1}$) determined by Young and coworkers (31, 32).

The current EAR for protein intake is $0.66 \text{ g} \cdot \text{kg}^{-1} \cdot \text{day}^{-1}$, and the RDA is $0.8 \text{ g} \cdot \text{kg}^{-1} \cdot \text{day}^{-1}$. Thus, a desirable amino acid pattern for adults includes at least 24 mg methionine plus Cys/g protein. Mixtures of proteins consumed in the United States actually contain a higher proportion of sulfur amino acids, about 35 mg methionine plus Cys/g protein. The RDA for sulfur amino acids (1.3 g/day for a 70-kg adult) is easily met in diets commonly consumed in the United States. Even the lowest methionine and Cys intakes reported in NHANES III (first percentile; 1.87 g for men and 1.4 g for women in the 31- to 50-year-old age bracket) exceeded the current RDA (29).

The RDAs for sulfur amino acids for pregnant and lactating women are 25 and $26 \text{ mg} \cdot \text{kg}^{-1} \cdot \text{day}^{-1}$. The RDAs for infants and children are $43 \text{ mg} \cdot \text{kg}^{-1} \cdot \text{day}^{-1}$ for 7- to 12-month-old infants, $28 \text{ mg} \cdot \text{kg}^{-1} \cdot \text{day}^{-1}$ for 1- to 3-year-old children, $22 \text{ mg} \cdot \text{kg}^{-1} \cdot \text{day}^{-1}$ for 4- to 8-year-old children, 22 and $21 \text{ mg} \cdot \text{kg}^{-1} \cdot \text{day}^{-1}$ for 9- to 13-year-old boys and girls, and 21 and $19 \text{ mg} \cdot \text{kg}^{-1} \cdot \text{day}^{-1}$ for 14- to 18-year-old boys and girls (29).

Despite the availability of food proteins that provide ample amounts of sulfur amino acids, it is likely that some persons have inadequate intakes, either because of inadequate intake of total protein or because of selection of a restricted variety of proteins that provide inadequate sulfur amino acids. Analysis of diets of long-term vegans living in California indicated an average protein intake of 64 g/day and a sulfur amino acid intake of 1.04 g (7.6 mmol)/day (27); this is equivalent to an intake of approximately $15 \text{ mg} \cdot \text{kg}^{-1} \cdot \text{day}^{-1}$ of sulfur amino acids and an amino acid pattern of 16 mg methionine plus Cys/g protein. This level of intake would meet the EAR, but not the RDA, for sulfur amino acids. Adults with higher-than-average requirements would be at risk of inadequate intake. Careful selection of plant proteins to ensure an adequate intake of sulfur amino acids may be very important for strict vegan adults and even more so for children fed a strict vegan diet.

Mixtures of proteins typically consumed in the United States supply about 40% of the total sulfur amino acids as Cys and 60% as methionine on a molar basis. This distribution would seem to allow optimal utilization of sulfur amino acids based on estimates of about 50% for the ability of Cys to replace methionine in the diet. In cases of limited ability to convert methionine to Cys (whether caused by hepatic dysfunction, inborn errors of methionine metabolism to Cys, or prematurity), one should consider the total amount of sulfur amino acids in the diet, the balance of Cys and methionine, and the adequacy of taurine.

Taurine

Although taurine is an end product of sulfur amino acid metabolism, it is usually obtained from the diet as well. Food taurine content has not been widely determined, but data from several reports (35–38) are summarized in Table 34.2. Taurine is present in most animal foods and is either absent or present in very low levels in most plant foods. Relatively high concentrations of taurine have been reported for some lower plants such as seaweeds (38, 39). Taurine-supplemented beverages have been popular for decades in Japan, where Taisho Pharmaceutical's Lipovitan is a favored drink. Since the mid-1990s, these taurine-supplemented beverages have become popular in many other countries, including the United States, and include Red Bull, Lipovitan, and Dark Dog, with 1000 mg/250-mL can, and Brute Force, with 1600 mg/can. Two studies of Red Bull demonstrated positive effects on mental performance and mood, but it is not clear that these effects are the result of taurine because this product also contains 80 mg of caffeine and 600 mg of glucuronolactone (40).

TABLE 34.2. TAURINE CONTENT OF SELECTED FOODS

FOOD	TAURINE CONTENT
Animal foods	
Poultry	89–2,245 μmol/100 g wet weight
Beef and pork	307–489 μmol/100 g wet weight
Processed meats	251–981 μmol/100 g wet weight
Seafood	84–6,614 μmol/100 g wet weight
Cow's milk	18–20 μmol/100 mL
Yogurt, ice cream	15–62 μmol/100 mL
Cheese	Not detected
Plant foods	
Most fruits, vegetables, seeds, cereals, grains, beans, peanuts	Not detected
Soybeans, chickpeas, black beans, pumpkin seeds, some nuts[a]	≤1–4 μmol/100 g wet weight
Seaweeds (marine algae)	1.5–100 μmol/100 g wet weight

[a]Low reported values should be regarded as upper limits because contamination of food or methodologic interference by compounds that coelute with taurine could account for these low concentrations of taurine.

Values from Laidlaw et al. (35), Pasantes-Morales et al. (36), Roe and Weston (37), and Kataoka and Ohnishi (38).

Analysis of the diets of strict vegans living in England yielded no detectable taurine, whereas the diets of omnivores contained 463 ± 156 (SE) μmol/day (26). The analyzed taurine intake of adults fed omnivorous diets in a clinical study center in the United States was 1000 to 1200 μmol/day (35). The wide range of taurine intakes from the diet is also illustrated by the cross-sectional study, involving 24 populations in 16 countries, by Yamori and colleagues (41). The highest median urinary taurine levels were found in men and women (2181 and 1590 μmol/day, respectively) in Beppu, Japan, whereas the lowest median urinary excretions of taurine were observed in men in St. John, Canada (192 μmol/day) and women in Moscow, Russia (128 μmol/day). The large variation in taurine excretion largely reflects the range of dietary intake and the contribution of seafood to taurine intake.

The taurine content of milk from lactating women was 413 ± 71 (SE) μmol/L for early milk (1–7 days) and 337 ± 28 μmol/L for later milk (>7 days) (42, 43). Taurine is added to infant formulas at levels comparable to those in human milk or at somewhat higher levels in formulas for premature infants (35). The mean taurine concentration of milk from lactating lacto-ovovegetarian women was only slightly lower than that of omnivores (43). The mean taurine content of milk of lactating vegan women is lower than that of lactating omnivores, but overlap of values between the two groups is still considerable, and the taurine concentration in milk of vegan mothers is about 30 times the level in the cow's milk–based infant formulas used before the mid-1980s (26).

Because strict vegan diets tend to be lower in total sulfur amino acid content and virtually free of taurine, adult vegans and particularly children consuming vegan diets are at somewhat greater risk of inadequate sulfur amino acid status. Human adults who consume a strict vegetarian diet have been reported to have lower plasma taurine concentrations and greatly reduced urinary taurine excretion compared with omnivores. However, vegans consuming little or no preformed taurine are healthy, and the children born to and nursed by vegan mothers have normal growth and development (26).

By general consensus, taurine is considered to be conditionally essential during infant development and probably for adults in some special circumstances. Because the brain and retina of human infants are not fully developed at birth and may be vulnerable to the effects of taurine deprivation, it has been judged prudent to supplement human infant formulas and pediatric feeding solutions with taurine (15, 39). During the 1980s, manufacturers of infant formulas began adding taurine to their products, and taurine is currently added to virtually all human infant formulas and pediatric parenteral solutions throughout the world (44). The taurine content of human milk has been used as a guideline for supplementation levels.

ABSORPTION, TRANSPORT, AND EXCRETION

Transporters and Transport Defects

Absorption of the products of protein digestion across the intestinal epithelium is highly efficient (~95–99%). Dietary methionine, a precursor of Cys, is transported by neutral amino acid transport systems ($B^{0,+}$, ASC, and L), and as methionine-containing peptides by peptide transport systems. Dietary Cys is absorbed as CySH, CySSCy, and as Cys-containing peptides by a variety of L-amino acid and peptide transport systems in the small intestinal mucosa. Transport of CySH is accomplished by neutral amino acid transporters including system B in the apical (brush border) membrane and system ASC in both the apical and basolateral plasma membranes of the intestinal mucosa cells; CySH uptake is largely sodium (Na^+) dependent. Cystine (CySSCy) is transported by system $b^{0,+}$, a Na^+-independent system that is present in the apical membranes of the intestinal mucosa and that serves cationic amino acids as well as zwitterionic amino acids. The Na^+-independent transporter LAT-2 (a subtype of system L) is responsible for the movement of cystine across the basolateral membrane of the enterocytes (45). Efficient absorption of taurine is facilitated by the β-amino acid or taurine transport system, which is a Na^+- and chloride-dependent carrier that serves taurine, β-alanine, and γ-aminobutyric acid and is present in the apical membrane of intestinal mucosa cells. The reabsorption of the taurine-conjugated bile acids secreted into the lumen of the bile occurs in the ileum, and this enterohepatic reabsorption plays an important role in taurine conservation.

Amino acids enter the plasma and circulate as free amino acids until they are removed by tissues. The liver removes a substantial proportion of the sulfur-containing amino acids from the portal circulation and uses them for synthesis of protein and GSH or for catabolism to taurine and sulfate. GSH is exported into plasma, and this Cys-containing tripeptide, as well as its metabolites, CysGly and γGluCys, can be a source of Cys to tissues. Hcy is not normally present in the diet, and only very low amounts are normally released from tissues into the plasma.

Cystinuria

Cystinuria is an inherited disorder of cystine and dibasic amino acid transport (46, 47). One cause of cystinuria is a defect in the gene that encodes the rBAT (related to $b^{0,+}$ amino acid transporter) protein, a subunit of the system $b^{0,+}$ transporter that is expressed by the kidney and small intestine (48–50). Urinary cystine excretion exceeding 1.2 mmol/day (~2.5 mmol Cys/day) is usually diagnostic of homozygous cystinuria (51). Cystine is very insoluble and can cause cystine stones if it is present above its aqueous solubility limit (250 mg/L or 1 mmol/L).

Cystinosis

Cystinosis is also a genetic disease caused by the lack of a functional cystine transporter. Cystinosis is caused by mutations in the gene that encodes cystinosin, a lysosomal membrane protein that transports cystine in a hydrogen ion–dependent manner (52). In patients with cystinosis, cystine from degraded proteins accumulates inside the lysosomes of cells.

Excretion

The reabsorptive epithelium of the kidney proximal tubule has transport systems similar to those of the absorptive epithelium of the intestine, and the kidney efficiently reabsorbs amino acids from the filtrate. Renal reabsorption of Cys and methionine is normally very high (>94%), and the loss of amino acids in the urine is normally negligible (46, 47). Urinary methionine excretion has been reported to be 22 to 41 µmol/day (26, 47). Urinary Cys excretion by adults has been reported as 63 to 285 µmol/day (26, 47).

Urinary excretion of extracellular Hcy is limited, even in persons with defective Hcy metabolism, owing to the extensive binding of plasma Hcy to proteins that limits filtration and the normally active renal reabsorption of free Hcy. Of the plasma Hcy filtered by the kidney, only about 1 to 2% is excreted in the urine (53). Normal urinary Hcy excretion ranges from 3.5 to 9.8 µmol/day (53). Higher levels of Hcy in urine are indicative of very high plasma tHcy concentrations and of an inborn error of metabolism. For example, Hcy excretion in urine of patients with $N^{5,10}$-methylenetetrahydrofolate reductase deficiency ranged from 15 to 667 µmol/day (54).

Unlike most amino acids, taurine is not usually completely reabsorbed, and fractional excretion may vary over a wide range. Normally, the kidneys regulate the body pool size of taurine and adapt to changes in dietary taurine intake by regulation of the proximal tubule brush border membrane transporter for taurine (β system). During periods of inadequate dietary intake of taurine or of its sulfur amino acid precursors, more taurine is reabsorbed from the filtrate because of enhanced taurine transporter activity, less taurine is excreted in the urine, and more of the tissue taurine stores are maintained. The renal taurine concentration seems to be the signal for changes in renal taurine transporter activity (55, 56). The intestinal uptake of taurine and the expression of the taurine transporter in the intestine do not respond to the level of dietary sulfur amino acids or taurine (57).

Consistent with variation in taurine intake, and with adaptive regulation of taurine reabsorption, urinary taurine levels vary widely. Urinary taurine levels of 250 µmol/day have been reported for adult vegans consuming diets with no preformed taurine, whereas excretion of taurine by adult omnivores is usually more than 600 µmol/day, with values higher than 1000 µmol/day not uncommon (26, 27, 47). Daily taurine excretions of less than 90 µmol/day have been reported for persons in Finland and Canada and of more than 2000 µmol/day for persons in Taiwan and Japan (41).

METHIONINE/HOMOCYSTEINE METABOLISM AND CYSTEINE FORMATION

Metabolic Pathways

Transmethylation

The essential amino acid, methionine, is activated by adenosine triphosphate to form S-adenosylmethionine in a reaction catalyzed by methionine adenosyltransferase (EC 2.5.1.6) (Fig. 34.3). Two isozymes of methionine adenosyltransferase exist: a liver-specific isozyme, encoded by gene *MAT1A*, that has a high Michaelis constant (K_m) for methionine and exists as a tetramer (MAT1) or dimer (MAT3), and a widely expressed, low-K_m form (MAT2) that is encoded by gene *MAT2A*. The unique liver isozyme allows the liver to respond to an influx of excess methionine with increased adenosylmethionine formation. Adenosylmethionine serves primarily as a methyl donor via reactions catalyzed by a variety of methyl transferases and involving a variety of acceptors. These S-adenosylmethionine–dependent methylations are essential for the biosynthesis of various cellular components including creatine, epinephrine, carnitine, phospholipids, proteins, DNA, and RNA.

S-Adenosylhomocysteine, the byproduct of these methyl transfer reactions, is hydrolyzed by S-adenosylhomocysteine hydrolase (EC 3.3.1.1), thus generating adenosine and Hcy. Although the equilibrium of S-adenosylhomocysteine hydrolase actually favors formation of S-adenosylhomocysteine, the reaction is normally driven forward by rapid removal of the products.

The Hcy generated by hydrolysis of S-adenosylhomocysteine has two likely metabolic fates, remethylation or transsulfuration. In remethylation, Hcy acquires a methyl group from N^5-methyltetrahydrofolate or from betaine to form methionine. In transsulfuration, the sulfur is transferred to serine to form Cys, and the remainder of the Hcy molecule is catabolized to α-ketobutyrate and ammonium.

Remethylation

The remethylation pathway allows methionine to be regenerated from Hcy using new methyl groups synthesized in the folate coenzyme system or using preformed methyl groups, both of which may subsequently be transferred to acceptors via S-adenosylmethionine–dependent methyltransferase reactions. The remethylation of Hcy by transfer of a methyl group from N^5-methyltetrahydrofolate is catalyzed by N^5-methyltetrahydrofolate–Hcy methyltransferase (EC 2.1.1.13), which is commonly called methionine synthase. Methionine synthase is widely distributed in mammalian tissues and contains methylcobalamin as an essential cofactor. The methyl group of N^5-methyltetrahydrofolate is synthesized de novo in the folate coenzyme system

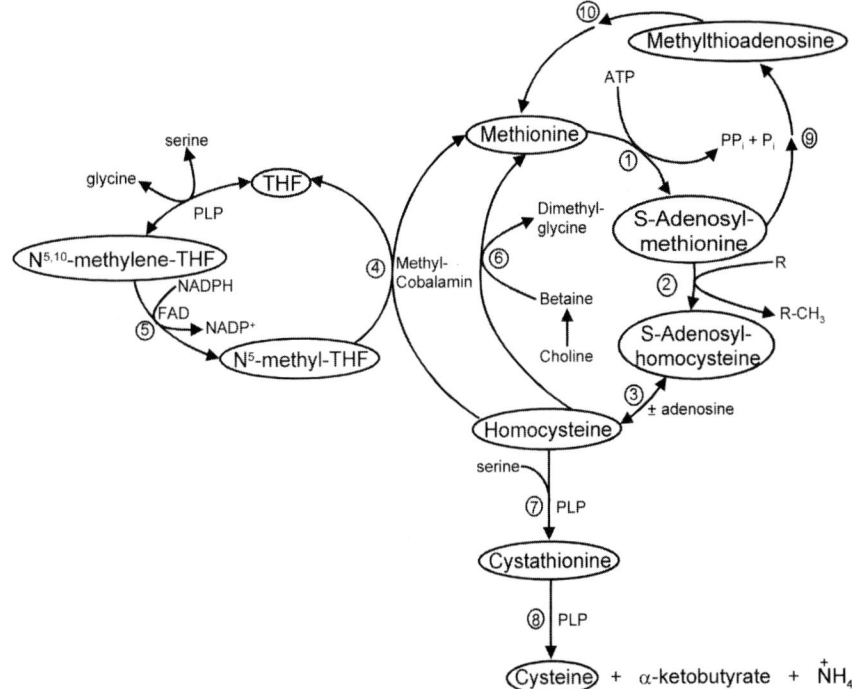

Figure 34.3. Methionine metabolism. Numbered reactions are catalyzed by the following enzymes: (1) methionine adenosyltransferase; (2) various methyltransferases; (3) adenosyl-homocysteine hydrolase; (4) N^5-methyltetrahydrofolate (methyl-THF)–homocysteine methyltransferase; (5) $N^{5,10}$-methylenetetrahydrofolate (methylene-THF) reductase; (6) betaine–homocysteine methyltransferase; (7) cystathionine β-synthase; (8) cystathionine γ-lyase; (9) enzymes involved in polyamine synthesis; and (10) enzymes involved in methylthioadenosine salvage pathway.

(see Chapter 28). The final step of N^5-methyltetrahydrofolate synthesis is the irreversible reduction of $N^{5,10}$-methylenetetrahydrofolate, which is catalyzed by the flavoenzyme, $N^{5,10}$-methylenetetrahydrofolate reductase (EC 1.1.1.68), using reduced nicotinamide-adenine dinucleotide (NADH) as the electron donor.

The other Hcy methyltransferase, betaine–Hcy methyltransferase (EC 2.1.1.5), is present only in liver, kidney, and lens of humans and requires betaine as the methyl donor (58). The betaine–Hcy methyltransferase may account for as much as half of the methionine synthesized in the liver (59). This reaction uses preformed methyl groups because betaine is obtained from the diet or derived from choline, which is either obtained from the diet or synthesized through successive S-adenosylmethionine–dependent methylations of phosphatidylethanolamine.

Transsulfuration

Although all cells are capable of transmethylation and remethylation, the catabolism of Hcy via transsulfuration is restricted. In the rat, transsulfuration occurs in liver, kidney, small intestine, and pancreas (59). Tissues that are not capable of transsulfuration require an exogenous source of Cys and also must export Hcy for further metabolism or removal by other tissues.

The transsulfuration of Hcy to Cys is catalyzed by two pyridoxal 5′-phosphate–(PLP-)dependent enzymes, cystathionine β-synthase (EC 4.2.1.22) and cystathionine γ-lyase (EC 4.4.1.1; cystathionase). Cystathionine β-synthase catalyzes the condensation of Hcy and serine to form cystathionine. The cystathionine is then hydrolyzed by cystathionine γ-lyase to form Cys and α-ketobutyrate plus ammonium. Thus, the

transsulfuration pathway is responsible both for the catabolism of Hcy derived from methionine and for the transfer of methionine sulfur to serine to synthesize Cys. As could be predicted, the overexpression of cystathionine β-synthase (on chromosome 21) in children with Down syndrome results in significantly reduced plasma levels of Hcy, methionine, S-adenosylhomocyst(e)ine, and S-adenosylmethionine and a significant increase in plasma cystathionine and Cys (60).

Regardless of the extent of remethylation, in the steady-state metabolic condition in physiologically normal persons, the intake of methionine sulfur is balanced by metabolism of an almost equivalent amount of Hcy sulfur through the transsulfuration pathway (61, 62). Although some methionine (via decarboxylated S-adenosylmethionine acting as a donor of aminopropyl groups) is used for polyamine synthesis, the methylthioadenosine that is a byproduct of this pathway is effectively recycled to methionine. The sulfur and methyl carbon of methionine and the carbon chain of ribose are reused in methionine synthesis by the methylthioadenosine salvage pathway (62, 63). Hence little sulfur is oxidized or lost during methionine metabolism, and essentially all methionine sulfur is transferred to Cys before oxidation or excretion of the sulfur atom.

Regulation of Remethylation Versus Transsulfuration

Response to Changes in Methionine Intake

The remethylation and transsulfuration pathways can be considered to be competing for available Hcy. Studies of whole-body methionine kinetics demonstrated that, in young men fed a diet with adequate methionine

(~14 mmol/day), about 17 mmol of Hcy was formed per day by transmethylation, and approximately 38% of this Hcy was remethylated to methionine, whereas 62% was catabolized by transsulfuration (32). In another study, transmethylation or Hcy formation decreased markedly in subjects fed a sulfur amino acid–free diet, from approximately 20 mmol/day in men on an adequate diet to 6 mmol/day in men on a sulfur amino acid–free diet; the percentage of Hcy remethylated to methionine increased from 36% in men on the adequate diet to 67% in men on the sulfur amino acid–free diet (64). As a result of decreased transmethylation or Hcy formation and the greater percentage remethylation of Hcy, transsulfuration or oxidation of methionine was reduced from 12 mmol/day in men fed the methionine-adequate diet to 2 mmol/day in subjects fed the sulfur amino acid–free diet. Women had slightly higher rates of transmethylation and remethylation but similar rates of transsulfuration (65).

Response to *S*-Adenosylmethionine as an Effector

The metabolism of Hcy by remethylation versus transsulfuration seems to be coordinated in response to cellular S-adenosylmethionine concentrations or the need to generate methionine methyl groups (66). S-Adenosylmethionine is both an allosteric inhibitor of $N^{5,10}$-methylenetetrahydrofolate reductase and an activator of cystathionine β-synthase. Hence, when the cellular S-adenosylmethionine concentration is low, the synthesis of N^5-methyltetrahydrofolate proceeds uninhibited, whereas cystathionine synthesis is suppressed. This results in the conservation of Hcy for methionine synthesis. Conversely, when the S-adenosylmethionine concentration is high, inhibition of N^5-methyltetrahydrofolate synthesis is accompanied by the diversion of Hcy through the transsulfuration pathway because of stimulated cystathionine synthesis. The outcome of this coordinate control is both the regulation of cellular S-adenosylmethionine concentration and the maintenance of a concentration of Hcy that is compatible with the need for methyl groups synthesized de novo.

Methionine-Sparing Effect of Cyst(e)ine

Cys is said to have a methionine-sparing effect by reducing methionine catabolism via the transsulfuration pathway, and this appears to occur with intakes of typical food proteins in which the ratio of methionine to Cys ranges from approximately 1:1 to 2:1 (67). Maximal sparing of methionine is about 64% as judged by observations in subjects consuming excess Cys and minimal methionine (68). The action of supplemental Cys when it is added to a sulfur amino acid–free diet or to a low-methionine diet may be explained at least partially by promotion of the incorporation of methionine into protein such that less methionine is catabolized (64, 69, 70). The action of Cys when it

is used to replace part of the dietary methionine, keeping total sulfur amino acid level the same, may be explained by a reduction in the hepatic concentrations of methionine and S-adenosylmethionine and hence less activation and reduced activity of hepatic cystathionine β-synthase. When the ratio of methionine to Cys of the diet was increased from 1:0 to 1:1 to 1:3, the ratio of metabolism of Hcy by remethylation versus transsulfuration increased from 0.75 to 1.3 to 1.9 (67). This sparing effect is largely the result of the "first-pass" metabolism of methionine in the splanchnic region and was not observed in studies in which methionine was administered intravenously (68). Less catabolism of Hcy by transsulfuration would result in an increase in the recycling of Hcy to methionine using methyl groups generated by the folate coenzyme system (see Chapter 28).

Response to Supplemental Betaine

Physiologically normal adult subjects given a control diet with a betaine supplement had increased rates of methionine transmethylation and transsulfuration (71), a finding suggesting that an increased dietary supply of methyl groups may increase methionine catabolism. A high dietary intake of betaine when coupled with a marginal intake of methionine could interfere with the normal coordinated regulation of remethylation versus transsulfuration by increasing S-adenosylmethionine concentration and stimulating methionine catabolism (71). Presumably, increased remethylation induced by betaine increases S-adenosylmethionine concentrations and results in inhibition of N^5-methyltetrahydrofolate–dependent remethylation and stimulation of Hcy catabolism.

Redox and Hormonal Regulation of Transsulfuration

Redox regulation of cystathionine β-synthase may provide a means to promote transsulfuration at the expense of remethylation, independently of methylation status, when the body has an increased need for Cys for GSH synthesis. Flux of Hcy through transsulfuration appears to be increased under oxidizing conditions, and this upregulation of transsulfuation has been associated with oxidation of the heme moiety in the N-terminal domain or targeted proteolysis of the C-terminal domain of cystathionine β-synthase (72, 73). The C-terminal domain is autoinhibitory and confers responsiveness of cystathionine β-synthase to its allosteric activator S-adenosylmethionine. Hepatic cystathionine β-synthase gene expression is increased by glucagon and glucocorticoids and is decreased by insulin (74, 75). Hormonal regulation of hepatic cystathionine β-synthase expression may serve to conserve methionine for protein synthesis in the fed state and to promote catabolism of the methionine/Hcy carbon chain to α-ketobutyrate, a gluconeogenic substrate, in the starved state.

Homocystinuria and Hyperhomocysteinemia

Metabolic Bases

An increase in plasma Hcy could result from an increased production rate (i.e., transmethylation), a decreased rate of removal by transsulfuration, a decreased rate of remethylation to methionine, or a decrease in the uptake and metabolism or excretion of Hcy by the kidney. Examples of the latter three mechanisms have been well established. Use of ninetieth percentile values as cutoffs has resulted in use of plasma fasting tHcy values greater than 14 to 16 μmol/L as indicators of hyperhomocysteinemia (21, 76). A lower cutoff for the normal range may be appropriate, however, because the frequency distribution of plasma tHcy concentrations is positively skewed (77), and improved vitamin status can decrease the 90% cutoff value to approximately 12 μmol/L.

Hyperhomocysteinemia frequently has a genetic basis. A milder form of $N^{5,10}$-methylenetetrahydrofolate reductase deficiency that results in approximately 50% residual enzyme activity in homozygotes is caused by a point mutation ($677C{\rightarrow}T$) in the $N^{5,10}$-methylenetetrahydrofolate reductase gene (78–80). Approximately 5% of subjects studied by Kang and associates (81) and 12% of those studied by Rozen and colleagues (82) were homozygous for this $677C{\rightarrow}T$ mutation in the $N^{5,10}$-methylenetetrahydrofolate reductase gene. Other genetic variants in the methylenetetrahydrofolate reductase gene have been identified (78). Heterozygosity for a gene coding for nonfunctional cystathionine β-synthase may cause hyperhomocysteinemia, but the incidence of heterozygosity for inborn errors is too small to account for a large proportion of the observed hyperhomocysteinemia.

Nutritional disorders that potentially lead to hyperhomocysteinemia, particularly in persons with underlying genetic predispositions, are deficiencies of folate, vitamin B_{12}, and vitamin B_6 (20, 83–85). Selhub and colleagues (20) estimated that 67% of the cases of hyperhomocysteinemia are at least partially the result of inadequate B-vitamin status. As noted earlier, the de novo synthesis of methionine methyl groups requires both vitamin B_{12} and folate coenzymes, whereas transsulfuration requires PLP (20, 21, 77, 84–87).

Severe forms of hyperhomocysteinemia result in excretion of HcySH, homocystine, and mixed disulfides of Hcy in the urine. Homocystinuria (urinary Hcy >10 μmol/24 hours) is rare and results from inborn errors of metabolism that are associated with severely elevated plasma tHcy concentrations. The most common inborn error of sulfur amino acid metabolism, and the most common cause of homocystinuria, is a lack of cystathionine β-synthase activity, which is commonly associated with plasma tHcy concentrations higher than 200 μmol/L in untreated patients. A second inborn error of metabolism that causes homocystinuria is a lack of $N^{5,10}$-methylenetetrahydrofolate reductase activity (see also Chapter 28).

This is the major known inborn error affecting folate metabolism and the second leading known cause of homocystinuria. Both diseases are inherited as autosomal recessive disorders; the incidence of cystathionine β-synthase deficiency is approximately ten times as high as that of $N^{5,10}$-methylenetetrahydrofolate reductase deficiency (see also Chapter 28). A third group of inborn errors giving rise to homocystinuria comprises those affecting various steps in synthesis of methylcobalamin, an essential cofactor for methionine synthase (see also Chapter 29).

Mild to moderate hyperhomocysteinemia has also been observed in patients with renal disease. Plasma tHcy is significantly increased in patients with moderate renal failure and rises steeply in terminal uremia (88, 89). The rise in plasma tHcy in patients with renal failure is thought to result from loss of renal parenchymal uptake and metabolism of plasma Hcy rather than from decreased urinary excretion of Hcy.

Certain drugs interfere with normal Hcy metabolism by causing secondary functional vitamin deficiencies. For example, theophylline is a vitamin B_6 antagonist, and valproate and carbamazepine have antifolate activity. These drugs can cause elevated plasma tHcy levels.

Untreated homocystinuria results in a wide range of neurologic and vascular disturbances. Apparent associations of mild hyperhomocysteinemia with cardiovascular diseases such as atherosclerotic and ischemic cardiovascular diseases, stroke, and venous thromboses have been reported (8, 9, 22, 77, 89–95). Additionally, epidemiologic studies have shown associations between hyperhomocysteinemia and neuropsychiatric disorders such as Alzheimer disease (see Chapter 88), developmental disorders such as neural tube defects, and complications of pregnancy such as placental abruption or infarction and unexplained pregnancy loss (10, 11, 92, 93). In populations of patients with atherosclerotic disease, mild hyperhomocysteinemia is observed about as frequently as hypercholesterolemia or hypertension. Hyperhomocysteinemia is now considered to be an independent risk factor for vascular disease of the coronary, cerebral, and peripheral arteries; an increase in plasma tHcy of only 5 μmol/L is estimated to result in a 50 to 80% increase in risk of cerebrovascular or coronary artery disease (81).

The basis of the association of hyperhomocysteinemia with vascular disease is not clear (9, 96–99). Hypotheses related to a direct adverse effect of Hcy (endothelial cell damage, oxidative damage, promotion of thrombogenesis via alterations in the coagulation and fibrinolytic systems, impaired regulation of vasoconstriction, stimulation of vascular smooth muscle cell proliferation) are currently being investigated. It is also possible that a decreased intracellular ratio of S-adenosylmethionine to S-adenosylhomocysteine or reduced availability of S-adenosylmethionine, either of which may be associated with hyperhomocysteinemia, interferes with essential methylation reactions and leads to the adverse effects associated with hyperhomocysteinemia.

Similarly, impaired methylation of proteins has been implicated as a possible cause of neural tube defects (100, 101).

Dietary Management

The goal of dietary treatment of homocystinuria is to decrease the biochemical abnormalities (reduce plasma Hcy, maintain normal concentrations of plasma methionine and Cys) and to minimize the development of clinical complications. Treatment of patients with inborn errors of transsulfuration (cystathionine β-synthase deficiency) usually involves restriction of dietary methionine intake with care to provide adequate Cys intake. In homocystinuria caused by inborn errors in the methionine remethylation pathway, the goal of dietary treatment is to maintain sufficient levels of methionine methyl groups without elevating the plasma Hcy concentration; this usually involves relatively high levels of B-vitamin supplementation (folate, vitamin B_{12}) to stimulate the N^5-methyltetrahydrofolate–dependent Hcy remethylation pathway, betaine or choline to stimulate the betaine-dependent Hcy remethylation pathway, and, in some cases, methionine supplementation to ensure sufficient availability of S-adenosylmethionine (102). Modest levels of vitamin supplementation (~0.6 mg folic acid, 0.4 mg cyanocobalamin, and 10 mg pyridoxine) have been shown to reduce plasma tHcy concentrations in some persons with mild hyperhomocysteinemia (77, 89, 103–105).

METABOLISM OF CYSTEINE

Pathways of Cysteine Metabolism

Cys, whether formed from methionine and serine via transsulfuration or supplied preformed in the diet, serves as a precursor for synthesis of proteins and several other essential molecules, as shown in Figure 34.4. These metabolites include GSH, coenzyme A, taurine, and inorganic sulfur.

At intakes near the requirement, a large proportion of available Cys is used for synthesis of proteins and of GSH (a tripeptide, γ-glutamylcysteinylglycine). In addition to the specific metabolic functions of GSH, GSH serves as a reservoir of Cys and as a means for transporting Cys to extrahepatic tissues (99). A large proportion of the sulfur amino acid intake is converted to GSH by the liver and is released into the circulation. γ-Glutamyl transpeptidase, an enzyme located on the outer surface of the plasma membrane of cells in a number of tissues, hydrolyzes GSH (or its disulfide) to yield CysGly (or its disulfide), which can be further degraded by peptidases to release Cys into the plasma. The normal human turnover of GSH is estimated to be 40 mmol/day (106, 107), approximately twice the typical sulfur amino acid intake of 20 mmol/day and six to seven times the average daily sulfur amino acid requirement for adults. This estimate suggests that the magnitude of turnover of the Cys pool as a result of GSH turnover may be about the same (~40 mmol/day) as that resulting from protein turnover in the body (32, 65).

Cys is also precursor for synthesis of coenzyme A and for production of taurine and inorganic sulfate. These three fates of Cys involve loss of the Cys moiety as such. Cys is substrate for coenzyme A synthesis in that it donates the cysteamine (decarboxylated CySH) moiety of the coenzyme A molecule and hence contributes the reactive sulfhydryl group. Very little is known about the rate of coenzyme A turnover. However, the identification of the pantothenate kinase gene *PANK2* as the gene responsible for Hallervorden-Spatz syndrome, which is characterized by the accumulation of Cys in the basal ganglia, has suggested

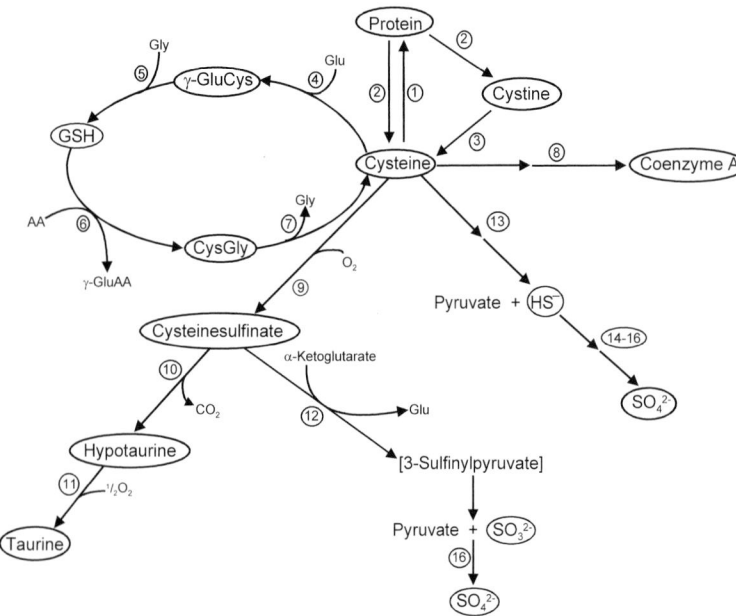

Figure 34.4. Pathways of cysteine metabolism. Numbered reactions are catalyzed by the following enzymes or pathways: (*1*) protein synthesis; (*2*) protein degradation; (*3*) glutathione (GSH) thioltransferase or nonenzymatic thiol disulfide exchange of cystine with GSH; (*4*) γ-glutamylcysteine synthetase; (*5*) GSH synthetase; (*6*) GSH transpeptidase; (*7*) dipeptidase; (*8*) pathway of coenzyme A synthesis; (*9*) cysteine dioxygenase; (*10*) cysteinesulfinate decarboxylase; (*11*) enzymatic or nonenzymatic oxidation of hypotaurine; (*12*) aspartate (cysteinesulfinate) aminotransferase; (*13*) cysteinesulfinate-independent or desulfhydration pathways of cyst(e)ine catabolism; (*14*) sulfide oxidase; (*15*) thiosulfate sulfurtransferase or GSH-dependent thiosulfate reductase; and (*16*) sulfite oxidase.

that coenzyme A turnover may consume a substantial amount of Cys (108, 109). The functions of coenzyme A are discussed in Chapter 27.

Both taurine and inorganic sulfur are products of Cys catabolism. As shown in Figure 34.4, there are several pathways for Cys catabolism. Cys catabolism may occur by desulfuration of CySH to yield pyruvate and reduced sulfur (often in the form of a persulfide such as thiocysteine, mercaptopyruvate, or thiosulfate). Cys desulfuration can be catalyzed by the β-cleavage of Cys by cystathionine γ-lyase, by action of cystathionine β-synthase, or by transamination of cysteine to β-mercaptopyruvate followed by desulfuration or transsulfuration by mercaptopyruvate sulfurtransferase (62). Levels of hydrogen sulfide (H_2S) and S-adenosylmethionine, a cystathionine β-synthase activator, were low and the level of Hcy was elevated in autopsied brain tissue from patients with Alzheimer disease compared with those of age-matched controls, consistent with a decrease in cystathionine β-synthase activity (110). Persons with a rare inborn error of metabolism in which β-mercaptopyruvate sulfurtransferase is deficient excrete the mixed disulfide of cysteine and β-mercaptolactate, a finding suggesting that transamination of cysteine to mercaptopyruvate occurs to some extent in humans (111). However, these patients excrete normal levels of urinary sulfate, a finding indicating that overall cysteine catabolism is not impaired. The reduced sulfur may be used in synthesis of molecules requiring a source of reduced sulfur, or it may be oxidized to thiosulfate (inner sulfur), sulfite, and finally sulfate. Although most of the inorganic sulfur is eventually oxidized to sulfate, mammals depend on the cysteinesulfinate-independent or desulfhydration pathways of Cys metabolism as a source of reduced forms of inorganic sulfur because they do not have the ability to reduce sulfate or sulfite to thiosulfate or sulfide.

In animals fed diets that provide protein or sulfur amino acids at levels near or above the requirement, the major pathway of Cys catabolism involves the oxidation of CySH to cysteinesulfinate by Cys dioxygenase (EC 1.13.11.20) (62, 112). Cys dioxygenase is expressed in high levels in liver, relative to other tissues, and Cys dioxygenase mRNA levels in liver of rats are not affected by the diet. Cys dioxygenase is rapidly degraded in liver of rats fed low-protein diets, thus keeping Cys dioxygenase activity very low. However, when rats are fed high levels of protein or sulfur amino acids, hepatic Cys levels increase and prevent the polyubiquitination of Cys dioxygenase and hence its degradation by the 26S proteasome. The regulation of Cys dioxygenase turnover allows a robust regulation of hepatic Cys dioxygenase in response to changes in dietary sulfur amino acid influx (113).

Cysteinesulfinate, formed by action of Cys dioxygenase on CySH, may be decarboxylated to hypotaurine, which is subsequently oxidized to taurine, or cysteinesulfinate may be transaminated (with α-ketoglutarate) to the enzyme-bound intermediate, β-sulfinylpyruvate, which gives rise to pyruvate and sulfite. Sulfite is further oxidized to sulfate by sulfite oxidase (EC 1.8.3.1). Thus, oxidation of CySH by Cys dioxygenase leads to both taurine and sulfate formation, with sulfate the dominant product.

In all catabolic pathways except that resulting in taurine formation, the carbon chain of Cys is released as pyruvate, the sulfur is released as inorganic sulfur, and the amino group is released as ammonium or is transferred to a keto acid acceptor. When taurine is the end product, only the carboxyl carbon of the Cys is released, and the other three carbons as well as the nitrogen and sulfur atoms remain in the end product. Thus, the distribution of Cys among its catabolic pathways potentially affects the utilization of amino acid carbon chains for energy, the net production of acid or fixed anions (sulfate), and the synthesis of essential metabolites (inorganic sulfur and taurine).

Human adults remain in sulfur balance, with sulfur excretion essentially equivalent to sulfur intake (14–28 mmol/day). Both sulfate and taurine are excreted in the urine. In studies of children and adults, free sulfate accounted for about 77 to 92%, ester sulfate for about 7 to 9%, taurine for about 2 to 6%, and Cys for about 0.6 to 0.7% of the total urinary sulfur excretion. Taurine excretion varies greatly with variation in taurine intake and can make up as much as 10% of total urinary sulfur. Other sulfur-containing compounds found in urine in trace amounts (<0.2% of total sulfur) include methionine, Hcy, cystathionine, N-acetylcysteine, mercaptolactate, mercaptoacetate, thiosulfate, and thiocyanate (47, 114). Nakamura and colleagues (115), in a study of young Japanese women, found that free sulfate, but not ester sulfate or taurine, was significantly correlated with urea excretion, a finding suggesting that free sulfate excretion is the best index of sulfur amino acid intake. Although taurine and sulfate can be regarded as end products of cellular Cys catabolism, both these compounds participate in conjugation reactions and have a variety of essential physiologic functions before their ultimate excretion.

Cysteine Oxidation and Taurine Synthesis in Humans

Taurine synthesis requires the presence of both Cys dioxygenase and cysteinesulfinate decarboxylase (EC 4.1.1.29). Significant expression of the Cys dioxygenase gene was indicated by the presence of mRNA for Cys dioxygenase in human liver, kidney, and lung (116). A low capacity to oxidize Cys to sulfate was observed in some patients with liver diseases or rheumatoid arthritis (117, 118) and inconsistently in patients with some chronic neurologic diseases (119, 120). These patients had elevated plasma ratios of Cys to sulfate because of higher Cys and lower sulfate concentrations, they excreted a smaller percentage of a dose of acetaminophen as the sulfate versus the glucuronide conjugate, or they had a lower sulfate concentration in synovial fluid, all consistent with impaired Cys oxidation.

The human liver has been reported to have a low activity of cysteinesulfinate decarboxylase (121). Nevertheless, human adults seem to have a significant ability to synthesize taurine. In vivo assessment of the ability of adults to synthesize taurine, based on incorporation of ^{18}O (from inhaled $^{18}O_2$) into taurine, resulted in conservative estimates of synthesis in the range of 200 to 400 μmol/day (122). These estimates are equivalent to 1 to 3% of the total sulfur amino acid intake and compare favorably with the mean taurine excretion of approximately 250 μmol/day observed in strict vegans consuming an essentially taurine-free diet (26, 27). Thus, the percentage of the sulfur amino acid intake or total urinary sulfur excretion that is represented by urinary taurine in humans fed taurine-free diets is similar to that observed in rats fed taurine-free diets (2–6%) (123). This similar pattern of metabolism between rats and humans seems to dispute the often-made statement that the rat has a high capacity for taurine synthesis whereas humans have a low capacity. It seems possible that a relatively high hepatic Cys dioxygenase activity in humans may permit high rates of Cys catabolism to cysteinesulfinate and that relatively high concentrations of cysteinesulfinate may allow adequate rates of taurine synthesis despite relatively low cysteinesulfinate decarboxylase activity.

ESSENTIAL FUNCTIONS OF CYSTEINE AND ITS METABOLITES

Synthesis of Protein and Glutathione

Cys, either preformed or synthesized from methionine and serine, is required for protein synthesis and hence for growth or nitrogen balance. Both the reactive sulfhydryl group of cysteinyl residues in proteins and the ability of these residues to form disulfide linkages play important roles in protein structure and function.

The Cys-containing tripeptide, GSH, has numerous essential functions in the body in addition to serving as a storage or circulating reservoir of Cys (124, 125). Because GSH has a reactive sulfhydryl group, it can readily form disulfides with itself (oxidized GSH or GSSG) or with other thiol compounds (GSSR). The ratio of GSH to GSSG in most cells is greater than 500, so GSH serves as a supply of reducing equivalents or electrons. GSH is involved in protection of cells from oxidative damage (see also Chapter 44) because of its role in reduction of hydrogen peroxide and organic peroxides via GSH peroxidases and because of its ability to inactivate free radicals by donating hydrogen to the radical. These processes result in oxidation of GSH to GSSG. GSSG and GSH can be interconverted via the GSH reductase reaction which uses oxidized NAD phosphate ($NADP^+$)/reduced NADP (NADPH) as the oxidant/reductant; hence GSH plays a role in maintenance of the cellular redox state. GSH is an important source of reducing equivalents for the intracellular reduction of cystine to

CySH. This reduction can occur by thiol-disulfide exchange or enzymatically by thioltransferase, with GSH providing the reducing equivalents.

GSH may participate in the transport of amino acids via the membrane-bound enzyme, γ-glutamyl transpeptidase. γ-Glutamyl transpeptidase, the same enzyme responsible for extracellular hydrolysis of GSH, catalyzes the transfer of the γ-glutamyl group of GSH to the α-amino group of an acceptor amino acid such as cystine or glutamine. The γ-glutamyl amino acid is transported into the cell, where the amino acid is released and the glutamyl moiety cyclizes to 5-oxoproline, which is then hydrolyzed to regenerate glutamate. The CysGly dipeptide that is the byproduct of γ-glutamyl transpeptidation can by hydrolyzed to Cys and glycine either extracellularly or intracellularly by dipeptidases; hence no net consumption of amino acids occurs as a result of this transport cycle.

GSH also serves as a cosubstrate for several reactions including certain steps in leukotriene synthesis and melanin polymer synthesis. GSH is the substrate for a group of enzymes, GSH S-transferases, that form GSH conjugates from a variety of acceptor compounds including various xenobiotics (126). These conjugates are normally degraded by the enzymes of the γ-glutamyl cycle to yield the cysteinyl derivatives that may be acetylated using acetyl coenzyme A to become mercapturic acids, which are excreted in the urine. This process is usually a detoxification and excretion process.

Functions of Inorganic Sulfur

Reduced sulfur is required for synthesis of iron-sulfur proteins and other compounds. Evidence suggests that H_2S serves as a neuromodulator and that production of H_2S by cystathionine β-synthase is activated in response to neuronal excitation (127, 128). H_2S acts to enhance NMDA receptor-mediated currents. Other observations indicate that H_2S may also function as a smooth muscle relaxant. Cystathionine γ-lyase, as well as cystathionine β-synthase, catalyzes the regulated production of H_2S in smooth muscle tissues (129, 130). Apparently, H_2S acts by opening potassium channels in vascular smooth muscle cells (131).

The activated form of sulfate, 3'-phospho-5'-phosphosulfate, serves as the substrate for a variety of sulfotransferase reactions. Many structural compounds are sulfated; in particular, the oligosaccharide chains of proteoglycans contain many sulfated sugar residues. In addition, many compounds of both endogenous and exogenous origin are excreted as sulfoesters; sulfoesters of steroid hormones and of the drug acetaminophen are examples. Inorganic sulfur is largely obtained from the metabolism of Cys in the body, but animal studies have suggested that dietary inorganic sulfate may improve growth, feed efficiency, and sulfation of cartilage proteoglycans when sulfur amino acid intake is insufficient (132).

Functions of Taurine

The only physiologic function of taurine that is well understood is its role in bile acid conjugation (39). Taurine conjugates are the major metabolites of taurine formed in vertebrates. Taurocholate is a very efficient bile acid because of the low pK_a of the sulfonic acid group, which faciliates its ionization and, hence, detergent action, solubility, slower reabsorption, and higher intraluminal concentration. Taurine also serves as a conjugation substrate for certain other compounds, such as all-*trans*-retinoic acid, thus increasing polarity, aqueous solubility, and, in most cases, clearance from the body.

Humans are able to conjugate bile acids with both taurine and glycine. In adults, the ratio of taurocholate and glycocholate is approximately 3:1, but this ratio varies from person to person and with changes in the hepatic concentration of taurine. In contrast, the human fetus and neonate are exclusive taurine conjugators. Glycine conjugation is not usually observed until about the third week of life, but it appears sooner in infants deprived of dietary taurine (133). Taurine supplementation resulted in lower cholesterol synthesis and higher bile acid excretion and fatty acid absorption in preterm infants with a gestational age of less than 33 weeks but not in older preterm or full-term infants (134). In men consuming a high-fat, high-cholesterol diet, oral supplementation with taurine (6 g/day) for 3 weeks resulted in a decrease in low-density lipoprotein cholesterol and total cholesterol (135).

Taurine is present in high concentrations in many human tissues ($\sim$25 μmol/g wet weight in retina and leukocytes), and numerous physiologic actions of taurine in various tissues have been studied (39, 56). Unfortunately, these actions are not well understood despite several decades of intensive work (15, 37, 49). Taurine is involved in osmoregulation and is an important organic osmolyte (136). The movement of taurine, as well as electrolytes, into or out of the cell is a major contributor to the volume regulation that accompanies an osmotic insult. A hypoosmotic insult (either an increase in cellular osmolality or a reduction in medium osmolality) triggers the release of taurine from the cell, whereas a hyperosmotic insult (a decrease in cellular osmolality or an increase in medium osmolality) leads to an elevation in tissue taurine content. Some of the actions of taurine may be caused by activation of osmotic-linked signaling pathways, such as enhanced gene expression, changes in the phosphorylation status of proteins, or cytoskeletal changes (137, 138).

Taurine has an antioxidant effect as judged by its ability to decrease the accumulation of oxidative markers (protein carbonyls or thiobarbituric acid reactive substances such as malondialdehyde that form during lipid peroxidation) and by the decrease in taurine in tissues of aged or diabetic animals (139, 140). The mechanism of this antioxidant effect of taurine is not clear. Taurine may minimize lipid peroxidation via its membrane-stabilizing activity or via its modulation of intracellular Ca^{2+} homeostasis and involvement in phospholipid-Ca^{2+} interactions. Taurine directly acts as an antioxidant in the removal of hypochlorite, a strong oxidant generated from peroxide and chloride by myeloperoxidase in activated neutrophils. The taurine chloramine thus formed is released from the neutrophils. Taurine chloramine acts as a potent antiinflammatory agent. Kontny and associates (141) reported that neutrophils isolated from the synovial fluid of patients with rheumatoid arthritis had an impaired ability to generate taurine chloramine compared with neutrophils from healthy volunteers. Taurine chloramine may act to downregulate the production of proinflammatory cytokines. The metabolic precursor of taurine, hypotaurine, also can function as an antioxidant.

Taurine is clearly involved in development, with substantial evidence supporting a crucial role of taurine during the prenatal and postnatal development of the central nervous and visual systems. The specific manner in which taurine participates in these events is not clear. Two high-affinity taurine transporters (TAUT-1 and TAUT-2) in rat brain have been cloned; TAUT-1 was associated with cerebellar Purkinje cells and with retinal photoreceptors and bipolar cells, whereas TAUT-2 was predominantly associated with glial cells (142). Lima and coworkers (143) demonstrated trophic effects of taurine on regenerating retina; taurine favored neuron proliferation and survival as well as neurite extension. Disruption of the Na^+-dependent taurine transporter gene in mice led to a loss of vision resulting from retinal degeneration (144). In primates deprived of taurine, retinal changes, impaired visual acuity, and degenerative ultrastructural changes in photoreceptor outer segments have been observed, with changes more severe in younger animals (39, 56, 145). The absence of immunostaining of taurine in the rod outer segments of the retina of light-adapted fish compared with intense staining in the dark-adapted state suggests a unique role of taurine in the visual cycle (146). Some human infants and children whose only nutrition was taurine-free parenteral infusion or taurine-devoid formulas have exhibited ophthalmoscopically and electrophysiologically detectable retinal abnormalities and immature brainstem auditory evoked responses (39, 56).

POSSIBLE CAUSES OF DEFICIENCY OF CYSTEINE OR TAURINE

Immaturity

Immaturity may be associated with a conditional requirement for both Cys and taurine. Preterm infants (<32 weeks' gestation) have a low capacity for transsulfuration (low cystathionine γ-lyase activity), low plasma Cys concentrations, elevated plasma cystathionine concentrations, and a low rate of GSH synthesis from methionine in erythrocytes (147, 148). These observations all suggest that transsulfuration may be insufficient to meet the Cys requirements of the very premature infant. Full-term, formula-fed infants have also been observed to have increased cystathionine and decreased taurine in urine, findings suggesting a limited capacity for transsulfuration even in term infants (149).

In addition to a limited capacity to convert methionine to Cys and hence to taurine (low synthetic rate), several other characteristics of premature infants contribute to their conditional requirement for taurine and/or Cys (15, 56). First, the premature infant may have a greater requirement for Cys as a result of more rapid growth and for taurine because of a likely role of taurine in development of the nervous and visual systems. The brain and retina of developing animals have high taurine concentrations, and morphologic and functional impairments have been observed in animals deprived of taurine during development. Second, premature infants are born with lower stores of taurine than are mature infants. Third, the β-amino acid transport system in the immature kidney does not adapt to poor taurine status by increasing reabsorption of taurine. The urinary taurine content of premature neonates is markedly elevated, with a fractional excretion ranging from 38 to 60% compared with a fractional excretion lower than 10% in term infants. Premature infants who received parenteral nutrition solutions devoid of taurine had high urinary taurine excretion rates despite very low plasma taurine values (55, 150, 151). By contrast, term neonates given a taurine-deficient parenteral nutrition solution can maintain plasma taurine concentrations by increased renal reabsorption of taurine, with as little as 1% of the filtered taurine load excreted.

Hepatic Dysfunction

Because liver is the major site for transsulfuration and taurine synthesis, hepatic dysfunction can have adverse effects on sulfur amino acid status. In published reports, patients with advanced forms of liver dysfunction or cirrhosis had low plasma taurine, Cys, and GSH concentrations, an elevated plasma cystathionine concentration, decreased urinary taurine excretion, a decreased ratio of urinary sulfate to total sulfur, and an increased urinary excretion of Cys and cystathionine (152, 153) (see Chapter 79). These patients appeared to have a decreased ability to metabolize methionine (to Cys, with cystathionine accumulation) and Cys (to taurine and inorganic sulfate, with thiosulfate, Cys, and N-acetylcysteine accumulation).

Total Parenteral or Enteral Nutrition

Patients receiving long-term total parenteral nutrition (TPN) have experienced adverse effects on their sulfur amino acid status, because of the route of administration and the composition of the TPN solutions. The amino acid mixtures used for TPN solutions usually contain little if any Cys, because CySH is rapidly converted to its disulfide, cystine, which is very insoluble in aqueous solution. Taurine is not routinely added to adult TPN solutions. Hence, patients receiving TPN must synthesize both Cys and taurine from the methionine provided by TPN. However, the synthesis of Cys and taurine from methionine is restricted when first-pass metabolism by the liver is bypassed with parenteral alimentation. In adult patients who were given parenteral alimentation solutions free of Cys by different routes, plasma Cys concentration dropped markedly when feeding was via the parenteral route, whereas it rose when feeding was switched to the oral route (154). The liver apparently removes much of the methionine on the first pass when solutions are administered by the oral route such that Cys synthesis and taurine synthesis from methionine are facilitated.

However, even enteral feeding including taurine may be marginal for ill patients. In a group of hospitalized male patients receiving long-term enteral nutrition, Cho and associates (155) found that, despite an average intake of 337 μmol taurine/day, the fasting serum and urinary taurine levels were decreased by 46 and 78%, respectively, in patients receiving enteral nutrition for 48 months compared with levels in patients receiving enteral nutrition for only 6 months. Boelens and colleagues (156) reported that patients with multiple trauma had low plasma taurine concentrations that were increased by glutamine supplementation, a finding suggesting that supplementation of enteral formulas with both taurine and glutamine would enhance taurine status.

Drug Metabolism

Various drugs and toxins are partially metabolized and excreted by conjugation with sulfate, GSH (mercapturic acid synthesis), or even taurine. Rats fed up to 1 g (6.6 mmol) of acetaminophen/100 g diet experienced dose-dependent inhibition of growth that was independent of hepatotoxicity and could be overcome by addition of methionine or Cys to the diet (106, 157). Lauterburg and Mitchell (106) found that therapeutic doses of acetaminophen (600 and 1200 mg or 4 and 8 mmol) administered to healthy adults markedly stimulated the rate of turnover of the pool of Cys available for the synthesis of GSH. Patients and volunteers with prolonged ingestion of acetaminophen in doses of 2 to 4 g (13–26 mmol)/day had a decreased urinary output of inorganic sulfate but no decrease in plasma sulfate concentrations (158). Subjects produced a maximum of 0.6 mmol/hour of acetaminophen sulfate, whereas total sulfur excretion was 7.5 to 26.7 mmol/24 hours (0.3–1.1 mmol/hour). A marginal sulfur amino acid intake accompanied by prolonged ingestion of high doses of drugs or toxins that are metabolized by sulfate and/or GSH conjugation could have adverse effects on both sulfur amino acid status and drug metabolism.

MEASURES OF TAURINE STATUS AND OF CYSTEINE AND/OR SULFUR AMINO ACID STATUS

Sulfur amino acid adequacy has generally been assessed by measures of nitrogen balance or growth. Although growth and nitrogen balance have been used to define the nutritional requirements for amino acids, they are not necessarily good indicators of whether sulfur amino acid intake is sufficient for optimal rates of production of GSH, inorganic sulfur, or taurine.

Plasma and blood taurine concentrations, plasma tCys concentration, and the plasma GSH concentration have been used as indicators of sulfur amino acid status. Normal values for these measures are discussed earlier in this chapter.

Because most of the sulfur from sulfur amino acids is excreted in the urine, primarily as inorganic sulfate, measures of total urinary sulfur or of urinary sulfate are useful indicators of sulfur amino acid intake and/or metabolism. The urinary taurine level can be used as an indicator of adequate taurine status because taurine excretion increases as plasma taurine concentration and/or taurine intake or biosynthesis increases.

TOXICITY

Large doses of CySH or cystine have been shown to be neuroexcitotoxic in several species. The effect of CySH seems to involve the N-methyl-D-aspartate subtype of the glutamate receptor for which cysteinesulfinate and cysteic acid are agonists (158–162). Single injections of CySH (0.6–1.5 g/kg) into 4-day-old rat pups resulted in massive damage to cortical neurons (162), permanent retinal dystrophy (163), atrophy of the brain (164), and hyperactivity (159). Cats fed a 5% cystine diet had no obvious immediate ill effects but exhibited acute neurotoxic symptoms after several months (165). The onset of symptoms in the cats was sudden, with rapid progression to a moribund state or death, usually within 48 hours. The morphologic changes observed in the retinas of cats fed the cystine-rich diets were comparable to those described in the retinas of young rodents treated with glutamate or certain other acidic or excitotoxic amino acids. It is not clear whether Cys or an acidic oxidized derivative (cysteinesulfinate or cysteic acid, each of which is an aspartate analog) is responsible for the cytotoxicity. These observations have given rise to concerns about administration of excess Cys to humans, especially to infants.

Studies in rodents have also demonstrated influences of dietary sulfur amino acids on lipid metabolism with 2 to 5% (by weight) L-cystine resulting in elevated plasma cholesterol concentration, increased hepatic cholesterol biosynthesis, and depressed plasma ceruloplasmin activity (166). Excess L-CySH (0.8 or 2% of diet by weight) did not result in an elevation in plasma cholesterol, whereas addition of 0.8% L-methionine did (148, 167).

Sturman and Messing (168) found no evidence of adverse effects of prolonged feeding of high-taurine diets (≤1 g or 8 mmol taurine/100 g diet) on adult female cats or their offspring. In fact, taurine may protect against toxic effects of some other compounds. Taurine addition to cat diets provided some protection against the adverse effects of the high level of cystine, a finding supporting a neuroprotective role of taurine against the excitotoxic damages in the mammalian nervous system (165). Studies in rodents have suggested that dietary taurine also has hypolipidemic and antiatherosclerotic effects (169, 170).

Although Hcy is not provided in any substantial amount by typical foods, certain types of diets (e.g., high methionine and low folate) can promote elevated Hcy levels (171). The mechanism by which Hcy (or Hcy sulfinic acid, a glutamate analog) exerts its toxic effects are not fully understood, but Hcy, like Cys, is readily oxidized, giving rise to reactive oxygen intermediates, and Hcy is neurotoxic. Its neurotoxicity seems to result from its effects on N-methyl-D-aspartate ionotropic glutamate receptors and metabotropic glutamate receptors and could possibly involve formation of Hcy sulfinic acid, a glutamate analog (172, 173).

REFERENCES

1. OsborneTB, Mendel LR. J Biol Chem 1915;20:351–78.
2. Mueller JH. Proc Soc Exp Biol Med 1921;19:161–3.
3. Jackson RW, Block, RJ. J Biol Chem 1932;98:465–77.
4. Womack M, Kemmerer KS, Rose WC. J Biol Chem 1937;121: 403–10.
5. Rose WC, Wixom RL. J Biol Chem 1955;216:763–73.
6. du Vigneaud VE. Trail of Research in Sulfur Chemistry and Metabolism and Related Fields. Ithaca, NY: Cornell University Press, 1952.
7. Carson NAJ, Neill DW. Arch Dis Child 1962;37:505–13.
8. Clarke R, Daly L, Robinson K et al. N Engl J Med 1991;324: 1149–55.
9. Robinson K, Mayer E, Jacobsen DW. Cleve Clin J Med 1994;61:438–50.
10. Steegers-Theunissen RPM, Boers GHJ, Trijbels FJM et al. Metabolism 1994;43:1475–80.
11. Wouters MCAJ, Boers GHJ, Blom HJ et al. Fertil Steril 1993; 60:820–5.
12. Tiedemann F, Gmelin L. Ann Physik Chem 1827;9:326–37.
13. Hayes KC, Carey RE, Schmidt SY. Science 1975;188: 949–51.
14. Sturman JA, Rassin DK, Gaull GE. Life Sci 1977;21:1–22.
15. Sturman JA. Physiol Rev 1993;73:119–47.
16. Mansoor MA, Bergmark C, Svardal AM et al. Arterioscler Thromb Vasc Biol 1995;15:232–40.
17. Andersson A, Isaksson A Brattstrom L et al. Clin Chem 1993; 39:1590–7.
18. Mansoor MA, Ueland PM, Svardal AM. Am J Clin Nutr 1994; 59:631–5.
19. Guttormsen AB, Schneede J, Fiskerstrand R et al. J Nutr 1994;124:1934–41.
20. Selhub J, Jacques PF, Wilson PWF et al. JAMA 1993;270: 2693–8.
21. Dalery K, Lussier-Cacan S, Selhub J et al. Am J Cardiol 1995;75:1107–11.
22. Nygard O, Vollset SE, Refsum H et al. JAMA 1995;274:1526–33.

23. Rasmussen K, Moller J, Lyngbak M et al. Clin Chem 1996;42:630–6.
24. Nygard Yap S, Naughten E. J Inherit Metab Dis 1998;21:738–47.
25. Trautwein EA, Hayes KC. Am J Clin Nutr 1990;52:758–64.
26. Rana SK, Sanders, TAB. Br J Nutr 1986;56:17–27.
27. Laidlaw SA, Shultz TD, Cecchino JT et al. Am J Clin Nutr 1988;47:660–3.
28. Malinow MR, Axthelm MK, Meredith MJ et al. J Lab Clin Med 1994;123:421–9.
29. Food and Nutrition Board, Institute of Medicine. Dietary Reference Intakes: Energy, Carbohydrate, Fiber, Fat, Fatty Acids, Cholesterol, Protein, and Amino Acids. Washington, DC: National Academy Press, 2002.
30. US Department of Agriculture. Agricultural Handbook No. 8. Washington, DC: Agriculture Research Service, United States Department of Agriculture, 1976–1986.
31. Young VR, Wagner DA, Burini R et al. Am J Clin Nutr 1991;54:377–85.
32. Storch KJ, Wagner DA, Burke JF et al. Am J Physiol 1988;255:E322–31.
33. FAO/WHO/UNI. Energy and Protein Requirements. WHO technical report no. 724. Geneva: World Health Organization, 1985.
34. Di Buono M, Wykes LJ, Ball RO et al. Am J Clin Nutr 2001;74:756–60.
35. Laidlaw SA, Grosvenor M, Kopple JD. JPEN J Parenter Enteral Nutr 1990;14:183–8.
36. Pasantes-Morales H, Quesada O, Alcocer L et al. Nutr Rep Int 1989;40:793–801.
37. Roe DA, Weston MO. Nature 1965;203:287–8.
38. Kataoka H, Ohnishi N. Agric Biol Chem 1986;50:1887–8.
39. Huxtable RJ. Physiol Rev 1992;72:101–63.
40. Seidl R, Peyrl A, Nicham R et al. Amino Acids 2000;19:635–42.
41. Yamori Y, Liu L, Ikeda, K et al. Hypertens Res 2001;24:453–7.
42. Rassin DK, Sturman JA, Gaull GE. Early Hum Dev 1978;2:1–13.
43. Kim ES, Cho KH, Park MA et al. Adv Exp Med Biol 1996;403:571–7.
44. Agostoni C, Carratu B, Boniglia C et al. J Am Coll Nutr 2000;19:434–8.
45. Segawa, H, Fukasawa Y, Miyamoto K. et al. J Biol Chem 1999;274:19745–51.
46. Paauw JD, Davis AT. Am J Clin Nutr 1994;60:203–6.
47. Martensson J, Hermansson G. Metabolism 1984;33:425–8.
48. Palacin M, Chillaron J, Mora C. Biochem Soc Trans 1996;24:856–63.
49. Mora C, Chillaron J, Calonge MJ et al. J Biol Chem 1996;271:10569–76.
50. Chillaron J, Estevez R, Mora C et al. J Biol Chem 1996;271:17761–70.
51. Sakhaee K. Min Electrolyte Metab 1994;20:414–423.
52. Kalatzis V, Antignac C. Pediatr Nephrol 2003:18:207–15.
53. Refsum H, Helland S, Ueland PM. Clin Chem 1985;31:624–8.
54. Erbe RW. Inborn errors of folate metabolism. In: Blakley, RL Whitehead VM, eds. Folates and Pterins, vol 3. New York: Wiley, 1986:413–65.
55. Jensen H. Biochem Biophys Acta 1994;1194:44–52.
56. Sturman JA, Chesney RW. Pediatr Nutr 1995;42:879–97.
57. Satsu H, Kobayashi Y, Yokoyama T et al. Amino Acids 2002;23:447–52.
58. McKeever MP, Weir DG, Molloy A et al. Clin Sci 1991;81:551–6.
59. Finkelstein JD. Am J Clin Nutr 2003;77:1094–5.
60. Finkelstein JD. Am J Clin Nutr 1998;68:224–5.
61. Pogribna M, Melnyk S, Pogribny I et al. Am J Hum Genet 2001;69:88–95.
62. Poole JR, Mudd SH, Conerly E et al. J Clin Invest 1975;55:1033–48.
63. Stipanuk MH. Annu Rev Nutr 1986;6:179–209.
64. Backlund PS Jr, Smith RA. J Biol Chem 1981;256:1533–5.
65. Storch KJ, Wagner DA, Burke JF et al. Am J Physiol 1990;258:E790–8.
66. Fukagama NK, Yu Y-M, Young VR. Am J Clin Nutr 1998;68:380–8.
67. Selhub J, Miller J. Am J Clin Nutr 1992;55:131–8.
68. Di Buono M, Wykes LJ, Ball RO et al. Am J Clin Nutr 2001;74:761–6.
69. Di Buono M, Wykes LJ, Cole DEC et al. J Nutr 2003;133:733–9.
70. Stipanuk MH, Benevenga NJ. J Nutr 1977;107:1455–67.
71. Storch KJ, Wagner DA, Young VR. Am J Clin Nutr 1991;54:386–94.
72. Taoka S, Lepore BW, Kabil O et al. Biochemistry 2002;41:10454–61.
73. Zou CG, Banerjee R. J Biol Chem 2003;278:16802–8.
74. Jacobs RL, Stead LM, Brosnan ME et al. J Biol Chem 2001;276:43740–47.
75. Ratnam S, Maclean KN, Jacobs RL et al. J Biol Chem 2002;277:42912–8.
76. Bostom AG, Jacques PF, Nadeau MR et al. Atherosclerosis 1995;116:147–51.
77. Ubbink JH, Becker PJ, Vermaak WJH et al. Clin Chem 1995;41:1033–7.
78. Rozen, R. Semin Thromb Hemost 2000;26:255–61.
79. Engbersen AMT, Franken DG, Bower GHJ et al. Am J Hum Genet 1995;56:142–50.
80. Jacques PF, Bostom AG, Williams RR et al. Circulation 1996;93:7–9.
81. Kang S-S, Wong PWK, Bock H-GO et al. Am J Hum Genet 1991;48:546–51.
82. Rozen R, Jacques P, Bostom A et al. Am J Hum Genet 1995;57S:A250.
83. Guttormsen AB, Schneede J, Ueland, PM et al. Am J Clin Nutr 1996;63:194–202.
84. Salles-Montaudon N, Parrot F, Balas D et al. J Nutr Health Aging 2003;7:111–6.
85. Ubbink JB, van der Merwe A, Delport R et al. J Clin Invest 1996;98:177–84.
86. Boushey CJ, Beresford SAA, Omenn GS et al. JAMA 1995;274:1049–57.
87. Schmitz C, Lindpaintner K, Verhoef P et al. Circulation 1996;94:1812–4.
88. Arnadotti M, Hultberg B, Nilsson-Ehle P et al. Scand J Clin Invest 1996;56:41–6.
89. Chauveau P, Chadefaux B, Conde M et al. Min Electrolyte Metab 1996;22:106–109.
90. Van der Put NMJ, Steegers-Theunissen RPM, Frosst P et al. Lancet 1995;346:1070–1.
91. den Heijer M, Koster R, Blom HJ et al. N Engl J Med 1996;334:759–62.
92. Mills JL, Scott JM, Kirke PN et al. J Nutr 1996;126:756S–60S.
93. Selhub J, Jacques PF, Bostom AG et al. N Engl J Med 1995;332:286–91.
94. Goddijn-Wessel TAW, Wouters, MGAJ, Van de Molen EF. Eur J Obstet Gynecol Reprod Biol 1996;66:23–9.

95. Kluijtmans LAJ, van den Heuvel LPWJ, Boers GHJ et al. Am J Hum Genet 1996;58:35–41.
96. Harpel PC, Zhang X, Borth W. J Nutr 1996;126;1285S–9S.
97. Blom HJ, Van der Molen EF. Fibrinolysis 1994;8[Suppl 2]:86–7.
98. Lentz SR, Sobey CG, Piegors DJ et al. J Clin Invest 1996;98:24–9.
99. Tsai JC, Wang H, Perrella MA et al. J Clin Invest 1996;97:146–53.
100. Moephuli SR, Klein NW, Baldwin MT et al. Proc Natl Acad Sci USA 1997;94:543–8.
101. Eskes TKAB. Eur J Obstet Gynecol Reprod Biol 1997;71:105–9.
102. Rosenblatt DS. Inherited disorders of folate transport and metabolism. In: Scriver CR, Beaudet AL, Sly WS et al, eds. The Metabolic and Molecular Bases of Inherited Disease, vol 3. 7th ed. New York, McGraw-Hill, 1995:3111-28.
103. Brattstrom LE, Israelsson B, Jeppsson JO et al. Scand J Clin Lab Invest 1988;48:215–21.
104. Ubbink JB, Vermaak WJH, van der Merwe A et al. J Nutr 1994;124:1927–33.
105. Kang S-S. J Nutr 1996;126:1273S–5S.
106. Lauterburg BH, Mitchell JR. J Hepatol 1987;4:206–211.
107. Fukagawa NK, Ajami AM, Young VR. Am J Physiol 1996;270:E209–14.
108. Gordon N. Eur J Paediat Neurol 2002;6:243–7.
109. Zhou B, Westaway SK, Levinson B et al. Nat Genet 2001;28:345–9.
110. Eto K, Asada T, Arima K et al. Biochem Biophys Res Comm 2002;293:1485–8.
111. Crawhall JC. Clin Biochem 1985;18:139–42.
112. Bella DL, Kwon YH, Stipanuk MH. J Nutr 1996;126:2179–87.
113. Stipanuk MH, Londono M, Hirschberger LL. FASEB J 2003;17:449.3.
114. Martensson J. Metabolism 1982;31:487–92.
115. Nakamura H, Kajikawa R, Ubuka T. Amino Acids 2002;23:427–31.
116. Koide T, Watanabe M, Shimada M. Acta Histochem Cytochem 1994;27:384.
117. Davies MH, Ngong JM, Pean A et al. J Hepatol 1995;22:551–60.
118. Bradley H, Gough A, Sokhi RS et al. J Rheumatol 1994;21:1192–6.
119. Heafield MT, Fearn S, Steventon GB et al. Neurosci Lett 1990;110:216–220.
120. Perry TL, Krieger C, Hansen S et al. Neurology 1991;41:1851.
121. Gaull GE, Rassin DK, Raiha NCR et al. J Pediatr 1977;90:348–55.
122. Irving CS, Marks L, Klein PD et al. Life Sci 1986;38:491–5.
123. Bella DL, Stipanuk, MH. Am J Physiol 1995;269:E910–7.
124. DeLeve LD, Kaplowitz N. Pharmacol Ther 1991;52:287–305.
125. Meister A. Pharmacol Ther 1991;51:155–94.
126. Hinchman CA, Ballatori N. J Toxicol Environ Health 1994;41:387–409.
127. Abe K, Kimura H. J Neurosci 1996;16:1066–1071.
128. Kimura H. Biochem Biophys Res Commun 2000;267:129–133.
129. Hosoki R, Matsuki N, Kimura H. Biochem Biophys Res 1997;237:528–31.
130. Sidhu R, Singh M, Samir G et al. Pharmacol Toxicol 2001;88:198–203.
131. Zhao W, Ahang J, Lu Y et al. EMBO J 2001;20:6008–16.
132. Salinas AE, Wong MG. Curr Med Chem 1999;6:279–309.
133. Brueton MJ, Berger HM, Brown GA et al. Gut 1978;19:95–8.
134. Wasserhess P, Becker M, Staab D. Am J Clin Nutr 1993;58:349–53.
135. Mizushima S, Nara Y, Sawamura M et al. Adv Exp Med Biol 1996;403:615–22.
136. Chiarla D, Giovannini I, Siegel, JH. Amino Acids 2003;24:89–93.
137. Schaeffer S, Takahashi K, Azuma J. Amino Acids 2000;19:527–46.
138. Schaeffer SW, Pastukh V, Solodushko V et al. Amino Acids 2002;23:395–400.
139. Eppler B, Dawson R, Jr. Biochem Pharmacol 2001;62:29–39.
140. DiLeo MAS, Santini SA, Cercone S et al. Amino Acids 2002;23:401–6.
141. Kontny E, Wojtecka-Lukasik E, Rell-Bakalarska K et al. Amino Acids 2002;23:415–8.
142. Pow DV, Sullivan R, Reye P et al. Glia 2002:37:153–68.
143. Lima L. Neurochem Res 1999;24:1333–8.
144. Heller-Stilb B, van Roeyen C, Rascher K et al. FASEB J 2002;16:231–3.
145. Militante JD, Lombardini JB. Nutr Neurosci 2002;5:75–90.
146. Omura Y, Inagaki M. Amino Acids 2000;19:593–604.
147. Miller RG, Jahoor F, Jaksic T. J Pediatr Surg 1995;30:953–8.
148. Vina J, Vento M, Garcia-Sala F et al. Am J Clin Nutr 1995;61:1067–9.
149. Martensson J, Finnstrom O. Early Hum Dev 1985;11:333–9.
150. Zelikovic I, Chesney RW, Friedman AL et al. J Pediatr 1990;116:301–6.
151. Helms RA, Christensen ML, Storm MC et al. J Nutr Biochem 1995;6:462–6.
152. Chawla RK, Berry CJ, Kutner MH et al. Am J Clin Nutr 1985;42:577–84.
153. Martensson J, Foberg U, Fryden A et al. Scand J Gastroenterol 1992;27:405–11.
154. Steglink LD, den Besten L. Science 1972;178:514–6.
155. Cho KH, Kim ES, Chen JD. Adv Exp Med Biol 2000;483:605–12.
156. Boelens PG, Houdijk APJ, de Thouars, HN et al. Am J Clin Nutr 2003;77:250–6.
157. McLean AEM, Armstrong GR, Beales D. Biochem Pharmacol 1989;38:347–52.
158. Blackledge HM, O'Farrell JO, Minton NA et al. Hum Exp Toxicol 1991;10:159–65.
159. Mathisen GA, Fonnum F, Paulsen RE. Neurochem Res 1996;21:293–8.
160. Santucci AC, Spincola L-J. Dev Brain Dysfunct 1994;7:230–6.
161. Porter RHP, Roberts PJ. Neurosci Lett 1993;154:78–80.
162. Zerangue N, Kavanaugh MP. J Physiol (Lond) 1996;493:419–23.
163. Pedersen OO, Lund-Karlsen R. Invest Ophthalmol Vis Sci 1980;19:886–92.
164. Lund-Karlsen R, Grofova I, Malthe-Sorenssen D et al. Brain Res 1981;208:167–80.
165. Imaki H, Sturman JA. Nutr Res 1990;10:1385–400.
166. Yang B-S, Wan Q, Kato N. Biosci Biotechnol Biochem 1994;58:1177–8.
167. Sugiyama K, Akai H, Muramatsu K. J Nutr Sci Vitaminol 1986;32:537–49.
168. Sturman JA, Messing JM. J Nutr 1992;122:82–8.
169. Murakami S, Yamagishi I, Asami Y et al. Pharmacology 1996;52:303–13.
170. Kamata K, Sugiura M, Kojima S et al. Eur J Pharmacol 1996;303:47–53.

171. Jakubowski H, Zhang L, Bardeguez A et al. Circ Res 2000;87: 45–51.
172. Brauer PR, Rosenquist TH. Dev Dyn 2002;224:222–30.
173. Shi Q, Savage JE, Hufeisen SJ et al. Exp Pharmacol Exp Ther 2003;305:131–42.

SELECTED READINGS

Dickinson DA, Forman HJ. Glutathione in defense and signaling: lessons from a small molecule. Ann NY Acad Sci 2002;973:488–504.

Herrmann W. The importance of hyperhomocysteinemia as a risk factor for diseases: an overview. Clin Chem Lab Med 2001;39: 666–74.

Militanta JD, Lombardini JB. Taurine: evidence of physiological function in the retina. Nutr Neurosci 2002;5:75–90.

Selhub J. Homocysteine metabolism. Annu Rev Nutr 1999;19: 217–46.

Stipanuk MH. Sulfur amino acid metabolism: pathways for production and removal of homocysteine and cysteine. Annu Rev Nutr 2004;24:539–77.

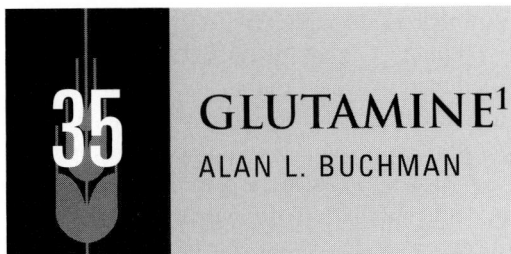

35 GLUTAMINE[1]
ALAN L. BUCHMAN

CHEMISTRY, BIOCHEMISTRY/BIOSYNTHESIS,
  AND GENETICS 563
ANALYTIC METHODS 563
DIGESTION, ABSORPTION, BIOAVAILABILITY,
  AND EXCRETION 563
TRANSPORT AND METABOLISM 564
CAUSES AND EFFECTS OF GLUTAMINE DEFICIENCY . . .564
IMPACT OF STRESS AND DISEASE ON NUTRIENT
  UTILIZATION 565
    Dietary Considerations and Requirements 565
    Glutamine Replacement Therapy 565
    Therapeutic Use of Glutamine in Pharmacologic
      Doses 566
SAFETY ISSUES AND INTERACTIONS WITH
  OTHER NUTRIENTS 568

Glutamine is classified as a nonessential amino acid because it can be synthesized from glutamate and glutamic acid by the enzyme glutamine synthetase. It may also be synthesized from arginine, although currently few data are available to support this occurrence in vivo (1). A significant amount of glutamine is extracted from the splanchnic circulation in humans, albeit less than in rats (2–5). A significant amount of the carbon fragments from the oxidation of exogenous glutamine enters the body's glucose pool (6). Glutamine stimulates crypt cell proliferation of ileal and colonic mucosa and, presumably, of jejunal epithelial cells as well in vitro (7). In humans, splanchnic extraction of glutamine is similar regardless of whether glutamine is provided enterally or parenterally, and therefore studies of supplemental parenteral and enteral glutamine can be considered together (5, 8). It remains unclear whether glutamine is *the* preferred fuel for the *human* small intestine. Data suggest that *glutamate*, rather than *glutamine*, may be the preferred fuel in the catabolic rat (9). Glutamate is more efficiently metabolized by the intestine than glutamine, and it enhances mucosal protein synthesis more than glutamine (9). Glutamine is a

precursor of purines, pyrimidines, nucleotides, urea, and ammonia. (10).

CHEMISTRY, BIOCHEMISTRY/BIOSYNTHESIS, AND GENETICS

The major source of glutamine (Fig. 35.1) entering the plasma compartment is muscle (11). Branched-chain amino acids, released from skeletal muscle during catabolism, are an important precursor of glutamine (12). Glutamine is the most abundant amino acid in the blood. The ligase, glutamine synthetase, catalyzes the synthesis of glutamine from glutamate and ammonia in the cytoplasm of perivenous hepatocytes, and its activity is the rate-limiting factor in glutamine synthesis. Increased plasma glutamine concentration, as during glutamine infusion, downregulates endogenous glutamine synthesis (13). Glutamate may also be amidated to glutamine.

Glutamine is a unique amino acid because it contains two nitrogen atoms. This characteristic must be taken into consideration in designing comparative amino acids when nitrogen balance is an outcome measure. Free glutamine is not stable in solution and decomposes to pyroglutamic acid and ammonia.

ANALYTIC METHODS

Amino acid concentrations in plasma, tissue, and other biologic samples may be determined using ion exchange chromatography. Automated equipment is available (14).

DIGESTION, ABSORPTION, BIOAVAILABILITY, AND EXCRETION

Approximately 60 to 90% of consumed glutamine is absorbed in humans (6, 15), with plasma glutamine concentration rising in a dose-dependent fashion (15). Of this, approximately 7% is converted to glucose (versus 10% from intravenously infused glutamine) (6). Stable isotope studies have shown that glutamine utilization is reduced approximately 20% in patients following extensive small intestinal resection (16). The splanchnic circulation is the primary source for glutamine uptake (17), although during conditions of acidosis, renal uptake significantly increases (18). Approximately 50% of enterally consumed glutamine

¹**Abbreviations:** **cAMP,** cyclic adenosine monophosphate; **GALT,** gut-associated lymphoid tissue; **ICU,** intensive care unit; **TPN,** total parenteral nutrition.

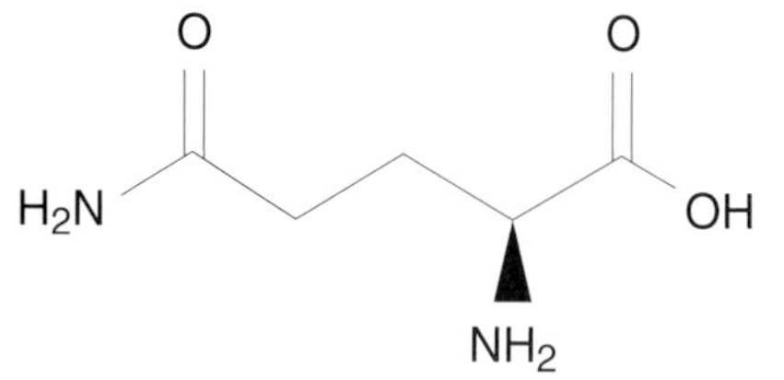

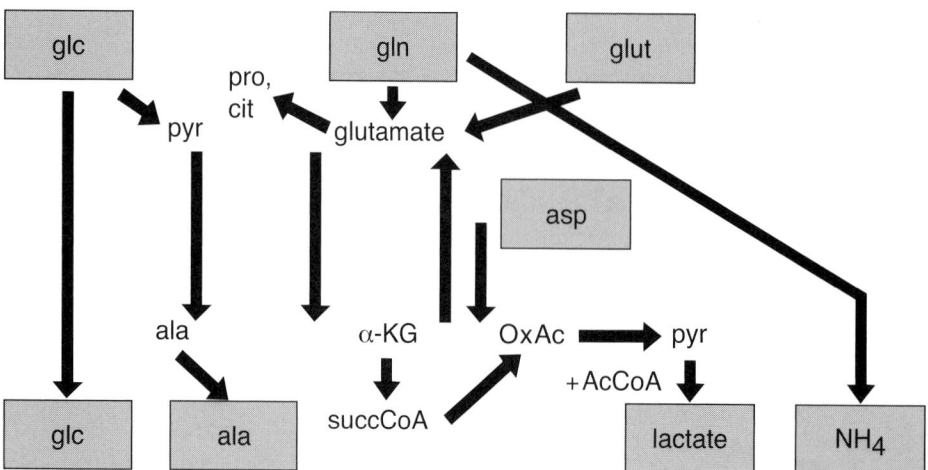

Figure 35.1. Chemical structure of glutamine.

escapes metabolism in the intestinal epithelium and enters the systemic circulation (15).

TRANSPORT AND METABOLISM

As with other amino acids, glutamine is transported by either sodium-dependent or sodium-independent mechanisms. Sodium-dependent transport uses the potential energy stored in sodium/potassium-adenosine triphosphatase to transport glutamine across the transmembrane electrochemical gradient. There exist several identified genes coding for sodium-dependent glutamine transport systems including systems ASC, $B^{0,+}$, y^+ L, A, and N. System N is especially important in the uptake of glutamine by hepatocytes (19), and therefore it may serve to regulate cytoplasmic glutamine concentration and potentially glutaminase activity (20). Sodium-independent transport systems include systems L, $b^{0,+}$ and n (21). Most of these transporters also mediate transmembrane movement of other amino acids in addition to glutamine.

Glutamine plays a central role in the regulation of gluconeogenesis and in ammonia detoxification via the urea cycle. The liver is the site of most glutamine metabolism. Urea synthesis occurs in the periportal areas, and glutamate

and excess ammonia are converted to glutamine in the perivenous sections. Glutamine is deaminated by the enzyme glutaminase to form glutamate, which, in turn, can be deaminated to form α-ketoglutarate, which enters the tricarboxylic acid cycle. The ammonia group from glutamate can also be used for asparate synthesis from oxaloacetate, and via aspartate, the nitrogen of glutamine can enter the urea cycle. Alanine, citruline, proline, and glutathione, as well as purine and pyrimidine nucleotides, may be produced from glutamine (22).

Animal studies have shown glutaminase activity may be upregulated to support gluconeogenesis during starvation (23) and chronic metabolic acidosis (24). Glutamine metabolism increases in chronic metabolic acidosis probably to effect greater ammonia secretion. Hepatic glutaminase activity appears to be upregulated by a mechanism dependent on cyclic adenosine monophosphate (cAMP) (25), and this activity is increased by medications such as glucagon that stimulate cAMP (26).

Although previous investigations found glutamine to be the preferred fuel for the small intestine (1), more recent studies have demonstrated that glutamate is interchangeable with glutamine as an intestinal fuel (27). Glutamine may be oxidized as a fuel and can be a primary energy substrate for enterocytes and lymphocytes (Fig. 35.2).

CAUSES AND EFFECTS OF GLUTAMINE DEFICIENCY

An important issue is whether glutamine deficiency occurs in humans. Animal model (primarily rat) investigations have shown that in most, but not all, cases (28–37), intestinal villus hypoplasia, increased intestinal permeability to macromolecules, decreased immunoglobulin A production

Metabolism of glutamine (gln) in intestinal cells

Figure 35.2. Glutamine metabolism in the enterocyte. AcCoA, acetyl coenzyme A; ala, alanine; asp, aspartate; cit, citrulline; glc, glucose; gln, glutamine; glut, glutamate; pyr, pyruvate; α-KG, α-ketoglutarate; OxAc, oxaloacetate; pro, proline; succCoA, succinyl coenzyme A. (From Alpers DH. Curr Opin Gastroenterol 2000;16:155–159, with permission.)

and changes in the number of gut–associated lymphoid tissue (GALT), and decreases in intestinal mucus gel secretion occur when animals experience systemic injury such as major trauma or sepsis or are provided with glutamine-free total parenteral nutrition (TPN) as an exclusive means of nutritional support.

Little evidence is available to support the notion of a glutamine deficiency state in humans other than decreased plasma glutamine concentration in a variety of conditions. It is therefore questionable whether a role exists for either glutamine replacement therapy or pharmacologic therapy with glutamine. Glutamine is one of the most abundant amino acids. Its plasma concentration often decreases postoperatively (38, 39), during sepsis (40), following multiple trauma (41), or in major burns (42), just as with many other amino acids, electrolytes, minerals, and trace elements. Decreased blood concentration is not necessarily indicative of a deficient state, although the decrease in serum glutamine concentration does correlate with the decrease in intestinal glutamine concentration (43). Critically ill patients may be unable to increase endogenous glutamine synthesis sufficiently to offset increased intracellular glutamine loss, primarily from skeletal muscle. Such intracellular concentrations of glutamine often do decrease in catabolic, critically ill patients. The decrease in plasma and serum amino acid concentration during critical illness is not specific to glutamine. However, the effects of such a decrease in plasma or serum glutamine concentration on disease diagnosis, treatment, and patient outcome are unclear, and, therefore, clinically significant glutamine deficiency in humans has yet to be identified.

Investigators have suggested that during TPN and the absence of luminal nutrients, intestinal atrophy develops. However, that observation appears to be a species-specific phenomenon. When human study subjects are provided with TPN as an exclusive source of nutrition for 2 weeks, intestinal *atrophy* does not occur. Jejunal villus height decreased in a group of normal volunteers provided with TPN, although it still remained normal. The decrease was related to *mild* hypoplasia, rather than *atrophy* (44). Electron microscopy showed normal microvilli after TPN. Increased permeability to lactulose and mannitol were observed during glutamine-free TPN, but this effect was unrelated to intestinal morphologic changes or plasma glutamine concentration. No subject developed diarrhea or signs of malabsorption. Investigations in patients have resulted in similar observations. For example, in a heterogeneous group of hospitalized patients who required TPN, Van der Hulst and associates (43) found that duodenal villus height decreased similarly to that observed by Buchman and colleagues (44) in the jejunum in that statistically significant (but clinically insignificant) changes were observed within the normal range of villus height after 10 to 14 days of glutamine-free TPN (45). Intestinal macromolecule permeability increased significantly, but if a single outlier is removed, no obvious difference appears to have occurred in intestinal permeability. Glutamine-supplemented TPN prevented these observed, albeit minor, intestinal changes. No intestinal morphologic data from "critically ill" patients have been reported, although morphologic changes do not occur acutely, and little evidence indicates that intestinal permeability increases as a result of "critical illness" alone (46). In addition, the clinical relevance of increased macromolecule permeability is unclear.

Investigators have proposed that intestinal atrophy leads to bacterial translocation and increased risk of sepsis, especially in critically ill patients, although Sedman and associates found that villus height was no different in patients who had documented bacterial translocation from villus height in patients who did not (47). Intestinal bacterial translocation, if it occurs and if it is clinically significant in humans (47), does not appear related to glutamine-induced morphologic changes in the intestine (48). However, glutamine also may play a role in the maintenance of normal intestinal immune function, which, in turn, most likely plays an important role in the prevention of bacterial translocation. Buchman and colleagues (49), as well as Van der Hulst and associates (50), demonstrated that glutamine–free TPN is not associated with intestinal immune dysfunction, as occurs in animal models (51). In both groups, intestinal immunoglobulin secretion and GALT remained normal and unchanged. The absence of such abnormalities in humans suggests that glutamine supplementation would be unlikely to prevent or reduce human intestinal bacterial translocation.

IMPACT OF STRESS AND DISEASE ON NUTRIENT UTILIZATION

Dietary Considerations and Requirements

Given that glutamine is currently considered a nonessential nutrient, no particular dietary requirements or adequate intake values have been set by the Food and Nutrition Board.

Glutamine Replacement Therapy

Although several studies showed improved nitrogen balance with glutamine supplementation, other measures of outcome did not always improve. Many studies did not have an isonitrogenous control because the presence of glutamine's two nitrogen atoms was not considered. In some investigations, nitrogen balance improved and plasma glutamine concentration increased with glutamine supplementation; however, muscle glutamine was not always repleted. This observation suggests that glutamine release from skeletal muscle may be a normal adaptation to catabolic stress (52). Glutamine may also be replaced under such conditions by increased intake of glutamine "homologs" including other amino and keto acids such as glutamic acid, aspartic acid, arginine, asparagine, and oxaloacetate (53). The substitution of glutamine for other amino acids in equivalent concentrations does not enhance visceral protein synthesis (54, 55). Intestinal glutaminase activity increases when increased glutamine supplementation is provided in rodent models (56). Glutamine metabolism is thus enhanced the more exogenous glutamine is provided.

Therapeutic Use of Glutamine in Pharmacologic Doses

Short Bowel Syndrome

Animal studies have suggested that glutamine supplementation may enhance intestinal adaptation following massive enterectomy, although investigations to demonstrate a similar effect in humans have been limited. Glutamine supplementation failed to enhance adaptation in a child with gastroschisis and necrotizing enterocolitis (57). An uncontrolled study of a "high-fiber" diet, growth hormone, and glutamine showed increased sodium, water, and energy absorption and decreased fecal weight (58). Two more recent placebo-controlled trials were unable to confirm these results. Scolapio and associates gave growth hormone (0.14 mg/kg/day), glutamine (oral, 0.63 mg/kg/day), and a complex carbohydrate diet to patients with short bowel syndrome (59). No improvement in carbohydrate or nitrogen absorption, magnesium loss, stool volume, or intestinal morphology was observed. (59, 60). However, significantly increased body weight (related to observed fluid retention and peripheral edema) and increased sodium and potassium absorption were found. Szkudlarek and colleagues provided growth hormone and glutamine (both oral and parenteral) or placebo for 28 days to patients who remained on their usual diet (61). No improvement in energy, fat, carbohydrate, nitrogen absorption, or decrease in fecal losses was observed. As in the study by Scolapio and associates, body weight, lean body mass, and sodium absorption all increased. This finding was most likely related to sodium and fluid retention associated with growth hormone use.

Glutamine-supplemented TPN (without growth hormone) may actually prevent fluid retention and extracellular fluid compartment expansion in patients after bone marrow transplantation and also in patients who have undergone radiation treatment with high-dose chemotherapy (62, 63). Therefore, it is possible that these positive effects of glutamine may have been masked in the previous studies in which growth hormone was also administered. Increased body weight and lean body mass have not been described in otherwise well-nourished patients with short bowel syndrome following glutamine supplementation (64).

Acute Pancreatitis and Inflammatory Bowel Disease

One study compared the use of glutamine-supplemented TPN with standard TPN in patients hospitalized with mild acute pancreatitis. Infectious complications, bacteremia, costs, and hospital stay were similar in both groups (65).

Five studies (one open-labeled study) were performed with glutamine supplementation in patients with Crohn disease. No benefit from glutamine supplementation in patients who received 15 to –30 g/day of glutamine supplementation was observed on disease activity, intestinal permeability, or nutritional parameters (66–70), although in the preliminary open-labeled study of Zoli and colleagues, a significant decrease in intestinal permeability was described (68). The pretreatment intestinal permeability in the patients studied, however, was greater than in virtually any other study, and the clinical significance of this observation is unclear. Such observations have not been replicated by other investigators (69).

The metabolism of glutamine to nitric oxide may actually increase intestinal and colonic inflammation rather than decrease it. In addition, glutamine supplementation stimulates T-cell function, which may also lead to increased inflammation. For example, Shinozaki and colleagues observed significantly increased colonic inflammation in a rodent model of ulcerative colitis in animals that received a diet supplemented with 24% glutamine (71). The least inflammation was observed in control animals. These data suggest the possibility that inflammatory bowel disease could worsen in patients who receive supplemental glutamine. Consistent with this concept is a study in children with Crohn disease whose pediatric Crohn disease activity index actually improved more in the control group than in the glutamine-supplemented group (70).

Glutamine suppositories (1 g/day for 21 days) were investigated in a unblinded study design in patients with ulcerative colitis after total colectomy with an ileal pouch who developed inflammation of the pouch (pouchitis) (72). Six of the ten patients who completed the trial had no recurrence of their pouchitis symptoms, although the follow-up period may have been too short for this conclusion to have validity.

Critical Care

Numerous studies have shown that although supplemental glutamine may maintain skeletal muscle glutamine concentration in some cases, net protein synthesis is not increased (73, 74). In addition, glutamine transport into and out of skeletal muscle is unaffected by supplementation (75). Although it has been hypothesized that glutamine is the preferred fuel for the human small intestine, enteral glutamine supplementation failed to improve the intestinal protein synthesis either in physiologically normal human volunteers made catabolic with corticosteroid therapy (76) or in critically ill patients (73).

Clinically significant improvements have been difficult to demonstrate with glutamine supplementation (77, 78). Several investigators reported that both parenteral and enteral glutamine supplementation led to decreased infectious complications and decreased duration of hospital stay in patients who required TPN, although the conclusions are controversial. Griffiths and associates reported that short-term (mean, 5 days) glutamine-supplemented TPN led to improved patient survival at 6 months in critically ill patients, although survival at 20 days was identical to that in controls (79). Decreased total hospital and intensive care unit (ICU) costs were lower in the glutamine-supplemented patients, although because patients in the glutamine group tended to die sooner than controls (8.5-day versus 13.5-day survival), the cost and length of their hospitalizations were naturally lower. Fewer patients in the glutamine-treated group died of multiorgan failure than the control group; however, the statistical analysis of this difference was not reported. A trend toward decreased length of stay in *control-group patients who survived* was reported, as well as an overall decreased ICU stay in control patients, but these differences were not statistically significant. Given the large number of correlations evaluated in this study, and the absence of the Bonferoni correction factor (a statistical correction that takes into account that the likelihood of a positive outcome is increased the more outcome variables are analyzed), it is difficult to conclude that 6-month survival was increased solely because of short-term glutamine supplementation. For most of the 6 months, the subjects ate uncontrolled diets at home. Other studies reported improved 6-month survival only in patients who received glutamine-supplemented TPN for at least 9 days (80) and no difference in 6-month survival following glutamine-supplemented enteral nutritional support (81). Patients who received glutamine-supplemented TPN had a similar number of hospital-acquired infections as controls (80, 82). Unfortunately, the study of Jones and associates (82) was unblinded (glutamine dipeptide was infused separately from TPN), the treatment group received significantly more protein than the control group, both groups received an unspecified amount of enteral feeding, and the data were not analyzed on an intent-to-treat basis. Furthermore, 30-day survival was not improved in patients who received glutamine-supplemented TPN. Patients who received glutamine also tended to develop renal insufficiency. No difference was observed in infection rate, nitrogen balance, plasma visceral protein concentration, ICU length of stay, or total length of hospitalization.

Some studies, however, have suggested that glutamine supplementation may be associated with decreased infection risk. Significantly reduced incidences of pneumonia, bacteremia, and sepsis within the first 2 weeks of injury were described in severely injured patients with multiple trauma who received a glutamine-supplemented enteral formula when compared with patients who received standard formula for at least 5 days (65, 83, 84). Conejero and colleagues reported that the development of nosocomial infections was decreased in patients who received a glutamine-supplemented enteral formula (84). However, development of multiorgan failure syndrome, ICU length of

stay, and mortality were not affected, the study was unblinded to the observers, and the data were not analyzed on an intent-to-treat basis. Glutamine-supplemented TPN has been shown to improve in vitro neutrophil bactericidal function in pediatric patients with burns and to decrease the incidence of bacteremia, although not clinical infections, in severely burned pediatric patients (79, 85). As a consequence, neither ICU stay nor total hospital stay was shortened.

Bone Marrow Transplantation, Radiation Therapy, and Chemotherapy

Glutamine-supplemented TPN has not been consistently associated with improvement in infections or gastrointestinal complications in patients receiving bone marrow transplantation, although some studies have reported decreased length of hospital stay in these patients (62, 86–90). Oral glutamine supplements have been studied in patients who have undergone chemotherapy and/or radiation therapy for various malignant diseases. In general, glutamine-supplemented TPN has had no effect on chemotherapy-associated toxicity (91, 92), although an open-labeled study, using primarily subjective measures of neurologic symptoms, found that patients who consumed an oral glutamine supplement had a reduction in the severity of their neuropathy following chemotherapy with paclitaxel (93). The reason for this observation is unclear. Oral glutamine supplementation has also been studied as a preventive therapy for mucositis, often seen with 5-flurouracil, methotrexate, and other chemotherapeutic agents, as well as with radiation therapy. Most studies have failed to show benefit (88, 94–99).

Peri-Operative and Postoperative Patients

Numerous studies have shown that plasma glutamine concentration falls immediately following surgery; however, glutamine-supplemented TPN and enteral nutrition have not been shown to decrease protein degradation either preoperatively or postoperatively (73, 100, 101). In fact, Rittler and colleagues found that colonic protein synthesis actually *decreased* in patients who received glutamine-supplemented TPN (101).

Few data support the hypothesis that glutamine supplementation is associated with decreased infection risk in general surgical patients. Diggory and colleagues found no difference in the number of patients who developed postoperative intraabdominal infection when glutamine-supplemented TPN was used preoperatively (102). Shortened hospital stay following major surgery was reported in two studies of patients who received glutamine supplementation (103, 104). Powell-Tuck and associates studied glutamine-supplemented TPN in 168 hospitalized patients who required TPN; most were preoperative patients (105). No differences in septic complications, TPN duration, length of stay, quality of life scores, overall mortality, 6-month mortality, ICU mortality, or cause of death were observed versus patients who received standard TPN.

Investigators have suggested that only the most severely ill and therefore most catabolic patients may benefit from glutamine supplementation. However, the evidence is not clear which, if any, patient groups would benefit from supplementation. For example, Lin and associates found that glutamine supplementation was of benefit only in less ill postoperative patients, and even then nitrogen balance failed to improve. The study's conclusion that glutamine-supplemented TPN improved immune response was flawed because the glutamine-supplemented patients had a higher CD4 count before TPN, and it persisted during the study (106). In addition, although blood culture and infection data were not reported, fever developed more often in the patients who received glutamine supplementation. This finding suggests a greater likelihood of either infection or inflammation. Similar observations were made in a group of patients who underwent resection of gastrointestinal malignant disease (107). Hospital stay was shorter in the glutamine-supplemented group, although there was no mortality in either group.

The potential mechanism for glutamine's effect on immunologic function has been evaluated only in two small studies. Aosasa and colleagues studied the in vitro effect of oral glutamine supplementation on the stimulation of mesenteric blood mononuclear cells from a group of patients with colorectal cancer (108). These investigators found that patients who received glutamine supplementation had lower tumor necrosis factor-α concentration in their mesenteric blood, although no difference (versus controls) was noted in the tumor necrosis factor-α or interleukin-10 concentration of peripheral blood. The investigators concluded that glutamine supplementation prevented mesenteric mononuclear cell activation and therefore would have blunted the systemic inflammatory response as *may* occur during sepsis. However, the story remains incomplete because other cytokines were not measured or reported, and the findings appeared unique to mesenteric blood; mucosal cytokine concentrations were not measured. In addition, the clinical significance of these observations, including the effect of glutamine supplementation on the in vivo systemic inflammatory response and patient progression to multiorgan failure, is unknown. In the second study, performed in patients in an ICU, the total lymphocyte count was actually greater in the control group (versus glutamine-supplemented patients), although the CD4:CD8 ratio increased in the glutamine-treated group (109).

SAFETY ISSUES AND INTERACTIONS WITH OTHER NUTRIENTS

Most short-term studies reported no safety concerns with intravenously infused glutamine in physiologically normal volunteers (46, 77, 92, 110–112). However, Hornsby-Lewis and colleagues found that glutamine supplementation in patients receiving TPN at home was associated with significantly elevated hepatic aminotransferases after 4 weeks, and these investigators were forced to stop their study prematurely (53). The reason for this observation is unknown, although a more recent preliminary study suggested that orally administered glutamine may precipitate or exacerbate hepatic encephalopathy and reaction time and is associated with electroencephalographic changes in patients who have otherwise stable cirrhosis (112). Therefore, liver function should be monitored in patients who receive glutamine supplementation, and this supplementation should not be provided to patients with hepatic insufficiency. Intravenous glutamine infusion may suppress lipolysis, although the clinical significance of this observation is unclear (15).

In vitro studies of peripheral lymphocytes from patients with Alzheimer dementia and from patients with Down syndrome showed significantly increased glutamine toxicity to lymphocytes versus physiologically normal controls, and similar observations have been made in otherwise healthy elderly persons (113). This heightened sensitivity to exogenous glutamine suggests the potential of a role for impaired glutamine metabolism in dementia and therefore of potential worsening of dementia with glutamine supplementation. Additional toxicity studies of glutamine supplementation in these patient groups as well as in elderly patients will be necessary before it can be deemed safe in these populations. Therefore, glutamine supplementation should be avoided in elderly persons.

Glutamine appears to be an essential amino acid for methylcholanthrene sarcoma growth in rats. However, two studies showed that glutamine (114) or glutamine precursor (115) supplementation did not stimulate tumor growth in animal models of fibrosarcomas and Yoshida ascites hepatoma. In addition, glutamine supplementation did not enhance mammary tumor growth in rats (116). However, theoretic issues remain with regard to glutamine's effects as a promotor (117). Longer-term studies will be necessary to determine whether glutamine promotes tumor growth in humans.

An extensive review by the Food and Nutrition Board concluded that glutamate supplementation has few side effects, the data on glutamine's adverse effects are controversial, and that data are insufficient to determine dose response assessment for either glutamate or glutamine (118).

CONCLUSION

Glutamine clearly illustrates the potentials pitfalls inherent in the extrapolation of animal data directly to the human organism (the "leap of faith" argument) (119). Until additional efficacy and safety data in humans are available, glutamine remains an important, but nonessential amino acid for humans. Routine supplementation should not be provided to patients outside a clinical trial.

REFERENCES

1. Windmueller HG, Spaeth AE. Arch Biochem Biophys 1976;175:670–6.
2. Windmueller HG, Spaeth AE. J Biol Chem 1978;253:69–76.
3. Van der Hulst RRWJ, Deutz NEP, Soeters PB et al. Clin Nutr 1993;12:10S–1S.
4. Darmaun D, Messing B, Just B et al. Metabolism 1991;40:42–4.
5. Hankard R, Goulet O, Ricour C et al. Pediatr Res 1994;36:202–6.
6. Haisch M, Fukagawa NK, Matthews DE. Am J Physiol 2000;278:E593–602.
7. Scheppach W, Loges C, Bartram P et al. Gastroenterology 1994;107:429–34.
8. Nurjhan N, Bucci A, Perriello G et al. J Clin Invest 1995;95:272–7.
9. Hasebe M, Suzuki H, Mori E et al. JPEN J Parenter Enteral Nutr 1999;23:78S–82S.
10. Smith RJ. Glutamine metabolism and its physiological importance. JPEN J Parenter Enteral Nutr 1990;14:40S–4S.
11. Nurjhan N, Bucci A, Perriello G et al. J Clin Invest 1995;95:272–77.
12. Darmaun D, Dechelotte P. Am J Physiol 1991;260:E326–9.
13. Perriello G, Nurjhan N et al. Am J Physiol 1997;272:E437–45.
14. Le Boucher J, Charret C, Coudray-Lucas C et al. Clin Chem 1997;43:1421–8.
15. Dechelotte P, Darmaun D, Rongier M et al. Am J Physiol 1991;260:G677–82.
16. Darmaun D, Messing B, Just B et al. Metabolism 1991;40:42–4.
17. Marliss EB, Aoki T, Pozefsky T et al. J Clin Invest 1971;50:814-7.
18. Tizianello A, DeFerrari G, Gariboto G et al. Clin Sci 1978;55:391–7.
19. Bode BP, Kaminski DL, Souba WW et al. Hepatology 1995;21:511–20.
20. Low SY, Salter M, Knowles RG et al. Biochem J 1993;295:617–24.
21. Bode BP. J Nutr 2001;131:2475S–85S.
22. Wu G. J Nutr 1998;128:1249–52.
23. Watford M, Vincent N, Zhan Z et al. J Nutr 1994;124:493–9.
24. Curthoys NP, Lowry OH. J Biol Chem 1973;248:162–8.
25. Watford M, Smith EM. Biochem Soc Trans 1989;17:175.
26. Lacey JH, Bradford NM, Joseph SK et al. Biochem J 1981;194:29–33.
27. Reeds PJ, Burrin DG. J Nutr 2001;131:2505S–8S.
28. Sitren HS, Bryant M, Ellis LM. JPEN J Parenter Enteral Nutr 1992;16:30S.
29. Bark T, Svenberg T, Theodorsson E et al. Clin Nutr 1994;13:79–84.
30. Scott T, Moellman J. JPEN J Parenter Enteral Nutr 1991;15:17S.
31. Wusteman M, Tate H, Weaver L et al. JPEN J Parenter Enteral Nutr 1995;19:22–7.
32. Spaeth G, Gottwald T, Haas W et al. JPEN J Parenter Enteral Nutr 1993;17:317–23.
33. Marks SL, Cook AK, Reader R et al. Am J Vet Res 1999;60:755–63.
34. Horvath K, Jami M, Hill ID et al. Gastroenterology 1994;106:A610.
35. Garrel DR, Bernier J, Jobin N. Clin Nutr 1999;18:S6.
36. Vanderhoff JA, Blackwood DJ, Mohammadpour BS et al. J Am Coll Nutr 1992;11:223–7.
37. Jacobs DO, Evans A, O'Dwyer ST et al. Surg Forum 1987;38:45–7.
38. Blomvist BI, Hammarqvist F, von der Decken A et al. J. Clin Nutr 1993;12:12S–3S.
39. Parry-Billings M, Baigrie RJ, Lamont PM et al. Arch Surg 1992;127:1237–40.
40. Planas M, Schwartz S, Arbos MA et al. JPEN J Parenter Enteral Nutr 1993;17:299–300.
41. Wernerman J, Hammarqvist F, Ali MR et al. Metabolism 1989;38:63–6.
42. Parry-Billings M, Evans J, Calder PC et al. Lancet 1990;336:523–5.
43. Van der Hulst RRWJ, Deutz NEP, Von Meyenfeldt MF et al. Clin Nutr 1994;13:228–33.
44. Buchman AL, Moukarzel AA, Bhuta S et al. JPEN J Parenter Enteral Nutr 1995;19:453–60.
45. Van der Hulst RRWJ, von Meyenfeldt MF, van Kreel BK et al. Lancet 1993;341:1363–5.
46. Wicks C, Somasundaram S, Bjarnason I et al. Lancet 1994; 344:837–40.
47. Sedman PC, Macfie J, Sagar P et al. Gastroenterology 1994;107:643–9.
48. Illig KA, Ryan CK, Hardy DJ et al. Surgery 1992;112:631–7.
49. Buchman AL, Mestecky J, Moukarzel A et al. J Am Coll Nutr 1995;14:656–61.
50. Van der Hulst RRWJ, Von Meyenfeldt MF, Tiebosch A et al. JPEN J Parenter Enteral Nutr 1997;21:310–5.
51. Alverdy JA, Aoys E, Weiss-Carrington P et al. J Surg Res 1992;52:34–8.
52. Karner J, Roth E, Ollenschlager G. Surgery 1989;106:893–900.
53. Hornsby-Lewis L, Shike M, Brown P et al. JPEN J Parenter Enteral Nutr 1994;18:268–73.
54. van Acker BAC, Hulsewe KWE, Wagenmakers AJM et al. Clin Nutr 1999;18:S18.
55. Hulsewe KWE, van Acker BAC, Wagenmakers AJM et al. Clin Nutr 1999;18:S42.
56. Kong S, Hall JC, Cooper D, et al. Biochim Biophys Acta 2000;1475:67–75.
57. Allen SJ, Pierro A, Cope L et al. J Pediatr Gastroenterol Nutr 1993;17:329–32.
58. Byrne TA, Morrissey TB, Ziegler TR et al. Surg Forum 1992;43:151–3.
59. Scolapio JS, Camilleri M, Fleming CR et al. Gastroenterology 1997;113:1074–81.
60. Scolapio JS, McGreevy K, Tennyson GS et al. Clin Nutr 2001;20:319–23.
61. Szkudlarek J, Jeppsen PB, Mortensen PB. Gut 2000;47:199–205.
62. Schloerb PR, Amare M. JPEN J Parenter Enteral Nutr 1993;17:407–13.
63. Scheltinga MR, Young LS, Benfell K et al. Ann Surg 1991;214:385–95.
64. Dias MCG, Faintuch J, Waitzberg DL et al. JPEN J Parenter Enteral Nutr 1999;S157.
65. Ockenga J, Borchert K, Rifai K et al. Clin Nutr 2002;21:409–16.
66. Akobeng AK, Miller V, Thomas AG et al. JPEN J Parenter Enteral Nutr 2000;24:196.
67. Cordum NR, Schloerb P, Sutton D et al. Gastroenterology 1996;110:A888.
68. Zoli G, Care M, Falco F et al. Gut 1995;37:A13.
69. Den Hond E, Hiele M, Peeters M et al. JPEN J Parenter Enteral Nutr 1999;23:7–11.
70. Akobeng AK, Miller V, Stanton J et al. J Pediatr Gastroenterol Nutr 2000;30:78–84.
71. Shinozaki M, Saito H, Muto T. Dis Colon Rectum 1997;40:59S–63S.

72. Wischmeyer P, Pemberton JH, Phillips SF. Mayo Clin Proc 1993;68:978–81.
73. Gore DC, Wolfe RR. JPEN J Parenter Enteral Nutr 2002;26:342–50.
74. Hammarqvist F, Sandgren A, Andersson K et al. Surgery 2001;129:576–86.
75. Gore DC, Wolfe RR. JPEN J Parenter Enteral Nutr 2003;27:307–14.
76. Bouteloup-Demange C, Claeyssens S, Maillot C et al. Am J Physiol 2000;278:G677–81.
77. Hulsewe KWE, van Acker BAC, Hameeteman W et al. Clin Nutr 1999;18:S25.
78. Tremel H, Kienle B, Weilemann LS et al. Gastroenterology 1994;107:1595–1601.
79. Griffiths RD, Jones C, Palmer TEA. Nutrition 1997;13: 295–302.
80. Griffiths RD, Allan KD, Andrews FJ et al. Nutrition 2002;18:546–52.
81. Hall JC, Dobb G, Hall J et al. JPEN J Parenter Enteral Nutr 2003;27:415S.
82. Jones C, Palmer TEA, Griffiths RD. Nutrition 1999;15: 108–15.
83. Houdjik APJ, Rijnsburger ER, Jansen J et al. Lancet 1998;352:772–6.
84. Conejero R, Bonet A, Grau T et al. Nutrition 2002;18:716–21.
85. Wischmeyer PE, Lynch J, Liedel J et al. Crit Care Med 2001;29:2075–80.
86. Ziegler TR, Young LS, Benfell K et al. Ann Int Med 1992;116:821–8.
87. Schloerb PR, Skikne BS. JPEN J Parenter Enteral Nutr 1999;23:117–22.
88. Anderson PM, Ramsay NKC, Shu XO et al. Clin Nutr 1997;16:33S–4S.
90. Jebb SA, Marcus R, Elia M. Clin Nutr 1995;14:162–5.
91. Richards EW, Long CL, Pinkston JA et al. FASEB J 1992;6:A1680.
92. Van Zaanen HCT, van der Lelie H, Timmer JG et al. Cancer 1994;74:2879–84.
93. Vahdat L, Papadopoulos K, Lange D et al. Clin Cancer Res 2001;7:1192–7.
94. Bozzetti F, Biganzoli L, Gavazzi C et al. Nutrition 1997;13:748–51.
95. Okuno SH, Woodhouse CO, Loprinzi CL et al. Am J Clin Oncol 1999;22:258–61.
96. Jebb SA, Osborne RJ, Maughan TS et al. Br J Cancer 1994;70:732–5.
97. Decker-Baumann C, Buhl K, Frohmuller S et al. Eur J Cancer 1999;35:202–7.
98. Skubitz KM, Andeson PM. J Lab Clin Med 1996;127:223–8.
99. Huang EY, Leung SW, Wang CJ et al. Int J Radiat Oncol Biol Phys 2000;46:535–9.
100. Van Acker BAC, Hulsewe KWE, Wagenmakers AJM et al. Am J Clin Nutr 2000;72:790–5.
101. Rittler P, Schiefer B, Demmelmair H et al. JPEN J Parenter Enteral Nutr 2003;27:S39.
102. Diggory T, Sedman P, Sagar P et al. Nutrition 1994;10:497.
103. Jiang ZM, Cao JD, Zhu XG et al. JPEN J Parenter Enteral Nutr 1999;23:62S–6S.
104. Morlion BJ, Stehle P, Wachtler P et al. Ann Surg 1998;227:302–8.
105. Powell-Tuck J, Jamieson CP, Bettany GEA et al. Gut 1999;45:82–8.
106. Lin MT, Kung SP, Yeh SL et al. Clin Nutr 2002;21:213–8.
107. Neri A, Mariani F, Piccolomini A et al. Nutrition 2001;17:967–9.
108. Aosasa S, Mochizuki H, Yamamoto T et al. JPEN J Parenter Enteral Nutr 1999;23:41S–4S.
109. Jensen GL, Miller RH, Talabiska DG et al. Am J Clin Nutr 1996;64:615–21.
110. Ogle CK, Ogle JD, Mao JX et al. JPEN J Parenter Enteral Nutr 1994;18:128–33.
111. Lowe DK, Benfeli K, Smith RJ et al. Am J Clin Nutr 1990;52:1101–6.
112. Oppong K, Al-Mardini H, Thick M et al. Gastroenterology 1995;108:A1138.
113. Peeters MA, Salabelle A, Attal N et al. J Neurol Sci 1995;133:31–41.
114. Klimberg VS, Souba WW, Salloum RM et al. J Surg Res 1990;48:319–23.
115. Le Bricon T, Cynober L, Baracos VE. Metabolism 1994;43:899–905.
116. Bartlett DL, Charland S, Torosian MH. Ann Surg Oncol 1995;2:71–6.
117. Chance WT, Lequin C, Fischer JE. JPEN J Parenter Enteral Nutr 1990;14:122–8.
118. Food and Nutrition Board, Institute of Medicine. Dietary Reference Intakes. Washington, DC: National Academy Press, 2002:10–94, 10–96 (prepublication issue).
119. Buchman AL. Am J Clin Nutr 2001;74:25–32.

36 ARGININE AND NITRIC OXIDE[1]

BENJAMIN M. CHIONGLO SY, ERIN E. DWEIK, AND RAED A. DWEIK

OVERVIEW OF ARGININE METABOLISM 571
ARGININE AND THE NITRIC OXIDE PATHWAY 572
    Nitric Oxide and Nitric Oxide Synthases 572
    Methylated Arginines 574
    The "Arginine Paradox" 575
SELECTED PHYSIOLOGIC AND PATHOLOGIC
    ROLES OF NITRIC OXIDE .576
    Vascular Effects 576
    Airway Effects 576
    Effects in Inflammation .576
EFFECTS OF ARGININE, METHYLATED ARGININES,
    AND NITRIC OXIDE IN SPECIFIC ORGAN SYSTEMS . .576
    Respiratory System 576
    Cardiovascular System .577
    Renal System and Hypertension 578
    Other Organ Systems 578
    SUMMARY 578

Until recently, this chapter would have focused on arginine synthesis and transport and its role in the urea cycle. Although these metabolic pathways are very important in the overall metabolism of arginine, recent advances in our understanding of the biology of nitric oxide (NO) shifted the attention to arginine catabolism, especially its role as a precursor for the production of NO. This shift started in the late 1980s when endothelial derived relaxing factor was identified as NO (1, 2). This discovery led to an exponential growth in our knowledge about NO and its role in human physiology and disease. Although NO has long been known as an atmospheric pollutant present in vehicle exhaust emissions, smog, and cigarette smoke, its clinical importance as a biologic mediator in animals and humans has been the focus of intensive research since the early 1990s.

NO is endogenously synthesized by NO synthases (NOSs) that convert L-arginine to L-citrulline, and NO is

produced (3). One of its major biologic roles is to activate soluble guanylate cyclase and to produce guanosine 3',5'-cyclic monophosphate (cGMP) in smooth muscle cells resulting in smooth muscle cell relaxation and vasodilation (4). Because of its highly reactive nature, NO is rapidly metabolized into more stable end products such as nitrite and nitrate (3, 5, 6).

Although the arginine-NO pathway represents only a fraction of the total arginine metabolism, it has attracted considerable attention because of the many versatile roles that NO plays in almost all organ systems. In this chapter, we review the various pathways of arginine metabolism with a particular focus on the arginine-NO pathway.

OVERVIEW OF ARGININE METABOLISM

Arginine or 2-amino-5-guanidinovaleric acid (Fig. 36.1) is a semiessential amino acid. Young mammals require arginine exogenously, whereas adults can synthesize it de novo. Plasma arginine levels, however, usually are dependent on dietary intake because the rate of endogenous arginine synthesis cannot increase in response to an inadequate supply (7, 8). The average arginine intake is 4 to 5 g/day (8, 9) and the normal arginine concentration in human plasma is around 95 to 250 umol/L (7). The kidney is the major site of endogenous arginine biosynthesis (from citrulline), which contributes to the plasma pool. Cell types with NOSs can reuse citrulline and synthesize arginine with the enzymes arginosuccinate synthase and arginosuccinate lyase (Fig. 36.2). The liver also synthesizes arginine, but this is primarily used in the urea cycle.

As outlined in Figure 36.2, arginine participates in various metabolic pathways:

- Arginine is a urea cycle (Krebs-Henseleit) intermediate in which it is cleaved (via arginase) into urea and ornithine. Urea allows for the excretion of excess nitrogen in mammals. Ornithine is used as a precursor of proline, glutamine, and polyamines, or it can be used to generate citrulline. Two types of arginase are recognized: cytosolic (type I), which is found in liver and is involved in the detoxification of ammonia and the urea cycle; and mitochondrial (type II), which is extrahepatic and is involved in the synthesis of ornithine, glutamine, and proline (10).

---

[1]**Abbreviations: ADMA,** asymmetric N^GN^G-dimethylarginine; **cGMP,** guanosine 3',5'-cyclic monophosphate; **DDAH,** dimethylarginine diamethylaminohydrolase; **ED,** erectile dysfunction; **iNOS,** inducible nitric oxide synthase; **L-NAME,** N^G-nitro-L-arginine methyl ester; **L-NMMA,** N^G-monomethyl-L-arginine; **NO,** nitric oxide; **NOS,** nitric oxide synthase; **PDE,** phosphodiesterase; **PRMT,** protein-arginine methytransferase; **SDMA,** symmetric N^GN^G-dimethylarginine.

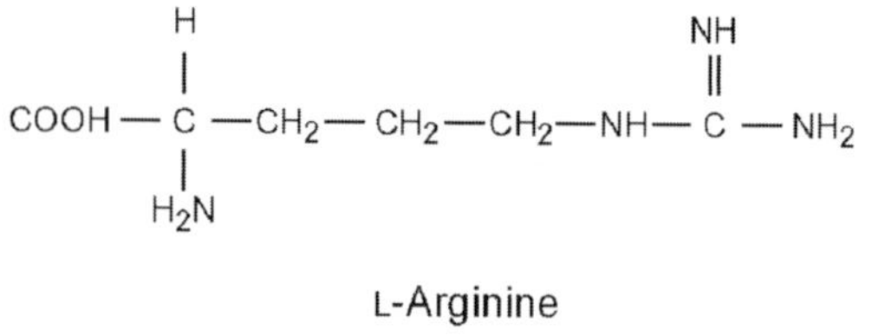

L-Arginine

Figure 36.1. Chemical structure of L-arginine.

- Arginine can be deaminated (via arginine deaminase) to citrulline (7, 10).
- Arginine can be used to synthesize creatine (via arginine-glycine amidinotransferase [AGAT] and guanidinoacetate n-methyltransferase [GMAT]) (7, 10).
- Arginine can be incorporated in the synthesis of proteins (in the form of methylated arginine derivatives) (7, 10).
- Arginine can be used as a precursor for the synthesis of NO (via the NOS isoenzymes) (4, 9, 11).

ARGININE AND THE NITRIC OXIDE PATHWAY

Nitric Oxide and Nitric Oxide Synthases

NO is produced by NOS (EC 1.14.13.39) (6, 11, 12) (Table 36.1; Fig. 36.3). These enzymes convert L-arginine to NO and L-citrulline in a reaction that requires oxygen and

reduced nicotinamide adenine dinucleotide phosphate, and the cofactors flavin adenine dinucleotide, flavin adenine mononucleotide, tetrahydrobiopterin, and calmodulin (6, 11, 12). Three NOSs (types I, II, and III) have been identified and are widely expressed in various tissues (5, 12). In general, NOS I and NOS III are constitutively expressed in neuronal and endothelial cells, respectively, and are dependent on increases in calcium to bind calmodulin, a process that results in enzyme activation and picomolar levels of NO production. NOS II (inducible NOS or iNOS) is regulated at the level of transcription and mRNA stability, is calcium independent, and produces nanomolar levels of NO. Regulation of NOS II expression varies in different cell types, but typically it is increased by cytokines such as interferon-γ (5, 6, 11–14).

NOS I is largely expressed in the brain. It is also found in the peripheral nervous system and in epithelial cells. It is otherwise known as bNOS (brain), cNOS (constitutive), bcNOS (a combination), or nNOS (neuronal). NO formed in the nervous system has been implicated in blood pressure regulation (reducing sympathetic vascular tone) and is also a neurotransmitter in the periphery in nonadrenergic, noncholinergic, or nitrergic (in reference to NO) nerves. NOS II, once induced, produces much higher levels of NO than that other two constitutive forms and has been implicated in

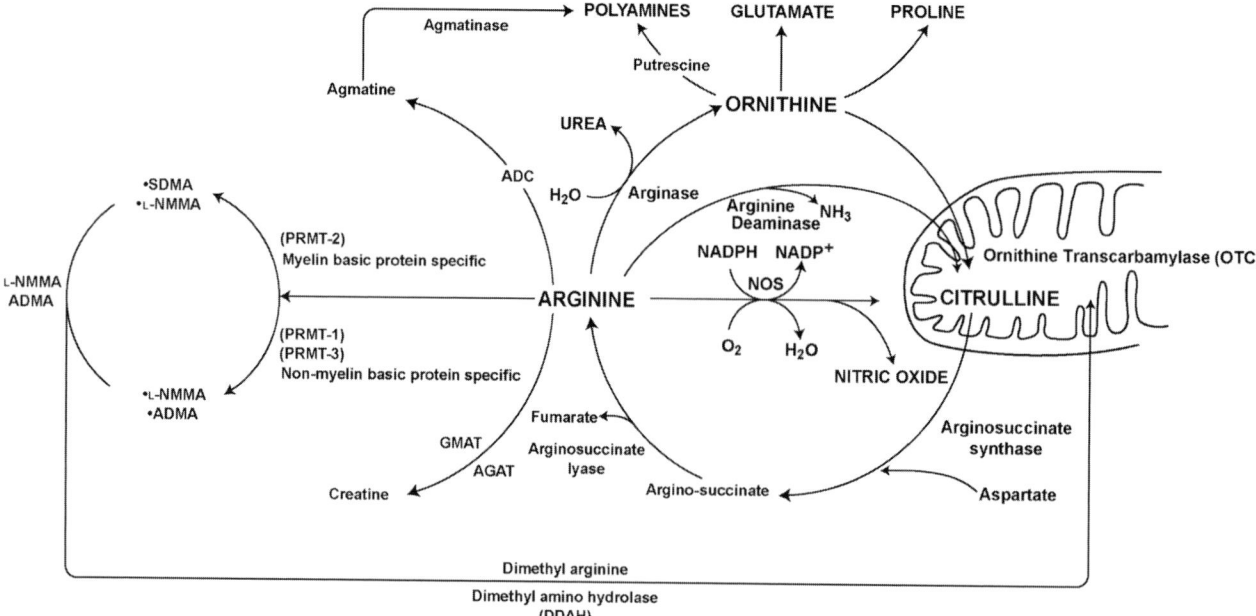

Figure 36.2. Metabolic pathways of arginine. Arginine is used for protein synthesis, as an intermediate in the urea cycle, as a precursor to glutamate, proline, and polyamines (via ornithine), and as a substrate for creatine and nitric oxide production. In the cytoplasm, arginine is hydrolyzed (via arginase) to urea and ornithine. Ornithine is transported into the mitochondria, where it is combined with carbamoyl phosphate to form citrulline (via ornithine transcarbamylase [OTC]). Citrulline combines with cytosolic aspartate to form arginosuccinate, which is cleaved to form fumarate and arginine. Arginine can also be directly deaminated to form citrulline. Methylated arginine residues (which are usually incorporated into proteins) are formed under the action of various methyltransferase enzymes (protein-arginine methyltransferase [PRMT]). These residues also serve as endogenous antagonists to arginine and may be converted back to citrulline as well (via dimethylarginine diamethylaminohydrolase [DDAH]). Finally, nitric oxide is formed (from arginine) by various nitric oxide synthases (NOS) in the presence of different cofactors (e.g., reduced nicotinamide adenine dinucleotide phosphate, heme, flavins) and oxygen as a cosubstrate. ADC, arginine decarboxylase; ADMA, asymmetric *N-N*-dimethylarginine; AGAT, arginine-glycine amidinotransferase; GMAT, guanidino acetate *N*-methyltransferase; LNMMA, *N*-monomethyl-L-arginine; SDMA, symmetric *N-N*-dimethylarginine

TABLE 36.1. NITRIC OXIDE SYNTHASE ENZYMES

NOS ISOFORMS	OTHER DESIGNATION	EXPRESSION	SOURCES	REGULATION	NITRIC OXIDE OUTPUT	CHROMOSOME
Type I	nNOS	Constitutive	Cytosol of neuronal cells	Calcium/CaM	Low (picomol)	12
Type II	iNOS	Inducible	Macrophages, vascular smooth muscle, vascular endothelium, myocardium, endocardium, hepatocytes, immune cells	Induced by cytokines, endotoxin, and oxidants	High (nanomol)	17
Type III	eNOS	Constitutive	Vascular endothelial cells, platelets, myocardium, endocardium, mast cells, neutrophils	Calcium/CaM	Low (picomol)	7

CaM, calmodulin; eNOS, endothelial nitric oxide synthase; iNOS, inducible nitric oxide synthase; nNOS, neural nitric oxide synthase; NOS, nitric oxide synthase,

the damaging effects of NO including its cytotoxic effects (on microbes and tumor cells, as well as normal cells), inflammation, allograft rejection, and the pathogenesis of diseases such as septic shock and asthma. NOS III is found in endothelial cells (eNOS). Like NOS I, it is calcium and calmodulin dependent. In vascular endothelium, NO serves as an endogenous vasodilator and inhibitor of platelet aggregation/adhesion. The relative deficiency of NO in the endothelium has been implicated in the pathogenesis of atherosclerosis and systemic and pulmonary hypertension. NO can also be formed nonezymatically, but the likely source of NO in biologic tissues is generated from enzymatic chemical reactions. Table 36.2 describes selected biologic functions of NO.

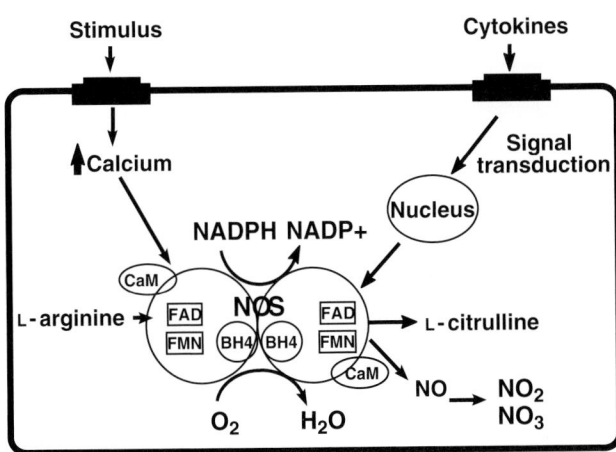

Figure 36.3. Formation of nitric oxide (NO) by nitric oxide synthases (NOS). NOS converts L-arginine to citrulline and NO in the presence of reduced nicotinamide adenine dinucleotide phosphate (NADPH) and molecular oxygen as cosubstrates. Flavoproteins (flavin adenine dinucleotide [FAD], flavin adenine mononucleotide [FMN]) and tetrahydrobiopterin (BH₄) are the other cofactors that the reaction requires. The N in NO comes form L-arginine, whereas the O comes from molecular oxygen; thus, oxygen is a cosubstrate in NO synthesis by NOS. CaM, calmodulin.

Once NO is formed, it diffuses into neighboring cells to exert its various functions. NO can also be detected in exhaled breath of all humans. One of its major biologic roles is to activate soluble guanylate cyclase and to produce cGMP in smooth muscle cells resulting in smooth muscle cell relaxation (4) (Fig. 36.4). As a free radical, NO has a short half-life. It is rapidly inactivated by hemoglobin, and this built-in feature of NO chemistry is probably the most important mechanism for keeping the action of NO localized (5, 13–15). NO is also inactivated by the free radical superoxide. Thus, scavengers of superoxide anion such as superoxide dismutase may protect NO, thus enhancing its potency and prolonging its duration of action. Interaction of NO with superoxide generates peroxynitrite ($ONOO^-$), which is a mediator of potent tissue damage (16) (Fig. 36.5).

Because of its highly reactive nature, once NO is produced it is rapidly metabolized into different more stable end products, depending on the local environment (5, 6, 12, 16–18):

- Reaction with oxygen (O_2) yields NO_2 (gas) or NO_2^- (solution).
- Reaction with superoxide anion (O_2^-) yields peroxynitrite anion ($ONOO^-$) that is further metabolized into nitrate (NO_3^-).
- Reacting with oxyhemoglobin yields methemoglobin and inorganic nitrate (NO_3^-).
- Reaction with thiols (R-SH) yields S-nitrosothiols (R-SNO). NO can react with –SH groups on amino acids, amines, organic acids, sugars, peptides, and proteins to yield the corresponding S-nitrosothiol.
- Reaction with heme iron yields nitrosyl-heme adducts (e.g., hemoglobin, myoglobin, cytochrome c, soluble guanylate cyclase). The binding affinity of hemoglobin for NO exceeds its binding affinity for carbon monoxide and is about 3,000 times that of hemoglobin's affinity to oxygen (5, 15).

TABLE 36.2. SELECTED BIOLOGIC FUNCTIONS OF NITRIC OXIDE

TARGET SYSTEM	BIOLOGIC FUNCTION	MECHANISM
Vascular system	Vascular smooth muscle relaxation	Increased cGMP formation
Brain	Neural messenger	Mediates the action of glutamate acting at *N*-methyl-D-aspartate receptors
Inflammatory system	Antiinflammatory effect	Decrease in lymphocyte (Th1) activation, scavenging superoxide
	Proinflammatory effect	Increase in leukocyte migration, indirect increase in Th2 lymphocytes and eosinophils, peroxynitrite-mediated tissue injury
Host defense	Participation in host defense	NO and/or its oxides (e.g., NO_2 [nitrogen dioxide], N_2O_3 [dinitrogen trioxide], and $ONOO^-$ [peroxynitrite]) can produce bactericidal and cytotoxic effects
Lungs (see also Table 36.3)	Bronchodilation	Functions as a neurotransmitter of the iNANC bronchodilator response
	Airway obstruction	Airway blood vessel dilatation and edema
	Vasodilation	Increased cGMP formation

cGMP, cyclic guanosine monophosphate; iNANC, inhibitory nonadrenergic noncholinergic; NO, nitric oxide; Th, T-helper.

The end products of NO metabolism may themselves exert some of the biologic function attributed to NO. Some of these metabolites (e.g., nitrosothiols) are thought to serve as biologic reservoirs that can release NO again when needed (5, 6, 12, 16–18). Figure 36.5 gives a simplified overview of NO products and actions.

Methylated Arginines

The identification and development of substances that inhibit NOS isoforms have been important strategies in understanding the physiologic and pathophysiologic roles of NO. Several arginine analogs have been developed for

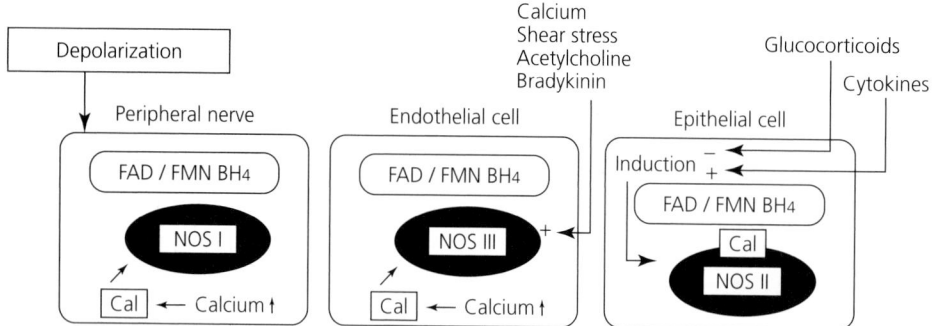

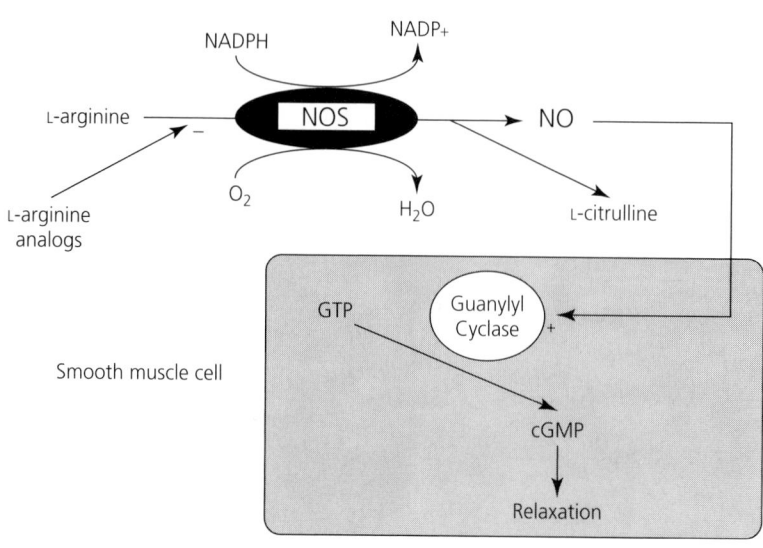

Figure 36.4. Arginine-nitric oxide synthase (NOS)-NO-cyclic guanosine monophosphate (cGMP) pathway. NOS I and NOS III are expressed in neuronal and endothelial cells and are dependent on increases in intracellular calcium to bind calmodulin (CaM) that result in enzyme activation. NOS II is calcium independent and binds CaM even at low calcium concentrations intracellularly. All NOSs can be inhibited by arginine analogs. NO activates guanylyl cyclase, leading to an increase in intracellular cGMP concentration, which then causes smooth muscle relaxation. BH_4, tetrahydrobiopterin; FAD, flavin adenine dinucleotide; FMN, flavin adenine mononucleotide; GTP, guanosine triphosphate.

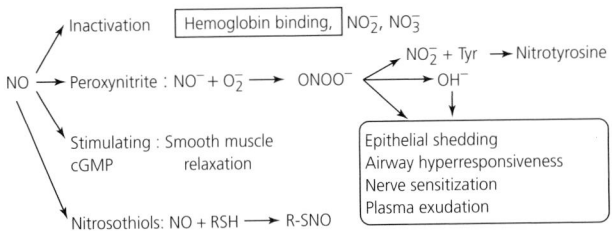

Figure 36.5. Simplified overview of nitric oxide (NO) products and actions. Once NO is formed, it (1) can be "inactivated" by hemoglobin, or by metabolism to nitrite (NO_2^-), and nitrate (NO_3^-) species; (2) can form peroxynitrite ($ONOO^-$) with superoxide anions (O_2^-); peroxynitrite generates hydroxyl radicals and results in nitrosylation of tyrosine (Tyr); (3) can cause smooth muscle relaxation by activation of guanylyl cyclase, which leads to an increase in intracellular cyclic guanosine monophosphate (cGMP); (4) or can be stored as nitrosothiols. RSH, thiols; R-SNO, S-nitrosothiols.

research and potential clinical applications, including N^G-monomethyl-L-arginine (L-NMMA), N^G-nitro-L-arginine (L-NOARG), N^G-nitro-L-arginine methyl ester (L-NAME), and N^G-iminoethyl-L-ornithine (L-NIO), all of which have been useful in revealing the role of endogenous NO in various processes (19).

As analogs of L-arginine, methylarginines act as false substrates for the NOS enzymes and therefore block the formation of endogenous NO (20, 21). By competitively inhibiting NO synthesis from L-arginine by NOS, these endogenous methylarginines can be potent vasoconstrictors. They have also been implicated in the pathogenesis of a variety of clinical conditions such as renal failure, hypertension, hyperlipidemia, and atherosclerosis (20–26). L-NMMA is the classic inhibitor of NOS, but asymmetric $N^G N^G$-dimethylarginine (ADMA) inhibition is equipotent. Symmetric $N^G N^G$-dimethylarginine (SDMA) has no effect on NOS. L-NMMA-induced inhibition of NOS can be overcome with the addition of arginine. Aside from NOS inhibition, all three methylarginines also compete with arginine for cationic amino acid transporters on the cell surface.

The presence of methylated arginine (Fig. 36.6) residues in various specialized proteins has been well documented, although their precise functions have remained unclear (20, 21). Subtypes of the protein-arginine methyltransferase enzyme (PRMT) have been identified (see Fig. 36.2) as being responsible for methylation of these arginine residues. The nonmyelin basic protein-specific enzyme (PRMT-1 and PRMT-3) is the major source of asymmetric methylarginines that inhibit NOS:L-NMMA and ADMA. The myelin basic protein-specific enzyme (PRMT-2) catalyzes the formation of L-NMMA and SDMA. ADMA and SDMA are the major circulating forms of endogenous methylarginines. Asymmetric methylarginines (L-NMMA and ADMA) can be hydrolyzed by dimethylarginine diamethylaminohydrolase (DDAH) to yield citrulline and monomethylamine or dimethylamine (22). DDAH does not hydrolyze SDMA. Overall, it appears that the synthesis and metabolism of endogenous methylarginines are highly regulated.

The "Arginine Paradox"

A peculiar concept in NO metabolism is the L-arginine paradox. It refers to the phenomenon that exogenous arginine causes NO-mediated effects even though, at physiologic state, NOS is already saturated with arginine, and its activity should not be affected by increasing arginine concentration. Both intracellular (0.1–1 mM) and extracellular (73–150 μM) arginine concentrations far exceed the apparent K_m (the half-saturating arginine concentration) of all NOSs (e.g., 2.9 μM for eNOS). Despite this, elevating plasma arginine levels enhances systemic and vascular NO production in a dose-dependent manner (7, 8, 27). This paradox is not fully understood, but several theories have been put forth to explain it based on our current understanding of arginine and NO metabolism (7, 8, 27):

- The compartmentalization of arginine in the cytoplasm—extracellular arginine—may be preferentially used by NOS within this microenvironment; it could also be that neither extracellular nor intracellular concentrations determine NOS activity but rather the amount of arginine transported across cell membranes. System y+ is the most important mechanism of arginine uptake in most cell types, and it has been shown that its expression is coinduced with iNOS, a finding indicating that arginine transport increases to support additional NO synthesis.
- L-Arginine induces insulin secretion, which, in turn, has vasodilatory properties.
- In disease states, this concept could be explained by the presence of endogenous NOS inhibitors, which competitively antagonize arginine (e.g., ADMA) and could be overcome with increasing arginine concentrations.
- L-citrulline, a NOS product, has inhibitory effects on NOS, so cells may need extra arginine to compete with citrulline.
- Arginase may compete with NOS for arginine (a substrate for both enzymes), thereby making less arginine available for NO production by NOS that could be overcome with increasing arginine concentrations.

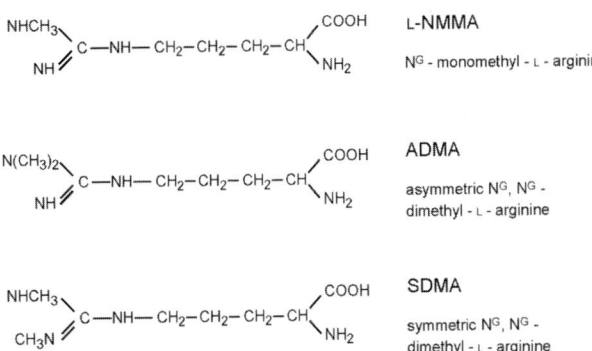

Figure 36.6. Chemical structures of endogenous methylarginines.

SELECTED PHYSIOLOGIC AND PATHOLOGIC ROLES OF NITRIC OXIDE

Vascular Effects

NO has a well-established role in the endothelial-dependent control of vascular tone and in mediating vascular smooth muscle relaxation in the pulmonary and systemic circulations. NO is a potent vasodilator in the bronchial circulation as well and may play an important role in regulating airway blood flow, as in the pulmonary circulation. NO may also modulate systemic vascular tone through its vasodilator property, and excess amounts of NO may cause the hypotension associated with sepsis. A diminution of NO within the lungs is implicated in pathologic states associated with pulmonary hypertension (28–30). NO also has antithrombotic functions, and exogenous NO given by inhalation is a selective pulmonary vasodilator and can improve ventilation-perfusion matching (31, 32).

Airway Effects

Similar to its effects on the vascular smooth muscle, NO can also promote bronchodilation by directly relaxing the smooth muscles of the airway. Produced continuously by the overlying airway epithelium, NO can diffuse easily into the bronchial smooth muscle and can result in smooth muscle relaxation through activation of cGMP (see Fig. 36.5). NO can also affect the bronchial tone indirectly as the neurotransmitter of the inhibitory nonadrenergic, noncholinergic bronchodilator nerves. NO generated by constitutive NOS in these nerves is thought to have bronchoprotective and bronchodilating effects (16, 19).

This dual effect of NO on the airway and the vascular smooth muscles suggests a potential role for NO in regulating ventilation-perfusion matching in the lung. It has long been known that oxygen is the major physiologic regulator of ventilation-perfusion matching in the lung, through vasoconstriction of pulmonary vessels in regions of low ventilation containing low oxygen levels (5). Studies suggest that oxygen regulation of pulmonary vascular tone may be mediated in part by NO (5). Studies in pulmonary endothelial cells, isolated pulmonary vascular rings, isolated perfused lungs, whole animals, and humans support an important role for NO in modulating the pulmonary vascular response to oxygen (5, 33, 34). Endogenous NO levels in the lung change rapidly in direct proportion to inspired oxygen, a finding that strongly supports a critical role for NO as mediator of ventilation-perfusion coupling in the lung. Because of the free diffusion of NO and the close proximity of airways to medium-sized pulmonary vessels that modulate pulmonary vessel tone (5), endogenous NO production in airways proximal to the alveolus may modulate pulmonary vasodilatation. Furthermore, hemoglobin in blood vessels may serve as a natural biologic sink for NO, by creating a continuous concentration gradient for NO to move toward perivascular myocytes and thus regulate blood flow.

Effects in Inflammation

NO can modulate acute and chronic inflammation, by producing both proinflammatory and antiinflammatory effects. NO is a highly reactive molecule/free radical and may have oxidant properties directly or in the form of the more noxious peroxynitrite. These properties give NO its bactericidal and cytotoxic effects and may participate in host defense by mediating antimicrobial activity and cytotoxicity for tumor cells (12, 19, 35). These same properties, however, may also promote an inflammatory response for NO (12, 19, 35). Many of the harmful effects of NO depend on the production of peroxynitrite, a potent oxidant and mediator of epithelial damage that results from the reaction of NO with superoxide anion. The generation of peroxynitrite from NO and superoxide radicals during inflammatory processes induces cell damage and release of inflammatory mediators. Peroxynitrite leads to nitrosylation of tyrosine residues on proteins, and nitrotyrosine may be detected immunocytochemically. Thus, NO and/or its oxides can nitrosate proteins or thiols altering protein functions and may cause inflammation by promoting irreversible lipid perooxidation and damage.

In contrast, NO can also have antiinflammatory properties. Although NO itself is a radical, many of the same chemical and physical properties of NO that allow it to exert oxidant effects can also result in antioxidant actions. The most effective protection against oxidant-mediated tissue damage is to scavenge the initiating radical. Because of its high reactivity with several reactive oxygen species and its ability to traverse membranes and lipoproteins, NO can effectively terminate radical species throughout all aspects of membrane and lipoprotein microenvironments (16, 19, 36), thus giving NO its antioxidant properties. For example, by reacting with superoxide to form peroxynitrite, NO may serve as scavenger of superoxide resulting in a net antioxidant effect. Thus, NO may exert antioxidant (antiinflammatory) or oxidant (inflammatory) effects, depending on the biochemical and physiologic conditions in the tissue milieu. When the oxidant load is high, NO may play an antioxidant role by scavenging superoxide and other reactive oxygen species. In an environment where the oxidant load is low, however, the highly reactive properties of NO give the molecule oxidant properties (16, 19, 36).

EFFECTS OF ARGININE, METHYLATED ARGININES, AND NITRIC OXIDE IN SPECIFIC ORGAN SYSTEMS

Respiratory System

All three types of NOS isoforms are present in the normal lung, with NOS II the predominant form. NOS I is found in nonadrenergic, noncholinergic nerves, NOS III is found in vascular endothelium in both the bronchial and pulmonary circulation, and NOS II is abundant in the airway

TABLE 36.3. FUNCTIONS OF NITRIC OXIDE IN THE LUNG

FUNCTION	POTENTIALLY BENEFICIAL EFFECTS	POTENTIALLY HARMFUL EFFECTS
Vasodilation	Vasodilation of pulmonary vessels improves ventilation-perfusion matching	Vasodilation of bronchial vessels increases airway edema and mucus secretion
Mucus secretion	Regulates mucociliary clearance and ciliary mobility	May directly stimulate mucus secretion from submucosal glands
Inflammation	Host defense: toxic effects on bacteria, viruses and parasites	Indirectly activates T-helper lymphocytes
	Antiinflammatory: scavenging oxidants (e.g., superoxide)	
Neurotransmission	Bronchodilation	Proinflammatory: through toxic metabolites (e.g., peroxynitrite)

epithelium. NO is known to be produced in both the upper and lower respiratory tract (in addition to the pulmonary circulation). A list of NO functions in the lung is provided in Table 36.3.

Increased levels of NO are detected in the exhaled breath of patients with asthma, a disease characterized by airway inflammation. This is related to the inflammatory cytokines, especially interferon-γ, inducing and maintaining the gene expression of NOS II in the airway epithelium, the major source of NO in the lung (16, 37). In addition to having increased levels of NOS II expression, airways of patients with asthma also have high levels of L-arginine, the NOS substrate and precursor of NO production (see Fig. 36.4) (16, 37). Administration of antiinflammatory drugs (e.g., corticosteroids) results in decrease in exhaled NO in these patients and decreases NOS II expression in the airway epithelium. Furthermore, because NO has both proinflammatory and antiinflammatory properties, it can modulate the underlying inflammation in asthma. Thus, the explanation for the elevated levels of NO in asthma turned out to be much more difficult than initially thought. NO could be involved in the pathogenesis of asthma by modifying bronchial hyperresponsiveness or the underlying airway inflammation, or it may be a simple overall marker of inflammation.

Cardiovascular System

Recently, interest in arginine and NO in the field of cardiovascular medicine has been considerable. Arginine seems to exert its effects mostly through the formation of NO, although it has NO-independent hemodynamic effects as well (38). NO-dependent actions include increased smooth muscle cell relaxation and endothelial cell proliferation as well as decreases in platelet aggregation, leukocyte adhesion, superoxide production, endothelin-1 release, and smooth muscle proliferation. NO-independent effects of arginine include increased plasmin generation or fibrinolysis, augmented release of insulin, growth hormone, and glucagon, decreased blood viscosity, decreased formation of fibrin, and decreased angiotensin-converting enzyme activity.

Long-term oral supplementation of dietary L-arginine decreased the surface area and the intimal thickness of atheromatous lesions in the thoracic aorta of hypercholesterolemic rabbits (39). This was associated with improved endothelium-dependent relaxation regardless of changes in cholesterol levels. In cholesterol-fed rabbits, L-arginine supplementation better reduced the progression of atherosclerotic plaques when compared with an hydroxymethylglutaryl–coenzyme A reductase inhibitor, lovastatin (40). This was attributed to an increase in systemic NO synthesis measured as urinary nitrate and cGMP. Platelet hyperaggregability in hypercholesterolemic persons was attenuated modestly by dietary L-arginine (41). This effect persisted up to 2 weeks after discontinuation of therapy and was most likely the result of endothelium or platelet-derived NO because of associated elevations in intraplatelet cGMP (subsequently reversed by the addition of a NOS antagonist, N-methyl-arginine). Intracoronary infusions of L-arginine significantly augmented coronary blood flow responses to acetylcholine in patients with microvascular angina but not in physiologically normal controls (42, 43). Impaired acetylcholine-induced endothelium-dependent vasodilatation of the coronary microcirculation was thought to be from defective synthesis and/or release of NO. Intravenous L-arginine has been shown to induce peripheral vasodilation in the diseased limb of patients with severe peripheral arterial occlusive disease (comparable to the effects seen with therapeutic doses of prostaglandin E₁, a prostaglandin used in the treatment of limb ischemia) (44). The L-arginine group also showed greater urinary nitrate and cGMP excretion rates, findings indicating that endogenous NO synthesis was enhanced during and after L-arginine infusion.

Dysregulation of endogenous NO production may contribute to the pathogenesis of heart failure (45, 46). Oral L-arginine has been shown to have beneficial effects in patients with moderate to severe heart failure (assessed by a quality-of-life questionnaire and a 6-minute walk test) (47). In addition, the limb blood flow during exercise and arterial compliance were significantly enhanced, and circulating levels of endothelin were reduced. NO thus seems to have favorable effects on vasodilation or vasorelaxation, angiogenesis (new vessel formation), and atherogenesis. The endothelial dysfunction in hyperhomocysteinemia may be mediated by the inhibitory effect of homocysteine on DDAH (see Fig. 36.2), which results in the accumulation of ADMA (48). In nonsmoking men, elevated levels of plasma ADMA may also predict acute coronary events (49).

Arginine and NO play an integral role in the pathogenesis of pulmonary hypertension. Pulmonary hypertension refers to a group of diseases characterized by high pulmonary artery pressures and pulmonary vascular resistance. It is a progressive disease that affects predominantly young and productive persons, is more common in female patients, and has a mean survival between 2 and 3 years from the time of diagnosis. The management of pulmonary hypertension is limited by poor understanding of its pathogenesis and by the lack of a selective pulmonary vasodilator. Discoveries in the NO field, however, are providing insights at both fronts. Patients with pulmonary hypertension have low levels of NO in their exhaled breath. In fact, the severity of pulmonary hypertension inversely correlates with NO levels estimated by measurement of NO reaction products in the lungs. Although this is a more complex issue than the simple lack of a vasodilator, replacement of NO seems to work well in treating the problem. Exogenous administration of NO gas by inhalation is probably the most effective and specific therapy for pulmonary hypertension. Although cost and unresolved technical difficulties in the delivery system of inhaled NO have prevented its widespread use so far, recent evidence suggests that other therapies for pulmonary hypertension may exert their beneficial effect at least in part through endogenous NO (28–31, 50). Dietary supplementation with L-arginine is also being explored as a very promising treatment option for this disease (51–54).

Renal System and Hypertension

The various isoforms of NOS are found throughout the kidney. Constitutive NOS (bNOS and eNOS) are distributed in the glomeruli and vasculature. iNOS is found in the juxtaglomerular apparatus and after immune stimulation, in the tubules. NO has a major role in the control of renal vascular tone. Generalized inhibition of NO has been shown to increase blood pressure and renal vascular resistance as well as to decrease renal blood flow and, subsequently, glomerular filtration rate (55). NO likely plays a role in the control of sodium balance. NO may control sodium excretion by directly acting on the tubules and by regulating medullary circulation (55). Increased levels of NO have been implicated in some forms of glomerular inflammation, sepsis, hypotension during hemodialysis, and renal allograft rejection. Elevated plasma ADMA levels may predict mortality in patients with end-stage kidney disease who are receiving hemodialysis (56).

L-Arginine infusions produced significant falls in mean blood pressures of human study subjects, and this was likely mediated in part by NOS, as evidenced by increases in plasma L-citrulline and expired NO (57). Conversely,

NO deficiency has been thought to be contributory to the pathogenesis of some persons with essential hypertension. Children of patients with essential hypertension are characterized by a reduced vasodilatory response to acetylcholine infusion linked to a defect in the NO pathway, a finding suggesting that an impairment in NO production precedes the onset of essential hypertension (58). NO deficiency in chronic renal failure is likely the result of reduced clearance of endogenous NO inhibitors (e.g., ADMA) and the reduced production of arginine from the kidney.

Other Organ Systems

Hematologic System

Patients with thrombotic thrombocytopenic purpura or hemolytic uremic syndrome were noted to have low levels of arginine and high levels of NO3- (the degradation product of NO) in plasma. The arginine concentration normalized on convalescence. Plasma levels of ADMA were noted to be elevated during active disease. This finding suggests that activation of NOS may play a role in the pathogenesis of thrombotic thrombocytopenic purpura and hemolytic uremic syndrome (59).

Endocrine System

Studies have suggested a glucose-induced impairment of DDAH activity, thus causing accumulation of ADMA in plasma and possibly contributing to vascular dysfunction in patients with diabetes (24). Furthermore, a correlation exists between insulin resistance and plasma ADMA levels (60). In thyroid disease, investigators have observed that plasma levels of arginine, ADMA, and SDMA are low in control subjects and in hypothyroid patients but elevated in those with hyperthyroidism (25). Free thyroxine levels were directly correlated with ADMA and were inversely correlated with NO concentrations.

Gastrointestinal Tract

The expression of iNOS was higher in collagenous and ulcerative colitis as compared with normal uninflamed bowel. In addition, L-NMMA administration reduced the output of NO, whereas L-arginine increased NO production in the gut lumen, a finding leading to the hypothesis that excess generation of NO may be the primary cause of diarrhea in this condition (61). Recent evidence suggests that acidified nitrite in the stomach can nitrosate thiols, forming S-nitrosothiols, and nitrosate amines, forming N-nitrosamines. However, the presence of excess nitrite in the acidic stomach environment also generates NO gas that has a protective effect on the gastric mucosa by improving blood flow and mucosal thickness (62). Investigators believe that this gastroprotective effect of NO generated from nitrite outweighs the potential carcinogenic risk of nitrosamines (also formed in the stomach from nitrite).

Reproductive System

An L-arginine-NO system has been demonstrated to be present in the uterus of pregnant rats. An L-arginine-NO-cGMP system in the uterus may be responsible for uterine smooth muscle relaxation during pregnancy. The inhibitory action of L-arginine and cGMP was considerably lower during delivery and post partum, a finding indicating that the NO system may contribute to the maintenance of uterine quiescence during pregnancy, when progesterone levels are elevated, but not during delivery (63). A reduction in basal release of NO has been implicated as a mediator of hypoxic fetoplacental vasoconstriction in the perfused human placental cotyledon in vitro (64). In preeclampsia, maternal endothelial dysfunction may precede clinical presentation and is associated with high serum ADMA levels (65).

Through the activation of cGMP, NO plays a major role in normal male erectile function by relaxing the vascular smooth muscle cells of the corpus cavernosum and improving penile blood flow. Pharmacologic amplification of this NO-cGMP cascade has revolutionized the treatment of men with erectile dysfunction (ED). This is achieved by medications that inhibit the phosphodiesterase (PDE) enzymes responsible for the intracellular hydrolysis of cGMP. This inhibition of PDE-5 stabilizes cGMP (the second messenger of NO), thus allowing a more sustained vasodilatory effect of endogenous NO and facilitating the NO-mediated penile erection (66). Men with ED, however, often also suffer from concomitant coronary artery disease and may be receiving treatment with oral nitrates. Because PDE-5 inhibitors may also potentiate the systemic vasodilatory effects of nitrates, the combination is contraindicated and may be lethal (67). Since the success of PDE-5 inhibitors in the treatment of ED, many dietary supplements that contain arginine have enjoyed tremendous popularity and use for this purpose. Numerous media outlets and alternative medicine publications seem to support the use of arginine as a NO precursor and a "safer" more natural alternative for ED (68–70). No studies to date, however, exist to support the claim that these supplements work better than placebo (70, 71). Adequate clinical trials are needed to evaluate the benefit of these dietary supplements in ED, especially because the placebo effect is approximately 25% (1 out of 4 benefit) based on past randomized trials of medications approved for ED by the US Food and Drug Administration (70).

Immune System

Dietary L-arginine has been reported to enhance wound healing and immunity. In the athymic mouse, L-arginine supplementation increases the number of T cells and augments delayed-type hypersensitivity (72). In sites of inflammation rich with macrophage infiltration, free arginine has been noted to be deficient. On the other side of the spectrum, it appears that excessive NO production (from iNOS) is responsible for the hypotension and refractory vasodilation frequently observed in severe septic shock (73). NO also seems to inhibit the positive inotropic and chronotropic response to β-adrenergic stimulation, thus resulting in myocardial depression. These and other findings have led to the experimental use of NOS inhibitors (e.g., L-NAME) and methylene blue (a guanylate cyclase inhibitor) to treat the refractory hypotension observed in sepsis (74). NO may mediate immunity to malaria, which seems to be associated with certain NOS II promoter polymorphisms that lead to increased endogenous NO production (75).

Table 36.4 summarizes the potential uses of arginine, NO, and their derivatives in the various organ systems.

TABLE 36.4. POTENTIAL CLINICAL USES OF ARGININE AND ITS DERIVATIVES

Respiratory	Inhaled NO is used as therapy for refractory hypoxemia
	Inhaled NO is used for persistent pulmonary hypertension of newborns
	Inhaled NO is used as therapy for pulmonary hypertension
	Inhaled NO has been used in high-altitude pulmonary edema
	Oral arginine has beneficial effects on hemodynamics and exercise capacity in patients with pulmonary hypertension
	Exhaled NO has been used as a marker for airway inflammation in asthma
Cardiovascular	Oral arginine improves coronary blood flow (in response to acetylcholine) in patients with coronary artery disease
	Arginine infusions improve peripheral circulation and improve symptoms of claudication
	Arginine infusion enhances functional performance in patients with severe congestive heart failure
	Arginine may have beneficial effects on preventing intimal lesions and xanthoma formation in atherosclerosis
	Oral arginine may reduce platelet hyperaggregability
Renal	Models of experimentally induced renal disease are improved with long-term dietary arginine supplementation (e.g., cyclosporin-induced, puromycin-induced)
	Acute arginine infusion reduces proteinuria in patients with chronic glomerulonephritis
	Oral arginine has favorable effects on lowering blood pressure in human volunteers
Immunologic	Oral arginine has been used to promote wound healing and reparative collagen synthesis
	NO synthase antagonists have been used to counteract the refractory hypotension observed in septic states

NO, nitric oxide.

This is by no means a comprehensive list. This is a rapidly evolving area with active research, and the list will likely change rapidly as new uses are identified and older ones are either proven or discarded.

SUMMARY

As a precursor of NO, polyamines, and other biologically important molecules, L-arginine plays versatile and key roles in nutrition and metabolism. Based on our current and expanding knowledge of its metabolic pathways, L-arginine offers great promise to improve our understanding of human health and disease in the future. Dietary L-arginine manipulation may represent a potentially novel nutritional strategy for preventing and treating a variety of diseases.

Although NO has long been known as an atmospheric pollutant, its clinical importance as a biologic mediator in animals and humans has been recognized only since the early 1990s. NO is present in virtually all mammalian organ systems and in exhaled human breath. NO is endogenously synthesized by NOSs, which convert L-arginine to L-citrulline. Once produced, NO is freely diffusible across membranes, thus allowing it to perform a wide array of functions. Because of its highly reactive nature, NO is rapidly metabolized into more stable end products. In addition to activating guanylate cyclase resulting in smooth muscle relaxation, NO is also involved in a variety of physiologic function including neurotransmission, host defense and bacteriostasis, airway and vascular smooth muscle relaxation, inflammation, mucociliary clearance, airway mucus secretion, and cytotoxicity.

Methylated arginine analogs competitively inhibit NO synthesis from L-arginine by acting as false substrates for the NOS enzymes and have been implicated in the pathogenesis of many clinical conditions.

A peculiar concept in arginine-NO metabolism is the arginine paradox, which refers to the phenomenon that exogenous arginine still causes NO-mediated effects despite the presence of more than saturating levels of arginine in the cells and the extracellular space.

Acknowledgment

Dr. Dweik is supported by National Institutes of Health grant HL68863. We would like to thank Jackie Pyle and Jennifer Duncan for critical review and help with the references.

REFERENCES

1. Ignarro LJ, Buga GM, Wood KS et al. Proc Natl Acad Sci USA 1987;84:9265–9.
2. Palmer RM, Ferrige AG, Moncada S. Nature 1987;327:524–6.
3. Stuehr DJ. Biochim Biophys Acta 1999;1411:217–30.
4. Moncada S, Higgs A. N Engl J Med 1993;329:2002–12.
5. Dweik RA, Laskowski D, Abu-Soud HM et al. J Clin Invest 1998;101:660–6.
6. Nathan C. FASEB J 1992;6:3051–64.
7. Wu G, Morris SM Jr. Biochem J 1998;336:1–17.
8. Boger RH, Bode-Boger SM. Annu Rev Pharmacol Toxicol 2001; 41:79–99.
9. Moncada S, Palmer, RM, Higgs EA. Biochem Pharmacol 1989; 38:1709–15.
10. Tapiero H, Mathe G, Couvreur P et al. Biomed Pharmacother 2002;56:439–45.
11. Nathan C, Xie QW. J Biol Chem 1994;269:13725–8.
12. Nathan C, Xie QW. Cell 1994;78:915–8.
13. Dweik RA, Laskowski D, Ozkan M et al. Am J Respir Cell Mol Biol 2001;24:414–8.
14. Dweik RA, Guo FH, Uetani K et al. Zhongguo Yao Li Xue Bao 1997;18:550–2.
15. Lancaster JR,Jr. Proc Natl Acad Sci USA 1994;91:8137–41.
16. Dweik RA, Comhair SA, Gaston B et al. Proc Natl Acad Sci USA 2001;98:2622–7.
17. Gaston B, Reilly J, Drazen JM et al. Proc Natl Acad Sci USA 1993;90:10957–61.
18. Gaston B, Sears S, Woods J et al. Lancet 1998;351:1317–9.
19. Ozkan M, Dweik RA. Clin Pulm Med 2001;8:199–206.
20. Leiper J, Vallance P. Cardiovasc Res 1999;43:542–8.
21. Tran CT, Leiper JM, Vallance P. Atherosclerosis 2003;4[Suppl]: 33–40.
22. Ogawa T, Kimoto M, Sasaoka K. J Biol Chem 1989;264:10205–9.
23. Smith CL, Birdsey GM, Anthony S et al. Biochem Biophys Res Commun 2003;308:984–9.
24. Lin KY, Ito A, Asagami T et al. Circulation 2002;106:987–92.
25. Hermenegildo C, Medina P, Peiro M et al. J Clin Endocrinol Metab 2002;87:5636–40.
26. Boger RH, Lentz SR, Bode-Boger SM et al. Clin Sci (Lond) 2001;100:161–7.
27. Maxwell AJ, Cooke JP. Curr Opin Nephrol Hypertens 1998;7: 63–70.
28. Kaneko FT, Arroliga AC, Dweik RA et al. Am J Respir Crit Care Med 1998;158:917–23.
29. Dweik R. Lancet 2002;360:886.
30. Ghamra ZW, Dweik RA. Cleve Clin J Med 2003;70[Suppl 1]:2S–8S.
31. Dweik RA. Cleve Clin J Med 2001;68:486, 488, 490, 493.
32. Dweik RA. Lancet 2002;360:886–7.
33. Nelin LD, Thomas CJ, Dawson CA. Am J Physiol 1996;271: H8–H14.
34. Gustafsson LE, Leone AM, Persson MG et al. Biochem Biophys Res Commun 1991;181:852–7.
35. Schmidt HH, Walter U. Cell 1994;78:919–25.
36. Rubbo H, Darley-Usmar V, Freeman BA. Chem Res Toxicol 1996;9:809–20.
37. Guo FH, Comhair SA, Zheng S et al. J Immunol 2000;164: 5970–80.
38. Wu G, Meininger CJ. J Nutr 2000;130:2626–9.
39. Cooke JP, Singer AH, Tsao P et al. J Clin Invest 1992;90: 1168–72.
40. Boger RH, Bode-Boger SM, Brandes RP et al. Circulation 1997; 96:1282–90.
41. Wolf A, Zalpour C, Theilmeier G et al. J Am Coll Cardiol 1997; 29:479–85.
42. Egashira K, Hirooka Y, Kuga T et al. Circulation 1996;94:130–4.
43. Palloshi A, Fragasso G, Piatti P et al. Am J Cardiol 2004;93: 933–5.
44. Bode-Boger SM, Boger RH, Alfke H et al. Circulation 1996; 93:85–90.
45. Seshadri N, Dweik RA, Laskowski D et al. Am J Cardiol 2003; 92:820–3.
46. Damy T, Ratajczak P, Shah AM et al. Lancet 2004;363:1365–7.
47. Rector TS, Bank AJ, Mullen KA et al. Circulation 1996;93:2135–41.
48. Stuhlinger MC, Tsao PS, Her JH et al. Circulation 2001;104: 2569–75.

49. Valkonen VP, Paiva H, Salonen JT et al. Lancet 2001;358: 2127–8.
50. Arroliga AC, Dweik RA, Kaneko FJ et al. Cleve Clin J Med 2000;67:175–8, 181–5, 189–90.
51. Mitani Y, Maruyama K, Sakurai M. Circulation 1997;96:689–97.
52. Nagaya N, Uematsu M, Oya H et al. Am J Respir Crit Care Med 2001;163:887–91.
53. Morris CR, Morris SM Jr, Hagar W et al. Am J Respir Crit Care Med 2003;168:63–9.
54. Fagan JM, Rex SE, Hayes-Licitra SA et al. Biochem Biophys Res Commun 1999;254:100–3.
55. Baylis C, Bloch J. Nephrol Dial Transplant 1996;11:1955–7.
56. Zoccali C, Bode-Boger S, Mallamaci F et al. Lancet 2001;358: 2113–7.
57. Mehta S, Stewart DJ, Levy RD. Chest 1996;109:1550–5.
58. Taddei S, Virdis A, Mattei P et al. Circulation 1996;94:1298–1303.
59. Herlitz H, Petersson A, Sigstrom L et al. Scand J Urol Nephrol 1997;31:477–9.
60. Stuhlinger MC, Abbasi F, Chu JW et al. JAMA 2002;287:1420–6.
61. Perner A, Andresen L, Normark M et al. Gut 2001;49:387–94.
62. Bjorne HH, Petersson J, Phillipson M et al. J Clin Invest 2004; 113:106–14.
63. Yallampalli C, Izumi H, Byam-Smith M et al. Am J Obstet Gynecol 1994;170:175–85.
64. Byrne BM, Howard RB, Morrow RJ et al. Placenta 1997;18: 627–34.
65. Savvidou MD, Hingorani AD, Tsikas D et al. Lancet 2003;361: 1511–7.
66. Goldstein I, Lue TF, Padma-Nathan H et al. N Engl J Med 1998; 338:1397–1404.
67. Zusman RM, Morales A, Glasser DB et al. Am J Cardiol 1999; 83:35C–44C.
68. McKay D. Altern Med Rev 2004;9:4–16.
69. Stanislavov R, Nikolova V. J Sex Marital Ther 2003;29:207–13.
70. Moyad MA. Urol Clin North Am 2002;29:11–22.
71. Klotz T, Mathers MJ, Braun M et al. Urol Int 1999;63:220–3.
72. Potenza MA, Nacci C, Mitolo–Chieppa D. Curr Drug Targets Immune Endocr Metab Disord 2001;1:67–77.
73. Symeonides S, Balk RA. Infect Dis Clin North Am 1999;13: 449–63.
74. Bakker J, Grover R, McLuckie A et al. Crit Care Med 2004;32: 1–12.
75. Hobbs MR, Udhayakumar V, Levesque MC et al. Lancet 2002; 360:1468–75.

PHYTOCHEMICALS[1]

RONALD L. PRIOR

MAJOR CLASSES OF FLAVONOIDS FOUND
  IN FOODS 583
    Flavonoid Analysis 584
FLAVONES 584
FLAVONOLS 584
    Chemistry, Dietary Sources, and Intakes 584
    Absorption and Metabolism 586
    Biologic Effects of Quercetin and Other
      Flavonols 587
FLAVANONES 587
    Chemistry, Dietary Sources, and Intakes 587
    Interactions of Grapefruit Juice and Drugs 587
FLAVAN-3-OLS (CATECHINS) 587
    Dietary Sources and Intakes 587
    Absorption and Metabolism 587
    Biologic Effects 588
PROANTHOCYANIDINS 588
    Chemistry, Dietary Sources, and Intakes 588
    Absorption and Metabolism 589
    Biologic Effects 589
ANTHOCYANINS 589
    Chemistry and Dietary Sources 589
    Absorption and Metabolism 590
    Biologic Effects 591
ISOFLAVONES 591
    Dietary Sources and Intakes 591
    Metabolism and Absorption 591
    Health Benefits of Soy Protein 592
OTHER PHYTOCHEMICALS 593

The term "phytochemical" refers to a broad and diverse group of compounds that are produced and accumulated in plants. Many of these compounds have potent biologic activities in mammalian systems, and some may have toxic effects when they are consumed at high enough levels. Interest in these compounds has developed because of compelling epidemiologic evidence that associates diets

rich in fruits, vegetables, and whole grains with improved health and decreased risk of chronic degenerative diseases. An indication of the interest in this area is reflected by the number of books and reviews that have been published in recent years related to this topic. Time and space will not permit a detailed treatise on all the phytochemicals, so readers are referred to several excellent reviews on the topic. Four widely respected books have been published based on proceedings of international phytochemical conferences: *Phytochemicals: A New Paradigm* (1), *Phytochemicals as Bioactive Agents* (2), *Phytochemicals in Nutrition and Health* (3), and *Phytochemicals: Mechanisms of Action* (4).

Flavonoids, a subclass of phytochemicals, constitute a large class of food constituents, many of which alter metabolic processes and may have a positive impact on health. Two books have been published that deal specifically with this group of phtochemical compounds: *The Flavonoids: Advances in Research Since 1980*, which appeared in 1988 (5) and *The Flavonoids: Advances in Research Since 1986*, which appeared in 1994 (6). Subsequently, a review was published in 2000 detailing some of the advances in flavonoid research since 1992 (7). Readers are also pointed to the classic reviews by the late Elliott Middleton, Jr (8–10) that very eloquently deal with the impact of plant flavonoids on mammalian biology, with emphasis on immunity, inflammation, and cancer. More recently, specific reviews dealing with flavonoids have been published by Beecher (11), as part of an international symposium on tea and human health, and by Havsteen (12), Lambert and Yang (13), and Yang and associates (14), dealing with the medical significance of flavonoids and cancer chemopreventive properties of tea and other polyphenolics.

The focus of this review is on the flavonoids. This chapter is not intended to be a comprehensive review of the literature, but merely to highlight recent research with some historical perspectives. Early research in the field of flavonoids was stimulated by the discovery of the French paradox, that is, the low cardiovascular mortality rate observed in Mediterranean populations in association with red wine consumption in spite of a high saturated fat intake (15). Further impetus for flavonoid research resulted from epidemiologic studies relating dietary intake to protection against various cancers (16, 17) and cardiovascular disease (18, 19).

---

[1]**Abbreviations: BCA,** black currant anthocyanin; **C3G,** cyanidin-3-glucoside; **DP,** degree of polymerization; **LDL,** low-density lipoprotein; **PAs,** proanthocyanidins; **PCs,** procyanidins; **USDA,** United States Department of Agriculture.

The study of flavonoids and their relevance to nutrition and health outcomes has been fraught with numerous limitations that have included a lack of appropriate analytic techniques, and of purified compounds or standards, particularly as required for developing any sort of database on the concentrations of these compounds in foods. Much of the early research on the biologic effects of flavonoids depended on the availability of pure compounds and the use of in vitro systems. As is apparent throughout this review, as we have learned more about the absorption and metabolism of flavonoids, it is evident that some flavonoids are modified during the absorption process, and thus the molecular structure found in target cells is much different from the parent compound in the food. Therefore, in vitro studies using the parent compound may be misleading if the bioactivities of the metabolite and parent compound differ. Results from in vitro studies need to be interpreted in light of this potential complication. In most cases, the true potential health benefits in vivo remain to be determined. Advances have been made such that we are now able to begin to produce databases of the food content of some of the phytochemicals. The work of the United States Department of Agriculture (USDA) under the USDA National Food and Nutrition Analysis Program established for the first time a database of flavonoids in foods, information that is posted on the USDA Nutrition Data Laboratory Web site (http://www.nal.usda.gov/fnic/foodcomp).

MAJOR CLASSES OF FLAVONOIDS FOUND IN FOODS

Flavonoids are perhaps the most important single group of phenolic compounds in plants. More than 5000 such compounds in plants were described by 1990. Flavonoid structure is based on a 2-phenyl-benzo[a]pyrane or flavane nucleus (Fig. 37.1). This nucleus is defined by having a system of two benzene rings (A and B), which are connected by an oxygen-containing pyrane ring (C). The flavonoids are further divided into subclasses based on the connection of the aromatic B ring to the heterocyclic ring, as well as the oxidation state and functional groups of the heterocyclic ring. Within each subclass, individual compounds are characterized by specific hydroxylation and conjugation patterns.

We consider specifically flavones, flavonols, flavanones, flavanols, proanthocyanidins (PAs), anthocyanins, and isoflavones. Flavonoids are widely distributed in nature,

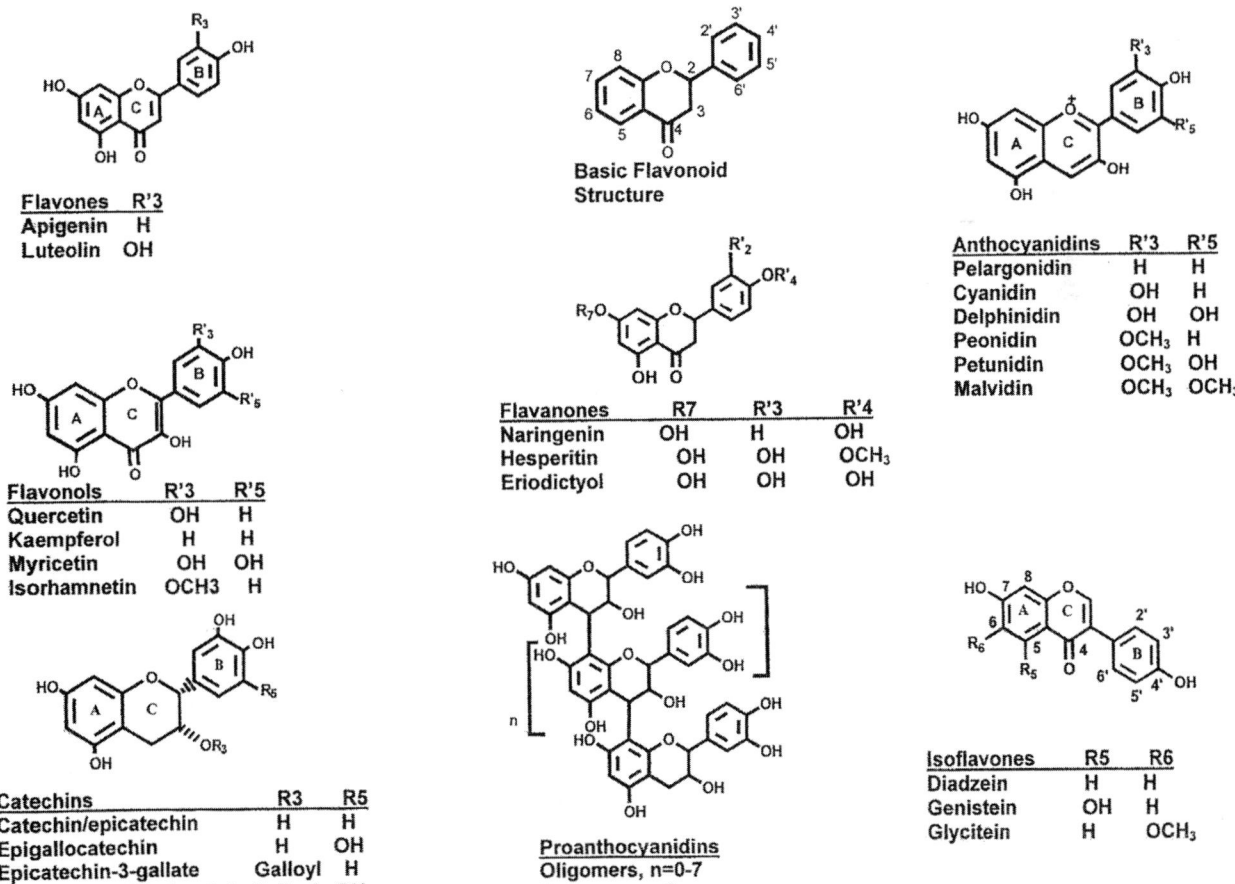

Figure 37.1. The basic flavonoid structure and structures of flavone, flavonols, flavanones, anthocyanidins, catechins, proanthocyanidins, and isoflavones. Most naturally occurring flavonoids are glycosides (with sugars), but the aglycones are shown in this figure. The flavans or flavan-3-ols include catechins and proanthocyanidins.

albeit not uniformly. As a result, specific groups of foods are often rich sources of one or more subclasses of these polyphenols. Concentrations of major compounds in each of the subclasses of flavonoids in selected foods are presented in Table 37.1.

Flavonoids are often used by botanists for taxonomic classification, and they may regulate plant growth, inhibit or kill many bacterial strains, inhibit important viral enzymes, and destroy some pathogenic protozoans. Yet their toxicity to animal cells is low (12). The content of flavonoids in foods is strongly influenced by variations in plant type, growing conditions, season, freshness, degree of ripeness, food preparation, and processing (20). Plant stressors can also have major effects on the levels of flavonoids in the plant.

Flavonoid Analysis

Because so many flavonoid compounds are present in plants, finding appropriate analytic methods and standards has been a challenge. Separation systems for flavonoids in foods have been oriented toward the measurement of several subclasses of the prominent flavonoids in a single food or procedures that quantify a single or a few subclasses in several foods. Methods that have been used have been summarized in a review (21). The most often used columns have been packed with reversed-phase C_{18} column material. Mobil phases employed have usually included acetonitrile and/or methanol in combination with water containing an acid. Anthocyanin analysis requires a higher acid concentration, usually 5% formic acid. Elution systems are usually binary, with an aqueous acidified polar solvent and a less polar organic solvent, such as methanol, which is acidified. Detection is usually with an ultraviolet-visible diode array detector. Anthocyanins have a very characteristic absorption in the 500- to 520-nm range. Isoflavonoids in foods are generally detected at wavelengths in the range of 236 to 280 nm; however, analyses in tissues and urine require the increased sensitivity provided by mass spectrometry specific ion detection. Flavanones and their glycosides and catechins are usually detected at 280 nm. Flavones, flavonols, and flavonol glycosides are usually detected at wavelengths of 365 to 370 nm.

Because of the lack of appropriate standards, early analytic work required hydrolysis of the flavonoid glycoside forms using relatively high concentrations of mineral acids (1–2 M) (22). However, these conditions may also degrade anthocyanidins (aglycone) and catechins. Thus, increased use of diode array detection occurs in tandem with a mass spectrometer for identification so digestion is not required.

Good analytic methods for analysis of PAs were not available until relatively recently (23). This procedure requires normal phase separation and fluorescence detection, although ultraviolet detection can be used but it is less specific. Because of the complexity of the chromatogram, it is also good to have a mass spectrometer

attached to the high-performance liquid chromatography system for identification of the individual peaks (24, 25).

FLAVONES

The basic flavane nucleus is the structural feature of the flavone (see Fig. 37.1). Among the flavones (~300 are known), apigenin and luteolin are present chiefly in grains, leafy vegetables, and herbs (see Table 37.1). Flavonols, which are discussed later, are 3-hydroxyflavones. Fewer research data are available on the flavones compared with the favonols.

Apigenin has been shown to have strong cytostatic and antiangiogenic effects in vitro (26). 2′,3′-Dihydroxyflavone, fisetin, apigenin, and luteolin inhibit the proliferation of normal and tumor cells as well as in vitro angiogenesis at half-maximal concentrations in the lower micromolar range (27). Apigenin suppressed 12-O-tetradecanoyl-phorbol-13-acetate–mediated tumor promotion in mouse skin (28).

FLAVONOLS

Chemistry, Dietary Sources, and Intakes

The flavonols (3-hydroxyflavones) are a subclass of flavonoids that are diverse in their chemical structure and characteristics (see Fig. 37.1). Quercetin, kaempferol, and myricetin are the most common flavonols. The flavonol quercetin (3,3′,4′,5,7-pentahydroxyflavone) is one of the most abundant and widely studied flavonoids. The availability of the pure compound made much of this early research possible. Its antioxidant effect is implied to be helpful for human health. Fruits, vegetables, and beverages such as tea and red wine are major sources of flavonols in the human diet (see Table 37.1). Dietary quercetin is primarily present in plants in its glycoside form. Data on the quercetin content of foodstuffs are limited, but available data suggest the following: a range of 0.2 to 25 mg quercetin/100 g wet weight in fruits; 0 to 10 mg/100 g in vegetables, with onions being especially high (20–60 mg/100 g); 0.4 to 1.6 mg/100 mL in red wine; 1.0 to 2.5 mg/100 mL in tea; and 0.2 to 2.3 mg/100 mL in fruit juices (29, 30). The daily consumption of flavonols is difficult to estimate because values depend on accurate assessment of eating habits and flavonol content in foods. The average dietary intake of quercetin in the Netherlands was estimated to be 16 mg/day (29). The overall flavonoid (flavonols and flavones) intake in a population of women in the United States was estimated to be 24.6±18.5 mg/day, of which quercetin was the major contributor (70.2%) (31). The mean intake of flavonoids (including flavonols, flavones, and flavanones) was estimated to be 24.2±26.7, 28.6±12.3, and 25.9 mg/day in the populations of Finland, Denmark, and the Netherlands, respectively (32–34). However, these authors did not include monomeric, oligomeric, and polymeric flavan-3-ols

TABLE 37.1. FLAVONOID CLASSES AND CONCENTRATIONS[a] OF MAJOR COMPOUNDS IN EACH CLASS IN SELECTED FOODS AND POSSIBLE HEALTH EFFECTS

CLASS (MAJOR COMPOUNDS)	CONCENTRATION	HEALTH EFFECTS (REFERENCE)
Flavones (apigenin, luteolin)		Anticancer effects (26, 28, 126)
Celery	5.9	
Celery hearts	22.6	
Peppers	1–7	
Spinach, raw	1.1	
Tea, green, brewed	0.3	
Flavonols (quercetin, kaempferol, myricetin, isorhamnetin)		Antioxidants in vivo (43, 48, 49)
Onions	15.4–38.7	
Kale	22.9–34.4	
Cocoa	20.1	
Broccoli	9.4	
Blueberries	3.9	
Spinach	4.9	
Blackberries	1.1	
Tea	3.8	
Celery	3.5	
Beans	3.1–3.4	
Lettuce	2.6	
Grapefruit	0.9	
Tomatoes	0.6	
Flavanones (hesperetin, naringenin, eriodictyol)		Antiinflammatory effects (127)
Lemons	49.8	Anticancer effects (127)
Lemon juice	18.4	Drug interactions (53, 54)
Oranges	43.9	
Grapefruit	54.5	
Flavan-3-ols (e.g., catechin, epicatechin, gallocatechin, epigallocatechin)[b]		Antioxidants in vivo
Tea, black	114	Anticancer effects in the gastrointestinal
Tea, green	133	tract (14, 63-66)
Chocolate	13.4–53.5	
Blackberries	18.7	
Apples	9.1	
Proanthocyanidins[c]		Prevention of low-density lipoprotein
Blueberries, cultivated	180	oxidation (76, 77)
Blueberries, low bush	332	Urinary tract infection factor: A type (83)
Cranberries	419	Antidiabetic effects (84, 85)
Apple	70–126	
Peaches	67	
Plums	215–257	
Sorghum, high-tannin	788	
Pinto beans, raw	796	
Pinto beans, simmered	26	
Red beans	457	
Kidney beans	564	
Hazelnuts	501	
Pecans	494	
Pistachios	237	
Almonds	184	
Anthocyanins (cyanidin, delphinidin, peonidin, petunidin, malvidin, pelargonidin)[d]		Vascular permeability (101)
Elderberry	1,550	Vision effects (102–107)
Chokeberry	1,486	Anticancer effects (109)
Blueberry	415	Angiogenesis (108)
Blackberry	317	
Cranberry	148	
Cherry	124	
Raspberry	96	
Strawberry	22	
Plum	20	
Nectarine	6	
Peach	5	
Red leaf lettuce	2	
Apple	1	

TABLE 37.1. FLAVONOID CLASSES AND CONCENTRATIONS^a OF MAJOR COMPOUNDS IN EACH CLASS IN SELECTED FOODS AND POSSIBLE HEALTH EFFECTS (continued)

CLASS (MAJOR COMPOUNDS)	CONCENTRATION	HEALTH EFFECTS (REFERENCE)
Isoflavones (genistein, diadzein)[e]		
Soy flour (full-fat, raw)	178	Cardiovascular effects (116, 117)
Soy flour (Textured)	149	Anti–breast cancer effects (110, 118, 119)
Soy fiber	44	Anti–prostate cancer effects (122)
Soy protein isolate	97	Bone health (125)
Soy cheese	31	
Soy milk	10	
Soy drink	7	
Natto (soybeans, boiled, fermented)	59	
Miso	43	
Miso soup mix, dry	60	
Infant formula, not reconstituted	25	
Instant beverage soy powder	110	
Tofu	23–33	

[a] Expressed as mg/100 g fresh weight of edible portion. Data from the US Department of Agriculture (USDA) Flavonoid database (http://www.nal.usda.gov/fnic/foodcomp/Data/Flav/flav.html) unless indicated otherwise. This table is not intended to be complete, and numbers presented are averages or ranges. Concentrations can vary considerably because of environmental, processing and other conditions. Readers are encouraged to refer to the original database for more complete information.

[b] Most foods containing proanthocyanidins contain monomeric flavan-3-ols.

[c] From data of Gu and colleagues (57) expressed as the total of all oligomers plus polymers (see the original publication for the breakdown of individual components).

[d] From data of Wu and colleagues (unpublished) expressed as total of all anthocyanins in various glycosylated forms.

[e] Data from USDA–Iowa State University Isoflavonoid database (http://www.nal.usda.gov/fnic/foodcomp/Data/isoflav/isoflav.html).

in their estimation. Apples were identified as a major dietary source of flavonoids in the epidemiologic studies. However, the extent of absorption of flavonoids such as quercetin is a critical issue relative to the many alleged health effects.

Absorption and Metabolism

Quercetin was originally assumed to be absorbed from the small intestine following cleavage of the β-glucoside linkage by colonic microflora (35). Hollman and coworkers (36) found that humans absorb quercetin as the aglycone but concluded that absorption was enhanced by conjugation with glucose. Although quercetin glycosides are subject to deglycosidation by enterobacteria for absorption in the large intestine, the small intestine can act as an effective absorption site for glucose-bound quercertin glucosides. This is because small intestinal cells possess a glucoside-hydrolyzing activity, and their glucose transport system is capable of participating in the absorption of quercetin glucoside. When a cell culture model for intestinal absorption was used, hydrolysis of quercetin glucosides accelerated quercetin absorption (37). Crespy and associates (38) found that quercetin, but not its glycosides, was absorbed from the rat stomach. Based on in vitro studies of Caco-2 cells, Walle and coworkers demonstrated a complete lack of absorption of the glucosides of quercetin, mainly resulting from effective efflux by the multidrug resistance protein 2 transporter (39, 40), but quercetin was readily absorbed. In subsequent studies in human subjects, Walle and colleagues (41) found that quercetin glucosides were

hydrolyzed in the small intestine by bacterial enzymes. Data suggest that β-glucosidases and also lactase phlorizin hydrolase in the small intestine may be capable of hydrolyzing quercetin glucosides, and these compounds are thus taken up as the aglycone and not as the intact glycosides (42). Despite some discrepancies in the literature, it seems that the absorption of quercetin glycosides from the diet depends largely on the type of sugar groups attached to their phenolic group. Glucose-bound glycosides are likely to be much more absorbable than others that are sugar bound (37). Hydrolysis to its aglycone by enterocytes or enterobacteria seems to be important for the effective absorption of quercetin glycosides in the intestinal tract.

The small intestine is also recognized as the site for metabolic conversion of quercetin and other flavonoids because it possesses enzymatic activity for glucuronidation and sulfation. The major circulating metabolites were glucuronide/sulfate conjugates of isorhamnetin (3'-O-methyl quercetin) and of quercetin. Glucuronides, sulfates, and their O-methylated derivatives accumulate as quercetin metabolites in the circulation after intake of a quercetin-rich diet (37, 43). Modulation of the intestinal absorption and metabolism may be beneficial for regulating the biologic effects of dietary quercetin (37).

Walle and associates (44) found that as much as 23 to 81% of a ^{14}C-quercetin dose was recovered as $^{14}CO_2$ in the expired air. Apparent absorption was quite high, ranging from 36 to 53% based on total radioactivity, and absorption of quercetin aglycone was calculated to be as high as 65 to 81% (41). Hollman and colleagues (45) found that absorption of quercetin in patients with an ileostomy was $52\pm5\%$ for quercetin glucosides from onions, $17\pm15\%$ for quercetin rutinoside, and $24\pm9\%$ for quercetin aglycone. Excretion of quercetin or its conjugates in urine in four separate studies ranged from 0.07 to 17.4% of intake (46). Fecal microflora can rapidly deconjugate the flavonols rutin, isoquercitrin, and a mixture of quercetin glucuronides. The main metabolite, 3,4-dihydroxyphenylacetic acid, appeared rapidly (within 2 hours) and was dehydroxylated to 3-hydroxyphenylacetic acid within 8 hours. Hydroxyphenylacetic acids were not methylated by colonic microflora in vitro (47).

Biologic Effects of Quercetin and Other Flavonols

Biologic effects of flavonols vary depending on the flavonol metabolites produced. Following intragastric quercetin (10 or 50 mg/kg) administration, quercetin glucuronide and/or sulfate conjugates were present in the plasma, and the plasma was more resistant to copper sulfate–induced lipid peroxidation than the control plasma on the basis of the accumulation of cholesterol ester hydroperoxides and the consumption of α-tocopherol (48). These results suggest that some conjugated metabolites of quercetin can act as effective antioxidants. Antioxidant activity of conjugated metabolites has also been observed in vitro (43, 49). Quercetin-3-glucuronide has been shown to suppress peroxynitrite-induced human low-density lipoprotein (LDL) degradation and lipoxygenase-dependent liposomal phospholipid peroxidation. In addition, quercetin-3-glucuronide was found to be effective in modulating angiotensin II–induced vascular smooth muscle cell hypertrophy through the inhibition of c-Jun N-terminal kinase activation, and its effect was comparable to that of quercetin (37). Numerous other in vitro effects have been reported (50, 51).

FLAVANONES

Chemistry, Dietary Sources, and Intakes

Flavanones (see Fig. 37.1) constitute the vast majority of all flavonoids in citrus fruits, including oranges, tangerines, mandarins, grapefruit, lemons, and limes (see Table 37.1). Overall, citrus flavonoids encompass a diverse set of structures, including numerous flavanone and flavone O- and C-glycosides and methoxylated flavones. Primary flavanones in citrus include hesperidin, naringin, narirutin, eriocitrin, neohesperidin, didymin, neoeriocitrin, and poncirin. Liquid chromatography mass spectrometry analyses of 12 dietary flavonoids in human urine showed that no flavonoid glycosides were excreted, and the citrus flavanones were excreted in higher amounts than the flavonols (42). Citrus flavonoids exhibit numerous in vitro and in vivo antiinflammatory and anticancer actions (52). These biologic properties are consistent with their effects on the microvascular endothelial tissue. Evidence suggests that the biologic

actions of the citrus flavonoids are possibly linked to their interactions with key regulatory enzymes involved in cell activation and receptor binding. The citrus flavonoids show little effect on normal, healthy cells and thus typically exhibit remarkably low toxicity in animals. The citrus flavonoids extend their influence in vivo through their induction of hepatic phase I and II enzymes and through the biologic actions of their metabolites (42, 52).

Interactions of Grapefruit Juice and Drugs

Phytochemicals in grapefruit juice have some apparently unique properties that can change the bioavailability of certain drugs and can alter drug action. The components of citrus juice responsible for clinical drug interactions have yet to be determined fully. Based on the flavonoid naringin's unique distribution in the plant kingdom, its abundance in grapefruit, and its ability to inhibit metabolic enzymes, naringin is likely to be one of the grapefruit components influencing drug metabolism. This phenomenon could also result from a complex synergy between flavonoids (naringin, naringenin), furanocoumarins (6',7'-dihydroxybergamottin, bergamottin) and sesquiterpen (nootkatone), which are all components of grapefruit. Grapefruit juice acts by inhibiting presystemic drug metabolism mediated by the cytochrome P450 enzyme CYP3A4 in the small intestine. This interaction appears to be more relevant if the CYP3A4 content is high and the drug has a strong first-pass degradation. A single glass of grapefruit juice can improve the oral bioavailability of a drug, thus either increasing its efficacy or enhancing its adverse effects, particularly if the therapeutic window is narrow (53, 54).

FLAVAN-3-OLS (CATECHINS)

Dietary Sources and Intakes

The major flavan-3-ols (see Fig. 37.1) are catechin, epicatechin, epicatechin-3-gallate, epigallocatechin, and epigallocatechin-3-gallate. Fruits, teas, and chocolate are common sources of the catechins (see Table 37.1). Arts and colleagues (55) estimated that the mean intake of flavan-3-ol monomers in the Netherlands was 50 mg/day, with tea being the major contributor (65.2–87.3%), followed by chocolate and apple. The daily intake of flavan-3-ol monomers from tea was estimated to be in the range of 12.7 to 34.2 mg/day/person for adults in the United States based on the data of Lakenbrink (56). The total intake of flavan-3-ol monomers is estimated to be 17.1 to 38.6 mg/day/person for adults in the United States after the contributions of flavan-3-ols from other foods are included (57).

Absorption and Metabolism

Approximately 1.68% of ingested catechins were present in the plasma, urine, and feces, and the apparent bioavailability of the gallated catechins was lower than that of the nongallated forms. Catechins were bioavailable; however, unless they were rapidly metabolized or sequestered, the catechins appeared to be absorbed in amounts that were small relative to intake (58).

Biologic Effects

Tea remains the most widely consumed drink in the world after water. Accumulating numbers of population studies suggest that consumption of green and black tea beverages may bring positive health effects. One hypothesis explaining such effects is that the high levels of flavonoids in tea can protect cells and tissues from oxidative damage by scavenging oxygen-derived free radicals. They may also function indirectly as antioxidants through the following: (a) inhibition of the redox-sensitive transcription factors, nuclear factor-κB and activator protein-1; (b) inhibition of "prooxidant" enzymes, such as inducible nitric oxide synthase, lipoxygenases, cyclooxygenases, and xanthine oxidase; and (c) induction of phase II and antioxidant enzymes, such as glutathione S-transferases and superoxide dismutases. Chemically, the flavonoids found in green and black tea are very effective radical scavengers. The tea flavonoids may therefore be active as antioxidants in the digestive tract or in other tissues after uptake. Human intervention studies with green and black tea demonstrate a significant increase in plasma antioxidant capacity in humans approximately 1 hour after consumption of moderate amounts of tea (1–6 cups/day). The effects of tea and green tea catechins on biomarkers of oxidative stress, especially oxidative DNA damage, appear very promising in animal models, but data on biomarkers of in vivo oxidative stress in humans are limited and are insufficient to draw firm conclusions (59–61). Animal studies provide an opportunity to assess the contribution of the antioxidant properties of tea polyphenols to the physiologic effects of tea administration in different models of oxidative stress. Most promising are the consistent findings in animal models of skin, lung, colon, liver, and pancreatic cancer that tea and tea polyphenol administration inhibit carcinogen-induced increases in the oxidized DNA base, 8-hydroxy-2′-deoxyguanosine (61).

Population studies of the association of high intakes of catechins with cancer incidence indicated that catechins derived primarily from fruits, (+)-catechin and (−)-epicatechin, tended to be inversely associated with upper digestive tract cancer, whereas catechins derived from tea were inversely associated with rectal cancer in postmenopausal women (62). Many epidemiologic, case-control, and cohort studies have investigated the effects of tea consumption on human cancer incidence (14, 63–65). A brief synopsis (66) of 30 studies aimed at examining tea consumption as a factor in the incidence of colon and rectal cancers from 12 countries and with data on consumption of both black and green tea did not provide consistent evidence to support the theory from animal studies and basic research that tea is a potent chemopreventive agent. The assessment of tea consumption in most of these studies was based on a single question and therefore may be subject to significant measurement error compared with more recent studies specifically aimed at assessing tea consumption (66).

In animal models of atherosclerosis, green and black tea administration resulted in modest improvements in the resistance of lipoproteins to ex vivo oxidation, although limited data suggest that green tea or green tea catechins inhibit atherogenesis (61). One epidemiologic study indicated that an increased intake of tea and flavonoids may contribute to the primary prevention of ischemic heart disease (33).

PROANTHOCYANIDINS

Chemistry, Dietary Sources, and Intakes

PAs, better known as condensed tannins, are oligomeric and polymeric flavan-3-ols (see Fig. 37.1). They are ubiquitous and are the second most abundant natural phenolic after lignin in plants. The flavan-3-ol units are linked mainly through the C4→C8 bond, but the C4→C6 bond also exists (both called B type) (see Fig. 37.1). The flavan-3-ol units can also be doubly linked by an additional ether bond between C2→O7 (A type). The size of PA molecules can be described by the degree of polymerization (DP) (24). Three common flavan-3-ols, which differ in their hydroxylation patterns, are found in PAs. The PAs consisting exclusively of (epi)catechin are procyanidins (PCs). PAs containing (epi)afzelechin or (epi)gallocatechin as subunits are named propelargonidins or prodelphinidins, respectively. Propelargonidins and prodelphinidins are less common in nature as compared with PCs. They are heterogeneous in their constituent units and coexist with the PCs (24, 25).

PAs are of great interest in nutrition and medicine because of their potent antioxidant capacity and possible protective effects on human health. PAs have been suggested to account for a significant fraction of polyphenols ingested in Western diet because of their ubiquitous existence. Studies have reported the content of other flavonoids in foods and their daily intake, but no data exist concerning the daily intake of oligomeric and polymeric flavan-3-ols because data on the PA content of foods have been lacking. Appropriate analytic methods have been developed for the measurement of PAs (57) such that a PA food database will be established as part of the USDA National Food and Nutrition Analysis Program (57). PAs are most prevalent in fruits and berries but are also found in chocolate (67) (see Table 37.1), a few cereals and beans, nuts, and cinnamon (57). The foods lacking PAs and those containing PAs have been surveyed (24, 25).

The initial calculation of average daily intake of oligomeric and polymeric PAs by Gu and associates (57) of 53.6 mg/day/person is higher than that of monomeric flavan-3-ols and is twice as high as the combined overall intake of other flavonoids, including flavonols, flavones, and flavanones. PAs are likely one of the major flavonoids ingested in the Western diet. Variations in PAs intake among individuals are expected to be large as a result of different eating habits. People who eat a medium-sized apple every day can easily ingest 100 mg of PAs daily. People who take dietary supplements, such as pine bark extract (Pycnogenol) or grape seed extracts, can ingest several hundreds of milligrams of PAs. The average daily intake of PAs for infants of 6 to 10 months is estimated to be 3.1 mg/day/kg body weight, which is four times higher than the average intake in adults of 20 years of age and older (0.77 mg/day/kg body weight) (57). Intake of PAs in 6- to 10-month-old infants increases markedly with the addition of fruits to the complementary foods. The daily intake of PAs for 10- to 24-month-old infants is expected to be even higher, because serving sizes are bigger and fresh fruits are introduced.

Absorption and Metabolism

Unlike the lower oligomers, PAs with a DP greater than 3 appear not to be absorbed directly in the gastrointestinal lumen (68, 69). These PAs were suggested to depolymerize into mixtures of epicatechin monomer and dimers in the acidic environment of the stomach. The resultant monomers and dimers are absorbed in the small intestine (70). Our observation on weaning pigs indicated that 8 to 15% of ingested polymers (DP >10) were depolymerized after 4 hours in the stomach with a concurrent increase of monomers, dimers, and trimers. Investigators have suggested that depolymerization is a slow process, and most PAs may transit into the small intestine intact (71). We noted that approximately 65% of the ingested PAs were degraded in the entire gastrointestinal lumen at 4 hours after eating. Major degradation of PAs takes place in the cecum and large intestine (Gu and Prior, unpublished data), where the colonic microflora may play an important role. Déprez and colleagues (72) reported that incubation of polymeric PCs with human colonic microflora in vitro in anoxic conditions led to a complete degradation of PCs after 48 hours. The degradation products included phenylacetic, phenylpropionic, and phenylvaleric acids with the monohydroxyl group mainly in the *meta-* or *para-* position. These phenolic acids have been suggested to be the major metabolites of oligomeric and polymeric PAs in healthy persons (73). Dimeric PCs can be detected in human plasma as early as 30 minutes after the consumption of a flavanol-rich food such as chocolate (74). However, no oligomers larger than the dimer have been detected in plasma.

Biologic Effects

PAs are of great interest in nutrition and medicine because of their potent antioxidant capacity and possible protective effects on human health in reducing the risk of chronic diseases such as cancer and cardiovascular diseases (75). In vitro studies have shown that PCs in chocolate inhibit human 5-lipoxygenase, decrease the LDL oxidative susceptibility (76, 77), inhibit platelet function (77), and promote transforming growth factor-β_1 homeostasis in peripheral blood mononuclear cells (78). PCs in grape seeds induce apoptotic death of human prostate carcinoma (79) and exhibit cytotoxicity toward MCF-7 breast cancer, A-427 lung cancer, and gastric adenocarcinoma cells, while enhancing the growth and viability of the normal cells (80).

PAs of different molecular size may differ in their physiologic effects. Mao and colleagues (81) studied the ability of the PCs to modulate interleukin-2 in vitro and found that higher oligomers inhibited interleukin-2 expression in stimulated cells, whereas the monomer had no effect. Tebib and associates (82) suggested that polymeric PAs were more effective than monomers in lowering blood cholesterol. The proposed mechanism is that PAs bind cholesterol in the intestine through hydrophobic association, which is more potent for PAs of higher DP. Different constituent flavan-3-ols and interflavan linkages in PAs may also influence their physiologic effects. In vitro studies have shown that PCs with the A-type interflavan linkage isolated from cranberries inhibit the adherence of uropathogenic *Escherichia coli* to the uroepithelial cell surfaces, whereas B-type PCs show no effects (83). In addition, the A-type polymers from cinnamon have insulin-like biologic activity (84), and cinnamon consumption (1–6 g) for 40 days by patients with type 2 diabetes lowered serum glucose, triglycerides, and total cholesterol concentrations (85).

ANTHOCYANINS

Chemistry and Dietary Sources

Anthocyanins (see Fig. 37.1) are water-soluble plant secondary metabolites responsible for the blue, purple, and red color of many plant tissues. They occur primarily as glycosides of their respective anthocyanidin chromophores, with the sugar moiety attached at the 3 position on the C ring or the 5 position on the A ring. The common anthocyanidins (aglycones) are cyanidin, delphinidin, petunidin, peonidin, pelargonidin, and malvidin. The differences in chemical structure of these six common anthocyanidins occur at the 3' and 5' positions (see Fig. 37.1). Aglycones are rarely found in fresh plant material. Several hundred anthocyanins are known, and they vary as follows: (a) in the number and position of hydroxyl and methoxyl groups on the basic anthocyanidin skeleton; (b) in the identity, number, and positions at which sugars are attached; and (c) in the extent of sugar acylation and the identity of the acylating agent (86). Common acylating agents are the cinnamic acids (caffeic, ρ-coumaric, ferulic, and sinapic). Acylated anthocyanins occur in some of the less common foodstuffs such as red cabbage, red lettuce, garlic, red-skinned potato, and purple sweet potato (87).

The chemistry and distribution of anthocyanins have been reviewed (88). Like other flavonoids, anthocyanins and anthocyanidins (the aglycone form) have antioxidant properties (89). The phenolic structure of anthocyanins (see Fig. 37.1) conveys marked antioxidant activity in model systems via donation of electrons or transfer of hydrogen atoms from hydroxyl moieties to free radicals. The cyanidin glycosides tend to have higher antioxidant capacity than peonidin or malvidin glycosides (89), likely because of the free hydroxyl groups on the 3' and 4' positions of cyanidin.

Cyanidin is the most common anthocyanidin, present in 90% of fruits (86, 90). Anthocyanin levels (mg/100 g fresh weight) range from 0.25 mg/100 g in the pear to 500 mg/100 g in the blueberry (90), and the fruits that are richest in anthocyanins (>20 mg/100 g fresh weight) are the very strongly colored (deep purple or black) berries (see Table 37.1).

Absorption and Metabolism

Anthocyanins are unique compared with other flavonoids in that they are absorbed intact as glycosides. The mechanism of absorption is not known. However, Passamonti and colleagues (91) found that anthocyanins can serve as ligands for bilitranslocase, an organic anion membrane carrier found in the epithelial cells of the gastric mucosa, and these investigators suggested that bilitranslocase could play a role in the bioavailability of anthocyanins. The addition of sucrose to elderberry juice led to reduced and delayed excretion of the anthocyanins (92), a finding suggesting that sugars may interfere with the anthocyanin transport mechanism. At least 13 different anthocyanins from seven different food sources have been observed to be absorbed intact and to be present in plasma or urine (86). In contrast to other flavonoids, the proportion of anthocyanins absorbed and excreted in the urine as a percentage of the intake seems to be quite small (93), perhaps much less than 0.1% of intake. Although no data are available on the exact amount of anthocyanins that are absorbed, together the plasma kinetic profile and the recovery of anthocyanins in the urine suggest that relatively small proportions are absorbed. However, urinary excretion does not provide an accurate measure of absorption, because metabolism and possible elimination in the bile may alter amounts excreted in the urine. Maximum plasma levels of total anthocyanins are reported in the range of 1 to 120 nmol/L with doses of 0.7 to 10.9 mg/kg in human studies (46, 94–96). The clearance of anthocyanins from the circulation is sufficiently rapid that by 6 hours, very little is generally detected in the plasma (96, 97). Rats seem to differ from the human in that in the rat, the aglycone (cyanidin) from cyanidin-3-glucoside (C3G) was detected in the jejunum (98), and protocatechuic acid, which may be produced by degradation of cyanidin, was present in the plasma at concentrations

eightfold higher than that of C3G. In the human, no cyanidin aglycone or protocatechuic acid has been observed in plasma or urine.

In studies by Cao and coworkers (96), the two major anthocyanins in elderberry (C3G and cyanidin 3-sambubioside) were detected as glycosides in human plasma and urine. Mulleder and colleagues (92) observed a greater urinary excretion of cyanidin-3-sambubioside than C3G (0.014 versus 0.004% of dose). The reduced excretion of C3G may be the result of increased degradation relative to cyanidin-3-sambubioside in the gastrointestinal tract (Wu and Prior, unpublished data). The complexity of the glycosidic pattern does not seem to noticeably affect absorption. Mazza and coworkers (99) suggested that acylated anthocyanins may be absorbed intact from blueberries, but these substances were not detected in plasma or urine in other reports. Most likely this is because they are present in low concentrations in the foods, and current methods are not sensitive enough to detect them. Most anthocyanins were excreted in urine during the first 4 hours after consumption (93, 96). Total elderberry anthocyanin excretion in the first 4 hours accounted for only 0.077 % of the dose.

Gut Metabolism

The metabolism of anthocyanins in the gut is an area that has largely been ignored up to this point. Felgines and coworkers (100) were among the first to report the presence of anthocyanins in gut contents of rats after adaptation to a diet containing blackberry anthocyanins. The blackberries contained primarily C3G, with a small amount of malvidin-3-glucoside (~1.9%). Recovery of cyanidin plus C3G in the total cecal contents was approximately 0.25%, whereas larger amounts of malvidin-3-glucoside were recovered in the cecum (~1.3%).

Tissue Metabolism

Wu and colleagues (93) identified four anthocyanin metabolites from elderberry in the urine: peonidin 3-glucoside, peonidin 3-sambubioside, peonidin monoglucuronide, and C3G monoglucuronide. However, Miyazawa and associates (95) were not able to detect conjugated or methylated anthocyanins in human plasma, but they did observe the presence of peonidin-3-glucoside in the liver of rats following the consumption of red fruit anthocyanins (C3G; C-3-diglucoside). The formation of the peonidin metabolites likely takes place in the liver through the catechol-O-methyl transferase reaction. Delphinidin would be the only other anthocyanidin that could undergo this methylation reaction because malvidin and petunidin already are methylated in the 3' position (see Fig. 37.1). Peonidin 3-glucoside was present in urine in rats fed a diet enriched with a lyophilized blackberry powder, and this finding likely resulted from hepatic methylation at the 3' hydroxyl moiety of C3G. Urinary recovery of C3G in either intact or methylated forms was approximately 0.26% of the ingested amount, whereas that of malvidin 3-glucoside was 0.67%. This result suggested that the structure of the aglycone moiety of anthocyanins could play an important role in their metabolism (100).

Biologic Effects

Vascular Permeability

Diabetic retinopathy can lead to blindness as a result of an abnormally high synthesis of connective tissue to repair leaking capillaries and to form new capillaries. Adult patients with diabetes who were treated with 600 mg/day of anthocyanins for 2 months significantly decreased the biosynthesis of connective tissue, especially polymeric collagen and structure glycoproteins in gingival tissue (101).

Effects on Vision

Early reports and some anecdotal information suggest that anthocyanins may improve night vision. Zadok and colleagues (102) assessed the effect of anthocyanins on three night vision tests in a double-blind, placebo-controlled, crossover study in which normal volunteers were given either 12 or 24 mg anthocyanins or a placebo, twice daily for 4 days. No significant effect was found on any of the three night vision tests. However, based on information presented earlier on dose and plasma levels, these doses would not be expected to produce measureable levels of anthocyanins in the plasma, and the length of treatment may have been insufficient to observe cumulative effects. In a double-blind, placebo-controlled, crossover study of healthy persons, Nakaishi and associates (103) studied the effects of oral intake of a black currant anthocyanin (BCA) concentrate on dark adaptation, video display terminal work-induced transient refractive alteration, and visual fatigue. Intake of BCA at three dose levels (12.5, 20, and 50 mg/subject, n = 12) appeared to bring about a dose-dependent lowering of the dark adaptation threshold with a significant difference at the 50-mg dose. In the assessment of subjective visual fatigue symptoms by questionnaire, significant improvement was recognized on the basis of statements regarding the eye and lower back after BCA intake. Muth and associates (104) failed to find an effect of bilberry anthocyanins on night visual acuity or night contrast sensitivity in subjects given 120 mg of anthocyanins daily for 21 days.

In a randomized, double-blind, placebo-controlled study, bilberry fruit extract (160 mg twice daily for 1 month) resulted in improvements in confirmed retinal abnormalities in 79% of the patients with either diabetic or hypertensive vascular retinopathy (105). Patients with type 2 diabetes and retinopathy who were given 480 mg of bilberry anthocyanins daily for 6 months showed improvement by the end of the trial period, as indicated by reduction of hemorrhage and alleviation of weeping exudates from the retina (106).

No consistent response seems to exist in terms of vision, based on the studies presented. Other studies using bilberry anthocyanins were reviewed by Upton (107). Dose and length of feeding are clearly factors affecting outcomes. Positive effects have been observed at intakes in the range of 300 to 600 mg/day taken over a period of several months. However, consumption of these levels of anthocyanins from foods will be difficult unless one consistently consumes some of the foods containing high concentrations of anthocyanins.

Other Effects

Although the published data are limited, fruits and berries may be protective through antioxidant mechanisms in preventing DNA damage, but they may also affect cell division, apoptosis, and/or angiogenesis (108). Hou (109) summarized some of the molecular mechanisms whereby anthocyanins may have cancer chemoprevention properties, including those related to antioxidants and induction of apoptosis in tumor cells.

ISOFLAVONES

Dietary Sources and Intakes

Isoflavonoids are found primarily in legumes. Soybeans are a rich source of the isoflavones genistein and daidzein. Harborne (5, 6) reported 180 kinds of isoflavone aglycones in 1975, but considerably more have been identified since that time. Genistein and daidzein and the daidzein metabolite equol are the common isoflavones of interest in human nutrition. Isoflavones have been considered as phytoestrogens because of their ability to function as ligands for the α- and β-estrogen receptors (110). In the United States, infants fed soy formula are the segment of the population that consumes the most soy. Most adults in the United States are not exposed to appreciable levels of soy foods (see Table 37.1). The opposite occurs in Asia, because Asians are more likely to consume relatively high levels of soy foods throughout life, except between birth and weaning, when breast-feeding or milk-based formula use is common (111). Japanese women show low incidence of, and mortality from, breast cancer and cardiovascular disease compared with white women. High soy intake may account for that observation, but it is not clear whether the effect results from soy protein itself or from isoflavones mixed in the soy protein (112).

Metabolism and Absorption

The metabolism of isoflavones in animals and humans is complex and involves both mammalian and gut microbial processes. Isoflavones are present predominantly as glucosides in most commercially available soy products. Evidence indicates that they are not absorbed in this form, and their bioavailability requires initial hydrolysis of the sugar moiety by bacterial β-glucosidases. After absorption, isoflavonoids are reconjugated predominantly to glucuronic acid and, to a lesser degree, to sulfate. Only a small portion of the free aglycone has been detected in blood, a finding demonstrating that the rate of conjugation is high. Extensive further metabolism of isoflavones (to equol and O-desmethylangolensin) by gut bacteria occurs. In vitro fermentation of daidzein and genistein with human fecal samples under anoxic conditions resulted in the production of dihydrodaidzein and equol from daidzein and of dihydrogenisten from genistein (113). In human study subjects, even those on controlled diets, large interindividual variation occurs in the metabolism of isoflavones, particularly in the production of the gut bacterial metabolite equol (from daidzein) (114, 115); 30 to 50% of adults do not excrete equol in the urine.

Health Benefits of Soy Protein

Dietary soy protein has been shown to have several beneficial effects on cardiovascular health. Some of the beneficial effects of soy appear to result from alterations in lipids, reductions in blood pressure, and decreases in lipid peroxidation, but experimental evidence also indicates possible favorable effects on vascular endothelial function. The best-documented effect of soy is on plasma lipid and lipoprotein concentrations, with reductions of approximately 10% in LDL cholesterol concentrations (116). Dietary soy protein improves flow-mediated arterial dilation in postmenopausal women but worsens that in men. Soy isoflavone extract improved systemic arterial compliance, an indicator of the extent of atherosclerosis (116). In 1999, the US Food and Drug Administration authorized a health claim stating that "25 grams of soy protein per day, as a part of a diet low in saturated fat and cholesterol, may reduce the risk of heart disease." To carry this claim, soy products must contain a minimum of 6.25 g of soy protein per serving and state the level of protein per serving, as well as its proportion of the recommended 25 g/day total protein. However, no definite experimental evidence exists currently to establish that the cardiovascular benefits of soy protein are accounted for by its isoflavones (116). In most studies, beneficial effects could not be attributed with certainty to soy isoflavones. If these components have any health-protecting effect in humans, it is small in comparison with the effect of soy protein itself. Data are currently insufficient to recommend the consumption of isoflavone supplements to lower plasma cholesterol levels (117).

Adlercreutz (118) concluded that a soy-containing diet in women is not, or is only slightly, protective with regard to breast cancer, but such a diet may be beneficial if consumed in early life before puberty or during adolescence, findings supporting results of immigrant and epidemiologic studies. Protective effects from soy and genistein against breast cancer in animal models were observed (110, 119). However, one potential caution for women with current or past breast cancer is that genistein and daidzein may stimulate existing breast tumor growth and may antagonize the effects of tamoxifen, and thus consumption of isoflavonoid containing foods may not be appropriate under these circumstances (120). Overall, Munro and colleagues indicated that, based on a review of the literature, the isoflavones as typically consumed in diets based on soy or containing soy products are safe (121).

Currently, although only limited epidemiologic data indicate that soy intake reduces prostate cancer risk, results from a pilot intervention trial suggest that isoflavones may be beneficial to patients with prostate cancer (122). Genistein, generally at levels much higher than found in soy, has been shown to inhibit carcinogenesis in animal models. A growing body of experimental evidence showed the inhibition of human cancer cells by genistein through the modulation of genes that are related to the control of cell cycle and apoptosis. Genistein also inhibits the activation of NF-κB and Akt signaling pathways, both of which are known to maintain a homeostatic balance between cell survival and apoptosis. Both in vivo and in vitro studies have shown that genistein may be effective in cancer chemoprevention (123).

Several dietary intervention studies examining the health effects of soy isoflavones alluded to the potential importance of equol in these effects by establishing that maximal clinical responses to soy protein diets are observed in people who are good "equol producers" (124). It is apparent that two distinct subpopulations of people with differential responses to soy isoflavones exist, and this situation may be a clue to the effectiveness of soy protein diets in cardiovascular, bone, and menopausal health. Setchell and colleagues (124) suggested that the failure to distinguish those subjects who are "equol producers" from "nonequol producers" in previous clinical studies may possibly explain the variance in reported data on the health benefits of soy.

Impressive data from the many studies on cultured bone cells and rat models of postmenopausal osteoporosis support a significant bone-sparing effect of the soy isoflavones genistein and daidzein. Translating this research to the clinic has been more challenging, and thus far only a few clinical studies have attempted to tease out the influence of phytoestrogens on bone from the many other components of the diet. Clinical studies thus far performed can be broadly divided into those that have assessed biochemical evidence of reduced bone turnover from measurement of surrogate markers of osteoblast and osteoclast activity and those that have examined changes in bone mineral density. Setchell and Lydeking-Olsen concluded from the literature reviewed that diets rich in isoflavone phytoestrogens may have bone-sparing effects in the long term, although the magnitude of the effect and the exact mechanisms of action are elusive or speculative at present (125).

OTHER PHYTOCHEMICALS

Other phytochemicals found in many fruits and vegetables include the following: (a) lignans, found in flax, rye, and some vegetables; (b) phenols (caffeic and ferulic acids) and phenolic acids (chlorogenic acid), found in many fruits and vegetables; (c) cyclic compounds, such as limonene found in citrus, and coumarins; (d) glucosinolates, indoles, and isothiocyanates, found in cruciferous vegetables such as broccoli, kale, and rutabaga; (e) saponins, found in soybeans and soy food; (f) ellagic acid; and (g) others. These phytochemicals are beyond the scope of this chapter, and readers are referred to some of the reviews cited for more information.

Acknowledgments

Appreciation is expressed to Dr. Liwei Gu and Dr. Xianli Wu for their assistance in reading and editing this chapter.

REFERENCES

1. Bidlack WR, Omaye ST, Meskin MS et al. Phytochemicals: A New Paradigm. Lancaster, PA: Technomic Publishing, 1998.
2. Meskin M. Phytochemicals as Bioactive Agents. Boca Raton, FL: CRC Press, 2000.
3. Meskin MS, Bidlack WR, Davies AJ et al. Phytochemicals in Nutrition and Health. Boca Raton, FL: CRC Press, 2002.
4. Meskin MS, Bidlack WR, Davies AJ et al. Phytochemicals: Mechanisms of Action. Boca Raton, FL: CRC Press, 2003.
5. Harborne JB, ed. The Flavonoids: Advances in Research Since 1980. London: Chapman & Hall, 1988.
6. Harborne JB, ed. The Flavonoids: Advances in Research Since 1986. London: Chapman & Hall, 1994.
7. Harborne JB. Phytochemistry 2000;55:481–504.
8. Middleton E Jr, Kandaswami C, Theoharides TC. Pharmacol Rev 2000;52:673–751.
9. Middleton E Jr, Kandaswami C. In: Harborne JB, ed. The Flavonoids: Advances in Research Since 1986. London: Chapman & Hall, 1994:619–52.
10. Middleton E Jr, Kandaswami C. Biochem Pharmacol 1992;43:1167–79.
11. Beecher GR. J Nutr 2003;133:3248S–54S.
12. Havsteen BH. Pharmacol Ther 2002;96:67–202.
13. Lambert JD, Yang CS. Mutat Res 2003;523–4:201–8.
14. Yang CS, Landau JM, Huang MT et al. Annu Rev Nutr 2001;21:381–406.
15. Nijveldt RJ, van Nood E, van Hoorn DEC et al. Am J Clin Nutr 2001;74:418–25.
16. Hertog MG, Hollman PC, Katan MB et al. Nutr Cancer 1993;20:21–9.
17. Hollman PC, Hertog MG, Katan MB. Biochem Soc Trans 1996;24:785–9.
18. Hertog MG, Feskens EJ, Hollman PC et al. Lancet 1993;342:1007–11.
19. Keli SO, Hertog MG, Feskens EJ et al. Arch Intern Med 1996;156:637–42.
20. Aherne SA, O'Brien NM. Nutrition 2002;18:75–81.
21. Merken HM, Beecher GR. J Agric Food Chem 2000; 48:577–99.
22. Merken HM. J Agric Food Chem 2001;49:2727–32.
23. Gu L, Kelm M, Hammerstone JF et al. J Agric Food Chem 2002;50:4852–60.
24. Gu L, Kelm MA, Hammerstone JF et al. J Agric Food Chem 2003;51:7513–21.
25. Gu L, Kelm MA, Hammerstone JF et al. J Mass Spectom 2003; 38:1272–80.
26. Engelmann C, Blot E, Panis Y et al. Phytomedicine 2002; 9:489–95.
27. Fotsis T, Pepper MS, Montesano R et al. Baillieres Clin Endocrinol Metab 1998;12:649–66.
28. Lin JK, Chen YC, Huang YT et al. J Cell Biochem 1997; 28–9[Suppl]:39–48.
29. Hertog MGL, Hollman PCH, Katan MB. J Agric Food Chem 1992;40:2379–83.
30. Hertog MGL, Hollman PCH, Putte B. J Agric Food Chem 1993;41:1242–6.
31. Sesso HD, Gaziano JM, Liu S et al. Am J Clin Nutr 2003; 77:1400–8.
32. Knekt P, Kumpulainen J, Jarvinen R et al. Am J Clin Nutr 2002; 76:560–8.
33. Geleijnse JM, Launer LJ, van der Kuip DAM et al. Am J Clin Nutr 2002;75:880–6.
34. Hertog MGL, Feskens EJM, Hollman PCH et al. Lancet 1993;342:1007–11.
35. Griffiths LA, Smith GE. Biochem J 1972;130:141–51.
36. Hollman PCH, De Vries JHM, Van Leeuwen SD et al. Am J Clin Nutr 1995;62:1276–82.
37. Murota K, Terao J. Arch Biochem Biophys 2003;417:12–7.
38. Crespy V, Morand C, Besson C et al. J Agric Food Chem 2002; 50:618–21.
39. Walgren RA, Karnaky KJ Jr, Lindenmayer GE et al. J Pharmacol Exp Ther 2000;294:830–6.
40. Walgren RA, Lin JT, Kinne RK et al. J Pharmacol Exp Ther 2000;294:837–43.
41. Walle T, Otake Y, Walle UK et al. J Nutr 2000;130:2658–61.
42. Rasmussen SE, Breinholt VM. Int J Vitam Nutr Res 2003; 73:101–11.
43. Morand C, Crespy V, Manach C et al. Am J Physiol 1998;275: R212–9.
44. Walle T, Walle UK, Halushka PV. J Nutr 2001;131:2648–52.
45. Hollman PC, van Trijp JM, Mengelers MJ et al. Cancer Lett 1997;114:139–40.
46. Prior RL. Am J Clin Nutr 2003;78:570S–8S.
47. Aura AM, O'Leary KA, Williamson G et al. J Agric Food Chem 2002;50:1725–30.
48. da Silva EL, Piskula MK, Yamamoto N et al. FEBS Lett 1998; 430:405–8.
49. Shirai M, Moon JH, Tsushida T et al. J Agric Food Chem 2001; 49:5602–8.
50. Graefe EU, Derendorf H, Veit M. Int J Clin Pharmacol Ther 1999;37:219–33.
51. Middleton E Jr, Kandaswami C, Theoharides TC. Pharmacol Rev 2000;52:673–751.
52. Manthey JA, Grohmann K, Guthrie N. Curr Med Chem 2001;8:135–53.
53. Lohezic-Le Devehat F, Marigny K, Doucet M et al. Therapie 2002;57:432–45.
54. Ameer B, Weintraub RA. Clin Pharmacokinet 1997;33:103–21.
55. Arts IC, Hollman PC, Feskens EJ et al. Eur J Clin Nutr 2001; 55:76–81.
56. Lakenbrink C. J Agric Food Chem 1999;47:4621–4.
57. Gu L, Kelm MA, Hammerstone JF et al. J Nutr 2004;134: 613–7.
58. Warden BA, Smith LS, Beecher GR et al. J Nutr 2001;131: 1731–7.
59. Rietveld A, Wiseman S. J Nutr 2003;133:3285S–92S.

60. Higdon JV, Frei B. Crit Rev Food Sci Nutr 2003;43:89–143.

61. Frei B, Higdon JV. J Nutr 2003;133:3275S–84S.

62. Arts ICW, Jacobs DR Jr, Gross M et al. Cancer Causes Control 2002;13:373–82.

63. Katiyar SK, Mukhtar H. J Cell Biochem 1997;64:59–67.

64. Yang CS, Landau JM. J Nutr 2000;130:2409–12.

65. Chung FL, Schwartz J, Herzog CR et al. J Nutr 2003;133:3268S–74S.

66. Arab L, Il'yasova D. J Nutr 2003;133:3310S–8S.

67. Keen CL. J Am Coll Nutr 2001;20:436S–9S, 440S–2S.

68. Déprez S, Mila I, Huneau JF et al. Antioxid Redox Signal 2001;3:957–67.

69. Donovan JL, Manach C, Rios L et al. Br J Nutr 2002;87:299–306.

70. Spencer JP, Chaudry F, Pannala AS et al. Biochem Biophys Res Commun 2000;272:236–41.

71. Rios LY, Bennett RN, Lazarus SA et al. Am J Clin Nutr 2002;76:1106–10.

72. Déprez S, Brezillon C, Rabot S et al. J Nutr 2000;130:2733–8.

73. Rios LY, Gonthier MP, Remesy C et al. Am J Clin Nutr 2003;77:912–8.

74. Holt RR, Lazarus SA, Sullards MC et al. Am J Clin Nutr 2002;76:798–804.

75. Schewe T, Kuhn H, Sies H. J Nutr 2002;132:1825–9.

76. Wan Y, Vinson JA, Etherton TD et al. Am J Clin Nutr 2001;74:596–602.

77. Murphy KJ, Chronopoulos AK, Singh I et al. Am J Clin Nutr 2003;77:1466–73.

78. Mao TK, Van De Water J, Keen CL et al. Exp Biol Med 2003;228:93–9.

79. Tyagi A, Agarwal R, Agarwal C. Oncogene 2003;22:1302–16.

80. Ye X, Krohn RL, Liu W et al. Mol Cell Biochem 1999;196:99–108.

81. Mao TK, Powell JJ, van de Water J et al. Int J Immunother 1999;15:23–9.

82. Tebib K, Besancon P, Rouanet JM. J Nutr 1994;124:2451–7.

83. Foo LY, Lu Y, Howell AB et al. J Nat Prod 2000;63:1225–8.

84. Anderson RA, Broadhurst CL, Polansky MM et al. J Agric Food Chem 2004;52:65–70.

85. Khan A, Safdar M, Khan MHA et al. Diabetes Care 2003;26:3215–8.

86. Prior RL. In: Meskin M, Bidlack WR, Davies AJ et al, eds. Phytochemicals: Mechanisms of Action. Boca Raton, FL: CRC Press, 2004:1–19.

87. Clifford MN. J Sci Food Agric 2000;80:1063–72.

88. Strack D, Wray V. In: Harborne JB, ed. The Flavonoids: Advances in Research Since 1986. London: Chapman and Hall, 1993.

89. Wang H, Cao G, Prior RL. J Agric Food Chem 1997;45:304–9.

90. Macheix J, Fleuriet A, Billot J. Fruit Phenolics. Boca Raton, FL: CRC Press, 1990.

91. Passamonti S, Vrhovsek U, Mattivi F. Biochem Biophys Res Commun 2002;296:631–6.

92. Mulleder U, Murkovic M, Pfannhauser W. J Biochem Biophys Methods 2002;53:61–66.

93. Wu X, Cao G, Prior RL. J Nutr 2002;132:1865–71.

94. Matsumoto H, Inaba H, Kishi M et al. J Agric Food Chem 2001;49:1546–51.

95. Miyazawa T, Nakagawa K, Kudo M et al. J Agric Food Chem 1999;47:1083–91.

96. Cao G, Muccitelli HU, Sanchez-Moreno C et al. Am J Clin Nutr 2001;73:920–6.

97. Bub A, Watzl B, Heeb D et al. Eur J Nutr 2001;40:113–20.

98. Tsuda T, Horio F, Osawa T. FEBS Lett 1999;449:179–82.

99. Mazza G, Kay CD, Cottrell T et al. J Agric Food Chem 2002;50:850–7.

100. Felgines C, Texier O, Besson C et al. J Nutr 2002;132:1249–53.

101. Boniface R, Robert AM. Klin Monatsbl Augenheilkd 1996;209:368–72.

102. Zadok D, Levy Y, Glovinsky Y. Eye 1999;13:734–6.

103. Nakaishi H, Matsumoto H, Tominaga S et al. Altern Med Rev 2000;5:553–62.

104. Muth ER, Laurent JM, Jasper P. Altern Med Rev 2000;5:164–73.

105. Perossini M, Guidi G, Chiellini S et al. Ottal Clin Ocul 1987;113:1173–90.

106. Orsucci PN, Rossi M, Sabbatini G et al. Clin Ocul 1983;5:377–81.

107. Upton R. Bilberry Fruit *Vaccinium myrtillus L.* Santa Cruz, CA: American Herbal Pharmacopoeia, 2001.

108. Prior RL, Joseph J. In: Bagchi D, Preuss HG, eds. Phytopharmaceuticals in Cancer Chemoprevention. Boca Raton, FL: CRC Press, 2004.

109. Hou DX. Curr Mol Med 2003;3:149–59.

110. Barnes S. Breast Cancer Res Treat 1997;46:169–79.

111. Badger TM, Ronis MJ, Hakkak R et al. J Nutr 2002;132:559S–65S.

112. Watanabe S, Uesugi S, Kikuchi Y. Biomed Pharmacother 2002;56:302–12.

113. Chang Y-C, Nair MG. J Nat Prod 1995;58:1892–6.

114. Rowland I, Faughnan M, Hoey L et al. Br J Nutr 2003;89:45S–58S.

115. Turner NJ, Thomson BM, Shaw IC. Nutr Rev 2003;61:204–13.

116. Clarkson TB. J Nutr 2002;132:566S–9S.

117. Demonty I, Lamarche B, Jones PJ. Nutr Rev 2003;61:189–203.

118. Adlercreutz H. J Steroid Biochem Mol Biol 2002;83:113–8.

119. Hakkak R, Korourian S, Shelnutt SR et al. Cancer Epidemiol Biomarkers Prev 2000;9:113–7.

120. de Lemos ML. Ann Pharmacother 2001;35:1118–21.

121. Munro IC, Harwood M, Hlywka JJ et al. Nutr Rev 2003;61:1–33.

122. Messina MJ. Nutr Rev 2003;61:117–31.

123. Sarkar FH, Li Y. Cancer Invest 2003;21:744–57.

124. Setchell KD, Brown NM, Lydeking-Olsen E. J Nutr 2002;132:3577–84.

125. Setchell KD, Lydeking-Olsen E. Am J Clin Nutr 2003;78:593S–609S.

126. Fotsis T, Pepper MS, Aktas E et al. Cancer Res 1997;57:2916–21.

127. Manthey JA, Grohmann K, Montanari A et al. J Nat Prod 1999;62:441–4.

38 CLINICAL MANIFESTATIONS OF NUTRIENT DEFICIENCIES AND TOXICITIES: A RESUME[1]

DOUGLAS C. HEIMBURGER, DONALD S. McLAREN, AND MAURICE E. SHILS

VITAMINS 595
  Vitamin A (Retinol) 595
  Vitamin D (Calciferol) 597
  Vitamin E (Tocopherol) .598
  Vitamin K (Phylloquinone) 598
  Thiamin (Vitamin B$_1$) .599
  Riboflavin 599
  Niacin 600
  Pyridoxine (Vitamin B$_6$) 601
  Biotin 601
  Vitamin B$_{12}$ (Cobalamin) 601
  Folic Acid 602
  Pantothenic Acid 602
  Vitamin C (Ascorbic Acid) 603
  Choline 603
ESSENTIAL FATTY ACIDS 603
  ω-6 Essential Fatty Acid Deficiency 603
  ω-3 Essential Fatty Acid Deficiency 604
MINERALS 604
  Calcium 604
  Phosphorus 604
  Potassium 605
  Magnesium 605
  Iodide (Iodine) 606
  Iron 606
  Copper 607
  Zinc 608
  Fluoride 608
  Selenium 609
  Chromium 609
  Molybdenum 609
  Manganese 609

Nutritional disorders result from an imbalance between the body's requirements for nutrients and energy sources and the supply of these substrates of metabolism. This imbalance may take the form of either deficiency or excess and may be attributable to inappropriate intake or to defective utilization or, frequently, a combination of both.

---

[1] **Abbreviations: DRI,** dietary reference intake; **HDN,** hemolytic disease of the newborn; **TPN,** total parenteral nutrition; **α-TTP,** α-tocopherol transfer protein.

Despite our extensive understanding of human nutritional requirements for maintenance of health, malnutrition continues to be one of the main causes of morbidity and mortality in developing countries, especially in young children. In technologically advanced societies, undernutrition resulting from dietary restriction no longer constitutes a major hazard to health, but it continues to occur in hospitalized patients and in other especially vulnerable groups. However, deficiency states continue to arise in patients with certain cultural or religious precepts, long-term alcohol or drug abuse, debilitating disease, or food faddism. Vigilance is needed to detect secondary undernutrition resulting from malabsorption, failure in transport, storage, or cellular utilization, excessive losses, or inactivation by genetic mutations of essential metabolic pathways that increase needs. The improper use of nutrient supplements, often because of ignorance about proper dosage or by failure of excretion through renal failure with continued nutrient intake, has been a major cause of toxicity (1).

This chapter is confined to a consideration of clinical manifestations of nutritional disorders related to vitamins, minerals, and essential fatty acids. It has been included because the chapters concerned with the individual nutrients do not uniformly discuss clinical aspects of deficiencies and excesses. Descriptions of clinical symptoms of deficiency of each nutrient are followed by brief consideration of who is likely to be at risk of deficiency and, if relevant, who is likely to be at risk of toxic levels.

VITAMINS

Vitamin A (Retinol)

Deficiency

The symptoms and signs of vitamin A deficiency have been studied in greater detail than those of any other nutritional deficiency disorder (2, 3). The eye is primarily involved, and the condition, given the general name of xerophthalmia, predominantly affects young children. Impaired dark adaptation or night blindness (i.e., decreased vision in dim light) is an early symptom and can be elicited by a careful history and some simple tests in a poorly illuminated room (4). Photopic and color vision, mediated by the retinal cones, is usually unaffected.

Dryness (xerosis) and unwettability of the bulbar conjunctiva follow. Conjunctival impression cytology is abnormal at this stage. Bitôt spot, a heaping up of desquamated cells most commonly seen in the interpalpebral fissure on the temporal aspect of the conjunctiva, is another sign (Fig. 38.1A). In older children and adults, Bitôt spots may be stigmata of past deficiency, or they may be entirely unrelated to vitamin A deficiency when local trauma is responsible. Corneal involvement, starting as a superficial punctate keratopathy (5) and proceeding to xerosis (Fig. 38.1B) and varying degrees of "ulceration" and liquefaction (keratomalacia) (Fig. 38.1C), frequently results in blindness. Punctate degenerative changes in the retina (xerophthalmic fundus) are rare signs of chronic deficiency usually seen in older children (6). Corneal scars may have many causes, but those that are bilateral in the lower and outer part of the cornea of a person with a history of past malnutrition and/or measles often signal earlier vitamin A deficiency.

Extraocular manifestations include perifollicular hyperkeratosis, an accumulation of hyperkeratinized skin epithelium around hair follicles most commonly seen on the lateral aspects of the upper arms and the thighs. This finding is also seen in starvation and has been attributed to a deficiency of B complex vitamins or essential fatty acids. Other changes, which include impaired taste, anorexia, vestibular disturbance, bone changes with pressure on cranial nerves, increased intracranial pressure, infertility, and congenital malformations, may occur (7).

Who Is at Risk of Deficiency? Because of limited placental transfer of fat-soluble vitamins, the liver content of vitamin A is low at delivery. However, when the mother has been ingesting an adequate amount of vitamin A, the milk intake of the nursing child, or the adequate content of the bottle formula, is an adequate source. In many developing countries, vitamin A intake of children is seriously limited; this causes millions of children to develop xerophthalmia each year, and many thousands go blind (8). International public health programs are underway to improve this situation (9).

Diseases that involve poor absorption of lipids including impaired pancreatic and/or biliary secretions, Crohn disease, celiac disease, radiation enteritis, ileal resection or damage, and various infections should lead to examination of the status of this vitamin as well as others.

Vitamin A deficiency is considered of public health importance if 15% or more of a defined population has a plasma retinol concentration of less than 0.7 μmol/L. Because circulating vitamin concentrations are reduced by conditions associated with inflammatory reactions or impaired retinal transport, a low level may be misleading. When measurements of indicators of inflammation, such as C-reactive protein and α_1-acid glycoprotein, are elevated, they may provide a basis for a corrective estimate (10, 11).

Toxicity (Hypervitaminosis A)

Most of the features relate to a rise in intracranial pressure: nausea, vomiting, headache, vertigo, irritability, stupor, fontanel bulging (in infants), papilledema, and pseudotumor cerebri (mimicking brain tumor) (12). Pyrexia and peeling of the skin also occur.

Chronic poisoning produces a bizarre clinical picture that is often misdiagnosed because of failure to consider excessive vitamin A intake (12). It is characterized by anorexia, weight loss, headache, blurred vision, diplopia, dry and scaling pruritic skin, alopecia, coarsening of the hair, hepatomegaly, splenomegaly, anemia, subperiosteal new bone growth, cortical thickening (especially bones of hands and feet and long bones of the legs), and gingival discoloration. The x-ray appearance may assist in making a correct diagnosis. Cranial sutures are widened in the young child.

Vitamin A and other retinoids are powerful teratogens in both pregnant experimental animals and women (12). Birth defects have been reported in the children of women receiving 13-*cis*-retinoic acid (isotretinoin) during pregnancy (13). An increased risk of birth defects is present in infants of women taking more than 10,000 IU/day of supplementary preformed vitamin A before the seventh week of gestation (14). Use of isotretinoin for treating acne is a serious risk factor for birth defects when this agent is taken by pregnant women.

Significant evidence indicates that long-term intake of larger-dose supplements of retinol is associated with increased risk of bone fractures in older Swedish men (15) and women (16), as well as in women in the United States (17).

Who Is at Risk of Excess/Toxicity? The tolerable upper limit of preformed vitamin A rises from 600 μg/day for infants progressively during growth to 2800 for adolescents up to 3000 μg for adults (see Chapter 19, Table 19.1 and Appendix Table A-2-f). The usual causes of hypervitaminosis A are prolonged consumption of vitamin A–containing supplements ("a little is good; a lot is better"); self- or physician-prescribed intake of preparations for skin abnormalities, or intake of liver that is very rich in vitamin A. Any one or all may lead to toxic symptoms. The physical form of retinol supplements is a major determinant of toxicity. Water-miscible, emulsified, and solid preparations of retinol are approximately ten times more toxic than oil-based retinol preparations (18).

Hypercarotenosis

Excessive intake of carotenoids can cause hypercarotenosis. Yellow or orange discoloration of the skin (xanthosis cutis, carotenoderma) affects areas where sebum secretion is greatest—nasolabial folds, forehead, axillae, and groin—and keratinized surfaces such as the palms and

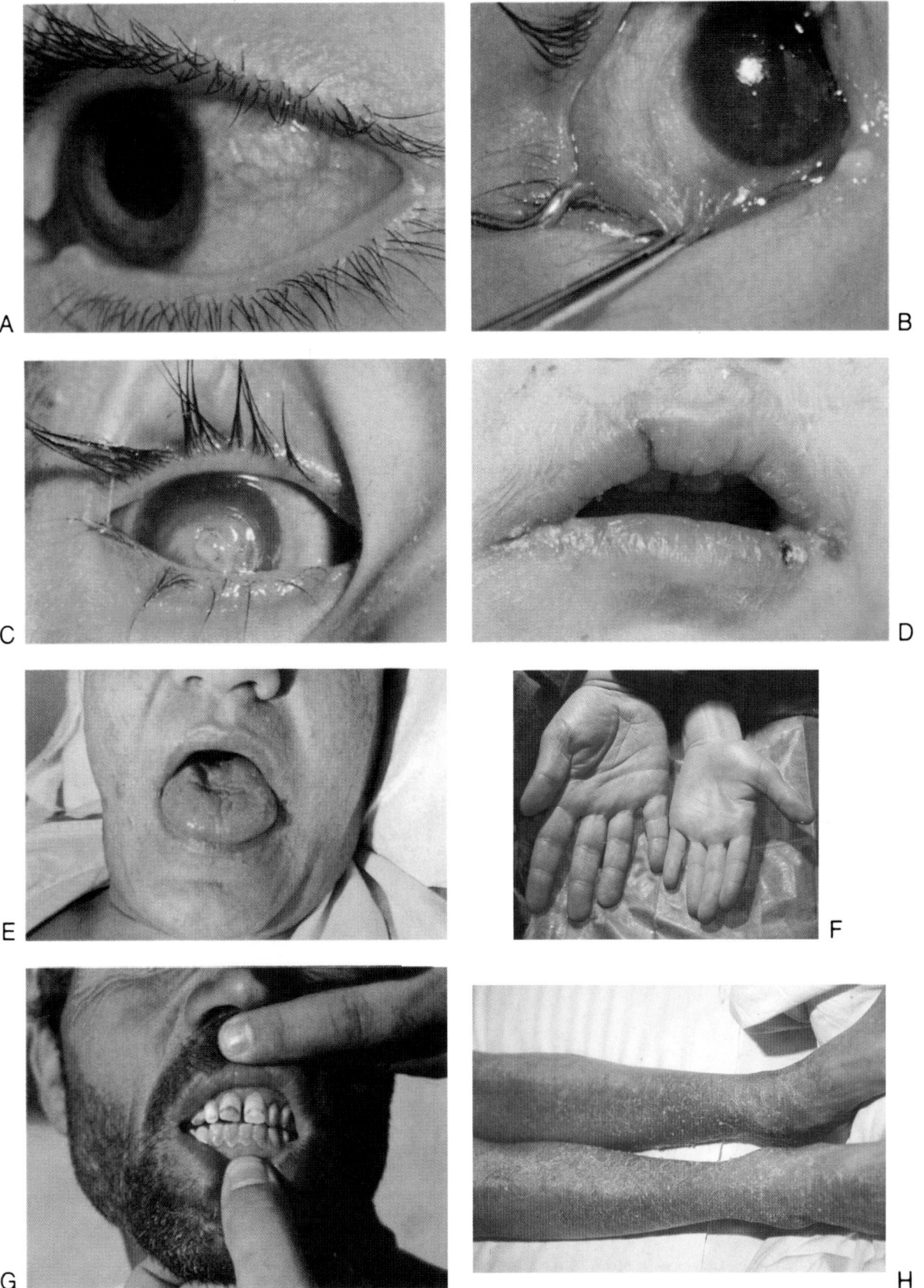

Figure 38.1. A. Vitamin A deficiency. Bitot spot in the temporal interpalpebral fissure. **B.** Vitamin A deficiency. Conjunctival and corneal xerosis. **C.** Vitamin A deficiency. Keratomalacia. **D.** Riboflavin deficiency. Cheilosis and angular stomatitis. **E.** Riboflavin deficiency. Magenta tongue. **F.** Palm of a woman with hypercarotenosis **(right),** compared with the palm of a person without hypercarotenosis **(left).** (From Mazzone A, Dal Canton A. Images in clinical medicine: hypercarotenemia. N Engl J Med 2002;346:821; copyright 2002, Massachusetts Medical Society; all rights reserved.). **G.** Fluorosis. Early stage with brown mottling that is most marked on upper central incisors. **H.** Zinc deficiency. Dermatitis in a patient with malabsorption. (Courtesy of DC Heimburger.)

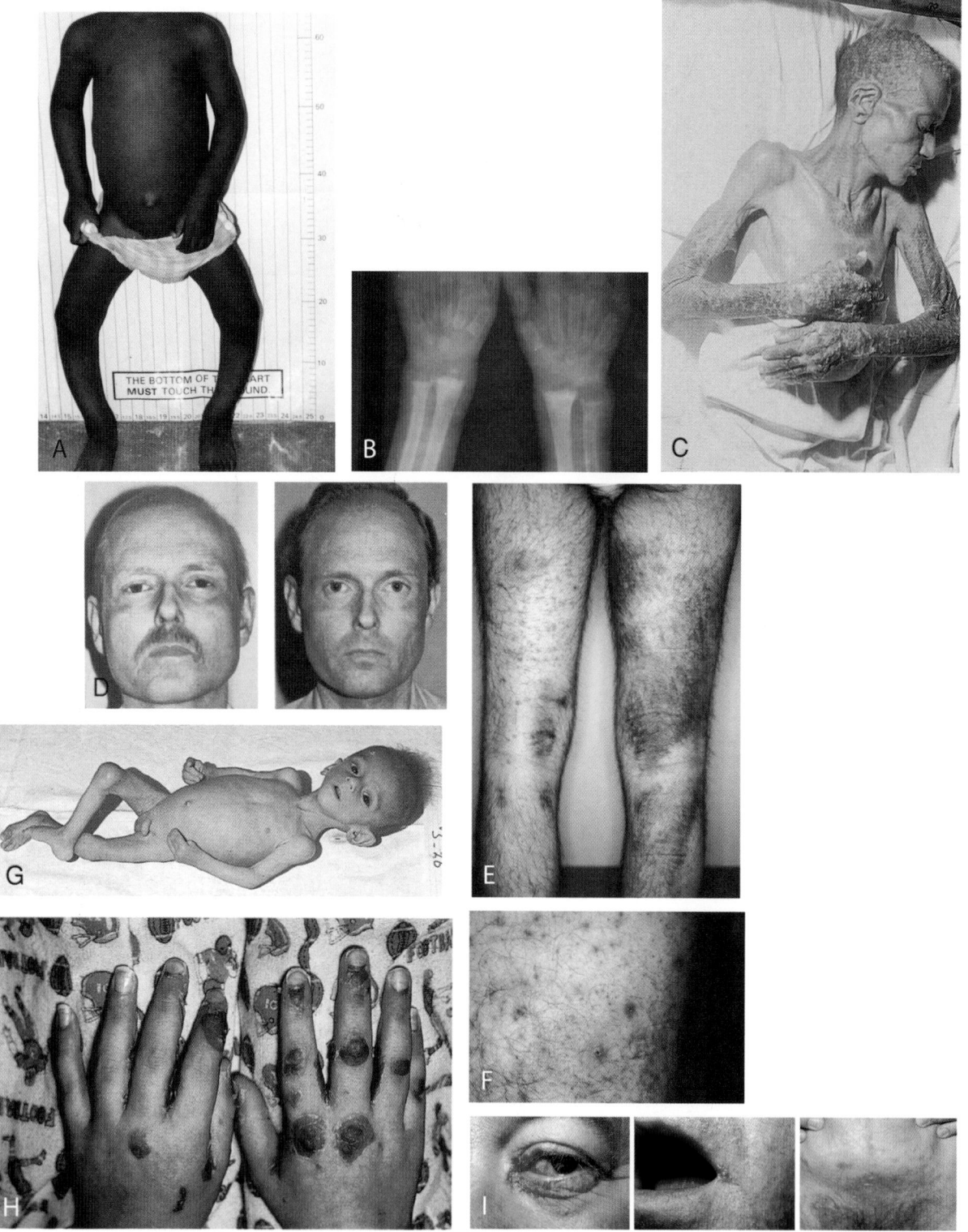

Figure 38.2. A. Rickets. Genu varum in a 30-month-old girl with nutritional rickets and progressive bowing of the legs since she began walking at the age of 11 months. (From Thacher TD. Images in clinical medicine: nutritional rickets. N Engl J Med 1999;341:576; copyright 1999, Massachusetts Medical Society; all rights reserved.). **B.** Rickets (same child as in *A*). Cupping and fraying of the metaphyses of the distal radius and ulna. **C.** Pellagra. Casal necklace, a broad band or collar of dermatitis, induced by exposure to sunlight, is a classic sign of pellagra. The patient was an elderly woman in Tanzania. **D.** Biotin deficiency. Adult with alopecia, dermatitis, and conjunctivitis who was receiving prolonged parenteral nutrition devoid of biotin **(left).** Slit-lamp examination revealed corneal lesions. All were corrected by inclusion of 60 μg of biotin daily **(right).** (From McClain CJ, Baker H, Onstad GR. Biotin deficiency in an adult during home parenteral nutrition. JAMA 1982;247:3116, with permission.) **E.** Scurvy. Large ecchymotic areas on the backs of the legs of a 46-year-old man. (From Kronauer CM, Bühler H. Images in clinical medicine: skin findings in a patient with scurvy. N Engl J Med 1995;332:1611; copyright 1995, Massachusetts Medical Society; all rights reserved.) **F.** Scurvy. A close-up view of the same patient as in *E* showing perifollicular hemorrhages, hyperkeratosis, and fragmented hairs. **G.** Hypocalcemia. The characteristic contraction of the hands (tetany) in this marasmic infant is associated with the presence of marked hypocalcemia often secondary to magnesium depletion. **H.** Zinc deficiency. Lesions on pressure areas on the back of the hands in a child receiving prolonged parenteral nutrition who had rapidly depleted zinc stores through loss of large volumes of intestinal contents following an intestinal fistula. Similar lesions occurred on the elbows and knees. Sterile pustules were present on the palms, and lesions were present about the mouth. All responded to increased zinc administration. (Courtesy of ME Shils.) **I.** Oculo-orogenital syndrome caused by deficiencies of pyridoxine and riboflavin in an alcoholic man. Findings included blepharoconjunctivitis **(left),** angular stomatitis **(middle),** a bright red and atrophic tongue, and dermatitis of the pubic area **(left).** (From Friedli A, Saurat J-H. Images in clinical medicine: oculo-orogenital syndrome—a deficiency of vitamins B$_2$ and B$_6$. N Engl J Med 2004;350:1130; copyright 2002, Massachusetts Medical Society; all rights reserved.)

soles (Fig. 38.1*F*). The sclerae and buccal membranes are not affected, a feature that distinguishes this condition from jaundice, in which these tissues are yellowed. No toxicity is apparent, and the discoloration gradually disappears with reduction of intake.

Vitamin D (Calciferol)

Deficiency

Vitamin D deficiency is manifested as rickets in children and osteomalacia in adults. Persons with those forms not resulting from primary vitamin D or calcium deficiency—previously termed metabolic rickets—also exhibit signs and symptoms of the underlying disease and hypocalcemia.

Rickets. The rachitic infant is restless and sleeps poorly. Craniotabes, softening of the bones of the skull and their ready depression on palpation, is often the earliest sign, but it must be present away from the suture lines to be diagnostic of rickets. Frontal bossing occurs, and the fontanels close late. Sitting, crawling, and walking are all delayed. If the disease is active when these activities occur, weight bearing results in bowing of the arms, knock-knees (genu valgum), or outward bowing (genu varum) (Fig. 38.2*A* and *B*). The characteristic x-ray appearance usually precedes clinical signs. Bone morphology is discussed elsewhere in this text.

Occasionally, stridor and intermittent sudden airway obstruction resulting from laryngospasm may present in infancy as a result of hypocalcemia accompanying biochemical and x-ray evidence of rickets but without the classic bony physical signs (19). A few instances of congenital cataract appear to be caused by vitamin D deficiency in the mother (20).

A recent review of rickets summarizes the world literature on factors increasing its prevalence in various areas and the need for a "safety net" of extra vitamin D for children as well as for pregnant women (21).

Osteomalacia. The main features of osteomalacia are bone pain and tenderness, skeletal deformity, and weakness of the proximal muscles. Muscle weakness is a subtle indicator of vitamin deficiency (22). In severe cases, all the bones are painful and tender, often enough to disturb sleep. Tenderness may be particularly marked over Looser zones (Milkman lines), usually occurring in the long bones, pelvis, ribs, and around the scapulae in a bilaterally symmetric pattern. These radiotranslucent zones are sometimes termed pseudofractures. True fractures of the softened bones are common. The proximal muscle weakness, the cause of which is uncertain, is more marked in some forms of osteomalacia than in others. Osteomalacia usually results in a waddling gait and in difficulty going up and down stairs. In elderly persons, it may simulate paraplegia; in younger persons, it may simulate muscular dystrophy.

Who Is at Risk of Deficiency? Today, vitamin D deficiency is likely to occur in those who make deliberate efforts to minimize direct ultraviolet light to the skin by the use of sunscreens or when the body is continuously covered by clothing. Elderly persons are particularly at risk because of decreased production of vitamin D in their skin, a frequent failure to consume milk and other good sources, and their tendency to stay indoors because of a variety of chronic conditions (23).

The increase in the population of immigrant religious Muslim women in Western countries who adhere to full clothing with veil coverage has resulted in vitamin D deficiency in them and in their children when these children are breast-fed for long periods (24).

As with the other fat-soluble vitamins, a variety of intestinal diseases that interfere with fat absorption will seriously decrease vitamin D availability and absorption, especially pancreatic and biliary obstruction, jejunal malabsorption, and gastric bypass surgery for obesity. Liver damage may decrease concentrations of the hydroxylating enzyme that forms calcidiol. See programs for vitamin D intake and sunlight exposure (21).

Toxicity (Hypervitaminosis D)

Some of the symptoms and signs are related to hypercalcemia and are common to all causes of that condition. Anorexia, nausea, vomiting, and constipation are usually present. Weakness, hypotonia, stupor, and hypertension are less common. Polyuria and polydipsia are caused by hypercalciuria. Renal colic resulting from stone formation may result. Radiography of the skeleton may assist in diagnosis. Epiphyseal bone density is increased in response to excessive calcium deposition.

Vitamin D excess has been reported to take two forms: mild and severe. In the mild form, the patient is usually 3 to 6 months of age, and the symptoms and signs are those already described. In the severe form, also seen in infants, in addition to the manifestations of hypercalcemia, patients have mental retardation, stenosis of the aorta and the pulmonary arteries, and a characteristic facial appearance termed elfin facies (25).

Who Is at Risk of Excess/Toxicity? The tolerable upper limit for vitamin D has been set at 1000 IU (25 μg) for infants and 2000 IU (50 μg) for children aged 1 to 18 years and for adults and pregnant and lactating women (see Appendix Table A-2-a-2). Because the skin destroys unabsorbed previtamin and vitamin D, increased sunlight irradiation does not cause excessive levels in the body. Persons at risk include those who use vitamin D–containing supplements in addition to large intakes of oily fish, fish oils, and fortified milk. Such a history should prompt a test of serum calcium concentrations because the hypercalcemia of excessive doses cause undesirable changes in kidney, bone, and the central nervous and cardiovascular systems.

Vitamin E (Tocopherol)

Deficiency

The Food and Nutrition Board has defined vitamin E requirements in terms of α-tocopherol. The molecular basis of two conditions in which vitamin E deficiency has long been known to figure prominently has been discovered (26). In spinocerebellar ataxias of the Friedreich type, patients have a defect in the α-tocopherol transfer protein (α-TTP), and in abetalipoproteinemia (Bassen-Kornzweig syndrome, acanthocytosis), patients have mutations in the gene coding for one subunit of the microsomal triglyceride transfer protein. Friedreich ataxia presents in childhood with progressive ataxia of gait, dysarthria, areflexia, extensor plantar signs, and impaired vibratory and positional sense. In abetalipoproteinemia, patients have steatorrhea, acanthocytes (erythrocytes with spiny projections of the membrane), retinitis pigmentosa–like changes in the retina, ataxia, and mental retardation.

Who Is at Risk of Deficiency? Vitamin E deficiency hardly ever occurs as a result of low dietary intake because of widespread distribution of tocopherols in foods, especially oils and fats. As noted earlier, genetic defects in α-TTP result in spinocerebellar ataxias. In addition to Friedreich ataxia, a similar neurologic abnormality (previously termed familial isolated vitamin E deficiency) exists, now termed ataxia with vitamin E deficiency. In addition to abetaliproteinemia (microsomal triglyceride transfer protein abnormality), a related condition is recognized, homozygous hypobetaliproteinemia (microsomal triglyceride transfer protein abnormality).

As in the case with other fat-soluble vitamins, vitamin E is malabsorbed to varying degrees in fat malabsorption syndromes (see Table 21.1 in Chapter 21). These conditions are responsive to oral or parenteral α-tocopherol supplements, depending on the state of the intestinal epithelium.

Toxicity

Reports that low-birth-weight infants receiving pharmacologic doses of vitamin E had a high incidence of sepsis and necrotizing enterocolitis (27) have not been confirmed. The tolerable upper limit of 1000 mg/day has been established for any form of α-tocopherol (see Appendix Table A-2-f). A meta-analysis reporting increased all-cause mortality in adults taking daily vitamin E supplements of 400 mg or more (28) has prompted discussion of whether the tolerable upper limit should be reduced.

Vitamin K (Phylloquinone)

Deficiency

Deficiency of vitamin K in the newborn is usually classified into three syndromes: early, classic, and late (29). The early form presents within 0 to 24 hours of birth, and the most common bleeding sites are the brain, the gut, and around the genitalia. Classic hemolytic disease of the newborn (HDN) presents on day 1 to 7, with the bleeding usually gastrointestinal, dermal, nasal, or from circumcision. The peak incidence of late HDN is from the third to the sixth week, and intracranial hemorrhage (rare in classic HDN) accounts for about 50% of the bleeding episodes at presentation. Late HDN may occur over weeks 2 to 12 and also commonly affects the skin and gastrointestinal tract. This deficiency led to the widespread intramuscular injection of small doses of phylloquinone to the newborn that has markedly reduced the incidence of HDN. The current recommendation is 0.5 to 1.0 mg (30).

Babies of mothers taking vitamin K antagonists during pregnancy were found to be at risk of congenital malformations (31). This led to the discovery of protein-bound α-carboxy-glutamate-containing proteins with vitamin K as the cofactor and to the new knowledge of the manifestations of dietary vitamin K deficiency as a risk for fractures (32). In adults, bleeding from vitamin K deficiency is most common in chronic liver disease, in obstructive jaundice, and in patients receiving anticoagulants or prolonged antibiotic therapy.

Who Is at Risk of Deficiency? The most common cause of vitamin K deficiency is treatment with oral anticoagulants; excessive anticoagulation often occurs with inadequate follow-up of prothrombin times/International Normalized Ratios. The excessive anticoagulation can be overcome and the desired International Normalized Ratio level achieved by lowering the anticoagulant dose or, if it is severely over the desired range, by infusion of phytonadione.

As with the other fat-soluble vitamins, low transfer of phylloquinone to the fetus occurs; in addition, when the vitamin K content of breast milk is low, this is an additional factor contributing to HDN. Inherited mutations leading to deficiencies of protein C (one of the vitamin K–dependent coagulation factors) have been shown to increase the risk of venous thromboembolism; by contrast, deficiency of protein Z (another vitamin K–dependent protein) has a significant association with arterial thrombosis, as manifested by low levels of this protein in the plasma of persons with previous ischemic stroke (33). Claims that bone loss in patients with Crohn disease or hip fracture in women on low-vitamin K diets may be related to vitamin K deficiency require more substantial evidence to establish causation.

Even though bacteria in the lower intestine produce vitamin K, its absorption is apparently limited. When significant impairment of absorption of ingested vitamin in various lipid malabsorption syndromes occurs, increased oral or parenteral phytonadione is indicated.

A recent US Food and Drug Administration regulation requires that vitamin K be included in the adult parenteral solutions used in parenteral nutrition; it has been required in pediatric solutions for many years.

Toxicity

The dietary reference intake (DRI) report on vitamin K states that "search of the literature revealed no evidence of toxicity associated with the intake of either phylloquinone or menaquinone forms of vitamin K. . . . A synthetic form of vitamin K, menadione, has been associated with liver damage . . . and therefore is no longer used therapeutically" (34).

Thiamin (Vitamin B$_1$)

Deficiency

Cardiovascular Beriberi. Cardiovascular beriberi (so-called wet beriberi) usually manifests as chronic high-output right- and left-sided heart failure with tachycardia, rapid circulation time, elevated peripheral venous pressure, sodium retention, and edema (35). A much less common acute fulminating form of heart failure (sometimes called shoshin) is characterized by severe metabolic lactic acidosis, intense dyspnea, thirst, anxiety, and cardiovascular collapse. Signs also include stocking-glove cyanosis, extreme tachycardia, cardiomegaly, hepatomegaly, and neck vein distention. Edema is usually absent (36).

Beriberi of the Nervous System

Cerebral Beriberi (Wernicke-Korsakoff Syndrome). Cerebral beriberi involves mental confusion accompanied by ophthalmoplegia resulting from paralysis of the sixth cranial nerve and leading to coma. Korsakoff psychosis consists of loss of memory for distant events, inability to form new ones, and loss of insight and initiative (37). The patient is alert and can converse, think, and solve problems. Response to thiamin is complete in only 25% of cases and partial in 50%. Ethanol is thought to have a direct part in neurotoxicity (38, 39). Wernicke encephalopathy is most likely to occur in patients with chronic alcoholism who have a high-carbohydrate diet without adequate thiamin replacement or in nonalcoholic depleted patients given glucose infusions without adequate thiamin. It is now also encountered as a complication of bariatric surgery (40).

Peripheral Neuropathy. The most characteristic features of peripheral neuropathy are symmetric footdrop, associated with marked tenderness of the calf muscles, and a mild disturbance of sensation over the outer aspects of the legs and thighs and in patches over the abdomen, chest, and forearms. Ataxia with loss of position and vibration sense, burning paresthesias in the feet, and amblyopia are less common.

Infantile Beriberi. Early manifestations of infantile beriberi are anorexia, vomiting, pallor, restlessness, and insomnia. The disease progresses typically to (a) an acute cardiac form in infants 2 to 4 months old, (b) a subacute aphonic form in those 5 to 7 months old, and (c) a chronic, pseudomeningeal form in those between 8 and 10 months of age. The acute form presents with dyspnea, cyanosis, a rapid, thready pulse, and other signs of acute heart failure. In the subacute form, aphonia or a characteristic hoarse cry, dysphagia, vomiting, and convulsions predominate. The chronic form is characterized by neck retraction, opisthotonos, edema, oliguria, constipation, and meteorism (41).

Subacute Necrotizing Encephalomyopathy (Leigh Disease). Subacute necrotizing encephalomyopathy may be related to a defect in thiamin metabolism. The onset is usually before 1 year of age. Hypoventilation and apnea, cranial neuropathies, and hypotonia are the most common features.

Who Is at Risk of Deficiency? Although thiamin is being incorporated into polished rice, fortified rice is unavailable to significant population groups in areas of Asia and Africa. With a high-carbohydrate intake from rice, pregnant and lactating women and their children are particularly vulnerable (42). An additional cause of insufficient intake is the loss of thiamin by thiaminases present in various forms in food such as raw fish, fish paste, certain ferns, and betel nut.

Clinically, thiamin deficiency remains a problem in patients with chronic alcoholism and in those with acquired immunodeficiency syndrome (42). Polyneuropathy and Wernicke syndrome are being increasingly observed after gastric bypass surgery for obesity (40, 43). Unfortunately, reports still occur of carelessness in the use of parenteral nutrition formulas when the complete formula is allowed to stand for hours after the thiamin-containing multivitamin solution is added and before it is infused into the patient; the bisulfite present with amino acids destroys the thiamin with time.

Possible Toxicity

Large doses of thiamin are routinely given to patients with alcoholism. Adverse effects, including sensitization of an anaphylactic nature, have been reported only rarely (44, 45). No anaphylactic reactions have been reported with multivitamins containing thiamin used in total parenteral nutrition (TPN) solutions.

Riboflavin

Deficiency

The skin and mucous membranes are affected in what is known as the oculoorogenital syndrome. Areas of skin involved are usually those containing many sebaceous glands, mainly the nasolabial folds, alae nasi, external ears, eyelids, scrotum in the male, and labia majora in the female (see Fig. 38.2I). These areas become reddened, scaly, greasy, painful, and pruritic. Photophobia, lacrimation, and conjunctival injection are also present. Plugs of inspissated sebum may accumulate in the hair follicles and may give the appearance known as dyssebacia, or sharkskin.

At the angles of the mouth, patients have painful fissures known as angular stomatitis when these lesions are active (see Fig. 38.1*D*). Vertical fissures of the vermilion surfaces of the lips constitute cheilosis. These and the angular lesions may become infected with *Candida albicans,* giving rise to the appearance known as perlèche. The tongue may be painful, swollen, and magenta (Fig. 38.1*E*). These mucocutaneous changes may also be seen in other nutrient deficiencies or in elderly edentulous persons with chronically moist angles of the mouth. Because deficiency is often multiple, it is rarely possible in clinical practice to demonstrate the precise cause.

Corneal neovascularization, so common in experimental animals, is rarely seen in humans. The hemopoietic and nervous systems are occasionally affected. Normocytic normochromic anemia, reticulocytopenia, leukopenia, thrombocytopenia from marrow hypoplasia, and peripheral neuropathies with hyperesthesia, altered temperature sensation, and pain have been reported (46).

Who Is at Risk of Deficiency? Because of the widespread distribution of riboflavin in many foods, healthy persons eating a well-balanced diet are not at risk. When the major sources of calories come from unfortified germ-free cereals (especially cornmeal) and fatty foods, deficiencies of riboflavin and other nutrients can occur.

Elderly persons with restricted income and who are either housebound or institutionalized and who, for one reason or another (e.g., lactose intolerance) refuse milk and its products and eat a restricted diet are at increased risk of deficiency (47). All persons with significant malabsorptive defects are at risk of depletion. Significant riboflavin depletion under certain dietary circumstances may potentiate niacin deficiency (see next section).

Some genetic mutations involve defects in riboflavin-containing enzymes that lead to metabolic problems (e.g., flavinadenine dinucleotide-dependent dehydrogenases for various acyl coenzyme As and low flavin mononucleotide pyridoxal phosphate because of a D-glucose-6-phosphate dehydrogenase deficiency). These situations usually respond to additional riboflavin.

Who Is at Risk of Excess/Toxicity?

No adverse effects have been noted with riboflavin intakes from food or supplements. In fact, single oral doses about 38 times the RDA given as a single bolus had no adverse effect (48).

Niacin

Deficiency

Pellagra affects primarily the skin, gastrointestinal tract, and nervous system and produces the "four D's" of dermatitis, diarrhea, dementia, and ultimately death. Dermatitis is usually the earliest and most prominent manifestation. It is symmetric and appears on parts exposed to sunlight or trauma. Erythema progresses to keratosis and scaling with pigmentation. The back of the hands, wrists, forearms, face, and neck (Casal necklace) are typically affected (Fig. 38.2*C*). The skin and mucous membrane changes of riboflavin deficiency are also commonly present (see earlier). The tongue often has a "raw beef" appearance, is bright red, swollen, and painful. Symptoms of gastritis, bouts of diarrhea, and signs of malabsorption suggest similar changes in the gastrointestinal tract.

Nervous system involvement is suggested in the early stages by periods of depression with insomnia, headaches, and dizziness. Later, tremulous movement or rigidity of the limbs occurs with loss of tendon reflexes, numbness, and paresis of the extremities. In profound deficiency, encephalopathy has been described resembling that of acute cerebral beriberi (see the earlier section on Thiamin) but responds to some extent to niacin. Mental disturbance is so prominent in some patients that a real danger exists that the true diagnosis may be missed and the patient be incarcerated in a mental institution.

Who Is at Risk of Deficiency? Historically, populations at risk of this deficiency have been those in economically deprived areas where the most available diets consisted of cornmeal without the germ, fatty foods, and restricted good protein sources, as in parts of the southern United States and Europe. The low tryptophan content of the diets combined with poor intake of riboflavin and vitamin B₆ led to minimum niacin formation from that amino acid, thus potentiating the deficiency. With the advent of the Works Project Administration in the 1930s with its jobs and other government support and then economic improvement with World War II, pellagra in the southern United States subsided significantly in association with the improved quality and amounts of food. In Latin America, the treatment of tortillas with an alkali in their preparation from cornmeal liberated the niacin from its bound form to an absorbable form, thus minimizing chances of deficiency.

Hartnup disease is caused by an autosomal recessive disorder that limits tryptophan (and some other amino acids) absorption in the intestine and kidney and causes varying degrees of niacin depletion; this condition responds to nicotinamide in relatively large doses. The tuberculosis drug isoniazid interferes with tryptophan conversion to niacin.

Who Is at Risk of Excess/Toxicity?

Side effects of megadoses of niacin (e.g., 1–3 g/day), which are effective in treating many dyslipidemias, include vasodilatation, flushing, pruritus, blistering of the skin with brown pigmentation, nausea, vomiting, and headache (49). Liver dysfunction manifest as elevated serum liver enzymes is reasonably common, and liver failure can occur. Diabetic patients also require special monitoring of glucose because niacin may worsen insulin resistance. Sustained-release forms of niacin are being used to minimize these effects.

Pyridoxine (Vitamin B$_6$)

Deficiency

Pyridoxine deficiency induced by poor intake in adults is rarely severe enough to produce signs or symptoms. Volunteers receiving a deficient diet and a pyridoxine antagonist became irritable and depressed. Seborrheic dermatitis affected the nasolabial folds, cheeks, neck, and perineum. Several subjects also developed glossitis, angular stomatitis, blepharitis, and peripheral neuropathy.

Pyridoxine deficiency can also be manifest as microcytic anemia, particularly in infants (50–52). An uncommon form of sideroblastic anemia, often severe, has been reported to respond in some instances to pyridoxine, but most cases appear to result from dependency rather than deficiency (53). An inherited error in the vitamin B$_6$–dependent enzyme cystathionine β-synthase leads to severe abnormalities at an early age.

Who Is at Risk of Deficiency? An uncommon familial syndrome termed pyridoxine-dependent seizures is manifest by the occurrence of status epilepticus at or shortly after birth. It is responsive to pyridoxine therapy.

Homocysteinuria is an inborn error of metabolism caused by a deficiency of a vitamin B$_6$–dependent cystathionine β-synthase resulting in very high plasma homocysteine levels with associated signs and symptoms, such as dislocation of the optic lens, skeletal abnormalities, neurologic disorders, and thrombembolism. One of the two forms of this disease is responsive to pyridoxine.

Certain drugs, including cycloserine, penicillamine, gentamycin, isoniazid, and L-dopa, bind with pyridoxal or pyridoxal phosphate and reduce the amount of pyridoxal phosphate coenzyme. Pyridoxine supplementation is routine when these drugs are administered. Pyridoxine supplementation may also ameliorate the hand-and-foot syndrome that can occur with capecitabine therapy.

Who Is at Risk of Excess/Toxicity?

Megadoses of pyridoxine (>200 mg/day) can cause sensory neuropathy, including progressive sensory ataxia and profound lower limb impairment of position and vibration sense (54). Touch, temperature, and pain perception are less affected. The tolerable upper limit for adults is 100 mg/day (see Appendix Table A-2-f).

Biotin

Deficiency

Biotin deficiency has occasionally been induced in patients who consumed large amounts of raw egg white over a prolonged period. Egg white contains avidin, which antagonizes the action of biotin. The skin of the face and hands becomes dry, shining, and scaling. The oral mucosa and tongue are swollen, magenta, and painful.

The most clear-cut cases of biotin deficiency occurred in children and adults maintained on long-term TPN in the early days before biotin was included in commercial vitamin formulations. An infant with short gut syndrome received TPN from 5 months of age. Five months later, the infant lost all body hair and developed a waxy pallor, irritability, lethargy, mild hypotonia, and an erythematous rash. Biotin deficiency was confirmed biochemically, and all signs were reversed by supplementation (55). Two adult patients receiving home parenteral nutrition after extensive gut resection developed hair loss that was reversed by 200 μg biotin given intravenously daily (56). Another adult with alopecia, rash, and metabolic acidosis responded to 60 μg of biotin added to parenteral fluids (Fig. 38.2D).

Who Is at Risk of Deficiency? Deficiency of the enzyme biotinidase results in decreased absorption of the vitamin from the intestinal tract and perhaps from the glomerular filtrate. The resulting biotin depletion has been termed secondary biotin deficiency. Treatment of enzyme-deficient persons with 50 to 150 μg/day overcomes the symptoms of deficiency.

Long-term anticonvulsant therapy may lead to biotin deficiency sufficient to impair amino acid metabolism (57). Reduced blood, liver, or urinary excretion has been reported in alcoholism, malabsorption syndromes, and protein-energy malnutrition.

Who Is at Risk of Excess/Toxicity?

No reports of adverse effects of biotin intake up to 200 mg orally or 20 mg intravenously have been published.

Vitamin B$_{12}$ (Cobalamin)

Deficiency

Deficiency may be primary or secondary, as in pernicious anemia.

Pernicious Anemia. Pernicious anemia, an autoimmune disorder resulting in a deficiency of intrinsic factor, is usually manifest after middle age, especially in persons with prematurely gray hair and blue eyes. A slight female preponderance exists. The most common complaints—those associated with anemia—ordinarily do not arise until the anemia is well advanced. Neurologic changes may long precede the hematologic changes. The tongue may be red, smooth, shining, and painful. Anorexia, weight loss, indigestion, and episodic diarrhea are all usually present. In advanced cases, patients usually have pyrexia, enlargement of the liver and spleen, and occasionally bruising resulting from thrombocytopenia. Older patients may present with congestive cardiac failure.

Distal sensory neuropathy with "glove and stocking" sensory loss, paresthesias, and areflexia may occur in isolation or more commonly together with a form of myelopathy known as subacute combined degeneration of the spinal cord. In this condition, the initial symptom is symmetric paresthesias of the feet or, occasionally, of the hands. A combination of weakness and loss of postural sense makes walking increasingly difficult. Psychiatric disturbances, especially mild dementia, may be the presenting or only feature. Visual loss from optic atrophy is not uncommon. Congenital lack of intrinsic factor presents before the age of 2 years with irritability, vomiting, diarrhea, weight loss, and megaloblastic anemia.

Primary Dietary Deficiency. When dietary lack or malabsorption is the cause of deficiency, megaloblastic anemia is usually the most prominent feature, but glossitis, optic atrophy, and subacute combined degeneration of the cord have also been described. Hyperpigmentation of the skin of the forearms has been reported. Megaloblastic anemia developed in an infant who was exclusively breast-fed by a vegan mother (58).

Who Is at Risk of Deficiency? Many other causes of vitamin B_{12} deficiency exist in addition to pernicious anemia, malabsorption, and long-term vegan diets. Numerous inherited disorders of cobalamin metabolism have signs or symptoms presenting early in children, such as failure to thrive, or with neurologic disorders that may not present until early adulthood. One genetic disorder involves failure to form the transport protein transcobalamin II that binds to vitamin B_{12} in the terminal ileum and transports it in the plasma to the cells. The effects of this deficiency present within the first 2 months of life and may be lethal. An absorption defect presenting between 1 and 2 years of age is the Grasbeck-Immerslund syndrome, with a low serum vitamin B_{12} level and megaloblastic anemia despite the presence of normal gastric juice and intestinal function.

Pancreatic insufficiency leads to a rise in intestinal pH and impaired digestion of haptocorrins. These changes result in a failure to transfer vitamin B_{12} to intrinsic factor and impaired vitamin B_{12} absorption in the ileum. Bariatric surgical procedures that bypass the stomach or duodenum often produce vitamin B_{12} deficiency. Resection or damage to the terminal ileum by surgery, radiation, or disease also markedly reduces vitamin B_{12} absorption. Both the blind loop syndrome and infestation by fish tapeworm cause vitamin B_{12} deficiency because of the uptake of the vitamin by microorganism flourishing in the loop and by the tapeworm in the intestine.

Deficiency in frail elderly persons may lead to neurologic symptoms in the absence of the megaloblastic anemia that usually serve as warning signs of deficiency (59). A possible factor in the neurologic symptoms is the combination of the hyperhomocysteinemia induced by the folate deficiency and increased serum methylmalonic acid from the vitamin B_{12} deficiency (60).

Folic Acid

Deficiency

The anemia of folic acid deficiency has morphologic features indistinguishable from those of vitamin B_{12} deficiency, but it develops much more rapidly. Subacute combined degeneration of the spinal cord does not occur, but about 20% of patients may have peripheral neuropathy. The tongue may be red and painful in the acute stage. In chronic deficiency, the tongue papillae atrophy, leaving a shiny, smooth surface. Hyperpigmentation of the skin similar to that occasionally seen in vitamin B_{12} deficiency has been noted.

Folic acid therapy before conception is now accepted as protective against neural tube defects in infants of families in which these abnormalities have previously arisen (61). Low plasma folate levels were associated with increased risk of early spontaneous abortion (62). Inadequate one-carbon metabolism in conditions associated with genetic mutations and hyperhomocysteinemia is described elsewhere in this text.

Who Is at Risk of Deficiency? Chronic alcoholism, usually associated with inadequate intake, interferes with folate metabolism (63). Malabsorption syndromes with one of multiple diseases of the small intestine place the patient at risk, in addition to certain drugs or inherited deficiencies (see Table 28.2, Chapter 28).

Who Is at Risk of Excess/Toxicity?

The required addition of 400-μg per serving of ready-to-eat cereals has raised the question of excess. Using data from the Food and Drug Administration, the Food and Nutrition Board of the Institute of Medicine stated: "it is unlikely that intake of folate added to foods or as supplements would regularly exceed 1000 μg for any of the life stage or gender groups" (64).

Administration of folate for megalobastic anemia should be given only after ruling out cobalamin deficiency as the primary cause, because folate administration may improve the hematologic manifestations of vitamin B_{12} deficiency without arresting its neurologic effects.

Caution should be exercised in the use of nitrous oxide anesthesia because of the possibility of the presence of a rare and severe methylene tetrahydrofolate reductase deficiency that may lead, as it did in the case of a child, to death associated with high homocysteine and low methionine blood levels (65, 66).

Pantothenic Acid

Deficiency

Researchers claimed that a "burning feet syndrome" in adult volunteers on a deficient diet responded to pantothenic acid. This distressing condition has rarely responded to this treatment. At present no certain clinical manifestation of dietary pantothenic acid deficiency exists.

Who Is at Risk of Deficiency? A genetic mutation encodes pantothenate-kinase2 (PANK2), a key regulatory enzyme in the biosynthesis of coenzyme A (67). The associated Hallevorden-Spatz syndrome is characterized by dystonia, parkinsonism, and iron accumulation in the brain (68). Acanthosis and a defect in plasma lipoproteins have been noted in association with these mutations (69). Despite speculation that supplemental pantothenate would compensate for partial enzyme deficiency (68), we are not aware of any published studies on this matter.

Patients with chronic alcoholism may be depleted of pantothenate because of interference with its metabolism. Patients with diabetes have increased vitamin excretion.

Vitamin C (Ascorbic Acid)

Deficiency

Infantile Scurvy (Barlow Disease). The onset of infantile scurvy, usually in the second half of the first year of life, is preceded by a period of fretfulness, pallor, and loss of appetite. Localizing signs are tenderness and swelling, most marked at the knees or ankles. These signs result from characteristic bone changes demonstrable by radiograph.

The infant often adopts the "pithed frog" position of maximum comfort, with the legs flexed at the knees and the hips partially flexed and externally rotated. The arms are less commonly involved. Hemorrhage and spongy changes in the gums are confined to the sites of teeth that have recently erupted or are about to do so. Bleeding may occur anywhere in the skin (the orbit is a frequent site) or from mucous membranes, including the renal tract. In infancy, intracranial hemorrhages are rapidly progressive if treatment is delayed, and death may occur. Petechiae and ecchymoses, usually found in the region of the bone lesions, are less common than in the adult. Microcytic hypochromic anemia is common, a normochromic normocytic picture less so. Older children may develop the perifollicular hemorrhages and hair changes seen in the adult.

Adult Scurvy. Early symptoms of adult scurvy are weakness, easy fatigue, and listlessness, followed by shortness of breath and aching bones, joints, and muscles, especially at night. These symptoms are followed by characteristic changes in the skin (70). Acne, indistinguishable from that of adolescence, precedes defects in the hairs of the body. These defects consist of broken and coiled ("corkscrew") hairs and a "swan-neck" deformity. Perifollicular hemorrhages and perifollicular hyperkeratosis are common, especially on the thorax, forearms, thighs, legs, and anterior abdominal wall (Fig. 38.2*E* and *F*).

Frank bleeding is a late feature of scurvy. The classic gum changes are only associated with natural teeth or buried

roots and are enhanced by poor dental hygiene and advanced caries. The interdental papillae become swollen and purple and bleed with trauma. In advanced scurvy, the gums are spongy and friable, bleeding freely. Secondary infection leads to loosening of the teeth and to gangrene. Patients who are edentulous or whose teeth are in good repair have little or no evidence of scorbutic gingivitis. Hemorrhage commonly occurs deep in muscles and into joints as well as over large areas of the skin in the form of ecchymoses. Multiple splinter hemorrhages may form a crescent near the distal ends of the nails. Old scars break down, and new wounds fail to heal. Bleeding into viscera or the brain leads to convulsions and shock; death may occur abruptly.

Who is at risk of excess/toxicity?

Chronic intake of vitamin C in excess of the adult tolerable upper limit of 2000 mg/day can cause diarrhea, kidney stones, and excess iron absorption.

Choline

The feeding of a choline-deficient diet restricted in methionine resulted in decreased choline stores in a large number of species ranging from rodents to baboons and caused liver dysfunction in most. Many also had growth retardation, renal dysfunction, hemorrhage, or bone abnormalities (71).

A low-choline diet ingested for 3 weeks by healthy men resulted in decreased plasma choline levels and some abnormal liver functions as indicated by a liver function test (72). In a placebo-controlled study of patients receiving parenteral feeding that compared a choline- and lipid-free formula plus placebo to a similar one with choline, liver chemistry studies became elevated, with evidence of liver steatosis. No changes in total bilirubin, hemoglobin, hematocrit, white cells, platelets, or other blood chemistry studies were noted (73). In a pilot study with patients receiving TPN, evidence indicated that a low-choline formula caused verbal and visual impairment (74).

However, evidence of a choline requirement in experimental laboratory animals occurred only in those with reduced dietary methionine. This finding is relevant because of the close relationships of choline, methionine, folate, and vitamin B_{12}. The human studies did not examine the role of added methionine or cysteine or of the vitamins that could have been inadequate. It is not certain whether these limited human experiments merit the inclusion of choline in the DRIs as an essential nutrient (see Appendix Table A-2-e).

ESSENTIAL FATTY ACIDS

ω-6 Essential Fatty Acid Deficiency

Growth retardation, sparse hair growth, branlike desquamation of the skin of the trunk, poor wound healing, and increased susceptibility to infection have been observed in infants receiving a formula deficient in essential fat or in children and adults receiving long-term, lipid-free parenteral nutrition (75). Sometimes, patients have only dry, flaky skin, but more advanced deficiency results in scaling, eczematoid dermatitis, usually starting on the nasolabial folds and eyebrows and spreading across the face and neck. Anemia and enlarged fatty liver have also been reported.

ω-3 Essential Fatty Acid Deficiency

The first human report of ω-3 EFA deficiency was of a 7-year-old girl with extensive gut resection who received TPN rich in ω-6 but very low in ω-3 fatty acids. Neurologic changes included paresthesias, weakness, inability to walk, pain in the legs, and blurred vision (76). These symptoms are reported to have responded to change of treatment, but it is possible that other deficiencies, including that of vitamin E, could have been responsible. Other possible cases have since been reported, and the subject has been reviewed (77). It now appears that the symptoms of the two kinds of fatty acid deficiency are quite distinct.

MINERALS

Calcium

Hypocalcemia

Symptoms and signs of underlying disorders are present in hypocalcemia. True hypocalcemia (i.e., subnormal ionized calcium) in clinical conditions is rarely caused by inadequate calcium ingestion but rather by a disorder of calcium metabolism involving the parathyroid gland, calcitriol, and, in infants and children, calcitonin. It affects the nervous system with depression and psychosis and progresses to dementia or encephalopathy. The most characteristic syndrome is tetany, consisting of the following: (a) paresthesias about the lips, tongue, fingers, and feet; (b) carpopedal spasm, resulting in Trousseau sign, a deformity that may be painful and prolonged (Fig. 38.2G); (c) generalized muscle aching; and (d) spasm of the facial muscles. At the earlier stage of latent tetany, neuromuscular irritability may be elicited by provocative tests. Chvostek sign is contraction of the facial muscles on light tapping of the facial nerve. Trousseau sign is carpopedal spasm induced by restriction of the blood supply to a limb by a blood pressure cuff applied for 3 minutes or less. Rarely, cataract is the earliest feature.

In about 80% of very-low-birth-weight infants, osteopenia can be diagnosed radiologically, and rickets is much less common (78). In the neonate and older infant, tetany may manifest as rhythmic, focal myoclonic jerks, sometimes followed by convulsions, cyanosis, and heart failure. Muscular spasms and laryngismus stridulus may occur in young children.

Osteoporosis. Calcium insufficiency, especially during growth, when bone mass is developing, and in later life is a risk factor for osteoporosis. It is common in elderly persons, especially in postmenopausal white women. Patients have bone deformity, localized pain, and fractures. Osteomalacia may coexist. The most common deformity is loss of height caused by vertebral collapse, which accounts for most of the pain. Fractures of the neck of the femur and Colles fracture above the wrist are most commonly precipitated by trauma, which may be trivial, in elderly persons with osteoporosis.

Calcium-Deficiency Rickets. True rickets can be produced by dietary calcium deficiency in the presence of normal vitamin D status (79). Such cases respond better to calcium therapy alone than to vitamin D supplementation alone (80).

Who Is at Risk of Deficiency? In clinical conditions, the most common cause of hypocalcemia is low serum albumin, reflecting decreased binding of calcium ions and without significance with respect to calcium metabolism. Aside from endocrinologically induced disturbances of calcium metabolism, a frequent cause of hypocalcemia is magnesium deficiency induced by intestinal malabsorption syndromes, renal wasting induced by hypoparathyroidism, genetic tubular defects, alcoholism, diabetes mellitus, and certain drugs such as cisplatins and long-term use of loop diuretics.

Failure to achieve optimal peak bone mass by young adulthood and subsequent intestinal and renal factors inducing calcium loss and poor physical activity all predispose to osteoporosis, especially in elderly persons.

Hypercalcemia

Hypercalcemia has a variety of causes including hyperparathyroidism and malignancy. It produces a symptom complex that is, to some extent, characteristic. Gastrointestinal symptoms include anorexia, nausea, vomiting, constipation, abdominal pain, and ileus. Renal system involvement produces polyuria, nocturia, polydipsia, stone formation, and sometimes hypertension and signs and symptoms of uremia. Muscle weakness and myopathy occur. Severe hypercalcemia, that causes psychosis, delirium, stupor, and coma, may be fatal.

Who Is at Risk of Excess/Toxicity? Hypercalcemia caused by excessive calcium intake is uncommon even in those ingesting large doses of calcium supplements. However, the combination of calcium supplements with sodium bicarbonate increases risk of nephrolithiasis.

Phosphorus

Hypophosphatemia

Hypophosphatemia (serum concentration <0.71 mmol/L, or 2.2 mg/dL) can occur with or without a significant decrease in total-body phosphate. Acute hypophosphatemia, without total-body phosphate depletion, occurs in any situation stimulating anaerobic glycolysis, such as infusion of hypertonic glucose (e.g., TPN), especially in cachectic patients without adequate phosphate replacement. This results in a rapid shift of phosphate into cells, thereby reducing serum phosphate and potentially depleting adenosine diphosphate levels and impairing multiple phosphate-requiring metabolic processes, including glycolysis. Marked hypophosphatemia (usually <0.30 mmol/L, or 0.93 mg/dL), for which cachectic patients are particularly at risk, can cause the refeeding syndrome, which consists of dramatic hyperglycemia, weakness, muscle paralysis, cardiorespiratory failure, and, unless treated promptly, death (81).

Total-Body Phosphate Depletion. Total-body phosphate depletion occurs with total-body nitrogen loss as the result of various diseases that lead to excessive loss of both in the stool (e.g., malabsorption, vitamin D deficiency) or in the urine (e.g., hyperparathyroidism, congenital or drug-induced renal tubular acidosis, severe potassium depletion). In the management of advanced renal disease, administration of phosphate-binding gels intended to reduce phosphate absorption in association with restricted phosphate in the diet may lead to symptomatic phosphate deficiency (82, 83).

Who Is at Risk of Deficiency? Because of the wide distribution of phosphate compounds in foods, phosphate depletion in healthy persons is very uncommon. Hypophosphatemia of both types mentioned earlier, however, is not uncommon in persons with serious clinical problems. Hyperventilation and respiratory alkalosis result in acute hypophosphatemia as intracellular pH rises, causing increased phosphofructokinase activity with phosphorylation of intracellular glucose. The resulting fall in intracellular phosphate causes plasma phosphate to enter the cell, thus depleting plasma levels. Acute hypophosphatemia also occurs after the infusion of glucose into cachectic patients on parenteral feeding, in diabetic patients with ketoacidosis who are given insulin, and in patents with chronic alcoholism during alcohol withdrawal and potassium infusions without accompanying phosphate administration.

Persons with X-linked hypophosphatemic rickets, autosomal dominant hypophosphatemic rickets, and osteogenic osteomalacia have both renal phosphate wasting and decreased phosphate absorption.

Who Is at Risk of Excess/Toxicity?

Chronic hyperphosphatemia (serum phosphorus >5 mg/dL) is a problem in advanced renal disease and in hypoparathyroidism. These conditions are potentially serious because of calcification of soft tissues.

Potassium

Deficiency

Potassium deficiency is usually the result of excessive losses in urine or stool, less commonly decreased intake, as in starvation or failure to give potassium in intravenous solutions, and losses in sweat, as in cystic fibrosis.

Severe hypokalemia (serum potassium <3 mmol/L, or <3 mEq/L) may cause muscle weakness leading to respiratory failure, paralytic ileus, hypotension, and tetany. Potassium-losing nephropathy results in polyuria with secondary polydipsia. Cardiac effects are particularly likely in patients receiving digitalis. The electrocardiogram is characteristic, with ST segment depression, increased U-wave amplitude, and T-wave amplitude less than that of U-wave amplitude in the same lead. Premature ventricular and atrial contractions and ventricular and atrial tachyarrhythmias occur.

Toxicity (Hyperkalemia)

Acute oliguric states are often responsible for hyperkalemia, but excessive ingestion or infusion may produce symptoms even in the presence of normal renal function. Cardiac toxicity, of serious import, starts with shortening of the QT interval of the electrocardiogram and tall, peaked T waves. Progressive toxicity with serum potassium levels greater than 6.5 mmol/L (>6.5 mEq/L) causes nodal and ventricular arrhythmias, widening of the QRS complex, PR interval prolongation and disappearance of the P wave, and, finally, degeneration of the QRS complex with ventricular asystole or fibrillation and death.

Magnesium

Deficiency

In depletion studies in humans as well as in clinical practice, when hypomagnesemia (defined as serum magnesium <1.5 mEq/L, <1.9 mg/dL) progresses to less than 1.0 mEq/L, it is often accompanied by hypocalcemia and hypokalemia.

The early symptoms and signs of both experimental and clinical deficiency are primarily neuromuscular: Trousseau and Chvostek signs, muscle fasciculations, tremor, muscle spasm, with later personality changes, anorexia, nausea, and vomiting. Despite the hypocalcemia present in severe magnesium deficiency, deep tendon reflexes are normal or depressed. Low dietary intake of magnesium was associated with impaired lung function and wheezing (84). Convulsion or coma in infancy is not infrequently associated with magnesium deficiency. In some clinical situations, serum magnesium may be within normal limits despite evidence of cellular or tissue depletion.

Who Is at Risk of Deficiency? Magnesium depletion in children and adults occurs from numerous conditions resulting in malabsorption of magnesium of various causes (inborn error or disease related) and from urinary wasting from genetic and disease-related disorders, nephrotoxic and loop diuretic drugs, diabetes, and severe phosphate and/or potassium depletion.

Toxicity (Hypermagnesemia)

Nausea and vomiting may appear in persons with serum magnesium levels greater than 3 mEq/L. At levels higher than 5 mEq/L, deep tendon reflexes disappear, and electrocardiographic abnormalities (prolonged PR interval, widening of QRS complex, and increased T-wave amplitude) occur. Hypotension, respiratory depression, narcosis, and ultimately cardiac arrest may occur with levels grater than 8 mEq/L.

Who Is at Risk of Excess/Toxicity? Hypermagnesemia is induced for therapeutic reasons in some clinical conditions, such as in the management of preeclampsia and eclampsia, in which high-dose magnesium sulfate is administered parenterally as the drug of choice in preventing convulsions. It is also given orally as a cathartic and with activated charcoal in the treatment of suspected drug overdose. Close medical supervision is required to prevent complications. Significant problems may occur with long-term ingestion of magnesium cathartics by persons with significant renal disease, with the escalating signs and symptoms noted earlier.

Iodide (Iodine)

Deficiency

Enlargement of the thyroid gland is the most common clinical sign of iodide deficiency. When it is the result of iodine lack, this condition is termed simple, colloid, endemic, or euthyroid goiter. It is more common in women and is often noted at the onset of puberty, during pregnancy, or at the menopause. Early on, the enlargement is soft, symmetric, and smooth; later, multiple nodules and cysts may appear. Most patients are euthyroid, a few have hyperthyroidism, and rarely hypothyroidism occurs.

Severe endemic goiter is often accompanied by cretinism. Endemic cretinism occurs in two distinct forms, the myxedematous and the neurologic, which may coexist (85). In most areas of the world, the neurologic form is by far the more common.

In recent years, attention has been focused on the effects of iodine deficiency in early life (86). It is responsible for a proportion of stillbirths, spontaneous abortions, congenital malformations, and neonatal deaths. Physical growth and mental development are impaired in early childhood.

Who Is at Risk of Deficiency? Persons living in areas where iodine has been leached from the soil surface are at risk. This deficiency is likely to occur in all mountainous regions as well as areas scoured by glaciation or heavy rainfall, as indicated by a very low iodine content of uniodized drinking water (87). In 1993, the World Health Organization estimated that about 1.6 billion people were at risk of iodine deficiency disorders (88). Under such conditions, ingestion of foods containing thyroid-inhibitory substances (goitrogens), such as cassava and millet, inhibit the ability of the thyroid gland to make the hormone.

Toxicity

Prolonged excessive intake of iodine leads eventually to iodide goiter and myxedema, especially in patients with preexisting Hashimoto thyroiditis.

Who Is at Risk of Excess/Toxicity? As indicated in the DRI data in Table 15.1 in Chapter 15, fairly large amounts of iodine are well tolerated by most persons; however, for some, the iodine load inhibits the thyroid's ability to make or release thyroid hormone, thus inducing hypothyroidism. Excess iodine may occur in radiocontrast media, sterilizing agents, and certain drugs (amiodarone).

Iron

Deficiency

Iron deficiency has its major impact on many systems via reduction in tissue oxygenation resulting from decreased hemoglobin concentration. The clinical picture depends on the rapidity of development of anemia and on its severity.

The typical microcytic hypochromic anemia of insidious onset manifests as increasing fatigue and slight pallor, best seen in the mucous membranes. Later, cardiorespiratory signs and symptoms include exertional dyspnea, tachycardia, palpitations, angina, claudication, night cramps, increased arterial and capillary pulsation, cardiac bruits, reversible cardiac enlargement, and, if cardiac failure occurs, basal crepitations, peripheral edema, and ascites. Neuromuscular involvement is evidenced by headache, tinnitus, vertigo, cramps, faintness, increased cold sensitivity, and retinal hemorrhage. Gastrointestinal symptoms include anorexia, nausea, constipation, and diarrhea. Low-grade fever, menstrual irregularity, urinary frequency, and loss of libido may occur.

Iron deficiency per se has certain characteristics not usually associated with other forms of anemia. Nonspecific glossitis with almost complete loss of filiform papillae is common. Angular stomatitis is less frequent. Spoon-shaped nails (koilonychia) are characteristic of long-standing iron deficiency. The Patterson-Kelly (Plummer-Vinson) syndrome is the association of iron deficiency anemia, glossitis, dysphagia, and achlorhydria, usually seen in middle-aged women, but much less commonly than was formerly the case. In severe cases, postcricoid webs and malignant change in this region may occur. Signs of deficiency of some B group vitamins are also often present. Pica (geophagia) is an occasional feature. Even mild iron deficiency is considered important in decreased work efficiency (89). In infants and young children, psychomotor development is impaired, but it improves after iron supplementation in anemic children (90).

Who Is at Risk of Deficiency? Iron deficiency exists without or with anemia (approximately in a ratio of 3:1 or 4:1 in the United States). The main causes are: low intake of bioavailable iron, particularly in those undergoing rapid growth, menstruation, or pregnancy; chronic blood loss, such as in ulcer disease, gastrointestinal malignancy or other gastrointestinal disorder; hookworm infestation; or schistosomiasis. Infection with *Helicobacter pylori* is associated with decreased iron stores and anemia. Blood lead levels are higher in iron-deficient children, and children with iron deficiency are at increased risk of lead poisoning. Bariatric surgery procedures that bypass the duodenum, where iron absorption mainly occurs, commonly lead to iron deficiency; routine supplementation is advisable (91, 92).

Toxicity

Acute iron poisoning causes vomiting, upper abdominal pain, pallor, cyanosis, diarrhea, drowsiness, and shock. Death may occur in children mistaking iron tablets for sweets.

Chronic toxicity (hemochromatosis, iron overload) affects many tissues. Diabetes, often the presenting feature, eventually develops in about 80% of patients. The skin is a characteristic slate-gray. The liver becomes enlarged and then cirrhotic, and hepatocellular cancer may develop in about 30% of patients with cirrhosis. Cardiomyopathy leads to heart failure in about 50% of patients, and mental aberrations may occur. Pituitary failure may cause testicular atrophy and loss of libido. Focal hemosiderosis damages the lungs and kidneys.

Who Is at Risk of Excess/Toxicity? Hereditary hemochromatosis is a common autosomal recessive disorder (three to five per thousand) in persons descended from Northern European, western and southern German, and northern Spanish ancestry. With the sequlae noted earlier, treatment includes vigorous phlebotomy to remove iron excess. Screening tests for iron excess are recommended beginning at the age of 20 years and repeated every few decades if negative in high risk groups.

Sub-Saharan hemochromatosis also appears to have a genetic basis, but it is usually associated with long-term diets high in iron derived from cooking pots or steel barrels used in preparation of fermented alcoholic beverages. Portal cirrhosis and diabetes are common.

Copper

Deficiency

The principal features of copper deficiency are hypochromic anemia (unresponsive to iron therapy), neutropenia, and osteoporosis. Early radiologic findings are osteoporosis of the metaphyses and epiphyses and retarded bone age. Typical findings are increased density of the provisional zone of calcification and cupping with sickle-shaped spurs in the metaphyseal region. Other skeletal abnormalities include periosteal layering and submetaphyseal and rib fractures.

Premature infants are especially vulnerable and have shown the following signs: pallor, decreased pigmentation of the skin and hair, prominent superficial veins, skin lesions resembling seborrheic dermatitis, failure to thrive, diarrhea, and hepatosplenomegaly. Some infants have features suggesting central nervous system damage, including hypotonia, apathy, psychomotor retardation, apparent lack of visual responses, and apneic episodes.

The most extreme form is seen in Menkes steely hair disease (93), a complex fatal X-linked disease of male infants in which both failure to absorb copper and then failure to form functional cuproteins occur. Interference with cross-linking of elastin and collagen because of dysfunction of lysyl oxidase is responsible for many of the features: premature rupture of the membranes leading to premature birth, lax skin and joints, elongation and dilatation of major arteries resulting in rupture and hemorrhage, subintimal thickening with partial occlusion of major arteries, hernias, and diverticula of bladder and ureters causing recurrent infection or rupture and osteoporosis. Lack of pigmentation of the skin and hair and abnormal spiral twisting (pili torti) and fragility of hair add to the characteristic appearance of affected babies. Neurologic development rarely progresses beyond 6 to 8 weeks, and even these functions are lost during the ensuing months. Ataxia is striking in mild cases. Parenteral copper increases serum copper and ceruloplasmin but does not improve the underlying disease.

Who Is at Risk of Deficiency? Copper depletion with signs and symptoms has been documented in infants recovering from malnutrition when copper is not included in the new diet, in some premature and low-birth-weight infants limited to milk diets, in malabsorptive diseases when the supplementation is not given, and, in previous years, in patients receiving prolonged TPN without added copper. Sterile copper salt solutions are available; occasionally, however, patients with biliary obstruction who excrete copper poorly may be mistakenly placed on copper-free solutions with resultant copper deficiency during prolonged feeding.

Who Is at Risk of Excess/Toxicity?

Acute poisoning has resulted from ingestion of solutions of copper salts or contaminated water supplies or dialysis fluid, especially in persons with biliary obstruction. In severe cases, evidence of hepatic or renal failure (or both) is found. Ceruloplasmin, a copper-containing protein that is also an acute-phase reactant, may rise two- or threefold higher than normal in various inflammatory conditions and in diabetes, cardiovascular disease, uremia, and trauma.

In Wilson disease (hepatolenticular degeneration), the Wilson protein, ATP7B, is deficient, commonly leading to cirrhosis, deposits in the brain (resulting in tremors, choreoathetoid movements, rigidity, dysarthria, and eventually dementia), anemia, and renal failure, with characteristic changes in the eye (the Kayser-Fleischer ring).

Indian child cirrhosis is a hereditary disease associated with rapid accumulation of copper in the liver when the diet is high in this ion. It occurs in children in the Indian subcontinent but also occurs in Indian children living elsewhere. It has been attributed to copper accumulation in the liver, and its development requires excessive copper ingestion (94, 95). Previously fatal, this disease can respond to chelation of copper that improves these patients' chances of survival.

Zinc

Deficiency

The first report of human zinc deficiency was from Iran and consisted of a syndrome of dwarfism, hypogonadism, anemia, hepatosplenomegaly, rough dry skin, and lethargy associated with geophagia (96). In a similar picture in Egypt, parasitism appears to play an important role. Hypogeusia (impaired taste) and growth retardation in otherwise healthy children have been found to respond to zinc supplementation in parts of North America (97). Zinc supplementation in pregnant women with relatively low plasma zinc levels was associated with higher infant birth weights and head circumferences (98).

Clinical cases of zinc deficiency have been reported with various manifestations, depending on the severity of depletion and other factors. In addition to those mentioned earlier they include dermatoses, immune deficiencies, glossitis, photophobia, lack of dark adaptation, and delayed wound healing. Precipitating factors include short bowel syndrome (Fig. 38.1H), alcoholism with pancreatic and liver disease, sickle cell anemia, certain chelating medications, the acrodermatitis enteropathica genotype, intestinal losses via fistula (Fig. 38.24), and inadequate amounts of zinc in parenteral nutrition fluids.

TPN with inadequate zinc supplementation has occasionally caused an acute deficiency syndrome consisting of diarrhea, mental depression, alopecia, and dermatitis, usually around the orbits, nose, and mouth (99). Severe loss of zinc through an intestinal fistula was responsible for

development of skin lesions about the mouth, palms (sterile pustules), and pressure points on hands and elbows in a 6-year-old child with non-Hodgkin lymphoma (Fig. 38.2H); the lesions responded rapidly to additional zinc.

Acrodermatitis enteropathica, an autosomal recessive disorder caused by a defect in zinc absorption, is characterized by extensive dermatitis, growth retardation, diarrhea, hair loss, and paronychia. The skin changes somewhat resemble those seen in kwashiorkor (100), but the skin changes of zinc deficiency have a typical appearance: the distribution is often acroorificial, commonly also involving the flexures and friction areas, and lesions may become generalized. Eczematoid, psoriaform, vesiculobullous, and pustular lesions may be present. The earliest skin lesions are bright reddish, nonscaly macules and patches.

Who Is at Risk of Deficiency? Persons, especially the young, who subsist primarily on foodstuffs low in zinc and high in phytate (that interferes with absorption) in areas in Asia, Africa, and the Eastern Mediterranean are at risk. Because zinc is lost in diarrhea, infections and parasitism affecting the gastrointestinal tract are additional and often important factors in infants and small children with marked stool losses. Malabsorptive disorders, radiation enteritis, and surgical loss of intestine with significant chronic diarrhea are significant risks, especially if food intake is poor.

Chelating drugs used in Wilson disease and in iron overload impair zinc absorption. As noted earlier, the rare genetic disorder acrodermatitis enteropathica produces zinc deficiency. Long-term use of TPN with inadequate zinc also represents a risk.

Who Is at Risk of Excess/Toxicity?

Ingestion of large amounts of zinc, usually from an acid food or drink from a galvanized container, or long-term consumption of high doses of zinc supplements, has caused vomiting and diarrhea. Accidental intravenous administration of 1.5 g has proven fatal. In addition to the causes of toxicity listed earlier, increased zinc fortification of various foods and supplements in the United States has resulted in increasing numbers of young children (and probably others) with an intake level that is rising toward the DRI's upper limit (101).

Fluoride

Deficiency

Fluorine has not been proved an essential element for humans, but it has a role in bone mineralization and hardening of tooth enamel. Areas with low fluorine content in the water supply have high rates of dental caries. Fluoridation of the water or use of supplemented tooth paste is associated with a significant fall in dental caries rates.

Toxicity (Fluorosis)

Fluorosis is associated with high levels (>10 ppm) in the drinking water. It is most evident in permanent teeth that develop during high fluorine intake. Deciduous teeth are affected only at very high levels. The earliest changes, chalky white, irregularly distributed patches on the surface of the enamel, become infiltrated by yellow or brown staining, giving rise to the characteristic "mottled" appearance (Fig. 38.1G). More severe fluorosis also causes pitting of the enamel. Long-term ingestion of very large amounts of fluoride (>5 mg/day) for years may lead to crippling skeletal fluorosis progressing from occasional stiffness or joint pain to chronic pain and osteoporosis of long bones. This rare condition is associated with drinking high-fluoride well water (102).

Selenium

Deficiency

Two syndromes have been described in areas of China where the soil is deficient in selenium. The first is Keshan disease, named for its place of origin, which consists of a highly fatal cardiomyopathy affecting mainly young children and women of childbearing age. Good response to selenium supplementation has been reported (103). The other, known as Kashin-Beck disease, features osteoarthritis during preadolescence or adolescence that results in dwarfing and joint deformities from cartilage abnormalities (104). However, the evidence for a role of selenium is now questionable; it may instead be related to iodine deficiency (105). Selenium deficiency was reported in patients receiving long-term TPN before the addition of selenium to TPN solutions became routine (106). Features included severe cardiomyopathy with localized necrosis, muscle pain and tenderness, dyschromotrichia, white fingernail beds, and macrocytosis.

Who Is at Risk of Deficiency? In most of the United States, selenium intake is more than adequate because of the widespread use of wheat products usually grown on soils high in selenium. In contrast, in New Zealand, where the soil is low in selenium, levels of plasma selenium and glutathione peroxidase are low. However, signs and symptoms of deficiency are rare there, except in persons with even more severely restricted intakes, such as those infused with selenium-deficient parenteral fluids over a period of time. Similar observations occurred in the United States in the period before selenium was added to TPN solutions; occasional patients developed cardiomyopathy with focal necrosis, muscle tenderness, and weakness, and some died.

Who Is at Risk of Excess/Toxicity?

Endemic selenosis, long recognized in animals, has been suspected in some human communities, most convincingly from China (107). The most frequently observed signs were loss of hair and nails. Skin lesions and polyneuritis were less certainly attributed to selenium toxicity. Alopecia and nail changes occurred from consumption of an over-the-counter supplement containing excessive amounts of selenium (108).

Who Is at Risk of Excess/Toxicity? Public health surveys carried out from 1936 to 1991 in seleniferous areas of the United States failed to establish any symptom specific for selenium poisoning (109). However, a few other countries, particularly China, have documented toxicities during periods of famine when there was emergency ingestion of seleniferous plants.

Chromium

Deficiency

Weight loss, peripheral neuropathy, and glucose intolerance that reversed with chromium therapy were reported in patients receiving prolonged TPN (110, 111).

Toxicity

Toxicity usually results from direct contact or inhalation in industry. Chrome ulcers on the hands or perforation of the nasal septum may result. Lung cancer can occur, but only after exposure to hexavalent compounds.

Molybdenum

Deficiency

An autosomal recessive molybdenum cofactor deficiency resulting in deficiencies of xanthine oxidase and sulfite oxidase was reported in more than 20 patients (112). Patients had severe brain damage and frequent convulsions, and about half failed to survive beyond early infancy.

Only one clear-cut case related to prolonged TPN has been reported to date (113), involving tachycardia, tachypnea, headache, night blindness, central scotomas, nausea, vomiting, lethargy, disorientation, and coma. These signs and symptoms were reversed by 300 μg/day of molybdenum, and the urinary excretion of abnormal amounts of methionine was dramatically decreased.

Toxicity

Elevated blood levels of molybdenum secondary to intakes of 10 to 15 mg/day were associated with hyperuricemia and a goutlike syndrome in Armenia in 1961 (114). However, other authors were unable to confirm this effect of molybdenum (34).

Manganese

Deficiency

One unsubstantiated case of human deficiency was reported to have occurred when manganese was inadvertently omitted from an experimental diet fed to a volunteer. Clinical signs included weight loss, transient dermatitis, nausea and vomiting, changes in hair color, and slow growth of hair (115).

Who Is at Risk of Deficiency? Because all species tested except humans have developed symptomatic experimental manganese deficiency characterized by reproductive failure, poor growth, and serious neurologic defects, manganese in very small amounts was recommended for inclusion in parenteral solutions and enteral feedings. As the result of more recent information about manganese contamination of parenteral fluids, the recommended levels for general use have been lowered.

Toxicity

Manganese toxicity is usually reported in persons who mine or refine ore. Initial signs include insomnia, depression, and delusions, followed by anorexia, arthralgias, and weakness. Eventually changes occur resembling parkinsonism or Wilson disease. Well water with high manganese content may be responsible for occurrence of a parkinsonian syndrome (116). Manganese accumulates in the basal ganglia of patients with biliary obstruction and cirrhosis of the liver, and investigators have suggested that this may be associated with the occurrence of encephalopathy in these patients (117). The excess manganese is associated with high signal intensity in the basal ganglion on a magnetic resonance imaging scan.

Who Is at Risk of Excess/Toxicity? The poisoning of exposed industrial workers has been noted earlier. Because the main route of excretion of manganese is the biliary system, the potential for excessive retention with intravenous feeding or oral intake of high levels escalates markedly when biliary obstruction is present and the warning sign of elevated bilirubin is not heeded. Even with normal liver function, high doses, especially in infants, can elevate blood levels. High signal intensity in the basal ganglia of the brain may occur in such children, and particularly in those with elevated bilirubin and high blood manganese levels. Cessation or marked reduction of manganese administration will reduce the abnormal signaling, as blood levels tend to fall over many weeks or months (118).

REFERENCES

1. Hathcock JN. Am J Clin Nutr 1997;66:427–37.
2. McLaren DS. Nutritional Ophthalmology. New York: Academic Press, 1980.
3. Sommer A, West KP Jr. Vitamin A Deficiency, Health, Survival and Vision. New York: Oxford University Press, 1996.
4. Sommer A, Hussaini G, Muhilal et al. Am J Clin Nutr 1980;33: 887–91.
5. Sommer A, Emran N, Tamba T. Am J Ophthalmol 1979;87: 330–3.
6. Teng KH. Ophthalmologica 1959;137:81–5.
7. International Vitamin A Consultative Group (IVACG). The Symptoms and Signs of Vitamin A Deficiency and Their Relationship to Applied Nutrition. Washington, DC: IVACG, 1981.
8. West KP Jr. J Nutr 2002;132[Suppl]:285S–66S.
9. Underwood BA, Smitasiri S. Annu Rev Nutr 1999;19:303–24.
10. Sommer A, Davidson FR. J Nutr 2002;132:2445–57.
11. Thurnham DO, McCabe GP, Northrop-Celwes CA et al. Lancet 2003;362:2052–8.
12. Hathcock JN, Hattan DG, Jenkins MY et al. Am J Clin Nutr 1990;52:183–202.
13. Lammer EJ, Chen DT, Hoar RM et al. N Engl J Med 1985; 313:837–41.
14. Rothman KJ, Moore LL, Singer MR et al. N Engl J Med 1995; 333:1369–73.
15. Michaelsson K, Lithel H, Vessly B et al. N Engl J Med 2003; 384:287–94.
16. Melhus H, Michaelsson K, Kindmark A et al. Ann Intern Med 1998;129:770–8.
17. Feskanich D, Singh V, Willett C et al. JAMA 2002;287:47–54.
18. Myrhe AM, Carlsen MH, Bohn SK et al. Am J Clin Nutr 2003; 78:1152–9.
19. Train JJA, Yates RW, Sury MRJ. BMJ 1995;310:48–9.
20. Blau EB. Lancet 1996;347:626.
21. Wharton B, Bishop N. Lancet 2003;362:1389–400.
22. Glenrup H, Mikkelsen K, Poulsen L et al. Calcif Tissue Int 2000;66:419–24.
23. Fahrleitner A, Dobnig H, Obernosterer A et al. J Gen Intern Med 2002;17:663–99.
24. Glenrup H, Mikkelsen K, Poulsen L et al. J Intern Med 2000;247:260–8.
25. Black JA, Bonham Carter JE. Lancet 1963;2:745–9.
26. Rosenberg RN. N Engl J Med 1995;333:1351–2.
27. Johnson L, Bowen FW Jr, Abbasi S et al. Pediatrics 1985;75: 619–38.
28. Miller ER 3rd, Pastor-Barriuso R, Dalal D, et al. Ann Intern Med 2005;142:37–46.
29. Shearer MJ. Lancet 1995;345:229–34.
30. American Academy of Pediatrics Committee on Fetus and Newborn. Pediatrics 2003;112:191–2.
31. Pettifor JM, Benson R. J Pediatr 1975;86:459–62.
32. Feskanich D, Weber P, Willett WC et al. Am J Clin Nutr 1999; 69:74–9.
33. Broze GJ, Jr. Lancet 2001;357:900.
34. Food and Nutrition Board, Institute of Medicine. Dietary Reference Intakes for Vitamin A, Vitamin K, Arsenic, Boron, Chromium, Copper, Iodine, Iron, Manganese, Molybdenum, Nickel, Silicon, Vanadium, and Zinc. Washington, DC: National Academy Press, 2001:187 (www.nap.edu/books/0309072794/html/index.html).
35. Campbell CH. Lancet 1984;2:446–9.
36. Jeffrey FE, Abelmann WH. Am J Med 1971;50:123–8.
37. Haas RH. Annu Rev Nutr 1988;8:483–515.
38. Editorial. Lancet 1990;2:912–3.
39. Victor M, Adams RD, Collins GH. The Wernicke-Korsakoff Syndrome. Oxford: Blackwell, 1971.
40. Seehra H, MacDermott N, Lascelles RG et al. BMJ 1996; 312:434.
41. Jelliffe DB. Infant Nutrition in the Tropics and Subtropics. 2nd ed. Geneva: World Health Organization, 1968.
42. Butterworth RF. Am J Clin Nutr. 2001;74:712–3.
43. Nakamura K, Roberson ED, Reilly LG et al. Am J Med 2003; 115:679–80.
44. Food and Nutrition Board, Institute of Medicine. Dietary Reference Intakes for Thiamin, Riboflavin, Niacin, Vitamin B$_6$,

Folate, Vitamin B$_{12}$, Pantothenic Acid, Biotin, and Choline. Washington, DC: National Academy Press, 2000:81 (www.nap.edu/books/0309065542/html/index.html).

45. Stephens JM, Grant R, Yeh CS. Am J Emerg Med 1992;10: 61–3.

46. Lopez R, Cole HS, Montoya MF et al. J Pediatr 1975;87:420–2.

47. Fanelli MI, Wotecki CE. Ann NY Acad Sci 1989;59:20–8.

48. Food and Nutrition Board, Institute of Medicine. Dietary Reference Intakes for Thiamin, Riboflavin, Niacin, Vitamin B$_6$, Folate, Vitamin B$_{12}$, Pantothenic Acid, Biotin, and Choline. Washington, DC: National Academy Press, 2000:115.

49. Hankes LV, Nicotinic acid and nicotinamide. In: Machlin LJ, ed. Handbook of Vitamins. New York: Marcel Dekker, 1984: 329–77.

50. Mueller JE, Vilter RW. J Clin Invest 1950;29:193–201.

51. Snyderman SE, Holt LE, Carretero R et al. Am J Clin Nutr 1953;1:200.

52. Bessey OA, Adam DJ, Hansen AE. Pediatrics 1957;20:33–44.

53. Weintraub LR, Conrad ME, Crosby WH. N Engl J Med 1966; 275:169–76.

54. Schaumberg H, Kaplan J, Windebank A et al. N Engl J Med 1983;309:445–8.

55. Mock DM, DeLorimer AA, Leberman WM et al. N Engl J Med 1981;304:820–3.

56. Innis SM, Allardyce DB. Am J Clin Nutr 1983;37:185–7.

57. Mock DM, Dyhen ME. Neurology 1997;49:1444–7.

58. Higginbottom MC, Sweetman K, Nyhan WL. N Engl J Med 1978;299:317–20.

59. Lindenbaum J, Healton EB, Savage DG et al. N Engl J Med 1988;318:1720–8.

60. Clarke R. Am J Clin Nutr 2001;73:151–2.

61. MRC Vitamin Study Research Group. Lancet 1991;338:131–7.

62. George L, Mills JL, Johansson ALV et al. JAMA 2002;288: 1867–73.

63. Suhja, Herlig AK, Stover PJ. Annu Rev Nutr 2001;21:255–82.

64. Food and Nutrition Board, Institute of Medicine. Dietary Reference Intakes for Thiamin, Riboflavin, Niacin, Vitamin B$_6$, Folate, Vitamin B$_{12}$, Pantothenic Acid, Biotin, and Choline. Washington, DC: National Academy Press, 2000:283.

65. Rothenberg SP, daCosta MP, Sequeira J et al. N Engl J Med 2004;350:134–42.

66. Erbe RW, Salis RJ. N Engl J Med 2003;349:5–6.

67. Zhou B, Westaway SK, Levinson B et al. Nat Genet 2001;28: 45–9.

68. Hayaflick J, Westaway SK, Levinson B et al. N Engl J Med 2003;348:33–40.

69. Ching KHL, Westaway SK, Levinson B et al. Neurology 2002; 58:1673–4.

70. Hodges RF, Hood J, Canham JE et al. Am J Clin Nutr 1971;24: 432–43.

71. Food and Nutrition Board, Institute of Medicine. Dietary Reference Intakes for Thiamin, Riboflavin, Niacin, Vitamin B$_6$, Folate, Vitamin B$_{12}$, Pantothenic Acid, Biotin, and Choline. Washington, DC: National Academy Press, 2000:396.

72. Zeisel SH, da Costa K-A, Franklin PD et al. FASEB J 1991; 5:2093–8.

73. Buchman AC, Ament ME, Sobel M et al. JPEN J Parenter Enteral Nutr 2001;25:260–8.

74. Buchman AL, Sobel M, Brown M et al. JPEN J Parenter Enteral Nutr 2001;25:30–5.

75. Fleming CR, Smith LM, Hodges RE. Am J Clin Nutr 1976;29: 976–83.

76. Holman RT, Johnson SB, Hatch TF. Am J Clin Nutr 1982;35: 617–23.

77. Anderson GJ, Connor WE. Am J Clin Nutr 1989;49:585–7.

78. Bentur L, Alon U, Berant M. Pediatr Rev Commun 1987;1: 291–310.

79. Bishop N. N Engl J Med 1999;341:602–4.

80. Thacher TD, Fischer PR, Pettifor JM et al. N Engl J Med 1999; 341:563–8.

81. Weinsier RL, Krumdieck CL. Am J Clin Nutr 1981;34:393–9.

82. Knochel JP. N Engl J Med 1985;313:447–9.

83. Berner YM, Shike M. Annu Rev Nutr 1988;8:121–48.

84. Britton J, Pavord I, Richards K et al. Lancet 1994;344:357–62.

85. Hetzel BS, Hay ID. Clin Endocrinol 1979;11:445–60.

86. Hetzel BS, Dunm JT. Annu Rev Nutr 1989;9:21–38.

87. Hetzel BS. The Story of Iodine Deficiency. Oxford: Oxford University Press, 1989.

88. World Health Organization. Global Prevalence of Iodine Deficiency Disorders. Geneva: World Health Organization/UNICEF/ICCIDD, 1993:1–80.

89. Andersen HT, Barkve H. Scand J Clin Lab Invest Suppl 1970;25:1–62.

90. Slotzfus RJ, Kvalsvig JD, Chwaya HN et al. BMJ 2001;323: 1389–96.

91. Skroubis G, Sakellaropoulos G, Pouggouras K et al. Obes Surg 2002;12:551–8.

92. Rhode BM, Shustik C, Christou NV et al. Obes Surg 1999; 9:17–21.

93. Danks DM. Annu Rev Nutr 1988;8:235–57.

94. Portmann B, Tanner MS, Mowat AP et al. Lancet 1978;2: 1338–40.

95. Tanner MS. Am J Clin Nutr 1998;1074S–81S.

96. Prasad AS. BMJ 2003;326:409–10.

97. Hambidge KM, Krebs NF, Walravens PA. Nutr Res 1985;1: 306–16.

98. Goldenberg RL, Tamura T, Neggers Y. JAMA 1995;274:463–8.

99. Younaszai HD. JPEN J Parenter Enteral Nutr 1983;7:72–4.

100. Golden MHN, Golden BE. Am J Clin Nutr 1981;34:900–8.

101. Arsenault JE, Brown KH. Am J Clin Nutr 2003;78:1011–7.

102. National Research Council. Health Effects of Ingested Fluoride. Washington, DC: National Academy Press, 1993.

103. Chen X, Yang G, Chen J et al. Biol Trace Elem Res 1980;2: 91–107.

104. Mo D. Pathology and selenium deficiency in Kashin-Beck disease. In: Combs GF Jr, Levander OA, Oldfield JE, eds. Selenium in Biology and Medicine. New York: Van Nostrand Reinhold, 1987:924–33.

105. Moreno-Reyes R, Mathieu F, Boelaert M et al. Am J Clin Nutr 2003;78:137–44.

106. Vinton NE, Dahlstrom KA, Strobel CT et al. J Pediatr 1987; 111:711–7.

107. Yang G, Wang S, Zhou R et al. Am J Clin Nutr 1983;37:872–81.

108. Centers for Disease Control. MMWR Morb Mortal Wkly Rep 1984;33:157–8.

109. Longnecker MP, Taylor PR, Levander OA et al. Am J Clin Nutr 1991;53;1288–94.

110. Jeejeebhoy KN, Chu RC, Marliss EB et al. Am J Clin Nutr 1977;30:531–8.

111. Verhage AH, Cheong WK, Jeejeebhoy KN. JPEN J Parenter Enteral Nutr 1996;20:123–7.

112. Rajagopalan KV. Annu Rev Nutr 1988;8:401–27.

113. Abumrad NN, Schneider AJ, Steele D et al. Am J Clin Nutr 1981;34:2551–9

114. Kovalski VV, Yatovaya GA, Shmavonyau DM. Zh Obshch Biol 1961;22:179.

115. Doisy EA Jr. Effects of deficiency in manganese upon plasma and cholesterol in man. In: Hoekstra WG, Suttie JW, Ganther

HE et al., eds. Trace Element Metabolism in Animals, vol 2. Baltimore: University Park Press, 1974:668–70.

116. Kondakis XG, Makris N, Leotsinidis M et al. Arch Environ Health 1989;44:175–8.

117. Krieger D, Krieger S, Jansen O et al. Lancet 1995;346:270–4.

118. Fell JME, Reynolds AP, Meadows N et al. Lancet 1996;347: 1218–21.

SELECTED READINGS

Food and Nutrition Board, Institute of Medicine. Dietary Reference Intakes. Washington, DC: National Academy Press. The volumes published to date are listed in Appendix Table A-2-a-1.

McLaren DS. A Colour Atlas, and Text of Diet-Related Diseases. New ed. London: Wolfe, 1992.

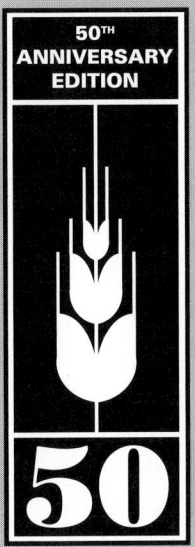

50TH ANNIVERSARY EDITION

50

PART III

NUTRITION IN INTEGRATED BIOLOGIC SYSTEMS

A. Intercellular Regulation: Tutorials / 617
B. Metabolic Regulation: Tutorials / 695

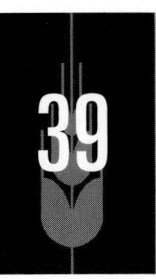

39

NUTRITIONAL REGULATION OF GENE EXPRESSION AND NUTRITIONAL GENOMICS[1]

ROBERT J. COUSINS

HISTORICAL PERSPECTIVE 615
GENOMIC ORGANIZATION AND REGULATION 615
GENE REGULATION BY NUTRIENTS 616
APPROACHES TO IDENTIFY GENES AND PROTEINS
    REGULATED BY INDIVIDUAL NUTRIENTS OR
    DIETARY PATTERNS 616
    Northern Analysis 617
    In Situ RNA Hybridization 618
    Solution Hybridization/RNase Protection Assays . .618
    Polymerase Chain Reaction 619
    Promoter Analysis 621
    Differential mRNA Display 621
    DNA Array Analysis 621
    Positional Cloning 622
    Polyacrylamide Electrophoresis of Proteins
        and Immunoblotting 622
    Immunohistochemistry and
        Immunocytochemistry 623
APPROACHES TO IDENTIFY AND MANIPULATE
    GENES REGULATED BY INDIVIDUAL NUTRIENTS
    OR DIETARY PATTERNS .623
    Transgenic Animals .623
    Gene Knockout (Null Mutation) Animals 624
    Inhibition of Gene Expression by RNA
        Interference 625
CONCLUSIONS 625

Gene expression is a term that has different interpretations. These are dictated by the context in which the term is used. For example, exhibited phenotypes for health and disease are manifestations of gene expression. Similarly, the mechanics and control factors for gene transcription and mRNA translation that influence which proteins are produced also constitute gene expression. From the standpoint of nutritional influences on gene expression, processes are envisioned in which dietary conditions, through either direct interaction of specific nutrients with transcription factors or mRNA binding proteins, or, more commonly, through indirect means (e.g., hormones or signaling systems), produce changes that define phenotypic expression. The technical approaches described in this tutorial chapter are central to all research in contemporary biologic science and are actively applied in the nutritional sciences.

HISTORICAL PERSPECTIVE

Although the classic experiments of Nobel laureates François Jacob and Jacques Monod in 1961 were conducted in bacteria, they demonstrated that genes, under nutrient control through an operon, influence synthesis of enzymes involved in the metabolism of that nutrient (1). Experiments with eukaryotic systems followed after the operon model was proposed. Classic experiments of particular note were those demonstrating that polyribosome formation depended on the presence of essential amino acids in the diet (2). In addition, inhibitors of mRNA synthesis (actinomycin D and cordycepin) and translation (cycloheximide) were used in animal experiments to study many nutrient-induced changes in gene expression. Salient examples include the iron-induced synthesis of ferritin (3), regulation of phosphoenolpyruvic-carboxykinase (PEPCK) by high carbohydrate intake and fasting (4), and biochemical and physiologic changes induced by vitamin D (5).

GENOMIC ORGANIZATION AND REGULATION

Our understanding of the complexity of genomic organization has advanced considerably since the early experiments on nutrient influences on gene expression. Basics of our understanding of gene expression, including activation of the gene to a transcribable structure followed by transcription, transcript processing and splicing, translocation to the cytoplasm, mRNA processing and translation and, for some proteins, posttranslational modification, continue to evolve and be described in exquisite detail (6, 7). Newly appreciated aspects of the human genome include about 35,000 genes in 3.1 gigabases of DNA sequence. Alternative splicing of RNA transcripts and RNA editing can produce at least 100,000 proteins. The major portion of these proteins is of unknown function (8). In comparison, the mouse genome also has about 35,000 genes within

---

[1]**Abbreviations: AGE,** agarose gel electrophoresis; C_T, threshold cycle; **ES,** embryonic stem; **MTF,** metal-responsive transcription factor; ^{32}**P,** phosphorus-32; **PCR,** polymerase chain reaction; **PEPCK,** phosphoenolpyruvic-carboxykinase; **Q-PCR,** quantitative real-time polymerase chain reaction; **RT,** reverse transcriptase; **siRNA,** small interfering RNA; **SNP,** single nucleotide polymorphism.

3 gigabases. Overall, mouse and human genes share similarities of about 85%. Similarity of human genes with other primates is 95 to 98%.

GENE REGULATION BY NUTRIENTS

Nutrient regulation of gene expression is a well-recognized research emphasis in contemporary nutritional science. It is difficult to separate direct effects of individual nutrients on gene expression from those produced indirectly through physiologically controlled mediators and modulating molecules that are responsive to the diet (Fig. 39.1). Consequently, experiments at the level of individual cells are essential to identify clearly direct effects of nutrients. However, interpretation of cell-level findings must be kept within an integrative context of the multiorgan system to appreciate fully how dietary components and patterns influence the expression of genes in various tissues. The way in which the diet, in concert with hormones, cytokines, and growth factors, interacts to influence the differential expression of specific genes has reached such a high level of awareness that a new term, nutritional genomics, has evolved to describe such research activities (9). Nutritional genomics includes all genetic factors, including epigenetic events, as they modulate individual genes and gene networks. It is one of a growing number of terms in general use (Table 39.1) and tends to replace the former nutrient-gene interactions. The latter is a narrow term that implies a direct interaction of a nutrient with a gene for which no examples currently exist. The closest examples of a nutrient-gene interaction are nutrient binding to a transcription factor for subsequent interaction with a response element of a gene and the methylation of specific genes by S-adenosylmethionine.

A generalized cell showing different modes of gene regulation by nutrients is illustrated in Figure 39.2. A "direct"

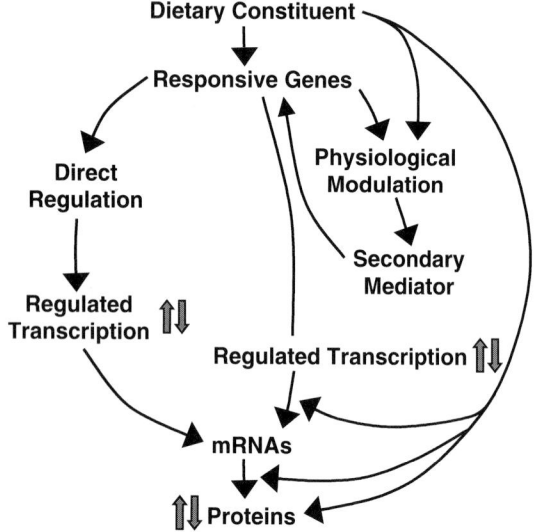

Figure 39.1. Generalized scheme showing direct and indirect actions of nutrients on regulation of gene expression.

effect of some nutrients (vitamins A, D, and E; zinc; n-3 fatty acids; and sterols) on gene transcription is shown in which, subsequent to ligand binding to a specific transcription factor, cytoplasmic to nuclear translocation of the complex occurs, and interaction through a specific domain of the factor with a response element sequence (specific nucleotide sequence) of the regulatory region produces a change in transcription rate of the gene. In some situations, more than one transcription factor is involved. An example of such complexity is the promoter for the gluconeogenic enzyme, PEPCK. Within the first 1 kb of upstream regulatory sequence (5′ from the transcription start site), five response-element sequences (cyclic adenosine monophosphate, glucocorticoid, insulin, peroxisome proliferators-activated receptor, and thyroid hormone), interact with at least ten transcription factors and provide multiple signals for PEPCK gene transcription (10). Such a direct effect has been described as a newtonian or linear mode of gene regulation (11). The direct interaction of response elements and transcription factors with nutrients has been documented. Examples include the sterol response element for sterol-regulated genes (12), the calcitriol receptor-response elements for vitamin D–regulated genes (13), the retinoic acid receptor-response element combinations for vitamin A–regulated genes (14, 15), fatty acids and some of their metabolites (16, 17), and the metal response elements for zinc-regulated genes (18) and associated transcription factors. Amino acid deprivation at the cellular level may activate transcription from specific defense genes through *cis*-acting nutrient-sensing response elements (19). The control of translation of specific mRNAs by iron (20) is another example of a "direct" nutrient effect on gene expression, in this case at the level of mRNA stability and translation efficiency, to increase the abundance of a protein.

Frequently, gene regulation by nutrients is more complex, where multiple and interconnected factors, including nutrient effects on signal transduction pathways, epigenetic effects on specific genes, mRNA splicing and translation, and posttranslational modifications, merge to define indirect effects on expression of a specific gene. Factors such as effects induced by hormones and cytokines, cellular redox, biologically active nonnutrient food components, and gene polymorphisms influencing nutrient utilization are modifiers of these nutrient effects and thus are more darwinian than newtonian. With this complexity, the genome can be viewed as flexible, with multiple pathways of regulation contributing to a phenotypic effect (11).

APPROACHES TO IDENTIFY GENES AND PROTEINS REGULATED BY INDIVIDUAL NUTRIENTS OR DIETARY PATTERNS

The following section describes some techniques and approaches investigators use to study the effect of nutrition on gene expression. Examples of these techniques from the contemporary literature concentrate on the results of

TABLE 39.1. GLOSSARY OF TERMS FREQUENTLY USED IN NUTRITIONAL REGULATION OF GENE EXPRESSION

cis-Acting	DNA elements on the same strand as a structural gene, usually upstream of the start site, to which transcription factors bind to initiate transcription	Polygenic	Disease or phenotypic characteristic caused by more than one gene

DNA array	Immobilized sequences of single-stranded DNA (probe) on a matrix that allows hybridization of mRNAs for quantitation of transcript abundance (also called gene chips or DNA chips)
	    Microarray (high-density array) = thousands of DNAs
	    Macroarray (low-density array) = numerous (usually <1000) DNAs
		Protein array	Antibodies or other proteins immobilized to a matrix, allowing abundance of specific proteins to be qualitatively detected or interacting proteins to be identified

		Proteomics	Proteome-wide analysis of protein regulation, expression, structure, posttranslational modification, interactions, and function
Epigenetic	Nonmutational modification of a gene, e.g., by methylation and histone changes that influence expression of a specific gene	Response element	Portion of a gene sequence that must be present for that gene to respond to a stimulus. Response elements are binding sites for transcription factors. Nutrients bind specific transcription factors that bind to DNA through specific response elements of a gene
Functional genomics	Relationship of genes, proteins, and regulatory networks to physiologic function		
Genomics	Study of the singular and/or collective roles that genes play in cellular processes as influenced by external factors. Prefixes such as chemo-, epi-, pharmaco-, or toxico- can define specialization in genomics	RNA interference (RNAi)	Use of short RNA molecules, frequently derived from double-stranded RNA, that, on introduction into cells and complementary hybridization to specific mRNA, decrease gene expression
Homolog	A gene that has the same evolutionary origin and function in two or more species	Single nucleotide polymorphism (SNP)	A single base substitution in a coding sequence of a gene. It frequently determines phenotypic differences in a population (human genome has about 10 million SNPs)
In silico	In or by means of computer simulation of complex biologic systems. The term is frequently used in microarray research in which extensive computational algorithms or comparisons are executed	Systems biology	Study of complex interactions of organ systems down to molecules
		trans-Acting factors	DNA-binding proteins (transcription factors) are *trans* because they are products of genes from other chromosomes that bind to regulatory elements. Transcription factors that bind some nutrients are *trans*-acting factors
Metabolomics	Global analysis of all metabolites in a complex system		
Monogenic	Disease or phenotypic characteristic produced by a single gene	Transcription factor	Proteins that bind regulatory regions of a gene and influence the transcription rate of the gene. The influence may be modified by protein-protein interactions
Nutritional genomics	Genomic studies that relate nutritional factors in regulation of genes that influence cellular processes genome wide		
Ortholog	A gene with similar function to a gene in an evolutionarily related species. Ortholog comparisons help predict gene function	Transcriptome	All transcribed mRNAs within a cell or tissue at a particular time

experiments with animals or human subjects fed diets that produce metabolic changes. Many of the techniques described use cellular DNA or RNA as the medium for analysis. Tissue RNA and DNA extraction procedures have evolved and, currently, guanidinium isothiocyanate–based methods (21), most with proprietary formulations, are almost universally used.

Northern Analysis

Northern analysis (Northern blotting) has been widely used in examining genes that are nutritionally regulated.

Northern analysis provides a semiquantitative estimate of relative static abundance of a specific mRNA (21, 22). The original method has been modified innumerable times. The method involves agarose gel electrophoresis (AGE) of the target RNA for separation by size, transfer to a filter (nylon or nitrocellulose), binding of the RNA to the filter by ultraviolet-induced cross-linking, and hybridization to a phosphorus-32 (^{32}P)–labeled DNA probe. Such probes are either cDNA fragments of cloned genes or oligonucleotides (oligomers, oligos) synthesized using DNA sequence information. Alternatively, probes for specific genes are commercially available, and

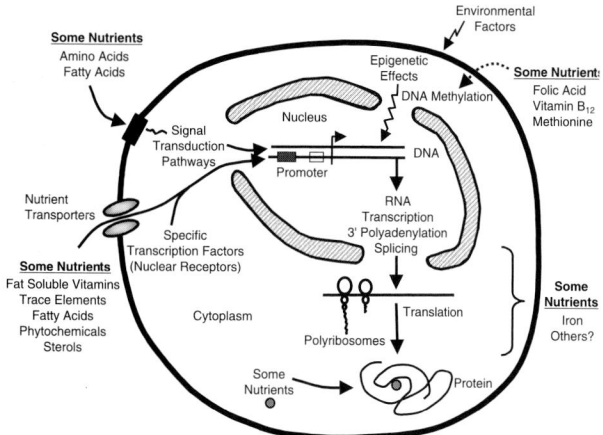

Figure 39.2. Regulation of gene expression by nutrients. Some nutrients, on cell uptake, are ligands for specific transcription factors (*trans*-acting), which are translocated to the nucleus for binding to specific DNA sequences (response elements) in regulatory regions (*cis*-acting) of specific genes. Some fat-soluble vitamins, trace elements, fatty acids, phytochemicals, and sterols exhibit this mode of action. Some nutrients activate transmembrane receptors, which use intracellular signaling pathways to initiate or modify gene expression. Single nucleotide polymorphisms and epigenetic changes can modify the expression of some genes. Nutrient effects on mRNA processing, editing, stability, and translation have been documented. Nutrients shown to have a direct effect on gene transcription include vitamin A (retinoic acid), vitamin D (calcitriol), zinc, n-3 polyunsaturated fatty acids, and specific sterols. In contrast, iron, and perhaps other nutrients, has a direct effect on gene regulation through control of translation or stability of specific mRNAs.

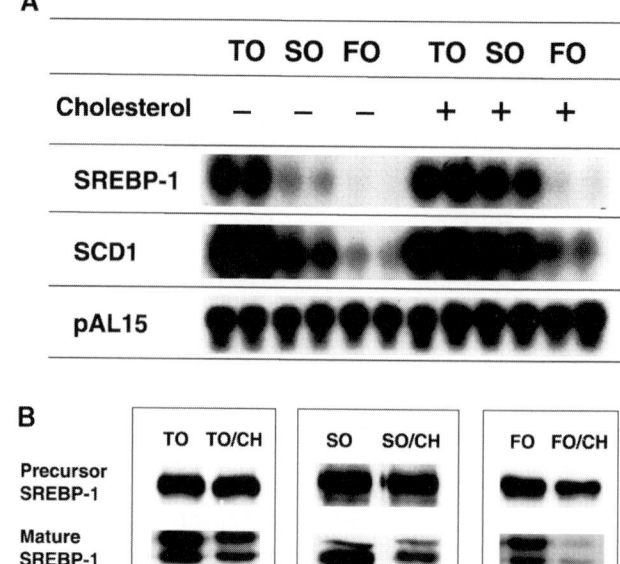

Figure 39.3. Northern analysis of mRNAs **(A)** and Western analysis of proteins **(B)**. Mice were fed diets with 5% fat as triolein (TO), soybean oil (SO), or fish oil (FO), and with (+) or without (−) 2% cholesterol (CH). **A.** Northern analysis of total liver RNA showing relative abundance of sterol regulatory element-binding protein-1 mRNA (SREBP-1), stearoyl-coenzyme A desaturase-1 mRNA (SCD1), and the normalizer mRNA (pAL15). **B.** Western (blot) analysis of membrane and nuclear fractions of liver showing the relative abundance of precursor and mature SREBP-1, respectively. (From Kim H-J, Miyazaki M, Ntambi JM. Dietary cholesterol opposes PUFA-mediated repression of the stearoyl-CoA desaturase-1 gene by SREBP-1 independent mechanism. J Lipid Res 2002;43:1750–7, with permission.)

most investigators are willing to share cDNAs for use as probes. Hybridization is detected by autoradiography or phosphorimaging instrumentation. Nonradioactive detection alternatives are not widely used. Intensity of the RNA-DNA hybridization is usually quantified by densitometry. A constitutively produced RNA (usually an unregulated housekeeping gene) should be concurrently examined as a control for equal loading of the RNA extracts for AGE and normalization. β-Actin and glyceraldehyde-3-phosphate dehydrogenase are frequently used as probes for normalization purposes. With RNAs of low abundance, it is frequently necessary to use poly(A)$^+$ RNA as the starting point for analysis in place of total RNA to enrich the mRNA pool. Ethidium bromide staining of RNA separated by AGE before transfer can also be used and provides a measure of RNA integrity (23). Results of typical Northern blot analyses are shown in Figure 39.3A. The influence of dietary cholesterol on polyunsaturated fatty acid–mediated changes in abundance of stearoyl-coenzyme A desaturase-1 mRNA and sterol regulatory element-binding protein-1 mRNA is shown (24). Such comparisons have a limited dynamic range of detection of RNA abundance compared with newer methods (discussed later). Northern analysis does provide qualitative information about transcript size and splicing.

In Situ RNA Hybridization

The technique of fluorescent in situ hybridization has received limited application in nutrition research. This allows qualitative estimation of the intracellular abundance of a specific mRNA in histologic sections using fluorescently labeled probes (25). It has the advantage of providing a cell-specific localization for the nutrient-responsive gene.

Solution Hybridization/RNase Protection Assays

Albeit not widely used, RNase protection assays provide an alternative to Northern analysis to estimate the relative abundance of a specific mRNA. Tissue RNA is hybridized with the ^{32}P-labeled antisense RNA probe and is treated with RNase to hydrolyze single-stranded RNA, and then protected ^{32}P-labeled RNA (hybridized RNA) is precipitated and separated by electrophoresis followed by autoradiography. Abundance is measured by densitometry. Once the assay has been established, the precipitated ^{32}P-labeled hybrid is measured directly by liquid scintillation counting for comparison of mRNA abundance (22).

Polymerase Chain Reaction

Polymerase chain reaction (PCR) has been applied to experiments focused on nutrition. PCR is a process that can provide multiple copies of a DNA or RNA sequence. Two oligonucleotide primers (a 5′ primer and a 3′ primer) that span the targeted sequence of interest must be synthesized (21). Availability of DNA sequence information allows the development of primers for most genes (http://www.ncbi.nlm.nih.gov). Reactants include the DNA, primers, *Taq* DNA polymerase, deoxynucleotides, and other components. Repeated sequential polymerase reactions in both directions of the target sequence under controlled temperatures with a thermocycler allow that sequence to be amplified as a double-stranded cDNA copy in sufficient quantity for further use. Frequently, the amplified DNA is cloned by standard methods and is purified by AGE.

Gene Polymorphism Detection

A major application of PCR is for identification of genetic polymorphisms. The number of single nucleotide polymorphisms (SNPs) in the human genome (3 billion bp) in databases is currently estimated at 10 million (http://snp.cshl.org; http://www.ncbi.nlm.nih.gov/SNP). SNPs have been documented in genes responsible for nutrient transport, utilization, and function. Some of these SNPs have health consequences, with those related to folic acid, iron metabolism, and vitamin D receptor function particularly evident (26–28). For example, in eight genes involved in iron metabolism, 96 SNPs have been detected (27).

Detection is a relatively straightforward procedure widely used in human genetics. DNA, usually from leukocytes, is extracted and is used as a template for PCR. Forward and reverse primers are constructed that are on either side of the polymorphic site in the sequence of the gene of interest using PCR as described earlier to amplify the intervening sequence. Appropriate restriction enzymes are then used to cleave the amplified sequence for subsequent AGE, visualizing, and archiving of the results. The method can be multiplexed, where more than one SNP is amplified, digested with appropriate restriction enzymes, and then separated with AGE, separately or collectively, depending on the fragment-resolving potential of the gel (28). Use of multiplex PCR for detection of two SNPs in the methylenetetrahydrofolate reductase (*MTHFR*) gene is shown in Figure 39.4.

The identification of SNPs is a powerful tool for identifying individuals with specific genomically based differences in nutrient utilization. Knowledge of the phenotypic effects of SNPs within the human genome is projected to become a factor in establishing dietary requirements for individual persons or groups sharing one or more common polymorphisms and in making dietary recommendations based on their individual SNP profiles and associated metabolic differences (29).

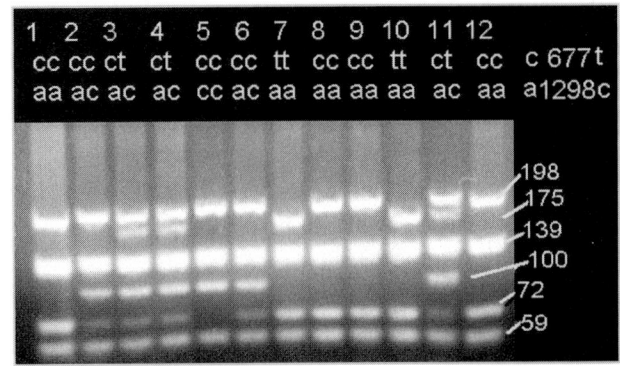

Figure 39.4. Polymerase chain reaction (PCR) for polymorphism detection. Multiplex PCR (described in ref. 28) was used to detect C677T and A1298C single nucleotide polymorphisms (SNPs) of the human methylenetetrahydrofolate reductase (*MTHFR*) gene simultaneously. Two primers spanning both polymorphic loci were used to amplify by PCR DNA extracted from lymphocytes. The PCR products were digested separately with appropriate restriction enzymes, pooled, separated by agarose gel electrophoresis, and visualized by ultraviolet illumination. The DNA fragments generated by PCR show that both SNPs are found within the 12 individual DNA samples, based on the presence or absence of restriction sites governed by each SNP examined. Numbers to the right are DNA size markers in base pairs (bp). The DNA bands represent C allele (198 bp) and T allele (175 bp) of C677T, and A allele (72 bp) and C allele (100 bp) of A1298C MTHFR SNPs. (Courtesy of Dr. Lynn B. Bailey and David R. Maneval, University of Florida, Gainesville, FL.)

Reverse Transcriptase Polymerase Chain Reaction

Reverse transcriptase PCR (RT-PCR) is used to produce cDNA copies of mRNA (21, 22). mRNA is first converted to cDNA with RT using a specific 3′ primer for the target mRNA. PCR is then performed with another specific primer to provide sufficient quantities of the DNA sequence of interest for purification and/or analysis by AGE. RT-PCR is semiquantitative at best, because the amplification process is exponential, and differences in mRNA levels encountered with nutritionally regulated genes are often not sufficiently large for the technique to be widely applicable for those applications. RT-PCR is applicable to the production of cDNAs for use as probes in Northern analysis experiments.

Competitive RT-PCR provides a measure of amplification efficiency and uses a third primer, which acts as a competitor of known concentration. It was described in the previous version of this chapter (30). Competitive RT-PCR was not widely applied in nutrition research despite its quantitative output. Newer PCR-based methodology has largely eliminated its use.

Quantitative Real-Time Reverse-Transcriptase Polymerase Chain Reaction

Northern analysis was the major technique used since the early 1980s to compare mRNA abundance. That task is being increasingly replaced by quantitative real-time RT-PCR (Q-PCR) methodology. Q-PCR is more attractive

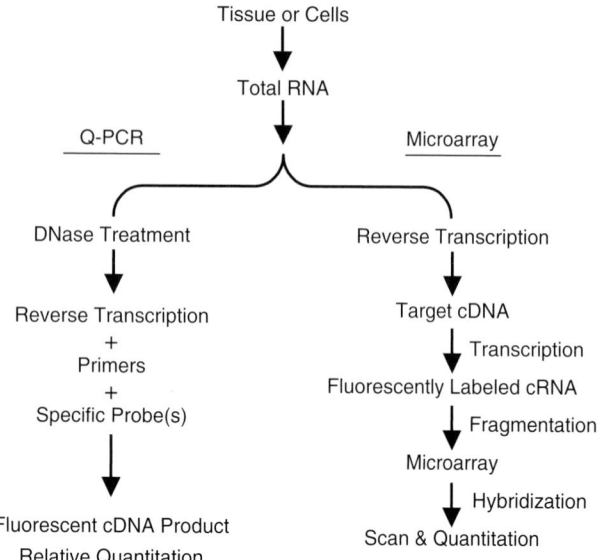

Figure 39.5. Abridged procedures used for quantitative real-time polymerase chain reaction (Q-PCR) and microarray analysis. Total RNA is extracted from tissue sample or isolated cells obtained by various methods, including laser capture microdissection of a tissue biopsy and purified leukocyte population prepared by density centrifugation. For Q-PCR, samples are treated with DNase to remove DNA contamination. RNAs for the two methods follow different analytic tracks to measure cellular abundance of a specific, individual mRNA (Q-PCR) or globally to measure 10^4 individual mRNAs (microarrays). Abundance is usually expressed on a relative basis.

because of sensitivity, dynamic range of quantitation (5-log range), applicability to small clinical samples, elimination of radioisotopes and decay of labeled probes, speed, and multiplexing of assays for different mRNAs using the same RNA sample. Q-PCR, as an evolving technology, has been frequently reviewed (22, 31–33). Reference RNA standards are now commercially available and will improve intralaboratory and interlaboratory consistency as this technology moves into the mainstream. A brief overview of steps in Q-PCR is shown in Figure 39.5. RNA for analysis is usually obtained from excised tissue, by laser capture microdissection (34), cultured cells, or blood cells.

Q-PCR is based on the combined reactions of reverse transcription and PCR (basically as described earlier) that are carried out in the same reaction tube to amplify stoichiometrically cDNAs produced from an mRNA population. In practice, the RNA is first rendered DNA free by DNase treatment. During PCR amplification, fluorophore-labeled probes in the reaction mixture generate a fluorescent signal. Through principles of fluorescence spectroscopy with appropriate wavelengths of excitation and emission, one or more fluorescent products can be monitored in real time. During the exponential phase of amplification, emitted fluorescence is proportional to the amount of PCR product accumulated relative to background (baseline) fluorescence. As the PCR cycle number increases, product fluorescence eventually reaches a threshold (e.g., ten times the standard deviation of the

baseline), and that cycle number (threshold cycle [C_T]) is used in developing the fold relationships among samples in the particular assay. Use of a standard curve can derive relative values for unknown samples. All values must be normalized to a housekeeping gene, as is done in Northern analysis. 18S ribosomal RNA is the most common normalizer for Q-PCR (22, 31, 32).

The relationship between C_T fluorescence and mRNA abundance is shown in Figure 39.6. Abundance of the target mRNA is less in samples with higher C_T values. Because the normalizer, 18S RNA, has comparable C_T values, the interpretation is that the difference in C_T for the target mRNA approximates the magnitude of the difference, with one C_T being about a twofold change. Details of calculating and expressing Q-PCR are available

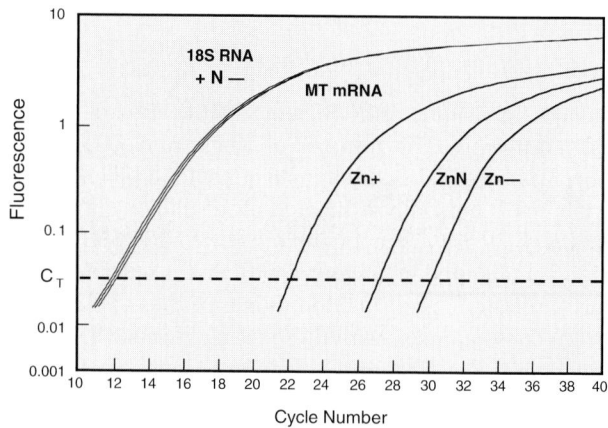

Figure 39.6. Analysis of mRNA abundance by quantitative polymerase chain reaction (Q-PCR). Influence of zinc on metallothionein (MT) mRNA abundance in human mononuclear cells (THP1 cells) as measured by Q-PCR. The cells were cultured to produce zinc-depleted (Zn–), zinc-normal (ZnN), or zinc-supplemented (Zn+) conditions, as described in reference 48. Total RNA was processed as outlined in Figure 39.5. The primers and probes used produce amplification plots for both 18S ribosomal mRNA and metallothionein mRNA. If the Q-PCR assay is multiplexed, only one PCR reaction is needed to measure both the normalizer (here 18S RNA) and experimental mRNAs (here MT mRNA) simultaneously for each sample. Multiplexing requires instrumental capabilities to detect fluorescence emission at two or more wavelengths. Without multiplexing, one PCR reaction is required to measure each RNA individually. When fluorescence is at ten times the standard deviation over background fluorescence, that is designated the threshold cycle (C_T). The C_T of 12 indicates a robust abundance of 18S RNA. Furthermore, the comparable C_T for the three groups of cells indicates zinc did not influence expression of 18S RNA (normalizer) because equal amounts of total RNA (2.5 ng) were used for each PCR reaction. MT mRNAs from the Zn+, ZnN, and Zn– cells produce C_T of 22, 27, and 30, respectively. Lower C_T values correspond to higher mRNA abundance because more mRNA allows fluorescent product to accumulate more rapidly with repeated PCR cycles. Each C_T represents a twofold change in relative abundance. In the example given here, the uniform 18S RNA and differing MT mRNA levels provide a relative difference in MT mRNA abundance of Zn– (8.0-fold relative decrease), ZnN (1.0), and Zn+ (32.0-fold relative increase) in the three cell groups. Detailed computations, including reference RNA use and standard curves, complete the analysis as described in references 31 to 33. (Data generated by Dr. Raymond K. Blanchard, University of Florida, Gainesville, FL.)

(31–33). A particularly attractive feature of Q-PCR is the small amount of starting material needed. The reactions mentioned earlier were derived from 2.5 ng of total RNA. By contrast, a Northern analysis would require at least 10 μg (10,000 ng) total RNA. Consequently, Q-PCR is amenable to extremely small sample sizes, including pediatric blood samples and samples collected in field conditions. One caveat is that heparin is a strong inhibitor of *Taq* DNA polymerase (35), and it should be avoided as an anticoagulant in blood used for Q-PCR experiments.

Promoter Analysis

Interaction between specific nutrients and transcription factors regulating expression of specific genes can be identified through promoter analysis. The approach taken to examine transcriptional regulation generally follows one of two techniques.

The first approach is a nuclear run-on experiment. This method is used to confirm regulation at the transcriptional level. The technique requires the generation of purified nuclei from cells or tissues. The nuclei are incubated in the presence of α-^{32}P uridine triphosphate to produce a radioactive RNA transcript. The transcripts of interest are then detected by hybridization to a specific probe. Because this ^{32}P uridine triphosphate is incorporated into mRNA only during transcription, any change in transcription rate as detected by ^{32}P incorporated into the nascent transcripts (that hybridize to the probe) in response to the nutrient is believed to reflect regulation at the level of transcription. Numerous genes, such as *PEPCK* (36), have been shown to be nutrient regulated through nuclear run-on assays. These experiments provide little information on mechanisms.

Another approach to promoter analysis enables determination of the specific sequences involved in gene regulation, but it requires sequence information about the genes of interest. In this technique, the promoter region, usually a few thousand bases (kb) of the 5′ flanking region, is excised with appropriate restriction enzymes and is ligated to a reporter gene. Most frequently, the chloramphenicol acyltransferase *(CAT)* or β-galactosidase *(β-Gal)* genes are used as reporters. The heterologous promoter-reporter construct must be transfected into a cell type of interest. Cell type is critical because transcription factor expression is cell specific. Reporter genes generate products that may be analyzed quantitatively. The approach has been used to examine regulation of certain nutritionally relevant genes (36–39). Promoter-reporter gene systems can be used as an in vitro model for screening the response of a promoter to specific nutrients, hormones, or phytochemicals. The regulation of stearoyl-coenzyme A desaturase-1 gene by polyunsaturated fatty acids using promoter-reporter constructs serves as an example of this potential (40). Using deletion analysis with restriction enzymes, the location of the nucleotide sequence of a promoter essential for nutrient regulation can be narrowed down and identified. Mutational analysis of the promoter can define the exact nucleotides needed for specific regulation. Frequently, the latter analysis shows that the response element (sequence) is not always completely uniform. Consequently, response elements are frequently reported as consensus sequences. Regulatory elements may not always be located upstream from the gene's start site. This situation complicates such experiments.

Differential mRNA Display

Differential mRNA display is an elegant approach to examine differential gene expression based on reverse transcription and PCR (30). It enables one to identify mRNAs that increase or decrease in response to multiple conditions. The technique has been applied to identify genes regulated or influenced by micronutrients (23, 41, 42). The method can provide valuable sequence information for previously unrecognized genes and about regulatory networks influenced by specific nutrients. The perfection of high-density DNA microarray technology has diminished the use of the method.

DNA Array Analysis

Much of the field of genomics, including nutritional genomics, is centered around DNA array technology. As with the earlier techniques of dot blotting and Northern analysis, arrays take advantage of nucleic acid hybridization principles to obtain an estimate of abundance of a particular RNA or DNA target. In the field of nutrition, two types of arrays are particularly relevant. The most common is the cDNA array, in which mRNA transcript abundance is estimated. The other is an array in which the DNA represents SNPs and other variants of the same genes.

Array technology frequently employs proprietary manufacturing methods to affix the DNA to a support wafer, slide, or membrane. Macroarrays are usually DNAs spotted onto membranes or slides. These arrays usually only have a limited number of DNA elements (probes) spotted (≤1000). The limited number of genes per array is a detracting feature and restricts the macroarray to specialized gene survey applications (e.g., apoptosis, cytokine expression, stress response). In contrast, the microarray can contain in excess of 30,000 DNA elements and thus can allow comparison of the entire genome simultaneously. The DNA elements are usually synthetic oligonucleotides of less than 30 bases in length that are chosen to be dissimilar to other genes and thus preclude cross-hybridization between gene probes. Multiple copies of the same DNA and mismatched DNA elements are included as controls. Photolithography is used to generate oligonucleotide microarrays. Methods of cDNA array production have been described (www.affymetrix.com). The general approach to the use of microarrays in a dual fluorescence detection system is outlined in Figure 39.7.

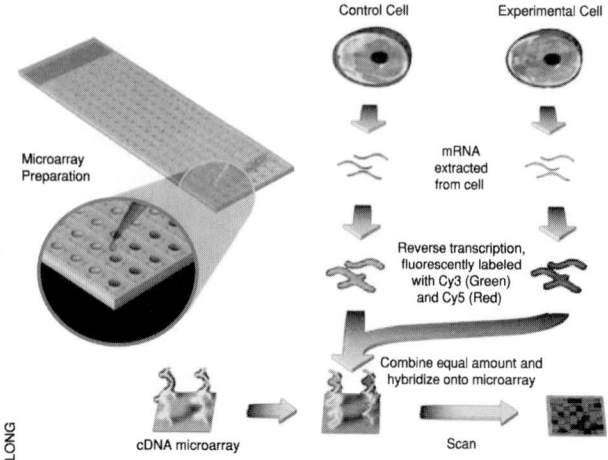

Figure 39.7. Microarray analysis. Steps for microarray analysis to compare transcript (mRNA) abundance in two RNA samples are shown. In this method, probes are used that provide different fluorescence emissions, so comparisons of a control and experimental group can be made using one array. More frequently, each experimental group has multiple chips with normalization among arrays achieved through internal standards. (From http://www.bioteach.ubc.ca/MolecularBiology/microarray/index.htm, with permission.)

Generalized mechanics of array use are shown in Figure 39.5. Microarrays are particularly attractive to applications in nutrition research. With completion of sequencing programs for the human and mouse genomes and the advancing state of completing the rat genome, the opportunity to define nutrient action on gene expression through the use of microarrays presents a new frontier. Transcriptome-wide studies of tissue-specific gene expression in human tissues, organs, cell, and cell lines have been completed (43, 44). Within the context of human nutrition research, microarray data using RNA from human blood cells show interesting specificities regarding cell type, but remarkably low intersubject variability (43). Data from multiple arrays require complex statistical analyses (e.g., cluster comparisons), and these have become an important focus in the fields of bioinformatics and biostatistics.

The numbers of nutritionally related literature citations in which DNA arrays have been used are increasing (9). Much of the earliest research was conducted with macroarrays with limited numbers of gene probes. Nevertheless, important gene-nutrient-disease relationships are among such citations. An early example of the power of microarrays was an analysis of genes influenced by caloric restriction and aging in mice that revealed defects in the expression of numerous β-oxidation enzymes (45, 46). Array results frequently generate new concepts. For example, zinc mediates the expression of some genes through zinc binding to the metal-responsive transcription factor 1 (MTF1) (47). Microarray experiments of human mononuclear cells showed that the *MTF1* gene is upregulated in zinc-deficient cells and that a homolog MTF2, a poorly characterized metal responsive transcription factor, is downregulated (48). The opposing responsiveness of *MTF1/MTF2* transcription factor genes to zinc has been suggested as potentially involved in regulation of zinc homeostasis in intact animals.

Microarray experiments are limited primarily by cost of the actual arrays, but many institutions and industrial facilities have the hardware and software to provide analyses on a "core facility" basis. Furthermore, as more array data are produced and are made publicly accessible at various Web sites (e.g., http://expression.gnf.org), data sharing is becoming a global activity in nutritional genomics.

Positional Cloning

An excellent nutritionally related example of positional cloning is that of the *ob* gene (49). This led to identification of a new peptide hormone, leptin, which, when secreted by adipocytes, regulates food intake and energy expenditure and influences type 2 diabetes in obese individuals. This research was based on observations of mutations in *ob* mice made in the 1960s.

The first requirement in this approach is to obtain genetic maps to identify the locus where the mutation of interest is located. In many cases, the chromosomal location of a mutation in the murine and human genomes is known. For genes that influence nutrition, phenotypic expression (i.e., development of obesity) is used to segregate the mutant gene through specific genetic crosses. Linkage studies position the gene relative to molecular markers or to known or identifiable areas of the genome. Establishing linkages to known genes helps greatly, particularly if they are "tightly linked" to the gene of interest. In the case of the *ob* gene, the region of chromosome 6 where the *ob* gene was located was identified by two flanking markers. Using this location information, the appropriate region of the DNA is cloned. Use of yeast artificial chromosomes, specific restriction enzyme digests, and specific crosses refine the location. Subsequent screening of restriction digests will yield smaller sections of DNA, some of which will hybridize to RNA from a tissue where the gene is expressed. Using this DNA as a probe, the mRNA of interest is identified, the cDNA sequence of the gene can then be established, and eventually, as in the case of leptin, the primary sequence of protein product deduced. Experiments of this type are extremely time consuming, and expertise in molecular genetics is essential. Nevertheless, the results of such endeavors have great benefit for understanding important aspects of nutrition.

Polyacrylamide Electrophoresis of Proteins and Immunoblotting

Extremely valuable information can be obtained by measuring specific gene products (proteins) related to altered phenotypic expression. For such purposes, proteins are most frequently separated by sodium dodecyl sulfate poly-acrylamide gel electrophoresis using any of the innumerable variations of the format (21). For identification of the proteins of interest, the proteins are electroblotted (transferred) to membranes (nitrocellulose, polyvinylidene fluoride, or nylon) from the polyacrylamide gel. Detection of the transferred proteins is most frequently by an immunologically based method. The process is referred to as Western blotting. Figure 39.3B shows a Western blot illustrating the effect of dietary fatty acids and cholesterol on the levels of precursor and mature sterol regulatory element-binding proteins in membrane and nuclear fractions of mouse liver (24).

Immunodetection methods afford investigators the opportunity to examine a specific protein from the thousands of tissue proteins transferred to the membrane. The spectrum of antibodies available for these applications from commercial sources is very substantial. Alternatively, many investigators working on newly identified or rare proteins use antibodies produced from chemically synthesized peptides, which correspond to a specific region of the intact protein that is likely to be highly antigenic. These peptides usually comprise 20 to 30 amino acids. Frequently, the amino acid sequence is deduced from the cDNAs of those genes in which the protein product has not been isolated and sequenced. This approach provides the opportunity to examine the nutritional regulation of proteins coded for by newly identified genes.

Small proteins or peptides used for production of antibodies are conjugated to enhance antigenicity. Antibodies are most frequently raised in rabbits, but goats and sheep are popular hosts. Immunization of chickens and recovery of antibodies from egg yolk is also gaining in popularity. Polyclonal antibodies are usually purified by protein A or G chromatography to obtain the immunoglobulin G fraction, and frequently are further selected by affinity chromatography where a support to which the protein or peptide antigen has been coupled is used to yield a monospecific immunoglobulin G. Monoclonal antibodies are also widely used in nutrition-related studies on gene expression. The availability of hybridoma facilities has greatly furthered the production of monoclonals. Protocols for incubating the blotted proteins on nitrocellulose with the primary antibody (immunoblot) vary widely. Options for detection via a secondary antibody center around colorimetric detection, binding of iodine-125–labeled protein A, or, most frequently, a very sensitive method in which the secondary antibody provides a luminescent signal detected by x-ray film or a fluorescence imager. For purposes of quantitation of the results from Western blots, the far greater dynamic range of fluorescence imaging increases sensitivity and makes it preferable to x-ray film. Furthermore, sensitivity of some immunodetection methods offers the opportunity to examine proteins present in low abundance. An example of antibody development, purification, and use in Western analysis is reported for zinc transporter 1 (50).

Immunohistochemistry and Immunocytochemistry

Advances in microscopy have dramatically increased the use of fluorescent antibodies for intracellular localization of specific proteins. Epifluorescence, confocal, and deconvolution microscopic techniques can all take advantage of fluorescently tagged antibodies and have been applied to proteins of nutritional interest. Flow cytometry can also be effectively used in nutritionally related research, particularly that focused on immunology (51).

APPROACHES TO IDENTIFY AND MANIPULATE GENES REGULATED BY INDIVIDUAL NUTRIENTS OR DIETARY PATTERNS

Transgenic Animals

The term transgenic refers to both overexpression and deletion of expression of a specific gene. However, transgenesis most frequently is used to describe the technique that results in overexpression of a structural gene. The transgenic overexpression technique involves production of a construct consisting of a promoter and structural gene. The promoter can be the gene's normal promoter (homologous) or a different promoter (heterologous). A purified sample of the construct is injected into fertilized eggs (usually murine or porcine), and, if the construct DNA becomes appropriately integrated into the genome, transgenic animals will be produced from those eggs after the eggs are returned to foster mothers for the full gestation period. Selective breeding can produce homozygous lines of animals carrying transgenes.

Transgenic animals have been used to address questions of nutritional interest. For example, the glucose transporter (GLUT4) was overexpressed in mice using the aP2 fatty acid binding protein promoter and a genomic DNA fragment containing the entire human GLUT4 gene as the construct (52). Overexpression of GLUT4 transporter protein resulted in higher glucose transport rates, lower glucose tolerance curves, and greater body fat than littermates (Fig. 39.8). Unfortunately, most transgenic mice strains do not exhibit such dramatic changes in phenotype or give unanticipated outcomes. Furthermore, both transgenics and the knockout technology described in the next section have some inherent characteristics that can influence interpretation of results derived from mice strains produced through these methods (53). The number of nutritionally relevant genes that have been overexpressed in transgenic mice is now extensive. Many strains of transgenic mice are available through the Jackson Laboratory (www.jax.org) and other specialized distributors.

The ability to introduce genes by recombinant adenovirus therapy has great potential for investigating genes of nutritional interest. For such purposes, investigators are not limited to use of mice. cDNA constructs with a viral promoter are prepared basically as described earlier and

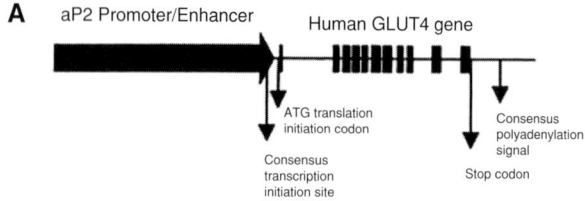

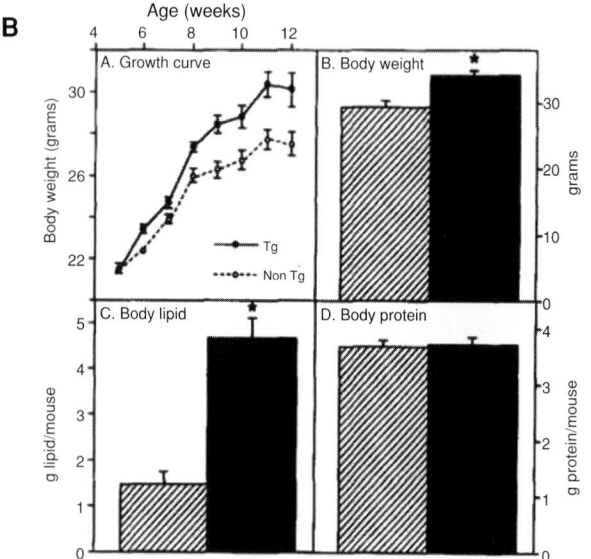

Figure 39.8. Overexpression of the human *GLUT4* gene in transgenic mice. **A.** The transgene construct consisting of the mouse aP2 fatty acid-binding promoter ligated to 6.3 kb of human genomic DNA that includes all 11 exons of the *GLUT4* transporter gene. **B.** Growth and body composition comparisons for control *(cross-hatched bars)* and *GLUT4* transgenic mice *(solid bars)* fed a normal diet. (From Shepherd PR, Gnudi L, Tozzo E et al. Adipose cell hyperplasia and enhanced glucose disposal in transgenic mice overexpressing GLUT4 selectively in adipose tissue. J Biol Chem 1993;268:22243–6, with permission.)

are administered intravenously. An example of this technology is the introduction of leptin cDNA into obese Zucker rats with adenovirus. This results in greatly increased lipid oxidation by adipocytes and a very rapid loss of body weight (54).

Gene Knockout (Null Mutation) Animals

Gene knockout technology provides the opportunity to delete expression of a specific gene (null mutation). As a result, the normal gene product is not produced. Null mutations produce phenotypes that run the gamut from lethality to no apparent effect. Consequently, the technology is not exactly the genetically engineered counterpart to spontaneous mutations that occur in laboratory animals and are propagated by selective breeding techniques. These usually result in altered function of the gene product. The *ob* gene mutation of mice (49) is an example of a spontaneous mutation.

The technique of creating a knockout animal model or null mutation is more correctly called "gene targeting by

homologous recombination." Animal cells are diploid; that is, each nucleus contains two copies (alleles) of a gene. The targeted gene is disrupted in one allele (produces heterozygotes with the null mutation). Two approaches to developing knockout mice are used (53). The original approach is to isolate the murine gene under investigation, identify the exons by mapping, delete part of an exon, and replace it with the gene encoding neomycin resistance (produces a marker for selection). An entire exon can also be deleted. This construct is the gene-targeting vector. The targeting vector is linearized and is transfected into embryonic stem (ES) cells by microinjection or electroporation. The transfected cells are then injected into blastocysts removed from pregnant mice and introduced into pseudopregnant mice. Chimeric pups are often identified by the agouti coat color provided by genes from the ES cells. Selective breeding to obtain a homozygous null mutant (–/–) genotype follows (21, 55). The second, and more recent, approach can provide cell type–specific targeting of a gene deletion. The gene is engineered to have lox P sites on either side, and, by ES cell technology, a transgenic line is created carrying the target gene and flanking lox P sites. Another transgenic strain is produced with a construct comprising the *CRe* recombinase gene and the Mx1 promoter, which can be activated by interferon-α. These strains are crossed and, when interferon-α is injected into offspring, the CRe gene product (CRe recombinase; a bacteriophage enzyme) acts at one of the lox P sites and deletes the target gene in a specific tissue or cell type in which the CRe gene product is produced (56, 57).

Knockout technology in animals has been applied exclusively to murine genes. In some cases, the animals die before term if a critical gene product is not produced or is sufficiently altered so there is loss of function. Numerous examples of this phenomenon have been reported. Deletion of the *C/EBPα* gene, which is required for energy (glucose) utilization, is an example of a lethal null mutation relevant to nutrition (58). In some instances, a gene may appear critical for nutrient metabolism (e.g., metallothionein for zinc metabolism), but, when deleted, may allow null mice to reproduce and develop normally, albeit with demonstrable metabolic abnormalities (59–62). Of note in this regard is that null mutation of the gene for MTF1, required for induction of metallothionein by zinc, results in lethality (63). Similarly, a null mutation in the cellular retinoic acid-binding protein 1 gene *(CRABP1)*, which is believed to be required for the function of vitamin A (retinol) via the metabolite retinoic acid, produces animals that appear to have a normal phenotype (64). These latter results indicate that, in some instances, another gene product provides the same phenotypic effect through redundancy of functional roles of specific genes or a gene family. Redundancy of function can obscure the unique function of the deleted gene. As with transgenic overexpressing mice, commercial suppliers may act as a resource for such animals.

An interesting extension of the knockout technology is to cross-breed transgenic mice and knockout mice. When this technique is skillfully applied, valuable insights into metabolic pathways and phenotypes can be produced. For example, breeding transgenic mice overexpressing apoliprotein A-I to apoliprotein E null mice produces increased high-density lipoproteins and increased atherosclerotic lesions (65). A mouse model with features of familial combined hyperlipidemia can be produced by crossing transgenic mice carrying the human apolipoprotein C-III to mice null for the low-density lipoprotein receptor (66). Similarly, the combined uses of transgenic overexpressing mice and knockout mice have many important contributions to understanding glucose homeostasis and thermogenesis (67, 68).

Inhibition of Gene Expression by RNA Interference

Antisense RNA technology has been used as a research tool for a limited number of genes of nutritional interest. The principle is that a small RNA sequence complementary (antisense) to a target mRNA can inhibit its translation and/or stimulate its degradation. The entire field has been extensively reviewed (69–71), is currently very active, and has considerable potential for research and commercial applications.

Early use of antisense RNA sequences for gene silencing employed short synthetic oligonucleotides transiently to inhibit the translation of specific mRNAs by hybridization. These oligonucleotides appear to be taken up by some tissues. The approach has been applied to inhibition of mRNAs for peptides involved in regulation of feeding behavior and body weight (72, 73). In these cases, antisense DNA sequences are introduced into specific areas of the brain.

The use of small interfering RNA (siRNA) has become widely accepted as an approach to gene silencing (74–76). Animals have retained an ancestral defense system that degrades double-stranded RNA using an RNase (i.e., Dicer) to RNA of 21 to 23 bp, called siRNA. These RNA strands bind to target mRNA and promote its degradation. A synthetic oligonucleotide can replace the siRNA. In practice, double-stranded RNAs (200–1000 bp) or short RNAs (20–25 bp) produced with commercially available reagents, expression vectors, and enzymes are available to accomplish gene silencing.

A disadvantage of the siRNA approach to gene suppression is that suppression is leaky; that is, inhibition of a specific gene is not 100%, as is the case with a knockout. Furthermore, the gene silencing achieved is frequently transient rather than stable. The technology has gained use for silencing genes of nutritional interest (75, 76). An advantage of siRNA for gene silencing is that it circumvents the issue of embryonic lethality that can occur with some genes in knockout mice. Some success has been achieved with heritable gene silencing (77), a finding suggesting siRNA could become an alternative to traditional knockout techniques. Of particular interest is the discovery that, in mammalian cells, siRNA can induce global upregulation of interferon-stimulated genes through the Jak-Stat pathway (78, 79). This property of siRNA technology may be a major complicating factor in interpretation of data from such experiments. Experiments with siRNA focused on nutrient metabolism and function must be carefully controlled because of this finding.

CONCLUSIONS

The area of nutrition and gene expression has developed rapidly and is now a recognized research discipline (nutritional genomics) in nutritional sciences. As our knowledge of animal and human genomes expands, the technologies described here, and new approaches still waiting to be developed, will have a profound impact on nutrition as a field and on our understanding of how diet and genetics influence phenotypic expression.

Acknowledgments

I express my appreciation to Dr. J. Bernadette Moore at the National Institutes of Health for her review of this chapter and valuable comments. Appreciation is expressed to the National Institute of Diabetes and Digestive and Kidney Diseases and Boston Family Endowment for long-term research support.

REFERENCES

1. Jacob F, Monod J. J Mol Biol 1961;3:318–56.
2. Baliga BS, Pronczuk AW, Munro HN. J Mol Biol 1968;34:199–218.
3. Zähringer J, Baliga BS, Munro HN. Proc Natl Acad Sci USA 1976;73:857–61.
4. Tilghman SM, Hanson RW, Reshef L et al. Proc Natl Acad Sci USA 1974;71:1304–8.
5. Zull JE, Czarnowska-Misztal E, DeLuca HF. Science 1965;149:182–4.
6. Lewin B. Genes VII. New York: Oxford University Press, 2000:1–990.
7. Alberts B, Johnson A, Lewis J et al, eds. Molecular Biology of the Cell. New York: Garland, 2002:1–1463.
8. Guttmacher AE, Collins FS. N Engl J Med 2002;347:1512–20.
9. Müller M, Kersten S. Nat Rev Genet 2003;4:315–22.
10. Savon SP, Hakimi P, Crawford DR et al. J Nutr 1997;127:276–85.
11. Greenspan RJ. Nat Rev Genet 2001;2:383–7.
12. Goldstein JL, Brown MS. Nature 1990;343:425–30.
13. Holick MF. Vitamin D. In: Shils ME, Shike M, Ross AC et al, eds. Modern Nutrition in Health and Disease. 10th ed. Baltimore: Lippincott Williams & Wilkins, 2004.
14. Ross AC. Vitamin A and carotenoids. In: Shils ME, Shike M, Ross AC et al, eds. Modern Nutrition in Health and Disease. 10th ed. Baltimore: Lippincott Williams & Wilkins, 2004.
15. Forman BM, Chen J, Evans RM. Proc Natl Acad Sci USA 1997;94:4312–7.
16. Kliewer SA Sundseth SS, Jones SA et al. Proc Natl Acad Sci USA 1997;94:4318–23.
17. Jump DB. J Biol Chem 2002;277:8755–8.
18. Cousins RJ. Annu Rev Nutr 1994;14:449–69.
19. Pan Y, Chen H, Siu F et al. J Biol Chem 2003;278:38402–12.

20. Theil EC, Eisenstein RS. J Biol Chem 2000;275:40659–62.

21. Ausubel FM, Brent R, Kingston RE et al, eds. Current Protocols in Molecular Biology, 4 vols. New York: John Wiley & Sons, 2001.

22. Reue K. J Nutr 1998;128:2038–44.

23. Blanchard RK, Cousins RJ. Proc Natl Acad Sci USA 1996;93: 6863–8.

24. Kim H-J, Miyazaki M, Ntambi, JM. J Lipid Res 2002;43:1750–7.

25. Cui L, Blanchard RK, Coy LM et al. J Nutr 2000;130:2726–32.

26. Fleet JC, Harris SS, Wood RJ et al. J Bone Miner Res 1995;10: 985–90.

27. Douabin-Gicquel V, Soriano N, Ferran H et al. Hum Genet 2001;109:393–401.

28. Yi P, Pogribny IP, James SJ. Cancer Lett 2002;181:209–13.

29. Fenech M. Food Chem Toxicol 2002;40:1113–7.

30. Cousins RJ. Nutritional regulation of gene expression. In: Shils ME, Olson JA, Shike M et al, eds. Modern Nutrition in Health and Disease. 9th ed. Baltimore: Williams & Wilkins, 1999: 573–84.

31. Bustin SA. J Mol Endocrinol 2002;29:23–39.

32. Livak KJ, Schmittgen TD. Methods 2001;25:402–8.

33. Ginzinger DG. Exp Hematol 2002;30:503–12.

34. Mikulowska-Mennis A, Taylor TB, Vishnu P et al. Biotechniques 2002;33:176–9

35. Johnson ML, Navanukraw C, Grazul-Bilska AT et al. Biotechniques 2003;35:1140–2, 1144.

36. Lamers WH, Hanson RW, Meisner HM. Proc Natl Acad Sci USA 1982;79:5137–41.

37. Jump DB Clarke SD MacDougald O et al. Proc Natl Acad Sci USA 1993;90:8454–8.

38. Levenson CW, Shay NF, Hempe JM et al. J Nutr 1994;124: 13–7.

39. Schoonjans K, Peinado-Onsurbe J, Lefebre A-M et al. EMBO J 1996;15:5336–48.

40. Waters KM, Miler CW, Ntambi JM. Biochim Biophys Acta 1997; 1349:33–42.

41. Moore JB, Blanchard RK, Cousins RJ. Proc Natl Acad Sci USA 2003;100:3883–8.

42. Inoue K, Matsuda K, Itoh M et al. Hum Mol Genet 2002;11: 1775–84.

43. Whitney AR, Diehn M, Popper SJ et al. Proc Natl Acad Sci USA 2003;100:1896–901.

44. Su AI, Cooke MP, Ching KA et al. Proc Natl Acad Sci USA 2002; 99:4465–70.

45. Lee CK, Klopp RG, Weindruch R et al. Science 1999;285: 1390–3.

46. Lee CK, Allison DB, Brand J et al. Proc Natl Acad Sci USA 2002;99:14988–93.

47. Lichtlen P, Wang Y, Belser T et al. Nucl Acids Res 2001;29: 1514–23.

48. Cousins RJ, Blanchard RK, Popp MP et al. Proc Natl Acad Sci USA 2003;100:6952–7.

49. Zhang Y, Proenca R, Maffei M et al. Nature 1994;372:425–32.

50. McMahon RJ, Cousins RJ. Proc Natl Acad Sci USA 1998;95: 4841–6.

51. Fraker PJ, King LE, Laakko T et al. J Nutr 2000;130: 1399S–406S.

52. Shepherd PR, Gnudi L, Tozzo E. J Biol Chem 1993;268: 22243–6.

53. Leiter EH. Diabetologia 2002;45:296–308.

54. Orci L, Cook WS, Ravazzola M et al. Proc Natl Acad Sci USA 2004;101:2058–63.

55. Majzoub JA, Muglia LJ. N Engl J Med 1996;334:904–7.

56. Gu H, Marth JD, Orban PC et al. Science 1994:265:103–6.

57. Kühn R, Schwenk F, Aguet M et al. Science 1995;269:1427–9.

58. Wang N, Fingold MJ, Bradely A et al. Science 1995;269: 1108–12.

59. Michalska AE, Choo KHA. Proc Natl Acad Sci USA 1993;90: 8088–92.

60. Masters BA, Kelly EJ, Quaife CJ et al. Proc Natl Acad Sci USA 1994;91:584–8.

61. Coyle P, Philcox JC, Rofe AM. Biochem J 1995;309:25–31.

62. Davis SR, McMahon RJ, Cousins RJ. J Nutr 1998;128:825–31.

63. Günes C, Heuchel R, Georgiev O et al. EMBO J 1998;17: 2846–54.

64. Gorry P, Lufkin T, Dierich A et al. Proc Natl Acad Sci USA 1994;91:9032–6.

65. Plump AS, Scott CJ, Breslow JL. Proc Natl Acad Sci USA 1994;91:9607–11.

66. Masucci-Magoulas L, Goldberg IJ, Bisgaier CL et al. Science 1997;275:391–4.

67. Magnuson MA, She P, Shiota M. J Biol Chem 2003;278: 32485–8.

68. Lowell BB, Bachman ES. J Biol Chem 2003;278:29385–8.

69. Hannon GJ. Nature 2002;418:244–51.

70. Elbashir SM, Harborth J, Lendeckel W et al. Nature 2001;411: 494–8.

71. Dillin A. Proc Natl Acad Sci USA 2003;100:6289–91.

72. Heilig M. Regul Pept 1995;59:201–5.

73. Hulsey MG, Pless CM, White BD et al. Regul Pept 1995;59: 207–14.

74. Birchler JA, Bhadra MP, Bhadra U. Curr Opin Genet Dev 2000; 10:211–6.

75. Jiang ZY, Zhou QL, Coleman KA et al. Proc Natl Acad Sci USA 2003;100:7569–74.

76. Zender L, Hutker S, Liedtke C et al. Proc Natl Acad Sci USA 2003;100:7797–802.

77. Carmell MA, Zhang L, Conklin DS et al. Nat Struct Biol 2003;10:91–2.

78. Sledz CA, Holko M, de Veer MJ et al. Nat Cell Biol 2003;5:834–9.

79. Moss EG, Taylor JM. Nat Cell Biol 2003;5:771–2.

SELECTED READINGS

Bartel DP. MicroRNAs: genomics, biogenesis, mechanism, and function. Cell 2004;116:281–97.

Guttmacher AE, Collins FS. Genomic medicine: a primer. N Engl J Med 2002;347:1512–20.

Hanson RW. New animal models for study of metabolism minireview series. J Biol Chem 2003;278:28357–8.

Müller M, Kersten S. Nutrigenomics: goals and strategies. Nat Rev Genet 2003;4:315–22.

Strohman R. Maneuvering in the complex path from genotype to phenotype. Science 2002;296:701–3.

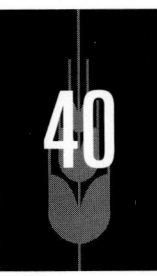

40 POLYMORPHISMS: EFFECT ON NUTRIENT UTILIZATION AND METABOLISM[1]

PATRICK J. STOVER AND CUTBERTO GARZA

HUMAN GENETIC VARIATION 627
    Prevalence of Human Genetic Variation 627
    Origin of Human Genetic Variation 628
    Haplotypes 630
    Transposable Elements .630
FUNCTIONAL CONSEQUENCES OF GENETIC
    VARIATION 631
    Genetic Variation and Gene Expression 631
    Genetic Variation and Protein Function 631
IDENTIFICATION OF GENETIC VARIATION
    THAT AFFECTS NUTRIENT METABOLISM
    AND UTILIZATION 632
    Candidate Gene Approaches 632
    Identification of Adaptive Genes 634

Metabolic impairments are integral components of chronic diseases, developmental anomalies, cancers, neurologic disorders, and most other pathologic processes. Often they precede anatomic and other signs of disease. Clinical investigations of inborn errors of metabolism provided some of the earliest and conclusive evidence that (a) metabolic impairments are heritable, (b) genes can modify nutrient utilization and metabolism, (c) metabolic impairments cause disease, and (d) the functional consequences of genetic mutations can be attenuated significantly by targeted nutritional therapies that compensate for and, less often, avoid genetically induced metabolic impairments. Phenylketonuria provides a classic paradigm that demonstrates the potential effectiveness of diet in modifying deleterious phenotypes that result from genetic mutations that alter metabolism. Phenylalanine-restricted diets lessen and may even prevent severe cognitive deficits in children who carry mutations in the phenylalanine hydroxylase gene (1). Inborn errors of metabolism are generally recessive and are relatively rare in most populations, and the initiation and/or progression of the associated disorders can be managed by diet or nutrition in some, but not all, cases.

Inborn errors of metabolism are typically monogenic disorders that follow mendelian modes of inheritance and therefore are well characterized with respect to their molecular and genetic bases. However, the most prevalent human metabolic disorders are complex polygenic diseases with contributions from multiple low penetrant susceptibility alleles, and the risks associated with these alleles are modifiable by both lifestyle and environmental factors including one or more dietary components. The genetic and biochemical causes of many cancers and chronic diseases, including cardiovascular disease and type 2 diabetes mellitus, remain unidentified. These disorders may not conform to classic mendelian inheritance patterns, and therefore genetic approaches based on "simple" linkage analyses are not always possible. Newer approaches capable of identifying susceptible genotypes are enabled by the availability of complete genome sequences from several mammalian species. Through comparative genomics, the origins and consequences of human genetic variation are decipherable, and allelic variants and interacting environmental risk factors that impair metabolic pathways and/or modify optimal dietary requirements can be inferred.

HUMAN GENETIC VARIATION

Prevalence of Human Genetic Variation

The primary sequence of the human genome contains approximately 3.1 billion nucleotide base pairs that are organized into 24 distinct chromosomes that range in size from 50 million to 250,000 million base pairs. The sequence of the human genome was obtained from five to ten persons of diverse ethnic and geographic backgrounds or ancestry (2). The human genome, including both nuclear and mitochondrial DNA, contains an estimated 25,000 genes that encode information required for the synthesis of all cellular proteins and functional RNA molecules. Fewer than 50% of human genes have known or putative functions assigned to them. Genes account for about 2% of the total human DNA primary sequence; the remaining DNA is termed noncoding and serves structural and/or regulatory or no known roles. The number of genes encoded within the genome does not limit the biologic complexity of the mammalian cell. A single gene can encode more than one RNA or protein product through

[1] **Abbreviations: ADH,** alcohol dehydrogenase; **ALDH,** aldehyde dehydrogenase; k_{cat}, maximal rate of product formation at infinite substrate concentration; **HFI,** hereditary fructose intolerance; K_m, Michaelis-Menten constant; **LD,** linkage disequilibrium; ^{me}C, methylcytosine; **SNP,** single nucleotide polymorphism.

posttranscriptional and posttranslational processing reactions including RNA editing, alternative splicing, and protein splicing or other modifications (e.g., differential phosphorylation). As a result of such processing and modification reactions, more than 100,000 proteins with distinct primary sequences can be derived from the human genome, and the number is greater when additional potential modifications are considered (3).

The primary nucleotide sequence of the genome is approximately 99.9% identical among humans (4). The 0.1% primary sequence variation among humans is referred to as polymorphism and constitutes one of the molecular bases for human phenotypic variation, including variations in human behavior, morphology, and susceptibility to disease. DNA sequence polymorphisms fall into several classes including single nucleotide polymorphisms (SNPs), microsatellite and macrosatellite repeat sequences, and viral insertions. SNPs are the most common variation in the primary sequence of human DNA; more than 10 million SNPs are estimated to be present in the human genome (5). SNPs are defined as nucleotide base pair differences in the primary sequence of DNA and can be single base pair insertions, deletions, or substitutions of one base pair for another. Nucleotide substitutions are the most common polymorphism; insertion/deletion mutations occur at one tenth the frequency (6). As of 2003, more than 3.7 million SNPs were identified. SNPs differ from mutations in that they are present in the germ line and therefore are heritable and by definition must have a prevalence of at least 1% in humans. SNPs contribute to susceptibility for common diseases and developmental anomalies, and polymorphic alleles have been identified that increase the risk of common disorders including neural tube defects, cardiovascular disease, cancers, hypertension, and obesity (7–9). SNPs also influence physiologic responses to environmental exposures including diet (10), pharmaceuticals (11), pathogens, and toxins (12), and therefore many SNPs have diagnostic value. High-density human SNP maps facilitate the identification of disease risk alleles through gene mapping studies of complex disease, including low penetrant alleles that make relatively small contributions to the initiation and or progression of the disorder (2).

Origin of Human Genetic Variation

Adaptive phenotypes arise in part through complex and reciprocal interactions among the genome and environmental exposures. Human genetic variation is a product of these interactions and is manifest through the formation and propagation of primary sequence alterations in DNA. Polymorphisms arise in populations through the sequential processes of genetic mutation followed by expansion of the mutant allele within the population, and environment can modify both these processes. The generation of primary sequence differences is a function of the DNA mutation

rate; the expansion of the mutation within a population is a function of effective population size, population demographic history, and the effect of the mutation on an organism's fitness (2).

Not all sequence variation has phenotypic consequences. DNA sequence that does not confer function can mutate freely without consequences, whereas changes in DNA sequences that encode information or function may alter physiologic process, and therefore the propagation and expansion of such sequences will be more constrained. DNA sequence that confers advantageous function is expected to be conserved and therefore shared at some level among species. Most human genetic variation present in noncoding regions, including those found in intronic and intergenic regions, is assumed to be selectively neutral and therefore a function of the DNA mutation rate (2), which is estimated to be 2.5×10^{-8} on average for autosomes in the germ line (6). The highest mutation rates for a human gene are approximately 1×10^{-5} per generation (13). Many factors contribute to DNA mutation rates. DNA replication and recombination do not occur with complete fidelity and thereby account for a significant portion of observable mutation rates. Polymerase error rates are enhanced by impairments in nucleotide biosynthesis that can result from nutrient deficiencies of iron and/or B vitamins including folic acid. For example, inhibition of deoxythimidine monophosphate synthesis results in the misincorporation of deoxyuridine triphosphate into DNA (14). Increased rates of uracil incorporation into DNA increase the rates of single point mutations as well as the frequency of DNA strand breaks. Purine and pyrimidine bases within DNA also undergo spontaneous chemical mutation; cytosine spontaneously deaminates to uracil with a frequency of 100 mutations/genome/day, and purine nucleotides undergo depurination mutations at a rate of 5000 mutations/genome/day. DNA repair systems are effective in detecting and correcting most of these mutations. Genotoxic xenobiotics, both natural products and synthetic chemicals, are present in the food supply and can modify DNA chemically and increase mutation rates. One class of natural compounds, aflatoxins (15), can dramatically increase DNA mutation rates, trigger cancers in somatic cells, and lead to localized cancer epidemics. Increased mutation rates have also been suggested to result from a lack of dietary antioxidants (16) or from excesses in prooxidant nutrients including iron (17); however, only mutations that occur in the germ line contribute to a species' heritable genetic variation.

DNA mutation rates and polymorphism frequency vary throughout the human genome. Such region-specific differences within the genome have been attributed to the frequency of DNA recombination as well as the mutagenic potential of specific nucleotide sequences. The most common genetic mutation within the human genome is the C to T transition (18). The sequence CpG is enriched in the promoter regions of mammalian genes and is recognized by DNA methylases, which convert the cytosine base (C) to methylcytosine (^{me}C). ^{me}C density within the genome is modifiable by dietary folic acid and one-carbon donors, and fetal methylation patterns established in utero can be metastable and can influence gene expression into adulthood [19]. Cytosine methylation influences the transcription rates of targeted genes by altering the affinity of DNA binding transcription factors and/or by enabling the recruitment of ^{me}C binding proteins that serve to silence gene transcription. DNA methylation usually is associated with gene silencing and is critical for the inactivation of imprinted genes and X chromosome inactivation. Methylated CpG sequences display increased rates of mutation [6], presumably because ^{me}C deaminates spontaneously to thymidine (T), whereas C deaminates to uracil. Uracil is recognized as foreign to DNA and is excised by the DNA repair enzymes, whereas T is not recognized as foreign. The sequence CpG is underrepresented in the human genome, and its frequency has decreased throughout evolution, consistent with that inherent instability [18]. DNA recombination rates also vary throughout the human genome, and sites of more frequent recombination may exhibit elevated mutation rates [2, 20].

Mutations that expand within a population contribute to genetic variation as polymorphisms, and this process is the basis for the molecular evolution of genomes. The fixation of a polymorphism within a population occurs through the process of genetic drift or natural selection. Drift is a stochastic process that results from chance assortment of chromosomes at meiosis. Only a few of all possible zygotes are generated or survive to reproduce [2]. Therefore, mutations can expand in the absence of selection through random fluctuations in the transmission of alleles from one generation to the next, resulting from the random sampling of gametes. Drift generally has a greater impact on allele frequencies in small populations expanding rapidly. Drift in static large populations is not usually as significant because of such populations' greater dilutional effect. Genetic drift, however, can have a greater than expected impact in large populations when they undergo bottlenecks (massive reductions in population) or founding events that have occurred during human migrations, such as populations that include groups such as the Old Order Amish, Hutterite, and Ashkenazi Jewish [2]. In these populations, rare disease alleles can expand rapidly and can increase the incidence of diseases such as breast cancer, Tay-Sachs disease, Gaucher disease, Niemann-Pick disease, and familial hypercholesterolemia [2].

It is assumed that most human genetic variations arose as a result of the neutral processes of mutation and genetic drift and are of no physiologic consequence. Comparative analyses of whole-genome sequence indicate that protein-coding sequences are, in general, conserved among mammalian species. However, the neutral theory of evolution cannot account for the proportion of amino acid substitutions observed in mammalian genomes [12, 20]. Rates of amino acid substitution vary markedly among proteins compared with rates of synonymous substitution among genes (changes in the coding region of genes that do not affect protein sequence) [20]. Patterns of genetic variation across the entire human genome are affected by demographic histories of populations, whereas variation at particular genetic loci is influenced by the effects of natural selection, mutation and recombination [2]. Mutations that change amino acid sequence can affect protein structure and function, and the resulting physiologic consequences can be beneficial, deleterious, or neutral and thereby may influence an organism's fitness in specific environmental contexts. Functional mutations that affect protein sequence or expression level are under constraint and are subject to both positive and negative selection. Darwinian selection favors the maintenance and expansion of favorable mutations (positive selection) and the elimination of mutations that are deleterious (negative selection). Natural selection, which is defined as the differential contribution of genetic variants to future generations, is the only evolutionary force that has adaptive consequences [21]. Selection increases rates of molecular evolution at defined loci within the genome, a finding indicating that not all genes are expected to evolve at the same rate. Comparison of mammalian genome sequences has permitted the identification of genes that have undergone accelerated evolution [12]. These rapidly evolving genes are assumed to enable adaptation and thus to have been positively selected [12]. Adaptive mutations expand within populations at accelerated rates relative to neutral mutations and replace a population's preexisting variation. The proportion of amino acid substitutions that result from positive selection is estimated to be 35 to 45% [20].

Comparison of mammalian genome sequences provides evidence that environmental exposures, including pathogens and dietary components, have been selective forces throughout evolution. These selective forces have influenced the generation of polymorphic alleles that alter the utilization and metabolism of dietary components and may be responsible for the generation of metabolic disease alleles across ethnically diverse human populations [2]. Such ethnic differences, however, are more likely the result of diverse environmental exposures of distinct genetic patterns because traits that are multigenic and quantitatively continuous exhibit greater variability within populations as opposed to between populations [3]. Genes associated with degenerate metabolic pathways or networks are genetically buffered and display greater genetic variation because mutations within these genes are likely to be less constrained and more tolerated [22]. Such genetic buffering likely increases tolerance for nutritional insults, a finding indicating that some metabolic disease can arise solely from extreme alterations in environmental exposures independent of genetic background (e.g., obesity).

Polymorphisms that result from positive selection are expected to arise from region-specific selective factors [2]. Therefore, the prevalence of specific functional polymorphisms may be associated with specific geographic or ethnic human populations to the degree that different selective pressures are operative across populations. Specific allelic variants may be adaptive only in certain environments and neutral or less favored in others (21). Both gene dosage and environment can influence the fixation and physiologic consequences associated with a polymorphic allele. For example, the relatively high prevalence of the E6V polymorphism in the β-globin gene likely is the result of an adaptation to the region-specific environmental challenge of the malaria parasite in African populations. The polymorphic allele confers resistance to malaria in heterozygote carriers, but it is also a recessive disease allele for sickle cell anemia. This disease allele apparently became fixed in the population because it enhanced fitness toward the region-specific environmental challenge of malaria in heterozygotes. Identifying and understanding the historic selection of gene variants will enable the discovery of human disease alleles that arose from nutritional challenges (2). In 1962, the "thrifty gene" hypothesis was proposed to account for the epidemic of obesity and type 2 diabetes that arises in traditional non-Western cultures that adopt Western style diets and lifestyles (13). The hypothesis states that repeated famine conditions selected for genotypes that were best adapted to an unpredictable and sometimes scant food supply by favoring mutations in genes that enabled the more efficient conversion of food into energy and fat disposition, genes such as insulin and leptin (13, 23). The putative adaptations also may have resulted in more efficient adaptations to fasting conditions (e.g., more rapid decreases in basal metabolism) and/or physiologic responses that facilitate excessive intakes in times of plenty. Adaptive alleles may be recessive disease alleles or may become disease alleles even in heterozygote individuals when the environmental conditions change profoundly, such as those brought about by the advent of civilization and agriculture, including alterations in the nature and abundance of the food supply (24–27).

Haplotypes

Alleles that are physically close with respect to primary DNA sequence usually do not segregate and are inherited together (3, 28). As a result of meiotic recombination, DNA sequence is inherited in "blocks" that average 25,000 base pairs (3). SNPs that are captured within these blocks are said to be in linkage disequilibrium (LD), which is defined as the nonrandom association of alleles at a nearby loci. LD is usually correlated with physical distance between loci as well as distance from the centromere, but it is also influenced by recombination frequency, which varies throughout the genome. Inherited blocks of genetic variation are referred to as haplotypes, and the size of the haplotype block is dependent on the number of meiotic recombination events within a population. Ancestral populations that maintain a high effective population size for long periods are expected to have shorter haplotypes and therefore lower LD because of the increased number of historic recombination and mutation events, both of which cause LD decay (23). Consistent with this notion, African populations have higher levels of genetic diversity compared with all other human populations whose founder groups likely exhibited less variability than the population from which they emerged and had less time to respond to their new environments. African patterns of LD are unique, and African populations exhibit a greater number of haplotypes and more divergent patterns of LD compared with non-African populations (2). LD in the Nigerian population extends an average distance of 5 kilobases, whereas European LD can extend nearly 60 kilobases, consistent with the increased absolute number of recombination events occurring in ancestral populations (2). Haplotype maps of human genetic variation are preferred for disease associational studies because of the reduced complexity compared with SNP maps (29). However, haplotype associations do not identify disease-causing mutations because of genetic hitchhiking (2) (polymorphisms that are in LD with a mutation that is under selection will change in frequency along with the site undergoing selection). Because disease alleles associated with risk can be geographically restricted, full characterization of SNP diversity and haplotype structure from ethnically diverse populations is critical for the identification of risk alleles that may be specific to small but identifiable subpopulations.

Transposable Elements

Approximately 50% of noncoding human DNA originates from the insertion of highly mobile repeat sequences termed transposable elements. The two types of transposable elements are retrotransposons and DNA transposons (30–32). Retrotransposons are classified by their size and include long interspersed nuclear elements, which encode all the necessary components to move within the genome, and short interspersed nuclear elements, which require other transposable elements for mobility. The most abundant short interspersed nuclear elements are the 280 base pair *Alu* elements; there are an estimated 1.4 million in the human genome, which account for about 10% of human genomic sequence. *Alu* elements are enriched in CpG sequences and display promoter activity that is usually silenced by CpG methylation; *Alu* transcripts cannot be translated because they lack an open reading frame. *Alu* elements can alter genome function and stability and are thought to be catalysts for organismal evolution (32). Because of their high abundance, *Alu* sequences can serve as nucleation sites for unequal intrachromosomal and interchromosomal homologous recombination events that lead to chromosomal aberrations including deletion and translocation events and therefore can be mutagenic.

Recent or de novo transposition events that occur within or near an existing gene can result in the elimination of that gene, can alter its expression, or can create a new gene. Whereas most *Alu* insertions are believed to be phenotypically silent or deleterious, others can impart new function that may be advantageous. *Alu*s can function as transcriptional silencers or activators. Some *Alu* elements have retinoic acid response elements and thereby can confer new forms of regulation to genes that neighbor the insertion site. Furthermore, *Alu* elements in gene promoters also can impart regulation by DNA methylation to that locus because they contain CpG sequences (19). More than 1200 *Alu* elements in the human genome integrated after early human migrations; a new *Alu* insertion occurs every 200 births (32). Therefore, current human populations are polymorphic for the presence or absence of these insertions (2). New *Alu* insertions directly cause approximately 0.1% of human genetic disorders including Apert syndrome, cholinesterase deficiency, and breast cancer. About 0.3% of human genetic disease results from *Alu*-mediated unequal homologous recombination events resulting in other inherited disorders including type 2 insulin-resistant diabetes and familial hypercholesterolaemia (32). *Alu*-mediated unequal homologous recombination events are inhibited by CpG methylation of the element.

FUNCTIONAL CONSEQUENCES OF GENETIC VARIATION

The metabolism of individual dietary components is affected by the activity, expression, and/or stability of the specific protein transporters and enzymes. Polymorphisms affect gene expression, as well as the physical and kinetic properties of cellular proteins, and thereby influence the rates of metabolic pathways and the steady-state concentration of reaction intermediates, some of which can be deleterious.

Genetic Variation and Gene Expression

Transcriptional regulatory sites have been suggested to be susceptible to genotype-by-environment interactions that drive the fixation of mutations through the process of natural selection (23). SNPs located within the promoter regions of genes, exons, introns, or noncoding exons potentially may alter the gene expression at the level of transcription or translation or alter mRNA splicing, processing, and/or stability. Transcription factor–DNA interactions are highly polymorphic within the human genome, and they influence both basal transcription rates and the magnitude of transcriptional responses that are elicited by signaling molecules. Two thirds of human polymorphisms identified in human promoter elements affect transcription rates by twofold or greater (23). The human genome may have more genetic variation that affects functional *cis*-regulatory sequences than variation that results in amino acid substitutions. Investigators have estimated that humans are heterozygous for 10,700 functional biallelic *cis*-regulatory

variants (23). *Cis*-regulatory polymorphisms influence the activity of both transcriptional activators and repressors that regulate the expression of metabolic enzymes and other regulatory proteins (23). Polymorphisms in the insulin 5′ promoter decreases insulin expression and increase the risk of type 1 diabetes mellitus (3, 33); the risk of type 2 diabetes mellitus is associated with polymorphisms in the calpain-10 gene promoter (3, 27, 34). Polymorphisms have been identified that affect the transcription of many metabolic and nutrient transport proteins including alcohol dehydrogenase, apolipoproteins, catalase, cytochrome P450 family members, glucokinase, lipase, and the vitamin D receptor (23). Retroviral polymorphisms have been identified that influence gene expression by altering promoter methylation status in mice, and the degree of silencing is dependent on folate and one-carbon nurtriture (19). However, no viral insertions have been identified in the human genome that affect transcription (25).

Genetic Variation and Protein Function

SNPs that change the amino acid sequence encoded within an mRNA transcript are referred to as nonsynonymous nucleotide substitutions. In general, conservative nonsynonymous substitutions that replace one amino acid with another of similar structural and chemical properties are more likely to be phenotypically silent. Nonconservative nonsynonymous substitutions that result from amino acid replacements may alter the physical or chemical properties of the polymorphic protein, for example, G$\underline{C}$C (ala) → G$\underline{T}$C(val), and are likely to have functional consequences for the organism. Likewise, nonsynonymous nucleotide substitutions that result in the formation or elimination of translational termination codons may affect protein structure and function. Insertion/deletion polymorphisms, from a single base pair to several million nucleotides, can result in a change of reading frame, which constitutes about 8% of human polymorphisms.

The rate of enzyme-catalyzed reactions, including nutrient transport and metabolism, is determined by the concentration of both enzyme (E) and substrate (S), and the intrinsic Michaelis-Menten kinetic properties (K_m and k_{cat}) of the enzyme (or transport protein).

$$E + S \leftrightarrow ES \leftrightarrow E + P$$

The Michaelis-Menten constant, K_m, refers to the affinity of E for S and is defined as the substrate concentration required for the enzyme to achieve one half maximal velocity. Formation of the ES complex requires productive collisions between the enzyme and substrate and is governed by the law of mass action. Therefore, the rate of an enzyme-catalyzed reaction is usually directly proportional to the molecular concentrations of the reacting substances (both E and S). Breakdown of the ES complex to product (P) is determined by k_{cat}, which refers to the maximal rate of product formation at infinite substrate concentration (all enzyme is present as an ES complex).

Genetic variation influences both the formation of the ES complex and the rate of P generation. Polymorphisms affect the formation of the ES complex by influencing the concentration of E or the affinity of E for S (K_m). SNPs influence the concentration of E by altering its rate of synthesis (gene expression or mRNA stability) or rate of degradation (protein stability and turnover). Nonsynonymous substitutions that affect the K_m alter the concentration of substrate required to drive the formation of ES. Therefore, SNPs that increase K_m result in the accumulation of metabolic intermediates in cells. SNPs also can influence k_{cat}, which is the rate of formation of product (P), by affecting the maximum rate of catalysis (conversion of S to P at infinite S concentration). Alterations in k_{cat} can influence rates of nutrient uptake or clearance of metabolic intermediates and overall net flux through a metabolic pathway in a substrate independent manner.

IDENTIFICATION OF GENETIC VARIATION THAT AFFECTS NUTRIENT METABOLISM AND UTILIZATION

Genomes that confer either nutrient requirements that cannot be met by the mother, or severe metabolic disruptions that impair basic physiologic processes, will be selected against in large part because of fetal loss and/or the failure to survive to reproduce. Some common SNPs in genes that encode metabolic enzymes are not in Hardy-Weinberg equilibrium (alleles are not inherited at the expected frequency) because the homozygous state reduces fetal viability (7, 10). Nearly 62% of all human conceptuses are not viable and do not survive to the twelfth week of gestation (35, 36). Genomes that survive gestation but confer atypical nutrient requirements or inefficient metabolism may encode one or more disease-causing alleles, and the penetrance of the disease allele may be modifiable by diet. High-dose vitamin therapy can rescue impaired metabolic reactions that result from genetic mutations and polymorphisms that decrease the affinity of substrates and cofactors for the encoded enzyme (K_m) (37). Polymorphic risk alleles that affect nutrient metabolism and utilization have been identified using candidate gene approaches, and more recently they have been inferred from nonbiased comparative genomic analyses.

Candidate Gene Approaches

Most polymorphisms that affect nutrient utilization or metabolism were discovered from epidemiologic or clinical studies, and many are disease alleles. Candidate genes are selected based on knowledge of metabolic pathways and predictions that their impairment results in metabolic phenotypes that either mirror a particular disease state or affect the concentration of a biomarker associated with chronic disease. The candidate gene approach has been successful in identifying many disease susceptibility alleles (Table 40.1) (37, 38), but it is limited by incomplete knowledge of transcriptional and metabolic networks capable of suggesting candidate genes for analyses and by

TABLE 40.1. EXAMPLES OF HUMAN GENE VARIANTS THAT AFFECT THE UPTAKE OR METABOLISM OF DIETARY COMPONENTS

FOOD COMPONENT	GENE	POLYMORPHIC ALLELE	REFERENCE
Vitamins			
Folate	MTHFR	A222V	(50)
	CBS	844ins68	(51)
	GCPII	H475Y	(52–54)
Vitamin B$_{12}$			
	MTR	N919G	(51)
	MTRR	I22M	(51)
Vitamin D	VDR	Many	(55)
Minerals			
Iron	HFE	C282Y	(56, 57)
Lipids			
	APOB	Many	(58, 59)
	APOC3	Many	(60)
	APOE	Many	(47)
Alcohol			
	ADH/ALDH2	Many	(42, 43)
Carbohydrate			
Lactose	LD	Promoter	(61)
Fructose	Aldolase B	Many	(45)
Detoxification/			
Oxidative Stress			
	NAT1/NAT2	Many	(62, 63)
	PON1	Q192R;L55M	(64)
	Mn-SOD	Ala(-9)Val	(65, 66)

inconsistent findings among studies. Furthermore, because many SNPs are in LD, it is not always possible to determine with certainty whether an individual SNP or allele is functional and disease causing or merely is a product of genetic drift. Some well-characterized alleles that affect nutrient metabolism are described in the following subsections.

One-Carbon Metabolism

One-carbon metabolism is required for purine, thymidylate, and methionine biosynthesis, and its pathways have been demonstrated to contain several polymorphic alleles that are associated with metabolic disruptions and specific pathologies. SNPs in the methylenetetrahydrofolate gene, *MTHFR* (A222V), and the methylenetetrahydrofolate dehydrogenase gene, *MTHFD1* (R653Q) (7), which encode folate-dependent enzymes, are associated with an increased risk of neural tube defects; the *MTHFR* (A222V) gene is protective against colon cancer in folate-replete subjects. These polymorphisms are not in Hardy-Weinberg equilibrium (7,39,40), consistent with evidence that the *MTHFR* A222V polymorphism is a risk factor for spontaneous miscarriage and decreased fetal viability (10). The MTHFR A222V variant protein has reduced affinity for riboflavin cofactors and is thermolabile, resulting in reduced cellular MTHFR activity (41). Carriers of the MTHFR A222V generally have lower red blood cell folate concentrations and require higher levels of dietary folate to reduce serum homocysteine levels. The polymorphism is prevalent in white and Asian populations, but it is nearly absent in African populations. The biochemical role of these polymorphisms in the etiology of neural tube defects and cancer is unknown.

Alcohol Metabolism

The metabolism of ethanol varies widely among human ethnic populations (42). Ethanol is oxidized to acetaldehyde by the enzyme alcohol dehydrogenase (ADH); acetaldehyde is subsequently oxidized to acetic acid by aldehyde dehydrogenase (ALDH). Three genes encode the class I ADH isozymes. The active enzyme is a heterodimer composed of subunits encoded by *ADH1*, *ADH2*, and *ADH3*. *ADH2* and *ADH3* are highly polymorphic; variations in *ADH2* show the greatest functional effects with respect to catalytic activity (Vmax), affinity of the protein for ethanol (Table 40.2), and rates of alcohol clearance from tissues. The ADH2 β1 variant predominates in white and African-Americans, whereas the ADH β2 variant predominates in Japanese and Chinese populations. The ADH β3 variant is mostly restricted to persons of African descent. The second enzyme in the pathway, ALDH, is also polymorphic. Populations of Asian descent carry a common dominant null allelic variant (E487K) and develop a "flush" reaction when consuming alcohol resulting from the accumulation of the metabolic intermediate acetaldehyde (43).

TABLE 40.2. KINETIC CHARACTERISTICS OF ALCOHOL METABOLIZING ISOZYMES ENCODED AT THE *ADH2* LOCUS

ADH GENOTYPE	ADH ISOZYME	K_m (μM)	Vmax (min^{-1})
ADH2*1	β1β1	50	9
ADH2*2	β2β2	900	400
ADH2*3	β3β3	36,000	300

ADH, alcohol dehydrogenase; K_m, Michaelis-Menten constant; Vmax, maximum velocity.

Data from Bosron WF, Li TK. Hepatology 1986;6:502–10.

Lactose Metabolism

The ability of mammals to metabolize the disaccharide lactose is dependent on the expression and activity of the enzyme lactase. The expression of lactase declines after weaning in most mammals, including most humans, and results in primary lactose intolerance. In some human populations, including humans of Northwest European descent and nomads of the African-Arabian desert region, lactase expression persists into adulthood. A polymorphism 14 kilobases upstream of the lactase transcriptional start site in a *cis*-acting transcriptional element is associated with the persistence of lactase expression throughout adulthood and confers resistance to primary lactose intolerance (44). This polymorphism is common in persons of Northern European descent, and its prevalence correlates with, but does not account fully for, lactase persistence. The benefits of milk consumption, both as a source of liquid in arid regions and for prevention of rickets and osteomalacia in regions of low solar irradiation, have been assumed to have driven the fixation of this polymorphism.

Fructose Metabolism

Hereditary fructose intolerance (HFI) is an autosomal recessive disorder of fructose metabolism resulting from impaired fructose-1,6-aldolase activity in the liver, which causes an accumulation of the toxic metabolic intermediate fructose-1-phosphate. Twenty-five allelic variants of aldolase B, which is the human liver isozyme, have been discovered that impair enzyme activity by altering K_m, k_{cat}, and/or protein stability (45). The prevalence of these variants differs throughout Europe; the L288 Δ C frameshift mutation is restricted to Sicilians. The accumulation of fructose-1-phosphate inhibits glycogen breakdown and glucose synthesis, resulting in severe hypoglycemia following ingestion of fructose. Affected persons are asymptomatic in the absence of fructose or sucrose consumption. Prolonged fructose ingestion in infants leads ultimately to hepatic and/or renal failure and death. The condition is manifested usually during infancy at weaning, when the child is introduced to fruits and vegetables, or when feeding is transferred from breast milk to foods with fructose containing sweeteners. Patients develop a strong distaste for sweet food and can avoid a recurrence of symptoms by remaining on a fructose- and

TABLE 40.3. CANDIDATE GENES/PATHWAYS THAT HAVE UNDERGONE ACCELERATED EVOLUTION IN PRIMATES

GENE	SPECIES	ADAPTIVE PRESSURE	REFERENCE
Lysozyme	Langur monkey	Digestion	(20, 48, 67)
Ribonuclease	Langur monkey	Digestion	(20, 48)
Cox4	Primates	?	(68)

PATHWAY		SPECIES	REFERENCE
Amino acid metabolism		Human, chimp	(12)
Amino acid transport		Chimp	(12)
Purine metabolism		Chimp	(12)

sucrose-free diet. The incidence of HFI intolerance has increased since the widespread use of sucrose and fructose as nutrients and sweeteners, because normally nonpenetrant "silent" aldolase B alleles now present as HFI disease alleles.

Iron Metabolism

Hereditary hemochromatosis is a recessive iron storage disease common in populations of European descent with an incidence of one in 300 persons. A common polymorphism in the *HFE* gene (C282Y), which encodes a protein that regulates iron levels, is associated with the disease phenotype in 60 to 100% of Europeans, although mutations in other genes are also associated with the phenotype. Iron storage diseases exist in Asia and Africa, where the *HFE* C282Y allele is essentially absent. The penetrance of the C282Y *HFE* allele for the iron overload phenotype varies widely among homozygotes, with some persons being asymptomatic. The *HFE* C282Y polymorphism expanded in human populations relatively recently and may have conferred unidentified selective advantages (46).

Lipid Metabolism

Apolipoprotein E is a polymorphic protein that that functions in lipid metabolism and cholesterol transport (47). Three common allelic variants are $\varepsilon2$, $\varepsilon3$, and $\varepsilon4$. The protein isoforms differ in both their affinity for lipoprotein particles and for low-density lipoprotein receptors. All human populations display apolipoprotein E polymorphism, but the relative distribution varies among populations; the frequency of the $\varepsilon4$ allele declines from Northern to Southern Europe. The $\varepsilon4$ allele increases the risk of late-onset Alzheimer disease and arteriosclerosis with low penetrance. Carriers of the $\varepsilon2$ allele tend to display lower levels of plasma total cholesterol, whereas carriers of the $\varepsilon4$ allele, which may be ancestral, display higher cholesterol levels.

Identification of Adaptive Genes

The acquisition of whole genome sequences is enabling comparative genomic approaches to identify allelic variants that may contribute to metabolic disease. Alleles that enable an organism to adapt to an unmet physiologic requirement or environmental challenge become fixed within a population as a result of positive selection, but they can become risk alleles in new or changing environments (12, 20, 21). Although this approach is in its infancy, genes and allelic variants involved in metabolism and nutrient transport (21), digestion (20, 48), amino acid metabolism (12), nucleotide metabolism (12), cation transport (12), and the *PPARG* gene (21) have been identified as rapidly evolving genes (Table 40.3). Accelerated genes become strong, nonbiased candidate genes for disease association studies, and modifying environmental risk factors can be inferred from the nutrients or metabolites that interact with the gene product under study. Although the success of this approach in identifying new genetic risk alleles remains to be demonstrated, it is reasonable to assume that both population genetics and candidate gene approaches will lead to the identification of functional human polymorphisms and will permit the elucidation of robust gene-by-nutrient interactions that will inform dietary approaches to prevent and/or manage complex metabolic disease.

REFERENCES

1. Koch R, Fishler K, Azen C et al. Biochem Mol Med 1997;60: 92–101.
2. Tishkoff SA, Verrelli BC. Annu Rev Genomics Hum Genet 2003;4:293–340.
3. Guttmacher AE, Collins FS. N Engl J Med 2002;347:1512–20.
4. Venter JC, Adams MD, Myers EW et al. Science 2001;291: 1304–51.
5. Cooper DN, Smith BA, Cooke HJ et al. Hum Genet 1985;69: 201–5.
6. Nachman MW, Crowell SL. Genetics 2000;156:297–304.
7. Brody LC, Conley M, Cox C et al. Am J Hum Genet 2002;71: 1207–15.
8. Hishida A, Matsuo K, Hamajima N et al. Haematologica 2003; 88:159–66.
9. Tishkoff SA, Williams SM. Nat Rev Genet 2003;3:611–21.
10. Stover PJ. Physiol Genomics 2004;16:161–5.
11. McCarthy JJ, Hilfiker R. Nat Biotechnol 2000;18:505–8.
12. Clark AG, Glanowski S, Nielsen R et al. Science 2003;302: 1960–3.
13. Diamond J. Nature 2003;423:599–602.
14. Blount BC, Mack MM, Wehr CM et al. Proc Natl Acad Sci USA 1997;94:3290–5.

15. Mishra HN, Das C. Crit Rev Food Sci Nutr 2003;43:245–64.
16. Ames BN. Mutat Res 2001;475:7–20.
17. Goswami T, Rolfs A, Hediger MA. Biochem Cell Biol 2002;80: 679–89.
18. Cooper DN, Krawczak M. Hum Genet 1989;83:181–8.
19. Waterland RA, Jirtle RL. Mol Cell Biol 2003;23:5293–300.
20. Wolfe KH, Li WH. Nat Genet 2003;33[Suppl]:255–65.
21. Akey JM, Zhang G, Zhang K et al. Genome Res 2002;12: 1805–14.
22. Kitami T, Nadeau JH. Nat Genet 2002;32:191–4.
23. Rockman MV, Wray GA. Mol Biol Evol 2002;19:1991–2004.
24. Wright AF, Carothers AD, Pirastu M. Nat Genet 1999;23: 397–404.
25. Wray GA, Hahn MW, Abouheif E et al. Mol Biol Evol 2003; 20:1377–419.
26. Inoue I, Nakajima T, Williams CS et al. J Clin Invest 1997;99: 1786–97.
27. Baier LJ, Permana PA, Yang X et al. J Clin Invest 2000;106: R69–73.
28. Wall JD, Pritchard JK. Nat Rev Genet 2003;4:587–97.
29. Gabriel SB, Schaffner SF, Nguyen H et al. Science 2002;296: 2225–9.
30. Van Blerkom LM. Am J Phys Anthropol 2003;37[Suppl]:14–46.
31. Brookfield JF. Curr Biol 2003;13:R846–7.
32. Batzer MA, Deininger PL. Nat Rev Genet 2002;3:370–9.
33. Todd JA. Bioessays 1999;21:164–74.
34. Horikawa Y, Oda N, Cox NJ et al. Nat Genet 2000;26:163–75.
35. Edmonds DK, Lindsay, KS, Miller JF et al. Fertil Steril 1982; 38:447–53.
36. Edwards RG. Int J Dev Biol 1997;41:255–62.
37. Ames BN, Elson–Schwab I, Silver EA. Am J Clin Nutr 2002;75: 616–58.
38. Young VR. J Nutr 2002;132:621–9.
39. Reyes-Engel A, Munoz E, Gaitan MJ et al. Mol Hum Reprod 2002;8:952–7.
40. Munoz-Moran E, Dieguez-Lucena JL, Fernandez-Arcas N et al. Lancet 1998;352:1120–1.
41. Kim YI. Nutr Rev 2000;58:205–9.
42. Bosron WF, Li TK. Hepatology 1986;6:502–10.
43. Loew M, Boeing H, Sturmer T et al. Alcohol 2003;29:131–5.
44. Swallow DM. Annu Rev Genet 2003;37:197–219.
45. Esposito G, Vitagliano L, Santamaria R et al. FEBS Lett 2002; 531:152–6.
46. Toomajian C, Kreitman M. Genetics 2002;161:1609–23.
47. Fullerton SM, Clark AG, Weiss KM et al. Am J Hum Genet 2000;67:881–900.
48. Zhang J, Zhang YP, Rosenberg HF. Nat Genet 2002;30:411–5.
49. Elliott R, Ong TJ. BMJ 2002;324:1438–42.
50. Bailey LB. J Nutr 2003;133:3748S–3753S.
51. Jacques PF, Bostom AG, Selhub J et al. Atherosclerosis 2003; 166:49–55.
52. Afman LA, Trijbels FJ, Blom HJ. J Nutr 2003;133:75–7.
53. Ordovas JM. Biochem Soc Trans 2002;30:68–73.
54. Devlin AM, Ling EH, Peerson JM et al. Hum Mol Genet 2000; 9:2837–44.
55. Uitterlinden AG, Fang Y, Bergink AP et al. Mol Cell Endocrinol 2002;197:15–21.
56. Griffiths W, Cox T. Hum Mol Genet 2000;9:2377–82.
57. Lee P, Gelbart T, West C et al. Blood Cells Mol Dis 2002;29: 471–87.
58. Bentzen J, Jorgensen T, Fenger M. Clin Genet 2002;61:126–34.
59. Hubacek JA, Pistulkova H, Skodova Z et al. Ann Clin Biochem 2001;38:399–400.
60. Brown S, Ordovas JM, Campos H. Atherosclerosis 2003;170: 307–13.
61. Poulter M, Hollox E, Harvey CB et al. Ann Hum Genet 2003;67: 298–311.
62. Hein DW. Mutat Res 2002;506–7:65–77.
63. Hein DW, Doll MA, Fretland AJ et al. Cancer Epidemiol Biomarkers Prev 2000;9:29–42.
64. Ferre N, Camps J, Fernandez-Ballart J et al. Clin Chem 2003; 49:1491–7.
65. Chistyakov DA, Savost'anov KV, Zotova EV et al. BMC Med Genet 2001;2:4.
66. Van Landeghem GF, Tabatabaie P, Kucinskas V et al. Hum Hered 1999;49:190–3.
67. Messier W, Stewart CB. Nature 1997;385:151–4.
68. Wu W, Goodman M, Lomax MI et al. J Mol Evol 1997;44: 477–91.

SUGGESTED READINGS

Cousins RJ. Nutrient and nutritional genomics. In: Shils ME, Shike M, Ross AC et al., eds. Modern Nutrition in Health and Disease, 10th ed. Baltimore: Lippincott Williams & Wilkins, 2005.
Guttmacher AE, Collins FS. Genomic medicine: a primer. N Engl J Med 2002;347:1512–20 (glossary of genetic terms).

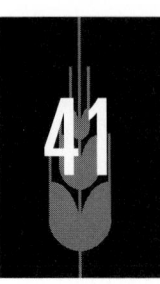

41 HORMONES AND GROWTH FACTORS[1]

IRWIN G. BRODSKY

INTESTINAL HORMONES AND GROWTH
   FACTORS 637
      Incretins 637
      Ghrelin 638
PANCREATIC HORMONES 638
      Insulin 638
      Glucagon 640
ADIPOSE TISSUE HORMONES 640
      Adiponectin 640
      Leptin 642
      Resistin 643
SKELETAL MUSCLE HORMONES 644
      Mechanogrowth Factor 644
HORMONES OF THE ENDOCRINE GLANDS 644
      Thyroid Hormones 644
      Cortisol 645
      Growth Hormone 646
      Testosterone 647
      Estrogen 648
NEURAL HORMONES 649
      Catecholamines .649
CARDIOVASCULAR HORMONES 650
      Angiotensin 650
      Natriuretic Peptides 651

UBIQUITOUS MULTITISSUE HORMONES AND
   GROWTH FACTORS 653
      Somatostatin 655

The metabolism of nutrients is a constant process for living organisms, but the consumption of food is episodic. The requirements for energy and macromolecules vary with physical activity and stresses. Hormones and growth factors provide many of the intercellular signals that move nutrients into and out of storage, alter the availability of stored nutrients for stresses, regulate the use of substrate for growth and reproduction, and redirect nutrients for wound repair.

The concept of endocrine signaling, in which a molecule is released from a hormone-producing cell to act on another cell in a remote location, was affirmed by Bayliss and Starling in 1902, when they described an intestinal extract that could produce remote effects on the pancreas to induce secretion of digestive juices. They coined the term hormone from the Greek *hormao* (to stir up) and named the first hormone that they discovered secretin. Since that time, a wealth of hormones and growth factors have been described that regulate the utilization of nutritional substrate.

Hormones and growth factors influence nutrients in varied ways. They modulate gene transcription, regulate membrane nutrient transporters, regulate intracellular signaling cascades, and control blood flow through nutritional vascular beds. This chapter describes the actions of key hormones and growth factors presently known to affect nutrient metabolism. Some hormones also affect the digestive process and intestinal nutrient absorption. Discussion of these is beyond the scope of this chapter. Likewise, the stresses of infection and inflammation result in the release of immune cytokines that affect nutrient metabolism directly and indirectly through their interaction with endocrine hormones. The discussion of cytokines is presented elsewhere in this text.

This chapter focuses on hormones and growth factors that affect macronutrient (glucose, fat, and protein) storage, release, utilization, and distribution after digestion (Table 41.1). In many cases, nutrient substrates reciprocally influence the production of hormones and growth

---

[1]**Abbreviations: AMP,** adenosine monophosphate; **AMPK,** AMP-sensitive kinase; **ANP,** atrial natriuretic peptide; **ATP,** adenosine triphosphate; **BNP,** brain or B-type natriuretic peptide; **cAMP,** cyclic adenosine monophosphate; **CNP,** C-type natriuretic peptide; **CTGF,** connective tissue growth factor; **DHT,** 5α-dihydrotestosterone; **DOPA,** dihydroxyphenylalanine; **EGF,** epidermal growth factor; **FGF,** fibroblast growth factor; **GIP,** alternately known as glucose-dependent insulinotropic polypeptide and gastric inhibitory polypeptide; **GLP-1,** glucagonlike polypeptide-1; **GLUT-4,** insulin-responsive glucose transporter; **HGF/SF,** hepatocyte growth factor/scatter factor; **hGH-V,** human growth hormone variant; **IGF-I,** insulinlike growth factor-I; **IRS,** insulin receptor substrates; **K$_{ATP}$,** ATP-sensitive potassium channels; **MGF,** mechanogrowth factor; **NGF,** nerve growth factor; **PC,** proprotein convertase; **PDGF,** platelet-derived growth factor; **PKA,** protein kinase A; **PPARα,** peroxisome proliferator activated receptor α; **PPARγ,** peroxisome proliferator activated receptor γ; **SS-14,** somatostatin 14; **SS-28,** somatostatin 28; **T$_3$,** triiodothyronine; **T$_4$,** thyroxine; **TFF,** trefoil factor; **TGF,** transforming growth factor; **TR,** thyroid hormone receptors; **VEGF,** vascular endothelial growth factor.

TABLE 41.1. EFFECT OF HORMONES ON NUTRIENT STORAGE AND BREAKDOWN[a]

HORMONE	APPETITE	GLYCOGEN SYNTHESIS	GLYCOGEN BREAKDOWN	FAT/TRIGLYCERIDE SYNTHESIS	FAT BREAKDOWN	PROTEIN SYNTHESIS	PROTEIN BREAKDOWN
GIP	↔	↔	↔	↑?	↓	↔	↔
GLP-1	↓	↔	↔	↔	↔	↔	↔
Ghrelin	↑↑↑	↔	↔	↔	↔	↔	↔
Insulin	↔?	↑	↓↓	↑	↓↓	↑	↓↓
Glucagon	↔	↓	↑↑	↔	↔	↔	↔
Adiponectin	↔	↔	↔	↓	↔	↔	↔
Leptin	↓↓	↔	↔	↓	↑	↔	↔
Resistin	↔	↓	↑	↔	↔	↔	↔
MGF	↔	↔	↔	↔	↔	↑	↔
Thyroid hormone	↑	↔	↑	↔	↑	↑	↑
Cortisol	↑	↑	↔	↑	↔	↓	↑
Growth hormone	↔	↔	↔	↓	↑↑	↑	↔
Testosterone	↔	↔	↔	↓?	↑	↑↑	↔
Estrogen	↔	↔	↔	↑	↑	↔	↔
Catecholamines	↔	↔	↑	↔	↑↑↑	↑	↔
Angiotensin	↔	↔	↔	↓	↔	↔	↔
Natriuretic peptides	↔	↔	↔	↔	↑	↔	↔
IGF-I	↔	↔	↔	↔	↔	↑	↔

↑, increased or stimulated; ↓, decreased or inhibited; ↔, no known effect; GIP, glucose-dependent insulinotropic polypeptide or gastric inhibitory polypeptide; GLP-1, glucagonlike polypeptide-1; IGF-I, insulinlike growth factor-I; MGF, mechanogrowth factor.
[a]Symbols represent direct effects of hormones on cells and tissues. See text for additional indirect effects of hormones not included in the table.

factors, and these effects will also be discussed as appropriate. The chapter is organized according to the physiologic site of hormone production.

INTESTINAL HORMONES AND GROWTH FACTORS

Incretins

Macronutrient concentrations are tightly regulated in healthy persons. Incretin hormones are intestinal hormones that initiate the process of nutrient distribution and storage before intestinal nutrient absorption is complete (1). This minimizes the excursions of nutrient blood concentrations after a meal and gives a head start to food storage.

Glucose is the nutrient most studied with regard to the incretin effect. Incretin hormone action can be measured as the ratio of the blood glucose response produced by oral ingestion of glucose to the blood glucose response produced by intravenous administration of an identical quantity of glucose. An incretin effect is demonstrated when blood glucose concentration increases to a smaller extent after oral glucose administration than after intravenous glucose administration.

The incretin effect is mediated, in large part, by the ability of the intestinal incretin hormones to augment glucose-induced insulin secretion. In essence, the incretin hormones sound a warning to the pancreatic β cells, notifying them of the impending absorption of nutrients and augmenting the insulin response to early increases in glucose concentrations after a meal.

Insulin is normally secreted in three phases (2). The cephalic phase produces a small increment in insulin through parasympathetic nerve stimulation of pancreatic β cells in response to mental recognition of food in advance of food ingestion. The first phase of insulin secretion occurs within the first 20 minutes of an increment in circulating glucose concentration and is particularly enhanced by incretin activity. The second phase of insulin secretion follows the first 20 minutes and produces the largest increase in insulin concentration of the three phases.

Clinical note: Diabetes is a disorder defined by elevated circulating glucose concentrations produced, in large part, by inadequate secretion of insulin. The most common form of diabetes, type 2 diabetes, is characterized by a decrease in insulin secretion that is only partial. Although the decrease in insulin is only partial, the first phase of insulin secretion is generally entirely absent in this disorder. Thus, agents such as incretins that enhance the first phase of insulin secretion would be attractive potential therapies for patients with type 2 diabetes.

The two most significant incretins are GIP (alternately known as glucose-dependent insulinotropic polypeptide and gastric inhibitory polypeptide) and glucagonlike polypeptide-1 (GLP-1). These hormones belong to the pituitary adenylate cyclase activating peptide/glucagon superfamily of hormones. The superfamily includes nine known hormones encoded on six genes (3). Their actions are mediated by G-protein coupled receptors with seven transmembrane regions. GIP and GLP-1 are secreted by the small intestine in response to the ingestion of glucose and fat. GIP slows gastric emptying, allowing gradual rather than abrupt nutrient absorption, and stimulates insulin secretion. It may also stimulate fat storage.

GLP-1 has additional effects to those of GIP. It stimulates production of several components of the insulin response apparatus, including elements of the glucose sensing pathway. Furthermore, it has trophic effects on islets in vitro, suggesting that it may serve as an islet growth factor. Its ability to suppress glucagon and consequently glucagon-induced hepatic glycogenolysis makes it more potent than GIP at minimizing postprandial glucose excursions. Reducing glucose excursions after a meal is particularly important in diabetes. Perhaps for this reason, GLP-1 has been more effective than GIP in experimental studies at restoring normal glucose metabolism in patients with type 2 diabetes.

Both GIP and GLP-1 are inactivated in vivo by dipeptidyl peptidase IV, a protease that cleaves amino terminus residues from the hormones. Much work in the pharmaceutical industry is now focused on developing treatments for type 2 diabetes that inhibit dipeptidyl peptidase IV or are analogs of GLP-1 resistant to dipeptidyl peptidase IV activity. A naturally occurring analog, exendin-4, has also been investigated for its therapeutic potential in type 2 diabetes.

Ghrelin

Ghrelin is a 28–amino acid peptide that was originally discovered as a natural secretagogue for growth hormone from the anterior pituitary. It was later noted that the primary endogenous source of ghrelin is the stomach. There is production in other areas of the intestine with a proximal-to-distal gradient, such that production is highest in the gastric fundus and lowest in the colon.

Ghrelin is the only known peptide produced by the gastrointestinal tract that increases appetite (4). Levels of ghrelin increase during fasting and correlate with appetite. Ghrelin levels decrease immediately after food consumption, suggesting that ghrelin serves as an appetite factor. Indeed, administration of ghrelin to humans acutely increases appetite and augments energy intake at a single meal by 28% (5). The hormone seems to receive some feedback from adipose tissue stores because ghrelin levels decrease with obesity and negatively correlate with fat cell size.

Clinical note: Gastric bypass surgery is the most effective long-term therapy known for superobesity. The majority of patients are able to lose more than 50% of their excess weight and keep it off for more than 10 years. This stands in stark contrast to most patients who lose weight with conventional dieting, in whom weight regain is the norm. Ghrelin levels are approximately 50% lower in patients who have undergone gastric bypass surgery when compared with their nonoperated obese counterparts (6). A decrease in ghrelin levels may be partly responsible for the long-term success of gastric surgery for weight loss.

PANCREATIC HORMONES

Insulin

The pancreas is well placed in the digestive tract for responding to the ingestion of food. It is a digestive organ with an exocrine component that secretes digestive enzymes. It also has an endocrine component organized in islands dispersed within the pancreatic ductal and acinar system known as the islets of Langerhans.

Insulin, the most extensively studied of the islet hormones, is an approximately 5800 MW hormone with two peptide chains: A (~2300 MW) and B (~3500 MW), coupled by two disulfhydryl linkages. The A chain tertiary structure is maintained by a third intrachain disulfhydryl linkage. Insulin is produced in the β cells of the islets of Langerhans as a prohormone, proinsulin, that contains a connecting peptide (clinically known as C peptide) between the A and B chains that is excised before secretion.

Clinical note: The C-peptide concentration is often used as a method of detecting endogenous insulin secretion in diabetic patients who inject insulin to control glucose. The C peptide is not present in manufactured insulin for clinical injection. Therefore, the presence of abundant C-peptide concentration may identify some patients taking insulin injections who continue to produce their own endogenous insulin and who can be treated without the injections.

Insulin promotes glucose storage as glycogen and inhibits degradation of glycogen. It promotes fat storage and inhibits the breakdown of lipid stores. It promotes protein synthesis and inhibits protein breakdown. Among these nutrients, there is a hierarchy of insulin requirements for their storage. Adipocytes inhibit lipolysis to maintain fat storage with very little insulin stimulation. In skeletal muscle, a lower insulin concentration is required to promote amino acid uptake and inhibit proteolysis than to promote glucose disposal.

Insulin signaling is mediated through a plasma membrane receptor that has two external chains (α chains) and two chains with transmembrane regions (β chains) (7–9). The β chains have tyrosine kinase activity. After insulin binding, the receptor undergoes tyrosine autophosphorylation. This initiates a phosphorylation cascade through tissue-specific insulin receptor substrates (IRS-1, IRS-2, IRS-3, and IRS-4) (10) and, subsequently, though two primary high-energy phosphate transfer systems (i.e., the ras system and the phosphatidyl inositol system). Several active products of these pathways mediate actions of insulin as diverse as stimulation of transmembrane nutrient transport, induction of DNA synthesis, induction of gene transcription, stimulation of protein synthesis, and inhibition of apoptosis.

Glucose uptake is stimulated when the phosphatidyl inositol system, through phosphatidyl inositol-3-kinase, produces inositol 3,4,5-triphosphate. Inositol 3,4,5-triphosphate, largely through protein kinase B/Akt, promotes the redistribution of the insulin-responsive glucose transporter, GLUT-4, from intracellular storage sites to the plasma membrane. GLUT-4 is primarily expressed in adipose and muscle tissues. An additional or alternate way in which insulin stimulates GLUT-4 translocation to the plasma membrane involves plasma membrane lipid raft-associated signaling pathways. In this alternate pathway, phosphorylation of Cbl

(Casitas B lineage) by the insulin receptor results in the activation of TC10 (isolated from teratocarcinoma cell line), a small Rho (*Ras* homolog) family guanosine triphosphate binding protein that stimulates intracellular F-actin rearrangement for GLUT-4 translocation.

Insulin stimulates fat storage through its contribution to adipocyte differentiation, its inhibition of lipolysis, and its stimulation of lipogenesis, although the latter is likely a minor effect in humans.

Insulin inhibits lipolysis in part by inhibiting the hormone-sensitive lipase translocation to the lipid droplet. Translocation of the lipase to the lipid droplet in the adipocyte is required for the liberation, by hormone-sensitive lipase, of free fatty acids from stored triglyceride. Analogous to its effect on glucose transport, insulin also promotes intracellular fatty acid transport by stimulating translocation of fatty acid binding proteins to the plasma membrane.

Insulin promotes protein storage primarily by inhibiting protein breakdown. One pathway mediating insulin inhibition of protein degradation is the insulin-degrading enzyme pathway (11). Insulin-degrading enzyme forms complexes with the 26S proteasome—the large intracellular complex responsible for the bulk of intracellular protein turnover. insulin-degrading enzyme, in the presence of insulin and after degrading insulin, inhibits the proteolytic activity of the proteasome. Insulin also promotes protein synthesis through its stimulation of protein kinase B/Akt and the mammalian target of rapamycin pathway. The latter pathway activates the enzyme p70 S6 kinase that has effects within the nucleus to promote transcription of ribosomal RNA and production of ribosomes, the structures responsible for mRNA translation and production of proteins. Most studies in adults indicate that the effect of insulin to inhibit protein degradation is a more prominent anabolic effect of insulin than its effect to promote protein synthesis.

Although insulin promotes nutrient storage, nutrients promote insulin production to begin the process. The β cells of the pancreatic islets respond exquisitely to their nutritional environment. Glucose phosphorylation by glucokinase to glucose-6-phosphate results in insulin secretion. Increased concentration of lipid in the islet β cell causes augmented insulin production, providing a reasonable mechanism by which the islet creates hyperinsulinemia as body fat content increases. It seems that glucose metabolism and subsequent adenosine triphosphate (ATP) production result in closure of ATP-sensitive potassium channels (K_{ATP}). The depolarization of the cell, in turn, induces intracellular calcium ion release from the endoplasmic reticulum to induce a first phase of insulin release after ingestion of nutrients in what some call the ion-dependent phase of insulin release. A second phase of insulin release follows approximately 20 minutes after the glucose influx in what seems to be an ion-independent process. Present evidence suggests that the second phase

results when accumulation of glucose metabolic byproducts in the islet β cell secondarily promotes fatty acid accumulation in the β cell and fatty acylation of proteins involved in insulin secretion (2). This hypothesized mechanism for second-phase insulin release is consistent with the augmentation of insulin secretion by increased islet fat content.

Thus, intestines absorbing nutrients, pancreatic islets, and nutrient storage depots form an exquisite axis of intercommunication. The nutrients themselves and intestinal incretins stimulate insulin secretion from the islet β cells. Insulin from the islet β cells enlarges the fat and glucose/glycogen storage depot (primarily in adipose tissue, muscle, and liver). Impaired storage of fatty acids or glucose results in increased islet content of these nutrients and compensatory increases in insulin secretion to produce hyperinsulinemia.

The benefit of maintaining a whole-body perspective on insulin as a food storage hormone has been illustrated by experiments in which insulin receptors have been selectively deleted from specific tissues. Disruption of the insulin receptor in selected tissues of mice has revealed a surprising ability of one tissue to compensate for disrupted insulin action in another (12, 13). Inability of insulin to promote glucose disposal in muscle produces compensatory increases in insulin secretion and storage of glucose in fat and liver. Inability of insulin to prevent output of glucose from the liver promotes increased disposal into muscle. The greatest impairment in glucose tolerance in mice seems to occur with impaired insulin action in pancreatic islets and in the brain. Insulin receptors in islets regulate postnatal islet development. Underdeveloped islets in animals lacking islet insulin receptors produce inadequate insulin concentrations for nutrient storage. Insulin receptors in the brain partly regulate nutrient intake, with absent receptors resulting in increased food intake, adiposity, and whole-body impairment of glucose disposal.

If there is a well-regulated system of intercommunication between pancreatic islets and storage depots of fat and glucose, why should increased food intake and adiposity produce impairment in glucose disposal rather than continued compensation by the islet to produce more insulin and induce more storage of these nutrients? Apparently, there are limits to how much lipid and glucose can be stored, although the limits seem to vary from one individual to another. When those limits are reached, resistance to the actions of insulin develops in insulin-sensitive tissues, a hallmark of type 2 diabetes. Humans with a condition known as lipodystrophy have very limited depots for fat storage, showing a well-muscled appearance because of a lack of subcutaneous fat. With a very minimal excess of energy intake above requirements, patients with lipodystrophy develop high levels of circulating glucose and triglyceride despite high compensatory levels of insulin. Excess nutrients may also be stored in the liver (14). It is common to encounter patients with type 2 diabetes or lipodystrophy who have what is called hepatic steatosis or fatty liver.

Clinical note: A family of medications known as thiazolidinediones stimulates the deposition of fat and glucose in the lower extremities. The increased capacity for fat and glucose storage they provide improves whole-body responsiveness to insulin and results in a decrease in circulating glucose and triglyceride levels in patients with type 2 diabetes.

Glucagon

Glucagon is the prototypical counterregulatory hormone—it counterregulates the actions of insulin. Glucagon is produced in the α cells of the pancreatic islet that are juxtaposed to the β cells producing insulin. The primary action of glucagon is to stimulate the production and release of glucose from the liver into the circulation (15). Thus, glucagon provides a first-line defense against low circulating blood glucose levels.

Glucagon is produced as a prohormone that is cleaved into its final form by one of three proprotein convertases (PC1-3). PC1-3 in intestinal cells produces glucagonlike peptides (see the section on GLP-1). PC2 in the α cells of pancreatic islets produces glucagon.

Glucagon coordinates the production of glucose by the liver through stimulation of glycogen breakdown, inhibition of glycogen synthesis, and stimulation of gluconeogenesis. Glucagon acts through the second-messenger cyclic adenosine monophosphate (cAMP). Glucagon stimulates a rhodopsinlike receptor at the liver cell surface that is associated with the adenylate cyclase enzyme capable of producing cAMP. The cAMP, in turn, stimulates protein kinase A (PKA), phosphorylase kinase, and glycogen phosphorylase. Glycogen phosphorylase mediates an enzymatic reaction in which a pyridoxal phosphate group transfers inorganic phosphate to the glucose molecule at the nonreducing end of a glycogen chain (nonreducing end merely indicates that the first carbon of glucose that can reduce copper in vitro is bound at the end of a glycogen chain in the typical α 1-4 linkage and cannot perform the reducing function; the nonreducing end of glucose is exposed at the end of the glycogen chain). Glucose is released from the glycogen chain as glucose-1-phosphate, converted to glucose-6-phosphate, and released into the circulation as glucose by the action of glucose-6-phosphatase, an enzyme also stimulated by glucagon.

The formation of cAMP by the action of glucagon, working through PKA, also phosphorylates the enzyme protein phosphatase 1. In its phosphorylated form, protein phosphatase 1 is inhibited and cannot dephosphorylate glycogen synthase to activate it for glycogen synthesis. Thus, glucagon can simultaneously cause glycogen breakdown by phosphorylating the phosphorylase kinase and phosphorylase while it stops glycogen synthesis by phosphorylating protein phosphatase 1. The net result is glucose release from the liver.

As glycogen stores diminish, glucose release from the liver is maintained by gluconeogenesis. Glucagon increases gluconeogenesis by stimulating the transcription of the phosphoenolpyruvate carboxykinase gene. The conversion of oxaloacetate to phosphoenolpyruvate is a rate-limiting step in the production of glucose by gluconeogenesis.

Glucagon can stimulate glycogen breakdown in muscle as well as liver. However, the bulk of the glucose entering the circulation from the action of glucagon comes from the liver.

Clinical note: Patients with type 1 diabetes experience frequent hypoglycemia from inadvertent overestimation of insulin dose requirements. Endogenous glucagon from pancreatic α cells helps defend against hypoglycemia, allowing recovery of normal glucose levels. Patients with type 1 diabetes are generally given a glucagon emergency kit for use in the event that endogenous defenses are inadequate to promote recovery from hypoglycemia and brain dysfunction occurs. A family member or friend must inject the glucagon intramuscularly. Recovery of glucose levels and brain function usually occurs within 10 to 15 minutes after administration of the glucagon.

ADIPOSE TISSUE HORMONES

Adipose tissue was once considered an inert storage depot for excess energy intake. Quite the contrary, adipose tissue is an extremely active endocrine organ (16). It produces unique hormones that govern nutrient storage. It also produces an abundance of cytokines and growth factors involved in inflammation and tissue repair. Of course, teleologically, it is reasonably important for the body to have some sense of its energy store before embarking on certain processes of reproduction, tissue repair, and tissue turnover. What better tissue to provide information about stored energy resources than fat tissue?

Adipose tissue produces cytokines such as tumor necrosis factor-α, interleukin-6, interleukin-1β, macrophage colony stimulating factor, interleukin-8, and complement system components, among others. The role of these factors, usually associated with immunity and inflammation, in adipose tissue functions is unknown. They may be involved in mobilizing nutrients, mediating an immune function, or both. The actions of immune cytokines on nutrients will be addressed in other chapters.

Growth factors are also produced within adipose tissue, generating questions regarding the role of adipose tissue in tissue regeneration and growth. Factors such as hepatocyte growth factor and fibroblast growth factors are discussed later in this chapter. The following paragraphs present information about hormones for which adipose tissue is the primary production site.

Adiponectin

Adiponectin has also been called adipocyte complement-related protein of 30 kDa (17). It is uniquely produced in adipose tissue and circulates at very high levels, nearly 1000 times the concentration of most other hormones, accounting for 0.01% of total plasma protein. Adiponectin has structural similarity to collagen VIII, collagen X, and the complement component C1q.

Adiponectin levels decrease as fat mass increases and increase as fat mass decreases (Figs. 41.1 and 41.2). Adiponectin accentuates sensitivity to insulin. It enhances tyrosine phosphorylation of the insulin receptor and of insulin receptor substrates in muscle. It decreases concentrations of circulating fatty acids and decreases levels of triglycerides in muscle and liver. The exact mechanism by which adiponectin achieves these effects is unknown. An adiponectin receptor has recently been identified (18). It has a structure distinct from other receptor families. There have been two isoforms identified. AdipoR1 is abundant in muscle, and AdipoR2 is expressed in liver. The adiponectin receptors activate the AMP-sensitive kinase (AMPK) and peroxisome proliferator activated receptor α (PPARα) signaling pathways (19). Because AMPK activity is stimulated when intracellular energy is low (i.e., when the ratio of AMP to ATP is high) and activates metabolic pathways that regenerate ATP, it seems that adiponectin is a hormone that replenishes cellular energy (20).

It is interesting to note that adiponectin levels parallel the activity of the peroxisome proliferator activated receptor γ (PPARγ) system. Dominant negative mutations decreasing PPARγ activity and polymorphisms decreasing

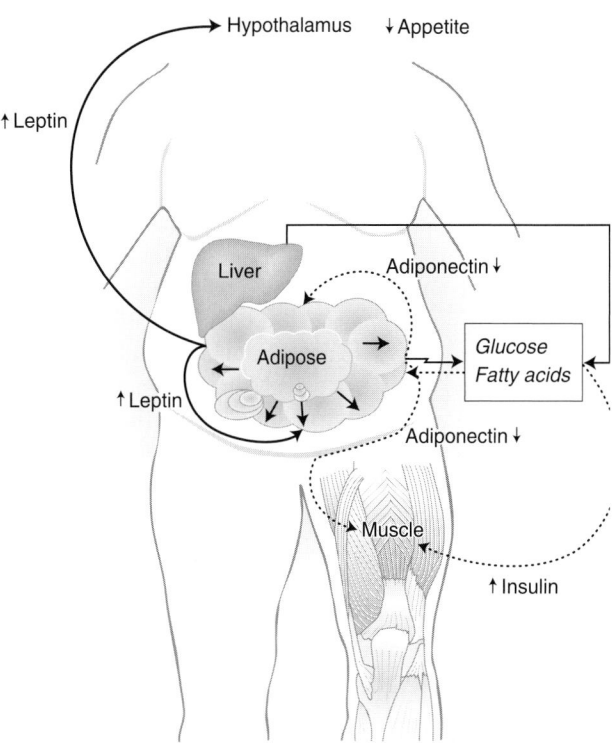

Figure 41.2. Hormonal response to weight gain. Adiponectin levels decrease, inhibiting substrate disposal. Leptin levels increase to blunt the appetite and the intake of additional substrate. Insulin levels increase to maintain modest substrate disposal in the face of tissue resistance to insulin action.

PPARγ activity decrease the concentrations of adiponectin. Agonists of the PPARγ receptor increase adiponectin levels. The PPARγ receptor is stimulated by a set of medications commonly used to treat insulin-resistant type 2 diabetes. These medications, termed thiazolidinediones, increase insulin sensitivity and are known to increase the proliferation of small adipocytes in peripheral subcutaneous fat depots. By contrast, the insulin resistance that accompanies type 2 diabetes and low levels of adiponectin is associated with fat storage in large adipocytes of the intraabdominal fat depot. Thus, high levels of adiponectin are associated not with fat storage but with the presence of peripheral fat storage capacity, a condition that enhances the response to the nutrient storage hormone insulin. Although adiponectin levels seem to increase and decrease with fat storage capacity and PPARγ activity, there is no evidence to date showing that adiponectin mediates the actions of the PPARγ system. On the contrary, PPARγ simulates the generation of new fat cells in peripheral fat to promote nutrient storage, whereas adiponectin steers metabolic pathways toward nutrient use and away from fat production. The apparent paradox may be reconciled if one speculates that the generation of new adipose tissue by PPARγ necessitates the replenishment of a high-energy state in the cell (i.e., high ATP) to facilitate new fat deposition. Under these conditions,

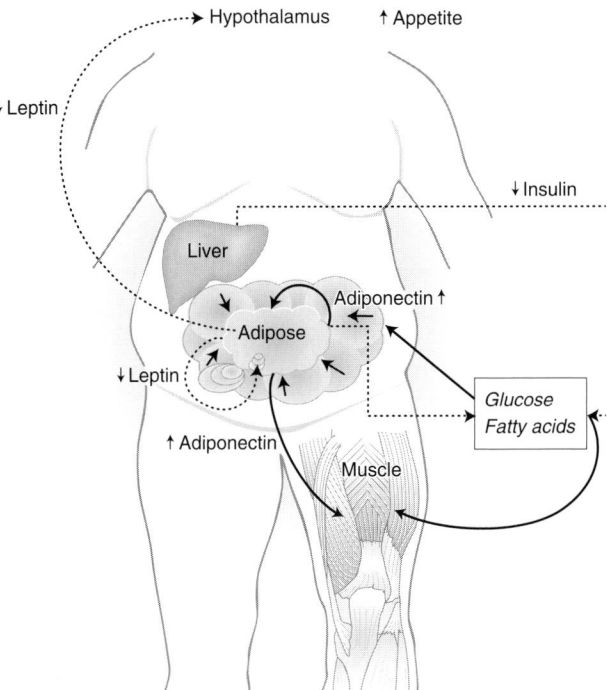

Figure 41.1. Hormonal response to weight loss. Adiponectin enhances disposal of substrates. Low leptin levels stimulate intake of additional substrate. Low insulin levels prevent deficiency of glucose and fat in the circulation.

nutrient uptake in fat and muscle will be enhanced and the insulin requirement to promote nutrient uptake will be reduced. In such a context, the decrease in insulin concentrations and the increase in insulin sensitivity seen with both PPARγ agonists and adiponectin make sense.

Adiponectin has certain additional actions that have implicated it as a protective agent for cardiovascular atherosclerosis. Adiponectin decreases adhesion molecules on vascular endothelium, decreases monocyte/macrophage adhesion to endothelium, prevents foam cell formation (i.e., the fat-laden macrophages found in atherosclerotic plaques), and inhibits proliferation of vascular smooth muscle cells.

To summarize, low levels of adiponectin are to be found when obesity and its associated health complications (type 2 diabetes, atherosclerotic disease) are present. High levels of adiponectin are found when one is lean, has ample capacity for nutrient storage and use, and has a low risk for atherosclerosis. The full spectrum of biochemical actions of adiponectin has yet to be defined.

Leptin

Leptin is a 16-kDa hormone with a structure similar to that of the immune cytokine interleukin-2 and, like adiponectin, it is produced primarily by adipose tissue. By contrast with adiponectin, leptin is secreted by adipose tissue in increasing amounts as fat mass increases. It is secreted to a greater degree by peripheral than by abdominal fat.

The coordinated function of leptin in vivo has been difficult to discern. There are leptin receptors on peripheral tissues such as muscle, liver, pancreatic islet, monocyte, lymphocyte, ovary, placenta, and testicular tissues. However, the effects of leptin on these tissues seem, at our present level of knowledge, to be subordinated to the more powerful effects of leptin on the central nervous system.

Two actions of leptin seem certain. First, leptin regulates body mass by inhibiting food intake. The discovery of leptin as the product of the *ob* gene occurred during crossbreeding experiments with the genetically obese *ob⁻/ob⁻* mouse. The absence of leptin in these mice was associated with hyperphagia and severe obesity. Leptin levels do not correlate with short-term satiety signals but rather with long-term appetite and maintenance of fat mass (21). As such, leptin may serve as a modulator of the degree of stimulation or inhibition of food intake by other short-term appetite regulators. The second major action of leptin is to regulate reproduction (22). Leptin stimulates the production of gonadotropin-releasing hormone in the hypothalamus, promoting fertility and possibly influencing the initiation of puberty. The presence of leptin is an important signal from adipose tissue to the brain that nutrient stores are sufficient both for the limitation of additional food intake and for the nutrient-demanding processes of pubertal development and reproduction.

Leptin's effect of modulating nutrient intake is mediated by its effects on several orexigenic (appetite stimulatory) and anorexigenic (appetite inhibitory) pathways. Leptin downregulates the production of the orexigenic neuropeptide Y, melanin-concentrating hormone, Agouti-related protein, and other orexins. Leptin upregulates anorexigenic factors like α-melanocyte stimulating hormone, corticotropin releasing hormone, and cocaine/amphetamine regulated transcript.

Although the ability of leptin to suppress appetite in the central nervous system may dominate its effect to limit the growth of body fat mass, there may be other peripheral pathways that contribute. Leptin can stimulate fat use by inhibiting lipogenesis, stimulating lipolysis, and stimulating fat oxidation. It seems to achieve this through stimulation of AMPK and related pathways (20). This phenomenon frames an unusual situation in which the hormone leptin, a signal of ample fat storage, stimulates a metabolic pathway (i.e., AMPK) that usually serves as a signal of intracellular energy deficiency. One may hypothesize that leptin simultaneously signals the adequacy of fat stores and limits their expansion, inhibiting food intake and wasting excess fat through stimulation of fat oxidation. In so doing, leptin seems to override the reliance of the AMPK pathway on low intracellular energy for its activity.

Several findings describe the role of leptin in the maintenance of fat mass in humans. Rare mutations in the leptin gene or the leptin receptor gene induce chronic hyperphagia and severe obesity. Parenteral administration of leptin to those with rare leptin mutations and leptin deficiency results in significant weight loss. Leptin levels decrease when humans are underfed, disproportionate to the degree of fat loss, suggesting that leptin signaling is important for communicating directional change in body nutrient stores as well as the nutrient mass itself. The decrease in leptin levels during underfeeding stimulates long-term food intake and the restoration of nutrient stores.

Although intuition would dictate that leptin levels would be low in obese humans as an explanation for chronically excessive food intake, the opposite is true. With the exception of the rare leptin mutations, the vast majority of obese humans exhibit elevated circulating leptin concentrations. The latter suggests that obesity in humans is associated with resistance to the effects of leptin on the brain appetite centers. This has limited the value of leptin as an agent for treating human obesity. Resistance to leptin is not generally caused by abnormalities in the leptin receptor, rather, it may be caused by impaired leptin transfer across the blood-brain barrier or decreased activity of downstream signaling pathways.

The effect of leptin on reproduction is multifaceted. Apart from its role in regulating gonadotropin-releasing hormone centrally, leptin may act locally to help embryo implantation in the endometrium, and the presence of leptin receptors on developing ovarian follicles suggests that it may have a role in oocyte maturation. After embryo implantation, trophoblasts, and ultimately placenta produce leptin. An abnormal increase in leptin during pregnancy may herald the onset of preeclampsia, although it is not known whether the change in leptin is the cause or the result of abnormal placental physiology. Finally, in the postpartum period, leptin is produced by mammary tissue and transferred to the milk. It is not certain whether the transfer of leptin from mammary tissue and blood into milk reflects the importance of leptin for lactation and neonatal physiology or reflects a leptin drain that signals the mother to increase nutrient intake during lactation.

Although the importance of leptin for maintenance of body mass and reproduction seems clear, there seem to be other functions of leptin that are less well understood. Leptin enhances the immune response through its stimulation of T-helper functions and its stimulation of mononuclear cells through trophic and secretory effects. Because immunity is partially dependent on nutrition, leptin may provide an important signal to the immune system of nutritional status. Whether high leptin levels in people with increased body fat produce a proinflammatory state is not clear.

Finally, leptin may also serve as a mediator of bone mass. A full understanding of the manner in which obesity preserves bone mass has been sought for some time. Leptin, a signal of fat mass adequacy, would be an attractive link between obesity and bone mass. The overall effect of leptin on bone mass of humans in vivo has not been determined. Leptin stimulates the sympathetic nervous system, which, in turn, induces bone loss. However, leptin is produced by osteoblasts, and in an autocrine manner, it promotes osteoblast proliferation, prevents osteoblast cell death, and enhances bone mineralization.

To summarize, in contrast with adiponectin, which signals available capacity for nutrient storage, leptin provides a signal to multiple tissues that ample food has been stored. Leptin also limits the expansion of fat mass by inhibiting additional food intake when the fat store is large and by allowing some wastage of fat through stimulation of fat oxidation. Leptin serves the important role of permitting body functions such as reproduction and pubertal development that are demanding in terms of their energy cost. Leptin promotes reproduction and puberty when nutrient stores are adequate and inhibits them via decreases in leptin concentration when nutrient stores are inadequate.

Resistin

Resistin is a cysteine-rich peptide hormone found generally as an oligomer and produced in adipocytes during their differentiation. However, the hormone seems to inhibit certain aspects of adipocyte differentiation. It is in a family of homologous resistinlike molecules found in varied tissues (23). Resistin was discovered when its transcript was found to be suppressed during adipocyte exposure to rosiglitazone, a thiazolidinedione drug that is an agonist of the adipogenic PPARγ intranuclear receptors. The thiazolidinedione drugs are, of course, those drugs

used to enhance insulin sensitivity in people with type 2 insulin-resistant diabetes mellitus.

Resistin gets its name from its ability to antagonize the actions of insulin, decreasing glucose uptake in adipocytes, muscle cells, and whole-body measurements. It is found in greater amounts in abdominal visceral adipose tissue (associated with insulin resistance) than in subcutaneous adipose tissue. Resistin production in adipose tissue increases during lipolytic conditions often associated with insulin resistance (e.g., growth hormone excess, insulin-deficiency with ketosis). Some animal studies suggest that its main effect, inducing insulin resistance, derives from its ability block the effect of insulin to suppress hepatic glucose-6-phosphatase, glycogenolysis, gluconeogenesis, and consequently overall hepatic glucose production (24, 25). Indeed, recent evidence in mice lacking the resistin gene indicates that resistin supports the production of gluconeogenic enzymes by the liver. The discovery of resistin during the study of thiazolidinedione drugs suggested that the ability of thiazolidinedione drugs to improve insulin sensitivity or diminish insulin resistance might be tied in part to their ability to suppress resistin production.

Although it has been tempting to identify resistin as the adipocyte-derived hormone that is responsible for insulin resistance and type 2 diabetes in individuals with a large fat mass, several findings should provoke caution in making such conclusions. Data are inconsistent regarding the relationship of resistin to the insulin resistance of obesity and type 2 diabetes in humans (26). They generally indicate that resistin increases with adiposity in humans but does not induce insulin resistance or diabetes. Resistin is produced in tissues other than adipose tissue, principally in bone marrow and macrophage/monocytes, in amounts greater than those from adipose tissue and in response to stimulation by proinflammatory immune cytokines and bacterial lipopolysaccharide. The latter suggests a relationship between resistin and inflammation. The primary function of resistin remains unknown at this time. In the final analysis, resistin may represent an agent promoting transfer of nutrients into circulation (e.g., inhibition of glucose uptake, promotion of hepatic glucose output), particularly during stress and inflammation.

A comment should be made about specific adipose depots and general physiologic patterns attributable to them. Long-term fat storage is primarily associated with peripheral subcutaneous fat. Hormones that signal the existence of stable fat storage (e.g., leptin) will be found predominantly in peripheral subcutaneous fat. Physiologic processes that require stable, long-lived fat stores (e.g., reproduction) are stimulated by such hormones. Hormones that promote long-term fat storage (e.g., insulin) act predominantly on the peripheral subcutaneous fat.

Rapid fat turnover and sensitive responses to lipolytic stimuli are associated with visceral abdominal fat. One can conceive of the visceral abdominal fat depot as an emergency depot or the adipose equivalent of short-term parking.

The visceral adipose depot produces hormones that counteract long-term nutrient storage and promote transfer of nutrients (i.e., glucose and fat) into the circulation (e.g., resistin, immune cytokines [tumor necrosis factor-α, interleukin-1, interleukin-6, interleukin-8, and others]). In counteracting long-term nutrient storage, hormones from the abdominal fat depot counteract the effect of insulin.

Clinical note: It logically follows that persons who accumulate fat predominantly in the abdominal visceral fat depot would have insulin resistance and those who store fat predominantly in the peripheral subcutaneous gluteofemoral (hip, buttock, thigh) area would retain insulin sensitivity. This pattern is what is usually observed clinically. Insulin-resistant type 2 diabetic patients have abdominal adiposity, and persons without insulin resistance have little abdominal fat compared with gluteofemoral fat. The correlation between body fat distribution and insulin resistance is also influenced by genetic and environmental factors.

SKELETAL MUSCLE HORMONES

Skeletal muscle has two primary functions. It is responsible for locomotion and for mechanical work. It is the body's largest protein depot, providing storage and release of amino acids.

Skeletal muscle responds to the actions of many hormones, growth factors, and nutrients. Skeletal muscle atrophy with export of amino acids into the circulation can result from the actions of immune cytokines (e.g., tumor necrosis factor-α, interleukin-6). Muscle growth can result from several circulating factors. Insulin inhibits muscle protein degradation. Growth hormone, insulinlike growth factor-I (IGF-I), and androgens increase muscle mass. Amino acids themselves, notably leucine, can stimulate muscle protein production. These factors circulate systemically and are not uniquely produced in muscle. Presumably, they foster muscle growth during ample nutrition and during sexual development.

Mechanogrowth Factor

Muscle growth is chiefly stimulated by exercise. The mechanism behind exercise-induced muscle growth remains poorly understood. However, one autocrine or paracrine mediator of exercise-induced muscle growth has been reported. A splice variant of IGF-I has been described that is smaller than IGF-I and is not glycosylated, giving it a shorter half-life. The IGF-I variant, known as mechanogrowth factor (MGF), or alternately as IGF-IEc, is produced by muscular stretch and contractile activity (27). Its overexpression in muscle produces an increase in muscle mass and an increase in the fiber size of the muscle fibers in which it is expressed. Electrical muscle depolarization is not required to induce MGF transcription. MGF does not use the IGF-I receptor to induce muscle growth. It has a unique binding protein that enhances its stability. MGF seems to recruit satellite muscle cells and induce factors essential for myocyte differentiation, augmenting production of new muscle after stretch, contractile activity, or muscle injury. Other IGF-I splice variants, such as IGF-IEa, seem to be produced later after muscle injury to promote the muscle protein synthesis required to complete muscle repair.

The discovery of MGF at least partly explains how exercise, muscle stretch, and muscle injury induce muscle growth. The response of MGF expression to exercise is smaller in elderly persons than in the young, perhaps explaining the tendency toward decreased muscle mass with aging. There seems to be synergy between growth hormone and exercise in the induction of MGF expression, suggesting that the response of muscle growth to exercise can be affected by other circulating anabolic hormones.

HORMONES OF THE ENDOCRINE GLANDS

Endocrine hormones are produced by discreet glands and act on tissues distant from their sites of production. In general terms, endocrine hormones orchestrate wholebody changes with unique responses in each of the several tissues on which they act. With regard to nutrients, endocrine hormones mediate patterns of nutrient disposal to coordinate anabolism, catabolism, growth, and stress responses.

Thyroid Hormones

The thyroid gland, a butterfly-shaped gland approximately 20 g, straddles the trachea at and just above the level of the sternal notch. It produces, stores, and secretes three hormones. Calcitonin is produced by neuroendocrine cells dispersed within the thyroid gland and inhibits calcium resorption from bone. Calcitonin will not be discussed in this chapter. Rather, the two classic thyroid hormones, thyroxine and triiodothyronine, also known as T_4 and T_3, respectively, are discussed here. Both are synthesized by the combination of two iodotyrosine molecules. When two molecules of diiodotyrosine combine, a molecule containing four iodine atoms, T_4, is produced. When a molecule of monoiodotyrosine and diiodotyrosine combine, a molecule with three iodine atoms, T_3, is produced. The T_3 molecule is the more biologically active of the two, and T_4 is converted to T_3 intracellularly by a 5'-deiodinase.

Thyroid hormone is necessary for growth and development in childhood. It is particularly important for the development of the central nervous system. Low levels of thyroid hormone in early development, including the period in utero, produce impaired growth and mental development. When this occurs in the setting of dietary iodine deficiency, the condition, called cretinism, is particularly severe because the thyroid glands of both the mother and the fetus show uncompensated dysfunction.

In adulthood, thyroid hormones enhance both synthesis and degradation of proteins. To view this function teleologically, the turnover of proteins promoted by thyroid hormone is required to prevent accumulation of unnecessary proteins and to create the new proteins needed for changing bodily requirements. The most remarkable example of the importance of this turnover function has been described in amphibians that require thyroid hormone to undergo metamorphosis. For tadpoles to become frogs, thyroid hormone must help them grow legs and lose their tails.

The enhancement of protein turnover is accompanied by an increase in oxygen consumption and the metabolic rate. An increased metabolic rate mediated by thyroid hormone is accompanied by increased heat generation (28). Part of the heat generation is attributable to heat produced by the metabolic reactions themselves, and part to the chemical inefficiencies created by the thyroid hormone–induced generation of uncoupling proteins (UCP-1, UCP-2, and UCP-3) that uncouple oxidative phosphorylation in the mitochondria. The purpose of the uncoupling of chemical energy production and the generation of heat is not certain, but it is speculated that it allows homeothermic animals to maintain a larger energy production capacity when the energy is not needed for mechanical or chemical work so that energy is rapidly available at other times when it is needed.

The metabolic requirements created by thyroid hormone action are supported by glucose production and fatty acid release. Increased concentrations of thyroid hormones produce increased glucose production by gluconeogenesis. Increased hepatic gluconeogenesis is supported by increased muscle glycogenolysis, glucose uptake, and glucose conversion to lactate (the cycling of glucose to lactate and back to glucose through gluconeogenesis is known as the Cori cycle) (29). Increased gluconeogenesis with high levels of thyroid hormone is likewise supported by increased amino acid release from muscle. By contrast, low levels of thyroid hormone decrease the rate of gluconeogenesis.

Increased thyroid hormone concentrations additionally produce increased fatty acid release. This is accomplished in two ways. High levels of thyroid hormone augment local release of catecholamines in the adipose tissue. Secondly, the lipolytic response to catecholamines is enhanced in the presence of high thyroid hormone concentrations. By corollary, the lipolytic response to catecholamines is diminished in the presence of low levels of thyroid hormone.

As expected, augmented oxygen consumption with elevated thyroid hormone levels requires greater cardiac output and peripheral circulation (30). High levels of thyroid hormone increase cardiac contractility, increase heart rate, and decrease peripheral arterial resistance.

The effects of thyroid hormone involve the induction of gene expression through thyroid hormone interaction with specific intranuclear receptors (31, 32). The thyroid receptors are related to those of the intranuclear receptor family associated with vitamin D_3, retinoic acid receptor, and glucocorticoid receptors (33). Thyroid hormone receptors are transcribed with at least nine variants because of alternative messenger RNA splicing. However, only four isoforms are known to be expressed. These are labeled thyroid hormone receptors (TR) $TR\alpha_1$, $TR\alpha_2$, $TR\beta_1$, and $TR\beta_2$. They mediate isoform-specific functions. Interaction of thyroid hormone with its receptor and binding of the complex to DNA most commonly causes derepression of genes, although suppression by thyroid hormone of thyrotropin secretion in pituitary thyrotrophs involves gene repression.

Clinical note: The clinical picture of thyroid hormone excess clearly reflects the increased rate of metabolic processes, the increased production of heat, and the increased production of catecholamines. Thyrotoxic patients are frequently heat intolerant, feeling warm and perspiring to dissipate heat when others in the same room feel comfortable. The heart rate is rapid. Thyrotoxic patients are often irritable and impatient. The effect of excess catecholamine sensitivity is seen as patients show a wide-eyed stare, a fine neuromuscular tremor, and rapid relaxation of neuromuscular reflexes. Appetite and food intake are often increased without a concomitant increase in accumulation of body fat. Although administration of excess thyroid hormone may seem attractive as a route to weight loss in obese patients, the long-term loss of skeletal muscle mass and function, cardiac muscle mass and function, and bone mass with chronically elevated thyroid hormone levels makes it inadvisable.

Patients with low levels of thyroid hormone show clinical features opposite of those of patients with high levels. Patients are cold intolerant. Skin is dry. Connective tissue proteins accumulate to produce weight gain and puffiness of tissues. Mental processes are slowed. The heart rate is slow. Relaxation of neuromuscular reflexes is slow. All of these abnormalities resolve with administration of thyroid hormone.

Cortisol

Cortisol is a steroid hormone produced in the adrenal gland cortex. The early discovery of its effects on glucose metabolism led to its being dubbed a glucocorticoid, in contrast to the mineralocorticoid aldosterone that regulates sodium and potassium handling. Cortisol coordinates the body's stress response. In so doing, it not only enhances acute physiologic responses but also prepares the body, under basal conditions, to respond to stress when the need arises. The general physiologic processes coordinated by cortisol include maintenance of vascular tone and blood flow distribution, preservation of glycogen stores, continuance of gluconeogenesis, determination of fat distribution (particularly promoting distribution within catecholamine-sensitive intraabdominal and truncal depots), maintenance of lipolysis, and perpetuation of proteolysis. All of these processes allow rapid mobilization of nutrients for preservation of normal physiology under stress.

The effect of cortisol on blood flow is to increase blood pressure and to enhance circulation to viscera rather than to peripheral tissues. Cortisol inhibits vasodilation of forearm arteries but enhances blood flow in the brain and renal arteries.

The effect of cortisol on glucose metabolism is to enhance both glucose storage and release into the circulation. Cortisol promotes hepatic glycogen synthesis and gluconeogenesis. It inhibits glucose uptake peripherally in skeletal muscle. Conceptually, cortisol redistributes glucose from peripheral use to visceral storage. By enhancing gluconeogenesis, it makes more glucose available for hepatic storage and makes more circulating glucose available for the central nervous system, the tissue most dependent on glucose for energy.

Cortisol promotes deposition of fat, in part through stimulation of lipoprotein lipase activity. Because there are greater numbers of glucocorticoid receptors in intraabdominal adipose than peripheral adipose tissue depots, cortisol promotes abdominal adiposity. Apart from the higher number of glucocorticoid receptors in abdominal adipose tissue, there may be increased local production of cortisol in abdominal fat by virtue of increased activity in abdominal fat of the 11-β-hydroxysteroid dehydrogenase-1 enzyme that converts inactive cortisone to cortisol (34, 35).

Intraabdominal fat has a greater sensitivity to catecholamine-induced lipolysis than peripheral subcutaneous fat. Therefore, the effect of cortisol to preferentially allocate fat to the abdominal depot has the tendency to increase the availability of circulating fatty acids under circumstances of stress with acute catecholamine release.

Cortisol induces protein breakdown and release of amino acids, particularly from muscle (36). Consistent with its role of increasing gluconeogenesis, there is also an increased transfer of nitrogen from branched-chain amino acids to alanine, a gluconeogenic amino acid. The increase in protein breakdown is, in large part, caused by the stimulation of components of the ubiquitin-proteasome system by cortisol. The proteasome is a large, barrel-shaped complex of approximately 2000 kDa in its active form that is responsible for the bulk of intracellular protein breakdown. The proteasome degrades proteins conjugated to the peptide ubiquitin by specific ubiquitin ligases. Cortisol increases the expression of ubiquitin ligases, including the muscle-specific ubiquitin ligases MuRF1 and atrogin-1/MAFbx (37, 38). The small peptides produced by proteasome degradation of larger proteins are further degraded to amino acids by tripeptidyl peptidase II, an extralysosomal peptidase. Cortisol increases tripeptidyl peptidase II expression. Cortisol is necessary for stimulation of protein breakdown during stress.

Cushing syndrome is a clinical condition of cortisol excess. It is associated with body protein wasting but not with significant increases in protein degradation. This suggests that cortisol may also inhibit protein synthesis. Indeed, glucocorticoids inhibit translation initiation through dephosphorylation of eukaryotic initiation factor 4E binding protein 1, and even more potently, through inhibition of the actions of the ribosomal S6 kinase, a stimulator of ribosome production (39). Although most of these effects have been described in skeletal muscle, it is clear that glucocorticoid excess also decreases the abundance of connective tissue, promoting loss of dermis and bone matrix. This is likely caused by the effect of glucocorticoids to decrease collagen synthesis, particularly collagen III.

Clinical note: Patients with adrenal gland insufficiency, whether by loss of pituitary stimulation of the adrenal cortex or by adrenal gland destruction (also known as Addison disease) generally have nonspecific symptoms. The most prominent features of the cortisol deficiency state are malaise and anorexia. However, under physiologic stress (e.g., infection, trauma), those with adrenal insufficiency become more severely ill than would be anticipated for the stress. They have hypotension, hypoglycemia, abdominal pain, and nausea with vomiting.

Patients with cortisol excess, Cushing syndrome, have weight gain with central adiposity. By contrast, with expansion of central nutrient stores, Cushing syndrome patients have peripheral muscle wasting, bone loss, and dermal wasting, resulting in purple intersecting striae in the skin.

Growth Hormone

Growth hormone is a peptide hormone, produced in the anterior pituitary gland, that inhibits glucose and fat storage but stimulates the accumulation of lean body mass. The primary action of growth hormone on nutrient metabolism seems to involve the stimulation of lipolysis and the oxidation of fat (Fig. 41.3). The latter has a sparing effect on both glucose and amino acid oxidation (40).

Growth hormone is a 22-kDa peptide that interacts with a cell-surface receptor belonging to the cytokine signaling receptor family. Growth hormone signaling is achieved through the tyrosine phosphorylation of nonreceptor Janus kinase 2 that associates with the growth hormone receptor. Subsequently, growth hormone stimulates several signaling cascades, including those of the signal transducer and activators of transcription, mitogen activated protein kinase, and phosphatidyl inositol 3' kinase pathways (41).

Growth hormone was named for its ability to enhance linear growth, particularly during puberty. In the late 1950s, it was noted that growth hormone does not directly stimulate growth of cartilage in vitro. The resulting speculation that an intermediary substance was induced by growth hormone and was ultimately responsible for augmenting cartilage growth led to the somatomedin hypothesis. The intermediary substance, the somatomedin, is

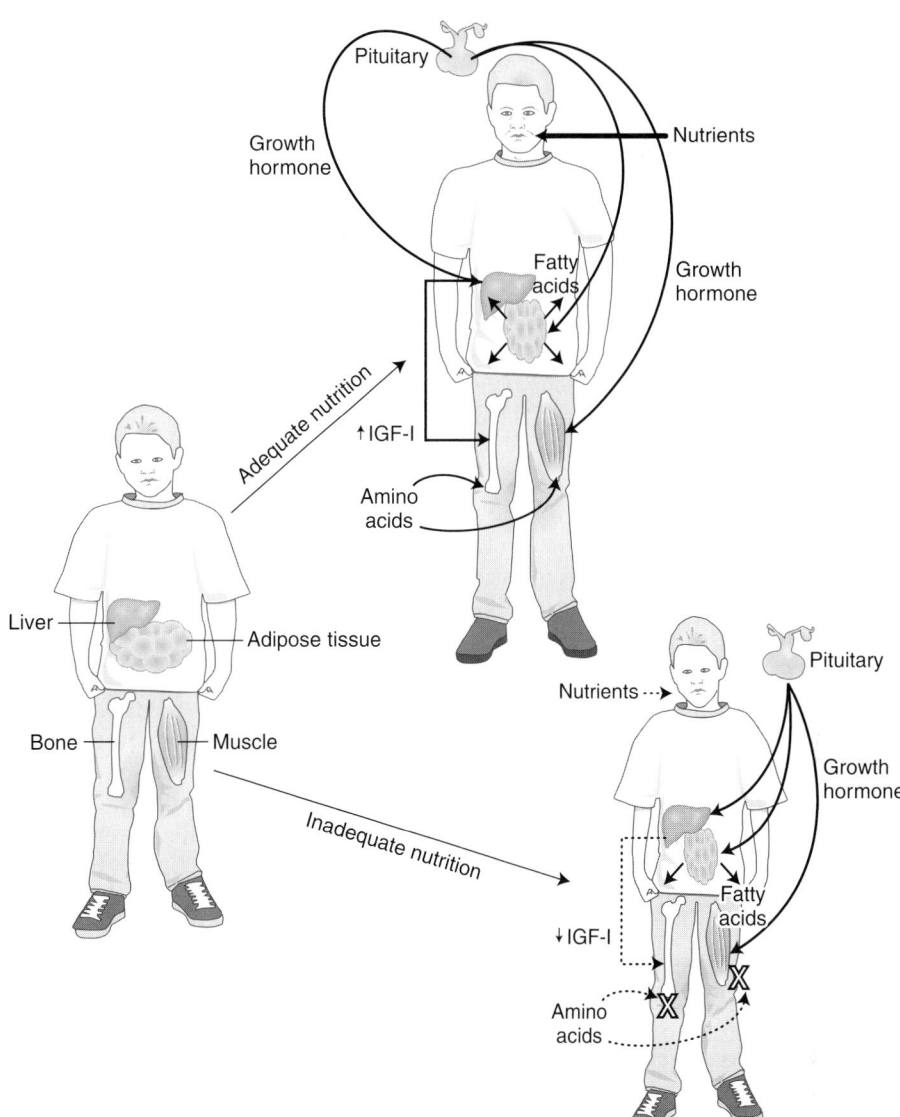

Figure 41.3. Growth: Effects of growth hormone. Growth hormone induces lipolysis with the mobilization of free fatty acids. In the context of adequate nutrition, growth hormone induces insulinlike growth factor-I (IGF-I), stimulating linear growth of bone and muscle. In the context of malnutrition, lipolysis continues but growth hormone cannot stimulate production of IGF-I.

IGF-I, a molecule with structural similarity to insulin that interacts with a receptor that has structural similarity to the insulin receptor.

Growth hormone induces IGF-I production by the liver, the source of 75% of circulating IGF-I. However, hepatic IGF-I production will only increase in response to growth hormone when nutrition is adequate. Starvation induces hepatic resistance to growth hormone induction of IGF-I.

Under circumstances of ample nutrient intake, growth hormone induces IGF-I production that in turn induces increased muscle and bone mass. Bone turnover is stimulated by growth hormone directly, but the bulk of chondrocyte stimulation and linear bone growth is mediated by IGF-I (42). The direct effect of growth hormone on adipocytes to increase lipolysis and on muscle to increase fat oxidation results in a decrease in fat mass. One can envision the pubertal situation in which growth hormone secretion increases and an adolescent loses his or her

"baby fat" while showing accelerated bone and muscle growth.

Under circumstances of inadequate nutrition, growth hormone secretion increases but IGF-I production is inhibited (43). The resulting lipolysis and oxidation of fat without growth of bone and muscle allow the sparing of glucose for central nervous system requirements and amino acids for the production of acute-phase (stress-related) proteins. It also allows for the sparing of muscle and visceral organ mass during chronic starvation while fat, a more energy dense and arguably more dispensable nutrient, is preferentially metabolized.

Testosterone

Testosterone is a steroid hormone produced in the testes, and to a much smaller extent, the ovaries, that is regulated by luteinizing hormone of the anterior pituitary. Levels of testosterone increase significantly during the male puberty and decline very gradually after age 35. Testosterone circulates bound to sex hormone binding globulin and must dissociate from it to initiate its intracellular actions.

Increased testosterone concentrations are associated with an increase in lean body mass and muscle mass during male puberty. Similarly, testosterone replacement therapy in hypogonadal men produces an increase in lean mass and an increase in skeletal muscle protein synthesis (44, 45). Conversely, testosterone decreases fat mass, particularly in the abdominal visceral fat depot. The response of adipose tissue to testosterone may be attributable to increased catecholamine-sensitive lipolysis or to inhibited triglyceride synthesis. However, the metabolic syndromes seen in men with mutations in aromatase (the enzyme that converts testosterone to estrogen) or mutations in estrogen receptors suggest that many of the effects of testosterone to decrease abdominal fat mass may be attributable to the conversion of testosterone to estrogen, a hormone that can cause fat redistribution to peripheral fat depots. Consistent with the benefits of peripheral fat storage capacity on insulin sensitivity and glucose metabolism, it may be the conversion of testosterone to estrogen by aromatase that produces improved insulin sensitivity in hypogonadal men who receive testosterone replacement. Men who cannot normally convert testosterone to estrogen retain abdominal fat and become markedly insulin resistant and diabetic (46).

Testosterone, through its conversion to estrogen, increases bone mass (47). Specifically, estrogen produced from testosterone increases spinal bone mass and spine growth. This is largely responsible for the truncal growth associated with puberty and the relatively short trunk-to-limb relative length in eunuchoidism. Men unable to produce estrogen from testosterone or to respond to the estrogen derived from testosterone have diminished spinal bone density. The sexual dimorphism in bone size with men having larger long bones than women derives from the direct effects of testosterone on periosteal bone apposition.

Testosterone acts primarily through the intracellular androgen receptor of the intranuclear receptor superfamily (48). Receptors in this family interact with DNA and coactivating or corepressing molecules to induce gene transcription (49). In some cells, testosterone is converted to 5α-dihydrotestosterone (DHT) by the enzyme 5α-reductase. DHT has greater affinity for the androgen receptor than testosterone, perhaps accounting for the required conversion of testosterone to DHT to promote certain testosterone actions. The expression of most male secondary sex characteristics (e.g., sex-dependent hair growth, male pattern alopecia, laryngeal growth) are DHT dependent.

One function of testosterone that does not seem to involve the intracellular testosterone receptor and DNA transcription is vasodilation (50). In particular, testosterone produces dilation of visceral arteries (e.g., coronary arteries, mesenteric arteries, pulmonary arteries, aorta) (51). The latter endothelium-independent effect of testosterone seems to be mediated by a direct effect of testosterone on ion channels, either those regulating potassium efflux from vascular smooth muscle or those regulating calcium influx.

The metabolic picture of testosterone action suggests that apart from its effect on male sexual characteristics and sexual function, testosterone causes growth of lean mass, muscle, and spinal bone. Abdominal fat mass is diminished by it, and insulin sensitivity is improved. Blood flow to visceral organs is enhanced.

Estrogen

Estrogens are a set of hormones associated with female sex characteristics. Estradiol is the predominant and most potent estrogen in women. It is produced in the ovaries. It and other estrogens are also produced in the periphery after conversion of androgens by aromatase.

Estrogen is vitally important for reproduction in women. It enhances uterine development, sustains growth of endometrium for embryonic implantation and pregnancy, and promotes mammary gland development for lactation. Estrogen actions are mediated by the estrogen receptor, an intracellular receptor with two subtypes, α and β (52). Like the androgen and progesterone receptors, the estrogen receptor moves to the nucleus to stimulate gene transcription after binding estrogen and forming a receptor homodimer. The homodimer binds to specific palindromic sequences on DNA.

Metabolically, estrogen promotes fatty acid turnover (53). It enhances both fatty acid release from adipose tissue and fatty acid uptake. The increased uptake of fatty acids promoted by estrogen does not result in increased oxidation of fat, however. Therefore, estrogen seems to promote a cycle in which the release of fatty acids from triglycerides and the reformation of triglycerides from fatty acids are both enhanced. These effects of estrogen make fatty acids more available in circulation and may allow women to divert fatty acids into oxidation more effectively than men when energy requirements change. This hypothesis would seem to be borne out by the finding that women derive a greater proportion of their energy from fat during exercise than men.

Estrogen by itself is not known to have any effect on glucose metabolism. However, there is a reciprocal relationship between oxidation of fat and oxidation of glucose. Thus, during exercise, the preferential oxidation of fat by women will spare glucose. Because estrogen is a female reproductive hormone, it is tempting to speculate that the effect of estrogen on fat metabolism would be supportive of pregnancy. Indeed, it is reasonable to believe that fat availability and glucose sparing would be helpful during the increased energy demands and fetal glucose use of pregnancy. This line of speculation is bolstered by examining the effects of other aspects of the hormonal milieu associated with pregnancy. At the time of embryonic implantation, high levels of progesterone, produced by the ovarian corpus luteum, accompany high levels of estrogen. Progesterone inhibits glucose uptake, contributing to a glucose-sparing, insulin-resistant environment. Exercise during the luteal phase of the menstrual cycle (i.e., during high progesterone) is associated with lower glucose use and insulin-stimulated glucose uptake than during the follicular phase of the menstrual cycle (i.e., low progesterone).

Later in pregnancy, placental hormones further inhibit maternal glucose uptake. Placental growth hormone, also called human growth hormone variant (hGH-V), suppresses pituitary growth hormone and is expressed in a continuous nonpulsatile manner. hGH-V works in concert with human placental lactogen to induce insulin resistance, diverting glucose and amino acids for fetal development. Although hGH-V and human placental lactogen actions induce insulin resistance, the major source of insulin resistance and diversion of glucose from maternal to fetal requirements in vivo seems to be placentally derived tumor necrosis factor-α, an immune cytokine produced in fat and placenta in increasing amounts over the course of pregnancy (54).

Clinical note: Insulin resistance induced by pregnancy can result in inappropriate hyperglycemia. This is known as gestational diabetes mellitus and resolves postpartum. Gestational diabetes seems to represent the effects of placental hormones to counterregulate insulin action superimposed on an underlying predisposition to diabetes among certain women. The predisposition is underscored by the findings that development of gestational diabetes predicts the onset of type 2 diabetes in 35 to 47% of women 15 years after the pregnancy, a rate that is approximately ten times that in women without a history of gestational diabetes. The likelihood of developing type 2 diabetes after gestational diabetes is proportional to pregravid obesity and weight gain after the birth of the first child.

NEURAL HORMONES

Catecholamines

Catecholamines are small molecules derived from the conversion of tyrosine to decarboxylated amines. Tyrosine is hydroxylated on its phenyl ring to produce dihydroxyphenylalanine (DOPA) by tyrosine hydroxylase. DOPA is decarboxylated, removing the first carbon to produce dopamine by DOPA decarboxylase. Subsequent hydroxylation of the second, β, carbon of dopamine by dopamine β hydroxylase produces norepinephrine. Methylation of norepinephrine on its α amine group by phenylethanolamine-N-methyltransferase produces epinephrine.

Catecholamines are produced in tissue of neuronal origin. They are produced by the adrenal gland medulla for export into the general circulation, the origin of the term adrenergic for this system of physiologic regulation. They are also produced at the nerve terminals of the sympathetic neuronal system and in central nervous system neurons. Catecholamines regulate many physiologic functions, enhancing, in general terms, physiologic functions such as the stress response, alertness, and exercise capacity (Fig. 41.4). The catecholamine response has been designated the fight or flight response to provide a colorful description of the augmented circulatory function, the enhanced release of nutrients into circulation, the augmented exercise capacity, the pupillary dilation, and the hyperalertness that catecholamines generate during fear.

The catecholamines most relevant to nutrient metabolism are epinephrine and norepinephrine. There are no well-understood direct effects of dopamine on nutrient production or use.

Catecholamines induce physiologic responses by interacting with a series of catecholamine receptors. These include the α adrenergic receptors α_1 and α_2, and β adrenergic receptors β_1, β_2, and β_3. The receptors are cell surface receptors, coupled to guanosine triphosphate binding proteins, that send signals via adenyl cyclase and the production of cAMP.

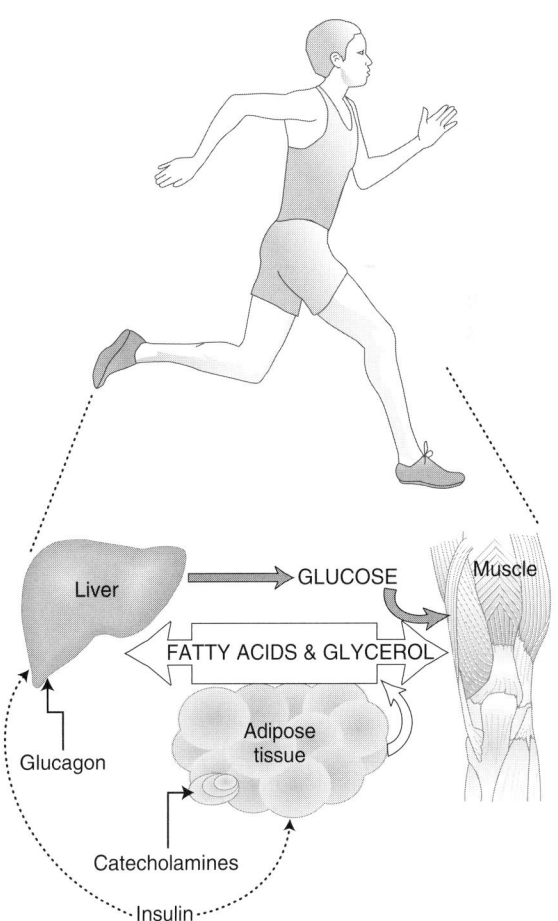

Figure 41.4. Exercise: Low levels of insulin facilitate the effects of glucagon to induce glycogen breakdown and hepatic glucose production and to facilitate effects of catecholamines to induce lipolysis for muscular activity.

The cardiovascular responses to epinephrine and norepinephrine are certainly important to metabolism and to controlling nutrient delivery among tissues, and use the broad range of catecholamine receptors. The α_1 receptors seem to mediate vasoconstriction and blood pressure responses. There are subtypes of α_1 receptors including α_1-A, B, and D. α_1-B and D may mediate central nervous system functions including pain perception. Likewise, α_2 receptors are expressed in at least three subtypes. α_2-A and α_2-C receptors are the classically understood presynaptic α_2 receptors that inhibit norepinephrine outflow and lower blood pressure. α_2-B receptors are postsynaptic and increase blood pressure. Stimulation of β_1 receptors augments heart rate. Stimulation of β_2 receptors augments peripheral blood flow.

Metabolically, catecholamines largely mobilize nutrients during stress. In this way, they join the other insulin counterregulatory hormones glucagon, cortisol, and growth hormone. The sympathetic nervous system can directly mediate these effects by augmenting the outflow of norepinephrine from nerve terminals at the level of target tissues or can indirectly mediate the effects by neurogenically stimulating the outflow of epinephrine from the adrenal medulla. The central nervous system may coordinate the metabolic effects of sympathetic nervous system activation by controlling the pattern of stimulation of adrenergic receptors in specific tissues such as liver, muscle, pancreatic islets, adipose tissue, and the adrenal medulla.

Catecholamines stimulate lipolysis, increasing the availability of fatty acids. They do so in adipocytes by stimulation of β_2 receptors. Activated receptors, in turn, stimulate hormone sensitive lipase by way of PKA activation. Release of free fatty acids from adipose tissue makes them available for muscle and other organs (55). Recent information indicates that catecholamines may also stimulate lipolysis in adipocytes through the AMPK pathway (20). Experiments with genetic disruption of the AMPK pathway result in elevation of catecholamine levels (56). Together, these findings may indicate that the AMPK pathway for lipolysis may be connected in a feedback loop with catecholamines, wherein inadequate AMPK-stimulated lipolysis results in increased catecholamine stimulation of the AMPK pathway.

Again, adipose tissue depots differ in their responsiveness to catecholamines. Abdominal adipose tissue shows greater lipolysis in response to catecholamine stimulation than peripheral subcutaneous adipose tissue in the gluteofemoral region. Abdominal adipose tissue, by corollary, is less responsive to the actions of insulin to inhibit lipolysis. Thus, those who store fat in abdominal depots have greater release of fatty acids into circulation than those who store fat in gluteofemoral depots. Because cortisol enhances abdominal fat storage, one can see how the elevation of glucocorticoids prepares the body for stress by readying the fat depot for rapid release of fatty acids when episodes of acute stress elicit elevation of catecholamine levels.

Apart from the effect of catecholamines of releasing fat into the circulation by stimulation of lipolysis in adipocytes, catecholamines can also increase fatty acid availability in skeletal muscle more directly by stimulating hydrolysis of intramuscular triglycerides. This, too, is mediated by PKA activation of hormone-sensitive lipase in skeletal muscle. Because muscular contraction itself can stimulate hormone-sensitive lipase in muscle, it is believed that the effects of muscular contractile activity and catecholamines are additive in mobilizing intramuscular fat.

Catecholamines increase glucose production by the liver. This seems to be mediated by both α and β adrenergic receptors. Although the subtypes responsible have not been entirely elucidated, responses in genetically altered mice suggest that the α1-b receptor may be particularly important in hepatic glycogen breakdown. The effect of epinephrine on augmenting glycogen breakdown in the liver, however, may be a less important contributor to hepatic glucose output than its effect of providing a substrate for gluconeogenesis. Gluconeogenesis accounts for about 60% of epinephrine-stimulated hepatic glucose output. Apart from providing a substrate for gluconeogenesis, epinephrine also produces a fatty acid influx to the liver. The fatty acids provide ATP, nicotinamide adenine dinucleotide, and stimulation of pyruvate carboxylase for gluconeogenesis.

Norepinephrine increases protein synthesis in muscle (57). This seems to be mediated by the β_2-adrenergic receptor and cAMP stimulation of PKA. Additionally, epinephrine may inhibit calcium-dependent protein degradation in muscle, a pathway primarily active during cellular injury or in muscular dystrophies. Taken together, catecholamines seem to have a qualitatively different effect on protein metabolism than fat and glucose metabolism in that catecholamines stimulate amino acid incorporation into muscle protein, an anabolic effect, whereas catecholamines induce glucose and fat mobilization, a catabolic effect.

CARDIOVASCULAR HORMONES

Angiotensin

The renin-angiotensin system is classically described as a hormonal system regulating blood pressure. In the classic concept, renin is produced by the kidney juxtaglomerular apparatus and converts hepatically derived angiotensinogen to angiotensin I. Angiotensin I is, in turn, converted in the lung to angiotensin II by angiotensin-converting enzyme. Angiotensin II has direct, potent vasoconstrictive effects mediated by the angiotensin II type 1 receptor. It also stimulates production of the mineralocorticoid aldosterone by the adrenal gland cortex zona glomerulosa. Aldosterone promotes sodium and fluid retention to further increase blood pressure.

The role of the angiotensin system in nutrient metabolism has been suggested by the finding that adipose tissue is a producer of virtually all components of the renin-angiotensin system, including angiotensinogen, renin, angiotensin-converting enzyme, and other yet-unidentified secreted heat-labile factors that promote aldosterone secretion from the adrenal cortex (58). Certainly this provides a potential connection between obesity and hypertension, two clinical conditions that coexist in the metabolic syndrome of insulin resistance. Equally interesting is the finding that angiotensin II inhibits adipocyte differentiation, an effect that is reversed by blockade of the angiotensin II type 1 receptor or in mice lacking the angiotensinogen gene (59). Because impaired adipose tissue development and fat storage capacity contribute to insulin resistance, it is possible that angiotensin II, locally produced in adipose tissue, induces insulin resistance. Some corroboration of this idea can be found in clinical trials showing that angiotensin-converting enzyme inhibitors and angiotensin II type 1 receptor blockers improve insulin sensitivity and decrease the risk of the development of diabetes (60). However, these findings should be viewed with caution. Some studies have failed to confirm the phenomenon, and the experimental and clinical studies designed to examine the relationship between the renin-angiotensin system and insulin resistance are often confounded by the variable effects of the hormones and hormone blockade on potassium, sex steroid effects, and the bradykinin system.

Natriuretic Peptides

The natriuretic peptides were identified, as their name implies, for their ability to augment sodium excretion in the urine, reversing hypervolemia. Three types of natriuretic peptides have been described. These include atrial natriuretic peptide (ANP), brain, or B-type, natriuretic peptide (BNP), and C-type natriuretic peptide (CNP). ANP was first noted as a secretory product of cardiac atria during stretch of atrial cardiac myocytes. Natriuretic peptides are primarily produced in cardiac atria and ventricles, but production has been discovered in extracardiac tissues such as lung, thymus, and gastric antrum.

Recent evidence suggests that natriuretic peptides have effects on lipolysis. ANP, and to a lesser extent BNP, have receptors on white adipocytes, including human adipocytes (61). It activates the guanyl cyclase pathway to produce cyclic guanosine monophosphate with subsequent activation of cyclic guanosine monophosphate–dependent protein kinase, hormone sensitive lipase, and perilipin A (62). Other ANP actions suggest that it responds to stress, including hypoxemia, oxidative injury, and burn stress, among others. Thus, its stimulation of lipolysis may be a stress response. Because it uses unique signaling pathways in adipocytes not stimulated by catecholamines or growth hormone, ANP may represent a distinct system by which nutrients are mobilized during stress.

UBIQUITOUS MULTI-TISSUE HORMONES AND GROWTH FACTORS

Many circulating growth factors are broadly produced and secreted in tissues. Their actions are most commonly on cells in close proximity to the cell of origin (paracrine) or on the cell of origin itself (autocrine) rather than at distant sites (hormones). Most are peptides. These agents are called growth factors not because they cause whole-body linear growth, although some, such as IGF-I, can promote whole-body growth. They are called growth factors because of their effects of promoting growth of cells locally within tissues. Generally, growth factors are present when tissues are being rearranged, such as during embryonic development or wound repair (63). They promote cell survival, migration, and proliferation. Many augment angiogenesis to provide new vasculature for the nourishment of newly developed or repaired tissue.

Among the ubiquitously produced growth factors is the widely studied IGF-I. IGF-1 has an insulinlike peptide structure and interacts with a cell-surface receptor that has substantial similarity to the insulin receptor. Approximately 75% of circulating IGF-I is produced in the liver as the result of growth hormone stimulation of the growth hormone receptor in hepatocytes. However, IGF-I is also ubiquitously produced in tissues, acting in a paracrine or autocrine manner, and producing a minority of circulating IGF-I. IGF-I is an important promoter of linear growth. However, the growth-promoting effects of IGF-I do not seem dependent on the high circulating concentrations of the hormone, because growth can occur normally even with very little hepatic production of IGF-I. This suggests either that the paracrine and autocrine actions of IGF-I are the most important for promotion of linear growth or that low circulating levels of hormone produced in nonhepatic tissues are sufficient for the endocrine actions of IGF-I (64).

Apart from its effect on linear growth, IGF-I is an important growth factor for protection against cellular injury. It inhibits programmed cell death (apoptosis) after cellular injury (65). IGF-I has been considered a promising clinical treatment for disorders involving tissue atrophy and death—disorders as varied as type 1 diabetes, with its loss of pancreatic islet β cells (66); burn injury, with its loss of gut integrity; aging, with its loss of muscle mass; and amyotrophic lateral sclerosis (Lou Gehrig disease), with its loss of motor neurons, among others (67, 68). The ability of IGF-I to sustain injured tissues may be a double-edged sword, because tumor cells often use IGF-I to sustain their own viability. Cancer biologists are pursuing interruption of IGF-I signaling as a potential treatment to induce death of cancer cells (69). Paradoxically, although IGF-I seems protective against cell death and loss of body mass, lifespan is greater when IGF-I is deficient or when IGF-I signaling pathways are interrupted (70, 71). Some evidence suggests that IGF-I activity makes the body more susceptible to damage from cellular oxidation reactions, with their resultant chemical radicals.

Several growth factors primarily affect epithelial cells, promoting their survival, migration, and reintegration to assist with wound healing or embryonic development. These include epidermal growth factor (EGF), transforming growth factor-α (TGF-α; a member of the EGF family), hepatocyte growth factor/scatter factor (HGF/SF) (72), and trefoil factors (TFFs; primarily intestinal growth factors) (73).

Other growth factors primarily stimulate rearrangement and reconstitution of connective tissue in embryonic development, organogenesis, or wound healing. They induce production of extracellular matrix and proliferation of blood vessels and smooth muscle cells. These include platelet-derived growth factor (PDGF) (74), fibroblast growth factors (FGFs), vascular endothelial growth factor (VEGF) (75, 76), and transforming growth factor-β (TGF-β) (77). VEGF, PDGF, and TGF-β all belong to a structural superfamily of glycoproteins containing a characteristic segment with eight regularly spaced cysteine amino acids (known as a cysteine knot region). Other potent stimulators of connective tissue growth are connective tissue growth factor (CTGF) (78), activin (a member of the TGF-β superfamily), and nerve growth factor (NGF; a member of the neurotrophin family that stimulates innervation but also fibroblast migration, matrix deposition, wound contraction, and epithelial proliferation).

The majority of peptide growth factors exert their effects through a family of receptors with many similarities. The EGF receptors, TGF-α receptors, HGF/SF receptors, PDGF receptors, VEGF receptors, and FGF receptors all have activity to phosphorylate themselves on tyrosine moieties (i.e., they show tyrosine autophosphorylation or tyrosine kinase activity). These receptors are said to belong to a receptor tyrosine kinase superfamily. When the growth factors bind their receptors, two or more of the receptors combine to form oligomers. After oligomerization, the receptors undergo autophosphorylation. Subsequently, the tyrosine-phosphorylated receptors interact with several intracellular signaling molecules that include a common structure known as an src homology 2 domain. The TGF-β receptor, different from the others, also contains a kinase, but it phosphorylates serine and threonine rather than tyrosine. It interacts with a specific set of signaling molecules known as SMADs (79).

The individual contributions of these growth factors to wound healing, their most important role after fetal development, is complex and difficult to unravel (63). It is helpful to recognize that wounds heal in three general stages. Initially, a clot forms. Platelets elaborate growth factors and recruit inflammatory cells to the wound. Roughly

3 days later, endothelial cells form new blood vessels in the wound and fibroblasts migrate into the wound to lay down a latticework of extracellular matrix. Epithelium (e.g., keratinocytes of a skin wound) proliferates at the edge of the wound. Finally, in about another 7 to 14 days, the epithelium migrates into the wound, covering it. Underlying fibroblasts develop smooth muscle characteristics to become myofibroblasts and cause contraction of the wound. Ordered, fibrillar collagen is laid down.

An amalgamation of studies from genetically modified animals either overexpressing or incapable of expressing individual growth factors yields the following rough estimate of growth factor contributions to the wound healing process. Platelets, in the early clot stage of the wound, release TGF-β, PDGF, and EGF. TGF-β serves to orchestrate the wound healing process (77). It inhibits migration of the epithelium in the early wound stages, preventing its covering the wound. However, it stimulates integrin formation at the membrane of the epithelium, promoting adherence of the epithelium later in the healing process. TGF-β, like many other immune cytokines that will be discussed elsewhere in this text, recruits inflammatory cells to the wound. Finally, TGF-β recruits fibroblasts to the wound. PDGF likewise recruits fibroblasts to the wound. EGF initiates epithelium proliferation.

In the second stage of wound repair, IGF, TGF-β, and PDGF enhance fibroblast growth. TGF-β, IGF-I, FGF-2 (one of 22 FGFs), activin, CTGF, and NGF promote matrix deposition. Angiogenesis is promoted by VEGF secreted by macrophages and by epithelium. HGF and TGF-α augment VEGF production by epithelium.

In the late stages of wound repair, TGF-β, IGF-I, activin, and CTGF continue to promote collagen deposition for scar formation. Additionally, EGF, FGF2, FGF7 (in skin; also called keratinocyte growth factor) (80), TGF-α, activin (80), and NGF promote reepithelialization.

Disruption of tissue integrity is, of course, a serious threat to health and survival. It is not surprising that the number of growth factors mediating wound repair are many and that there seems to be some redundancy in their function. Because these growth factors work locally on wound repair, their potential clinical uses will likely also require local administration. Systemic administration of these growth factors would require caution for their potential effects to promote inflammation, augment scar formation, and induce the growth of cells that might exhibit tumor behavior.

Clinical note: Ulceration of the feet is a serious complication of diabetes mellitus. It may occur because of breakdown of skin in areas of pressure induced by peripheral nerve dysfunction and loss of sensation. It may also occur because of peripheral arterial disease and loss of circulation. Becaplermin is a clinically available gel containing the PDGF isoform PDGF-BB. It is applied to the foot ulcers of diabetic patients to hasten healing.

Somatostatin

Although many ubiquitous growth factors serve as paracrine and autocrine stimulators of cellular growth, initiating positive stimulation peptide cascades, one peptide family serves as a universal inhibitor of peptide secretion—the somatostatin family. Somatostatin was originally identified as an inhibitor of growth hormone secretion (somatotropin release inhibitory factor) secreted by the hypothalamus. Subsequently, somatostatin production was identified in a broad range of tissues (81). It is secreted as either a 14- or a 28-amino-acid peptide (SS-14, SS-28). SS-14 is the primary form secreted in the central nervous system and pancreatic islets. SS-28 is the primary form secreted in the intestine.

Somatostatin is the ligand for a family of five G-protein couple receptors (82, 83). Receptor variation among tissues is responsible for the varied actions of somatostatin among tissues, but all responses are inhibitory to peptide secretion. In the intestine, somatostatin inhibits the secretion of several other hormones, including gastrin, secretin, vasoactive intestinal peptide, and cholecystokinin. It results in inhibition of gastric secretions, pancreatic exocrine secretions, and slowing of gastrointestinal motility. In pancreatic islets, it inhibits secretion of both insulin and glucagon. In peripheral tissues, somatostatin can inhibit the secretion of growth factors such as IGF-I and VEGF, slowing angiogenesis and tissue remodeling.

Metabolically, somatostatin excess, as seen in rare somatostatin-secreting tumors, produces mild glucose intolerance. This is likely caused by the competing effects of the effect of somatostatin to inhibit the secretion of growth hormone, glucagon, and insulin.

REFERENCES

1. Vahl T, D'Alessio D. Curr Opin Clin Nutr Metab Care 2003;6: 461–8.
2. Aizawa T, Sato Y, Komatsu M. Diabetes 2002;51:S96–8.
3. Sherwood NM, Krueckl SL, McRory JE. Endocr Rev 2000;21: 619–70.
4. Flier JS, Maratos-Flier E. N Engl J Med 2002;346:1662–3.
5. Wren AM, Seal LJ, Cohen MA et al. J Clin Endocrinol Metab 2001;86:5992.
6. Cummings DE, Weigle DS, Frayo RS et al. N Engl J Med 2002; 346:1623–30.
7. Saltiel AR, Pessin JE. Trends Cell Biol 2002;12:65–71.
8. Saltiel AR. N Engl J Med 2003;349:2560–2.
9. Pessin JE, Saltiel AR. J Clin Invest 2000;106:165–9.
10. Sesti G, Federici M, Hribal ML et al. FASEB J 2001;15: 2099–111.
11. Bennett RG, Hamel FG, Duckworth WC. Endocrinology 2000;141:2508–17.
12. Kitamura T, Kahn CR, Accili D. Annu Rev Physiol 2003;65: 313–32.
13. Okamoto H, Accili D. J Biol Chem 2003;278:28359–62.
14. Gavrilova O, Marcus-Samuels B, Graham D et al. J Clin Invest 2000;105:271–8.
15. Jiang G, Zhang BB. Am J Physiol Endocrinol Metab 2003;284: E671–8.
16. Guerre-Millo M. J Endocrinol Invest 2002;25:855–61.
17. Diez JJ, Iglesias P. Eur J Endocrinol 2003;148:293–300.
18. Yamauchi T, Kamon J, Ito Y et al. Nature 2003;423:762–9.
19. Yamauchi T, Kamon J, Minokoshi Y et al. Nat Med 2002;8: 1288–95.
20. Ruderman NB, Saha AK, Kraegen EW. Endocrinology 2003; 144:5166–71.
21. Jequier E. Ann NY Acad Sci 2002;967:379–88.
22. Apter D. Ann NY Acad Sci 2003;997:64–76.
23. Steppan CM, Brown EJ, Wright CM et al. Proc Natl Acad Sci USA 2001;98:502–6.
24. Rajala MW, Obici S, Scherer PE et al. J Clin Invest 2003;111: 225–30.
25. Hotamisligil GS. J Clin Invest 2003;111:173–4.
26. Janke J, Engeli S, Gorzelniak K et al. Obes Res 2002;10:1–5.
27. Goldspink G. Biochem Soc Trans 2002;30:285–90.
28. Silva JE. J Clin Invest 2001;108:35–7.
29. Dimitriadis GD, Raptis SA. Exp Clin Endocrinol Diabetes 2001; 109[Suppl 2]:S225–39.
30. Kahaly GJ, Kampmann C, Mohr-Kahaly S. Thyroid 2002;12: 473–81.
31. Viguerie N, Langin D. Curr Opin Clin Nutr Metab Care 2003;6: 377–81.
32. Zhang J, Lazar MA. Annu Rev Physiol 2000;62:439–66.
33. Lazar MA. J Clin Invest 2003;112:497–9.
34. Masuzaki H, Paterson J, Shinyama H et al. Science 2001;294: 2166–70.
35. Masuzaki H, Flier JS. Curr Drug Targets Immune Endocr Metabol Disord 2003;3:255–62.
36. Hasselgren PO. Curr Opin Clin Nutr Metab Care 1999;2:201–5.
37. Wray CJ, Mammen JM, Hershko DD et al. Int J Biochem Cell Biol 2003;35:698–705.
38. Glass DJ. Nat Cell Biol 2003;5:87–90.
39. Shah OJ, Kimball SR, Jefferson LS. Am J Physiol 2000;278: E76–82.
40. Moller N, Norrelund H. Horm Res 2003;59[Suppl 1]:62–8.
41. Herrington J, Smit LS, Schwartz J et al. Oncogene 2000;19: 2585–97.
42. Olney RC. Med Pediatr Oncol 2003;41:228–34.
43. Scacchi M, Ida Pincelli A, Cavagnini F. Front Neuroendocrinol 2003;24:200–24.
44. Brodsky IG, Balagopal P, Nair KS. J Clin Endocrinol Metab 1996;81:3469–75.
45. Bhasin S, Woodhouse L, Storer TW. J Endocrinol 2001;170: 27–38.
46. Maffei L, Murata Y, Rochira V et al. J Clin Endocrinol Metab 2004;89:61–70.
47. Riggs BL, Khosla S, Melton LJ III. Endocr Rev 2002;23: 279–302.
48. Lee HJ, Chang C. Cell Mol Life Sci 2003;60:1613–22.
49. Heinlein CA, Chang C. Endocr Rev 2002;23:175–200.
50. Orshal JM, Khalil RA. Am J Physiol 2004;286:R233–49.
51. Wynne FL, Khalil RA. J Endocrinol Invest 2003;26:181–6.
52. McDonnell DP, Norris JD. Science 2002;296:1642–4.
53. Nielsen S, Guo Z, Albu JB et al. J Clin Invest 2003;111:981–8.
54. Kirwan JP, Hauguel-De Mouzon S, Lepercq J et al. Diabetes 2002;51:2207–13.
55. Horowitz JF, Klein S. Am J Clin Nutr 2000;72:558S–63.
56. Viollet B, Andreelli F, Jorgensen SB et al. Biochem Soc Trans 2003;31:216–9.
57. Navegantes LC, Migliorini RH, do Carmo Kettelhut I. Curr Opin Clin Nutr Metab Care 2002;5:281–6.
58. Ehrhart-Bornstein M, Lamounier-Zepter V, Schraven A et al. Proc Natl Acad Sci USA 2003;100:14211–6.

59. Ailhaud G, Fukamizu A, Massiera F et al. Int J Obes Relat Metab Disord 2000;24[Suppl 4]:S33–5.

60. Padwal R, Laupacis A. Diabetes Care 2004;27:247–55.

61. Dessi-Fulgheri P, Sarzani R, Rappelli A. Nutr Metab Cardiovasc Dis 2003;13:244–9.

62. Sengenes C, Bouloumie A, Hauner H et al. J Biol Chem 2003; 278:48617–26.

63. Werner S, Grose R. Physiol Rev 2003;83:835–70.

64. Butler AA, Yakar S, LeRoith D. News Physiol Sci 2002;17:82–5.

65. Butt AJ, Firth SM, Baxter RC. Immunol Cell Biol 1999;77: 256–62.

66. George M, Ayuso E, Casellas A et al. J Clin Invest 2002;109: 1153–63.

67. Kaspar BK, Llado J, Sherkat N et al. Science 2003;301:839–42.

68. Torres-Aleman I. Mol Neurobiol 2000;21:153–60.

69. Baserga R, Peruzzi F, Reiss K. Int J Cancer 2003;107:873–7.

70. Longo VD, Finch CE. Science 2003;299:1342–6.

71. Holzenberger M, Dupont J, Ducos B et al. Nature 2003;421: 182–7.

72. Zhang YW, Vande Woude GF. J Cell Biochem 2003;88:408–17.

73. Taupin D, Podolsky DK. Nat Rev Mol Cell Biol 2003;4:721–32.

74. Heldin C-H, Westermark B. Physiol Rev 1999;79:1283–316.

75. Ferrara N, Gerber HP, LeCouter J. Nat Med 2003;9:669–76.

76. Shibuya M. Cell Struct Funct 2001;26:25–35.

77. Govinden R, Bhoola KD. Pharmacol Ther 2003;98:257–65.

78. Moussad EE, Brigstock DR. Mol Genet Metab 2000;71:276–92.

79. Roberts AB, Russo A, Felici A et al. Ann NY Acad Sci 2003; 995:1–10.

80. Beer HD, Gassmann MG, Munz B et al. J Invest Dermatol Symp Proc 2000;5:34–9.

81. Barnett P. Endocrine 2003;20:255–64.

82. Patel YC. Front Neuroendocrinol 1999;20:157–98.

83. Moller LN, Stidsen CE, Hartmann B et al. Biochim Biophys Acta 2003;1616:1–84.

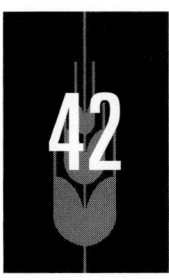

42 CYTOKINES AND EICOSANOIDS[1]

JOSEPH G. CANNON

OVERVIEW 655
CYTOKINES 655
    History 655
    General Characteristics 656
    Integrated Responses 661
    Therapy 664
EICOSANOIDS 665
    History 665
    Synthesis 666

OVERVIEW

Contrary to common assumption, infection-induced "illness" is usually *not* caused by microbes or toxins that "damage" normal physiologic processes. The signs and symptoms that we usually experience are similar for many types of infection: They are induced by our own endogenously produced signaling molecules, particularly cytokines and eicosanoids. These molecules trigger antimicrobial immune responses and regulate physiologic adaptations that make the internal environment less favorable to pathogen growth. Although their actions are most noticeable during infection, cytokines and eicosanoids are critical for normal growth and development as well. Because dozens of eicosanoids and more than 100 cytokines exist, a detailed description of each one is not possible in this chapter. Instead, the general characteristics of cytokines and eicosanoids are described, and the mutual regulation between these signaling pathways is highlighted. Nevertheless, three cytokines—interleukin-1β

(IL-1β), tumor necrosis factor-α (TNF-α), and IL-6—and one eicosanoid—prostaglandin E_2 (PGE_2)—receive particular attention because of their extensive cross-regulation and their important influences on whole-body metabolism, nutritional status, and body composition. A first encounter with cytokine biology can be disconcerting because of the inconsistent and confusing nomenclature. The extended historical section is intended to provide some perspective on these idiosyncrasies.

CYTOKINES

History

Historical preludes to cytokine therapy can be traced to separate cases of erysipelas (*Streptococcus pyogenes* infection), occurring within a year of each other, but on opposite sides of the Atlantic Ocean. In 1883, Viennese psychiatrist Julius Wagner von Jauregg noticed that a patient recovered from severe mental illness (resulting from neurosyphilis) after contracting erysipelas (1). In this preantibiotic era, Wagner-Jauregg began infecting patients suffering from "untreatable" neurosyphilis with microbes that were either benign or controllable with the drugs of the time. The best results were obtained when the infection induced fever, a finding prompting Wagner-Jauregg to focus on malaria infections, which induced multiple febrile episodes and could be controlled with quinine.

Meanwhile, in 1884, a New York man with a massive, inoperable sarcoma of the neck went into remission after an erysipelas infection. This case inspired surgeon William Coley to begin treating sarcomas with local injections of heat-killed streptococci (2). Coley noted that the tumors became pale and soft, a finding indicating degeneration of the vasculature and connective tissue, but a fever was not necessary for tumor regression.

Although bacterial proteins or toxins were suspected to be the causative agents in these therapies, some investigators were beginning to consider the possibility that infection-induced factors from the patient's own white blood cells could play a role. In 1922, Alexis Carrel and Albert Ebeling published observations that fibroblast growth was enhanced when cocultured with leukocytes. These investigators remarked that "Leucocytes may be regarded as mobile unicellular glandular bodies which set free their

---

[1] **Abbreviations: bFGF,** basic fibroblast growth factor;
cAMP, cyclic adenosine monophosphate; **COX,** cyclooxygenase;
CSF, colony-stimulating factor; **GM-CSF,** granulocyte-macrophage-colony-stimulating factor; **gp,** glycoprotein; **IFN,** interferon;
IL, interleukin; **IL-1Ra,** interleukin-1 receptor antagonist;
LTA_4, LTB_4, and **LTC_4,** leukotrienes A_4, B_4, and C_4;
MAPK, mitogen-activated protein kinase; **NF-κB,** nuclear factor-κB;
NSAID, nonsteroidal antiinflammatory drug; **15-PGDH,**
15-hydroxyprostaglandin dehydrogenase; **PGE_2,** prostaglandin E_2;
PGH_2, prostaglandin H_2; **PGI_2,** prostacyclin; **RCS,** rabbit aorta-contracting substance; **SOCS,** suppressors of cytokine signaling;
SRS, slow-reacting substance; **STAT,** signal transducer and activator of transcription; **sTNFR,** soluble tumor necrosis factor receptor; **TGF-β,**
transforming growth factor-β; **T_H1** and **T_H2,** T-helper type 1 and 2
cells; **TNF-α,** tumor necrosis factor-α; **TXA_2,** thromboxane A_2.

secretions in the humors of the organism. But little is known of the nature and functions of the substances they secrete" (3). We now call these substances cytokines, and many of the reactions induced by Wagner-Jauregg's and Coley's therapies (including fever, stimulation of antibacterial immune responses, connective tissue breakdown, tumor cell killing, and vascular remodeling) can be attributed to the actions of cytokines including, but not limited to, IL-1, TNF, and interferon (IFN).

A first challenge in characterizing such host-derived substances involved separating them from ubiquitous bacterial contaminants, such as endotoxin. It was not until 1948 that a satisfactory demonstration was made that fever could be produced by a white cell product (originally called endogenous pyrogen) devoid of any such contamination.

A second challenge was presented by the finding that these substances exist at very low concentrations, but have very high specific activities. As Carrel and Ebeling so presciently stated, cytokine "glands" (leukocytes) are mobile; thus miniscule, but concentrated, doses of cytokines can be delivered to a local tissue environment. Isolation and purification procedures yielded biologically active preparations, but they were of such infinitesimal mass that the molecular characteristics could not be determined with certainty. Interferon was named in the early 1950s without any clear knowledge of "its" molecular characteristics (several IFNs are now known). The same was true for colony-stimulating factors (CSFs) that promoted hematopoiesis, and various growth factors that stimulated proliferation and/or differentiation of cells not originating in the bone marrow. The term "lymphokine" was coined in 1969 (4), in reference to factors secreted by lymphocytes (-kine, Greek "to set in motion"). However, the term did not fully represent the true variety of cellular sources and targets for these factors, hence the more general term "cytokine" was introduced in 1974 (5).

Although unsuspected at the time of discovery, each factor was capable of multiple biologic activities. For example, macrophage extracts were studied in numerous laboratories. Some investigated a fever-inducer called endogenous pyrogen, others isolated a protein influencing protein, glucose, and lipid metabolism called leukocyte endogenous mediator, and still others investigated a promoter of lymphocyte proliferation called lymphocyte activating factor. By the late 1970s, these investigators began to realize that their macrophage products shared similar biochemical characteristics and suspected that they could, in fact, all be studying the same molecule. Identical situations were occurring with extracts from lymphocytes and other cellular sources. Some researchers sought to establish a more generic nomenclature that did not narrowly define a factor by a single biologic activity. Therefore, although specific amino acid sequences and molecular structures were still not known, IL-1 and IL-2 were defined in 1979 as macrophage and T-cell products, respectively, with molecular weights and isoelectric points

that fell within specified ranges and met other rather general biochemical and functional criteria (6). Subsequent cloning of these molecules confirmed the multiple (pleiotropic) activities originally reported for the purified extracts.

In ensuing years, other cytokines with activity-based names were assigned IL numbers. Nevertheless, many pleiotropic cytokines retained original activity-based names that do not adequately indicate their biologic roles (most of these cytokines have acronyms, and it is often best not to worry about what the acronym represents). A nomenclature subcommittee of the International Union of Immunological Societies attempted to impose order in the numbering process. However, as the number of interleukins advanced beyond 20, some investigators unilaterally assigned IL numbers to their discoveries without consultation with the subcommittee. This resulted in completely different proteins appearing in published papers and databases with the same IL number and, conversely, different IL numbers applied to proteins that ultimately proved to be "functionally related" (7).

The *functional* relationship between cytokines is a particularly thorny issue with regard to nomenclature. The human and murine cytokines originally named IL-1 had identical biologic activities, but they turned out to have an amino acid sequence homology of only 24% (similarities in their three-dimensional conformations enabled them to bind to the same receptors). Actually, both humans and mice made both forms of IL-1, so Greek suffixes were applied to differentiate IL-1α from IL-1β. A third cytokine with a similar degree of sequence homology was called IL-1γ for a time. However, it bound to a different receptor and mediated a different spectrum of biologic activities; hence it was given a separate IL designation, IL-18. Recent genomic mapping has identified more genes encoding proteins with homologies ranging from 13 to 52% with the known forms of IL-1, resulting in a current total of ten *sequence*-related members of the IL-1 family. Additional sequence-based cytokine families are emerging, adding additional stress to nomenclature. Thus, the Greek suffixes (α, β, γ, and so forth) may be supplanted by family suffixes (F1, F2, F3, and so forth). It has yet to be established whether some of these genes are translated into biologically significant amounts of protein or whether they have any functional relationship with other members of their families (7).

General Characteristics

Cytokines are basically intercellular signaling proteins, usually ranging in molecular weight between approximately 8 and 30 kDa, that bind to multiunit receptors expressed on the surface of target cells. In contrast to classic hormones that serve as negative feedback signals in the maintenance of homeostasis, cytokines can be considered as feedforward signals that direct the transition to a new physiologic state (i.e., they can reset a homeostatic set point) (8). Such transitions can be permanent, as in growth and development, or they can be temporary, as in host defense adaptations to infection, sleep/wake cycles, or the reproductive transitions of the menstrual cycle and pregnancy.

Virtually all nucleated cells can produce cytokines, although white blood cells (leukocytes) are major sources, and endothelial cells, fibroblasts, and smooth muscle cells merit specific mention. Production of some cytokines is constitutive in some tissues, but more often, cytokines are induced by microbes, toxins, radiation, extremes in oxygen tension, cellular deformation, degraded extracellular matrix and, very importantly, by other cytokines.

Most cytokines are synthesized de novo before they are secreted in response to a stimulus. Thus, regulation of cytokine secretion can take place at the transcription, translation, and export stages of the process. The extensive post-transcriptional control that exists for many cytokines often means that mRNA expression is an insufficient measure of cytokine involvement in a biologic response.

Less commonly, cytokines are preformed and stored in granules. For example, TNF-α stored in mast cells can be rapidly released by immunoglobulin E or substance P; IL-16 stored in cytotoxic T cells can be released by histamine or serotonin. Some preformed cytokines exist as latent forms in extracellular matrices (9), including basic fibroblast growth factor (bFGF) in skeletal muscle and transforming growth factor-β (TGF-β) in bone. When the matrices are disrupted, these cytokines are released and become biologically active. bFGF promotes repair of overloaded muscle fibers by attracting and stimulating muscle precursor cells and fibroblasts. TGF-β moderates the bone resorptive activities of osteoclasts. TGF-β also circulates in a latent form that can be activated by blood clotting, hyperthermia, or changes in pH.

Figure 42.1 is a Venn diagram presenting a general summary of some of the immunologic activities modulated by IL-1 through IL-18 (and other selected cytokines). Alternative Venn diagrams could be drawn that group cytokines in subsets based on any number of other considerations, such as their metabolic activities or their influences on vascular function. Two main points are illustrated by this figure. First, most cytokines modulate more than one biologic process (i.e., they are pleiotropic), and second, many different cytokines can modulate the same process (i.e., they are redundant). In many cases, this redundancy can be explained by the mechanisms involved in receptor binding and signal transduction.

Receptor Interactions and Signal Transduction

Each cytokine binds to the extracellular segment of a specific receptor subunit (designated the α subunit). However, this binding event alone is usually insufficient to initiate intracellular signal transduction. The cytokine must also

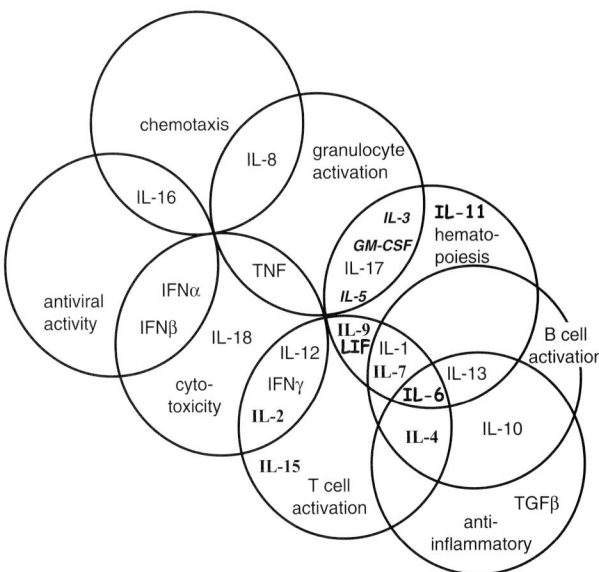

Figure 42.1. Venn diagram summarizing some immunologic responses modulated by cytokines. The diagram illustrates that each response is stimulated by several cytokines (redundancy), and each cytokine is capable of stimulating several different responses (pleiotropism). Various typefaces other than Ariel fonts indicate cytokine families that share common β or γ receptor subunits.

bind the extracellular segment of one or more additional receptor subunits (β and γ subunits, Fig. 42.2A)(10). The close association of these subunits assembles their intracellular segments and other cytosolic proteins into functional protein kinases that phosphorylate additional intracellular domains on the receptor subunits and other cytosolic proteins (Fig. 42.2B). These initial events can cause dimerization of signal tranducers and activators of transcription (STATs) (10) or set off cascades involving several generations of kinases such as mitogen-activated protein kinases (MAPKs; Fig. 42.3, events 1–3) (11). The result can be activation and translocation of transcription factors (e.g., STATs and nuclear factor-κB [NF-κB]) into the nucleus, where they bind to DNA recognition sites and initiate expression of multiple genes (see Fig. 42.3, event 4). Alternatively, the products of signaling cascades can interact with untranslated regions on mRNA, thus regulating stability and translation of the message into protein (see Fig. 42.3, event 5) (12).

Some gene products give rise to cellular responses such as proliferation, differentiation, apoptosis, expression of receptors, or secretion. Others gene products impose negative feedback on the intracellular activation pathway (see Fig. 42.3, event 6). Examples include IκB, which binds and inhibits NF-κB; and suppressors of cytokine signaling (SOCS) that can interfere with early receptor-associated phosphorylation events (13). This negative feedback automatically shuts off (or resets) the signaling pathways after a cytokine-induced cellular response has been accomplished.

The multiunit receptor structure provides one mechanism for cytokine redundancy. For example, IL-6, IL-11,

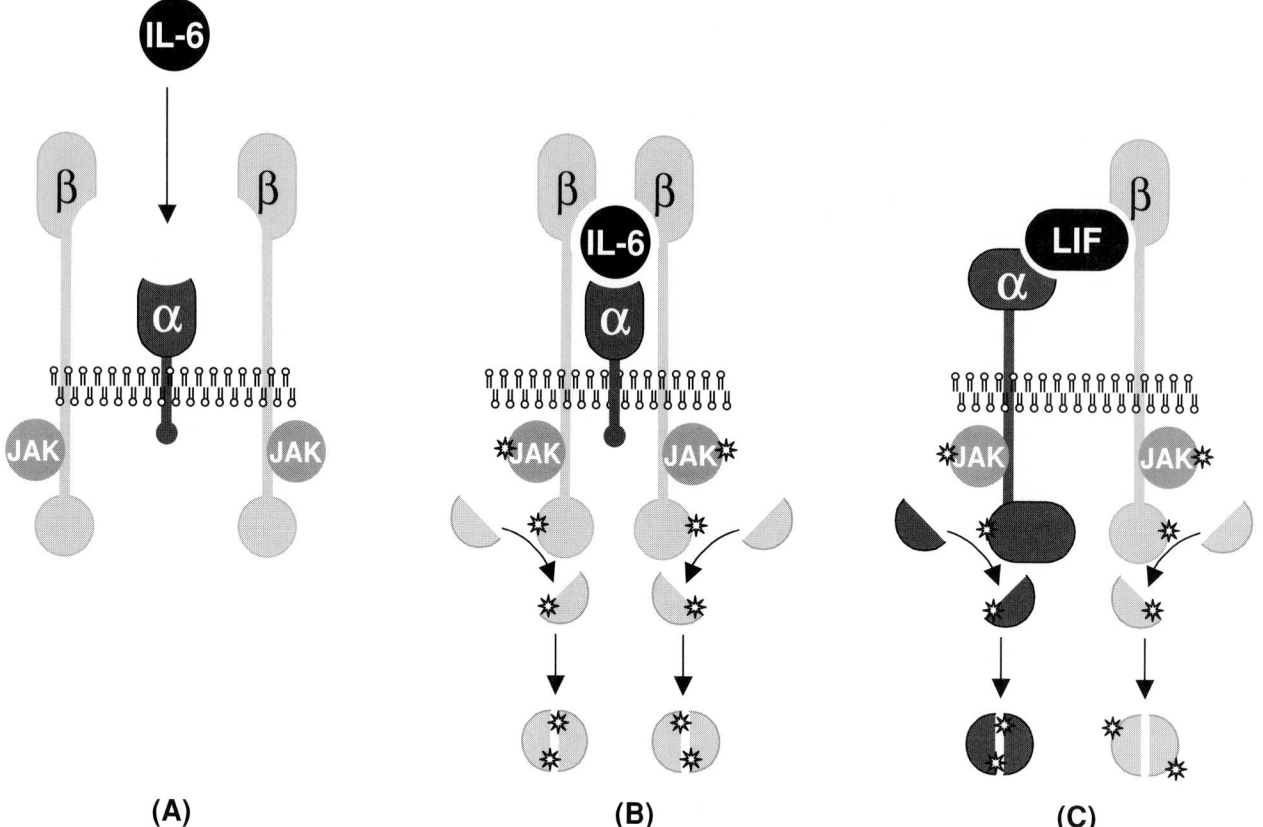

Figure 42.2. A–C. Cytokine receptor structure and function. A cytokine links two or more receptor subunits together, assembling the intracellular domains and recruiting cytosolic proteins (e.g., the JAK structures shown) into functional kinases that initiate intracellular signal transduction (including signal tranducer and activator of transcription [STAT] phosphorylization, indicated by *stars,* and dimerization, as shown). JAKs are a family of kinases named for Janus, the Roman god of doorways. Mitogen-activated protein kinase and other pathways are also activated, but are not shown.

leukemia inhibitory factor (LIF), and several other cytokines each bind different α receptor subunits, but they all bind a common 130-kDa glycoprotein (gp130) β subunit (14). As a result, they all activate signaling pathways characteristic of the common subunit in addition to individualized signaling dictated by the kinases associated with the α subunit for each cytokine (see Fig. 42.2C). These cytokines induce fever and hepatic protein synthesis, and promote hematopoiesis to greater or lessor degrees. Another common β subunit is the 120 kDa protein shared by IL-3, IL-5, and granulocyte-macrophage CSF (GM-CSF). The various common β subunits tend to be expressed rather generally among many different types of cells, whereas the α subunits are often more restricted. For example, neutrophils express α subunits for only GM-CSF, and monocytes express α subunits for GM-CSF and IL-3, whereas basophils and eosinophils express α subunits for GM-CSF, IL-3, and IL-5 (15). These cytokines stimulate degranulation, respiratory burst, antibody-mediated killing, and hematopoiesis.

Redundancy ensures that an inability to produce any one cytokine will not threaten the loss of an important biologic response. However signaling through a common

receptor subunit has an "Achilles heel" with serious clinical consequences. IL-2, IL-4, IL-7, IL-9, and IL-15 all bind a common γ receptor subunit, and all mediate T-cell development and/or activation (10). Mutations in the gene encoding this γ subunit can disrupt T-cell development and can render affected persons extremely susceptible to infection, a clinical condition known as severe combined immunodeficiency. These patients must be isolated from the normal microbe-laden environment, and they have a poor prognosis unless bone marrow can be successfully transplanted. Current research is directed at transferring the gene encoding the common γ subunit into the patient's own bone marrow cells.

In contrast to the receptor structures described so far, one subset of cytokines—the chemokines—bind to serpentine membrane proteins that associate with cytosolic G proteins. The chemokine family consists of more than 40 members including IL-8, the only one with an IL designation; most of the rest have rather cryptic acronyms (16). Each is a relatively small (~5–10 kDa) protein with characteristic cysteine-disulfide bonds. The chemokines direct recruitment of leukocytes to the site of an injury or infection by activating adhesion molecules that promote leukocyte

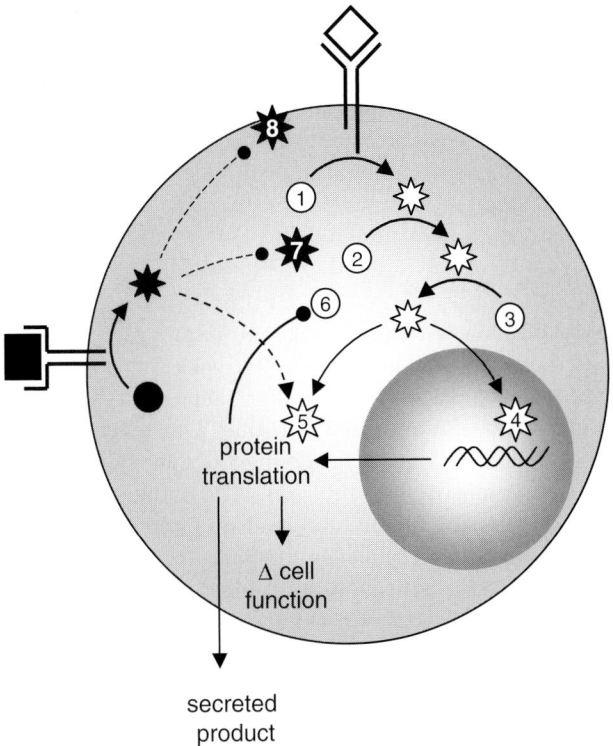

Figure 42.3. Cytokine-receptor binding triggers intracellular phosphorylation cascades (events 1–3) that lead to activation of transcription (event 4), regulation of translation (event 5), and synthesis of negative feedback inhibitors (event 6). A second cytokine can alter the activity of the first by activating phosphatases (event 7) and metalloproteases (event 8) that interrupt the cascades and cleave receptor subunits of the first cytokine. In this and all other figures, *arrowheads* denote stimulation, and *blunt ends* indicate inhibition.

extravasation. They also establish chemical concentration gradients used by leukocytes to home in on the injury or infection (hence the name chemokine).

Cytokine Language

Classic protein hormones generally have a distinct organ source and induce a consistent biologic response in specific target tissues. We often think in terms of a "binary" (increase or decrease) signal delivered by these hormones, although this is not necessarily true. In contrast, any one cytokine can have many cellular sources in many tissues and can act on diverse targets. Moreover, the biologic action of any one cytokine can be radically altered by the presence of other cytokines. It is possible for a cytokine to have little or no effect on a target cell response by itself, but it may amplify the action of a second cytokine and inhibit the action of a third (17). Therefore, the signals delivered are the net result of several cytokines, like the assembly of several letters into a word. One cytokine can influence the activity of another by the following means:

1. Altering cytokine receptor synthesis, thus modulating target cell sensitivity. As an example, IL-1 increases the expression of IL-2 receptors on lymphocytes.

2. Changing the conformation or phosphorylation state of cytokine receptors already expressed on the membrane of a target cell. IL-1β and TNF-α alter epidermal growth factor receptor function in this way (18).

3. Activating intracellular regulatory signaling factors that target the untranslated regions on mRNA that has been transcribed in response to another cytokine. This modifies mRNA stabilization and/or translation and thus alters protein synthesis (see the *dashed pathway* leading to event 5 in Fig. 42.3). This includes cytokine-induced cytokine synthesis: IL-1β, IL-6, IL-8, TNF-α, GM-CSF, and probably many other cytokines are regulated in this manner (12).

4. Binding the same α subunit as another cytokine, but not activating additional subunits necessary for signal transduction, thus acting as a competitive inhibitor. IL-1 receptor antagonist (IL-1Ra) is the only naturally occurring example of this form of inhibition known at this time (19). Alternatively, different cytokines may bind separate α subunits, but compete for shared β or γ subunits. This type of competition exists for IL-3, IL-5, and GM-CSF, but the biologic consequences are subtle. The latency or duration of the target cell response may be altered somewhat by the receptor binding kinetics for each cytokine (15).

5. Inducing expression of membrane-bound "decoy" receptors (20). These receptor subunits often have a higher affinity for a cytokine than functional α subunits, but do not assemble with appropriate β and/or γ subunits and therefore do not transduce an intracellular signal. Such decoys exist for several cytokines, including IL-1, IL-10, IL-13, IL-18, and TNF-α.

6. Activating a phosphatase that interferes with (terminates) a kinase cascade initiated by a different cytokine (see Fig. 42.3, event 7).

7. Stimulating synthesis of an inhibitory cytosolic protein (e.g., SOCS) that inactivates an intracellular signaling pathway activated by another cytokine (13).

8. Inducing the release of cytokine receptor subunits from a target cell, resulting in decreased receptor density on the cell. Furthermore, these shed receptors can intercept a cytokine before it can bind to membrane-associated receptors. The shedding of these soluble receptors is a modulatory mechanism for most cytokines.

Soluble Receptors

Receptor subunit shedding is accomplished through several different mechanisms (9). First, membrane-bound metalloproteases can be activated to cleave the extracellular domain of the receptor from the membrane (see Fig. 42.3, event 8). Second, alternatively spliced forms of mRNA can encode receptor subunits lacking membrane anchorage domains that are secreted from the cells. Third (and less regulated or specific), receptors can be cleaved by extracellular proteases released by neighboring inflammatory cells.

Soluble receptors often inhibit cytokine-mediated biologic responses, but not always. A soluble receptor with a relatively low affinity for a cytokine can act as a chaperone, protecting the cytokine from proteolytic cleavage or glomerular filtration until the cytokine is transferred to a membrane-associated receptor with a higher affinity. Soluble TNF receptors (sTNFR) extend biologic half-life for TNF-α via this mechanism.

Alternatively, some receptor subunits do not contain cytosolic domains directly involved with kinase activation and do not need to be anchored in the membrane to participate in cytokine signaling. For example, the IL-6/IL-6Rα complex joins two identical gp130 β subunits containing the intracellular domains necessary for initiating signal transduction. The IL-6/IL-6Rα complex can perform its linkage function regardless of whether it is embedded in the membrane or not (Fig. 42.4A). Association with soluble (s-) IL-6Rα not only extends IL-6 biologic half-life, but also allows IL-6 to influence a wide variety of cells that express gp130 even though they do not express IL-6Rα. In contrast, the soluble β subunit, s-gp130, is inhibitory because IL-6/s-gp130 complexes cannot assemble the necessary intracellular signaling structures (Fig. 42.4B). α Receptors that do possess intracellular domains involved in signaling cannot transduce a signal in their soluble forms (Fig. 42.4C).

The circulating concentrations of soluble receptors are usually in the ng/mL range, making them far easier to detect than the low pg/mL concentrations of the cytokine ligands themselves. In addition, leukocyte activation usually increases the shedding rate, thus making soluble receptor concentrations useful indicators of leukocyte activation in clinical studies.

Cytokine Systems

Cytokines are often conceptualized in groups or systems, based on their cooperative roles in generating a particular type of biologic response and/or their primary cellular sources. Integrating several cytokines into functional networks helps to reduce overwhelming numbers of cytokines into comprehensible paradigms. The monocyte-derived cytokines IL-1β, TNF-α, and IL-6 are often characterized as "inflammatory" cytokines for their regulatory roles in fever, leukocyte activation, local blood flow, edema, and pain. They also mediate widespread metabolic changes, termed the acute-phase response (described in detail later).

The microbial and humoral environment modifies the development of naive helper T cells into subsets with characteristic cytokine secretion profiles (21). T-helper type 1 cells (T_H1) produce a spectrum of cytokines, including IL-2 and IFN-γ, that bias an immune response in favor a

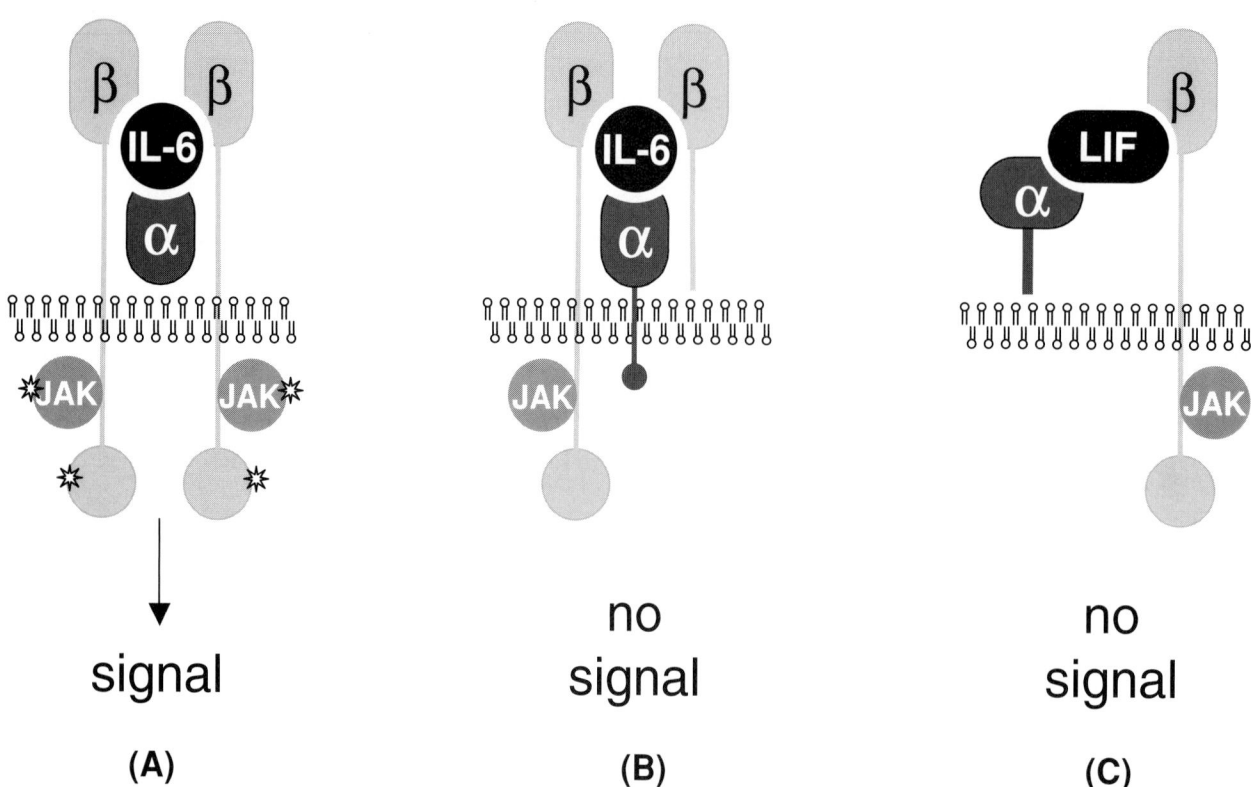

Figure 42.4. Soluble cytokine receptors, **A.** α Subunits lacking intracellular domains involved in signaling can be shed from a cell and retain their functional role in receptor assembly **B.** β Subunits can also be shed, but they cannot contribute to functional receptor assembly because they lack necessary intracellular domains **C.** α Subunits that do possess intracellular signaling domains lose functionality when shed.

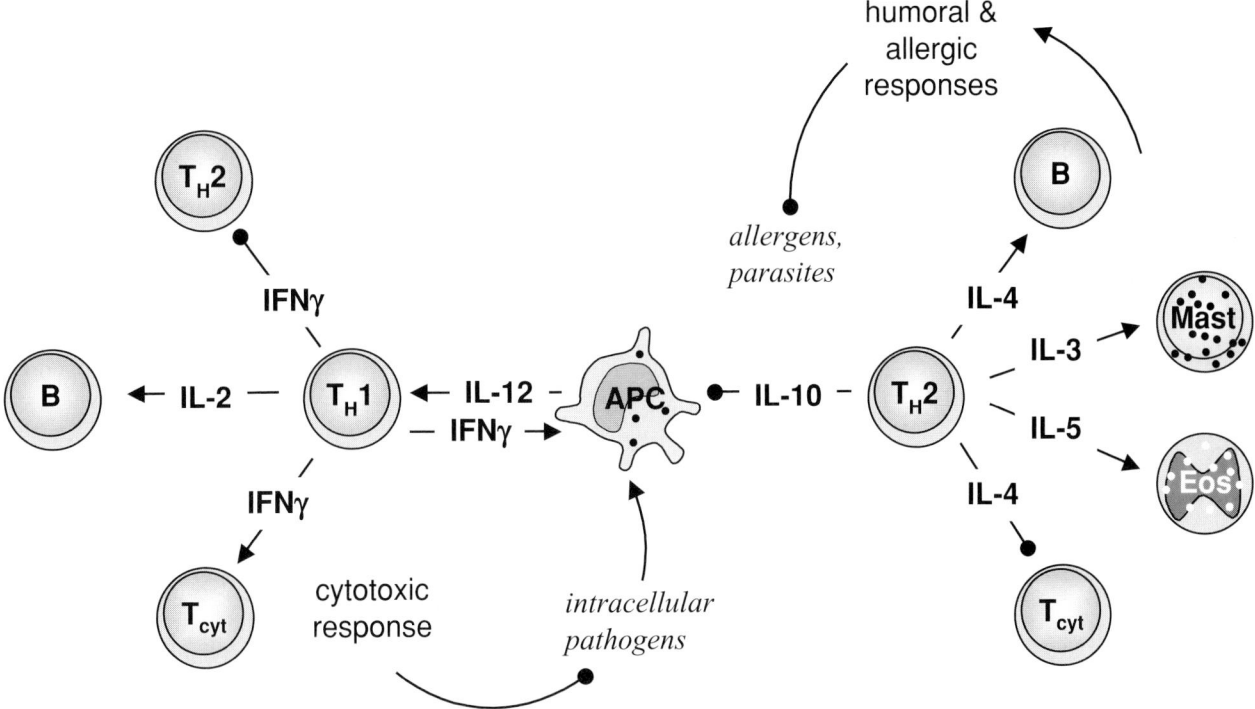

Figure 42.5. The effector mechanisms activated in an immune response are biased toward a cytotoxic response or a humoral response, depending on the balance of T-helper 1 (T$_H$1) versus T$_H$2 cytokines. APC, antigen-presenting cells; Eos, eosinophil; IFN, interferon; IL, interleukin; T$_{cyt}$, cytotoxic T cell.

cytotoxic response. In contrast, type 2 helper cells (T$_H$2 cells) produce IL-4, IL-5, IL-10, and other cytokines that promote humoral immunity and allergic responses. The helper T subsets are mutually inhibitory: IFN-γ from T$_H$1 cells inhibits T$_H$2 cells, and IL-4 from T$_H$2 cells inhibits T$_H$1 cells (Fig. 42.5). The paradigm has proven to be useful in many situations, but it cannot accurately represent all immunologic conditions (22). For example, differences in human helper T cells are less clear-cut than murine cells. Thus, T$_H$1 and T$_H$2 phenotypes are probably best considered to be the extremes on each end of a spectrum.

Integrated Responses

Human Cytokine Dynamics

Endotoxin (cell wall fragments from gram-negative bacteria) induces essentially the same acute responses as an actual infection, but with fewer attendant risks. Consequently, human host defense mechanisms, including cytokine dynamics, have been investigated extensively in response to this stimulus (23). Plasma TNF-α reaches maximal concentrations within 90 minutes after a bolus intravenous injection (Fig. 42.6A). This rapid appearance suggests that release of presynthesized intracellular stores is an important contributing mechanism in TNF-α appearance. Plasma IL-6 and IL-1β reach peak concentrations after approximately 2 to 3 hours (Fig. 42.6B and C). The latency suggests that de novo synthesis is the

primary mechanism responsible for the appearance of these cytokines.

In the first few hours, fever, hypercortisolemia and myalgia are triggered by cytokine-induced PGE$_2$ (24), an eicosanoid described in detail later. PGE$_2$ not only promulgates cytokine action, but also inhibits TNF-α synthesis and IL-1β secretion (25). Thus, it provides one of several negative feedback signals that keep the inherently destructive inflammatory response from causing undue harm to the host. As shown in Figure 42.6A, taking ibuprofen (a PGE$_2$ synthesis inhibitor) before the endotoxin infusion eliminates PGE$_2$-mediated negative feedback and results in higher circulating concentrations of TNF-α.

TNF-α, IL-6, and IL-1β synthesis and secretion are induced directly by endotoxin and are augmented further by the autocrine and paracrine actions of endotoxin-induced TNF-α and IL-1β. This positive feedback augmentation of IL-6 production can be interrupted by blocking TNF-α or IL-1β activity. As shown in Figure 42.6B, the peak IL-6 concentration can be suppressed by about two thirds if sTNFR is infused before the endotoxin (*dashed line*).

In vitro studies have shown that IL-1Ra does not effectively inhibit IL-1β activity until it reaches molar excesses of approximately 100-fold. Such concentrations are readily attained in vivo, but not before IL-1β has had an opportunity to act unopposed (see Fig. 42.6C).

Although IL-6 is temporally associated with the proinflammatory cytokines TNF-α and IL-1β, it is actually an

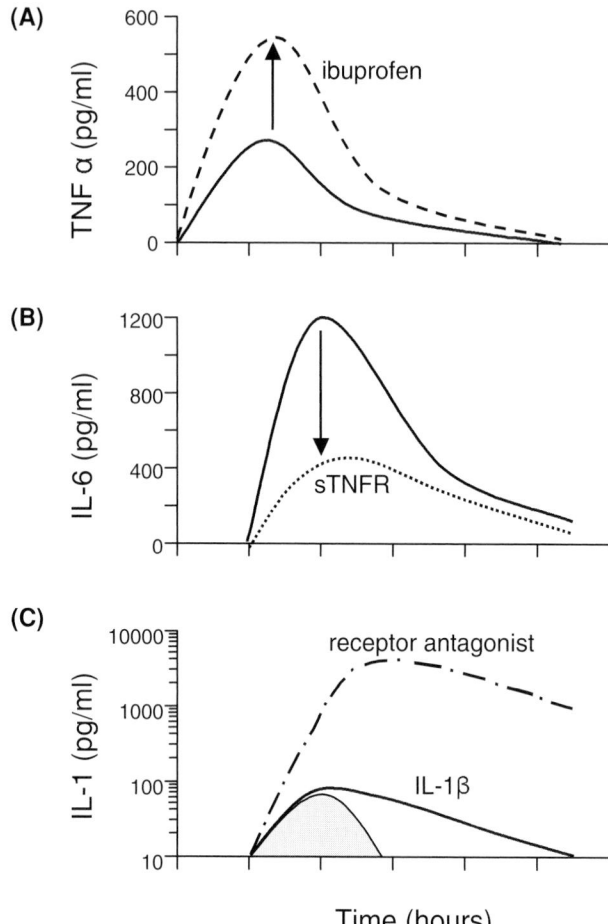

Figure 42.6. Circulating cytokine concentrations induced by intravenous injection of bacterial endotoxin. These idealized responses are based on data from references 24 and 62 to 65. **A.** The *solid line* depicts the normal tumor necrosis-α (TNF-α) response to endotoxin. Blocking prostaglandin E₂ synthesis with ibuprofen removes endogenous negative feedback inhibition of TNF-α synthesis, resulting in higher concentrations. **B.** The *solid line* depicts the normal interleukin-6 (IL-6) response. Blocking TNF-α activity with soluble TNF receptor (sTNFR) interrupts a positive feedback influence on IL-6 synthesis and results in lower concentrations. **C.** The **bottom panel** depicts the appearance of IL-1β (*solid line*) and IL-1 receptor antagonist (IL-1Ra) (*interrupted line*). The shaded area represents the temporal "window of activity" for IL-1β before IL-1Ra reaches sufficient concentrations to compete successfully for IL-1 receptors.

*anti*inflammatory cytokine. IL-6 inhibits synthesis of TNF-α and IL-1β, providing negative feedback control of TNF-α and IL-1β (Fig. 42.7). This is reinforced by the previously mentioned negative feedback signal, PGE₂, which *augments* IL-6 production. IL-6 also induces IL-1Ra, sTNFR, and hepatic production of acute-phase proteins, including antiproteases (α₁-proteinase inhibitor) and antioxidants (ceruloplasmin) that protect host tissues from the destructive, nonspecific proteases and reactive oxygen species released by inflammatory leukocytes as part of the antimicrobial response. IL-1β and TNF-α also induce production of acute-phase proteins, sometimes in synergy with IL-6. Because IL-6 is antiinflammatory, and

the functions of IL-1β and TNF-α transcend inflammation, these cytokines would be better described as acute-phase cytokines rather than as inflammatory cytokines.

Fever and Iron

Seemingly disparate actions of an individual cytokine can work together in a coordinated manner to promote host defense. For example, IL-1β activates fever-inducing mechanisms in the brain, inhibits hepatic transferrin synthesis, and stimulates ferritin synthesis in cells distributed throughout the body. These actions work in concert to make a host's internal environment more hostile to an invading microorganism. The survival of a bacterium within a host (and hence its virulence) depends on its ability to extract nutrients from the surrounding environment. Many of the more virulent bacteria secrete iron-binding siderophores and express specialized receptors for uptake of iron/siderophore complexes (26). Because of its low aqueous solubility, virtually all iron in the body is bound, and its distribution depends on the relative concentration of extracellular binding proteins (transferrin) versus intracellular

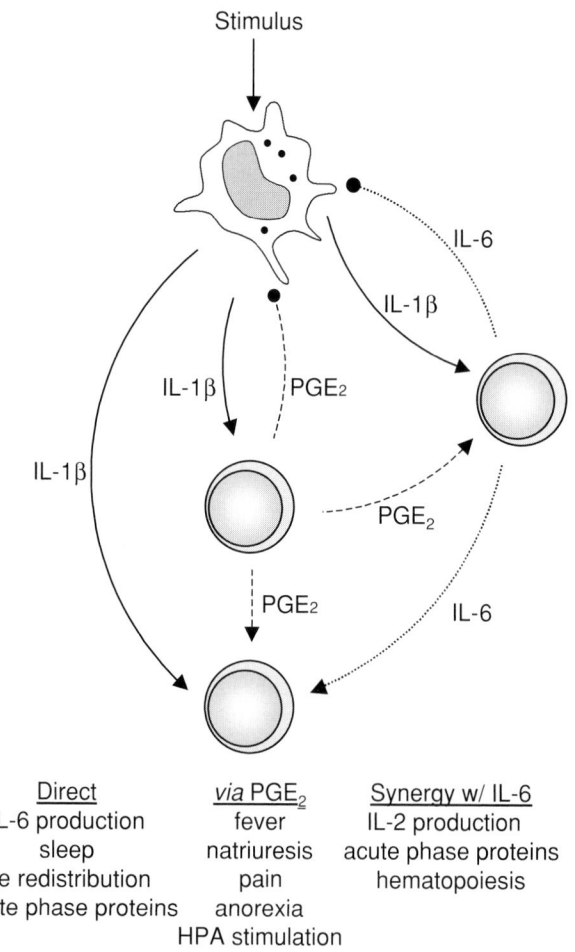

Figure 42.7. Local feedback regulation of prostaglandin E₂ (PGE₂) *(dashed lines)* and interleukin-6 (IL-6) *(dotted lines)* on IL-1β synthesis, secretion, and action. HPA, hypothalamic-pituitary-adrenal axis.

binding proteins (ferritin). During infection, IL-1β inhibits production and release of transferrin while stimulating synthesis of ferritin. The net result is a *redistribution* of iron from extracellular to intracellular compartments (not to be confused with iron *deficiency*), thus rendering this nutrient less accessible to bacteria (27). Furthermore, the elevated temperature resulting from IL-1–induced fever inhibits bacterial synthesis of iron-binding siderophores and thus reduces bacterial capacity to extract iron from host extracellular fluids (28).

Cytokine-Modulated Behavior

Loss of appetite, pain, fatigue, and sleepiness are familiar sensations associated with an injury or infection. They all discourage physical activity and comprise another set of coordinated mechanisms induced by acute-phase cytokines.

TNF-α and IL-1β modulate pain indirectly by inducing local production of PGE₂, which, in turn, increases neuronal sensitivity to painful stimuli. They also influence neurons directly by increasing expression of receptors for kinins and excitatory amino acids (29). Furthermore, IL-1β induces release of the pain-inducing neuropeptide substance P. In vivo, sTNFR and anti-TNF-α antibodies decrease the transmission of painful signals, apparently by inhibiting the activity of TNF-α produced by the neurons themselves. TNF-α–mediated neuromodulation may involve activation of MAPK pathways (30).

Both IL-1β and TNF-α promote non–rapid eye movement sleep (31). They are constitutively expressed in the brain, and their concentrations rise and fall in synchrony with the sleep-wake cycle. Both cytokines alter sleep-associated neuronal activity in the anterior hypothalamus and basal forebrain by increasing neuronal calcium ion concentrations. IL-1β may upregulate expression of neuronal receptors for somnogenic neuropeptides such as growth hormone releasing hormone.

The acute-phase cytokines act at several sites to depress food intake (32). For example, IL-1β increases the firing rates of glucose-sensitive neurons in the ventromedial hypothalamus and modulates the function of receptors for neuropeptide Y, cholecystokinin, glucagon, and other mediators of ingestive behavior. Peripherally, several cytokines inhibit gastric acid secretion and gastrointestinal motility. IL-1β also stimulates synthesis and release of the anorexic hormone leptin from adipocytes.

Pain, sleepiness, and loss of interest in food all discourage mobility. The potential adaptive value to the individual includes conservation of energy substrates (to be redirected to activated immune cells) and reduced physical strain on a damaged organ or tissue (facilitating healing). The potential adaptive value to a population is reduced spread of a contagious disease by an infected individual. However, the interruption in dietary nutrient intake is itself a challenge to the host that requires metabolic adjustments.

Protein, Carbohydrate, and Lipid Metabolism

Skeletal muscle protein breakdown, hyperglycemia, and hypertriglyceridemia often accompany severe infection. IL-1β and TNF-α can induce these conditions in vivo, but direct actions of these cytokines on relevant tissues in vitro is inconsistent (33). Some of the metabolic alterations seem to be indirectly affected by cytokines, via altered secretion of regulatory hormones including cortisol, epinephrine, insulin, and glucagon. However, the mechanisms underlying these indirect actions are not well understood, either. For example, intravenous injection of IL-1β can increase plasma insulin concentrations, but application of IL-1β to isolated pancreatic islets inhibits insulin release. IL-1β and TNF-α probably affect numerous endocrine and neuroendocrine cells that interact in a complex network to regulate metabolic processes. Furthermore, these cytokines induce secretion of many other cytokines that affect endocrine tissues.

The change in endocrine milieu promotes release of amino acids from "storage" (i.e., proteolytic breakdown of skeletal muscle). Subsequent deamination of glutamine to glutamate provides fuel for activated leukocytes. Liberated amino acids are also channeled into hepatic synthesis pathways and are recycled into the acute-phase proteins, which increase dramatically (some up to 1000-fold) in the bloodstream during infection (34). Some of these acute-phase proteins have direct antimicrobial properties (complement, C-reactive protein), whereas others promote wound repair (fibrinogen) or protect the host from reactive oxygen species and proteases, as described earlier (Fig. 42.8). C-reactive protein may also contribute to feedback regulation of cytokine activity because it stimulates IL-1Ra release and sIL-6R shedding (35).

Hypertriglyceridemia is another hallmark of infection mediated by coordinated, pleotropic actions of cytokines (36). TNF-α, IL-1β, IL-6, and the IFNs increase hepatic fatty acid synthesis, increase lipolysis in adipocytes (fatty acid mobilization), and decrease lipoprotein lipase activity (fatty acid clearance). The net result is high circulating concentrations of very-low-density lipoproteins that bind bacterial toxins and neutralize viruses and parasites. Lipoprotein infusions can actually reduce mortality in animal models of sepsis.

Neuroendocrine Regulation

The acute-phase cytokines stimulate hypothalamic release of corticotropin-releasing hormone, leading to pituitary secretion of adrenocorticotropic hormone, and ultimately, adrenal secretion of cortisol (see Fig. 42.8) (37). Cortisol feeds back on cytokine synthesis and action at several levels. It associates with cytosolic receptors that move into the nucleus and bind regulatory elements on DNA, inhibiting transcription of mRNA for the cytokines while increasing gene expression for IκB, the feedback inhibitor of NF-κB (an important transcription factor for many cytokine-induced cellular responses). Cortisol/receptor complexes

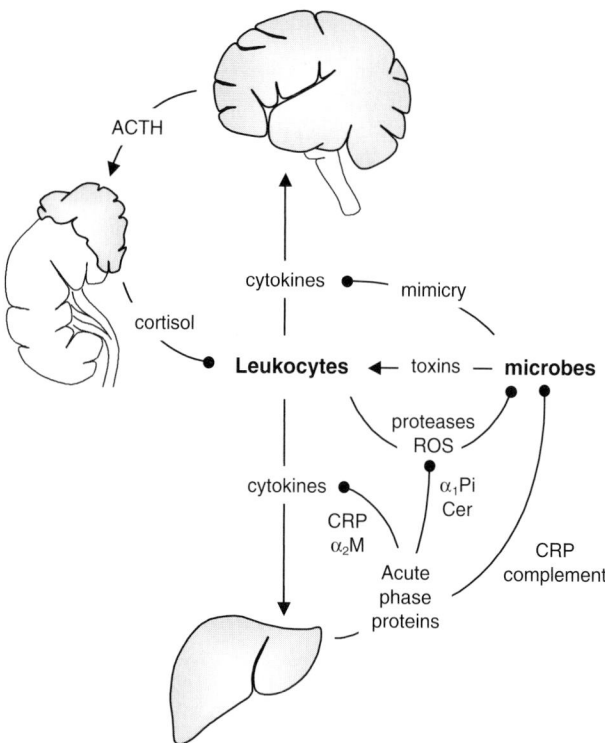

Figure 42.8. Systemic feedback regulation of IL-1β, IL-6, and TNF production and action via the hypothalamic-pituitary-adrenal axis and the liver. In viral infections, the microbes attempt to evade cytokine-mediated host defenses by producing factors that mimic cytokine regulatory proteins (66), including soluble receptors for IL-1β and TNF-α, and homologs for IL-10 (which inhibit production of IL-1β and TNF α). ACTH, adrenocorticotropic hormone; Cer, ceruloplasmin; CRP, C-reactive protein; α₂M, α₂-macroglobulin; α₁Pi, α₁-protease inhibitor; ROS, reactive oxygen species.

also bind untranslated regions on mRNA, thus causing destabilization and/or repressed translation of cytokine-induced message. Cortisol also promotes synthesis of IL-1Ra and shedding of cytokine receptors.

Cytokines in the Brain

The hypothalamus is a principal target for cytokine actions (38), but how a cytokine arising from a peripheral infection can affect this immunologically privileged brain tissue has been a conundrum. A protein the size of a cytokine should not be able to pass through the tight endothelial blood-brain barrier, but several mechanisms that bypass this barrier have been identified: (a) an anatomic breach in the barrier at the organum vasculosa of the lamina terminalis; (b) cytokine-receptor interactions on the luminal side of an endothelial cell, triggering secretion of a second messenger (notably PGE_2) on the brain side; (c) facilitated transport through endothelial cells; and (d) cytokine-stimulated neural impulses, especially through afferent vagal fibers and afferent neurons arising from lymph nodes, that ultimately induce cytokine synthesis by microglial and neuronal cells in the brain.

Cytokines in the Reproductive Tract

Women are generally more resistant to infection than men, but they also tend to be more susceptible to autoimmune diseases. This increased immune activity is the result, in part, of differential influences of estradiol, progesterone, and testosterone on leukocyte function, including cytokine production (39). Testosterone generally has suppressive influences on IL-1β and TNF-α secretion and receptor expression, whereas estradiol and progesterone have more complicated biphasic dose-response influences on cytokine synthesis and receptor expression.

Ovulation and implantation are essentially inflammatory processes that seem to involve IL-1 and other cytokines. During the menstrual cycle, plasma and endometrial concentrations of IL-1β and endometrial expression of IL-1 receptors are higher in the luteal phase than in the follicular phase. Follicle rupture requires coordinated release of proteolytic enzymes, whereas trophoblast implantation into maternal decidua requires extracellular matrix remodeling, increased vascular permeability, phagocytosis, cellular proliferation, and differentiation. These are all cytokine-modulated events.

From an immunologic point of view, pregnancy is an acquired maternal tolerance of a fetal allograft requiring downregulation of cytotoxic T-cell–mediated rejection processes. The endocrine milieu of pregnancy shifts cytokine profiles away from T_H1, toward a dominance of T_H2. Recurrent spontaneous abortions have been associated with elevated IFN-γ and TNF-α and abnormally low IL-10. Meanwhile, the elevated circulating IL-1β and IL-6 concentrations that occur during pregnancy may promote nonspecific host defense mechanisms.

Whereas reproductive steroids modulate cytokine production, reciprocal regulation also exists: Cytokines modulate steroid hormone synthesis in the ovaries and testes. Moreover, the concentrations of acute-phase cytokines achieved during infection inhibit pituitary luteinizing hormone secretion and block ovulation. The adaptive value of this action could be to limit reproductive capacity during times of infection, famine, or other environmental stress that could compromise a pregnancy and lead to weakened offspring.

Therapy

In contrast to the nonspecific cytokine-inducing methods of Wagner-Jauregg and Coley, modern cytokine therapy involves the selective application of individual recombinant cytokines or cytokine inhibition by specific antibodies or soluble receptors. Cytokine-based interventions are currently under study for a wide range of diseases, including cancer, septic shock, and chronic inflammatory diseases such as rheumatoid arthritis.

Cancer

Intense research is currently focused on the use of cytokines, or cytokine inhibitors, in the treatment of patients with cancer (40, 41). In animal models, various cytokines have been shown to (a) kill or inhibit tumor cells directly (e.g., TNF-α), (b) activate T-cell and natural killer cell–mediated cytotoxicity against tumors (e.g., IL-2, IL-12, IFN-γ), (c) inhibit the ability of a tumor to establish vasculature (several chemokines), or (d) restore the bone marrow after chemotherapy (IL-1, IL-11). Some clinical success has been achieved with cytokine therapy, but toxicity to the patient and unexpected hematologic reactions are recurring problems. Combination therapies are under investigation (e.g., IL-2 plus IL-12) that may have synergistic antitumor activity at lower doses that lack side effects. Alternatively, chimeras composed of cytokines fused to antibodies against tumor-specific antigens are under study (42). These constructs have the potential to concentrate the cytokine in the tumor, thus increasing the antitumor activity and reducing distal side effects.

Septic Shock

Septic shock has been characterized as a modern disease, a consequence of improved critical care for normally fatal injuries. Advancements in wound treatment, fluid replacement, and cardiorespiratory support give patients a better chance of surviving an initial trauma. However, these patients can be at an increased risk of severe infection, especially if the protective barrier of the skin is breached to a significant extent (e.g., severe burn injuries). A massive release of TNF-α, IL-1β, and other cytokines can occur, triggering widespread vascular permeability, vasodilation, and intravascular coagulation. This can ultimately lead to shock, organ failure, and death.

Anticytokine strategies have included intravenous infusion of IL-1Ra, monoclonal antibodies directed against TNF-α, and chimeric constructs of sTNFR fused to the Fc region of immunoglobulin G. Although phase II trials have been promising, larger phase III trials have often failed to demonstrate increased survival for patients treated with anticytokine regimens (43). Some of the problems may be related to timing (relative to onset of infection): Treatment *after* IL-1β and TNF-α have been released may be too late if these cytokines have already triggered the multiple kinin, eicosanoid, and cellular effector mechanisms involved in shock.

Other reasons for phase III trial failures may have been related to patient selection. Post hoc analyses of some trials have indicated that perhaps anticytokine therapy was beneficial for subsets of patients, that is, protecting the most severe cases and/or those with high circulating cytokine concentrations from cardiovascular collapse. However, anticytokine treatment may have inhibited important antimicrobial mechanisms in patients who had a moderate cytokine response and therefore increased their risk of fatality through infection. If this is true, then one challenge for future anticytokine therapy is to devise very rapid cytokine analyses that can identify the appropriate patients for treatment.

Rheumatoid Arthritis

Rheumatoid arthritis is characterized by synovial cell proliferation along with cartilage and bone damage. The pathogenesis is complex, involving activated T cells, abnormal antibodies, and complement activation. Anti–TNF-α, sTNFR, and IL-1Ra therapies can reduce the rate of tissue destruction and can relieve clinical signs and symptoms, but these treatments can also increase the risk of serious infection (44). As with septic shock, determining an optimal anticytokine dose that diminishes inappropriate catabolic activities without seriously compromising host defense remains a challenge. In rheumatoid arthritis, careful screening of patients for concurrent infection or use of immunosuppressive drugs including glucocorticoids seems necessary.

EICOSANOIDS

History

Like cytokines, the eicosanoids were targets of clinical intervention long before their molecular characteristics were understood (45). Through the centuries, myrtle leaves, poplar extracts, and willow tree bark have been used to relieve pain and fever. By the nineteenth century, the active substances in these botanicals—salicylates—were isolated, and synthetic forms were produced. Notably, acetylsalicylic acid or aspirin (a, acetyl; spirin, from *Spiraea*, the genus of natural sources of salicylates) came on the market in 1899. Aspirin and other nonsteroidal antiinflammatory drugs (NSAIDs) inhibit synthesis of many eicosanoids, but this concept would not be understood for another 70 years.

In the early 1930s, semen was found to contain lipids that relaxed isolated uterine smooth muscle in vitro and increased blood pressure when it was injected intravenously into animals (46). The term "prostaglandin" arose from the assumption that the prostate gland was the source of these lipids. Ensuing discoveries revealed that the term prostaglandin was too restrictive, because these lipids were actually produced by a wide variety of tissues throughout the body (reminiscent of the problems with cytokine nomenclature). At about the same time, other bioactive lipids were isolated, including slow-reacting substance (SRS), which caused a delayed, sustained contraction of isolated smooth muscle (in contrast to the immediate, transient effect of histamine), and rabbit aorta-contracting substance (RCS) (47).

In the 1970s, the biosynthetic pathway for prostaglandins was elucidated, including the isolation of a key enzyme in this process, cyclooxygenase (COX). This led to the discovery that aspirin-like drugs blocked the enzymatic activity of COX (45). During this same period, other products of COX, including thromboxanes (the major bioactive components of RCS) and prostacyclins, were characterized. Furthermore, the COX-*in*dependent synthesis pathways for leukotrienes (the bioactive components of SRS) were characterized (47).

Synthesis

Prostaglandins, prostacyclins, thromboxanes, and leukotrienes are all 20-carbon molecules known collectively as eicosanoids (48), a term of Greek etymology meaning 20. The synthetic pathways for several important eicosanoids are shown in Figure 42.9. The first step involves liberating arachidonic acid from membrane phospholipids through a reaction catalyzed by cytosolic phospholipase A_2, an enzyme expressed in practically all cells (49). Its enzymatic activity is upregulated via phosphorylation triggered by mechanical stresses, by increases in cytosolic calcium ion concentrations, or by cytokines including IL-1β and TNF-α. In addition, transcription of phospho-

lipase A_2 is increased by IL-1β and TNF-α and is inhibited by glucocorticoids. Once liberated, arachidonic acid can be processed along the COX or the lipoxygenase pathway (or metabolized in other ways outside the scope of this chapter).

Cyclooxygenase Pathway

The COX enzyme exists in two isoforms (50). Both transform arachidonic acid to prostaglandin H_2 (PGH_2; the subscript for this and all other eicosanoids denotes the number of double bonds in the molecule). Most cells contain COX-1, which is constitutively expressed and supports basal production of prostaglandins that maintain blood flow and provide cytoprotection. The expression of COX-2 is induced and is restricted to certain types of cells. The stimuli for COX-2 expression are the factors relevant to that cell's function, such as shear stress (endothelial cells), sodium concentrations (kidney macula densa cells), gonadotropins (granulosa cells), bacterial toxins and cytokines (neurons, monocytes, and macrophages).

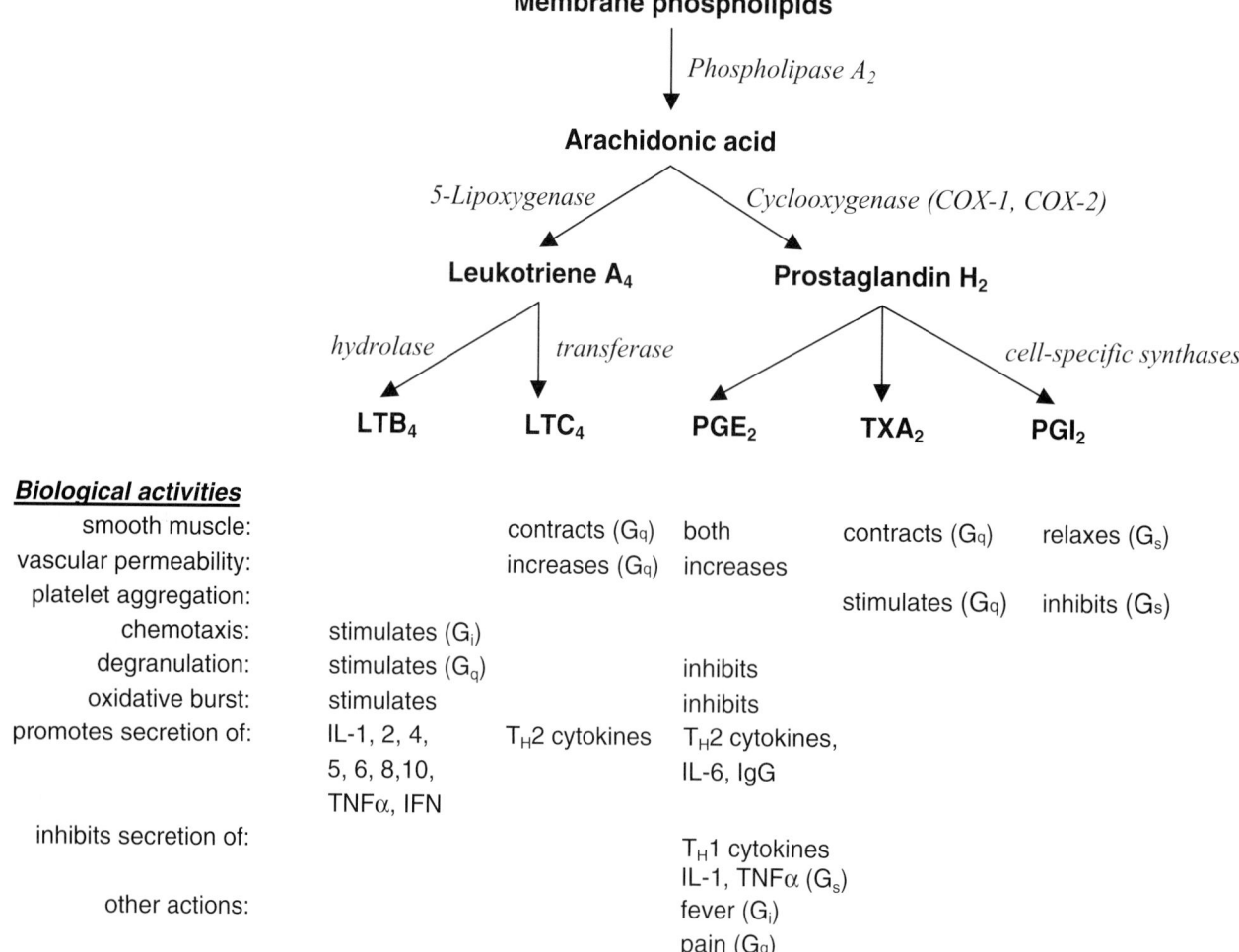

Figure 42.9. Major pathways of eicosanoid synthesis and summary of eicosanoid activities. See text for details.

The cell-specific production of biologically active end products of both COX-1 and COX-2 is determined by downstream enzymes that are segregated to various types of cells. For example, platelets contain thromboxane A_2 (TXA_2) synthase, whereas endothelial cells express prostacyclin (PGI_2) synthase. This enzyme compartmentalization is the basis for the opposing roles of platelets and endothelial cells in vascular homeostasis. Endothelium-derived PGI_2 maintains blood flow under normal conditions by inhibiting platelet aggregation and relaxing vascular smooth muscle (vasodilation). In response to vascular injury, activated platelets release TXA_2, causing vasoconstriction and platelet aggregation, which plugs injured vascular walls and reduces blood loss. Other synthases not shown in Figure 42.9 exist in mast cells (which produce PGD_2, a bronchoconstrictor) and in uterine tissue (producing $PGF_{2\alpha}$, which causes uterine smooth muscle contraction).

Tissue-specific actions of eicosanoids also depend on the location and function of specific eicosanoid receptors (48). These receptors are all serpentine proteins that associate with one of three types of cytosolic G proteins: G_s proteins increase cytosolic concentrations of cyclic adenosine monophosphate (cAMP) in target cells (often associated with relaxation); G_i proteins decrease cAMP production, and G_q increases cytosolic calcium ion concentrations (often associated with constriction). As shown in Figure 42.9, the type of G-protein a receptor associates with can account for *some* common bioactivities among the eicosanoids, but several receptors have multiple isoforms that bind to various G proteins, so eicosanoid action cannot be predicted simply by G-protein associations.

Because most cells express PGE synthase, PGE_2-mediated signaling is widespread. Four PGE_2 receptors exist, so this prostaglandin induces a diverse set of responses. Peripherally, PGE_2 increases the sensitivity of neurons to painful stimuli (hyperalgesia). Centrally, PGE_2 causes neuronal hyperexcitability, transforming nonpainful afferent signals into painful sensations (allodynia). Cytokine-induced PGE_2 in the hypothalamus is a critical link in resetting the thermoregulatory set point leading to fever. PGE_2 also augments bradykinin- and histamine-induced vasodilation and vascular permeability. Thus, inhibiting synthesis of this eicosanoid can reduce all four of the cardinal signs of inflammation: dolor (pain), calor (heat), rubor (redness), and tumor (swelling). PGE_2 also induces several metalloproteases responsible for the breakdown of connective tissue.

For all these reasons, drugs that block prostaglandin synthesis are prescribed for degenerative inflammatory diseases such as arthritis. Steroidal antiinflammatory drugs (glucocorticoids) inhibit both COX-1 and COX-2 enzyme *synthesis* (51). In contrast, NSAIDs compete with arachidonic acid for binding to the active site of COX and therefore inhibit enzyme *activity* (50). Although binding is reversible for most NSAIDs, aspirin actually causes a covalent modification to the enzyme. Acetaminophen inhibits COX in the central nervous system, thus blocking pain and fever, but has little effect on peripheral inflammation. The reason for this is uncertain; perhaps oxidants released by leukocytes within a local inflammatory site interfere with the ability of acetaminophen to bind the enzymatic site in COX (52). Older NSAIDs inhibit both COX-1 and COX-2, but recently developed NSAIDs selectively inhibit COX-2.

Although inhibiting prostaglandin production can reduce destruction of arthritic joints or other chronically inflamed tissues, this inhibition can *cause* destruction elsewhere. By increasing mucus and bicarbonate secretion, prostaglandins protect the gastric mucosa from acidic erosion. That is why aspirin and other nonspecific COX inhibitors can cause serious gastrointestinal damage, including ulcers (53). The newer COX-2–specific inhibitors avoid these gastrointestinal side effects because they block the COX-2 activity of leukocytes in areas of inflammation, but they have no effect on the production of mucosa-preserving prostaglandins by the COX-1 enzymes in the gastrointestinal tract.

PGE_2 and PGI_2 help to preserve renal blood flow during periods of cardiovascular stress, such as heat stress or hemorrhage, by counterbalancing sympathetic- and angiotensin II–mediated vasoconstriction. Nonselective NSAIDs have been implicated in cases of acute ischemic renal injury (54). Because glomerular, macula densa, and mesangial cells express both COX isoforms, COX-2 inhibitors may present less risk. However, they still have the potential to diminish prostaglandin-mediated renal protection, which may have adverse consequences for the elderly and patients with renal disease.

One may ask how low-dose aspirin therapy can reduce the risk of inappropriate blood clots in cardiovascular disease if it irreversibly inhibits COX and therefore blocks downstream production of *both* PGI_2 and TXA_2. The reason is a differential regeneration of COX by endothelial cells, compared with platelets. Nucleated endothelial cells can synthesize new COX protein and can resume producing PGI_2 fairly soon (hours). In contrast, the anuclear platelets are incapable of synthesizing new enzyme proteins, so TXA_2 production cannot resume until new platelets are produced by the bone marrow (days). COX-2 inhibitors may be counterproductive in reducing the risk of occlusive cardiovascular events because endothelial cell production of PGI_2 is diminished by these drugs without any concomitant reductions in TXA_2 production (platelets express only COX-1) (55). In fact, one COX-2–specific drug has been withdrawn from the market for this reason (55a).

Prostaglandin activity depends on the balance between synthesis and clearance (or metabolic deactivation). A key enzyme involved in deactivating PGE_2, PGI_2, $PGF_{2\alpha}$, and other eicosanoids is the ubiquitously expressed enzyme 15-hydroxyprostaglandin dehydrogenase (15-PGDH) (56). As shown in Table 42.1, IL-1β and TNF-α inhibit 15-PGDH while inducing synthetic enzymes, thereby promoting increased concentrations of PGE_2 in a coordinated

TABLE 42.1. PROINFLAMMATORY AND ANTIINFLAMMATORY MEDIATOR INFLUENCES ON ENZYMES INVOLVED IN PROSTAGLANDIN METABOLISM

	IL-1β AND TNF-α	IL-10	GLUCOCORTICOIDS
Phospholipase A_2	Induce	Inhibit	Inhibit
Cyclooxygenase-2	Induce	Inhibit	Inhibit
Prostaglandin E synthase	Induce	Not reported	Inhibit
15-Hydroxyprostaglandin dehydrogenase	Inhibit	Antagonizes IL-1β and TNF-α	Variable, depending on dose and cell type

IL, interleukin; TNF, tumor necrosis factor.

manner. The influences of two important antiinflammatory agents, IL-10 and glucocorticoids, are also summarized in Table 42.1.

Lipoxygenase Pathway

An alternative fate of arachidonic acid is conversion to leukotriene A_4 (LTA$_4$) by the enzyme 5-lipoxygenase (57). The name "leukotriene" is derived from the findings that 5-lipoxygenase is restricted primarily to leukocytes, and the eicosanoids produced by this enzyme all have a characteristic structure containing three adjacent double bonds (with a fourth elsewhere). The activity of 5-lipoxygenase is stimulated posttranslationally by GM-CSF and is inhibited by PGE$_2$. (Other arachidonic acid–derived eicosanoids exist, such as lipoxins, but they are not covered here because of space limitations).

LTA$_4$ is the precursor for several other leukotrienes, as shown in Figure 42.9. LTB$_4$ is formed by the hydrolysis of LTA$_4$, and LTC$_4$ is formed by the transfer of a peptide side chain (Cys-Glu-Gly) to the carbon backbone (58). Additional leukotrienes (D$_4$ and E$_4$, not shown) are produced by successive cleavage of Gly and Glu from LTC$_4$ by peptidases.

The C, D, and E products are known collectively as cysteinyl leukotrienes and are the active components of SRS, which was originally isolated from lung perfusates in early studies of asthma and hypersensitivity reactions. Cysteinyl leukotrienes act on smooth muscle and vascular endothelium. They are important mediators of bronchoconstriction and edema formation associated with these diseases (59).

The first antiasthma drugs were based on an herb called khellin, which was extracted from the seeds of a plant native to eastern Mediterranean regions and used for centuries as a muscle relaxant (60). Once the active component was isolated and structural analogs were produced, it was discovered that they acted by competing with LTC$_4$ and LTD$_4$ for receptor occupancy on target cells. Although these original receptor antagonists were relatively weak and were never adopted for routine clinical use, they set the precedent for several current medications that also act by way of receptor antagonism (although inhibitors of the leukotriene synthesis enzymes also exist).

NSAIDs can affect the lipoxygenase pathway in two ways. First, inhibition of COX tends to shunt arachidonic acid in the direction of leukotriene synthesis. Second, PGE$_2$ synthesis is blocked, which normally inhibits 5-lipoxygenase activity. For persons with abnormally high LTC synthase activity, taking NSAIDs can lead to bronchoconstriction resulting from excessive production of cysteinyl leukotrienes, a condition known as aspirin-induced asthma (61).

REFERENCES

1. Whitrow M. Med Hist 1990;34:294–310.
2. Wiemann B, Starnes CO. Pharmacol Ther 1994;64:529–64.
3. Carrel A, Ebeling AH. J Exp Med 1922;36:645–59.
4. Dumonde DC, Wolstencroft RA, Panayi GS et al. Nature 1969;224:38–42.
5. Cohen S, Pierluigi PE, Yoshida T. Cell Immunol 1974;12:150–9.
6. Aarden LA, Brunner TK, Cerottini JC et al. J Immunol 1979;123:2928–9.
7. Eberl M. Trends Immunol 2002;23:341–2.
8. Cannon JG. News Physiol Sci 2000;15:298–303.
9. Fernandez-Botran R. Crit Rev Clin Lab Sci 1999;36:165–224.
10. Taniguchi T. Science 1995;268:251–5.
11. Garrington TP, Johnson GL. Curr Opin Cell Biol 1999;11:211–8.
12. Clark A. Arthritis Res 2000;2:172–4.
13. Yasukawa H, Sasaki A, Yoshimura A. Annu Rev Immunol 2000;18:143–64.
14. Taga T, Kishimoto T. Annu Rev Immunol 1997;15:797–819.
15. Lopez AF, Elliott MJ, Woodcock J et al. Immunol Today 1992;13:495–500.
16. Wuyts A, Proost P, Van Damme J. Interleukin-8 and other CXC chemokines. In: Thomson A, ed. The Cytokine Handbook. San Diego: Academic Press, 1998:271–312.
17. Roberts AB, Anzano MA, Wakefield LM et al. Proc Natl Acad Sci USA 1985;82:119–23.
18. Bird TA, Saklatvala J. J Immunol 1989;142:126–33.
19. Dinarello CA. Blood 1996;87:2095–147.
20. Mantovani A, Bonecchi R, Martinez FO et al. Int Arch Allergy Immunol 2003;132:109–15.
21. Mosmann TR, Cherwinski H, Bond MW et al. J Immunol 1986;162:2348–57.
22. Gor DO, Rose NR, Greenspan NS. Nat Immunol 2003;4:503–5.
23. Santos AA, Wilmore DW. Shock 1996;6:S50–6.
24. Michie HR, Majzoub JA, O'Dwyer ST et al. Surgery 1990;108:254–61.
25. Williams JA, Shacter E. J Biol Chem 1997;272:25693–9.
26. Neilands JB. J Biol Chem 1995;270:26723–6.

27. Weinberg ED. Physiol Rev 1984;64:65–102.
28. Kluger MJ. Physiol Rev 1991;71:93–127.
29. Sorkin LS, Wallace MS. Surg Clin North Am 1999;79:213–29.
30. Schafers M, Svensson CI, Sommer C et al. J Neurosci 2003;23: 2517–21.
31. Krueger JM, Majde JA. Ann NY Acad Sci 2003;992:9–20.
32. Plata-Salaman CR. Ann NY Acad Sci 1998;856:160–70.
33. Chang HR, Bistrian B. JPEN J Parenter Enteral Nutr 1998;22: 156–66.
34. Gabay C, Kushner I. N Engl J Med 1999;340:448–54.
35. Jones SA, Novick D, Horiuchi S et al. J Exp Med 1999;189: 599–604.
36. Grunfeld C, Feingold KR. Nutrition 1996;12:S24–6.
37. Besedovsky HO, del Rey A. Endocr Rev 1996;17:64–102.
38. Turnbull AV, Rivier CL. Physiol Rev 1999;79:1–71.
39. Cannon JG. Ann NY Acad Sci 1998;856:234–42.
40. Maini A, Morse PD, Wang CY et al. Anticancer Res 1997;17: 3803–8.
41. Oppenheim JJ, Murphy WJ, Chertov O et al. Clin Cancer Res 1997;3:2682–6.
42. Penichet ML, Morrison SL. J Immunol Methods 2001;248: 91–101.
43. Abraham E. Intensive Care Med 1999;25:556–66.
44. Weisman MH. J Rheumatol 2002;29[Suppl 65]:33–8.
45. Vane JR, Botting RM. Am J Med 1998;104:2S–8S.
46. Kurzrok R, Lieb CC. Proc Soc Exp Biol Med 1930;28:268–72.
47. Samuelsson B. Am J Respir Crit Care Med 2000;161:S2–S6.
48. Funk CD. Science 2001;294:1871–5.
49. Serhan CN, Haeggstrom JZ, Leslie CC. FASEB J 1996;10: 1147–58.
50. Smith WL, DeWitt DL, Garavito RM. Annu Rev Biochem 2000; 69:145–82.
51. Goppelt-Struebe M. Biochem Pharmacol 1997;53:1389–95.
52. Lippincott JB. Analgesic–antipyretic and antiinflammatory agents. In: Drug Facts and Comparisons. St. Louis: Kluwer, 1993:631.
53. Levi S, Shaw-Smith C. Br J Rheumatol 1994;33:605–12.
54. Khan KNM, Paulson SK, Verburg KM et al. Kidney Int 2002; 61:1210–9.
55. Mukherjee D. Biochem Pharmacol 2002;63:817–21.
55a. Fitzgerald GA. N Engl J Med 2004;351:1709–11.
56. Tai H-H, Ensor CM, Tong M et al. Prostaglandins Lipid Med 2002;68–69:483–93.
57. Bigby TD. Mol Pharmacol 2002;62:200–2.
58. Crooks SW, Stockley RA. Int J Biochem Cell Biol 1998;30: 173–8.
69. Barnes PJ, Chung KF, Page CP. Pharmacol Rev 1998;50: 515–96.
60. Edwards AM, Howell JBL. Clin Exp Allergy 2000;30:756–74.
61. Babu KS, Salvi SS. Chest 2000;118:147–1476.
62. Granowicz EV, Santos AA, Poutsiaka DD. Lancet 1991;338: 1423–4.
63. Spinas GA, Bloesch D, Keller U et al. J Infect Dis 1991;163: 89–95.
64. Suffredini AF, Reda D, Banks SM et al. J Immunol 1995;155: 5038–45.
65. van der Poll T, Coyle SM, Levi M et al. Blood 1997;89:3727–34.
66. Alcami A. Nat Rev 2003;3:36–50.

SELECTED READINGS

Aggarwal BB, Puri RK, eds. Human Cytokines: Their Role in Disease and Therapy. Cambridge: Blackwell Science, 1995.

Gallin J, Goldstein I, Snyderman R, eds. Inflammation: Basic Principles and Clinical Correlates, 2nd ed. New York: Raven Press, 1992. and 3rd ed. Philadelphia: Lippincott Williams & Wilkins, 1999 (the third edition complements, but does not supplant the second edition).

Ibelgaufts H. Cytokines Online Pathfinder Encyclopaedia. http://www .copewithcytokines.de/cope.cgi, 2003.

Majno G, Joris I. Cells, Tissues and Disease. Cambridge: Blackwell Science, Cambridge, 1996.

Thomson A, ed. The Cytokine Handbook. San Diego: Academic Press, 1998.

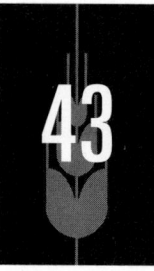

43 NUTRITION AND THE IMMUNE SYSTEM[1]
GABRIEL FERNANDES, CHRISTOPHER A. JOLLY, AND RICHARD A. LAWRENCE

INTERACTION OF NUTRIENTS AND THE
 IMMUNE SYSTEM 670
DEVELOPMENT OF THE IMMUNE SYSTEM
 (HEMATOPOIESIS) 670
 B Cells 671
 T Cells 673
INNATE AND ADAPTIVE IMMUNITY 674
 B-Cell Signaling and Activation 674
 T-Cell Signaling and Activation 675
 Programmed Cell Death (Apoptosis) 676
ROLE OF NUTRIENTS IN INNATE AND
 ADAPTIVE IMMUNITY .677
 Innate Immunity 677
 Adaptive Immunity .679
CONCLUDING SUMMARY .680

INTERACTION OF NUTRIENTS AND THE IMMUNE SYSTEM

The sciences of nutrition and immunity are intimately linked to each other and are currently facilitating the understanding of cellular and molecular mechanisms involved in maintaining a healthy and disease-free life span. In recent years, nutrition research and immunologic studies have been extremely valuable in understanding human growth and development, maintenance of proper health, disease prevention, and disease control. The nutrients in foods are chemical components that (a) provide fuel and energy for regulation and maintenance of physiologic processes and (b) promote growth and repair of body tissues. The role of nutrition in the immune system was studied initially, in the early 1970s, by Fernandes and Good and colleagues (1–4), Walford and associates (5, 6), and Fraker and colleagues (7).

[1]**Abbreviations: APC,** antigen-presenting cell; **BCR,** B-cell receptor; **CD,** cluster of differentiation; **CLA,** conjugated linoleic acid; **DC,** dendritic cell; **DHA,** docosahexaenoic acid; **DP,** double-positive (cell); **EPA,** eicosapentaenoic acid; **HIV,** human immunodeficiency virus; **HSC,** hematopoietic stem cell; **Ig,** immunoglobulin; **IL,** interleukin; **ITAM,** immunomodulatory tyrosine-based activating motif; **ITIM,** immunomodulatory tyrosine-based inhibitory motif; **MHC,** major histocompatibility complex; **NK,** natural killer (cell); **SP,** single-positive (cell); **TCR,** T-cell receptor; **Th,** T-helper (cell); **TNF,** tumor necrosis factor.

Since then, numerous investigations on the influence of both macronutrients and micronutrients on both cellular and humoral immunity have been conducted, mostly in rats and mice. The immune system requires nutrients to produce and distribute normal healthy immune cells throughout the body (hematopoiesis, see next section), to combat invasive pathogenic microorganisms (innate and adaptive immunity), and to discriminate between self- and nonself-antigens (adaptive immunity). Collectively, these functions serve to protect the integrity of the host organism. The immune system is a highly intricate, delicately regulated network of cells that are intimately involved in both innate and adaptive immune responses. The tools of immunology and molecular biology provide a resourceful approach to investigate the role of various dietary components in maintaining the optimal function of immune cells, not only to prevent infection, but also possibly to protect against the occurrence of cardiovascular disease, cancer, age- and autoimmune-related disorders, and acquired immunodeficiency syndrome in humans.

The immune system is fully equipped to recognize and to respond constantly, not only to viral and other infectious agents, but also to a large number of invading foreign antigens. New sources of antigens are regularly infused into the body by absorption of a variety of common food products and liquids. Besides allergenic food substances, insults from carcinogens, food preservatives (e.g., nitrate and nitrite), or polycyclic aromatic hydrocarbons ingested in charred foods, vegetables, or fruits may initiate the activation of immune responses (8). In this chapter, we provide a concise review of recent advances in understanding innate and adaptive immunity including B- and T-cell development, signaling, activation, and the demise of immune cells by apoptosis. The second half of the chapter focuses on the role of selected key nutrients in innate and adaptive immunity.

DEVELOPMENT OF THE IMMUNE SYSTEM (HEMATOPOIESIS)

All blood cells are derived from hematopoietic stem cells (HSCs) by differentiation. Populations of cells at various stages in development of the different branches are present in all tissues supporting hematopoiesis. As the progeny of these cells pass through progressive stages, they become more and more restricted in the number of cell types that they can produce. These cells are spoken of as being committed to a given cell lineage or range of lineages.

In the early fetal development of the mouse, nucleated erythrocytes with embryonic forms of hemoglobin appear in the yolk sack. These cells are incapable of producing other hematopoietic lineages (9), but they may have a greater lineage potential when injected directly into a newborn liver (10). Generation of all blood cell types including lymphocytes is initiated at about 9 to 10 days post coitus in the splanchopleural aorta-gonad-mesenepheros (Sp/AGM) (11). These cells are capable of long-term repopulation of lethally irradiated adults giving rise to all the lineages of blood cells (12, 13). These multipotent cells then colonize the liver at about 11 days post coitus, and hematopoiesis takes place there until shortly before birth. Just before birth, the spleen becomes the primary site for hematopoiesis. Thereafter, hematopoiesis in the spleen gradually declines to very low levels over 2 to 4 weeks while concomitantly this process increases in the bone marrow.

B Cells

Advances in our understanding of B-cell development and function have recently been described (14). The intermediate stages that stem cells pass through on their way to becoming B cells have been described in terms of expression of a variety of cell-surface and internal proteins, some with known functions and others whose roles are still unclear. The B-cell development pathway is defined by isolation and culture of intermediate stages and documentation of their progression to later stages. For example, uncommitted HSCs generate more committed progeny expressing interleukin (IL)-7Rα that, in turn, produce B-lineage–restricted cells expressing CD45R/B220 (CD is cluster of differentiation), but not CD19, which is characteristic of later B-cell stages. Thus, a scheme can be constructed for B-cell development on which the influence of mediators such as transcription factors, cytokines (Table 43.1), and gene mutations can be tested. The appearance of processes known to occur during B-cell development such as rearrangement of the D-J (diversity-joining) region and immunoglobulin (Ig) heavy-chain expression can also be incorporated into this scheme (14). As hematopoiesis is initiated, the earlier stages of the B-cell lineage predominate, then successively later stages of B-cell development predominate until birth (15).

B cells produced in the liver during gestation are distinctly different in some respects from those produced in the bone marrow of the adult mouse. Fetal cells lack the enzyme terminal deoxynucleotide transferase (TdT) (16), which catalyzes nontemplate-dependent addition of nucleotides at the D-J and V-D (variable-diversity) junctions of the Ig heavy-chain gene locus (17).

In the adult mouse, the bone marrow is the primary source of B cells. Bone marrow contains a mixture of cells at various stages of commitment to the blood cell lineages. The least committed cells, capable of producing any of the blood cells, are termed "lineage negative" HSCs. This fraction makes up less than 5% of HSCs or 1/30,000th of the bone marrow cells. When successively transferred into recipient mice devoid of nucleated blood cell precursors these cells are capable of repopulating all blood cell lineages in two successive transfers. Another population of HSCs, termed common lymphoid progenitor (CLP) cells, can generate B, T, natural killer (NK), and a subset of dendritic cells (DCs). These cells lack a panel of lineage markers but express the IL-7Rα chain and lower levels of c-kit and make up about 1/3000th of bone marrow cells.

Distinct stages of B-cell development can be defined by function or phenotype. Functionally, the earliest cells require contact with nonlymphoid adherent cells present in bone marrow, known as stromal cells, and IL-7 for growth in culture (18), whereas later stages can grow without cell contact but still require cytokines (19). Adhesion molecules such as CD44 and VLA-4 that interact with hyaluronate and VCAM-1 appear to explain at least part of the dependence on stromal cells (20). Stromal cells also produce IL-7 (18), which is critical for proliferation. The phenotype of developing B cells can be identified using specific surface or intracellular markers detected by the binding of fluorescent antibodies to these markers, followed by fluorescence microscopy or flow cytometry. Some examples are CD45Ra (T200) and RA3-6B2, which is highly stage restricted (21). However, even these highly restricted markers can be present on other cell types including certain stages or subsets of NK cells and DCs. Multiparameter/multicolor flow cytometry with additional antibodies can differentiate many of these intermediate stages (19).

After their formation in the bone marrow, B cells migrate to the spleen, where they undergo further maturation in the red pulp; then they enter the splenic follicle region, where they form a pool of cells that circulates from the spleen to the periphery. Cell migration is dependent on the interaction of receptors on the cell surface with chemokines. T-cell–dependent immune responses result in the formation of anatomically distinct structures in the spleen and lymph nodes called germinal centers. Germinal centers contain large numbers of rapidly cycling B cells, marked by their ability to bind peanut agglutinin (PNA) and their lack of surface (s)IgD (22). Many of these cells have a low level of expression of BCL-2 and elevated expression of FAS and are therefore destined for apoptosis (see later) unless they receive strong B-cell receptor (BCR) signaling (23). Lack of IgD expression results in a decrease of surface BCR expression of at least tenfold. Cells with increased affinity for antigen generated by a process called hypermutation arethus favored.

TABLE 43.1. CYTOKINES AFFECTED BY NUTRITION[a]

CYTOKINE	SOURCE	TARGET	FUNCTION
GM-CSF	Th cells	Progenitor cells	Growth and differentiation of monocytes and dendritic cells
IL-1α	Monocytes	Th cells	Costimulation
IL-1β	Macrophages	B cells	Maturation and proliferation
	B cells	NK cells	Activation
	Dendritic cells	various	Inflammation, acute-phase response, fever
IL-2	Th1 cells	Activated T and B cells, NK cells	Growth, proliferation, activation
IL-4	Th2 cells	Activated B cells	Proliferation and differentiation
		Macrophages	IgG$_1$ and IgE synthesis
		T cells	MHC class II proliferation
IL-5	Th2 cells	Activated B cells	IgA synthesis proliferation and differentiation
IL-6	Monocytes	Activated B cells	Differentiation into plasma cells
	Macrophages	Plasma cells	Antibody secretion
	Th2 cells	Stem cells	Differentiation
	Stromal cells	Various	Acute-phase response
IL-7	Marrow stroma	Stem cells	Differentiation into progenitor B and T cells
	Thymus stroma		
IL-8	Macrophages	Neutrophils	Chemotaxis
	Endothelial cells		
IL-10	Th2 cells	Macrophages	*Cytokine production*
		B cells	Activation
IL-12	Macrophages	Activated Tc cells	Differentiation into CTL (with IL-2)
	B cells	NK cells	Activation
IFN-α	Leukocytes	Various	*Viral replication*
			MHC I expression
IFN-γ	Th1 cells,	Various	*Viral replication*
	Tc cells, NK cells	Macrophages	MHC expression
		Activated B cells	Ig class switch to IgG$_{2a}$
		Th2 cells	*Proliferation*
		Macrophages	Pathogen elimination
TGF-β	T cells, monocytes	Monocytes, macrophages	Chemotaxis
		Activated macrophages	IL-1 synthesis
		Activated B cells	IgA synthesis
		Various	*Proliferation*
TNF-α	Macrophages, mast cells, NK cells	Macrophages	Cell adhesion molecule and cytokine expression
		Tumor cells	Cell death
TNF-β	Th1 and Tc cells	Phagocytes	Phagocytosis, nitric oxide production, cell death
		Tumor cells	

CTL, cytotoxic T lymphocyte; GM-CSF, granulocyte-macrophage colony-stimulating factor; IFN, interferon; Ig, immunoglobulin; IL, interleukin; MHC, major histocompatibility complex; NK, natural killer; TGF, transforming growth factor; TNF, tumor necrosis factor.
[a]Cytokines listed in bold letters are known to be affected by one or more nutrients as indicated in the text. Italics indicates a major function of this cytokine shown to be affected by nutrition.

Adapted from http://microvet.arizona.edu/Courses/MIC419/Tutorials/cytokines.html.

B-Cell Subsets

Distinct populations of B cells can be distinguished by their phenotype and anatomic location (24). Immature B cells shortly after exiting the bone marrow are found in the spleen and are membrane (m) mIgM$^+$mIgD$^-$ cells. Whereas most of these cells are eliminated by apoptosis with a half-life of 2 to 3 days, some of them, called conventional or B-2 B cells, reach a longer-lived recirculating compartment in which they have a half-life of approximately 30 days. These mature B cells, typically mIgD^{++}mIgM$^+$, comprise more than 95% of naive B cells found in the peripheral lymph nodes and are the precursors for the T-helper (Th)–cell–dependent B-cell responses to most foreign protein antigens. Cells of another subset, termed B-1 B cells, are distinct from B-2 B cells in their expression of CD5, CD11b, CD43, and high levels of sIgM and low levels of sIgD, B220, CD21, and CD23 (25).

The origin of these B-1 B cells is uncertain; some investigators suggest that they are derived from precursors in the fetal liver as long-lived products of a separate lineage of B cells that emerged and stabilized during the neonatal period (26). B-1 B cells are found in large numbers in the peritoneal and pleural cavities, where they constitute a high percentage of total B cells, and in spleen, where they constitute a much lower percentage of B cells. They are characterized by their ability to produce self-reactive antibodies to branched carbohydrates, glycolipids, and glycoproteins including phosphorylcholine, phosphatidyl-choline, the Thy-1 glycoprotein, and bacterial cell wall constituents (27). These so-called natural autoantibodies are not pathogenic, but their biologic function is not known for certain. At least some of them are thought to be important for clearance of senescent cells or proteins, and some may provide initial immunity to common bacterial or viral pathogens (28). One of the major roles of B cells is to produce various Igs that are essential for eliminating infection. The production of antigen-specific antibodies by B cells is central to successful vaccination.

Another B-cell subset found in the periphery comprises the memory B cells. Memory B cells are produced during T-cell–dependent immune responses. These cells are very long-lived or self-regenerating, and they probably only arise from antigen-stimulated follicular B cells in the germinal center. Their Ig genes are isotype switched (IgM to IgG$^+$), and these B cells continue to express CD45R/B220 and a low surface density of BCR (29). When they are challenged with a previously encountered antigen, memory B cells are capable of rapid, high-level production of high-affinity antibodies (30). This memory or recall response is also a hallmark of successful vaccination and provides long-term protection to the vaccinated host.

T Cells

Unlike B cells, most circulating T cells develop in the thymus (Fig. 43.1). Bone marrow cells entering the thymus from the circulation undergo a course of differentiation and selection to become T cells. Advances in our understanding of this process have recently been fully described (31). This cycle occurs continuously from about the midgestational period throughout adulthood in mammals. Some T cells also develop in the intestinal epithelium but do not circulate outside of the intestines. T cells that develop in the thymus are also rigorously screened there to eliminate T cells expressing useless or potentially harmful T-cell receptors (TCRs) in a process that has been labeled repertoire selection. The cells entering the thymus from the bone marrow are called DN1 or TN1 cells, and they are capable of differentiating into all the subsets of T cells, as well as NK cells (32). At this stage, their cell-surface phenotype is c-*kit*$^+$, Thy-1^{low}, CD44^{high}, CD25$^-$, and CD24^{low} and their TCR genes are not yet rearranged.

The next stage of development is called DN2 or TN2 (33). In this stage, the cell population expands rapidly, and TCR gene rearrangement also begins with rearrangement of the TCRγ, TCRδ, and TCRβ loci, but the TCRα locus remains inaccessible to rearrangement. From this point, development of T cells branches into αβ and γδ T cells, depending on the rearrangements that have occurred. γδ T-cell development proceeds with little additional proliferation and downregulation of CD25 and CD24 surface markers. In contrast, the T cells that have rearranged

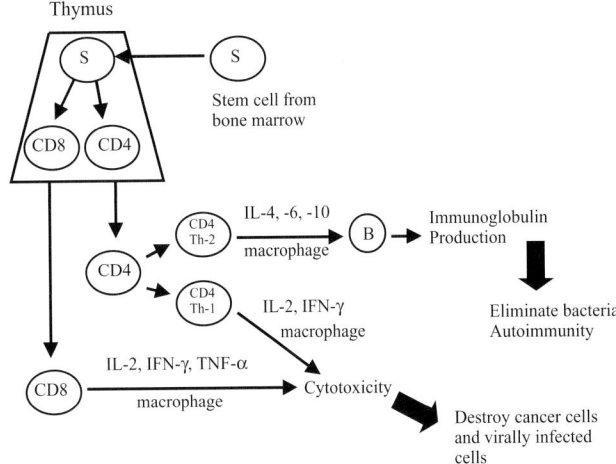

Figure 43.1. T-lymphocyte development and effector function. Stem cells from the bone marrow travel to the thymus and develop into either CD4 or CD8 receptor positive T lymphocytes. In the periphery, the CD4 T lymphocytes are activated by antigen-presenting cells (B cells, macrophages, and dendritic cells) and differentiate into either a T-helper (Th)-1 or Th-2 phenotype defined by their cytokine profiles. Th-2 CD4 T-lymphocytes produce primarily IL-4, IL-6, and IL-10 cytokines, which stimulate B lymphocytes to produce immunoglobulins (Ig), which are important in eliminating extracellular organisms such as bacteria. If the T lymphocytes are inappropriately activated, autoantibodies could be produced, leading to the development of autoimmunity. Alternatively, Th-2 CD4 T lymphocytes produce primarily IL-2 and interferon-γ (IFN-γ), which propagate cytotoxicity or cell-mediated immunity. Cytotoxicity is important in destroying cancer cells and cells infected with intracellular organisms such as viruses. The CD8 T lymphocyte produces primarily IL-2, IFN-γ, and tumor necrosis factor-α (TNF-α), which enhances cytotoxic responses. The macrophage plays an important role in various aspects of the immune response by processing and presenting antigen to T lymphocytes. This diagram is not inclusive of all aspects of the immune response, but it focuses on the elements discussed in this review.

TCRβ begin a complex pathway called β selection. In the DN3 stage, the cells are fully committed to the T-cell lineage (34). They stop proliferating, and TCRβ, γ, and δ gene rearrangement proceeds very efficiently.

The cell lineages then progress through DN4 and immature single-positive (ISP) cells to the double-positive (DP) cells expressing CD8$^+$CD4$^+$CD3^{low} (35). TCRβ, γ, and δ rearrangement is stopped and TCRα rearrangement is begun, CD25 is downregulated, and CD4 and CD8 become expressed. Those DP cells that do not rearrange TCR to allow interaction with major histocompatibility complex (MHC) molecules will die within about 3 days. Only about 5% of DP cells meet these criteria, and about 30% of this population in the spleen dies each day.

DP T cells that survive the selection process then branch once more into two lineages. Those with TCRs that recognize MHC class II molecules tend to develop as CD4$^+$ helper/regulatory T cells, whereas those with TCRs that recognize MHC class I molecules develop into CD8$^+$ cytotoxic T cells. After commitment to the CD8 or CD4 SP lineages, T cells continue to mature and eventually leave the thymus to fulfill their roles in the periphery. This T-cell maturation process involves not only downregulation of one coreceptor (CD4 or CD8) and expression of the other, but also the expression of many other effector genes specific to the T-helper (Th, CD4+) or T-cytotoxic (CD8+) phenotype, and suppression of those genes not needed. These effector genes are first expressed early in the maturation process (36). Once these SP T cells have matured, they still must receive survival signals to enable their prolonged survival. Mature T cells finally leave the thymus in a noncoordinated fashion between 7 and 14 days after positive selection (37).

In addition to the SP CD8 and CD4 T cells are other T cells that arise during the developmental stages. One of these is the NKT cell, a type similar to NK cells in many ways including expression of surface markers (38). However, unlike ordinary T cells, these NKT cells are capable of producing high levels of IL-4 and interferon-γ on encountering antigen, and they therefore may be important in controlling autoimmunity and tumors as well as infectious diseases. Most NKT cells bind the nonclassic class I MHC relative, CD1d (39). NKT cells first appear approximately 6 days after birth in mice and increase 12- to 14-fold by 5 to 6 weeks of age, when they comprise about 0.6 to 0.7 % of thymocytes. Although they recognize a class I MHC-type ligand, most are CD4$^+$ or DN.

Other types of NKT cells exist at much lower abundance and vary in their surface markers, TCR repertoire, CD1d dependence, NK1.1 expression, and tissue localization. Although NKT cells generally require all the genetic functions of αβT cells and depend on the presence of pTα (40), they probably represent a separate lineage because several mutations that affect their development do not have much effect on conventional αβT-cell development, and vice versa (41, 42). These NKT cells are capable of producing a combination of Th2 cytokines and NK cell-like cytolytic functions, and, like NK cells, their prodution depends on IL-15/IL-15R and lymphotoxin (LT)/LTβR signals (40, 43).

Another type of T cells, termed regulatory T (Treg) cells and which are potent suppressors of organ-specific autoimmunity, has also been identified (44). These cells constitute about 5% of mature thymic CD4 SP cells (45). Regulatory T cells appear to arise from CD4 SP cells during the time of negative selection and maturation in the thymus and require IL-2 for their development or survival or both (46). These cells express the transcription factor Foxp3 (Scurfin), which antagonizes conventional T-cell activation responses. Mutant mice lacking this gene develop lethal autoimmunity (47). Deficiency of certain nutrients such as folate and other vitamins causes selective T-cell dysfunction and disruption of the maturation process.

INNATE AND ADAPTIVE IMMUNITY

Innate immunity is mediated by monocyte/macrophage cell lineages. During infection, these cells alone are actively involved in clearing infectious agents. Monocytes can differentiate into multiple effector cell types. Macrophages are important for bacterial clearance, glial cells are important for brain function, osteoclasts are important in bone remodeling, and Kupffer cells are important in liver homeostasis.

Adaptive or acquired immunity refers to antigen-specific immunity that develops over a longer period. It involves humoral and cell-mediated immunity produced by B and T lymphocytes, respectively. Adaptive immunity enables the host to respond to specific pathogenic organisms and to retain memory of those organisms for subsequent responses.

The generation of an immune response involves a series of interactions between lymphocytes and mononuclear cells, including cell-cell communications, generation of immunoreactive molecules, mitotic division, Ig synthesis and secretion, and expression of several cell-surface markers not found on resting lymphocytes. An effective immune response requires balanced functioning of T-helper (CD4) and T-cytotoxic (CD8) subsets of thymic-dependent T lymphocytes, antibody-producing B lymphocytes (Ig$^+$), macrophages, and NKs, and the interplay of various enhancing or inhibiting cytokines.

B-Cell Signaling and Activation

Signaling Pathways

As one component of the adaptive immune response, humoral immunity provides immediate and long-term protection from a wide variety of infectious agents. Infection results in signaling and recruiting antigen-specific B cells, leading to an adaptive immune response. B-cell signaling and activation have recently been fully described (48). The BCR signaling complex involves a membrane bound form of Ig (mIg), which interacts with and binds specific antigens, and a noncovalently associated heterodimer composed of Ig-α (CD79a) and Ig-β (CD79b), which acts as a signaling subunit for the BCR complex (49). The α/β heterodimer is associated with the heavy-chain constant region of the mIg in a 1:1 ratio (50). These complexes segregate in the membrane as BCR oligomers in an Ig isotype-specific manner. The α/β heterodimers associated with all classes of mIg are the same except for differences in glycosylation (51). Both Ig-α and Ig-β contain a region in their cytoplasmic tail region referred to as an immune-receptor tyrosine-based activation motif (ITAM), characterized by six conserved amino acid residues (52, 53). Such motifs are also found on the cytoplasmic regions of TCR signaling components, certain Fc receptors, and CD22. Cross-linking of these receptors induces tyrosine kinase activity and the mobilization of intracellular calcium (53). These motifs function as one means of communicating a BCR signaling event into one or more of several intracellular signaling pathways. The α/β heterodimer is essential for B-cell development from precursors (54), and the mIg signaling is essential for the survival of B cells in the periphery (55).

On antigen binding to BCR, the complexes associate rapidly into cholesterol-rich lipid rafts in the cell's plasma membrane (56). These lipid rafts also contain high concentrations of the activating kinase Lyn, a member of the Src family kinase (SFK). Early activation events initiate a cascade of kinase recruitment and activation through transphosphorylation and cross-phosphorylation that culminates in binding of adaptor proteins such as the B-cell linker protein (BLNK) and the B-cell cytoplasmic adaptor protein (BCAP) (57). Although these proteins have no known intrinsic enzymatic activity, they possess binding domains that allow assembly of the calcium initiation complex (58, 59). Sustained high levels of cytoplasmic calcium result in the activation of nuclear factors NF-ATc and NF-B. The protein kinase C (PKC) enzyme pathway (60), the phosphoinositol (PI)-3K/Akt pathway (also called protein kinase B, PKB, pathway) (54), and the Ras/mitogen-activated protein kinase (Ras/MAPK) pathways are also activated (61). These pathways regulate gene expression, cell survival, and cell proliferation. They are complex, multistep pathways with numerous control points, and their relative contributions depend on the stimulus applied.

Modulators of B-Cell Receptor Signaling

Several cell-surface proteins regulate the BCR signaling complex. Specifically, CD19 and CD22 both associate with the sIgM and may affect both the basal survival of the B cell and the activation signals received through the BCR (62). CD19 enhances the B-cell response, and CD22 acts as a negative regulator of the response. Coligation of the BCR and CD19 with C3d-coupled antigen results in an approximately 1000-fold decrease in the amount of antigen required for threshold activation of the B cell (63). CD19 is phosphorylated by the SFK Lyn, which is transphosphorylated and activated as well. When CD19 is coligated with the BCR, it acts as a transmembrane adaptor protein and recruits PI-3K and Btk, thus upregulating the subsequent calcium response. The Lyn that is activated by CD19 phosphorylates CD22, causing it to bind SHP-1 at its immunomodulatory tyrosine-based inhibitory motif (ITIM) (64). It is postulated that CD22 may target the ITAMs of Igα/Igβ, Lyn, Syk, CD19, and PLCγ. Thus, CD22 is activated through CD19 activation and serves to temper the CD19-mediated enhancement of the BCR response.

FcγRIIb is the Fc receptor for IgG on B cells (64). It is a glycoprotein with a ligand binding extracellular domain and a cytoplasmic ITIM motif, and it binds with low affinity to IgG. When the FcγRIIb is coligated with the BCR, the tyrosine in the ITIM is phosphorylated, creating an SH2 recognition site that recruits SH2-domain–containing inositol S-phosphatase (SHIP) (65). SHIP then hydrolyzes $PI(3,4,5)P_3$ to $PI(3,4)P_2$, thus interfering with the binding of molecules such as Btk and phospholipase C (PLC), which are involved in calcium responsiveness. Coligation of FcγRIIb also decreases phosphorylation of CD19 and recruitment of PI-3K to the membrane. Because formation of IgG complexes is a feature of the late primary or memory B-cell response, it is unlikely that FcγRIIb affects initial activation of naive B cells. It most likely serves to maintain peripheral B-cell tolerance and control ongoing immunity and self-reactivity.

T-Helper–Mediated B-Cell Response

Although B cells can respond to some antigens independent of T-cell stimulation, they respond to T-cell stimulation to produce affinity-matured immunity when they respond to most protein antigens. On the initial encounter with foreign protein antigens, the DCs of the innate immune system are activated. They migrate to the T-cell zones of the draining lymph nodes and act as antigen-presenting cells (APCs). There they attract naive T cells using CCR7 and CCR4 ligands and "screen" for TCRs with the appropriate pMHC specificity (66). Activated effector Th cells then expand clonally (67) and migrate to the T/B borders of secondary lymphoid organs to participate in the regulation of B-cell development (68). Antigen-specific naive B cells recruited in the early stages of inflammation relocate to the T/B border, and this increases the likelihood of their contact with cognate Th cells (69). The B cells that recognize antigen and internalize it then process and present this antigen on their surface as peptide/MHC (70), functioning as APCs to acquire T-cell help. B cells are then stimulated to differentiate into short-lived plasma cells (71), which produce large amounts of antibody, and long-lived memory B cells (72), which are available for rapid response in future encounters with the antigen. As discussed later, both nutrient deficiencies and age-related changes have the potential to alter B-cell functions and, in particular, T-cell functions.

T-Cell Signaling and Activation

The activation of naive T cells is a very complex and involved process that has recently been described in detail (73). This complexity serves to enhance the specificity of the response and maintain tolerance to self-antigens. TCR stimulation is a necessary but not sufficient condition for T-cell activation. The action of costimulatory molecules is required, and many interacting receptors and modulators can either enhance or inhibit T-cell activation. The TCR consists of α/β or γ/δ heterodimers associated with up to six other invariant proteins coded by four genes. The exact number of chains is not known with certainty (74). Among these other proteins are ε/γ and ε/δ noncovalently linked heterodimers of the CD3 complex and either a disulfide-linked homodimer of the ζ chain or a disulfide-linked heterodimer of the ζ chain and the γ chain of the high-affinity IgE Fc receptor (75). The α/β heterodimer is largely extracellular, with only five amino acid residues in the cytoplasmic domain, which is insufficient to couple them to signal transducers in the cytoplasm. This signal-transducing function is supplied by the CD3 and ζ chain components of the TCR complex (76). These chains contain the ITAM sequences that are typical of many different receptors on several different types of cells (76).

The mechanism of signaling from the CD3 and ζ chains after antigen has bound to the α/β chains is not well understood. Some evidence suggests a cross-linking or dimerization model, whereas other evidence argues for allosteric changes (77). There is also a suggestion that the CD3 and ζ chains may allow other cell-surface molecules such as CD2, CD4, or CD8 to interact with the TCR to form a larger receptor complex (78). Within seconds after binding of MHC-associated antigen to the TCR, tyrosines on the ITAMs are phosphorylated (79). This phosphorylation is mediated by protein tyrosine kinases (PTKs) of the Src and Syk families and persists for hours (80). These PTKs, in turn, phosphorylate other proteins and activate effector molecules downstream through the MAPK and other signaling pathways. This cascade of events results in the stimulation of cytokine production and the appearance of new cell-surface molecules that facilitate the role of the T cell in recruiting and activating B cells (i.e., humoral immunity) and promoting destruction of invading organisms (i.e., cell-mediated immunity) (81, 82).

Protein phosphorylation is influenced not only by phosphorylases but also by phosphatases. Phosphatases are expressed at high levels on all hematopoietic cells, with the exception of mature erythrocytes, and catalyze the hydrolysis of phosphate bonds, resulting in dephosphorylation. T cells possess several phosphatases such as the membrane-bound CD45 (leucocyte common antigen or T200), CD148, PTPaseα (LRP), and the cytosolic T-cell phosphatases, PEP, SHP-1, and SHP-2 (83). The best characterized of these is CD45. Various isoforms of CD45 are expressed differentially according to the cell's maturity and activation state (84). Studies with CD45 deficient cells suggest that its target may be the negative regulatory site of Lck. Removal of a phosphate from this site results in a conformational change in Lck that allows it to become activated by transautophosphorylation of tyrosine in its activation loop (85). PTPases can also remove phosphate from such activation sites and thereby negatively regulate signaling activity. After the successful completion of the immune response, excess T-cell populations are eliminated by apoptosis, as discussed in the following section.

Programmed Cell Death (Apoptosis)

As has been recently described in detail (86), an important part of the flexibility essential to the adaptive immune system and control of self-tolerance is regulation of the number and specificity of immune cells by survival or death (87–90). This is accomplished by expression of certain proteins within or on the surface of the cells that initiate a sequence of events leading to the death of the cell. This type of cell death has been named apoptosis, from the Greek meaning to "fall off," as in leaves falling from a tree during the annual dormant phase (91). This term is used to distinguish this natural programmed death from the accidental or toxin-induced death, termed necrosis. This term has become associated with a specific pathway involving the action of proteases called caspases and a distinctive morphology of the cells as they progress through the various stages of apoptosis. Molecular programs have also been defined that result in necrotic death of cells (92).

At several points during the development of lymphocytes from stem cells, as discussed earlier, large numbers of cells bearing receptors of varying selectivity are produced, and then those that are useful are selected to survive, whereas the remaining cells are eliminated by apoptosis. As one example, during the development of thymocytes, the TCR genes become rearranged in a somewhat random fashion. Those rearrangements that yield receptors with a useful range of affinity for the MHC-antigen complex result in survival of the respective T cells, and those that do not result in cell death. The selection of these cells is based on the strength of the TCR signal. If there is no TCR stimulation, the cells will undergo what has been termed death by neglect (93). This effectively eliminates cells whose TCR rearrangement has not resulted in MHC-antigen recognition. In T cells receiving a low level of TCR stimulation, this death by neglect is antagonized, and this event is called positive selection. Thus, T cells with a minimum threshold level of MHC recognition are selected for survival (94). Those T cells whose TCR signal is excessively strong will receive a proapoptotic signal that is termed negative selection. Negative selection prevents the appearance of strongly autoreactive lymphocytes in the periphery (93).

In the periphery, it is necessary to limit the proliferation of mature thymocytes that have been stimulated and performed their function. This regulation must, however, be antigen specific because some T cells may be undergoing expansion in response to an invasion at the same time that others, responding to a different antigen, have accomplished their purpose and need to be checked. The term "propriocidal regulation" is used to refer to the mechanisms that have been developed to accomplish this purpose. This apoptosis is triggered by the level of cell cycling and the level of antigen restimulation (89). Cell death can occur actively by antigen-stimulated apoptosis or passively by lymphokine (survival signal) withdrawal. Initiation of active cell death requires more than activation and proliferation of T cells. Strong restimulation by antigen while in the activated state after the initial antigen stimulation is required (95). Thus, the initial response to an invading antigen is not compromised, but continued stimulation by the same antigen, which is most likely to occur with self-antigens, is prevented by eliminating these cells. The biologic function of antigen-stimulated (activation-induced) apoptosis seems to be to promote tolerance to self and thereby avoid the development of autoimmunity.

As active cell death prevents overreaction during an immune response, passive cell death or lymphokine withdrawal eliminates excess activated T cells after a successful immune response is completed. This is similar to the death by neglect that occurs during T-cell development. When the signal for activated T lymphocytes, typically IL-2, is turned off as a result of reduced antigen stimulation, the T cells undergo apoptosis (96). The exact steps involved are unknown at the present time (97).

Some activated T cells from an immune response persist without continued antigen exposure as memory cells. These cells are thought to escape apoptosis by some means (98). Another hypothesis is that these memory T cells do not escape apoptosis but are continually replaced by an antigen dependent low-level proliferation of CD8$^+$ T cells that is probably maintained by IL-15 (99). Thus, a balance of a reduced rate of death and proliferation results in a constant fraction of memory T cells over time.

B cells and DCs are also regulated by apoptosis. Apoptosis in B cells is similar in many respects to that in T cells. B cells undergo a series of expansions and apoptotic contractions in the bone marrow during their development (100). B cells undergo selection in which nonproductive rearrangements of the Ig genes and B cells that express BCRs directed at self-antigens are eliminated by apoptosis (101). In mature B cells, receptors of the TNFR family such as Fas and CD40 regulate the balance of cell survival and cell death (102). B-cell activation requires not only BCR ligation but also ligation with CD40L, expressed on activated T cells, to prevent B-cell apoptosis (103). Although DCs are known to undergo natural turnover in the mouse (104), the mechanisms are not yet well defined.

ROLE OF NUTRIENTS IN INNATE AND ADAPTIVE IMMUNITY

In general, deficiency in any nutrient will result in the impairment of most adaptive and innate immune responses. Furthermore, replenishing nutrient levels to normal physiologic levels will, for the most part, restore appropriate immune function. A key issue in today's society, in which nutrient supplementation is extremely popular, is what effects specific nutrients have on various aspects of adaptive and innate immunity, when these nutrients are consumed in excess. The following discussion focuses primarily on the current literature, examining single nutrient studies, because in multivitamin or mineral supplementation designs it is difficult to attribute the immune outcome to a specific nutrient. The majority of the current literature in nutritional immunology examines nutrient impact on T-lymphocyte functions. This focus is primarily because the T cell is a key immunoregulatory cell involved in controlling both the type and the extent of

an immune response. In addition, it is relatively easy to obtain significant numbers of T cells from the spleens of rodents and the peripheral blood of humans. A significant body of literature also addresses the impact of nutrients on monocyte/macrophages, DCs, and NK cells. Of the many nutrients our bodies need daily, vitamins E, A, and D, dietary fat, including n-3 (ω-3) fatty acids and conjugated fatty acids, and minerals such as selenium and zinc have been most intensively studied. Dietary (caloric) restriction has also received significant attention because of its potent antiaging effect in many experimental models. A key concept is that consuming nutrients in excess can often be as detrimental as not consuming enough. The following discussion focuses on recent findings for a few key nutrients and indicates what is currently known about their potential mechanisms of action in the immune system. Whenever possible, recent key reviews will be cited for the reader wanting more in-depth information.

Innate Immunity

Monocytes and Macrophages

Dietary Restriction. In general, calorie restriction (food restriction) has been shown to prolong life span and improve immune function in long-lived strains of mice and rats (105). Either calorie restriction or provision of n-3 fatty acids has been shown to delay the onset of diseases such as autoimmune disorders in short-lived autoimmune disease–prone mice (106). However, young mice fed a calorie-restricted diet were more susceptible to sepsis from experimentally induced peritonitis. Interestingly, macrophage function was reduced in healthy mice following peritonitis, whereas macrophage function was greatly increased in well-fed mice and survival was prolonged (107). The latter outcome is supported by additional evidence showing enhanced prostaglandin and proinflammatory cytokine production in the activated peritoneal macrophages of young calorie-restricted mice (108).

n-3 Fatty Acids. The n-3 fatty acids eicosapentaenoic acid (EPA) and docosahexaenoic acid (DHA) (see Chapter 5) derived from fish oil are known to act as antiinflammatory agents (109). n-3 fatty acids inhibit the production of macrophage-derived IL-12 (110), nitric oxide (111), tumor necrosis factor-α (TNF-α) (112), and IL-6 (113) in vitro and in vivo. Some of these effects, such as decreased IL-6 production, may result from n-3 fatty acid–dependent changes in prostaglandin production (114). The suppressive effects of fish oil on macrophage function may have additional health benefits including decreasing the loss of bone mass by inhibiting osteoclasts (bone macrophage-like cells) and delaying heart disease by altering the lipid composition of arterial plaques (115) and cholesterol flux in a macrophage-like monocytic cell line (116).

Conjugated Fatty Acids. Conjugated linoleic acid (CLA) has been shown to be beneficial in preventing cachexia in lipopolysaccharide-injected mice, which was correlated with reduced nitric oxide production by macrophages in vitro and reduced TNF-α production in vivo (117).

Vitamin A. Retinoic acid has been shown to delay the onset of autoimmune disease in mice (118), and it may even be beneficial in viral infections because retinoic acid can inhibit human immunodeficiency virus (HIV) replication in macrophages in vitro (119). Retinoic acid may also be important in generating monocytes from progenitors in the bone marrow (119) and subsequently in assisting the differentiation of monocytes into macrophages (120) or DCs (121).

Vitamin D. Studies in vitamin D receptor knockout mice have revealed that vitamin D is important in macrophage functions such as chemotaxis, although phagocytosis was normal, but it does not appear to play a role in the generation of monocytes (122). Treatment of macrophages with vitamin D in vitro enhanced the phagocytic uptake of bacteria (123). Vitamin D is also known to regulate bone resorption and increase blood calcium levels by regulating osteoclast activity, a cell type of the monocyte/macrophage cell lineage (124).

Vitamin E. A human study has shown that vitamin E supplementation can reduce the risk of respiratory tract infections in the elderly (125). The macrophage is the likely target (126). Vitamin E–dependent regulation of macrophage function may also be important in the development of heart disease (127). Vitamin E supplementation prevented macrophage accumulation in the aorta of rabbits fed a diet high in saturated fat and cholesterol (atherogenic diet) (128). However, some vitamin E isomers are cytotoxic to macrophages and other cell types in vitro (129), a finding suggesting that caution in the use of supplemental vitamin E is warranted.

Zinc. Zinc has been shown to regulate cytokine gene expression selectively in macrophages. Zinc increased the expression of macrophage colony-stimulating factor (130) and decreased the expression of TNF-α, IL-1β, and IL-8 genes (131).

Selenium. Selenium reduced the production of nitric oxide by activated murine macrophages (132), and selenium deficiency increased nitric oxide production in a macrophage-like cell line (133).

Natural Killer Cells

Most of the studies examining the impact of nutrients on NK cell activity have centered on how nutrients affect the ability of NK cells to kill tumor cells.

Vitamin A. A lack of vitamin A, even marginal deficiency, resulted in a lower number and percentage of NK cells in both young and old rats (134), concomitant with reduced cytolytic activity in standard NK cell assays. These changes were reversed by retinoic acid. Aging vitamin A–marginal rats with low NK cells had, conversely, an increased number of NKT cells, associated with reduced

CD4+ T cells and a lower CD4:CD8 ratio (135). Feeding a diet with elevated levels of vitamin A resulted in increased NK and reduced NKT cells, compared with age-matched controls, a finding indicating reciprocal regulation of these cell types by vitamin A (135). In vitamin A–deficient mice (136) and rats with low NK cells (137), blood granulocytes were significantly increased.

n-3 Fatty Acids. Both increases and decreases in NK cell activity have been observed in human and rodent studies in which n-3 polyunsaturated fatty acids have been fed (138). These differences are likely the result of the modulating impact of other factors. For example, some n-3 fatty acids were more potent than others at inhibiting human NK cell activity (139), and the ratio of polyunsaturated to saturated fatty acid in the diet was a determinant of whether NK cell activity was increased or decreased in rodents (140).

Conjugated Fatty Acids. Supplementing healthy men with CLA isomers was tested on NK cell function, but it was without an effect (141).

Zinc. Zinc supplementation at a level to return plasma zinc status to physiologic levels (12–16 umol/L) resulted in restoration of normal NK cell function. Physiologically relevant levels of zinc supplementation in elderly persons resulted in increased NK cell activity (142). When zinc was added to NK cells in vitro at concentrations higher than normal physiologic levels, NK cell activity was inhibited (143). Thus, too much zinc may have a similar negative effect as zinc deficiency. An important mechanism by which zinc increases NK cell activity is by increasing the interaction between NK cell receptors and MHC I receptors on target cells (144).

Dendritic Cells

The literature examining the impact of nutrients on DC function is limited, but it has been expanding rapidly as it has become appreciated that DCs may serve as the key link between innate and adaptive immunity (145).

Vitamin A. Vitamin A may be important in regulating the production of a sufficient number of DCs. Retinoic acid added in vitro helped to induce the differentiation of murine myeloid (progenitor) bone marrow cells into the DC phenotype (146) and, similarly in human cells, of peripheral blood mononuclear cells of the DC phenotype (147). In T cells, the effects of retinoic acid favored the production of IL-12 (121), which would increase a cell-mediated type of immune response by T cells.

Vitamin D. Vitamin D and several analogs have been shown to inhibit the ability of DCs to stimulate naive T cells (148). This inhibitory effect may be specific to T-cell stimulation for the generation of a Th-1 type of response, because DCs cultured with vitamin D exhibited increased IL-10 secretion, which would favor an antibody-mediated (Th-2) response (149). This specific downregulation of cell-mediated immunity may be important in regulating autoimmune diseases such as such as some forms of diabetes (150). A more comprehensive examination of the effects of vitamin D on DC gene expression was conducted by Griffin and colleagues using gene microarray profiling (151).

Vitamin E. Supplementation of tumor-bearing mice with α-tocopherol succinate, an esterified derivation of vitamin E, increased the immunotherapeutic effects of DC-dependent slowing of tumor growth (152).

Adaptive Immunity

T and B Cells

The majority of the literature in nutrition immunology has focused on T cells more than B cells. However, in many animal models, Ig levels, a reflection of B- and T-cell function, have been measured in response to different dietary regimens. Whether these effects represent a direct effect of diet on B-cell function or are indirect through modulating T-cell function is not clear, and therefore the impact of diet on T-cell and B-cell function is considered together. Very few studies have examined the impact of diet on B-cell function directly.

Dietary Restriction. Many data show that dietary restriction delays the onset of autoimmune diseases and aging, in part by preventing disease and age-associated changes in T-cell function (153, 154). Dietary restriction is known to decrease proinflammatory cytokine, chemokine, and adhesion molecule expression on T lymphocytes and gene expression in transgenic mice (153, 155–157).

n-3 Fatty Acids. n-3 fatty acids are well-known and widely studied dietary components because of their antiinflammatory effects (109, 158, 159). Several reviews have described the effects of n-3 fatty acids in humans (160) and in animal models (161) and have discussed their potential mechanism of action (162). Of the n-3 fatty acids, EPA and DHA derived from fish oil have received the most attention because they are considered to be the most potent at delaying the onset of autoimmune disease in rodents (163). n-3 fatty acids have also prevented bone loss in ovariectomized mice, in which they decrease proinflammatory cytokines (164). Although the antiinflammatory effects of n-3 fatty acids are beneficial, consuming an excess of n-3 fatty acids may be detrimental and may possibly exacerbate certain types of infectious diseases. For example, mice fed a high intake of n-3 fatty acids were rendered more susceptible to *Listeria monocytogenes* infection (165).

In general, n-3 fatty acids are thought to exert their effects by reducing T-cell IL-2 production and subsequent cell proliferation. This effect has been shown fairly consistently in rodents (158, 166), humans ranging from young adults to the elderly (160, 167), and in vitro (168). Evidence from human feeding trials showed that the antiinflammatory effects of dietary fish oil using purified n-3 fatty acids (EPA and DHA) on T-cell function were negligible when

humans consumed less than 2 g/day (169). Another variable that affects the potency of n-3 fatty acids is the amount of n-3 fatty acid that is incorporated into T-cell membranes (170), which is also dependent on the intake of competing fatty acids in other dietary fats. Although both EPA and DHA can reduce T-cell proliferation, the cytokines and genes they regulate may be different, as has been shown in vitro (171–173).

Some studies have begun to examine which T-cell subset is most affected by dietary fish oil. Dietary fish oil inhibited antigen-driven murine CD4 T-cell proliferation both in vitro (174) and in vivo (175). Dietary n-3 fatty acids may also inhibit the proliferation of murine CD8 T cells, in addition to CD4 T cells, but the relative impact of n-3 fatty acids appears to be dependent on the type of stimuli used (176) and on whether costimulatory accessory cells are present (177). The mechanism by which dietary fish oil inhibits the proliferation of CD4 T cells in this murine model appears to be by inducing apoptosis in CD4 T cells expressing the Th-1 phenotype (178). Similar results have been shown in vitro in the Jurkat human T-cell line (179). Increased apoptosis may result from alterations in lipid raft formation and subsequent CD28 receptor function (180). Currently, two consistent mechanisms have been proposed by which fish oil–derived n-3 fatty acids such as DHA may function. The first, as mentioned earlier, is by changing the membrane lipid microenvironment and formation of lipid rafts, as observed both in vitro and in vivo (181), which, in turn, may recruit appropriate signaling molecules into close proximity. Another mechanism, which also may be a result of altered lipid raft formation, is a reduction in the activity of the MAPKinase signaling pathway, as shown in vitro (182).

Conjugated Fatty Acids. CLA has been shown to have effects similar to those of n-3 fatty acids on cytokine production. However, CLA appears to increase T-cell proliferation in mice (183). In humans, CLA has been shown to improve the production of protective antibodies against hepatitis B without any significant change in cytokine production (141). Although these studies have yielded slightly different results depending on the model used, the commonality is that dietary CLA inhibited immune-mediated disease in mice (183) and decreased viral infectivity in pigs (184). However, CLA does not seem to help replenish the immune system once an animal has become immunodepleted (185). Treatment with CLA also resulted in a reduced number of B cells, whereas it enhanced IgA and IgM antibody production (186). Which specific isomers of CLA are the most immunopotent is not yet clear.

Vitamin A. Retinoic acid has been shown to decrease the severity of autoimmune disease in mice (187). Susceptibility to infection may be related to the association of vitamin A deficiency with an increased production of IL-10, which favored the Th-2 phenotype and decreased Th-1 responses in mice (188). The IL-10 producing Th-2 regulatory cells then may downregulate not only Th-1 responses but ultimately may prevent appropriate antibody responses as well (188). In children with very low plasma retinol levels, inflammatory cytokine production was elevated as compared with that in children without severe deficiency (189). The ability of vitamin A to boost immunity in mice may be indirect by increasing APC function (190). Mechanistically, retinoic acid increased T-cell function by increasing IL-2Rα expression (191) and IL-2 secretion (192). In addition, T-cell functioning may be improved through alterations in T-cell development in the thymus (193). Alternatively, as alluded to earlier, retinoic acid may regulate T-cell function indirectly by altering MHC expression on APCs or other target cells (194). Vitamin A supplementation may not have a benefit in all infectious diseases because vitamin A supplementation was shown to have no impact on herpes simplex virus infectivity (195) or HIV disease progression (196).

Vitamin D. Vitamin D can exert antiinflammatory effects leading to suppressed experimental autoimmune encephalitis, systemic lupus erythematosus, type 1 diabetes (197, 198), inflammatory bowel disease (198), and murine allergic airway disease (199). Several different analogs of vitamin D have been developed as immunomodulators as well (200). The immunoregulatory properties of vitamin D may be exerted indirectly by altering accessory cell function, as in DCs (150), or by directly altering T-cell function. Vitamin D has been shown to modulate integrin receptor-mediated T-cell homing (201) and to repress CD95 ligand receptor expression (202), which may inhibit T-cell apoptosis. In primary T-cell cultures, vitamin D inhibited Th-1 cytokine production but did not alter Th-2 cytokine production in CD4 cells (203), whereas in other experimental cultures vitamin D increased both Th-1 and Th-2 cytokine production (204). The discrepancy in some of these studies may be explained by observations showing that the effect of vitamin D on T-cell function is dependent on the differentiation and activation status of the T cell (205). Although CD8 T cells have the highest expression of the vitamin D receptor, CD8 T cells are not needed for vitamin D to inhibit experimental autoimmune encephalomyelitis (206). Vitamin D may also have a direct effect on B cells because recent evidence indicates that IgE production in activated B cells is inhibited (207). Recently, heterogeneous nuclear ribonucleoprotein has been shown to inhibit vitamin D–induced gene expression (208), which may explain why some T cells are resistant to immunoregulation by vitamin D.

Vitamin E. Vitamin E (α-tocopherol) is best known for its antioxidant capability and for protecting the immune system against oxidative damage. Examples include protecting T cells from lead-induced toxicity (209) and B cells from hydrogen peroxide promoted viral transformation (210). Vitamin E is thought to be important in downregulating allergic inflammation by suppressing IL-4 expression (211) and may prevent pathologic deletion of T cells by blocking apoptosis (212). Blocking apoptosis may

be an important mechanism in the ability of vitamin E to increase the proliferation of naive T cells in aged mice (213). Memory T cells, which become predominant during aging, were not affected by vitamin E (213), and this finding may explain why adding vitamin E had no apparent effect in bulk aged T-cell cultures in vitro (214). A unique application of taking advantage of vitamin E's immunoregulatory properties is seen in coating a hemodialyzer with vitamin E; this abated the spontaneous release of IL-4 and IL-10 by the CD4+ T cells and of IL-12 and IL-18 by the peripheral blood mononuclear cells of patients undergoing dialysis (215).

Zinc. Two reviews provide an excellent detailed explanation of the role of zinc on T-cell–dependent immune function (216, 217). In general, zinc deficiency is associated with a decline in most aspects of immune function. Zinc deficiency renders people more susceptible to infections. Conversely, zinc supplementation in humans has shown benefit in immune responses to bacterial (218) and viral infections (219). However, zinc could also have deleterious effects on immune function because it can also serve to promote oxidative damage. In a study in healthy persons, zinc supplementation did not have a negative effect on T-cell function in general (220). This is especially important because zinc can modulate gene expression in the thymus, where T cells mature (131, 221), and thereby affect subsequent T-cell production (222).

Selenium. Most research on selenium and T-cell function has examined selenium deficiency (223). Selenium appears beneficial in Th-1–type immune responses against intracellular pathogens (224). Evidence from a clinical study suggests that increasing selenium intake may be beneficial in polioviral infections in humans (225).

CONCLUDING SUMMARY

Nutritional status has been found to affect all the major cell lineages involved in immune function. Food restriction has been reported to decrease inflammation and preserve immune function during aging, but it has also been reported to decrease resistance to sepsis in young animals. n-3 and conjugated fatty acids such as CLA have been shown to decrease inflammation and to influence the production of a number of cytokines and prostaglandins. The fat-soluble vitamins A, D, and E have many effects on the immune system, ranging from the maturation of various cell lineages to cell functions such as phagocytosis and apoptosis. These various effects may be mediated through alterations of cytokine and receptor expression. The trace elements zinc and selenium are also known for their effects on immune cells. Adequate zinc levels are necessary for NK cell function, and zinc regulates cytokine expression in macrophages and enhances T-cell function. The effects of selenium are less well characterized and appear most closely to be related to its antioxidant capacity.

Acknowledgments

We wish to acknowledge support from National Institutes of Health grants AG023648, AG014541, and AG020239 (G.F.) and AG020651 (C.A.J.) for our work. We are also grateful to Dr. Catharine Ross for her helpful suggestions.

REFERENCES

1. Fernandes G, Yunis EJ, Smith J et al. Proc Soc Exp Biol Med 1972;139:1189–96.
2. Fernandes G, Yunis EJ, Good RA. Proc Natl Acad Sci USA 1976;73:1279–83.
3. Fernandes G, Yunis EJ,Good RA. Nature 1976;263:504–7.
4. Good RA, Fernandes G, Yunis EJ et al. Am J Pathol 1976;84: 599–614.
5. Gerbase-DeLima M, Liu RK, Cheney KE et al. Gerontologia 1975;21:184–202.
6. Weindruch R, Walford R. The Retardation of Aging and Disease by Dietary Restriction. Springfield, IL: Charles C Thomas, 1988:436.
7. Fraker PJ, Haas SM, Luecke RW. J Nutr 1977;107:1889–95.
8. Fernandes G. Curr Opin Immunol 1989;2:275–81.
9. Moore MA, Metcalf D. Br J Haematol 1970;18:279–96.
10. Yoder MC, Hiatt K, Dutt P et al. Immunity 1997;7:335–44.
11. Medvinsky AL, Samoylina NL, Muller AM et al. Nature 1993; 364:64–7.
12. Muller AM, Medvinsky A, Strouboulis J et al. Immunity 1994;1: 291–301.
13. Medvinsky A, Dzierzak E. Cell 1996;86:897–906.
14. Hardy RR. B-lymphocyte development and biology. In: Paul WE, ed. Fundamental Immunology. 5th ed. Philadelphia: Lippincott Williams & Wilkins, 2003:159–94.
15. Strasser A, Rolink A, Melchers F. J Exp Med 1989;170: 1973–86.
16. Li YS, Hayakawa K, Hardy RR. J Exp Med 1993;178:951–60.
17. Desiderio SV, Yancopoulos GD, Paskind M et al. Nature 1984; 311:752–5.
18. Hayashi S, Kunisada T, Ogawa M et al. J Exp Med 1990;171: 1683–95.
19. Hardy RR, Carmack CE, Shinton SA et al. J Exp Med 1991; 173:1213–25.
20. Miyake K, Underhill CB, Lesley J et al. J Exp Med 1990;172: 69–75.
21. Johnson P, Greenbaum L, Bottomly K et al. J Exp Med 1989; 169:1179–84.
22. Przylepa J, Himes C, Kelsoe G. Curr Top Microbiol Immunol 1998;229:85–104.
23. Zhang X, Li L, Choe J et al. Cell Immunol 1996;173:149–54.
24. Hardy RR, Hayakawa K. Annu Rev Immunol 2001;19:595–621.
25. Martin F, Kearney JF. Curr Opin Immunol 2001;13:195–201.
26. Berland R, Wortis HH. Annu Rev Immunol 2002;20:253–300.
27. Hayakawa K, Carmack CE, Hyman R et al. J Exp Med 1990; 172:869–78.
28. Ochsenbein AF, Fehr T, Lutz C et al. Science 1999;286:2156–9.
29. Hayakawa K, Ishii R, Yamasaki K et al. Proc Natl Acad Sci USA 1987;84:1379–83.
30. Romano TJ, Mond JJ, Thorbecke GJ. Eur J Immunol 1975;5: 211–5.
31. Rothenberg EV, Yui MA, Telfer JC. T-cell developmental biology. In: Paul WE, ed. Fundamental Immunology. 5th ed. Philadelphia: Lippincott Williams & Wilkins, 2003:259–302.
32. Res P, Martinez-Caceres E, Cristina Jaleco A et al. Blood 1996; 87:5196–206.
33. Michie AM, Carlyle JR, Schmitt TM et al. J Immunol 2000;164: 1730–3.
34. Anderson G, Moore NC, Owen JJ et al. Annu Rev Immunol 1996;14:73–99.
35. Ceredig R, Rolink T. Nat Rev Immunol 2002;2:888–97.
36. Matechak EO, Killeen N, Hedrick SM et al. Immunity 1996;4: 337–47.
37. Scollay R, Godfrey DI. Immunol Today 1995;16:268–73; discussion 273–4.
38. Wilson SB, Byrne MC. Curr Opin Immunol 2001;13:555–61.
39. Matsuda JL, Naidenko OV, Gapin L et al. J Exp Med 2000;192: 741–54.
40. Eberl G, Fehling HJ, von Boehmer H et al. Eur J Immunol 1999;29:1966–71.
41. Gadue P, Morton N, Stein PL. J Exp Med 1999;190:1189–96.
42. Walunas TL, Wang B, Wang CR et al. J Immunol 2000;164: 2857–60.
43. Elewaut D, Brossay L, Santee SM et al. J Immunol 2000;165: 671–9.
44. Shevach EM. Annu Rev Immunol 2000;18:423–49.
45. Itoh M, Takahashi T, Sakaguchi N et al. J Immunol 1999;162: 5317–26.
46. Papiernik M, de Moraes ML, Pontoux C et al. Int Immunol 1998;10:371–8.
47. Hori S, Nomura T, Sakaguchi S. Science 2003;299:1057–61.
48. McHeyzer-Williams M. B-cell signaling mechanisms and activation. In: Paul WE, ed. Fundamental Immunology. 5th ed. Philadelphia: Lippincott Williams & Wilkins, 2003:195–226.
49. Reth M, Wienands J. Annu Rev Immunol 1997;15:453–79.
50. Schamel WW, Reth M. Immunity 2000;13:5–14.
51. Venkitaraman AR, Williams GT, Dariavach P et al. Nature 1991;352:777–81.
52. Reth M. Nature 1989;338:383–4.
53. Sanchez M, Misulovin Z, Burkhardt AL et al. J Exp Med 1993; 178:1049–55.
54. Kurosaki T. Annu Rev Immunol 1999;17:555–92.
55. Lam KP, Kuhn R, Rajewsky K. Cell 1997;90:1073–83.
56. Guo B, Kato RM, Garcia-Lloret M et al. Immunity 2000;13: 243–53.
57. Leo A, Schraven B. Curr Opin Immunol 2001;13:307–16.
58. Beals CR, Clipstone NA, Ho SN et al. Genes Dev 1997;11: 824–34.
59. Peng SL, Gerth AJ, Ranger AM et al. Immunity 2001;14:13–20.
60. Dorn GW 2nd, Mochly-Rosen D. Annu Rev Physiol 2002;64: 407–29.
61. Wienands J. Immunobiology 2000;202:120–33.
62. Fujimoto M, Bradney AP, Poe JC et al. Immunity 1999;11: 191–200.
63. Dempsey PW, Allison ME, Akkaraju S et al. Science 1996;271: 348–50.
64. Doody GM, Justement LB, Delibrias CC et al. Science 1995; 269:242–4.
65. D'Ambrosio D, Fong DC, Cambier JC. Immunol Lett 1996;54: 77–82.
66. Cyster JG. Science 1999;286:2098–102.
67. McHeyzer-Williams LJ, Panus JF, Mikszta JA et al. J Exp Med 1999;189:1823–38.
68. Bishop GA, Hostager BS. Curr Opin Immunol 2001;13:278–85.
69. Reif K, Ekland EH, Ohl L et al. Nature 2002;416:94–9.
70. Watts C. Annu Rev Immunol 1997;15:821–50.
71. Calame KL. Nat Immunol 2001;2:1103–8.
72. McHeyzer-Williams MG, Ahmed R. Curr Opin Immunol 1999;11:172–9.
73. Weiss A, Samelson LE. T-lymphocyte activation. In: Paul WE, ed. Fundamental Immunology. 5th ed. Philadelphia: Lippincott Williams & Wilkins, 2003:321–64.

74. Weiss A. Annu Rev Genet 1991;25:487–510.
75. Orloff DG, Ra CS, Frank SJ et al. Nature 1990;347:189–91.
76. Wegener AM, Letourneur F, Hoeveler A et al. Cell 1992;68: 83–95.
77. Goldsmith MA, Weiss A. Proc Natl Acad Sci USA 1987;84: 6879–83.
78. Dianzani U, Shaw A, al-Ramadi BK et al. J Immunol 1992;148: 678–88.
79. Qian D, Griswold-Prenner I, Rosner MR et al. J Biol Chem 1993;268:4488–93.
80. Irving BA, Weiss A. Cell 1991;64:891–901.
81. Weiss A, Imboden JB. Adv Immunol 1987;41:1–38.
82. Samelson LE. Annu Rev Immunol 2002;20:371–94.
83. Veillette A, Latour S, Davidson D. Annu Rev Immunol 2002; 20:669–707.
84. Bottomly K, Luqman M, Greenbaum L et al. Eur J Immunol 1989;19:617–23.
85. Cahir McFarland ED, Hurley TR, Pingel JT et al. Proc Natl Acad Sci USA 1993;90:1402–6.
86. Chan FK, Lenardo MJ. Programmed cell death. In: Paul WE, ed. Fundamental Immunology. 5th ed. Philadelphia: Lippincott Williams & Wilkins, 2003:841–64.
87. Lenardo M, Chan KM, Hornung F et al. Annu Rev Immunol 1999;17:221–53.
88. Ashton-Rickardt PG, Bandeira A, Delaney JR et al. Cell 1994; 76:651–63.
89. Lenardo MJ. Nature 1991;353:858–61.
90. Page DM, Roberts EM, Peschon JJ et al. J Immunol 1998;160: 120–33.
91. Kerr JFR, Wyllie AH, Currie AR. Br J Cancer 1972;26:239–57.
92. Holler N, Zaru R, Micheau O et al. Nat Immunol 2000;1: 489–95.
93. von Boehmer H, Teh HS, Kisielow P. Immunol Today 1989;10: 57–61.
94. Jameson SC, Hogquist KA, Bevan MJ. Annu. Rev Immunol 1995;13:93–126.
95. Zheng L, Trageser CL, Willerford DM et al. J Immunol 1998; 160:763–9.
96. Razvi ES, Jiang Z, Woda BA et al. Am J Pathol 1995;147:79–91.
97. Chao DT, Korsmeyer SJ. Annu Rev Immunol 1998;16: 395–419.
98. Sprent J, Tough DF. Science 2001;293:245–8.
99. Ku CC, Murakami M, Sakamoto A et al. Science 2000;288: 675–8.
100. Norvell A, Mandik L, Monroe JG. J Immunol 1995;154: 4404–13.
101. Sandel PC, Monroe JG. Immunity 1999;10:289–99.
102. Rathmell JC, Townsend SE, Xu JC et al. Cell 1996;87:319–29.
103. Choi MS, Boise LH, Gottschalk AR et al. Eur J Immunol 1995; 25:1352–7.
104. Ingulli E, Mondino A, Khoruts A et al. J Exp Med 1997;185: 2133–41.
105. Fernandes G, Venkatraman J, Turturro A et al. J Clin Immunol 1997;17:85–95.
106. Fernandes G, Bysani C, Venkatraman JT et al. J Immunol 1994; 152:5979–87.
107. Sun D, Muthukumar AR, Lawrence RA et al. Clin Diagn Lab Immunol 2001;8:1003–11.
108. Stapleton PP, Fujita J, Murphy EM et al. Nutrition 2001;17: 41–5.
109. Fernandes G, Jolly CA. Nutr Rev 1998;56:S161–9.
110. Zhang M, Fritsche KL. Br J Nutr 2004;91:733–9.
111. Komatsu W, Ishihara K, Murata M et al. Free Radic Biol Med 2003;34:1006–16.
112. Freedman SD, Weinstein D, Blanco PG et al. J Appl Physiol 2002;2:2169–76.
113. MooNY, Pestka JJ. J Nutr Biochem 2003;14:717–26.
114. Bagga D, Wang L, Farias-Eisner R et al. Proc Natl Acad Sci USA 2003;100:1751–6.
115. Thies F, Garry JM, Yaqoob P et al. Lancet 2003;361:477–85.
116. Lada AT, Rudel LL, St Clair RW. J Lipid Res 2003;44:770–9.
117. Yang M, Cook ME. Lipids 2003;38:21–4.
118. Perez de Lema G, Lucio-Cazana FJ, Molina A et al. Kidney Int 2004;66:1018–28.
119. Hanley TM, Kiefer HL, Schnitzler AC et al. J Virol 2004;78: 2819–30.
120. Chen Q, Ross AC. Exp Cell Res 2004;297:68–81.
121. Mohty M, Morbelli S, Isnardon D et al. Br J Haematol 2003; 122:829–36.
122. O'Kelly J, Hisatake J, Hisatake Y et al. J Clin Invest 2002;109: 1091–9.
123. Chandra G, Selvaraj P, Jawahar MS et al. J Clin Immunol 2004; 24:249–57.
124. Suda T, Ueno Y, Fujii K et al. J Cell Biochem 2003;88:259–66.
125. Meydani SN, Leka LS, Fine BC et al. JAMA 2004;292:828–36.
126. Beharka AA, Wu D, Serafini M et al. Free Radic Biol Med 2002;32:503–11.
127. Devaraj S, Harris A, Jialal I. Nutr Rev 2002;60:8–14.
128. Koga T, Kwan P, Zubik L et al. Atherosclerosis 2004;176: 265–72.
129. McCormick CC, Parker RS. J Nutr 2004;134:3335–42.
130. Kanekiyo M, Itoh N, Kawasaki A et al. J Cell Biochem 2002;86: 145–53.
131. Bao B, Prasad AS, Beck FW et al. Am J Physiol Endocrinol Metab 2003;285:E1095–102.
132. Kim SH, Johnson VJ, Shin TY et al. Exp Biol Med (Maywood) 2004;229:203–13.
133. Prabhu KS, Zamamiri-Davis F, Stewart JB et al. Biochem J 2002;366:203–9.
134. Dawson HD, Li NQ, DeCicco KL et al. J Nutr 1999;129: 1510–7.
135. Dawson HD, Ross AC. J Nutr 1999;129:1782–90.
136. Kuwata T, Wang IM, Tamura T et al. Blood 2000;95:3349–56.
137. Zhao Z, Ross AC. J Nutr 1995;125:2064–73.
138. Kelley DS. Nutrition 2001;17:669–73.
139. Thies F, Nebe-von-Caron G, Powell JR et al. J Nutr 2001;131: 1918–27.
140. Robinson LE, Clandinin MT, Field CJ, Breast Cancer Res Treat 2002;73:145–60.
141. Albers R, van der Wielen RP, Brink EJ et al. Eur J Clin Nutr 2003;57:595–603.
142. Mocchegiani E, Muzzioli M, Giacconi R et al. Mech Ageing Dev 2003;124:459–68.
143. Ibs KH, Rink L. J Nutr 2003;133:1452S–6S.
144. Vales-Gomez M, Erskine RA, Deacon MP et al. Proc Natl Acad Sci USA 2001;98:1734–9.
145. Kapsenberg ML. Nat Rev Immunol 2003;3:984–93.
146. Hengesbach LM, Hoag KA. J Nutr 2004;134:2653–9.
147. Almand B, Clark JI, Nikitina E et al. J Immunol 2001;166: 678–89.
148. van Halteren AG, Tysma OM, van Etten E et al. J Autoimmun 2004;23:233–9.
149. Adorini L, Penna G, Giarratana N et al. J Steroid Biochem Mol Biol 2004;89–90:437–41.
150. Adorini L, Penna G, Giarratana N et al. J Cell Biochem 2003; 88:227–33.
151. Griffin MD, Xing N, Kumar R. J Steroid Biochem Mol Biol 2004;89–90:443–8.

152. Ramanathapuram LV, Kobie JJ, Bearss D et al. Cancer Immunol Immunother 2004;53:580–8.

153. Jolly CA. J Nutr 2004;134:1853–6.

154. Fernandes G, Venkatraman JT. Dietary n-3 polyunsaturated fatty acids modulate T-lymphocyte activation: clinical relevance in treating diseases of chronic inflammation. In: Klurfeld DM, ed. Human Nutrition: A Comprehensive Treatise. New York: Plenum Press, 1993:91–120.

155. Muthukumar A, Sun D, Zaman K et al. J Clin Immunol 2004;24:471–80.

156. Fernandes G, Chandrasekar B, Troyer DA et al. Proc Natl Acad Sci USA, 1995;92:6494–8.

157. Venkatraman J, Meksawan K. J Nutr Biochem 2002;13:479.

158. Chapkin RS, McMurray DN, Jolly CA. Dietary n-3 polyunsaturated fatty acids modulate T-lymphocyte activation: clinical relevance in treating diseases of chronic inflammation. In: Keen CL, ed. Nutrition and Immunology: Principles and Practice. Totowa NJ: Humana Press, 2000:121–34.

159. Fernandes G. Clin Immunol Immunopathol 1994;72:193–7.

160. Calder PC. Lipids 2003;38:343–52.

161. Anderson M, Fritsche KL, J Nutr 2002;132:3566–76.

162. Ma DW, Seo J, Switzer KC et al. J Nutr Biochem 2004;15: 700–6.

163. Jia Q, Shi Y, Bennink MB et al. J Nutr 2004;134:1353–61.

164. Sun D, Krishnan A, Zaman K et al. J Bone Miner Res 2003;18:1206–16.

165. Irons R, Anderson MJ, Zhang M et al. J Nutr 2003;133:1163–9.

166. Jolly CA, Muthukumar A, Avula CP et al. J Nutr 2001;131: 2753–60.

167. Kew S, Mesa MD, Tricon S et al. Am J Clin Nutr 2004; 79:674–81.

168. Stulnig TM. Int Arch Allergy Immunol 2003;132:310–21.

169. Miles EA, Banerjee T, Dooper MM et al. Br J Nutr 2004;91: 893–903.

170. Kew S, Banerjee T, Minihane AM et al. Am J Clin Nutr 2003; 77:1278–86.

171. Verlengia R, Gorjao R, Kanunfre CC et al. J Nutr Biochem 2004;15:657–65.

172. Jolly CA, Muthukumar A, Reddy Avula CP et al. Cell Immunol 2001;213:122–33.

173. Jolly CA, Fernandes G. J Clin Immunol 1999;19:172–8.

174. Pompos LJ, Fritsche KL. J Nutr 2002;132:3293–300.

175. Anderson MJ, Fritsche KL. J Nutr 2004;134:1978–83.

176. Arrington JL, Chapkin RS, Switzer KC et al. Clin Exp Immunol 2001;125:499–507.

177. Chapkin RS, Arrington JL, Apanasovich TV et al. Clin Exp Immunol 2002;130:12–8.

178. Switzer KC, McMurray DN, Morris JS et al. J Nutr 2003;133: 496–503.

179. Siddiqui RA, Jenski LJ, Harvey KA et al. Biochem J 2003; 371:621–9.

180. FaNYY, McMurray DN, Ly LH et al. J Nutr 2003;133:1913–20.

181. FaNYY, Ly LH, Barhoumi R et al. J Immunol 2004;173: 6151–60.

182. Madani S, Hichami A, Cherkaoui-Malki M et al. J Biol Chem 2004;279:1176–83.

183. O'Shea M, Bassaganya-Riera J, Mohede IC. Am J Clin Nutr 2004;79:1199S–206S.

184. Bassaganya-Riera J, Pogranichniy RM, Jobgen SC et al. J Nutr 2003;133:3204–14.

185. Turini ME, Boza JJ, Gueissaz N et al. Eur J Nutr 2003;42: 171–9.

186. Yamasaki M, Chujo H, Hirao A et al. J Nutr 2003;133:784–8.

187. Kinoshita K, Yoo BS, Nozaki Y et al. J Immunol 2003;170: 5793–8.

188. Stephensen CB, Jiang X, Freytag T. J Nutr 2004;134:2660–6.

189. Jason J, Archibald LK, Nwanyanwu OC et al. Clin Diagn Lab Immunol 2002;9:616–21.

190. Hoag KA, Nashold FE, Goverman J et al. J Nutr 2002;132: 3736–9.

191. Gorgun G, Foss F. Blood 2002;100:1399–403.

192. Ertesvag A, Engedal, N, Naderi S et al. J Immunol 2002;169: 5555–63.

193. Garcia AL, Ruhl R, Herz U et al. Immunology 2003;110:180–7.

194. Vertuani S, De Geer A, Levitsky V et al. Cancer Res 2003;63: 8006–13.

195. Baeten JM, McClelland RS, Corey L et al. J Infect Dis 2004; 189:1466–71.

196. Fawzi W, Msamanga G, Antelman G et al. Clin Infect Dis 2004;38:716–22.

197. Gregori S, Giarratana N, Smiroldo S et al. Diabetes 2002;51:1367–74.

198. Deluca HF, Cantorna MT. FASEB J 2001;15:2579–85.

199. Matheu V, Back O, Mondoc E et al. J Allergy Clin Immunol 2003; 112:585–92.

200. Van Etten E, Decallonne B, Verlinden L et al. J Cell Biochem 2003;88:223–6.

201. Topilski I, Flaishon L, Naveh Y et al. Eur J Immunol 2004;34: 1068–76.

202. Cippitelli M, Fionda C, Di Bona D et al. J Immunol 2002;168: 1154–66.

203. Staeva-Vieira TP, Freedman LP. J Immunol 2002;168:1181–9.

204. Rausch-Fan X, Leutmezer F, Willheim M et al. Int Arch Allergy Immunol 2002;128:33–41.

205. Mahon BD, Wittke A, Weaver V et al. J Cell Biochem 2003;89: 922–32.

206. Meehan TF, DeLuca HF. Proc Natl Acad Sci USA 2002;99: 5557–60.

207. Heine G, Anton K, Henz BM et al. Eur J Immunol 2002;32: 3395–404.

208. Chen H, Hewison M, Hu B et al. Proc Natl Acad Sci USA, 2003;100:6109–14.

209. Fernandez-Cabezudo MJ, Hasan MY, Mustafa N et al. Free Radic Res 2003;37:437–45.

210. Chen C, Reddy KS, Johnston TD et al. J Surg Res 2003;113: 228–33.

211. Li-Weber M, Giaisi M, Treiber MK et al. Eur J Immunol, 2002; 32:2401–8.

212. Li-Weber M, Weigand MA, Giaisi M et al. J Clin Invest 2002; 110:681–90.

213. Adolfsson O, Huber BT, Meydani SN. J Immunol 2001;167: 3809–17.

214. Douziech N, Seres I, Larbi A et al. Exp Gerontol 2002;37: 369–87.

215. Libetta C, Zucchi M, Gori E et al. Kidney Int 2004;65:1473–81.

216. Fraker PJ, King LE. Annu Rev Nutr 2004;24:277–98.

217. Walker CF, Black RE. Annu Rev Nutr 2004;24:255–75.

218. Raqib R, Roy SK, Rahman MJ et al. Am J Clin Nutr 2004;79: 444–50.

219. Langkamp-Henken B, Bender BS, Gardner EM et al. J Am Geriatr Soc 2004;52:3–12.

220. Bonham M, O'Connor JM, Alexander HD et al. Br J Nutr 2003; 89:695–703.

221. Moore JB, Blanchard RK, Cousins RJ. Proc Natl Acad Sci USA 2003;100:3883–8.

222. Hosea HJ, Rector ES, Taylor CG. Br J Nutr 2004;91:741–7.

223. Saito Y, Yoshida Y, Akazawa T et al. J Bio Chem 2003;278: 39428–34.

224. Kidd P. Altern Med Rev 2003;8:223–46.

225. Broome CS, McArdle F, Kyle JA et al. Am J Clin Nutr 2004;80: 154–62.

SELECTED READINGS

Abbas A, Lichtman A, Pober J, eds. Cellular and Molecular Immunology. Philadelphia: WB Saunders, 1991.

Calder PC, Gill HA, Field CJ, eds. Nutrition and Immune Function. Cambridge, MA: CAB International, 2002.

Gershwin ME, Keen CL, German JB, eds. Nutrition and Immunology: Principles and Practice. Totowa, NJ: Humana Press, 2000.

Hughes DA, Bendich A, Darlington LG, eds. Diet and Human Immune Function. Totowa, NJ: Humana Press, 2004.

Paul WE, ed. Fundamental Immunology. 5th ed. Philadelphia: Lippincott Williams & Wilkins, 2003.

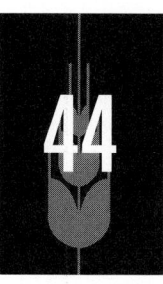

44 OXIDANT DEFENSE IN OXIDATIVE AND NITROSATIVE STRESS[1]

JAMES A. THOMAS

RADICALS AND NONRADICALS IN OXIDATIVE STRESS . .685
    Oxygen Species 685
    Nitrogen Species 687
EFFECTS OF OXIDANTS ON MACROMOLECULES 688
    Carbohydrates 688
    Nucleic Acids 688
    Proteins 688
    Lipids 689
CELLULAR ANTIOXIDANTS 689
    The Glutathione and Protein Sulfhydryl
       Redox Cycle 690
    Vitamin E and Membrane Peroxidation 691
    Enzymes as Antioxidants in Cells 692
PLASMA ANTIOXIDANTS 692
HUMAN DISEASE AND OXIDATIVE STRESS 692
    Cancer 692
    Cataracts and Eye Injury 693
    Reperfusion Injury 693
    Arthritis and Rheumatic Disorders 693
    Amyotrophic Lateral Sclerosis 693
    Viral Autoimmune Disease 693

Oxidative and nitrosative stress have been implicated in human disease as a result of either cellular damage or alterations in normal cell signaling pathways. Eukaryotic cells have multiple protective mechanisms against the damaging effects of oxidative and nitrosative stress. For the most part, these are quite effective in minimizing cell damage. Dietary constituents play an important role by providing protective agents, ranging from antioxidant vitamins and minerals to food additives that may enhance the action of natural antioxidants. Indeed, at least part of the beneficial effect of a diet high in fruits and vegetables is thought to derive from the variety of plant antioxidants that may act as beneficial supplements in humans. On the other hand, materials such as pesticides, polyunsaturated lipids, and a variety of plant- and microorganism-derived toxins might produce prooxidant effects in humans. This chapter describes our current understanding of the molecules contributing to oxidative and nitrosative stress at the cellular level and to the antioxidant systems that function at the cellular and organism level. Other chapters in this volume present more detailed information about individual vitamins and minerals and their potential participation in oxidative stress.

Oxidative stress was first defined as a disturbance in the equilibrium status of prooxidant/antioxidant systems in intact cells (1), and recently nitrosative stress has been understood in similar terms. This definition of oxidative/nitrosative stress implies that cells have intact prooxidant/antioxidant systems that continuously generate and detoxify a variety of oxidants resulting from the generation of reduced oxygen and nitrogen species by aerobic metabolism. When the prooxidant systems outbalance the antioxidant systems, oxidative damage may accumulate in lipids, proteins, carbohydrates, and nucleic acids, ultimately leading to cell death in severe oxidative stress. Oxidative stress may directly alter the antioxidant systems by inducing or repressing the proteins that participate in these systems and by depleting cellular stores of antioxidant materials such as glutathione, vitamin E, carotenoids, and other antioxidant molecules.

A disturbance in prooxidant/antioxidant systems results from myriad different oxidative radical and nonradical molecules generated during radiation, xenobiotic metabolism of environmental pollutants and administered drugs, and challenges to the immune system in human disease or in abnormal immune function, and even from normal cell signaling events. A radical species is specifically understood to be any atom that contains one or more orbital electrons with unpaired spin states. The radical may be a very small molecule such as oxygen or nitric oxide (NO), or it may be a part of a large biomolecule such as a protein, carbohydrate, lipid, or nucleic acid. Some radical species are very reactive with other biomolecules, and others, such as the normal triplet state of molecular oxygen, are relatively inert.

RADICALS AND NONRADICALS IN OXIDATIVE STRESS

Oxygen Species

Radicals of oxygen (superoxide anion, hydroxyl radical, and peroxy radicals) and reactive nonradical oxygen species such as hydrogen peroxide and singlet oxygen, as well as

---

[1]**Abbreviations: ADP,** adenosine diphosphate; **cGMP,** cyclic guanosine monophosphate; **LDL,** low-density lipoproteins; **NADH,** reduced nicotinamide adenine dinucleotide; **NADPH,** reduced nicotinamide adenosine dinucleotide phosphate; **NO,** nitric oxide; **pKa,** ionization constant.

carbon, nitrogen, and sulfur radicals, constitute the variety of reactive molecules that can pose an oxidative stress to cells (2, 3). It has been estimated that a maximum of 5% of the total oxygen metabolism of liver tissue results in the production of partially reduced oxygen species such as those shown in Figure 44.1. This represents a significant stress in itself, but extracellular sources of these molecules may be even more significant sources of oxidative stress. Therefore, considerable attention centers on the identification of oxyradical-generating processes.

Atmospheric oxygen, although a radical, is not particularly reactive with biologic molecules because the two orbital electrons participating in oxidation reactions have the same spin state. The spin restriction imposed by this electronic configuration prevents rapid reactions with compounds that could easily react without the spin restriction. Any process that produces a one-electron-reduction of oxygen produces the more reactive radical called superoxide anion. Subsequent reduction of superoxide anion or other partially reduced forms of oxygen can form singlet oxygen, a much more reactive form with paired electrons. Reaction of singlet oxygen does not have the same spin state restriction. It has been identified in tissues under oxidative stress.

Superoxide anion is generated continuously by several cellular processes, including the microsomal and mitochondrial electron transport systems. In addition, xanthine dehydrogenase/oxidase and other cellular oxidases may be important sources of this molecule. Myeloid cells have a special role in the production of superoxide anion because they contain a plasma membrane–bound electron transfer complex, reduced nicotinamide adenosine dinucleotide phosphate (NADPH) oxidase, that reduces oxygen with NADPH to produce copious amounts of superoxide anion (4). The products of this reaction are essential for effective bacterial killing. Absence of this enzyme activity is responsible for an inherited human condition called chronic granulomatous disease, which is characterized by recurrent infections.

The universal presence of superoxide dismutase in both cytoplasm and mitochondria ensures that much of the superoxide anion is rapidly converted into hydrogen peroxide. Superoxide anion is not a particularly reactive molecule, and it can diffuse to a considerable distance from its site of production. It may combine with other reactive species, such as NO, produced by macrophages, to yield a more reactive species. It can be transported across membranes (by an anion transport mechanism), and in the vicinity of membranes it may be protonated to $HO_2\cdot$, becoming a much more reactive substance.

Hydrogen peroxide is generated by the same sources that produce superoxide anion because both enzymatic (superoxide dismutase) and nonenzymatic destruction of superoxide anion produces hydrogen peroxide. Other specific enzymes also produce hydrogen peroxide directly. These include peroxisomal enzymes associated with fatty acid metabolism and cytoplasmic enzymes responsible for the oxidation of a variety of cell metabolites. Hydrogen peroxide can diffuse over considerable distances and may pass membranes readily in this process. Thus, pools of hydrogen peroxide equilibrate rapidly.

Hydrogen peroxide and superoxide anion can occur in the extracellular space and in blood plasma as a result of the membrane-associated reaction in myeloid cells such as neutrophils and macrophages (4). The membrane-associated NADPH-oxidase produces superoxide anion that rapidly dismutes to hydrogen peroxide as well.

In the presence of a transition cation such as iron or copper, superoxide anion can give rise to the highly reactive hydroxyl radical species ($HO\cdot$ by the Haber-Weiss reaction (see the following equation) (5, 6). Some forms of bound iron are more efficient than free iron in this process. Other complexes of iron prevent its participation in these reactions.

Haber-Weiss reaction:

$$O_2\cdot^- + H_2O_2 \rightarrow O_2 + HO^- + HO\cdot$$

Iron-catalyzed Haber-Weiss reaction:

$$Fe^{III} + O_2\cdot^- \rightarrow Fe^{II} + O_2$$

$$Fe^{II} + H_2O_2 \rightarrow Fe^{III} + HO^- + HO\cdot$$

The hydroxyl radical is considered to be a principal actor in the toxicity of partially reduced oxygen species because it is very reactive with all kinds of biologic macromolecules, producing products that cannot be regenerated by cell metabolism (Fig. 44.2). The rate of reaction of the hydroxyl radical is controlled by diffusion, and it reacts near its site of production. Therefore, damage by this radical is very site specific.

Peroxyl radicals occur during the oxidation of lipids in oxidative stress, and they are associated with the action of prostaglandin H synthase in prostaglandin synthesis (7).

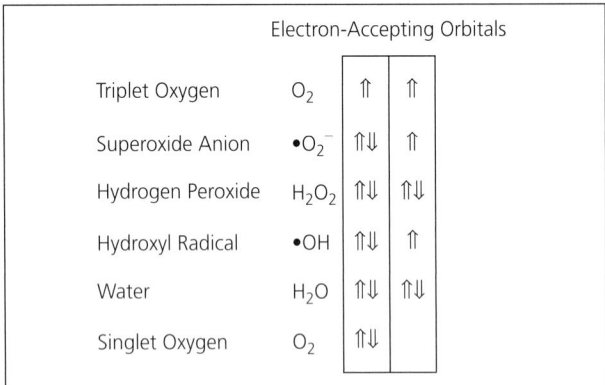

Figure 44.1. Molecular species of oxygen in oxidative stress. Each relevant orbital electron is indicated by an *arrow* showing its spin state. Each molecular species (except for singlet oxygen) is obtained by a one electron reduction of the one above it in the table. In intact cells singlet oxygen is formed by oxidation of one of the partially reduced states of oxygen.

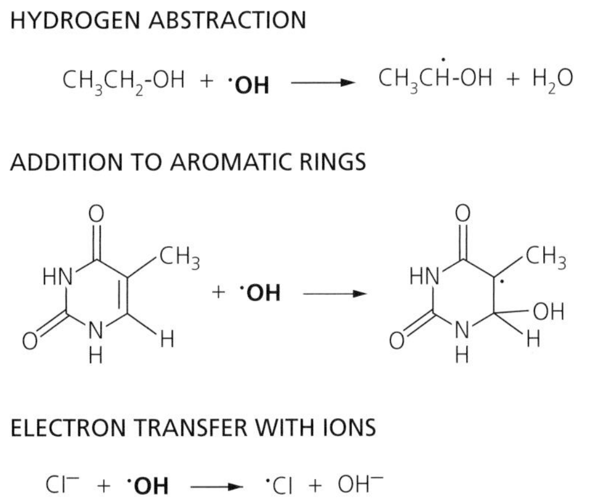

HYDROGEN ABSTRACTION

$$CH_3CH_2\text{-}OH + \cdot OH \longrightarrow CH_3\overset{\cdot}{C}H\text{-}OH + H_2O$$

ADDITION TO AROMATIC RINGS

ELECTRON TRANSFER WITH IONS

$$Cl^- + \cdot OH \longrightarrow \cdot Cl + OH^-$$

Figure 44.2. Reaction of hydroxyl radicals with biologic molecules.

These radicals are formed by a one-electron transfer from a carbon-centered radical to oxygen (reaction 1 in the following equation). The peroxyl radical species, which are not very reactive, may diffuse a considerable distance. One particularly good target of this radical is the sulfhydryl group (thiols) found in glutathione and many proteins. The reaction generates the thiyl radical (reaction 2 in the following equation) (8).

(1) $R\text{-}CH_2\cdot + O_2 \rightarrow R\text{-}CH_2\text{-}OO\cdot$

(2) $R\text{-}S^- + ROO\cdot \rightarrow \quad \cdot R\text{-}S\cdot + ROO^-$

thiolate	thiyl
anion	radical

The variety of oxygen species described above indicates the complexity of the reactions that can result from an oxidative stress. Factors such as the site of production, the availability of transition metals, and the action of enzymes determine the fate of each radical species and its availability for reaction with cellular molecules. The H_2O_2 concentration under steady state conditions in the liver has been estimated to be 10^{-7} to 10^{-9} M, whereas superoxide anion may be 10^{-11} M.

Nitrogen Species

NO is an important oxidative biologic signaling molecule that was first discovered in smooth muscle relaxation, neurotransmission, and immune regulation (9). Several different forms of the NO synthase enzyme (Fig. 44.3A) generate the nitrogen-based radical by a five-electron oxidative reaction with arginine as its substrate. This enzyme is found in both constitutive and inducible forms in many different cell types, and its activity is highly regulated by calcium ion and other factors. The reaction uses flavin and pterin molecules to catalyze the synthetic reaction, and calcium sensitivity may be imparted by calmodulin. Because NO synthase is highly active in macrophages and neutrophils, these cells are rich sources of both superoxide

anion (produced by the NADPH oxidase enzyme complex) and NO. During the oxidative burst, triggered during inflammatory processes, NO and superoxide anion may react together to produce significant amounts of a much more oxidatively active molecule, peroxynitrous acid (peroxynitrite at a neutral pH) (10) (Fig. 44.3B). Peroxynitrite is a strong oxidant that attacks protein cysteines and methionines. It also reacts with protein tyrosines by adding an NO_2 to the ring of these amino acids. The protein modifications that result from peroxynitrite production may provide explanations for some of the observed biologic effects of NO. Another reaction product of NO produces a metabolically reversible modification of protein thiols that plays a role in signal transduction (Fig. 44.3C). A one-electron oxidation of the thiol to an S-nitrosylated thiol is mediated by the intermediate reaction of NO with oxygen to produce the oxidizing N_2O_3 species. The N_2O_3 directly oxidizes a thiol by forming an S-nitrosylated adduct. The role of this protein modification in signaling is of increasing interest in nitrosative stress.

Production of NO can trigger the production of cyclic guanosine monophosphate (cGMP) through NO-mediated stimulation of the guanylate cyclase enzyme; it can produce adducts with various cellular thiols, that is, glutathione and protein thiols, generating S-nitrosothiols (see Fig. 44.3C); it can cause nitration of protein tyrosine residues through

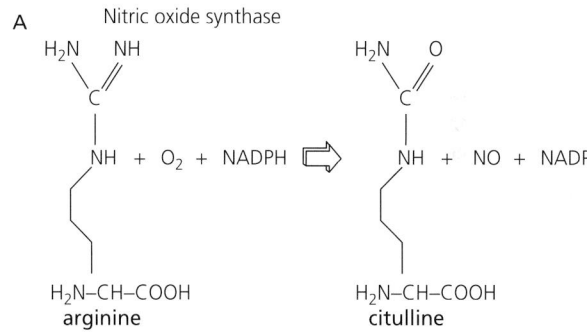

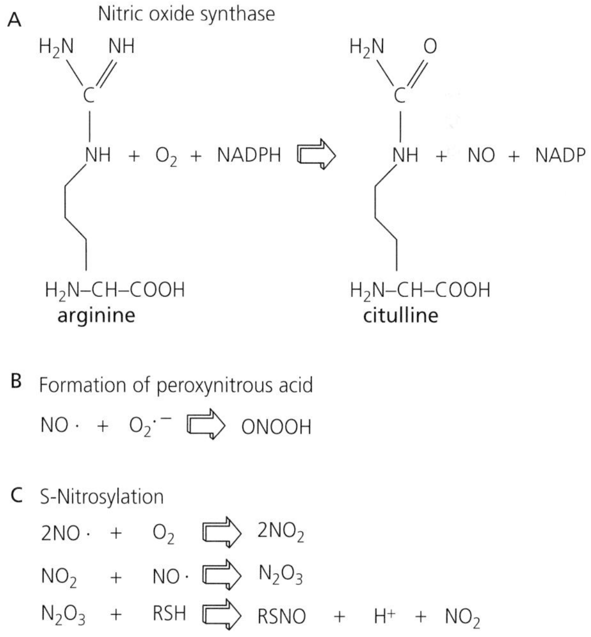

Figure 44.3. Formation and reactions of nitric oxide. **A.** The reaction catalyzed by nitric oxide (NO) synthase. The exact stoichiometry of the reaction is not known. The five electron reaction generates NO and oxidizes reduced nicotinamide adenine dinucleotide phosphate (NADPH) in the process. **B.** Formation of peroxynitrite as a simple addition product of superoxide anion and NO. No oxidation or reduction is necessary. **C.** Oxidative chemistry responsible for direct S-nitrosylation of sulfhydryl groups.

direct nitration reactions; and it can increase oxidative stress through the generation of peroxynitrite. Some evidence also indicates that copious amounts of NO may even act as an antioxidant. These ideas suggest that the ratio of superoxide anion to NO and oxygen determines the metabolic and cellular effects attributed to the generation of these oxidative species.

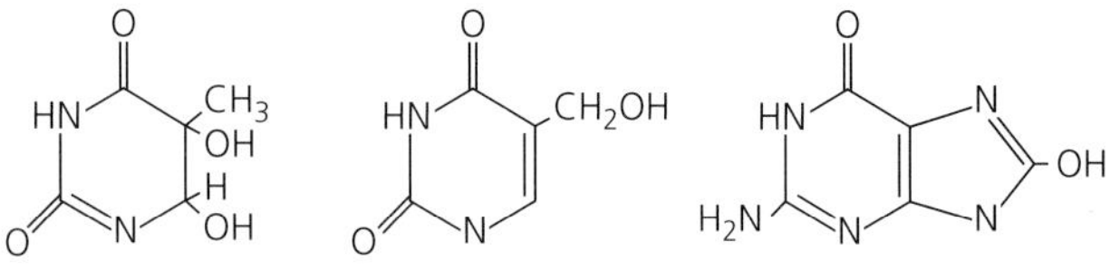

EFFECTS OF OXIDANTS ON MACROMOLECULES

Carbohydrates

Hydroxyl radicals react with carbohydrates by randomly abstracting a hydrogen atom from one of the carbon atoms, producing a carbon-centered radical (12). This leads to chain breaks in important molecules such as hyaluronic acid (Fig. 44.4) in a process involving intermediates such as peroxyl radicals. In the synovial fluid surrounding joints, an accumulation and activation of neutrophils during inflammation produces a significant amount of oxyradicals. This phenomenon apparently accounts for a significant decrease in the synovial fluid of affected joints.

Nucleic Acids

Nucleic acids are pentose-phosphate polymers that can undergo reactions with hydroxyl radicals such as those depicted for hyaluronic acid (see Fig. 44.4) (13). In addition, there are several important examples of modifications to the base portion of the polymer (Fig. 44.5). In fact, these base modifications may be responsible for the genetic defects produced by oxidative stress. Recently, 8-hydroxy guanosine has generated considerable interest

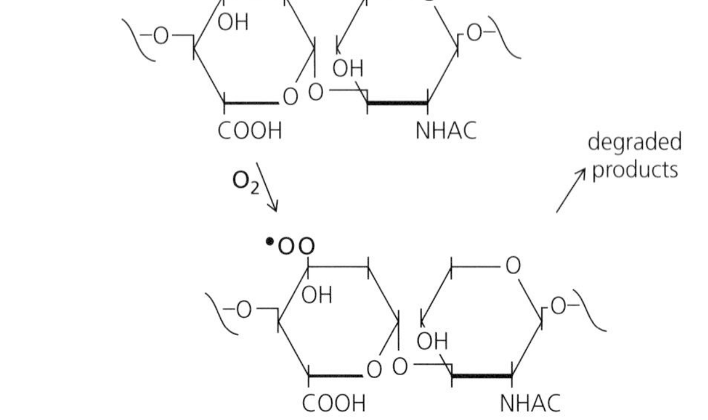

Figure 44.5. Selected modified bases found in DNA after oxidative stress.

as a product of hydroxyl radical attack on DNA that can be used to estimate DNA damage in humans (14, 15). In humans, oxidative damage to DNA has been estimated as 104 hits per cell per day. Estimation of modified bases in urine is a useful means of assessing the amount of DNA damage in an animal. Products such as 8-hydroxy guanosine, thymidine glycol, and uric acid are used for these estimates. DNA damage has also been estimated by chain breaks and base modifications in cultured cells under oxidative stress. An important metabolic effect of DNA damage is the rapid induction of polyadenosine diphosphate ribose synthesis (adenosine diphosphate [ADP] ribosylation) in nuclei, resulting in extensive depletion of cellular reduced nicotinamide adenine dinucleotide (NADH) pools. ADP ribosylation has been associated with repair of damaged DNA.

Proteins

Proteins have many reactive sites that can be damaged during oxidative stress, but interest has centered on three measurable events. First, aggressive radicals such as the hydroxyl radical can fragment proteins in plasma, and the fragmented products of specific proteins, if known, can be detected (16). This fragmenting is associated with reactions at specific amino acids such as proline (Fig. 44.6A) and histidine (17). Second, proteins may contain metal binding sites that are especially susceptible to oxidative events through interaction with the metals. These reactions usually produce irreversible modifications in amino acids that may be involved in metal ion binding, for example, histidine. These modifications may produce signal sequences that are recognized by specific cellular proteases that degrade such proteins (18, 19). Finally, many intracellular proteins have "reactive" sulfhydryl groups on specific cysteine residues (see Cellular Antioxidants) that can be oxidized to S-glutathiolated or S-nitrosylated forms that are easily reduced again by metabolic processes (20). Similarly, some proteins have a "reactive" methionine that can undergo a reversible modification to methionine sulfoxide (Fig. 44.6B) (21, 22). The disulfide and sulfoxide forms of these two amino acids may actually serve a protective role because the metabolic reversibility of the protein modification effectually detoxifies the oxidative species that caused the modification.

Figure 44.4. Reaction of hydroxyl radicals with polysaccharides (hyaluronic acid).

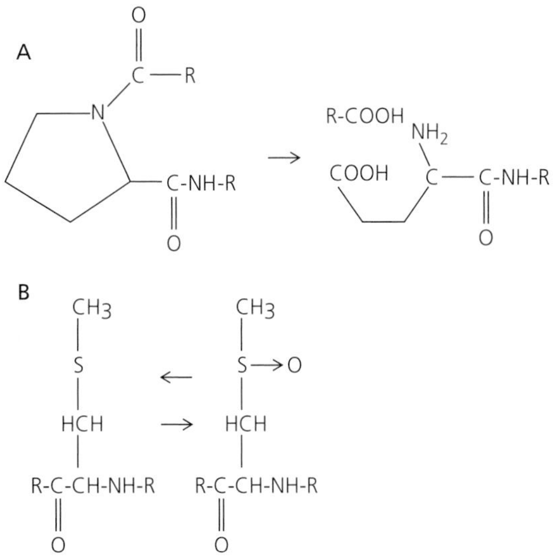

Figure 44.6. Methionine and proline oxidation. **A.** The reaction shows the irreversible oxidation of proline in a peptide. The results are a break in the polypeptide chain and the introduction of new carboxyl groups that can be measured to quantitate these events. **B.** The reaction demonstrates the reversible oxidation/reduction of methionine as it occurs in several proteins. The reduction is an enzymatic process that requires a reduced thiol such as glutathione.

Lipids

Lipid peroxidation of polyunsaturated lipids is a facile process. This oxidation affects materials that are prevalent in dietary constituents, seriously affecting the flavor of foods. In intact cells, polyunsaturated lipids are major constituents of cellular membranes (23, 24), where peroxidation of membrane lipid seriously impairs membrane function. Most membrane lipid peroxidation occurs as a result of oxidative stress in intact cells, but some dietary material may be directly incorporated into cell structures (25). Lipid peroxidation is a radical-initiated chain reaction that is self-propagating in cellular membranes. As a result, isolated oxidative events may have profound effects on membrane function. The reactions of this process are depicted in Figure 44.7.

The products of lipid peroxidation are easily detected in blood plasma and have been used as a measure of oxidative stress. The most commonly measured product is malondialdehyde (see Fig. 44.7). In addition, the unsaturated aldehydes produced from these reactions have been implicated in modification of cellular proteins and other materials (26). The peroxidized lipid can produce peroxy radicals and singlet oxygen by the reactions discussed earlier. Vitamin E is particularly effective as an antioxidant in lipid peroxidizing systems.

CELLULAR ANTIOXIDANTS

The most effective antioxidant in oxidative stress is dependent on the specific molecules causing the stress, that is, superoxide anion, lipid peroxides, iron-generated hydroxyl

STEPS OF LIPID PEROXIDATION

(INITIATION) LIPID + $R^{\bullet}/O^{\bullet}H$ → $LIPID^{\bullet}$

(PROPAGATION) $LIPID^{\bullet}$ + O_2 → $LIPID\text{-}OO^{\bullet}$

$LIPID\text{-}OO^{\bullet}$ + LIPID → LIPID-OOH + $LIPID^{\bullet}$

(TERMINATION) $LIPID^{\bullet}$ + $LIPID^{\bullet}$ → LIPID-LIPID

$LIPID\text{-}OO^{\bullet}$ + $LIPID^{\bullet}$ → LIPID-OO-LIPID

(SCAVENGING) $LIPID^{\bullet}$ + VIT E → LIPID + VIT $E^{\bullet}$

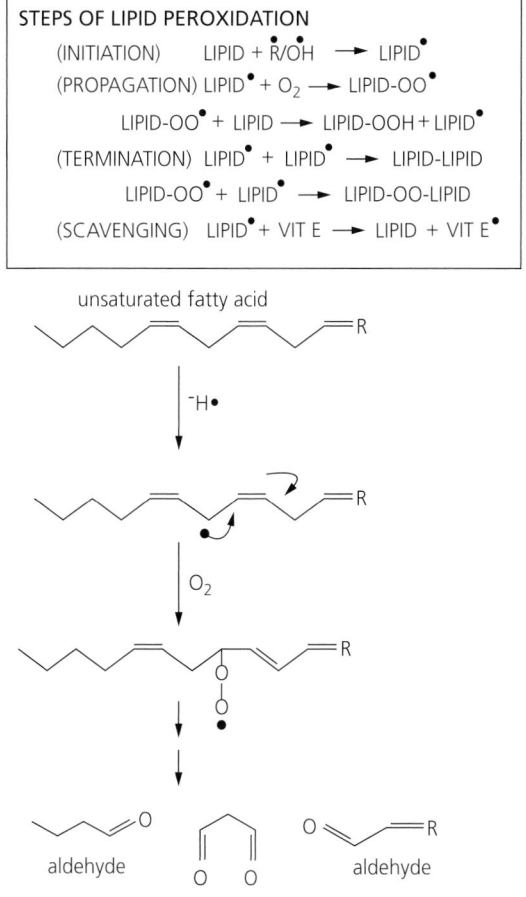

Figure 44.7. Reactions of lipid peroxidation.

radical, and so on, and the cellular or extracellular location of the source of these molecules. As an example, damage to a cell membrane occurs from both internally and externally generated oxidative stress. This damage is most effectively prevented by vitamin E, which reacts with peroxyl and hydroxyl radicals; by carotenoids, which react with singlet oxygen; and possibly by membrane-bound proteins. The chain-breaking antioxidant function of vitamin E in membranes results from its close association with polyunsaturated components of the membrane (27). It can be regenerated by reaction with cytoplasmic vitamin C and glutathione, or by membrane-bound quinols. Vitamin C is subsequently reduced by glutathione through the glutathione cycle described later. Thus, a specific attack on membranes results in the participation of at least three different antioxidants. Similarly, when oxidative stress occurs in plasma, a variety of different antioxidants participate in the response. Many plasma proteins are affected by the process, causing either irreversible or reversible loss of functional protein activity. A good example is the oxidation of methionine residues in α1-protease inhibitor (an inhibitor of elastase). The modification can be reversed by a specific reductase enzyme that restores that activity of the inhibitor (21) (see Fig. 44.6).

The Glutathione and Protein Sulfhydryl Redox Cycle

The low-molecular-weight thiol, glutathione, and "reactive" protein sulfhydryls (exposed cysteines in many proteins) are primary participants in cellular antioxidant systems. Glutathione (Fig. 44.8A) is abundant (3–10 mM) in cytoplasm, nuclei, and mitochondria and is the major soluble antioxidant in these cell compartments (28). Reactive protein sulfhydryls are abundant both in soluble proteins and in membrane-bound proteins (29).

The sulfur atom in sulfhydryl groups easily accommodates the loss of a single electron (reaction 1 in the following equation), and the lifetime of radical species of sulfur, that is, a thiyl radical, may be significantly longer than that of many other radicals generated during stress. Sulfhydryl groups also partially ionize at cellular pH values, producing the more reactive nucleophile thiolate anion (reaction 2). The ionization constant (pKa) of the sulfhydryl group of glutathione is 9.3, and many other sulfhydryl groups, especially those on proteins, may have considerably lower pKas as a result of local electronic effects on the functional group. The thiolate anion is responsible for the reactivity of thiols with a variety of foreign materials in conjugation reactions during xenobiotic metabolism. Thus, the reactions of the sulfhydryl groups during oxidative stress include examples in which both sulfur radicals and thiolate anions are important.

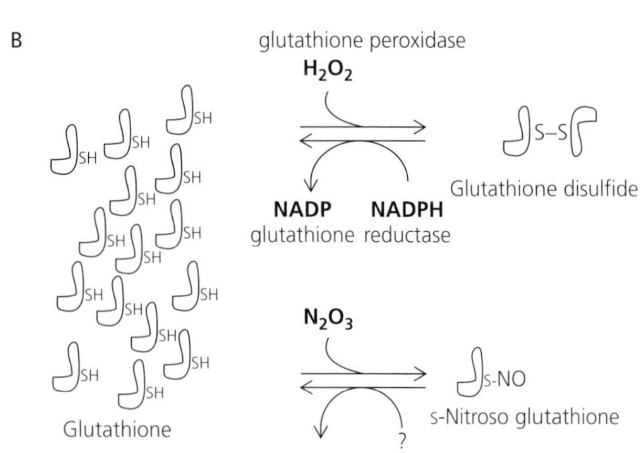

(1) Glutathione-SH → glutathione-$\dot{\text{S}}$·

Protein-SH → protein-$\dot{\text{S}}$·

(2) R-SH → R-S^- + H+

Protein-SH → protein-S$^-$

The reactions of the glutathione oxidation cycles are shown in Figure 44.8B. The two-electron oxidation/reduction of glutathione is primarily mediated by glutathione peroxidase and glutathione reductase enzymes. The primary cellular glutathione peroxidase is a selenium-containing enzyme that uses hydrogen peroxide to produce glutathione disulfide. There is a family of peroxidases, and some of these enzymes may also use lipid peroxides rather than hydrogen peroxide as the oxidant. Thus, glutathione can detoxify both soluble and lipid peroxides. Glutathione disulfide is subsequently reduced by glutathione reductase using NADPH as the reductant. Cellular NADPH, produced by the pentose-P pathway and other cytoplasmic sources, provides the major source of reducing power for detoxifying many peroxides.

S-nitrosylated glutathione (see Fig. 44.8B) is a one-electron oxidation product of glutathione that is also in rapid equilibrium with the total glutathione pool. In cells, the glutathione pool is maintained at a very reduced state, and only minor amounts of glutathione disulfide and S-nitrosylated glutathione have been observed, even under oxidative or nitrosative stress.

The concentration of cellular glutathione has a major effect on its antioxidant function because it acts as a trap for numerous oxidants produced by both oxidative and nitrosative stress. Its concentration varies considerably as a result of nutrient limitation, exercise, oxidative stress, and aging. Under oxidative conditions, the concentration of glutathione can be considerably diminished through conjugation to xenobiotics and by secretion of both the glutathione conjugates and glutathione disulfide from the affected cells. A considerable amount of glutathione may also become protein-bound during severe oxidative stress. The rate of glutathione synthesis may be compromised in aging, leading to a decrease in the total pool of this antioxidant. Recently, compounds that can both increase and decrease the glutathione concentration when administered to animals have been discovered (30). Some of these compounds may provide the means to modify glutathione concentration in humans in the future. Experiments have already shown beneficial effects of augmenting the glutathione concentration in autoimmune disease.

One of the primary antioxidant roles of the intracellular glutathione pool is protection of protein sulfhydryls. These reactive amino acids must be kept in a reduced state to function in their various unique roles inside cells. Figure 44.9 shows some of the potential oxidative reactions that may affect protein sulfhydryls during oxidative and nitrosative stress. Two readily reversible oxidized forms are currently of great interest for their potential roles in the signal

Figure 44.8. A. Structure of glutathione. **B.** Reversible oxidative formation of both disulfides and S-nitrosylated thiols. NADP, nicotinamide adenine dinucleotide phosphate (NADPH, reduced form).

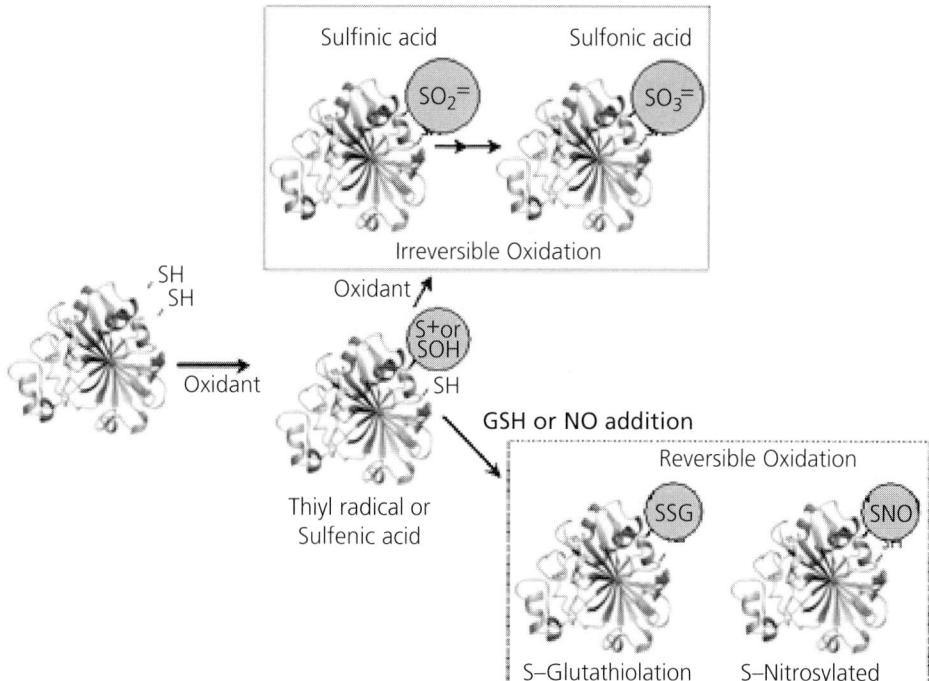

Figure 44.9. Oxidative reactions of protein sulfhydryls, exemplified by two surface cysteines in carbonic anhydrase III. Several oxidants may participate in these reactions, including both partially reduced oxygen species and derivatives of nitric oxide (NO). Partially oxidized protein cysteines are either trapped by glutathione (GSH) or NO or are more fully oxidized to less easily reversed acidic forms of cysteine.

transduction effects of oxidative and nitrosative stress. These are shown in Figure 44.9 as the S-glutathiolated and S-nitrosylated forms of carbonic anhydrase III, a protein with two reactive cysteines that has been studied extensively. These two protein forms are only transient in cells because multiple enzymic and nonenzymic reactions readily reduce the oxidized form back to the free sulfhydryl. The most abundant and highly studied enzymes responsible for reduction of S-glutathiolated and S-nitrosylated proteins are thioredoxin and glutaredoxin (31, 32). These two proteins contain a unique active-site dithiol sequence that can efficiently reduce proteins.

When the glutathione concentration is not sufficient to trap oxidized protein sulfhydryls, irreversible oxidation to the sulfinic and sulfonic acid may result. Investigators have recently found that protein sulfinic acids are normally present in otherwise healthy animals. These acids occur to the extent of about 5% of the total exposed sulfhydryls. In aging and under glutathione-depleting conditions, this sulfhydryl damage is increased at least twofold. Thus, it is suspected that damage to protein sulfhydryls is a consequence of inadequate glutathione protection. It should be mentioned here that protein-protein disulfides are not found to any great extent in intracellular proteins, although these modifications are abundant in extracellular proteins.

Vitamin E and Membrane Peroxidation

Vitamin E refers to a family of related compounds (tocopherols) that have hydroxylated aromatic rings (chromanol rings) and isoprenoid side chains. The molecule is highly lipophilic and resides almost exclusively in cell membranes,

where the chromanol ring may be at the surface of the membrane and the isoprenoid chain may be inserted into the bilayer (33). Because lipid peroxidation occurs on unsaturated fatty acid chains that reside within the lipid bilayer, and the chromanol ring is the active radical quenching part of the vitamin, the function of vitamin E as an antioxidant must involve considerable movement of the lipids and vitamin E to promote molecular interaction (34). The reactions in which a chromanol ring can participate in these processes are shown in Figure 44.10. This figure shows that

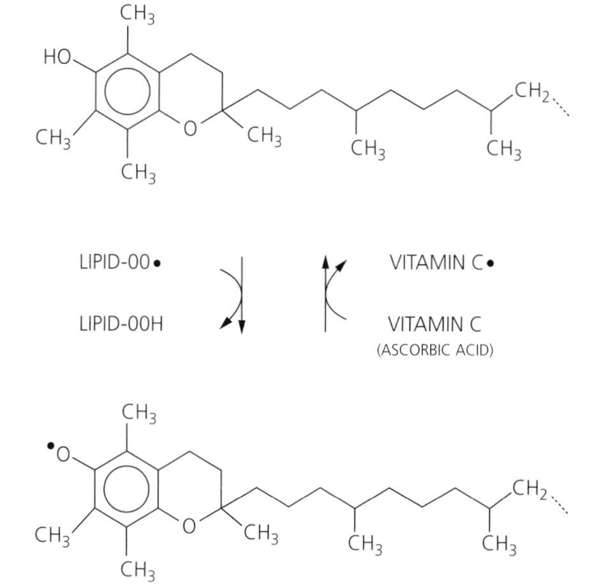

Figure 44.10. Oxidation of vitamin E by lipid radicals and reduction by vitamin C.

vitamin E is a chain reaction–breaking antioxidant because it quenches the intermediate in the chain reaction. The ascorbate radical formed in this process reacts rapidly with the reduced glutathione pool or with a specific vitamin C reductase enzyme.

Enzymes as Antioxidants in Cells

Superoxide dismutase is one of the most important enzymes that function as cellular antioxidants (35). It is present in cell cytoplasm (copper-zinc enzyme) and in mitochondria (manganese enzyme) to maintain a low concentration of superoxide anion. It catalyzes the dismutation of superoxide anion in the following manner.

$$2 \, O_2 \cdot^- + 2 \, H^+ \rightarrow O_2 + H_2O_2$$

The absence of this enzyme is lethal. However, too much may also be detrimental because an excess of this enzyme may produce hydrogen peroxide at a rate that is toxic to cells during oxidative stress. The amount of superoxide dismutase is controlled by specific redox-sensitive genes in cells (36). There is also an extracellular form of superoxide dismutase in plasma, lymph, and synovial fluid that is different from the intracellular forms of the enzyme (37). This enzyme may function at cell surfaces.

Catalase is a heme protein that catalyzes the reaction shown in the following equation, in which hydrogen peroxide is detoxified. It is usually found in peroxisomes, except in cells such as erythrocytes, which do not contain these organelles (38). In that case, catalase is a cytoplasmic enzyme. Catalase provides a protective role that is similar to that of glutathione peroxidase because both are important means of removing hydrogen peroxide. The relative contribution of catalase and glutathione peroxidase to hydrogen peroxide detoxification may be quite variable (39).

$$2 \, H_2O_2 \rightarrow O_2 + 2 \, H_2O$$

PLASMA ANTIOXIDANTS

Human plasma contains little catalase, superoxide dismutase, glutathione, or glutathione peroxidase, but some small molecules and protein constituents contribute to the antioxidant properties of this important fluid. Plasma has been studied with the use of artificially generated oxidants and with natural oxidants such as cigarette smoke. Plasma ascorbate is among the first compounds that become oxidized in stress (40, 41). Other materials may become oxidized only when ascorbate is depleted. Oxidation affects thiol groups (mostly on proteins), bilirubin, urate, and vitamin E. Bilirubin (bound to albumin) and uric acid, both considered to be waste products in plasma, are potentially good scavengers of oxyradicals. Transport into and out of erythrocytes may provide additional antioxidant potential because the reductive processes of these cells are quite vigorous.

The most important antioxidant proteins of plasma include ceruloplasmin, albumin, transferrin, haptoglobin, and hemopexin. The first three proteins may sequester iron and copper ions in forms that prevent their participation in reactions that generate the aggressive hydroxyl radical. Haptoglobin and hemopexin bind free heme, a source of iron that can participate in lipid oxidation reactions.

A second aspect of oxidative stress in plasma fractions is the oxidation of lipid particles such as low-density lipoproteins (LDLs) (42). These materials contain proteins and lipids that are good targets for oxidation, and the oxidized forms of LDLs are strongly implicated in fatty lesions (atheromas) in artery walls. Oxidation of LDLs causes a fragmentation of the apoprotein B component of these particles while also producing a variety of lipid peroxidation products, including adducts between lipid and apoprotein B. LDL particles contain a significant amount of vitamin E that serves as a primary antioxidant.

HUMAN DISEASE AND OXIDATIVE STRESS

The role of oxidative stress in human disease has been a subject of intense interest in recent years. The human immune response makes extensive use of many of the oxidative molecules discussed here, generating both superoxide anion and NO as an integral part of the response to foreign materials. It is clear that this defense system is a two-edged sword that also increases the oxidative risk to its human host. Other foreign materials, including some medications, also generate oxidative stress during metabolic events associated with their detoxification or excretion. The following paragraphs are summaries of research that points to the potential importance of oxidative stress in specific human diseases.

Cancer

Radicals of different kinds are potentially involved in both initiation and promotion in multistage cancer development (43, 44). In this process, DNA is damaged and the cellular antioxidant systems are modified as a result of the expression of different genetic components in precancerous and tumor cells. Because specific genes are apparently controlled by oxidation/reduction switching of important gene regulatory proteins, the effect of oxidative stress may be manifested directly by alterations in these specific proteins (36, 44). Conversely, base modifications (Fig. 44.5) may also cause an altered response by certain genes during oxidative stress. Free radical scavengers function as inhibitors at both the initiation and the promotion stage of carcinogenesis, thus protecting cells from the oxidative damage that occurs (45). In tumors the enzymes involved in antioxidant systems are altered, that is, tumors are low in manganese superoxide dismutase and possibly the copper-zinc enzyme, whereas glutathione peroxidase, reductase, and S-transferase are increased. In keeping with an increase in glutathione metabolism, one also finds increased glucose 6-P dehydrogenase, a source of NADPH for the glutathione and protein S-thiolation cycles (Fig. 44.9).

Some of the effective quinone-type anticancer drugs are promoters of oxyradical production (46). It may be that these drugs are effective in part because of their ability to generate oxidative species that cause DNA, membrane, or enzyme damage in tumor cells.

Cataracts and Eye Injury

The crystallins, major proteins of the eye lens, are long-lived proteins that are abundant in methionine and cysteine. As discussed earlier, these amino acids are sensitive to oxidation, and much work has suggested that oxidation of these proteins is involved in the development of opacities in the lens (47, 48). The lens is a highly susceptible target because it is continually exposed to the effects of light and certain oxidizing metabolic products. It has a high concentration of glutathione and glutathione reductase, and evidence indicates that glutathione decreases substantially in lens lesions. The vitreous humor of the eye also contains hyaluronic acid that is depolymerized when exposed to oxyradicals. Dietary vitamin E has been shown to help prevent eye damage in infants exposed to high oxygen concentrations.

Reperfusion Injury

Growing evidence shows that oxyradicals can mediate tissue injury during ischemia and reperfusion (49). The accumulation of neutrophils in the damaged tissue produces a significant amount of oxidant stress to the surviving tissue cells, leading to irreversible injury to those cells as a result of the massive generation of superoxide anion and other neutrophil products (50). Much of this damage is preventable by inhibitors of oxyradical generation and by materials that destroy the radicals after generation, that is, superoxide dismutase or mannitol.

Arthritis and Rheumatic Disorders

These diseases are characterized by inflammatory responses, in which extensive tissue damage can occur through oxidative stress (51). In rheumatoid arthritis, the effects of oxyradicals on the function of synovial fluid have been well documented (see Fig. 44.4). In addition, extensive cellular damage results in the release of clastogenic factors, and typical cellular damage products are detected in urine. Thus, materials such as peroxidized lipid or modified bases from cellular DNA have been found in patients who have these diseases. Investigators have postulated that antigens may be created by oxyradical attack on biomolecules, thereby instigating development of autoimmune antibodies and a continuing inflammatory response in affected tissue.

Amyotrophic Lateral Sclerosis

The motor neuron degeneration that is characteristic of this disease has been related to genetic defects in the superoxide dismutase gene (52). Many patients with the familial form of this disease have defective superoxide dismutase enzymes. The mutations in the protein occur in many different locations, and apparently all can be related to a loss of the enzyme activity. Because nonhereditary forms of this disease do not contain these lesions, the exact role of oxidative stress in motor neuron degeneration is unclear.

Viral Autoimmune Disease

The autoimmune disease caused by the retroviruses is characterized by a loss of specific circulatory immune cells and a depression of the glutathione content of virus-infected cells (53). Investigators have suggested that glutathione deficiency is permissive for the replication of the AIDS virus and that supplementation with agents that can increase glutathione is preventive for virus replication (54, 55). It has also been suggested that part of this effect may result from the oxidation/reduction control of certain transcription factors, including NFκB.

REFERENCES

1. Sies H. Oxidative stress: introductory remarks. In: Sies H, ed. Oxidative Stress. Orlando, FL: Academic Press, 1985:1–10.
2. Cardenas E. Annu Rev Biochem 1989;58:79–110.
3. Slater TF. Biochem J 1984;222:1–15.
4. Badwey JA, Karnovsky ML. Curr Top Cell Regul 1986;28: 183–208.
5. Halliwell B, Gutteridge JMC. Biochem J 1984;219:1–14.
6. Sutton HC. J Free Radic Biol Med 1985;1:195–202.
7. Marnett LJ. Carcinogenesis 1989;8:1365–73.
8. Willson RL. Organic peroxy free radicals as ultimate agents in oxygen toxicity. In: Sies H, ed. Oxidative Stress. Orlando, FL: Academic Press, 1985:41–72.
9. Bredt DS, Snyder SH. Annu Rev Biochem 1994;63:175–95.
10. Radi R, Beckman JS, Bush KM et al. J Biol Chem 1991;266: 4244–50.
11. Gow AJ, Buerk DG, Ischiropoulos H. J Biol Chem 1997;272: 2841–5.
12. von Sonntag C. Adv Carbohydr Chem Biochem 1980;37:7–77.
13. Shulte-Frohlinde D, von Sonntag C. Radiolysis of DNA and model systems in the presence of oxygen. In: Sies H, ed. Oxidative Stress. Orlando, FL: Academic Press, 1985:11–37.
14. Fraga CG, Shigenaga JP, Degan P et al. Proc Natl Acad Sci USA 1990;87:4533–7.
15. Floyd RA. FASEB J 1990;4:2587–97.
16. Wolff SP, Garner A, Dean RT. Trends Biochem Sci 1986;11:27–31.
17. Dean RT, Wolff SP, McElligott MA. Free Radic Res Commun 1989;7:97–103.
18. Stadtman ER. Free Radic Biol Med 1990;9:315–25.
19. Davies KJA. J Biol Chem 1987;262:9895–901.
20. Thomas JA, Poland B, Honzatko R. Archiv Biochem Biophys 1995;319:1–9.
21. Brot H, Weissbach H. Arch Biochem Biophys 1983;223:271–81.
22. Levine RL, Mosoni L, Berlett BS, et al. Proc Natl Acad Sci USA 1997;93:15036–40.
23. Gutteridge JMC. Lipid peroxidation; some problems and concepts. In: Halliwell B, ed. Oxygen Radicals and Tissue Injury. Bethesda, MD: FASEB, for Upjohn, 1988:9–19.
24. Gardner HW. Free Radic Biol Med 1989;7:65–86.

25. Wills ED. The role of dietary components in oxidative stress in tissues. In: Sies H, ed. Oxidative Stress. Orlando, FL: Academic Press, 1985:197–20.
26. Witz G. Free Radic Biol Med 1989;7:333–49.
27. Pascoe GA, Reed DJ. Free Radic Biol Med 1989;6:209–24.
28. Meister A. J Biol Chem 1988;263:17205–8.
29. Ziegler DM. Annu Rev Biochem 1985;54:305–30.
30. Anderson ME, Meister A. Anal Biochem 1989;183:16–20.
31. Jung CH, Thomas JA. Arch Biochem Biophys 1996;335:61–72.
32. Gravina SA, Mieyal JJ. Biochemistry 1993;32:3368–76.
33. Niki E, Yamamoto Y, Takahashi M et al. Ann NY Acad Sci 1989;570:23–31.
34. Wayner DDM, Burton GW, Ingold KU et al. Biochim Biophys Acta 1987;924:408–19.
35. Fridovich I. J Biol Chem 1989;264:7761–4.
36. Storz G, Tartaglia LA, Ames BN. Science 1990;248:189–94.
37. Marklund SL. Proc Natl Acad Sci USA 1982;79:7634–8.
38. Jones DP. Arch Biochem Biophys 1982;214:806–14.
39. Thayer WS. FEBS Lett 1986;202:137–40.
40. Halliwell B, Gutteridge JMC. Arch Biochem Biophys 1990;280: 1–8.
41. Stocker R, Glazer AN, Ames BN. Proc Natl Acad Sci USA 1987;84:5918–22.
42. Steinbrecher UP, Zhang H, Lougheed M. Free Radic Biol Med 1990;9:155–68.
43. Sun Y. Free Radic Biol Med 1990;8:583–99.
44. Abate C, Patel L, Raucher FJ et al. Science 1990;249:1157–61.
45. Ito N, Hirose M. Adv Cancer Res 1989;53:247–303.
46. Powis G. Free Radic Biol Med 1989;6:63–101.
47. Bloemendal H. CRC Crit Rev Biochem 1982;14:1–38.
48. Mandel K, Chakrabarti B, Thomson J, et al. J Biol Chem 1987; 262:8096–102.
49. Simpson PJ, Fantone JC, Lucchesi BR. Myocardial ischemia and reperfusion injury: oxygen radicals and the role of the neutrophil. In: Halliwell B, ed. Oxygen Radicals and Tissue Injury. Bethesda, MD: FASEB, for Upjohn, 1988:63–80.
50. Warren JS, Yabroff KR, Mandel DM et al: Free Radic Biol Med 1990;8:163–72.
51. Halliwell B, Gutteridge JMC. Free Radicals in Biology and Medicine. 2nd ed. Oxford: Clarendon Press, 1989:422–38.
52. Deng HX, Hentati A, Tainer JA et al. Science 1993;261:1047–51.
53. Staal FJT, Roederer M, Israelski R et al. AIDS Res Hum Retroviruses 1992;8:20–9.
54. Staal FJ, Roederer M, Herzenberg LA et al. Proc Natl Acad Sci USA 1990;87:9943–7.
55. Kalebic T, Kinter A, Poli G et al. Proc Natl Acad Sci USA 1991; 88:986–90.

SELECTED READINGS

Gitler C, Danon A, eds. Cellular Implications of Redox Signaling. London: Imperial College Press, 2003.

Halliwell B, Gutteridge JMC. Free Radicals in Biology and Medicine. 2nd ed. Oxford: Clarendon Press, 1989.

Packer L, ed. Methods in Enzymology: Oxygen Radicals in Biological Systems, part C. San Diego: Academic Press, 1994.

Packer L, ed. Methods in Enzymology: Oxygen Radicals in Biological Systems, part D. San Diego: Academic Press, 1994.

Sies H, ed. Oxidative Stress: Oxidants and Anti-oxidants. London: Academic Press, 1991.

Tarr M, Samson R, eds. Oxygen Free Radicals and Tissue Injury. Boston: Birkhauser, 1993.

Weir EK, Archer SL, Reeves JT, eds. Nitric Oxide and Radicals in the Pulmonary Vasculature. Armonk, NY: Futura Publishing, 1996.

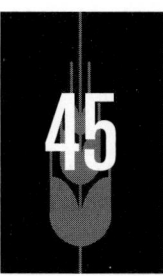

NUTRITION AND THE CHEMICAL SENSES[1]
RICHARD D. MATTES

CHEMOSENSORY SYSTEMS 696
    Gustation 696
    Olfaction 697
    Chemesthesis 697
ASSESSMENT OF CHEMOSENSORY FUNCTION 697
    Threshold Sensitivity 697
    Scaling (Intensity) and Identification 697
    Time Intensity 698
    Hedonics 698
CHEMOSENSORY DISORDERS 698
    Manifestations 698
    Prevalence 699
    Etiology and Management 699
    Health Implications 699
RELATIONSHIPS BETWEEN NUTRITION AND
THE CHEMICAL SENSES 700
    Effects of Nutritional Status on
       Chemosensory Function 700
    Effects of the Chemical Senses on Food Choice
       in Healthy Humans with Special Reference to
       Propylthiouracil Tasting, Aging, and Smoking . . .701
    Effects of the Chemical Senses on
       Nutrient Utilization 702
    Chemical Senses and Diet in Selected
       clinical Populations 702

Taste, smell, and chemesthesis (chemically mediated irritancy) are distinguished from the other human senses (vision, audition, somesthesis) by their transduction of information conveyed by chemical signals from the external and internal environments into electrical signals that can be interpreted and responded to by the central nervous system. The chemical senses are often considered the minor senses, but they have been integral to survival throughout human evolution, and they continue to play vital roles with nutritional implications. One function is to detect and protect against exposure to toxins. Olfaction is a distant sense in that it allows identification of potentially spoiled or unwholesome foods in the environment by the volatile compounds they release. It also contributes to ingestive decisions through detection of volatile compounds released in the oral cavity during mastication. Taste is a more intimate sense requiring contact between foodstuffs and specialized end organs in the oral cavity. The chemesthetic sense contributes information by both mechanisms. Some stimuli, fortunately many toxins, are inherently unpleasant or aversive (e.g., fecal odors, bitter tastes) and elicit rejection responses. Others may acquire negative connotations through associative learning in which an item's sensory properties become linked to a postingestive adverse event (e.g., gastrointestinal distress). Subsequent exposures to such items then result in avoidance. However, both mechanisms can be, and routinely are, overridden through experiences that allow selected foods containing toxic substances (e.g., ethanol, caffeine) to be safely ingested in moderation despite their chemosensory signature. However, the chemical senses are not a fully reliable system to ensure food safety. Approximately 76 million cases of food poisoning occur annually (1), in large part because of a failure of the chemical senses to detect a problematic toxin.

Second, the sensory properties of foods remain a primary determinant of food choice and a modulator of postingestive processes. Taste, in particular, has been linked with nutritive components in the diet. Teleologic arguments have been made that sensitivity to sweetness aids carbohydrate detection and consumption, salt taste is related to electrolyte balance, sourness facilitates avoidance of strong acids, bitterness enables toxin detection and rejection, and umami is a signal for protein sources, and evidence suggests the possibility of a true taste mechanism for dietary fat with particular sensitivity for essential fatty acids (2). Evidence is also available that correction of specific nutrient imbalances (e.g., calcium [3, 4], thiamin [5], amino acids [6]) by exploratory ingestive behavior is guided by chemosensory input. Cultural culinary practices have exerted mixed effects on diet quality. Clay application to foods for the purpose of improving sensory appeal may bind toxins and release essential minerals (7). However, the development of beriberi in Eastern countries is directly related to the preference for and widespread adoption of white rice. Generally, where food availability and cost are not limiting factors, purchasing and ingestive decisions are more strongly determined by sensory factors

---

[1]**Abbreviations: AIDS,** acquired immunodeficiency syndrome; **HIV,** human immunodeficiency virus; **LFA,** learned food aversion.

than by health concerns (8–10). Less well recognized is the fact that sensory stimulation modulates the digestion of foods and the absorption and utilization of nutrients. This role was documented by Pavlov in 1902 through evidence that sensory exposure stimulated gastric motility and acid secretion (11), but the mechanisms and functions of these processes are only now being systematically examined.

Third, the chemical senses add to the quality of life. It has been argued that sensory variety is inherently pleasant to humans, and foods provide a rich source of sensory stimulation. Not inconsequently, the appeal of sensory variety promotes diet diversity and balance. The extent to which extremes in variety exposure result in beneficial or undesired health outcomes is not well defined. Monotonous diets have long been proposed for weight management. Actual prescriptions have varied across foods or food groups (e.g., cabbage diet or very high-protein diet) and generally are effective at promoting weight loss. However, often losses are not maintained, in part because of low acceptability and compliance. More recently, there has been concern that variety may promote positive energy balance. Variety within a meal promotes greater intake (12), but this has limited carryover to subsequent meals (13), in which compensation may occur. Very limited data suggest an inverse association between dietary variety and energy intake (14), but depending on the food groups assessed, this may result in positive (entrees) or negative (vegetables) correlations with body weight. Nevertheless, concern about the influence of variety on energy balance contributed to a decision to omit the long-standing recommendation to consume a varied diet from the 2000 dietary guidelines (15).

Despite widespread recognition of the important roles played by the chemical senses in health and survival, understanding of the basic mechanisms of these senses remains limited, as does knowledge of their role in health promotion or disease remediation. Given the established association between diet and health and the knowledge that food choice is largely, if not primarily, guided by sensory factors (8–10), work in these areas holds great public health and clinical promise.

CHEMOSENSORY SYSTEMS

The three chemosensory systems are distinct anatomically, have different functional characteristics, and contribute unique information. Thus, they may vary independently (e.g., a loss of olfaction does not necessarily result in an alteration of taste). Together with the other senses, they define the flavor of a food. Colloquially, taste and flavor are often, inappropriately, used interchangeably. Olfaction is the predominant contributor to flavor, but variation in any one source of input will alter the overall perceived flavor of a food, much as the loss of a single piece can alter the appearance of a jigsaw puzzle. Variability may be

innate or acquired. The prevalence of innate selective olfactory and gustatory deficits in individuals with otherwise normal senses of smell and taste is high (>50% of the population) (16). The incidence of acquired selective losses resulting from, for example, disease or medication use is not known. Temporary losses attributable to perceptual adaptation following exposure to selected sensory stimuli (17) or acute illness (18) is common. These conditions contribute to individual perceptual variability and virtually ensure that no food is experienced in quite the same way by any two individual persons. Thus, the notion that some food or beverage is of high sensory quality in any absolute sense is illogical. Nonetheless, the fundamental properties of the chemosensory systems are generally applicable.

Gustation

In mammals, the peripheral gustatory system is composed of specialized epithelial cells located on the tongue, soft palate, pharynx, epiglottis, larynx, and upper third of the esophagus. On the tongue, taste cells coalesced in onion-shaped taste buds occur in fungiform, foliate, and circumvallate papillae. The total number of taste buds on a tongue can range from 3000 to 12,000, with a mean of about 5000. Still, taste cells comprise less than 1% of the lingual epithelium. There is a weak but significant association between taste bud number and taste sensitivity (19). Taste receptor cells have rapid turnover times (mean, ~10 days) rendering them highly sensitive to various toxic insults such as chemotherapy or radiotherapy.

Fungiform papillae are mushroom-shaped structures (appearing as red bumps) on the anterior two thirds of the tongue. Approximately 20% of all taste buds are in the fungiform papillae. Taste receptor cells in fungiform papillae receive innervation from the chorda tympani nerve (lingual branch of the facial nerve [cranial nerve VII]). Foliate papillae appear as two to nine folds on the posterior lateral margins of the tongue and contain an average of 120 to 140 taste buds per papillae. Taste buds in the foliate papillae comprise about one third of the oral total. These structures are innervated anteriorly by the chorda tympani nerve and by the glossopharyngeal nerve posteriorly. Eight to twelve circumvallate papillae are arranged in a V-shaped configuration on the posterior dorsal tongue. Each papilla is surrounded by a trench where 200 to 700 taste buds, arranged in tiers on the lower two thirds of the papillae, face the opposing wall of the trench. Taste buds in these structures account for about 50% of the total. Innervation of these taste cells is provided by the glossopharyngeal nerve. The relatively small numbers of taste buds on the epiglottis are innervated by the superior laryngeal branch of the vagus nerve. The greater superficial petrosal nerve subserves taste buds on the soft palate (20, 21). Interneural interactions are considerable. Activity of one may normally inhibit another, and when the former is damaged, the other may compensate and thus prevent a loss of perceptual sensitivity. Unilateral damage to the chorda tympani nerve results in the loss of taste function on the half of the anterior two thirds of the tongue, but patients are often unaware of this loss (22). The concept of a tongue map with regional specificity for different taste qualities is not correct (23).

The prevailing view is that taste is composed of four primary qualities: sweet, salty, sour, and bitter. Two additional qualities have been proposed as primary qualities but do not yield unique singular sensations. Umami is the better accepted of the two. The prototypical stimulus is monosodium glutamate, and taste quality reports include soapy, salty, or bitter. Although tactile cues may be the primary mechanism for detection of dietary fat, accumulating data support the possibility of a taste component for fatty acids as well (2).

Olfaction

Olfactory stimuli consist of volatile molecules. They reach the olfactory epithelium via orthonasal (through the anterior nares) and retrosasal (through the posterior nares of the nasopharynx) routes. A 1- to 2-cm^2 patch of olfactory epithelium is located at the apex of the superior turbinate, although receptor cells are also intermixed with respiratory epithelial cells over a wider area (24, 25). There are about 10^7 receptor cells and about 900 genes coding for different types of receptors (26). This large anatomic investment results in the ability to detect more than 10,000 distinct odors. Little evidence exists for odor primary qualities. The receptors are located on cilial membrane surfaces of the primary olfactory neurons exposed to nasal mucus and the passing air stream. These first-order neurons are unique in two respects. First, they are in direct contact with both the external environment and the central nervous system. Second, they are capable of regeneration. Given the primacy of their location and susceptibility to damage by volatile environmental toxins, the latter characteristic reflects the importance of the sense and undoubtedly accounts for the preservation of function over much of the life cycle. Turnover of primary olfactory neurons occurs in 10 to 15 days.

Chemesthesis

Sensitivity to chemical irritants (e.g., capsaicin, the burning compound in chili peppers) in the oral and nasal cavities is mediated by elements of the somatosensory system. This subpopulation of fibers is often referred to as the trigeminal sense or common chemical sense. The primary somatosensory pathway in the nose and mouth is the trigeminal nerve. Its association with taste and olfaction is so close that these senses may be viewed as an integrated system (27).

ASSESSMENT OF CHEMOSENSORY FUNCTION

Human chemosensory systems have multiple dimensions, and each provides unique functional information. Several rapid screening tests for different attributes have been published (28–31), but they serve primarily as a means to identify patients requiring more extensive evaluation. Because olfactory abnormalities are more common than taste disorders, most commercially available tests focus on olfactory assessment (32–35). Descriptions of more complete assessments are also available (36–39), but there is no widely accepted standard protocol for diagnosis of chemosensory disorders. Generally, testing should be tailored to the nature of the complaint. In addition to a detailed history and relevant clinical tests, the sensory assessment may include measures of one or more of the following attributes: threshold sensitivity, scaling (intensity) and identification, time intensity, and hedonics.

Threshold Sensitivity

Taste and odor threshold sensitivities are not innate, invariant characteristics of an individual. They are the lowest concentrations of a stimulus that can be detected (detection threshold) or recognized (quality recognition threshold) under a given set of conditions at better than an arbitrarily defined level of probability. Generally, thresholds are lower for stimuli in water as compared with more chemically complex foods. The criterion for performance is typically set at 50%, although this may be increased or decreased depending on the consequences of overdiagnosis and underdiagnosis. Thresholds are strongly influenced by numerous environmental and methodologic factors such as patient motivation, education, recent use of oral care products, the number and concentrations of test stimuli, and test instructions. Thus, testing is not a simple practice. Thresholds are an index of sensory system sensitivity but hold little predictive power for suprathreshold sensory responsiveness, hedonics, or food choice.

Scaling (Intensity) and Identification

Intensity ratings reflect the strength of sensation elicited by suprathreshold stimulus concentrations. Generally, a graded series of stimuli is presented in random order in duplicate. A pause or rinse is used between stimuli presentations to avoid adaptation and fatigue effects. For taste and somatosensation, stimulation may be through whole-mouth application (e.g., sipping and swishing a solution) or by regional application to explore the functional status of the various gustatory nerves. For the latter, stimuli may be presented with a cotton-tip applicator. By manipulating the route of olfactory stimulation (orthonasal versus retronasal), it is possible to determine the source of olfactory complaints more accurately. This involves having patients rate stimuli after sniffing or holding them in their oral cavity with the nose open and pinched.

The degree to which chemical irritants (e.g., capsaicin, piperine) interact with taste and odor compounds and influence food flavor is poorly characterized. Although alterations of chemesthesis are not common, because irritants may modify the overall flavor impact of a food, chemesthetic assessment as part of a full evaluation may provide useful clinical information. Most odorants have a pungent quality that complicates evaluation of olfactory function. Independent assessment of the olfactory and trigeminal systems may be accomplished by exploiting the fact that the source of irritation can be localized, whereas this is not the case with olfaction. To differentiate the two, a blank is presented to one nostril and a true stimulus to the other simultaneously. The patient indicates which contains the stimulus. Graded concentrations can be present in this manner to determine threshold or intensity functions.

Time Intensity

The foregoing measures represent integrated information and fail to recognize that the time course of sensation following chemosensory stimulation varies across stimuli and for a given stimulus in different media. Sensation parameters that vary include onset time, rate of appearance, time to maximal intensity, rate of extinction, and total duration. Temporal properties can markedly alter the appeal of foods.

Hedonics

Assessments of food acceptability rely on higher-order processing of intensity and quality information from the periphery. Commonly evaluated hedonic dimensions include, but are not limited to, the preferred frequency of stimulus intake, the preferred concentration of the stimulus in a medium, and preference for stimuli with a characteristic quality.

Hedonic responses to the odors, tastes, and irritants of foods reflect innate and acquired characteristics. Knowledge of innate taste and odor preferences is rudimentary. Compelling data indicate that the appeal of sweetness and saltiness is congenital, although, for the latter, a postnatal lag of about 6 months occurs before it is apparent (40). Data are less clear for responses to sour, bitter, glutamate, and fat, but they suggest that the former two are unpleasant and the latter two are pleasant. Human neonates consistently exhibit a preferential orientation to breast and amniotic fluid odors suggesting early olfactory preferences (41). However, in light of evidence that maternal diet can influence the sensory qualities of amniotic fluid and breast milk (42), it is not clear whether such early preferences are innate or are attributable to fetal conditioning. The basis for the appeal of dietary fats has not been established. Differential sucking responses to formulas with varying fat content among newborns have been small and inconsistent (43, 44), as have heritability estimates for fat preferences and intake in children and adults (45, 46).

The resistance of immigrants to abandon the flavor principles of their native diet underscores the importance of culture and learning on flavor preferences. Multiple mechanisms are likely involved, including exposure effects and associative learning. Studies with children and adults demonstrate a direct association between frequency of exposure to novel items and their acceptance ratings (47). However, quality specificity occurs; sweet and salty novel foods gain in acceptability more readily than do sour or bitter items (48). Exposure frequency can also modify responses to familiar foods. Reduced sensory exposure to dietary salt and fat leads to a heightened preference for foods with lower salt and fat levels, respectively, compared with ratings from persons with similar intakes but higher sensory exposure (18, 49). Preliminary evidence suggests that hedonic shifts based on restricted sensory exposure require about 8 to 12 weeks to develop. The extent to which desired shifts in preferred levels of dietary constituents facilitate long-term compliance with therapeutic diets (e.g., reduced sodium or fat) has not been determined.

The flavors of foods also acquire positive and negative properties as a result of their association with metabolic cues stemming from ingestion. Illness following ingestion of a food can lead to subsequent rejection of that and related items based on their sensory characteristics. Approximately one fourth of the population has such a food aversion (50). Conditioned preferences have been shown in animals, but they have been more difficult to demonstrate in humans.

Whether early hedonic responses are innate or learned, the limited available data do not indicate that they are predictive of preferences later in life. This finding has been documented for selected food constituents such as sugar (51) and salt (52), as well as for diets. Changes in flavor preferences are marked over the life cycle, as exemplified by the early rejection of bitter or spicy foods, yet items with these qualities (e.g., coffee, alcohol, chili peppers) become highly preferred. Indeed, family studies of food preferences generally reveal a low-order association between parents and children, with a stronger relationship among peers (53).

CHEMOSENSORY DISORDERS

Manifestations

Disorders may present as a loss, diminution, distortion, or, rarely, heightened sensation. Losses are termed ageusia (taste) or anosmia (smell) and may be complete or quality specific. Approximately one third of patients reporting to taste and smell centers are anosmic. Ageusia is rare, accounting for less than 1% of patient complaints. Hypogeusia and hyposmia (the most common disorders) are diminutions of sensation that may be generalized or quality specific. Dysgeusia and dysosmia (parosmia) are taste and smell distortions in which patients experience inappropriate and/or unpleasant sensations to common stimuli. A variant of this problem is phantom tastes or smells, which are persistent and often objectionable sensations in the absence of obvious stimuli. This type of condition may be especially problematic with respect to quality of life. Olfactory and gustatory agnosia refers to an inability to identify or classify odor and taste stimuli, respectively. Hyperosmia and hypergeusia are terms for heightened sensation and are rarely encountered.

These disorders may occur alone or in combination. Most patients with a primary chemosensory complaint report that both taste and smell are affected, but this is confirmed in fewer than 10% of cases. Most have only an olfactory disturbance. This finding likely stems from patient confusion over their reduced ability to sense the odorous volatile compounds released from food in the oral cavity via retronasal stimulation. Because the oral cavity is the source of such olfactory stimuli, the sensation they evoke is often incorrectly referred to as a taste.

Prevalence

The prevalence of chemosensory abnormalities in the general population in the United States has been estimated at 3.2 million adults (54), but this is an underestimate because it excludes institutionalized patients who likely have a high prevalence of disorders. In addition, data have not been systematically collected, in part because of a lack of standardized evaluation criteria, low awareness by health care workers who therefore do not solicit information on these senses when evaluating patients, and incomplete reporting by many affected persons who do not view the problem as life-threatening. However, nearly everyone experiences at least a mild transient abnormality (e.g., reduced olfactory ability associated with a cold), and in some persons, the problem is severe and chronic.

Etiology and Management

Chemosensory disorders have multiple causes (28, 55, 56). References of implicated pathologic features, medications, and toxins have been published (28, 57–59), but more than half of these cases can be ascribed to one of three causes. Most frequently, they are associated with upper respiratory tract infection (15–25% of patients). Symptoms may appear suddenly and be persistent, or they may manifest gradually and spontaneously remit. No known treatment exists for abnormalities attributable to viral infection. Damage to peripheral and/or central structures following head trauma accounts for approximately 10 to 20% of patient visits. Aside from surgical reconstruction to facilitate odorant access to the olfactory epithelium, no known treatments exist for chemosensory abnormalities stemming from head trauma. Five to 40% of patients recover olfactory function spontaneously, and the prognosis may be somewhat better for taste. Nasal or sinus disease resulting in obstruction of pathways for odorants to the olfactory epithelium accounts for another 15 to 20%

of cases. Surgical procedures and steroid sprays to reduce swelling have proven effective in some patients (60, 61). Another 15 to 20% of patient complaints are classified as idiopathic. Most chemosensory disturbances related to pathologic processes and medications resolve when the underlying illness is effectively treated or the offending medication is discontinued. Marked nutrient imbalances may adversely affect taste and smell, but are rarely the primary cause. If a nutrient deficiency is not a contributory factor, nutrient supplementation holds little promise of efficacy.

Health Implications

Abnormalities of taste and/or smell can increase the risk of environmental toxin exposure, compromise the quality of life, and adversely affect diet and nutritional status. Among patients presenting at clinical taste and smell centers, approximately 75% report decreased enjoyment of food, and about half adopt compensatory eating patterns. The latter response can be problematic if it involves less healthful dietary choices such as reliance on a limited array of foods or increased use of salt or fat. Fifteen to 20% of patients with a primary taste or smell complaint experience an increase or decrease of body weight exceeding 10% of their predisorder weight (62). Approximately half gain weight because of increased intake as a means to derive the missed sensory pleasure foods provide or as an attempt to mask an unpleasant sensation. Others decrease intake because food has lost its appeal or is believed to exacerbate an unpleasant sensation. At present, no set of patient or symptom characteristics provides a reliable predictor of a specific dietary response.

Should a chemosensory disorder adversely modify diet quality, dietary intervention must be individualized. To do so requires integration of the environmental and physiologic factors influencing food choice. Because disorders may be lifelong, recommendations must be appropriate for long-term adherence. High doses of selected nutrients (zinc, vitamin B_6, vitamin B_{12}) have generally not proven effective (55, 63), and they may pose additional health risks. Flavor fortification has been proposed as a remedy for patients with diminished function (64). However, to date, this has been shown to improve the palatability and intake of a limited set of foods only (65). This approach would not be applicable to patients with a total loss of function or sensory distortions or those reducing intake for nonsensory reasons (e.g., cachexia). It also poses a risk of rendering foods unpalatable to patients with lesser sensory decrements when applied in group settings. Nevertheless, when individualized, this approach may hold promise (66, 67). It may also prove useful to manipulate food attributes not affected by the chemosensory abnormality such as temperature, appearance, and texture (68). The efficacy of such an approach remains largely untested.

RELATIONSHIPS BETWEEN NUTRITION AND THE CHEMICAL SENSES

A reciprocal relationship exists between nutrient intake and chemosensory function. Peripheral gustatory and olfactory tissues are composed of specialized epithelial cells with relatively high metabolic requirements. Provision of adequate nutrients is vital for proper function. The functional status of these sensory systems can influence food intake. Despite long-standing recognition of this association, little is known about the nutrient requirements of these tissues (69).

Effects of Nutritional Status on Chemosensory Function

Vitamin A

Vitamin A deficiency leads to increased keratinization of the oral and nasal epithelia. In addition, decreased mucopolysaccharide synthesis leads to reduced cleansing of the perireceptor area and drying of the epithelia. Blockage of stimulus access to chemosensory receptors ensues. Vitamin A depletion results in a gradual loss of taste in rats (70) that is reversible with vitamin repletion. Chemosensory deficits are not a common feature of vitamin A deficiency in areas where this problem is endemic; however, hypogeusia and hyposmia have been reported in physiologically normal adults made vitamin A deficient as well as in patients with cirrhosis, acute viral hepatitis, and malabsorption disorders who were depleted of the vitamin (71). Supplementation with vitamin A reverses these chemosensory losses. It is important to recognize the role of zinc in maintaining normal plasma vitamin A levels, especially among patients with liver disorders. Zinc administration may also be effective at reducing taste deficits in patients with alcoholic cirrhosis (72). Vitamin A deficiency should be confirmed before supplementation is initiated.

B Vitamins

Studies in dogs reveal that diet-induced deficiencies of niacin, riboflavin, pyridoxine, pantothenic acid, and folic acid result in noninflammatory lesions of the oral mucosa, especially on the dorsal tongue surface (73). Papillary atrophy and degeneration are also observed, particularly on the anterior tongue, although in niacin deficiency, the entire tongue surface may be involved. The fungiform papillae are the most severely affected. No abnormalities have been noted in the circumvallate papillae. Pathologic changes progressively worsen with successive deficiency trials. Replacement therapy results in prompt restoration of the epithelium. Improvement is apparent in 2 to 3 days and is complete within a week. Recovery of connective tissue is slower. Distinct lesions are apparent with specific vitamin deficiencies, and these identifiable lesions are superimposed with multiple deficiencies.

Findings similar to those reported in dogs have been observed in humans (74). In addition, deficiencies of pyridoxine, riboflavin, and cobalamin may lead to peripheral neuropathies. However, this has been reported only in case studies involving severe deficiency (75). Although repletion of pyridoxine has reportedly corrected chemosensory disturbances in patients with subclinical pellagra (75), high levels of pyridoxine have also been associated with peripheral neuropathy (76). In such patients, nonspecific axonal degeneration has been observed with a loss of sensory nerve action potentials in response to an electromyogram. Thus, indiscriminate use of high levels of B vitamins to treat chemosensory disorders is inappropriate.

Vitamin E

A direct association, but no causal relationship, between plasma vitamin E concentration and papillary atrophy was reported in one study of elderly patients with atrophic glossitis (77). No data link vitamin E status to subjective reports of chemosensory function.

Copper

Reversible hypogeusia has been reported in persons with low ceruloplasmin levels during treatment with penicillamine (78). However, it is not clear that the effect of penicillamine is copper specific. The drug also binds zinc, nickel, and other cations, and zinc has also been reported to improve taste sensitivity in patients treated with this medication. Administration of penicillamine to patients with Wilson disease does not lead to chemosensory complaints.

Iodine

Diminutions of taste and olfactory sensitivity or dysgeusias have been documented in hypothyroid patients (79). The reported incidence of sensory complaints in such patients ranges from a few percent to more than 80%. This may be attributable to the generally slow onset of symptoms and the consequent lack of subjective awareness. Replacement hormone therapy generally results in correction of the chemosensory disorder. Treatment of hyperthyroid patients with antithyroid agents (e.g., methimazole, methylthiouracil) has also led to partial or complete loss of taste and smell that resolves on cessation of drug use.

Iron

Hypogeusia has been reported in patients with iron deficiency anemia (80). Normalization of iron status with oral iron supplements (50–100 mg/day) leads to restoration of taste within 2 weeks in most patients and improvement in others. Cravings and pica have been associated with iron depletion, but no evidence indicates that this is related to shifts of chemosensory function.

Zinc

Marked zinc deficiency may lead to chemosensory abnormalities (i.e., hypogeusia, hyposmia, distortions) that resolve with zinc repletion (81). Whether sensory disturbances reported by patients with pathologic features involving negative zinc balance or altered zinc metabolism (e.g., acute infectious hepatitis, chronic cirrhosis of the liver, Crohn disease, chronic renal disease) are attributable to the change in zinc status or to other factors remains largely unresolved. Double-blind crossover studies (82, 83) have not supported a causal role for zinc in most patients with chemosensory complaints. Evidence that levels of zinc recommended for use in patients with chemosensory abnormalities (i.e., 100 mg/day) may lead to anemia, neutropenia, and impaired immune function (84) indicates that this therapeutic approach must be used with caution.

Effects of the Chemical Senses on Food Choice in Healthy Humans with Special Reference to Propylthiouracil Tasting, Aging, and Smoking

It is widely recognized by health care professionals (10) and workers in the food industry (8) that food choice is primarily guided by sensory factors. However, it has been extremely difficult to link this observation to indices of chemosensory function. Three examples in which higher or lower chemosensory sensitivity are hypothesized to alter food choice and nutritional status underscore this point. The first involves genetically based differences in sensitivity to the bitter compound propylthiouracil. Because bitterness is generally viewed as unpleasant, it has been hypothesized that foods with bitter tastes would be less acceptable to very sensitive "supertasters" than to nontasters, and this would result in differential disease risk. Theoretically, nontasters would be at increased risk of goiter and alcoholism because of greater acceptance of bitter goitrogen-inducing foods and alcohol, respectively, whereas supertasters would be at increased risk of cancer because of lower intake of bitter phytochemical-rich cruciferous vegetables. However, neither situation has been substantiated, for various reasons. First, as noted, some bitter foods have positive nutritive value, so an innate rejection response would not necessarily optimize diet wholesomeness or quality. Second, the acceptability of bitter foods can be modified by dietary experience. Overtly bitter items such as coffee and wine are highly regarded. Third, bitter foods are commonly modified by processing and by culinary practices to improve their appeal. Fourth, responsiveness to bitterness may change over the life cycle or as a result of health changes or medication use. Finally, bitterness has multiple transduction mechanisms, so sensitivity to one bitter compound may not translate to equal sensitivity to other bitter compounds in foods.

Aging is a second example in which widely held assumptions about a close link between chemosensory ability and diet must be carefully evaluated. Statistically significant declines in taste and especially smell sensitivity have been reported in many, but not all, studies of elderly persons (85). These declines are typically small in absolute magnitude and of slow onset. Further, they are highly variable, a finding suggesting that they are not a biologic imperative. To reconcile these observations with the high level of complaints of diminished sensory abilities by elderly persons requires consideration of more subtle aspects of sensory function and testing. Elderly persons exhibit slower recovery following adaptation to a stimulus, reduced retronasal olfaction (a large component of food flavor), and compromised ability to discriminate stimuli in complex foods. These measures are not generally included in standard chemosensory testing regimens. Increased use of medications and a higher prevalence of health disorders that may influence sensory function may also contribute to the belief that aging is associated with marked declines in chemosensory function. Changes are more profound in institutionalized elderly persons, who likely have poorer health (86). Finally, age-related decrements in memory, cognition, and testing skills can result in poorer testing. The decline in taste bud number with age is not closely correlated with taste function because only a small number of buds may provide the full range of sensory experience (much as a small patch of skin can convey temperature information as well as a larger area), and losses of sensation in one area of the oral cavity are compensated by receptive structures in other areas (87). The nutritional implications of age-related chemosensory changes are uncertain (88, 89). They are poorly correlated with diet quality (90, 91). This may stem from adjusted flavor expectations. Decreased sensitivity to selected qualities does not necessarily translate into reduced flavor appreciation, just as red-green color blindness does not preclude appreciation of visual art. Indeed, diminished sensitivity to less pleasant chemosensory stimuli may aid food acceptance by improving flavor profiles (92) and by reducing neophobic responses to less familiar foods introduced for health benefits.

Third, smoking is commonly presumed to alter chemosensory function and, as a consequence, ingestive behavior. However, the preponderance of evidence indicates that smoking has little effect on taste. Studies of taste thresholds before and immediately after smoking a cigarette (93, 94), or following 2-week periods of enforced increased and decreased smoking frequency (95), reveal no significant differences. Comparisons of long-term smokers and nonsmokers, controlling for recent use, have yielded mixed findings (96–98). Perceived intensity ratings also show little difference between smokers nonsmokers (100). Studies of taste hedonics have focused on sweetness and have yielded mixed findings (99, 100).

Early work on olfaction showed no significant general elevation of thresholds (93, 101). Small but significant differences in perceived intensity ratings (102, 103) and odor identification (101) have been reported more recently. Whether the effects are attributable to smoking is questioned by evidence that smokers have elevated thresholds for other sensory modalities (e.g., audition [104]) presumably unaffected by smoking status. Cigar and pipe smoking has not altered test performance. At present, no evidence supports a causal role for smoking-related chemosensory changes in the lower body weight of smokers or their increase in weight on cessation of smoking.

Effects of the Chemical Senses on Nutrient Utilization

A role of sensory stimulation in the digestion, absorption, and utilization of nutrients has been recognized for a century, but it remains poorly characterized. Processes that occur as food passes through the gastrointestinal tract are initiated by sensory, especially chemosensory, stimulation. These preabsorptive or cephalic phase responses (105) are generally smaller in magnitude than those occurring during the digestive, absorptive, and postingestive periods and are transient. They may peak within 4 to 5 minutes of sensory exposure and return to baseline in 10 to 15 minutes. Examples of such responses are listed in Table 45.1 (106–117). Their primary function may be to modulate food digestion and nutrient absorption and utilization. They may hold positive and negative health implications. Bypassing the chemosensory systems by infusion of glucose (118), blocking the acute-phase insulin response to glucose ingestion by somatostatin infusion (119), and infusing insulin only 15 minutes after meal initiation in patients with type I diabetes (120) resulted in greater postprandial glycemic responses. Thus, sensory stimulation aids glucose tolerance. In contrast, oral exposure to dietary fat promotes a prolonged postprandial triacylglycerol elevation (121). This is largely the result of an effect on lipid absorption, but influences on de novo hepatic lipid synthesis and/or decreased lipid clearance may also be involved.

TABLE 45.1. HUMAN CEPHALIC PHASE RESPONSES

SYSTEM (REFERENCE)	INCREASED RESPONSE
Salivary (106)	Flow
Gastric (107–109)	Acid gastrin and gut peptide secretion, motility
Intestinal (88, 109–111)	Lipase, amylase, trypsin, chymotrypsin, total digestive enzyme secretion, gut peptides, lipid absorption
Pancreatic endocrine (112–114)	Insulin, glucagon, pancreatic polypeptide
Thermogenic (115)	Heat production
Cardiovascular (116)	Heart rate, cardiac output, resistance of mesenteric vasculature
Renal (117)	Volume (decreased osmolality) to hypotonic stimulus

Chemical Senses and Diet in Selected Clinical Populations

Cancer

Changes of chemosensory function (sensitivity and preferences) are frequently reported by patients with untreated cancer. Systematic study of these complaints has failed to identify any consistent pattern of change with respect to the nature of the sensory complaint (e.g., quality specific versus general loss, loss versus distortion) and the site, severity, or duration of disease. Similarly, no clear association between sensory function and anorexia has been established in this patient population (122, 123). Antineoplastic treatment may be more problematic for the sensory systems than the cancer. Radiotherapy involving gustatory and olfactory tissues results in a profound loss of function caused by damage to the sensory end organs as well as supporting tissues (e.g., salivary glands) (124). Bitter and salty tastes are often more severely affected than sweet and sour tastes. Impairment is first apparent following an accumulated dose of approximately 20 Gy. A total dose of 60 to 70 Gy may lead to elevated thresholds (i.e., decreased sensitivity) that persist for years (123), whereas suprathreshold function may be less severely affected (125). An association exists between loss of sensory function and weight among patients with head and neck cancer who are receiving radiotherapy. Altered chemosensory function may also result from chemotherapy regimens, but the impact of these changes on diet is less clear (126).

It is commonly argued that learned food aversions (LFAs) contribute to anorexia and weight loss in cancer patients. In patients with untreated cancer, the incidence of aversions is about 50%, but following the onset of either chemotherapy or radiotherapy, approximately 50 to 55% of patients form new LFAs. High-protein items are particularly problematic, but any item, including water, may be targeted (127). Typically, treatment-related aversions are specific (a mean of three to four items per individual) and transient (often less than 1 month in duration); consequently they hold little dietary significance. Several approaches aimed at preventing the formation of LFAs have been explored. First, patients may be counseled to refrain from eating before treatments, but evidence that LFAs may form toward items consumed the day before or following treatment indicates that such advice is often not practical. Antiemetics administered to reduce the adverse side effects of treatments (the purported conditioning stimulus) have also proven ineffective. One approach that appears promising involves exposing patients to a nutritionally inconsequential food just before their first treatment. This may interfere with the formation of LFAs toward wholesome foods in the patient's customary diet. Such an approach has reduced the incidence of treatment-related LFAs by more than 30% (128).

Diabetes

Disturbances of taste and smell in patients with diabetes have long been recognized (129) and may affect more than 60% of patients. The most consistent sensory changes involve alterations in glucose taste thresholds among patients with non–insulin-dependent diabetes as well as their nondiabetic first-degree relatives. This finding suggests a general abnormality of glucose receptors. However, complications of hyperglycemia probably also contribute because the severity of hypogeusia increases with progressing neuropathy (130). Macrovascular disease and peripheral neuropathy have also been implicated in olfactory disturbances (131, 132). Despite considerable speculation, no association between chemosensory changes and food choice has been objectively documented (133).

Human Immunodeficiency Virus Infection

Changes of chemosensory function in persons infected with human immunodeficiency virus (HIV) may stem from opportunistic infections, oral disease, medication use, and/or neurologic complications. No clear association has emerged with fatigue, age, or lymphocyte count. The severity of olfactory complications, most notably odor identification ability, is directly related to the progression of disease. The most marked olfactory changes are present in patients with acquired immunodeficiency syndrome (AIDS) dementia complex (134). Few changes of taste have been reported (135). The limited available data do not support a substantive role for chemosensory disturbances in the loss of appetite associated with infection, although this has not been evaluated in patients with AIDS (136).

Hypertension

The view that sodium intake is related to hypertension has prompted studies of salt taste in various high-risk populations including different classes of hypertensive patients (e.g., low versus high renin, salt sensitive versus salt insensitive) and normotensive children of hypertensive patients. Small differences between some of these groups and control subjects on isolated measures of salt taste (i.e., recognition thresholds) have been noted. However, the preponderance of work has failed to reveal any meaningful associations (137, 138). Further, no clear evidence indicates a heightened preference for salt by hypertensive patients. Normotensive and hypertensive persons exhibit a comparable increment in hedonic responses to reduced-salt foods following adherence to a diet restricted in sensory exposure to the salty taste.

Liver Disease

Altered chemosensory acuity is a common finding in patients with acute and chronic liver disease, although the association between subjective and objectively measured changes is weak (139). Appetite is also often poor, and investigators have hypothesized that diminished perception of sweetness and heightened awareness of bitterness contribute to reduced food appeal and intake (140). However, changes of sensory function are not well correlated with food preferences (139). Repletion of vitamin A in deficient patients improves chemosensory function (71), as does liver transplantation (141). Zinc supplementation has yielded mixed success.

Obesity

Although small differences in sensory responses to aqueous solutions of taste stimuli or experimentally prepared foods have been noted between obese and lean persons (142, 143), the preponderance of evidence fails to support an association between body weight and chemosensory responses (144–146). Differences in the importance and nature of food and flavor preferences are reported more consistently (147) and may lead to erroneous assumptions about sensory function. Given the paucity of data indicating that sensory responses among obese persons actually influence their eating behavior, assumptions that sensory factors play an etiologic role in the onset or maintenance of obesity are not currently appropriate.

Renal Disease and Dialysis

Patient complaints of diminished chemosensory sensation are supported by evidence that taste detection and recognition thresholds are elevated in patients with chronic uremia, as well as in patients undergoing intermittent dialysis or continuous ambulatory peritoneal dialysis (148–150). Concomitant low levels of zinc in some studies and improved sensory function with zinc supplementation (151, 152) prompted hypotheses that this may be the underlying cause. However, additional data showed no correlation between zinc status and sensory measures (148, 153, 154) and a lack of therapeutic efficacy of zinc supplementation (155, 156). There may be a subset of patients with compromised zinc status who will benefit from supplementation, but many patients will require alternative approaches. Some reports showed that dialysis has no effect or that it exacerbates or improves sensory deficits (149, 153, 154, 157). The lack of consistency among reports calls into question a role for accumulating uremic toxins, fatigue, cognitive impairment, or anticoagulants. Renal transplantation can improve chemosensory function, but it may require an extended period (i.e., up to 1 year) (158). The limited published data on hedonic shifts associated with uremia and dialysis are inconsistent (157, 159, 160). The influence of sensory changes on food selection and nutritional status remains poorly characterized.

REFERENCES

1. Mead PS, Slutsker L, Dietz V et al. Emerg Infect Dis 1999; 5:607–25.
2. Mattes RD. Food Aust 2003;55:510–4.
3. Richter C, Eckert J. Endocrinology 1937;21:50–4.
4. Leshem M, Del Cacho S, Schulkin J. Physiol Behav 1999; 67: 555–9.
5. Rozin P. J Comp Physiol Psychol 1969;69:126–32.
6. Naito-Hoopes M, McArthur L, Gietzen D. Physiol Behav 1993; 53:485–94.
7. Johns T, Duquette M. Am J Clin Nutr 1991;53:448–56.
8. Giese J. Mod Food Tech 1994;48:106–16.
9. Glanz K, Basil M, Maibach E et al. J Am Diet Assoc 1998;98: 1118–26.
10. National Dairy Council. Dietary Guidelines and Children's Nutrition: A Survey of Health Care Professionals. Rosemont, IL: National Dairy Council, 1995.
11. Pavlov V. The Work of the Digestive Glands. London: Charles Griffin, 1902:76–92.
12. Rolls ET. J Neurophysiol 1996;75:1970–81.
13. Hetherington M, Rolls B, Burley,V. Appetite 1989;12:57–68.
14. McCrory M, Fuss P, McCallum J et al. Am J Clin Nutr 1999; 69:440–7.
15. US Department of Agriculture (USDA). Nutrition and Your Health: Dietary Guidelines for Americans. Home and Garden Bulletin no. 232. Washington, DC: Department of Health and Human Services, 2000.
16. Amoore JE. Chem Sens 1977;2:267–81.
17. Dalton P. Chem Sens 2000;25:487–92.
18. Mattes RD. Am J Clin Nutr 1993;57:373–81.
19. Delwiche JF, Buletic Z, Breslin PAS. Percept Psychophys 2001; 63:761–76.
20. Sandick B, Cardello AV. Chem Sens 1981;6:197–214.
21. Mistretta CM. Gerontology 1984;3:131–6.
22. Lehman CD, Bartoshuk LM, Catalanotto CF et al. Physiol Behav 1995;57:943–51.
23. Bartoshuk LM. Taste. In: Atkinson RC, Herrenstein RJ, Lindzey G et al, eds. Stevens' Handbook of Experimental Psychology. 2nd ed. New York: Wiley, 1988:5–26.
24. Nakashima T, Kimmelmann CP, Snow JP. Arch Otolaryngol 1984;110:641–6.
25. Leopold D, Hummel T, Schwob J et al. Laryngoscope 2000; 110:417–21.
26. Sullivan SL. Neuroreport 2002;13:A9–10.
27. Green BG. Food Qual Pref 2002;14:99–109.
28. Mott AE, Leopold DA. Med Clin North Am 1991; 75: 1321–53.
29. Davidson T, Murphy C. Arch Otolaryngol Head Neck Surg 1997;123:591–4.
30. Hummel T, Nesztler C, Kallert S et al. Chem Sens 2001;26:118.
31. Duff K, McCaffrey RJ, Solomon GS. Clin Neurosci 2002; 14:197–201.
32. Yoshida M. Bull Fac Sci Eng Chuo Univ 1984;27:343–53.
33. Kobal G, Hummel T, Sekinger B et al. Rhinology 1996;34: 222–6.
34. Hummel T, Sekinger B, Wolf S et al. Chem Sens 1997;22: 39–52.
35. Doty RL. The Smell Threshold Test: Administration Manual. Haddon Heights, NJ: Sensonics, 2000.
36. Cain WS. Ear Nose Throat J 1989;68:322–8.
37. Leopold D. Chem Sens 2002;27:611–5.
38. Shusterman D. Chem Sens 2002;27:551–64.
39. Heckmann S, Habiger S, Wichmann M et al. Chem Sens 2003;28:e24.

40. Beauchamp GK, Cowart BJ, Moran M. Dev Psychobiol 1986; 19:17–25.
41. Varendi H, Porter RH, Winberg J. Acta Paediatr 1996; 85: 1225–7.
42. Mennella JA, Beauchamp GK. Olfactory preferences in children and adults. In: Laing DG, Doty RL, Breipohl W, eds. The Human Sense of Smell. Berlin: Springer-Verlag, 1992:167–80.
43. Chan S, Pollitt E, Leibel R. Infant Behav Dev 1979;2:201–8.
44. Nysenbaum AN, Smart JL. Early Hum Dev 1982;6:205–13.
45. Falciglia GA, Norton PA. J Am Diet Assoc 1994;94:154–8.
46. Oliveria SA, Ellison RC, Moore LL et al. Am J Clin Nutr 1992;56:593–98.
47. Pliner P, Pelchat M, Grabski M. Appetite 1993;20:111–23.
48. Mattes RD. Physiol Behav 1994;6:1229–36.
49. Bertino M, Beauchamp GK, Engelman K. Am J Clin Nutr 1982;36:1134–44.
50. Mattes RD. Physiol Behav 1991;50:499–504.
51. Beauchamp GK, Moran M. Appetite 1984;5:291–305.
52. Beauchamp GK, Cowart B, Moran M. Dev Psychobiol 1986; 19:17–25.
53. Borah-Giddens J, Falciglia GA. J Nutr Ed 1993;25:102–7.
54. Hoffman H, Ishii E, Macturk R. Ann NY Acad Sci 1998; 855: 716–22.
55. Deems DA, Doty RL, Settle G et al. Arch Otolaryngol 1991;117:519–28.
56. Nordin S, Murphy C, Davidson TM et al. Laryngoscope 1996; 106:739–44.
57. Schiffman SS. Drugs influencing taste and smell perception. In: Getchell TV et al, eds. Smell and Taste in Health and Disease. New York: Raven Press, 1991:845–50.
58. Doty RL, Bartoshuk LM, Snow JB Jr. Causes of olfactory and gustatory disorders. In: Getchell TV et al, eds. Smell and Taste in Health and Disease. New York: Raven Press, 1991:449–62.
59. Rankin KM, Mattes RD. Toxic agents, chemosensory function, and diet. In: Massaro EJ, ed. Handbook of Human Toxicology. Boca Raton, FL: CRC Press, 1997:347–67.
60. Lildholdt T, Rundcrantz H, Bende M et al. Arch Otolaryngol Head Neck Surg 1997;123:595–600.
61. Wolfensberger M, Hummel T. Chem Sens 2002;27:617–22.
62. Mattes RD, Cowart BJ. J Am Diet Assoc 1994;94:50–6.
63. Gibson R, Smit Vanderkooy PD, MacDonald AC et al. Am J Clin Nutr 1989;49:1266–73.
64. Shiffman SS. J Nutr 2000;130:927S–30S.
65. Griep M, Mets T, Massart D. Br J Nutr 2000;83;105–13.
66. Schiffman SS. Food Rev Int 1998;14:321–33.
67. Mathey MF, Seibelink E, deGraaf C et al. J Gerontol 2001;56:200–5.
68. Cassens D, Johnson RD, Keelan S. Natl Rev 1996;51S–4S.
69. Gershoff SN. The role of vitamins and minerals in taste. In: Maller O, Kare MR, eds. The Chemical Senses and Nutrition. New York: Academic Press, 1977.
70. Reifen R, Orly A, Weiser H et al. Metabolism 1998;47:1–2.
71. Garrett-Laster M, Russell RM, Jacques PF. Hum Nutr Clin Nutr 1984;38C:203–14.
72. Weismann K, Christensen E, Dreyer V. Acta Med Scand 1979;205:361–6.
73. Afonsky D. Ann NY Acad Sci 1960;85:362–7.
74. Afonsky D, Changsha H. Oral Surg Oral Med Oral Pathol 1950;3:1299–327.
75. Green RF. JAMA 1971;218:1303.
76. Schaumburg H, Kaplan J, Windebank A et al. N Engl J Med 1983;309:445–8.
77. Drinka PJ, Langer EH, Voeks SK et al. J Am Coll Nutr 1993; 12:14–20.

78. Henkin RI, Keiser HR, Jaffe IR et al. Lancet 1967;2:1268.
79. Mattes RD, Heller AD, Rivlin RS. Abnormalities in suprathreshold taste function in early hypothyroidism in humans. In: Meiselman HL, Rivlin RS, eds. Clinical Measurement of Taste and Smell. New York: Macmillan, 1986.
80. Osaki T, Ohshima M, Tomita Y et al. J Oral Pathol Med 1996;25:38–43.
81. Henkin RI. Biol Trace Elem Res 1984;6:263–80.
82. Henkin RI, Schecter PJ, Friedewald WT et al. Am J Med Sci 1976;272:285–99.
83. Gibson RS, Vanderkooy PDS, MacDonald AC et al. Am J Clin Nutr 1989;49:1266–73.
84. Fosmire GJ. Am J Clin Nutr 1990;51:225–7.
85. Murphy C, Cain WS, Hegsted DM. Nutrition and the Chemical Senses in Aging: Recent Advances and Current Research Needs. New York: Annals of the New York Academy of Sciences, 1989.
86. Spitzer ME. J Gerontol 1988;43:71–4.
87. Kveton JF, Bartoshuk LM. Laryngoscope 1994;104:25–9.
88. Mattes RD. J Am Diet Assoc 2002;102:192–5.
89. Kim W, Hur M, Cho M et al. Nutr Res 2003;23:723–34.
90. Griep MI, Verleye G, Franck AH et al. Eur J Clin Nutr 1996;50:816–25.
91. De Jong N, De Graf C, VanStaveren A. Physiol Behav 1996;60:1453–62.
92. Drewnowski A. Nutr Rev 2001;59:163–9.
93. Pangborn RM, Trabue IM, Barylko-Pikielna N. Percept Psychophys 1967;2:529–32.
94. Krut LH, Perrin MJ, Bronte-Stewart B. BMJ 1961;1:384–7.
95. Pangborn RM, Trabue IM. Percept Psychophys 1973;1:139–44.
96. Sinnot JJ, Rauth JE. J Gen Psychol 1937;17:151–3.
97. Krut LH, Perrin MJ, Bronte-Stewart B. BMJ 1961;1:384–8.
98. McBurney DH, Moskat LJ. Percept Psychophys 1975;18:71–3.
99. Perkins KA, Epstein LH, Stiller RL et al. Pharmacol Biochem Behav 1990;35:671–6.
100. Pomerleau C, Garcia A, Drewnowski A. et al. Pharmacol Biochem Behav 1991;40:995–9.
101. Moncrieff RW. Am Perfumer 1957;72:40–3.
102. Ahlström R, Berglund B, Berglund U et al. Am J Otolaryngol 1987;8:1–6.
103. Frye RE, Schwartz BS, Doty RL. JAMA 1990;263:1233–6.
104. Berglund B, Nordin S. Chem Sens 1992;17:291–306.
105. Brand JG, Cagan RH, Naim M. Annu Rev Nutr 1982;2:249–76.
106. Richardson CT, Feldman M. Am J Physiol 1986;250:G85–91.
107. Feldman M, Richardson CT. Gastroenterology 1986;90:428–33.
108. Katschinski M, Dahmen G, Reinshagen M et al. Gastroenterology 1992;103:383–91.
109. Wisén O, Björvell H, Cantor P et al. Regul Pept 1992;39:43–54.
110. Novis BH, Banks S, Marks IN. Scand J Gastroenterol 1971;6:417–22.
111. Behrman HR, Kare MR. Proc Soc Exp Biol Med 1968;129:343–6.
112. Teff KL, Engelman K. Am J Physiol 1996;270:R1371–9.
113. Louis-Sylvestre J, LeMagnen J. Neurosci Biobehav Rev 1980;4:43–6.
114. Teff K, Devine J, Engelman K. Physiol Behav 1995;57:1089–95.
115. Diamond P, Brondel L, LeBlac J. Am J Physiol 1985;248:E75–9.
116. Vatner SF, Patrick TA, Higgins CB et al. J Appl Physiol 1974;36:524–9.
117. Akaishi T, Shingai T, Miyaoka Y et al. Chem Sens 1991;16:277–81.
118. Teff K. Appetite 2000;34:206–13.
119. Calles-Escandon J, Robbins D. Diabetes 1987;36:1167–72.
120. Kraegen EW, Chisholm DJ, McNamara ME. Horm Metab Res 1981;13:365–7.
121. Mattes RD. J Nutr 2001;131:1491–6.
122. Trant AS, Serin J, Douglass HO. Am J Clin Nutr 1982;36:45–58.
123. Carson, JAS, Gormican A. J Am Diet Assoc 1977;70:361–5.
124. Mossman KL. Br J Cancer 1986;53:9–11.
125. Schwartz LK, Weiffenbach JM, Valdez IH et al. Physiol Behav 1993;53:671–7.
126. Bruera E, Carraro S, Roca E et al. Cancer Treat Rep 1984;68:873–6.
127. Mattes RD, Curran WJ, Alavi J et al. Cancer 1992;70:192–200.
128. Mattes R. Nutr Cancer 1994;21:13–24.
129. Settle RG. Diabetes mellitus and the chemical senses. In: Meiselman HL, Rivlin RS, eds. Clinical Measurement of Taste and Smell. New York: Macmillan, 1986.
130. Abbasi AA. Geriatrics 1981;36:73–8.
131. Weinstock RS, Wright HN, Smith DU. Physiol Behav 1993;53:17–21.
132. Le Floch J-P, Le Lièvre G, Labroue M et al. Diabetes Care 1993;16:934–7.
133. Tepper B, Hartfiel L, Schneider S. Physiol Behav 1996;60:13–8.
134. Brody D, Serby M, Etieene N et al. Am J Psychiatry 1991;148:248–50.
135. Graham C, Graham B, Barlett J et al. Physiol Behav 1995;58:287–93.
136. Mattes RD, Wysocki CJ, Graziani A et al. Laryngoscope 1995;105:862–6.
137. Mattes RD. J Chronic Dis 1984;37:195–208.
138. Mattes RD, Falkner B. Chem Sens 1989;14:673–9.
139. Madden A, Bradbury W, Morgan M. Hepatology 1997;26:40–8.
140. Deems R, Deems M, Friedman L et al. Appetite 1993;20:209–16.
141. Bloomfield R, Graham B, Schiffman S et al. Physiol Behav 1999;66:203–7.
142. Rodin J, Moskowitz HR, Bray GA. Physiol Behav 1976;17:591–7.
143. Drewnowski A, Brunzell JD, Sande K et al. Physiol Behav 1985;35:617–22.
144. Spitzer L, Rodin J. Appetite 1981;2:293–329.
145. Frijters JER, Rasmussen-Conrad EL. J Gen Psychol 1982;107:233–47.
146. Pangborn RM, Bos KEO, Stern JS. Appetite 1985;6:25–40.
147. Drewnowski A. Int J Obesity 1985;9:201–12.
148. Burge JC, Park HS, Whitlock CP et al. Kidney Int 1979;15:49–53.
149. Conrad P, Corwin J, Katz L et al. Nephron 1987;47:115–8.
150. Middleton RA, Allman-Frainelli, MA. J Nutr 1999;129:122–5.
151. Mahajan SK, Prasad AS, Lambujon J et al. Am J Clin Nutr 1980;33:1517–21.
152. Atkin-Thor E, Goddard BW, O'Nion J et al. Am J Clin Nutr 1978;31:1948–51.
153. Vreman HJ, Venter C, Leegwater J et al. Nephron 1980;26:163–70.

154. Ciechanover M, Peresecenschi G, Aviram A et al. Nephron 1980;26:20–2.

155. Zetin M, Stone RA. Clin Neurol 1980;13:20–5.

156. Henkin RI, Schechter PJ, Friedewald WT et al. Am J Med Sci 1976;272:285–99.

157. Bellisle F, Dartois A-M, Kleinknecht C et al. J Am Diet Assoc 1990;90:951–4.

158. Mahajan SK, Abraham J, Migdal SD et al. Transplantation 1984;38:599–602.

159. Shepherd R, Farleigh CA, Atkinson C et al. Appetite 1987; 9:79–88.

160. Shapera MR, Moel DI, Kamath SK et al. J Am Diet Assoc 1986;86:1359–65.

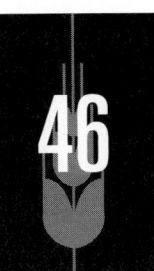

46 CONTROLS OF FOOD INTAKE[1]

GERARD P. SMITH

MEALS AND THE CONTROLS OF FOOD INTAKE 707
CONTROLS OF MEAL SIZE .708
    Peripheral Controls from the Gut 708
    Peripheral Controls from the Pancreatic Islets 710
    Peripheral Controls from Adipose Tissue 710
    Peripheral Controls from the Gonads 711
    Interactions among Peripheral Controls 711
    Leptin and Central Peptides 712
    Neuropeptide Y 712
    Conditioned Orosensory Controls 713
    Direct and Indirect Controls 713
CONTROLS OF MEAL NUMBER 714
    Effective Stimuli 714
    Central and Peripheral Mechanisms 715
GENETICS OF HYPERPHAGIA 715
FOOD AND DRUGS 716
    Ethanol 716
    Sugars and Amphetamine 716
TRANSLATION BETWEEN ANIMAL
    AND HUMAN RESEARCH 716
CONCLUSION 717

Eating is how animals acquire energy. The amount of energy acquired is a function of the amount and kinds of food ingested. Thus, food intake is one term in the fundamental energy equation:

$$\text{Intake of energy} - \text{Expenditure of energy} = \text{Storage of energy}$$

---

[1] **Abbreviations: AGRP,** agouti-related peptide; **α-MSH,** α-melanocyte-stimulating hormone; **CART,** cocaine and amphetamine-regulated transcript; **C75,** inhibitor of fatty acid synthase; **CCK,** cholecystokinin; **CCK_1,** receptor subtype 1 of the cholecystokinin receptors; **DA,** dopamine; **db/db mouse,** mouse that has a null mutation of the leptin receptor ($Lepr^{db}/Lepr^{db}$); **fa/fa rats,** rats with a genetic mutation of the leptin receptor that reduces transport of the receptor to the cell surface and signaling efficiency ($Lepr^{fa}/Lepr^{fa}$), also known as Zucker rats; **fa(f)/fa(f) rats,** rats with a null mutation of the leptin receptor ($Lepr^{faf}/Lepr^{faf}$), also known as Koletsky rats; **FAS,** fatty acid synthase; **GLP-1,** glucagonlike peptide-1; **MC_4 receptor,** subtype 4 of melanocortin receptors; **MCH,** melanin-concentrating hormone; **NTS,** nucleus tractus solitarius; **NPY,** neuropeptide Y; **ob/ob mouse,** mouse that does not synthesize normal leptin (Lep/Lep); **P,** postnatal day; **POMC,** proopiomelanocortin; **PVN,** paraventricular hypothalamic nucleus.

The major site of energy storage is white adipose tissue. Changes in the mass of adipose tissue are produced by inverse changes of intake and expenditure: fat mass increases most when intake increases and expenditure decreases; fat mass decreases most when intake decreases and expenditure increases. These relationships among intake, expenditure, and storage of energy are referred to as *nutritional homeostasis*.

Nutritional homeostasis is the framework in which the controls of eating have been investigated since Curt Richter's seminal observations in the 1930s. Richter demonstrated that when a nutritional deficit was produced by imposing a dietary deficiency, intake of a normal diet increased until the deficit was abolished (1). This was the critical demonstration of a specific nutritional control functioning homeostatically, and it was considered an experimental model of nutritional deficiencies that occurred in animals and humans eating deficient diets because of ecologic constraints. This idea, derived from specific and identifiable deficiencies, was then stretched to cover the increased eating that occurred after periods of food deprivation.

The cycles of metabolic depletion and repletion that control intake in the service of nutritional homeostasis, however, do not occur when access to food and water is unlimited and environmental temperature and health are stable. Despite the absence of metabolic depletion and repletion, the amount and kind of food ingested under these conditions vary widely as a result of the palatability of the diet, diurnal and estrogenic rhythms, ecologic constraints, such as patchiness of food and predator density, social stimuli, conditioned stimuli, and cognitive, cultural, religious, and aesthetic stimuli in humans. The biologic and medical importance of eating under these conditions is widely acknowledged; the fact that nutritional homeostatic controls do not account for this eating is not. Thus, nutritional homeostatic controls are important, but they are only one of many controls of eating (2), and as diet-induced obesity shows, nutritional homeostatic controls are inadequate to prevent hyperphagia and obesity when rodents and humans have easy access to palatable food.

MEALS AND THE CONTROLS OF FOOD INTAKE

Food intake is determined by the size and number of meals. The size of meals affects nutrient partitioning: long-term ingestion of large meals increases fat storage more than the ingestion of the same number of calories in more frequent, small meals (3), and abnormally large meals characterize all the monogenic obesities in rodents and humans in which meal size has been measured (see the later discussion on the genetics of hyperphagia). Therefore, the analysis of the controls of food intake consists of identifying the relevant stimuli and neural and endocrine mechanisms that initiate eating (the number of meals) and that maintain and stop eating after it begins (the size of meals).

CONTROLS OF MEAL SIZE

The size of meals is determined by the brain's integration of peripheral and central mechanisms that maintain eating and those that stop it. Analysis of this integration consists of (a) identifying the kind, potency, and sites of sensory stimuli provided by the food eaten, (b) specifying the peripheral mechanisms that transmit peripheral signals to the brain, and (c) determining the molecular mechanisms of the central networks in the brain that process the sensory information and integrate it into a command for starting or stopping eating. The sites of the peripheral controls of meal size are the mouth, stomach, small intestine, pancreatic islets, adipose tissue, and gonads.

Peripheral Controls from the Gut

The controls from the gut are activated by chemical and mechanical stimuli of ingested food contacting the mucosal surface of the gut from the mouth to the end of the small intestine during each meal. The importance of these controls was demonstrated by comparing meal size when rats sham fed a diet with meal size when rats ate the diet normally. The most common form of sham feeding in

rats consists of draining ingested liquid food out of a chronic gastric fistula. This prevents food from accumulating in the stomach or emptying into the duodenum (Fig. 46.1). Rats *always* ate significantly *more* nutrient liquids during sham feeding than during real feeding (4). The larger intake during sham feeding demonstrated the importance of two kinds of peripheral feedback control. The first was positive from the mouth: Orosensory stimulation *alone* was sufficient to maintain eating during sham feeding, and the rate of eating was a function of the concentration of orosensory stimuli, such as sucrose and corn oil (4). The second was negative from the stomach and small intestine. The evidence for negative-feedback control was that when the postingestive effects of food were eliminated by sham feeding, intake increased significantly. When prior experience with the diet, hours of food deprivation, phase of the diurnal and estrogenic rhythms, and environmental temperature were held constant, meal size was determined by the brain's integration of the potencies of the peripheral positive and negative feedbacks (Fig. 46.2).

Mechanisms of Positive-Feedback Control

When food contacts the surfaces of the tongue and palate, the sensory information is used by the brain to continue or to stop eating. This neural decision is based on the stimuli of the food and prior experience with eating it. Some food stimuli (e.g., sweet) are intrinsically acceptable, and some (e.g., bitter) are intrinsically aversive. Most of these decisions to eat or not to eat, however, are based on prior experience with acceptable stimuli. If that experience produced sickness, the previously acceptable stimuli are rejected, and eating stops. Conversely, if prior experience was nonaversive or

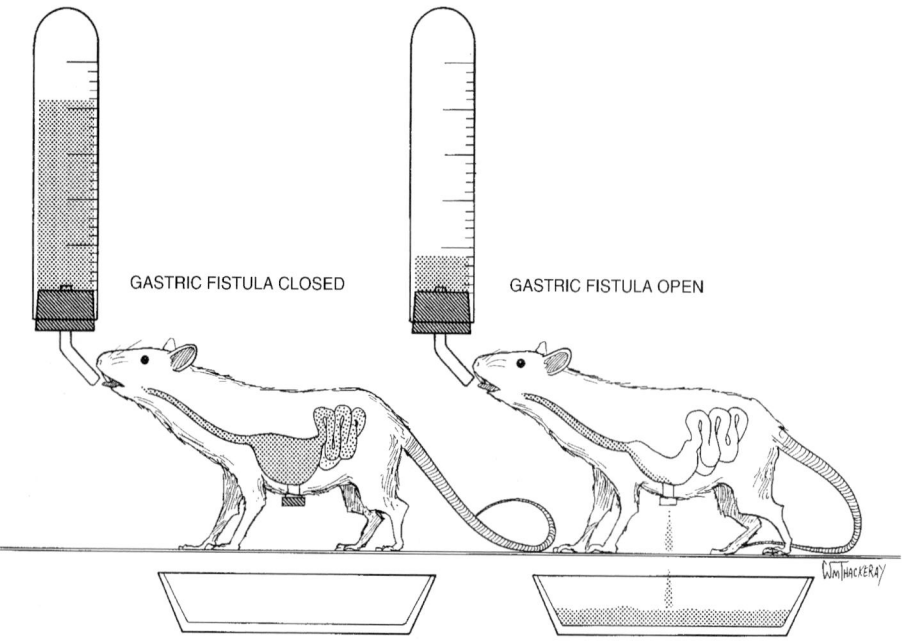

GASTRIC FISTULA CLOSED   GASTRIC FISTULA OPEN

Figure 46.1. Chronic gastric fistula rat preparation for sham feeding. When the cannula is opened during a test **(right),** ingested food drains out of the stomach so the postingestive negative-feedback effects of food are minimized or eliminated. Outside the test situation, the cannula is closed with a screw cap **(left),** ingested food is digested and absorbed normally, and the rat maintains normal nutrition and body weight. (From Smith GP, Gibbs J, Young RC. Fed Proc 1974;33:1146–9, with permission.)

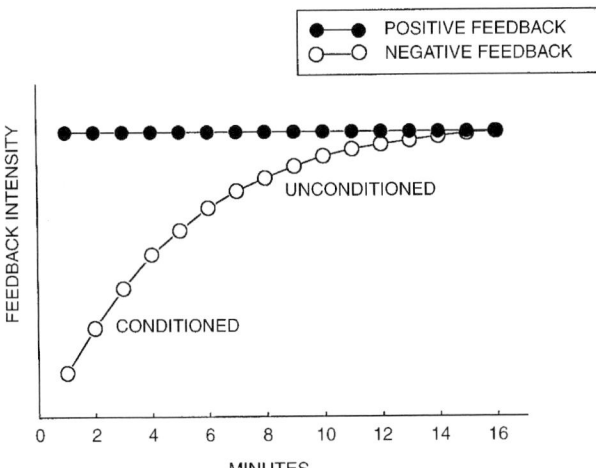

Figure 46.2. Temporal interaction of positive-feedback effects from the mouth and negative-feedback effects from the stomach and small intestine produced by ingested carbohydrate solutions during a scheduled meal. Eating stops and the meal ends when the central potencies of the peripheral feedbacks are judged to be equal by a comparator function of the brain. The negative-feedback effect early in the meal is a conditioned orosensory effect, but the negative feedback during the later part of the meal is unconditioned. The positive-feedback effect can be unconditioned but is usually conditioned. (From Smith GP, Davis JD, Greenberg D. In: Bray GA, Ryan DH, eds. Molecular and Genetic Aspects of Obesity. Pennington Medical Center Nutrition Series, vol 5. Baton Rouge, LA: Louisiana State University Press, 1996:161–74, with permission.)

positive, eating continues. Decisions based on the effects of prior experience are the result of learned associations between oral stimuli and other oral or postingestive stimuli (see the later section on Conditioned Orosensory Controls).

Once the decision to continue occurs, oral stimuli stimulate eating and produce positive feedback. The potency of positive feedback is determined by the concentration of adequate oral stimuli. These include monosaccharides, disaccharides, and polysaccharides, fatty acids, oils, and textural stimuli. Orosensory stimuli are transduced into neural activity of the gustatory afferent fibers of cranial nerves VII, IX, and X and the sensory fibers of the trigeminal nerve. All these afferent fibers project directly to the rostral nucleus tractus solitarius (NTS) in the hindbrain. Orosensory stimuli also stimulate olfactory receptors through the retronasal route, and the olfactory fibers project first to the forebrain and then to the hindbrain.

The positive-feedback potency of oral stimuli is modulated by the duration of food deprivation and by prior experience. When deprivation is long (e.g., overnight), an orosensory stimulus is more potent than when deprivation is 3 hours or less. Potency is also increased when prior experience has produced a conditioned preference for the orosensory stimuli (see the later discussion of Conditioned Orosensory Controls).

Dopamine (DA) and opioids are the main transmitters in the brain that mediate the positive-feedback potency of orosensory stimuli, particularly sweet taste (5), but evidence

indicates that excitatory amino acids, cannabanoids, and neuropeptide Y (NPY) are probably also involved.

In addition to the central mechanisms of positive feedback, a peripheral cholinergic mechanism that can be blocked by peripheral atropinization is necessary for the positive-feedback effect of orosensory stimuli during sham feeding (6). Neither the site of this peripheral cholinergic mechanism nor how it interacts functionally with the central mechanisms of positive feedback is known.

The positive feedback of orosensory stimuli is what drives eating during a meal. It is one aspect of the rewarding effect of food. Deeper understanding of the neural mechanisms that mediate the rewarding effect of food is important in itself, is probably relevant to hyperphagia in obesity and binge eating in a variety of eating disorders in humans, and is likely to provide information about the common mechanisms underlying the similarities between ingesting sugars and self-administering psychostimulant drugs (see the later section on Food and Drugs).

Mechanisms of Negative-Feedback Control

The stomach is one site of negative-feedback control of meal size (Fig. 46.3). Investigators have used a reversible pyloric cuff to isolate the postingestive negative-feedback effect of food stimuli to the stomach by preventing food stimuli from emptying into the small intestine during a meal. When postingestive food stimuli are restricted to the stomach, meal size is normal under a variety of conditions, but if gastric negative feedback is abolished by removing the food from the stomach, intake increases (4). The adequate stimulus for gastric negative feedback is volume, not nutrients (7). Volume produces distention that is monitored by mechanoreceptors of afferent fibers of the abdominal vagus nerve (8), but the importance of this vagal afferent input for gastric negative feedback is controversial. It is possible that spinal visceral afferent fibers and locally released bombesin-like peptides are involved in gastric negative feedback, but their physiologic importance has not been demonstrated.

The small intestine also provides significant postingestive negative-feedback control of meal size. The adequate stimuli are protein and its digestive products, monosaccharides, and fatty acids. All these stimuli act preabsorptively on receptors in the mucosa of the small intestine. Thus, negative feedback from the small intestine, like negative feedback from the stomach, is a sensory effect of ingested food.

The digestion products of ingested food stimulate preabsorptive receptors on vagal afferent terminals and on endocrine cells. The endocrine cells release numerous peptides. Glucagon was the first to be scrutinized for negative-feedback effects on eating (9), and peptide YY and glucagonlike peptide-1 (GLP-1) are the most recent (10). However, cholecystokinin (CCK) released from the small intestine is the *only* peptide that has been demonstrated to

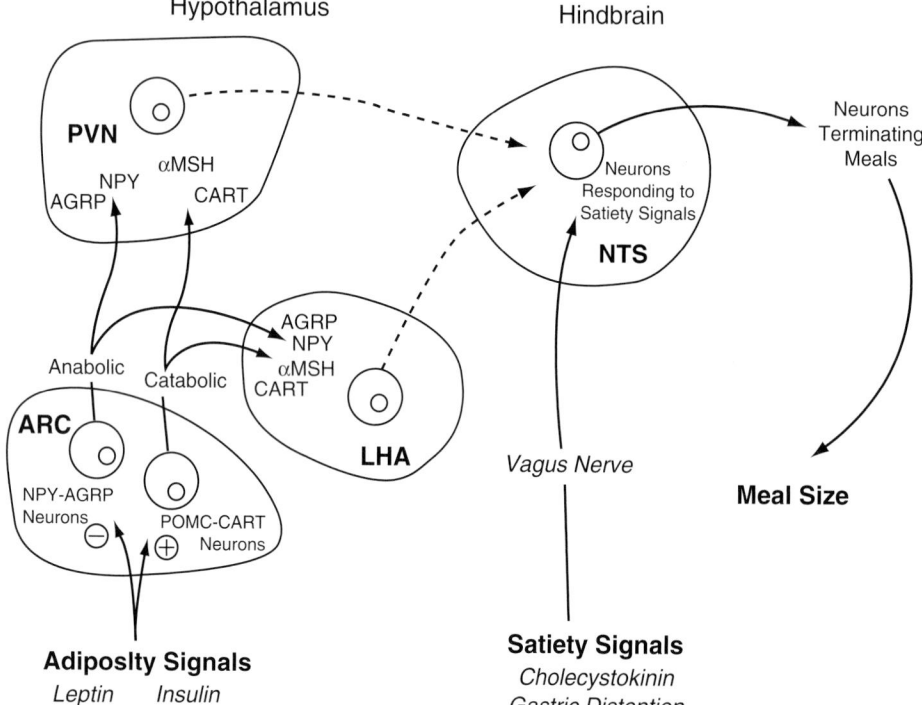

Figure 46.3. Schematic diagram of the relationship of some of the peripheral and central mechanisms of the control of meal size. Satiety signals arising in the periphery, such as gastric distention and cholecystokinin (CCK) are relayed by vagal afferent nerves to the nucleus of the solitary tract in the hindbrain. Leptin and insulin, the two circulating adiposity signals, enter the brain and interact with receptors in the arcuate nucleus (ARC) and other brain areas. These adiposity signals inhibit medial ARC neurons that synthesize neuropeptide Y (NPY) and agouti-related peptide (AgRP) and stimulate lateral ARC neurons that synthesize proopiomelanocortin (POMC), the precursor of α-melanocyte-stimulating hormone (α-MSH), and cocaine and amphetamine-related transcript (CART). These ARC neurons, in turn, project to other hypothalamic areas, including the paraventricular nuclei (PVN) and the lateral hypothalamic area (LHA). Catabolic signals from the PVN, possibly mediated by corticotrophin-releasing factor and oxytocin, and anabolic signals from the LHA are integrated with peripheral satiety signals in the nucleus tractus solitarius (NTS) to control meal size. (From Porte D Jr, Baskin DG, Schwartz MW. Nutr Rev 2002; 60:S20–9, with permission.)

have a negative-feedback effect under physiologic conditions in a number of animals and humans (11). CCK acts through a paracrine mode in the rat to stimulate afferent terminals of vagal mechanoreceptors in the small intestine. Thus, these vagal afferent terminals are a site of peripheral integration of mechanical and chemical stimulation (8).

Peripheral Controls from the Pancreatic Islets

Preabsorptive products of intraluminal digestion not only stimulate negative-feedback mechanisms from the small intestine, but also stimulate the release of glucagon, insulin, and amylin from the pancreatic islets. These pancreatic hormones have negative-feedback effects on meal size (12). Glucagon's negative-feedback effect is more clearly established than that of insulin. The liver is the site of action for glucagon, and hepatic vagal afferent fibers mediate the satiating effect under some conditions. In contrast, the area postrema, a circumventricular organ that lies on top of the fourth cerebral ventricle, is the site of action of the inhibitory effect of amylin.

The peripheral negative-feedback effects of insulin and amylin are produced by their release during a meal. Both

peptides also decrease eating through a central action that results from their cumulative release over time and is discussed in the next section.

Peripheral Controls from Adipose Tissue

In 1953, Kennedy proposed that fat mass exerted an inhibitory control on eating (13). This lipostatic hypothesis postulated that the plasma concentration of a hormone or other humoral signal that was directly correlated with the mass of fat provided inhibitory control of food intake and body weight by acting on the ventromedial region of the hypothalamus. Kennedy suggested that loss of this inhibitory control was the cause of the marked hyperphagia and obesity observed after bilateral lesions of the ventromedial hypothalamus.

Woods and colleagues proposed pancreatic insulin as the inhibitory signal (14). Although insulin was not produced by adipose tissue, its basal concentration was correlated with fat mass in humans and animals. This finding satisfied one of the criteria for the signal.

How did the basal concentration of insulin affect the brain to decrease eating? Insulin entered the brain by a specific transport mechanism in the wall of cerebrovascular capillaries, and it produced neuronal effects by binding to specific receptors on nerve cells in the ventromedial hypothalamus and other brain regions. A key part of the evidence was that infusions of insulin into the third ventricle near the ventromedial hypothalamus decreased meal size, but when these same infusions were given peripherally, they had no effect (15).

If the identification of insulin as an adiposity signal was the result of physiologic insight, the identification of the second adiposity signal, leptin, was the result of a systematic search by Leibel and Friedman to identify the mutant gene responsible for the hyperphagia and obesity of the ob/ob mouse. The mutant gene (*Lep^{ob}*) was found on mouse chromosome 6 (16). Positional cloning techniques demonstrated that the *Lep* gene encoded for a peptide that was secreted by fat cells into the circulation. The peptide was called leptin for its hoped-for ability to produce thinness. Normal leptin was not synthesized in the ob/ob mouse. The lack of leptin caused the hyperphagia and obesity in the ob/ob mouse because peripheral administration of leptin reversed the syndrome completely.

When leptin was tested in db/db mice, however, leptin had no effect on the hyperphagia or obesity. The failure of the db/db mouse to respond to leptin was explained by the discovery that the db/db mouse had a null mutation of the gene for the leptin receptor (*Lepr^{db}*) on chromosome 4 (17, 18).

These results stimulated investigation of the role of endogenous leptin in rodents and humans. Leptin was shown to be important in the increased intake and gain of body weight that occurred after 24 to 48 hours of food deprivation. Deprivation decreased plasma leptin to very low levels; the increased food intake during refeeding restored body weight and plasma leptin to normal. The importance of the low concentration of leptin to the increased intake during refeeding was demonstrated by administering leptin peripherally or into the third ventricle of the brain during refeeding. Such leptin treatment decreased intake. Similar results were obtained with insulin (15).

Although the results during refeeding suggested a role for low plasma leptin or insulin in the increased eating after food deprivation, it did not provide insight into the problem of hyperphagia and obesity in animals or humans who develop obesity in the context of easy access to palatable foods. As fat mass increases in diet-induced obesity, plasma leptin and insulin increase, but hyperphagia and weight gain continue. Thus, as the plasma concentrations of endogenous leptin and insulin increase over time, their inhibitory effects on food intake decrease. This phenomenon is referred to as *leptin* or *insulin resistance*. It is important that the resistance is not permanent; significant weight loss abolishes it.

Although the mechanisms of resistance are not known, Banks and colleagues recently reported that high concentrations of triglycerides decrease the transport of leptin across the blood-brain barrier (19). Furthermore, when drug treatment lowered the concentration of triglycerides, leptin transport increased. These results suggest new approaches to the treatment of leptin resistance.

Leptin is just one of several peptides (adipokines) secreted by adipocytes. Others include tumor necrosis factor-α, acylation-stimulating protein, adiponectin, angiotensinogen, and resistin (20, 21). Some evidence indicates that tumor necrosis factor-α decreases food intake (22), and the others may affect intake through actions on energy expenditure, nutrient partitioning, and insulin resistance. The role of adipokines in the control of food intake deserves more experimental attention.

Fatty acid synthase (FAS), a key enzyme for the synthesis of long-chain fatty acids, is present in adipose tissue, brain, liver, and lung. Inhibitors of this enzyme, such as C75, decrease food intake and block the usual homeostatic increases of central neuropeptides, such as NPY, and of plasma fatty acids and ketones to decreased food intake and low plasma concentrations of leptin (23–25). This results in substantial loss of body weight in mice with genetic obesity (*Lep^{ob}/Lep^{ob}*) and diet-induced obesity . The body weight loss is the result of loss of adipose tissue and fat in the liver. Decreased intake does not account for all the weight loss; C75 also produces a significant increase in energy expenditure apparently by increasing fatty acid oxidation (26).

The anorexic and energy expenditure effects of C75 have been observed mainly after peripheral administration, but the same effects also occur after central administration into the third or lateral ventricle (27, 28). The suggested mechanisms of the central effects of C75 include hypothalamic malonyl-coenzyme A (29, 30), hypothalamic adenosine monophsophate–activated protein kinase (28), and increased glucose metabolism by the brain (31). Although the effects of inhibitors of FAS are interesting for the development of new anorectic drugs, the implication of this work for the physiologic control of meal size and meal initiation is not clear.

Peripheral Controls from Gonads

Ovarian estrogen is the other peripheral hormonal negative-feedback control of eating (32). Plasma estrogen has a 4- to 5-day rhythm in rodents. It peaks on the evening of proestrus and then declines to basal levels. During the 24 hours after estrogen peaks, estrogen decreases food intake by decreasing meal size. The satiating effect of estrogen is mediated through estrogen receptor-α (33). In contrast to the inhibitory effect of leptin, melanocortin 4 receptors (MC$_4$) are not necessary for the inhibitory effect of estrogen (34). Testosterone has little or no effect on food intake (35).

Interactions among Peripheral Controls

Meal size is determined by the brain's integration of the potencies of the peripheral positive and negative feedbacks stimulated by the ingestion of food (see Fig. 46.2). These preabsorptive controls from the gut are fundamental because they are stimulated directly by the food that is eaten during every meal. Their potency is a function of the concentration and volume of the ingested and digested food. If volume and concentration of the food being eaten were the only determinants of the potencies of the peripheral feedbacks, however, the size of the meal of a specific food would be constant and predictable. That is not the case—the size of a meal of a specific food varies widely because the potencies of the gut feedbacks are modulated by other factors, such as the duration of deprivation, prior experience with the food, the difficulty of access to the food, adiposity signals, and phase of the diurnal or estrogenic rhythm.

For example, the potency of orosensory positive feedback is increased by food deprivation. This is probably the result of increased release of NPY (see later) and increased release of DA in the nucleus accumbens of the brain (5). The potency of the orosensory positive feedback is also increased when a rat has learned a conditioned flavor-flavor or flavor-nutrient preference. This learned increased potency of orosensory positive feedback is also accompanied by increased release of accumbens DA.

The potency of postingestive negative feedback from the small intestine mediated by the release of intestinal CCK is increased by leptin, insulin, and estrogen (11). Estrogen also increases the inhibitory effect of glucagon (36). The inhibitory potency of CCK, however, is decreased in the dark phase of the diurnal cycle (4).

The finding that the central effects of adiposity signals, such as leptin and insulin, exert most, if not all, of their effect on meal size by increasing the potency of the negative-feedback effect of peripheral CCK released by the food eaten is relevant to the traditional distinction of short-term signals that control the size of a single meal and long-term signals that control meal size over many meals and thus have an important effect on body weight. This is usually discussed as if these two controls of meal size were acting through parallel and separate central neural systems. This is no longer coherent, however, because *the effects of long-term controls on meal size cannot be measured in the absence of the peripheral feedbacks stimulated by the ingested food* (see the later section on direct and indirect controls). Thus, the effects of long-term controls and their central peptide or amine mechanisms on meal size can be expressed only through their modulation of the potencies of the peripheral feedbacks from the gut (37–39).

Leptin and Central Peptides

The analysis of how leptin decreased eating uncovered a new central network of peptide controls of eating (40, 41). Although the receptors for leptin are widespread throughout the brain, the arcuate nucleus in the ventromedial hypothalamus is a nodal point for leptin's action. Leptin

stimulates a lateral population of arcuate neurons containing proopiomelanocortin (POMC) and cocaine and amphetamine-regulated transcript (CART) that inhibit intake; leptin inhibits a medial population of arcuate neurons that contain NPY and agouti-related peptide (AGRP) that stimulate eating (see Fig. 46.3). Recent neurophysiologic evidence suggests that leptin's excitatory and inhibitory effects on these two populations of neurons involve rapid changes in the number of excitatory and inhibitory synapses and postsynaptic currents on NPY and POMC neurons (42).

α-Melanocyte-stimulating hormone (α-MSH) released by POMC neurons acts on MC_4 receptors in the hypothalamus and probably in the hindbrain (43). Stimulation of MC_4 receptors is necessary for leptin's inhibition of food intake, because when a specific antagonist blocks the MC_4 receptor, leptin does not inhibit food intake. Furthermore, MC_4 knockout mice are hyperphagic and obese despite high levels of circulating leptin.

Identification of the functional relationships of these peptides for mediating the decreased intake produced by leptin sparked anatomic investigations that used immunocytochemical techniques to trace connections from NPY-AGRP neurons to orexin and melanin-concentrating hormone (MCH) neurons in the lateral hypothalamus and projections of NYP-AGRP neurons and POMC neurons to the paraventricular hypothalamic nucleus (PVN) in the anteromedial hypothalamus and to the hindbrain, especially in the region of the NTS.

Corticotropin-releasing factor (CRF) is also involved in the inhibitory effect of leptin. The role of other peptides, such as orexin A, GLP-1, ghrelin, apolipoprotein-4, MCH, syndecan, and mahogony protein, in the action of leptin is not clear.

Neuropeptide Y

Leptin's inhibitory effect on NPY neurons is an important mediator of leptin's inhibitory effect on food intake. When the plasma concentration of leptin is reduced by food deprivation, NPY expression increases, and NPY stimulates eating during the refeeding period until the concentration of leptin becomes normal and NPY expression is inhibited. Disinhibition of NPY also stimulates eating when leptin's inhibitory action is blocked by mutations of leptin synthesis (ob/ob mouse) or mutations of the leptin receptor (db/db mouse, fa/fa rat, and fa(f)/fa(f) rat; see the later discussion of the Genetics of Hyperphagia). The evidence for this is that genetic knockout of NPY reduced the hyperphagia of ob/ob mice and administration of an NPY antagonist abolished the hyperphagia of fa/fa rats (44).

The stimulation of eating by NPY also occurs during a spontaneous meal (45) when plasma leptin's action is normal and food deprivation has not occurred. This stimulation is produced by NPY neurons in the arcuate nucleus that project to the PVN and release NPY there. NPY increases intake primarily by increasing meal size, although it can also initiate eating (see the later section on Controls of Meal Number). NPY increases meal size by increasing the potency of orosensory positive feedback without changing the potency of postingestive negative feedback. Central DA and opioids mechanisms are necessary for the increased potency of orosensory positive feedback produced by NPY. The opioid mediation of the effect of NPY depends on connections between the forebrain and hindbrain, because blockade of opioid function in the NTS blocks the stimulating effect of NPY on eating (46).

These results with NPY are a good example of how it is possible to do a top-down analysis of the functional meaning of a central peptide from its effect on intake, to an effect on meal size, to changes of the potency of peripheral feedbacks, to the central site of release and action, and to some of other neural systems required for its action. This demonstrates that the report of a peptide stimulating or inhibiting food intake is not the end, but the beginning, of an investigation of effects and mechanisms at behavioral, neural, and neurochemical levels of analysis. Until the numerous central peptides and amines reported to increase or decrease food intake have been characterized in this manner, their relative importance in the normal controls of eating will not be known, their specific contribution to pathologic hyperphagia cannot be assessed, and their therapeutic potential will be obscure (9).

Conditioned Orosensory Controls

As successful omnivores, rats and humans forage, discriminate foods from water and poisons, and learn preferences and aversions by associating taste or flavors with postingestive stimuli through Pavlovian conditioning. Thus, learning about eating goes on all the time because every meal provides a large number of orosensory and postingestive stimuli for association.

Conditioned Preferences

Two kinds of conditioned preference exist: (a) flavor-flavor and (b) flavor-postingestive nutrient (47). The flavor-postingestive nutrient associations appear to be more potent than the flavor-flavor associations. Conditioned preferences based on flavor-postingestive associations reveal the ability of the rat to detect and discriminate specific postingestive stimuli and to use them to form associations with flavors. The site and adequate stimulus of these postingestive mechanisms are unknown and are under active investigation.

Central dopaminergic and opioid systems that mediate orosensory positive feedback have been investigated as mediators of conditioned preferences. Central dopaminergic mechanisms, particularly those mediated by D_1 receptors, are important in the acquisition and expression of conditioned preferences, but central opioid mechanisms are apparently not involved (5).

Conditioned Aversions

Associations between tastes or flavors and an aversive or toxic postingestive stimulus form conditioned aversions (48). For example, conditioned aversions occur in rats eating an imbalanced diet of amino acids (49) and in humans undergoing chemotherapy for cancer (50).

The most common experimental procedure for producing a conditioned taste aversion is to pair the ingestion of sucrose with toxic doses of lithium chloride. Formation of the conditioned taste aversion reverses the hedonic response to sucrose from unconditioned preference to learned aversion. This qualitative hedonic change results from alterations of the processing of sucrose in the amygdala and gustatory cortex of the forebrain, rather than from changes in the hindbrain or in the transduction of orosensory stimuli in the mouth (51).

Conditioned Orosensory Negative Feedback

Conditioned orosensory negative feedback occurs during the first 5 minutes of a liquid meal. It results from prior association between the orosensory stimuli and postingestive stimuli during real feeding. The most important postingestive stimulus is the osmolality of liquid foods. The higher the osmolality, the stronger the conditioned negative feedback will be (52). The association is acquired within two meals during real feeding, and it extinguishes within two or three sham-fed meals. This conditioned negative feedback decreases intake to prevent the aversive effect of loading the small intestine with hypertonic gastric contents ("dumping syndrome"). It probably depends on stimulation of small intestinal osmoreceptors, and this information is carried to the brain by vagal afferent fibers.

Direct and Indirect Controls

The stimulation of eating by NPY in the hypothalamus depends on opioid mechanisms in the hindbrain. This illustrates the fundamental point that the neural integration of eating depends on reciprocal connections between the forebrain and the caudal brainstem. This has been established by the analysis of eating in the chronic decerebrate rat (53).

Chronic decerebration cuts all the connections between the caudal brainstem and forebrain (Fig. 46.4), and these rats never initiate eating despite being able to walk around, climb, and groom themselves. Despite this total lack of spontaneous eating, the decerebrate rat eats if milk or other liquid food is infused into its mouth through a chronically implanted oral catheter. Ingestion continues until the decerebrate rat is satiated and allows the infused liquid to drip out of its mouth.

Thus, the chronic decerebrate rat, like neurologically intact rats, eats meals. The only controls of meal size that function in the decerebrate rat are the afferent nerves that

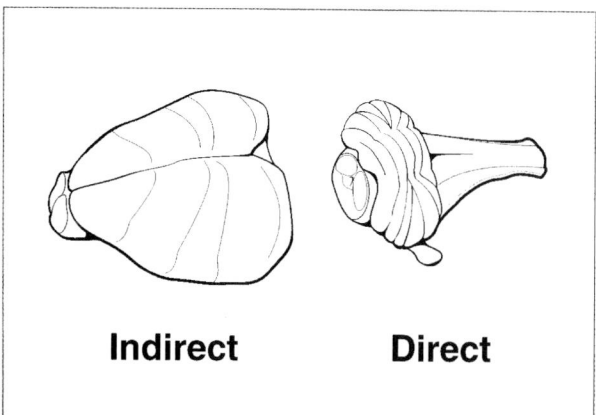

Indirect   **Direct**

Figure 46.4. Schematic illustration emphasizing that chronic decerebration disconnects the forebrain **(left)** from the caudal brainstem **(right).** The feedback controls from mouth, stomach, and small intestine that are activated by direct contact with preabsortive food stimuli project directly to the caudal brainstem behind the disconnection. The caudal brainstem has sufficient neural complexity to integrate these *direct controls* of meal size. In contrast, all other controls of meal size do not share these two characteristics of the direct controls, and they consititute the *indirect controls* of meal size. The decrebrate rat does not respond to *indirect controls* because they are dependent on intact connections between the forebrain and caudal brainstem. When the connections are intact in the normal rat, eating is the integrated action of *indirect* and *direct controls* of meal size.

mediate the peripheral feedbacks from the mouth, stomach, and small intestine and enter the hindbrain behind the decerebrating lesion, and this anatomic fact allows them to influence the amount eaten. The decerebrate rat, however, is not capable of integrating internal metabolic changes, environmental contingencies, or prior experience into its control of eating because these controls depend on the reciprocal connections between the forebrain and hindbrain that were cut by the decerebrating lesion.

All the controls of meal size in the decerebrate rat are the result of *direct* peripheral stimulation of receptors in the mucosa of the mouth, stomach, and small intestine. These peripheral stimuli are carried to the hindbrain by afferent fibers that project *directly* to the hindbrain. These are the *direct controls* of eating. All the other controls of eating are *indirect controls* (2, 37, 38). They include the controls necessary for nutritional homeostasis, the inhibitory effects of peptides related to the size of the fat mass, learning about eating, and the effects of the diurnal and estrogens rhythms. The finding that *direct* and *indirect controls* depend on the same final common motor output of the hindbrain for eating movements is the neurologic constraint that makes it impossible to measure the function of the *indirect controls* in the absence of *direct controls*. The effect of the *direct controls*, however, can be measured in the absence of indirect controls in the decerebrate rat because they are the only controls that function after the disconnection of the forebrain from the caudal brainstem.

CONTROLS OF MEAL NUMBER

Effective Stimuli

The external stimuli for the controls of meal initiation are extracted from the ecologic structure of the environment by learning: Lights, odors, places, and other environmental stimuli associated with access to food become conditioned stimuli for the initiation of eating in animals (54). Once a conditioned stimulus is perceived, the difficulty of obtaining food affects the number of times eating is initiated (55). In humans, effective stimuli for meal initiation include work and family schedules and various kinds of cultural events (56).

Although learned external stimuli associated with prior experience of finding and eating food dominate the initiation of eating in complex environments, three internal stimuli may be involved when rats live alone in a cage: (a) a decrease of activity-independent metabolic rate, (b) a pattern of small changes of plasma glucose concentration, and (c) the amount of food consumed in the last meal.

The decrease of metabolic rate is correlated with the initiation of eating, but it is not clear that it is causal (57). In contrast, a probably causal relationship between a pattern of changes of plasma glucose and the initiation of eating has been demonstrated in rats eating alone (58). The pattern consists of an approximately 12% decrease in plasma glucose beginning about 10 minutes before a meal. While plasma glucose is returning to baseline, rats begin to eat. If food is not available while the plasma glucose is returning to normal, eating does not begin, and the next meal is not initiated until the same pattern of changes of plasma glucose appears hours later. Although this pattern of changes of plasma glucose is sufficient to initiate eating under these isolated conditions, it is not necessary because the presentation of food or its conditioned stimulus initiates eating in the absence of these changes.

The correlation between glucodynamics and meal initiation has also been observed in humans when they are studied after less than a day of loss of some time cues. The correlation was not observed, however, in humans isolated for weeks from temporal and other environmental cues (59).

The size of a meal determines the interval until the next meal begins under some (54), but not all (60), conditions. It has been assumed that this relationship depends entirely on the postabsorptive metabolic effects of the ingested food. This assumption is not correct because sham feeding after 3 hours of deprivation produces an intermeal interval that is about half of that produced by a normal meal in rats (4). Given the marked effects of this orosensory, preabsorptive mechanism, the relative importance of preabsorptive and postabsorptive effects of a meal on the postprandial intermeal interval and the initiation of the next meal is an open question.

Central and Peripheral Mechanisms

Central administration of catecholamines (norepinephrine and DA) and peptides, such as opioids, NPY, galanin, orexins, CART, MCH, and AGRP, can initiate eating. Ghrelin, a peptide released from the stomach before a meal, also initiates eating. Unlike the other peptides that act centrally, ghrelin not only acts centrally, but also acts peripherally by stimulating vagal afferent fibers. It is not known which of these candidate molecules mediates the initiation of eating in response to specific external or internal stimuli.

Eating may also be initiated by the decay of the inhibitory action of postingestive negative-feedback mechanisms that terminate a meal. For example, if gastrin-releasing peptide is administered peripherally within 15 minutes after a meal ends, the initiation of the next meal is delayed (61).

Woods argued that the autonomic and metabolic changes that occur just before a meal are important for the metabolism and distribution of the ingested food. These visceral changes are learned, and they are proposed to be crucial for dealing with the digestive and metabolic load of a large meal (3). It is possible that the mechanisms for initiating eating also integrate these visceral changes.

GENETICS OF HYPERPHAGIA

The first decade of applying molecular genetic techniques to monogenic syndromes of obesity and hyperphagia in rodents has been very productive. Extensive and detailed information exists about specific mutations and their associated syndromes (62, 63). It is now clear that mutations of central or peripheral controls of food intake can produce obesity.

How does a genetic mutation express a behavioral phenotype such as hyperphagia? The frequent answer is that mutation of gene x causes hyperphagia. This assumes that the relationship between gene and behavior is linear, even homuncular. The expression of a behavioral phenotype, however, is subject to epigenetic factors during embryogenesis and development. Furthermore, in the case of a behavioral phenotype, such as hyperphagia, the expression of a genetic mutation is measured by changes in the *range* of adequate stimuli and motor responses, not by the presence or absence of the behavior. Phenotypic expression of genes for the controls of eating is analog, not digital.

It is interesting that all monogenic hyperphagias in which meals have been measured are characterized by bigger meals, rather than by more frequent meals. The magnitude of the hyperphagia depends on the genetic background in which the mutation occurs and the diet that the mutant rodent eats. The effect of genetic background on expression shows that the effect of genetic mutations is modified by other genes. The effect of different diets shows that the expression of hyperphagia in mutant rodents is through the effect of the mutation on the potency of positive and negative feedbacks produced by the diets.

It is axiomatic that the precision of the measure of the phenotype is a major limiting factor of the power of the experimental analysis of treatments of monogenic hyperphagia. For example, attempts to rescue the hyperphagia that occurs in mice with mutations of the leptin receptor have been considered successful because the amount eaten in 24 hours by the rescued mice was significantly less than the amount eaten by the mutant mice (64). However, 24-hour intakes are crude measures of hyperphagia. What needs to be shown is that the genetic rescue restored the normal size of meals and the normal diurnal pattern of meals on this and other diets.

Investigation of monogenic heterozygote mutations, such as $+$/Lep^{ob} and $+$/$Lepr^{db}$, has revealed an incomplete dominance pattern of expression (65). Heterozygote ob mice have decreased circulating leptin, and heterozygote db mice have increased circulating leptin relative to fat mass. Both heterozygotes have increased fat mass compared with normal and increased body weight gain on a high-fat diet. This pattern of expression is important for the analysis of the genetic controls of eating in these rodents, and it suggests that the search for the genetic basis of hyperphagia and obesity in humans requires the evaluation of the heterozygote state of candidate genes.

Hyperphagia and obesity in monogenic mutations are frequently apparent immediately after weaning in rodents and in early childhood in humans. Recent work has measured meal size before weaning in rats and found increased meal size as early as postnatal day (P) 12 in rats with a mutation of the leptin receptor ($Lepr^{fa}$/$Lepr^{fa}$). In humans with leptin deficiency, the hyperphagia becomes less severe in adolescence than it was in early childhood (63). Determining the earliest age at which hyperphagia occurs is the best time to investigate candidate mechanisms for the expression of the hyperphagia because it eliminates secondary changes in mechanisms resulting from the prolonged presence of hyperphagia and obesity.

An example of this strategy was carried out in the fa/fa rat. Hyperphagia occurs as early as P12 in this mutant when the pup eats independently away from the dam (66). Given the importance of NPY for the hyperphagia in adult fa/fa rats, its importance for the hyperphagia on P12 was investigated. The results were consistent with the hypothesis: NPY mRNA in the arcuate nucleus of the hypothalamus was expressed more in the mutant than in the wild type pup as early as P2 (67); this is 10 days before hyperphagia appeared. Furthermore, indirect evidence showed increased NPY release in the mutant pups on P12, the day hyperphagia appeared, but not on P10 or P11 (68).

Another reason to carry out developmental experiments is the recent evidence of the neurotrophic effect of leptin in the ob/ob mouse (69). Leptin deficiency in that mutant decreased the number of fibers from the arcuate nucleus to other hypothalamic nuclei involved in the control of food intake. This anatomic deficiency was rescued by daily treatment with leptin from P4 to P12. When leptin was given for 20 days to adult mutants, however, it did not increase the density of the projection fibers from the arcuate nucleus.

Preweaning leptin treatment had prolonged functional effects because it reduced food intake on P32 to levels that were intermediate between wild-type and untreated mutant mice. This is a model system in which to evaluate optimal neonatal treatment with systemic injections of a genetically deficient hormone for amelioration of severe hyperphagia and obesity.

The neurotrophic and anorexic effects of leptin are separate because leptin decreased food intake in preweaning and adult ob/ob mice, whereas it had a neurotrophic effect only in the first and second postnatal weeks. The inhibition of food intake in adult ob/ob mice is correlated with changes in the synaptic density of arcuate neurons (42), but not in changes of the number of their projected fibers.

FOOD AND DRUGS

Ethanol

Ethanol is on the borderland of food and drugs. Drinking ethanol, like eating food, occurs in bouts, and its pathology takes a similar form of excessive intake and binge drinking. Over the past decade, there has been increasing interest in investigating the effect of peptides that produce significant changes in food intake and meal size on the intake of alcohol-preferring rats. The early results are not straightforward (70). A melanocortin agonist, CCK-8 (an octapeptide form of CCK) and CRF decreased intake of ethanol and food. Leptin, conversely, increased intake of ethanol under conditions in which it decreased food intake. In contrast to its robust stimulation of food intake, NPY's effect on ethanol intake was inconsistent.

Devazepide, a specific antagonist of the CCK_1 receptor that mediates the inhibitory effect of CCK on meal size, increases meal size and ethanol intake. This finding implicates endogenous CCK in the negative-feedback control of ethanol intake. Further work in this area is likely to be productive.

Sugars and Amphetamine

Hyperphagia in obese or normal-weight people with bulimia nervosa or binge-eating disorder is not explained by nutrient homeostasis (2). The difficulty of effective treatment, the frequent relapse of people apparently motivated to change their pathologic eating, and the deleterious secondary effects on health comprise a profile similar to the problems of drug addiction. Is there a common mechanism for the rewarding and motivating effects of foods and addictive drugs? Recent experiments with sugars and amphetamine suggest that there is.

A relationship between sucrose and amphetamine was investigated in rats that had spontaneous differences in sucrose intake. High-intake rats pressed levers more often for 20% sucrose than did low-intake rats (71). High-intake rats also had a larger release of DA from the nucleus accumbens after peripheral administration of amphetamine than low-intake rats (72).

Further support for a common DA mechanism for sucrose and amphetamine came from experiments in which amphetamine was administered repetitively. After repetitive administration, rats become sensitized to amphetamine in the sense that the behavioral response to the same dose of amphetamine increased markedly. Rats sensitized to amphetamine consumed more 10% sucrose in daily 1-hour tests for 5 days than nonsensitized rats (73). Furthermore, the relationship was reciprocal: When rats had access to 10% sucrose and chow for 12 hours alternating with deprivation for 12 hours for 21 days, their locomotor response to amphetamine was significantly increased compared with the response of rats without that dietary experience (74). This evidence of cross-sensitization between amphetamine and sucrose complements the evidence of signs of dependency to ingested glucose (75).

These results are heuristic. They suggest that DA release in the accumbens is a common mechanism for increasing the motivating and rewarding effect of psychostimulant drugs and sucrose, a potent orosensory stimulant for the control of eating. The results are also preliminary. Other food stimuli and other sites and transmitters in the brain that have been thought important for the mediation of the motivating and rewarding effect of drugs need to be investigated.

TRANSLATION BETWEEN ANIMAL AND HUMAN RESEARCH

The preceding parts of this chapter describe what we have learned from research in rodents. How much of this has been translated into knowledge about humans? The short answer is, "A lot." Some of the progress has been the result of direct translation of monogenic obesity from rodents to humans (63). Five Pakistani subjects from three unrelated families and one subject from a Turkish family were described with severe, early-onset hyperphagia and obesity resulting from mutations of the *OB* gene that result in undetectable levels of circulating leptin. Daily leptin treatment for up to 4 years reversed the syndrome. These patients also responded to leptin when they were adults (76). These impressive therapeutic effects of leptin in subjects with mutation of the *LEP* gene is in marked contrast to the minimal or absent effects of leptin treatment in people with diet-induced obesity who have high levels of circulating leptin (77, 78). These effects in humans are the counterpart of the results in rodents: Peripherally administered leptin reverses hyperphagia and obesity in the ob/ob mouse, but it has no significant effect in mice with diet-induced obesity (79, 80).

Mutations of the MC_4 receptor are another example of monogenic obesity in humans. Recall that genetic knockout of these receptors in mice produced hyperphagia and early-onset obesity (81). Farooqi and colleagues (82) found mutations of the MC_4 receptor in 5.8% of 500 subjects who were obese before they were 10 years old.

The pattern of transmission of the mutation was incomplete dominance because obesity was more severe in homozygous subjects than in heterozygous subjects.

The penetrance of the phenotype was incomplete. Approximately one third of relatives with heterozygous mutations did not have obesity.

Subjects with a mutation of MC_4 ate significantly more after overnight deprivation than controls. The hyperphagia of these subjects was less than that previously reported in subjects with leptin deficiency. This difference suggests that some of the effects of leptin on food intake are mediated by non-MC_4 mechanisms.

In a related study, 24 of 469 (5.1%) severely obese adults had mutations or polymorpisms of the MC_4 receptor (83). Using a questionnaire and interviews to assess binge eating in a subset of these subjects, the investigators found that all 20 carriers reported binge eating, but only 17 of 120 obese noncarriers reported it. This association between binge eating and MC_4 mutations, however, was not replicated (84).

Direct translation of CCK, a molecular negative-feedback mechanism (11), has also been achieved. The satiating effect of CCK has been demonstrated in humans, and the effect is physiologic because it occurs with concentrations of CCK that are in the range observed during a meal (85). Furthermore, patients with bulimia nervosa with a history of frequent binge eating release less CCK during a large meal than do physiologically normal patients (86). The smaller release of CCK means that the negative feedback produced by CCK is less than normal, and this probably contributes to the binge meals in these patients.

Some of the progress in human research does not depend on results in rodents, however, but rather exploits human sensitivity to verbal, cognitive, and social cues. When instructed "to eat as much as you want," bulimic patients ate significantly more than physiologically normal persons (87). The effect of verbal instructions demonstrates the potency of cognitive control of eating in humans.

The range of stimuli that increase eating in humans is impressive. Stimuli include the expectations of the occasion, prior experience with the cuisine, learned food preferences, the number of people eating together and the purpose of the gathering, the size of portions, and the décor of restaurants (88). The efficacy of these cognitive and cultural stimuli makes the point that new controls emerge in humans because they think and talk about food, and they use it for a variety of purposes beyond nutritional homeostasis. Although the analysis of the mechanisms of these learned stimuli remains to be done, they are *indirect controls,* and their effects on meal size must be produced by changing the potency of the peripheral gut feedbacks stimulated by the food eaten.

CONCLUSION

Our understanding of the controls of food intake has increased considerably since the last edition of this book. Peptide mechanisms for the increased food intake that follows food deprivation have been clarified: Reductions in the circulating concentrations of leptin and insulin disinhibit central orexic peptides, such as NPY, and decrease stimulation of anorexic peptides, such as α-MSH. Both these central effects increase intake. Increased intake continues until the concentrations of leptin and insulin are normal.

The importance of the various central and peripheral peptides has been delineated by the use of specific antagonists, monogenic mutations, and transgenic knockouts. Immunocytochemical and microinjection techniques have provided an anatomic outline of the brain's network for the homeostatic increase of intake after deprivation.

The progress in understanding the control of intake after food deprivation highlights the problem of diet-induced obesity in rodents and humans. Increased intake of preferred diets, usually high-fat diets, occurs despite increased concentrations of leptin and insulin produced by the enlarging mass of adipose tissue. Thus, the negative-feedback system that accounts for the homeostatic effect of deprivation on food intake is not able to control intake of a palatable diet that can be obtained easily. Unfortunately, this is just the environmental condition in which obesity thrives.

The failure of the negative-feedback system to prevent diet-induced obesity has not been explained, but resistance to the effects of leptin and insulin on the brain appears to be involved. It is also likely that the increased orosensory positive feedback provided by the palatable diet stimulates intake.

It is clear that the pattern of eating affects the metabolism and nutrient partitioning of ingested food. A few large meals increase adiposity more than frequent small meals when total caloric intake is equivalent. In addition, increased meal size, rather than increased meal number, characterizes all monogenic obesities in rodent and humans in which meals have been investigated.

Meal size is under numerous controls. The importance of feedback control from the gut during a meal has been demonstrated. Food stimuli act preabsorptively to produce positive feedback from the mouth and negative feedback from the stomach, small intestine, and pancreatic islets. The orosensory stimulation is encoded into afferent nerve activity. The postingestive stimuli are encoded into peptides that stimulate afferent nerves, or the stimuli act on afferent terminals directly. All this sensory information projects to the caudal brainstem, where central processing begins. Through a poorly understood mechanism, the brain compares the relative potency of the positive and negative feedbacks. Eating continues as long as positive-feedback potency exceeds negative-feedback potency. When they become equal, eating stops. Thus, meal size results from the central integration of the gut feedbacks. All other signals, such as leptin, insulin, NPY, and estrogen, and all other procedures, treatments, or mutations that change meal size produce their effects by changing the central potency of the feedbacks from the gut that are activated by the food eaten during the meal. Significant electrophysiologic, pharmacologic, and neurochemical evidence for this functional interaction exists.

Learning produced by Pavlovian conditioning exerts a pervasive and prominent control of intake in rodents and humans. Conditioned preferences, aversions, and orosensory negative feedback produce significant changes in meal size. Learning about the time and place of availability of food dominates the initiation of eating and the number of meals. Thus, eating is rarely an unconditioned response to metabolic deficits.

Despite this considerable progress, research on the development of the controls of eating from birth to puberty lags. This is unfortunate because such research is exactly what is required to deal with the epidemic of obesity that has spread to children and the continuing problems posed by eating disorders that usually begin around puberty. Mechanistic knowledge of the controls of eating during development would have early and possibly prolonged preventive effects that no amount of adult research can deliver.

Acknowledgments

I thank Professors Timothy Moran, Anthony Sclafani, and Stephen Woods for constructive criticism of the penultimate draft of this manuscript. Marcia Miller, the librarian at the Westchester Division, provided expert bibliographic assistance.

REFERENCES

1. Richter CP. Harvey Lect 1943;38:63–103.
2. Smith GP. Nutrition 2000;16:814–20.
3. Woods SC. Appetite 2002;38:161–5.
4. Smith GP. Pregastric and gastric satiety. In: Smith GP, ed. Satiation: From Gut to Brain. New York: Oxford University Press, 1998:10–39.
5. Smith GP. Accumbens dopamine is a physiological correlate of the rewarding and motivating effects of food. In: Stricker E, Woods SC, eds. Handbook of Behavioral Neurobiology. New York: Kluwer Press, 2004:15–42.
6. Lorenz D, Nardi P, Smith GP. Pharmacol Biochem Behav 1978; 8:405–7.
7. Eisen S, Davis JD, Rauhofer E et al. Am J Physiol 2001;281: R1201–14.
8. Schwartz GJ. Nutrition 2000;16:866–73.
9. Smith GP. Neuropeptides 1999;33:323–8.
10. Stanley S, Wynne K, Bloom S. Am J Physiol 2004;286:G693–7.
11. Smith GP. Cholecystokinin: a molecular negative-feedback control of eating. In: Pfaff D, Arnold AP, Etgen AM et al., eds. Hormones, Brain, and Behavior. New York: Academic Press, 2002: 143–52.
12. Geary N. Neuropeptides 1999;33:400–5.
13. Kennedy GC. Proc R Soc Lond Biol 1953;140:578–92.
14. Woods SC, Lotter EC, McKay LD et al. Nature 1979;282:503–5.
15. Benoit SC, Clegg DJ, Seeley RJ et al. Recent Prog Horm Res 2004;59:267–85.
16. Zhang Y, Proenca R, Maffei M. Nature 1994;372:425–32.
17. Tartaglia LA, Dembski M, Weng X et al. Cell 1995;83:1263–71.
18. Chua SC Jr, Chung WK, Wu-Peng XS et al. Science 1996;271: 994–6.
19. Banks WA, Coon AB, Robinson SM et al. Diabetes 2004;53: 1253–60.
20. Shuldiner AR, Yang R, Gong DW. N Engl J Med 2001;345: 1345–6.
21. Rajala MW, Scherer PE. Endocrinology 2003;144:3765–73.
22. Plata-Salaman CR. Int J Obes Relat Metab Disord 2001;25 [Suppl 5]:48S–52S.
23. Loftus TM, Jaworsky DE, Frehywot GL et al. Science 2000;288:2379–81.
24. Kumar MV, Shimokawa T, Nagy TR et al. Proc Natl Acad Sci USA 2002;99:1921–5.
25. Cha SH, Hu Z, Lane MD. Biochem Biophys Res Commun 2004;317:301–8.
26. Thupari JN, Kim EK, Moran TH et al. Am J Physiol 2004;287: E97–104.
27. Clegg DJ, Wortman MD, Benoit SC et al. Diabetes 2002;51: 3196–201.
28. Kim EK, Miller I, Aja S et al. J Biol Chem 2004;279:19970–6.
29. Loftus TM, Jaworsky DE, Frehywot GL et al. Science 2000;288: 2379–81.
30. Hu Z, Cha SH, Chohnan S et al. Proc Natl Acad Sci USA 2003;100:12624–9.
31. Wortman MD, Clegg DJ, D'Alessio D. Nat Med 2003;9:483–5.
32. Geary N. Peptides 2001;22:1251–63.
33. Geary N, Asarian L, Korach KS et al. Endocrinology 2001;142: 4751–7.
34. Polidori C, Geary N. Peptides 2002;23:1697–1700.
35. Wu-Peng S, Rosenbaum M, Nicolson M et al. Obes Res 1999;7: 586–92.
36. Geary N, Asarian L. Am J Physiol 2001;281:R1290–4.
37. Smith GP. Neurosci Biobehav Rev 1996;20:41–6.
38. Smith GP. Prog Brain Res 2000;122:173–86.
39. Woods SC. Am J Physiol 2004;286:G7–13.
40. Flier JS. Cell 2004;116:337–50.
41. Saper CB, Chou TC, Elmquist JK. Neuron 2002;36:199–211.
42. Pinto S, Roseberry AG, Liu H et al. Science 2004;304:110–5.
43. Yang YK. Obes Rev 2003;4:239–48.
44. Beck B. Neurosci Biobehav Rev 2001;25:143–58.
45. Kalra SP, Dube MG, Sahu A et al. Proc Natl Acad Sci USA 1991; 88:10931–5.
46. Kotz CM, Glass MJ, Levine AS et al. Am J Physiol 2000;278: R499–503.
47. Sclafani A. Int J Obes Relat Metab Disord 2001;25[Suppl 5]: 13S–6S.
48. Houpt TA. Nutrition 2000;16:827–36.
49. Gietzen DW, Magrum LJ. J Nutr 2001;131:851S–5S.
50. Mattes RD, Arnold C, Boraas M. Cancer 1987;60:2576–80.
51. Selcher JC, Weeber EJ, Varga AW et al. Neuroscientist 2002; 8:122–31.
52. Davis JD, Smith GP, Singh B. Am J Physiol 2000;278:R383–9.
53. Grill HJ, Kaplan JM. Front Neuroendocrinol 2002;23:2–40.
54. Strubbe JH, Woods SC. Psychol Rev 2004;111:128–41.
55. Collier G, Johnson DF, Mathis C. J Exp Anal Behav 2002;78: 31–61.
56. de Castro JM, Stroebele N. Clin Geriatr Med 2002;18:685–97.

57. Nicolaidis S, Even P. Ann NY Acad Sci 1989;575:86–104.
58. Campfield LA, Smith FJ. Physiol Rev 2003;83:25–58.
59. Green J, Pollak CP, Smith GP. Physiol Behav 1987;41:141–7.
60. Collier G, Johnson DF, Mitchell C. Physiol Behav 1999;67: 339–46.
61. Rushing PA, Gibbs J. Peptides 1998;19:1439–42.
62. Chua SC Jr. Behav Genet 1997;27:277–84.
63. Farooqi IS, O'Rahilly S. Recent Prog Horm Res 2004;59: 409–24.
64. Kowalski TJ, Liu SM, Leibel RL et al. Diabetes 2001;50: 425–35.
65. Chung WK, Belfi K, Chua M et al. Am J Physiol 1998;274: R985–90.
66. Kowalski TJ, Ster AM, Smith GP. Am J Physiol 1998;275: R1106–9.
67. Kowalski TJ, Houpt TA, Jahng J et al. Physiol Behav 1999; 67:521–5.
68. Ster AM, Kowalski TJ, Dube MG et al. Physiol Behav 2003;78: 517–20.
69. Bouret SG, Draper SJ, Simerly RB. Science 2004;304:108–10.
70. Thiele TE, Navarro M, Sparta DR et al. Neuropeptides 2003;37: 321–37.
71. Brennan K, Roberts DC, Anisman H et al. Psychopharmacology (Berl) 2001;157:269–76.
72. Sills TL, Crawley JN. Eur J Pharmacol 1996;303:177–81.
73. Avena NM, Hoebel BG. Pharmacol Biochem Behav 2003;74: 635–9.
74. Avena NM, Hoebel BG. Neuroscience 2003;122:17–20.
75. Colantuoni C, Rada P, McCarthy J et al. Obes Res 2002;10: 478–88.
76. Licinio J, Caglayan S, Ozata M et al. Proc Natl Acad Sci USA 2004;101:4531–6.
77. Heymsfield SB, Greenberg AS, Fujioka K et al. JAMA 1999; 282:1568–75.
78. Hukshorn CJ, van Dielen FM, Buurman WA et al. Int J Obes Relat Metab Disord 2002;26:504–9.
79. Frederich RC, Hamann A, Anderson S et al. Nat Med 1995;1: 1311–4.
80. Widdowson PS, Upton R, Buckingham R et al. Diabetes 1997; 46:1782–5.
81. Weide K, Christ N, Moar KM et al. Physiol Genomics 2003; 13:47–56.
82. Farooqi IS, Yeo GS, O'Rahilly S. N Engl J Med 2003;349:606–9.
83. Branson R, Potoczna N, Kral JG et al. N Engl J Med 2003;348: 1096–103.
84. Hebebrand J, Geller F, Dempfle A et al. Mol Psychiatry 2004;9: 796–800.
85. Degen L, Matzinger D, Drewe J et al. Peptides 2001;22:1265–9.
86. Devlin MJ, Walsh BT, Guss JL et al. Am J Clin Nutr 1997;65: 114–20.
87. Walsh BT, Kissileff HR, Cassidy SM. Arch Gen Psychiatry 1989; 46:54–8.
88. Stroebele N, de Castro JM. Nutrition 2004;20:821–38.

SELECTED READINGS

Benoit SC, Clegg DJ, Seeley RJ et al. Insulin and leptin as adiposity signals. Recent Prog Horm Res 2004;59:267–85.

Flier JS. Obesity wars: molecular progress confronts an expanding epidemic. Cell 2004;116:337–50.

Sclafani A. Psychobiology of food preferences. Int J Obes Relat Metab Disord 2001;25[Suppl 5]:13S–6S.

Smith GP. Accumbens dopamine is a physiological correlate of the rewarding and motivating effects of food. In: Stricker E, Woods SC, eds. Handbook of Behavioral Neurobiology. New York: Kluwer Press, 2004:15–42.

Strubbe JH, Woods SC. The timing of meals. Psychol Rev 2004;111: 128–41.

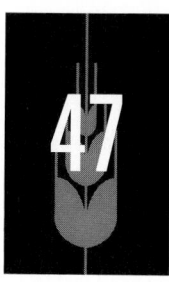

47 PHYSICAL ACTIVITY, FITNESS, AND HEALTH[1]

GARY R. HUNTER

DEFINITION OF FITNESS 721
SUBSTRATE UTILIZATION DURING WORK 721
MUSCLE FIBER TYPES 723
FORCE GENERATION 723
CARDIORESPIRATORY FITNESS (AEROBIC FITNESS) . . .723
AGING 724
INTERACTION OF FITNESS AND PHYSICAL ACTIVITY
    FOR MORTALITY AND RISK OF DISEASE 724
PHYSICAL ACTIVITY AND WEIGHT MAINTENANCE 725
HOW MUCH PHYSICAL ACTIVITY IS REQUIRED? 725
HIGH-INTENSITY EXERCISE AND ENERGY
    EXPENDITURE 726
EXERCISE TRAINING AND RESTING ENERGY
    EXPENDITURE 727
IMPROVED FUNCTION IN PHYSICAL ACTIVITY 727
EXERCISE TRAINING AND WEIGHT LOSS MAY
    BREAK THIS FEEDBACK LOOP 727

This chapter reviews the complex interactions between exercise training and activity-related energy expenditure (AEE) and the independent effects each has on health maintenance and the risk of disease. Obviously, physical training and AEE are related. Persons who do exercise training will also expend energy in physical activity. However, it is possible to expend relatively large amounts of AEE that is of insufficient intensity to create a training effect; that is, no increased fitness occurs. For example, low- to moderate-intensity activities such as slow walking and gardening can increase AEE substantially if done often and long enough, but they will have little effect on cardiorespiratory or strength fitness. Because intense training and AEE are interrelated, it is difficult to separate their effects on health maintenance and risk of disease. The problem is compounded for several reasons. First,

both cardiorespiratory fitness and strength fitness have a strong genetic basis (1), and it is often difficult to separate the genetic from the training-induced component of fitness. Second, fitness is actually more than one entity; different kinds of fitness have markedly different physiologic effects on the body. Persons who are fit to run a marathon will not necessarily be fit to compete in Olympic weight lifting, whereas persons who are fit to throw the discus will not necessarily be fit to run the mile. Third, regular AEE is difficult to measure, and most available techniques are imprecise, restrictive of free-living involvement, or very expensive. Fourth, body composition, as well as fat distribution, influences risk of disease but, in turn, is affected by exercise training and AEE. Before discussing the interactive effects of exercise training and physical activity, it is of interest to review some of the more important early findings that lay the groundwork for our understanding of the physiologic effects of AEE and fitness training.

In 1813, the carbon dioxide that was exhaled by men exercising to fatigue was measured by the Englishman William Prout (2). He showed that carbon dioxide production eventually reached a plateau during moderate-intensity exercise and introduced the concept of steady-state exercise, that is, exercise in which heart rate and oxygen uptake increase to a level that is then maintained. During the middle part of the nineteenth century, Edward Smith, a British physician, used a closed circuit respiratory system to conduct experiments on himself (2). He determined the relative carbon dioxide production for doing hard physical labor, similar to that required by prisoners, and found that carbon dioxide production increased 66% above resting during a 7.5-hour work period. He also found that urea production in four prisoners doing the same amount of work did not account for this dramatic increase in carbon dioxide production, a finding suggesting that protein metabolism was not responsible for the majority of AEE as previously proposed by Liebeg (2). This led to further work by two Germans, Adolf Eugen Fick and Johannes Wislicenus (2). They determined that the urea production during mountain climbing was similar to what would be expected at rest and concluded that protein metabolism could not be the primary fuel during work (2). Himwich and Rose (3) first demonstrated the importance of fat as a fuel in 1927 with their description of respiratory quotients of dogs at rest and during exercise in both fed and starvation states.

---

[1]**Abbreviations: AEE,** activity-related energy expenditure; **ADP,** adenosine diphosphate; **ATP,** adenosine triphosphate; **H^+,** hydrogen ion; **HDL,** high-density lipoprotein; **LDH,** lactate dehydrogenase; **LDL,** low-density lipoprotein; **MET,** metabolic equivalent; **NAD,** nicotinamide adenosine dinucleotide; **NADH,** reduced nicotinamide adenosine dinucleotide; **P_i,** inorganic phosphate; **^{31}P MRS,** phosphorus-31 magnetic resonance spectroscopy.

A.V. Hill's findings (for which he received a Nobel Prize in 1922) on heat production during exercise paved the way for a more comprehensive understanding of engergetics during exercise (2). During 1923 and 1924, W.O. Fenn demonstrated that more heat is produced when a muscle is shortened than during static contractions (4). In 1925, Meyerhof linked lactate production to muscle contraction. This finding, coupled with the discovery that adenosine triphosphate (ATP) (5) is used to drive the muscle under normal circumstances, further improved our understanding of energetics during muscle contraction. Finally, the development of Scholander's micrometer gas analyzer in 1947 allowed measurement of relatively small quantities of carbon dioxide and oxygen in expired gas with a great degree of accuracy (2). This device gave a new generation of exercise physiologists a tool for accurate measurement of energy expenditure during exercise.

Our understanding of muscle function and structure was also increasing during this period. Ranvier distinguished red and white muscle fibers in 1873, and Knoll reported variations in muscle fiber size in 1891 (6). Utilization of histochemical and physiologic techniques allowed the identification and description of different muscle fiber types during the first half of the twentieth century (6). In 1954, the sliding filament theory of muscle contraction was proposed independently by A.F. Huxley and Niedergerke and by H.E. Huxley (not related to A.F. Huxley) and Hanson (5). Before 1962, few studies reported results of the analyses of muscle from living humans. Development of microscopic methods of analysis in 1936 by Hevesy and Levi and a special biopsy needle by Bergstrom in 1962 (7) heralded a wave of study concerning the function and structure of human skeletal muscle. More recently, the advent of phosphorus-31 magnetic resonance spectroscopy (^{31}P MRS) in 1980 by Chance and associates allowed for the first time the study of metabolism during exercise in human muscle in vivo (8).

DEFINITION OF FITNESS

Because most of the scientific literature concerning the interaction of fitness and wellness is confined to cardiorespiratory endurance (aerobic fitness will be considered synonymous with cardiorespiratory endurance) and muscular strength, this chapter focuses on these two components of fitness. Cardiorespiratory fitness is defined as ability of the cardiovascular and respiratory systems to supply oxygen to the working muscles during sustained hard dynamic exercise (9). Cardiorespiratory fitness is normally evaluated by measuring maximum oxygen uptake (VO_2max) during a progressive graded exercise test on a treadmill or bicycle ergometer. Muscular strength is defined as the maximum force or tension that can be generated by a muscle and is normally measured by determining how much weight a person can lift in a certain movement or by how much force or torque a person can

exert during an isometric (no movement at the affected joint) or isokinetic (constant velocity) contraction.

SUBSTRATE UTILIZATION DURING WORK

It is beyond the scope of this chapter to go into any detailed description of the biochemical energy transfer during exercise. However, it is necessary to review this important matter briefly (10). Cleavage of the terminal phosphate from ATP to adenosine diphosphate (ADP) provides the energy for work in muscle (ATP $\xrightarrow{\text{myosin ATPase}}$ ADP + P_i [inorganic phosphate] + energy). Only a small amount of ATP is stored in the cell, so intense muscular contractions lasting more than a few milliseconds require energy sources for replacing phosphate to ADP. The most immediate source of energy for maintaining ATP levels during work is the creatine kinase reaction (ADP + creatine phosphate $\xrightarrow{\text{creatine kinase}}$ ATP + creatine) and, to a smaller extent, the myokinase reaction (2ADP $\xrightarrow{\text{Myokinase}}$ ATP + adenosine monophosphate). These reactions occur almost instantaneously, so ATP and creatine phosphate are normally considered to be one high-energy phosphate pool that is available for very high-intensity muscular contractions. Although quantitatively more than ATP, only a small amount of creatine phosphate is stored in muscle; therefore, muscular contractions that continue for more than a few seconds depend on other sources of energy for maintaining ATP levels.

The breakdown of glucose or glycogen to pyruvate during glycolysis can supply energy at a somewhat slower rate. The energy yield from anaerobic or fast glycolysis is relatively small (glucose + P_i + 2ADP + 2NAD$^+$ [nicotinamide adenosine dinucleotide] $\Rightarrow$ 2 pyruvate + 2ATP + 2NADH [reduced NAD] + 2H$_2$O). It also cannot continue at a high rate longer than a few seconds unless NADH is oxidized (loses its hydrogen ion [H$^+$]). This can occur for a short time by the lactate dehydrogenase (LDH) catalyzed conversion of pyruvic acid to lactic acid (pyruvate + NADH + H$^+$ $\xrightarrow{\text{LDH}}$ lactate + NAD$^+$). The temporary storage of hydrogen ion in this conversion of pyruvic acid to lactate is a convenient way for the disappearance of end products of fast glycolysis. The lactate can rapidly diffuse into the bloodstream, where it can be used by other muscle fibers (especially type I muscle fibers) or heart muscle and can be fuel to resynthesize ATP. However, as the level of lactate and H$^+$ increase in the muscle and blood, fatigue sets in, and exercise must slow or stop. Fatigue is probably caused by multiple factors, but increased acidity is believed to inactivate certain enzymes that are involved in energy transfer in skeletal muscle. Glycolysis in which the end product is lactate is termed anaerobic or fast glycolysis.

A much greater production of ATP occurs during aerobic or slow glycolysis. Lactate is not formed because NADH$^+$ is transported to the mitochondria (assuming sufficient mitochondria and oxygen exist in the muscle fiber), thus freeing NAD^+ for further reaction during glycolysis. The H^+ is used to generate energy during electron transport. Pyruvate is also transported to the mitochondria, where it is converted to acetyl-coenzyme A and is used to generate further substrate for electron transport generation of ATP. The complete breakdown of glucose to water and carbon dioxide during slow glycolysis generates 36 to 38 ATP per glucose molecule versus the 2 net ATP generated during anaerobic glycolysis. However, aerobic glycolysis is relatively slow and requires oxygen and high mitochondrial density. During high-intensity exercise such as running a quarter mile, some muscle fibers may be activated that have low mitochondrial density, and sufficient oxygen may not be available in all skeletal muscle mitochondria to complete the oxidation of pyruvate to water and carbon dioxide, thus increasing the dependence on fast glycolysis. Figure 47.1 illustrates the relative estimated contributions of different energy systems for endurance events of different duration.

Fat oxidation also occurs in skeletal muscle during muscle contractions. Both intracellular triglyceride and triglyceride stored in fat cells can be used as a source of fatty acids. After entering the mitochondria, fatty acids are broken down in a series of reactions called β-oxidation to numerous acetyl-coenzyme A and H^+ molecules. A large number of net ATP (147 ATP molecules for an 18-carbon fatty acid) can then be formed through the Krebs cycle and electron transport.

Protein is an additional fuel during exercise. From 5 to 15% of energy expended during exercise is estimated to be obtained from the oxidation of amino acids, especially the amino acids leucine, isoleucine, valine, glutamine, and aspartate. Removal of nitrogen by transamination can occur in both muscle tissue and liver. Once the nitrogen-containing group is removed from the amino acid, the remaining "carbon skeleton" is normally very similar to one of the reactive compounds active in energy transfer. For example, after losing its nitrogen-containing group and gaining a double bond, alanine forms pyruvic acid. Numerous different factors influence the rates of fuel used.

Composition of recent diet is a very important factor. A high-carbohydrate diet will increase the storage of glycogen in skeletal muscle and will thus increase the rate of use of carbohydrate as a fuel (2). Conversely, a diet high in fat will increase storage of myocellular lipid and will increase rate of fat oxidation during exercise. For example, consumption of an isocaloric diet that included 35% fat in the 3 days following a long-duration training run increased intramuscular lipid stores about 45% more than an isocaloric diet that included only 10% fat (11). Consistent with the concept that low fat intakes may be detrimental to endurance performance, a 7-day isocaloric diet that consisted of 38% fat before a treadmill run resulted in exhaustion after 91 minutes, whereas a diet that included 15% fat resulted in exhaustion after only 76 minutes (12). Exercise intensity also affects substrate oxidation rates. Generally, the more intense the exercise, the more dependent muscle fibers are on carbohydrate metabolism. For example, a well-nourished person consuming a mixed diet would obtain about 55% of the energy from oxidation of carbohydrate while running at 65% of VO_2max and about 85% of energy from oxidation of carbohydrate while running at 80% of VO_2max.

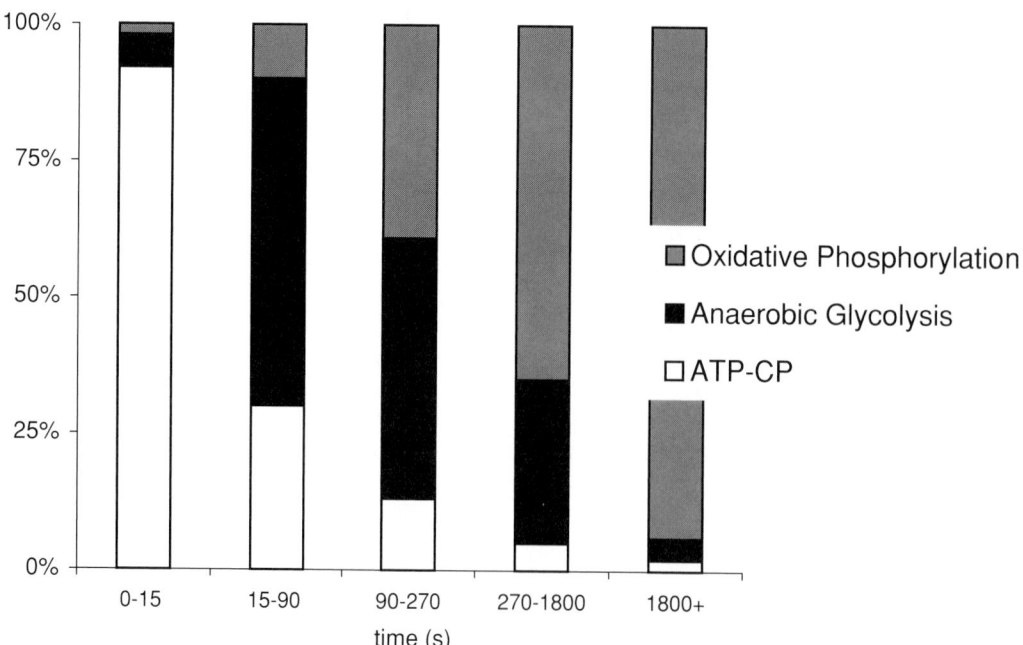

Figure 47.1. Approximate contributions of different energy systems for endurance events of different duration. ATP-CP, adenosine triphosphate–creatine phosphate.

Exercise training, especially long slow-distance endurance training, will increase the ability of skeletal muscle to use fat as a fuel and can have a glycogen-sparing effect in long-duration exercise such as the marathon (13). Exercise duration also plays a role with fat oxidation, by gradually increasing as exercise duration increases.

MUSCLE FIBER TYPES

Two major fiber types, type I and type II, have been identified in human muscle. Type I muscle fibers (slow-twitch muscle fibers) have slower contraction velocities but are more fatigue resistant than type II (fast-twitch muscle fibers). Type I muscle fibers have more mitochondria, oxidative enzyme activity, myoglobin levels, lipid stores, and capillarization than type II muscle fibers. Type II muscle fibers have greater glycolytic capacity and are capable of greater force and power production. Two main subcategories of type II muscle fiber exist: type IIa (fast-twitch glycolytic oxidative) and type IIb (fast-twitch glycolytic). Type IIa muscle fibers have metabolic characteristics more similar to those of type I muscle fibers, whereas type IIb fibers primarily depend on glycolysis for generating ATP.

Fiber type may also be related to insulin resistance and blood pressure. Type I muscle fiber distribution is related to improved glucose removal and reduced blood pressure, perhaps because of differences in microcirculation (14). It is also possible that type II muscle fiber distribution and oxidative enzyme activity may be linked to weight gain and obesity (14). Type II muscle fibers also require more ATP to generate force than type I muscle fibers, thus making persons who have increased type II muscle fiber distribution less economical at doing work. Table 47.1 summarizes differences in muscle fiber type.

FORCE GENERATION

Several factors can affect generation of force within a muscle. Force production is proportional to the number of myosin cross-bridges that are attached to actin filaments at any one time. A greater amount of calcium ion in a myofibril (domain within a muscle fiber containing the contractile components myosin and actin) results in more myosin cross-bridge heads binding to actin filaments and thus more tension within the muscle. The amount of calcium ion released from the sarcoplasmic reticulum is related to how frequently the innervating motor neuron stimulates the muscle. Thus, increased activation of a motor neuron will result in increased force developed in that motor neuron's motor unit (motor neuron and all muscle fibers it innervates). Peak force for a motor unit will normally be achieved at a neural action potential frequency of about 50 Hz (a lower frequency for slow motor units and a higher frequency for fast motor units). In addition, the number of motor units that are activated will result in an increase in the number of muscle fibers activated and thus more force production.

A larger muscle cross-sectional area will increase the total number of myosin cross-bridge heads available to bind with actin filaments and the potential for maximum force production. Anatomic structure can also influence force production. When we measure human strength, we are measuring maximal force output at the end of a lever system (e.g., the hand during an arm curl). The ratio of the length of these levers and attachment point of the muscle's tendon to bone (e.g., forearm length to elbow's axis of rotation in relation to distance of attachment of the biceps brachii and brachialis to the axis of rotation) will affect the application of force at the end of the lever system.

Other factors probably affect maximal force production, including angle of muscle pennation (pennate muscle fibers extend at an angle from the tendon as the barbs do from a feather), with more acute pennation angle increasing force that can be exerted. Fiber type also influences strength and power production; type II muscle fibers have greater strength and power production potential than type I muscle fibers. Because creatine kinase and myokinase activity are related to strength independent of muscle size and both seem to be increased in strength-trained persons, it is probable that high-energy phosphate availability in the myofibril can be limiting to expression of maximal force (15).

CARDIORESPIRATORY FITNESS (AEROBIC FITNESS)

Mode of exercise, heredity, state of training, gender, and age can all affect a person's VO_2max. This parameter is generally evaluated during some kind of progressive exercise

TABLE 47.1. TYPICAL FIBER TYPE VARIATIONS

TYPE I: SLOW-TWITCH	TYPE IIA: FAST-TWITCH OXIDATIVE-GLYCOLYTIC	TYPE IIB OR TYPE IIX: FAST-TWITCH GLYCOLYTIC
Many mitochondria	Intermediate mitochondria	Few mitochondria
High oxidative capacity	Moderate to high oxidative capacity	Low oxidative capacity
Efficient	Inefficient	Inefficient
Fatigue resistant	Intermediate	Quick to fatigue
Low power	High power	High power
Slow contraction and relaxation	Fast contraction and relaxation	Fast contraction and relaxation

task in which large muscle groups are being exercised. Treadmill walking or running will result in the highest VO_2max for most persons. Because slightly lower peak values of oxygen uptake will normally be found for other activities such as riding a bicycle ergometer, many exercise physiologists believe that VO_2max values for a particular type of exercise should be defined as peak oxygen uptake, if it is likely that a higher value could have been obtained with another test modality.

VO_2max is normally reported in absolute values (liters of oxygen per minute) or relative to body mass (milliliters of oxygen per kilogram of body weight per minute). When cardiorespiratory fitness is being used to evaluate someone's ability to move his or her body mass (i.e., during walking or running), the relative value is normally used. However, estimates of physiologic capacity will be confounded by variations in fat mass when adjustments are made with body mass because fat mass increases the body mass but does not contribute markedly to oxygen uptake during the exercise. Adjustment for fat free mass (milliliters of oxygen per kilogram of fat-free mass per minute) is often done when one wishes to adjust aerobic capacity relative to physiologically active fat-free mass.

Not only will training increase VO_2max, but it will also increase it to a greater extent in the training modality in which the person trains. For example, those who train on a bicycle will often increase their peak oxygen uptakes while cycling, so their peak oxygen uptake in that modality is higher than while running, even though an untrained person's peak oxygen uptake while cycling is normally only 85 to 90% of peak oxygen uptake while running.

Numerous studies have been done to determine the proportion of a person's VO_2max that results from hereditary factors and training (2). Little doubt exists that training can be increased much more in some persons than in others. The genetic effect of aerobic fitness is probably about 40%, although the genetic effect for physical work capacity for relatively long-duration activities is probably a little more than 50% (2). A properly administered aerobic endurance training program to an untrained person will increase VO_2max about 20% over 12 to 16 weeks, although some persons will improve less than 10% and others as much as 50%. Aerobic capacity in women is typically about 10 to 30% lower than in men. This difference occurs even among trained athletes. Table 47.2 illustrates typical VO_2max values for various groups.

AGING

After the age of about 30 years, both cardiorespiratory fitness and strength fitness decline at a rate of about 1% per year (2, 15). The rate of decline in fitness can be decreased but not stopped despite continuing activity levels at high levels. The decline in cardiorespiratory fitness is related to reduced central and peripheral function. Maximum heart rate declines at a rate of about 1 beat/year and is the main contributor to reduced maximum cardiac output. Loss of muscle mass, peripheral blood flow capacity, and capacity of skeletal muscle to generate ATP from oxidative processes also occur.

The primary cause for the decline in strength fitness is an age-related atrophy of skeletal muscle, defined as sarcopenia. Skeletal muscle sarcopenia is characterized by some atrophy of both type I and type II muscle fibers. However, sarcopenia occurs more rapidly in type II than in type I muscle fibers. Muscle fiber necrosis, muscle fiber type grouping (a shift from a heterogeneous to a more homogeneous muscle fiber distribution), and increased intramuscular content of adipose and connective tissues also occur with aging (15, 16) and probably contribute to a decrease in muscle quality (strength per unit area of muscle) with age. Power (time-rate of doing work) decreases proportionally more than strength as we age. Preferential type II muscle fiber atrophy accounts for some of the accelerated loss of power with age because the maximum velocity of shortening and power production are higher in type II than in type I muscle fibers. The decreased strength and power production also appear to result from impaired excitation-contraction coupling, because calcium release and dihydropyridine receptor expression both decline with age (15). Adults appear to lose only 5 to 10% of their muscle mass between the ages of 30 and 50 years, but they can lose an additional 30 to 40% between the ages of 50 and 80 years.

INTERACTION OF FITNESS AND PHYSICAL ACTIVITY FOR MORTALITY AND RISK OF DISEASE

Debate continues to surround the relative contributions of exercise fitness and physical activity to overall wellness and well-being. Both physical activity (defined as any body movement produced by contraction of skeletal muscle

TABLE 47.2. TYPICAL MAXIMUM OXYGEN UPTAKE VALUES IN HEALTHY PERSONS[a]

AGE GROUP	UNTRAINED	TRAINED	ELITE ENDURANCE ATHLETES
Young men (20–30 y)	40–45	57–62	75–85
Older men (50–60 y)	33–38	47–53	58–64
Young women (20–30 y)	32–36	45–52	63–70
Older women (50–60 y)	25–30	36–42	45–52

[a] In milliliters of oxygen per kilogram of body weight/minute.

that substantially increases energy expenditure) and cardiorespiratory fitness are inversely related to all-cause mortality in men and women (1, 17, 18). The risk of pancreatic cancer has even been shown to be dramatically reduced, especially in overweight persons (19).

A dose-response relationship appears to exist, with the most physically active or fit persons experiencing mortality rates less than one half those of the least physically active or fit (17). However, it is unclear whether the favorable effects of the physical activity are obtained entirely by increased energy expenditure or whether further favorable health-related effects can be obtained by participation in physical activity of sufficient intensity to create a training effect.

Several studies suggest that intense vigorous activity gives some advantage over light- to moderate-intensity physical activity (17). For example, reviews suggest that insulin insensitivity, dyslipidemia, and hypertension are more strongly affected by training that affects cardiorespiratory fitness (20).

However, the whole problem is complicated because visceral adiposity is strongly related to an adverse lipid profile, increased blood pressure, insulin insensitivity, cardiovascular disease, diabetes, and mortality (21). Of course, both more active and more fit persons have lower visceral fat levels (22, 23). Few studies have evaluated the independent effects of physical activity, aerobic fitness, and visceral adiposity on risk of developing cardiovascular disease and diabetes, although available population studies suggest that metabolic changes associated with weight loss may be primarily responsible for decreased incidence of cardiovascular disease found in more active men (24). Lara Castro and colleagues (unpublished data from our laboratory), using the best current techniques for measurement of physical activity (combination of doubly labeled water and indirect calorimetry), aerobic fitness (VO_2max), and visceral fat (computed tomography), showed that visceral fat is adversely related to insulin sensitivity and blood lipids independent of physical activity and aerobic fitness. Although not as strongly related, physical activity was independently related to total cholesterol and low-density lipoprotein (LDL) cholesterol, whereas cardiorespiratory fitness was independently related to high-density lipoprotein (HDL) cholesterol and insulin sensitivity. Consistent with these results, Thompson and associates (25) suggested that relatively high-intensity physical activity ($\geq 75\%$ VO_2max) may be necessary to improve glucose metabolism, and prolonged exercise is necessary to produce changes in LDL cholesterol. In any event, it is probable that both physical activity of low- to moderate-intensity and cardiorespiratory fitness training have positive independent effects on risk of disease. However, some of the positive effects of participation in physical activity and cardiorespiratory training may be mediated through their effects on visceral adiposity (26, 27).

PHYSICAL ACTIVITY AND WEIGHT MAINTENANCE

Whether persons gain or lose weight is totally dependent on the balance between caloric intake and caloric expenditure. Studies have shown that total energy expenditure is related to obesity and subsequent weight gain. This is particularly problematic as we age because both resting energy expenditure and AEE decline with age. The decrease is even more pronounced in AEE (15). A review by Westerterp (28) indicated that daily AEE decreases from 35% of the total energy expenditure at age 20 years to 25% at age 90 years. Decreased AEE can have a major adverse effect on weight maintenance; several studies have shown that persons who are physically active are more successful in maintaining weight than those who are less physically active (15). In fact, in a doubly labeled water study, investigators demonstrated that 77% of the differences in weight gain between gainers and maintainers was accounted for by AEE (29). The rest of the weight gain was presumably caused by increased energy intake in the gainers.

HOW MUCH PHYSICAL ACTIVITY IS REQUIRED?

It is very difficult to quantitate the amount of physical activity that is needed to prevent weight gain, for several reasons. First, it is difficult to measure physical activity accurately. Questionnaires and records have only limited accuracy. Doubly labeled water is very expensive and therefore is not available for large-scale studies. In addition, dietary assessment has limited validity, and factors such as culture, social, work, and home environment may affect both eating and exercising habits. Studies using doubly labeled water to measure energy expenditure and thus to estimate the amount of time that would need to be spent in moderate-intensity exercise suggest that about 80 minutes per day would be needed to prevent weight gain (29, 30). The 2002 International Society for the Study of Obesity First Stock Conference consensus report on physical activity recommended 60 to 90 minutes per day of moderate-intensity exercise or lesser amounts of vigorous intensity activity for maintaining weight (31). Moderate-intensity exercise is defined as exercise that is 3 to 4 metabolic equivalents (MET). A MET is an increment of resting metabolic rate. For example, an individual exercising at 4 METs would be exercising at an intensity that is four times resting energy expenditure. The recommendation of 60 minutes/day of exercise at 3 to 4 METs is double that recommended as a minimum for health by numerous prestigious organizations including the American College of Sports Medicine, the US Centers for Disease Control, and the US Surgeon General. These groups claim, and the literature supports them, that significant increases in overall health can be obtained with as little as 30 minutes per day of moderate-intensity exercise, and that it is difficult to persuade people to exercise even 30 minutes per day. However, at least 80 minutes per day of moderate-intensity exercise (one study suggests as much as 101 minutes) may be needed to prevent weight gain if dietary restriction is not practiced (Fig. 47.2) (15). Because many persons will not have the time or motivation to participate in 100 minutes per day or even 80 minutes per day of physical activity, weight maintenance may entail dietary restraint as well as an active lifestyle. It is evident that the relationship between physical activity and well-being should be considered a continuum, with some physical activity better than none, and further increases in physical activity associated with increased health until some ceiling effect is reached above which further improvements in health are not obtained, probably in excess of 80 to 100 minutes of moderate-intensity exercise.

It is obvious that increased energy expenditure, especially the most variable component of energy expenditure (AEE) may be beneficial for weight maintenance. Because low- to moderate-intensity exercise is believed to be more easily tolerated by the general population, recent efforts for increasing physical activity have focused on low- to moderate-intensity exercise (23). However, high-intensity exercise may be important to exercise programs, adding components that cannot be achieved solely with low- to moderate-intensity exercise. For example, Kraus and colleagues (32) found that exercise equivalent to walking or jogging 12 miles per week was associated with some improvements in blood lipid profile. However, Kraus and associates (32) also found that higher levels (20 miles per week) of high-intensity exercise (jogging at 65 to 80 % peak oxygen uptake) was necessary to increase HDL cholesterol. In addition, relatively short-duration high-intensity exercise training is related to greater decreases in subcutaneous skinfolds than longer duration low-intensity exercise

training that produced more than twice the energy expenditure. The high-intensity training must have been associated either with an increase in muscle or an increase in energy expenditure during nontraining time (23).

HIGH-INTENSITY EXERCISE AND ENERGY EXPENDITURE

Besides the possible relationship between cardiorespiratory fitness and increased HDL cholesterol and insulin sensitivity, high-intensity exercise training appears to have certain potential advantages for increasing total energy expenditure and decreasing the likelihood of gaining metabolically harmful visceral fat (23). First, much more energy can be burned in a short period during high-intensity exercise. This occurs for two reasons. First, the volume of work is much greater than in low-intensity exercise. A person will burn more energy in running 3 miles in 30 minutes than he or she would burn while walking 1.5 miles in 30 minutes. In fact, the ratio of energy expended to work is approximately linear as long as the work is performed at the same relative intensity. Second, as the intensity of most exercise tasks increases, efficiency or economy decreases. Running is one of the few activities in which this does not seem to occur. The magnitude of the variation can be quite large, increasing more than 300% over a wide spectrum of exercise intensities. For example, 22% more energy is required to bicycle at 100 watts for 30 minutes than to bicycle at 50 watts for 60 minutes, whereas 12 times as much energy is required to complete one bench press at 80% maximum strength compared with one bench press at 20% of maximum (23). Although a definitive answer to what causes the inverse relationship between exercise intensity and efficiency is unknown, it probably can at least be partly

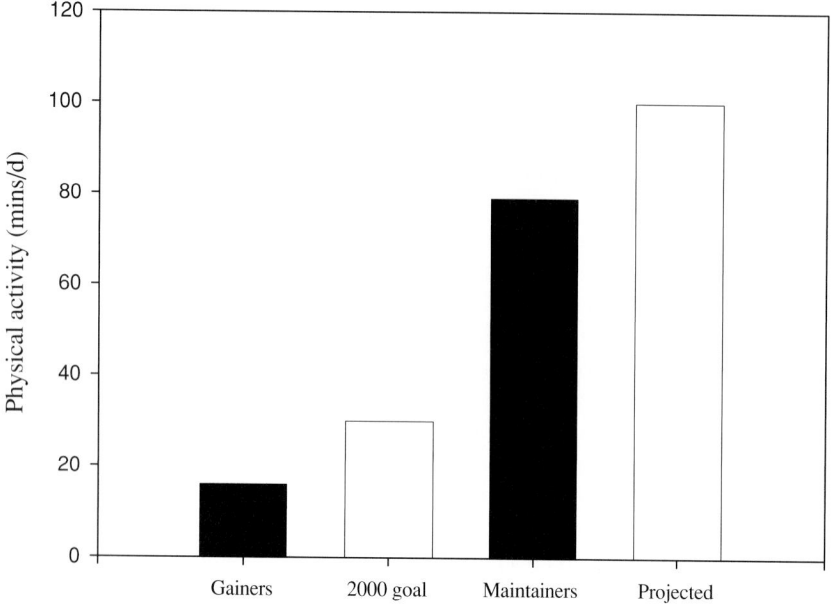

Figure 47.2. Estimated time necessary to prevent weight gain (minutes/day). Based on difference in energy expenditure between groups of maintainers and gainers, maintainers would have to restrict energy intake to maintain weight. If no dietary restriction were present in maintainers (differences in activity-related energy expenditure accounting for all of the difference in time spent in physical activity between the gainers and maintainers), 101 minutes instead of 79 minutes of moderate-intensity exercise would be needed to maintain weight (group-labeled projected). (Adapted from Weinsier RL, Hunter GR, Desmond RA et al. Am J Clin Nutr 2002;75:499–504, with permission.)

explained by the increased dependence of inefficient fast-twitch muscle fibers (type II) as the intensity of exercise increases (33).

EXERCISE TRAINING AND RESTING ENERGY EXPENDITURE

High-intensity exercise may have some effect on resting energy expenditure. Cross-sectional studies have demonstrated that athletes who participate in high-intensity exercise training have resting energy expenditures that are 5 to 20% higher than nonathletes even after adjusting for fat-free mass (23). In addition, a single bout of cardiorespiratory exercise of at least 70% of VO$_2$max will increase resting energy expenditure for up to 48 hours (23). Increases in sympathetic nervous system activity (34) and increased protein turnover (23) are likely factors in contributing to this transient increase in resting energy expenditure.

Bodybuilders have resting energy expenditures that are 5 to 31% higher than would be expected for young men and women of similar age and body mass (23). In addition, strength training programs of 4 to 6 months in untrained persons result in increases in fat-free mass of between 2 and 6 pounds (15). This increase in fat-free mass is normally associated with an increase in resting energy expenditure of 5 to 10%. The increase in fat-free mass and hence in resting energy expenditure can occur with a relatively small investment in time of as little as 30 minutes of training twice a week (23).

IMPROVED FUNCTION IN PHYSICAL ACTIVITY

The ability to be physically active reaches a peak in the early 30s and thereafter declines with age. This decline occurs in both cardiorespiratory fitness and strength

fitness. The decline cannot be prevented by being physically active, as evidenced by progressive declines in performance of highly trained athletes with age (15). Numerous factors probably cause this decrease including decreases in lung function, maximal heart rate and cardiac output, muscle size, muscle quality, and metabolic capacity of skeletal muscle, as well as increases in fat mass (2, 15). Of course, decreases in physical activity with age account for some of the age-related decline in function. In fact, one half or more of the decline probably is caused by declines in quantity and intensity of physical activity (2). This situation creates a positive feedback loop that can lead to progressively lower physical activity levels and weight gain: (a) decreased physical activity leads to both a reduction in functional fitness (cardiorespiratory and strength) and weight gain; (b) decreased functional fitness and the increased work required to move additional weight (from weight gain) during physical activity lead to increased difficulty in being physically active and a reduction in energy expended in physical activity; and (c) further reductions in physical activity lead to further reductions in functional fitness.

EXERCISE TRAINING AND WEIGHT LOSS MAY BREAK THIS FEEDBACK LOOP

Diet-induced weight loss is associated with a decrease in exercise difficulty as measured by heart rate, ventilation, and perceived exertion during activities such as walking, climbing stairs, and bicycling (35). These decreases in difficulty of being physically active occur despite a lack of change in exercise training. The measures of difficulty are also related to increased physical activity, a finding suggesting that a weight loss–induced decrease in difficulty

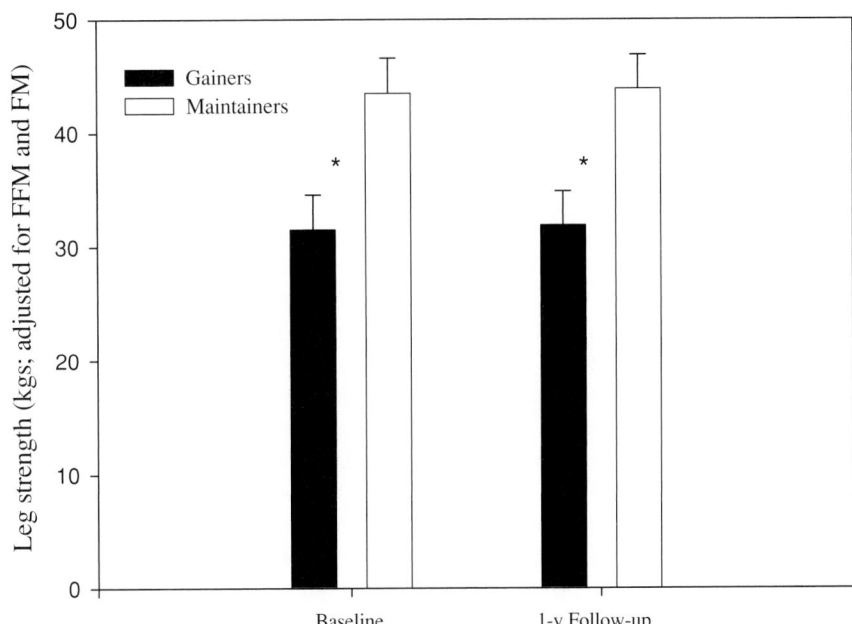

Figure 47.3. Leg strength in premenopausal women who gained and maintained weight over 1 year. FM, fat mass; FFM, fat-free mass. (Adapted from Weinsier RL, Hunter GR, Desmond RA et al. Am J Clin Nutr 2002;75:499–504, with permission.)

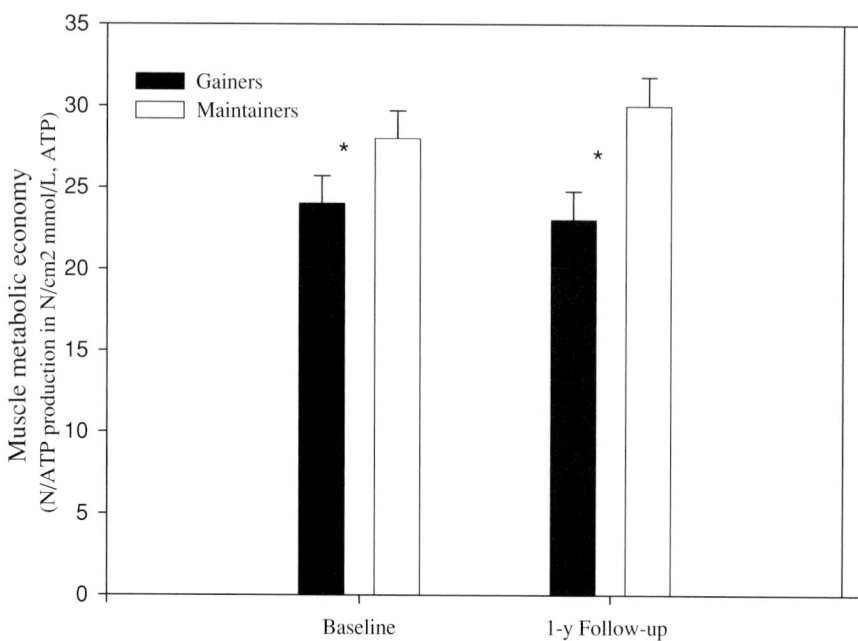

Figure 47.4. Muscle metabolic economy (as measured by phosphorus-31 magnetic resonance spectroscopy) in women who gained and women who maintained weight over 1 year. (From unpublished data from our laboratory.)

may be beneficial in increasing physical activity. Because most persons who lose weight also gain it back within a few years, it is obvious that other interventions are also required.

Training-induced improvements in functional fitness may decrease the rate of weight gain. Cardiorespiratory fitness (VO_2max and endurance time) are negatively related to weight gain over 1 year. In addition, women who maintain weight over 1 year are stronger (Fig. 47.3) and have better muscle metabolic economy (produce more force per unit of ATP) (Fig. 47.4) than women who gain weight. Muscle metabolic economy, VO_2 max, and quadriceps strength all are independently related to a low rate of weight gain, a finding suggesting that training that increases VO_2max, strength, and muscle metabolic economy can be protective of weight gain.

Quadriceps isometric strength and ^{31}P MRS–measured muscle oxidative capacity (postexercise ADP recovery rate × volume of muscle/body weight) are independently related to time to exhaustion on an endurance test (36). The results were similar when whole-body VO_2 max was substituted for muscle oxidative capacity. Both strength and aerobic capacity independently influence walking endurance for a maximal task of approximately 6 to 7 minutes (a modified Bruce treadmill protocol to exhaustion). It is not unusual that oxidative capacity is related to an endurance task of this duration. However, it is interesting to observe that strength is independently related to endurance. One possible explanation for a relationship between physical strength and endurance performance is that less muscle activation would be needed to perform a task when a muscle is stronger (23), hence decreasing reliance on inefficient fast-twitch muscle fibers and delaying fatigue.

Resistance training improves whole-body exercise economy, including running even in trained runners (15). Ease of performing daily tasks, such as standing from a chair and carrying a simulated box of groceries, as measured by normalized electromyography and heart rate response is improved while performing daily tasks following 16 weeks of resistance training (15). This finding suggests that improved exercise economy and strength may make it easier to be physically active. Stronger persons probably can do work more economically and thus with less difficulty. This can then assist in increasing physical activity and the likelihood of weight maintenance. Specifically after training, muscle fibers are larger and stronger and are capable of more force. Therefore more work can be accomplished by low threshold, efficient fatigue-resistant (type I) motor units, thus decreasing the need to activate less efficient, fatigable type II motor units (23). This contention is further supported by the finding that not only are weight maintainers stronger than weight gainers, but also women who regularly participate in large amounts of physical activity (>60 minutes/day) have more leg strength and muscle maximal creatine kinase activity than women who regularly participate in low levels of physical activity (<20 minutes/day) (15).

Existing data suggest that weight maintenance programs should include some combination of high- and low- to moderate-intensity physical activity. The low-intensity exercise, if this is preferred by the participant, may be done more frequently, and it will be the exercise in which the majority of energy is expended. Much of the low-intensity exercise may not consist of formalized exercise training but may involve efforts to increase daily free living activity. Increasing use of stairs instead of elevators, walking or bicycling short to moderate distances rather than driving, and using a push lawn mower rather than a riding lawn mower are examples of ways to increase physical activity without large increases in time commitment. However, some minimum amount of high-intensity exercise may be needed to elevate AEE and resting energy expenditure, to improve fitness, and thus to decrease exercise difficulty. It is not known what combination of high- and low-intensity exercise will be most productive. It will probably vary depending on the individual's available time and tolerance for high-intensity exercise.

Acknowledgments

This chapter is in memory of Dr. Roland L. Weinsier, a good friend, colleague, and nutrition scientist. This work is supported in part by National Institues of Health grants R01 DK49779 and R01 DK51684.

REFERENCE

1. Blair SN, Yiling C, Holder JS. Med Sci Sports Exerc 2001; 33:379S–99S.
2. McArdle WD, Katch FI, Katch VL. Exercise Physiology. Philadelphia: Lippincott Williams & Wilkins, 2001.
3. Rose MI, Himwich HE. Am J Physiol 1927;81:485–6.
4. Ford LE. Muscle Physiology and Cardiac Function. Traverse City, MI: Cooper Publishing Group, 2000.
5. Huxley AF. The Origin of Force in Skeletal Muscle: Energy Transfer in Biological Systems. New York: Ciba Foundation, 1975:271–99.
6. Pette D, Staron RS. Rev Physiol Biochem Pharmacol 1990;116: 1–76.
7. Bergstrom J. Scand J Clin Lab Invest 1962;68:1-110.
8. Chance B, Eleff S, Leigh GS. Proc Nat Acad Sci USA 1980; 77:7430–4.
9. Howley ET. Med Sci Sports Exerc 2001;33:364S–9S.
10. Houston ME. Biochemistry Primer for Exercise Science. Champaign, IL: Human Kinetics, 1995.
11. Larson DE, Newcomer BR, Hunter GR. Am J Physiol 2004; 282:E95–106.
12. Muoio DM, Leddy JJ, Horvath PJ et al. Med Sci Sports Exerc 1994;26:81–8.
13. Hargreaves M. Exerc Sport Sci Rev 1997;25:21–39.
14. Bassett DR Jr. Med Sci Sports Exerc 1994;26:957–66.
15. Hunter GR, McCarthy JP, Bamman MM. Sports Med 2004; 34:329–48.
16. Lexell J. J Gerontol A Biol Sci Med Sci 1995;50:11–6.
17. Lee IM, Paffenbarger RS Jr. Exerc Sport Sci Rev 1996;24: 135–71.
18. Kohl HWI. Med Sci Sports Exerc 2001;33:472S–83S.
19. Michaud DS, Giovannucci E, Willett WC et al. JAMA 2001;286:921–9.
20. Shephard RJ. Med Sci Sports Exerc 2001;33:400S–18S.
21. Despres J-P, Lemarche B. Physical activity and the metabolic complications of obesity. In: Claude Bouchard, ed. Physical Activity and Obesity. Champaign, IL: Human Kinetics, 2000: 331–54.
22. DiPietro L. Exerc Sports Sci Rev 1995;23:275–303.
23. Hunter GR, Weinsier RL, Bamman MM et al. Int J Obes 1998;22:489–93.
24. Williams PT. Med Sci Sports Exerc 2001;33:611S–21S.
25. Thompson PD, Crouse SF, Goodpaster B et al. Med Sci Sports Exerc 2001;33:438S–45S.
26. Hunter GR, Kekes-Szabo T, Snyder S et al. Med Sci Sports Exerc 1997;29:362–9.
27. Hunter GR, Kekes-Szabo T, Treuth MS et al. Int J Obes 1996; 20:860–5.
28. Westerterp KR. Curr Opin Clin Nutr Met Care 2000;3:485–8.
29. Weinsier RL, Hunter GR, Desmond RA et al. Am J Clin Nutr 2002;75:499–504.
30. Schoeller DA, Shay K, Kushner RF. Am J Clin Nutr 1997;66: 551–6.
31. Saris WHM, Blair SN, van Baak MA et al. Obes Rev 2003;4: 101–14.
32. Kraus WE, Houmard JA, Duscha BD et al. N Engl J Med 2002;347:1483–92.
33. Hunter GR, Newcomer BR, Larson-Meyer DE et al. Muscle Nerve 2001;24:654–61.
34. Poehlman ET, Danforth E. Am J Physiol 1991;261:E233–9.
35. Hunter GR, Weinsier RL, Zuckerman PA et al. Int J Obes 2004(in press).
36. Larew K, Hunter GR, Larson-Meyer EE et al. Med Sci Sports Exerc 2003;35:230–6.

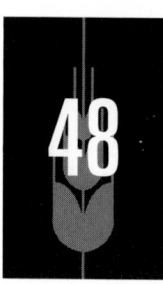

48

METABOLIC CONSEQUENCES OF STARVATION[1]

L. JOHN HOFFER

DEFINITIONS 730
PROLONGED FASTING 731
   Carbohydrate Metabolism 731
   Ketosis 732
   Protein and Energy Metabolism 733
   Weight Loss 734
   Other Metabolic Effects 734
   Nutritional Modifications of Fasting Metabolism . .734
   Survival 735
PROTEIN DEFICIENCY 735
   Minimum Protein Requirement 735
   Protein Intakes above and below the
      Requirement Level 735
   Kwashiorkor 736
PROTEIN-ENERGY DEFICIENCY 737
   Composition of Weight Loss 737
   Adaptation 737
   Survival 740
MECHANISMS OF ADAPTATION TO STARVATION 741
   Energy Metabolism 741
   Protein Metabolism 741
CACHEXIA 742
CHRONIC ENERGY DEFICIENCY 742
CALORIE RESTRICTION AND LIFE EXTENSION 743
REFEEDING 743

Starvation is the physical condition brought about by inadequate consumption, absorption, or retention of protein or dietary energy from carbohydrate and fat. The disease eventually caused by starvation is *protein-energy malnutrition*. This chapter explains the physiology of starvation, which occurs both as a disease and in a nonpathologic form during therapeutic weight reduction. The usual cause of pathologic starvation is a general reduction of food consumption, so it is commonly complicated by deficiencies of micronutrients as well as macronutrients (1, 2).

The physiology of starvation is central to human nutrition and is important for understanding many aspects of metabolism and medicine. Chapter 57 deals with the clinical aspects of protein-energy malnutrition. This chapter summarizes what is known about the metabolic features of protein and energy insufficiency, as studied, for the most part, in humans. The aim is to establish links between nutritional physiology and areas of applied clinical nutrition covered in other chapters in the text, including, among others, protein and energy metabolism, body composition, and nutritional assessment.

DEFINITIONS

Many terms are used to describe starvation. In this chapter, "starvation" refers to states of negative protein or energy balance and their physiologic effects. A "fast" or "total fast" is a unique form of starvation in which all food energy is excluded. Some authors consider any diet restricted to only a few nutrients as a fast, such as a "juice fast." The term fast is also commonly applied to the normal condition of any person after the overnight sleep (i.e., the period before breakfast). Terms such as starvation, inanition, emaciation, wasting, and cachexia have, in the past, been used synonymously to describe the malnourished condition of famine victims, underfed prisoners, or patients with chronic disease and important weight loss. In recent years, the term cachexia has been used, along with cytokine-induced malnutrition (3), to refer to the body protein loss caused by persistent low-grade inflammation or metabolic stress (4). Advancing age is associated with loss of muscle mass and function, termed sarcopenia (5, 6). Although it is potentially modifiable by diet and lifestyle, sarcopenia is not considered as a form of starvation in this chapter.

Starvation takes different forms. Prolonged fasting is characterized by ketone body production and, at least in its initial phase, increased body protein catabolism (7). Contrary to what is sometimes written, ketosis is neither sensitive nor specific as an indicator of starvation. Mild ketonuria is normal for lean, healthy adults after the overnight fast or while consuming a carbohydrate-restricted diet. Because ketosis is prevented or abolished by carbohydrate intakes as low as 100 g/day (8), it is not present in most starving persons.

[1] **Abbreviations: ADP,** adenosine monophosphate; **ATP,** adenosine triphosphate; **BMI,** body mass index; **CED,** chronic energy deficiency; **CR,** calorie restriction; **FFM,** fat-free mass; **IGF,** insulinlike growth factor; **N,** nitrogen; **REE,** resting energy expenditure; **SIRS,** systemic inflammatory response syndrome; **T₄,** thyroxine; **T₃,** triiodothyronine; **UCP,** uncoupling protein.

PROLONGED FASTING

Carbohydrate Metabolism

A description of carbohydrate metabolism during prolonged fasting best proceeds from the last meal before the fast begins. Characteristic of the fed state are increased blood concentrations of glucose, triglycerides, amino acids, and their metabolites. The digestion and absorption of carbohydrate and amino acids stimulate insulin secretion, which regulates their disposition within the tissues by stimulating glycogen, triglyceride, and protein synthesis. Glucagon levels are unchanged or are decreased by carbohydrate consumption, whereas protein consumption stimulates secretion of both insulin and glucagon (7). Glucagon stimulates liver glycogen breakdown and increases hepatic glucose output, thereby maintaining a normal blood glucose level in the presence of concurrent insulin-induced glucose uptake by the peripheral tissues.

The fed state ends after the last nutrient has been absorbed and the transition to endogenous fuel consumption begins. The condition that exists after an overnight fast is convenient for study and is termed the basal or postabsorptive state. It is characterized by the release, interorgan transfer, and oxidation of fatty acids and the net release of glucose from liver glycogen and amino acids from muscle; all these processes result from the relatively low circulating insulin level that prevails in this situation. The body's predominant postabsorptive fuel is fat, even in the context of a high-carbohydrate diet. As indicated by the typical nonprotein respiratory quotient of 0.8, fat oxidation accounts for two thirds of the body's postabsorptive resting energy expenditure (REE) (9).

Under postabsorptive conditions, glucose disappears into the tissues at a rate of 8 to 10 g/hour, replacing the body's free glucose pool of approximately 16 g every 2 hours (10). Glucose is normally the brain's only fuel, and reduction in blood glucose below a critical level promptly impairs consciousness and, if prolonged, may lead to neuron death. Given the brain's fixed and high metabolic requirement—approximately half the total glucose production rate—no room for error exists in the delivery of adequate amounts of glucose from the liver into the circulation. The blood glucose concentration of healthy persons is closely regulated by several physiologic control systems, chief of which are the insulin and glucagon systems.

In the period that follows disposition of a meal, continuing removal of glucose by the tissues progressively lowers the blood glucose concentration. Insulin levels fall in parallel, automatically slowing glucose removal from the circulation by reducing glucose transport by muscle and fat cells, while simultaneously stimulating hepatic glycogenolysis and inhibiting hepatic glycogen synthesis, thereby ensuring continued release of glucose from the liver into the bloodstream.

Hepatic gluconeogenesis (the synthesis of glucose molecules from lactate, amino acids, and glycerol) proceeds continuously, even in the fed state (11). Early in the postabsorptive period, approximately half the glucose appearing in the circulation is derived from gluconeogenesis, and the other half is derived from glycogenolysis (10, 12). Their precise relative contributions to the circulating glucose pool depend on the carbohydrate and protein content of the preceding diet, because these factors, respectively, determine the size of the liver's glycogen store and the amount of substrate reaching the liver for gluconeogenesis (13). As a fast is extended, the glucose molecules derived from gluconeogenesis increasingly pass directly into the circulation rather than being sequestered in glycogen, and the liver gradually releases its entire glycogen store into the circulation.

A fast longer than 12 to 24 hours reduces insulin levels further, and this mobilizes free fatty acids and glycerol from adipose tissue triglycerides and amino acids from muscle (14). Their delivery to the visceral organs provides energy and substrate for protein synthesis and hepatic gluconeogenesis. Plasma glucagon concentrations stay constant or increase; this lowers the insulin-glucagon ratio and activates the liver to oxidize the increased amounts of fatty acids now being delivered to it. Once activated in this way, the liver's fatty acid oxidation rate is determined by the rate at which fatty acids are delivered (15). Thus, along with diminished conversion of glucose and glucose precursors to acetyl-coenzyme A (the entry substrate for the Krebs cycle), acetyl-coenzyme A production resulting from fatty acid oxidation increases. Some of the acetyl-coenzyme A produced from fatty acid oxidation is completely oxidized to carbon dioxide through the intrahepatic Krebs cycle, serving as the liver's predominant energy source (16), but most of it is oxidized only as far as the four-carbon molecule, acetoacetic acid, which interconverts with its oxidoreduction partner, β-hydroxybutyric acid, and, to a lesser extent, is irreversibly decarboxylated to acetone. These three molecules are termed the ketone bodies.

A fast longer than 2 or 3 days completely depletes the liver's approximately 80-g glycogen reserve (12, 17) and about half the glycogen in muscle (17, 18). Gluconeogenesis neither increases or decreases and consequently accounts for an increasing fraction of the liver's glucose output into the circulation (12, 19), which decreases by 40 to 50% within the first few days of fasting (12, 20). Once the liver's glycogen supply is completely gone, all glucose oxidized in the body is synthesized, via gluconeogenesis, from two types of precursor: (a) glycerol and the glucogenic amino acids; and (b) lactate and pyruvate, three-carbon intermediates that are themselves the products of glycolysis and hence represent recycled glucose molecules (21). The oxidation rate of preformed carbohydrate is now zero, and, as proof of this, the nonprotein respiratory quotient is 0.7 (9).

Despite the marked reduction in hepatic glucose release, serum glucose concentrations decrease only moderately, because tissue glucose uptake and metabolism are also reduced. Only part of this reduction in glucose metabolism results from reduced terminal glucose oxidation in muscle and fat, and none of it is caused by a slower rate of lactate and pyruvate reconversion to glucose (the Cori cycle). Indeed, in a whole-body tracer study, no significant change in the rate of the Cori cycle could be demonstrated after several weeks of fasting (22). An important reason for reduced tissue glucose utilization early in fasting, and the main reason for it during prolonged fasting, is reduced brain glucose uptake and metabolism resulting from a progressive switch to ketone bodies as an alternative fuel (16). This phenomenon was demonstrated in a study of persons who fasted on a short-term basis in which a combination of positron emission tomography and arterial-internal jugular vein sampling was used to measure glucose metabolism and β-hydroxybutyrate consumption. After 3.5 days of fasting, glucose consumption by the brain decreased by 25% (440–340 kcal/24 hours), and ketone body extraction increased correspondingly (14–145 kcal/24 hours) (23).

Ketosis

Ketogenesis is the cardinal sign of prolonged fasting, but even in the fed state, small amounts of acetoacetic acid are produced and oxidized in the liver (24). Under normal nutritional conditions, acetoacetate oxidation furnishes only 2 to 3% of the body's total energy requirement (16), and circulating ketone body concentrations are almost unmeasurably low (25). Starvation ketosis is arbitrarily defined as being present when the blood acetoacetate concentration rises to 1.0 mmol/L and β-hydroxybutyrate to 2 to 3 mmol/L; this typically occurs by day 2 or 3 of fasting (16). Ketone bodies are usually absent from overnight fasting urine, but mild ketonuria is not abnormal in thin persons, especially women, and is an indication of a relatively low basal insulin state (26, 27). After being released into the blood, acetoacetic acid and β-hydroxybutyric acid dissociate to form water-soluble anions. Acetone is volatile, and after 3 or 4 days of fasting, its characteristic sweet odor is detectable in the breath.

The rate of free fatty acid delivery to the liver is one of two major determinants of its ketone body synthesis rate. The other is the liver's maximum rate of fatty acid β-oxidation, which is limited by the availability of adenosine monophosphate (ADP) generated from adenosine triphosphate (ATP) turnover (28). All mitochondria oxidize ketone bodies, and ketone body oxidation accounts for 30 to 40% of the body's total energy use during the first 4 to 7 days of a total fast. However, after approximately 2 weeks of fasting, free fatty acids replace ketone bodies as the main fuel of muscle (10). The mechanism governing this late change in muscle fuel selection is not understood. Ketogenesis reaches its maximum rate as early as 3 days of fasting, but blood ketone body levels continue to rise, because muscle ketone body oxidation decreases and renal

tubular reabsorption increases. By week 3, a steady circulating ketone body concentration is reached that is approximately double the level that existed after 3 to 5 days. The brain uses ketone bodies in proportion to their delivery to it, so brain ketone body oxidation steadily increases over this period, and brain glucose oxidation decreases yet further. After 3 to 5 weeks of fasting, brain glucose uptake is globally reduced by approximately 50% (29). Moreover, by this time only 60% of the glucose taken up by the brain is oxidized to carbon dioxide and water; the other 40% is metabolized no further than to pyruvate and lactate, which return to the liver for use in gluconeogenesis (30). This combined adaptation of reduced terminal oxidation and increased local Cori cycling reduces irreversible glucose oxidation in the brain by 75%, with an equivalent reduction in the body's requirement for gluconeogenesis from amino acids and glycerol.

Biologic Significance of Ketosis

Mention of ketosis or ketoacidosis (ketosis sufficient to reduce the serum bicarbonate concentration but still within its normal buffering capacity) brings diabetes mellitus to mind. In the most severe form of diabetes, destruction of the β cells of the pancreas produces nearly total insulin deficiency. The results are mobilization of fatty acids and a priming of the liver for ketone body production and gluconeogenesis, as occurs in simple fasting (15, 31). When carbohydrate is ingested in this setting, little of the resulting blood glucose is removed by muscle and adipose tissue, and the blood glucose concentration rises to high levels, greatly exceeding the renal threshold for glucose reabsorption. This causes glycosuria and osmotic diuresis that depletes the body of water and extracellular fluid. In prolonged fasting by nondiabetic persons, ketone body levels seldom rise higher than 6 to 8 mmol/L, but they rise much higher in diabetic ketoacidosis, imposing an acid load too great for the body's buffering system to absorb and causing a dangerous fall in pH (ketoacidemia).

It is often reported in the popular media that ketone bodies are toxic and the ketonuria associated with dietary carbohydrate restriction "damages the kidneys." This claim has no scientific basis. Perhaps it arose because ketone bodies partially inhibit urinary excretion of urate (10), and this—especially in the setting of extracellular volume depletion, which increases renal tubular urate reabsorption (32, 33)—raises the serum urate concentration. An attack of gout may thus occur in susceptible persons during total fasting or severe carbohydrate restriction. The possibility has been raised that hyperketonemia during pregnancy could adversely affect the fetal brain (27) or could predispose to congenital malformations (34). It is true that the rapid glucose utilization characteristic of late pregnancy predisposes to fasting hypoglycemia, hypoinsulinemia, mild ketosis, and ketonuria (35) and that ketone bodies are used as fuel by fetal tissues. However, no plausible mechanism has been advanced to explain why this would be toxic, and the observational evidence linking ketonuria with adverse fetal outcomes is unconvincing. It nevertheless remains a common practice to counsel pregnant women to avoid periods of prolonged fasting (27).

Why does diabetic ketoacidosis evolve into life-threatening metabolic acidosis, whereas the ketosis of simple fasting is mild and clinically benign? One possibility is that high ketone body concentrations stimulate insulin secretion in physiologically normal persons, partially restraining lipolysis and ketogenesis (25, 35, 36). Against this, at least as a sole explanation, is the uncommon but well-known syndrome of nondiabetic ketoacidosis, which typically occurs in persons who, following an alcoholic drinking binge with little or no food consumption, develop protracted vomiting and ketoacidemia as severe as diabetic ketoacidosis but with a normal or only moderately increased blood glucose concentration (37, 38). Nondiabetic ketoacidosis also occurs rarely in pregnancy. As with alcoholic nondiabetic ketoacidosis, gestational nondiabetic ketoacidosis occurs in a setting of fasting, hypoglycemia, and volume depletion or metabolic stress (39).

Two features that distinguish severe ketoacidosis from the benign ketoacidosis of fasting are volume depletion and hypermetabolism. Volume depletion worsens existing ketoacidosis (and worsens hyperglycemia) by reducing blood flow to the kidneys and brain, thus reducing brain and renal ketone body oxidation and preventing ketone body elimination in the urine (38). Fasting is normally a hypometabolic state, whereas uncontrolled diabetes and hypermetabolic volume depletion are characterized by hyperglucagonemia and increased norepinephrine secretion. These hormones increase free fatty acid delivery to the liver (40, 41) and potentially increase its rate of energy consumption and hence its ketogenic capacity (28) under conditions in which volume depletion decreases glomerular filtration and renal tubular sodium reabsorption, reducing the kidney's rate of energy consumption and ketone body oxidation (38). The net effect is a large increase in circulating ketone bodies. In nondiabetic fasting persons, a stress-induced increase in blood glucose normally stimulates insulin release and restrains lipolysis, hepatic glucose release, and ketogenesis (25), but in severely volume-depleted states, this does not always happen, presumably because hyperadrenergic states inhibit insulin secretion (38). The development of severe nondiabetic ketoacidosis in a setting of fasting and hypermetabolism is consistent with observations made in the preinsulin era. Before 1922, the only treatment that extended the life of insulin-dependent diabetic patients was a diet low in carbohydrate, to prevent hyperglycemia, and low in energy, to reduce the metabolic rate and hence the maximum rate of ketone body synthesis (42).

In summary, prolonged fasting is characterized by a low blood glucose concentration, physiologic hypoinsulinemia, and moderate ketosis, whereas uncontrolled insulin-dependent diabetes is characterized by a high blood glucose concentration, volume depletion, hypermetabolism, and severe ketosis, all of which are the direct or indirect result of severe insulin lack. Unlike diabetic ketoacidosis, fasting ketosis is physiologic and is a manifestation of appropriate metabolic regulation. It does not evolve into a severe condition similar to diabetic ketoacidosis, except, potentially, in a setting of severe volume depletion and metabolic stress.

Protein and Energy Metabolism

Muscle proteolysis is normally restrained by circulating insulin, but as insulin levels fall in the postabsorptive state, amino acids are released from muscle and are taken up by the splanchnic organs for use in gluconeogenesis and protein synthesis. In extended fasting, insulin levels fall lower yet, further releasing muscle proteolysis. The loss of skeletal muscle from the body is considerable. During the first 7 to 10 days of fasting, whole-body nitrogen (N) loss is in the range of 10 to 12 g/day, excreted chiefly as urinary urea. Because protein is 16% N and the lean tissues are 75 to 80% water, the loss from the body of 10 to 12 g/day N is equivalent to the loss of 1 to 2 kg/day of lean tissue (43, 44). If this rate of body N loss were to continue, the body's lean tissue reserve would be lethally depleted within 3 weeks of fasting. Instead, an adaptation takes effect after 7 to 10 days of fasting, which, by the end of 2 to 3 weeks, reduces the rate of N loss to less than one half of the rate during the first several days. This incompletely understood adaptation is all the more remarkable when it is considered that one half of urinary N by this time is in ammonium, excreted to buffer the protons generated by ketoacid production (7, 45). When ammonium excretion is reduced to normal by providing an exogenous buffer, body N losses in prolonged "adapted" fasting are close to the "obligatory" rate of N loss considered to reflect the maximum attainable efficiency of endogenous protein turnover (46–49).

Plasma branched-chain amino acid concentrations approximately double during the first 1 to 3 days of fasting, and their release from whole-body proteins and subsequent oxidation increase by variable amounts (50, 51). Urinary excretion of 3-methylhistidine, an indicator of contractile protein breakdown, also increases in the first few days of fasting (50, 52). By 7 to 10 days, the initial increase in amino acid turnover is superseded, in most (50, 53), although not all (51), studies, by a reduction of tracer-measured leucine or lysine (54) appearance in a setting of continued important urinary N loss and leucine oxidation. By the fourth week, when N excretion has greatly diminished, plasma leucine turnover is reduced even further (55, 56), and urinary 3-methylhistidine excretion falls to less than the prefasting rate (55).

The protein-sparing adaptation that occurs in prolonged fasting is the result of reduced net amino acid release from muscle (10, 57). The high rate of muscle catabolism characteristic of the early phase of fasting is caused by reduced protein synthesis (the consequence of absent exogenous amino acids and the lowered insulin level, because insulin normally stimulates protein synthesis) and the loss of insulin's restraint of muscle proteolysis (14, 58). What reverses this catabolic process after approximately 2 weeks of fasting? Most authorities regard the shift in the muscle metabolism from ketone body oxidation to fatty acid oxidation (and the resulting rise in blood ketone bodies) as crucial and argue that as ketone bodies increasingly displace glucose as the brain's fuel, the body no longer needs to convert so much muscle protein into new glucose molecules.

Missing from this explanation, however, is identification of the signal that "tells" muscle that it can now reduce its net protein catabolic rate (7). Some observations suggest that hyperketonemia has a direct protein-sparing effect on skeletal muscle (59, 60), but a clear demonstration of this is lacking (51). It is also possible that the process by which muscle metabolism switches from ketone body oxidation to fatty acid oxidation after 2 weeks of fasting is in some way responsible for the reduction in muscle proteolysis. An important role of free fatty acids in muscle protein sparing has been shown in persons who fast on a short-term basis (61). It is conceivable that increased muscle fatty acid oxidation spares the branched-chain amino acids (which have structural similarity to fatty acids), and that the branched-chain amino acids (or their metabolites) somehow mediate a reduction in proteolysis (7). This hypothesis is supported by evidence that these molecules, particularly leucine, have protein-sparing effects (62). Finally, ketone bodies could stimulate a rise in peripheral insulin that is too slight to be detected (25, 35, 36), but that, nevertheless, exerts a protein-sparing effect.

Weight Loss

Weight loss and body N loss occur at a rate that is roughly in direct proportion to existing body weight and lean body mass (63, 64), but the pattern is highly variable. Nonobese men with free access to water may lose 4 kg over the first 5 days of fasting and a further 3 kg over the next 5 days (44, 65), whereas obese men lose about 50% more than this. In one extreme case, a patient initially weighing 245 kg lost 32 kg after 30 days of fasting (63).

Water, not fat, accounts for most of the early weight loss of total fasting (66). Approximately 65% of the total water lost from the body during the first 3 days is extracellular (65). This rapid mobilization of extracellular water and sodium is partly the result of the lack of dietary sodium and partly the result of the low insulin state, which reduces insulin-mediated renal tubular sodium reabsorption (67). A rapid loss of intracellular water also occurs, owing to the dissolution of lean tissues (19–25 g water/g N), liver glycogen (2–3 g water/g glycogen [68]), and, to a

lesser extent, muscle glycogen (3–4 g water/g glycogen [69]) (43). However, after 3 days, all glycogen has disappeared from the liver, and by 2 weeks, extracellular fluid balance has stabilized (63). Consequently, weight loss slows greatly, now exclusively the result of lean tissue and adipose tissue loss, both of which are themselves slowed by adaptive protein sparing and reduced energy expenditure. Weight loss by a 3-week fasting, moderately obese person is typically approximately 350 g/day. The daily negative N balance of approximately 4 g is equivalent to the loss of 125 g hydrated lean tissue. Adipose tissue is approximately 85% pure fat (70–72), so the daily negative energy balance of approximately 1700 kcal is equivalent to the daily loss of approximately 200 g adipose tissue. The rate of weight loss continues to slow as the lean tissue mass diminishes, in keeping with a first-order kinetic process.

Other Metabolic Effects

REE decreases within days of initiating a total fast; indeed, sleeping energy expenditure has been reported to decrease within the first 48 hours (73). A small *increase* in REE is sometimes observed early in fasting (74, 75), presumably because of the catecholamine stimulation that occurs if extracellular volume depletion is not prevented by generous sodium provision (76). After 2 weeks, REE has decreased by approximately 15% (77), and by 3 to 4 weeks, it has decreased by 25 to 35% below normal (65). The early reduction in REE is adaptive, being far too rapid to be explained entirely by the loss of metabolically active tissues. The further reduction in REE that occurs as fasting continues is due to the body's decreasing metabolic mass.

Serum albumin concentrations remain normal both in short-term and prolonged fasting, but concentrations of the rapidly turning over liver secretory proteins, transthyretin (thyroid-binding prealbumin) and retinol-binding protein, promptly fall, as occurs even with simple carbohydrate restriction (78, 79). Ketonemia and extracellular volume depletion increase serum urate concentrations (10, 32). Serum total bilirubin typically increases by 50% after 24 hours of fasting and is twice normal after 48 hours, but it remains constant thereafter (80). Gastric emptying slows after 4 days of fasting (81). Mild chronic ketosis activates fetal hemoglobin production, and this may lead to a detectable increase in circulating fetal hemoglobin in some situations (82). In therapeutic fasts lasting longer than 4 weeks, postural hypotension and nausea often occur. Other metabolic effects and medical complications of prolonged fasting are described in older clinical reviews (10, 63, 83).

Nutritional Modifications of Fasting Metabolism

Carbohydrate provision reduces the early protein catabolic phase of fasting, whereas fat has no such protein-sparing effect (9, 53). As little as 100 to 150 g/day of glucose prevents the ketonuria of fasting and reduces urea N excretion and extracellular volume loss by one half (84). The important protein-sparing effect of carbohydrate occurs in the first 7 to 10 days of a fast. When provided later, even large amounts of carbohydrate reduce N loss only marginally below the low rate to which adaptation has already brought it by this time (8, 85). By contrast, protein consumption has little effect on net body protein loss in the first 7 to 10 days of fasting, but after 2 or more weeks of continuous high-quality protein feeding in doses of 50 to 80 g/day, N balance improves and may even return to zero (86, 87). When protein is introduced in the late, adapted phase of a total fast, N balance abruptly turns positive even though energy balance is strongly negative (55, 88). This finding illustrates the operation of the mechanisms entrained to minimize body N loss during prolonged fasting, which increase the efficiency with which endogenous proteins are turned over and the avidity with which dietary protein is retained.

Survival

The usual determinant of survival during prolonged fasting is the size of the body's initial fat store (89). Adults who were initially of normal body weight die after approximately 60 days of continuous fasting (90), a time span consistent with complete loss of body fat but only about one third of the lean tissues (89). Fatty acids need to be instantly available in prolonged fasting because the brain depends on ketone bodies and glucose for energy, and fatty acids provide both the substrate for ketone body synthesis and the fuel to drive hepatic gluconeogenesis, an energy-using process (13). Fasting therefore should be considered especially hazardous for persons with low fat stores even if their lean tissue stores are ample (91).

Obese persons have tolerated fasts of astonishing length (92, 93). The longest monitored fast on record was by a 27-year-old man whose starting weight was 207 kg. He lost 60% of his body weight after 382 days of uninterrupted fasting (94). Despite such spectacular experiences, total fasts longer than about 4 weeks are potentially dangerous even for obese persons. Although reduced to a minimum, lean tissue loss does not cease. In cases of extremely prolonged fasting in which lean tissue loss was measured, critical levels of depletion were observed (93). Acute thiamin deficiency is a devastating preventable complication of prolonged fasting (95) and refeeding after it (96).

PROTEIN DEFICIENCY

Minimum Protein Requirement

A state of pure protein deficiency comes about when protein intake is less than the minimum requirement level, but intake of the other essential nutrients, including energy, remains adequate. Protein deficiency rarely occurs in clinical medicine in the absence of energy deficiency. Its effects are of interest, however, because they bear on the definition of minimum protein or essential amino acid requirements (46, 97–99).

The normal response to a reduction in protein intake is an adaptive reduction of amino acid catabolism commensurate with the lower intake, so that, after a few days, zero N balance is restored. The protein intake below which a person cannot correspondingly reduce amino acid catabolism, and hence reestablish N equilibrium, is conventionally considered to define his or her minimum protein requirement (46, 98). Although easy to state, this definition can be difficult to apply in practice. N balance turns negative whenever protein intake is reduced, but it typically returns to zero after a few days, either with no adverse consequence or after a certain amount of body protein has been jettisoned. Was the protein intake that produced this adaptive response "deficient"? For example, the nineteenth-century German physiologist Voit concluded that the protein requirement of physiologically normal men was 120 g/day after observing that their N balance became negative for the first few days after their protein intake was reduced below this level. However, as has been pointed out (97), Voit's subjects did not *require* a daily ration of 120 g of protein daily; they were merely *habituated* to it.

To account for this phenomenon, terms such as adaptation or normal adaptation have been used to describe normal homeostatic adjustments to changes in protein intake that occur *at or above* the minimum requirement, and terms such as pathologic adaptation or accommodation have been used to describe metabolic changes that restore N equilibrium only by means of important lean tissue sacrifice and at a physiologic cost. *Adaptation* is thought of as an aspect of normal homeostasis, whereas *accommodation* implies that homeostasis has been reestablished at the expense of a physiologic compromise with adverse health implications (100).

Protein Intakes above and below the Requirement Level

Adaptive responses to changes in protein consumption *above* the minimum requirement are different from those made when protein intake is *below* the minimum requirement. Amino acids in excess are toxic and cannot be stored, so any surfeit consumption obliges the body promptly to catabolize the equivalent amount of amino acids. Under equilibrium conditions, body N loss precisely equals N intake, a metabolic agenda that calls for "zero" metabolic efficiency. The kinetic properties of the enzymes that catabolize the amino acids are such that transamination and oxidation increase linearly with increasing tissue concentration (101). Surfeit amino acid consumption increases free amino acid pool sizes, and this automatically increases their catabolism (102, 103). In confirmation of this understanding, whole-body leucine oxidation is generally found to be proportional to its plasma concentration (104).

The agenda is different when protein intake falls below the requirement level. In this situation, the body conserves dietary amino acids efficiently, both by reducing proteolysis and by increasing protein synthesis from dietary and endogenous amino acids. These adaptations reduce the size of the free amino acid pools and limit the increase that normally occurs in the fed state, thereby minimizing "overflow" catabolism. Amino acid catabolism is also minimized by reducing the amounts or specific catalytic activities of key amino acid degradative enzymes (100, 105).

In quantitative terms, the major decision whether tissue amino acids will be catabolized or deposited in newly synthesized proteins occurs in the fed state (106). The opportunity to modulate endogenous amino acid oxidation continues throughout the periods between meals, however, and, indeed, it is difficult to conceive of an adaptive process aimed at improving the efficiency of dietary amino acid utilization that is not measurably in effect in the basal period preceding meal consumption. Leucine oxidation is a measure of whole-body amino acid catabolism, and most studies confirm that the increased or decreased leucine oxidation evoked by high or low protein intakes, and even different meal patterns, extends into the period between meals (107–110).

Consumption of a severely protein-deficient diet for 7 to 10 days reduces whole-body amino acid turnover (48, 111) and the rate of albumin synthesis, even though the serum albumin concentration does not change (112). Urinary N excretion falls until, after an adaptation period of from 4 to 7 days, it reaches a pseudosteady-state (and highly reproducible) rate of 37 mg/kg body weight (46). The other sources of body N loss (feces, sweat, and skin desquamation) are unaffected by short-term variations in protein intake (46, 47, 112). Urinary N excretion after short-term adaptation to complete protein deprivation (with normal nonprotein energy provision) is termed "endogenous" or "obligatory" urinary N and is considered to indicate the maximum efficiency with which endogenous protein can be turned over to conserve the body's active protein store (46–49).

No one questions that minimum human protein and essential amino acid requirements exist (46, 98). Determining precisely what they are requires the demonstration that prolonged intake of these nutrients at less than a specific level has adverse physiologic consequences. Practical and ethical considerations make this almost impossible, so the question of what constitutes the true minimum protein requirement for optimum health continues to be debated, despite more than a century of research (97). The adult average minimum requirement for high-quality protein is currently taken to be 0.6 kg/kg normal body weight. It was determined by measuring the lowest protein intake at which zero N balance is attained by normal persons consuming a diet adequate in all other nutrients, including energy (98).

In a clinical study to determine whether dietary protein restriction slows the progression of chronic renal disease, patients with this disease consumed a diet containing only 0.4 g protein/kg/day for several months (113). The results, after 6 months, were weight loss and reduced serum transferrin concentrations but no change in serum albumin (113). Energy supplementation failed to induce weight regain, a finding suggesting that at least some of the weight loss experienced by the study participants was from their lean tissue stores and hence a manifestation of protein deficiency.

The most detailed protein restriction study carried out to date was one in which healthy elderly women were randomly allocated to diets providing either surfeit (0.92 g/kg) or inadequate (0.45 g/kg) daily protein with adequate energy (114, 115). After 9 weeks, the body weight of the protein-restricted women was maintained, and their N balance was only slightly negative, findings indicating successful accommodation to their deficient protein intake. Unlike the control subjects who consumed adequate protein, their active cell mass was reduced, and their muscle function and immune status were impaired (114). Protein restriction had no effect on basal plasma leucine concentration, on proteolysis or protein synthesis (as measured in the fed state either per kilogram of body weight or fat-free mass [FFM]), or on urinary 3-methylhistidine excretion (115). Serum concentrations of the liver secretory proteins, albumin, retinol-binding protein, and transferrin, remained normal (114). This study provides evidence that plasma transthyretin (prealbumin), retinol-binding protein, and transferrin concentrations, often taken as indicators of the adequacy of protein nutrition, appear to be more sensitive to carbohydrate and total energy intake than they are to protein nutrition per se (78, 79).

Kwashiorkor

Kwashiorkor, or edematous hypoalbuminemic malnutrition of infants, differs importantly from the predominant form of childhood protein-energy malnutrition, known as marasmus. Children with marasmus have poor linear growth and are fat and muscle depleted, while lacking the fluid accumulation, fatty liver, and skin and hair changes that occur in kwashiorkor. Kwashiorkor has been thought to be caused by subsistence on a protein-deficient, high-carbohydrate diet. According to this view, the high carbohydrate intake stimulates insulin secretion and drives scarce dietary amino acids into the insulin-responsive muscles at the expense of the liver (116). This reduces hepatic albumin synthesis, causes hypoalbuminemia and edema, and reduces lipoprotein synthesis in a setting of hepatic lipogenesis from dietary carbohydrate, thus causing fatty liver. Adult variants have been postulated when malnourished hospitalized patients receive prolonged intravenous dextrose without amino acids (117). Although attractive, this understanding of kwashiorkor is incomplete and lacks a clear clinical or metabolic formulation. More sophisticated, but nevertheless, still incomplete explanations have been proposed (118–120). It appears that hypoalbuminemia usually occurs in the malnourished child or adult for the same reasons as in physiologically normal persons, as part of the negative acute-phase response to infection or injury. This response lowers serum albumin concentrations by redistributing albumin into the extravascular space and by increasing its catabolism (121, 122). A current focus of research in this area is inflammation-induced oxidant stress in the context of antioxidant micronutrient deficiency, including deficiency of the sulfur amino acids, which are precursors of the important intracellular antioxidant, glutathione (123–125). Further complexity is introduced by observations in humans (126) and rats (127) that protein-energy malnutrition may itself induce a low-grade inflammatory state.

Nevertheless, the results of field research (128), a case report of kwashiorkor seemingly resulting from pure protein deficiency (129), and tracer data indicating that protein restriction reduces albumin synthesis (112, 130) support the clinical impression that hypoalbuminemia develops more rapidly and profoundly in the presence of inadequate protein nutrition, and that it will persist if adequate protein is not provided (131, 132).

PROTEIN-ENERGY DEFICIENCY

The most common form of starvation results from insufficient food consumption and hence combines the features of energy deficiency, protein deficiency, and in all likelihood deficiencies of certain micronutrients (97, 133). Protein-energy deficiency may broadly be considered as combining the hypometabolic adaptation of energy deficiency with the reduced whole-body protein turnover characteristic of severe or chronic protein deficiency, but its manifestations are more variable.

Composition of Weight Loss

The most detailed study of the effects of chronic human energy and protein deficiency was carried out between 1944 and 1946 in an experiment in which 32 healthy young men volunteered to live on the campus of the University of Minnesota while they consumed a diet of approximately 1600 kcal/day, or about two thirds of their normal energy requirement (134).

The Minnesota volunteers lost an average of 23% of their initial body weight and more than 70% of their body fat. Muscle was also lost: in all, 24% of the lean tissue mass (termed "active tissue mass" in the study) was lost, and this accounted for 60% of the total weight loss. Total weight loss actually underestimated the sum of fat and lean tissue losses, because the extracellular fluid volume increased. In extreme cases (and especially in the presence of other diseases associated with water retention), the increase in extracellular volume that occurs in this setting causes obvious

fluid swelling within the skin and other interstitial tissues, called "hunger edema."

Adaptation

As with fasting, weight loss is most rapid in the early phase of starvation. It often finally slows to zero even when there is no change in the starvation diet. This occurred for the Minnesota volunteers after 24 weeks. This lifesaving adaptation involves the reestablishment of fat (energy) and lean tissue (protein) homeostasis.

Energy Expenditure

The REE of the Minnesota volunteers decreased by 40% after 24 weeks of starvation, thus coming approximately into line with their low energy intake. This decrease was partly adaptive, but mostly it was caused by their diminished lean tissue mass, which is responsible for most of the processes that involve energy expenditure (135). Total energy expenditure also decreased substantially, because smaller meals evoke a smaller thermic effect of food, and a lighter body demands less work of moving (136) and allows physical tasks to be performed with greater energy efficiency (137). Moreover, the volunteers reduced their voluntary physical activity by more than half, a form of adaptation observed in other studies of chronic starvation (138–140) and in some (141, 142), but not all (143), short-term starvation studies. Nonvolitional or purposeless movements, known as "fidgeting," can contribute substantially to daily energy expenditure (144), so reduction in this kind of activity will also conserve energy during prolonged starvation. Such adjustments, when successful, bring starving persons back into energy equilibrium.

It is common when attempting to identify the factors responsible for changes in energy metabolism to divide the measured REE by body weight or FFM, on the assumption that a change in REE/FFM indicates a change in cellular metabolic activity. This is incorrect. The FFM is inhomogeneous with respect to its energy-using elements (145, 146), and in starvation, body substance is lost unequally from the different compartments of FFM: skeletal muscle bears the brunt of the loss, whereas the highly metabolically active central lean tissues are relatively spared (146, 147). As a consequence, REE/weight and REE/FFM increase as weight and FFM decrease (146, 148). In studies that adjusted for FFM appropriately using covariate analysis, adjusted REE was indeed found to be reduced in adapted starving patients (149, 150), a finding confirming that an important component of the reduction of REE in starvation is indeed the result of metabolic adaptation.

Lean Tissue Loss

The energy-restricted person is able to reestablish zero energy balance by jettisoning lean tissue mass, but he or

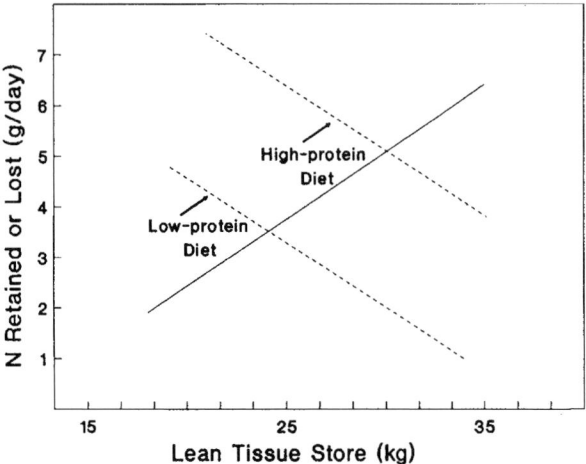

Figure 48.1. A hypothetic scheme to account for adaptation to starvation in the adult. A first-order (linear) relationship exists between the amount of lean tissue and the rate at which it is depleted. This is indicated by the *solid line*. An *inverse* relationship exists between the amount of lean tissue and the efficiency of retention of protein in the diet. This relationship is affected by the concentration of protein in the diet, resulting in a family of curves (*dashed line*). As starvation progresses and the lean tissue store diminishes, the rate of protein depletion slows as the amount of protein retained from each meal increases. At the crossover point, a new equilibrium is established, and lean tissue loss ceases. The "price" paid to achieve this physiologic adaptation is a diminished lean tissue store. This scheme illustrates that a high-protein diet may permit protein equilibrium after only moderate lean tissue wasting; a low-protein diet may also be compatible with protein equilibrium, but the cost, in terms of protein wasting, will be greater.

she cannot afford to lose so much of it that the adverse consequences become intolerable. N equilibrium is reestablished by a process that can be separated conceptually into two components: decreased endogenous N loss and increased efficiency of dietary protein retention (Fig. 48.1). As starvation proceeds, the rate of lean tissue loss is approximately proportional to the amount of lean tissue remaining; this means that its rate of loss automatically slows as the lean tissue mass decreases (151). Also apparent are adaptations of cellular metabolism that reduce the rate of endogenous amino acid oxidation (102) and increase the efficiency with which exogenous proteins are retained from the diet. The phenomenon of increased avidity of retention of dietary protein in starvation has long been recognized (152–154). Net body protein loss continues until the slowing of endogenous protein loss matches the increasing efficiency of dietary protein retention and a new state of protein equilibrium is established (see Fig. 48.1).

Protein Turnover

Few studies of whole-body protein turnover have been carried out in chronically starved nonobese persons. From the results of these studies (115, 155), animal studies, and extrapolations from the literature on therapeutic weight reduction and short-term protein deficiency, one may

tentatively conclude that adaptation to starvation reduces protein turnover in many tissues (103, 112, 156, 157). It also appears that the major influence on protein turnover is protein intake itself. Thus, very-low-energy (500 kcal/day) reducing diets that include generous amounts of high-quality protein maintain protein turnover (56, 107, 158), whereas fasting (55, 56) or low-energy diets low in good-quality protein reduce it (53, 158).

As with energy expenditure, the contribution of diminished lean tissue mass to the slowing of whole-body protein turnover during starvation cannot be indicated simply by dividing a whole-body turnover parameter by body weight or FFM. Protein turnover proceeds at different rates in the different lean tissue compartments (159), which are depleted to different extents during starvation (146, 147). In studies of chronic protein-energy starvation, whole-body protein turnover per kilogram of FFM may be higher than in physiologically normal adults, owing to a disproportionately greater loss of slowly turning over skeletal muscle protein than of rapidly turning over central proteins (147, 160).

Determinants of Lean Tissue Conservation

Because the starving person is often obliged to sacrifice a certain amount of protein to reestablish zero energy and N balance, protein loss can be regarded as a survival mechanism (161). However, energy intake is only one of several factors that influence the rate of N is loss during starvation and the total amount of lean tissue that needs to be sacrificed to reestablish N equilibrium. These factors include energy balance, protein intake, protein nutritional state, biologic individuality, and possibly obesity.

Energy Balance. The Minnesota volunteers consumed close to the amount of protein regarded as safe for physiologically normal adults (0.75 g/kg body weight), but they still lost a large amount of their lean tissue store. Many studies have shown that N balance at a constant protein intake is improved by an increase and is worsened by a decrease in energy intake (116, 162, 163). The predominant energy source (carbohydrate or fat) is immaterial (164). Because it is the amount of dietary energy in surplus or in deficit after accounting for expenditure, energy balance is probably the specific physiologic variable that when negative worsens N balance and when positive improves it (165, 166).

Protein Intake. N balance is improved by an increased protein intake over a wide range of energy intakes from deficient to maintenance (116, 167). When the lean tissues are depleted, the efficiency of retention of the protein in a given meal becomes greater. A meal high in protein therefore permits greater absolute protein retention than one low in protein. As illustrated in Figure 48.1, a high-protein starvation diet may be associated with protein equilibrium after only moderate lean tissue wasting, whereas a low-protein diet is associated with greater lean tissue wasting, even though equilibrium is ultimately reestablished. Most, but not all (87), studies have shown that a protein intake of 1.5 g protein/kg normal body weight during starvation maintains N balance (86) or FFM (168) better than lower intakes.

Stage of Starvation. Prior protein depletion increases the efficiency of N retention at any protein and energy intake (55). This occurs partly because a smaller mass of active body protein requires less amino acid replacement than a larger one and partly because of cellular adaptations, as described in a later section. The influence of protein-nutritional status is implicit in the scheme shown in Figure 48.1, in which a given lean tissue mass (as indicated on the horizontal axis) has an important effect on endogenous protein loss and the avidity of dietary protein retention.

Exercise. Physical exercise maintains or mitigates loss of muscle mass during starvation (138, 169).

Obesity. Investigators have often claimed that obesity confers a sparing effect on protein loss during fasting and starvation (66, 170). In my view, this is not established, given the confounding effect differences in body stature, physical activity, and protein intake have on N loss in starvation, the paucity of controlled data, and the absence of a plausible biologic mechanism for an obesity-specific protein-sparing phenomenon in starvation (171). An analysis of the composition of weight loss by weight-reducing obese patients failed to show slower loss of FFM in the more obese patients (172). This finding is not surprising, because some of the protein lost from the body during weight reduction by obese persons is obligatory: a lighter body frame needs less muscle to support it. Moreover, approximately 15% of the weight of adipose tissue is FFM that is lost from the body as the fat mass decreases (70–72). It is therefore predictable that, to the extent lean tissue mass is increased in severely obese persons, their rate of N and FFM loss will, if anything, be faster than in less obese persons (63, 173). Finally, unlike in obesity, the lean tissue mass of moderately energy-restricted persons of normal weight is well maintained (174–176), presumably because of their high level of physical activity (169), generous protein intake, and only modest adipose tissue unloading.

Other Factors. When weight loss continues in spite of conditions conducive to adaptation, attention should be directed to correctable factors such as malabsorption, the adequacy of micronutrient provision (133, 177, 178), or a supervening catabolic state. These factors are considered in more detail in a later section, but even when all of them are controlled or considered, the variation in individual responses to starvation is wide (179).

Characteristics of Successful Adaptation

Pathologic adaptation "succeeds" when metabolic adjustments and lean tissue sacrifice reestablish energy and N equilibrium. The organism survives, but at a metabolic and functional cost (112). The most apparent deficits are the loss of insulating fat and muscle with its associated loss of physical power. A hypometabolic state of unwellness is induced reminiscent of (but not identical to) hypothyroidism (180). Starving patients are hypothermic and do not mount an appropriate thermic response to environmental cold (181). The loss of muscle diminishes the body's protein reserve, and this, together with slower protein turnover in the remaining muscle (182), reduces the body's options for protein remodeling in response to changing metabolic needs. Starving persons mount a blunted rise of protein turnover and a smaller catabolic response during metabolic stress (183).

In addition to the loss of muscle, deficits in central protein function occur. The anatomic and functional consequences of severe human starvation are covered in clinical depictions (134, 184, 185) and medical reviews (2, 186–188). These include anemia, altered heart muscle mass and function (189, 190), decreased respiratory muscle function and reduced ventilatory drive (191, 192), impaired healing of skin ulcers (193), altered gut anatomy and function (194), altered drug metabolism (195), bone loss (196, 197), and immunodeficiency (198).

Weight-stable anorexia nervosa in an otherwise healthy person provides a conceptual paradigm of successful pathologic adaptation to starvation (199). More complex examples can be observed daily in any outpatient chronic disease clinic and in segments of the population of many parts of the world. The defining metabolic features of successful adaptation are a less than critical total lean tissue depletion, weight stability, a normal plasma albumin level (in the absence of dehydration), a normal peripheral blood total lymphocyte count, and intact delayed cutaneous hypersensitivity (200).

Failed Adaptation

This situation should be suspected when a starving patient develops a catabolic state, as indicated by fever or a rapid heart rate. However, these responses to tissue injury or invasion may be blunted in starvation, and their absence does not rule out a catabolic stimulus, nor does it exclude other factors that can reverse the adapted state. A more reliable sign of stress-induced protein wasting is an inappropriate rise in serum urea concentration and urinary urea excretion. The simplest indicator of the reversal of accommodation from any cause is the resumption of weight loss in a previously weight-stable, malnourished patient or failure to *gain* weight despite the development of edema. Either situation indicates that new lean tissue loss is occurring. The presence of factors that impair adaptation should alert the clinician to the possibility. They include further diminution of food intake, worsening of the primary disease or the development of one of its complications, the onset of a new disease that imposes a metabolic stress, or the administration of a treatment that alters protein or energy metabolism (132).

Catabolic Stress. The hypermetabolic, catabolic response to severe infection, trauma, or traumatic major surgery reverses the adaptation to starvation (3, 200, 201) (see Chapters 89 and 91), as does the less intense inflammatory condition of cachexia, described later in this chapter.

Mineral Deficiency. Mineral deficiencies, particularly those of potassium (177), phosphorus (177), zinc (202, 203), and presumably magnesium, prevent maximal protein-sparing and an appropriate anabolic response to refeeding.

Metabolic Disease or the Administration of Hormones or Antimetabolites. Hyperthyroidism, pheochromocytoma, glucagonoma, poorly controlled diabetes mellitus, and states of glucocorticoid excess (204) cause protein wasting. The presence of any of these diseases or its new development in starving patients calls for attention to the patient's nutritional status. In any of these situations, protein-energy malnutrition may rapidly develop, or the previously successful adaptation to existing starvation may be reversed. Some evidence reveals that the efficiency of protein metabolism remains abnormal even with appropriate insulin treatment of insulin-dependent diabetes (205). Such persons may be at increased risk of protein depletion during starvation.

Food Restriction too Severe. The most common maladaptation to starvation should not be described as maladaptation at all, but is merely the consequence of food deprivation so severe that adaptation is impossible. The result is continuous weight loss until death supervenes.

Clinical Significance of Serum Albumin

Hypoalbuminemia is an important predictor of an adverse clinical outcome, but it is neither a sensitive nor a specific marker of protein deficiency or protein-energy malnutrition (121,122). Knowledge of the serum albumin concentration is, nevertheless, invaluable in nutritional assessment. First, a normal serum albumin concentration in a volume-replete patient rules out the presence of an acute-phase response with failed adaptation to starvation and portends a favorable clinical outcome. Second, hypoalbuminemia, whatever its cause, almost always occurs in a clinical context of anorexia and inadequate food intake and therefore alerts the clinician of the need for a comprehensive nutritional assessment.

Survival

The Minnesota study demonstrated that total weight loss tracks lean tissue loss relatively closely in starving persons whose initial body composition is normal. About half of the total protein in the human body is structural (mostly collagen). The other half is found within the lean tissues, which make up nearly half of total body weight in health and are the source of the N lost from the body in starvation (206). Investigators usually consider that a 50% or greater depletion of the body's lean tissues is incompatible with survival (2, 90, 207). Body mass index (BMI, body weight in kilograms divided by the square of height in

meters) is a better predictor of the certainty of death than body weight. Data analyzed by Henry (208) suggested that death is certain when the BMI falls to less than approximately 13 in men and 12 in women, but subsequent experience indicated that a BMI of 10 is compatible with life in mature adults, and even lower BMIs have been tolerated by young adults (209). One fifth of starving adults more than 25 years of age and nearly one half of those less than 25 years old who were admitted to a medical unit in Somalia had a BMI less than 12. Survival with a BMI this low is rare in affluent countries, where advanced starvation typically occurs in elderly persons suffering from a primary medical or surgical condition. This finding further confirms the importance of the interaction among malnutrition, age, and disease in causing starvation-related death.

In developed countries, where severe malnutrition is almost always associated with a primary medical or surgical disease, the proximate causes of death are infectious pneumonia (related to decreased ventilatory mechanical function and drive, lung stasis, and ineffective cough), skin breakdown with local and systemic infection (related to inactivity, skin thinning, and edema), sepsis spreading from intravenous infusion catheters, diarrhea with dehydration, and synergistic worsening of the primary disease. Contributing to all these causes is starvation-induced immunodeficiency, itself the result of decreased mobilizable protein stores, hypothermia, and micronutrient deficiencies (1,2). In some patients, death is attributed to a cardiac arrhythmia (134, 210).

In summary, it appears that the nature and tempo of the primary disease are strong, but far from sole, determinants of death in moderate, in-hospital starvation. As lean tissue depletion approaches and exceeds about 40%, death directly resulting from starvation becomes increasingly more certain, manifesting a thermodynamic law that is unaffected by the number of diagnostic procedures, operative interventions, or antibiotic combinations administered to the patient, unless these interventions are combined with nutrition therapy (211).

Descriptions of needless death from starvation evoke feelings of dismay in most commentators. Particularly moving are the writings of Fliederbaum, whose observations in the Warsaw ghetto constitute probably the best clinical description of the effects of severe starvation ever published (185):

> . . . boys and girls from blooming like roses change into withered old people. One of the patients said, "Our strength is vanishing like a melting wax candle." Active, busy, energetic people are changed into apathetic, sleepy beings, always in bed, hardly able to get up to eat or to go to the toilet. Passage from life to death is slow and gradual, like death from physiological old age. There is nothing violent, no dyspnea, no pain, no obvious changes in breathing or circulation. Vital functions subside simultaneously. Pulse rate and respiratory rate get slower and it becomes more and more difficult to reach the patient's awareness, until life is gone. People fall asleep in bed or on the street and are dead in the morning. They die during physical effort, such as searching for food, and sometimes even with a piece of bread in their hands.

MECHANISMS OF ADAPTATION TO STARVATION

The foregoing discussion deals with nutritional factors that affect the physiologic adaptation to starvation. This section focuses on the biochemical mechanisms that could mediate this adaptation.

Energy Metabolism

The adaptive reduction in REE during energy restriction is caused by alterations in the peripheral metabolism of thyroxine (T_4), the hormone secreted by the thyroid gland, to its more active metabolite, triiodothyronine (T_3), and perhaps, to a lesser extent, by changes in sympathetic nervous system activity (86, 151, 180, 212, 213). Serum T_4 levels and those of thyrotropin (the pituitary hormone that regulates T_4 secretion) remain normal, but serum T_3 decreases within a few days (or even hours) of initiating a starvation diet. Serum levels of an inactive metabolite, reverse T_3, rise (214, 215). Both energy intake and, specifically, the amount of carbohydrate consumed affect this conversion process, apparently through their effect on insulin secretion (180, 216, 217). Although an association exists between decreased circulating T_3 and lowered REE during starvation, its precise nature is not well understood (86, 180), nor is T_3 the only modulating factor. Thus, a carbohydrate-free diet that provides maintenance energy reduces T_3 levels, but REE does not decrease (218). Poorly controlled diabetes mellitus is associated with decreased serum T_3 levels, but the metabolic rate is increased (219).

As long as volume depletion is prevented (76), catecholamine secretion and turnover decrease in uncomplicated starvation. The blood pressure, heart rate, and core temperature of starving patients are reduced, as is their thermic response to cold or to a norepinephrine infusion. Pupil size, an indicator of basal sympathetic tone, is diminished (134, 139, 181). As with T_4 to T_3 conversion, both energy balance and carbohydrate intake, at least in part because of their effect on insulin release, appear to be important regulators of these effects. The thyroid and catecholamine effects are interconnected (161). T_3 increases the number of tissue norepinephrine receptors, and in its absence, the number decreases (220).

Plasma concentrations of leptin, a cytokinelike hormone released by adipocytes, decrease importantly both in short- and long-term energy restriction, while also reflecting the magnitude of the body fat store in states of energy equilibrium (221, 222). Leptin is regulated by insulin levels (221). The acute fall in circulating leptin caused by carbohydrate restriction could mediate the reduction of serum T_3 and the increase in reverse T_3 that occurs in this situation, findings suggesting a role for leptin in the regulation of energy expenditure (223).

The uncoupling proteins (UCPs) are transporters that allow protons to leak into the mitochondrial matrix by channels separate from the ones that drive ADP conversion to ATP. Their effect is to dissipate as heat some of the free energy that would otherwise be stored in new ATP molecules. Recognition that UCP1 mediates the thermogenic function of brown adipose tissue fueled speculation that the other UCPs (particularly UCP3, which is mainly expressed in muscle) could be involved in the regulation of whole-body energy expenditure. It now appears that their role is to protect mitochondria from excessive oxygen free radical formation in situations of local oxygen accumulation and ATP repletion (or rather, ADP absence), to regulate ATP-dependent reactions, or (in the case of UCP3) to transport fatty acid anions, rather than to mediate adaptive reductions and increases in energy expenditure in response to starvation and overfeeding (224, 225).

Protein Metabolism

Our understanding of the way in which hormones govern the adaptation to starvation remains rudimentary (217, 226). T_3 is involved in regulating muscle metabolism, but its precise effects in starvation remain poorly defined (180, 227). T_3 levels decrease early in starvation (as reverse T_3 levels increase), and T_3 administration to fasting obese persons increases body N loss (180), findings suggesting that the reduction of T_3 is important, at least permissively, for successful adaptation. However, the relationship between T_3 and N balance that is apparent in total fasting studies is less clear in patients consuming hypocaloric diets (86).

Insulin stimulates protein synthesis and inhibits its breakdown in muscle and in liver, and insulin lack reduces protein synthesis and increases proteolysis (14, 57). Whereas protein synthesis in the splanchnic tissues increases in response to amino acid provision even in low insulin states, muscle protein synthesis requires both insulin and a supply of amino acids (228). Insulin levels are typically reduced in starvation (175, 229), and although they are not low enough to induce ketosis, it is likely that the combination of a relatively low insulin state and reduced dietary amino acid delivery curtails muscle protein synthesis (103) and, secondarily, proteolysis (227). The combination of reduced insulin action and a diminished amino acid supply could be expressed both directly on the cells and indirectly, by diminishing the peripheral action of thyroid hormone (227).

Protein or energy restriction and catabolic states reduce circulating concentrations of the protein anabolic peptide hormone, insulinlike growth factor-I (IGF-I). This occurs despite increased serum concentrations of growth hormone, which normally stimulates IGF-I release (217, 230). Structurally related to insulin, IGF-I stimulates net protein synthesis in cultured cells and in isolated muscle in a manner similar to that of insulin (14). Much information about IGF-I and its nutritional interactions is now available (231–233). Despite the complexity of IGF-I's autocrine and paracrine functions and its numerous plasma binding proteins (IGFBPs), it is clear that IGF-I plays an important role in the adaptation of protein metabolism to altered nutritional states, by acting in concert with insulin and thyroid hormone (234, 235).

IGF-I is synthesized in many tissues, but most of the IGF-I found in the bloodstream has been released there by the liver, where it circulates as part of a large ternary complex with IGFBP-3 (232). Serum total IGF-I corresponds closely to the serum IGFBP-3 concentration (232). The IGF-I–IGFBP-3 complex is too large to leave the circulation, but IGF-I complexes with other binding proteins, notably IGFBP-I, which are smaller and readily enter the extracellular space; their presumed role is to deliver IGF-I from the circulation to its tissue receptors (230, 232). The circulating half-life of the IGF-I–IGFBP-3 complex is more than 12 hours, and its plasma concentration changes only sluggishly, whereas circulating IGFBP-I turns over very rapidly, its human serum levels increase dynamically by as much as sevenfold (236) in response to short-term fasting or pathologic insulin deficiency, and levels rapidly decrease following glucose or food consumption or in response to insulin administration in diabetic persons. These changes result both from changes in hepatic release and from clearance from the circulation (232).

Both energy and protein intake affect IGF-I levels. When dietary energy is severely restricted, the amount of carbohydrate eaten becomes a major determinant of the circulating IGF-I response to growth hormone stimulation (230, 237). In the rat, short-term protein restriction reduces hepatic IGF-I mRNA (238) and increases IGF-I clearance from the circulation (233). Serum IGF-I levels decrease and IGFBP-I levels increase in protein-restricted persons (230, 239). A specific role for IGFBP-2 in the metabolic adaptation to protein restriction has been suggested (238, 239).

In summary, the level and quality of protein intake appear to be the key external regulators of the adaptation of protein metabolism to starvation, because the resulting amino acids provide the substrate for body protein synthesis. Both energy restriction and protein restriction evoke an intricate, coordinated hormonal response, mediated by insulin, growth hormone, IGF-I, and thyroid hormone, that reorganizes amino acid traffic to bring about an orderly adaptation to the altered nutritional environment (240). Under favorable conditions, this adaptation progressively reduces the maintenance protein requirement until it matches protein intake. The adaptation is partly automatic (because the lean tissue mass has decreased) and partly regulated, given that a lower rate of protein synthesis and breakdown in the remaining lean tissues allows for more efficient processing of dietary protein and recycling of endogenous amino acids.

CACHEXIA

Patients with severe tissue injury develop a hypermetabolic response termed the systemic inflammatory response syndrome (SIRS), defined as the presence of two or more of the following: fever (or profound hypothermia), tachycardia, tachypnea, and leukocytosis (or increased numbers of band forms) (241). Other defining features of the SIRS are changes in acute-phase serum protein concentrations (242), anorexia, increased energy expenditure, increased whole-body protein turnover, and protein wasting (241). Protein wasting may be regarded as the metabolic cost of rapidly mobilizing amino acids for wound healing and synthesis of immune cells and proteins (243).

A milder inflammatory condition is common in general medical and surgical wards. This syndrome, described as cytokine-induced malnutrition (3) and cachexia (4), occurs in chronic infection (244), inflammatory disease, neoplastic disease associated with continuous involuntary weight loss (245), and in many forms of end-organ disease including chronic renal failure and end-stage heart disease (246–248). Its features are changes in acute-phase serum protein concentrations (242) (some of which, e.g., C-reactive protein, fibrinogen, and ferritin, are increased, whereas others, e.g., transferrin, transthyretin, and albumin, are decreased), the anemia of chronic disease (249), anorexia, and the partial nullification of a previously successful adaptation to starvation.

Some investigators have argued that cachexia should not be regarded as a form of malnutrition, because it is neither caused by inadequate nutritional intake nor cured by supplemental nutrition (250). However, unlike SIRS, in which protein catabolism dominates, inadequate food intake (combined with failed adaptation) is the most important contributor to lean tissue loss in the common cachectic syndromes. Cytokine inhibition of anabolic signals hinders nutritional rehabilitation, and the constitutional symptom of fatigue limits mobility and the muscular exercise needed to maintain or rebuild lean tissues (251). Nevertheless, protein and energy balance can be maintained in many cases if an appropriate nutritional and exercise strategy is implemented (245, 252–254).

CHRONIC ENERGY DEFICIENCY

It is easy to recognize starving patients in a clinic or hospital ward (132, 255, 256), but determining the minimum acceptable food intake and corresponding nutritional state can be difficult in societies where food scarcity and low body weight are common (161, 207, 257). To address this, a form of adapted protein-energy starvation called adult chronic energy deficiency (CED) has been defined (258, 259). This stable but undernourished condition is compatible with gainful employment, pregnancy, and other aspects of daily life. CED is defined as a subnormal BMI classified into three grades of severity: grade I, 17.0 to 18.4; grade II, 16.0 to 16.9; and grade III, less than 16 (258).

BMI reflects the body's fat store both in obesity and underweight. A BMI between 20 and 25 is generally regarded as normal (46). In the United States, Hungary, or Brazil, fewer than 5% of adults have a BMI less than 18.5, whereas 10% of Chinese adults, 20% of Congolese adults, 25% of Pakistani or Philippino adults, and nearly 50% of Indian adults are in this category (258, 259). Only grades II and III CED are associated with an increasing probability of days of illness, reduced physical work capacity, poorer reproductive function, and poorer lactation performance. Decreased voluntary physical activity has been shown only in grade III CED. These observations suggest that a BMI of 17.0 to 18.5 may be compatible with normal function (260). Appreciable numbers of physiologically normal persons, especially young adults, whose BMI is in this range could be incorrectly labeled as malnourished (258, 259).

CED in active young adults living in poor countries could be like the condition of successfully adapted protein-energy malnutrition in anorexia nervosa or the wasting that commonly accompanies certain chronic diseases. The BMI of the Minnesota volunteers fell from 21.4 to 16.3 after 6 months of starvation (134). If one subtracts their 1.8 kg of additional extracellular fluid, the BMI becomes 16.0, a value associated with disability in CED. Conversely, the BMI of severely malnourished patients in one detailed study (128) was 17.5. In that study, undernutrition was diagnosed from a combination of features that included serum albumin and urinary creatinine for height in addition to body weight for height.

In summary, it appears that young adults lacking intercurrent disease can tolerate a BMI as low as 17 without physiologic dysfunction, despite their lack of nutritional reserves. Even a BMI less than 17, although associated with disability, can be tolerated in well-adapted CED. This is in marked contrast to much medical experience, which dictates that weight loss more than 10% lower than normal is sufficient to identify malnutrition (261). At the other extreme, a BMI greater than 18.5 does not rule out severe malnutrition, because fat and extracellular fluid mass can greatly affect body weight. Evidently, better criteria than body weight or BMI alone are required to identify dangerous protein or protein-energy starvation. The best criteria currently available are ones that point to failed adaptation to starvation: continuing weight loss, functional disability, and hypoalbuminemia, the last indicating the presence of a catabolic state (4, 262, 263). It is not usually difficult to distinguish a normal state from CED in persons with low but stable body weight. The physiologically normal person will report normal appetite and food intake, will have a normal level of physical function, and will be found to have adequate muscle mass on physical examination.

CALORIE RESTRICTION AND LIFE EXTENSION

A nutritional intervention called calorie restriction (CR) prolongs the life span of many species and has been suggested as a strategy for delaying human aging (264, 265). CR has been described as "undernutrition without malnutrition," because caged rodents whose energy intake is restricted well below ad libitum levels live longer, appear healthier, have a lower spontaneous incidence of certain cancers, and are resistant to certain carcinogens (265).

Mechanisms by which CR could delay aging include the following: reduced oxygen utilization within individual tissues with a corresponding reduction in oxygen free radical production (266–268); altered turnover rate or increased apoptosis of certain cells, thus limiting the accumulation of age-related adverse cellular changes, possibly mediated by reduced IGF-I production; and the prevention of deleterious secondary effects of excessive adipose tissue accumulation (269, 270). Some beneficial effects could be governed by specific signals. The extended life span of yeast cells partially starved of glucose depends on the induction of a single histone deacetylase, Sir2 (271), which has homologs in higher organisms (272).

Short-term CR studies involving persons whose initial BMI was normal indicate that moderate restriction of energy (but not protein or other nutrients) can reduce the BMI to approximately 20 without important muscle loss, reduction in physical activity, or physiologic dysfunction (174, 176, 273, 274). The low-normal BMI, lowered blood pressure, improved blood lipid profile, and increased insulin effectiveness that result from CR (275) are consistent with epidemiologic data predicting a greater life expectancy (276, 277).

REFEEDING

The refeeding syndrome may develop in severely wasted patients during the first week of nutritional repletion (96, 201, 278–280). Expansion of the extracellular fluid volume is rapid and considerable, frequently producing dependent edema. This is caused by increased sodium intake combined with the antinatriuretic effect of insulin, whose levels increase in response to increased carbohydrate consumption. This aspect of the syndrome can be minimized by limiting sodium and carbohydrate intake during refeeding (131). Carbohydrate refeeding can stimulate enough glycogen synthesis to lower serum phosphate and potassium concentrations. Refeeding also increases REE, and, when combined with protein, stimulates N retention, new cell synthesis, and cellular rehydration (131, 281). Depletion of phosphate, potassium, magnesium, and vitamins occurs commonly in this setting (201, 278), and unless mineral status is judiciously monitored during refeeding, acute deficiencies, especially of phosphorus and potassium, will develop. Mild deficiencies may merely prevent an anabolic response to refeeding (177, 178, 202). Left-sided heart failure may occur, especially in predisposed patients (279). The ingredients for heart failure are an abrupt increase of intravascular volume, increased REE (which increases demands for cardiac output), an atrophic left ventricle with a poor stroke volume (134, 282), and myocardial deficiencies of potassium, phosphorus, or magnesium.

Cardiac arrhythmias may occur (283). Acute thiamin deficiency is a potential hazard.

REE returns toward normal as the result of two processes. First, the hypometabolic state of adapted starvation rapidly reverses, thus causing an important increase in REE within the first week of refeeding (281, 284), and second, REE increases as the lean tissue mass is rebuilt.

Circulating IGF-I, which is reduced in all forms of starvation, increases rapidly within days to a week of refeeding in concert with improving N balance (230, 239, 285). Because T_3 potentiates growth hormone–induced expression of mRNA for IGF-I (234) and stimulates IGF-I release from the liver (286), this effect could be mediated by insulin-stimulated rises in T_3 (227).

The specific changes in body composition induced by refeeding are determined by the existing metabolic state and body composition, and, importantly, by the composition of the refeeding diet (287–289). A diet high in sodium and carbohydrate predisposes to large increases in extracellular volume and edema. A low-protein, high-energy diet brings about fat gain but no increase in the lean tissue mass (131). A high-protein diet (e.g., 2 g/kg body weight/day) can arrest ongoing N losses even when energy balance is negative (290). A high-energy, high-protein diet will replete both fat and lean tissue stores at a rate that can be predicted with reasonable accuracy from the resulting energy and N balances, both of which can be measured or estimated. Activity stimulates muscle accretion. Malnourished patients who are inactive will increase their central protein stores—an important benefit—but will not regain muscle mass unless they exercise (288, 291, 292). Cachexia can reduce or prevent lean tissue gain, even in the presence of a positive energy balance, which merely induces fat accumulation.

Several features of the refeeding process were illustrated by a clinical trial in which two protein levels were sequentially provided to severely starved men (131). When the diet was generous in energy (2250 kcal/day) but low in protein (27 g/day), the patients' weight, body fat, and serum cholesterol increased but N balance remained nearly zero; their serum albumin, blood hematocrit, and urinary creatinine excretion failed to increase even after 45 days of refeeding. When the protein content of the diet was increased to 100 g/day, daily N balance became strongly positive. After 45 days on this diet, BMI had increased to normal, serum albumin was nearly normal, and creatinine excretion had increased by 40%. Ninety days of the 100-g protein diet were required before serum albumin, BMI, and blood hemoglobin levels were fully normalized.

In general, the steps in refeeding severely malnourished patients are as follows. After fluid and electrolyte disorders have been normalized and are maintained, if necessary, by continuing supplementation, a mixed diet is provided at the estimated maintenance energy level to establish tolerance and to avoid the refeeding syndrome. Even at this level of energy provision, N balance will become positive (167). Energy intake is then increased to create a positive energy balance to promote fat regain and to accelerate protein accretion. A generous protein intake (1.5–2.0 g/kg dry body weight) promotes the most rapid repletion of body protein at any energy level (167). Protein intakes greater than this confer no additional advantage to the adult and could be harmful (209).

REFERENCES

1. Golden MHN, Jackson AA. Chronic severe undernutrition. In: Olson RE, Brosquist HP, Chichester CO et al, eds. Present Knowledge in Nutrition. Washington, DC: Nutrition Foundation, 1984:57–67.
2. Rivers JPW. The nutritional biology of famine. In: Harrison GA, ed. Famine. Oxford: Oxford University Press 1988:57–106.
3. Beisel WR. Am J Clin Nutr 1995;62:813–9.
4. Kotler DP. Ann Intern Med 2000;133:622–34.
5. Rosenberg IH. J Nutr 1997;127:990S–1S.
6. Doherty TJ. J Appl Physiol 2003;95:1717–27.
7. Cahill GF Jr. Clin Endocrinol Metab 1976;5:397–415.
8. Aoki TT, Muller WA, Brennan MF et al. Am J Clin Nutr 1975; 28:507–11.
9. Lusk G. The Science of Nutrition. Philadelphia: WB Saunders, 1928.
10. Felig P. Starvation. In: DeGroot LJ, Cahill GF Jr, Odell WD et al, eds. Endocrinology. New York: Grune & Stratton 1979: 1927–40.
11. Radziuk J, Pye S. Diabetes Metab Res Rev 2001;17:250–72.
12. Rothman DL, Magnusson I, Katz LD et al. Science 1991;254: 573–6.
13. Jungas RL, Halperin ML, Brosnan JT. Physiol Rev 1992;72: 419–48.
14. Kettelhut IC, Wing SS, Goldberg AL. Diabetes Metab Rev 1988;4:751–72.
15. Foster DW, McGarry JD. N Engl J Med 1983;309:159–69.
16. Owen OE, Caprio S, Reichard GA Jr et al. Clin Endocrinol Metab 1983;12:359–79.
17. Hultman E, Nilsson LH. Nutr Metab 1975;18 [Suppl 1]:45–64.
18. Sugden MC, Sharples SC, Randle PJ. Biochem J 1976;160: 817–9.
19. Landau BR, Wahren J, Chandramouli V et al. J Clin Invest 1996;98:378–85.
20. Nair KS, Woolf PD, Welle SL et al. Am J Clin Nutr 1987;46: 557–62.
21. Katz J, Tayek JA. Am J Physiol 1998;275:E537–42.
22. Streja DA, Steiner G, Marliss EB et al. Metabolism 1977;26: 1089–98.
23. Hasselbalch SG, Knudsen GM, Jakobsen J et al. J Cereb Blood Flow Metab 1994;14:125–31.
24. Endemann G, Goetz PG, Edmond J et al. J Biol Chem 1982; 257: 3434–40.
25. Balasse EO, Fery F. Diabetes Metab Rev 1989;5:247–70.
26. Haymond MW, Karl IE, Clarke WL et al. Metabolism 1982;31: 33–42.
27. Rudolf MC, Sherwin RS. Clin Endocrinol Metab 1983;12: 413–28.
28. Halperin ML, Cheema-Dhadli S. Diabetes Metab Rev 1989; 321–36.
29. Redies C, Hoffer LJ, Beil C et al. Am J Physiol 1989;256: E805–10.
30. Owen OE, Morgan AP, Kemp HG et al. J Clin Invest 1967;46: 1589–95.

31. McGarry JD, Woeltje KF, Kuwajmi M et al. Diabetes Metab Rev 1989;5:271–84.

32. Weinman EJ, Eknoyan G, Suki WN. J Clin Invest 1975;55: 283–91.

33. Feinstein EI, Quion-Verde H, Kaptein EM et al. Am J Nephrol 1984;4:77–80.

34. Eriksson UJ. Diabetes Metab Rev 1995;11:63–82.

35. Laffel L. Diabetes Metab Res Rev 1999;15:412–26.

36. Robinson AM, Williamson DH. Physiol Rev 1980;60:143–87.

37. Fulop M. Diabetes Metab Rev 1989;5:365–78.

38. Halperin ML, Cherney DZI, Kamel KS. Ketoacidosis. In: DuBose TD Jr, Hamm LL, eds. Acid-Base Disorders: A Companion to Brenner and Rector's The Kidney. Philadelphia: WB Saunders, 2002:67–82.

39. Mahoney CA. Am J Kidney Dis 1992;20:276–80.

40. Schade DS, Eaton RP. Diabetes 1979;28:5–10.

41. Miles JM, Haymond MW, Nissen SL et al. J Clin Invest 1983; 71:1554–61.

42. Bliss M. The Discovery of Insulin. Toronto: McLelland & Stewart, 1982.

43. Reifenstein EC Jr, Albright F, Wells SL. J Clin Endocrinol 1947;5:367–95.

44. Krzywicki HJ, Consolazio CF, Matoush LO et al. Am J Clin Nutr 1968;21:87–97.

45. Sapir DG, Chambers NE, Ryan JW. Metabolism 1976;25: 211–20.

46. FAO/WHO/UNU Expert Consultation. Energy and Protein Requirements. Technical report series no. 724. Geneva: World Health Organization, 1985.

47. Crim MC, Munro HN. Proteins and amino acids. In: Shils ME, Olson JA, Shike M, eds. Modern Nutrition in Health and Disease. 8th ed. Philadelphia: Lea & Febiger 1994:3–35.

48. Lariviere F, Kupranycz D, Chiasson J-L et al. Am J Physiol 1992;263:E173–9.

49. Raguso CA, Pereira P, Young VR. Am J Clin Nutr 1999;70: 474–83.

50. Lariviere F, Wagner DA, Kupranycz D et al. Metabolism 1990; 39:1270–7.

51. Umpleby AM, Scobie IN, Boroujerdi MA et al. Eur J Clin Invest 1995;25:619–26.

52. Giesecke K, Magnusson I, Ahlberg M et al. Metabolism 1989; 38:1196–200.

53. Vazquez JA, Morse EL, Adibi SA. J Clin Invest 1985;76: 737–43.

54. Henson LC, Heber D. J Clin Endocrinol Metab 1983;57: 316–9.

55. Hoffer LJ, Forse RA. Am J Physiol 1990;258:E832–40.

56. Winterer J, Bistrian BR, Bilmazes C et al. Metabolism 1980;29: 575–81.

57. Abumrad NN, Williams P, Frexes-Steed M et al. Diabetes Metab Rev 1989;5:213–26.

58. Jefferson LS. Diabetes 1980;29:487–96.

59. Palaiologos G, Felig P. Biochem J 1976;154:709–16.

60. Nair KS, Welle SL, Halliday D et al. J Clin Invest 1988;82: 198–205.

61. Norrelund H, Nair KS, Nielsen S et al. J Clin Endocrinol Metab 2003;88:4371–8.

62. May ME, Buse MG. Diabetes Metab Rev 1989;5:227–45.

63. Drenick EJ. Weight reduction by prolonged fasting. In: Bray GA, ed. Obesity in Perspective: John E. Fogarty International Center for Advanced Study in the Health Sciences. DHEW publication no. NIH 75–708. Bethesda, MD: National Institutes of Health, 1973:341–60.

64. Contaldo F, Presto E, Di Biase G et al. Int J Obes 1982;6: 97–100.

65. Drenick EJ. The effects of acute and prolonged fasting and refeeding on water, electrolyte, and acid-base metabolism. In: Maxwell MH, Kleeman CR, eds. Clinical Disorders of Fluid and Electrolyte Metabolism. New York: McGraw-Hill, 1980: 1481–501.

66. Van Itallie TB, Yang M-U. N Engl J Med 1977;297:1158–61.

67. Hood VL. Fluid and electrolyte disturbances during starvation. In: Kokko JP, Tannen RL, eds. Fluids and Electrolytes. Philadelphia: WB Saunders, 1986:712–41.

68. Nilsson LH. Scand J Clin Lab Invest 1973;32:317–23.

69. Olsson K-E, Saltin B. Acta Physiol Scand 1970;80:11–8.

70. Grande F, Keys A. Body weight, body composition and calorie status. In: Goodhart RS, Shils ME, eds. Modern Nutrition in Health and Disease. 6th ed. Philadelphia: Lea & Febiger, 1980:3–34.

71. Garrow JS. Am J Clin Nutr 1982;35:1152–8.

72. Waki M, Kral JG, Mazariegos M et al. Am J Physiol 1991;261: E199–203.

73. Weyer C, Vozarova B, Ravussin E et al. Int J Obes 2001;25: 593–600.

74. Elia M. Effect of starvation and very low calorie diets on protein-energy interrelationships in lean and obese subjects. In: Scrimshaw N, Schurch B, eds. Protein-Energy Interactions. Lausanne, Switzerland: Nestlé Foundation, 1992:249–84.

75. Zauner C, Schneeweiss B, Kranz A et al. Am J Clin Nutr 2000; 71:1511–5.

76. Welle S. Am J Clin Nutr 1995;62:1118S–22S.

77. Tracey KJ, Legaspi A, Albert JD et al. Clin Sci 1988;74:123–32.

78. Shetty PS, Watrasiewicz KE, Jung RT et al. Lancet 1979;2:230–2.

79. Hoffer LJ, Bistrian BR, Young VR et al. Metabolism 1984;33: 820–5.

80. Barrett PVD. JAMA 1971;217:1349–53.

81. Corvilain B, Abramowicz M, Fery F et al. Am J Physiol 1995; 269:G512–7.

82. Peters A, Rohloff D, Kohlmann T et al. Blood 1998;91: 691–4.

83. Stunkard AJ, Rush J. Ann Intern Med 1974;81:526–33.

84. Gamble JL. Harvey Lect 1947;43:247–73.

85. O'Connell RC, Morgan AP, Aoki TT et al. J Clin Endocrinol Metab 1974;39:555–63.

86. Gelfand RA, Hendler R. Diabetes Metab Rev 1989;5:17–30.

87. Vazquez JA, Kazi U, Madani N. Am J Clin Nutr 1995;62: 93–103.

88. Bolinger RE, Luker BP, Brown RW et al. Arch Intern Med 1966;118:3–8.

89. Leiter LA, Marliss EB. JAMA 1982;248:2306–7.

90. Elia M. Clin Nutr 2000;19:379–86.

91. Friedl KE, Moore RJ, Martinez-Lopez LE et al. J Appl Physiol 1994;77:933–40.

92. Thomson TJ, Runcie J, Miller V. Lancet 1966;2:992–6.

93. Barnard DL, Ford J, Garnett ES et al. Metabolism 1969;18: 564–9.

94. Stewart WK, Fleming LW. Postgrad Med J 1973;49:203–9.

95. Devathasan G, Koh C. Lancet 1982;2:1108–9.

96. Crook MA, Hally V, Panteli JV. Nutrition 2001;17:632–7.

97. Carpenter KJ. Protein and Energy: A Study of Changing Ideas in Nutrition. New York: Cambridge University Press, 1994.

98. Panel on Macronutrients, Subcommittees on Upper Reference Levels of Nutrients and Interpretation and Uses of Dietary Reference Intakes, Standing Committee on the Scientific Evaluation of Dietary Reference Intakes. Dietary Reference

Intakes for Energy, Carbohydrate, Fiber, Fat, Fatty Acids, Cholesterol, Protein, and Amino Acids (Macronutrients). Washington, DC: Food and Nutrition Board, Institute of Medicine, National Academy Press, 2002.

99. Pencharz PB, Ball RO. Annu Rev Nutr 2003;23:101–16.
100. Young VR, Marchini JS. Am J Clin Nutr 1990;51:270–89.
101. Krebs HA. Adv Enzymol Regul 1972;10:397–420.
102. Young VR, Moldawer LL, Hoerr R et al. Mechanisms of adaptation to protein malnutrition. In: Blaxter K, Waterlow JC, eds. Nutritional Adaptation in Man. London: John Libbey, 1985:189–217.
103. Eisenstein RS, Harper AE. J Nutr 1991;121:1581–90.
104. Young VR, Meredith C, Hoerr R et al. Amino acid kinetics in relation to protein and amino acid requirements: the primary importance of amino acid oxidation. In: Garrow JS, Halliday D, eds. Substrate and Energy Metabolism in Man. London: John Libbey, 1985:119–34.
105. Millward DJ, Rivers JPW. Eur J Clin Nutr 1988;42:367–93.
106. Hamadeh MJ, Hoffer LJ. Am J Physiol 2001;280:E857–66.
107. Hoffer LJ, Bistrian BR, Young VR et al. J Clin Invest 1984;73:750–8.
108. Quevedo MR, Price GM, Halliday D et al. Clin Sci 1994;86:185–93.
109. Forslund AH, Hambraeus L, Olsson RM et al. Am J Physiol 1998;275:E310–20.
110. Arnal MA, Mosoni L, Boirie Y et al. Am J Physiol 2000;278:E902–9.
111. Hoerr RA, Matthews DE, Bier DM et al. Am J Physiol 1993;264:E567–75.
112. Waterlow JC. Annu Rev Nutr 1986;6:495–526.
113. Ihle BU, Becker G, Whitworth JA et al. N Engl J Med 1989;321:1773–7.
114. Castaneda C, Charnley JM, Evans WJ et al. Am J Clin Nutr 1995;62:30–9.
115. Castaneda C, Dolnikowski GG, Dallal GE et al. Am J Clin Nutr 1995;62:40–8.
116. Munro HN. General aspects of the regulation of protein metabolism by diet and hormones. In: Munro HN, Allison JB, eds. Mammalian Protein Metabolism, vol 1. New York: Academic Press, 1964:381–481.
117. Latham MC. Protein-energy malnutrition. In: Brown ML, ed. Present Knowledge in Nutrition. Washington, DC: International Life Sciences Institute, Nutrition Foundation, 1990:39–46.
118. Jelliffe DB, Jelliffe EF. Pediatrics 1992;90:110–3.
119. Mayatepek E, Becker K, Gana L et al. Lancet 1993;342:958–60.
120. Golden MH. Br Med Bull 1998;54:433–44.
121. Franch-Arcas G. Clin Nutr 2001;20:265–9.
122. Ballmer PE. Clin Nutr 2001;20:271–3.
123. Becker K, Leichsenring M, Gana L et al. Free Radic Biol Med 1995;18:257–63.
124. Badaloo A, Reid M, Forrester T et al. Am J Clin Nutr 2002;76:646–52.
125. Manary MJ, Leeuwenburgh C, Heinecke JW. J Pediatr 2000;137:421–4.
126. Dulger H, Arik M, Sekeroglu MR et al. Mediators Inflamm 2002;11:363–5.
127. Ling PR, Smith RJ, Kie S et al. Am J Physiol 2004;287:R801–08.
128. Barac–Nieto M, Spurr GB, Lotero H et al. Am J Clin Nutr 1978;31:23–40.
129. Lunn PG, Morley CJ, Neale G. Clin Nutr 1998;17:131–3.
130. Jackson AA, Phillips G, McClelland I et al. Am J Physiol 2001;281:G1179–87.
131. Barac-Nieto M, Spurr GB, Lotero H et al. Am J Clin Nutr 1979;32:981–91.
132. Hoffer LJ. Can Med Assoc J 2001;165:1345–9.
133. Golden BE, Golden MH. Eur J Clin Nutr 1992;46:697–706.
134. Keys A, Brozek J, Henschel A et al. The Biology of Human Starvation. Minneapolis: University of Minnesota Press, 1950.
135. Ravussin E, Lillioja S, Anderson TE et al. J Clin Invest 1986;78:1568–78.
136. Foster GD, Wadden TA, Kendrick ZV et al. Med Sci Sports Exerc 1995;27:888–94.
137. Rosenbaum M, Vandenborne K, Goldsmith R et al. Am J Physiol 2003;285:R183–92.
138. Prentice AM, Goldberg GR, Jebb SA et al. Proc Nutr Soc 1991;50:441–58.
139. Shetty PS, Kurpad AV. Eur J Clin Nutr 1990;44[Suppl 1]:47–53.
140. Toth MJ. Curr Opin Clin Nutr Metab Care 1999;2:445–51.
141. Leibel RL, Rosenbaum M, Hirsch J. N Engl J Med 1995;332:621–8.
142. Rosenbaum M, Hirsch J, Murphy E et al. Am J Clin Nutr 2000;71:1421–32.
143. Heyman MB, Young VR, Fuss P et al. Am J Physiol 1992;263:R250–57.
144. Levine JA, Schleusner SJ, Jensen MD. Am J Clin Nutr 2000;72:1451–4.
145. Weinsier RL, Schutz Y, Bracco D. Am J Clin Nutr 1992;55:790–4.
146. McClave SA, Snider HL. Curr Opin Clin Nutr Metab Care 2001;4:143–7.
147. Soares MJ, Piers LS, Shetty PS et al. Clin Sci 1994;86:441–6.
148. Ravussin E, Bogardus C. Am J Clin Nutr 1989;49:968–75.
149. Luke A, Schoeller DA. Metabolism 1992;41:450–6.
150. Scalfi L, Di Biase G, Coltorti A et al. Eur J Clin Nutr 1993;47:61–7.
151. Grande F. Man under caloric deficiency. In: Dill DB, ed. Handbook of Physiology, Section 4: Adaptation to the Environment. Washington DC: American Physiological Society, 1964:911–37.
152. Lusk G. Physiol Rev 1921;1:523–52.
153. Smith SR, Pozefsky T, Chhetri MK. Metabolism 1974;23:603–18.
154. Hamadeh MJ, Schiffrin A, Hoffer LJ. Am J Physiol 2001;281:E341–8.
155. Waterlow JC. Annu Rev Nutr 1995;15:57–92.
156. Rennie MJ, Harrison R. Lancet 1984;1:323–5.
157. Wykes LJ, Fiorotto M, Burrin DG et al. J Nutr 1996;126:1481–8.
158. Garlick PJ, Clugston GA, Waterlow JC. Am J Physiol 1980;238:E235–44.
159. Tessari P, Garibotto G, Inchiostro S et al. J Clin Invest 1996;98:1481–92.
160. Kurpad AV, Regan MM, Raj T et al. Am J Clin Nutr 2003;77:101–8.
161. Shetty PS. Nutr Res Rev 1990;3:49–74.
162. Elwyn DH, Gump FE, Munro HN et al. Am J Clin Nutr 1979;32:1597–611.
163. Pellett PL, Young VR. The effects of different levels of energy intake on protein metabolism and of different levels of protein intake on energy metabolism: a statistical evaluation from the published literature. In: Scrimshaw N, Schurch B, eds. Protein-Energy Interactions. Lausanne, Switzerland: Nestlé Foundation, 1992:81–121.
164. Munro HN. Physiol Rev 1951;31:449–88.
165. Kinney JM, Elwyn DH. Annu Rev Nutr 1983;3:433–66.
166. Goranzon H, Forsum E. Am J Clin Nutr 1985;41:919–28.
167. Shaw SN, Elwyn DH, Askanazi J et al. Am J Clin Nutr 1983;37:930–40.

168. Piatti PM, Monti F, Fermo I et al. Metabolism 1994;43:1481–7.
169. Ballor DL, Poehlman ET. Int J Obes 1994;18:35–40.
170. Elia M, Stubbs RJ, Henry CJ. Obes Res 1999;7:597–604.
171. Hoffer LJ, Bistrian BR. J Obes Weight Reduction 1984;3: 35–47.
172. Donnelly JE, Jacobsen DJ, Whatley JE. Am J Clin Nutr 1994; 60:874–8.
173. Henry RR, Wiest-Kent TA, Scheaffer L et al. Diabetes 1986; 35:155–64.
174. Velthuis-te Wierik EJM, Westerterp KR, van den Berg H. Int J Obes 1995;19:318–24.
175. Friedl KE, Moore RJ, Hoyt RW et al. J Appl Physiol 2000;88: 1820–30.
176. Weyer C, Walford RL, Harper IT et al. Am J Clin Nutr 2000;72: 946–53.
177. Rudman D, Millikan WJ, Richardson TJ et al. J Clin Invest 1975;55:94–104.
178. Knochel JP. Adv Intern Med 1984;30:317–35.
179. Passmore R, Strong JA, Ritchie FJ. Br J Nutr 1958;12:113–22.
180. Danforth E Jr, Burger AG. Annu Rev Nutr 1989;9:201–27.
181. Golden MHN. Marasmus and kwashiorkor. In: Dickerson JWT, Lee MA, eds. Nutrition and the Clinical Management of Disease. London: Edward Arnold, 1988:88–109.
182. Millward DJ. Proc Nutr Soc 1979;38:77–88.
183. Tomkins AM, Garlick PJ, Schofield WN et al. Clin Sci 1983;65:313–24.
184. Helweg-Larsen P, Hoffmeyer H, Kieler J et al. Acta Med Scand Suppl 1952;144:1–460.
185. Fliederbaum J. Clinical aspects of hunger disease in adults. In: Winick M, ed. Hunger Disease: Studies by the Jewish Physicians in the Warsaw Ghetto. New York: John Wiley & Sons, 1979:11–44.
186. Owen OE. Starvation. In: DeGroot LJ, Besser GM, Cahill GF Jr, et al, eds. Endocrinology. Philadelphia: WB Saunders, 1989:2282–93.
187. Grant JP. Clinical impact of protein malnutrition on organ mass and function. In: Blackburn GL, Grant JP, Young VR, eds. Amino Acids: Metabolism and Medical Applications. Boston: John Wright, 1983:347–58.
188. Mora RJF. World J Surg 1999;23:530–5.
189. de Simone G, Scalfi L, Galderisi M et al. Br Heart J 1994;71: 287–92.
190. Cooke RA, Chambers JB. Br J Hosp Med 1995;54:313–7.
191. Baier H, Somani P. Chest 1984;85:222–5.
192. Pingleton SK. Clin Chest Med 2001;22:149–63.
193. Thomas DR. Nutrition 2001;17:121–5.
194. Stacher G. Scand J Gastroenterol 2003;38:573–87.
195. Speerhas R. Cleve Clin J Med 1995;62:73–5.
196. Schurch MA, Rizzoli R, Slosman D et al. Ann Intern Med 1998;128:801–9.
197. Spence LA, Weaver CM. Am J Clin Nutr 2003;133:850S–1S.
198. Woodward B. Nutr Rev 1998;56:S84–S92.
199. Wade S, Bleiberg F, Mosse A et al. Am J Clin Nutr 1985;42: 275–80.
200. Bistrian BR. Nutritional assessment of the hospitalized patient: a practical approach. In: Wright RA, Heymsfield S, eds. Nutritional Assessment. Boston: Blackwell Scientific Publications, 1984:183–205.
201. McMahon MM, Farnell MB, Murray MJ. Mayo Clinic Proc 1993;68:911–20.
202. Wolman SL, Anderson GH, Marliss EB et al. Gastroenterology 1979;76:458–67.
203. Khanum S, Alam AN, Anwar I et al. Eur J Clin Nutr 1988;42: 709–14.

204. Garrel DR, Delmas PD, Welsh C et al. Metabolism 1988;37: 257–62.
205. Hoffer LJ. J Nutr 1998;128:333S–6S.
206. James HM, Dabek JT, Chettle DR et al. Clin Sci 1984; 67: 73–82.
207. James WPT, Ferro-Luzzi A, Waterlow JC. Eur J Clin Nutr 1988;42:969–81.
208. Henry CJK. Eur J Clin Nutr 1990;44:329–35.
209. Collins S. Nat Med 1995;1:810–4.
210. Isner JM, Roberts WC, Heymsfield SB et al. Ann Intern Med 1985;102:49–52.
211. Kotler DP, Tierney AR, Wang J et al. Am J Clin Nutr 1989;50: 444–7.
212. Palmblad J, Levi L, Burger A et al. Acta Med Scand 1977; 201:15–22.
213. Fricker J, Rozen R, Melchior J-C et al. Am J Clin Nutr 1991; 53:826–30.
214. Engler D, Burger AG. Endocr Rev 1984;5:151–84.
215. Bianco AC, Salvatore D, Gereben B et al. Endocr Rev 2002;23:38–89.
216. Spaulding SW, Chopra IJ, Sherwin RS et al. J Clin Endocrinol Metab 1976;42:197–200.
217. Becker DJ. Annu Rev Nutr 1983;3:187–212.
218. Phinney SD, Bistrian BR, Wolfe RR et al. Metabolism 1983;32:757–68.
219. Pittman CS, Suda AD, Chambers JB Jr et al. Metabolism 1979;28:333–8.
220. Bilezikian JP, Loeb JN. Endocr Rev 1983;4:378–88.
221. Coleman RA, Herrmann TS. Diabetologia 1999;42:639–46.
222. Prentice AM, Moore SE, Collinson AC et al. Nutr Rev 2002;60:S56–S67.
223. Rosenbaum M, Murphy EM, Heymsfield SB et al. J Clin Endocrinol Metab 2002;87:2391–4.
224. Garvey WT. J Clin Invest 2003;111:438–41.
225. Rousset S, Alves-Guerra MC, Mozo J et al. Diabetes 2004;53: 130S–5S.
226. Crim MC, Munro HN. Protein-energy malnutrition and endocrine function. In: DeGroot LJ, Cahill GF Jr, Odell WD et al, eds. Endocrinology. New York: Grune & Stratton, 1979: 1987–2000.
227. Millward DJ. Clin Nutr 1990;9:115–26.
228. Nygren J, Nair KS. Diabetes 2003;52:1377–85.
229. Hoogwerf BJ, Laine DC, Greene E. Am J Clin Nutr 1986;43: 350–60.
230. Clemmons DR, Underwood LE. Annu Rev Nutr 1991;11: 393–412.
231. Jones JI, Clemmons DR. Endocr Rev 1995;16:3–34.
232. Bach LA, Rechler MM. Diabetes Rev 1995;3:38–61.
233. Ketelslegers J-M, Maiter D, Maes M et al. Metabolism 1995;44:50–7.
234. Tollet P, Enberg B, Mode A. Mol Endocrinol 1990;4:1934–42.
235. Fryburg DA, Barrett EJ. Diabetes Rev 1995;3:93–112.
236. Shishko PI, Dreval AV, Abugova IA et al. Diabetes Res Clin Pract 1994;25:1–12.
237. Snyder DK, Clemmons DR, Underwood LE. J Clin Endocrinol Metab 1989;69:745–52.
238. Strauss DS, Takemoto CD. Endocrinology 1990;127:1849–60.
239. Smith WJ, Underwood LE, Clemmons DR. J Clin Endocrinol Metab 1995;80:443–9.
240. Millward DJ, Rivers JPW. Diabetes Metab Rev 1989;5: 191–211.
241. Davies MG, Hagen PO. Br J Surg 1997;84:920–35.
242. Gabay C, Kushner I. N Engl J Med 1999;340:448–54.
243. Bistrian BR. J Nutr 1999;129:290S–4S.

244. Langhans W. Nutrition 2000;16:996–1005.
245. Laviano A, Meguid MM, Rossi-Fanelli F. Lancet Oncol 2003;4: 686–94.
246. Bistrian BR. Am J Kidney Dis 1998;32:S113–S117.
247. Anker SD, Coats AJ. Chest 1999;115:836–47.
248. Thomas DR. Clin Geriatr Med 2002;18:883–91.
249. Ganz T. Blood 2003;102:783–8.
250. Mitch WE. J Clin Invest 2002;110:437–9.
251. Franssen FM, Wouters EF, Schols AM. Clin Nutr 2002;21: 1–14.
252. Pennington CR. Proc Nutr Soc 1997;56:393–407.
253. Lucia A, Earnest C, Perez M. Lancet Oncol 2003;4:616–25.
254. Zinna EM, Yarasheski KE. Curr Opin Clin Nutr Metab Care 2003;6:87–93.
255. Jeejeebhoy KN, Detsky AS, Baker JP. JPEN J Parenter Enteral Nutr 1990;14:193S–6S.
256. Detsky AS, Smalley PS, Chang J. JAMA 1994;271:54–8.
257. Garby L. World Rev Nutr Diet 1990;61:173–208.
258. Shetty PS, James WP. FAO Food Nutr Paper 1994;56:1–57.
259. James WPT, Ralph A. Eur J Clin Nutr 1994;48[Suppl 3]: 1S–202S.
260. Borgonha S, Shetty PS, Kurpad AV. Indian J Med Res 2000; 111:138–46.
261. ASPEN Board of Directors and the Clinical Guidelines Task Force. JPEN J Parenter Enteral Nutr 2002;26:1SA–138SA.
262. Okabe K. Intern Med 1993;32:837–42.
263. American Dietetic Association. J Am Diet Assoc 1994; 94:902–7.
264. Heilbronn LK, Ravussin E. Am J Clin Nutr 2003;78:361–9.
265. Hursting SD, Lavigne JA, Berrigan D et al. Annu Rev Med 2003;54:131–52.
266. Ramsey JJ, Harper ME, Weindruch R. Free Radic Biol Med 2000;29:946–68.
267. Weinert BT, Timiras PS. J Appl Physiol 2003;95:1706–16.
268. Li D, Sun F, Wang K. Biochem Biophys Res Commun 2003; 309:457–63.
269. Barzilai N, Gabriely I. J Nutr 2001;131:903S–6S.
270. Poehlman ET, Turturro A, Bodkin N et al. J Gerontol A Biol Sci Med Sci 2001;56A:45–54.
271. Anderson RM, Bitterman KJ, Wood JG et al. Nature 2003; 423:181–5.
272. Hekimi S, Guarente L. Science 2003;299:1351–4.
273. Walford RL, Mock D, Verdery R et al. J Gerontol A Biol Sci Med Sci 2002;57A:B211–B224.
274. Fontana L, Meyer TE, Klein S et al. Proc Natl Acad Sci USA 2004;101:6659–63.
275. Roth GS, Ingram DK, Lane MA. Ann NY Acad Sci 2001; 928:305–15.
276. Willett WC, Dietz WH, Colditz GA. N Engl J Med 1999; 341:427–34.
277. Lee IM, Blair SN, Allison DB et al. J Gerontol A Biol Sci Med Sci 2001;56A:7–19.
278. Solomon SM, Kirby DF. JPEN J Parenter Enteral Nutr 1990; 14:90–7.
279. Foxx-Orenstein A, Jensen GL. Nutr Rev 1990;48:406–13.
280. Mehler PS. Hospital Practice 1996;31:109–13.
281. Grande F, Anderson JT, Keys A. J Appl Physiol 1958;12:230–8.
282. Webb JG, Kiess MC, Chan-Yan CC. Can Med Assoc J 1986; 135:753–8.
283. Fisler JS. Am J Clin Nutr 1992;56:230S–4S.
284. Obarzanek E, Lesem MD, Jimerson DC. Am J Clin Nutr 1994;60:666–75.
285. Donahue SP, Phillips LS. Am J Clin Nutr 1989;50:962–9.
286. Ikeda T, Fujiyama K, Hoshino T et al. Ann Nutr Metab 1990;34:8–12.
287. Heymsfield SB, Casper K. Am J Clin Nutr 1988;47:900–10.
288. Loprinzi CL, Schaid DJ, Dose AM et al. J Clin Oncol 1993; 11:152–4.
289. Royall D, Greenberg GR, Allard JP et al. JPEN J Parenter Enteral Nutr 1995;19:95–9.
290. Hoffer LJ. Am J Clin Nutr 2003;78:906–11.
291. Russell JD, Mira M, Allen BJ et al. Am J Clin Nutr 1994;59: 98–102.
292. Gray-Donald K, Payette H, Boutier V. J Nutr 1995;125: 2965–71.

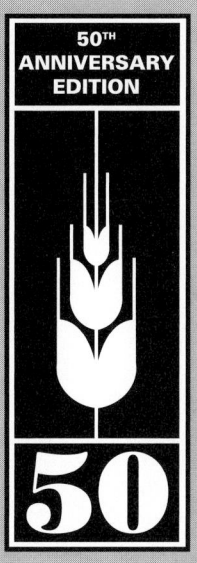

50TH ANNIVERSARY EDITION

50

PART IV

NUTRITION NEEDS AND ASSESSMENT DURING THE LIFE CYCLE

BODY COMPOSITION AND ANTHROPOMETRY[1]

STEVEN B. HEYMSFIELD AND RICHARD N. BAUMGARTNER

ASSESSMENT COMPONENTS .751
    Steady-State Relations 751
    Balance 753
    Function 754
ANTHROPOMETRY 754
BODY COMPOSITION MODELS 754
    Atomic 754
    Molecular 754
    Cellular 755
    Tissue-System 756
    Whole-Body 756
    Features of the Model 757
    Measurements 757
    Reference Values 765
CLINICAL APPLICATIONS 766
AGING AND ANTHROPOMETRIC INDICES 766
EVALUATING AND CONTROLLING ERROR
    SOURCES 767
CONCLUSION 768

A person's body composition reflects his or her total lifetime nutrient and energy balance. Maintaining optimum health requires the maintenance of adequate tissue levels of essential nutrients and a source of energy. More than 40 syndromes develop if tissue levels of these are either too low or too high (1). Anthropometry is the science of estimating or predicting body composition based on measurements of weight, stature, body circumferences, and subcutaneous fat thicknesses. This chapter describes methods for predicting protein and energy stores from anthropometry because most patients seen for clinical evaluation have a disorder of protein-energy balance (2, 3). This is prefaced by a discussion of the principles underlying energy and protein balance and body composition models.

---

[1]**Abbreviations: BCM,** body cell mass; **BIA,** bioimpedance analysis; **BMI,** body mass index; **D_b,** body density; **DXA,** dual-energy x-ray absorptiometry; **FFM,** fat-free mass; **R,** bioelectric resistance; **RMR,** resting metabolic rate; **TBF,** total body fat; **TBW,** total body water.

ASSESSMENT COMPONENTS

Steady-State Relations

The concept of steady-state relations between energy exchange and protein stores is important because disruptions result in disordered body composition and associated pathologic features. The difference between energy intake and expenditure affects three main body composition components, the small storage carbohydrate glycogen pool, the larger structural and functional protein pool, and the variable lipid or fat storage pool (Fig. 49.1). Taken together with associated water and minerals, the collective energy compartment is reflected by and changes parallel with body mass. Body weight is therefore a fundamental measurement in nutritional assessment because it is an indirect marker of protein mass and energy stores.

The consequences of weight change depend on initial body composition. Weight loss in a frail elderly patient with sarcopenia (low muscle mass), whether voluntary or involuntary, conveys very different risks than weight loss in a middle-aged overweight patient with adequate muscle mass. Weight loss involves the depletion of body nutrient stores. The excessive depletion of protein stores, whether from wasting or cachexia, results in the loss of specific cellular and tissue functions, with consequences ranging from loss of cell-mediated immunity to cognitive impairment. Conversely, weight loss in an overweight or obese person with adequate protein stores mainly consists of loss in fat mass, which improves certain cellular and tissue functions, for example by reducing levels of oxidative stress and improving insulin sensitivity and glucose and lipid metabolism.

A major portion of tissue function can be attributed to proteins that are activated by energy derived from metabolism of organic fuels (4). As an organic compound, protein is also a metabolic fuel, and, under conditions of weight stability, oxidation of amino acids provides about 15% of daily energy requirements (5). The energy-producing reactions take this general form:

$$\text{Fuel} + O_2 \rightarrow \text{high energy intermediate} \rightarrow CO_2 + H_2O + \text{heat} + \text{urea} \quad (1)$$

Urea is not metabolized further and is excreted unchanged in urine. During periods of nutritional deprivation, approximately half the total body protein mass can

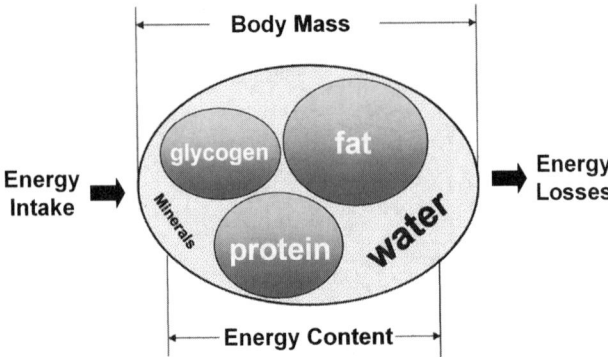

Figure 49.1. Interrelations between energy intake, output, and stores. (Data from Heymsfield SB, Baumgartner RN, Pan S-F. Nutritional assessment of malnutrition by anthropometric methods. In: Shils ME, Olson JA, Shike M, eds. Modern Nutrition in Health and Disease. 9th ed. Baltimore: Williams & Wilkins, 1999:903–21; and Heymsfield SB, Hoffman DJ, Testolin C et al. Evaluation of human adiposity. In: Björntorp ed. International Textbook of Obesity. Chichester, UK: John Wiley & Sons, 2001:85–97.)

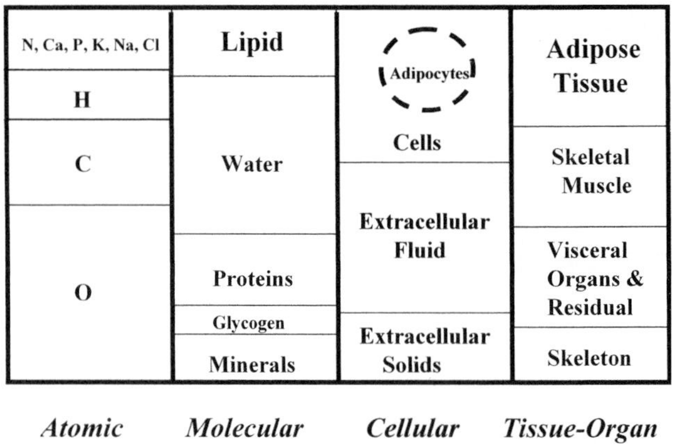

N, Ca, P, K, Na, Cl	Lipid	Adipocytes	Adipose Tissue
H		Cells	
C	Water		Skeletal Muscle
		Extracellular Fluid	
O	Proteins		Visceral Organs & Residual
	Glycogen	Extracellular Solids	
	Minerals		Skeleton

Atomic   Molecular   Cellular   Tissue-Organ

Figure 49.2. The first four of the five levels of human body composition. Components related to "fatness" are identified by bold enclosure. ECS and ECF are extracellular and intracellular solids, respectively. (From Bistrian BR, Blackburn GL, Vitale J et al. JAMA 1976;235:1567–70, with permission.)

be used as metabolic fuel (6). A greater loss of protein is incompatible with survival. Therefore, when food intake is less than nutrient losses, amino acids from proteins are oxidized to provide energy, various tissue functions are altered, and, ultimately, protracted negative protein balance results in a rapid rate of lean tissue depletion and death. The extent to which this occurs depends on the availability of other nonprotein energy stores.

The main sources of nonprotein energy are glycogen and fat or triglyceride. Glycogen is stored primarily in liver and skeletal muscle (7). Glycogen stores are small (<400 g), and carbohydrate oxidation on a usual diet in the United States accounts for about 50% of daily energy production (5).

Fat is found almost entirely within adipocytes or fat cells (8). A small amount of lipid is also present within muscle and liver cells (9). Fat stores vary widely in humans, with fatty acid oxidation representing about 35% of energy production in the average US diet (5). Both glycogen and fat are oxidized in reactions similar to that for protein (Equation 1), except urea is produced only with amino acid oxidation.

The sum of protein, glycogen, and fat constitutes total body energy content. These fuels account for more than 90% of the nonaqueous portion of body weight (10). Generalizations can be made on how body weight, protein, glycogen, fat, and energy stores relate to each other. Glycogen and protein are both solubilized by water and electrolytes. About 2 to 4 g water will bind to 1 g of either glycogen or protein (11). Changes in glycogen or protein balance are thus associated with greater changes in body weight than can be attributed to loss of the actual chemical component. For example, oxidation and loss of 100 g glycogen would result in approximately a 0.5-kg reduction in body weight.

The main remaining chemical components exclusive of fat are minerals, found primarily in the skeleton (8, 10).

The total fat-free portion of body weight thus consists of protein, glycogen, water, and minerals (Fig. 49.2). In healthy adults, the steady-state fractional contribution of three of these components to total fat-free mass (FFM) is reasonably constant: protein = 0.195, water = 0.725, and mineral = 0.08, respectively. Glycogen levels vary throughout the day and represent a fraction of FFM in the range of 0.01 to 0.02. With long-term weight loss, the change in FFM is approximately the same as the relative reduction in protein (1). Acute changes in body weight and FFM may also reflect alterations in glycogen and fluid balance.

Fat maintains a relatively constant, although more complex relation to fat-free components. Figure 49.3 shows a plot of total body fat(TBF)/height^2 versus body weight/height^2 in 414 women. Fat was measured in the women using a four component model (8). The ratio body weight/height^2, referred to as body mass index (BMI, kg/m^2), is

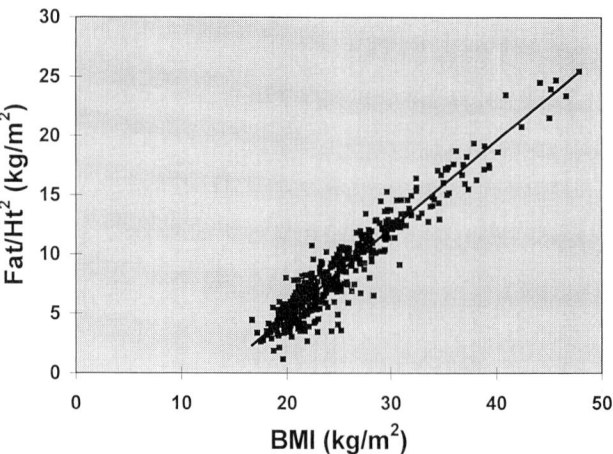

Figure 49.3. Relationship between total body fat (measured by four component model [8]) adjusted for stature and body mass index (BMI) in 414 healthy women (R^2 = 0.91, p < .001).

discussed later in more detail. Two important points are related to this figure. First, the intercept for zero TBF is a BMI of approximately 13, which represents a woman without any fat and minimal protein stores, a condition incompatible with survival. Second, the slope of the regression line (i.e., the change in fat adjusted for stature/the change in body weight adjusted for stature) of approximately 0.74 indicates that body weight added above a BMI of about 13 is predicted to be about three fourths fat and one fourth FFM. The composition of "excess weight," however, may differ between men and women and vary with race, age, and disease (12). Figure 49.4 shows how the relationship between BMI and percentage of body fat changes with age in healthy women and men. With increasing age, any measured BMI corresponds to a higher level of body fat, owing to the slow, age-related loss of muscle mass, or "sarcopenia" (13, 14).

In summary, body weight is a general, indirect marker of protein mass and energy stores. A loss or gain in body weight is usually assumed to reflect proportional changes in protein and energy stores. How this relationship varies with gender, race, and age, and particularly in relation to disease, is important for correct interpretation of anthropometric measurements used to estimate or predict fat and protein stores, as described in later sections of this chapter.

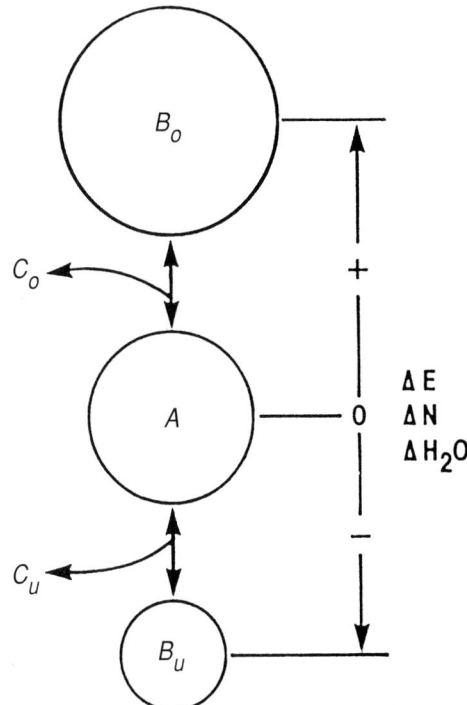

Figure 49.5. Model depicting changes in metabolic balance and body composition in protein-energy malnutrition and obesity. Point A is the range of body composition and tissue function found in health. Weight is stable, and balances of energy, nitrogen (N), and water are zero. Disease causes negative metabolic balance, weight loss, and changes in body composition and tissue function. Point B_u is the minimal range of body composition and tissue function that is compatible with survival. The course of a patient moving between points A and B_u may be interrupted by a complication related to malnutrition, and this is indicated by point C_u. Positive balance leads to obesity, and a similar set of end points, B_o and C_o, is designated.

Balance

Body composition is in a dynamic state over time. Both total body protein mass and energy content decline between meals as a result of obligatory amino acid oxidation and metabolism of other fuels (7, 15). The result is negative protein and energy balance. With food intake, balance becomes positive, and total body protein and energy content increase. Over a typical day, net protein and energy balance are zero, and body weight remains constant. These relations are depicted in Figure 49.5, in which point A represents an optimal state in which long-term balance is zero and health risks are minimal (1). If the individual at point A develops an acute or chronic illness, then food intake may be inadequate to replace nutrient losses, so net energy and nitrogen balance become negative and body weight is lost. If the condition persists and balance remains negative, the subject ultimately approaches the point at which survival is no longer possible (B_u). Loss of functional proteins and other essential nutrients results in the clinical complications described at the beginning of this chapter and shown in Figure 49.5 as C_u. Clinically significant abnormalities in

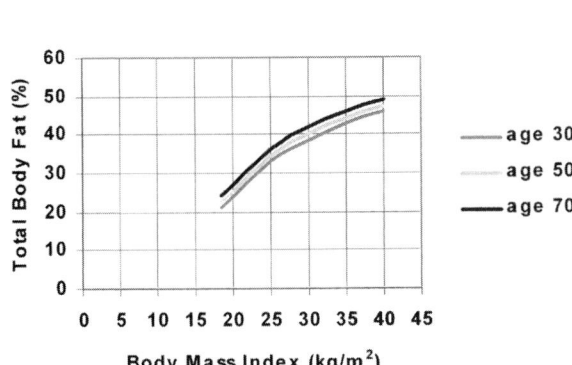

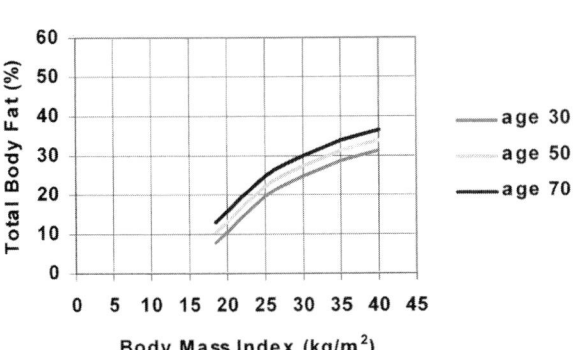

Figure 49.4. Total body fat, expressed as a percentage of body weight, versus body mass index in females (**upper panel**) and males (**lower panel**). The regression lines were developed based on the formula of Gallagher and associates [#6] (39).

physiologic function and loss of total body protein are seen in most hospitalized patients who lose more than 20% of their preillness body weight (16).

Conversely, overeating relative to nutrient utilization results in positive balance and, if sustained, causes weight gain (B_o). The maximum survivable body weight is approximately 500 kg or a body BMI of approximately 150. As with undernutrition, obesity is associated with complications (C_o). The discovery that adipose tissue does not function merely as a storage organ for excess energy, but also acts as an endocrine organ that participates with the brain and other peripheral tissues to regulate metabolism as well as immune function, has revolutionized the understanding of the mechanisms that underlie the health complications of obesity.

Figure 49.5 embodies the main aims of nutritional assessment: to define the patient's status relative to points A, B, and C, and four specific questions:

1. What is the patient's body weight and body composition status relative to arbitrarily defined "normal" or "healthy" values for gender, age, and race?
2. If the patient is determined to be either undernourished or overnourished, what are the mechanisms leading to either negative or positive nutrient balance?
3. Is the patient at risk of developing health complications as a result of their altered nutritional status?
4. With nutritional treatment is balance altered, and, over time, is the patient's weight and body composition moving toward the healthy range?

Function

An important assumption of nutritional assessment is that body composition is an indirect measure of cellular function. Body composition estimates are usually highly correlated with specific functional tests. For example, anthropometric midarm muscle area is strongly correlated with forearm grip strength (17). However, body composition should not be assumed equivalent to tissue function; the two are different types of biologic measurements that serve different purposes but can, under certain conditions, be used in exchange for one another. An example in which mass and function can dissociate is the case of a patient with cardiomyopathy. Massive enlargement of the heart muscle is possible, yet the capacity of the myocardium to generate force and eject blood into the systemic circulation is severely impaired. The distinction between body composition estimates and cellular function indices should be kept in mind when evaluating the results of a patient's anthropometric and biochemical evaluations (16).

ANTHROPOMETRY

Anthropometry was originally developed in the late nineteenth century by anthropologists to quantify variation in human form across age, gender, and racial groups. Its use

for assessing nutritional status was first realized in the late nineteenth century by Richer, who used skinfold thickness as an index of fatness (18). The modern era of nutritional anthropometry began with the studies of Matiegka during World War I (19). Matiegka's interest in the physical efficiency of soldiers led him to develop methods of anthropometrically subdividing the human body into muscle, fat, and bone. Anthropometric techniques are now widely used in many areas of human biologic research (20–22).

The purpose of nutritional anthropometry is to quantify the amount and distribution of the major nutritionally relevant components of body weight. A full appreciation of anthropometric measurements requires an understanding of human body composition and its organizational levels. Human body composition can be studied at five levels: I, atomic; II, molecular; III, cellular; IV, tissue-system; and V, whole-body (8). The first four levels and their major components are shown in Figure 49.2. Accurate methods have been developed for estimating components at each of these levels. It is important to understand the merits and limitations of these methods because anthropometric techniques are usually developed using one or more of these as the reference standard.

BODY COMPOSITION MODELS

Atomic

The first level of body composition consists of 11 elements that comprise more than 99.5% of body weight. The primary elements are oxygen, hydrogen, carbon, nitrogen, and calcium. Triglycerides stored in adipose tissue are composed of carbon, hydrogen, and oxygen in proportions of approximately 76.7, 12.0, and 11.3%, respectively; protein is 16.1% nitrogen; and bone mineral is about 39.8% calcium (23–28). These stable elemental proportions allow the calculation of TBF, protein, and mineral masses from measurements of elemental masses. Whole-body measurements at this level are generally made by in vivo neutron activation analysis methods (24–27). Anthropometric methods, however, are available for estimating total body nitrogen, calcium, and potassium at the atomic level based on prediction equations developed by statistical regression of anthropometric measurements on these elemental measurements (25).

Molecular

The second level of body composition consists of the major molecular components that comprise body weight, particularly water, protein, glycogen, mineral (osseous and nonosseous), and lipid that can be quantified in vivo (23). Total body lipid includes triglycerides, sphyngomyelin, phospholipids, steroids, fatty acids, and terpenes. The term "total body fat," however, generally refers to triglycerides, which are the primary storage lipids in humans and comprise nearly 90% of the total lipid component. TBF can be estimated using a two-component model in which the molecular level is simplified to body weight = TBF + FFM. Several two-component methods are used to estimate either TBF or FFM, including underwater weighing, total body potassium, and total body water (TBW) (23). Each method relies on one or more assumptions that relate measurable body composition quantities to the unknown component of interest. As an example, FFM can be estimated from TBW, as measured by isotope dilution analysis, by assuming that FFM has an average hydration of 73% (i.e., TBW/FFM = 0.73 or FFM = TBW/0.73). TBF can then be calculated as the difference between body weight and estimated FFM. The assumption that FFM is 73% water has been shown to be valid across a wide range of species, including humans (28, 29).

Another commonly applied two-component method is underwater weighing, which is based on the relatively stable densities of fat (0.9007 g/cm^3) and FFM (1.100 g/cm^3). In this method, body density (D_b) is measured by immersing the subject in a specially designed water tank and using Archimedes principle of buoyancy or water displacement. Newer methods using air displacement have also been developed (30). TBF is then estimated from D_b and body weight using the following equation:

$$Body\ mass/D_b = TBF/0.9007 + FFM/1.100 \quad (2)$$

Which, by algebraic rearrangement, gives the following:

$$TBF = (4.95/D_b - 4.50) \times body\ mass \quad (3)$$

However, the assumption of a constant FFM density of 1.100 g/cm^3 causes some model error as FFM density actually varies, although within a relatively narrow range. To avoid this model error, three-, four-, and/or five-component models were developed for measuring TBF with improved accuracy (31).

Dual-energy x-ray absorptiometry (DXA) has emerged as an increasingly popular method of estimating three molecular level components: TBF, total body bone mineral (TBBM) and lean soft tissue mass (LST), where FFM = TBBM + LST. This method is based on the differential attenuation of photons at low and high energy levels within a scanning x-ray beam. Elements of low atomic weight, such as hydrogen, minimally attenuate photons, whereas elements such as calcium are highly attenuating. The ratio of high to low energy attenuation is specific to each element and therefore to each molecular component. As the x-ray beam scans a person's body on a pixel-by-pixel basis, the quantities of mineral, fat, and lean soft tissue are calculated for each pixel based on the measured attenuation ratios and calibration equations. The values for all pixels scanned are then summed to estimate these molecular level components for the whole body. Various studies have established that DXA estimates are highly precise and generally accurate. The main limitation is that the accuracy of the DXA method is influenced by the thickness of the energy absorbing tissues in the path of the x-ray beam. Thus, accuracy decreases when scanning either very thin subjects, such as infants, or thick subjects, such as obese adults (32–33).

The molecular level of body composition is important in nutritional assessment because fat and FFM are the major components in which energy stores are distributed. Fat has an energy density of 9.4 kcal/g, and all but 1 to 2 kg is metabolically available during periods of protracted negative energy balance. Protein and glycogen have respective energy densities of 5.65 and 4.1 kcal/g. Assuming that the proportions of protein and glycogen are relatively normal in FFM, the metabolically available energy from FFM is 1.02 kcal/g (34, 35). Accordingly,

$$Total\ body\ energy\ content\ (kcal) = [9.4 \times total\ fat\ (g)] + [1.02 \times FFM(g)] \quad (4)$$

Half of the energy contained within FFM can usually be used as fuel during long-term semistarvation (35). The estimation of TBF and FFM thus allows the calculation of total body energy content and thereby changes in energy balance over time.

FFM is generally accepted as an index of protein stores, and changes over time are assumed to represent alterations in protein balance. Resting oxygen consumption, carbon dioxide production, and heat production (i.e., energy expenditure) are all highly correlated with FFM, and FFM accounts for approximately 50 to 80% of the individual variation in energy expenditure (36). Thus, resting metabolic rate (RMR, kcal/day) is commonly estimated from FFM using prediction equations such as (37):

$$RMR\ (kcal/day) = 370 + 21.6 \times FFM\ (kg) \quad (5)$$

where FFM is in kilograms. Such equations have always been recognized as being somewhat imprecise, specifically at the extremes of body weight. Recently, Müller and colleagues (38) published new equations for children and adolescents and adults that may provide somewhat better accuracy across a range of BMIs for use in white populations (see Appendix Table A-10-f). Anthropometric methods are available for estimating TBW, FFM, and TBF at the molecular level (20, 21, 23, 25, 39–41).

Cellular

The cellular level of body composition consists of three main components: cells, extracellular fluid, and extracellular solids (8). Measurement techniques are available for quantifying extracellular fluid and solids, although total cell weight or the weight of specific cell groups is difficult to quantify in vivo. A widely used model of body composition at this level was suggested by Moore and his colleagues (40). Total cell mass was considered to be composed of two components: fat (a molecular level component) and fat-free, or body cell mass (BCM), the component responsible for most of the body's metabolic processes.

Moore and associates proposed that total body potassium, or exchangeable potassium, which is approximately equivalent in amount, could be used to estimate BCM because the potassium concentration of intracellular fluid is relatively constant at 150 mmol/L, and the ratio of intracellular fluid to solids is approximately 4:1 (i.e., intracellular fluid = BCM × 0.80). BCM could then be calculated using these relations combined with an estimate of either total body or exchangeable potassium (i.e., BCM = [total body potassium/150] × [1/0.80] or total body potassium × 0.0083). The equation for body weight according to Moore and his colleagues was thus equal to fat + BCM + extracellular fluids and solids.

Cells are the main functional components, and quantification of BCM enables investigators to explore important physiologic and functional relations. At present, several anthropometric equations can be used to predict BCM at the cellular level (40).

Tissue-System

The tissue-system level of body composition consists of the major tissues and organs. Body weight at this level is equal to the sum of adipose tissue, skeletal muscle, bone, and visceral organ masses.

Human adipose tissue is often assumed to be on average of 80% lipid, 14% water, 5% protein, and less than 1% mineral, and a density of 0.92 g/cm^3 at body temperature (42). In truth, there is actually large variation in adipose tissue composition. Level of adiposity, age, gender, and heredity all play important roles in determining adipose tissue composition, notably fat content.

Adipose tissue is distributed into subcutaneous, visceral, and interstitial anatomic compartments. Subcutaneous adipose tissue is generally defined as that between the fascia of skin and the muscles. Visceral adipose tissue is defined as that surrounding the organs, or viscera, in the thorax, abdomen, and pelvis. Interstitial adipose tissue is interspersed between cells within a tissue, particularly skeletal muscle. The proportions of total adipose tissue in these compartments are not constant and are under hormonal and genetic control, with metabolic properties of adipose tissue varying among different anatomic locations (43). Men, elderly persons, and obese subjects tend to have a higher percentage of total adipose tissue in the visceral compartment than women, young, and lean subjects, respectively (43, 44). Obese, elderly, and physically inactive subjects tend to have a higher proportion of interstitial adipose tissue (45). This component is also increased in many muscle diseases, such as Duchene muscular dystrophy. Weight gain or loss is associated with different relative rates of adipose tissue change in these compartments as well as from different subcutaneous sites (46). This differential loss of adipose tissue is important when interpreting anthropometric measurements. A strong positive correlation exists between the amount of visceral adipose tissue and the health risks of obesity.

Skeletal muscle is the largest component within the adipose tissue-free body mass, accounting for approximately half of adipose tissue-free body mass in healthy adults (8, 9). Skeletal muscle consists of muscle tissue, nerves, and tendons. Approximately 20% of adipose tissue-free skeletal muscle is protein, and muscle is the largest tissue reservoir of amino acids (6). Depletion of up to 75% of skeletal muscle mass is possible during prolonged semistarvation (6). Skeletal muscle mass decreases with age after about 45 years, with greater losses in men than women (47). This age-related loss leads to a state of deficient muscle mass, or sarcopenia, in many elders in which protein stores are insufficient for an adequate response to the physiologic stresses posed by acute or chronic illnesses. Sarcopenia is accordingly associated with age-related impairment of thermogenesis and immunocompetency, functional limitation and disability, and increased risk of falls and bone fractures, and sarcopenic elders are particularly vulnerable to weight loss (48). In about 10% of elders, a condition known as sarcopenic obesity may develop in which muscle mass is reduced in the presence of excess adipose tissue mass (49). Careful evaluation of body composition is needed for these persons because the excess mass of adipose tissue may obscure their low muscle mass and vulnerability to weight loss.

The response of visceral organs to semistarvation is variable. Organs decrease in weight at different rates during uncomplicated semistarvation. For example, liver mass decreases rapidly in rodents with underfeeding, whereas heart weight decreases at about the same rate as body weight (46). The pattern of visceral organ changes in protein-energy malnutrition associated with physiologic stress may differ from that of uncomplicated underfeeding. An example is the severe weight loss that often accompanies metastatic malignant disease. Cancer cachexia in both animals and humans is accompanied by preservation of some visceral organs despite loss of body weight and atrophy of skeletal muscles (50). The preservation of visceral organs with physiologic stress may represent an adaptive response to injury or infection that is the anatomic counterpart to increased synthesis of serum acute-phase reactants.

Magnetic resonance imaging and computed tomography are used by investigators to quantify total body and regional adipose tissue and skeletal muscle (8, 23). Imaging and ultrasonic techniques can also be used to estimate visceral organ and skeletal weights. Skeletal muscle and adipose tissue are important components in nutritional assessment because they are readily estimated by anthropometric techniques. At present, many anthropometric equations can be used to predict total and visceral adipose tissues, skeletal muscle, and bone mass at the tissue-system level (8, 51, 52).

Whole-Body

The whole-body level of body composition includes the main anthropometric dimensions of weight, stature, circumferences, breadths, and skinfold thicknesses. Other whole-body measures include body weight, volume, density, and electrical impedance.

Features of the Model

The five-level model has several important features. First, the model is consistent as a whole and each component is distinct (8). Connections between components are important in relation to anthropometric methods, however. An example is a group of related components at atomic to tissue-system levels, calcium, bone mineral, extracellular solids, skeleton, and bone breadths. Each of these components is distinct, and yet all five are linked because they are different constituents or dimensions of the human skeleton (8).

Second, steady-state relations exist between many components at the same or different levels (8). Steady-state as defined here means a stable relation between components over a specified time interval, usually months or years. Some steady-state relations were described earlier, such as the hydration of FFM = 0.73 and intracellular potassium concentration = 150 mmol/L. These quantitative associations are important in developing body composition models that relate a known component to an unknown component of interest. The steady-state relations are particularly important in the field of anthropometry because all anthropometric measurements are at the whole-body level, and yet they are used primarily to infer information about the first four body composition levels. It is important to understand how steady-state relations are altered by gender, age, race, and disease and thus change the quantitative associations established between anthropometric dimensions and other body components. The following is a summary of anthropometric methods in the context of the five-level model.

Measurements

The anthropometric measurements generally used for nutritional assessment include body weight, stature, skinfolds, circumferences, and bone breadths. These whole-

body measurements can be used in indices or prediction equations to estimate the values of components at the other four levels (Table 49.1). The following discussion groups the various anthropometric measurements and techniques into three categories: (a) body weight and stature; (b) estimates of fatness and energy stores; and (c) lean tissue indices, protein mass, and functional components.

Body Weight and Stature

Body weight is the sum of all components at each level of body composition. As described earlier, body weight is a rough measure of total body energy stores, and changes in weight parallel energy and protein balance. A significant correlation exists (r = 0.6, $p < 0.05$) between loss of body weight and change in total body protein in seriously ill adults (14).

Body weight usually varies less than ±0.1 kg/day in healthy adults. A loss in weight of more than 0.5 kg/day either indicates negative energy or water balance or a combination of the two. Clinically significant weight loss is considered a relative decrease in weight of more than 10% over a time interval of less than 6 months (1).

The severity of weight loss in an individual person is determined by two factors: the rate of weight change over time and the total reduction in weight. The rate of weight loss in total starvation is approximately 0.4 kg/day, and survival is sustained to about 70% of desirable (i.e., ideal) body weight (1). Semistarvation, the more typical cause of negative energy balance in patients, results in a more gradual loss in weight compared with that in total starvation. In patients with chronic disease, the weight change may occur over years or decades. The minimal survivable body weight in humans is between 48 and 55% of desirable body weight or a BMI of approximately 13 (i.e., point B_u in Fig. 49.5). Body weight at this point consists of less than 5% metabolically available fat (1). Exhaustion of the remaining usable fat mass results in rapid depletion of lean tissue and death.

The absolute body weight and rate of change in weight have prognostic value, and two aspects are recognized. The first is that an absolute body weight of less than 55 to

TABLE 49.1. SOME CHARACTERISTIC COMPONENTS AT LEVELS I TO IV AND RELATED ANTHROPOMETRIC MEASURES AT LEVEL V

CHARACTERISTIC COMPONENTS				ANTHROPOMETRIC MEASURES AT LEVEL V				
LEVEL I	LEVEL II	LEVEL III	LEVEL IV	BW	STATURE	CIRCUMFERENCES	SKINFOLDS	BREADTHS SKELETAL
TBC	Fat	Fat cells	Adipose tissue	X		X	X	
TBO	TBW	BCM + ECF	ATFW	X		X	X	
TBCa, TBP	Mo	ECS	Bone, skeleton	X	X			X
TBN, TBK	Pro, Ms	BCM	Muscle + viscera	X	X	X	X	
TBNa, TBCl	MS	ECF	Blood + ISF	X	X			

ATFW, adipose tissue-free body weight; BCM, body cell mass; BW, body weight; TBW, total body water; ECF, extracellular fluid; ECS, extracellular solids; ISF, interstitial fluid; Pro, protein; Mo, bone mineral; MS, soft tissue mineral; TBC, TBCa, TBCl, TBK, TBN, TBNa, TBO, TBP: total body carbon, calcium, chloride, potassium, nitrogen, sodium, oxygen, and phosphorus, respectively; TBW, total body weight; levels I to V: atomic, molecular, tissue-system, and whole-body levels of body composition, respectively.

60% of desirable places the subject at or near the survival limits of starvation (1). Further negative balance could not be tolerated for long. The second aspect is that a significant reduction in body weight from preillness weight (between 10 and 20%) over a time interval of less than about 6 months places the patient at risk of developing functional impairment of multiple organ systems and an adverse clinical outcome.

Studley was among the first to associate weight loss with disease outcome (53). In 1936, this pioneering investigator made the classic observation that marked weight loss before surgical procedures for peptic ulcer resulted in a higher postoperative mortality rate relative to that in weight-stable patients. Modern workers have identified weight loss as a major determinant of prognosis in many disease states and conditions, such as survival time in patients with carcinoma of the colon and chronic obstructive lung disease (54, 55). Seltzer and his colleagues found a 19-fold increase in mortality in adult patients undergoing elective surgery who lost more than 10 lb body weight preoperatively compared with patients with no or small weight loss (56).

Hirsch and associates observed a 21% preoperative weight loss in patients who died postoperatively compared with a 12% preoperative weight loss in survivors (57).

An important study by Windsor and Hill refined Studley's classic observation by demonstrating that the postoperative patients with weight loss who are at the highest risk of complications are those who also have clinically obvious impairment in organ function (58). Postoperative patients with clinically apparent organ impairment in this study also had significant abnormalities of a variety of measured physiologic functions and a reduced weight of total body protein. Summarizing this and other studies from his laboratory, Hill concluded that a weight loss of less than 10% of preillness body weight is usually not associated with functional abnormalities; a weight loss of between 10 and 20% of preillness body weight is accompanied by functional abnormalities in some patients; and a weight loss of more than 20% of preillness body weight is associated with protein-energy malnutrition and multiple functional abnormalities in almost all patients (14). Weight loss is thus an important indirect index of multiple physiologic functions the underlying severity of disease and a guide to a patient's prognosis.

Body weight is measured longitudinally to establish the effectiveness of nutritional therapy. A change in weight reflects energy, protein, and water balance.

Measurement. In the hospital, body weight should be measured within ±0.1 kg on a calibrated physician's scale. Special scales should be used in bedridden or wheelchair-bound patients. Edema, if present, should be recorded with the weight. The general procedure is to obtain a morning weight following evacuation of the bladder. The weight of the hospital gown can be subtracted from the total weight if the desired goal is nude weight. When com-

paring the patient's weight with standard values, the patient's attire is usually presented in a footnote on the table. Serial weights should be measured on the same or a carefully calibrated scale. Intake and output records may be useful in interpreting the significance of changes in weight.

Height is usually measured by a sliding bar attached to the physician's scale, although more accurate techniques are used for research purposes. Height can be estimated in bedridden patients using knee height or arm span prediction equations (Table 49.2) (59–62). Knee height is measured in the sitting position with an anthropometric caliper. The bottom of the patient's foot is placed flat on the floor and forms a right angle with the knee. The heel is raised, and the caliper blade is placed under the heel. The caliper's movable blade is then lowered to the top of the thigh at a minimum of 2 inches posterior to the kneecap. Methods for recumbent measurement of knee height are also available. Arm span is defined as the distance between the tips of the longest finger of each hand with subjects standing erect against the wall and both arms fully stretched horizontally (60, 62).

Interpretation. Interpretation of body weight as an index of available energy supply must be used with caution in four conditions:

1. Edema and ascites cause a relative increase in extracellular fluid and may mask loss in chemical or cellular components.
2. Massive tumor growth or organomegaly can mask loss in fat or lean tissues such as skeletal muscle.
3. Lean tissue and cellular atrophy are partially masked by residual fat and connective tissue in obese patients undergoing rapid or severe weight loss. Patients may still be overweight and yet suffer severe protein-energy malnutrition and also be at increased risk of adverse health outcomes secondary to semistarvation.
4. Large changes in energy intake cause corresponding changes in glycogen mass and bound water over several days. Similarly, large changes in sodium intake are associated with brief periods of fluid readjustment and body weight change.

For these reasons, and also to provide a more complete characterization of body composition, anthropometric methods are used to assess body weight further. These methods are described under two general headings as they relate to nutritional assessment: measures of fat stores and measures of lean tissues. Reference tables provide a standard weight for height, and in some cases an adjustment is made for frame size (see Appendix Tables A-12 and 14 to 16).

Fat

Although fat refers specifically to a chemical component at the molecular level of body composition, this section as a

TABLE 49.2. RECOMMENDED EQUATIONS FOR PREDICTING STATURE IN ADULTS AND CHILDREN[a]

GROUP	AGE GROUP	EQUATION	REFERENCE
White men	18–60	Stature = 1.88(knee height) + 71.85	49
	17–67	Stature = 2.3(knee height) + 51.1	50
	60–80	Stature = 2.08(knee height) + 59.01	51
	17–67	Stature = 2.30(knee height) − 0.63(age) +54.9	50
	17–67	Stature = 0.762(arm span) + 40.7	50
Black men	18–60	Stature = 1.79(knee height) + 73.42	49
	60–80	Stature = 1.37(knee height) + 95.79	51
White women	18–60	Stature = 1.87(knee height) − 0.06(age)+70.25	49
	22–71	Stature = 1.84(knee height) + 70.2	50
	22–71	Stature = 1.91(knee height) − 0.098(age)+71.3	50
	60–80	Stature = 1.91(knee height) − 0.17(age)+75.0	50
	22–71	Stature = 0.693(arm span) + 50.3	50
Black women	18–60	Stature = 1.86(knee height) − 0.06(age)+68.1	49
	60–80	Stature = 1.96(knee height) + 58.72	51
White boys	6–18	Stature = 2.22(knee height) + 40.54	49
Black boys	6–18	Stature = 2.18(knee height) + 39.6	49
Chinese boys	4–16	Stature = 0.92(arm span) + 10.84	52
White girls	6–18	Stature = 2.15(knee height) + 43.21	49
Black girls	6–18	Stature = 2.02(knee height) + 46.59	49
Chinese girls	4–16	Stature = 0.93(arm length) + 10.34	52

[a] Arm span, knee height, and stature in cm; age in years.

whole relates to the following five-level sequence: atomic, carbon; molecular, fat; cellular, fat cells; tissue-system, adipose tissue; and whole-body, anthropometric dimensions (e.g., skinfolds and circumferences) (see Table 49.1). Anthropometric measurements are well suited for estimating fatness because the subcutaneous adipose is readily accessible and measurable. Although more accurate and reproducible methods of estimating fatness exist, anthropometric methods are the simplest, safest, most practical, and least costly of the available techniques.

The amount of fat in healthy subjects varies greatly, with relatively small amounts in some highly trained athletes and relatively large amounts during the later stages of pregnancy. During protracted undernutrition, all but a small amount of TBF can be used as metabolic fuel (1). Two factors determine the adequacy of fat: the amount of total body triglyceride present and energy balance. Very little fat is sufficient if the person is healthy and in zero energy balance. In contrast, a small amount of fat in the presence of marked negative energy balance implies a limited survival time. The usual practice is to compare fat values from an individual patient with reference standards and also to follow trends over time. During nutritional therapy, the measurement of fat provides an indirect guide to energy balance.

Measurement and Interpretation. Four methods of assessing fatness are available: (a) the single skinfold method, (b) the limb fat area method, (c) TBF (or adipose tissue) calculated from multiple anthropometric measurements, and (d) TBF from the difference between body weight and FFM predicted from anthropometry and bioelectric impedance measurements. The fourth method is indirect, depending on the primary estimation of TBW or

FFM, as discussed further later in the section on bioimpedance analysis (BIA). Skinfold thicknesses are additionally used to describe the anatomical variation in subcutaneous fat thickness, or "fat pattern," and waist circumference is used as an index of the amount of visceral adipose tissue. The measurements common to these techniques are now briefly reviewed, and the interested reader should consult additional references for added details (20–22).

Skinfolds represent a double layer of subcutaneous tissue, including a small and relatively constant amount of skin and variable amounts of adipose tissue, and they are measured with specially design calipers. The caliper should be a rugged and light instrument, and jaw pressure should be maintained at 10 g/mm^2 throughout the measurement range. The contact surface area of the jaws can vary between 30 and 100 mm^2, and the jaws on some calipers remain parallel as they are opened wider. The essential technique is to pinch and elevate a skinfold at specific anatomic sites using the thumb and fingers and to measure the thickness of the fold with the calipers. These measurements are correlated with, but are not directly representative of, the actual thickness of subcutaneous adipose tissue. It is important to make repeated measurements because errors will occur. Standardized measuring techniques and methods for optimizing precision should be carefully followed (20–22). Skinfold measurements are not accurate in massively obese patients, and they are not useful for predicting amounts of intraabdominal adipose tissues. Commonly measured skinfold thicknesses include: biceps, triceps, subscapular, suprailiac, thigh, and calf (1).

The absolute skinfold thickness can be used directly for comparison with reference tables and for longitudinal follow-up (see Appendix Tables A-16 and A-17 and subdivisions). The limitation of evaluating one skinfold thickness is that a single measurement is a relatively poor predictor of the absolute amount and rate of change in TBF because (a) large interindividual differences exist in fat distribution, (b) as TBF changes, each skinfold site responds differently relative to changes in TBF, and (c) the relationship between skinfold thickness and TBF is complex (e.g., an exponential relationship exists between subcutaneous skinfold thickness and TBF and between subcutaneous fat and visceral fat) (51, 63). Other factors that limit a single skinfold thickness as a measure of fatness include changes in the composition of adipose tissue with age and nutritional status; variation in skinfold distribution and compressibility with age; and the inclusion of a small amount of nonadipose tissues (e.g., skin) in the measurement (1, 21, 51). The final consideration is that the day-to-day variability in measuring the same skinfold is large, even when the rigorous procedures are followed. Measuring skinfold thickness should therefore be considered a qualitative measure of the amount and rate of change in TBF. The advantages are ease and rapidity of measurement, especially in bedridden patients.

Standardized methods have been developed for measuring body circumferences, or girths, on the limbs and trunk that can be also used to estimate body fatness and grade body fat distribution. Body circumferences are useful in that, unlike skinfold thicknesses, they can always be measured, even in extremely obese subjects. They reflect internal as well as subcutaneous adipose tissue, but they are also influenced by variation in muscle and bone. As a result, the interpretation of circumference measurements, and especially circumference ratios, is often not straightforward. As for all anthropometric variables, body circumferences should be measured with close attention to standardized procedures (19). Flexible, inelastic cloth, and steel tapes are recommended. The tape measure should be durable, should resist stretching, and have an accuracy of ± 0.1 cm.

The most useful circumferences for grading or predicting body fat and for describing adipose tissue distribution are upper arm, chest, waist or abdomen, hip or buttocks, proximal or midthigh, and calf (20). Waist or abdomen circumferences are usually very highly correlated with total fat mass and percentage of body fat in men ($r > 0.85$); in women, hip or thigh circumferences may have slightly higher correlations. Correlations of upper arm, thigh, and calf circumferences with measures of body fat are somewhat lower, and these circumferences tend to be more strongly influenced by variation in appendicular skeletal muscle. Waist circumference and ratios of waist to hip or thigh circumference are widely used to grade or estimate visceral adiposity, which is recognized as the main aspect of adipose tissue distribution that is associated with increased risk of chronic disease (64). Waist circumference is now used in conjunction with BMI to classify persons into risk levels for chronic disease. Risks are increased for BMIs greater than 25 kg/m^2 when waist circumference is greater than 108 cm in men and 88 cm in women (65). Zhu and colleagues (66) also developed cutpoints for grading chronic disease risk specifically from waist circumference. Their analysis indicated that a waist circumference greater than 100 cm in men and 93 cm in women was associated with a disease risk equivalent to a BMI greater than 30 kg/m^2, indicating the need for clinical weight loss.

Combining a limb skinfold thickness with a corresponding circumference allows calculation of limb fat areas using the following general equation:

$$\text{Fat area (cm}^2) = \frac{[\text{C} \times \text{SF}]}{2} - \frac{[\pi \times (\text{SF})^2]}{4} \quad (6)$$

where C is a limb circumference measurement (i.e., upper arm, midthigh, calf), and SF is a skinfold measurement taken at the same level as the circumference measurement following standard methods. Most of the problems related to a single skinfold measurement also occur with the limb fat area. The advantage generally ascribed to area calculations is that the result includes the contribution of limb circumference; two limbs with equal skinfolds but unequal circumferences will have different amounts of fat.

Many prediction equations are available for calculating TBF from measured skinfold thicknesses, circumferences, body weight, and stature. All the present methods in use are "descriptive" in that measured anthropometric dimensions are converted to TBF or other components using statistically derived equations in the absence of an underlying theory or mechanism. In contrast, some body composition methods are based on theoretic or mechanistic models (e.g., BCM is calculated from exchangeable potassium using a model that assumes a constant intracellular potassium concentration). All descriptive methods, including anthropometry, share in common the following: development in a well-defined subject group, use of a criterion method for estimating TBF, and a prediction model formulated using regression analysis. Some methods, for convenience and speed, are based only on gender, body weight, stature, and circumferences (67, 68). As all prediction formulas are population specific, they should be cross-validated in new subject groups before application. Ideally, the fat-prediction formula would be used in a group similar to the population on whom it was developed.

A good example and most widely applied TBF prediction formula was developed by Durnin and Womersley using underwater weighing as the criterion for fat estimation (69) (Table 49.3). The sample consisted of 209 white men and 272 women who were less than 68 years of age and on average were normal or slightly overweight. Once TBF is known, it can be subtracted from body weight to provide a value for FFM.

TABLE 49.3. CALCULATION OF FAT AND FAT-FREE BODY MASS ACCORDING TO THE METHOD OF DURNIN AND WOMERSLEY

1. Determine the patient's age and weight (kg)
2. Measure the following skinfolds in mm: biceps, triceps, subscapular, suprailiac
3. Compute the sum (Σ) of these skinfolds
4. Compute the logarithm of Σ
5. Apply one of the following age- and sex-specific equations to compute body density (D, g/mL)

AGE RANGE (Y)	MEN	WOMEN
17–19	D = 1.1620 − 0.0630 × (logΣ)	D = 1.1549 − 0.0678 × (logΣ)
20–29	D = 1.1631 − 0.0632 × (logΣ)	D = 1.1599 − 0.0717 × (logΣ)
30–39	D = 1.1422 − 0.0544 × (logΣ)	D = 1.1423 − 0.0632 × (logΣ)
40–49	D = 1.1620 − 0.0700 × (logΣ)	D = 1.1333 − 0.0612 × (logΣ)
50+	D = 1.1715 − 0.0779 × (logΣ)	D = 1.1339 − 0.0645 × (logΣ)

6. Fat mass (kg) is then calculated as: FM = Body weight (kg) × [4.95/D − 4.5]
7. Fat-free mass (FFM) (kg) = Weight (kg) − Fat mass (kg)

A literature search will turn up many fat-prediction formulas that are applicable in specific populations and that vary in use of measurement type (i.e., circumferences and skinfolds) and anatomic location. Some examples of methods in current use for female subjects are presented in Table 49.4. In most of these formulas, the dependent (i.e., predicted) variable is D_b. These methods were developed using underwater weighing as a reference for D_b estimation and anthropometric dimensions along with other covariates such as age were set in regression models as independent variables. The anthropometric "predicted" density can be converted to percentage of fat using traditional two component body composition models, as outlined in Table 49.4.

The advantages of calculating TBF are that (a) more than one skinfold site is usually included in the calculation and (b) the result (in kilograms) can be used directly to calculate energy reserves as fat. The latter values can then be integrated with estimates of energy balance calculations, thus providing a more physiologic description of the patient's nutritional state. A cautionary note is that, as with all prediction equations, results are most accurate on populations on which the equation was derived. The accuracy of the Durnin-Womersley equation and those presented in Table 49.4 is unknown in patients with severe weight loss, and the techniques should not be applied when a gross distortion in body habitus or obvious fluid accumulation is present (69). As emphasized by Damon and Goldman, skinfold thicknesses describe, but do not measure, TBF (70). The error of prediction of TBF from skinfolds may be considerable in some persons even when group means are accurate. More accurate methods of measuring fat are therefore usually applied in research studies of body composition.

It is customary to express TBF estimates as a percentage of body weight. A problem in interpreting this approach is

TABLE 49.4. ANTHROPOMETRIC EQUATIONS THAT PREDICT BODY DENSITY IN THE FEMALE POPULATION[a]

AUTHORS (DATE; REF.)	EQUATION	n	MEAN OR RANGE	r	SEE
Katch & McArdle (1973; 106)	Density = 1.09246 − [0.00049 (scapula SF)] − [0.00075 (iliac SF)] + [0.00710 (ED)] − [0.00121 (thigh C)]	69	25.6 ± 6.4%	0.84	0.0086 (3.6%)
Jackson et al. (1980; 107)	Density = 1.1470 − [0.0004293 (chest SF + midaxillary SF + triceps SF + subscapular SF + abd SF + suprailiac SF + thigh SF)] + [0.00000065 (7SF)^2] − [0.00009975 (A) − [0.000621415 (gluteal C)]	249	4–44%	0.87	0.0079 (3.6%)
Wright et al. (1980; 108)	Density = [1.051 (biceps C)] − [1.522 (forearm C)] − [0.879 (neck C)] + [0.326 (abd$_2$ C)] + [0.597 (thigh C)] + 0.707	181	2–37%	0.73	(4.1%)
Hodgdon & Beckett (1984; 67)	Density = −(0.35004 [log$_{10}$ (waist C + hip C − neck C)] + (0.22100 [log$_{10}$ (H)]) + 1.29579	214	10–47%	0.80	0.0080 (3.7%)
Vogel et al. (1988; 109)	% Body fat = [0.173 (hip C)] + (105.328 [log$_{10}$ (Wt)]) − 0.515 (H)] − [1.574 (forearm C)] − [0.533(neck C)] − [0.200 (wrist C)] − 35.6	266	5–50%	0.77	(3.9%)
Tran & Weltman (1989; 110)	Density = 1.168297 − [0.00284 (abd C)] + [0.0000122098 (abd^2)] − [0.000733128 (hip C)] + [0.000510477 (H)] − [0.00021616 (A)]	400	35.9 ± 7.7%	0.89	0.0095 (4.2%)

[a] A, age (y); Abd, average waist and abdomen at naval (cm); C, circumference (cm); ED, elbow diameter (cm); H, height (cm); SF, skinfold (mm); Wt, weight (kg). Correlations are show for test group samples unless otherwise specified. The interested reader should consult original source for information regarding application of specific equation.

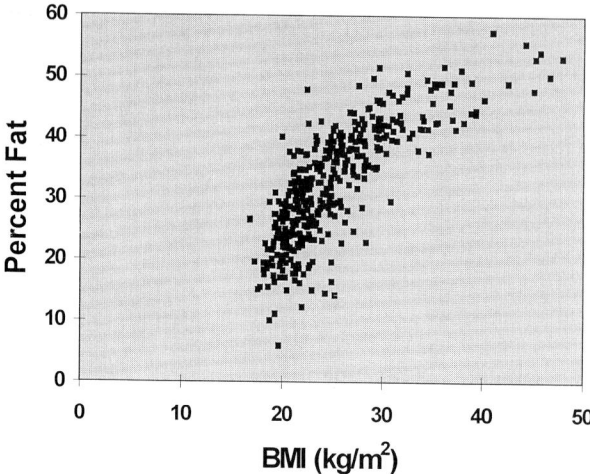

Figure 49.6. Percentage of body weight as fat in 413 healthy women versus body mass index (BMI). Fat was measured by four component model (8).

that, as a person gains or loses weight, both fat and FFM change. Additionally, the relationship between body fat and body weight has a nonzero intercept (see Fig. 49.3). The result is that a curvilinear relationship exists among TBF, expressed as a percentage of body weight, and body weight or BMI (see Fig. 49.6). These complex relationships can result in some confusing situations, such as when a severely obese patient loses a relatively large amount of weight and yet the percentage of fat change is relatively small. A highly trained athlete and a severely malnourished patient may have an equivalent percentage of body weight as fat. They could also have a similar absolute fat weight. To overcome these difficulties, Van Itallie and colleagues suggested calculating a fat (or FFM)-stature index similar to BMI as follows: fat/height^2 (71). A low or high "fat mass index" would then represent a reduced or increased actual fat mass relative to stature, respectively. For example, fat mass index in a malnourished patient would be lower than in a highly trained athlete, even though both had an equivalent percentage of body weight as fat. This is because the athlete with a similar percentage of body weight as fat would have a much larger absolute fat mass and also a much larger FFM and greater body weight than the malnourished patient.

Lean Tissues

Lean tissues refer in general to the following sequence of components at the five levels of body composition: atomic: nitrogen, potassium, and calcium; molecular: FFM, water, and protein; cellular: BCM; tissue-system: skeletal muscle, skeleton, and visceral organs; whole-body: anthropometric measurements (e.g., skinfolds/circumferences) (see Table 49.1). These various components are associated with the major portion of whole-body metabolic activity and biologic functions.

Semistarvation. Semistarvation results in negative balances of energy, protein, water, and minerals, a reduction in FFM and BCM, and atrophy of tissues and organs (1, 72). Not all lean components change at the same rate during periods of negative balance. At the molecular level, cellular proteins are depleted rapidly, and connective tissue proteins are lost at a slower rate (1). Similarly, at the cellular level, rapid changes can occur in BCM, whereas extracellular fluid is lost more slowly or may even increase in volume (72). Organs and tissues also differ in their rate of weight loss during semistarvation. Liver mass decreases rapidly and brain weight changes very little if at all in uncomplicated semistarvation; liver and other visceral organs may be preserved in chronic catabolic conditions such as metastatic malignant diseases (50). Skeletal muscle is a major reservoir of amino acids for acute-phase protein synthesis and can decrease by up to 75% in weight during protein-energy malnutrition (6). The malnourished patient with a reduced body weight therefore has a different composition at each of the five levels compared with his or her normally nourished counterpart. This explains why anthropometric equations developed in physiologically normal subjects may not predict a specific component with equal accuracy in an undernourished seriously ill patient.

In anthropometrically assessing the severity of malnutrition, an important goal is to define the amount and rate of change in total body or skeletal muscle protein (6). The main anthropometric indices used for this assessment are FFM (molecular level) and limb muscle areas (tissue-system level). Because lower limits compatible with survival are known for both types of measurement, the severity of protein-energy malnutrition is usually judged as the patient's value relative to the normal range on the one hand and the minimal range on the other (1). In terms of prognostic value, these measurements will provide some index of potential survival time; given the patient's anthropometric FFM or muscle index and nitrogen balance, progression toward or away from potentially lethal starvation can be established. During nutritional therapy and follow-up, the anthropometric FFM indices are used as measures of nitrogen balance, and specific details regarding interpretation are presented in the following paragraphs.

Measurement and Interpretation. Measuring FFM is accomplished by anthropometric methods, such as those described earlier in the section on fat. The same cautions in measurement technique and selection of patients noted in the earlier discussion of fat also apply to FFM. With regard to interpretation, in theory multiplying FFM (in grams) by 0.195 and 1.02 provides the amount of total body protein in grams and metabolizable energy in kilocalories. Of the metabolizable energy in the healthy subject, about half of that in FFM is available during prolonged periods of semistarvation (1). When combined with balance data and information on TBF, these bedside calculations often provide an interesting insight into a patient's course. Unfortunately, the information needed for accurate prediction of total body protein cannot be derived from anthropometric FFM because of the changes in body hydration and variability of skinfold measurements described earlier. A large tumor burden or organomegaly of any cause may also add mass (as water, protein, and mineral) to FFM that is metabolically unavailable. In patients without serious derangements in body composition, FFM can be used to calculate RMR as presented earlier in Equation 5. This FFM-based calculation of RMR is largely independent of sex and age although evidence is accumulating that ethnic RMR differences exist even after controlling for body composition (36).

Calculating the amount of limb muscle tissue from anthropometric data requires only two measurements: the limb circumference and the corresponding skinfold thickness. The midportion of the upper limb is usually studied, and little additional information is gathered by also measuring thigh and calf muscle areas (46). Calf muscle measurement would, of course, be useful in subjects whose upper extremities are burned, amputated, edematous, or immobilized by casts or traction devices. The upper arm muscles tend to atrophy slightly more rapidly during semistarvation than the muscles of the thigh or calf, but the differences are not large (46). Equations for estimating limb muscle area from anthropometry take the following general form:

$$\text{Muscle area (cm}^2) = [C - \pi \times SF]^2/4\,\pi \quad (7)$$

where C is a limb circumference (e.g., upper arm, midthigh, calf), and SF is a skinfold taken at the same level as the circumference using standardized methods.

The primary application of limb muscle measurements is to obtain a measure of the amount and rate of change in skeletal muscle protein. The following three factors should therefore be considered:

1. The mass of a skeletal muscle represents a three-dimensional measurement (i.e., volume), whereas limb muscle area and circumference are two- and one-dimensional indices, respectively (1, 46). As the muscle changes volume, the corresponding proportional changes in muscle area and circumference will be smaller than the change in volume. For example, a 50% decrease in muscle volume will correspond to a theoretic decrease in muscle area and circumference of 37 and 21%, respectively. As a rule, the relative change in muscle area will be larger than the change in muscle circumference.

2. The equations for calculating limb muscle indices are based on simple theoretic assumptions regarding arm geometry (1, 46). Actually, the calculated arm muscle area overestimates the amount of skeletal muscle by 15 to 25% in relatively young, nonobese subjects. Half of this overestimate results from the inclusion of bone in the calculated area, and the remainder results from

errors in the assumptions and the inclusion of nonmuscle tissue (e.g., neurovascular bundle) in the result (73). Two methods of correcting this overestimate of muscle area are available. The first is to express results as a percentage of standard, because the standard value will also contain these 'nonskeletal muscle' components. The second approach is to calculate bone-free arm muscle area by subtracting a constant value (10 cm^2 for men; 6.5 cm^2 for women) from the arm muscle area estimate obtained by the general equation. Studies by Forbes and Baumgartner and their colleagues suggested that arm muscle area assumptions are also inaccurate in obese and elderly subjects, respectively (74, 75). Martin and colleagues developed an anthropometric prediction formula for total body skeletal muscle mass, although the accuracy of this method in monitoring changes in muscle mass and associated protein content has not been reported (52). Further studies are therefore needed to improve our understanding of the relationship between anthropometric muscle estimates at the whole-body level of body composition and actual skeletal muscle mass at the tissue-system level.

3. Atrophic skeletal muscle differs in chemical composition from normal tissue. Per gram of muscle, the amounts of water, total lipid, and collagen are increased, whereas the noncollagen proteins are reduced. Thus, the concentration of functional proteins per unit arm muscle area or circumference is relatively lower in the atrophied muscle. Another chemical consideration is that muscle size can abruptly change by ±5 to 10% in response to rapid changes in muscle glycogen as a result of the water-binding properties of glycogen (46).

Thus, both anthropometric FFM and muscle indices are truly indirect markers of the active protein component of body weight. The two lean tissue indices should be considered approximate bedside guides to the amount of total body protein. Despite their approximate nature, anthropometric muscle estimates correlate with more complex methods of estimating skeletal muscle (e.g., total limb muscle area versus total body skeletal muscle volume by magnetic resonance imaging; Fig. 49.7) over the broad biologic range of muscle mass in humans.

Small changes in total body protein cannot be detected by anthropometry, and nitrogen balance and other techniques must be used for this assessment.

Bioimpedance Analysis

Nutritional assessment using anthropometry is now increasingly augmented through the additional measurement of BIA. This technique is used to predict body composition based on the electrical conductive properties of the human body. The ability of the body to conduct an electric current is the result of the presence of free ions, or electrolytes, in the body water. The amount of electricity

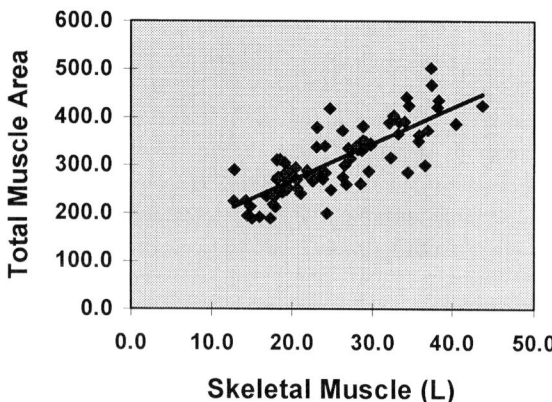

Figure 49.7. Correlation between total limb muscle area (sum of arm, calf, and thigh muscle areas in cm²) and total body skeletal muscle volume in L by whole-body magnetic resonance imaging in healthy subjects. N = 79, Total muscle area (cm²) = 7.6 × Skeletal muscle (L) + 115.4, R² = 0.6423, p < 0.001.

that can be conducted is determined mainly by the total volume of electrolyte-rich fluid in the body. Measures of bioelectric conductivity are therefore proportional to TBW and to body composition components with high water concentrations such as the FFM and skeletal muscle mass. As a result, these methods predict TBW, FFM, and total body skeletal muscle mass. TBF must be derived as the difference between body weight and predicted FFM (76).

Many factors other than the amount and electrolyte concentration of body water, however, influence measurements of electrical conductivity. These include body temperature, distribution of fluids between intracellular and extracellular spaces, body proportions or "geometry," the amounts and structures of different conductive, as well as nonconductive, tissues, and technical issues such as correct calibration and application of the equipment. The net result is that exact functional relationships between measurements of bioelectric conductivity and TBW or other fat-free components cannot be derived from either physiochemical models or experimentally. Thus, relationships between conductivity measurements and body composition components are established indirectly by statistical calibration against criterion measures (e.g., estimates of TBW from deuterium dilution analysis or FFM from DXA) in a sample of subjects (76).

Measurement and Interpretation. The most commonly used BIA method injects a high-frequency, low-amplitude alternating electric current (50 kHz at 500 to 800 μA) into the body using distally placed electrodes and measures the voltage drop caused by resistance with proximal electrodes. Conventionally, surface gel electrodes are used with standardized placements on the right ankle and hand, although other electrode arrangements have been described that allow estimation of segmental (e.g., arm or leg) electrical properties (76). Stainless steel contact electrodes are also now used in some systems in place of the conventional gel electrodes.

The amount of resistance measured (R) is inversely proportional to the volume of electrolytic fluid in the body. It is also dependent on the proportions or "geometry" of this volume (i.e., ratio of length [L] to cross-sectional area [A], or R α L/A). These relationships have led to the use of the simple formula $V = \rho L^2/R$ as the theoretic basis of most BIA applications, where V is conductive volume (e.g., TBW), L is a measure of body length (usually stature), R is measured resistance, and ρ is an estimate of the "specific resistivity" of the conductive material (76).

The validity of this simple formula has certain limitations. The formula is accurate only for a cylindric conductor with uniform cross-sectional area and homogenous composition (e.g., a wire). The human body could be described as a series of roughly cylindric conductors with variable cross-sectional area and heterogeneous, highly structured composition. The value of ρ is influenced by all these factors and consequently cannot be deduced directly. As a result, equations for predicting body composition must be developed based on independent measurements of resistance, stature, and other anthropometric variables, and TBW or FFM in a sample of subjects. Least-squares regression techniques are applied to the data to derive an equation of the basic form:

$$V \text{ (i.e., TBW or FFM)} = a + bS^2/R + e \quad (8)$$

where a is intercept, b is slope, and e is residual error or unexplained variation in V caused by random measurement errors and/or misspecification of the parameters (a and b) in the equation. It is not possible to interpret the parameter b in this equation as an estimate of ρ in the formula $V = \rho L^2/R$, unless the intercept (a) and residual error (e) approach zero. These conditions are rarely, if ever, met for the reasons given earlier. BIA prediction equations usually include additional parameters for age, gender, body circumferences, and skinfold thickness. Thus, this method can be considered a supplement to anthropometry for predicting body composition in patients. Some equations for predicting TBW, FFM and total body skeletal muscle mass are given in Table 49.5 (77–79).

TABLE 49.5. EQUATIONS FOR PREDICTING BODY COMPOSITION FROM BIOELECTRIC IMPEDANCE AND ANTHROPOMETRY

Males 12–80 y[a]
   TBW = 1.203 + 0.176(Weight) + 0.449(Stature²/R)
   FFM = −10.678 + 0.262(Weight) + 0.652(Stature²/R)
Females 12–80 y[a]
   TBW = 3.747 + 0.113(Weight) + 0.45(Stature²/R) + 0.015(R)
   FFM = −9.529 + 0.168(Weight) + 0.696(Stature²/R) + 0.016(R)
Adults 18–86 y[b]
   Total skeletal muscle mass = 5.102 + 0.401(Stature²/R)
     + 3.825(gender) −0.071(age)

Weight (kg); Stature (cm); R, resistance (ohms); TBW, total body water; FFM, fat-free mass. TBF, total body fat = Weight – FFM.
[a]Data from reference 77.
[b]Data from reference 78.

Similar to anthropometric prediction methods, BIA equations tend to lose accuracy when applied to subjects who do not resemble those included in the sample from which the equations were developed. Thus, their generalizability may be limited and all equations should be prevalidated in a subsample against an accepted reference method before general extension to an entire study population. In clinical application, the user should be aware that large disturbances in body fluid distribution between intracellular and extracellular compartments, for example edema or ascites, may affect the accuracy of BIA equations for predicting body composition. Conversely, methods have been developed that take advantage of the sensitivity of BIA to alterations of body water distribution in patients with various disorders (80).

Reference Values

Body Weight

The patient's body weight is evaluated using two reference sources. The first reference values are those of the patient, and these include a "usual weight" by history or previous measured weight. This is important because many obese patients who lose weight during an illness and are thus potentially malnourished will still be overweight by conventional standards. The second reference source is the healthy population. In this approach, the individual person's actual body weight is compared with that of a gender-, stature-, and age-appropriate reference or desirable body weight (see Appendix Tables A-12, A-14, and A-15 and their subdivisions). The subject's actual body weight is expressed as a percentage of desirable. The normal range for desirable body weight varies among different sources, but it usually is set between 90 and 120%. A body weight below or above these levels is consistent with undernutrition and obesity, respectively.

Another method of comparing the patient's weight with that of a reference population is to calculate a body weight (BW)-stature (S) index (81). Most weight-stature indices in present use take the form W/S^p (69). The term p indicates how stature is to be scaled. The main assumptions of weight-stature indices are that they are independent of height, represent an indirect index of body composition, correlate with health outcomes, and can be generalized across different populations.

The use of BMI, calculated as $BW/height^2$, has gained wide acceptance as a weight-stature index for use in diagnosing both protein-energy malnutrition and obesity (82–84). Most of the assumptions of weight-stature indices are fulfilled by BMI, although several limitations should be noted. First, although the correlation between BMI and TBF is relatively strong (r = 0.5 to 0.8), individual variation is large and some subjects can be misclassified as undernourished or obese (81). For example, some athletic subjects have a large skeletal muscle mass and a high BMI but are not obese. Thus, man with a BMI of 27 can have

TBF ranging from 10 to 31% of body weight (85). This variability in percentage of body fat may also increase in old age (86). In studies such as these, some of the observed error may be in the reference method for estimating body fat. BMI may also have a small stature dependence because persons with short legs for their height have higher BMI values independent of fatness (82). Finally, Gallagher and colleagues, using a four-component model as the criterion for body fat estimation, reported that BMI as a measure of fatness in their healthy cohort was age and sex dependent but independent of ethnicity in their African-American and white adults (87). Figure 49.4 shows how the relationship between BMI and body fat changes with age, as noted earlier.

Generally accepted BMI ranges for classifying patients as normal, overweight, and obese are presented in Table 49.6 (88) (see also Appendix Tables A-13 and A-18 and their subdivisions). Table 49.6 also gives three BMI levels for grading chronic protein-energy malnutrition that are less well accepted (89). The diagnosis of protein-energy malnutrition or obesity and of their associated risks is often multifactorial and may require additional estimates including body composition, energy expenditure, organ and tissue function, and biochemical markers.

Fat and Lean

Two methods are used to process anthropometric data other than body weight. The first method is to express the individual person's values relative to a healthy reference population. This method provides the anthropometric component used to assess whether and to what extent the patient is malnourished. The anthropometric reference tables present the results of large surveys and usually describe the general population. Reference data are now available for estimates from bioelectric impedance. The data in Appendix Tables A-15-e-1, 2, and 3 were adapted from Chumlea and associates and are based on data from the Third National Health and Nutrition Examination Survey (79). The estimates of TBW, percentage of fat, and FFM in these tables were derived from bioelectric resistance (R) measurements using standard prediction equations.

TABLE 49.6. BODY MASS INDEX AND GRADES OF OBESITY AND PROTEIN-ENERGY MALNUTRITION

BODY MASS INDEX	GRADE
<16	Grade III protein-energy malnutrition
16.0–16.9	Grade II protein-energy malnutrition
17.0–18.5	Underweight (grade I protein-energy malnutrition)
18.5–24.9	Normal
25–29.9	Overweight
30–34.9	Class I obese
35–39.9	Class II obese
>40	Class III severe obesity

The reference tables usually present data in three forms: (a) as a mean value; (b) as mean and standard deviation (SD); and (c) as percentiles. Describing a population in terms of mean and SD assumes that the measurement under study is symmetrically (normally) distributed. If data fit this model, then the mean ±2 SD includes 95% of the population. An abnormal value is more than 2 SD above or below the mean. Some tables provide only a mean, and the patient's value is then expressed as a percentage of the standard or reference value. A weakness of this approach is that tables of this type do not provide the observer with a method of determining whether the result is within the normal range. The second type of table includes the SD, or 95% range of the healthy population, thus indicating whether and to what degree the patient's results are abnormal. The third mode of expression is in terms of percentiles (e.g., see Appendix Tables A-12 to A-16, and A-18-b). The advantage of expressing results as a percentile rather than as a percentage of standard is that the reference population need not be symmetrically distributed. Often anthropometric surveys of populations produce "skewed" distributions, and therefore the easiest option is to present results in percentiles (90). In this approach, the values of the subject exactly in the middle of the group are at the fiftieth percentile. If the patient's value is between the fifth and the ninety-fifth percentile, the result is considered normal; a result below or above these respective values is abnormal.

No simple method of judging the severity or potential morbidity of protein-energy malnutrition from anthropometric data is available. Studies in adults have not yet clearly defined the "risk" of a subnormal anthropometric index, especially for results falling just below the normal range. Combining anthropometric data with the results of other components of the nutritional assessment provides some measure of potential morbidity (91).

The second method of expressing anthropometric data is in terms of the individual person's total body energy content, TBF, and FFM. When estimated energy and nitrogen balance are combined with these body composition data, a whole spectrum of potential calculations is possible. Of course, these are approximations, but their application in teaching and solving simple clinical questions often proves useful.

CLINICAL APPLICATIONS

Suggested applications of anthropometry are the following:

1. Weight and height should be recorded in the chart of every hospitalized patient. Weight indices, such as recent weight loss, should be added to the data base for all patients who have a history of weight change. The weight of all patients undergoing short-term nutritional support should be measured daily.
2. The uses of one skinfold measurement, limb fat area, and limb muscle area are helpful:

   a. When body weight is an invalid index of energy reserves because of edema or massive tumor burden. The upper limb is usually not affected by dependent edema.
   b. When body weight is unmeasurable because of immobilizing devices, such as a cast or respirator.
   c. When patients are seen for nutritional consultation or are seen at rounds removed from the bedside. Anthropometric estimates provide a quantitative description of what is usually visible at the bedside. Although weight alone is useful in this regard, two patients of the same height and weight may differ in body composition.
   d. During the initial evaluation of hospitalized patients who are prescribed short-term nutritional support. Although changes in fat and lean tissue will most likely not be detected over a 1- to 2-week period, the baseline anthropometric data will become a permanent component of the nutritional data base. This information will then be available if a future reevaluation is needed.

3. TBF and FFM are useful indices:

   a. In patients who are undergoing long-term nutritional follow-up over months or years. Limb muscle area measurements, preferably of the upper arm, should also be included in this group to complete the body composition data base.
   b. In groups of subjects forming the basis of nutritional studies, when a more critical assessment of body composition is often useful and more accurate techniques of evaluating body composition are not available.
   c. In estimating RMR based on FFM.
   d. For teaching purposes, when the interrelations of metabolic balance, body composition, and nutritional therapy are the subject of discussion.

AGING AND ANTHROPOMETRIC INDICES

Body composition changes throughout the adult life span, and this must be considered when evaluating anthropometric indices (92). Height declines and, assuming body weight remains unchanged, there is more fat and less FFM in an elderly person than in a younger one of the same sex (92–94). Most of the loss in FFM can be accounted for by a decrease in skeletal muscle (95). A summary of how body composition changes with age and how anthropometric measures are affected is presented in Table 49.7.

Because of these changes in body size, shape, and composition of the FFM, investigators now advocate geriatric-specific anthropometric and bioimpedance body composition prediction equations (96–98).

A difficult problem in the elderly is estimation of height, especially in wheelchair-bound, bedridden, or kyphotic

TABLE 49.7. EFFECTS OF AGING ON BODY COMPOSITION AND ANTHROPOMETRIC MEASUREMENTS

ANTHROPOMETRIC MEASUREMENT	AGE-EFFECT
Weight	The average population value increases until the fifth decade and then plateaus or declines
Height	The average population value decreases by 0.5 to 1.5 cm per decade after maturity; the rate of decline is sex and race dependent
Fat	Fat increases as a percentage of body weight up to about 50 y and then plateaus or declines in old age after 70 y; redistribution occurs from limb to truncal subcutaneous sites and from subcutaneous to internal, visceral, and interstitial sites
FFM	FFM decreases after age 40 y owing to decreases in skeletal muscle and bone; rates of loss in muscle are higher in men and accelerate after age 70 y; rates of loss in bone are higher in women and accelerate during menopause; the mass of visceral organs decreases slightly in old age; the hydration of FFM becomes more variable
Skinfolds	The compressibility of skinfolds changes with age owing to a loss in elastic recoil of skin and an increase in the viscoelastic recovery time; skinfolds in the elderly are often pendulous and difficult to measure additionally owing to loss of underlying muscle tone
Circumferences	Pendulous skinfolds can make circumferences more difficult to measure in the elderly; it is more difficult to locate bony landmarks in the obese

FFM, fat-free mass.

persons. Specialized approaches such as recumbent anthropometry may be useful in hospitalized or nursing home patients (99). Another useful approach is to measure knee height or arm span (see Table 49.2) to predict adult stature. Knee height and arm span undergo little change with age in adults and provide estimates of stature that are difficult to obtain by conventional methods. The estimated value for height can then be used in calculating other assessment indices and for comparison of these results to height-adjusted reference values. Alternatively, knee height can be used in place of stature in indices such as fat/knee height[2] (100).

Anthropometric measurements may be useful in diagnosing malnutrition in hospitalized elderly subjects. Lansey and colleagues examined 47 consecutive geriatric patients admitted to an acute care facility and found that approximately 45% of the patients had two anthropometric measures (i.e., midarm circumference and muscle area; subscapular and triceps skinfold) less than the fifth percentile, indicating severe malnutrition (101). In contrast, only 28% of patients were at less than 90% of ideal body weight. Anthropometric measurements may therefore supplement and be more sensitive than body weight and stature in the evaluation of malnutrition in hospitalized elderly patients.

Anthropometric measures may also predict disability and mortality in elderly populations. Rolland and associates reported that the simple measurement of calf circumference predicted self-reported disability in a population of elderly women (102). Campbell and colleagues reported that low arm muscle area and triceps skinfold thickness were associated with significantly increased mortality risk in 758 subjects who were more than 70 years old (103). The Mini-Nutritional Assessment, which is now widely used to screen elderly patients for malnutrition, incorporates midarm and calf circumferences and BMI (104).

EVALUATING AND CONTROLLING ERROR SOURCES

As with all measurements, anthropometric evaluations include error. In this section, we provide an introductory discussion on anthropometric error sources. The interested reader is referred to comprehensive reviews for an advanced discussion of this important topic (8, 20, 22).

Error can be considered in the context of the fundamental body composition methodology equation as shown in Figure 49.8. The equation in the figure indicates that

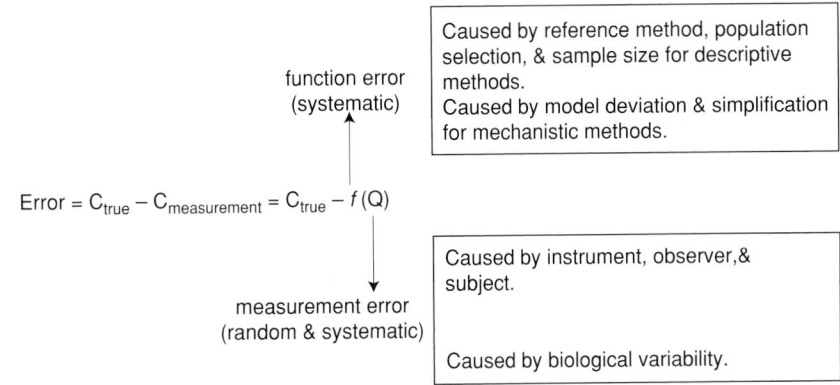

$$\text{Error} = C_{\text{true}} - C_{\text{measurement}} = C_{\text{true}} - f(Q)$$

function error (systematic)

Caused by reference method, population selection, & sample size for descriptive methods.
Caused by model deviation & simplification for mechanistic methods.

measurement error (random & systematic)

Caused by instrument, observer, & subject.

Caused by biological variability.

Figure 49.8. Sources of error in anthropometric methods.

error in the estimation of a body composition component (e.g., TBF) from anthropometric measurements is a function of two main errors sources, measurement of a quantity (Q) and mathematic function (i.e., descriptive or mechanistic). The figure also notes that errors of measurement may be either or both systematic (nonrandom) and random. Errors resulting from misspecification of mathematical functions are always systematic. The following discussion first considers measurable quantity errors and then proceeds to an overview of mathematic function errors.

A subject's anthropometric dimensions can be evaluated at a single point in time or on repeated occasions over time. Measurement error is the main concern with a single evaluation and measurement error combined with normal biologic variation must be considered with repeated measurements. Measurement error can be caused by instrument error and observer error. Methods of minimizing instrument error are reviewed in earlier sections. In summary, these mainly resolve to the correct choice of appropriate measurement instruments and accurate calibration. Observer error is related to three factors: precision, reliability, and accuracy.

Accuracy is the level of agreement between the measured value and the "true" dimension. Accuracy of an anthropometric dimension is usually established by comparison to a reference method. For example, subcutaneous adipose tissue thickness estimated using a skinfold caliper can be compared with corresponding estimates by computed tomography or magnetic resonance imaging. Of course, any such analysis also includes instrument and observer errors. In clinical situations, measurements by an anthropometrist are usually compared with those of a designated "expert" (20).

Precision, as distinct from accuracy, defines the quality of a measurement in terms of being sharply defined or exact. In this sense, precision refers to the scale of measurement; for example, a skinfold measured to the nearest 1 mm is more precise than one measured to the nearest 0.5 cm. A highly precise measurement (e.g., body weight measured to the nearest gram) is not necessarily accurate if the weight scale used is improperly calibrated. The definition of precision overlaps to some extent with that of reliability. Reliability is the degree to which a measurement is replicable using the same instrument by the same or a different observer (105). The linkage to precision comes in that it is difficult for a measurement to be precise or exact if it is unreliable.

The precision of an anthropometric measurement can be quantified as the variability among repeated measurements over a short time in the same subject (22). One way of expressing precision is the technical error of measurement, which is the standard deviation of repeated measurements on the same subject by the same or different observers. The technical error of measurement, which is expressed in the same units as the measured quantity, can

also be expressed in percent as a coefficient of variation (i.e., SD/mean × 100) (20).

Reliability is also referred to as "reproducibility" or "repeatability" (105). Reliability, as distinct from precision, is more commonly expressed in terms of the intraclass correlation among repeated measurements, sometimes called the reliability coefficient. Measures of reliability often include both measurement error and physiologic variation.

The total variation of an anthropometric measurement monitored over time includes measurement variation and biologic variation. Biologic variation occurs even in the healthy person as weight and fluid balance fluctuate over time. This aspect of measurement variability is the difference between total anthropometric dimension variation over time and that caused by measurement error. Some measures, such as stature, are extremely stable in adults, whereas others, such as selected skinfold thicknesses, are moderately variable over time. In practice, this biologic component of variability is often included in estimates of the reliability on anthropometric measurements.

Anthropometric dimensions are often used directly, as for example triceps skinfold thickness as a measure of fatness. Mathematically transforming an anthropometric measurement to a component estimate involves error sources. The validity of an anthropometric method in this context is the degree to which it accurately measures or predicts a specific component. Descriptive or type I methods are population specific, and error may arise when applying the prediction formula to a new subject group or outside the original subject range for age, weight, and stature. Mechanistic or type II methods include model error. For example, calculation of arm muscle area from triceps skinfold and midarm circumference is based on a simple geometric model. Actual arm muscle area may deviate from the assumed model, and this introduces error into the component estimate. Both types of error are nonrandom or systematic.

Anthropometry is applied widely in evaluating a single subject or whole populations. Professionals who apply anthropometry in their clinical work or research should fully comprehend the nature of anthropometric error sources and apply procedures to maximize the quality of their measurements. A good policy is to set up an evaluation program for the anthropometrists (20). An approach such as suggested in these reports will help to maintain a high-quality measurement standard.

CONCLUSION

Anthropometry is one of the oldest approaches to quantifying body composition, and it is the most practical to apply in field and clinical settings. The severity, response to nutritional treatment, and aspects of subject malnutrition risk can be established using relatively simple and easily acquired anthropometric measurements. For these reasons, anthropometry is an indispensable tool for the practitioner of clinical nutrition.

REFERENCES

1. Heymsfield SB, Baumgartner RN, Pan S-F. Nutritional assessment of malnutrition by anthropometric methods. In: Shils ME, Olson JA, Shike M, eds. Modern Nutrition in Health and Disease. 9th ed. Baltimore: Williams & Wilkins, 1999:903–21.

2. Bistrian BR, Blackburn GL, Vitale J et al. JAMA 1976;235:1567–70.

3. Bistrian BR, Blackburn GL, Hallowell E. JAMA 1974;230:858.

4. Crim MC, Munro HN. The proteins and amino acids. In: Shils ME, Olson JA, Shike M, eds. Modern Nutrition in Health and Disease. 8th ed. Philadelphia: Lea & Febiger, 1994:3–35.

5. Garrow JS. Obesity and Related Diseases. Edinburgh: Churchill Livingstone, 1988.

6. Heymsfield SB, C, Smith J. Am J Clin Nutr 1982;35:1192–9.

7. Stryer L. Biochemistry. 4th ed. New York: WH Freeman, 1995:582.

8. Heymsfield SB, Baumgartner RN, Ross R. Evaluation of total and regional body composition. In: Bray GA, Bouchard C, James WPT, eds. Handbook of Obesity. New York: Marcel Dekker, 1998.

9. Machann J, Haring H, Schick F et al. Diabetes Obes Metab 2004;6:239–48.

10. International Commission on Radiologic Protection: Report of the Task Group on Reference Man: Adopted by the Commission in October. New York: Pergamon Press, 1974.

11. Heymsfield SB, Stevens V, Noel R. Am J Clin Nutr 1982;36:131–42.

12. Forbes GB. Nutr Rev 1987;45:225–31.

13. Gallagher D, Heymsfield SB, Heo M et al. Am J Clin Nutr 2000;72:694–701.

14. Pietrobelli A, Allison DB, Heshka S et al. Int J Obes Relat Metab Disord 2002;26:1339–48.

15. Heymsfield SB, Casper K, Funfar J. Am J Cardiol 1987;60:75G–81G.

16. Hill GJ. JPEN J Parenter Enteral Nutr 1992;16:197–218.

17. Klidjian AM, Foster KJ, Kammerling RM. BMJ 1980;281:899–901.

18. Richer P. Nouv Inconogr Salpetriere 1890;3:20–6.

19. Matiegka J. Am J Phys Anthropol 1921;3:223–30.

20. Lohman TG, Roche AF, Martorell R, eds. Anthropometric Standardization Reference Manual. Champaign, IL: Human Kinetics, 1988.

21. Himes JH. Anthropometric Assessment of Nutritional Status. New York: Wiley-Liss, 1991.

22. Norton K, Olds T, eds. Anthropometrica: A Textbook of Body Measurement for Sports and Health Courses. Sydney, Australia: UNSW Press, 1996.

23. Heymsfield SB, Wang Z, Baumgartner RN et al. Annu Rev Nutr 1997;17:527–58.

24. Ellis KJ, Shypailo R, Schoknecht P et al. J Radioan Nucl Chem 1995;195:139–44.

25. Ellis KJ. Biol Trace Elem Res 1990;26–27:385–400.

26. Dilmanian FA, Weber DA, Yasumura S et al. Performance of the neutron activation systems at Brookhaven National Laboratory. In: Yasumura S, McNeill KG, Woodhead AD et al., eds. Advances in In Vivo Composition Studies. New York: Plenum Press, 1990.

27. Ellis KJ. Whole-body counting and neutron activation analysis. In: Roche AF, Heymsfield SB, Lohman TG, eds. Human Body Composition. Champaign, IL: Human Kinetics, 1996;45–62.

28. Wang Z, Deurenberg P, Heymsfield SB. Ann NY Acad Sci 2000;904:306–11.

29. Wang Z, Deurenberg P, Wang W et al. Am J Physiol 1999;276:E995–E1003.

30. Elia M, Stratton R, Stubbs J. Proc Nutr Soc 2003;62:529–37.

31. Wang Z, Pi-Sunyer FX, Kotler DP et al. Am J Clin Nutr 2002;76:968–74.

32. Testolin CG, Gore R, Rivkin T et al. J Appl Physiol 2000;89:2365–72.

33. Pietrobelli A, Formica C, Wang Z et al. Am J Physiol 1996;271:E941–51.

34. Merrill AL, Watt BK, eds. Energy Value of Foods. Washington, DC: US Government Printing Office, 1973.

35. Heymsfield SB, Casper K. JPEN J Parenter Enteral Nutr 1987;11:36S–41S.

36. Ravussin E, Bogardus C. Am J Clin Nutr 1989;49:968–75.

37. Cunningham JJ. Am J Clin Nutr 1991;54:963–9.

38. Müller MJ, Bosy-Westphal A, Klaus S et al. Am J Clin Nutr 2004;80:1379–90.

39. Ellis KJ, Yasumura S, Vartsky D et al. J Lab Clin Med 1982;99:917.

40. Moore FD, Olesen KH, McMurray JD et al., eds. The Body Cell Mass and Its Supporting Environment. Philadelphia: WB Saunders, 1963.

41. Chumlea WC, Guo SS, Zeller C et al. Kidney Int 2001;59:2250–8.

42. Snyder WM, Cook MJ, Nasset ES et al. Report of the Task Group on Reference Man. Oxford: Pergamon Press, 1975.

43. Kissebah AH, Freedman DS, Peiris AN. Med Clin North Am 1989;73:111–38.

44. van der Kooy K, Seidell JC. Int J Obes Relat Metab Disord 1993;17:187–96.

45. Song MY, Ruts E, Kim J et al. Am J Clin Nutr 2004;79:874–80.

46. Heymsfield SB, McManus CB III, Seitz SB et al. Anthropometric assessment of adult protein-energy malnutrition. In: Wright RA, Heymsfield SB, eds. Nutritional Assessment. Boston: Blackwell Scientific Publications, 1984;27–82.

47. Janssen I, Heymsfield SB, Wang ZM et al. J Appl Physiol 2000;89:81–8.

48. Evans W. J Nutr 1997;127:998S–1003S.

49. Baumgartner RN. Ann NY Acad Sci 2000;904:437–48.

50. Heymsfield SB, McManus CB. Cancer 1985;55:238–43.

51. Sjostrom L. Int J Obes Relat Metab Disord 1991;15:19–30.

52. Martin AD, Spenst LF, Drinkwater DT et al. Med Sci Sports Exerc 1990;22:729–33.

53. Studley HO. JAMA 1936;106:458–60.

54. Nixon DW, Heymsfield SB, Cohen AB et al. Am J Med 1980;68:683–90.

55. Vandenbergh E, Van de Woestijne KP, Gyselen A. Am Rev Respir Dis 1967;195:556–66.

56. Seltzer MH, Slocum BA, Cataldi-Betcher ML. JPEN J Parenter Enteral Nutr 1982;6:218.

57. Hirsch S, de Obaldia N, Petermann M et al. J Am Coll Nutr 1992;11:21–4.

58. Windsor JA, Hill G. Ann Surg 1988;207:290–6.

59. Chumlea WC, Guo S, Steinbaugh ML. J Am Diet Assoc 1994;94:1385–8.

60. Han TS, Lean ME. Int J Obes Relat Metab Disord 1996;20:21–7.

61. Chumlea WC, Guo SS. J Gerontol 1992;47:M197–203.

62. Cheng JC, Leung SS, Lau J. Clin Orthop 1996;323:22–30.

63. Schreiner PJ, Terry JG, Evans GW et al. Am J Epidemiol 1996;144:335–45.

64. Björntorp P. Obes Res 1993; 1:206–22.

65. Lemieux S, Prud'homme D, Bouchard C et al. Am J Clin Nutr 1996;64:685–93.

66. Zhu S-K, Wang Z, Heshka S et al. Am J Clin Nutr 2002;76:743–9.

67. Hodgdon JA, Beckett MB. Prediction of Percent Body Fat for U.S. Navy Men from Body Circumferences and Height. Report no. 84–11. San Diego: Naval Health Research Center, 1984.

68. Hodgdon JA, Beckett MB. Prediction of Percent Body Fat for U.S. Navy Women from Body Circumferences and Height. Report no. 84–92. San Diego: Naval Health Research Center, 1984.

69. Durnin JV, Womersley J. Br J Nutr 1974;32:77–9.

70. Damon A, Goldman RF. Hum Biol 1964;36:32–44.

71. Van Itallie TB, Yang MU, Heymsfield SB et al. Am J Clin Nutr 1990;52:953–9.

72. Keys A, Brozek J, Henschel A et al., eds. The Biology of Human Starvation. vols 1 and 2. Minneapolis: University of Minnesota Press, 1950.

73. Knapik JJ, Staab JS, Harman EA. Med Sci Sports Exerc 1996;28:1523–30.

74. Forbes GB, Brown MR, Griffiths HJL. Am J Clin Nutr 1988; 47:929–31.

75. Baumgartner RN, Rhyne RL, Garry PJ et al. J Nutr 1993;123 [Suppl]:444–8.

76. Baumgartner RN. Electrical impedance and TOBEC. In: Roche AF, Lohman TG, Heymsfield SB, eds. Human Body Composition: Methods and Findings. Champaign, IL: Human Kinetics, 1996.

77. Sun SS, Chumlea WC, Heymsfield SB et al. Am J Clin Nutr 2003;77:331–40.

78. Janssen I, Heymsfield SB, Baumgartner RN et al. J Appl Physiol 2000;89:465–71.

79. Chumlea WC, Guo SS, Kuczmarski RJ et al. Int J Obes Relat Metab Disord 2002;26:1596–609.

80. Roos AN. Tetrapolar Body Impedance Reflects Clinical Important Alterations in Total Body Water. The Hague: CIP-Data, Koninklijke Bibliotheek, 1993.

81. Cole TJ. Weight-stature indices to measure underweight, overweight, and obesity. In: Himes JH, ed. Anthropometric Assessment of Nutritional Status. New York: Wiley-Liss, 1991.

82. Garn SM, Leonard WR, Hawthorne VM. Am J Clin Nutr 1986;44:996–7.

83. James WPT, Ferro-Luzzi A, Waterlow JC. Eur J Clin Nutr 1988;42:969–81.

84. Luke A, Durazo-Arvizu R, Rotimi C et al. Am J Epidimiol 1997;145:620–8.

85. Smalley KJ, Knerr AK, Kendrick ZV et al. Am J Clin Nutr 1990;52:405.

86. Baumgartner RN, Heymsfield SB, Roche AF. Obes Res 1995;3: 73–96.

87. Gallagher D, Visser M, Sepúlveda D et al. Am J Epidemol 1996; 143:228–39.

88. World Health Organization. Obesity: Preventing and Managing the Global Epidemic of Obesity. Report of the WHO Consultation of Obesity. Geneva: World Health Organization, 1997.

89. McLaren DS. A fresh look at anthropometric classification schemes in protein-energy malnutrition. In: Himes JH, ed. Anthropometric Assessment of Nutritional Status. New York: Wiley-Liss, 1991.

90. Galen RS, Gambino SR. Beyond Normality: The Predictive Value and Efficiency of Medical Diagnoses. New York: John Wiley & Sons, 1975.

91. Jeejeebhoy KN, Detsky AS, Baker JP. JPEN J Parenter Enteral Nutr 1990;14:193S–6S.

92. Baumgartner RN. Prog Food Nutr Sci 1993;17:223–60.

93. Forbes G. Human Body Composition: Growth, Aging, Nutrition and Activity. New York: Springer-Verlag, 1987.

94. Baumgartner RN, Stauber PM, McHugh D et al. J Gerontol A Biol Sci Med Sci 1995;50:M307–16.

95. Gallagher D, Ruts E, Visser M et al. Am J Physiol 2000;279: E366–75.

96. Baumgartner RN, Heymsfield SB, Lichtman S et al. Am J Clin Nutr 1991;53:1345–9.

97. Goran MI, Toth MJ, Poehlman ET. J Am Geriatr Soc 1997;45: 837–43.

98. Roubenoff R, Baumgartner RN, Kiel DP et al. J Gerontol A Biol Sci Med Sci 1997;52A:M128–36.

99. Chumlea WC, Guo SS, Vellas B et al. J Gerontol A Biol Sci Med Sci 1995;50A:45–51.

100. Roubenoff R, Wilson PW. Am J Clin Nutr 1993;57:609–13.

101. Lansey S, Waslien C, Mulvihill M et al. Gerontology 1993;39: 346–53.

102. Rolland Y, Lauwers-Cances V, Cournot M et al. J Am Geriatr Soc 2003;51:1120–4.

103. Campbell AJ, Spears GFS, Brown JS et al. Age Ageing 1990;19: 131–5.

104. Guigoz Y, Vellas B, Garry PJ. Nutr Rev 1996;54:59S–65S.

105. Last SM. A Dictionary of Epidemiology. New York: Oxford University Press, 1983.

106. Katch VI, McArdle WD. Hum Biol 1973;45:445–53.

107. Jackson AS, Pollack ML, Ward A. Med Sci Sports Exerc 1980; 12:175–82.

108. Wright HF, Dotson CO, Davis PO. US Navy Med 1980;71: 15–26.

109. Vogel JA, Kirkpatrick JW, Fitzgerald PI et al. US Army Research Institute of Environmental Medicine. Technical Report T17–88. Natick, MA: US Army Research Institute of Environmental Medicine,1988.

110. Tran ZU, Weltman A. Med Sci Sports Exerc 1989;21: 101–4.

111. Heymsfield SB, Hoffman DJ, Testolin C et al. Evaluation of human adiposity. In: Björntorp, ed. International Textbook of Obesity. Chichester, UK: John Wiley & Sons, 2001:85–97.

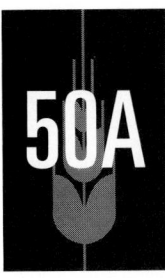

50A NUTRITION DURING PREGNANCY[1]

R. ELAINE TURNER

CURRENT PUBLIC HEALTH OBJECTIVES RELATED
  TO PREGNANCY AND NEONATAL HEALTH 771
PRECONCEPTIONAL HEALTH 771
MATERNAL PHYSIOLOGIC CHANGES DURING
  PREGNANCY 773
WEIGHT GAIN 773
ENERGY AND NUTRIENT NEEDS 774
  Energy 774
  Protein 774
  Carbohydrate 775
  Fat 775
  Fat-Soluble Vitamins 775
  Water-Soluble Vitamins and Choline 775
  Water and Electrolytes .776
  Macrominerals 777
  Trace Minerals 777
DIETARY RECOMMENDATIONS AND ADEQUACY
  OF MATERNAL DIETS 778
OTHER DIETARY AND LIFESTYLE FACTORS 779
  Alcohol 779
  Smoking 779
  Illicit Drugs 779
  Caffeine 779
  Herbal and Other Dietary Supplements 779
  Exercise 780
NUTRITION-RELATED COMPLICATIONS AND
  PROBLEMS 780
  Gastrointestinal Problems 780
  Low Birth Weight 780
  Gestational Diabetes Mellitus 781
  Hypertensive Disorders . . . . . , ...781
  Neural Tube Defects 781
SUMMARY 781

Optimal nutrition is integral to a healthy pregnancy, which can be described as "without physical or psychological pathology in the mother or fetus and results in the delivery of a healthy baby" (1) Although the influence of poor nutritional status on adverse pregnancy outcomes was documented early in the twentieth century, retrospective studies considering the effects of food shortages during World War II clearly identified the influence of diet on pregnancy outcome (2). Nutrition can affect the mother's health and risk of pregnancy complications; it also affects the growth and development of the fetus, the risk of birth defects, and health at delivery.

CURRENT PUBLIC HEALTH OBJECTIVES RELATED TO PREGNANCY AND NEONATAL HEALTH

Maternal health and infant health are important predictors of the future health of the nation's citizens. As identified in *Healthy People 2010*, a major public health goal is to "improve the health and well-being of women, infants, children, and families" (3). Current issues related to maternal and child health include morbidity and mortality of pregnant and postpartum women, fetal, perinatal, and infant mortality, birth outcomes, prevention of birth defects, and access to preventive care. *Healthy People 2010* objectives related to maternal and infant health are summarized in Table 50A.1 along with baseline data. Improvements in nutrition and prenatal care are major elements in progress toward achieving these objectives.

PRECONCEPTIONAL HEALTH

Nutritional status before pregnancy is a key factor in overall maternal health and in the risk of birth defects. Women who are contemplating pregnancy can make dietary and lifestyle changes that will reduce the risk of poor pregnancy outcome. Folic acid supplements before and during the early stages of pregnancy reduce the risk of neural tube defects (NTDs) and other birth defects. Ideally, all women of childbearing age should be consuming 400 μg/day of folic acid in addition to folate provided through foods (4) because nearly one half of all pregnancies in the United States are unplanned (5). Women contemplating pregnancy are more likely to take periconceptional folic acid (6). For women who are planning a pregnancy and

---

[1] **Abbreviations: AI,** adequate intake; **BEE,** basal energy expenditure; **BMI,** body mass index; **DHA,** docosahexaenoic acid; **DRI,** dietary reference intake; **EAR,** estimated average requirement; **EER,** estimated energy requirement; **FAS,** fetal alcohol syndrome; **GDM,** gestational diabetes mellitus; **IOM,** Institute of Medicine; **IUGR,** intrauterine growth restriction; **LBW,** low birth weight; **NTD,** neural tube defect; **PKU,** phenylketonuria; **RDA,** recommended dietary allowance; **TEE,** total energy expenditure; **UL,** tolerable upper intake level.

TABLE 50A.1. SELECTED HEALTHY PEOPLE 2010 OBJECTIVES FOR MATERNAL AND INFANT HEALTH

OBJECTIVE	BASELINE DATA	2010 TARGET
5-8. (Developmental) Decrease the proportion of pregnant women with gestational diabetes		
16-1. Reduce fetal and infant deaths		
16-1a. Fetal deaths at ≥20 wk of gestation	6.8/1,000 live births	4.1/1,000
16-1b. Fetal and infant deaths during perinatal period	7.5/1,000 live births	4.5/1,000
16-1c. All infant deaths (within 1 y)	7.2/1,000 live births	4.5/1,000
16-1d. Neonatal (within 28 d)	4.8/1,000 live births	2.9/1,000
16-1e. Postneonatal (28 d–1 y)	2.4/1,000 live births	1.2/1,000
16-4. Reduce maternal deaths	7.8/100,000 live births	3.3/100,000
16-5. Reduce maternal illness and complications of pregnancy		
16-5a. Maternal complications during hospitalized labor and delivery	31.2/100 deliveries	24/100
16-6. Increase in the proportion of pregnant women who receive early and adequate prenatal care		
16-6a. Care beginning in first trimester	83% of live births	90%
16-6b. Early and adequate prenatal care	74% of live births	90%
16-9. Reduce cesarean births among low-risk women		
16-9a. Women giving birth for the first time	18%	15%
16-9b. Prior cesarean birth	72%	63%
16-10. Reduce low birth weight and very low birth weight		
16-10a. Low birth weight	7.6%	5.0%
16-10b. Very low birth weight	1.4%	0.9%
16-11. Reduce preterm births		
16-11a. Total preterm births	11.6%	7.6%
16-11b. Live births at 32–36 wk of gestation	9.6%	6.4%
16-11c. Live births at <32 wk of gestation	2.0%	1.1%
16-12. (Developmental) Increase the proportion of mothers who achieve a recommended weight gain during their pregnancies		
16-15. Reduce the occurrence of spina bifida and other neural tube defects	6 new cases/10,000 live births	3 new cases/10,000
16-16. Increase the proportion of pregnancies begun with an optimum folic acid level		
16-16a. Consumption of at least 400 μg/d of folic acid by nonpregnant woman aged 15–44 y	21%	80%
16-16b. Median RBC folate level among nonpregnant women aged 15–44 y	160 ng/mL	220 ng/mL
16-17. Increase reported abstinence in past month from substances by pregnant women		
16-17a. Alcohol	86%	94%
16-17b. Binge drinking	99%	100%
16-17c. Cigarette smoking	87%	99%
16-17d. Illicit drugs	98%	100%
16-18. (Developmental) Reduce the occurrence of fetal alcohol syndrome (FAS)		
19-13. Reduce anemia among low-income pregnant women in their third trimester	29%	20%
19-14. (Developmental) Reduce iron deficiency among pregnant women		
27-6. Increase smoking cessation during pregnancy	14%	30%

From US Department of Health and Human Services. Healthy People 2010. 2nd ed. With Understanding and Improving Health and Objectives for Improving Health. 2 vols. Washington, DC: US Government Printing Office, 2000.

who have not been taking folic acid, supplementation should begin at least 1 month before conception (7). Women following vegan or other strict vegetarian diets should also take supplemental vitamin B_{12} because the status of this vitamin is another risk factor for NTDs (4).

Preconceptional iron status is important to reducing risk for iron deficiency and anemia during pregnancy. Studies are lacking on the effectiveness of prepregnancy iron supplementation on iron depletion during pregnancy (1); nonetheless, women with a history of anemia can take steps to improve their iron status. Multivitamin and mineral supplementation may help to improve nutritional sta-

tus in women who are following inappropriate diets, avoiding numerous foods or groups of foods, underweight, trying to lose weight, or abusing alcohol.

Achieving a healthy weight before pregnancy can improve chances of conception, can improve pregnancy outcome, and may improve lactation (8). Women who are obese at the start of pregnancy are at greater risk of hypertension and gestational diabetes mellitus (GDM) and of experiencing induced labor and cesarean section. Obese women may also have more difficulty initiating breastfeeding (1). Infants born to women who were obese before pregnancy are at increased risk of macrosomia, low

Apgar scores, shoulder dystocia, and childhood obesity. In addition, pregnancy obesity has also been linked to an increased risk of spina bifida, omphalocele, heart defects, and multiple anomalies (9). Physical activity can help to improve weight and nutritional status; however, the amount of physical activity needed daily for weight management, chronic disease risk reduction, and enhanced physical fitness varies (10, 11).

Management of preexisting chronic disease is another important element of preconception planning. Women with hypertension are at risk of maternal, fetal, and neonatal morbidity and mortality (12).

Diabetes increases the risk of birth defects, especially defects of the heart and central nervous system, although the exact mechanism is unclear (13). Increased risk of birth defects was not found among women with diabetes who took multivitamins during the periconceptional period (13).

Approximately 3000 to 4000 women of childbearing age in the United States have phenylketonuria (PKU) without severe mental retardation (14). To prevent mental retardation and microcephaly in the infant, pregnant women with PKU must resume a low-protein, amino acid-modified diet during pregnancy. Ideally, women with PKU should resume the diet before conception to regain control of blood phenylalanine and then maintain continued tight control throughout pregnancy.

MATERNAL PHYSIOLOGIC CHANGES DURING PREGNANCY

Numerous anatomic, biochemical, and physiologic changes occur during pregnancy to maintain a healthy environment for the growing fetus without compromising the mother's health. Many of these changes begin in the early weeks of pregnancy, and together they regulate maternal metabolism, promote fetal growth, and prepare the mother for labor, birth, and lactation. A review of the physiologic changes during pregnancy sets the stage for understanding the changes in nutrient requirements that accompany pregnancy.

Maternal plasma volume begins to expand near the end of the first trimester, with a total increase in volume of 45 to 50% by 34 weeks' gestation. Red blood cell production is stimulated, with a total increase in red cell mass of about 33%. Hematocrit levels decline until the end of the second trimester, by which time red cell synthesis is synchronized with plasma volume increase. Declining concentrations of plasma proteins and other nutrients are expected as a result of the expansion of blood volume.

Cardiac output increases approximately 40% during pregnancy. Elevated cardiac output occurs in response to increased tissue demands for oxygen and is accompanied by an increase in stroke volume. The size of the heart increases by about 12%, probably owing to the increased blood volume and cardiac output. Systemic blood pressure declines slightly during pregnancy, with most of the change occurring in diastolic pressure (5–10 mm Hg). Diastolic pressure returns to prepregnancy levels near term.

Respiratory changes support increased maternal and fetal requirements for oxygen. As the uterus enlarges, the diaphragm is elevated, which reduces lung capacity by about 5%, and residual volume is reduced by about 20%. Tidal volume increases as pregnancy progresses, resulting in increased alveolar ventilation and more efficient gas exchange. Respiration rate increases only slightly.

The kidneys increase slightly in both length and weight during pregnancy, and the ureters elongate, widen, and become more curved. Glomerular filtration rate increases by about 50%, and renal plasma flow rate increases by 25 to 50%. Renin levels increase early in the first trimester and continue to rise until term. Most pregnant women are resistant to the pressor effects of the resulting elevation of angiotensin II levels, but enhanced renin secretion may help to explain preeclampsia. A marked increase in excretion of glucose, amino acids, and water-soluble vitamins occurs, probably because the higher glomerular filtration rate presents higher levels of nutrients than the tubules can reabsorb.

Changes along the gastrointestinal tract support the increased demand for nutrients during pregnancy. Appetite increases, although initially this may be offset by nausea and vomiting. Motility of the gastrointestinal tract is reduced by increased levels of progesterone, which, in turn, decrease the production of motilin, a hormone that stimulates smooth muscle in the gastrointestinal tract. Elongation in gastrointestinal transit time occurs largely in the third trimester of pregnancy and is not accompanied by a change in gastric emptying time (15). Gallbladder emptying time is reduced and often incomplete.

The basal metabolic rate rises by the fourth month of gestation and is usually increased by 15 to 20% by term. An elevated basal metabolic rate reflects the increased demand for and consumption of oxygen. Most (50–70%) of the energy needs of the fetus are provided by glucose, with about 20% coming from amino acids, and the remainder from fat. Use of fatty acids for fuel is enhanced in the mother to conserve glucose for use by the fetus.

WEIGHT GAIN

Optimal birth weight is influenced by maternal weight gain. In 1990, the Institute of Medicine (IOM) released weight gain recommendations for pregnancy (16). These recommendations, based on prepregnancy body mass index (BMI), reflect the total gestational weight gain and rate of weight gain associated with best pregnancy outcome (Table 50A.2)

Poor weight gain is associated with poor fetal growth and risk of preterm delivery (17). Carmichael and Abrams found that a marked acceleration or deceleration of gain toward the end of pregnancy was associated with lower

TABLE 50A.2. WEIGHT GAIN RECOMMENDATIONS

PREPREGNANCY BODY MASS INDEX (kg/m²)	RECOMMENDED TOTAL GAIN (kg)	RECOMMENDED RATE OF GAIN[a] (kg/wk)
<19.8	12.5–18	0.5
19.8–26.0	11.5–16	0.4
>26.0–29.0	7–11.5	0.3
>29.0	≥7	

[a]Second and third trimesters.

From Institute of Medicine. Nutrition During Pregnancy. Part I: Weight Gain. Washington, DC: National Academy Press, 1990.

gestational age and a risk of spontaneous preterm delivery (17). Low weight gain during pregnancy is also associated with NTDs; if weight gain in the first trimester (when NTD formation occurs) is minimal, it is more likely that lowered weight gain may be a consequence of carrying an NTD-affected fetus (18).

Excessive weight gain affects infant growth, body fatness in childhood, and the potential for postpartum weight retention and future obesity. Women who are overweight or obese are more likely than women of normal weight to gain more weight than is recommended (19), and exceeding of recommendations was found to be more likely in low-income women (20). Excessive gestational weight gain is further associated with postpartum weight retention and future overweight or obesity (21).

Ideally, weight gain recommendations should be individualized to promote best outcomes while reducing risk for excessive postpartum weight retention and reducing the risk of later chronic disease in the child. Unfortunately, approximately 50% of women receive no prenatal advice or inappropriate advice regarding gestational weight gain (22). Cogswell and associates (23) found that among those who received advice, 14% were advised to gain less than recommended, while 22% were advised to gain more than recommended, and the odds of being advised to gain more than recommended were higher in women with high BMI (>26.0 kg/m²). When no advice on gestational weight gain was given, pregnant women tended to gain outside the IOM recommendations. Consideration of a woman's attitude toward pregnancy and weight gain is crucial to the success of counseling about weight gain (24).

ENERGY AND NUTRIENT NEEDS

To support the growth of the fetus and the health of the mother, requirements for energy and for most vitamins and minerals are higher during pregnancy. Since 1997, the IOM has released a series of reports defining dietary reference intakes (DRIs) for vitamins, minerals, macronutrients, and energy. These reports expand and replace the 1989 *Recommended Dietary Allowances*. See the Appendix for specific DRI values.

Energy

Energy is needed to support basal energy expenditure (BEE), physical activity, the thermic effect of food, and, in pregnant women, growth of the fetus and deposition of maternal tissues. BEE increases because of the enhanced metabolism of the uterus and fetus and the increased work of the heart and lungs. Increased BEE represents the major component of increased energy requirements. Studies estimate the cumulative increase in BEE at 106 to 180 kcal/day, although variation among subjects is substantial (11). Late in pregnancy, the fetus uses approximately 56 kcal/kg/day, which represents about one half of the increment of BEE.

The theoretic energy cost of energy deposition can be estimated from the amount of protein and fat deposited (11). Mean total energy deposition is 39,862 kcal (180 kcal/day). Analysis of studies employing the doubly labeled water method show a median change in total energy expenditure (TEE) of 8 kcal/gestational week. The estimated energy requirement (EER) for pregnancy is thus derived from the sum of TEE for a nonpregnant woman plus 8 kcal/gestational week plus 180 kcal/day for energy deposition. This increase in recommended energy intake is suggested only for the second and third trimesters because TEE changes little in the first trimester, and weight gain is minimal. Thus, during the second trimester, an additional 340 kcal/day greater than nonpregnant energy requirements is recommended. This increase climbs to 452 kcal/day extra in the third trimester.

The EER is higher than values published in the 1989 *Recommended Dietary Allowances* (25). In 1989, an additional 300 kcal/day was recommended for the second and third trimesters of pregnancy. However, this publication predated studies of TEE using the more reliable doubly labeled water method. The EER values are consistent with a study by Butte and colleagues, which found a negligible increase in energy requirements in the first trimester and increases of 350 and 500 kcal/day in the second and third trimesters, respectively (26). Ultimately, the best method for assessing the adequacy of energy intake is to monitor gestational weight gain. The recommended balance of energy sources during pregnancy is the same as for nonpregnant women: 10 to 35% as protein, 45 to 65% as carbohydrate, and 20 to 35% of kcal as fat (11).

Protein

Protein is a major structural component of all cells in the body. Proteins also function as enzymes, in membranes, as transport carriers, as hormones, and as precursors for important molecules including nucleic acids, hormones, and vitamins. During pregnancy, whole-body protein turnover increases, and substantial amounts of protein are accumulated by the growth of the fetus, uterus, blood volume, placenta, amniotic fluid, and maternal skeletal muscle (11). Considering protein deposition over the last two trimesters, the recommended dietary allowance (RDA) increases by 25 g/day. For a reference woman weighing 57 kg, this is an additional 0.27 g/kg/day, for a total of 1.1 g/kg/day during pregnancy. Although the 1989 RDA for protein for nonpregnant women was the same as the current RDA (0.8 g/kg/day), the recommended increment for pregnancy was 10 g/day.

Carbohydrate

The primary role of carbohydrates is to provide energy to cells in the body, particularly the brain and nervous system, red blood cells, white blood cells, and the kidney medulla. In pregnancy, the fetus uses glucose as its major energy source. The transfer of glucose from mother to fetus is estimated at 17 to 26 g/day. By the end of pregnancy, all this glucose is thought to be used by the fetal brain (11). The estimated average requirement (EAR) for carbohydrate increases to 135 g/day, which translates to an RDA for carbohydrate for pregnant women of 175 g/day.

Fat

Fat is a major source of energy for the body and aids in the absorption of fat-soluble vitamins and carotenoids. Some studies have shown lower maternal concentrations of arachadonic acid in plasma and red blood cell phospholipids (11). However, no evidence indicates that supplementation with n-6 fatty acids has any effect on fetal growth and development. The developing brain accumulates large amounts of docosahexaenoic acid (DHA) during prenatal and postnatal development, continuing through the first 2 years of life. Fetal tissue has active desaturases to allow DHA formation from α-linolenic acid. There is no evidence of physiologic benefit to the infant of increasing DHA intake during pregnancy if the diet meets n-3 and n-6 requirements. Therefore, adequate intake (AI) values for essential fatty acids during pregnancy are based on median intakes among pregnant women in the United States: 13 g/day for linoleic acid and 1.4 g/day for α-linolenic acid.

Fat-Soluble Vitamins

Vitamin A is important for regulation of gene expression and for cell differentiation and proliferation, particularly for the development of the vertebrae and spinal cord, the limbs, heart, eyes, and ears. Direct studies of vitamin A status are lacking, but the increase in maternal requirement of 50 μg/day is estimated based on the amount of vitamin A assumed to be accumulated by the fetal liver (27).

Excess retinol intake is a known human teratogen. The most critical period for damage appears to be in the first trimester, and the primary birth defects seen are those derived from cranial neural crest cells. The threshold for risk remains controversial (28–30); however, teratogenicity was used as the critical adverse effect for women of childbearing

age in determining the tolerable upper intake level (UL) of 3000 μg/day.

The main function of vitamin D is to maintain serum calcium and phosphorus concentrations by enhancing gastrointestinal absorption. Vitamin D is also a potent antiproliferative and prodifferentiation hormone. In pregnancy, vitamin D supplementation increases the circulating concentration of $25(OH)D_3$ and may improve neonatal handling of calcium (31). Because only a small amount of $25(OH)D_3$ is transferred from mother to fetus, the AI (5 μg/day) was not increased for pregnancy. The AI for pregnancy is half of the 1989 RDA of 10 μg/day, and several studies suggest the AI is too low, especially for dark-skinned women, and those living in environments with little sun exposure (32, 33). The UL for vitamin D is 50 μg/day for both pregnant and nonpregnant women. However, Hollis and Wagner argued that no evidence exists in humans for ill effects on a developing fetus from doses as high as 2.5 mg/day (33).

Vitamin E is a chain-breaking antioxidant that prevents propagation of lipid peroxidation, especially for polyunsaturated fatty acids within membrane phospholipids and in plasma lipoproteins. α-Tocopherol also inhibits protein kinase activity in cellular proliferation and differentiation. Blood concentrations of α-tocopherol increase during pregnancy, and the rate of placental transfer appears constant. In the absence of reports of vitamin E deficiency during pregnancy, the RDA for pregnant women is the same as for nonpregnant women (34).

Vitamin K is used as a coenzyme in the synthesis of certain proteins involved in blood coagulation and bone metabolism. Data on vitamin K status during pregnancy are very limited, and no data exist on vitamin K content of fetal tissue (27). Thus, the AI for vitamin K is based on median intake and is the same for pregnant and nonpregnant women.

Water-Soluble Vitamins and Choline

Thiamin participates as a coenzyme in the metabolism of carbohydrate and branched-chain amino acids. An increased requirement of about 30% during pregnancy is based on increased growth in maternal and fetal compartments along with a small increase in energy utilization (4).

Riboflavin acts as a coenzyme in numerous oxidation-reduction reactions. Riboflavin is also needed for biosynthesis of niacin-containing coenzymes, for formation of pyridoxal-5-phosphate, and for reduction of 5,10-methylenetetrahydrofolate. Additional requirements for riboflavin in pregnancy are based on increased growth and energy utilization, along with lower urinary excretion of riboflavin (4).

Niacin is required for the formation of nicotinamide-adenine dinucleotide and nicotinamide-adenine dinucleotide phosphate and as such is involved with oxidation of energy sources and biosynthesis of fatty acids and steroids. A small increment in niacin intake is considered adequate to cover increased energy utilization and growth (4).

The coenzyme form of vitamin B_6 is involved in the metabolism of amino acids, glycogen, and sphingoid bases. Vitamin B_6 coenzymes catalyze the first step in heme synthesis and are involved in the *trans*-sulfuration pathway from homocysteine to cysteine. Indicators of vitamin B_6 status in plasma and blood decrease throughout pregnancy, and during the second and third trimesters, fetal blood concentrations of pyridoxal phosphate are higher than in the mother (4). It is estimated that the fetus and placenta accumulate about 25 mg of vitamin B_6, but this is only an increased need of 0.1 mg/day averaged over the course of gestation.

Folate functions as a coenzyme for single-carbon transfers in the metabolism of nucleic and amino acids. DNA synthesis depends on a folate coenzyme (for pyrimidine nucleotide biosynthesis), and thus folate is required for normal cell division. Folate requirements increase substantially during pregnancy because of a higher rate of single-carbon transfer reactions, especially in nucleotide synthesis and cell division. Folate is also transferred to the fetus in substantial amounts. When intake is inadequate, maternal serum and erythrocyte folate concentrations decline, and megaloblastic changes may occur (4). A controlled metabolic study found that 600 μg/day of dietary folate equivalents was adequate to maintain normal folate status (35), and thus, a value of 600 μg/day was set as the RDA for pregnancy. Folate demonstrates most clearly the advancement of science between the 1989 RDAs and the DRIs. The 1989 publication makes no mention of any link between folate status and the risk of NTDs, a link that is well-established today. The 1989 values were 180 μg/day for nonpregnant women and 400 μg/day for pregnant women. Although many women will need folic acid supplementation to meet the current RDA for pregnancy, supplementation should be approached cautiously because the UL is only 1000 μg/day.

Vitamin B_{12} functions as a coenzyme in the metabolism of odd-chain-length fatty acids and in methyl transfer reactions. Adequate vitamin B_{12} is essential for normal blood formation and neurologic function. During pregnancy, absorption may decrease, and serum total vitamin B_{12} concentrations decline in the first trimester more than would be expected solely from hemodilution (4). The placenta appears to concentrate vitamin B_{12} and then to transfer it to the fetus, so serum vitamin B_{12} concentrations in the newborn are about twice the level found in the mother. Based on liver content, the fetus accumulates 0.1 to 0.2 μg/day, which necessitates a slight increase in the RDA (4). Because only newly absorbed vitamin B_{12} is readily transported across the placenta, pregnant women who follow vegan diets will need a supplemental source of vitamin B_{12}.

Pantothenic acid is a component of coenzyme A and phosphopantetheine. Little information is available on pantothenic acid use and status during pregnancy. Usual intakes in the United States and Canada appear to support healthy outcomes, and therefore the AI is set at 6 mg/day for pregnancy (4).

Biotin coenzymes function in biocarbonate-dependent carboxylations. These reactions include the formation of malonyl-coenzyme A and carboxylation of pyruvate for the tricarboxylic acid cycle or glucose formation. Degradation of leucine and formation of D-methylmalonyl-coenzyme A also depend on biotin (4). Animal studies support the idea that biotin deficiency is teratogenic (36). Although studies have raised questions about biotin status during pregnancy, evidence to set a different AI for pregnant women was insufficient. Mock and colleagues found that biotin status, as indicated by urinary excretion of 3-hydroxyisovaleric acid, decreased during pregnancy (37), and increased excretion of this acid could be reversed with biotin supplementation (38).

Choline serves as a precursor to acetylcholine, phospholipids, and betaine. Although choline is synthesized in the body, this synthesis may be inadequate under certain conditions, and thus an AI for choline of 425 mg/day for women was set. In animals, large amounts of choline are delivered to the fetus, and maternal stores decline. Extrapolating from animal data, it is estimated that intake of 3000 mg of choline is needed for fetal and maternal tissues. Thus, the AI for pregnancy is 450 mg/day.

Water and Electrolytes

Water is a solvent for biochemical reactions, is essential for maintaining vascular volume, serves as the medium for transport of nutrients and waste, and helps to control body temperature. The AI for women, 2.7 L/day, is based on a median intake of total water from fluids (~80% of total water) and foods (20% of total water intake) (39). Total water accumulation of 6 to 9 L occurs during pregnancy, with about 1.8 to 2.5 L as intracellular fluid. Plasma osmolality decreases by 8 to 10 mOsm/kg during gestation and stays low until term. The AI for total water intake is based on median intake during pregnancy: 3.0 L/day. In 1989, water recommendations were based on energy intake, with a recommendation for adults of 1 mL/kcal consumed under average conditions of energy expenditure and environmental exposure; the suggested increase for pregnancy was only 30 mL/day.

Sodium and chloride are required for maintenance of extracellular volume and serum osmolality. Sodium is the principal cation of extracellular fluid, and chloride is the principal anion in extracellular fluid. Chloride is also important for production of gastric acid. Although substantial changes in both intracellular and extracellular fluid volumes occur during pregnancy, the amount of additional electrolytes needed to maintain fluid balance does not justify different sodium or chloride requirements for pregnancy.

Potassium is the major extracellular cation in the body and has a great influence on neural transmission, muscle contraction, and vascular tone. The AI for potassium is based on the level of intake that reduces blood pressure and risk of kidney stones. For adults, the AI is 4.7 g/per day. Cumulative gain of potassium during pregnancy is unknown, with estimates ranging from 3.9 to 12.5 g (39). Progesterone may help to conserve potassium. Because the overall accretion is relatively small, the AI for pregnancy is the same as for nonpregnant women. The potassium AI is substantially higher than the 1989 estimated minimum requirement of 1600 to 2000 mg/day and is supported by studies of mineral intake and hypertension (40).

Macrominerals

Calcium contributes to the strength of bones and teeth, and it mediates vascular contraction, vasodilation, muscle contraction, nerve transmission, and glandular secretion. Approximately 25 to 30 g of calcium is transferred to the fetus, with the majority of calcium accretion occurring in the third trimester. Generally, the increase in fetal demand for calcium is met by increased maternal absorption, which occurs in response to increased maternal $1,25(OH)2D_3$ (31). Results of supplementation studies suggest that fetal bone accretion is less when maternal calcium intake is low. When undernourished pregnant women were supplemented with 300 or 600 mg/day, bone mineral density in the neonate was higher than in infants born to unsupplemented mothers, but no changes were noted in mothers' bone mineral density (41). Because of the increased efficiency of absorption during pregnancy, if intake is sufficient for maximizing bone accretion when a woman is not pregnant, then intake does not need to be increased in pregnancy.

Phosphorus is an essential component of all tissues and has structural (phospholipids, nucleotides, nucleic acids) and regulatory functions. A term infant has approximately 17 g of phosphorus, the majority (88%) of which is in bone and water (31). Maternal changes that enhance calcium absorption also increase absorption of phosphorus, and this enhanced absorption covers the increased requirement for phosphorus, leaving the RDA for pregnant women the same as for nonpregnant women. Because of the increased efficiency of phosphorus absorption during pregnancy, the UL for pregnant women (3500 mg/day) is less than for nonpregnant women (4000 mg/day).

Magnesium is a required cofactor for more than 300 different enzymes. A newborn contains approximately 750 mg of magnesium, 60% of which is in the skeleton (42).

Considering the amount of lean tissue accretion along with enhanced bioavailability, the RDA for pregnancy rises by 40 mg/day (31).

Trace Minerals

Chromium potentiates the action of insulin in vivo and in vitro. Several reports suggested that chromium is depleted throughout pregnancy (27). Older studies showed that tissue levels in the newborn decline after birth, a finding suggesting the need for deposition during pregnancy, but an accurate prediction of chromium needs has not been determined. To date, studies have not convincingly associated adverse effects with excess chromium intake from food or supplements, so a UL has not been determined.

Copper is a component of metalloenzymes that act as oxidases in the reduction of molecular oxygen. The EAR is based on estimates of the amount of copper that must be accumulated during pregnancy to account for copper in the fetus and products of pregnancy (27). A full-term infant contains about 13.7 mg of copper, primarily in the liver. This, combined with copper accumulated in the placenta and maternal tissues, translates into an RDA of 1000 μg/day.

Fluoride is mainly associated with calcified tissues. It also inhibits the initiation and progression of dental caries and stimulates new bone development. Fluoride crosses the placenta and is incorporated into primary teeth. Data from prospective, randomized double-blind trials do not support an association between low caries level and prenatal fluoride exposure (43), and so supplementation during pregnancy is not supported. In fact, fluoride balance is maintained at intakes similar to those in nonpregnant women, so no increase in AI is recommended (31). Excess fluoride intake during pregnancy is not associated with increased susceptibility to fluorosis.

Iodine is an essential component of thyroid hormones that regulate key biochemical reactions including protein synthesis and enzymatic activity. Thyroid hormone is important to myelination of the central nervous system and is most active in the perinatal periods. Lack of iodine is particularly damaging to the developing brain. Iodine deficiency disorders include mental retardation, hypothyroidism, and goiter. Cretinism is an extreme form of neurologic damage from fetal hypothyroidism that results in gross mental retardation and varying degrees of short stature, deaf/mutism, and spasticity (27).

The requirement of iodine in pregnancy is based on the iodine content of the newborn thyroid gland (50–100 μg), an amount that almost completely turns over each day. It is estimated that fetal uptake of iodine is 75 μg/day. Prenatal exposure to excess iodine results in goiter and hypothyroidism in the newborn.

Iron is a component of proteins in four major classes: heme proteins, iron-sulfur proteins, proteins for iron storage and transport, and other iron-containing or iron-activated enzymes (27). Lack of iron during pregnancy is associated with perinatal maternal mortality when anemia is severe, and even moderate iron deficiency anemia is associated with a twofold higher risk of maternal death. Maternal anemia is also associated with premature delivery, low birth weight (LBW), and perinatal mortality (44), although large epidemiologic studies showing increased perinatal mortality have been criticized for measuring maternal hemoglobin only at delivery (27). Physiologic factors cause maternal hemoglobin concentration to rise shortly before delivery. Iron deficiency limits the expansion of maternal red blood cell mass, whereas elevated hemoglobin concentration probably reflects decreased plasma volume and is often associated with maternal hypertension and eclampsia (27).

Fetal requirements for iron appear to be met at the expense of maternal iron stores; however, iron supply to the fetus may be suboptimal in severe maternal anemia. The net iron cost of pregnancy is estimated at 700 to 800 mg— this considers basal losses (250 mg), fetal and placental deposition (320 mg), and increase in hemoglobin mass (500 mg), along with blood loss at delivery and the amount of iron that reverts to maternal stores (27). Bioavailability of iron approaches 25% during the second and third trimester, giving an overall requirement of 6.4 mg/day in the first trimester, 18.8 mg/day in the second, and 22.4 mg/ day in the third trimester. Because bioavailability from a vegetarian diet is substantially lower, iron requirements in vegetarians are estimated to be 1.8 times higher than for nonvegetarians (27). Most women will require supplemental iron to meet the RDA (45). Supplemental iron can contribute to gastrointestinal side effects, and large doses may impair zinc absorption if both are consumed in the fasting state.

Manganese is essential for the formation of bone and in the metabolism of amino acids, cholesterol, and carbohydrates. Data on manganese in pregnancy are limited. The manganese concentration in fetal tissues ranges from 0.35 to 9.27 µg/g dry weight (27). Problems associated with manganese deficiency during pregnancy in animals have not been seen in humans.

Molybdenum is a cofactor for a limited number of enzymes: sulfite oxidase, xanthine oxidase, and aldehyde oxidase, which are involved in the catabolism of sulfur amino acids and heterocyclic compounds. No direct data are available on molybdenum requirements for pregnancy, so the RDA for pregnant women (50 µg/day) was extrapolated from values in nonpregnant women using a median weight gain of 16 kg (27). The UL for adults, 2 mg/day, is based on adverse reproductive effects of excess molybdenum intake in animal studies.

Selenium-containing proteins defend against oxidative stress, regulate thyroid hormone action, and regulate the redox status of vitamin C and other molecules. Selenium intake during pregnancy should allow enough accumulation by the fetus to saturate selenoproteins (34). Using an estimated selenium content of 250 µg/kg body weight, a 4-kg fetus would contain would contain 1000 µg. This translates to an additional requirement of 4 µg/day.

Zinc has catalytic, structural, and regulatory functions. Nearly 100 enzymes depend on zinc, representing all six enzyme classes (27). It is estimated that maternal and fetal tissues accumulate progressively more zinc over the course of pregnancy, with a value of 0.73 mg/day in the final quarter of pregnancy. Animal and human evidence suggests that maternal zinc deficiency can lead to prolonged labor, intrauterine growth retardation, teratogenesis, and embryonic or fetal death (46). Scholl and associates found that pregnant women with zinc intake less than 6 mg/day had a high incidence of premature deliveries (47). Goldenberg and colleagues (48) reported that supplementation of African-American women of low socioeconomic status with zinc above a baseline level of 13 mg/day increased birth size and gestational age at delivery; however, a large study of Peruvian women found no effect of supplementation above their dietary intake of 7 mg/day on pregnancy duration or size at birth (49). However, a subsequent study using a higher dose of zinc (25 md/day) showed beneficial effects on fetal femoral length and cardiac patterns (50, 51).

The requirement for zinc may be up to 50% higher for vegetarians, especially when the major food staples have a high ratio of phytate to zinc (e.g., grains, legumes). Excess zinc has been linked to premature deliveries and stillbirth in case reports, but detailed studies are lacking for determining a different UL for pregnant women.

DIETARY RECOMMENDATIONS AND ADEQUACY OF MATERNAL DIETS

Dietary choices of pregnant women need to support the increased nutritional needs as indicated earlier. Because the requirement of increased energy (~14–18% greater than nonpregnant needs) is less than the increased need for most nutrients, food choices must be nutrient dense. Nutrient needs increase the most for iron (50%), folate (50%), iodine (47%), vitamin B_6 (46%), zinc (38%), and protein (38%). Iron supplementation during pregnancy has consistently been supported by scientific societies and public health agencies (45), and continued supplementation with folic acid is needed by most women to meet the RDA. The need for dietary supplementation with other nutrients is less well documented.

Most studies of dietary intake during have focused exclusively on low-income populations and/or have compared results with RDA values instead of the newer and more appropriate comparison standard for groups, the EAR (52). Turner and associates found that when comparing food intake of middle- to upper-income pregnant women with the EAR values for selected nutrients (thiamin, riboflavin, niacin, vitamin B_6, vitamin B_{12}, vitamin C, magnesium, iron, zinc, selenium, and protein), median intake of the study population was less than the EAR only for iron and magnesium (45, 53). The probability of nutrient intake less than the EAR was 0.20 for selenium, 0.21 for vitamin B_6, 0.31 for zinc, 0.53 for magnesium, and 0.91 for iron. Ideally, early prenatal visits should assess the adequacy of the maternal diet and make recommendations for supplementation as needed (54). The recommendations of the US Department of Agriculture food guide pyramid for 2200 or 2800 kcal/day will meet all the nutrient needs of pregnant women, with the exception of iron and folate (55, 56). The DRI's are given in Appendix Tables A-2d to A-2h.

OTHER DIETARY AND LIFESTYLE FACTORS

Alcohol

In the United States, more than 500,000 fetuses are exposed to alcohol each year (57). Most of these exposures are to low levels of alcohol intake and usually early in pregnancy. However, approximately 3% of pregnant women continue to drink either frequently (seven or more drinks/week) or in binges (five or more drinks per occasion). Alcohol use can cause numerous adverse effects on the fetus, the most severe outcomes being mortality and fetal alcohol syndrome (FAS) (58). However, the specific amount of alcohol exposure required to cause FAS has not been determined. Dose, timing, duration of exposure, genetic factors, and protective factors are all contributors (58). Studies suggest that approximately nine to ten of every 1,000 live births are negatively affected by alcohol consumption during pregnancy.

According the IOM, the diagnosis of FAS requires (a) confirmed maternal exposure, (b) the presence of a characteristic pattern of facial anomalies, (c) growth retardation, (d) and central nervous system neurodevelopmental abnormalities (59). The characteristic facial features include short palpebral fissures, epicanthal folds, midface hypoplasia, depressed wide nasal bridge, anteverted nares, long hypoplastic philtrum, and a thin upper vermilion border (60). Central nervous system abnormalities can include decreased head size, brain structure abnormalities, impaired fine motor skills, hearing loss, poor tandem gait, and poor hand-eye coordination. Growth retardation typically continues after delivery and often persists into adolescence (61).

The only preventive measure for FAS and milder versions of the disorder known as partial FAS is the complete abstinence from alcohol during pregnancy. Longitudinal data suggest that deficits in height, weight, head circumference, palpebral fissues, and skinfold thickness are apparent even among light drinkers consuming up to 1.5 drinks/week (62).

Smoking

Cigarette smoking during pregnancy is linked to preterm delivery, spontaneous abortion, and LBW. Carbon monoxide and nicotine from cigarettes increase fetal carboxyhemoglobin and reduce placental blood flow, thus limiting oxygen delivery to the fetus (1). In 2000, nearly 12% of births to US mothers who smoked were LBW (<2500 g), whereas 7.2% of births to nonsmoking women were LBW. Even light smoking (fewer than five cigarettes/day) is associated with LBW (63). Cigarette smoking during pregnancy declined in 2000 to 12.2%, and has fallen 37% since 1989 (64). Smoking rates are higher for older teens and women in their early 20s, and white, non-Hispanic women with less than a high school education (63).

Illicit Drugs

In addition to alcohol and tobacco, illicit drugs such as marijuana, cocaine, and heroin can have devastating effects on a developing fetus. During 1996 to 1998, 6.4% of nonpregnant women and 2.8% of pregnant women reported use of illicit drugs (65). Marijuana accounted for 75% of the illicit drug use, and more than half of pregnant women also used cigarettes and alcohol. Although it is often difficult to isolate the effects of an illicit drug from concurrent use of alcohol and/or tobacco, marijuana and cocaine have been linked to reduced fetal growth (1). Cocaine use has also been associated with premature labor and spontaneous abortion. Exposure to heroin and other opiates leads to a withdrawal syndrome that affects the central nervous, autonomic, and gastrointestinal systems (66). Although most outcomes of prenatal illicit drug use are limited to the early postnatal period (67), results are emerging from longitudinal studies that suggest longer-term effects on language function (67) and academic achievement (68).

Caffeine

The need to restrict or eliminate caffeine intake during pregnancy remains controversial. Caffeine is metabolized more slowly in pregnant woman and passes readily through the placenta to the fetus. High caffeine intake has been shown to be teratogenic in animal studies and has been linked to LBW in humans, although some studies suggest that this association occurs most often in combination with smoking. Epidemiologic studies investigating a link between caffeine intake and the risk of spontaneous abortion have been inconclusive. In a case-control study in Sweden, Cnattingius and associates (69) found a progressive increase in risk for spontaneous abortion with increasing caffeine intake in early pregnancy. This effect was noticeable only for nonsmoking women. Given that most caffeine-containing foods are low in nutritional value (e.g., coffee, tea, colas, and other soft drinks), it is prudent for pregnant women to limit their caffeine consumption.

Herbal and Other Dietary Supplements

Although many pregnant women benefit from supplementation with vitamins and/or minerals to achieve the recommended nutrient intakes in pregnancy, less is known about benefits or risks of herbal and other dietary supplements. Very few studies have examined the efficacy and safety of alternative therapies during pregnancy (70), and so it is most prudent to consider these remedies as suspect until proven safe. Remedies promoted to pregnant women are often for easing gastrointestinal distress (71). Although ginger shows promise for relieving the nausea and vomiting of early pregnancy (72), other botanical therapies such as red raspberry, peppermint, and wild yam have not been formally studied.

Many herbal products have been identified as potentially unsafe for use during pregnancy (1). Safety issues range from potential embryotoxicity to the more likely hormonal effects and drug interactions (73). Given the lack of premarket requirements for proof of safety and efficacy for dietary supplements, pregnant women should discuss such supplements with their health care provider before continuing to use them. Unfortunately, sometimes advice of the health care provider carries its own risks. Finkel and Zarlengo reported a case of a woman advised by her obstetrician to drink a tea made from blue cohosh, an herb used in Native American medicine to induce labor (74). Two days after delivery, the infant suffered a stroke, and the cocaine metabolite benzoylecgonine was detected in the infant's urine and in the mother's bottle of blue cohosh. It was not known whether benzoylecgonine is also a metabolite of blue cohosh or whether the supplement was contaminated with cocaine or if toxicologic testing may have identified a cross-reacting substance. Other reports of contaminants found in supplements have surfaced, including a finding of the alkaloid colchicine in placental blood of patients using a commercially available ginkgo biloba product (75).

Exercise

Exercise can be beneficial for pregnant women and should be encouraged in the absence of contraindications (76). Exercise helps to prevent excessive weight gain, promotes faster delivery, and hastens recovery (11). Exercise may also help to reduce the risk of GDM (77) and can be a helpful adjunct to therapies directed at controlling blood glucose. Epidemiologic studies have suggested a link between strenuous physical activities and growth retardation and preterm delivery, although findings are not consistent. Generally, a wide variety of physical activities can be maintained during pregnancy. Those to be avoided include sports with a high potential for contact, activities with a high risk of falling, vigorous racquet sports with a risk of abdominal trauma, scuba diving, and any exercise in the supine position after the first trimester (76). Women who continue a regular exercise program need to be sure to maintain adequate energy, nutrient, and fluid intake throughout pregnancy (1), along with adequate weight gain. The *Dietary Guidelines for Americans* recommends that pregnant women obtain 30 or more minutes daily of moderate-intensity physical activity unless medical or obstetric complications exist (10).

NUTRITION-RELATED COMPLICATIONS AND PROBLEMS

Gastrointestinal Problems

Among the most common problems during early pregnancy are nausea and vomiting. So-called morning sickness affects 50 to 70% of pregnant women (78). Early nausea is

associated with gastric dysrhythmias and hormonal changes that slow gastrointestinal motility (79). Studies in humans and animals associated reduced energy intakes in early pregnancy with higher placental weight, leading to the hypothesis that secretion of human chorionic gonadotropin and thyroxine results in morning sickness and decreased energy intake, which, in turn, lowers maternal secretion of anabolic hormones (78). Suppressing maternal tissue synthesis may favor nutrient partitioning to the developing placenta.

Management of nausea and vomiting depends on the severity of symptoms; most women with mild episodes are helped by eating smaller, more frequent meals, avoiding offending odors, and drinking adequate fluids (80). In a small study, Jednak and colleagues found that meals high in protein reduced nausea and gastric dysrhythmia to a greater extent than meals higher in carbohydrate or fat (79), although other sources suggest high-carbohydrate meals instead (1).

Heartburn is another common gastrointestinal complaint experienced by approximately two thirds of pregnant women. The main factor in heartburn is lowered pressure across the lower esophageal sphincter caused by increased progesterone secretion. Serious reflux complications are rare during pregnancy (81). Heartburn is generally relieved by eating smaller, more frequent meals, avoiding lying down after eating, elevating the head while sleeping, and avoiding known irritants (1).

Constipation resulting from slowed gastrointestinal motility can be aggravated by high-dose iron supplements. Including generous amounts of fiber, adequate fluids, and regular exercise can help to relieve constipation (1).

Low Birth Weight

Infants who are born with LBW (<2500 g) can be divided into two categories: those born too early and those with intrauterine growth restriction (IUGR). In developed countries, about 50% of all LBW infants are born preterm, whereas in developing countries most are affected by IUGR. Approximately 7 to 8% of live births in the United States are LBW; this statistic may be as high as 25% in South Asia (82). LBW is the risk factor most closely associated with neonatal death; therefore, improving birth weight has a significant effect on infant mortality.

Poor nutrition is a known cause of LBW, especially in developed countries. Other contributing factors include smoking, infections, hypertension, and environmental factors. In the United States, it is estimated that 20 to 30% of LBW is attributable to smoking and its impact on IUGR. Low weight gain in either the second or third trimester increases the risk of IUGR, as does low prepregnancy BMI and young age (1). Longitudinal studies are beginning to shed light on the influence of birth weight on cognitive function and the future risk of chronic disease (78, 83). Consistent, early prenatal care can help to improve nutrition and identify patterns of weight gain that pose a risk of LBW.

Gestational Diabetes Mellitus

GDM affects approximately 4% of all pregnant women (84). Numerous risk factors are associated with increased incidence of GDM, the strongest of these are age, prepregnancy weight, family history of diabetes mellitus, and ethnicity. Maternal complications associated with GDM include higher rates of hypertensive disorders, cesarean delivery, recurrent GDM, and future development of type 2 diabetes. For the fetus, GDM increases the risk of macrosomia, hyperbilirubinemia, hypoglycemia, and erythremia. Macrosomia (usually defined as a birth weight >4000 g) is the most common fetal complication and is associated with high prepregnancy BMI and previous GDM (85).

Diabetes and nutrition counseling, along with intensive self-monitoring of blood glucose and insulin therapy, are effective in reducing the negative outcomes associated with GDM (86). Saldana and colleagues found that impaired glucose tolerance and GDM were more likely in women with higher fat and lower carbohydrate intakes (87).

Hypertensive Disorders

Hypertension in pregnancy is classified into one of five categories: chronic (preexisting) hypertension, preeclampsia, chronic hypertension with superimposed preeclampsia, gestational hypertension, and transient hypertension (12). Gestational hypertension is defined as hypertension (blood pressure >140 mm Hg systolic or 90 mm Hg diastolic) without proteinuria occurring after 20 weeks' gestation. Transient hypertension is the retrospective diagnosis resulting from gestational hypertension that is resolved by 12 weeks postpartum.

Preeclampsia is defined as hypertension with proteinuria (>300 mg/24 hours) after 20 weeks' gestation. It is more common in nulliparous women, women carrying multiple fetuses, women with hypertension for at least 4 years, a family history of preeclampsia, hypertension in previous pregnancy, and renal disease (12). Preeclampsia may progress to eclampsia, a condition marked by seizures that is life-threatening to both mother and infant. Preeclampsia affects 3 to 5% of pregnancies in the United States and is associated with substantial risks including fetal IUGR, death, preterm delivery, and maternal renal failure, seizures, pulmonary edema, stroke, and death (88). Currently, the cause of preeclampsia is unknown, and accurate screening tests are not available.

Preeclampsia is thought to be a two-stage disease (89): reduced placental perfusion is followed by hypertension and proteinuria. In addition to these maternal features, reduced perfusion extends to virtually all organs and is caused by vasoconstriction, microthrombi formation, and reduced circulating plasma volume. Endothelial dysfunction is also present and appears to predate clinical symptoms. Roberts and associates hypothesized that reduced perfusion interacts with other maternal factors such as obesity, black race, insulin resistance, thrombophilias, and hyperhomocysteinemia to produce the disorder (89).

Because of an increased incidence of preeclampsia noted in women of low socioeconomic status, nutritional factors have long been suggested as contributing to the disorder. Energy intake, macronutrient balance, n-3 fatty acids, calcium, sodium, zinc, iron, magnesium, and folate have all been studied for causal or preventive roles; however, conclusive links between nutrient intake and preeclampsia have not been found. Future directions for research include the role of nutrients in the inflammatory response, in insulin resistance, and in oxidative stress, all thought to be contributing factors to the development of preeclampsia (89).

Neural Tube Defects

NTDs are the most common major congenital malformations of the central nervous system and represent varying degrees of disturbance of the embryonic process of neuralation. NTDs include anencephaly, meningomyelocele, meningocele, and craniorachischisis. Neuralation is the first organogenetic process to be initiated and completed (4). The process begins approximately 21 days after conception and is completed by day 28.

The etiology of NTDs includes heredity, probably related to multiple genes influenced by environmental factors. The relationship between folate and NTDs was first suggested by Hibbard in 1964 (4). Observational studies show a reduced risk of NTDs with increased dietary folate intake (90, 91). Studies of folic acid supplements generally support a 70 to 80% risk reduction with 400 μg/day of folic acid (4). The mechanism by which folate could reduce NTDs is still unknown; improved folate status may overcome deficiency in production of proteins or DNA at the time of neural tube closure.

As a result of the accumulated evidence, the US Public Health Service recommended in 1992 that all women capable of becoming pregnant consume 400 μg/day of folic acid, a recommendation echoed in the 1998 DRI report on water-soluble vitamins (4). In an effort to improve folic acid intake, mandatory fortification of enriched cereal grains began in 1998. The required level of fortification (1.4 mg folic acid/kg grain) was estimated to increase folic acid intake by 100 μg/day. Data from population-based surveillance systems show a reduction in the estimate number of NTD-affected pregnancies from 4000 in 1995 to 1996 to 3000 in 1999 to 2000 (92).

SUMMARY

Healthy outcomes for both mother and baby can result from good nutrition, healthy lifestyle choices, adequate weight gain, and early prenatal care. Prenatal care is important for nutrition assessment, evaluation of risk factors, and follow-up to ensure optimal outcomes. Early screening can identify physiologic or psychologic problems and initiate appropriate therapy. As the nation works toward reaching the objectives set in *Healthy People 2010,* researchers need to continue to identify nutritional intervention strategies that are effective at improving pregnancy outcomes (93).

REFERENCES

1. Kaiser LL, Allen L, American Dietetic Association. J Am Diet Assoc 2002;102:1479–90.
2. Shabert JK. Nutrition during pregnancy and lactation. In: Mahan LK, Escott-Stump S, eds. Krause's Food, Nutrition, and Diet Therapy. 11th ed. Philadelphia: WB Saunders, 2004:182–213.
3. US Department of Health and Human Services. Healthy People 2010. 2nd ed. With Understanding and Improving Health and Objectives for Improving Health. 2 vols. Washington, DC: US Government Printing Office, 2000.
4. Food and Nutrition Board, Institute of Medicine. Dietary Reference Intakes for Thiamin, Riboflavin, Niacin, Vitamin B_6, Folate, Vitamin B_{12}, Pantothenic Acid, Biotin, and Choline. Washington, DC: National Academy Press, 1998.
5. Henshaw SK. Fam Plann Perspect 1998;30:24–9, 46.
6. Rosenberg KD, Gelow JM, Sandoval AP. Pediatrics 2003;111:1142–5.
7. Czeizel AE. Curr Opin Obstetr Gynecol 1995;7:88–94.
8. Norman RJ, Clark AM. Reprod Fertil Dev 1998;10:55–63.
9. Watkins ML, Rasmussen SA, Honein MA et al. Pediatrics 2003;111:1152–8.
10. US Department of Health and Human Services and US Department of Agriculture. Dietary Guidelines for Americans. 6th ed. Washington, DC: US Government Printing Office, 2005.
11. Food and Nutrition Board, Institute of Medicine. Dietary Reference Intakes for Energy, Carbohydrate, Fiber, Fat, Fatty Acids, Cholesterol, Protein, and Amino Acids. Washington, DC: National Academy Press, 2002.
12. Chobanian AV, Bakris GL, Black HR et al. Hypertension 2003;42:1206–52.
13. Correa A, Botto L, Liu Y et al. Pediatrics 2003;111:1146–51.
14. Brown AS, Fernhoff PM, Waisbren SE et al. Genet Med 2002;4:84–9.
15. Chiloiro M, Darconza G, Piccioli E et al. J Gastroenterol 2001;36:538–43.
16. Institute of Medicine. Nutrition During Pregnancy. Part I: Weight Gain. Washington, DC: National Academy Press, 1990:27–233.
17. Carmichael SL, Abrams B. Obstet Gynecol 1997;89:865–73.
18. Shaw GM, Todoroff K, Carmichael SL et al. Int J Epidemiol 2001;30:60–5.
19. Strychar IM, Chabot C, Champagne F et al. J Am Diet Assoc 2000;100:353–6.
20. Schieve LA, Cogswell ME, Scanlon KS. Matern Child Health J 1998;2:111–6.
21. Linne Y, Dye L, Barkeling B et al. Int J Obes Relat Metab Disord 2003;27:1516–22.
22. Kleinman RE, ed. Pediatric Nutrition Handbook. 5th ed. Elk Grove Village, IL: American Academy of Pediatrics, 2004:167–90.
23. Cogswell ME, Scanlon KS, Fein SB et al. Obstet Gynecol 1999;94:616–22.
24. DiPietro JA, Millet S, Costigan KA et al. J Am Diet Assoc 2003;103:1314–9.
25. Food and Nutrition Board, Institute of Medicine. Recommended Dietary Allowances. 10th ed. Washington, DC: National Academy Press, 1989.
26. Butte NF, Wong WW, Treuth MS et al. Am J Clin Nutr 2004;79:1078–87.
27. Food and Nutrition Board, Institute of Medicine. Dietary Reference Intakes for Vitamin A, Vitamin K, Arsenic, Boron, Chromium, Copper, Iron, Manganese, Molybdenum, Nickel, Silicon, Vanadium, and Zinc. Washington, DC: National Academy Press, 2001.
28. Voyles LM, Turner RE, Lukowski MJ et al. J Am Diet Assoc 2000;100:1068–70.
29. Rothman KJ, Moore LL, Singer MR et al. N Engl J Med 1995;333:1369–73.
30. Miller RK, Hendricks AG, Mills JL et al. Reprod Toxicol 1998;12:75–88.
31. Food and Nutrition Board, Institute of Medicine. Dietary Reference Intakes for Calcium, Phosphorus, Magnesium, Vitamin D, and Fluoride. Washington, DC: National Academy Press, 1997.
32. Nesby-O'Dell S, Scanlon K, Cogswell M et al. Am J Clin Nutr 2002;76:187–92.
33. Hollis BW, Wagner CL. Am J Clin Nutr 2004;79:717–26.
34. Food and Nutrition Board, Institute of Medicine. Dietary Reference Intakes for Vitamin C, Vitamin E, Selenium, and Carotenoids. Washington, DC: National Academy Press, 2000.
35. Caudill MA, Cruz AC, Gregory JF et al. J Nutr 1997;127:2363–70.
36. Zempleni J, Mock DM. Proc Soc Exp Biol Med 2000; 223:14–21.
37. Mock DM, Stadler DD, Stratton SL et al. J Nutr 1997;127:710–6.
38. Mock DM, Quirk JG, Mock NI. Am J Clin Nutr 2002;75:295–9.
39. Food and Nutrition Board, Institute of Medicine. Dietary Reference Intakes for Water, Potassium, Sodium, Chloride, and Sulfate. Washington, DC: National Academy Press, 2004.
40. Svetkey LP, Sacks FM, Obarzanek E et al. J Am Diet Assoc 1999;99:96S–104S.
41. Specker B. J Nutr 2004; 134:691S–5S.
42. Prentice A. J Nutr 2003;133[Suppl]:1693S–9S.
43. Leverett DH, Adair SM, Vaughan BW et al. Caries Res 1997;31:174–9.
44. Allen LH. Am J Clin Nutr 2000;71[Suppl]:1280S–4S.
45. Turner RE, Langkamp-Henken B, Littell RC et al. J Am Diet Assoc 2003;103:461–6.
46. King JC. Am J Clin Nutr 2000;71[Suppl]:1334S–43S.
47. Scholl TO, Hediger ML, Schall JI et al. A J Epidemiol 1993;137:1115–24.
48. Goldenberg RL, Tamura T, Neggers Y et al. JAMA 1995;274:463–8.
49. Caulfield LE, Zavaleta N, Figueroa A et al. J Nutr 1999;129:1563–8.
50. Merialdi M, Caulfield LE, Zavaleta N et al. Obstet Gynecol Surv 2005;60:13–5.
51. Merialdi M, Caulfield LE, Zavaleta N et al. Am J Obstet Gynecol 2004;190:1106–12.
52. Barr SI, Murphy SP, Poos MI. J Am Diet Assoc 2002;102:780–8.
53. Turner RE, Langkamp-Henken R, Littell R. J Am Diet Assoc 2003;103:563.
54. Institute of Medicine. Nutrition During Pregnancy. Part II: Nutrient Supplements. Washington, DC: National Academy Press, 1990.
55. US Department of Agriculture. Food Guide Pyramid: A Guide to Daily Food Choices. Home and Garden Bulletin no. 252.

Washington, DC: US Dept of Agriculture, Human Nutrition Information Service, 1992.

56. Shaw A, Fulton L, Davis C et al. Using the Food Guide Pyramid: A Resource for Nutrition Educators. http://www.nal.usda.gov/fnic/Fpyr/guide.pdf. Accessed July 1, 2004.

57. Centers for Disease Control and Prevention. MMWR Morb Mortal Wkly Rep 2002;51:273–6.

58. Lupton C, Burd L, Harwood R. Am J Med Genet 2004;127C:42–50.

59. Stratton K, Howe C, Battaglia F. Fetal Alcohol Syndrome: Diagnosis, Epidemiology, Prevention and Treatment. Washington, DC: National Academy Press, 1996:17–20.

60. Stoler JM, Holmes LB. Am J Med Genet 2004;127C:21–7.

61. Day NL, Leech SL, Richardson GA et al. Alcohol Clin Exp Res 2002;26:1584–91.

62. Day NL, Richardson GA. Am J Med Genet 2004;127C:28–34.

63. Ventura SJ, Hamilton BE, Mathews TJ et al. Pediatrics 2003;111:1176–80.

64. Mathews TJ, Menacker F, MacDorman MF. Natl Vital Stat Rep 2002;50:1–28.

65. Ebrahim SH, Gfroerer J. Obstet Gynecol 2003;101:374–9.

66. Chiriboga CA. Neurologist 2003;9:267–79.

67. Bandestra ES, Vogel AL, Morrow CE et al. Subst Use Misuse 2004;39:25–59.

68. Goldschmidt L, Richardson GA, Cornelius MD et al. Neurotoxicol Teratol 2004;26:521–32.

69. Cnattingius S, Signorello LB, Anneren G et al. N Engl J Med 2000;343:1839–45.

70. Murphy PA. Obstet Gynecol 1998;91:149–55.

71. Westfall RE. Complement Ther Nurs Midwifery 2004;10:30–6.

72. Fisher-Rasmussen W, Kjaer SK, Dahl C et al. Eur J Obstet Gynecol Reprod Biol 1990;38:19–24.

73. Rousseaux CG, Schachter H. Birth Defects Res 2003;68:505–10.

74. Finkel RS, Zarlengo KM. N Engl J Med 2004;351:302–3.

75. Petty HR, Fernando M, Kindzelskii AL et al. Chem Res Toxicol 2001;14:1254–9.

76. American College of Gynecologists and Obstetricians. Obstet Gynecol 2002;99:171–3.

77. Dye TD, Knox KL, Artal R. Am J Epidemiol 1997;146:961–5.

78. Huxley RR. Obstet Gynecol 2000;95:779–82.

79. Jednak MA, Shadigian EM, Kim MS et al. Am J Physiol 1999;277:G855–61.

80. American Dietetic Association. Pregnancy Nutrition: Good Health for You and Your Baby. New York: John Wiley & Sons, 1998.

81. Richter JE. Gastroenterol Clin North Am 2003;32:235–61.

82. Ramakrishnan U. Am J Clin Nutr 2004;79:17–21.

83. Richards M, Hardy R, Kuh D et al. BMJ 2001;322:199–203.

84. American Diabetes Association. Diabetes Care 1998;21[Suppl]:560–1.

85. Van Wootten W, Turner RE. Am J Diet Assoc 2002;102:241–3.

86. Langer O, Rodriguez DA, Xenakis MJ et al. Am J Obstet Gynecol 1994;83:362–6.

87. Saldana TM, Siaga-Riz AM, Adair LS. Am J Clin Nutr 2004;79:479–86.

88. Solomon CG, Seely EW. N Engl J Med 2004;350:641–2.

89. Roberts JM, Balk JL, Bodnar LM et al. J Nutr 2003;133[Suppl]:1684S–92S.

90. Shaw Gm, Schaffer D, Verlie EM et al. Epidemiology 1995;6:219–26.

91. Werler MM, Shapiro S, Mitchell AA. JAMA 1993;269:1257–61.

92. Centers for Disease Control and Prevention. MMWR Morb Mortal Wkly Rep 2004;53:362–5.

93. Jackson AA, Bhutta ZA, Lumbiganon P. J Nutr 2003;133[Suppl]:15895–915.

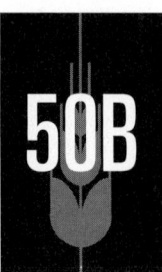

50B LACTATION[1]

MARY FRANCES PICCIANO AND SHARON S. MCDONALD

PREVALENCE OF BREAST-FEEDING 785
    Throughout the World 785
    In the United States 785
MAMMARY GLAND AND REGULATION
    OF MILK SECRETION 786
COMPOSITION OF HUMAN MILK 786
    Nutritional Factors 787
    Bioactive Components 790
IMPACT OF LACTATION ON THE INFANT 791
    Nutritional Status 791
    Brain Development 791
    Overweight and Obesity 792
    Human Immunodeficiency Virus 792
    Morbidity 793
IMPACT OF LACTATION ON THE MOTHER 793
    Breast and Ovarian Cancers 793
    Osteoporosis 794
    Fertility 794
FUTURE RESEARCH DIRECTIONS 795

Human milk, a complex food, provides both nutrition and bioactive components that confer benefits for the growth, development, and health of infants. Although the recommended duration of exclusive breast-feeding varies from a low of 4 months to a high of 6 months, national and international professional and health organizations acknowledge that exclusive breast-feeding is the preferred method of infant feeding. For example, the American Academy of Pediatrics (AAP) recommends exclusive breast-feeding for both term and preterm infant feeding for approximately the first 6 months after birth and continued breast-feeding along with complementary foods for at least 12 months and thereafter for as long as mutually

desired (1). The World Health Organization (WHO) similarly recommends exclusive breast-feeding for 6 months, with introduction of complementary foods and continued breast-feeding for up to 2 years (2). The Canadian Paediatric Society, Dieticians of Canada, and Health Canada, however, recommend exclusive breast-feeding for at least the first 4 months of life, followed by continuation of breast-feeding along with complementary foods for up to 2 years and beyond (3). In the United States, 2010 target health objectives are to increase the proportion of mothers who breast-feed (any breast-feeding) their babies to 75% in the early postpartum period, 50% at 6 months, and 25% at 1 year, compared with 64, 29, and 16%, respectively, in 1998 (the baseline year) (4). Few contraindications to breast-feeding exist. Generally, women who test positive for human immunodeficiency virus (HIV), have active and untreated tuberculosis, or use either illegal drugs or certain prescribed drugs, such as chemotherapeutic drugs for cancer treatment, should not breast-feed (4). In developing countries, however, a safe alternative to breast-feeding may not be available, and evaluation of the relative risks of infant feeding choices may be necessary.

Human milk is a unique food that provides much more than nutrition for the infant. In addition to macronutrients and micronutrients, an impressive body of evidence indicates that human milk contains a host of other components—including antiinflammatory agents, immunoglobulins, antimicrobials, antioxidants, oligosaccharides, cytokines, hormones, and growth factors—that have biologic activities related to development, metabolic regulation, inflammation, and pathogenesis. The combined effects of these bioactive components may result in the observed protection that human milk provides breast-feeding infants against infectious diseases, allergic disorders, and chronic diseases with an immunologic basis (5).

This chapter summarizes information on the prevalence of lactation, its physiologic aspects, and the composition of human milk. In addition, it highlights the possible beneficial impact of lactation on both the breast-fed, full-term infant and the breast-feeding mother and suggests directions for future lactation research.

---

[1]**Abbreviations: AA,** arachidonic acid; **ALA,** α-linolenic acid; **AAP,** American Academy of Pediatrics; **BMD,** bone mineral density; **DHA,** docosahexanoic acid; **HIV,** human immunodeficiency virus; **IDDM,** insulin-dependent diabetes mellitus; **IQ,** intelligence quotient; **LA,** linoleic acid; **LC-PUFA,** long-chain polyunsaturated fatty acid; **NHANES-III,** Third National Health and Nutrition Examination Survey; **OR,** odds ratio; **RR,** relative risk; **TGF-β1,** transforming growth factor-β1; **UNICEF,** United Nations Children's Fund; **WHO,** World Health Organization.

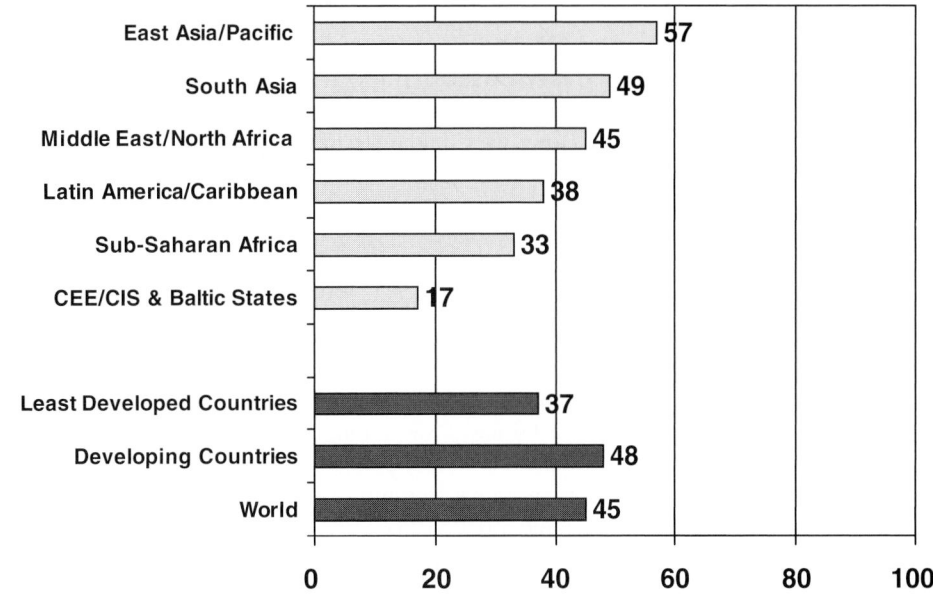

Figure 50B.1. Exclusive breast-feeding rate (<4 months), 1995 to 2000. (Data from United Nations Children's Fund (UNICEF). Breastfeeding and Complementary Feeding. Geneva: World Health Organization, 2001. http://www.childinfo .org/eddb/brfeed/current1.htm. Accessed January 26, 2004.)

Source: UNICEF, 2001

PREVALENCE OF BREAST-FEEDING

Throughout the World

Collection and evaluation of data on the prevalence of exclusive breast-feeding are carried out by international organizations such as WHO and the United Nations Children's Fund (UNICEF), which obtain information from national and regional surveys and studies on breast-feeding prevalence and duration. Data from the WHO Global Data Bank on Breastfeeding, for estimated rates for exclusive breast-feeding of infants 0 to 4 months of age, indicate the highest rate for the Southeast Asia Region (49%), followed by the Eastern Mediterranean Region (39%), the Region of the Americas (29%), and the African Region (18%) (6). UNICEF data, presented in Figure 50B.1 (7), also show the highest rates of exclusive breast-feeding for Asia (East Asia/Pacific, 57%; South Asia, 49%). The lowest rate of 17% was found for Central and Eastern Europe/ Commonwealth of Independent States. Because the regional

groupings differ somewhat between WHO and UNICEF, an exact comparison of the data is difficult. However, findings clearly demonstrate that, worldwide, fewer than one half of infants less than 4 months of age are exclusively breast-fed, and in the least developed countries, the proportion drops to almost one third.

In the United States

The prevalence of breast-feeding in the United States has been estimated by several large, relatively recent surveys, including the Ross Laboratories Mothers Survey and the Third National Health and Nutrition Examination Survey (NHANES-III). The Ross Laboratories Mothers Survey is a large national survey, initiated in 1954 and expanded considerably since then, that is designed to determine patterns of milk feeding during infancy. Prevalence data from this survey for any breast-feeding (Fig. 50B.2) and exclusive breast-feeding (Fig. 50B.3), compared in the hospital

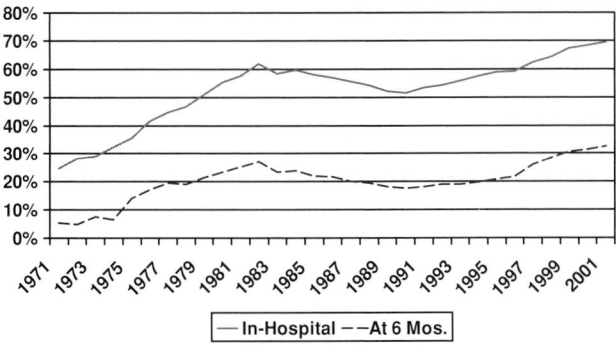

Figure 50B.2. Breast-feeding rates in the hospital and at 6 months of age by year, 1971 to 2001. (Data from Ryan AS, Wenjun Z, Acosta A. Pediatrics 2002;110:1103–9.)

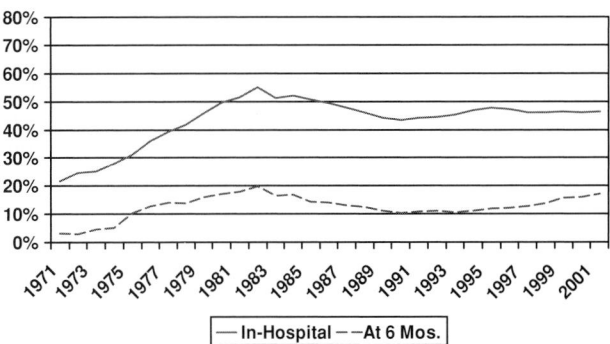

Figure 50B.3. Exclusive breast-feeding rates in the hospital and at 6 months of age by year, 1971 to 2001. (Data from Ryan AS, Wenjun Z, Acosta A. Pediatrics 2002;110:1103–9.)

(postpartum) and at 6 months, show similar trends (8). Breast-feeding increased from low levels in the 1950s and 1960s to a high point in 1982 and then declined throughout the 1980s, but it increased through the 1990s. In 2001, prevalence data for any breast-feeding were higher than the 1980s peak values; 69.5% of mothers breast-fed in the hospital, and 32.5% were still breast-feeding at 6 months. Both in-hospital and 6-month breast-feeding were more common among white and Hispanic women than among black women (8). Other data support differences in prevalence of breast-feeding among ethnic groups. Results from NHANES-III (1988–1994) indicated that the proportions of infants ever breast-fed and exclusively breast-fed at 4 months, respectively, were 60 and 23% among whites, 26 and 9% among blacks, and 54 and 20% among Mexican Americans (9). Although certain subgroups in NHANES-III met the Healthy People 2010 goal of 75% for breast-feeding initiation—mother graduated from college (82%), head of household graduated from college (80%), income greater than 350% of the poverty-income ratio (75%)—none met the goals for breast-feeding at either 6 months or 12 months (10).

MAMMARY GLAND AND REGULATION OF MILK SECRETION

The mature breast of nonpregnant, nonlactating women has a treelike pattern of branching ducts that extends from the nipple to the edges of the fat pad. Alveolar clusters exist in a dynamic state, with growth and complexity increasing and decreasing in response to the hormonal changes of the menstrual cycle. During pregnancy, lobular alveolar complexes expand dramatically in response to progesterone, prolactin, and placental lactogen. Secretory differentiation occurs around midpregnancy (stage 1 lactogenesis), but milk secretion is inhibited by the high progesterone levels (11, 12).

Lactogenesis and lactation are regulated through complex endocrine system control mechanisms that coordinate the actions of various hormones, including the reproductive hormones prolactin, progesterone, placental lactogen, oxytocin, and estrogen (11, 13). Although it is known that progesterone suppresses active milk secretion during lactogenesis 1, hormonal regulation during this stage is not well understood (13). After parturition, lactogenesis 2, also called secretory activation, is initiated through progesterone withdrawal, combined with high levels of prolactin; this results in secretion of colostrum ("early milk") and then milk. Initiation of lactogenesis 2 does not require infant suckling, but suckling must begin by 3 to 4 days postpartum to maintain milk secretion. Prolactin, required to maintain milk production after lactation is established, is released into the circulation from the anterior pituitary in response to suckling. During lactation, release of prolactin is mediated by a transient decline in the secretion of dopamine, an inhibiting factor, from the hypothalamus. Because plasma prolactin levels do not correlate with rate of milk secretion, investigators have

suggested that prolactin may be a permissive factor for milk secretion, rather than a regulatory factor (13).

A diagram of an alveolar complex, the milk-secreting unit of the human breast, is shown in Figure 50B.4 (14). It consists of a layer of epithelial cells surrounded by various supporting structures, including myoepithelial cells, vasculature, and a stroma that contains adipocytes, fibroblasts, and plasma cells. To produce milk, four integrated secretory processes take place in the alveolar complex. These are as follows: exocytosis of milk protein, lactose, and other components of the aqueous phase via Golgi-derived secretory vesicles; fat synthesis and secretion via milk fat globules; secretion of ions, water, and glucose; and transcytosis of immunoglobulins and other substances from the interstitial spaces. Milk is secreted into the alveolar lumina and stored there until ejection by contraction of the myoepithelial cells (12). Although milk secretion is a continuous process, the amount produced is regulated primarily by infant demand. Suckling causes neural impulses to be sent to the hypothalamus; this triggers oxytocin release from the posterior pituitary. Oxytocin brings about contraction of the myoepithelial cells and thus forces milk into the ducts of the nipple so it is available for the infant. This response (let-down) also can be triggered simply by seeing the infant or hearing the infant cry. When milk is removed from the breast after parturition, milk volume increases significantly within several days postpartum. During lactation, the typical daily volume of milk transferred to the infant increases from 0.50 mL on day 1, to 500 mL by day 5, to 650 mL by 1 month, and to 750 mL by 3 months. Most women are capable of secreting considerably more milk than needed by a single infant. When milk is not removed by either infant suckling or other means, involution of the mammary epithelium occurs, and milk secretion stops within 1 to 2 days.

COMPOSITION OF HUMAN MILK

Human milk is a remarkably complex biologic fluid. It is composed of thousands of constituents that are dispersed throughout various phases, including an aqueous phase with true solutions (87%), colloidal dispersions of casein molecules (0.3%), emulsions of fat globules (4%), fat globule membranes, and live cells. The constituents of human milk can be broadly categorized according to their physical and/or physiologic properties (Table 50B.1) (15). Milk composition changes substantially as early milk develops the characteristics of mature milk, which are evident by day 10 of lactation. For example, lactose increases; sodium, potassium, and chloride decrease; total lipids increase; the immune factors lactoferrin and secretory immunoglobulin A decrease; and oligosaccharides decrease. Representative values for early and mature human milk constituents are listed in Table 50B.2 (16). Both the composition and volume of human milk secreted are influenced to some degree by factors such as genetic individuality, maternal

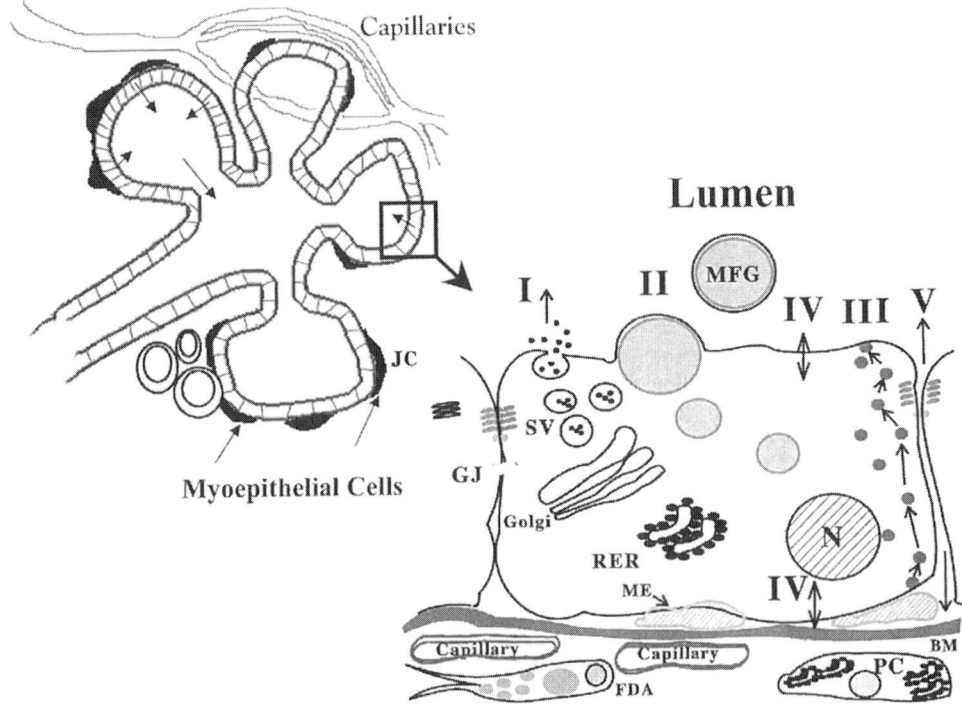

Figure 50B.4. Diagram of the mammary alveolus and alveolar epithelial cell showing pathways for milk secretion. Milk is secreted by alveolar epithelial cells into the lumen and is then expressed through the ducts by contract of myoepithelial cells (ME). The alveolus is surrounded by a well-developed vasculature and a stroma that includes extracellular matrix components, fibroblasts, and adipocytes. The region **inside the box** is expanded to show key structural and transport properties of alveolar cells. *I,* Exocytotic secretion of milk proteins, lactose, calcium, and other aqueous-phase milk components. *II,* Formation of cytoplasmic lipid droplets that move to the apical membrane to be secreted as membrane-bound milk fat globule (MFG). *III,* Vesicular transcytosis of proteins such as immunoglobulins from the intersttiial space. *IV,* Transporters for the movement of monovalent ions, water, and glucose across the apical and basal membranes of the cell. *V,* Transport of plasma components and leukocytes through the paracellular pathway (open only during pregnancy, involution, and in inflammatory states such as mastitis). BM, basement membrane; FDA, fat-depleted adipocyte; GJ, gap junction; JC, junctional complex; N, nucleus; PC, plasma cell; RER, rough endoplasmic reticulum; SV, secretory vesicle. (Redrawn from McManaman JL, Neville MC. Adv Drug Del Rev 2003;55:629–41, with permission.)

nutrition (particularly fatty acids, B vitamins, selenium, and iodine), and stage of lactation. The mammary gland is able to actively extract most nutrients from the circulation, independently of maternal regulatory systems, so milk may contain adequate levels of nutrients even during inadequate maternal intake. However, persistent maternal deficiencies may result in inadequate micronutrient concentrations in the milk. Although most constituents of human milk, including nutrients, are in fact bioactive, nutritional factors are grouped separately in the following discussion.

Nutritional Factors

Macronutrients

The protein constituents of human milk provide essential amino acids for growth, protective factors (e.g., immunoglobulins, lysozymes, lactoferrin), carriers for vitamins (e.g., folate-, vitamin D-, and vitamin B_{12}-binding proteins) and for hormones (e.g., thyroxine- and corticosteroid-binding proteins), enzymatic activity (e.g., amylase, bile-salt stimulated lipase), and other biologic activities (e.g., insulin, epidermal growth factor). Although the total protein content of human milk is the lowest among species, it is easily

digestible, and evidence indicates that nitrogen utilization from human milk for deposition of lean body mass is exceptionally high (17). The nonprotein nitrogen fraction of human milk comprises more than 200 compounds, including free amino acids, carnitine, taurine, amino sugars, nucleic acids, nucleotides, and polyamines. Maternal nutrition possibly may alter both the total protein and nonprotein nitrogen constituents of human milk; however, consequent effects on the nursing infant have not been investigated (18).

Human milk lipids, the major energy-yielding fraction (45–55% of total kcal), are the most variable constituents in human milk. Circulating lipids, a reflection of maternal diet and adipose stores, are the main substrates for human milk fat. The characteristic features of human milk lipids are reviewed elsewhere (19). Human milk is a rich source of linoleic acid (LA) and α-linolenic acid (ALA), both essential fatty acids, as well as their long-chain polyunsaturated fatty acid (LC-PUFA) derivatives, arachidonic acid (AA) and docosahexanoic acid (DHA). Because fat digestion is not yet fully developed in the newborn, several enzymes join forces to aid in digestion of milk lipids. These include the following: lingual lipase, which initiates hydrolysis in the

TABLE 50B.1. CONSTITUENTS IN HUMAN MILK

CATEGORY	REPRESENTATIVE CONSTITUENTS	CATEGORY	REPRESENTATIVE CONSTITUENTS
Proteins	α-Lactalbumin	Water-soluble vitamins	Biotin
	β-Lactoglobulin		Choline
	Caseins		Folate
	Cytokines		Inositol
	Enzymes		Niacin
	Growth factors		Pantothenic acid
	Hormones		Riboflavin
	Lactoferrin		Thiamin
	Lysozyme		Vitamin B_{12}
	Secretory immunoglobulin		Vitamin B_6
	A/other immunoglobulins		Vitamin C
Nonprotein Nitrogens	α-Amino	Major minerals and ions	Bicarbonate
	Creatine		Calcium
	Creatinine		Chloride
	Glucosamine		Citrate
	Nucleic acids		Magnesium
	Nucleotides		Phosphate
	Polyamines		Potassium
	Urea		Sodium
	Uric acid		Sulfate
Carbohydrates	Lactose	Trace minerals	Chromium
	Oligosaccharides		Cobalt
	Glycopeptides		Copper
	Bifidus factors		Fluoride
Lipids	Fat-soluble vitamins		Iodine
	(A, D, E, K)		Iron
	Carotenoids		Manganese
	Fatty acids		Molybdenum
	Phospholipids		Nickel
	Prostaglandins		Selenium
	Sterols/hydrocarbons		Zinc
	Triglycerides	Cells	Epithelial
			Leukocytes
			Lymphocytes
			Macrophages
			Neutrophils

Data from Picciano MF. Pediatr Clin North Am 2001;48:53–67.

stomach; gastric lipase; pancreatic lipase; and bile salt-dependent lipase, which is a constituent of human milk.

Lactose, a disaccharide, is a major human milk constituent and the primary carbohydrate (20); variability results mainly from maternal individuality. Milk lactose increases rapidly in early lactation. Glucose also is present in human milk, but in relatively small quantities. In addition, human milk also contains amylase, an enzyme that can aid in carbohydrate digestion, nucleotide sugars, glycolipids, glycoproteins, and oligosaccharides, which inhibit the growth and function of certain pathogens (21).

Micronutrients

In general, the vitamin content of human milk is related to maternal intake and/or vitamin nutritional status. If maternal status is low, milk vitamin concentrations also are low, but they increase if maternal intake increases; if maternal status is adequate, milk vitamin concentrations also are adequate and are less affected by maternal intake (20). In contrast to vitamins, mineral concentrations in human

milk generally do not correlate well with maternal intake, with the exception of selenium and iodine.

Human milk contains the fat-soluble vitamins A, D, K, and E, as well as certain carotenoids (α-carotene, β-carotene, lutein, cryptoxanthin, lycopene) that have varying degrees of biologic activity. The vitamin A content of human milk is influenced more by maternal intake than by vitamin A status (22). Retinyl esters in chylomicrons and plasma retinol-binding protein–retinol are the sources of vitamin A for human milk synthesis. The retinyl esters are directly related to maternal intake, whereas retinol-binding protein–retinol is relatively constant, regardless of maternal vitamin A liver stores. Human milk vitamin D content is somewhat related to maternal vitamin D status. If maternal plasma levels fall to critically low levels—as a result of restricted intake of vitamin D–rich foods and inadequate sunlight exposure—transfer of the vitamin to milk can be limited. However, milk content is not very responsive to increased maternal intake, and, at best, human milk contains only low amounts of vitamin D (23). Thus, the AAP recommends that all breast-fed infants receive a daily supplement

TABLE 50B.2. REPRESENTATIVE VALUES FOR CONSTITUENTS OF HUMAN MILK

CONSTITUENT (per liter)[a]	EARLY MILK	MATURE MILK	CONSTITUENT (per liter)[a]	EARLY MILK	MATURE MILK
Energy (kcal)		653–704	Water-soluble vitamins		
Carbohydrate			Vitamin C (mg)		100
Lactose (g)	20–30	67	Thiamin (μg)	20	200
Glucose (g)	0.2–1.0	0.2–0.3	Riboflavin (μg)		400–600
Oligosaccharides (g)	22–24	12–14	Niacin (mg)	0.5	1.8–6.0
Total nitrogen (g)	3.0	1.9	Vitamin B_6 (mg)		0.09–0.31
Nonprotein nitrogen (g)	0.5	0.45	Folate (μg)		80–140
Protein nitrogen (g)	2.5	1.45	Vitamin B_{12} (μg)		0.5–1.0
Total protein (g)	16	9	Pantothenic acid (mg)		2.0–2.5
Casein (g)	3.8	5.7	Biotin (μg)		5–9
β-Casein (g)	2.6	4.4	Fat-soluble vitamins		
κ-Casein (g)	1.2	1.3	Vitamin A (mg)	2	0.3–0.6
α-Lactalbumin (g)	3.62	3.26	Carotenoids (mg)	2	0.2–0.6
Lactoferrin (g)	3.53	1.94	Vitamin K (μg)	2–5	2–3
Serum albumin (g)	0.39	0.41	Vitamin D (μg)		0.33
Serum immunoglobulin A (g)	2.0	1.0	Vitamin E (mg)	8–12	3–8
Immunoglobulin M (g)	0.12	0.2	Minerals		
Immunoglobulin G (g)	0.34	0.05	Macronutrient minerals		
Total lipids (%)	2	3.5	Calcium (mg)	250	200–250
Triglyceride (% total lipids)	97–98	97–98	Magnesium (mg)	30–35	30–35
Cholesterol[b] (% total lipids)	0.7–1.3	0.4–0.5	Phosphorus (mg)	120–160	120–140
Phospholipids (% total lipids)	1.1	0.6–0.8	Sodium (mg)	300–400	120–250
Fatty acids (weight %)	88	88	Potassium (mg)	600–700	400–550
Total saturated	43–44	44–45	Chloride (mg)	600–800	400–450
C12:0		5	Micronutrient minerals		
C14:0		6	Iron (mg)	0.5–1.0	0.3–0.9
C16:0		20	Zinc (mg)	8–12	1–3
C18:0		8	Copper (mg)	0.5–0.8	0.2–0.4
Monounsaturated		40	Manganese (μg)	5–6	3
C18:1 ω-9	32	31	Selenium (μg)	40	7–33
Polyunsaturated	13	14–15	Iodine (μg)		150
Total ω-3	1.5	1.5	Fluoride (μg)		4–15
C18:3 ω-3	0.7	0.9			
C22:5 ω-3	0.2	0.1			
C22:6 ω-3	0.5	0.2			
Total ω-6	11.6	13.06			
C18:2 ω-6	8.9	11.3			
C20:4 ω-6	0.7	0.5			
C22:4 ω-6	0.2	0.1			

[a]All values are expressed as per liter of milk with the exception of lipids, which are expressed as a percentage on the basis of either milk volume or weight of total lipids.
[b]The cholesterol content of human milk ranges from 100 to 200 mg/L in most samples of human milk after day 21 of lactation.
From Picciano MF. Pediatr Clin North Am 2001;48:263–4, with permission.

of 200 IU vitamin D/day (24). The vitamin K content of human milk does not correlate well with maternal dietary intake; some studies report, however, that maternal vitamin K supplementation with pharmacologic doses (5 or 20 mg/day) significantly increases vitamin K concentrations in milk and improves vitamin K status of breast-fed infants (15). Infants are born with low tissue stores of vitamin K and thus normally receive a prophylactic dose at birth to reduce the risk of hemorrhagic disease (25). Most of the vitamin E in human milk is in the form of α-tocopherol (83%); small quantities of β-, γ-, and δ-tocopherols also are present. Some data indicate that vitamin E concentration in human milk can be increased only through supplementation with large amounts of the vitamin (25).

Water-soluble vitamins in human milk include vitamin C, thiamin (B_1), riboflavin (B_2), niacin, vitamin B_6 (pyroxidine

and related compounds), vitamin B_{12} (cobalamin), folate, and biotin. Their concentrations in human milk all are dependent on maternal diet. Vitamin B_{12} deficiencies have been reported in infants nursed by mothers who follow a strict vegetarian diet. Although vitamin B_{12} supplementation resolves the deficiency-related abnormalities, some evidence suggests that lasting neurodisability may result (26). It appears that preferential use of folate by the mammary gland over the maternal hematopoietic system occurs. For example, lactating women in the United States whose diets furnished approximately 80% of the recommended amount of folate showed a decrease of folate stores between 3 and 6 months to maintain milk folate secretion (27).

Human milk contains the major minerals calcium, phosphorous, magnesium, sodium, and potassium as well as various trace minerals, including iron, copper, zinc, manganese, selenium, and iodine. The concentrations of major minerals in human milk generally do not correspond to their values in maternal serum. In fact, increased maternal bone resorption for calcium, phosphorus, and magnesium, accompanied by decreased urinary excretion, appears to provide the necessary amounts of these minerals for milk production, independent of maternal dietary intake (23). Although the amounts of iron, copper, and zinc in human milk are relatively low, regardless of maternal intake, high bioavailability of human milk iron and zinc has been reported (15). The iron provided by human milk plus a full-term infant's stored iron is adequate for breastfed infants for about the first 6 months after birth. Unlike most minerals, the concentrations of selenium and iodine

in human milk are dependent on maternal diet and can vary widely by geographic region. For example, the milk iodine content in iodine-sufficient areas is approximately ten times that of milk in areas where iodine deficiency disorders, which include brain damage and mental retardation, are prevalent. Maternal iodine supplementation can be effective in preventing iodine deficiency disorders (28).

Bioactive Components

Some of the numerous known bioactive components of human milk, including several nutrients, and their possible functions are outlined in Table 50B.3 (21, 29). Generally, these components fall into two functional categories: those

TABLE 50B.3. POSSIBLE FUNCTIONS OF BIOACTIVE FACTORS IN HUMAN MILK

BIOACTIVE FACTORS	POSSIBLE FUNCTION
Proteins (nonenzymatic)	
Immunoglobulins (e.g., IgA, IgM, IgG)	Immune protection through specific antigen-targeted antiinfective activity
Lactoferrin	Antimicrobial, antiviral, immunomodulatory activity, antiinflammatory
Lysozyme	Antimicrobial, immunomodulatory activity
κ-Casein	Antimicrobial
Cytokines (e.g., IL-10, TNF-α, interferon-γ)	Modulated maturation and functions of the immune system
Carbohydrates	
Oligosaccharides	Antimicrobial
Glycoconjugates	Antimicrobial, antiviral
Free fatty acids (produced from triglycerides during digestion)	Antimicrobial, antiviral, antiprotozoan
Vitamins	
A	Antiinflammatory
C	Antiinflammatory
E	Antiinflammatory
Nucleotides	Enhanced T-cell maturation, natural killer cell activity, and antibody response to certain vaccines
Enzymes	
Bile salt-dependent lipase	Production of free fatty acids with antibacterial/antiviral/antiprotozoan activity
Catalase	Antiinflammatory
Glutathione peroxidase	Antiinflammatory
PAF factor:acetylhydrolase	Protection against necrotizing enterocolitis
Antienzymes	
α_1-Antitrypsin	Inhibition of inflammatory proteases
α_1-Antichymotrypsin	Inhibition of inflammatory proteases
Prostaglandins	Possible cytoprotection in intestine of newborn
Cells (e.g., macrophages, polymorphonuclear cells, lymphocytes)	Antimicrobial, production of lymphokines/cytokines, enhancement of other protective agents, modulation of maturation and function of immune system
Growth/development-related substances	
Erythropoietin	Stimulation of erythropoiesis in newborns
Insulin	Neonatal glycemia effects
Prolactin	Help in regulation of development of neuroendocrine, reproductive, and immune system functioning
Adrenal steroids	Stimulation of organ maturation
GnRH	Increase in ovarian GnRH receptors in newborns
GHRH	Possible regulation of GH secretion in newborns
TRH	Possible regulation of TSH secretion in newborns
TSH	Possible regulation of T_3/T_4 secretion in newborns
EGF	Stimulation of gastrointestinal tract growth, acceleration of gut closure
TGF-α	Stimulation of gastrointestinal tract growth
IGFs	Stimulation of gastrointestinal tract growth, possible systemic growth effects

EGF, epidermal growth factor; GH, growth hormone; GnRH, gonadotropin-releasing hormone; GHRH, growth hormone–releasing hormone; IGF, insulinlike growth factor; IL, interleukin; PAF, platelet-activating factor; T_3, triiodothyronine; T_4, thyroxine; TGF-α, transforming growth factor-α; TRH, thyroid-releasing hormone; TSH, thyroid-stimulating hormone.

Data from Hamosh M. Pediatr Clin North Am 2001;48:69–86; and Grosvenor CE, et al. Endocr Rev 1992;14:710–28.

that protect the infant from disease, either by direct actions on microorganisms or by modulating immune function and antiinflammatory activity; and those that may help to stimulate and regulate growth, development, and maturation of the gut, immune system, and neuroendocrine systems in the newborn. Some components may act through more than one mechanism. For example, lactoferrin, a glycosylated protein that is present in greater amounts in early milk than in mature milk, has broad-spectrum antimicrobial action; it shows antiviral activity against herpes simplex virus, cytomegalovirus, and HIV; it exhibits various immunomodulating activities; and it possesses antiinflammatory activity, carried out through scavenging iron as well as several other processes (21). Data indicate that many hormones and growth factors in human milk survive the gut, are absorbed into the circulation of the infant, and carry out important functions. These bioactive substances include agents from numerous systems, including the pituitary, pancreas, hypothalamus, thyroid, parathyroid, gut, adrenal gland, and gonads (29, 30). Although knowledge regarding the specific influences of individual agents on the neonate is still scant, recent studies, which demonstrated that factors in human milk play a necessary signaling role in the postnatal development of the anterior pituitary gland, may provide a prototype for future research (30). Much remains to be learned about the functions of human milk constituents, both known constituents and those that likely are yet to be discovered.

IMPACT OF LACTATION ON THE INFANT

Nutritional Status

Human milk, which provides an appropriate balance of nutrients in forms that are readily digestible and bioavailable, provides optimal nutrition for the newborn. When the mother is well nourished, exclusive breast-feeding can meet all the infant's nutrient requirements for approximately 6 months, except possibly for vitamin D in some populations (31) and for iron in infants with low birth weights, who have inadequate body stores of iron (32). After 6 months of age, exclusively breast-fed infants require complementary iron-fortified weaning foods, to prevent iron deficiency. Dewey recently estimated the amounts of nutrients from complementary foods required by exclusively breast-fed infants ages 6 to 8 months, 9 to 11 months, and 12 to 23 months in developed countries (33). These foods represented 29, 55, and 71% of total energy needs, respectively, reflecting the decreased intake of human milk with age. For several nutrients (vitamin A, folate, vitamin B_{12}, selenium), the amount needed from complementary foods before 12 months was estimated to be close to zero. For other nutrients, however, the amounts ranged from 3% (iodine) and 16% (vitamin C) to 96% (vitamin D) and 97% (iron), with values ranging from 56 to 88% for the majority of essential nutrients (33).

Observational studies have reported a slower rate of weight and length gain in exclusively breast-fed infants compared with formula-fed infants (33, 36). Evidence indicates that breast-fed infants self-regulate their energy intake at a lower level than formula-fed infants, and thus the growth pattern of the former may better reflect normal physiologic response to adequate intake (33, 36).

Brain Development

Studies that investigated cognitive outcome in relation to breast-feeding versus formula feeding have been the focus of several critical reviews (37–39). Jain and colleagues (37) used defined criteria based on epidemiologic principles to evaluate 40 publications published between 1929 and 2000. These investigators determined that many studies had methodologic flaws; only nine studies controlled for both socioeconomic factors and stimulation/interaction of the child, considered to be critical confounding factors. Although 27 studies found that breast-feeding promotes intelligence, only two studies satisfied all defined criteria, and only one of these two studies found a significant effect of breast-feeding on intelligence. An earlier evaluation of 24 studies published after 1970 reported that four of the six studies that met the evaluators' methodologic standards found up to a five intelligence quotient (IQ) point advantage for breast-fed infants (38). Metaanalysis of 20 studies, after adjustment for covariates, indicated a mean benefit of 3.16 IQ points for breast-fed infants; benefits increased with duration of breast-feeding (39). However, the metaanalysis did not interpret results based on the quality of the study and thus represents a pooled estimate from a group of heterogeneous studies (37). Findings from several large recent cohort studies not included in the critical reviews support a duration-related benefit of breast-feeding on cognitive development in childhood (40, 41) as well as adulthood (42), findings suggesting potential long-term effects. For children exclusively breast-fed for more than 6 months, compared with those never breast-fed, adjusted verbal IQ at 6 years of age was 3.56 points higher in one study (40), and at 5 years of age was 8.2 points higher for girls and 5.8 points higher for boys in another study (41). An evaluation of two independent samples of young adults, a mixed-gender group (mean age, 27.2 years) and an all-male group (mean age, 18.7 years), that used different intelligence tests for each group demonstrated significant associations between duration of breast-feeding and measured adult intelligence in both groups. For the mixed-gender group, mean measured IQ increased from 99.4 for 1 month or less of breast-feeding to 104.4 for more than 9 months of breast-feeding (42).

Investigators suggested that the positive link between breast-feeding and cognitive development may be partly the result of the long-chain fatty acids DHA and AA, which are present in high concentration in breast milk but not in infant formulas (43, 44). Both DHA and AA are important for the development of the central nervous system, including the rapid growth of the brain, that takes place in the fetus during the last trimester and in the neonate during the first several postnatal months (44, 45). Although humans can synthesize DHA and AA from precursor fatty acids present in both infant formula and human milk, this capacity is limited in premature infants (43). A recent study that examined the effect of supplementing pregnant and lactating women with cod liver oil (high in DHA and other LC-PUFAs) versus corn oil (high in LA) reported that children of mothers in the group receiving cod liver oil had higher mental processing scores at 4 years of age than children of mothers in the group receiving corn oil (106.4 versus 102.3), and the benefit was significantly associated with maternal intake of DHA (44). However, it is also recognized that human milk contains numerous bioactive factors other than LC-PUFAs, including oligosaccharides, growth factors, and hormones, that could potentially influence cognitive development (38, 43).

Overweight and Obesity

Breast-feeding may indirectly reduce the risk of overweight by facilitating self-regulation of energy intake or by activating regulatory systems that maintain energy balance (47, 48). This effect of breast-feeding was explored in numerous studies over the past decades (47, 49). An evaluation of 18 studies conducted from 1976 through 1999 concluded that the protective effect of breast-feeding on later obesity remained controversial. Breast-feeding was directly associated with later body fatness in two studies and was inversely associated in four studies, whereas the remaining 12 studies found insignificant effects; control for confounders, however, varied across studies (49). In a later review of 11 studies, nine of which were published between 1999 and 2002, eight studies showed a lower risk of overweight in children who had been breast-fed, after adjustment for possible confounding factors (47). Recently published results indicated that infants either formula fed from birth or breast-fed for less than 3 months were three times more likely to be obese at age 6 years compared with infants breast-fed for more than 3 months; differences in prevalence of both overweight and obesity between the groups increased significantly after age 4 years (48). One recent study found no association between breast-feeding and body mass index in adulthood (50), whereas another reported a small, but not statistically significant, protective effect against increased body mass index at age 33 years (51). Overall, the data seem to indicate a beneficial but relatively small effect (47).

Human Immunodeficiency Virus

A recent report from the AAP summarized the information available on breast-feeding transmission of HIV-1 (53). HIV-1, hepatitis B, hepatitis C, cytomegalovirus, and human T-cell leukemia virus-1 all have been isolated from human milk (52). The viral load in breast milk of HIV-positive mothers varies widely. To illustrate, analysis of human milk from 145 HIV-1–infected lactating women over the first 3 months postpartum found that HIV-1 was shed intermittently, the viral load could differ between breasts in the same woman at any given sampling, and the viral load was undetectable in approximately one third of samples (54). Estimates of HIV transmission to breast-fed infants are 12 to 14% when mothers already have HIV infection during pregnancy, but 29% when mothers acquire HIV infection just before or during the breast-feeding period, possibly because of higher blood levels of virus in the latter group (53, 55).

Complete avoidance of breast-feeding by HIV-infected mothers is the only way to prevent transmission to the infant. Avoidance of breast-feeding is recommended when replacement feeding is accessible, acceptable, affordable, sustainable, and safe, normally the case in the United States and other developed countries (53, 55, 56). In many developing countries, however, replacement feeding may not be affordable for most HIV-infected mothers, and safe preparation of replacement foods may be impossible because of the lack of clean water. For example, a study in India that examined early postpartum rates of hospitalization of infants born to 148 HIV-infected mothers reported that 29% of infants receiving replacement feeding were hospitalized; no breast-fed infants were hospitalized. Reasons for hospitalization included gastroenteritis (13 infants), sepsis/acute respiratory infection (five infants), sepsis (three infants), jaundice (three infants), and dermatitis (one infant) (57). When the use of replacement feeding is problematic, HIV-infected women face the difficult choice of subjecting their infants to either increased risk of HIV through breast-feeding or increased risk of morbidity and mortality from infectious diseases and malnutrition (55, 57). Some evidence suggests that exclusive breast-feeding for the first few months of life, followed by a relatively rapid transition to replacement feeding, may be an alternative for HIV-infected mothers (56). In a recent prospective study, the cumulative probabilities of HIV infection at 6 months of age for infants exclusively breast-fed for 3 months or more, infants never breast-fed, and infants partially breast-fed were 0.094, 0.094, and 0.261, respectively (58). The mechanism through which exclusive breast-feeding may be safer than partial breast-feeding is not clear, although entry of HIV into bowel tissues damaged by contaminated fluids and foods has been proposed (58). Currently, the WHO recommends that, when replacement feeding is not an option, exclusive breast-feeding is recommended during the first months of life, after which it should be discontinued as soon as feasible. In addition, HIV-infected mothers should receive information about the known risks and benefits of various feeding alternatives as well as guidance about how to select the best approach for their circumstances (56).

Morbidity

Considerable epidemiologic evidence supports a beneficial effect of breast-feeding on morbidity—and, in some cases, mortality—in infancy, as a result of its protection against various illnesses, infections, and allergic reactions, including gastrointestinal disease, lower respiratory tract infections, ear infections, and asthma (59–61). More limited evidence suggests that breast-feeding also may protect against less common illnesses such as urinary tract infections and infant botulism (59, 60). A pooled analysis of mortality data from three developing countries, where poor sanitation often prevails, found that infants not breast-fed had a greater risk of dying of either diarrhea (relative risk [RR] = 6.1) or acute respiratory infection (RR = 2.4) in the first 6 months of life (61). Similarly, a recent study in India reported that the mortality risks for diarrhea (RR = 3.94) and acute respiratory infection (RR = 2.40) were greater for infants either partially or not breast-fed than for infants exclusively breast-fed (62). Data from the National Maternal and Infant Health Survey indicated that breast-feeding also decreases the incidence of diarrhea and respiratory illnesses in developed countries such as the United States, where clean water and good sanitation are the norm (63). One US study reported inverse associations between risk of neonatal respiratory tract infections in girls and either exclusive breast-feeding (odds ratio [OR] = 0.5) or partial breast-feeding (OR = 0.6); no associations, however, were found for infections in boys (64). Findings in Australia indicated that predominant breast-feeding for less than 6 months was significantly associated with two or more hospital, doctor, or clinic visits (OR = 2.07) or hospital admission (OR = 2.65) because of wheezing lower respiratory illness; in addition, predominant breast-feeding for less than 2 months or partial breast-feeding for less than 6 months increased the risk of upper respiratory infection (65). These effects of breast milk are likely to be mediated by several of the many bioactive compounds present in human milk. A recent study reported that milk concentration of transforming growth factor-β1 (TGF-β1) was inversely associated with infant wheeze. Risk of wheeze was significantly decreased (OR = 0.22) for long breast-feeding duration/medium-high concentration of TGF-β1 compared with short breast-feeding duration/low concentration of TGF-β1 (66).

Some evidence suggests that breast-feeding also may protect against chronic diseases that develop later in childhood and in adolescence, particularly diseases with an immunologic basis (67, 68). Most studies, summarized in a recent review, examined whether breast-feeding influences the risk of insulin-dependent diabetes mellitus (IDDM), celiac disease, childhood cancer, and inflammatory bowel disease (68). IDDM is an autoimmune disease with an etiology that includes both genetic and environmental factors. A large body of literature suggests that formula feeding in the first 3 to 6 months after birth increases the risk of later IDDM development. Investigators have proposed that early exposure to cow's milk results in formation of antibodies to a peptide fragment of bovine serum albumin, a cow's milk protein. The antibodies may cross-react with receptors on the pancreatic β-cell surface, because the structure of the peptide fragment is homologous with the structure on pancreatic islet cell antigens, thus resulting in sensitization and a possible first step in IDDM development. It is not clear, however, whether the increased IDDM risk in formula-fed children results from the introduction of foreign proteins, from the absence of protective compounds provided by breast-feeding, or from a combination of these (68). Celiac disease also is an autoimmune disease; genetic susceptibility and dietary exposure to gluten both contribute to its development. Children with IDDM are at increased risk of celiac disease. Data suggest that, to reduce risk of celiac disease, infants should be breast-fed while gluten is introduced and for several months afterward. Although longer duration and exclusivity of breast-feeding have been associated with later onset of celiac disease, the accumulated evidence is inconclusive (68). Numerous studies have investigated a possible association between breast-feeding and childhood cancer, with some investigators studying groups of cancers such as leukemias and lymphomas and others studying all cancers. Overall, the results have been mixed; some studies showed an increased risk for formula-fed children, and others showed no significant association with formula feeding (67). Similarly, findings have been inconclusive in studies that examined the possible influence of breast-feeding on the risk of inflammatory bowel diseases such as colitis and Crohn disease, which usually do not present until the teens or adulthood (68).

IMPACT OF LACTATION ON THE MOTHER

Just as for the infant, evidence indicates that breast-feeding has several direct health benefits for the mother. These include the following: an increased rate of uterine contraction after childbirth and a consequent reduced risk of postpartum blood loss; a reduced risk of breast cancer, particularly premenopausal breast cancer; a reduced risk of ovarian cancer; and a possible reduced risk of spinal and hip fractures after menopause. In addition, the amenorrhea and decreased fertility that generally accompany lactation can contribute to effective family planning efforts during breast-feeding (69).

Breast and Ovarian Cancers

Several reviews have focused on the numerous epidemiologic studies that investigated a possible link between breast-feeding and breast cancer risk (70–72). The findings from both a qualitative literature review (71) and a metaanalysis of appropriate published studies (72) suggest that breast-feeding reduces risk, especially among pre-menopausal women, and that risk reduction is directly related to lifetime duration of breast-feeding. For ever breast-feeding versus never breast-feeding, the metaanalysis (random effects model) reported adjusted ORs of 0.84, 0.76, and 0.83 for all women, nonmenopausal women, and menopausal women, respectively, and noted that various studies adjusted for different covariates (72). For all women, breast-feeding longer than 12 months reduced breast cancer risk by 28% (not adjusted for covariates), compared with breast-feeding for 0 to 6 months. A more recent reanalysis of data from 47 epidemiologic studies in 30 countries reported a RR of 0.96 for ever breast-feeding versus never breast-feeding, and breast cancer risk decreased by 4.3% for every 12 months of breast-feeding. Risk reduction did not differ significantly by menopausal status, age, parity, ethnicity, or various other personal characteristics (70). Several biologic mechanisms for a protective effect of breast-feeding on breast cancer have been proposed, including the following: delay in reestablishing ovulation, which reduces exposure to reproductive hormones; removal of estrogens through breast fluid; physical changes in the mammary epithelial cells that accompany milk production (maximum differentiation); and production of growth factors during lactation such as TGF-β1, shown to be a negative growth factor in human breast cancer cells (71–73).

Epithelial ovarian cancers, which account for approximately 90% of all ovarian cancers, have significant histologic differences, findings suggesting that these cancers may have heterogeneous causes. Some evidence indicates that reproduction-related risk factors are inversely related to risk for nonmucinous tumors (e.g., serous, endometrioid, clear cell) but not for mucinous tumors (74–76). One recent multiethnic, case-control study reported that, compared with never breast-feeding, ever breast-feeding lowered the risk of all types of epithelial ovarian cancer, except for invasive mucinous tumors. In addition, duration of breast-feeding was significantly associated with decreased risk of nonmucinous tumors (RR = 0.4 for >16 months), but not mucinous tumors (RR = 0.9 for >16 months) (74). In another study, ever breast-feeding was associated with significant decreased risk only for endometrioid/clear cell tumors (RR = 0.4), and the risk decreased with breast-feeding duration (75). Some other investigations, however, did not find significant differences in risk among histologic types of epithelial ovarian cancer in relation to breast-feeding practices (76, 77). Suppression of ovulation, which results in less chronic trauma to the ovarian epithelium, has been proposed as one potential mechanism through which breast-feeding may reduce ovarian cancer risk (75).

Osteoporosis

Calcium resorbed from the bones of the lactating woman is the primary source of calcium in human milk (78, 79),

and evidence indicates that increasing calcium intake through either diet or supplementation does not prevent the resorption (23, 80, 81). However, studies consistently show that the skeletal calcium lost during lactation is rapidly regained after weaning (78, 79). The recovery of bone mineral density (BMD) after weaning appears to be influenced by the duration of lactation and postpartum amenorrhea, and recovery varies among skeletal sites (78). For example, greater BMD increases have been found in the lumbar spine than in the femoral neck during the first 6 months after weaning (78, 82). Bone recovery is complete for most women and occurs even with multiple and closely spaced pregnancies and periods of lactation (82, 83). A study that measured BMDs for 30 grand multiparous Finnish American women who had borne at least six children and breast-fed each child for at least 6 months found that repeated pregnancies and lactation, without a recovery interval, was not associated with either lowered BMD or osteoporosis or osteopenia in these women. Moreover, women with ten or more children did not have lower BMDs than women who had six to nine children (83). In general, duration of lactation does not appear to be associated with increased fracture risk or with osteoporosis later in life (78).

Fertility

Breast-feeding is accompanied by a period of amenorrhea and infertility that results from suckling-induced suppression of ovarian activity. Suckling interferes with the normal pulsatile secretion pattern of hypothalamic gonadotrophin-releasing hormone and, consequently, with the secretion of luteinizing hormone and follicle-stimulating hormone, gonadotrophins stimulated by gonadotrophin-releasing hormone. Normal secretion of follicle-stimulating hormone returns early in lactation, and ovarian follicles may develop; luteinizing hormone secretion, however, remains suppressed by suckling. Because ovarian follicles do not produce normal levels of estradiol while luteinizing hormone remains suppressed, ovulation also is suppressed by suckling, and lactational amenorrhea is the result (84). In fact, the Bellagio consensus of 1988 postulated that full or nearly full breast-feeding during lactational amenorrhea provides approximately 98% protection from pregnancy in the first 6 months after childbirth (85). This estimate of contraceptive efficacy has been confirmed by prospective studies of lactating women in both developing and developed countries (86, 87). A study of more than 4000 mother-infant pairs reported that, for full breast-feeding, cumulative pregnancy rates during lactational amenorrhea ranged from 0.9 to 1.2% in the first 6 months postpartum, but they increased to 6.6 to 7.4% at 12 months postpartum (86). A decline in sucking stimulus appears to be the critical factor that determines when postpartum ovulation will resume (84). Thus, supplementation with formula or solid foods during breast-feeding may hasten the return of fertility.

FUTURE RESEARCH DIRECTIONS

It is clear that breast-feeding provides optimal nutrition and other health benefits for the newborn as well as health benefits for the lactating mother. What is not yet clear is the extent of these benefits and the mechanisms responsible. For example, the regulatory mechanisms that govern both the transition from colostrum to mature milk and the changes in nutrient composition of milk during lactation are unknown. In addition, little is known about either the synthesis and regulation of already identified bioactive components in milk or their relation to maternal diet. In fact, it is likely that many more bioactive components will be identified in human milk, and extensive research will be essential to investigate not only their origins but also their specific roles in contributing to potential health benefits for the infant. It is difficult to isolate and purify large quantities of bioactive components from human milk. However, because many of these components are proteins, it is possible that they could be produced for research purposes through recombinant methods (88).

Comprehensive, carefully designed prospective studies that rigorously adjust for confounding variables must be carried out to define possible existing relationships between breast-feeding, especially duration of breast-feeding, and specific outcomes for infants, including cognitive development, risk of overweight or obesity in childhood and adulthood, and risk of acute disease in infancy as well as chronic disease in childhood and beyond. Likewise, research must focus on clarifying associations between breast-feeding and consequences for maternal health. For example, can breast-feeding influence genetic susceptibility with regard to a woman's risk of hormone-related cancers? In all studies, identifying the biologic mechanisms underlying any observed relationships between breast-feeding and outcomes in infants and women is paramount. Clearly, controlled clinical trials that randomize mother-infant pairs to either breast-feeding or no breast-feeding are not possible because of ethical considerations, and alternative trial designs must be developed. One trial randomized an intervention that included advice about breast-feeding, with standard practices as the control, by cluster assignment of maternity hospitals and affiliated clinics. Assessment of the degree of breast-feeding and the occurrence of gastrointestinal tract infection, respiratory tract infection, and atopic eczema demonstrated that, for infants at the intervention sites, both duration of breast-feeding and exclusive breast-feeding increased, and the risk of gastrointestinal tract infection and eczema disease decreased (89).

It is reasonable to expect that breast-feeding recommendations may differ depending on whether the infant is at increased risk of disease because of environmental factors, genetic susceptibility, or maternal factors (e.g., viral infection) and on whether the mother is at increased risk of acute disease, as are malnourished or HIV-infected mothers, or for chronic diseases such as hormone-related cancers. Finding answers to the many questions regarding the potential short-term and long-term health benefits of breast-feeding, for both mother and infant, will help to determine how best to optimize these benefits for mother-child pairs in various circumstances, whether in developing or developed countries.

REFERENCES

1. American Academy of Pediatrics, Work Group on Breastfeeding. Pediatrics 1997;100:1035–9.
2. World Health Organization. The Optimal Duration of Breast-feeding: Results of a WHO Systematic Survey. Geneva: World Health Organization, 2001. http://www.who.int/inf-pr-2001/en/note2001-07.html. Accessed January 26, 2004.
3. Canadian Paediatric Society, Dieticians of Canada, Health Canada. Nutrition for Healthy Term Infants: Statement of the Joint Working Group. Ottawa: Minister of Health, 1998. http://www.hc-sc.gc.ca/dca-dea/publications/pdf/infant_e.pdf. Accessed January 8, 2004.
4. US Department of Health and Human Services. Healthy People 2010: With Understanding and Improving Health and Objectives for Improving Health. 2nd ed. Washington, DC: US Government Printing Office, 2000.
5. Newburg DS. Adv Exp Med Biol 2001;501:1–592.
6. World Health Organization. Global Data Bank on Breastfeeding. Geneva: World Health Organization, 2003. http://www.who.int/nut/db_bfd.htm. Last updated September 3, 2003. Accessed January 26, 2004.
7. United Nations Children's Fund (UNICEF). Breastfeeding and Complementary Feeding. Geneva: World Health Organization, 2001. http://www.childinfo.org/eddb/brfeed/current1.htm. Accessed January 26, 2004.
8. Ryan AS, Wenjun Z, Acosta A. Pediatrics 2002;110:1103–9.
9. Li R, Grummer-Strawn L. Birth 2002;29:251–7.
10. Li R, Ogden C, Ballew C et al. Am J Public Health 2002;92:1107–10.
11. Neville MC, Morton J. J Nutr 2001;131:3005S–8S.
12. Neville MC. Pediatr Clin North Am 2001;48:13–34.
13. Neville MC, McFadden TB, Forsyth I. J Mammary Gland Biol Neoplasia 2002;7:49–66.
14. McManaman JL, Neville MC. Adv Drug Del Rev 2003;55:629–41.
15. Picciano MF. Pediatr Clin North Am 2001;48:53–67.
16. Picciano MF. Pediatr Clin North Am 2001;48:263–4.
17. Motil KJ, Sheng HP, Montandon CM, Wong WW. J Pediatr Gastroenterol Nutr 1997;24:10–7.
18. Institute of Medicine. Nutrition During Lactation. Washington, DC: National Academy Press, 1991.
19. Jensen RG. Lipids 1999;34:1273–1.
20. Jensen RG. Handbook of Milk Composition. San Diego: Academic Press, 1995:919.
21. Hamosh M. Pediatr Clin North Am 2001;48:69–86.
22. Haskell MJ, Brown KH. J Mammary Gland Biol Neoplasia 1999;4:243–57.
23. Food and Nutrition Board, Institute of Medicine. Dietary Reference Intakes for Calcium, Phosphorus, Magnesium, Vitamin D, and Fluoride. Washington, DC: National Academy Press, 1997.
24. Gartner LM, Greer FR, Section on Breastfeeding and Committee on Nutrition. Pediatrics 2003;111:908–10.
25. Institute of Medicine. Nutrition During Pregnancy. Washington, DC: National Academy Press, 1990.

26. von Schenck U, Bender-Götze C, Koletzko B. Arch Dis Child 1997;77:137–9.

27. Mackey AD, Picciano MF. Am J Clin Nutr 1999;69:285–92.

28. Delange F. Proc Nutr Soc 2000;59:75–9.

29. Grosvenor CE, Picciano MF, Baumrucker CR. Endocr Rev 1992;14:710–28.

30. Nusser KD, Frawley LS. Is milk a conduit for developmental signals? In: Newburg DS, ed. Bioactive Components of Human Milk. New York: Kluwer Academic/Plenum Press, 2001;71–7.

31. Greer FR. Pediatr Clin North Am 2001;48:415–24.

32. Griffin IJ, Abrams SA. Pediatr Clin North Am 2001;48:401–14.

33. Dewey KG. Pediatr Clin North Am 2001;48:87–104.

34. Whitehead RG, Paul AA. Proc Nutr Soc 2000;59:17–23.

35. Centers for Disease Control and Prevention, National Center for Health Statistics. CDC Growth Charts: United States. May 30, 2000. http://www.cdc.gov/growthcharts/. Accessed January 26, 2004.

36. Kramer MS, Guo T, Platt RW et al. Pediatrics 2002;110:343–7.

37. Jain A, Concato J, Leventhal JM. Pediatrics 2002;109:1044–53.

38. Drane DL, Logemann JA. Paediatr Perinatol Epidemiol 2000; 14:349–56.

39. Anderson JW, Johnstone BM, Remley DT. Am J Clin Nutr 1999;70:525–35.

40. Oddy WH, Kendall GE, de Klerk NH et al. Paediatr Perinatol Epidemiol 2003;17:81–90.

41. Quinn PJ, O'Callaghan M, Williams GM et al. J Paediatr Child Health 2001;37:465–9.

42. Mortensen EL, Michaelsen KF, Sanders SA et al. JAMA 2002; 287:2365–71.

43. Heird WC. Pediatr Clin North Am 2001;48:173–88.

44. Helland IB, Smith L, Saarem K et al. Pediatrics 2003;111:e39–e44.

45. Herrara E. Placenta 2002;23[Suppl A]:9S–19S.

46. Ogden CL, Flegal KM, Carroll MD et al. JAMA 2002;288: 1728–32.

47. Dewey KG. J Hum Lact 2003;19:9–18.

48. Bergmann KE, Bergmann RL, von Kries R et al. Int J Obes 2003;27:162–72.

49. Butte NF. Pediatr Clin North Am 2001;48:189–206.

50. Martin RM, Davey Smith G, Mangtani P et al. Arch Dis Child 2002;87:F193–F201.

51. Parsons TJ, Power C, Manor O. Arch Dis Child 2003;88:793–4.

52. Georgeson JC, Filteau SM. AIDS Patient Care STDs 2000;14: 533–9.

53. Read JS, Kline MW, Boyle RJ et al. Pediatrics 2003;112: 1196–205.

54. Willumsen JF, Newell M-L, Filteau SM et al. AIDS 2001;15: 1896–8.

55. Weinberg GA. Birth 2000;27:199–205.

56. World Health Organization. New Data on the Prevention of Mother-to-Child Transmission of HIV and Their Policy Implications: Conclusions and Recommendations. WHO technical consultation on behalf of the UNFPA/UNICEF/WHO/UNAIDS Inter-Agency Task Team on Mother-to Child Transmission of HIV, Geneva, 11–13 October 2000. Geneva: World Health Organization, 2001. http://www.unaids.org/en/resources/publications.asp.

57. Phadke MA, Gadgil B, Bharucha KE et al. J Nutr 2003;133: 3153–7.

58. Coutsoudis A, Pillay K, Kuhn L et al. AIDS 2001;15:379–87.

59. Oddy WH. Breastfeed Rev 2001;9:11–8.

60. Heinig MJ. Pediatr Clin North Am 2001;48:105–23.

61. WHO Collaborative Study Team on the Role of Breastfeeding on the Prevention of Infant Mortality. Lancet 2000;355:451–5.

62. Arifeen S, Black RE, Antelman G et al. Pediatrics 2001;108: e67–e74.

63. Raisler J, Alexander C, O'Campo P. Am J Public Health 1999;89: 25–30.

64. Sinha A, Madden J, Ross-Degnan D et al. Pediatrics 2003;112: e303–e7.

65. Oddy WH, Sly PD, de Klerk NH et al. Arch Dis Child 2003;88: 224–8.

66. Oddy WH, Halonen M, Martinez FD et al. J Allergy Clin Immunol 2003;112:723–8.

67. Villalpando S, Hamosh M. Biol Neonate 1998;74:177–91.

68. Davis MK. Pediatr Clin North Am 2001;48:125–41.

69. Labbock MH. Pediatr Clin North Am 2001;48:143–58.

70. Collaborative Group on Hormonal Factors in Breast Cancer. Lancet 2002;360:187–95.

71. Lipworth L, Bailey LR, Trichopoulos D. J Natl Cancer Inst 2000;92:302–12.

72. Bernier MO, Plu-Bureau G, Bossard N et al. Hum Reprod Update 2000;6:374–86.

73. Newcomb PA, Egan KM, Titus-Ernstoff L et al. Am J Epidemiol 1999;150:174–82.

74. Tung K-H, Goodman MT, Wu AH et al. Am J Epidemiol 2003; 158:629–38.

75. Titus-Ernstoff L, Perez K, Cramer DW et al. Br J Cancer 2001; 84:714–21.

76. Purdie DM, Siskind V, Bain CJ et al. Am J Epidemiol 2001;153: 860–4.

77. Modugno F, Ness RB, Wheeler JE. Ann Epidemiol 2001;11: 568–74.

78. Kalkwarf HJ, Specker BL. Endocrinology 2002;17:49–53.

79. Kovacs CS. J Clin Endocrinol Metab 2001;86:2344–8.

80. Kalkwarf HJ, Specker BL, Ho M. J Clin Endocrinol Metab 1999;84:464–70.

81. Prentice A, Jarjou LMA, Stirling DM et al. J Clin Endocrinol Metab 1998;83:1059–66.

82. Karlsson C, Obrant KJ, Karlsson M. Osteoporosis Int 2001;12: 828–34.

83. Henderson PH III, Sowers M, Kutzko KE et al. Am J Obstet Gynecol 2000;182:1371–7.

84. McNeilly A. J Mammary Gland Biol Neoplasia 1997;2:291–8.

85. Kennedy KI, Rivera R, McNeilly AS. Contraception 1989;39: 477–95.

86. World Health Organization Task Force on Methods for the Natural Regulation of Fertility. Fertil Steril 1999;72:431–40.

87. Kennedy KI, Visness CM. Lancet 1992;339:227–30.

88. Lönnerdal B. Nutrition 2000;16:509–11.

89. Kramer MS, Chalmers B, Hodnett ED et al. JAMA 2001;285: 413–20.

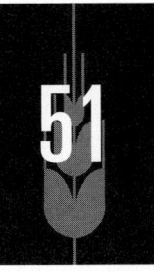

51 INFANCY AND CHILDHOOD[1]

WILLIAM C. HEIRD AND ARTHUR COOPER

NUTRIENT NEEDS OF THE NORMAL INFANT
  AND CHILD 797
    Energy 798
    Protein 801
    Minerals 801
    Trace Minerals and Vitamins 802
    Water and Electrolytes .802
FEEDING THE INFANT 803
    Breast-Feeding 803
    Formula Feeding 803
FEEDING THE OLDER INFANT 804
    Infant Formula versus Bovine Milk 805
    Complementary Feeding 806
FEEDING THE TODDLER 807
    Reduced Food Intake 807
    Self-Selection of Diet 807
    Self-Feeding 807
    Eating Habits 807
FEEDING DURING LATER CHILDHOOD 808
NUTRIENT NEEDS OF THE LOW-BIRTH-WEIGHT
  INFANT 809
    Goals of Nutritional Management 809
    Energy Requirements 812
    Protein Requirements 812
    Fat Requirements 813
    Carbohydrate Requirements 813
    Fluid and Electrolyte Requirements 814
    Mineral Requirements .814
    Vitamin Requirements .815
DELIVERY OF NUTRIENT REQUIREMENTS TO
  LOW-BIRTH-WEIGHT INFANTS 815
ROLE OF HUMAN MILK IN FEEDING THE
  LOW-BIRTH-WEIGHT INFANT 816

The nutritional requirements of infants and children reflect this population's unique needs for growth and developmental changes in organ function and body composition

---

[1] **Abbreviations: AI,** adequate intake; **DRI,** dietary reference intake; **EAR,** estimated average requirement; **EER,** estimated energy requirement; **LBW,** low birth weight; **PC,** physical activity level; **RDA,** recommended dietary allowance; **TEE,** total energy requirement; **UL,** tolerable upper intake level.

as well as their maintenance needs. Moreover, because the metabolic rate of infants and children is greater and the turnover of nutrients more rapid than those of the adult, the unique nutrient needs for growth and development are superimposed on higher maintenance requirements than those of the adult. In addition, the potential impact of intake during early life on later development and health must be considered. Finally, provision of these greater needs, particularly to the smaller members of this population, is hindered by their lack of teeth as well as by their limited digestive and metabolic processes.

In this chapter, the nutrient needs of normal infants and children as well as factors of importance in meeting these needs are discussed, as are the nutritional needs of low-birth-weight (LBW) infants and ways of providing these needs. The nutrient needs of infants and children with acute or chronic diseases that affect nutrient needs and/or management are discussed in Chapters 55 to 61. Chapter 61 also includes a general discussion of approaches to providing the nutritional needs of compromised infants and children as well as a detailed discussion of parenteral nutrition in infants and children.

NUTRIENT NEEDS OF THE NORMAL INFANT AND CHILD

For details on the definitions, bases, and rationale for the dietary reference intakes (DRIs), see Chapter 104 and Appendix Tables A-1-a through A-1-h. In the pediatric age group, certain nutrients lack an estimated average requirement (EAR) definition, owing to the limited data available. In those cases, recommended intakes are based on the adequate intake (AI). The EAR of a specific nutrient is the amount of that nutrient that results in some predetermined physiologic end point. In infants, the major point usually is maintenance of satisfactory rates of growth and development and/or prevention of specific nutrient deficiencies. The EAR is usually defined experimentally, often over a relatively short period and in a relatively small study population. Thus, the EAR by definition, meets the needs of roughly half the population in which it was established but not necessarily the needs of the other half. For some, it may be excessive, whereas for others, it may be inadequate.

The recommended dietary allowance (RDA) of a nutrient, conversely, is the intake of an essential nutrient deemed by a scientifically knowledgeable group to meet the "requirement" of most healthy members of a population. RDAs are useful for assessing nutrient intakes of individual persons; that is, usual intake of a nutrient at or above its RDA has a low probability of being inadequate. RDAs are less useful for assessing the adequacy of the nutrient intake of a group.

In recognition of the lack of a valid EAR for many nutrients and the uncertainty of an RDA based on limited information, the latest recommendations of the Food and Nutrition Board of the Institute of Medicine are designated DRIs (1–6). The DRIs include RDAs for those nutrients for which an EAR has been established, and an RDA therefore can be determined reliably as well as other "reference intakes."

The AI is the observed intake of a specific nutrient by a group of healthy persons. Thus, a mean intake of a nutrient at or above the AI has a low probability of being inadequate. The content of specific nutrients in the average volume of milk consumed by healthy, normally growing, breast-fed infants is considered an adequate intake of most nutrients for infants less than 6 months of age. This definition is consistent with national and international recommendations for exclusive breast-feeding for the first 6 months of life (7, 8). For the 7- to 12-month-old infant, the AI of many nutrients is set at the amount of the nutrient in the average volume of human milk plus the average amount of complementary foods consumed by healthy, normally growing 7- to 12-month-old infants. The AIs of other nutrients for the 7- to 12-month-old infant are extrapolated from that of the 0- to 6-month-old infant or that of the older child or adult. An EAR for a few nutrients has been established for the 7- to 12-month old as well as for older infants and children, either directly or by extrapolation from EARs of adults or older children. For these, an RDA can be (and has been) established.

The tolerable upper intake level (UL) is the highest daily intake of a specific nutrient that has not been associated with adverse effects when consumed regularly. It is not a recommended level of intake but, rather, an aid for avoiding excessive intakes and adverse effects secondary to such intakes.

The most recent reference intakes of various nutrients, proposed by the Food and Nutrition Board of the Institute of Medicine, for infants and children less than 8 years of age are summarized in Table 51.1 and in Appendix Tables A-2-d-1 through A-2-e and A-2-g. ULs of those nutrients for which such a value has been established are summarized in Table 51.2 and in Appendix Tables A-2-f and A-2-g. The DRIs of some nutrients for the 0- to 6-month old infant, the 7- to 12-month-old infant, the 1- to 3-year-old child, and the 4- to 8-year-old child are discussed briefly in the sections that follow.

Energy

Per unit of body weight, the normal infant and young child require at least twice as much energy as the adult, that is, 80 to 100 versus 30 to 40 kcal/kg/day. This greater need reflects primarily the infant's higher resting metabolic rate and special needs for growth and development.

The estimated energy requirement (EER) of the infant and young child proposed by the Food and Nutrition Board (5), that is, the energy intake predicted to maintain energy balance, is based on analysis of total energy expenditure (TEE) data obtained by the doubly labeled water method (TEE = 88.6 × weight − 99.4) plus an allowance for energy deposition incident to growth as determined from measurements of weight gain and body composition of normally growing infants and young children (9).

Equations for predicting the EER (kcal/day) of infants and children under 3 years of age are as follows:

0 to 3 months, (88.6 × weight of infant − 99.4) + 175

4 to 6 months, (88.6 × weight of infant − 99.4) + 56

7 to 12 months, (88.6 × weight of infant − 99.4) + 22

1 to 3 years, (88.6 × weight of child − 99.4) + 22

The EER of the infant less than 6 months of age determined in this way is very close to the mean energy intake of exclusively breast-fed infants.

The EER of the 3- to 8-year-old child also is based on TEE measured by the doubly labeled water method plus an allowance for growth (20 kcal/day) and an adjustment for physical activity level. For this age group, the equation predicting TEE differs between boys and girls and includes age, height, and weight. This is adjusted for physical activity level (PC, 1.0 for sedentary to 1.42 for boys or 1.56 for girls if very active). For 3- to 8-year-old boys, the equation for EER (kcal/day) is as follows:

$$EER = 88.5 - 61.9 \times age\ [y] + PC \\ \times (26.7 \times weight\ [kg] + 903 \times height\ [m]) + 20$$

For girls, it is as follows:

$$EER = 135.3 - 30.8 \times age\ [y] + PC \\ \times (10 \times weight\ [kg] + 934 \times height\ [m]) + 20$$

With respect to the source of energy, no evidence indicates that either carbohydrate or fat is superior, provided total energy intake is adequate. Sufficient carbohydrate to avoid ketosis and/or hypoglycemia is required (~5.0 g/kg/day), as is enough fat to avoid essential fatty acid deficiency (0.5–1.0 g/kg/day of linoleic acid plus a smaller amount of α-linolenic acid).

The AIs of carbohydrate and fat proposed by the Food and Nutrition Board (5), for the 0- to 6-month-old infant, that is, 60 g/day (~10 g/kg/day) and 31 g/day (~5 g/kg/day), respectively, are based on the carbohydrate and fat contents of an average intake of human milk. Those for the 7- to 12-month-old infant, that is, 95 g/day (~10.5 g/kg/day)

TABLE 51.1. DAILY REFERENCE INTAKES OF NUTRIENTS FOR NORMAL INFANTS

NUTRIENT	REFERENCE INTAKE PER DAY			
	0–6 mo (6 kg)	7–12 mo (9 kg)	1–3 y (13 kg)	4–8 y (22 kg)
Energy (kcal (kJ)/24 h)	550 (2,310)	750 (3,013)	1,074 (4,494)	See text
Fat (g/24 h)	31[a]	30[a]	—	—
Linoleic acid (g/24 h)	4.4[a]	4.6[a]	7[a]	10[a]
α-Linolenic acid (g/24 h)	0.5[a]	0.5[a]	0.7[a]	0.9[a]
Carbohydrate (g/24 h)	60[a]	95[a]	130[a]	130[a]
Protein (g/24 h)	9.3[a]	11[b]	13.7[b]	21[b]
Electrolytes and minerals				
Calcium (mg/24 h)	210[a]	270[a]	500[a]	800[a]
Phosphorus (mg/24 h)	100[a]	275[a]	460[b]	500[b]
Magnesium (mg/24 h)	30[a]	75[a]	80[b]	130[b]
Sodium (mmol/24 h)	5[a]	6[a]	42[a]	53[a]
Chloride (mmol/24 h)	5[a]	16[a]	42[a]	53[a]
Potassium (mmol/24 h)	10[a]	18[a]	77[a]	97[a]
Iron (mg/24 h)	0.27[a]	11[b]	7[b]	10[b]
Zinc (mg/24 h)	2[a]	3[b]	3[b]	5[b]
Copper (μg/24 h)	200[a]	220[a]	340[b]	440[b]
Iodine (μg/24 h)	110[a]	130[a]	90[b]	90[b]
Selenium (μg/24 h)	15[a]	20[a]	20[b]	30[b]
Manganese (mg/24 h)	0.003[a]	0.6[a]	1.2[a]	1.5[a]
Fluoride (mg/24 h)	0.01[a]	0.5[a]	0.7[a]	1.0[a]
Chromium (μg/24 h)	0.2[a]	5.5[a]	11[a]	15[a]
Molybdenum (μg/24 h)	2[a]	3[a]	17[b]	22[b]
Vitamins				
Vitamin A (μg/24 h)	400[a]	500[a]	300[b]	400[b]
Vitamin D (μg/24 h)	5[a]	5[a]	5[a]	5[a]
Vitamin E (mg α-TE/24 h)	4[a]	5[a]	6[b]	7[b]
Vitamin K (μg/24 h)	2.0[a]	2.5[a]	30[a]	55[a]
Vitamin C (mg/24 h)	40[a]	50[a]	15[b]	25[b]
Thiamin (mg/24 h)	0.2[a]	0.3[a]	0.5[b]	0.6[b]
Riboflavin (mg/24 h)	0.3[a]	0.4[a]	0.5[b]	0.6[b]
Niacin (mg NE/24 h)	2[a]	4[a]	6[b]	8[b]
Vitamin B$_6$ (μg/24 h)	0.1[a]	0.3[a]	0.5[b]	0.6[b]
Folate (μg)	65[a]	80[a]	150[b]	200[b]
Vitamin B$_{12}$ (μg/24 h)	0.4[a]	0.5[a]	0.9[b]	1.2[b]
Biotin (μg/24 h)	5[a]	6[a]	8[a]	12[a]
Pantothenic acid (mg/24 h)	1.7[a]	1.8[a]	2[a]	3[a]
Choline (mg/24 h)	125[a]	150[a]	200[a]	250[a]
Water (L/24 h)	0.7[a]	0.8[a]	1.3[a]	1.7[a]

*RDA
[a]Adequate intake (e.g., for infants <6 mo of age, this is the mean intake of normal breast-fed infants).
[b]Recommended dietary allowance.
Data from references 1 to 6.

and 30 g/day (~3.3 g/kg/day), respectively, are based on the average consumption of carbohydrate and fat from human milk plus complementary foods. An EAR for carbohydrate for the older child was established by extrapolation from adult requirements. It is 100 g/day for both the 1- to 3-year-old child (8.3 g/kg/day) and the 4- to 8-year-old child (5 g/kg/day). The RDA is 130 g/day (10.8 and 6.5 g/kg/day, respectively, for the younger and older child). AIs for fat beyond a year of age were not determined.

The AIs of n-6 polyunsaturated fatty acids (primarily linoleic acid) and n-3 polyunsaturated fatty acids (primarily α-linolenic acid) proposed for the 0- to 6-month-old infant, based on the average consumption of these fatty acids by exclusively breast-fed infants, are 4.4 g/day (~0.73 g/kg/day)

and 0.5 g/day (~83 mg/kg/day), respectively (5). Those for the 7- to 12-month-old infant, based on the average consumption of these fatty acids from human milk plus complementary foods, are 4.6 g/day (~0.5 g/kg/day) and 0.5 g/day (~56 mg/kg/day), respectively (5). AIs of these fatty acids for the 1- to 3-year-old child and the 4- to 8-year-old child are based on the median intakes of these fatty acids by children of these age groups reported by the Continuing Survey of Food Intake by Individuals. They are 7 and 10 g/day (0.58 and 0.5 g/kg/day), respectively, for n-6 polyunsaturated fatty acids and 0.7 and 0.9 g/day (58 and 45 mg/kg/day), respectively, for n-3 polyunsaturated fatty acids. On average, AIs of these two fatty acid groups account for 5 to 7% and 0.5 to 1.0% of the EER, respectively.

TABLE 51.2. TOLERABLE UPPER INTAKE LEVELS OF NUTRIENTS FOR INFANTS AND YOUNG CHILDREN

NUTRIENT	INTAKE PER DAY			
	0–6 mo (6 kg)	7–12 mo (9 kg)	1–3 y (13 kg)	4–8 y (22 kg)
Energy (kcal (kJ)/24 h)	ND	ND	ND	ND
Fat (g)	ND	ND	ND	ND
Carbohydrate	ND	ND	ND	ND
Protein (g/24 h)	ND	ND	ND	ND
Electrolytes and minerals				
Calcium (mg/24 h)	ND	ND	2,500	2,500
Phosphorus (g/24 h)	ND	ND	3	3
Magnesium (mg/24 h)	ND	ND	65	110
Sodium (mg/24 h)	ND	NA	65	83
Chloride (mg/24 h)	ND	ND		
Potassium (mg/24 h)	ND	ND	ND	ND
Iron (mg/24 h)	40	40	40	40
Zinc (mg/24 h)	4	5	7	12
Copper (μg/24 h)	ND	ND	1,000	3,000
Iodine (μg/24 h)	ND	ND	200	300
Selenium (μg/24 h)	45	60	90	150
Manganese (mg/24 h)	ND	ND	2	3
Fluoride (mg/24 h)	0.7	0.9	1.3	2.2
Chromium (μg/24 h)	ND	ND	ND	ND
Molybdenum (μg/24 h)	ND	ND	300	600
Vitamins				
Vitamin A (μg/24 h)	600	600	600	900
Vitamin D (μg/24 h)	25 (1,000 IU)		50 (2,000 IU)	50 (2,000 IU)
Vitamin E (mg α-TE/24 h)	ND	ND	200	300
Vitamin K (μg/24 h)	ND	ND	ND	ND
Vitamin C (mg/24 h)	ND	ND	400	650
Thiamin (mg/24 h)	ND	ND	ND	ND
Riboflavin (mg/24 h)	ND	ND	ND	ND
Niacin (mg/24 h)	ND	ND	10	15
Vitamin B_6 (μg/24 h)	ND	ND	30	40
Folate (μg)	ND	ND	300	400
Vitamin B_{12} (μg/24 h)	ND	ND	ND	ND
Biotin (μg/24 h)	ND	ND	ND	ND
Pantothenic acid (mg/24 h)	ND	ND	ND	ND
Choline (mg/24 h)	ND	ND	1	1
Water (L/24 h)	ND	ND	ND	ND

ND, data insufficient to establish a tolerable upper intake level for normal persons.

Data from references 1 to 6.

There is concern that infants may also require a preformed intake of at least some of the longer-chain, more unsaturated derivatives of linoleic and α-linolenic acids (e.g., arachidonic and docosahexaenoic acids). These fatty acids are present in human milk but, until recently, were not present in formulas. Further, the contents of these fatty acids in plasma and erythrocyte lipids are lower in infants fed unsupplemented formulas versus breast-fed infants (10, 11) or infants fed supplemented formulas. The brain content of docosahexaenoic, but not arachidonic acid also is lower in infants fed unsupplemented formula than in breast-fed infants (12, 13). However, the results of functional outcome studies of breast-fed versus formula-fed infants and infants fed formulas with and without arachidonic and docosahexaenoic acid are inconclusive (14–16). Overall, these studies provide little evidence that the absence of these fatty acids in term infant formulas is problematic, provided intakes of both linoleic and α-linolenic

acid are adequate (17). Moreover, no convincing evidence indicates that the amounts of long-chain polyunsaturated fatty acids in available supplemented formulas pose safety concerns, and a strong argument can be made for the likelihood that some infants may benefit from the supplemented fatty acids.

The requirements for carbohydrate and fat, including long-chain polyunsaturated fatty acids, amount to no more than 30 kcal (125.5 kJ)/kg/day, or only about a third of infant and young child's EER. Whether the remainder should be composed predominantly of carbohydrate, predominantly of fat, or of equicaloric amounts of each is not known. Human milk and most currently available formulas contain roughly equicaloric amounts of each. Because a higher percentage of energy as carbohydrate will increase osmolality and a higher percentage as fat may exceed the infant's ability to digest and absorb fat, roughly equicaloric amounts of each seem reasonable.

In concert with the recommendation that the dietary fat intake of the general population be reduced to improve cardiovascular health, it has been suggested that this guideline be applied to infants and young children. However, because fat is a major source of energy as well as the only source of essential fatty acids, concern exists that such diets could limit growth. Thus, groups responsible for making recommendations for infants and young children have not endorsed this recommendation for children less than 2 years of age (18). However, there is little reason not to reduce intake of cholesterol and saturated fat. The acceptable macronutrient distribution range of fat suggested for the 1- to 3-year-old child by the Panel on Macronutrients of the Food and Nutrition Board (5) is 30 to 40% of energy. The range suggested for the 4- to 8-year-old child is 25 to 35% of energy (5–10% of n-6 and 0.6 to 1.2% as n-3 fatty acids).

Until recently, few actual data were available concerning the growth of infants and young children receiving "low-fat" diets, but an ongoing study in Finland suggests that the fear of growth failure with such diets may be overrated (19). In this study of more than a thousand infants, half of whose parents received dietary counseling to limit saturated fat and cholesterol intakes and half of whom did not, growth of the two groups did not differ. Interestingly, although energy and fat intake of the intervention group was somewhat lower than that of the control group, the mean fat intake of both groups was close to 30% of total energy. The intervention group also had lower serum cholesterol concentrations at 3 years of age or on termination of the study.

Protein

The protein needs of the infant and young child per unit of body weight also is greater than those of the adult, a finding reflecting primarily the infant's and young child's additional needs for growth. The AI of protein established by the Food and Nutrition Board (5) for the 0- to 6-month-old infant, 9.3 g/day or approximately 1.5 g/kg/day (assuming a mean weight of 6 kg), is based on the observed mean protein intake of infants fed principally with human milk.

EARs for protein intake were established for the 7- to 12-month old infant as well as the 1- to 3-year-old and 4- to 8-year-old child (5). These values are based on maintenance protein needs plus the additional need for protein deposition as determined by measurements of body composition of normally growing infants and children, assuming an efficiency of deposition of dietary protein intake of 56%. The EAR for the 7- to 12-month-old infant is 0.98 g/kg/day. That for the 1- to 3-year-old child is 0.86 g/kg/day, and that for the 4- to 8-year-old child is 0.76 g/kg/day. Because the calculated coefficient of variation is approximately 12%, RDAs are 1.24 × EAR: 1.2 g/kg/day for the 7- to 12-month-old infant, 1.05 g/kg/day for the 1- to 3-year-old child, and 0.95 g/kg/day for the 4- to 8-year-old child.

TABLE 51.3. DIETARY REFERENCE INTAKES (mg/kg/d) OF ESSENTIAL AMINO ACIDS FOR INFANTS AND CHILDREN

AMINO ACID	0–6 mo[a]	7–12 mo[b]	1–3 y[b]	4–8 y[b]
Aromatic amino acids	120	61	46	38
Isoleucine	78	36	28	25
Leucine	139	71	56	47
Lycine	95	66	51	43
Sulfur amino acids	52	32	25	21
Threonine	65	36	27	22
Tryptophan	25	10	7	6
Valine	77	42	32	27

[a] Adequate intake.
[b] Recommended dietary allowance.

The required intake of protein is a function of its amino acid composition and digestibility. It also follows that the overall quality of a specific protein can be improved by supplementing it with the lacking (or limiting) indispensable amino acids. An example is soy protein, which, in the native state, has insufficient methionine but when fortified with methionine approaches or equals the overall quality of human milk protein (20).

AIs of the essential amino acids for the 0- to 6-month-old infant are set at the amounts of each in the amount of human milk protein equal to the AI of protein. For the 7- to 12-month-old infant, 1- to 3-year-old child, and 4- to 8-year-old child, EARs of the essential amino acids are based on the pattern of these amino acids in body protein and the EAR of protein. The AIs of the essential amino acids for the 0- to 6-month-old infant and the EARs of the older infant and young child are shown in Table 51.3.

Minerals

Calcium accounts for 1 to 2% of the weight of the adult, and approximately 99% of this is in teeth and bones. Accretion of calcium during infancy and early childhood ranges from 60 to 100 mg/day in children between 2 and 5 years of age to 100 to 160 mg/day between 6 and 8 years of age. Because the percentage of absorption is quite variable, an adequate intake obviously is important. The AIs of calcium set by the Food and Nutrition Board for the 0- to 6-month-old infant and the 7- to 12-month-old infant are based, respectively, on the amount of calcium in the average intake of principally breast-fed infants and the average intakes of calcium from human milk plus complementary foods (3), that is, 210 and 270 mg/day, respectively. Calcium absorption of formula-fed infants is less than that of breast-fed infants, but the calcium content of formulas is higher; thus, calcium retention of breast-fed and formula-fed infants differs minimally, if at all. The AI of calcium for the 4- to 8-year-old child, 800 mg/day, is based on balance studies showing that an intake of 800 to 900 mg/day results in a mean calcium accretion of 174 mg/day. There being no similar balance data for the 1- to 3-year-old child, the AI of this age group, 500 mg/day, is based on extrapolation from the AI of the 4- to 8-year-old child. Assuming 20% retention, this intake should result in accretion of approximately 100 mg/day.

The AI of phosphorus is 100 mg/day for the 0- to 6-month-old infant and 275 mg/day for the 7- to 12-month-old infant (3). These values are based on the average intake of the 0- to 6-month-old breast-fed infant and the combined intake of breast milk and complementary foods of the 7- to 12-month-old infant. EARs of phosphorus were established for the 1- to 3-year-old child and the 4- to 8-year-old child, based on factorial estimates; these are 380 and 405 mg/day, respectively. RDAs (EAR × 1.20) are 460 and 500 mg/day, respectively.

Trace Minerals and Vitamins

DRIs have been established for all trace minerals except arsenic, boron, nickel, silicon, and vanadium, as well as for all vitamins (2, 4). These values are summarized in Table 51.1 and in Appendix Tables A-2-e and A-2-g. Those of major importance are iron, zinc, and vitamin D.

Although the normal infant, in theory, has sufficient stores of iron at birth to meet requirements for 4 to 6 months, iron deficiency during infancy is quite common. This probably reflects the marked variability in both iron stores and iron absorption among infants. Despite the low iron content of human milk, the Food and Nutrition Board set the AI of iron for the 0- to 6-month-old infant at the intake of iron by the principally breast-fed infant (4), that is, 0.27 mg/day. Moreover, the iron content of human milk is much more bioavailable than that of formulas. For this reason, only iron-fortified formulas are recommended. The EARs of iron for the 7- to 12-month-old infant, the 1- to 3-year-old child, and the 4- to 8-year-old child are based on a factorial approach accounting for obligatory losses as well as increases in hemoglobin mass, tissue iron, and storage iron. Assuming 10% bioavailability for the 7- to 12-month-old infant and 18% for the 1- to 8-year old child, EARs were set at 6.9, 3, and 4.1 mg/day, respectively, for the 7- to 12-month-old infant, the 1- to 3-year-old child, and the 4- to 8-year-old child. RDAs are 11, 7, and 10 mg/day, respectively.

Zinc is a component of as many as 100 enzymes with quite diverse functions (e.g., RNA polymerases, alcohol dehydrogenase, carbonic anlydrase, alkaline phosphatases). It also is important for the structural integrity of proteins and in regulation of gene transcription. Because of its participation in such a wide range of vital metabolic processes, symptoms of deficiency, even mild deficiency, are quite diverse. A primary feature of deficiency is impaired growth velocity, which can occur with only modest degrees of restriction and circulating zinc concentrations that are indistinguishable from normal. Other features of deficiency include alopecia, diarrhea, delayed sexual maturation, eye and skin lesions, and impaired appetite. Because of these diverse features of deficiency

and the lack of reliable clinical or functional indicators of zinc status, adequate zinc intake is of primary importance.

As for other nutrients, the AI of zinc for the 0- to 6-month-old infants is based on the mean zinc intake of exclusively breast-fed infants (4). Because the zinc concentration of human milk falls from about 4 mg/L at 2 weeks postpartum to approximately 1.0 mg/L at 6 months postpartum, the AI, 2 mg/day, reflects an average intake of human milk of 0.78 L and a zinc concentration of 2.5 mg/L. EARs of zinc for the 7- to 12-month-old infant, the 1- to 3-year-old child, and the 4- to 8-year-old child are based on factorial analysis or extrapolation from the adult EAR, both of which are similar (2.5 mg/day for the 7- to 12-month-old infant and the 1- to 3-year-old child; 4 mg/day for the 4- to 8-year-old child). RDAs reflect a coefficient of variation or 10% (i.e., 1.2 × EAR).

The major function of vitamin D is to maintain serum calcium and phosphorus concentrations within the normal range by enhancing their absorption from the small intestine. Vitamin D is present in very few foods naturally; rather, it is synthesized from sterols in skin by the action of sunlight. With even limited sunlight exposure, neither the breast-fed infant nor the formula-fed infant requires vitamin D. However, some infants and children who live in northern latitudes or whose exposure to sunlight is otherwise limited (e.g., use of sun blocks or avoiding sunlight to prevent cancer; extensive clothing for religious or modesty reasons) require supplemental vitamin D. The AIs established by the Food and Nutrition Board, 200 IU/day for the 0- to 6-month old and 7- to 12-month-old infant as well as the 1- to 3-year-old and 4- to 8-year-old child, are based on the assumption that no vitamin D is obtained by exposure to sunlight (3). These intakes maintain normal serum 25-hydroxy vitamin D values and are not associated with evidence of vitamin D deficiency. Although available infant formulas provide as much as 400 IU/day, this amount is not thought to be excessive.

Water and Electrolytes

The AI of water for the normal infant is based on the average fluid intake of the predominantly breast-fed 0- to 6-month-old infant (~700 mL/day) and the average intake of human milk and complementary foods (including juices and other fluids) by the 7- to 12-month-old infant (~800 mL/day). However, because of higher obligate renal, pulmonary, and dermal water losses, as well as a higher overall metabolic rate, the infant is more susceptible to development of dehydration, particularly with vomiting and/or diarrhea. Thus, provision of 150 mL/kg/day is often recommended. Intakes of electrolytes by breast-fed and formula-fed infants as well as by children between 1 and 8 years of age fed conventional foods appear to approximate the DRIs of each (see Table 51.1).

FEEDING THE INFANT

The DRIs are for individual nutrients. However, these nutrients are not provided individually but, rather, as components of the diet. For the infant, who experiences considerable growth as well as developmental advances, providing the foods necessary to meet specific needs for all nutrients can sometimes be challenging. Some of the most important issues in meeting this challenge are discussed in the sections that follow.

Breast-Feeding

Human milk is uniquely adapted to the human infant's needs and, hence, breast-feeding is the preferred form of feeding the infant. Human milk contains bacterial and viral antibodies that are thought to provide local gastrointestinal immunity against organisms entering the body via this route. These antibodies probably account, at least partially, for the lower prevalence of diarrhea as well as otitis media, pneumonia, bacteremia, and meningitis during the first year of life in infants who are exclusively breast-fed versus formula-fed for the first 4 to 6 months of life (7, 8). Some evidence also indicates that breast-fed infants may have a lower frequency of food allergies as well as a lower incidence of chronic diseases in later life.

The psychologic advantages of breast-feeding for both mother and infant are well recognized. The mother is personally involved in the nurturing of her baby, and this results both in a feeling of being essential and a sense of accomplishment while the infant is provided with a close and comfortable physical relationship with the mother.

The first 2 weeks after birth are crucial for establishing successful breast-feeding. Daily weight gains of the infant, although important for ascertaining the volume of milk produced, should not be overly emphasized during this time. Further, supplemental bottle feedings to achieve weight gain may compromise attempts at breast-feeding and, therefore, should be limited.

Except in the case of mothers who are seropositive for human immunodeficiency virus, in whom breast-feeding increases the risk of transmitting the virus to the infant, there are no adverse consequences of breast-feeding the healthy term infant. Allergens to which the infant is sensitized can be conveyed in the milk, but the presence of such allergens is rarely a valid reason to stop breast-feeding. Rather, an attempt should be made to identify the offending allergen and remove it from the mother's diet.

Maternal contraindications to breast-feeding also are few. Markedly inverted nipples may be troublesome, as may fissuring or cracking of the nipples, but the latter can usually be avoided by preventing engorgement. Mastitis also may be alleviated by continued and frequent nursing on the affected breast to keep it from becoming engorged, but local heat applications and antibiotics may occasionally be necessary. Acute maternal infection may be a contraindication to breast-feeding if the infant does not have the same infection; otherwise, there is no need to stop nursing unless the condition of either the mother or the infant necessitates it. If the mother's condition does not permit breast-feeding, the breast may be emptied and the milk given to the infant by bottle or cup. Mothers with septicemia, active infections, or breast cancer should not breast-feed. Substance abuse and severe neuroses or psychoses may also be contraindications to breast-feeding.

Formula Feeding

Objective studies of growing infants less than 4 to 6 months of age show minimal, if any, differences in rate of growth, blood constituents, metabolic performance, or body composition between breast-fed infants and infants fed modern iron-supplemented formulas. Thereafter, growth of the formula-fed infant usually is somewhat more rapid than that of the breast-fed infant. Such investigations attest to the ability of both breast milk and modern infant formulas to support normal growth and development of the infant. Thus, the mother who is unable or does not wish to nurse her infant need not have a lesser sense of accomplishment or affection for her baby than the nursing mother. Moreover, the quality of attachment and mothering and the degree of security and affection provided the infant need not be different with formula-feeding versus breast-feeding. Further, the clear economic advantages and microbiologic safety of breast-feeding are of lesser importance for affluent, developed societies with ready access to a clean water supply and refrigeration than for less developed and less affluent societies. Thus, a reasonable and conservative approach is to allow the mother to make an informed choice of how she wishes to feed her infant and support her in that decision. As stated by Fomon and associates (21): "In industrialized countries, any woman with the least inclination toward breast-feeding should be encouraged to do so, and all assistance possible should be provided. At the same time, there is little justification for attempts to coerce women to breast-feed. No woman in an industrialized country should be made to feel guilty because she elects not to breast-feed her infant."

The nutrient content of infant formulas marketed in the United States is regulated by the Infant Formula Act and is enforced by the Food and Drug Administration. Most industrialized and many developing countries have similar regulations. All formulas must contain minimum amounts of all nutrients known or thought to be required by infants, and increasing emphasis is being placed on avoiding specified maximum amounts of each. The most recent recommendations for the minimum and maximum nutrient contents of term infant formulas marketed in the United States are shown in Table 51.4 (22). The minimum recommended amount of each nutrient is greater than the amount of that nutrient in human milk and, hence, greater than the DRI of that nutrient for infants less than 1 year of age (see Table 51.1).

TABLE 51.4. LIFE SCIENCES RESEARCH OFFICE RECOMMENDATIONS FOR TERM INFANT FORMULAS[a]

	MINIMUM	MAXIMUM
Energy (kcal/dL)	63	71
Fat (g)	4.4	6.4
Linoleic acid (%)	8	35
α-Linolenic acid (%)	1.75	4
Ratio linoleic acid: α-linolenic acid	16:1	6:1
Carbohydrate (g)	9	13
Protein (g)	1.7	3.4
Electrolytes and minerals		
Calcium (mg)	50	140
Phosphorus (mg)	20	70
Magnesium (mg)	4	17
Sodium (mg)	25	50
Chloride (mg)	50	160
Potassium (mg)	60	160
Iron (mg)	0.2	1.65
Zinc (mg)	0.4	1.0
Copper (μg)	60	160
Iodine (μg)	8	35
Selenium (μg)	1.5	5
Manganese (μg)	1.0	100
Fluoride (μg)	0	60
Chromium	0	0
Molybdenum	0	0
Vitamins		
Vitamin A (IU)	200	500
Vitamin D (IU)	40	100
Vitamin E (mg α-tocopherol)	0.5	5.0
Vitamin K (μg)	1	25
Vitamin C (mg)	6	15
Thiamin (μg)	30	200
Riboflavin (μg)	80	300
Niacin (μg)	550	2,000
Vitamin B_6 (μg)	30	130
Folate (μg)	11	40
Vitamin B_{12} (μg)	0.08	0.7
Biotin (μg)	1	15
Pantothenic acid (μg)	300	1,200
Other ingredients		
Carnitine (mg)	1.2	2.0
Taurine (mg)	0	12
Inositol (mg)	4	40
Choline (mg)	7	30
Bycleotides (mg)	0	16

[a] Amounts/100 kcal, unless indicated otherwise.

Adapted from Raiten DJ et al (22).

Numerous formulas are available for feeding the normal infant. The composition of the most commonly used formulas is shown in Table 51.5. Most are available in ready-to-use, concentrated liquid, and powdered forms. Powdered formulas are somewhat lower in cost and are used with increasing frequency.

The most commonly used formulas contain various mixtures of bovine milk proteins. The protein concentration of all formulas is about 1.5 g/dL. Thus, the infant who receives a sufficient volume to provide the EER, approximately 90 or approximately 135 mL/kg/day, receives a protein intake of about 2.0 g/kg/day. This is about 50% more

than the intake of the breast-fed infant and, hence, the recent AI of protein for the 0- to 6-month-old infant; it is about 70% more than the RDA of protein for the 7- to 12-month-old infant.

Unmodified bovine milk protein has a whey-to-casein ratio of 18:82, whereas modified bovine milk protein can have a variety of ratios; historically, the most common has been 60:40. Both modified and unmodified bovine milk proteins appear to be equally efficacious for the normal term infant, but the lower curd tension of the whey-predominant proteins is thought to be preferable. Formulas containing soy protein as well as formulas containing partially hydrolyzed bovine milk proteins are available for feeding infants who are intolerant of bovine milk or soy protein (Table 51.6).

Although lactose-free bovine milk formulas are available, the major carbohydrate of the most commonly used formulas is lactose. The most commonly used soy protein formulas contain either sucrose or a glucose polymer. Thus, these formulas or lactose-free bovine milk protein formulas are useful for the infant with either transient or congenital lactase deficiency.

The fat content of both bovine milk and soy protein formula usually comprises about 50% of the nonprotein energy. In general, intestinal absorption of the blend of vegetable oils present in current formulas is at least 90%. Formulas supplemented with the long-chain polyunsaturated fatty acids, docosahexaenoic acid and arachidonic acid, have become available.

The electrolyte, mineral, and vitamin contents of most formulas are similar and, when fed in adequate amounts, provide the DRIs for minerals and vitamins. Both iron-supplemented (~12 mg/L) and nonsupplemented (~1 mg/L) formulas are available, but iron-supplemented formulas are recommended.

FEEDING THE OLDER INFANT

The goal of both breast-feeding and formula-feeding is to deliver enough nutrients to support adequate growth. Exclusive breast-feeding is thought to do so for the first 6, certainly the first 4, months of life, whereas exclusive formula-feeding can do so for at least the first year of life. As a rule of thumb, the normal term infant's weight should double by 4 to 5 months of age and triple by 12 months of age.

By 6 months of age, the infant's capacity to digest and absorb a variety of dietary components as well as to metabolize, use, and excrete the absorbed products of digestion is near the capacity of the adult (23). Moreover, the infant is more active, has good head control, and is beginning to sit alone and to explore his or her surroundings. Hence, during this interval, diet plays a variety of roles other than delivery of nutrients. With the eruption of teeth, the role of diet in development of dental caries must be considered (24). The long-term effects of inadequate or excessive intakes during infancy also must be considered, as must

TABLE 51.5. NUTRIENT CONTENT OF COMMON FORMULAS[a]

COMPONENT	SIMILAC[b]	ENFAMIL[c]	GOOD START[d]
Energy (kcal/L)	676	680	676
Protein (g)	2.07 (52% casein, 48% whey)	2.1 (40% casein; 60% whey)	2.4 (100% whey)
Fat (g)	5.4 (high-oleic safflower, coconut, and soy oils)	5.3 (palm olein, soy, coconut, and high-oleic sunflower oils)	5.1 (palmolein, soy, coconut, and high-oleic safflower oils)
Carbohydrate (g)	10.8 (lactose)	10.7 (lactose)	11.0 (lactose, corn maltodextrin)
Electrolytes and minerals			
Calcium (mg)	78	78	64
Phosphorus (mg)	42	53	36
Magnesium (mg)	6.1	8	7.1
Iron (mg)	1.8	1.8	1.5
Zinc (mg)	0.75	1	0.8
Manganese (μg)	5	15	7.1
Copper (μg)	90	75	80.5
Iodine (μg)	6.1	10	12
Selenium (μg)	—	—	—
Sodium (mg)	24	27	24
Potassium (mg)	105	107	101
Chloride (mg)	65	63	65.5
Vitamins			
Vitamin A (IU)[d]	300	2,094	302
Vitamin D (IU)	60	60	60
Vitamin E (IU)	1.5	2	2
Vitamin K (μg)	8	8	8.0
Thiamin (μg)	100	80	60
Riboflavin (μg)	150	140	141
Vitamin B$_6$ (μg)	60	60	75
Vitamin B$_{12}$ (μg)	0.25	0.3	0.25
Niacin (μg)	1,050	1,000	750
Folic acid (μg)	15	16	15
Pantothenic acid (μg)	450	500	453
Biotin (μg)	4.4	3	2.2
Vitamin C (mg)	9	12	9
Choline (mg)	16	12	12
Inositol (mg)	4.7	6	18

[a] Amount/100 kcal unless noted otherwise.
[b] Ross Laboratories, Columbus, OH.
[c] Mead-Johnson Nutritionals, Evansville, IN.
[d] Carnation Nutritional Products, Glendale, CA.

the psychosocial role of foods during development and the impact of feeding practices during this period on subsequent feeding behavior.

These considerations are the basis for most of the recommendations for feeding during the second 6 months of life, particularly for the formula-fed infant, whose nutrient needs during this period can be met with reasonable amounts of currently available infant formulas. The exclusively breast-fed infant, however, requires additional nutrients (e.g., iron) after 4 to 6 months of age.

Infant Formula versus Bovine Milk

Although current recommendations are to avoid intake of bovine milk, particularly low-fat or skim milk, before at least a year of age, a recent survey shows that many infants older than 6 months of age and even some younger infants are fed homogenized bovine milk rather than infant formula (25). The consequences of these practices are not known with certainty. Bovine milk contains roughly three

times as much protein and about twice as much sodium as the most commonly used infant formulas, but less than half as much linoleic acid. Ingestion of bovine milk also increases intestinal blood loss and thus may contribute to the development of iron deficiency anemia (26). The protein and sodium intakes of infants fed skim rather than whole bovine milk are even higher, the iron intake is equally low, and the intake of linoleic acid is very low.

Whether the high protein and sodium intakes of infants fed either whole or skim milk result in adverse health effects is not known at the present time. The low iron intake is clearly undesirable but can be compensated for by supplementation. The low intake of linoleic acid may be more problematic. Although signs and symptoms of essential fatty acid deficiency appear to be uncommon in infants fed either whole or skim milk, I am not aware of systematic research on this possibility. Moreover, biochemical evidence of essential fatty acid deficiency without overt signs and symptoms has been reported in both younger and older infants fed formulas with a low content

TABLE 51.6. NUTRIENT CONTENT (AMOUNT/100 kcal) OF SOY FORMULAS AND HYDROLYZED FORMULAS

COMPONENT	ISOMIL[a,b]	PROSOBEE[c]	NUTRAMIGEN[c]	ALIMENTUM[a]
Energy (kcal/L)	676	680	680	676
Protein (g)	2.45 (soy protein isolate; L-methionine)	2.5 (soy protein isolate; L-methionine)	2.8 (casein hydrolysate)	2.75 (casein hydrolysate)
Fat (g)	5.3 (soy high-oleic safflower; coconut oils)	5.3 (palm-olein; soy; coconut and high-oleic sunflower oils)	5.0 (corn oil)	5.5 (67% LCT; 33% MCT)
Carbohydrate (g)	10.3 (corn syrup; sucrose)	10.6 (corn syrup solids)	11 (corn syrup solids; modified cornstarch)	10.2
Electrolytes and Minerals				
Calcium (mg)	105	104	94	105
Phosphorus (mg)	75	82	63	75
Magnesium (mg)	7.5	11	11	7.5
Iron (mg)	1.8	1.8	1.8	1.8
Zinc (mg)	0.75	1.2	1	0.75
Manganese (μg)	25	25	25	8
Copper (μg)	75	75	75	75
Iodine (μg)	15	15	15	15
Selenium (μg)	—	—	—	—
Sodium (mg)	44	35	47	44
Potassium (mg)	108	120	108	120
Chloride	62	80	85	80
Vitamins				
Vitamin A (IU)	300	294	294	300
Vitamin D (IU)	60	60	50	45
Vitamin E (IU)	1.5	2	2	3
Vitamin K (μg)	11	8	8	15
Thiamin (μg)	60	80	80	60
Riboflavin (μg)	90	90	90	90
Vitamin B_6 (μg)	60	60	60	60
Vitamin B_{12} (μg)	0.45	0.3	0.3	0.45
Niacin (μg)	1,350	1,000	1,000	1,350
Folic acid (μg)	15	16	16	15
Pantothenic acid (μg)	754	500	500	754
Biotin (μg)	4.5	3	3	4.5
Vitamin C (mg)	9	12	12	9
Choline (mg)	8	8	12	8
Inositol (mg)	5	6	17	5

LCT, long-chain triglyceride; MCT, medium-chain triglyceride.
[a] Ross Laboratories, Columbus, OH.
[b] Isomil-SF (sucrose free) has similar composition with exception that glucose polymers are substituted for corn syrup and sucrose.
[c] Mead Johnson Nutritionals, Evansville, IN.

of linoleic acid (27). In contrast, infants who are breast-fed or fed formulas with a high linoleic acid content earlier in life may have sufficient body stores to limit the consequences of a low intake later.

Resolving the issues concerning the use of bovine milk in feeding the infant is important for economic as well as health reasons. Because the cost of bovine milk is considerably less than that of infant formula, replacing formula with homogenized bovine milk before a year of age obviously has important economic advantages for most families. In addition, if the various food assistance programs could provide homogenized bovine milk rather than formula to infants, even infants older than 6 months of age, the programs' current funds would permit expansion of benefits to many more needy infants. Clearly, this cannot be considered without further data concerning the consequences of feeding bovine milk.

Complementary Feeding

Complementary foods (i.e., the additional foods, including formulas or bovine milk, given to the breast-fed infant) or replacement foods (i.e., food other than formula given to formula-fed infants) should be introduced in a stepwise fashion to both breast-fed and formula-fed infants, beginning about the time the infant is able to sit unassisted, usually between 4 and 6 months of age (28). Iron-supplemented cereals are usually the first such foods given. Vegetables and fruits are introduced next followed, shortly, by meats and, finally, eggs. Historically, the order in which foods are introduced has received considerable attention. However, this is no longer considered crucial, and many now recommend introducing meats, a good source of iron and zinc, as one of the first complementary foods. It is important that only one new food be introduced at a time and that additional new foods be spaced by at least 3 days both to allow detection of any adverse reactions to each newly introduced food and to allow the infant to become familiar with the taste and texture of the new food. New foods may be introduced even more slowly if there is a family history of food or other allergies.

Either home-prepared or manufactured complementary or replacement foods can be used. Many commercial products are fortified with one or more nutrient (e.g., iron, zinc, some vitamins) and are available in different consistencies to match the infant's ability to tolerate larger size particles as he or she matures.

Prepared dinners and soups containing a meat and one or more vegetables are quite popular. However, the protein content of these products is not as high as that of strained meat. Puddings and desserts also are popular items, but, aside from their milk and egg content, they are poor sources of nutrients other than energy; thus, intakes of these should be limited. Moreover, intake of egg-containing products generally should be delayed, especially if there is a family history of food or other allergies, until after the infant has demonstrated tolerance of eggs (either a mashed hard boiled egg yolk or a commercial egg yolk preparation).

Historically, juices have been considered a necessary item in the infant's diet. However, aside from their vitamin content, they provide minimal nutrients other than energy that may interfere with adequate intakes of other nutrients. Considering this, current recommendations are to limit juice intake to 4 oz (120 mL)/day. Sweetened flavored drinks, of course, should be avoided (29).

Although feeding practices vary widely during the latter half of the first year of life, most recent surveys indicate that infants fed according to current practices receive adequate intakes of most nutrients (30).

FEEDING THE TODDLER

By the end of the first year of life, most infants have adapted to a schedule of three meals a day plus about two snacks. Although considerable latitude in the diet of each infant should be permitted to allow for personal idiosyncrasies and family habits, parents should be given an outline of the basic daily dietary needs. Equally important, they should be aware of what to expect in terms of eating behavior as the child matures.

Reduced Food Intake

Toward the end of the first year of life, the rate of growth decreases, and the child's intake, accordingly, also decreases or fails to increase as rapidly as it did during the first year of life. Further, it is not unusual for the child to have temporary periods of not being interested in certain foods or, indeed, in any food. Failure to expect and recognize these changes in eating behavior often results in attempts to force feed. The child naturally rebels, and feeding problems ensue. Because preventing problems is more effective than correcting them, the changing pattern

of food habits during the second year of life should be explained to parents before it is apparent, and parents should be reassured that the child's lack of interest in food is probably temporary and that attempts to force feed not only are futile but also are likely to result in more severe feeding problems.

Self-Selection of Diet

Children's strong likes or dislikes of particular foods become apparent after about a year of age and, if possible and practicable, should be respected. For example, the virtues of some nonessential foods (e.g., spinach) probably have been overemphasized, and conflicts about such foods certainly should not be allowed to occur. Often, a food that is refused when it is first offered will be accepted when it is offered again a few days or weeks later. It may be necessary to offer other foods repeatedly before they are accepted. Conversely, if basic staples such as milk and cereal are consistently rejected, alternative forms of these basic staples (e.g., cheese, yogurt, breads) should be offered.

Children tend to select diets that, over several days, are well balanced (30). Thus, the child may be permitted a wide choice of foods, as long as he or she eats adequately over the longer period. Normally, the child determines the quantity of a given food or an entire meal that will be eaten. At this age, eating habits, particularly food likes and dislikes, also may be influenced by older children in the family. Thus, because eating patterns and habits developed in the first 2 years of life may persist for several years, such influences should be monitored closely.

Self-Feeding

Infants should be permitted to participate in feeding themselves as soon as they seem physically able to do so, usually long before a year of age. By approximately 6 months of age, most can hold a bottle and, within another 2 to 3 months, a cup. Zwieback, graham crackers, or other hand-held foods can be introduced by the age of 7 to 8 months. Between 10 and 12 months of age, most infants can hold a spoon and direct it to the mouth. Mothers often inhibit this important learning process because it is messy, but it also is an important aspect of the infant's overall development and should be encouraged, certainly tolerated. By the end of the second year of life, infants should be largely responsible for feeding themselves. However, because the risk of aspiration is reasonably high until approximately 4 years of age, children younger than this should not be given foods that are easily aspirated (e.g., grapes, nuts, chunks of cheese and meat) unless a responsible adult is present.

Eating Habits

Because eating habits formed in the first and second years of life may affect those of subsequent years, it is important that these habits be as "optimal" as possible. Feeding difficulties frequently result from excessive parental insistence on eating and subsequent anxiety of the parents as well as the child if this insistence is not heeded. The child's negative reactions often result from undue mealtime stress, the correction of which requires improvement in parent-child relations. Other factors that disturb eating are too much confusion at mealtime, insufficient time for eating, voiced food dislikes by other members of the family, and poorly prepared, unattractively served food. A comfortable chair of proper height with a footrest is important for the smaller child's ease at the table.

The child's appetite should be respected; if his or her desire for food is below average at times, there should be no pressure to eat more. Adults should understand that eating habits are taught better by example than by formal explanation.

FEEDING DURING LATER CHILDHOOD

By 2 years of age, a child's diet should not differ from that of the rest of the family. All known required nutrients can be supplied by a varied diet selected according to current food guidelines (see later). Recent recommendations from the Institute of Medicine and from the Dietary Guidelines for Americans Committee recommend that the fat content of children's diet should move progressively from the high-fat content of human milk (~50%) to the 20 to 35% range recommended for adults. Because humans do not require saturated fat, this should be kept to the minimum compatible with a balanced diet, which is usually between 6 and 10% of calories. Similarly, cholesterol should be no more than 100 mg/1000 kcal, with polyunsaturated fatty acids supplying 7 to 8% of energy and monounsaturated fatty acids between 12 and 13% (32). In the absence of well-documented individual or family risk factors, systematic fat or cholesterol restrictions are not recommended at this age. Some studies have shown, however, that as long as total energy intake and essential nutrient intake remain adequate, these restricted diets may support normal growth, even in young children (19).

The Dietary Guidelines for Americans is revised every 5 years and constitutes the basis from which the Food Guide Pyramid is developed as an educational tool (Table 51.7). The aim of the guidelines is to ensure that the population reaches the RDA for all nutrients, according to the Institute of Medicine's DRI recommendations. The guidelines are the basis from which the Food Guide Pyramid is developed as an educational tool. The pyramid will be revised in 2005, following the issue of the 2005 Dietary Guidelines. In the current pyramid, the numbers of servings from each food group needed for well-balanced 1600, 2200, and 2800 kcal/day diets are shown in Table 51.8. The 1600 kcal/day diet is appropriate for the moderately active 4- to 6-year-old child. For the 2- to 4-year-old child, serving sizes of all food groups except milk should be reduced by about one third.

TABLE 51.7. FOOD GUIDELINES

FOOD GROUP	SERVINGS/DAY	SERVING SIZE
Grain	6–11	1 slice bread ½ cup rice (cooked) ½ cup pasta
Fruit	2–4	¼ medium melon 1 whole fruit ¾ cup juice ½ cup canned fruit ½ cup berries, grapes
Vegetables	3–5	½ cup raw or cooked 1 cup leafy
Milk	2–3	1 cup milk, yogurt 2 oz cheese
Meat	2–3	2–3 oz lean, cooked ½ cup dried beans[a] 1 egg[a]
Fats/Sweets	Limit	

[a]These amounts are equal to 1 oz lean meat; 2 servings are equal to 1 meat serving.

The 2200 kcal/day diet is appropriate for most modestly active 6- to 10-year-old children. Active teenage boys may require 2800 kcal/day or even more, the same as suggested for active adults. The higher energy intakes are achieved primarily by more servings of the various food groups.

Although these guidelines are useful and can be used to design appropriate diets for all children older than 2 years of age, the variation in energy needs among children of the same age is considerable. The level of activity is a major determinant of the amount of energy needed (see earlier). Another is the variability in energy expenditure among seemingly similar groups of children, which can vary by as much as 15 to 20%. Thus, even those children whose diets are based on the food guidelines must be followed closely to ensure that growth is adequate but not excessive.

As children become older and more independent, increasing numbers of meals are eaten away from home, often at establishments where adherence to the food guidelines is difficult, if not impossible. An obvious solution is to limit such occasions. However, this approach is likely to be resisted by the child. Moreover, with the increasing number of mothers in the work force, many family meals are either

TABLE 51.8. SERVINGS OF VARIOUS FOOD GROUPS NEEDED TO PROVIDE DIFFERING DAILY ENERGY INTAKES

Food Group	SERVINGS NEEDED FOR DAILY ENERGY INTAKES		
	1,600 kcal	2,200 kcal	2,800 kcal
Bread	6	9	11
Fruits	2	3	4
Vegetables	3	4	5
Meat	5 oz	6 oz	7 oz
Milk	2–3	2–3	2–3
Total Fat (g)	53	73	83
Added Sugar (tsp)	6	12	18

eaten at the same type of establishment or purchased there for consumption at home.

NUTRIENT NEEDS OF THE LOW-BIRTH-WEIGHT INFANT

Approximately 7% of all infants born in the United States each year weigh less than 2500 g at birth, and, over the past few decades, their survival has improved steadily. Today, at least 75% of even the smallest such infants (i.e., those weighing less than 1000 g at birth) survive, and survival of larger LBW infants approaches 100% (34). These increasing numbers of surviving LBW infants must be fed, thus heightening awareness of the problems encountered in meeting their nutritional needs.

The practical importance of adequate early nutritional management of the LBW infant can be illustrated by considering the energy metabolism of the fasted infant (35). As in the adult, energy to meet ongoing needs during fasting is derived from endogenous stores of various nutrients. Although hepatic glycogen stores are used initially, these are quite limited and, hence, are soon depleted. Fat stores then become the major source of endogenous energy, although protein stores also are used to provide amino acids from which glucose can be synthesized (i.e., gluconeogenesis) for use by tissues having an absolute requirement for glucose. Therefore, if hydration is adequate, the available endogenous stores of fat and protein are the ultimate determinants of the length of time a fasting infant can survive.

As illustrated in Table 51.9, the body content of both protein and fat, particularly fat, increases throughout gestation (36). Thus, an infant weighing 3500 g at birth has more extensive endogenous nutrient reserves than one weighing 2000 g, and an infant weighing 1000 g has very limited reserves. Assuming on-going energy needs of 50 kcal/kg/day, the 1000-g infant who receives no exogenous nutrient intake has sufficient endogenous reserves to survive for only 4 to 5 days, the 2000-g infant has sufficient reserves to survive for approximately 12 days, and the term infant has sufficient reserves to survive for approximately

a month (35). Provision of glucose intravenously (e.g., 7.5 g/kg/day, the amount provided by 150 mL/kg/day of a 5% glucose solution or 75 mL/kg/day of a 10% glucose solution), theoretically, will prolong survival of the 1000-, 2000-, and 3500-g infant, respectively, by 7, 18, and 50 days (35).

These theoretic calculations agree generally with clinical observations concerning the LBW infant's susceptibility to starvation and, hence, the necessity for careful attention to early nutritional management. In addition to this very practical role of nutrition in preventing starvation, suboptimal nutrition at any time during the period of cellular proliferation of various organ systems, particularly the central nervous system, may result in nonrecoupable cellular deficits (37). If so, the prematurely born infant, whose brain would have grown considerably during the last trimester of intrauterine life, may be particularly vulnerable to inadequate nutrition. Although the period of cellular proliferation of the entire human brain encompasses at least the first 18 months of life (38) and cellular deficits apparently can be reversed if adequate nutrition is provided before the end of this period (39), little is known concerning the duration of cellular proliferation within specific regions of the brain. This uncertainty, coupled with the persistently high incidence of neurodevelopmental deficits in surviving LBW infants (40, 41), suggests that better nutritional management may not only decrease mortality but also improve neurodevelopmental outcome.

Goals of Nutritional Management

The most generally accepted goal for nutritional management of the LBW infant is to provide sufficient amounts of all nutrients to support, at a minimum, continuation of intrauterine rates of growth and nutrient retention (42). Thus, the LBW infant's minimal requirements for various nutrients are usually assumed to be the amounts necessary to allow their accumulation at intrauterine rates (see Table 51.9). This concept figures prominently in the recommended nutrient intakes for LBW infants (42–45) proposed by a variety of groups (Table 51.10), as well as the recommended

TABLE 51.9. INTRAUTERINE ACCRETION RATES OF VARIOUS NUTRIENTS DURING THE LAST TRIMESTER OF PREGNANCY

	ACCUMULATION DURING VARIOUS STAGES OF GESTATION[a]		
Component	26–30 wk	30–34 wk	34–38 wk
Weight (g)	600	750	930
Protein (g)	68	97	126
Fat (g)	60	95	145
Water (g)	459	539	627
Calcium (g)	3.4	5.12	8.7
Phosphorus (g)	2.2	3.3	5.4
Magnesium (mg)	93	131	193
Sodium (mEq)	46	53	64
Potassium (mEq)	25	31	39
Chloride (mEq)	35	37	37

[a] Body weight increases from 880 g at 26 wk to 1480 g at 30 wk, 2230 g at 34 wk, and 3160 g at 38 wk.

Adapted from Ziegler EE, O'Donnell AM, Nelson SE et al. Growth 1976;40:329–40, with permission.

TABLE 51.10. COMPARISON OF RECOMMENDATIONS FOR NUTRIENT INTAKES OF LOW-BIRTH-WEIGHT INFANTS

	AMERICAN ACADEMY OF PEDIATRICS COMMITTEE ON NUTRITION (1985)	ESPGAN COMMITTEE ON NUTRITION (1987)	CONSENSUS GROUP (1993)	HEALTH CANADA (1995)
Water (mL/kg/d)	150	138–185	150–200	120–200
Energy (kcal/kg/d)	120	130 (110–165)	120	105–135
Protein (g/kg/d)	3.5–4.0	2.7–3.7	3.6–3.8 (BW, <1,000 g)	3.5–4.0 (BW, <1000 g)
			3.0–3.6 (BW, >1,000 g)	3.0–3.6 (BW, >1000 g)
Carbohydrate (g/kg/d)	10.8–15.6	8.4–16.8	Lactose 3.8–11.8	7.5–15.5
			Oligomers 0–8.4	
Fat (g/kg/d)	5.4–7.2	4.3–8.5		4.5–6.8
	LA, 0.48	LA, 0.6–1.7	LA, 0.5–2	LA, 4.5%E
		ALA, > 0.06	ALA, 0.13–0.5	ALA, 1%E
		LA/ALA, 5–15	LA/ALA, 5–15	—
Sodium (mEq/kg/d)	2.5–3.5	1.2–2.8	2.0–3.0	2.5–4.0
Chloride (mEq/kg/d)	—	1.9–3.0	2.0–3.0	2.5–4.0
Potassium (mEq/kg/d)	2.0–3.0	2.8–4.7	2.0–3.0	2.5–3.5
Calcium (mg/kg/d)	200–250	84–168	120–230	160–240
Phosphorus (mg/kg/d)	110–125	60–104	60–140	108.5–118
Magnesium (mg/kg/d)	—	7.2–14.4	8–15	4.8–9.6
Zinc (μg/kg/d)	>600	660–1,320	1,000	508–812
Manganese (μg/kg/d)	>6	1.8–9.0	7.6	0.54–1.1
Copper (μg/kg/d)	108	108–144	120–150	69–120
Iron (mg/kg/d)	2–3	1.8	2.0	2–4
Iodine (μg/kg/d)	6	12–54	30–60	31–62
Selenium (μg/kg/d)	—	—	1.3–3.0	3.2–4.9
Chromium (μg/kg/d)	—	—	0.1–0.5	0.05–0.1
Molybdenum (μg/kg/d)	—	—	0.3	0.2–0.4
Vitamin A (IU/100 kcal)	75–225	270–450	583–1,250	167–375
Vitamin K (μg/100 kcal)	4	4–15	6.7–8.3	—
Thiamin (μg/100 kcal)	> 40	20–250	150–200	33–42
Riboflavin (μg/100 kcal)	>60	60–600	200–300	300–383
Niacin (μg/100 kcal)	>250	800–5,000	3,000–4,000	8.6 NE/5,000 kJ
Pyridoxine (μg/100 kcal)	>35	35–250	125–175	15 μg/g protein
Pantothenic acid (μg/100 kcal)	>300	>300	1,000–1,500	667–1,083
Vitamin B_{12} (μg/100 kcal)	>0.15	>0.15	0.25	0.15 μg/d
Biotin (μg/100 kcal)	>1.5	>1.5	3–5	1.25
Folic acid (μg/100 kcal)	33	>60	21–42	50 μg/d
Vitamin C (mg/kg/d)	35	7–40	15–20	6–10
Vitamin D (IU/d)	400	800–1,600	400	400
Vitamin E (IU/d)	>1.1	0.6–10	5–10	0.5–0.9 mg/kg
Taurine (mg/kg/d)	—	—	4.5–9.0	—
Inositol (mg/kg/d)	—	—	32.4–81	—
Carnitine (mg/kg/d)	—	—	2.9	—
Choline (mg/kg/d)	—	—	14.4–28.1	—

ALA, α-linolenic acid; BW, body weight; ESPGAN, European Society for Pediatric Gastroenterology and Nutrition; LA, linoleic acid; NE, niacin equivalents.

composition of formulas (46) designed for feeding the hospitalized LBW infant (Table 51.11).

Opposing views concerning the goals for nutritional management of LBW infants include, on the one hand, concern that failure to provide human milk will deprive the infant of factors needed for optimal development of the gastrointestinal tract and immune system and, on the other, the desire to produce the most rapid growth rate possible, thereby permitting the roughly 10 to 15% of body weight usually lost over the first several days of life to be recouped more rapidly and also possibly reducing the duration and, hence, the cost of hospitalization. Proponents of the former view advocate feeding human milk because of its demonstrated and theoretic nonnutritional benefits, such as enhanced maternal-infant bonding, protection against infection and necrotizing enterocolitis, and better neurodevelopmental outcome. They also point out that the lower protein content of human milk is less likely to overwhelm the LBW infant's limited capacity to catabolize excess protein. Proponents of the latter view stress the potential advantages of catch-up growth and point out that protein intakes well in excess of those from human milk do not appear to tax the LBW infant's ability to catabolize protein.

Ongoing findings of a multicenter study begun in the early 1980s in England (47) provide some insight into this

TABLE 51.11. LIFE SCIENCES RESEARCH OFFICE RECOMMENDATIONS FOR LOW-BIRTH-WEIGHT INFANTS[a,b]

NUTRIENT (UNITS)	MINIMUM	MAXIMUM
Energy (kcal 100 mL)	67	94
Protein (g/100 kcal)	2.5	3.6
Total fat (g/100 kcal)	4.4	5.7
Linoleic acid (% of total fatty acids)	8	25
α-Linolenic acid (% of total fatty acids)	1.75	4.0
Linoleic acid: α-linolenic acid	6:1	16:1
Total carbohydrate (g/100 kcal)	9.6	12.5
Lactose (g/100 kcal)	4	12.5
Oligosaccharides (g/100 kcal)	c	c
Medium-chain triglycerides (% of total fatty acids)	c	50
Docosahexaenoic acid (% of total fatty acids)	c	0.35
Arachidonic acid (% of total fatty acids)	c	0.6
Arachidonic acid: docosahexaenoic acid	1.5:1	2:1
Eicosapentaenoic acid (% of docosahexaenoic acid)	c	30
Myristic acid (% of total fatty acids)	c	12
Lauric acid (% of total fatty acids)	c	12
Minerals		
Calcium (mg/100 kcal)	123	185
Calcium:Phosphorus	1.7:1	2:1
Phosphorus (mg/100 kcal)	82	109
Magnesium (mg/100 kcal)	6.8	17
Iron (mg/100 kcal)	1.7	3.0
Zinc (mg/100 kcal)	1.1	1.5
Manganese (μg/100 kcal)	6.3	25
Copper (μg/100 kcal)	100	250
Iodine (μg/100 kcal)	6	35
Sodium (mg/100 kcal)	39	63
Potassium (mg/100 kcal)	60	160
Chloride (mg/100 kcal)	60	160
Selenium (μg/100 kcal)	1.8	5.0
Fluoride (μg/100 kcal)	c	25
Chromium (μg/100 kcal)	c	c
Molybdenum (μg/100 kcal)	c	c
Vitamins		
Vitamin A (μg RE/100 kcal)	204	380
Vitamin D (IU/100 kcal)	75	270
Vitamin E (mg α-tocopherol/100 kcal)	2	8
Vitamin E (mg): polyunsaturated fatty acid (g)	>1.5:1	c
Vitamin K (μg/100 kcal)	4	25
Vitamin B_1 (thiamin) (μg/100 kcal)	30	250
Vitamin B_2 (riboflavin) (μg/100 kcal)	80	620
Vitamin B_3 (niacin) (μg/100 kcal)	550	5,000
Vitamin B_6 (pyridoxine) (μg/100 kcal)	30	250
Vitamin B_{12} (cobalamin) (μg/100 kcal)	0.08	0.7
Folic acid (μg/100 kcal)	30	45
Pantothenic acid (μg/100 kcal)	300	1,900
Biotin (μg/100 kcal)	1.0	37
Vitamin C (ascorbic acid) mg/100 kcal	8.3	37
Taurine (mg/100 kcal)	5	12
Other		
Carnitine (mg/100 kcal)	2	5.9
Nucleotides (mg/100 kcal)	c	c
Choline (mg/100 kcal)	7	23
Inositol (mg/100 kcal)	4	44

[a] Appropriate nutrient concentration in a specific formulation depends on numerous factors including total composition, potential renal solute load, osmolality, and various nutrient ratios.

[b] The maximum is based on the absence of adverse effects, either in clinical studies or at the maximum amount in current domestic formulas as reported by manufacturers. In some instances, this will underestimate the amounts fed without adverse effects because the panel did not review data on manufacturing practices.

[c] No value given.

Adapted from Klein CJ (46).

long-standing controversy. In this study, infants whose mothers elected to provide milk for feeding their infants were assigned randomly to receive supplements of either banked human milk or formula, and infants whose mothers elected not to provide milk were assigned randomly, at some centers, to receive either a preterm formula or banked human milk and, at others, to receive a preterm or term formula. Infants fed human milk, either as the sole diet or with formula, had a lower incidence of both necrotizing enterocolitis and infections during the neonatal period (48). In addition, although developmental indices at 18 months (49) and 7 years of age (50) were higher in infants assigned to the preterm versus the term formula (i.e., higher versus lower intakes of protein and other nutrients) during the neonatal period, those infants assigned to banked human milk versus preterm formula did not differ, and those assigned to banked human milk that provided less protein than term formula were less adversely affected than those who received term formula (51). Moreover, neurodevelopmental indices of infants fed their own mother's milk during hospitalization showed a neurodevelopmental advantage at 7 to 8 years of age (52).

Energy Requirements

It is usually assumed that LBW infants require approximately 120 kcal/kg/day, 75 kcal/kg/day for resting expenditure and the remainder for specific dynamic action (10 kcal/kg/day), replacement of inevitable stool losses (10 kcal/kg/day), and growth (25 kcal/kg/day). The usual allotment for resting needs (75 kcal/kg/day) includes the basal requirement (50–60 kcal/kg/day), as well as additional allotments for activity and response to cold stress. However, LBW infants are relatively inactive, and, with careful control of environmental temperature, energy expenditure in response to cold stress is minimal. Most studies in relatively inactive infants maintained in a strictly thermoneutral environment suggest that the resting energy requirement (i.e., the basal requirement plus requirements for activity and response to cold stress) is little more than 60 kcal/kg/day (53–56). Fecal losses of nutrients, especially fat, are inevitable in the fed LBW infant. The extent of these losses is a function of the infant's stage of development and the nature of the fat intake (see the later discussion of fat requirements), but infants fed either human milk or modern formulas rarely experience stool fat losses exceeding 10% of the fat intake, or 5% of the nonprotein energy intake.

The energy requirement for growth includes two components: the energy cost of synthesizing new tissue, which is included in the measurement of resting expenditure; and the energy value of stored nutrients. Values of 3 to 6 kcal/g weight gain have been quoted for the latter component. Because deposition of calorically dense fat tissue requires more calories than deposition of lean body mass, such a range is not surprising. The calculated energy value of tissue deposited by the normally growing fetus between the thirtieth and thirty-eighth weeks of gestation is 2.0 to 2.5 kcal/g (see Table 51.9), whereas the calculated energy value of tissue deposited by the normally growing term infant between birth and 4 months of age is approximately 4.5 kcal/g (57). Although the energy requirements of LBW infants vary considerably, an energy intake of 120 kcal/kg/day seems to be adequate for most LBW infants (see Table 51.10).

Protein Requirements

Several studies, some conducted as early as 1947, have shown a direct relationship between protein intake and deposition of lean body mass as well as between solute intake and deposition of extracellular fluid (58–60). A protein intake of approximately 3 g/kg/day appears to support intrauterine rates of weight gain and nitrogen retention (61, 62). Conversely, higher intakes are usually well tolerated and support greater rates of weight gain and nitrogen retention (63, 64). The protein, of course, must provide sufficient amounts of all essential amino acids (65). The minimum and maximum contents of each recommended by the Life Sciences Research Office Expert Panel on Nutrient Contents of Preterm Infant Formulas (45) are shown in Table 51.12. These values are based on the amounts of essential amino acids in human milk protein if fed at the minimum and maximum amounts recommended (see Table 51.11).

Current formulas for LBW infants contain modified bovine milk protein (60% whey proteins and 40% caseins), but little evidence suggests that this protein is more efficacious than unmodified bovine milk protein (18% whey proteins and 82% caseins), particularly with respect to growth (66).

Most LBW infants currently are fed either "fortified" human milk or an LBW infant formula, both providing protein intakes of 3.2 to 3.6 g/kg/day. Despite these protein intakes, which support intrauterine rates of protein accretion and growth, 90% of infants who weigh less than 1250 g at birth weigh less than the tenth percentile of intrauterine growth standards at discharge (34, 67), a finding

TABLE 51.12. MINIMUM AND MAXIMUM CONTENTS OF ESSENTIAL AMINO ACIDS (mg/100 kcal) RECOMMENDED FOR PRETERM INFANT FORMULAS BY THE LIFE SCIENCES RESEARCH OFFICE PANEL ON NUTRIENT CONTENTS OF PRETERM INFANT FORMULAS

AMINO ACID	MINIMUM	MAXIMUM
Histidine	53	76
Isolelucine	129	186
Leucine	252	362
Lysine	182	263
Sulfur amino acids	85	123
Aromatic amino acids	196	282
Threonine	113	163
Tryptophan	38	55
Valine	132	191
Arginine	72	104

Adapted from Klein CJ (46).

TABLE 51.13. COMPOSITION (AMOUNT/100 kcal) OF STANDARD FORMULAS FOR LOW-BIRTH-WEIGHT INFANTS

COMPONENT	SIMILAC SPECIAL CARE[a]	ENFAMIL PREMATURE[b]
Energy (kcal/L)	806	810
Protein (g)	2.73 (bovine milk; whey)	3 (bovine milk; whey)
Fat (g)	5.43 (50% medium-chain triglycerides; 20% soy oil; 20% coconut oil)	5.1 (40% medium-chain triglycerides; 40% soy oil; 20% coconut oil)
Carbohydrate (g)	10.7 (40% lactose; 60% glucose polymers)	11.1 (50% lactose; 50% glucose polymers)
Electrolytes and minerals		
Calcium (mg)	181	165
Phosphorus (mg)	91	83
Magnesium (mg)	12.4	6.8
Iron (mg)	0.4[c]	0.25
Zinc (mg)	1.5	1.5
Manganese (mg)	12.4	6.3
Copper (μg)	252	125
Iodine (μg)	6.2	25
Selenium (μg)	—	—
Sodium (mg)	43	40
Potassium (mg)	131	101
Chloride (mg)	84	85
Vitamins		
Vitamin A (IU)	1,250	1,250
Vitamin D (IU)	150	272
Vitamin E (IU)	4	6.3
Vitamin K (μg)	12	8
Thiamin (μg)	250	200
Riboflavin (μg)	620	300
Vitamin B_6 (μg)	250	150
Vitamin B_{12} (μg)	0.55	0.25
Niacin (μg)	5,000	4,000
Folic acid (μg)	37	35
Pantothenic acid (μg)	1,900	1,200
Vitamin C (mg)	37	20
Biotin (μg)	37	4
Choline (mg)	10	12
Inositol (mg)	6	17

[a] Ross Laboratories, Columbus, OH.
[b] Mead Johnson Nutritionals, Evansville, IN.
[c] Iron content of low-iron formula.

illustrating the inadequacy of these intakes to support sufficient catch-up growth. For this reason, more recent recommendations for protein intake of LBW infants approach 4 g/kg/day (46). Unfortunately, formulas and human milk fortifiers providing these higher recommended intakes are not available (Table 51.13).

In recognition of the finding that most LBW infants remain growth retarded at discharge, "postdischarge" formulas have been introduced. These provide more protein and somewhat more energy than standard term infant formulas with the intent of supporting continued catch-up growth after hospital discharge. Based on the limited data available, these formulas support some catch-up growth, but this appears to be true for only a short time after discharge (68–71). However, the growth advantage achieved during this period persists through 18 months of age.

Fat Requirements

Fat accounts for about half of the nonprotein energy content of human milk and most infant formulas, including those designed for LBW infants. Most of this fat is needed solely as a source of energy, because the two essential fatty acids, linoleic acid and α-linolenic acid, comprise a relatively small proportion of total fat calories ($\sim$3–5%). Evidence indicates that two long-chain unsaturated fatty acids, arachidonic acid and docosahexaenoic acid, may be conditionally essential in LBW infants, because these infants' ability to synthesize them from precursor fatty acids may be very limited (72–74). These fatty acids accumulate in the retina and brain during development and play a key role in maturation of the central nervous system. They are present in human milk in variable concentrations and have been recently added to infant formulas.

Carbohydrate Requirements

The central nervous system and the hematopoietic tissue are dependent primarily on glucose as a metabolic fuel that, in the term infant and adult, can be produced from either exogenously administered protein or endogenous protein stores (i.e., gluconeogenesis). However, exogenous glucose is necessary to prevent hypoglycemia, particularly in preterm infants.

Carbohydrates, like fat, comprise approximately half of the nonprotein energy content of both human milk and LBW infant formulas. Although the predominant carbohydrate of human milk is lactose, LBW infant formulas usually contain a mixture of lactose and glucose polymers (see Table 51.13). Even though development of intestinal lactase activity lags behind development of other disaccharidases, most viable infants tolerate lactose quite well.

Fluid and Electrolyte Requirements

Recommended water intakes of LBW infants range from 138 to 200 mL/kg/day (see Table 51.10). These include allotments for insensible water loss, obligatory renal losses, other losses, and growth, all of which are quite variable and are affected by numerous physiologic factors (e.g., body temperature, ambient temperature, ambient humidity, activity, and respiratory rate).

Insensible water loss varies considerably among LBW infants. Moreover, both pulmonary and cutaneous components of insensible water loss are related inversely to ambient humidity. Under usual nursery conditions, the insensible water loss of term infants is approximately 30 mL/kg/day, but the very small infant's altered skin permeability to water may result in much greater cutaneous losses. Phototherapy also increases insensible water losses (75). Nursing the infant in relatively high humidity, in contrast, tends to decrease cutaneous losses as well as pulmonary losses. In general, the insensible water losses of LBW infants usually are at least twofold greater than those of the term infant, and those of the most immature LBW infants may be severalfold greater.

Obligatory renal water losses of LBW infants also are quite variable. Although even very immature infants can regulate the volume of urine excreted according to the solute load and the available water, both renal concentrating and diluting mechanisms are somewhat limited (76). In general, allowance for a urinary volume of 50 to 60 mL/kg permits excretion of the usual range of solute loads at urine concentrations of 150 to 450 mOsm/L, which are easily achieved, even by a very immature kidney.

In unfed infants, fluid losses via the gastrointestinal tract are minimal, but, in fed infants, approximately 10% of the fluid intake is lost in stool. Infants receiving phototherapy experience even greater stool losses of water (75).

The fluid requirement for growth is a function of both the rate of growth and the water content of the newly synthesized tissue. The water content of tissue deposited during the last trimester of gestation is approximately 70% (see Table 51.9), whereas the water content of the tissue deposited by the term infant between birth and 4 months of age is only 40 to 45% (57). An estimate of 50 to 60% for the growing LBW infant seems reasonable.

The water requirements for insensible (30–60 mL/kg/day) and obligatory (50–60 mL/kg/day) losses, as well as for growth (10–20 mL/kg/day), are reduced by the endogenously produced water of oxidation (i.e., ~12 mL/kg/day). Thus, the LBW infant, like the term infant, seems to have a minimum water requirement of about 100 mL/kg/day; however, the very immature infant and the infant undergoing phototherapy may require much more. In general, a fluid intake of 140 mL/kg/day is well tolerated by most infants after the first few days of life. Intakes greater than this amount are thought to increase the likelihood of developing patent ductus arteriosus (77).

Recent recommendations for sodium, chloride, and potassium intakes of LBW infants are 2.0 to 3.0 mEq/kg/day of each. These intakes should replace obligatory losses and support reasonable rates of growth. The quantities of potassium and chloride present in the volumes of both human milk and commonly used formulas usually ingested are sufficient to provide the recommended amounts. However, the sodium content of human milk (~1.2 mEq/100 kcal), even if completely absorbed, may be low.

Mineral Requirements

Early studies of calcium and phosphorus needs of infants, including LBW infants, were directed toward defining the intakes necessary to prevent hypocalcemia. Because this condition develops more commonly in infants fed formulas with a high content of phosphorus relative to calcium (i.e., a low calcium-to-phosphorus ratio), the ratio of calcium to phosphorus intake rather than the absolute intake of either was emphasized. Experience has shown that a ratio of roughly 1.5 to 2.0 is satisfactory.

The amount of calcium retained during the latter part of normal intrauterine growth is approximately 5 mmol (200 mg)/kg/day (see Table 51.9). The calcium content of human milk is sufficient to provide only about 10% of this amount. Thus, if the LBW infant's requirement for calcium is assumed to be the amount necessary to support continuation of the intrauterine rate of accumulation, human milk obviously contains inadequate calcium. The phosphorus content of human milk also is somewhat low. Moreover, LBW infants fed unsupplemented human milk have less dense skeletons radiographically than those fed formulas containing large amounts of calcium, and many develop rickets or fractures (78, 79). Thus, LBW infants fed human milk, including those fed their own mother's milk, require supplemental calcium and phosphorus for optimal skeletal mineralization. The calcium content of modern preterm infant formulas appears to be adequate.

The LBW infant has more limited stores of iron than the term infant and is therefore more susceptible to the development of iron deficiency, especially during periods of rapid growth. It has been estimated that iron stores in the LBW infant may be depleted by the second or third month of life, rather than by the fourth or fifth month, as is estimated for the term infant. Additional risk for iron deficiency in the LBW stems from frequent blood drawing needed for medical care. Thus, it is recommended that the LBW infant receive iron supplements or iron-fortified formulas as early as possible. Iron supplementation, in turn, may increase the infant's need for vitamin E, especially when formulas high in polyunsaturated fatty acids are fed (see later). In addition, the bactericidal properties of the iron-binding proteins of human milk (i.e., lactoferrin and lactoglobulin) are abolished if they are saturated with iron (80). Current LBW infant formulas contain moderate amounts of polyunsaturated fats, ample vitamin E, and 0.37 to 1.88 mg/100 kcal of iron (see Table 51.13).

Little information is available concerning the LBW infant's requirements for other trace minerals. In general, the recommended intakes of these minerals are based either on the amounts provided by human milk or the amounts that accumulate in utero during the last trimester of pregnancy. The amounts listed in Table 51.10 appear to be adequate.

A zinc intake of 500 µg/100 kcal, assuming 50% absorption from the gastrointestinal tract, should allow accumulation of zinc at the intrauterine rate. The concentration of zinc in human milk is approximately 3 to 5 mg/L; thus, it provides minimally adequate zinc to allow accumulation at the intrauterine rate. In contrast, the zinc content of human milk is absorbed more efficiently than that of bovine milk (81). The recommended copper intake (see Table 51.10) is approximately the amount present in human milk and may not allow accumulation of copper at the intrauterine rate. Thus, some recommend a higher copper intake. Because hepatic stores of copper are quite large, this probably is not necessary.

Vitamin Requirements

Recommendations concerning either requirements or advisable allowances of vitamins for LBW infants are based largely on recommendations for term infants, and these appear to be reasonable. Infants fed sufficient amounts of either human milk or currently available formulas to produce adequate growth receive sufficient amounts of all vitamins, although human milk alone may not provide the full vitamin D requirement. Because consumption of sufficient volumes of formula to satisfy vitamin requirements may not be attained for several weeks, a supplement containing vitamins A, C, and D is often recommended. In addition, the LBW infant may have special needs for vitamin E.

Vitamin E functions as an antioxidant to prevent peroxidation of polyunsaturated fatty acids in cell membranes, and inadequate intake results in erythrocyte hemolysis (82). Because the polyunsaturated fatty acid content of all membranes is related to intake of these fatty acids, infant formulas containing vegetable oils with a high polyunsaturated

fatty acid content impose a greater vitamin E requirement. Such formulas, therefore, should have a higher vitamin E content. In general, the aim should be to provide at least 1 IU of vitamin E per gram of polyunsaturated fatty acids, that is, a ratio of vitamin E to polyunsaturated fatty acid of 1. This may need to be reevaluated now that formulas supplemented with long-chain polyunsaturated fatty acids are available; however, these fatty acids comprise no more than 1% of the total fat content.

LBW infants fed formulas containing polyunsaturated fats and given therapeutic doses of iron also have a greater incidence of erythrocyte hemolysis and lower serum vitamin E levels than infants fed formulas containing less iron and polyunsaturated fats (83). Thus, the relationship between the vitamin E and iron contents of the formula and the relationship between the vitamin E and polyunsaturated fat contents of the formula are important. For this reason, careful attention must be given to vitamin E intake if iron supplements are given.

Large doses of vitamin E have been recommended to prevent both retrolental fibroplasia (83) and bronchopulmonary dysplasia (85). However, it is not clear that these recommendations are warranted, particularly considering the potential toxicity of the large doses often recommended.

DELIVERY OF NUTRIENT REQUIREMENTS TO LOW-BIRTH-WEIGHT INFANTS

Delivering the recommended nutrient levels to LBW infants, particularly those weighing less than 1250 to 1500 g at birth, is usually a challenging task. Concurrent illnesses, inadequate sucking and swallowing, delayed gastric emptying, and poor intestinal motility, among other factors, make delivery by the enteral route frequently impossible, particularly during the early neonatal period. In very sick LBW infants during the first few days of life, a limited goal may be the delivery, via the parenteral route, of at least 60 kcal/kg/day, and 2.5 g/kg/day of amino acids, plus the necessary electrolytes, minerals, and vitamins (86, 87).

Within reason, every infant should be given a trial at conventional feeding, that is, tolerated intermittent nipple or gavage feedings of either human milk or a standard formula plus intravenous supplementation. If adequate nutrients cannot be delivered in this way, a trial of continuous nasogastric or, perhaps, transpyloric feedings is warranted. Tolerated enteral feedings delivered conventionally or by continuous infusion also can be supplemented by intravenous infusions of appropriate mixtures of glucose, amino acids, and lipid. In the event that enteral feedings are not tolerated, parenteral administration of a balanced nutritional mixture is indicated. A regimen that provides 75 kcal/kg/day plus amino acids (3.0 g/kg/day), electrolytes, minerals, and vitamins can be delivered by peripheral vein infusion without imposing an unreasonable fluid load. Such a regimen certainly maintains existing body composition and may support some growth; hence, it is particularly applicable for infants who are likely to tolerate enteral intake within a brief period. Use of a central vein catheter allows delivery of a more concentrated nutrient mixture and is particularly useful in situations associated with prolonged intolerance of enteral feedings.

ROLE OF HUMAN MILK IN FEEDING THE LOW-BIRTH-WEIGHT INFANT

Growth rates of LBW infants fed human milk are lower than those of infants fed LBW formulas (89), and their plasma albumin and transthyretin concentrations are often very low (90). This may be observed even when LBW infants are fed their own mother's milk, which has substantially higher protein content than term human milk (88). In addition, the calcium and phosphorus content of human milk does not support the higher requirements of the LBW infant.

In contrast to the nutritional limitations of human milk for the LBW infant, its immunologic properties are a distinct advantage. These properties (i.e., cellular as well as humoral components) confer passive immunity and enhance immunologic maturation, and they may offer protection against infections and, perhaps, necrotizing enterocolitis. Recent studies show that the incidence of both infection and necrotizing enterocolitis is lower in infants fed either banked human milk or their own mother's milk. These advantages far outweigh the nutritional limitations of human milk, which, in any case, can be overcome by use of commercial human milk fortifiers (91, 92).

REFERENCES

1. Food and Nutrition Board, Institute of Medicine. Dietary Reference Intakes for Vitamin C, Vitamin E, Selenium, and Carotenoids. Washington, DC: National Academy Press, 2000.
2. Food and Nutrition Board, Institute of Medicine. Dietary Reference Intakes for Thiamin, Riboflavin, Niacin, Vitamin B_6, Folate, Vitamin B_{12}, Pantothenic Acid, Biotin, and Choline. Washington, DC: National Academy Press, 1998.
3. Food and Nutrition Board, Institute of Medicine. Dietary Reference Intakes for Calcium, Phosphorus, Magnesium, Vitamin D, and Fluoride. Washington, DC: National Academy Press, 1997.
4. Food and Nutrition Board, Institute of Medicine. Dietary Reference Intakes for Vitamin A, Vitamin K, Arsenic, Boron, Chromium, Copper, Iodine, Iron, Manganese, Molybdenum, Nickel, Silicon, Vanadium, and Zinc. Washington, DC: National Academy Press, 2001.
5. Food and Nutrition Board, Institute of Medicine. Dietary Reference Intakes for Energy, Carbohydrate, Fiber, Fat, Fatty Acids, Cholesterol, Protein, and Amino Acids. Washington, DC: National Academy Press, 2002.
6. Food and Nutrition Board, Institute of Medicine, Dietary Reference Intakes for Water, Potassium, Sodium, Chloride, and Sulfate. Washington, DC: National Academy Press, 2004.
7. American Academy of Pediatrics Work Group on Breastfeeding. Pediatrics 1997;100:1035–9.
8. World Health Organization. Infant and Young Child Nutrition: Global Strategy for Infant and Young Child Feeding. April 16, 2002. Available at: http://www.who.int/gb/EB_WHA/PDF/WHA55/ea5515.pdf
9. Butte NF, Hopkinson JM, Wong WW et al. Pediatr Res 2000;47:578–85.
10. Ponder DL, Innis SM, Benson JD et al. Pediatr Res 1992;32:683–8.
11. Agostoni C, Riva E, Bell R et al. J Am Coll Nutr 1994;13:658–64.
12. Farquaharson J, Jamieson EC, Abbasi KA et al. Arch Dis Child 1995;72:198–203.
13. Makrides M, Neumann MA, Byard RW et al. Am J Clin Nutr 1994;60:189–94.
14. Jorgensen MH, Hernell O, Lund P et al. Lipids 1996;31:99–105.
15. Auestad N, Montalto MB, Hall RT et al. Pediatr Res 1997;41:1–10.
16. Carlson SE, Ford AJ, Werkman SH et al. Pediatr Res 1996;39:882–8.
17. Gibson RA, Chen W, Makrides M. Lipids 2001;36:873–83.
18. Committee on Nutrition, American Academy of Pediatrics. Pediatrics 1992;89:525–7.
19. Niinikoski H, Lapinleimu H, Viikari J et al. Pediatrics 1997;99:687–94.
20. Fomon SJ, Thomas LN, Filer LJ et al. Acta Pediatr Scand 1973;62:33–45.
21. Fomon SJ. Recommendation for feeding normal infants. In: Fomon SJ, ed. Nutrition of Normal Infants. St Louis: Mosby, 1993:455–8.
22. Raiten DJ, Talbot JM, Waters JH. J Nutr 1998;128:2059S–293S.
23. Montgomery RK. Functional development of the gastrointestinal tract the small intestine. In: Heird WC, ed. Nutritional Needs of the Six- to Twelve-Month-Old Infant. New York: Raven Press, 1991:1–17.
24. Mandel ID. The nutritional impact on dental caries. In: Heird WC, ed. Nutritional Needs of the Six- to Twelve-Month-Old Infant. New York: Raven Press, 1991:89–107.
25. Devaney B, Ziegler P, Pac S et al. J Am Diet Assoc 2004;104 [Suppl 1]:14S–21S.
26. Committee on Nutrition, American Academy of Pediatrics. AAP News 1992;8:18–22.
27. Crawford MA, Stassam AG, Stevens PA. Prog Lipid Res 1981;20:31–40.
28. Committee on Nutrition, American Academy of Pediatrics. Complementary feeding. In: Kleinman RE, ed. Pediatric Nutrition Handbook. 5th ed. Elk Grove Village, IL: American Academy of Pediatrics, 2004:103–15.
29. Committee on Nutrition, American Academy of Pediatrics. Pediatrics 2001;107:1210–13.
30. Butte NF, Cobb K, Dwyer J et al. J Am Diet Assoc 2004;104:442–54.
31. Davis CM. Am J Dis Child 1928; 36:651–79.
32. National Cholesterol Education Program. Pediatrics 1992;89 [Suppl]:525.
33. Center for Nutrition Policy and Promotion Committee. Tips for Using the Food Guide Pyramid for Young Children 2 to 6 Years Old. Program aid 1647. Washington, DC: US Department of Agriculture, 1999.
34. Lemons JA, Bauer CR, Oh W et al. Pediatrics 2001;107:E1.
35. Heird WC. Nutritional support of the pediatric patient including the low birth weight infant. In: Winters RW, Greene HC, eds. Nutritional Support of the Seriously Ill Patient. New York: Academic Press, 1983:157–79.
36. Ziegler EE, O'Donnell AM, Nelson SE et al. Growth 1976;40:329–40.
37. Fish I, Winick M. Exp Neurol 1969;25:534–70.
38. Dobbing J, Sands J. Early Hum Dev 1970;3:79–83.

39. Winick M, Rosso P, Waterlow J. Exp Neurol 1970;26:293–300.
40. Hack M, Horbar JD, Malloy MH et al. Pediatrics 1991;87:587–97.
41. Saigal S, Stoskopf BL, Streiner DL et al. Pediatrics 2001;108: 407–15.
42. American Academy of Pediatrics Committee on Nutrition. J Pediatr 1985;75:976–86.
43. Aggett PJ, Haschke F, Heine F et al. Committee on Nutrition. Acta Paediatr Scand 1991;80:887–96.
44. Consensus Group. In: Tsang RC, Lucas A, Uauy R et al., eds. Nutritional Needs of the Preterm Infant: Scientific Basis and Practical Guidelines. Baltimore: Williams & Wilkins, 1993.
45. Health Canada. Can Med Assoc J 1995;152:1765–85.
46. Klein CJ. J Nutr 2002;132:1395S–577S.
47. Lucas A, Gore SM, Cole TJ et al. Arch Dis Child 1984;59:722–30.
48. Lucas A, Cole TJ. Lancet 1990;336:1519–23.
49. Lucas A, Morley R, Cole TJ. Lancet 1990;335:1477–81.
50. Lucas A, Morley R, Cole TJ. BMJ 1998;317:1481–7.
51. Lucas A, Morley R, Cole TJ et al. Arch Dis Child 1994;70: F141–6.
52. Lucas A, Morley R, Cole TJ et al. Lancet 1992;339:261–4.
53. Whyte RK, Haslam R, Vlainic L et al. Pediatr Res 1983;17: 891–8.
54. Reichman BL, Chessex P, Putet G et al. Pediatrics 1982;69: 446–51.
55. Schulze KF, Stefanski M, Masterson J et al. J Pediatr 1987;110: 753–9.
56. Van Aerde J, Sauer P, Heim T et al. Pediatr Res 1985;13:215–20.
57. Fomon SJ. Pediatrics 1967;40:863–70.
58. Gordon HH, Levine SZ, McNamara H. Am J Dis Child 1947;73: 442–52.
59. Kagan BM, Stanicova V, Felix NS et al. Am J Clin Nutr 1972;25: 1153–67.
60. Davidson M, Levine SZ, Bauer CH et al. J Pediatr 1967;70: 694–713.
61. Zlotkin SH, Bryan MH, Anderson GH. J Pediatr 1981;99: 115–20.
62. Kashyap S, Forsyth M, Zucker C et al. J Pediatr 1986;108: 955–63.
63. Kashyap S, Schulze KF, Forsyth M et al. J Pediatr 1988;113: 713–21.
64. Kashyap S, Schulze KF, Ramakrishnan R et al. Pediatr Res 1994; 35:704–12.
65. Heird WC, Kashyap S. Protein and amino acid requirements. In: Polin RA, Fox WW, eds. Fetal and Neonatal Physiology. 2nd ed. Philadelphia: WB Saunders, 1998:654–64.
66. Kashyap S, Okamoto E, Kanaya S et al. Pediatrics 1987;79: 748–55.
67. Ehrenkranz RA, Younes N, Lemons JA et al. Pediatrics 1999; 104:280–9.
68. Cooke RJ, Griffin IJ, McCormick K et al. Pediatr Res 1998;3: 355–60.
69. Cooke RJ, Embleton ND, Griffin IJ et al. Pediatr Res 2001;49: 719–22.
70. Carver JD, Wu, PYK, Hall RT et al. Pediatrics 2001;107:683–9.
71. Lucas A, Fewtrell MS, Morley R et al. Pediatrics 2001;108: 703–11.
72. Uauy RD, Hoffman DR, Birch EE et al. J Pediatr 1994;124: 612–20.
73. Clandinin M, Van Aerde J, Antonson D et al. Pediatr Res 2002; 51:187A–8A.
74. O'Connor DL, Hall R, Adamkin D et al. Pediatrics 2001;108: 359–71.
75. Oh W, Kareoki H. Am J Dis Child 1972;124:130–2.
76. Aperia A, Broberger O, Herin P et al. Acta Paediatr Scand Suppl 1983;305:61–5.
77. Bell EF, Warburton D, Stonestreet BS et al. N Engl J Med 1980; 302:598–604.
78. Steichen JJ, Gratton TL, Tsang RC. J Pediatr 1980;96:528–34.
79. Greer FR, McCormick A. J Pediatr 1988;112:961.
80. Bullen JJ, Rogers HJ, Leigh L. BMJ 1972;1:69–75.
81. Sanstrom B, Cedeblad A, Lonnerdal B. Am J Dis Child 1983; 37:726–9.
82. Oski FA, Barness LA. J Pediatr 1967;70:211–20.
83. Williams ML, Shoot RJ, O'Neal PL et al. N Engl J Med 1975; 292:887–90.
84. Mintz-Hittner H, Godio LB, Rudolph AJ et al. N Engl J Med 1981;305:1366–71.
85. Ehrenkranz RA, Bonta BW, Ablow RC et al. N Engl J Med 1978;299:564–9.
86. Anderson TL, Muttart CR, Bieber MA et al. J Pediatr 1979;94:947–51.
87. Kashyap S, Heird WC. Protein requirements of low birthweight, very low birthweight, and small for gestational age infants. In: Räihä, NCR, ed. Protein Metabolism during Infancy. Nestlé Nutrition Workshop Series, vol 33. New York: Raven Press, 1994:133–51.
88. Atkinson SA, Anderson GH, Bryan MH. Am J Clin Nutr 1980; 33:811–5.
89. Gross SJ. N Engl J Med 1983;308:237–41.
90. Kashyap S, Schulze KF, Forsyth M et al. Am J Clin Nutr 1990; 52:254–62.
91. Schanler RJ, Hurst NM. Semin Perinatol 1994;18:476–84.
92. Schanler RJ, Burns PA, Abrams SA et al. Pediatr Res 1992;31: 583–6.

52 ADOLESCENCE[1]

MARGARITA S. TREUTH AND IAN J. GRIFFIN

NUTRITIONAL REQUIREMENTS 818
    Energy 818
    Protein, Carbohydrates, and Fats 820
    Micronutrients 820
SPECIAL NUTRITIONAL PROBLEMS 823
    Effect of Nutrition during Adolescence on Adult
        Morbidity and Mortality 823
    Physical Activity 824
    Eating Disorders 825
    Pregnancy 826
SUMMARY 827

Adolescence is a time of rapid developmental change at multiple levels. Physically, adolescents have marked increases in height and weight, shifts in fat distribution, and the emergence of secondary sex characteristics (1, 2). The growth spurt during adolescence involves all skeletal and muscular tissues and most organs and systems of the body, except the brain and head (3). Although substantial variability exists, increases in growth occur in girls between 10 and 12 years and in boys 2 years later (4). Studies of children enrolled in the Fels Longitudinal Study demonstrated that growth in stature ended by a mean age of 17.3 years in girls and 21.2 years in boys (5). However, a great deal of variability in growth was noted in these children. Linear growth (stature) is often the preferred marker of continuing growth and development because, unlike weight, increases in linear growth cannot occur after growth ceases. Many factors affect the normal nutritional needs of adolescents, including puberty onset, changes in body composition, physical activity, and the onset of menstruation in girls (4). The changes in body composition include a relative increase in body fat compared with boys, who have a higher proportional increase in fat-free mass.

Biologic development is accompanied by changes in the ways in which young people think and see themselves and the world around them. This interaction of physical, psychosocial, and cognitive development has profound effects for the well-being of young people and for their successful transition to adulthood. Some adolescent girls are more vulnerable to the psychosocial consequences of biologic changes than are others. For example, in a culture that extols thinness as the standard for beauty, it is not surprising that normal physical changes (e.g., gaining weight, broadening of hips) among girls have been associated with declines in self-esteem (6). Conversely, adolescent boys may have other social stressors. This chapter focuses on the nutritional requirements of the adolescent.

As adolescents bridge that period between childhood and adulthood, nutritional assessment should be carried out as described elsewhere (see Chapter 49). Growth should also be carefully assessed, as in children. If significant concerns exist, assessment of pubertal development may be appropriate.

NUTRITIONAL REQUIREMENTS

The report from the Food and Nutrition Board of the National Institute of Medicine is entitled *Dietary Reference Intakes for Energy, Carbohydrate, Fiber, Fat, Fatty Acids, Cholesterol, Protein, and Amino Acids* (2) (see Chapter 104). These dietary reference intakes (DRIs) recommend similar ranges for children and adults, except a higher proportion of fat for infants and younger children. These new DRIs include three additional reference values, namely the estimated average requirement (EAR), the adequate intake (AI), and the tolerable upper intake level (UL). Because adolescents differ in their rates of physical growth, the timing of the growth spurt, physiologic maturation, and physical activity levels (PALs), the nutritional needs of adolescents also vary.

Energy

Energy balance is achieved when energy intake equals energy expenditure. Weight gain results when intake exceeds expenditure, and the converse is true for weight loss. In adolescents who are in a rapid period of growth, additional energy is required for growth.

---

[1]**Abbreviations: AI,** adequate intake; **BMD,** bone mineral density; **BMI,** body mass index; **CATCH,** Children's Activity Trial; **CDC,** Centers for Disease Control and Prevention; **CSFII,** Continuing Study of Food Intake of Individuals; **DRI,** dietary reference intake; **EAR,** estimated average requirement; **NHANES,** National Health and Nutrition Examination Surveys; **NHLBI,** National Heart, Lung and Blood Institute; **PAL,** physical activity level; **RDA,** recommended dietary allowance; **UL,** tolerable upper intake level.

The most recent report from the Institute of Medicine contains the DRIs for energy. The estimated energy requirement is defined as the dietary energy intake that is predicted to maintain energy balance in a healthy adult of a defined age, gender, weight, height, and level of physical activity consistent with good health (2). Requirements for adolescents differ from those of adults in that energy requirements increase because of growth and developmental changes. Therefore, the committee developed prediction equations specifically for adolescents based on a comprehensive review of the scientific data. The report (2) has equations for both adolescent girls and boys 9 through 18 years of age. For adolescents, an extra 25 kcal/day was added for energy deposition to the estimated energy requirement. This was based on the rates of weight gain of children enrolled in the Fels Longitudinal Study (7) and the rates of protein and fat deposition for adolescents (8). During adolescence, fat deposition is higher in girls than in boys, and that difference may influence the nutritional requirements.

The estimated energy requirement equations use age, weight, height, the extra for energy deposition, and physical activity. The four levels of activity are sedentary, low active, active, and very active, based on PALs derived from previous doubly labeled water studies. These four PALs are given different physical activity coefficients (PA coefficients) in the equation. Thus, to estimate the energy requirements, the activity group the adolescent belongs to must also be estimated. Because of the differences between boys and girls in growth and fat deposition, gender-specific equations were developed. These equations are as follows (2):

Boys: Estimated Energy Requirement
$$= 88.5 - 61.9 \times Age[y] + PA$$
$$\times (26.7 \times Weight[kg] + 903 \times Height[m])$$
$$+ 25 \ (kcal/day \ for \ Energy \ Deposition);$$

Girls: Estimated Energy Requirement
$$= 135.3 - 30.8 \times Age[y] + PA$$
$$\times (10.0 \times Weight[kg] + 934 \times Height[m])$$
$$+ 25 \ (kcal/day \ for \ Energy \ Deposition).$$

For example, a male adolescent 14 years of age, with a weight of 51.0 kg, height of 1.64 m, and a sedentary PAL, would have an estimated energy requirement of 2090 kcal/day. The same adolescent who had a high active PAL would have an estimated energy requirement of 3283 kcal/day. An adolescent girl 14 years of age, with a weight of 49.4 kg, height of 1.60 m, and a sedentary PAL, would have an estimated energy requirement of 1718 kcal/day. If this female adolescent increased her PAL to high active, her estimated energy requirement would be 2831 kcal/day. These examples are useful to illustrate the marked differences in requirements between an adolescent classified as either sedentary or a with high PAL. If one wishes to predict an adolescent's energy requirements accurately, it is clear that the PAL

level must be determined correctly. Otherwise, a mismatch between intake and expenditure could lead to either undernutrition or overnutrition. Choosing the appropriate PAL level (and therefore the PA coefficient) is probably the most difficult challenge and limitation of using these equations.

Several studies have assessed energy expenditure and activity in children and adolescents, as measured by the doubly labeled water technique (9, 10). Total absolute energy expenditure increases with age during adolescence. PALs of adolescents are highly variable because of the large variability in lifestyles. The 1985 report of the Food and Agriculture Organization/World Health Organization/United Nations University noted PALs of 1.6 to 1.73 in adolescent boys and girls 11 to 14 years of age, and 1.5 to 1.65 in adolescents 15 to 18 years of age (11). The review by Torun and colleagues (12) also included PALs in older children. The range from several studies in PALs for boys 6 to 13 years of age was 1.71 to 1.86, with a mean of 1.79±0.06. Correspondingly, for girls, the range was 1.69 to 1.90, with a mean of 1.80±0.12. For adolescents more than 14 years old, the mean for boys was 1.84±0.05 (range, 1.79–1.88), and for girls it was 1.69± 0.03 (range, 1.67–1.69) (12).

The new DRIs make a recommendation of a PAL of 1.6 to prevent excess weight gain (2). This means that to move from a very sedentary (PAL of 1.4) to an active lifestyle (PAL >1.6), children and adolescents must participate in moderately intense activity a total of 60 minutes per day. Longitudinal studies are needed to monitor PALs and normal growth patterns.

Dietary intake plays a major role in the growth patterns of adolescents. Several changes in the adolescents diet over the last few decades have led to an increased concern over the nutritional content of the diet. One change has been the increase in soft drink consumption. Troiano and associates (13) reported that the mean percentage of energy from total fat (33.5%) and saturated fat (12.2%) decreased in youth ages 2 to 19 years enrolled in the third National Health and Nutrition Examination Surveys (NHANES III). Soft drinks contributed 8% of energy in adolescents, with beverages contributing 20 to 24% of energy across all ages (13). The prevalence of soft drink consumption among 6 to 17 year olds was reported to be 37% in the Nationwide Food Consumption Survey 1977/1978 and increased to 56% in the combined Continuing Survey of Food Intakes by Individuals 1994/1996, and the Supplemental Children's Survey 1988 (14). The mean intake increased from 5 to 12 fl oz/day. This increase was largely the result of an increase in the home consumption, but increases from other sources (e.g., fast-food restaurants, vending machines) were also found (14). National survey data also revealed that by age 13 years, more carbonated soft drinks were consumed than 100% fruit juice, milk, or fruit drinks (15). Another change has occurred in the school environment. Specifically, school vending machines and à la carte availability of foods also have changed, and both can play a role in the energy intake of adolescents. In seventh grade students, snack vending machines were negatively correlated with fruit consumption (16). In addition, à la carte availability was positively associated with total and saturated fat intake (16). The home environment has also been explored as influencing dietary intake. Adolescents from higher-income families had higher intakes of polyunsaturated fat, protein, calcium, and folate, and intakes of total fat, saturated fat, and cholesterol decreased as parents' education levels increased (17). In another study (18), inadequate daily consumption of fruits and vegetables was reported in 40% of adolescents from low socioeconomic backgrounds. Results from the National Longitudinal Study of Adolescent Health (19) revealed that at home, parental presence at the evening meal was associated with higher consumption of fruits and vegetables. The authors (19) also indicated that approximately 20% of adolescents skip breakfast each day. In the Growing Up Today Study of more than 14,000 children, the longitudinal relationship of skipping breakfast and weight change was evaluated (20). Cross-sectionally, skipping breakfast was associated with overweight. However, body mass index (BMI) decreased in overweight children who reported never eating breakfast compared with overweight children who ate breakfast nearly every day (20). By contrast, skipping breakfast in children of normal weight was associated with a greater gain in weight over time than in adolescents who ate breakfast nearly every day; however, this was not statistically significant (20). These findings are interesting in that the already overweight child who skipped breakfast over time would have a lower total daily energy intake, leading to a lower BMI over time, than the overweight child who consumed breakfast.

These changes in the adolescents diet over time warrant attention. The data from the Youth Risk Behavior Survey from 1999 recommended (among other things) that efforts to promote healthy weight management should emphasize increasing fruit and vegetable consumption (21). It has also been suggested that to promote low-fat foods in the school cafeteria to adolescents, the taste, availability, and labeling of these low-fat foods need to be addressed (22). Both the school and the home environment could potentially serve as modifiers of the adolescent's intake.

Protein, Carbohydrates, and Fat

Protein requirements for adolescents have been provided by the newest DRIs (see Appendix Table A-2-d-7). The acceptable distribution range for protein (2) is between 10 and 30% of the total calories for children and adolescents 4 to 18 years of age. The recommended dietary allowance (RDA) for men and women is 0.8 g/kg weight. The EAR

for protein is 27 and 44 g/day for boys 9 to 13 and 14 to 18 years of age, respectively (2). For girls, the EAR is 28 g/day for 9 to 13 year olds and 38 g/day for 14 to 18 year olds.

Carbohydrate, including sugars and starches, are needed for energy. The acceptable distribution range for carbohydrate (2) is between 45 and 65% of the total caloric intake. The recent RDA (2) for carbohydrates is set at 130 g/day for children and adolescents. Previously, the estimate was also 130 g/day (4). This level is typically exceeded, except in those on high-protein, low-carbohydrate diets. The median intake that is age dependent is 200 to 330 g/day for men and 180 to 230 g/day for women.

The acceptable distribution range for fat (2) is between 25 and 55% of the total caloric intake for children 4 to 18 years of age. Fat requirements are specific to two types of polyunsaturated fatty acids, both of which are essential in humans. These include an ω-3 fatty acid (α-linolenic acid) and an ω-6 fatty acid (linoleic acid). AI of these polyunsaturated fatty acids are set at 1.6 and 1.1 g/day of α-linolenic acid for men and women, respectively. The acceptable distribution for children and adolescents is 5 to 10% of fat calories for linoleic acid and 0.6 to 1.2% for α-linolenic acid (2). Because fat is a major source of energy for the body, the intake of fat needs to be adequate only for energy needs.

Micronutrients

The rapid growth that occurs during adolescence leads to high mineral requirements in nonpregnant adolescents. During the peak of the adolescent growth spurt, requirements for calcium, iron, and zinc may be two to three times the average requirement during the second decade of life (Table 52.1). For some minerals, such as iron and zinc, this requirement can be met both by mobilizing stores and from the diet. However, in the case of calcium, no calcium

TABLE 52.1. DAILY INCREMENTS IN BODY CONTENT DUE TO GROWTH

MINERAL	SEX	AVERAGE FOR AGE 10–20 Y (mg)	AT PEAK OF GROWTH SPURT PERIOD (mg)
Calcium	M	210	400
Iron	M	0.57	1.1
Nitrogen	M	320	610
Zinc	M	0.27	0.50
Magnesium	M	4.4	8.4
Magnesium	F	2.3	5.0
Calcium	F	110	240
Iron	F	0.23	0.9
Nitrogen	F	160	360
Zinc	F	0.18	0.31

From Food and Nutrition Board, Institute of Medicine. Iron. In: Dietary Reference Intakes for Vitamin A, Vitamin K, Arsenic, Boron, Chromium, Copper, Iodine, Iron, Manganese, Molybdenum, Nickel, Silicon, Vanadium and Zinc. Washington, DC: National Academy Press, 2000.

stores are available that can be used to support bone mineralization, and the adolescent's requirements must be met entirely from dietary sources. Pubertal changes during the adolescent period increase sexual dimorphism, and it is not surprising that mineral requirements begin to differ between boys and girls, either because of changes in body composition or because of additional mineral losses (especially iron) associated with the onset of menses. Daily increments in mineral content vary during adolescence and are highest during the period of peak growth velocity (see Table 52.1).

Calcium

More than 99% of total body calcium resides in the skeleton. Because adolescence is a time of very rapid expansion of bone mass, it is not surprising that calcium requirements are higher during adolescence than at any other time of the life cycle.

Bone mineral accretion during adolescence is a significant contribution factor to total bone mineral content, with 92% of peak bone mass present by the end of the eighteenth year of life (23). Peak bone mass, in turn, is an important modifier of the long-term fracture risk and the risk of osteoporosis; approximately half this mass is deposited during the adolescent years. Optimizing calcium intake during adolescence would be expected to increase bone mineralization and reduce fracture risk, and this is supported by the literature.

Elegant stable isotope studies have demonstrated that the period of peak bone mineral deposition in girls occurs about 8 months before menarche (24). Many studies have examined the effect of increasing calcium intake in preadolescent girls (typically 7–12 years old) on bone mineralization either using calcium supplements (25–27) or dietary interventions such as increasing consumption of milk or other calcium-rich foods (28). The overall consensus is that increasing calcium intakes to more than 1000 mg/day enhances bone mineralization, and the effect appears to persist beyond the time of the intervention (29). Bone mineralization occurs more slowly in adolescents, and whether dietary calcium intake is so critical at this time has been less clear, although cross-sectional data suggest that it may be (30). Higher milk consumption during childhood and adolescence in associated with increased bone mineral density (BMD) in women after the menopause (31). One study (32) addressed the effect of calcium supplementation in older adolescent girls. One hundred girls with calcium intakes less than 800 mg/day were studied. This calcium intake is similar to the mean calcium intake of girls age 14 to 18 years old from the NHANES III dietary survey (33). Eligible subjects were at least 1 year beyond the menarche and in good health. They were randomized to receive 1000 mg/day calcium as calcium carbonate or placebo for 12 months. Calcium-supplemented girls had

greater accretion of total body BMD and lumbar spine BMD than the controls. Of particular interest, little benefit was seen in girls who were within 2 years of the menarche. Girls between 2 and 4 years after the menarche showed an almost doubling of BMD in response to the calcium supplementation (32). Although these results need confirmation, and it is unclear whether these benefits persist, they are encouraging. They suggest a second window of opportunity in which increased calcium intake may significantly increase peak BMD. In addition to the premenarche period, a further opportunity may exist after the menarche, perhaps 2 to 4 years later.

The current AI of calcium is 1300 mg/day for children aged 14 to 18 years, with insufficient evidence to determine differential requirements between the genders (33). This is very similar to the previous recommended dietary intake from 1989 (34). Because the Institute on Medicine believed there was insufficient evidence to set an RDA for calcium, individuals should aim to meet the AI (33). However, the NHANES III dietary survey estimates that the average calcium intakes in girls aged 14 to 18 years is only 753 mg/day, and less than 5% of girls met the AI for calcium. For boys, the situation was somewhat better, with an average calcium intake of 1025 mg/day. Approximately one fourth of boys achieved the AI for calcium. The most important dietary source of calcium is milk, which provides 46% of the calcium intake of boys 12 to 18 years old, and 43% for girls (35). Cheese provides an addition 16 to 19% of calcium intake and bread approximately 7%. Other foods provide relatively little calcium (35).

Optimizing calcium intake is important throughout the entire life cycle. However, in terms of maximizing peak BMD a prime time is immediately before the menarche. The data of Rozen (32) suggest that a second opportunity may occur between 2 and 4 years after the menarche. Whether this period can overcome inadequate calcium intake earlier is not known, nor is the relative importance of the different time periods. However, these data underline the importance of encouraging calcium intake during the adolescent period.

Iron

Adolescence is a particularly common time for the development of iron deficiency anemia in the United States. Looker and colleagues (36) estimated that 9% of girls aged 12 to 15 years are anemic (hemoglobin <12 g/dL [37]), as are 11% of girls aged 16 to 19 years. In contrast, 1% or less of boys the same age are anemic (36).

Sexual differences in mineral requirements are particularly apparent for iron. Girls have increased iron losses associated with the onset on menses, which significantly increases iron requirements. However, this is partially offset by the differences in body composition between the genders, because the increase in total body iron that occurs during adolescence is significantly greater in boys than in girls. Most (85%) of total body iron is in the form of hemoglobin, and approximately 10% is myoglobin. During adolescence, differences in body composition develop; boys have a greater increase in muscle mass than girls. This results in an increased requirement for myoglobin (found in muscle) and hemoglobin (because muscle has a relatively larger blood supply than adipose tissue). One estimate is that growth in boys requires 42 mg of iron/kg body weight, compared with 31 mg/kg in girls (38). Iron requirements for boys may be greater than for girls during early adolescence. However, at the end of adolescence, as the growth rate slows in boys and menstrual losses persist in girls, the requirements for girls exceed those of boys (see Table 9-10 in reference 39).

The 1989 RDA for iron in adolescents was 15 mg/day for girls and 12 mg/day for boys (34). The more recent DRIs are very similar: 15 mg/day for girls aged 14 to 18 years and 11 mg/day for boys of the same age (39). These later requirements were estimated using a factorial approach taking into account the following:

- Iron requirement for tissue growth
- Iron requirement for expansion of circulating hemoglobin
- Basal iron losses
- Menstrual losses in girls
- Differences in blood volume between boys and girls
- Iron absorption of 18%

Iron absorption in preadolescents appears to be greater in girls than in boys after correcting for iron status (40). Whether the same is true in adolescents in not known.

When comparing iron intakes in a population, the most appropriate reference intake to use is the EAR: 7.7 mg/day for boys and 7.9 mg/day for girls. Table 52.2 illustrates the Iron intake from food estimated by the NHANES III dietary survey, Total Diet Study, and Continuing Study of Food Intake of Individuals (CSFII) (39).

Although iron intakes are somewhat different between the surveys, it is clear that iron intakes are significantly greater in boys, and 5 to 10% of girls fail to meet the EAR for iron. Ready-to-eat cereal provides between 20 and 26% of the iron intake for children aged 12 to 18 years (35), bread provides about 14%, and beef 9% (35).

Given the high incidence of iron deficiency anemia in adolescent girls, the US Centers for Disease Control and Prevention (CDC) has made recommendations for the prevention of iron deficiency anemia in this age group (37), which include the following:

- Encouraging a diet high in iron-rich foods
- Screening of all women of childbearing age for anemia every 5 to 10 years
- Screening of high-risk women (low iron intakes, high menstrual losses) annually

TABLE 52.2. IRON INTAKE FROM FOOD ESTIMATED BY THE THIRD NATIONAL HEALTH AND NUTRITION EXAMINATION SURVEYS DIETARY SURVEY, TOTAL DIET STUDY, AND CONTINUING STUDY OF FOOD INTAKE OF INDIVIDUALS

AGE	PERCENTILE	NHANES III[a] (mg/d)	TOTAL DIET SURVEY (mg/d)	CSFII (mg/d)
Males 14–18 y (EAR = 7.7 mg/d)				
	Fifth	10.3	6.4	10.6
	Tenth	11.6	7.9	12.2
	Fiftieth	18.1	12.7	19.3
	Mean	20.0	16.5d	20.7
Females 14–18 y (EAR = 7.9 mg/d)				
	Fifth	6.6	3.7	7.4
	Tenth	7.5	5.1	8.5
	Fiftieth	11.6	9.2	12.7
	Mean	12.2	12.3	13.5

CSFII, Continuing Study of Food Intake of Individuals; EAR, estimated average requirement; NHANES III, Third National Health and Nutrition Examination Surveys.
[a]Intake from food *and* supplements.

From Food and Nutrition Board, Institute of Medicine. Iron. In: Dietary Reference Intakes for Vitamin A, Vitamin K, Arsenic, Boron, Chromium, Copper, Iodine, Iron, Manganese, Molydbenum, Nickel, Silicon, Vanadium and Zinc. Washington, DC: National Academy Press, 2000.

If anemia is diagnosed, girls should be treated with 60 to 120 mg/day of oral iron for 2 to 3 months (37), and they should be given dietary counseling to increase iron intake from foods (37). If anemia does not improve after 4 weeks, further investigation is required (37). No specific screening is required for adolescent boys.

Although not directly mentioned by the CDC, another high-risk group for iron deficiency anemia may be adolescent athletes. Between 16% (41) and 34% (42) may have low iron stores. Reasons for this may include decreased iron intake, increased red cell destruction, or, in some cases, occult gastrointestinal bleeding (42).

Zinc

Zinc deficiency was first described in humans by Prasad in the 1960s (43). He described boys in Iran, and later in Egypt, with delayed puberty and short stature. The Iranian boys had very low zinc intakes, pica (geophagia), hepatosplenomegaly, and iron deficiency anemia. Their anemia responded to iron therapy, and the remaining symptoms resolved when their diet was improved during hospital admission (44). Subsequently, similar findings were described in Egyptian boys, who were more extensively studied (45). They were shown to have low plasma, hair and red cell zinc concentration, increased zinc-65 turnover, and reduced zinc excretion in the urine and feces (43). Zinc supplementation led to rapid improvements in growth, clinical status, and normalization of plasma zinc and serum alkaline phosphate concentrations (43, 44). Severe zinc deficiency is known to cause the clinical features of acrodermatitis enteropathica (46), with dermatitis, diarrhea, alopecia, poor growth, delayed sexual development, thymic atrophy, and immune dysfunction.

As noted previously, adolescence is a time of rapid growth in bone mass and lean muscle mass. Because 60% of total body zinc is present in skeletal muscle, and a further 30% is found in the bone, zinc requirements during adolescence are relatively high. Indeed, the 1989 RDAs of 15 mg/day for boys and 12 mg/day for girls were higher than for any other group, except lactating women (34). The more recent DRIs quote somewhat lower RDAs: 11 mg/day for boys and 9 mg/day for girls (39). Once again, these values were calculated using a factorial approach based on estimates of intestinal, urinary, and integumentary losses, menstrual or seminal losses, the requirement for growth, and an estimate of zinc absorption of 40% (39). The EAR is 8.5 mg/day for boys and 7.3 mg/day for girls (39), and these requirements are compared with estimated zinc intakes in Table 52.3, derived from values for zinc intake from food estimated by the NHANES III dietary survey, Total Diet Study, and CSFII (39).

TABLE 52.3. ZINC INTAKE FROM FOOD ESTIMATED BY THE THIRD NATIONAL HEALTH AND NUTRITION EXAMINATION SURVEYS DIETARY SURVEY, TOTAL DIET STUDY, AND CONTINUING STUDY OF FOOD INTAKE OF INDIVIDUALS

AGE	PERCENTILE	NHANES III[a] (mg/d)	TOTAL DIET SURVEY (mg/d)	CSFII (mg/d)
Males 14–18 y (EAR = 8.5 mg/d)				
	Fifth	8.6	5.0	8.4
	Tenth	9.6	6.2	9.6
	Fiftieth	14.8	11.5	14.3
	Mean	15.8	15.1	15.0
Females 14–18 y (EAR = 7.3 mg/d)				
	Fifth	5.2	2.6	5.5
	Tenth	6.2	3.7	6.3
	Fiftieth	9.0	7.4	9.5
	Mean	9.8	9.5	9.9

CSFII, Continuing Study of Food Intake of Individuals; EAR, estimated average requirement; NHANES III, Third National Health and Nutrition Examination Surveys.
[a]Intake from food *and* supplements.

From Food and Nutrition Board, Institute of Medicine. Iron. In: Dietary Reference Intakes for Vitamin A, Vitamin K, Arsenic, Boron, Chromium, Copper, Iodine, Iron, Manganese, Molybdenum, Nickel, Silicon, Vanadium and Zinc. Washington, DC: National Academy Press, 2000.

Once again, it is apparent that intake is lower in girls than in boys, and that more girls than boys have intakes below the EAR. Important dietary sources of zinc for children aged 12 to 18 years include beef (~25% of intake), milk (12%), ready-to-eat cereal (7.5–10.7%), cheese (6–7%), poultry (5%), and breads (5%) (35).

Vitamin Requirements

Fat-Soluble Vitamins. No evidence indicates that adolescence is a period of unusually high requirements for any of the fat-soluble vitamins. Requirements for vitamin A (47), vitamin K (48), vitamin E (49), and vitamin D (50) increase steadily through childhood into adolescence, and they are typically extrapolated from adult values. Adolescence is a period of increased bone formation and calcium absorption, partly because of changes in vitamin D metabolism (51), although this does not appear to be associated with an increase in vitamin D requirements (50).

Water-Soluble Vitamins. Very little data on the requirements for water-soluble vitamins exist, and current recommendations are typically extrapolated from adult data, such as for riboflavin (52), niacin (53), vitamin B_6 (54), folate (55), vitamin B_{12} (56), and vitamin C (57). One study of adolescents in Taiwan suggests that the current recommendations for vitamin B_6 intake appear appropriate (58).

As adolescent girls enter puberty, they should increase their folate intake to reduce the risk of neural tube defects in their children, as should every women of childbearing age (see Chapter 50).

A study of postpartum adolescents (14–19 years old) (59) demonstrated a decline in red cell folate between 4 and 12 weeks after delivery. This change was seen both in lactating and nonlactating adolescents (59). Supplementation with 300 μg/day folate was sufficient to prevent this decrease (59). The Institute of Medicine recommended that lactating women increase their folate intake by about 130 μg/day to replace the folate lost in breast milk (55). It is unclear whether this level of supplementation would have been as adequate.

SPECIAL NUTRITIONAL PROBLEMS

Effect of Nutrition during Adolescence on Adult Morbidity and Mortality

Obesity is one factor that is linked to adult-onset diseases. The analysis of the National Health Examination Survey (cycles II and III) and the first, second, and third NHANES found that the prevalence of obesity increased the greatest from 1988 to 1991 (13). Among children (ages 6–11 years) and adolescents (12–17 years), 22% were defined as overweight based on the eighty-fifth percentile for BMI, and 10.9% were defined as obese based on the ninety-fifth percentile for BMI (13).

The prevalence of children with a BMI higher than the ninety-fifth percentile has increased from 4% in 1974 to 15% in 2000 (60). Several studies have shown the prediction of adult obesity from indicators of adiposity at younger ages (54, 55). Adolescence is a key time period, because the probability of overweight at age 35 years was predicted most accurately from a BMI at age 18 (62). In addition, the risk of adult obesity was greatest at any age in obese and nonobese children if at least one parent was obese (61). Thus, tracking of obesity to adulthood is evident, as well as the familial predisposition to obesity.

Childhood obesity has also been shown to be a predictor of development of syndrome X (63). In the Bogalusa Heart Study, childhood BMI and insulin values were predictors of adult clustering of risk factors (63). Not only has obesity risen in the United States, but also the rate of type 2 diabetes mellitus has increased from 4.9% in 1990 to 6.5% in 1998, corresponding to a 30% increase (64). In the Growing Up Today Study, Gillman and colleagues (65) reported that higher birth weight predicted increased risk of overweight in adolescence. In addition, maternal gestational diabetes was also associated with increased overweight in adolescence. As noted (65), their results only partially support a causal role of altered maternal-fetal glucose metabolism in the initiation of obesity in adolescents.

Increasing evidence indicates that adolescents are presenting with what has been traditionally adult-onset diseases. These include hypertension, cardiovascular disease, and type 2 diabetes. The Bogalusa Heart Study provided the research community with a wealth of information on childhood metabolic factors and their relation to metabolic diseases of adulthood (63, 66–70). In the Bogalusa cohort of white and black young adults, the Framingham risk score (used to identify early risk for coronary artery disease) was related to carotid artery intimal-medial thickness (68). One article found that childhood low-density lipoprotein cholesterol and BMI predicted carotid artery intimal-medial thickness in young adults (69). (Carotid intimal-medial thickness is a quantitative measure of atherosclerosis that is predictive of subsequent myocardial infarction and stroke.) In another article, Freedman and associates (67) reported that high adult carotid artery intimal-medial thickness was seen only among overweight children (defined as greater than the ninety-fifth percentile) who became obese adults. Another study in Finland reported that the risk factor profile during adolescence predicted adult carotid artery intimal-medial thickness, independent of other cardiovascular risk factors (71). These studies suggest that adolescents with several risk factors such as obesity, dyslipidemia, and elevated blood pressure are at increased risk of developing atherosclerosis.

Another childhood and adolescent dietary component that has marked potential to influence adult disease is calcium. Inadequate calcium intake will affect bone calcium accumulation during adolescence and will then be a determinant of osteoporosis during adulthood.

Physical Activity

The CDC recommends that students in kindergarten to grade 12 (ages 5–18 years) have comprehensive, daily physical education. Federal guidelines recommend that children participate in at least 60 minutes/day of moderate physical activity (72). The newest guidelines for 2004 from the National Association for Sport and Physical Education recommend that children spend at least 60 minutes/day and up to several hours of physical activity daily. Physical activity has been shown to decline during adolescence (73, 74). Only 60% of high school students are enrolled in physical education classes, and only 25% take daily physical education (74). In adolescents, certain ethnic groups (non-Hispanic black) also have lower moderate to vigorous physical activity compared with whites (75). A precipitous drop in physical activity in white and African-American girls during adolescence was reported from the National Heart, Lung and Blood Institute (NHLBI) Growth and Health Study (73). By age 17, the study found a 100% decline in physical activity in African-American girls and a 64% decline in white girls. The factors related to this decline included ethnicity, parental education, pregnancy, cigarette smoking, and BMI (73). Sallis (76) estimated that between the ages of 10 and 17 years, the estimated decline could be between 1.8 and 2.7%/year for boys and between 2.6 and 7.4%/year for girls. One study of more than 4000 children from ages 8 to 16 years showed that approximately 20% of US children do not exercise vigorously more than twice per week, with rates higher in girls (26%) than in boys (17%) (77).

Insufficient levels of physical activity in US children may lead to increases in adiposity. Several studies have suggested that reduced physical activity plays a significant role in the etiology of childhood obesity (78, 79). Interventions have been developed to combat this increased obesity and lack of physical activity in adolescents. One intervention study, Children's Activity Trial (CATCH), was designed to alter physical activity in children. The original CATCH study was successful in modifying physical activity and dietary behaviors. In the follow-up study of these children during their adolescent years at grade 8, information regarding PAL and BMI was obtained (80). The children in the intervention schools maintained significantly higher PALs than control children; however, no differences in BMI were found. Thus, the original CATCH study was successful in terms of activity, and these effects continued without further intervention (80). At present, an NHLBI-sponsored, multisite intervention study, Trial of Adolescent Activity in Girls, is under way designed to prevent the decline in physical activity in adolescent girls. Interventions targeting adolescent boys and certain minorities are certainly warranted.

Studies have evaluated the determinants of physical activity and fitness in adolescents (81, 82), but they are not well understood (76, 83). Fitness is also an important variable because low fitness is a significant predictor of cardiovascular disease and mortality in men and women (84). Data from the 1990 Youth Risk Behavior Survey showed that low activity was associated with a negative health behavior, specifically lower fruit and vegetable consumption, greater television watching, smoking, failure to wear a seat belt, and low perception of academic performance (81). In adolescent girls enrolled in the Penn State Young Women's Health Study, fruit consumption, circulating β-carotene, and α-tocopherol were positively correlated with fitness (82). In this same cohort, girls with the lowest body fat had a better ratio of total cholesterol to high-density lipoprotein cholesterol, higher β-carotene, and reported a higher consumption of fruits and dietary fiber (82).

Increased evidence indicates that environmental factors play a role in promoting and supporting physical activity (85, 86). Environmental determinants of physical activity patterns were evaluated in US adolescents enrolled in the 1996 National Longitudinal Study of Adolescent Health (75). Participation in daily physical education programs, use of community recreation centers, and high family income were associated with increased physical activity. Maternal education was inversely associated with high inactivity. The authors pointed out that physical activity was associated with environmental factors, whereas inactivity was associated with sociodemographic factors, stressing the importance of exploring other environmental factors that may affect inactivity (75). Certainly, continuation of these positive health behaviors (fitness, physical activity, consumption of fruits and vegetables/fiber) should be encouraged into adulthood to reduce the risk of later disease.

Eating Disorders

Adolescence is a time when eating disorders emerge (see also Chapter 87). These disorders include anorexia nervosa, bulimia, and a wide range of unhealthy food restriction practices, such as dieting and other patterns of binging behavior (87). Binge eating disorder is characterized by eating large quantities of food, binge eating episodes, and feeling distressed about binge eating. Bulimia nervosa is characterized by recurrent episodes of overeating, engaging in methods to control shape and weight, specific behavior (binge and compensate) to control weight or body shape at least twice a week in the past 2 months, and preoccupation with body shape and weight. Anorexia nervosa is characterized by a refusal to maintain body weight over minimal normal weight for age and height (<85%), intense fear of gaining weight or becoming fat, disturbances in the way one's body, weight, or shape is experienced, and amenorrhea in postmenarcheal girls and women.

The estimates for the United States are that 0.5 to 1% of adolescent girls between ages 12 and 18 years meet the diagnostic criteria established by the American Psychiatric Association for anorexia nervosa (88). However, the rates are higher for those exhibiting subclinical problems such as excessive exercising, strict dieting, and occasional binging and purging (88). The general medical complications of anorexia include hypothermia, edema, hypotension, bradycardia, renal failure, and failure of menarche. Two risk periods, early adolescence (13–14 years of age) and late adolescence (17–19 years of age), have been identified (89). Girls tend to be at higher risk for development of these disorders. The family environment has been considered to be highly important in the development of disordered eating in adolescent girls (90–92). Pubertal development has also been linked to eating and body image problems (93). Negative perceptions of the adolescent's parent-adolescent relationship were associated with higher diet scores and lower body image (88). Involvement in sports that put restrictions on weight (distance running, figure skating, gymnastics, wrestling) is one risk factor for boys. Assessment tools for disorded eating have been developed for both genders (94).

The Youth Risk Behavior Surveillance System evaluated weight loss practices in adolescents (21, 95, 96). Kann and associates (95) reported in 1993 that 40% of high school students were attempting to lose weight. In 2002, Lowry and colleagues (21) reported that of the high school students participating in the 1999 Youth Risk Behavior Survey, 43% were attempting to lose weight and 19% were trying to maintain their current weight. Other studies (97–99) have documented that between 14 and 40% of adolescents diet, with 30 to 46% reporting having been on a diet. Lowry and colleagues (21) evaluated the associations among physical activity, fruit and vegetable consumption, and smoking with weight management goals and practices of high school students who participated in the 1999 Youth Risk Behavior Survey. Among the students trying to lose weight or trying to maintain their current weight, 32% of girls and 17% of boys used unhealthy weight control methods such as fasting, diet pills, laxatives, and vomiting to try to lose weight.

Factors that explain weight reduction behavior have been the subject of investigation (96, 97, 100). Self-esteem was shown to be a good predictor of weight reduction behaviors, including diet frequency, diet pill use, and purging (96). Adolescents strongly believe that greater levels of self-worth and social confidence would be attained with weight loss (96, 101). Whether self-esteem is related to changes in weight or obesity over time has also been investigated (97, 100). In adolescents followed over a 3-year period, low self-esteem was not related to obesity over time (100). In a sample of more than 10,000 16 to 24 year olds, changes in global self-esteem was not related to overweight status over a 7-year period (100). Gender differences may also play a role in weight reduction behavior.

Girls tend to value physical attractiveness more than boys, so changes in their appearance have a greater impact on their self-concept and feelings of self-worth. In a study of young adolescents, Koff and colleagues (102) found that higher levels of body satisfaction were associated with higher reported self-esteem, particularly among girls. Studies of overweight adolescent girls suggest that low self-esteem is strongly correlated with negative perceptions of physical appearance (103–106).

Addressing the nutritional consequences of eating disorders should be a public health priority. Ponton (87) stressed the importance of linking both prevention programs and treatment programs and noted the importance of developing appropriate messages, especially to those at highest risk. High-risk populations such as middle school girls should be screened. Interventions should be tailored to these high-risk populations and should be culturally acceptable and age appropriate (87).

Pregnancy

The United States has the highest adolescent birth rate of all developed countries (4). The revised population-based birth rates are lower based on the 2000 census (1991–1999 data) compared with the 1990 census (107). Specific to teens, the summary of the vital statistics for 2001 indicates that the birth rate for teen mothers continues to fall (108). This rate dropped 5% from 2000 to 2001, and it has dropped 26% since 1991. This decline was more rapid for teens aged 15 to 17 years than for teens 18 to 19 years old. The actual current rate is 45.9 births per 1000 (108). The overall infant mortality rate (6.9/1000 live births) has remained unchanged since 2000.

One of the most important predictors of infant mortality is birth weight. Several studies have reported that adolescent girls have a high risk of delivering premature and low-birth-weight infants, who have high mortality within the first year of life (109–111). Low- or very low-birth-weight infants are more likely to be born to younger teenagers (112, 113). These infants are also likely to be at risk for physical neglect and abuse (113). Pregnant African-American adolescents had a higher incidence of low-birth-weight infants compared with overall US data (114). In addition, the low birth weight of the infants was related to low prepregnancy BMI, inadequate weight gain, and smoking history in their pregnant African-American adolescent mothers (115). One study (116) found no differences in abnormal deliveries between adolescent and older pregnant women and noted that good prenatal care was the likely factor of this positive finding. One intervention that included five structured home visits during pregnancy was successful in reducing adverse neonatal events but was not effective in improving infant vaccination or knowledge (117).

Pregnant adolescents require additional energy during their second and third trimesters, especially considering that some adolescents are still growing (118). Suggested weight gain during pregnancy depends on the initial weight of the adolescent and varies from 15 to 40 lb (119). Previously, the Institute of Medicine report recommended that weight gains be based on preconception weight (underweight, normal weight, overweight). For adolescents, the recommendation was for an intake at the upper end of the ranges. In contrast, the more recent DRIs (120) provide equations to estimate the energy requirements for the pregnant adolescent 14 to 18 years of age. The estimated energy requirement during pregnancy is composed of the total energy expenditure, a change in total energy expenditure of 8 kcal/week of pregnancy, and the energy deposition during pregnancy (180 kcal/day). This estimate is for the second and third trimesters only, because total energy expenditure remains fairly constant during the first trimester. As with pregnancy in adults, protein requirements increase, as well as requirements for vitamins (118). Pregnant adolescents may also require additional zinc, calcium, and iron supplementation (118).

Maternal growth during pregnancy in adolescents has been studied (121–125), but whether growth of the adolescent while pregnant has adverse effects on the adolescent or the fetus is controversial (126). Some studies have shown adverse outcomes (121, 122), and others have not (123). Small changes in stature and weight have been reported for adolescents with successive pregnancies (124, 125). In a prospective study of pregnant adolescent girls enrolled in the Camden Study, maternal growth during pregnancy was prevalent and was associated with increased gestational weight gain (126). Certainly, the nutritional needs of the adolescent who is still growing must be considered as well as the nutritional needs of the developing fetus.

As reviewed by Lenders and associates (127), adolescents have inadequate diets, and they lack adequate knowledge of appropriate nutrition during pregnancy. The studies discussed in this paragraph examined the energy intakes and dietary quality of pregnant adolescents and the fetal outcomes (128–130). In the Camden study that enrolled adolescents, Scholl (130) reported that high levels of ferritin in the third trimester were associated with extremely preterm deliveries and maternal infection. In pregnant adolescents in Guam, inadequate consumption of nutrients, specifically calcium, folate, vitamin E, magnesium, and iron, were reported (128). It is possible that pregnant adolescents compete with the developing fetuses for certain nutrients, and the growth of each may be hindered (119). Bone development is one such example. Bone loss in pregnant adolescent girls was greater than in grown women, but the amount of bone loss was consistent with the amount needed for fetal mineralization and the amount needed for continued maternal skeletal growth (131). Chang and colleagues (129) evaluated the effect of maternal dairy intake on fetal femur development in infants born to African-American adolescents 13 to 18 years of age. Consumption of less than two servings of dairy products daily was negatively related to fetal femur growth (129).

Social factors have been associated with poor birth outcomes (4, 132). These include poverty, low education, unmarried status, crowding, drug use, and inadequate prenatal care. Pregnant adolescent girls appear to have slightly lower perceived quality of life (133). Depression is common among pregnant and postpartum adolescents; in one study (134), 42% of pregnant adolescents aged 12 to 18 years reported depressive symptoms. Stress and social support appeared to be important mediators of this condition (134). It is clear that both the nutritional needs and other important social factors need to be addressed in the pregnant adolescent. A protocol for assessing and managing a normal adolescent pregnancy has been developed to include many of these issues (135).

Other diseases that during adolescence occur are not discussed here. The reader is referred to Chapter 76 for a discussion of inflammatory bowel diseases, Chapter 77 for celiac disease, and Chapter 65 for information on juvenile diabetes mellitus.

SUMMARY

Adolescent growth affects the energy requirements and nutritional needs during the adolescent years. Increased energy intake is needed; however, many adolescents consume an intake that is beyond their needs. The result is obesity during adolescence that may result in the development of typically adult-onset diseases. Poor nutritional status during adolescence can be related to adult disease.

Adolescence is an important time, in that behaviors learned at this age may translate into adulthood. In addition, the incidence of adult disease such as type 2 diabetes, seen in adolescents, is a compelling reason to incorporate healthy dietary and physical activity practices in our youth. Maintenance of body weight and composition is highly important in terms of health consequences for children. Many social, political, economic, and environmental changes have occurred in the past few decades that have made our society conducive to overweight and the undesirable future health consequences for children and adolescents. As stated by St-Onge and colleagues (136), certainly it is "imperative that interventions occur early in childhood and adolescence in an attempt to prevent or reverse the possible adverse health effects of overweight and poor eating habits." In addition, the health consequences of inadequate intake of micronutrients (calcium and others) give an indication that these factors deserve equal intervention.

REFERENCES

1. National Research Council and Institute of Medicine. Adolescent development and the biology of puberty: summary of a workshop on new research. In: Kipke M, ed. Forum on Adolescence. Washington, DC: National Academy Press, 1999.

2. Food and Nutrition Board, Institute of Medicine. Energy, Carbohydrate, Fiber, Fat, Fatty Acids, Cholesterol, Protein, and Amino Acids. Washington, DC: National Academy Press, 2002.

3. Tanner JM. Growth at Adolescence. 2nd ed. Oxford: Blackwell Scientific Publications, 1972.

4. American Academy of Pediatrics. Pediatrics 1999;103:516–20.

5. Roche AF, Davila GH. Pediatrics 1972;50:874–80.

6. Allen KM, Thombs D, Mahoney CA et al. J Sch Health 1993;63:176–81.

7. Baumgartner RN, Roche AF, Himes JH. Am J Clin Nutr 1986;43:711–22.

8. Haschke F. Body composition during adolescence. In: Body Composition Measurements in Infants and Children: Report of the 98th Ross Conference on Pediatric Research. Columbus, OH: Ross Laboratories, 1989:76–83.

9. Livingstone MB, Coward WA, Prentice AM et al. Am J Clin Nutr 1992;56:343–52.

10. Wong WW. J Am Coll Nutr 1994;13:332–7.

11. Food and Agriculture Organization/World Health Organization/United Nations University (FAO/WHO/UNU). Energy and Protein Requirements. Report of a Joint FAO/WHO/UNU Expert Consultation. Technical Report Series No. 724. Geneva: World Health Organization, 1985.

12. Torun B, Davies PSW, Livingstone MBE et al. Eur J Clin Nutr 1998;50:S37.

13. Troiano RP, Briefel RR, Carroll MD et al. Am J Clin Nutr 2000;72:1343S–53S.

14. French SA, Lin BH, Guthrie JF. J Am Diet Assoc 2003;103:1326–31.

15. Rampersaud GC, Bailey LB, Kauwell GP. J Am Diet Assoc 2003;103:97–100.

16. Kubik MY, Lytle LA, Hannan PH et al. Am J Public Health 2033;93:1168–73.

17. Xie B, Gilliland FD, Li YF et al. Prev Med 2003;36:30–40.

18. Neumark-Sztainer D, Story M, Resnick MD et al. Prev Med 1996;25:497–505.

19. Videon TM, Manning CK. J Adolesc Health 2003;32:365–73.

20. Berkey CS, Rockett HRH, Gillman MW et al. Int J Obes 2003;27:1258–66.

21. Lowry R, Galuska DA, Fulton JE et al. J Adolesc Health 2002:31:133–44.

22. Shannon C, Story M, Fulkerson JA et al. J Sch Health 2002;72:229–34.

23. Teegarden D, Proulx WR, Martin BR et al. J Bone Miner Res 1995;10:711–5.

24. Abrams SA, O'Brien KO, Stuff JE. J Clin Endocrinol Metab 1996;81:2017–20.

25. Lee WT, Leung SS, Wang SH et al. Am J Clin Nutr 1994;60:744–50.

26. Dibba B, Prentice A, Ceesay M et al. Am J Clin Nutr 2000;71:544–9.

27. Lloyd T, Andon MB, Rollings N et al. JAMA 1993;270:841–4.

28. Bonjour JP, Carrie AL, Ferrari S et al. J Clin Invest 1997;99:1287–94.

29. Dibba B, Prentice A, Ceesay M et al. Am J Clin Nutr 2002;76:681–6.

30. Chan GM. Am J Dis Child 1991;145:631–4.

31. Sandler RB, Slemenda CW, LaPorte RE et al. Am J Clin Nutr 1985;42:270–4.

32. Rozen GS, Rennert G, Dodiuk-Gad RP et al. Am J Clin Nutr 2003;78:993–8.

33. Food and Nutrition Board, Institute of Medicine. Calcium. In: Dietary Reference Intakes for Calcium, Phosphorus, Magnesium,

Vitamin D and Fluoride. Washington, DC: National Academy Press, 1997:71–145.

34. Subcommittee on the Tenth Edition of the RDAs. Recommended Dietary Allowances. 10th ed. Washington, DC: National Academy Press, 1989.

35. Subar AF, Krebs-Smith SM, Cook A et al. Pediatrics 1998;102: 913–23.

36. Looker AC, Dallman PR, Carroll MD et al. JAMA 1997;277: 973–6.

37. Yip R. MMWR 1998;47:1–29.

38. Hepner R. Nutrient Requirements in Adolescence. Cambridge, MA: MIT Press, 1976.

39. Food and Nutrition Board, Institute of Medicine. Iron. In: Dietary Reference Intakes for Vitamin A, Vitamin K, Arsenic, Boron, Chromium, Copper, Iodine, Iron, Manganese, Molydbenum, Nickel, Silicon, Vanadium and Zinc. Washington, DC: National Academy Press, 2000:290–393.

40. Woodhead JC, Drulis JM, Nelson SE et al. Pediatr Res 1991; 29:435–9.

41. Brown RT, McIntosh SM, Seabolt VR et al. J Adolesc Health Care 1985;6:349–52.

42. Nickerson HJ, Holubets MC, Weiler BR et al. J Pediatr 1989; 114:657–63.

43. Prasad AS, Miale A, Farid Z et al. J Lab Clin Med 1963;61: 537–49.

44. Prasad AS. Metabolism of zinc and its deficiency in human subjects. In: Prasad AS, ed. Zinc Metabolism. Springfield, IL: Charles C Thomas, 1966:250–303.

45. Prasad AS. Am J Clin Nutr 1991;53:403–12.

46. Aggett PJ. J Inherit Metab Dis 1983;6[Suppl 1]:39–43.

47. Food and Nutrition Board, Institute of Medicine. Vitamin A. In: Dietary Reference Intakes for Vitamin A, Vitamin K, Arsenic, Boron, Chromium, Copper, Iodine, Iron, Manganese, Molydbenum, Nickel, Silicon, Vanadium and Zinc. Washington, DC: National Academy Press, 2000:82–161.

48. Food and Nutrition Board, Institute of Medicine. Vitamin K. In: Dietary Reference Intakes for Vitamin A, Vitamin K, Arsenic, Boron, Chromium, Copper, Iodine, Iron, Manganese, Molydbenum, Nickel, Silicon, Vanadium and Zinc. Washington, DC: National Academy Press, 2000:161–98.

49. Food and Nutrition Board, Institute of Medicine. Vitamin E. In: Dietary Reference Intakes for Vitamin C, Vitamin E, Selenium, and Carotenoids. Washington, DC: National Academy Press, 2000:186–324.

50. Food and Nutrition Board, Institute of Medicine. Vitamin D. In: Calcium, Phosphorus, Magnesium, Vitamin D, and Fluoride. Washington, DC: National Academy Press, 1997:250–87.

51. Aksnes L, Aarskog D. J Clin Endocrinol Metab 1982;55: 94–101.

52. Food and Nutrition Board, Institute of Medicine. Riboflavin. In: Thiamin, Riboflavin, Niacin, Vitamin B_6, Folate, Vitamin B_{12}, Pantothenic Acid, Biotin and Choline. Washington, DC: National Academy Press, 1998:87–122.

53. Food and Nutrition Board, Institute of Medicine. Niacin. In: Thiamin, Riboflavin, Niacin, Vitamin B_6, Folate, Vitamin B_{12}, Pantothenic Acid, Biotin and Choline. Washington, DC: National Academy Press, 1998:123–49.

54. Food and Nutrition Board, Institute of Medicine. Vitamin B_6. In: Thiamin, Riboflavin, Niacin, Vitamin B_6, Folate, Vitamin B_{12}, Pantothenic Acid, Biotin and Choline. Washington, DC: National Academy Press, 1998:150–95.

55. Food and Nutrition Board, Institute of Medicine. Folate. In: Thiamin, Riboflavin, Niacin, Vitamin B_6, Folate, Vitamin B_{12}, Pantothenic Acid, Biotin and Choline. Washington, DC: National Academy Press, 1998:196–305.

56. Food and Nutrition Board, Institute of Medicine. Vitamin B_{12}. In: Thiamin, Riboflavin, Niacin, Vitamin B_6, Folate, Vitamin B_{12}, Pantothenic Acid, Biotin and Choline. Washington, DC: National Academy Press, 1998:306–57.

57. Food and Nutrition Board, Institute of Medicine. Vitamin C. In: Dietary Reference Intakes for Vitamin C, Vitamin E, Selenium, and Carotenoids. Washington, DC: National Academy Press, 2000:95–185.

58. Chang SJ, Hsiao LJ, Hsuen SY. J Nutr 2003;133:3191–4.

59. Keizer SE, Gibson RS, O'Connor DL. Am J Clin Nutr 1995;62: 377–84.

60. Ogden CL, Flegal KM, Carroll MD et al. JAMA 2002;288: 1728–32.

61. Whitaker RC, Wright JA, Pepe MS et al. N Engl J Med 1997; 337:869–73.

62. Guo SS, Huang C, Maynard LM et al. Int J Obes Relat Metab Disord 2000;24:1628–35.

63. Srinivasan SR, Myers L, Berenson GS. Diabetes 2002;51:204–9.

64. Centers for Disease Control and Prevention. Diabetes Care 2000;23:1278–83.

65. Gillman MW, Rifas-Shiman S, Berkey CS et al. Pediatrics 2003;111:E221–6.

66. Berenson GS. Am J Cardiol 2002;90:3L–7L.

67. Freedman DS, Dietz WH, Tang R et al. Int J Obes Relat Metab Disord 2004;28:159–66.

68. Kieltyka L, Urbina EM, Tang R et al. Atherosclerosis 2003;170: 125–30.

69. Li S, Chen W, Srinivasan SR et al. JAMA 2003;290:2271–6.

70. Nicklas TA, Yang SJ, Baranowski T et al. Am J Prev Med 2003; 25:9–16.

71. Raitakar IT, Juonala M, Kahonen M et al. JAMA 2003;290: 2277–83.

72. US Department of Agriculture, US Department of Health and Human Services. 5th ed. Washington, DC: US Government Printing Office, 2000.

73. Kimm SYS, Glynn NW, Kriska AM et al. N Engl J Med 2002;347:709–15.

74. United States, Department of Health and Human Services (USDHHS), Public Health Service. MMWR 1997;46:1.

75. Larsen RG, McMurray RG, Popking BM. Pediatrics 2000;105: E83.

76. Sallis JF, Hovell MF, Hofstetter CR et al. Soc Sci Med 1992;34: 25–32.

77. Andersen RE, Crespo, CJ, Bartlett, SJ et al. JAMA 1998;279: 938.

78. Berkowitz, RI, Agras WS, Korner AF et al. J Pediatr 1985;106: 734.

79. Eck LH, Klesges RC, Hanson CL et al. Int J Obes 1992;16:71.

80. Nader PR, Stone EJ, Lytle LA et al. Arch Pediatr Adolesc Med 1999;153:695–704.

81. Pate RR, Heath GW, Dowda M et al. Am J Public Health 1996; 86:1577–81.

82. Lloyd T, Chinchilli VM, Rollings N et al. Am J Clin Nutr 1998;67:624–30.

83. King AC, Blair SN, Bild DE et al. Med Sci Sports Exerc 1992; 24:221S–36S.

84. Blair SN, Kampert JB, Kohl HW et al. JAMA 1996;276:204–10.

85. King AC. Med Sci Sports Exerc 1994;26:1405–12.

86. King AC, Jeffery RW, Fridinger F et al. Health Educ Q 1995;22:499–511.

87. Ponton LE. Disordered eating. In: DiClemente RJ, Hansen WB, Ponton LE, eds. Handbook of Adolescent Health Risk Behavior. New York: Plenum Press, 1996:83–108.

88. Archibald AB, Graber JA, Brooks-Gunn J. J Res Adolesc 1999; 9:395–415.

89. Halmi K. Psychosomatics 1984;24:111–29.

90. Humphrey LL. J Am Acad Child Adolesc Psychiatry 1987;26: 248–55.

91. Humphrey LL. J Am Acad Child Adolesc Psychiatry 1988;27: 544–551.

92. Leung F, Schwartzman A, Steiger H. Int J Eat Disord 1996;20: 367–75.

93. Graber JA, Brooks-Gunn J, Paikoff RL et al. Dev Psychol 1994; 30:823–34.

94. Lewinsohn P, Seeley J, Moerk K et al. Int J Eat Disord 2002;32: 426–40.

95. Kann L, Warren CW, Harris WA et al. MMWR CDC Surveill Summ 1995;44:1–56.

96. Thombs DL, Mahoney CA, McLaughlin ML. J Nutr Educ 1998;30:107–13.

97. French SA, Jeffery RW. Health Psychol 1994;13:195–212.

98. Leon GR, Perry CL, Mangelsdorf C et al. J Youth Adolesc 1989;18:273–82.

99. Rosen JC, Gross J. Health Psychol 1987;6:131–47.

100. Gortmaker SL, Must A, Perrin JH et al. N Engl J Med 1993; 329:1008–12.

101. Allen KM, Thombs D, Mahoney CA et al. J Sch Health 1993; 63:176–81.

102. Koff E, Rierdan J, Stuggs M. et al. J Early Adolesc 1990;10: 56–8.

103. Brooks-Gunn, Petersen AC, eds. Girls at Puberty: Biological and Psychosocial Perspectives. New York: Plenum Press: 127–154.

104. Adami G, Gandolfo P, Campostano A. Int J Eat Disord 1998; 24:299–306.

105. Geller J, Johnston C, Madsen K. Cogn Ther Res 1997;21:5–24.

106. Whadden T, Brown G, Foster G. Int J Eat Disord 1991;10: 407–14.

107. Hamilton BE, Sutton PD, Ventura SJ. Natl Vital Stat Rep 2003;51:1–94.

108. MacDorman MF, Minino AM, Strobino DM et al. Pediatrics 2002;110:1037–52.

109. McAnarney ER. Am J Dis Child 1987;141:1053–59.

110. Adelson PL, Frommer MS, Pym MA et al. Am J Public Health 1992;16:238–44.

111. Cooper LG, Leland NL, Alexander G. Soc Biol 1995;42:22–35.

112. Chandra PC, Schiavello HJ, Ravi B et al. Int J Gynecol Obstet 2002;79:117–23.

113. Elfenbein DS, Felice ME. Pediatr Clin North Am 2003;50: 781–800.

114. Chang SC, O'Brien KO, Nathanson MS et al. J Pediatr 2003;143:250–7.

115. Chang SC, O'Brien KO, Nathanson MS et al. J Nutr 2003;133:2348–55.

116. Mahfouz AAR, El-Said MM, Al-Erian RAG et al. Eur J Obstet Gynecol 1995;59:17–20.

117. Quinlivan JA, Box H, Evans SF. Lancet 2003;361:893–900.

118. Wahl R. Pediatr Ann 1999;28:107–1.

119. Gutierrez Y, King JC. Pediatr Ann 1993;22:99–108.

120. Institute of Medicine, National Academy of Sciences. Nutrition during Pregnancy. Washington, DC: National Academy Press, 1990.

121. Beal VA. Am J Clin Nutr 1981;34[Suppl]:691–696.

122. Frischanco AR, Matos J, Leonard WR et al. Am J Phys Anthropol 1985;66:247–61.

123. Garn SM, Petzold AS. Am J Dis Child 1983;137:365–8.

124. Garn SM, Lavelle M, Pesick SD et al. Am J Dis Child 1984;138: 32–4.

125. Sukanich AC, Rogers KD, McDonald HM. Pediatrics 1986;78: 31–6.

126. Scholl TO, Hediger ML, Cronk CE et al. Horm Res 1993; 39[Suppl 3]:59–67.

127. Lenders CM, McElrath TF, Scholl TO. Curr Opin Pediatr 2000;12:291–6.

128. Pobocik RS, Benavente JC, Boudreau NS et al. J Am Diet Assoc 2003;103:611–4.

129. Chang SC, O'Brien KO, Nathanson MS et al. Am J Clin Nutr 2003;77:1248–54.

130. Scholl TO. Obstet Gynecol 1998;92:161–6.

131. Sowers MF, Scholl T, Harris L et al. Obstet Gynecol 2000;96: 189–93.

132. McAnarney ER, Hendee WR. JAMA 1982;262:74–77.

133. Drescher KM, Monga M, William P et al. Am J Obstet Gynecol 2003;188:1231–3.

134. Barnet B, Joffe A, Duggan AK et al. Arch Pediatr Adolesc Med 1996;150:64–9.

135. Rees JM, Lederman SA. Adolesc Med State Art Rev 1992;3: 439–57.

136. St-Onge MP, Keller KL, Heymsfield SB. Am J Clin Nutr 2003; 78:1068–73.

53 ADULTHOOD[1]
DOUGLAS C. HEIMBURGER

DIETARY REFERENCE INTAKES 830
    Defining Needs and Avoiding Toxicities 830
    Toward Optimizing Health 830
MALNUTRITION 830
    Distinguishing Malnutrition from Disease 830
    Protein-Energy Malnutrition 832
    Micronutrient Malnutrition 834
NUTRITIONAL ASSESSMENT 835
    Nutritional History 835
    Physical Examination 835
    Laboratory Studies 835
    Integrated Nutritional Assessment Scores 840
    Functional Assessment .841

DIETARY REFERENCE INTAKES

Defining Needs and Avoiding Toxicities

The current US and Canadian standards for adequate intakes (AIs) of healthy persons by age and gender of both macronutrients and micronutrients have been developed and published by the Food and Nutrition Board, Institute of Medicine, as dietary reference intakes (DRIs) in a series of volumes beginning in 1997 (1–5). Like the 1989 report on recommended dietary allowances (RDAs) (6), the DRIs are reference values that apply to the healthy general population. Unlike earlier reports that specified only RDAs, the DRIs also contain estimated average requirements (EARs), AIs, and tolerable upper intake levels (ULs). The EAR is the nutrient intake estimated to meet the requirement as defined by a specific indicator in 50% of individuals. The EAR serves as a basis for establishing the RDA if data are sufficient to set it at two standard deviations above the EAR. Similar to the goal of the older RDAs, this is the estimated daily nutrient intake sufficient to meet the requirements of nearly all (97–98%) the persons considered. The AI is nutrient intake that

appears to sustain a defined nutritional state; it exceeds the EAR, and in some cases the RDA, for the nutrient. The UL is the maximum level of intake that is unlikely to incur a risk of adverse health effects; it is established when sufficient data are available. The DRIs for men and women (19 years or older) published to date, together with the criteria (e.g., methods, rationale) used for developing them, are compared with the 1989 RDAs in Table 53.1. Appendix Tables A-2-a through A-2-h contain key graphics, summary text, and all the DRIs and ULs published to date for all nutrients by age and gender.

Toward Optimizing Health

Previous editions of the RDAs focused only on dietary intakes required to prevent deficiencies. By contrast, the new DRI volumes incorporate many data reviewing pertinent literature on levels of intake that may promote long-term health and prevent diseases. This broadened scope is most relevant for antioxidant nutrients, energy, lipids, cholesterol, dietary fiber, calcium, and folate because substantial evidence has emerged in recent years on the effects of varying intakes of these nutrients on risks for heart disease, cancer, obesity, osteoporosis, congenital neural tube defects, and other conditions. Choline is listed as an essential nutrient for the first time (2). The DRIs for energy are adjusted for weight, height, age, gender, and physical activity level to assist in achieving and maintaining appropriate body weights, of relevance to the increasing prevalence of obesity. Whereas the 1989 RDAs suggested lower calcium requirements for adults than for adolescents, the DRIs recommend higher levels for elderly persons than for younger adults, with a view to maintaining optimal bone density. Further details on the evidence supporting these health effects are provided in the chapters covering the respective nutrients.

MALNUTRITION[2]

Distinguishing Malnutrition from Disease

One of the principal challenges that faces nutrition practitioners is to distinguish underlying disease from malnutrition and to separate their effects on patient outcome. It is

---

[1]**Abbreviations: AI,** adequate intake; **BMI,** body mass index; **BUN,** blood urea nitrogen; **DRI,** dietary reference intake; **EAR,** estimated average requirement; **INI,** Instant Nutritional Index; **LOM,** Likelihood of Malnutrition; **PEM,** protein-energy malnutrition; **RDA,** recommended dietary allowance; **SGA,** Subjective Global Assessment; **TLC,** total lymphocyte count; **UL,** tolerable upper intake level; **UNA,** urinary nitrogen appearance; **UUN,** urinary urea nitrogen; **WBC,** white blood cell.

[2] This section was adapted, with permission, from Heimburger DC, Weinsier RL. Handbook of Clinical Nutrition. 3rd ed. St. Louis: Mosby, 1997; and Weinsier RL, Heimburger DC. Am J Clin Nutr 1997;66:1063–4.

TABLE 53.1. RECOMMENDED DIETARY ALLOWANCES FOR ADULTS: COMPARISON OF 1989 VALUES AND DIETARY REFERENCE INTAKES (1997–2002)[a]

NUTRIENT	1989 RDA (REFERENCE 6)		DRI RDA (REFERENCES 1–5)		DRI CRITERION
	MEN	WOMEN	MEN	WOMEN	
Energy (kcal)	AEA[b] 2,300–2,900	AEA[b] 1,900–2,200	Wide ranges of EER[b] based on weight, height, age, gender, and PAL[b]		Doubly labeled water studies
Carbohydrate (g)	≥250 (>50% kcal)	≥250 (>50% kcal)	130 (AMDR 45–65% kcal)	130 (AMDR 45–65% kcal)	Average minimum amount of glucose used by the brain
Dietary fiber (g)	None	None	AI[b] 38–30	AI[b] 25–21	Coronary heart disease protection
Total fat (% of total calories)	≤30%	≤30%	20–35%	20–35%	AMDR[b]
n-6 Polyunsaturated fatty acids (g)	None	None	AI[b] 17–14	AI[b] 12–11	Median population intakes
n-3 Polyunsaturated fatty acids (g)	None	None	AI[b] 1.6	AI[b] 1.1	Median population intakes
Saturated fat (% of total calories)	≤10%	≤10%	None	None	No absolute requirement for saturated fatty acids
Protein and amino acids (g)	58–63 (0.8 g/kg)	46–50 (0.8 g/kg)	56 (AMDR 10–35% kcal)	46 (AMDR 10–35% kcal)	Nitrogen equilibrium
Vitamin A (μg RAE)	1,000	800	900	700	Adequate vitamin A stores
Thiamin (mg)	1.5–1.2	1.1–1.0	1.2	1.1	Biochemical measures
Riboflavin (mg)	1.7–1.4	1.3–1.2	1.3	1.1	Biochemical measures
Niacin (mg)	19–15	15–13	16	14	Urinary excretion of niacin metabolites
Vitamin B_6 (mg)	2.0	1.6	1.3–1.7	1.3–1.5	Plasma pyridoxal phosphate
Vitamin B_{12} (μg)	2.0	2.0	2.4	2.4	Serum vitamin B_{12}, maintenance of hematologic status
Folate (μg DFE[b])	200	180	400	400	Plasma and red blood cell folate, plasma homocysteine
Vitamin C (mg)	60	60	90	75	Antioxidant protection
Vitamin E (mg)	10	8	15	15	Antioxidant protection (prevent peroxide-induced hemolysis)
Vitamin D (μg)	10–5	10–5	AI[b] 5–15	AI[b] 5–15	Serum 25(OH) vitamin D
Vitamin K (μg)	70–80	60–65	AI[b] 120	AI[b] 90	Intakes of health persons
Calcium (mg)	1,200–800	1,200–800	AI[b] 1,000–1,200	AI[b] 1,000–1,200	Calcium retention and balance, and bone mineral density
Chromium (μg)	ESAI[b] 50–200	ESAI[b] 50–200	AI[b] 35–30	AI[b] 25–20	Intakes of health persons
Copper (μg)	ESAI[b] 1,500–3,000	ESAI[b] 1,500–3,000	900	900	Human depletion/repletion studies
Iron (mg)	10	15–10	8	18–8	Factorial analysis
Magnesium (mg)	350	280	400–420	310–320	Magnesium balance, decreased absorption with aging
Phosphorus (mg)	1,200–800	1,200–800	700	700	Serum inorganic phosphate
Selenium (μg)	70	55	55	55	Antioxidant protection (maximum glutathione peroxidase synthesis)
Zinc (mg)	15	12	11	8	Factorial analysis

DRI, dietary reference intake.

[a] When listed as ranges, values for younger adults precede the hyphens, and those for older adults follow them.

[b] Values listed are recommended dietary allowances (RDAs) except where noted as AI (adequate intake), AEA (average energy allowance), EER (estimated energy requirement), PAL (physical activity level), AMDR (acceptable macronutrient distribution range), ESAI (estimated safe and adequate daily dietary intakes), RAE (retinol activity equivalents), or DFE (dietary folate equivalents).

widely appreciated that the findings associated with one can confound detection of the other, and it is generally acknowledged that the two interact in such a way that either improvement or deterioration in one influences the course of the other. The challenge lies in proving that in the presence of significant and life-threatening diseases such as those that result in hospitalization in Western countries, malnutrition independently worsens outcome, and nutritional support improves it.

The prevalence of malnutrition in hospitalized general medical and surgical patients was reported as 44% by Bistrian and colleagues in 1976 (7), 48% by Weinsier and associates in 1979 (8), 38% by Coats and colleagues in a 1988 cohort (9), and 45 to 62% by Naber and colleagues in 1997 (10). That these rates changed little over the years does not necessarily indicate a failure of physicians to prevent or to treat malnutrition. Rather, the rates may simply reflect the interrelatedness of disease and malnutrition, so patients admitted to a hospital with underlying disease either have a higher likelihood of malnutrition or their diseases share signs in common with malnutrition. The 1979 study by Weinsier and colleagues showed nutritional deterioration in 69% of patients during the course of hospitalization (8). In 1997, Naber and associates found no increase and, by some criteria, a decrease in the prevalence of malnutrition. This change is encouraging and may suggest that once patients are admitted, malnutrition is more likely to be recognized and clinicians are more likely to provide nutritional support.

Among patients admitted to US hospitals, it is likely that malnutrition and underlying disease states are inextricably interwoven, and only in unusual circumstances, such as self-imposed malnutrition as in anorexia nervosa, is malnutrition clearly separable from other diseases. One could ask whether nutrition specialists have furthered their cause by trying to separate the adverse effects of underlying disease from those of malnutrition. For instance, reduced levels of circulating proteins such as albumin do not necessarily indicate malnutrition, as many have been taught. Rather, they represent responses to the hypermetabolic, stressed state or liver failure, which, in turn, increases the risk of malnutrition (11). In fact, a consensus report on nutritional support in clinical practice concluded that all current nutrition assessment techniques are affected by illness and injury, and their validity as measures of nutritional risk (and hence clinical outcome) independently has not been proven (12).

Of greater importance than discerning the independent contribution of malnutrition to the hospital course is the potential impact of nutritional support on reducing medical complications, regardless of the origin. Advances in nutritional support techniques and education of health care professionals have contributed greatly to the quality of patient care, thus perhaps decreasing the likelihood of developing malnutrition during hospitalization. Reviews and consensus reports have summarized the impact of nutritional support in patients with various diseases (12, 13). Regardless of whether medical complications are a direct result of the malnutrition or the disease, evidence is mounting that nutritional support, in certain instances, is beneficial. Major challenges in demonstrating the impact of improved nutrition support on disease outcomes include the ethical difficulty of conducting randomized clinical studies with fed and non-fed groups and the variability of published studies in terms of numbers and types of patients and types and durations of nutritional support (12).

Protein-Energy Malnutrition

The two classic types of protein-energy malnutrition (PEM), marasmus and kwashiorkor, are mainly prevalent in developing countries. As the end-stage of starvation resulting from energy deprivation, there is little dispute that marasmus occurs in patients with severe chronic illnesses in developing countries. However, overlaps among the manifestations of acute and chronic diseases and those of kwashiorkor (e.g., hypoalbuminemia) have generated debate over whether kwashiorkor exists in developed countries, where food supplies are relatively stable and abundant (11). Clearly, hypoalbuminemia alone does not signify kwashiorkor, nor do low-protein diets alone cause it. However, when defined as hypoalbuminemia accompanied by other physical findings, such as poor skin integrity (pressure sores, skin breakdown, or failure of wounds to heal), edema unexplained by other conditions, and hair changes such as easy pluckability, we believe that the diagnosis of kwashiorkor is warranted. Likewise, although it is inappropriate to assign the diagnosis of marasmus to all patients with weight loss, it applies appropriately to patients who have starved sufficiently to consume virtually all available fat stores. Even more important than the labels we give them, however, is the selective approach required to manage the two: whereas the hypermetabolism and catabolism of kwashiorkor warrant aggressive feeding, the severe starvation of marasmus requires gradual refeeding to avoid life-threatening complications of the refeeding syndrome (14).

Table 53.2 compares the clinical and laboratory features of marasmus and kwashiorkor, and Table 53.3 offers minimum criteria for their diagnosis. Marasmus and kwashiorkor can occur singly or in combination, as marasmic kwashiorkor. Kwashiorkor can occur rapidly, whereas marasmus is the end result of a gradual wasting process that passes through stages of underweight and then mild, moderate, and severe cachexia.

Marasmus

Marasmus is the state in which virtually all available body fat stores have been exhausted because of starvation. Illnesses that produce marasmus in developed countries are chronic and indolent, such as cancer, acquired immunodeficiency

TABLE 53.2. COMPARISON OF MARASMUS AND KWASHIORKOR

	MARASMUS	KWASHIORKOR
Clinical setting	↓ Energy intake	↓ Protein intake during stress state
Time course to develop	Months or years	Weeks
Clinical features	Starved appearance	Well-nourished appearance
	Weight <80% standard for height	Easy hair pluckability
	Triceps skinfold <3 mm	Edema
	Midarm muscle circumference <15 cm	
Laboratory findings	Creatinine-height index <60% standard	Serum albumin <2.8 g/dL
		Total iron-binding capacity <200 μg/dL
		Lymphocytes <1,500/mm^3
		Anergy
Clinical course	Reasonably preserved responsiveness to shortterm stress	Infections
		Poor wound healing, decubitus ulcers, skin breakdown
Mortality	Low, unless related to underlying disease	High

From Heimburger DC, Weinsier RL. Handbook of Clinical Nutrition. 3rd ed. St. Louis: Mosby, 1997, with permission.

syndrome, and chronic pulmonary disease. Marasmus is easy to detect because of the patient's emaciated appearance. Diminished skinfold thickness reflects the loss of fat reserves; reduced arm muscle circumference with temporal and interosseous muscle wastage reflects the resorption of protein throughout the body, including vital organs such as the heart, liver, and kidneys.

The laboratory picture in marasmus is relatively unremarkable. Urinary creatinine excretion is low, reflecting the loss of muscle mass noted on clinical examination. Occasionally, the serum albumin level is reduced, but it does not usually drop below 2.8 g/dL in uncomplicated cases. Despite a morbid appearance, immunocompetence, wound healing, and the ability to handle short-term stress are reasonably well preserved.

Marasmus is a chronic, fairly well adapted form of starvation rather than an acute illness; it should be treated

TABLE 53.3. MINIMUM DIAGNOSTIC CRITERIA FOR MARASMUS AND KWASHIORKOR

MARASMUS	KWASHIORKOR[a]
Triceps skinfold <3 mm	Serum albumin <2.8 g/dL
Midarm muscle circumference <15 cm	At least one of the following:
	Poor wound healing, decubitus ulcers, or skin breakdown
	Easy hair pluckability[b]
	Edema

[a] The findings used to diagnose kwashiorkor must be unexplained by other causes.
[b] Tested by pulling from the top (not the sides or back) of the head a lock of hair *firmly* grasped between the thumb and forefinger. An average of three or more hairs removed easily and painlessly is considered abnormal hair pluckability.

From Heimburger DC, Weinsier RL. Handbook of Clinical Nutrition. 3rd ed. St. Louis: Mosby, 1997, with permission.

cautiously, in an attempt to reverse the downward trend gradually. Although nutritional support is necessary, overly aggressive repletion can result in severe, even life-threatening metabolic imbalances such as hypophosphatemia and cardiorespiratory failure. When possible, enteral nutritional support is preferred; treatment started slowly and increased gradually allows readaptation of metabolic and intestinal functions.

Kwashiorkor

Kwashiorkor (or hypoalbuminemic malnutrition [15], hypoalbuminemic stress syndrome, or protein dysmetabolism [11], as some prefer to call it) results mainly from acute, critical illnesses such as trauma and sepsis or from other illnesses typically seen in intensive care units. The physiologic stress produced by these illnesses increases protein and energy requirements at a time when intake is often limited. A now-classic situation in which kwashiorkor develops is in the acutely stressed patient who receives only 5% dextrose solutions for a period as short as 2 weeks. Although the etiologic mechanisms are not clear, the fact that the adaptive response of protein sparing normally seen in starvation is blocked by the stress state and by carbohydrate infusion may be an important factor.

In its early stages, the physical findings of kwashiorkor are few and subtle. Fat reserves and muscle mass may be normal or even above normal, giving the deceptive appearance of adequate nutrition. Signs that support the diagnosis of kwashiorkor include easy hair pluckability, edema, skin breakdown, and poor wound healing. The major sine qua non in the diagnosis is severe reduction of levels of serum proteins such as albumin (<2.8 g/dL) and transferrin (<150 mg/dL) or iron-binding capacity (<200 μg/dL). Cellular immune function is depressed, reflected by lymphopenia (<1500 lymphocytes/mm^3 in adults and older children) and lack of response to "recall" skin test antigens (anergy).

The prognosis of adult patients with full-blown kwashiorkor is guarded, even with aggressive nutritional support. Surgical wounds often dehisce (fail to heal), pressure sores develop, gastroparesis and diarrhea can occur with enteral feeding, the risk of gastrointestinal bleeding from stress ulcers is increased, host defenses are compromised, and death from overwhelming infection may occur despite antibiotic therapy. Unlike treatment in marasmus, aggressive feeding is often necessary to restore better metabolic balance rapidly.

Marasmic Kwashiorkor

Marasmic kwashiorkor, the combined form of PEM, can develop when the cachectic or marasmic patient is subjected to an acute stress such as surgery, trauma, or sepsis, superimposing kwashiorkor onto chronic starvation. If kwashiorkor predominates, vigorous nutritional therapy is indicated. It is important to determine the major component of PEM so the appropriate nutritional plan can be developed because the starved, unstressed hypometabolic patient is at risk for the complications of overfeeding, and the stressed, hypermetabolic patient is more likely to suffer the consequences of underfeeding.

Physiologic Characteristics of Hypometabolic and Hypermetabolic States

The metabolic characteristics and nutritional needs of hypermetabolic patients who are stressed from injury or infection are considerably different from those of hypometabolic patients who are unstressed but chronically starved. In both cases, nutritional support is important, but misjudgments in selecting the appropriate approach may have untoward consequences.

The hypometabolic patient is typified by the relatively unstressed but mildly catabolic and chronically starved person who, with time, will develop marasmus. The hypermetabolic patient stressed from injury or infection is catabolic (experiencing rapid breakdown of body mass) and is at high risk of developing kwashiorkor if nutritional needs are not met and/or the illness does not resolve quickly. As shown in Table 53.4, the two states are distinguished by differing alterations in metabolic rate, rates of protein breakdown (proteolysis), and rates of gluconeogenesis. These differences appear to be mediated largely by alterations in cytokines and counterregulatory hormones—tumor necrosis factor, interleukin-1, catecholamines (epinephrine and norepinephrine), glucagon, and cortisol—that are relatively reduced in hypometabolic patients and increased in hypermetabolic patients. Although insulin levels are also elevated in stressed patients, insulin resistance in the target tissues inhibits the exertion of insulin's anabolic actions.

TABLE 53.4. PHYSIOLOGIC CHARACTERISTICS OF HYPOMETABOLIC AND HYPERMETABOLIC STATES

PHYSIOLOGIC CHARACTERISTICS	HYPOMETABOLIC, NONSTRESSED PATIENT (CACHECTIC, MARASMIC)	HYPERMETABOLIC, STRESSED PATIENT (KWASHIORKOR RISK)
Cytokines, catecholamines, glucagon, cortisol, insulin	↓	↑
Metabolic rate	↓	↑
Proteolysis, gluconeogenesis	↓	↑
Urea excretion	↓	↑
Fat catabolism, fatty acid utilization	↑	↑
Adaptation to starvation	Normal	Abnormal

From Heimburger DC, Weinsier RL. Handbook of Clinical Nutrition. 3rd ed. St. Louis: Mosby, 1997, with permission.

Micronutrient Malnutrition

The same illnesses and reductions in nutrient intake that lead to PEM can produce deficiencies of vitamins and minerals. Deficiencies of nutrients having small body stores (such as the water-soluble vitamins) or lost through external secretions (such as zinc in diarrhea fluid or burn exudate) are probably quite common. If levels of these nutrients were measured more routinely, deficiencies would probably be diagnosed more frequently.

In my experience, deficiencies of vitamin C, folic acid, and zinc are common in hospitalized patients. For instance, signs of scurvy such as corkscrew hairs on the lower extremities are found fairly frequently in chronically ill and/or alcoholic patients hospitalized for acute illnesses. The diagnosis can be confirmed with plasma vitamin C levels. Folic acid intakes and blood levels are often less than optimal even among healthy persons; when illness, alcoholism, poverty, or poor dentition is present, deficiency is common. Low blood magnesium and zinc levels are also prevalent in patients with malabsorption syndromes such as inflammatory bowel disease. Patients with zinc deficiency often exhibit poor wound healing, decubitus ulcer formation, and impaired immunity. Thiamin deficiency is a common complication of alcoholism, but it may be seen less commonly than the foregoing deficiencies because of the frequent use of therapeutic doses of thiamin after patients are admitted for alcohol abuse.

Hypophosphatemia develops in hospitalized patients with remarkable frequency, generally because of rapid intracellular shifts of phosphate in patients with cachexia or alcoholism who are receiving intravenous glucose (especially in total parenteral nutrition) or taking antacids without phosphate replacement. The adverse clinical sequelae are numerous, and some, such as acute cardiopulmonary failure, can be life-threatening (see Chapter 10). Chapter 8 covers additional electrolyte abnormalities.

NUTRITIONAL ASSESSMENT

Because the interaction between illness and nutritional status is complex, many physical and laboratory findings are a reflection of underlying disease as well as of nutritional status. Therefore, the nutritional evaluation of a patient requires an integration of the history, physical examination, anthropometrics, and laboratory studies. This approach helps to detect nutritional problems while avoiding the conclusion that an isolated finding such as hypoalbuminemia, which can be caused by the underlying illness, indicates a nutritional problem when it may not. As with any medical discipline, clinical nutrition has a specialized history review, physical examination, and laboratory approach, all of which are important to a complete nutritional assessment.

Nutritional History

The nutritional history is directed toward identifying underlying mechanisms that put patients at risk of nutritional depletion or excess. These mechanisms, outlined in Table 53.5, include inadequate intake, impaired absorption, decreased utilization, increased losses, and increased requirements of nutrients. To focus the standard review of systems on nutritional issues, the symptoms and signs listed in Table 53.6 should be explored. Persons with the characteristics listed in Table 53.7 are at high risk of nutritional deficiencies.

Obtaining a dietary history is also an important part of nutritional assessment. Of the many types of diet histories (16), those most commonly used are the following: dietary recalls, generally covering 24 hours; food records, in which patients write down everything consumed during a 1- to 7-day period; and food frequency questionnaires, in which patients estimate how often they consume the foods and beverages identified on a list (17). Various computer programs permit rapid estimation of nutrient intake from these questionnaires or records (18, 19). Each method has advantages and disadvantages, such as labor intensity, cost, and accuracy. For instance, 24-hour dietary recall is the most feasible method of dietary assessment during an initial patient visit, but it may not reflect usual intakes because the particular 24-hour period is not representative of broader patterns and/or because of imprecision of memory. Multiday food records provide a reasonable way to obtain a qualitative estimate of nutrient intakes, especially in follow-up patient visits, but the act of recording intake invariably influences food choices, thus making these records potentially unrepresentative of broader patterns. Sometimes combinations of the various methods work best. For routine nutritional assessment in the clinic or hospital setting, a 24-hour dietary recall provides an adequate overview of the patient's dietary pattern to determine whether further detailed evaluation is necessary, and

3- or 4-day food records are helpful in follow-up outpatient visits. In the course of the entire medical history, however, it is important to elicit information concerning the areas noted in Tables 53.5 and 53.6 (e.g., presence of alcoholism, dental disease, drug use, malabsorption, weight loss) to identify potential nutrient deficiencies not elicited by the dietary recall.

Physical Examination

The nutritional physical examination begins with assessment of body mass, using anthropometric methods that provide information on muscle mass and fat reserves. Body mass index (BMI, weight in kilograms/height in meters squared) is the universal reference standard for normal body weight (20). Although BMI does not distinguish between lean and fat mass, adults with BMIs greater than 25 kg/m² are considered overweight, and those with BMIs greater than 30 are generally obese and at increased risk of comorbid conditions. Persons with BMIs lower than 18.5 are generally considered underweight, and BMIs lower than 15 indicate severe cachexia or marasmus. Physical examinations of muscle mass on the extremities, interosseous areas of the chest, and the temporal area of the face can indicate cachexia. The most practical measurements to distinguish muscle and fat mass are triceps skinfold and midarm muscle circumference.

Physical findings that suggest vitamin, mineral, and protein-energy deficiencies and excesses are outlined in Table 53.8. Most of them are not specific for individual nutrient deficiencies, and they must be integrated with the historical, anthropometric, and laboratory findings to make a diagnosis. For example, the finding of follicular hyperkeratosis isolated to the back of one's arms is a fairly common, normal finding. Conversely, if it is widespread in a person who consumes little fruits and vegetables and/or smokes regularly (increasing ascorbic acid requirements), vitamin C deficiency is a possible cause. Similarly, easily pluckable hair may be a consequence of recent chemotherapy, but in a hospitalized patient who has poorly healing surgical wounds and hypoalbuminemia, and who has not received chemotherapy, easily pluckable hair suggests kwashiorkor.

Laboratory Studies

Numerous laboratory tests used routinely in clinical medicine can yield valuable information about a patient's nutritional status if one adopts a slightly different approach to their interpretation. For example, abnormally low levels of serum albumin, low total iron-binding capacity, and anergy may each have a separate explanation. Collectively, and in the clinical setting of a hypermetabolic, acutely ill patient who is edematous and has easily pluckable hair and inadequate protein intake, they indicate kwashiorkor. Commonly used laboratory tests for assessment of nutritional status are outlined in Table 53.9. Because none of them is specific for

TABLE 53.5. NUTRITIONAL HISTORY SCREEN, BY MECHANISMS OF DEFICIENCY AND MEDICAL CONDITIONS

MECHANISM OF DEFICIENCY	HISTORY	CONDITIONS	DEFICIENCIES TO SUSPECT
Inadequate intake	Weight loss	AIDS, cancer, depression, gastrointestinal obstruction or dysmotility (e.g., gastroparesis), aging, neurologic disease, hyperemesis gravidarum	Calories, protein, multiple nutrients
	Alcohol abuse, substance abuse		Calories, protein, thiamin, niacin, folate, pyridoxine, riboflavin
	Avoidance of fruit, vegetables, grains		Vitamin C, thiamin, niacin, folate
	Avoidance of meat, dairy products, eggs		Protein, vitamin B_{12}
	Isolation, poverty, food idiosyncrasies	Poor dentition, gingivitis	Various nutrients
	Eating disorder	Anorexia or bulimia nervosa	Calories, protein, multiple nutrients
		Constipation, hemorrhoids, diverticulosis	Dietary fiber
		Hospitalization, NPO (nothing by mouth) status	Calories, protein, multiple nutrients
Inadequate digestion and/or absorption	Maldigestion (diarrhea, steatorrhea, weight loss)	Pancreatic insufficiency, cystic fibrosis, cholestasis, intestinal bacterial stasis or overgrowth	Calories, protein, vitamins A, D, K, calcium, magnesium, zinc
		Disaccharidase deficiency (e.g., lactase)	Calories, protein
	Malabsorption (diarrhea, steatorrhea, weight loss)	Short bowel syndrome, radiation enteritis, inflammatory bowel disease, Whipple's disease	Vitamins A, D, K, protein, calcium, magnesium, zinc
		AIDS, gluten enteropathy (celiac sprue), tropical sprue, intestinal lymphoma	Calories, protein, iron, various nutrients
		Parasites (fish tapeworm)	Iron, vitamin B_{12}
		Pernicious anemia	Vitamin B_{12}
		Surgery:	
		Gastrectomy	Vitamin B_{12}, iron, folate
		Intestinal resection	Vitamin B_{12}, iron, others as in malabsorption
	Drugs (antacids, anticonvulsants, cholestyramine, laxatives, neomycin, alcohol)		See Chapter 97
Decreased utilization, impaired metabolism		Chronic liver disease	Calories, protein, vitamins A, D, E, K, B_{12}, thiamin, folate, pyridoxine
		Chronic renal disease	Calories, vitamin D, water-soluble vitamins
		Inborn errors of metabolism	Various nutrients
	Drugs (corticosteroids, anticonvulsants, antimetabolites, oral contraceptives, isoniazid, alcohol)		See Chapter 97
Abnormal losses	Alcohol abuse		Magnesium, zinc
	Blood loss		Iron
	Centesis (ascitic, pleural fluid)		Protein
		Diabetes, uncontrolled	Calories (glycosuria)
	Diarrhea		Protein, zinc, magnesium, electrolytes
		Draining abscesses, wounds	Protein, zinc
		Protein-losing enteropathy	Protein
		Nephrotic syndrome	Protein, zinc
	Peritoneal or hemodialysis		Protein, water-soluble vitamins, zinc
Increased requirements	Fever		Calories
	Physiologic demands (infancy, adolescence, pregnancy, lactation)		Various nutrients
	Cigarette smoking		Vitamins C and E, folate, β-carotene
		Hyperthyroidism	Calories
		Surgery, trauma, burns, infection	Calories, protein, vitamin C, zinc
		Chronic lung disease	Calories

From Heimburger DC, Weinsier RL. Handbook of Clinical Nutrition. 3rd ed. St. Louis: Mosby, 1997, with permission.

TABLE 53.6. NUTRITIONAL REVIEW OF SYSTEMS

General
  Usual adult weight
  Current weight
  Prepubertal weight
  Maximum and minimum weights
  Weight 1 and 5 years ago
  Recent changes in weight (include time periods)
  Recent changes in appetite or food tolerance
  Presence of weakness, fatigue, fever, chills, night sweats
  Recent changes in sleep habits, daytime sleepiness
  Edema and/or abnormal swelling
Gastrointestinal tract
  Abdominal pain, nausea, vomiting
  Diarrhea (consistency, frequency, volume, color, presence of
    cramps, food particles, fat drops)
  Constipation or other changes in bowel habits
  Difficulty or pain with swallowing (solids versus liquids,
    intermittent versus continuous)
  Early satiety
  Indigestion or heartburn
  Food intolerance or preferences
  Oral lesions (aphthous ulcers, dental problems), sore tongue
    or gums
Neurologic
  Confusion or memory loss
  Difficulty with night vision
  Gait disturbance
  Loss of position sense
  Numbness, paresthesias, and/or weakness
Skin
  Rash or dryness of skin
  Hair loss, recent change in texture

Adapted from Newton J, Halsted CH. Clinical and functional assessment of adults. In Shils ME, Olson JA, Shike M et al., eds. Modern Nutrition in Health and Disease. 9th ed. Baltimore: Williams & Wilkins, 1999:897.

TABLE 53.7. THE HIGH-RISK PATIENT

Underweight (weight-for-height <80% of standard) and/or
  recent loss of 10% or more of usual body weight
Poor intake: anorexia, food avoidance (e.g., psychiatric
  condition), or "NPO" status (nothing allowed by mouth) for
  more than about 5 days
Protracted nutrient losses: malabsorption, enteric fistulas,
  draining abscesses or wounds, renal dialysis
Hypermetabolic states: sepsis, protracted fever, extensive
  trauma or burns
Long-term use of alcohol or drugs with antinutrient or
  catabolic properties: steroids, antimetabolites (e.g.,
  methotrexate), immunosuppressants, antitumor agents
Poverty, isolation, and/or advanced age

From Heimburger DC, Weinsier RL. Handbook of Clinical Nutrition. 3rd ed. St. Louis: Mosby, 1997, with permission.

a nutritional problem, tips are provided in the table to help avoid assigning nutritional significance to tests that may be abnormal as a result of nonnutritional conditions.

Assessment of Body Composition

The serum creatinine level reflects muscle mass to a certain extent, with values less than 0.6 mg/dL suggesting muscle wasting. Because the rate of formation of creatinine from creatine phosphate in skeletal muscle is constant, the amount of creatinine excreted in the urine each 24 hours also reflects skeletal muscle mass. However, it rarely yields information that cannot be obtained by physical examination. Dual-energy x-ray absorptiometry (DXA), which is now universally used to measure bone density, can also measure lean and fat mass when appropriate software is used. However, although this technique is a valuable research tool, its use to assess body composition for clinical purposes is rarely justified.

Assessment of Circulating ("Visceral") Proteins

The visceral compartment is composed of proteins that act as carriers, binders, and immunologically active proteins.

The serum proteins that may be used to assess nutritional status include albumin, total iron-binding capacity (or transferrin), thyroxine-binding prealbumin (or transthyretin), and retinol-binding protein. Because they have differing synthesis rates and half-lives (the half-life of albumin is about 21 days, whereas that of retinol-binding protein is closer to 12 hours), some of these proteins reflect changes in nutritional status more quickly than others.

Levels of circulating proteins are influenced by their rates of synthesis and catabolism, by "third spacing" (loss into interstitial spaces), and in some cases by external loss. Although adequate intake of calories and protein is necessary to achieve optimal circulating protein levels, the levels do not sensitively reflect protein intake. A drop in the serum level of, for instance, albumin or transferrin often accompanies significant physiologic stress, as from infection or injury, and is not necessarily an indication of malnutrition or poor intake. For example, a low serum albumin level in a burned patient with both hypermetabolism and increased dermal losses of protein may not indicate malnutrition. In contrast, adequate nutritional support of the patient's calorie and protein needs is critical for the return of circulating proteins to normal levels as the stress resolves. Thus, low values by themselves do not define malnutrition but often point toward an increased risk of malnutrition resulting from the hypermetabolic stress state. It is not unusual for protein levels to remain low despite aggressive nutritional support, as long as significant physiologic stress persists. However, if they do not rise after the underlying illness has resolved, the patient's protein and calorie needs should be reassessed to ensure that intake is sufficient.

Assessment of Protein Catabolic Rate Using Urinary Urea Nitrogen

Because urea is a major byproduct of protein catabolism, the amount of urea nitrogen excreted each day can be used to estimate the rate of protein catabolism, and to determine whether protein intake is adequate to offset it.

TABLE 53.8. PHYSICAL FINDINGS OF NUTRITIONAL DEFICIENCIES

CLINICAL FINDINGS	CONSIDER DEFICIENCY OF[a]	CONSIDER EXCESS OF	FREQUENCY[b]
Hair, nails			
Flag sign (transverse depigmentation of hair)	Protein		Rare
Easily pluckable hair	Protein		Common
Sparse hair	Protein, biotin, zinc	Vitamin A	Occasional
Corkscrew hairs and unemerged coiled hairs	Vitamin C		Common
Transverse ridging of nails	Protein		Occasional
Skin			
Scaling	Vitamin A, essential fatty acids, biotin Zinc (hyperpigmented)	Vitamin A	Occasional
Cellophane appearance	Protein		Occasional
Cracking (flaky paint or crazy pavement dermatosis)	Protein		Rare
Follicular hyperkeratosis	Vitamins A, C		Occasional
Petechiae (especially perifollicular)	Vitamin C		Occasional
Purpura	Vitamins C, K		Common
Pigmentation, scaling of sun-exposed areas	Niacin		Rare
Yellow pigmentation sparing sclerae (benign)		Carotene	Common
Poor wound healing, decubitus ulcers	Protein, vitamin C, zinc		Common
Eyes			
Papilledema		Vitamin A	Rare
Night blindness	Vitamin A		Rare
Perioral			
Angular stomatitis	Riboflavin, pyridoxine, niacin		Occasional
Cheilosis (dry, cracking, ulcerated lips)	Riboflavin, pyridoxine, niacin		Rare
Oral			
Atrophic lingual papillae (slick tongue)	Riboflavin, niacin, folate, vitamin B_{12}, protein, iron		Common
Glossitis (scarlet, raw tongue)	Riboflavin, niacin, pyridoxine, folate, vitamin B_{12}		Occasional
Hypogeusesthesia, hyposmia	Zinc		Occasional
Swollen, retracted, bleeding gums (if teeth present)	Vitamin C		Occasional
Bones, joints			
Beading of ribs, epiphyseal swelling, bowlegs	Vitamin D		Rare
Tenderness (subperiosteal hemorrhage in children)	Vitamin C		Rare
Neurologic			
Headache		Vitamin A	Rare
Drowsiness, lethargy, vomiting		Vitamins A, D	Rare
Dementia	Niacin, vitamin B_{12}, folate		Rare
Confabulation, disorientation	Thiamin (Korsakoff's psychosis)		Occasional
Ophthalmoplegia	Thiamin, phosphorus		Occasional
Peripheral neuropathy (e.g., weakness, paresthesias, ataxia, foot drop, and decreased tendon reflexes, fine tactile sense, vibratory sense, and position sense)	Thiamin, pyridoxine, vitamin B_{12}	Pyridoxine	Occasional
Tetany	Calcium, magnesium		Occasional
Other			
Parotid enlargement	Protein (consider also bulimia)		Occasional
Heart failure	Thiamin ("wet" beriberi), phosphorus		Occasional
Sudden heart failure, death	Vitamin C		Rare
Hepatomegaly	Protein	Vitamin A	Rare
Edema	Protein, thiamin		Common

[a] In this table, "protein deficiency" is used to signify kwashiorkor.
[b] These frequencies are an attempt to reflect our experience in the setting of a US medical practice. Findings common in other countries but virtually unseen in usual medical practice settings in the United States (e.g., xerophthalmia and endemic goiter) are not listed.

From Heimburger DC, Weinsier RL. Handbook of Clinical Nutrition. 3rd ed. St. Louis: Mosby, 1997, with permission.

TABLE 53.9. LABORATORY TESTS FOR NUTRITIONAL ASSESSMENT

Section A:

TEST (NORMAL VALUES)	NUTRITIONAL USE	CAUSES OF NORMAL VALUE DESPITE MALNUTRITION	OTHER CAUSES OF ABNORMAL VALUE

Serum albumin (3.5–5.5 g/dL)	2.8–3.5: Compromised protein status
	 <2.8: Possible kwashiorkor
	 Increasing value reflects positive protein balance
		Dehydration
		
		 Infusion of albumin, fresh frozen plasma, or whole blood
			LOW
			 Common:
			   Infection and other stress, especially with poor protein intake
			   Burns, trauma
			   Congestive heart failure
			   Fluid overload
			   Severe liver disease
			 Uncommon:
			   Nephrotic syndrome
			   Zinc deficiency
			   Bacterial stasis/ overgrowth of small intestine

Total iron-binding capacity (TIBC) 270–400 µg/dL	<200: Compromised protein status, possible kwashiorkor Increasing value reflects positive protein balance More labile than albumin	Iron deficiency	LOW Similar to albumin HIGH Iron deficiency
Prothrombin time <2 s beyond control value	Prolongation: Vitamin K deficiency		PROLONGED Anticoagulant therapy (warfarin) Severe liver disease

Serum creatinine 0.6–1.6 mg/dL	<0.6: Muscle wasting resulting from calorie deficiency
	 Reflects muscle mass
			HIGH
			 Despite muscle wasting:
			   Renal failure
			   Severe dehydration

24-h urinary creatinine 500–1,200 mg/d (standardized for height and sex)	Low value: Muscle wasting resulting from calorie deficiency	>24-h collection Decreasing serum creatinine	LOW Incomplete urine collection Increasing serum creatinine Neuromuscular wasting

Section B:

TEST (NORMAL VALUES)	NUTRITIONAL USE	OTHER CAUSES OF ABNORMAL VALUE

24-h urinary urea nitrogen (UUN) <5 g/d (depends on level of protein intake)	Determine level of catabolism (as long as protein intake is ≥10 g below calculated protein loss or <20 g total, but at least 100 g carbohydrate is provided)
	   5–10 g/d = mild catabolism or normal fed state
	   10–15 g/d = moderate catabolism
	   >15 g/d = severe catabolism
	 Estimate protein balance
	   Protein balance = protein intake – protein loss
	   where protein loss (protein catabolic rate) =
	     [24-h UUN (g) + 4] × 6.25
	 Adjustments required in burned patients and others with large nonurinary nitrogen losses and in patients with fluctuating BUN levels (e.g., renal failure)	

Blood urea nitrogen (BUN) 8–23 mg/dL	<8: Possibly inadequate protein intake
	 >12: Possibly adequate, even excessive, protein intake
	 If serum creatinine is normal, use BUN
	 If serum creatinine is elevated, use BUN/creatinine ratio
		LOW
		 Severe liver disease
		 Anabolic state
		 Syndrome of inappropriate antidiuretic hormone
		 HIGH
		 Despite poor protein intake:
		   Renal failure (use BUN/ creatinine ratio)
		   Congestive heart failure
		   Gastrointestinal hemorrhage

From Heimburger DC, Weinsier RL. Handbook of Clinical Nutrition. 3rd ed. St. Louis: Mosby, 1997, with permission.

Total protein loss and protein balance can be calculated from the urinary urea nitrogen (UUN) as follows:

$$\text{Protein catabolic rate (g/day)}$$
$$= [\text{24-hour UUN (g)} + 4] \times 6.25$$

The value of 4 g added to the UUN represents a liberal estimate of the unmeasured nitrogen lost in the urine (e.g., creatinine and uric acid) and in sweat, hair, skin, and feces. The factor 6.25 adjusts for the grams of protein represented by each gram of nitrogen. When protein intake is small (e.g., less than about 20 g/day), the equation indicates both the patient's protein requirement and the severity of the catabolic state (see Table 53.9). More substantial protein intakes can raise the UUN because some of the ingested or infused protein is catabolized and converted to UUN. Thus, at lower protein intakes the equation is useful for estimating requirements, and at higher protein intakes it is useful for assessing protein balance (the difference between intake and catabolism):

$$\text{Protein balance (g/day)}$$
$$= \text{Protein intake} - \text{Protein catabolic rate}$$

As noted in Table 53.9, changes in the concentration of blood urea nitrogen (BUN) or in body water content during the 24-hour period of urine collection can confound interpretation of the UUN. Misleading results are particularly likely in patients who are receiving intermittent renal dialysis and who have rapid changes in BUN during the UUN collection, as well as in patients undergoing diuresis. If changes in BUN and body weight (as a reflection of changes in fluid status) are determined from measurements taken at the beginning and the end of the urine collection, the UUN can be corrected with the calculation shown here. This calculation yields a more accurate estimation of the protein catabolic rate, called urinary nitrogen appearance (UNA), as follows:

$$\text{UNA (g)} = \text{UUN (g)} + \frac{(\Delta\text{BUN} \times 10)(W_m)(BW) + (\text{BUN}_m \times 10)(\Delta W)}{1000}$$

where . . .

ΔBUN = change in BUN (mg/dL) during the urine collection (final BUN minus initial BUN)

BUN_m = mean BUN (mg/dL) during the urine collection [(final BUN plus initial BUN)/2]

ΔW = change in weight (kg) during the urine collection (final weight minus initial weight)

W_m = mean weight (kg) during the urine collection [(final W plus initial W)/2]

BW = assumed body water as a proportion of body weight:
   normal value is 0.5 for women and 0.6 for men;
   subtract 0.05 for marked obesity or dehydration;
   add 0.05 for leanness or edema

To make a corrected calculation of the patient's rate of protein breakdown, the value for UNA is substituted for UUN in the original protein catabolic rate equation. Under most situations, the standard UUN calculation is reliable as long as both BUN and body water content are stable during the urine collection, even if they are abnormal. Under these circumstances, ΔBUN and ΔW equal zero, and UNA equals UUN.

Another common cause of a spuriously high UUN is gastrointestinal hemorrhage. Because no accurate way exists to correct for this condition in calculating the protein catabolic rate, UUN measurements should be postponed in patients with such hemorrhage.

Assessment of Protein Intake Using Blood Urea Nitrogen

As dietary protein intake increases, the BUN level generally rises, unless the patient is unusually anabolic and is using all available amino acids for protein synthesis. The converse is also true: BUN levels generally fall when protein intake is reduced. Thus, when the BUN is high and no other causes, such as renal insufficiency, dehydration, or gastrointestinal hemorrhage, are present, dietary protein intake is likely to be excessive. If the BUN is low (e.g., <8 mg/dL), it suggests low and possibly inadequate protein intake. Nondietary causes of low and high BUN levels are outlined in Table 53.9.

Assessment of Immune Status Using Total Lymphocyte Count

Derived arithmetically from the total white blood cell (WBC) and differential count (total lymphocyte count [TLC] = WBC × % lymphocytes), the TLC can reflect the immunocompromise associated with kwashiorkor. However, it is of little use in following the course of nutritional status because many medical conditions affect it and because of significant fluctuation in both total WBC and differential counts from day to day.

Assessment of Vitamin and Mineral Status

The use of laboratory tests to confirm suspected micronutrient deficiencies is desirable because the physical findings for these deficiencies are often equivocal and nonspecific. Low blood micronutrient levels can predate more serious clinical manifestations and may also indicate drug-nutrient interactions. Useful assays for micronutrient assessment are covered in the chapters on the respective nutrients.

Integrated Nutritional Assessment Scores

Various investigators have combined the parameters used in nutritional assessment to form quantitative scores reflecting nutritional status. Some of these scores were developed mainly for research purposes, and others have potential applicability to patient care. Weinsier and colleagues constructed a Likelihood of Malnutrition (LOM) score based on the following: body weight, triceps skinfold thickness, and midarm muscle circumference; serum folate, vitamin C, and albumin; and absolute lymphocyte count and hematocrit (8). The LOM suggested that 48% of medical patients were malnourished on hospital admission, 69% of patients hospitalized longer than 2 weeks demonstrated further decline in six nutritional parameters, and worsening of the LOM score was associated with longer hospitalization and increased mortality. Twelve years later, fewer admitted medical patients had a high LOM score, and patients had shorter hospital stays (9).

The Prognostic Nutritional Index, developed by Mullen and Buzby and their associates from serum albumin, serum transferrin, delayed hypersensitivity, and triceps skinfold measurements, correlated with postoperative complications and mortality (21, 22). The Instant Nutritional Index (INI) developed by Seltzer and colleagues identified available parameters intended to alert the practitioner to a more thorough nutritional assessment. In the INI, the serum albumin level and the absolute lymphocyte count correlated with the incidence of hospital infection (23, 24); a subsequent study added weight loss to the INI (25). Forse and Shizgal assessed the validity of seven parameters frequently used for nutritional assessment: weight for height, serum total protein and albumin level, midarm muscle area, triceps skinfold thickness, creatinine/height index, and hand grip strength (26). Weight for height correlated best with body cell mass (r = 0.82), whereas the creatinine/height index had the worst correlation (r = 0.37). All parameters had wide confidence intervals. Multiple linear regression predicted malnutrition with only 11% false-negative results but with 32% false-positive results. Finally, patients categorized as severely malnourished by a Nutrition Risk Index based on serum albumin and history of weight loss benefited from preoperative parenteral nutrition, whereas those with mild or borderline malnutrition did not (27).

Because these composite nutritional indices combine key elements of the history, physical examination, and laboratory values detailed earlier, they can be useful in nutritional assessment. However, like the parameters that comprise them, they correlate with, and are thus limited and potentially confounded by, the patient's underlying illness. They are best suited to comparisons of patient groups, such as in screening patients admitted to the hospital or in testing differences among groups cross-sectionally or longitudinally in research settings.

The Subjective Global Assessment (SGA) provides an integration of historical and physical data that allows the clinician to make a bedside assessment of nutritional status (28). The historical features include (a) weight change during the preceding 6 months and 2 weeks, (b) changes in dietary intake, (c) gastrointestinal symptoms, (d) functional capacity, and (e) the assumed metabolic demand of the underlying disease. Physical findings, rated on a four-point

scale, include loss of subcutaneous fat, muscle wasting in the quadriceps and deltoid muscles, and the presence of ankle and sacral edema and ascites. Laboratory values are not included. Patients are categorized as follows: A, well nourished; B, moderately (or suspected of being) malnourished; or C, severely malnourished. Weight loss, poor dietary intake, loss of subcutaneous tissue, and muscle wasting are weighted most heavily. Conversely, the presence of ascites, edema, or a large tumor mass reduces the significance of body weight. Patients fall into category B if they have had at least a 5% weight loss in the preceding 2 weeks, together with reduction in dietary intake and mild loss of subcutaneous tissue. Patients in category C demonstrate obvious physical signs of malnutrition with ongoing weight loss, an overall decline of at least 10% of their normal weight, and changes in the other parameters. Ottery adapted the SGA for use in outpatient settings, by using forms that are partially completed by the patient, and called it the Patient-Generated SGA (www.accc-cancer.org/publications/pgsga.pdf).

Functional Assessment

Investigators have shown some interest in measures of functional status that predict the downstream effects of nutritional aberrations. Among these is skeletal muscle function, which, in the alert and cooperative patient, can be assessed by testing grip strength with a hand dynamometer (29). Hand grip strength was found to be a sensitive predictor of complications in patients undergoing major abdominal surgery (30), especially when age- and sex-derived standards were used (31). Hill and Windsor also described a bedside technique in which the patient squeezes the clinician's index and middle fingers for at least 10 seconds. However, the determination of strength impairment, which is subjectively based on the patient's age, sex, and body habitus, makes this assessment questionably reproducible (32).

REFERENCES

1. Food and Nutrition Board, Institute of Medicine. Dietary Reference Intakes For Calcium, Phosphorus, Magnesium, Vitamin D, and Fluoride. Washington, DC: National Academy Press, 1999. (www.nap.edu/books/0309063507/html/index.html).
2. Food and Nutrition Board, Institute of Medicine. Dietary Reference Intakes For Thiamin, Riboflavin, Niacin, Vitamin B$_6$, Folate, Vitamin B$_{12}$, Pantothenic Acid, Biotin, and Choline. Washington, DC: National Academy Press, 2000. (www.nap.edu/books/0309065542/html/index.html).
3. Food and Nutrition Board, Institute of Medicine. Dietary Reference Intakes for Vitamin C, Vitamin E, Selenium, and Carotenoids. Washington, DC: National Academy Press, 2000. (www.nap.edu/books/0309069351/html/index.html).
4. Food and Nutrition Board, Institute of Medicine. Dietary Reference Intakes for Vitamin A, Vitamin K, Arsenic, Boron, Chromium, Copper, Iodine, Iron, Manganese, Molybdenum, Nickel, Silicon, Vanadium, and Zinc. Washington, DC: National Academy Press, 2002. (www.nap.edu/books/0309072794/html/index.html).

5. Food and Nutrition Board, Institute of Medicine. Dietary Reference Intakes for Energy, Carbohydrate, Fiber, Fat, Fatty Acids, Cholesterol, Protein, and Amino Acids (Macronutrients). Washington, DC: National Academy Press, 2002. (www.nap.edu/books/0309085373/html/index.html).

6. Food and Nutrition Board, Institute of Medicine. Recommended Dietary Allowances. 10th ed. Washington, DC: National Academy Press, 1989.

7. Bistrian BR, Blackburn GL, Hallowell E et al. J Am Med Assoc 1976;235:1567–70.

8. Weinsier RL, Hunker EM, Krumdieck CL et al. Am J Clin Nutr 1979;32:418–26.

9. Coats KG, Morgan SL, Bartolucci AA et al. J Am Diet Assoc 1993;93:27–33.

10. Naber THJ, Schermer T, de Bree A et al. Am J Clin Nutr 1997;66:1232–9.

11. Seres DS, Resurreccion LB. Nutr Clin Pract 2003;18:297–301.

12. Klein S, Kinney J, Jeejeebhoy K et al. JPEN J Parenter Enteral Nutr 1997;21:133–56.

13. Heyland DK, Dhaliwal R, Drover JW et al. JPEN J Parenter Enteral Nutr 2003;27:355–73.

14. Heimburger DC, Weinsier RL. Handbook of Clinical Nutrition. 3rd ed. St. Louis: Mosby, 1997.

15. Bistrian BR. Nutritional assessment. In: Goldman L, Ausiello D, eds. Cecil Textbook of Medicine. 22nd ed. Philadelphia: Elsevier, 2004:1312–5.

16. Kipnis V, Midthune D, Freedman L et al. Public Health Nutr 2002;5:915–23.

17. Cade J, Thompson R, Burley V et al. Public Health Nutr 2002;5:567–87.

18. Nutrition Analysis Tool. http://nat.crgq.com/.

19. USDA Interactive Healthy Eating Index. http://www.usda.gov/cnpp/ihei.html

20. Expert Panel on the Identification, Evaluation, and Treatment of Overweight in Adults. Am J Clin Nutr 1998;68:899–917.

21. Buzby GP, Mullen JL, Matthews DC et al. Am J Surg 1980;139:160–7.

22. Mullen JL, Buzby GP, Waldman MT et al. Surg Forum 1979;30:80–2.

23. Seltzer MH, Bastidas JA, Cooper DM et al. JPEN J Parenter Enteral Nutr 1979;3:157–9.

24. Seltzer MH, Fletcher HS, Slocum BA et al. JPEN J Parenter Enteral Nutr 1981;5:70–2.

25. Seltzer MH, Slocum BA, Cataldi-Betcher E et al. JPEN J Parenter Enteral Nutr 1982;6:218–21.

26. Forse RA, Shizgal HM. Surgery 1980;88:17–24.

27. Veterans Affairs Total Parenteral Nutrition Cooperative Study Group. N Engl J Med 1991;325:525–32.

28. Detsky AS, McLaughlin JR, Baker JP. JPEN J Parenter Enteral Nutr 1987;11:8–13.

29. Vaz M, Thangam S, Prabhu A et al. Br J Nutr 1996;76:9–15.

30. Klidjian AM, Archer TJ, Foster KJ et al. JPEN J Parenter Enteral Nutr 1982;6:119–21.

31. Webb AR, Newman LA, Taylor M et al. JPEN J Parenter Enteral Nutr 1989;13:30–3.

32. Hill GL, Windsor JA. Nutrition 1995;11[Suppl]:198–201.

54 THE ELDERLY[1]

CONNIE WATKINS BALES AND CHRISTINE SEEL RITCHIE

NUTRITIONAL NEEDS OF THE ELDERLY 843
   Current Nutritional Status in the Population 843
   Standards For Assessment of Dietary Adequacy:
     Dietary Reference Intakes 843
   Age-Related Determinants of Nutritional
     Requirements and Reported Status 844
NUTRITIONAL ASSESSMENT 853
   Dietary Assessment 853
   Biochemical Assessment 853
   Clinical and Anthropometric Assessments 854
   Nutrition Indices 854

As a result of the convergence of "successful aging" and declining birth rates in most developed countries, the proportion of the population that is elderly is at an all time high (13% in the United States) and growing steadily. By the year 2030, this "graying" effect will peak, with an estimated 20% of the population being elderly (>65 years of age). This same trend prevails worldwide; the global average life span has increased from 49.5 years in 1972 to more than 63 years at present. The elderly as a group have an increased susceptibility to a number of age-related chronic diseases that may be delayed or ameliorated by nutritional intervention (1), including cardiovascular disease (CVD), neurologic disease, hypertension, diabetes, and some types of cancer. The use of medical therapies tends to escalate with age; thus, dietary interventions to preserve health in the elderly may help to reduce future health care expenditures in this population. Older adults have more complex health problems, make more outpatient visits, and are hospitalized more often than other population subgroups. Thus, defining and meeting the unique nutritional needs of older adults, in terms of both basal requirements and the

prevention or delay of chronic diseases linked to diet, will be an important challenge for the field of nutrition in the coming decades.

NUTRITIONAL NEEDS OF THE ELDERLY

Current Nutritional Status in the Population

Only a few large representative surveys have compared the dietary intakes of older individuals to indicators of their nutritional needs (e.g., recommended dietary allowances [RDAs]) or in some other way measured dietary adequacy (2). The major sources of representative dietary data are the large, national cross-sectional studies, including the Nationwide Food Consumption Surveys, the National Health Interview Surveys, the Continuing Survey of Food Intakes by Individuals (CSFII), and the National Health and Nutrition Examination Surveys (NHANES) studies (NHANES-I–III). A few longitudinal studies have provided diet data, including the Baltimore Longitudinal Study of Aging (3), the New Mexico Aging Process Study (4), the Framingham study (5), the Health, Aging, and Body Composition Study (6), and a 20-year follow-up study by Flynn and co-workers (7); however, most longitudinal studies examine relatively small population samples who may not be representative of the general elderly population. Although countless other small studies of specific nutrients within subgroups of the elderly have been reported, conclusions concerning nutritional status of the elderly in this chapter will reply primarily on the national studies unless otherwise indicated.

Standards for Assessment of Dietary Adequacy: Dietary Reference Intakes

Nutrient requirements expressed as RDAs have traditionally been published approximately every 10 years by the Food and Nutrition Board of the Institute of Medicine. In the period from 1997 to 2002, this group developed and released an updated set of recommendations, which have been published in stages as they were completed (see Chapter 104 and Appendix Tables A-2-a through A-2-k). Updated dietary reference intakes (DRIs), including RDAs, adequate intakes (AIs), estimated average requirements, and tolerable upper intake levels (ULs), as appropriate, are now available for all recognized essential nutrients,

---

[1]**Abbreviations: AI,** adequate intake; **BMD,** bone mineral density; **BMI,** body mass index; **Ca,** calcium; **Cr,** chromium; **CSFII,** Continuing Survey of Food Intakes by Individuals; **Cu,** copper; **CVD,** cardiovascular disease; **DRI,** dietary reference intake; **EGRAC,** erythrocyte glutathione reductase activity coefficient; **Fe,** iron; **IGF,** insulinlike growth factor; **Mg,** magnesium; **MNA,** Mini Nutritional Assessment; **NHANES,** National Health and Nutrition Examination Surveys; **RDA,** recommended dietary allowance; **Se,** selenium; **SGA,** Subjective Global Assessment; **TEE,** total energy expenditure; **UL,** tolerable upper intake level; **Zn,** zinc.

TABLE 54.1. DIETARY REFERENCE INTAKES FOR ADULTS AGED 51 YEARS OLD OR OLDER

GENDER AND AGE (y)	PROTEIN[a] (g)	CARBOHYDRATE (g)	FIBER (TOTAL)[b] (g)	FAT[c] (g)	
				LINOLEIC ACID[b]	α-LINOLENIC ACID[b]
Men					
51–70 y	56	130	30	14	1.6
>70 y	56	130	30	14	1.6
Women					
51–70 y	46	130	21	11	1.1
>70 y	46	130	21	11	1.1

[a] 0.80 g/kg/d.
[b] Adequate intakes (AIs) represent the recommended average daily intake level based on observed or experimentally determined approximations. AIs are used when information to determine a recommended dietary allowance is insufficient.
[c] There is no dietary reference intake for total fat, because of insufficient data. AIs are given in this table for essential fatty acids.

including macronutrients, vitamins, and minerals. In general, these new standards focus more on health maintenance and the prevention of chronic diseases and metabolic disorders than previous recommendations, which mainly targeted the prevention of nutritional inadequacies. Of particular relevance to aging populations is the new age category of older than 70 years. In previous RDAs, the oldest age category was older than 51 years; even so, many of the recommendations for this broad age group were based on extrapolations from studies of younger persons. Although not complete, the literature now provides numerous published studies of older subjects. These findings were used whenever available to develop the new, more age-specific DRIs for older adults. Tables 54.1 and 54.2 show the RDAs (or AIs when RDAs are not available) for adults more than 51 years of age.

Age-Related Determinants of Nutritional Requirements and Reported Status

The actual requirements for some, but certainly not all, nutrients are changed by metabolic and physiologic changes during the aging process; some of the changes increase and some decrease requirements, as noted in Table 54.3. A host of social, economic, and psychologic factors can affect dietary intakes and thus can determine whether nutritional needs are actually met. Although the incidence of frank nutritional deficiencies in the elderly is

generally low, the increased risk of malnutrition and of subclinical deficiencies in this population and its high-risk subgroups is considerable.

Macronutrient Needs

Calorie and protein-calorie malnutrition are not common in free-living elderly populations but may be routinely encountered in high-risk subgroups. Rates of protein-calorie malnutrition ranging from 30% to more than 50% are reported in elderly nursing home residents (8). Undernutrition is also a problem in the homebound elderly (9). However, an excess of body weight resulting from overeating and reduced activity can also produce a host of detrimental effects on the health and quality of life of the elderly (10, 11). Clearly, energy balance and dietary adequacy present many complex considerations for this age group (12).

Energy. Requirements for energy decrease with age because of reductions in metabolic rate, loss of lean body mass, and a diminution of energy expenditure for physical activity (13). Food intake and calorie (energy) intakes also decrease with age. This finding is consistent in both cross-sectional studies (e.g., NHANES-II and III, CSFII, National Health Interview Surveys) and longitudinal studies spanning 2 decades or more (e.g., Baltimore Longitudinal Study of Aging). Whereas men consume more calories than women, their caloric intakes decline more precipitously

TABLE 54.2. DIETARY REFERENCE INTAKES FOR ADULTS AGED 51 YEARS OLD OR OLDER

GENDER AND AGE (y)	VITAMIN A (μg RETINOL ACTIVITY EQUIVALENT)	VITAMIN D[a] (μg)	VITAMIN E (mg)	VITAMIN K[a] (μg)	VITAMIN C (mg)	THIAMIN (mg)	RIBOFLAVIN (mg)	NIACIN (mg)
Men								
51–70 y	900	10	15	120	90	1.2	1.3	16
>70 y	900	15	15	120	90	1.2	1.3	16
Women								
51–70 y	700	10	15	90	75	1.1	1.1	14
>70 y	700	15	15	90	75	1.1	1.1	14

[a] Adequate intakes (AIs) represent the recommended average daily intake level based on observed or experimentally determined approximations. AIs are used when information to determine a recommended dietary allowance is insufficient.

with age (2). Early decreases in caloric intake (e.g., before age 60 years) generally do not have a detrimental effect, because they are offset by the aforementioned decrements in energy requirements. As noted in a later section, overweight and excessive adiposity can present serious health risks for older adults and may occur despite the reduction in food intake with age. However, in later life, low energy and food intake can become a health concern, in terms of both overall body mass maintenance and intake of other essential nutrients. In the CSFII study, the median energy intake of women aged 70 to 79 years and more than 80 years, was only 1358 and 1296 kcal, respectively. In NHANES-III, between the decades of the 20s and the 80s, mean energy intakes are reduced by more than 1200 kcal in men and about 600 kcal in women. Inadequate intakes of energy and low body mass index (BMI) are linked with functional decline and failure to thrive in the elderly (14). Low food intakes also jeopardize the adequacy of other nutrients by limiting their consumption; food choices may be poor when appetites falter (see Chapter 96).

The Institute of Medicine (15) recently released recommendations for macronutrients (see Table 54.1) and provided formulas for calculation of total energy expenditures (TEE). A gradual reduction in TEE occurs with age, assumed to be about 7 and 10 kcal/year for women and men, respectively. A report from the Health, Aging, and Body Composition study assessed the TEE-derived energy requirements of subjects 70 to 79 years of age using the doubly labeled water technique and confirmed the 2002 DRIs for energy in this elderly age group (16).

Protein. Total protein intake steadily declines with age. For example, in NHANES-III, protein intakes in white women declined from more than 65 g/day in those less than 50 years old to a mean of 52 g/day in those more than 80 years of age. In most cases, the amount of protein intake remains sufficient to meet the needs of healthy elderly populations (17); however, because the lowest intakes predominate in the oldest age groups, protein insufficiency may be a concern in some high-risk persons, especially when health problems or other stressors are manifest and certainly when institutionalization occurs.

Study of adult protein requirements has been considerable since the 1970s; however, the results of studies comparing the protein requirements of elderly versus young adults have not always been in agreement. A meta analysis by Rand and associates (18) considered data from 19 studies in 235 adult subjects and concluded that although the young tended to have lower median requirements than older subjects, this difference was not significant. The current RDA for protein is not changed with age and is 0.80 g/kg/day. In close agreement, the study by Rand and colleagues (18) led to a recommended protein intake for all healthy adults of 0.83 g good-quality protein/kg/day.

Fat. A major fuel source for the body, fat also aids in the absorption of fat-soluble vitamins and other dietary components. Saturated fatty acids, monounsaturated fatty acids, and cholesterol are not required because they can be synthesized by the body. The reader is referred to Table 54.1 and to Chapter 5. Total gastrointestinal transit time and fat absorption are unchanged with aging (19, 20). Likewise, no age-related change occurs in the amount of fat intake recommended. The dietary intake of fat declines with age, and the percentage of calories coming from fat in the diet also declines after age 60 years (NHANES-III) and reaches its lowest value in the oldest age groups. Intakes of cholesterol are also reduced with age (2).

Carbohydrate and Fiber. Carbohydrates (sugars, starches) provide an energy source for all cells in the body. The RDA for carbohydrate is 130 g/day for adults of all ages; a certain minimum intake is necessary to provide glucose as an energy source for the brain. Absolute intakes of carbohydrate decrease with age as energy intakes gradually decline. However, because of the reduction in fat intakes with age, the percentage of dietary calories coming from carbohydrate increases slightly.

Fiber intakes are generally lower than recommended in all segments of the population, and this is true for the elderly as well. Although the National Cancer Institute recommends an intake of 20 to 30 g/day, distribution data showed that intakes are substantially lower; 50% of women consume fewer than 13 g/day, and 50% of men consume fewer than 17 g/day. (2). Although according to NHANES-III, fiber intake does not decline significantly

FOLACIN (μg)	VITAMIN B_6 (mg)	VITAMIN B_{12} (μg)	CALCIUM[a] (mg)	MAGNESIUM (mg)	IRON (mg)	ZINC (mg)	COPPER (μg)	CHROMIUM[a] (μg)	SELENIUM (μg)
400	1.7	2.4	1,200	420	8	11	900	30	55
400	1.7	2.4	1,200	420	8	11	900	30	55
400	1.5	2.4	1,200	320	8	8	900	20	55
400	1.5	2.4	1,200	320	8	8	900	20	55

TABLE 54.3. PHYSIOLOGIC AND METABOLIC FACTORS THAT CAN ALTER NUTRIENT NEEDS IN THE ELDERLY

FACTOR OR CONDITION	EFFECT ON REQUIREMENTS
Atrophic gastritis	IR for folate, calcium, vitamin K, vitamin B$_{12}$, and iron via reduced absorption
Reduced skin synthesis; impaired renal activation; reduced gut response to 1,25(OH)$_2$D$_3$	IR for vitamin D, calcium
Retention of vitamin A; altered hepatic metabolism	DR for vitamin A
Age-related elevation of homocysteine	Possible IR for folate and vitamin B$_{12}$
Menopause; cessation of menstrual period	DR for iron for women
Poor fluid balance regulation	Could be IR or DR for fluids; monitoring required
Decreased total energy expenditure; reduced lean body mass; reduced activity	DR for calories; IR for nutrient density
Decreased immunocompetence with aging	Possible IR for iron, zinc, other nutrients

DR, decreased requirement; IR, increased requirement.

with age (21), increasing dietary fiber intake more toward the recommended level could play an important role in the prevention of age-related chronic diseases such as diabetes (22) and cancer (23).

Fluid. Appropriate hydration is essential for good health and is sometimes a special concern in the elderly. Traditionally, the concern has been about dehydration (24). However, more recently, the potential negative effects of excessive water consumption have also been noted, including dilutional hyponatremia (water intoxication) and increased nocturia (25). The findings of Lindeman and co-workers (26) supported the recommendation that consumption of six glasses of fluid a day is adequate for healthy elderly people except during stressful situations likely to increase fluid loss (e.g., severely hot weather, heavy exertion). The DRIs for water, potassium, sodium, chloride, and sulfate have recently become available (27).

Vitamin and Mineral Requirements

Vitamin A. The requirement for this vitamin does not appear to increase with age. In fact, experimental evidence shows that body retention of vitamin A is enhanced with age, probably as a result of decreased clearance from the periphery (28, 29). Liver stores are well maintained with age, and the possibility of excessive accumulation exists in persons who consume large amounts of vitamin A from supplements and fortified foods (30). Results from NHANES-III indicated an upward shift with age in the dietary intakes of this vitamin. Vitamin A intakes were found to increase with age in both men and women until

the age of 80 years (2). Concerns exist about the vitamin A content of multivitamin supplements, as well as fortified foods, especially because the daily value used in food labeling for this vitamin (1500 μg) is not based on current, but rather older, dietary recommendations (30, 31). The accumulation of this vitamin with age and the ease of exceeding the UL (3000 μg) are of particular concern because there is evidence linking high levels of vitamin A with increased risk of osteoporotic fractures, specifically hip fractures, in men and women (32, 33). The current RDA for men (900 retinol activity equivalent [RAE]) and women (700 RAE) was adjusted downward from the 1989 version, in part because of these concerns about vitamin A retention (see Chapter 19). Recommendations about supplements for the elderly as well as food fortification may also need to be adjusted.

Vitamin D. The role of vitamin D in bone health via the regulation of calcium (Ca) and phosphorus metabolism is well recognized and is particularly critical in the later years of life as bone mineral density (BMD) continues to decline. In addition, inadequate vitamin D status has been linked with muscle weakness, functional impairment, and increased risk of falls and fractures (34, 35), and it has been reported that the use of supplemental vitamin D may reduce the risk of falls in healthy elderly persons (36). A risk allele for sarcopenia (age-related loss of muscle mass) associated with a vitamin D receptor genotype was recently identified (37).

Certain age-related changes contribute to an increased requirement for vitamin D in older adults, including decrements in skin photosynthesis, impaired renal conversion of 25-hydroxyvitamin D to the active form, and reduced gut responsiveness to 1,25(OH)$_2$D. An age-related decrease occurs in the rate of skin conversion of 7-dehydrocholesterol to vitamin D$_3$; compared with adults in their 20s, persons who are more than 60 years old have a dramatic reduction in the rate of production of vitamin D$_3$ in skin (38). In addition, concerns about cancer and skin damage may lead to reduced opportunities for vitamin D$_3$ synthesis because of sun avoidance, increased use of clothing to cover the skin, and use of sun block (39); situations of being "homebound" may also limit the necessary exposure of skin to ultraviolet light in older adults. Direct evidence from animal studies (40) and supporting evidence in humans (41) indicates a reduced ability of the aging kidney to dihydroxylate 25-hydroxyvitamin D to the active 1,25-dihydroxyvitamin D (calcitriol) form. Evidence also indicates that intestinal absorption of vitamin D is adversely affected with aging, apparently via increased resistance of the duodenal Ca transport mechanism to the stimulatory action of 1,25(OH)$_2$D (42, 43) during Ca insufficiency.

Clearly, vitamin D is a high-risk nutrient for older adults. Poor vitamin D status results in decreased Ca absorption; it leads to secondary hyperparathyroidism and osteomalacia, aggravates osteoporosis, and enhances the likelihood of falls and fractures. The intake of the nutrient from dietary sources is difficult to augment because only a few common foods (e.g., oily fish, fortified foods) provide important amounts of the vitamin. Some dairy products are vitamin D fortified; however, intake of dairy products may not be optimal because of preferences or concerns about lactose intolerance. A 20-year follow-up to the Framingham study indicated a high prevalence of problems with vitamin D status, as indicated by low plasma 25(OH)D concentrations, that was associated with season of examination and was inversely related to age and time spent indoors (44).

In response to the increased risk of vitamin D insufficiency with age, the AI reference values for dietary intakes were increased in the latest version of the RDAs to 10 μg/day for ages 51 to 70 years; the AI for ages 71 years and older is 15 μg/day. This amount of vitamin D may not be sufficient for some persons, particularly if they do not have sun exposure (45), or if they are at high risk of osteoporosis. Supplements of 20 μg of vitamin D have been shown to help prevent the loss of BMD in the femoral neck of postmenopausal women (46). Elderly persons can absorb pharmacologic doses of the vitamin equally well as younger subjects (47); supplements of 10 to 20 μg have been recommended for persons at risk of deficiency (45, 48).

Vitamin E. Vitamin E is the generic term for a group of tocopherol and tocotrienol compounds, with α-tocopherol having the highest biologic activity. The most widely accepted metabolic function of this vitamin is that of general lipid antioxidant, and it plays a critical role in protecting biologic membranes. A considerable amount of evidence, direct and indirect, argues for a mechanistic link between vitamin E and the prevention of chronic diseases, although more evidence will be needed before the recommended intake can be revised based on this premise (49). The RDA for vitamin E is 15 mg/day for persons older than 50 years, an increase from the recommendation in 1989 (see Chapter 21). However, no evidence indicates that either absorption or utilization for the vitamin changes with age (49).

The consumption of vitamin E is often less than the recommended amount, possibly because of efforts among adults to cut intakes of fatty foods as protection against atherosclerosis. The best sources of the vitamin include vegetable oils, nuts, peanut butter, and whole grains. Additionally, underreporting of consumption of lipid-rich foods may exaggerate the magnitude of the deficient intake. Nonetheless, dietary consumption of vitamin E has been found to be less than that recommended in several studies of older adults (4, 17, 50). Although frank deficiency of vitamin E is extremely rare, low intakes could be a concern in the elderly because of its link with nervous system function. Numerous reports in the literature indicate that vitamin E plays a role in the function of the central nervous system, probably by protection from oxidative damage.

Vitamin K. The role of vitamin K in the synthesis of numerous blood coagulation factors has long been established. More recently, vitamin K was found to function as a cofactor for the enzyme catalyzing the posttranslational conversion of protein-bound glutamyl residues to γ–carboxyglutamyl residues, essential for the formation of γ-carboxyl–containing proteins in bone, including osteocalcin. Several recent studies linked poor intake of vitamin K and/or levels of undercarboxylated osteocalcin with low BMD and increased risk of hip fracture in women. Szulc and colleagues (51) reported an inverse correlation of bone density in elderly women with the amount of undercarboxylated osteocalcin in their serum; these same investigators reported an increased risk of hip fracture in elderly women with more serum undercarboxylated osteocalcin (52). Likewise, Feskanich and associates (53) found an association of low vitamin K intake with risk of hip fracture in a large prospective cohort study (the Nurses' Health Study) of women aged 38 to 63 years.

Reported intakes of vitamin K are generally adequate and tend to be higher in older adults because of an increased intake of vegetable sources (54). The AI for vitamin K was increased from the 1989 recommendation in the latest version of dietary standards; however, present evicence is insufficient to establish an age-related alteration in the vitamin K requirement. One metabolic study of induced subclinical vitamin K deficiency indicated that older adults may be less likely to show signs of a deficit (decreased urinary excretion of γ-carboxyglutamic acid) than younger subjects (55). However, the role of vitamin K in bone health needs more exploration with regard to recommended intakes for older adults, especially postmenopausal women, who are generally more susceptible to loss of BMD. Recent reports indicate that to support maximal osteocalcin γ-carboxylation, vitamin K intakes may need to exceed the current AI levels in both women (56) and men (57).

Vitamin C. Vitamin C is a potent antioxidant that performs its protective role by scavenging free radicals via a nonenzymatic mechanism; it is also essential for wound healing via its role in connective tissue formation and for several aspects of the immune response, including lymphocyte proliferation, natural killer cell activity, and chemotaxis. Ascorbate intakes are highly variable among different groups of older adults. Most elderly populations consume generous amounts of foods high in the vitamin, such as fruits and vegetables, and have adequate status (2); however, some groups, such as those who are edentate (58), have dementia (59), and/or are nursing home residents (60), have been shown to have low intakes of the vitamin.

Because the absorption and metabolism of vitamin C are not changed with aging, observations of low serum levels in some elderly subjects are attributed to low intakes, chronic disease, or other stressors (49). Although no direct evidence indicates an increased need for ascorbic acid to prevent age-related deficits, certain health promotion benefits may accrue to older persons when they maintain generous stores, including protection against cataracts (61), heart disease (62), and oxidative stress (63). Moreover, in any at-risk population with low vitamin C intakes or high metabolic requirements for the vitamin (such as smokers), correction of an inadequacy will likely convey substantial health benefits (62, 64).

Thiamin, Riboflavin, and Niacin. These B vitamins function as coenzymes in energy metabolism, including certain important biologic redox reactions and thus, along with other functional roles, are essential for the oxidation of energy fuel molecules. Because energy expenditures decline with age, it could be expected that the requirement for one or more of these nutrients would decrease with age. To date, however, no indication exists that the requirements for these nutrients are different in the elderly.

Intakes and status for these vitamins in older populations are more variable. A substantial subgroup of elderly persons has poor thiamin status, as indicated by erythrocyte transketolase activity or thiamin pyrophosphate levels (65, 66). This is most likely the result of poor intakes, but laboratory status is not always correlated with reported intakes. Thiamin status can also be impaired by long-term alcohol consumption. As indicated in data from NHANES-III, mean intakes of thiamin for persons 50 years and older exceed the RDA.

The best sources of riboflavin are milk and dairy products; thus, some elderly persons are at risk of low intake because of avoidance or unavailability of good dietary sources (meats and cereals are also good sources). Low intakes of the vitamin are often prevalent in elderly populations (29, 67) and can be endemic when milk and meat are lacking from the diet (68). The most recent NHANES results showed mean intakes that exceeded current RDAs (69). However, a study in the United Kingdom (70) indicated that 41% of free-living and 35% of institutionalized people who are more than 65 years old had evidence of biochemical riboflavin deficiency as indicated by erythrocyte glutathione reductase activity coefficient (EGRAC). Madigan and co-workers (71) conducted a similar study in Northern Ireland and reported abnormal EGRAC levels in 49% of subjects, despite presumably adequate intakes of riboflavin. Boisvert and colleagues (72) monitored EGRAC in riboflavin-deficient subjects who were more than 60 years old and who were gradually repleted with riboflavin and found a dietary requirement similar to that of young adults. Based partly on this finding, the riboflavin requirement for older adults is thought to be maintained at the same level as younger adults.

Niacin intakes are generally adequate in most elderly persons, and mean intakes exceeded RDAs for all ages of adult men and women in NHANES-III (69). However, pockets of special concern may exist; Lee and Frongillo (73) reported lower intakes of 19 nutrients, including niacin and riboflavin, in elderly persons with food insecurity who participated in NHANES-III. As previously noted, requirements for this nutrient are assumed to be unchanged with age.

Folate. The role of folate as a coenzyme for single-carbon transfers is critical for a host of functions related to the metabolism of nucleic and amino acids, including homocysteine. Thus, although no physiologic evidence indicates an increase in the folate requirement with age (74), inadequate folate status could contribute to the risk of chronic disease in the elderly via promotion of hyperhomocysteinemia (75). The metabolism of homocysteine is described in detail in Chapters 28 and 34. Poor folate status can also contribute to procarcinogenic changes in DNA and increased risk of cognitive dysfunction. In addition to dietary inadequacies, other factors that could contribute to a folate deficiency include genetic polymorphisms, malabsorption syndromes, alcohol intake, and adverse effects of antifolate medications such as methotrexate (76).

In part because of new information concerning the role of folate in the metabolism of homocysteine (77) and other essential functions, general recommendations for folate intake are higher in the current version of the DRIs; the current RDA for folate is 400 μg/day (increased from 1989). Although folate status as measured by serum or erythrocyte levels has not been shown to decline with aging (78), dietary intakes of the vitamin have previously been found to be marginal in the elderly. Previous assessment of dietary intakes (NHANES-III, phase I data collected from 1988 to 1991; 1997 CSFII) indicated that substantial numbers of adults were not meeting the current RDA (400 μg) for folate (2, 79). This finding was confirmed in numerous other studies and could be attributed to insufficient intakes of vegetables and fruits to provide the amounts recommended (17). However, in the late 1990s, folate fortification of grains was mandated by the Food and Drug Administration, with the intent of repletion of women of childbearing age and thus reduction of the risk of neural tube birth defects. The bioavailability of the synthetic form of folate found in supplements and fortified foods (85–100%) is considerably higher than that of naturally occurring food folate (~50%). As a result, folate intakes of all adults, including the elderly, have increased substantially. In fact, because of the relatively high use of supplements in this age group, as well as their consumption of ready-to-eat breakfast cereals, concern exists that their daily intakes may exceed the UL for folate of 1000 μg/day. One of the most serious concerns in this case would be the masking of a vitamin B_{12} deficiency by high folate consumption, because vitamin B_{12} deficiency is more common than folate deficiency in this age group. Thus, when folate supplements are given, a multivitamin that includes vitamin B_{12} should also be recommended (76). However, in populations not receiving fortified foods or supplements, especially high-risk groups such as nursing home patients (80), inadequate folate intakes and biochemical status continue to be a risk.

Vitamin B₆. The function of vitamin B_6 (pyridoxine and related compounds) is as a coenzyme in the metabolism of amino acids, glycogen, and sphingoid bases (see Chapter 26). The need for vitamin B_6 is increased with age, as reflected in the newest version of RDAs; the RDAs for adults aged more than 51 to 70 years and more than 70 years are the highest within the adult category. The mechanism for this increase is not fully understood, because absorption seems unaffected by age; thus, presumably, the requirement relates to some other alteration in metabolism (81).

Intakes of pyridoxine in elderly populations are sometimes suboptimal (65, 82); results from the 1997 CSFII showed that substantial numbers of adults older than age 50 years (52–66%) are not meeting the dietary recommendations for vitamin B_6 (79). Several high-risk subgroups of the population have low biochemical status (based on pyridoxal 5'-phosphate levels), including those with dementia (83), stroke (84), and rheumatoid arthritis (85), as well as patients admitted to a nursing home (80). Bates and colleagues (86) studied elderly men and women participating in the National Diet and Nutrition Survey in the United Kingdom and found that 48% of community-dwelling and 75% of institutionalized elderly persons had inadequate plasma pyridoxal 5'-phosphate levels.

Vitamin B₁₂. Vitamin B_{12} is required as a coenzyme for essential methyl transfer reactions; it is also required for normal blood formation and neurologic function (see Chapters 29 and 92). No evidence indicates a change in absorption or other aspects of vitamin B_{12} metabolism as a result of aging per se (87). However, in 10 to 30% of persons 50 years old and older, low stomach acid secretion caused by atrophic gastritis seriously impaired the absorption of this vitamin (88, 89). Thus, persons with reduced vitamin B_{12} absorption are at risk of deficiency, which can include hematologic conditions (macrocytic megaloblastic anemia) and neurologic changes (e.g., paresthesia, sensory loss, ataxia, dementia, psychiatric disorders, impaired memory). Early intervention is essential to correct these deficiencies. Moreover, as noted in Chapter 29, vitamin B_{12} deficiency should be avoided because marginal status can lead to higher plasma homocysteine concentrations and can thereby increase the risk of vascular disease.

Biochemical evidence of low vitamin B_{12} status is commonly detected among elderly persons (90–92). This deficiency is not likely to be caused by dietary inadequacy, except in the rare instance of a total vegan diet, because B_{12} is found exclusively (and widely) in animal foods. Intakes of the vitamin are generally quite adequate in older adults, as found most recently in NHANES-III (2). The most likely underlying cause of low status is the malabsorption resulting from inadequate pepsin activity and gastric acid production (93, 94). In addition to age-related atrophic gastritis, other causes of protein-bound vitamin B_{12} malabsorption can include gastric resection, gastric infection with *Helicobacter pylori*, and the widespread use

of medications that suppress gastric acid secretion (88). Persons who have a defect in absorbing vitamin B_{12} should obtain the recommended intake of the vitamin from synthetic and fortified food sources. A very small (~2%) proportion of the elderly has pernicious anemia and cannot absorb the vitamin in any form and must receive vitamin B_{12} injections.

In the 1989 RDAs, the recommendation for vitamin B_{12} for the two oldest age categories (>51–70 years and >71 years) is the same as for younger adults (65). However, because it is usually unknown whether an older adult has impaired vitamin B_{12} absorption, it is recommended that for persons more than 51 years of age, most of the requirement should be met by taking supplements containing vitamin B_{12} or by eating fortified food products (65, 17). The amount of vitamin B_{12} in supplements and food products is expressed as a percentage of the daily value (total daily value = 6 μg/day), which is not the RDA but is higher, based on the 1968 RDA (88).

Calcium. Although adequate Ca intake may be linked to the prevention of numerous chronic illnesses, it is the role of Ca in bone health and osteoporosis that is the most important consideration for nutritional requirements in the elderly (see Chapters 9, 84, and 86). Osteoporosis affects 25% of white women who are more than 50 years old and causes more than 1.5 million fractures within that population each year (95); it is thus a major determinant of health quality in older adults. However, the amounts of Ca needed to promote bone health may also have beneficial effects in the prevention of colon cancer (96) and hypertension (97).

The need for Ca increases with age because of several factors. Ca absorption is reduced with age in both men (98) and women (99). Reasons include achlorhydria (present in 10–30% of those >50 years old), and the previously noted decline in gut responsiveness to active vitamin D. It is recognized that BMD loss beginning at age 40 years occurs at a rate of 0.5 to 1.0% per year in both sexes, with a transient acceleration in women after menopause. Based on balance data from Spencer and collaborators (100) indicating the amount of Ca required for maximum retention, the AI reference value for Ca for those who are more than 51 years of age has been increased from 800 mg/day (1989 RDA) to 1200 mg/day. Correction of low Ca intakes has been demonstrated to preserve BMD (101) and to reduce fracture rates (102). Ca can enhance the effectiveness of hormone replacement therapy (103) and can partially offset the acceleration of bone loss (104), but it cannot totally compensate for perimenopausal BMD loss. This is an unfortunate finding, because the use of hormone replacement is no longer considered a safe option for many women (105).

Ca intakes are lower than recommended levels for much of the adult population, including the elderly (82). The primary source of this nutrient is dairy products, but a minimum of three servings a day is needed to meet the Ca needs of most older adults; this goal is often not met. NHANES-III confirms a significant decline in Ca intakes with age (2). In this national survey, investigators found that 70 to 75% of men and 87% of women had low Ca intakes; even accounting for the combined intakes of diet and supplements in subjects who took them, the rates of deficient intake were at 60 and 66% for men and women, respectively (106). The discrepancy between the need for Ca and the amount of Ca consumed is probably the most disparate observed for any of the essential micronutrients. Efforts to remedy shortages of Ca intake in all older adults, and especially women, are urgently needed.

Magnesium. Magnesium (Mg) is required as a cofactor for a host of essential reactions, including those involving adenosine triphosphate and guanosine triphosphate. It stabilizes DNA and RNA and is required for normal muscle and nerve function, as well as bone structure. With age, absorption of the mineral tends to decrease, and urinary Mg excretion increases (107, 108). As noted in Chapter 11, Mg depletion is common in diabetes mellitus. A diet suboptimal in Mg would therefore present special concerns and has often been observed in older persons (107, 109). Conversely, hypermagnesemia may be a concern in elderly persons who, because of chronic constipation, ingest Mg laxatives regularly. The RDA for Mg (see Table 54.2) increases at age 31 years but is not changed thereafter.

Along with vitamin D and Ca, Mg is a nutrient that is known to be essential for bone health. Because the role of Mg was recognized more recently than that of Ca, to date only limited numbers of studies have explored the relationship of its dietary consumption with BMD; however, several of these studies found a positive correspondence (110–112). Significant reductions in serum Mg and BMD have been reported in women with postmenopausal osteoporosis compared with age-matched controls (113). Tucker and colleagues (109) reported a direct relationship of Mg intake (past and present) with BMD at a hip site (men and women) and in the forearm (men) in a follow-up of Framingham Heart Study subjects. Animal studies of Mg deficiency have also supported the role of this mineral in bone health; Mg-deficient rats have bone loss that is attributed to accelerated bone resorption (114). In addition, a study by Stendig-Lindberg and associates (115) demonstrated a beneficial effect of Mg supplements on BMD and fracture rates in a 2-year trial of postmenopausal women.

Iron. The role of iron (Fe) in oxygen transport to the tissues as a component of hemoglobin is well recognized; Fe is also required for numerous other essential functions, including immune response (see Chapter 12). The effect of age on Fe requirements, apart from that caused by impaired absorption resulting from atrophic gastritis, is apparently not large, because Fe stores are thought to increase with age (116). In fact, investigators have suggested that increased Fe stores could be associated with

the development of age-related diseases by promoting oxidative changes (117); specific evidence links Fe accumulation with disordered glucose regulation (118), insulin resistance (119), and CVD in persons carrying hemochromatosis gene mutations (120). The question for nutritionists is whether dietary Fe intake directly influences the size of Fe stores. Despite considerable study (121, 122), this question has not been fully resolved. Most recently, Garry and colleagues (116) found no association between heme and nonheme Fe intake and Fe stores as indicated by serum ferritin levels in both cross-sectional and longitudinal assessments of elderly men and women. These investigators concluded that increasing dietary Fe in the diet will not overwhelm absorption and lead to an accumulation of the mineral. However, in this same study, Fe stores in women were linked both to age and the intake of supplemental Fe (>18 mg/day).

Although the RDA for women less than 50 years of age is higher than for men, recommendations after that age do not differ by gender because the extra Fe loss in menses is no longer a factor in the female requirement. The current RDA is 8 mg/day, a slight decrease from the 1989 RDA, which was 10 mg/day. An inadequate amount of dietary Fe can still be a cause for concern. Fe is generally adequate in the diets of healthy populations (82, 106), but it may be inadequate in certain high-risk subgroups, including the homebound elderly (123). For those persons with poor Fe absorption caused by low gastric acidity, marginal Fe status could be precipitated if the dietary Fe sources are mainly nonheme. Heme-Fe absorption does not require stomach acid and thus is unaffected by atrophic gastritis (81).

Although the prevalence of anemia increases with age, it is not considered a normal finding in older persons (124). Anemia is strongly associated with numerous negative health outcomes, including cardiovascular complications, functional impairment, chronic fatigue, and decreased muscle strength (125), and it needs appropriate diagnosis and intervention. Fe deficiency anemia is just one of several nutritional anemias and may occur concomitantly with the anemia of chronic disease, thus making it difficult to diagnose (126). Nutritrional deficiency anemias can also result from inadequacies of folate, vitamin B_{12}, and protein or energy, although Fe deficiency anemia is the most common nutritional type. When Fe deficiency is present, treatment with Fe sulfate (325 mg three times/day) is generally recommended. The reticulocyte response should be obvious in 1 week; if not, intravenous Fe should be considered (124).

Fe deficiency can also cause impairments in cell-mediated and innate immunity, thus increasing susceptibility to infections. Ahluwalia and colleagues (123) recently demonstrated that among older women who were homebound and Fe deficient based on multiple Fe status tests, 40 to 50% had impaired T-cell proliferation upon stimulation, and 25% had a decline in respiratory burst.

Zinc. Zinc (Zn) has numerous essential catalytic, structural, and regulatory functions; it is required for more than 200 metalloenzymes and also for gene expression via Zn finger proteins (see Chapter 13). The immunoregulative role of Zn is particularly important for the elderly because immune function declines with age (127, 128), especially T-cell response and function, effects similar to those of a Zn deficit (129). The effects of a mild to moderate Zn deficiency could result in subtle impairments in resistance to infection and response to immunizations and thereby could contribute to increased susceptibility to illness in elderly persons (128).

The impact of aging on Zn requirements is not well understood. Studies of the effect of aging on Zn absorption yielded equivocal results (130, 131), as did investigations of age effects on Zn balance (132, 133). Thus, there is little direct evidence suggesting that the Zn requirements of the elderly are different from those of younger adults; however, increased physiologic demands (e.g., decrements in immune function, wound healing) known to be age related suggest that Zn metabolism in aging could be compromised.

Several studies found evidence linking Zn deficits to functional and biochemical impairments in older subjects (134–136), a result that would imply that the baseline Zn status of many elderly individuals is suboptimal. As already noted, considerable evidence supports the role of Zn status in the immunocompetence of older adults. Cross-sectional studies showed a relationship between Zn status indicators and immunity (128, 137), and problems with immune function are reported in Zn deficiency. For example, Kreft and associates (138) reported impaired response to a diphtheria vaccination in elderly patients who were undergoing hemodialysis and who had Zn deficiency. Numerous Zn supplementation studies showed beneficial effects on immune function and reduced susceptibility to infections in elderly subjects (135, 139). Girodan and co-workers (140) showed beneficial effects of a trace element supplement (Zn and selenium [Se]) on resistance to infections and antibody response to influenza vaccine.

Other potential functions of Zn are less well explored. Elderly patients with pressure ulcers are more likely to have low serum Zn levels (141), and, in some cases, Zn has been shown to enhance wound healing. This is likely the result of correction of a deficiency state; large-dose supplementation with Zn for pressure ulcers could have adverse effects (142). Prasad and colleagues (143) showed that elderly men who were marginally Zn deficient increased serum testosterone levels when they took a Zn gluconate supplement for 3 to 6 months. Zn may also be protective of the retina (144). High-dose Zn supplementation should be avoided because it can induce copper (Cu) deficiency and/or immune suppression. For repletion of Zn deficiency, a low dose (~40–50 mg/day) is recommended unless the patient is being regularly monitored for Cu status (129).

Low dietary intakes of Zn are commonly reported (82). NHANES-III data indicated that persons more than age 70 years were among the populations most likely to have inadequate Zn intakes (145). Despite the previously noted findings, which seemingly point to high risk of marginal Zn status in the elderly, the current RDA for persons who are more than 51 years old is the same as for younger adults and is lower than the 1989 RDA; this change in the RDA needs to be noted when reviewing the results of dietary studies using the 1989 RDA as a standard. The dilemma regarding specific age effects is the result, in part, of the difficulties in documenting human Zn status (146). Serum Zn levels do not consistently reflect Zn nutriture; likewise, other indicators of Zn status have not be found to be fully reliable (147). Some uncertainty also exists about whether serum Zn levels change with age (148, 149). The potential to enhance immune function and thus to improve resistance to infection by correcting a marginal, although difficult to document, Zn deficiency (150, 151) merits continued study, as do certain other important potential roles of Zn in the health of the elderly.

Copper. Cu is another divalent trace mineral with numerous essential catalytic functions; Cu metalloenzymes include superoxide dismutase, lysyl oxidase, dopamine β-hydroxylase, and cytochrome C-oxidase (see Chapter 14). The RDA for Cu for persons who are more than 51 years old is the same as for younger adults. Cu intakes are not always adequate in adults, including the older population (152, 153), although overt deficiency signs are rare (147). An exception is noted in institutionalized elderly persons receiving long-term tube feedings; in these persons, Cu deficiency accompanied by hematologic effects (anemia) has been reported (154). Chronic Zn supplementation, as noted in the previous section, can also cause Cu deficiency, owing to competitive inhibition of Cu absorption. As is the case with Zn, the assessment of Cu is difficult because the serum level is not a reliable index of status (155).

As previously noted by the specified RDA, to date, evidence is insufficient to support an age affect on Cu requirements (146), but several areas of study in Cu metabolism may have implications for the elderly in the future. Cu insufficiency has been linked with CVD (156) and also with osteoporosis (153, 157, 158). In addition, Cu homeostasis is apparently disrupted in Alzheimer disease such that certain patients with this disease have elevated serum Cu levels (159, 160). In one study (161), patients with Alzheimer disease had Cu levels that were correlated with poor neurologic performance.

Chromium. For decades, investigators have recognized that chromium (Cr) plays an essential role in glucose and insulin metabolism (see Chapter 17B). Cr is thought to exert this role by increasing insulin binding, number of receptors, and receptor internalization so that insulin sensitivity is enhanced. The mineral has been found to improve glucose and insulin regulation in both hypoglycemic and hyperglycemic subjects (162), although not in every case (163). In a study conducted by Amato and coworkers (164), supplementation with Cr picolinate supplementation did not appear to improve insulin sensitivity in nonobese, healthy men and women aged 63 to 77 years. Yet numerous studies have demonstrated beneficial effects on insulin sensitivity and glucose tolerance, as well as serum lipid profiles and body composition (162).

Dietary intakes of Cr in the United States are often less than the recommended amount, particularly in elderly persons (129, 164). The dietary recommendation for Cr intake is currently expressed as an AI (see Table 54.2), is lower than the 1989 recommendation, and is not different according to age. However, considerable indirect evidence indicates that Cr requirements could change with aging, including decreases in levels of the mineral in serum, hair, and sweat (165). Moreover, the suggestion that a deficiency of Cr leads to impaired glucose tolerance (166) is of particular interest because it is known that insulin sensitivity and glucose tolerance decline with age (167). Persons with type 2 diabetes have lower plasma levels of Cr (168).

Selenium. The functions of this essential trace element include defense against oxidative stress, regulation of thyroid hormones action, and regulation of the redox status of vitamin C and other molecules (see Chapter 16). Se absorption and utilization do not appear to be affected by aging; adults who are more 51 years of age are thought to have the same Se requirement as younger adults (55 μg/day); this RDA is lower than the 1989 recommendation of 70 μg.

In some elderly persons, serum Se levels are lower than normal (129, 148). However, no pathologic conditions related to Se insufficiency have been reported in the United States. Although frank Se deficiency has long been linked with cardiomyopathy in areas of the world that have Se-poor soil and in patients receiving total parenteral nutrition without Se, studies of the possible role of a mild Se deficiency on CVD and cardiomyopathy in the elderly for the most part have not yet been conducted (169). The potential roles of Se in host defense mechanisms and in certain cancers also need further study (129).

Use of Nutritional Supplements

Compared with the general population, larger proportions of elderly persons use vitamin and other nutrient supplements. The rate of use among older persons in the United States is estimated at 31 to 56%, based on data from NHANES-III (106). Use of vitamins tends to be higher than for minerals (17). Supplement use is more likely in women than men and in whites compared with blacks, but it seems similar between the age decades of the 60s and the 80s (142, 170). In the past, many studies showed that the choice to take a nutritional supplement did not seem linked to severity of health problems but rather was more likely to occur in elderly persons with strong health-seeking behaviors (171). The real benefits of nutritional supplements may

be more in health promotion than in the prevention of overt deficiency. McKay and colleagues (172) found that a multivitamin and mineral supplement improved the status of B vitamins and reduced the plasma levels of homocysteine in 80 healthy adults aged 50 to 87 years who were already consuming a folate-fortified diet. Supplements have also been shown to improve antioxidant status (173) and immune function (174, 175).

In a recent review article (176), it was suggested that all adults should take a multivitamin and mineral supplement, and the elderly should take two. However, the type and amount of nutrients contained in any supplement should be carefully considered, for the elderly, as well as for other adults. In this same article, the possibilities that excessive vitamin A could increase the risk of hip fractures or that Fe could aggravate hemochromatosis were noted. Thus, it may be better for the elderly person to take one multivitamin along with extra vitamins B_{12} and D. Fe supplements, unless given to remedy an anemic condition, may not be a wise recommendation for older adults who are otherwise healthy. The risk may be particularly important for those who are homozygous or heterozygous for mutations of the hemochromatosis-associated gene because even relatively modest amounts of supplemental Fe could increase the likelihood of diabetes and CVD (4). Other concerns, previously noted, could be that large intakes of folate could mask certain symptoms of a vitamin B_{12} deficiency. Supplementation with Zn as a single nutrient, especially at high doses, can have adverse effects that include interfering with Cu nutriture and impairment of immune functions (128, 129). Except in the case of a documented deficiency of a single nutrient, it is generally best to rely on a multivitamin and mineral supplement. In contrast, the amount of Ca contained in a multitype supplement is too low (generally <200 mg) to be physiologically important; if supplemental Ca is needed, an additional Ca supplement should be taken.

Nutritional Factors that Increase the Risk of Poor Health Outcomes

Nutritional Frailty. The progressive decrease in food intake with age increases the importance of high micronutrient density in the diets of older adults. Whereas calorie needs decline with age, the requirements for other nutrients generally do not decrease (exceptions are vitamin A, Fe in women). Dietary nutrient density, unfortunately but not unexpectedly, is not any higher in older adults compared with young; in fact, the added complications of chronic illness and the side effects of medications and various medical interventions for ongoing chronic conditions (e.g., special diets, surgery, chemotherapy) decrease the likelihood that dietary intakes of essential nutrients will be fully adequate on a regular basis.

Elderly persons may be at nutritional risk because of numerous factors, including sociodemographic factors (limited income, lack of social support, living arrangements), depression, poor functional status, and poor oral health (177–179). The burden of one or more chronic medical conditions may take its toll on nutritional and functional status and may contribute to an overall decline (180, 181). Institutionalization is almost always linked with increased nutritional risk. Essama-Tjani and colleagues (80) studied dietary intakes and blood levels of folate in elderly subjects entering a nursing home and found a drop in folate plasma and red blood cell levels during the first year of institutionalization.

Risk of Obesity and Excess Abdominal Adiposity. In contrast to the stereotypical profile of nutritional frailty, many elderly persons are at risk because of the metabolic frailty that results from excessive body fat. Little question exists that being overweight (BMI >25 to 29.9) or obese (BMI >30) has significant detrimental effects on the health and quality of life of older adults (10, 11). Overweight and obesity are associated with CVD, diabetes, hypertension, and some forms of cancer, as well as increased use of health care resources (182), surgical complications, and functional disabilities (183). The longer the duration of the overweight or obesity, the more profound the effects will be. As visceral adiposity increases with age, it leads to glucose intolerance, hyperinsulinemia, and hypertriglyceridemia (184–186). In addition, overweight and obesity contribute to functional decline in older adults (187–189). Being overweight has also been linked with poor nutritional status in rural elderly women (190).

NUTRITIONAL ASSESSMENT

Dietary Assessment

The assessment of dietary intake has some unique considerations in the case of older adults, particularly for frail or disabled persons. Conventionally accepted methods of dietary assessment may be difficult to implement, owing to time and effort burdens on the patient and/or caregiver, cognitive limitations and the lack of a proxy source for dietary information, and, in the case of the institutionalized patient (e.g., hospital, nursing home), shortage of staff time for data collection (Table 54.4). Although methods such as food records (191) and weighed food intake assessments (192) are effective, they are often impractical

TABLE 54.4. SPECIAL CONCERNS FOR DIETARY ASSESSMENT OF THE ELDERLY

Poor short-term memory can affect 24-hour recall and food frequency type data collection.

Cognitive impairment and the need for a dependable proxy may limit data availability from high-risk persons.

The need for more time may increase the burden on the patient and/or the evaluator.

If the patient has health problems, and other difficulties are sporadic, it may be difficult to obtain representative information without multiple sampling.

except in a research context. The collection of dietary data from some elderly subjects, particularly the oldest old and those with memory and/or cognitive problems, may be affected in terms of time and cost by the need for patience and additional resources (193). Extra time may be required for interviews, and confirmatory or supplementary information may need to be sought from a caregiver or proxy. For this age group, methods that rely solely on memory (e.g., 24-hour recall) may not be as accurate as information enriched by an ongoing record or checklist that can be completed as soon as a meal is eaten (193). For all these reasons, the collection of dietary information may be more costly for this than for younger age groups.

Biochemical Assessment

Markers of Protein Status

Albumin. Albumin is one of the most abundant and commonly measured serum proteins. When albumin production and degradation are in equilibrium, it has a half-life of 18 days. With aging, serum albumin levels decline slightly (0.8 g/L/decade in persons >60 years of age), but factors other than age per se have never been completely excluded in these studies. Despite the relationship demonstrated between albumin and morbidity and mortality, current evidence does not support the use of serum albumin as the sole marker of nutritional status (194, 195). Chronic inflammation, advanced liver disease, heart failure, nephrotic syndrome, and protein-losing enteropathy all can result in hypoalbuminemia. Furthermore, very few data reveal improvement in serum albumin outcomes following repletion because of the time necessary for improvement (196).

Prealbumin (Transthyretin). Prealbumin (or transthyretin) is a transport protein for thyroxine. Prealbumin has a half-life of 2 days and superior sensitivity to albumin in evaluating acute nutritional change. Although aging does not affect prealbumin levels in healthy persons, a decrease may occur in very old men (>90 years). Prealbumin levels usually increase by 10 mg/L every day with good nutritional repletion (197). An increase of less than 20 mg/L in 1 week indicates either inadequate nutritional support or poor response by the patient and poor prognosis.

Insulinlike Growth Factor-I. Insulinlike growth factor (IGF-I) is a peptide produced by the liver under the stimulation of growth hormone. IGF-I levels drop rapidly during starvation. Nutritional repletion leads to a rapid return to normal levels. IGF-I has a very short half-life of 2 to 4 hours and a relatively small body pool, such that it is a very sensitive indicator of nutritional changes. Low IGF-I levels in hospitalized older adults are associated with an increase in morbidity, specifically the occurrence of life-threatening complications (198).

C-Reactive Protein. To date, no study has shown a major role for C-reactive protein in the evaluation of nutritional status in older adults. Because visceral protein levels are often influenced by the degree of systemic inflammation present, adjustment of visceral protein levels according to C-reactive protein level may be a reasonable way to address the visceral protein-inflammation relationship while using these indicators to evaluate nutritional status. More studies will be required before this approach can be routinely advocated.

Clinical and Anthropometric Assessments

The detection of poor nutrition requires attention to early subtle clues (see Chapters 49 and 96). Advanced deterioration may eventually become apparent from the clinical course, but at this point intervention may be less successful. Fatigue, weakness, changes in ability to taste or smell, gastrointestinal complaints (poor appetite, oral problems, nausea, vomiting, diarrhea, constipation), and changes in mental or emotional status (199) may all suggest undernutrition. Overnutrition (and, in particular, increased fat mass with decreased muscle mass) may be masked by relatively normal weight (13).

Anthropometric Assessment

Weight. In older adults, serial measurement of body weight offers the simplest indicator of nutritional adequacy and of change in nutritional status. Obtaining regular body weights is not always easy, particularly in frail patients. If the patient cannot stand on an upright balance beam scale, a chair or bed scale should be used, and all scales should be regularly calibrated. If weight loss is noted, the measurement should be confirmed by a repeat weighing (18). Care should also be used when ascertaining height for calculation of BMI; whenever possible, the patient's height before age 50 years should be used as the reference height, to avoid the effects of kyphosis resulting from osteoporosis (200). Low body weight often is defined as less than 80% of the recommended body weight.

Weight Loss. Clinically significant weight loss is considered a decrease in weight exceeding 2% of baseline body weight in 1 month, 5% in 3 months, or 10% in 6 months (201). The Omnibus Budget Reconciliation Act of 1987 stipulates that nursing home patients are considered to have meaningful weight loss if they have lost 5% of usual body weight in 30 days or 10% 6 months. As little as 5% weight loss over a 3-year period has been shown to be associated with increased mortality among community-dwelling older adults (202).

Stable weight parameters may not indicate normal muscle and fat mass. Many older adults with normal or increased body weight have marked reduction in fat-free mass and/or excesses in fat mass (203). Hence, tools to measure body fat and fat-free mass may be important to assess risk for insulin resistance (in the case of excess fat mass) or functional decline.

Measurement of Body Fat. Although body fat is best measured with dual-energy x-ray absorptiometry or computed tomography, in most settings, this approach is impractical and costly. Surrogate measures for total body fat include BMI, waist circumference, and sagittal diameter (using an abdominal caliper at the level of the iliac crest). These measures correlate well with total body fat but correlate less well with visceral fat stores (204). Skin fold measurements have also been used to estimate total body adipose tissue. Although skin fold measurements correlate strongly with total body adipose tissue, these measurements do not correlate with visceral adipose tissue. This is in part because, in both men and women, the fraction of total adipose tissue sequestered in the subcutaneous tissue decreases with age. Dual-energy x-ray absorptiometry and computed tomography provide a better indication of visceral fat stores (205).

Measurement of Muscle Mass. Skeletal muscle atrophy, or sarcopenia, is very common in older adults and is strongly associated with disability, independent of morbidity (206). Skeletal muscle mass can be measured anthropometrically. Arm muscle area calculated by triceps skin fold and mean arm circumference measures correlates well with arm muscle area measured by computed tomography. The average error for a given patient is 7 to 8% but requires a relatively complex equation for conversion:

$$([(MAC - \pi \times TSF)2/4\,\pi] - 10 \text{ and}$$
$$[(MAC - \pi \times TSF)2/4\,\pi] - 6.5)$$

where MAC is mean arm circumference and TSF is triceps skinfold thickness (207). A more reliable approach to muscle mass measurement could include dual-energy x-ray absorptiometry, computed tomography, and magnetic resonance imaging (208).

Nutrition Indices

Nutrition indices often used in frail, older adults include the Mini Nutritional Assessment (MNA) and the Subjective Global Assessment (SGA). The MNA is a validated tool with a positive predictive value for detecting undernutrition of 97%. The sensitivity and specificity of this tool have been shown to be 96 and 98%, respectively. The MNA incorporates several domains, including functional status, lifestyle, diet, self-perception of health, and anthropometric indices, and it has been shown to be predictive of adverse clinical events and mortality among older hospitalized patients (209). The SGA includes history and physical examination and allows a clinical grading of nutritional status (210, 211). Features in the SGA are weight loss in the previous 6 months and in the previous 2 weeks, dietary intake in relation to the patient's usual pattern, the presence of significant gastrointestinal symptoms, functional capacity, metabolic demands of underlying disease, the loss of subcutaneous fat (back part of upper arm, thorax), muscle wasting (quadriceps femoris, deltoideus), and the presence of edema (ankle, sacral). Judgment of nutritional status using the SGA is largely based on subjective assessment rather than on detailed measurements. Neither the MNA or the SGA addresses overnutrition or the existence of micronutrient deficiencies in the presence of excess fat or calorie intake. Identifying better markers of nutrition risk in the context of overnutrition is an area of active investigation.

Acknowledgments

CWB was supported by National Institutes of Health grants HL57354 and AG22132 and acknowledges the excellent editorial assistance of Melissa Orenduff.

REFERENCES

1. Fried LP. Epidemiol Rev 2000;22:95–106.
2. Wakimoto P, Block G. J Gerontol A Biol Sci Med Sci 2001; 56:65–80.
3. Hallfrisch J, Tobin JD, Muller DC et al. J Gerontol 1988;43: M64–8.
4. Garry PJ, Goodwin JS, Hunt WC et al. Am J Clin Nutr 1982; 36:319–31.
5. Dawber TR, Meadors GF, Moore FE Jr. Am J Public Health 1951;41:279–86.
6. Holvoet P, Kritchevsky SB, Tracy RP et al. Diabetes 2004;53: 1068–73.
7. Flynn MA, Nolph GB, Baker AS et al. J Am Coll Nutr 1992; 11:660–72.
8. Ritchie CS, Bales CW. Sarcopenia and nutritional frailty: diagnosis and intervention. In: Bales CW, Ritchie CS, eds. Handbook of Clinical Nutrition and Aging. Totowa, NJ: Humana Press, 2004:309–333.
9. Ritchie CS, Burgio KL, Locher JL et al. Am J Clin Nutr 1997; 66:815–8.
10. Rossner S. Obes Rev 2001;2:183–8.
11. Kotz CM, Billington CJ, Levine AS. Clin Geriatr Med 1999; 15:391–412.
12. Ritz P. Public Health Nutr 2001;4:561–8.
13. Roubenoff R, Hughes VA, Dallal GE et al. J Gerontol A Biol Sci Med Sci 2000;55:M757–60.
14. Markson EW. Clin Geriatr Med 1997;13:639–52.
15. Food and Nutrition Board, Institute of Medicine. Dietary Reference Intakes for Energy, Carbohydrate, Fiber, Fat, Fatty Acids, Cholesterol, Protein, and Amino Acids. Washington, DC: National Academy Press, 2002.
16. Blanc S, Schoeller DA, Bauer D et al. Am J Clin Nutr 2004; 79: 303–10.
17. Foote JA, Giuliano AR, Harris RB. J Am Coll Nutr 2000; 19: 628–40.
18. Rand WM, Pellett PL, Young VR. Am J Clin Nutr 2003;77: 109–127.
19. Brauer PM, Slavin JL, Marlett JA. Am J Clin Nutr 1981; 34: 1061–70.
20. Russell RM. Am J Clin Nutr 1992;55[Suppl]:1203S–7S.
21. Bialostocky K, Wright JD, Kennedy-Stephenson J et al. Vital Health Stat 2002;11:245.
22. Meyer KA, Kushi LH, Jacobs DR Jr et al. Am J Clin Nutr 2000; 71:921–30.
23. Dreosti IE. Ann NY Acad Sci 1998;854:371–7.
24. Weinberg AD, Minaker KL. JAMA 1995;274:1552–6.
25. Morley J. J Geriatr 2000;55A:M359–60.
26. Lindeman RD, Romero LJ, Liang HC et al. J Geriatr 2000; 55A:M361–5.
27. Food and Nutrition Board, Institute of Medicine. Dietary Reference Intakes for Water, Potassium, Sodium, Chloride, and Sulfate. Washington, DC: National Academy Press, 2004.
28. Krasinski SD, Cohn JS, Schaefer EJ et al. J Clin Invest 1990; 85:883–92.
29. Russell RM. Am J Clin Nutr 2000;72[Suppl]:529S–32S.
30. Penniston KL, Tanumihardjo SA. J Am Diet Assoc 2003;103: 1185–7.
31. Clinical Nutrition Service, Warren Grant Magnuson Clinical Center, National Institutes of Health Web site. Facts about Dietary Supplements: Vitamin A and Carotenoids. http//www.cc.nih.gov/home.cgi. National Institutes of Health, 2003. Accessed March 16, 2004.
32. Feskanich D, Singh V, Willett WC et al. JAMA 2002;287:47–54.
33. Melhus H, Michaelsson K, Kindmark A et al. Ann Intern Med 1998;129:770–8.
34. Janssen HCJP, Samson MM, Verhaar HJJ. Am J Clin Nutr 2002; 75:611–5.
35. Pfeifer M, Begerow B, Minne HW. Osteoporosis Int 2002;13: 187–94.
36. Bischoff-Ferrari HA, Dawson-Hughes B, Willett WC et al. JAMA 2004;291:1999–2006.
37. Roth SM, Zmuda JM, Cauley JA et al. J Gerontol Biol Sci 2004; 59A:10–15.
38. MacLaughlin J, Holick MF. J Clin Invest 1985;76:1536–8.
39. Matsuoka LY, Wortsman J, Dannenberg MJ et al. J Clin Endocrinol Metab 1992;75:1099–103.
40. Friedlander J, Janulis M, Tembe V et al. J Bone Miner Res 1994;9:339–45.
41. Tsai KS, Heath H 3rd, Kumar R et al. J Clin Invest 1984; 73:1668–1672.
42. Wood RJ, Fleet JC, Cashman K et al. Endocrinology 1998; 139:3843–8.
43. Pattanaungkul S, Riggs BL, Yergey AL et al. J Clin Endocrinol Metab 2000;85:4023–7.
44. Jacques PF, Felson DT, Tucker Kl et al. Am J Clin Nutr 1997; 66:929–36.
45. Holick MF. Am J Clin Nutr 2004;79:362–371.
46. Dawson-Hughes B, Harris SS, Krall EA et al. Am J Clin Nutr 1995;61:1140–5.
47. Clemens TL, Zhou XY, Myles M et al. J Clin Endocrinol Metab 1986;63:656–60.
48. Gennari C. Public Health Nutr 2001;4:547–59.
49. Food and Nutrition Board, Institute of Medicine. Dietary Reference Intakes for Vitamin C, Vitamin E, Selenium, and Carotenoids. Washington, DC: National Academy Press, 2000.
50. Ryan AS, Craig LD, Finn SC. J Gerontol 1992;47:M145–50.
51. Szulc P, Chapuy MC, Meunier PJ et al. Bone 1996;18:487–8.
52. Szulc P, Arlot M, Chapuy MC et al. J Bone Miner Res 1994; 9:1591–5.
53. Feskanich D, Weber P, Willett WC et al. Am J Clin Nutr 1999; 69:74–9.
54. Booth SL, Pennington JA, Sadowski JA. J Am Diet Assoc 1996; 96:149–54.
55. Ferland G, Sadowski JA, O'Brien ME. J Clin Invest 1993; 91: 1761–8.
56. Booth SL, Martini L, Peterson JW et al. J Nutr 2003; 133: 2565–9.
57. Binkley NC, Krueger DC, Kawahara TN et al. Am J Clin Nutr 2002;76:1055–60.
58. Sheiham A, Steele JG, Marcenes W et al. J Dent Res 2001; 80:408–13.

59. Charlton KE, Rabinowitz TL, Geffen LN et al. J Nutr Health Aging 2004;8:99–107.

60. Lowik MR, Hulshof KF, Schneijder P et al. J Am Diet Assoc 1993;93:167–72.

61. Leske MC, Chylack LT Jr, Wu SY. Arch Ophthalmol 1991; 109:244–51.

62. Fletcher AE, Breeze E, Shetty PS. Am J Clin Nutr 2003;78: 999–1010.

63. Jacob RA, Sotoudeh G. Nutr Clin Care 2002;5:66–74.

64. Richardson TI, Ball L, Rosenfeld T. Postgrad Med J 2002; 78:292–4.

65. Food and Nutrition Board, Institute of Medicine. Dietary Reference Intakes for Thiamin, Riboflavin, Niacin, Vitamin B$_6$, Folate, Vitamin B$_{12}$, Pantothenic Acid, Biotin, and Choline. Washington, DC: National Academy Press, 1998.

66. Wilkinson TJ, Hanger HC, Elmslie J et al. Am J Clin Nutr 1997; 66:925–8.

67. Powers HJ. Am J Clin Nutr 2003;77:1352–60.

68. Boisvert BA, Castaneda C, Mendoza I et al. Am J Clin Nutr 1993;58:85–90.

69. Alaimo K, McDowell MA, Briefel RR et al. Adv Data 1994; 258:1–28.

70. Bates CJ, Prentice AM, Cole TJ et al. Br J Nutr 1999;82:7–15.

71. Madigan SM, Tracey F, McNulty H et al. Am J Clin Nutr 1998; 68:389–95.

72. Boisvert WA, Mendoza I, Castaneda C et al. J Nutr 1993; 123:915–925.

73. Lee JS, Frongillo EA Jr. J Nutr 2001;131:1503–9.

74. Bailey LB, Cerda JJ, Bloch BS et al. J Nutr 1984;114:1770–6.

75. Wilmink AB, Welch AA, Quick CR et al. J Vasc Surg 2004;39: 513–6.

76. Rampersaud GC, Kauwell GP, Bailey LB. J Am Coll Nutr 2003; 22:1–8.

77. Kuller LH, Evans RW. Circulation 1998;98:196–9.

78. Rosenberg IH. Folate. In: Hartz SC, Russell RM, Rosenberg IH, eds. Nutrition in the Elderly: The Boston Nutritional Status Survey. London: Smith–Gordon, 1992:135–9.

79. U.S. Department of Agriculture, Agriculture Research Service. Data Tables: Results from USDA's 1994–96 Continuing Survey of Food Intakes by Individuals and 1994–96 Diet and Health Knowledge Survey, ARS Food Surveys Research Group. http//www.barc.usda.gov/bhnrc/foodsurvey/home.htm.

80. Essama-Tjani JC, Guilland JC, Potier de Courcy G et al. J Am Coll Nutr 2000;19:392–404.

81. Russell RM. J Nutr 2001;131[Suppl]:1359S–61S.

82. Marshall TA, Stumbo PJ, Warren JJ et al. J Nutr 2001;131: 2192–6.

83. Miller JW, Green R, Mungas DM et al. Neurology 2002; 58:1471–5.

84. Kelly PJ, Kistler JP, Shih VE et al. Stroke 2004;35:12–5 (Epub 2003 Dec 04).

85. Chiang EP, Bagley PJ, Selhub J et al. Am J Med 2003;114:283–7.

86. Bates CJ, Pentieva KD, Prentice A et al. Br J Nutr 1999;81: 191–201.

87. van Asselt DZ, van den Broek WJ, Lamers CB et al. J Am Geriatr Soc 1996;44:949–53.

88. Ho C, Kauwell GP, Bailey LB. J Am Diet Assoc 1999;99:725–7.

89. Scarlett JD, Read H, O'Dea K. Am J Hematol 1992;39:79–83.

90. Morris MS, Jacques PF, Rosenberg IH et al. J Nutr 2002; 132:2799–803.

91. Joosten E, van den Berg A, Riezler R. Am J Clin Nutr 1993; 58:468–76.

92. Wright J, Bialostosky K, Gunter E et al. Vital Health Stat 1998; 11:1–78.

93. Carmel R, Sinow RM, Siegel ME et al. Arch Intern Med 1988; 148:1715–9.

94. Saltzman JR, Russell RM. Gastroenterol Clin North Am 1998; 27:309–4.

95. Bryant RJ, Cadogan J, Weaver CM. J Am Coll Nutr 1999; 18[Suppl]:406S–12S.

96. Garland C, Shekelle RB, Barrett-Connor E et al. Lancet 1985; 1:307–9.

97. McCarron DA, Morris CD, Young E et al. Am J Clin Nutr 1991;54[Suppl]:215S–19S.

98. Bullamore JR, Wilkinson R, Gallagher JC et al. Lancet 1970; 2:535–7.

99. Heaney RP, Recker RR, Stegman MR. J Bone Miner Res 1989; 4:469–75.

100. Spencer H, Kramer L, Lesniak M et al. Clin Orthop 1984; 184:270–80.

101. Dawson-Hughes B, Dallal GE, Krall EA et al. N Engl J Med 1990;323:878–83.

102. Recker RR, Hinders S, Davies KM et al. J Bone Miner Res 1996;11:1961–6.

103. Nieves JW, Komar L, Cosman F et al. Am J Clin Nutr 1998; 67:18–24.

104. Macdonald HM, New SA, Golden MH et al. Am J Clin Nutr 2004;79:155–65.

105. Anonymous. FDA Consum 2003;37:36–7.

106. Ervin R, Wright J, Kennedy-Stephenson J. Vital Health Stat 1999;11:1–14.

107. Lowik MR, van Dokkum W, Kistemaker C et al. Magnes Res 1993;6:223–32.

108. Martin BJ. Aging (Milano) 1990;2:291–6.

109. Tucker KL, Hannan MT, Chen H et al. Am J Clin Nutr 1999; 69:727–36.

110. New SA, Bolton-Smith C, Grubb DA et al. Am J Clin Nutr 1997;65:1831–9.

111. New SA, Robins SP, Campbell MK et al. Am J Clin Nutr 2000; 71:142–51.

112. Tranquilli AL, Lucino E, Garzetti GG et al. Gynecol Endocrinol 1994;8:55–8.

113. Reginster JY, Strause L, Deroisy R et al. Magnesium 1989;8:106–9.

114. Rude RK, Gruber HE, Norton HJ et al. J Nutr 2004;134:79–85.

115. Stendig-Lindberg G, Tepper R, Leichter I. Magnes Res 1993; 6:155–63.

116. Garry PJ, Hunt WC, Baumgartner RN. J Am Coll Nutr 2000; 19:262–9.

117. Vaquero MP. J Nutr Health Aging 2002;6:147–53.

118. Tuomainen TP, Nyyssonen K, Salonen R et al. Diabetes Care 1997;20:426–8.

119. Fernandez-Real JM, Ricart-Engel W, Arroyo E et al. Diabetes Care 1998;21:62–8.

120. Tuomainen TP, Kontula K, Nyyssonen K et al. Circulation 1999;100:1274–9.

121. Hallberg L, Hulten L, Gramatkovski E. Am J Clin Nutr 1997; 66:347–56.

122. Fleming DJ, Jacques PF, Dallal GE et al. Am J Clin Nutr 1998; 67:722–33.

123. Ahluwalia N, Sun J, Krause D et al. Am J Clin Nutr 2004;79: 516–21.

124. Thomas DR. J Gerontol A Biol Sci Med Sci 2004;59:M238–41.

125. Cesari M, Pennix BW, Lauretani F. J Gerontol A Biol Sci Med Sci 2004;59:M249–54.

126. van Tellingen A, Kuenen JC, de Kieviet W et al. Neth J Med 2001;59:270–9.

127. Goodwin JS. Nutr Rev 1995;53:S41–4; discussion S44–6.

128. Bogden JD. J Nutr Health Aging 2004;8:48–54.
129. McClain CJ, McClain M, Barve S et al. Clin Geriatr Med 2002; 18:801–18.
130. Couzy F, Kastenmayer P, Mansourian R et al. Am J Clin Nutr 1993;58:690–4.
131. Hunt JR, Gallagher SK, Johnson LK et al. Am J Clin Nutr 1995; 62:621–32.
132. Hallfrisch J, Powell A, Carafelli C et al. J Nutr 1987;117: 48–55.
133. Wood RJ, Zheng JJ. Am J Clin Nutr 1997;65:1803–9.
134. Bales CW, DiSilvestro RA, Currie KL et al. J Am Coll Nutr 1994; 13:455–62.
135. Prasad AS, Fitzgerald JT, Hess JW et al. Nutrition 1993;9: 218–24.
136. Boukaiba N, Flament C, Acher SA. Am J Clin Nutr 1993;57: 566–72.
137. Bogden JD, Oleske JM, Munves EM et al. Am J Clin Nutr 1987;46:101–9.
138. Kreft B, Fischer A, Kruger S et al. Biogerontology 2000;1: 61–6.
139. High KP. Clin Infect Dis 2001;33:1892–900.
140. Girondan F, Blache D, Monget AL et al. J Am Coll Nutr 1997; 16:357–65.
141. Gengenbacher M, Stahelin HB, Scholer A et al. Aging Clin Exp Res 2002;14:420–3.
142. Houston DK, Johnson MA, Daniel TD et al. Int J Vitam Nutr Res 1997;67:183–91.
143. Prasad AS, Mantzoros CS, Beck FW et al. Nutrition 1996; 12:344–8.
144. Ugarte M, Osborne NN. Prog Neurobiol 2001;64:219–49.
145. Briefel RR, Bialostosky K, Kennedy-Stephenson J et al. J Nutr 2000;130[Suppl]:1367S–73S.
146. Food and Nutrition Board, Institute of Medicine. Dietary Reference Intakes for Vitamin A, Vitamin K, Arsenic, Boron, Chromium, Copper, Iodine, Iron, Manganese, Molybdenum, Nickel, Silicon, Vanadium, and Zinc. Washington, DC: National Academy Press, 2001.
147. Failla ML. Proc Nutr Soc 1999;58:497–505.
148. Savarino L, Granchi D, Ciapetti G et al. Exp Gerontol 2001;36: 327–39.
149. Madaric A, Ginter E, Kadrabova J. Physiol Res 1994;43: 107–11.
150. Cakman I, Kirchner H, Rink L. J Interferon Cytokine Res 1997;17:469–72.
151. Fortes C, Forastiere F, Agabiti N et al. J Am Geriatr Soc 1998; 46:19–26.
152. Ma J, Betts NM. J Nutr 2000;130:2838–43.
153. Klevay LM. J Am Coll Nutr 1998;17:322–6.
154. Masugi J, Amano M, Fukuda T. Ann Intern Med 1994;121: 386.
155. Milne DB. Am J Clin Nutr 1998;67[Suppl]:1041S–5S.
156. Saari JT. Can J Physiol Pharmacol 2000;78:848–55.
157. Conlan D, Korula R, Tallentire D. Age Ageing 1990;19: 212–4.
158. Strause L, Saltman P, Smith KT et al. J Nutr 1994;124: 1060–4.
159. Squitti R, Pasqualetti P, Cassetta E et al. Neurology 2003; 60:2013–4.
160. Christen Y. Am J Clin Nutr 2000;71:621S–9S.
161. Squitti R, Lupoi D, Pasqualetti P et al. Neurology 2002;59: 1153–61.
162. Anderson RA. J Am Coll Nutr 1997;16:404–10.
163. Offenbacher EG, Rinko CJ, Pi–Sunyer FX. Am J Clin Nutr 1985;42:454–61.
164. Amato P, Morales AJ, Yen SS. J Gerontol A Biol Sci Med Sci 2000;55:M260–3.
165. Davies S, McLaren Howard J, Hunnisett A et al. Metabolism 1997;46:469–73.
166. Brown RO, Forloines-Lynn S, Cross RE et al. Dig Dis Sci 1986; 31:661–4.
167. Harris MI, Flegal KM, Cowie CC et al. Diabetes Care 1998; 21:518–24.
168. Ekmekcioglu C, Prohaska C, Pomazal K et al. Biol Trace Elem Res 2001;79:205–19.
169. Witte KK, Clark AL, Cleland JG. J Am Coll Cardiol 2001; 37:1765–74.
170. Subar AF, Block G. Am J Epidemiol 1990;132:1091–2101.
171. Payette H, Gray-Donald K. Am J Clin Nutr 1991;54:478–88.
172. McKay DL, Perrone G, Rasmussen H et al. J Nutr 2000; 130:3090–6.
173. Girodon F, Galan P, Monget AL et al. Arch Intern Med 1999; 159:748–54.
174. Bogden JD, Bendick A, Kemp FW et al. Am J Clin Nutr 1994; 60:437–47.
175. Chandra R. Lancet 1992;340:1124–7.
176. Fletcher RH, Fairfield KM. JAMA 2002;287:3127–9.
177. Morley JE. Am J Clin Nutr 1997;66:760–73.
178. Morley JE J Gerontol Med Sci 2001;56:81–8.
179. Ritchie CS, Joshipura K, Silliman RA. J Gerontol Med Sci 2000; 55:M366–71.
180. Black SA, Rush RD. J Am Geriatr Soc 2002;50:1978–86.
181. Fried LP, Guralnik JM. J Am Geriatr Soc 1997;45:92–100.
182. Wolf AM, Colditz GA. Obes Res 1998;6:97–106.
183. Davison KK, Ford ES, Cogswell ME et al. J Am Geriatr Soc 2002;50:1802–9.
184. Sowers JR. Am J Med 2003;115[Suppl]:37S–41S.
185. Jensen GL, Rogers J. J Am Diet Assoc 1998;98:1301–11.
186. Kissebah AH. Diabetes Res Clin Pract 1996;30[Suppl]: 25–30.
187. Fine JT, Colditz GA, Coakley EH et al. JAMA 1999;282: 2136–42.
188. Coakley EH, Kawachi I, Manson JE et al. Int J Obes Relat Metab Disord 1998;22:958–65.
189. Jensen GL, Friedman JM. J Am Geriatr Soc 2002;50:918–23.
190. Ledikwe JH, Smiciklas-Wright H, Mitchell DC et al. Am J Clin Nutr 2003;77:551–8.
191. Persson M, Elmstahl S, Westerterp KR. Eur J Clin Nutr 2000; 54:789–96.
192. Bingham SA, Cassidy A, Cole TJ et al. Br J Nutr 1995; 73: 531–50.
193. van Staveren WA, de Groot LCPGM, Blauw YH et al. Am J Clin Nutr 1994;59[Suppl]:221–3.
194. Robinson MK, Trujillo EB, Mogensen KM et al. JPEN J Parenter Enteral Nutr 2003;27:389–95.
195. Sullivan DH, Bopp MM, Roberson PK. J Gen Intern Med 2002;17:923–32.
196. Omran ML, Morley JE. Nutrition 2000;16:131–40.
197. Clemmons DR, Underwood LE, Dickerson RN et al. Am J Clin Nutr 1985;41:191–8.
198. Sullivan DH, Carte WJ. J Am Coll Nutr 1994;13:184–91.
199. Fabiny AR, Kiel DP. Clin Geriatr Med 1997;4:737–51.
200. Thomas DR, Ashmen W, Morley JE et al. J Gerontol Med Sci 2000;55A:M725–34.
201. Zawada ET Jr. Postgrad Med 1996;100:207–22.
202. Newman AB, Yanez D, Harris T et al. J Am Geriatr Soc 2001; 49:1309–18.
203. Gallagher D, Ruts E, Visser M et al. Am J Physiol Endocrinol Metab 2000;279:E366–75.

204. Harris TB, Visser M, Everhart J et al. Ann NY Acad Sci 2000;904:462–73.
205. Heymsfield SB, Nunez C, Testolin C et al. Eur J Clin Nutr 2000;54[Suppl]:26S–32S.
206. Baumgartner RN, Koehler KM, Gallagher D et al. Am J Epidemiol 1998;147:744–63.
207. Heymsfield SB, McManus C, Smith J et al. Am J Clin Nutr 1982;36:680–90.
208. Hansen RD, Raja C, Aslani A et al. Am J Clin Nutr 1999; 70:228–33.
209. Donini LM, Savina C, Rosano A et al. J Nutr Health Aging 2003;7:282–93.
210. Detsky AS, Smalley PS, Chang J. JAMA 1994;271:54–58.
211. Sacks GS, Dearman K, Replogle WH et al. J Am Coll Nutr 2000;19:570–7.

SUGGESTED READINGS

Ho C, Kauwell GP, Bailey LB. Practitioners' guide to meeting the vitamin B_{12} recommended dietary allowance for people aged 51 years and older. J Am Diet Assoc 1999;99:725–7.

Holick MF. Vitamin D: importance in the prevention of cancers, type 1 diabetes, heart disease, and osteoporosis. Am J Clin Nutr 2004;79: 362–371.

McClain CJ, McClain M, Barve S et al. Trace metals and the elderly. Clin Geriatr Med 2002;18:801–818.

Russell RM. The aging process as a modifier of metabolism. Am J Clin Nutr 2000;72[Suppl]:529S–32S.

Wakimoto P, Block G. Dietary intake, dietary patterns, and changes with age: an epidemiological perspective. J Gerontol A Biol Sci Med Sci 2001;56:65–8.

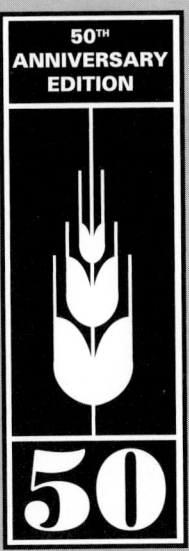

50TH ANNIVERSARY EDITION

50

PART V

PREVENTION AND MANAGEMENT OF DISEASE

A. Pediatric and Adolescent Disorders / 861
B. Disorders of Metabolism / 1004
C. Prevention and Management of Cardiovascular Disease / 1067
D. Disorders of the Alimentary Tract / 1115
E. Prevention and Management of Cancer / 1260
F. Prevention and Management of Skeletal and Joint Disorders / 1314
G. Psychiatric, Behavioral, and Neurological Disorders / 1353
H. Nutrition in Surgery, Infection, and Trauma / 1381
I.   Other Systemic Disorders / 1436
J.   Drug-Nutrient Interaction / 1539
K. Systems of Nutritional Support / 1554

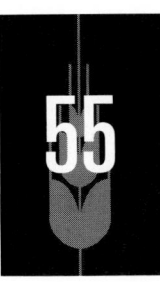

55 MALNUTRITION AMONG CHILDREN IN THE UNITED STATES: THE IMPACT OF POVERTY[1]

ROBERT KARP

MALNUTRITION IN THE CONTEXT OF POVERTY ..... .861
DEFINING POVERTY .... .861
CONSEQUENCES OF LIVING IN POVERTY .... .862
  "Microsocial" and "Macrosocial"
    Environments .... .862
  The Working Poor .... .863
IMPACT OF POVERTY ON NUTRITIONAL
  STATUS .... .863
  Impact of Poverty on Growth .... .863
  Impact of Poverty on Micronutrient Status ..... .864
  Impact of Poverty on Overnutrition .... .864
  Impact of Poverty on Food Insecurity .... .864
HOW POVERTY LEADS TO MALNUTRITION .... .865
  Impact of Food Cost on Food Selection
    and Nutritional Status .... .865
  Impact of Food Culture on Food Selection
    and Nutritional Status .... .866
IMPACT OF POVERTY ON LEARNING
  AND BEHAVIOR .... .866
UNDERNUTRITION AND LEARNING FAILURE .... .867
  A Historical Perspective: Heredity,
    Environment, or Nutrition? .... .867
HOW NUTRITION AND ENVIRONMENT INTERACT
  TO AFFECT LEARNING .... .867
  Environment as Cofactor .... .868
ECOLOGY OF POVERTY, MALNUTRITION,
  AND LEARNING FAILURE .... .868
  Child Development: A Theory of Trajectories ..... .868
NUTRITION-DRUG INTERACTIONS AND
  THEIR EFFECTS .... .870
  Drug Abuse Is Increased by Poverty .... .870
  Prevalence and Consequences of Drug,
    Alcohol, and Tobacco Use .... .870
IMPORTANCE OF PUBLIC POLICY: KEEPING
  NUTRITIOUS FOOD AVAILABLE TO
  THE POOR .... .871
  Effective Interventions .... .872
SUMMARY .... .872

[1] Abbreviations: BMI, body mass index; CNS, central nervous system; FAS, fetal alcohol syndrome; NHANES, National Health and Nutrition Examination Study; PRWORA, Personal Responsibility and Work Opportunity Reconciliation Act; WIC, Women, Infants, and Children.

MALNUTRITION IN THE CONTEXT OF POVERTY

In 2002, as many as 12.1 million (16.7%) of all children in the United States lived in families with incomes below the poverty level. Children less than 6 years old were particularly vulnerable to living in poverty. Almost 49% of children living with a single mother were in poverty as compared with 9.7% of children in married-couple families (1, 2). These rates of child poverty are substantially higher than those of other industrial democracies (3).

Persistent poverty leads to the consequences of malnutrition and learning failure (4). Data from the National Longitudinal Survey of Youth of 5300 children born between 1979 and 1988 substantiated the impact of poverty lasting more than 10 years. Children in families living at or below an average of one half the poverty level for 10 years were 2.9 times as likely to experience "wasting," defined as less than the tenth percentile for weight –for length adjusted for sex, as compared with children living in income-secure families with an averaged 10-year income of greater than three times the poverty level. Children living in families with a 10-year average income between twice and one times the poverty level were 1.9 times as likely to be wasted as children living in income-secure families. By contrast, children with a single year of poverty had 1.3 times the likelihood of wasting than children in income-secure homes (4).

Some effects of poverty are direct. Nutritious food is simply too expensive to purchase without support. Other effects are indirect; behavioral adjustments to chronic poverty are likely to affect nutritional status adversely (4). This chapter shows how the powerful environment created by poverty affects food intake, nutritional status, behavior, and intellectual performance of children concomitantly in an interactive model (e.g., each variable affects outcome depending on levels or characteristics of the others) (5, 6). These consequences contribute to ongoing cycles of poverty and malnutrition (7).

DEFINING POVERTY

Since the mid-1960s, the US government has used the following absolute definition of poverty: an income three times the value of a low-cost diet for a family unit (8). This definition originated with a need to provide economic support for the miner's widow or an incapacitated worker and

TABLE 55.1. POVERTY LEVEL FOR FAMILIES OF DIFFERENT SIZES IN 2003

SIZE OF FAMILY UNIT	INCOME LEVEL (DOLLARS)
1	8,980
2	12,120
3	15,260
4	18,400
5	21,540

Data from Proctor B, Dalaker J. US Census Bureau, Poverty in the United States: 2002, Current Population Reports, P60–222, Washington, DC: US Government Printing Office, 2003.

assumed economic dependence. Using this definition in 2002, 34.6 million people (12.1% of the total population of the United States) were living below the poverty threshold. Of these people, 14.1 million (4.9% total) were considered to be in "severe poverty." Income levels for families of different sizes are shown in Table 55.1 (1). Although children living in single-parent homes are highly vulnerable to poverty, substantial numbers of poor children live in two-parent homes with one or both parents working. As noted, over 9% of families with two parents and two children live below the poverty level (2).

The absolute definition of poverty is not adjusted for resources provided to the family, the cost of living in different localities, or the cost of going to work (e.g., transportation, clothing, or day care). "Welfare-reliance" is no longer accepted as an appropriate response to poverty. The Personal Responsibility and Work Opportunity Reconciliation Act (PRWORA) of 1996 calls for "work-reliance" to promote economic independence (9). To this end, the National Academy of Science suggested using a relative definition of poverty that calculates the sum of earned income plus support and then credits the family for expenses necessary to work, such as health care, clothing, day care, transportation, and their own education (8). Poverty-level incomes are adjusted for the cost of living in specific localities. For example, the proposed changes would convert the poverty status of a three-person family in a large New England city with a working low-income parent and minimal support for rent, heat, or food from "nonpoor" to "poor." By contrast, a family living in similar conditions in the rural Midwest and receiving substantial support would be reclassified from "poor" to "nonpoor."

Recalculating the percentage of family income from employment or from unearned income has no effect on the absolute number of families classified as "poor." It does, however, equalize the percentage of families who work across the economic spectrum with an almost identical percentage of families who work at all levels of family income. In Boston, families living below the poverty level cannot survive without working (10). Otherwise, their children will starve (9). Vozoris and colleagues provided similar data for poor families in Toronto, Canada (11).

CONSEQUENCES OF LIVING IN POVERTY

"Microsocial" and "Macrosocial" Environments

Living in poverty means having inadequate social as well as economic resources in the environment (11). Children live in the world of their parents and the institutions that serve families directly. This is the "microsocial" environment proximal to children's experience (5), including being at home with parents or babysitters, in day care, preschool, or school, at the library, or with police in the neighborhood.

For the casual observer, failure to nurture children within the microsocial environments that are characteristic of poverty is seen as the *cause* rather than the *consequence* of poverty (12, 13). The beliefs held by many people in the United States about the cause of poverty distinguish between the people who deserve support and those who do not, based on how well the poor harbor their resources and behave. This view fails to recognize that, for the poor, behavior is shaped by the power of a macrosocial environment they are unable to change, distal from the experiences of children and family (5, 6, 12–14). For families living in persistent poverty, the schools, health care system, and opportunities for work fail the family and indirectly affect their children's welfare. The greatest impact of poverty, therefore, is the creation of a powerful environment seemingly out of the control of those living in it (14). What may seem irrational or even self-destructive from the perspective of those living outside such a powerful environment may seem perfectly appropriate and effective from within (12–14).

Malnutrition, like most child health problems in the United States, wrote Weitzman and Moss (15), is not distributed evenly through the population. It disproportionately affects and clusters among children living in social adversity:

> Low birth weight, infant mortality, deaths due to unintentional injuries, HIV infection, asthma, lead poisoning, iron deficiency anemia, abuse, under and over nutrition, school failure, mental health problems, and [dental] caries all are more common among children who live in poverty, are minorities, and who have parents with low educational achievement (15).

No cause-and-effect relationship between environment or nutrition and developmental or health outcome should be assumed. Rather, a covariate, interactive model is suggested (5, 6). Chronic poverty affects all outcomes including measures of long-term health and development. Social environments, including parenting and educational opportunity, are intermediary variables where:

POVERTY negatively affects SOCIAL ENVIRONMENT, which negatively affects OUTCOMES.

As shown in Figure 55.1, the elements associated with living in poverty in the United States—malnutrition, learning failure, lack of social support, poor self-esteem, and dysfunctional or ineffective parental behavior—feed on

MALNUTRITION and THE CYCLE OF POVERTY

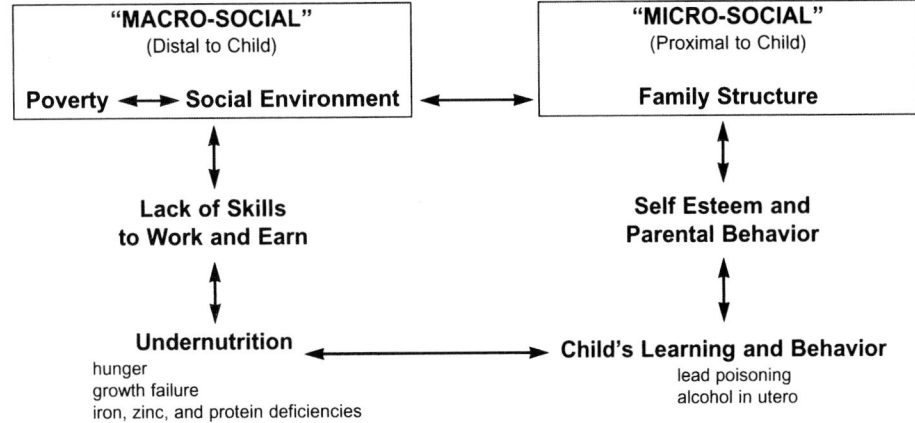

Figure 55.1. Malnutrition and the cycle of poverty. (From Karp RJ. The dimensions of poverty among children in the United States: an exposition of causes and consequences. Epilogue to the Curriculum for Poor and Underserved Children of the Ambulatory Pediatric Association, 2002. http://www.servingtheunderserved .org.html. Copyright 2002 Ambulatory Pediatric Association, with permission.)

© 2002, Ambulatory Pediatric Association

themselves to regenerate poverty, from one generation to the next.

The Working Poor

Under the recently enacted PRWORA regulations, after 2 years on public assistance, recipients must work. Families that have been on assistance for more than 5 years are ineligible for cash aid. The 2002 reauthorization of PRWORA called for more stringent work requirements, but it also allotted more funds for low-income child care on the federal and state level (9). Even before PRWORA, however, the poor were just as likely to be employed as the affluent, albeit with work that often did not pay sufficiently well to provide for the necessities of life (8). Success in transforming a "welfare-reliant" to "work-reliant" low-income workforce, therefore, requires implementation of a complete package of increased expectation and increased support (8, 9, 16).

IMPACT OF POVERTY ON NUTRITIONAL STATUS

In 1965, D. B. Jelliffe (17) described four overlapping types of malnutrition found in communities. These were (a) caloric undernutrition, (b) specific nutrient deficiencies, (c) caloric overnutrition, and (d) nutrient imbalance. Jelliffe defined nutrient imbalance as the pathologic state resulting from a disproportion among essential nutrients, with or without the absolute deficiency of any specific nutrient (17). Using a sample of 9698 children, 2 to 16 years of age, from the third National Health and Nutrition Examination Study (NHANES III) (1988–1994), Nead and associates (18) found 13.7% to have a body mass index (BMI, defined as weight in kilograms divided by the square of the height in meters) between the eighty-fifth and ninety-fifth percentiles for age, with an additional 10.2%

having a BMI greater than the ninety-fifth percentile for age. Using an "abnormal two of three" rule for measures of erythrocyte protoporphrin level, percentage of iron saturation, and ferritin level, these authors found that the prevalence of iron deficiency increased from 2.1% for children with a BMI lower than the eighty-fifth percentile to 5.3% for those with a BMI between the eighty-fifth and the ninety-fifth percentile, and 5.5% for children with a BMI greater than the ninety-fifth percentile. This sample was weighted to include a sufficient number of African-American and Mexican-American children, and the data were adjusted for levels of family income and education.

Impact of Poverty on Growth

As Garn and Clark (19) pointed out, "The dimensions of poverty are spelled out in the growth of children." The impact of poverty on the growth of individual children may be either direct or indirect. Growth retardation may reflect a spectrum of problems ranging from inadequate income for food, to ineffective (20) or frankly abusive parenting (21), or to chronic illness (22). The prevalence of growth retardation as seen in communities of children, however, is a measure of the health and well-being of the community itself (23). Failures in the macrosocial environment include the lack of educational resources for mothers and children, inadequate day care, insufficient support for housing and other necessities, the absence of a national policy for provision of food for families with children, and the lack of access to preventive and therapeutic medicine. After 5 years of age, height for age is the single most important indicator of child's well-being. Hardships too small to measure individually accumulate over time (23).

Both undernutrition and overnutrition in early life affect the metabolic milieu of the fetus and infant. Abundant data now show the theory proposed by David Barker (24) to be correct, namely, that early experiences with nutritional deprivation program later responses to abundance. As explained by Krishnaswamy and colleagues (25):

> [T]he fetus in a malnourished womb has to adapt to a limited supply of nutrients thereby changing its physiology, function, and metabolism. Such "programmed" changes may trigger a number of diseases in later life when dietary intakes and lifestyles differ greatly from the deprivation experienced in utero.

Although Barker focused on undernutrition (low birth weight and poor weight gain in the first year of life), obesity in infancy and early childhood may contribute to the consequences he described (24).

Impact of Poverty on Micronutrient Status

Both national surveys (4, 19, 26) and those conducted in small communities (27, 28) show that micronutrient deficiencies are a common phenomenon among extremely poor children. Deficient intake and biochemical measures of micronutrient status, based solely on income, are found for folate (26, 29–32), ascorbic acid, and several of the B vitamin group (31). Although the earlier literature showed vitamin A deficiencies associated with poverty (31), more recent data from NHANES III showed no associations between household income and serum retinol concentration in children (33). NHANES data for 1999 to 2000 were used to calculate a healthy eating index, a summary checklist scoring from 0 to 10 for ten elements of nutritional quality, which showed significant differences between families with incomes below the poverty level and those families with greater than 1.84 times the poverty income in five of the ten categories. Those with the higher level incomes "... had an average variety score of 8.2, while people with household income below the poverty threshold had an average score of 7" (34).

Although substantial declines have been shown in the prevalence of iron deficiency with use of iron-fortified formulas, continued iron deficiency exists in the most vulnerable populations. As Sherry, Mei, and Yip (35) pointed out, our limited progress in elimination of iron deficiency is not from a lack of scientific knowledge about the prevalence, causes, or consequences of iron deficiency, but results from limited implementation of effective intervention strategies and from ineffective communication tools.

Impact of Poverty on Overnutrition

Obesity and nutrient imbalance are the predominate forms of malnutrition among families living at or just above the poverty level (19). The impact of heredity is most striking when both parents are obese or both are lean. When one parent is obese and one is lean, however, the realities of socioeconomic status have greater influence in determining whether children maintain normal body weight or become obese. In poorer populations, the tendency is for fathers and sons to be leaner than mothers and daughters, with the opposite phenomenon in

middle- and upper-income families (19). At the lowest income levels, for families living well below the poverty level, leanness is the rule for everyone (19, 36). Hofferth and Curtin (36) showed that the relationship of poverty with obesity is not linear. Rather, as they wrote, "Children in families whose income ranges from 100 and 300% of poverty are more likely to be overweight (22–23%) than children from either higher- or lower-income families (12% each)." This finding may reflect an early but not yet adequate rise from economic deprivation (37). These phenomena belie the possibility that obesity is a determinant rather than a consequence of poverty.

As Jean Mayer wrote in an earlier edition of this text (38):

> [P]opulations which expect to be subjected at regular intervals to scarcity of food may consider a certain measure of obesity as desirable, indeed as necessary for survival.

The curvilinear relationship between poverty and obesity in families is shown in Figure 55.2.

Impact of Poverty on Food Insecurity

Food insecurity is defined as an uncertainty of having enough food to meet basic needs for all household members because of insufficient money or other resources for food (39). During the period from 1998 to 2000, an average of 613,000 children in 275,000 households (16.1%) were hungry as a result of "resource-restrained hunger." Child hunger was ten times more prevalent in households with incomes below 185% of the official poverty line and three times more prevalent among racial and ethnic minorities (39). The prevalence of food insecurity in households with children was more than double that in households without children (16.1 versus 7.7% in 2001). Children being raised by a single mother were particularly vulnerable (39). The Children's Sentinel Nutrition Assessment Program conducted surveys in six cities in the United States during the period from 1998 to 2004 seeking to determine the interaction between household food security and children's health (40). Among their findings

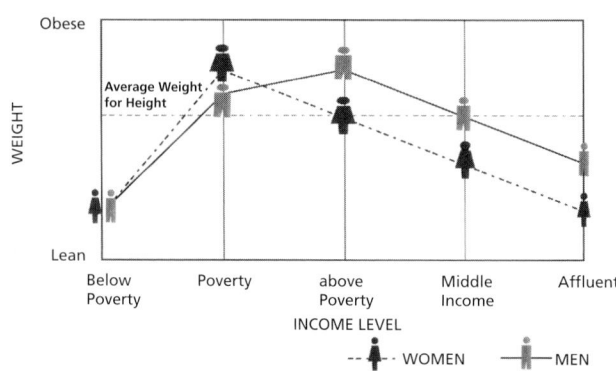

Figure 55.2. Both deprivation and secure substantial incomes are associated with leanness, whereas obesity is common among those of midlevel poverty, especially when it is associated with food insecurity. (From Garn SM, Clark DC. Pediatrics 1975;56:306–19, with permission.)

were a 90% higher chance that infants and toddlers in food-insecure households were in fair or poor health than comparable children in food-secure households. Eligible infants who did not receive Women, Infants, and Children (WIC) benefits were almost twice as likely to be reported in fair or poor health. Moreover, children in food-insecure families receiving housing subsidies were only half as likely to be underweight as those whose families did not receive housing subsidies. Families that had had their food stamp benefits reduced or terminated were more than twice as likely to experience child food insecurity (40).

In a survey conducted in Minneapolis of 2303 children for whom at least one parent was an immigrant from Latin America, Kersey and colleagues (41) found that Latino children were 22.2 times as likely to live in a food-insecure home than non-Latino children in that same community. Moreover, 3.3 times as many Latino children whose parents reported hunger were likely to show laboratory evidence of iron deficiency than children whose parents did not report hunger (41).

Although food insecurity in adults is consistently associated with obesity, the effect of food insecurity on the prevalence of obesity in childhood remains uncertain. Food insecurity is associated with obesity in adolescent girls in poor white families. Whereas the prevalence of obesity is higher in black and Hispanic families at all income levels, food insecurity does not seem to increase the levels of obesity among poor children in these communities (42). Although substantial hereditary contributions to obesity exist (see Chapter 63), endemic poverty, food insecurity, and both low (24) and high birth weights (25) must also be considered as risk factors. As suggested by primate data, food insecurity is only one element of an environment likely to promote obesity as mediated through a universal stress response (43).

HOW POVERTY LEADS TO MALNUTRITION

Impact of Food Cost on Food Selection and Nutritional Status

The Engels phenomenon describes the changes in food consumption likely to occur with decreased income or increased cost for food or other necessities (44–46). With chronic poverty, food selection narrows to those items providing the most energy at the lowest cost (44). Over time, micronutrients disappear from the diet, and specific nutrient deficiencies follow. The relationship between income and expenses for necessities at all income levels is shown in Figure 55.3.

As shown in Figure 55.3, poorer workers' increased earnings do not generate discretionary income until the total of income from earnings plus supplementation reaches poverty level (44, 46–48). By contrast, affluent persons have more than enough income to cover the costs of necessities, and every new dollar is spent on something

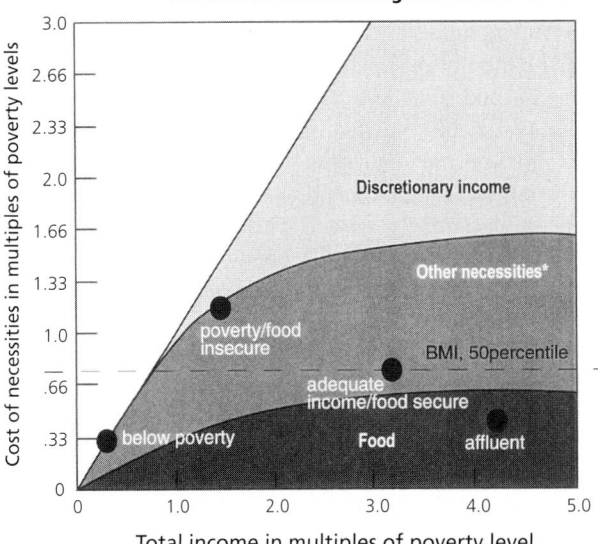

Figure 55.3. Engel curves. (From Karp R. The problem of changing food habits: 1. How habits are formed. In: Karp RJ, ed. Malnourished Children in the United States: Caught in the Cycle of Poverty. New York: Springer, 1993:194–211, with permission.)

of their own choosing, not necessarily food, housing, or other necessities of life. The observation derives from a description of eating patterns of English workers from the midnineteenth century by Freidrich Engels (45):

> The habitual food of an individual working man naturally varies according to his wage. The better paid workers, especially those in whose families every member is able to earn something, have good food as long as this state of things last; meat daily and bacon and cheese for supper. Where wages are less, meat is used only two or three times a week, and the proportion of bread and potatoes increases. Descending gradually, we find animal food reduced to a small piece of bacon cut up with potatoes; lower still, even this disappears, and there remain only bread, cheese, porridge, and potatoes, until on the lowest round of the ladder, among the Irish, potatoes form the sole food (45).

Evidence of iron deficiency anemia following a rise in food costs (49), growth retardation associated with high housing costs (28, 47), and a gradient of food selection by income (50) provide examples of the Engels phenomenon at work among inner-city poor children in today's society.

Several contemporary studies have shown the impact of living at poverty level incomes and below on nutritional status (10, 47). Bhattacharya and colleagues (47) interpolated data from the Consumer Expenditure Survey and from NHANES III showing increases in fuel expenditure in colder weather of about $9 for every 10°F decrement for both families living in poverty and those with midlevel and higher incomes. By contrast, the associated change in expenditure for wealthier families was an $11 increase for each 10°F decrement. Poor families decreased food expenditure by 9% for each 10°F decrement. A "Health Rating Index" applied to the diet histories (34) showed that both quality of food consumed and nutritional status deteriorated among poorer children, with increases in the prevalence of anemia and vitamin deficiency. These results, however, did not reach statistical significance.

Vozoris and colleagues (11), in a study of a single community in Toronto, showed that the cost of basic needs for food and housing competed with each other. Welfare-dependent families had insufficient total income for food when they attempted to live without rental support. As these investigators wrote, "Living in rent-geared-to-income housing afforded substantial financial advantage, but the welfare income of single-person households was still insufficient to meet basic needs." Drewnowski and Specter (48) reviewed data from several national and international surveys to make an essential point consistent with the Engel phenomenon. Spending less on food leads to high-fat, energy-dense diets that are similar in composition to those consumed by low-income groups (49). Such diets are more affordable than health-prudent diets based on lean meats, fish, fresh vegetables, and fruit (50).

Krebs-Smith and colleagues (29) compared the daily food intake of children from the poorest families (household incomes <$10,000/year) with that of children from the wealthiest families (>$50,000/year). These investigators showed that 59.6% of the poorest children consumed less than one serving of fruit each day as compared with 46.5% of children from the wealthiest. Moreover, the diet of poor children was less likely to contain the recommended five servings of fruit and vegetables (16.3 versus 24.5%), whereas only a minority of children in the United States meets the new standard, regardless of income, of three to five servings of fruits and of vegetables each day (29).

Using confirmatory biochemical markers to avoid overdiagnosing iron deficiency as the cause of anemia, NHANES II, conducted from 1976 to 1980, showed that 20.6% of children 1 to 2 years of age from families living below the poverty level had iron deficiency (51). This finding compared with 6.7% for nonpoor children. For children 3 to 4 years of age, the difference was 9.7% compared with 2.5%. Older children take in more calories and thus more iron. These differences by economic status then disappear until girls reach adolescence, when iron requirements increase. As shown in NHANES II, the differences, which are highly significant, were 8.2% for poor and 2.8% for nonpoor teenage girls (51). Data from NHANES III separated by socioeconomic level are not yet available. As noted earlier, however, children living in poverty continue to be at risk of malnutrition of all forms.

Impact of Food Culture on Food Selection and Nutritional Status

Parental beliefs and practices have a profound effect on the quantity and variety of food that is brought into the family as well as the allocation to each member (23). As Gopalan (23) wrote:

[D]ifferences in the nature of intra-familial distribution of food, in particular in infant feeding and child-rearing practices, between the families and between communities can result in important differences with nutritional status (especially of children) between households, and between communities with nearly similar overall levels of dietary inadequacy.

The use of convenience foods, characteristic of contemporary food consumption patterns in the United States, illustrates how the Engels phenomenon affects the poor. Cheaper convenience foods have lower nutrient density (high fat or sugar content) compared with nutritious foods that people with higher incomes can afford to purchase (44). For some parents—the homeless or indigent, those living in motel rooms or in migrant labor camps—there may be no alternative to convenience foods. These parents may be quite willing to purchase nutritious foods and to prepare and distribute them to their children but are hampered by their circumstances. Their indigenous food preferences may be unique, and their preferred nutritious food choices may be unavailable (10, 11, 50). Moreover, adjustments to chronic poverty may serve to establish cultural norms. Food preferences formed in childhood last a lifetime (44) and affect the likelihood of malnutrition.

IMPACT OF POVERTY ON LEARNING AND BEHAVIOR

The other important long-term effects of early nutritional deprivation are on learning and behavior. No direct cause-and-effect relationship should be assumed between either nutrition or environment and developmental outcome (5, 6). Rather, nonlinear relations exist between nutrition and environment such that the effect of one factor on an outcome depends on the level or characteristic of the other. A seminal work illustrating nutrition-environment interaction was the study by Winick and colleagues (52) of variably undernourished Korean orphans who were reared in good home environments. Long-term consequences of undernutrition depended on the level of preadoption malnutrition of the child. In this as well as other studies, nutrition and environment are shown to combine to affect developmental outcomes (5, 53, 54).

Malnutrition has direct effects on neurodevelopment, however, as with growth retardation (53, 54), iron deficiency (55, 56), and lead poisoning (6, 57). These effects substantially increase the risk of school failure and social dysfunction (5, 6). The relation of nutritional deficiencies to neurodevelopment and developmental outcomes depends on which nutrients, what aspects of neurodevelopment, and during what time period the nutritional deficiency is occurring (5, 6). Moreover, these outcomes depend on what covaries with nutritional deficiencies and what interventions are taken after the nutritional insult. Simply addressing undernutrition (iron deficiency and/or growth retardation) or lead poisoning alone without a multisystem approach to intervention is a certain prescription for failure (5, 6, 53–56). As the National Research Council reported (6):

> The longstanding debate about the importance of nature versus nurture, considered as independent influences, is overly simplistic and scientifically obsolete. ... The important questions now concern how environments influence the expression of genes and how genetic makeup, combined with children's previous experiences, affects their ongoing interactions with their environments during the early years and beyond.

UNDERNUTRITION AND LEARNING FAILURE

Although measures of socioeconomic status are too broad to use in labeling the capability of persons within any of these groups (5, 6) in the United States, children from the poorest and least educated families consistently perform poorly on measures of cognitive ability. This section addresses links between nutrition and the environmental experience that underlie education. How children experience their environment predicts the effects of poverty better than family income or parental educational level alone.

A Historical Perspective: Heredity, Environment, or Nutrition?

At the turn of the twentieth century, examples of transgenerational mental retardation were widely represented by two socially dysfunctional families—the Jukes of New York State and the Kallikaks of central New Jersey (58). The use of their family histories (e.g., heredity) illustrates the failings of a main-effect model—heredity *or* environment *or* nutrition— as *the* cause of learning failure (5–7, 58). Subsequently, it was recognized that there are sensitive periods in a child's development during which malnutrition affects intellectual achievement (5–7). By the 1960s, nutrition, separate from environment, was shown to affect cellular and metabolic changes in developing neural tissues, and attempts were then made to use nutritional influences, rather than multifactorial explanations, for behavioral consequences. As shown by Karp and Qazi (59), the Kallikaks were affected by alcohol in utero (fetal alcohol syndrome [FAS]), and their alcoholism was most likely reinforced by the environment in which they lived.

In 1969, Winick and Rosso suggested (60) that retarded mental development was caused by the permanent cellular changes induced by early undernutrition, following a model of

"POVERTY" → "brain growth" and/or central nervous system (CNS) effects → LEARNING FAILURE and recurrent poverty.

The model was supported by the observation of marked decreases in brain weight and DNA content in infants dying of protein-energy malnutrition, with decreased head circumference and developmental delay in survivors (60). Oski (61) was among the first to suggest that learning problems associated with iron deficiency were mediated by the lack of iron availability for the formation of specific structures and/or key enzyme systems in the CNS. His case-controlled studies of children from impoverished north central Philadelphia found that intellectual performance was directly linked to iron status after controlling for other factors. Oski postulated that behavior is affected by (a) deficiencies in iron-catalyzed CNS monoamine and cytochrome oxidase systems, (b) decreased iron stores in brainstem nuclei, and (c) effects on the γ-aminobutyric acid system in the CNS (55, 60, 61). This theory was supported by the work of Pollitt (62), who wrote, "even at the very early stages of iron deficiency, a decrement in iron-dependent dopamine D2 receptors alters dopamine neurotransmission in the cortex, which in turn, impairs cognitive function."

Neurotransmitter activity in the CNS operates in parallel with the severity of iron deficiency, that is, the decease in hemoglobin levels (56). This has been demonstrated by studies in Latin America that have shown minimal effects on learning with mild iron depletion (decreased ferritin level) and iron deficiency without anemia (decreased serum iron and percentage of saturation). From this perspective, learning failure occurs only in the last phase of iron deficiency in the presence of anemia. The inability to transport oxygen limits a child's ability to sustain motor activity (56), which is critical for learning by exploration and repetition.

Although Idjradinata and Pollitt (55) provided data suggesting that the effects of iron deficiency are reversible with the provision of iron, the preponderance of evidence is that the consequences of iron deficiency in infancy are irreversible (56). These consequences may be a function of the critical phase of development at which they occur and/or of intrinsic effects of iron itself. At the conclusion of a long series of investigations, Lozoff and colleagues (56) provided support for the importance of providing adequate iron in the second 6 months of life to prevent the long-standing consequences of iron deficiency.

As appealing and elegant as the simple model seems, as shown by numerous studies in developing countries (53, 54) as well as in the United States (63), a more appropriate conceptualization is that the *interaction* between nutrition and environment is more important than either entity taken alone (5–7).

HOW NUTRITION AND ENVIRONMENT INTERACT TO AFFECT LEARNING

Parallel to the direct effects of malnutrition on the CNS, malnutrition also contributes to learning failure by affecting transitions, transactions, and the way children experience their environment (5, 6). Because of the transitional nature of learning, cumulative learning failure results when critical phases in neurodevelopment are missed. Malnourished children are often developmentally unprepared to benefit from age-appropriate educational experiences

(5–7, 53, 54). The interactions between malnourished children and their adult caregivers fail to satisfy the emotional needs of either the children or the adults. Malnourished infants and children's lack of attention and unresponsiveness to social stimuli, along with their inability to elicit responses from others, undermine the enthusiasm of parents and teachers alike. These children are "temperamentally different from well nourished ones and will be treated so during the toddler and preschool years" (65). These consequences of malnutrition affect children's ability to learn—to receive, process, comprehend, and transmit information and concepts—differently from well-nourished peers. This phenomenon is called the "experience of environment" (5). Learning experiences throughout life and the likelihood of reward for success are affected.

Unless parents living in poverty are taught how to respond to the special needs of malnourished children, the children's learning and nutrition will continue to cycle downward. Working with poor children in Providence, Rhode Island, Sameroff and colleagues (65) recognized that the variability in outcome of birth weight in medically compromised infants was a function of the "cluster effects" of multiple consequences of poverty. The transactional model for learning described above derives from their work.

Environment as Cofactor

The effects of malnutrition must always be considered in the context of the particular social environment, whether or not evidence of direct toxicity exists (5–7). Ineffective relationships within families and between parents and children affect the growth of poor children. Other family members are frequently undernourished (7). The pattern of single parenthood without a support system is common (13). Medical, social, and educational resources are often inadequately available and underused (12–15). Delayed entry into school and poor attendance are likely (63). Often, the reduced somatic growth used to define malnutrition reflects the concomitant effects of iron and zinc deficiency, inadequate caloric intake (5, 6), exposure to lead (6, 57), and exposure to alcohol and drugs in utero (66).

Successful interventions therefore must target both the nutritional and social environment. Rivera and associates (67) reviewed data for several generations of an ongoing rural Mexican support program that augmented health care, nutrition, and maternal education on rates of anemia and growth. Using a crossover design to preclude any children and families from being denied services, these investigators found that children in the intervention group had hemoglobin concentrations of 11.2 g/dL as compared with 10.75 g/dL in children not yet receiving treatment. A statistically significant age- and length-adjusted height difference of 1.1 cm 1 year after entry was reported (67).

Grantham-McGregor and Ani (53) in Jamaica reported on long-term follow-up of 127 children, identified as undernourished from 9 to 24 months of life, who were assigned at random to receive nutrition support, psychosocial support, both, or neither. The growth and developmental outcomes for these children were compared with one another as well as with a fifth group of 32 well-nourished children included in the original study as controls and an outside control group of 32 children from the same community as the poorly nourished group. Children receiving either the supplementation alone or the stimulation alone did better then the group receiving neither nutrition nor support. However, neither of the single-intervention groups did as well with respect to their immediate and long-term developmental scores as the group of children receiving both supplementation and stimulation. Nevertheless, all groups of growth-retarded children remained developmentally behind children who were normally nourished in infancy.

Similarly, Galler and Barrett (54) followed-up previously undernourished Barbadian children over a 20-year period. These investigators suggested that even with combined nutrition and psychosocial support, children who fail to grow in the first year of life are likely to experience attention problems as they mature. From these studies, they concluded that "behavioral deficits arising from prenatal and [early] childhood malnutrition are much more permanent than physical ones" (54). The emphasis, therefore, must be on prevention of undernutrition prenatally and in early life.

ECOLOGY OF POVERTY, MALNUTRITION, AND LEARNING FAILURE

In developed countries, the prevalence and consequences of malnutrition in young children are related so closely to chronic poverty that one can only rarely distinguish the consequences of these disorders from the consequences of living in the milieu in which undernutrition occurs. Giving food and micronutrients to the nutritionally and socially deprived child without correcting the environment in which the undernutrition occurs is unlikely in the long run to change greatly anything related to learning. Rather, the combination of social and nutritional intervention is more effective than either social or nutritional interventions taken alone (5–7, 53, 54).

Child Development: A Theory of Trajectories

The probability of success or failure of a child's future development is derived from the cumulative experience of success or failure of the past. As described by Pollitt (68), a trajectory for achievement in life is predicted, although not determined, by past experiences. With optimal origins, the trajectory of development in utero is likely to be high with ready achievement of developmental milestones. Within this hypothetically ideal environment, a stronger base is provided for a newborn infant who is fortunate enough to be the result of a no-risk pregnancy than would be provided for an infant born after a problematic pregnancy affected by hypertension, nutrient deficiency, or lead or alcohol exposure. Infants encountering multiple risks during gestation are likely to reach developmental milestones at older ages. Expectations diminish along with achievement.

Similarly, the trajectory of development during the first year of life for a privileged child is likely to be high. There will be a stronger foundation for future success for a 1-year-old child with good nutrition, no exposure to toxins, and responsive, sensitive, stimulating parents. This child is more likely to reach a higher level of development than the toddler with a problematic first year characterized by undernutrition, lead poisoning, or unresponsive, insensitive, or unstimulating parents.

Unfortunately, the longer the string of failures is, the less likely it is that the child will encounter a positive experience or be able to take advantage of that experience. Malnutrition in young children can lead to growth failure and iron deficiency. Lead poisoning often occurs simultaneously. Both growth failure and iron deficiency, in turn, can accentuate the impact of lead on child development. As stated in a report from the Institute of Medicine (69):

> Deficits in brain growth and central nervous system development resulting from early malnutrition can compromise early learning, which can then become a risk for decreased economic opportunities and poverty.

This phenomenon, however, is not predetermined. Neither biology nor environment is destiny (5). Simply stated, the *probability* of future success builds on past success, and the *probability* of future failure builds on past failure, whereas each failure increases the *probability* of encountering later failure, and each success increases the *probability* of later success. Thus, links between one negative experience and another can be disrupted by one or more positive experiences. The cluster of poverty effects that burden poor families can be shed, often one at a time (65). The mother can obtain training in parental skills. The child can have a warm and caring nursery school teacher. Effective medical care can limit, although not eliminate, the consequences of malnutrition and lead poisoning (7, 16).

An important question to consider is whether malnutrition and lead poisoning create unique effects that limit the resilience of affected children. A crisis in development occurs in the fourth grade, when children who have not developed the ability to process information fail in school (70). Higher levels of cognitive function are expected. No longer do children read to demonstrate an ability to decode symbols and say words. They must read to learn to obtain information, to process that information, and to apply it to accomplishing a task. Similarly, children must have their numeric abilities in place to process mathematic information and use it to solve problems. The most complex challenge for 9- and 10-year-old children in fourth grade is the mathematics problem with information provided in words.

The processing must cross boundaries of past learning. As Ramey and colleagues (71) showed, success in early childhood intervention can only be assumed when the fourth grade "ceiling" is passed.

What will be seen in school, as shown in Figure 55.4, is a distinct difference in developmental score or intelligence quotient between advantaged and disadvantaged children. The social environment mediates the impact of nutrition on developmental outcome (5). This occurs in three ways:

1. Passive: An infant is born into a poor family that is less likely to be able or willing to provide nutritious food and/or a supportive home environment. The child is more likely to become iron deficient, lead poisoned, or growth retarded.
2. Reactive: The child is likely to become an inactive or oppositional student. Teachers and other caregivers in the setting of poverty are more likely to be unresponsive or hostile, and a hostile child is more likely to elicit negative-punitive discipline, which, in turn, only increases the child's hostility and the likelihood of more negative discipline. The probability of failure in the school environment increases.
3. Active: The child's characteristics influence the nature of his or her subsequent environment. There is a selection (not necessarily conscious) of specific environments by children, with potential consequences that follow. A child with oppositional characteristics is more likely to select into environments that have other children with these same characteristics, thus reinforcing

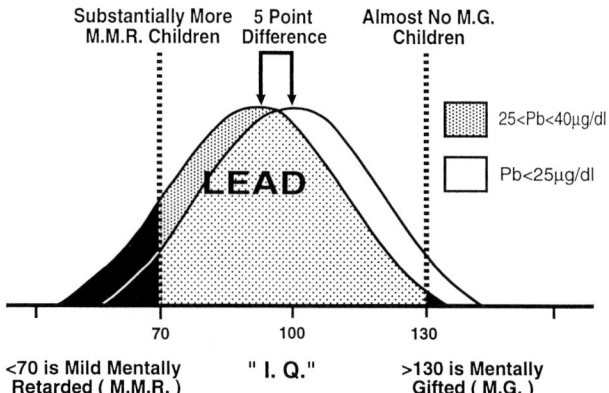

Impact of mild to moderate malnutrition on intellectual development in a community of children

Figure 55.4. A downward shift in mean "IQ" score of 5 points may have very little effect on the life of an affected individual, but the effect on the community is severe. Classes for the mentally gifted (M.G.) where children have an "IQ" 2 standard deviations above the mean (>130) are emptied while the small change at the mean causes the classes for children who are mildly mentally retarded (M.M.R.)—"IQ" 2 standard deviations below the mean (<70)—to become full to capacity. (From Harris P, Clark M, Karp RJ. The prevention of lead poisoning (:in) Karp RJ (ed) Malnourished Children in the United States: Caught in the Cycle of Poverty. New York: Springer, 1993:91–100, with permission.)

the original oppositional tendencies. The child who fails in school may achieve success in the "underground economy" of life on the streets, where oppositional behavior and delinquency become measures of success in the hard life of inner-city youth (12). The trajectory for success in the dominant society points downward.

NUTRITION-DRUG INTERACTIONS AND THEIR EFFECTS

Drug Abuse Is Increased by Poverty

Chronic poverty affects a sustained, disproportionate use of both legal (tobacco and alcohol) (72) and illegal (marijuana, cocaine, and heroin) addictive, mood-altering substances (73). Alcohol, tobacco, and other drugs of abuse affect nutritional status in direct relation to the duration of use (74). In some populations living in seemingly hopeless circumstances, the prevalence and consequences of alcoholism are disproportionately high (75). These include Native Americans living in desolate reservations (an estimated 25% of infants are born with FAS), poor whites in decaying industrial cities (10% of school children with FAS in one town [59]), and inner-city black families.

Particularly problematic is drug use during pregnancy. Among women of childbearing age, poverty engenders chronic depression (76), thus increasing the risk of drug and alcohol abuse during pregnancy, with the concomitant increased risk of teratogenesis (77). As illustrated by studies of alcoholic mothers and children, variability in outcome for children exposed to drugs in utero is substantial (78). To an extent that is not yet well determined, maternal nutrition and alcohol intake contribute to these differences (74, 75). Besides the severe consequences to the fetus from exposure to illicit drugs, there are risks from alcohol consumption and smoking tobacco during pregnancy, which are both better defined and more widespread (78). Moreover, for people living in poverty, illicit drug use is unusual in a woman who neither smokes nor drinks alcohol.

Prevalence and Consequences of Drug, Alcohol, and Tobacco Use

Socioeconomic differences in usage patterns for illicit drugs vary according to pressures from peers, law enforcement officers, educational efforts, and simple experimentation with new drugs. Data on prevalence for illegal drugs are highly suspect, and studies of effects must always be read cautiously. The occurrence of status offenses—behaviors permitted by adults but forbidden to adolescents, including alcohol and tobacco use, or considered criminal in adults but delinquent in youth, including drug use—are ubiquitous in society. The incidence of drug, alcohol, and tobacco use among teenagers is similar across the social and economic spectrum (79).

Differences in outcome, however, are strikingly dissimilar, with arrest, incarceration, and continued drug use more likely among the poor (13). Health measures are affected by chronicity of drug use, bingeing behavior, nutritional status, and aging (74). Hepatic dysfunction associated with chronic alcoholism alters the detoxification process for other drugs of abuse as well as for environmental pollutants and allows toxic metabolites to reach the fetus. A contemporary view, reported by Lieber (74), is that "at cellular, biochemical and molecular levels, the nutritional and toxic effects of alcohol converge." Thus, polydrug abuse concomitant to aging of mothers creates a nutrient-deprived environment in utero for the fetus that, in turn, increases the risk of teratogenic consequences of drug exposure on the growing fetus. The consequences of alcohol and other drug use are highly influenced by nutritional status and hepatic function. Specific alcohol-nutrition interactions likely to increase the in utero effect include the following: (a) a decrease in gastric alcohol dehydrogenase with age, thus allowing higher blood alcohol levels; (b) maternal and fetal loss of zinc and magnesium; (c) maternal decreased intake of essential nutrients, including both antioxidants and B vitamins; and (d) failure in maternal hepatic degradation of alcohol and other potentially toxic substances that allows potentially toxic substances and metabolites to affect the fetus (74). A model for teratogen [x] malnutrition effects, derived from the work of Lieber (74), can be found in Chapter 60 of the ninth edition of this text (75).

Alcohol produces a characteristic dysmorphism deriving from altered CNS growth and function. Children with FAS show midface hypoplasia, short palpebral fissures, and increased distance from the base of the nose to the upper lip, absent philtrum, and narrow vermilion border of the upper lip (59, 75). These children have concomitant growth retardation at birth, with failure to catch up, and persistent neurodevelopmental problems. Infants born to drinking mothers have CNS depression and withdrawal syndrome (75). Alcohol-related problems subsequent to birth are common, even without the full FAS, because drinking severely hampers parental effectiveness. Among pregnant women in 2002, 9.1% used alcohol, and 3.1% admitted to binge drinking (72).

Growth retardation is the principal in utero consequence of smoking tobacco, and it is directly proportional to the number of cigarettes smoked each day (78). The decrease in mean birth weight for infants born to tobacco-smoking mothers is approximately 200 g, with a concomitant increase in infant morbidity and mortality greater than could be expected from a simple shift to the left in birth weight versus mortality curves (78). The pattern of growth retardation tends to be symmetric, all anthropometric measures—weight, length, and head circumference—are affected equally. This pattern has been associated with failure to achieve catch-up growth and developmental delay.

The effects of smoking on the fetus include (a) placental arterial spasm, (b) carbon monoxide binding of hemoglobin,

(c) decreased maternal intake, and (d) reduced levels of ascorbic acid from the oxidative stress of passive as well as active smoking (78). In the United States, tobacco use is now common only among those with limited education and limited income. The prevalence of cigarette smoking decreases with increasing levels of education. Among adults 18 years old or older in 2002, college graduates were the least likely to report smoking cigarettes (14.5%) compared with 35.2% of adults who lacked a high school diploma (78).

Like alcohol, smoking promotes malnutrition in two ways: first, the diets of smokers are of lower nutritional value than those of nonsmokers; and second, smoking has direct antinutrient effects, including reductions in vitamin C levels with passive smoking (80). Steinberg (81) suggested that decreased intake and increased utilization of antioxidant nutrients (vitamins C and E and carotenoids) accelerate oxidation of low-density lipoprotein cholesterol and unfavorably alter the balance between clotting and antithrombotic activity.

Marijuana use is widespread in society; use by women of childbearing age ranges from 10 to 25% (72). In 2002, an estimated 2.0 million persons (0.9%) were current cocaine users. Among youths aged 12 to 17 years, 11.6% were current illicit drug users: 8.2% used marijuana, 4.0% used prescription-type drugs, 1.2% used inhalants, 1.0% used hallucinogens, and 0.6% used cocaine (72).

Cocaine is a powerful sympathomimetic that affects both placental function and the fetus directly throughout pregnancy. The principal effects of cocaine use by the mother on the fetus are symmetric growth retardation with reduced head circumference and premature delivery. Roizen and colleagues (82), in a study of 98 cocaine-exposed infants, showed significant developmental delay in these children as compared with nonexposed controls. This delay, however, was predicted by the growth retardation concomitant to premature delivery and from living in homes with drug-affected mothers or relatives, rather than from cocaine exposure per se (82). Moreover, with respect to postnatal development (82, 83) and growth (84), the social milieu in which cocaine use occurs and concomitant alcohol and tobacco use during pregnancy may be of more importance than the cocaine use alone. Again, these findings must be judged cautiously and in the context of the environment in which it occurs. Fortunately, the use of crack cocaine is diminishing among inner-city youth.

IMPORTANCE OF PUBLIC POLICY: KEEPING NUTRITIOUS FOOD AVAILABLE TO THE POOR

In his biographic essay on the life of Joseph Goldberger, Sebrell wrote (85):

> Goldberger was well aware that pellagra was a problem of poverty and that only improvement in economic conditions would eradicate the disease...he could see the great economic and social advantages

to be gained if the cycle could be broken and disease prevented long enough for the stronger healthier people to help themselves by improving their own food supply.

Malnutrition, as part of a "poverty syndrome," occurs in some poor families when society accepts the legitimacy of poverty and malnutrition (23). There is more to chronic poverty than lack of income, but mass poverty and a nation's economic policy and the politics of entitlement are the direct causes of malnutrition in society. "In fact," writes Rosen, "the poor are not dysfunctional operators in a limited resource base but are highly adaptive actors in an essentially dysfunctional economic system" (12). The results of policies that nurture and nourish children yield remarkable improvements in health and social stability.

The prevalence of malnutrition will depend on the depth of poverty to which society allows those with the least income and resources to sink (16). Failed or inadequate public policy predicts the prevalence of the consequences of poverty, which include malnutrition. Which poor families are affected, however, depends on family characteristics. Parents in affected families often lack the skills to nourish and nurture children. To resolve the problem of malnourished children in the United States, resources must be made available to provide nutritious food and to address the multiple, interdependent problems faced by poor families. Support for the poorest in society begins with a broad base of support for everyone (16, 86, 87). Otherwise, noted Chamberlin (86), "for every family whose functioning is improved by some kind of intensive intervention, several more medium-risk families will take their place as their life circumstances change."

In the United States, provision of food stamps, school lunches, breakfasts, and the special WIC program have improved nutritional status both by providing nutritious food and by allowing the purchase of a higher-quality diet with the same amount of money budgeted for food, thus effectively reversing the Engels phenomenon (44). These supports are often referred to as "welfare," implying an unearned benefit to the recipient. Actually, the benefit for these programs is to everyone by creating a healthy population able to learn, work, and earn. These programs do not create "welfare dependence" because supplemental programs provide essential food to working families and their children. Contemporary food programs have never been shown to be a detriment to work. Rather, they are an alternative to the bread lines and soup kitchens of a post-Victorian era (87, 88).

Childhood malnutrition in the context of poverty predicts various end points: learning failure, social dysfunction, and increased risks of drug use, delinquency, birth defects, and chronic illness later in life. Although it is incorrect to maintain that any form of malnutrition is the solitary cause of the phenomenon of recurrent poverty, ignorance, dysfunction, and disease, malnutrition in the context of poverty is a significant contributor to a self-sustaining system of learning failure, poverty, and malnutrition

(5–7). These unfortunate outcomes are contingent on chronic poverty and are concomitant to malnutrition. Yet, the poor in the United States often live in social environments that are harsh and hostile rather than supportive, with substandard schools and an inadequate system of health care (4, 13, 15). Eliminating poverty includes the provision of food and structures of opportunity within which the poor can adapt and cope. Poor people must be treated as real people, not as caricatures of a defective culture. These calls for the investment of human and monetary resources may seem unrealistic, but the political unacceptability of effective policies should not cause us to "turn to politically acceptable formulas which provide no real solutions" (12).

Effective Interventions

A long-term commitment to ensuring the availability of nutritious food is an important first step in prevention and treatment of malnutrition and its consequences among children and adults living in poverty. Promoting good nutrition *plus* addressing multiple developmental risks must inform public policy. The need, therefore, is to develop model programs capable of increasing awareness and knowledge. Successful programs for nutrition awareness and knowledge address cost, culture, and behavior by (a) creating consortia of community-based organizations, (b) forming focus groups, (c) developing programs unique to targeted communities, (d) preparing material that promotes use of new foods, (e) holding cooking classes, and (f) evaluating the effectiveness of their intervention.

A study evaluating the Michigan Farmers' Market Nutrition Program showed that both educational interventions and direct interventions (coupons for fruit and vegetables) had positive effects on fruit and vegetable consumption. A combination of both education and coupons had the maximal effect, by increasing fruit and vegetable consumption and by changing participants' attitudes (89).

With respect to food costs and availability, supplemental programs (WIC and food stamps) are particularly effective in maintaining high-quality diets. These programs provide nutritious food and allow money saved to raise the quality of food purchases. Supplemental food programs have a substantial impact on nutrition in pregnancy and limit weight gain for older children and adults. A study of low-income households, both food-secure and food-insecure households, revealed that food assistance programs lower the risk of overweight in low-income children, particularly girls in food-insecure households (89). Unfortunately, these resources are being limited in a society promoting self-sufficiency as a cure-all for the ills of the poor.

A general recommendation for the sake of a healthy US society is to follow the example of other industrial democracies and take advantage of the wealth generated by a free-market economy to maintain the general well-being, including good nutrition, of our people. Successful interventions include earned income tax credits, supplemental programs for food, housing, day care, transportation, and health care. At times, direct subsidies are needed (90).

SUMMARY

It is necessary to challenge the notion that either societal neglect or aberrant personal behavior constitutes the single cause of the multiple problems faced by poor children and their families. An emphasis on the dichotomy between failed public policy, on the one hand, and seemingly dissolute parental behaviors, on the other, leads only to a politicization of poor people's problems. It does not advance any coherent or effective strategies for prevention or treatment of the consequences to children of living in poverty.

Poverty implies insufficient income to obtain adequate goods and services to be able to work and become self-supporting. The escape from poverty is enhanced by generous support for food, housing, education, transformation, day care and health care, which are necessary to achieve a level of income at which formerly poor people have a discretionary "income of opportunity" to participate fully in society. The results of policies that nurture and nourish children yield remarkable improvements in health and social stability.

Support for the poorest in society begins with a broad base of support for everyone and an appreciation of how chronic poverty affects the way in which poor children and families appreciate their experiences in life. It is unfortunate that interventions on behalf of the poor are seen as hostile to economic development. As Nobel laureate economist Amaryta Sen argued, in the end eliminating poverty and its consequences enhances, rather than hinders, economic development (87, 88).

Acknowledgments

The assistance of Cindy Cheng in preparation of this chapter is greatly appreciated. I also thank Ann Gray, Alan Meyers and Theodore Wachs for their thoughtful comments, and Dorcas Gelabert for the composition of the figures.

REFERENCES

1. Proctor B, Dalaker J. US Census Bureau, Poverty in the United States: 2002, Current Population Reports, P60–222, Washington, DC: US Government Printing Office, 2003.

2. US Bureau of the Census. www.census.gov/hhes/poverty C CRS P60–222

3. Rainwater L, Smeeding T. A Comparative Study of Children's Wealth. Luxembourg Income Study (LIS) working paper no. 127. Syracuse, NY: Syracuse University, 1995.

4. Miller J, Korenman S. Am J Epidemiol 1994;78:75–7.

5. Wachs TD. Necessary but Not Sufficient: The Respective Roles of Single and Multiple Influences on Individual Development. Washington, DC: American Psychological Association, 2002.

6. Shonkoff JP, Phillips DA, eds. From Neurons to Neighborhoods: The Science of Early Child Development. Committee on

Integrating the Science of Early Childhood Development. Washington, DC: National Academy Press, 2000.

7. Sewell TE, Price VD, Karp RJ. The ecology of poverty undernutrition and learning failure. In: Karp RJ, ed. Malnourished Children in the United States: Caught in the Cycle of Poverty. New York: Springer, 1993:24–30.

8. Citro CF, Michael RT, eds. Measuring Poverty: A New Approach. Washington, DC: National Academy Press, 1995.

9. LoPrest P. Assessing the New Federalism. Discussion paper 99–02. Washington, DC: Urban Institute, 1999.

10. Edin K, Lein L. Making Ends Meet: How Single Mothers Survive Welfare and Low-Wage Work. New York: Russell Sage Foundation, 1977.

11. Vozoris N, Davis, B, Tarasuk V. Can J Public Health 2002;93: 36–4.

12. Rosen D. Failure of response to poverty. In: Karp RJ, ed. Malnourished Children in the United States: Caught in the Cycle of Poverty. New York: Springer, 1993:250–2.

13. Wilson JW. The Truly Disadvantaged: The Inner-City, The Underclass and Public Policy. Chicago: University of Chicago Press, 1987.

14. Bloom BS. Stability and Social Change in Human Characteristics. New York: Wiley 1964.

15. Weitzman M, Moss ME. Ambul Pediatr 2001:162–6.

16. Karp RJ. The Dimensions of Poverty among Children in the United States: An Exposition of Causes and Consequences. Epilogue to the Curriculum for Poor and Underserved Children of the Ambulatory Pediatric Association, 2002. http://www.servingtheunderserved.org.html.

17. Jelliffe DB. The Assessment of Nutritional Status of the Community. World Health Organization monograph series no. 53. Geneva: World Health Organization, 1965.

18. Nead KG, Halterman JS, Kaczorowski JM et al. Pediatrics 2004; 114:104–8.

19. Garn SM, Clark DC. Pediatrics 1975;56:306–19.

20. Pollitt E. Fed Proc 1975;34:1593–7.

21. Karp R, Snyder E, Fairorth et al. J Fam Pract 1984;18: 731–5.

22. Bithony WG, Dubowitz HG. Organic concomitants of nonorganic failure to thrive: implications for research. In: Drotar D, ed. New Directions in Failure to Thrive. New York: Plenum Press, 1986:47–56.

23. Gopalan C. Undernutrition: measurement and implication. In: Osmani SR, ed. Nutrition and Poverty. New York: Oxford University Press, 1992:17–48.

24. Barker DJP. BMJ 1995;311:171–4.

25. Krishnaswamy K, Naidu AN, Prasad Reddy GA. Nutr Rev 2002; 60:35S–9S.

26. US Department of Agriculture, Human Nutrition Information Service. Nationwide Food Consumption Survey: Continuing Survey of Food Intakes by Lndividuals, Low-Income Women 19–50 years and Their Children 1–5 Years, 1 Day, 1986. NFCS, CFSII report no. 86–2. Hyattsville, MD: US Department of Agriculture, 1987.

27. Scholl TO, Karp RJ, Theophano J et al. Public Health Rep 1987; 102:278–83.

28. Meyers A, Frank D, Roos N et al. Arch Pediatr Adolesc Med 1995;149:1079–84.

29. Krebs-Smith SM, Cook DA, Subar AF et al. Arch Pediatr Adolesc Med 1996;150:81–6.

30. Alaimo K, McDowell MA, Breifel RR et al. Dietary Intake of Vitamins and Minerals, and Fiber of Persons Age 2 Months and over in the United States: Third National Health and Nutrition Examination Survey, Phase I, 1989–1991. Advance Data from

Vital Statistics no. 258. Hyattsville, MD: National Center for Health Statistics, 1994.

31. Johnson RK, Guthrie H, Smicklas-Wright H et al. Public Health Rep 1994;109:414–20.

32. Scholl TO, Johnson WG. Am J Clin Nutr 2000;1[Suppl]: 1295S–303S.

33. Ballew C, Bowman BA, Sowell AL et al. Am J Clin Nutr 2001; 73:586–93.

34. Bastiotis PB, Carlson A, Gerrior SA et al. Fam Econ Nutr Rev 2004;16:39–48.

35. Sherry B, Mei Z, Yip R. Pediatrics 2001;107:677–82.

36. Hofferth SL, Curtin S. Food programs and obesity among US children. Paper presented at Annual Meeting of Association for Public Policy Analysis and Management Nov 6–8, 2003. http://www.gwu.edu/~labor/papers/hofferth.pdf

37. Kumanyika SK. Ann Intern Med 1993;119:650–4.

38. Mayer J. Obesity. In: Goodhart RS, Shils ME, eds. Modern Nutrition in Health and Disease. 6th ed. Philadelphia: Lea & Febiger, 1980:721.

39. Nord M, Bickel G. Measuring Children's Food Insecurity in US Households, 1995–1999. Food Assistance and Nutrition research report no. 25. Washington, DC: Food and Rural Economics Division, Economic Research Service, US Department of Agriculture, 2000.

40. Neault N, Cook J. The Safety Net in Action: Protecting the Health and Nutrition of Young American Children. Report from a multi-site children's health study. Boston: Children's Sentinel Nutrition Assessment Program, 2004.

41. Kersey M, Geppert J, Cutts DB. Pediatr Res 2003;53:580.

42. Alaimo K, Olson CM, Frongillo EA. Arch Pediatr Adolesc Med 2001;155:1161–7.

43. Gohil BJ, Rosenblum LA, Coplan JD et al. CNS Spectrums 2001;47:581–9.

44. Karp R. The problem of changing food habits: 1. How habits are formed. In: Karp RJ, ed. Malnourished Children in the United States: Caught in the Cycle of Poverty. New York: Springer, 1993:194–211.

45. Engels F. The Conditions of the Working Class in England. London: Penguin Books, 1845 (republished in 1987).

46. Immink MDC. Purchasing power and food consumption behavior: how poverty level is defined. In: Sanjur D, ed. Social and Cultural Perspectives in Nutrition. Engelwood Cliffs, NJ: Prentice-Hall, 1982:91–122.

47. Bhattacharya J, DeLeire T, Haider S et al. Am J Public Health 2003;93:1149–54.

48. Drewnowski A, Specter S. Am J Clin Nutr 2004;79:6–16.

49. Karp RJ, Fairorth J, Kanofsky P et al. Public Health Rep 1978; 93:456–9.

50. Groth MV, Fagt S, Brondsted C. Eur J Clin Nutr 2001;55: 959–66.

51. Pilch SM, Senti FR. Assessment of the Iron Nutritional Status of the US Population Based on Data Collected in the Second National Health and Nutrition Examination Survey. Contract no. FDA 223–83–2384. Bethesda, MD: FASEB, 1984.

52. Winick M, Meyer K, Harris R. Science 1975;190:1173–5.

53. Grantham-MacGregor S, Ani C. J Nutr 2001;131[Suppl]: 649S–68S.

54. Galler JR, Barrett LR. Ambul Child Health 2001;7:85–95.

55. Idjradinata P, Pollitt E. Lancet 1993;341:1–4.

56. Lozoff B, De Andraca I, Castillo M. Pediatrics 2003;112:846–54.

57. Harris P, Clark-Golden M, Karp R. Preventing lead poisoning. In: Karp RJ, ed. Malnourished Children in the United States: Caught in the Cycle of Poverty. New York: Springer, 1993:91–100.

58. Kevles D. In the Name of Eugenics. New York: Knopf, 1986.

59. Karp RJ, Qazi QH. Fetal alcohol syndrome. In: Karp RJ, ed. Malnourished Children in the United States: Caught in the Cycle of Poverty. New York: Springer, 1993:101–8.

60. Winick M, Rosso P. Pediatr Res 1969;3:181–4.

61. Oski FA. Am J Dis Child 1979;133:315–22.

62. Pollitt L. Annu Rev Nutr 1993;13:521–37.

63. Karp RJ, Martin R, Sewell T, et al. Clin Pediatr 1992;32:336–40.

64. Barret S. Nutr Rev 1986;44[Suppl]:224–36.

65. Sameroff A, Seifer R, Barocas R et al. Pediatrics 1987;79: 3453–50.

66. Russell M. The epidemiology of alcohol. In: Estes NJ, Heinemann ME, eds. Alcoholism: Development, Consequences and Interventions. St Louis: CV Mosby, 1986:31–52.

67. Rivera JA, Barquera S, Gonzalez-Cossio T et al. J Nutr Rev 2004; 62:149S–57S.

68. Pollitt E. J Nutr 2000;130[Suppl 2]:350S–3S.

69. National Research Council and Institute of Medicine. New findings on poverty and child health and Nutrition: summary of a research briefing. In: Bridgeman A, Philips D, eds. Board on Children, Youth and Families, Commission on Behavioral and Social Sciences and Education. Washington, DC: National Academy Press, 1998.

70. Hirsch ED. Am Educator 2000;24:4–9.

71. Ramey CT, Campbell FA. Poverty, early childhood education, and academic competence: the ABECEDARIAN project. In: Huston C, ed. Children in Poverty. New York: Cambridge University Press, 1992.

72. Office of Applied Studies. Results from the 2002 National Survey on Drug Use and Health: National Findings. NHSDA Series H–22, DHHS publication no. SMA 03–3836. Rockville, MD: US Department of Health and Human Services, 2002.

73. Jacobson JL, Sokol RJ, Martier SS et al. J Pediatr 1994;124: 757–64.

74. Leiber CS. Am J Clin Nutr 1993;58:430–42.

75. Karp R. Malnutrition among children in the United States: the impact of poverty. In: Shils ME, Shike M, Olson JA et al., eds. Modern Nutrition in Health and Disease. 9th ed. Baltimore: Lippincott Williams & Wilkins, 1999.

76. Streissguth AP. Fetal Alcohol Syndrome. Medford, NJ: Paul H. Brookes, 2003.

77. Sidel R. Women and Children Last: The Plight of Poor Women in Affluent America. New York: Viking Penguin, 1986.

78. Berlin CM Jr. Pediatr Rev 1991;12:232–7.

79. Schwartz J, Weiss S. Am J Clin Nutr 1994;59:110–4.

80. Alderman EM, Friedman SB. Pediatr Ann 1995;24:186–91.

81. Steinberg D. N Engl J Med 1995;346:36–8.

82. Roizen NJ, Martinez S, Kime K et al. Arch Pediatr Adolesc Med Abstr 1996;150:16.

83. Hurt H, Giannetta J, Brodsky NL et al. J Pediatr 2001;138:911–3.

84. Beeghly M, Frank DA, Rose-Jacobs R et al. Neurotoxicol Teratol 2003;252:23–38.

85. Sebrell WH. Joseph Goldberger. J Nutr 1955;55:3–12.

86. Chamberlin RW. Pediatr Rev 1992;13:64–71.

87. Sen AK. Poverty and Famine: An Essay on Entitlement and Deprivation. New York: Oxford University Press, 1983.

88. Sen AK. The Political Economy of Hunger. WIDER Studies in Developmental Economics. New York: Oxford University Press, 1995.

89. Anderson J Bybee DI, Brown RM et al. J Am Diet Assoc 2001; 101:195–202.

90. Jones S. Arch Ped Adolesc Med 2003;157:780–4.

91. Primus W. The Safety Net Delivers: The Effects of Government Benefit Programs in Reducing Poverty. Washington, DC: Center on Budget and Policy Notes, 1997.

SELECTED READINGS

Nord M, Bickel G. Measuring Children's Food Insecurity in US Households, 1995–1999.

Food Assistance and Nutrition research report no. 25. Washington, DC: Food and Rural Economics Division, Economic Research Service, US Department of Agriculture, 2000.

Shonkoff JP, Phillips DA, eds. From Neurons to Neighborhoods: The Science of Early Child Development. Committee on Integrating the Science of Early Childhood Development. Washington, DC: National Academy Press, 2000.

Wachs TD. Necessary but Not Sufficient: The Respective Roles of Single and Multiple Influences on Individual Development. Washington, DC: American Psychological Association, 2002.

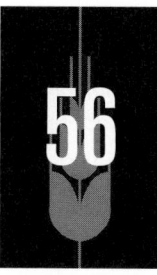

56 PEDIATRIC FEEDING PROBLEMS

RICHARD KATZ, RAMASAMY MANIKAM, AND LINDA SCHUBERTH

CLASSIFICATION AND DIAGNOSIS 876
ASSESSMENT 877
    History 877
    Physical Examination 877
    Anthropometry 877
    Behavioral Observation .878
    Environment 879
TREATMENT 879
SUMMARY 880

This chapter addresses issues in pediatric feeding disorders and offers insight into the nature of a surprising yet relatively common pediatric problem. Assessment techniques are outlined, as is the scope of interventions and organizational principles necessary to treat children with feeding problems effectively.

Undernutrition is a major problem in the world and certainly a major contributor to disease and poor growth in vulnerable populations. Prolonged undernutrition affects the physical health and the mental and social development of children. In addition, it exacts a heavy cost to their families and society at large. Although insufficient food availability is an important cause of undernutrition, the ability or willingness to consume available foods is another major factor. This chapter focuses on the latter causes of undernutrition, also known as feeding disorders.

Feeding disorders is a term used to describe children experiencing difficulty in consuming adequate nutrition by mouth (impaired feeding), those who eat too much (hyperphagia), and those who eat inappropriate items (pica). The term is often mistaken for eating disorders such as anorexia and bulimia, although feeding problems and pica in young children have been identified as risk factors for adolescent bulimia and anorexia nervosa (1).

Most healthy children learn to accept and consume a well-balanced, healthful diet to sustain growth and health (2). They develop the capacity for self-regulation and adapt to a variety of parental and environmental changes. Satter (3) expanded this concept and outlined the role of the child and the parent during feeding. However, biologic, personal, and social factors can interfere with the principle of self-regulation.

Nearly 25% of infants and children are affected by feeding disorders. This rate increases to nearly 80% for children with developmental disabilities. Further breakdown of the prevalence indicates that 52% of toddlers are not consistently hungry at mealtimes, 42% end meals after a brief session, 35% are picky eaters, and 33% show food selectivity (4). Severe feeding problems, however, are noted in children (3–10%) (5), particularly those with physical disabilities (26–90%), as well as with medical illness and prematurity (10–49%) (6–8).

The consequences of undernutrition on growth and development are well documented (9–11) and cause substantial morbidity and mortality. Feeding disorders affect the whole family, resulting in "bonding failure," disordered attachments, and behavior problems. Two thirds of a caregiver's waking time may be spent in attending to a child with disordered feeding (12), and this intense involvement of a primary caregiver with the feeding-disordered child takes away time from other family and household duties.

Feeding disorders have multiple causes, including medical, nutritional, behavioral, psychologic, and environmental factors (9, 10). Table 56.1 presents examples of common childhood feeding disorders. Children with developmental disabilities, medical conditions, and severe behavior problems are unlikely to outgrow their feeding problems without intervention. Therefore, it is important that caregivers and care providers recognize a child's feeding problem early and have an evaluation performed to offer early intervention to arrest the problem.

Children's feeding progresses from biologic, maturational learning and a nurturing social environment. Thus, feeding disorders should be conceptualized as biopsychosocial problems. Interactions among the three mechanisms pose a challenge to the differential diagnosis, evaluation, and treatment. Most persistent feeding difficulties in children have an underlying structural, neurologic, physiologic condition or disorder associated with it.

Feeding is a complex task requiring a sequential progression of a repertoire of skills to be successful. Guidance to families based on developmental progressions observed in healthy children would be inappropriate for children with cerebral palsy, failure to thrive, syndromic disorders, and muscular and neuromuscular problems. Poor coordination of oral structures may interfere with the ability to

TABLE 56.1. COMMON FEEDING DISORDERS

Total food refusal
Food refusal by volume
Food refusal by texture
Food refusal by type
Bottle dependency
Lengthy meals
Maladaptive behaviors

move food in the mouth, chew, or swallow in a safe and effective manner. Delayed motor skills may interfere with self-feeding.

Successful feeding is often gauged as a metric for parent-infant bonding. The ability to feed one's child successfully is often perceived by parents as an element of a "good and nurturing parent." Successful feeding relationships provide satisfaction to the parent and a sense of accomplishment to the child, thus establishing a mutually satisfying relationship between parent and child. A successful feeding transaction between parent and child often is contingent on the ability of both to give, read, and interpret the other's cues. Neurologic impairment may interfere with the ability to give clear hunger or satiety cues.

Children usually refuse food after a negative experience, such as pain or discomfort. When food is presented, the pain memory returns, and the child refuses to eat. Parents need to know that this is an expected response to pain, discomfort, or stress. It is important not to characterize this situation as a "bad" or "difficult" child or to suggest that "it is all in his or her head." Problems are often worsened by caregiver mismanagement. Even then, it is important not to blame parents for the situation. In most cases, the caregivers feel guilty about their contribution to the child's feeding problems. They need assurance that a few changes (e.g., to make a meal time pleasant; Table 56.2) in their behaviors may improve their child's eating behaviors.

Children with feeding disorders are a heterogeneous group. They range from those without medical problems to those who have gastrointestinal tract disorders, systemic illness, developmental delay, and physical disabilities. Forty-five percent of normally developed children have mealtime problems (13). Most of these children's feeding concerns were reported as poor appetite, and in 23% of these cases, the children were of normal weight and height.

Feeding disorders include a variety of feeding behaviors and characteristics. These behaviors can be categorized into ability (unable to perform) and motivational deficits (unwilling) (14). A child with low energy or fine motor deficits may not feed himself or herself. A child reported as having poor appetite and reduced consumption may have swallow dysfunction, taste aversion, texture sensitivity, dental problems, recurring ear infections, or many other disorders. A child with severe gastroesophageal reflux may actively gag and/or vomit to relieve the discomfort. Total food refusal is uncommon in physiologically normal, healthy children, except during illness or transiently when they are emotionally upset. However, a comprehensive assessment is still necessary to rule out physical causes of food refusal.

CLASSIFICATION AND DIAGNOSIS

Children with feeding disorders can broadly be divided into three categories. These are children who are healthy, children who have digestive disorders, and children who have special needs. Feeding difficulty in healthy children often is transitional and resolve spontaneously. However, in some children, the problem persists and may require professional care. Suboptimal calorie intake, food selectivity by type, disruptive mealtime behaviors, and excessive meal duration are commonly seen feeding problems in healthy children.

Diagnosing medical disorders in children with feeding difficulties is a challenge, especially in infants and toddlers, who are unable to report on their conditions. Table 56.3 lists examples of medical conditions commonly seen in children with complex feeding difficulties. In most cases, a team of experienced professionals from several disciplines, including gastroenterology, nutrition, occupational and/or speech therapy, and psychology, is necessary to establish a differential diagnosis of the presenting symptoms, to specify the cause or function. Members of a multidisciplinary team perform the following functions: the physician treats underlying medical causes; the dietitian determines calories needed, appropriate foods, and required nutrients; the occupational or speech therapist deals with seating and positioning, utensils, and oral motor issues; the psychologist works to eliminate the child's inappropriate feeding behaviors and to overcome resistance and motivates the child to accept the foods presented, in

TABLE 56.2. OPTIMIZING THE FEEDING ENVIRONMENT

Quiet room
Meal set up before child brought to feeding area
All equipment and reinforcers in position
Proper seated positioning of child
Developmentally appropriate utensils
Child alert to focus in feeding
Stable routine and schedules

TABLE 56.3. MEDICAL CONDITIONS SEEN IN FEEDING PROBLEMS

Anatomic abnormalities
Severe constipation
Aspiration
Dysphagia
Reflux
Abdominal pain
Motility disorders

addition to teaching and training the parent to be an effective feeder. All referral concerns, no matter how simple or unimpressive, should be addressed. This will allay caregiver concerns and avert a more serious problem. Prognosis with early intervention is very favorable for most cases. Early intervention increases the effectiveness of therapy.

ASSESSMENT

The process of understanding the cause of feeding disorders involves noting symptoms, identifying behaviors, and determining the predisposing, precipitating, and perpetuating factors. Child characteristics such as temperament, recurrent illness, low resilience and parent characteristics of depression or poor coping ability can act as predisposing factors. Precipitating factors include acute illness, injury, pain, and child abuse. Perpetuating factors include continued pain, discomfort, and reinforcement derived from behaviors. Identification of these factors has strong treatment implications.

When assessing children with feeding disorders, five major areas should be evaluated: history, physical examination, nutritional assessment, anthropometric assessment, and behavioral observation.

History

A detailed history helps to formulate the nature of the problem, especially for the conditions that affect nutritional status and feeding care. Focus should also be on the child's developmental level and the caregiver's understanding and knowledge of appropriate feeding regimen, texture, volume, and feeding methods. The possible effects of medication on a child's feeding include depressed appetite, nausea, gastrointestinal irritation, and constipation. Some medications and their effects on the gastrointestinal system and the potential for feeding difficulties are presented in Table 56.4.

A profile of the child's feeding history should include the onset, course, frequency, intensity, duration, and variability of feeding behaviors across time, settings, and personnel. A profile of the caregiver's temperament, knowledge of child development and feeding practices, his or her own feeding history, attitude toward the child, coping skills, and resources should also be gathered. The role of the family, particularly the primary feeder, be it the mother, father, grandparent,

baby sitter, or, day care worker, is paramount in the management of feeding difficulties. In a normal feeding situation, the parent decides what to serve the child, and the child eats to satisfaction. Caregiver disorders, temperament, knowledge, resources, and motivation can profoundly affect feeding sessions. A high prevalence of psychiatric disturbances has been reported in caregivers of children with feeding disorders (1).

A determination whether the child's feeding pattern is normal for age and developmental levels should be made. Often, children's behaviors of concern to parents are developmental variations, such as poor self-feeding or messy eating at 1 year of age. Caregivers who fail to understand developmental variations become anxious and devise novel feeding techniques, thereby often creating a conflict between parent compulsion and child capacity. Variability in eating between meals is common in children between the ages of 2 and 5 years. They are active, easily distracted, and resistant to being confined in a high chair for very long. They demand independence and control and insist on certain utensils and foods. In fact, weight gain slows down, and children of this age do not require the same number of calories that they did as infants. The slope in the National Center for Health Statistics growth chart reflects this decrease in growth velocity.

Physical Examination

A thorough physical examination should be conducted to rule out organic causes. Any organ or system of the body, especially the gastrointestinal system, can act as a precipitating factor for feeding problems.

Nutritional assessment of the child's dietary intake is critical: dietary information can be used to determine calories consumed and the nutritional balance of the diet. Diet history should include both current and past practices and feeding patterns. Dietary information can be obtained through caregiver recall; however, this method may be inaccurate. Children's feeding varies between meals and days. Assessing a single meal or a day's calorie count does not reveal the child's true nutritional status. Therefore, analysis of a 5- to 7-day food log provides the most valid estimate of the child's true intake variations in food types eaten and amounts consumed. Nutritional strategies given to families should consider family preferences, resources, culture, ethnicity, and education, Parents should be reassured if their children are receiving adequate nutrition and are following their growth curve, no matter how small or thin these children may appear.

Anthropometry

Measurements of height, weight, and weight/height ratio are indispensable in determining nutrition and growth status. Much can be learned about the child's growth and development by plotting serial points of these values. A thorough analysis of the serial points can help to establish

TABLE 56.4. MEDICATIONS CAUSING INTERFERING SIDE EFFECTS

MEDICATION	POSSIBLE GASTROINTESTINAL EFFECTS
Iron	Nausea, vomiting, pain
Amoxicillin	Nausea, vomiting
Nonsteroidal antiinflammatory drugs	Mucosal injury
Psychotropic agents	Lethargy, dysphagia

the onset, course, and precipitating and perpetuating factors of the feeding problem. Children below the fifth percentile should not be assumed to have a problem. Weight gain should be a concern only if the child's growth velocity falters and falls off the growth curve. However, even well-nourished children often need assistance because they may exhibit feeding behaviors that interfere with routines and are a source of stress and concern for caregivers.

Feeding disorders in healthy children usually manifest as restricted food variety, inappropriate food consistency, insufficient calories, and disruptive mealtime behaviors. Children who missed the opportunity to experience foods and textures at certain developmental stages, the "critical" or "sensitive" periods, are more resistant to new foods and higher textures. Texture difficulty, in the absence of oral-motor dysfunction, can result from poor oral strength, dental problems, or avoidance because of an aversive experience of gagging and choking. Food diaries may show that the parent serves large portion sizes, inappropriate food consistency, or large quantities of liquids during meals.

Feeding disorders in children with medical problems are complex because they interact with behavioral and social factors and thus make differential diagnoses more challenging. The most common clinical symptoms suggestive of medical conditions are dysphagia, gastroesophageal reflux, and diarrhea and constipation. Gastrointestinal disorders interfere with the process of consumption, retention, digestion, absorption, and elimination (Table 56.5) and result in weight loss, lethargy, illness, and feeding disorders.

In some cases, children with seemingly functional disorders may later reveal underlying organic causes of the feeding disorder. For example, delayed gastric emptying without evidence of systemic disease may develop in healthy children (15). Similar findings of latent physical problems without clinical evidence was identified by Staiano and colleagues (16) in their study of upper gastrointestinal tract motility in children with progressive muscular dystrophy. It is not uncommon for symptoms of a motility disorder, food allergy, and lactose intolerance to emerge once children are taught to eat a larger volume and an increased variety of foods. Presumably, the child had been self-regulating and avoiding the "toxic" substance through food refusal. Most often, a

TABLE 56.6. SYMPTOMS OF DYSPHAGIA

Drooling
Chewing difficulty
Packing food
Gagging
Coughing

diagnostic evaluation is needed to confirm presumed clinical diagnoses.

Dysphagia can be caused by the following: oral-motor malformation and malfunction at the oral stage; incoordination at the pharyngeal stage; and achalasia, stenosis, and dysfunctional peristalsis at the esophageal stage of eating. Dysphagia may be a sign of an underlying disorder, and it may be difficult to diagnose by clinical evaluation alone. Table 56.6 presents a list of varied symptoms in children with dysphagia. Manipulation of food properties can help with swallowing. Examples are given in Table 56.7.

Emesis is a common presenting symptom in children with gastrointestinal tract disorders, food allergy, conditioned aversion, rumination, or other underlying disorders. Most common, however, is gastroesophageal reflux. Symptoms of reflux are presented in Table 56.8. Children with such symptoms should be referred to a gastroenterologist for diagnosis and therapy.

Behavioral Observation

Observation of feeding is of tremendous value and provides direct evidence and insight into the feeding problem. The child's feeding behavior affects the caregiver's attitude toward the child and feeding methods, just as the parent's temperament and feeding techniques affect the child's response to the feeding situation. Observation of the parent-child dyad in clinic may not represent their natural behaviors. Videotaping of home meal sessions, when possible, offers a more realistic performance. Observation should focus on child temperament, tactile responses, motor control, oral integrity, coordination, suck-swallow competency, positioning, and signs of pain and discomfort. A physician may observe the visible portion of the feeding anatomy to assess its function and clear the patient for oral feeding safety; speech and occupational therapists may conduct feeding trials to explore oral motor functioning, positioning, sensation, swallow efficiency, muscle strength, suck-swallow-breathing coordination, and self-feeding skills; psychologists may carry out

TABLE 56.5. GASTROINTESTINAL DISORDERS AFFECTING THE PROCESS OF NUTRITION ASSIMILATION

Consumption: appetite, dysphagia, aspiration, craniofacial abnormalities
Retention: emesis, diarrhea
Digestion: food allergy, lactose intolerance
Absorption: celiac disease, dumping syndrome
Elimination: constipation, Hirshprung disease

TABLE 56.7. FOOD PROPERTY MANIPULATION IN DYSPHAGIA

Temperature: hot or cold (stimulates swallowing)
Taste: sweet, spicy, sour, salty (stimulates swallowing)
Texture: graduated hierarchy
Consistency: formed

TABLE 56.8. SYMPTOMS OF GASTROESOPHAGEAL REFLUX

Vomiting	Coughing
Frequent swallowing	Regurgitation
Dental erosion	Food refusal
Stricture	Barrett esophagus
Anemia	Bleeding
Stridor	Hoarseness
Arching	Posturing

observations on behavioral issues. Important elements of parent-child behaviors to be observed during meal trials are presented in Table 56.9.

Environment

Environmental factors are given little importance in feeding disorders. Yet, overwhelming evidence indicates their significance in the development, maintenance, and exacerbation of feeding problems (13, 17). Thus, planned assessment and observation of the feeding environment during the assessment phase are important. The child's natural feeding environment can provide critical information in understanding the parents' priorities, available resources, and settings that affect the child's feeding behaviors. Children do not eat for nutritional value. Rather, they are motivated by taste, smell, color, and social reinforcement. Functional analysis to determine their likes and dislikes will reveal why children accept some foods, eat well at certain meals, or eat with one caregiver and not another.

TABLE 56.9. PARENT-CHILD INTERACTION

PARENT: POSITIVE BEHAVIORS	PARENT: NEGATIVE BEHAVIORS
Affectionate	Distant, depressed, underinvolved
Enthusiastic	Passive
Supportive	Overindulgent, controlling, critical
Expressing pleasure	Harsh, irritable
Reinforcing	Using physical punishment, punitive
Calm, reassuring	Fostering anxiety
Interpreting the child's cues correctly	Promoting dependency
Coping with stress and frustration	Losing control
Setting limits effectively	Too permissive
CHILD: POSITIVE BEHAVIORS	CHILD: NEGATIVE BEHAVIORS
Demonstrating anger, joy, warmth	Uncommunicative, demanding
Pleasant	Passive, withdrawn
Cooperative	Stubborn
Accepting limits	Out-of-control
Playing with parents	Uncooperative, having temper outburst

TREATMENT

Treatment is fairly straightforward in many cases once the origin and functional causes of the feeding disorder have been identified. Gastroenterologists have developed many noninvasive techniques for the evaluation of gastrointestinal functions (18). Medical treatment is extensive for organically based feeding difficulties. Occasionally, hospitalization may be needed for objective clinical observation when initial assessment does not provide the answer to the problem or when caregiver report and child status are incongruent. In many cases, management using alternative routes of delivering nutrition may be needed. Enteral feedings should be considered in children who cannot take in sufficient calories by mouth, as well as those who tire easily from the effort to chew and swallow, consume undue amounts of caregiver time, become ill frequently, are in a medically unsafe condition, or cannot consume liquid. Children with severe malnutrition and failure to thrive may also benefit from enteral feeding.

Applied behavior analysis has been successfully applied in treating feeding problems including disruptive mealtime behaviors (19), food refusal (20, 21), and food preference (22). Feeding disorders in children that result from behavioral and caregiver mismanagement can be effectively treated using applied behavioral techniques. Table 56.10 presents ideas on how to improve mealtime behaviors in a child who is a picky eater. Initial treatment should always be aimed at making changes to the feeding routine, schedules, feeding environment, and caregiver feeding skills. What occurs outside feeding sessions, including sleep deprivation, poor bowel habits, lethargy, and irritability, can significantly affect children's feeding behaviors. Intervention should be focused on teaching the parent to understand the child's temperament, to set limits, and to facilitate the child's internal regulation of feeding (23). This includes dietitians' instructions about foods with good nutritional values, food preparation and storage techniques, and tube feeding management, and this approach should always be attempted before more intrusive treatment procedures.

TABLE 56.10. STRATEGIES TO IMPROVE MEALTIME BEHAVIORS OF PICKY EATERS

Cut down on grazing.
Keep junk foods out of view.
Caregivers should model eating novel foods.
Offer small amounts at each serving.
Present the same novel food for 10 to 20 meals.
Make the foods attractive.
Food consistency should suit the child.
Add condiments and sauces that the child likes.
Add other foods to boost calories, such as grated cheese.
Aim for high-density, low-volume foods.
Reinforce appropriate feeding behaviors.

As part of the therapeutic process, the occupational or speech therapist often manipulates parts of the oral-facial region to raise sensory awareness, to strengthen muscles, and to reduce effort with proper positioning. The therapist may adjust food taste, temperature, texture, and consistency (24), to assist in swallowing. As noted by Martin (23), strong flavors stimulate salivation and swallowing, hot or cold temperatures stimulate the swallowing response, and thick liquids make it easier to form a bolus and swallow.

In most cases, effective therapeutic techniques and maneuvers exist to treat pediatric feeding problems. However, prioritizing target behaviors and the methods used to treat these conditions are complex and at times cause conflict among members of the feeding team and with the family's goals. Such conflicts are unavoidable; however, a cohesive team with mutual respect for each other can achieve consensus and can then present their findings and recommendations for caregiver input.

SUMMARY

Feeding disorders are surprisingly common. The incidence of feeding disorders will continue to rise as sick children survive with advances in medical technology. Feeding disorders occur for medical, sensory, physical, personal, social, and environmental reasons. These factors rarely operate independently. Prolonged feeding problems have grave consequences for the child's physical, cognitive, and social health, and they lead to caregiver stress and family dysfunction. The multifactorial origin of feeding disorders demands a multidisciplinary feeding team to treat the whole child and his or her caregivers effectively.

Enteral feeding should be reserved for children who are unsafe oral feeders and for those who are very malnourished and require an immediate boost. Even when a child is receiving enteral feedings, nonnutritive and nutritive stimulation should be initiated at the earliest possible opportunity. Caregiver education and training are indispensable to maintenance and generalization, as well as to

avoid regression and the revolving-door phenomenon. Most children with feeding disorders can be effectively treated, in the absence of an active medical problem, by an experienced feeding team.

REFERENCES

1. Marchi M, Cohen P. J Am Acad Child Adolesc Psychiatry 1990; 29:112–7.
2. Davis CM. Can Med Assoc J 1939;41:257–61.
3. Satter E. J Pediatr 1990;117:181–9.
4. Reau NR, Senturia YD, Lebailly SA et al. J Dev Behav Pediatr 1966;17:49–53.
5. Lindberg L, Bohlin G, Hagekull B. Int J Eat Disord 1991;10: 395–405.
6. Reilley S, Skuse D, Problete X. J Pediatr 1996;129:877–82.
7. Douglas JE, Bryon M. Arch Dis Child 1985;75:304–8.
8. Thommessen M, Heidberg A, Kasse BF et al. Acta Paediatr 1991;80:527–33.
9. Riordan MM, Iwata BA, Wohl KM et al. Appl Res Ment Retard 1980;1:95–112.
10. Babbitt RL, Hoch TA, Coe DA, et al. J Dev Behav Pediatr 1994; 15:278–91.
11. Barett DE, Radke-Yarrow M, Klein RE. Dev Psychol 1984; 18:541–56.
12. Chase HP, Martin HP. N Engl J Med 1970;282:933–9.
13. Linscheid TR. Psychological problems in early life, early life conditions and chronic diseases. In: Magrab PR, ed. Chronic Diseases. Baltimore: University Park Press, 1978:191–218.
14. Manikam R, Perman J. J Clin Gastroenterol 2000;11:34–46.
15. Cucchiara S. Int Semin Paediatr Gastroenterol Nutr 1998;7:1–8.
16. Staiano A, Giudice ED, Romano A et al. J Pediatr 1992;121: 720–4.
17. Palmer S, Horn S. Feeding problems in children. In: Palmer S, Ekvall S, eds. Pediatric Nutrition in Developmental Disorders. 6th ed. Springfield, IL: Charles C Thomas, 1978:107–29.
18. O'Brian F, Azrin NH. J of Appl Behav Anal 1972;5:389–99.
19. Sloane HN. Dinner's Ready: A Behavior Guide. Fountain Valley, CA: Telesis, 1983.
20. Ahearn WH, Kerwin ME, Eicher PS et al. J Appl Behav Anal 1996;29:321–32.
21. Thompson RJ, Palmer S. J Nutr Educ 1974;6:63–6.
22. Chatoor I, Hirsch R, Persinger M. Infant Young Child 1997;9: 12–22.
23. Martin AW. Dysphagia 1991;16:129–34.
24. Birch LL, Fisher JA. Pediatr Clin North Am 1995;42:931–54.

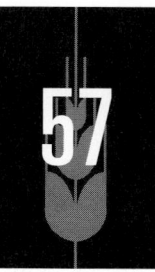

PROTEIN-ENERGY MALNUTRITION[1]

BENJAMIN TORÛN

HISTORICAL BACKGROUND 881
ETIOLOGY AND EPIDEMIOLOGY 882
   Magnitude of the Problem 882
   Causes 882
   Age of the Host 883
PATHOPHYSIOLOGY AND ADAPTIVE RESPONSES 883
   Energy Mobilization and Expenditure 883
   Protein Breakdown and Synthesis 884
   Endocrine Changes 884
   Hematology and Oxygen Transport 885
   Other Physiologic and Metabolic Changes 886
FACTORS LEADING TO KWASHIORKOR 887
DISRUPTION OF ADAPTATION 889
DIAGNOSIS 889
   Classification of Protein-Energy Malnutrition 889
   Mild and Moderate Protein-Energy
      Malnutrition 891
   Severe Protein-Energy Malnutrition 891
PROGNOSIS AND RISK OF MORTALITY 895
TREATMENT 896
   Severe Protein-Energy Malnutrition 896
   Mild and Moderate Malnutrition 905
PREVENTION AND CONTROL 905
   Food Availability 905
   Reducing Infections 906
   Education 906

Protein-energy malnutrition (PEM) results when the body's needs for protein and energy fuels are not satisfied by the diet. It is accompanied by deficiency of several micronutrients, and its clinical characteristics are conditioned by the relative severity of energy, protein, and micronutrient deficit, the duration and cause of the deficiencies, the age of the host, and the association with infectious diseases. Severe PEM can become manifest as *marasmus*, a nonedematous syndrome characterized by gradual emaciation associated with near starvation and pre-dominant energy deficit, or as *kwashiorkor*, a syndrome characterized by bipedal edema that progresses rapidly, associated with predominant protein deficiency and varying degrees of energy deficit. *Marasmic kwashiorkor* combines edema and emaciation associated with chronic energy deficiency and chronic or acute protein deficit. Milder forms of the disease result in weight loss, growth retardation, and several forms of functional impairment.

The origin of PEM can be *primary*, when it is the result of inadequate food intake, or *secondary*, when it is the result of other diseases that lead to low food ingestion, inadequate nutrient absorption or utilization, increased nutritional requirements, and/or increased nutrient losses. Its onset can be relatively fast, as in starvation resulting from abrupt withholding of food, or gradual. This chapter discusses *primary PEM* of a relatively gradual onset, in which the metabolic alterations and clinical characteristics of protein and/or energy deficits predominate. PEM secondary to other diseases and the metabolic and clinical manifestations of starvation and of specific vitamin and mineral deficiencies are described in other chapters.

HISTORICAL BACKGROUND

It has long been recognized that inadequate food intake produces weight loss and growth retardation and, when severe and prolonged, leads to body wasting and emaciation. It has taken longer to understand the nature of the edematous forms of PEM, partly because they could be found among children who were not starving. Descriptions of the disease in the early part of the twentieth century paid special attention to dermatologic signs and led to the belief that the disease was caused by tropical parasites or a vitamin deficiency (1–7). The real nature of the disease was studied more carefully after Cicely Williams' descriptions in the mid-1930s of "kwashiorkor" (8, 9). This term, used by the Ga tribe in the Gold Coast (now Ghana) for "the disease the deposed baby gets when the next one is born," suggested that the disease could be associated with inadequate diet during the weaning period. Other pediatricians who worked in tropical countries in the 1930s showed that the edematous disease could be cured by feeding milk or other high-protein foods (10, 11). In the 1940s, researchers showed that most patients had low concentrations of serum proteins, and that this could also be related to the quality of dietary proteins (12).

[1] **Abbreviations: AIDS,** acquired immunodeficiency syndrome; **BMI,** body mass index; **D/W,** dextrose in water; **HIV,** human immunodeficiency virus; **ORS,** oral rehydration solution; **PEM,** protein-energy malnutrition; **WHO,** World Health Organization.

The nature and importance of this disease gained worldwide recognition in the 1950s, partly owing to publications such as those of Brock and Autret (13), Autret and Behar (10), and Trowell, Davies, and Dean (11). By then, more than 40 names had been given to this clinical syndrome (11). Some of them, such as "síndrome policarencial de la infancia" (infantile pluricarential syndrome), indicated that young children were mainly affected and that a deficit of various nutrients was involved. Others, such as "Mehlnahrschade" ("damage by cereal flours"), "starch edema," and "sugar babies" indicated that it was caused by the intake of foods with high carbohydrate and low protein contents. Today, the more comprehensive term of "protein-energy (or protein-calorie) malnutrition" is universally accepted (14), and its severe forms are called "marasmus," "kwashiorkor," and "marasmic kwashiorkor." The term "malnutrition" is usually used in lay language for PEM.

Prevention and treatment of PEM continue having high priority. Prevalence has remained high around the world, with outbursts of severe PEM since the mid-1980s, associated with draughts, famines, and civil strife in regions of Africa, Asia, Europe, and the Americas. Inadequate understanding of metabolic adaptation and disruption resulted in inappropriate treatment and high mortality rates in many centers (15).

Studies done since the 1960s have shown that marasmus and kwashiorkor have distinct metabolic features, that some manifestations, such as anemia and reduced physical activity, are partly the result of adaptive mechanisms, that the immune response of severely malnourished patients is impaired, that free radicals may play a role in kwashiorkor, and that physical and emotional stimulation are important elements in treating malnourished children. These findings are the basis of current therapeutic measures that have reduced mortality rates and improved the dietary management of mild, moderate, and severe PEM.

ETIOLOGY AND EPIDEMIOLOGY

PEM is the most important nutritional disease in developing countries because of its high prevalence and relationship with child mortality rates, impaired physical growth, and inadequate social and economic development. Most deaths of children 6 to 59 months old in developing countries are attributable to the potentiating effects of moderate and severe malnutrition on infections (16). Malnutrition is especially associated with increased risk of death from diarrhea and acute lower respiratory infections (17, 18), and nutritional interventions reduce the risk (19). Conversely, infections are a major factor in the etiology of PEM as a result of increased nutrient demands, greater nutrient losses, and disruption of metabolic equilibrium. In industrialized countries, primary PEM is seen mainly among young children of the lower socioeconomic groups, elderly persons who live alone, and adults addicted to alcohol and drugs. Some cases of kwashiorkor have been reported in association with diet faddism and nutritional ignorance (20).

Magnitude of the Problem

Prevalence of stunting, an indicator of child malnutrition, has decreased gradually in the last 25 years (21). Yet, there are still about 800 million undernourished people in the world, and child malnutrition remains a major public health problem in developing countries; in some of these countries, severe malnutrition is the most common reason for pediatric hospitalization. Around 27% of the children younger than the age of 5 years in the developing world are underweight, 32% are stunted, and 10% are wasted, based on a deficit of more than 2 standard deviations below the World Health Organization (WHO)/US National Center for Health Statistics reference values for weight for age, height for age and weight for height, respectively. This prevalence ranges from 8% underweight, 16% stunted, and 3% wasted in Latin America and CEE/CIS/Baltic states to 46% underweight, 44% stunted, and 15% wasted in South Asia (22).

Causes

Social, economic, biologic, and environmental factors may be underlying causes for the insufficient food intake or ingestion of foods with proteins of poor nutritional quality that lead to PEM.

Social and Economic Factors

Poverty that results in low food availability, overcrowded and unsanitary living conditions, and improper child care is a frequent cause of PEM. *Ignorance*, by itself or associated with poverty, leads to poor infant- and child-rearing practices, misconceptions about the use of certain foods, inadequate feeding conducts during illnesses, and improper food distribution among family members. A decline in the practice and duration of breast-feeding, combined with *inadequate weaning practices* when breast milk is withdrawn or when it can no longer provide sufficient dietary energy and protein to the infant, is associated with growing rates of infantile PEM. *Social problems* such as child abuse, maternal deprivation, abandonment of the elderly, alcoholism, and drug addiction can result in PEM. *Cultural and social practices* that impose food taboos, some food and diet fads, particularly popular among adolescents and women, and the migration from traditional rural settings to urban slums can also contribute to, or precipitate, the appearance of PEM.

Biologic Factors

Maternal malnutrition before and/or during pregnancy is more likely to produce an underweight newborn baby (22, 23). Intrauterine malnutrition can be compounded after birth by insufficient food to satisfy the infant's needs for catch-up growth, resulting in PEM. A recent study demonstrated that low birth weight was a predictor of wasting in Africa, Asia, and Latin America (24).

Infectious diseases are major contributing and precipitating factors in PEM. Diarrheal disease, measles, acquired immunodeficiency syndrome (AIDS), tuberculosis and other infections frequently result in negative protein and energy balance resulting from anorexia (reduced food intake), vomiting, decreased absorption (increased nutrient losses), and catabolic processes (increased requirements and metabolic losses). Intestinal parasites have little or no effect unless the infection is extensive and causes anemia or diarrhea (25).

Diets with low concentrations of proteins and energy, as occur with overdiluted milk formulas or bulky vegetable foods that have low nutrient densities, can lead to PEM in young children whose gastric capacity does not allow the ingestion of large amounts of food and in elderly persons with anorexia or difficulty in eating without assistance. Diets poor in protein and rich in carbohydrates are particularly likely to produce kwashiorkor.

Environmental Factors

Overcrowded and/or unsanitary living conditions lead to frequent infections. This is an important cause of PEM, especially among weanlings who develop severe or frequent episodes of diarrhea. *Agricultural patterns, droughts, floods, wars, and forced migrations* lead to cyclic, sudden, or prolonged food scarcities and can cause PEM among whole populations. Postharvest losses of food resulting from bad storage conditions and inadequate food distribution systems contribute to PEM, even after periods of agricultural plenty.

Age of the Host

PEM can affect all age groups, but it is more frequent among *infants* and *young children* whose growth increases nutritional requirements, who cannot obtain food by their own means, and who, when living under poor hygienic conditions, frequently become ill with diarrhea and other infections. Infants who are weaned prematurely from the breast or who are breast-fed for a prolonged time without adequate complementary feeding practices become malnourished for lack of adequate energy and protein intake. The long-term intake of insufficient food can result in marasmus, which is the most common form of severe PEM before 1 year of age. Kwashiorkor is more frequent after 18 months of age and typically occurs in children with diets consisting of starchy gruels, diluted cereal-based beverages, and vegetable foods rich in carbohydrates but almost devoid of proteins of good nutritional quality (i.e., lacking one or more essential amino acid). The appearance of edema is frequently preceded or accompanied by acute diarrhea or other infectious disease.

Most often, the severe protein deficit is associated with chronic dietary energy deficit and results in the combined form of marasmic kwashiorkor.

Older children usually have milder forms of PEM because they can cope better with social and food availability constraints. Infections and other precipitating factors become less severe, and early survival may imply a natural selection of the more fit. *Pregnant and lactating women* can also have PEM resulting from the increases in nutritional requirements. However, the consequences of the dietary deficiencies affect mainly the growth, nutritional status, and survival rates of their fetuses, newborn babies, and infants. *Elderly persons* who are unable to care properly for themselves tend to suffer from PEM. Gastrointestinal alterations can be an important contributing factor.

Adolescents, *men*, and *nonpregnant, nonlactating women* usually have the lowest prevalence and the mildest forms of the disease because of greater opportunities to obtain food and cultural practices that protect the productive members of the family. Severe PEM occurs as a primary disorder in conditions of extreme privation and famine and in situations of social or chemical dependency without adequate support, as may be the case with mental patients, prisoners, persons with alcoholism, and drug addicts. It is more frequently secondary to other illnesses, such as chronic infections, cancer, AIDS, malabsorption, and liver and endocrine diseases. In such cases, both the malnutrition and the underlying cause must be treated.

PATHOPHYSIOLOGY AND ADAPTIVE RESPONSES

PEM develops gradually in weeks or months. This allows a series of metabolic and behavioral adjustments that result in decreased nutrient demands and a nutritional equilibrium compatible with a lower level of cellular nutrient availability. If the supply of nutrients becomes persistently lower, the patient can no longer adapt and may even die. Metabolic disruptions can be caused by severe nutrient deficit, complications (e.g., infections), or inadequate treatment (e.g., abrupt administration of large amounts of dietary energy or protein). Patients whose PEM develops slowly, as is usually the case in marasmus, are better adapted to their current nutritional status and maintain a less fragile metabolic equilibrium than those with more acute PEM, as in kwashiorkor of rapid onset.

Energy Mobilization and Expenditure

A decrease in energy intake is quickly followed by a decrease in energy expenditure, accounting for shorter periods of play and physical activity in children (26) and for longer rest periods and less physical work in adults (27). When the decrease in energy expenditure cannot compensate for the insufficient intake, body fat is mobilized, with a decrease in adiposity and weight loss (28). Lean body mass diminishes at a slower rate, mainly as a consequence of muscle protein catabolism with increased efflux of amino acids, primarily alanine, that contribute to the energy sources. As the cumulative energy deficit becomes more severe, subcutaneous fat is markedly reduced, and protein catabolism leads to muscular wasting. Visceral protein is preserved longer, especially in the marasmic patients.

In marasmus, these alterations in body composition lead initially to increased basal oxygen consumption (i.e., basal metabolic rate) per unit of body weight, and it decreases in more severe stages (29). In kwashiorkor, the severe dietary protein deficit leads to an earlier visceral depletion of amino acids that affects visceral cell function and reduces oxygen consumption; therefore, basal energy expenditure decreases per unit of lean or total body mass.

Blood glucose concentration remains normal, mainly at the expense of gluconeogenic amino acids and glycerol from fats, and it falls in severe PEM or when complicated by serious infections or fasting.

Protein Breakdown and Synthesis

The poor availability of dietary proteins reduces protein synthesis (30). Adaptations lead to the sparing of body protein and the preservation of essential protein-dependent functions. The gradual and inevitable loss of body protein as a result of long-term dietary protein deficit is primarily from skeletal muscle. Table 57.1 illustrates some enzymatic changes that favor muscle protein breakdown and liver protein synthesis, as well as energy mobilization from fat depots (31). Some visceral protein is lost in the early development of PEM but then becomes stable until the nonessential tissue proteins are depleted; the loss of visceral protein then increases, and death may be imminent unless nutritional therapy is successfully instituted.

Under normal conditions, about 75% of the free amino acids that enter the body pool from dietary and tissue proteins are recycled or reused for protein synthesis, and 25% are broken down for other metabolic purposes. When protein intake is reduced, there is not so much a decrease in total nitrogen or amino acid turnover as an adaptive increase to 90 to 95% in the proportion that is recycled for synthesis and a proportional decrease in amino acid catab-

olism (30, 32). The latter markedly reduces urea synthesis and urinary nitrogen excretion.

The half-lives of several proteins increase. The rate of albumin synthesis decreases initially, but after a time lag of a few days the rate of breakdown also falls, and its half-life increases. In addition, a shift of albumin from the extravascular to the intravascular pool assists in maintaining adequate levels of circulating albumin in the presence of reduced synthesis. When protein depletion becomes too severe, the adaptive mechanisms fail, and the concentration of serum proteins, and especially albumin, decreases. The ensuing reduction in intravascular oncotic pressure and outflow of water into the extravascular space contribute to the development of the edema of kwashiorkor.

Endocrine Changes

Hormones are important in the adaptive metabolic processes. However, circulating levels of hormones do not always explain endocrine changes in PEM, because cellular responses to hormonal stimulation may also be altered. Table 57.2 summarizes the main changes in hormonal activity seen in patients with severe energy or protein deficiencies. These changes contribute to the maintenance of energy homeostasis through increased glycolysis and lipolysis, increased amino acid mobilization, preservation of visceral proteins through increased breakdown of muscle proteins, decreased storage of glycogen, fats, and proteins, and decreased energy metabolism. These effects can be summarized as follows (Fig. 57.1; the numbers in the following list refer to the numbers in Fig. 57.1): (1) The decreased food intake tends to reduce plasma concentrations of glucose and free amino acids, which, in turn, reduce insulin secretion and increase glucagon and epinephrine release; the latter further reduces insulin secretion; (2) the low plasma amino acid levels, seen mainly in kwashiorkor, also stimulate the secretion of human growth hormone and reduce somatomedin activity; this produces a further increase in growth hormone levels because of the absence of feedback inhibition; the increased levels of growth hormone and epinephrine influence the reduction

TABLE 57.1. SELECTED ENZYME ACTIVITY CHANGES IN PROTEIN-ENERGY MALNUTRITION

CELLS	ENZYME ACTIVITY[a]
Muscle and leukocytes	↓Aldolase
	↓Amino acid dehydrogenases
	↓Pyruvic kinase
	↑Aminotransferases
Liver	↓Phenylalanine hydroxylase
	↓Urea cycle enzymes
	↑Amino acid activating enzymes

[a]↑, ↓, increase or decrease in activity.

Adapted from Viteri FE. Primary protein-energy malnutrition: Clinical, biochemical, and metabolic changes. In: Suskind RM, ed. Textbook of Pediatric Nutrition. New York: Raven Press, 1981, with permission.

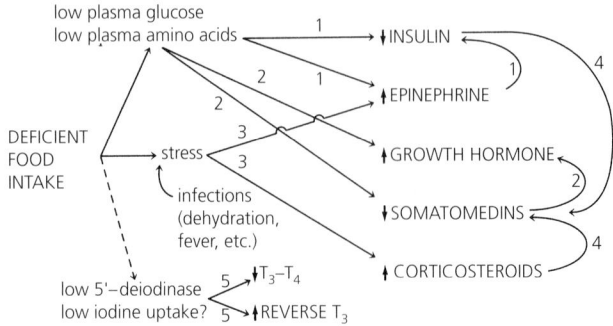

Figure 57.1. Endocrine adaptive functions in severe protein-energy malnutrition related to energy and protein metabolism. See text for an explanation of the numbered events.

TABLE 57.2. SUMMARY OF SELECTED HORMONAL CHANGES USUALLY SEEN IN SEVERE PROTEIN-ENERGY MALNUTRITION AND THEIR MAIN METABOLIC EFFECTS

HORMONE	INFLUENCED IN PEM BY	HORMONAL ENERGY DEFICIT	ACTIVITY IN PROTEIN DEFICIT	EFFECTS OF ABNORMALITY IN PEM
Insulin	Low food intake ($\downarrow$Glucose) ($\downarrow$Amino acids)	Decreased	Decreased	$\downarrow$Muscle protein synthesis $\downarrow$Lipogenesis $\downarrow$Growth
Growth hormone	Low protein intake ($\downarrow$Amino acids) Reduced somatomedin synthesis	Variable	Increased	$\uparrow$Visceral protein synthesis $\downarrow$Urea synthesis $\uparrow$Lipolysis $\downarrow$Glucose uptake by tissues
Somatomedins (insulinlike growth factors)	Low protein intake	Variable	Decreased	$\downarrow$Muscle and cartilage protein synthesis
	Low circulating insulin High circulating cortisol			$\downarrow$Collagen synthesis $\downarrow$Lipolysis $\downarrow$Growth $\uparrow$Production of growth hormone
Epinephrine	Stress of food deficiency, infections ($\downarrow$Glucose)	Normal but can increase	Normal but can increase	$\uparrow$Lipolysis $\uparrow$Glycogenolysis inhibits insulin secretion
Glucocorticoids	Stress of hunger	Increased	Normal or increased	$\uparrow$Muscle protein catabolism
	Fever ($\downarrow$Glucose)			$\uparrow$Visceral protein turnover $\uparrow$Lipolysis $\uparrow$Gluconeogenesis $\downarrow$Somatomedin-dependent actions of growth hormone
Renin-aldosterone	$\downarrow$Blood volume $\uparrow$Extracellular potassium? $\downarrow$Serum sodium?	Normal	Increased	$\uparrow$Sodium retention and $\uparrow$Water retention contribute to appearance of edema
Thyroid hormones	$\downarrow$5'-Deiodinase ($\uparrow$Reverse T_3)	T_4 normal or decreased; T_3 decreased	T_4 usually decreased; T_3 decreased	$\downarrow$Glucose oxidation $\downarrow$Basal energy expenditure $\uparrow$Reverse T_3
	Defect in iodine uptake?			
Gonadotropins	Low protein intake? Low energy intake?	Decreased	Decreased	Delayed menarche

$\downarrow$, low or reduced; $\uparrow$, high or increased; PEM, protein-energy malnutrition; T_3, triiodothyronine; T_4, thyroxine.

of urea synthesis, thereby favoring amino acid recycling; (3) the stress induced by the low food intake and further amplified by fever, dehydration, and other manifestations of the infections that frequently accompany PEM also stimulates epinephrine release and corticosteroid secretion, more so in marasmus than in kwashiorkor, probably because of the greater severity in energy deficit that characterizes marasmus; resistance to the peripheral action of insulin increases, probably from the increase in plasma free fatty acid concentration resulting from the lipolytic activity of growth hormone, glucocorticoids, and epinephrine; (4) the low levels of circulating insulin and high levels of circulating cortisol may further reduce the secretion of somatomedins; and (5) a decrease in the activity of 5'-monodeiodinase reduces the production of 3,5,3' triiodothyronine with a concomitant increase in the inactive reverse triiodothyronine; thyroxine levels are also reduced, possibly by a decrease in iodine uptake by the thyroid; the

reduction in active thyroid hormone levels decreases thermogenesis and oxygen consumption, leading to energy conservation.

The secretion of hormones involved in nonvital growth-related functions, such as gonadotropins, decreases; the functional capacities of the hypothalamic-pituitary axis and adrenal medulla are preserved, thus allowing endocrine and metabolic responses to stress conditions. Some investigators have postulated that the evolution of PEM into either kwashiorkor or marasmus may be partly related to differences in adrenocortical response, whereby the better response will preserve visceral proteins more efficiently and lead to the better-adapted syndrome of marasmus (33).

Hematology and Oxygen Transport

The reduction in hemoglobin concentration and red cell mass that almost always accompanies severe PEM is, at least

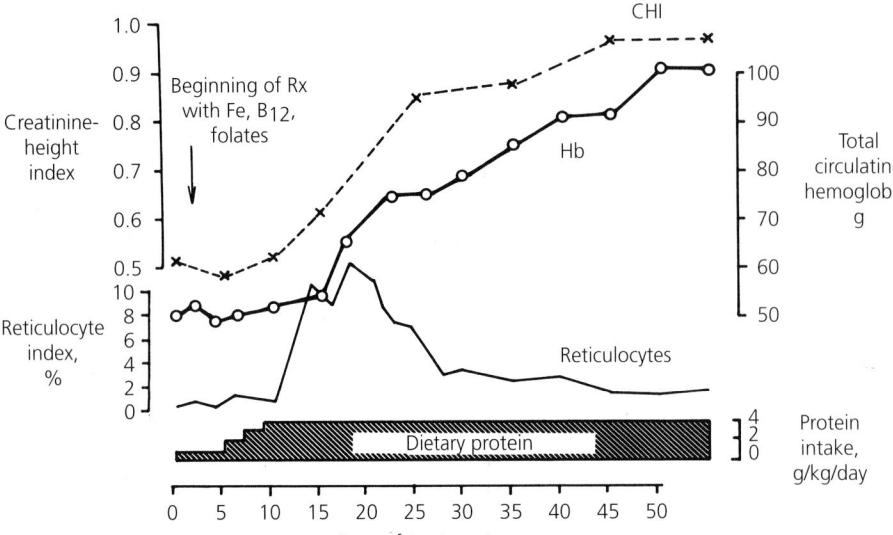

Figure 57.2. Hematologic response of a child with severe protein-energy malnutrition. Treatment with iron, folic acid, and vitamin B_{12} began on day 2; dietary energy and proteins were increased gradually to 150 kcal and 4 g protein/kg/day on day 9. No reticulocyte or hemoglobin response occurred until lean body mass, assessed by the creatinine-height index, began increasing.

in part, an adaptive phenomenon related to tissue oxygen needs (34). The reduction in lean body mass and the lower physical activity of malnourished patients lead to lower oxygen demands. The simultaneous decrease in dietary amino acids results in reduced hematopoietic activity, which spares amino acids for synthesis of other, more necessary body proteins. As long as the tissues' needs for oxygen are satisfied by the existing capacity for oxygen transport, this should be considered an adaptive response and not "functional" anemia (i.e., with tissue hypoxia). When tissue synthesis, lean body mass, and physical activity begin improving with dietary treatment, there is a rise in oxygen demands calling for accelerated hematopoiesis. If iron, folic acid, and

vitamin B_{12} are not available in sufficient amounts, functional anemia with tissue hypoxia will develop.

Figure 57.2 shows that the administration of hematinics to a severely malnourished patient will not induce a hematopoietic response until dietary treatment produces an increase in lean body mass. Figure 57.3 shows that the reticulocyte response is related to the amount of protein intake when erythropoietic substances are not limiting (31). The severely malnourished patient may have relatively high body iron stores (35) and retains the ability to produce erythropoietin and reticulocytes in response to acute hypoxia (36, 37). Nevertheless, these patients are prone to develop functional, severe anemia if there is a superimposed dietary deficiency of iron or folic acid, or chronic blood loss, as in hookworm infection.

Other Physiologic and Metabolic Changes

Not all pathophysiologic changes lead to advantageous adjustments. Certain functions are affected, and some nutrient reserves decrease, thus making malnourished persons more susceptible to injuries that a well-nourished person can withstand with little repercussion.

Cardiovascular and Renal Functions

Cardiac output, heart rate, and blood pressure decrease, and central circulation takes precedence over peripheral circulation (38, 39). Cardiovascular reflexes are altered, leading to postural hypotension and diminished venous return. In severe PEM, peripheral circulatory failure comparable to hypovolemic shock may occur. Hemodynamic compensation occurs primarily from tachycardia, rather than from increased stroke volume. Renal plasma flow and glomerular filtration rates may be reduced as a consequence of the decreased cardiac output, but water clearance and the ability to concentrate and acidify urine appear unimpaired (40, 41).

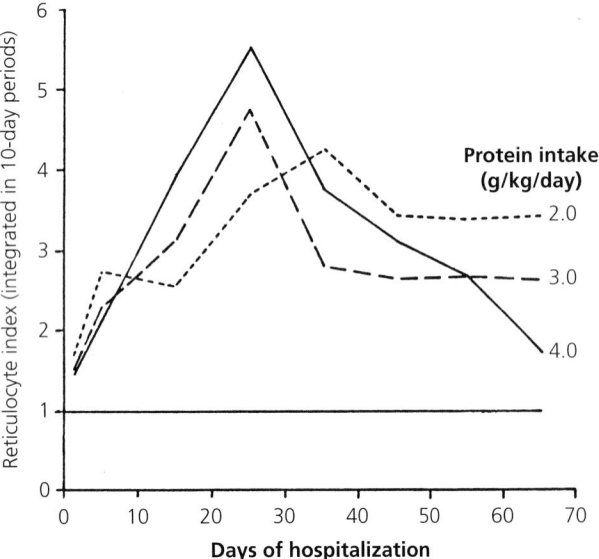

Figure 57.3. Reticulocyte response of children treated for severe protein-energy malnutrition with different amounts of dietary energy and hematinics. (From Viteri FE. Primary protein-energy malnutrition: Clinical, biochemical, and metabolic changes. In: Suskind RM, ed. Textbook of Pediatric Nutrition. New York: Raven Press, 1981, with permission.)

Immune System

The major defects seen in severe PEM seem to involve T lymphocytes and the complement system (42). A marked depletion of lymphocytes from the thymus and atrophy of the gland occur. In addition, cells from the T-lymphocyte regions of the spleen and lymph nodes are depleted, probably owing to a decrease in thymic factors (43). Alteration in monokine metabolism, particularly decreased activity of interleukin-1, may contribute to the low proliferation of T cells in severe malnutrition (44). The production of several complement components, the functional activity of the complement system assessed by both the classic and alternative pathways, and the opsonic activity of serum are depressed in severe PEM (45). These deficiencies may explain the high susceptibility of severely malnourished patients to gram-negative bacterial sepsis. Phagocytosis, chemotaxis, and intracellular killing are also impaired, partly because of the defects in opsonic and complement functional activities. The B-lymphocyte areas of spleen and lymph nodes and the circulating levels of B cells and immunoglobulin are relatively normal, but there may be defects in antibody production, such as secretory immunoglobulin A (42).

The overall consequences of all these alterations in severe PEM are greater predispositions to infections and to severe complications of otherwise less important infectious diseases. The defects in immune functions disappear with nutritional rehabilitation, except perhaps when they are the result of intrauterine malnutrition (43).

Monokines

Monokines and cytokines are peptide/glycoprotein mediators of the body's response to injury. They are synthesized primarily by activated monocytic and phagocytic cells lining the liver and spleen. These peptides activate neighboring tissue in a paracrine fashion and also enter the circulation to exert more distant effects. The most extensively characterized monokines are interleukin-1 and cachectin or tumor necrosis factor.

Macrophages from children with severe edematous PEM have decreased activity of interleukin-1 (44). In addition to the immunologic alterations mentioned previously, this may contribute to the poor febrile response and low leukocyte count in infections (46). Conversely, serum levels of tumor necrosis factor seem to be increased in severe malnutrition (47). This change could be associated with the anorexia and the muscle wasting and lipid abnormalities of PEM.

Electrolytes

Total body potassium decreases in PEM because of the reduction in muscle proteins and loss of intracellular potassium. The low insulin action and diminished intracellular energy substrates reduce the availability of adenosine triphosphate and phosphocreatine. This process probably alters the cellular exchange of sodium and potassium, leading to potassium loss and increased intracellular sodium (48). Water accompanies the sodium influx, and although total body intracellular water is decreased because of the loss in lean body mass, intracellular overhydration may occur. These alterations in cell electrolytes and energy sources may explain, at least in part, the increased fatigability and reduced strength of skeletal muscle.

Gastrointestinal Functions

Impaired intestinal absorption of lipids and disaccharides and a decreased rate of glucose absorption occur in severe protein deficiency. The greater the protein deficit, the greater is the functional impairment. A decrease in gastric, pancreatic, and bile production is also observed, with normal to low enzyme and conjugated bile acid concentrations (49, 50). These alterations further impair the absorptive functions. Nevertheless, the ingestion of nutrients in high therapeutic amounts usually allows for their uptake in sufficient quantity to permit nutritional recovery (51). Malnourished persons, however, are prone to diarrhea because of these alterations and possibly also because of irregular intestinal motility and gastrointestinal bacterial overgrowth. Diarrhea aggravates the malabsorption and can further impair nutritional status. Malabsorption disappears with nutritional recovery unless there is an underlying food or nutrient intolerance unrelated to primary PEM.

Nervous System and Cognitive Functions

Persons who suffer severe PEM at an early age may have decreased brain growth, nerve myelination, neurotransmitter production, and velocity of nervous conduction. The long-term functional implications of these alterations have not been clearly demonstrated, because environmental and social support can improve behavior and the cognitive state of malnourished children (52, 53). In contrast, a recent study indicated that after controlling for psychosocial adversity, malnutrition at 3 years of age was associated with poorer cognition at that age and at 11 years, and children with more severe malnutrition at age 3 had a 15-point deficit in intelligence quotient at age 11 (54). It seems that the severity, timing, and duration of nutritional deprivation, the quality of nutritional rehabilitation, emotional, and psychosocial support, and the degree of care and affective stimulation provided by family members and caretakers will influence a developing child's behavior and cognitive functions.

FACTORS LEADING TO KWASHIORKOR

The metabolic factors leading to kwashiorkor are not yet fully understood. Severe dietary protein deficiency, especially when accompanied by a less severe energy deficit as in nonstarving persons, is an important causal factor of edematous PEM. Lack of some vitamins and minerals usually present in protein foods of animal origin is another important factor. The changes in body reserves and micronutrient requirements during infancy may explain, at least in part, some age-related epidemiologic features of marasmus and kwashiorkor.

Other factors, such as overloading a severely malnourished person with carbohydrates and the metabolic stress induced by infections, may contribute to the appearance of kwashiorkor with its characteristic edema, hypoalbuminemia, and enlarged fatty liver. Some investigators postulated that the evolution of PEM into either kwashiorkor or marasmus may be partly related to differences in adrenocortical response, whereby a greater response preserves visceral proteins more efficiently and leads to the better-adapted syndrome of marasmus (33). Others proposed that kwashiorkor results from aflatoxin poisoning (55, 56), but a more recent study in mice counters this hypothesis (57).

Another theory is related to the production of toxic free radicals and their safe disposal (58, 59). Among the factors that would increase free radicals are infections, toxins, sunlight, trauma, and catalysts such as iron. Formation of free radicals is decreased by the antioxidant function of vitamins A (or β-carotene), C, and E, by ceruloplasmin and transferrin that bind free iron and favor its oxidation, and by zinc-metallothionein, which acts as a free radical sink. Free radicals and the peroxides they generate are removed through reactions catalyzed by enzymes in which glutathione and trace minerals play an important role, such as copper-zinc and manganese superoxide dismutase and selenuim glutathione peroxidase. Compared with well-nourished or marasmic children, patients with kwashiorkor have lower levels of glutathione and of the enzymes responsible for maintaining glutathione in the reduced state (60–62). Other studies have confirmed that children with kwashiorkor have lower plasma concentrations of antioxidants, higher concentrations of biomarkers of oxidant-induced tissue damage, and an improvement in these biochemical findings with nutritional recovery and disappearance of clinical symptoms (63–65). The toxic effects of free radicals are probably involved in the cell damage leading to the alterations seen in kwashiorkor, such as edema, fatty liver, and skin lesions. An association between congestive heart failure in kwashiorkor and selenium deficiency has also been reported (66). However, the free-radical theory has not been firmly established and must be subjected to the test of animal experiments. Nevertheless, it has drawn attention to factors and processes in the pathogenesis of severe PEM that have previously been neglected, and it may have important implications for treatment (67, 68).

When there is a severe lack of food, endocrine adjustments mobilize fatty acids from adipose tissue and amino acids from muscle tissue; plasma protein concentration remains normal, and hepatic gluconeogenesis is enhanced.

An increase in carbohydrate intake when protein intake is very low can produce a breakdown of those adjustments, as follows:

1. Carbohydrate intake induces insulin release and a reduction in the production of epinephrine and cortisol.
2. Lipolysis decreases and the action of insulin is enhanced because of the suppression of the inhibitory effects of free fatty acids on the peripheral action of insulin.
3. Muscle protein breakdown is reduced, and the body pool of free amino acids decreases. The decreased supply of muscle amino acids to the other organs results in less visceral protein synthesis.
4. The decreased synthesis of plasma proteins in the liver, particularly albumin, reduces intravascular oncotic pressure. Plasma water decreases and accumulates in extravascular tissues, tissue pressure rises, and cardiac output diminishes. This contributes to the appearance or increase of edema.
5. Increased hepatic fatty acid synthesis from the excess carbohydrate, impaired lipolysis, and reduced production of apoβ-lipoproteins for lipid transport lead to fatty infiltration of the liver and hepatomegaly.

Infections in undernourished children also can precipitate the onset of kwashiorkor. The process by which this occurs has not been satisfactorily explained, but the following mechanisms may be involved:

1. Infections may divert the meager amino acid pool to the production of globulins and acute-phase reactant proteins, instead of albumin and transport proteins.
2. The increase of acute-phase reactant proteins that are proteinase inhibitors, such as α_1-antitrypsin and α_1-antichymotrypsin, may impair muscle protein breakdown.
3. Impaired production and utilization of ketone bodies for energy during infections may lead to the use of more amino acids for gluconeogenesis.
4. Protein catabolism and nitrogen losses are enhanced by many viral and febrile infections, probably through increased epinephrine and cortisol actions. Regardless of the mechanisms involved, protein losses during severe infections can amount to as much as 2% of muscle protein per day (69).
5. Leukocytes stimulated by infectious organisms produce large quantities of superoxide and hydrogen peroxide. These are released into the surrounding medium and contribute to the production of kwashiorkor, according to the free-radical theory.

The pathogenesis of edema in severe PEM has aroused much discussion. It is an important issue because of the key role of edema in the diagnosis of kwashiorkor and because it may give clues about the patient's dietary background and other precipitating factors of the disease. The edema of kwashiorkor has been classically linked to hypoalbuminemia through a reduction in colloid osmotic pressure of the plasma, which leads to outflow of fluid from the capillaries into the interstitial space. However, an overlap in serum albumin levels is noted between edematous and nonedematous PEM in children and adults; experimental studies in dogs fed a low-protein diet showed that many animals with plasma albumin concentrations lower than 20 g/L did not have edema, whereas almost all edematous dogs had albumin levels lower than that value (70). Furthermore, the edema of kwashiorkor is reduced after treatment with protein-free or low-protein diets that contain potassium and other minerals and moderate amounts of carbohydrates. All this suggests that hypoalbuminemia may be a necessary but not a sufficient cause of edema, and that some other factors may be needed, at least in some cases (67). These factors include potassium deficiency, which promotes water and sodium retention (71), excessive administration of water and sodium, and extravasation of fluid resulting from increased capillary permeability in infection.

A theory that became widely accepted for the production of edema in severe PEM involved a reduction in renal blood flow and glomerular filtration rate resulting from decreased plasma volume and decreased cardiac output as consequence of hypoalbuminemia; the decrease in renal blood flow and glomerular filtration rate would result in sodium retention and production of renin and aldosterone, which, in turn, would increase the tubular reabsorption of sodium and water, leading to edema (72). However, evidence about the changes in plasma volume in kwashiorkor is conflicting, and aldosterone activity may increase in children with marasmus as well as in children with edema (73, 74). Other theories include an increase in ferritin that stimulates production of antidiuretic hormone by the posterior pituitary (75, 76), energy deficiency that does not allow adequate function of the sodium pump and restoration of intracellular potassium (77), and leakiness of cell membranes caused by the damaging effects of free radicals (58, 59, 61). It is possible that the pathogenesis of edema in PEM is not a single entity and that it differs in accordance with the multiple nutritional deficiencies, the age of the patients, and other concomitant conditions. Nevertheless, hypoproteinemia, especially hypoalbuminemia, is an essential component.

DISRUPTION OF ADAPTATION

When the supply for tissue and cell energy can no longer be maintained by patients with severe energy deficiency, serious decompensation occurs causing hypoglycemia, hypothermia, impaired circulatory and renal functions, acidosis, coma, and death. These events can occur within a few hours. Metabolic decompensation resulting from severe protein deficiency, in addition to the changes discussed in the onset of kwashiorkor, may include the following: hemorrhagic diathesis and jaundice caused by

failure by the liver to synthesize several clotting factors and transport proteins; various degrees of renal failure with acidosis and water and sodium retention; decreased cardiac work, pulmonary congestion, and increased susceptibility to pulmonary infections; coma; and death.

A high-carbohydrate, low-protein diet is not the only iatrogenic cause of serious metabolic disruption in patients who have or are prone to develop edematous PEM. The abrupt administration of too much protein to patients with edematous PEM can also have serious, life-threatening consequences. When such patients have been eating minute amounts of protein or none at all, and they are suddenly fed large amounts of proteins or given large transfusions of plasma or blood, they may experience a rapid increase in intravascular protein concentration and entry of extracellular fluid into the vascular compartment leading to cardiovascular insufficiency and pulmonary edema. In fact, premature introduction of a high-energy or high-protein diet may be fatal to a severely malnourished patient (15, 78–81).

DIAGNOSIS

The clinical, biochemical, and physiologic characteristics of PEM vary according to the severity of the disease, the patient's age, the presence of other nutritional deficits and infections, and the predominance of energy or protein deficiency.

Classification of Protein-Energy Malnutrition

The classification scheme shown in Table 57.3 is useful for the diagnosis and treatment of PEM and for the application and evaluation of public health measures. *Severity* is determined mainly by anthropometry, because other clinical findings and biochemical indexes usually do not show changes unless the disease is well advanced. More accurate measurements, such as assessment of body composition, are not practical or feasible in most of the settings in which primary PEM occurs, and they are usually used for research rather than for clinical purposes. The so-called functional indicators are not as yet well standardized, can be influenced by deficits of more than one single nutrient, or may be too complex to measure routinely (82). Classification of the *course* or *duration* of the disease as acute, chronic, or acute with a chronic background is also done

TABLE 57.3. CLASSIFICATION OF PROTEIN-ENERGY MALNUTRITION ACCORDING TO SEVERITY OF DISEASE, ITS COURSE OR DURATION, AND PREDOMINANT NUTRIENT DEFICIENCY

SEVERITY	COURSE	MAIN DEFICIT
Mild	Acute	Energy
Moderate	Chronic	Protein
Severe	Both	Both

TABLE 57.4. CLASSIFICATION OF SEVERITY OF CURRENT ("WASTING") AND PAST OR CHRONIC ("STUNTING") PROTEIN-ENERGY MALNUTRITION IN INFANTS AND CHILDREN, BASED ON WEIGHT FOR HEIGHT AND ON HEIGHT FOR AGE[a, b]

	NORMAL	MILD	MODERATE	SEVERE
Weight for height (deficit = wasting)	90–110 (±1 Z)[b]	80–89 (−1.1 to −2 Z)	75–79 (−2.1 to −3 Z)	<75, or with edema (<−3 Z)
Height for age (deficit = stunting)	95–105 (±1 Z)	90–94 (−1.1 to −2 Z)	85–89 (−2.1 to −3 Z)	<85 (<−3 Z)

[a]Expressed as percentage relative to the median National Center for Health Statistics standard (87, 88).
[b]In parentheses, standard deviations from the National Center for Health Statistics median, or Z scores (88).

by anthropometry to assess current nutritional status and degree of growth retardation in children. Dietary history is useful, especially in adults, as are dietary surveys in population groups. The relative contributions of dietary *protein and energy deficits* in the mild and moderate forms of PEM are assessed mainly by the individual person's dietary history or the population's dietary habits and food availability. Clinical characteristics and biochemical data confirm the diagnosis in severe PEM.

Anthropometric Measurements

The choice of anthropometric measurements depends on their simplicity, accuracy, and sensitivity, on the availability of measuring instruments, and on the existence of reference standards for comparison.

To allow international comparisons, it is sensible to use the same standard of reference for various populations. International or universal standards based on reliable anthropometric data can be used for the following reasons: (a) most children have similar growth potentials, regardless of ethnic background (83, 84); (b) the relationship of various anthropometric measurements, especially weight and height, is relatively constant in normal, healthy persons of all age groups; (c) the reference standards are merely for purposes of comparison and do not necessarily represent and ideal or a target; and (d) the interpretation of the comparison (i.e., the values that separate "normal" from "deficient" and further divide the latter into "mild," "moderate," and "severe" forms) is a matter of judgment that comes into play when deciding whether the expected normal value for a given population should be 100%, 90%, or another proportion of the standard. Setting different cutoff points relative to a single standard is more practical than constructing local standards that, in a country with heterogeneous population groups, may pose the same problem as a "foreign" commonly used reference. At present, the WHO recommends the data from the US National Center for Health Statistics as reference for weight and height (85) (see Appendix Tables A-14-a to A-14-e).

The best anthropometric assessment of nutritional status and PEM is based on measurements of weight and height or length, and records of age, to calculate two indexes: *weight for height,* as an index of current nutritional status; and *height for age,* as an index of past nutritional history. Deficient height for age may represent a

short period of growth failure at an early age or a longer period at a later age. Waterlow suggested the terms *wasting* for a deficit in weight for height and *stunting* for a deficit in height for age (86). Patients may then fall into four categories: (a) normal, (b) wasted but not stunted (suffering from acute PEM), (c) wasted and stunted (suffering from acute and chronic PEM), and (d) stunted but not wasted (past PEM with present adequate nutrition, or "nutritional dwarfs"). The intensity of wasting and stunting can be graded by calculating weight as a percentage of the reference median weight for height, and height as a percentage of the reference median height for age, as follows:

$$\% \text{ weight for height (or height for age)} = \text{observed weight (or height)/reference weight for patient's height (or reference height for patient's age)} \times 100$$

The use of centiles or standard deviations from the mean, instead of percent deviations from the median, is statistically more adequate. However, percent deviations are easier to understand by the general public and to calculate by field workers. The grading shown in Table 57.4 is suggested for most countries, although some may find it convenient to use different cutoff points for specific groups. For example, the normal height for age in populations that are genetically short could be less than 95% of the reference. Color-coded charts and graphs have been devised to simplify the measurements and their interpretation (87, 88).

The *body mass index* (BMI, or Quetelet index), weight/height^2, is recommended for adolescents and adults (Table 57.5). In adolescents, interpretation of BMI must take into account sexual maturation (89). In general, the diagnosis of PEM in adolescent boys and girls can be based on a BMI *below 15.0 at ages 11 to 13 years* and *below 16.5 at ages 14 to 17 years*. The corresponding values for *severe* PEM would be *below 13.5* and *below 14.5*, respectively.

TABLE 57.5. CLASSIFICATION OF INTENSITY OF PROTEIN-ENERGY MALNUTRITION IN MEN AND WOMEN

BODY MASS INDEX	PROTEIN-ENERGY MALNUTRITION
≥18.5	Normal
17.0–18.4	Mild
16.0–16.9	Moderate
<16.0	Severe

Based on the classification proposed for chronic energy deficiency in James WPT, Ferro-Luzzi A, Waterlow JC. Eur J Clin Nutr 1988;42:969–81.

The use of deficit in weight for age does not differentiate between a truly underweight child (current PEM) and one who is short in stature but well proportioned in weight (past PEM); furthermore, the information about chronologic age is not always reliable. However, the classification of PEM as grades I (75–90% of reference weight for age), II (60–74%), and III (<60%), is useful in public health and epidemiologic studies, because it indicates the proportion of children in a population group who at some time in their lives have had malnutrition (90).

Use of the upper arm circumference has been advocated under field conditions without access to a weighing scale. It is not a sensitive index, but it allows one to differentiate between a moderately to severely malnourished child and one in better nutritional condition.

Mild and Moderate Protein-Energy Malnutrition

The main clinical feature of mild and moderate PEM is weight loss. A decrease in subcutaneous adipose tissue may become apparent. When PEM is chronic, children show growth retardation in terms of height (stunting). Groups of populations in whom PEM is highly prevalent or "endemic" show slow weight gains, as illustrated in Figure 57.4.

Physical activity and energy expenditure of children decrease (28, 91–93), and other functional indicators of behavior may be altered. These include low physical activity at play and school, reduced attention span, and varying degrees of apathy. In adults, mild to moderate PEM results in leanness with reduction in subcutaneous tissue. The most common change in body composition is a reduc-

tion of adiposity to less than 12 and 20% in men and women, respectively. Capacity for prolonged physical work is reduced, but this change is usually apparent only in persons engaged in intense, energy-demanding occupations (27, 94). Malnourished pregnant women tend to have babies with low birth weights.

Biochemical alterations are not consistent in mild and moderate PEM. Laboratory data related to low protein intakes may include low urinary excretion of creatinine, leading to a low creatinine-height index in children (95), low urinary urea nitrogen and hydroxyproline excretions, altered plasma patterns of free amino acids with a decrease in branched-chain essential amino acids, slight decreases in serum transferrin and albumin, and a reduced number of circulating lymphocytes.

Severe Protein-Energy Malnutrition

The diagnosis is principally based on dietary history and clinical features. Marasmus is usually associated with severe food shortage, prolonged semistarvation, early weaning, or infrequent feeding of infants, and kwashiorkor is associated with late weaning and poor protein intakes. Chronic or recurrent diarrhea and infections are common features.

Marasmus

Generalized muscular wasting and absence of subcutaneous fat give the patient with severe, nonedematous PEM a "skin and bones" appearance (Figs. 57.5 and 57.6). Marasmic patients frequently have 60% or less of the

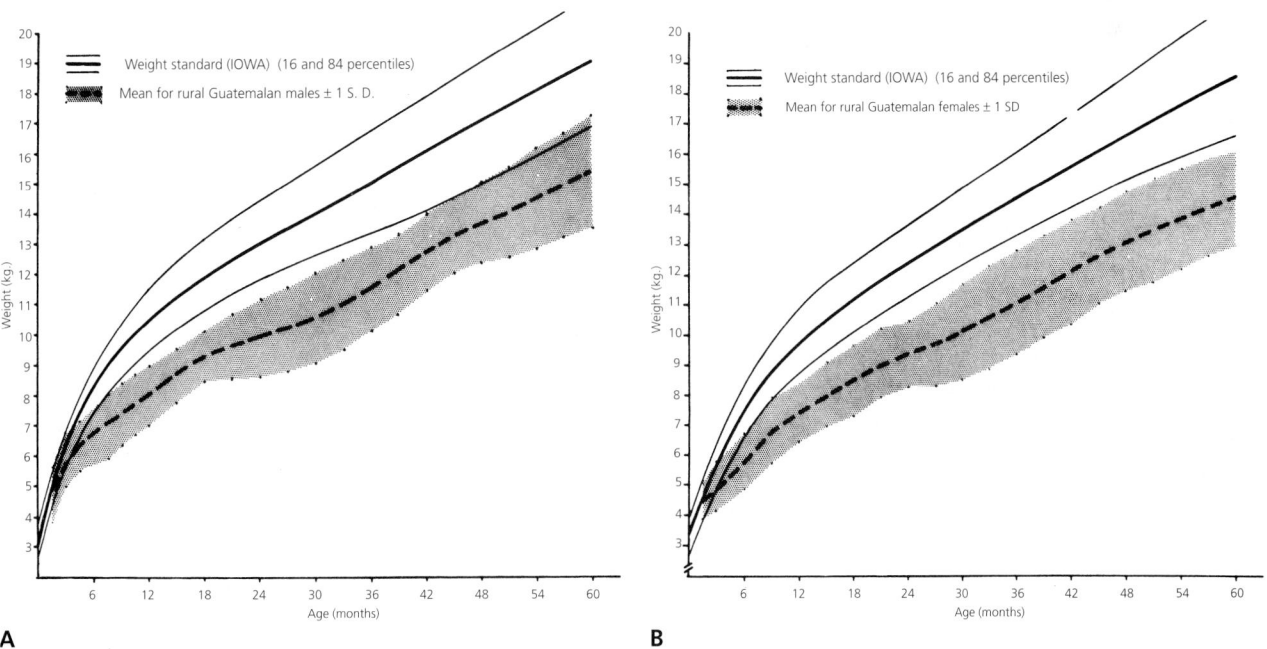

Figure 57.4. Pattern of weight gain, from birth to 5 years, in 431 boys **(A)** and 436 girls **(B)** from low-income families in rural Guatemala. (From INCAP. Evaluación nutricional de la polación de Centro América y Panamá: Guatemala. Guatemala: Instituto de Nutrición de Centro América y Panamá, 1969, with permission.)

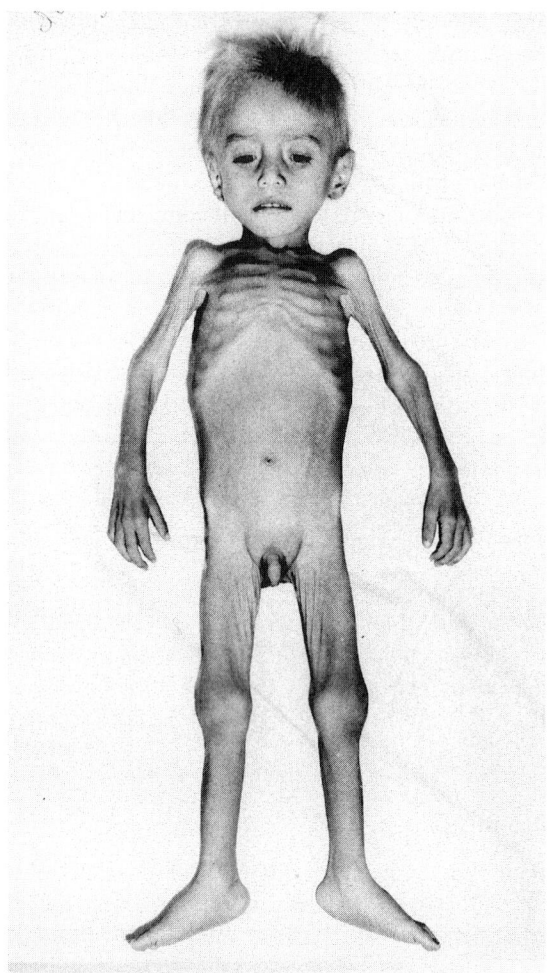

Figure 57.5. Marasmus in a 21-month-old child. (From Viteri FE. Primary protein-energy malnutrition: Clinical, biochemical, and metabolic changes. In: Suskind RM, ed. Textbook of Pediatric Nutrition. New York: Raven Press, 1981, with permission.)

weight expected for their height, and children have marked retardation in longitudinal growth. The hair is sparse, thin, and dry, without its normal sheen; it is easily pulled out without causing pain. The skin is dry, thin with little elasticity, and wrinkles easily. Patients are apathetic but usually aware and have a look of anxiety on their face. These features and the sunken cheeks caused by disappearance of the Bichat fat pads, which are among the last subcutaneous adipose depots to disappear, give the marasmic child's face the appearance of a monkey's or an old person's face.

Some patients are anorexic, whereas others are ravenously hungry, but they seldom tolerate large amounts of food, and they vomit easily. Diarrhea may be present. Patients have marked weakness, and children frequently cannot stand without help. Heart rate, blood pressure, and body temperature may be low, but tachycardia may be present. Hypoglycemia can occur, especially after fasting for 6 or more hours, and is often accompanied by hypothermia of 35.5°C or less. The viscera are usually

small. Abdominal distention may be present. The lymph nodes are easily palpable.

Differential diagnosis must be made from the secondary PEM of AIDS and other body-wasting diseases. Dietary history plays an important role.

Common complicating features are acute gastroenteritis, dehydration, respiratory infections, and eye lesions resulting from hypovitaminosis A. Systemic infections lead to septic shock or intravascular clotting with high mortality rates.

Kwashiorkor

The predominant feature is soft, pitting, painless edema, usually in the feet and legs, but extending to the perineum, upper extremities, and face in severe cases (Fig. 57.7). Most patients have skin lesions, often confused with pellagra, in the areas of edema, continuous pressure (e.g., at the buttocks and back), or frequent irritation (e.g., in the perineum and thighs). The skin may be erythematous, and it glistens in the edematous regions with zones of dryness, hyperkeratosis, and hyperpigmentation, which tend to become confluent. The epidermis peels off in large scales, exposing underlying tissues that are easily infected. Subcutaneous fat is preserved, and some muscle wasting may be present. Weight deficit, after accounting for the weight of edema, is usually not as severe as in marasmus. Height may be normal or retarded, depending on the chronicity of the current episode and on past nutritional history.

The hair is dry, brittle, and without its normal sheen, and it can be pulled out easily without causing pain. Curly hair becomes straight, and the pigmentation usually changes to dull brown, red, or even yellowish white. Alternating periods of poor and relatively good protein intake can produce alternating bands of depigmented and normal hair, which have been termed the "flag sign" (Fig. 57.8).

Patients may be pale, with cold and cyanotic extremities. They are apathetic and irritable, cry easily, and have an expression of misery and sadness. Anorexia (sometimes necessitating nasogastric tube feeding), postprandial vomiting, and diarrhea are common. These conditions improve without specific gastrointestinal treatment as nutritional recovery progresses. Hepatomegaly with a soft, round edge caused by severe fatty infiltration is usually present. The abdomen is frequently protruding because of distended stomach and intestinal loops. Peristalsis is irregular and frequently slow. Muscle tone and strength are greatly reduced. Tachycardia is common. Both hypothermia and hypoglycemia can occur after short periods of fasting.

Differential diagnosis must be made from other causes of edema and hypoproteinemia and from secondary PEM resulting from impairment in protein absorption or metabolism.

The same complications occur as in marasmus, but diarrhea and respiratory and skin infections are more frequent and severe. Serious, fatal infections may occur, often without fever, tachycardia, respiratory distress, or

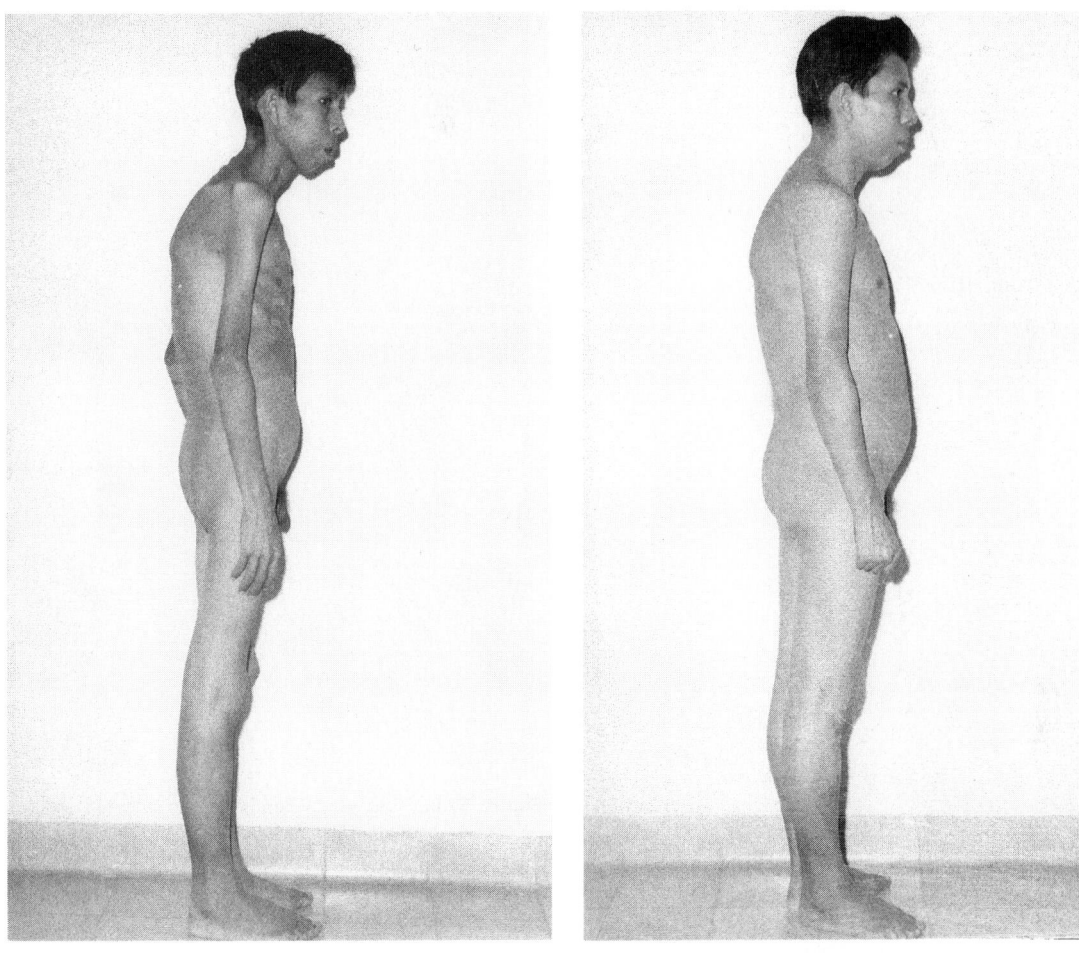

Figure 57.6. A. Marasmic protein-energy malnutrition in a 29-year-old man. **B.** The same patient after 3 months of treatment.

appropriate leukocytosis. The most common causes of death are pulmonary edema with bronchopneumonia, septicemia, gastroenteritis, and water and electrolyte imbalances.

Marasmic Kwashiorkor

This form of edematous PEM combines clinical characteristics of kwashiorkor and marasmus. The main features are the edema of kwashiorkor, with or without its skin lesions, and the muscle wasting and decreased subcutaneous fat of marasmus (Figs. 57.9 and 57.10). When edema disappears during early treatment, the patient's appearance resembles that of marasmus. Biochemical features of both marasmus and kwashiorkor are seen, but the alterations of severe protein deficiency usually predominate.

Biochemical and Histopathologic Features

The most common biochemical findings are the following: (a) serum concentrations of total proteins, and specially albumin, are markedly reduced in edematous PEM, and they are normal or moderately low in marasmus; (b) hemoglobin and hematocrit are usually low, more so in

kwashiorkor than in marasmus; (c) the ratio of nonessential to essential amino acids in plasma is elevated in kwashiorkor and is usually normal in marasmus; (d) serum levels of free fatty acids are elevated, particularly in kwashiorkor; (e) blood glucose level is normal, or it is low after fasting 6 or more hours; (f) urinary excretions of creatinine, hydroxyproline, 3-methylhistidine, and urea nitrogen are low. Edematous children have markedly reduced urinary creatinine excretions in relation to their height, leading to a low creatinine-height index (95), whereas marasmic children may have a normal or somewhat low index.

Plasma levels of other nutrients vary and tend to be moderately low. They do not necessarily reflect the body stores. For example, serum iron and retinol may be normal with almost depleted body stores, or in kwashiorkor they may be relatively low with adequate stores because of alterations in the transport proteins, transferrin, and retinol-binding protein.

Many other biochemical changes have been described in severe PEM; some of them are discussed in the earlier section on pathophysiology and adaptive responses. Others are listed in Table 57.6. Although these changes

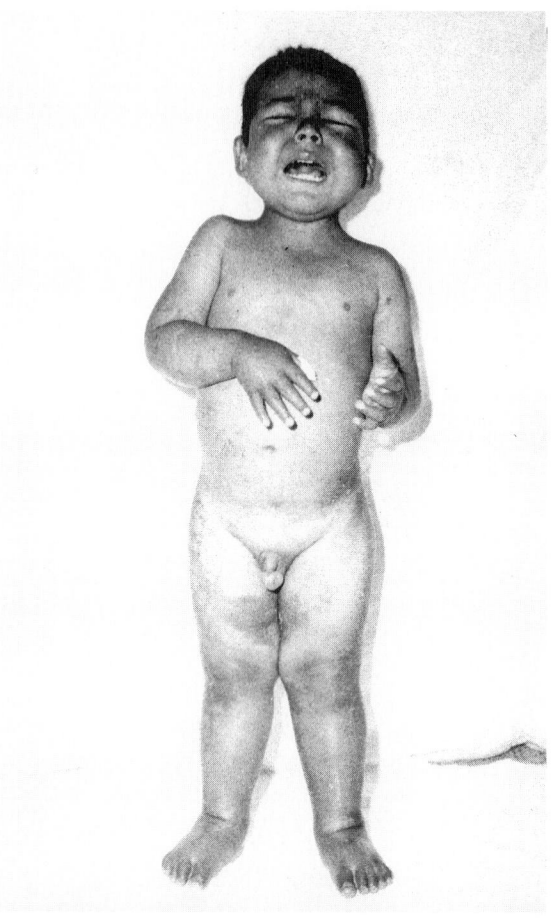

Figure 57.7. Kwashiorkor in a 36-month-old child.

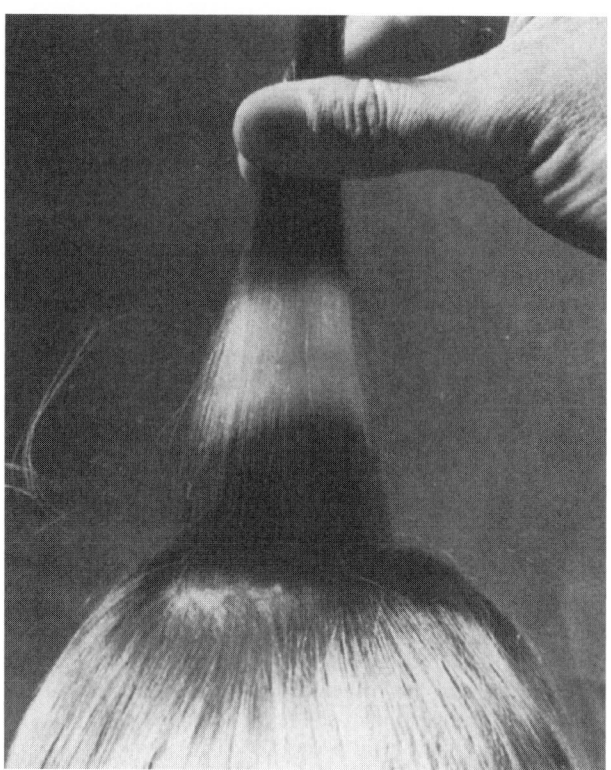

Figure 57.8. "Flag sign": Bands of depigmented and normal hair caused by alternating periods of poor and relatively good protein intake. (From Torun B, Viteri FE. Protein-energy malnutrition. In: Warren KS, Mahmoud AAF, eds. Tropical and Geographic Medicine. 2nd ed. New York: McGraw-Hill, 1990, with permission.)

have little practical importance in diagnosing the disease, they allow better understanding of the pathophysiologic modifications.

Body protein decreases at a slow rate, most of it from muscle, and the greater loss of adipose tissue results in a

relative increase of total body water (i.e., per unit of body mass), mainly as intracellular water. In severe protein deficiency (kwashiorkor), extracellular water also increases. The intracellular concentrations of potassium and magnesium decrease, and that of sodium increases, although the

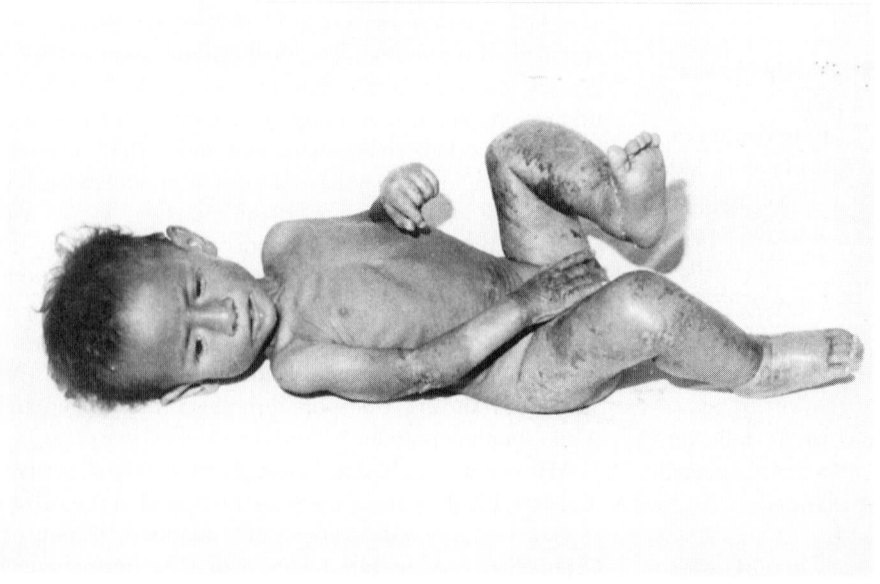

Figure 57.9. Marasmic kwashiorkor in a 22-month-old child. Note the edema in the lower part of the body, the emaciated upper part, and the skin lesions. (From Torun B, Viteri FE. Protein-energy malnutrition. In: Warren KS, Mahmoud AAF, eds. Tropical and Geographic Medicine. 2nd ed. New York: McGraw-Hill, 1990, with permission.)

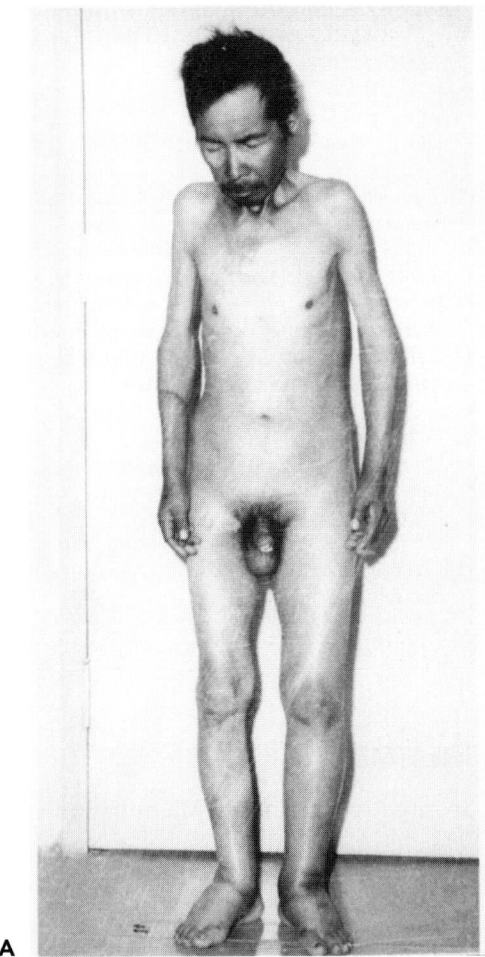
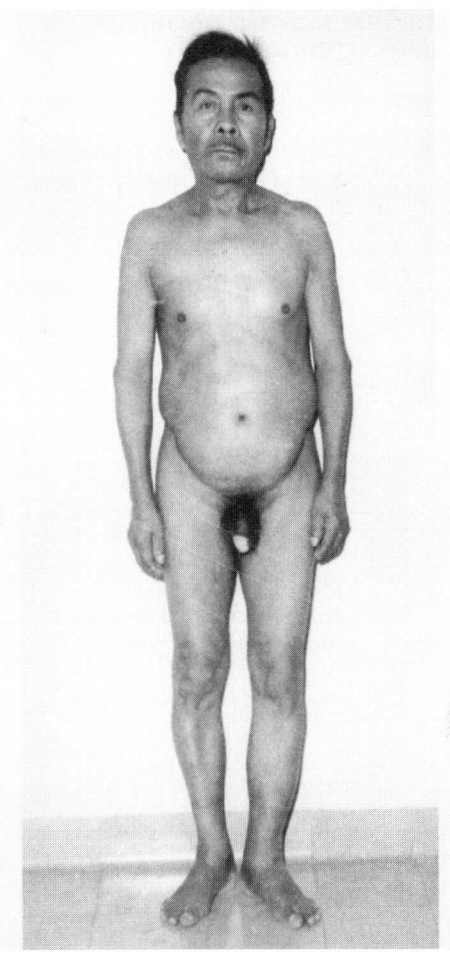

A   **B**

Figure 57.10 A. Edematous protein-energy malnutrition in a 46-year-old man. **B.** The same patient after 3 months of treatment.

serum concentrations of electrolytes do not necessarily reflect these alterations (96).

Histopathologic studies show nonspecific atrophy, mainly in tissues with greater cell turnover rates, such as intestinal mucosa, red bone marrow, and testicular epithelium; intestinal villi are flattened, and enterocytes lose their columnar appearance. Patients with marasmus have generalized atrophy of skeletal muscle. The skin changes consist of dermal atrophy, ecchymosis, ulcerations, and hyperkeratotic desquamation, seen primarily in areas subjected to irritation and not necessarily restricted to exposed areas, as in pellagra. The liver in persons with kwashiorkor is enlarged with fatty infiltration; periportal fat appears first and advances centripetally as severity increases. Other histologic analyses, special staining techniques, and electron microscopy reveal more alterations, not all of which result specifically from primary PEM. All do reflect generalized atrophy, however. Lesions resulting from superimposed infections and other nutrient deficiencies often are evident macroscopically and on histopathologic examination. These changes usually revert to normal with nutri-

tional recovery, although some residual lesions may persist for some time.

PROGNOSIS AND RISK OF MORTALITY

Treatment of mild and moderate PEM corrects the acute signs of the disease, but children's catch-up growth in height may take a long time or may never be achieved. These children have been deprived not only of food but also of opportunities for development, and they may have missed the critical periods for harmonic physical, mental, and social maturation. Weight for height can be restored easily, but the child may remain stunted, and a small body size may influence his or her maximal working capacity as an adult. Many severely malnourished children appear to have residual behavioral and mental problems in terms of creativity and social interaction. However, the causal roles of malnutrition and a poor living environment are difficult to disassociate, and no irrefutable evidence indicates that the damage cannot be corrected in a good, stimulating environment.

Patients with severe PEM are at a high risk of mortality. Table 57.7 lists the characteristics that generally indicate a

TABLE 57.6. ADDITIONAL SELECTED BIOCHEMICAL CHANGES OBSERVED IN PROTEIN-ENERGY MALNUTRITION

	MARASMUS	EDEMATOUS PROTEIN-ENERGY MALNUTRITION
Body composition		
Total body water	High	High
Extracellular water	High	Higher
Total body potassium	Low	Lower
Total body protein	Low	Low
Serum or plasma		
Transport proteins[a]	Normal or low	Low
Branched-chain amino acids	Normal or low	Low
Tyrosine-phenylalanine ratio	Normal or low	Low
Enzymes (in general)[b]	Normal	Low
Transaminase	Normal or high	High
Liver		
Fatty infiltration	Absent	Severe
Glycogen	Normal or low	Normal or low
Urea cycle and other enzymes[c]	Low	Lower
Amino acid synthesizing enzymes	High	Not as high

[a] For example, transferrin, ceruloplasmin, retinol-, cortisol-, and thyroxine-binding proteins, α- and β-lipoproteins.
[b] For example, amylase, pseudocholinesterase, alkaline phosphatase.
[c] For example, xanthine oxidase, glycolic acid oxidase, cholinesterase.

From Torun B, Viteri FE. Protein-energy malnutrition. In: Warren KS, Mahmoud AAF, eds. Tropical and Geographic Medicine. 2nd ed. New York: McGraw-Hill, 1990, with permission.

poor prognosis and demand closer surveillance. Malnutrition increases the risk of death in children admitted to hospital (97), and a recent study of more than 8000 Kenyan children showed that wasting and kwashiorkor were among the six prognostic indicators of deaths that occurred within 48 hours of admission (98). The other five indicators were part of those listed in Table 57.7, which are associated with the life-threatening complications that often accompany severe malnutrition: jaundice, severe anemia, respiratory distress, neurologic and consciousness alterations, and hypothermia.

Mortality rates among children with severe PEM are associated with the quality of treatment. In many parts of the world, median case fatality has remained unchanged at 20 to 30% since the mid-1950s, with the highest levels (40–60%) among those with edematous PEM, resulting from outmoded and faulty case management (15). Among severely malnourished adults with mean BMI of 13.1 treated in an emergency war zone center in Somalia, mortality rates were 34 and 22% for edematous and marasmic patients, respectively, and as high as 52% when high-protein diets were used to treat edematous patients (80). Low mortality rates of 5% or less for both edematous and nonedematous children and adults are attainable with adequate treatment.

TABLE 57.7. CHARACTERISTICS THAT INDICATE POOR PROGNOSIS IN PATIENTS WITH PROTEIN-ENERGY MALNUTRITION

- Age <6 months
- Deficit in weight for height >30%, or in weight for age >40%
- Signs of circulatory collapse: cold hands and feet, weak radial pulse, diminished consciousness
- Stupor, coma, or other alterations in awareness
- Infections, particularly bronchopneumonia or measles
- Petechiae or hemorrhagic tendencies (purpura usually associated with septicemia or a viral infection)
- Dehydration and electrolyte disturbances, particularly hypokalemia, and severe acidosis
- Persistent tachycardia, signs of heart failure, or respiratory difficulty
- Total serum proteins <30 g/L
- Severe anemia (<50 g hemoglobin/L) with clinical signs of hypoxia
- Clinical jaundice or elevated serum bilirubin
- Extensive exudative or exfoliative cutaneous lesions or deep decubitus ulcerations
- Hypoglycemia
- Hypothermia

TREATMENT

Severe Protein-Energy Malnutrition

Patients with uncomplicated PEM should be treated outside the hospital whenever possible. Hospitalization increases the risk of cross-infections, and the unfamiliar setting may increase apathy and anorexia in children, thereby making feeding more difficult. Severely malnourished children with signs of a poor prognosis (see Table 57.7) or other life-threatening complications, and those who live under social conditions that do not permit adequate medical and nutritional treatment as outpatients, must be hospitalized. Treatment strategy can be divided into three stages: (a) resolving life-threatening conditions, (b) restoring nutritional status without disrupting homeostasis, and (c) ensuring nutritional rehabilitation.

Resolving Life-Threatening Conditions

On admission, the child with severe PEM is often a medical emergency at a high risk of death. Initial treatment must address life-threatening conditions. If necessary, nutritional rehabilitation may be delayed until those conditions are resolved.

Fluid and Electrolyte Disturbances. The assessment of dehydration is not always easy in severe PEM. Useful signs and symptoms are history of watery diarrhea or vomiting, thirst, low urinary output, weak and rapid pulse, low blood pressure, cool and moist extremities, and a declining state of consciousness. Other signs, such as sunken eyeballs and decreased skin turgor, may be present in well-hydrated severely malnourished patients, whereas typical signs of hypovolemia may not be evident in edematous patients; irritability and apathy that often accompany severe PEM complicate assessment of mental awareness. Treatment differs from that in well-nourished patients because dehydrated patients with severe PEM usually have the following: (a) hypoosmolality with moderate hyponatremia; (b) mild to moderate metabolic acidosis, which disappears when the patient receives energy-containing food or glucose in oral or intravenous rehydration solutions; (c) high tolerance to hypocalcemia, partly because the acidosis produces a relative increment in ionized calcium and partly because hypoproteinemia makes less protein available to bind calcium ions; (d) decreased body potassium without hypokalemia; and (e) decreased body magnesium, with or without hypomagnesemia.

Whenever possible, patients should be rehydrated by mouth or through a nasogastric tube. As first choice for severely malnourished patients, administer an oral rehydration solution (ORS) with less sodium (45 mmol/L) and more potassium (40 mmol/L) than the solutions commonly used to treat better-nourished dehydrated patients (99, 100), such as ReSoMal shown in Table 57.8. When commercial or ready-made ReSoMal is not available, a comparable solution can be prepared based on the traditional WHO-ORS salts in one of the following ways:

1. If the mineral mix shown in Table 57.9 to complement locally prepared therapeutic diets is available, dissolve 40 mL or 6.25 g of the mineral mix, plus one packet WHO-ORS salts, plus 50 g sugar in 2 L of water.
2. If the mineral mix is not available, dissolve one packet WHO-ORS salts, plus 45 mL of 10% potassium chlo-

TABLE 57.8. COMPARISON OF MODIFIED ORAL REHYDRATION SOLUTION FOR SEVERELY MALNOURISHED CHILDREN (ReSoMal) WITH STANDARD WORLD HEALTH ORGANIZATION SOLUTION (mmol IN 1 L OF WATER)[a, b]

	CONCENTRATION (mmol/L)	
COMPONENT	MODIFIED SOLUTION (ReSoMal)	STANDARD SOLUTION (WHO-ORS)
Glucose	125	110
Sodium	45	90
Potassium	40	20
Chloride	70	80
Citrate	7	10
Magnesium	3	—
Zinc	0.3	—
Copper	0.045	—
Water	1,000 mL	1,000 mL
Osmolarity	300	310

WHO-ORS, World Health Organization oral rehydration solution.
[a]When ready-made ReSoMal is not available, it can be prepared diluting *one* packet of standard WHO-ORS salts, plus *40 mL* (or *6.25 g*) of the mineral mix shown in Table 57.9, plus *50 g* sucrose in *2 L* of water (~320 mmol/L) (based on WHO recommendations in reference 103).
[b]1 mmol glucose = 180 mg; 1 mmol Na = 23.0 mg; 1 mmol K = 39.1 mg; 1 mmol Cl = 35.5 mg; 1 mmol citrate = 207.1 mg; 1mmol Mg = 24.3 mg; 1 mmol Zn = 65.4 mg; 1 mmol Cu = 63.5 mg.

TABLE 57.9. MINERAL MIX FOR COMPLEMENTATION OF LIQUID FOODS AND FOR PREPARATION OF ReSoMal WHEN MIXED WITH STANDARD WORLD HEALTH ORGANIZATION ORAL REHYDRATION SOLUTION AND SUGAR[a]

SALT	AMOUNT (g)	CATIONS (mmol)
Potassium chloride	89.5	1,514 potassium[b]
Tripotassium citrate	32.4	
Magnesium chloride·6H$_2$O	30.5	150 magnesium
Zinc acetate·2H$_2$O	3.3	15 zinc
Copper sulfate·7H$_2$O	0.56	3.5 copper
Total dry salts	156.26	

[a]Add water to make 1,000 mL of concentrated mineral mix solution that can be stored at room temperature, or prepare packets with 3.12 g of dry mineral mix. Add 20 mL of the concentrated solution or one packet to each liter of modified oral rehydration solution or liquid food (calculated from World Health Organization recommendations in reference 103).
[b]1 mmol K = 39.1 mg; 1mmol Mg = 24.3 mg; 1 mmol Zn = 65.4; 1 mmol Cu = 63.5 mg.

ride solution, plus 50 g sugar in *2* L of water (81); this solution will not have mangnesium, zinc, and copper, which are not indispensable to rehydrate critically ill, severely malnourished patients, but it will provide sodium, potassium, and carbohydrate in concentrations equivalent to those in ReSoMal.

When neither the mineral mix nor a 10% potassium chloride solution is available, *standard WHO-ORS solution can be used* to rehydrate severely malnourished patients, as has been the successful practice in many hospitals and nutrition rehabilitation centers.

The ORS should be given in small quantities (a teaspoonful or sips from a cup) every few minutes at a slower rate than customary for better-nourished children, to provide 70 to 100 mL/kg body weight over a period of 12 hours (100, 101). Start with about 10 mL/kg/hour during the first 2 hours for children with mild to moderate dehydration, and up to 30 mL/kg/hour for those with severe dehydration. An additional 50 to 100 mL should be given after each loose stool to children less than 2 years old, and twice as much to older children. Breast-feeding should continue approximately every half-hour. *Patients must be evaluated every hour.* As soon as hydration improves (usually after 4–6 hours), small amounts of liquid diet containing or supplemented with potassium, calcium, magnesium, and other minerals (e.g., with the mineral mix shown in Table 57.9) should be offered every 2 to 3 hours. If the condition is improving but signs of dehydration are still present after 12 hours, another 70 to 100 mL/kg can be given over the next 12 hours. Proper rehydration should allow a diuresis of at least 200 mL in 24 hours in children and 500 mL in adults, or micturition every 2 to 3 hours. If signs of overhydration appear (e.g., puffy eyelids, increased edema, filled jugular veins, accelerated respiratory rate), only breast milk or liquid diet should be given.

Children who vomit frequently or cannot be fed orally must be rehydrated by *nasogastric tube*, giving 3 to 4 mL of ORS solution/kg slowly or drop by drop every half-hour. If the patient has repeated vomiting or increasing abdominal distention, give the fluid more slowly and in smaller portions. If hydration does not improve after 4 hours, begin intravenous rehydration. When vomiting ceases and hydration improves, give ORS by mouth and, if the child tolerates oral solutions for the next 2 hours, remove the nasogastric tube.

Intravenous fluids must be used when patients have repeated vomiting or persistent abdominal distention, as well as in severe dehydration with hypovolemia and impending shock. Hypoosmolar solutions (200–280 mOsm/L) must be used. Potassium (when urinating) and sodium should not exceed 6 and 3 mmol/kg/day, respectively, and glucose must provide at least 63 to 126 kJ (15–30 kcal)/kg/day. Solutions that have been successfully used include a 1:1 mixture of 10% dextrose in water (D/W), with isotonic saline (i.e., 5% glucose in 0.5 normal saline) or with Darrow solution, a 1:2:3 mixture of 0.17 sodium lactate:isotonic saline:10% D/W, or Hartmann solution (Ringer lactated solution). One of these should be infused *during the first hour* at a rate of 10 to 30 mL/kg, depending on the patient's condition. After that, 5% glucose in 0.2 normal saline (800 mL of 5% D/W, 20 mL of 50% D/W, and 200 mL of isotonic saline), or a 1:2:6 mixture of lactate:isotonic saline:5% glucose with 50 mL of 50% D/W added to each 500 mL, should be infused at a rate of 5 to 10 mL/kg/hour, based on hourly evaluations of the patient, until oral therapy is initiated. When the patient is urinating, 2 g potassium chloride (27 mmol potassium) is added to each liter of the infusion solution.

Increases in pulse and respiratory rate with weight gain after accounting for weight of excreta, pulmonary rales, and appearance or exacerbation of edema indicate overhydration. Increases in pulse and respiratory rate with weight loss, low urine output, and continuing losses from diarrhea and vomiting suggest insufficient fluid therapy.

Patients with severe hypoproteinemia (<30 g/L), anuria, and signs of hypovolemia or impending circulatory collapse should be given 10 mL plasma/kg in 1 to 2 hours, followed by 20 mL/kg/hour of a mixture of two parts of 5% dextrose and one part of isotonic saline for 1 or 2 hours. This will increase plasma protein concentration by about 5 to 10 g/L and will help to prevent the rapid exit of water from the intravascular compartment. If diuresis does not improve, the dose of plasma can be repeated 2 hours later. Further treatment is similar to that of well-nourished patients. Unless the patient is at risk of imminent death, only plasma tested to be negative for human immunodeficiency virus (HIV) should be used.

Hypocalcemia may occur secondary to magnesium deficiency. When the patient has symptoms of hypocalcemia and serum magnesium determinations are not available, it is essential not only to give calcium infusion but also to give magnesium intravenously or intramuscularly. When the serum concentration of calcium rises to normal level or the symptoms of hypocalcemia disappear, calcium infusion may be discontinued. Intramuscular or oral magnesium supplementation should follow the initial parenteral magnesium until normal levels of serum and urine magnesium concentrations are achieved. If no laboratory facilities are available, a general therapeutic guideline is to give a 50% solution of magnesium sulfate intramuscularly in doses of 0.5, 1, and 1.5 mL for patients who weigh less than 7 kg, between 7 and 10 kg, and more than 10 kg, respectively. The dose can be repeated every 12 hours until there is no recurrence of the hypocalcemic symptoms, followed by oral magnesium at a dose of 0.25 to 0.5 mmol mg (0.5–1 mEq) kg/day.

Infections. Malnourished patients are particularly prone to infections, which are frequently the immediate cause of death in severe PEM. Paradoxically, clinical manifestations may be mild, without fever, tachycardia, and leukocytosis. Antigen-antibody reactions are often impaired, and skin tests such as tuberculin often give false-negative results. Given the high mortality rate from infections, it is safer to assume that all ill and severely malnourished patients have a bacterial infection and to treat them with antibiotics to cover both gram-positive and gram-negative microorganisms; the latter are particularly common in PEM. When septicemia is suspected, a broad-spectrum antibiotic or a combination of antibiotics is usually given intravenously. Other supportive treatment may also be necessary, such as treatment for respiratory distress, hypothermia, and hypoglycemia.

Drug metabolism may be altered and detoxification mechanisms may be compromised in severe PEM as a result of delayed absorption, abnormal intestinal permeability, reduced protein binding, changes in the volume of distribution, decreased conjugation or oxidation in the liver, and decreased renal clearance (102, 103). For example, in malnourished children, the half-lives of chloramphenicol (104), sulfadiazine (105), and gentamicin (102) are increased, and their clearance is decreased. To reduce the risk of potential toxicity, including the possibility of absorbing drugs normally not absorbed by a healthy intestine, treatment for intestinal parasites, which is rarely urgent, should be deferred until nutritional rehabilitation is under way.

Every child should be vaccinated against measles on admission, because of the high mortality rates associated with this disease in severe PEM. Because seroconversion may be impaired at this early stage of treatment, a second dose of vaccine should be given before discharge.

Hemodynamic Alterations. Cardiac failure may develop in severe anemia, during or after administration of intravenous fluids, or shortly after the introduction of high-protein and high-energy feedings or of a diet with high sodium content, leading to pulmonary edema and frequent secondary pulmonary infection. These alterations may be the result of impaired cardiac function, sudden expansion of the intravascular fluid volume, severe hypoxia, or impaired membrane function. Diuretics such as furosemide (10 mg intravenously or intramuscularly, repeated as necessary) should be given, and other supportive measures should be taken. Many clinicians advocate the use of digoxin (0.03 mg/kg intravenously, every 6–8 hours). *The use of diuretics to accelerate the disappearance of edema in kwashiorkor is contraindicated.*

Severe Anemia. The routine use of blood transfusions endangers the patient; hemoglobin levels will improve with proper dietary treatment supplemented with hematinics. Therefore, blood transfusions should be given only in cases of severe anemia with less than 40 g hemoglobin/L, less than 12% packed cell volume (hematocrit), or with clinical signs of hypoxia or impending cardiac failure. When no resources are available to screen the blood supply for HIV, transfusions should be used only in life-threatening situations. Whole blood (10 mL/kg) can be used in marasmic patients, but it is better to use packed red blood cells (6 mL/kg) in edematous PEM. The transfusion should be given slowly, over 2 to 3 hours, and repeated if necessary after 12 to 24 hours. If there are signs of heart failure, 2.5 mL blood/kg should be withdrawn before the transfusion is started and at hourly intervals so the total volume of blood transfused equals the volume of anemic blood removed.

Hypothermia and Hypoglycemia. Body temperature lower than 35.5°C and plasma glucose concentration less than 3.3 mmol/L (60 mg/dL) can result from impaired thermoregulatory mechanisms, reduced fuel substrate availability, or severe infection. Asymptomatic hypoglycemia can be treated (and prevented) by feeding small volumes of glucose- or sucrose-containing diets and solutions every 2 to 3 hours, day and night. Severe symptomatic hypoglycemia must be treated intravenously with 10 to 20 mL of 50% glucose solution followed by oral or nasogastric administration of 25 to 50 mL of 10% glucose solution at 2-hour intervals for 24 to 48 hours.

Body temperature usually rises in the hypothermic patient after frequent feedings of glucose-containing diets or solutions. Patients must be closely monitored when external heat sources such as heavy clothing, heat lamps, and radiators are used to reduce the loss of body heat, because patients may rapidly become hyperthermic. It is best to keep the seminude patients in an ambient temperature of 30 to 33°C. Treatment must also be given as for hypoglycemia and systemic infection.

Severe Vitamin A Deficiency. Severe PEM is often associated with vitamin A deficiency. A large dose of vitamin A should be given on admission, because ocular lesions can develop as a result of increased demands for retinol when adequate protein and energy feeding begins. Water-miscible vitamin A as retinol should be given orally or intramuscularly on the first day at a dose of 52 to 105 μmol (15,000–30,000 μg or 50,000–100,000 IU) for infants and preschool children, or 105 to 210 μmol (30,000–60,000 μg or 100,000–200,000 IU) for older children and adults, followed by 5.2 μmol (1500 μg or 5000 IU) orally each day for the duration of treatment. The initial dose should be repeated for 2 more days in symptomatic patients. Corneal ulcerations should be treated with ophthalmic drops of 1% atropine solution and antibiotic ointments or drops until the ulcerations heal.

Homeostatic Restoration of Nutritional Status

Nutritional treatment should start as soon as measures to control life-threatening conditions have been established. The slow onset and progression of the disease allow metabolic adjustments to the severely malnourished state, and the reversal of those adjustments during the early stages of nutritional treatment must be gradual, to avoid deleterious metabolic disruptions. Thus, nutritional rehabilitation must start slowly and progress gradually, as summarized in Table 57.10. Intravenous alimentation is not justified in primary PEM and can increase mortality rates (106, 107).

Initially, the diet must provide energy and protein in amounts lower than daily maintenance requirements, followed by progressing increments. It is best to begin with a liquid formula fed orally or by nasogastric tube, divided equally into six to 12 feedings per day, depending on the patient's age and condition. This frequent feeding of small volumes must be given around the clock to avoid fasting for more than 4 hours, to prevent vomiting, and to reduce the risk of hypoglycemia and hypothermia. For older children and adults, the liquid formula can be partly substituted

---

TABLE 57.10. GENERAL PRINCIPLES FOR DIETARY MANAGEMENT OF SEVERE MALNUTRITION

- Start feeding as soon as life-threatening conditions have been addressed.
- Begin feeding liquid foods in small volumes at short intervals.
- Begin with small amounts of high-quality protein and dietary energy, and increase them gradually.
- Supplement the diet with electrolytes, minerals, and vitamins (see below for iron).
- Do not give iron during the first week of dietary treatment.
- Do not interrupt breast-feeding.
- Administer abundant fluids (≥I mL/4 kJ or 1 kcal).
- Help patients to eat, but do not force them.
- When necessary, feed through a nasogastric tube.
- Do not use intravenous alimentation.
- Evaluate patients at least once daily.
- Involve parents and other relatives in care and feeding.
- Add nutritious semisolid and solid foods based on the patient's age and progress.
- Increase the amount of food and nutrient concentration as the patient progresses and appetite improves.
- Add locally available, culturally acceptable, nutritious foods before discharge.
- Show parents how to prepare nutritious foods and diets using ingredients available at home.

with solid foods that have a high concentration of good-quality, easily digestible nutrients. The same diet can be used for marasmic and edematous patients, although the marasmic patient may require larger amounts of dietary energy after 1 or 2 weeks of dietary treatment, which can be provided by adding vegetable oil to increase the diet's energy density. Diets that derive as much as 60 to 75% of their energy from fats are usually well tolerated; although patients may have some steatorrhea without profuse diarrhea, 85% or more of the fat is usually absorbed (51).

The protein source must be of high biologic value and easily digested. Cow's milk is frequently available, and although intestinal lactase activity decreases in severe PEM, milk is usually well tolerated and can be safely advocated (108, 109). Goat's, ewe's, buffalo's, and camel's milk can also be used. Human milk, mare's milk, and ass's milk, however, have very low protein concentrations. Eggs, meat, fish, soy isolates, and some vegetable protein mixtures are also good protein sources. Most vegetable proteins are 10 to 20% less digestible than animal proteins, thus making it necessary to feed larger amounts. The low energy density of skim milk and vegetable protein sources can be increased adding sugar and vegetable oil; the latter will also provide essential fatty acids.

The diet must be supplemented to provide daily about 5 to 8 mmol potassium and 0.5 to 1 mmol magnesium (1–2 mEq)/*kg body weight*, and 150 to 300 μmol zinc and 40 to 50 μmol copper. Sodium content should be low, especially for patients with edematous PEM. This can be accomplished by adding to the diet appropriate amounts of a mineral mix, like that shown in Table 57.9. Additional supplements should include daily doses of 5.2 μmol (1500 μg or 5000 IU) vitamin A, 1.2 mmol (0.3 mg) folic acid, and other vitamins and trace elements in the doses provided by most proprietary preparations, which should be higher than the daily recommended allowances for well-nourished persons of the corresponding age. Supplemental calcium to provide

about 15 mmol (600 mg)/day should be given when nondairy diets are used. Administration of supplemental iron (1–2.1 mmol or 60–120 mg/day) should begin *1 week after* starting dietary therapy. Earlier administration of iron will not elicit a hematologic response (see Fig. 57.2), it may facilitate bacterial growth in the organism, and it may produce metabolic disturbances according to the free-radical theory.

Therapeutic Dietary Regimens. To avoid the danger of initial excessive intakes of protein and energy by hungry patients, two types or therapeutic regimens have been successfully used: (a) structured increments in nutrient delivery and (b) sequential administration of two formulations with different nutrient concentrations.

Structured Increments. Each day, a fixed amount of food is offered, with gradual increments in protein and energy concentrations at 2-day intervals, to reach optimal therapeutic levels (around three to four times the protein requirement and 1.5 times to twice the energy requirement) by the seventh day. A practical way to achieve this is based on preparing a liquid food with high concentrations of proteins and energy and diluting it with different amounts of water every 2 days. Table 57.11 gives examples to prepare high-protein, high-energy liquid formulations using different food protein sources, and Table 57.12 shows a dilution scheme to treat infants and young children with increasing amounts of protein and energy. The intervals for dietary increments can be extended to 3 or 4 days in extremely malnourished children, especially if their plasma protein concentration is less than 30 g/L. The energy density of the diet of marasmic patients who are not gaining weight at an adequate rate (an average of at least 5 g/kg/day) by the second week should be increased at 5- to 7-day intervals by adding vegetable oil, as shown in Table 59.12.

Additional water must be given immediately after or between meals to provide at least 1 mL of total fluids for each 4 kJ or 1 kcal of dietary energy. Electrolytes, vitamins, and minerals must be given daily for the duration of

TABLE 57.11. EXAMPLES OF FORMULATIONS FOR HIGH-PROTEIN (3–4 g/100 mL), HIGH-ENERGY (565–905 kJ OR 135–145 kcal/100 mL) LIQUID FOODS USED AS THE BASIS FOR STRUCTURED DIETARY TREATMENT OF SEVERE PROTEIN-ENERGY MALNUTRITION

FOOD USED AS PROTEIN SOURCE	AMOUNT (g OR mL)	CEREAL FLOUR OR SUGAR (g)[a]	SUGAR (g)	OIL (mL)[b]	WATER (mL)
Cow's milk, dried, whole	130	50	50	40	1,000
Cow's milk, dried, skim	100	50	50	70	1,000
Cow's, goat's or camel's milk, fluid	1,000	50	50	40	—
Buffalo's or ewe's (sheep's) milk, fluid	650	50	50	40	350
Yogurt (from cow's or goat's milk, whole)	1,000	50	50	40	—
Eggs, soft or hard boiled, liquefied	300[c]	—	200	60	750
Incaparina vegetable mix, flour[d]	140	—	100	55	1,000
Commercial soy protein formulas, powder	250	—	—	10	1,000

[a]First choice: precooked rice, corn or other cereal flour, or heat-popped ground rice. If not available, substitute with either 50 g sugar or 20 mL vegetable oil; this will diminish total protein concentration by about 0.5 g/100 mL.
[b]When cereal flour is used, one half of the vegetable oil can be substituted with isoenergetic amounts of sugar, where 1 mL oil = 2.2 g sugar.
[c]About six medium-sized chicken eggs.
[d]High-protein-quality mix developed by INCAP (58% corn flour + 38% cottonseed flour + 4% mixture of vitamins, minerals, and lysine), which provides 1,360 kJ (325 kcal) and 27.5 g protein per 100 g of dry flour.

TABLE 57.12. EXAMPLE OF A STRUCTURED DIETARY THERAPEUTIC REGIMEN FOR CHILDREN, BASED ON GRADUALLY DECREASING DILUTIONS OF THE HIGH-ENERGY, HIGH-PROTEIN FOODS SHOWN IN TABLE 57.11[a]

DAYS FROM BEGINNING OF TREATMENT	PROPORTIONS OF FOODS SHOWN IN TABLE 57.11 + WATER PROPORTIONS	VOLUME (mL)	ADDITIONAL SUGAR (g/100 mL)	ADDITIONAL OIL (mL/100 mL)	FOOD VOLUME PER MEAL (mL/kg/meaL) EVERY 2 h	EVERY 3 h	100 mL PROVIDES PROTEIN (g)	ENERGY (kcal)
1–2	1 + 2	33 + 67	10	—	8.3	12.5	1–1.2	75–85
3–4	1 + 1	50 + 50	10	—	8.3	12.5	1.5–2	105–115
5–6	3 + 1	75 + 25	5	—	8.3	12.5	2.3–3	120–130
7–8	Undiluted	100 + 0	—	—	8.3	12.5	3–4	135–145
FOR MARASMIC PATIENTS WITHOUT ADEQUATE WEIGHT GAIN[b]								
13–17	Undiluted	100 + 0	—	2.5	Ad libitum		3–4	160–170
18–22	Undiluted	100 + 0	—	5	Ad libitum		3–4	185–195
23–27	Undiluted	100 + 0	—	7.5	Ad libitum		3–4	210–220
28–32, etc.	Undiluted	100 + 0	—	10, etc.	Ad libitum		3–4	235, etc.

[a]Formulas should initially be fed at a volume of 100 mL/kg/day. They must be supplemented with appropriate amounts of vitamins, minerals, and electrolytes, or adding to each liter of diet 20 mL of the mineral mix in Table 57.9 and a vitamin mix. After 8 days, the undiluted formula can be fed to satiety (ad libitum). *Additional water must be given* after or between feedings, to provide each day at least 1 mL of total fluids per 4 kJ or 1 kcal in the diet.
[b]Marasmic patients may require more dietary energy when weight gain is <5 g/kg/day. Half a teaspoonful (2.5 mL) of vegetable oil should be added for every 100 mL of liquid diet at 5-day intervals.

treatment, as described earlier. Severely weak or anorexic patients must be fed by nasogastric tube until appetite and strength to eat are restored.

The structured and gradual increment in nutrient ingestion prevents the risk of excessive intake by ravenous patients in the first 2 to 4 days of treatment, when complications or death resulting from acute metabolic imbalance are more likely to occur. By providing food with high protein and energy density after the first week of treatment,

this approach also prevents a slow and prolonged recovery in young children whose small gastric capacity can limit the amount of food they eat.

Two-Step Regimen. This option, which is particularly useful for emergency and relief conditions, is advocated by several international organizations. It consists of two liquid foods called F-75 and F-100 prepared from commercial powder formulations (99) or the ingredients shown in Tables 57.13 and 57.14. Other formulations with

TABLE 57.13. EXAMPLES TO PREPARE 1 L OF A LIQUID FOOD SIMILAR TO F-75[a] USING LOCALLY AVAILABLE INGREDIENTS (100 mL WILL PROVIDE ~375 kJ [75 kcal] AND 1.1–1.2 g PROTEIN)

FOOD USED AS PROTEIN SOURCE	AMOUNT (g OR mL)	CEREAL FLOUR (E.G., RICE, CORN) (g)[b]	SUGAR (g)	OIL (mL)	WATER (mL)	MINERAL MIX (mL)[c]	VITAMIN MIX (mg)[d]
Cow's milk, dried, whole	35	50	50	20	1,000	20	150
Cow's milk, dried, skim	25	50	50	30	1,000	20	150
Cow's, goat's or camel's milk, fluid	250	50	50	20	750	20	150
Buffalo's or ewe's (sheep's) milk, fluid	175	50	50	20	825	20	150
Yogurt (from cow's or goat's milk, whole)	275	50	50	20	725	20	150
Eggs, soft or hard boiled, liquefied	100[e]	—	100	20	950	20	150
Incaparina vegetable mix, flour[f]	50	—	100	20	1,000	20	150
Commercial soy protein formulas, powder	85	—	50	10	1,000	20	150

[a]F-75 formula suggested by the World Health Organization (as noted in reference 103).
[b]If precooked flour or heat-popped rice is not available, add 50% more of the food protein source (e.g., 52 g instead of 35 g of whole dried milk) plus an additional 25 g sugar *or* 10 mL vegetable oil. When additional fluid milk or yogurt is used, the volume of additional water must be reduced by the same amount to make a total volume of 1,000 mL.
[c]See Table 57.9.
[d]Can be substituted with a proprietary multivitamin product at an age-related dose.
[e]About two medium-sized chicken eggs.
[f]High-protein-quality mix developed by INCAP (58% corn flour +38% cottonseed flour +4% mixture of vitamins, minerals and lysine), which provides 1,360 kJ (325 kcal) and 27.5 g protein per 100 g of dry flour.

TABLE 57.14. EXAMPLES TO PREPARE 1 L OF A LIQUID FOOD SIMILAR TO F-100[a] USING LOCALLY AVAILABLE INGREDIENTS (100 mL WILL PROVIDE ~420 kJ [100 kcal] AND 2.8–2.9 g PROTEIN)

FOOD USED AS PROTEIN SOURCE	AMOUNT (g OR mL)	CEREAL FLOUR (E.G., RICE, CORN) (g)[b]	SUGAR (g)	OIL (mL)	WATER (mL)	MINERAL MIX (mL)[c]	VITAMIN MIX (mg)[d]
Cow's milk, dried, whole	90	50	50	20	20	150	1,000
Cow's milk, dried, skim	70	50	50	40	20	150	1,000
Cow's, goat's or camel's milk, fluid	700	50	50	20	20	150	300
Buffalo's or ewe's (sheep's) milk, fluid	450	50	50	20	20	150	550
Yogurt (from cow's or goat's milk, whole)	800	50	50	15	20	150	200
Eggs, soft or hard boiled, liquefied	250[e]	—	100	25	20	150	800
Incaparina vegetable mix, flour[f]	100	—	100	30	20	150	1,000
Commercial soy protein formulas, powder	190	—	—	—	20	150	1,000

[a] F-100 formula suggested by the World Health Organization (as noted in reference 103).
[b] If precooked flour or heat-popped rice is not available, add 20% more of the food protein source (e.g., 108 g instead of 90 g of whole dried milk) plus an additional 25 g sugar *or* 10 mL vegetable oil. When additional fluid milk or yogurt are used, the volume of additional water must be reduced by the same amount to make a total volume of 1,000 mL.
[c] See Table 57.9. All formulas satisfy calcium requirements, except for the egg-based preparation.
[d] Can be substituted with a proprietary multivitamin product at an age-related dose.
[e] About five medium-sized chicken eggs.
[f] High-protein-quality mix developed by INCAP (58% corn flour +38% cottonseed flour +4% mixture of vitamins, minerals and lysine), which provides 1,360 kJ (325 kcal) and 27.5 g protein per 100 g of dry flour.

locally available foods have also been successfully used in international relief work (110, 111).

F-75 provides 375 kJ (75 kcal) and about 1 g protein/100 mL, and it is given during the initial phase of treatment in amounts restricted to 105 to 135 mL/kg/day for young children, equivalent to 330 to 425 kJ (80–100 kcal)/kg/day. When the patient improves and appetite returns, usually after 1 week of treatment, F-100 (420 kJ and 2.9 g protein/100 mL) is fed to satiety (ad libitum). Twenty milliliters of the mineral mix in Table 57.9 and a multivitamin mix are added to each liter of the F-75 and F-100 diets. Iron supplements should also be given when F-75 is switched to F-100. If an appropriate vitamin mix is not available, a proprietary vitamin supplement and other minerals must be given daily in the doses described earlier for the duration of the treatment.

A variation of this regimen employs a ready-to-use food with higher energy density than commercial F-100, in which 25% of the dried skim milk in F-100 is replaced with peanut butter, and the protein and other nutrient composition per megajoule is similar (112, 113). The two-step regimen is easier to prepare and follow, especially for emergency and field conditions, but it is more costly when it relies on commercial F-75, F-100, or ready-to-use food formulations.

Appetite and Catch-up Weight Gain. The attitude of the person who feeds the patient is important to overcome the patient's lack of appetite. Patience and loving care are needed gently to coax malnourished children to eat all the diet. The appearance, color, and flavor of the foods also play a role on appetite and food acceptance.

The initial response to the diet is either no change in weight or a decrease caused by loss of edema (Fig. 57.11) accompanied by large diuresis. After 5 to 15 days is a period of rapid weight gain or catch-up, which is usually slower in marasmus than in kwashiorkor. In children, the rate of catch-up weight gain generally is ten to 15 times that of a nutritionally normal child of the same age, and it can be as high as 20 to 25 times greater. However, some children only show a four- or fivefold increase in catch-up. Low weight gains are most often associated with insufficient energy intakes (e.g., because of inadequately prepared formula, insufficient amounts of formula given at each feeding, too few feedings per day, anorexia, or lack of patience of the person who feeds the child) or with overt or asymptomatic infections; urinary infections and tuberculosis are the most commonly seen asymptomatic diseases.

Treatment of Older Children and Adults. The physiologic changes and principles of management of children with severe PEM also apply to older children and adults. Clinical and dietary history, as well as laboratory tests, are particularly important to identify underlying causes and to include them in the therapeutic program. Complications and life-threatening conditions must be treated as described for children.

Initial dietary treatment should provide average energy and protein requirements for the patient's age (~190 kJ [45 kcal] and 0.75 g protein/kg/day for adolescents, and 160 kJ [38 kcal] and 0.6 g protein/kg/day for adults), followed by a gradual increase to about 1.5 times the energy and three to four times the protein requirements when

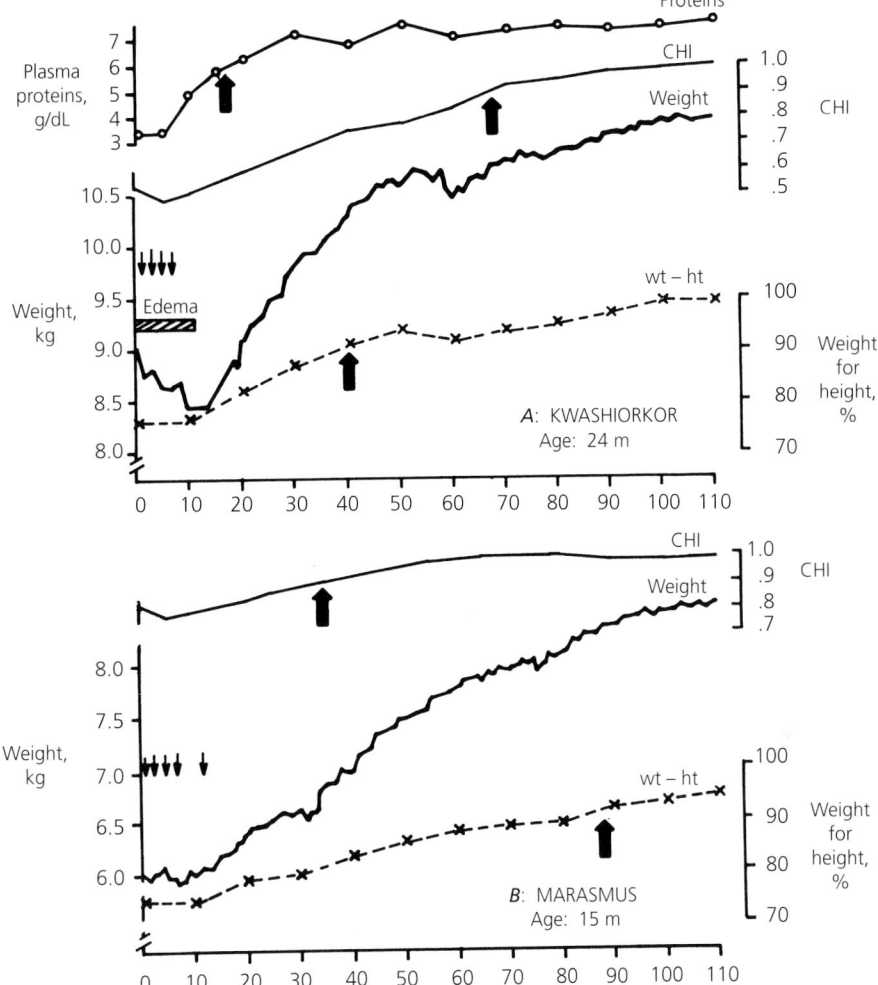

Figure 57.11. Weight gain and improvement in weight for height, creatinine-height index (CHI), and plasma protein concentration of two children treated at INCAP for kwashiorkor (child *A*) and marasmus (child *B*). The *thin, downward arrows* indicate gradual increments in dietary proteins and energy. The *thick, upward arrows* indicate the day when the lower limit of normal values was reached. The marasmic child had a normal plasma protein concentration on admission. Weight for height was calculated for child *A* on admission, after correcting for the weight of edema. Dietary energy was reduced on days 60 and 80 for child *A* and on day 100 for child *B*.

edema disappears, steady weight gain is established, and other clinical features improve. Among edematous adults, mortality rates are significantly lower and weight gain is faster when the diet contains 8.5% of energy from protein (~2.1 g protein/420 kJ or 100 kcal) compared with diets that provide twice as much protein (80). Weight gains of 5 to 6 g/kg/day represent the lower end of the spectrum of reasonable catch-up for adults (80). Minerals and vitamins must be given in amounts at least twice greater than the recommended daily allowances, following the same schedule as for children. Except for pregnant women, a single dose of 210 μmol (60 mg or 200,000 IU) retinol should be given.

The liquid diets described for infants and young children can be given, especially to weak and anorexic patients. However, adults and adolescents are often reluctant to eat anything other than habitual foods, and liquid diets must be prescribed as a medicine, rather than as a food. When appetite improves, a diet should be given based on local foods with a good protein content, such as combinations of rice or maize with chicken, fish, meat, or powdered milk, and with added sugar and fats (e.g., vegetable oil, peanut butter, lard, butter) to increase energy

density, plus vitamins and minerals. A wide variety of foods should be provided in amounts to satisfy the appetite, taking into account the patient's inclinations and taboos. The liquid diet with vitamins and minerals should be given between meals and at night.

Ensuring Nutritional Rehabilitation

This last stage of treatment begins when the patient is without serious complications, eating satisfactorily, and gaining weight, usually 2 to 3 weeks after admission. It may start in the hospital and continue on an outpatient basis, preferably at a nutrition rehabilitation center or similar facility that gives daytime care. When no such facility is available, the hospital must continue to provide care until the patient is ready for discharge. The importance of continuing the high-energy, high-protein diet until full recovery has taken place must be clearly explained to the child's mother or caretaker. If this can be done at home, the patient can continue treatment there with regular follow-up in a nutrition clinic or its equivalent or by home visits by trained personnel.

Introduction of Traditional Foods. When edema has disappeared, the skin lesions are notably improved, the patient becomes active and interacts with the environment, the appetite is restored, and adequate rates of catch-up growth have been achieved, other foods, especially those available at home, are gradually introduced into the diet *in addition to the high-energy, high-protein formula*. For children, a daily minimum intake of 3 to 4 g of protein and 500 to 625 kJ (120–150 kcal)/kg of body weight (or more in marasmus) must be ensured. To achieve this goal, the energy density of solid foods must be increased with oil, and protein concentration and quality must be high, using animal proteins, soybean protein preparations, and good vegetable protein mixtures in appropriate combinations (113–116), *in addition to the liquid formula*, as in the following examples:

1. One part of a dry pulse or its flour (e.g., black beans, soybeans, kidney beans, cowpeas) and three parts of a dry cereal or flour (e.g., corn, rice, wheat); fat or oil should be added to the mashed or strained pulse during or after cooking in amounts equal to the weight of the dry pulse or flour and to the cereal preparations in amounts of 10 to 30 mL oil/100 g dry cereal product, depending on the type of preparation.
2. Four parts of dry rice and one part of fresh or dry fish; fat or oil should be added in amounts equal to 20 to 40% of the dry weights.

The food can be served as separate dishes, or the parts can be mashed or blended and fed as paps to infants and young children. Lipid-rich pastes with high energy density resist bacterial contamination (116, 117). The diet must be supplemented with minerals and vitamins as described for the initial dietary treatment until full nutritional rehabilitation is achieved.

Emotional and Physical Stimulation. Malnourished children need affection and tender care from the beginning of treatment. This requires patience and understanding by the hospital staff and the relatives. *Involvement of parents or relatives must be encouraged.* Hospital wards should be brightly colored and cheerful, preferably with music. As soon as the child can move without assistance and is willing to interact with the staff and other children, he or she must be encouraged to explore, to play, and to participate in activities that involve body movements. Relatively small increments in physical activity through active play during the course of nutritional rehabilitation result in faster longitudinal growth and accretion of lean body tissues (118, 119). Parents should be encouraged to stimulate and teach their children by playing and talking. Toys and play materials can often be made from discarded local articles.

Adult patients should exercise regularly with gradual increments in cardiorespiratory workload.

Treatment of Diarrhea and Other Health Problems. Mild diarrhea often disappears without specific treatment as nutritional status improves. However, persistent or recurrent diarrhea can contribute to the development of a new episode of PEM. Treatment is determined by the underlying cause of diarrhea, usually repeated intestinal infections, excessive bacterial flora in the upper gut that ferment food substrates and deconjugate bile salts, intestinal parasitic infestations (particularly giardiasis, cryptosporidiosis, and trichiuriasis), and intolerance to food components. The apparent high prevalence of lactose malabsorption and intolerance in PEM is often founded on inadequate diagnostic procedures. When intolerance to milk or other food is suspected, the diet should be modified, taking care to preserve its nutritional quality and density. Before branding a patient intolerant to a given food, the food should be reintroduced into the diet, and adequate diagnostic tests should be done to confirm the diagnosis.

Other minor complications, such as intestinal parasites, must be treated. Children should be vaccinated against infectious diseases.

Criteria for Recovery. Premature termination of treatment increases the risk of recurrence of malnutrition. The most practical criterion of recovery is catch-up in weight, and almost all fully recovered patients should reach the weight expected for their height or a normal BMI (see Fig. 57.11). Repletion of body protein is best assessed through body composition indicators, such as the creatinine-height index. When body composition cannot be assessed, as a general guideline dietary therapy should continue for 1 month after the patient reaches a normal weight (Tables 57.4 and 57.5) without clinical signs of edematous PEM or for 15 days after the marasmic patient reaches that weight. Some patients, however, apparently remain underweight because they are in the lower end of the normal distribution curves of weight for height or BMI. If they continue growing at a normal rate and have no functional impairments, treatment can be terminated after 1 month of adequate dietary intake and weight gain (or, in adults, weight stabilization). Specific treatment of other nutritional problems (e.g., iron deficiency) sometimes must be prolonged beyond discharge for PEM.

Before being discharged, patients or their parents must be taught about the causes of PEM, with emphasis on rational and nutritious use of household foods, personal and environmental hygiene, appropriate immunizations, and early treatment, including dietary management, of diarrhea and other diseases. Adolescents and adults can be discharged when they are eating well and gaining weight, they have a reliable source of nutritious food outside the hospital, and other problems have been diagnosed and treatment begun. Supplementary feeding should continue as an outpatient until the BMI is greater than 15.0, 16.5, and 18.5, respectively, for adolescents 11 to 13 years old, adolescents 14 to 17 years old, and adults.

Mild and Moderate Malnutrition

The less severe forms of PEM should be treated in an ambulatory setting, by supplementing the home diet with easily digested foods that contain proteins of high biologic value, a high energy density, and adequate amounts of micronutrients. In some instances, therapy can be achieved merely by instructing the adult patient about adequate eating habits and a better use of food resources or by instructing mothers in improved child-feeding practices and in more nutritious culinary habits. It is almost always necessary, however, to provide both nutritious food supplements and instructions for their use.

The quantity of food supplements will vary depending on the degree of malnutrition and the relative deficit of proteins and energy. As a general guideline, the goal should be to provide a total intake, including the home diet, of *at least* twice the protein and 1.5 times the energy requirements. For preschool children, this would signify a daily intake of about 2 to 2.5 g of high-quality protein and 500 to 625 kJ (120–150 kcal)/kg of body weight, and for infants less than 1 year old, about 3.5 g protein and 625 kJ (150 kcal)/kg/day.

The ingestion of the food supplement by the malnourished person must be ensured. This is more likely to occur if the food is appetizing to both the child and the mother, if it is ready made or easy to prepare, if additional amounts are provided to feed other children living in the same household, and if it does not have an important commercial value outside the home that would make it easy and profitable for the family to sell the item for cash. A substitution effect on the home diet (i.e., a decrease in the usual food intake) is almost always unavoidable, but it can be reduced by using low-bulk supplements with high protein and energy concentrations. Special attention should be given to avoid a decrease in breast-feeding. The supplements for breast-fed infants should be paps or solid foods that will not quench the infant's thirst and thus not change the infant's demand or the mother's attitude toward lactation.

Adequate amounts of vitamins and minerals must be ensured, although mild deficiencies can be overcome by the micronutrients in the food or by use of fortified vehicles such as iron-enriched bread or sugar fortified with retinol.

PREVENTION AND CONTROL

Rates of malnutrition have declined rapidly in countries that have reduced poverty and have invested in health, nutrition, education, and the social sector (120). The strategies for preventing malnutrition must follow a multisectoral approach that involves food production, distribution, and availability (food security), preventive medicine, education, social development, and economic improvement. At a national or regional level, effective control and prevention can be achieved only through sustained long-term

political commitments and actions aimed at eradicating the underlying causes of malnutrition. Physicians, nutritionists, health personnel, social workers, and educators can and must play an active role.

When resources are limited, a profile of risk factors is useful to set priorities. The most likely victims of malnutrition are children less than 2 years of age from low socioeconomic strata whose parents have misconceptions concerning the use of foods, who come from broken or unstable families, whose families have a high prevalence of alcoholism, who live under poor sanitary conditions in urban slums and rural areas or in regions frequently subject to droughts or floods, and whose societal beliefs prohibit the use of certain nutritious foods. Other highly vulnerable groups are preschool-aged children, pregnant adolescents, and multiparous women who are socially and economically deprived.

The presence of a malnourished child in a family indicates that something is wrong in that family and suggests that other members of the household may also be at risk of malnutrition. Therefore, actions and preventive measures must not be restricted to the index case, but should include the prevention of nutritional deterioration of other family members, especially siblings and pregnant and lactating women. Similarly, a high prevalence of children with malnutrition or growth retardation indicates that the entire community is at some risk of impaired nutrition.

Food Availability

Foods of animal origin are the best protein sources, but they tend to be expensive, not always available, or prohibited by religious practices. Under such circumstances, staple vegetable foods can be complemented with other culturally acceptable vegetable foods combined in proportions that result in good essential amino acid complementation and improve the biologic value of dietary protein. For example, corn and black bean combinations that provide proteins in a proportion of about 60:40, equivalent to about three parts of dry corn and one part of dry beans, have an excellent amino acid composition and permit adequate growth and function (121). The same is true of a series of other combinations of grains and pulses (114). The relatively low nitrogen digestibility of these vegetable sources must be considered when recommending the amounts to be eaten. Energy density can be increased adding sugar and oil or other fats.

It is often necessary to convince parents about the safety of using foods that, in some cultures, are fed only to adults and older children. This is especially true of foods used to complement mother's milk or to wean infants from the breast. Breast-fed infants from populations at risk of PEM should start receiving at 6 months of age—or earlier, if weight gain is not satisfactory—commercial preparations of cooked rice, oat, or wheat, or home-made paps prepared by mashing boiled rice, bread soaked in about 50% water, or cooked corn products (e.g., tamale, tortilla). After 6 months

TABLE 57.15. PAPS TO COMPLEMENT BREAST MILK, USING COMMON FOODS AND BASED ON COMBINATIONS OF LEGUME WITH A CEREAL OR POTATO AND VEGETABLE OIL

	A	B	C	D
Cooked beans (g) (60% water)[a]	25	25	25	25
Corn dough (g) (57% water)[a]	75	—	—	—
White bread (g) (50% water)[a]	—	75	—	—
Boiled rice (g) (55% water)[a]	—	—	75	—
Boiled potatoes (g) (33% water)[a]	—	—	—	75
Water (mL)	25	25	25	25
Vegetable oil (mL)	10	10	10	15
Protein (g/100 g)[b]	3.6	4.8	3.4	2.2
Energy (kcal/100 g)[b]	176	176	183	147

[a]In parentheses: proportion of water added to prepare 100 g.
[b]Protein and energy content of 100 g of pap, ready to eat.

Modified from unpublished observations by FE Viteri, B Garcia, and B Torun. Black beans (Phaseolus vulgaris) cooked, mashed, and strained. Corn dough cooked with limestone, according to Guatemalan customs. White bread soaked in equal weight of water.

of age, fish, egg, or minced meat, or one part of a cooked pulse (e.g., kidney beans, soybeans, chick peas) should be added for every three parts of rice, corn, or bread to provide a better protein mixture. If the child is underweight, 1 teaspoon of vegetable oil or 2 teaspoons of sugar can be added to every 2 to 3 ounces of pap. Paps based on a pulse, such as black beans (Phaseolus vulgaris), a cereal, and vegetable oil can be fed to babies as young as 3 months of age without intestinal discomfort and without decreasing breast milk intakes. Examples of such paps are shown in Table 57.15.

Children who are fully weaned or only occasionally breast-fed must receive adequate amounts of energy- and protein-rich staples and, ideally, animal foods to satisfy their nutritional needs and allow adequate growth. It is also important to convince parents that food should not be withheld when a child has diarrhea, because in many developing countries children less than 5 years of age have loose stools 15 to 20% of the time. It has been shown that many local foods of vegetable origin that are rich in fiber can be safely used and may even shorten the duration of diarrhea (122).

Reducing Infections

The risk of infections must be reduced because of the interaction of infection with nutrition. High priority must be given to immunizations, sanitary measures to reduce fecal contamination, and early oral rehydration and feeding of children with diarrhea.

Education

Girls and women should be specially targeted in educational and developmental programs (22). Education programs must also be devised for community leaders, civic action groups, and the community as a whole. Such programs must emphasize promotion of breast-feeding, appropriate use of weaning foods, nutritional alternatives using traditional foods, home food security, personal and environmental hygiene, feeding practices during illness and convalescence, and early treatment of diarrhea and other diseases. Personal and communal involvement should be pursued through commitments to apply the recommendations. Toward this aim, it is important that all educational programs incorporate the community's own assessment of their nutritional problems and their feelings toward personal participation in solving these problems.

REFERENCES

1. Patron-Correa JP. Rev Med Yucatan (Mexico) 1908;3:89–96.
2. Normet L. Bull Soc Pathol Exot 1926;19:207–13.
3. Kerandel J. Bull Soc Pathol Exot 1926;19:302–11.
4. McConnell RE. Uganda Annual Medical Sanitation Report (Appendix 2). Entebbe: Government Printer, 1918.
5. Procter RAW. Kenya Med J 1927;3:264.
6. Mann WL, Helm JB, Brown CJ. JAMA 1920;75:1416–8.
7. Payne GC, Payne FK. Am J Hyg 1927;7:73–83.
8. Williams CD. Arch Dis Child 1932;8:423–33.
9. Williams CD. Lancet 1935;2:1151–2.
10. Autret M, Behar M. Síndrome policarencial infantil (Kwashiorkor) and Its Prevention in Central America. FAO Nutrition Studies no. 113. Rome: Food and Agriculture Organization, 1954.
11. Trowell HC, Davies JNP, Dean RFA. Kwashiorkor. London: Edward Arnold, 1954.
12. Hegsted DM, Tsongas AG, Abbott DB et al J Lab Clin Med 1946;31:261–84.
13. Brock JF, Autret M. Kwashiorkor in Africa. FAO Nutrition Studies no. 8. Rome: Food and Agriculture Organization, 1952.
14. Jelliffe DB. J Pediatr 1959;54:227–56.
15. Schofield C, Ashworth A. Bull World Health Org 1996;74: 223–9.
16. Pelletier DL, Frongillo EA, Schroeder DG et al. Bull World Health Org 1995;73:443–8.
17. Rice AL, Sacco L, Hyder A, Black RE. Bull World Health Org 2000;78:582–94.
18. Duke T, Michael A, Mgone J et al. Bull World Health Org 2002;80:16–25.
19. Lambrechts T, Bryce J, Orinda V. Bull World Health Org 1999; 77:582–94.
20. Liu T, Howard RM, Mancini AJ et al. Arch Dermatol 2001;137: 630–63.
21. de Onis M, Frongillo EA, Blossner M. Bull World Health Org 2000;78:1222–333.
22. UNICEF: The State of the World's Children 2004: Girls, Education and Development. New York: UNICEF, 2004.
23. de Onis M, Blossner M, Villar J. Eur J Clin Nutr 1998;52[Suppl 1]: 5S–15S.
24. Fernandez ID, Himes JH, de Onis M. Bull World Health Org 2002;80:282–91.
25. Chagas C, Keusch GT, eds. The interaction of parasitic diseases and nutrition. Pontificiae Academiae Scientiarum Scripta Varia no. 61. Vatican: Pontifical Academy of Sciences, 1986.
26. Torun B. Short and long-term effects of low or restricted energy intakes on the activity of infants and children. In: Schurch B,

Scrimshaw NS, eds. Activity, Energy Expenditure and Energy Requirements of Infants and Children. Lausanne: International Dietary Energy Consultancy Group, 1990:335–59.

27. Viteri FE, Torun B. Bol Sanit Panam 1975;78:58–74.

28. Torun B, Viteri FE. UN Univ Food Nutr Bull 1981;Suppl 5:229–41.

29. Viteri FE, Alvarado J. Rev Col Med (Guatemala) 1970;21: 175–230.

30. Waterlow JC, Garlick PJ, Millward JD. Protein Turnover in Mammalian Tissues and in the Whole Body. Oxford: North Holland, 1978.

31. Viteri FE. Primary protein-energy malnutrition: Clinical, biochemical, and metabolic changes. In: Suskind RM, ed. Textbook of Pediatric Nutrition. New York: Raven Press, 1981: 189–215.

32. Tomkins AM, Garlick PJ, Schofield WN et al. Clin Sci 1983;65: 313–24.

33. Reddy V. Protein-energy malnutrition: An overview. In: Harper AE, Davis GK, eds. Nutrition in Health and Disease and Industrial Development. New York: Alan R. Liss, 1981:227–35.

34. Viteri FE, Alvarado J, Luthringer DG et al. Vitam Horm 1968; 26:573–615.

35. Caballero B, Solomons NW, Batres R et al. J Pediatr Gastroenterol Nutr 1985;4:97–102.

36. MacDougall LG, Moodley G, Eyberg C et al. Am J Clin Nutr 1982;35:229–35.

37. Wickramasinghe SN, Mary-Cotes P, Gill DS et al. Br J Haematol 1985;60:515–24.

38. Viart P. Am J Clin Nutr 1977;30:334–48.

39. Heymsfield SB, Bethel RA, Ansley JD et al. Am Heart J 1978; 95:584–94.

40. Paniagua R, Santos D, Muñoz R et al. Pediatr Res 1980;14: 1260–2.

41. Mahakur AC, Mishra AC, Panda SN et al. J Assoc Physicians India 1983;31:79–81.

42. Keusch GT. Malnutrition, infection and immune function. In: Suskind RM, Lewinter-Suskind L, eds. The Malnourished Child. Nestlé Nutrition Workshop Series vol 19. New York: Raven Press, 1990:37–59.

43. Chandra RK. Am J Clin Nutr 1991;53:1087–101.

44. Bhaskaram R, Siwakumar B. Arch Dis Child 1986;61:182–5.

45. Keusch GT, Torun B, Johnson RB et al. J Pediatr 1984;105: 434–6.

46. Kauffman CA, Jones RG, Kluger MJ. Am J Clin Nutr 1986;44: 449–52.

47. Cerami A, Ikeda Y, LeTrang N et al. Immunol Lett 1985;11:173–5.

48. Nichols BL, Alvarado J, Hazlewood CF et al. J Pediatr 1972;80: 319–30.

49. Viteri FE, Schneider R. Med Clin North Am 1974;58: 1487–505.

50. Torun B, Solomons NW, Viteri FE. Arch Latinoam Nutr 1979; 29:445–94.

51. Torun B. Nutrient absorption in malnutrition. In: Chagas C, Keusch GT, eds. The Interactions of Parasitic Diseases and Nutrition. Pontificiae Academiae Scientiarum Scripta Varia no. 61. Vatican: Pontifical Academy of Sciences, 1986:81–94.

52. Winick M. J Pediatr Gastroenterol Nutr 1987;6:833–5.

53. Kretchmer N, Beard JL, Carlson L. Am J Clin Nutr 1996;63: 997S–1001S.

54. Liu J, Raine A, Venables PH et al. Arch Pediatr Adolesc Med 2003;157:593–600.

55. Hendrickse RG. Trans R Soc Trop Med Hyg 1984;78:427–35.

56. Coulter JBS, Suliman GI. Eur J Clin Nutr 1988;42:787–96.

57. Kocalas CN, Coskun T, Yurdakov M et al. Hum Exp Toxicol 2003;22:155–8.

58. Golden MHN. The consequences of protein deficiency in man and its relationship to the features of kwashiorkor. In: Blaxter KL, Waterlow JC, eds. Nutritional Adaptation in Man. London: John Libby, 1985:169–88.

59. Golden MHN, Ramdath D. Proc Nutr Soc 1987;46:53–68.

60. Jackson AA. Trans R Soc Trop Med Hyg 1986;80:911–3.

61. Golden MHN, Ramdath D, Golden BE. Free radicals and malnutrition. In: Dreosti IE, ed. Trace Elements, Micronutrients and Free Radicals. Clifton, NJ: Humana Press, 1990.

62. Becker K, Leichsenring M, Gana L et al. Free Radic Biol Med 1995;18:257–63.

63. Lenhartz T, Ndasi R, Anninos A et al. J Pediatr 1998;132: 879–81.

64. Reid M, Badaloo A, Forrester T et al. Am J Physiol 2000;278: E405–12.

65. Fechner A, Bohme C, Gromer S et al. Pediatr Res 2001;49: 237–43.

66. Manar MJ, MacPherson GD, McCardle F et al. Acta Paediatr 2001;90:950–2.

67. Waterlow JC. Protein Energy Malnutrition. London: Edward Arnold, 1992.

68. Badaloo A, Reid M, Forrester T et al. Am J Clin Nutr 2002;76: 646–52.

69. Powanda MC. Am J Clin Nutr 1977;30:1254–68.

70. Weech AA. Bull NY Acad Med 1939;15:63–91.

71. Walter SJ, Shore AC. Clin Sci 1988;75:621–8.

72. Klahr S, Alleyne GAO. Kidney Int 1973;3:129–41.

73. Migeon CJ, Beitins IZ, Kowarski A et al. Plasma aldosterone concentration and aldosterone secretion rate in Peruvian infants with marasmus and kwashiorkor. In: Gardner LI, Amacher P, eds. Endocrine Aspects of Malnutrition. Santa Ynez, CA: Kroc Foundation, 1973:399–424.

74. Beitins IZ, Graham GG, Kowarski A et al. J Pediatr 1974;84: 444–51.

75. Srikantia SG, Gopalan C. Am J Appl Physiol 1959;14:829–33.

76. Srikantia SG, Mohanham S. J Clin Endocrinol 1970;31:312–4.

77. Golden MHN. Lancet 1982;1:1261–5.

78. Torun B, Viteri FE. Rev Col Med (Guatemala) 1976;27:43–62.

79. Golden BE, Corbett M, McBurney R et al. Trans R Soc Trop Med Hyg 2000;94:12–3.

80. Collins S, Myatt M, Golden B. Am J Clin Nutr 1998;68:193–9.

81. Deen JL, Funk M, Guevara V et al. Bull World Health Org 2003;81:237–43.

82. Benjamin DR. Pediatr Clin North Am 1989;36:139–61.

83. Habicht JP, Martorell R, Yarborough C et al. Lancet 1974; 1:611–5.

84. Graitcer PL, Gentry EM. Lancet 1981;2:297–9.

85. World Health Organization. Measuring Change in Nutritional Status. Geneva: World Health Organization, 1983.

86. Waterlow JC. Classification and definition of protein-energy malnutrition. In: Beaton GH, Bengoa JM, eds. Nutrition in preventive medicine. Geneva: World Health Organization, 1976.

87. Nabarro D, McNab S. J Trop Med Hyg 1980;83:21–33.

88. Torun B, Samayoa C. Un sistema sencillo para evaluar el estado nutricional de niños, con participación comunitaria. In: Proceedings of the 9th Latin American Congress of Nutrition. San Juan, PR, 1991:159.

89. World Health Organization. Physical Status: The Use and Interpretation of Anthropometry. Technical Report Series no. 854. Geneva: World Health Organization, 1995.

90. Gomez F, Ramos-Galvan R, Frenk S. Adv Pediatr 1955;7: 131–69.

91. Rutishauser IHE, Whitehead RG. Br J Nutr 1972;28:145–52.

92. Viteri FE, Torun B. Nutrition, physical activity and growth. In: Ritzen M, Aperia A, Hall K et al, eds. The Biology of Normal Human Growth. New York: Raven Press, 1981:265–73.

93. Spurr GB, Reina JC. Eur J Clin Nutr 1988;42:819–34.

94. Viteri FE, Torun B, Immink MDC et al. Marginal malnutrition and working capacity. In: Harper AE, Davis GK, eds. Nutrition in Health and Disease and International Development. New York: Alan R. Liss, 1981:277–83.

95. Viteri FE, Alvarado J. Pediatrics 1970;46:696–706.

96. Parra A, Garza C, Garza Y et al. J Pediatr 1973;82:133–42.

97. Man WD, Weber M, Palmer A et al. Trop Med Int Health 1998;3:678–86.

98. Berkley JA, Ross A, Mwangi I et al. BMJ 2003;326:361–6.

99. World Health Organization. Management of Severe Malnutrition: A Manual for Physicians and Other Senior Health Workers. Geneva: World Health Organization, 1999.

100. World Health Organization. Management of a Child with a Serious Infection or Severe Malnutrition: Guidelines for Care at the First Referral Level in Developing Countries. Geneva: World Health Organization, 2000.

101. World Health Organization. A Manual for the Treatment of Diarrhea: Programme for the Control of Diarrhea Disease. WHO/CDD/SER/80.1 Rev. 1 1990. Geneva: World Health Organization, 1990.

102. Krishnaswamy K. Clin Pharmacokinet 1989;17[Suppl 1]:68–88.

103. Mehta S. Drug metabolism in the malnourished child. In: Suskind RM, Lewinter-Suskind L, eds. The Malnourished Child. Nestlé Nutrition Workshop Series vol 19. New York: Raven Press, 1990;329–38.

104. Mehta S, Nain CK, Kalso HK et al. Indian J Med Res 1981;74:244–50.

105. Mehta S, Naim CK, Sharma B et al. Pharmacology 1980;21:369–74.

106. Janssen F, Bouton JM, Vuye A et al. JPEN J Parenter Enteral Nutr 1983;7:26–36.

107. Weinsier RL, Krumdieck CL. Am J Clin Nutr 1981;34:393–9.

108. Solomons NW, Torun B, Caballero B et al. Am J Clin Nutr 1984;40:591–600.

109. Torun B, Solomons NW, Caballero B et al. Am J Clin Nutr 1984;40:601–10.

110. Briend A, Lacsala R, Kamnadji J et al. Lancet 1999;353:1767–8.

111. Collins S, Sadler K. Lancet 2002;360:1824–30.

112. Briend A. Br J Nutr 2001;85[Suppl 2]:175S–9S.

113. Diop HI, Dossou NI, Ndour MM et al. Am J Clin Nutr 2003;78:302–7.

114. Torun B, Young VR, Rand WM, eds. UN Univ Food Nutr Bull 1981;Suppl 5.

115. Khanum S, Ashworth A, Huttly SRA. Lancet 1994;344:1728–31.

116. Manary MJ, Ndekha MJ, Ashorn P et al. Arch Dis Child 2004;89:557–61.

117. Briend A. Ann Med Interne (Paris) 2000;151:629–34.

118. Torun B, Schutz Y, Bradfield RB et al. Effect of physical activity upon growth of children recovering from protein-calorie malnutrition (PCM). In: Proceedings of the 10th International Congress of Nutrition. Kyoto: Victory-sha Press, 1976;247–9.

119. Torun B, Viteri FE. Eur J Clin Nutr 1994;48[Suppl 1]:S186–90.

120. Dayrit MA. Bull World Health Org 1998;76[Suppl 2]:80–4.

121. Torun B. Alimentación de niños con desnutrición proteínico-energética y diarrea, con énfasis en las experiencias del INCAP. In: Pan American Health Organization Meeting on Feeding of Children Ill with Diarrhea. Washington, DC: Pan American Health Organization, 1983.

122. Viteri FE, Torun B, Arroyave G et al. Food Nutr Bull 1981;Suppl 5:202–9.

123. Torun B, Chew F. Trans R Soc Trop Med Hyg 1991;85:12–7.

124. INCAP: Evaluación nutricional de la población de Centro América y Panamá: Guatemala. Guatemala: Instituto de Nutrición de Centro América y Panamá, 1969.

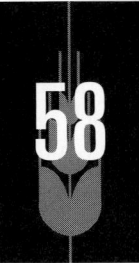

58 INHERITED METABOLIC DISEASE: AMINO ACIDS, ORGANIC ACIDS, AND GALACTOSE[1]

LOUIS J. ELSAS II AND PHYLLIS B. ACOSTA

GENETIC PERSPECTIVE 909
GENETIC DISORDERS BENEFITED BY
   NUTRITION SUPPORT 910
GENERAL PRINCIPLES OF GENETIC DISEASE
   MANAGEMENT 913
AROMATIC AMINO ACIDS .916
   Biochemistry 916
SULFUR-CONTAINING AMINO ACIDS 928
   Biochemistry 928
ORGANIC ACIDS 932
   Biochemistry 932
   Glutaric Acidemia Type I 945
AMMONIA 946
   Biochemistry 946
GALACTOSE 950
   Biochemistry 950

[1] **Abbreviations: ARG**, arginine; **ASA**, argininosuccinic lyase deficiency; **ATP**, adenosine triphosphate; **BCAA**, branched-chain amino acid; **BCKA**, branched-chain α-ketoacid; **BCKAD**, branched-chain α-ketoacid dehydrogenase; **BH$_4$**, tetrahydrobiopterin; **CH$_3$-B$_{12}$**, methylcobalamin; **CIT**, citrulline; **CNS**, central nervous system; **CoA**, coenzyme A; **CβS**, cystathionine β-synthase; **DHPR**, dihydropteridine reductase; **DNPH**, dinitrophenylhydrazine; **EEG**, electroencephalogram; **ETF**, electron transfer factor; **FAA**, fumarylacetoacetate; **FAH**, fumarylacetoacetic acid hydrolase; **G/G**, homozygous for galactose-1-phosphate uridyl transferase alleles; **GA-I**, glutaric acidemia type I; **GAL**, galactose; **GALT**, galactose-1-phosphate uridyl transferase; **GC/MS**, gas chromatography/mass spectrometry; **GCD**, glutaryl-coenzyme A dehydrogenase; **GLU**, glucose; **GLY**, glycine; **HMG-CoA**, 3-hydroxy-3-methylglutaryl- coenzyme A; **ILE**, isoleucine; **IVA**, isovaleric acid; **IVD**, isovaleryl-coenzyme A dehydrogenase; **IQ**, intelligence quotient; **IVG**, isovalerylglycine; **L-DOPA**, L-3,4-dihydroxyphenylalanine; **LEU**, leucine; **LYS**, lysine; **MAT**, methionine-S-adenosyltransferase; **MET**, methionine; **MMA**, methylmalonic acidemia; **MPKUCS**, Collaborative Study of Maternal Phenylketonuria; **MS/MS**, tandem mass spectrometry; **MSUD**, maple syrup urine disease; **NTBC**, 2-(2-nitro-4-trifluoromethylbenzoyl)-1, 3-cyclohexanedione; **OHIVA**, hydroxyisovaleric acid; **ORN**, ornithine; **OTC**, ornithine transcarbamylase; **PAH**, phenylalanine hydroxylase; **PHE**, phenylalanine; **PKU**, phenylketonuria; **p-OHPPAD**, 4-hydroxyphenylpyruvic acid dioxygenase; **PPA**, propionic acidemia; **RDA**, recommended dietary allowance; **SAM**, S-adenosylmethionine; **THR**, threonine; **TPP**, thiamin pyrophosphate; **TRP**, tryptophan; **TYR**, tyrosine; **UCD**, urea cycle defect; **UCED**, urea cycle enzyme defect; **UDP**, uridine diphosphate; **VAL**, valine; **δ-ALA**, δ-aminolevulinic acid.

GENETIC PERSPECTIVE

Geneticists approach the general subject of nutrition and the specific requirement for nutrients with the view that the recommended dietary allowance (RDA) (1) for an essential nutrient is not optimum for all individuals. Rather, individuals in a population have genetically determined variations in their nutrient requirements that extend over a wide range. This concept arose historically from two older scientific disciplines: human biochemical genetics and nutrition science. The former discipline originated with Sir Archibald Garrod's Croonian lectures of 1908. Garrod defined four "inborn errors of metabolism" as blocks in the normal flow of metabolic processes. Biochemical and clinical expression of these metabolic blocks demonstrated patterns of inheritance consistent with Mendel's predictions for transmission of single genes with a large effect on the phenotype. Thus arose the concept that genes controlled metabolism and that disease states were created by blocks in this metabolic flow, yielding accumulated precursors and deficient products.

Today, we recognize that "inborn errors" are discontinuous traits resulting from variations in the structure and function of enzymes or protein molecules. The amino acid sequences of enzymes and their quantity are dictated by genes. The control of enzyme function is predicated by molecular regulation through gene transcription, posttranscriptional processing of RNA, translation, posttranslational modification, and protein turnover. More than 8000 monogenic human disorders are cataloged and available. Of these, about 300 have a defined biochemical basis (2). The extent of normal variation in genes controlling enzyme activity suggests that about 30% of our population is heterozygous for common alleles (3). Within this continuous diversity, mutations produce discontinuous, relatively rare traits that are expressed as disease under normal environmental conditions.

Mutant gene frequencies vary in populations; for example, mitochondrial branched-chain α-ketoacid dehydrogenase (BCKAD) deficiency (maple syrup urine disease, MSUD) occurs in one of approximately every 185,000 newborns worldwide, but occurs in one of 176 in an inbred Mennonite population (4). The mutation is one of a few that are not private to individual families. The Mennonite mutation is in the E1α gene and changes a tyrosine

(TYR) at position 194 to asparagine (Y302N). In the homozygous state, it produces extreme toxicity due to accumulated branched-chain α-ketoacids (BCKAs) if affected newborns are fed the RDA for branched-chain amino acids (BCAAs). However, normal development is expected if dietary isoleucine (ILE), leucine (LEU), and valine (VAL) are restricted to 20 to 40% of the RDA during rapid growth (5), and much less is required during stable growth.

Considerable human variation occurs in the structure and activity of enzymes involved in the catabolism of essential amino acids, but only a few are so impaired that ingestion of the RDA creates severe disease. Population-based newborn screening and dietary intervention are now applied through public health programs to many rare inborn errors for which newborn screening predicts genetic susceptibility given a normal diet (6). By contrast to these relatively rare inborn errors, all humans lack the enzyme that converts L-gulono-α-lactone to ascorbic acid, but scurvy does not occur if sufficient vitamin C is ingested and absorbed (7). Thus, the frequency of genetic susceptibility given a "normal" diet ranges from rare to common and extends to the metabolism of amino acids, nitrogen, carbohydrates, lipids, purines, pyrimidines, minerals, and vitamins.

GENETIC DISORDERS BENEFITED BY NUTRITION SUPPORT

More than 300 genetic disorders have been reported in which toxic manifestations relate to accumulation, deficiency, or overproduction of normally occurring substrates and products of metabolic flow. In many of them, modification of the dietary supply will alleviate the manifestations. In a large number, however, irreversible damage has already occurred by the time symptoms appear. Optimum management of these disorders depends on identifying affected subjects while they are presymptomatic or before irreversible disease has occurred. Because the disorders are heritable, genetic markers are present from the moment of conception, and thus the genetic power of prediction and prevention is applicable. In practice, a number of disorders can be detected in the fetus in the tenth to sixteenth week of gestation by studies on chorionic villus or amniotic fluid cells. Prenatal diagnosis can be made in the ninth to twelfth week of gestation through the use of chorionic villus biopsy (8). Teratogenic sequelae of an inborn error in a pregnancy, such as birth defects in children of mothers with phenylketonuria (PKU), may be prevented by strict control of blood phenylalanine (PHE) before conception and throughout pregnancy. Other inherited metabolic alterations are detected postnatally in the presymptomatic infant by analysis of blood, urine, erythrocytes, leukocytes, or cultured skin fibroblasts for impaired enzymes, accumulated substrates, or products of alternate metabolic pathways.

A selective search for presymptomatic genetic disease is often undertaken when there is a family history of inherited disease. Selective screening for inherited disease is also initiated for relatively common symptoms such as failure to thrive in childhood. Early treatment has proven effective for many diseases such as PKU, galactosemia, isovaleric acidemia, homocystinuria, MSUD, argininosuccinic aciduria, and citrullinemia. Irreversible brain damage occurs if treatment is not initiated in PKU before the second week of life. In MSUD, galactosemia, isovaleric acidemia, and disorders of the urea cycle, irreversible damage to the brain may occur within the first week of life, whereas disorders of fatty acid oxidation may remain undetected for weeks until an intermittent infection produces lethal hypoglycemia. To prevent this, population-wide nonselective screening of newborns has been instituted for PKU, galactosemia, homocystinuria, tyrosinemia, disorders of fatty acid oxidation, and some urea cycle enzyme defects (UCEDs). Some states are also screening for organic acidemias such as branched-chain ketoaciduria (MSUD), isovaleric acidemia and other disorders of LEU catabolism, propionic acidemia (PPA), methylmalonic acidemia (MMA), and glutaric acidemia. Thus, speed in diagnosis and treatment is of the utmost importance in preventing a poor outcome in newborns with these inherited metabolic disorders.

In the future, population-based presymptomatic detection will be extended to other disorders. However, before screening is initiated as a public health program, several criteria should be fulfilled (Table 58.1). Knowledge of pathogenesis, preventability, and availability of therapy must precede initiation of routine screening programs. Table 58.2 lists genetic disorders in which modification of nutrient intake has been used. Effectiveness in preventing clinical sequelae is experimental in some of the therapies listed.

Although many patients with inherited disorders benefit from nutrition support, each would require a chapter for adequate discussion. Thus, this chapter emphasizes

TABLE 58.1. CRITERIA FOR NONSELECTIVE NEWBORN SCREENING

1	The disorder produces a high burden to the affected individual, yet is preventable.
2	Methods for screening retrieval, diagnosis, and management must be practical and available to the population as a whole.
3	Inheritance and pathogenesis of the disease should be understood.
4	Benefit-to-cost ratio of the program should be greater than one.
5	Patients' rights should be protected (including confidentiality and informed consent).
6	False-negative laboratory screening results should not occur.
7	False-positive laboratory screening results should be minimized.

TABLE 58.2. NUTRITION TREATMENT OF GENETIC DISORDERS

DISORDER	THERAPY
Abetalipoproteinemia	Medium-chain triglycerides; vitamins A, D, E, and K parenterally or in excess orally
Acrodermatitis enteropathica	Supplement zinc sulfate
Adenine phosphoribosyltransferase	Purine restriction; avoid alkali; allopurinol
Alkaptonuria (ochronosis)	Restrict phenylalanine and tyrosine; supplement ascorbic acid
Anemia, hypochromic, sideroblastic	Supplement pyridoxine
Argininemia	Restrict protein; supplement essential amino acids and ornithine
Argininosuccinic aciduria	Restrict protein; supplement essential amino acid, L-carnitine, arginine, benzoic acid, and phenylbutyrate or phenylacetate
β-Methylcrotonylglycinuria	Restrict leucine; supplement L-carnitine
β-Methylglutaconic aciduria type I	Restrict leucine; supplement L-carnitine
β-Sitosterolemia	Restrict plant sterols
Biotinidase deficiency	Supplement biotin
Carbamylphosphate synthetase deficiency	Restrict protein; supplement essential amino acids, L-carnitine, arginine, benzoic acid, and phenylbutyrate or phenylacetate
Chediak-Higashi syndrome	Supplement ascorbic acid
Chloride diarrhea	Supplement chloride
Chylomicronemia	Restrict fat, medium-chain triglycerides
Citrullinemia	Restrict protein; supplement L-carnitine, essential amino acids, arginine, and phenylbutyrate or phenylacetate
Combined hyperlipidemia	Restrict energy, carbohydrates, and saturated fatty acids; nicotinic acid, mevinolin, and cholestyramine therapy
Cystathioninuria	Supplement pyridoxine
Cystic fibrosis	Supplement enteric enzymes (trypsin, lipase, chymotrypsin)
Cystinosis	Supplement alkali, phosphate, and vitamin D; cysteamine to reduce cystine
Cystinuria	Alkali, hyperhydration, D-penicillamine
Diabetes insipidus	Water, low-solute diet, vasopressin
Diabetes mellitus	Insulin, controlled diet
Dibasic aminoaciduria	Restrict protein; supplement arginine
Ehlers-Danlos syndrome, lysyl hydroxylase defect	Supplement ascorbic acid
Fatty acid oxidation defects (mitochondrial)	Restrict fat; supplement glycine and L-carnitine; avoid fasting
Folic acid reductase deficiency	Supplement N^5-formyltetrahydrofolic acid
Folic acid transport defect	Supplement parenteral folate
Fructose intolerance	Fructose-free diet
Fructose malabsorption	Fructose-free diet
Fructose-1, 6-diphosphate deficiency	Reduce fructose intake; frequent glucose; supplement folate
Galactokinase deficiency	Galactose-restricted diet
Galactosemia	Galactose-restricted diet; aldose reductase inhibition
Gaucher disease, type I	Intravenous β-glucocerebrosidase
Glucose-galactose malabsorption	Restrict glucose and galactose; supplement fructose
Glucose-6-phosphate dehydrogenase deficiency	Avoid fava beans and drugs that cause erythrocyte hemolysis
Glutaric acidemia type I	Restrict lysine and tryptophan; supplement L-carnitine and riboflavin
Glutaric acidemia type II	Restrict fat and protein; supplement L-carnitine and riboflavin
Glycogen storage	
Type I (glucose-6-phosphatase deficiency)	Frequent feeding, supplement complex starch (liver transplantation)
Type III (amylo-1,6-glucosidase deficiency)	Frequent feeding, high protein
Type VI (phosphorylase deficiency)	Frequent feeding
Type VIII (phosphorylase kinase deficiency)	Avoid fasting; high protein
Glutamate-aspartate transport defect	Glutamine supplement
Gout	Restrict purine; allopurinol
Gyrate atrophy of the choroid and retina	Restrict arginine and protein; supplement essential amino acids
Hartnup disease	Supplement nicotinamide
Hereditary methemoglobinemia	Supplement ascorbate, riboflavin, and methylene blue
Histidinemia	None
Homocystinuria	
Cystathionine β-synthase deficiency	Restrict methionine; supplement cysteine; augment block with pyridoxine; provide alternate routes with folate and betaine
N^5,N^{10}-methylenetetrahydrofolate reductase deficiency	Supplement folic acid
3-Hydroxy-3-methylglutaryl-CoA lyase deficiency	Restrict leucine and fat
Hydroxykynureninuria	Supplement nicotinic acid
Hyperbeta-alaninemia	Supplement pyridoxine

(continued)

TABLE 58.2. NUTRITION TREATMENT OF GENETIC DISORDERS (continued)

DISORDER	THERAPY
Hypercholesterolemia	Restrict saturated fatty acids and cholesterol; supplement fiber, mevinolin, nicotinic acid, and cholestyramine
Hyperphenylalaninemia	
Dihydropteridine reductase deficiency	Restrict phenylalanine; carbidopa, 5-hydroxytryptophan, tetrahydrobiopterin
Biopterin biosynthetic blocks	Carbidopa, 5-hydroxytryptophan, tetrahydrobiopterin
Hyperornithinemia-hyperammonemia-homocitrullinuria syndrome	Restrict protein; supplement essential amino acids
Hypertriglyceridemia	Restrict carbohydrate; reduce weight
Hypophosphatemia	Supplement vitamin D and phosphorus
Isovaleric acidemia	Restrict leucine; supplement L-carnitine and glycine
Ketoacidosis of infancy	Supplement alkali and glucose
Lactic acidosis, intermittent	
Pyruvate dehydrogenase deficiency	Supplement thiamine; provide high-fat, low-carbohydrate diet; alkali
Pyruvate carboxylase deficiency	Supplement thiamine and biotin; alkali; frequent feeds
Lactose intolerance	Lactose restriction
Lipoprotein lipase deficiency	Supplement with essential fatty acids and medium-chain triglycerides; low-fat diet
Lysine intolerance (hyperlysinemia)	Restrict protein; supplement citrulline
Maple syrup urine disease	Restrict isoleucine, leucine, and valine; supplement thiamine
Methionine malabsorption	Restrict methionine; supplement cysteine
Methylmalonic aciduria	
Defective reduction or transport of cobalamin	Supplement parenteral megadoses of B_{12}, oral betaine, and OH-B_{12}
Impaired cobalamin methylation	Supplement parenteral megadoses of B_{12}, oral betaine, and OH-B_{12}
Impaired synthesis of 5'-deoxyadenosylcobalamin	Supplement parenteral megadoses of B_{12}, oral betaine and OH-B_{12}
Methylmalonyl-CoA mutase/racemase deficiency	Restrict isoleucine, methionine, threonine, and valine; supplement L-carnitine
Multiple carboxylase deficiency	Supplement biotin
Niemann-Pick disease type C	Restrict cholesterol; mevinolin, cholestyramine
Nonketotic hyperglycinemia	Restrict protein; supplement energy; benzoic acid, dextromethorphan
Ornithine transcarbamylase deficiency	Restrict protein; supplement L-carnitine, arginine, benzoic acid, and phenylbutyrate or phenylacetate
Orotic aciduria	Supplement uridine
Oxalosis	Supplement water (liver and kidney transplantation), pyridoxine, and magnesium orthophosphate
Periodic paralysis	
Hypokalemic	Restrict carbohydrate; potassium salts, sodium chloride
Hyperkalemic	Increase carbohydrates
Peroxisome dysfunction	Supplement docosahexaenoic acid, bile acid, steroids, vitamin K
Phenylketonuria	Restrict phenylalanine; supplement tyrosine
Porphyria, acute intermittent	High glucose; hematin infusions for feedback control
Pseudohypoparathyroidism	Supplement calcium and vitamin D
Prolidase deficiency	L-Proline, $MgCl_2$, vitamin C
Propionic acidemia	Restrict isoleucine, methionine, threonine, and valine; supplement biotin and L-carnitine
Pyridoxine dependency with seizures	Parenteral pyridoxine; supplement oral pharmacologic B_6
Pyroglutamic aciduria	Restrict protein; alkali
Pyruvate dehydrogenase deficiency, partial	Restrict carbohydrate; supplement thiamine and energy (lipids); ketogenic diet
Refsum disease	Restrict phytanic acid; diet low in dairy and ruminant fats
Sucrose-isomaltose malabsorption	Restrict sucrose; ingestion of sucrase-isomaltase containing *Streptomyces cerevisiae*
Tryptophanuria with dwarfism	Nicotinic acid
Tyrosinemia type Ia	2-(2-Nitro-4-trifluoromethylbenzoyl)-1,3-cyclohexanedione); restrict phenylalanine and tyrosine; high-energy diet; liver transplantation
Tyrosinemia with keratosis and corneal dystrophy (type II)	Restrict phenylalanine and tyrosine
Tyrosinemia type III	Restrict phenylalanine and tyrosine
Valinemia	Restrict valine
Vitamin A defect (β-carotene 15, 15'-dioxygenase)	Supplement vitamin A
Vitamin B_{12} defect (conversion of B_{12} to precursor of 5'-deoxyadenosyl-B_{12} and methyl B_{12})	Supplement vitamin B_{12}

(continued)

TABLE 58.2. NUTRITION TREATMENT OF GENETIC DISORDERS (continued)

DISORDER	THERAPY
Vitamin D-dependent rickets	Supplement 1,25 dihydroxy D
Vitamin K-dependent coagulation defects (factors VII, IX, and I; protein C, protein S deficiency)	Supplement vitamin K
Williams-Beuren syndrome	Restrict calcium and vitamin D
Wilson disease	Restrict copper; D-penicillamine
Xanthinuria	Restrict purine; supplement allopurinol, fluids, and alkali
Xanthurenic aciduria	Pyridoxine

disorders for which population-based screening, retrieval, diagnosis, and nutrition support are available to prevent their irreversible, severe pathologic problems.

GENERAL PRINCIPLES OF GENETIC DISEASE MANAGEMENT

Specific enzymes produced under the direction of individual genes catalyze specific reactions as noted in the following genetic and metabolic sequences. Substrate A is transported unchanged into the cell. A is converted to D through intermediates B and C using enzymes AB, BC, and CD:

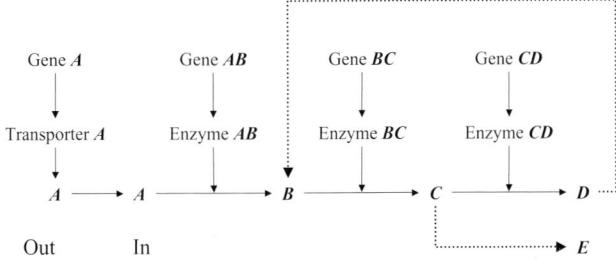

If enzyme CD were genetically impaired, at least six pathophysiologic consequences could occur:

1. Deficiency of product D. For example, in PKU, when PHE is not hydroxylated to form TYR, not only is accumulated PHE toxic, but also TYR becomes an essential nutrient. TYR must be supplemented to maintain proper growth in the dietary management of PKU.
2. Loss of feedback control. If product D normally functions in feedback control of enzyme AB, overproduction of an intermediate product may occur because D is not present in amounts necessary to regulate production of intermediates B and C. An example of this phenomenon is acute intermittent porphyria, in which heme is deficient and does not exert feedback control on δ-aminolevulinic acid (δ-ALA) and porphobilinogen synthesis, with consequent excess accumulation and neuropathic sequelae.
3. Accumulation of C, the immediate precursor of the blocked reaction. In MSUD, toxic BCKAs accumulate

because they can neither be decarboxylated and transacylated to their coenzyme A (CoA)-acyl acid derivatives nor completely reaminated by their BCAA precursors. The consequence in the neonate is severe central nervous system (CNS) depression and apnea, stupor, coma, and death. If the neonate survives, permanent encephalopathy ensues if the child is not treated by diet restriction within the first week of life.

4. Accumulation of A or B, remote precursors of the blocked reaction sequence CD. If the preceding reactions are freely reversible, a precursor, in addition to the one immediately before the block, will accumulate. This process is illustrated in MSUD by increased LEU, ILE, and VAL, which are formed by reamination of the accumulating BCKAs: α-ketoisocaproic, α-keto-β-methylvaleric, and α-ketoisovaleric acids, respectively.
5. Increased production of alternative products (E) through little-used metabolic pathways. As illustrated in Figure 58.1, when PHE accumulates because of impaired PHE hydroxylase (PAH), phenylpyruvic, phenylacetic, and phenyllactic acids are produced in larger-than-normal amounts through existing pathways that normally do not function at physiologic concentrations of cellular PHE.
6. Inhibition of alternate pathways by accumulated substrate. For example, neurotransmitter synthesis may be depressed in PKU owing to increased blood PHE that competitively inhibits TYR hydroxylase and tryptophan (TRP) hydroxylase in the CNS. Another example is type I tyrosinemia. The accumulation of succinylacetone inhibits δ-ALA dehydratase (Fig. 58.2) and results in secondary accumulation of δ-ALA, attacks of acute porphyria with peripheral neuropathy, hypertension, and bizarre behavior.

Twelve approaches to therapy of inherited metabolic disease are discussed here. The choice of therapy depends on the mechanisms producing disease. Several therapeutic approaches may be tried sequentially or used simultaneously, depending on the acuteness of the disease process.

1. Enhancing anabolism and depressing catabolism. This involves the use of high-energy feeds, appropriate

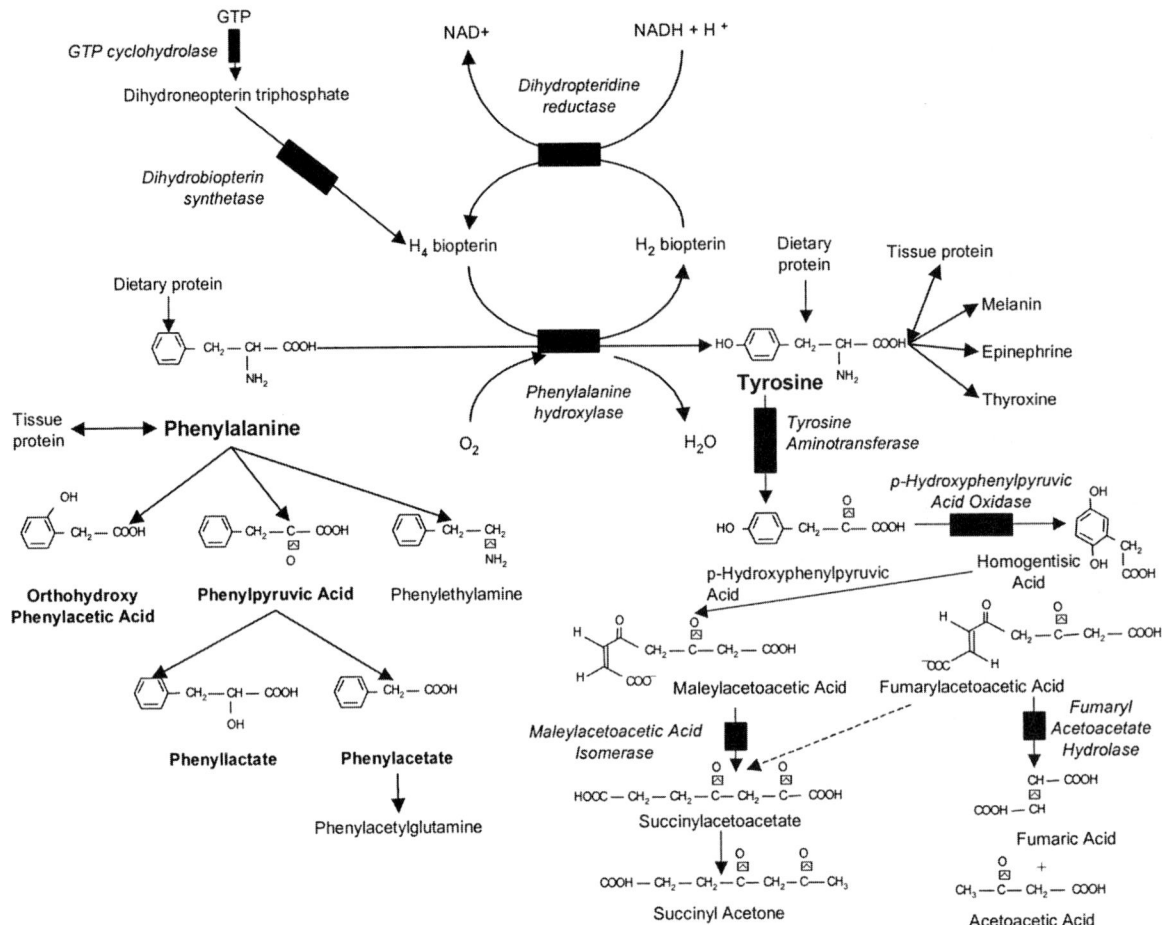

Figure 58.1. Metabolism of aromatic amino acids. The metabolic flow and nutrient interaction in disorders of phenylalanine and tyrosine are diagrammed. The *black bars* represent impaired enzymes in biopterin biosynthesis, phenylketonuria, and tyrosinemia. GTP, guanosine triphosphate; NAD, nicotinamide adenine dinucleotide (NADH is the reduced form).

amino acid mixtures, and occasionally the administration of insulin. A catabolic state must be prevented. This therapeutic maneuver should be common to all inborn errors involving catabolic pathways. However, caution must be exercised to use high-energy feeds primarily during the acute presentation, but not chronically, to prevent overweight or obesity.

2. Correcting the primary imbalance in metabolic relationships. This correction involves using both dietary restriction to reduce accumulated substrate(s) that are toxic and provision of products that may be deficient. For example, in PAH deficiency, PHE is restricted and TYR is supplemented.

3. Enhancing excretion of accumulated substances that are overproduced. The kidney can aid as a dialysis organ in removing accumulated toxic precursors. Maintaining diuresis with hydration is a critical component of therapy.

4. Providing alternative metabolic pathways to decrease accumulated toxic precursors in blocked reaction sequences. There are many examples, for instance the accumulated ammonia in enzyme defects of the urea

cycle is reduced by removing nitrogen through administration of therapeutic amounts of phenylbutyric or phenylacetic acid to form phenylacetylglutamine from glutamine. Similarly, in isovaleric acidemia, innocuous isovalerylglycine (IVG) is formed from accumulating isovaleric acid (IVA) if supplemental glycine (GLY) is provided to drive GLY-*N*-transacylase. IVG is then excreted in the urine. Betaine is used to drive methylation of homocysteine to methionine (MET) in cystathionine β-synthase (CβS) deficiency.

5. Using metabolic inhibitors to lower overproduced products. For example, allopurinol inhibits xanthine oxidase and decreases overproduction of uric acid in gout, lovastatin and compactin suppress hydroxymethylglutaryl CoA reductase and reduce excess cholesterol biosynthesis in familial hypercholesterolemia, and 2-(2-nitro-4-trifluoromethylbenzoyl)-1,3-cyclohexanedione) (NTBC) inhibits *p*-hydroxyphenylpyruvic acid dioxygenase (*p*-OHPPAD) and thus succinylacetone production in type I tyrosinemia.

6. Supplying products of blocked secondary pathways. In cystic fibrosis, the exocrine pancreas does not function

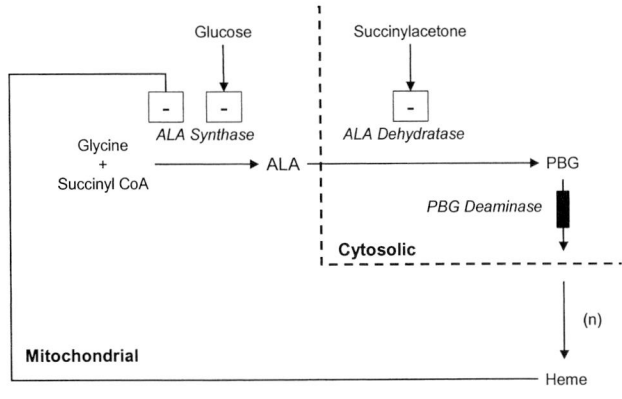

Negative feedback or inhibition.

ALA = δ-aminolevulinic acid; PBG, porphobilinogen

Figure 58.2. Inhibition site in heme biosynthesis of relevance to diagnosis and treatment of tyrosinemia type I. The *black bar* represents the partial block in acute intermittent porphyria with resultant overproduction of δ-aminolevulinic acid (δ-ALA) and porphobilinogen (PBG) with decreased heme biosynthesis. In type I tyrosinemia, succinylacetone is produced and inhibits δ-ALA dehydratase with accumulation of δ-ALA alone, which is neurotoxic. δ-ALA accumulation can be reduced by addition of excess dietary glucose and by hematin infusions that negatively control δ-ALA synthase at levels of both enzyme and gene expression.

in a normal manner to produce and secrete digestive enzymes. Administration of these pancreatic enzymes partially corrects this insufficiency and may prevent the sequelae of fat-soluble vitamin deficiency in the newborn and young child.

7. Stabilizing altered enzyme proteins. The rate of biologic synthesis and degradation of holoenzymes depends on their structural conformation. In some holoenzymes, saturation by coenzyme increases their biologic half-life, and thus overall enzyme activity at the equilibrium produced by mutant proteins. This therapeutic mechanism is exemplified in homocystinuria and MSUD. Pharmacologic intake of vitamin B_6 in homocystinuria or vitamin B_1 in MSUD increases intracellular pyridoxal phosphate or thiamin pyrophosphate (TPP) and will increase the specific activity of CβS or BCKAD complex, respectively (9–12). Another approach is to provide chemical chaperones to stabilize mutant proteins. For example, excess intravenous infusion of D-galactose has increased defective α-galactosidase in the cardiac variant of Fabry disease (13).

8. Replacing deficient coenzymes. A variety of vitamin-dependent disorders are caused by blocks in coenzyme production and are "cured" by lifetime pharmacologic intake of a specific vitamin precursor. This mechanism presumably involves overcoming a partially impaired enzyme reaction by mass action. If reactions are impaired that are required to produce methylcobalamin (CH_3-B_{12}) and/or adenosylcobalamin, homocystinuria or MMA (or both) will result. Daily intake of milligram quantities of vitamin B_{12} may cure both disorders (14). In biotinidase deficiency,

the coenzyme biotin is not released from its covalently bound state. Reviews of "vitamin-dependency syndromes" have been published (10, 11).

9. Artificially inducing enzyme production. If the structural gene or enzyme is intact, but suppressor, enhancer, or promoter elements are not functional, abnormal amounts of enzyme may be produced. It should be possible to "turn on" or "turn off" the structural gene and enable normal enzymatic production to occur. In the acute porphyria of type I tyrosinemia, excessive δ-ALA production may be reduced by suppressing transcription of the δ-ALA synthase gene with excess glucose (GLU) and hematin (see Fig. 58.2). In type I tyrosinemia, the overproduction of succinyl acetone may be "turned off" by blocking an earlier enzyme *p*-OH-phenylpyruvate oxidase with the drug (NBTZ).

10. Replacing enzymes. Many attempts to replace deficient enzymes by plasma infusion and microencapsulation have been tried with limited success. Recently the use of polyethylene glycol coating of adenosine deaminase significantly prolonged the biologic half-life of this enzyme in treating severe combined immunodeficiency (15). The engineering of β-glucosidase with a high mannan receptor site enables intravenous use of Ceredase to treat type I Gaucher disease. Human α-galactosidase A replacement therapy in Fabry disease reverses substrate storage in the lysosome (13). Recombinant human α-glucosidase can prevent progression and improve cardiac and muscle function in Pompe disease (16).

11. Transplanting organs. Liver transplantation in a host of inherited metabolic disorders benefits systemic metabolism with the return of organ function replacing deficient enzyme activity (17, 18). Bone marrow and kidney transplantations are also of benefit.

12. Correcting the underlying defect in DNA so that the body can manufacture its own functionally normal enzymes. The DNA for many proteins that are functionally deficient, such as adenosine deaminase, hypoxanthine-guanine phosphoribosyl transferase, ornithine transcarbamylase (OTC), and the LDL cholesterol receptor have been cloned, and retroviral constructs containing their cDNA transfected into dividing somatic cells from affected individuals. Human gene therapy is currently contemplated for these inborn errors, although several technical problems in the toxicity of vectors, gene stability, and gene expression must be solved first. Other molecular approaches such as homologous recombination to correct mutant sequences or inhibit RNA for dominant disorders producing antagonism to the normal allele are also future possibilities (19, 20).

Nutrition management remains a principal component in treating all of these inherited disorders, and some practical considerations for nutrition support should be considered.

Foremost is the need to maintain normal growth, which cannot be achieved without adequate intake of energy, amino acids, and nitrogen. Energy requirements are greater than normal when intact protein is restricted and free amino acids supply protein equivalent (21). Free amino acids administered in one daily dose are oxidized to a much greater extent than those in the same dose divided and administered throughout the day (22). Nitrogen balance was improved considerably when free amino acids were ingested in several doses throughout the day with intact protein, rather than in one dose (23). If adequate energy and amino acids cannot be ingested to support normal growth through oral feeds, then nasogastric, gastrostomy, or parenteral feeds should be used. Failure to adapt nutrient intake to the individual needs of each patient can result in mental retardation, metabolic crises, neurologic crises, growth failure, and with some inherited metabolic diseases, death. When specific amino acids or nitrogen require restriction, total deletion of the toxic nutrient for one to three days in the presence of excess energy intake is the best approach to initiating therapy. Longer deletion or overrestriction may precipitate deficiency of the amino acid(s) or nitrogen. Because the most limiting nutrient in the diet determines growth rate, overrestriction of an amino acid, nitrogen, or energy will result in further intolerance of the toxic nutrient(s).

Diet restrictions to correct imbalances in metabolic relationships require the use of elemental medical foods. These medical foods must be accompanied by small amounts of intact protein that supply the restricted amino acid(s). Intact proteins seldom supply more than 50%, and often supply much less, of the protein requirements of patients. Nitrogen-free foods that provide energy are limited in their range of nutrients. Consequently, care must be taken to provide all nutrients required in adequate amounts (1).

Elemental medical foods consist of small molecules that often provide an osmolality that exceeds the physiologic tolerance of the patient. Abdominal cramping, diarrhea, distention, nausea, and vomiting result from hyperosmolar feeds. Aside from gastrointestinal distress, more serious consequences can occur, such as hypertonic dehydration, hypovolemia, hypernatremia, and death. Osmolalities of selected medical foods intended for inherited diseases of amino acid metabolism have been published (24).

AROMATIC AMINO ACIDS

Inborn errors of the aromatic amino acids were historically the first to respond to nutrition support. PKU was discovered in 1933, and the prevention of its resultant mental retardation by diet intervention is classic.

Biochemistry

The essential amino acid PHE is used for tissue protein synthesis and hydroxylation to form TYR. The hydroxylation reaction requires PAH, O_2, tetrahydrobiopterin (BH_4), dihydropteridine reductase (DHPR), and nicotinamide adenine dinucleotide + H^+ (see Fig. 58.1). The normal adult uses only 10% of the RDA for PHE for new protein synthesis, and approximately 90% is hydroxylated to form TYR. The growing child uses 60% of the required PHE for new protein synthesis, and 40% is hydroxylated to form TYR. Mass spectrometry and stable isotope studies of patients with PKU provide information on other pathways available for PHE metabolism. These alternative pathways (see Fig. 58.1) are minor in the metabolism of PHE at 50 μmol/L concentration in the plasma of normal individuals. However, byproducts become apparent when PHE is not hydroxylated to TYR and accumulates to more than 500 μmol/L (25).

TYR is the normal immediate product of PHE and is essential to five pathways (see Fig. 58.1), including synthesis of protein, catecholamines, melanin pigment, and thyroid hormones. TYR also provides energy when catabolized through p-OHPPAD to fumarate and acetoacetate. Enzymes required in this latter degradative pathway include TYR aminotransferase, p-OHPPAD, homogentisic acid oxidase, and fumarylacetoacetic acid hydrolase (FAH) (see Fig. 58.1).

Phenylketonuria

PKU is a group of inherited disorders of PHE metabolism caused by impaired PAH activity. The disease is expressed at 3 to 6 months of age and is characterized by developmental delay, microcephaly, abnormal electroencephalogram (EEG), eczema, musty odor, and hyperactivity. If not treated before 2 weeks of age, the metabolic imbalance produces mental retardation that is worsened with increasing time to treatment. The defect in metabolism in classic PKU is associated with less than 2% of the activity of normal PAH, and these classic mutations are now defined (26). The enzyme is expressed primarily in liver.

Molecular Biology. Five of the most frequent mutations in a US clinic include I65T, R408W, Y414C, L348V, and IVS10nt546, which account for more than 50% of mutant PAH alleles. Genotypes with R408W and IVS10nt546 result in more severe PAH impairment, whereas Y414C and I65T have relatively mild phenotypes (26). Heterozygous parents for classic PKU have 50% enzyme activity, and in the absence of known DNA changes, can be identified by increased ratios of midday semifasting PHE squared to TYR (P^2/T) in vivo (27).

The genetic bases for disorders of PAH followed localization of the PAH gene to chromosome 12q22-q24.1 and cloning of the gene, which has 90 kilobases (kb), 13 exons, and 12 introns (Table 58.3). Four hundred and forty-nine different mutations have been identified that cause the "PKU phenotype," and these involve deletions in coding frames, missense mutations, and intron splice site mutations. Ethnic variation occurs in the type and frequency of PAH mutations (25). Cloning of the PAH gene and identification of different mutations have assisted in genotyping probands, counseling families, and predicting the amount of dietary PHE that will be required (26). Immediate and

TABLE 58.3. CHROMOSOMAL LOCATION, GENE SIZE, NUMBER OF EXONS, NUMBER OF MUTATIONS, TISSUE DISTRIBUTION OF GENES, AND GENOTYPE/PHENOTYPE CORRELATIONS

ENZYME	CHROMOSOMAL LOCATION	GENE SIZE (kb)	NUMBER OF MUTATIONS	TISSUE DISTRIBUTION	GENOTYPE/ PHENOTYPE CORRELATION
Enzymes of Amino Acid Metabolism					
Phenylalanine hydroxylase	12q22-q24.1	>90	449	Liver, kidney	Genotype broadly predicts metabolic and clinical phenotype
Dihydropteridine reductase	4p15.1-p16.1		21	Liver, fibroblasts, erythrocytes, leukocytes, platelets	?
Guanorine triphosphate cyclohydrolase	14q22.1-q22.2	30	42	Liver	None
6-pyruvoyltetrahydropterin synthase	11q22.3-q23.3	?	>28	Liver, erythrocytes	Genotype associated with phenotype
Pterin-4 α-carbinolamino dehydratase	10q22		7	Lymphocytes, scalp hair root cells	Mild phenotypes
Fumarylacetoacetate hydrolyase	15q23-q25		34	Liver, renal tubules, lymphocytes, erythrocytes	Genotype not clearly associated with phenotype
Maleylacetoacetate isomerase	14q24.3	?	3	Liver, fibroblasts, kidney	?
Tyrosine aminotransferase	16q22.1	10.9	15	Liver, kidney	None
4-hydroxyphenylpyruvate dioxygenase	12q24-qter	21	?	Liver	?
Cystathiomne β-synthase	21q22.3	30	30	Liver, fibroblasts, brain, phytohemagglutinin-stimulated lymphocytes, amniotic fluid cells, chorionic villus cells	Genotype associated with phenotype I278T - B_6 responsive T353M - African, non-B_6 responsive G307S - Celtic, non-B_6 responsive
Enzymes of Organic Acid Metabolism					
Branched-chain α-ketoacid dehydrogenase complex					
E1α (decarboxylase)	19q13.3	55	12	Liver, fibroblasts, leucocytes, muscle	Y393W (Mennonite) (classical phenotype)
E1β (stabilizes E1 α)	6q1.4	100	4	Liver, fibroblasts, leucocytes, muscle	11bp del → stop
E2 (transacylase)	1p31	68	6	Liver, fibroblasts, leucocytes, muscle	E163X R183P, common in Ashkenazi?
E3 (lipoamide dehydrogenase)	7p22	20	10	Liver, fibroblasts, leucocytes, muscle	Affects pyruvate and α-ketoglutarate dehydrogenases as well
E1α kinase (inactivating)	16p13.12	40	2	Liver, fibroblasts, leucocytes, muscle	Inhibited by-tumor neaosis factor-α and produces cancer cachexia
E1α phosphatase (activating)	?	?	?	Liver, fibroblasts, leucocytes, muscle	Actives branchedchain α-ketoacid dehydrogenase complex
Isovaleryl-CoA dehydrogenase	15q14-q15	2.1–4.6	20	Liver, fibroblasts	Genotype not associated with phenotype
3-Methylcrotonyl-CoA carboxylase	?	?	?	Fibroblasts, lymphocytes	Genotype associated with phenotype
3-Methyfglutaconyl-CoA-hydratase (type 1)	?	?	?	Fibroblasts, lymphocytes	?
3-Hydroxy-3-methyl-glutaryl-CoA lyase	1p35.1.36.1	?	?	Liver	Genotype associated with phenotype

(continued)

TABLE 58.3. CHROMOSOMAL LOCATION, GENE SIZE, NUMBER OF EXONS, NUMBER OF MUTATIONS, TISSUE DISTRIBUTION OF GENES, AND GENOTYPE/PHENOTYPE CORRELATIONS (continued)

Glutaryl-CoA dehydrogenase	19p13.2	7	>90	Liver, kidney, fibroblasts, leukocytes, amniotic fluid cells, chorionic villus cells	None between genotype and clinical severity Specific mutations correlate with severity of organic aciduria
Propionyl-CoA carboxylase				Heart, kidney, liver cells	None
α-subunit	13q32	100	?		
β-subunit	3q13.3q22	?	?		
Methylmalonyl-CoA mutase	6p12-p21.2		22	Kidney, liver, placenta cells	Genotype associated with phenotype
Enzymes of Nitrogen Metabolism					
Mitochondrial					
Carbamylphosphate synthetase 1	2q35	122	>32	Liver, intestine, kidney (trace)	Genotype associated with phenotype
N-acetylglutamate synthetase	17q21.31	?	?	Liver, intestine, kidney (trace), spleen	Genotype associated with phenotype
Ornithine transcarbamylase	Xp21.1	73	>230	Liver, intestine, kidney (trace)	Genotype associated with phenotype
Cytosol					
Argininosuccinate synthetase	9q34.1 (many pseudogenes) 7cen-q11.2	53	14	Liver, kidney, fibroblasts, brain (trace)	Genotype associated with phenotype
Argininosuccinate lyase	?		12	Liver, kidney, brain, fibroblasts	Genotype associated with phenotype
Arginase	6q23	13	2	Liver, erythrocytes, lens, brain (trace)	Genotype associated with phenotype
Enzymes of Galactose Metabolism					
Galactose-4-epimerase	1p36-35	4	9	Erythrocytes, fibroblasts, liver	Unclear
Galactokinase	17p24	7.3	13	Liver	Cataracts only
Galactose-1-phosphate uridyltransferase	9p13	4.3	>150	Erythrocytes, leukocyte, fibroblasts, intestinal mucosa, liver	Genotype associated with phenotype Q188R (white) S135L (black) Δ5 kg (Ashvenazim)

CoA, coenzyme A.

lifelong avoidance of excess PHE in the diet continues to be the principal therapy of PKU.

Several investigators have recently reported oral 6-R-1-erythro-5,6,7,8-tetrahydrobiopterin responsiveness within 24 to 48 hours at doses of 5 to 10 mg/kg in patients with selected mild mutations in the PAH gene (28–32). A hypothesis has been proposed whereby oral administration of BH_4 makes it possible for the mutant enzymes to suppress their low binding affinity for BH_4, enabling this subset of PAH mutations to perform the PHE hydroxylation reaction (32). Although certain genotypes, such as those containing L485, may respond with increased PAH gene expression, other missense mutations may have effects on increased catalysis or increased PAH stability. Further studies are required to determine the best practice for BH_4 use, and entry into a research protocol is advised.

Other forms of PKU may result from defects in other enzymes involved in the overall reaction. DHPR, an enzyme normally present in many tissues, reduces the quinonoid form of dihydrobiopterin to BH_4 (see Fig. 58.1). The gene for DHPR is located on chromosome 4p15.1-p16.1. Several other types of PKU result from defects in the synthesis of BH_4 (see Fig. 58.1) (see Table 58.3). In addition to functioning as a coenzyme for PAH, BH_4 is also required by TYR hydroxylase and TRP hydroxylase (see Fig. 58.1). Because these enzymes produce essential neurotransmitters, defects in biopterin synthesis are associated with progressive neurologic disease unless BH_4, L-3,4-dihydroxyphenylalanine (L-DOPA), and serotonin are replaced (33).

Although the precise pathogenesis of mental retardation in classic PKU is not known, accumulation of PHE or its catabolic byproducts, deficiency of TYR or its products, or all four circumstances will produce CNS damage if PHE accumulates in plasma above normal concentrations during critical periods of brain development. The pathologic consequence varies with the time in brain development at which the chemical insult occurs. Deficient myelination and abnormalities in brain proteolipids and/or proteins occur in late gestation and during the first 6 to 9 months of life (34). During this period, oligodendroglia migration may also be impaired, resulting in irreversible brain damage later in childhood. Protein synthesis in the brain is also depressed, probably owing to competitive inhibition by high PHE concentrations on blood-brain barrier transport with consequent imbalance in intraneuronal amino acid concentrations (35). In the mature brain, neurodegeneration (36), behavioral difficulties, and prolonged performance times may result from depressed neurotransmitter synthesis. Impairment of these neuropsychological functions in the mature brain may be reversible when PHE returns toward normal concentrations in cells and blood (37, 38).

Screening. The disorders of PHE metabolism require identification, diagnosis, and appropriate therapy before clinical expression of the disease. Nutrition and possibly other therapy should be instituted before the third week of life. Thus, a tetrapartite public health program involving screening, retrieval, diagnosis, and treatment must be coordinated and efficient to prevent mental retardation. A screening test of dried blood on filter paper using the bacterial inhibition assay (39) or, more recently, tandem mass spectrometry (MS/MS) (40) detects potential cases in the newborn population. The actions taken in retrieval depend on the concentration of blood PHE, days of age, and protein intake at the time of screening.

Protein ingestion may not be required for a positive PKU screen, but quantitative normal concentrations during the first 48 hours of life are needed for comparison (41). Almost all infants with PKU have blood PHE concentrations above normal during the first day of life, even before the first feeding if they have classic PKU mutations (26). Neonates with PAH gene mutations resulting in less severely impaired PAH may take longer to develop an elevated blood PHE concentration. Some infants with a relatively mild elevation of blood PHE have serious neuropathology that is progressive because of a defect in synthesis of BH_4.

Newborn screening in all 50 states, in conjunction with aggressive, rapid approaches to retrieval and diagnosis, has led to early institution of diet therapy and prevention of mental retardation (41). With the present early infant discharge from the newborn nursery and the increase in breast-feeding, lower PHE concentrations of 121 to 242 μmol/L (2 to 4 mg/dL) are considered positive and follow-up is initiated (42). Approximately one in 14,000 white newborns in the United States is affected with PKU (43), whereas one in 132,000 newborns in the black population is affected (44). For non-PKU hyperphenylalaninemia without tyrosine elevation, the estimated incidence is one in 48,000 for all newborns (43).

Diagnosis. If the follow-up screening test yields blood PHE levels above 242 μmol/L (4 mg/dL), all plasma amino acids should be quantitated by ion-exchange chromatography with the infant on a known PHE intake from intact protein sources. A precise diagnosis is necessary to establish the mode of therapy.

Differential diagnosis requires several laboratory procedures. These include ion-exchange chromatography or MS/MS to determine plasma PHE, TYR, and other amino acid concentrations; urinary organic analysis by gas chromatography/MS (GC/MS) genotyping of parents and proband (25, 26, 45); and assays of erythrocyte DHPR and urinary biopterin (46). For families with an affected child, prenatal diagnosis is available through direct mutational analysis of fetal cell DNA for known PAH genes, or indirect restriction fragment length polymorphism analysis of PAH in parents and proband for unknown fetal PAH genes (25). Because PAH is not expressed in cultured amniotic fluid cells and because PHE concentrations do not increase in amniotic fluid until the last trimester, prenatal diagnosis was not possible before molecular techniques became available.

Treatment. Patients with plasma PHE concentrations above 250 μmol, plasma TYR concentrations below 50 μmol, and normal BH_4 and DHPR require prompt treatment with a PHE-restricted, TYR-supplemented diet. The objective of nutrition support of the child with classic PKU is to maintain blood PHE concentrations that will allow optimum growth and brain development by supplying adequate energy, protein, and other nutrients while restricting PHE and supplementing TYR intake.

Therapy of the child with biopterin-deficient forms of hyperphenylalaninemia requires administration of BH_4 and use of the PHE-restricted, TYR-supplemented diet in combination with L-DOPA and carbidopa (46). Serotonin that is derived from TRP may improve behavior because TRP hydroxylase is also impaired by diminished BH_4 (33).

Initiation of Nutrition Support of Classic Phenylketonuria. Blood PHE concentration at the time of diagnosis may be rapidly lowered by feeding the infant a 20-kcal/oz (67 kcal/dL) PHE-free formula (47). A minimum of 120 kcal/kg/day intake is necessary. Within a mean of 4 days (SD ± 3), blood PHE concentration should decrease to treatment range on a PHE-free formula. Treatment should be initiated in hospitalized infants to enable adequate parental information transfer and to monitor blood amino acid concentrations daily. Laboratory results should be available promptly to prevent precipitation of PHE deficiency and to enable rapid replacement of blood PHE and TYR to optimum concentrations.

If the infant or child is not hospitalized for initiation of nutrition support or if only weekly blood PHE concentrations are obtained, 48 hours of a PHE-free formula followed by a maintenance formula containing adequate PHE should be prescribed. Blood PHE concentration will decrease to treatment range within a mean of 10 days (SD ± 5) with this approach (47). Blood PHE concentrations should be between 60 and 300 μmol no later than the third week of life.

Chronic Care. Long-term care of the patient with classic PKU dictates that medical food and intact protein provide all nutrients in required amounts.

Nutrient Requirements. Table 58.4 outlines the PHE, TYR, protein, energy, and fluid to offer. A prescription

TABLE 58.4. APPROXIMATE DAILY REQUIREMENTS FOR SELECTED NUTRIENTS[a] BY INFANTS AND CHILDREN WITH SELECTED INHERITED DISORDERS OF AMINO ACID AND ORGANIC ACID METABOLISM

NUTRIENT	UNIT	AGE						
		0–6 mo	6–12 mo	1–4 y	4–7 y	7–11 y	11–15 y	15–19 y
Energy	kcal/kg[b]	150–100	140–85	—	—	—	—	—
	kcal/d (range)	—	—	1,300 (900–800)	1,700 (1,300–2,300)	2,400 (1,650–3,300)	2,200–2,700 (1,500–3,700)	2,100–1,800 (1,200–3,900)
Fluid	mL/kg[b]	160–135	145–120	95	90	75	50–55	50–65
Protein	g/kg	3.5–3.0	3.0–2.5	—	—	—	—	—
	g/d	—	—	30	35	40	50–55	50–65
Carbohydrate	g/d	$\dfrac{\text{kcal} \times 0.35 \text{ to } 0.30}{4}$	$\dfrac{\text{kcal} \times 0.50 \text{ to } 0.60}{4}$					
Fat	g/d	$\dfrac{\text{kcal} \times 0.50}{9}$		$\dfrac{\text{kcal} \times 0.25 \text{ to } 0.35}{9}$				
Linoleic acid	g/d	$\dfrac{\text{kcal/d} \times 0.0}{9}$						
α-Linolenic acid	g/d	$\dfrac{\text{kcal/d} \times 0.006}{9}$						
Isoleucine,[c]								
MSUD	mg/kg	90–30	90–30	85–20	80–20	30–20	30–20	30–10
PPA/MMA[c]	mg/kg	100–70	90–60	80–50	70–40	60–30	50–25	40–20
Leucine,[c] MSUD	mg/kg	100–60	75–40	70–40	65–35	60–30	50–30	41–15
Isovaleric acidemia[c]	mg/kg	150–70	130–70	100–60	90–50	80–40	70–30	60–25
Lysine, GA-I[c]	mg/kg	100–70	90–40	80–30	75–25	65–25	60–20	55–15
Methionine,[c] homocystine,								
HCU	mg/kg	35–20	35–15	30–10	20–10	20–10	20–10	10–5
PPA/MMA	mg/kg	50–30	45–25	40–20	35–15	30–10	25–10	20–10
Phenylalanine,[c]								
PKU	mg/kg	70–20	50–15	40–15	35–15	30–15	30–15	30–10
Tyrosinemias[c]	mg/kg	95–45	90–35	85–30	80–25	70–20	70–20	65–15
Threonine,[c]								
PPA/MMA	mg/kg	80–50	70–40	60–30	55–25	50–25	45–25	40–25
Tyrosine,[c] PKU	mg/kg	350–300	300–250	230	175	140	110–120	110–120
Tyrosinemias	mg/kg	95–45	75–30	60–30	50–25	40–20	30–15	30–10
Tryptophan,[c] GA-I	mg/kg	40–10	30–10	20–10	15–8	10–6	8–5	8–4
Valine,[c] MSUD	mg/kg	95–40	60–30	85–30	50–30	30–25	30–20	30–15
PPA/MMA[c]	mg/kg	85–50	80–45	75–45	70–40	60–30	60–30	50–30

GA-I, glutaric acidemia type I; MMA, methylmalonic acidemia; MSUD, maple syrup urine disease; PKU, phenylketonuria; PPA, propionic acidemia.
[a] All known essential amino acids, essential fatty acids, minerals, and vitamins must be provided in adequate amounts.
[b] At least 1.5 mL of fluid should be offered for each kilocalorie of energy ingested by the infant and 1 mL/kcal by children and adults.
[c] After 1 to 3 days of deleting appropriate amino acids, introduce those amino acids at the maximum noted for age. Monitor plasma concentrations frequently, and modify amino acid prescription appropriately.

must be written that is individualized to the age, specific genotype (26), growth rate, and energy needs of each patient. Weekly adjustments in the diet prescription are necessary during the first 6 months of life, based on hunger, growth, development, and laboratory analyses of plasma PHE and TYR concentrations. The prescribed PHE should maintain the 3- to 4-hour postprandial plasma PHE concentration between 60 and 300 μmol (48). PHE is an essential amino acid (49) and cannot be deleted from the diet without producing death. Excess restriction produces growth failure, rashes, bone changes, and mental retardation (50).

The infant with classic PKU requires 20 to 50 mg PHE per kilogram body weight for growth, with younger infants requiring the larger amount (51). The PHE requirement declines rapidly between 3 and 6 months of age as growth rate declines. Requirements for PHE in the 6- to 12-month-old patient with classic PKU may decrease to 15 mg/kg/day, but they vary considerably (see Table 58.4). Frequent monitoring of blood PHE and TYR concentrations and of intake is required to prevent excess intake when growth rate decelerates and to prevent inadequate intake when growth rate is at its peak, as in early infancy and during the prepubertal and pubertal growth spurts.

TYR is an essential amino acid for individuals with PKU. For this reason, plasma TYR concentrations must be monitored; if they are low, L-TYR supplements are given. To supply adequate TYR intake to patients with PKU, about 10% of protein prescribed should be as TYR. TYR supplements alone will not prevent mental retardation in classic PKU (52).

Protein requirements are increased above the RDA when a free amino acid mix is the primary protein source rather than intact protein (53). Thus, recommendations for protein for nutrition support exceed the RDA. A mean protein intake 24% above the 1989 RDA for age was associated with greater PHE tolerance and growth in infants with PKU than was found when mean protein intake was near the RDA (54). Recommendations for energy and fluid intake (see Table 58.4) are the same as those for normal individuals (1).

Minerals and some vitamins often must be considerably greater than the RDA for age (1) to prevent deficiency in patients on elemental diets (55, 56). See Table 58.5 for recommended mineral and vitamin intakes.

TABLE 58.5. RECOMMENDED DIETARY ALLOWANCES FOR MINERALS AND VITAMINS BY INFANTS AND CHILDREN

NUTRIENT	RECOMMENDED INTAKE FOR AGE						
	0–<6 mo	0–<12 mo	1–<4 y	4–<7 y	7–<11 y	11–<15 y	15–<19 y
Minerals							
Calcium (mg)	400	600	800	800	1,300	1,300	1,300
Chloride (mEq)	8–20	11–34	14–43	20–60	26–79	40–120	40–120
Chromium (μg)	0.2	5.5	11	15	20	25	25
Copper (mg)	0.20	0.22	1.0–1.5	1.5–2.0	2.0–2.5	2.0–3.0	2.0–3.0
Iodine (μg)	40	50	70	90	120	150	150
Iron (mg)[a]	10	15	15	10	10	18	18
Magnesium (mg)	50	75	150	200	250	410	410
Manganese (mg)	0.3	0.6	1.0–1.5	1.5–2.0	2.0–3.0	2.5–5.0	2.5–5.0
Molybdenum (μg)	2.0	3.0	17	22	22	43	45
Phosphorus (mg)	300	500	800	800	1,250	1,250	1,200
Potassium (mEq)	9–24	11–33	14–42	20–60	26–77	39–117	39–117
Selenium (μg)	15	20	20	30	40	55	55
Sodium (mEq)	5–15	11–33	14–42	20–59	26–78	39–117	39–117
Zinc (mg)	5	5	10	10	10	15	15
Vitamins							
A (μg RE)	400	500	400	500	700	1,000	1,000
D (μg)	5	5	5	5	5	5	5
E (mg α-TE)	6	7	6	7	11	15	15
K (μg)	5	10	15	20	30	45	65
Ascorbic acid (mg)	40	50	45	45	45	75	90
Biotin, (μg)	35	50	65	85	120	120	120
B_6 (mg)	0.3	0.6	0.9	1.3	1.6	1.8	2.0
B_{12} (μg)	0.5	1.5	2.0	2.5	3.0	3.0	3.0
Choline (mg)	125	150	200	250	375	550	550
Folate (μg)	65	80	150	200	300	400	400
Niacin equiv (mg)	6	8	9	11	16	18	18
Pantothenic acid (mg)	2.0	3.0	3.0	3.0	4.0	5.0	5.0
Riboflavin (mg)	0.4	0.6	0.8	1.0	1.4	1.6	1.7
Thiamin (mg)	0.3	0.5	0.7	0.9	1.2	1.4	1.4

[a] Iron needs of patients with phenylketonuria may be greater than recommended dietary allowances. See references 55 and 90.
[b] Niacin needs of patients with phenylketonuria are greater than recommended dietary allowances. See reference 56.

Adapted from Trumbo P, schlicker S, yates AA et al. J Am Diet Assoc. 2002; 102:1621–30, with permission.

Phenylalanine-Free Medical Foods. Adequate amino acids and nitrogen cannot be obtained from intact protein without ingesting excess PHE (intact proteins contain 2-9% PHE by weight) (57). Thus, special elemental medical foods are used to provide protein, minerals, and vitamins. Formulations, composition of major nutrients, and sources of these products are given in Appendix Table A-25-a.

Intact Proteins. Serving lists are available to simplify the PHE-restricted diet for families and professional persons guiding them (see Appendix Table A-25-b). The lists are similar to diabetic exchange lists in that foods of similar PHE content are grouped together and can be exchanged one for another within a list to vary the diet. Portion sizes of foods in each list may be found in reference 58.

Diet plans for infants with PKU using different medical foods may be found in Appendix Table A-25-c. By 4 years of age, patients with some genotypes might require as much as 25 mg/kg/day and others as little as 15 mg/kg. Periflex, Phenex-2, Phenyl-Free 2, Phenyl-Free 2 HP, XP Maxamaid, or XP Maxamum are available medical foods for patients more than 1 year of age (see Appendix Table A-25-a) (58–60).

Management Problems. Management problems described for children with PKU occur in other children with inherited disorders of metabolism. Principles described here apply to children with other disorders as well but are not reiterated in other sections.

Maintenance of an adequate intake of protein and energy is important for the infant and child with PKU, although PHE must be restricted. Excess energy intake may lead to obesity (61) that is difficult to correct, and weight loss results in elevation of plasma PHE concentrations. Nutrition support must be aggressive, and if intake fails to meet the prescription, a nasogastric or gastrostomy tube should be placed to achieve anabolism. This is extremely important in disorders of BCAAs and nitrogen metabolism. Amino acids and nitrogen are obtained from medical foods; therefore, the amount of medical food offered must be varied to provide needs. Nonprotein sources of energy such as corn syrup (57), Modular and Protein-Free Diet Powder (Mead Johnson Nutritionals, Evansville, IN) (60), Polycose Glucose Polymers, Pro-Phree (Ross Products Division, Abbott Laboratories, Columbus, OH) (58), Duocal (Scientific Hospital Supplies, Ltd, Gaithersburg, MD) (59), sugar, and pure fats (57) can be added to maintain energy intake and to satisfy the child's hunger without affecting blood PHE concentrations.

Various factors may influence blood PHE concentrations. Those that may elevate blood PHE concentration include acute infections or trauma with concomitant tissue catabolism, excessive or inadequate PHE intake, and inadequate protein or energy intake. Any infection should be promptly diagnosed and appropriately treated. The best approach to nutrition support during short-term infections is to decrease the intake of PHE and increase the intake of fluids and carbohydrates through the use of Pedialyte with added Polycose powder (Ross Products Division, Abbott

Laboratories, Columbus, OH); fruit juices; high-carbohydrate, protein-free beverages; and soft drinks that do not contain caffeine.

Excess PHE intake is the most common cause of elevated blood PHE concentration in the older child and adult with PKU. This condition may be caused by overprescription, misunderstanding of the diet by the caretaker, or dietary noncompliance. Frequent evaluations of blood PHE concentration with accompanying accurate diet diaries for calculation of intake are used to determine the dietary PHE prescription. By monitoring urinary organic acids, increases or decreases in ketone excretion aid in differentiating between inadequate calories and excess PHE intake, respectively.

PHE deficiency associated with inadequate PHE intake has three specific stages of development (62). The first stage is characterized biochemically by decreased blood and urine PHE. Clinically, the child may appear normal, lethargic, or anorectic and may fail to gain length or weight. In the older child, increases in blood alanine and β-hydroxybutyric and acetoacetic acidemia result from muscle alanine production and β-lipolysis. In the second stage, blood PHE concentrations increase as a result of muscle protein degradation, although blood TYR may be low. BCAA concentrations may increase with decreases in other plasma amino acids. Aminoaciduria appears because of renal tubular malabsorption. In this stage, body protein stores are catabolized, energy sources are depleted, and active membrane transport functions are impaired. Eczema is common. In the third stage of PHE deficiency, blood PHE concentration is below normal, as are those of other amino acids. Accompanying clinical manifestations include failure to grow, osteopenia, anemia, sparse hair, and, finally, death if the deficiency is not corrected by supplemental dietary PHE and TYR.

Insufficient protein intake results in an inadequate supply of essential amino acids and/or nitrogen for growth. When protein synthesis is decreased, PHE is no longer used for growth and accumulates in the blood. If catabolism occurs because of a prolonged lack of nitrogen and/or amino acid intake, the blood PHE concentration increases because tissue protein contains some 5.5% PHE. In instances of protein insufficiency, medical food intake should be increased to supply the required nitrogen and/or essential amino acids.

Energy, the first requirement of the body, is necessary for growth. When energy is provided as carbohydrate and fat, and if adequate nitrogen is available, nonessential amino acids may be synthesized from their ketoacid precursors. Further, carbohydrate ingestion leads to insulin secretion, and insulin promotes amino acid transport into the cell and consequent protein synthesis (63). When energy intake is inadequate, tissue catabolism occurs to meet energy needs. Such catabolism releases PHE, leading to an elevated blood PHE concentration. Sufficient energy must be provided through generous use of nonprotein and low-protein foods to ensure a normal growth rate.

A low blood PHE concentration (<25 μmol/L) may lead to a depressed appetite (64), decreased growth (65), and if prolonged, mental retardation (48). Low blood PHE concentrations are often caused by inadequate prescription of PHE. In such cases, the prescription for PHE can be increased by the addition of measured amounts of intact protein.

Assessment of Nutrition Support. Along with biweekly assessment of growth through measurement of length, weight, and head circumference and evaluation of development, the adequacy of PHE and TYR intake is determined by twice-weekly quantitation of plasma PHE and TYR concentrations during the first 6 months and weekly thereafter until the child is 1 year of age. The first year is the period of most rapid growth and of greatest vulnerability to nutrition insult. After 1 year of age, weekly blood tests suffice for monitoring the diet. If plasma PHE concentrations exceed 300 μmol/L (5 mg/dL), the prescription for PHE is decreased and frequent blood tests are done until plasma PHE concentrations are between 60 and 300 μmol/L.

For blood tests to be of use in adjusting the prescription, laboratory analyses must be both accurate and prompt. Fluorimetric, ion exchange, high-performance liquid chromatography, or MS/MS methods are quantitative and are preferred to the Guthrie bioassay test to monitor plasma PHE and TYR concentrations. If properly instructed, parents may be given responsibility for obtaining the specimens on filter paper or in microcapillary tubes and mailing them to a central laboratory.

A record of food ingested before blood sampling for PHE and TYR measurement is essential and should be kept by the child's caregiver. The correlation between the child's intake of PHE, TYR, protein, and energy; the child's clinical status; and the plasma PHE and TYR concentrations is considered when the diet is altered.

Results of Therapy. Early diagnosis and treatment (before 2 weeks of age) of infants with PKU with a nutritionally adequate, PHE-restricted, TYR-supplemented diet promote normal growth and prevent mental retardation. A national study showed that mean height, weight, head circumference, and intelligence quotient (IQ) scores of early-treated children were the same as those of normal children at 4 years of age (66, 67). Trefz and colleagues (45) reported that when blood PHE concentration was maintained below 360 μmol/L, there was no difference in mean IQ by genotype of 9-year-old children.

The semisynthetic nature of the PHE-restricted diet has led to questions concerning its adequacy. Mean serum carnitine (total and free) of treated patients was in the reference range when patients were fed medical foods containing carnitine (68, 69). Medical foods containing increased amounts of L-TYR have alleviated the problem of low plasma TYR concentrations (70, 71). After an overnight fast, the concentrations of plasma GLY were elevated in patients, one group of whom received a GLY-free medical food (Periflex, Scientific Hospital Supplies, Inc, Gaithersburg, MD) (72).

Treated patients with PKU often have below-normal concentrations of transthyretin when fed the RDA for protein (73). Arnold and colleagues (74) and Acosta and colleagues (61) reported a positive correlation between height and plasma transthyretin with concentrations less than 200 mg/L associated with poor linear growth.

Depressed plasma concentrations of total cholesterol have been reported in treated children and untreated adults with PKU (75–77). Pregnant women with PKU whose serum cholesterol concentrations failed to increase during early gestation often had a spontaneous abortion (78), possibly because of an inadequate hormonal response to pregnancy. Castillo and colleagues (79) reported inhibition of brain and liver 3-hydroxy-3-methylglutaryl-CoA reductase and mevalonate-5-pyrophosphate decarboxylase in experimental hyperphenylalaninemia. According to Artuch and colleagues (80), elevated plasma PHE concentrations resulted in decreased serum ubiquinone 10 concentrations. However, Hargreaves and colleagues (81) found no difference in mononuclear cell coenzyme Q_{10} concentrations among control, treated, and untreated patients with PKU. Lower-than-normal plasma and erythrocyte docosahexaenoic acid concentrations and higher-than-normal n-6 series fatty acid concentrations have been found in patients undergoing therapy for PKU (82, 83). The significance of these differences is unclear, but they appear to be diet related (84, 85).

Iron deficiency has been reported in children undergoing therapy for PKU despite intakes greater than the RDA (86, 87). A poor selenium status has been found in children with PKU who were receiving medical foods without added selenium (88). Patients with PKU and low selenium concentrations had elevated concentrations of T4 and rT3, which decreased significantly with selenium supplementation (89). Plasma retinol concentrations of children with PKU are often below those of normal subjects (73), but are within reference ranges with adequate medical food intake (90).

Bone changes were reported as early as 1956 in treated children with PKU. Preschool children with plasma PHE concentrations within treatment range had normal bone mineralization (91–94). Greeves and colleagues (95) reported that 25% of patients with PKU, most of whom were more than 8 years of age, had a history of fractures compared with 18% of normal siblings. Untreated PKU mice (PAH[enu-2]) had reduced mean femur weight compared with treated and control mice, and shorter mean femur length than control mice. Femur strength was greater in treated mice compared with control mice (96). Elevated serum prolactin concentrations in patients with poorly controlled PKU resulted in a high prevalence of menstrual irregularities in the girls (97). As blood PHE concentration increased in older patients under poor dietary control, values for bone mineral content and bone density were always lower than control values. Amino acid imbalances, inadequate protein intake, the need for phosphorus to buffer organic acids made from excess dietary PHE, and inadequate estrogen because of excess prolactin secretion could have contributed to bone abnormalities (98).

Mean plasma concentrations of immunoglobulin A and immunoglobulin M were significantly lower in patients with PKU undergoing therapy (99) than in normal children.

Diet Discontinuation. In the past, certain clinicians suggested that the diet might be discontinued at 4, 6, or 12 years of age with no adverse effects (100–103). Investigators have questioned this possibility because studies have shown significant differences in performance and intelligence in children (104, 105) and neurologic function in adults who discontinued the diet and those who remained on the diet (36, 105). Severe agoraphobia (106), reversible by a return to the PHE-restricted diet, has also been reported in adults. Vitamin B_{12} deficiency resulting in hematologic changes and neurologic disease occurs in off-diet patients who refuse foods of animal origin but fail to ingest PHE-free medical foods (107, 108). Vegan-type methylmalonic aciduria from vitamin B_{12} deficiency is the most likely pathophysiologic mechansim.

In studies using the patient as his or her own control, elevated plasma PHE concentrations prolonged the performance time on neuropsychologic tests of higher integrative function, reduced the mean power frequency of the EEG, and decreased urinary dopamine excretion and plasma L-DOPA in older treated patients with PKU (109, 110). A correlation was found between high plasma PHE concentrations, prolonged performance time on neuropsychologic tests, and decreased urinary dopamine in ten patients. In a study of eight additional patients, statistically significant decreases were found in the mean power frequency of the EEG and in plasma L-DOPA when plasma PHE concentration increased (110). EEG slowing occurred in PKU heterozygotes at concentration changes of blood PHE that are induced by aspartame ingestion (150 μmol/L) (37). These effects were reversible and correlated in the reverse direction when plasma PHE concentration was reduced. Severe neurologic deterioration occurred in several off-diet patients with PKU (36, 105). Reversal of most of the symptoms occurred in a patient who returned to a PHE-restricted, medical food–containing diet (36).

Maternal Phenylketonuria. Pregnant women with PKU who are untreated at conception and during gestation have children with intrauterine growth retardation, microcephaly, and congenital anomalies, often severe and incompatible with life. Mental retardation is common in children of mothers whose plasma PHE concentration is higher than the normal range (111). The pathogenesis of the fetal damage is uncertain but is believed to be related to elevated maternal blood PHE concentration (112) because PHE is actively transported across the placenta to the fetus (113). Fetal plasma PHE concentrations are one and one half to two times those of maternal blood (114). Such elevated fetal plasma PHE concentrations are again concentrated twofold to fourfold by the fetal blood-brain barrier (115). Intraneuronal PHE concentrations of 600 μmol

interfere with brain development by one or more of the several previously described mechanisms, including abnormal oligodendroglial migration and/or myelin and other protein synthesis (116). Thus, it is extremely important to maintain normal plasma PHE concentrations in the reproductive female with PKU before conception and throughout gestation. Surviving children of untreated women fail to grow and develop normally. In fact, Kirkman (117) predicted that if the fertility of these women is normal and they are not treated with dietary control of PHE intake, the incidence of PKU-related mental retardation could return to the prescreening level after only one generation.

In 1984, the Collaborative Study of Maternal Phenylketonuria (MPKUCS) was initiated to answer questions related to diet and reproductive outcome in women with PKU (118). Results of the MPKUCS support the premise that a PHE-restricted diet, plasma PHE concentrations lower than 360 μmol/L, and the gestational age at which it is initiated affect reproductive outcome (119).

Nutrition Support of Maternal Phenylketonuria. The PHE-restricted diet should be initiated at least 3 months before a planned pregnancy by women who have PKU, if they have previously discontinued the diet. The objectives of therapy for pregnant women with PKU are a healthy mother and a normal, healthy newborn. To obtain adequate protein and fat storage in early pregnancy to support third-trimester fetal growth, careful attention must be paid to diet and nutrition status. Although the plasma PHE concentration most likely to yield the best reproductive outcome is unknown, one group of investigators suggests that these objectives may be achieved by a PHE-restricted diet that maintains plasma PHE concentration between 60 and 180 μmol/L (120). Plasma PHE concentrations below 60 μmol/L may lead to maternal muscle wasting and poor fetal growth. The recommended PHE intake to prescribe for initiating therapy is given in Appendix Table A-25-d (121). Other indices of nutrition status should be in the normal range for pregnant women. After initiation of diet with the minimum recommended PHE prescription (see Appendix Table A-25-d), the plasma PHE concentration should be monitored twice weekly to maintain the targeted plasma PHE concentration.

Even after the plasma PHE concentration is stabilized in the treatment range, frequent changes in the individualized diet prescription are required as pregnancy progresses, based on concentrations of plasma PHE, TYR, and other amino acids and on weight gain. PHE and TYR requirements of each pregnant woman depend on genotype, age, state of health, and trimester of pregnancy (78, 121). About midpregnancy, PHE tolerance increases considerably.

As noted for the child with PKU, the amount of protein prescribed (see Appendix Table A-25-d) exceeds the RDA because of the use of free amino acids as the primary source of protein equivalent. A PHE-free medical food (see Appendix Table A-25-a) is used to provide most of the protein prescribed, and nitrogen-free foods, such as pure

TABLE 58.6. RECOMMENDED WEIGHT GAIN DURING PREGNANCY FOR WOMEN PHENYLKETONURIA

WEIGHT STATUS AT CONCEPTION	RECOMMENDED WEIGHT GAIN	
	First Trimester (kg)	Total (kg)
Normal weight	1.6	15.5–16.0
Underweight	2.3	12.5–18.0
Overweight	0.9	7.0–11.5

Data from the Subcommittee on Nutritional Status and Weight Gain During Pregnancy, 1990.

sugars and fats, are used to supply the remaining energy needs. A protocol is available that suggests an approach to planning and evaluating nutrition support for the pregnant woman with PKU (121).

Birth measurements of neonates of women with PKU are negatively correlated with maternal plasma PHE concentrations and positively correlated with maternal energy and protein intakes and weight gain during pregnancy. The plasma PHE concentration of the pregnant woman with PKU is negatively correlated with total protein intake (122), suggesting that total protein intake should minimally be at the amount recommended in Appendix Table A-25-d for better control of plasma PHE.

Appropriate maternal weight gain is related to height and prepregnancy weight and is greater for underweight than for normal-weight women (123). Data in Table 58.6 describe recommended pregnancy weight gain for underweight, normal-weight, and overweight women.

Two families of fatty acids, linoleic (C18:2, n-6) and α-linolenic (C18:3, n-3), are essential for humans (124). Adequate intakes of linoleic and α-linolenic acids are suggested to be 1.3 and 1.4 g/day, respectively, during pregnancy (1). Women in the MPKUCS who had a good reproductive outcome had a greater fat intake throughout pregnancy than women with a poor outcome (78).

Whether the poor outcome was caused by inadequate essential fatty acids is not clear. Because some of the medical foods are devoid of or contain very little fat and essential fatty acids (see Appendix Table A-25-a), the fat used to supply 30 to 40% of energy in the diet should be obtained from cooking and salad oils, margarines, salad dressing, and shortenings with either unhydrogenated canola or soybean oil as the first ingredient (125).

PHE-free medical foods that provide the prescribed protein equivalent (nitrogen × 6.25) for the pregnant woman with PKU also provide the required amounts of minerals and vitamins. Therefore, a prenatal vitamin capsule containing vitamins A and D should not be prescribed for women ingesting adequate amounts of PHE-free medical food. In fact, supplementation may provide vitamin A at levels approaching those that are teratogenic (126). However, those women who do not ingest adequate medical food before and during gestation should be given supplements of folic acid and vitamin B_{12} to help decrease the incidence of congenital heart defects in children (127).

Monitoring Nutrition Support. Ongoing monitoring of women with PKU involves measuring plasma concentrations of PHE and TYR, maternal weight gain, concentrations of other plasma amino acids, transthyretin, ferritin, and zinc. Because pregnant women with PKU are at risk for premature delivery, they should be treated as high-risk patients, even if their plasma PHE concentrations are in the targeted treatment range. Multiple ultrasound studies, beginning at 16 to 20 weeks' gestation, may be requested to monitor fetal head size and intrauterine growth patterns. A level II ultrasound to scan for heart defects and other malformations may also be ordered.

Tyrosinemias

Several known disorders of TYR metabolism (Table 58.7) may be amenable to nutrition support (see Fig. 58.1).

TABLE 58.7. INHERITED DISORDERS PRODUCING INCREASED PLASMA TYROSINE

DESIGNATION	ENZYME DEFECT	CLINICAL FEATURES
Hepatorenal tyrosinemia (type Ia)	Fumarylacetoacetate hydrolyase	Cirrhosis Renal Fanconi syndrome Acute porphyria (succinylacetone) Hepatocellular carcinoma
Hepatorenal tyrosinemia (type Ib)	Maleylacetoacetate isomerase	Liver failure Fanconi syndrome Psychomotor retardation (no succinylacetone)
Oculocutaneous tyrosinemia (type II)	Hepatic cytosol tyrosine aminotransferase	Eye and skin disorders with variable mental retardation Hydroxyphenylpyruvic acidemia
Primary p-OHPPAD deficiency (type IIIa)	p-OHPPAD	Neurologic abnormalities Mental retardation
Hawkinsinuria (type IIIb)	p-OHPPAD	Metabolic acidosis Microcephaly
Transient neonatal (type IIIc)	p-OHPPAD	Prematurity, possibly benign
Tyrosinosis (Medes)	Possibly type Ia	Myasthenia (possibly acute porphyric attack)

p-OHPPAD, 4-hydroxyphenylpyruvic acid dioxygenase.

Precise biochemical diagnosis is important because disorders such as liver disease, scurvy, and prematurity may produce increases in blood TYR that are not caused by permanent specific enzyme defects in TYR metabolism.

Seven clinical forms of hereditary tyrosinemia have been reported (see Table 58.7). Type Ia is caused by a primary defect of hepatic FAH with the production of an abnormal metabolite, succinylacetone (128). The gene for FAH has been localized to chromosome 15q23-25 (see Table 58.3) (128). Succinylacetone is formed from the accumulated substrate fumarylacetoacetate (FAA) (see Fig. 58.1). FAA, at subapoptotic doses, has been reported to induce spindle disturbances and segregational defects in both rodent and human cells, leading to the speculation that FAA functions as a thiol-reacting and organelle/mitotic spindle disturbing agent (129). If maleylacetoacetic acid isomerase is functional, succinylacetone is also formed from maleylacetoacetate. Succinylacetone is extremely toxic and is associated with impaired active transport function and disordered hepatic enzymes, including p-OHPPAD and δ-ALA dehydratase (128). Decreased activity of both hepatic and erythrocyte δ-ALA dehydratase has been reported in these patients and is postulated to be the mechanism for development of acute porphyric-like episodes (see Fig. 58.2) (128). Using the drug NTBC to inhibit p-OHPPAD activity has prevented acute porphyric episodes and decreased rates of progression of cirrhosis and Fanconi syndrome (130).

Tyrosinemia type Ia is characterized by a generalized renal tubular impairment with hypophosphatemic rickets, progressive liver failure producing cirrhosis and hepatic cancer, hypertension, episodic behavioral and peripheral nerve deficiencies, and elevated concentrations of blood PHE and TYR with succinylacetone and δ-ALA excretion in urine (128). The most common mutant allele is a splice donor site gain in intron 12 (IVS12G A+5). Many other missense and nonsense mutations are known (see Table 58.3). Reversion of the IVS12 mutation to normal in noncancerous hepatic nodules is described. FAH is expressed in amniotic and chorionic villus cells, and prenatal diagnosis is available by biochemical or molecular techniques (128).

Tyrosinemia type Ib, believed to be caused by a deficiency of maleylacetoacetate isomerase, has been reported in one infant (128). Liver failure, renal tubular disease, and progressive psychomotor retardation occurred before death at 1 year of age. Succinylacetone did not accumulate. If this is confirmed, the pathophysiology of tyrosinemia type I will require reevaluation.

Tyrosinemia type II is characterized by greatly elevated concentrations of blood and urine TYR and increases in urinary phenolic acids, N-acetyltyrosine, and tyramine. A deficiency of hepatic cytosolic TYR aminotransferase has been demonstrated (128). Characteristic physical findings include stellate corneal erosions and plaques and bullous lesions of the soles and palms. Persistent keratitis and hyperkeratosis occur on the fingers and palms of the hands and on the soles of the feet (131). These skin abnormalities

respond to restriction of dietary PHE and TYR. Intracellular crystallization of TYR is thought to cause these inflammatory responses. Mental retardation may occur. The TYR aminotransferase gene is located on human chromosome 16q22.1 (see Table 58.3). Missense, deletions, nonsense, and splice site mutations are known.

Three clinical subsets of type III tyrosinemia result from dysfunctions of p-OHPPAD (see Fig. 58.1 and Table 58.7). The most severe is type IIIa with no hepatic p-OHPPAD. Neurologic abnormalities, including seizures, ataxia, and mental retardation, have been reported in untreated patients with type IIIa (132). Hawkinsinuria (type IIIb) is named for the 2- L-cysteinyl 5-1,4-dihydroxycyclohexenyl-acetic acid that presumably is formed from an intermediate of impaired p-OHPPAD reaction. Metabolic acidosis and failure to thrive with a "swimming pool"-like odor are described. PHE and TYR restriction improves the critical condition.

Type IIIc is neonatal tyrosinemia, associated with increased plasma and urinary concentrations of TYR and its metabolites. It occurs in 0.2 to 10% of neonates (128). Short-term protein restriction to 1.5 to 2.0 g/kg body weight/day has lowered plasma TYR concentrations in most patients within 4 weeks of life. Whether added ascorbate will stabilize and increase the activity of p-OHPPAD in this disorder is not clear. Persistence of hypertyrosinemia in this disorder may lead to impaired mental function (133), and short-term diet and ascorbate therapy are recommended.

Diagnosis. Differential diagnosis, imperative for institution of appropriate therapy, requires quantitation of plasma amino acids by ion-exchange chromatography and of urinary organic acids by GC/MS. The more severe tyrosinemia type I may not be detected by newborn screening using the bacterial inhibition assay because newborn blood TYR may not be above 8 mg/dL (440 μmol/L). If blood TYR is above 8 mg/dL (440 μmol/L) at 14 days of age, we evaluate renal tubular and hepatic function as well as urine by organic acid analysis for the presence of p-hydroxyphenyl acids and succinylacetone. Prenatal diagnosis of hereditary tyrosinemia type I has been made by measurement of succinylacetone in amniotic fluid (134), by measurement of FAH activity in cultured amniotic fluid cells, and by molecular analyses. Tyrosinemia type II results in a marked increase in urinary p-OH-phenylacids and blood TYR (128). It increases with increasing age of the infant, whereas type IIIc decreases. Hawkinsinuria is measured by its ninhydrin reaction using ion-exchange chromatography.

Treatment. Therapy of the hereditary tyrosinemias requires a firm diagnosis because the approaches to treatment between types are different. The objective of nutrition support for the hereditary tyrosinemias is to provide a biochemical environment that allows normal growth and development of intellectual potential. Nutrition management alone will prevent pathophysiologic changes only in types II and III, for which the prognosis is excellent. Plasma PHE concentration should be maintained between 40 and 80 μmol/L, and plasma TYR concentration between 50 and 150 μmol/L. NTBC therapy in tyrosinemia type Ia, with concomitant nutrition management to maintain plasma TYR concentration at less than 500 μmol/L (135), has prevented acute porphyria episodes, decreased rates of progression of cirrhosis and Fanconi syndrome, greatly improved the survival of patients, and reduced the need for liver transplantation during early childhood. The homeostatic effects of NTBC on succinylacetone production also decreases but does not eliminate the risk for hepatocarcinoma.

Renal impairment, if present, must also be treated in tyrosinemia type Ia. Generalized renal tubular failure may result in metabolic acidosis, hypophosphatemia, rickets, and hypokalemia unless replacement of bicarbonate, phosphate, 1,25-dihydroxycholecalciferol, and potassium is instituted. Rapid treatment of infections is required to prevent a catastrophic catabolic state with overproduction of succinylacetone.

Many of the porphyric symptoms are caused by overproduction of δ-ALA secondary to the inhibitory effect of succinylacetone on δ-ALA dehydratase and/or decreased heme biosynthesis (see Fig. 58.2). Parenteral nutrition with 20 to 25% dextrose solution may control these acute porphyric attacks (136). Continued or progressive loss of energy-requiring functions that involve loosely bound heme to heme-protein (plasma membrane transporters, cytochrome P-450) may be caused by rapid turnover and insufficient heme biosynthesis (see Fig. 58.2). Infusions of hematin have produced transient decreases in δ-ALA and have improved acute attacks of intermittent porphyria, but this invasive therapy is not recommended unless NTBC is unavailable (137, 138). Hepatocellular carcinoma, however, will not be prevented and will require liver transplantation to prevent metastases (128). The drug NTBC, which inhibits the activity of *p*-OHPPAD in the treatment of tyrosinemia type I, reduces the need for liver transplantation, and diet therapy is an indicated adjunct to drug therapy (135). There is an excellent mouse model (139). It is not clear whether newborn or infant treatment of tyrosinemia type I with diet and NTBC will prevent hepatocarcinoma. Follow-up of liver α-fetoprotein and enzymes, as well as hepatic sonography, is indicated. Hepatic transplantation may be required.

Nutrient Requirements. A prescription that recommends daily amounts of PHE, TYR, protein, energy, and fluid should be written. The prescription for PHE and TYR is based on blood analyses correlated with intake that indicate the child's requirement and/or tolerance for each amino acid (see Table 58.4).

Because a large portion of PHE is normally hydroxylated to form TYR, PHE must also be restricted in the diet of patients with tyrosinemia. PHE requirements appear to be greater for children with tyrosinemia than for children with PKU. In general, the more distal the block is in the catabolic pathway, the more normal the amino acid requirement is.

TYR needs of children with tyrosinemia have been inadequately described and will vary with the metabolic state of the child and the accumulation of succinylacetone. If plasma TYR is inadequately controlled in NTBC-treated patients, symptoms of tyrosinemia type II occur (135).

Because the primary protein source used for infants is a free amino acid mix, the recommended intake is greater than for normal infants (53). For tyrosinemia type Ia, when NTBC is administered, energy needs are similar to those of normal infants (1).

Medical Foods Free of Phenylalanine and Tyrosine. Adequate protein cannot be obtained from intact protein without ingesting excess PHE and TYR (proteins contain, by mass, 1.4 to 5.8% TYR). Thus, special medical foods are used that contain no PHE or TYR. Several medical foods free of PHE and TYR are available to provide protein: Tyrex-1 Amino Acid Modified Medical Food with Iron; XPHEN, TYR Analog; Tyrex-2 Amino Acid-Modified Medical Food and XPHEN, TYR Maxamaid (see Appendix Table A-25-a). Formulations, composition of major nutrients, and sources of medical foods are given in Appendix Table A-25-a.

Serving Lists. Serving lists are available for the PHE- and TYR-restricted diet (see Appendix Table A-25-b). Portion sizes of individual foods in each list are given in reference 58.

Initiation of Nutrition Support. The most rapid decline of blood TYR concentration at the time of diagnosis may be obtained by feeding a 20 kcal/oz (67 kcal/dL) PHE- and TYR-free formula with no added sources of PHE and TYR. Total energy intake above 120 kcal/kg/day is required to prevent a catabolic phase. Laboratory results of blood PHE and TYR concentrations should be rapidly available or deficiency of PHE and TYR (140) could be precipitated. Catabolism, caused by inadequate intake of energy, PHE, or TYR, is particularly undesirable in treating tyrosinemia type I because a catabolic phase with overproduction of succinylacetone will worsen the clinical state. Intact protein sources containing 20 to 70 mg PHE and 60 to 80 mg TYR/kg body weight/day are usually required after 3 to 4 days of total restriction in the newborn period in the patient with tyrosinemia type II or III. Patients with tyrosinemia type Ia may tolerate more dietary PHE and TYR if managed with NTBC.

Assessment of Nutrition Support. Frequency of assessment is dictated by the type of tyrosinemia and the clinical course of the patient. In tyrosinemia type I, vital signs, height, weight, head circumference, neurologic examination, and development are documented weekly for the first 3 months, biweekly for the second 3 months, and monthly between 6 months and 1 year of life. Plasma amino acids are quantitated by ion-exchange chromatography or MS/MS, and succinylacetone and *p*-hydroxyphenyl organic acids by GC/MS. Additional laboratory studies include urinary δ-ALA, blood and urine assessment of renal losses (HCO$_3$, K$^+$, Na$^+$), and liver status (α-fetoprotein and liver function tests). Clinical status, dietary intake, and laboratory data should be monitored and correlated in managing tyrosinemia type Ia at intervals indicated previously. Application for eventual liver transplantation should be initiated within the first year of life for patients with type Ia tyrosinemia.

Outcomes of Nutrition Support. Outcomes to date have been variable with tyrosinemia type Ia (128). Some of this variation is caused by the lack of clear diagnostic criteria in the past to delineate the various types of tyrosinemia. Early detection and diagnosis using GC/MS, PHE and TYR restriction, hematin infusions, and early replacement of renal tubular losses bring success at early ages in patients with treated tyrosinemia type Ia. Although NTBC may be the ultimate treatment for tyrosinemia type Ia, institution of the treatment immediately after birth may be necessary to prevent hepatocellular carcinomas, and hepatic transplantation will be required if liver nodules progress on hepatic sonography or if liver α-fetoprotein rises suddenly (130). The PHE- and TYR-restricted diet has been successful in several patients with tyrosinemia types II and III, with rapid resolution of clinical signs and symptoms (128). Neonatal tyrosinemia requires early but transient protein restriction. The efficacy of oral ascorbate at 50 mg/day is unclear. Controlled outcome data are not yet available.

SULFUR-CONTAINING AMINO ACIDS

The biochemistry and nutrition requirements for sulfur-containing amino acids have been largely elucidated in humans by studies of inherited blocks in their metabolic pathways.

Biochemistry

Intact protein contains approximately 0.3 to 5.0% MET. Some dietary MET is used by the body for tissue protein synthesis, but the majority is utilized through the transsulfuration pathway to form adenosylmethionine, adenosylhomocysteine, homocysteine, cystathionine, a-ketobutyrate, cysteine, and their derivatives (Fig. 58.3). The first step in the transsulfuration pathway is the synthesis of S-adenosylmethionine (SAM), a reaction catalyzed by MET-S-adenosyltransferase (MAT). Impaired MAT results in hypermethioninemia and variable clinical expression from sulfurous breath odor to mental retardation. The hepatic isoform of MAT only is deficient (141). In this reaction, the adenosyl portion of adenosine triphosphate (ATP) is transferred to MET. Biologically important compounds that obtain their methyl group from SAM include creatine, choline, phosphatidylcholine, methylated DNA and RNA, and epinephrine. Decarboxylated SAM is the source of the three carbon moieties of spermidine and spermine. S-adenosylhomocysteine is formed as an intermediary product in this pathway and is hydrolyzed to homocysteine.

Homocysteine has four possible pathways open to it. Homocysteine reacts with serine in the presence of CβS, found in liver and brain, to form cystathionine (see Fig. 58.3). CβS requires pyridoxal phosphate as a coenzyme. Homocysteine can also be remethylated to form MET through two different enzymatic reactions. In one reaction, the methyl group is derived from betaine and is catalyzed by betaine-homocysteine methyltransferase. The second reaction requires N^5-methyltetrahydrofolate as a methyl donor to CH_3-B_{12} (see Fig. 58.3) and is catalyzed by 5-methyltetrahydrofolate-homocysteine methyltransferase. Finkelstein (142) used an in vitro system that approximated in vivo conditions in rat liver to measure the simultaneous product formation by the three enzymes that use homocysteine. In this control system, 5-methyltetrahydrofolate-homocysteine methyltransferase, betaine homocysteine methyltransferase, and CβS accounted for 27%, 27%, and 46% of the homocysteine consumed, respectively. The fourth pathway open to homocysteine is spontaneous oxidation to homocystine (see Fig. 58.3). This reaction occurs inside cells only when homocysteine is present in abnormal amounts. It is essentially irreversible because the disulfide bond of homocystine is covalent. Homocystine is not further metabolized. CβS metabolizes most homocysteine with high affinity to cystathionine, using serine as a cosubstrate and pyridoxal phosphate as a stabilizing active coenzyme. Cystathionine is then hydrolyzed to cysteine and α-ketobutyrate. The enzyme cystathioinnase, which also uses pyridoxal phosphate as a coenzyme, is required for this reaction (see Fig. 58.3). A deficiency of cystathioninase results in cystathioninuria, which has no pathologic consequence. α-Ketobutyrate is converted to propionyl CoA, which is carboxylated to methylmalonyl CoA and isomerized to succinyl CoA, a Krebs-cycle intermediate. L-Cysteine is catabolized to pyruvate, NH_3, and H_2S.

Homocystinuria

Defects in the function of CβS or 5-methyltetrahydrofolate-homocysteine methyltransferase result in classical homocystinuria. Impaired activity of the latter enzyme may be caused by failure to synthesize CH_3-B_{12} from vitamin B_{12} or by a deficiency in 5, 10- methylenetetrahydrofolate reductase, as well as by mutations in the apoenzyme CβS. Several different defects impair the uptake, transfer, and conversion of dietary vitamin B_{12} to CH_3-B_{12} (10, 143).

The most common form of homocystinuria is caused by a deficiency of CβS. The human CβS locus has been mapped to chromosome 21q-22.3 (144). The gene has been cloned, and more than 90 mutations are characterized in expression systems. Although phenotypes vary for the same genotype, some mutations respond to vitamin B_6 (I278T, P145L, A114V) and others do not (G307S) (145). Severely impaired enzyme function produces accumulation of plasma homocyst(e)ine and MET and decreased

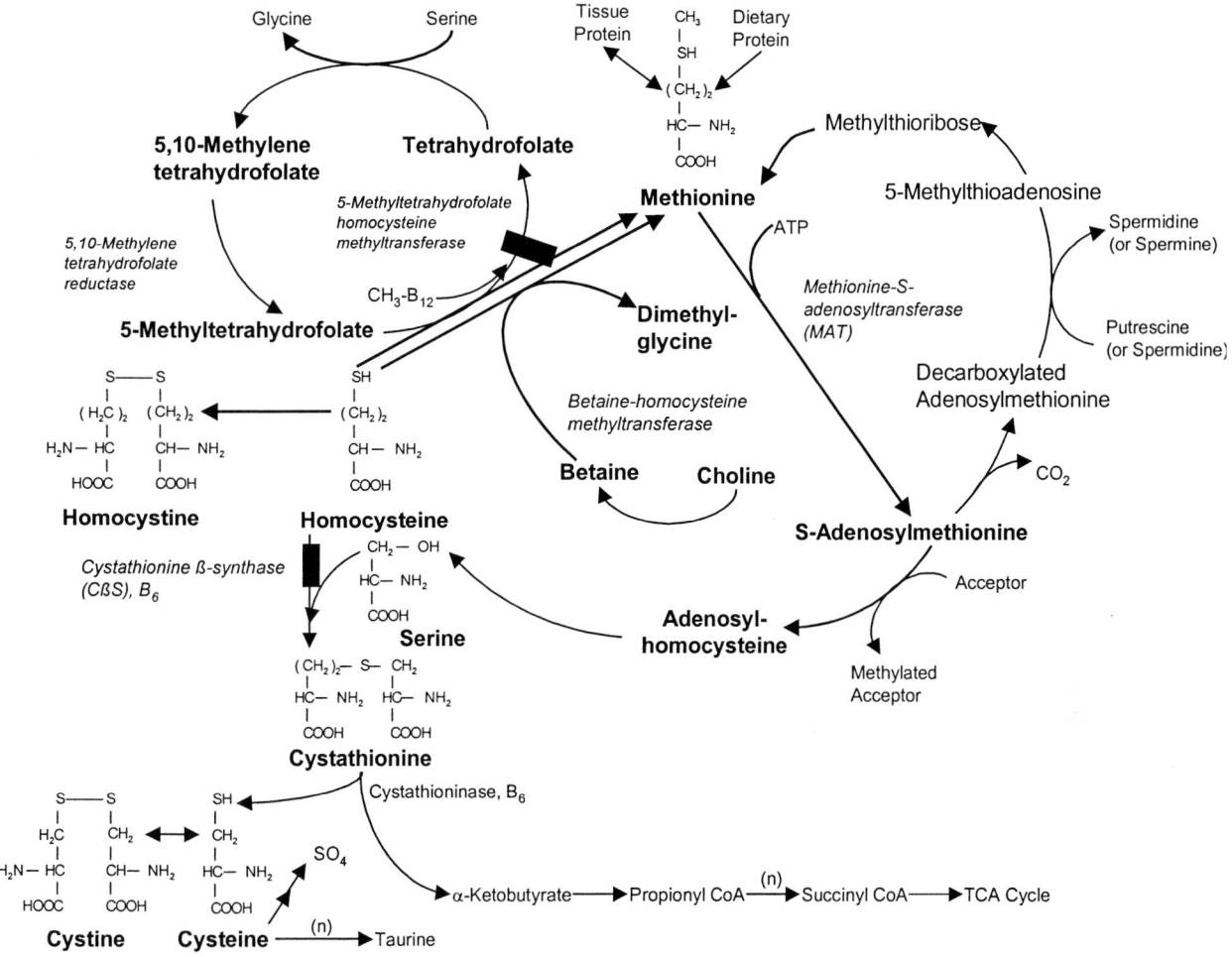

Figure 58.3. Metabolic pathways of sulfur amino acids. The *black bars* represent impaired reactions in three inherited metabolic disorders resulting in hyperhomocyst(e)inemia. CoA, coenzyme A; TCA, tricarboxylic acid.

cyst(e)ine in cells and physiologic fluids. If this biochemical circumstance is not treated early in life, skeletal changes, dislocated lenses, intravascular thromboses, osteoporosis, malar flushing, and, in some patients, mental retardation will occur.

The skeletal changes and dislocated lenses are presumably caused by a structural defect in collagen formation produced by α-homocystine interaction with aldose groups on collagen (141) or by irreversible inhibition of lysyl oxidase by homocysteine thiolactone (146). Intravascular thromboses may occur at any age and have been found in coronary, renal, carotid, and intracranial arteries. The natural history of homocystinuria caused by CβS deficiency has been clarified in a large series of patients (147). Heterozygosity for some mutations in CβS (and/or in tetrahydrofolate reductase) may predispose patients to development of premature occlusive arterial disease (148).

It is not known to what degree the mental retardation seen in homocystinuria is attributable to a metabolic sequela, such as a deficiency of cystathionine in myelin formation, or results from multiple small cerebrovascular thromboses. Mental deficiency may occur with severely impaired CβS as a consequence of multiple cerebral-arteriolar obstructions if homocystinemia is not controlled by diet.

Screening. CβS deficiency is inherited as an autosomal-recessive disease. Accurate estimates of the incidence for homocystinuria are not available, but newborn screening in 13 countries found one case in 344,000 infants screened (141). Homocystinuria occurs in many ethnic groups, but has a higher frequency in persons of Irish descent than in other ethnic groups, one in 58,000 (141). This finding may be a bias of ascertainment because of the original description of and continued screening for this disorder in the Irish population. Vitamin B₆–responsive mutations in CβS are probably not ascertained by neonatal screening for elevated blood MET concentrations.

Selective screening uses the inexpensive urinary nitroprusside reaction. In this reaction, excessive amounts of reduced homocysteine and cysteine form a stable red color with nitroprusside. This selective screening test for sulfur amino acids should be included in the evaluation of any patient with an unknown cause of arterial thrombosis, dislocated lens, marfanoid habitus, or mental retardation. This test result is also positive in cystinuria and should be included as a screen for patients with nephrolithiasis.

In a large survey of patients with homocystinuria caused by CβS deficiency, only 13% had a response to vitamin B_6 (141). Most of these patients had "leaky mutations" with residual CβS activity and disease that was expressed in adolescence or young adulthood rather than early childhood. Response to vitamin B_6 occurs in several mutations, with some residual enzyme activity. The mechanism involves stabilizing CβS to biologic degradation (141). The more residual enzyme activity present, the more dramatic the response to vitamin B_6. Hypermethioninemia may not be present in the newborn if CβS activity exceeds 15% of normal. Some patients with CβS deficiency have no activity in the fibroblasts, yet appear to have a B_6 response (145).

Diagnosis. Positive results in a newborn screen by bacterial inhibition assay for MET must be followed by an assay of plasma amino acids using ion-exchange chromatography or MS/MS because many environmental as well as genetic variations cause neonatal hypermethioninemia. With a CβS defect, homocystine, cysteine-homocysteine, and MET are all elevated in plasma and increase with increased protein intake (see Fig. 58.3). Demonstration of significantly decreased CβS, folate, CH_3-B_{12}, or homocysteine methyltransferases is necessary to confirm the diagnosis and implement appropriate therapy. MET may be elevated in the absence of homocystinemia in liver disease and in specific impairment of SAM. By contrast, in defects of homocysteine remethylation to MET, MET is low or normal, whereas homocysteine concentrations are elevated. Hyperhomocysteinemia caused by disorders of cobalamin methylation to CH_3-B_{12} or the two homocysteine methyltransferases will not be detected by nonselective newborn screening for elevated blood MET. Similarly, B_6-responsive mild CβS deficiency is missed by newborn screening. Thus, selective screening using urinary nitroprusside reaction or plasma amino acid analysis is indicated for all children or adults with ectopic lens, unexplained vascular occlusions, marfanoid habitus, and mental delay.

Management of CH_3-B_{12} deficiency or impaired methyl transfer with homocystinuria does not include MET-restricted diets. Rather, pharmacologic amounts of vitamin B_{12}, folate, choline, or betaine are added depending on the primary defect. Liver biopsy specimens, transformed lymphoblasts, or cultured skin fibroblasts express CβS and are used to confirm the most common cause of homocystinuria, and molecular screening and sequencing of the CβS gene are useful in predicting management. Prenatal diagnosis can be provided by direct enzyme assay of amniotic fluid cells or by DNA analysis if the mutations are known (141, 145).

Treatment. If homocystinuria is caused by CβS deficiency expressed in the newborn, the clinical objectives are (a) to prevent the development of skeletal and ocular abnormalities, (b) to prevent intravascular thromboses, and (c) to ensure normal intellectual development.

Pharmacologic doses of pyridoxine should be tried in all patients with hypermethioninemia and homocystinemia (141, 145). Some mutations are known to be responsive (see Table 58.3). In newborns and early childhood, 25 to 100 mg/day should be tried for 4 weeks before MET restriction. Older children and adults should be given oral pyridoxine (1 g/day). Pyridoxine's effect on plasma MET and homocystine concentrations is monitored weekly on a constant protein intake. Because enzyme stabilization is the most common mechanism of vitamin responsivity, weeks may be required for a biochemical response to occur. If the plasma MET and homocysteine concentrations are reduced, the amount of pyridoxine should be gradually lowered until the minimum dose required to maintain biochemical normality is reached. Doses of 25 to 750 mg/day have been required for some patients. Excess vitamin B_6 for prolonged periods may cause peripheral neuropathy (149) and liver injury (150); consequently, if vitamin B_6 is not helpful, it should be discontinued. Betaine supplements (6 g/day) will help maintain postprandial plasma homocysteine concentrations in the near-normal range in vitamin B_6-responsive individuals (151).

Patients whose condition does not respond completely to pyridoxine will require a MET-restricted diet supplemented with L-cysteine. Cysteine becomes an essential amino acid in homocystinuria (see Fig. 58.3). If plasma folate concentrations are below normal owing to excess use in remethylating homocysteine to MET, folate should be added as a supplement.

Betaine is used as adjunctive therapy in B_6 nonresponsive patients. Doses required range from 120 to 150 mg/kg/day and are divided into three doses per day. Total plasma homocyst[e]ine should be followed as the parameter of effective therapy because both free MET and free homocysteine in plasma may decrease to normal while total plasma homocyst[e]ine remains elevated and in concentrations that increase risks of vascular occlusion (152).

Nutrient Requirements. In prescribing and implementing nutrition care plans for infants and children with homocystinuria caused by CβS deficiency, one must consider energy, protein, MET, cysteine, folate, vitamins B_6 and B_{12}, betaine, and fluid needs. Younger infants have a greater MET requirement per kilogram of body weight than older infants. Suggested daily MET intakes range from 35 mg/kg in the young infant to 5 mg/kg in the 15- to 19-year-old patient. Suggested beginning energy, protein, MET, and fluid intakes for infants and children of different ages are given in Table 58.4. If the medical food mixture provides more than 24 kcal/oz, extra fluid should be offered between feedings to prevent dehydration.

Calcium cystinate, a soluble form of L-cystine, should supplement the MET-restricted diet at all ages. The young infant should be offered 300 mg/kg body weight. This amount may be decreased to 200 mg/kg at 6 months of age and 100 mg/kg at 3 years of age and thereafter. The calcium cystinate should be mixed with the MET-free medical food to provide even distribution throughout the day. Older children can sprinkle it in applesauce or other low-protein solids.

Methionine-Free Medical Foods. Several medical foods have been developed as protein sources for patients with homocystinuria. Formulations, composition of major nutrients, and sources of these products are given in Appendix Table A-25-a.

Serving Lists. MET may be provided for the young infant by addition of specified amounts of proprietary infant formula to the MET-free medical foods. As growth and development proceed, intact protein-containing foods should be added at the usual ages. The MET requirement is small, and most foods contain moderate amounts in relation to the requirement (57). Because of this, the amount of intact protein that can be ingested is small. To provide variety to the MET-restricted diet, serving lists have been prepared (58). Average MET, cystine, protein, and energy contents of these lists are given in Appendix Table A-25-e. Sample diets for a neonate are given in Appendix Table A-25-f.

Assessment of Nutrition Support. After the introduction of the diet and stabilization, plasma MET and cystine concentrations should be monitored twice weekly until 3 months of age. Weekly monitoring is suggested until 6 months of age and twice monthly thereafter if blood MET concentrations are stable. Because free MET and homocystine in plasma may revert to normal while total plasma homocyst[e]ine remains elevated, the latter test is recommended when the free MET is normal or the free homocystine is not measurable. After a diet change, plasma MET and cysteine should be measured after 3 days have elapsed. A 3-day diet diary before each blood sample is necessary to evaluate plasma MET and cysteine. Plasma MET should be maintained between 15 and 45 μmol in 2- to 4-hour postfeeding plasma. Little or no homocystine should be present in blood and urine. Total plasma homocyst[e]ine should approach 10 μM/L. Growth and development as well as clinical evaluation of the pulses, skeletal growth, and ocular lenses are routinely assessed.

Results of Nutrition Support. In a retrospective study of 629 patients with CβS deficiency, MET restriction initiated neonatally prevented mental retardation, decreased the frequency of lens dislocation, and reduced the incidence of seizures. Pyridoxine treatment of late-detected vitamin B$_6$–responsive patients decreased the rate of thromboembolic events (147). Hispanic male twins born at 38 weeks' gestation with homocystinuria grew well during the entire first year of life while on nutrition support. The protein intake of these two patients averaged 3.7 g/kg/day during the first 6 months of life and 2.6 g/kg/day during the second 6 months. Energy intake averaged 131 kcal/kg during the first 6 months and 100 kcal/kg during the second 6 months. Patients with poorly controlled plasma homocysteine concentrations may have excessive growth in height. Optimal metabolic control may prevent overgrowth (153, 154).

Cysteine deficiency manifested as abnormally low plasma cystine concentrations, elevated plasma MET, and weight loss in a 3-year-old boy with homocystinuria who received 32 mg/kg/day of L-cysteine was reported (155). The Hispanic twins referred to above received 58 to 118 mg cystine/kg/day, which resulted in plasma cystine concentrations of 19 to 30 μmol/L. Up to 150 mg L-cystine/kg/day may be required to maintain normal plasma cystine concentrations.

Elevated plasma copper and ceruloplasmin concentrations were found in 15 patients with homocystinuria, compared with values found in age- and gender-matched normal controls. No relationship to plasma homocysteine could be found (156). The twins mentioned above had elevated serum copper concentrations of 151 and 144 μg/dL at about 13 months of age. Low plasma selenium concentration (about 15 μmol/L) and erythrocyte glutathione peroxidase activity (about 3 U/g Hgb) were found in a child with homocystinuria treated with a medical food free of selenium (157). Administration of 50 μg selenium (in selenium-enriched yeast) every other day was required to maintain normal indices of selenium status. The twins mentioned above ingested, on average, 26 μg selenium (as sodium selenite) daily throughout the first year of life. Serum selenium concentrations ranged between 60 and 72 μg/L, very similar to values reported for normal human milk–fed babies (158).

Vitamin A absorption tests were carried out in eight untreated patients with homocystinuria by measuring the elevation in serum after administration of vitamin A alcohol (retinol). The explanation proposed for the resulting subnormal serum vitamin A elevation was that retinol was oxidized by -SH groups excreted into the gut (159). Of the eight plasma retinol values obtained on the twins studied, one was less than 20 μg/dL and five were between 20 and 30 μg/dL. According to parental report, vitamin A intake was always more than adequate (1.20-5.58 times the RDA for age). Serum transthyretin concentrations were all less than 20 mg/dL (marginal), and two of the four values obtained were less than 15 mg/dL (deficient).

Fasting serum folate concentrations in eight untreated patients with homocystinuria were found to be abnormally low (4 ng/mL compared with 8 ng/mL in control subjects). Two of these subjects were treated with 20 mg/day folate, which led to a decrease in urinary homocystine excretion (160). Severe folate deficiency was found in an untreated infant with homocystinuria who was receiving diluted boiled cow's milk for an episode of gastroenteritis. Excessive use of 5-methyltetrahydrofolate in the remethylation of homocysteine to form MET is proposed as a reason for folate deficiency in untreated patients (161). The twins in our study had adequate hemoglobin concentrations after 4 months of age, and mean corpuscular volume was normal.

Termination of Nutrition Support. Most clinicians who treat individuals with homocystinuria believe that patients should be kept on the diet indefinitely. Termination of diet after growth is achieved may lead to thromboembolisms and ciliary muscle laxity with lens dislocation. Yap and colleagues (162) reported that appropriate homocysteine-lowering therapy significantly reduced the vascular risk in patients with homocystinuria. When initiation or maintenance of nutrition support is not possible, acetylsalicylic acid (1 g/day) and dipyridamole (100 mg/day) increase platelet survival time and decrease thrombotic events (163). Pharmacologic doses of vitamin E may reduce oxidative stress and platelet activation in patients with homocystinuria (164). Vitamin B_6 in pharmacologic doses should be continued in vitamin B_6–responsive patients.

Reproductive Performance. Fewer conceptions are reported for both men and women whose condition does not respond to vitamin B_6 than for those whose condition does. Children of male patients do not suffer excess losses and are generally reported to be normal. A study showed that higher rates of fetal loss occurred in presumptive heterozygous fetuses carried by CβS-deficient mothers than occurred in physiologically normal women (147). Good reproductive outcome has recently been reported in children of a woman with tight metabolic control during pregnancy (165). Whether hypermethioninemia, homocysteinemia, or other metabolic variations in MET metabolism are teratogenic is as yet unclear, but a teratogenic mechanism as defined for maternal PKU is possible. In addition, folate-responsive neural tube defects may involve hyperhomocyst(e)inemia as a pathophysiologic mechanism.

Carrier State. Heterozygotes for CβS deficiency may be at risk for premature vascular occlusion. The physician's duty to diagnose, inform, and treat extended family members of probands with CβS deficiency awaits further definition of this risk and outcomes of intervention (166).

ORGANIC ACIDS

Several essential amino acids contribute to the synthesis of the acyl groups of organic acids. Among these are the BCAAs, ILE, LEU, and VAL; the sulfur amino acid MET; the hydroxy amino acid threonine (THR); and the dibasic amino acids lysine (LYS) and TRP (see Fig. 58-3; Fig. 58.4).

Biochemistry

The BCAAs, ILE, LEU, and VAL are essential nutrients. In the newborn, 75% of the amounts ingested is used for protein synthesis. That present in excess of need for synthetic purposes is degraded through many steps to provide energy (see Fig. 58.4). When acetyl-CoA and succinyl-CoA are not formed from the appropriate BCAA, they are not available to enter the tricarboxylic acid cycle to yield energy because the organic acids are excreted in the urine. The initial step in catabolism is reversible transamination, requiring a specific transaminase and the coenzyme pyridoxal phosphate. The second step is irreversible oxidative decarboxylation, which uses the BCKAD complex. This complex is located in the inner mitochondrial membrane and requires the coenzymes TPP, lipoic acid, CoA, and NAD^+ (167–171). Figure 58.4 diagrams this overall reaction. At least six proteins are involved, E1α, E1β, E2, E3, a kinase, and phosphatase.

Isovaleryl-CoA, synthesized from α-ketoisocaproic acid by BCKAD, is catalyzed to 3-methylcrotonyl-CoA by isovaleryl-CoA dehydrogenase (IVD), a mitochondrial enzyme that requires flavoprotein and uses electron transfer factor (ETF) (see Fig. 58.4). Mutations in the gene for IVD result in isovaleric acidemia (see Table 58.3) (172). According to Xu and colleagues (173), some 14% of α-ketoisocaproate is catabolized to hydroxymethylbutyrate in homogenized rat and human liver by a cytosolic α-ketoisocaproate dehydrogenase. However, no in vivo data to support this pathway have been published.

3-Methylcrotonyl-CoA is carboxylated at the 4-carbon by 3-methylcrotonyl-CoA carboxylase to form 3-methylglutaconyl-CoA (see Fig. 58.4). This enzyme, associated with the inner mitochondrial membrane, contains covalently bound biotin. Mutations in the gene for 3-methylcrotonyl-CoA carboxylase result in 3-methylcrotonylglycinuria (see Table 58.3).

3-Methylglutaconyl-CoA hydratase, presumably located in the mitochondria, hydrates 3-methylglutaconyl-CoA to 3-hydroxy-3-methylglutaryl-CoA (HMG-CoA). HMG-CoA is cleaved by HMG-CoA lyase to acetoacetic acid and acetyl-CoA (see Fig. 58.4). Mutations in the gene for 3-methylglutaconyl-CoA hydratase result in 3-methylglutaconic aciduria, whereas mutations in the gene for HMG-CoA lyase result in hydroxymethylglutaric aciduria (see Table 58.3).

Complete catabolism of ILE through its major degradative pathway results in the synthesis of acetyl-CoA and succinyl-CoA (see Fig. 58.4). After synthesis of 2-methylbutyryl-CoA by BCKAD, this organic acid is catalyzed by a dehydrogenase to tiglyl-CoA, which is acted on by a hydratase to form 2-methyl-3-hydroxybutyryl-CoA. This compound is used by a dehydrogenase to form 2-methylacetoacetyl-CoA. Mitochondrial acetoacetyl-CoA thiolase interconverts 2-methylacetoacetyl-CoA to acetyl-CoA plus propionyl-CoA. Propionyl-CoA + HCO_3^-, in the presence of ATP, biotin, and Mg+, is acted on by propionyl-CoA carboxylase to form D-methylmalonyl-CoA. The biotin molecule is responsible for the transfer of the carboxyl group. Isolated deficiency of the propionyl-CoA carboxylase, caused by mutations in the genes encoding its nonidentical α- and β-subunits (see Table 58.3), results in PPA (174).

Methylmalonyl-CoA racemase converts D-methylmalonyl-CoA to L-methylmalonyl-CoA, which is isomerized

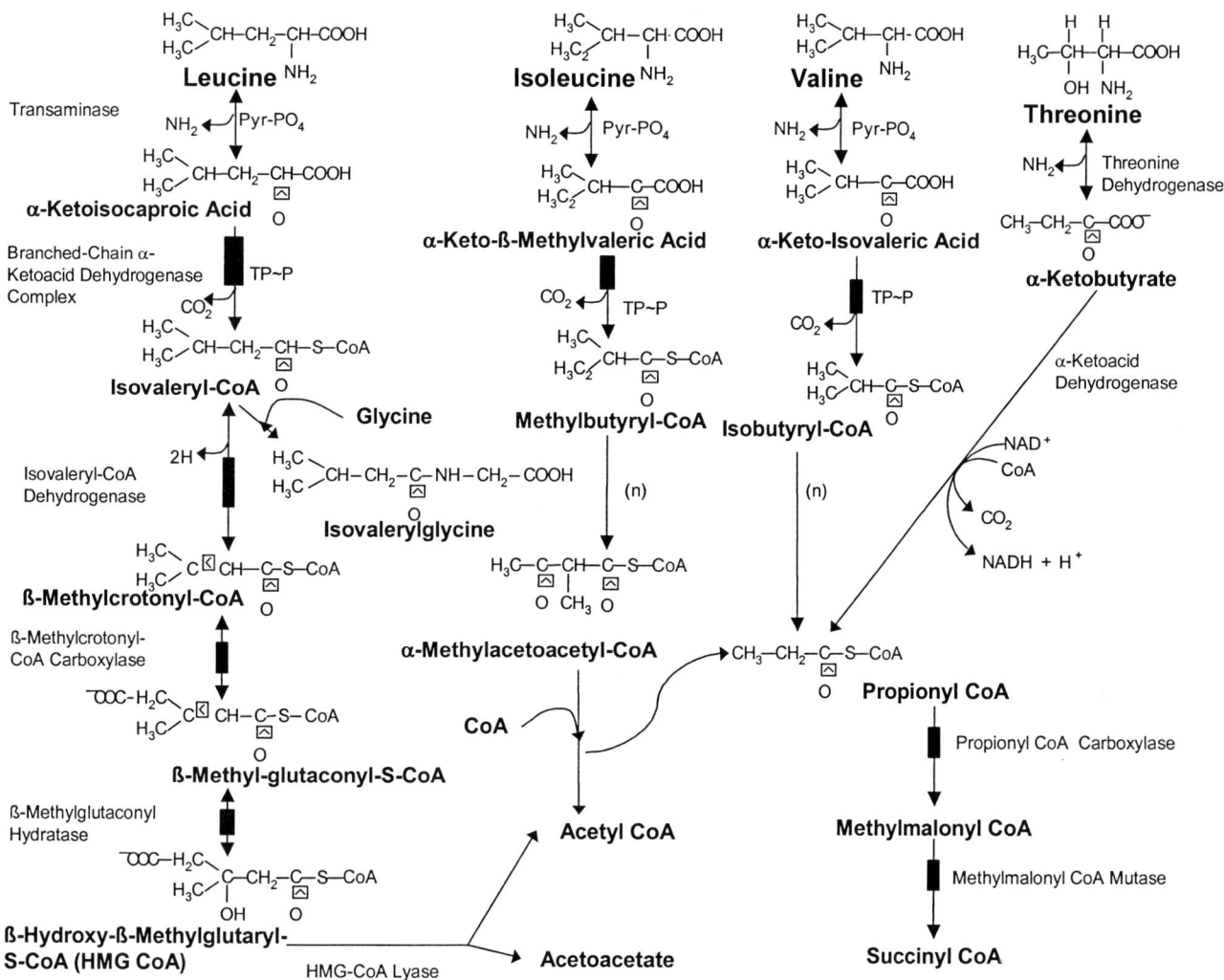

Figure 58.4. Metabolism of branched-chain amino acids and threonine. The *black bars* indicate sites of enzyme defects. (n), several steps.

to succinyl-CoA by methylmalonyl-CoA mutase. This dimer contains 1 mol of tightly bound adenosylcobalamin per mole of subunit. Mutations in the gene encoding for methylmalonyl-CoA mutase, as well as those encoding for mitochondrial glutathionylcobalamin reductase and adenosylreductase, result in MMA (see Table 58.3 and Fig. 58.4). Cytosolic cobalamin reductase/β-ligand transferase deficiency results in homocystinuria and MMA (174).

After synthesis of isobutyryl-CoA from 2-ketoisovaleric acid by BCKAD (see Fig. 58.4), it is acted on by a dehydrogenase, followed by a hydratase, a deacylase, and two further dehydrogenases to form propionyl-CoA (174).

Two other amino acids, MET and THR, as well as odd-chain fatty acids, thymine, uracil, and the side-chain of cholesterol, are catabolized to propionyl-CoA (see Figs. 58.3 and 58.4). The transamination of MET becomes most prominent when plasma MET concentrations exceed 350 μmol/L and seems to function as a spill-over pathway that accounts for only a minor portion of total MET catabolism (175). However, even in the fasting state with plasma

MET concentrations in the normal range, some MET is transaminated and decarboxylated to form 3-methylthiopropionate (176, 177), and the α-ketobutyrate formed via the transsulfuration pathway is also used to synthesize propionyl-CoA (see Fig. 58.3).

The major pathway of THR catabolism is via oxidation of the hydroxyl group by a specific dehydrogenase to form α-amino-β-ketobutyrate, which subsequently forms acetyl-CoA + GLY. Another lesser-used pathway of catabolism is via serine (THR) dehydrogenase and deamination to form α-ketobutyrate (178), which is acted on by α-ketoacid dehydrogenase to form propionyl-CoA (179) (see Fig. 58.4). Energy, normally obtained from the oxidation of succinyl-CoA in the tricarboxylic acid cycle, is lost in the urine as propionic acid and methylmalonic acid in PPA and MMA, respectively.

Two essential amino acids contained in food and body protein, LYS and TRP, are precursors of glutaric acid (Fig. 58.5). The metabolism of TRP does not resemble that of any other metabolite (178). Its principal degradative pathway occurs in the liver and leads to the formation of nicotinic acid, usually classified as a vitamin, and many byproducts that accumulate under normal circumstances. TRP metabolism also leads to serotonin. The initial reaction in the main pathway is oxygenation to form formylkynurenine. The enzyme, TRP oxygenase, contains an iron porphyrin. The formate of N-formylkynurenine is handled as a C_1 fragment by the H_4 folate system. Kynurenine is a branch point; the main pathway continues with a mixed-function oxygenase that includes flavin adenine dinucleotide and uses nicotinamide adenine dinucleotide or nicotinamide adenosine dinucleotide phosphate as the cosubstrate in the synthesis of 3-hydroxykynurenine. One side branch splits off the bulk of the side chain as alanine through the action of the pyridoxal phosphate enzyme kynureninase, and another side branch removes the α-amino group by transamination (also using pyridoxal phosphate), but the keto group forms a Schiff base with the aromatic amine to form the stable aromatic compound kynurenate. Kynurenate has recently been found to be in the brain, where it antagonizes the effects of excitatory amino acids. 3-Hydroxykynurenine is also a branch point. The main pathway now

uses the kynureninase that caused a branch earlier to remove alanine but to produce 3-hydroxyanthranilate. The branch is again caused by transamination, which also results in a quinoline ring to form xanthurenic acid. A third oxygenase cleaves 3-hydroxyanthranilate to an unstable intermediate, 2-amino-3-carboxymuconic 6-semialdehyde. This unstable intermediate cyclizes to a Schiff base to form quinolinate. An enzyme, picolinic carboxylase, exists that competes with the formation of quinolinate. It decarboxylates the intermediate to one that forms picolinate. Most of the decarboxylated material is caught by a dehydrogenase, however, that converts the aldehyde to an acid and leads through α-ketoadipate and glutaryl CoA to acetoacetyl-CoA (see Fig. 58.5).

LYS is one of two essential amino acids that have an α-amino group that does not equilibrate with the body pool of amino groups; the other is THR. The amino group of LYS is transferred to other amino acids, but the reverse does not occur. Most degradation of LYS occurs by a unique pathway in which a secondary amine is formed between the ϵ-amino group and the carbonyl group of α-ketoglutarate. The product, saccharopine, is formed by an enzyme that reduces the

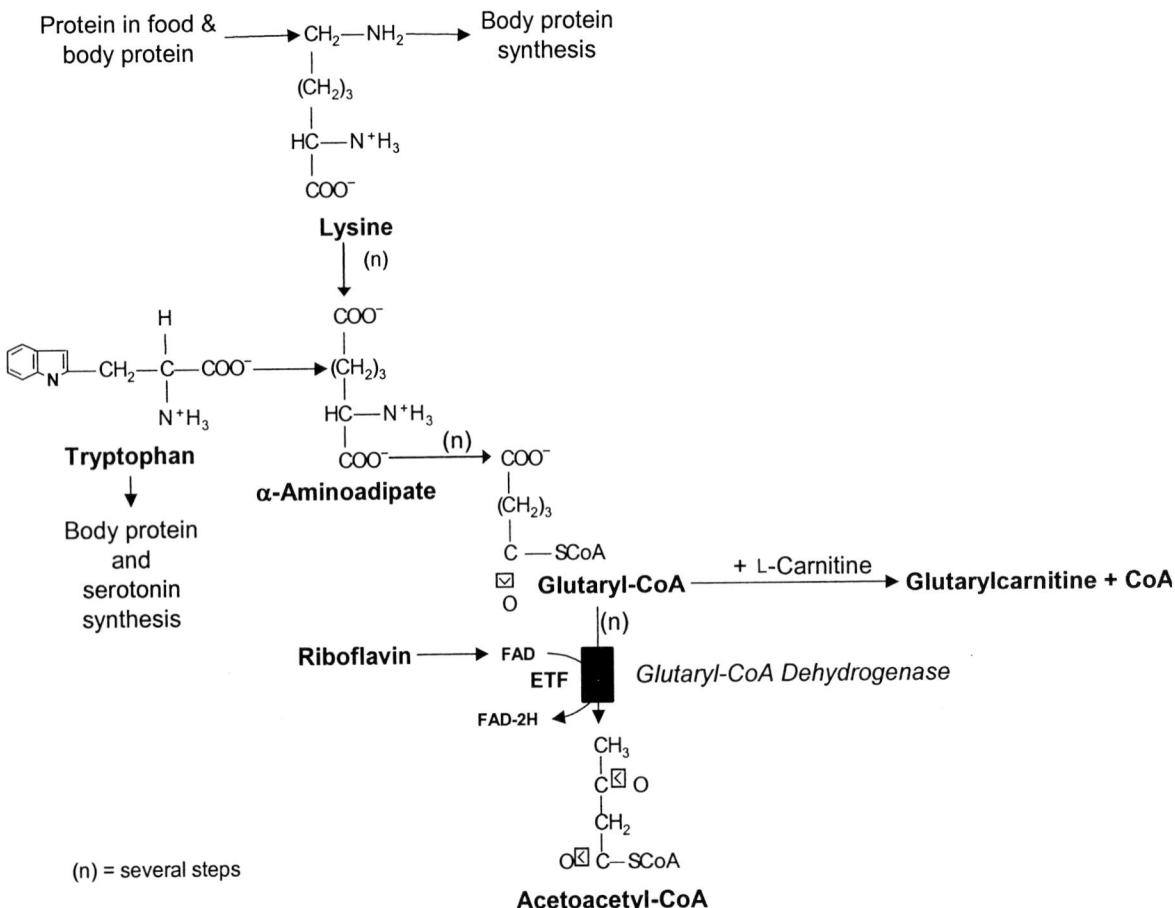

Figure 58.5. Metabolism of lysine and tryptophan. The *black bar* indicates the site of the enzyme defect in glutaric acidemia type I. L-Carnitine enhances urinary excretion of glutaric acid. ETF is the electron transfer factor that, when impaired, may cause glutaric aciduria and the accumulation of other substrates using ETF. CoA, coenzyme A; FAD, flavin adenine dinucleotide.

hypothetical Schiff base with nicotinamide adenosine dinucleotide phosphate. Normally, saccharopine does not accumulate but is oxidized by another dehydrogenase that splits the linkage on the other side of the bridge nitrogen. The sum of the reduction-oxidation reactions is effectively a transamination yielding glutamate and α-aminoadipic semialdehyde. The latter can form a Schiff base, but with the double bond on the side of the nitrogen atom away from the carboxylate. This compound can be oxidized by another dehydrogenase to become α-aminoadipate. A transamination converts this homolog of glutamate to the corresponding α-ketoadipate. In a reaction analogous to the oxidation of α-ketoglutarate to succinyl CoA, glutaryl-CoA is formed (see Fig. 58.5). Another oxidation introduces a double bond, forming glutaconyl CoA, which is decarboxylated to crotonyl CoA. This unsaturated fatty acyl CoA is an intermediate in the normal oxidation of fatty acids, and subsequent reactions of the material derived from LYS are those of fatty acid oxidation leading to acetoacetyl-CoA (178).

Branched-Chain α-Ketoaciduria (Maple Syrup Urine Disease)

MSUD is a group of inherited disorders of ILE, LEU, and VAL metabolism. These disorders result from several different gene mutations that impair various components of the multienzyme BCKAD (Fig. 58.6; see Table 58.3). These genes are E1α, E1β, E2, and E3 (167). E1α is inactivated by a kinase and activated by its phosphatase (see Table 58.3). The BCKAD-specific kinase and phosphate have not been cloned, nor do they have chaperonin proteins involved in their mitochondrial assembly process. Almost all mutations in these proteins that produce MSUD are private. The only one common among Mennonites is the one in the E1α protein, and it is a substitution of asparagine for TYR at amino acid 393 (Y393N) (see Table 58.3). Although most mutant enzymes are immunologically present, one reported patient had absent branched-chain acyl transferase (E2) as a cause of thiamin-resistant MSUD (169, 180, 181). An autosomal-recessive mode of inheritance was found in all reported cases, supporting nuclear rather than mitochondrial origin of these proteins. The cellular mechanisms involved in assembling the products of these nuclear genes into a multienzyme complex in mitochondria are of considerable clinical and fundamental importance and are still unresolved.

Infants with MSUD appear normal at birth and are clinically well until after they eat a protein-containing feed. The most severely impaired enzymes may produce

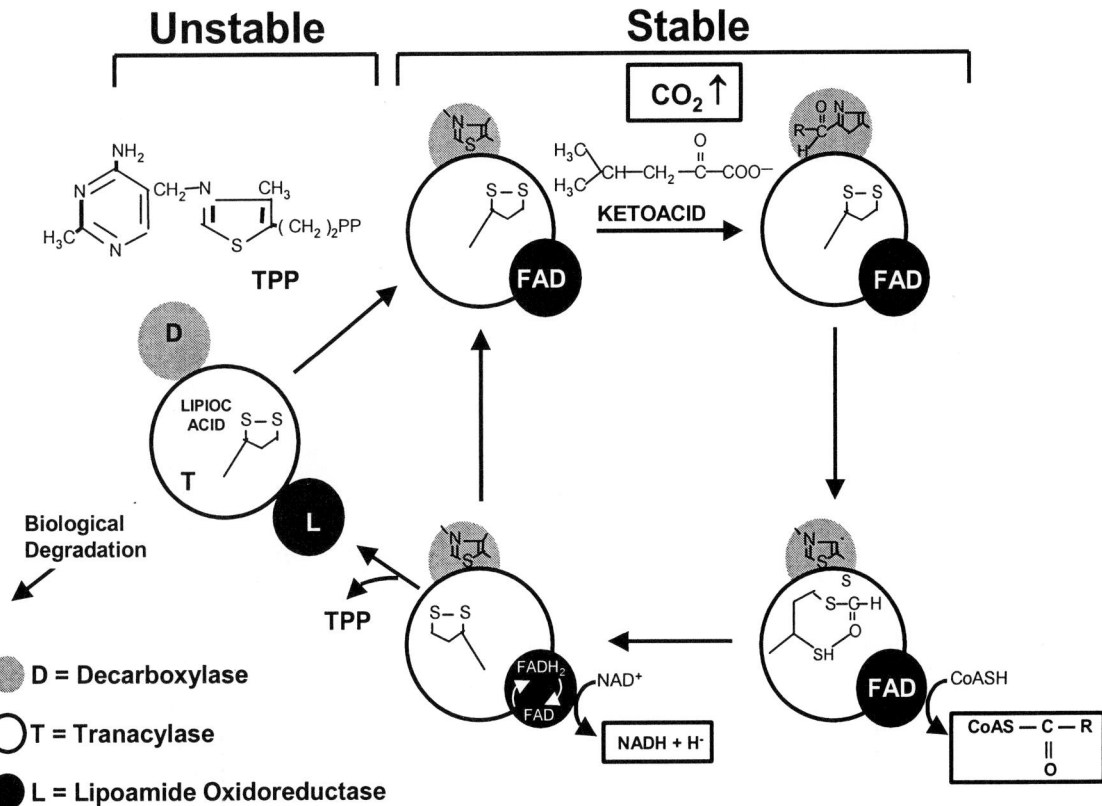

Figure 58.6. Model for stabilization of branched-chain α-ketoacid dehydrogenase by thiamin pyrophosphate. The multienzyme complex branched-chain α-ketoacid dehydrogenase has a configuration that is more stable to degradation when thiamin pyrosphosphate (TPP) binding sites on its decarboxylase moiety are occupied. FAD and NAD, flavin and nicotinamide adenine dinucleotide.

seizures, apnea, and death within 10 days of birth. The disorder is characterized by elevated blood, urine, and cerebrospinal fluid concentrations of the BCKAs, their amino acid precursors, and the pathognomonic alloisoleucine. Progressive neurologic dysfunction and production of fragrant urine with the odor of burnt sugar (caramel) or maple syrup follow. The sweet smell may only be evident in earwax, easily sensed after otoscopic examination. Neurologic impairment in the newborn is manifested by poor sucking, irregular respiration, rigidity alternating with periods of flaccidity, opisthotonos, progressive loss of Moro reflex, and seizures.

Several variants covering a spectrum of impaired mitochondrial BCKAD complexes have been reported. Clinical manifestations are expressed intermittently on protein loading or with febrile illness in patients with partial enzyme activity between 5 and 20% of normal. Patients with 3 to 30% BCKAD complex activity express an intermediate form of the disease. A thiamin-responsive form with expression similar to the intermediate form has been described (167). Whole-body LEU-1-^{13}C oxidation to ^{13}CO$_2$ may be the best method of ascertaining total body needs because peripheral cells may not reflect liver and renal BCKAD function (169, 170).

Untreated patients with classic MSUD (less than 2% BCKAD complex activity) who survive beyond early infancy have retarded physical and mental development (180, 181). Early diagnosis and therapy lead to normal growth and development (5). If death occurs in the first few days of life, few unique abnormalities are seen in the brain. With prolonged survival, deficient myelination is thought to be caused by enzymes involved in myelin formation, inhibition of amino acid transport, and inhibition by BCKAs of oxidative phosphorylation (180, 181). Jouvet and colleagues (182) reported that increased concentrations of BCKAs, in particular of α-ketoisocaproic acid, induced apoptosis in glial and neuronal cells in culture and in vivo after intracerebral injection into the developing rat brain.

Screening. Because apnea and death may be the first clinical manifestations of the classic disorder, newborn screening, retrieval, and initiation of therapy are urgent, and all four processes must be completed within the first week of life. Nonselected screening of the newborn population is currently in progress (in some states) using a bacterial-inhibition or MS/MS assay for blood LEU concentrations (183). Bedside screening in selected children uses the urinary dinitrophenylhydrazine (DNPH) reaction for branched-chain α-ketoaciduria. This reaction can also be used to monitor dietary progress. International newborn screening indicates that the incidence of MSUD is about one in 185,000 (183).

Diagnosis. Any infant with a blood LEU concentration greater than 4 mg/dL (305 μmol/L) on the newborn screening test should be immediately evaluated. Most infants with the classic disease have more than 8 mg/dL

(610 μmol/L) LEU at 72 hours of age. Diagnosis is confirmed using ion-exchange chromatography to quantitate plasma ILE, LEU, VAL, and alloisoleucine and GC/MS to identify urinary BCKAs. The extent of enzyme impairment should be determined on cultured cells such as dermal fibroblasts to enable future prenatal diagnosis, because prenatal monitoring is available if the cellular phenotype is confirmed in fibroblasts cultured from the patient's skin (184). However, total body LEU oxidation using stable isotopes and the ^{13}CO$_2$ breath test is the most reliable diagnostic tool for establishing dietary needs, including thiamin responsivity (170). Except in Mennonites, molecular analysis is useful only for research purposes.

Treatment. Relatively little help in managing MSUD has resulted from advances in mutation analysis except for the role of pharmacologic coenzymes. When TPP saturates its site on E1α, the biologic turnover of BCKAD is decreased (see Fig. 58.6). Increasing thiamin ingestion increases intracellular TPP, and the TPP binding sites on the decarboxylase (E1) moiety of the BCKAD complex become saturated. When these TPP binding sites are occupied, the multienzyme complex undergoes a conformational change that makes it more resistant to chymotrypsin and heat degradation. The biologic half-life of the enzyme and overall activity are increased when a new equilibrium of enzyme synthesis and degradation is reached. This model has been tested and is supported by clinical, functional, and structural studies (169, 171, 184, 185) (see Fig. 58.6).

Although hemodialysis with nitrogen-free dialysate or exchange transfusion may be required when diagnosis is delayed, if screening, retrieval, and diagnosis are completed within 8 to 10 days of life, these actions are seldom necessary. Because hemodialysis superimposes iatrogenic risk and prolongs a catabolic phase, it is not recommended. BCAA-free orogastric feeding of protein and energy should begin as soon as the diagnosis is made. The objective is to produce anabolism in the infant and thereby prevent accumulation of neurotoxic BCKAs (186). If orogastric feeding is not acceptable, gastrostomy or a central line for hyperalimentation with dextrose and lipid should be initiated for initial care of classic MSUD during the neonatal period. Except during illness, restricting protein intake to 1.5 g/kg/day may be adequate therapy for those with 20% or more of enzyme activity.

Long-term therapy for MSUD is dietary. The objective of long-term nutrition support in the child with MSUD is to maintain plasma concentrations of BCAAs that will allow maximal development of intellect while supplying adequate energy, protein, and other nutrients for optimal growth. Plasma concentrations of BCAAs (3–4 hours after a meal) should be maintained within the following ranges: ILE, 40 to 90 μmol/L; LEU, 80 to 200 μmol/L; and VAL, 200 to 425 μmol/L. ILE deficiency results in skin lesions that resemble acrodermatitis enteropathica (187, 188). With a deficiency of ILE or VAL, the plasma concentration of LEU remains elevated. With deletion of the BCAAs, plasma ILE returns to normal first, followed by VAL. If adequate dietary ILE and VAL are then added to maintain normal plasma concentrations, plasma LEU concentration returns to normal in 5 to 10 days (189).

The objectives of nutrition support are met by using a combination of medical foods (see Appendix Table A-25-a) and intact protein (see Appendix Table A-25-f). Most patients with MSUD who have detectable BCKAD multienzyme complex by immunoassay respond to oral thiamin administration of 100 to 1000 mg daily (169, 170, 185). Supraphysiologic amounts of oral thiamin should be added for at least a 3-month trial period because it stabilizes the enzyme complex (see Fig. 58.6). Increased residual specific activity of mitochondrial membrane-bound enzymes may require this prolonged period because of the biologic half-life of this subcellular organelle. During this period, decreased sensitivity to dietary BCAAs is usually observed, and more can be added to the diet. Evaluation of total body LEU oxidation before and during thiamin administration gives direct evidence for responsivity (170). In classic MSUD, thiamin is only an adjunct therapy, and dietary restriction of ILE, LEU, and VAL is needed.

Orthoptic liver transplantation resulted in a clear increase in whole-body BCKA oxidation to at least the level of MSUD variants. These patients no longer required BCAA restriction, and the risk of metabolic decompensation during catabolism was abolished (190).

Nutrient Requirements. Data in Table 58.4 outline the suggested amounts of BCAAs, protein, energy, and fluid to offer the infant or child with MSUD. Because the BCAAs are essential, they cannot be deleted from the diet without producing growth failure and death. In planning nutrition support of the infant or child with MSUD, a prescription should be written that includes recommended amounts of BCAAs, protein, energy, and fluid for the day. Frequent adjustments in the diet prescription are necessary, and are needed daily during the first few weeks and biweekly during the first 6 months of life, based on appetite, growth, development, and laboratory analyses of plasma BCAAs and BCKAs. Because LEU residues are more prominent than ILE and VAL in most proteins, supplemental free L-ILE and L-VAL may be necessary in the newborn period and beyond to prevent deficiency of these two essential amino acids. However, competition between the free BCAAs at the intestinal cell can cause imbalances in plasma amino acids (191).

Requirements for ILE, LEU, and VAL vary considerably depending on age, type and extent of enzyme defect, growth rate, and state of health. Younger infants normally have greater requirements per unit of body weight than older infants. A rapid decline occurs in requirements for BCAAs between 3 and 6 months of age. Careful monitoring of plasma concentrations and intake of BCAAs is required to prevent excess intake when growth rate declines and to provide adequate intake when growth is accelerated, as in early infancy, during prepuberty and puberty, and during the last half of gestation. Successful pregnancy has occurred in two adults with MSUD (192, 193).

The recommended protein intake for infants with MSUD (see Table 58.4) is greater than that for normal infants and children because the primary protein source consists of free amino acids (21). The recommended energy intake after the initial acute period is somewhat higher for normal infants and children because the ketoacids of the BCAAs cannot be used for energy synthesis (see Table 58.4) (1). During the neonatal acute period, up to 170 kcal/kg/day may be required (194).

Medical Foods Free of Branched-Chain Amino Acids. Adequate protein cannot be obtained from ordinary foods without ingesting more BCAAs than are required in classic MSUD. The BCAA content of foods as a percentage of protein ranges from approximately 3.5 to 8.5% (57). Because of the BCAA content of most proteins, medical foods are used that are formulated from amino acids free of BCAAs. In the United States, several products are available that provide protein. Formulations, major nutrient composition, and sources of these products are given in Appendix Table A-25-a.

Equivalent Lists. Equivalent lists of foods are available to assist in providing variety and needed intact protein in the diet (58). The lists are similar to diabetic exchange lists in that foods of similar LEU content are grouped together and may be exchanged for one another within the same list. The average ILE, LEU, VAL, protein, and energy contents of these lists are given in Appendix Table A-25-g.

Initiation of Nutrition Support. A rapid decline in plasma ILE and VAL can be achieved at the time of diagnosis by feeding formula free of BCAAs. However, the plasma LEU will continue to increase over the first 4 days of life, even if dietary BCAA restriction is implemented at birth (189). MSUD is not expressed at birth in most patients, and infants whose screening results are positive are treated at 7 to 14 days of life. In our experience, branched-chain ketoacidosis can be averted by high energy intake with no added BCAAs over a 72-hour period if instituted between 8 and 11 days of age. There is an association among the degree of α-ketoisocaproic acid excretion, LEU elevation, and clinical outcome (195). Laboratory results of plasma BCAAs should be rapidly available to prevent the predicted deficiency in ILE and VAL. When replacement is begun, these two amino acids may be added as free L-amino acids to increase their ratio to LEU in intact protein. High-energy intake of 140 to 170 kcal/kg of body weight during this period prevents catabolism of body protein. If the osmolality of formula permits, protein at 3.0 to 3.5 g/kg should be offered. This regimen will lower the concentrations of BCAAs to near-normal ranges. If deficiency of either ILE or VAL occurs, plasma LEU concentrations will remain elevated as a function of muscle catabolism or decreased protein synthesis.

The LEU required at birth may decrease from 70 to 40 mg/kg/day at 2 years. Medical foods designed for MSUD should be used for therapy; however, to prevent deficiency of the essential amino acids ILE and VAL, solutions of these two BCAAs are added back to the formula. See Appendix Table A-25-h for sample diets for an infant.

Assessment of Nutrition Support. Frequency of assessment is dictated by the clinical course and the response of plasma amino acids. Monitoring of therapy should use three combined approaches. Ion-exchange or MS/MS should be used daily to quantitate plasma amino acid concentrations for approximately 3 weeks after birth; these help to determine requirements for the individual BCAAs. Urine can be evaluated at bedside for decline in the DNPH reaction, much like Clinitest was used to monitor diabetic ketoacidosis. Quantitation of organic acids by GC/MS can detect a decline in BCKAs and the presence of β-lipolysis.

After requirements are established, plasma amino acid concentrations are determined approximately every 2 weeks to ensure that the child has not outgrown the prescription. Samples should be obtained at midday before the noon feeding. We have found organic acid analysis of urine to be helpful. BCKAs decrease under optimum dietary conditions. If energy or a specific amino acid is overrestricted, evidence of β-lipolysis (acetoacetic acid, β-OH-butyric acid) is found.

After hospital discharge, daily testing of urine with DNPH by a parent at home screens rapidly for ketoaciduria. As a rule, preventive clinical evaluation of the child for cryptogenic infections before overt ketoacidosis occurs is more effective than trying to treat the child after a catabolic phase has produced its attendant ketoacidosis. If the urine DNPH results are positive, a blood sample should be collected on filter paper for LEU assay and the urine should be further analyzed by GC/MS to differentiate ketonuria from branched-chain α-ketonuria. With a diet history, a physician's examination, and laboratory analyses, one can usually differentiate among overrestriction, intercurrent infection, or diet underrestriction as a cause for BCKA. Every effort should be made to maintain plasma BCAAs in the normal range. A plasma LEU concentration greater than 600 μmol/L is associated with clinically significant a-ketoacidemia and the appearance of ataxia (195). Changes suggesting dysmyelination were found in the white matter, cerebral hemispheres, brainstem, mesencephalon, thalamus, and globus pallidus of patients with chronically elevated concentrations of BCAAs and BCKAs (196).

Episodes of infection and trauma can evoke catabolism of tissue protein and increase plasma concentrations of BCAAs. Clinical improvement is rapid if some BCAAs are administered along with an amino acid mix that provides 150 to 200 kcal/kg per day. Parenteral amino acid solutions free of BCAAs have also caused a rapid decline in plasma BCAAs during infection with concomitant clinical

improvement (197). During and after surgery, intravenous GLU administration is important to prevent hypoglycemia (198).

Outcome of Nutrition Support. Patients diagnosed at 5 days of age or less had IQs (97 ± 13 SD) greater than those of physiologically normal siblings or parents (5). Factors influencing IQ were age at the time of diagnosis, neonatal condition, and long-term metabolic control.

The first attempt to manage an 8-month-old infant with MSUD used pure amino acids totaling approximately 50 g daily, oil and sugar to yield 1500 kcal/day, and mineral and vitamin mixtures. Plasma concentrations of BCAAs decreased significantly and the maple syrup odor disappeared from the urine. During the diet trial, length and weight increased from the third to the fiftieth percentile (199).

Nutrition support of a neonate with BCKA was subsequently described (200). Plasma amino acids were measured as a basis for diet changes. Approximate protein intake ranged from 3.5 to 3.0 g/kg/day, and energy intake was about 125 kcal/kg/day between 3 and 8 months of age. At birth, the infant was at the tenth percentile for length and weight; during the first year of life, length increased toward the fiftieth percentile, but weight remained at about the tenth percentile. Anemia, with a hemoglobin of 85 g/L, was present from 1 to 3 months of age. At 55 weeks of age, the patient had a developmental quotient of 97, which is in the normal range.

Experience with seven patients with MSUD, three of whom died, was reported (201). The surviving patients received an amino acid mix free of BCAAs to which corn oil (43% of energy), dextrimaltose (45% of energy), minerals, and vitamins were added. Protein and energy intake was not reported. Linear growth of one patient by 1 year of age was considerably below the tenth percentile. Three of the four surviving patients had weights below the tenth percentile; length/height percentiles were not given.

A number of other investigators have reported poor growth in treated children with BCKA (202–207). Except for Henstenburg and colleagues (207), who indicated that mean protein and energy intakes were 78 and 86% of RDA, respectively, few investigators reported protein or energy intake. However, intakes of both protein and energy by children with MSUD have been reported to be below those of comparably aged normal children (208). Whether failure to thrive is caused by the underlying disease or by iatrogenic dietary effects is unclear. Some investigators reported normal growth when adequate protein and energy were fed (199, 200). Because of competitive inhibition of mitochondrial oxidative phosphorylation between BCKAs and pyruvate, there may be a need for a greater energy intake than that recommended by the Institute of Medicine (1).

Selenium deficiency has been found in treated patients with MSUD receiving selenium-free medical food (209). Folic acid deficiency was reported in an infant after about

4 months on a synthetic diet (210). Acidosis occurred in an infant treated with an amino acid mix in which several amino acids were provided as the HCl salt (211).

Termination of Nutrition Support. Patients with classic MSUD are unable to terminate the diet, even if they respond to thiamine. The occurrence of death in variants with intermittent MSUD suggests the need for some form of ongoing therapy in even these relatively stable patients. The BCKAs are relatively acute neurotoxins and probably interfere with oxygen consumption and ATP production in the medullary reticular substance of the brain (167).

Isovaleric Acidemia

This disorder was first described in 1967 and was identified by the urinary excretion of IVA (212). Subsequently, a deficiency of IVD was defined in cultured skin fibroblasts (213). Although a deficiency of electron transfer protein is also reported, mutations in the apoenzyme are specific for isovaleryl CoA as substrate. IVD deficiency results in a block in the catabolism of LEU at the step after BCKAD complex (see Fig. 58.4). The IVD gene was assigned to chromosome 15q14-q15 (214) (see Table 58.3), and molecular heterogeneity is defined and five classes are proposed on the basis of the effects of various mutations of the IVD gene (214, 215). Class I has normal-sized IVD and missense mutations. Classes II, III, and IV have reduced-size proteins, and class V has no immunologically detectable IVD. IVA, 3-hydroxyisovaleric acid (OHIVA), and the adduct IVG accumulate in body fluids. Gas-liquid chromatography and mass spectrometry can identify these compounds in body fluids, and the enzyme is quantifiable in cultured dermal fibroblasts (172, 213).

The phenotypic abnormalities result from the toxic accumulation of free IVA. An alternate pathway producing IVG using GLY-*N*-acylase reduces the accumulation of the toxic precursors. Thus, clinical differences in phenotype are caused by the degree of impaired IVD and epigenetic phenomena, such as the degree of detoxification available to this alternative pathway (172, 216, 217). Carnityl adducts offer an additional alternate pathway for detoxifying free isovaleric acidemia (218, 219).

Despite molecular advances in understanding the mutations affecting IVD, two disease forms continue to be clinically useful classifications: the acute form and the chronic intermittent form (172). Patients with the acute form of isovaleric acidemia are generally normal full-term infants. Within the first days of life, poor feeding, tachypnea, vomiting, and a characteristic "sweaty feet" odor (caused by IVA) of the blood and urine are frequently noted. Diarrhea, lethargy, hypotonia, and tremors may also be found. Some cases do not respond to treatment; the patients may become cyanotic or comatose, and death often results. The exact cause of death is frequently unknown. Severe metabolic acidosis, hyperammonemia, CNS hemorrhage,

cardiac arrest, and sepsis are some probable causes. Infants whose conditions are detected early and respond to treatment survive the neonatal period and develop appropriately. If acute neonatal disease is prevented, the condition progresses into the chronic intermittent type of isovaleric acidemia.

In thechronic intermittent form, babies are normal at birth. During late infancy, they may develop episodes of vomiting, acidosis, stupor, and coma. A sweaty-feet odor is usually present, and a transient alopecia is occasionally seen. These episodes may begin as early as 2 weeks of age, and the frequency of attacks seems to decrease with age. Urinary tract and upper respiratory infections frequently trigger these episodes, as do excessive intake of protein and aspirin. Many children affected by the intermittent form prefer fruits and vegetables over meat and milk. The degree of enzyme (IVD) impairment and the capacity of the alternate IVG-producing pathway, as well as intake, probably produce these clinically different presentations (172).

Several patients with either the acute or the chronic form of isovaleric acidemia have had moderate to severe hematologic abnormalities, including leukopenia and thrombocytopenia, with pancytopenia being the most common. Isovaleric acidemia inhibits granulopoietic progenitor cell proliferation in bone marrow cultures and may account for the neutropenia often seen in isovaleric acidemia (220). In one instance, transfusion of packed red cells and platelets prevented further complications. Depressed hemoglobin concentrations were also seen in several patients. Transient alopecia seems to be more common with the chronic intermittent form than with the acute form of the disease and may be nutritionally related. Hyperammonemia (up to 1200 μmol) has also been reported during neonatal crises (172).

Screening. Several states now screen for isovaleric acidemia using MS/MS (see Fig. 58.4). As newborn screening and diagnosis of isovaleric acidemia expand to all states, the incidence of this disorder will become known.

Diagnosis. Because IVG is excreted during both remission and ketotic attacks, measurement of urinary IVG by GC/MS is the best method of diagnosis. Normal 3- to 5-year-old unaffected children have no detectable urinary IVG (less than 2 mg/day). Affected children of the same age excrete from 40 to 250 mg/day. During ketotic episodes, urinary 3-OHIVA, 4-OHIVA, and methylsuccinic acid are excreted in large quantities as well (172).

Diagnosis is confirmed by measuring the impaired ability of skin fibroblasts cultured from affected individuals to oxidize LEU-2-^{14}C to $^{14}CO_2$ (213, 221). A more complicated assay using mitochondria and 1-^{14}C-IVA has also been used (222). High-field proton nuclear magnetic resonance is a promising new technique for the rapid diagnosis of isovaleric acidemia because it can readily detect IVG in a small sample of urine (223).

Prenatal diagnosis is available by combined organic acid analysis of amniotic fluid and enzyme assay of cultured amniotic fluid cells. A heterozygote for IVD has been detected prenatally (224).

Treatment. During acute ketotic attacks, parenteral fluid therapy and correction of the metabolic acidosis are indicated as adjuncts to high energy intake and L-carnitine and GLY therapy. Serum and urine IVA concentrations are monitored during ketotic attacks. GC/MS analysis is the most accurate means of determining serum and urinary IVA. A special method of GC/MS allows separate quantitation of the two isomers, IVA and 2-methylbutyric acid. Serum IVA ranges from 0.1 to 84 mg/dL (172) depending on the patient's clinical status. A simple and rapid method of determining 4-OHIVA concentrations in the plasma has recently been devised (225); however, elevations of this metabolite lag at least 36 hours behind the maximum plasma concentrations of IVA, which limits its use clinically. Monitoring urinary IVG provides a good parameter of nutrition therapy. Titration of IVG with free GLY to a stable optimum level is desirable. However, excess GLY over free substrate (IVA) may inhibit IVG production. When LEU restriction is optimal and the patient is stable, about 90 mg GLY/kg/day is optimal. During acute disease, a higher intake (300 to 600 mg/kg/day) of GLY may be necessary until infection or dietary LEU indiscretions are removed (226).

Nutrient Requirements. A low-protein diet of 1.2 to 1.5 g/kg/day in infants improves clinical symptoms, and many patients restrict protein by choice (172). This represents only 60% of the RDA. Protein restriction alone is therefore not the best mode of therapy because over-restriction of essential BCAAs (ILE, VAL) is inevitable if LEU is adequately restricted in intact protein.

LEU restriction and the use of pharmacologic doses of GLY have been reported. In six patients with isovaleric acidemia, GLY therapy resulted in decreased IVA in plasma and urine (172). Urinary IVG simultaneously increased, often twofold to threefold. Clinical improvement occurred that was characterized by increased growth, control of acidosis, and resolution of pancytopenia with GLY supplements and protein restriction over a 2-week period.

GLY used to remove IVA through an alternative pathway is a prototype for nutrition detoxification of accumulated substrates in inborn errors of metabolism (226, 227). The ubiquitous enzyme GLY-N-acylase has a broad range of substrates that accumulate in other inborn errors of metabolism and might also be amenable to this approach. The relative amounts of GLY required to optimize removal of IVA (or other substrates for the GLY-N-acylase reaction) need careful evaluation and will change with the clinical condition of the patient (226).

Some evidence exists supporting substrate inhibition of the reaction when excess GLY is added under stable conditions. The optimal dose of supplemental GLY was determined for a 9-year-old white girl with isovaleric acidemia who was well and who maintained a LEU intake of 54 ± 3.6 mg/kg/day. Supplementation with GLY below or above the range of 50 to 150 mg/kg resulted in a 50% decrease in IVG excretion. Urinary IVA excretion was consistent throughout the study. No β-OHIVA was detected in plasma or urine. The results of this study indicated that (a) the optimal dose of GLY for this patient under these stable clinical and nutrition conditions was 50 to 150 mg/kg; (b) an optimal dose of GLY should be quantitated for specific ages, clinical states, degree of enzyme activity, and LEU intake in the treatment of isovaleric acidemia; and (c) GLY supplements above 300 mg/kg/day increased plasma and urinary concentrations of GLY, but resulted in decreased IVG excretion, as if this substrate inhibited GLY-N-acylase when concentrations of its cosubstrate, isovaleryl CoA, were controlled (226).

Systemic carnitine deficiency has been demonstrated in several patients with isovaleric acidemia (228). Although plasma levels of carnitine were low in these patients, the acylcarnitine ester—isovaleryl carnitine—was increased, especially during illness (228, 229). Relative deficiency of muscle carnitine and use of carnitine as an adduct for isovaleric acidemia are two reasons for treating with extra L-carnitine. The relative therapeutic value of L-carnitine has been compared with that of GLY in the treatment of isovaleric acidemia in a 4.5-year-old black boy (229). Administration of GLY plus LEU resulted in the excretion of more IVA as IVG than when LEU was administered alone. LEU plus L-carnitine increased isovaleryl carnitine excretion from a pretreatment level of 7 μmol/24 hours to a posttreatment level of 1470 μmol/24 hours. Large doses of carnitine are needed in the range of 100 to 200 mg/kg/day to accomplish this therapeutic excretion, whereas 100 to 150 mg/kg/day of GLY will suffice. Smaller doses of carnitine supplements are recommended to prevent deficiency.

Medical Foods Free of Leucine. Four medical foods free of LEU have been designed specifically for the nutrition support of patients with isovaleric acidemia and other disorders of LEU catabolism. Formulations, major nutrient composition, and sources of these medical foods are given in Appendix Table A-25-a.

Outcome of Nutrition Support. A male infant with isovaleric acidemia, treated from the neonatal period with a medical food designed for MSUD with added L-ILE and L-VAL, and whole protein to supply essential restricted LEU, had normal growth and development. Height and weight were between the twenty-fifth and fiftieth percentile. Head circumference was at the fiftieth percentile. On average, the diet supplied 2.5 to 3.0 g protein/kg/day and 100 mg LEU/kg/day. L-Carnitine and GLY were not a part of the diet regimen (230).

Growth of a male infant diagnosed prenatally with isovaleric acidemia has been reported. At birth the infant was breast-fed ad libitum, and 250 mg GLY/kg/day were administered. In spite of the low protein intake from human milk and the GLY supplement, the patient became acidotic and began to vomit and hyperventilate at 3 days of age. Breast-feeding was discontinued, and a LEU-free diet providing 125 kcal/kg supplemented with 380 mg GLY/kg/day was begun. His clinical status improved rapidly. Dietary LEU at 45 mg/kg/day with GLY at 250 mg/kg/day and protein at 2.0 g/kg was introduced at 5 days of age. At 2 years of age, the patient was developmentally normal and was higher than the ninety-fifth percentile for height and weight. Diet at 2 years of age supplied the following per kilogram: 46 mg LEU, 1.7 g protein, and 72 kcal. Only one hospitalization for vomiting and dehydration was required during the 2-year period (226).

Outcomes in nine patients with isovaleric acidemia managed by protein restriction (1.5 to 2.0 g/kg in infancy, 0.8 to 1.5 g/kg thereafter) and 250 mg GLY/kg/day have been reported (231). Because all of the patients had secondary carnitine deficiency (total serum carnitine 19 ± 3 μmol/L), diets of four of the children were supplemented with 50 mg/kg/day L-carnitine, and in these, serum carnitine concentrations returned to normal (51 ± 5 μmol/L). Actual height, weight, and head circumference of patients were not reported, although growth velocities were stated to be normal after diet initiation. Developmental quotients or IQ scores of the five subjects in whom diet was initiated during the neonatal period ranged from 49 to 115.

Food refusal has been reported in a patient with isovaleric acidemia (232). Both physiologic and behavioral components to feeding problems were reported. The physiologic component involved altered serotonin metabolism. Any factor such as hyperammonemia or a high-carbohydrate, low-protein diet that stimulates the transport of TRP, a precursor of serotonin, into the brain could lead to anorexia. A low-TRP diet was suggested as one alternative to the treatment of anorexia.

Of 11 reported French patients with isovaleric acidemia, eight were alive after the neonatal period. LEU restriction and GLY supplementation were used to manage patients. Six of eight surviving patients had normal development (233).

Other Organic Acidemias

Other disorders resulting in organic acidemia that are now screened for during the newborn period in some states using MS/MS are described in Table 58.8. This table includes the trivial name of the disorder, the enzyme defect, presenting clinical and laboratory symptoms, diagnostic studies, nutrition support during diagnostic workup and illness, long-term therapy, and outcomes. Data in Table 58.4 describe ranges of recommended intakes for major nutrients. Recommendations for mineral and vitamin intakes are presented in Table 58.5.

3-Methylcrotonylglycinuria. 3-Methylcrotonylglycinuria, caused by deficiency of 3-methylcrotonyl-CoA carboxylase (see Fig. 58.4), has a wide spectrum of clinical symptoms. Some neonates may present with severe hypotonia and seizures, whereas other infants may present at a later age with hypotonia and without severe metabolic acidosis. Some infants may be only mildly delayed with hypoglycemia, failure to thrive, respiratory failure, and hemiparesis during febrile illness. Some patients may not present until adulthood with fatigue, weakness, myopathy, and fatty liver with elevated liver enzymes. Presymptomatic detection using abnormal acylcarnitine profiles by MS/MS is now occurring. Some patients are asymptomatic (172). Treatment with L-carnitine, prevention of fasting, and essential LEU restriction usually results in normal development (see Table 58.8).

3-Methylglutaconic Aciduria. At least four types of this disorder are known. Type I, with a deficiency of 3-methylglutaconyl-CoA hydratase (see Fig. 58.4), has diverse and nonspecific clinical symptoms. The major urinary metabolites are 3-methylglutaconic and 3-hydroxyisovaleric acids. L-Carnitine supplementation and essential LEU restriction may be beneficial (see Table 58.8) (172). The other three types do not respond to diet intervention.

3-Hydroxy-3-Methylglutaric Aciduria. One-third of patients with 3-hydroxy-3-methylglutaryl-CoA lyase deficiency (see Fig. 58.4) present in the neonatal period, and two-thirds present between 3 and 11 months of age with severe hypoglycemia and metabolic acidosis (but with little or no ketosis), hyperammonemia, vomiting, and hypotonia, which may progress to coma and death. The symptoms resemble those of Reye syndrome. Treatment by restriction of essential LEU and fat, avoidance of fasting, and L-carnitine supplementation generally leads to normal development (see Tables 58.4 and 58.8). 3-Hydroxy-3-methylglutaryl-CoA lyase deficiency is a disorder of BCAA (LEU) metabolism; its diagnosis is from the major abnormal metabolites in urine, 3-hydroxy-3-methylglutaric, 3-methylglutaconic, and 3-hydroxyisovaleric acids. This disorder is also one of ketone body metabolism (172).

Propionic Acidemia

Isolated deficiency of propionyl-CoA carboxylase (see Figs. 58.3 and 58.4) results in the accumulation of propionate in blood and of 3-hydroxypropionate, methylcitrate, tiglyglycine, and unusual ketone bodies in urine (174). Two complementation groups, *pccA* and *pccBC* , have been defined among propionyl-CoA carboxylase-deficient patients. These groups correspond to mutations affecting genes coding for the α- and the β-subunits, respectively, of the carboxylase apoprotein. Clinically, the disorder is characterized by severe metabolic ketoacidosis, which often appears in the neonatal period and requires vigorous alkali therapy; restriction of essential ILE, MET, THR, VAL, and odd-chain fatty acids; prevention of fasting and

TABLE 58.8. ORGANIC ACIDEMIAS FOR WHICH NEWBORN SCREENING OCCURS BY TANDEM MASS SPECTROMETRY IN SOME STATES

DISORDER (ENZYME DEFECT)	PRESENTING SYMPTOMS CLINICAL	PRESENTING SYMPTOMS LABORATORY	DIAGNOSTIC STUDIES	NUTRITION SUPPORT DURING DIAGNOSIS AND ACUTE ILLNESS	LONG-TERM THERAPY	NUTRITION ASSESSMENT	OUTCOME
3-Methylcrotonyl-CoA (3-methylcrotonyl-CoA carboxylase, MCC) (181)	Variable Neonatal onset: irritability drowsiness, difficulty feeding, vomiting, rapid respirations, apnea, seizures, spasms, coma, death, if untreated lacer onset: hypotonia some patients have no clinical symptoms	Metabolic acidosis Hypoglycemia Later onset: mild metabolic acidosis	Identification of blood and urinary 3-methyl-crotonylglycine Evaluation of MCC activity in cells, MCC mutation analysis	Delete dietary LEU 1–2 d only Administer IV L-carnitine. Vigorous fluid replacement Correct metabolic acidosis and electrolyte abnormalities Provide adequate energy to suppress catabolism (125–150% RDA for age) If necessary, give IV glucose, lipid, and L-amino acids free of LEU Return to oral medical food and complete diet as rapidly as tolerated	Restrict LEU; Administer L-carnitine and glycine Prevent fasting See Table 58–4 for recommended nutrient Intakes	Plasma LEU, L-carnitine, GLY, IVG, serum transthyretin, ferritin Bone radiographs of lumbar vertebrae Urinary isovaleryl-glycine, β-hydroxyisovaleric acid Cation/anion gap Dietary intakes of LEU, protein, energy, minerals, vitamins Growth	Normal growth and development with neonatal diagnosis and excellent therapy with LEU restriction, L-carnitine, and GLY
3-Methylglutaconic aciduria type 1 (3-methyl-glutaconyl-CoA hydratase) (181)	Coma, psychomotor retardation and/or speech retardation may be present	Metabolic acidosis on fasting may be present Hypoglycemia on fasting may be present	Identification of 3-methylgtutaconic acid Assay of hydratase activity in fibroblasts	Delete dietary LEU 1–2 d only Administer IV L-carnitine Vigorous fluid replacement Correct metabolic acidosis and electrolyte abnormalities Provide adequate energy to suppress catabolism (125–150% RDA for age) If necessary, give IV glucose, lipid, and L-amino acids free of LEU Return to oral medical food and complete diet as rapidly as tolerated	Restrict LEU; administer L-carnitine and glycine Prevent fasting See Table 58–4 for recommended nutrient Intakes	Plasma LEU, L-carnitine, GLY, IVG, serum transthyretin, ferritin Bone radiographs of lumbar vertebrae Urinary isovaleryl-glycine, β-hydroxyisovaleric acid Cation/anion gap Dietary intakes of LEU, protein, energy, minerals, vitamins Growth	Normal growth and development with neonatal diagnosis and excellent therapy with LEU restriction, L-carnitine, and GLY
3-Hydroxy-3-methylglutaric aciduria (3-hydroxy-	Babies appear normal at birth, but symptoms	Metabolic acidosis with very low blood pH	Quantification of urinary 3-hydroxy-	Rapid intervention is required Limit exogenous protein	Restrict LEU and fat Administer	Plasma LEU, carnitine (free) Serum	Normal growth and development with

Disorder (enzyme)	Clinical features	Laboratory findings	Diagnosis	Treatment	Monitoring	Outcome
3-methylglutaryl-CoA lyase, 3-HMG-CoA lyase (181)	appear during the first week of life, infancy, or childhood. Vomiting, hypotonia, lethargy, seizures, and/or coma in 10% of cases, death. Symptoms similar to Reye syndrome	Severe hypoglycemia, Hypoketonemia, Hypoketonuria, Hyperammonemia and/or elevated transaminases may be present	3-methylglutaric acid, 3-methyl-glutaconate, 3-hydroxyiso-valerate, plasma 3-methylglutaryl-carnitine. Analysis of enzyme activity in fibroblasts and mutation analysis	intake 1–2 d only. Limit fat intake. Administer L-carnitine. Vigorous replacement of fluids. Correct severe metabolic acidosis and electrolyte abnormalities. Provide adequate energy to suppress endogenous protein catabolism (125–150% RDA for age). Suspect concurrent sepsis: have a low threshold to treat after obtaining appropriate cultures. L-carnitine. Prevent fasting. See Table 58-4 for recommended nutrient intakes	transthyretin, ferritin. Urinary 3-methyl-glutaric acid. Dietary Intake of LEU, protein, fat, energy, minerals, vitamins. Growth	early and lifelong therapy
Propionic acidemia (propionyl-CoA carboxylase, PCC) (182)	Refusal to feed, Vomiting, Dehydration, Lethargy, Hypotonia, Seizures, Coma, Developmental retardation, Osteoporosis, Hepatomegaly may be present	Severe metabolic acidosis, EEG abnormalities, Hyperammonemia, Hyperglycinemia, Neutropenia, anemia, and thrombocyto-penia may be present	Measurement of plasma propionate, urinary 3-hydroxypro-pionate, methyl-citrate, tiglyl-glycine. Analysis of PCC activity and mutations in cultured fibroblasts	Rapid intervention is required. Limit exogenous protein Intake 1–2 d only. Administer L-carnitine. Vigorous replacement of fluids. Correct severe metabolic acidosis and electrolyte abnormalities. Provide adequate energy to suppress endogenous protein catabolism (125–150% RDA for age). Suspect concurrent sepsis: have a low threshold to treat after obtaining appropriate cultures. Restrict ILE, MET, THR, VAL, linoleic acid, odd-chain fatty acids. Prevent fasting. Administer L-carnitine. See Table 58–4 for recommended nutrient intakes. Avoid breads with calcium or sodium propionate, butter, cream, olive oil, chicken fat, men-haden oil	Plasma ILE, MET, THR, VAL, GLY. Blood ammonia. Cation/anion gap. Urinary metabolites of propionate. serum transthyretin, ferritin. Bone radiographs of lumbar vertebrae. Dietary intake of ILE, MET, THR, VAL, protein, energy, minerals, vitamins. Growth	Normal growth with early therapy. Neurologic outcome improved
Methylmalonic aciduria (methylmalonyl-CoA mutase° or-, MMA) (182)	Hypertonia, Areflexia, lethargy, Failure to thrive, Recurrent vomiting	Acidosis, Ketosis, Ketonuria, Hyperammonemia, Hyperglycinemia, Hypoglycemia	Urinary methylmalonic acid and/or MMA in blood by MS/MS. Fibroblast studies	Rapid intervention is required. Limit exogenous protein intake 1–2 d only. Administer L-carnitine. Vigorous replacement of. Restrict ILE, MET, THR, VAL, linoleic acid, odd-chain fatty acids	Plasma ILE, MET, THR, VAL, GLY. Blood ammonia. Cation/anion gap. Urinary metabolites of propionate	Normal growth with early therapy. Neurologic outcome improved

(continued)

943

TABLE 58.8. ORGANIC ACIDEMIAS FOR WHICH NEWBORN SCREENING OCCURS BY TANDEM MASS SPECTROMETRY IN SOME STATES (continued)

DISORDER (ENZYME DEFECT)	PRESENTING SYMPTOMS		DIAGNOSTIC STUDIES	NUTRITION SUPPORT DURING DIAGNOSIS AND ACUTE ILLNESS	LONG-TERM THERAPY	NUTRITION ASSESSMENT OUTCOME
	CLINICAL	LABORATORY				
	Dehydration Severe mental retardation or death if untreated Coma, hepatomegaly, muscular hypotonia, and respiratory distress may be present	Hyperuricemia Neutropenia Thrombocytopenia Pancytopenia	of enzymes Measure total plasma homocysteine, free methionine, and homocystine	fluids Correct severe metabolic acidosis and electrolyte abnormalities Provide adequate energy to suppress endogenous protein catabolism (125–150% RDA for age) Suspect concurrent sepsis: have a low threshold to treat after obtaining appropriate cultures	Prevent fasting Administer L-carnitine See Table 58-4 for recommended nutrient intakes	and methylmalonate Serum transthyretin, ferritin Bone radiographs of lumbar vertebrae Dietary intake if ILE, MET, THR, VAL, protein, energy, minerals, vitamins Growth
Methylmalonic acidemia (cobalamin reductase adenosyltransferase)	Lethargy Failure to thrive Recurrent vomiting Dehydration Respiratory distress Muscular hypotonia, developmental retardation, hepatomegaly, coma may be present	Metabolic acidosis Ketonemia/ketonuria Hyperammonemia, leukopenia, thrombocytopenia, hypoglycemia may be present	Urinary methylmalonic acid and/or MMA in blood by MS/MS Fibroblast studies of enzymes Measure total plasma homocysteine, free methionine, and homocystine	Rapid intervention is required Limit exogenous protein intake 1–2 d only Administer L-carnitine Vigorous replacement of fluids Correct severe metabolic acidosis and electrolyte abnormalities Provide adequate energy to suppress endogenous protein catabolism (125–150% RDA for age) Suspect concurrent sepsis: have a low threshold to treat after obtaining appropriate cultures	1–2 mg OH cobalamin daily Modest protein restriction.	Plasma ILE, MET, THR, VAL, GLY Blood ammonia Cation/anion gap Urinary metabolites of proplonate and methylmalonate Serum transthyretin, ferritin Bone radiographs of lumbar vertebrae Dietary intake if ILE, MET, THR, VAL, protein, energy, minerals, vitamins Growth

CoA, coenzyme A; EEG, electroencepahlographic; GLY, glycine; ILE, isoleucine; IV, intravenous; LEU, leucine; MET, methionine; MCC, 3-methylcrotonyl-coenzyme Acarboxylase; MMA, methylmalonic acid; MS, mass spectrometry; PCC, propionyl-coenzyme A carboxylase; RDA, recommended dietary allowance; THR, threonine; VAL, valine.

weight loss (234); L-carnitine supplementation; and adequate energy for growth to cover that lost in the urine as propionylcarnitine (see Tables 58.4 and 58.8). Appendix Table A-25-i supplies average contents of ILE, MET, THR, VAL, protein, and energy in servings lists for PPA and MMA. Actual food lists with portion sizes may be found in reference 58. Medical foods available for PPA and MMA are given in Appendix Table A-25-a. Overrestriction of ILE in the diet may result in acrodermatitis enteropathicalike cutaneous lesions in patients with either PPA or MMA (235). Sample diets for an infant with PPA or MMA are given in Appendix Table A-25-j. Oral antibiotic therapy to reduce gut propionate production may also prove useful. Screening of almost 1,000,000 newborns for PPA or MMA with MS/MS resulted in finding one of 65,000 infants affected (236).

Foods containing odd-chain fatty acids that must be deleted from the diets of patients with PPA or MMA include some fish oils (menhaden, mullet, tuna); chicken fat; olive oil; lard (237); the fat of ruminants (238), including butterfat and cream; and any food to which propionate is added to retard spoilage. Dupont and Mathias (239) reported γ-oxidation of ^{14}C-linoleate into methylmalonate to be 20 times greater than from ^{14}C-palmitate.

North and coworkers (240) reported that no deaths had occurred in their cohort of patients with PPA. Growth and nutrition status were improved with the use of medical foods and gastrostomy tube feedings. However, hypotonia and cognitive delay were still present in all children. Pancreatitis, acute or chronic, has been reported as a complication of all organic acidemias (241). Suppression of granulopoietic progenitor cell proliferation (220, 242) and pancytopenia (243) have been reported in patients with organic acidemias. A successful pregnancy has been reported in a woman with PPA (192).

Thomas and colleagues (244) suggested that the energy needs of patients with PPA were below those of normal children. Feillet and colleagues (245), who used intact protein restriction without use of medical foods (free amino acids), found resting energy expenditure to be about 20% reduced in patients with MMA or PPA. deKoning and colleagues (246) found higher resting energy expenditure in patients fed adequate medical food than in those fed none, perhaps because of higher lean body mass. Yannicelli and colleagues (247) found normal growth in seven infants and children with PPA or MMA when they were fed energy at 98% of RDA and protein at 115% of the recommendations of the Food and Agriculture Organization, World Health Organization, and United Nations University.

Methylmalonic Acidemia

Neonatal or infantile metabolic acidosis is the clinical hallmark of isolated methylmalonyl-CoA mutase deficiency (see Figs. 58.3 and 58.4). Cells from some apomutase-deficient children have no functional mutase (designated mut^0); cells from others contain a structurally altered mutase with reduced affinity for adenosylcobalamin and with reduced stability (mut^-) (174). Such children have MMA that does not respond to cobalamin supplementation but can be treated with the same diet and medical therapy as PPA. Mild mutase deficiency may be unmasked in infancy by prolonged breast-feeding by a vegan mother (248). Differential diagnosis may include B_{12} deficiency caused by many environmental (e.g., vegan diets) or transport defects (e.g., intrinsic factor deficiency, ileitis, rare transporter defects). In these situations, MMA and aciduria are accompanied by homocystinemia and homocystinuria caused by CH_3-B_{12}. as well as adenosylcobalamin deficiency (see Fig. 58.3).

Progressive renal insufficiency occurs in patients with poorly controlled conditions and true MMA (249). Combined liver-kidney transplantation has proven beneficial in such patients with end-stage renal failure (250).

Pregnancy in a woman with late-onset MMA was reported to have a normal outcome. At 3 years of age, the child was developing normally (251). Early onset MMA often results in early death in spite of aggressive therapy with diet, L-carnitine, gastrostomy feeding, and metronidazole (252). See Appendix Table A-25-h for average values for food lists and reference 58 for portion sizes of foods in each list. Table 58.4 provides suggested nutrient intakes by age, and Appendix Table A-25-a lists appropriate medical foods available.

Glutaric Acidemia Type I

Deficiency of glutaryl-CoA dehydrogenase (GCD) (see Fig. 58.5) causes glutaric acidemia type I (GA-I), a disorder characterized by macrocephaly at birth and dystonia and dyskinesia appearing during the first years of life, chemically by excretion of glutaric and 3-hydroxyglutaric acids in urine, and pathologically by neuronal degeneration of the caudate and putamen. Computed tomography and magnetic resonance imaging scans often show frontotemporal atrophy and/or arachnoid cysts before the onset of symptoms. GCD deficiency is inherited as an autosomal recessive trait. More than 60 pathogenic mutations have been identified in the GCD gene (19p13.2), and because no one mutation is prominent outside of inbred groups, most GA-I patients are heterozygous for two different mutant alleles (253). The exact cause of the pathophysiology of GA-I is not known, but may be attributable to toxic effects of glutaric acid, quinolinic acid, or 3-hydroxyglutaric acid or an abnormality in γ-aminobutyric acid metabolism. The incidence of GA-I is not known, but may be as high as one in 30,000 live births with an increased prevalence in an old-order Amish community. Striatal damage and neurologic phenotype do not develop in all patients, and there is evidence that early supplementation with L-carnitine, vigorous treatment of intercurrent infections with fluids,

GLU, and insulin; dietary restriction of essential LYS and TRP; and prevention of fasting may prevent their development (254, 255). There are some genotype/phenotype relationships to outcome. In the Ontario mutation (IVS-1 + 5ntG → T), treatment from birth, after prenatal diagnosis, failed to prevent acute neurologic episodes in early childhood (256). Table 58.4 describes recommended nutrient intakes, Appendix Table A-25-a outlines appropriate medical foods, Appendix Table A-25-k gives average nutrient values of serving lists, and portion sizes of foods in the lists may be found in reference 58. See Appendix Table A-25-l for sample diets for an infant with GA-I.

Prenatal diagnosis is possible and is based on demonstrating increased concentrations of glutaric acid in amniotic fluid, deficiency of GCD in cultured amniocytes or (probably) material obtained by chorionic villus sample, or in appropriate families, by mutation analysis (253).

AMMONIA

Nutrition management of disorders involving ammonia fixation and urea production uses traditional rules for treating inborn errors of metabolism. Three essential rules are restricting the toxic precursor, adding deficient product, and encouraging alternative pathways for nitrogen excretion. Further, an anabolic state should be maintained to promote growth and prevent catabolism of lean body mass. Study of the biologic variation imparted on ammonia fixation and the urea cycle by heritable mutations in these biochemical reactions has greatly increased our

understanding of the normal physiology, biochemistry, and molecular biology of human nitrogen metabolism (257).

Biochemistry

Central dogma holds that ammonia is converted to urea in the liver through the Krebs-Henseleit cycle (Fig. 58.7) and excreted in the urine. The first three enzymes of the cycle and *N*-acetylglutamate synthetase are mitochondrial. *N*-acetylglutamate synthetase catalyzes the conversion of acetyl-CoA plus glutamate to *N*-acetylglutamate, an essential cofactor for carbamylphosphate synthesis. Carbamylphosphate synthetase I catalyzes the conversion of ammonia, ATP, and bicarbonate to carbamylphosphate. OTC uses carbamylphosphate and ornithine (ORN) as cosubstrates to form citrulline (CIT), which is exported from mitochondria to the cytoplasm, where cytosolic reactions are linked to those three mitochondrial functions. CIT and aspartate form argininosuccinic acid, a reaction catalyzed by argininosuccinic acid synthetase. Fumarate is cleaved from argininosuccinic acid by argininosuccinic acid lyase, yielding arginine (ARG). Urea is then formed by the action of arginase, regenerating cytosolic ORN, which is transported back into the mitochondria to react with OTC.

Urea Cycle Enzyme Deficiencies

Disorders of the urea cycle are a group of inherited defects in these six enzymes that produce urea (see Fig. 58.7) (257). With the exception of OTC deficiency, all

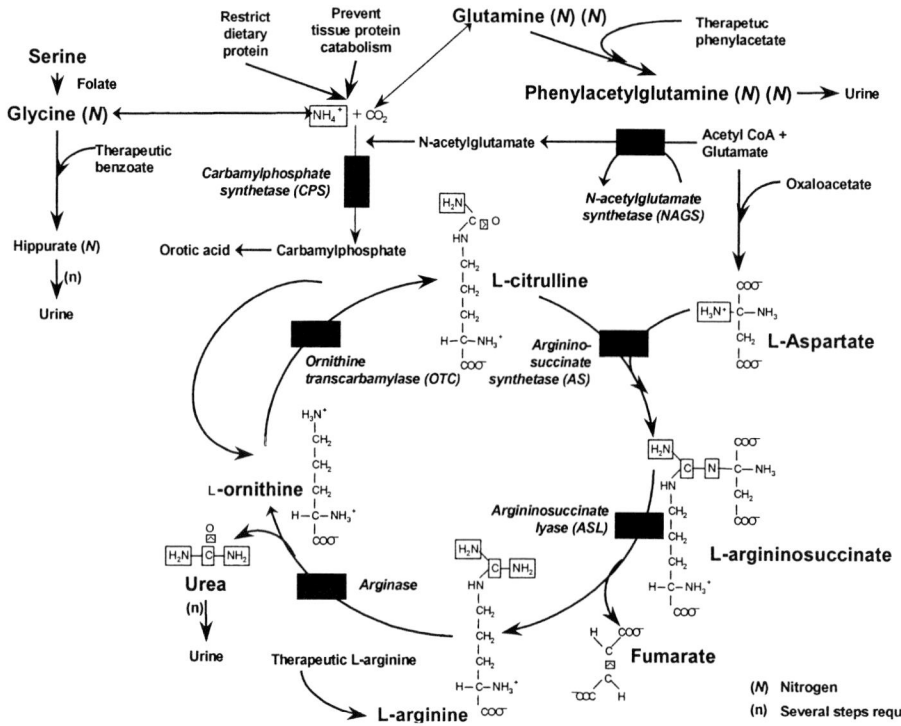

Figure 58.7. Inborn errors in the urea cycle and nutrition approaches to their management. Ammonia fixation and urea production are metabolically cycled with inherited blocks producing hyperammonemia indicated by *black bars*. Important nitrogen molecules and the biochemical origins are outlined in *boxes*. Mitochondrial enzymes in urea synthesis are carbamylphosphate synthetase, *N*-acetylglutamate synthetase, and ornithine transcarbamylase. Use of benzoate, phenylacetate, and phenylbutyrate is indicated to provide alternate pathways for nitrogen excretion. Dietary arginine is added to provide urea cycle substrate distal to genetically impaired reactions. Restriction of dietary protein and addition of dietary energy to prevent protein catabolism are also indicated.

have an autosomal-recessive mode of inheritance. OTC deficiency is inherited as an X-linked dominant trait that is usually lethal in male patients. Many of the genes for these enzymes have been localized to the human genome, cloned, and had mutations defined. OTC, a 73-kb gene containing ten exons, is located on Xp21.1. More than 230 mutations have been defined with some genotype/phenotype relationships (258). For example, the generation of stop codons from R109X and R109Q results in no residual liver enzyme and severe neonatal presentation. By contrast, the R129-to-histidine mutation also present in the spf-ash mouse model of OTC deficiency has a milder phenotype and residual liver enzyme activity (259). Carbamylphosphate synthetase is located on 2q35, argininosuccinic acid synthetase on 9q34, argininosuccinic acid lyase on 7q11, and arginase on 6q23. All are primarily expressed in liver, and all of these genes have defined mutations in their respective disorders (see Table 58.3) (257, 258, 260, 261). Argininosuccinic acid synthetase has several pseudogenes that confound DNA analysis (257). In OTC deficiency, defects in the protein include disordered mitochondrial uptake and immunologically absent protein in this organelle (259). Arginase has two genes with differential expression in liver and erythrocytes. In addition to these defects in ureagenesis, a seventh cause of hyperammonemia is the hyperammonemia, homocitrullinemia, hyperornithinemia syndrome, which is caused by defective mitochondrial uptake of ORN (262).

Hyperammonemia is a biochemical manifestation of all disorders of the urea cycle. Other biochemical characteristics of each defect follow: carbamylphosphate synthetase I defect causes decreased plasma CIT; OTC deficiency results in orotic aciduria and X-linked patterns of transmission; argininosuccinate synthetase deficiency is associated with increased plasma CIT accompanied by orotic aciduria; argininosuccinate lyase deficiency (ASA) causes increased argininosuccinate in plasma and urine; and arginase deficiency has increased ARG in plasma and urine. Clinical features in the newborn suggesting urea cycle defects (UCDs) occur with protein ingestion. In increasing order of severity, these defects include poor feeding, vomiting, lethargy, hypotonia, stupor, bleeding diatheses, convulsions, coma, shock, and death (257, 263). Mental retardation occurs in survivors of these disastrous newborn episodes, but successful control of hyperammonemia in the newborn may prevent this sequela.

Clinical Phenotypes. Hyperammonemia and its clinical sequelae of vomiting, lethargy, and coma relate to excessive protein intake, catabolism, or valproate therapy (264) and are observed in all the UCEDs. However, biochemical and phenotypic manifestations differ in the individual enzyme deficiencies. In ASA, a specific hair abnormality, trichorrhexis nodosa, is evident. This condition is related to ARG deficiency and the relatively high ARG content of normal hair protein. Hair reverts to normal with ARG supplementation. Adult siblings with ASA may

have little to no clinical manifestations despite identical mutations. In patients with defects in one of the first four enzymes, ARG deficiency is also associated with progressive degeneration of the CNS and a peculiar rash with control of hyperammonemia through protein restriction alone (265, 266).

Each enzyme defect has a spectrum of clinical manifestations ranging from death in the newborn period to cyclical vomiting and migraine in adolescence. For example, the typical male patient with OTC deficiency has less than 5% activity and dies in the neonatal period. A surviving male child with the late-onset form of OTC deficiency has immunologically present OTC with a decreased affinity for ORN, a shift of pH optimum, and 25% of normal activity under physiologic conditions (267). Mutational analyses of the OTC gene have differentiated neonatal from late-onset phenotypes (257, 259).

Enzymatic evidence for genetic heterogeneity comes from kinetic studies in fibroblasts of patients with argininosuccinic acid synthetase deficiency. Early biochemical studies showed that enzymes from patients with citrullinemia all showed decreased binding of CIT and/or aspartate, but the residual argininosuccinic acid synthetase had a distinct and different curve of activity in each patient (268). Analyses of RNA in citrullinemic patients showed heterogeneity, and more than 20 different mutations are now defined (257).

Expression of the Heterozygous State for Ornithine Transcarbamylase Deficiency. The female heterozygote of OTC deficiency may have mild protein intolerance manifested clinically by migraine in adults and by cyclic vomiting with intermittent hyperammonemia in children. When protein or ammonium chloride loads were administered to 15 children with migraine and cyclic vomiting, nine had abnormally high baseline plasma ammonium levels; the tests produced marked hyperammonemia in eight, and six developed migraine symptoms. Enzyme assay in seven girls with cyclical vomiting showed three with deficient OTC activity. Heterozygous female patients with OTC deficiency may be asymptomatic or as severely affected as hemizygous male patients (269).

Screening. Nonselected screening of all newborns for UCDs was routinely conducted in Massachusetts using a bacterial auxotroph that required ARG. Nine of 700,000 newborns were found to be homozygous-affected or heterozygous for ASA (270). Problems associated with analysis of ammonia in blood are described by Barsotti (271). This method can be readily adopted in offices and hospitals for selective screening. Its lack of use in this country is related to cost and demand. Several states now screen for citrullinemia and argininosuccinic aciduria using MS/MS.

The true incidence of UCDs is not known because population-based screening has not been conducted, and many undiagnosed deaths may be caused by these disorders. The overall incidence is underestimated at one in 30,000 live births (272).

Diagnosis. Hyperammonemia in association with other characteristic biochemical and clinical findings is diagnostic of specific disorders in the urea cycle (257). The enzyme defect can be inferred from metabolites (in addition to ammonia) that accumulate in blood and urine: orotic acid in the urine in OTC deficiency; and CIT, argininosuccinic acid, and ARG in the plasma and urine in argininosuccinate synthetase deficiency, ASA, and arginase deficiency, respectively. Carbamylphosphate synthetase or the rare N-acetylglutamate synthetase deficiency is suggested by exclusion of these four enzymopathies and requires liver biopsy with enzyme analyses for diagnosis (273). Hyperammonemia can also be caused by acute or chronic liver diseases, galactosemia, neonatal Niemann-Pick disease type IC, tyrosinemia type I, hereditary fructose intolerance, Reye syndrome, asparaginase treatment, PPA, lysinuric protein intolerance, hyperornithinemia, isovaleric acidemia, MMA, long-term use of parenteral amino acids, and a wide range of infectious agents in infancy. Definitive diagnosis depends on clinical acumen followed by appropriate laboratory studies (263). A suggested algorithm for differential diagnosis of UCEDs is given in Figure 58.8. A suspected UCED is a medical emergency and requires immediate intervention.

Treatment. The treatment of inherited urea cycle enzymopathies can be divided into short- and long-term therapy and depends on the specific diagnosis (274). Valproate therapy should be avoided in patients with UCEDs because its use may enhance hyperammonemia (264).

Short-Term Therapy. We prefer to begin orogastric perfusion with high energy intake (150 kcal/kg/day) but no protein. Pro-Phree or Protein-Free Diet Powder is useful for this approach (see Appendix Table A-25-a). L-ARG (350–500 mg/kg/day) should be added to this formulation. Sodium benzoate (300 mg/kg/day) can successfully reduce acute hyperammonemia in the neonatal period by conjugation of benzoic acid with GLY to form hippurate. Phenylbutyric acid or phenylacetic acid (500 mg/kg/day) is also given to form phenylacetylglutamine, which is excreted in the urine, eliminating from the body two nitrogen atoms per molecule (see Fig. 58.7 and Appendix Table A-25-m).

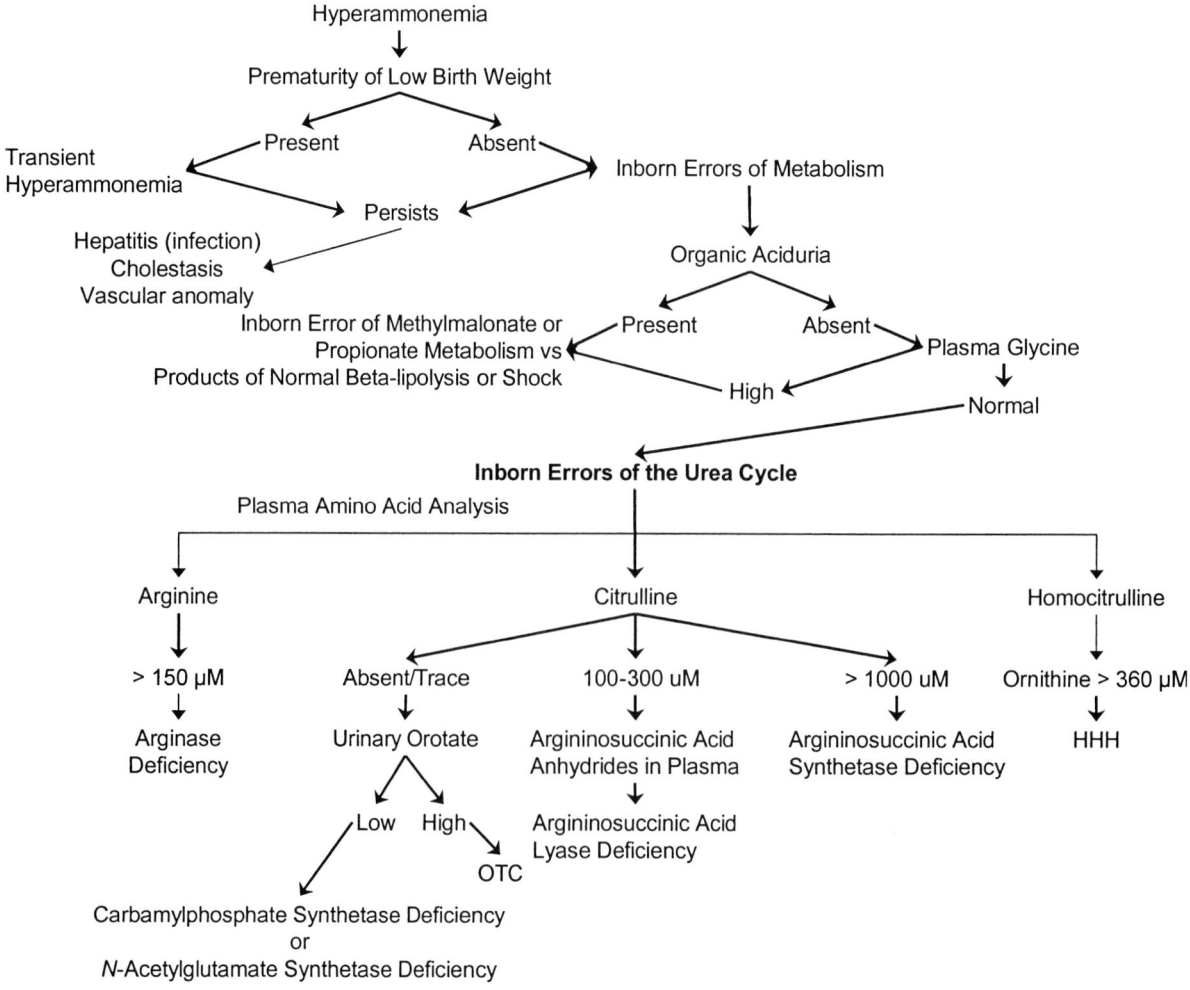

Figure 58.8. Algorithm for differential diagnosis of urea cycle disorders. HHH, hyperornithinemia, homocitrullinemia, and hyperammonemia, OTC, ornithine transcarbamylase.

Urinary potassium loss is enhanced by the excretion of hippurate and phenylacetylglutamine. Consequently, plasma potassium concentrations should be monitored and supplements given if needed.

Hemodialysis may be useful in the presence of coma in reducing plasma ammonium concentrations. Peritoneal dialysis for 7 days in a male neonate with OTC deficiency removed 50 times more ammonia than a single exchange transfusion did. However, peritoneal dialysis includes risks such as *Candida peritonitis* and continued catabolism. If dialysis is used, parenteral L-ARG HCl and sodium phenylbutyrate should be given as well. Continued intravenous protein-free energy is also recommended.

A priority of newborn therapy is to force the neonate into an anabolic phase with high-energy feedings. Peripheral venous hyperalimentation with 10 to 20% GLU and lipid (2 to 4 g/kg) may be necessary if gavage is not tolerated. As gavage feedings are increased, peripheral alimentation should be decreased. After 2 to 3 days of no-protein, high-energy, L-ARG HCl- and benzoate-supplemented feedings, blood ammonia levels should revert to near normal. Cautious addition of 1.0 to 1.5 g/kg/day of protein is then necessary.

Long-Term Therapy. The objectives of therapy in a child with a UCD are to maintain plasma concentrations of ammonia as close to normal as possible and to supply protein and other essential amino acids and nutrients that will allow maximal intellectual development and optimal growth. Four major approaches are used in treating individuals with UCDs (see Fig. 58.7): (a) reducing precursors of ammonia (protein intake), (b) correcting ARG deficiency, (c) enhancing alternate mechanisms of waste nitrogen loss, and (d) accelerating renal excretion of accumulated intermediates (276, 277).

Methods used to reduce ammonia precursors include protein restriction, prevention of body protein catabolism, and use of essential and semiessential amino acids. Any time that intake of protein or essential amino acids is severely restricted, precursors for synthesis of carnitine (LYS, MET), glutathione (cysteine, glutamate), and taurine (cysteine) may be limiting. Restricted MET intake may result in a decrease in the available pool of labile methyl groups required for synthesis of important metabolic compounds.

L-ARG base supplementation is required in all of the UCEDs except arginase deficiency. To maintain normal or slightly elevated plasma ARG concentrations, 100 to 500 mg/kg of body weight daily is used (275). L-ARG can then produce ORN for ammonia fixation and drive the cycle to CIT and argininosuccinate (see Fig. 58.7). These two amino acids are poorly absorbed by the kidney and allow nitrogen loss. Acceleration of renal excretion of accumulated intermediates in the impaired cycle is sought. ARG supplementation increases CIT and argininosuccinic acid excretion in argininosuccinic acid synthetase and ASA, respectively.

Waste nitrogen urinary loss can be enhanced by the use of sodium benzoate, phenylacetate, or phenylbutyrate (275) (see Fig. 58.7). GLY conjugates with benzoate via GLY-*N*-acylase, which leads to excretion of a nearly stoichiometric quantity of nitrogen as hippurate (see Fig. 58.7). Toxicity is low on 200 to 500 mg/kg/day. Folate must be administered to provide a source of one-carbon fragments for synthesis of GLY from serine to prevent GLY depletion. Pyridoxine is necessary for transamination. Pantothenic acid (4 mg/L) in tissue culture media enhanced CoA and hippurate concentrations to a greater extent than smaller or greater amounts (278). Phenylbutyrate and phenylacetate increase urinary nitrogen excretion as phenylacetylglutamine. The suggested dose is 500 mg/kg of body weight. This efficient alternative pathway removes two molecules of nitrogen per molecule of phenylacetylglutamine and requires monitoring of protein intake to prevent deficiency. Excess use of these nitrogen-binding drugs can lead to nitrogen deficiency and poor growth.

Catabolism during a febrile illness or because of poor appetite may lead to life-threatening elevations in blood ammonia. In addition to prompt diagnosis and treatment of the infection, decreased protein intake (0 g for 1–2 days), increased energy intake, and peritoneal dialysis may all be required. Gastrostomy feedings may be required to ensure adequate intake and prevent inadequate growth or catabolism.

In planning nutrition support of the infant or child with a UCED, a formal prescription should be written that includes recommended amounts of protein, energy, fluid, and L-ARG, and drugs that enhance nitrogen loss. The prescription for protein should be based on the specific diagnosis, degree of impaired urea cycle, and blood ammonia concentrations and correlated with various parameters of growth, including rates of height and weight increase and hair, nails, teeth, and skin changes.

Protein intakes suggested in Appendix Table A-25-n are based on amounts required to cover obligatory nitrogen losses and growth needs (279) and are modified based on unpublished data from ten infants with one of four different enzyme defects diagnosed within the first 10 days of life. Intakes may need to be increased if the child does not grow adequately on the recommended intake or if sodium benzoate, phenylacetate, or phenylbutyrate is administered. Overrestriction of protein may lead to catabolism and impaired renal activity to excrete NH_4+. TRP intake should be at the minimal requirement for growth to prevent excess serotonin synthesis that suppresses appetite (280).

Energy intakes recommended in Appendix Table A-25-n are somewhat higher than those for normal infants and children to provide ketoacid precursors from carbohydrate for synthesis of nonessential amino acids and to prevent protein degradation. Carbohydrate should not provide more than 50% of the energy because of frequently elevated plasma triacylglycerol concentrations.

In any situation in which protein-restricted diets are fed, L-carnitine supplements may be necessary. Recommended amounts of supplemental L-carnitine are 50 to 100 mg/kg/day. L-Carnitine supplements are reported to lower blood ammonium concentrations (281, 282). Citrate deficiency has been reported in patients with ASA, and supplementation was recommended (283, 284).

Medical Foods for Urea Cycle Disorders. Nutrition support of UCEDs requires restricting nitrogen intake, which is best accomplished by providing about two-thirds the prescribed protein in the form of essential amino acids only. Formulation, composition, and sources of medical foods for UCEDs are given in Appendix Table A-25-a. Cyclinex-1 and Cyclinex-2 contain 25 mg of L-carnitine per gram of protein.

Serving Lists. Serving lists of food containing intact protein are available to simplify protein-restricted diets for professionals and for families (see Appendix Table A-25-b). Portion sizes of foods in each list may be found in reference 58. Appendix Table A-25-o provides a sample diet for an infant with a UCED.

Assessment of Nutrition Support. Frequency of assessment is in part dictated by the clinical course of the patient. Blood ammonia concentrations should be monitored routinely and maintained at less than 50 μM. Plasma concentrations of amino acids should be monitored and maintained in the normal range. Plasma albumin and globulin concentrations are indices of protein status and should be evaluated frequently. Plasma transthyretin and retinol-binding protein have shorter half-lives than albumin and can provide information on protein status at an earlier stage in deficiency than albumin can. Caretakers should provide diet diaries and records of health status in tandem with blood for ammonia and plasma amino acid determinations. Growth and development should be routinely assessed. If evidence of protein deficiency occurs or growth is not maintained, increased protein intake is necessary.

Results of Nutrition Support. Results of therapy in infants with complete or near-complete enzyme deficiencies have been less than optimal, with delayed death and below-normal development. If serious brain swelling and coma are prevented in the neonatal period or if the onset of disease expression is delayed, physical growth and mental development are more nearly normal with nutrition and pharmacologic support (257, 285–287). If diagnosis is anticipated and treatment is begun during the neonatal period in affected siblings with citrullinemia or argininosuccinic acidemia, a relatively normal outcome is observed even with severe enzyme defects (288). Female patients with symptomatic OTC deficiency have fewer hyperammonemic episodes and a reduced risk of further cognitive decline if treated with a protein-restricted diet and drugs that enhance waste nitrogen excretion (285, 289, 290). A successful pregnancy outcome has been reported in a woman with ASA (291).

GALACTOSE

Biochemistry

Because lactose from milk is the principal carbohydrate and energy source for infants and young children, galactose (GAL) maintains a central metabolic role in human nutrition. Lactose is hydrolyzed in the intestine by lactase to GLU and GAL, and 0.5 to 1.0 mg GAL/kg/min is produced endogenously (292). GAL is converted to GLU-1-phosphate (GLU-1-P) and energy through the Leloir pathway. This occurs primarily in the liver, where GAL becomes GLU through four evolutionarily conserved catalytic processes (Fig. 58.9). First, GAL enters cells by a permease. Then GAL is phosphorylated to GAL-1-phosphate (GAL-1-P) by galactokinase. Classic galactosemia is caused by impaired GAL-1-P uridyl transferase (GALT). GALT is highly conserved from *Escherichia coli* to humans in its catalytic structure and function. There are two dissociation reactions by which uridine diphosphate (UDP) GLU binds and releases GAL-1-P. Then the UMP-GALT complex binds GAL-1-P, releases UDP-GAL, and frees GALT for a subsequent set of bimolecular reactions. UDP-GAL and UDP-GLU are important precursors for glycoproteins and glycolipids; UDP-GAL and UDP-GLU are interconverted by epimerase (see Fig. 58.9).

Galactosemia

Elevated blood GAL levels may occur because of deficient functioning of galactokinase, GALT, or UDP-GAL-4-epimerase (293) (see Fig. 58.9). Patients with galactokinase deficiency produce excess galactitol and galactonic acid through alternate pathways and have only cataracts without hepatocellular dysfunction. Galactokinase deficiency does not produce the acute hepatotoxic manifestations or the

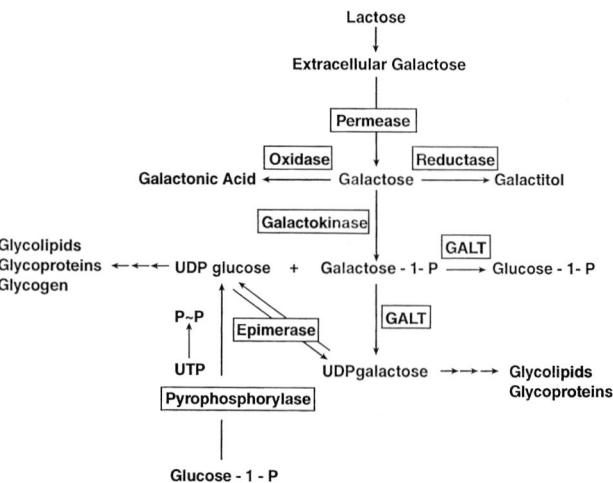

Figure 58.9. Metabolic blocks in galactose metabolism that lead to galactosemia. Classic galactosemia is caused by galactose-1-phosphate uridyl transferase (GALT) deficiency. ATP, adenosine triphosphate; UDP; uridine diphosphate.

accumulation of GAL-1-P seen with GALT deficiency. Several variants with different degrees of function and structure have been described for mutant GALT (294). This gene locus is on chromosome 9p (293). The cDNA and gene for GALT have been accurately sequenced, and many different mutations have been identified (295–298). A common missense mutation, Q188R, alters the UMP-GALT complex and prevents the second dissociation reaction (298).

Galactosemia caused by deficiency of GALT leads to an accumulation of GAL-1-P that is toxic and competes with GLU-1-P for the production of UDP-GLU through the pyrophosphorylase reaction (see Fig. 58.9). This leads to deficient UDP-GLU and UDP-GAL and reduced post-translational production of glycoproteins and glycolipids (299–307). GALT-deficient patients were found to have defective galactosylation of serum transferrin (300–303) and follicle-stimulating hormone (304). After treatment, the proportion of truncated glycans decreased and the proportion of disialylated biantennary complex type increased, returning almost, but never completely, to normal (302). In GALT-deficient yeast, gene transfer of the pyrophosphorylase enables them to grow on GAL, and a similar UDP-hexose deficiency was recently reported in human galactosemia cells (306, 307).

Clinical symptoms of the GALT defect appear early in infancy. Acute hepatotoxicity may appear with the start of human milk or feeding of proprietary infant formulae that contain lactose. Prolonged neonatal jaundice at 4 to 10 days of age is common. Hyperbilirubinemia and hyperammonemia is exacerbated by toxic injury to liver cells. Bleeding diatheses, *E. coli* sepsis, and shock are catastrophic events that may occur during the neonatal period unless GAL is withheld. Therefore, rapid screening, retrieval, diagnosis, and treatment are essential for population-based newborn screening programs if the clinical sequelae of neonatal galactosemia are to be prevented. Other relatively minor symptoms occur. About 10% of infants with GALT deficiency are born with cataracts. Anemia from various causes is present in about 40% of untreated patients. Lethargy, hypotonia, food refusal, vomiting, and diarrhea are also common symptoms in infancy. Localized *E. coli* infections may present after therapy is initiated.

Retarded mental and physical growth occur in most of the untreated patients who survive (308). The pathophysiology of galactosemia remains unclear, but early diet therapy clearly prevents neonatal sepsis, shock, and bleeding. Some effects of GALT deficiency may occur during embryogenesis (309). Cataracts occur in about 45% of untreated children and are thought to result from formation and accumulation of galactitol in the lens of the eye, which is impermeable to efflux. Galactitol creates an osmotic gradient that allows glutathione to efflux and results in decreased concentrations of lens glutathione. When glutathione concentrations are decreased, glutathione peroxidase is inactivated, and hydrogen peroxide accumulates to toxic levels. Hydrogen peroxide denatures lens protein, producing lenticular cataracts (293). Hepatomegaly occurs in nearly all cases of GALT deficiency, and cirrhosis develops in untreated patients. Liver damage results in decreased synthesis of liver coagulants and albumin and a decrease in a wide range of liver functions. Because of decreased albumin synthesis and proteinuria, ascites and generalized edema occur in about 36% of untreated patients. The albumin synthesized by untreated patients with galactosemia contains large amounts of GAL, whereas albumin of normal individuals is free of GAL (310). Untreated or poorly controlled patients are extremely susceptible to infection with gram-negative organisms, probably as a direct result of inhibition by GAL-1-P of posttranslational processing of secreted or membrane-bound proteins (307). GAL-1-P also impairs active renal tubular transport. This results in generalized aminoaciduria, galactosuria, and glucosuria, and loss of phosphate, potassium, and bicarbonate. On rare occasions, hypoglycemia occurs. Causes include reduced glycogen stores attributable to depressed UDP-GLU concentrations and hyperinsulinemia that may result from GAL stimulation of pancreatic cells.

Despite early diagnosis and removal of GAL during the neonatal period, some patients with classic (G/G, homozygous for galactose-1-phosphate uridyl transferase alleles) galactosemia have long-term poor outcomes including infertility in female patients, growth failure, dyspraxic speech, ataxia, and mental retardation (308, 311). The risk factors for premature ovarian failure in female patients with GALT deficiency have been described as (a) the patient's molecular genotype for GALT, (b) alternate pathways for GAL metabolism, and (c) the patient's nutrition environment at diagnosis and during treatment (312). The enigmatic outcome may be of intrauterine origin and has been associated with severe mutations in GALT. For example, the Q188R mutation in exon 6 is prevalent among white people. Homozygosity for this mutation is a risk factor for both dyspraxic speech and ovarian failure (312, 313). By contrast, the S135L mutation in exon 5 of the GALT gene is associated with good outcomes in patients treated from birth, is prevalent in black patients, and has differential expression in different organs (314). Other variant mutations, such as the Duarte variant (N314D), when associated with G alleles such as E203K may return structural integrity and function to the dimeric GALT protein and produce a good clinical outcome (294, 315, 316). More than 150 mutations have been defined to date in patients with galactosemia (295). A breath test that quantifies total body oxidation of D-GAL to CO_2 and thus includes liver function of GALT may be the best predictor of outcome (312).

Screening. GALT deficiency of clinical importance to the neonate is found in approximately one in 8000 births. The most common screening method used is the Beutler fluorescent test for galactosemia (317). This procedure consists of incubating eluted erythrocytes from dried blood on filter paper with a mixture of UDP-GLU, GLU-6-P dehydrogenase, and nicotinamide adenine dinucleotide phosphate. Erythrocytes from physiologically normal persons containing GALT and phosphoglucomutase produce GLU-1-P, GLU-6-P, and fluorescent reduced nicotinamide adenine dinucleotide phosphate through the added (linked) reaction of excess GLU-6-P dehydrogenase. If heat has inactivated this reaction (e.g., in summer), GLU-1-P is added to differentiate between heat inactivation that included endogenous phosphoglucomutase and GALT deficiency alone (true galactosemia).

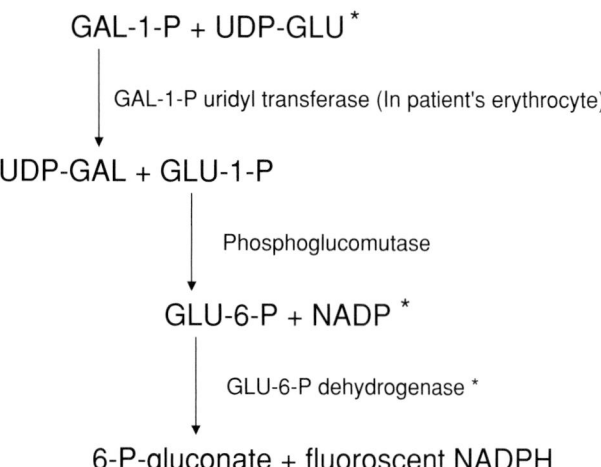

GAL-1-P + UDP-GLU *

↓ GAL-1-P uridyl transferase (In patient's erythrocyte)

UDP-GAL + GLU-1-P

↓ Phosphoglucomutase

GLU-6-P + NADP *

↓ GLU-6-P dehydrogenase *

6-P-gluconate + fluoroscent NADPH

* Added to reaction

Positive screening results occur with classic (G/G) GALT deficiency and with variants of GALT that are thermolabile, such as the Duarte/galactosemia compound heterozygote. Confirmation of positive Beutler screening test results requires quantitative enzyme activity and quantitation of erythrocyte GAL and GAL-1-P content. A combined analysis of the GALT biochemical phenotype and molecular genotype is important for diagnosis, therapy, prognosis, and genetic counseling (294, 313). A test of total body oxidation of GAL to expired CO_2 is the method of choice for prognosis (312).

Diagnosis. Patients with positive Beutler test results should have all lactose removed from their diets immediately while enzyme diagnosis and family workup proceed. Fresh, sterile heparinized blood should be sent to a central laboratory experienced in enzyme, analyte, and molecular analyses. Both the patient and the parents should be evaluated by the center for biochemical phenotype and molecular genotype. Diagnosis of galactosemia is accomplished through measurement of activity of GALT in erythrocytes, erythrocyte GAL-1-P content, and molecular analysis of the GALT gene for prevalent mutations. No activity occurs in individuals homozygous for the classic disease (G/G), whereas heterozygotes (G/N) have approximately one-half normal activity. Because the Q188R allele occurs in 70% of

white people with G/G galactosemia, it is important to identify (298, 299, 313). The Duarte allele (N314D) has a characteristic isozyme pattern when erythrocytes are studied by isoelectric focusing for the GALT enzyme. The need for therapy in patients with an activity of 25% or less of GALT, as in compound heterozygotes for Duarte/galactosemia alleles, has not been established. However, GAL should be restricted in any infant with any mutant genotype if erythrocyte GAL-1-P is more than 2 mg/dL, urinary galactitol exceeds 20 mmol/mol creatinine, or hepatotoxicity is present.

GALT is expressed in cultured amniotic fluid cells and chorionic villi. Thus, GALT deficiency can be detected prenatally by both direct enzyme assay and DNA analysis if the mutations are known (318). Amniotic fluid of a fetus with galactosemia has recently been found to have an elevated concentration of galactitol. Assessment of the galactitol content of amniotic fluid by GC/MS provides an ancillary method for prenatal diagnosis and may be related to enigmatic outcome (319).

Treatment. Objectives of therapy in galactosemia are to ameliorate or prevent symptoms while providing adequate energy and nutrients for normal growth and development. Treatment should begin as early in life as possible and consists of removal of all sources of lactose and GAL from the diet of patients with no enzyme activity. Patients with 5 to 10% of normal GALT activity may tolerate small amounts of GAL found in muscle meats, fruits, and vegetables.

Nutrient Requirements. Energy and nutrient requirements of infants and children with well-controlled galactosemia are the same as those for normal individuals of the same age, gender, and physical activity level. Whether above-normal energy and protein intakes prevent the linear growth retardation seen in children with poorly controlled galactosemia is not known. Because of poor bone mineralization in patients with GALT deficiency (320, 321), calcium recommendations are given in Table 58.5.

Formulas. Human milk contains 6 to 8% lactose, cow's milk 3 to 4% lactose, and many proprietary infant formulas 7% lactose. These milks must be replaced by a powdered formula free of bioavailable GAL (Isomil Soy Formula with Iron powder, Ross Products Division, or Prosobee powder, Mead Johnson Nutritionals). Both ready-to-feed and concentrated liquid Isomil and Prosobee contain carrageenan, which contains 27% GAL; thus, they are not recommended for infants with GALT deficiency.

Powdered formulas containing soy protein isolate have about 14 mg GAL/L in the form of raffinose and stachyose, oligosaccharides that contain GAL. At one time it was thought that these oligosaccharides yielded free GAL on hydrolysis in the intestine. It is now believed that the human intestine has no enzymes to hydrolyze these oligosaccharides. Thus, they may be safely used for feeding infants and children with galactosemia. Isomil 2 Advance powder (Ross Products Division) and Next Step Follow-up

Prosobee Lipil Formula powder (Mead Johnson Nutritionals) may be used by children and adults who require a GAL-free formula. Casein hydrolysates such as Alimentum (Ross Products Division), Nutramigen, and Pregestimil (Mead Johnson Nutritionals) have been treated to remove lactose but may still contain small amounts of GAL (<37 mg/L). Liquid Alimentum also contains carrageenan. Alimentum powder contains xanthan gum as a stabilizer, and although the casein hydrolysate contains less than 37 mg/L GAL, the xanthan gum provides no bioavailable GAL. Lactose-free infant formulas may contain as much as 75 mg GAL/L and should be avoided for infants with GALT deficiency. Data in Appendix Table A-25-p describe foods allowed in and excluded from the GAL-restricted diet. The breath test that quantitates $[1-^{13}C]$ GAL to $^{13}CO_2$ provides information on whole-body GAL oxidation and may be used to determine the amount of GAL that can be safely fed (322, 323).

Free Galactose in the Diet. Milk and milk products are well-known sources of lactose and casein. Less well known is that different forms of casein and cheeses contain GAL in various amounts (324–326). Based on studies by botanists and plant physiologists that began in the early 1950s, it is clear that cereals, fruits, legumes (dried beans and peas), nuts, seeds, tubers, and vegetables contain GAL. But many believe that the GAL in these foods is in linkages resistant to human digestive enzymes. Many fruits and vegetables, however, contain free (soluble) GAL in amounts ranging from less than 0.5 mg/100 g to 35.4 mg/100 g fresh weight (327). Ten of 12 baby foods had detectable amounts of free GAL, with applesauce and squash containing the largest amounts (328). GAL has also been found in fermented cocoa beans (329).

Oral loads of raffinose and stachyose were administered to one patient with GALT deficiency (330). No changes were observed in erythrocyte GAL-1-P, the analyte used to monitor diet compliance. Soybean formula was fed to a 14-year-old patient with GALT deficiency, and an insignificant change in GAL-1-P was found (331). These observations led clinicians to suggest that legumes could be used freely in the diets of patients with GALT deficiency, although explicit warning of the possible release of absorbable free GAL in the small intestine by bacteria when the patient had diarrhea had been given (330). The GALT-deficient mouse given a chow diet containing 1.75% of GAL-containing carbohydrates excreted significant amounts of GAL, galactonate, and galactitol in the urine, suggesting the digestion and absorption of bound GAL (332). Ingestion of legumes over a 5-year period led to a 21 to 100% increase in erythrocyte GAL-1-P in four patients with GALT deficiency, whereas of four patients who did not receive legumes, three had decreases in GAL-1-P of 17%, 19%, and 23%, and one had an increase of 37% (333). Chickpea flour contains 110 mg free GAL per 100 g flour (334). Free GAL in six types of cooked legumes ranged from 42 to 444 mg/100 g dry

beans (335). Many legumes, cereals, fruits, nuts, seeds, and vegetables have not yet been analyzed for free GAL. Until such analyses are conducted, we will not know the extent of free GAL in foods.

Free and Bound Galactose in Food and Drugs. Free GAL is present in abundance in the lactulose that is used to treat hyperammonemia. Caution to exclude this medication in neonates is emphasized. Bound GAL is present in lactose, arabinogalactans I and II, feruloylated GAL, galactan, glycolipids, galactinol, galactopinitols, and rhamnogalacturonans I and II (335). Lactose is found in milk and dairy products and as an extender in many over-the-counter and prescription drugs (336). Hash-browned potatoes and some other prepared foods contain added lactose, and some chefs sprinkle meat with lactose before frying for faster and better browning (335). Calcium lactobionate, the active ingredient in Neocalglucon, a liquid calcium supplement, is a substrate of β-galactosidases (337) and yields free GAL.

Organ meats such as brain, kidney, liver, pancreas, and spleen contain galactosylcerebrosides, gangliosides, and lactosyl sulfatide. These compounds are constantly turned over in living organisms. In patients with GALT deficiency, the free GAL liberated is metabolized to GAL-1-P or other metabolites such as galactitol (338). Glycoproteins found in muscle meats contribute significant amounts of GAL to the diet (339). Commercial meats, prepared for infant consumption, contain microgram amounts of free and bound GAL per 100 g (340).

Enzymes that Degrade Compounds Containing Bound Galactose. α-Galactosidases, enzymes that digest carbohydrates with GAL in α-linkages, are found in human tissues and are probably responsible for the degradation of human galactosylcerebrosides, galactosylsulfatides, and gangliosides. α-Galactosidases also appear to be distributed in many plant tissues (335). α-Galactosidases digest carbohydrates with GAL in a-linkages. Bean-O is an α-galactosidase isolated from *Aspergillus niger* and marketed by AkPharma, Inc, as a food enzyme that reduces gas formation from many vegetables. α-Galactosidases can hydrolyze the terminal GAL attached to digalactosyldiacylglycerol, yielding GAL and monogalactosyldiacylglycerol (335).

β-Galactosidases are found in many foods, including apples and pears, peppers, tomatoes, and cocoa beans (335). The human intestine also contains β-galactosidases (341). The β-galactosidases in the human intestine digest lactose, but also have heterogenous activity on compounds with GAL in β-1,4 linkages (341). β-Galactosidase preparations from *E. coli* release GAL from ferulic acid and from monogalactosyldiacylglycerols (335). Galactolipids in foods are hydrolyzed by human pancreatic lipolytic enzymes and duodenal contents (342).

Results of Nutrition Support. Treatment of patients with GALT deficiency, although lifesaving, may not result in complete freedom from the sequelae of the disorder.

Infants diagnosed and treated early who maintain excellent dietary control have better intellectual function than those who have poor control or are diagnosed late (308). Control is defined on the basis of erythrocyte GAL-1-P concentrations and is considered excellent if consistently below 2 mg/dL (343). Patients may have difficulty with language, abstract thinking, visual perception, ovarian failure, and cataracts despite early diagnosis and good dietary control (344–346). These clinical deficits may be related to intrauterine damage from intrauterine accumulation of GAL-1-P or galactitol and/or maternal GAL transported into the vulnerable fetus (309, 312). Embryonic membranes are constantly synthesized and degraded and require GAL and UDP-GAL. GAL (i.e., milk) restriction in at-risk pregnant women is generally advised, although little change in outcome has been observed (308). This may be because many fruits, vegetables, and legumes contain free GAL, making restriction of all exogenous GAL impossible (335).

The recent observations that UDP-GLU and UDP-GAL are deficient in cells from patients with galactosemia offers a most likely reason for poor outcome despite adequate lactose restriction (299–305, 312, 347). Unfortunately, uridine supplements have not been helpful in therapy (348, 349). This is to be expected if irreversible damage to the number of ovarian cells present at birth has occurred.

Bone mineralization of both female and male patients with galactosemia was below that of normal age-, gender-, and ethnicity-matched subjects (320, 321). Bone mineralization was positively correlated with calcium intake and in women was improved in those who received estrogen (320). Many patients with GALT deficiency fail to ingest adequate calcium to maintain appropriate bone density (350).

A recently described mouse knockout for GALT has no acute hepatotoxicity or apparent ovarian failure. The mouse model differs from that for humans in that it has no aldose reductase and does not overproduce galactitol (see Fig. 58.9). Thus, a pathologic effect of polyol production and treatment using aldose reductase inhibitors is of considerable research interest for future therapeutic intervention (351).

Assessment of Nutrition Support. Evaluation of growth, development, lens development, liver function, erythrocyte GAL-1-P concentrations, and urinary galactitol excretion are necessary to determine the adequacy of diet intervention. Urinary galactonate may be of use in determining the body GAL burden (352).

Diet Termination. Although some investigators have recommended liberalizing the GAL-restricted diet at 12 to 13 years of age, this is not warranted because the potentially damaging effects of accumulated galactitol and GAL-1-P in the lens, liver, kidney, and brain remain. Women with galactosemia must continue treatment with GAL exclusion to reduce possible in utero damage to their future children (353). Diet termination is not recommended.

REFERENCES

1. Trumbo P, Schlicker S, Yates AA et al. J Am Diet Assoc 2002;102:1621–30.
2. McKusick VA, ed. Mendelian Inheritance in Man: Catalog of Autosomal Dominant, Recessive, and X-linked Phenotypes. 11th ed. Baltimore: Johns Hopkins University Press, 1994.
3. Harris H, ed. The Principles of Human Biochemical Genetics. 3rd ed. Amsterdam: North Holland Publishing, 1980.
4. National Newborn Screening Reports: 1992, 1993. McLean, VA: National Maternal and Childhealth Clearinghouse, 1992, 1993.
5. Kaplan P, Mazur A, Field M et al. J Pediatr 1991;119:46–50.
6. Elsas LJ. Newborn screening. In: Rudolph AM, ed. Pediatrics. 20th ed. New York: Appleton-Century Crofts, 1994.
7. Burns JJ. Am J Med 1959;26:740.
8. Lipson MH, Kraus J, Rosenberg LE. J Clin Invest 1980;66:188–93.
9. Elsas LJ, Danner DJ. Ann NY Acad Sci 1982;378:404–21.
10. Elsas LJ, McCormick DB. Vitam Horm 1987;43:103–44.
11. Elsas LJ, McCormick D. Vitam Horm 1987;44:145.
12. Fowler B. Eur J Pediatr 1998;157[Suppl 2]:S60–6.
13. Desnick RJ, Brady R, Barranger J et al. Ann Intern Med 2003;138:338–46.
14. Baumgartner ER, Wick H, Linnell JC et al. Helv Paediatr Acta 1979;34:483–96.
15. Hershfield MS, Buckley RH, Greenberg ML et al. N Engl J Med 1987;316:589–96.
16. Van den Hout JM, Reuser AJ, de Klerk JB et al. J Inherit Metab Dis 2001;24:266–74.
17. Burdelski M. Pediatr Transplant 2002;6:361–3.
18. Kayler LK, Merion RM, Lee S et al. Pediatr Transplant 2002;6:295–300.
19. Elsas LJ. Inborn errors of metabolism. In: Bennett JC, Plum F, eds. Cecil's Textbook of Medicine. 22nd ed. Philadelphia: WB Saunders, 2004.
20. Fraites TJ Jr, Schleissing MR, Shanely RA et al. Mol Ther 2002;5:571–8.
21. Pratt EL, Snyderman SE, Cheung MW et al. J Nutr 1955;56:231–51.
22. Herrmann ME, Brosicke HG, Keller M et al. Eur J Pediatr 1994;153:501–3.
23. Schoeffer A, Herrmann ME, Broesicke HG et al. J Nutr Med 1994;4:415–8.
24. Martin SB, Acosta PB. J Am Diet Assoc 1987;87:48–52.
25. Scriver CR, Kaufman S. The hyperphenylalaninemias. In: Scriver CR, Beaudet AL, Sly WS et al., eds. The Metabolic and Molecular Bases of Inherited Disease. 8th ed. New York: McGraw-Hill, 2001:1667–724.
26. Eisensmith RC, Martinez DR, Kuzmin AI et al. Pediatrics 1996;97:512–6.
27. Griffin RF, Elsas LJ. J Pediatr 1975;86:512–7.
28. Kure S, Hou DC, Ohura T et al. J Pediatr 1999;135:375–8.
29. Lassker U, Zschocke J, Blau N et al. J Inherit Metab Dis 2002;25:65–70.
30. Muntau AC, Roschinger W, Habich M et al. N Engl J Med 2002;347:2122–32.
31. Trefz FK, Aulela-Scholz C, Blau N. Eur J Pediatr 2001;160:315.
32. Erlandsen H, Stevens RC. J Inherit Metab Dis 2001;24:213–30.

33. Blau N, Thöny B, Cotton RGH et al. Disorders of tetrahydrobiopterin and related biogenic amines. In: Scriver CR, Beaudet AL, Sly WS et al., eds. The Metabolic and Molecular Bases of Inherited Disease. 8th ed. New York: McGraw-Hill, 2001: 1725–76.

34. Dobbing J. The later development of the brain and its vulnerability. In: Davis JA, Dobbing J, eds. Scientific Foundations of Paediatrics. London: Heinemann, 1981.

35. Pardridge WM, Choi TB. Fed Proc 1986;45:2073–8.

36. Villasana D, Butler IJ, Williams JC et al. J Inherit Metab Dis 1989;12:451–7.

37. Krause W, Halminski M, McDonald L et al. J Clin Invest 1985; 75:40–8.

38. Epstein CM, Trotter JF, Averbook A et al. Electroencephalogr Clin Neurophysiol 1989;72:133–9.

39. Guthrie R, Susi A. Pediatrics 1963;32:338–43.

40. Zytkovicz TH, Fitzgerald EF, Marsden D et al. Clin Chem 2001;47:1945–55.

41. Pass K, Levy H. Impact of Early Discharge on Screening for Inborn Errors of Metabolism. Washington, DC: MCH CORN Clearinghouse, 1995.

42. Doherty LB, Rohr R, Levy HL. Pediatrics 1991;87:240–4.

43. NIH Consensus Statement. 2000;17:1–33.

44. Fernhoff PM, Fitzmaurice N, Milner J et al. South Med J 1982; 75:529.

45. Trefz FK, Burgard P, Konig T et al. Clin Chim Acta 1993;217: 15–21.

46. Kaufman S. J Inherit Metab Dis 1985;8[Suppl 1]:20–7.

47. Acosta PB, Wenz E, Williamson M. J Am Diet Assoc 1978;72: 164.

48. Smith I, Beasley MG, Ades AE. Arch Dis Child 1990;65: 472–8.

49. Rose WC. Nutr Abstr Rev 1957;27:631–47.

50. Hanley WB, Linsao L, Davidson W et al. Pediatr Res 1970;4: 318–27.

51. Acosta PB. The contribution of therapy of inherited amino acid disorders to knowledge of amino acid requirements. In: Wapnir RA, ed. Congenital Metabolic Disease: Diagnosis and Treatment. New York: Marcel Dekker, 1985.

52. Batshaw ML, Valle D, Bessman SP. J Pediatr 1981;99:159–60.

53. Jones BJM, Lees R, Andrews J et al. Gut 1983;24:78–84.

54. Acosta PB, Yannicelli S. Acta Paediatr Suppl 1994;407:66–7.

55. Acosta PB, Stepnick-Gropper S, Clarke-Sheehan N et al. JPEN J Parenter Enteral Nutr 1987;11:287–92.

56. Lewis J, Loskill S, Bunker ML et al. Fed Proc 1974;33:666A.

57. Pennington JAT, ed. Bowes and Church's Food Values of Portions Commonly Used. 17th ed. Philadelphia: Williams & Wilkins, 1998:316–82.

58. Acosta PB, Yannicelli S, eds. Nutrition Support Protocols. 4th ed. Columbus, OH: Ross Products Division, 2001.

59. SHS North America. Metabolic Products. Easy Reference Guide. Gaithersburg, MD: SHS North America, 2003:1–73.

60. Mead Johnson Nutritional Division. Pediatric Products Handbook. Evansville, IN: Mead Johnson, 2004.

61. Acosta PB, Yannicelli S, Singh RH et al. J Am Diet Assoc 2003; 103:1167–73.

62. Umbarger B, Berry HK, Sutherland BS. JAMA 1965;193:128–34.

63. Elsas LJ, Macdonell RC Jr, Rosenberg LE. J Biol Chem 1971;246:6452–9.

64. Nakagawa I, Takahashi T, Suzuki T et al. J Nutr 1962;77:61.

65. Sibinga MS, Friedman CJ, Steisel IM et al. Dev Med Child Neurol 1971;13:63–70.

66. Holm VA, Kronmal RA, Williamson M et al. Pediatrics 1979;63: 700–7.

67. Azen CG, Koch R, Friedman EG et al. Am J Dis Child 1991; 145:35–9.

68. Schulpis KH, Nounopoulos C, Scarpalezou A et al. Acta Paediatr Scand 1990;79:930–4.

69. Acosta PB. Phenylalanine Hydroxylase Deficiency Managed by Analog XP. Columbus, OH: Ross Products Division, Abbott Laboratories, 1992.

70. Francois B, Diels M, de la Brassinne M. J Inherit Metab Dis 1989;12:332–4.

71. Acosta PB, Yannicelli S, Marriage B et al. J Am Coll Nutr 1999; 18:102–7.

72. Buist NRM, Prince AP, Huntington KL et al. Acta Paediatr Suppl 1994;407:75–7.

73. Acosta PB, Greene C, Yannicelli S et al. Int Pediatr 1993;8: 6–16.

74. Arnold GL, Vladutiu CJ, Kirby RS et al. J Pediatr 2002;141: 243–6.

75. Acosta PB, Alfin-Slater RB, Koch R. J Am Diet Assoc 1973; 63:631–5.

76. Galluzzo CR, Ortisi MT, Castelli L et al. J Inherit Metab Dis 1985;8[Suppl 2]:129.

77. Schulpi KH, Scarpalezou A. Clin Pediatr 1989;28:466–9.

78. Acosta PB, Michals-Matalon K, Austin V et al. Nutrition findings and requirements in pregnant women with phenylketonuria. In: Platt LD, Koch R, de la Cruz F, eds. Genetic Disorders and Pregnancy Outcome. New York: Parthenon Publishing Group, 1997:21–32.

79. Castillo M, Zafra MF, Garcia-Peregrin E. Neurochem Res 1988;13:551–5.

80. Artuch R, Colome C, Vilaseca MA et al. J Inherit Metab Dis 2001;24:359–66.

81. Hargreaves IP, Heales SJ, Briddon A et al. J Inherit Metab Dis 2002;25:673–9.

82. Galli C, Agostoni C, Mosconi C et al. J Pediatr 1991;119:562–7.

83. Sanjurjo P, Perteagudo L, Rodriguez-Soriano J et al. J Inherit Metab Dis 1994;17:704–9.

84. Poge AP, Baumann K, Muller E. J Inherit Metab Dis 1998;21: 373–81.

85. Acosta PB, Yannicelli S, Singh R et al. J Pediatr Gastroenterol Nutr 2001;33:253–9.

86. Bodley JL, Austin VJ, Hanley WB et al. Eur J Pediatr 1993;152: 140–3.

87. Gropper SS, Trahms C, Cloud HH et al. Int Pediatr 1994;9: 237–43.

88. Zachara BA, Wasowicz W, Gromadzinska J et al. Biomed Biochim Acta 1987;46:S209–13.

89. Calomme MR, Vanderpas JB, Francois B et al. Experientia 1995;51:1208–15.

90. Acosta PB, Yannicelli S. Biol Trace Elem Res 1999;67:75–84.

91. Al Qadreh A, Schulpis KH, Athanasopoulou H et al. Acta Paediatr 1998;87:1162–6.

92. Carson DL, Greeves LG, Sweeney LE et al. Pediatr Radiol 1990;20:598–9.

93. Hillman L, Schlotzhauer C, Lee D et al. Eur J Pediatr 1996;155 [Suppl 1]:S148–52.

94. McMurry MP, Chan GM, Leonard CO et al. Am J Clin Nutr 1992;55:997–1004.

95. Greeves LG, Carson DJ, Magee A et al. Acta Paediatr 1997;86: 242–4.

96. Yannicelli S, Medeiros DM. J Inherit Metab Dis 2002;25:347–61.

97. Schulpis KH, Papakonstantinou E, Michelakakis H et al. Clin Endocrinol (Oxf) 1998;48:99–101.

98. Klibanski A, Neer RM, Beitins IZ et al. N Engl J Med 1980; 303:1511–4.

99. Gropper SS, Chaung HC, Bernstein LE et al. J Am Coll Nutr 1995;14:264–70.

100. Holtzman NA, Welcher DW, Mellits ED. N Engl J Med 1975; 293:1121–4.

101. Hudson FP. Arch Dis Child 1967;42:198–200.

102. Horner FA, Streamer CW, Alejandrino LL et al. N Engl J Med 1962;266:79.

103. Holtzman NA, Kronmal RA, van Doorninck W et al. N Engl J Med 1986;314:593–8.

104. Seashore MR, Friedman E, Novelly RA et al. Pediatrics 1985; 75:226–32.

105. Thompson AJ, Smith I, Brenton D et al. Lancet 1990;336: 602–5.

106. Waisbren SE, Levy HL. J Inherit Metab Dis 1991;14:755–64.

107. Aung TT, Klied A, McGinn J et al. J Inherit Metab Dis 1997;20:603–4.

108. Hanley WB, Feigenbaum A, Clarke JTR et al. Lancet 1993;342: 99.

109. Krause W, Epstein C, Averbook A et al. Pediatr Res 1986;20: 1112–6.

110. Elsas LJ, Trotter JF. Changes in physiological concentrations of blood phenylalanine produce changes in sensitive parameters of human brain function. Dietary Phenylalanine and Brain Function. Boston: Birkhauser, 1987:187–95.

111. Lenke RR, Levy HL. N Engl J Med 1980;303:1202–8.

112. Levy HL. Enzyme 1987;38:312–20.

113. Kudo Y, Boyd CAR. J Inherit Metab Dis 1990;13:617–26.

114. Hanley WB, Clarke JT, Schoonheyt W. Clin Biochem 1987;20: 149–56.

115. Kirby ML, Miyagawa S. J Inherit Metab Dis 1990;13:634–40.

116. Okano Y, Chow IZ, Isshiki G et al. J Inherit Metab Dis 1986;9: 15–24.

117. Kirkman HN. Appl Res Ment Retard 1982;3:319–28.

118. Koch R, Friedman EG, Wenz E. J Inherit Metab Dis 1986;9 [Suppl 2]:159–68.

119. Platt LD, Koch R, Hanley WB et al. Am J Obstet Gynecol 2000;182:326–33.

120. Smith I, Glossop J, Beasley M. J Inherit Metab Dis 1990;13: 651–7.

121. Matalon K, Acosta PB, Castiglioni L et al., eds. Protocol for nutrition support of maternal PKU. Bethesda, MD: National Institute of Child Health and Human Development, 1998.

122. Michals K, Acosta PB, Austin V et al. Eur J Pediatr 1996;155 [Suppl 1]:S165–8.

123. Subcommittee on Nutritional Status and Weight Gain During Pregnancy. Washington, DC: National Academy Press, 1990.

124. Innis SM. Prog Lipid Res 1991;30:39–103.

125. Hunter JE. Am J Clin Nutr 1990;51:809–14.

126. Rothman KJ, Moore LL, Singer MR. N Engl J Med 1995;333: 1369–73.

127. Matalon KM, Acosta PB, Azen C et al. Ment Retard Dev Disabil Res Rev 1999;5:122–4.

128. Mitchell GA, Grompe M, Lambert M et al. Tyrosinemia and related disorders. In: Scriver CR, Beaudet AL, Sly WS et al., eds. The Metabolic and Molecular Bases of Inherited Disease. 8th ed. New York: McGraw-Hill, 2001:1777–806.

129. Jorquera R, Tanquay RM. Hum Mol Genet 2001;10:1741–52.

130. Lindstedt S, Holme E, Lock EA. Lancet 1992;340:813–7.

131. Macsai MS, Schwartz TL, Hinkle D et al. Am J Ophthalmol 2001;132:522–7.

132. Cerone R, Holme E, Schiaffino MC et al. Acta Paediatr 1997; 86:1013–5.

133. Mamunes P, Prince PE, Thornton NH et al. Pediatrics 1976; 57:675–80.

134. Gagne R, Lescault A, Grenier A et al. Prenat Diagn 1982;2: 185–8.

135. Holme E, Lindstedt S. Clin Liver Dis 2000;4:805–14.

136. Shemin D. Harvey Lect 1954–55;50:258.

137. Sassa S, Granick S. Proc Natl Acad Sci USA 1970;67:517–22.

138. Rank JM, Pascual-Leone A, Payne W. J Pediatr 1991;118: 136–9.

139. Grompe M, Lindstedt S, al Dhalimy M et al. Nat Genet 1995; 10:453–60.

140. Cohn RM, Yudkoff M, Yost B et al. Am J Clin Nutr 1977;30: 209–14.

141. Mudd SH, Levy HL, Kraus JP. Disorders of transsulfuration. In: Scriver CR, Beaudet AL, Sly WS et al., eds. The Metabolic and Molecular Bases of Inherited Disease. 8th ed. New York: McGraw-Hill, 2001:2007–56.

142. Finkelstein JD. J Nutr Biochem 1990;1:228–37.

143. Rosenblatt DS, Fenton WA. Inherited disorders of folate and cobalamin transport and metabolism. In: Scriver CR, Beaudet AL, Sly WS et al., eds. The Metabolic and Molecular Bases of Inherited Disease. 8th ed. New York: McGraw-Hill, 2001: 3897–34.

144. Kraus JP. Eur J Pediatr 1998;157[Suppl 2]:S50–3.

145. Kraus JP. J Inherit Metab Dis 1994;17:383–90.

146. Liu G, Nellaiappan K, Kagan HM. J Biol Chem 1997;272: 32370–7.

147. Mudd SH, Skovby F, Levy HL. Am J Hum Genet 1985;37: 1–31.

148. Boers GHJ, Smals AGH, Trijbels FJM et al. N Engl J Med 1985;313:709–15.

149. Schaumburg H, Kaplan J, Windebank A et al. N Engl J Med 1983;309:445–8.

150. Yoshida I, Sakaguchi Y, Nakano M et al. J Inherit Metab Dis 1985;8:91.

151. Matthews A, Johnson TN, Rostami-Hodjegan A et al. Br J Clin Pharmacol 2002;54:140–6.

152. Singh RH, Kruger WD, Wang L et al. Genet Med 2004;6:90–5.

153. Fritzer-Szekeres M, Blom HJ, Boers GH et al. Biochim Biophys Acta 1998;1407:1–6.

154. Topaloglu AK, Sansaricq C, Snyderman SE. Pediatr Res 2001; 49:796–8.

155. Sansaricq C, Garg S, Norton PM et al. Acta Paediatr Scand 1975;64:215–8.

156. Dudman NPB, Wilcken DEL. Clin Chim Acta 1983;127: 105–13.

157. Spooner RJ, Fell GS, Halls DJ et al. Clin Nutr 1986;5:29–32.

158. Smith AM, Picciano MF, Milner JA. Am J Clin Nutr 1982; 35:521–6.

159. Carey MC, Donovan DE, Fitzgerald O. Am J Med 1968;45: 7–25.

160. Carey MC, Fennelly JJ, Fitzgerald O. Am J Med 1968;45: 26–31.

161. Wagstaff J, Korson M, Kraus JP et al. J Pediatr 1991;118: 569–72.

162. Yap S, Naughten ER, Wilcken B et al. Semin Thromb Hemost 2000;26:335–40.

163. Marcus AJ. N Engl J Med 1983;309:1515–7.

164. Davi G, Di Minno G, Coppola A et al. Circulation 2001;104: 1124–8.

165. Yap S, Barry-Kinsella C, Naughten ER. Br J Obstet Gynaecol 2001;108:425–8.

166. Kang SS, Wong PW, Malinow MR. Annu Rev Nutr 1992;12: 279–98.

167. Chuang DT, Shih VE. Maple syrup urine disease (branched-chain ketoaciduria). In: Scriver CR, Beaudet AL, Sly WS et al.,

eds. The Metabolic and Molecular Bases of Inherited Disease. 8th ed. New York: McGraw-Hill, 2001:1971–2006.

168. Danner DJ, Armstrong N, Heffelfinger SC et al. J Clin Invest 1985;75:858–60.

169. Ellerine NP, Herring WJ, Elsas LJ et al. Biochem Med Metab Biol 1993;49:363–74.

170. Elsas LJ, Ellerine NP, Klein PD. Pediatr Res 1993;33:445–51.

171. Heffelfinger SC, Sewell ET, Elsas LJ et al. Am J Hum Genet 1984;36:802–7.

172. Sweetman L, Williams JC. Branched-chain organic acidurias. In: Scriver CR, Beaudet AL, Sly WS et al., eds. The Metabolic and Molecular Bases of Inherited Disease. 8th ed. New York: McGraw-Hill, 2001:2125–64.

173. Xu M, Nakai N, Ishigure K et al. Biochem Biophys Res Commun 2000;276:1080–4.

174. Fenton WA, Gravel RA, Rosenblatt DS. Disorders of propionate and methylmalonate metabolism. In: Scriver CR, Beaudet AL, Sly WS et al., eds. The Metabolic and Molecular Bases of Inherited Disease. 8th ed. New York: McGraw-Hill, 2001:2165–93.

175. Tangerman A, Wilcken B, Levy HL et al. Metabolism 2000;49: 1071–7.

176. Steele RD, Benevenga NJ. J Biol Chem 1978;253:7844–50.

177. Kaji H, Niioka T, Kojima Y et al. Res Commun Chem Pathol Pharmacol 1987;56:101–9.

178. Coomes MH. Amino acid metabolism II: metabolism of the individual amino acids. In: Devlin TM, ed. Textbook of Biochemistry with Clinical Correlation. 5th ed. New York: Wiley-Liss, 2002:779–824.

179. Baretz BH, Tanaka K. J Biol Chem 1978;253:4203–13.

180. Elsas LJ, Pask BA, Wheeler FB et al. Metabolism 1972;21: 929–44.

181. Elsas LJ, Danner D, Lubitz D et al. Metabolic consequences of inherited defects in branched-chain alpha-ketoacid dehydrogenase: mechanisms of thiamine action. In: Walser M, Williamson GR, eds. Metabolism and Clinical Implications of Branched-Chain Amino Acids and Ketoacids. New York: Elsevier, 1981:369–82.

182. Jouvet P, Rustin P, Taylor DL et al. Mol Biol Cell 2000;11: 1919–32.

183. Jones PM, Bennett MJ. Clin Chim Acta 2002;324:121–8.

184. Elsas LJ, Priest JH, Wheeler FB et al. Metabolism 1974;23: 569–79.

185. Fernhoff PM, Lubitz D, Danner DJ et al. Pediatr Res 1985;19: 1011–6.

186. Thompson GN, Francis DEM, Halliday D. J Pediatr 1991; 119:35–41.

187. Giacoia GP, Berry GT. Am J Dis Child 1993;147:954–6.

188. Koch SE, Packman S, Koch TK et al. J Am Acad Dermatol 1993;28:289–92.

189. Di George AM, Rezvani I, Garibaldi LR et al. N Engl J Med 1982;307:1492–5.

190. Wendel U, Saudubray JM, Bodner A et al. Eur J Pediatr 1999; 158[Suppl 2]:S60–4.

191. Szmelcman S, Guggenheim K. Biochem J 1966;100:7–11.

192. van Calcar SC, Harding CO, Davidson SR et al. Am J Med Genet 1992;44:641–6.

193. Grunewald S, Hinrichs F, Wendel U. J Inherit Metab Dis 1998; 21:89–94.

194. Hammersen G, Wille L, Schmidt H et al. Monogr Hum Genet 1978;9:84–9.

195. Snyderman SE, Goldstein F, Sansaricq C et al. Pediatr Res 1984;18:851–3.

196. Treacy E, Clow CL, Reade TR et al. J Inherit Metab Dis 1992; 15:121–35.

197. Berry GT, Heidenreich R, Kaplan P et al. N Engl J Med 1991; 324:175–9.

198. Delaney A, Gal TJ. Anesthesiology 1976;44:83–6.

199. Dent CE, Westall RG. Arch Dis Child 1961;36:259–68.

200. Westall RG. Am J Dis Child 1967;113:58–9.

201. Snyderman SE, Norton PM, Roitman E et al. Pediatrics 1964;34:454–72.

202. Schwartz JF, Kolendrianos ET. Dev Med Child Neurol 1969; 11:460–70.

203. Dickinson JP, Holton JB, Lewis GM et al. Acta Paediatr Scand 1969;58:341–51.

204. Gaull GE. Biochem Med 1969;3:130–49.

205. Committee for Improvement of Hereditary Disease Management. Can Med Assoc J 1976;115:1005–13.

206. Parsons HG, Carter RJ, Unrath M et al. J Inherit Metab Dis 1990;13:125–36.

207. Henstenburg JD, Mazur AT, Kaplan PB. J Am Diet Assoc 1990; 90:A32.

208. Gropper SS, Naglak MC, Nardella M et al. J Am Coll Nutr 1993;12:108–14.

209. Lombeck I, Kasperek K, Feinendegen LE et al. Monogr Hum Genet 1978;9:114–7.

210. Levy HL, Truman JT, Ganz RN et al. J Pediatr 1970;77:294–6.

211. Foreman JW, Yudkoff M, Berry G et al. J Pediatr 1980;96:62–4.

212. Budd MA, Tanaka K, Holmes LB et al. N Engl J Med 1967;277: 321–7.

213. Rhead WJ, Tanaka K. Proc Natl Acad Sci USA 1980;77:580–3.

214. Kraus JP, Matsubara Y, Barton D et al. Genomics 1987;1:264–9.

215. Shigematsu Y, Sudo M, Momoi T et al. Pediatr Res 1982;16: 771–5.

216. Truscott RJ, Malegan D, McCairns E et al. Clin Chim Acta 1981;110:187–203.

217. Lehnert W, Niederhoff H. Eur J Pediatr 1981;136:281–3.

218. Fries MH, Rinaldo P, Schmidt-Sommerfeld E et al. J Pediatr 1996;129:449–52.

219. Itoh T, Ito T, Ohba S et al. Tohoku J Exp Med 1996;179:101–9.

220. Hutchinson RJ, Bunnell K, Thoene JG. J Pediatr 1985;106: 62–5.

221. Dubiel B, Dabrowki C, Wetts R et al. J Clin Invest 1983;72: 1543–52.

222. Ikeda Y, Tanaka K. J Biol Chem 1983;258:1077.

223. Lehnert W, Hunkler D. Eur J Pediatr 1986;145:260–6.

224. Blaskovics ME, Ng WG, Donnell GN. J Inherit Metab Dis 1978;1:9–11.

225. Shigematsu Y, Kikawa Y, Sudo M et al. Clin Chim Acta 1984; 138:333–6.

226. Naglak M, Salvo R, Madsen K et al. Pediatr Res 1988;24:9–13.

227. Bartlett K, Gompertz D. Biochem Med 1974;10:15–23.

228. Stanley CA, Hale DE, Shiteman DEH et al. Pediatr Res 1983; 17:269A.

229. Roe CR, Millington DS, Maltby DA et al. J Clin Invest 1984;74: 2290–5.

230. Lott IT, Erickson AM, Levy HL. Pediatrics 1972;49:616–8.

231. Berry GT, Yudkoff M, Segal S. J Pediatr 1988;113:58–64.

232. Hyman SL, Porter CA, Page TJ et al. J Pediatr 1987;111: 558–62.

233. Rousson R, Guibaud P. J Inherit Metab Dis 1984;7 [Suppl]:10–2.

234. Sbai D, Narcy C, Thompson GN et al. Am J Clin Nutr 1994;59: 1332–7.

235. De Raeve L, de Meirleir L, Ramet J et al. J Pediatr 1994;124: 416–20.

236. Chace DH, DiPerna JC, Kalas TA et al. Clin Chem 2001;47: 2040–4.

237. Schlenk H. Fed Proc 1972;3:1431A.

238. Mulder H, Walstra P, eds. The Milk Fat Globule. Emulsion Science as Applied to Milk Products and Comparable Foods. Farnham Royal, Bucks, England: Commonwealth Agricultural Bureau, 1974:25–32.

239. Dupont J, Mathias MM. Lipids 1969;4:478–83.

240. North KN, Korson MK, Gopal YR et al. J Pediatr 1995;126: 916–22.

241. Kahler SG, Sherwood WG, Woolf D et al. J Pediatr 1994;124: 239–43.

242. Inoue S, Krieger I, Sarnaik A et al. Pediatr Res 1981;15:95–8.

243. Stork LC, Ambruso DR, Wallner SF et al. Pediatr Res 1986; 20:783–8.

244. Thomas JA, Bernstein LE, Greene CL et al. J Am Diet Assoc 2000;100:1074–6.

245. Feillet F, Bodamer OA, Dixon MA et al. J Pediatr 2000;136: 659–63.

246. deKoning TJ, van Hagen CC, Carbasius-Weber E et al. J Inherit Metab Dis 2002;25:46.

247. Yannicelli S, Acosta PB, Velazquez A et al. Mol Genet Metab 2003;80:181–8.

248. Ciani F, Poggi GM, Pasquini E et al. Clin Nutr 2000;19:137–9.

249. Baumgartner ER, Viardot C. J Inherit Metab Dis 1995;18: 138–42.

250. van't Hoff WG, Dixon M, Taylor J et al. J Pediatr 1998;132: 1043–4.

251. Diss E, Iams J, Reed N et al. Am J Obstet Gynecol 1995;172: 1057–9.

252. van der Meer SB, Poggi F, Spada M et al. J Pediatr 1994;125: 903–8.

253. Goodman SI, Frerman FE. Organic acidemias due to defects in lysine oxidation: 2-ketoadipic acidemia and glutaric acidemia. In: Scriver CR, Beaudet AL, Sly WS et al., eds. The Metabolic and Molecular Bases of Inherited Disease. 8th ed. New York: McGraw-Hill, 2001:2195–204.

254. Baric I, Zschocke J, Christensen E et al. J Inherit Metab Dis 1998;21:326–40.

255. Hoffmann GF, Zschocke J. J Inherit Metab Dis 1999;22: 381–91.

256. Greenberg CR, Reimer D, Singal R et al. Hum Mol Genet 1995;4:493–5.

257. Brusilow SW, Horwich AL. Urea cycle enzymes. In: Scriver CR, Beaudet AL, Sly WS et al., eds. The Metabolic and Molecular Bases of Inherited Disease. 8th ed. New York: McGraw-Hill, 2001:1909–64.

258. Azevedo L, Stolnaja L, Tietzeova E et al. Mol Genet Metab 2003;78:152–7.

259. Tuchman M. Hum Mutat 1993;2:174–8.

260. Haberle J, Schmidt E, Pauli S et al. Hum Mutat 2003;21:444.

261. Haberle J, Schmidt E, Pauli S et al. Hum Mutat 2003;21:593–7.

262. Valle D, Simell O. The hyperornithinemias. In: Scriver CR, Beaudet AL, Sly WS et al., eds. The Metabolic and Molecular Bases of Inherited Disease. 8th ed. New York: McGraw-Hill, 2001:1857–98.

263. Leonard JV, Morris AA. Semin Neonatol 2002;7:27–35.

264. Oechsner M, Steen C, Sturenburg HJ et al. J Neurol Neurosurg Psychiat 1998;64:680–2.

265. Kline JJ, Hug G, Schubert WK et al. Am J Dis Child 1981;135: 437–42.

266. Cederbaum SD, Shaw KN, Valente M. J Pediatr 1977;90: 569–73.

267. Levin B, Abraham JM, Oberholzer VG et al. Arch Dis Child 1969;44:152–61.

268. Kennaway NG, Harwood PJ, Ramberg DA et al. Pediatr Res 1975;9:554–8.

269. Legras A, Labarthe F, Maillot F et al. Crit Care Med 2002;30: 241–4.

270. Levy HL, Coulombe JT, Shin V. The New England experience. In: Bickel H, Guthrie R, Hammersen G, eds. Neonatal Screening for Inborn Errors of Metabolism. Berlin: Springer-Verlag, 1980.

271. Barsotti RJ. J Pediatr 2001;138:S11–9.

272. Summar M, Tuchman M. J Pediatr 2001;138:S6–10.

273. Steiner RD, Cederbaum SD. J Pediatr 2001;138:S21–9.

274. Summar M. J Pediatr 2001;138:S30–9.

275. Batshaw ML, MacArthur RB, Tuchman M. J Pediatr 2001;138: S46–54.

276. Berry GT, Steiner RD. J Pediatr 2001;138:S56–60.

277. Leonard JV. J Pediatr 2001;138:S40–4.

278. Palekar A. Pediatr Res 2000;48:357–9.

279. FAO/WHO/UNU Expert Consultation on Energy and Protein Requirements. Geneva: World Health Organization, 1985: 71–112.

280. Hyman SL, Coyle JT, Parke JC. J Pediatr 1986;108:705–9.

281. Ohtani Y, Ohyanagi K, Yamamoto S et al. J Pediatr 1988;112: 409–14.

282. Ohtsuka Y, Griffith OWL. Biochem Pharmacol 1991;41: 1957–61.

283. Iafolla AK, Gale DS, Roe CR. J Pediatr 1990;117:102–5.

284. Renner C, Sewell AC, Bervoets K et al. Eur J Pediatr 1995; 154:909–14.

285. Maestri NE, Brusilow SW, Clossold DB et al. N Engl J Med 1996;335:855–9.

286. Maestri NE, Clissold D, Brusilow SW. J Pediatr 1999;134: 268–72.

287. Nicolaides P, Liebsch D, Dale N et al. Arch Dis Child 2002;86: 54–6.

288. Sanjurjo P, Rodriguez-Soriano J, Vallo A et al. Eur J Pediatr 1991;150:730–1.

289. Burlina AB, Ogier H, Korall H et al. Mol Genet Metab 2001; 72:351–5.

290. Scaglia F, Zheng Q, O'Brien WE et al. Pediatrics 2002;109: 150–2.

291. Mardach MR, Roe K, Cederbaum SD. J Inherit Metab Dis 1999;22:102–6.

292. Wilson O, Schfert W, Ballatore W et al. Pediatr Res 1995;37: 323A.

293. Holton JB, Walter JH, Tyfield LA. Galactosemia. In: Scriver CR, Beaudet AL, Sly WS et al., eds. The Metabolic and Molecular Bases of Inherited Disease. 8th ed. New York: McGraw-Hill, 2001:1553–8.

294. Elsas LJ, Langley S, Steele E et al. Am J Hum Genet 1995;56: 630–9.

295. Elsas LJ, Lai K. Genet Med 1998;1:40–8.

296. Flach JE, Reichardt JK, Elsas LJ. Mol Biol Med 1990;7:365–9.

297. Leslie ND, Immerman EB, Flach JE et al. Genomics 1992;14: 474–80.

298. Lai K, Willis AC, Elsas LJ. J Biol Chem 1999;274:6559–66.

299. Elsas LJ, Fridovich-Keil J, Leslie ND. Int Pediatr 1993;8: 101–9.

300. Kadhom N, Baptista J, Brivet M et al. Biochem Med Metab Biol 1994;52:140–4.

301. Wolfrom C, Raynaud N, Kadhom N et al. J Inherit Metab Dis 1993;16:78–90.

302. Charlwood J, Clayton P, Keir G. Glycobiology 1998;8:351–7.

303. Stibler H, von Dobeln V, Kristiansson B et al. Acta Paediatr 1997;86:1377–8.

304. Prestoz LLC, Couto AS, Shin YS et al. Eur J Pediatr 1997;156: 116–20.

305. Lai KW, Cheng LY, Cheung ALM. Cell Tissue Res 2003;311: 417–25.
306. Lai K, Elsas LJ. Biochem Biophys Res Commun 2000;271: 392–400.
307. Lai K, Langley SD, Khwaja FW et al. Glycobiology 2003;13: 285–94.
308. Waggoner DD, Buist NR, Donnell GN. J Inherit Metab Dis 1990;13:802–18.
309. Irons M, Levy HL, Pueschel S et al. J Pediatr 1985;107:261–3.
310. Urbanowski JC, Cohenford MA, Levy HL et al. N Engl J Med 1982;306:84–6.
311. Schweitzer S, Shin Y, Jakobs C et al. Eur J Pediatr 1993;152: 36–43.
312. Guerrero NV, Singh RH, Manatunga A et al. J Pediatr 2000; 137:833–41.
313. Elsas LJ, Langley S, Paulk EM et al. Eur J Pediatr 1995;154: S21–27.
314. Lai K, Langley SD, Singh RH et al. J Pediatr 1996;128:89–95.
315. Elsas LJ, Dembure PP, Langley S et al. Am J Hum Genet 1994; 54:1030–6.
316. Fridovich-Keil JL, Langley SD, Mazur LA et al. Am J Hum Genet 1995;56:640–6.
317. Beutler E, Baluda MC. J Lab Clin Med 1966;68:137–41.
318. Elsas LJ. Prenat Diagn 2001;21:302–3.
319. Jakobs C, Kleijer WJ, Allen J et al. Eur J Pediatr 1995;154: S33–6.
320. Kaufman FR, Loro ML, Azen C. J Pediatr 1993;123:365–70.
321. Rubio-Gozalbo ME, Hamming S, van Kroonenburgh MJ et al. Arch Dis Child 2002;87:57–60.
322. Berry GT, Nissim I, Gibson JB et al. Eur J Pediatr 1997;156 [Suppl 1]:S43–9.
323. Berry GT, Singh RH, Mazur AT et al. Pediatr Res 2000;48: 323–8.
324. Harvey CD, Jenness R, Morris HA. J Dairy Sci 1981;64: 1648–54.
325. Hettinga DH, Miah AH, Hammond EG et al. J Dairy Sci 1970; 53:1377–80.
326. Reynolds LM, Henneberry GO, Baker BE. J Dairy Sci 1959;42: 1463–71.
327. Gross KC, Acosta PB. J Inherit Metab Dis 1991;14:253–8.
328. Gropper SS, Gross KC, Olds SJ. J Am Diet Assoc 1993;93:328.

329. Cerbulis J. Arch Biochem Biophys 1954;49:442–50.
330. Gitzelmann R, Auricchio S. Pediatrics 1965;36:231.
331. Koch R, Acosta PB, Ragsdale N et al. J Am Diet Assoc 1963;43: 212.
332. Ning C, Reynolds R, Chen J et al. Pediatr Res 2000;48: 211–7.
333. Holton JB. Galactosemia. In: Schaub J, Van Hoof J, Vis HL, eds. Inborn Errors of Metabolism. New York: Raven Press, 1991.
334. Lineback DR, Ke CH. Cereal Chem 1975;52:334–47.
335. Acosta PB, Gross KC. Eur J Pediatr 1995;154:S87–92.
336. Kumar A, Weatherly MR, Beaman DC. Pediatrics 1991;87: 352–60.
337. Harju M. Milchwissenschaft 1990;456:411–5.
338. Segal S. Int Pediatr 1992;7:75–82.
339. Wiesmann UN, Rose-Beutler B, Schluchter R. Eur J Pediatr 1995;154:S93–6.
340. Weese SJ, Gosnell K, West P et al. J Am Diet Assoc 2003;103: 373–5.
341. Asp NG. Biochem J 1971;121:299–308.
342. Andersson L, Bratt C, Arnoldsson KC et al. J Lipid Res 1995;36:1392–400.
343. Donnell GN, Bergren WR, Perry G et al. Pediatrics 1963;31: 802–10.
344. Kaufman FR, Xu YK, Ng WG. J Pediatr 1988;112:754–6.
345. Shield JPH, Wadsworth EJK, MacDonald A et al. Arch Dis Child 2000;83:248–50.
346. Webb AL, Singh RH, Kennedy MJ et al. Pediatr Res 2003;53: 396–402.
347. Ng WG, Kaufman FR, Donnell GN. J Inherit Metab Dis 1989;12:257–66.
348. Gibson JB, Reynolds RA, Palmieri MJ et al. Metabolism 1995;44:597–604.
349. Manis FR, Cohn LB, McBride-Chang C et al. J Inherit Metab Dis 1997;20:549–55.
350. Rutherford PJ, Davidson DC, Matthai SM. J Hum Nutr Diet 2002;15:39–42.
351. Berry GT. Eur J Pediatr 1995;154:S53–64.
352. Wehrli SL, Berry GT, Palmieri M et al. Pediatr Res 1997;42: 855–61.
353. Komrower GA. J Inherit Metab Dis 1982;5[Suppl 2]:96–104.

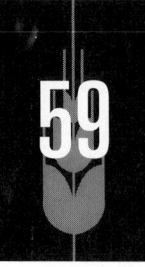

INHERITED METABOLIC DISEASES: DEFECTS OF β-OXIDATION[1]

JERRY VOCKLEY AND DEBORAH L. RENAUD

ENZYMES OF β-OXIDATION .962
    Mitochondria 962
    Peroxisomes 963
DEFECTS OF FATTY ACID METABOLISM 964
    Mitochondria 964
    Peroxisomes 968
DIAGNOSIS OF DEFECTS OF FATTY ACID
    METABOLISM 969
    Mitochondria 969
    Peroxisomes 970
GENETICS OF DEFECTS OF FATTY ACID
    METABOLISM 971
SUDDEN INFANT DEATH AND DEFECTS OF FATTY
    ACID METABOLISM 971
TREATMENT OF DEFECTS OF FATTY ACID
    METABOLISM 972
    Mitochondria 972
    Peroxisomes 973

β-Oxidation, which results in sequential cleavage of two carbon units from fatty acids, represents an important source of energy for the body during times of fasting and metabolic stress. Free fatty acids released into the blood via catabolism of fat stores or from dietary sources are metabolized in two intracellular compartments: the peroxisomes and the mitochondria.

Peroxisomes (sometimes referred to as microbodies) are subcellular organelles bounded by a single lipid bilayer membrane (1). They are ubiquitously distributed in tissues but are particularly abundant in liver and kidney (2). All peroxisomal proteins are encoded in the nuclear genome and are transported to the organelle posttranslationally. This process is mediated by at least three mechanisms (3–6). The most common is the presence of a serine-lysine-leucine amino acid motif at the carboxy terminus of the protein. This peroxisomal targeting signal (PTS1), present in more than 95% of proteins destined for the peroxisomal matrix, binds to the cytosolic receptor protein Pex5p. A second mechanism uses an amino terminus targeting signal (PTS2), which binds to the receptor protein Pex7p (5, 6). PTS2 enzymes include thiolase, phytanoyl-coenzyme A (CoA) hydroxylase, and alkyl-dihydroxyacetone phosphate synthetase (6). The PTS-receptor complexes are stabilized and are transported to the peroxisomal membrane, where they interact with the docking machinery and are then translocated into the peroxisomal matrix. The receptors are recycled to the cytoplasm. A series of Pex proteins involved in these processes has been identified and characterized (5, 6). An internal amino acid motif (mPTS), consisting of positively charged amino acids adjacent to at least one hydrophobic domain, targets proteins to the peroxisomal membrane (5).

Mitochondria are more complex structures than peroxisomes and are bounded by two lipid bilayer membranes (the inner and outer mitochondrial membranes). The intermembrane space constitutes a distinct compartment within the mitochondria, whereas the space bounded by the inner mitochondrial membrane is known as the matrix. Mitochondria are unique organelles in animals in that they contain their own unique genetic information (7). The mitochondrial genome is composed of a circular DNA molecule encoding several protein subunits that constitute part of the electron transfer chain complexes as well as genes for specific tRNA molecules necessary for mitochondrial protein translation. Human sperm cells are nearly devoid of mitochondria, whereas human oocytes contain numerous mitochondria. Genes on the mitochondrial chromosome therefore are inherited strictly from the mother by both sexes and can be passed on to subsequent generations only by females (7). This leads to the characteristic pattern of maternal inheritance seen in disorders associated with defects in the mitochondrial genome.

---

[1]**Abbreviations: ACD,** acyl-coenzyme A dehydrogenase (**LCAD, MCAD, SCAD, VLCAD,** long-, medium-, short, and very-long-chain acyl-coenzyme A dehydrogenase, respectively); **AFLP,** acute liver failure of pregnancy; **ATP,** adenosine triphosphate; **CoA,** coenzyme A; **CPT,** carnitine palmitoyl transferase; **DHA,** docosahexanoic acid; **ETF,** electron transfer flavoprotein; **FAD,** flavin adenine dinucleotide; **GA,** glutaric aciduria; **HELLP,** hemolysis, elevated liver enzymes, low platelet; **HMG,** hydroxymethyl glutaryl; **LCHAD,** long-chain 3-hydroxyacyl-coenzyme A dehydrogenase; **MADD,** multiple acyl-coenzyme A dehydrogenation disorder; **MCT,** medium-chain triglyceride; **MRI,** magnetic resonance imaging; **PTS,** peroxisomal targeting signal; **SCHAD,** short-chain 3-hydroxyacyl-coenzyme A dehydrogenase; **SCOT,** succinyl-coenzyme A: 3-ketoacid coenzyme A transferase; **SIDS,** sudden infant death syndrome; **S/MCHAD,** short-/medium-chain 3-hydroxyacyl-coenzyme A dehydrogenase; **TFP,** trifunctional protein; **X-ALD,** X-linked adrenoleukodystrophy.

Most proteins found in the mitochondria are nuclear encoded and thus are inherited in a standard mendelian fashion. In general, they are synthesized in a larger precursor form containing information in an amino terminal signal peptide necessary for targeting the proteins to the mitochondria (8–18). These signal sequences are usually removed after import of the protein into the mitochondrion. More than one targeting signal may be necessary to direct the imported protein to the correct mitochondrial space or membrane. Peroxisomes and mitochondria arise by division of previously existing organelles and are randomly distributed to daughter cells on cellular division.

Mitochondrial fatty acid oxidation is predominantly responsible for the oxidation of fatty acids of carbon length 20 or less, whereas the peroxisomal pathway is physiologically more relevant for longer-chain fatty acids (19, 20). Mitochondrial β-oxidation is a complex process involving transport of activated acyl-CoA moieties into the mitochondria and sequential removal of two-carbon acetyl-CoA units (21). The pathway of mitochondrial fatty acid oxidation is initiated by activation of fatty acids to acyl-CoA esters in the cytosol. The fatty acids are then transferred across the mitochondrial membrane bound to carnitine. Within the mitochondrial matrix, the fatty acids are converted back to acyl-CoA. The four steps of the β-oxidation cycle then sequentially remove two carbons until the acyl-CoA (n carbons) is fully converted to n/2 acetyl-CoA molecules. In peripheral tissues, the acetyl-CoA is terminally oxidized in the Krebs cycle for adenosine triphosphate (ATP) production. In the liver, the acetyl-CoA from fatty acid oxidation is used via the 3-hydroxy-3-methylglutaryl-CoA pathway for synthesis of ketones, 3-hydroxybutyrate, and acetoacetate, which are then exported for final oxidation by brain and other tissues.

At least 25 enzymes and specific transport proteins are responsible for carrying out the steps of mitochondrial fatty acid metabolism, some of which have only recently been recognized (Fig. 59.1 and Table 59.1) (22, 23). Of these, defects in at least 22 have been shown to cause disease in humans (21). The first of these disorders was identified in 1973 (24, 25), and most were identified in the mid-1990s. Fatty acid oxidation in peroxisomes uses a different set of enzymes (see Fig. 59.1 and Table 59.2) (26, 27). Although this system functions optimally for fats of carbon chain lengths between 12 and 16, its role in oxidation of fats longer than 20 carbons may be physiologically more relevant because these molecules are not well used as substrates by the mitochondrial enzymes of β-oxidation. Activation of fatty acids to fatty acyl-CoAs is probably coincident with transport into peroxisomes (28). Following a series of enzymatic steps resulting in shortening of the acyl-CoA moiety in two-carbon unit increments to a minimum of six carbons, reaction products can be exported from the peroxisome as acylcarnitines. They are also available for use in intraperoxisomal anabolic pathways such as cholesterol synthesis. β-Oxidation in peroxisomes involves fewer enzymes than

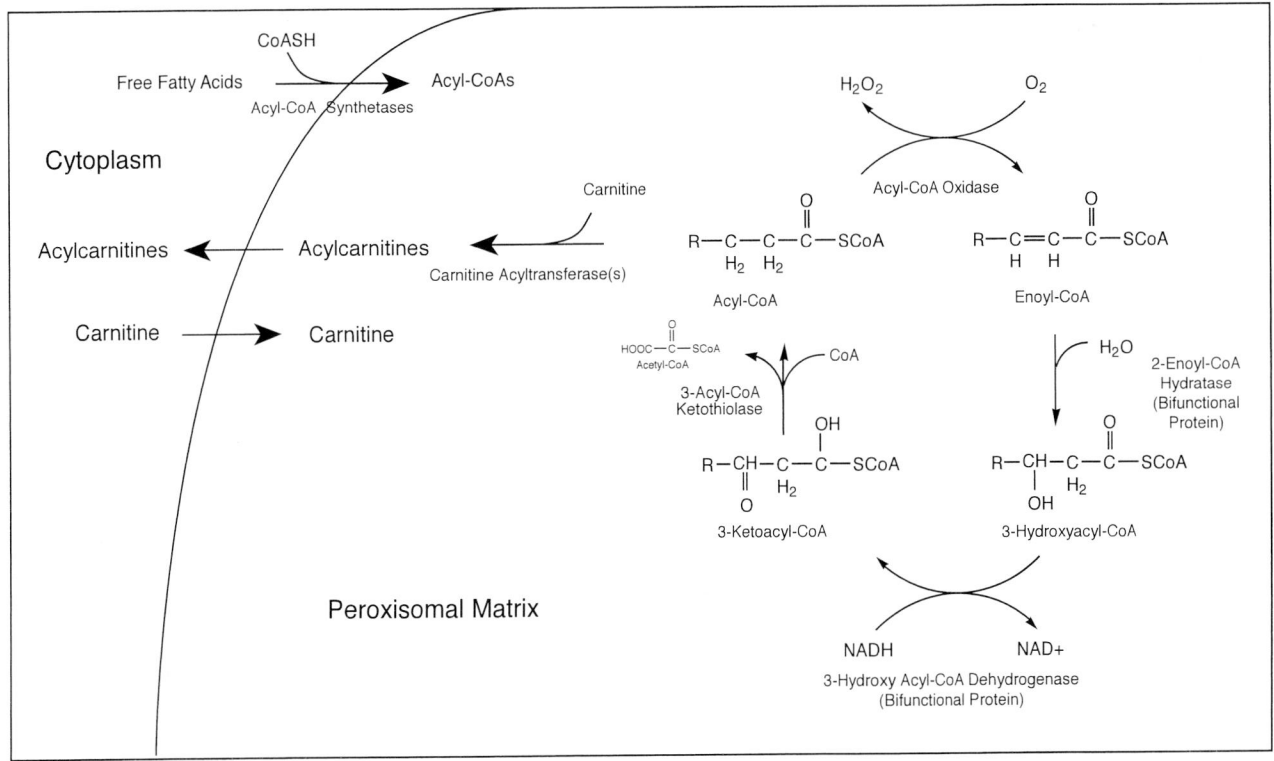

Figure 59.1. β-Oxidation of fatty acids in the peroxisome.

TABLE 59.1. ENZYMES INVOLVED IN MITOCHONDRIAL FATTY ACID OXIDATION

ENZYME	PROVEN CLINICAL DISORDER
Fatty acid activation	
Acyl-CoA synthetase	No
Carnitine cycle	
Plasma membrane carnitine transporter	Yes
CPT I	Yes
Carnitine/acylcarnitine translocase	Yes
CPT II	Yes
Mitochondrial β-Oxidation spiral	
Very-long-chain acyl-CoA dehydrogenase (membrane)	Yes
LCAD (matrix)	No
MCAD	Yes
SCAD	Yes
Trifunctional protein	
Long-chain 2-enoyl CoA hydratase	Yes
Long-chain 3-hydroxyacyl-CoA dehydrogenase	Yes (isolated)
Long-chain 3–ketoacyl-CoA thiolase	Yes
Crotonase (short-chain 2-enoyl-CoA hydratase)	No
SCHAD	Yes
Short-chain 3-ketoacyl-CoA thiolase	Possible
Enzymes of β-Oxidation of unsaturated fats	
Long-chain Δ^3, Δ^2-enoyl-CoA isomerase	No
Short-chain Δ^3, Δ^2-enoyl-CoA isomerase	No
2, 4-Dienoyl-CoA reductase	Possible
Enzymes of ketone body production	
HMG-CoA synthase	Yes
HMG-CoA lyase	Yes
D-3-hydroxybutyrate dehydrogenase	Yes

CoA, coenzyme A; CPT, carnitine palmitoyl transferase; HMG, hydroxymethyl glutayl; LCAD, MCAD, SCAD, long-, medium-, short-, and very-long-chain acyl coenzyme A dehydrogenase; SCHAD, short-chain 3-hydroxy acyl-coenzyme A dehydrogenase.

in mitochondria, and defects in most of them have been identified as causes of human disease. However, abnormalities of peroxisomal biogenesis leading to multiple enzymatic deficiencies represent a much more common type of defect in humans.

TABLE 59.2. ENZYMES OF PEROXISOMAL β-OXIDATION

Acyl-CoA synthetases
Acyl-CoA oxidases (straight-chain and branched-chain)
Bifunctional protein
    2-Enoyl-CoA hydratase
    3-Hydroxyacyl-CoA dehydrogenase
3-Ketoacyl-CoA thiolases
Carnitine acyltransferases
2-Methyl-CoA racemase
Enzymes of β-oxidation of unsaturated fats
    2,4-Dienoyl-CoA reductase
    3/2-Enoyl-CoA isomerase
    2-Enoyl-CoA hydratase
    2,5-Enoyl-CoA reductase
    3,5/2,4-Dienoyl-CoA isomerase

CoA, coenzyme A.

ENZYMES OF β-OXIDATION

Mitochondria

Free fatty acids are transported through the blood after intestinal absorption or mobilization from endogenous stores by the use of albumin as a carrier protein or in the form of triacylglycerols in lipoprotein complexes (29). Transport of free fatty acids intracellularly and through the cytoplasm is probably accomplished by a specific transport process; however, the mechanism of this step is not well characterized (30, 31). Before undergoing β-oxidation, free fatty acids must be activated to their corresponding acyl-CoA thioesters. Long-chain specific acyl-CoA synthetases can be found in various subcellular locations but are thought to arise from a single gene product (32). Short- and medium-chain carboxylic acids directly enter the mitochondrial matrix where they are activated. In contrast, long-chain fats are activated in the cytoplasm and require active transport into mitochondria. Transport of long-chain acyl-CoAs requires at least two enzymes, a transporter protein and the use of carnitine as an intermediate carrier molecule. Carnitine is itself transported intracellularly by a specific transporter protein (33, 34). Two carnitine transporters have been described, one specific to liver and a second with a more ubiquitous distribution including kidney, muscle, and fibroblasts (35). Long-chain acyl-CoAs are conjugated to carnitine by carnitine palmitoyl transferase I (CPT I) (29, 36). This enzyme is located on the inner aspect of the outer mitochondrial membrane. Tissue-specific isoforms of this enzyme probably exist. Long-chain acylcarnitines are then passed to carnitine palmitoyl transferase II (CPT II) in the inner mitochondrial membrane by a translocase (37).

Once present in the mitochondrial matrix, acyl-CoAs of all chain lengths undergo a series of enzymatic reactions resulting in the release of the two-carbon unit acetyl-CoA and a new acyl-CoA molecule that is two carbons shorter. The first step in this cycle is the dehydrogenation of the acyl-CoA to 2-enoyl-CoA. This reaction is catalyzed by a family of related enzymes, the acyl-CoA dehydrogenases (ACDs) (38–41). Four different members of this family are active in β-oxidation: very-long, long-, medium-, and short-chain acyl-CoA dehydrogenases (VLCAD, LCAD, MCAD, and SCAD, respectively), which differ in their chain length specificity. The role of LCAD in fatty acid β-oxidation is unclear (42–45). It is present in much lower concentrations than VLCAD in tissues where the two have been separated, and thus it would appear to play a minor role in the flux of fatty acids through β-oxidation. LCAD, however, has significant activity toward long, branched-chain substrates, unlike VLCAD, and thus may be more important in their metabolism (43, 45). A new enzyme with maximal activity toward palmitoyl-CoA has recently been described, but its physiologic role is as yet unknown (46).

The ACDs differ from most other dehydrogenases because they use electron transfer flavoprotein (ETF) as a final electron acceptor and thus can channel electrons directly into the ubiquinone pool of the electron transport machinery by way of ETF:ubiquinone oxidoreductase (ETF dehydrogenase) (47–49). The ACDs are homotetramers (except VLCAD, which is a homodimer) synthesized in a larger precursor form in the cytoplasm from nuclear encoded transcripts and then transported into mitochondria (50). Once inside the mitochondrial matrix, the leader peptide is removed by a specific protease, and the mature subunits assemble into the active homotetramer. One molecule of flavin adenine dinucleotide (FAD) is noncovalently attached to each ACD subunit. cDNAs for each of these proteins have been cloned, and sequence analysis shows that they are approximately 30 to 35% conserved, a finding suggesting evolution from a common primordial gene (41, 51–53). Three other members of this gene family are involved in branched-chain amino acid metabolism rather than in fatty acid oxidation (54–57).

The 2-enoyl-CoA moieties produced from longer-chain fatty acids by the ACDs are hydrated to 3-hydroxy-acyl-CoAs. These, in turn, undergo 2,3 dehydrogenation to 2-ketoacyl-CoAs, followed by cleavage of the thioester bond. This releases acetyl-CoA and completes one turn of the recursive β-oxidation cycle. The exact mechanism of these steps varies for substrates of differing chain length. The mitochondrial trifunctional protein (TFP) contains 2-enoyl-CoA hydratase, 3-hydroxy-acyl-CoA dehydrogenase, and 3-ketoacyl-CoA thiolase activities for longer-chain acyl-CoA substrates (58–61). This complex is an octamer consisting of four α and four β subunits. Long-chain 3-hydroxyacyl-CoA dehydrogenase (LCHAD) and 3-enoyl-CoA hydratase activities reside on the β subunit, whereas 3-ketoacyl-CoA thiolase activity resides on the β subunit. Evidence suggests that VLCAD and TFP, both associated with the inner mitochondrial membrane, may interact with the acylcarnitine transport and respiratory chain complexes to allow channeling of substrate directly from one enzyme to the next with ultimate release of shortened acyl-CoAs into the mitochondrial matrix when utilization by VLCAD is no longer efficient (62, 63). In contrast, individual proteins that catalyze these reactions for shorter-chain substrates have single activities. These proteins include a short/medium-chain 3-hydroxyacyl-CoA dehydrogenase (S/MCHAD), a short-chain enoyl-CoA hydratase (also called crotonase), and distinct medium- and short-chain 3-ketoacyl-CoA thiolase (23, 64–70). An additional enzyme originally designated as a short-chain 3-hydroxyacyl-CoA dehydrogenase has more recently been shown to have maximal activity towards steroid intermediates as substrates and probably does not play a role in fatty acid oxidation (71–73). The substrate specificities of many of these enzymes overlap, and additional enzymes with yet different substrate optima likely exist for some steps of β-oxidation (74, 75). Enzymes catalyzing several additional sets of reactions are necessary for the complete oxidation of unsaturated fatty acyl-CoA molecules, including a 2,4-dienoyl-CoA reductase (76) and a Δ^3, Δ^2-enoyl-CoA isomerase (45). In odd-chain (carbon number) fatty acid oxidation, the final three-carbon intermediate propionyl-CoA is metabolized by propionyl-CoA carboxylase.

Ketone bodies are produced exclusively in the liver from acetyl-CoA generated by β-oxidation (see Fig. 59.1). Hydroxymethyl glutaryl (HMG)-CoA synthase forms 3-hydroxy-3-methylglutaryl-CoA (HMG-CoA) from acetoacetyl-CoA and acetyl-CoA. Acetyl-CoA and acetoacetate are then produced by cleavage of HMG-CoA by HMG-CoA lyase (77–80). Finally, acetoacetate is reduced to D-3-hydroxybutyrate by D-3-hydroxybutyrate dehydrogenase within mitochondria (81, 82).

Several alternative metabolic pathways become important when mitochondrial β-oxidation is impaired. Peroxisomal β-oxidation allows continued metabolism of longer-chain fats, whereas ω-oxidation in the cytosol (which proceeds from the opposite end of the fatty acid) results in the production of the characteristic dicarboxylic acids often present in these disorders. In addition, deacylation of acyl-CoA by cytosolic thioesters and conjugation of acyl-CoAs to glycine and carnitine become important mechanisms of CoA scavenging and detoxification, respectively.

Peroxisomes

The β-oxidation cycle in peroxisomes differs from mitochondria in several important ways (26, 83, 84). First, the peroxisomal cycle results in chain shortening rather than complete oxidation of fatty acids. Second, ATP production in peroxisomes is less efficient because electrons produced by peroxisomal oxidases are donated directly to molecular oxygen for hydrogen peroxide production rather than to the respiratory chain. Third, carnitine plays a role in the export of chain-shortened fatty acids from the peroxisome but is not involved in fatty acid uptake (84).

Four peroxisomal half ABC transporters have been described in recent years including ALDP, ALDRP, PMP70 and PMP69. The best characterized of these half transporters is ALDP, which catalyses the uptake of VLCFA-CoAs. X-linked adrenoleukodystrophy (X-ALD) is caused by mutations in the *ALD* gene coding for ALDP (84). The activation of fatty acids to fatty acyl-CoAs is accomplished by acyl-CoA synthetases in the peroxisomal membrane (85). The first step of the β-oxidation cycle in the peroxisomal matrix is oxidation by straight-chain acyl-CoA oxidase (also called palmitoyl-CoA oxidase), leading to production of an enoyl-CoA (84, 86). Additional oxidases can perform similar reactions using 2-methyl branched-chain acyl-CoAs and CoA intermediates of bile acids as substrates (branched-chain acyl-CoA oxidases). Because the branched-chain acyl-CoA oxidases are stereospecific, 2-methyl-CoA racemase converts (2R)-methyl fatty acids to their (2S) diastereomers for oxidation (87–90). The second and third steps of the β-oxidation cycle are carried out by a bifunctional protein complex containing enoyl-CoA hydratase and 3-hydroxyacyl-CoA dehydrogenase activities associated with the inner aspect of the peroxisomal membrane (91, 92). Peroxisomal specific 3-ketoacyl-CoA thiolases catalyze the final step of the cycle, producing acetyl-CoA and regenerating an acyl-CoA (84, 93). Multiple carnitine acyltransferases with different chain-length specificities catalyze the conversion of acetyl-CoA and acyl-CoAs to acetyl-carnitine and acyl-carnitines, thus facilitating their export from the peroxisome (85). The chain-shortening step of the synthesis of docosahexanoic acid (DHA) (C22:6) is achieved by a single cycle of peroxisomal β-oxidation (85). Additional enzymes involved in the metabolism of unsaturated long-chain fats in peroxisomes include organelle-specific 2,4-dienoyl-CoA reductase, 3/2-enoyl-CoA isomerase, 2-enoyl-CoA hydratase, 2,5-enoyl-CoA reductase, and 3,5/2,4-dienoyl-CoA isomerase.

DEFECTS OF FATTY ACID METABOLISM

Mitochondria

Defects of the Carnitine Cycle

Deficiencies of several steps of the carnitine cycle have been described. These include defects of a specific plasma membrane carnitine transporter protein, CPT I and II, and the carnitine-acyl-carnitine translocase. A single report of two patients with defects in fatty acid oxidation and uptake in fibroblasts has been published (94). Both defects were more dramatic with oleate than with palmitate as substrate, and both resolved with treatment of the fibroblasts with digitonin, which permeabilizes cellular but not mitochondrial membranes. Thus, a defect in cellular fatty acid uptake is likely, although the affected gene remains unidentified.

Deficiency of the plasma membrane carnitine transporter represents a true primary carnitine deficiency (35, 95–102). Carnitine is freely filtered by the kidney and must be reabsorbed from the proximal tubules to preserve plasma levels. Because the transporter for carnitine is deficient in kidney as well as in muscle and liver, tissues whose carnitine content is highest, this defect results in defective renal reabsorption and reduced tissue storage of carnitine. This leads to a deficiency of carnitine in end organs and an impairment of long-chain fatty acid metabolism. Patients with carnitine transporter deficiency can present with severe hypoglycemia and dilated cardiomyopathy in infancy or childhood. Alternatively, they may show onset of hypertrophic cardiomyopathy, progressive muscle weakness, and muscle lipid storage in the first year of life. A mixed picture of these findings can also occur. Fetal hydrops secondary to this disorder has been reported (95, 103). Plasma carnitine levels are extremely low or undetectable in these children, but levels rise dramatically with supplementation with pharmacologic doses of carnitine (100 mg/kg/day of body weight). Patients' symptoms also show dramatic resolution with therapy. Outcome for these children is likely to be good if the diagnosis is promptly made and therapy is instituted (104). Carnitine transporter deficiency can be diagnosed by uptake studies using cultured fibroblast, or by direct molecular analysis of the OCTN2 gene. No common mutations have been described to date.

Deficiency of liver CPT I has been reported. The disease is generally characterized by episodic hypoketotic hypoglycemia beginning in infancy and multiorgan system failure (105–111). Approximately 20 cases have been reported. Muscle and cardiac symptoms are not present. In one case, an apparently healthy girl aged 2 years 9 months developed hepatomegaly and coma following a viral illness and died (109). Organic aciduria is not prominent in this disorder, but hyperammonemia may be present. Plasma carnitine is normal or elevated, with a high free fraction. Elevated levels of creatine kinase were seen in sibs from one family. Analysis of samples from patients with CPT I deficiency revealed normal CPT I levels in muscle, but low activity in other tissues including liver (105, 106). Molecular analysis of patients with CPT I deficiency identified mutations in the CPT1A gene including a common mutation leading to deficiency in the Hutterite population (112, 113). Patients with isolated muscle CPT I deficiency have not been reported date. Patients thus far have not responded well to therapy with carnitine, but presymptomatic treatment in subsequent affected sibs and infants identified through expanded newborn screening programs may change this observation. Diagnosis is based on enzymatic and mutation analysis.

Deficiency of carnitine-acylcarnitine translocase was initially reported in newborns who had a nearly uniform poor outcome (108, 114, 115). Patients have presented with severe hypoketotic hypoglycemia and cardiac arrhythmias and/or hypertrophy. All have had a grossly elevated ratio of acylcarnitine to free carnitine, whereas dicarboxylic aciduria was reported in one. One child died at 36 months of age following a prolonged course of progressive muscle weakness (108). He had episodes of coma associated with intercurrent illness and fasting that left him profoundly weak for 2 to 3 weeks following recovery. Another patient died at 8 days of age of a pulmonary hemorrhage probably secondary to liver failure (114). Mild hyperammonemia was present in both cases. Organic aciduria was not prominent. Two sibs died at age 2 months of liver failure after presentation at age 2 days (115). Carnitine supplementation did not appear to improve clinical symptoms in either patient. More recently, patients with a more benign clinical course have been identified who have responded well to modest carnitine supplementation and dietary therapy (37, 114–117). It appears that this group of patients has a higher level of residual enzyme activity than the more severely affected patients. Specific diagnosis of this disorder can be made via direct enzyme or molecular analysis.

CPT II deficiency is the most common of this group of disorders. It classically presents in late childhood or early adulthood as episodes of recurrent exercise- or stress-induced myoglobinuria (118). These can be severe enough occasionally to lead to acute renal failure. Patients are typically well between episodes. They have no tendency to develop hypoglycemia. Weakness and muscle pain are uncommon findings. The characteristic diagnostic findings in these patients are a low total plasma carnitine level with increased acylcarnitine fraction and no dicarboxylic aciduria. Long-chain acylcarnitines may, in fact, be elevated (107). A more severe variant of CPT II deficiency similar in symptoms to CPT I deficiency was also reported (107, 119). In these patients, the presenting symptoms were neonatal hypoglycemia, hepatomegaly, and cardiomyopathy. A severe reduction of CPT II activity was found in all tissues tested including liver, heart, muscle, and fibroblasts, whereas CPT I activity was normal. This decrease in CPT II activity was in the same range as seen with the later-onset form of the disease. Plasma carnitine was not increased. Mutations in the cDNA for CPT II have been described, and expression studies of mutant CPT II alleles suggest that the level of residual function of the mutant enzyme may be responsible for determining the clinical phenotype (119–121). Carnitine supplementation does not benefit the severe form of CPT II deficiency (122). Familial phenotypic variation has been reported (123). A common mutation has been reported to account for half of mutant alleles in the late-onset form of the disease (120, 124). A common coding polymorphism has also been reported in the CPT II coding region that may predispose to clinical symptoms under some (unknown) circumstances. Occasional families with apparent autosomal dominant transmission of partial CPT II deficiency have been described, and at least one case appears to be related to a mutation on one CPT II allele (123, 125). It is unknown why these patients exhibit symptoms, although a dominant negative effect on tetramer assembly and modifying gene effects have been postulated (123, 126).

Defects of Acyl-Coenzyme A Dehydrogenases

The first patient with VLCAD deficiency presented with ventricular fibrillation and respiratory arrest at 2 days of age and exhibited massive dicarboxylic aciduria (127). Plasma glucose and ammonia levels were not reported. She has been treated with a low-lipid diet and carnitine supplementation. Despite the dramatic neonatal presentation, the patient recovered and is reported to be well at 2 years of age, without muscle or cardiac abnormalities. The patient's older sibling died suddenly at 2 days of age and showed hepatic steatosis at necropsy. It is now clear that VLCAD deficiency is commonly associated with early-onset cardiac

and skeletal myopathy, although hypoketotic hypoglycemia, hyperammonemia, and hepatocellular failure also occur (128). Recurrent rhabdomyolysis and myopathy beginning in adolescence have also been described (129). 3-Hydroxy-dicarboxylic acids or saturated dicarboxylic acids may be present in the urine (127, 130). Cloning of the gene for VLCAD has allowed identification of a variety of genetic defects, but no common mutations have emerged (53, 131–134). Investigators disagree about the correlation of specific genotypes with phenotype, although mutations apparently leading to late-onset disease have been reported (23, 44, 135–137). Newborn screening for this disorder is possible by tandem mass spectrometry (138).

Putative LCAD deficiency has been reported, but all the patients originally categorized as LCAD deficient subsequently were proven to have a deficiency of VLCAD instead (139–141). Thus, no known patients with bona fide LCAD deficiency exist.

Patients with SCAD deficiency have been described (142–149). Clinical findings have included episodes of intermittent metabolic acidosis, neonatal hyperammonemic coma, neonatal acidosis with hyperreflexia, multicore myopathy, and infantile-onset lipid storage myopathy with failure to thrive and hypotonia. Hypoglycemia is a rare finding in this disorder. The characteristic metabolites of ethylmalonic and methylsuccinic acids of SCAD deficiency were also detected in persons with normal SCAD activity in fibroblasts (149). Subsequently, investigators demonstrated that the presence of one of two relatively common variants of SCAD (625 G>A and 511 C>T) predisposes to excessive ethylmalonic acid production (150, 151). These polymorphisms subtly affect the function of the purified proteins encoded by these variants, but both are still active (152). Most recently, it was shown that only one of ten patients identified on the basis of elevated ethylmalonic acid excretion, neuromuscular symptoms, and deficient SCAD activity in fibroblasts carried two pathogenic mutations (149). The remaining patients were double heterozygous for a pathogenic mutation and the previously identified 625 G>A variation, homozygous for one of the variations (625 G>A or 511 C>T), or double heterozygous for both. One patient previously identified as SCAD deficient had no mutations or polymorphisms in the SCAD gene, and retesting of his fibroblasts showed normal SCAD activity. Thus, it appears that the standard fibroblast assay is not suitable for diagnosis of this disorder. The presence of the common polymorphisms can lead to elevated butyrylcarnitine in newborn screening blood tests, but this result is not high enough to confuse with apparent complete deficiency (153). SCAD deficiency in mice has been shown to affect the electroencephalographic pattern of these mice during sleep (154). The full clinical spectrum of this deficiency and the clinical relevance of the common polymorphisms remain to be defined.

MCAD deficiency has emerged as one of the most common inborn errors of metabolism in certain populations, and it has been extensively reviewed (20, 23, 155, 156). The most frequent clinical presentation is one of intermittent hypoketotic hypoglycemia with onset in the second year of life (20, 38). Mild hyperammonemia and coma may or may not be present. These findings often lead to the nonspecific diagnose of Reye syndrome. The patient is usually well between attacks. Dicarboxylic aciduria is extensive during the attacks, but it can be undetectable by routine means when the patient is well. Similarly, microvesicular and macrovesicular hepatic steatosis, muscle weakness, and lipid excess in muscle present during the acute illness may resolve between acute episodes. Most patients who die of MCAD deficiency do so after having survived an initial episode (20). Thus, recurrent Reye syndrome–like episodes should trigger suspicion of this disorder. Sudden death in a previously healthy child has been described in numerous cases of MCAD deficiency. This can occur as early as the first day of life, and it has been seen in a previously healthy adult who was under calorie restriction after abdominal surgery. In the appropriate age range, such deaths are often misascribed to sudden infant death syndrome (SIDS). Autopsy usually demonstrates the characteristic microvesicular and macrovesicular steatosis and should suggest the diagnosis. Analysis of the acylcarnitine and acylglycine profile from a bile specimen, as well as enzyme assay in cultured fibroblast (which may be recovered from deep tissues such as the fascia lata of the thigh up to 48 hours post mortem), may be helpful in proving it. Finally, completely asymptomatic persons have been identified in the course of family studies of patients. The diagnosis of MCAD deficiency in asymptomatic persons has been made possible by dramatic advances in laboratory techniques based on the identification of alternate metabolites that accumulate in various bodily fluids (157–159).

Remarkable progress has been made in recent years in our understanding of the molecular mechanisms responsible for MCAD deficiency. Following cloning of the cDNA for MCAD, several groups simultaneously reported that a single common mutant allele was responsible for up to 90% of mutant alleles in patients with this disorder (160, 161). The substitution of a G for an A residue at position 985 (985 A>G) results in the replacement of a lysine by a glutamic acid residue and production of an unstable protein (162). Furthermore, screening of newborn blood samples has revealed a high carrier frequency for this disorder in some populations. Allele frequencies for the 985 A>G mutation range from one in 20 in northern European populations to less than one in 100 in Asian and some southern European populations. In the United States, the estimated carrier frequency for all mutations in whites is one in 60 (163). This translates into a predicted disease frequency of one in 15,000. MCAD deficiency is much less frequent in the African and Asian populations. The public health issues surrounding a disease with potentially such a high frequency have been vigorously debated. The predicted incidence for MCAD based on these studies is similar to or greater than that for phenylketonuria, a disorder screened for in all 50 states in the United States. Thus, a strong feeling exists among some groups that newborn screening for MCAD deficiency is warranted (164–171).

Deficiency of Other β-Oxidation Enzymes

Patients with a deficiency of 3-hydroxyacyl-CoA dehydrogenase (LCHAD) tend to fall into two clinical subclasses (172–178). One group presents primarily with symptoms of cardiomyopathy, myopathy, and hypoglycemia. Peripheral neuropathy and recurrent myoglobinuria may be present (74, 179–181). These patients are deficient in all three enzymatic activities of the TFP. The other group has hepatocellular disease with hypoglycemia with or without pigmentary retinopathy. Cholestasis and fibrosis may also be present (182). Considerable overlap in these groups has been described, however, and LCHAD deficiency has also been reported in patients with recurrent Reye syndrome–like symptoms and in sudden infant death (183). Milder cases with adolescent onset of recurrent rhabdomyolysis have been reported (184). In a large series of patients with isolated LCHAD deficiency, the mean age of clinical presentation was 5.8 months, with seven presenting in the neonatal period (185). Thirty-nine patients presented with hypoketotic hypoglycemia, whereas 11 presented with chronic problems, consisting of failure to thrive, feeding difficulties, cholestatic liver disease, and/or hypotonia. Most patients presenting with an acute metabolic derangement were determined in retrospect to also have some symptomatology. Mortality in this series was high, with 38% dying within 3 months of diagnosis. Morbidity in the surviving patients was also high, with recurrent metabolic crises and muscle problems despite therapy. In a recent series of 21 patients with TFP deficiency, nine presented with rapidly progressive clinical deterioration. Six of these patients had hypoketotic hypoglycemia. The remaining 12 patients presented with nonspecific, chronic symptoms, including hypotonia (100%), cardiomyopathy (73%), failure to thrive, or peripheral neuropathy. Ten patients presented in the neonatal period. Mortality was high (76%) and was mostly attributable to cardiac disease. Two patients who were diagnosed prenatally died despite treatment (178).

Defects in the α subunit destabilize the TFP, resulting in the multiple enzymatic deficiencies seen in some patients (186–188). A common G to C mutation at nucleotide position 1528 (1528 G>C) accounts for approximately 60% of mutant alleles identified thus far (187). Heterozygosity for TFP α–subunit deficiency has been implicated as a potential risk factor in the development of fatty liver of pregnancy or hemolysis, elevated liver enzymes, low platelet (HELLP) syndrome (see later). Mutations in the β subunit of TFP have been less well characterized, but they can also lead to destabilization of TFP (188). The reasons for the clinical heterogeneity in this disorder remain to be elucidated (189). Patients with primary defects in respiratory chain function can have a secondary decrease of LCHAD activity and/or a less specific decrease in fibroblast oxidation of radiolabeled palmitate. Thus, care must be taken to differentiate these patients appropriately from those with primary LCHAD deficiency.

Three patients have been reported with a deficiency of short-chain 3-hydroxyacyl-CoA dehydrogenase (SCHAD) deficiency (70, 190). The first was a 16-year-old, previously healthy girl who developed episodic myoglobinuria at age 13 years. At age 16 years, she developed a flu-like illness with generalized weakness, hypoketotic hypoglycemia, and lethargy. She subsequently died of a cardiac arrhythmia. Dicarboxylic aciduria and 3-hydroxydicarboxylic aciduria were present acutely. An older brother died at age 8 years of encephalopathy after a 6-year history of intermittent episodes of irritability, ataxia, and mild mental retardation. She had 35% of normal SCHAD activity in muscle compared with controls with a preservation of activity with long-chain substrates. A second patient presented with episodic vomiting, dehydration, and hyperammonemia beginning at age 13 months (70). Urine findings during acute episodes included elevated 3-hydroxybutyrate and acetoacetate, along with dicarboxylic acids and 3-hydroxydicarboxylic acids of chain length C6 to C14. Urinary carnitine was increased and was mostly conjugated. A final patient presented with a complex clinical picture complicated by the presence of a concurrent chromosomal abnormality but showed biochemical findings similar to those of the second patient. Only the last patient exhibited hypoglycemia. SCHAD activity in isolated mitochondria from the latter two patients was reduced to about 5% of normal (70).

Three patients with deficiency of mitochondrial 3-ketoacyl-CoA thiolase were originally described with developmental delay and muscle weakness, one of whom died of a Reye syndrome–like illness with urine metabolite findings suggestive of a defect in mitochondrial 3-ketoacyl-CoA thiolase (69). Definitive enzyme testing was not performed. Since then, more than 30 patients have been identified with mutations in this gene, also known as short-chain 3-ketoacyl-CoA thiolase. Most have had a presentation of recurrent episodes acidosis exacerbated by intercurrent illness, but with a characteristic persistence of the presence of ketone bodies in blood and urine when well (67, 80, 191–195). Hypoglycemia has not been common. A single patient with medium-chain 3-ketoacyl-CoA thiolase deficiency had metabolic acidosis, liver dysfunction, and rhabdomyolysis associated with vomiting and dehydration (67).

One patient has been reported to have a potential defect in the enzyme 2,4-dienoyl-CoA reductase (196). This patient presented in the newborn period with persistent hypotonia. She was found to have elevated lysine and decreased carnitine in plasma. 2-*trans*,4-*cis*-Decadienenoylcarnitine was identified in plasma and urine, and reduced activity of 2,4-dienoyl-CoA reductase was found in liver and muscle. The patient died at 4 months of age of respiratory acidosis. Confirmation of the clinical significance of these biochemical abnormalities awaits the identification of additional patients.

Multiple Acyl-Coenzyme A Dehydrogenation Disorder

Abnormalities of ETF or ETF:ubiquinone oxidoreductase (ETF dehydrogenase) deficiency lead to an in vivo deficiency of all the dehydrogenases that use ETF as an electron acceptor (48, 197–199). This group includes the ACDs discussed earlier, as well as isovaleryl-CoA dehydrogenase, 2-methylbutyryl-CoA dehydrogenase, isobutyryl-CoA dehydrogenase, glutaryl-CoA dehydrogenase, dimethylglycine dehydrogenase, and sarcosine dehydrogenase, enzymes involved in the intermediate metabolism of branched-chain amino acids, tryptophan, lysine, and choline. Accumulation of intermediate compounds related to blockages in all of these pathways is seen. Because of the presence of glutaric acid in the urine of some patients, this disorder is frequently referred to as glutaric aciduria type II (GA II), to distinguish it from a primary deficiency of glutaryl-CoA dehydrogenase (GA I). Clinical manifestations of multiple acyl-CoA dehydrogenation disorder (MADD) are extremely heterogeneous (200). A neonatal form can be seen with severe hypotonia, dysmorphic features, and cystic kidneys. These infants also exhibit metabolic acidosis and hypoglycemia. Milder variants are common, presenting with nonspecific neurologic signs, lipid storage myopathy, fasting hypoketotic hypoglycemia, and/or intermittent acidosis. In some patients, only fasting hypoketotic hypoglycemia or intermittent acidosis is seen and can be of late onset (201–207). In these cases, the organic acid profile in times of illness is usually dominated by ethylmalonic and adipic acids, leading to the alternate name of ethylmalonic-adipic aciduria for this disorder. Structural brain abnormalities are common, including agenesis of the cerebellar vermis, hypoplastic temporal lobes, and focal dysplasia of cerebral cortex (201, 202, 205, 206). Neuronal migration abnormalities may be present. A riboflavin-responsive form of MADD has been reported, including one patient with leukodystrophy (204, 206, 208, 209).

Analysis of fibroblasts from patients with MADD has revealed defects in both protein subunits of ETF and in ETF dehydrogenase (210). Cell lines with and without immunologically cross-reactive material have been described. cDNAs for both subunits of ETF and ETF dehydrogenase have been cloned, and direct mutational analysis has revealed a variety of defects in patients (211). Thus far, correlation of the mutation identified with severity of clinical symptoms has not been possible.

Riboflavin-Responsive Defects of Fatty Acid Metabolism

Riboflavin is the precursor to FAD, an essential cofactor for the ACDs, ETF, and ETF dehydrogenase. Several patients with biochemical abnormalities suggestive of β-oxidation defects have been described who respond with clinical improvement to pharmacologic doses of riboflavin (100–200 mg/kg/day). One of these groups clinically resembles multiple dehydrogenase deficiency and appears to represent a variant of ETF or ETF dehydrogenase with an as yet undefined defect in interaction with FAD. Increasing intramitochondrial concentrations of FAD by administration of riboflavin apparently allows enough cofactor binding to restore activity. A second set of patients with a picture of late-onset lipid storage myopathy and muscle weakness showing some level of hepatic dysfunction has been described. Again, these patients appear to respond to therapy with riboflavin, but their defect remains undefined. Marked clinical heterogeneity within each group has been documented.

Deficiencies of Ketone Body Production

Deficiency of HMG-CoA lyase, which is also active in the metabolism of leucine, presents with hypoketotic hypoglycemia with hyperammonemia and acidosis (80). Identification of hydroxymethylglutaric acid in the urine is diagnostic. Succinyl-CoA: 3-ketoacid CoA transferase (SCOT) functions in conjunction with mitochondrial acetoacetyl-CoA thiolase to generate ketones in extrahepatic tissues. SCOT deficiency presents as persistent ketonuria in the first 1 to 2 years of life, whereas acetoacetyl-CoA thiolase deficiency presents with variable clinical symptoms and exaggerated ketoacidosis in response to minor physiologic stress (81, 82, 212). Hypoglycemia is unusual in both disorders. It is seen, however, in another rare inborn error of metabolism, HMG-CoA synthetase deficiency (78). HMG-CoA synthase deficiency has been reported in a child who presented with fasting hypoketotic hypoglycemia.

Multiple Defects in Energy Metabolism

Inborn errors of fatty acid metabolism show considerable variation in the severity of symptoms. This is often ascribed to the differential effects of specific mutations on gene/enzyme function, but such genotype/phenotype correlations are usually imprecise. In addition, in some patients with clinical and biochemical findings consistent with a defect in energy metabolism (especially recurrent hypoglycemia or rhabdomyolysis), it is ultimately impossible to arrive at a precise enzymatic diagnosis. In this situation, the identification of concurrent partial defects in β-oxidation with or without partial deficiencies in other energy metabolism pathways has been reported (126, 213). The apparent development of symptoms consistent with reductions in energy metabolism related to the compound effects of these partial defects has been termed synergistic heterozygosity. Based on the relatively high frequencies of known disorders of energy metabolism, this may represent a previously unrecognized, relatively common mechanism of disease of potentially great clinical relevance.

Pregnancy-Induced Symptoms in β-Oxidation Defects

To date, 61 reported LCHAD-deficient patients have been born following pregnancies complicated by a variety of complications (23, 214–219). In 21 of these pregnancies, acute liver failure of pregnancy (AFLP) or HELLP syndrome occurred. The 1528 G>C mutation was present on at least one allele of the TFP α-subunit gene in all 12 affected infants in whom molecular genetic studies were done. These clinical complications, however, are not limited to carriers of LCHAD mutations; they also occur in other disorders of fatty acid oxidation. Three patients with CPT I deficiency, one patient with carnitine-acylcarnitine translocase deficiency, one patient each with MCAD and SCAD deficiency, and more than one patient with complete TFP deficiency were born to mothers who developed liver disease during pregnancy (220–225). Thus, it seems reasonable to suggest that pregnancies complicated by AFLP or HELLP syndrome should trigger an evaluation for a β-oxidation defect in the baby following delivery.

Peroxisomes

Defects of Peroxisomal Biogenesis

Defects of peroxisomal biogenesis with a resulting failure to import all or a subset of matrix enzymes are far more common than single enzyme deficiencies. Apparent absence or significant reduction in the number of peroxisomes has been demonstrated in four disorders historically considered to be distinct: Zellweger syndrome, neonatal adrenal leukodystrophy, infantile Refsum disease, and pipecolic acidemia (1, 226). It is now clear that these are related disorders that form a spectrum of clinical severity from the early lethal phenotype seen in Zellweger syndrome to the later-onset symptoms of infantile Refsum disease and pipecolic acidemia. Zellweger syndrome was the first disorder of peroxisomal biogenesis to be identified (227). Classic findings include characteristic dysmorphic facial features and other malformations accompanied by severe neurologic dysfunction with hypotonia, seizures, and ultimate deterioration. Liver function is abnormal, as is that of the gastrointestinal tract, leading to failure to thrive. Neuronal heterotopia and renal cortical cysts are seen pathologically. Proximal limb shortening may be present. Death usually occurs within the first year of life. Although peroxisomes were originally believed to be absent, peroxisomal ghosts have been identified. These consist of peroxisomal membranes containing typical membrane proteins but devoid of their contents. This finding results from defective import of PTS1 and PTS2 matrix enzymes. These peroxisomal enzymes are mislocalized to the cytosolic compartment (5, 6). This results in severe impairment of cholesterol synthesis, bile acid metabolism, β-oxidation of very-long-chain fats and branched-chain fats, ether phospholipid synthesis, and phytanic acid and pipecolic acid metabolism.

Neonatal adrenoleukodystrophy and infantile Refsum disease can present in the first 6 months of life similarly to Zellweger syndrome, but with slightly later onset of symptoms (228, 229). These disorders, along with pipecolic acidemia, can also appear in early childhood (<3 years of age) with findings of psychomotor retardation (228–230), ophthalmologic abnormalities, and other neurologic deficits including neurosensory impairment and nystagmus. Biochemical findings in patients with neonatal adrenoleukodystrophy, infantile Refsum disease, and pipecolic acidemia are similar to those of Zellweger syndrome, but they may be more subtle. Rhizomelic chondrodysplasia punctata, characterized by abnormal facies, developmental delay, cataracts, abnormal calcifications of epiphyses, and severe proximal limb shortening, results from failure to import PTS2-associated enzymes in response to mutations in the *PEX7* gene (6).

Understanding of the molecular basis for deficient peroxisomal biogenesis in this group of disorders is evolving rapidly. Complementation analysis of fibroblasts from these patients reveals that at least ten to 12 separate genes are affected (231–233). Some of the complementation groups are rare and are identified only in patients with the Zellweger phenotype thus far (231, 233). Patients in the remaining complementation groups may exhibit any of the clinical phenotypes. Patients with the Zellweger spectrum phenotypes clinically have also been shown to have single enzyme deficiencies (231, 234). Peroxisomal assembly is not disrupted in these patients.

Disorders of Single Enzymes

X-ALD is the most common disorder involving peroxisomal β-oxidation, affecting one in 20,000 males (27). Initial biochemical studies originally characterized an impaired ability to activate fatty acids to their acyl-CoA esters and suggested that this was a disorder of an acyl-CoA synthetase. More recent molecular data, however, have identified defects in an ATP-binding transporter located in the peroxisomal membrane as being responsible for this disorder (235). The reason that this defect affects the activity of acyl-CoA synthetase remains to be elucidated. Regardless, patients show a severely impaired ability to metabolize very-long-chain fatty acids in the peroxisomes. Several clinical phenotypes have been associated with defects in this locus (232, 234–240). Classic cerebral childhood adrenoleukodystrophy is the most common of these and accounts for 50% of cases. Boys are usually well until the second half of the first decade of life when progressive

quadriplegia, blindness and dementia develop. Death generally occurs within 5 years of onset of symptoms. In 30% of patients, a later-onset disorder designated adrenomyeloneuropathy is seen. Here, male patients experience progressive spastic paraparesis with peripheral neuropathy beginning in the second or third decade of life. Up to 30% of women who are carriers of X-ALD also show a similar picture beginning at about age 30 years. Finally, some boys and men with a defect in this gene show only adrenal insufficiency (which also accompanies almost 90% of adrenoleukodystrophy and adrenomyeloneuropathy). There may be great clinical heterogeneity within families.

The remaining defects in peroxisomal β-oxidation are relatively rare, with only a handful of reported cases each. Deficiency of acyl-CoA oxidase is characterized by early-onset seizures, developmental delay, and hypotonia similar to neonatal adrenoleukodystrophy and is often referred to as pseudoneonatal adrenoleukodystrophy (241). Dysmorphic features are not seen. Hepatic peroxisomes are present, and isolated elevation of very-long-chain fatty acids is found in blood and urine. Ten patients have been described to date (242). Peroxisomal bifunctional protein deficiency also presents with a Zellweger-like phenotype. An accumulation of very-long-chain fatty acids, bile acid intermediates, and branched-chain fatty acids is present but with normal plasmalogen synthesis, which distinguishes this disorder from a peroxisomal biogenesis defect. (242–247). Patients with isolated deficiency of one of the components of the bifunctional protein have also been described (242). 2-Methylacyl-CoA racemase deficiency presents with adult-onset sensory motor neuropathy and pigmentary retinopathy (242).

Classic Refsum disease resulting from deficiency of phytanic acid oxidase is not a defect of peroxisomal β-oxidation per se, but it deserves mention because of the confusing nomenclature. Clinical findings include retinitis pigmentosa, cerebellar ataxia, and peripheral neuropathy, with onset of symptoms varying from childhood to the fifth decade of life (248). Patients have no cognitive impairment, dysmorphic features, or hepatomegaly. This disorder is characterized by accumulation of phytanic acid in blood and tissues, whereas other peroxisomal enzyme functions are normal.

DIAGNOSIS OF DEFECTS OF FATTY ACID METABOLISM

Mitochondria

Diagnosis of defects of mitochondrial fatty acid metabolism requires a high level of suspicion in the appropriate clinical settings (Table 59.3). This is crucial because in many instances, the biochemical abnormalities that may suggest a defect of β-oxidation often resolve along with clinical symptoms. Thus, patients with unexplained hypoglycemia, acidosis, hyperammonemia, myopathy with or

TABLE 59.3. FINDINGS SUGGESTIVE OF A DEFECT IN MITOCHONDRIAL β-OXIDATION

Hypoketotic hypoglycemia with fasting or stress
Reye syndrome (especially recurrent)
Hypotonia and/or muscle weakness
Peripheral neuropathy
Coma
Sudden death in infancy or childhood
Cardiomyopathy
Unexplained metabolic acidosis with or without
   hyperammonemia
Hyperuricemia
Recurrent myoglobinuria
Elevated serum creatine kinase
Dicarboxylic aciduria
Carnitine deficiency

without recurrent myoglobinuria, or progressive neuropathy should be considered candidates for one of these disorders. All cases of Reye syndrome, patients with Reye syndrome–like symptoms, or "SIDS" or unexplained sudden or near death in childhood should be evaluated for a defect in fat metabolism. When a patient presents with such a clinical picture, it is critical to obtain blood and urine samples acutely for appropriate analysis, because biochemical findings may disappear when the patient is well. Because routine organic acid analysis is often normal when patients are not in an acute crisis, these patients should be more extensively evaluated if a diagnosis is not immediately obvious. This is best done in a referral center by a specialist trained in the evaluation of these patients. Plasma free and total carnitine levels can often suggest whether a deficiency is primary or secondary (Table 59.4) (21, 23, 155, 249).

Laboratory clues to the diagnosis of one of these disorders include dicarboxylic aciduria or 3-hydroxy dicarboxylic aciduria, hypoglycemia in the presence of little or no ketosis, mild lactic acidosis, and mild hyperammonemia. Hyperuricacidemia is a useful sign if present, but it is nonspecific. Myoglobin in blood or urine and elevated plasma creatine kinase levels can be seen when muscle involvement is present. Highly sensitive techniques, using mass spectrometry, have been developed for the detection of minute quantities of intermediates that are specific for certain fatty acid oxidation disorders. These intermediates

are often not detectable by routine organic acid analysis (157, 158). All patients with a suspected defect in fatty acid metabolism should receive an echocardiogram because of the high incidence of cardiomyopathy in many of these disorders. A fasting test with or without a subsequent challenge test with medium-cahin triglycerides (MCTs) or long-chain triglycerides may induce excretion of a diagnostic metabolite, but it should be undertaken only in a hospital setting by someone with experience in performing such tests. An MCT loading test must only be performed after specifically excluding the diagnosis of MCAD deficiency, because catastrophic consequences can result in patients with MCAD deficiency. Direct DNA mutational analysis is readily available for the common A to G985 mutation responsible for MCAD deficiency (160). Specific enzyme analysis can be performed for many of these defects on cultured fibroblasts and/or liver or skeletal muscle. Newborn screening for MCAD deficiency has been suggested, but it remains controversial (164, 250).

Newborn screening for many disorders of β-oxidation, using tandem mass spectroscopy of dried blood samples collected before discharge from the nursery, has been implemented in several states and is being evaluated in others (164–171, 250). Such screening remains controversial; opponents have raised concerns about cost-to-benefit ratios. It is clear, however, that presymptomatic identification of these patients can, in many instances, prevent catastrophic events, especially sudden death. Savings in medical expenses related to evaluation of children who would have been identified by newborn screening must also be considered (251–254). It seems likely that such screening will be widely implemented in the near future.

Peroxisomes

Diagnosis of defects of peroxisomal β-oxidation is more straightforward than for mitochondrial defects because clinical symptoms and biochemical abnormalities are not intermittent. Clinical findings suggestive of a defect of peroxisomal biogenesis or an isolated defect in β-oxidation are summarized in Table 59.5. It is important to consider these diagnoses in the setting of unexplained seizures and/or developmental delay, especially if accompanied by hypotonia. The relative concentrations of key metabolites in these disorders are outlined in Table 59.6. Screening of

TABLE 59.4. PLASMA CARNITINE LEVELS IN DEFECTS OF β-OXIDATION

ENZYME DEFECT	TOTAL CARNITINE	FREE CARNITINE	FREE/TOTAL CARNITINE
Carnitine transporter	Very Low	Low	Normal
CPT I	Normal or high	High	High
Translocase and CPT II	Low	Very low	Low
VLCAD, LCAD, MCAD, SCAD, LCHAD, SCHAD, ETF and ETF dehydrogenase, 2,4-dienoyl-CoA reductase	Low	Low	Normal or low

CoA, coenzyme A; CPT, carnitine palmitoyl transferase; ETF, electron transfer flavoprotein; LCAD, MCAD, SCAD, VLCAD, long-, medium-, short-, and very-long-chain acyl coenzyme A dehydrogenase; SCHAD, short-chain 3-hydroxy acyl-CoA dehydrogenase.

TABLE 59.5. FINDINGS SUGGESTIVE OF A DEFECT IN PEROXISOMAL β-OXIDATION

Neurologic and/or intellectual features
  Developmental delay or regression
  Seizures
  Hypotonia
  Peripheral neuropathy
  Neuronal migration defects
  Demyelination
Dysmorphic features
  Large anterior fontanelle
  High forehead
  Epicanthal folds
Rhizomelic chondrodysplasia
Hepatomegaly and/or hepatic failure
Renal cysts
Adrenal insufficiency
Ophthalmologic abnormalities
  Optic atrophy
  Cataracts
  Retinopathy
Hearing impairment
Failure to thrive

plasma and/or urine for very-long-chain fatty acids, pipecolic acid, phytanic acid, and pristanic acid will identify most patients. The measurement of plasma very-long-chain fatty acids should not be used to exclude hemizygosity for X-ALD in females (234). Additional investigations can include quantitation of bile acid and cholesterol synthesis intermediates, red blood cell membrane plasmalogen level, and the presence or absence of peroxisomes in cultured skin fibroblasts. Finally, specific enzyme analysis on cultured skin fibroblasts as well as complementation analysis can be performed to identify the precise nature of the defect in a patient. Molecular mutational analysis remains largely a research tool.

GENETICS OF DEFECTS OF FATTY ACID METABOLISM

All the defects of mitochondrial fatty acid metabolism identified thus far and all the peroxisomal orders except X-ALD are inherited in an autosomal recessive fashion.

The recurrence risk for subsequent siblings is therefore 25%. X-ALD is inherited as an X-linked trait. Affected males are hemizygous for one abnormal gene, whereas carrier women are heterozygous for one normal and one mutant allele. Thus, carrier women face a 50% risk to have an affected male or carrier female with each pregnancy. There may be great clinical heterogeneity within families, and persons with the severe childhood-onset and less severe myeloneuropathy forms may be present in the same family. To explain this, it has been proposed that one or more additional autosomal genes may be responsible for modulating the clinical severity of this disorder.

SUDDEN INFANT DEATH AND DEFECTS OF FATTY ACID METABOLISM

The role of mitochondrial β-oxidation defects in SIDS bears special mention. It is necessary to be precise when discussing the issue of SIDS. Because the definition of SIDS includes the presence of normal autopsy findings, many patients with defects of β-oxidation will be eliminated from this population by careful microscopic study of muscle, heart, and liver. Unfortunately, not all deaths reported as "SIDS" receive the same level of scrutiny, and thus cases of β-oxidation disorders may still be represented. In addition, some disorders of β-oxidation can clearly present with minimal or no tissue changes, thus making postmortem diagnosis far more difficult. An early claim that 15 to 17% of cases of SIDS are caused by defects of β-oxidation has been tempered by additional data, but it is likely that approximately 1 to 3% of unexplained sudden deaths in infancy and childhood are related to such disorders (255–257). Because of this high frequency, and because of the lack of reliable autopsy findings, all children who die suddenly of unexplained causes (whether or not they are infants) should be evaluated for possible metabolic defects, including disorders of β-oxidation. Postmortem examination should include analysis of blood, urine, or vitreous humor for organic acids and acylglycines and/or acylcarnitines. Tissues samples of liver, skeletal muscle, and heart should be rapidly frozen and stored at −70°C for future enzymatic analysis, and a skin fibroblast

TABLE 59.6. RELATIVE CONCENTRATION OF SPECIFIC METABOLITES IN PEROXISOMAL DISORDERS

ENZYME DEFECT	VLCFA	PHYTANIC ACID	PIPECOLIC ACID	PRISTANIC ACID	BILE ACID INTERMEDIATES	PLASMALOGENS
Peroxisomal biogenesis defects	High	High	High	High	High	Low
Rhizomelic chondrodysplasia punctata	Normal	Very high	Normal	Normal	Normal	Low
X-linked adrenoleukodystrophy	High	Normal	Normal	Normal	Normal	Normal
Straight-chain acyl-CoA oxidase deficiency	High	Normal	—	Normal	Normal	—
D-Bifunctional protein deficiency	High	—	—	High	High	—
2-Methylacyl-CoA racemase deficiency	Normal	Normal to mildly elevated	—	Very high	Very high	—

CoA, coenzyme A, VLCFA, very-long-chain fatty acids.

culture should be started when possible. Only with such an intense effort to determine a diagnosis in these cases can accurate counseling be presented to the family regarding recurrence risks and can asymptomatic siblings be identified. Investigators have suggested that newborn screening for MCAD deficiency could reduce the incidence of SIDS, but this remains to be substantiated (164, 250).

TREATMENT OF DEFECTS OF FATTY ACID METABOLISM

Mitochondria

Current clinical practice includes diverse approaches to the dietary treatment primarily focused on manipulation of dietary fat intake and frequency of food intake, and the effectiveness of therapies and techniques has largely been reported on a case-by-case basis. The avoidance of fasting by prescribing increased frequency of meals is a simple, preventive measure to ensure a constant supply of glucose. Minimizing the need to mobilize fatty acids for energy from adipose tissue may reduce the accumulation of toxic fatty acid metabolites, which when elevated can cause vomiting, lethargy, coma, and possibly death (258, 259). The optimal prescribed time limit between meals is not well established and may vary for infants, children, and adults with fatty acid oxidation disorders (260, 261). A regimen of restricted fat and high carbohydrate intake has generally been recommended in effort to reduce demands for lipolysis (262). Prescribed fat restrictions are variable, but typical calories from dietary fat are 30% or less (261). Increased caloric intake from carbohydrates may be necessary during intercurrent illness because of increased metabolic demands on the body. This need can be met via oral or nasogastric tube administration of an appropriate formula intravenous fluid if oral intake is inadequate. Intravenous infusion of glucose (8–10 mg/kg/minute) can be used when oral intake is interrupted or during acute episodes associated with infection (260, 261).

Supplementation of the diet with uncooked cornstarch can ameliorate the effects of fasting intolerance in affected persons. This provides a sustained release source of glucose, thereby preventing hypoglycemia and lipolysis (179, 263). Cornstarch is usually initiated at 8 months of age, when pancreatic enzymes are first able to function at full capacity for appropriate absorption (264). Dosing starts at 1.0 to 1.5 g/kg and can be gradually increased to 1.75 g/kg by 2 years of age (179).

Carnitine supplementation has long been used in the treatment of disorders of β-oxidation on the rationale that it allows repletion of the intramitochondrial carnitine pool and accelerates the removal of toxic fatty acid intermediates (262). Its use, however, remains controversial and of unproven value except in carnitine transporter deficiency (260, 265). Carnitine supplementation has been reported to normalize plasma carnitine levels and to increase urinary

excretion of acyl-carnitine esters; however, it does not always prevent the accumulation of toxic medium-chain free fatty acids in plasma, prevent spontaneous episodes of hypoglycemia, or reduce symptoms of lethargy, hypoglycemia, and vomiting (258, 259, 266). Conversely, short periods of carnitine supplementation have been suggested to increase ketogenesis and to reduce symptoms during periods of fasting hypoglycemia (267). Concern over the arrhythmogenic potential of long-chain acylcarnitine intermediates remains (268). Recommended doses range from 50 mg/kg/day in children to 150 mg/kg/day in adults (261).

Fat restriction along with supplementation of dietary fat with an alternate fat form is commonly used in patients with defects in β-oxidation, but there are limited published studies demonstrating the therapeutic benefit of this approach. Use of MCT oil as a lipid substrate emphasizes fatty acid oxidation pathways not affected by long-chain fat defects because it is composed of shorter-length fatty acids (C8:0 and C10:0 acids) that are not dependent on carnitine for entry into the mitochondria for subsequent oxidation (269, 270). Ingestion of 15 to 18% of total energy from MCT oils is commonly recommended (261). Augmentation of diet with essential fatty acids (at 1–2 % of total energy intake) is often used to reduce the risk for essential fatty acid deficiency (270, 271). Flaxseed, canola, walnut, or safflower oils are used for this purpose (261). Recent data from LCHAD- or TFP-deficient patients suggested the use of a diet providing age-appropriate protein, while limiting long-chain fatty acid intake to 10% of total calories. In addition, ingestion of 10 to 20% of calories as MCTs and a daily multivitamin and mineral supplement that includes all the fat-soluble vitamins were also recommended. The diet should be supplemented with vegetable oils as part of the 10% total long-chain fatty acid intake to provide essential fatty acids (272). On this diet, no correlation was found between plasma acylcarnitines and level of carnitine supplementation, and most patients were healthy, with no episodes of metabolic decompensation.

DHA deficiency may develop in patients with LCHAD deficiency, and it has been hypothesized as a cause for retinal degeneration in these patients (273). Use of the anaplerotic odd-chain triglyceride triheptanoic acid has recently been reported to be of value in the therapy of long-chain fat defects, and it appears to show promise (274). Riboflavin (200 mg/kg/day) may be useful in some patients with MADD and defects in riboflavin metabolism (200).

Commercially available medical foods provide formulations composed of modified fats, concentrated proteins, and multivitamins (275); however, no medical formulas have been designed specifically to meet the complete nutritional needs of patients with fatty acid oxidation disorders. Formulas that contain a high percentage of calories from MCT oil have been suggested for use to manage patients with long-chain fatty acid oxidation disorders.

When prescribed in conjunction with sufficient essential fatty acid supply, this approach can theoretically meet the essential nutrient needs of patients. Other strategies include a combination of available formulas to produce a diet high in complex carbohydrates, low in fat, and adequate in vitamin and mineral content (261). No clinical studies have been performed to assess the long-term efficacy of these formulas for the unique requirements of patients with fatty acid oxidation disorders.

Peroxisomes

Treatment of patients with defects in peroxisomal β-oxidation has been problematic. Therapy for X-ALD has received the most attention. Several inhibitors of very-long-chain fatty acid synthesis have been used in an attempt to control excess accumulation of very-long-chain fatty acids in patients. These include oleic acid, glycerol trioleate, and glycerol trierucate. The first extensive therapeutic trial to address the efficacy of "Lorenzo's oil" (primarily glycerol trierucate) employed a diet that provided 10% of calories as fat, with less than 10 to 15 mg of C26:0 fatty acid/day (276). In addition, 1.7 g/kg body weight/day of glycerol trioleate oil and 0.3 g/kg body weight/day of glycerol trierucate were also given, along with 10 to 15 mL of safflower oil and 2 g fish oil (to avoid a deficiency of essential fatty acids). Using this regimen, very-long-chain fatty acid levels were normalized in patients with either adrenoleukodystrophy or adrenomyeloneuropathy, but little or no clinical improvement could be documented (276). A more recent study showed similar results (277). This study, however, raised significant safety concerns about Lorenzo's oil and prompted a recommendation not to prescribe Lorenzo's oil routinely in patients with X-ALD who already have neurologic deficits (277). Results of concurrently conducted studies in Europe and the United States on the preventive effect of Lorenzo's oil in presymptomatic patients with X-ALD have recently been presented but are not yet published (H. Moser, personal communication). Prospective evaluation of boys with biochemically proven X-ALD, aged less than 6 years at enrollment and with normal neurologic examinations and magnetic resonance imaging (MRI) scans, was performed. Lorenzo's oil delayed the onset of neurologic and MRI abnormalities in the group of patients whose plasma C26:0 concentrations normalized on treatment. The protective effect was partial; 24% of patients in this group developed neurologic or MRI abnormalities. Twelve patients with X-ALD treated with lovastatin for 3 to 12 months had an initial decline in very-long-chain fatty acids that was variably sustained. No conclusion about clinical efficacy was possible from this small study (278).

Bone marrow transplantation has shown the most promise for boys with the childhood cerebral form. Short-term (279–281) and long-term (282) stabilization of clinical findings and MRI abnormalities have been demonstrated in patients when bone marrow transplantation is performed early in the course of the disease. In the most recent study, two patients received peripheral blood stem cell transplantation (281). There continues to be no effective treatment for boys with advanced disease. Therapy for the other single-enzyme defects of peroxisomal β-oxidation has not been reported.

Treatment of the disorders of peroxisomal biogenesis has been difficult because of the multisystemic involvement and the numerous metabolic pathways affected in these patients. In addition to reduction of very-long-chain fatty acid intake, patients may benefit from reduction of phytanic acid intake (<10 mg/day), as in adult Refsum disease (248). Dairy products, ruminant fats, and ruminant meats are the prime dietary sources of phytanic acid. Green vegetables, originally excluded from the diet, are no longer believed to contribute significantly to the physiologic phytanic acid load. Unfortunately, limited information is available on many food items. Because it is difficult to reduce dietary intake to less than 10 to 20 mg/day, it may be necessary to supplement with an artificial liquid formula. Benefits in uncontrolled studies have been reported for supplementation of patients with oral formulations of ether lipids, cholic (100 mg/day) and deoxycholic acids (100 mg/day), and docosahexenoic acid (250 mg/day) (283–285). Five patients with peroxisomal biogenesis disorders whose DHA levels were normalized with supplementation (200–600 mg/day) were found to have some clinical improvement in vision and muscle tone. Progression in myelination on MRI scans was noted during DHA supplementation (286).

The largest reported series to date describes 20 patients treated with DHA ethyl ester (100–500 mg/day) for 6 weeks to 9 years. All patients received an age-appropriate diet, limiting green leaves and white fat in meat, and supplemented with vitamins A, D, E, and K. Liver function studies improved in all patients, and very-long-chain fatty acid levels decreased in 18 of 20 patients. An improvement in vision was observed in 12 of 20 children. Muscle tone was believed to be subjectively ameliorated in 13 of 20. Progression in myelination on MRI scans was observed in nine of the 12 patients for whom data were available (287). The improvement in vision noted with normalization of blood DHA levels may be related to the role of DHA in the visual pathway. DHA-containing phospholipids bilayers within the retina optimize the kinetics of the metarhodopsin II–G-protein-coupled signaling pathway (288). Correction of DHA deficiency in patients with peroxisomal biogenesis defects should be initiated as early as possible. Detailed prospective studies to evaluate the effectiveness of treatment in these patients are needed.

REFERENCES

1. Lazarow PB, Moser HW. Disorders of peroxisome biogenesis. In: Scriver C, Beaudet AL, Sly W et al, eds. The Metabolic and Molecular Basis of Inherited Disease. 7th ed. New York: McGraw-Hill, 1995:2287–324.

2. Molzer B, Bernheimer H, Budka H et al. J Neurol Sci 1981;51: 301–10.

3. Purdue PE, Lazarow PB. J Biol Chem 1994;269:30065–8.

4. Subramani S. Annu Rev Cell Biol 1993;9:445–78.

5. Purdue PE, Lazarow PB. Annu Rev Cell Dev Biol 2001;17: 701–52.

6. Brosius U, Gartner J. Cell Mol Life Sci 2002;59:1058–69.

7. Wallace DC. Sci Am 1997;277:40–7.

8. Hartl F-U, Pfanner N, Nicholson DW et al. Biochim Biophys Acta 1989;988:1–45.

9. Glick B, Schatz G. Annu Rev Genet 1991;25:21–44.

10. Glick B. Methods Cell Biol 1991;34:389–99.

11. Glick B, Beasley E, Schatz G. Trends Biochem Sci 1992;17: 453–9.

12. Horwich AL, Kalousek F, Rosenberg LE. Proc Natl Acad Sci USA 1985;82:4920–33.

13. Horwich AL, Kalousek F, Mellman I et al. EMBO J 1985;4: 1129–35.

14. Horwich AL, Kalousek F, Fenton WA et al. Cell 1986;44:451–9.

15. Rosenberg LE, Fenton WA, Horwich AL et al. Ann NY Acad Sci 1987;488:99–108.

16. Koehler CM. FEBS Lett 2000;476:27–31.

17. Pfanner N, Meijer M. Curr Biol 1997;7:R100–3.

18. Lithgow T. FEBS Lett 2000;476:22–6.

19. Wanders RJA. Single peroxisomal enzyme deficiencies. In: Scriver C, Beaudet AL, Sly W et al, eds. The Metabolic and Molecular Basis of Inherited Disease. 8th ed. New York: McGraw-Hill, 2001:3219–56.

20. Roe CR, Ding J. Mitochondrial fatty acid oxidation disorders. In: Scriver C, Beaudet AL, Sly W et al, eds. The Metabolic and Molecular Basis of Inherited Disease. 8th ed. New York: McGraw-Hill, 2001:2297–326.

21. Vockley J, Whiteman DA. Neuromuscul Disord 2002;12: 235–46.

22. Saudubray JM, Martin D, de Lonlay P et al. J Inherit Metab Dis 1999;22:488–502.

23. Bennett M, Rinaldo P, Strauss A. Crit Rev Clin Lab Sci 2000; 37:1–44.

24. Engel AG, Angelini C. Science 1973;173:899–902.

25. DiMauro S, DiMauro PMM. Science 1973;182:929–31.

26. Hashimoto T. Ann NY Acad Sci 1982;386:5–12.

27. Moser HW, Smith KD, Moser AB. X-linked Adrenoleukodystrophy. In: Scriver C, Beaudet AL, Sly W et al, eds. The Metabolic and Molecular Basis of Inherited Disease. 7th ed. New York: McGraw-Hill, 1995:2325–49.

28. Krisans SK, Mortensen RM, Lazarow PB. J Biol Chem 1980; 255:9599–607.

29. McGarry JD, Foster DW. Annu Rev Biochem 1980;49: 395–420.

30. Stremmel W, Strohmeyer G, Borchard F et al. Proc Natl Acad Sci USA 1985;82:4–8.

31. Stremmel W, Strohmeyer G, Berk PD. Proc Natl Acad Sci USA 1986;83:3584–8.

32. Abe T, Fujino T, Fukuyama R et al. J Biochem 1992;111:123–8.

33. Bremer J. Physiol Rev 1983;63:1420–80.

34. Martinuzzi A, Vergani L, Rosa M et al. Biochim Biophys Acta 1991;1095:217–22.

35. Treem WR, Stanley CA, Finegold DN et al. N Engl J Med 1988;319:1331–6.

36. Murthy MSR, Pande SV. Proc Natl Acad Sci USA 1987;84: 378–82.

37. Pande SV. Proc Natl Acad Sci USA 1975;72:883–7.

38. Iafolla AK, Thompson RJ, Roe CR. J Pediatr 1994;124:409–15.

39. Ikeda Y, Dabrowski C, Tanaka K. J Biol Chem 1983;258: 1066–76.

40. Ikeda Y, Tanaka K. J Biol Chem 1983;258:1077–85.

41. Matsubara Y, Indo Y, Naito E et al. J Biol Chem 1989;264: 16321–31.

42. Kurtz DM, Rinaldo P, Rhead WJ et al. Proc Natl Acad Sci USA 1998;95:15592–7.

43. Battaile KP, McBurney M, VanVeldhoven PP et al. Biochim Biophys Acta 1998;1390:333–8.

44. Mathur A, Sims HF, Gopalakrishnan D et al. Circulation 1999; 99:1337–43.

45. Lea WP, Abbas AS, Sprecher H et al. Biochim Biophys Acta 2000;1485:121–8.

46. Zhang J, Zhang W, Zou D et al. Biochem Biophys Res Commun 2002;297:1033–42.

47. Beckmann JD, Frerman FE. Biochemistry 1985;24:3922–5.

48. Frerman FE. Biochem Soc Trans 1988;16:416–8.

49. Frerman F. Prog Clin Biol Res 1990;321:69–77.

50. Ikeda Y, Keese S, Fenton WA et al. Arch Biochem Biophys 1987;252:662–74.

51. Matsubara Y, Ito M, Glassberg R et al. J Clin Invest 1990;85: 1058–64.

52. Kelly D, Kim J, Billadello J et al. Proc Natl Acad Sci USA 1988;85:4068–72.

53. Aoyama T, Souri M, Ueno I et al. Am J Hum Genet 1995;57: 273–83.

54. Vockley J, Parimoo B, Tanaka K. Am J Hum Genet 1991;40: 147–57.

55. Rozen R, Vockley J, Zhou L et al. Genomics 1994;24:280–7.

56. Willard J, Vicanek C, Battaile KP et al. Arch Biochem Biophys 1996;331:127–33.

57. Gibson KM, Burlingame TG, Hogema B et al. Pediatr Res 2000;47:830–3.

58. Uchida Y, Izai K, Orii T et al. J Biol Chem 1992;267:1034–41.

59. Carpenter K, Pollitt RJ, Middleton B et al. Biochim Biophys Res Commun 1992;183:443–8.

60. Kamijo T, Aoyama T, Miyazaki J et al. J Biol Chem 1993;268: 26452–60.

61. Kamijo T, Aoyama T, Komiyama A et al. Biochem Biophys Res Commun 1994;199:818–25.

62. Yao KW, Schulz H. J Biol Chem 1996;271:17816–20.

63. Parker A, Engel P. Biochem J 2000;345:429–35.

64. Barycki JJ, O'Brien LK, Bratt JM et al. Biochemistry 1999;38: 5786–98.

65. Barycki JJ, O'Brien LK, Birktoft JJ et al. Protein Sci 1999;8: 2010–8.

66. Vredendaal P, Vandenberg IET, Malingre HEM et al. Biochem Biophys Res Commun 1996;223:718–23.

67. Kamijo T, Indo Y, Souri M et al. Pediatr Res 1997;42:569–76.

68. Abe H, Ohtake A, Yamamoto S et al. Biochim Biophys Acta 1993;1216:304–6.

69. Bennett MJ, Sherwood WG. Clin Chem 1993;39:897–901.

70. Bennett MJ, Weinberger MJ, Kobori JA et al. Pediatr Res 1996;39:185–8.

71. He XY, Merz G, Yang YZ et al. Biochim Biophys Acta 2000; 1484:267–77.

72. He XY, Merz G, Mehta P et al. J Biol Chem 1999;274: 15014–9.

73. He XY, Schulz H, Yang SY. J Biol Chem 1998;273:10741–6.

74. Jackson S, Kler RS, Bartlett K et al. J Clin Invest 1992;90: 1219–25.

75. Hiltunen JK, Qin Y. Biochim Biophys Acta 2000;1484:117–28.

76. Helander HM, Koivuranta KT, Horellikuitunen N et al. Genomics 1997;46:112–9.

77. Fukao T, Song XQ, Mitchell GA et al. Pediatr Res 1997;42: 498–502.

78. Thompson GN, Hsu BYL, Pitt JJ et al. N Engl J Med 1997;337:1203–7.

79. Mitchell GA, Robert MF, Hruz PW et al. J Biol Chem 1993;268:4376–81.

80. Mitchell GA, Fukao T. Inborn errors of ketone body metabolism. In: Scriver C, Beaudet AL, Sly W et al, eds. The Metabolic and Molecular Basis of Inherited Disease. 8th ed. New York: McGraw-Hill, 2001:2327–56.

81. Kassovskabratinova S, Fukao T, Song XQ et al. Am J Hum Genet 1996;59:519–28.

82. Song XQ, Fukao T, Mitchell GA et al. Biochim Biophys Acta 1997;1360:151–6.

83. Vandenbosch H, Schutgens RBH, Wanders RJA et al. Annu Rev Biochem 1992;61:157–97.

84. Wanders RJ, Vreken P, Ferdinandusse S et al. Biochem Soc Trans 2001;29:250–67.

85. Ramsay RR. Am J Med Sci 1999;318:28–35.

86. Van Veldhoven PP, Vanhove G, Assselberghs S et al. J Biol Chem 1992;267:20065–74.

87. Schmitz W, Albers C, Fingerhut R et al. Eur J Biochem 1995;231:815–22.

88. Van Veldhoven PP, Croes K, Asselbergh S et al. FEBS Lett 1996;388:80–4.

89. Van Veldhoven PP, Croes K, Asselbergh S et al. Biochim Biophys Acta 1997;1347:62–8.

90. Schmitz W, Conzelmann E. Eur J Biochem 1997;244:434–40.

91. Palosaari PM, Vihinen M, Mantsala PI et al. J Biol Chem 1991;266:10750–3.

92. Palosaari PM, Hiltunen JK. J Biol Chem 1990;265:2446–9.

93. Hijikata M, Wen JK, Osumi T et al. J Biol Chem 1990;265:4600–6.

94. Al Odaib A, Shneider BL, Bennett MJ et al. N Engl J Med 1998;339:1752–7.

95. Steenhout P, Elmer C, Clercx A et al. J Inherit Metab Dis 1990;13:69–75.

96. Bennett MJ, Hale DE, Pollitt RJ et al. Clin Cardiol 1996;19:243–6.

97. Tein I, Bukovac SW, Xie ZW. Arch Biochem Biophys 1996;329:145–55.

98. Tein I, Xie ZW. Clin Chim Acta 1996;252:201–4.

99. Pons R, Carrozzo R, Tein I et al. Pediatr Res 1997;42:583–7.

100. Lamhonwah AM, Tein I. Biochem Biophys Res Commun 1998;252:396–401.

101. Nezu JI, Tamai I, Oku A et al. Nat Genet 1999;21:91–4.

102. Lamhonwah AM, Tein I. Biochem Biophys Res Commun 1999;264:909–14.

103. Shapira Y, Glick B, Harel S et al. Pediatr Neurol 1993;9:35–8.

104. Lamhonwah AM, Olpin SE, Pollitt RJ et al. Am J Med Genet 2002;111:271–84.

105. Demaugre F, Bonnefont J-P, Mitchell G et al. Pediatr Res 1988;24:308–11.

106. Demaugre G, Bonnefont J-P, Cepanec C et al. Pediatr Res 1990;27:497–500.

107. Hug G, Bove KE, Soukup S. N Engl J Med 1991;325:1862–4.

108. Stanley CA, Sunaryo F, Hale DE et al. J Inherit Metab Dis 1992;15:785–9.

109. Vianey-Saban C, Mousson B, Bertrand C et al. Eur J Pediatr 1993;152:334–8.

110. Britton CH, Schultz RA, Zhang B et al. Proc Natl Acad Sci USA 1995;92:1984–8.

111. Ijlst L, Mandel H, Oostheim W et al. J Clin Invest 1998;102:527–31.

112. Gobin S, Bonnefont JP, Prip-Buus C et al. Hum Genet 2002;111:179–89.

113. Prasad C, Johnson JP, Bonnefont JP et al. Mol Genet Metab 2001;73:55–63.

114. Pande SV, Brivet M, Slama A et al. J Clin Invest 1993;91:1247–52.

115. Pande SV, Murthy M. Biochimi Biophys Acta 1994;1226:269–76.

116. Roschinger W, Muntau A, Duran M et al. Clin Chim Acta 2000;298:55–68.

117. Stanley CA, Hale DE, Berry GT et al. N Engl J Med 1992;327:19–23.

118. Angelini C, Trevisan C, Isaya G et al. Clin Biochem 1987;20:1–27.

119. Taroni F, Verderio E, Fiorucci S et al. Proc Natl Acad Sci USA 1992;89:8429–33.

120. Taroni F, Verderio E, Dworzak F et al. Nat Genet 1993;4:314–20.

121. Bonnefont JP, Taroni F, Cavadini P et al. Am J Hum Genet 1996;58:971–8.

122. Elpeleg ON, Joseph A, Gutman A. J Pediatr 1994;124:160–1.

123. Vladutiu GD, Bennett MJ, Fisher NM et al. Muscle Nerve 2002;26:492–8.

124. Taggart RT, Smail D, Apolito C et al. Hum Mutat 1999;13:210–20.

125. Vladutiu GD, Bennett MJ, Smail D et al. Mol Genet Metab 2000;70:134–41.

126. Vockley J, Rinaldo P, Bennett MJ et al. Mol Genet Metabol 2000;71:10–8.

127. Bertrand C, Largilliere C, Zabot MT et al. Biochim Biophys Acta 1993;1180:327–9.

128. Aoyama T, Souri M, Ushikubo S et al. J Clin Invest 1995;95:2465–73.

129. Ogilvie I, Pourfarzam M, Jackson S et al. Neurology 1994;44:467–73.

130. Aoyama T, Uchida Y, Kelley RI et al. Biochem Biophys Res Commun 1993;191:1369–72.

131. Orii KO, Aoyama T, Souri M et al. Biochem Biophys ResCommun 1995;217:987–92.

132. Andresen BS, Bross P, Vianeysaban C et al. Hum Mol Genet 1996;5:461–72.

133. Strauss AW, Powell CK, Hale DE et al. Proc Natl Acad Sci USA 1995;92:10496–500.

134. Andresen BS, Vianeysaban C, Bross P et al. J Inherit Metab Dis 1996;19:169–72.

135. Andresen BS, Olpin S, Poorthuis B et al. Am J Hum Genet 1999;64:479–94.

136. Straussberg R, Strauss AW. Pediatr Neurol 2002;27:136–7.

137. Takusa Y, Fukao T, Kimura M et al. Mol Genet Metabol 2002;75:227–34.

138. Wood JC, Magera MJ, Rinaldo P et al. Pediatrics 2001;108:110–2.

139. Hale DE, Batshaw ML, Coates PM et al. Pediatr Res 1985;19:666–71.

140. Tream WR, Stanley CA, Hale DE et al. Pediatrics 1991;87:328–33.

141. Yamaguchi S, Indo Y, Coates PM et al. Pediatr Res 1993;34:111–3.

142. Amendt B, Green C, Sweetman L et al. J Clin Invest 1987;79:1303–9.

143. Coates PM, Hale DE, Finocchiaro G et al. J Clin Invest 1988;81:171–5.

144. Bhala A, Willi SM, Rinaldo P et al. J Pediatr 1995;126:910–5.

145. Sewell AC, Herwig J, Bohles H et al. Eur J Pediatr 1993;152:922–4.

146. Turnbull DM, Bartlett K, Stevens DL et al. N Engl J Med 1984;311:1232–6.

147. Gregersen N, Winter VS, Corydon MJ et al. Hum Mol Genet 1998;7:619–27.

148. Tein I, Haslam RHA, Rhead WJ et al. Neurology 1999;52: 366–72.

149. Corydon M, Vockley J, Rinaldo R et al. Pediatr Res 2001; 49:18–23.

150. Kristensen MJ, Kmoch S, Bross P et al. Hum Mol Genet 1994;3:1711.

151. Corydon MJ, Gregersen N, Lehnert W et al. Pediatr Res 1996; 39:1059–66.

152. Nguyen T, Riggs C, Babovic-Vuksanovic D et al. Biochemistry 2002;41:11126–33.

153. Nagan N, Kruckeberg KE, Tauscher AL et al. Mol Genet Metabol 2003;78:239–46.

154. Tafti M, Petit B, Chollet D et al. Nat Genet 2003;34:320–5.

155. Rinaldo P, Raymond K, Al-Odaib A et al. Curr Opin Pediatr 1998;10:615–21.

156. Vockley J. Mayo Clin Proc 1994;69:249–57.

157. Rinaldo P, O'Shea JJ, Coates PM et al. N Engl J Med 1988;319: 1308–13.

158. Millington DS, Tereca N, Chace DH et al. The role of tandem mass spectrometry in the diagnosis of fatty acid oxidation disorders. In: Coates PM, Tanaka K, eds. Progress in Clinical and Biological Research: New Developments in Fatty Acid Oxidation. New York: Wiley-Liss, 1992:339–54.

159. Chace DH, Hillman SL, Vanhove JLK et al. Clin Chem 1997; 43:2106–13.

160. Matsubara Y, Narisawa K, Shigeaki M et al. Biochem Biophys Res Comm 1990;171:498–505.

161. Andresen BS, Bross P, Udvari S et al. Hum Mol Genet 1997;6: 695–707.

162. Yokota I, Saijo T, Vockley J et al. J Biol Chem 1992;267: 26004–10.

163. Matsubara Y, Narisawa K, Tada K et al. Lancet 1991;338:552–3.

164. Ziadeh R, Hoffman EP, Finegold DN et al. Pediatr Res 1995;37:675–8.

165. Carpenter KH, Wilcken B. J Inherit Metab Dis 1999;22:840–1.

166. Wilson CJ, Champion MP, Collins JE et al. Arch Dis Child 1999;80:459–62.

167. Chace DH, Adam BW, Smith SJ et al. Clin Chem 1999;45: 1269–77.

168. Green A, Pollitt RJ. J Inherit Metab Dis 1999;22:572–9.

169. Ciske JB, Hoffman G, Hanson K et al. WMJ 2000;99:38–42.

170. Wiley V, Carpenter K, Wilcken B. Acta Paediatr Suppl 1999; 88:48–51.

171. Chace DH, DiPerna JC, Naylor EW. Acta Paediatr Suppl 1999; 88:45–7.

172. Hale DE, Thorpe C, Braat K et al. The L-3-hydroxyacyl-CoA dehdrogenase deficiency. In: Tanaka K, Coates PM, eds. Progress in Clinical and Biological Research: Fatty Acid Oxidation: Clinical, Biochemical and Molecular Aspects. New York: Alan R. Liss, 1990:503–10.

173. Pollitt RJ. Clinical and biochemical presentations in 20 cases of hydroxydicarbocylic aciduria. In: Tanaka K, Coates PM, eds. Progress in Clinical and Biological Research: Fatty Acid Oxidation: Clinical, Biochemical and Molecular Aspects. New York: Alan R. Liss, 1990:495–502.

174. Hagenfeldt L, van Dobein U, Holme E et al. Pediatrics 1990;116:387–92.

175. Wanders RJA, Ijlst L, van Gennip AH et al. J Inherit Metab Dis 1990;13:311–4.

176. Rocchiccioli F, Wanders RJA, Aybourg P et al. Pediatr Res 1990;28:657–62.

177. Wanders RJA, Ijlst L, Duran M et al. J Inherit Metab Dis 1991;14:325–8.

178. den Boer MEJ, Dionisi-Vici C, Chakrapani A et al. J Pediatr 2003;142:684–9.

179. Vici CD, Burlina AB, Bertini E et al. J Pediatr 1991;118:744–6.

180. Bertini E, Dionisivici C, Garavaglia B et al. Eur J Pediatr 1992;151:121–6.

181. Ibdah JA, Tein I, Dionisivici C et al. J Clin Invest 1998;102: 1193–9.

182. Odievre MH, Sevin C, Laurent J et al. Acta Paediatr 2002;91: 719–22.

183. Pons R, Roig M, Riudor E et al. Pediatr Neurol 1996;14: 236–43.

184. Miyajima H, Orii KE, Shindo Y et al. Neurology 1997;49: 833–7.

185. den Boer ME, Wanders RJ, Morris AA et al. Pediatrics 2002; 109:99–104.

186. Brackett JC, Sims HF, Rinaldo P et al. J Clin Invest 1995;95:2076–82.

187. Ijlst L, Wanders RJ, Ushikubo S et al. Biochim Biophys Acta 1994;1215:347–50.

188. Ushikubo S, Aoyama T, Kamijo T et al. Am J Hum Genet 1996;58:979–88.

189. Ijlst L, Uskikubo S, Kamijo T et al. J Inherit Metab Dis 1995; 18:241–4.

190. Tein I, Devivo DC, Hale DE et al. Ann Neurol 1991;30:415–9.

191. Yamaguchi S, Sakai A, Fukao T et al. Pediatr Res 1993;33: 429–32.

192. Wakazono A, Fukao T, Yamaguchi S et al. Hum Mutat 1995; 5:34–42.

193. Fukao T, Yamaguchi S, Orii T et al. J Clin Invest 1992;89:474–9.

194. Fukao T, Yamaguchi S, Orii T et al. Hum Mutat 1995;5:113–20.

195. Fukao T, Song XQ, Yamaguchi S et al. Hum Mutat 1997;9: 277–9.

196. Roe CR, Millington DS, Kodo NN et al. J Clin Invest 1990;85: 1703–7.

197. Frerman FE, Goodman SI. Proc Natl Acad Sci USA 1985;82: 4517–20.

198. Colombo I, Finocchiaro G, Garavaglia B et al. Hum Mol Genet 1994;3:429–35.

199. Freneaux E, Sheffield VC, Molin L et al. J Clin Invest 1992;90:1679–86.

200. Frerman F, Goodman S. Defects of electron transfer flovoprotein and electron transfer flavoprotein-ubiquinone oxidoreductase: glutaric acidemia type II. In: Scriver C, Beaudet AL, Sly W et al, eds. The Metabolic and Molecular Basis of Inherited Disease. 8th ed. New York: McGraw-Hill, 2001:2357–65.

201. Takanashi J, Fujii K, Sugita K et al. Pediatr Neurol 1999;20: 142–5.

202. Stockler S, Radner H, Karpf EF et al. J Pediatr 1994;124: 601–4.

203. Mongini T, Doriguzzi C, Palmucci L et al. Eur Neurol 1992; 32:170–6.

204. Gregersen M, Rhead W, Christensen E. Riboflavin responsive glutaric aciduria type II. In: Tanaka K, Coates PM, eds. Progress in Clinical and Biological Research: Fatty Acid Oxidation: Clinical, Biochemical, and Molecular Aspects. New York: Alan R. Liss, 1990:477–94.

205. Wilson GN, de Chadarevian JP, Kaplan P et al. Am J Med Genet 1989;32:395–401.

206. de Visser M, Scholte HR, Schutgens RB et al. Neurology 1986;36:367–72.

207. Curcoy A, Olsen RKJ, Ribes A et al. Mol Genet Metab 2003;78: 247–9.

208. Rhead W, Roettger V, Marshall T et al. Pediatr Res 1993;33: 129–35.

209. Uziel G, Garavaglia B, Ciceri E et al. Pediatr Neurol 1995;13: 333–5.

210. Loehr JP, Goodman SI, Frurman FE. Pediatr Res 1990;27: 311–5.

211. Colombo I, DiDonato S, Volta M et al. Prog Clin Biol Res 1992; 375:561–6.

212. Pretorius CJ, Son GGL, Bonnici F et al. J Inherit Metab Dis 1996;19:296–300.

213. Vladutiu G. Muscle Nerve 2000;23:1157–9.

214. Treem WR, Rinaldo P, Hale DE et al. Hepatology 1994;19: 339–45.

215. Isaacs JD, Sims HF, Powell CK et al. Pediatr Res 1996;40: 393–8.

216. Treem WR, Shoup ME, Hale DE et al. Am J Gastroenterol 1996;91:2293–300.

217. Tyni T, Ekholm E, Pihko H. Am J Obstet Gynecol 1998;178: 603–8.

218. Ibdah JA, Bennett MJ, Rinaldo P et al. N Engl J Med 1999; 340:1723–31.

219. Ibdah JA, Dasouki MJ, Strauss AW. J Inherit Metab Dis 1999; 22:811–4.

220. Chalmers RA, Stanley CA, English N et al. J Pediatr 1997;131: 220–5.

221. Bonnefont JP, Haas R, Wolff J et al. J Child Neurol 1989;4: 198–203.

222. Innes AM, Seargeant LE, Balachandra K et al. Pediatr Res 2000;47:43–5.

223. Nelson J, Lewis B, Walters B. J Inherit Metab Dis 2000;23:18–9.

224. Walter JH. J Inherit Metab Dis 2000;23:229–36.

225. Matern D, Hart P, Murtha A et al. J Pediatr 2001;138:585–8.

226. Wanders RJA, Schutgens RBH, Barth PG. J Neuropathol Exp Neurol 1995;54:726–39.

227. Zellweger H. Dev Med Child Neurol 1987;29:821–9.

228. Thomas GH, Haslam RH, Batshaw ML et al. Clin Genet 1975;8:376–82.

229. Gatfield PD, Taller E, Hinton GG et al. Can Med Assoc J 1968;99:1215–33.

230. Al-Essa MA, Chaves-Carballo E, Ozand PT. Pediatr Neurol 1999;21:826–9.

231. Moser AB, Rasmussen M, Naidu S et al. J Pediatr 1995;127: 13–22.

232. Moser HW. Mol Genet Metab 1999;68:316–27.

233. Suzuki Y, Shimozawa N, Imamura A et al. J Inherit Metab Dis 2001;24:151–65.

234. Moser AB, Kreiter N, Bezman L et al. Ann Neurol 1999;45: 100–10.

235. Mosser J, Lutz Y, Stoeckel ME et al. Hum Mol Genet 1994;3: 265–71.

236. Scotto JM, Hadchouel M, Odievre M et al. J Inherit Metab Dis 1982;5:83–90.

237. Ulrich J, Herschkowitz N, Heitz P et al. Acta Neuropathol 1978;43:77–83.

238. Schaumburg HH, Powers JM, Raine CS et al. Neurology 1977;27:1114–9.

239. Griffin JW, Goren E, Schaumburg H et al. Neurology 1977;27: 1107–13.

240. Budka H, Sluga E, Heiss WD. J Neurol 1976;213:237–50.

241. Poll-The BT, Roels F, Ogier H et al. Am J Hum Genet 1988;42: 422–34.

242. Clayton PT. Biochem Soc Trans 2001;29:298–305.

243. Wanders RJ, van Roermund CW, Schelen A et al. J Inherit Metab Dis 1990;13:375–9.

244. Clayton PT, Lake BD, Hjelm M et al. J Inherit Metab Dis 1988;11[Suppl 2]:165–8.

245. Watkins PA, Chen WW, Harris CJ et al. J Clin Invest 1989; 83:771–7.

246. Wanders RJ, van Roermund CW, Brul S et al. J Inherit Metab Dis 1992;15:385–8.

247. Moller G, van Grunsven EG, Wanders RJ et al. Mol Cell Endocrinol 2001;171:61–70.

248. Steinberg D. Refsum Disease. In: Scriver C, Beaudet AL, Sly W et al, eds. The Metabolic and Molecular Basis of Inherited Disease. 7th ed. New York: McGraw-Hill, 1995:2351–69.

249. Vockley J, Singh RH, Whiteman DA. Curr Opin Clin Nutr Metab Care 2002;5:601–9.

250. Lemieux B, Giguere R, Cyr D et al. Pediatrics 1993;91: 986–8.

251. Koeberl DD, Young SP, Gregersen N et al. Pediatr Res 2003; 54:219–23.

252. Matern D, He M, Berry SA et al. Pediatrics 2003;112:74–8.

253. Schulze A, Lindner M, Kohlmuller D et al. Pediatrics 2003;111: 1399–406.

254. Wilcken B, Wiley V, Hammond J et al. N Engl J Med 2003;348: 2304–12.

255. Pollitt RJ. J Inherit Metab Dis 1989;12[Suppl 1]:215–30.

256. Harpey J-P, Charpentier C, Paturneau-Jouas M. Biol Neonate 1990;58[Suppl 1]:70–80.

257. Bennett MJ, Ragni MC, Hood I et al. Ann Clin Biochem 1992; 29:541–5.

258. Schmidt-Sommerfeld E, Penn D, Kerner J et al. J Pediatr 1989; 115:577–82.

259. Tream WR, Stanley CA, Goodman SI. J Inherit Metab Dis 1989;12:112–9.

260. Catzeflis C, Bachmann C, Hale DE et al. Eur J Pediatr 1990; 149:577–81.

261. Solis J, Singh R. J Am Diet Assoc 2002;102:1800–3.

262. Kerner J, Hoppel C. Annu Rev Nutr 1998;18:179–206.

263. Fernandes J, Smit G. The glycogen storage diseases. In: Fernandes J, Saudubray J, Van den Berghe C, eds. Inborn Error of Metabolic Diseases: Diagnosis and Treatment. 3rd ed. New York: Springer-Verlag, 2001:88–101.

264. Hayde M, Widhalm K. Eur J Pediatr 1990;149:630–3.

265. Howat AJ, Bennett MJ, Variend S et al BMJ 1985;290:1771–3.

266. Rinaldo P, Schmidtsommerfeld E, Posca AP et al. J Pediatr 1993;122:580–4.

267. Nyhan W, Ozand P. Disorders of fatty acid oxidation. In: Atlas of Metabolic Diseases. London: Chapman and Hall Medical, 1998:223–30.

268. Bonnet D, Martin D, de Lonlay P et al. Circulation 1999;100: 2248–53.

269. Pollitt RJ. J Inherit Metab Dis 1995;18:473–90.

270. Gillingham M, Van Calcar S, Ney D et al. J Inherit Metab Dis 1999;22:123–31.

271. Uauy R, Treen M, Hoffman DR. Semin Perinatol 1989;13: 118–30.

272. Gillingham MB, Connor WE, Matern D et al. Mol Genet Metabol 2003;79:114–23.

273. Harding CO, Gillingham MB, van Calcar SC et al. J Inherit Metab Dis 1999;22:276–80.

274. Roe CR, Sweetman L, Roe DS et al. J Clin Invest 2002;110: 259–69.

275. Acosta P, Yannicelli S. The Ross Metabolic Formula System Nutrition Support Protocols. Columbus, OH: Ross Products Divisions, 2001.

276. Aubourg P, Adamsbaum C, Lavallardrousseau MC et al. N Engl J Med 1993;329:745–52.

277. van Geel BM, Assies J, Haverkort EB et al. J Neurol Neurosurg Psychiatry 1999;67:290–9.

278. Pai GS, Khan M, Barbosa E et al. Mol Genet Metab 2000;69: 312–22.

279. Loes DJ, Stillman AE, Hite S et al. AJNR Am J Neuroradiol 1994;15:1767–71.

280. Suzuki Y, Isogai K, Teramoto T et al. J Inherit Metab Dis 2000;23:453–8.

281. Baumann M, Korenke GC, Weddige–Diedrichs A et al. Eur J Pediatr 2003;162:6–14.

282. Shapiro E, Krivit W, Lockman L et al. Lancet 2000;356:713–8.

283. Setchell KD, Bragetti P, Zimmer–Nechemias L et al. Hepatology 1992;15:198–207.

284. Martinez M. Prog Clin Biol Res 1992;375:389–97.

285. Martinez M, Pineda M, Vidal R et al. Neurology 1993;43: 1389–97.

286. Martinez M, Vazquez E. Neurology 1998;51:26–32.

287. Martinez M. J Mol Neurosci 2001;16:309–16, discussion 17–21.

288. Litman BJ, Niu SL, Polozova A et al. J Mol Neurosci 2001;16: 237–42, discussion 79–84.

60 CHILDHOOD OBESITY[1]

WILLIAM H. DIETZ

DEFINITION 979
    Use of the Body Mass Index 979
    Changes in Body Fat and Fat Distribution
       with Age 979
EPIDEMIOLOGY 980
    Prevalence 980
    Critical Periods for the Onset of Childhood
       Overweight 981
    Role of the Physical Environment 981
    Role of the Behavioral Environment 982
CLINICAL EFFECTS 983
    Syndromes Associated with Childhood
       Overweight 983
    Consequences of Overweight in Childhood 983
    Clinical Assessment 984
TREATMENT 985
    Education 985
    Dietary Modification 985
    Alterations in Activity .986
    Behavior Modification .987
    Alternative Therapies .987
    Outcome 988
PREVENTION 988

DEFINITION

Use of the Body Mass Index

Because weight and height change throughout childhood, the cutoff points of any measure used to define obesity must be age and gender dependent. The ideal anthropometric measure of fatness is one that correlates reasonably well with fat as a percentage of body weight. Among children and adolescents, weight for height, body mass index (BMI; weight in kilograms/height[2] in meters), and triceps skinfold demonstrate comparable correlation coefficients with fat as a percentage of body weight, measured by underwater weighing (1). Despite similar correlation coefficients, variants of weight for height and triceps skinfold

thickness probably capture different aspects of body fat. Although triceps skinfold thickness measures fat directly, it only does so at one location in the body. Furthermore, because body fat redistributes centrally during adolescence, the triceps skinfold thickness decreases even as body fat increases. Weight and height measures do not determine fatness directly, but use of an index such as BMI removes most of the weight and height covariance and thereby more directly measures the effect of increased fat on weight.

Convenient algorithms (2, 3) exist to screen children and adolescent patients for overweight (Fig. 60.1). One algorithm begins with a BMI greater than or equal to the ninety-fifth percentile for age and gender, using tables derived from representative surveys of the US population (4), or a BMI greater than or equal to 30.0. An international growth chart has also been proposed to compare populations around the world (5). If the BMI exceeds the ninety-fifth percentile for age or gender, or if it is greater than or equal to 30, an in-depth medical assessment is warranted. Although a BMI greater than or equal to 30 in a young adult is the criterion used to identify obesity, and a BMI greater than or equal to the ninety-fifth percentile is roughly equivalent to a BMI of 30 in a young adult, we use overweight rather than obesity in this chapter to refer to children and adolescents whose BMI is greater than or equal to the ninety-fifth percentile for age and gender. The meaning of the terms obesity or overweight to patients and their families has not been carefully tested. However, our clinical experience suggests that the term overweight is more acceptable.

In children and adolescents, selection of the BMI greater than or equal to the ninety-fifth percentile as a screening tool reduces the measure's sensitivity, but increases its specificity (6, 7). Use of the BMI greater than or equal to the ninety-fifth percentile for children or adolescents of the same age and gender therefore minimizes the likelihood that overweight will be overdiagnosed and thereby lead to excessive concern about weight when a significant problem does not exist.

Changes in Body Fat and Fat Distribution with Age

The BMI and triceps skinfold do not change synchronously with age. In girls after the first year of life, the

---

[1] **Abbreviations: ACT,** energy spent on activity; **BMI,** body mass index; **NHANES,** National Health and Nutrition Examination Survey; **RMR,** resting metabolic rate; **TEE,** total energy expenditure; **TEF,** thermic effects of food.

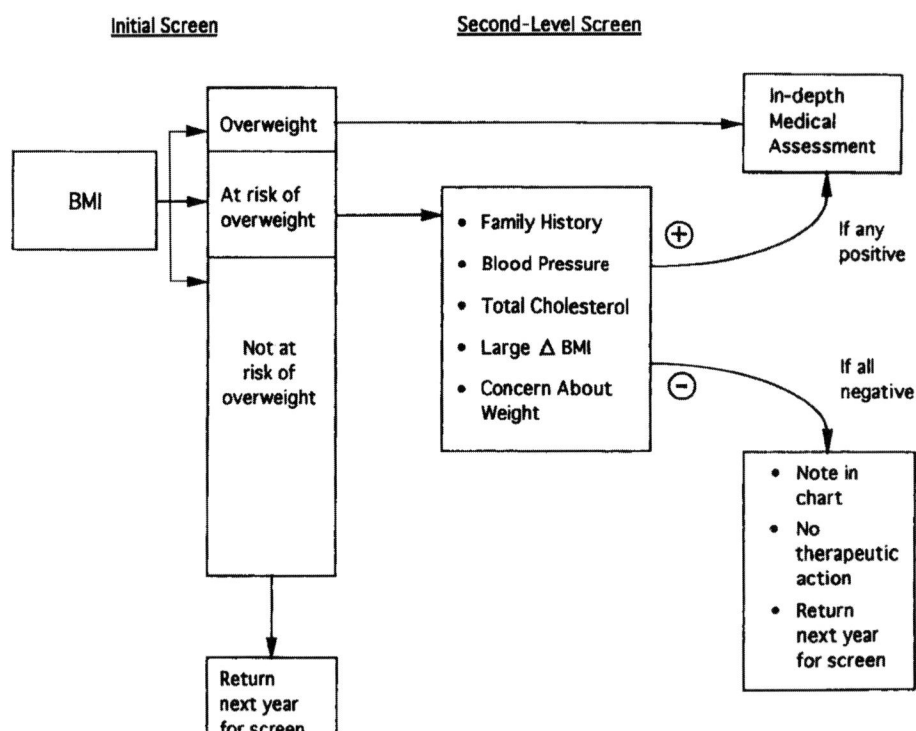

Figure 60.1. A convenient algorithm (2) exists to screen patients for obesity. The algorithm begins with a body mass index (BMI) greater than or equal to the ninety–fifth percentile for age and gender, using tables derived from representative surveys of the US population (4) or a BMI greater than or equal to 30. If the BMI exceeds the ninety–fifth percentile for age and gender or if it is greater then 30 BMI units, an in-depth medical assessment is warranted.

triceps skinfold thickness remains stable, and it begins to increase in early adolescence (8). Female adolescence is characterized by a body fat increase from a mean of 17% to 25% of body weight. In boys, changes in fatness are more complex. The triceps skinfold decreases at approximately 4 years of age, increases immediately before puberty, and then decreases during the adolescent growth spurt. Male adolescence is characterized by a decline in body fat from a mean of 18% to 11% of body weight.

Changes in BMI with age are similar for both genders. BMI rises between birth and 9 months of age, declines to a nadir at 4 to 5 years of age (9), and then rises through adolescence. The period at which BMI begins to increase after the nadir has been called adiposity rebound, but it is more appropriately described as the period of BMI rebound.

The pattern of fat distribution also changes with age and differs for boys and girls. In both genders during adolescence, body fat redistributes from peripheral to central sites (10, 11). In girls, more fat is deposited in gluteal than abdominal regions. In boys, fat tends to be deposited more centrally.

Changes in adipocyte numbers tend to parallel changes in body fatness that occur from early childhood. Adipocyte replication occurs as body fat increases, regardless of whether the increase in body fat is normal or excessive (12, 13). Adipocyte size increases in early infancy and remains relatively constant until puberty, when another small increase occurs. Factors that control the regionalization of body fat and adipocyte replication throughout childhood remain unclear.

EPIDEMIOLOGY

Prevalence

Repeated measures in representative surveys of the US population indicate that the prevalence of overweight among children and adolescents in the United States has increased rapidly since the 1980s. Between 1984 and 2000, when the National Health and Nutrition Examination Survey II (NHANES II) and current continuous NHANES examinations were completed, and based on age- and gender-specific BMIs greater than or equal to the ninety-fifth percentiles of the Centers for Disease Control and Prevention growth charts, the prevalence of overweight doubled in children aged 6 to11 years and increased threefold in adolescents aged 12 to 19 years (14). Approximately 15% of children and adolescents in the United States are now overweight. The prevalence of overweight among boys and girls is comparable, but it is greater among 6- to 11-year-old and 12- to 19-year-old African-American and Mexican-American than among white boys and girls (14).

The factors that account for the rapid shifts in the prevalence of childhood obesity remain uncertain. However, the rapid increases cannot be accounted for by shifts in the gene pool. Therefore, the increases in prevalence can only reflect shifts in the environment that promote food intake or inactivity. Dietary patterns changed substantially over the last 20 years. For example, more than 40% of a family's income spent on food is spent on food consumed outside the home (15). Because more parents are working, family meals have declined. Soft drink consumption has almost doubled since 1971 (16), and our analyses of data from the Continuing Survey of Food Intake of Individuals indicates that soft drinks now supply approximately 11% of an adolescent's usual caloric intake. A greater variety of products is available in supermarkets (17). Portion size has increased dramatically (18). Although each change has been associated with increased caloric intake, or in some cases obesity, and logical explanations exist for how these changes could cause obesity, clear causal linkages have not been established. Nonetheless, because most of these practices increase short-term caloric intake, they are reasonable targets for dietary efforts aimed at prevention or treatment.

Over the same period, physical activity patterns also appear to have changed. For example, fewer than one third of children who live within 1 mile of school walk to school (19, 20), although, historically, walking to school was the norm. Furthermore, although 25% of all trips are less than 1 mile, 75% are made by car (21). Since the 1980s, sedentary behavior appears to have increased. Data from the National Longitudinal Survey of Youth suggest that the median amount of television viewed by children and adolescents increased from approximately 2 hours/day in 1963 to 1970 (22) to almost 5 hours/day in 1990 (23). In 1990, more than 30% of children watched 5 or more hours of television daily (23). Nonetheless, the relative contributions of diet and inactivity to the increases in prevalence of obesity remain unclear.

Critical Periods for the Onset of Childhood Overweight

A critical period for the development of overweight is defined as a developmental stage in which physiologic alterations increase the later prevalence of obesity (24). Fetal life and adolescence appear to be critical periods for the onset of overweight in children and adolescents. Several groups appear at risk for overweight or its complications as a consequence of intrauterine developments. Low-birth-weight infants appear to have an increased risk of hypertension and cardiovascular disease as adults (25). However, it is not clear that adults born with low birth weights have an increased prevalence of overweight in adulthood, although visceral fat may be increased (26). However, children with increased birth weights are consistently at increased risk for the development of later overweight (27). Studies of infants of diabetic mothers provide a provocative example of this relationship. Infants of diabetic mothers are fatter at birth than infants of non-diabetic mothers. By 1 year of age, the differences in fatness apparent at birth are no longer present (28). By 5 to 6 years, children of mothers diabetic during their pregnancy have an increased prevalence of overweight that persists through age 18 years (29).

A second period in childhood that has previously been considered a critical period is the period of adiposity rebound. This period is more appropriately termed the period of BMI rebound, because it represents the period when BMI increases after a nadir at 4 to 6 years of age. Children with a BMI rebound before 4 to 6 years are at increased risk of an increased BMI in later life (30, 31). However, it has not yet been demonstrated that early BMI rebound is associated with greater fatness at the time of rebound or that the increased BMI that follows is associated with increased body fatness. Furthermore, BMI at rebound may predict subsequent BMI better than the time of rebound (32).

Adolescence, particularly in girls, represents a second critical period for the development of overweight. Longitudinal data suggest that the risk that adolescent overweight will persist into adulthood is threefold greater in adolescent girls than boys (33). Overweight present in adolescence increases the risk of all-cause and cardiovascular mortality in men and in cardiovascular morbidity in men and women that appears independent of adult weight (34).

Regardless of age of onset, fatness appears increasingly canalized with age (35, 36). Estimates suggest that 25 to 80% of overweight children remain overweight as adults (37, 38). Adults who were overweight in early childhood appear to account for a disproportionate percentage of morbidly obese adults (38, 39).

The mechanisms that act to entrain overweight and its complications at these periods remain unclear. The relationship between early fetal undernutrition and morbidity may be mediated by fetal adaptations to stress such as hypercortisolism (40). Whether fetal undernutrition also leads to increased body fat or enhances the likelihood of comorbidities of overweight remains unclear. Increased body fatness in infants of diabetic mothers may entrain either the number of fat cells, central regulation of fatness by the hypothalamic-pituitary-adrenal axis, or adipocyte factors concerned with body fat regulation. Factors that operate in early childhood to increase the severity of subsequent overweight remain less certain. Early childhood may represent the first important period in life when social forces begin to affect activity and diet. Entrainment of these behaviors could disproportionately affect the onset and persistence of later overweight. As indicated earlier, major changes in body fat and fat distribution occur in both genders in adolescence. Excessive body fat increases during female adolescence appear to increase the risk of persistent body fat increases. In men, the risks of adult disease entrained by adolescent overweight may reflect the central redistribution of fat that occurs at adolescence (10, 11).

Role of the Physical Environment

Childhood overweight has been associated with several variables within the physical environment, including season, region, and population density (41). Overweight among children and adolescents was more prevalent in winter and spring than in summer and fall. In early studies (41), childhood overweight was more prevalent in the northeastern United States, followed in descending order by the midwest, south, and west. Within each region, overweight was more prevalent in densely settled urban areas than in areas with lower population densities. However, our reanalyses of the same variables in NHANES III failed to replicate the earlier findings, which suggested that in the 25 years between these studies, the country became much more homogenous with respect to overweight or factors that affect it.

Role of the Behavioral Environment

Family Environment

Familial and behavioral variables have also been associated with childhood overweight. Children of obese parents have an increased risk of overweight (8). Overweight is most prevalent among single children and is less prevalent among children from large families (42).

The role of socioeconomic class in the genesis of childhood overweight remains unclear. Although an early study demonstrated an inverse relationship of overweight with socioeconomic class (43), other studies have shown either a direct (44) or no significant relationship (45). Several data sources suggest that overweight may determine, rather than result from, socioeconomic class in young adults (46, 47). The effect of social class on the prevalence of childhood overweight has not been examined in more recent representative surveys of the US population. Children who are the victims of parental neglect (48) and children who suffer from increased psychosocial problems (49, 50) also appear at increased risk for the development of overweight.

Diet

Energy balance results when energy intake equals energy expenditure. Energy expenditure can be characterized as TEE = RMR + TEF + ACT where TEE is total daily energy expenditure, RMR is resting metabolic rate, TEF is thermic effects of food, and ACT is energy spent on activity. Overweight occurs when energy intake exceeds energy expenditure. The only discretionary components of energy balance are food intake and the ACT.

The absence of a clear relationship of dietary intake with the development of childhood overweight derives in part from the difficulties inherent in the accurate measurement of dietary intake. For example, overweight children rarely gain more than 5 extra kg/year. Based on the presumptions that all excess weight is fat, that the cost of synthesis of adipose tissue is minimal, and that 1 kg of adipose tissue contains 150 to 200 g of water (50, 51), the daily caloric excess necessary to gain 5 kg of adipose tissue annually approximates 100 kcal/day (Table 60.1).

Comparisons of reported dietary intake with energy expenditure measured by the doubly labeled water method

TABLE 60.1. CALORIC EXCESS NECESSARY TO GAIN 5 KG OF ADIPOSE TISSUE PER YEAR

Adipose tissue = 20% H_2O
1 g fat = 9 kcal/g
1 kg adipose = 800 g fat = 7200 kcal
5 kg adipose tissue = 36,000 kcal/365 d = 98 kcal/d

emphasize the imprecise measurements of the minor caloric imbalances necessary to generate overweight. For example, careful dietary records collected from adolescents of normal weight and from overweight adolescents underestimated measured energy expenditure by 20 and 40%, respectively (52). Although younger children may provide more accurate estimates of food intake (53, 54), dietary records still cannot provide the valid caloric intakes necessary to establish the source of caloric imbalance. Nonetheless, dietary records may help individual patients to identify foods that are the appropriate target of therapy or eating patterns that could be modified to reduce caloric intake.

Because dietary records to establish caloric intake are inaccurate, studies of patterns of eating or food consumption may represent a more fruitful approach to examine the role of diet in the genesis of childhood overweight. Such studies have just begun. The increased caloric density of fat and the possibility that individual differences in fat oxidation account for a differential susceptibility to weight gain (55, 56) suggest that reduced dietary fat intake is an appropriate target for preventive efforts.

Breast-feeding appears the most important dietary factor consistently associated with a lower prevalence of childhood overweight (57–59). The mechanism by which breast-feeding reduces the risk of overweight appears uncertain, and it may reflect increased insulin (60) and/or insulin-related growth factors among formula-fed infants or increased sensitivity to the infant's satiety cues among breast-fed infants.

Activity

Energy expenditure includes energy spent on RMR, TEF, and ACT. Although an initial report demonstrated that maternal obesity appeared related to reduced energy expenditure in infants (61), subsequent studies failed to reveal significant differences in energy expenditure between infants born of normal and overweight mothers (62). Furthermore, TEE at age 12 weeks failed to predict changes in body fat that had occurred by 9 months and 2 years of age (63).

Studies of RMR in overweight and nonoverweight children (64) and adolescents (65) have consistently shown an elevated RMR in overweight subjects, even after normalization for fat-free mass. Although the TEF was lower in overweight than in nonoverweight children, no differences were observed after weight reduction (66). Furthermore, no significant differences in TEF have been observed between overweight and nonoverweight adolescents (67).

Reduced ACT could also increase susceptibility to overweight in children and adolescents. For example, vigorous physical activity declines markedly in girls during adolescence and may increase the risk of onset of overweight during this period (68, 69). An extensive compendium of doubly labeled water studies indicated that ACT, calculated from TEE measured with doubly labeled water and RMR, gradually increases throughout childhood (70). If reduced ACT represented a risk factor for the development of overweight, the incidence of overweight should be inversely related to ACT. However, increases with age in ACT suggest that alterations in activity do not adequately account for the increased risk of adolescent overweight. Nonetheless, reductions in the energy spent on RMR, TEF, or ACT could predispose persons or subgroups to an increased risk for the development of overweight. Our prospective data in girls as they enter and complete adolescence have failed to substantiate reductions in energy expenditure as risks for excess weight gain (70a).

Inactivity

Decreased activity in adolescents (68, 69) and adults (71) in the United States has focused attention on inactivity as a potential cause of overweight. Activity within populations, measured by time of participation in specific activities, may have an effect on the prevalence of overweight independent of the effect of inactivity, measured by television time (72). If inactivity was the reciprocal of activity, the effects of activity and inactivity on overweight prevalence would not be independent. These data also suggest that inactivity may be better understood as a sedentary behavior rather than as a function of energy expenditure.

The principal sedentary behavior in the United States is television viewing. Data from 1990 suggested that approximately one third of 10- to 15-year-old children in the United States viewed more than 5 hours of television per day (23). Television viewing occupies more time on an annual basis than any other behavior except sleep. Television viewing has been linked with a variety of adverse health outcomes (73), including overweight (22, 23). Furthermore, the relationship between television viewing and overweight may be causal (22). Television viewing is associated with reduced activity, although the metabolic rate may not be lower than when children engage in other sedentary activities such as reading (74). Television viewing is also associated with increased food intake, and the foods consumed are those advertised on television (75).

Several data sources are consistent with the view that the concurrence of inactivity with other behaviors may contribute to the adverse effects of inactivity on overweight. For example, although television viewing is a sedentary activity, it has been significantly associated with increased fat intake (74). Studies of adolescents have demonstrated significant relationships between inactivity and other adverse health practices, such as smoking, consumption of less healthy foods, or increased fat intake (76, 77).

CLINICAL EFFECTS

Syndromes Associated with Childhood Overweight

Table 60.2 includes most clinical syndromes associated with childhood and adolescent overweight (78). Even in specialty clinics that deal with childhood obesity, syndromes associated with overweight are rare and are readily identified by physical examination because of short stature, dysmorphic features, gonadal dysfunction, or ocular anomalies.

Because childhood overweight is generally accompanied by an increase in linear growth (79), short stature in association with overweight should prompt a careful search for other characteristics associated with potential clinical syndromes. Other features common to more than one syndrome include ocular (Alstrom-Hallgren syndrome [80], Bardet-Biedl syndrome [81], pseudohypoparathyroidism), hand (Carpenter syndrome, Cohen syndrome, Bardet-Biedl syndrome, Prader-Labhart-Willi syndrome [82, 83], pseudohypoparathyroidism), or menstrual abnormalities (Cushing syndrome [84], hypothalamic dysfunction [85], Bardet-Biedl syndrome, polycystic ovary disease [86], Prader-Labhart-Willi syndrome, Turner syndrome).

Consequences of Overweight in Childhood

Many of the consequences of childhood overweight resemble those in adults, but they occur less frequently. Several are unique to childhood-onset overweight.

Among the most prevalent consequences of overweight in children is discrimination by their peers. Young children learn to associate overweight with other undesirable characteristics. For example, children as young as age 6 consistently rank overweight children as less desirable candidates as friends than children with any other handicap (87).

TABLE 60.2. CLINICAL SYNDROMES ASSOCIATED WITH CHILDHOOD OBESITY

Alstrom-Hallgren syndrome
Carpenter syndrome
Cohen syndrome
Cushing syndrome
Growth hormone deficiency
Hyperinsulinemia
Hypothalamic dysfunction or tumor
Hypothyroidism
Laurence-Moon-Biedl syndrome
Polycystic ovary disease
Prader-Labhart-Willi syndrome
Pseudohypoparathyroidism
Turner syndrome

As children grow older, discrimination becomes more institutionalized. Among adolescents, college acceptance rates for overweight girls are lower than those for nonoverweight girls who have comparable academic credentials (88). As adults, girls overweight in late adolescence and early adulthood complete fewer years of education, marry significantly less frequently, and have lower family incomes and increased poverty rates (46).

Orthopedic problems unique to childhood occur more frequently among the overweight. Slipped capital femoral epiphysis occurs among children with a prevalence of approximately three per 100,000 persons per year (89), but most children with this problem are overweight (90). The disease probably reflects the susceptibility of the femoral head epiphysis to the increased stress of weight bearing. The disease may present only with hip pain or a limp. Blount disease (91), or bowed tibia with a consequent deformity of the medial aspect of the proximal tibial metaphysis, occurs more often among overweight children. Blount disease reflects the effects of increased weight bearing on cartilaginous bone, with compensatory tibial overgrowth. Surgery may be necessary to correct the deformity. Minor injuries such as ankle sprains may resolve more slowly or may become chronic in overweight children and adolescents, and they may account for persistent extremity pain.

Although cardiovascular consequences of childhood overweight occur less frequently than they do in adults, precursors of adult disease are present in childhood. More than 60% of overweight 5- to 10-year-old children have at least one additional cardiovascular disease risk factor, and 25% have two or more (92). Acanthosis nigricans, increased pigmentation of the skin of the neck and axillae, may be a consequence of increased friction between skinfolds, but it may also indicate abnormal glucose tolerance and hyperinsulinemia (93). However, acanthosis nigricans and glucose intolerance may only reflect the increased BMI associated with both abnormalities (94). Because of rapid increases in the prevalence of overweight, type 2 diabetes mellitus in some locations now accounts for almost 50% of all new cases of diabetes in adolescents (95). Glucose intolerance may occur in up to 25% of overweight children and adolescents (96). Hyperlipidemia is frequent among overweight children, and the lipoprotein pattern is characterized by elevated levels of low-density lipoproteins and decreased levels of high-density lipoproteins (97, 98).

Hepatic abnormalities occur in a sizeable fraction of overweight children (99). These abnormalities generally consist of modest elevations of liver enzymes and may reflect hepatic steatosis (99, 100). In severely overweight patients, hepatic steatosis may progress to cirrhosis. Weight loss can normalize liver enzymes. As in adults, overweight may also be associated with cholecystitis (101). A more common cause of abdominal pain is gastroesophageal reflux caused by the increased intraabdominal pressure of visceral or subcutaneous abdominal fat.

The two most serious and urgent complications of childhood and adolescent overweight are sleep apnea (102) and pseudotumor cerebri. Severe sleep apnea invariably occurs in association with snoring, and parents may describe apneic episodes. Long apneic episodes are associated with hypoxia and may trigger a fatal cardiac arrhythmia. Up to 50% of children with pseudotumor cerebri may be overweight (103), although the role that excess weight plays in the pathophysiology of pseudotumor cerebri remains unclear. Optic nerve compression may produce visual field cuts. Rapid weight reduction is essential for both problems.

Clinical Assessment

Few causes or consequences of overweight occur without signs or symptoms. Therefore, a careful history and physical examination are crucial to exclude underlying associated syndromes or to identify complications of overweight.

History

A careful history of the age of onset of overweight may help to identify underlying risk factors that may predispose to the persistence of the disease. Such factors include gestational diabetes in the mother or early childhood onset of overweight. Questions regarding discrimination at school may help to engage the child's or adolescent's interest and participation in the therapeutic process. A family history of severe overweight or associated hypertension, diabetes, or cardiovascular morbidity heightens concern about future comorbidities in the pediatric patient and helps to establish the level of family concern regarding medical complications of overweight.

Although the dietary history cannot be used to establish a valid caloric intake, a 24-hour recall and a brief series of quantitative questions about the consumption of juice, milk, soft drinks, fast food, and snacks of high caloric density such as candy bars, chips, cookies, ice cream, or frozen yogurt may identify foods that can be reduced or eliminated from the diet. Questions about time spent outdoors, participation in vigorous activities, and time spent viewing television are essential to establish activity levels and to identify potential approaches to reduce inactivity or increase vigorous activity.

The review of systems should include questions that address the principal morbidities outlined earlier. Headaches or visual changes may indicate the presence of pseudotumor cerebri or the rare hypothalamic tumor. Snoring in association with daytime somnolence suggests possible sleep apnea. Dyspnea on exertion provides a functional measure of activity and the activity restriction imposed by excess weight. Abdominal pain may be functional and may result from school avoidance, but it may also indicate the presence of gastroesophageal reflux or cholecystitis. Irregular menstrual periods or amenorrhea may indicate polycystic ovary disease. Hip pain or a limp suggests imminent or acute slipped capital femoral epiphysis.

Physical Examination

The physical examination should begin with the calculation of BMI and comparison of the child's BMI with the Centers for Disease Control and Prevention BMI charts to establish the severity of overweight. Inspection and measurement of the triceps skinfold thickness will help to establish whether the excess weight represents body fat or increased frame size. Blood pressure determination with an appropriate-size cuff and use of age-appropriate standards is essential.

Short stature or dysmorphic features should prompt careful exclusion of syndromes associated with childhood overweight. Inspection of the skin may reveal the violaceous striae that characterize Cushing syndrome or acanthosis nigricans. A careful fundoscopic examination should be performed to exclude papilledema suggestive of increased intracranial pressure. Enlarged tonsils may contribute to sleep apnea. If a tonsillectomy is warranted, careful postoperative care is essential because overweight children are at high risk of postoperative obstruction from peripharyngeal swelling that follows a tonsillectomy. Abdominal tenderness may reflect cholecystitis or cholelithiasis. Limited hip flexion may be the only indication of slipped capital femoral epiphysis. In younger children, bowed extremities require radiologic examination to exclude the possibility of early Blount disease.

Laboratory Assessment

Routine tests should include serum cholesterol levels to exclude the possibility of hyperlipidemia, liver enzymes levels to identify hepatic steatosis, and urinalysis to exclude glucosuria. Abnormal liver function tests in a child with a history of abdominal pain or a family history of gallbladder disease require an ultrasound examination of the abdomen to exclude cholelithiasis. Fasting glucose and insulin levels may help to clarify the risk of diabetes mellitus in a child or adolescent with acanthosis nigricans, although precise cutoff points for prediabetes in children and adolescents have not been established. A history consistent with sleep apnea warrants a sleep study to determine the frequency and severity of apneic episodes. Sex hormones, luteinizing hormone, and follicle-stimulating hormone may be helpful adjunct measures in girls with signs or symptoms of polycystic ovary disease. Laboratory studies not suggested by the history or physical examination are rarely helpful.

TREATMENT

Family involvement in the treatment of childhood and adolescent overweight is crucial (3, 104, 105), because pediatric patients rarely purchase, prepare, or serve their own food. Such involvement is implicit in the therapeutic approaches described later.

Regardless of the severity of overweight, the first consideration for any overweight person is weight maintenance. For some children, weight maintenance for 1 year may be the only step necessary to achieve ideal weight for height. However, aggressive therapy must be considered from the outset for the morbidly obese adolescent who is 200% of ideal weight. Although dietary therapy is necessary to reduce weight, increased levels of activity may be essential to maintain weight after weight loss.

Education

Education of the overweight child or adolescent rarely succeeds as an isolated intervention. However, several principles are useful in the treatment of children and families. Use of the US Department of Agriculture's food guide pyramid to guide food choices may help to reduce dietary fat intake (106). Furthermore, use of labels to establish fat and caloric content will help families to purchase foods lower in fat and calories.

Dietary Modification

Reduced caloric intake must remain the cornerstone of weight-reduction therapy because it is easier to achieve a caloric deficit by reduced food intake than by increased activity. The most useful function of a dietary history is to identify foods that can be altered or eliminated.

Low-Fat Diets

Reductions in dietary fat represent the first step toward the modification of dietary intake. According to the current recommendation of the American Academy of Pediatrics, dietary fat intake should approximate 30% of calories for children older than the age of 2 years. Several caveats accompany this recommendation. First, although no comparable studies in children have been done, reductions in dietary fat in the absence of reduced caloric intake may only achieve modest weight loss in adults (107). Even though anecdotal reports suggest that excessive concerns about the effects of dietary fat have led to growth failure in young children (108), concerns about the effect of caloric restriction on the growth of the population become moot when the risks of persistent overweight exceed the minor adverse effects of diet.

A second alternative for children and young adolescents is the Stoplight Diet (109). This approach classifies foods as green, yellow, and red, according to whether the food can be consumed freely, with caution, or only on rare occasions. The Stoplight Diet has been used repeatedly and effectively in weight-reduction studies of 8- to12-year-old children. According to one study, increases in fruit and vegetable intake may cause greater reductions in fat and carbohydrate intake than efforts to decrease high-fat or high-carbohydrate foods (110).

The manner in which dietary modifications are introduced may be as important as the dietary modification itself. It is considerably easier to modify the intake of a food that can be counted, such as soft drinks per day, than to follow a generic instruction to reduce the percentage of calories from fat. Children also appear to respond better when foods that families can eat are emphasized, such as fruits and vegetables, rather than when foods are restricted (105). This observation is consistent with the finding that children and adolescents for whom specific diets were recommended lost less weight than children and adolescents on less specific diets (111). Both observations suggest that results of therapy are likely better when children and families have more control over their dietary choices.

Use of Highly Restrictive Diets

Severely obese adolescents whose weight is 200% or more in excess of ideal or children or adolescents with diabetes, sleep apnea, or another major complication of excess body weight may require more aggressive dietary interventions such as the protein modified fast. The protein modified fast should be used cautiously in patients with renal or cardiac disease, but it may have a highly beneficial effect in patients with liver disease that results from hepatic steatosis. Before the diet is started, it is essential to determine whether the candidate for the diet is capable of weight maintenance for an 8- to 12-week period. If weight maintenance is impossible before the diet is started, the patient is more likely to have a relapse after the diet is discontinued.

The protein modified fast consists of a carbohydrate-free diet that contains 2.0 to 2.5 g protein/kg ideal body weight/day provided as meat or other high-quality protein, supplemented daily with 30 mEq potassium chloride, 800 mg calcium, and a multivitamin with minerals (78, 112). Vegetables low in carbohydrate may be consumed ad libitum. Fluid intake should be maintained at 48 oz of noncaloric fluids daily. Ketosis appears within 48 to 72 hours after the initiation of the diet and can be used to monitor dietary adherence. The diet should be continued for several months. Weight loss is most rapid in the first 2 weeks and thereafter averages 0.5 to 1.0 kg weekly. Patients should be seen frequently during the diet to monitor adherence, to identify potentially adverse effects, and to provide ongoing family support. Blood counts, liver function tests, amylase, albumin levels, and ketonuria should be monitored monthly. At the termination of the diet, carbohydrates should be reintroduced over several weeks.

Complications of the protein modified fast include malaise during the transition to ketosis, orthostatic hypotension, and diarrhea or constipation. Although gallbladder disease may occur in association with fat-free diets, this complication is rare in children and adolescents following the protein modified fast, perhaps because the fat in a meat-based diet causes gallbladder contraction and thereby reduces biliary sludging. Nonetheless, if a patient develops abdominal pain with weight reduction, an ultrasound scan of the abdomen is essential to exclude cholelithiasis or pancreatitis.

Alterations in Activity

Increased Activity

Increased activity during weight reduction may have several benefits. Increased activity in association with a low-calorie diet may increase the rate of weight loss, and in adults it decreases many obesity-associated comorbidities, regardless of the effects of activity on weight (113). In addition, increased activity levels may increase the likelihood of weight maintenance after weight loss (114). Despite widespread interest in physical activity as a weight-control strategy, the dose of physical activity necessary to prevent overweight in children and adolescents has not been established. The *Dietary Guidelines for Americans* recommend 1 hour/day of moderate physical activity for children and adolescents (115), but no studies have yet demonstrated that this dose reduces the incidence of overweight or achieves weight maintenance. The International Consensus Conference on Physical Activity Guidelines for Adolescents suggested that adolescents participate in three or more sessions per week of moderate to vigorous activity that last 20 minutes or more (116). However, recommendations for vigorous activity are not appropriate for massively obese adolescents, who may achieve maximal energy expenditure with walking. For this group, simple increases in activity should be the goal.

Increased activity among overweight preadolescents increases TEE and is not apparently counterbalanced by reduced activity in other areas (117). As in adults (118), fat loss is likely to depend on the person's capacity for fat oxidation, the exercise intensity, and the quantity of fat in the diet.

How activity is increased may contribute to the long-term success of the intervention. For example, lifestyle activities chosen by the child may accomplish more sustained weight loss than structured exercise programs that provide fewer choices (119), perhaps because children are more likely to participate in an activity that they choose. Furthermore, when children make a choice, they may feel more responsible for the decision to change (120).

Reduced Inactivity

Both increased activity and reduced inactivity may have beneficial effects on weight changes in the population. Long-term effects of increased activity and reduced inactivity on weight reduction have only recently been carefully examined. When the effect on weight of increased activity was compared with reduced inactivity, 4-month and 1-year weight losses were significantly greater for the group reinforced for reduced inactivity than in the group reinforced for increased activity (120). Furthermore, attitudes toward high-intensity activity were more positive among children reinforced for decreased sedentary activity than among those reinforced for increased activity. More recently, two school-based interventions demonstrated that the strategy of reduced television time was associated with reduced rates of overweight (121) or decreased rates of weight gain (122). These data emphasize that reduced television time represents an important weight-control strategy and demonstrate again that reduced inactivity under circumstances in which children choose the alternative activity is more effective than when children are reinforced for the activity itself. The major challenge in the use of reduced television time as a weight-control strategy is to identify incentives for parents to control television time.

Behavior Modification

The most critical treatment issue is whether the family is prepared to make the behavioral changes necessary to control the child's weight. The provider should not assume that the family views the child's overweight with a high degree of concern. It is often helpful to initiate care with open-ended questions about the family's level of concern, previous attempts to control the child's weight, and the outcome of prior attempts. If the family is not concerned about the child's weight, and the child does not have a substantial weight problem or adverse weight-related health effects, it may be more appropriate for the provider to inform the family about the risks and consequences of overweight and to indicate his or her availability should the family become concerned. If the family is concerned, the provider should explore the family's interest and confidence in their ability to change some of the factors related to the child's weight. Solutions that originate with the family are more likely to succeed than those that originate with the provider (123).

Behavior modification is not an additional therapeutic endeavor but rather constitutes the mechanism by which changes in diet and activity are effected. As indicated earlier (3) and in repeated studies by Epstein and colleagues (104), parental involvement in children's weight-reduction programs is essential.

The major components of behavior modification include contracting, self-monitoring, and social reinforcement and modeling (104). Contracts reinforce adherence to the weight-reduction regimen or provide incentives for weight loss. Self-monitoring involves careful daily observation of diet and activity. Social reinforcement and modeling involve teaching children and parents how to model diet and activity-related behaviors for other family members. The capacity to choose among alternatives appears to have a highly beneficial effect on adherence and should constitute a central consideration in the design of weight-reduction programs for children and adolescents.

Other therapies aimed at the modification of family behaviors, such as family therapy, have not been studied as intensively. One reason is that such interventions are not as readily quantified. Likewise, because studies of behavior modification have focused most intensively on children younger than 12 years of age, the effectiveness of this intervention in other age groups has not been established.

Alternative Therapies

Therapies for morbid obesity in adolescents, as in adults, are associated with a high relapse rate. For example, virtually all patients studied as inpatients in various studies of hypocaloric diets regained weight after discharge from the study. Substantial numbers of patients may not be able to initiate hypocaloric diets or may be so incapacitated by their weight that movement is impossible. For these patients, more aggressive therapies, such as pharmacotherapy or bariatric surgery, may be warranted. Unfortunately, experience with these therapies in adolescents is limited.

Pharmacotherapy

Few pharmacotherapy trials in adolescents have been reported. Adverse events associated with the use of phentermine and fenfluramine emphasize the caution with which drugs should be used in the treatment of children and adolescents, particularly because drug therapy may be required for long periods or even for a lifetime. Since the removal of fenfluramine from the market, orlistat and sibutramine have been approved for use in adults (124), but not in children or adolescents. A trial of sibutramine in adolescents has been published (125), and although the drug caused more weight loss than the placebo, the net effects were modest. Therefore, pharmacotherapy must be reserved for morbidly obese adolescents, but only after more conservative approaches have failed and only with informed consent under a research protocol that has been approved by an institutional review board. Adolescents and their physicians must retain realistic expectations regarding the response to therapy. Based on weight losses achieved in adults, the current drugs will not achieve the massive weight reduction necessary for the morbidly obese patient to achieve ideal body weight.

Surgery

An expert committee has recommended that bariatric surgery be reserved for adolescents with a BMI greater than or equal to 40 with a major complication of overweight, such as type 2 diabetes mellitus, sleep apnea, or pseudotumor cerebri or adolescents with a BMI greater than or equal to 50 with a less urgent complication of overweight (126). Additional criteria include failure of at least 6 months of organized attempts at weight management, physiologic maturity, agreement to avoid pregnancy for at least 1 year postoperatively, and capacity to provide informed consent to surgical management. Only three reports have been published regarding the use of surgery to treat obesity in the pediatric age group (127–129). These studies suggested that mean weight loss is in excess of 30 kg, depending on operation type of operation and patient gender. These results may underestimate the effects of surgery, because weight gains in some of the operative patients would have continued unabated without intervention. Surgery is probably not warranted for patients with Prader-Labhart-Willi syndrome, most of whom promptly would regain any lost weight. Acute complications of surgery include anastomosis leaks and wound infections and may occur in a substantial number of patients (129). Long-term complications include anemia. Nonetheless, weight losses have been sustained in most patients for more than 7 years.

Outcome

Childhood and adolescent onset overweight appears to account for 25 to 30% of adult cases of obesity. Furthermore, overweight present in male and female adolescents appears associated with a risk of adult morbidity and mortality independent of the effect of adolescent weight on adult weight. These observations suggest that effective treatment of overweight children and adolescents may exert a substantial effect on the morbidity and mortality of adult obesity.

Children also appear more responsive to weight-reduction therapies than adults. For example, Epstein and associates (104) showed that the long-term effects of a family-based program of diet and activity promoted by behavior modification could still be demonstrated 10 years later. These results indicate that children should be targeted for an increased proportion of resources and efforts aimed at weight control in the US population.

PREVENTION

The high prevalence of overweight children and adolescents indicates that efforts must focus on prevention as well as treatment. Although few successful models have been published, several effective strategies can be implemented in primary care and community settings. These include promotion of breast-feeding (57–59), control of the amount of time that children watch television (120–122), and physical activity (113). Published evidence-based recommendations have been published that describe community strategies that increase physical activity (130). Although an evidence-based review has also considered community and school-based strategies for weight control in children and adolescents, evidence is insufficient to warrant a recommendation, largely because too few studies have been done or the outcome measures were not consistent across studies (D. Katz, personal communication).

Major prevention challenges include the lack of reimbursement for counseling in primary care and the lack of effective strategies to increase breast-feeding rates or to reduce television time. Efforts to address overweight that are limited to primary care settings will not likely be successful unless complementary strategies are employed in other settings. For example, efforts to reduce television time may not succeed unless alternatives are available for children after school. Efforts to increase physical activity may not succeed unless schools restore physical education programs. Finally, none of these efforts are likely to succeed without resources necessary to develop and implement comprehensive efforts that integrate clinical, school-based, and community efforts to improve nutrition and to increase physical activity among children and adolescents.

REFERENCES

1. Roche AF, Siervogel RM, Chumlea WC et al. Am J Clin Nutr 1981;34:2831–8.
2. Himes JH, Dietz WH. Am J Clin Nutr 1994;59:307–16.
3. Barlow SE, Dietz WH. Obesity Evaluation and Treatment: Expert Committee Recommendations. http://www.pediatrics.org/cgi/content/full/102/3/e29.
4. http://www.cdc.gov/growthcharts.
5. Cole TJ, Bellizzi MC, Flegal KM et al. BMJ 2000;320:1240–3.
6. Himes JH, Bouchard C. Int J Obes 1989;13:183–93.
7. Mei Z, Grummer-Strawn LM, Pietrobelli A et al. Am J Clin Nutr 2002;75:978–85.
8. Garn SM, Clark DC. Pediatrics 1976;57:443–55.
9. Rolland-Cachera M-F, Deheeger M, Guilloud-Bataille M et al. Ann Hum Biol 1987;14:219–29.
10. Goran MI, Kaskoun M, Shuman WP. Int J Obes 1995;19:279–83.
11. Mueller WH. Soc Sci Med 1982;16:191–6.
12. Malina RM, Bouchard C. Adipose tissue changes during growth. In: RM Malina, C Bouchard, eds. Growth, Maturation, and Physical Activity, Champaign, IL: Human Kinetics Books, 1991:133–49.
13. Knittle JL, Timmers K, Ginsberg-Fellner F et al. J Clin Invest 1979;63:239–46.
14. Ogden CL, Flegal KM, Carroll MD et al. JAMA 2002;288:1728–32.
15. Putnam JJ. Allshouse JE. Food Consumption, Prices and Expenditures 1970–97. US Department of Agriculture Statistical Bulletin no. 965. Washington, DC: US Government Printing Office, 1999.
16. Life Sciences Research Office. Third Report on Nutrition Monitoring in the United States, Executive Summary. Washington, DC: US Government Printing Office, 1995.
17. Food Institute Report. New Products Slip a Trifle in '97. Fairlawn, NJ: American Institute of Food Distributors, 1998.
18. Young LR, Nestle M. Am J Public Health 2002;92:246–9.
19. Tracking Healthy People 2010. Washington, DC: US Department of Health and Human Services, 2000:22–3.
20. Bricker SK, Kanny D, Mellinger-Birdsong M et al. Morb Mortal Wkly Rep 2002;51:704–5.
21. Schimek P. Unpublished observations.
22. Dietz WH, Gortmaker SL. Pediatrics 1985;75:807–12.
23. Gortmaker SL, Must A, Sobol AM et al. Arch Pediatr Adolesc Med 1996;150:356–62.
24. Dietz WH. Am J Clin Nutr 1994;59:955–9.

25. Barker DJP, Hales CN, Fall CHD et al. Diabetologia 1993; 36:62–7.
26. Law CM, Barker DJP, Osmond C et al. J Epidemiol Comm Health 1992;46:184–6.
27. Whitaker RC, Dietz WH. J Pediatr 1998;132:768–76.
28. Vohr BR, Lipsitt LP, Oh W. J Pediatr 1980;97:196–9.
29. Pettit DJ, Baird HR, Aleck KA et al. N Engl J Med 1983;308: 242–5.
30. Rolland-Cachera M-F, Deheeger M, Bellisle F et al. Am J Clin Nutr 1984;39:129–35.
31. Siervogel RM, Roche AF, Guo S et al. Int J Obes 1991;15: 479–85.
32. Dietz WH. Lancet 2000;356:2027–8.
33. Braddon FEM, Rodgers B, Wadsworth MEJ et al. BMJ 1986; 293:299–303.
34. Must A, Jacques PF, Dallal GE et al. N Engl J Med 1992;327: 1350–5.
35. Crisp AH, Douglas WB, Ross JM et al. J Psychosom Res 1970;14:313–20.
36. Serdula MK, Ivery D, Coates RJ et al. Prev Med 1993;22: 167–77.
37. Lloyd JK, Wolff OH, Whelen WS. BMJ 1961;2:145–8.
38. Freedman DS, Kettel-Kahn L, Dietz WH et al. Pediatrics 2001;108:712–8 .
39. Rimm IJ, Rimm AA. Am J Public Health 1976;66:479–81.
40. Barker DJP. BMJ 1995;311:171–4.
41. Dietz WH, Gortmaker SL. Am J Clin Nutr 1984;39:619–24.
42. Ravelli GP, Belmont L. Am J Epidemiol 1979;109:66–70.
43. Stunkard A, d'Aquili E, Fox S et al. JAMA 1972;221:579–84.
44. Garn SM, Clark DC. Pediatrics 1975;56:306–19.
45. Lissau-Lind-Sorensen I, Sorensen TIA. Int J Obes 1992;16: 169–75.
46. Gortmaker SL, Must A, Perrin JM et al. N Engl J Med 1993; 329:1008–12.
47. Sargent JD, Blanchflower DG. Arch Pediatr Adolesc Med 1994;148:681–7.
48. Lissau I, Sorensen TIA. Lancet 1994;343:324–7.
49. Mellbin T, Vuille J-C. Acta Paediatr Scand 1989;78:568–75.
50. Martinsson A. Acta Med Scand 1967;182:795–803.
51. Bjorntorp P, Hood B, Martinsson A. Acta Med Scand 1966; 180:123–7.
52. Bandini LB, Schoeller DA, Dietz WH. Am J Clin Nutr 1990;52: 421–5.
53. Bandini LG, Cyr H, Must A et al. Am J Clin Nutr 1997;65 [Suppl]:1138S–41S.
54. Livingstone MBE, Prentice AM, Coward WA et al. Am J Clin Nutr 1992;56:29–35.
45. Flatt JP. Ann NY Acad Sci 1987;499:104–23.
56. Zurlo F, Lillioja S, Esposito-Del Puente A et al. Am J Physiol 1990;259:E650–7.
57. Dietz WH. JAMA 2001;285:2506–7.
58. Hediger ML, Overpeck MD, Kuczmarski RJ et al. JAMA 2001;285:2453–60.
59. Gillman MW, Rifas-Shiman SL, Camrago CA Jr et al. JAMA 2001;285:2461–7.
60. Lucas A, Sarson DL, Blackburn AM et al. Lancet 1980;1: 1267–9.
61. Roberts SB, Savage J, Coward WA et al. N Engl J Med 1988;318:461–6.
62. Davies PSW, Wells JCK, Fieldhouse CA et al. Am J Clin Nutr 1995;61:1026–9.
63. Davies PSW, Day JME, Lucas A. Int J Obes 1991;15:727–31.
64. Maffeis C, Schutz Y, Micciolo R et al. J Pediatr 1993;122: 556–62.
65. Bandini LG, Schoeller DA, Dietz WH. Pediatr Res 1990;27: 198–203.
66. Maffeis C, Schutz Y, Pinelli L. Eur J Clin Nutr 1992;46:577–83.
67. Bandini LG, Schoeller DA, Edwards J et al. Am J Physiol 1989; 256:E357–67.
68. Wolf AM, Gortmaker SL, Cheung L et al. Am J Public Health 1993;83,1625–7.
69. Heath GW, Pratt M, Warren CW et al. Arch Pediatr Adolesc Med 1994;148:1131–6.
70. Food and Nutrition Board, Institute of Medicine. Dietary Reference Intakes for Macronutrients. Washington, DC: National Academy Press, 2003:Appendix I, Table I–2.
70a. Bandini LG, Must A, Phillips SM et al. Am J Clin Nutr (in press).
71. Centers for Disease Control. Morb Mortal Wkly Rep 1993;42: 576–9.
72. Ching PLYH, Willett WC, Rimm EB et al. Am J Public Health 1996;86:25–30.
73. Dietz WH, Strasburger VC. Curr Prob Pediatr 1991;21:8–31.
74. Dietz WH, Bandini LG, Morelli JA et al. Am J Clin Nutr 1994;59:556–63.
75. Robinson TN, Killen JD. J Health Ed 1995;26[Suppl]:91–8.
76. Lytle LA, Kelder SH, Perry CL et al. Health Ed Res 1995;10: 133–46.
77. Raitakari OT, Porkka KVK, Taimela S et al. Am J Epidemiol 1994;140:195–205.
78. Dietz WH, Robinson TN. Pediatr Rev 1993;14:337–44.
79. Forbes GB. J Pediatr 1977;91:40–2.
80. Alstrom-Hallgren, Goldstein JL, Fialkow PJ. Medicine (Baltimore) 1973;52:53–71.
81. Green JS, Parfrey PS, Harnett JD et al. N Engl J Med 1989; 321:1002–9.
82. Holm VA, Sulzbacher SJ, Pipes PL. Prader-Willi Syndrome. Baltimore: University Park Press,1981.
83. Greenswag LR, Alexander RC. Management of Prader-Willi Syndrome. New York: Springer-Verlag, 1988.
84. Magiakou MA, Mastorakos G, Oldfield EH et al. N Engl J Med 1994;331:629–36.
85. Dunger DB, Wolff OH, Leonard JV et al. Lancet 1980;1: 1277–81.
86. McKenna TJ. N Engl J Med 1988;318:558–62.
87. Richardson SA, Hastorf AH, Goodman N et al. Am Sociol Rev 1961;26:241–7.
88. Canning H, Mayer J. N Engl J Med 1966;275:1172–4.
89. Kelsey JL, Keggi KJ, Southwick WO. J Bone Joint Surg Am 1970;52:1203–16.
90. Kelsey JL, Acheson RM, Keggi KJ. Am J Dis Child 1972;124: 276–81.
91. Dietz WH, Gross WL, Kirkpatrick JA Jr. J Pediatr 1982; 101:735–7.
92. Freedman DS, Dietz WH, Srinivasan SR et al. Pediatrics 1999; 103:1175–82.
93. Richards GE, Cavallo A, Meyer WJ III et al. J Pediatr 1985; 107:893–7.
94. Nguyen TT, Keil MF, Russell DL et al. J Pediatr 2001;138: 474–80.
95. Fagot-Campagna A, Pettitt DJ, Engelgau MM et al. J Pediatr 2000;136:664–72.
96. Sinha R, Fisch G, Teague B et al. N Engl J Med 2002;346: 802–10 .
97. Freedman DS, Burke GL, Harsha DW et al. JAMA 1985;254: 515–20.
98. Lauer RM, Lee J, Clarke WR. Pediatrics 1988;82:309–18.
99. Strauss RS, Barlow SE, Dietz WH. J Pediatr 2000;136:727–33.

100. Mallory GB Jr, Fiser DH, Jackson R. J Pediatr 1989;115:892–7.

101. Baldridge AD, Perez-Atayde AR, Graeme-Cook F et al. J Pediatr 1995;127:700–4.

102. Crichlow RW, Seltzer MH, Jannetta PJ. Digest Dis 1972;17:68–72.

103. Weisberg LA, Chutorian AM. Arch Dis Child 1977;131:1243–8.

104. Epstein LH, Valoski A, Wing RR et al. JAMA 1990;264:2519–23.

105. Epstein LH. Int J Obes 1996;20[Suppl 1]:14S–21S.

106. Kennedy E, Goldberg J. Nutr Rev 1995;53:111–26.

107. Sheppard L, Kristal AR, Kushi LH. Am J Clin Nutr 1991;54:821–8.

108. Pugliese MT, Weyman-Daum M, Moses N et al. Pediatrics 1987;80:175–82.

109. Epstein LH, Squires S. The Stoplight Diet for Children. Boston: Little, Brown, 1988.

110. Epstein LH, Gordy CC, Raynor HA et al. Obes Res 2001;9:171–8.

111. Haddock CK, Shadish WR, Klesges RC et al. Ann Behav Med 1994;16:235–44.

112. Dietz WH, Schoeller DA. J Pediatr 1982;100:638–44.

113. National Institutes of Health. Clinical Guidelines on the Identification, Evaluation, and Treatment of Overweight and Obesity in Adults. Washington, DC: Department of Health and Human Services, 1998.

114. McGuire MT, Wing RR, Klem ML et al. Int J Obes 1998;22:572–7.

115. United States Department of Agriculture and Department of Health and Human Services. Dietary Guidelines for Americans. 5th ed. Home and Garden Bulletin no. 232. Washington, DC: United States Department of Agriculture and Department of Health and Human Services, 2000.

116. Sallis JF, Patrick K. Pediatr Exerc Sci 1994;6:302–14.

117. Blaak EE, Westerterp KR, Bar-Or O et al. Am J Clin Nutr 1992;55:777–82.

118. Tremblay A, Almeras N. Int J Obes 1995;19[Suppl 4]:97S–101S.

119. Epstein LH, Wing RR, Koeske R et al. Behav Ther 1982;13:651–65.

120. Epstein LH, Valoski AM, Vara LS et al. Health Psychol 1995;14:109–15.

121. Gortmaker SL, Peterson K, Wiecha J et al. Arch Pediatr Adolesc Med 1999;153:409–18.

122. Robinson TN. JAMA 1999;282:1561–7.

123. Bodenheimer T, Lorig K, Holman H et al. JAMA 2002;288:2469–75.

124. Yanovski SZ, Yanovski JA. N Engl J Med 2002;346:591–602.

125. Berkowitz RI, Wadden TA, Tershakovec AM et al. JAMA 2003;289:1805–12.

126. Inge T, Krebs N, Garcia V et al. Pediatrics 2004;114:217–23.

127. Soper RT, Mason EE, Printen KJ et al. J Pediatr Surg 1975;10:51–8.

128. Greenstein RJ, Rabner JG. Obes Surg 1995;5:138–44.

129. Strauss RS, Bradley LJ, Brolin RE. J Pediatr 2001;138:499–504.

130. Task Force on Community Preventive Services. Am J Prev Med 2002;22:67–72.

SELECTED READINGS

Epstein LH, Valoski A, Wing RR et al. JAMA 1990;264:2519–23.

Dietz WH, Robinson TN. Pediatr Rev 1993;14:337–44.

Barlow SE, Dietz WH. Obesity Evaluation and Treatment: Expert Committee Recommendations. Http://www.pediatrics.org/cgi/content/full/102/3/e29.

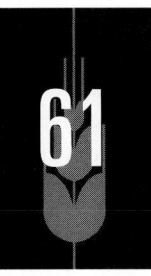

61 NUTRITIONAL MANAGEMENT OF INFANTS AND CHILDREN WITH SPECIFIC DISEASES OR OTHER CONDITIONS[1]

ARTHUR COOPER AND WILLIAM C. HEIRD

SPECIFIC DISEASES AND/OR OTHER CONDITIONS
  REQUIRING NUTRITIONAL MANAGEMENT 991
    Cystic Fibrosis 991
    Congenital Heart Disease 992
    Gastrointestinal Disorders 992
    Acute Diarrhea 992
    Crohn's Disease 994
    Short Bowel Syndrome 995
    Human Immunodeficiency Virus Infection/
      Acquired Immunodeficiency
      Syndrome 996
    Other Conditions 996
  GENERAL APPROACH TO NUTRITIONAL THERAPY 996
  PARENTERAL NUTRITION .997
    Route of Administration 997
    The Nutrient Infusate .997
    Use of Parenteral Lipid Emulsions 999
    Weaning Infants from Total Parenteral Nutrition .1001
    Home Parenteral Nutrition 1001

SPECIFIC DISEASES AND/OR OTHER CONDITIONS REQUIRING NUTRITIONAL MANAGEMENT

Cystic Fibrosis

Cystic fibrosis is characterized by progressive deterioration of pulmonary and pancreatic function. The former may increase nutrient requirements somewhat, but probably affects nutrition more by adversely affecting intake, particularly during acute exacerbations and in older children with severe pulmonary disease. Pancreatic insufficiency severely limits the absorption of fat, a major energy source of most diets. Thus, the cause of malnutrition in infants and children with this disease can be both primary (i.e., inadequate nutrient intake) and secondary (i.e., fecal losses of protein, and particularly, of fat). The latter cause usually can be controlled with appropriate pancreatic enzyme replacement because there does not seem to be a primary defect in energy metabolism associated with the disease (1).

Traditionally, a high-protein, low-fat diet has been advocated for patients with cystic fibrosis. However, with appropriate pancreatic enzyme replacement, most patients can maintain a reasonable nutritional status with a normal diet. Younger patients usually have a very good appetite, but with advanced pulmonary disease, appetite usually decreases. In many patients with advanced disease, intakes of both protein and energy, but especially energy, are far lower than recommended. From time to time, the theoretic possibility of essential fatty acid deficiency secondary to poor fat absorption is mentioned. However, unless the intake of essential fatty acids is quite low, this is rarely a significant problem, except in infants with meconium ileus who undergo surgical resection of the distal ileum (2).

There is some concern that malnutrition may hasten deterioration of pulmonary function, and an increasing body of evidence supports this concern (3–5). Further, it is clear that acute improvement of nutritional status improves muscle strength (6). Thus, attempts either to improve nutritional status or to prevent even minimal deterioration of nutritional status are warranted, particularly because it seems that early intervention may prevent malnutrition and improve long-term growth (7). Unfortunately, eating behaviors in infants, toddlers, and school-age children with cystic fibrosis may not be sufficient to meet the additional dietary requirements imposed by the disease (8, 9). In such cases, use of pharmacologic adjuncts, for example, the growth hormone megestrol acetate, may be effective in enhancing weight gain. However, weight gain and improvement of other anthropometric indices may significantly underestimate the extent of malnutrition in affected children (10–12).

In recent years, high-fat formulas have been advocated for patients with chronic pulmonary disease. The rationale, supported adequately by fact, is that oxidation of fat produces less carbon dioxide than oxidation of carbohydrate, and hence a high-fat intake imposes less stress on the already-compromised pulmonary system. This obviously is an important consideration in patients who require mechanical ventilation or who have severely compromised pulmonary function. One product based on this principle (Pulmocare®, Ross Laboratories, Columbus, OH) is available for patients with pulmonary disease. Although designed for adults, the product is used in pediatric patients; however, it should be noted that its

Abbreviations: AIDS, acquired immunodeficiency syndrome;
EFA, essential fatty acid; **HIV,** human immunodeficiency virus;
LBW, low birth weight.

sodium content is quite high. Finally, attention must be given to adequate supplementation of fat-soluble vitamins, particularly vitamin K, which may be deficient in patients with cystic fibrosis (13).

Although it is clear that much progress has been made in the medical and nutritional management of cystic fibrosis in recent years, much more remains to be done (14). A recent Consensus Report on Nutrition for Pediatric Patients with Cystic Fibrosis, from the Cystic Fibrosis Foundation and the North American Society for Pediatric Gastroenterology and Nutrition, details current recommendations in greater depth than is possible here (15).

Congenital Heart Disease

Chronic protein-energy malnutrition, manifested chiefly by growth failure, also is a common finding in infants with congenital heart disease, particularly those with conditions associated with congestive heart failure. Although not studied extensively, the nutrient needs of patients with heart disease do not seem to be much greater, if at all, than those of infants or children without heart disease. Rather, in most patients, the cause of the accompanying malnutrition can be traced to inadequate intake. In some patients, this is a result simply of poor appetite; in others, it seems to be the result of excessive tiring during feeding. In addition, fluid and sodium intakes frequently are restricted as a part of treatment and the use of diuretics is common. Either practice, of course, may limit growth even if intake of protein and energy is adequate.

The most common form of nutritional therapy for infants with congenital heart disease is use of a high-nutrient-density formula, thereby reducing the volume that must be ingested. Tube feedings via either a nasogastric or a gastrostomy tube are frequently necessary, particularly in infants whose disease is sufficiently severe to cause excessive tiring during feeding. In general, if sufficient nutrients are delivered, most such patients will grow at a reasonably normal rate.

Gastrointestinal Disorders

Malnutrition is endemic among infants and children with gastrointestinal disorders. The cause usually is loss of nutrients secondary to the specific derangement in gastrointestinal function, either diarrhea or vomiting. However, both diarrhea and vomiting are frequently treated by withholding all nutrients except water and electrolytes. This practice, of course, contributes to the development of malnutrition.

Acute Diarrhea

Acute diarrhea caused by most common organisms rarely persists for more than 4 to 5 days. During this time, the major goal of therapy is to ensure a normal state of hydration. This can be accomplished with use of oral rehydra-

tion solution, modified oral rehydration solution for malnourished children, and/or special formulas (Table 61.1), each with its own advantages and disadvantages (16). Hospitalization and intravenous fluid therapy may be necessary, particularly if fever and/or vomiting accompany the diarrhea.

What to feed and whether to feed the child with acute diarrhea have been subjects of considerable controversy for many years, and both remain unresolved. In general, stool output is greater in the patient who is fed, but this does not mean necessarily that feeding should be proscribed. In most patients, at least some nutrient intake is possible; however, the nature of this intake must be selected carefully taking into account the probable etiology of the diarrhea. The approach that we follow is outlined later; other approaches, of course, may be equally successful, particularly in undeveloped countries where hospital resources may be limited, necessitating use of a liquid milk-based diet, and/or a dry, solid, ready-to-use food that can be eaten without adding water, thereby minimizing the risk of bacterial contamination (17). A recent Working Group Report from the First World Congress of Pediatric Gastroenterology, Hepatology, and Nutrition summarizes the latest advances in this field (18).

In general, the etiology of most acute diarrhea is either bacterial or viral. Thus, a stool culture to detect the specific pathogen is indicated. In most developed countries, the recognized enteropathogenic bacteria (*Salmonella*, *Shigella*, and enteropathogenic *Escherichia coli*) are infrequent causes of diarrhea. Rather, the causative organism of most acute bacterial diarrheas is one of the many toxicogenic strains of most gram-negative organisms. Thus, a routine stool culture, unless it suggests a predominant organism, usually is not helpful. Conversely, because the pathogenesis of toxicogenic bacterial diarrhea (i.e., a secretory diarrhea resulting from stimulation of the adenylate cyclase system, as occurs in cholera [19]) is different from that of viral diarrhea (i.e., an osmotic diarrhea secondary to inhibition of glucose transport as described for rotavirus [20]), testing the stool for pH and the presence of reducing substances can be very helpful. In general, a low pH (<6.0) and the presence of reducing substances suggest a viral etiology. The stool must be tested, of course, after a period of adequate intake of a reducing sugar (e.g., a 5% glucose solution or a rehydration solution); in addition, the water content of the stool rather than any solid matter should be tested.

If the etiology of the diarrhea seems to be viral, a carbohydrate-free formula (see Table 61.1) usually is well tolerated. However, such formulas result in ketosis and sometimes hypoglycemia; thus, some carbohydrate intake is necessary. In the hospitalized child, this can be provided intravenously. Most who do not require hospitalization usually will tolerate at least some sugar intake by the enteral route. In general, 0.5 g of glucose or sucrose per ounce of formula, provided intake is adequate but not excessive, is

TABLE 61.1. COMPOSITION (AMOUNT/100 kcal) OF SPECIAL FORMULAS FOR INFANTS WITH DERANGED INTESTINAL FUNCTION

COMPONENT	RCF[a][b]	PREGESTAMIL[c]	NUTRAMIGEN[c]	PORTAGEN[c]	ALIMENTUM[a]	PEDIASURE[a]
Protein (g)	4.95 (Soy protein isolate)	2.8 (Casein hydrolysate cyst(e)ine, tyrosine, tryptophan)	2.8 (Casein hydrolysate, cyst(e)ine, tyrosine, tryptophan)	3.5 (Sodium caseinate)	2.75 (Casein hydrolysate, cyst(e)ine, tyrosine, tryptophan)	3.0 (Low-lactose whey protein and sodium caseinate)
Fat (g)	8.91 (Soy and coconut oils)	5.6 (MCTs, corn, soy, high-oleic safflower oils)	3.9 (Corn and soy oils)	4.8 (MCTs, corn oil)	5.54 (MCTs, safflower and soy oils)	5.0 (MCTs, soy and high-oleic safflower oils)
Carbohydrate (g)	0	10.3 (Corn syrup solids, modified corn starch, dextrose)	13.4 (Corn syrup solids, modified corn starch)	11.5 (Corn syrup solids, sucrose)	10.2 (Sucrose, modified tapioca starch)	11.0 (Hydrolyzed cornstarch, sucrose)
Calcium (mg)	173	94	94	94	105	97
Phosphorus (mg)	124	63	63	70	75	80
Magnesium (mg)	12.4	10.9	10.9	20	7.5	20
Iron (mg)	0.37	1.88	1.88	1.88	1.8	1.4
Zinc (mg)	1.2	0.94	0.78	0.94	0.75	1.2
Manganese (μg)	50	31	31	125	30	250
Copper (μg)	124	94	94	156	75	100
Iodine (μg)	25	7	7	7	15	9.7
Selenium	3.5	2.3	2.3	—	2.8	2.3
Sodium (mg)	73	39	47	55	44	38
Potassium (mg)	180	109	109	125	118	131
Chloride (mg)	103	86	86	86	80	101
Vitamin A (IU)	500	380	310	780	300	257
Vitamin D (IU)	100	75	63	78	45	51
Vitamin E (IU)	5.0	3.8	3.1	3.1	3.0	2.3
Vitamin K (IU)	25	18.8	15.6	15.6	15	3.8
Thiamin (mg)	100	78	78	156	60	270
Riboflavin B$_2$	150	94	94	188	90	210
Vitamin B$_6$	100	63	63	210	60	260
Vitamin B$_{12}$	0.75	0.31	0.31	0.62	0.45	0.6
Niacin (μg)	2,230	1,250	1,250	2,100	1,350	1,690
Folic acid (μg)	25	15.6	15.6	15.6	15	37
Pantothenic acid	1,240	470	470	1,050	750	1,000
Vitamin C (mg)	13.6	11.7	8.1	8.1	9.0	10
Biotin (mg)	7.5	7.8	7.8	7.8	4.5	32
Choline (mg)	13	13.3	13.3	13.3	8	30
Inositol (mg)	8	4.7	4.7	4.7	5	8

MCT, medium-chain triglyceride; RCF, Ross Carbohydrate Free.
[a] Ross Laboratories, Columbus, OH.
[b] Note that this formula contains no carbohydrate, which accounts for the markedly different nutrient content of it versus the others shown.
[c] Mead Johnson Nutritional Division, Evansville, IN.

well tolerated and prevents ketosis and/or hypoglycemia. If this preparation is tolerated, the amount of carbohydrate can be increased daily or every other day as tolerance for carbohydrate increases. Once full carbohydrate content (i.e., approximately 2 g/oz) is tolerated, the patient usually can be switched to a carbohydrate-containing formula.

If the etiology of the diarrhea is a toxicogenic bacterium, feeding usually does not affect the volume of stool output. In many cases, in fact, a glucose-electrolyte solution seems to decrease the volume of stool output. In such patients, therefore, decisions concerning feeding must be based on clinical experience.

The tendency to avoid feedings containing lactose in all infants with diarrhea, regardless of etiology, probably is unnecessary. If stool pH is normal when the child is first seen and reducing substances are not present, lactase deficiency is an unlikely contributor to the diarrhea.

In a small number of patients, the acute episode of diarrhea does not resolve in the usual 4 to 5 days. In these, nutritional management becomes a much more important consideration. Although most infants can tolerate a 4- to 5-day period with little or no nutritional intake, few can tolerate a period of more than 2 weeks without becoming malnourished and developing secondary intestinal changes caused by both persistent diarrhea and malnutrition. Such infants are much more likely to develop secondary deficiencies of mucosal hydrolases (e.g., lactase deficiency, and less commonly, sucrase deficiency) and also monosaccharide intolerance. In these infants, management without hospitalization is much more difficult. Choice of formula again must be made on the basis of the suspected or culture-proven etiology of the diarrhea; in addition, the much greater likelihood of secondary mucosal hydrolase deficiencies must be taken into account. If small volumes of a particular formula are reasonably well tolerated, it frequently is possible to deliver sufficient amounts to meet nutritional needs by use of a continuous infusion technique (20). In small infants, of course, this usually requires hospitalization.

Many other congenital and/or acquired forms of chronic diarrhea (e.g., abetalipoproteinemia, celiac disease), if not managed appropriately, frequently result in the same secondary changes in mucosal function. Celiac disease (gluten-sensitive enteropathy), in particular, recently has been recognized to be far more common than was previously thought (21, 22). Strict adherence to a gluten-free diet is the cornerstone of therapy, although compliance is problematic, especially among adolescents diagnosed through mass screening, who may lack the typical symptoms (23). Fortunately, oat cereals recently have been found to be a safe substitute for gluten-rich cereals, for example, wheat, rye, and barley, and may facilitate management of children with this condition (24). A gluten-free diet is important for reasons other than symptom management. Bone mineral density is consistently lower in patients with celiac disease than in normal children, but can be improved through strict avoidance of gluten-containing foodstuffs (25, 26). Again, a recent Working Group Report from the First World Congress of Pediatric Gastroenterology, Hepatology, and Nutrition describes the current approach to treatment of these patients (27).

Crohn's Disease

Crohn's disease (regional enteritis) is another condition associated with chronic diarrhea and growth failure (28). The etiology of this chronic inflammatory disease of the full intestinal wall (but it can involve any area of the alimentary canal) remains uncertain. Anti-inflammatory agents, for example, corticosteroids, 5-aminosalicylate derivatives, have been the mainstay of conservative therapy, but are associated with an unacceptably high incidence of side effects in children. The observation that patients prepared for surgical management of complications related to Crohn's disease, for example, intestinal obstruction, perforation, abscesses, and fistulas, experienced improvement in symptoms led to the use of elemental and semielemental diets as a primary treatment. Although the precise mechanism of this improvement is unknown, it is clear that elemental enteral nutrition may achieve treatment results in children, although not in adults, that are comparable to those obtained with anti-inflammatory agents (29). Nutritional management of Crohn's disease in children has been reviewed recently, and, once again, a recent Working Group Report from the First World Congress of Pediatric Gastroenterology, Hepatology, and Nutrition outlines the challenges that remain in the treatment of pediatric patients with this illness (30, 31).

Nutritional management of other chronic diarrheas, in general, is similar to that described earlier and must be coordinated with the usual medical management of these conditions. Although diet is a major aspect of the therapy of most chronic diarrheas, a detailed discussion of this aspect of therapy is beyond the scope of this chapter.

Most acute episodes of vomiting are of short duration and present few nutritional problems. However, chronic vomiting accompanies a number of conditions. The most common of these conditions intrinsic to the gastrointestinal tract is gastroesophageal reflux. To some extent, this condition is physiologic in infancy; however, it assumes pathologic significance if it results in failure to thrive and/or recurrent pulmonary aspiration. Clinical practice guidelines for evaluation and treatment of gastroesophageal reflux in infants and children have recently been published by the North American Society of Pediatric Gastroenterology and Nutrition (32).

In the early stages, nutritional management of this condition includes maintaining the patient in an upright position during and immediately after feeding and reassuring caregivers that the persistent vomiting is causing no harm so long as the infant is gaining weight normally and is not having respiratory symptoms. Although a prone position during sleep reduces the frequency of gastroesophageal reflux, it is associated with a higher rate of sudden infant death syndrome, and therefore should be avoided. In formula-fed infants with vomiting, a 1- to 2-week trial of a hypoallergenic formula is warranted. Thickening agents, for example, rice cereal, do not decrease the episodes of reflux, but may decrease the episodes of vomiting. In children and adolescents, left-sided positioning and elevation of the head of the bed during sleep, and abstinence from caffeine, chocolate, spicy foods, tobacco, and alcohol, may help reduce symptoms. Histamine receptor antagonists and proton pump inhibitors may also relieve pain and promote healing. Prokinetic agents, for example, cisapride, may also be used in symptomatic treatment, but their use must be balanced against the potential risk of cardiac arrhythmias. If either growth failure or a decrease in weight for height develops despite optimal medical management, remedial nutritional therapy is indicated, that is, feedings delivered continuously into the duodenum or jejunum to minimize the risk of further reflux. In many patients, corrective surgery, that is, Nissen fundoplication, is necessary.

Short Bowel Syndrome

Functionally, short bowel syndrome can be considered in the same way as chronic diarrhea. In this condition, the alterations of gastrointestinal motility, secretion, digestion, and absorption are secondary to massive small intestinal loss rather than to bacterial and/or viral invasion and the secondary effects of these organisms and malnutrition. In general, the severity of the short bowel syndrome is related inversely to the length of the remaining intestinal segment; however, loss of the ileocecal valve, which acts as a physiologic sphincter to slow transit time and prevent backwash ileitis, also increases severity (33, 34). Specific symptoms also result from removal of specific segments of intestine. Because disaccharidase activity is greater in jejunal cells and because cholecystokinin and other intestinal hormones are secreted by jejunal sites, removal of the jejunum results in more severe carbohydrate malabsorption, and perhaps in decreased biliary and pancreatic secretions as well as deranged motility. Ileal loss, conversely, results in loss of both bile salt uptake and absorption of vitamin B_{12}. In general, the ileum's potential for adaptation seems to be inferior to that of the jejunum. Thus, loss of jejunum usually is better tolerated than loss of the ileum.

The early phase of the short bowel syndrome immediately after massive resection usually is associated with massive fluid and electrolyte losses, making effective enteral alimentation impossible. Thus, during both this phase and the early part of the intermediate phase, the majority of the nutrient requirements must be provided parenterally.

As the remaining small bowel gradually adapts, enteral intake usually can be advanced, but this must proceed slowly. In general, continuous feeding via either an indwelling nasogastric or a gastrostomy tube is better tolerated during this phase than is bolus feeding (35). In addition, elemental formulas (see Table 61.1) generally are better tolerated than nonelemental formulas.

Eventually, maximum adaptation is achieved and more complex proteins and carbohydrates can be introduced. Even during this final phase, however, frequent small feedings may be necessary. During all phases, pharmacologic manipulations (e.g., cholestyramine to chelate bile acids, loperamide and/or paregoric to slow transit time, antibiotics to eradicate significant bacterial overgrowth) may provide symptomatic as well as physiologic improvement.

The pace of recovery from short bowel syndrome is dependent on a number of factors. The length of residual intestine is more important than the presence of an intact ileocecal valve, whereas early use of breast milk and/or amino acid–based formulas, particularly those supplemented with glutamine and/or long-chain fatty acids, are thought by some to stimulate mucosal growth and accelerate the pace of intestinal adaptation (36–40).

Adaptation proceeds by two mechanisms, hypertrophy of the remaining bowel and hyperplasia of the intestinal mucosa, which act synergistically to increase the total intestinal surface area. Conversely, bacterial overgrowth may slow the pace of intestinal adaptation (41). Prompt restoration of intestinal continuity and early feeding both exert a protective effect on hepatic function that may slow development of total parenteral nutrition–associated cholestasis and ultimately secondary biliary cirrhosis, a major source of morbidity and mortality during the intermediate and late phases of intestinal adaptation (39, 42). Regardless, once cholestasis is well established, most often by systemic infections, reversal via timely weaning from parenteral nutrition or via pharmacologic (cholecystokinin-octapeptide) and/or surgical (biliary irrigation) means must be considered to prevent progression to cirrhosis, hepatic failure, and death (43–45).

Despite these advances, recovery from short bowel syndrome is ultimately dependent on the affected infant's achieving sufficient growth that caloric requirements decrease from the 115 to 125 kcal/kg/day needed to support the more rapid rate of growth in early infancy to the 80 to 90 kcal/kg/day required to support growth after the first birthday. In other words, complete weaning from parenteral support is unlikely to occur until the total intestinal surface area has increased sufficiently to allow the infant's gradually decreasing energy requirements to be met through enteral support alone. For patients in whom optimal medical management fails, surgical bowel lengthening procedures, that is, the Bianchi and serial transverse enteroplasty procedures, and in severe cases, small intestinal transplantation (combined with liver transplantation for patients with end-stage liver disease) may be required.

Once more, a recent Working Group Report from the First World Congress of Pediatric Gastroenterology, Hepatology, and Nutrition discussed the problems facing those who care for infants and children with short bowel syndrome and related conditions, for example, congenitally or functionally short guts (46).

Human Immunodeficiency Virus Infection/Acquired Immunodeficiency Syndrome

Maintenance of nutritional status is essential to delay the progression of human immunodeficiency virus (HIV) disease from latent infection to immune compromise. Antiretroviral therapy and supportive care of this chronic illness constitute the definitive therapy of HIV/acquired immunodeficiency syndrome (AIDS), but nutritional support is critical to the integrity of the body cell mass, which is adversely affected by HIV wasting syndrome, a major component of the disease. Without adequate nutritional support, wasting leads to malnutrition, which predisposes to superinfection, further worsening nutritional status. In addition, in advanced disease states, gastrointestinal derangements may further compromise adequate nutrient intake. It is hardly surprising given these synergistic elements that approximately 90% of all children with HIV/AIDS are malnourished at some time during the course of their disease (47, 48).

The malnutrition associated with HIV/AIDS is multifactorial. Oral, gingival, and esophageal lesions, for example, ulcers, periodontitis, and thrush, can make eating a distasteful and painful experience. Gastritis, nausea, vomiting, and abdominal pain, caused by either infection or irritation from medications, can adversely affect appetite. Pancreatitis, which typically presents with vomiting, is a known side effect of dideoxyinosine and pentamidine. Chronic diarrhea may also cause ongoing nutrient loss. Finally, encephalopathy, which may be present in as many as one third of patients with advanced disease (49), can also cause an inadequate energy intake. However, even those HIV-infected children with grossly normal dietary intakes seem to gain weight more slowly than do uninfected controls (50). Although this may be caused at least in part by mucosal damage and impaired absorption resulting from either HIV or enteric pathogens, impaired energy use has also been implicated as a possible cause (51).

Nutritional support of children with HIV/AIDS should begin with oral dietary supplements. An energy intake of as much as 50% more than the estimated requirement of normal children may be required for adequate weight gain. If these intakes fail to support relatively normal growth, enteral formula supplements may be considered. In selected refractory cases, gastrostomy tube insertion (percutaneous, laparoscopic, or surgical) may be necessary to achieve sufficient intake. This has the added advantage that distasteful medications also can be delivered via this route (52, 53). Megestrol acetate may stimulate appetite in HIV-infected children for whom gastrostomy tube insertion is not an option (54). Growth hormone also has been used in selected patients with some success. Total parenteral nutrition should be considered only if all other options fail.

The benefits of nutritional support in HIV/AIDS are not limited merely to prevention of growth failure. Recent evidence indicates that nutritional intervention may restore intestinal absorption and increase CD4 cell numbers (55). Thus, children at risk for failure to thrive, that is, children with a history of pneumonia, maternal illicit drug use during pregnancy, lower CD4 cell count, exposure to antiretroviral therapy by 3 months of age, and measurable viral load, should be candidates for nutritional support (56). As before, a recent Working Group Report from the First World Congress of Pediatric Gastroenterology, Hepatology, and Nutrition focused on modern concepts and future directions in the management of HIV disease in infants and children (57).

Other Conditions

Although a full discussion of the nutritional management of children with critical illnesses, developmental disabilities, and feeding disorders is beyond the scope of this chapter, recent studies address each of these complex problems. Critically ill pediatric patients on mechanical ventilatory support should be nourished with enteral or parenteral diets high in protein and fat but low in carbohydrate (58). Nutritional management of children with developmental disabilities may decrease disability-related morbidity (59). Finally, hospitalized infants and young children may be no less subject to feeding disorders than they are to inadequate nutrition, and are best managed using a multidisciplinary team (60).

GENERAL APPROACH TO NUTRITIONAL THERAPY

Accurate determination of nutritional status obviously is the first step in all types of nutritional therapy. However, assessment of the nutritional status of infants is difficult (61). In part, this is because there is no precise definition of malnutrition, and in part because the earliest changes of malnutrition are subtle adaptations that tend to ameliorate the effects of malnutrition. Nonetheless, some objective evaluation of nutritional status should be applied to every child who is a potential candidate for nutritional therapy. If for no other reason, this evaluation provides a baseline for monitoring the results of therapy.

Many anthropometric and biochemical assessment techniques are available; their specific advantages, disadvantages, and limitations have been discussed extensively (61). In general, no single test or combination of tests is ideal. Indeed, clinical judgment, based on knowledge of the disease process and the status of the body's nutritional reserves, seems to be as reliable as any of the commonly used "objective" tests (62). In our experience, assessment of weight in relation to length or height is one of the most useful indices of nutritional status. A child who falls below the tenth percentile on this standard curve, regardless of either weight for age or height (length) for age, can be assumed to be malnourished and in need of nutritional therapy. However, although weight for length or height is easier to use, body mass index for age recently has been advocated because it reflects changes in the weight for stature relation with age (63).

The situation of the child whose weight is appropriate for length or height (i.e., the wasted child) but whose weight and height are low for age (i.e., the stunted child) is more problematic (64). There is no convincing evidence that such a child is malnourished and in need of aggressive nutritional intervention. Conversely, an attempt to permit the child to achieve his or her growth potential is warranted. This usually requires both a nutritional history and a more extensive medical evaluation, including evaluation of endocrinologic status.

In general, the approach advocated for nutritional management of the low-birth-weight (LBW) infant (see Chapter 51) is equally applicable to any malnourished infant or child—indeed, for any infant or child with an underlying condition predisposing to development of malnutrition. Initially, particularly in less severely affected children, attempts should be made to increase nutrient intake by conventional means. If this approach is unsuccessful, one of several commercially available supplements may be used. However, these often replace usual food intake and may not achieve the desired result of increased total intake. Moreover, most of the products currently available were designed for adults and are not optimal for pediatric patients. One exception is Pediasure® (Ross Laboratories, Columbus, OH) (see Table 61.1).

If conventional foods are not tolerated, use of special formulas or supplements, and perhaps delivery by tube, either as a bolus or continuously, are the next steps. The choice of both formula and method of delivery must be dictated by the patient's underlying condition. Tube feedings can be given throughout the day or only during part of the day (e.g., at night), depending on the patient's age, condition, and nutritional status. If the patient's condition (e.g., pulmonary disease) makes use of an indwelling nasal tube inadvisable, a gastrostomy tube, inserted percutaneously, laparoscopically, or surgically, should be considered. If gastrointestinal tolerance of even elemental formulas is severely limited, parenteral nutrients may be used, either as the sole source of nutrition or as a supplement to tolerated enteral nutrient combinations.

PARENTERAL NUTRITION

The now-widespread use of parenteral nutrition usually is considered to be one of the major contributing factors to the current reasonably low mortality of infants born with surgically correctable lesions of the gastrointestinal tract (e.g., omphalocele, gastroschisis, intestinal atresias) as well as of infants with short bowel syndrome and intractable diarrhea (65). Although the role of parenteral nutrient delivery in decreasing the mortality and morbidity of other groups of pediatric patients (e.g., LBW infants) is less clear, the technique is used in a wide variety of pediatric patients. Moreover, despite the many hazards of the technique, most agree that the obvious anabolism that can be achieved with parenteral delivery of nutrients is preferable to the inevitable continuation of catabolism if delivery of adequate nutrients by other routes is impossible. This is particularly true if careful attention is paid to every aspect of the technique, thereby minimizing its hazards and maximizing its benefits.

Route of Administration

Parenteral nutrients can be infused by either central vein or peripheral vein. An energy intake of 70 to 80 kcal/kg/day can be provided consistently and safely by the peripheral venous route, but for obvious reasons, the duration of this type of delivery is limited. Much greater intakes (100–120 kcal/kg/day) can be delivered for a longer period by the central venous route. Acceptable intakes of all other nutrients are possible by either route.

Although the advantages and disadvantages of these two routes of delivery are frequently discussed, both are efficacious when used in the appropriate circumstances. In general, the time that parenteral nutrients are likely to be required and the nutrient needs of the patient should be the determining factors for choosing one route of administration over the other. If it is likely that parenteral nutrients will be required for more than approximately 10 days, central venous delivery usually is preferable.

In LBW infants, the infusate frequently is delivered by umbilical vessel catheters. Although this route of delivery is convenient, it cannot be recommended. The flow characteristics of the umbilical vessels do not permit sufficient dilution of the nutrient infusate to circumvent intimal damage. In addition, the incidence of thrombosis with umbilical catheters is quite high. Further, malposition of these catheters can result in severe consequences. Moreover, the incidence of sepsis seems to be greater when nutrients are delivered by umbilical vessels than when delivered by either central or peripheral vein.

The Nutrient Infusate

The nutrient infusate should include a nitrogen source as well as sufficient energy (glucose and lipid), electrolytes, minerals, and vitamins. Suitable infusates for both central vein and peripheral vein delivery are shown in Table 61.2. Although these are acceptable for most infants and children, modification may be required to reflect the specific needs of individual patients.

TABLE 61.2. COMPOSITION OF SUITABLE PARENTERAL NUTRITION INFUSATE(S)

COMPONENT	AMOUNT/kg/d
Amino acids	3.0–4.0 g
Energy	60–120 kcal
Glucose[a]	15–30 g
Lipid[b]	0.5–3.0 g
Electrolytes and minerals	
Sodium (as chloride)	2–4 mEq
Potassium (as phosphate and chloride)[c]	2–4 mEq
Calcium (as gluconate)	1.5–2.0 mmol
Magnesium (as sulfate)	0.25 mEq
Phosphorus (as potassium phosphate)[c]	1.5 mmol
Trace minerals	See Table 61.4
Vitamins	See Table 61.5
Volume	100–150 mL

[a] For peripheral vein infusion, glucose concentration should not exceed 10 to 12.5%.
[b] Lipid must be infused separately (see text).
[c] Potassium, as phosphate, should be limited to 2.5 mEq/kg/d (approximately 1.7 mmol phosphate) unless chemical monitoring suggests the need for more phosphate; if only additional potassium is required, it should be provided as the chloride salt.

Crystalline amino acid mixtures usually are used as the nitrogen source of parenteral nutrition infusates. Several such mixtures are available (Table 61.3); all contain most essential amino acids (exceptions are cystine and tyrosine, which are either unstable or insoluble in aqueous solution) and varying amounts of nonessential amino acids. An amino acid intake of 3.0 to 4.0 g/kg/day is recommended. Higher intakes, although tolerated by most infants, are more likely to result in elevated plasma amino acid concentra-

tions and azotemia. Some advocate amino acid intakes of less than 2.5 g/kg/day for the LBW infant, particularly during the initial few days of therapy when nonprotein energy intake is low (because of glucose and lipid intolerance). Recent studies suggest that there is no reason to advocate this practice, even if concomitant energy intake is quite low (66).

Glucose is the preferred nonlipid parenteral energy source; however, the ability of some infants to metabolize it is limited. Many infants, particularly during the early period of parenteral nutrition, develop hyperglycemia and osmotic diuresis with concomitant urinary loss of electrolytes when the amount of glucose infused exceeds tolerance. Careful, continuous administration of small doses of insulin seems to alleviate the problem of glucose intolerance in LBW infants, thereby permitting administration of much greater glucose intakes (67).

Most LBW infants tolerate 5 to 7% solutions of dextrose (3.5–5.0 mg/kg/min or 17–25 kcal/kg/day) if volume is limited to 100 mL/kg/day), even during the first few days of life; thus, in very small and/or unstable infants, it is wise to begin parenteral nutrition with these lower glucose intakes and increase the intake as the infant's tolerance for glucose improves. In older, more stable infants, an initial glucose intake of 15 g/kg/day (about 50 kcal/kg/day) usually is well tolerated. This intake can be delivered easily by the peripheral route without exceeding a glucose concentration of 10%. With central venous delivery, much greater intakes (i.e., 25–30 g/kg/day or 85–102 kcal/kg/day) are eventually tolerated. Even in the most stable patients, however, these higher intakes should be achieved gradually with daily increments of no more than 5 g/kg/day. In

TABLE 61.3. AMINO ACID CONTENT (mg/2.5 g) OF COMMERCIALLY AVAILABLE AMINO ACID MIXTURES

AMINO ACID	AMINOSYN[a]	AMINOSYN-Pf[a]	TRAVASOL (B)[b]	NOVAMINE[c]	FREAMINE III[d]	TROPHAMINE[d]
Isoleucine	180	191	120	124	175	204
Leucine	235	297	155	174	228	350
Lysine	180	170	145	198	182	204
Methionine	100	45	145	124	132	83
Phenylalanine	110	107	155	174	140	121
Threonine	130	129	105	124	100	104
Tryptophan	40	45	45	41	38	50
Valine	200	161	115	162	165	196
Histidine	75	79	109	147	71	121
Cystine	0	0	0	<12	<6	<8
Tyrosine	11	16	10	9	0	58
Taurine	0	18	0	0	0	6
Alanine	320	175	518	353	178	133
Aspartic acid	0	132	0	74	0	79
Glutamic acid	0	206	0	124	0	125
Glycine	320	96	518	174	350	92
Proline	215	204	104	147	280	171
Serine	105	124	0	100	148	96
Arginine	245	308	258	247	238	304

[a] Abbott Laboratories, North Chicago, IL.
[b] Clintec, Deerfield, IL.
[c] Kabi-Vitrum, Franklin, OH.
[d] B. Braun, Irvine, CA.

all patients, close monitoring of glucose tolerance is necessary as glucose intake is being increased (see later). Once achieved, the higher intakes usually are well tolerated so long as the patient's condition remains stable.

Electrolyte requirements vary from patient to patient; thus, the amounts suggested in Table 61.2 should not be interpreted as absolute requirements. Adjustments are often necessary and should be made on the basis of close monitoring (see later).

The amounts of calcium and phosphorus required for optimal skeletal mineralization, that is, 100 to 120 and 60 to 75 mg/kg/day, respectively, in the normally growing LBW infant, usually cannot be incorporated into the parenteral nutrition infusate because of the chemical incompatibility of calcium and phosphate. In general, the amounts suggested in Table 61.2 are compatible and cause no problems over the short term. However, if parenteral nutrition is required for weeks to months, skeletal mineralization may be inadequate. This is particularly true for the LBW infant.

The addition of trace minerals to the infusate is recommended if exclusive parenteral nutrition is likely to exceed 7 to 10 days. Suggested intakes (68) are given in Table 61.4. Many advocate including zinc and copper from the outset.

Parenteral vitamin requirements also are not known with certainty. Obviously, the usual dietary reference intakes may not apply when administration is by the parenteral route. Recommended parenteral intakes are given in Table 61.5 (68). Currently, however, a multivitamin preparation that provides the recommended intakes of all vitamins is not available. Intakes provided by the most commonly used pediatric multivitamin mixture also are shown in Table 61.5.

TABLE 61.4. RECOMMENDED PARENTERAL INTAKES (AMOUNT/kg/d) OF TRACE MINERALS[a]

TRACE MINERAL[a]	PRETERM INFANTS	TERM INFANTS AND CHILDREN[b]
Zinc (μg)	400	250 (5,000)
Copper (μg)	20	20 (300)
Selenium (μg)	2.0	2.0 (30)
Chromium (μg)	0.2	0.2 (5)
Manganese (μg)	1.0	1.0 (50)
Molybdenum (μg)	0.25	0.25 (5)
Iodide (μg)	1.0	1.0 (1)
Iron[c]		

[a] If parenteral nutrients are used as a supplement for tolerated enteral feedings or as sole source of nutrients for fewer than 4 weeks, only zinc and perhaps copper are needed.
[b] Maximum recommended intake per day is shown in parentheses.
[c] Iron dextran (1–2 mg/L) has been used safely in adults, but reported experience in children, particularly infants, is limited. Estimated requirements, based on the assumption that 10% of the recommended enteral intake is absorbed, are 100 and 200 μg/kg/d, respectively, for the term and preterm infant.

From Greene HL, Hambidge KM, Schanler R et al. Am J Clin Nutr 1988;48:1324–42, with permission.

TABLE 61.5. SUGGESTED PARENTERAL INTAKES OF VITAMINS

VITAMIN	PRETERM INFANTS[a] (AMOUNT/kg/d)	TERM INFANTS AND CHILDREN[b] (AMOUNT/d)
A (μg)	500	700
E (mg)	2.8	7
K (μg)	80	200
D (μg)	4 (160 IU)	10
Ascorbic acid (mg)	25	80
Thiamin (mg)	0.35	1.2
Riboflavin (mg)	0.15	1.4
Pyridoxine Cl (mg)	0.18	1.0
Niacin (mg)	6.8	17
Pantothenate (mg)	2.0	5
Biotin (μg)	6.0	20
Folate (μg)	56	140
B_{12} (μg)	0.3	1.0

[a] Total daily dose should not exceed that recommended for term infants and children. A dose of 2 mL reconstituted MVI-Pediatric (Armour Pharmaceutical Co, Chicago, IL) provides the following intakes (amount/kg/day): Vitamin A, 280 mg; vitamin E, 2.8 μg; vitamin K, 80 μg; vitamin D, 4 μg (160 IU); ascorbic acid, 32 mg; thiamin, 0.48 mg; riboflavin, 0.56 mg; pyridoxine, 0.4 mg; niacin, 6.8 mg; pantothenate, 2.0 mg; biotin, 8.0 μg; folate, 56 μg; vitamin B_{12}, 0.4 μg.
[b] These amounts are provided by one vial of reconstituted MVI-Pediatric.

From Greene HL, Hambidge KM, Schanler R et al. Am J Clin Nutr 1988;48:1324–42, with permission.

Use of Parenteral Lipid Emulsions

Infants who receive fat-free parenteral nutrition, particularly LBW infants and nutritionally depleted infants, develop classical essential fatty acid (EFA) deficiency very quickly (i.e., days) when growth and/or regrowth is initiated (69). Thus, use of lipid emulsions to prevent this deficiency, which becomes apparent biochemically (i.e., a ratio of eicosatrienoic to arachidonic acid of >0.25) before clinical signs appear, is desirable. Parenteral lipid emulsions also are a useful source of energy. Emulsions of either soybean oil (Intralipid®, Chicago, IL; Kabi-Vitrum, Stockholm, Sweden; Travamulsion®, Travenol Laboratories, Chicago, IL; Liposyn III®, Abbott Laboratories, Chicago, IL) or a mixture of safflower and soybean oils (Liposyn II®, Abbott Laboratories) are available in both 10% and 20% concentrations. A dose of only 0.5 g/kg/day of soybean oil emulsion is sufficient to prevent classic EFA deficiency; because the linoleic acid content of the emulsion of soy and safflower oils is even greater, a smaller dose may be sufficient. The linolenic acid content of the latter emulsion is somewhat lower but probably is adequate, although not optimal.

All infants, including LBW infants, probably can tolerate the small dose of parenteral lipid emulsion necessary to prevent EFA deficiency. However, the ability of an individual infant to tolerate a larger dose is quite variable. In general, the ability to metabolize intravenous fat emulsions is related directly to maturity (70), but the stressed and/or malnourished patient (i.e., the small-for-gestational-age LBW infant and the nutritionally depleted older child) also may have difficulty metabolizing these preparations (71).

Administration of doses of fat emulsion in excess of the infant's ability to metabolize it results in accumulation of triglycerides in the blood stream. This, in turn, may decrease pulmonary diffusion capacity, presumably secondary to accumulation of small lipid droplets within the pulmonary capillaries (72). It also results in recruitment of the reticuloendothelial system for lipid clearance, and hence in lipid accumulation in these cells (73). This lipid accumulation is a likely explanation for the impaired host defense mechanisms reported in patients receiving lipid emulsions (74). Metabolism of the infused lipid results in increased serum concentrations of free fatty acids, which compete with bilirubin and other substances for binding to albumin (75). Thus, administration of large doses of lipid emulsion may be hazardous for infants with pulmonary disease, infection, and/or hyperbilirubinemia.

Considering the difficulties of monitoring serum concentrations of both triglycerides and free fatty acids, it probably is wise to limit the dose of lipid emulsion given to patients who are likely to be intolerant to 0.5 to 1.0 g/kg/day, at least initially. In most other patients, a dose of 3 g/kg/day or more usually is well tolerated; however, even in these patients, it is wise to begin with a smaller dose (e.g., 1–1.5 g/kg/day) and increase the dose slowly. In LBW infants, administration of lipid emulsion should be initiated with a relatively low dose (0.5 g/kg/day) and increased gradually to a maximum dose of 3 g/kg/day. In all patients, the emulsion should be infused continuously throughout the day.

The 20% soybean oil emulsion seems to be cleared more rapidly than the 10% emulsion, and therefore is less likely to cause hypertriglyceridemia (76). Hyperphospholipidemia and hypercholesterolemia, both of which occur routinely in patients receiving the 10% soybean emulsion, do not occur with use of the 20% emulsion (76). The explanation presumably is the lower phospholipid–triglyceride ratio of the 20% versus the 10% emulsion.

Because the size of the lipid particles of the emulsions (0.4–0.5 μm) exceeds the pore size of an effective filter (0.22 μm), filters should not be used for the infusion of fat emulsions. Nor should the emulsions be mixed directly with other components of the infusate. This practice, which seems to be relatively common, may not destroy the emulsion but it certainly inhibits detection of chemical incompatibilities within the complicated infusate (e.g., precipitation of calcium phosphate). The potential hazards of the latter possibility are compounded by the fact that filters cannot be used.

Complications of TPN. TPN is associated with a number of complications, both catheter (or infusion)-related and metabolic.

Catheter (infusion)-related complications include vein catheter insertion, pneumothorax, hemothorax, injury to an artery and/or hematoma at the time of catheter insertion. Thrombosis, dislodgment, perforation, infusion leaks (peri-

cardial, pleural, mediastinal) and infections also may occur reported during use of central vein catheters. The most common infusion-related problem is infection. Phlebitis and soft tissue sloughs are the most frequent complications of peripheral vein infusions. All of these complications can be controlled but it is difficult to prevent them entirely. Careful attention to care of the central catheter, including frequent dressing changes, is particularly important for controlling infection. Careful frequent observation of the infusion site is necessary to prevent infiltration of infusates delivered by peripheral vein as well as to insure proper long-term function of central vein catheters.

Metabolic complications result either from the limited metabolic capacity of the patient for the various components of the nutrient infusate or from the infusate itself. The metabolic complications most commonly observed and their probable causes are listed in Table 61.6. One of the more troublesome of these is the occurrence of abnormal plasma amino acid patterns with use of many of the currently available amino acid mixtures (77). Cyst(e)ine and tyrosine, both of which are thought to be essential amino acids for the newborn, and perhaps for all patients receiving parenteral nutrients, are unstable and/or only sparingly soluble; hence, none of the currently marketed mixtures contains appreciable amounts of these amino acids (see Table 61.3). Further, all result in very low plasma

TABLE 61.6. METABOLIC COMPLICATIONS OF TOTAL PARENTERAL NUTRITION AND THEIR PROBABLE ETIOLOGIES

COMPLICATION	PROBABLE ETIOLOGY
Disorders related to metabolic capacity of patient	
Hyperglycemia	Excessive intake (either excessive concentration or infusion rate), change in metabolic state (e.g., infection, surgical stress)
Hypoglycemia	Sudden cessation of infusion
Azotemia	Excessive nitrogen intake
Electrolyte disorders	Excessive or inadequate intake
Mineral disorders	Excessive or inadequate intake
Vitamin disorders	Excessive or inadequate intake
Essential fatty acid deficiency	Failure to provide essential fatty acids
Hyperlipidemia	Excessive intake, change in metabolic state (e.g., stress, sepsis)
Disorders related to infusate components	
Metabolic acidosis	Use of hydrochloride salts of amino acids (e.g., cysteine)
Hyperammonemia	Inadequate arginine intake
Abnormal plasma aminograms	Amino acid pattern of nitrogen source
Hepatic disorders	Unknown; suggested etiologies include prematurity, malnutrition, sepsis, inadequate stimulation of bile flow, toxic effects of amino acids, specific amino acid deficiency, excessive amino acid and/or carbohydrate intake, and nonspecific response to lack of feeding

cyst(e)ine and tyrosine concentrations (77). Many available mixtures also have large amounts of only a few nonessential amino acids (e.g., glycine) rather than a mixture of all nonessential amino acids (see Table 61.3); thus, extremely high plasma concentrations of the amino acid(s) present in excess are commonly seen.

Whether these abnormal plasma amino acid patterns are hazardous, or even undesirable, is not known. However, considering the well-known relationship between abnormally high plasma amino acid concentrations and mental retardation in infants with inborn errors of metabolism (e.g., phenylketonuria) as well as the relationship between inadequate intake of a specific amino acid and a low plasma concentration of that amino acid, normalization of plasma amino acid patterns seems warranted. Some of the newer amino acid mixtures (e.g., TrophAmine, B. Braun, Irvine, CA) accomplish this to a large extent (78).

Although some of the metabolic complications are unavoidable, many can be controlled by careful monitoring and appropriate adjustment of the infusate. A suggested monitoring schedule is given in Table 61.7. The monitoring required to ensure safe and efficacious use of lipid emulsions is the most problematic. The most common practice (i.e., inspection of the plasma for turbidity) may not reliably detect elevated plasma triglyceride and free fatty acid concentrations (79). For this purpose, actual chemical determinations are required. Because this usually is not practical, a reasonable compromise is to observe the plasma frequently (at least three times per day initially) for evidence of lipid accumulation (primarily triglyceride) and to measure triglyceride and free fatty acids less frequently. Careful monitoring is particularly important while the lipid dose is being increased, while the infant is unstable, and when a change in the infant's condition occurs. If turbidity of the plasma is observed, the rate of infusion should be decreased or the infusion stopped completely until the turbidity clears. Usually, infusion can then be resumed at a lower rate. Once the desired dose of intravenous fat is achieved, serum turbidity should be checked once per day (unless the patient becomes unstable) and actual determinations of serum triglyceride and free fatty acid concentrations should be made weekly.

Weaning Infants from Total Parenteral Nutrition

In most infants, administration of parenteral nutrients need not interfere with introducing enteral feedings as soon as they are likely to be tolerated. Once started, the volume of enteral feedings can be advanced as tolerated by the infant and the volume of the parenteral nutrition infusate can be decreased. During the period of combined enteral and parenteral nutrition, care should be taken to ensure both that nutrient requirements are met as nearly as possible and that tolerance for both fluids and nutrients is not exceeded. This requires careful attention to the total (parenteral plus enteral) intake and frequent adjustment downward of the parenteral intake as enteral intake increases.

Home Parenteral Nutrition

Today, most patients who require parenteral nutrients for a long period of time leave the hospital and receive this therapy at home. Considering the many difficulties of in-hospital parenteral nutrition (see earlier), the potential problems of total parenteral nutrition at home seem formidable. Nonetheless, both patients who can tolerate some enteral intake and patients who can tolerate only parenteral nutrients have been treated successfully at home for several months to years. In many cases, sufficient nutrients can be administered during only a portion of the day, allowing the older patient to pursue reasonably normal daytime activities and the younger patient (as well as his or her parents) to sleep with little danger of accidental disconnection of the infusion system. Small portable infusion pumps are available such that the necessary apparatus can be enclosed in vests, backpacks, and so on, allowing even the patient who requires constant infusion of parenteral nutrients to pursue a reasonably normal life. Obviously, home parenteral nutrition is more likely to be successful for the older child, adolescent, or adult. However, with careful patient (and parent) selection, young infants also can be managed quite successfully at home.

TABLE 61.7. SUGGESTED MONITORING SCHEDULE DURING TOTAL PARENTERAL NUTRITION

VARIABLES TO BE MONITORED	SUGGESTED FREQUENCY (per wk)[a]	
	INITIAL PERIOD[a]	LATER PERIOD[a]
Growth variables		
Weight	7	7
Length	1	1
Head circumference	1	1
Metabolic variables		
Plasma electrolytes	3–4	2
Plasma calcium, magnesium, phosphorus	2	1
Blood acid-base status	3–4	1
Blood urea nitrogen	2	1
Plasma albumin	1	1
Liver function studies	1	1
Serum lipids[b]		
Hemoglobin	2	2
Urinary glucose	2–6/d	2/d
Variables for detection of infection		
Clinical observations (activity, temperature, etc)	Daily	Daily
White blood cell count	As indicated	As indicated
Cultures	As indicated	As indicated

[a] Initial period is the time during which the desired energy intake is being achieved or the time(s) of metabolic instability.
[b] See text.

In general, the catheter used for home total parenteral nutrition is the Broviac catheter, which can be used for several months, and frequently for years. Standard nutrient infusates are obtained from the hospital pharmacy or from a number of commercial concerns and are stored in a small home refrigerator. Catheter care is managed by the patient or by a family member after careful training before patient discharge.

All of the usual metabolic and catheter-related complications of parenteral nutrition can occur at home as well as in the hospital. However, patients who can be managed successfully with home parenteral nutrition usually have reached the point at which requirements are reasonably stable. Thus, less frequent monitoring is sufficient. Nonetheless, successful home parenteral nutrition, particularly for the young pediatric patient, requires frequent outpatient visits as well as frequent telephone contact. Some commercial home parenteral nutrition services include frequent home visits by a nurse.

Overall, administration of parenteral nutrients at home has been much more successful than initially envisioned. Certainly, the practice improves the quality of life for patients who require long-term parenteral nutrition. However, it must be remembered that the purpose of parenteral nutrition is to provide the necessary nutrients transiently while the compromised gastrointestinal function necessitating use of parenteral nutrition recovers. Some patients may never be able to survive without parenteral nutrition, but attempts to increase enteral intake must continue. In our experience, this is not always the case; rather, discharge from the hospital often is viewed as the goal of therapy, and once achieved, attempts to increase the tolerance of enteral intake slows or stops. It is important that this attitude not become more common.

REFERENCES

1. Bines JE, Truby HD, Armstrong DS et al. J Pediatr 2002;140: 527–33.
2. Lai H–C, Kosorok MR, Laxova A et al. Pediatrics 2000;105: 53–61.
3. Zemel BS, Jawad AF, FitzSimmons S et al. J Pediatr 2000;137: 374–80.
4. Peterson ML, Jacobs DR, Milla CE. Pediatrics 2003;112:588–92.
5. Konstan MW, Butler SM, Wohl MEB et al. J Pediatr 2003;142: 624–30.
6. Mansell AL, Andersen JC, Muttart CR et al. J Pediatr 1984;109: 700–5.
7. Farrell PM, Kosorok MR, Rock MJ et al. Pediatrics 2001;107: 1–13.
8. Stark LJ, Mulvihill MM, Jelalian E et al. Pediatrics 1997;99: 665–71.
9. Powers SW, Patton SR, Byars KC et al. Pediatrics 2002;109(5). Available at: http://www.pediatrics.org/cgi/content/full/109/5/e75.
10. Hardin DS, Ellis KJ, Dyson M et al. J Pediatr 2001;139:636–42.
11. Eubanks V, Koppersmith N, Wooldridge N et al. J Pediatr 2002; 140:439–44.
12. McNaughton SA, Shepard RW, Greer RG et al. J Pediatr 2000; 136:188–94.
13. Wilson DC, Rashid M, Durie PR et al. J Pediatr 2001;138:851–5.
14. Couper R, Belli D, Durie P et al. J Pediatr Gastroenterol Nutr 2002;35:S213–33.
15. Borowitz D, Baker RD, Stallings V. J Pediatr Gastroenterol Nutr 2002;35:246–59.
16. Alam NH, Hamadani JD, Dewan N et al. J Pediatr 2003;143: 614–9.
17. Diop EHI, Dossou NI, Ndour MM et al. Am J Clin Nutr 2003; 78:302–7.
18. Udall JN, Bhutta ZA, Firmansyah A et al. J Pediatr Gastroenterol Nutr 2002;35:S173–9.
19. Sack RB. Bacterial and parasitic agents of acute diarrhea. In: Bellanti JA, ed. Acute Diarrhea: Its Nutritional Consequences in Infancy. New York: Raven Press, 1983:53–65.
20. Hamilton JR. Viral enteritis: A cause of disordered small intestinal epithelial renewal. In: Lebenthal E, ed. Chronic Diarrhea in Children. New York: Raven Press, 1984:269–76.
21. Hill I, Fasano A, Schwartz R, et al. J Pediatr 2000;136:86–90.
22. Hoffenberg EJ, MacKenzie T, Barriga KJ et al. J Pediatr 2003; 143:308–14.
23. Fabiani E, Taccari LM, Ratsch I-M et al. J Pediatr 2000;136: 841–3.
24. Hoffenberg EJ, Haas J, Drescher A et al. J Pediatr 2000;137: 361–6.
25. Kalayci AG, Kansu A, Girgin N et al. Pediatrics 2001;108(5). Available at: http://www.pediatrics.org/cgi/content/full/108/5/e89.
26. Mora S, Borera G, Beccio S et al. J Pediatr 2001;139:516–21.
27. Hill ID, Bhatnagar S, Cameron DJS et al. J Pediatr Gastroenterol Nutr 2002;35:S78–S88.
28. Sentongo TA, Semeao EJ, Piccoli DA et al. J Pediatr Gastroenterol Nutr 2000;31:33–40.
29. Hueschkel RB, Menache CC, Megerian JT et al. J Pediatr Gastroenterol Nutr 2000;31:8–15.
30. Ruemmele FM, Roy CC, Levy E et al. J Pediatr 2000;136: 285–91.
31. Buller H, Chin S, Kirschne B et al. J Pediatr Gastroenterol Nutr 2002;35:S151–8.
32. Rudolph CD, Mazur LJ, Liptak GS et al. J Pediatr Gastroenterol Nutr 2001;32[Suppl 2]:S1–S31.
33. Wilmore DW. J Pediatr 1972;80:88–95.
34. Cooper A, Floyd TF, Ross AJ et al. J Pediatr Surg 1984;19: 711–8.
35. Parker P, Stroop BS, Greene H. J Pediatr 1981;99:360–4.
36. Kurkchubasche AG, Rowe MI, Smith SD. J Pediatr Surg 1993; 28:1069–71.
37. Sondheimer JM, Cadnapaphornchai M, Sontag M et al. J Pediatr 1998;132:80–4.
38. Bines J, Francis D, Hill D. J Pediatr Gastroenterol Nutr 1998; 26:123–8.
39. Andorsky DJ, Lund DP, Lillehei CW et al. J Pediatr 2001;139: 27–33.
40. Kollman KA, Lien EL, Vanderhoof JA. J Pediatr Gastroenterol Nutr 1999;28:41–5.
41. Kaufman SS, Loseke CA, Lupo JV et al. J Pediatr 1997;131: 356–61.
42. Farrell MK, Balistreri WF. Clin Perinatol 1986;13:197–212.
43. Sondheimer JM, Asturias E, Cadnapaphornchai M. J Pediatr Gastroenterol Nutr 1998;27:131–7.
44. Teitelbaum DH, Han-Markey T, Schumacher RE. J Pediatr Surg 1995;30:1082–95.
45. Cooper A, Ross AJ, O'Neill JA et al. J Pediatr Surg 1985;20: 772–4.
46. Walker–Smith J, Barnard J, Bhutta Z et al. J Pediatr Gastroenterol Nutr 2002;35:S98–S105.

47. McKinney RE, Robertson WR, and the Duke Pediatric AIDS Clinical Trials Unit. J Pediatr 1993;123:579–82.

48. Miller TL, Evans S, Orav EJ et al. Am J Clin Nutr 1993;57:588–92.

49. Falloon F, Eddy J, Pizzo PA. J Pediatr 1989;144:1–30.

50. Miller TL Evans SE, Vasquez I et al. Pediatr Res 1997;41:85A.

51. Miller TL, Orav EJ, Colan S et al. Am J Clin Nutr 1997;66:660–4.

52. Henderson RA, Saavedra JM, Perman JA et al. J Pediatr Gastroenterol Nutr 1994;18:429–34.

53. Miller TL, Awnetwant EL, Evans S et al. Pediatrics 1995;96:696–702.

54. Clarick RH, Hanekom WA, Yogev R et al. Pediatrics 1997;99:354–7.

55. Guarino A, Spagnuolo MI, Giocomet V et al. J Pediatr Gastroenterol Nutr 2002;34:366–71.

56. Miller TL, Easley KA, Zhang W et al. Pediatrics 2001;108:1287–96.

57. Jirapinyo P, Brewster D, Succi RCDM et al. J Pediatr Gastroenterol Nutr 2002;35:S134–42.

58. Coss–Bu JA, Klish WJ, Walding D et al. Am J Clin Nutr 2001;74:664–9.

59. Schwarz SM, Corredor J, Fisher-Medina J et al. Pediatrics 2001;108:671–6.

60. Rommel N, DeMeyer A–M, Feenstra L et al. J Pediatr Gastroenterol Nutr 2003;37:75–84.

61. Cooper A, Heird WC. Am J Clin Nutr 1982;35:1132–41.

62. Baker JP Detsky AS, Wesson DE et al. N Engl J Med 1982;306:969–72.

63. Flegal KM, Wei R, Ogden C. Am J Clin Nutr 2002;75:761–6.

64. Waterlow JC. Br Med J 1972;3:566–9.

65. Heird WC. Justification of total parenteral nutrition. In: Yu VYH, MacMahon RA, eds. Intravenous Feeding of the Neonate. London: Edward Arnold, 1992:166–75.

66. Kashyap S, Heird WC. Protein requirements of low birthweight, very low birthweight, and small for gestational age infants. In: Räihä NCR, ed. Protein Metabolism During Infancy. Nestlé Nutrition Workshop Series, vol 33. New York: Raven Press, 1995:133–51.

67. Collins JN, Hoope M, Brown K et al. J Pediatr 1991;118:921–7.

68. Greene HL, Hambidge KM, Schanler R et al. Am J Clin Nutr 1988;48:1324–42.

69. Paulsrud JR, Pensler L, Whitten CF et al. Am J Clin Nutr 1972;25:897–904.

70. Shennan AT, Bryan MD, Angel A. J Pediatr 1977;91:134–7.

71. Park W, Paust H, Br`sicke H et al. JPEN J Parenter Enteral Nutr 1986;10:627–30.

72. Greene HL, Hazlett D, Demree R. Am J Clin Nutr 1976;29:127–35.

73. Friedman Z, Marks MH, Maisels J et al. Pediatrics 1978;61:694–8.

74. Loo LS, Tang JP, Kohl S. J Infect Dis 1982;146:64–70.

75. Odell GTB, Cukier JO, Ostrea EM Jr et al. J Lab Clin Med 1977;89:29–307.

76. Haumont D, Deckelbaum RJ, Richelle M et al. J Pediatr 1989;115:787–93.

77. Winters RW, Heird WC, Dell RB et al. Plasma amino acids in infants receiving parenteral nutrition. In: Green HL, Holliday MA, Munro HN, eds. Clinical Nutrition Update: Amino Acids. Chicago: American Medical Association, 1977:147–54.

78. Heird WC, Dell RB, Helms RA et al. Pediatrics 1987;80:401–8.

79. Schreiner RL, Glick MR, Nordschow CW et al. J Pediatr 1979;94:197–200.

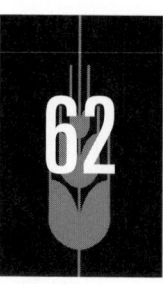

METABOLIC SYNDROME: DEFINITION, RELATIONSHIP TO INSULIN RESISTANCE, AND CLINICAL UTILITY[1]

GERALD M. REAVEN

INDIVIDUAL COMPONENTS OF THE METABOLIC
  SYNDROME 1006
    Waist Circumference 1006
    Fasting Plasma Glucose Concentration 1007
    Blood Pressure 1008
    Dyslipidemia 1009
  CONCLUSION 1010

From the late 1930s to 1949, Himsworth and colleagues initiated a series of elegant experiments that produced the first evidence of the importance of insulin resistance in human disease (1–5). Their research efforts were focused on the link between resistance to insulin action and the pathogenesis of what is now referred to as type 2 diabetes, using a straightforward experimental approach to demonstrate that "diabetes mellitus is a disease in which the essential lesion is a diminished ability of the tissue to utilize glucose. The high blood sugar is a controlled and compensatory phenomenon, the object of which is to facilitate the utilization of glucose by the tissues." The results of their experiments clearly questioned the conventional wisdom at that time (and for many more years) that "all cases of human diabetes could be explained by a deficiency of insulin" and suggested, "a state of diabetes might result from inefficient action of insulin as well as from a lack of insulin." Furthermore, they proposed that diabetes could be subdivided into two categories "according to which of these disorders predominates into insulin sensitive and insulin insensitive types."

As prescient as Himsworth's findings were, the view that diabetes was one disease, secondary to an absolute deficiency of insulin, remained relatively unchallenged until 1960, when Yalow and Berson introduced the insulin immunoassay (6). When they used this specific measurement of plasma insulin concentration to compare nondiabetic subjects with patients with type 2 diabetes, these investigators concluded "that the tissues of the maturity-onset diabetic do not respond to his insulin as well as the tissue of the nondiabetic responded to his insulin." To use Himsworth's terminology, Yalow and Berson provided evidence that patients with maturity-onset (type 2) diabetes were insulin insensitive.

Although the findings of Yalow and Berson provided substantial evidence that such a thing as insulin resistance existed, the importance of a defect in insulin action in playing a role in human disease continued to be debated until the introduction in the following decade of specific methods with which to quantify insulin-mediated glucose disposal (7, 8). Once these methods were available, investigators demonstrated over the next several years that most patients with either impaired glucose tolerance or type 2 diabetes were insulin resistant (7–11), and the presence of insulin resistance in normoglycemic persons predicted the development of type 2 diabetes (12, 13). Thus, approximately 40 years later, there was general agreement that "insulin insensitivity," as defined by Himsworth, is a characteristic defect in patients with type 2 diabetes.

The importance of insulin resistance in the pathophysiology of type 2 diabetes is no longer an issue. However, it has become apparent since the mid-1980s that the clinical implications of this defect in insulin action extend far beyond its role in the etiology of states of glucose intolerance. A phenomenon that is not widely appreciated is that values of insulin-mediated glucose disposal vary six- to eightfold in apparently healthy persons (14, 15), and significant numbers of patients with normal glucose tolerance are as insulin resistant as patients with type 2 diabetes (16). Insulin-resistant, nondiabetic persons are able to secrete the amount of insulin needed to maintain normal or near-normal glucose tolerance. However, the combination of insulin resistance and compensatory hyperinsulinemia is hardly benign. For example, the more insulin resistant and hyperinsulinemic a person is, the greater the stimulation of hepatic triglyceride (TG) synthesis, and the higher the plasma TG concentration will be (17–19). Plasma high-density lipoprotein cholesterol (HDL-C) concentrations are significantly lower in insulin resistant/hyperinsulinemic persons, and both a high TG concentration and a low HDL-C concentration are independently related to insulin

---

[1] **Abbreviations: ADMA,** asymmetric dimethylarginine; **ATP III,** Adult Treatment Panel III; **BMI,** body mass index; **CVD,** cardiovascular disease; **FCR,** fractional catabolic rate; **FFA,** free fatty acid; **IFG,** impaired fasting glucose; **HDL-C,** high-density lipoprotein cholesterol; **LDL,** low-density lipoprotein; **NHANES,** National Health and Nutrition Examination Survey; **TG,** triglyceride; **VA-HIT,** Veterans Affairs HDL Intervention Trial; **VLDL-TG,** very-low-density triglyceride; **WC,** waist circumference.

TABLE 62.1. HALLMARKS OF SYNDROME X: INCREASED CARDIOVASCULAR DISEASE RISK INSULIN RESISTANCE

Compensatory hyperinsulinemia
Some degree of glucose intolerance
Essential hypertension
↑ Plasma triglyceride concentration
↓ High-density lipoprotein concentration

resistance/hyperinsulinemia (20). Evidence also indicates that the prevalence of insulin resistance/hyperinsulinemia is increased in patients with essential hypertension (21, 22). Because the risk of cardiovascular disease (CVD) is increased in association with all three of the abnormalities associated with insulin resistance (23–25)—high TG, low HDL-C, and hypertension—it seemed apparent that type 2 diabetes was not the only clinical syndrome likely to develop in insulin-resistant persons. In 1988, the findings listed in Table 62.1 were subsumed under the rubric of syndrome X (26), with the suggestion that this cluster of related abnormalities significantly increased the risk of CVD.

The concept of Syndrome X was introduced to emphasize that type 2 diabetes was not the only clinical syndrome related to insulin resistance, and this notion is shown schematically in Figure 62.1. As indicated in this figure, not all insulin-resistant persons develop type 2 diabetes. Indeed, most them continue to secrete enough insulin to prevent gross decompensation of glucose tolerance, but they develop the manifestations of syndrome X. Persons with the cluster of abnormalities comprising syndrome X (see Table 62.1) remain at risk to develop type 2 diabetes, but

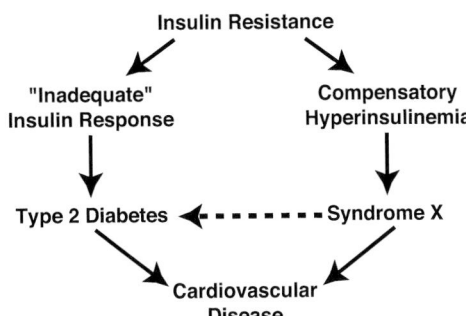

Figure 62.1. Schematic relationship between insulin resistance, the plasma insulin response to the defect in insulin action, and risk of cardiovascular disease. Type 2 diabetes develops when the magnitude of the pancreatic β-cell response is not able to overcome the insulin resistance (an "inadequate" insulin response). Most insulin-resistant persons are able to maintain normal, or near-normal, glucose tolerance by secreting large amounts of insulin. However, they are at increased risk of developing the cluster of abnormalities related to insulin resistance listed in Table 62.1 (syndrome X). Although patients with syndrome X remain at increased risk of developing type 2 diabetes, most of them are able to maintain the degree of hyperinsulinemia needed to prevent frank decompensation of glucose homeostasis. However, irrespective of whether an insulin-resistant person is classified as having type 2 diabetes or syndrome X, he or she is at increased risk of cardiovascular disease.

more to the point, they are at greatly increased risk of CVD. In other words, it does not matter whether insulin-resistant persons develop type 2 diabetes or the manifestations of syndrome X; they are at increased risk of CVD.

The number of abnormalities and clinical syndromes more likely to occur in insulin-resistant persons continues to grow, and the insulin resistance syndrome now seems to be a more appropriate term than syndrome X to designate the protean manifestations associated with insulin resistance (27, 28).

At the same time that the clinical consequences of insulin resistance were realized to extend far beyond type 2 diabetes and CVD, the report of the Adult Treatment Panel III (ATP III) of the National Cholesterol Education Program (29) formally acknowledged the importance as CVD risk factors of abnormalities associated with insulin resistance/compensatory hyperinsulinemia. Specifically, the ATP III recognized as CVD risk factors what the panel referred to as a "constellation of lipid and non-lipid risk factors of metabolic origin," substituted the term metabolic syndrome for syndrome X, and reaffirmed the view that "this syndrome is closely related to insulin resistance." Table 62.2 lists the five criteria selected by the ATP III to identify individuals with the metabolic syndrome (obesity, elevated blood pressure, impaired fasting glucose [IFG], and high TG and low HDL-C concentrations) and reflects the panel's view that insulin resistance is at the root of the problem. However, although the two terms, syndrome X and the metabolic syndrome, are often used synonymously, they represent two entirely different concepts. As indicated earlier, syndrome X was introduced to provide a physiologic construct to account for the interrelationship of insulin resistance, hyperinsulinemia, glucose intolerance, hypertension, and high TG and low HDL-C concentrations and to suggest that this cluster of related abnormalities had not been sufficiently recognized as increasing CVD risk. It

TABLE 62.2. NATIONAL CHOLESTEROL EDUCATION PROGRAM EXPERT PANEL ON DETECTION, EVALUATION, AND TREATMENT OF HIGH BLOOD CHOLESTEROL IN ADULTS (ADULT TREATMENT PANEL III) CRITERIA FOR DIAGNOSING THE METABOLIC SYNDROME[a]

Abdominal obesity
   Men: Waist circumference >40 inches
   Women: Waist circumference >35 inches
Fasting glucose ≥110 <126 mg/dL
Blood pressure ≥130/85 mm Hg
Triglycerides ≥150 mg/dL
High–density lipoprotein cholesterol
   Men <40 mg/dL
   Women <50 mg/dL

[a]The metabolic syndrome is present when three or more of these five criteria are met.

From National Cholesterol Education Program Expert Panel on Detection, Evaluation, and Treatment of High Blood Cholesterol in Adults (Adult Treatment Panel III). JAMA 2001;285:2486–97, with permission.

was not meant to represent a diagnostic category. In contrast, the report of the ATP III began with the basic premise that certain CVD risk factors are associated with insulin resistance/compensatory hyperinsulinemia, and it established specific criteria to be used in making a clinical diagnosis of the metabolic syndrome. The purpose of diagnosing the metabolic syndrome is to identify individuals at increased CVD risk, and with this added information to initiate lifestyle changes that will help to decrease this risk. The remainder of this chapter consists of a consideration of each of the five components of the metabolic syndrome as defined by the ATP III, as well as a discussion of the potential advantages and disadvantages of making this diagnosis.

INDIVIDUAL COMPONENTS OF THE METABOLIC SYNDROME

To identify a patient as having the metabolic syndrome, the ATP III stated that any three of the five criteria listed in Table 62.2 must be satisfied. The five variables listed in Table 62.2 appear to have been selected because they tend to cluster together, and they have all been associated with increased CVD risk. However, the rationale for choosing the numeric upper limit for each of the five components is less clear and is certainly not derived from outcome data. Although this issue is crucial, the suggested cutpoints for each criteria are not considered, but rather the focus is on the five individual components, and each is evaluated in terms of its (a) relationship with insulin resistance and (b) its role in increasing CVD risk.

Waist Circumference

The inclusion of a measure of excess adiposity (waist circumference [WC]) as one of the ATP III criteria for identifying persons with the metabolic syndrome is interesting in that, as distinguished from the other criteria, it is not a consequence of insulin resistance. Instead, obesity appears to be a lifestyle variable that, along with physical inactivity, has an adverse effect on insulin-mediated glucose disposal (30–32) (see Chapters 63 and 64), thereby increasing chances that the abnormalities and clinical syndromes associated with insulin resistance/compensatory hyperinsulinemia will develop. Not all insulin-resistant persons are overweight or obese, nor are all overweight or obese persons insulin resistant (30–34). To have a mechanistic view of how the metabolic syndrome develops, it is necessary that obesity be viewed as a contributor to insulin resistance/hyperinsulinemia, rather than a consequence of the defect in insulin action. This distinction is not meant to minimize the important role that the current epidemic of obesity plays in increasing the prevalence of the metabolic syndrome as diagnosed by ATP III criteria, but rather to emphasize that obesity increases the likelihood that a person will be insulin resistant and hyperinsulinemic,

although insulin resistance/hyperinsulinemia does not make it more likely that a person will become obese.

Although WC may be more closely related to insulin resistance and its consequences than generalized obesity as estimated by body mass index (BMI), its superiority as a clinical tool can be questioned. At the simplest level, the values of the two variables were highly correlated in a recent analysis (35) of data from approximately 20,000 participants in the National Health and Nutrition Examination Surveys (NHANES) from 1988 to 1994 and from 1999 to 2000. More specifically, the r-values were greater than 0.9 in every subgroup analyzed, and they were essentially identical irrespective of gender, age, or ethnicity.

Height and weight are routinely measured in most health care facilities, and the BMI is easily calculated by referring to simple tables. In contrast, the following paragraph describes how WC should be measured according to the NHANES protocol (36):

> The subject stands and the examiner, positioned at the right of the subject, palpates the upper bone to locate the iliac crest. Just above the uppermost lateral border of the right iliac crest, a horizontal mark is drawn, and then crossed with a vertical mark on the midaxillary line. The measuring tape is placed in a horizontal plane around the abdomen at the level of this marked point on the right side of the trunk. The plane of the tape is parallel to the floor and the tape is snug, but does not compress the skin. The measurement is made at normal minimal inspiration.

To the best of my knowledge, data are not available on the reproducibility of measurements of WC within any given clinical setting (let alone from site to site) when this precise protocol has been followed. It also seems reasonable to express skepticism concerning the likelihood that measurements of WC will be performed with this same degree of seriousness, and in a uniform manner, in health centers throughout the United States. Assuming this to be the case, it would seem necessary to provide strong evidence that measuring the WC provides a more sensitive approach than does calculation of BMI to identify insulin-resistant persons at increased risk to develop CVD. Perhaps the most compelling evidence that this is probably not the case comes from the results presented by the European Group for the Study of Insulin Resistance (37). These investigators evaluated the relationship between insulin-mediated glucose disposal, as measured by the euglycemic clamp technique, and obesity in more than 1100 nondiabetic volunteers, and they reported that the magnitude of the correlation between insulin resistance and obesity was not increased when the ratio of waist-to-hip girth was substituted for BMI as the marker of obesity.

In summary, it appears that (a) BMI and WC are tightly correlated, (b) legitimate questions can be raised concerning the ability to measure WC as accurately as height and weight, and (c) results of specific measures of insulin-mediated glucose disposal suggest that the relationship between insulin resistance and adiposity as assessed by BMI is not improved by taking abdominal circumference into consideration. If the goal of the ATP III is to obtain a measure of obesity to help identify insulin-resistant persons at increased risk of CVD, it can be argued that measurement of BMI is a simpler and more effective way to accomplish that task. Finally, and perhaps of greatest importance, is that as important as abdominal obesity may be in decreasing insulin sensitivity and increasing CVD risk, the level of excess adiposity at which these adverse consequences will develop is less in many ethnic groups of non-European ancestry (38). Indeed, a recent report from a World Health Organization expert consultation team emphasized that the level at which the adverse consequences of obesity occur varies as a function of ethnic group (38). Although the ATP III considered the issue of ethnicity, they concluded that evidence was not sufficient to warrant varying the WC criteria for different ethnic groups. Indeed, if obesity were to be used as a diagnostic criterion, rather than as a variable that increased the likelihood of insulin resistance, the upper limit of normal would have to be almost tailor made for each ethnic group. The difficulty in accomplishing this task is self-evident.

Fasting Plasma Glucose Concentration

The American Diabetes Association proposed that IFG be used to describe persons with a fasting plasma glucose concentration of 110 to 126 mg/dL (39) and that these persons be considered prediabetic. Because a fasting glucose concentration greater than 126 mg/dL is diagnostic of diabetes, a disease known to increase CVD risk, it seems likely that the selection of IFG by the ATP III to aid in the diagnosis of the metabolic syndrome stemmed from the creation of this diagnostic criteria by the American Diabetes Association. Although substantial epidemiologic evidence indicates that the higher the plasma glucose concentration, the more likely a person is to develop type 2 diabetes, it is not so clear that the use of IFG provides a particularly effective way either to identify the presence of insulin resistance or to predict CVD risk. Because values of insulin-mediated glucose disposal are distributed continuously throughout the nondiabetic population (15), there is no objective cutpoint to decide who is sufficiently insulin resistant to be at increased risk of an adverse outcome. One way to approach this issue is to quantify insulin action at baseline and to assess the clinical outcome of apparently healthy persons over time. This has been done on two occasions (40, 41), and the results indicated that the clinical syndromes associated with the defect in insulin action occurred primarily in the upper third of the population in terms of insulin resistance. When this definition was applied to a population of apparently healthy subjects, the results (Figure 62.2A) showed that only 27 out of 490 persons (5.5%) had IFG, and 17 of these 27 (63%) were in the insulin-resistant tertile (42). As shown in Table 62.3, these findings translate to a test with high specificity, but very low sensitivity. The results in Figure 62.2B show that the

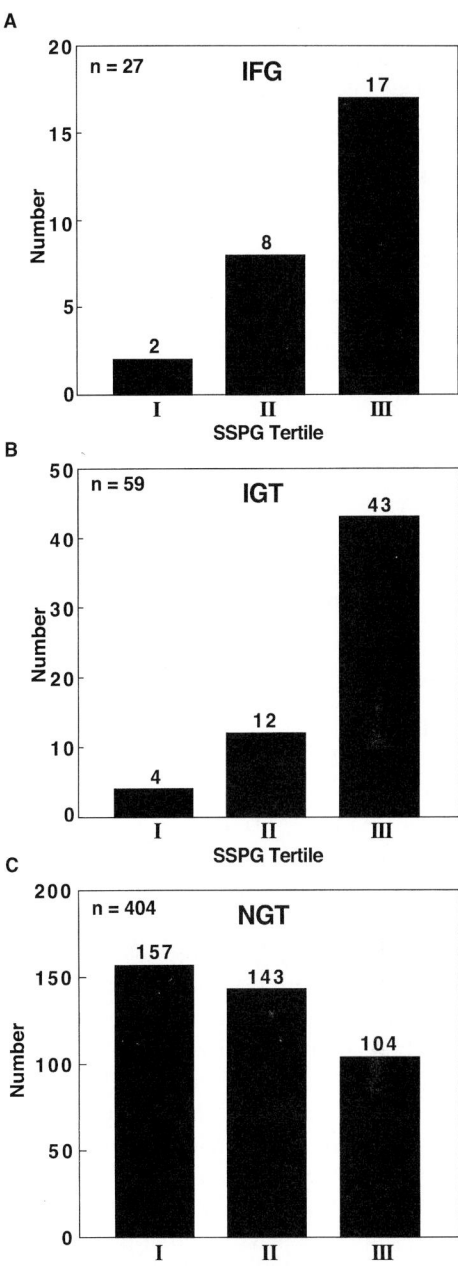

Figure 62.2 A–C. Frequency distribution of 443 apparently healthy persons defined as having impaired fasting glucose (IFG), impaired glucose tolerance (IGT), or normal glucose tolerance (NGT) as a function of their steady-state plasma glucose (SSPG) concentration during the insulin suppression test. SSPG tertile 1 represents the third of the population that was most insulin resistant, SSPG tertile I the third that was most insulin sensitive. (Adapted from Tuan C-Y, Abbasi F, Lamendola C et al. Am J Cardiol 2003;92:606–10, with permission.)

presence of impaired glucose tolerance (plasma glucose concentration greater than 140 mg/dL and less than 200 mg/dL 120 minutes after a 75-g oral glucose challenge) provides a criterion that was approximately threefold more sensitive than IFG in identifying insulin-resistant persons. Furthermore, the results of the DECODE Study Group (43) showed that post–glucose challenge plasma glucose concentrations

TABLE 62.3. SENSITIVITY AND SPECIFICITY OF PLASMA GLUCOSE MEASUREMENTS IN IDENTIFYING INSULIN-RESISTANT PERSONS

METABOLIC VARIABLE	SENSITIVITY	SPECIFICITY
Impaired fasting glucose	0.10	0.97
Impaired glucose tolerance	0.26	0.95

Adapted from Tuan C-Y, Abbasi F, Lamendola C et al. Am J Cardiol 2003;92:606–10, with permission.

were superior to fasting values in predicting CVD risk. However, perhaps the most crucial findings are those in Figure 62.2C, indicating that approximately 25% of persons with normal glucose tolerance were in the most insulin-resistant tertile. It is apparent from these findings that the presence of IFG occurs too infrequently to be very useful in the diagnosis of the metabolic syndrome, and significant numbers of normal glucose-tolerant persons are sufficiently insulin resistant to be at increased risk of CVD.

Blood Pressure

The relationship among insulin resistance, essential hypertension, and CVD risk is complex; it cannot be discussed in detail in the context of this chapter, but it has recently been reviewed (44). Focusing initially on the relationship between insulin resistance/hyperinsulinemia and blood pressure, evidence indicates that (a) patients with essential hypertension as a group are insulin resistant and hyperinsulinemic (21, 22), (b) normotensive first-degree relatives of patients with essential hypertension are relatively insulin resistant and hyperinsulinemic as compared with a matched control group without a family history of hypertension (45–47), and (c) hyperinsulinemia, as a surrogate estimate of insulin resistance, has been shown in population-based studies to predict the eventual development of essential hypertension (48–50). These findings provide substantial support for the view that insulin resistance/hyperinsulinemia plays a role in the pathogenesis of essential hypertension, but probably no more than 50% of patients with essential hypertension are insulin resistant (51). Thus, just as there are insulin-resistant persons who do not develop essential hypertension, not all patients with essential hypertension are insulin resistant.

Although substantial evidence indicates that essential hypertension is more likely to develop in insulin-resistant/

hyperinsulinemic persons, understanding of the causal relationship between the changes in insulin metabolism and blood pressure regulation is less clear, and it requires addressing the issue of differential insulin sensitivity. The abilities of insulin to stimulate muscle glucose disposal and to inhibit adipose tissue lipolysis are highly correlated within the same person, and muscle and adipose tissue insulin resistance can exist at the same time that many, if not all, of the other tissues in that person retain normal insulin sensitivity (52). For example, insulin infusions increase renal sodium retention in persons with insulin-resistant muscle and adipose tissue (53). Furthermore, sodium and water retention in response to an increase in sodium intake occurs primarily in insulin-resistant persons (54), and salt sensitivity is largely confined to normotensive and hypertensive insulin-resistant persons (54–56). Finally, the compensatory hyperinsulinemia associated with insulin resistance can stimulate sympathetic nervous system activity in insulin-resistant persons and can lead to various changes that increase the likelihood of essential hypertension (57, 58). The abilities of insulin to enhance renal sodium retention and to stimulate sympathetic nervous system activity normally may not be the only explanations for an increased prevalence of essential hypertension in insulin-resistant persons, but these characteristics certainly contribute to this phenomenon and provide examples of the importance of differential tissue insulin sensitivity in the etiology of the clinical syndromes that are increased in prevalence in insulin-resistant persons.

Finally, in the context of discussing the metabolic syndrome, the relationship between blood pressure and CVD requires further attention. More specifically, it is necessary briefly to review observations indicating that the subset of patients with essential hypertension who are also insulin resistant is at the greatest risk of CVD (59–61). For example, patients with essential hypertension with electrocardiographic evidence of ischemic changes are somewhat glucose intolerant and hyperinsulinemic as compared with either a normotensive control group or patients with essential hypertension whose electrocardiograms are entirely normal (59). Not surprisingly, measurement of insulin-mediated glucose disposal demonstrated that patients with essential hypertension and ischemic electrocardiographic changes were insulin resistant, and the results in Table 62.4 show that that the dyslipidemic changes associated with

TABLE 62.4. MEAN (±SEM) LIPID AND LIPOPROTEIN CONCENTRATIONS (mmol/L)

GROUP	C	LDL-C	HDL-C	TG
Control (n = 25)	5.0 ± 0.2	3.1 ± 0.2	1.4 ± 0.1	1.2 ± 0.1
Normal ECG (n = 24)	4.8 ± 0.2	3.0 ± 0.2	1.3 ± 0.1	1.2 ± 0.1
Abnormal ECG (n = 29)	5.3 ± 0.2	3.4 ± 0.2	1.1 ± 0.1[a]	1.8 ± 0.1[a]

C, cholesterol; ECG, electrocardiogram; HDL-C, high-density lipoprotein cholesterol; LDL-C, low-density lipoprotein cholesterol; n, number; TG, triglyceride.
[a]Significantly different from control, $p < .05$.
Adapted from Sheu WH-H, Jeng C-Y, Shieh S-M et al. Am J Hypertens 1992;5:444–8, with permission.

insulin resistance/hyperinsulinemia were present in these persons as compared with normotensive persons or hypertensive patients with normal electrocardiograms.

The link between the dyslipidemia present in insulin-resistant/hyperinsulinemic patients with essential hypertension and CVD is consistent with results of two reports from the Copenhagen Male Study. In the first publication (60), Jeppesen and colleagues showed that the development of CVD in persons with high TG and low HDL-C concentrations was independent of differences in baseline systolic or diastolic blood pressure. In contrast, the higher either systolic ($p < .001$) or diastolic ($p < .03$) blood pressure was at the beginning of the study, the greater was the incidence of CVD in those men without the dyslipidemic changes associated with insulin resistance.

In a second study (61), 2906 participants in the Copenhagen Male Study were divided into three groups on the basis of their fasting plasma TG and HDL-C concentrations. Men whose plasma TG and HDL-C concentrations were in the upper third or lower third, respectively, of the whole population, were assigned to the high TG–low HDL-C group. At the other extreme, a low TG–high HDL-C group was composed of those persons whose plasma TG and HDL-C concentrations were in the lower third and upper third, respectively, of the study population for these two lipid measurements. The intermediate group consisted of those participants whose lipid values did not qualify them for either of the two extreme groups. The investigators then defined the interaction between the TG–HDL-C group and CVD in patients with essential hypertension. The results indicated that CVD risk was not increased in patients with hypertension in the absence of high TG and low HDL-C concentrations, and the group at greatest risk was that with high blood pressure and high TG and low HDL-C concentrations.

Jeppesen and associates (60, 61) used high plasma TG and low HDL-C concentrations as markers of insulin resistance, without necessarily suggesting that these specific changes in lipoprotein metabolism were the entire explanation for the increased risk of CVD in this subset of the population with essential hypertension. No reason exists to suspect that the hyperinsulinemia, glucose intolerance, dyslipidemia, procoagulant state, and endothelial dysfunction associated with insulin resistance will not contribute to the increased CVD risk in those patients with essential hypertension who are also insulin resistant (27, 28).

Changes in endothelial function that are likely to contribute further to increased CVD risk also vary as a function of differences in insulin-mediated glucose disposal in patients with essential hypertension. For example, the first step in the process of atherogenesis is the binding of mononuclear cells to the endothelium (62), and evidence indicates that the adherence to cultured endothelial cells of mononuclear cells isolated from patients with hypertension is directly related to their degree of insulin

resistance (63). However, the relationship between insulin resistance and binding of isolated mononuclear cells to endothelium is similar in normotensive (r = 0.86) and hypertensive (r = 0.74) volunteers in that the more insulin resistant an person is, irrespective of blood pressure status, the greater will be the adherence of their isolated mononuclear cells to endothelium ($p < .001$).

Similar findings were observed when the relationship between plasma asymmetric dimethylarginine (ADMA) concentration and insulin-mediated glucose disposal was evaluated (64). Plasma concentrations of ADMA, an endogenous inhibitor of nitric oxide synthase, have been shown to be predictive of CVD in several clinical syndromes (65), and a highly significant relationship ($p < .001$) between insulin-mediated glucose disposal and plasma ADMA concentrations exists (64) in apparently healthy volunteers (r = 0.73), as well as in patients with essential hypertension (r = 0.74). Thus, as was the case with the binding of isolated mononuclear cells to endothelium, plasma ADMA concentrations are increased to a similar degree in insulin-resistant persons, whether they are normotensive or hypertensive.

Dyslipidemia

The dyslipidemic components of the metabolic syndrome are probably the features linked most closely with both insulin resistance and CVD risk. The ability of a low HDL-C concentration to predict CVD risk has been known for many years (24), and although questions have been raised concerning the role of an increase in TG concentrations as an "independent" CVD risk factor (66), evidence certainly exists in support of that notion (24, 25) (see Chapter 67). Furthermore, although not cited as one of the criteria for diagnosing the metabolic syndrome, the atherogenic lipoprotein profile associated with insulin resistance also includes a decrease in low-density lipoprotein particle diameter (small, dense LDL) and the postprandial accumulation of TG-rich remnant lipoproteins (67, 68), and these changes have been shown to increase CVD risk (69, 70). Furthermore, evidence from both the Helsinki Heart Study and the Veterans Affairs HDL Intervention Trial (VA-HIT) study demonstrates that the use of gemfibrozil, an agent that lowers plasma TG and raises HDL-C concentrations, is able to decrease CVD risk significantly (71, 72). Of particular interest in this context is the recent analysis of the VA-HIT data indicating that patients who had the highest plasma insulin concentrations at baseline, and were presumably insulin resistant, benefited the most from gemfibrozil treatment (73). Consequently, abundant information suggests that the dyslipidemic criteria proposed by the ATP III are the abnormalities most characteristic of insulin resistant/hyperinsulinemic subjects, highly predictive of CVD risk, and when these conditions are treated, the incidence of CVD is consequently decreased.

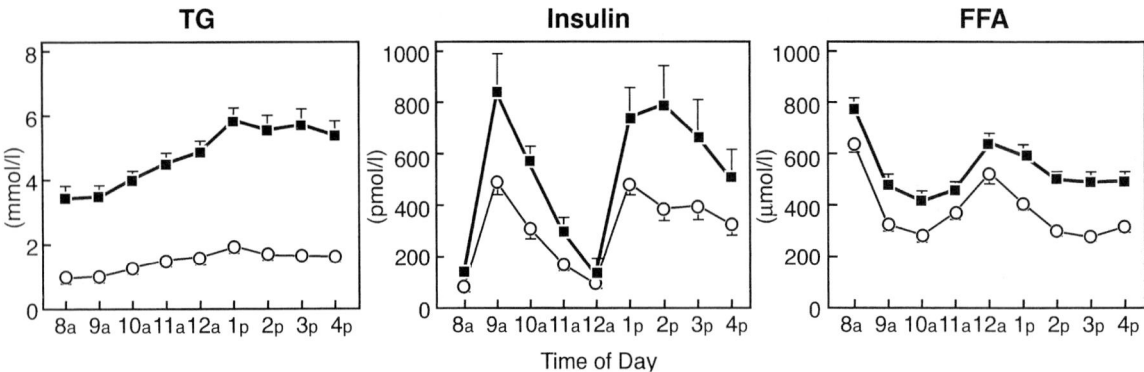

Figure 62.3. Plasma triglyceride (TG), insulin, and free fatty acid (FFA) concentrations measured at hourly intervals in apparently healthy persons, selected on the basis of being either insulin resistant and hypertriglyceridemic (*filled squares*) or insulin sensitive with normal plasma TG concentrations (*open circles*). Breakfast (containing 20% of estimated daily caloric requirements) was given at 8 AM, and lunch (containing 40% of estimated daily caloric requirements) was given at noon. (Data from Jeng C-Y, Fuh MM-T, Sheu WH-H et al. Endocrinol Metab 1994;1:15–21.)

Hypertriglyceridemia is the central feature of the dyslipidemia associated with insulin resistance/hyperinsulinemia (17–19), and its development is another example of the importance of the concept of differential tissue insulin sensitivity. Resistance to insulin-mediated glucose by muscle leads to higher day-long plasma insulin concentration, and free fatty acid (FFA) concentrations are increased as a consequence of resistance to the antilipolytic effect of insulin at the level of the adipose tissue (74). The combination of increased plasma concentrations of both FFA and insulin acts on a normally insulin-sensitive liver to increase hepatic very-low-density TG (VLDL-TG) synthesis and secretion, leading to hypertriglyceridemia (17–19). The results shown in Figure 62.3 provide an example of the difference in day-long plasma TG, insulin, and FFA concentrations seen when insulin-resistant, hypertriglyceridemic persons are compared with insulin-sensitive subjects with normal plasma TG concentrations (74, 75). Figure 62.3 also provides a dramatic depiction of the degree to which the postprandial accumulation of TG-rich lipoproteins occurs in insulin-resistant persons once fasting plasma TG concentrations increase.

Furthermore, once the plasma TG plasma pool is expanded, the rate of transfer, catalyzed by cholesteryl ester transfer protein, of cholesteryl ester from HDL to VLDL will also increase (76); the higher the VLDL pool size, the greater the transfer rate from HDL to VLDL, and the lower the ensuing HDL-C concentration will be. Evidence also indicates that the fractional catabolic rate (FCR) of apoprotein A-I is increased in patients with primary hypertriglyceridemia (77), hypertension (78), and type 2 diabetes (79). In type 2 diabetes, investigators have shown that the greater degree of hyperinsulinemia is, the lower the HDL-C concentration will be (79). Investigators have also demonstrated in nondiabetic persons that the higher the apoprotein A-I FCR is, the lower the HDL-C concentration will be (80). Thus, it is likely that insulin resistance and hyperinsulinemia contribute to a low HDL-C concentration indirectly by being responsible for the increase in VLDL pool size and directly by increasing the FCR of apoprotein A-I.

CONCLUSION

Perhaps the single point that deserves the most emphasis is that insulin resistance is not a disease, but rather the description of a physiologic state that greatly increases the chances that a person will develop certain closely related abnormalities and associated clinical syndromes (27, 28), including an increase in CVD. The original goal of introducing the notion of syndrome X was not only to emphasize that insulin resistance was a fundamental abnormality in patients with type 2 diabetes, but also to highlight the connections among insulin resistance, its associated cluster of abnormalities, and increased CVD. In contrast, the notion of the metabolic syndrome, as defined by the ATP III, represents an effort to make a clinical diagnosis. Consequently, its value must be considered not in pathophysiologic terms, but as a pragmatic approach to obtain a better clinical outcome. Thus, the finding that obesity is a variable that contributes to insulin resistance, and not a consequence of the defect in insulin action, does not necessarily detract from its use as one of the criteria with which to make a diagnosis of the metabolic syndrome. However, the possibility that the measure of obesity listed in Table 62.2 may be less than ideal, or that the values for abdominal obesity may be most applicable to persons of European ancestry, seems to decrease its clinical utility substantially. Similarly, what is the value of including as a one of the criteria for making a diagnosis of the metabolic syndrome a fasting plasma glucose concentration that applies to only approximately 5% of an apparently healthy population? However, the most fundamental question relates to the clinical utility of deciding whether or not a person has the metabolic syndrome.

Imagine two men, identical in that neither satisfies the WC and fasting glucose criteria proposed by the ATP III, but both meet the blood pressure and plasma TG levels required for a diagnosis of the metabolic syndrome. However, only one of them has an HDL-C concentration low enough to qualify as the third criterion necessary for a positive diagnosis of the metabolic syndrome. Are these persons fundamentally different? Would the treatment options differ in any substantive way? A very persuasive argument can be made that both men are likely to be insulin resistant, but more important, the therapeutic interventions appropriate to decrease CVD risk would be the same. These considerations are not to question the relationship between the five ATP III criteria and increased CVD risk. Indeed, the most obvious advantage of the publicity that has surrounded the ATP III definition of the metabolic syndrome is to draw attention to the finding that insulin resistance and its associated abnormalities represent important CVD risk factors.

Consistent with the clinical example discussed earlier, the appearance of any one of the criteria in Table 62.2 that reflects a metabolic outcome of insulin resistance is sufficient to increase the likelihood that a person is at a substantially increased risk of CVD. A patient with essential hypertension and hypertriglyceridemia is at increased CVD risk, irrespective of WC, fasting glucose level, or HDL-C concentration, and the absence of a positive diagnosis of the metabolic syndrome in this instance is of relatively little clinical relevance. If the greatest benefit of the concept of the metabolic syndrome is to point out that insulin resistance/hyperinsulinemia leads to a cluster of abnormalities that increase CVD risk, the greatest potential drawback is to focus attention on whether or not a given person meets the proposed diagnostic criteria. The important clinical information will be derived from seeing and responding appropriately to the "trees" (individual CVD risk factors) and paying less attention to whether they are part of an arbitrarily defined "forest" (the metabolic syndrome).

REFERENCES

1. Himsworth HP. Lancet 1939;2:1–6.
2. Himsworth HP. Lancet 1939;2:65–8.
3. Himsworth HP. Lancet 1939;2:118–32.
4. Himsworth HP. Lancet 1939;2:171–5.
5. Himsworth HP. Lancet 1949;1:465–73.
6. Yalow RS, Berson SA. J Clin Invest 1960;39:1157–75.
7. Shen S-W, Reaven GM, Farquhar JW. J Clin Invest 1970;49: 2151–60.
8. DeFronzo RA, Tobin JD, Andres R. Am J Physiol 1979;237: E214–23.
9. Ginsberg H, Olefsky JM, Reaven GM. Diabetes 1974;23:674.
10. Ginsberg H, Kimmerling G, Olefsky JM et al. J Clin Invest 1975;55:454.
11. Reaven GM. Am J Med 1983;74:3.
12. Warram JH, Martin BC, Krowlewski AS et al. Ann Intern Med 1990;113:909–15.
13. Lillioja S, Mott DM, Spraul M et al. N Engl J Med 1993;329: 1988–92.
14. Hollenbeck CB, Reaven GM. J Clin Endocrinol Metab 1987;64: 1169–73.
15. Yeni-Komshian H, Carantoni M, Abbasi F et al. Diabetes Care 2000;23:171–5.
16. Reaven GM, Hollenbeck CB, Chen Y-DI. Diabetologia 1989; 32:52.
17. Reaven GM, Lerner RL, Stern MP et al. J Clin Invest 1967;46: 1756–67.
18. Olefsky JM, Farquhar JW, Reaven GM. Am J Med 1974;57: 551–60.
19. Tobey TA, Greenfield M, Kraemer F et al. Metabolism 1981;30: 165–71.
20. Laws A, Reaven GM. J Intern Med 1992;231:25–30.
21. Ferrannini E, Buzzigoli G, Bonadona R. N Engl J Med 1987; 317:350–7.
22. Shen D-C, Shieh S-M, Fuh M et al. J Clin Endocrinol Metab 1988;66:580–3.
23. Kannel WB. JAMA 1996;275:1571–6.
24. Castelli WP, Garrison RJ, Wilson PWF et al. JAMA 1986;256: 2385–7.
25. Austin MA, Hokanson JE, Edwards KI. Am J Cardiol 1998;81: 7B–12B.
26. Reaven GM. Diabetes 1988;37:1595–607.
27. Reaven GM. Curr Atheroscler Rep 2003;5;364–71.
28. Einhorn D, Reaven GM, Cobin RH et al. Endocr Pract 2003;9: 237–52.
29. National Cholesterol Education Program Expert Panel on Detection, Evaluation, and Treatment of High Blood Cholesterol in Adults (Adult Treatment Panel III). JAMA 2001;285: 2486–97.
30. Olefsky JM, Reaven GM, Farquhar JW. J Clin Invest 1974;53: 64–76.
31. Bogardus C, Lillioja S, Mott DM et al. Am J Physiol 1985; 248:E286–91.
32. Abbasi F, Brown BWB, Lamendola C et al. J Am Coll Cardiol 2002;40:937–43.
33. McLaughlin T, Abbasi F, Lamendola C et al. Circulation 2002;106:2908–12.
34. McLaughlin T, Abbasi F, Cheal K et al. Ann Intern Med 2003; 139:802–9.
35. Ford ES, Mokdad AH, Giles WH. Obes Res 2003;11:1223–31.
36. Centers for Disease Control and Prevention. Third National Health and Nutrition Examination Survey (NHANES III 1988–1994) Reference Manuals and Reports. Hyattsville, MD: US Public Health Service, 1994.
37. Ferrannini E, Natali A, Bell P et al. J Clin Invest 1997;100: 1166–73.
38. World Health Organization Expert Consultation. Lancet 2004;363:157–63.
39. Expert Committee on the Diagnosis and Classification of Diabetes Mellitus. Diabetes Care 2002;25[Suppl 1]:5S–20S.
40. Yip J, Facchini FS, Reaven GM. J Clin Endocrinol Metab 1998;83:2773–6.
41. Facchini FS, Hua N, Abbasi F et al. J Clin Endocrinol Metab 2001;86:3574–8.
42. Tuan C-Y, Abbasi F, Lamendola C et al. Am J Cardiol 2003;92: 606–10.
43. DECODE Study Group, on behalf of the European Diabetes Epidemiology Group. Arch Intern Med 2001;161:397–404.
44. Reaven GM. J Clin Endocrinol Metab 2003;88:2399–403.
45. Ferrari P, Weidmann P, Shaw S et al. Am J Med 1991;91:589–96.
46. Facchini F, Chen Y-DI, Clinkingbeard C et al. Am J Hypertens 1992;5:694–9.
47. Allemann Y, Horber FF, Colombo M et al. Lancet 1993;341: 327–31.
48. Skarfors ET, Lithell HO, Selinus I. J Hypertens 1991;9:217–23.

49. Lissner L, Bengtsson C, Lapidus L et al. Hypertension 1992;20: 797–801.

50. Taittonen L, Uhari M, Nuutinen M et al. Am J Hypertens 1996; 9:193–9.

51. Zavaroni I, Mazza S, Dall'Aglio E et al. J Intern Med 1992;231: 235–40.

52. Reaven GM. Am J Kidney Dis 1997;30:928–31.

53. Skott P, Vaag A, Bruum NE et al. Diabetologia 1991;34:275–81.

54. Facchini FS, DoNascimento C, Reaven GM et al. Hypertension 1999;33:1008–12.

55. Sharma AM, Schorr U, Distler A. Hypertension 1993;21:273–9.

56. Zavaroni I, Coruzzi P, Bonini L et al. Am J Hypertens 1995;8: 855–8.

57. Reaven GM, Lithell H, Landsberg L. N Engl J Med 1996;334: 374–81.

58. Facchini FS, Riccardo A, Stoohs A et al. Am J Hypertens 1996;9: 1013–7.

59. Sheu WH-H, Jeng C-Y, Shieh S-M et al. Am J Hypertens 1992;5: 444–8.

60. Jeppesen J, Hein HO, Suadicani P et al. Hypertension 2000;36: 226–39.

61. Jeppesen J, Hein HO, Suadicani P et al. Arch Intern Med 2001; 161:361–6.

62. Ross R. N Engl J Med 1986;314 488–500.

63. Chen N-G, Abbasi F, Lamendola C et al. Circulation 1999;100: 940–3.

64. Stuhlinger MC, Abbasi F, Chu JW et al. JAMA 2002;287:1420–6.

65. Vallance P. Lancet 2002;358:2096–7.

66. Hulley SH, Roseman RH, Bawol RD et al. N Engl J Med 1980;302:1383–9.

67. Reaven GM, Chen Y-DI, Jeppesen J et al. J Clin Invest 1993; 92:141–6.

68. Jeppesen J, Hollenbeck CB, Zhou M-Y et al. Arterioscler Thromb Vasc Biol 1995;15:320–4.

69. Austin MA, Breslow JL, Hennekens CH et al. JAMA 1988;260: 1917–21.

70. Patsch JR, Miesenbock T, Hopferwieser T et al. Arterioscler Thromb 1992;2:1336–45.

71. Manninen V, Tenkanen L, Koskinen P et al. Circulation 1992;85: 37–45.

72. Rubins HB, Robins SJ, Collins D et al. N Engl J Med 1999;341: 410–8.

73. Robins SJ, Rubins HB, Fass FH et al. Diabetes Care 2003; 26:1513–7.

74. Abbasi F, McLaughlin T, Lamendola C et al. J Clin Endocrinol Metab 2000;85:1251–4.

75. Jeng C-Y, Fuh MM-T, Sheu WH-H et al. Endocrinol Metab 1994;1:15–21.

76. Swenson TL. Diabetes Metab Rev 1991;7:139–53.

77. Fidge N, Nestel P, Ishikawa T et al. Metabolism 1980;29: 643–53.

78. Chen Y-DI, Sheu WH-H, Swislocki ALM et al. Hypertension 1991;17:386–93.

79. Golay A, Zech L, Shi M-Z et al. J Clin Endocrinol Metab 1987; 65:512–8.

80. Brinton EA, Eisenberg S, Breslow JL. Arterioscler Thromb 1994;14:707–20.

SELECTED READINGS

Einhorn D, Reaven GM, Cobin RH et al. American College of Endocrinology position statement the insulin resistance syndrome. Endocr Pract 2003;9:237–52.

Facchini FS, Hua N, Abbasi F et al. Insulin resistance as a predictor of age-related diseases. J Clin Endocrinol Metab 2001;86:3574–8.

Reaven GM. Role of insulin resistance in human disease. Diabetes 1988; 37:1595–607.

Reaven GM. Insulin resistance/compensatory hyperinsulinemia, essential hypertension, and cardiovascular disease. J Clin Endocrinol Metab 2003;88:2399–403.

Reaven GM. The insulin resistance syndrome. Curr Atheroscler Rep 2003;5;364–71.

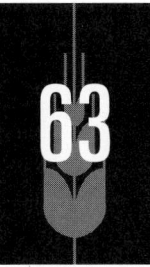

63 OBESITY: ETIOLOGY[1]

JAMES O. HILL, VICTORIA A. CATENACCI, AND HOLLY R. WYATT

DEFINING THE PROBLEM 1013
    Body Mass Index 1013
    Fat Distribution: Waist Circumference 1013
EPIDEMIOLOGY OF OBESITY 1014
    Changes in Obesity Rates Over Time 1015
    Effect of Gender 1015
    Effect of Race 1016
    Effect of Socioeconomic Status 1016
    Effect of Age 1016
    Childhood Obesity 1016
OBESITY AS A DISORDER OF ENERGY BALANCE 1016
    Components of Energy Balance 1017
    Consequences of Energy Imbalance 1018
    Does Energy Balance Differ Between Obese
       and Nonobese Persons? 1019
GENETIC, MEDICAL, ENVIRONMENTAL, AND
    BEHAVIORAL INFLUENCE ON REGULATION
    OF ENERGY BALANCE AND DEVELOPMENT
    OF OBESITY 1019
    Genetic Influences on Obesity 1019
    Medical Disorders Causing Obesity 1021
    Environmental and Behavioral Influences
       on Obesity 1023
DEVELOPMENT OF OBESITY WITHIN SOCIETIES:
    THE ONSET OF THE OBESITY EPIDEMIC 1026
    Obesity as a Societal Issue 1026
    Obesity as a Threat to Public Health 1026
    Economic Consequences of Obesity 1027
SUMMARY 1027

Whether or not obesity develops within an individual depends on a complex interaction among genetic, environmental, and behavioral factors, all acting on energy balance (i.e., energy intake, energy expenditure, or energy storage). Obesity has existed in the population throughout recorded history, but only in recent generations has it increased to an extent that US public health experts are calling it an epidemic (1). This rapid increase in the prevalence of obesity within society has captured the interest not just of health care professionals but of the media, employers, schools, private industry, and policy makers. Because of the association between obesity and many other chronic diseases, obesity has become the public health issue of our time. This chapter deals with the reasons that obesity develops within individual persons and within societies.

DEFINING THE PROBLEM

Obesity is a condition of excess body fat. However, because of the difficulty in obtaining accurate measures of body fatness in the population, measures of height and body weight have been widely used to identify overweight and obesity. Obesity is currently defined using body mass index (BMI).

Body Mass Index

BMI is calculated as weight (kg)/height squared (m^2) and is independent of sex. Table 63.1 shows selected BMI units. BMI is significantly correlated with total body fat content and as such serves as an easily determined surrogate for body fat content (2). BMI is now internationally accepted as a means of identifying overweight and obesity. Table 63.2 shows the generally agreed on classes of relative body weight based on BMI. The BMI classification scheme is based on data obtained from epidemiologic studies evaluating the relationship between BMI and morbidity and mortality, and it provides a way to identify persons who are at increased risk of developing adiposity-related complications (3–5). The risks of developing type 2 diabetes, heart disease, and cancer all increase as BMI increases, with the lowest risk generally seen at BMIs of 22 to 25 kg/m^2. Mortality increases gradually above a BMI of 25 kg/m^2 with a sharper increase above a BMI of 30 kg/m^2. This J-shaped curve of all-cause mortality compared with BMI is shown in Figure 63.1 (6).

Fat Distribution: Waist Circumference

BMI is a good, but not perfect, surrogate for body fatness. Some persons with an "obese" BMI may have a normal amount of body fat and a large muscle mass, whereas others

[1]**Abbreviations: BMI,** body mass index; **BMR,** basal metabolic rate; **CI,** confidence interval; **MC₄,** melanocortin subtype 4; **NEAT,** non–exercise-associated thermogenesis; **NHANES,** National Health and Nutrition Examination Surveys; **PAEE,** physical activity–related energy expenditure; **REE,** resting energy expenditure; **RMR,** resting metabolic rate; **TEE,** total energy expenditure; **TEF,** thermic effect of food; **WHO,** World Health Organization.

TABLE 63.1. SELECTED BODY MASS INDEX UNITS CATEGORIZED BY INCHES (cm) AND POUNDS (kg)

HEIGHT IN INCHES (cm)	BMI 25 kg/m² WEIGHT IN POUNDS (kg)	BMI 27 kg/m² WEIGHT IN POUNDS (kg)	BMI 30 kg/m² WEIGHT IN POUNDS (kg)
58 (147.32)	119 (53.98)	129 (58.51)	143 (64.86)
59 (149.86)	124 (56.25)	133 (60.33)	148 (67.13)
60 (152.40)	128 (58.06)	138 (62.60)	153 (69.40)
61 (154.94)	132 (59.87)	143 (64.86)	158 (71.67)
62 (157.48)	136 (61.69)	147 (66.68)	164 (74.39)
63 (160.02)	141 (63.96)	152 (68.95)	169 (76.66)
64 (162.56)	145 (65.77)	157 (71.21)	174 (78.93)
65 (165.10)	150 (68.04)	162 (73.48)	180 (81.65)
66 (167.64)	155 (70.31)	167 (75.75)	186 (84.37)
67 (170.18)	159 (72.12)	172 (78.02)	191 (86.64)
68 (172.72)	164 (74.39)	177 (80.29)	197 (89.36)
69 (175.26)	169 (76.66)	182 (82.56)	203 (92.08)
70 (177.80)	174 (78.93)	188 (85.28)	207 (93.89)
71 (180.34)	179 (81.19)	193 (87.54)	215 (97.52)
72 (182.88)	184 (83.46)	199 (90.27)	221 (100.25)
73 (185.42)	189 (85.73)	204 (92.53)	227 (102.97)
74 (187.96)	194 (88.00)	210 (95.26)	233 (105.69)
75 (190.50)	200 (90.72)	216 (97.98)	240 (108.86)
76 (193.04)	205 (92.99)	221 (100.25)	246 (111.58)

BMI, body mass index.

with a "normal" BMI may have excess adiposity and reduced muscle mass. In most cases, these exceptions are obvious, but measuring the circumference of the waist can provide an additional check. Waist circumference is highly correlated with the amount of intraabdominal or visceral fat, which in many studies is an independent predictor of increased risk for diabetes, hypertension, dyslipidemia, and ischemic heart disease (7). The combination of waist circumference and BMI can be useful in assessing health risk. An elevated BMI with a low waist circumference may indicate that BMI overestimates risk in a particular person, and a low BMI with a high waist circumference may indicate the opposite. The National Institute of Health Expert Panel on the Identification, Evaluation, and Treatment of Overweight and Obesity in Adults proposed that men with a waist circumference greater than 102 cm (40 in) and women with a waist circumference greater than 88 cm (35 in) are at increased risk

of metabolic diseases (6). Waist circumference is also valuable in evaluating the health risks of persons in the overweight category (with a BMI of 25–30 kg/m²). Overweight persons with a high waist circumference, predictive of high visceral fat, are at much higher risk of metabolic disorders of excessive body fat than overweight persons without an elevated waist circumference. Table 63.2 shows disease risk relative to normal weight and waist circumference. Although waist circumference is an easily measured surrogate for visceral fat, computed tomography and magnetic resonance imaging techniques exist for its accurate measurement.

EPIDEMIOLOGY OF OBESITY

Since the mid-1980s, the prevalence of obesity has increased steadily and markedly in both Westernized and non-Westernized countries, and there are no indications

TABLE 63.2. DISEASE RISKᵃ RELATIVE TO NORMAL WEIGHT AND WAIST CIRCUMFERENCE

	BMI kg/m²	OBESITY CLASS	WAIST CIRCUMFERENCE MEN ≤102 cm (≤40 in) WOMEN ≤88 cm (≤35 in)	WAIST CIRCUMFERENCE MEN >102 cm (>40 in) WOMEN >88 cm (>35 in)
Underweight	<18.5		—	—
Normalᵇ	18.5–24.9		—	—
Overweight	25.0–29.9		Increased	High
Obesity	30.0–34.9	I	High	Very high
	35.0–39.9	II	Very high	Very high
Extreme obesity	≥40	III	Extremely high	Extremely high

BMI, body mass index.
ᵃDisease risk for type 2 diabetes, hypertension, and cardiovascular disease.
ᵇIncreased waist circumference can also be a marker for increased risk even in persons of normal weight.

Adapted from National Institutes of Health, National Heart, Lung and Blood Institute. Clinical guidelines on the identification, evaluation and treatment of overweight and obesity in adults: the evidence report. Obes Res 1998;6[Suppl 2]:51S, with permission.

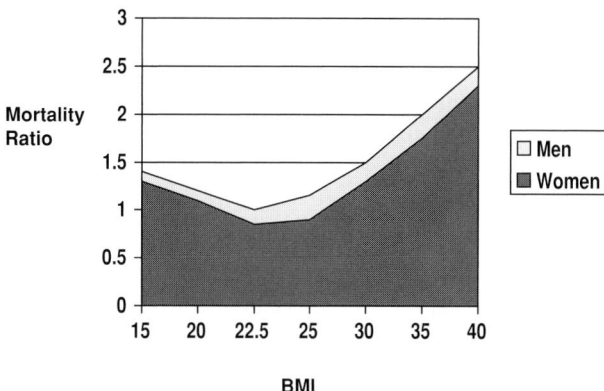

Figure 63.1. J-shaped curve of all-cause mortality compared with body mass index (BMI).

that this trends is abating. For the first time in history, most US adults are overweight or obese (8), and as such they have substantially increased morbidity and mortality from hypertension, stroke, coronary artery disease, dyslipidemia, type 2 diabetes, sleep apnea, and numerous other conditions. Higher BMI also increases all-cause mortality.

Changes in Obesity Rates Over Time

Our most accurate data about changes over time in overweight and obesity rates come from the National Health and Nutrition Examination Surveys (NHANES). The NHANES program of the National Center for Health Statistics, Centers for Disease Control and Prevention, includes a series of cross-sectional nationally representative health examination surveys beginning in 1960. In these surveys height and weight of a large representative sample of the population are taken. Each cross-sectional survey provides a national estimate for United States population at the time of the survey, enabling an examination of trends over time in population. Previous national surveys include the National Health Examination Survey (NHES I, 1960–1962) and the first, second, and third NHANES surveys (NHANES I, 1971–1974; NHANES II, 1976–1980; and NHANES III, 1988–1994). Beginning in 1999, NHANES became a continuous survey without a break between cycles, and the data for the first 2 years of the continuous NHANES (1999–2000) were published in 2002 (9). Review of the NHANES data reveals that the prevalence of obesity was relatively constant from 1960 to 1980, then increased as reported in NHANES III (1988–1994). The most recent data from NHANES 1999–2000 show further increases for both men and women in all age groups and in all racial and ethnic groups studied. According to NHANES 1999–2000, an estimated 64% of persons in the United States are overweight (BMI 25–30) or obese (BMI >30). This represents a prevalence that is 8% higher than the age-adjusted overweight estimates obtained from

NHANES III (1988–1994) and 17% higher than in NHANES I (1971–1974). Among adults 20 to 74 years old, the estimated prevalence of obesity (BMI >30) doubled between NHANES II and NHANES 1999–2000 from approximately 15 to 31%. These data are presented graphically in Figure 63.2.

In addition, data from the Behavioral Risk Factor Surveillance System as analyzed by Sturm (10) indicate that the prevalence of clinically severe obesity is increasing much faster than that of mild obesity. Between 1986 and 2000, the prevalence of a self-reported BMI of 40 or greater (~100 lb [45 kg] overweight) quadrupled from about one in 200 adults in the United States to one in 50; the prevalence of a BMI of 50 or greater increased by a factor of 5, from about one in 2000 to one in 400. In contrast, obesity (BMI >30) roughly doubled during the same period, from about one in ten to one in five. Thus, the published increases in overweight and obesity may underestimate the consequences for the health care system because obesity-related comorbidities are much higher among severely obese persons.

Effect of Gender

Obesity affects both men and women, although with some notable sex differences. More men than women are in the overweight category, but more women than men are in the obese category (11). Overweight and obesity prevalence differences between men and women vary greatly across racial and ethnic groups. In data from NHANES 1999–2000 (9), obesity rates are similar in white men (27.3%) and women (30.1%), but obesity rates are much higher in African-American women (49.7%) than in African-American men (28.1%). Similarly, obesity rates are 39.7% in Hispanic women and

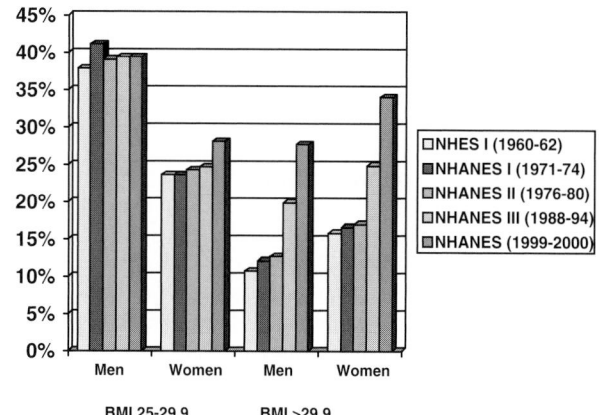

Figure 63.2. Age-adjusted prevalence of overweight and obesity for US adults ages 20 to 74 years, 1960 to 2000. BMI, body mass index; NHES, National Health Examination Survey; NHANES, National Health and Nutrition Examination Surveys. (Data from Flegal KM, Carroll MD, Ogden CL et al. Trends in the age-adjusted and age-specific prevalence of obesity for adults aged 20–74 years, 1960–2000. JAMA 2002; 288:1723–7.)

TABLE 63.3. PREVALENCE OF OVERWEIGHT AND OBESITY BY AGE, SEX, AND RACIAL OR ETHNIC GROUP: UNITED STATES

| SEX | AGE (y)[a] | SAMPLE SIZE (NO.) | | | | PREVALENCE OF OVERWEIGHT (BMI ≥25) (%) | | | |
		ALL[b]	NON-HISPANIC WHITE	NON-HISPANIC BLACK	MEXICAN-AMERICAN	ALL[b]	NON-HISPANIC WHITE	NON-HISPANIC BLACK	MEXICAN-AMERICAN
Both	≥20	4,115	1,831	794	1,105	64.5	62.3	69.6	73.4[c]
Men	≥20	2,043	946	374	538	67.2	67.4	60.7	74.7
	20–39	666	276	125	184	60.5	61.0	52.6	67.5
	40–59	595	262	127	157	70.0	69.9	63.9	79.1
	≥60	782	408	122	197	74.1	74.3	69.1	79.6
Women	≥20	2,072	885	420	567	61.9	57.3	77.3[c]	71.9
	20–39	640	249	140	180	54.3	49.0	70.8[c]	61.6
	40–59	653	249	141	193	66.1	61.0	81.5[c]	79.3
	≥60	779	387	139	194	68.1	65.8	81.7[c]	77.5

BMI, body mass index.

[a] Estimated prevalences for ages ≥20 years were age-standardized by the direct method to the 2000 US Census population using age groups 20 to 30, 40 to 50, and ≥60 years old.

[b] Includes racial or ethnic groups not shown separately.

[c] Significantly different from non-Hispanic whites, $p < .05$ (with Bonferroni correction).

Adapted from Flegal KM, Carroll MD, Ogden CL et al. Trends in the age-adjusted and age-specific prevalence of obesity for adults aged 20–74 years, 1960–2000. JAMA 2002;288:1723–7, with permission.

only 28.9% in Hispanic men. These data are presented in Table 63.3. Body fat distribution also differs between sexes, with men more predisposed to visceral (abdominal) obesity.

Effect of Race

In NHANES 1999–2000, the prevalence of overweight and obesity in men varied little by racial or ethnic group, and no significant differences were reported among groups. Among women, non-Hispanic black women had a higher prevalence of both overweight (77 versus 57%) and obesity (50 versus 33%) than non-Hispanic white women. Mexican-American women had a prevalence that was intermediate between the other two groups. Some groups of Native Americans (e.g., the Pima Indians of Arizona) have even higher rates of obesity. Evidence indicates that these racial differences persist even after controlling for socioeconomic status (12).

Effect of Socioeconomic Status

In developed countries, an inverse relationship exists between socioeconomic status and obesity (12). Among men in the United States, an inconsistent relationship exists between socioeconomic status and obesity, whereas an inverse relationship is noted among women (13). There is also a clear trend for the prevalence of obesity to decrease with increasing levels of education. In 1999 an 11% difference in prevalence as reported between those who had less than a high school education (25.3%) and those who had a college education or more (14.3%) (11). Although the prevalence of obesity differs by socioeconomic status, the increases over time seem to be similar in all socioeconomic groups.

Effect of Age

The prevalence of obesity rises steadily from age 20 to age 60 years, at which time it peaks. After age 60 years, obesity rates begin to decline (12). Investigators have suggested that the increased mortality associated with obesity is selectively weaning the obese from the elderly population, thereby decreasing prevalence of obesity (11).

Childhood Obesity

Overweight and obesity are increasing in children at even more rapid rates than in adults. Data from NHANES III (1988–1994) showed that 10 to 15% of children and adolescents (ages 6–17 years) in the United States are overweight, defined as a BMI in the ninety-fifth percentile for age and gender from the revised National Health Statistics growth charts (14). These values represent a doubling of the rates of overweight observed for children and adolescents in earlier studies. Childhood obesity portends obesity in adulthood, as well as an increased risk of obesity-related diseases (15). Investigators have estimated that 30% of adults become obese during childhood, and about 80% of obese adolescents become obese adults (16). Obesity-related disorders including type 2 diabetes, hypertension, gallbladder disease, hyperlipidemia, orthopedic complications, sleep apnea, and nonalcoholic steatohepatitis are now seen with increasing frequency in the pediatric population (17). Prevention and treatment of childhood obesity are discussed in detail in Chapter 60.

OBESITY AS A DISORDER OF ENERGY BALANCE

Obesity can develop only as a result of an imbalance between energy intake and energy expenditure (i.e., positive energy balance). Understanding the etiology of obesity requires understanding the complex ways in which positive energy balance can occur. Both energy intake and energy expenditure are influenced by genetic factors and by many factors within the environment in which we live. Further, changes in energy expenditure can influence energy intake and vice versa. Because of this complexity, the development of obesity cannot be attributed simply to excessive energy intake or low energy expenditure. High energy intake leads to obesity only if it is not matched by high energy expenditure, and low energy expenditure leads to obesity only if it is not matched by low energy intake.

Energy balance can be illustrated in the following equation below, often called the energy balance equation. The equation states that any change in body weight (ΔBody weight) must be caused by a difference between energy intake (E_{in}) and energy expenditure (E_{out}).

$$E_{in} - E_{out} = \Delta\text{Body weight}$$

The first law of thermodynamics states that energy can be neither created nor destroyed. Energy balance in the body occurs when the energy content of food consumed is matched by the amount of energy expended. For body weight to change, energy imbalance must occur. When intake is lower than expenditure, negative energy balance occurs, and body energy stores are reduced. When energy intake exceeds expenditure, positive energy balance occurs, and body energy stores are increased.

Factors that affect the etiology of obesity must affect one or more components of energy balance. This is why an understanding of energy balance is essential for an understanding of how obesity develops.

Components of Energy Balance

Energy Intake

We take in energy in the foods we eat. The major macronutrient sources of dietary energy are fat, carbohydrate, protein, and alcohol. Humans regulate their food intake in a complex way that is incompletely understood. After consumption of food, satiety signals are generated in the periphery from the mouth, from the rest of the gastrointestinal system, and as a consequence of peripheral metabolic processes involved in digestion and absorption of nutrients. Signals from the periphery are monitored by a sophisticated neural system that is incompletely understood. Many hormones and peptides, deriving both from the periphery and from the central nervous system, appear to be involved in the food intake regulatory system. Neural peptides such as α-melanocyte-stimulating hormone, agouti-related peptide, neuropeptide Y, and melanocyte concentrating hormone are known to influence eating behavior (18). In addition, gut peptides such as cholecystokinin, gastrin-releasing peptide, glucagon-like peptide-1, bombesin, insulin, and ghrelin can also modify

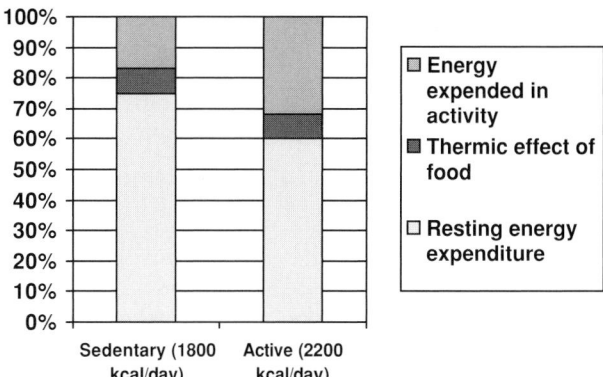

Figure 63.3. Components of total energy expenditure TEE in sedentary and active persons.

feeding behaviors (18). Longer range signals of satiety may be related to body energy stores (e.g., body fat, glycogen). Leptin is a hormone secreted from adipocytes as fat cell size increases and may serve as a signal within the brain to decrease food intake and increase energy expenditure (19).

Energy Expenditure

Total energy expenditure (TEE) is the sum of resting energy expenditure (REE), thermic effect of food (TEF) and physical activity–related energy expenditure (PAEE). The components of TEE and a comparison of TEE in sedentary and active persons are shown in Figure 63.3.

Resting Energy Expenditure. The majority of human energy expenditure is through the body's metabolism at rest, called REE. REE comprises 60 to 80% of TEE in most people. REE is the energy required by the body to maintain basic physiologic functions such as pumping blood, making hormones, and maintaining body temperature. Basal metabolic rate (BMR) is the theoretic minimum level of energy expended by the body to sustain life. REE is the body's energy expenditure measured during rest in the fasted state. REE is slightly (~3%) higher than BMR because of the energy required for arousal. REE is in general related to lean body mass, primarily organ and muscle mass. The resting energy requirements of different organs and tissues differ dramatically and are shown in Table 63.4. In adults, lean organs account for almost 75% of REE, although they constitute only 10% of body weight. Skeletal muscle consumes approximately 20% of REE and comprises 40% of body weight. Adipose tissue normally comprises 20% of body weight but consumes only 5% of REE. To illustrate this point, take the example of a physiologically normal 70-kg man. His 300-mg kidney would consume approximately 360 kcal/day, whereas the 15 kg of adipose tissue consumes a total of only 80 kcal/day. REE is generally higher in obese persons than in lean persons because of an increase in lean body mass (organ mass and muscle mass) in addition to the increase in adipose tissue in the obese (20).

TABLE 63.4. CONTRIBUTION OF DIFFERENT ORGANS AND TISSUES TO ENERGY EXPENDITURE

	WEIGHT		METABOLIC RATE	
ORGAN OR TISSUE	kg	(% OF TOTAL)	kcal/kg/d	(% OF TOTAL)
Kidneys	0.3	(0.5)	440	(8)
Brain	1.4	(2.0)	240	(20)
Liver	1.8	(2.6)	200	(21)
Heart	0.3	(0.5)	440	(9)
Muscle	28.0	(40.0)	13	(22)
Adipose tissue	15.0	(21.4)	4	(4)
Other (skin, gut, bone, etc.)	23.2	(33.0)	12	(16)
Total	70.0	(100)		(100)

Adapted from Matthews DE. Proteins and amino acids. In: Shils ME, Olson JA, Shike M et al., eds. Modern Nutrition in Health and Disease. 9th ed. Baltimore: Lippincott Williams & Wilkins, 1999:11–48, with permission.

Physical Activity Energy Expenditure. PAEE is the component of energy expenditure that is most under voluntary control because it is influenced most strongly by the amount of physical activity. PAEE is the most variable component of energy expenditure and can easily range from 10% of TEE in sedentary persons to 40% of TEE in highly active persons. PAEE includes volitional activities such as daily activities and exercise and nonvolitional behaviors such as spontaneous muscle contractions, maintenance of posture, and fidgeting. Although obese and lean persons expend the same amount of energy during activities in which the body weight is supported, obese persons expend more energy than lean persons during weight-bearing activities because of the increased work involved in carrying more weight. Physical activity provides the greatest source of flexibility in the energy expenditure system, and it is the component through which large changes in energy expenditure can be achieved.

Thermic Effect of Food. TEF is the increase in energy expenditure associated with digestion, absorption, and storage of ingested macronutrients, usually 7 to 10% of the total caloric content of the meal. The energy cost of a meal is associated with the macronutrient composition of food consumed, with the TEF higher for carbohydrate and protein than for fat. The reason for this finding is that the process for energy storage of ingested fat is very efficient, whereas for carbohydrate and protein, additional energy is needed for conversion to an appropriate storage form (e.g., glucose to glycogen, amino acids to protein). Whether or not obese persons have a systematically lower TEF than lean persons is a matter of great controversy. Certainly, data suggest that this is the case, but supposed differences are very small and are of questionable importance in body weight regulation. If such differences are present, it is not clear whether they existed before the development of obesity and thus may have contributed to weight gain or whether they arise as a consequence of the obese state (21). A reduction in TEF in the obese person could be related to increased insulin resistance and blunted sympathetic nervous system activity that is often associated with obesity (22).

Energy Stored in the Body. The body stores energy as protein, carbohydrate, and fat. The body has very limited storage capacity for both protein (in muscle and organs) and carbohydrate (as glucose and glycogen). The capacity for the body to store fat in adipose tissue depots is virtually unlimited. Because of their high energy density and hydrophobic nature, triglycerides are a fivefold better fuel per unit mass than glycogen. A lean adult has approximately 35 billion adipocytes, each containing 0.4 to 0.6 μg of triglyceride. Triglycerides liberate 9.3 kcal/g when oxidized; by comparison, glycogen stored in the liver and muscle produces 4.1 kcal/g when oxidized. Triglycerides are stored very compactly inside the fat cell, thereby accounting for 85% of its weight. Thus, total storage capacity of adipose tissue in lean persons is approximately 80,000 to 130,000 kcal. In obese persons, triglyceride stores can increase tremendously because of both increased adipocyte size and increased adipocyte cell number. The total body stores of glycogen and protein (as muscle) in an average 70-kg man are approximately 1800 and 110,000 kcal, respectively, in a person of normal weight. However, the body can mobilize only approximately half its protein stores for fuel before life-threatening loss of lean tissue occurs. Thus, adipose tissue represents an effective mechanism for storing fuel and permits survival during periods of food deprivation. The duration of survival during starvation depends on the amount of body fat mass; in lean men, death occurs after approximately 60 to 90 days. In contrast, obese persons have undergone prolonged therapeutic fasts ingesting only noncaloric fluids, vitamins, and minerals for more than a year without consequences (23).

Consequences of Energy Imbalance

The average person consumes close to 1 million calories per year, yet many persons are able to maintain a remarkable state of equilibrium. Even a slight perturbation in energy balance would lead to dramatic weight gain or loss. An error in matching intake to expenditure of only 5% would result in a change of 15 kg over the course of a year. Short-term overfeeding and underfeeding studies suggest that energy expenditure is affected when energy intake is altered. During food restriction, energy expenditure declines, attenuating the loss of body weight that results from the negative energy balance (24). During overfeeding, some increase in energy expenditure occurs to mitigate the increase in body weight that would occur as a result of positive energy balance (25). The changes in energy expenditure are much greater with underfeeding than with overfeeding, a finding suggesting the body has a strong ability to defend against loss of body weight and a much weaker ability to defend against body weight gain.

Negative Energy Balance Results in Weight Loss

An energy deficit of approximately 3500 kcal is needed to lose 1 lb of body weight. Approximately 75 to 85% of weight lost by dieting is composed of fat, and 15 to 25% is fat-free mass. There is regional heterogeneity in the distribution of fat loss, with loss of subcutaneous adipose tissue generally preceding the loss of muscle mass and visceral fat (26). Most of the loss in fat is caused by a decrease in lipid content of existing adipocytes; however, long-term fat loss may decrease the number of fat cells as well.

Positive Energy Balance Results in Weight Gain

When energy intake exceeds energy expenditure, a state of positive energy balance is reached, and excess calories are stored in the body. The composition of weight gain during positive energy balance is predominately fat (~70–80%), with some gain in lean body mass (20–30%). Not all excess energy is stored in the body during overfeeding. Another way of saying this is that efficiency of storage of excess energy is not 100%. It is generally accepted that efficiency of storage of excess nutrients is somewhere between 60 and 90% (27, 28). Efficiency of storage of excess energy seems to be influenced by characteristics of the subjects (i.e., genetics) and by the composition of the diet overconsumed. Bouchard and colleagues (29) found that twins responded with similar amounts of body weight gain when they were overfed, a finding suggesting that genes influence the efficiency of storage during overfeeding.

Horton and associates (30) demonstrated differences in efficiency of storage of excess fat versus excess carbohydrate. They overfed 16 men isoenergetic amounts (50% above energy requirements) of fat and carbohydrate for 14 days each. Fat overfeeding had minimal effects on fat oxidation and TEE, leading to efficient storage of 90 to 95% of the total excess energy consumed. In contrast, carbohydrate overfeeding produced progressive increases in carbohydrate oxidation and TEE and decreases in fat oxidation. This resulted in storage of only 75 to 85% of excess energy during fat overfeeding. Thus, carbohydrate overfeeding was associated with a lower storage efficiency than fat overfeeding.

Does Energy Balance Differ Between Obese and Nonobese Persons?

Results from a large number of studies suggest that TEE is similar between lean and obese persons, after taking differences in body composition into account (31). The lack of difference is probably the result of the opposing effects of the additional energy cost of weight-bearing activities in subjects with greater body mass and the greater REE caused by increased fast mass versus the decreased likelihood of physical activity associated with carrying additional fat mass. In addition, studies using indirect calorimetry have shown that obese persons clearly consume more calories than lean persons. In "diet-resistant" patients who fail to lose weight despite claiming strict adherence to low-calorie diets, defects in REE or TEE have not been found (32). These patients underestimate their food intake and consume twice as many calories as recorded in daily food records (33). Although energy metabolism in obese subjects at a steady weight does not seem defective, the role of alterations in energy metabolism in the development of obesity and the response to dieting are less clear.

GENETIC, MEDICAL, ENVIRONMENTAL, AND BEHAVIORAL INFLUENCE ON REGULATION OF ENERGY BALANCE AND DEVELOPMENT OF OBESITY

Most people regulate their body weight within a defined range that is likely determined by genetic factors. Some investigators have described regulation of body weight as a "set point" model, in which each individual person has a preferred level of body weight to defend. However, the gradual weight gain over time of the population suggests this may not be the best description.

A better model may be a "settling point." This model would predict that an individual person within a constant environment with constant genetic factors would defend a specific body weight level. However, if either genes or environmental factors change, the level of body weight defended would change. This model is a better fit with data suggesting that as the environment has changed over the past few decades, the long-term body weight of the population has increased.

Genetic Influences on Obesity

Several lines of evidence show strong genetic influences on body weight.

Family Studies

Within any given environment, a certain degree of variation in body weight exists among individuals. It is estimated that up to 40% of variation in BMI is explained by genetic factors (34). BMI is highly correlated among first-degree family members, with an increased relative risk for the development of obesity for a first-degree relative of an obese person. Family studies demonstrate that obese parents produce the highest proportion of obese children (35). However, in these nuclear family studies that examine sibling-sibling and sibling-parent correlations, it is difficult to separate genetic factors from the effect of the environment.

Adoption studies provide another approach for estimating heritability based on the similarity of adoptive childrens' body weight to that of both their adoptive and biologic parents. These studies suggest a stronger role for genetics than for environment in predicting future weight. The BMI of the biologic parents is much more strongly correlated with the adult weight of the adoptive child than is the BMI of the adoptive parents (35).

Twin studies have been an integral part of the research into the genetics of obesity, and they provide stronger support for the effect of genetic factors on BMI. BMI has been shown to be similar between twins, with the strongest correlation in monozygotic twin pairs. The observation holds true whether twins were raised separately or apart.

Single-Gene Defects

Although several single genes causing obesity have been identified in rodents (36), only a few monogenic causes of obesity have been described in humans. The gene whose contribution is thought to be most prevalent is the melanocortin-4 receptor gene (*MC4R*) (37). *MC4R* mutations have been suggested as the most frequent single-gene cause of obesity, and they are estimated to be present in about 4% of patients with severe obesity (19). The MC_3 and MC_4 receptors are involved in suppression of food intake by α-melanocyte-stimulating hormone; deficiency of the MC_4 receptor leads to massive obesity in humans. A much rarer form of obesity has been described with mutations in proopiomelanocortin (38), the precursor for the peptides that act on the MC_4 receptor. Perhaps the best known single-gene mutation involves the recently isolated hormone leptin. Leptin is a 167-amino acid protein produced by fat cells and is thought to be critical in the regulation of body fat and body weight. Leptin signals the brain through leptin receptors about the size of adipose stores. Mutations in genes for leptin (39) and the leptin receptor have also been associated with obesity (40). However, very few individuals with these defects have been identified. Treatment of leptin-deficient (but not leptin receptor–deficient) children leads to weight loss. The peroxisome proliferator-activator-γ receptor (41) is important in the control of fat cell differentiation and proliferation. Defects in the proliferator-activator-γ receptor have been reported to cause modest obesity that begins later in life. Another defect described is in the prohormone convertase-1 (42).

In one family, defects in this gene, and in a second gene were associated with obesity. Members of the family with only the prohormone convertase-1 defect were not obese, a finding suggestive that the interaction of the two genes led to obesity. These genes illustrate the potentially powerful effect that specific genes can have on obesity; however, these disorders are at present extraordinarily rare.

Polygenic Interactions

An additional 250 genes, markers, and chromosomal regions have been linked with obesity, but the clinical importance of each association is not yet known (43). It is likely that obesity is a highly polygenic and complex disorder, resulting from the input of multiple genes, with additional interactions between genes and environment and genes and behavior. In addition, the increased global prevalence of obesity could not be driven by changes in the gene pool, because substantial changes take thousands of years to accumulate and affect the phenotype of a population. Rather, it is more likely that acute changes in behavior and environment have contributed to the rapid increase in obesity and that genetic factors may be important in differing individual susceptibilities to these changes (31).

Genes and Energy Balance

Genes can affect each component of energy balance. Although the majority of research has focused on genetic influences on food intake, genes can also affect each component of energy expenditure and the efficiency with which body mass is gained or lost during periods of energy imbalance.

Energy Intake. As discussed previously, numerous neuropeptides and gut-derived peptides have been implicated in the regulation of appetite and hunger. Genetic differences among individuals in levels or activity of these peptides and hormones or their receptors could potentially affect energy intake and body weight. Genes may also influence preference for certain foods or for certain macronutrients.

Energy Expenditure. Each component of energy expenditure could be influenced by genetics. Ravussin and Bogardus (44) showed genetic influences on resting metabolic rate (RMR). Investigators have suggested genetic influences on TEF. Genes may also influence the energy expended in physical activity. In addition, genetic variations may underlie individual differences in non–exercise-associated thermogenesis (NEAT). Levine and colleagues (45) investigated the physiologic basis of interindividual variation in weight gain in response to overeating by measuring changes in energy storage and expenditure in 16 nonobese volunteers overfed 1000 kcal/day for 8 weeks. Two thirds of the increases in total daily energy expenditure resulted from increased NEAT, which is associated with fidgeting, maintenance of posture, and other physical activities of daily life. Changes in NEAT accounted for the tenfold differences in fat storage that occurred and directly predicted resistance to fat gain with overfeeding. These results suggest that as humans overeat, activation of NEAT dissipates excess energy to preserve leanness, and failure to activate NEAT may result in ready fat gain. At present, the genetic basis of NEAT remains undefined, but NEAT may be extremely important in determining the response to the environmental factors that lead to obesity.

Storage Efficiency. Genetic influences on how much weight is lost or gained during periods of positive or negative energy balance likely exist. Such differences could result from differences in substrate oxidation or differences in how much excess energy is stored as (or comes from) fat versus protein during periods of energy imbalance. Positive or negative energy balance produces changes in body weight in everybody; the extent of body weight changes may be partially determined by genetic factors.

Medical Disorders Causing Obesity

True medical disorders causing obesity are rare; however, the prevalence of eating disorders in the obese suggests some role for these disorders in the development and maintenance of obesity. In addition, several drugs used commonly in the population may contribute to weight gain and difficulty in losing weight.

Congenital Causes of Obesity

Prader-Willi Syndrome. Prader-Willi syndrome results from an abnormality on chromosome 15q11.2 that is transmitted paternally and produces infantile myotonia, mental retardation, hypogonadism, overeating, and obesity. This syndrome has an incidence of one per 10,000 to 15,000 live births, and massive obesity usually develops in the first year of life.

Down Syndrome. Trisomy 21 is a genetic disorder with either a complete or a partial extra chromosome 21. The prevalence of Down syndrome is one in 600 to 800 live births. The obesity predisposition in Down syndrome has been suggested to result from a reduced metabolic rate (46).

Bardet-Biedel Syndrome. Bardet-Biedel syndrome is a rare autosomal recessive disorder with early-onset, modest obesity. Patients also have mental retardation, polydactyly, hypogonadism, and congenital heart defects. This syndrome has genetic heterogeneity, with abnormalities described on five different chromosomes.

Alstrom Syndrome. Alstrom syndrome is associated with truncal obesity that has onset between the ages of 2 and 5 years, normal intelligence quotient, and hypogonadism in male but not female patients.

Cohen Syndrome and Carpenter Syndrome. Both Cohen syndrome and Carpenter syndrome are autosomal recessive syndromes of obesity associated with craniofacial abnormalities.

Neuroendocrine Disorders

Cushing Syndrome. A common feature of Cushing syndrome is progressive centripetal obesity, usually involving the face, neck (leading to a buffalo hump and obscuring the clavicles), trunk, abdominal mesentery, and mediastinum. The extremities are usually spared and may be wasted. In contrast to adults, children with Cushing syndrome have generalized obesity accompanied by a decrease or cessation in linear growth (47).

Hypothalamic Disorders. Injury to the vetromedial or paraventicular regions of the hypothalamus or the amygdala, regions of the brain responsible for integrating metabolic information regarding nutrient stores with afferent sensory information about food availability, leads to hyperphagia and obesity. Hypothalamic obesity can be caused by trauma, tumors, inflammatory diseases, surgery, or increased intracranial pressure.

Hypothyroidism. People with hypothyroidism may gain weight because of a general slowing of metabolic activity. The weight gain associated with hypothyroidism is usually modest (5–10 kg), with marked obesity uncommon (47).

Polycystic Ovary Syndrome. More than 50% of women with polycystic ovary syndrome are obese. Features of this syndrome include oligomenorrhea, hirsutism, polycystic ovaries, insulin resistance, and increased ovarian production of testosterone. The factors responsible for this association are not well understood (47).

Growth Hormone Deficiency. Adults deficient in growth hormone have increased subcutaneous and visceral fat and decreased lean body mass. The gradual decline in growth hormone with age may in part explain the increase in visceral fat with age (47).

Drug-Related Causes

Medications Associated with Weight Gain. Medications are a significant source of iatrogenic overweight and obesity. Weight gain associated with medications is an important cause of treatment noncompliance and may increase morbidity and mortality from obesity-related disorders. Many antipsychotic agents (especially clozapine and olanzapine, but not ziprasidone) are associated with weight gain. A recent review by Aronne and Segal (48) discussed several psychotropic drugs with side effects of weight gain. The weight gain associated with clozapine was associated with a 37% increase in the incidence of type 2 diabetes. Antidepressants vary considerably in terms of their weight gain potential; tricyclic antidepressants and monoamine oxidase inhibitors are more likely to cause weight gain than selective serotonin reuptake inhibitors and some of the newer agents such as bupropion. The mood stabilizer lithium causes weight gain in one third to two thirds of patients, which can range from 5 to 15 kg over 2 years. Most antiepileptic drugs, with the exeptions of topiramate, lamotrigine, and felbamate, are associated with weight gain. When used for the treatment of seizure disorders, both valproate and neurontin have substantial weight gain potential. These authors concluded that it is critical to weigh patients regularly, to determine whether medication regimens are contributing to weight gain, and to consider alternative agents that do not promote weight gain or that cause weight loss.

Other classes of drugs associated with weight gain are (a) steroid hormones (corticosteroids and hormonal contraceptives), (b) antidiabetic agents (insulin, sulfonylureas, and thiazoladenediones) (c) antihistamines, (d) antihypertensive agents (α- and β-blockers), and (e) protease inhibitors. The degree of weight gain with these drugs is generally not sufficient to produce true obesity, except in patients treated with high-dose corticosteroids (47). However, the possibility of weight gain as a side effect should be discussed with the patient before the treatment is started. For patients who are already overweight, alternate agents that do not promote weight gain should be considered. Drugs that may promote weight gain and their therapeutic alternatives are shown in Table 63.5.

Cessation of Smoking. Weight gain is common when people discontinue smoking. The prevalence of smoking has declined over the same period that the rates of overweight and obesity have increased. Flegal and colleagues (49) analyzed data on current and past weight and smoking status for a national sample of 5247 adults 35 years of age or older who participated in NHANES III, conducted from 1988 through 1991. These investigators found that the weight gain over a 10-year period that was associated with the cessation of smoking (i.e., the gain among smokers who

quit that was in excess of the gain among continuing smokers) was 4.4 kg for men and 5.0 kg for women. In addition, they estimated that smoking cessation within the past 10 years increased the odds ratio of obesity 2.4-fold in men and 2.0-fold in women. Although the health benefits are undeniable, smoking cessation may nevertheless be associated with a small increase in the prevalence of overweight.

Eating Disorders

Night Eating Syndrome. Night eating syndrome is a well known pattern of disordered eating in the obese. It is defined as consumption of at least 25%, and often more than 50%, of daily energy intake between the evening meal and the next morning. It is related to sleep disturbances and may be related to sleep apnea, in which nocturnal awakenings are common.

Binge Eating Disorder. Binge eating disorder is a psychiatric illness characterized by uncontrolled episodes of eating that usually occur in the evening. It is estimated that 10 to 25% of obese persons experience binge eating episodes, whereas only 3% meet the diagnosis of binge eating disorder (50). These patients may respond to drugs that modulate serotonin release or reuptake.

Progressive Hyperphagic Obesity. A few obese persons become overweight in childhood and then have relentless weight gain, often reaching 300 pounds by age 30 years. Because an intake of approximately 22 kcal is required to maintain each extra kilogram of body weight,

TABLE 63.5. DRUGS THAT MAY PROMOTE WEIGHT GAIN AND THERAPEUTIC ALTERNATIVES

DRUGS THAT MAY PROMOTE WEIGHT GAIN	DRUGS THAT ARE WEIGHT NEUTRAL OR PROMOTE WEIGHT LOSS
Psychiatric/neurologic medications	Alternative psychiatric/neurologic medications
Antipsychotic drugs	Antipsychotic drugs
Olanzapine, clozapine	Ziprasidone, risperidone, quetiapine
Antidepressants	Antidepressants
SSRIs, TCAs, MAOIs	Bupropion, nefazodone
Antiepileptic drugs	Antiepileptic drugs
Gabapentin, valproate, carbamazepine	Topiramate, lamotrigine
Lithium	Alternatives to steroid hormones
Steroid hormones	Barrier contraceptive methods
Hormonal contraceptives	NSAIDs
Corticosteroids	Weight loss
Progestational steroids	Alternative antidiabetic agents
Antidiabetic agents	Metformin
Insulin	Acarbose, miglitol
Sulfonylureas	Orlistat, sibutramine
Thiazolidinediones	Decongestants, inhalers
Antihistamines	Alternative antihypertensive agents
Antihypertensive agents	ACE inhibitors, calcium channel blockers
α- and β-Adrenergic blockers	
Protease inhibitors[a]	

ACE, angiotensin-converting enzyme; MAOI, monoamine oxidase inhibitor; NSAID, nonsteroidal antiinflammatory drug; SSRI, selective serotonin reuptake inhibitor; TCA, tricyclic antidepressant.
[a] May cause weight gain, but less than the drugs they replace.

From Aronne LJ, Segal KR. Weight gain in the treatment of mood disorders. J Clin Psychiatry 2003;64[Suppl 8]:22–9. Copyright 2003, Physicians Postgraduate Press; reprinted by permission.

energy requirements increase year by year, and thus weight gain must be the result of progressive increases in caloric intake.

Environmental and Behavioral Influences on Obesity

It clear that nongenetic factors can influence our behavior, which, in turn, can have a major influence on whether or not obesity develops. We make choices about what and when to eat and about our physical activity patterns that have a big impact on energy balance. A summary of environmental factors providing a constant pressure toward positive energy balance and an increase in body fat mass is shown in Figure 63.4.

Environmental and Behavioral Influences on Energy Expenditure

Resting Metabolic Rate. RMR can be affected by behaviors that produce negative energy balance, such as food restriction. Whether or not RMR can be influenced by physical activity is controversial; some studies suggest that long-term exercise can increase RMR, and some suggest that this is not the case (51). The extent to which differences in RMR caused by differences in physical activity affect the development of obesity is unclear. Very little evidence suggests that differences in RMR (for whatever reason) play a role in development of obesity.

Thermic Effect of Food. Similarly, TEF can be influenced by amount and composition of food eaten and possibly by physical activity level (52). However, little indication exists that differences in TEF play a major role in development of obesity.

Physical Activity Energy Expenditure. The biggest impact of the environment on energy expenditure is through PAEE. Although some genetic influences on desire

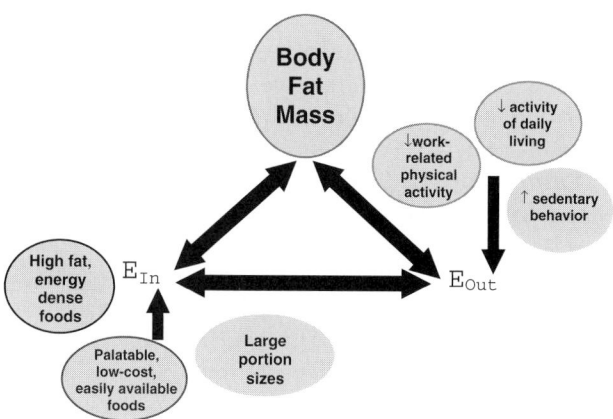

Figure 63.4. Environmental factors providing a constant pressure toward positive energy (E) balance and an increase in body fat mass. (From Hill JO, Wyatt HR, Melanson EL. Genetic and environmental contributions to obesity. Med Clin North Am 2000;84:333–46. Copyright 2000, with permission from Elsevier.)

to engage in physical activity may exist, the influence of the environment on this component of energy expenditure is clearly strong. A low level of physical activity decreases TEE and, unless matched by a decrease in energy intake, causes weight gain. Restriction of activity in rodents produces weight gain, and animals in zoos tend to be heavier than animals in the wild. Several observations illustrate the importance of energy expenditure in the origin of weight gain. Estimates of average recorded energy intake in Britain declined substantially as obesity rates escalated. These results suggest that levels of physical activity have declined even faster and reduced energy expenditure is more important in causing obesity (53). A 1983 study of almost 900 middle-aged men in the Netherlands found that despite an average weight gain of 3.5 kg over 10 years, daily energy intake decreased by approximately 450 calories during the same time period (54). A prospective study from Finland also demonstrated a 225 kJ/day decline in work-related physical activity from 1982 to 1992 (55).

Cross-sectional and population studies have also shown a negative relationship between level of physical activity and BMI. Cross-sectional analysis of both baseline and follow-up data from NHANES I revealed that recreational physical activity was inversely related to body weight. The estimated relative risk of major weight gain for those in the low activity level at the follow-up survey compared with those in the high activity level was 3.1 (95% confidence interval [CI], 1.6–6.0) in men and 3.8 (2.3–6.5) in women. In addition, the relative risk for persons whose activity level was low at both the baseline and follow-up surveys was 2.3 (0.9–5.8) in men and 7.1 (2.2–23.3) in women (56). In NHANES III, low levels of physical activity and recreation were strongly related to subsequent weight gain, with men and women in the lowest tertile of activity level almost four times as likely to gain weight (57).

In our affluent society, labor-sparing devices in the home and workplace reduce energy expenditure. Although it has not been definitively documented, it is intuitively obvious that improvements in technology over the past several decades have probably reduced energy expenditure required for daily living to a fraction of what it was centuries ago. Modes of mechanized transportation of people (cars, escalators, elevators) and information (computers, telephones, faxes) have replaced walking, horseback riding, and biking. Data from the National Personal Transportation Survey in the United States showed that between 1990 and 1995, the number of annual walking trips had declined by 12.4%, whereas the number of daily car trips had increased a nearly identical amount of 12.3% (58). Television, video games, and the Internet have replaced more active entertainment and leisure time activities in many adults and children. The average child watches 28 hours of television per week (59). Use of automated equipment in the household (central heat, washing machines) has decreased the energy required in preparing food and maintaining a comfortable home. Physical activity in the workplace has also been reduced as a result of computers, automated equipment, and electronic mail. Increased concern with crime limits walking and playing outside in some areas. Fewer than 25% of US adults report engaging in regular physical activity during leisure time, defined as 3 times a week for a minimum of 20 minutes (60).

Environmental and Behavioral Influences on Energy Intake

The environment can influence the amount and composition of the food we eat. Obtaining data on trends in total energy intake is difficult, and available data are problematic because they rely on self-reported energy intake, which is notoriously unreliable. However, the available data suggest either a slight increase or a modest decline in total energy intake since the 1970s and 1980s (61, 62). Several factors in the environment may affect energy intake. These include diet composition, portion size, convenience, variety, and cost.

Diet Composition

Dietary Fat. Diets high in fat have been suggested to increase the risk of obesity. Sedentary animals given ad libitum high-fat diets gain weight and become obese as compared with those given a low-fat diet (35). Studies in humans also support the role of dietary fat in the development of obesity. Because subjects tend to eat a constant weight of food on both high-fat and low-fat diets, high-fat diets seem to increase the risk of overeating (35). The epidemiologic literature on the relationship between fat intake and body weight was critically reviewed by Lissner and Heitmann (63). Although the data were not entirely consistent, these investigators concluded that the greater the amount of dietary fat humans consume, the greater their body weight. In addition, it appears that a reduction in dietary fat without intentional restriction of energy intake causes weight loss. Astrup and colleagues performed a metaanalysis to evaluate the efficacy of ad libitum low-fat diets in reducing body weight in persons who did not have diabetes. They included data from 16 trials, enrolling 1910 individuals. Low-fat intervention groups showed a greater weight loss than control groups (3.2 kg, 95% CI, 1.9–4.5 kg; $p < .0001$) and a greater reduction in energy intake (1138 kJ/day, 95% CI, 564–1712 kJ/day; $p = .002$) (64).

Energy Density. The effect of dietary fat on energy intake is difficult to separate from an effect of energy density (65). Because foods higher in fat provide more energy per gram (9 kcal/g) than carbohydrate or protein (both ~4 kcal/g), some investigators have suggested that the energy density of the diet, rather than the dietary fat, is responsible for increased energy intake and weight gain (66, 67). Although fat content is a major determinant of energy density, water content is also important, and the combination of fat and water content explains 99% of the

variance in energy density (68). In general, energy-dense foods are highly palatable but not very satiating, so they may be more easily overconsumed (69). Studies have shown that energy intake increases as energy density increases even when the dietary fat content is maintained at a constant level (67). However, no data are available on how the energy density of food has changed over time, nor do data correlate energy density with obesity (24).

Sugar. Sugar is often implicated in development of obesity, but definitive data are lacking. Generally, an inverse relationship exists between fat and sugar intake, a finding suggesting that high sugar intake should be associated with low fat intake and reduced energy intake. However, refined products with high sugar and low water content are high in energy density and could promote food intake. Ludwig and associates (70) suggested that consumption of high levels of sugar, particularly in soft drinks, could affect food intake and increase the chances of developing obesity. More data are needed to determine the specific relationship between sugar content of foods and total energy intake.

Carbohydrate Intake. Dietary carbohydrates (particularly carbohydrates with a high glycemic index) have been implicated in the development of obesity (71). However, data on the percentage of dietary calories consumed as carbohydrate over time are conflicting. Hallfrisch and colleagues evaluated dietary records from 105 men in the Baltimore Longitudinal Study and found that the percentage of calories consumed as carbohydrate increased from 39% in the 1960s to 44% in the 1980s (72). In contrast, data from the Framingham cohort showed no changes in the percentage of dietary calories obtained from carbohydrate between the 1950s and the 1980s (73).

Fruit and Vegetable Intake. Perez (74) analyzed data from the first half of cycle 1.1 of the Canadian Community Health Survey, collected from September 2000 through February 2001. Multivariate linear regression was used to model the associations between eating fruit and vegetables and health behaviors, while controlling for other influences. When other influences are taken into account, the frequency of eating fruits and vegetables is positively related in both sexes to being physically active, not smoking, and not being overweight.

Larger Portion Sizes. Since the mid-1980s, portion sizes have exploded, with the advent of supersizing and ever larger baked goods and candy bars. The US population associates quantity with quality, so restaurants and food manufacturers are providing larger and larger quantities as evidence of value. The greater energy content of larger food portions could be contributing to the increasing prevalence of overweight and obesity. Young and Nestle (75) determined marketplace portion sizes, identified changes in these sizes with time, and compared these marketplace portions with federal standards as defined by the US Department of Agriculture and the Food and Drug Administration. These investigators found that most marketplace portions exceed standard serving sizes by at least a factor of 2 and sometimes eightfold. In addition, portions have increased over time. For example portion sizes at fast food chains are often two to five times larger than the original size. Although research is insufficient to implicate portion size definitively as a contributor to overeating and obesity, it is reasonable to think that this may be the case.

Dietary Variety. Before the twentieth century, refined sugars and flours were luxury items used only on special occasions. Our current diet consists of numerous highly palatable snacks and desserts produced from fats, refined sugars, and starches. The aggressive and sophisticated marketing of the food industry targets children and adolescents with appealing images of sweetened cereals, candies, cookies, and high-calorie beverages. Studies have suggested that a high variety of sweets, snacks, condiments, entrees, and carbohydrates coupled with a low variety of vegetables promotes long-term increases in energy intake and body fatness. McCrory and colleagues (76) evaluated 71 healthy men and women who provided accurate reports of dietary intake and completed a body-composition assessment. These investigators found that dietary variety was positively associated with energy intake within each of ten food groups. In a multiple regression analysis controlled for age and sex, dietary variety of sweets, snacks, condiments, entrees, and carbohydrates (as a group) was positively associated with body fatness, whereas variety from vegetables was negatively associated.

Low Cost and Availability. Ready access to inexpensive, highly palatable foods induces excess consumption. In the past, the process of obtaining food required energy expenditure: hunting, farming, or at the very least the act of preparing and cooking the food. Now, a staggering variety of premade foods are easily available, and dining outside the home has become more prevalent. US market data show an inverse correlation between energy density and cost, with hamburgers and French fries severalfold less expensive than fresh fruits and vegetables on a per calorie basis (77). The extent to which these factors promote overeating deserves further study.

Economics of Diet and Physical Activity

Food has become cheap, and physical activity has become expensive. Economic reasons for this situation exist.

Economic Factors Influencing Diet. The average person in the United States spends only about 10.7% (78) of net income on food. Food with high levels of fat and sugar is particularly cheap. A recent article by Drewnowski and Specter (77) explored the relationships among fat and sugar consumption, energy density of food, and energy costs of food and came to the following conclusions. First, the rates of obesity in the United States follow a socioeconomic gradient, such that the highest obesity rates are associated with the lowest incomes and levels of education.

Second, an inverse relation exists between energy density of food and energy cost of food, such that energy-dense foods composed of fats and sugars are lower in cost. Third, the high energy density and palatability of sweets and fats are associated with higher energy intakes. Fourth, poverty and food insecurity are associated with lower food expenditures and lower-quality diets. This economic approach suggests that food choices and diet are influenced by economic resources and food costs. Low-cost, energy-dense diets are likely to be highly palatable, to contain added sugars and fats, and to promote the development of obesity and overweight.

Economic Factors Influencing Physical Activity. In contrast, technologic advances have eliminated a great deal of physical activity from our lives. Few occupations require manual labor, so adults have little physical activity on the job. Similarly, elimination of physical education from many schools ensures that most children have little physical activity at school. Technologic changes have also produced labor-saving devices to reduce physical activity in the home and entertainment advances that increase the amount of our free time we spend in sedentary pursuits such as watching television, playing video games, and watching movies. Because little physical activity occurs in daily living, obtaining adequate physical activity requires money (gym membership, home exercise equipment) and time.

Early Environmental Factors

Prenatal Influences. Environmental factors very early in life may affect subsequent body weight. Several studies found that men and women born small for gestational age were more likely to have a higher BMI, a higher waist-to-hip circumference ratio, the metabolic syndrome, and coronary artery disease than those who were of normal size at birth (79--82). The reason for this observation is not clear, but it has been hypothesized that fetal undernutrition and impaired fetal development may have long-term effects on organ function (83). Maternal smoking and diabetes also increase the risk of being overweight as children and adults (84, 85).

Breast-Feeding. Evidence suggests that having been breast-fed could be protective against obesity (86–89). A German cross-sectional study of more than 9000 children found a protective effect of breast-feeding in the first year of life on the risk of overweight and obesity at age 5 to 6 years (86). The protective effect followed a dose-response relationship and was not explained by social class or lifestyle. A US survey of more than 15,000 children (89) aged 9 to 14 years and their mothers found that among subjects who had been only or mostly fed breast milk, compared with those only or mostly fed formula, the odds ratio for being overweight was 0.78 (95% CI, 0.66–0.91), after adjustment for age, sex, sexual maturity, energy intake, time watching television, physical activity, mother's BMI, and other variables reflecting social, economic, and lifestyle factors. However, other recent cohort studies (90–92) have found no effect. The reason for these contradictory findings are unclear but may be related to differences in the methods used for ascertaining exposure to breast milk, differences in the methods used for measuring and adjusting for confounders, the selection of disparate end points for the measurement of obesity, and the statistical power of the studies (93). According to Clifford (93), "the possibility remains that even if the effect of breast feeding on future obesity is small the public health impact can be tremendous," and future research is needed to address this question. Alternatively, mothers who breast-feed their infants may be more vigilant about other aspects of the environment that could affect weight gain.

Childhood and Parental Obesity. Both childhood obesity and parental obesity affect the risk of becoming obese as an adult. Among children who were obese during childhood, the chance of obesity in adulthood ranged from 8% for 1 or 2 year olds without obese parents to 79% for 10 to 14 year olds with at least one obese parent. After adjustment for parental obesity, the odds ratios for obesity in adulthood associated with childhood obesity ranged from 1.3 (95% CI, 0.6–3.0) for obesity at 1 or 2 years of age to 17.5 (7.7–39.5) for obesity at 15 to 17 years of age. After adjustment for the child's obesity status, the odds ratios for obesity in adulthood associated with having one obese parent ranged from 2.2 (95% CI, 1.1–4.3) at 15 to 17 years of age to 3.2 (1.8–5.7) at 1 or 2 years of age. The authors of the study concluded that obese children younger than 3 years of age and whose parents are not obese are at low risk of obesity in adulthood, but among older children, obesity is an increasingly important predictor of adult obesity, regardless of whether the parents are obese. Parental obesity more than doubles the risk of adult obesity among both obese and nonobese children less than 10 years of age (94). Weight in adolescence is an even better predictor of adult weight (95).

DEVELOPMENT OF OBESITY WITHIN SOCIETIES: THE ONSET OF THE OBESITY EPIDEMIC

Obesity as a Societal Issue

The marked increase in the prevalence of obesity since the mid-1980s cannot be attributed to changes in the gene pool and must be largely a result of alterations in environmental factors. It is probable that both an increase in food consumption (energy intake) and a decline in physical activity (energy expenditure) play a role. Obesity is a chief contributor to preventable death in the United States and poses a major public health challenge.

Consequences of an Ancient Metabolism in a Modern World

Genes involved in the regulation of body weight are estimated to have evolved 200,000 to 1 million years ago, at a time when environmental factors controlling habitual physical activity and food acquisition were dramatically different (96). The rapid increase in the global prevalence of obesity occurred in a time too short for a change in gene pool, a finding suggesting that factors in the environment are promoting weight gain. Humans evolved in an environment of paucity in which high levels of physical activity were necessary for survival and food acquisition. Starvation, not obesity, was a serious threat. Physiologic mechanisms were useful to oppose weight loss but not weight gain. The abilities to conserve and store energy were critical for survival; inefficient energy storage and excessive nonessential physical activity were maladaptive. Over time, the modern environment changed to one with endless varieties of inexpensive, plentiful, palatable, energy-dense foods and ever-increasing technologic advances designed to decrease physical activity. As a result, our current environment has an extraordinary strong and sustained propensity to promote positive energy balance and obesity. Our physiology has not developed to oppose these environmental pressures, so the recent increase in the prevalence of obesity in the population can be attributed to a mismatch between our physiology and our environment.

Worldwide Rates of Obesity

Other developed countries are experiencing similar increases in obesity. In the United Kingdom and other countries in Europe, approximately 15% of men and 20% of women are obese (97). Obesity has also increased in Southeast Asia, Japan, and China and occurs in more than 60% of men and 75% of women in urban Samoa (98). Less-developed countries also show increases in obesity as they become more affluent (99). The World Health Organization (WHO) estimated that numbers of obese adults worldwide increased 50% from 1995 to 2000, bringing total numbers to approximately 300 million. The relationship between economic development and obesity is apparent. The WHO categorizes countries according to economic development, and the frequency of obesity in the population is related to the degree of economic development. As economies grow from "least developed" to "developing" to "economy in transition" to "developed market economy," the obesity prevalence increases from 1.8 to 4.8% to 17.1 to 20.4%, respectively (11). Overall, in countries with the poorest economies, obesity is rare except in the highest socioeconomic groups.

Obesity as a Threat to Public Health

Obesity becomes a disease when excess body fat reaches levels associated with increased morbidity and mortality. The increases in overweight and obesity raise critical questions about the implications of these trends for health outcomes. The WHO consultation on obesity designated obesity as the major unmet public health problem worldwide (99). Obesity is an important risk factor for many serious medical complications that lead to impaired quality of life, considerable morbidity, and premature death. Using the relative hazards associated with an elevated BMI in six large US studies, the national distribution of adult BMI, the estimates of adult population size, and total deaths from the same period, Allison and colleagues calculated that the annual number of deaths attributable to obesity was 280,000 (100). Efforts are urgently needed to combat the obesity epidemic and to reverse the current prevalence trends.

Economic Consequences of Obesity

Accompanying the increase in the prevalence of obesity are the economic costs related to this ever more widespread condition. This burden results primarily from the associated morbidity and mortality associated with excess body weight. Estimates of the direct medical costs of obesity in the United States were approximately $70 billion in 1995, representing approximately 7.2% of national health care costs (101). The economic costs to the nation of lost wages and productivity related to obesity are comparable to those associated with smoking. Obese workers take increased amounts of sick leave and have higher numbers of disability claims (102, 103). It is estimated that paid sick leave and disability insurance cost US businesses more than $3 billion in 1996 (103).

SUMMARY

The current obesity epidemic can be attributed, in large part, to a "modern" environment that discourages physical activity and encourages the consumption of supersized portions of energy-dense foods. Traditional approaches that have emphasized education and individual responsibility alone are unlikely to be effective. Most people know what they must do to lose weight permanently or prevent weight gain, but they are unable to implement the needed lifestyle changes. Thus, efforts toward the prevention of obesity must both aid individual persons in maintaining cognitive controls over their weight and target the environment for change. Successful prevention will require public policy initiatives to enhance safe and easy access for physical activity and to facilitate low-calorie food choices. Strategies for the prevention of obesity should involve public and private sector partnerships among community leaders, school administrators, employers, healthcare providers, and governmental agencies.

REFERENCES

1. Flegal KM. Med Sci Sports Exerc 1999;31[Suppl]:509–14S.
2. Gallagher D Heymsfield SB, Heo M et al. Am J Clin Nutr 2000; 72:694.
3. Troiano RP, Frongillo EA Jr, Sobal J et al. Int J Obes Relat Metab Disord 1996;20:63.
4. Calle EE, Thun MJ, Petrelli JM et al. N Engl J Med 1999; 341:1097.
5. Manson JE, Willet WC, Stampfer MJ et al. N Engl J Med 1995; 333:677.
6. National Institutes of Health, National Heart, Lung, and Blood Institute. Obes Res 1998;6[Suppl 2]:51S.
7. Kissebah AH, Vydelingum N, Murray R et al. J Clin Endocrinol Metab 1982;54:254.
8. National Center for Health Statistics, Centers for Disease Control and Prevention. Web site www.cdc.gov/nchs/products/pubs/pubd/hestats/obese/obse99.htm. Accessed 9/03.
9. Flegal KM, Carroll MD, Ogden CL et al. JAMA 2002;288: 1723–7.
10. Sturm R. Arch Intern Med 2003;163:2146–8.
11. Zimmerman RL. Clin Fam Pract 2002;4:229–47.
12. Allison DB, Saunders SE. Med Clin North Am 2000;84:305–33.
13. Sobal J, Stunkard AJ. Psychol Bull 1989;105:260–275.
14. Flegal KM, Troiano RP. Int J Obes Relat Metab Disord 2000; 24:807.
15. Guo SS, Huang C, Maynard LM et al. Int J Obes Relat Metab Disord 2000;24:1628.
16. Pi Sunyer FX. Obesity. In: Shils ME, Olson JA, Shike M et al., eds. Modern Nutrition in Health and Disease, 9th ed. Baltimore: Lippincott Williams & Wilkins, 1999:1395–1418.
17. Barlow SE, Dietz WH. Pediatrics 1998;102:E29.
18. Tritos NA, Maratos-Flier E. Neuroendocrine control of energy balance. In: Eckel RH, ed. Obesity: Mechanisms and Clinical Management. Baltimore: Lippincott Williams & Wilkins, 2003:128–46.
19. Eckel RH. Obesity: disease or physiologic adaptation. In: Eckel RH, ed. Obesity: Mechanisms and Clinical Management. Baltimore: Lippincott Williams & Wilkins, 2003:3–30.
20. Ravussin E, Burnand B, Schutz, Y et al. Am J Clin Nutr 1982; 35:566.
21. Segal KR, Lacayanga I, Dunaif A et al. Am J Physiol 1989;256: E573.
22. de Jonge L, Bray GA. Obes Res 1997;5:622.
23. Stewart WK, Fleming LW. Postgrad Med J 1973;49:203.
24. Hill JO, Donahoo WT. Environmental influences on obesity. In: Eckel RH, ed. Obesity: Mechanisms and Clinical Management. Baltimore: Lippincott Williams & Wilkins, 2003:75–90.
25. Levine JA, Eberhardt NL, Jensen MD. Science 1999;283:212.
26. Keys A, Brozek J, Henschel A et al. Body Fat. In: Biology of Human Starvation, vol 1. Minneapolis, MN: University of Minnesota Press, 1950:161–83.
27. Diaz EO, Prentice AM, Goldberg GR et al. Am J Clin Nutr 1992;56:641–55.
28. Jebb SA, Prentice AM, Goldberg GR et al. Am J Clin Nutr 1996;64:259–66.
29. Bouchard C, Tremblay A, Despres JP et al. N Engl J Med 1990; 322:1477.
30. Horton TJ, Drougas H, Brachey A et al. Am J Clin Nutr 1995; 62:19–29.
31. Goran MI. Med Clin North Am 2000;84:347–85.
32. Skov AR, Toubro S, Buemann B et al. Clin Physiol 1997;17:279.
33. Lichtman SW, Pisarska K, Berman ER et al. N Engl J Med 1992;327:1893.
34. Bouchard C, Petrusse L. Annu Rev Nutr 1993;13:337.
35. Hill JO, Wyatt HR, Melanson EL. Med Clin North Am 2000; 84:333–46.
36. Comuzzie AG, Allison DB. Science 1998;280:1374–7.
37. Farooqi IS, Yeo GS, Keogh JM et al. J CLin Invest 2000; 106:271.
38. Krude H, Biebermann H, Luck W et al. Nat Genet 1998; 19:155.
39. Montague CT, Farooqi IS, Whitehead JP et al. Nature 1997; 387: 903.

40. Clement K, Vaisse C, Lahlou N et al 1998;392:398.

41. Ristow M, Muller-Wieland D, Pfeiffer A et al. N Engl J Med 1998;339:953.

42. Jackson RS, Creemers JW, Ohagi S et al. Nat Genet 1997; 16:218.

43. Bouchard C, Petrusse L. Annu Rev Nutr 1993;13:337.

44. Ravussin E, Bogardus C. Am J Clin Nutr 1989;49:968–75.

45. Levine JA, Eberhardt NL, Jensen, MD. Science 1999;283:212.

46. Allison DB, Pietrobelli A, Faith MS et al. Genetic influences on obesity. In: Eckel RH, ed. Obesity: Mechanisms and Clinical Management. Baltimore: Lippincott Williams & Wilkins, 2003: 31–74.

47. Bray GF. Clin Fam Pract 2002;4:249–75.

48. Aronne LJ, Segal KJ. J Clin Psychiatry 2003;64[Suppl 8]:22–9.

49. Flegal KM, Troiano RP, Pamuk ER et al. N Engl J Med 1995; 333:1214–6.

50. McGuire MT, Jeffery RW, French SA. Clin Fam Pract 2002;4: 319–31.

51. Speakman JR, Selman C. Proc Nutr Soc 2003;62:621–34.

52. Denzer CM, Young JC. Int J Sport Nutr Exerc Metab 2003;13: 396–402.

53. Prentice AM, Jebb SA. BMJ 1995;311:437.

54. Kromhout D. Am J Clin Nutr 1983;37:287.

55. Fogelholm M, Mannisto S, Vartianen E et al. Int J Obes Relat Metab Disord 1996;20:1097–104.

56. Williamson DF, Madans J, Anda RF et al. Int J Obes Relat Metab Disord 1993;17:279–86.

57. US Department of Health and Human Services. Physical Activity and Health: A Report of the Surgeon General. Atlanta, GA: US Department of Health and Human Services, 1996.

58. Hu PS, Young JR 1995 US Personal Transportation Survey. Washington, DC: US Department of Transportation, 1995.

59. Brownell KD, Wadden TA. J Consult Clin Psychol 1992;60: 505–17.

60. US Department of Health and Human Services. Surgeon General's Report on Nutrition and Health. Washington, DC: US Department of Health and Human Services, 1988.

61. Ernst ND, Obarzanek E, Clark MB et al. J Am Diet Assoc 1997;97:47S–51S.

62. Federation of American Societies for Experimental Biology LS Research Office. Food Consumption and Nutrient Intake: Third Report in Nutrition Monitoring in the United States. Washington, DC: US Government Printing Office, 1995:148–9.

63. Lissner L, Heitmann BL. Eur J Clin Nutr 1995;49:79A–90A.

64. Astrup A, Grunwald GK, Melanson EL et al. Int J Obes Relat Metab Disord 2000;24:1545-52.

65. Hill JO, Peters JC. Science 1998;280:1371–4.

66. Rolls BJ, Bell EA. Eur J Clin Nutr 1999;53:166S–73S.

67. Stubbs RJ, Harbon CG, Murgatroyd PR et al. Am J Clin Nutr 1995;62:316–29.

68. Grunwald GK, Seagle HM, Peters JM. Br J Nutr 2001;86: 265–76.

69. Drewnowski A. Nutr Rev 1998;56:347–53.

70. Ludwig DS, Peterson KE, Gortmaker SL. Lancet 2001;357: 505–8.

71. Ludwig DS. J Nutr 2000;130:280S–2S.

72. Hallfrisch J, Muller D, Drinkwater D et al. J Gerontol 1990;45: M186–91.

73. Posner BM, Franz MM, Quatromoni PA et al. J Am Diet Assoc 1995;95:171–9.

74. Perez CE. Health Rep 2002;13:23–31.

75. Young LR, Nestle M. J Am Diet Assoc 2003;103:231–4.

76. McCrory MA, Fuss PJ, McCallum JE et al. Am J Clin Nutr 1999;69:440–7.

77. Drewnowski A, Specter SE. Am J Clin Nutr 2004;79:6–16.

78. Putnam JJ, Allshouse JE. Food consumption, prices and expenditures, 1970–1997. USDA Statistical Bulletin 965. Washington, DC: US Department of Agriculture, Food and Rural Economic Division, Economic Research Service, 1999.

79. Barker DJ, Winter PD, Osmond C et al. Lancet 1989;2:577.

80. Barker DJ, Hales CN, Fall CH et al. Diabetologia 1993; 36:62.

81. Valdez R, Athens MA, Thompson GH et al. Diabetologia 1994; 37:624.

82. Phillips DI, Barker DJ, Hales CN et al. Diabetologia 1994; 37:150.

83. Barker DJ. Eur J Clin Nutr 1992;46[Suppl 3]:3S.

84. Power C, Jefferis BJ. Int J Epidemiol 2002;31:413.

85. Dabelea D, Hanson RL, Lindsay RS et al. Diabetes 2000;49: 2208.

86. von Kries R, Koletzko B, Sauerwald T et al. Adv Exp Med Biol 2000;478:29.

87. Bergmann KE, Bergmann RL, Von Kries R et al. Int J Obes Relat Metab Disord 2003;27:162–72.

88. Toschke AM, Vignerova J, Lhotska L et al. J Pediatr 2002;141: 764–9.

89. Gillman MW, Rifas-Shiman SL, Camargo CA Jr et al. JAMA 2001;285:2461–7.

90. Li L, Parsons TJ, Power C. BMJ 2003;327:904–5.

91. Victora CG, Barros F, Lima RC et al. BMJ 2003;327:901.

92. Hediger ML, Overpeck MD, Kuczmarski RJ et al. JAMA 2001; 285:2453–60.

93. Clifford TJ. BMJ 2003;327:879–80.

94. Whitaker, RC, Wright, JA, Pepe, MS et al. N Engl J Med 1997; 337:869.

95. Braddon FEM, Rodger, B, Wadsworth MEJ et al. BMJ 1986; 293:299.

96. Bessessen DB. Obesity. In: McDermott MT, ed. Endocrine Secrets. Philadelphia: Hanley and Belfus, 2002:81–97.

97. Kopelman PG. Nature 2000;404:635.

98. International Diabetes Institute, World Health Organization. The Asia-Pacific Perspective: Redefining Obesity and Its Treatment. Geneva: World Health Organization, 2000:155 (www.idi.org.au).

99. World Health Organization. Obesity: Preventing and Managing the Global Epidemic. WHO Technical Report, Series 894. Geneva: World Health Organization, 2000.

100. Allison DB, Fontaine KR, Manson JE et al. JAMA 1999;282: 1530–8.

101. Colditz GA. Med Sci Sports Exerc 1999;31:663S–7S.

102. Burton WN, Chen CY, Schultz AB et al. J Occup Environ Med 1998;40:786.

103. Thompson D, Edelsberg J, Kinsey KL et al. Am J Health Promot 1998;13:120.

SELECTED READINGS

Eckel RH, ed. Obesity: Mechanisms and Clinical Management. Baltimore: Lippincott Williams & Wilkins, 2003.

Hill JO, Peters JC. Environmental contributions to the obesity epidemic. Science 1998;280:1371–4.

Jensen M, ed. Obesity. Med Clin North Am 2000;84.

Moran RF, ed. Clin Fam Pract 2002;4.

National Institutes of Health, National Heart, Lung, and Blood Institute. Clinical guidelines on the identification, evaluation, and treatment of overweight and obesity in adults: the evidence report. Obes Res 1998;6[Suppl 2]:51S.

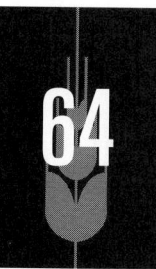

64 OBESITY: MANAGEMENT[1]

THOMAS A. WADDEN, KIRSTIN J. BYRNE, AND STEPHANIE
KRAUTHAMER-EWING

ASSESSMENT OF THE OBESE INDIVIDUAL 1029
   Physical Assessment 1029
   Psychosocial Evaluation 1030
   Assessment of Eating and Activity Habits 1031
   Weight Loss Readiness .1031
SELECTING TREATMENT: AN ALGORITHM 1031
   Dietary Intervention 1031
   Balanced-Deficit Diets .1032
   Low-Calorie Diets 1032
   Portion-Controlled Servings and
      Meal Replacements 1032
   Low-Fat and Low-Energy-Density Diets 1033
   Low-Carbohydrate, High-Protein Diets 1033
   Diets Based on the Glycemic Index 1034
   Very-Low-Calorie Diets 1034
   Summary 1034
PHYSICAL ACTIVITY FOR WEIGHT CONTROL 1034
   Exercise and Short-Term Weight Loss 1035
   Exercise and Long-Term Weight Control 1035
   Programmed Versus Lifestyle Activity 1035
   Exercise Target for Maintaining Weight Loss 1035
   Benefits of Physical Activity 1036
BEHAVIOR THERAPY 1036
   Components of Behavioral Treatment 1036
   Structure of Behavioral Treatment 1037
   Results of Behavioral Treatment 1037
   Improving the Behavioral Maintenance
      of Weight Loss 1038
PHARMACOLOGIC TREATMENT OF OBESITY 1038
   Medications Approved by the US
      Food and Drug Administration 1038
   Future Medications 1039
SURGICAL TREATMENT OF OBESITY 1039
   Other Surgical Procedures 1040
   Dietary and Behavioral Counseling 1040
CONCLUSIONS 1040

The Diabetes Prevention Program recently provided compelling evidence of the health benefits of modest weight loss and increased physical activity (1). This randomized controlled trial enrolled more than 3200 overweight or obese persons with impaired glucose tolerance. Participants in a lifestyle intervention group who lost 7 kg of initial weight and exercised more than 150 minutes/week reduced their risk of developing type 2 diabetes by 58% over a 3- to 4-year period compared with control participants. The lifestyle intervention also was superior to treatment with metformin (i.e., 850 mg twice daily). These data, together with other findings (2, 3), leave little doubt of the health benefits of modest weight loss.

This chapter provides an overview of the assessment and treatment of obesity. Diet and exercise interventions are reviewed in detail, with lesser attention to pharmacologic and surgical therapies because of their lesser use. The chapter is written with the knowledge that far greater effort must be devoted to the prevention of obesity if we are to control the epidemic that now confronts the United States and other industrialized nations.

ASSESSMENT OF THE OBESE INDIVIDUAL

In 1998, an expert panel convened by the National Heart, Lung, and Blood Institute (NHLBI) conducted an extensive review of the health complications of obesity and of the safety and efficacy of treatments for this disorder (4). The panel proposed a classification scheme, shown in Table 64.1, that has implications for both risk assessment and treatment.

Physical Assessment

The first step of assessment is determination of the body mass index (BMI), calculated as weight in kilograms divided by height in meters squared (i.e., kg/m^2). As shown in Table 64.1, overweight is defined by a BMI of 25.0 to 29.9 and is associated with increased risks of morbidity (particularly type 2 diabetes) but not mortality (5). The table shows three classes of obesity, the third of which is characterized by a BMI greater than 40 and is referred to as extreme obesity. The greater the degree of obesity, the greater the risk of mortality (5).

The second step of assessment is measurement of the waist circumference, which provides an estimate of body

[1]Abbreviations: **BMI**, body mass index; **FDA**, US Food and Drug Administration; **GI**, glycemic index; **LCD**, low-calorie diet; **NAASO**, North American Association for the Study of Obesity; **NHLBI**, National Heart, Lung, and Blood Institute; **VLCD**, very-low-calorie diet.

TABLE 64.1. CLASSIFICATION OF OVERWEIGHT AND OBESITY BY BODY MASS INDEX, WAIST CIRCUMFERENCE, AND ASSOCIATED DISEASE RISK

			DISEASE RISK RELATIVE TO NORMAL WEIGHT AND WAIST CIRCUMFERENCE	
WEIGHT CATEGORY	BMI	OBESITY CLASS	MEN <102 cm (<40 in) WOMEN <88 cm (<35 in)	MEN >102 cm (>40 in) WOMEN >88 cm (>35 in)
Underweight	<18			
Normal	18.5–24.9			
Overweight	25.0–29.9		Increased	High
Obesity	30.0–34.9	I	High	Very high
	35.0–39.9	II	Very high	Very high
Extreme obesity	>40.0	III	Extremely high	Extremely high

BMI, body mass index.

fat distribution (in lieu of computed tomography or magnetic resonance imaging). Excess fat in the upper body (particularly the intraabdominal cavity) is associated with an increased risk of hypertension, type 2 diabetes, dyslipidemia, and other complications compared with the same amount of fat carried in the lower body (4, 6). Upper body obesity is suggested by a waist circumference greater than 35 inches (88 cm) in women and greater than 40 inches (102 cm) in men (4). Table 64.1 shows that upper body obesity compounds the risk of health complications in the presence of a BMI of 25.0 to 34.0.

Persons with a disease risk equal to or greater than "high," as determined by the table, are advised to have a thorough medical examination with appropriate laboratory tests to determine whether they have already developed conditions that require treatment. Some diseases (e.g., hypertension, diabetes) further contribute to the increased mortality risk associated with obesity (5). A history and physical examination should identify (a) the number, type, and severity of existing comorbid conditions; and (b) how to coordinate treatment of these conditions with weight loss. The following table summarizes diseases and behaviors identified as additional risks by a joint expert panel convened by the NHLBI and the North American Association for the Study of Obesity (NAASO) (Table 64.2) (7).

Assessment also should identify contraindications to weight reduction, which is inappropriate for pregnant or lactating women, as well as for persons with a terminal illness, recent myocardial infarction, cholelithiasis, osteoporosis, and other conditions (8).

Psychosocial Evaluation

Whenever possible, the physical examination should be complemented by an evaluation of potential behavioral and psychosocial complications, as described by Wadden and Phelan (9). Of these, depression and binge eating are the most common. Population studies have shown that obesity is associated with an increased risk of major depression and suicidal ideation in women but not men (10). The gender difference is probably attributable to the greater importance of weight and shape in women than men. Among obese women who seek weight reduction, approximately 10 to 15% can be expected to report symptoms of moderate or severe depression (11). Thirty percent of severely obese women suffer from significant depression (12). Depression can be assessed by paper-and-pencil tests such as the Beck Depression Inventory II (13) or more informally by inquiring about the patient's mood, enjoyment of work and leisure activities, sleep patterns, and energy level. Obese persons with significant

TABLE 64.2. OBESITY COMORBIDITIES CONVEYING INCREASED RISK

- Cigarette smoking
- Hypertension (systolic blood pressure of ≥140 mm Hg or diastolic blood pressure of ≥90 mm Hg) or current use of antihypertensive agents
- High-risk LDL cholesterol (serum concentration ≥160 mg/dL); a borderline high-risk LDL-cholesterol (130–159 mg/dL) plus two or more other risk factors also confers high risk

- Low HDL cholesterol (serum concentration <35 mg/dL)
- IFG (fasting plasma glucose between 110 and 125 mg/dL). IFG is considered by many authorities to be an independent risk factor for cardiovascular (macrovascular) disease, thus justifying its inclusion among risk factors contributing to high absolute risk. IFG is well established as a risk factor for type 2 diabetes.

- Family history of premature CHD (myocardial infarction or sudden death experienced by the father or other male first-degree relative at or before 55 years of age, or experienced by the mother or other female first-degree relative at or before 65 years of age)
- Age ≥45 y for men or age ≥55 y for women (or postmenopausal)

HDL, high-density lipoprotein; IFG, impaired fasting glucose; LDL, low-density lipoprotein.

depression should be provided appropriate treatment (cognitive behavior therapy and/or pharmacotherapy) before undertaking weight reduction.

Approximately 15 to 25% of obese persons who seek weight reduction suffer from binge eating disorder, in which they consume objectively large amounts of food in a short period of time (i.e., 2 hours) and experience loss of control during these episodes (14). These persons, however, do not purge, which distinguishes this disorder from bulimia nervosa. Binge eating is frequently associated with symptoms of depression and negative body image, which may require treatment if severe (14). Binge eating disorder can be assessed by the Questionnaire on Weight and Eating Patterns (15), a self-report test that should be followed by a brief interview to confirm that the patient consumes a large amount of food and experiences loss of control. Although specific cognitive behavioral therapies have been developed for the treatment of binge eating disorder, the condition responds favorably to a structured weight loss program (as described later).

Assessment of Eating and Activity Habits

Eating and activity habits should be assessed to determine their contribution to the patient's obesity (9). The assessment should provide a sketch of the individual's daily eating pattern, calorie intake, problem eating, and physical activity. A key task is to determine the number of meals and snacks consumed daily. More formal methods can be used to assess food intake, including a 24-hour dietary recall or the Block Food Frequency Questionnaire (16).

Physical activity can be assessed by inquiring about the number of blocks walked, flights of stairs climbed, and hours of television watched. This provides an estimate of the individual's lifestyle activity (17). Programmed or purposeful activity can be assessed by inquiring about the patient's frequency of walking (or jogging) and participation in other aerobic or anaerobic activities (9). More formal assessment can be conducted using a pedometer to determine the number of steps walked daily, or an accelerometer, which also assesses the intensity of activity. Evaluation of eating and activity habits typically continues throughout treatment. Patients in behavioral weight loss programs record daily their food intake and physical activity.

Weight Loss Readiness

The patient's interest in pursuing weight control also must be determined. For persons who are unmotivated to lose weight, prevention of weight gain, with medical treatment of comorbid conditions, is an appropriate goal (7). In addition, the practitioner should try to illuminate factors associated with the patient's lack of motivation, including previous failed efforts. With patients who seem motivated to reduce, the practitioner should help them set realistic expectations for changes in weight, health, and appearance. Practitioners should remind patients at every opportunity that a 5 to 10% weight loss is a successful loss, associated with improvements in health and well-being (1–3).

SELECTING TREATMENT: AN ALGORITHM

In 2000, the NHLBI-NAASO panel issued the Practical Guide to the Identification, Evaluation, and Treatment of Overweight and Obesity in Adults (7). This document includes a treatment algorithm, shown in Table 64.3, that recommends interventions based on the individual's BMI and cardiovascular risk factors. Persons who have a BMI of 25.0 to 29.9 but do not have two or more risk factors are encouraged to prevent weight gain. However, patients who fall in this BMI range and have two or more risk factors are advised to lose weight by using a program of diet, exercise, and behavior therapy. This tripartite approach, often referred to as lifestyle modification, is recommended for all persons who need to reduce and induces a loss of approximately 10% of initial weight in 4 to 6 months (4, 7). Pharmacotherapy is an option for persons with a BMI greater than 30 (or a BMI greater than 27 with comorbid conditions) who are not successful with lifestyle modification alone. Bariatric surgery may be appropriate for persons with a BMI greater than 40 or for persons with a BMI of greater than 35 who have significant comorbid conditions.

Dietary Intervention

Dietary intervention remains the cornerstone of weight reduction efforts (18). This is because obese persons typically find it easier to reduce their food intake than to increase their physical activity in order to induce a negative energy balance. Dozens of reducing diets are available, but

TABLE 64.3. A GUIDE TO SELECTING TREATMENT

TREATMENT	BODY MASS INDEX CATEGORY				
	25–26.9	27–29.9	30–35	35–39.9	>40
Diet, exercise, and behavior therapy	With comorbidity	With comorbidity	+	+	+
Pharmacotherapy		With comorbidity	+	+	+
Surgery				With comorbidity	+

they all vary on two principal dimensions: calorie content and macronutrient balance. Calorie content is by far the more important for weight loss (18). The lower the calorie intake, the greater the energy deficit and the resulting weight loss. If a person is in negative energy balance, the relative balance of carbohydrate and fat has little impact on weight loss (19). This has been shown in inpatient studies of isocaloric diets that systematically manipulated fat and carbohydrate content (20).

Reducing diets are frequently categorized on the basis of their calorie content. Very-low-calorie diets (VLCDs) provide fewer than 800 kcal/day, whereas low-calorie diets (LCDs) contain 800 to 1500 kcal/day. The term hypocaloric balanced-deficit diet is often used to describe plans that provide more than 1500 kcal/day of conventional foods, with an appropriate balance of macronutrients (19).

The NHLBI/NAASO panel recommends that overweight persons (BMI of 25.0 to 29.9) with two or more cardiovascular risk factors consume a mildly hypocaloric balanced-deficit diet (7). A reduction of 300 to 500 kcal/day may be adequate. By contrast, persons with a BMI greater than 35 often require a deficit of 500 to 1000 kcal/day, as induced by an LCD (4, 7). Greater caloric restriction induces more rapid weight loss, considering that these persons must lose more weight to reach a 10% goal. Portion-controlled meal plans and VLCDs are options for persons who are not successful with an LCD of conventional foods.

Balanced-Deficit Diets

Balanced-deficit diets prescribe a balanced profile of foods and nutrients, similar to that recommended for the general population to promote health (19). They are relatively low in fat (<30% of calories), high in carbohydrate (>55% of calories), moderate in protein (10–15% of calories), high in fiber (25–30 g/day), and very low in alcohol. Most overweight men and obese women who reduce their intake by only 500 kcal/day would continue to consume more than 1500 kcal/day (which places them above the range of an LCD). Reducing servings from the Food Guide Pyramid (21) provides a simple method of consuming a balanced-deficit diet.

Balanced-deficit diets potentially are easy to adhere to because they require only small changes in eating habits, traditionally achieved by cutting out hidden sources of fat and sugar (19). Their disadvantage, as viewed by some dieters, is the relatively slow rate of weight loss. A diet of 1500 to 1800 kcal/day will induce a loss of less than 0.5 kg/week in most obese women and of 0.5 to 1.0 kg in men.

Low-Calorie Diets

LCDs are similar to balanced-deficit diets in macronutrient distribution. In clinical practice, diets providing fewer than 1000 kcal/day of conventional foods are rarely prescribed because of concerns that they cannot provide adequate

levels of macronutrients, vitamins, and minerals (19). Table 64.4 provides an example of a LCD (7).

More than 30 randomized trials have shown that LCDs, providing 1000 to 1500 kcal/day, produce losses of approximately 8 to 10% of initial weight in 16 to 26 weeks of treatment (4). Two points, however, should be noted. First, in most studies patients consumed a diet of their own choosing but were instructed to keep daily diaries in which they recorded their food and calorie intake. Such record keeping is essential for reducing on an LCD of conventional foods (4). Second, in many studies, patients also attended weekly group or individual weight-loss sessions, as described later. Most patients require this support to lose 8 to 10% of initial weight (22, 23).

Portion-Controlled Servings and Meal Replacements

Several studies have demonstrated the benefits of LCDs that provide portion-controlled servings of conventional foods or of liquid meal replacements (23). Portion-controlled diets

TABLE 64.4. LOW-CALORIE STEP 1 DIET

NUTRIENT	RECOMMENDED INTAKE
Calories[a]	Approximately 500–1,000 kcal/d reduction from usual intake
Total fat[b]	30% or less of total calories
Saturated fatty acids[c]	8–10% of total calories
Monounsaturated fatty acids	≤15% of total calories
Polyunsaturated fatty acids	≤10% of total calories
Cholesterol[c]	<300 mg/d
Protein[d]	~15% of total calories
Carbohydrate[e]	≥55% of total calories
Sodium chloride	No more than 100 mmol/d (~2.4 g sodium or ~6 g sodium chloride)
Calcium[f]	1,000–1,500 mg
Fiber[e]	20–30 g

[a] A reduction in calories of 500 to 1,000 kcal/d will help achieve a weight loss of 1 to 2 lb/wk.
[b] Fat-modified foods may provide a helpful strategy for lowering total fat intake, but will only be effective if they are also low in calories and if there is no compensation by calories from other foods.
[c] Patients with high blood cholesterol levels may need to use the step 2 diet to achieve further reductions in low-density lipoprotein cholesterol levels; in the step 2 diet saturated fats are reduced to less than 7% of total calories and cholesterol levels to less than 200 mg/d. All of the other nutrients are the same as in step 1.
[d] Protein should be derived from plant sources and lean sources of animal protein.
[e] Complex carbohydrates from different vegetables, fruits, and whole grains are good sources of vitamins, minerals, and fiber. A diet rich in soluble fiber, including oat bran, legumes, barley, and most fruits and vegetables, may be effective in reducing blood cholesterol levels.
[f] During weight loss, attention should be given to maintaining an adequate intake of vitamins and minerals. Maintenance of the recommended calcium intake of 1,000 to 1,500 mg/d is especially important for women who may be at risk of osteoporosis.

From the National Heart, Lung, and Blood Institute and the North American Association for the study of Obesity (NAASO). Practical Guide to the Identification, Evaluation, and Treatment of Overweight and Obesity in Adults. Bethesda, MD: National Institutes of Health, 2000.

provide patients with a fixed amount of food with a known calorie content, an approach that facilitates adherence to the target calorie goal. By contrast, obese persons underestimate their calorie intake by 30 to 50% when instructed to consume a diet of self-selected foods (24). Jeffrey and colleagues (25), for example, showed that patients who were prescribed a conventional diet of 1000 kcal/day lost 7.7 kg in 6 months. Those who were prescribed the same number of calories, but who were given the actual foods for five breakfasts and five dinners per week, lost a significantly greater 10.1 kg.

Similarly favorable results were obtained with a popular liquid meal replacement (i.e., SlimFast). Ditschuneit and colleagues (26) showed that patients who replaced two meals and two snacks per day (with liquid shakes and snack bars) lost 8% of initial weight in the first 3 months, compared with a loss of only 1.5% for patients who were prescribed the same number of calories (i.e., 1200–1500 kcal) but consumed a self-selected diet of conventional foods. Five additional randomized controlled trials, reviewed by Heymsfield and colleagues (27), confirmed the superiority of liquid meal replacements, although persons prescribed this approach lost an average of only 2.5 kg more than persons who consumed a conventional reducing diet.

In an open-label study, patients in the Ditschuneit trial who continued to replace one meal and one snack per day achieved a loss of 11% of initial weight at 27 months and 8% at 51 months (28). These findings suggest that long-term use of a meal replacement may significantly improve the maintenance of weight loss (28). Randomized controlled trials are needed to confirm this hypothesis.

Low-Fat and Low-Energy-Density Diets

Both LCDs and VLCDs (reviewed later) focus principally on caloric restriction that, although effective in the short term, may be associated over time with reports of hunger and deprivation as well as with weight regain (19). These findings have led several investigators to propose an alternative strategy that reduces fat intake while allowing ad libitum intake of carbohydrates.

Two principal findings have emerged from studies of ad libitum low-fat diets. First, decreasing fat intake alone induces smaller weight loss than restricting both fat and total calorie intake (18). Schlundt and colleagues (29), for example, found that patients who were instructed to eat 25 g/day of fat with ad libitum intake of carbohydrate lost 4.6 kg in 20 weeks, compared with a significantly greater loss of 8.8 kg for patients who were prescribed the same fat goal as part of a diet of 1200 to 1500 kcal/day. The second finding, contrary to expectations, is that long-term weight losses have generally not been superior with ad libitum low-fat diets (29, 30). At 9 to 12 months' follow-up, patients in the Schlundt low-fat group maintained a loss of only 2.6 kg, compared with 5.6 kg for patients who

consumed the LCD (29). Jeffrey and colleagues (30) obtained comparable findings. More encouraging results were reported by Toubro and Astrup (31). Two years after having lost an average of 13.6 kg, patients who were assigned to a low-fat ad libitum diet during the maintenance period regained only 5.4 kg, compared with a gain of 11.3 kg for patients prescribed a LCD.

Energy density

Low-fat diets are typically low in energy density, the latter term referring to the energy (i.e., calories) in a given weight (grams) of food. Although replacing fat (9 kcal/g) with carbohydrate or protein (4 kcal/g) is the most common method of reducing energy density, other methods include adding fiber or water to foods (19). Water, in particular, increases the weight of food without increasing caloric content. This is potentially important in view of findings that food intake seems to be regulated, at least in the short term, by the weight of food ingested rather than by the energy content (32, 33). In laboratory studies, both lean and obese persons ate a constant weight of food, even when the fat content and energy density of the diet were systematically manipulated. In one study (32), for example, participants ate the same weight of food and reported comparable satiety when they consumed a high-fat/high-energy-density diet that provided 3000 kcal/day, compared with a low-fat/low-energy-density diet that contained 1570 kcal/day.

With obese persons, long-term studies are needed to determine whether patients gradually compensate for low energy density by eating a greater weight of food (and thus more calories). Further studies similar to that of Turbo and Astrup (31) are needed to determine whether this approach produces better maintenance of weight loss than a traditional LCD.

Low-Carbohydrate, High-Protein Diets

Low-carbohydrate, high-protein diets, as recommended by Atkins (34), are currently very popular in the United States and some other Western nations. During the weight loss induction phase, the Atkins plan allows ad libitum consumption of protein and fat, while limiting carbohydrate intake to 20 g. This approach has been roundly criticized because of its provision of large amounts of saturated fat (which may increase cardiovascular risk), as well as its deficiencies in fiber, vitamins and minerals, and essential carbohydrate (i.e., approximately 100 g/day of glucose required by the brain) (19). Proponents (34) argue that low-carbohydrate, high-protein diets satisfy appetite and are associated with reductions in insulin and triglyceride levels, all of which they believe are exacerbated by high carbohydrate intake.

Four randomized controlled trials of low-carbohydrate diets have been conducted in adults. A study of severely obese patients, many of whom had diabetes or metabolic syndrome, found that those who consumed a low-carbo-hydrate diet for 6 months, compared with a low-fat diet, lost more weight (5.8 versus 1.9 kg, respectively) and had greater improvements in triglyceride levels and insulin sensitivity (35). Differences in weight loss were not significant at 1 year (5.1 versus 3.1 kg) because those on the low-fat diet lost additional weight from months 7 to 12 (36). However, the low-carbohydrate diet was still associated with significantly greater improvements in triglycerides and, in patients with type 2 diabetes, with significantly greater reductions in HbA_{1c}. A second study similarly found significantly greater weight losses on a low-carbo-hydrate diet than on a low-fat diet at 6 months (6.9 kg versus 3.2 kg, respectively), but differences between groups were not significant at 1 year (4.3 versus 2.5 kg, respectively) because of weight regain in both groups (37). Patients on the low-fat diet had significantly greater improvements in LDL cholesterol at 6 months (but not 12 months), whereas low-carbohydrate-treated patients had significantly greater increases in HDL cholesterol at both times. Two additional 6-month trials both found significantly larger weight losses in persons who received the low-carbohydrate diet (38, 39), as did a study of obese adolescents (40).

Results of these studies suggest that low-carbohydrate, high-protein diets are effective in inducing weight loss and seem to be safe for short-term use. Additional studies are needed of long-term (>2 years) changes in both weight and health to determine the ultimate safety and efficacy of this approach. Although low-carbohydrate diets may be appropriate for inducing weight loss, current health guidelines suggest that, after losing weight, patients should decrease their consumption of saturated fat and increase that of fruits and vegetables (19).

Diets Based on the Glycemic Index

The glycemic index (GI) describes changes in blood glucose resulting from consumption of a defined amount of carbohydrate (usually 50 g) in a test food relative to changes after consumption of the same amount of carbohydrate from either glucose or white bread (41). The GI was first developed as a tool to assist patients with diabetes, but recently has been suggested as method for treating (or preventing) obesity (42). The premise is that foods that trigger a rapid, high peak in blood glucose (high-GI foods), with a subsequent surge in insulin secretion, cause a rapid decrease in blood glucose, below levels before eating. This is purported to result in a more rapid return of hunger compared with that seen with foods that produce a more moderate blood glucose response (42, 43). Poor appetite regulation is thought to increase energy consumption and, eventually, body weight.

A recent study of obese adolescents showed that a GI-based diet was associated with significantly greater weight loss than a low-fat diet, although changes in both groups were very modest (42). Further study is needed to determine whether dieters can readily learn the complexities of GI-based diets and whether this approach has short- or long-term benefits in adults (19).

Very-Low-Calorie Diets

VLCDs provide fewer than 800 kcal/day (44). They may be consumed as a liquid (shake) or as servings of lean meat, fish, or fowl (referred to as a protein-sparing modified fast). In either case, they provide approximately 70 to 100 g/day of dietary protein to preserve lean body mass. VLCDs appear to be safe when supplemented with vitamins and minerals and provided to appropriately selected patients under careful medical supervision (44, 45). They are, however, associated with an increased risk of gallstones, which can be reduced by taking ursodeoxycholic acid or aspirin (46). VLCDs are typically limited to persons with a BMI greater than 30, in whom the greater risk of health complications may justify the greater intensity and cost of treatment (approximately $3,000 for 6 months).

VLCDs induce losses of approximately 15 to 20% of initial weight in 12 to 16 weeks, losses nearly double the size of those produced by a conventional LCD. At least seven randomized trials have compared the short- and long-term results of these two approaches (47–53). The majority found no significant differences in weight loss 1 or more years after treatment because of greater weight regain in VLCD-treated participants. This approach would be more attractive if there were effective methods of maintaining the large weight losses induced. Pharmacotherapy may be an option with some patients (54).

Summary

This review has shown that there are numerous dietary options for inducing weight loss, all of which are supported by short-term randomized controlled trials. As a result, the choice of a particular approach depends, in part, on personal preferences. As a general rule, a portion-controlled diet will induce weight loss faster than a traditional LCD, as will a high-protein, low-carbohydrate diet. Rapid weight loss, however, may not be an important consideration for some persons. Moreover, the ultimate benefit of a reducing diet must be judged by long-term, not short-term, changes in weight and health (19). At present, there are not adequate long-term data (i.e., more than 2 years) to recommend one approach over another.

PHYSICAL ACTIVITY FOR WEIGHT CONTROL

A joint panel of the American College of Sports Medicine and the Centers for Disease Control and Prevention recommended that all adults (regardless of weight) engage in at least 30 minutes of moderately vigorous physical activity most days of the week (55). This is the amount and intensity of activity believed to improve cardiovascular health (56). Exercise is of particular benefit to obese persons, whether or not they are trying to lose weight. This section discusses the effects of exercise on weight control and describes methods of increasing physical activity.

Exercise and Short-Term Weight Loss

Physical activity alone, in absence of caloric restriction, produces minimal weight loss. As reviewed by Wing (57), walking four times per week for 45 to 60 minutes per bout produces a loss of only 2 to 3 kg during 16 to 52 weeks of treatment. Similarly, adding a walking program to an LCD only marginally increases weight loss (by 2–3 kg) during a 16- to 26-week behavioral program (57). These findings indicate that the weight-reducing benefits of exercise should not be overstated. The principal benefits of exercise are maintaining (not inducing) weight loss and improving health (56, 58).

Exercise and Long-Term Weight Control

Long-term physical activity seems to be crucial for maintaining weight loss, as suggested by the results of several case series, including the National Weight Control Registry (59). Participants in the Registry have lost at least 14 kg and maintained the loss for more than 1 year. These persons report expending approximately 2800 kcal/week, the equivalent of walking more than 1 hour/day for 7 days/week.

The results of randomized trials have yielded mixed results (57). Some studies have shown superior maintenance of weight loss 1 or more years after treatment, whereas others have found no difference between participants randomly assigned to exercise or no-exercise conditions. The difference between the studies seems to be attributable to exercise adherence (60). In several of the trials, persons who were assigned to the physical activity condition did not continue to exercise once treatment ended (60). This has led investigators to examine methods of facilitating long-term exercise adherence.

Programmed Versus Lifestyle Activity

Programmed activity consists of regularly scheduled bouts of running, swimming, or other aerobic activity that is usually undertaken at a relatively high intensity level (i.e., 60–80% of maximum heart rate) for a discrete period of time (i.e., 30–60 minutes) (56). Programmed activity may also include strength (or weight) training, which is essential to maintaining muscle tone and mass (56). By contrast, lifestyle activity involves increasing energy expenditure throughout the day by activities such as walking rather than riding, using stairs rather than escalators, and discarding energy-saving devices such as TV remote controls (56). The principal goal is to increase energy expenditure without concern for the intensity of activity.

Programmed activity

Two approaches may improve adherence to programmed activity. The first is to break exercise into several short (i.e., 10 minutes) bouts rather than one long bout (i.e., 40 minutes). Jakicic and colleagues (61) found that obese persons who were assigned to short bouts (i.e., 10 minutes) of activity reported exercising more minutes per week than those in a long-bout (i.e., 40 minutes) condition. In addition, there was a trend for those in the former group to lose more weight. The second approach is to have patients exercise at home rather than at a health club or similar facility. Perri and colleagues (62) showed that adherence to a walking program and maintenance of weight loss were significantly better at 1 year and beyond in patients who were assigned to walk at home, compared with those who participated in a supervised on-site program. Others have obtained similar results (63). Home exercise is associated with fewer barriers, including costs, travel, and time (56). The use of home exercise equipment, such as a treadmill, also may improve adherence and long-term weight loss (64).

Lifestyle activity

Lifestyle activity has numerous potential advantages over programmed exercise, including reducing patients' negative attitudes toward exercise (56). In addition, recent studies have shown that physical activity need not be as vigorous as once thought in order to improve fitness and reduce mortality. Moderately vigorous activity, requiring 4.5 metabolic equivalents, may be sufficient to reduce mortality, and can be achieved, for example, by brisk walking (56).

Epstein and colleagues found that lifestyle activity was associated with significantly better maintenance of weight loss in obese children than was programmed exercise (65). A study of obese women found that both lifestyle activity and programmed exercise, when combined with a 1200 kcal/day diet, produced a loss of approximately 8.5 kg during a 16-week behavioral program (17). Equivalent improvements were observed between groups in cardiorespiratory fitness, as well as in lipids and lipoproteins. There was also a (nonsignificant) trend in this pilot study for lifestyle activity to be associated with better maintenance of weight loss 1 year after treatment (Fig. 64.1). Thus lifestyle activity seems to provide an excellent alternative for obese persons who report that they "hate to exercise."

Exercise Target for Maintaining Weight Loss

Recent studies indicate that to achieve the best maintenance of weight loss, patients need to expend approximately 2500 kcal/week, the equivalent of walking approximately 1 hour/day most days of the week (64, 66). Most persons will have to increase both their lifestyle and programmed activity to achieve the high rates of energy expenditure (i.e., 2800 kcal/week) reported by participants in the National Weight

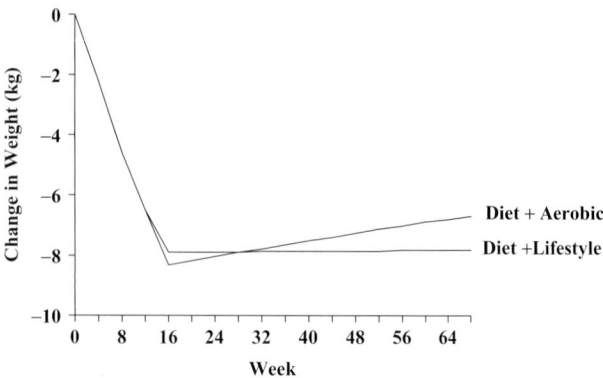

Figure 64.1. Mean changes in body weight in participants assigned to diet plus lifestyle activity and diet plus programmed aerobic activity. The difference between groups at week 68 approached statistical significance (*p* < .07) (From Andersen RE, Wadden TA, Bartlett SJ et al. Effects of lifestyle activity vs. structured aerobic exercise in obese women: a randomized trial. JAMA 1999; 281:335–40, with permission.)

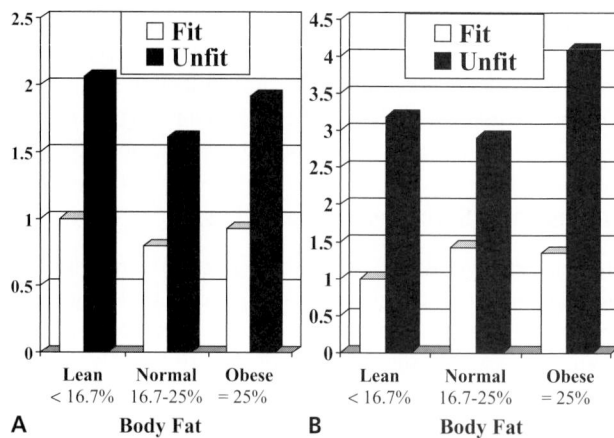

Figure 64.2. Relative risk fore all-cause mortality **(A)** and cardiovascular disease **(B)** and all-cause mortality by stratum of percentage of body fat and cardiorespiratory fitness level in 21,925 men followed for 176,742 person-years of observation (428 deaths, 144 from cardiovascular disease). Relative risks are adjusted for age (single year), examination year, smoking status, alcohol intake, and parental history of coronary heart disease. Unfit men *(black bars)* were the least fit 20% in each age group, and all other men were classified as fit. (From Blair SN, Leermakers EA. Exercise and weight management. In: Wadden TA, Stunkard AJ, eds. Handbook of Obesity Treatment. New York: Guilford Press, 2002:283–300, with permission.)

Control Registry (59). Pedometers provide a reliable and inexpensive method of tracking walking that occurs in both lifestyle and programmed activity. A reasonable goal is to increase the number of steps walked daily by 1000 per month until the patient walks at least 5000 steps/day more than at baseline (equal to ~2 additional miles/day). Some investigators have set a target of 10,000 steps/day (67).

Benefits of Physical Activity

Exercise has other benefits in addition to facilitating the maintenance of weight loss. It minimizes the loss of fat-free mass that typically occurs with weight loss (68). Strength training in particular may maintain or even increase muscle mass, and thus prevent a reduction in resting energy expenditure (69). In addition, regular exercise improves lipid levels and insulin sensitivity (56).

Perhaps the most important benefit of regular physical activity is improved fitness, which seems to be associated with a reduced risk of cardiovascular disease, regardless of body weight (56). Lee and colleagues (70) examined nearly 22,000 men divided into lean, normal, and obese groups based on body composition. Men were further divided into fit and unfit groups on the basis of results of a maximal exercise test performed on a treadmill. As shown in Figure 64.2, fitness was a stronger predictor of cardiovascular disease and all-cause mortality than was fatness. Fat but fit men had a significantly lower risk of health complications than did lean men who were unfit. Thus, overweight and obese persons should be encouraged to improve their fitness regardless of the effect that activity has on their weight.

BEHAVIOR THERAPY

Behavior therapy provides patients a set of principles and techniques for achieving their diet and exercise goals. Treatment relies on a functional analysis that examines antecedent events, behaviors, and consequences (the ABC model) associated with eating (23). Such analysis identifies events (e.g., times, places, events, people) that are associated with inappropriate eating (and activity) behaviors, as well as the cognitive and emotional consequences of these behaviors. The analysis identifies opportunities for intervention, as described later.

Components of Behavioral Treatment

Behavioral treatment has several distinguishing characteristics (71). First, it is goal oriented. It specifies very clear goals in terms that can be easily measured. This is true whether the goal is walking five times per week or decreasing the number of self-critical comments. Specific goals allow a clear assessment of progress. Second, treatment is process oriented. It is more than helping people decide what they want to accomplish; it helps them identify how to do so. Patients are encouraged to identify the specific behavior they wish to adopt and when, where, and how (and with whom) they will practice it. When the behavior is not adopted, attention is devoted to finding new strategies or to removing barriers. This skill-building philosophy views weight management as a set of skills to be learned, similar to playing a musical instrument.

The behavioral treatment of obesity has evolved into a "package" that includes several components, such as self-monitoring, stimulus control, slowing eating, problem solving, relapse prevention, and cognitive restructuring. This approach has been summarized in several manuals, including the Diabetes Prevention Program (1) and the

LEARN Program for Weight Management 2000 (72). Given the availability of such manuals, as well as reviews of the literature, we briefly review here only two components of behavioral treatment: self-monitoring and stimulus control.

Self-monitoring

Self-monitoring is the cornerstone of behavioral treatment (71). Patients keep detailed records of their food intake, physical activity, and weight throughout treatment. In the initial weeks, they record daily the types, amounts, and caloric values of foods eaten. Record keeping can be used with virtually any plan, ranging from a low-carbohydrate diet to a VLCD. Recording is increased over time to include information about times, places, and feelings associated with eating. Several studies have shown that recording food intake correlates with long-term weight loss (23, 71).

Stimulus control

Stimulus control techniques teach patients to manage cues associated with inappropriate eating (71). Chief among these are avoiding high-risk venues such as fast-food restaurants, all-you-can-eat buffets, convenience stores, and certain aisles of the grocery store. At home, patients are taught to store foods out of sight, to serve modest portion sizes, to keep serving dishes off the table, and to clean plates immediately after eating (to decrease nibbling on leftovers). Positive cues are used to increase physical activity. These might include placing a treadmill in a frequently used room (i.e., the bedroom rather than the basement), leaving walking shoes at the front door, or keeping an activity calendar on the refrigerator.

Structure of Behavioral Treatment

Patients typically attend behavioral treatment weekly for an initial period of 16 to 26 weeks (23, 71). This time-limited approach provides a clear starting and finishing line that helps people pace their efforts. In hospital and university clinics, therapy is usually provided to groups of 10 to 20 persons (during 60–90 minute sessions) by registered dietitians, behavioral psychologists, exercise specialist, or related health professionals. Group sessions provide a combination of social support and friendly competition (71). A recent study showed that group treatment induced significantly greater weight loss (~2 kg) than individual counseling (73). The weekly weigh-in seems to be a major motivator for participants, who compare weight losses (either formally or informally) with each other.

Treatment visits are usually conducted following a structured curriculum, such as that provided by the LEARN Program (72) or the Diabetes Prevention Program (1). The practitioner typically reviews patients' completion of their food and activity records, helps them identify strategies to cope with problems identified, and then introduces a new topic for the week. Lecturing is held to a minimum in favor of participants asking questions or discussing their progress in completing assignments. Visits conclude with discussion of homework for the coming week.

Results of Behavioral Treatment

Table 64.5 summarizes the results of behavioral treatment from 1974 to 2002, as determined from randomized controlled trials published in four journals: *Addictive Behaviors*, *Behavior Research and Therapy*, *Behavior Therapy*, and *Journal of Consulting and Clinical Psychology*. Only studies representative of standard behavioral treatment are included in the table. No interventions prescribed a diet providing fewer than 900 kcal/day (71).

The data indicate that patients currently treated by a comprehensive group behavioral approach lose approximately 10.7 kg (~10–12% of initial weight) in 30 weeks of treatment (71). In addition, about 80% of patients who begin treatment complete it. Thus, behavior therapy yields very favorable results as judged by the criteria for success (i.e., a 10% reduction in initial weight) proposed by the National Heart, Lung, and Blood Institute (4). A comparison of early (i.e., 1974) and more recent (1996–2002) studies reveals that weight losses have more than doubled over the past 25 years as treatment duration has increased threefold. The rate of weight loss, however, has remained constant at about 0.4 to 0.5 kg/week.

Weight regain is a problem after virtually all dietary and behavioral interventions (71). As shown in Table 64.5, patients treated with behavior therapy for 20 to 30 weeks typically regain about 30 to 35% of their lost weight in the year after treatment. Weight regain slows after the first year, but by 5 years, 50% or more of patients are likely to have returned to their baseline weight (71).

TABLE 64.5. SUMMARY OF BEHAVIOR THERAPY FOR OBESITY

	1974	1985–1987	1991–1995	1996–2002[a]
Number of studies	15	13	5	9
Sample size	53.1	71.6	30.2	28.0
Initial weight (kg)	73.4	87.2	94.9	92.2
Length of treatment (wk)	8.4	15.6	22.2	31.4
Weight loss (kg)	3.8	8.4	8.5	10.7
Loss/wk (kg)	0.5	0.5	0.4	0.4
Attrition (%)	11.4	13.8	18.5	21.2
Length of follow-up (wk)	15.1	48.3	47.7	41.8
Loss at follow-up (kg)	4.0	5.3	5.9	7.2

[a] All studies sampled were published in the following four journals: *Addictive Behaviors*, *Behavior Therapy*, *Behavior Research and Therapy*, and *Journal of Consulting and Clinical Psychology*. All values, except for number of studies, are weighted means; thus, studies with larger sample sizes had a greater impact on mean values than did studies with smaller sample sizes.

Data from Despres JP. Effects of rimonabant in the reduction of major cardiovascular risk factors. Presented at the American College of Cardiology, March 9, 2004.

Improving the Behavioral Maintenance of Weight Loss

Obesity is increasingly recognized as a chronic disorder that requires long-term care (4). When considered from this perspective, the long-term results of obesity treatment are not entirely surprising. Few practitioners, for example, would expect 30 weeks of antihypertensive medication to provide adequate control of blood pressure 1 year, or even 1 month, after medication was terminated (74). The same holds true of the treatment of type 2 diabetes. In both cases, continuous, long-term care is needed. When long-term treatment, in the form of behavior therapy, is similarly applied to obesity, the maintenance of weight loss improves significantly. There are several methods of providing continued care, including on-site treatment, telephone, and Internet/e-mail.

Several studies have demonstrated the benefits of patients continuing to attend weight maintenance classes after completing an initial 16- to 26-week weight-loss program (75, 76). Perri and colleagues (76), for example, found that persons who attended every-other-week group maintenance sessions for the year after weight reduction maintained 13.0 kg of their 13.2 kg end-of-treatment weight loss, whereas those who did not receive such therapy maintained only 5.7 kg of a 10.8-kg loss. Maintenance sessions seem to provide patients the support and motivation needed to continue to practice weight control skills, such as keeping food records and exercising regularly (71).

Long-term contact also may be provided by telephone or mail. Perri and colleagues (77) demonstrated that therapist contact by either of these modalities significantly improved weight maintenance, compared with no further intervention. When scheduling telephone calls, the same therapist optimally should contact the patient on each occasion. A study in which patients were contacted by staff members unknown to them failed to produce weight maintenance results superior to those of a no-contact group (78).

More recently, investigators have explored the internet and e-mail as methods of providing behavioral treatment, both short and long term. Two studies by Tate and colleagues found that patients who were prescribed a behavioral weight control program lost approximately 4 to 5 kg in 6 to 12 months of treatment (79, 80). Although Internet interventions do not seem to be as effective as traditional in-clinic programs, they provide a low-cost and convenient method of reaching the millions of people who need weight control. Further research is likely to improve the efficacy of this approach.

PHARMACOLOGIC TREATMENT OF OBESITY

Pharmacotherapy is recommended as an adjunct to lifestyle modification for persons with a BMI greater than 30 (or 27 in the presence of health complications) who are unable to reduce by diet and exercise alone (4). Medications may increase short-term weight loss by facilitating the patient's dietary adherence. Perhaps of greater value, pharmacotherapy potentially could improve the maintenance of weight loss if patients took weight loss medications on a long-term basis (i.e., >1 year) in the same manner that antihypertensive or antidiabetic agents are taken (74, 81).

Medications Approved by the US Food and Drug Administration

To be prescribed long-term, weight loss medications must be both safe and effective. Two agents, sibutramine (Meridia) and orlistat (Xenical), currently are approved by the US Food and Drug Administration (FDA) "for weight loss and the maintenance of weight loss." Sibutramine is a combined serotonin-norepinephrine reuptake inhibitor that seems to act on receptors in the hypothalamus that affect satiation (i.e., feelings of fullness) (82). In randomized trials, diet plus sibutramine (provided as 10–15 mg/day, in the morning) produced a 7% reduction in initial weight at 1 year, compared with 2% for patients treated by diet plus placebo (83, 84). Losses of 10 to 15% were achieved when sibutramine was combined with a more intensive program of diet and exercise modification, suggesting that behavior therapy may improve the effects of weight loss medication (85, 86). Patients studied by James and colleagues maintained a 10% loss of initial weight at 2 years that was associated with significant improvements in low-density lipoprotein and high-density lipoprotein cholesterol.

Sibutramine

Sibutramine is associated with small increases in heart rate (i.e., 4–5 beats/minute) and blood pressure (i.e., 1–2 mm Hg), and thus should not be used in patients with uncontrolled hypertension or cardiovascular disease (82). Moreover, vital signs must be monitored regularly in all patients to identify the small minority of persons who may have marked increases (i.e., >10%) in blood pressure or heart rate. Sibutramine also is not recommended for use in combination with several medications, including selective serotonin reuptake inhibitors for depression (82).

Orlistat

Orlistat is a gastric lipase inhibitor that blocks the absorption of about one third of the fat contained in a meal (82, 83). The undigested fat is passed in stool, leading to the loss of approximately 150 to 180 kcal/day. In addition, orlistat requires patients to eat a low-fat diet. If they consume more than 20 g of fat per meal, or a total of 70 g/day, they increase the risk of adverse gastrointestinal events that include oily stools, flatus with discharge, and fecal urgency. Thus, patients are negatively reinforced to eat a low-fat diet, which may further reduce their energy intake. Because orlistat is not centrally absorbed, it may be taken by patients who use selective serotonin reuptake inhibitors and other central nervous system agents (82). Patients on orlistat are advised to take a multivitamin supplement that includes fat-soluble vitamins. This is to guard against small reductions in serum levels of vitamins A, D, E, and K that may occur (82).

In randomized trials, diet plus orlistat (provided as 120 mg, three times daily, at mealtime) induced a 10% reduction in initial weight at 1 year, compared with a loss of 6% for diet alone (83, 87). Patients who remained on the drug for an additional year maintained a loss of 8% of weight at the end of this time. A recent 4-year trial revealed a 6.4% loss at the end of this time and a significant reduction in the development of type 2 diabetes in persons with impaired glucose tolerance (88). Weight loss with orlistat also is associated with significant improvements in cardiovascular risk factors (83, 87, 88).

Phentermine

Several other medications are approved by the FDA for short-term use (i.e., 6–12 weeks), the best known of which is phentermine (Ionamin, Fastin, and Adipex) (82, 83, 89). It is a norepinephrine releaser (prescribed as 15–30 mg, in the morning) that seems to target hypothalamic cells that affect hunger. The medication was approved by the FDA in 1959, when long-term studies of safety or efficacy were not required (89). The longest study, a 9-month placebo-controlled trial, observed a loss of approximately 12 kg, compared with 4 kg for placebo (90). The most common side effects of phentermine include insomnia, dry mouth, restlessness, and constipation (82). At the time of this writing, phentermine is the most widely prescribed weight loss medication, largely because it is cheaper than sibutramine and orlistat but seems to have comparable efficacy (82). Although many practitioners use phentermine on a long-term basis (off label), it should be reiterated that there are no long-term safety or efficacy data to support such use.

Future Medications

The next decade will witness an intensified search for medications that decrease energy intake and/or increase energy expenditure (83, 89). This search was accelerated in 1994 by the discovery of leptin, a hormone released from adipose tissue that signals receptors in the hypothalamus concerning the state of the body's energy needs (91). Leptin deficiency is associated with hyperphagia and marked weight gain. Initial hypotheses that most obese persons would have reduced leptin levels proved incorrect (92), and the provision of recombinant leptin was associated with only modest weight loss (93) (such that the manufacturer is unlikely to seek approval from the FDA).

Nonetheless, leptin has unlocked the key to the neurohumoral regulation of body weight and has revealed several targets for pharmacologic intervention, including agents that block neuropeptide y, which stimulates eating,

as well as those that stimulate the melanocortin 4 receptor, which inhibits food intake (82, 83). The two agents in the most advanced stages of investigation (at the time of this writing) are axokine and rimonabant. Axokine is a truncated form of ciliary neurotrophic factor that shares similarities with leptin (94). Despite initially promising results, a 1-year randomized trial of axokine observed a loss of only 2.8 kg, attributable to a majority of patients developing antibodies to the drug (82). Greater efficacy has been reported with rimonabant, an antagonist of the cannabinoid CB1 receptor, which is the target of Δ 9-tetrahydrocannabinoid, the active component of marijuana (82, 95). A recent 1-year trial showed that rimonabant was associated with a loss of 8% of initial weight, compared with 1% for placebo, and with substantial reductions in lipids (96). The medication also seems to be effective in reducing cigarette smoking and in preventing the weight gain usually associated with such efforts. Further research on the genetics of body weight regulation is likely to identify further targets for weight regulation.

SURGICAL TREATMENT OF OBESITY

Surgical treatment is an increasingly popular option for patients with a BMI greater than 40 (or >35 in the presence of comorbid conditions) (4), and was sought by approximately 125,000 persons in 2004. The most widely used procedure in the United States is the Roux-en-Y gastric bypass, pioneered by Mason and Ito (97). The operation creates a small (20–30 mL) gastric pouch at the base of the esophagus to limit intake. In addition, the stomach and part of the intestine (duodenum) are bypassed by anastomosing the pouch to a limb of the jejunum (98, 99). The operation, which is increasingly performed laparoscopically, results in a loss of approximately 30% of initial weight 1 to 2 years after surgery, with excellent maintenance of weight loss a decade or more later (100).

Gastric bypass is associated with the near-elimination of type 2 diabetes and with improvements in cardiovascular risk factors, sleep apnea, physical mobility, and quality of life (98–100). Risks of the operation include a perioperative (i.e., 30 days) mortality rate of approximately 0.5 to 1.0%, resulting from pulmonary embolus, anastomotic leaks, and wound infections (98, 99). Expected side effects in the first several months after surgery include vomiting, as patients adjust to their smaller gastric pouch, and "dumping," which is characterized by nausea, flushing, bloating, and extreme diarrhea after consumption of refined carbohydrates (98). (Thus, patients are negatively reinforced to avoid these foods.) Nutritional considerations include the need for patients to consume adequate amounts of protein, as well as to monitor vitamin B_{12} and iron levels (98). Menstruating women should take two iron sulfate tablets (325 mg/day) as long as they continue to menstruate. Magnesium and calcium levels also should be monitored and may require supplementation.

Other Surgical Procedures

The gastric bypass has largely replaced vertical banded gastroplasty, which also creates a small gastric pouch to limit intake but does not alter the gastrointestinal tract (98). Several randomized trials found that the gastric bypass produced greater long-term weight loss than gastroplasty (98, 100), perhaps because of the slight malabsorption associated with the former procedure, as well as its more favorable effects on ghrelin, a gut peptide that increases before mealtime and is associated with reports of hunger (101). The gastric bypass seems to be associated with long-term suppression of ghrelin, potentially contributing to patients' reduced appetite.

Laparoscopic adjustable gastric banding is currently considered the procedure of choice in Europe, Australia, and South America principally because of its extremely low mortality rate (i.e., ~0.1%) (102). A small pouch (i.e., 30 mL) and small stoma are created immediately below the esophagus using a silicone band, the circumference of which can be adjusted by injecting saline into a subcutaneously implanted port (98, 102). Some trials have reported weight losses as great as 25 to 30%, although smaller reductions were observed in a US study (103), thus dampening enthusiasm for the procedure in this country. Randomized trials that include an economic analysis are needed to compare laparoscopic adjustable gastric banding with the older gastric bypass. Similar studies are needed to assess the efficacy of the biliopancreatic diversion, pioneered by Scopinaro and colleagues (104).

Dietary and Behavioral Counseling

Our research team believes that all candidates for bariatric surgery should receive both preoperative and postoperative counseling from a multidisciplinary team that includes a registered dietitian and mental health specialist (12). Approximately 30% of candidates for bariatric surgery suffer from depression or other psychiatric complications that are poorly controlled (12). In addition, many have a limited understanding of the dietary changes required with surgery. Postsurgical consultation with a dietitian is required to ensure that patients understand the progression from liquid to pureed to conventional foods, as well as foods that should be avoided (i.e., refined carbohydrates). Many patients appear to enjoy and benefit from monthly support groups after surgery. The behavioral evaluation and care of surgical patients has been described elsewhere (12).

CONCLUSIONS

This review has shown that there are several effective options for inducing losses of 8 to 10% of initial weight and that losses of this size are associated with significant improvements in health (1–3). Improving the maintenance of weight loss remains the greatest challenge faced by behavioral and pharmacologic interventions. At present, only bariatric surgery is associated with durable long-term weight loss, but this procedure is appropriate for only a small minority of persons who are obese.

The treatment of obesity is likely to improve with increased research on body weight regulation, as well as efforts to translate findings from clinical trials into interventions for primary care and community practice. However, far greater resources and efforts must be devoted to the prevention of obesity if we are to halt the progression of this epidemic, let alone reverse it. Our best hope for prevention may lie with children and adolescents (105). Efforts should be devoted to improving meals and snacks served at schools, to providing more opportunities for physical activity at school and at home, and to educating youth about the importance of diet, activity, and a healthy body weight. Ultimately, we must tackle what Brownell has referred to as a "toxic environment" that explicitly encourages the consumption of supersized servings of high-fat, high-sugar foods while implicitly discouraging physical activity as a result of sedentary work and leisure habits (106). Changing this environment will require public policy initiatives, as were needed, for example, to reduce cigarette smoking and to increase seat belt use. Although behavioral, pharmacologic, and surgical treatment can assist those who already are obese, a pressing need exists for large-scale environmental interventions that will reduce the number of persons who require such treatments.

Acknowledgments

Preparation of this chapter was supported in part by grant DK065018 from the National Institute of Diabetes Digestive and Kidney Disease.

REFERENCES

1. Diabetes Prevention Program Research Group. N Engl J Med 2002;346:393–403.
2. Tuomilehto J, Lindstrom J, Eriksson JG et al. N Engl J Med 2001;344:1343–50.
3. Gregg EW, Williamson DF. The relationship of intentional weight loss to disease incidence and mortality. In: Wadden TA, Stunkard AJ, eds. Handbook of Obesity Treatment. New York: Guilford Press, 2002:125–43.
4. National Heart, Lung, and Blood Institute. Obes Res 1998;6: 51S–210S.
5. Manson JE, Willett WC, Stampfer MJ et al. N Engl J Med 1995;333:677–85.
6. Lapidus L, Bengtsson C, Larsson B et al. Br Med J 1984;289: 1257–61.
7. National Heart, Lung, and Blood Institute and North American Association for the Study of Obesity (NAASO). Practical Guide to the Identification, Evaluation, and Treatment of Overweight and Obesity in Adults. Bethesda, MD: National Institute of Health, 2000.
8. Atkinson RL. Medical evaluation of the obese patient. In: Wadden TA, Stunkard AJ, eds. Handbook of Obesity Treatment. New York: Guilford Press, 2002:173–85.
9. Wadden TA, Phelan S. Behavioral assessment of the obese patient. In: Wadden TA, Stunkard AJ, eds. Handbook of Obesity Treatment. New York: Guilford Press, 2002:186–226.

10. Carpenter KM, Hasin DS, Allison DB et al. Am J Public Health 2000;90:251–7.
11. Wadden TA, Anderson DA, Foster GD et al. Arch Fam Med 2000;9:854–60.
12. Wadden TA, Sarwer DB, Womble LG et al. Surg Clin North Am 2001;81:1001–24.
13. Beck AT, Steer RA. Manual of the Beck Depression Inventory. New York: Psychological Cooperation, 1987.
14. Stunkard AJ, Allison KC. Int J Obes Relat Metab Disord 2003;27:1–12.
15. Spitzer RL, Yanovski S, Wadden T et al. Int J Eat Disord 1993;13:137–53.
16. Block G, Woods M, Potosky A et al. J Clin Epidemiol 1990;43:1327–35.
17. Andersen RE, Wadden TA, Bartlett SJ et al. JAMA 1999;281:335–40.
18. Astrup A. Best Pract Res Clin Endocrinol Metab 1999;13:109–20.
19. Melanson K, Dwyer J. Popular diets for treatment of overweight and obesity. In: Wadden TA, Stunkard AJ, eds. Handbook of Obesity Treatment. New York: Guilford Press, 2002:249–75.
20. Golay A, Allaz AF, Morel Y et al. Am J Clin Nutr 1996;63:174–8.
21. US Departments of Agriculture and Health and Human Services. Dietary Guidelines for Americans. Washington, DC: US Government Publishing Office, 2000.
22. Wadden TA, McGuckin BG, Rothman RA et al. J Gastrointest Surg 2003;7:452–63.
23. Wing RR. Behavioral treatment of obesity. In: Wadden TA, Stunkard AJ, eds. Handbook of Obesity Treatment. New York: Guilford Press, 2002:301–16.
24. Bandini LG, Schoeller DA, Cyr HN et al. Am J Clin Nutr 1990;52:421–5.
25. Jeffrey RW, Wing RR, Thornson C et al. J Consult Clin Psychol 1993;61:1038–42.
26. Ditschuneit HH, Fletcher-Mors M, Johnson TD et al. Am J Clin Nutr 1999;69:198–204.
27. Heymsfield SB, van Mierlo CA, van der Knaap HC et al. Int J Obes Relat Metab Disord 2003;27:537–49.
28. Fletchner-Mors M, Ditschuneit HH, Johnson TD et al. Obes Res 2000;8:399–402.
29. Schlundt DG, Hill JO, Pope-Cordle J et al. Int J Obes Relat Metab Disord 1993;17:623–9.
30. Jeffery RW, Hellerstedt WL, French S et al. Int J Obes Relat Metab Disord 1995;19:132–7.
31. Toubro S, Astrup A. BMJ 1997;314:29–34.
32. Rolls BJ, Bell EA. Eur J Clin Nutr 1999;53:S166–73.
33. Rolls B, Barnett RA. Volumetric. New York: Harper Collins, 2000.
34. Atkins RC. Dr. Atkins' New Diet Revolution. 2nd ed. New York: Avon Books, 1999.
35. Samaha FF, Iqbal N, Seshadri P et al. N Engl J Med 2003;348:2074–81.
36. Stern L, Iqbalo N, Seshadri P et al. Ann Intern Med 2004;140:778–85.
37. Foster GD, Wyatt HR, Hill JO et al. N Engl J Med 2003;348:2082–90.
38. Brehm BJ, Seeley RJ, Daniels SR et al. J Clin Endocrinol Metab 2003;88:1617–23.
39. Yancy WS, Olsen MK, Guyton JR et al. Ann Intern Med 2004;140:769–77.
40. Sondike SB, Copperman N, Jacobson MS. J Pediatr 2003;142:253–8.
41. Wolever TM, Jenkins DJ, Jenkins AL et al. Am J Clin Nutr 1991;54:846–54.
42. Ludwig DS, Majzoub JA, Al-Zahrani A et al. Pediatrics 1999;103:E26.
43. Melanson KJ, Westerterp-Plantenga MS, Saris WH et al. Am J Physiol 1999;277:R337–45.
44. National Task Force on the Prevention and Treatment of Obesity. JAMA 1993;270:967–74.
45. Wadden TA, Berkowitz RI. Very-low-calorie diets. In: Fairburn CG, Brownell KD, eds. Eating Disorders and Obesity. New York: Guilford Press, 2001:529–33.
46. Broomfield PH, Chopra R, Sheinbaum RC et al. N Engl J Med 1988;319:1567–72.
47. Miura J, Arai K, Ohno M et al. Int J Obes 1989;13:73S–7S.
48. Ryttig KR, Flaten H, Rossner S. Int J Obes Relat Metab Disord 1997;21:574–9.
49. Torgerson JS, Lissner L, Lindroos AK et al. Int J Obes Relat Metab Disord 1997;21:987–94.
50. Wadden TA, Foster GD, Letizia KA. J Consult Clin Psychol 1994;62:165–71.
51. Wadden TA, Sternberg JA, Letizia KA et al. Int J Obes 1989;13:39S–46S.
52. Wing RR, Blair E, Marcus M et al. Am J Med 1994;97:354–62.
53. Wing RR, Marcus MD, Salata R et al. Arch Intern Med 1991;151:1334–40.
54. Apfelbaum M, Vague P, Ziegler O et al. Am J Med 1999;106:179–84.
55. Pate RR, Pratt M, Blair SN et al. JAMA 1995;273:402–7.
56. Blair SN, Leermakers EA. Exercise and weight management. In: Wadden TA, Stunkard AJ, eds. Handbook of Obesity Treatment. New York: Guilford Press, 2002:283–300.
57. Wing RR. Med Sci Sports Exerc 1999;31:S547–52.
58. Pronk NP, Wing RR. Obes Res 1994;2:587–99.
59. Klem ML, Wing RR, McGuire MT et al. Am J Clin Nutr 1997;66:239–46.
60. Wadden TA, Vogt RA, Foster GD et al. J Consult Clin Psychol 1998;66:429–33.
61. Jakicic JM, Wing RR, Butler BA et al. Int J Obes Relat Metab Disord 1995;19:893–901.
62. Perri MG, Martin AD, Leermakers EA et al. J Consult Clin Psychol 1997;65:278–85.
63. King AC, Haskell WL, Young DR et al. Circulation 1995;91:2596–604.
64. Jakicic JM, Winters C, Lang W et al. JAMA 1999;282:1554–60.
65. Epstein LH, Wing RR, Koeske R et al. Behav Ther 1982;13:651–65.
66. Jeffery RW, Wing RR, Sherwood NE et al. Am J Clin Nutr 2003;78:684–9.
67. Yamanouchi K, Shinozaki T, Chikada K et al. Diabetes Care 1995;18:775–8.
68. Ballor DL, Poehlman ET. Int J Obes Relat Metab Disord 1994;18:35–40.
69. Wadden TA, Vogt RA, Foster GD et al. J Consult Clin Psychol 1998;66:429–33.
70. Lee CD, Blair SN, Jackson AS. Am J Clin Nutr 1999;69:373–80.
71. Wadden TA, Butryn ML. Endocrinol Metab Clin North Am 2003;32:981–1003.
72. Brownell KD. The LEARN Program for Weight Management 2000. Dallas, TX: American Health Publishing, 2000.
73. Renjilian DA, Perri MG, Nezu AM et al. J Consult Clin Psychol 2001;69:717–21.
74. Bray GA. Ann Intern Med 1993;119:707–13.

75. Perri MG, Corsica JA. Improving the maintenance of weight lost in behavioral treatment of obesity. In: Wadden TA, Stunkard AJ, eds. Handbook of Obesity Treatment. New York: Guilford Press, 2002:357–79.

76. Perri MG, McAllister DA, Gange JJ et al. J Consult Clin Psychol 1988;56:529–34.

77. Perri MG, Shapiro RM, Ludwig WW. J Consult Clin Psychol 1984;52:404–13.

78. Wing RR, Jeffery RW, Hellerstedt WL. Ann Behav Med 1996;18:172–6.

79. Tate DF, Wing RR, Winett RA. JAMA 2001;285:1172–7.

80. Tate DF, Jackvony EH, Wing RR. JAMA 2003;289:1833–6.

81. Stunkard AJ. Life Sci 1982;30:2043–55.

82. Thearle M, Aronne LJ. Endocrinol Metab Clin North Am 2003;32:1005–24.

83. Yanovski SZ, Yanovski JA. N Engl J Med 2002;346:591–602.

84. Arterburn DE, Crane PK, Veenstra DL. Arch Intern Med 2004;164:994–1003.

85. James WP, Astrup A, Finer N et al. Lancet 2000;356:2119–25.

86. Wadden TA, Berkowitz RI, Sarwer DB et al. Arch Intern Med 2001;161:218–27.

87. Sjöstron L, Rissanen A, Andersen T et al. Lancet 1998;352:167–72.

88. Torgerson JS, Hauptman J, Boldrin MN et al. Diabetes Care 2004;27:155–61.

89. Bray GA, Greenway FL. Endocrinol Rev 2000;20:805–75.

90. Munro JF, McCuish AC, Wilson EM et al. Br Med J 1968;i:352–6.

91. Zhang Y, Proenca R, Maffei M et al. Nature 1994;372:425–32.

92. Considine RV, Sinha MK, Heiman ML et al. N Engl J Med 1996;334:292–5.

93. Heymsfield SB, Greenberg AS, Fujioka K et al. JAMA 1999;282:1568–75.

94. Ettinger MP, Littlejohn TW, Schwartz SL et al. JAMA 2003;289:1826–32.

95. Colombo G, Agabio R, Diaz G et al. Life Sci 1998;63:PL113–7.

96. Despres JP. Effects of rimonabant in the reduction of major cardiovascular risk factors. Presented at the American College of Cardiology. March 9, 2004.

97. Mason EE, Ito C. Ann Surg 1969;170:329–39.

98. Latifi R, Kellum JM, De Maria EJ et al. Surgical treatment of obesity. In: Wadden TA, Stunkard AJ, eds. Handbook of Obesity Treatment. New York: Guilford Press, 2002:339–56.

99. Brolin RE. JAMA 2002;288:2793–6.

100. Albrecht RJ, Pories WJ. Best Pract Res Clin Endocrinol Metab 1999;13:149–72.

101. Cummings DE, Shannon MH. J Clin Endocrinol Metab 2003;88:2999–3002.

102. O'Brien PE, Dixon JB. Arch Surg 2003;138:908–12.

103. Pender JR, Pories WJ. Surgical treatment of obesity. Psychiatr Clin North Am (in press).

104. Scopinaro N, Gianetta E, Adami GF et al. Surgery 1996;119:261–8.

105. Wadden TA, Brownell KD, Foster GD. J Consult Clin Psychol 2002;70:510–25.

106. Brownell KD, Horgen KB. Food Fight: The Inside Story of the Food Industry, America's Obesity Crisis, and What We Can Do about It. New York: McGraw-Hill, 2003.

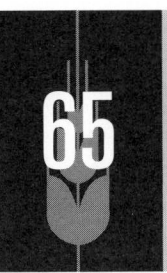

65

DIABETES MELLITUS: MEDICAL NUTRITION THERAPY[1]

JAMES W. ANDERSON

HISTORICAL OVERVIEW 1043
CLASSIFICATION 1044
EPIDEMIOLOGY 1045
DIAGNOSIS 1045
BODY FUEL REGULATION .1046
    Role of Hormones 1046
    Energy Stores 1046
    Fed State 1047
    Fasting State 1047
METABOLIC DERANGEMENTS 1048
DIABETIC COMPLICATIONS 1048
    Acute Problems 1048
    Short-Term Complications 1049
    Long-Term Complications 1049
    Atherosclerosis 1050
GOALS OF MEDICAL NUTRITION THERAPY 1050
NUTRITIONAL PLAN 1051
    Carbohydrates 1051
    Proteins 1052
    Fats 1053
    Fiber 1053
    Sweeteners 1054
    Alcohol 1056
    Micronutrients 1056
SPECIAL NUTRITIONAL CONSIDERATIONS 1056
    Children 1056
    Elderly Persons 1057
    Pregnancy 1057
    Renal Disease 1058
    Dyslipidemia 1058
WEIGHT MANAGEMENT 1059
    Weight-Loss Approaches 1059
    Weight Maintenance .1060
PHYSICAL ACTIVITY 1061
NUTRITION AND PHARMACOTHERAPY 1061
    Insulin Therapy 1061

    Oral Antidiabetes Drug Therapy 1062
NUTRITIONAL ASSESSMENT AND EDUCATION 1063
INSTRUCTION IN MEAL PLANS 1063
    General Guidelines 1063
    Carbohydrate Counting 1063
    Food Exchanges 1063
CONCLUSION 1064

Diabetes mellitus is occurring at epidemic rates in the United States (1) and in most parts of the world (2, 3). The number of adults with diabetes in the world is projected to increase from 135 million in 1995 to 300 million in 2025 (4). In the United States, approximately 20 million people have diabetes and approximately 15 million have impaired fasting glucose levels. Of special concern is the emergence of type 2 diabetes in adolescents (5), closely linked to the fourfold increase in prevalence of obesity in children and teens in the past 30 years (6). Diabetes is the fifth leading cause of death in the United States, and the estimated costs for medical expenditures and lost productivity for diabetes in the United States are more than $132 billion annually (7).

Lifestyle changes—physical activity and healthy nutrition practices—are vital for persons with diabetes to maintain quality of life and longevity. Medical nutrition management is the cornerstone for treatment of all persons with diabetes because appropriate dietary practices decrease all of the risks and complications associated with diabetes and can potentially restore normal life expectancy. Weight management is the most important therapeutic goal for obese persons with diabetes. Central to glycemic level, lipid level, and weight management are high-carbohydrate, high-fiber, low-animal-fat diets (8, 9). Because of their high risk for cardiovascular disease (10), persons with diabetes should develop a prevention strategy for normalizing serum lipids and minimizing other risk factors such as overweight, physical inactivity, hypertension, and oxidative stress. Health care team members counsel diabetic persons to empower them to manage their diabetes and lifestyle for maintenance of optimal health.

HISTORICAL OVERVIEW

Ancient civilizations in Egypt, Greece, Rome, and India recognized diabetes and the effect of dietary intervention. The Roman Aretaeus, AD 70, noted polydipsia and polyuria

---

[1] **Abbreviations: ADA,** American Diabetes Association; **BMI,** body mass index; **DHA,** decosahexanoic acid; **DKA,** diabetic ketoacidosis; **EPA,** eicosapentaenoic acid; **FDA,** US Food and Drug Administration; **GDM,** gestational diabetes mellitus; **GI,** glycemic index; **HDL,** high-density lipoproteins; **LDL,** low-density lipoprotein; **MR,** meal replacement; **MUS,** monounsaturated; **NIDDM,** non–insulin-dependent diabetes mellitus; **VLDL,** very-low-density lipoprotein.

TABLE 65.1. NUTRITIONAL RECOMMENDATIONS[a] FOR PERSONS WITH DIABETES: 1930 TO 2004

NUTRIENT	1930	1955	1970	1990	2004
Carbohydrate, total (g/d)	70	176	225	290	295
Percentage energy (%)	14	35	45	58	59
Simple (g/d)	40	71	112	130	115
Complex (g/d)	30	105	113	160	180
Fat, total (g/d)	153	99	82	60	60
Percentage of energy (%)	69	45	37	27	27
Saturated (g/d)	87	46	35	14	16
Monounsaturated (g/d)	50	37	31	26	28
Polyunsaturated (g/d)	9	11	13	17	16
Cholesterol (mg/d)	1,060	690	550	<200	<200
Protein (g/d)	85	101	90	75	70
Percentage of energy (%)	17	20	18	15	14
Dietary fiber (g/d)	8	15	20	40	35

[a]Values for 2000 kcal/d diet.

Data from Anderson JW, Randles KM, Kendall CWC et al. J Am Coll Nutr 2004;23:5–17; and Anderson JW. Nutritional management of diabetes mellitus. In: Shils ME, Olson JA, Shike M et al., eds. Modern Nutrition in Health and Disease. 9th ed. Baltimore: Williams & Wilkins, 1999:1365–94.

and named the condition diabetes, meaning to flow through. Thomas Willis, a London physician, later introduced the term mellitus or honey-like after noting the sweet taste of urine. Early dietary recommendations were based on theory rather than on scientific fact. As today, debate raged on the amount of carbohydrate allowed. Champions of low-carbohydrate, high-fat diets argued that excess sugar present in blood and urine required a restriction in carbohydrate. Proponents of high-carbohydrate diets argued that dietary carbohydrate was needed to replace that lost in urine. Universally agreed on, and still relevant today, was that diabetes is best treated by energy-restricted diets (11).

Frederick M. Allen of New York developed the famous "Allen Starvation Treatment" of diabetes in 1912. Using 1000-kcal diets containing 10 g carbohydrate, he sustained the lives of a few young men until insulin became available. Thus, just before the discovery of insulin, diabetes was treated with low-carbohydrate semistarvation regimens. Over the years, many sources of carbohydrate were identified as therapeutic including milk, vegetables, rice, potatoes, and oatmeal. Even after insulin was discovered in 1921, most Western diabetes specialists used low-carbohydrate, high-fat diets to treat lean persons with diabetes. The few clinicians to report that high-carbohydrate, low-fat diets benefited diabetic persons included Geylin in 1935, Sansum in 1926, and Kempner in 1958 (12).

Recent scientific data analyzed by numerous international diabetes associations and expert panels support recommendations of a generous carbohydrate, fat-restricted diet (9). Table 65.1 outlines major changes in nutrition recommendations in the United States over 70 years. The recommended carbohydrate intake has increased steadily since 1930 and has recently reached a plateau. Recommended total fat intake has steadily declined, whereas protein intake has remained about the same. Recommended fiber intake has increased dramatically.

CLASSIFICATION

Diabetes mellitus can result from a variety of genetic, metabolic, and acquired conditions eventuating in hyperglycemia. Metabolic derangements in the metabolism of glucose and profound abnormalities in metabolism of fat, protein, and other substances characterize the pathology of diabetes. Current research recognizes that diabetes mellitus has several antecedents, although each type has a similar outcome once established. A heterogeneous disorder both genetically and clinically, all classifications of diabetes have in common hyperglycemia, attributable to either insulin insufficiency or insulin resistance. The traditional classification segregates hyperglycemic conditions into these groups: insulin-dependent diabetes mellitus (IDDM or type 1), non–insulin-dependent diabetes mellitus (NIDDM or type 2), other specific types of diabetes and gestational diabetes mellitus (GDM) (Table 65.2). In the past decade, a new variant of diabetes in adults has been characterized; this has been termed latent autoimmune diabetes in adults or type 1.5 diabetes. Latent autoimmune diabetes in adults usually develops in nonobese persons who are more than 35 years old and who have specific types of serum antibodies (13). These observations point to the complex interaction of genetic and environmental factors that play roles in all forms of diabetes (14).

Type 1 diabetes accounts for approximately 5% of diabetes and is manifested by insulin deficiency caused by destruction of the pancreatic β cells. Type 2 diabetes accounts for about 90% of diabetes and is characterized by two primary defects: insulin resistance (diminished tissue

TABLE 65.2. ETIOLOGIC CLASSIFICATION OF DIABETES MELLITUS AND PREDIABETES

Diabetes
 I. Type 1 diabetes (β-cell destruction with lack of insulin)
 II. Type 2 diabetes (insulin resistance with relative insulin deficiency)
 III. Other specific types: Genetic defects of β-cell function; genetic defects of insulin action; diseases of the exocrine pancreas; endocrinopathies (e.g., acromegaly); drug- or chemical-induced; infectious; immune-mediated diabetes from other uncommon conditions; genetic syndromes sometimes associated with diabetes (e.g., Down syndrome)
 IV. Gestational diabetes mellitus

Prediabetes
 I. Impaired fasting glucose: fasting plasma glucose concentrations 100 to 125 mg/dL (5.6–6.9 mmol/L) or
 II. Impaired glucose tolerance: plasma glucose value 140 to 199 mg/dL (7.8–11.1 mmol/L) at 2 hours after glucose load

From American Diabetes Association. Diabetes Care 2004;27:5S–10S, with permission.

sensitivity to insulin) and impaired β-cell function (delayed or inadequate insulin release). Other causes account for the remaining 5% of diabetes in the United States (3).

The onset of gestational diabetes typically occurs between the twenty-fourth and twenty-eighth weeks of pregnancy, when the body's demand for insulin is dramatically increased. In the United States it affects from 4 to 7% of all pregnancies, depending on the diagnostic criteria (15). Nutritional intake and glycemic control influence the outcome of pregnancy and fetal health.

People with impaired fasting glucose or impaired glucose tolerance are also considered to have prediabetes, indicating that they are at high risk for developing diabetes in the future. Prediabetes is one risk factor for developing diabetes, along with obesity, lack of physical activity, and age. Because the onset of overt diabetes can be delayed by diet and exercise, these patients should be counseled about lifestyle measures when they have a single fasting glucose value greater than or equal to 100 mg/dL (8).

EPIDEMIOLOGY

Estimates that 20 million persons have diagnosed or undiagnosed diabetes and 15 million persons have impaired fasting glucose in the United States are based on estimates for 1999 to 2000 (16), annual rates of increase (17), and the lowering of the criteria for impaired fasting glucose (18). In 1999 to 2000, the National Health and Nutrition Examination surveys reported that the prevalence of total diabetes (diabetes, undiagnosed diabetes, and impaired fasting glucose) was significantly higher in men (17.6%) than in women (12.5%) (16). The prevalence of total diabetes increased with age from 10 to 39 years (3.8%) to greater than or equal to 60 years (33.9%). Total diabetes was less common in non-Hispanic whites (13.1%) than in Mexican Americans (18.8%) and non-Hispanic blacks (21.1%) (16). In the United States, the prevalence of diabetes is highest among Native Americans; adult Pima Indians have rates of approximately 50%, the highest in the world (3).

The prevalence of type 1 diabetes is very different from that of type 2 diabetes. In Sweden the annual incidence, or development of new cases, of type 1 diabetes is very high, with rates that are about twice those in the United States and 100 times those in Peru. In the United States, the prevalence, or number of persons with the condition, of type 1 diabetes for persons less than 20 years old is approximately 1.7 per 1000 with a total number of children and adults with type 1 diabetes of approximately 750,000 (19). Because of its heritability, about 50% of persons in whom type 1 diabetes develops have a family history of the condition. The incidence rates of type 1 diabetes around the world seem to be increasing slightly, but not at the epidemic rates observed for type 2 diabetes (20).

The prevalence of type 2 diabetes varies enormously from ethnic group to ethnic group within a country and around the world. Some Chinese populations have very low rates, whereas the residents of the Nauru in the South Pacific have rates approaching those of the American Pima Indians (3). Genetic and environmental factors contribute to the development of type 2 diabetes. The inheritability of type 2 diabetes is very strong, with approximately 80% of persons having two parents with type 2 diabetes developing the disease during their lifetime. Some ethnic groups, such as Pima Indians and Nauru residents, have very high risks for type 2 diabetes, whereas others, such as Mapuche Indians and Bantus, have very low rates. The emerging epidemic of type 2 diabetes in developed and developing countries seems related to the unmasking of a genetic disposition to type 2 diabetes by lifestyle factors—adopting a Western-type diet and decreased physical activity (3, 21).

DIAGNOSIS

Classic symptoms such as polydipsia, polyuria, and rapid weight loss associated with gross and unequivocal elevation of blood glucose (≥200 mg/dL or 11.1 mmol/L) make the diagnosis of diabetes mellitus (Table 65.3). A fasting plasma glucose level greater than or equal to 126 mg/dL (7.0 mmol/L) on two occasions is diagnostic of diabetes (18). The oral glucose tolerance test may be used to screen for diabetes but is not recommended for routine clinical use (22). The hemoglobin A_{1c} is a convenient screening test for diabetes and may be obtained when the fasting plasma glucose value is measured. When the hemoglobin A_{1c} is greater than mean + 2 standard deviations, the presence of diabetes is likely and should be confirmed with repeat fasting plasma glucose values (22).

GDM is defined as glucose intolerance that is first detected during pregnancy. Recommendations for screening, diagnostic criteria, and clinical management are all controversial topics (15, 23). Furthermore, GDM may be one of the strongest risk factors for subsequent development of overt diabetes, and thus should serve as a strong indicator for lifestyle counseling (23). The criteria for

---

TABLE 65.3. CRITERIA FOR DIAGNOSIS OF DIABETES MELLITUS[a]

1. Symptoms of diabetes plus casual plasma glucose values of ≥200 mg/dL (11.1 mmol/L). Casual is defined as any time of day without regard to time since last meal. Classic symptoms of diabetes include polydipsia, polyuria, and unexplained weight loss.
2. Fasting plasma glucose value ≥126 mg/dL (7.0 mmol/L). Fasting is defined as no energy intake for at least 8 hours.
3. 2-hour postload plasma glucose value of ≥200 mg/dL during an oral glucose tolerance test.

[a] In the absence of unequivocal hyperglycemia, these criteria should be confirmed by a second measurement on a different day. The oral glucose tolerance test is not recommended for routine clinical use.

Adapted from American Diabetes Association. Diabetes Care 2004;27:5S–10S, with permission.

TABLE 65.4. DIAGNOSIS OF GESTATIONAL DIABETES MELLITUS

	mg/dL	mmol/L
100-g oral glucose load		
Fasting plasma glucose value	95	5.3
1-h value	180	10.0
2-h value	155	8.6
3-h value	140	7.8
75-g oral glucose load		
Fasting plasma glucose value	95	5.3
1-h value	180	10.0
2-h value	155	8.6

Adapted from American Diabetes Association. Diabetes Care 2004; 27:5S–10S, with permission; see reference for details.

diagnosis are listed in Table 65.4, and the timing and selection of testing procedures are given in detail elsewhere (15, 23, 24).

BODY FUEL REGULATION

Role of Hormones

Glucose homeostasis is orchestrated by an exquisite interplay of pancreatic and gut hormones (Table 65.5). The pancreatic β cells produce insulin and amylin. Insulin is the hormone primarily responsible for the metabolism and storage of the body fuels that are ingested. The pancreas sustains a basal level of insulin release and secretes additional insulin in response to increased blood glucose after a meal. Amino acids and gut hormones enhance postprandial insulin secretion. Ingested nutrients stimulate perhaps half of the postmeal insulin release, and the additional insulin response is facilitated by gut hormones. Glucagon-like peptide-1, produced by the L cells of the distal ileum and colon, seems responsible for about 80% of this incremental insulin response, whereas gastric inhibitory peptide, produced by the K cells of the duodenum and jejunum, seems responsible for the remaining 20% (25, 26). The postprandial secretion of insulin promotes glucose, amino acids, and fat uptake by tissues (primarily liver, adipose, and muscle tissue) where the glucose is used or stored. Insulin production decreases as the blood glucose level decreases. Amylin, also synthesized in the pancreatic β cells, is cosecreted with insulin and acts to delay gastric emptying, inhibit glucagon secretion, and decrease food intake (3, 27). Glucagon, the third pancreatic hormone, is secreted by the pancreatic α cells in response to decreased blood glucose levels and under conditions of stress (3). The balance between insulin and glucagon levels is vital for normal glucose homeostasis, fatty acid metabolism, and protein preservation. Of interest, most of these pancreatic and gut hormones inhibit food intake and enhance satiety (fullness after a meal) or satiation (lack of hunger between meals) (28). Only ghrelin from the stomach and duodenum acts to stimulate food intake (29). Cholecystokinin, another gut hormone acting to stimulate contraction of the gallbladder, also delays gastric emptying and decreases food intake.

Insulin is the main signal to the body for the fed or fasting states. After a large meal, high serum insulin levels stimulate fuel and energy storage. After an overnight fast, low serum insulin levels permit mobilization of fuel and energy from storage depots. Glucagon facilitates fuel and energy release with low blood insulin levels. Under stressful circumstances, hypoglycemia, or trauma, glucagon and other counterregulatory hormones, which oppose or counter insulin action, are released. These counterregulatory hormones—glucagon, catecholamines, glucocorticoids, and growth hormone—act specifically to decrease glucose use, to promote glucose production, and to mobilize fatty acids. During fasting, exercise, and stress, fatty acids emerge as major sources of energy (3).

Energy Stores

A healthy 70-kg man stores approximately 70 g liver glycogen, 200 g muscle glycogen, and 30 g glucose in body fluids (1200 kcal). Available glucose stores can meet energy needs for only 12 to 18 hours. However, adipose tissue

TABLE 65.5. PANCREATIC AND GUT HORMONES AFFECTING METABOLISM AND FOOD INTAKE

HORMONE (REFERENCE)	SOURCE	GLUCOSE EFFECTS	GUT EFFECTS	APPETITE/FOOD INTAKE
Insulin (3)	Pancreas: β cells	Stimulates glucose metabolism		Decreases
Amylin (27)	Pancreas: β cells	Inhibits glucagon release	Delays gastric emptying	Decreases
Glucagon (3)	Pancreas: α cells	Stimulates glucose release		
Glucagon-like peptide-1 (26)	Intestine and colon: L cells	Enhances insulin release, inhibits glucagon release	Delays gastric emptying	Decreases
Gastric inhibitory peptide (25)	Duodenum and jejunum: K cells	Enhances insulin release		
Ghrelin (29)	Stomach			Increases
Peptide YY (122)	Intestine and colon: L cells			Decreases
Cholecystokinin (123)	Duodenum and jejunum: I cells		Delays gastric emptying	Decreases

triglycerides typically represent energy deposits of 120,000 kcal, 100 times the glucose energy reserves. During starvation or stress, fatty acids are released for energy. Body proteins, skeletal and visceral structures, and other vital components are unavailable for energy except under conditions of prolonged starvation or severe stress (3, 11).

Fed State

A multifaceted system of hormones, nervous tissue, and digestive tissue is necessary to sustain the fed individual. This state commences as food travels down the digestive tract and is broken down by various enzymes into smaller units, such as amino acids, peptides, sugars, glycerol, and fatty acids. Next, these nutrients are absorbed by the small intestine and then transported further. The portal blood carries amino acids and sugars to the liver. Lymph carries lipids as chylomicrons from the small intestine to the circulatory system, where it is transported to numerous tissues (11).

Pancreatic β cells release insulin in response to perfusion by blood enriched with glucose, amino acids, pancreatic hormones, and other secretagogs. The same action of glucose also decreases production of glucagon. In response to the release of insulin, nutrients are taken up and stored in cells and tissues. Insulin stimulates glycogen synthesis, aerobic and anaerobic glycolysis, protein synthesis, and fatty acid syntheses in the liver. Insulin inhibits glycogenolytic, gluconeogenic, proteolytic, and lipolytic processes. After activation by phosphorylation, glucose enters glycogen depots, generates energy in glycolytic and Kreb cycle pathways, and yields precursors for fatty acid and protein synthesis. Other simple sugars enter the glycogen pool, generate energy, or become precursors for synthetic processes. Amino acids enter precursor pools for protein synthesis (3, 11).

Muscle and adipose tissue receive a large percentage of glucose and amino acids released after large meals. High serum insulin concentrations specifically stimulate the transport of glucose and amino acids into muscle cells and glucose into adipose tissue. In muscle cells, under the influence of insulin, glucose enters glycogen depots and generates energy while amino acids serve as precursors for protein synthesis. Insulin also facilitates the conversion of glucose products to fatty acids for storage as triglycerides in fat cells. Most other tissues are freely permeable to glucose as well as amino acids and use the nutrients for glycogen formation, energy, and protein synthesis (3, 11).

Gut, liver, and other tissues handle ingested fat differently from glucose and amino acids. Gut hydrolyzes fats to fatty acids, glycerol, cholesterol, phospholipids, and other constituents. Short- and medium-chain fatty acids are absorbed and enter the portal vein for use in the liver. Long-chain fatty acids, cholesterol, and phospholipids are repackaged by gut mucosa and enter the lymphatics as chylomicrons, which enter the superior vena cava through the thoracic duct. In the systemic circulation, chylomicrons release fatty acids for use by liver, muscle, fat, and other cells (3, 11).

High serum insulin levels affect lipid metabolism in several ways. Insulin stimulates synthesis of lipoprotein lipases, which are secreted onto capillary membranes. These lipases extract fatty acids from triglyceride-rich circulating lipoproteins and facilitate entry of fatty acids into various tissues. In the fed state, a large proportion of these fatty acids is extracted by adipose tissue and is incorporated into triglyceride storage. Liver cells exposed to generous amounts of insulin extract fatty acids from chylomicrons and repackage them as very-low-density lipoprotein (VLDL) particles, which are secreted into the systemic circulation. VLDLs also deliver fatty acids to adipose tissue for deposition (3, 11).

Fasting State

When levels of nutrients in the blood are decreased, after 12 hours or longer without food intake, the individual is said to be in the postabsorptive, or fasting, state. This phase commences as nutrients cease to move from the intestines to the liver, accompanied by a gradual decrease in serum insulin concentrations and an increase in serum glucagon levels. When the insulin-to-glucagon ratio decreases, the liver switches enzyme machinery from glucose use to glucose production through gluconeogenesis and glycogenolysis. After 12 hours of fasting, half the liver glycogen is depleted. During longer starvation, hepatic glycolytic rates and activities of key glycolytic enzymes decrease over 48 to 96 hours and then stabilize, whereas hepatic gluconeogenesis rates and key gluconeogenic enzyme activity increase. After 72 hours of fasting, the liver has low glycolytic rates and has retooled for maximal gluconeogenesis (11).

The brain, other nervous tissues, red blood cells, and renal medulla have ongoing requirements for glucose for energy, whereas other tissues begin using fatty acids and ketones for energy. Low serum insulin levels permit lipolysis in adipose tissue; fatty acids are released at rates required for energy by various tissues. Lipolysis is further stimulated by high serum concentrations of glucagon and catecholamines. The liver burns fatty acids to meet energy needs and to fuel gluconeogenesis. Ketones are hepatic byproducts of fatty acid oxidation. Glucogenic amino acids released by muscles and other tissues are major substrates for active gluconeogenesis. When glycogen reserves of the liver and muscle are exhausted, most tissues are dependent on fatty acids and ketones to meet their energy needs (11).

High levels of free fatty acids decrease the number of insulin receptors on various tissues and act in other ways to block insulin action. Because of low serum insulin and high serum free fatty acids, glucose and other amino acids are not transported into muscle cells. Protein synthesis stops, and proteolysis is activated with amino acids released into circulation. Glucocorticoids also foster release of amino acids to support gluconeogenesis in the liver (11).

During a short-term fast, serum insulin and glucagon orchestrate changes in fuel homeostasis resulting in a steady supply of glucose to the brain and other glucose-dependent tissues while mobilizing free fatty acids to meet the energy needs of other tissues. After a 7- to 10-day fast, the brain develops the capacity to use ketones for fuel and the need to convert amino acids to glucose abates, allowing adjustment to long-term fasting with sparing of skeletal and visceral proteins (11).

METABOLIC DERANGEMENTS

Diabetes resembles fasting, especially regarding the responses of the liver, muscle cells, and adipose tissues. With low serum ratios of insulin to glucagon and high levels of fatty acids, the liver produces glucose, whereas other tissues use fatty acids and ketones instead of glucose. Muscle cells and adipose tissue respond by using ketones and fatty acids. Although these resemblances between fasting and diabetes are striking, pathologically low serum insulin levels disrupt the efficiency seen during fasting (11).

With low insulin levels, key glycolytic enzyme activities decrease. Glucose use decreases to levels far below those seen during fasting. Concurrently, hepatic gluconeogenic enzyme activities and gluconeogenic rates increase. Bombarded with free fatty acids, the liver increases gluconeogenesis, secreting large amounts of VLDLs and accumulating fatty acids in droplet form. A long-term toxic effect of diabetes is the accumulation of 25% more lipid than normal. In the diabetic state, the liver oxidizes these fatty acids and produces acetone, acetoacetate, and β-hydroxybutyrate (11).

Muscle cells and adipose tissue also show major metabolic changes in diabetes. Muscle glycogen almost disappears, and muscle protein is broken down to support gluconeogenesis. Cardiac and skeletal muscles meet their energy needs from ketones and fatty acids. Fat cells actively release fatty acids under the lipolytic stimuli of glucagon, catecholamines, and insulin deficiency (11).

Non–insulin-dependent tissues respond to diabetes totally differently. Hexokinase, the key stimulus of glucose use, is increased in jejunal mucosa, the renal cortex, and the peripheral nerves of diabetic animals. In hyperglycemia, glucose use increases and sugars accumulate. Excess glucose accumulation leads to tissue damage. Diabetic rats have 30% more total body glycogen than nondiabetic rats. Glycogen accumulates in renal tubules to values 50 times higher than in nondiabetic rats. Glycogen accumulation may contribute to tubular dysfunction and susceptibility to damage from x-ray dyes. Unimpeded entry of glucose into many tissues increases cellular glucose, producing linkage of glucose to tissue proteins (glycosylation). The diabetic state damages non–insulin-dependent tissues, including glomeruli, retinal vessels, nerves, and circulating blood cells (11).

DIABETIC COMPLICATIONS

Acute Problems

Diabetes can first become manifest with either symptomatic hyperglycemia or a medical emergency caused by severe hyperglycemia, ketoacidosis, or severe hyperlipidemia. Most symptoms of diabetes are related to hyperglycemia or accumulation of glucose in various tissues. As hyperglycemia develops, people have increased polyuria, thirst, lack of energy, irritability, blurred vision, and weight loss. Adults usually develop these symptoms over weeks to months, whereas children may develop them in hours or days. If hyperglycemia goes undetected or if stress or illness intervenes, the person will develop stupor or coma.

The most frequent complication for diabetic persons who are treated with insulin is hypoglycemia. Levels of blood glucose below normal are characteristic of this complication. Insulin administration may cause a decreased blood glucose concentration, which necessitates the replenishment of circulating glucose. Otherwise, the functioning of the brain will be permanently altered. Hypoglycemia may be triggered by missed or late meals, consumption of food in insufficient quantities, consumption of alcohol without food, or physical work. Some symptoms of hypoglycemia are confusion, headaches, deficient coordination, irritability, shakiness, anger, sweating, and even coma or death. Patients should be taught to check the blood glucose level to confirm the presence of hypoglycemia for appropriate treatment. Desired treatment for hypoglycemia for adults is 10 to 20 g of carbohydrates administered to raise the blood glucose level to between about 50 and 100 mg/dL.

Persons with type 1 diabetes are vulnerable to diabetic ketoacidosis (DKA) characterized by hyperglycemia and ketonemia, which results either from insulin deficiency or from stress. Both a hyperglycemic nonketotic state and ketoacidosis can be fatal. Vigorous therapy includes insulin, fluids, and electrolytes. DKA is most frequently caused by the lack of patient education or by the patient's inadequate compliance with instructions. Symptoms of DKA include nausea and confusion. Therapy for DKA includes administration of electrolytes, fluids, and insulin because untreated DKA can result in a coma or death (11).

In adults with type 2 diabetes, the hyperglycemic nonketotic state, characterized by plasma glucose values exceeding 750 mg/dL without significant ketonemia, is likely to develop. These patients may be protected from ketoacidosis by circulating insulin in spite of low-normal or low levels. The hyperglycemic nonketotic condition can be precipitated by excessive sugar intake, dehydration, heat exposure, illness, or drug therapy. Impaired renal function, hyperosmolarity, lack of ketosis, and/or problems with the central nervous system may occur as part of this

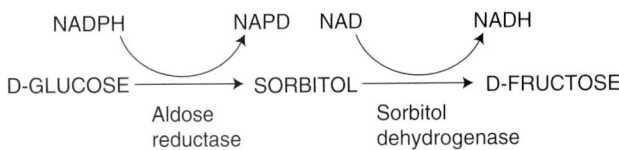

Figure 65.1. Polyol pathway. NAD, nicotinamide adenine dinucleotide (NADH, reduced form); NAPD, nicotinamide adenine dinucleotide phosphate (NADPH, reduced form).

condition. Usually, the hyperglycemic nonketotic state is seen in persons with type 2 diabetes. In addition, these people have decreased, but not completely deficient, insulin levels released from the pancreas. The hyperglycemic nonketotic state is often caused by dehydration or by diabetes associated with a coexisting illness. Symptoms of this condition include dehydration, hypotension, decreased mental ability, confusion, seizures, and coma. Therapy for the hyperglycemic nonketotic state includes insulin therapy and electrolyte and fluid replacement, as well as treating the basic causes (11).

Severe hypertriglyceridemia can be a serious medical emergency. Serum triglycerides exceed 2000 mg/dL and may be accompanied by neurologic symptoms, skin lesions, or abdominal symptoms from pancreatitis. Treatment includes intravenous fluids or a clear liquid diet to lower serum triglycerides, insulin to control hyperglycemia, and appropriate therapy for other medical problems (11).

Short-Term Complications

Sustained hyperglycemia alters glucose metabolism in virtually every tissue. Non–insulin-dependent cells are particularly vulnerable because sugar alcohols (polyols) accumulate and proteins are glycosylated. Most tissues gradually convert glucose to polyols, which are used slowly. Hyperglycemia causes high intracellular glucose, leading to rapid formation of polyols (Fig. 65.1), which accumulate rapidly but are degraded slowly. Sorbitol and fructose, the major polyols, accumulate and cause cell distention and toxicity. Blurred vision, for example, is caused by distention of the lens. Polyol accumulation can alter the function of peripheral nerves (3).

Excess glucose affects production of glycoproteins, proteins containing sugar side chains (Fig. 65.2). The condensation reaction between glucose and an amino acid component of protein has two stages: (a) the aldehyde group of glucose links to the amino group of an amino acid forming an aldimine (Schiff base), and (b) the unstable aldimine releases glucose or undergoes an Amadori rearrangement to form

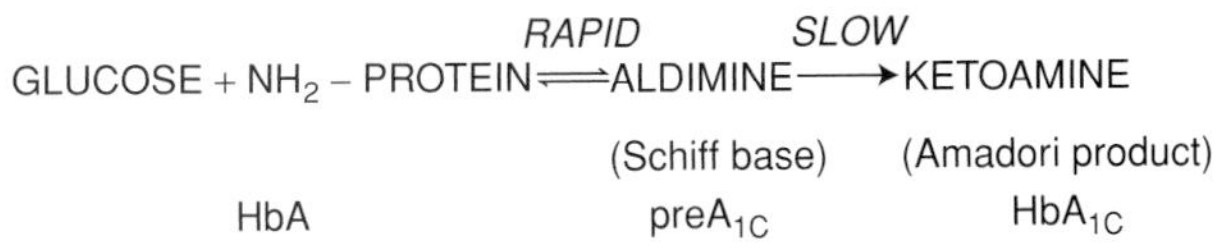

$$\text{GLUCOSE} + \text{NH}_2 - \text{PROTEIN} \underset{\text{}}{\overset{\textit{RAPID}}{\rightleftharpoons}} \text{ALDIMINE} \overset{\textit{SLOW}}{\longrightarrow} \text{KETOAMINE}$$

	(Schiff base)	(Amadori product)
HbA	preA$_{1C}$	HbA$_{1C}$

Figure 65.2. Pathway for nonenzymatic glycosylation. HbA, hemoglobin A.

the stable ketoamine linkage. This process, occurring spontaneously without enzyme action, is termed nonenzymatic glycosylation. Hemoglobin, serum albumin, and many other proteins are glycosylated. In diabetes, glycosylation is related to the magnitude and duration of hyperglycemia (3).

The sugar content of hemoglobin, the best-characterized glycoprotein, is normally less than 6%. In diabetes, the percentage of glycosylated hemoglobin can exceed 25% of total hemoglobin. When erythrocytes are incubated with glucose, the hemoglobin A$_{1c}$ level doubles within hours. Most glucose is attached by the unstable aldimine linkage, which can be dissociated if erythrocytes are incubated in low-glucose solutions. Long-term exposure to high glucose levels causes the formation of irreversible ketoamine linkages that persist until the cell is degraded. Thus, hemoglobin A$_{1c}$ measurements reflect glycemic control over the previous 6 to 8 weeks. In patients with excellent glycemic control, hemoglobin A$_{1c}$ concentrations are normal. Poor diabetic control yields hemoglobin A$_{1c}$ values exceeding 9%. The degree of glycosylation of circulating proteins, hormones, lipoproteins, plasma membranes of cells, basement membranes, and other proteins in diabetes has not been determined. This may contribute to basement membrane thickening, vascular permeability, microcirculation defects, and functional abnormalities of erythrocytes, leukocytes, and platelets (3).

Hyperglycemia induces a host of other metabolic derangements. Glycogen accumulates in non–insulin-dependent tissues. Increased flux of glucose through insulin-insensitive pathways such as mucopolysaccharide synthesis leads to abnormalities of mucopolysaccharides, possibly contributing to atherosclerosis. Hyperglycemia alters the orderly formation of glycoproteins in the kidney and other tissues, contributing to diabetic glomerulosclerosis. Many short-term problems of hyperglycemia can be avoided by maintaining satisfactory plasma glucose concentrations, and in some cases, derangements can be reversed by good glycemic control (3).

Long-Term Complications

The pathogenesis of the long-term manifestations of diabetes is still under intense study and remains poorly understood. Metabolic, genetic, and other factors affect major diabetic complications: retinopathy, nephropathy, and neuropathy. Chronic hyperglycemia accelerates the development of these complications. Long-term complications cannot be prevented, but risks can be lowered with good diabetic control. The Diabetes Control and Complication Trial was a landmark study in type 1 diabetes documenting that improved control decreases the development of diabetic retinopathy, nephropathy, and neuropathy (30).

Pirart (31) carefully documented the prevalence of diabetic complications among 4,400 diabetic patients. After 25 years, most patients had complications of some type; however, complications were less frequent in patients who maintained fairly good glycemic control than in those who had maintained poor diabetic control. Individual genetic tendencies toward complications also affect their frequency. Some diabetic patients develop complications at an accelerated rate despite reasonable glycemic control, whereas others show little tendency toward these complications.

The Diabetes Control and Complication Trial was a carefully controlled clinical study conducted by the National Institute of Digestive and Kidney Disease in the United States. The study shows that keeping the blood glucose levels as close to normal as possible slows the onset and progression of eye, kidney, and nerve diseases caused by diabetes. Over a 7-year period, the study compared the effects of a standard treatment regimen with an intensive treatment regimen. The study showed that lowering blood glucose concentrations reduced the risk for diabetic retinopathy by 76%, reduced the risk for diabetic nephropathy by 50%, and reduced the risk for diabetic neuropathy by 60% (30).

Atherosclerosis

Atherosclerosis is the most common complication of diabetes. Diabetic men have a twofold to threefold higher risk of coronary heart disease, stroke, and peripheral vascular disease, whereas diabetic women have a threefold to four-fold higher risk than matched nondiabetic people. Mechanisms responsible for accelerated atherosclerosis are not understood, and many interacting factors contribute. Reducing the risk of vascular disease requires improved glycemic control, avoidance of cigarette smoking, normal blood pressure, and desirable serum lipoprotein levels. Hypertension is the major risk factor for coronary heart disease in type 1 diabetes. Diabetic patients, particularly women, develop hypertension more frequently than the general population. Hypertension-related factors may act synergistically with arterial wall abnormalities, cellular dysfunction, lipoprotein abnormalities, and platelet derangements to accelerate atherosclerosis (32).

Lipoprotein abnormalities play a major role in atherosclerosis. Serum low-density lipoprotein (LDL) abnormalities, decreased serum high-density lipoproteins (HDL), and increased serum triglycerides contribute to accelerated atherosclerosis in diabetes. LDL may be glycosylated or altered in other ways to enhance atherogenicity in diabetes. Many lipoprotein alterations in diabetes increase the risk of atherosclerosis (32).

In addition to hypertension and lipoprotein derangements, diabetic persons have an increased prevalence of other cardiovascular risk factors: elevated serum insulin, elevated fibrinogen and von Willebrand factor, platelet function abnormalities, glycosylation of proteins throughout the body, leukocyte abnormalities contributing to vascular endothelial dysfunction and coagulation, macrophage dysfunction leading to foam cell formation, and increased susceptibility to oxidation of LDL and HDL dysfunction.

The nutrition plan focuses on reducing the risk of atherosclerosis by promoting desirable weight maintenance, reducing saturated/trans fat intake, achieving optimal serum lipoprotein levels, and reducing other cardiovascular risk factors (33, 34).

GOALS OF MEDICAL NUTRITION THERAPY

Medical nutrition therapy is pivotal in the management and care of diabetes patients. Goals for nutrition management for persons with diabetes are listed in Table 65.6. These are modified from those of the American Diabetes Association (ADA) (35) to emphasize the important role of weight management in obese persons with type 2 diabetes (9). Specific guidelines are specific to the diabetic individual, whereas general guidelines apply to all people. The first and preeminent goal is achieving and maintaining near-normal blood glucose levels by balancing food intake with insulin (either endogenous or exogenous) or antidiabetes agents. Optimizing glucose use, normalizing glucose production, and enhancing insulin sensitivity will also regulate safe levels of fatty acids, ketones, and amino acids. Immoderate hyperglycemia, as well as ensuing hypoglycemia, is hazardous and should be minimized by diet. Of equal or greater importance for the obese diabetic person is attaining and maintaining a desirable body weight (8). Important for all diabetic persons is achieving and maintaining optimal serum lipid levels.

Nutrition measures to retard development of atherosclerosis include maintaining desirable body weight; sustaining a diet high in dietary fiber, soy protein, antioxidants, and water-soluble vitamins; and having a diet low in fat, saturated fat, and cholesterol (8, 36, 33). Regardless of the type of diabetes present, utmost consideration must be given to individual preferences, cultural or social mores, and ability to understand and follow the prescribed diet.

General goals give consideration to the provision of variety, balance, and moderation. *Dietary Guidelines for Americans* (37) and the *Food Guide Pyramid* (38) summarize and illustrate nutritional guidelines and nutrient needs for all healthy Americans and can be used by people with diabetes and their family members (35). Optimal

---

TABLE 65.6. GOALS FOR NUTRITION THERAPY OF DIABETES

Specific
   Achieve physiologic blood glucose levels
   Attain and maintain desirable body weight
   Maintain desirable plasma lipid levels
   Reduce likelihood of specific diabetic complications
   Retard development of atherosclerosis
General
   Consume a health-promoting selection of nutrients
   Maintain energy needs in a timely manner
   Address special requirements (e.g., pregnancy)
   Tailor for therapeutic needs (e.g., renal disease)

selection of nutrients is addressed through food-value exchanges, allowing individual preferences to reign yet including foods from each of the food groups. Energy needs are met through the distribution of meals throughout the day with allowances for snacks when indicated. Meal distribution and close monitoring of blood glucose levels prevent hyperglycemic or hypoglycemic episodes of undue frequency. Eliminating excessive calorie and fat intake is indicated for attainment and maintenance of desirable body weights for adults, especially in persons with NIDDM. However, provision of adequate calories is crucial for normal growth and development rates in children and adolescents, increased metabolic needs during pregnancy and lactation, and recovery from catabolic illnesses. Medical nutrition therapy aims at the reduction and prevention of complications of diabetes during short-term illnesses and exercise-related problems, and of long-term complications such as renal disease, hypertension, and atherosclerotic cardiovascular disease. Special tailoring is needed for existing complications such as renal failure (39).

NUTRITIONAL PLAN

Across the international community there is surprising agreement on the nutrition recommendations for persons with diabetes (9). To develop recommendations for this chapter, all of these recommendations were considered. The strongest scientific support for recommendations comes from a quantitative assessment of the clinical trial evidence. Thus the recommendations presented in Table 65.7 represent the carbohydrate, protein, fat, and fiber data and weight management guidelines emerging from these analyses. These analyses and the international community

TABLE 65.7. NUTRITION RECOMMENDATIONS FOR PERSONS WITH DIABETES (9)

CATEGORY	RECOMMENDATION
Weight management	Attain and maintain desirable body weight (body mass index ≤25)
Carbohydrate (% of energy)	55–65%
Polysaccharides	Emphasize whole grains, legumes, vegetables
Monosaccharides and disaccharides	Use in moderation
Glycemic index	Incorporate into exchanges and teaching material
Fiber, total	25–50 g/d (15–25 g/1,000 kcal)
Protein (% of energy)	12–16%
Total fat (% of energy)	<30%
Saturated fatty acids/trans fatty acids (% of energy)	<10%
Monounsaturated fatty acids	12–15%
Polyunsaturated fatty acids	<10%
Cholesterol (mg/d)	<200 mg/d

From Anderson JW, Randles KM, Kendall CWC et al. J Am Coll Nutr 2004;23:5–17, with permission.

recommend achieving a desirable body weight and increased dietary fiber intake (9). In contrast, the ADA recommends modest weight loss and fiber intake as recommended for the general population (40).

Carbohydrates

Carbohydrate should provide 55 to 65% of energy intake (9). Greater amounts, up to 70%, are tolerated in research studies and by highly committed persons but are not generally recommended for most persons with diabetes. Simple carbohydrates, although not as severely restricted in the past, should make up less than one third of total carbohydrate intake. Unrefined carbohydrates, with natural fiber intact, have distinct advantages over highly refined versions because of their other benefits, such as a lower glycemic index, greater satiety, and cholesterol-lowering properties.

Amount

About 1980, the American and the British Diabetes Associations finally relinquished the antiquated strategy of carbohydrate-restricted diets for persons with diabetes, aiming instead for a diet restricted in fat but higher in complex carbohydrate and dietary fiber (12). This action was followed by the introduction of similar recommendations in many other countries (9). The enthusiasm for high-carbohydrate, high-fiber diets has waned somewhat, but these diets still have the strongest scientific basis for recommendation (9). Under certain circumstances, especially with low fiber intakes, high-carbohydrate, low-fat diets can worsen blood glucose control, increase serum triglyceride concentrations, and lower HDL cholesterol concentrations. The fiber content of the diet seems critical in preventing these problems (41). The popularity of the "Mediterranean diet" has led some to recommend lower carbohydrate and higher monounsaturated (MUS) fat intakes to favorably alter serum lipid concentrations and reduce risk for oxidation of LDL. However, only a few controlled studies support this recommendation, and the effect of higher fat intakes on obesity in type 2 diabetes is a major concern (9).

Glycemic Response

Carbohydrates in foods have traditionally been classified as either simple (sugars) or complex (starches). Simple carbohydrates, monosaccharides, and disaccharides from commonly used foods raise blood glucose concentrations more than many complex carbohydrates that are rich in fiber. The glycemic response to 50 g glucose is much greater than the response to a variety of foods providing 50 g starch. Our analysis of recommendations from nine expert diabetes panels and the evidence-based analysis lead us to recommend that added sugars (such as the high-fructose corn syrup widely used as a sweetener) should be used in moderation or should not exceed 40 g/day (9).

Complex carbohydrates, polysaccharides in different forms, also evoke different glycemic responses. Bread and potatoes raise blood glucose levels much more than beans and pasta (42). Jenkins and colleagues introduced the term glycemic index to describe these responses comparing test foods to the glycemic response from a reference food such as bread or glucose (43). Many factors influence the glycemic response to foods. Sipping 50 g glucose slowly over a several-hour period produces a much smaller increase in blood glucose than rapid intake of the same amount. Eating three apples takes 15 minutes, whereas their juice can be consumed in 1.5 minutes. Differences in fiber content and ingestion time influence the resultant glycemic response. Fat, protein, water-soluble fiber, and other factors influence gastric emptying time. Food form makes a major impact on digestion time; bread can be digested more rapidly than pasta. Methods of processing and cooking foods, and in the case of fruit, degree of ripeness, influence the glycemic response. Foods with higher ratios of the amylopectin to the amylose form of starch are digested more rapidly than those with low ratios (11).

Fiber is only one of many components of food that influence the glycemic response. Beans have lower glycemic indices than any other group of carbohydrate-rich foods. The low glycemic response to beans is probably related to their high soluble fiber content, food form (usually eaten as cooked rather than in bakery products), and naturally occurring starch blockers (inhibitors of digestive enzymes responsible for hydrolysis of starch). Finally, fiber fermentation products such as short-chain fatty acids are absorbed from the colon into the portal vein; in the liver they may directly affect glucose metabolism (44).

Low-glycemic-index (GI) foods are healthy choices for persons with diabetes or dyslipidemia. Metaanalyses of eight randomized, controlled clinical trials document that lower-GI diets compared with higher-GI diets significantly decrease fasting plasma glucose and hemoglobin A_{1c} or fructosamine values in diabetic persons. The high-GI diets also decreased serum LDL cholesterol and triglycerides while increasing HDL cholesterol values (9). Because of the substantial evidence (9) that lower-GI foods offer many advantages over higher-GI foods, we recommend that GI information be incorporated into exchanges and teaching material. The GIs of selected starchy foods are presented in Table 65.8.

Proteins

The adult recommended daily allowances of 0.8 g/kg body weight of protein provides for metabolic and nutritional needs. Although current ADA recommendations allow 15 to 20% energy intake as protein (45), we recommend a more conservative 12 to 16% of total energy needs as protein (9). Persons with diabetes, on average, consume more protein than nondiabetic persons (46), and excessive protein intake has been linked to diabetic nephropathy

TABLE 65.8. GLYCEMIC INDEX RANKING OF SELECTED STARCHY FOODS

HIGHER: GI >90[a]	INTERMEDIATE: GI 70–90	LOWER: GI <70
Most dry cereals	Oat bran	All bran cereals
Most breads	Whole-wheat bread	Oatmeal, muesli, pumpernickel bread
Most crackers	Most muffins	Most pasta
White rice, boiled	Long-grain rice	Barley
Most cakes	Most cookies	
Most potatoes	New potatoes	Yams
Pancakes and waffles	Sweet corn	Most dry beans and lentils

GI, glycemic index.
[a] Using bread as 100 for reference (124).

Data from Anderson JW. Nutritional management of diabetes mellitus. In: Shils ME, Olson JA, Shike M et al., eds. Modern Nutrition in Health and Disease. 9th ed. Baltimore: Williams & Wilkins, 1999:1365–94; and Foster-Powell K, Holt SHA, Brand-Miller JC. Am J Clin Nutr 2002;76:5–56.

(39, 47). According to current guidelines, in the presence of diabetic nephropathy, protein should not exceed 0.8 g/kg or approximately 10% of total calories (45).

At present, there is insufficient evidence supporting a protein allowance higher or lower than that for the general population. High-biologic-value protein should be given consideration, although protein should be included from both animal and vegetable sources. With the onset of nephropathy, protein intake should be no greater than the recommended daily allowance of 0.8 g/kg. Ten percent of daily calories should be sufficiently restrictive and is recommended for persons with evidence of nephropathy (48). Higher amounts (more than 12%) are likely in diets with greater emphasis on vegetable sources of protein, particularly the cereals and legumes, which are recommended for diabetes from other considerations. Further work is required to establish whether a higher protein intake is acceptable from the renal point of view if it comes mainly from vegetable sources (39).

Soy Protein

Soy protein offers many advantages related to cardiovascular health, weight management, insulin sensitivity, and bone health (49, 39). Current research indicates that soy protein diets reduce hyperfiltration and albuminuria in persons with diabetes, and substituting soy protein for animal protein should be considered as a preventive measure for diabetic persons (50, 51, 52). Soy protein acts to lower serum total and LDL cholesterol and triglyceride values while increasing HDL cholesterol values (53). Soy protein–containing meal replacements seem to facilitate more rapid weight loss than meal replacements with casein and decrease visceral adipose tissue more than casein (54, 55). Soy protein intake also increases insulin sensitivity in type 2 diabetes (56). Because of these documented and potential health benefits for diabetic persons, we recommend that our clients with diabetes consume 10 g soy protein twice daily.

Fats

Amount

Fat intake generally should not exceed 30% of energy. Most importantly, the sum of saturated and trans fatty acids, because of their atherogenic potential, should be held at a maximum of 10% of energy needs. Polyunsaturated fats, with their tendency to lower HDL cholesterol values and their susceptibility to oxidation, should also be held under 10%. However, up to 35% of energy from fat can be used for nonobese persons with acceptable serum triglyceride values if the additional fat comes from MUS sources such as olive, or less recommended, canola oil. Cholesterol intake, although less influential than saturated fats on serum lipid values, should be less than 200 mg/day. These recommendations are consistent with those of the American Heart Association and other groups (33, 9).

Dr. Elliott P. Joslin, in 1928, stated that "with an excess of fat diabetes begins and from an excess of fat diabetics die" (57). The weight of scientific evidence still supports this prescient observation. Excessive fat intake contributes to obesity, insulin resistance, hypertension, and atherosclerotic cardiovascular disease. Maintenance of serum lipids is one of the most important goals in diabetes management. Hyperlipidemia, common in persons with type 2 diabetes, is a major risk factor for cardiovascular disease. Epidemiologic evidence indicates that high-fat diets contribute to atherosclerosis. Intake of high-fat diets cause insulin resistance and impaired intracellular glucose metabolism. High-fat diets decrease the number of insulin receptors in several tissues, decreasing glucose transport into muscle and adipose tissue and decreasing activities of insulin-stimulated processes. Glycogen synthesis rates, glycogen accumulation, and glucose oxidation are also lower with high-fat diets (9).

Type

Monounsaturated Fats. The role of MUS fats in the diabetic diet has been critically examined over the past 15 years (58). In individualizing the diet to the person with diabetes, MUS fats can be substituted for carbohydrates, allowing the sum of carbohydrates and MUS fats to provide 60 to 70% of energy intake (45). Garg (58) performed a meta-analysis of clinical trials in which MUS-fat diets, providing 22 to 33% of energy from MUS fats, were compared with higher-carbohydrate diets, providing 49 to 60% of energy from carbohydrates. The fiber content of the diets was not provided in this review but was in the moderate range of about 25 g/day (59). The high-MUS-fat diets were associated with significantly lower serum triglycerides and higher HDL cholesterol values than the high-carbohydrate diets. In this analysis, plasma glucose values tended to be lower on the high-MUS-fat diet than the high-carbohydrate diet. These short-term studies with median durations of 2 weeks were not designed to assess body weight changes, and no differences were noted in body weight (58). These studies indicate that MUS fats can be substituted for carbohydrate in the diet without adverse effects on serum lipids or glycemic control. The long-term effect of increasing the percentage of energy intake from fats on body weight is unknown.

ω-3 Fatty Acids. Certain essential fatty acids of the ω-3 class lower serum cholesterol moderately and serum triglyceride levels markedly (60). These ω-3 fatty acids, popularly known as fish oils, may also decrease platelet aggregation, which may potentially reduce the cardiovascular disease risk in diabetes. Twice weekly intake of fish decreases risk for coronary heart disease in nondiabetic persons and, presumably, in diabetic persons as well (61). Intake of less than or equal to 3 g fish oil daily significantly lowers serum triglyceride values without affecting glucose metabolism (62). When type 2 diabetic subjects use either 4 g/day eicosapentaenoic acid (EPA) or 4 g/day decosahexanoic acid (DHA), serum glucose values may increase and serum triglyceride values decrease significantly (63). Because most fish oil preparations provide only 200 mg DHA and 300 mg EPA per gram intake of 3 g/day fish oil, providing only 600 mg of DHA and 900 mg of EPA seems unlikely to significantly impair glucose homeostasis.

Fat Substitutes. Olestra, a sucrose polyester, is a recent fat substitute approved by the US Food and Drug Administration (FDA). Although the release of this food ingredient has generated considerable attention, the general experience indicates that it is well tolerated by most consumers; gastrointestinal side effects probably will limit overuse by persons who do not tolerate it well. Olestra is a nondigestible fat made from sucrose bonded with eight long-chain fatty acids into a molecule too large to be hydrolyzed in the small intestine. It currently is available in potato chips and similar snack foods. Incorporating Olestra into the diets of overweight persons is associated with weight loss (64). Another product, Simplesse, is made from the protein of egg whites and milk. Manufactured by a microparticulation process, it imparts a creamy smooth sensation much like that of fat. Because this product is a protein, it contains only 1.5 kcal/g instead of 9 kcal/g in actual fats. Oattrim is another product produced from oat bran. Clinical tests indicate that this product is useful in decreasing glycemic responses and in lowering serum cholesterol concentrations in nondiabetic subjects. Controlled studies using these fat substitutes in the diabetic diet are needed to establish their potential usefulness. If results are positive, fat substitutes may foster improved dietary fat compliance in the diabetic population (35).

Fiber

Dietary fiber has emerged as a major dietary component in the management of diabetes. It has therapeutic value and may reduce the prevalence of diabetes (44). In 1960, Trowell reported diabetes to be rare among African hospital patients (65). Walker then postulated that increased cereal fiber intake might prevent the development of diabetes (66). Walker and colleagues documented that healthy Bantu school children in South Africa had lower glycemic responses than urban children, and these differences were related to dietary fiber intake (67). Trowell speculated that prolonged intake of fiber-depleted starch promoted the development of diabetes and formulated the dietary fiber hypothesis of the etiology of diabetes (68). The therapeutic value of fiber in diabetes emerged in 1976 when the Oxford group (69) reported that fiber supplements reduced postprandial glycemic responses, and we (70) reported that high-fiber diets decreased the insulin requirements of lean persons with diabetes. Many others confirmed that either fiber-supplemented diets or high-fiber diets benefited diabetic persons (9, 44). The detrimental effects of high fat intakes on blood glucose and lipid values and the beneficial effects of a high-carbohydrate, high-fiber, low-fat diet are well documented (71). As illustrated in Table 65.9, high-carbohydrate, high-fiber diets have a significant and favorable effect on all aspects of glucose metabolism and on most serum lipoprotein levels.

Current recommendations from international diabetes bodies are that diabetic persons consume 25 to 35 g/day (9). Recently the US National Academy of Sciences Institute of Medicine made the following recommendations for daily fiber intake: men 50 years old or less, 38 g; more than 50 years old, 30 g; women 50 years old or less, 25 g; more than 50 years old, 21 g (72). Because of the specific benefits of increased fiber intake for persons with diabetes (9, 44), we recommend intake of approximately 35 g/day or 15 to 25 g/1000 kcal. This level of fiber intake can easily be achieved using high-carbohydrate, high-fiber exchanges (Table 65.10) or ADA exchanges (Table 65.11), with an emphasis on higher-fiber choices such as whole-grain breads, high-fiber cereals, generous intakes of fruits and vegetables, and regular use of legumes. Because of the specific benefits of soluble fiber on postprandial hyperglycemia as well as serum cholesterol and LDL cholesterol values, generous amounts of soluble fiber from oats, beans, fruits, and vegetables are recommended (73).

TABLE 65.9. META-ANALYSIS DATA FOR HIGH-FIBER DIETS[a]

PARAMETER	NUMBER OF SUBJECTS	WEIGHTED AVERAGE PERCENT CHANGE
Fasting plasma glucose	141	−14.3*
Postprandial plasma glucose	47	−13.6*
Average daily plasma glucose	37	−12.5*
Hemoglobin A$_{1c}$	79	−6.0*
Total serum cholesterol	146	−19.3*
LDL cholesterol	71	−16.4*
HDL cholesterol	91	−6.3
Fasting serum triglycerides	119	−12.8*

HCHF, high-carbohydrate, high-fiber; HDL, high-density lipoprotein; LDL, low-density lipoprotein; MCLF, moderate-carbohydrate, low-fiber.
[a]Comparison of changes in 12 clinical trials comparing HCHF diets with MCLF diets. Changes are those for HCHF diets minus MCLF diets. All values except HDL cholesterol were significantly lower with HCHF diets than with MCLF diets. Measurements available from 12 trials for fasting plasma glucose but only three trials for postprandial and average plasma glucose values. The number of subjects is listed.
Data from Anderson JW, Randles KM, Kendall CWC et al. J Am Coll Nutr 2004;23:5–17.
* Significantly different from MCLF diets

Sweeteners

Traditionally, persons with diabetes have been advised to curtail the intake of foods that aggravate hyperglycemia, increase serum triglyceride concentrations, and foster additional weight gain. Often, these same foods contain excessive amounts of fat and calories contributing to poor metabolic control. Much of the focus has been on the limitation of refined sweets and processed foods. Recently, the ADA and others have eased their restrictions on the use of sweets in the diet (9). However, this should not be construed as a recommendation to increase the amount of sweets consumed in the total diet. It merely illustrates that various foods may be included as they fit into a well-balanced meal plan. It is still wise to limit the consumption of sugar in patients with diabetes to that recommended for the general population. It is worth pointing out that this represents a major change in eating habits for many people. Up to 25 g of added sucrose may be allowed, provided that it is part of a diet low in fat and high in fiber and that it substitutes for an isocaloric amount of fat or high-GI

TABLE 65.10. HIGH-CARBOHYDRATE, HIGH-FIBER EXCHANGE LIST

FOOD GROUP	ENERGY (kcal)	CARBOHYDRATE (g)	PROTEIN (g)	FAT (g)	FIBER (g)
Starches	70	15	2	—	2
Cereals	90	20	3	—	4
Proteins	50	—	8	2	—
Beans	95	17	7	—	5
Vegetables	25	5	1	—	2
Fruits	60	15	—	—	2.5
Skim milk	85	12	8	—	—
Fats	45	—	—	5	—

TABLE 65.11. AMERICAN DIABETES ASSOCIATION EXCHANGE LISTS[a]

FOOD GROUP	ENERGY (kcal)	CARBOHYDRATE (g)	PROTEIN (g)	FAT (g)
Starch/bread	80	15	3	Trace
Meat and substitutes				
Lean	55	—	7	3
Medium-fat	75	—	7	5
High-fat	100	—	7	8
Vegetables	25	5	2	—
Fruit	60	15	—	—
Milk				
Skim	90	12	8	Trace
Low-fat	120	12	8	5
Whole	150	12	8	8
Fat	45	—	—	5

[a] Multiplying the grams of carbohydrate and protein by 4 in the starch/bread and skim milk lists will not yield the total number of calories given for these two lists. These exchanges contain less than 1 g of fat per serving, and the term trace is used to make teaching easier. Dietitians may wish to use 1 g of fat in their calculations to achieve the total caloric value for the exchange group.

food or other nutritive sweeteners. There would be no strong reason to recommend fructose in preference to sucrose within this limit (11).

There are two basic categories of sweeteners: nutritive (calorie-containing) and nonnutritive (noncaloric). Nutritive sweeteners, such as fructose found in fruits, and common sugar alcohols, the polyols, in modest amounts are acceptable in the diabetic meal plan. Fructose as a natural component of foods is sweeter than other sugars and is metabolized without the use of insulin, thus producing less hyperglycemia. Although fructose may increase an already-high blood glucose level in persons with poorly controlled diabetes, its effect is minimal in those with adequate diabetes control. When substituting fructose for sucrose or glucose it lowers the average blood glucose levels, producing a glycemic response of only 20 and 33%, respectively. When we incorporated 50 to 60 g fructose per day in a prudent diet for 14 diabetic men for a 24-week period, no adverse effects were noted in plasma glucose, hemoglobin A_{1c}, cholesterol, triglycerides, lactate, or uric acid concentrations. Inclusion of fruits containing fructose in accordance with the Dietary Guidelines for Americans, two to four servings per day according to calorie and activity level, should provide balance and variety in the diabetic person's diet (11).

The polyols (sorbitol, mannitol, xylitol, lactitol, and maltitol) are formed by the partial hydrolysis and hydrogenation of edible starches. Polyols also produce a lower glycemic response than do sucrose and other carbohydrates. There seem to be no significant advantages of the polyols over other nutritive sweeteners. Excessive amounts of polyols may, however, have a laxative effect (74).

Alternative sweeteners, noncaloric, are an acceptable means of decreasing excessive amounts of refined sugars in the diet. Although adequately safe, to avoid excesses of any one type, using a variety of different sweeteners is recommended for persons who elect to use them. Each sweetener has its distinctive tastes, advantages, and risks.

Saccharin, aspartame, acesulfame-K, and sucralose are approved for use by the FDA. The FDA also determines an acceptable daily intake for approved additives, including nonnutritive sweeteners. Nonnutritive sweeteners approved by the FDA are safe to consume by all people with diabetes. Saccharin, one of the first artificial sweeteners, is a petroleum derivative with potential associations of bladder cancer when ingested in excessive quantities. Although the typical diet certainly would not exceed a moderate amount, it is recommended that pregnant women avoid saccharin and that children not exceed two cans of saccharin-sweetened soft drinks daily. Aspartame is a dipeptide containing aspartic acid and phenylalanine. Aspartame is present in a large variety of foods and is contraindicated only for those persons with phenylketonuria. Its use is limited to foods that do not rely on heat exposure in processing or baking. Acesulfame potassium, a derivative of acetoacetic acid, is approved for broad product applications. Sucralose tastes like sugar because it is made from sucrose. Like the other sweeteners, sucralose does not affect the blood glucose level. Intake of artificial sweeteners should be limited to established safe levels. Practical resources are available to assist in counseling patients with diabetes in regard to sweeteners (74).

Diabetic Foods

So-called "diabetic" specialty foods are not recommended for people with diabetes or for anyone else. No evidence indicates that the foods or drinks offer any advantage to people with diabetes when compared with conventional products. They often contain large amounts of sorbitol or fructose and similar energy to the conventional equivalent. The term diabetic when attached to a food for promotional purposes has been interpreted by patients and relatives as meaning freely available and even therapeutically beneficial. The main arguments for use of these products relate to risks of dental caries and of becoming overweight. Reduced-sugar products labeled diabetic are usually more expensive; ordinary reduced-sugar products should be used. There also is a risk of hypoglycemia if reduced-sugar foods are taken inadvertently by insulin-treated patients (11).

Alcohol

A moderate intake of alcohol is associated with a decrease in the incidence of diabetes (75). Furthermore, the incidence of coronary heart disease is lower in diabetic persons who drink moderate amounts of alcohol compared with nondrinkers (75). Because of its potential hypoglycemic effects, heavy alcohol use is not recommended in the diabetic population. However, if it is included in the diet, it should be limited to no more than two drinks per day for men and no more than one drink per day for women. One drink would consist of a 1.5-oz shot of distilled spirits (i.e., whiskey, scotch, vodka, gin, rum), a 4-oz glass of wine, or a 12-oz beer. Alcohol does not require insulin to be metabolized; it is directly absorbed from the stomach, duodenum, and jejunum. The liver is the site of alcohol metabolism and oxidation. Excessive alcohol enters the general circulation, exerting its effects on the central nervous system.

In diabetic persons, alcohol induces fasting hypoglycemia by inhibition of gluconeogenesis. If consumed, it should be ingested with a meal. Alcohol may provoke hypertriglyceridemia. Impaired judgment from alcohol intake may disrupt otherwise stable eating patterns and insulin dosage. Alcoholic beverages provide 7 kcal/g, similar to fat, and are metabolized similarly. This may result in excessive energy intake without corresponding nutritive value. For insulin-dependent diabetes, the caloric value should be counted in the meal plan. In the non–insulin-dependent diabetic diet, alcohol is best substituted as a fat exchange (one alcoholic beverage = two fat exchanges). Additional calories from mixers must be included. Inquiry regarding the use of alcohol should be part of a thorough assessment of a diabetic patient. People may not be aware of the effects of alcohol and should be provided with at least the following guidelines: (a) potential or current intake should be discussed with the physician and nutrition counselor, (b) alcohol should be consumed slowly and with food to lessen hypoglycemic episodes, (c) identification should be worn indicating diabetic diagnosis because the symptoms of insulin reaction are similar to those of intoxication, (d) drinking to the extent of impaired judgment and operating a motor vehicle should be avoided, (e) persons with poorly controlled diabetes should abstain from alcohol use, and (f) pregnant women, whether diabetic or not, should not consume alcohol (11, 45).

Micronutrients

Nutrition supplements are widely used by nondiabetic and diabetic persons (76). Minerals commonly mentioned in relationship to diabetes are chromium, magnesium, and vanadium (45). Chromium deficiency has been related hypothetically to the development of diabetes in humans for many years, but persuasive studies in Western people are not available (77). The use of herbs and dietary supplements for prevention and treatment of diabetes has attracted interest for centuries. Yeh and colleagues (78) performed a systematic literature review and analysis of clinical trial results for 36 herbs and nine vitamin/mineral supplements involving more than 4500 subjects. They concluded that there is insufficient evidence to draw definitive conclusions about individual herbs and supplements for use in diabetes, but they seem to be safe. Chromium was the most widely studied supplement, and four of eight studies showed favorable outcomes, whereas the remaining four failed to show significantly positive outcomes. The best evidence available for efficacy of herbal products was for American ginseng and *Coccinia indica* (ivy gourd). Vanadium, nopal, and several herbs have preliminary support. In my practice, for inquiring persons with strong risk factors for diabetes or impaired fasting glucose values, I recommend daily intake of chromium 200 μg, vanadium 20 to 100 μg, and vitamin E 400 mg. For persons with diabetes, I recommend an inexpensive multivitamin to minimize serum homocysteine levels and 1000 to 1500 mg calcium (79, 80).

SPECIAL NUTRITIONAL CONSIDERATIONS

Children

Type 1 Diabetes

Diabetic children have unique needs. It is important to address their fears and their level of understanding and to assess the family support. Each stage of childhood requires revision of the diabetic management plan. Both child and parent should participate in the learning process. As therapy progresses, children should be allowed to assume increased responsibility for their management goals. Restoring the sense of wellness, of "feeling good," is the primary goal. Eliminating the hallmark signs of diabetes such as polydipsia, polyuria, and polyphagia; preventing ketoacidosis, hypoglycemia, and hyperglycemia are specific preliminary objectives to be covered with the child and caregiver. Adequate growth should be monitored and can be documented and plotted on standardized charts appropriate for the child's age and gender several times yearly, especially during the initial learning phase. An individualized plan including adequate nutrition with consideration for preferences and eating habits and normal-for-age levels of physical activity are the cornerstones of a child's diabetes management.

A generous carbohydrate and fiber intake coupled with limited fat intake provides the same advantages for children as for adults with diabetes (9). During periods of rapid growth or increased energy requirements, more carbohydrates may be added. Consistent levels of food intake are more important than carbohydrate distribution for the insulin-dependent diabetic child. Three meals each providing approximately 20 to 25% (65% total) of energy needs with an additional three snacks using the remaining 35% of energy needs is appropriate. The dietitian may develop a meal plan based on the child's food preferences and daily schedule, then insulin doses are tailored to achieve good glycemic control.

Simple guidelines should be provided regarding the appropriate glycemic range and increasing snack intake for increased physical activities. Self-monitoring of blood glucose is extremely important in preventing hypoglycemic or hyperglycemic episodes experienced with physical activity, changes in meal intake, and sedentary or sick days. By trial and error the child and caregiver will learn which variables require adjustment or closer monitoring. Autonomy and acceptance are tools necessary in the development of a healthy well-adjusted adult without physical or psychosocial limitations. Periodic nutritional reassessment is needed to adjust requirements for growth and physical activity. Changes in insulin dosage and meal planning should evolve as the child matures (40).

Type 2 Diabetes

Newly recognized, type 2 diabetes in children and adolescents is increasing at an alarming rate (5, 81). This seems largely related to the fourfold increase in obesity among American children in the past 3 decades. If diabetes is recognized in the asymptomatic individual, lifestyle changes directed at weight loss is the initial therapy. If the child has symptomatic hyperglycemia, oral agent therapy should be considered. Although no oral agents have been approved by the FDA for use in children, metformin is often used for initial pharmacotherapy. Effective medical nutrition management of the adolescent with diabetes requires that the primary care provider and dietitian forge a partnership with the patient and the parent. Usually the goal is for the adolescent to assume major responsibilities for lifestyle activities, with the parent serving in an empowering role.

Elderly Persons

Diabetes is a major chronic problem for a growing elderly population. The prevalence of diabetes, diagnosed and undiagnosed, is approximately 19% for Americans older than age 60, with another 15% having impaired fasting glucose (16). Diabetic persons older than age 65 have a relative risk of mortality that is approximately 1.5-fold higher than that of nondiabetic persons. Factors that contribute to glucose intolerance and development of diabetes in the elderly population include decreased physical activity, intake of less complex carbohydrate and of a higher percentage of energy from fat, and increased adiposity with decreased lean body mass. Other illnesses or medications may contribute to the development of diabetes in the elderly population.

Because elderly persons have multiple defects including impaired insulin secretion, decreased action of insulin to suppress hepatic glucose output, and peripheral insulin resistance, treatment should first focus on increasing sensitivity to insulin through nutrition and physical activity. Considerations for oral agent use include age, body mass index (BMI), and renal function. When oral agents lose effectiveness, a daily dose of long-acting insulin is usually added. Goals for blood glucose control are tailored to each individual's circumstances.

Eating a nutritious diet providing adequate energy from a variety of foods is extremely important. Fat intake should be less than 30% of energy, with limits in saturated fat and cholesterol. The generous carbohydrate intake can include simple and complex carbohydrates rich in dietary fiber. Fruits, juices, and sweeteners usually do not need to be limited if fat guidelines are followed. Usually a multivitamin supplement and 1200 mg calcium daily should be recommended (40). The antidiabetes agent or insulin regimen usually can be adjusted to allow persons to follow meal plans that suit their preferences or circumstances. Special teaching skills and involvement of the patient are required to optimize learning for elderly persons with diabetes. Nutrition counselors need to use a positive attitude, patience, and praise to enable elderly persons to change lifelong dietary and exercise habits successfully.

Pregnancy

Pregnancy changes eating habits, exercise patterns, the emotional state, insulin sensitivity, and hormone secretions. These changes alter glucose control and insulin requirements. In the nondiabetic woman, as placental and ovarian hormones decrease insulin sensitivity, more insulin is secreted to maintain satisfactory glucose levels. However, approximately 5 to 10% of women lack the pancreatic reserve to meet this challenge and develop gestational diabetes. This condition usually abates after delivery, but these women are much more likely to develop diabetes during subsequent pregnancies or later in life, particularly if they are obese (15, 23). For all diabetic women, the reduction of maternal, fetal, and perinatal risks requires excellent glucose control during the preconception period (for women with diabetes or impaired fasting glucose) and throughout the pregnancy and postpartum period (82).

Insulin requirements change dramatically during pregnancy. To sustain a healthy fetus, the diabetic woman must adjust her nutrient intake and insulin dose to control glucose levels and avoid ketosis. During the first half of pregnancy, insulin requirements may decrease by 20 to 30% because of decreased food intake and increased glucose uptake by the fetus and placenta. During the second half of pregnancy, insulin requirements often increase by 60 to

100% above prepregnancy levels because of placental hormone production and insulin resistance related to other factors. After delivery and removal of the placenta, insulin requirements decrease precipitously; much smaller doses are required the week after delivery, but insulin requirements gradually increase to prepregnancy levels by 6 weeks after delivery. Proper adjustment of insulin therapy during pregnancy and the postpartum period requires careful blood glucose monitoring (82, 83).

Pregnant women have lower fasting glucose levels than nonpregnant women; normal fasting blood glucose is 55 to 65 mg/dL. This level normally peaks at 140 mg/dL 1 hour after a meal; the 24-hour average level is 80 to 85 mg/dL. To ensure the best possible outcome, normal glucose levels are the goal for diabetic pregnant women. Goals during pregnancy include meeting the nutrition needs of both mother and fetus while maintaining excellent blood glucose control. Specifically, these goals are to achieve glucose control before gestation and during the early weeks of pregnancy to reduce the risks of congenital malformations; to provide energy intake for appropriate weight gain (a range of 6.8–18.1 kg [15–40 lb], based on prepregnancy BMI) to meet increased protein needs; to provide carbohydrate to minimize ketosis, meeting the needs of the fetus and placenta; to optimize tissue sensitivity to insulin; and, during the critical 3 to 4 weeks before delivery, to maintain excellent glucose control to reduce neonatal risk and fetal macrosomia (82, 83).

Requirements for most nutrients increase with pregnancy and are similar for diabetic and nondiabetic women. Folic acid supplements, 400 μg/day, are recommended and the need for iron should be assessed. Protein requirements are met by providing a minimum of 0.75 g/kg body weight plus 10 g (40). In general the percentage energy from carbohydrate, protein, and fat during pregnancy can parallel that of the nonpregnant diabetic person. During the first trimester, most women should gain 0.9 to 1.8 kg (2–4 lb); this can be achieved by increasing energy intake by 419 kJ (100 kcal)/day. During the second and third trimesters, a gain of about 1 lb/week depending on prepregnancy BMI is the goal. This is achieved by increasing energy intake by 15%, or 1256 kJ (300 kcal)/day (40, 83).

Gestational Diabetes

The prevalence of GDM varies from 0.15 to 12.3% of pregnant women, depending on the location, ethnicity, and screening procedure (82). This makes it the most common medical disorder occurring during pregnancy. It seems to occur only rarely in women younger than 20 years of age. Although most of these women return to normal glucose tolerance after delivery, 40 to 60% of them may develop NIDDM in 15 to 20 years. Those who maintain a reasonable body weight and exercise on a regular basis have been shown to have a decreased incidence of developing NIDDM. From the twenty-fourth to the twenty-eighth week of pregnancy, the body's need for insulin increases dramatically. Risks for GDM include occurrence of GDM during an earlier pregnancy, delivery of a previous macrocosmic infant (>9 lb birth weight), a family history of diabetes, and maternal obesity (>120% of ideal body weight) (15, 23).

Renal Disease

Renal disease is a major complication that affects 30 to 50% of type 1 and more than 20% of persons with type 2 diabetes. Diabetic nephropathy is accompanied by proteinuria, decreased glomerular filtration rate, and hypertension. Development of microalbuminuria, urine protein of 40 to 300 mg per 24 hours, is the forerunner of overt nephropathy. Hypertension accelerates the development and progression of renal disease, whereas poor glycemic control and high protein intakes may contribute to the development and progression of nephropathy (84).

Protein restriction in management of chronic renal failure is discussed elsewhere. High protein intakes are proposed to lead to renal damage in diabetic persons by various mechanisms. Extensive protein feeding increases glomerular filtration rate, renal blood flow, single nephron glomerular filtration rate, and transcapillary hydraulic pressure in laboratory animals (85). Unlimited protein intake is inappropriate in patients with diabetic nephropathy. Protein restriction decreases the progression of chronic renal failure in nondiabetic persons and perhaps in diabetic nephropathy. At present, it seems prudent to restrict protein intake to 0.8 g/kg body weight/day for persons with established diabetic nephropathy with appropriate adjustments for proteinuria and careful clinical monitoring (40). Carbohydrate should provide at least 50% of energy intake, and saturated fat and cholesterol intake should be restricted. Recent research indicates that substitution of soy protein for animal protein may decrease the risk of developing diabetic nephropathy. Furthermore, substituting soy protein for animal protein may reduce proteinuria and slow progression of nephropathy. Further research is required to rigorously test this "soy protein for diabetic nephropathy" hypothesis (39).

Dyslipidemia

Most diabetic persons have lipoprotein abnormalities. There are multiple abnormalities of VLDL, LDL, and HDL composition, function, and metabolism (86, 80). Hypertriglyceridemia and low HDL cholesterol values are seen more commonly in diabetic than nondiabetic persons (80). Hypertriglyceridemia seems to confer a higher risk of atherosclerotic cardiovascular disease on diabetic than on nondiabetic persons. Low HDL cholesterol values are another major risk factor (87).

To minimize the risk of atherosclerotic cardiovascular disease, the following goals or desirable fasting values for diabetic persons are recommended: total cholesterol less than 170 mg/dL, LDL cholesterol less than 100 mg/dL, triglycerides less than 150 mg/dL, and HDL cholesterol for men greater than 45 mg/dL and for women greater than 55 mg/dL (33). Because abnormally low HDL cholesterol levels are difficult to increase by dietary or pharmacologic measures, reducing the LDL cholesterol to achieve ratios of LDL-to-HDL cholesterol of less than 2.2 for men and less than 1.8 for women is recommended.

The diabetes nutrition plan outlined in this chapter and elsewhere is the basic approach for most hyperlipidemic persons. Good glycemic control, attaining and maintaining a desirable body weight, regular exercise, and moderation in alcohol intake—practices recommended for all diabetic persons—reduce hyperlipidemia. The approach to hyperlipidemia can focus on management of elevated LDL cholesterol, elevated triglycerides, decreased HDL cholesterol, or combinations of these disorders.

Elevations of LDL cholesterol occur with the same frequency in diabetic as in nondiabetic persons; treatment is similar. A high-carbohydrate (50–65% of energy), high-fiber (25 g/1000 kcal), low-fat (~25% of energy with <8% saturated fat), low-cholesterol (<200 mg/day) diabetes diet is the first step. This diet should include generous amounts of soluble dietary fiber from oat and bean products. Including a soluble fiber intake of 4 to 6 g/day without other changes in the diet can decrease LDL cholesterol by approximately 7 to 10%. If these levels of soluble fiber cannot be achieved with foods, psyllium products or capsules can be included (73). The second step is daily inclusion of 10 g soy protein twice daily to achieve another LDL cholesterol reduction of 7 to 10% (53). The third step is inclusion of approximately 3 g plant stanols in the form of gel capsules (e.g., Benecol) to obtain an LDL cholesterol reduction of 10 to 15% (36). These dietary measures can reduce serum LDL cholesterol values by 25 to 30% (88). When desirable LDL cholesterol levels are not achieved with dietary interventions, hydroxymethyl-glutaryl coenzyme A reductase inhibitors (commonly called statins) are usually the pharmacologic agents of choice (89, 90).

Hypertriglyceridemia is more common in diabetic persons, especially in type 2 diabetes, than in nondiabetic persons and carries a greater risk of atherosclerosis. Almost all patients can be managed effectively with a high-fiber, high-carbohydrate diet if they lose weight and decrease their fat intake to a satisfactorily low level (41). Persistently elevated triglyceride levels usually are the result of excessive dietary fat intake; triglyceride levels plummet when patients are hospitalized and receive a low-fat diet. Sometimes excessive alcohol or simple sugar intake aggravates hypertriglyceridemia. Fibric acid derivatives and nicotinic acid are pharmacologic choices for a patient whose condition is not responding adequately to diet (89). Persons with type 2 diabetes commonly have decreased HDL cholesterol levels (91). Performing regular physical activity such as walking 2 to 3 miles daily and not smoking are important lifestyle practices for increasing HDL cholesterol. Dietary measures

for decreasing serum triglycerides and the regular use of oat and soy products may increase HDL cholesterol by 10 to 20%. HDL cholesterol usually decreases when intensive nutritional measures are used. However, most people cannot increase HDL cholesterol levels by more than 5 to 10 mg/dL by these lifestyle measures. Pharmacologic considerations include nicotinic acid, fibric acids (87), and statins (if the LDL cholesterol value is >100 mg/dL) (92).

WEIGHT MANAGEMENT

About 75% of persons with type 2 diabetes in the United States are obese. Weight gain and obesity seem to be major contributors to the development and maintenance of type 2 diabetes in 60 to 90% of persons. Achieving and maintaining a desirable body weight through diet and exercise is the treatment of choice. Antidiabetes drugs and insulin are important adjunctive measures, but they cannot be substituted for exercise and a diet appropriate in energy, fat, complex carbohydrate, and fiber (8).

Weight-Loss Approaches

The health care team sets the stage for effective weight loss by being empathetic and supportive while continuing to emphasize the detrimental effects of overeating on diabetes and health. However, the obese individual must make a commitment to losing weight before nutrition counseling will be effective. Our team offers a variety of weight-loss programs, as outlined in Table 65.12. These interventions support the fact that achieving and maintaining a desirable body weight (BMI <25) is task one for management of the overweight or obese individual with diabetes (8).

All persons with diabetes should be counseled by a dietitian or nutritionist about a diabetes diet; overweight and obese persons should have specific counseling related to lifestyle changes. Irrespective of the nutrition intervention, increased physical activity is important for preserving health and for weight loss and maintenance. Everyone can increase their physical activity, and counselors should work with the individual on finding ways to achieve this goal. For example, water aerobics is appropriate for older persons with arthritis. Additionally, setting goals for fruit and vegetable intake should be done for all persons. These foods are rich in nutrients and phytochemicals that enhance insulin sensitivity, lower blood pressure, improve vascular reactivity, decrease oxidative stress, and assist in weight loss and maintenance. Low-intensity nutrition counseling provides the stimulus for a small percentage of persons to lose weight, especially men and those with newly diagnosed diabetes. We counsel our diabetic clients to avoid the popular low-carbohydrate, high-fat diets because of their potential thrombotic and atherogenic effects (93).

Recommending meal replacement (MR) use is one of the most cost-effective approaches for facilitating weight

TABLE 65.12. NUTRITION APPROACHES TO OVERWEIGHT AND OBESITY IN DIABETES: EXPECTED WEIGHT LOSSES OF DIABETIC PERSONS AFTER 6 MONTHS WITH DIFFERENT INTERVENTIONS[a]

CATEGORY	BMI[b]	TREATMENT CONSIDERATIONS	EXPECTED WEIGHT LOSS (%)[c]	REFERENCES
Overweight	25–29.9	a. RD counsel about lifestyle changes	3–5	(95, 96)
		b. Recommend 2 MR[d] per day	6–9	(55, 95)
		c. Refer to community program	6	(98)
Class 1 obesity	30–34.9	a. RD counsel about lifestyle changes	3–5	(95, 96)
		b. Recommend 2 MR[d] per day	6–9	(55, 95)
		c. Refer to intensive LED program	14–17–21	(8, 9)[d]
		d. Consider pharmacotherapy	6–10	(55, 96)
Class 2 obesity	35–39.9	a. Refer to intensive LED program	14–17–21	(8, 9)[d]
		b. Consider pharmacotherapy	6–10	(55, 96)
		c. Consider pharmacotherapy	6–10	(55, 96)
Class 3 obesity	≥40	a. Refer to intensive LED program	14–17–21	(8, 9)[d]
		b. Consider pharmacotherapy	6–10	(55, 96)
		c. Refer for bariatric surgery	25	(106)

BMI, body mass index; LED, low-energy diet; MR, meal replacement; RD, registered dietitian.
[a] Estimates are based on recent literature and unpublished experience (Anderson JW).
[b] BMI is calculated as kg/m^2.
[c] Weight loss expressed as a percentage of initial body weight.
[d] MR-meal replacements
[e] Unpublished weight loss data for diabetic subjects; the intervention is similar to the recent report using medically supervised LEDs and weekly behavioral sessions (101).

loss for nondiabetic and diabetic persons (55, 94, 95). MRs are inexpensive, easy to use, widely available, and available in many forms. In our practice we usually recommend cans of liquid meal replacements such as SlimFast (96). For most persons, we recommend use of one MR at breakfast with or without fresh fruit and one MR for lunch with salad, vegetables, and possibly fruit. Community programs are popular and can be effective for overweight or modestly obese persons (97, 98). Responses of diabetic persons to self-help programs such as Weight Watchers have not been documented.

The most effective intervention program for modestly to moderately obese persons is a medically supervised, intensive behavioral program using weekly education sessions. Most of these programs use shakes and prepackaged entrees as MR and may include fruits and vegetables (55, 99, 100, 101). Currently, diabetic persons who enroll in our program (Health Management Resources) are losing an average of 48 pounds (17.4% of initial body weight) in an average of 19 weeks. These weight losses are slightly less than the 56 pounds (20.8%) lost in an average of 24 weeks by nondiabetic persons treated concurrently in the same manner (Anderson JW, unpublished observations).

Pharmacotherapy is a modest to moderate adjunct to lifestyle intervention for diabetic and nondiabetic obese persons (96, 102, 103). Because all diabetic persons who are older than age 40 have a high risk for coronary heart disease (33, 34), use of agents that increase heart rate and blood pressure should be done cautiously. Orlistat is a safe and modestly effective agent for diabetic persons (103), and sibutramine has moderate effectiveness in diabetes but blood pressure must be monitored (104). Bupropion SR, although not approved for use in obesity, may also have efficacy in diabetes (96).

Recent approaches using laparoscopic or minimally invasive approaches have significantly decreased the risk for bariatric surgery for morbidly obese diabetic and nondiabetic persons. Currently, the roux-en-Y gastric bypass procedures are the most effective approaches for facilitating weight loss and maintenance (105). Diabetic persons show dramatic improvements or remissions in their diabetic conditions (106). Although intensive low-energy diets are the safest treatment for moderately and severely obese persons, bariatric surgery is another option. With diabetes as a comorbidity, diabetic persons with moderate obesity (BMI, 35–40) may be considered for bariatric surgery if intensive low-energy diets are not effective.

Weight Maintenance

Weight loss is not the cure for obesity. This chronic condition requires a long-term maintenance program and access to lifelong counseling about lifestyle changes important in weight maintenance. After nonsurgical weight-loss programs, long-term weight maintenance, as a percentage of initial weight loss, is reported to be about 36% at 2 years and about 5% at 5 years (107). Most obese persons who complete community weight-loss programs, behavioral modification programs, and very-low-calorie programs regain all the weight they lost within 2 to 5 years. Newer very-low-energy diet programs that stress physical activity, use the best available behavioral techniques, and facilitate achievement of desirable body weights are obtaining better long-term weight maintenance. Obese persons completing our HMR Weight Management Program at the University of Kentucky are maintaining about 63% of their initial weight loss at 2 years after completing the weight-loss phase. Recent data indicate that graduates of the University of Kentucky program are maintaining about 20% of their weight loss at 7 years; approximately 25% are maintaining a loss of at least 10% of their initial weight (i.e., maintaining more than 10 kg of weight loss) (100). Several recent studies document that the more weight that persons lose initially, the more weight loss they maintain long term (107). The best predictors of good weight maintenance are low fat intakes and good levels of physical activity, such as walking 20 miles/week (108). Much further development is required to enable formerly obese people to maintain desirable weights for long periods (99).

PHYSICAL ACTIVITY

Routine physical activity is health-promoting for all people. Exercise is important for weight management, enhanced physical and psychologic fitness, better work capacity, improved body composition, and increased HDL cholesterol values. Exercise offers even greater benefits for persons with type 1 or 2 diabetes. Regular physical activity has these favorable effects for diabetic persons: sense of well-being, weight control, improved blood lipoprotein values, lower blood pressure, decreased insulin requirements, and a lower risk for atherosclerotic cardiovascular disease (109). Physical activity provides both short- and long-term benefits to the diabetic patient. However, persons with diabetes are at greater risk of suffering complications from exercise, so several precautions must be taken. For most people, after assessment for potential risks related to exercise, an effective program can be established.

Many of the benefits of exercise relate to the glucose and insulin effects. Acutely, physical activity increases glucose uptake by muscles about 15-fold above resting levels; increased insulin sensitivity is maintained for 24 to 72 hours after exercising (109). Maintaining the exercise regimen sustains this enhanced insulin sensitivity on a long-term basis (110). Moderate-intensity activity combined with dietary changes that decrease body weight seem to have the greatest long-term advantages. Aerobic training may improve endothelial function of vessels to reduce the risk of cerebrovascular disease (111). Anaerobic exercise and aerobic exercise both have benefits. However, a combination of these modes may have the greatest effects on insulin sensitivity (112). Physical activity also produces its beneficial effects by reducing hemoglobin A_{1c} by about 10 to 20% (113). Exercise and lower body weight must be sustained to maintain these benefits.

Because highly intense exercise may have some negative consequences for this population, moderately intense exercise is usually recommended (114). Specifically, exercise that produces a target heart rate of 60 to 80% of the maximum heart rate is often recommended. Aerobic exercise that uses large muscles throughout the whole body is preferred. Walking 6000 to 10,000 steps per day may be one of the best modes of exercise. Light jogging, aerobics classes, biking, and swimming are also good examples. Low-load resistance exercise can be used in addition.

Several recommendations are important to follow to prevent exercise-induced complications. Hypoglycemia is one of the most common risks. These tips are helpful for preventing hypoglycemia: check blood glucose levels before and after exercising, consume 15 to 30 g carbohydrate every 30 minutes of exercise, warm up and cool down properly, decrease premeal insulin by 20 to 50% and decrease long-acting insulin, avoid injecting short-acting insulin in an extremity that will be vigorously exercised, consume snacks after exercise, and wear an identification bracelet. Before beginning an exercise program, diabetic persons should be evaluated for coronary heart disease, peripheral neuropathy, and foot problems. Diabetic retinopathy should be treated and stabilized before recommending a moderate exercise program. Patients with neuropathy may require a podiatry examination and use of special shoes or orthotic devices (109). For most persons with diabetes, regular physical activity should be included in the treatment plan because the potential disadvantages are far outweighed by the health and well-being benefits.

NUTRITION AND PHARMACOTHERAPY

Insulin Therapy

Although insulin replacement therapy has been used for more than 80 years, the physiologic replacement of insulin for diabetic persons remains an elusive goal. In lean, non-diabetic adults, insulin is secreted into the portal system in the basal state at a rate of approximately 0.75 U/hour. After the intake of food, the increase in blood glucose and gastrointestinal hormones triggers a five- to tenfold increase in insulin secretion rates. Basal plus food-related insulin secretion totals approximately 40 U/day for lean, nondiabetic adults. Although various human insulins are available, this physiologic response cannot be mimicked.

Both diet and exercise have major effects on insulin sensitivity in type 1 and type 2 diabetic persons (Fig. 65.3). High-carbohydrate, high-fiber diets increase insulin

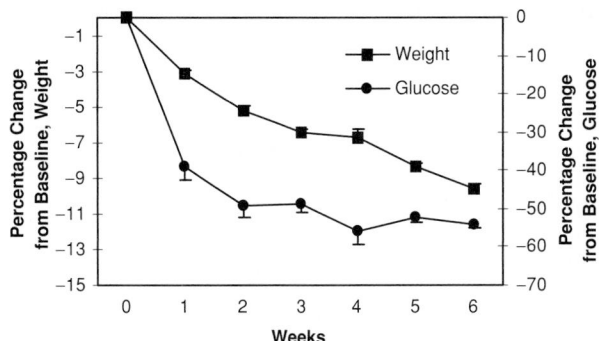

Figure 65.3. Reduction in insulin doses and blood glucose values with weight reduction for obese type 2 diabetic subjects on very-low-energy diets. Values are expressed as percentage of baseline values. Baseline fasting plasma glucose values were 252 mg/dL. Mean values are from ten studies including 152 subjects. (Modified from Anderson JW, Kendall CWC, Jenkins DJA. J Am Coll Nutr 2003;22:331–9, with permission.)

sensitivity and decrease insulin requirements, whereas high-fat diets have opposite effects (9). In one case, a slender 38-year-old farmer required 57 U/day insulin for good glycemic control on a conventional high-fat (37% of energy), low-carbohydrate (43% of energy), low-fiber diet in 1974. After 16 years of good adherence to a high-carbohydrate (~60% of energy), high-fiber (~45 g/day), low-fat (<25% of energy) diet, he takes 36 U/day insulin to maintain fairly good control as an outpatient. Regular physical activity seems to act in a similar manner by increasing skeletal muscle sensitivity to insulin. In another case, when a family practice physician trains for marathons by running more than 60 miles/week, he requires only 20 U/day of insulin, but when not in training he requires about 50 U/day.

These two case studies indicate that algorithms based on body weight are limited in their accuracy. The farmer had a 37% reduction in insulin dose related to diet without change in body weight or physical activity. The physician required 250% the insulin dose while in his busy practice than when in training for marathons without significant changes in body weight. Likewise, algorithms for premeal insulin doses used for carbohydrate counting are better based on total insulin dose of the individual than on body weight. For example, if someone takes 50 U/day insulin, about 40% or 20 U is related to basal insulin needs and should be provided as longer-acting insulins. The remaining 30 U are assigned to short-acting insulins before meals and snacks. If the person consumes 2400 kcal/day and 300 g carbohydrate, one can make an estimate that the carbohydrate to insulin ratio is 10:1 and initiate carbohydrate counting and premeal insulin on this basis. Properties of some insulin preparations are compared in Table 65.13.

Oral Antidiabetes Drug Therapy

Since 1995, numerous new antidiabetes agents have allowed the tailoring of therapy to the presumed pathologic

TABLE 65.13. USUAL TIMING OF INSULIN ACTION

TYPE	ONSET	PEAK	USUAL EFFECTIVE DURATION
Long-acting			
Glargine (Lantus)	1.1 h	No peak	24 h
Human Ultralente	6–10 h	10–16 h	18–20 h
Intermediate-acting			
Human NPH	2–4 h	4–10 h	10–16 h
Human Lente	3–4 h	4–12 h	12–18 h
Fast-acting			
Human regular	0.5–1 h	2–3 h	3–6 h
Ultrafast-acting			
Lispro (Humalog)	<15 min	0.5–1.5 h	2–4 h
Aspart (Novolog)	5–10 min	1–3 h	3–5 h
Mixtures of shorter-acting and longer-acting 70/30, 75/25, 50/50	Varies	Varies	Varies

TABLE 65.14. OVERVIEW OF ANTIDIABETES AGENTS COMMONLY USED IN THE UNITED STATES

CLASS	DRUG	DAILY DOSE, mg	DURATION OF ACTION
Sulfonylureas	Glyburide	2.5–20	12–24 h
	Glipizide	2.5–40	12–24 h
	Glipizide XL[a]	2.5–20	24 h
	Glimepiride	1–8	16–24 h
Secretagoges[b]	Nateglinide	180–360	4–6 h
	Rapliginide	0.5–16	4–6 h
Biguanide	Metformin	250–2,550	~4 wk
Thiazolidinediones	Rosiglitazone	2–8	~4 wk
	Piaglitizone	15–45	~4 wk
α-Glucosidase inhibitors	Acarbose	150–300	~4 h
	Miglitol	75–300	~4 h

[a]XL, extended-release preparation.
[b]Nonsulfonylurea insulin secretagoges.

Data from DeFronzo RA. Ann Intern Med 1999;131:281–303; and package inserts.

defects in type 2 diabetes. Four organs play major roles in the pathophysiology of type 2 diabetes: pancreas, with decreased insulin secretion; muscle, with decreased insulin sensitivity; liver, with unchecked glucose production; and gut, with more rapid absorption of glucose. The major classes of agents are listed in Table 65.14. The sulfonylurea agents act mainly to enhance glucose-stimulated insulin release but also to enhance insulin sensitivity. The nonsulfonylurea secretagogs act predominantly on the pancreatic β cells to stimulate postprandial insulin release. Metformin inhibits hepatic gluconeogenesis and acts to enhance the sensitivity of liver and peripheral tissues to insulin. The α-glucosidase inhibitors competitively inhibit the enzymes involved in hydrolysis of oligosaccharides and disaccharides in the small intestine, and thus slow the absorption of glucose. The thiazolidinediones act to enhance insulin sensitivity of liver, muscle, and other tissues. The thiazolidinediones bind to perioxime proliferators-activated receptor γ and have a variety of effects in different tissues. The oral agents are adjunctive to diet in the management of type 2 diabetes, and unfortunately most of these agents—except the α-glucosidase inhibitors and metformin—may be associated with weight gain (115).

Diet and exercise retain central importance in the management of type 2 diabetes. Our experience indicates that approximately three fourths of patients with type 2 diabetes treated with insulin, sulfonylureas, or the combination can be managed with diet and exercise alone. Whether insulin or sulfonylureas are used or not, overeating is the major cause of hyperglycemia in type 2 diabetes; a mildly energy-restricted diet generous in complex carbohydrate and fiber and restricted in fat almost universally improves glycemic control as it facilitates weight loss (8).

The insulin secretagogs and α-glucosidase inhibitors are given before meals and usually do not produce hypoglycemia. If postprandial hypoglycemia results, the doses should be reduced. The sulfonylureas can produce hypoglycemia, and sometimes the timing of doses needs to be altered to reduce hypoglycemic episodes. When people start diets that are moderately restricted in energy, the doses of these three classes of agents are usually reduced or the agent is discontinued (116). Metformin has a weight-neutral effect, and doses do not need to be altered when the individual initiates a weight-loss program. Rapid weight gain is sometimes seen after initiating thiazolidinediones, and this possibility should be explored in persons who report unexplained weight gains of 20 to 50 pounds.

NUTRITIONAL ASSESSMENT AND EDUCATION

A thorough nutritional assessment of the diabetic individual involves evaluating these and other elements: age; type of diabetes; medical history of problems such as hypertension, dyslipidemia, and renal disease; current medications such as Coumadin; social history of environment and resources; behavioral assessment for capacity and willingness to change lifestyle habits; BMI, waist circumference and desirable body weight; presence of physical handicaps; serum lipid profile; and current diabetes medical treatment regimen. Current eating habits should be assessed by a diet history or food records. The nutrition management plan is developed based on this and other information shared at the nutrition counseling sessions.

Every person with diabetes should receive training about the general management of their diabetes and specific nutrition education and counseling. The social and cultural importance of eating behavior has often been neglected, and the degree of difficulty involved in making permanent changes to entrenched eating habits is still greatly underestimated. Many diabetic persons consider diet to be the most traumatic aspect of their treatment. Adherence to diabetes diets has been notoriously poor, and full goals are probably attained by rather few patients. All people should, with guidance, be able to make significant improvements in their nutrition practices, but few will be willing or able to achieve the full goals, and certainly not overnight. Finding the right balance at which nutritional goals are desirable, beneficial, and attainable is critical. The dietary goals should continue to be presented consistently by all members of the diabetes care team. It is important to identify the types of situations that make nutritional adherence difficult for a particular person. This involves the following:

1. Effectively communicate to health care team members that nutrition intervention is an important component of intensive therapy. Many physicians and nurses are not certain that nutritional counseling is cost-effective for optimizing glycemic control.
2. Individualize the diet to include lifestyle and food preferences and expand counseling beyond nutritional requirements. Social and environmental influences greatly affect choices; the individual patient needs to

have options for addressing these situations. "Ideal" meal plans that are generic for all patients often are never implemented.
3. Persons with type 1 diabetes especially should be taught how to estimate portion sizes; patients adjusting insulin doses to match intake need be able to identify portions and/or grams of carbohydrate.
4. During the initial stages of intervention, food records are an important aid in adjusting medication and food intake.
5. For persons implementing intensive therapy, remind them that although they may "cover" any food with insulin, there are considerable risks for weight gain if this causes increased caloric consumption (8).

INSTRUCTION IN MEAL PLANS

General Guidelines

Although use of food exchange lists have a long tradition in medical nutrition therapy of diabetes, many additional approaches are now widely used (117). Simplified systems of nutrition education should be considered for certain persons. Instead of using formal exchange lists, general nutrition recommendations may be made. Guidelines for optimal food choices are available (118). The US Department of Agriculture Food Guide Pyramid or Dietary Guidelines for Americans (37) and booklets or pamphlets are suitable for some patients (117). Some persons prefer specific menu plans.

Carbohydrate Counting

Carbohydrate counting is an effective method for allowing diabetic persons to obtain needed nutrition while attaining the desired blood glucose values. This approach focuses on carbohydrate intake because carbohydrates have the most significant effect on blood glucose levels (117). Persons with an insulin pump, with multiple daily injections of insulin, or who desire more choices in food selection are good candidates for this method. There are several methods of carbohydrate counting. Each has advantages and disadvantages that should be considered for each individual. The individual needs to feel comfortable with the math involved and satisfied with the resulting blood glucose levels obtained. Carbohydrate counting can involve difficult or simple math. More complex math allows the patient greater freedom when choosing a food plan (119).

Food Exchanges

The ADA and American Dietetic Association Exchange Lists for Meal Planning (120) are still widely used for meal planning. We developed the High-Carbohydrate, High-Fiber Exchange Lists (121) to follow this pattern. See Tables 65.10 and 65.11. Exchange-based nutrition

TABLE 65.15. WORKSHEET FOR DEVELOPING 2000-kcal DIETS

EXCHANGE	SERVINGS	ENERGY (kcal)	CARBOHYDRATE (g)	PROTEIN (g)	FAT (g)
Starch/bread	8	640	120	24	Trace
Meat and substitutes	3	165	—	21	9
Vegetables	7	175	35	14	—
Fruit	7	420	10	—	—
Milk	2	180	24	16	Trace
Fat	10	450	—	—	50
Total	—	2,030	284	75	59
Target	—	2,000	290	75	60

plans provide flexibility and choice while maintaining consistency from day to day. Exchange groups include foods of similar nutrient composition; all serving sizes or portions in one exchange provide similar amounts of energy, carbohydrate, protein, and fat. Using an exchange diet, an individual chooses a certain number of items from each food group daily. Because each exchange group includes many different foods, the diet can be quite varied.

Step-by-Step Guide to an Exchange Diet

1. Estimate energy requirements. Numerous equations are available. We use this approximation at the bedside to estimate energy requirements. Middle-aged men require a daily intake of 11 to 13 kcal/lb plus about 500 kcal for every hour of active aerobic activity; middle-aged women require a daily intake of 10 to 12 kcal/lb plus about 400 kcal for every hour of active aerobic activity. For weight reduction, subtract 500 kcal/day for a weight loss of 1 lb/week.
2. Calculate the desired energy intake for each macronutrient based on caloric level. If one is following suggested guidelines, carbohydrate would be calculated at 50 to 65% of energy needs, protein at 12 to 16%, and fat at less than 30%. For example, with an intake of 2000 kcal/day the macronutrient breakdown might be as follows: carbohydrate, 57% = 1160 kcal; protein, 15% = 300 kcal; and fat, 27% = 540 kcal/day (see Table 65.15).
3. Convert kilocalories to grams by dividing by the appropriate conversion factors: protein and carbohydrate are each 4 kcal/g, fat is 9 kcal/g. Using the earlier example, the grams are as follows: carbohydrate, 290 g; protein, 75 g; and fat, 60 g.
4. Distribute the grams of carbohydrate, protein, and fat into exchange lists tailored to the eating pattern of the individual. Much greater compliance is ensured if the diet is based on cultural, ethnic, and personal eating habits. Begin by estimating servings of starch/bread, vegetables, fruit, and milk to meet the carbohydrate goal. Add the meat and meat substitutes required to meet the protein goal. Finally, add the fat exchanges. In tailoring personal exchange plans, vegetarian, nondairy, or other dietary preferences can be accommodated.
5. Assign exchanges to the meal/snack plan. We routinely develop meal plans to include three meals and an evening snack. For most persons taking insulin, midmorning and midafternoon snacks also are needed. Distribute energy intake according to these guidelines: The three main meals should provide at least 65% of energy intake, whereas snacks provide up to 35%. Breakfast has 20 to 30%, the noon meal 20 to 35%, and the evening meal 25 to 40% of energy intake. Snacks provide 0 to 15% each at midmorning, midafternoon, and evening. Insulin-treated persons should be taught methods of increasing their food intake in response to exercise or hypoglycemia.
6. Finally, calculate the fiber content of the diet. The exchange worksheet diet provides approximately 21 g fiber from starches/breads if one serving of whole grain cereal and beans are included, 14 g from vegetables, and 18 g from fruits, for a total of 51 g fiber or 25 g/1000 kcal (121).

CONCLUSION

An individualized nutrition plan is vital to the successful management of diabetes. The diabetic individual and the health care team integrate the nutrition plan into the daily schedule of activities to match the available insulin. The diet, physical activities, levels of stress, and available insulin (endogenous or exogenous) change daily. The diabetic individual needs information, education, motivation, and experience to respond to these changes. The health care team should provide education, encouragement, and coaching in an empathetic manner to help the diabetic individual integrate diet, exercise, and medication to achieve blood glucose goals from day to day. Both short-term and long-term considerations affect the nutrition plan. Feeling good and avoiding trouble, although desirable attributes, should not lull the diabetic individual or the health care team into accepting undesirable nutrition practices. Achieving good glycemic control, maintaining a desirable body weight, having optimal serum lipoprotein levels, and reducing risks for metabolic, microvascular, and atherosclerotic complications are the key goals of the diabetes nutrition plan.

Acknowledgment

The assistance of Katy Patterson is greatly appreciated.

REFERENCES

1. Mokdad AH, Ford ES, Bowman BA et al. JAMA 2003;289:76–9.
2. James PT, Leach R, Kalamara E et al. Obes Res 2001;9: 228S–33S.
3. Alberti KGMM, Zimmet P, DeFronzo RA et al. International Textbook of Diabetes. 2nd ed. New York: John Wiley & Sons, 1997:1–1827.
4. King H, Aubert RE, Herman WH. Diabetes Care 1998;21: 1414–31.
5. Pinhas-Hamiel O, Standifer D, Hamiel D et al. Arch Pediatr Adolesc Med 1999;153:1063–7.
6. Ogden CL, Flegal KM, Carroll MD et al. JAMA 2002;288: 1728–32.
7. American Diabetes Association. Diabetes Care 2003;26: 917–32.
8. Anderson JW, Kendall CWC, Jenkins DJA. J Am Coll Nutr 2003;22:331–9.
9. Anderson JW, Randles KM, Kendall CWC et al. J Am Coll Nutr 2004;23:5–17.
10. Gu K, Cowie CC, Harris MI. JAMA 1999;281:1291–7.
11. Anderson JW. Nutritional management of diabetes mellitus. In: Shils ME, Olson JA, Shike M et al., eds. Modern Nutrition in Health and Disease. 9th ed. Baltimore: Williams & Wilkins, 1999:1365–94.
12. Anderson JW. The role of dietary carbohydrate and fiber in the control of diabetes. In: Stollerman GH, ed. Advances in Internal Medicine. Chicago: Year Book, 1980:67–96.
13. Palmer JP, Hirsch IB. Diabetes Care 2003;26:536–8.
14. Scheuner MT, Raffel LJ, Rotter JL. Geentics of diabetes. In: Alberti KGMM, Zimmet P, DeFronzo RA et al., eds. International Textbook of Diabetes. 2nd ed. New York: John Wiley & Sons, 1997:37–88.
15. Kjos SJ, Buchanan TD. N Engl J Med 1999;341:1749–56.
16. Cowie CC, Rust KF, Byrd-Holt D et al. MMWR Morb Mortal Wkly Rep 2003;52:833–7.
17. Mokdad AH, Ford ES, Bowman BA et al. Diabetes Care 2001; 24:412.
18. American Diabetes Association. Diabetes Care 2004;27:S5–S10.
19. Karvonen MJ. Diabetes Metab Rev 1997;13:275–91.
20. American Diabetes Association. Diabetes 2001 Vital Statistics. Alexandria, VA: American Diabetes Association, 2001:1–134.
21. Hu FB, Manson JE, Stampfer MJ et al. NEngl J Med 2001;345: 790–7.
22. Barr RG, Nathan DM, Meigs JB et al. Ann Intern Med 2002; 137:263–72.
23. Kim C, Newton KM, Knopp RH. Diabetes Care 2002;25: 1862–8.
24. American Diabetes Association. Diabetes Metab 2004;27: S88–S90.
25. Drucker DJ. Diabetes Care 2003;26:2929–40.
26. Perfetti R, Merkel P. Eur J Endocrinol 2000;143:717–25.
27. Fineman MS, Koda JE, Shen LZ et al. Metabolism 2002;51: 636–41.
28. Woods SC. Am J Physiol Gastrointest Liver Physiol 2004;286: G7–G13.
29. Cummings DE, Weigle DS, Frayo RS et al. N Engl J Med 2002;346:1623–30.
30. The Diabetes Control and Complications Trial Research Group. N Engl J Med 1993;329:977–86.
31. Pirart J. Diabetes Metab 1977;3:97–107.
32. Bierman EL. Arterioscler Thromb Vasc 1992;12:647–56.
33. Krauss RM, Eckel RH, Howard BV et al. Circulation 2000; 102: 2296–311.
34. Grundy SM. Circulation 2002;105:2696–8.
35. American Diabetes Association. Diabetes Care 2002;25:202–12.
36. Anderson JW. JAMA 2003;290:531–3.
37. US Department of Agriculture and US Department of Health and Human Services. Publication no. 232. Washington, DC: US Department of Agriculture, 2000:1–215.
38. US Department of Agriculture. Home and Garden Bulletin 252. Washington, DC: US Department of Agriculture, 1992.
39. Jenkins DJA, Kendall CWC, Marchie A et al. Am J Clin Nutr 2003;78:610S–6S.
40. American Diabetes Association. Diabetes Care 2004;27:S36–S46.
41. Anderson JW. Curr Atheroscler Rep 2000;2:536–41.
42. Jenkins DJ, Kendall CW, Augustin LS et al. Am J Clin Nutr 2002;76:266S–73S.
43. Jenkins DJA, Wolever TMS, Taylor RH et al. Am J Clin Nutr 1981;34:362–6.
44. Anderson JW, Akanji AO, Randles KM. Treatment of diabetes with high fiber diets. In: Spiller GA, ed. Dietary Fiber in Human Nutrition. Boca Raton, FL: CRC Press, 2001:363–90.
45. American Diabetes Association. Diabetes Care 2004;27:S1–S150.
46. Anderson JW. Med Exerc Nutr Health 1993;2:65–8.
47. Brenner BM, Meyer TW, Hostetter TH. N Engl J Med 1982; 307:652–9.
48. Henry RR. Diabetes Care 1994;17:1502–13.
49. Anderson JW, Hanna TJ. Soy foods and health promotion. In: Watson T, ed. Vegetables, Fruits, and Herbs in Health Promotion. Boca Raton, FL: CRC Press, 2001:117–34.
50. Stephenson TJ. Therapeutic benefits of a soy protein rich diet in the prevention and treatment of nephropathy in young persons with type 1, insulin-dependent diabetes mellitus. PhD thesis. Lexington, KY: University of Kentucky, 2001:1–238.
51. Teixeira SR, Tappenden KA, Carson L et al. J Nutr 2004;134: 1874–80.
52. Azadbakht L, Shakerhosseini R, Atabak S et al. Eur J Clin Nutr 2003;57:1292–4.
53. Anderson JW, Johnstone BM, Cook-Newell ME. N Engl J Med 1995;333:276–82.
54. Anderson JW. SCANs Pulse 2004;23:8–9.
55. Anderson JW, Luan J, Hoie LH. Adv Ther 2004;21:61–75.
56. Jayagopal V, Albertazzi P, Kilpatrick ES et al. Diabetes Care 2002;25:1709–14.
57. Joslin EP. The Treatment of Diabetes. 4th ed. Philadelphia: Lea & Febiger, 1928.
58. Garg A. Am J Clin Nutr 1998;67:577S–82S.
59. Garg A, Grundy SM, Unger RH. Diabetes 1992;41:1278–85.
60. Connor WE. Ann Intern Med 1995;123:950–2.
61. Burr ML, Fehily AM, Gilbert JF. Lancet 1989;2:757–61.
62. Friedberg CE, Heine RJ, Janssen MJFM et al. Diabetes Care 1998;21:494–500.
63. Woodman RJ, Mori TA, Burke V et al. Am J Clin Nutr 2002; 76:1007–15.
64. Eldridge AL, Cooper DA, Peters JC. Obes Rev 2002;3:17–25.
65. Trowell HC. Non-infective Diseases. London: Edward Arnold, 1960.
66. Walker ARP. S Afr Med J 1961;35:114–5.
67. Walker ARP, Walker BF, Richardson BD. Lancet 1970;2:51–2.
68. Trowell HC. Diabetes 1975;24:762–6.
69. Jenkins DJA, Leeds AR, Gassull MA. Lancet 1976;2:172–4.
70. Kiehm TG, Anderson JW, Ward K. Am J Clin Nutr 1976;29: 895–9.

71. O'Dea K, Traianedes K, Ireland P et al. J Am Diet Assoc 1989; 89:1076–86.

72. Panel on Dietary Reference Intakes for Macronutrients and National Academy of Sciences. *http://www4* nationalacademies org news nsf/isbn 2002.

73. Anderson JW, Allgood LD, Turner C et al. Am J Clin Nutr 1999;70:466–73.

74. Henkel J. FDA Consumer 2003;1–5.

75. Howard A, Arnsten JH, Gourevitch MN. Ann Intern Med 2004;140:211–9.

76. Egede LE, Ye X, Zheng D et al. Diabetes Care 2002;25:324–9.

77. Althuis MD, Jordan NE, Ludington EA et al. Am J Clin Nutr 2002;76:148–55.

78. Yeh GY, Eisenberg DM, Kaptchuk TJ et al. Diabetes Care 2003;26:1277–94.

79. Anderson JW, Gowri MS, Turner J et al. J Am Coll Nutr 1999; 18:451–61.

80. Diwadkar VA, Anderson JW, Bridges SR et al. P Soc Exp Biol Med 1999;222:178–84.

81. American Diabetes Association. Diabetes Care 2000;23:381–9.

82. Persson B, Hanson U, Lunell N-O. Diabetes and pregnancy. In: Alberti KGMM, Zimmet P, DeFronzo RA, et al., eds. International Textbook of Diabetes Mellitus. 2nd ed. New York: John Wiley, 1997:1135–49.

83. Gavin LA, Lyons L, Kitzmiller JL. Type 1 diabetes mellitus in pregnancy. In: DeFronzo RA, ed. Current Therapy of Diabetes Mellitus. St. Louis: Mosby, 1998:228–36.

84. Anderson JW, Blake JE, Turner J et al. Am J Clin Nutr 1998; 68:1347S–53S.

85. Mackenzie HS, Brenner BM. Am J Kidney Dis 1998;31: 161–70.

86. Gowri MS, Van der Westhuyzen DR, Bridges SR et al. Arterioscler Thromb Vasc 1999;9:2226–33.

87. Rubins HB, Robins SJ, Collins D et al. NEngl J Med 1999; 341:410–8.

88. Jenkins DJA, Kendall CWC, Marchie A et al. JAMA 2003; 290:502–10.

89. Kreisberg RA, Oberman A. J Clin Endocrinol Metab 2003;88:2445–61.

90. Snow V, Aronson MD, Hornbake ER et al. Ann Intern Med 2004;140:644–9.

91. Robins SJ, Rubins HB, Faas FH et al. Diabetes Care 2003;26:1513–7.

92. Hurst RT, Lee RL. Ann Intern Med 2003;129:824–34.

93. Anderson JW, Konz EC, Jenkins DJA. J Am Coll Nutr 2000; 19:578–90.

94. Heymsfield SB, van Mierlo C, van der Knaap HCM et al. Int J Obes 2003;27:537–49.

95. Yip I, Go VLW, DeShields S et al. Obes Res 2001;9:341S–7S.

96. Anderson JW, Greenway FL, Fujioka K et al. Obes Res 2002;10:633–41.

97. Heshka S, Greenway F, Anderson JW et al. Am J Med 2000; 109:282–7.

98. Heshka S, Anderson JW, Atkinson RL et al. JAMA 2003;289: 1799–805.

99. Daly A, Konz EC, Soler N et al. J Am Diet Assoc 2000;100:1456 (letter).

100. Anderson JW, Vichitbandra S, Qian W et al. J Am Coll Nutr 1999;18:620–7.

101. Reynolds LR, Konz EC, Frederich RC et al. Diabetes Obes Metab 2002;4:270–5.

102. Haddock CK. Int J Obes 2003;26:262–73.

103. Myles JM, Leiter L, Hollander PA et al. Diabetes Care 2002; 25:1123–8.

104. McNulty SJ, Ur E, Williams GMSSG. Diabetes Care 2003; 26:125–31.

105. Higa KD, Boone KB, Ho T. Obes Surg 2000;10:509–13.

106. Pories WJ, MacDonald KG Jr, Morgan EJ et al. Am J Clin Nutr 1992;55:582S–5S.

107. Anderson JW, Konz EC, Frederich RC et al. Am J Clin Nutr 2001;74:579–84.

108. Klem ML, Wing RR, McGuire MT et al. Am J Clin Nutr 1997;66:239–46.

109. Baraz L, Schneider SH. Clin Diabetes 1994;94–8.

110. Borghouts LB, Keizer HA. Int J Sports Med 2000;21:1–12.

111. Fuchsjager-Mayri G, Pleiner J, Weisinger GF et al. Diabetes Care 2002;25:1795–1801.

112. Kitamura I, Takeshima N, Tokudome M et al. Geriatr Gerontol Int 2003;3:47–52.

113. Dunstan DW, Daly RM, Owen N et al. Diabetes Care 2002; 25:1729–36.

114. Sato Y, Nagasaki M, Nakai N et al. Exp Biol Med 2003;228: 1208–12.

115. DeFronzo RA. Ann Intern Med 1999;131:281–303.

116. Reynolds LR, Anderson JW. Endocr Pract 2004;19:153–9.

117. Holler HJ, Pastors JG. Diabetes Medical Nutrition Therapy: A Professional Guide to Management and Nutrition Education Resources. Alexandria, VA: American Dietetic Association and American Diabetes Association, 1997.

118. Mann JI, Lewis-Barned NJ. Dietary management of diabetes mellitus in Europe and North America. In: Alberti KGMM, Zimmet P, DeFronzo RA, et al., eds. International Textbook of Diabetes Mellitus. 2nd ed. New York: John Wiley, 1997:759–71.

119. Gillespie SJ, Kulkarni KD, Daly AE. J Am Diet Assoc 1998; 98:897–905.

120. American Diabetes Association and American Dietetic Association. Exchange Lists for Meal Planning. Alexandria, VA: American Diabetes Association, 1995.

121. Anderson JW, Gustafson NJ. Dr. Anderson's High-Fiber Fitness Plan. Lexington, KY: University Press of Kentucky, 1994.

122. Batterham RL, Cohen MA, Ellis SM et al. N Engl J Med 2003; 349:941–8.

123. Konturek SJ, Konturek JW, Pawlik T et al. J Physiol Pharmacol 2004;55:137–54.

124. Foster-Powell K, Holt SHA, Brand-Miller JC. Am J Clin Nutr 2002;76:5–56.

SELECTED READINGS

American Diabetes Association, National Institute of Diabetes and Digestive and Kidney Disease. Prevention or delay of type 2 diabetes. Diabetes Care 2004;27:S47–S54.

American Diabetes Association. Nutrition principles and recommendations in diabetes. Diabetes Care 2004;27:S36–S46.

Anderson JW, Akanji AO, Randles KM. Treatment of diabetes with high fiber diets. In: Spiller GA, ed. Dietary Fiber in Human Nutrition. Boca Raton, FL: CRC Press, 2001:363–90.

Anderson JW, Kendall CWC, Jenkins DJA. Importance of weight management in type 2 diabetes: review with meta-analysis of clinical studies. J Am Coll Nutr 2003;22:331–9.

Anderson JW, Randles KM, Kendall CWC et al. Carbohydrate and fiber recommendations for individuals with diabetes: a quantitative assessment and meta-analysis of the evidence. J Am Coll Nutr 2004; 23:5–17.

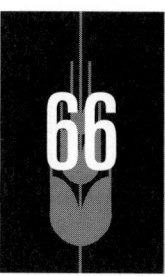

66 NUTRIENT AND GENETIC REGULATION OF LIPOPROTEIN METABOLISM[1]
MARGO A. DENKE

HISTORY OF DIET AND LIPOPROTEIN METABOLISM . .1067
GENETIC DISORDERS OF LIPOPROTEIN METABOLISM 1067
    High Total Cholesterol .1067
    High Triglycerides 1069
    Low Cholesterol and Triglyceride Levels 1071
    Miscellaneous Genetic Defects in Lipoprotein
        Metabolism 1073
FUTURE DIRECTIONS IN UNDERSTANDING
   NUTRIENT AND GENETIC REGULATION
   OF LIPOPROTEIN METABOLISM 1074
    Effects of Drugs on Lipoprotein Metabolism 1074
    Speculations on Thrifty Phenotype and the
        Dyslipidemia of Insulin Resistance 1074

HISTORY OF DIET AND LIPOPROTEIN METABOLISM

In the last century, the genetics of lipoprotein metabolism has been unraveled piece by piece. By their very nature, the initial discoveries of genetic differences in lipoprotein metabolism relied heavily on case reports of rare and often dramatic presentations of disease. What clinician would not take note of a child with milky plasma presenting with acute pancreatitis, or a child dying of congestive heart failure because of aortic root obstruction caused by cholesterol accumulation? The premature deaths of these patients required a search for the cause, and the search began by investigating the health of family members. The defect was characterized as autosomal dominant or recessive according to the family history of the proband; consanguinity was queried. The development of assays for cholesterol, triglycerides, lipoproteins, and later apoproteins and enzymes further characterized the disorder. The role of diet was one of therapy: in disorders in which increases in serum chylomicrons were the major manifestation, severe restrictions

in dietary fat were prescribed; in disorders attributable to cholesterol excess, low-animal-product diets were prescribed. Dietary therapy never normalized the disorder, but it reduced symptomatic disease.

Although diet as a therapy is helpful in only a few monogenic disorders, in physiologically normal persons, diet plays a fundamental role in lipid metabolism. Dietary intake of saturated fat and dietary cholesterol increases total and low-density lipoprotein (LDL) cholesterol levels by reducing LDL receptor expression. The population response to a cholesterol-lowering diet is consistent and predictable. The influence of diet is not diminished by concomitant lipid-lowering drug therapy. No single heritable pathway explains the cholesterol-raising effects of diet (1). The reader is referred to a review of lipoprotein metabolism and the effects of diet on serum lipoprotein levels in Chapter 67.

In this tutorial chapter, we first discuss specific monogenic disorders of lipoprotein metabolism and the role that diet plays in expression of disease. In a departure from previous formats, disorders will be classified not by the enzyme/apoprotein involved but by the alterations seen in plasma lipoprotein levels. The reasons for this will become apparent—some mutations express a different disorder in the heterozygous state compared with the homozygous state. Tables are included to show clinical information regarding these disorders—because these are rare disorders, the approximate incidence is provided as a relative guide of how likely it is that the reader will encounter a patient with this genetic abnormality. The chapter concludes with mention of two different genetic sites of action of drug therapy and brief speculations regarding how new advances in the field of gene expression proving that maternal nutrition alters gene expression may explain how fetal nutrition exposure may alter the risk for chronic disease.

GENETIC DISORDERS OF LIPOPROTEIN METABOLISM

High Total Cholesterol

Cholesterol levels in the population do not follow a gaussian distribution. There is a significant "tail to the right", with some persons having very high cholesterol levels. Most of these persons had very high rates of premature coronary disease.

---

[1]**Abbreviations: ABC,** adenosine triphosphate–binding cassette; **Apo,** apoprotein; **ARH,** autosomal recessive hypercholesterolemia; **CETP,** cholesterol ester transfer protein; **FH,** familial hypercholesterolemia; **HDL,** high-density lipoprotein; **IDL,** intermediate-density lipoprotein; **LCAT,** lecithin cholesterol acyltransferase; **LDL,** low-density lipoprotein; **LPL,** lipoprotein lipase; **PPAR,** peroxisome proliferator–activated receptor; **SREBP,** sterol regulatory element–binding protein; **VLDL,** very-low-density lipoprotein.

After the characterization of lipoproteins, the increases in total cholesterol level were characterized as increases in LDL (by far the most common), increases in high-density lipoproteins (HDLs), or increases in the cholesterol content of triglyceride-rich lipoproteins [chylomicrons, very-low-density lipoproteins (VLDLs), or intermediate-density lipoproteins (IDLs)]. This latter cause is discussed later in disorders of triglycerides.

Genetic Causes of High LDL Cholesterol

LDL is the primary carrier of serum cholesterol, typically containing 65 to 70% of the total cholesterol in plasma. As can be assumed from its name, LDL is defined by its density characteristics. Every LDL has one molecule of Apo B-100. All genetic conditions causing elevations in LDL cholesterol carry a high risk for premature atherosclerotic disease (Table 66.1). Three major categories of defects have been defined: defects in Apo

B-100 (familial defective Apo B) defects in the LDL receptor (familial hypercholesterolemia [FH]), and defects in a phosphotyrosine binding protein that permits internalization of the LDL-LDL receptor complex (ARH). Although the primary cause of hypercholesterolemia is genetic, cholesterol-lowering diets in these patients in general achieve a greater percentage reduction in LDL than is seen in the normal population.

Familial Defective Apoprotein B. Apo B-100 is a ligand for the LDL receptor. Multiple mutations occurring in the ligand binding areas of Apo B, reducing binding to the LDL receptor, have been identified (2, 3).

Familial Hypercholesterolemia. Clearance of LDL is primarily mediated by LDL receptors (4). The LDL receptor gene encodes for a receptor protein of 110,000 daltons. A cysteine-rich domain binds both Apo B-100 and Apo E. Once LDL is bound to the receptor, the complex is internalized and dissociates. The LDL receptor returns

TABLE 66.1. GENETIC CAUSES OF HIGH TOTAL CHOLESTEROL

DISORDER	ESTIMATED INCIDENCE	TYPICAL LIPIDS	ASSOCIATED FINDINGS	GENE DEFECT	DIETARY AND OTHER THERAPY
Heterozygous familial hypercholesterolemia	1:500	Adult LDL cholesterol >250 mg/dL; children LDL 150–400 mg/dL; cord blood LDL > 100 mg/dL is suggestive of the disease	Tendon xanthoma, xanthelasma, corneal arcus may develop by age 20 Premature coronary disease	Mutation in LDL receptor gene; severity of lipid defect is due to specifics of the mutations	Restriction of dietary saturated fat and dietary cholesterol; respond to statin drug therapy because the one normal allele produces some LDL receptors
Homozygous familial hypercholesterolemia	1:1 million	Childhood LDL cholesterol level >400	Planar, tendon, and tuberous xanthoma by age 6; coronary disease as early as 18 mo of age	Mutation in LDL receptor gene; severity of lipid defect is due to specifics of the mutations	Restriction of dietary saturated fat and dietary cholesterol; respond to apheresis to selectively remove LDL; liver transplant achieves an 80% reduction in LDL by providing hepatic LDL receptors; after liver transplant use of satin therapy provides an additional 50% reduction in LDL
Familial defective Apo B	1:500	Adult LDL cholesterol >190 mg/dL	Tendon xanthoma xanthelasma Premature coronary disease	Variations in Apo B gene impairing binding to LDL receptor	Restriction of dietary saturated fat and dietary cholesterol; respond to statin drug therapy because particles with normal Apo B sequence are more rapidly cleared
Autosomal recessive hypercholesterolemia	<40 kindreds described	Average LDL 480 mg/dL compared with homozygous FH controls 625 mg/dL	Tendon xanthoma Premature coronary disease	Defect in ARH gene leads to defective internalization of LDL bound to the LDL receptor	Restriction of dietary saturated fat and dietary cholesterol; unlike homozygous FH, these patients respond to statin drug therapy

Apo, apoprotein; FH, familial hypercholesterolemia; LDL, low-density lipoprotein.

to the cell membrane, and the lipoprotein is degraded by cellular lysosomes. Some but not all mutations in the LDL receptor gene lead to expression of FH (5). Several classes of defects in the LDL receptor gene are associated with FH. Class 1 mutations create a null allele where no immunoprecipitatable LDL receptor protein is identified. Class 2 mutations, which account for half of the clinical mutations in FH, create a membrane protein that is synthesized but not transported to the Golgi in a timely manner; degradation occurs. Class 3 mutations create a receptor that has a binding defect. Class 4 mutations create a receptor that cannot internalize the LDL and move it to the Golgi, and class 5 mutations create receptors that do not recycle. Rare promoter mutations in the LDL receptor gene have also been described.

Autosomal Recessive Hypercholesterolemia. Rare patients have presented with what seemed to be homozygous FH. When their fibroblasts were assayed for LDL receptors, a normal number were found. Absence of the phosphotyrosine-binding domain protein, autosomal recessive hypercholesterolemia (ARH), explains the defect (6). ARH functions as an adapter protein, combining with the LDL-LDL receptor complex to permit its endocytosis. Absence of ARH causes an internalization defect; the clinical consequences are similar to the complete absence of LDL receptors.

Genetic Causes of High High-Density Lipoprotein Cholesterol

Much rarer than isolated increases in LDL cholesterol levels are isolated increases in HDL cholesterol levels (Table 66.2).

Cholesterol Ester Transfer Protein Deficiency. Cholesterol ester transfer protein (CETP) shuttles cholesterol esters between plasma lipoproteins. Primarily, CETP controls clearance of cholesterol ester from HDL. Deficiency in CETP leads to an increase in HDL size because the HDL cannot download its cholesterol esters. CETP is an example in which high levels of HDL are not necessarily protective against coronary disease—the high HDL in CETP deficiency indicates a defect in cholesterol transport. Regarding the risk for coronary disease, the benefits of CETP deficiency remain unclear. Some have speculated that if the deficiency is compensated for by higher HDL particle number (in men this corresponds to an HDL >60), the defect seems protective against coronary artery disease (7). Others speculate that the failure to identify living Japanese elderly persons with the mutation indicates a failure of the mutation to protect against coronary disease.

Hepatic Lipase Polymorphisms. Hepatic lipase seems to have two primary functions: conversion of VLDL to IDL and IDL to LDL, and degradation of HDL. Frank deficiency of this enzyme is a rare cause of hypertriglyceridemia, discussed later. Polymorphisms in the hepatic lipase gene explain the higher HDL cholesterol levels observed in African-Americans compared with white Americans (8).

High Triglycerides

Triglycerides in lipoproteins are derived from two sources: exogenous (from dietary fat) and endogenous (from hepatic production or release from adipose tissue). The monogenic disorders of chylomicron metabolism comprise the first descriptions of dietary links to lipids. Even today, dietary therapy remains the primary treatment.

TABLE 66.2. GENETIC CAUSES OF HIGH HIGH-DENSITY LIPOPROTEIN CHOLESTEROL

DISORDER	ESTIMATED INCIDENCE	TYPICAL LIPIDS	ASSOCIATED FINDINGS	GENE DEFECT	DIETARY AND OTHER THERAPY
CETP deficiency	In Japan, heterozygotes account for 8% of the population, 1% having a null mutation and 7% having a functional but defective enzyme	Homozygous TG 56–381 mg/dL LDL 31–131 mg/dL HDL 98–248 mg/dL Heterozygotes TG 43–229 mg/dL LDL 52–191 mg/dL HDL 41–104 mg/dL	None	Mutations in CETP gene; null mutation results in more extreme lipid disturbance	Unstudied; because a defect in reverse cholesterol transport is seen, a cholesterol-lowering diet should show benefits
Hepatic lipase polymorphisms	Common; ethnic distribution	African Americans have HDL cholesterol levels 10 mg/dL higher than white Americans	None	Polymorphism in hepatic lipase gene reduces rate of enzyme degradation	None

CTEP, cholesterol ester transfer protein; HDL, high-density lipoprotein; LDL, low-density lipoprotein; TG, triglyceride.

TABLE 66.3. GENETIC CAUSES OF HIGH TRIGLYCERIDES WITH FASTING CHYLOMICRONEMIA

DISORDER	ESTIMATED INCIDENCE	TYPICAL LIPIDS	ASSOCIATED FINDINGS	GENE DEFECT	DIETARY AND OTHER THERAPY
Homozygous familial lipoprotein lipase deficiency	1:1 million	Serum triglycerides 1,500–4,500 or higher	Presents in childhood, often in the first year of life. Eruptive xanthomas, hepatomegaly, and splenomegaly from triglyceride accumulation in organs occurs; all regresses with dietary therapy Normal lifespan if dietary therapy initiated	Mutations in LPL gene causing markedly reduced or absent enzyme activity	Restrict dietary fat to <20 g/d; this will provide maintenance of TG levels below 2,000 mg/dL; supplemental vitamin E is not required because Apo B–containing lipoproteins are present
Apoprotein C-II deficiency	<20 kindreds described	Serum triglycerides 1,500–4,500 or higher	Presents later in life than homozygous familial lipoprotein lipase deficiency (age 13–60 y) No association with premature atherosclerosis	Mutations in Apo C-II gene lead to absent or nonfunctional Apo C-II	Restrict dietary fat to <20 g/d; supplemental vitamin E is not required because Apo B–containing lipoproteins are present Acute pancreatitis can be treated using transfusion of plasma from normal people, supplying Apo C-II and temporarily correcting the abnormality

Apo, apolipoprotein; LPL, lipoprotein lipase; TG, triglyceride.

Genetic Causes of Fasting Chylomicronemia

Impaired removal of absorbed dietary fat from the circulation results in significant disease (9). The severity of the clinical presentation is directly linked to the magnitude of the hypertriglyceridemia. Dietary therapy plays a clear and ever important role in controlling disease (Table 66.3).

Familial Lipoprotein Lipase Deficiency. Mutations in the lipoprotein lipase gene leading to low or absent enzyme activity have been described. The clinical condition of lipoprotein lipase deficiency is rare because manifestation of the complete syndrome requires homozygosity for two defective genes. Some mutations lead to detectable levels of lipoprotein lipase (LPL) in plasma, but the enzyme lacks activity. The role of restricting dietary fat is essential—endogenously produced triglycerides can be cleared from smaller VLDL particles by alternative pathways, including hepatic lipase. VLDL cholesterol levels remain elevated, however, because the major pathway for clearance of VLDL is via lipoprotein lipase.

Apolipoprotein C-II Deficiency. Apo C-II is a necessary cofactor for the action of lipoprotein lipase. Apo C-II is found on the apoprotein coat of chylomicrons and VLDL; it is thought that Apo C-II induces a conformational change in LPL, resulting in its activation. A small proportion of patients presenting with familial chylomicronemia have normal lipoprotein lipase activity but a deficiency in Apo C-II (10).

Genetic Causes of Hypertriglyceridemia Without Fasting Chylomicronemia

Table 66.4 lists genetic causes of hypertriglyceridemia, including conditions in which the defect only manifests in the postprandial state.

Partial Lipoprotein Lipase Deficiency. LPL activity is upregulated in adipose tissue after a meal. In people who are heterozygous for LPL deficiency, the rate of clearance of postprandial lipoproteins is reduced; particles are eventually removed, and fasting lipids are often normal. Because triglyceride-rich lipoproteins are known to be atherogenic, it is speculated that the delay in clearance of postprandial lipids will increase the risk for atherosclerotic disease (11).

Dysbetalipoproteinemia or Type III Hyperlipoproteinemia. Receptor recognition for removal of triglyceride-rich remnants (chylomicron remnants and VLDL remnants) requires the presence of Apo E. Apo E is acquired by chylomicrons during peripheral metabolism (12). Three Apo E isoforms, E2, E3, and E4, have been identified; the isoforms differ in a single amino acid substitution. E3 binds normally to the receptor, E4 is more avid than E3, and E2 is less avid. Patients with the E4 isoform have higher LDL levels than those with other isoforms; the increase in LDL is thought to be the result of the enhanced rate of clearance of remnants. Patients with the E2 isoform have lower levels of LDL. As a consequence of delayed

TABLE 66.4. GENETIC CAUSES OF HIGH TRIGLYCERIDES WITHOUT FASTING CHYLOMICRONEMIA

DISORDER	ESTIMATED INCIDENCE	TYPICAL LIPIDS	ASSOCIATED FINDINGS	GENE DEFECT	DIETARY AND OTHER THERAPY
Partial lipoprotein lipase deficiency	1:35	Heterozygotes have TG 120–520 mg/dL and HDL levels 30–45 mg/dL; some have near normal levels	None	Mutations in LPL gene causing markedly reduced or absent enzyme activity	Not formally studied; restrictions in dietary fat and avoidance of high-fat splurges would be expected to reduce TG levels
Dysbeta-lipoproteinemia type III	1:5,000	Total cholesterol averages 450 mg/dL with TG 700 mg/dL; direct measurements of LDL will be disproportionately low (e.g., 120 mg/dL) and this LDL includes IDL particles; most TG-rich lipoproteins are β-VLDL	Palmar xanthomas, tuberous and tuberoeruptive xanthomas. Premature atherosclerosis	Several mutations in the Apo E gene create either a dominant or a recessive Apo E2 isoform to be secreted	Weight loss can cause remission of the overt lipoprotein disorder; high-fat meals worsen dyslipidemia Reduced-fat diet reduces chylomicron production, improving fasting lipids
Hepatic lipase deficiency	<20 kindreds described	Most have TG 200–450 mg/dL; normal and very high have been observed β-VLDL is present HDL high but ranges from 31–132 mg/dL	None	Defective hepatic lipase gene leading to absence of hepatic lipase activity	Not formally studied

Apo, apoprotein; HDL, high-density lipoprotein; IDL, intermediate-density lipoprotein; LDL, low-density lipoprotein; TG, triglyceride; VLDL, very-low-density lipoprotein.

clearance, patients homozygous for the E2 isoform have an abnormal lipoprotein, β-VLDL. β-VLDL is a remnant lipoprotein derived from either chylomicron or hepatic VLDL; its longer residence time causes the lipoprotein to be abnormally enriched in cholesterol.

Manifestation of the lipid disorder, type III, with equal elevations in cholesterol and triglycerides, typically requires an additional factor besides E2/E2 homozygozity including diabetes, estrogen deficiency, or hypothyroidism.

Various mutations in the Apo E gene cause the E2 and E4 isoforms; these mutations can be dominant or recessive. The Apo E4 isoform has been associated with a higher risk for developing Alzheimer disease (13).

Hepatic Lipase. Hepatic lipase is the enzyme responsible for catabolizing triglyceride-rich remnants in the liver; in particular, hepatic lipase is responsible for converting VLDL to IDL and IDL to LDL. The role of hepatic lipase in HDL metabolism is discussed earlier. Hepatic lipase deficiency is a rare cause of fasting hypertriglyceridemia. Homozygosity for a specific mutation that leads to inactivation of enzymatic activity is required (14).

Low Cholesterol and Triglyceride Levels

Despite the primary focus on the harm of increases in cholesterol levels, low cholesterol levels, resulting from a defect in lipoprotein metabolism, often cause disease. Mutations associated with low lipid levels are listed in Table 66.5.

Genetic Causes of Low Cholesterol Levels

Abetalipoproteinemia (Microsomal Transfer Protein Deficiency). Abetalipoproteinemia was first described in 1950; the delay in identifying this disorder was likely the result of misdiagnosis as celiac disease. Patients would present with malabsorption and chronic diarrhea, as seen with celiac disease; later on in their illness they would develop ataxia, atypical pigmentation of the retina, star-shaped erythrocytes (acanthocytosis), and low serum cholesterol levels with near absence of particles in the B-globulin fraction. Although a defect in the Apo B gene had been suspected for some time, the Apo B gene is normal in patients with abetalipoproteinemia. The defect seems to be in the microsomal triglyceride transfer protein that is involved in assembly, processing, and secretion of Apo B–containing lipoproteins (15). Without this microsomal transfer protein, patients with abetalipoproteinemia cannot manufacture a circulatable form of Apo B. Thus, no chylomicrons, VLDL, or LDL appears in plasma. The defect is not fatal because Apo E–rich HDL takes over as the primary cholesterol carrier.

Fat malabsorption is significant; lysosomal hypertrophy in enterocytes may compensate for polyunsaturated fatty acid absorption. Sufficient vitamin A can be absorbed when supplemented in normal amounts, but vitamin E deficiency is a significant, ongoing clinical problem in these patients. Vitamin E absorption requires chylomicron as a carrier to the liver and LDL as a carrier to the periphery.

TABLE 66.5. GENETIC CAUSES OF LOW CHOLESTEROL AND TRIGLYCERIDES

DISORDER	INCIDENCE	TYPICAL LIPIDS	ASSOCIATED PHYSICAL FINDINGS	GENE DEFECT	DIETARY AND OTHER THERAPY
Abetalipoproteinemia	<120 cases described	Total cholesterol <50 mg/dL TG range from 2–45 mg/dL	Malabsorption presenting in childhood; acanthocytosis, retinopathy, and peripheral neuropathy if vitamin E supplementation is not initiated	Autosomal recessive; defect in microsomal transferase gene leading to an inability to secrete Apo B	Restrict long-chain dietary TG to <15 g/d Medium-chain TG can be used as a calorie source if needed 1,000–2,000 mg/d concentrated vitamin E in infants and 5,000–10,000 mg/d in older children and adults
Homozygous hypobetalipoproteinemia	<10 kindreds	Total cholesterol in the 33–42 mg/dL range TG range from 60–100 mg/dL	Malabsorption presenting in childhood; acanthocytosis, retinopathy and peripheral neuropathy if vitamin E supplementation is not initiated	Autosomal-dominant Truncations in Apo B gene	Restrict long-chain dietary TG to <15 g/d Medium-chain TG can be used as a calorie source if needed; supplement with 1,000–2,000 mg/d concentrated vitamin E in infants and 5,000–10,000 mg/d in older children and adults
Heterozygous hypobetalipoproteinemia	1:3,000	Total cholesterol in the 40–180 mg/dL range TG range from 615–150 mg/dL	Rare cases reported with acanthocytosis, impaired fat malabsorption Neurologic disease is less advanced than in homozygotes	Truncations in Apo B gene	Heterozygous people can develop neurologic deficits from vitamin E deficiency Recommend supplementation with 400–800 mg/d; fat restriction recommended if malabsorption is present

Apo, apoprotein; TG, triglyceride.

If high doses of vitamin E are not provided to these patients, pigmentary retinal degeneration and large sensory neuron degeneration occurs (16).

Hypobetalipoproteinemia. Hypobetalipoproteinemia is the result of a defect in the Apo B gene. Because of multiple different mutations, a truncated message is formed from the Apo B gene (17). A patient with heterozygous hypobetalipoproteinemia typically has an LDL cholesterol level half that of an unaffected family member. Disease related to vitamin E deficiency can occur in these patients; vitamin E supplementation is recommended (18).

Genetic Causes of Low High-Density Lipoprotein

Very low HDL levels have been associated with a variety of defects in the apoproteins and enzymes that form HDL (Table 66.6). HDL is created in the plasma when nascent Apo A-1 discs become spheric as they acquire cholesterol esters for their cores. Lecithin cholesterol acyltransferase (LCAT) catalyzes the esterification of free cholesterol to cholesterol ester; LCAT activity is essential for the formation of spheric HDL (19). Defective Apo A-1 leads to a failure to form these initial nascent discs; deficiency in LCAT results in formation of HDL. A defective membrane transporter allowing cholesterol to be removed from tissues also results in low HDL. Many disorders of HDL metabolism are associated with premature coronary disease.

Familial Lecithin Cholesterol Acyltransferase Deficiency. Familial LCAT deficiency is the absence of LCAT activity (20). Corneal opacities, anemia, proteinuria, mild hypoalbuminemia, and dyslipidemia occur. The anemia is the result of altered red blood cell membrane lipids. The renal lesion consists of abnormal lipid deposition in the mesangial area, glomeruli, and interstitial membranes; LDL particles are not always detected, so an immune complex– and complement-mediated mechanism for renal dysfunction is postulated.

Fish Eye Disease. Fish eye disease is the result of a partial deficiency of LCAT activity; the partial deficiency limits the abnormalities to corneal opacifications that occur later in life. The corneal opacifications are the result of deposition of LCAT substrates (free cholesterol and phospholipids) on the cornea.

Apo A1 Deficiency. The Apo A1 gene is on chromosome 11q23 with a cluster of other lipid genes: Apo C-III

TABLE 66.6. GENETIC CAUSES OF LOW HIGH-DENSITY LIPOPROTEIN CHOLESTEROL

DISORDER	INCIDENCE	TYPICAL LIPIDS	ASSOCIATED PHYSICAL FINDINGS	GENE DEFECT	DIETARY AND OTHER THERAPY
Familial LCAT deficiency	<40 kindreds	Total cholesterol 89–185, TG 110–723, HDL 0–12 mg/dL	Corneal opacities Normochromic normocytic anemia Proteinuria with increased risk for renal failure by age 40–50 y	Defect in LCAT gene leading to absent or markedly reduced LCAT enzyme	Not determined
Partial LCAT deficiency (fish eye disease)	<15 kindreds	Total cholesterol 185–253, TG 60–408, HDL 0–7 mg/dL	Corneal opacities	Gene defect in LCAT leading to normal measurable LCAT levels but ineffective ability to esterify free cholesterol in HDL	Not determined
Apo A1 deficiency	<20 kindreds	HDL cholesterol levels 0–30 mg/dL with majority <10 mg/dL	Corneal opacities Diffuse palmar xanthoma	Multiple distinct mutations in Apo A1 gene leading to reduced Apo A1 levels	Not determined
Tangier disease	<70 kindreds	Total cholesterol 18–177, TG 40–580, HDL 0–9 mg/dL	Corneal opacities Yellow/orange tonsils Hepatosplenomegaly	Defects in *ABC1* gene, prevent formation of HDL	LDL levels are low, but clearance of TG-rich lipoproteins is defective Low-fat diets are recommended

ABC, adenosine triphosphate–binding cassette; Apo, apoprotein; HDL, high-density lipoprotein; LCAT, lecithin cholesterol acyltransferase; TG, triglyceride; VLDL, very-low-density lipoprotein.

and Apo A-IV. Disorders in this gene sequence commonly present with corneal opacifications and premature heart disease. Multiple mutations in the Apo A1 gene have been reported, but not all seem related to an increased risk for heart disease. Some mutations are in a region that results in abnormal LCAT activation, whereas others are associated with amyloidosis (21). The folding of Apo A1, and how this is altered by the mutation, seems to explain the effect (22).

Tangier Disease. Cholesterol accumulation in macrophages is characteristic of Tangier disease. Mutations in the adenosine triphosphate–binding cassette (ABC) transporter explain the defect (23). In contrast with many low-HDL conditions in which Apo A1 production is reduced, in Tangier disease Apo A1 catabolism is increased (24).

Miscellaneous Genetic Defects in Lipoprotein Metabolism

Two rare, heritable conditions also deserve mention (Table 66.7).

Phytosterolemia

Plant sterols are absorbed through the same enterocyte transporter that absorbs cholesterol. In contrast with cholesterol, which is esterified in the enterocyte and shuttled into chylomicrons, phytosterols are transported back out

into the intestinal lumen. Two half-transporters, ABC G5 (25) and ABC G8 (26), members of the ABC family, are responsible for removing phytosterols. Defects in either half-transporter cause phytosterolemia. In this condition, hyperabsorption of phytosterols is the result of the inability of normally absorbed phytosterols to be "kicked out" of the intestinal cells; the phytosterols find their way into the plasma circulation. Cholesterol and phytosterols are removed by the body through biliary excretion. ABC G5 and ABC G8 transporters are also present in the liver and further impair elimination of phytosterols into the bile.

Lp(a)

Lp(a) is a distinct particle complex formed from LDL bound to Apo (a) by a single disulfide bond (27). The complex is larger than LDL, higher in lipid content, and slightly lower in density. It is difficult to quantify what percentage of LDL particles are of the Lp(a) type because the amount of Apo(a) attached to a single Apo B varies according to its genetically determined size. The complex seems poorly cleared by the LDL receptor; it has been postulated that the kidney is the site of removal (28). The rate of synthesis of Apo (a) determines Apo a concentration. Measurements of Lp(a) are difficult to perform, and wide interindividual and intraindividual variations makes conclusions regarding the effectiveness of interventions on Lp(a) difficult (29).

TABLE 66.7. GENETIC CAUSES OF MISCELLANEOUS LIPID DISORDERS

DISORDER	INCIDENCE	TYPICAL LIPIDS	ASSOCIATED PHYSICAL FINDINGS	GENE DEFECT	DIETARY AND OTHER THERAPY
Lp(a)	Quantitative genetic trait	Range of Lp(a) 0.2–200 mg/dL; determinant of concentration is rate of synthesis	Premature coronary disease	Number of Kringle IV repeats in Apo (a) gene correlates with levels; frequency distribution of these repeats varies among ethnic populations	Not well-controlled studies; particles are heterogeneous and variation is high
Phytosterolemia	<40 kindreds	Sitosterol levels 14–65 mg/dL, normal is 0.2–1.0 mg/dL Half of patients have increases in total cholesterol >250 mg/dL, and some have low HDL	Tendon xanthoma Tuberous xanthoma Premature coronary disease		Reduce dietary cholesterol and plant sterols Eliminate all vegetable oils from the diet, as well as nuts, seeds, wheat germ, shellfish, chocolate, olives, and avocados

Apo, apoprotein; HDL, high-density lipoprotein.

FUTURE DIRECTIONS IN UNDERSTANDING NUTRIENT AND GENETIC REGULATION OF LIPOPROTEIN METABOLISM

As the sophistication of our understanding of genetics improves, a few mechanisms by which genes can alter multiple pathways of lipid metabolism have been described (Table 66.8).

Effects of Drugs on Lipoprotein Metabolism

Sterol Regulatory Element Binding Protein Mutations and Human Immunodeficiency Virus Therapy

Sterol regulatory element–binding proteins (SREBPs) are membrane-bound transcription factors regulated by sterols. Once activated, SREBPs bind to specific promoter elements found on several target genes. The single act of upregulating SREBP is capable of affecting changes in the transcription rate of multiple target genes, causing pleiotropic effects. Recently, the acquired insulin resistance, lipodystrophy, and dyslipidemia observed in acquired immunodeficiency syndrome patients taking antiretroviral drugs were linked to the ability of these drugs to activate SREBP-1c (30).

Peroxisome Proliferator–Activated α-Receptor Activation

The presence of peroxisome proliferator–activated receptor (PPARs) on genes results in promotion of their transcription. Fibrates, a class of drugs used in lipid management, activate PPAR-α, resulting in a multiple effects on lipid metabolism, including lowering triglyceride levels and at the same time raising the HDL level (31).

Speculations on Thrifty Phenotype and the Dyslipidemia of Insulin Resistance

An association between low birth weight and future development of coronary disease has been noted (32). The "thrifty phenotype" hypothesis (33) suggests that in states of poor maternal nutrition, the neonate adapts its regulation of energy to survive. Support for a genetic adaptation has been bolstered by the recent discovery that gene transcription can be suppressed or activated by DNA methylation. It is presumed that the methylation of DNA impairs or enhances the

TABLE 66.8. EXAMPLES OF DRUGS THAT ALTER LIPOPROTEIN METABOLISM VIA TRANSCRIPTIONAL FACTORS AFFECTING FUNCTION OF MORE THAN ONE GENE

DISORDER	INCIDENCE	TYPICAL LIPIDS CHANGE	MECHANISM
Human immunodeficiency virus lipodystrophy	Patients taking antiretroviral drugs	High triglycerides, high cholesterol, low HDL	Drugs increase activation of SREBP-1c–containing genes
Dyslipidemia	Patients taking fibrates	Low triglycerides, high HDL	Drugs increase activation of PPARα–containing genes

HDL, high-density lipoprotein; PPAR, peroxisome proliferator—activated receptor; SREBP, sterol regulatory element–binding protein.

unraveling of DNA sequences required for transcription. Fetal DNA methylation can occur in utero, and the pattern of methylation can be modified by nutrient intake, notably folate (34). Approximately 1% of human DNA is methylated, accounting for 70 to 80% of all CpG dinucleotides that are susceptible to methylation. The observed association between small birth weight and methylation of the insulin-like growth factor II gene may account for the insulin resistance often seen in adulthood (35, 36). This insulin resistance leads to a characteristic dyslipidemia of high triglycerides and low HDL. Whether this mechanism can prove the thrifty phenotype hypothesis has yet to be determined.

REFERENCES

1. Denke MA, Adams-Huet B, Nguyen AT. JAMA 2000;284:2740–7.
2. Chatterton JE, Schlapfer P, Butler E et al. Biochemistry 1995; 34:9571.
3. Hansen PS. Dan Med Bull 1998;45:370–82.
4. Goldstein JL, Hobbs HH, Brown MS. Familial hypercholesterolemia. In: Scriver CR, Beaudet AL, Sly WS et al., eds. The Metabolic and Molecular Bases of Inherited Disease. 8th ed. New York: McGraw-Hill, 2001:2863–913.
5. Jensen HK. Dan Med Bull 2002;49:318–45.
6. Cohen JC, Kimmel M, Polanski A et al. Curr Opin Lipidol 2002; 14:121–7.
7. Barter PJ, Brewer HB Jr, Chapman MJ et al. Arterioscler Thromb Vasc Biol 2003;23:160–7.
8. Guerra RG, Wang SM, Grundy SM et al. Proc Natl Acad Sci USA 1997;94:4532.
9. Santamarina-Fojo S. Endocrinol Metab Clin North Am 1998;27:551–67.
10. Breckenridge WC, Little JA, Steiner G et al. N Engl J Med 1978; 298:1265.
11. Evans V, Kastelein JJ. Cardiovasc Drug Ther 2002;16:283–7.
12. Mahley RW, Rall SC. Type III hyperlipoproteinemia (dysbetalipoproteinemia): the role of apolipoprotein E in normal and abnormal lipid metabolism. In: Scriver CR, Beaudet AL, Sly WS et al., eds. The Metabolic and Molecular Bases of Inherited Disease. 8th ed. New York: McGraw-Hill, 2001:2835–62.
13. Mahley RW, Rall SC Jr. Annu Rev Genomics Hum Genet 2000; 1:507–37.
14. Connelly PW, Hegele RA. Crit Rev Clin Lab Sci 1998;35: 547–72.
15. Hussain MM, Iqbal J, Anwar K et al. Front Biosci 2003; 8:s500–6.
16. Hegele RA, Angel A. Can Med Assoc J 1985;132:41.
17. Schonfeld G. J Lipid Res 2003;44:878–83.
18. Linton MF, Faresee RV Jr, Yhoung SG. J Lipid Res 1993;34: 292.
19. Dobiasova M, Frohlich JJ. Clin Chim Acta 1999;286:257–71.
20. Kuivenhoven JA, Pritchard H, Hill J et al. J Lipid Res 1997; 38:191–205.
21. Sorci-Thoolmas MD, Thomas MJ. Trends Cardiovasc Med 2002;12:121–8.
22. Marcel YL, Kiss RS. Curr Opin Lipidol 2003;14:151–7.
23. Oram JF. Trends Molec Med 2002;8:168–73.
24. Assmann G, von Eckardstein A, Brewer HB Jr. Familial analphalipoproteinemia: Tangier disease. In: Scriver CR, Beaudet AL, Sly WS et al, eds. The Metabolic and Molecular Bases of Inherited Disease. 8th ed. New York: McGraw-Hill, 2001: 2937–60.
25. Lee MH, Lu K, Hazard S et al. Nat Genet 2001:27:27–83.
26. Berge KE, Tian, H, Graf GA et al. Science 2000;290:1771–5.
27. Hobbs HH, Whyite AL. Curr Opin Lipidol 1999;10:225–36.
28. Kronenberg F, Trenkwalder E, Lingenhel A et al. J Lipid Res 1997;38:1755.
29. Albers JJ, Marcovina SM. Curr Opin Lipidol 1994;5:417.
30. Miserez AR, Muller PY, Spaniol V. AIDS 2002;16:1587–94.
31. Fruchart JC, Duriez P, Staels B. Curr Opin Lipidol 1999;10: 245–57.
32. Barker DJB, ed. Fetal and Infant Origins of Adult Disease. London: BMJ Books, 1992.
33. Hales CN, Barker DJP. Diabetologia 1992;35:595–601.
34. Frisco S, Choi SW. J Nutr 2002;132:2382S–7S.
35. Bird A. Genes Dev 2002;21:16–21.
36. Tycko B, Efstratiadis A. Nature 2002;417:913–4.

SELECTED READINGS

Bachmann C, Berthold K. Genetic Expression and Nutrition. New York: Lippincott Williams & Wilkins, 2002.
Scriver CR, Beaudet AL, Sly WS et al., eds. The Metabolic and Molecular Bases of Inherited Disease. 8th ed. New York: McGraw-Hill, 2001.

67 NUTRITION IN THE MANAGEMENT OF DISORDERS OF SERUM LIPIDS AND LIPOPROTEINS[1]

SCOTT M. GRUNDY

RELATION OF LIPOPROTEINS TO ATHEROSCLEROTIC
   CARDIOVASCULAR DISEASE 1076
PUBLIC HEALTH PREVENTION OF
   ATHEROSCLEROTIC CARDIOVASCULAR DISEASE ..1077
HYPERCHOLESTEROLEMIA 1077
   Causes 1077
   Management 1082
   Chylomicronemia 1087
ATHEROGENIC DYSLIPIDEMIA 1088
   Causes 1089
   Management 1090

This chapter outlines the major abnormalities of serum cholesterol and other disorders of serum lipids and lipoproteins. These can be conveniently divided into three categories: hypercholesterolemia, chylomicronemia, and atherogenic dyslipidemia. Hypercholesterolemia occurs in varying degrees from mild to severe and is characterized by high serum levels of low-density lipoproteins (LDLs). Chylomicronemia consists of a marked elevation of chylomicrons, with or without high very-low-density lipoprotein (VLDL) levels. Finally, atherogenic dyslipidemia is a disorder characterized by multiple lipoprotein abnormalities occurring simultaneously in a single person. These three abnormalities are the focus of this chapter.

RELATION OF LIPOPROTEINS TO ATHEROSCLEROTIC CARDIOVASCULAR DISEASE

There is a growing recognition that high serum cholesterol levels and related disorders of serum lipoproteins promote the development of atherosclerosis, which, in turn, is a precursor of atherosclerotic cardiovascular disease (ASCVD). This evidence derives from animal models, surveys of different populations, findings of premature ASCVD in persons with genetic forms of hyperlipidemia, investigations in laboratory animals, and clinical trials (1, 2). Controlled clinical trials of cholesterol-lowering therapy (3–7) provide irrefutable evidence that high serum cholesterol levels predispose to ASCVD; these trials, moreover, demonstrate conclusively that reducing serum cholesterol levels decreases the incidence of ASCVD.

The major cholesterol-carrying lipoprotein of serum is LDL. LDL contains a nonpolar core composed mostly of cholesterol ester. It is held in solution in serum by apolipoprotein B-100 (ApoB-100). In clinical practice, LDL is measured by its cholesterol content (LDL-C). It appears to be the most atherogenic of all lipoproteins. For this reason, LDL-C has been identified as the primary target of lipid-lowering therapy by the US National Cholesterol Education Program (NCEP) (1, 2). Circulating LDL can penetrate into the arterial wall, where it can initiate the process of atherosclerosis. On entrance into the subendothelial space of the arterial wall, LDL is modified in several ways. Modified LDL initiates an inflammatory response that culminates in atherosclerotic plaque. Steps in inflammatory atherogenesis include macrophage infiltration and engulfment of lipid, followed by smooth muscle formation and collagen deposition. Lipid-rich areas of advanced plaques are susceptible to rupture, which can precipitate an acute coronary syndrome (e.g., myocardial infarction).

LDL is considered to be the *primary* risk factor for ASCVD because it appears to be required for the initiation and progression of atherosclerotic plaques. Nonetheless, in the presence of some elevation of serum LDL, other risk factors can accelerate the rate of atherogenesis. These factors include cigarette smoking, hypertension, and diabetes. In the absence of some LDL elevation, these risk factors generally are not accompanied by significant rates of ASCVD (8); however, when LDL levels begin to rise, the process of atherogenesis is accelerated. The precise mechanisms whereby other risk factors promote atherosclerosis have not been determined with certain. Likely, multiple mechanisms are involved for each risk factor.

LDL is not the only atherogenic lipoprotein. Another category includes several species of triglyceride-rich

---

[1] **Abbreviations: Apo B,** apolipoprotein B; **ASCVD,** atherosclerotic cardiovascular disease; **BMI,** body mass index; **CETP,** cholesterol ester transfer protein; **CHD,** coronary heart disease; **ERT,** estrogen replacement therapy; **FCR,** fractional catabolic rate; **FDB,** familial defective apolipoprotein B-100; **FFA,** free fatty acid; **FH,** familial hypercholesterolemia; **HDL,** high-density lipoprotein; **HDL-C,** high-density lipoprotein cholesterol; **HTGL,** hepatic triglyceride lipase; **LDL,** low-density lipoprotein; **LDL-C,** low-density lipoprotein cholesterol; **LPL,** lipoprotein lipase; **MTP,** microsomal lipid transfer protein; **NCEP,** National Cholesterol Education Program; **PPAR,** peroxisome proliferation activator receptor; **TGRLP,** triglyceride-rich lipoprotein; **TZD,** thiazoladinedione; **VLDL,** very-low-density lipoprotein.

lipoproteins (TGRLPs) (2). Those TGRLPs produced by the liver are VLDLs. They also contain cholesterol ester and ApoB and appear to promote atherogenesis independently of LDL. Another TGRLP is the chylomicron, which carries the triglyceride of newly absorbed fat. Chylomicrons may not be atherogenic, but some investigators believe that after removal of excess triglyceride, the chylomicron "remnant" has some potential to produce atherosclerosis. Finally, another species of lipoprotein is high-density lipoprotein (HDL). This lipoprotein also contains cholesterol, but HDL does not promote atherosclerosis; in fact, high serum levels of HDL may protect against ASCVD in several ways (2).

PUBLIC HEALTH PREVENTION OF ATHEROSCLEROTIC CARDIOVASCULAR DISEASE

The US public, as well as populations of other developed nations, carries a heavy burden of ASCVD. The development of atherosclerosis is a slow but progressive process throughout life. Two strategies exist for the prevention of ASCVD. The public health strategy is aimed at *primary prevention* of atherosclerosis. This aim is best achieved by reducing the risk factors for ASCVD in the public at large (2). Based on five large cohort studies conducted in the United States, Stamler and associates (9) concluded that "for individuals with favorable levels of cholesterol and blood pressure who do not smoke and do not have diabetes, MI (myocardial infarction), or ECG (electrocardiogram) abnormalities, long-term mortality is much lower and longevity is much greater. A substantial increase in the proportion of the population at lifetime low risk could contribute decisively to ending the CHD [coronary heart disease] epidemic." In agreement, an international study known as INTERHEART, reported that nine preventable risk factors account for 90% of all heart attacks:

- Smoking
- Abnormal cholesterol
- Diabetes
- High blood pressure
- Stress
- Abdominal obesity
- Sedentary lifestyle
- Eating too few fruits and vegetables
- Abstaining from alcohol

The INTERHEART study assessed 15,152 people who had had a first heart attack and 14,820 controls who had not, but who were from the same age group, gender, and city. The nine major risk factors were found to be the same across ethnic groups and in different areas of the world (10).

Risk factor reduction includes (a) prevention or cessation of cigarette smoking, (b) consumption of risk-reducing ("heart-healthy") foods, (c) weight control, and (d) regular physical activity. In the United States, smoking has declined, but it still remains well above an acceptable

level. Foods that are mostly heart healthy are consumed by a portion of the public, but many people continue to eat in ways that promote atherosclerosis. Worse, obesity has become epidemic in the US public and threatens to wipe out much of the reduction in ASCVD that has been achieved since the 1980s. Moreover, the public as a whole continues to be too sedentary, and those who do perform optimal amounts of exercise may do so sporadically. A final component of the public health strategy is for adults to be checked on a regular basis for risk factors (serum lipoproteins and blood pressure). Some persons are genetically susceptible to developing risk factors, and clinical intervention may be required at some stage of life. Although this chapter emphasizes the clinical management of lipid risk factors, nutrition is crucial in the primordial prevention of risk factors for reducing the burden of ASCVD in the public.

HYPERCHOLESTEROLEMIA

The term *hypercholesterolemia* is used in the context of this chapter has an isolated elevation of serum LDL-C. The NCEP (1, 2) classifies LDL-C according to the degree of severity, as shown in Table 67.1. In the current review, this classification is modified slightly and is expressed in terms of hypercholesterolemia. According to this latter classification, hypercholesterolemia can be divided into mild, moderate, and severe. Lower ranges of serum LDL-C can be separated into optimal and near optimal. Optimal levels of LDL-C are those associated with minimal risk for ASCVD. Near-optimal LDL-C levels, although higher than optimal, are typically accompanied by relatively low rates of ASCVD, except when other risk factors are present.

Causes

Optimal Low-Density Lipoprotein Cholesterol Levels

Serum LDL-C levels lower than 100 mg/dL (2.6 mmol/L, or total cholesterol levels typically lower than 160 mg/dL, 4.1 mmol/L) are considered optimal (2). Within this range, atherosclerosis develops at a very slow rate; consequently,

TABLE 67.1. CLASSIFICATION OF SERUM LOW-DENSITY LIPOPROTEIN CHOLESTEROL

CLASSIFICATION CATEGORY	LOW-DENSITY LIPOPROTEIN-CHOLESTEROL (mg/dL)	HYPERCHOLESTEROLEMIA
"Optimal"	<100	
Near optimal	100–129	
Borderline-high	130–159	Mild
High	160–189	Moderate
Very high	>190	Severe

the risk for ASCVD is very low. Optimal serum cholesterol levels are often present in children and young adults, but they also are common in middle-aged and older persons in various populations around the world (e.g., rural Asia). In these latter populations, intakes of saturated fatty acids and cholesterol typically are very low, daily physical activity is high, and body fat content is low; this combination of dietary and life habits apparently keeps serum cholesterol levels in the optimal range throughout life. The very low rates of atherosclerotic disease in these populations appear to demonstrate the benefit of keeping serum cholesterol levels low (8). Some investigators have suggested that very low serum cholesterol levels in these populations can be explained by genetic factors; even if so, cholesterol rises when changes in eating and exercise habits change, even in populations that historically have expressed very low cholesterol levels (11).

Not only does an elevated serum LDL-C promote atherogenesis, but also restoration of LDL-C levels to the optimal range markedly reduces the risk of ASCVD, even in persons who already have advanced atherosclerotic disease (3, 4, 6). For example, in patients who have established ASCVD, reducing serum cholesterol levels to near the optimal range decreases the rate of recurrent myocardial infarction (3, 4, 6). Similar risk reduction follows a therapeutic lowering of serum cholesterol levels in hypercholesterolemic patients who have not yet developed ASCVD (5, 7). Other clinical studies (12), in which coronary arteries were visualized directly by angiography, revealed that reducing serum LDL-C retards progression of coronary atherosclerosis. Therefore, an elevation of LDL-C contributes to the initiation and progression of coronary atherosclerosis; but of equal importance, elevated LDL-C plays a critical role later in the course of atherosclerotic disease by predisposing to acute coronary events, such as myocardial infarction. Thus, a growing recognition exists that optimal cholesterol levels convey substantial protection against development of ASCVD.

Near-Optimal Low-Density Lipoprotein Cholesterol Levels

The NCEP (1, 2) defines an LDL-C range of 100 to 129 mg/dL as near optimal. Although near-optimal levels of LDL-C may still promote atherogenesis, compared with optimal levels, premature ASCVD (i.e., onset of ASCVD before age 65 years), is relatively uncommon in this LDL-C range in the absence of other ASCVD risk factors (13). For most adults in the United States who live in an urbanized setting, it is unrealistic to expect cholesterol levels to remain throughout life at optimal levels (e.g., LDL-C <100 mg/dL). Serum LDL-C levels in a somewhat higher range, but still near optimal, can be produced by small incremental increases in dietary saturated fatty acids and cholesterol, a modest excess in body fat, and failure to maintain vigorous physical activity (14). Premature ASCVD

nonetheless is relatively uncommon in people who have near-optimal LDL-C concentrations, provided they avoid cigarette smoking and maintain normal blood pressure (13). It is a major goal of the NCEP to bring about a change in serum cholesterol levels in the US public so a greater proportion of the population achieves and sustains cholesterol concentrations in this near-optimal zone (15). At present, almost half of all US adults have LDL-C levels lower than 130 mg/dL (2, 16). Fortunately, serum cholesterol levels in the general public have been declining since the 1980s (16); as a result, a larger fraction of the population has near-optimal LDL-C concentrations, compared with the past.

Dietary Prevention of Hypercholesterolemia: Maintenance of Optimal or Near-Optimal LDL-C Levels. An important public health goal for adults of the general population is to keep LDL-C levels in a safer range (<130 mg/dL), that is, to prevent the development of hypercholesterolemia. The reduction in intakes of saturated fatty acids and cholesterol that has occurred since the 1980s in the United States has increased the proportion of the general population with desirable cholesterol levels. Table 67.2 compares current macronutrient intakes in the US public (17) with intakes currently recommended by government-sponsored panels (15, 18). If population mean intakes of saturated fatty acids and cholesterol could be reduced to recommended levels, a greater proportion of the population would achieve LDL-C levels in the optimal or near-optimal range.

Another cause of higher cholesterol levels is being overweight. Investigators have estimated that the gain of weight that typically occurs with aging accounts for a rise in serum cholesterol of approximately 25 mg/dL (14). The average US adult gains about 10 kg (22 lb) between ages 20 and 50 years. A significant increase in serum cholesterol levels is one consequence of this weight gain (19, 20). Thus,

TABLE 67.2. CURRENT MACRONUTRIENT INTAKES IN THE UNITED STATES PUBLIC

	RECOMMENDED INTAKE[a]	CURRENT AMERICAN INTAKE[b]
	PERCENTAGE OF TOTAL CALORIES (%)	
Total fat	20–35	33–35
Cholesterol-raising fatty acids:		
Saturated	<10	11–15
Trans	≈1[c]	2–5
Monounsaturated fatty acids	10–15	≈14
Polyunsaturated fatty acids	<10	≈6
Carbohydrate	55	≈50
Protein	15	≈15
Cholesterol (mg/d)	<300	250–350

[a]Recommended macronutrient intakes (13, 16).
[b]Values approximated from existing data (15).
[c]Trans fatty acids should be kept as low as feasible.

weight control, particularly reduction in the amount of weight gained with aging, is an important goal in the public health prevention of hypercholesterolemia. The gain of weight with aging results from two factors: (a) decline of metabolic rate with aging and (b) reduction in physical activity. The decline of metabolic rate results largely from a decrease in muscle mass (21), which likewise is caused in part by a reduction in physical activity. Although increased physical activity that does not produce weight loss does not significantly lower cholesterol levels, maintenance of a high level of exercise sufficient to prevent weight gain contributes to lower serum cholesterol levels. In the majority of persons, however, maintenance of a moderate level of physical activity is not enough to prevent an increase in body weight with aging; some reduction in caloric intake is also required.

In spite of the success among US residents in reducing serum cholesterol levels through a decrease in the intake of saturated fatty acids and cholesterol, the public has not been successful in weight control. Obesity has increased progressively in the United States. Table 67.3 shows the proportion of the population within each category of body mass index (BMI) (22). A normal BMI is 25 kg/m². In this category, cholesterol levels are at their lowest (20, 21). Persons with BMIs in the ranges of 25 to 29.9 kg/m² and greater than or equal to 30 kg/m² are called overweight and obese, respectively. As noted in Table 67.3, most persons in the United States fall into the overweight/obese range. Obesity stands in the way of achieving desirable serum cholesterol levels for many persons.

Mild Hypercholesterolemia

About 25% of US adults have mild hypercholesterolemia (LDL-C, 130 to 159 mg/dL) (2). These levels are called borderline high by the NCEP. In middle-aged adults with mild hypercholesterolemia, the risk of ASCVD in the short term (5–10 years) is increased by about 1.5 times above that accompanying serum cholesterol levels in the desirable range (13). Analyses suggest that, over a lifetime, the risk differential is even greater; that is, in the presence of mild hypercholesterolemia, the long-term (30–40 years) risk is three to four times greater than that associated with desirable cholesterol levels (23, 24).

TABLE 67.3. DISTRIBUTION OF BODY MASS INDEXES IN THE UNITED STATES PUBLIC

WEIGHT CATEGORY	BODY MASS INDEX[a] (kg/m²)	MEN (%)	WOMEN (%)
Normal	<25	31.2	38.4
Overweight	25–29.9	41.2	42.8
Obese	≥30	27.6	33.2

[a]Distribution of body mass indexes estimated from the data of Hedley et al. (22).

In the majority of persons, several causative factors underlie mild hypercholesterolemia (14). Those implicated include (a) diets high in cholesterol, (b) diets high in cholesterol-raising fatty acids (saturated fatty acids and *trans*-fatty acids), (c) increases in body weight with aging, (d) aging per se, (e) genetic factors, and (f) loss of estrogens in postmenopausal women. Each of these factors is worthy of some attention. If a greater portion of the public is going to achieve desirable cholesterol levels, it will be necessary to modify several of these factors. The effects of two factors—genetics and aging pre se—cannot be mitigated short of treatment with cholesterol-lowering drugs; however, the other factors can be changed by modifying life habits.

Genetic Contribution to Mild Hypercholesterolemia. Some people appear to be unusually susceptible to higher serum cholesterol levels. In addition, the broad range of serum cholesterol concentrations in the general population suggests variability in genetic susceptibility. Genetic epidemiologists (25) have calculated that about 50% of the variation in cholesterol levels in the general population can be explained by polymorphism in the genes that influence serum total cholesterol and LDL-C.

Genetic factors potentially regulate LDL-C levels at multiple control points. A discussion of these sites of control requires that we examine the origins and fates of serum LDL. LDL is derived from the catabolism of TGRLPs, which, in turn, are produced by the liver. The liver secretes TGRLP (e.g., VLDL) that contains mainly triglycerides in its core and three apolipoproteins in the surface coat: Apo B-100, Apo C, and Apo E. VLDL triglycerides are hydrolyzed by lipoprotein lipase (LPL), degrading VLDL to smaller TGRLP called VLDL remnants, whereas most Apo Cs are lost from VLDL particles during this process. VLDL remnants can either be take up by the liver (via LDL receptors) or be converted to LDL. Hepatic triglyceride lipase (HTGL) on the hepatic sinusoidal surface probably hydrolyzes the remaining triglycerides in VLDL remnants and causes the conversion of VLDL to LDL. The only apolipoprotein of LDL is Apo B-100, and it is Apo B-100 that is recognized by LDL receptors (26). Most LDL particles are removed via LDL receptors on liver cells (26). The synthesis of each of the factors that influence LDL levels is under genetic control and is subject to modification by genetic aberration.

One factor influencing LDL levels is the rate of formation of lipoproteins by the liver. Most lipoproteins made by the liver are rich in triglycerides; hence they are secreted as VLDL. The amount of hepatic triglyceride available for incorporation into VLDL may influence the rate of VLDL secretion. In cultured hepatocytes, supplying more fatty acids for triglyceride synthesis increases the number of VLDL particles secreted by the cells (27). The transfer of triglycerides into newly forming VLDL particles is mediated by microsomal lipid transfer protein (MTP) (28). This protein shuttles both triglyceride and phospholipid into

VLDL particles. In patients with a congenital absence of MTP, VLDL particles do not mature; affected persons consequently manifest an absence of Apo B–containing lipoproteins in the circulation (abetalipoproteinemia) (28). The rate of formation of Apo B-100 itself could affect the rate of VLDL secretion. At the other extreme, high serum levels of both cholesterol and triglycerides (combined hyperlipidemia) could result from excessive synthesis and secretion of Apo B-100 by the liver (29). Unfortunately, available methodology limits precise measurements of these key parameters of Apo B-100 kinetics (30). Whether the availability of cholesterol in the liver influences the rate of VLDL secretion also remains to be determined. In laboratory animals, high doses of drugs that inhibit cholesterol synthesis also reduce VLDL secretion rates, but whether the usual doses of these drugs used in humans have this same effect is uncertain. In summary, multiple factors under genetic control undoubtedly affect the assembly and secretion of hepatic VLDL. Because LDL is derived from VLDL, secretion rates of VLDL can influence LDL levels (14, 29). Consequently, a genetic aberration leading to overproduction of Apo B–containing lipoproteins by the liver may be one cause of hypercholesterolemia.

Rates of removal of LDL from the circulation also influence LDL-C levels. The process of clearance of LDL has been extensively studied. Most circulating LDL particles are removed via LDL receptors that are located on liver cells (26). LDL receptors specifically bind Apo B-100. Variation in the number of LDL receptors expressed on liver cells is a major determinant of serum LDL-C levels. A critical factor controlling the expression of hepatic LDL receptors is the amount of cholesterol in the liver cell (26). When the cholesterol content of the liver rises, synthesis of LDL receptors is reduced. Much of the detailed molecular mechanism responsible for the link between hepatic cholesterol content and LDL-receptor synthesis has been elucidated (31). Increased availability of cholesterol in the liver has the opposite effect, namely, it suppresses LDL-receptor activity. Steady-state amounts of cholesterol in the liver cells depend on synthesis rates of cholesterol, secretion rates of cholesterol into bile, and conversion rates of cholesterol into bile acids (14). All these metabolic pathways are under genetic regulation, and genetic polymorphism of multiple proteins regulating these pathways could enhance availability of intracellular cholesterol and hence LDL-receptor expression (31). Future research may uncover various genetic polymorphisms in the complex system of LDL-receptor regulation that lead to higher LDL-C levels. Genetic polymorphism probably accounts for much of the variability in LDL-C levels in the US public, and some polymorphisms undoubtedly underlie the development of mild hypercholesterolemia.

Rise of Cholesterol Levels with Age. In the United States, between ages 20 and 50 years, the average serum total cholesterol concentration rises by about 40 to 50 mg/dL

(2, 14). About half of this increase apparently results from increasing body weight, but another portion seems to be linked to aging per se (32, 33). The aging process is accompanied by delayed clearance of LDL from the circulation; presumably, the complex mechanisms regulating LDL-receptor function become less efficient with aging. For example, cholesterol disposal by the liver may be slightly retarded with age, thus leading to an increased hepatic cholesterol content. Alternatively, the synthesis of LDL receptors may become sluggish, causing a decrease in LDL-receptor expression. However, a curious observation has been made: serum cholesterol levels do not rise progressively from middle age into older age (2). Most of the increase in serum cholesterol levels occurs between ages 20 and 50 years; thereafter, LDL-C levels plateau or even decline somewhat. This finding suggests that external factors, such as weight gain, play a central role in the age-related increase in serum cholesterol levels.

Obesity and the Rise of Cholesterol with Aging. A strong correlation exists between changes in serum cholesterol concentrations and changes in body weight from young adulthood into middle age (19, 20). Most of the weight gain in adults occurs between ages 20 and 50 years; during this same period, serum cholesterol concentrations rise. Although epidemiologic studies indicate that serum cholesterol levels rise with aging even in persons who show little weight gain (19, 20), those who gain more weight manifest greater increments in serum cholesterol. The increase of serum cholesterol with aging occurs in both VLDL and LDL fractions (19, 20); this combined change further suggests an obesity effect. This is because the major influence of obesity on lipoprotein metabolism is on the input pathway (34, 35), and isotope kinetic studies suggest that obesity induces overproduction of hepatic VLDL (34, 35). Consequently the rise in LDL-C levels with increasing body weight is likely to be secondary to increased secretion of VLDL, followed by increased conversion of VLDL to LDL. Thus, it is not surprising that both VLDL and LDL levels rise concomitantly with increasing obesity.

Cholesterol-Raising Fatty Acids. Two classes of dietary fatty acids can raise serum cholesterol levels: saturated fatty acids (36), and *trans*-monounsaturated fatty acids (37, 38) (see Chapter 5 for a detailed discussion of fatty acids). Increments in total cholesterol levels that are induced by these fatty acids occur largely in the LDL fraction. Specifically, these fatty acids elevate LDL-C concentrations relative to other nutrients: polyunsaturated fatty acids, *cis*-monounsaturated fatty acids, and carbohydrates (36). Because these last nutrients do not raise LDL-C levels, they are called neutral. Although saturated fatty acids as a class raise serum LDL levels, as compared with neutral nutrients, even the different types of saturates differ in their influence on LDL-C levels. The saturated fatty acid present in the largest quantities in the diet is palmitic acid (C16:0). As shown in a review of the literature, palmitic acid is a potent cholesterol-raising fatty acid (36). Another saturated acid, myristic acid (C14:0), is present in lesser amounts in the diet, but it appears to be even more potent than palmitic acid in elevating serum LDL-C (39). Investigations have revealed that a shorter species of long-chain saturated fatty acid, lauric acid (C12:0) (39), and the medium-chain fatty acids, C10:0 and C8:0 (41), also raise serum LDL-C levels, although somewhat less so than palmitic acid. Still another saturated fatty acid, stearic acid (C18:0), does not increase LDL-C levels as compared with the effect of unsaturated fatty acids (42, 43). This fatty acid seemingly is rapidly converted into oleic acid (C18:1) once it enters the body (44). Hence, stearic acid, like oleic acid, is a neutral fatty acid with respect to its effects on LDL-C levels.

Although the saturated fatty acids comprise most of the cholesterol-raising fatty acids in the diet, studies indicate that *trans*-monounsaturated fatty acids also increase LDL levels (37, 38, 45). *Trans*-fatty acids are produced by hydrogenation of vegetable oils. The *trans* configuration of their double bonds gives them structural properties similar to those of saturated fatty acids, and this may explain their ability to raise serum LDL concentrations. In the US diet, *trans*-fatty acids account for only about one fourth as much energy intake compared with saturated fatty acids. However, their role as a contributor to mild hypercholesterolemia is nonetheless significant and should not be discounted.

The mechanisms whereby cholesterol-raising fatty acids elevate the serum LDL-C remain to be fully elucidated. However, investigations in animal models point to a suppression of LDL-receptor activity as the primary site of action (46). One hypothesis holds that these fatty acids interfere with the esterification of cholesterol in the liver (47), likely by interfering with the esterifying enzyme, acyl-coenzyme A:cholesterol acyltransferase. If saturated fatty acids retard the formation of cholesterol esters in the liver, more unesterified cholesterol will be left available to activate suppression of LDL-receptor activity. Other mechanisms also have been proposed to explain the action of saturated fatty acids to raise cholesterol levels, but most data support the concept that by one means or another they suppress the activity of LDL receptors.

Dietary Cholesterol. In many animal models, high intakes of cholesterol exert a powerful hypercholesterolemic action (48, 49). The mechanism of this response seems straightforward. When the diet is enriched with cholesterol, hepatic cholesterol content rises, and this, in turn, downregulates LDL-receptor synthesis. The same mechanism presumably pertains in humans. However, humans are less susceptible to the hypercholesterolemic action of dietary cholesterol than are many animal models (50). Increasing dietary cholesterol apparently fails to induce such marked rises in unesterified cholesterol concentrations in the human liver, for several possible reasons. First, less than half of human dietary cholesterol is absorbed, and this limits its availability to the liver. Moreover, humans

may be more efficient in esterifying cholesterol in hepatocytes or secreting it into bile; both mechanisms would reduce the amount of unesterified cholesterol in liver cells. In spite of these protective mechanisms, increasing the amount of cholesterol in the diet definitely raises LDL-C concentrations in many people, and a relatively high intake of cholesterol in the US diet contributes to the common occurrence of mild hypercholesterolemia in the general population.

Rise of Cholesterol after the Menopause. Loss of estrogens after the menopause leads to an increase of serum cholesterol levels in many women (2, 14). Estrogens stimulate LDL-receptor synthesis in several animal models (51), and the same response presumably occurs in humans. After the menopause and with loss of estrogens, LDL-receptor activity falls. This decline in receptor function and consequent rise in LDL-C levels can be reversed by estrogen replacement therapy (ERT) after the menopause (52).

Moderate Hypercholesterolemia

Moderate hypercholesterolemia describes total cholesterol levels in the range of 240 to 300 mg/dL, and more specifically, serum LDL-C levels in the range from 160 to 219 mg/dL (1, 2). These higher cholesterol levels produce a still greater increment in ASCVD risk. Approximately 20% of US adults have moderate hypercholesterolemia (2). The causes of moderate elevations of LDL-C are similar to those of mild hypercholesterolemia, except genetic factors play an increasingly dominant role. For most people with moderate hypercholesterolemia, modifying the diet alone will not reduce cholesterol levels to the desirable range; instead, the responsible genetic factors will maintain some elevation in LDL. Studies from our laboratory have identified several different patterns of LDL metabolism that underlie a rise in LDL-C from a range of mild to moderately elevated LDL-C (14, 53). These patterns include (a) a higher rate of formation of LDL, (b) a lower fractional clearance rate for LDL, and (c) an enrichment of LDL particles with cholesterol ester. The mechanisms underlying each of these factors are examined briefly.

Overproduction of Low-Density Lipoproteins. In patients with moderate hypercholesterolemia, two potential mechanisms underlie overproduction of LDL: (a) an increased input of VLDL particles and (b) a reduced uptake of VLDL remnants by the liver (14, 53). Both changes produce increased conversion of VLDL to LDL. Isotope kinetic studies (53) suggest that either mechanism can occur in persons with moderate hypercholesterolemia. These mechanisms seemingly can be distinguished by differences in fractional catabolic rates (FCRs) for LDL. In persons who have overproduction of VLDL particles, input rates for LDL are high, whereas FCRs for LDL are relatively low. Low FCRs for LDL occur because LDL receptors are relatively overloaded with an excess of lipoprotein particles, thus reducing the fractional clearance of LDL. Conversely, in persons who have decreased uptake of VLDL remnants, high rates of input of LDL are combined with increased FCRs for LDL. High inputs of LDL result from an increased fractional rate of conversion of VLDL to LDL, whereas high FCRs for LDL can be explained by an increased availability of LDL receptors; the latter occurs because of reduced uptake of VLDL remnants by LDL receptors. Our studies (52) suggest that the first pattern, that is, overproduction of lipoprotein particles, probably occurs because of heightened genetic sensitivity to the effects of mild obesity. The mechanism for the second type, that is, reduced remnant uptake and increased conversion of VLDL to LDL, has not been determined.

Reduced Clearance of Low-Density Lipoproteins. Another pattern of LDL metabolism responsible for moderate hypercholesterolemia is a reduced fractional clearance of LDL. This abnormality presumably reflects a decreased availability of LDL receptors (14, 52). Some of the dietary or acquired factors listed before can suppress the synthesis of LDL receptors. In patients with moderate hypercholesterolemia, however, genetic factors presumably come increasingly into play. The regulation of LDL-receptor expression is complex, and the genetic aberrations underlying a moderately reduced synthesis of LDL-receptors have not been elucidated. A few persons may have mutations in the gene encoding for LDL receptors (54), although such mutations usually produce severe hypercholesterolemia. Polymorphisms in other genes that indirectly influence LDL receptor synthesis are more likely candidates to explain moderate hypercholesterolemia, but few of these polymorphisms have been discovered.

Cholesterol-Enriched Low-Density Lipoproteins. Some persons have moderately elevated serum LDL-C concentrations because their LDL particles contain excessive amounts of cholesterol ester (14, 55). The reasons for this compositional change are not known. Cholesterol ester-enriched LDL particles are more likely to occur in persons who have relatively low FCRs for LDL; in such persons, the slow clearance of LDL may allow more time for cholesterol esters to enter LDL particles through the action of cholesterol ester transfer protein (CETP) (56, 57). In patients without a reduced clearance rate for LDL, an increased serum concentration of CETP may account for cholesterol ester-enriched LDL particles (57).

Severe Hypercholesterolemia

A small portion of the population has severe hypercholesterolemia, defined as serum LDL-C levels of 220 mg/dL or higher. Most patients with severe hypercholesterolemia have a reduced activity of LDL receptors, although the elevation in LDL-C concentrations may be accentuated in some persons by overproduction of lipoproteins by the liver or by enrichment of LDL particles with cholesterol (14, 53). Almost certainly, genetic factors play the predominant role

in the development of severe hypercholesterolemia; in most patients of this type, however, the precise genetic defects have not been elucidated.

A few severely hypercholesterolemic patients have mutations in the gene encoding for the LDL receptor. This genetic abnormality produces the condition called familial hypercholesterolemia (FH) (26). Affected patients can have either heterozygous FH or homozygous FH, depending on whether one or both alleles for the LDL-receptor gene are defective. Heterozygous FH occurs in one in 500 people, whereas homozygous FH is present once in 1,000,000 people. LDL-C is elevated to approximately twice normal levels in heterozygous FH and is fourfold elevated in homozygous FH. A related disorder is called familial defective Apo B-100 (FDB) (58, 59). This form of hypercholesterolemia is characterized by a defect in the structure of Apo B-100 such that it fails to bind normally to LDL receptors; consequently, the clearance of LDL from the circulation is retarded. Patients with FDB can have either moderate or severe hypercholesterolemia.

Management

Two general approaches to clinically elevated levels of LDL-C are *therapeutic lifestyle change* and *drug therapy.* Before exploring specific conditions that require clinical management of persons with elevated LDL-C, both lifestyle and drug modalities can be reviewed.

Lifestyle Therapies

Dietary Fat and Cholesterol. Diet composition can be modified to conform to the NCEP cholesterol-lowering diet (1, 2) (Table 67.4). The essential features of this diet are intakes of saturated fatty acids of less than 7% (*trans*-fatty acids should be kept as low as feasible), dietary cholesterol less than 200 mg/dL, and total fat 25 to 35%, with the balance of fatty acids coming from unsaturated fatty acids (monoene-to-polyene fatty acid ratio of approximately 2:1). Most persons with mild hypercholesterolemia in the United States exceed the recommendations for intake of saturated fatty acids and cholesterol. Reductions in nutrient intake to achieve the goals of the NCEP cholesterol-lowering diet

TABLE 67.4. NATIONAL CHOLESTEROL EDUCATION PROGRAM CHOLESTEROL-LOWERING DIET

NUTRIENT	PERCENT OF TOTAL CALORIES
Total fat	25–35
Saturated fatty acids[a]	<7
Monounsaturated fatty acids	11–17
Polyunsaturated fatty acids	<10
Carbohydrates	≥59–60
Protein	15
Cholesterol	<200 mg/d

[a] *Trans* fatty acids should be kept as low as feasible.

can be expected to produce a decrease in serum LDL-C levels of about 10% (59, 60).

About two thirds of saturated fatty acids in the US diet come from animal fats. Sources of animal fat include milk fat and meat fat. Milk fat is more hypercholesterolemic than meat fat because of its higher content of cholesterol-raising fatty acids (43). The remainder of saturated fatty acids in the diet comes from vegetable fats. Among the latter, the tropical oils (i.e., palm oil, coconut oil, and palm kernel oil) have a very high content of saturated fatty acids. Other vegetable oils have a lower content, but they still contribute some saturated fat to the diet. In recent years in the United States, the use of tropical oils by the food industry has decreased. A further reduction in saturated fatty acids in the US diet must come mainly through decreasing use of animal fats. Replacement of fatty meats, including fatty cuts of steak, hamburger, and processed meats, with leaner products is one appropriate way to decrease intake of saturated fatty acids. Replacement of traditional milk-based products (whole milk, butter, cream, ice cream, and cheese) with low-fat or fat-free milk products likewise will reduce consumption of saturated fatty acids. The goal for the general US public is to decrease dietary saturated fatty acids by at least one third.

Because *trans*-fatty acids are now known to belong to the category of cholesterol-raising fatty acids, these, too, must be reduced to achieve the goals of the Step I diet. Estimates of intakes of *trans*-fatty acids in the United States are variable, ranging from 2 to 5% of total calories; the average intake is about 3% of total calories. This percentage can be cut in half by avoidance of hard margarine as spreads and baked products containing shortenings. At present, commercially produced bakery goods and snack foods tend to be rich in *trans*-fatty acids. Thus, to promote cholesterol lowering, the food industry should make an effort to decrease the *trans* content of food products by modifying the types of fats used in their manufacture.

Numerous dietary reports have advocated low intakes of dietary fats (15–25% of total calories). Most of the fat calories in this diet should come from vegetable oils. Currently, there is a dispute over what is the most desirable percentage of calories from fat in the diet. Some investigators favor a higher fat content, such as 30 to 35% fat (61), whereas others advocate a lower intake, such as 15 to 20% fat (62). The argument in favor of a lower percentage of dietary fat is that lower-fat diets may promote weight reduction. Certainly, reducing the intake of animal fats without replacement will decrease the total caloric intake and thus promote weight reduction. Whether intakes of vegetables oils should be reduced is problematic. Maintaining a moderate intake of vegetable oils will help to sustain a relatively low level of serum triglycerides and a high level of HDL-cholesterol (HDL-C) (61). Assigning a higher priority to reducing the intake of high-sugar foods seems preferable to decreasing the intake of vegetable oils. The current recommendation of consuming 25 to 35% of total

calories mostly in the form of vegetable oils seems reasonable (1, 2).

A reduction in animal fats will also decrease cholesterol intake. This, too, will help to reduce serum LDL-C levels. Intakes of cholesterol are typically divided about equally among eggs, milk-based products, and meats. The current intake of cholesterol can be cut by one third to one half by keeping the intake of foods containing egg yolks low, by using low-fat or fat-free milk products, and by decreasing the intake of meat fats.

Low-Density Lipoprotein–Lowering Dietary Options. Other dietary factors can be employed to enhance LDL-C lowering beyond reducing saturated fatty acids, dietary cholesterol, and *trans*-fatty acids. One such class of factors consists of the plant stanols and sterols (see Chapter 6). These products, which typically are consumed in the esterified form in margarines, interfere with cholesterol absorption. An intake of approximately 2 g/day of stanol or sterol will reduce LDL-C levels by about 10% (63). In addition, nutritional studies have shown that higher intakes of soluble fiber and soy protein will produce incremental reductions in LDL-C levels (1, 2).

Obesity. The rise of body weight with aging contributes importantly to raising LDL-C levels (14, 19, 20). Consequently, weight reduction in people who are overweight also helps to restore serum LDL-C to a lower range. For many persons, reducing the intake of cholesterol and cholesterol-raising fatty acids isnot sufficient to obtain serum cholesterol levels in the near-optimal range, without concurrent weight reduction. Effective weight reduction usually requires a combination of calorie control and increased exercise. Many people with elevated LDL-C levels fall into the overweight category and on average consume about 300 calories/day more than is needed to maintain their BMI in a normal (or acceptable) range (19, 20). Eliminating this excess of calories should not be difficult for most people, but effective weight reduction requires a combination of continuous attention to body weight, a moderate reduction of food intake, and increased exercise. These simple rules can be followed for weight reduction in overweight/obese persons:

- Achieve a normal range BMI by losing 10% of body weight yearly until a normal BMI has been attained
- For the overweight category (BMI 25–29.9 kg/m^2), reduce caloric intake by 300 calories/day
- For the obese category (BMI ≥30 kg/m^2), reduce caloric intake by 500 calories/day

Certain foods should be a priority as targets for caloric restriction. Highest on the list for elimination are animal fats (milk fat and meat fat); their removal not only will decrease total caloric intake, but at the same time will lower serum cholesterol levels. To achieve weight loss, the animal fats removed from the diet must not be replaced by calories from other sources. Second on the priority list are high-sugar foods, such as soft drinks, desserts, candies, and cookies. High-sugar products, advertised as low in fat, have become popular in the United States. The increased use of these foods has offset much of the benefit derived from reduction in high-fat foods. Therefore, to achieve weight reduction, high-sugar foods must be curtailed as well. Third on the list are high-starch foods, such as breads, potatoes, rice, and pasta. When less desirable sources of calories of the first and second type are removed, care must be taken not to replace them with excessive intakes of high-starch foods. The same holds for replacement with vegetable oils. Although oils such as olive oil, canola oil, and soy bean oil produce a favorable lipoprotein pattern, when compared with saturated fatty acids, excess consumption of these oils provides excess calories and can prevent weight reduction.

Physical Activity. A second approach to weight reduction is to increase physical activity. Restoration of caloric balance required for desirable weight can be achieved in part through increased caloric expenditure associated with exercise. Suitable exercises include regular walking, swimming, biking, and competitive supports (2, 63). For purposes of caloric expenditure, aerobic exercise is preferable to weight training. The latter, however, is also useful in older persons to maintain muscle mass, to improve musculoskeletal function, and to prevent falls (63). The institution of an appropriate regimen of regular exercise that will expend excess calories is therefore an integral element in the management of elevated LDL-C. Examples of moderate exercise regimens that can assist in achieving and sustaining weight reduction are listed in Table 67.5.

Other Antiatherogenic Nutrients. An important question is whether some nutrients will reduce the risk of ASCVD independently of the caloric content and their effects on LDL-C levels. The one category of foods that can be safely increased is fruits and colored vegetables (65). These products are relatively low in calories and are rich in other nutrients; the latter include antioxidants

along with fiber, phytoestrogens, phytosterols, polyphenols, carotenoids, indoles, quinones, and organosulfur compounds. Epidemiologic studies and investigations in laboratory animals suggest that many of these substances may protect against ASCVD, stroke, or cancer (64). There also is interest in the possibility that supplemental antioxidants, especially vitamin E and vitamin C, will give added protection against ASCVD or cancer (67). Although studies of several types support this possibility, a benefit of antioxidant supplements has not been proved through controlled clinical trials. In fact, recent clinical trials do not support the efficacy of antioxidant supplements for reducing ASCVD events over a period of 5 years (68). In many persons with hypercholesterolemia, elevated blood pressure is a concomitant risk factor. A reduction in salt intake combined with an increased consumption of potassium derived from fruits and vegetables may reduce the risk of ASCVD by decreasing blood pressure (69).

Maximal Therapeutic Lifestyle Change. Through a combination of dietary and lifestyle change, it should be possible to achieve substantial risk reduction for ASCVD, short of drug therapy. The features of maximal lifestyle change are shown in Table 67.6. Any person who enters clinical management for risk factor reduction should be urged to adopt these changes, whether drug therapy is employed or not. These changes target several risk factors besides elevated LDL-C, and, in addition, changes in lifestyle factors will reduce the risk of ASCVD though other mechanisms. Thus, smoking cessation in smokers will reduce the risk of ASCVD events by at least 20 to 30%, and perhaps more (70, 71). Reductions in intakes of saturated fatty acids and cholesterol will lower LDL-C levels by at least 10% in most people (2). Additional LDL-C lowering can be obtained by adding plant stanol/sterols (2 g/day) and 5 to 10 g/day of viscous fiber to the diet. Weight reduction in overweight or obese persons will produce further LDL-C lowering. A moderate dose of a bile acid sequestrant can achieve a 10 to 15% lowering of LDL-C; although bile acid sequestrants are listed among drugs for LDL lowering, they are nonsystemic agents and can be used as part of lifestyle change. Maximal lifestyle change further can target blood pressure to achieve additional risk reduction. The impact of lifestyle change has been detailed in recent national guidelines for blood pressure management (72). Weight reduction lowers blood pressure, as does moderation of alcohol intake. The same is true for a reduction of dietary salt and increased intakes of fruits and vegetables. Finally, regular physical activity appears to reduce the risk of ASCVD independently of other lifestyle changes; the mechanisms underlying this benefit likely are multiple.

Drug Therapies

The major LDL-lowering drugs currently available are 3-hydroxy-3-methylglutaryl (HMG)-CoA reductase inhibitors

---

TABLE 67.5. EXAMPLES OF MODERATE PHYSICAL ACTIVITY

Brisk walking (3–4 mph) for 30–40 min
Swimming: laps for 20 min
Bicycling for pleasure or transportation, 5 mi in 30 min
Volleyball (noncompetitive) for 45 min
Raking leaves for 30 min
Moderate lawn mowing (push a powered mower) for 30 min
Home care: heavy cleaning
Basketball for 15–20 mins
Golf: pulling a cart or carrying clubs
Social dancing for 30 mins

From National Cholesterol Education Program (NCEP) Expert Panel on Detection, Evaluation, and Treatment of High Blood Cholesterol in Adults (Adult Treatment Panel III). Third report of the National Cholesterol Education Program (NCEP) Expert Panel on Detection, Evaluation, and Treatment of High Blood Cholesterol in Adults (Adult Treatment Panel III) final report. Circulation 2002;106:3143–421, with permission.

TABLE 67.6. MAXIMAL NONDRUG THERAPY AND APPROXIMATE ASCVD RISK REDUCTION*

THERAPEUTIC TARGET	LIFESTYLE CHANGE	APPROXIMATE LDL-C REDUCTION	APPROXIMATE SBP REDUCTION	APPROXIMATE ASCVD RISK REDUCTION
Cigarette smoking	Complete smoking cessation			≥20%
Saturated fat	Reduce saturated fat to <7% of calories	8–10%		>8–10%
Dietary cholesterol	Reduce dietary cholesterol to <200 mg/d	3–5%		>3%
Plant stanols/sterols	Add plant stanols/sterols 2 g/d	6–10%		>6%
Dietary fiber	Viscous fiber 5–10 g/d	3–5%		>3%
Bile acid sequestrants	Low-dose bile acid sequestrants	10–15%[a]		>10%
Weight reduction	Weight reduction 10-lb weight loss	5–8%	5–10 mm Hg	>5% (LDL-C) >5% (SBP)
		Total LDL–C lowering 25–35%		
Physical activity	Moderate exercise 30 min/d		4–9 mm Hg	>10% (some due to BP change)
Dietary salt	Reduction of dietary salt <2 g/d		2–8 mm Hg	>5%
Other nutrients	Increased fruits and vegetables (e.g., DASH diet) 5 servings/d		8–14 mm Hg	>10%
Alcohol	Moderation of alcohol intake		2–4 mm Hg	>3%
			Total BP lowering >10 mm Hg	≥10% reduction in ASCVD including stroke
				Total ASCVD risk reduction >40%

ASCVD, atherosclerotic cardiovascular disease; BP, blood pressure; LDL-C, low-density lipoprotein cholesterol; SBP, systolic blood pressure.
[a] Low dose bile acid sequestrant is a nonsystemic agent that can be classified as a drug.

Data from National Cholesterol Education Program (NCEP) Expert Panel on Detection, Evaluation, and Treatment of High Blood Cholesterol in Adults (Adult Treatment Panel III). Third report of the National Cholesterol Education Program (NCEP) Expert Panel on Detection, Evaluation, and Treatment of High Blood Cholesterol in Adults (Adult Treatment Panel III) final report. Circulation 2002;106:3143–421; and Chobanian AV, Bakris GL, Black HR et al. Hypertension 2003;42:1206–52.

(statins), bile acid sequestrants, and ezetimibe. The essential characteristics of these drugs are briefly reviewed in the following sections.

3-Hydroxy-3-methylglutaryl-Coenzyme A Reductase Inhibitors (Statins). Six statins are available for treatment of elevated LDL-C; the standard doses of these statins are listed in Table 67.7 (73, 74). At these doses, LDL-C levels are reduced by approximately 30 to 40%. These drugs inhibit cholesterol synthesis in the liver and thereby raise the activity of LDL-receptors. All statins are

TABLE 67.7. LOW-DENSITY LIPOPROTEIN CHOLESTEROL AVERAGE REDUCTION WITH STANDARD DOSES OF CURRENTLY AVAILABLE STATINS

DRUG	DOSE (mg/d)	LOW-DENSITY LIPOPROTEIN REDUCTION (%)
Atorvastatin	10[a]	39
Lovastatin	40[a]	31
Pravastatin	40[a]	34
Simvastatin	20–40[a]	35–41
Fluvastatin	40–80	25–31
Rosuvastatin	5–10[b]	39–45

[a] All these are available at doses up to 80 mg.
[b] Doses available up to 40 mg.

identical in mechanism but differ in dose-response curves. The major side effect of statins is myopathy, which can occasionally occur at high doses of statins or in persons who are susceptible to this side effect. Many controlled clinical trials (2–7) have documented that LDL lowering using statin therapy reduces the risk of major ASCVD events.

Bile Acid Sequestrants. Three bile acid sequestrants can be used in clinical practice: cholestyramine, colestipol, and colesevelam. These agents interfere with the absorption of bile acids by the intestine; this action enhances conversion of cholesterol into bile acids in the liver, reduces hepatic cholesterol content, and enhances the activity of LDL receptors (75). These drugs lower LDL-C by about 15%. The major side effects of bile acid sequestrants are gastrointestinal, notably constipation. Colesevelam may produce less constipation than the other sequestrants. One major clinical trial (76, 77) documents the efficacy of sequestrants for reducing the risk of CHD.

Ezetimibe. This drug inhibits the absorption of cholesterol in the intestine (78). It thereby reduces LDL-C by about 15 to 20%. Although experience with this drug is limited, to date it has not been associated with significant side effects. No clinical trials are available to document its efficacy for reducing the risk of ASCVD events.

Combined Drug Therapy. When two LDL-lowering drugs are combined, the reduction of LDL-C levels is greater than obtained with either drug alone (79). In clinical practice, a bile acid sequestrant or ezetimibe has increasingly been used in combination with statins to obtain an approximately 50% reduction in LDL-C levels.

Estrogens. In postmenopausal women, consideration is often given to ERT. Estrogens partially restore LDL-receptor activity that normally declines after the menopause (52). ERT thus can reduce serum LDL-C levels by 10 to 15%. Although ERT can lower LDL-C levels, it is no longer recommended as a treatment for high LDL-C levels. This is because recent clinical trials suggested that the side effects of ERT may outweigh any of the benefits of ERT for reduction of risk for ASCVD (2). If ERT is indicated for other clinical reasons, such is a judgment call of a qualified clinician. However, the modest benefits of ERT on serum lipoproteins do not justify their use for this purpose because of the associated risk.

Treatment Algorithm for Elevated Low-Density Lipoprotein Cholesterol

The NCEP (2, 80) provides treatment algorithms for elevated LDL-C (Table 67.8). Management of elevated LDL-C is predicated on initial assessment of risk for ASCVD, which will define type and intensity of treatment. This table shows treatment goals and suggested cholesterol levels for initiating therapeutic lifestyle changes and drug therapy. Persons can be categorized into three risk categories: (a) *high risk* (established CHD and CHD risk equivalents [2, 80]), (b) *moderate-to-moderately high risk* (multiple [2+] risk factors), and (c) *lower risk* (zero to one [0–1] risk factor). Definitions of risk factors and risk status are included in Table 67.8. CHD risk equivalents include noncoronary forms of clinical atherosclerotic disease, diabetes, and multiple (2+) CHD risk factors with 10-year risk for CHD greater than 20%.

High Risk. The goal for LDL-lowering therapy in high-risk patients is an LDL-C level lower than 100 mg/dL. Current NCEP guidelines suggest that lifestyle change be initiated for all high-risk patients, and LDL-lowering drugs should be considered when the LDL-C levels are higher than 100 mg/dL. In addition, for *very high-risk* patients, physicians have a therapeutic option to reduce LDL-C to less than 70 mg/dL. Factors that qualify a person for the *very high-risk* status are the presence of established CHD plus the following: (a) multiple major risk factors, especially diabetes; (b) severe and poorly controlled risk factors, especially continued cigarette smoking; (c) multiple risk factors of the metabolic syndrome, especially elevated triglyceride greater than or equal to 200 mg/dL plus non–HDL-C greater than or equal to 130 mg/dL with low HDL-C (<40 mg/dL); and (d) acute coronary

TABLE 67.8. ADULT TREATMENT PANEL LOW-DENSITY LIPOPROTEIN CHOLESTEROL GOALS AND CUTPOINTS FOR THERAPEUTIC LIFESTYLE CHANGES AND DRUG THERAPY IN DIFFERENT RISK CATEGORIES AND PROPOSED MODIFICATIONS BASED ON RECENT CLINICAL TRIAL EVIDENCE

RISK CATEGORY	LDL-C GOAL	INITIATE THERAPEUTIC LIFESTYLE CHANGES	CONSIDER DRUG THERAPY[g]
CHD[a] or CHD Risk Equivalents[b] *High Risk*	<100 mg/dL (optional goal: <70 mg/dL)	≥100 mg/dL[f]	≥100 mg/dL[h] (<100 mg/dL: consider drug options)[h]
2+ Risk Factors[c] (10-year risk 10–20%) *Moderately High Risk*	<130 mg/dL[e]	≥130 mg/dL[f]	≥130 mg/dL (100–129 mg/dL; consider drug options)[i]
2+ Risk Factors[c] (10-year risk <10%) *Moderate Risk*	<130 mg/dL	≥130 mg/dL	>160 mg/dL
0–1 Risk Factor[d]	<160 mg/dL	≥160 mg/dL	≥190 mg/dL (160–189 mg/dL: LDL-lowering drug optional)

CHD, coronary heart disease; LDL-C, low-density lipoprotein cholesterol.

[a] CHD includes a history of myocardial infarction, unstable angina, stable angina, coronary artery procedures (angioplasty or bypass surgery), or evidence of clinically significant myocardial ischemia.

[b] CHD risk equivalents include clinical manifestations of noncoronary forms of atherosclerotic disease (peripheral arterial disease, abdominal aortic aneurysm, and carotid artery disease [transient ischemic attacks or stroke of carotid origin or >50% obstruction of a carotid artery]), diabetes, and 2+ risk factors with 10-year risk for hard CHD >20%.

[c] Risk factors include cigarette smoking, hypertension (blood pressure, >140/90 mm Hg or on antihypertensive medication), low HDL-C (<40 mg/dL), family history of premature CHD (CHD in male first-degree relative, <55 years; CHD in female first-degree relative, <65 years), and age (men, ≥45 years; women, ≥55 years)

[d] Almost all people with 0–1 risk factor have a 10-year risk <10%, and 10-year risk assessment in people with 0–1 risk factor is thus not necessary.

[e] Optional LDL-C goal <100 mg/dL.

[f] Any person at high risk or moderately high risk who has lifestyle-related risk factors (e.g., obesity, physical inactivity, elevated triglyceride, low high-density lipoprotein cholesterol [HDL-C], or metabolic syndrome) is a candidate for therapeutic lifestyle changes to modify these risk factors regardless of LDL-C level.

[g] When LDL-lowering drug therapy is employed, it is recommended that intensity of therapy be sufficient to achieve at least a 30 to 40% reduction in LDL-C levels.

[h] If baseline LDL-C is <100 mg/dL, institution of an LDL-lowering drug is optional, depending on clinical judgment. If a high-risk person has high triglycerides or low HDL-C, combining a fibrate or nicotinic acid with an LDL-lowering drug can be considered.

syndromes. The optional goal of achieving LDL-C lower than 70 mg/dL does not apply to persons who are not at high risk.

Moderately High Risk. Persons who at moderately high risk are those with multiple (2+) risk factors and a 10-year risk of CHD of 10 to 20%. Risk is determined by Framingham risk scoring (1, 2). Persons with a 10-year risk by Framingham risk scoring of more than 20% are placed in the high-risk category; for these persons, the LDL-C goal is less than 100 mg/dL. For moderately high-risk persons, the LDL-C goal is less than 130 mg/dL. LDL-lowering dietary therapy is universally advocated for patients with an LDL-C greater than the goal level. When the 10-year risk is 10 to 20%, drug therapy should be considered if the LDL-C level is greater than the goal level (i.e., ≥130 mg/dL) after a trial of dietary therapy. An optional goal for patients whose 10-year risk is close to 20% is an LDL-C of less than 100 mg/dL.

Moderate Risk. Persons with multiple (2+) risk factors and a 10-year risk for CHD of less than 10% can be said to be at *moderate risk*. The LDL-C goal for this category is less than 130 mg/dL, and dietary therapy can be initiated for those persons whose LDL-C level is greater than or equal to 130 mg/dL. However, an LDL-lowering drug need not be considered unless the LDL-C level is greater than or equal to 160 mg/dL on maximal dietary therapy.

Lower Risk. Finally, most persons with one risk factor or no risk factors have a 10-year risk of less than 10%; that is, they are at *lower risk*. For these persons, clinical management and dietary therapy are recommended when the LDL-C level is greater than or equal to 160 mg/dL. The goal is to reduce LDL-C concentrations to less than 160 mg/dL. If the LDL-C is greater than or equal to 190 mg/dL after an adequate trial of dietary therapy, consideration should be given to adding a cholesterol-lowering drug. When serum LDL-C ranges from 160 to 189 mg/dL, introduction of a cholesterol-lowering drug is optional, depending on clinical judgment.

Other Lipid Targets. Although LDL-C is the primary target of lipid-lowering therapy, other lipid parameters may sometimes become targets for intervention. For example, non–HDL-C, which equates to (VLDL + LDL-C), is a secondary target of treatment in patients with elevated triglycerides (≥200 mg/dL). For patients with high triglycerides, the non–HDL-C goal is 30 mg/dL higher than the LDL-C goal. Non–HDL-C is included as a secondary target of therapy to take into account the atherogenic potential associated with chylomicron and VLDL remnant lipoproteins in patients with hypertriglyceridemia (see the next section). Although the potential benefit of HDL-raising therapy has evoked considerable interest, current documentation of risk reduction through controlled clinical trials is not sufficient to warrant setting a specific value as the goal for raising HDL-C.

Chylomicronemia

Chylomicrons are lipoproteins that carry newly absorbed dietary fat into the circulation. These lipoproteins derive their triglycerides from dietary fat. When fat enters the intestinal tract, it is hydrolyzed by pancreatic lipase into fatty acids and monoglycerides. The uptake of these lipids into intestinal mucosal cells is facilitated by biliary products—the bile salts and phospholipids. Following uptake by enterocytes, fatty acids and monoglycerides are resynthesized into triglycerides. These triglycerides are transferred into newly formed chylomicron particles by MTP (29, 30).

The core of chylomicron particles is composed almost exclusively of triglycerides, but a small amount of cholesterol ester, derived from newly absorbed cholesterol, also is present. The major apolipoprotein of chylomicrons is Apo B-48. In addition, Apo Cs (CII and CIII), and Apo As (AI and AIV) are present on chylomicrons. These lipoproteins are secreted into the lymphatic circulation, where they pass via the thoracic duct into the systemic circulation. When chylomicrons distribute into the peripheral microcirculation, they come into contact with the enzyme LPL located on the surface of capillary endothelial cells. LPL hydrolyzes the triglycerides of chylomicrons and releases their free fatty acids (FFAs) into the circulation. Much of LPL is located in the capillary beds of adipose tissue; consequently, many of the newly released FFAs are taken up directly by adipocytes, where they recombine to form triglycerides for storage. Lesser amounts of FFAs enter the systemic circulation, where they can be taken up either by liver or muscle. Muscle cells also express LPL, and its activity in the capillaries of muscle tissue facilitates FFA uptake by myocytes. When the lipolysis of triglycerides is almost complete, a residual lipoprotein, termed a *chylomicron remnant*, is released from LPL, reenters the circulation, and is removed by the liver. Chylomicron remnants are cholesterol-enriched lipoproteins, and some investigators believe that they have atherogenic potential.

Type I Hyperlipoproteinemia

Lipoprotein Lipase Deficiency. A lipoprotein pattern consisting of increased chylomicrons with relatively normal VLDL concentrations is called *type I hyperlipoproteinemia* (81). Mutations in the LPL gene can cause a deficiency of enzyme activity. This defect leads to type I hyperlipoproteinemia (81). The severity of the resulting hypertriglyceridemia depends on the nature of the defect, that is, whether the LPL gene is functionally absent or has only diminished function. A few patients are homozygous for severe defects, and they develop severe chylomicronemia when their diet contains appreciable amounts of fat. Molecular biology studies have uncovered many of defects in the LPL gene responsible for this form of hyperlipidemia (82).

Patients who have a complete absence of LPL activity manifest severe chylomicronemia from birth (83). Depending on the level of fat intake, plasma triglyceride levels can vary from 1000 to 10,000 mg/dL. When plasma triglycerides exceed 2000 mg/dL, the risk of acute pancreatitis increases greatly. Pancreatitis can occur even in infants with severe chylomicronemia. In LPL-deficient patients, increases in triglycerides are predominantly in chylomicrons; VLDL triglycerides generally are not strikingly elevated. This lack of severely elevated VLDL triglycerides probably reflects a relatively low output of VLDL particles by the liver. An increase in circulating chylomicrons alone probably does not promote the development of atherosclerosis. This may be because chylomicrons are very large lipoproteins and seemingly do not penetrate the arterial wall.

Apolipoprotein CII Deficiency. Apo CII is an apolipoprotein that activates LPL. Rare patients have a genetic deficiency of Apo CII (83, 84). As a result, LPL remains nonfunctional, and chylomicron triglycerides cannot be hydrolyzed. Affected patients have severe chylomicronemia similar to those with LPL deficiency. They, too, have the pattern of type I hyperlipoproteinemia.

Type V Hyperlipoproteinemia

Type V hyperlipoproteinemia is characterized by high serum levels of both chylomicrons and VLDL (83, 85). In contrast to early manifestations of the genetic deficiencies of LPL and Apo CII, type V hyperlipoproteinemia typically makes its appearance later in life (85). Two defects in triglyceride metabolism appear to underlie this disorder (86). One is an overproduction of VLDL particles by the liver. This defect typically is secondary to obesity and/or insulin resistance. The other is a delay in lipolysis of TGRLP. Of interest, an excess of circulating VLDL particles resulting from overproduction can be one cause of a lipolytic "defect" for TGRLP. This is because the lipolytic system becomes "saturated" with excess TGRLP, causing their retention in serum (83). Elevations of chylomicrons in type V hyperlipoproteinemia can be explained in part by this mechanism. In addition, the inherent activity of LPL may be low in many patients with this condition (87). This added defect exacerbates the accumulation of both VLDL and chylomicrons in the serum.

Management

In patients with type I hyperlipoproteinemia, LPL activity is absent because of mutations in the LPL gene or the Apo CII gene. No triglyceride-lowering drugs are available that overcome these defects. The only effective management of these forms of chylomicronemia is to reduce dietary fat. Intakes of fat should be reduced to less than 10% of total calories. Triglycerides containing medium-chain fatty acids can be partially substituted for long-chain fatty acids because medium-chain fatty acids are not absorbed into chylomicrons; their use thus does not induce chylomicronemia. The purpose of treatment of severe chylomicronemia is to lessen

the danger of acute pancreatitis, not to decrease the risk of ASCVD.

In type V hyperlipoproteinemia, very-low-fat diets also should be employed. Such diets are necessary to reduce the severity of chylomicronemia. Moreover, weight reduction in obese patients combined with increased physical activity will lessen overproduction of VLDL by reducing hepatic lipid overload. However, in many patients with type V hyperlipoproteinemia, changes in eating and exercise habits alone are not sufficient to control the severe hypertriglyceridemia effectively. Such patients require triglyceride-lowering drugs. The fibric acids comprise one class of effective drugs (88). Available fibric acids include clofibrate, gemfibrozil, fenofibrate, and bezafibrate. Gemfibrozil and fenofibrate are the agents currently employed in the United States. All the fibric acids have a similar mechanism of action. Recent studies show that fibric acids act mainly by binding to nuclear receptors called perioxisomal proliferation activating receptors-α (PPARs-α) (89). Activation of these receptors initiates a cascade of reactions that elicit changes in Apo CIII and LPL; synthesis of Apo CIII in liver is reduced, and synthesis of LPL in peripheral tissues is increased. In addition, fibrates may increase the oxidation of fatty acids in the liver. All these changes tend to lower serum concentrations of TGRLP. Most patients with type V hyperlipoproteinemia require fibric acids for effective control of hypertriglyceridemia. Reduction of chylomicronemia lessens the risk of acute pancreatitis; decreasing VLDL levels also may reduce the likelihood of developing ASCVD, although this latter benefit has not been proven.

Another agent that can be employed in type V hyperlipoproteinemia is nicotinic acid. At low intakes, nicotinic acid acts as a vitamin (see Chapter 25); in high doses, it becomes a triglyceride-lowering drug. The precise mechanism of action for nicotinic acid is not known, although it appears to act in the liver to reduce the formation of VLDL (90). This action often is sufficient to control severe hypertriglyceridemia. Although nicotinic acid is highly effective as a triglyceride-lowering drug, side effects occur all too often. For example, nicotinic acid can worsen insulin resistance and can raise glucose levels in diabetic patients (91). Nicotinic acid also has other side effects including gastrointestinal irritation, hepatotoxicity, flushing and itching of the skin, and hyperuricemia. For these reasons, nicotinic acid is used less frequently in the treatment of type V hyperlipoproteinemia than are the fibric acids. However, in other conditions discussed subsequently, nicotinic acid therapy may be useful.

ATHEROGENIC DYSLIPIDEMIA

A third major category of lipoprotein abnormalities can be called atherogenic dyslipidemia (92). This form of dyslipidemia is characterized by a constellation of lipoprotein abnormalities that often occur together. Four components typically make up atherogenic dyslipidemia: (a) mild hyper-cholesterolemia; (b) mild to moderate hypertriglyceridemia; (c) small, dense LDL particles; and (d) low HDL-C. Atherogenic dyslipidemia generally does not result from a single metabolic defect, but from the coexistence of several defects. Five categories of causation for atherogenic dyslipidemia are recognized: (a) obesity, (b) diets high in cholesterol-raising fatty acids; (c) physical inactivity, (d) aging, and (e) genetics (92). These causes resemble the categories of factors underlying hypercholesterolemia; however, among them, obesity and physical inactivity tend to predominate as causes of atherogenic dyslipidemia, whereas a diet high in cholesterol-raising fatty acids and aging more commonly stand out as causes of hypercholesterolemia. A different pattern of genetic aberration also tends to be present in patients with atherogenic dyslipidemia compared with patients with predominant hypercholesterolemia.

Causes

The major causes of atherogenic dyslipidemia may simultaneously be responsible for other nonlipid risk factors, notably hypertension, non–insulin-dependent diabetes mellitus, and a prothrombotic state. The coexistence of these several risk factors can be called the syndrome of multiple metabolic risk factors, or simply the *metabolic syndrome* (2, 93, 94) (see also Chapter 62). Obesity usually is present in patients with the metabolic syndrome and is often the predominant cause. As indicated before, obesity leads to high levels of FFAs that overload the liver with lipid, and excess hepatic lipid predisposes to atherogenic dyslipidemia (95). This sequence also causes insulin resistance, which predisposes to non–insulin-dependent diabetes mellitus. It also can raise blood pressure, and it may induce a prothrombotic state (93, 94). These multiple actions of obesity that initiate the metabolic syndrome are commonly augmented by lack of exercise, aging, diet, and genetic factors. Because of the concurrence of several metabolic risk factors in the metabolic syndrome, it is difficult to identify the relative contributions of each risk factor to atherogenesis. Nonetheless, evidence exists that each is atherogenic; and when the impact of all the risk factors is summed, together they substantially raise the risk of ASCVD.

Some investigators postulate that the underlying condition responsible for the metabolic syndrome is a state of insulin resistance (96). This condition represents a generalized metabolic disorder in which fatty acids displace glucose as the preferred energy source. One important cause of insulin resistance is tissue uptake of excess fatty acids derived from adipose tissue (95). The metabolic result of this overloading of tissues with lipids is an inhibition of insulin action at the cellular level; this leads secondarily to hyperinsulinemia. A state of disordered metabolism, which has been called insulin resistance, thus is commonly present

in patients exhibiting multiple metabolic risk factors including atherogenic dyslipidemia (93, 94). The following discussion briefly reviews the causes and features of each component of atherogenic dyslipidemia.

Elevated Apolipoprotein B

Most persons having the other components of atherogenic dyslipidemia also manifest high levels of Apo B. The increase in Apo B is partitioned between VLDL and LDL. The higher LDL-Apo B is usually accompanied by some increase in LDL-C. Serum levels of LDL-C levels frequently are in the range of 130 to 159 mg/dL (mild hypercholesterolemia). Because some elevation of LDL is prerequisite for atherogenesis, a rise in LDL concentrations into the mildly elevated range usually is present when patients with atherogenic dyslipidemia develop premature ASCVD. The causes of mild hypercholesterolemia are described earlier. In patients with atherogenic dyslipidemia, obesity often is a major contributing cause of elevated serum LDL, but the other factors considered before also can play a role.

Mild to Moderate Hypertriglyceridemia

Most people with atherogenic dyslipidemia have some elevation in plasma triglycerides (2). Two categories of triglyceride elevation can be present: mild hypertriglyceridemia (triglycerides, 150–199 mg/dL) or moderate hypertriglyceridemia (200–500 mg/dL). Elevations of serum triglycerides occur mostly in the VLDL fraction. The usual cause of mild to moderate hypertriglyceridemia is an increased hepatic production of VLDL secondary to obesity (97,98). Production rates of VLDL triglycerides can be further enhanced by decreased physical inactivity or by a diet high in carbohydrates. Overproduction of VLDL triglycerides often unmasks mild defects in lipolysis; this combination of abnormalities frequently elevates serum triglycerides into hypertriglyceridemic range (97). Mild lipolytic defects may be of genetic origin, possibly from mild abnormalities in the expression of LPL. As already noted, insulin resistance, which is common in patients with atherogenic dyslipidemia, is accompanied by overproduction of Apo CIII (99), an apolipoprotein that inhibits the activity of LPL (100).

An important question is whether an elevation of VLDL particles directly promotes the development of atherosclerosis. To address this question, it must be recognized that VLDL particles are not homogenous in size or composition. At least two varieties of VLDL should be distinguished: (a) newly secreted VLDL and (b) VLDL remnants. VLDL remnants consist of partially catabolized VLDLs; some of their triglycerides have been hydrolyzed, and they have acquired more cholesterol esters. In fact, in fasting serum, most VLDL particles are remnants. Growing evidence indicates that VLDL remnants have an atherogenic potential comparable to that of LDL (2). In contrast, newly secreted

VLDLs may not be atherogenic. The atherogenicity of VLDL remnants is most striking in type III hyperlipoproteinemia (101); in this condition, catabolism of VLDL remnants is curtailed because of a genetic defect in the structure of Apo E that impairs binding of VLDL remnants to hepatic LDL receptors (101). Because of their slow removal from the circulation, remnants in type III hyperlipoproteinemia accumulate excessive amounts of cholesterol esters; this excess cholesterol content apparently makes then highly atherogenic.

Small, Dense Low-Density Lipoprotein Particles

Another feature of atherogenic dyslipidemia is an abnormality in LDL particle size, specifically, the presence of abnormally small, dense LDL particles (92). Small LDL particles frequently occur in patients with premature ASCVD (102–104). They may have greater atherogenic potential than normal-sized LDLs. The reasons for the unusually high atherogenicity of small LDL particles could be several. For example, small, dense LDL particles could enter the arterial wall more readily than larger LDLs. Moreover, they appear to be more sensitive to oxidation than larger LDLs (105); this, too, could enhance their atherogenicity. In spite of these possibilities, it is difficult to define the degree of increased risk accompanying small LDL particles quantitatively; this is mainly because of the common association between small LDLs with other components of atherogenic dyslipidemia and other risk factors of the metabolic syndrome (93, 94).

Low High-Density Lipoprotein Cholesterol

The fourth component of atherogenic dyslipidemia is a low HDL-C level. In particular, a tight link exists among elevated triglycerides, small LDL particles, and low HDL-C concentrations (104). Prospective epidemiologic studies reveal a strong inverse relation between low HDL-C levels and the risk of ASCVD (106–109). This inverse correlation may have several explanations. First, HDL may directly retard atherogenesis by blocking the atherogenic action of LDL; second, a low HDL level can be a marker for the presence of other components of atherogenic dyslipidemia; and third, a low HDL concentration commonly denotes the presence of the nonlipid risk factors in the metabolic syndrome (110). These several links may explain why low HDL levels have been reported to be such a strong predictor of ASCVD (106–109).

The underlying causes of low HDL-C are the same as for other causes of atherogenic dyslipidemia: obesity, lack of exercise, aging, diet, and genetics. Increasing obesity causes a progressive fall in HDL-C concentration (19, 20). Sedentary life habits lower HDL levels; these low levels can be reversed by regular and vigorous exercise (111). Both obesity and lack of exercise increase insulin resistance, and investigators have reported that insulin resistance is commonly present in patients having low HDL-C levels

(112). One dietary pattern resulting in low HDL levels is a low-fat, high-carbohydrate diet (113, 114). Cigarette smoking also reduces serum HDL levels (115). Finally, genetic polymorphism accounts for about 50% of the variation in serum HDL-C levels in the general population (116, 117); therefore, genetic factors probably contribute to many cases of low serum HDL levels.

There is genetic control over many key metabolic pathways affecting HDL-C levels. For instance, multiple genetic factors contribute to higher serum triglyceride levels. Higher serum triglycerides, in turn, are accompanied by lower HDL-C concentrations (118); triglycerides in TGRLP exchange for cholesterol esters in HDLs, and thereby lower HDL-C levels. One factor that is under genetic control and that affects both triglycerides and HDL-C levels is LPL; a reduced activity of LPL often is present in patients with low HDL levels (119, 120). Another determinant of HDL levels is HTGL activity. In this case, increased activity of HTGL commonly accompanies reduced serum HDL-C levels (110, 120). Polymorphisms in the HTGL gene account for about half of the genetic contribution to the variation in HDL-C concentrations (117, 121). Current evidence suggests that increased HTGL activity degrades HDL particles and promotes HDL catabolism (122). Enhanced catabolism of HDLs also may occur from high activity of CETP (123); this protein promotes transfer of cholesterol ester from HDL to TGRLP. Genetic polymorphism of the CETP gene accounts for about 20% of the variability of CETP levels in plasma (125). Studies of apolipoprotein kinetics (125, 126) have revealed that an increased catabolism of HDL is responsible for most cases of low serum HDL-C levels; accelerated HDL catabolism may be secondary to increased serum triglycerides, reduced activity of LPL, increased activity of HTGL, and increased activity of CETP. All these changes can be influenced by genetic polymorphism, although acquired factors, such as insulin resistance, also may contribute. Finally, a reduced production of Apo AI may be another cause of low HDL-C levels (126); production rates of Apo AI likewise appear to be under genetic control (117). Thus, low HDL-C concentrations, which are often part of the syndrome of atherogenic dyslipidemia, appear to be determined in part by polymorphism in a few key genes regulating HDL metabolism and in part by external influences on these genes. When patients become insulin resistant, genetic influences magnify the impact on HDL metabolism.

Management

The strategy for management of atherogenic dyslipidemia is based on its twofold origin. First, a generalized metabolic disorder—a state of insulin resistance—commonly is present in dyslipidemic patients. However, because the severity of particular components of atherogenic dyslipidemia is modified by genetic factors, treatment must be directed toward (a) lessening of insulin resistance and, when necessary, (b) direct therapeutic modification of individual components of the metabolic syndrome.

Insulin Resistance. Reduction of insulin resistance is best brought about by caloric restriction and increased physical activity (93, 94). Both changes in life habits will lower serum insulin levels and will dampen the lipid abnormalities characteristic of atherogenic dyslipidemia. Therefore, weight control and increased physical activity are the foundations of the management of atherogenic dyslipidemia. Interest in the use of drugs designed specifically to reduce insulin resistance (insulin-sparing drugs) has been growing. One drug of this type is metformin. Its primary site of action appears to be the liver. The precise biochemical target of metformin action is not known. One consequence of its action, however, is a reduction in hepatic glucose production, which reduces insulin resistance (127). Associated with this change can be a reduction in triglyceride levels (128). Unfortunately, metformin does not completely correct the metabolic abnormalities characteristic of the insulin resistance state, and hence dyslipidemia is only partially improved.

The thiazoladinediones (TZDs) are another class of drugs that can modify cellular metabolism and lessen insulin resistance. Among these, piaglitazone and rosiglitazone currently are in clinical use. The TZDs appear to act by binding to the nuclear receptor, PPAR-γ (129). The biochemical consequences of this action are not fully understood. One response, however, appears to be an inhibition of FFA release from adipose tissue. This action alone should reduce the availability of lipid for accumulation in liver and skeletal muscle; TZDs also may act directly on liver and skeletal muscle to affect metabolic processes favorably. These actions result in a decrease in plasma insulin levels, a finding that indicates a reduction in insulin resistance (130). Reports have noted that treatment of patients with TZDs improves atherogenic dyslipidemia (131). However, insulin resistance is only partially corrected by TZDs, and serum lipid patterns usually remain abnormal, although improved.

Available data indicate that effective weight reduction and increased physical activity exercise are as effective in correcting insulin resistance as are drugs (132, 133). In some patients, insulin-sparing agents may be a useful adjunct, but the efficacy of current agents probably is too weak to normalize the serum lipid pattern in most patients. The foundations of treatment of atherogenic dyslipidemia therefore are weight reduction and physical activity. Unfortunately, in many patients, changes in life habits are not enough to normalize serum lipids, either because they are not adequately employed or because they alone are insufficient. In such patients, it becomes necessary to turn to lipid-lowering drugs to normalize the lipoprotein profile.

Low-Density Lipoprotein Cholesterol: Primary Target of Lipid-Lowering Therapy. As indicated previously, the primary therapeutic target for lipid modification in atherogenic dyslipidemia is an elevation of serum LDL-C (2, 80). A reduction in intake of cholesterol-raising fatty acids and cholesterol will produce some decrease in LDL-C concentrations. The goals of LDL-lowering depend on a patient's absolute risk of ASCVD and are outlined earlier, in the sections on management of hypercholesterolemia. In patients at high risk or very high risk, LDL-lowering drugs usually are required (2, 80). The statins are first-line therapy in higher-risk patients with atherogenic dyslipidemia. Many patients enrolled in the statin trials (4, 134) had a lipoprotein pattern characteristic of atherogenic dyslipidemia; the marked reduction in acute coronary events in patients in the CARE study who received pravastatin therapy reveals the benefit of aggressive lowering of LDL-C levels.

Secondary Targets of Lipid-Lowering Therapy. These targets include serum triglycerides, VLDL-C, and Apo B. A simple approach is to identify non–HDL-C as *the* secondary target of lipid lowering therapy. Non–HDL-C (total cholesterol minus HDL-C) equals the cholesterol content of LDL+VLDL. Non–HDL-C is highly correlated with total Apo B levels. Therefore, in patients with elevated triglyceride (≥150 mg/dL), non–HDL-C can be a secondary target of treatment, *after* LDL-C. The goals for non–HDL-C are 30 mg/dL higher than those for LDL-C (see Table 67.8). For many patients with atherogenic dyslipidemia, the question arises whether addition of a triglyceride-lowering drug will provide further benefit if it is combined with one of the statins. Available drugs to use in combination with statins are fibric acids and nicotinic acid. Their use is attractive because of reports that these drug combinations can markedly improve the lipoprotein pattern (135). However, the incremental benefit of combined drug therapy over statins alone has never been documented in clinical trials designed to quantify risk reduction. Until such trials are carried out, it remains uncertain whether combined drug therapy, in spite of its theoretic benefits, is advantageous in patients with mild to moderate hypertriglyceridemia. If a fibrate is used in combination with statins, the drug should be fenofibrate, because gemfibrozil carries too high a risk of severe myopathy.

Small Low-Density Lipoprotein Particles. Another component of atherogenic dyslipidemia consists of small LDL particles. Treatment with statins certainly will reduce the concentration of small, dense LDL particles in the circulation, which itself should reduce risk of atherogenic dyslipidemia. The addition of a triglyceride-lowering drug to statin therapy will result in conversion of smaller LDL particles into larger particles (136). This is one theoretic benefit of combined drug therapy. Should it be shown through future clinical trials that combined drug therapy is advantageous, one mechanism of benefit may be through a change in the size of LDL particles.

Low High-Density Lipoprotein Cholesterol. The final component of atherogenic dyslipidemia is a low HDL-C level. Modest elevations of HDL-C levels can be brought about by statins and fibric acids. Their use in combination produces moderate increases (136, 137). However, the best available agent for raising HDL-C levels is nicotinic acid (138, 139). The combination of a statin plus nicotinic acid leads to a particularly striking increase in HDL-C concentrations. In spite of this beneficial response, many patients are unable to tolerate nicotinic acid because of its side effects. Certainly, in very-high-risk patients, an effort can be made to lower LDL-C concentrations maximally and to raise HDL-C levels by combined drug therapy. Alternatively, if it seems unacceptable to combine a triglyceride-lowering drug with a statin, then the prudent approach may be to offset the risk of a low HDL-C level partially by more effectively lowering the LDL-C level by using a higher dose of statin.

REFERENCES

1. Expert Panel on Detection, Evaluation, and Treatment of High Blood Cholesterol in Adults. JAMA 2001;285:2486–97.
2. National Cholesterol Education Program (NCEP) Expert Panel on Detection, Evaluation, and Treatment of High Blood Cholesterol in Adults (Adult Treatment Panel III). Circulation 2002;106:3143–421.
3. Scandinavian Simvastatin Survival Study Group. Lancet 1994;344:1383–9.
4. Sacks FM, Pfeffer MA, Moye LA et al. N Engl J Med 1996;335:1001–9.
5. Shepherd J, Cobbe SM, Ford I et al. N Engl J Med 1995;333:1301–7.
6. Heart Protection Study Collaborative Group. Lancet 2002;360:7–22.
7. Sever PS, Dahlof B, Poulter NR. Lancet 2003;361:1149–58.
8. Grundy SM, Wilhelmsen L, Rose R. Eur Heart J 1990;11:462–71.
9. Stamler J, Stamler R, Neaton JD et al. JAMA 1999;282:2012–8.
10. Yusuf S. Lancet 2004;364:937.
11. Benfante R. Hum Biol 1992;64:791–805.
12. Brown BG, Zhao X-Q, Bardsley J et al. J Intern Med 1997;241:283–94.
13. Stamler J, Wentworth D, Neaton JD. JAMA 1986;256:2823–8.
14. Grundy SM. Arterioscler Thromb 1991;11:1619–35.
15. National Cholesterol Education Program. Circulation 1991;83:2154–232.
16. Johnson CL, Rifkind BM, Sempos CT et al. JAMA 1993;269:3002–8.
17. Federation of American Societies for Experimental Biology, Life Sciences Research Office. Prepared for the Interagency Board for Nutrition Monitoring and Related Research. Third Report on Nutrition Monitoring in the United States, vol 1. Washington, DC: US Government Printing Office, 1995.
18. US Departments of Agriculture and Health and Human Services. Nutrition and Your Health: Dietary Guidelines for Americans. 5th ed. Home and Garden Bulletin no. 232. Washington, DC: US Department of Agriculture, 2000.
19. Denke MA, Sempos CT, Grundy SM. Arch Intern Med 1993;153:1093–103.
20. Denke MA, Sempos CT, Grundy SM. Arch Intern Med 1994;154:401–10.
21. Tzankoff SP, Norris AH. J Appl Physiol 1978;45:536–9.
22. Hedley AA, Ogden CL, Johnson CL et al. JAMA 2004;291:2847–50.
23. Law MR, Wald NJ, Wu T et al. BMJ 1994;308:363–6.
24. Law MR, Wald NJ, Thompson SM. BMJ 1994;308:367–73.
25. Perusse L, Despres J, Tremblay A et al. Arteriosclerosis 1989;9:308–18.
26. Goldstein JL, Hobbs HH, Brown MS. Familial hypercholesterolemia. In: Scriver CR, Beaudet AL, Sly WS et al., eds. The Metabolic and Molecular Bases of Inherited Diseases. 8th ed. New York: McGraw-Hill, 1995:1981–2030.
27. Dixon JL, Furukawa S, Ginsberg HN. J Biol Chem 1991;266:5080–6.
28. Wetterau JR, Aggerbeck LP, Bouma M–E et al. Science 1992;258:999–1001.
29. Grundy SM: J Lipid Res 1984;25:1611–8.
30. Grundy SM, Vega GL. What is Meant by Overproduction of Apo B–containing Lipoproteins? In: Malmendier CL, Alaupovic P, Brewer HB Jr, eds. Hypercholesterolemia, Hypocholesterolemia, Hypertriglyceridemia. New York: Plenum Press, 1992:213–22.
31. Horton JD, Goldstein JL, Brown MS. J Clin Invest 2002;109:1125–31.
32. Grundy SM, Vega GL, Bilheimer DW. Arteriosclerosis 1985;5:623–30.
33. Ericsson S, Eriksson M, Vitols S et al. J Clin Invest 1991;87:591–6.
34. Kesaniemi YA, Beltz WF, Grundy SM. J Clin Invest 1985;76:586–95.
35. Egusa G, Beltz WF, Grundy SM et al. J Clin Invest 1985;76:596–603.
36. Grundy SM, Denke MA. J Lipid Res 1990;31:1149–72.
37. Mensink RP, Katan MB. N Engl J Med 1990;323:439–45.
38. Judd JT, Clevidence BA, Muesing RA et al. Am J Clin Nutr 1994;59:861–8.
39. Zock PL, de Vries JHM, Katan MB. Arterioscler Thromb 1994;14:567–75.
40. Denke MA, Grundy SM. Am J Clin Nutr 1992;56:895–8.
41. Cater NB, Heller HJ, Denke MA. Am J Clin Nutr 1997;65:41–5.
42. Bonanome A, Grundy SM. N Engl J Med 1988;318:1244–8.
43. Denke MA, Grundy SM. Am J Clin Nutr 1991;54:1036–40.
44. Bonanome A, Bennett M, Grundy SM. Atherosclerosis 1992;94:119–7.
45. Zock PL, Katan MB. J Lipid Res 1992;33:399–410.
46. Dietschy JM, Turley SD, Spady DK. J Lipid Res 1993;34:1637–59.
47. Daumeri CM, Woollett LA, Dietschy JM. Proc Natl Acad Sci USA 1992;89:10797–801.
48. McGill HC Jr, McMahan CA, Kruski AW et al. Arteriosclerosis 1981;1:3–12.
49. Rudel LL, Parks JS, Bond MG. Ann NY Acad Sci 1985;454:248–53.
50. Grundy SM, Barrett-Connor E, Rudel LL et al. Arteriosclerosis 1988;8:95–101.
51. Ma PT, Yamamoto T, Goldstein JL et al. Proc Natl Acad Sci USA 1986;83:792–6.
52. Denke MA. Am J Med 1995;99:29–35.
53. Vega GL, Denke MA, Grundy SM. Circulation 1991;84:118–28.
54. Arca M, Vega GL, Grundy SM. JAMA 1994;271:453–9.
55. Vega GL, Grundy SM. Arterioscler Thromb Vasc Biol 1996;16:517–22.
56. Tall AR. J Lipid Res 1993;34:1255–74.
57. Tato F, Vega GL, Tall AR et al. Arterioscler Thromb Vasc Biol 1995;15:112–20.
58. Vega GL, Denke MA, Grundy SM. J Clin Invest 1986;78:1410–14.

59. Innerarity TL, Mahley RW, Weisgraber KH et al. J Lipid Res 1990;31:1337–49.
60. Denke MA, Grundy SM. Arch Intern Med 1994;154:317–25.
61. Katan MB, Grundy SM, Willett WC. N Engl J Med 1997;337:563–6.
62. Connor WE, Connor SL. N Engl J Med 1997;337:562–3.
63. Katan MB, Grundy SM, Jones P et al. Mayo Clin Proc 2003;78:965–78.
64. US Department of Health and Human Services. Physical Activity and Health: A Report of the Surgeon General. Atlanta, GA: US Department of Health and Human Services, Centers for Disease Control and Prevention, National Center for Chronic Disease Prevention and Health Promotion, 1966.
65. US Department of Agriculture and Department of Health and Human Services. Nutrition and Your Health: Dietary Guidelines for Americans. 3rd ed. Home and Garden Bulletin no. 232. Washington, DC: US Department of Agriculture, 1990.
66. Committee on Comparative Toxicity of Naturally Occurring Carcinogens, National Research Council. Carcinogens and Anticarcinogens in the Human Diet: A Comparison of Naturally Occurring and Synthetic Substances. Washington, DC: National Academy Press, 1996.
67. Jialal I, Devaraj S. J Nutr 1996;126:1053S–7S.
68. Heart Protection Study Collaborative Group. Lancet 2002;360:23–33.
69. Appel LJ, Moore TJ, Obarzanek E et al. N Engl J Med 1997;336:1117–24.
70. Jousilahti P, Vartiainen E, Korhonen HJ et al. J Cardiovasc Risk 1999;6:293–8.
71. Critchley J, Capewell S. Cochrane Database Syst Rev 2004;1:CD003041.
72. Chobanian AV, Bakris GL, Black HR et al. Hypertension 2003;42:1206–52.
73. Endo A. J Lipid Res 1992;33:1569–82.
74. Grundy SM. N Engl J Med 1988;319:24–33.
75. Grundy SM. Bile acid resins: mechanisms of action. In: Pharmacological Control of Hyperlipidemia. Barcelona: JR Prous Science Publishers, 1986:3–19.
76. Anonymous. JAMA 1984;251:351–64.
77. Anonymous. JAMA 1984;251:365–74.
78. Davidson MH. Expert Rev Cardiovasc Ther 2003;1:11–21
79. Bilheimer DW, Grundy SM, Brown MS et al. Proc Natl Acad Sci USA 1983;80:4124–8.
80. Grundy SM, Cleeman JI, Merz CN et al. Circulation 2004;110:227–39
81. Fredrickson DS, Levy RI, Lees RS. N Engl J Med 1967;276:34–42, 94–103, 148–56, 215–25, 273–81.
82. Santamarina-Fojo S, Dugi KA. Curr Opin Lipidol 1994;5:117–25.
83. Brunzell JD. Familial lipoprotein lipase deficiency and other causes of the chylomicronemia syndrome. In: Scriver CR, Beaudet AL, Sly WS et al., eds. Metabolic and Molecular Bases of Inherited Diseases. 6th ed. New York: McGraw-Hill, 1989:1116–250.
84. Breckenridge WC, Little JA, Steiner G et al. N Engl J Med 1978;298:1265–73.
85. Nikkila E. Familial lipoprotein lipase deficiency and related disorders of chylomicron metabolism. In: Stanbury JB, Wyngaarden JB, Fredrickson DS et al., eds. The Metabolic Basis of Inherited Disease. 5th ed. New York: McGraw-Hill, 1983:622–42.
86. Kesaniemi YA, Grundy SM. JAMA 1984;251:2542–7.
87. Brunzell JD, Hazzard WR, Porte D Jr et al. J Clin Invest 1973;52:1578–85.
88. Grundy SM, Vega GL. Am J Med 1987;83:9–20.
89. Staels B, Vu-Dac N, Kosykh VA et al. J Clin Invest 1995;95:705–12.
90. Grundy SM, Mok HYI, Zech L et al. J Lipid Res 1981;22:24–36.
91. Garg A, Grundy SM. JAMA 1990;264:723–6.
92. Grundy SM. Circulation 1997;95:1–4.
93. Grundy SM, Brewer HB Jr, Cleeman JI et al. Circulation 2004;109:433–8.
94. Grundy SM, Hansen B, Smith SC Jr et al. Circulation 2004;109:551–6.
95. Grundy SM. Endocrine 2000;13:155–65.
96. Reaven GM. Am Heart J 1991;121:1283–8.
97. Grundy SM, Mok HY, Zech L et al. J Clin Invest 1979;63:1274–83.
98. Grundy SM. Metabolism of very low density lipoprotein–triglycerides in man. In: Gotto AM, Smith LC, Allen B eds. Atherosclerosis V. New York: Springer-Verlag, 1980:586–90.
99. Damerman M, Sandkuijl LA, Halaas JL et al. Proc Natl Acad Sci USA 1993;90:4562–6.
100. Aalto–Setala K, Fisher EA, Chen X et al. J Clin Invest 1992;90:1889–900.
101. Mahley RW, Rall SC Jr. Annu Rev Genomics Hum Genet 2000;1:507–37
102. Austin MA, King M-C, Vranizan KM et al. Circulation 1990;82:495–506.
103. Austin MA, Breslow JL, Hennekens CH et al. JAMA 1988;260:1917–21.
104. Austin MA, Hokanson JE, Brunzell JD. Curr Opin Lipidol 1994;5:395–403.
105. de Graaf J, Hak-Lemmers HLM, Hectors MPC et al. Arterioscler Thromb 1991;11:298–306.
106. Miller NE, Thelle DS, Forde OH et al. Lancet 1977;1:965–8.
107. Gordon T, Castelli WP, Hjortland MC et al. Am J Med 1977;62:707–14.
108. Assman G, Schulte H, Oberwittler W et al. New aspects in the prediction of coronary artery disease: the Prospective Cardiovascular Munster Study. In: Fidge NH, Nestel PJ, eds. Atherosclerosis VII. Amsterdam: Elsevier Science, 1986:19–24.
109. Gordon DJ, Probstfeld JL, Garrison RJ et al. Circulation 1989;79:8–15.
110. Vega GL, Grundy SM. Curr Opin Lipidol 1996;7:209–16.
111. Durstine JL, Haskell WL. Exerc Sport Sci Rev 1994;22:477–521.
112. Karhapaa P, Malkki M, Laakso M. Diabetes 1994;43:411–17.
113. Ettinger WH. Med Clin North Am 1989;73:1525–30.
114. Mensink RP, Katan MB. Lancet 1987;1:122–5.
115. Craig WY, Palomaki GE, Haddow JE. BMJ 1989;298:784–8.
116. Heller DA, de Faire U, Petersen NL et al. N Engl J Med 1993;328:1150–66.
117. Cohen JC, Wang Z-F, Grundy SM et al. J Clin Invest 1994;94:2377–84.
118. Schaefer EJ, Levy RI, Anderson DW et al. Lancet 1978;2:391–3.
119. Nikkila EA, Taskinen M-R, Rehunen S et al. Metabolism 1978;27:1661–71.
120. Blades B, Vega GL, Grundy SM. Arterioscler Thromb 1993;13:1227–35.
121. Guerra R, Wang JP, Grundy SM et al. Proc Natl Acad Sci USA 1997;94:4532–7.
122. Groot PHE, Scheek LM, Jensen H. Biochim Biophys Acta 1983;751:393–400.
123. Tato F, Vega GL, Grundy SM. Arterioscler Thromb Vasc Biol 1995;15:446–51.

124. McPherson R, Grundy SM, Guerra R et al. J Lipid Res 1996; 37:1743–8.

125. Brinton EA, Eisenberg S, Breslow JL. J Clin Invest 1991;87: 536–44.

126. Gylling H, Vega GL, Grundy SM. J Lipid Res 1992;33:1527–39.

127. Widen EI, Eriksson JG, Groop LC. Diabetes 1992;41:354–8.

128. DeFronzo RA, Goodman AM, Multicenter Metformin Study Group. N Engl J Med 1995;333:541–9.

129. Forman BM, Chen J, Evans RM. Proc Natl Acad Sci USA 1997; 94:4312–7.

130. Nolan JJ, Lukvik B, Beerdsen P et al. N Engl J Med 1994;331: 1188–93.

131. Tan MH, Johns D, Strand J et al. Diabet Med 2004;21:859–66.

132. Niskanen I, Uusitupa M, Sarlund H et al. Int J Obes 1996;20: 154–60.

133. Perseghin G, Price TB, Petersen KF et al. N Engl J Med 1996;335:1357–62.

134. Ballantyne CM, Olsson AG, Cook TJ et al. Circulation 2001; 104:3046–51.

135. Vega GL. Endocrinol Metab Clin North Am 2004;33:525–44 vi.

136. Vega GL, Ma PT, Cater NB et al. Am J Cardiol 2003;91: 956–60.

137. East C, Bilheimer DW, Grundy SM. Ann Intern Med 1988;109: 25–32.

138. Vega GL, Grundy SM. Arch Intern Med 1994;154:73–82.

139. Martin-Jadraque R, Tato F, Mostaza JM et al. Arch Intern Med 1996;156:1081–8.

SELECTED READINGS

Chobanian AV, Bakris GL, Black HR et al. Joint National Committee on Prevention, Detection, Evaluation, and Treatment of High Blood Pressure. National Heart, Lung, and Blood Institute; National High Blood Pressure Education Program Coordinating Committee. Seventh report of the Joint National Committee on Prevention, Detection, Evaluation, and Treatment of High Blood Pressure. Hypertension 2003;42:1206–52.

Grundy SM, Hansen B, Smith SC Jr et al. Clinical management of metabolic syndrome: report of the American Heart Association/National Heart, Lung, and Blood Institute/American Diabetes Association conference on scientific issues related to management. Circulation 2004;109:551–6.

Mensink RP, Katan MB. Effect of dietary *trans* fatty acids on high-density and low-density lipoprotein cholesterol levels in healthy subjects. N Engl J Med 1990;323:439–45.

National Cholesterol Education Program (NCEP) Expert Panel on Detection, Evaluation, and Treatment of High Blood Cholesterol in Adults (Adult Treatment Panel III). Third Report of the National Cholesterol Education Program (NCEP) Expert Panel on Detection, Evaluation, and Treatment of High Blood Cholesterol in Adults (Adult Treatment Panel III) final report. Circulation 2002;106:3143–421.

US Department of Agriculture and US Department of Health and Human Services. Nutrition and Your Health: Dietary Guidelines for Americans. 5th ed. Home and Garden Bulletin no. 232. Washington, DC: US Department of Agriculture, 2000.

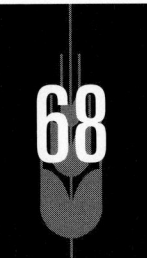

68   NUTRITION, DIET, AND HYPERTENSION[1]

THEODORE A. KOTCHEN AND JANE MORLEY KOTCHEN

SODIUM CHLORIDE 1095
OBESITY 1098
INSULIN RESISTANCE 1098
POTASSIUM 1099
CALCIUM 1099
MAGNESIUM 1100
ALCOHOL 1101
LIPIDS 1101
PROTEIN 1102
CARBOHYDRATE 1102
OVERALL DIET 1102
PRIMARY PREVENTION AND TREATMENT
        OF HYPERTENSION 1103
PUBLIC HEALTH IMPLICATIONS 1103

Between 1971 and 1991, national health examination surveys documented a downward trend of blood pressure levels and prevalence of hypertension in the United States (1). Adoption of healthier lifestyles may have contributed to this favorable trend. However, between 1991 and 2000, the prevalence of hypertension in the United States increased by 3.7%, and more than half of this increase was attributed to an increased prevalence of obesity (2). Hypertension continues to be a major risk factor for cardiovascular disease (3). As many as 58 million people in the United States have elevated blood pressure (systolic blood pressure >140 mm Hg and/or diastolic blood pressure >90 mm Hg) or are taking antihypertensive medications (2).

Blood pressure–associated risks ensue incrementally and progressively over a wide range of blood pressure levels, and a critical value of blood pressure above which persons are classified as "hypertensive" is arbitrary. Furthermore, even among normotensive persons, blood pressure level is predictive of morbidity and mortality from stroke, heart disease, and renal impairment (3). Although categorization of

persons as hypertensive or normotensive provides pragmatic guidelines for medical intervention, it insufficiently addresses blood pressure–related risks. Indeed, between 30 and 40% of all blood pressure–related cardiovascular disease events occur in persons with average blood pressures lower than currently defined hypertensive levels but greater than 120/80 mm Hg. A recent consensus report recommended that the goal of treating hypertensive patients is to maintain blood pressure levels at less than 140/90 mm Hg; however, in patients with hypertension and diabetes or renal disease, the goal blood pressure is less than 130/80 mm Hg. Further, this consensus report recommends that persons with a systolic blood pressure of 120 to 139 mm Hg or a diastolic blood pressure of 80 to 89 mm Hg should be considered "prehypertensive" and require health-promoting lifestyle modifications to prevent cardiovascular disease (3).

This chapter reviews evidence that specific nutrients and interactions among nutrients influence blood pressure. Figure 68.1 presents a schematized, incomplete compilation of highly interrelated physiologic factors that contribute to regulation of arterial pressure. As discussed later, many of these factors have been implicated as potential mechanisms by which specific nutrients affect blood pressure. An understanding of the relationship between diet and blood pressure has important implications not only for the treatment of hypertension but also for developing population-based strategies to decrease the long-term risk of cardiovascular disease.

SODIUM CHLORIDE

A high sodium chloride (NaCl) intake convincingly contributes to elevated arterial pressure in numerous genetic and acquired models of experimental hypertension. The chimpanzee is phylogenetically close to the human, and in a carefully controlled study, the addition of NaCl to the usual diet of the chimpanzee (a fruit and vegetable diet that is low in sodium and high in potassium) over 20 months resulted in a significant elevation of blood pressure (4). Blood pressure did not increase in control animals maintained on their usual diets. Despite individual variation, blood pressures increased progressively with progressive increases in dietary NaCl, and at the highest NaCl intake studied, systolic and diastolic pressures increased by 33 and

---

[1]**Abbreviations: CRR,** corticotropin-releasing hormone; **Dahl-R rat,** Dahl salt-resistant rat; **Dahl-S rat,** Dahl salt-sensitive rat; **DASH,** Dietary Approaches to Stop Hypertension; **NaCl,** sodium chloride; **NHANES,** National Health and Nutrition Examination Surveys; **PTH,** parathyroid hormone; **SHR,** spontaneously hypertensive rat; **TONE,** Trial of Non-pharmacologic Intervention in the Elderly.

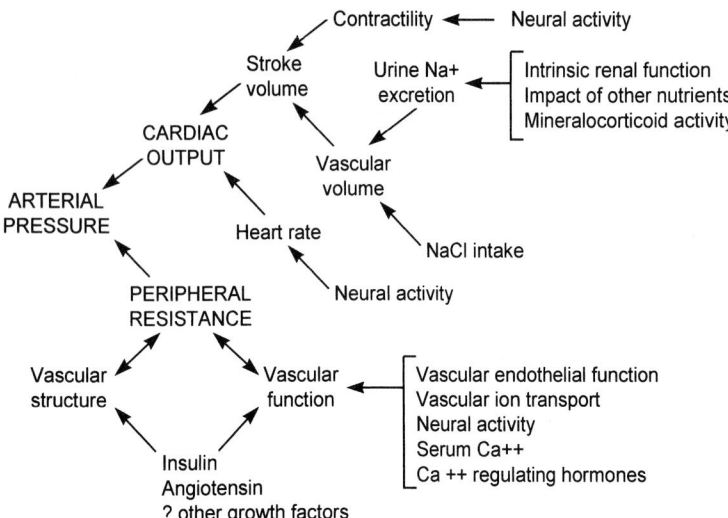

Figure 68.1. Interrelated physiologic factors that contribute to the regulation of arterial pressure. Arterial pressure is determined by cardiac output and peripheral vascular resistance, and cardiac output is determined by stroke volume and heart rate. Cardiac contractility and vascular volume determine stroke volume. Structural and functional changes in the vasculature affect vascular resistance, and increased vascular resistance induces structural and functional changes in the vasculature. Factors that contribute to the regulation of myocardial contractility, vascular volume, and vascular structure and function are also noted.

10 mm Hg, respectively. These increases were completely reversed within 6 months of cessation of the high NaCl intake. Animal studies (as well as limited epidemiologic and clinical observations) also suggested that diets high in NaCl may have deleterious cardiovascular consequences independent of blood pressure, such as cerebral arterial disease and stroke, left ventricular hypertrophy, renal vascular disease, and glomerular injury (5, 6).

In the human, evidence for an association between NaCl intake and blood pressure is provided by both observational and intervention studies (7–11). The effect of NaCl on blood pressure increases with age, with the height of the blood pressure, and, in normotensive persons, with a family history of hypertension (12). There may also be a modest association between higher NaCl intake and higher blood pressure in children and adolescents (13), and results of a randomized trial suggested that a high NaCl intake during the first 5 weeks of life is associated with higher blood pressures during adolescence (14). Increased sodium concentrations in drinking water have been reported to increase blood pressure in neonates (15).

Among populations, the prevalence of hypertension is related to NaCl intake. The Intersalt study described the relationship between blood pressure and 24-hour urine sodium excretion in more than 10,000 persons in 52 centers around the world (16, 17). Two principal findings of this study were as follows: (a) a difference of 100 mEq/day in sodium intake is associated with a 3 to 6 mm Hg difference in systolic blood pressure, and (b) lowering the sodium intake by 100 mEq/day attenuates the rise of systolic blood pressure in persons between the ages of 25 and 55 years by 10 mm Hg.

Based on results of acute NaCl depletion or acute NaCl loading protocols (depending on criteria for the definition of NaCl sensitivity), approximately 30 to 50% of hypertensive persons and a smaller percentage of nor-

motensive persons are estimated to be NaCl sensitive; that is, arterial pressure is decreased by NaCl depletion and/or increased by NaCl loading (18, 19). In short-term intervention trials of the effects of moderate NaCl restriction on blood pressure, the overall reduction of blood pressure is relatively small. As reviewed in two metaanalyses, reduction of blood pressure by NaCl restriction is more prominent in hypertensive (4.9/2.9–3.7/0.9 mm Hg) than in normotensive (1.7/1.0–1.0/0.1 mm Hg) persons (20, 21). This modest reduction of blood pressure in normotensive persons led some investigators to question recommendations for reducing NaCl intake in the general population. However, many of the trials included in the metaanalyses were of short duration (<2 weeks), and the full impact of NaCl reduction on blood pressure may increase over time. It has been estimated that these small reductions of blood pressure in the population would reduce risks of stroke by 15% and coronary heart disease by 6% (22).

The anion accompanying sodium is important in determining the magnitude of the blood pressure increase in response to high dietary intake of NaCl. The full expression of NaCl-sensitive hypertension depends on concomitant administration of both sodium and chloride (23). In both experimental models of NaCl-sensitive hypertension and in the human, blood pressure is not increased by high dietary sodium intake with anions other than chloride, and a high chloride intake without sodium has less effect on blood pressure than NaCl. The failure of nonchloride sodium salts to produce hypertension may be related to their failure to expand plasma volume. In usual diets, however, sodium is generally consumed as NaCl.

Blood pressure responses to NaCl may be modified by other components of the diet. Both epidemiologic evidence and clinical evidence suggest that dietary intake of potassium or calcium lower than the recommended dietary allowances potentiates NaCl sensitivity of blood pressure (24, 25). Conversely, high dietary intake of potassium or calcium prevents or attenuates the development of NaCl-induced hypertension in several animal models.

Genetic Influences

Within a population, overall blood pressure responses to NaCl restriction may mask individual variability. Experimental models of hypertension and increasing information in the human provide convincing evidence for genetic susceptibility and genetic resistance to the effects of dietary NaCl on arterial pressure. For example, different strains of rats are either sensitive or resistant to the effect of NaCl intake on blood pressure, such as Dahl salt-sensitive (Dahl-S) rats and Dahl salt-resistant (Dahl-R) rats. In an intercross of normotensive Brown Norway and Dahl-S rats, based on results of a total genome scan, salt sensitivity of blood pressure is reportedly linked to a specific region on chromosome 18 (26). Further, in a consomic animal model, substitution of Brown Norway chromosome 13 on the background of an inbred Dahl-S rat nearly abolishes the rise of arterial pressure observed with a high-salt diet (27). Genetically altered mice with knockout genes for γ-melanocyte-stimulating hormone, atrial natriuretic peptide and its receptor, the prostaglandin receptor EP2, or the bradykinin receptor, all exhibit salt-sensitive hypertension (28). The relevance of these observations to human hypertension remains to be determined.

In humans, a familial resemblance in the change of blood pressure in response to salt restriction has been described, and a phenotype of haptoglobin may be a marker of NaCl sensitivity (29). In the United States, larger proportions of both normotensive and hypertensive African-Americans are NaCl sensitive, compared with whites (30). Reasons for this are not entirely clear but may in part be genetic. Clinically, evidence indicates heritability of sodium excretion, levels of hormones that regulate sodium excretion, and salt sensitivity of blood pressure in both whites and African-Americans. African-Americans excrete sodium less efficiently than whites; plasma renin activity tends to be suppressed in African-Americans, and low plasma renin may be a surrogate marker for salt sensitivity of blood pressure (31). Investigators have estimated that more than 50% of African-American hypertensive persons in the United States are salt sensitive; the prevalence of diuretic-sensitive (and presumably salt-sensitive) blood pressures approaches 75% (32). Some studies have addressed the potential role of specific genetic polymorphisms in salt sensitivity of blood pressure in humans (33). Among the most frequently studied polymorphisms include the following: α-adducin Gly460Trp, angiotensin-converting enzyme I/D, angiotensinogen M235T, G protein β-3 C825T; aldosterone synthase gene, and 11-β-hydroxysteroid dehydrogenase type2 G534A. Results among studies have been inconsistent, in part reflecting genetic heterogeneity among populations and heterogeneity in the method of salt sensitivity testing.

Physiologic Mechanisms

Several interrelated blood pressure control mechanisms may contribute to blood pressure elevations induced by NaCl (Fig. 68.1). Experimental and clinical evidence suggests that a genetically determined decreased capacity to excrete sodium contributes to NaCl-induced elevations of arterial pressure in the susceptible host (34). The Dahl-S rat is a well-characterized genetic model of low-renin, NaCl-sensitive hypertension associated with insulin resistance. In this model, the pressure natriuresis curve (inflow pressure versus sodium excretion) from the isolated kidney is shifted to the right; that is, the kidney of the NaCl-sensitive animal requires a greater pressure to excrete sodium than the kidney from the Dahl-R rat. Similarly, in the human, several, but not all, investigators reported that NaCl-sensitive hypertensive patients retain more sodium in response to a NaCl load than NaCl-resistant patients (35). In humans, several rare monogenic forms of hypertension resulting from an impaired capacity to excrete sodium have been described (36).

Nitric oxide is a vascular endothelium–derived vasodilator. In the normal rat, nitric oxide activity increases in response to a high NaCl intake, perhaps facilitating natriuresis and blood pressure homeostasis, and impaired nitric oxide synthase activity may contribute to NaCl sensitivity of blood pressure (37). Pharmacologic inhibition of nitric oxide synthesis shifts the pressure-natriuresis relationship to higher levels of arterial pressure and produces hypertension (34); conversely, long-term treatment with arginine shifts the pressure-natriuresis relationship to lower pressures and prevents development of hypertension in the Dahl-S rat and the spontaneously hypertensive rat (SHR).

Increased sympathetic nervous system activity and impaired baroreflex function may also contribute to NaCl-sensitive hypertension in experimental animals and in humans (38–40). In the Dahl-S rat, dietary NaCl loading potentiates the increment of vascular resistance in response to neural stimulation and increases the rate of basal firing of the splanchnic nerve. A high NaCl intake increases vascular reactivity to norepinephrine in the prehypertensive Dahl-S rat. A high-NaCl diet also exacerbates impairment of baroreceptor reflex control of heart rate in the Dahl-S rat, whereas in the Dahl-R rat, a high-NaCl diet enhances afferent discharge of aortic baroreceptors and augments sympathoinhibitory responses to volume expansion. In the normotensive rat, dog, and rabbit, impaired baroreflex function renders the animal susceptible to NaCl-induced blood pressure elevations.

NaCl sensitivity of blood pressure is also associated with alterations of ion transport in vascular smooth muscle that favor vasoconstriction (41). Based primarily on studies in circulating blood cells, most evidence suggests that active membrane sodium transport is suppressed by high NaCl intake and that suppression of sodium transport by a high-NaCl diet may be less prominent in circulating cells of hypertensive persons than of normotensive persons. Hypertension is also associated with increased red blood cell lithium/sodium countertransport and decreased sodium-potassium/2 chloride cotransport; increased red cell lithium/sodium countertransport may be a marker for NaCl sensitivity of blood pressure. Dietary NaCl loading has been reported to increase intracellular calcium in lymphocytes of NaCl-sensitive humans. Based on nuclear magnetic resonance spectroscopy studies of the intracellular ionic consequences of NaCl loading, patients with salt-sensitive hypertension have an exaggerated increase in intracellular sodium and, in contrast to non–salt-sensitive persons, elevation of cytosolic free calcium and suppression of intracellular pH and magnesium levels (42). These ionic alterations may contribute to increased peripheral resistance. More recently, in African-Americans, but not in whites, salt sensitivity of blood pressure has been shown to be positively associated with intracellular concentrations of sodium and calcium in erythrocytes and with the ratios of intracellular sodium to intracellular potassium and intracellular calcium to intracellular magnesium (43).

Reduction of dietary sodium to 60 mEq/day has been shown to increase arterial compliance, to reduce arterial stiffness, and to lower arterial pressure in older persons with primarily systolic hypertension (44). Investigators have suggested that NaCl dependence of arterial pressure in these persons can be attributed to multiple mechanisms that underlie arterial compliance and vascular resistance (45). NaCl activates tissue angiotensin II and sodium pump ligands, affects endothelial and vascular cell function, and affects arterial structural remodeling, which results in arterial stiffening. Platelet reactivity increases with a high dietary NaCl intake, possibly as a consequence of increased intracellular calcium, and this may be a mechanism by which NaCl contributes to occlusive stroke independent of blood pressure (46).

OBESITY

An association between obesity and hypertension has been amply documented. Data from cross-sectional studies indicate a direct linear correlation between body weight (or body mass index) and blood pressure (3, 47–49). Centrally located body fat is a more important determinant of blood pressure elevation than peripherally located body fat in both women and men. In longitudinal studies, a direct correlation exists between change in weight and change in blood pressure over time, even when dietary salt intake is held constant (43). The proportion of the prevalence of hypertension attributable to obesity is an important public health question. Investigators have estimated that 60% of

hypertensive adults are more than 20% overweight, and hypertension is detectable in about 30% of overweight children (50). The high prevalence of overweight combined with the corresponding increase in risk of developing high blood pressure led to estimates that 20 to 30% of hypertension can be attributed to this exposure. The increasing prevalence of hypertension in the United States in recent years has been attributed at least in part to the increasing prevalence of obesity (2, 51, 52). In addition, blood pressure levels of US children have increased in the past decade, and this may also be attributable, at least in part, to an increased prevalence of overweight (53).

A reduction of blood pressure by weight loss has been clearly documented in short-term trials in both hypertensive and normotensive persons. Based on pooling results of controlled dietary intervention trials, investigators have estimated that a mean change in body weight of 9.2 kg is associated with a 6.3 mm Hg change in systolic blood pressure and a 3.1 mm Hg change in diastolic blood pressure (49).

Obesity-related hypertension has been variously ascribed to hypervolemia and increased cardiac output without an appropriate reduction of peripheral resistance, to increased sympathetic nervous system activity, and to insulin resistance (54).

INSULIN RESISTANCE

Obesity is associated with resistance to insulin-stimulated glucose uptake and hyperinsulinemia, and weight loss increases insulin sensitivity (55). Depending on the populations studied and the methodologies for defining insulin resistance, approximately 25 to 50% of nonobese, nondiabetic hypertensive persons are also insulin resistant (56, 57). Higher insulin levels have been reported to be associated with an increased risk of hypertension in both African-Americans and whites (58). The constellation of insulin resistance, reactive hyperinsulinemia, increased serum triglyceride concentrations, decreased high-density lipoprotein cholesterol, and hypertension has been designated syndrome X. Independent of obesity, centripetal distribution of body fat is also associated with insulin resistance and elevated blood pressure. Insulin resistance is also associated with alterations in the blood clotting cascade that accentuate thrombosis by increasing coagulation and inhibiting fibrinolysis. In both women and men, centripital obesity is predictive of coronary heart disease, independent of body mass index, and waist-to-hip ratio may be a better predictor of cardiovascular risk than body mass index (56).

Increasing evidence suggests that insulin resistance is associated with salt sensitivity of blood pressure in both normotensive and hypertensive persons (55, 56, 59). Like patients with salt-sensitive hypertension, even in the absence of hypertension, obese persons and/or persons with type

2 diabetes mellitus reportedly also have elevated intracellular calcium and suppressed intracellular magnesium levels, and these ionic alterations may contribute to insulin resistance (59, 60).

Syndrome X may in part be heritable; however, in the rat, simple carbohydrate feeding (sucrose, glucose, or fructose) also results in insulin resistance, dyslipidemia, and increased blood pressure (55). Sucrose feeding also potentiates development of hypertension in the SHR, in a rat model of adrenal regeneration hypertension, and in normotensive rats fed high-NaCl diets. Although certain putative mechanisms have been proposed, it is unclear whether insulin resistance and hyperinsulinemia actually cause hypertension. Putative mechanisms include antinatriuretic effect of insulin, increased sympathetic nervous system activity, augmented vasoconstriction in response to norepinephrine and angiotensin, impaired endothelium-dependent vasodilatation, and stimulation of vascular smooth muscle growth by insulin.

POTASSIUM

Potassium loading prevents or ameliorates development of hypertension in several animal models of genetic and NaCl-induced hypertension (24). Conversely, in both Dahl-S and Dahl-R rats on a high-NaCl diet, a low potassium intake results in blood pressure elevation and renal vascular remodeling (increased wall-to-lumen ratio), indicating increased renal vascular resistance (61).

In societies with high potassium intakes, both mean blood pressure and the prevalence of hypertension tend to be lower than in societies with low potassium intakes (24, 62). Several large surveys have demonstrated a significant inverse correlation between potassium intake and blood pressure among persons within a population; this inverse association is more prominent in those on a high-NaCl diet (16, 24). However, in some studies, after adjusting for other variables (e.g., age, weight, consumption of alcohol, fiber, magnesium), dietary potassium was not found to be independently associated with blood pressure (63), and not all surveys documented an association between potassium intake and either level of blood pressure or prevalence of hypertension. Failure to observe this association may be related to insufficient sample sizes. The urine sodium-to-potassium ratio appears to be a stronger correlate of blood pressure than either sodium or potassium alone (16, 24, 62, 64); in children, the rise of blood pressure with age is directly related to the urine sodium-to-potassium ratio (65).

In 1928, Addison reported that a high potassium intake has an antihypertensive effect in humans (66). Metaanalyses of clinical trials concluded that oral potassium supplements significantly lower both systolic and diastolic blood pressures (67, 68). The magnitude of the blood pressure lowering effect is greater in hypertensive than in normotensive persons and is more pronounced with a longer duration of supplementation. The effect of a high potassium intake on blood pressure is also more pronounced in blacks than in whites and in persons consuming a high-NaCl diet (24, 68). Increased intake of potassium has been reported not to affect blood pressure in hypertensive men on a low-NaCl diet (69); however, reduced sodium and increased potassium and magnesium intake lowered blood pressure in men and women with mild to moderate hypertension (70). Conversely, potassium depletion induced either by a low-potassium diet or by diuretics is associated with blood pressure elevation (71, 72).

Proposed mechanisms by which a high dietary intake of potassium may lower blood pressure include a natriuretic effect of potassium, inhibition of renin release, antagonism of the pressor response to angiotensin II, direct vasodilatation, augmentation of endothelium-dependent vasodilatation, decreased production of the vasoconstrictor thromboxane, and increased production of the vasodilator kallidin (24).

Dietary potassium may affect morbidity and mortality, independent of an effect on blood pressure. Unrelated to changes of blood pressure, a high-potassium diet was reported to decrease stroke mortality in the stroke-prone SHRs and to decrease renal damage in several rat models of hypertension (73, 74). Similarly, in a prospective clinical study, the 12-year risk of stroke death was associated with potassium intake, independent of blood pressure (65). In a prefecture in Japan, introducing a diet with a low sodium-to-potassium ratio was associated with a reduced 10-year stroke mortality rate (75).

CALCIUM

More than 80 studies have reported that blood pressure is lowered by increasing dietary calcium in experimental models of hypertension (76). This effect of calcium on blood pressure may be more pronounced in models of salt-sensitive hypertension (77).

Within and among human populations, as with potassium, there "is an inverse association between dietary calcium intake and blood pressure, and low calcium intake is associated with an increased prevalence of hypertension" (25, 78). Data from both epidemiologic reports and animal studies suggest a threshold for calcium intake below which arterial pressure increases (79), and a low calcium intake may amplify the effects of a high-NaCl diet on blood pressure. In the human, diets with less than 600 mg calcium/day are most clearly associated with hypertension (80). Based on results of two published metaanalyses including 23 and 66 populations, weak but statistically significant inverse correlations were observed for association of dietary calcium with both systolic and diastolic blood pressures (80, 81). However, because of the size of the estimate, the heterogeneity among studies, the difficulty of assessing calcium intake, and the possibility of confounding and publication bias, the authors concluded that increasing calcium intake to more than the recommended dietary alllowance is not recommended for the prevention or treatment of high blood pressure. Dietary calcium is also inversely related to systolic blood pressure in young children (82).

Most clinical trials evaluating the effect of increased dietary calcium on blood pressure supplemented diets with 1000 to 1500 mg/day of elemental calcium. Reductions of blood pressure were modest and inconsistent, and no gradient of calcium effect or threshold intake level was identified. Two metaanalyses of randomized clinical trials showed a small, statistically significant reduction of systolic, but not diastolic, blood pressure (83, 84). As with the data in the observational studies, results of these clinical trials do not justify recommending calcium supplementation to the general population for prevention or treatment of hypertension.

Within a population, it may be possible to identify subgroups more likely to be responsive to calcium. For example, calcium supplementation may preferentially lower blood pressure in patients with NaCl-sensitive hypertension and low-renin hypertension, whereas calcium may actually increase blood pressure in patients with high- renin or renin-dependent hypertension (25). During pregnancy, calcium supplementation has been reported to reduce both systolic and diastolic blood pressure (85). Despite earlier evidence to the contrary (86), results of a randomized, multicenter trial indicate that calcium supplementation during pregnancy does not prevent preeclampsia or pregnancy-associated hypertension (87). Calcium supplementation more convincingly lowers blood pressure in persons consuming low-calcium diets (88, 89).

Considerable speculation exists about mechanisms by which dietary calcium may affect blood pressure (89). Calcium has a natriuretic effect, which may explain the apparent greater sensitivity of patients with NaCl-sensitive hypertension to the blood pressure–lowering effect of calcium. Conversely, in both the human and the intact rat, NaCl loading increases urinary calcium excretion and serum parathyroid hormone (PTH) and 1,25-dihydroxyvitamin D concentrations. Hypercalcuria, decreased plasma ionized calcium concentrations, and increased plasma concentrations of PTH and 1,25-dihydroxyvitamin D have been observed in experimental models of NaCl-sensitive hypertension and in patients with low-renin hypertension (90). Investigators have hypothesized that PTH results in vasoconstriction by influencing neural activity and/or vasoactive hormones either directly or indirectly via changes in serum calcium. Other studies have emphasized a role for vitamin D, especially in NaCl-related hypertension.

Conceivably, NaCl-sensitive hypertension may be a calcium-losing state, resulting in secondary hyperparathyroidism (76, 89, 90). Calcium supplementation may reduce blood pressure by correcting this calcium deficiency and the associated hyperparathyroidism. Alternatively, alterations of calcium metabolism and calcium-regulating hormones may be epiphenomena of NaCl loading that are not causally related to the development of hypertension.

Other putative mechanisms by which high dietary calcium intake may lower blood pressure include decreased calcium influx into vascular smooth muscle cells and increased capacity of these cells to extrude calcium, potential vasoactive effects of calcium-regulating hormones (PTH, 1,25-dihydroxyvitamin D, calcitonin gene–related peptide), and modulation of sympathetic nervous system activity.

MAGNESIUM

Relatively little information is available concerning dietary magnesium and blood pressure. High magnesium intakes lower blood pressure in rat models of hypertension, and in the rat, blood pressure increases in response to magnesium deprivation (91, 92).

In the human, as with calcium, evidence suggests an association between lower magnesium in the diet and higher blood pressures (25). Since the early 1900s, the availability of magnesium-rich foods has declined, and consumption of processed foods that have lost magnesium has increased. Investigators have proposed that subclinical magnesium deficiency has developed in industrialized countries, and this has paralleled the increased prevalence of hypertension (93). Conversely, persons consuming vegetarian diets, which are usually high in magnesium and fiber content, tend to have lower blood pressures than nonvegetarians, a finding raising the possibility that dietary magnesium is inversely related to blood pressure. However, in one cross-sectional study of 9- to 10-year-old girls, after adjusting for dietary fiber, a significant inverse association between magnesium intake and blood pressure was no longer discerned (94). In older persons, diets high in both magnesium and potassium are associated with lower blood pressures (70). Limited evidence suggests that dietary intake of magnesium is lower in hypertensive persons than in normotensive persons; in one prospective study, lower calcium (<400 versus >800 mg/day) and lower magnesium (<200 versus >300 mg/day) intake predicted a risk of subsequent hypertension (95). In another prospective study, dietary magnesium, potassium, and fiber were each significantly associated with lower risk of hypertension when considered separately; however, when these nutrients were considered simultaneously, only dietary fiber had an inverse association with hypertension (96).

Limited information is available about the effects of magnesium supplementation on blood pressure in hypertensive persons, and the results are inconsistent. At best, the overall hypotensive response to magnesium supplementation is small and may become more apparent in trials of more than 6 months' duration (97, 98). The capacity of magnesium to lower blood pressure appears to be greater in hypertensive persons who are hypomagnesemic and/or are taking diuretics (99, 100). A recent metaanalysis of trials conducted with both hypertensive and normotensive persons reported dose-dependent blood pressure reduction from magnesium supplementation (101). However, the authors concluded that this relationship should be confirmed by adequately powered trials with sufficiently high doses of magnesium supplements.

A plausible physiologic rationale exists for an effect of magnesium on blood pressure. Magnesium decreases vascular tone and contractility, possibly by decreasing cellular uptake of calcium and thereby decreasing cytosolic calcium (25). In addition, magnesium administration in endothelial cells and in humans stimulates production of prostaglandin I_2, a vasodilator, when serum magnesium is raised acutely. Conversely, magnesium deficiency is associated with resistance to insulin-stimulated glucose uptake and enhanced vascular contractility.

ALCOHOL

Observational studies suggest a J-shaped relationship between alcohol consumption and blood pressure (102–104). Light drinkers (one to two drinks per day) have lower blood pressures than teetotalers (105), whereas in comparison with nondrinkers, a small but significant elevation of blood pressure is seen in persons consuming three or more drinks per day (a standard drink contains approximately 14 g of ethanol and is defined as a 12-ounce glass of beer, a 6-ounce glass of table wine, or 1.5 ounces of distilled spirits). These higher blood pressures are not related to potentially confounding variables such as age and body mass. The assumption is that alcohol is a vasodilator at low doses but a vasoconstrictor at higher doses.

The contribution to the prevalence of hypertension attributed to consuming more than two drinks of alcohol per day has been estimated to be 5 to 7%; the contribution in men is greater than in women, although in women the risk of hypertension increases progressively with alcohol intake in excess of 20 g/day. In controlled studies, reduction of alcohol consumption has been associated with a reduction of 4 to 8 mm Hg in systolic blood pressure and a lesser reduction of diastolic pressure. Blood pressure of normotensive persons may also decrease in response to a reduction of alcohol consumption. A metaanalysis of 15 randomized, controlled trials reported a relationship between mean percentage of alcohol reduction and mean blood pressure reduction, and the effects of the intervention were enhanced in participants with higher baseline blood pressures (106).

The mechanism by which alcohol may affect blood pressure has not been established. In both the rat and the human, alcohol ingestion augments sympathetic nervous system activity (105). Alcohol also stimulates corticotropin-releasing hormone (CRR) and cortisol secretion, and CRR appears to stimulate sympathetic neural activity. In physiologically normal subjects, it has been reported that dexamethasone inhibits both the augmented neural discharge and blood pressure increment in response to alcohol infusion (107). This observation suggests that the alcohol-induced elevation of blood pressure is related to CRR-mediated sympathetic activation. Additionally, short-term administration of alcohol results in an early rise in serum magnesium level followed by a transient decrease in PTH, associated with transient hypocalcemia and hypercalcuria and followed by a late rise in PTH. What relation, if any, this may have to alcohol-induced increases of blood pressure is not clear.

LIPIDS

Both animal and human data suggest that polyunsaturated n-3 and n-6 fatty acids play a role in blood pressure regulation (108). In experimental models of hypertension, both linoleic acid (a long-chain n-6 polyunsaturated fatty acid) and fish oil (rich in eicosapentaenoic and docosahexaenoic acids, both n-3 fatty acids) attenuate the development of renin-dependent hypertension (109). Limited epidemiologic evidence suggests a direct association between diets high in saturated fats and blood pressure, and many populations with low mean blood pressure levels consume diets low in total fat and saturated fatty acids (110). Conversely, diets high in n-3 fatty acids may be associated with lower blood pressures (111). Several trials have failed to show a significant blood pressure effect by varying the dietary content of fat or by exchanging polyunsaturated fatty acids for saturated fatty acids, and there is ongoing debate whether reducing saturated fat and/or increasing polyunsaturated fat in the diet lowers blood pressure (112). Limited evidence suggests that linoleic acid–enriched diets reduce blood pressure in normotensive and hypertensive persons.

Results of a metaanalysis of 31 controlled trials showed a small, statistically significant reduction of blood pressure by fish oil (3.0/1.5 mm Hg) at an overall mean dose of 4.8 g of n-3 fatty acids (or approximately ten capsules) per day (113). In these trials, little or no effect was reported among healthy normotensive persons; however, hypertensive patients showed a dose-response hypotensive effect of fish oil. A more recent metaanalysis of 90 randomized trials concluded that high intake of fish oil (median dose, 3.7 g/day) reduced blood pressure by 2.1./1.6 mm Hg (114). The blood pressure reductions were larger in hypertensive persons and in those older than 45 years. Fish oil also had a moderate effect on blood pressure in hypercholesterolemic patients and in patients with atherosclerotic cardiovascular disease. The authors concluded that fish oil is unlikely to benefit healthy person for the prevention or treatment of hypertension, given the uncertainty of response and the large dose required to elicit small changes in blood pressure. Despite some earlier evidence to the contrary, one randomized, controlled trial concluded that fish oil in doses that reduce blood pressure in hypertensive persons does not adversely affect insulin sensitivity or glucose metabolism (115).

In contrast to n-3 polyunsaturated fatty acids, results of clinical trials show little or no evidence that saturated fats and n-6 polyunsaturated fats have an independent effect on blood pressure beyond changing body weight (116, 117). The blood pressure reductions attributed to n-3 fatty acids may be related to alterations of prostaglandin metabolism, alterations of vascular endothelial function, increased vascular responsiveness to pressor agents, and inhibition of vascular smooth muscle proliferation.

PROTEIN

Several observational studies, including the Intersalt study, suggested that blood pressure level is inversely associated with dietary protein and fiber consumption (16, 118, 119). However, limited clinical intervention trials showed no evidence that amount or type of protein in the diet affects blood pressure (105). Conceivably, specific amino acids could affect neurotransmitters or humoral substances that control blood pressure. For example, acute administration of tryptophan or tyrosine (either peripherally or directly into the central nervous system) reduces blood pressure in experimental animals, possibly via effects on neuronal pathways involved in blood pressure control (118).

CARBOHYDRATE

As discussed earlier, simple carbohydrate feeding induces insulin resistance. In the rat, high dietary intake of glucose, sucrose, or fructose may increase arterial pressure in the normotensive animal, may augment NaCl sensitivity of blood pressure, and may potentiate development of hypertension in several experimental models (55). However, in the human, no evidence indicates that manipulating the carbohydrate content of the diet affects blood pressure.

OVERALL DIET

In general, results of both observational and intervention studies demonstrate that lacto-ovo vegetarian diets consumed by acculturated persons are associated with a decreased prevalence of hypertension and lower blood pressure levels than omnivorous diets (120–123). A strict lacto-ovo vegetarian diet consists of a relatively low intake of saturated fat, a high ratio of polyunsaturated to saturated fat, and a high intake of fruits, vegetables, and other fiber. Dietary intakes of carbohydrate, potassium, magnesium, and calcium tend to be increased, and dietary protein is lower than that in omnivores.

The specific nutrients responsible for the blood pressure reduction associated with vegetarian diets have not been defined. Although vegetarians tend to be slimmer, the lower blood pressure appears not to be totally accounted for by body weight. Results of randomized controlled dietary trials suggest that the hypotensive effect of a vegetarian diet is

also not the result of the absence of meat protein per se (122). Substituting animal fat with starch and sugar appears not to lower blood pressure, whereas blood pressure is lowered by replacing fat with vegetable products, including vegetable oils (120). The effect of dietary fiber on blood pressure remains an unresolved issue (124); carefully controlled studies with different types of fiber are needed. Additionally, vegetables are a primary source of vitamin C, and several observational studies suggest an inverse correlation between plasma vitamin C levels and blood pressure; however, the limited available clinical trial data do not demonstrate a convincing blood pressure reduction with increased consumption of vitamin C (125).

Based on a review of data from the third National Health and Nutrition Examination Surveys (NHANES III), the southern region of the United States, which includes the "stroke belt," has dietary patterns that may contribute to the high prevalence of hypertension and cardiovascular disease in that region (126). Compared with other regions of the United States, residents in the south reported the highest sodium consumption and the lowest consumption of potassium, calcium, and magnesium. Also based on NHANES data, a diet low in sodium, alcohol, and protein is associated with lower systolic blood pressure and pulse pressure. Potassium intake was associated with lower systolic and diastolic blood pressure. In addition, the age-related increases in systolic blood pressure were attenuated by higher calcium and protein intakes (127).

The Dietary Approaches to Stop Hypertension (DASH) trial was a randomized multicenter study that evaluated the effects of three dietary patterns over 8 weeks on blood pressure in 459 adults with high-normal blood pressure or mild hypertension (128). The dietary interventions were as follows: (a) control diet, with potassium, calcium, and magnesium levels close to the twenty-fifth percentile of US consumption; (b) a diet rich in fruits and vegetables; and (c) a "combination" diet rich in fruits, vegetables, and low-fat dairy products. NaCl content was equivalent in all three diets (8 g/day). Systolic and diastolic blood pressures were significantly reduced by the fruit and vegetable diet (-2.8 and -1 mm Hg, respectively) and, compared with controls, were reduced even more by the combination diet (-5.5 and -3.0 mm Hg, respectively).

In a subsequent trial, the DASH-Sodium trial, the effects of reduced sodium intake in the context of the DASH diet and a more typical US diet were examined. Three levels of sodium intake (50, 100, and 150 mEq/day) were evaluated for 30 days each in 412 persons consuming either the DASH diet or a control diet. Highly significant decreases in blood pressure were observed with decreased sodium intake in participants following either diet. Overall, the combined effects of the DASH-low-sodium diet lowered systolic and diastolic blood pressure by 8.9 and 4.5 mm Hg, respectively, compared with the high-sodium phase of the control diet (129). The effect of sodium reduction was especially pronounced in hypertensive persons, African-Americans, women, and persons older than 45 years of age (130). Further, the DASH diet steepened the slope of the relationship between mean arterial pressure and urinary sodium excretion, a finding suggesting a natriuretic action of the DASH diet (131).

PRIMARY PREVENTION AND TREATMENT OF HYPERTENSION

In children, a strong correlation exists between obesity and blood pressure, and a direct association is found between changes in body weight and change in blood pressure (132). In addition, blood pressures in the young tend to track over time, and a large proportion of obese children become obese adults. Prevention of obesity, beginning in childhood, would seem important for the primary prevention of hypertension and cardiovascular disease.

Several trials have tested the efficacy of preventing hypertension in adults through altered dietary intake. In one trial, approximately 200 subjects with diastolic blood pressures in the high-normal ranges (80–89 mm Hg) were assigned to either a control group or a combined intervention consisting of weight loss, sodium restriction, moderate alcohol restriction, and moderate isotonic physical activity (133). Subjects were followed over a 5-year period. Nine percent of intervention subjects developed hypertension, compared with 19% of control subjects ($p < 0.027$). In a second prevention trial, 841 men and women between the ages of 25 and 49 years with diastolic blood pressures between 78 and 89 mm Hg were assigned to one of five groups: (a) control, (b) reduced calories, (c) reduced sodium, (d) reduced calories and sodium, and (e) reduced sodium and increased potassium (134). Calorie counseling reduced mean diastolic and systolic blood pressures at 6 months (2.8 and 5.1 mm Hg, respectively) and 3 years (1.8 and 2.4 mm Hg). Somewhat unexpectedly, the combination of calorie and sodium counseling was less effective than calorie counseling alone. The other interventions did not significantly affect blood pressure.

The Trial of Hypertension Prevention was designed to evaluate nonpharmacologic interventions in the primary prevention of hypertension in men and women with diastolic blood pressures ranging from 80 to 89 mm Hg. Different groups of subjects were exposed to different interventions. In phase I (which included 2182 subjects), stress management or dietary supplementation for 6 months with calcium, magnesium, potassium, or fish oil did not significantly reduce systolic or diastolic blood pressure, compared with controls; however, blood pressure was reduced by weight reduction and, to a lesser extent, by modest salt restriction over an 18-month period (135, 136). Phase II was designed to test the effects of weight loss and sodium restriction, alone and in combination, on blood pressure over 3 to 4 years in overweight adults with high-normal blood pressures. Both weight loss and reduction of sodium

intake, individually and in combination, lowered systolic and diastolic blood pressures in the short term (6 months), although the effects of the two interventions were not additive. Beyond 6 months, the interventions were less effective in maintaining both weight loss and sodium restriction, and although their impact on blood pressure (although still significant) lessened, hypertension incidence was reduced. After 7 years of follow-up, the incidence of hypertension was 18.9% in the weight-loss group and 40.5% in its control group, and it was 22.4% in the sodium-reduction group and 32.0% in its control group (137).

In a randomized controlled Trial of Non-pharmacologic Intervention in the Elderly (TONE), sodium reduction alone, weight loss alone, and the combined intervention of sodium reduction and weight loss were shown to lower blood pressure effectively and safely in older persons with hypertension (138). At the end of TONE follow-up (just over 2 years), 43% of participants in the combined-intervention group were no longer taking medication compared with 25% in the usual-care group. Forty-eight months after the end of TONE, 23% of the patients in the combined-intervention group versus 7% of the usual-care group were not taking medication (139).

The impact of dietary intervention on blood pressure is most pronounced in persons with hypertension. With appropriate dietary modifications, it may be possible to treat hypertensive patients with fewer drugs and with lower doses; in a significant percentage of hypertensives, particularly patients with mild hypertension, dietary modifications may totally obviate the need for drug therapy (140–143). Among overweight adults who are taking antihypertensive medications, a comprehensive lifestyle intervention (including the DASH diet, sodium reduction, weight loss, and exercise) has been shown to improve blood pressure control as well as to lower total and low-density lipoprotein cholesterol (144). In hypertensive persons whose blood pressures have been controlled with medications, weight loss or NaCl restriction more than doubles the likelihood of maintaining normal blood pressure after withdrawal of drug therapy. The following lifestyle modifications have been recommended as adjunctive or definitive therapy for hypertension: weight reduction if overweight; aerobic exercise; limited NaCl and alcohol intake; maintenance of adequate dietary potassium, calcium, and magnesium intake; smoking cessation; and reduced dietary saturated fat and cholesterol intake for overall cardiovascular health (3).

PUBLIC HEALTH IMPLICATIONS

Recent evidence of increased levels of blood pressure associated with an increased prevalence of overweight and obesity accentuates the need for broad population-based strategies to address dietary intake. In addition, recommendations for dietary changes have been extended to include children with blood pressures in the high-normal or prehypertensive ranges (145). Observational and interventional studies in humans, supported by findings from animal studies, provide a clear rationale for the following population-based recommendations to optimize the effect of diet on blood pressure: reduce NaCl intake; control body weight; consume adequate amounts of potassium, calcium, and magnesium; and moderate alcoholic beverage intake. Blood pressure–lowering interventions applied to the entire community would result in a small downward shift in the blood pressure distribution, which would have a substantial impact on preventing hypertension and reducing the burden of blood pressure–related cardiovascular disease (3, 128, 146). A strong rationale exists for a population-based educational approach to blood pressure control through diet. A population-based approach reaches children during years when lifestyles and dietary preferences are established. It also reinforces recommended dietary changes for hypertensive persons. We found that educational efforts directed to an entire community significantly decreased blood pressure levels and improved control of high blood pressure (147).

Investigators have estimated that 20 to 30% of hypertension can be attributed to overweight (3, 49). The strength of the associations between body weight and blood pressure and between change in weight and change in blood pressure over time indicates that weight reduction in overweight persons and avoidance of obesity should be key strategies for both prevention and treatment of hypertension. The National High Blood Pressure Education Program Working Group on High Blood Pressure in Children and Adolescents recommended weight reduction as the primary therapy for obesity-related hypertension and prehypertension in children (145).

Opinion is divided concerning a recommendation on NaCl restriction for the entire population (3, 148). Arguments for this recommendation include the following: current NaCl intake exceeds the physiologic need; the tendency for blood pressure to increase with high NaCl intake occurs over the entire population; although relatively large differences in dietary NaCl have a relatively small impact on blood pressure within and across populations, these blood pressure differences may significantly affect the overall incidence of cardiovascular disease; within a population, a certain percentage of persons may be particularly susceptible to the effect of dietary NaCl on blood pressure; and identification of NaCl-sensitive persons is not practical. Arguments against the recommendation for reduction of NaCl consumption for the entire population include the following: limited or no proven blood pressure reduction for a large segment of the population; little evidence that reduction of NaCl intake affects cardiovascular disease end points (e.g., stroke, heart attack, and kidney disease); and potential adverse health consequences of NaCl restriction.

Despite these reservations, it is generally recommended that excessively high intake of dietary NaCl be avoided.

Current estimates of NaCl intake in the United States are in the range of 8 to 10 g/day. As an example of a specific guideline, the US Dietary Guidelines Advisory Committee and the American Heart Association recommended that dietary NaCl be restricted to no more than 6.0 g/day, and more rigorous NaCl restriction may be recommended for hypertensive persons. Others have also recommended more rigorous NaCl restriction for the general population (149). Admittedly, in the absence of long-term, convincing clinical trial data with cardiovascular end points, these recommendations are based on the secondary end point of blood pressure. However, because of the well-documented relationship of blood pressure with cardiovascular end points, the recommendation for modest salt restriction in the general population seems prudent. In the absence of blatant salt-losing disorders, no convincing evidence indicates that reduction in salt intake to 6.0 g/day has any long-term, adverse health consequences; nevertheless, this concern has been raised. Alderman and associates reported an increased incidence of myocardial infarction over an average 3.8-year follow-up in drug-treated hypertensive men with the lowest levels of sodium excretion (<4 g NaCl/day) at entry (150). The design of this observational study makes it impossible to exclude the influence of such potentially confounding variables as severity of underlying disease, presence of other cardiovascular disease risk factors, and usual long-term NaCl consumption. An analysis of NHANES data suggests that a high sodium intake is strongly and independently associated with an increased risk of cardiovascular disease and all-cause mortality in overweight persons (151).

Recommendations about other nutrients should also be considered. Because of the strong association of alcohol intake with blood pressure, a recommendation to restrict alcohol intake to two drinks per day would seem reasonable, particularly in persons with hypertension. Low intake of potassium, calcium, or magnesium has been associated with higher levels of blood pressure, and the effects of a high NaCl intake on blood pressure may be amplified by diets low in both potassium and calcium. Furthermore, dietary deficiencies of these ions may be associated with other disorders such as calcium deficiency and osteoporosis. The National Academy of Science recommendations for calcium consumption are 1300 mg/day for adolescents (ages 9–18 years), 1000 mg/day for adults less than 50 years of age, and 1200 mg/day for those more than 50 years old. Although serum cholesterol and hence cardiovascular disease risk may be modified by dietary fat intake, information is currently insufficient to make recommendations about dietary intake of lipids or carbohydrates for the prevention or treatment of hypertension.

Strategies for the prevention and treatment of hypertension should address overall cardiovascular disease risk, not simply elevated blood pressure. Dietary recommendations should be incorporated into a comprehensive program that also addresses other cardiovascular disease risk factors such as elevated serum cholesterol concentrations, cigarette smoking, and a sedentary lifestyle. In developing recommendations, the potential impact of changing the intake of a single nutrient on the dietary content and/or bioavailability of a wide range of nutrients should also be considered.

Recently issued US Department of Agriculture guidelines emphasize healthier food choices and increased physical activity for all US residents. The population is advised as follows: consume a variety of foods; control caloric intake; maintain a desirable weight; increase daily intake of fruits, vegetables, whole grains, and low-fat or nonfat dairy products; reduce salt intake (less than 2300 of mg/day of sodium). Fruits and vegetables are cited as potassium-rich foods. The guidelines specifically mention adopting a diet such as the DASH diet (151). For those who drink, the recommendation is to use alcoholic beverages in moderation. In addition, the National Cancer Institute and others have promoted "Five a Day for Better Health," the recommendation that US residents consume five fruits and vegetables a day as a tangible way to improve dietary intake. The US Department of Agriculture has made major changes in nutritional standards for reimbursable school breakfasts and lunches. These changes require decreased salt and fat in the foods provided in schools. In addition, federal support exists for nutritional education programs in schools for children and for food service employees. Finally, federally mandated food labeling permits persons to assess their nutritional intake accurately and to modify it more readily.

REFERENCES

1. Burt VL, Cutler JA, Higgins M et al. Hypertension 1995;26: 60–69.
2. Hajjar IJ, Kotchen TA. JAMA 2003;290:199–206.
3. National High Blood Pressure Education Program/National Institutes of Health. The Seventh Report of the Joint National Committee on Detection, Evaluation, and Treatment of High Blood Pressure. National Institutes of Health publication no. 03-5233. Bethesda, MD: National Institutes of Health, 2003.
4. Denton D, Weisinger R, Mundy N et al. Nat Med 1995;l: 1009–16.
5. Antonios TF, MacGregor GA. Clin Exp Pharmacol Physiol 1995;22:180–4.
6. Aviv A. Arch Intern Med 2001;161:507–10.
7. Law MR, Frost CD, Wald NJ. BMJ 1991;302:811–5.
8. Frost CD, Law MR, Wald NJ. BMJ 1991;302:815–8.
9. Law MR, Frost CD, Wald NJ. BMJ 1991;302:819–24.
10. Weinberger MH. The effects of sodium on blood pressure in humans. In: Laragh JH, Brenner BM, eds. Hypertension: Pathophysiology, Diagnosis, and Management. 2nd ed. New York: Raven Press, 1995:2703–14.
11. Simpson FO. Blood pressure and sodium intake. In: Laragh JH, Brenner BM, eds. Hypertension: Pathophysiology, Diagnosis, and Management. 2nd ed. New York: Raven Press, 1995: 273–81.
12. Overlack A, Ruppert M, Kolloch R et al. Hypertension 1993;22: 331–8.
13. Simons-Morton DG, Obarzanek E. Pediatr Nephrol 1997;11: 244–9.
14. Geleijnse JM, Hutman A, Witteman JCN et al. Hypertension 1997;29:913–7.
15. Pomeranz A, Dolfin T, Korzets Z et al. J Hypertens 2002;20: 203–207.
16. Intersalt Cooperative Research Group. BMJ 1988;297:319–28.
17. Elliott P, Stamler J, Nichols R et al. BMJ 1996;312:1249–53.
18. Weinberger MH, Miller JH, Luft FC et al. Hypertension 1986;8[Suppl II]:127–34.
19. Sullivan JM, Prewitt EL, Ratts TE. Am J Med Sci 1988;295: 370–7.
20. Cutler JA, Follmann D, Elliott P et al. Hypertension 1991; 17[Suppl I]:27–33.
21. Midgley JP, Matthew AG, Greenwood CM et al. JAMA 1996; 275:1590–7.
22. Cook NR, Cohen J, Hebert P et al. Arch Intern Med 1995;155: 701–9.
23. Boegehold M, Kotchen TA. Hypertension 1991;17[Suppl I]: 158–61.
24. Morris RC, Sebastian A. Potassium responsive hypertension. In: Laragh JH, Brenner BM, eds. Hypertension: Pathophysiology, Diagnosis, and Management. 2nd ed. New York: Raven Press, 1995:2715–26.
25. Harlan WR, Harlan LC. Blood pressure and calcium and magnesium intake. In: Laragh JH, Brenner BM, eds. Hypertension: Pathophysiology, Diagnosis, and Management. 2nd ed. New York: Raven Press, 1995:1143–54.
26. Cowley AW, Stoll M, Greene AS et al. Physiol Genomics 2000;2:107–15.
27. Cowley AW, Roman RT, Kaldunski ML et al. Hypertension 2001;37:456–61.
28. Reudelhuber TL. J Clin Invest 2003;111:1115–16.
29. Miller JZ, Weinberger MB, Christian JC et al. Am J Epidemiol 1987;126:822–30.
30. Weinberger MB, Miller JZ, Fineberg NS et al. Hypertension 1987;10:443–6.
31. Grim CE, Luft FC, Weinberger MB et al. Aust NZ J Med 1984; 14:453–7.
32. Freis ED, Reda DJ, Materson BJ. Hypertension 1988;12: 244–50.
33. Beeks E, Dessels AGH, Kroon AA et al. J Hypertens 2004;22: 1243–49.
34. Cowley AW, Roman RJ. JAMA 1996;275:1581–9.
35. Gill JR, Gullner HG, Lake CR et al. Hypertension 1988;11: 312–9.
36. Lifton RP, Gharavi AC, Geller DS. Cell 2001;104:545–56.
37. Tolins JP, Shultz PJ. Kidney Int 1994;46:230–6.
38. Reddy RS, Baylis C, Kotchen TA. Am J Physiol 1990;260: R32–8.
39. Sullivan JM. Hypertension 1991;17[Suppl I]:61–8.
40. Shimamoto H, Shimamoto Y. J Hypertens 1992;10:855–61.
41. Rusch NJ, Kotchen TA. Vascular smooth muscle regulation by calcium, magnesium and potassium in hypertension. In: Swales JD, ed. Textbook of Hypertension. London: Blackwell Scientific Publications, 1994:188–99.
42. Resnick LM, Gupta RK, DiFabio B et al. J Clin Invest 1994;94: 1269–76.
43. Wright JT, Rahman M, Scarpa A et al. Hypertension 2003;42: 1087–92.
44. Gates PE, Tanaka H, Hiatt WR et al. Hypertension 2004;44: 35–41.
45. Bagrov AY, Lakatta EG. Hypertension 2004;44:22–24.
46. Aviv A. Arch Intern Med 2001;161:507–510.
47. Kannell W, Brand N, Skinner J et al. Ann Intern Med 1967;67: 48–59.

48. Chiang BN, Perlman LV, Epstein RH. Circulation 1969;39:403–21.

49. MacMahon SW, Cutler J, Brittan E et al. Eur Heart J 1987;8 [Suppl B]:57–70.

50. Sorof J, Daniels S. Hypertension 2002;40:441–47.

51. Flegal KM Carroll MD, Ogden CL et al. JAMA 2002;288:1723–27.

52. Mokdad AH, Bowman BA, Ford ES et al. JAMA 2001;286:1195–200.

53. Munter P, He J, Cutler JA et al. JAMA 2004;291:2107–13.

54. Krieger DR, Landsberg L. Obesity and hypertension. In: Laragh JH, Brenner BM, eds. Hypertension: Pathophysiology, Diagnosis, and Management. 2nd ed. New York: Raven Press, 1995:2367–88.

55. O'Shaughnessy IM, Kotchen TA. Curr Opin Cardiol 1993;8:757–64.

56. Kotchen TA, Kotchen JM, O'Shaughnessy IM. Curr Opin Cardiol 1996;11:483–9.

57. Reaven G. J Clin Endocrinol Metab 2003;88:2399–403.

58. He J, Klag MJ, Caballero B et al. Arch Intern Med 1999;159:498–503.

59. Zavaroni I, Coruzzi P, Bonini L et al. Am J Hypertens 1995;8:855–88.

60. Sowers JR. Am J Physiol 2004;286:H1597–602.

61. Resnick LM, Gupta R, Bhargava KR et al. Hypertension 1991;17:951–7.

62. Khaw KT, Barrett-Conner E. Circulation 1985;77:653–61.

63. Ascherio A, Rimm EB, Giovannucci EL et al. Circulation 1992;86:1475–84.

64. McCarron D, Morris C, Henry H et al. Science 1984;224:1392–8.

65. Khaw KT, Barrett-Conner E. N Engl J Med 1987;316:235–40.

66. Addison W. Can Med Assoc J 1928;18:281–5.

67. Cappuccio FP, MacGregor GA. J Hypertens 1991;9:465–73.

68. Whelton PK, He J. Semin Nephrol 1999;19:494–9.

69. Grimm RH, Neaton JD, Elmer PJ et al. N Engl J Med 1990;322:569–74.

70. Geleijnse JM, Witteman JC, den Breeijen JH. J Hypertens 1996;14:737–41.

71. Lawton WJ, Fita AE, Anderson EA et al. Circulation 1990;81:173–84.

72. Krishna GC, Kapoor SC. Ann Intern Med 1991;115:77–83.

73. Tobian L, MacNeil D, Johnson MA et al. Hypertension 1984;6 [Suppl I]:170–6.

74. Liu DT, Wang MX, Kincaid-Smith P et al. Clin Exp Hypertens 1994;16:391–414.

75. Yamori Y, Horie R. Health Rep 1994;6:181–8.

76. Hatton DC, McCarron DA. Hypertension 1994;23:513–30.

77. Butler TV Cameron J, Kirchner KA. Am J Hypertens 1995;8:615–21.

78. Cutler JA, Brittain E. Am J Hypertens 1990;3:137S–46S.

79. McCarron DA, Hatton D. JAMA 1996;275:1128–9.

80. Cappuccio FP, Elliott P, Allender PS. Am J Epidemiol 1995;9:935–45.

81. Pryer J, Cappuccio FP, Elliott P. J Hum Hypertens 1995;9:597–604.

82. Gillman MW, Oliveria SA, Moore LL et al. JAMA 1992;267:2340–3.

83. Bucher HC, Cook RJ, Guyatt GH et al. JAMA 1996;275:1016–22.

84. Allender PS, Cutler JA, Follmann D et al. Ann Intern Med 1996;124:825–31.

85. Bucher HC, Guyatt GH, Cook RJ et al. JAMA 1996;275:1113–7.

86. Belizan JM, Villar J, Gonzalez L et al. N Engl J Med 1991;325:1399–405.

87. Levine RJ, Hauth JC, Curet LB et al. N Engl J Med 1997;337:69–76.

88. Gillman MW, Hood MY Moore LL et al J Pediatr 1995;127:186–92.

89. McCarron DA, Hatton D, Roullet JB et al. Can J Pharmacol 1994;72:937–44.

90. Resnick LM. Ionic disturbances of calcium and magnesium metabolism in essential hypertension. In: Laragh JH, Brenner BM, eds. Hypertension: Pathophysiology, Diagnosis, and Management. 2nd ed. New York: Raven Press, 1995:1169–91.

91. Rayssiguier Y Mbega JD, Durlach V et al. Magnes Res 1992;5:139–46.

92. Summanen JU, Vuorela HJ, Hiltunen RK. J Pharm Sci 1994;83:249–51.

93. Durlach J, Bara M, Guiet-Bara A. Magnesium 1985;4:5–15.

94. Simon JA, Obarzanek E, Daniels SR et al. Am J Epidemiol 1994;139:130–40.

95. Witteman JCM, Willett WC, Stampfer MJ et al. Circulation 1989;80:1320–7.

96. Ascherio A, Rimm EB, Giovannucci EL et al. Circulation 1992;86:1475–84.

97. Whelton P, Klag M. Am J Cardiol 1989;63:26G–30G.

98. Witteman JCM, Grobbee DE, Derkx FHM et al. Am J Clin Nutr 1994;60:129–235.

99. Lind L, Lithell H, Pollare T et al. Am J Hypertens 1991;4:674–9.

100. Zemel PC, Zemel MB, Urberg M et al. Am J Clin Nutr 1990;5:665–9.

101. Jee SH, Miller ER, Guallar E et al. Am J Hypertens 2002;15:691–6.

102. Witteman JCM, Willett WC, Stampfer MJ et al. Am J Cardiol 1990;65:633–7.

103. Klatsky AL. Blood pressure and alcohol intake. In: Laragh JH, Brenner BM, eds. Hypertension: Pathophysiology, Diagnosis, and Management. 2nd ed. New York: Raven Press, 1995:2649–68.

104. Klag MJ, He J, Whelton PK et al. Hypertension 1993;22:365–70.

105. Victor RG, Hansen J. N Engl J Med 1995;332:1782–3.

106. Xin X, He J, Frontini MG et al. Hypertension 2001;38:1112–7.

107. Randin D, Vollenweider P, Tappy L et al. N Engl J Med 1995;332:1733–7.

108. Pietinen P. Ann Med 1994;26:465–8.

109. Reddy SR, Kotchen TA. J Am Coll Nutr 1996;15:92–6.

110. Sacks FM. Nutr Rev 1989;47:291–300.

111. Knapp HR. Nutr Rev 1989;47:301–13.

112. Iacono JM, Dougherty PM. Blood pressure and fat intake. In: Laragh JH, Brenner BM, eds. Hypertension: Pathophysiology, Diagnosis, and Management. New York: Raven Press, 1990:257–76.

113. Morris M, Sacks F, Rosner B. Circulation 1993;88:523–33.

114. Geleijnse JM, Giltay EJ, Grobbee DE et al. J Hypertens 2002;20:1493–99.

115. Toft I, Bonaa KH, Ingebretsen OC et al. Ann Intern Med 1995;123:911–8.

116. Beilin LJ. Ann NY Acad Sci 1993;683:35–45.

117. Morris MC. J Cardiovasc Risk 1994;1:21–30.

118. Obarzanek E, Velletri PA, Cutler JA. JAMA 275:1598–603.

119. He J, Whelton PK. Clin Exp Hypertens 1999;21:785–96.

120. Moore TJ, McKnight JA. Endocrinol Metab Clin North Am 1995;24:643–55.

121. Rouse IL, Beilin U. Hypertensive disease and kidney structure. In: Laragh JH, Brenner BM, eds. Hypertension: Pathophysiology,

Diagnosis, and Management. New York: Raven Press, 1990: 241–56.

122. Beilin LJ, Burke V. Clin Exp Pharmacol Physiol 1995;22: 195–8.

123. Melby CL, Toohey ML, Cebrick J. Am J Clin Nutr 1994;59: 103–9.

124. Swain JF, Rouse IL, Curley CB. N Engl J Med 1990;322: 147–52.

125. Ness AR, Khaw KT, Bingham S et al. J Hypertens 1996;14: 503–8.

126. Hajjar I, Kotchen TA. J Nutr 2003;133:211–14.

127. Hajjar I, Grim CE, George V et al. Arch Intern Med 2001;161: 598–93.

128. Appel LJ, Moore TJ, Obarzanek E et al. N Engl J Med 1997;336:1117–24.

129. Sacks FM, Svetky LP, Vollmer WM et al. N Engl J Med 2001;344:3–10.

130. Vollmer WM, Sacks FM, Ard J et al. Ann Intern Med 2001;135: 1019–28.

131. Akita S, Sacks FM, Svetky LP et al. Hypertension 2003;42: 8–13.

132. Kotchen JM, Holley J, Kotchen TA. Semin Nephrol 1989;9: 296–303.

133. Stamler R, Stamler J, Gosch FC et al. JAMA 1989;262:1801–7.

134. Hypertension Prevention Trial Research Group. Arch Intern Med 1990;150:153–62.

135. Trials of Hypertension Prevention Collaborative Research Group. JAMA 1992;267:1213–20.

136. Yamamoto ME, Applegate WB, Klag MJ et al. Ann Epidemiol 1995;5:96–107.

137. He J, Whelton PK, Appel LJ et al. Hypertension 2000;35: 544–9.

138. Whelton PK, Appel LJ, Espeland MA et al. JAMA 1998;279: 839–46.

139. Kostis JB, Wilson AC, Shindler DM et al. Am J Hypertens 2002;15:732–34.

140. Langford HG, Davis BR, Blaufox D et al. Hypertension 1991; 17:210–7.

141. Treatment of Mild Hypertension Research Group. Arch Intern Med 1991;151:1413–23.

142. Ramsay LE, Yeo WW, Chadwick IG et al. Br Med Bull 1994;50: 494–508.

143. Beilin LJ. J Hypertens 1994;12:71S–81S.

144. Miller ER, Erlinger TP, Young DR et al. Hypertension 2002;40:612–18.

145. Fourth Report on the Diagnosis, Evaluation, and Treatment of High Blood Pressure in Children and Adolescents. Pediatrics 2004;11:555–76.

146. Cook NR, Cohen J, Hebert P et al. Arch Intern Med 1995;155: 701–9.

147. Kotchen JM, McKean HE, Thayer ST et al. JAMA 1986;255: 2177–82.

148. Swales JD. Blood Press 1992;1:201–4.

149. He FJ, MacGregor GA Hypertension 2003;42:1093–99.

150. Alderman MH, Madhavan S, Cohen H et al. Hypertension 1995;25:1144–52.

151. He J, Whelton PK, Appel LJ et al. Hypertension 2000;35: 544–9.

152. US Department of Agriculture. http://www.healthierus.gov/dietary guidelines/.

69 CONGESTIVE HEART FAILURE[1]

JOHN R. HOYLE AND FREDERIC R. KAHL

HEART FAILURE DEFINITION AND NOMENCLATURE . .1108
EPIDEMIOLOGY AND PUBLIC HEALTH FEATURES 1109
PATHOPHYSIOLOGY 1109
CLINICAL RECOGNITION .1109
CAUSES 1110
MANAGEMENT 1110
    Medical Therapy 1111
    Interventional and Surgical Therapy 1112
    Nutritional Management 1112

HEART FAILURE DEFINITION AND NOMENCLATURE

The signs and symptoms of congestive heart failure (CHF) generally reflect reduced exercise tolerance leading to fatigue and volume (salt and water) overload accounting for shortness of breath and peripheral edema. Heart failure is a syndrome caused by a wide variety of disorders of the cardiovascular system affecting the myocardium, the cardiac valves, the coronary circulation, and the pericardium. The definitions of heart failure have undergone changes as our understanding of the syndrome has progressed. Heart failure can be viewed as a clinical syndrome resulting from abnormal cardiovascular function, often caused by structural heart disease, in which the circulatory function of the heart is inadequate to meet the metabolic needs of the body and leads to impaired exercise tolerance. The syndrome further is characterized by neurohumoral activation of the renin-angiotensin-aldosterone axis and the sympathetic nervous system, which promote the signs and symptoms of the condition and, when chronic, are counterregulatory. The result is further cardiac dysfunction leading to a negative spiral of deteriorating cardiac function and worsening symptoms. Finally, heart failure is characterized by an increased risk of both atrial and ventricular arrhythmias and an increased risk of complications of these rhythm disturbances including sudden cardiac death (1).

Cardiac dysfunction is commonly caused either by derangements in cardiac contractility leading to systolic dysfunction or by abnormalities in cardiac filling producing diastolic dysfunction. Accordingly, assessment of both systolic and diastolic function is important as the initial step in the clinical evaluation of patients suspected of having CHF. An evaluation of cardiac contractility is essential, and if the ejection fraction measured by a variety of methods (echocardiography, radioisotope angiography, contrast angiography, or cardiac magnetic resonance imaging) is less than 40%, then CHF may be attributed to systolic dysfunction. If systolic function is normal or near normal, diastolic function can be assessed usually by echocardiographic techniques to define the presence of abnormal cardiac filling properties characteristic of diastolic dysfunction. The pathophysiology of CHF in patients with either systolic or diastolic dysfunction indicates both differences and similarities in the two conditions. Likewise, the clinical presentation and natural history of systolic and diastolic dysfunction share similar patterns in some respects and differ in others (2).

Once heart failure is characterized as resulting from either systolic or diastolic dysfunction, other grading systems have been proposed to indicate the clinical severity.

The New York Heart Association (NYHA) four-point scale is a venerable and still useful system for evaluating the severity of symptoms (3, 4). A patient with NYHA class I symptoms has a history of heart failure but is currently asymptomatic and is not limited by symptoms on effort. NYHA class II indicates a patient with symptoms of heart failure (fatigue and shortness of breath) only at levels of more than ordinary activity. NYHA class III refers to a patient with symptoms of heart failure that occur at levels of less than ordinary activity. NYHA class IV represents a patient with symptoms of heart failure that occur at rest. This clinical scaling system has been useful in assessing prognosis in patients with heart failure as well as in determining treatment and resources needed for management.

Another approach to classification of heart failure was published in 2001 under the American College of Cardiology/American Heart Association Guidelines for the Evaluation and Management of Heart Failure in the Adult and emphasizes the stages of progression of the heart failure syndrome (5). Stage A indicates a patient at high risk of developing CHF but who does not yet have evidence of

---

[1]**Abbreviations: AB,** aldosterone blocking agent; **ACEI,** angiotensin-converting enzyme inhibitor; **ARB,** angiotensin II receptor blocker; **BB,** β-blocker; **CCB,** calcium channel blocking agent; **CHF,** congestive heart failure; **NYHA,** New York Heart Association.

structural heart disease (e.g., a patient with hypertension and diabetes but with no evidence of systolic or diastolic dysfunction). Stage B refers to a patient with structural heart disorder predisposing to the development of heart failure but who is still asymptomatic (e.g., a patient with a prior myocardial infarction or asymptomatic left ventricular dysfunction or valvular heart disease). Stage C indicates a patient with structural heart disease and past or current symptoms of heart failure (fatigue, shortness of breath). Stage D refers to a patient with end-stage heart disease who requires intensive specialized treatments to address symptoms of heart failure (such treatments could be circulatory assist devices, intravenous medications, heart transplantation, or home hospice care).

EPIDEMIOLOGY AND PUBLIC HEALTH FEATURES

CHF is a major public health issue in the United States because it is common and is characterized by high mortality and morbidity. Statistics indicate a prevalence of 4.8 million persons, and it is estimated that about 500,000 new cases are identified each year (6). Patients with CHF require considerable medical resources and account for about 15 million outpatient visits and 6.5 million days of hospitalization each year; the cost of providing care exceeds 20 billion dollars per year (7, 8). Mortality is substantial, and the risk of death approaches 50% in 5 years; mortality rates in patients with myocardial infarction complicated by CHF are as high as 21% in 1 year (9). The Framingham study reports that the lifetime risk of developing CHF is one in five for both men and women (10).

The prevalence of heart failure increases with age, and it is the leading diagnosis for hospitalized patients aged 65 years and older. Secular trends indicate that hospital discharge and deaths attributable to heart failure have increased by more than 100% since the mid-1980s. Moreover, it is anticipated that the established trend of increasing CHF prevalence will continue in the next decade by a two- to threefold factor as a result of the aging of the public and increased survival of patients with various forms of heart disease (8).

PATHOPHYSIOLOGY

Left ventricular failure leads to release of a variety of neurohormonal mediators, which attempt to maintain the cardiac output. Decreased renal perfusion results in increased plasma renin levels, which subsequently elevate circulating angiotensin II, aldosterone, and norepinephrine concentrations. Angiotensin II is a potent vasoconstrictor, but it has later deleterious effects in CHF as a result of apoptosis of cardiomyocytes (11), increased collagen deposition and fibrosis in the myocardium (12), and, potentially, induction of an anorexic effect (11). Aldosterone production results in increased salt and water retention, contributing to fluid overload; medications countering these effects have been

shown to improve survival in patients with NYHA class III heart failure (13). Additional mediators, such as endothelin, have potent vasoconstrictive properties and portend an adverse prognosis in heart failure (11).

Release of inflammatory mediators, such as tumor necrosis factor-α and interleukins, can be caused by β-adrenergic receptor stimulation by elements of the sympathetic nervous system. These inflammatory mediators worsen left ventricular contraction and promote apoptosis of the cardiomyocytes. Further, they promote cytokine secretion and also worsen anorexia. Clinically, an increase in circulating levels of these mediators has been associated with a worse prognosis (11). Therapy with β-blockers (BBs) and angiotensin-converting enzyme inhibitors (ACEIs) likely attenuates these adverse effects.

CLINICAL RECOGNITION

The hallmarks of CHF are decreased exercise tolerance and a tendency to volume overload with retention of salt and water. This latter phenomenon results from neurohumoral activation of the renin-angiotensin-aldosterone axis and the sympathetic nervous system that leads to renal adjustments to promote sodium retention as well as fluid retention (14).

Fluid retention increases pulmonary congestion and can lead to shortness of breath (dyspnea) under a variety of conditions. Shortness of breath may initially develop only with exertion (NYHA class II), but with disease progression can occur at rest (NYHA class IV). If the pulmonary congestion occurs at night, when the patient finds it necessary to elevate the head with two or more pillows to become comfortable, the patient has orthopnea. The patient may also have alarming episodes of breathlessness at night, described as paroxysmal nocturnal dyspnea. At times, the pulmonary congestion resulting from fluid overload can be manifest as airway obstruction and may clinically appear to be asthma: this is termed cardiac asthma. Pulmonary congestion can be recognized by a variety of signs on physical examination. If it is severe, the respiratory rate is increased, and signs of hypoxia are evident, with peripheral cyanosis of skin, mucous membranes, and nails. The excess fluid in the lungs causes audible crackles heard with the stethoscope when the patient inhales; these are called rales. At times, the fluid accumulation in the lungs and chest cavity can be extreme, leading to a large pleural effusion, which can be recognized on physical examination as well. Finally, audible wheezing is not uncommon, especially in the patient with advanced CHF, and it can be detected with and without the stethoscope.

Fluid retention can also occur in the periphery and takes the form of peripheral edema. Usually, this involves the ankles and lower legs at first, and it may be transitory. As the heart failure worsens, the edema becomes more permanent and more severe and is known as pitting edema; it can advance up the legs and cause massive swelling. The external genitalia in women and men are very susceptible to large amounts of fluid accumulation in advanced heart failure, and this condition can be disabling and alarming to both patient and caregiver. The fluid accumulation can involve the abdominal cavity, with substantial accumulations of fluid called ascites; this usually is seen in advanced CHF. The liver and spleen can also be affected with substantial fluid accumulation within these organs; the liver in particular can enlarge enormously. At times, this causes discomfort, and liver function itself may become impaired, leading to jaundice and other findings of advanced liver disease.

The volume overload leads to an increase in intravascular volume, particularly on the venous side, and engorgement of the veins is not uncommon. Increase in jugular venous pressure resulting from congestion is common and is used as an index of the severity of the heart failure. The increased intravascular volume may affect the heart secondarily, and auscultatory findings that reflect this include an audible atrial filling sound (the S_4) and an audible ventricular filling sound (the S_3); at times, murmurs reflecting the incompetence of the mitral or tricuspid valve may become apparent in a patient with decompensated heart failure.

In advanced heart failure, in which the metabolic and nutritional needs of the body are not being met, patients can have loss of muscle mass, bone marrow function, renal function, and liver function leading to cachexia, anemia, renal failure, and liver failure. These patients clearly have end-stage CHF with secondary multiorgan dysfunction, which causes substantial morbidity and leads to early death (15, 16).

Wide variation exists in clinicians' ability to detect the various clinical signs of heart failure (17). The chest x-ray study is very helpful in detecting pulmonary congestion, and a blood test that measures a protein released by the heart, brain natriuretic peptide, has become useful in confirming the CHF diagnosis (18).

CAUSES

Multiple conditions are responsible for the development of CHF. The most important conditions are ischemic heart disease, dilated cardiomyopathy, primary valvular heart disease, hypertensive heart disease, and congenital heart disease. Ischemic heart disease leads to heart failure in several ways and produces both systolic and diastolic dysfunction. Myocardial infarction, chronic ischemia, ventricular remodeling, arrhythmias, and acquired structural defects (ventricular septal defect, mitral regurgitation, ventricular aneurysm) represent common causes. Conditions that are risk factors for ischemic heart disease, such as hypertension and diabetes mellitus and obesity, are independent risk factors (10, 19–21).

Cardiomyopathy, which can be classified as dilated, hypertrophic, or restrictive, can lead to heart failure. The cause of cardiomyopathy in many cases is not known and is classified as idiopathic; however, some cases are related to myocarditis, infiltrative diseases such as hemachromatosis and amyloidosis, postpartum cardiomyopathy, human immunodeficiency virus infection, connective tissue disorders, substance abuse, and treatment with chemotherapeutic agents (doxorubicin) (22).

CHF in patients with chronic compensated heart failure can be exacerbated by a variety of causes including acute myocardial ischemia, hypertension, atrial fibrillation and other cardiac arrhythmias, and treatment with negative inotropic agents, such as certain calcium channel blocking agents (CCBs), BBs, and antiarrhythmic agents. Other conditions that can lead to decompensated CHF include superimposed infection, acute renal failure, anemia, poorly controlled diabetes, thyroid dysfunction, and excessive alcohol intake. Nonsteroidal antiinflammatory agents have been associated with worsening heart failure. Additionally, noncompliance with dietary sodium and fluid restrictions and noncompliance with a medication program controlling the heart failure syndrome can lead to worsening symptoms and the need for acute care of heart failure (23).

MANAGEMENT

The management of patients with heart failure or those at risk of developing heart failure is complex and involves multiple strategies including patient education, access to medical care, nonpharmacologic and pharmacologic treatment programs, and cardiac interventional and surgical treatments.

In asymptomatic patients, the general treatment plan is designed to forestall the development of symptoms, to prevent harmful ventricular remodeling, and to reduce the risk of adverse chronic neurohumoral activation. Control of coronary risk factors is exceedingly important in this approach because ischemic heart disease is such an important cause of heart failure. When patients become symptomatic, these prevention strategies are supplemented by treatment strategies, which aim to reduce symptoms and to decrease the risk of death. Practical goals of treatment are to maintain functional capacity at the highest achievable level and to reduce the rate of readmission to the hospital for heart failure exacerbation (24, 25).

Nonpharmacologic therapy begins with education of the patient and family regarding outpatient management. Restriction of sodium and fluid represents an important component of management for all patients; exercise programs are also helpful in the setting of chronic heart failure. Patients should be instructed regarding activities that can lead to cardiac decompensation such as excessive alcohol intake, dietary indiscretion regarding salt, certain medications (nonsteroidal antiinflammatory agents), and the importance of blood pressure and weight control. Home blood pressure cuffs and monitoring and daily weight measurement and monitoring are extremely helpful in the practical management of patients with heart failure. Effective follow-up and access to medical care, either from the treating physician or in a structured heart failure outpatient management program, are also beneficial (26).

Patients with heart failure should be alert to signs and symptoms of myocardial ischemia and cardiac arrhythmias because both can occur suddenly and can lead to worsening heart failure. Effective management of diabetes and hypertension is also important in heart failure management because poor blood glucose and blood pressure control can lead to more severe heart failure. In this regard, it is important for the treating physicians to be aware that certain medical options for both blood pressure control and diabetes management can themselves worsen heart failure and should be avoided.

Medical Therapy

Specific treatments for heart failure are advancing rapidly and are based on large randomized control trials (27, 28). The one exception of testing of efficacy by randomized control trials is the use of diuretics, which have been a mainstay in the treatment of CHF for many decades. The main role of diuretics is to promote excretion of excess sodium and water and to manage volume overload. Multiple diuretic options are available to the caregiver, including oral and intravenous formulations of various classes of diuretic agents. The most commonly prescribed agents include thiazide diuretics, loop diuretics, and aldosterone blocking agents (ABs), which can be used intermittently, on a long-term basis, and in combination with each other. Diuretic therapy is generally effective in relieving symptoms of volume overload, but it may lead to increased activation of the renin-angiotensin-aldosterone and sympathetic nervous systems and may paradoxically promote adverse neurohumoral activation. Diuretic therapy may also lead to metabolic abnormalities involving potassium and uric acid, and it may impair carbohydrate metabolism (29).

ACEIs are currently indicated in all patients with symptomatic and asymptomatic heart failure resulting from left ventricular dysfunction. These drugs lead to arterial and venous vasodilation and ameliorate the increased activation of the renin-angiotensin-aldosterone and sympathetic nervous systems. The ACEIs also act to prevent adverse remodeling of the left ventricle, which leads to worsened pump performance and further neurohumoral activation. Because of these various actions, ACEIs reduce symptoms and have shown improved survival in patients with CHF, regardless of symptoms. Side effects of ACEIs include orthostatic hypotension, worsening renal function, hyperkalemia, and cough. Monitoring of potassium and renal function is important in patients receiving ACEIs (30, 31).

Angiotensin II receptor blockers (ARBs) comprise another class of agents that block the renin-angiotensin-aldosterone and sympathetic nervous systems, promote balanced arterial and venous vasodilation, and improve

symptoms in patients with heart failure resulting from systolic dysfunction. Randomized control trials have shown ambiguous results regarding a survival benefit of ARBs. Currently, the role of ARBs is in the management of heart failure in patients who are not able to use ACEIs, and, in some cases of refractory heart failure, ARBs are used in combination with ACEIs in an effort to control symptoms. Like ACEIs, ARBs can cause orthostatic hypotension and worsening renal function and hyperkalemia (32).

BBs have been shown in multiple randomized control trials to improve survival in patients with left ventricular dysfunction, regardless of cause. These agents ameliorate the adverse effects of chronic neurohumoral activation and stabilize symptoms in heart failure. The use of BBs in patients with heart failure is to some extent counterintuitive because BBs are known to worsen heart failure in some patients. The type of BB, a small starting dose, and slow upward titration of the dose reduce this effect considerably. BBs have multiple side effects including bradycardia, hypotension, fatigue, and depression, which need to be closely monitored in this population of patients (33).

ABs have been shown also to control symptoms and to improve survival in patients with CHF resulting from systolic dysfunction; these drugs are particularly useful in patients with more severe stages of heart failure (NYHA class III or IV). They ameliorate excessive neurohumoral activation and are believed to reduce myocardial fibrosis; the risk of sudden death in actively treated patients in AB trials was decreased. Side effects of ABs include hyperkalemia and deterioration of renal function; gynecomastia is an uncommon side effect (34, 35).

Digitalis glycosides have been used to manage heart failure for centuries, and the role of these agents has been controversial. The now-completed DIG randomized control trial indicated no significant survival benefit, and symptomatic benefit was modest. In patients with heart failure, digitalis now appears to be reserved for those who have received intensive medical therapy (diuretics, ACEIs, BBs, ABs) and who are still symptomatic. Side effects of digitalis glycosides are numerous and include arrhythmias, loss of appetite, nausea and vomiting, and, rarely, gynecomastia (36).

CCBs appear to have a modest role in CHF management. CCBs such as verapamil, diltiazem, and nifedipine are well known to worsen symptoms. However, two second-generation CCBs, amlodipine and felodipine, were studied in randomized control trials in patients with heart failure and did not demonstrate any survival benefit, but these drugs were tolerated without worsening symptoms and accordingly may have a role in the CHF patient with hypertension despite ACEIs, BBs, and ABs (37).

Antiarrhythmic agents have been studied in randomized control trials, and trials with encainide, flecainide, moricizine, D-sotalol showed increased mortality in patients treated with these agents. Proarrhythmia effects and decreased survival seem to be common properties of antiarrhythmic agents and are especially notable in patients with severely reduced left ventricular function. Amiodarone may be the exception to this observation and appears to be effective in patients with atrial fibrillation, CHF, and systolic dysfunction (38, 39).

Anticoagulant agents have been considered as a means to reduce the risk of thromboembolic events in patients with systolic dysfunction. The data on patients in sinus rhythm are unconvincing. However, it would seem reasonable to consider long-term anticoagulant therapy with warfarin in patients with heart failure and systolic dysfunction who also have atrial fibrillation, a history of systemic or pulmonary embolism, or evidence of ventricular clot by echocardiographic evaluation (40).

Interventional and Surgical Therapy

Electrophysiologic treatments are important options in the overall management of patients with CHF and systolic dysfunction. Because the risks of sudden death and of ventricular arrhythmias are high in these patients, treatments to reduce these events have been developed and studied in randomized control trials. Drug-based antiarrhythmic therapy has not been shown to be effective and may actually increase mortality. Use of implanted automatic defibrillators has also been studied in patients with reduced ejection fraction and has shown a survival benefit by reducing the risk of sudden cardiac death (41, 42). Patients with prolonged electrical depolarization on the electrocardiogram, identified as a wide QRS complex, benefit from electrophysiologic treatment. The functional consequence of this abnormal electrical activation of the ventricles is dyssynchronous mechanical contraction. Correction of this defect can be achieved by biventricular pacemaker therapy, which effects electrical and mechanical resynchronization of the ventricles in patients with systolic dysfunction, heart failure, and a wide QRS complex. In these selected patients, biventricular pacemaker therapy has been shown to improve symptoms (43, 44). Advances in electrophysiologic device therapy continue, and combined automatic defibrillator-biventricular pacemaker therapy is already feasible.

Surgical and interventional therapies are particularly effective when the underlying cause of heart failure (either systolic or diastolic) can be shown to be ischemic heart disease. Symptoms can be improved with revascularization strategies (percutaneous coronary artery intervention or coronary artery bypass surgery) appropriate to the coronary artery disease pattern identified by cardiac catheterization. In patients who have coronary artery disease and left ventricular aneurysm, resection of the aneurysmal segment may lead to symptomatic benefit (45). In patients with cardiomyopathy resulting from an enlarged left ventricle, partial left venticulectomy to achieve left ventricular volume reduction may be beneficial. In patients with significant mitral or aortic valve disease, valve repair or valve replacement may be beneficial. In cases of mitral stenosis, mitral regurgitation, aortic stenosis, and aortic regurgitation, a classic indication for valve surgery is the presence or development of CHF. Patients with aortic stenosis and CHF appear to derive substantial benefit, with improvement of symptoms and left ventricular function after valve surgery. Patients with mitral regurgitation have represented a treatment challenge because instances of worsening left ventricular function and heart failure have been reported after mitral valve replacement. Contemporary surgical treatment of mitral regurgitation that relies on mitral valve repair (not replacement) and maintenance of the integrity of the papillary muscles has resulted in substantially improved clinical benefit, even in patients with left ventricular dysfunction noted preoperatively (46).

Nutritional Management

Definitive nutritional management of patients with CHF has remained elusive. Although many randomized, controlled trials have examined drug therapies for left ventricular dysfunction, few clinical studies have evaluated specific nutritional interventions. An American Heart Association dietary guideline examined the role of nutrition in reducing cardiovascular disease risk, but this publication had limited recommendations for CHF (47). However, although published data supporting particular nutritional therapies may be lacking, our level of understanding of the nutritional requirements of patients with CHF has increased. Therefore, clinical assessment of the patient in heart failure should, after initial stabilization of the acute hemodynamic problems, include a nutritional analysis and a multidisciplinary approach to treatment.

Nutritional Deficiencies

The wasting associated with chronic heart failure (cardiac cachexia) has been recognized since the time of Hippocrates (48), and it has been associated with a poor prognosis in CHF (49). The origin of the cachexia is likely multifactorial, stemming from decreases in physical activity and increased metabolic demands in the setting hemodynamic compromise. Further, dietary vitamin and micronutrients become depleted, with resulting deleterious effects.

Chronic heart failure represents a catabolic state. The failing ventricle stimulates a barrage of neuroendocrine and inflammatory mediators that increase cardiac output and overall metabolic demand. Up to 70% of daily energy in patients with CHF is used in maintaining the resting metabolic rate. This increased expenditure is largely in the form of increased cardiac and ventilatory work (11). Further, increased resting peripheral oxygen consumption is higher because of decreased cardiac output. Neuroendocrine activation (mediated by norepinephrine and growth hormone) of catalytic enzymes depletes fat stores. A loss of muscle mass occurs early in the course of the disease and worsens with progression of heart failure (50). Bone density is also decreased through low levels of vitamin D and secondary hyperparathyroidism (50, 51).

In addition to increased metabolism and tissue loss, vitamin and mineral stores can become compromised by (and contribute to) worsening heart failure. Malabsorption of such critical nutrients as fat-soluble vitamins has been described, potentially resulting from gut edema. Selenium deficiency has been implicated in cardiomyopathies (both idiopathic and peripartum) in the developing world, whereas thiamin (vitamin B₁) deficiency can induce a reversible form of high-output heart failure (50). Diuretic use can result in the depletion of important electrolytes, such as potassium and magnesium, which can predispose to ventricular arrhythmias.

Nutritional and Nonpharmacologic Management

Because 60% of the heart failure in the general population of the United States may be attributed to coronary artery disease (52), dietary and lifestyle practices that lower the incidence of atherosclerosis represent practical measures of prevention (see Chapter 67). The American Heart Association guidelines emphasize diets high in vegetables, fruit, and low-fat dairy products, as well as limitations on sodium (<2 g/day) and alcohol consumption (47). Sodium restriction in patients with heart failure is indicated when symptoms develop or worsen and is particularly important in the management of edema accompanying heart failure. These guidelines certainly are useful in reducing the risk of onset of CHF, but the daily energy requirements in patients with existing heart failure remain poorly defined (53). In fact, up to 50% of patients hospitalized with heart failure reportedly are malnourished (54).

Dietary indiscretion, however, chiefly in the form of increased sodium and fluid intake, remains a common and preventable cause of hospitalization in patients with CHF. Therefore, traditional recommendations have included, in addition to sodium restriction, fluid restriction (<1200 mL of water, depending on disease severity) and restriction of saturated fats (55).

However, following these recommendations can be difficult for patients, particularly the elderly, and compliance with the numerous clinical instructions from providers remains poor (56). Multidisciplinary care, provided by teams consisting of a primary care provider, a nurse coordinator, a dietitian, a nurse specializing in heart failure, and a cardiologist, has proven to reduce readmissions for CHF and to improve the quality of life for patients. Consultation with a dietitian experienced in cardiovascular disease is useful for counseling patients regarding dietary measures to help manage the symptoms of heart failure. Reports showed that compliance rates improved using individualized treatment plans, consisting of diet and exercise monitoring and titration of medications by nurses specializing in heart failure (under the direction of a cardiologist). This team approach to the care of heart failure was accomplished at similar cost to traditional methods of management (56–58).

Although team management approaches and careful dietary instructions can improve outcomes, specific dietary supplements to improve the overall course of heart failure have not been examined in large-scale clinical trials. Deficiency of micronutrients and vitamins can contribute to heart failure. An excellent review of the role in heart failure played by deficiencies of various micronutrients was prepared by Witte and colleagues and included data regarding calcium, vitamin D, copper, selenium, thiamin, ubiquinone (coenzyme Q10), and carnitine (50). Increased surveillance for nutrient deficiencies is particularly advised for patients who are taking diuretics. Renal thiamin excretion is augmented by diuretic use, and thiamin deficiency has been found to be significantly more frequent in patients with CHF who are receiving long-term diuretic therapy. Additionally, in small observational studies, thiamin replacement resulted in improved cardiac ejection fraction as assessed by echocardiography (59). Selenium and copper balance have also been implicated in symptomatic cardiovascular disease, but the significance of deficiencies of these micronutrients in patients with cardiomyopathy and heart failure has been controversial (60). However, particularly in patients receiving large doses of diuretics on a long-term basis, prevention of micronutrient deficiency with routine multivitamin supplementation would be reasonable (50).

Obesity has been associated with various adverse effects on cardiac function, and the probability of heart failure increases with long-standing, morbid obesity (58). Therefore, weight loss involving increased physical activity and attention to a diet that emphasizes fruits, vegetables, and low-fat dairy products can be beneficial. Dietary interventions can augment the effects of pharmacologic therapy, thereby decreasing cardiovascular events. Clinicians should mention to all patients with heart disease, including those with CHF, that even small reductions in weight and blood pressure decrease the risk of stroke and coronary heart disease (47). Additionally, maintenance of diets high in fruits and vegetables can reduce deficiencies of potassium, magnesium, and calcium. These electrolytes tend to be depleted by loop diuretics such as furosemide and predispose patients to complex cardiac arrhythmias. Careful monitoring of electrolyte levels should be included in the management of all patients with heart failure who are treated with long-term diuretics. Foods high in ω-3 fats, particularly fatty fish such as salmon, but also flaxseed and canola oil and nuts, may also be beneficial. Although large-scale trials involving patients with heart failure are lacking, evidence has linked ω-3 fats to a cardioprotective effect and a reduction in the incidence of sudden death (47).

In patients with advanced CHF and cachexia, nourishment can be difficult, given the heightened metabolism of these persons. Nutritional and vitamin supplements may become necessary in the presence of poor oral intake. Calories and overall fat intake can be increased, because weight loss in late-stage heart failure is associated with an ominous prognosis (58).

REFERENCES

1. Young JB. The heart failure syndrome. In: Mills R, Young JB, eds. Practical Approaches to The Treatment of Heart Failure. Baltimore: Williams & Wilkins, 1998.
2. Konstam MA. J Card Fail 2003;9:1–3.
3. Criteria Committee of the New York Heart Association. Nomenclature and Criteria for Diagnosis. 9th ed. Boston: Little, Brown, 1994.
4. Goldman L, Hashimoto B, Cook EF et al. Circulation 1981;64:1227–34.
5. Hunt SA, Baker DW, Chin MH et al. Circulation 2001;104:2996–3007.
6. Ansari M, Massie BM. Am Heart J 2003;146:1–4.
7. Fonarow GC, Horwich TB. Rev Cardiovasc Med 2003;4:8–17.
8. Adams KF, Baughman KL, Dec WG et al. J Card Fail 1999;5:357–82.
9. Hellermannn JP, Jocobsen SJ, Gersh BJ et al. Am J Med 2002;113:324–30.
10. Lloyd-Jones DM, Larson MG, Leip EP et al. Circulation 2002;106:3068–72.
11. Berry C, Clark AL. Eur Heart J 2000;21:521–32.
12. Kitzman DW. Heart failure and cardiomyopathy. In: Abrams WB, Beers MH, Berkow B, eds. The Merck Manual of Geriatrics. 3rd ed. Whitehouse Station, NJ: Merck Research Laboratories, 2000:900–14.
13. Weber KT. N Engl J Med 2001;345:1689–97.
14. Armstrong PW. Heart 2000;84[Suppl I]:I15–7.
15. Stuthers AD. Heart 2000;84:334–8.
16. Task Force on Heart Failure of the European Society of Cardiology. Eur Heart J 1995;16:741–51.
17. Badgett RG, Lucey CR, Mulrow CD. JAMA 1997;277:1712–9.
18. Bhatia VV, Nayyar PP, Dhindsa SS. J Postgrad Med 2003;49:182–5.
19. Kenchaiah S, Evans JC, Levy D et al. N Engl J Med 2002;347:305–13.
20. Kannel WB. J Clin Epidemiol 2000;53:229–35.
21. Grossman E, Messerli F. Ann Intern Med 1996;125:305–10.
22. Lutton SR, Ratliff NB, Young JB. Cardiomyopathy and myocardial failure. In: Topol E, ed. Textbook of Cardiovascular Medicine. 2nd ed. Philadelphia: Lippincott Williams & Wilkins, 2002.
23. Jain P, Massie BM, Gattis WA et al. Am Heart J 2003;145[Suppl]:3S–17S.
24. Jessup M, Brozena S. N Engl J Med 2003;348:2007–2018.
25. Deedwania PC. Arch Intern Med 2000;160:1585–94.
26. McAllister FA, Lawson FM, Teo KK et al. Am J Med 2001;110:378–84.
27. Nohria A, Lewis E, Stevenson LW. JAMA 2002;287:628–40.
28. Klein L, O'Connor CM, Gattis WA. Am J Cardiol 2003;91[Suppl 9A]:18F–40F.
29. Gomberg-Maitland M, Baran DA, Fuster V. Arch Intern Med 2001;161:342–52.
30. Garg R, Yusuf S for the Collaborative Group on ACE Inhibitor Trials. JAMA 1995;273:1450–6.
31. Flather MD, Yusuf S, Kober L et al. Lancet 2000;355:1575–81.
32. Jong P, Demers C, McKelvie RS. J Am Coll Cardiol 2002;39:463–70.
33. Foody J, Farrell MH, Krumholz HM. JAMA 2002;287:883–9.
34. Pitt B, Zannad F, Remme WJ et al. N Engl J Med 1999;341:709–17.
35. Brown NJ. Circulation 2003;107:2512–8.
36. Digitalis Investigators Group. N Engl J Med 1997;336:525–33.
37. Packer M, O'Conner CM, Ghali JK et al. N Engl J Med 1996;335:1107–4.
38. Maggioni AP. Heart 2001;85:97–103.
39. Middlekauf HR, Wiener I, Stevenson WG. Am J Cardiol 1993;72:75F–81F.
40. Koniaris L, Goldhaber SZ. J Am Coll Cardiol 1998;31:745–8.
41. Englestein E. Am J Cardiol 2003;91:62F–73F.
42. Moss AJ, Zareba W, Hall WJ et al. N Engl J Med 2002;346:877–83.
43. Saxon LA, De Marco T. J Am Coll Cardiol 2001;38:1971–3.
44. Abraham WT, Fisher WG, Smith L et al. N Engl J Med 2002;346:1845–53.
45. Baumgartner WA. J Am Coll Surg 2001;192:345–55.
46. Bishay ES, McCarthy PM, Cosgrove DM et al. Eur J Cardiothorac Surg 2000;17:213–21.
47. Krauss RM, Eckel, RH, Howard B et al. Circulation 2000;102:2284–99.
48. Katz AM, Katz PB. Br Heart J 1962;24:257–62.
49. Adigun AQ, Ajayi AA. Eur J Heart Fail 2001;3:359–63.
50. Witte KK, Clark AL, Cleland JG. J Am Coll Cardiol 2001;37:1765–74.
51. Shane E, Mancini D, Aaronson K et al. Am J Med 1997;103:197–207.
52. He J, Ogden LG, Bazzano LA et al. Arch Intern Med 2001;161:996–1002.
53. Toth MJ, Gottlieb SS, Fisher ML et al. Metabolism 1997;46:1294–98.
54. Freeman LM, Roubenoff R. Nutr Rev 1994;52:340–7.
55. Silver MA. J Am Coll Cardiol 2003;42:1224–25.
56. Kasper EK, Gerstenblith G, Hefter G et al. J Am Coll Cardiol 2002;39:471–80.
57. Rich MW, Beckham V, Wittenberg C et al. N Engl J Med 2995;333:1190–5.
58. Colonna P, Sorino M, D'Agnostino C et al. Am J Cardiol 2003;91[Suppl]:41F–50F.
59. Shimon I, Almog S, Vered Z et al. Am J Med 1995;98:485–90.
60. da Cunha S, Filho FM, da Cunha Bastos VL et al. Arq Bras Cardiol 2002;79:460–5.

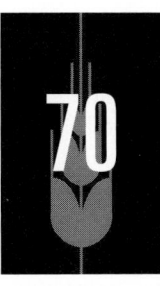

70   ALIMENTARY TRACT IN NUTRITION[1]
SAMUEL KLEIN, STEVEN M. COHN, AND DAVID H. ALPERS

GASTROINTESTINAL TRACT STRUCTURE 1115
    Substructures and Cells .1115
    Esophagus 1116
    Stomach 1117
    Small Intestine 1118
    Colon 1119
    Rectum 1120
VASCULATURE 1120
ENTERIC NERVOUS SYSTEM AND MOTILITY 1121
GASTROINTESTINAL HORMONES 1125
INTEGRATED RESPONSE TO A MEAL 1126
    Regulation of Food Intake 1126
    Stimuli-Evoked Responses 1127
    Mouth 1127
    Esophagus 1128
    Stomach 1128
    Duodenum 1129
    Biliary System 1131
    Pancreas 1131
NUTRIENT ABSORPTION .1132
    Fluid and Electrolytes 1132
    Lipid 1133
    Carbohydrate 1135
    Protein 1137
    Minerals 1138
    Vitamins 1139
INTESTINAL MICROFLORA 1139
IMMUNE SYSTEM 1140

The alimentary tract is a tubular structure that extends from the posterior oropharynx to the anus. Its primary function is to digest and absorb ingested nutrients. The purpose of this chapter is to review the structural and functional components of the alimentary tract and to describe the interactions of these components in response to a meal. Gastrointestinal (GI) tract flora and the GI immune system will also be reviewed briefly because of their importance in overall gut function.

GASTROINTESTINAL TRACT STRUCTURE

Substructures and Cells

The structure of the GI tract is reviewed briefly, with a consideration of the localization of numerous cells and substructures that are critical for its function. The GI tract consists of four contiguous segments: the esophagus, stomach, small intestine, and colon (Fig. 70.1). The wall of each segment contains four distinctive layers: the mucosa, submucosa, muscularis propria, and serosa or adventitia (Fig. 70.2). The mucosa is composed of three distinct layers: the epithelium, lamina propria, and muscularis mucosae. The epithelial layer forms a barrier between the lumen and the underlying tissues. Many of the different region-specific secretory, absorptive, and barrier functions of the alimentary tract are accounted for by differences in the type and distribution of various differentiated epithelial cell populations along the length of the gut. Thus, the epithelium shows the greatest degree of variability among different regions of the GI tract. The lamina propria is a connective tissue space between the epithelium and the thin layer of muscle fibers, the muscularis mucosae, which forms the lower boundary of the mucosa. The lamina propria contains many cells involved in immunologic functions, including immunoglobulin (Ig)–secreting plasma cells, macrophages, and lymphocytes. In addition, abundant lymphoid nodules that often extend through the muscularis mucosae into the underlying submucosa are present. Subepithelial fibroblasts produce collagen and many other extracellular matrix components that underlie the basal lamina of the epithelium. These fibroblasts and the extracellular matrix that they secrete have an important role in regulating cell proliferation and differentiation events within the overlying epithelium.

The mucosal epithelium contains numerous enteroendocrine cells, in addition to cells that serve secretory, absorptive, and barrier functions. The enteroendocrine cells, found in gastric, intestinal, and colonic epithelium, are characterized by their polygonal shape, broad base,

[1]**Abbreviations: ATPase,** adenosine triphosphatase; **bicarbonate,** HCO₃⁻; **CCK,** cholecystokinin; **Cl,** chloride; **CNS,** central nervous system; **EC,** enterochromaffin cells; **ECL,** enterochromaffinlike; **ENS,** enteric nervous system; **GALT,** gut-associated lymphoid tissue; **GI,** gastrointestinal; **GIP,** glucose-dependent insulinotropic peptide; **GLP,** glucagonlike peptide; **GRP,** gastrin-releasing peptide; **Ig,** immunoglobulin; **K,** potassium; **LCT,** long-chain triglyceride; **MCT,** medium-chain triglyceride; **Na,** sodium; **NO,** nitric oxide; **PYY,** peptide YY; **SCFA,** short-chain fatty acid; **VIP,** vasoactive intestinal polypeptide.

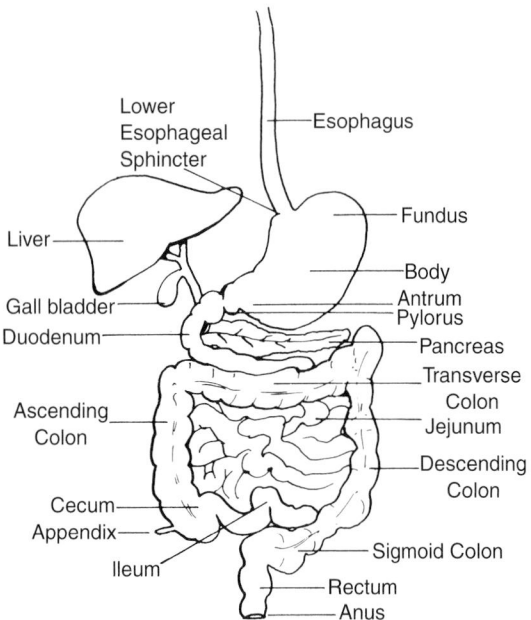

Figure 70.1. Anatomy of the stomach, small intestine, and large intestine. The duodenum is located in the retroperitoneal space and bends around the head of the pancreas. The jejunum lies within the peritoneal cavity and begins at the ligament of Trietz. Jejunal bowel loops are predominately located in the left and middle upper abdomen. The proximal ileum lies in the middle abdominal region. The distal ileum lies in the right lower quadrant and joins the colon at the ileal cecal valve. The *cutout* reveals the duodenum and the ligament of Trietz that lie behind the transverse colon.

and numerous basilar membrane-bound secretory granules. Enteroendocrine cells are joined to other adjacent cells in the epithelium via junctional complexes located near the apical pole. The regulatory peptides or bioamine products stored in the basally located secretory granules

are secreted through the basolateral membrane and act through paracrine or endocrine mechanisms as mediators of GI secretion, absorptive function, and motility in response to luminally and/or basolaterally derived signals.

The submucosa extends from the mucosa to the muscularis externa and contains numerous small to moderate-sized veins, arteries, and lymphatic channels surrounded by connective tissue. Ganglion cells and autonomic nerve fibers of the Meissner plexus are also found in the submucosa. Fibers of this submucosal plexus together with the myenteric plexus form the enteric nervous system (ENS), which regulates and coordinates numerous intestinal functions including motility. Additionally, scattered lymphoid aggregates or nodules may be found in this layer of the gut wall.

The muscularis propria is organized into two layers of muscle: an inner circular layer, in which muscle cells circle the intestine, and an outer longitudinal layer, in which muscle cells run parallel with the long axis of the intestine. In the upper esophagus, skeletal muscle fibers interdigitate with smooth muscle fibers, whereas the muscularis of the remaining alimentary tract is composed entirely of smooth muscle.

Esophagus

The adult esophagus is approximately 25 cm long and extends from the posterior oropharynx at the level of the cricoid cartilage to just below the diaphragmatic hiatus, where it enters the stomach at the esophagogastric junction. The esophageal mucosa is lined with a thick incompletely keratinized stratified squamous epithelium that provides protection against abrasion during passage of a swallowed food bolus and against refluxed stomach acid. The lamina propria contains occasional lymphoid aggregates and

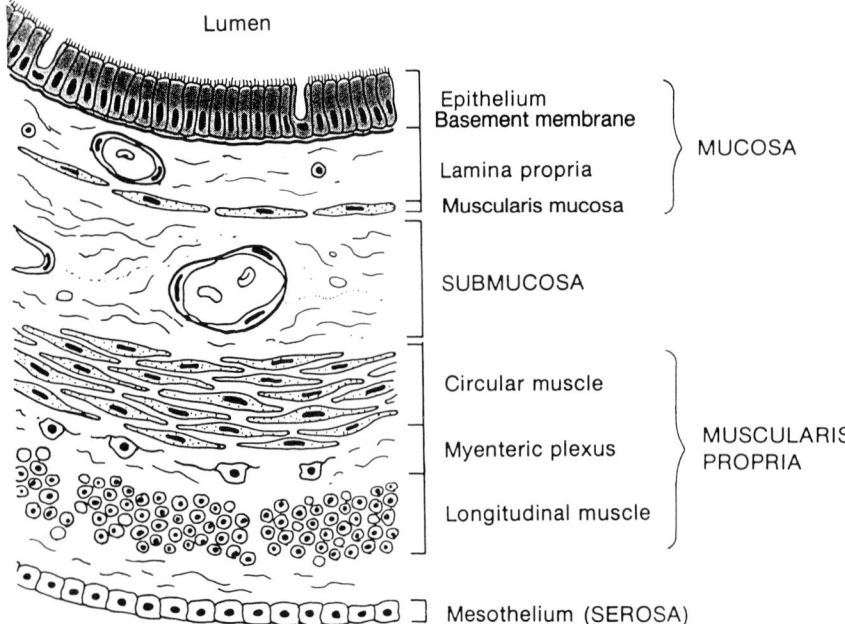

Figure 70.2. Schematic organization of the wall of the gastrointestinal tract. (From Yamada T, Alpers DH, Owyang C et al., eds. Textbook of Gastroenterology. 2nd ed. Philadelphia: JB Lippincott, 1991:142, with permission.)

mucosal glands that secrete neutral mucus. Submucosal glands that secrete acidic mucus extend through the lamina propria and muscularis mucosae and are most abundant in the upper half of the esophagus.

In the upper esophagus, skeletal muscle fibers blend with the smooth muscle fibers found throughout the rest of the esophagus. The upper esophageal sphincter consists of a thickened band of oblique muscle. These skeletal muscle fibers are under voluntary control and are involved in regulating the initial passage of a swallowed bolus into the upper esophagus. The remaining smooth muscle of the muscularis is innervated by parasympathetic fibers originating from the vagus nerve. A thickened band of circular smooth muscle adjacent to the esophagogastric junction forms the lower esophageal sphincter. Contraction of this specialized region of smooth muscle, coupled with the abrupt angulation of the esophagus as it passes through the diaphragmatic hiatus, where it joins the gastric cardia, provides a mechanism for preventing reflux of the acid contents of the stomach into the esophagus.

Stomach

The stomach is an asymmetric organ that extends from the gastroesophageal junction in the cardia to the duodenum (Fig. 70.3). The upper portion of the stomach that lies under the left hemidiaphragm is called the fundus. The gastric body comprises the largest portion of the stomach and extends to the angularis, where the stomach abruptly bends. The gastric antrum lies between the angularis and the pylorus. The pyloric sphincter is a round band of muscle that forms the opening of the stomach into the duodenum. The flat glandular mucosa of the stomach changes to the villus epithelium seen in the duodenum at the pylorus.

The entire stomach is lined by a simple columnar epithelium. The mucosa contains numerous invaginating gastric pits or foveolae that form glands at their bases. Each glandular unit is composed of three regions: the upper pit region, lined by surface mucus-secreting cells; a narrow isthmus or neck, containing the proliferative zone

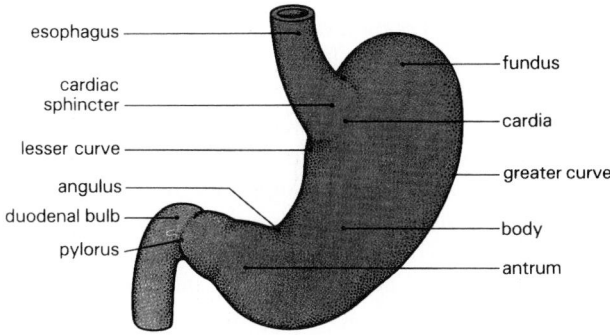

Figure 70.3. Regional organization of the stomach and proximal duodenum. (From Yamada T, Alpers DH, Owyang C et al., eds. Textbook of Gastroenterology. 2nd ed. Philadelphia: JB Lippincott, 1991:1304, with permission.)

and many immature undifferentiated cells and mucous neck cells; and a basilar gland that contains three cell types—parietal cells, chief cells, and enteroendocrine cells. The majority of the gastric body and fundus is lined by oxyntic mucosa, consisting of fundic-type glands responsible for secretion of acid pepsinogens, and intrinsic factor. These glands contain abundant parietal cells in the upper half of the gland. Chief cells predominate near the base of the glands in fundic-type mucosa. The cardiac glands, found in the first 3 to 4 cm adjacent to the esophagogastric junction, are primarily mucus-secreting glands with few parietal or chief cells. Pyloric glands in the prepyloric antrum are coiled and are remarkable for their fairly long foveolae and increased population of enteroendocrine cells.

Surface mucous cells form a uniform population of columnar epithelial cells lining the surface mucosa and gastric pits. These cells secrete a glycoprotein-rich neutral mucous layer that protects the epithelium from the acid environment of the stomach. Surface mucous cells are constantly shed into the gastric lumen and are replaced by replication of undifferentiated cells within the neck or isthmus region of each gastric gland that differentiate during migration up the foveola and onto the gastric mucosal surface.

Parietal cells secrete hydrochloric acid and are located in the middle and basilar portions of the gastric glands. These cells are large with clear or acidophilic cytoplasm and abundant mitochondria. These cells have well-developed intracellular canaliculi containing a microvillus border that greatly expands the apical surface available for acid secretion. Receptors for histamine, gastrin, and acetylcholine are located at the basolateral surface and regulate parietal cell secretory function. Hydrogen/potassium (K)–adenosine triphosphatase (ATPase), the enzyme that secretes hydrogen ions into the lumen, is located on the canalicular membrane. Intrinsic factor, a binding protein for vitamin B_{12}, is secreted by parietal cells.

Chief cells or zymogenic cells are found near the base of the gastric glands. These cells contain an extensive basilar rough endoplasmic reticulum and supranuclear zymogen granules, reflecting their role in the production of pepsinogens and other proteases. Pepsinogens are synthesized and secreted by these cells into the gastric lumen. Hydrochloric acid in the lumen catalyzes the conversion of the proenzyme pepsinogen to the active pepsins that begin digestion of proteins to lower-molecular-weight polypeptides.

Enteroendocrine cells are most abundant in the prepyloric antrum, and secrete many different neuropeptides and regulatory molecules that are discussed later. Gastrin-secreting G cells predominate in the antrum, enterochromaffin cells (ECs) are found throughout the gastric mucosa and secrete serotonin and either substance P or motilin, glucagon-secreting A cells are found in the proximal third of the stomach, and somatostatin-secreting D cells can be found in both the upper third of the stomach

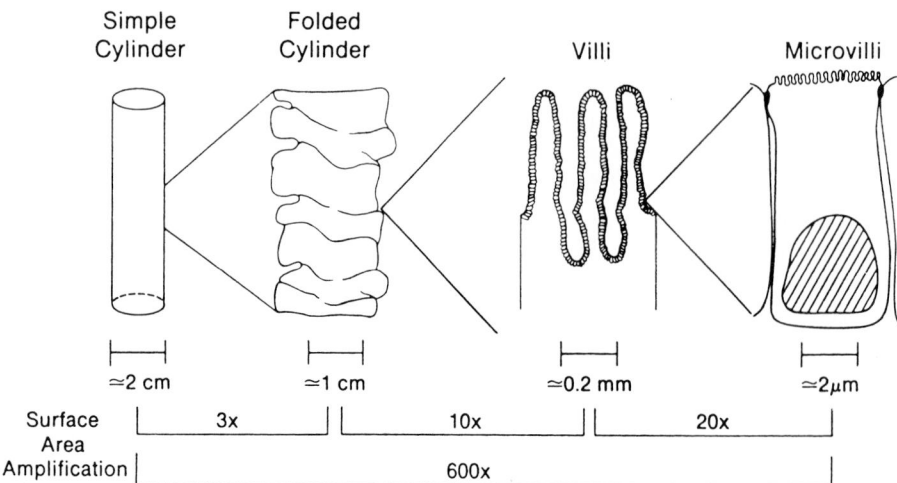

Figure 70.4. The surface area of intestinal surface area is expanded by the presence of intestinal folds (plicae conniventes) and villi. Microvilli further expand the surface area of epithelial cells in contact with luminal contents. These structural features taken together expand the surface area of the small intestine by approximately 600-fold. (From Yamada T, Alpers DH, Owyang C et al., eds. Textbook of Gastroenterology. 2nd ed. Philadelphia: JB Lippincott, 1991: 327, with permission.)

and the antrum but not in the midstomach. This complex web of enteroendocrine signals is important in integrating responses to both luminal conditions and basolateral signals.

Small Intestine

The small intestine extends from the gastric pylorus to the ileocecal valve and is divided into three regions, the duodenum, the jejunum, and the ileum.

Duodenum

The duodenum is approximately 30 cm in length and is fixed in place, molded around the head of the pancreas. Histologically, the duodenum is characterized by the presence of abundant submucosal Brunner glands that secrete alkaline mucus. The first portion of the duodenum, known as the bulb, is attached to a mesentery that is attached to the posterior wall of the peritoneal cavity. The second (descending), third (transverse), and fourth (ascending) portions of the duodenum are retroperitoneal in location. Bile and pancreatic secretions enter the second portion of the duodenum from the common bile duct at the ampulla (papilla) of Vater. The junction of the duodenum and the jejunum is defined by the position of the ligament of Treitz, where the duodenum reenters the peritoneal cavity. There is no change in the histologic appearance of the small intestine at this transition.

Jejunum and Ileum

The jejunum and ileum are mobile because of their attachment to an extensive mesentery. The proximal two fifths of the small intestine beyond the ligament of Treitz is defined as jejunum, whereas the distal three fifths are ileum. The jejunum has a larger diameter, more prominent folds, and longer villi than the ileum. The ileum is characterized by the presence of abundant lymphoid follicles (Peyer patches) in the submucosa.

The length of the jejunum and ileum in adults ranges from 320 to 846 cm. Several structural features of the small intestine amplify the mucosal surface area available for nutrient absorption to more than 200 m², which is larger than a doubles tennis court (Fig. 70.4). Magnification of the surface area is achieved by a series of folds and invaginations. First, the cylinder of the intestine is heaped up into circular folds (plicae circulares) involving both submucosa and mucosa. These folds are particularly prominent in the jejunum. Second, the mucosal surface is further expanded by the presence of numerous villi, long fingerlike projections of mucosa containing an arteriole, vein, and central draining lacteal. Third, the apical surface of each small intestinal epithelial cell along the villi is covered by microvilli, providing thousands of hills and valleys for surface expansion. The presence of folds, villi, and microvilli increase the surface area to 600 times that of the surface area present in a simple cylinder.

Epithelium

The simple columnar epithelium that lines the small intestine is composed of four principal differentiated cell types—absorptive enterocytes, goblet cells, Paneth cells, and enteroendocrine cells. Cells are joined to adjacent cells by junctional complexes that regulate the paracellular movement of fluid and macromolecules (see the fluid and electrolytes section). Absorptive enterocytes are responsible for digestion of dipeptides, tripeptides, and disaccharides, and for nutrient absorption. The microvilli of absorptive enterocytes are supported by a central core of actin filaments that join with a dense terminal web of actin and myosin filaments oriented parallel to the apical surface of the enterocyte. The apical surface is covered by a glycoprotein-rich glycocalyx. Many enterocyte-encoded proteins important for digestive function are present at the apical surface, including dipeptidases, disaccharidases, enterokinase, and intestinal alkaline phosphatase. Goblet cells are flask-shaped cells with large apical vesicles that store and secrete mucus. Mucus secreted by the goblet cell forms a viscous gel that functions both as a lubricant and to protect the surface epithelium against adherence of invading pathogens. Goblet cells also secrete small cysteine-rich proteins that participate in the defense against certain parasites, including nematodes. Paneth cells reside at the base of the intestinal crypts and produce proteins involved in antibacterial defenses, including lysozyme and a variety of defensins.

Enteroendocrine cells contain a large number of neuroendocrine mediators (see the section on gastrointestinal hormones). The distribution of individual enteroendocrine cell subpopulations within the epithelium differs along the length of the small intestine. Although enteroendocrine cells arise from the same stem cell as the other differentiated cell types found in the small intestine, they have a much longer half-life than enterocytes or goblet cells. Thus, their migration onto and along the intestinal villi is uncoupled from the migration of the other epithelial cell types in the intestine.

Renewal

Under normal physiologic circumstances, cells within the intestinal epithelium are continuously and rapidly replaced by migration of cells onto the villus from several adjacent crypts of Lieberkühn or intestinal glands (Fig. 70.5). The four principal differentiated cell types of the small intestinal epithelium are all derived from multipotent stem cell(s) located near the base of each intestinal crypt. These

crypt stem cells divide rarely to produce a daughter stem cell (self renewal) as well as a more rapidly replicating transit cell. Transit cells, in turn, undergo four to six rapid cell divisions in the proliferative zone located in the lower half of each crypt, and their progeny subsequently differentiate during a bipolar migration away from this zone. Goblet cells and enterocytes undergo terminal differentiation as they are rapidly translocated upward from the zone of proliferation to the apical extrusion zone (a process lasting 48 to 72 hours) located adjacent to the villus tip, where they undergo apoptosis and are sloughed into the lumen. Paneth cells arise during downward migration to the crypt base, and enteroendocrine cells differentiate during migration from the zone of proliferation in either direction. Cell renewal, migration, and differentiation are interrelated processes that are regulated at multiple levels.

Colon

Structure

The colon is approximately 100 to 150 cm in length, extending from the ileocecal valve to the proximal rectum (see Fig. 70.1). The colon consists of the cecum, ascending colon, hepatic flexure, transverse colon, splenic flexure, descending colon, and sigmoid colon. The terminal ileum enters the cecum on its posteromedial border at the ileocecal valve. The cecum is a large blind pouch approximately 7.5 to 8.5 cm in diameter that projects from the

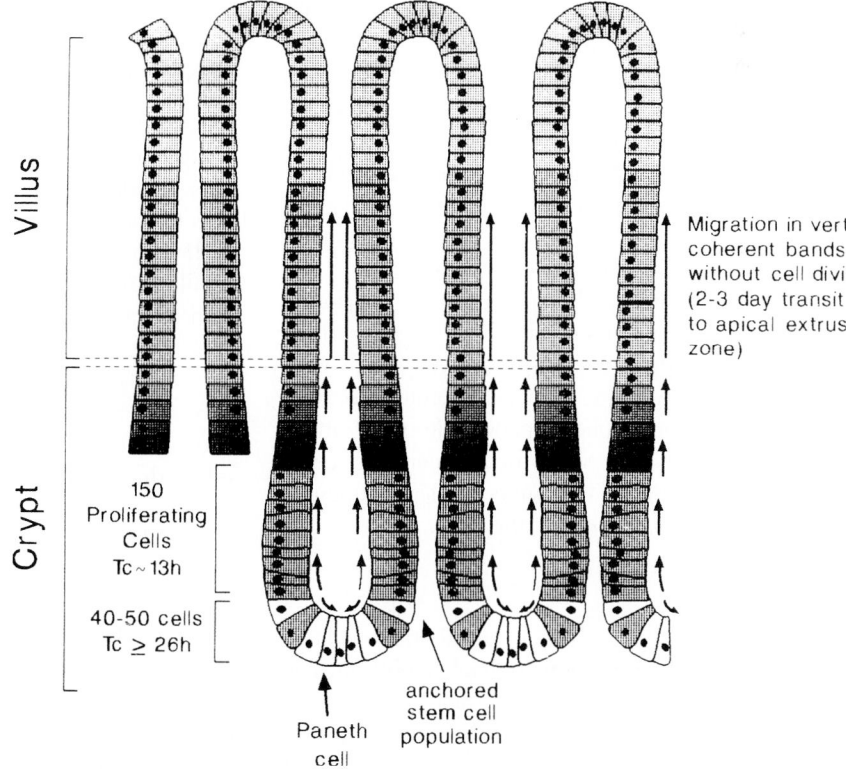

Figure 70.5. Schematic organization of the epithelium in the adult mouse small intestine. The small intestinal crypt contains approximately 250 cells. The lower five cell positions contain 40 to 50 cells that have an average cycle time (Tc) of 26 hours or longer. This region includes Paneth cells and is postulated to include undifferentiated, anchored stem cells at the fifth cell position above the base. The undifferentiated cells divide asymmetrically to give rise to proliferating transit cells (Tc ~13 hours) that migrate upward toward the villus and subsequently differentiate into enterocytes, goblet cells, and enteroendocrine cells. Paneth cells differentiate during downward translocation to the crypt base. Senescent cells are extruded near the villus tips. (From Yamada T, Alpers DH, Owyang C et al., eds. Textbook of Gastroenterology. 2nd ed. Philadelphia: JB Lippincott, 1991:1561, with permission.)

Villus

Crypt

150 Proliferating Cells Tc ~ 13h

40-50 cells Tc ≥ 26h

Migration in vertical coherent bands without cell division (2-3 day transit to apical extrusion zone)

Paneth cell

anchored stem cell population

antimesenteric side of the ascending colon. The appendix extends from a narrow opening in the base of the cecum. The diameter of the colon diminishes progressively; the sigmoid colon is approximately 2.5 cm in diameter and is the narrowest portion of the colon. The omentum is attached to the transverse colon on its anterior superior edge. The ascending colon, descending colon, rectum, and posterior surface of the hepatic and splenic flexures are fixed retroperitoneal structures. The cecum, transverse, and sigmoid colon are intraperitoneal and therefore lack a complete serosal layer.

Epithelium

Three principal differentiated epithelial cell types are present in the adult colonic epithelium: absorptive colonocytes, goblet cells, and enteroendocrine cells. As found in the small intestine, all these cell lineages appear to be derived from a common epithelial stem cell precursor. Undifferentiated cells, replicating cells, and enteroendocrine cells predominate near the base of each colonic gland (crypt). Cells belonging to each of the principal cell lineages differentiate as they migrate away from the zone of proliferation toward the surface epithelium. The average life span of goblet cells and absorptive cells, from their birth deep in the crypt to the point at which they are sloughed into the lumen, is approximately 6 days. As in the small intestine, some enteroendocrine cell subtypes appear to have a much longer life span than goblet cells or absorptive colonocytes.

As absorptive colonocytes differentiate during their migration up the crypt, they develop short microvilli and clear apically oriented vesicles containing a fibrillar glycoprotein-rich secretory product that may contribute to a glycocalyx. These apical vesicles are lost, and microvilli elongate and increase in number as the maturing absorptive cells emerge onto the surface epithelium. At this point, alkaline phosphatase activity appears on the brush border and the basolateral membranes have acquired a considerable amount of sodium $(Na^+)/K^+$-ATPase activity, reflecting their function in water and electrolyte transport.

Many different enteroendocrine cell types are found within the colonic epithelium, including L cells, which contain both enteroglucagon and peptide YY (PYY); cells that secrete only PYY; EC_1 cells, which secrete serotonin, substance P, and leu-enkephalin; pancreatic polypeptide-secreting cells; and rare somatostatin-secreting cells. Enteroendocrine cells are more numerous in the appendix and the rectum than in the rest of the colon.

Other Layers

The inner circular muscle fibers form a continuous layer around the colon. The outer longitudinal smooth muscle fibers are condensed into three bands (taeniae coli) equidistant around the circumference of the colon. Haustra are the bulging sacculations that form between adjacent taeniae coli. The serosa is a mesothelial-derived cell layer that covers the peritoneal aspects of the colonic wall. Therefore, regions of the ascending colon, the descending colon, and the rectum that do not lie within the peritoneal cavity have no outer serosal layer.

Appendix

The appendix is similar in histologic organization to the rest of the colon. The mucosa of the appendix consists of deep folds lined with a columnar epithelium forming simple tubular or forked glands. This epithelium contains abundant goblet cells and enteroendocrine cells. Numerous lymphoid nodules are found in the lamina propria. The normal histologic architecture of the adult appendix is often replaced by fibrous scar tissue as a result of subclinical bouts of appendicitis.

Rectum

The rectum is approximately 12 to 15 cm in length and extends from the sigmoid colon to the anal canal following the curve of the sacrum (see Fig. 70.1). The rectal wall consists of mucosal, submucosal, inner circular, and outer longitudinal muscular layers. There is no serosal layer in the rectum. The anal canal is approximately 3 cm long. The anal verge is the junction between anal and perianal skin. Anal epithelium (anoderm) lacks hair follicles, sebaceous glands, and sweat glands. The dentate line is the true mucocutaneous junction located just above the anal verge. A 6- to 12-mm transitional zone exists above the dentate line, where the squamous epithelium of the anoderm becomes cuboidal and then columnar epithelium.

VASCULATURE

Blood and lymphatic vessels provide the transportation system for delivering absorbed nutrients to other body tissues. In addition, the arterial blood supply provides nutrients to the alimentary tract itself. In the small intestine, each villus contains a single arteriole that breaks into a capillary network at the villus tip before anastomosing with a draining venule. Each villus contains a lymphatic vessel (lacteal) that drains into a submucosal plexus connected to larger lymphatics. In the colon, arterioles pass between crypts to the epithelial cell surface and form a network of capillaries around the crypts. Lymphatic vessels in the colon do not extend higher than the base of the crypts.

Blood from the small intestine and colon drain into the portal vein that delivers absorbed water-soluble nutrients directly to the liver, where these nutrients can be metabolized or released directly into the hepatic veins and ultimately into the systemic circulation. Bile salts absorbed in the terminal ileum travel through the portal vein to the liver, where they can be secreted back into the small intestine, providing an enterohepatic circulation for bile salt recycling, which is critical for normal bile salt homeostasis and fat absorption. Intestinal lymphatic vessels, which are closely associated with arteries supplying the alimentary tract, carry absorbed fat-soluble nutrients to the thoracic duct, which drains into the left subclavian vein and the systemic circulation.

Adequate intestinal blood flow is critical because it provides the oxygen necessary for intestinal cell survival. Therefore, GI tract blood flow is carefully regulated by metabolic, vascular, and hormonal factors to ensure adequate tissue oxygenation. Food ingestion increases intestinal blood flow and oxygen requirements.

ENTERIC NERVOUS SYSTEM AND MOTILITY

Many GI tract motor patterns have been described and involve complicated interactions between a series of stimulatory and inhibitory impulses from the ENS to GI smooth muscle. Intestinal smooth muscle consists of circular and longitudinal muscle layers, so the interaction of muscular contraction between layers determines the pattern of motility. The two most important motility patterns are the migrating myoelectric complex and peristalsis, which are programmed by the ENS.

The migrating myoelectric complex, the major complex motility pattern in mammals, is cyclical and passes from the stomach to the terminal ileum. During digestion this complex consists of irregular contractions that promote mixing and propulsion over moderate distances, modulated by distention and by chemical and mechanical stimulation of the mucosa. Sleeve contractions facilitate mixing of core and peripheral intestinal fluid contents and enhance nutrient contact with intestinal mucosa. During interdigestive periods, the migrating myoelectric complex consists of coordinated activity that empties the stomach and sweeps down the intestine. The frequency of interdigestive ring contraction waves varies with location. Contractions occur at a rate of three per minute in the stomach and 11 to 12 per minute in the duodenum, and decrease progressively down the small intestine to seven per minute in the ileum. The functional role of these interdigestive movements is to clear the gut for the next meal. The migrating myoelectric complex also includes sleeve contractions, which are also rhythmic, and their periodicity decreases along the small intestine.

The regulation of peristalsis, the smallest unit of the propulsive reflex, is one of the simplest of the programmed motor activities of the ENS but is still quite complex (Fig. 70.6). There are two components of the reflex, orad contraction and caudad relaxation, the combination of which moves intestinal contents in a caudad direction. The propulsive movement is the end result of contractions and relaxations of the longitudinal and circular external muscles and of the muscularis mucosae. The circular muscle has the major role in mixing and propulsion by ring contractions that decrease the diameter of the intestine, whereas the longitudinal muscle creates shortening of the segment by sleeve contractions with little alteration in luminal diameter. Excitatory and inhibitory motor neurons supply the muscle, and inhibitory reflexes modulate these activities by monitoring luminal contents. Multiple chemical mediators are involved in this reflex (Fig. 70.7; Table 70.1).

The presence of luminal nutrients can increase absorption by feedback regulation of intestinal motility. Fat or carbohydrate in the ileum and colon stimulate the release

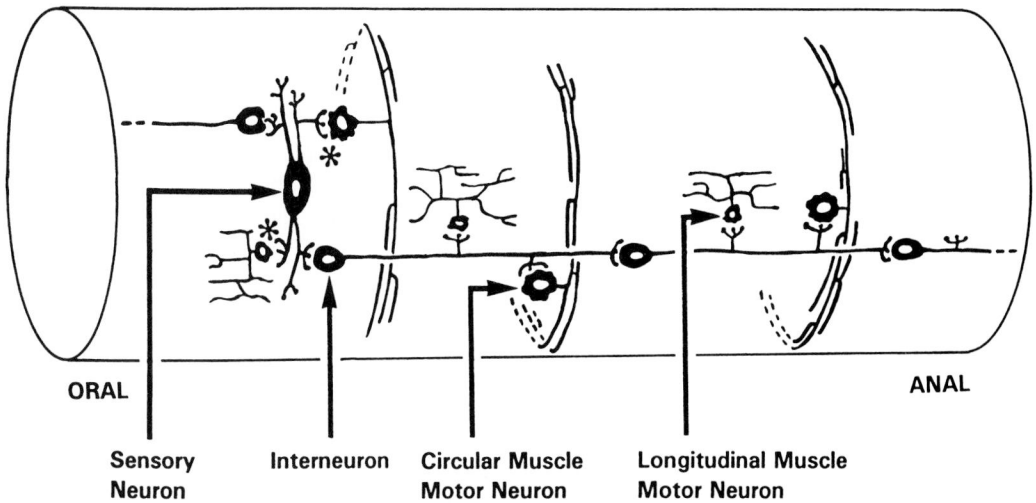

ORAL   **ANAL**

Sensory   Interneuron   Circular Muscle   Longitudinal Muscle
Neuron   Motor Neuron   Motor Neuron

Figure 70.6. The pathways for propulsive reflexes in the intestine. A short segment of intestine is represented, on which the descending inhibitory reflex pathway and the first connections of the ascending pathway are depicted. They provide outputs to ascending and descending interneurons and monosynaptic connections to motor neurons *(asterisk)*. The interneurons form descending and ascending chains and provide outputs to motor neurons. In the descending pathway, some neurons excite the longitudinal muscle, and some neurons inhibit the circular muscle. Ascending reflex pathways supply inputs to excitatory longitudinal muscle motor neurons and excitatory circular muscle motor neurons. (From Yamada T, Alpers DH, Owyang C et al., eds. Textbook of Gastroenterology. 2nd ed. Philadelphia: JB Lippincott, 1991:15, with permission.)

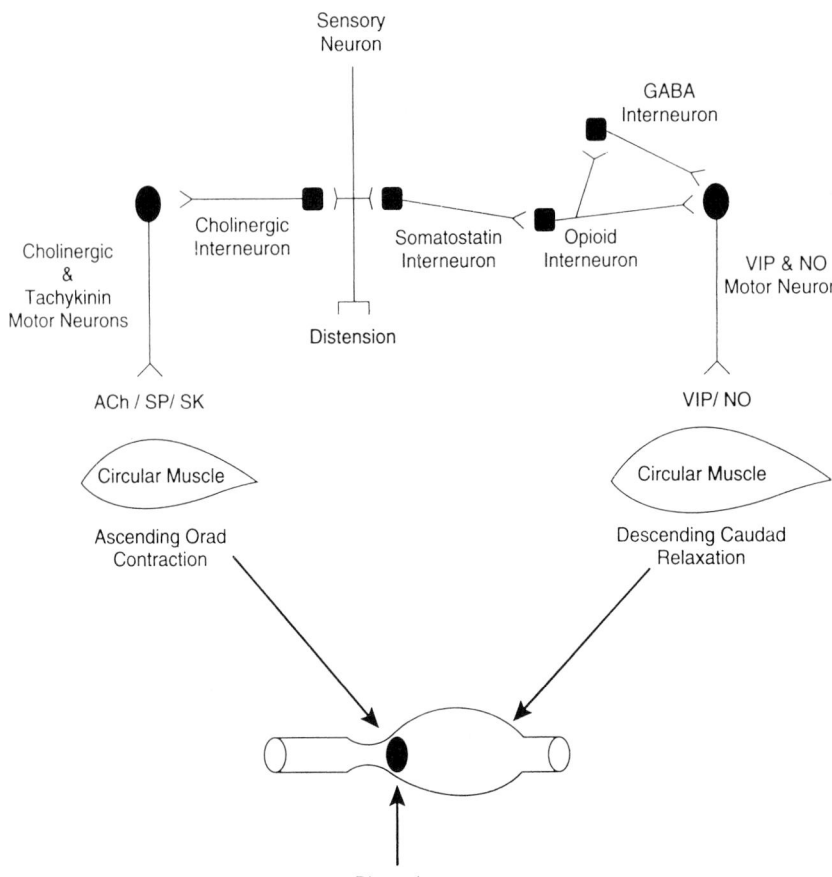

Figure 70.7. Regulation of peristaltic reflex by neurons of the myenteric plexus. The reflex has two components: ascending or orad contraction and descending or caudad relaxation. The stimulus (i.e., distention or mucosal stimulation) is relayed by sensory neurons to cholinergic interneurons coupled to vasoactive intestinal peptide (VIP) and nitric oxide synthase (NOS) neurons caudad and acetylcholine (Ach) and tachykinin (SP, SK) neurons orad. Somatostatin, opioid, and γ-aminobutyric acid (GABA) neurons exert a modulatory influence on VIP and NOS neurons. (From Yamada T, Alpers DH, Owyang C et al., eds. Textbook of Gastroenterology. 2nd ed. Philadelphia: JB Lippincott, 1991:105, with permission.)

of PYY from ileal and colonic endocrine cells. PYY then enters the systemic circulation, and inhibits gastric emptying and slows down small intestinal transit. Thus, this ileal and colonic brake mechanism enhances absorption by increasing the contact time between luminal nutrients and intestinal mucosa.

The ENS is able to regulate such complex and diffuse motility functions by its vast network throughout the GI tract. The ENS consists of approximately 100 million nerve cell bodies (neurons) and their processes that are embedded in the wall of the GI tract. These neurons lie in clusters (ganglia) and are segregated largely into two layers: (a) the myenteric ganglia, which form a continuous plexus between the circular and longitudinal muscle layers of the muscularis propria and extend from the upper esophagus to the internal anal sphincter; and (b) the submucous plexus, which is located in the submucosa and is especially prominent in the small and large intestines. The processes from these ganglia form dense networks and innervate the muscularis propria, muscularis mucosae, epithelium, and other structures. There are also nonganglionated plexuses that supply all of the layers of the tubular GI tract accompanying the arteries that supply the gut wall.

The ENS has many different types of neurons (Table 70.2). Moreover, these neurons may differ in function in different regions of the digestive tract. Excitatory motor neurons innervate the longitudinal and circular smooth muscle and muscularis mucosae. In addition, they innervate enteric endocrine cells and Peyer patches. Secretomotor neurons in the small and large intestine and gallbladder regulate water and electrolyte secretion. In the stomach, they stimulate acid secretion. Interneurons are present in all regions of the gut, but their characteristics vary more than those of other neuron types. They are present as a chain within the myenteric plexus that runs from mouth to anus. Intrinsic reflex pathways that control gut movement, blood flow, and secretion are activated by sensory neurons that respond to mechanical and chemical stimuli and to distension. These neurons are now known as intrinsic primary afferent neurons. Intrinsic primary afferent neurons are multiaxonal and connect to other intrinsic primary afferent neurons, to motor neurons, and to interneurons. They differ from extrinsic sensory neurons because their responses can be modified by synapses at the cell body.

The ENS is connected to the central nervous system (CNS) by transmission along axons in both directions, from GI tract to brain and from brain to ENS. The connections are largely through the vagus nerve and pathways leaving the spinal cord. Most vagal fibers (more than 90%) are afferent fibers that interact with neurons in the

TABLE 70.1. GASTROINTESTINAL HORMONES

PEPTIDE	ACTION	SITE OF RELEASE	RELEASER
Endocrine			

Gastrin	Stimulates:
	  Gastric acid secretion
	  Growth of gastric oxyntic
	  gland mucosa
		Antrum (duodenum)	Peptides
			Amino acids
			Distention
			Vagal stimulation

CCK	Stimulates:
	  Gallbladder contraction
	  Pancreatic enzyme secretion
	  Pancreatic bicarbonate secretion
	  Growth of exocrine pancreas
	Inhibits gastric emptying
		Duodenum
		Jejunum
			Peptides
			Amino acids
			Fatty acids >8C
			  in length

Secretin	Stimulates:
	  Pancreatic bicarbonate secretion
	  Biliary bicarbonate secretion
	  Growth of exocrine pancreas
	  Pepsin secretion
	Inhibits:
	  Gastric acid secretion
	  Trophic effect of gastrin
		Duodenum	Acid

GIP	Stimulates insulin release Inhibits gastric acid secretion	Duodenum Jejunum	Glucose Amino acids Fatty acids
Peptide YY	Ileal brake	Ileum	Fatty acids Glucose
Motilin[a]	Stimulates gastric and duodenal motility	Duodenum Jejunum	Unknown

Pancreatic
  polypeptide[a]
	Inhibits:
	  Pancreatic bicarbonate secretion
	  Pancreatic enzyme secretion
		Pancreas	Protein

Enteroglucagon[a]	Unknown	Ileum	Glucose Fat
Neurocrine			
VIP	Relaxes sphincters Relaxes gut circular muscle Stimulates intestinal secretion Stimulates pancreatic secretion	Mucosa and smooth muscle of GI tract	
Bombesin or GRP	Stimulates gastrin release	Gastric mucosa	
Substance P	Mediates pain reflexes	Spinal afferent neurons	Afferent nerve input

Enkephalins,
  endomorphins,
  dynorphins
	Stimulates smooth muscle
	  contraction
	Inhibits intestinal secretion
		Mucosa and smooth
		  muscle of GI tract
			Unknown

Paracrine			

Somatostatin	Inhibits:
	  Gastrin release
	  Other peptide hormone release
	  Gastric acid secretion
		GI mucosa
		Pancreatic islets
			Acid
			Vagus inhibits
			  release

GLP-1, GLP-2	Increase proliferation, decrease apoptosis, decrease motility	GI endocrine cells	Nutrient ingestion
Insulinlike growth factor-I	Increase proliferation	Gut mucosal cells	Nutrient ingestion
Histamine[b]	Stimulates gastric acid secretion	Oxyntic gland mucosa ECL cell	Unknown
Epidermal growth factor	 Unknown proliferation, mucosal barrier	Decrease gastric acid, increase gland cells	Gut mucosal, salivary

Leptin-NPY	Regulates food intake at
	  hypothalamus, decreases NPY
	  release
		Adipose tissue, chief
		  cells
			CCK, gastric volume,
			  glucose, cytokines

Ghrelin	Increases food intake, GH release	Gastric endocrine cells	Fasting

CCK, cholecystokinin; GH, gorwth hormone; GI, gastrointestinal; GIP; glucose-dependent insulinotropic peptide; GLP, glucagonlike peptide; GRP, gastrin-releasing peptide; NPY, neuropeptide Y; VIP, vasoactive intestinal polypeptide.
[a]Unknown physiologic function.
[b]Histamine is an amine, not a peptide.

From Furness JB, Clerc N, Vogalis F et al. The enteric nervous system and its extrinsic connections. In: Yamada T, Alpers DH, Kaplowitz N et al., eds. Textbook of Gastroenterology. 4th ed. Philadelphia: Lippincott Williams & Wilkins, 2003:12–34; and from Hasler WL. Motility of the small intestine and colon. In: Yamada T, Alpers DH, Kaplowitz N et al., eds. Textbook of Gastroenterology. 4th ed. Philadelphia: Lippincott Williams & Wilkins, 2003:220–47.

TABLE 70.2. TYPES OF NEURONS IN THE ENTERIC NERVOUS SYSTEM

LOCATION	FUNCTION	CHEMICAL TRANSMITTER
Circular muscle	Excitatory motor neurons	Ach, tachykinins
	Inhibitor motor neurons	NO, ATP, VIP, PACAP
Longitudinal muscle	Excitatory motor neurons	Ach, tachykinins
	Inhibitory motor neurons	NOS, VIP, GABA
Muscle layers	Primary sensory neurons	ChAT, calbindin, tachykinins
	Interneurons (sensorimotor reflex, MMC)	ChAT, 5-HT, somatostatin
	Secretomotor (gut endocrine cells, gastric glands)	Not known
Submucosa	Secretomotor/vasodilator	Ach (type 1), VIP/GAL (type 2)
	Secretomotor (not vasodilator)	Ach
	Intrinsic primary afferent neurons	Tachykinins (presumed)

Ach, acetylcholine; ChAT, choline acetyltransferase; GABA, γ-aminobutyric acid; GAL, galanin; 5-HT, 5-hydroxytryptamine; MMC, migrating myoelectric complex; NO, nitric oxide; NOS, nitric oxide synthase; PACAP, pituitary adenylate cyclase-activating peptide; VIP, vasoactive intestinal polypeptide.

Adapted from Furness JB, Clerc N, Vogalis F et al. The enteric nervous system and its extrinsic connections. In: Yamada T, Alpers DH, Kaplowitz N et al., eds. Textbook of Gastroenterology. 4th ed. Philadelphia: Lippincott Williams & Wilkins, 2003:17.

nucleus tractus solitarius in the midbrain. Because there are relatively few efferent vagal fibers compared with the large number of ENS neurons, the vagus functions more to initiate activity of the integrated circuits in the ENS rather than to coordinate gut function by direct signaling. Efferent centers in the spinal cord can receive efferent signals from the CNS, which are relayed to the ENS. In addition, the spinal centers can process afferent signals from the gut.

The vagal and spinal components comprise the extrinsic branches of the autonomic nervous system, including

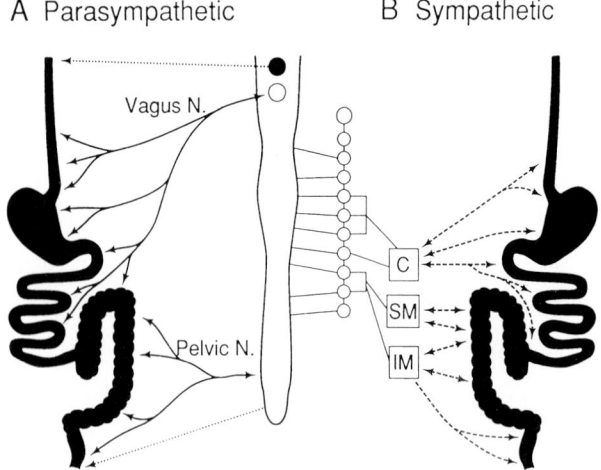

Figure 70.8. The extrinsic branches of the autonomic nervous system. **A.** Parasympathetic. *Dashed lines* indicate cholinergic innervation of the striated muscle in the esophagus and external anal sphincter. *Solid lines* indicate afferent and preganglionic innervation of the remaining gastrointestinal tract. **B.** Sympathetic. *Solid lines* denote the afferent and preganglionic efferent pathways between the spinal cord and the prevertebral ganglia. C, celiac; IM, inferior mesenteric; SM, superior mesenteric. *Dotted lines* indicate the afferent and postganglionic efferent innervation. (From Johnson LR, Alpers DH, Jacobson ED et al., eds. Physiology of the Gastrointestinal Tract, vol 1. 3rd ed. New York: Raven Press, 1994:451, with permission.)

the parasympathetic and sympathetic systems (Fig. 70.8). The striated muscles in the upper esophagus and external anal sphincter are directly innervated by cholinergic fibers, whereas the remaining gut is innervated by a variety of neural mediators, including acetylcholine, gut peptides, and nitric oxide (NO). These preganglionic fibers form synapses with the enteric plexuses, which in turn are connected with smooth muscle, secretory, and endocrine cells. The sympathetic nervous system contains preganglionic connections between prevertebral ganglia and the spinal cord, but the gut itself is innervated by postganglionic connections, mediated largely by epinephrine and norepinephrine. These postganglionic fibers innervate the plexuses of the ENS, as do the parasympathetic fibers, but the sympathetic fibers also directly innervate blood vessels, smooth muscle layers, and mucosal cells.

The sympathetic nervous system affects intestinal secretion, blood flow, and motility. The sensory fibers that accompany the sympathetic nerves (intestinofugal neurons) are primary sensory neurons that are not part of the autonomic nervous system, and are not really "sympathetic" sensory nerves. Sympathetic efferent neurons inhibit motility by decreasing contractile activity and by constricting sphincters. These various effects can be relayed along the gut to other regions before returning to the region of the initial stimulus by means of prevertebral ganglia connections. Examples of these inhibitory reflexes include slowing of gastric emptying by acidity or hypertonicity in the upper small intestine.

Intestinal smooth muscle is of the unitary type and is characterized by spontaneous activity, including active tension to stretching, and by activity that is not initiated by nerves but modulated by them. The circular muscle is innervated by both excitatory and inhibitory motor neurons and forms a thick syncytium surrounding the submucosa. Contraction shortens the radius but increases the length of each fiber, and in turn, of the syncytium. In contrast, the longitudinal muscle layer surrounding the circular muscle is thin, is shortened by contraction (with enlarged radius), and is only innervated by excitatory neurons. Electrical slow waves derive from the muscle itself and trigger action potentials, which lead to contractile activity. Action potentials in intestinal smooth muscle are propagated through gap junctions from cell to cell, creating an electrical syncytium.

GASTROINTESTINAL HORMONES

The mucosa of the GI tract contains an abundance of regulatory substances that are critical for the precise coordination of activities necessary to handle a meal. These substances are mostly peptides that communicate by endocrine, neurocrine, and paracrine pathways (Fig. 70.9; Table 70.1), not all of them mutually exclusive. Endocrine peptides are hormones released from sensory cells in the intestine in response to a mechanical or chemical stimuli and enter the bloodstream to act on a distant target organ. Gut neurocrine peptides are produced within the ENS and are located in nerves within the gut itself. Most of these peptides are also produced by the brain and represent a gut-brain axis. Paracrine peptides (and histamine) are produced by intestinal cells and act on adjacent or nearby cells. This can occur either by direct cellular extension to other cells, or by release of the peptide (or histamine) into the mucosa (e.g., somatostatin, histamine) or into the intestinal lumen (e.g., monitor peptide, cholecystokinin [CCK]-releasing peptide, trefoil peptides).

Some of the hormones listed in Table 70.1 may be especially important in the response to a meal (e.g., gastrin, CCK, secretin, motilin, glucose-dependent insulinotropic peptide [GIP], somatostatin, peptide NPY, leptin, ghrelin)

and all three major macronutrients (protein, carbohydrate, fat) are responsible for the release of these substances. Others hormones are also released in response to a meal, but do not act at the level of intestinal mucosal cells or the hypothalamic satiety centers (e.g., insulin, glucagon) and will not be considered further here. Because the coordination of function in the upper intestinal tract is so crucial, involving the stomach, duodenum, pancreas, and gallbladder, it is not surprising that these sites are most important in the release of GI hormones.

The specificity and coordination of action of GI hormones is dependent on three major factors: the multiple functions of each hormone, the paracrine actions between neuroendocrine and mucosal cells, and the regulatory functions of the ENS. Most GI hormones have multiple actions and mediate both stimulatory and inhibitory functions (e.g., gastrin, CCK, secretin, GIP, vasoactive intestinal polypeptide [VIP], enkephalins) (Table 70.1). Other GI hormones or amines are solely stimulatory (e.g., histamine, motilin, gastrin-releasing peptide [GRP], monitor peptide, CCK-releasing peptide), or inhibitory (e.g., somatostatin, pancreatic polypeptide). Thus, release of these hormones has the potential to create multiple effects on GI organs, coordinated in time. The presence of multiple cells in the mucosa, each possessing receptors to many of the GI hormones, also helps to create specificity of response. For example, in isolated cell systems, CCK stimulates acid production. However, CCK injected into the intact animal does not stimulate acid production because of the greater effect of CCK on the D cell producing somatostatin, an inhibitor of acid secretion, than on the parietal cell that produces acid. Gastrin, conversely, has the reverse effects on those two mucosal cells. In this

Figure 70.9. Three mechanisms of communication mediate responses in the gastrointestinal (GI) tract. The three mechanisms of communication that mediate responses are endocrine, neurocrine, and paracrine. For the endocrine mechanism, sensory cells respond to stimuli by releasing transmitters that travel by way of the blood to their target cells or tissues. There are many examples of endocrine sensory cells through the gastrointestinal tract that respond to either mechanical or chemical stimuli to release their hormones. Some types of endocrine cells respond to changes in pH or osmolality, whereas others respond to changes in specific nutrients. For the neurocrine mechanisms, the sensing and transmissions to the target tissue are completely mediated by nerves and neurotransmitters. Nerves sense stimuli such as nutrients, pH, and osmolality in the luminal contents, as well as movement of the contents and distention of the gut lumen. (From Raybould H, Pandol SJ. Integrated Response to a Meal. Undergraduate Teaching Project, Unit 29. Bethesda, MD: American Gastroenterological Association, 1995, with permission.)

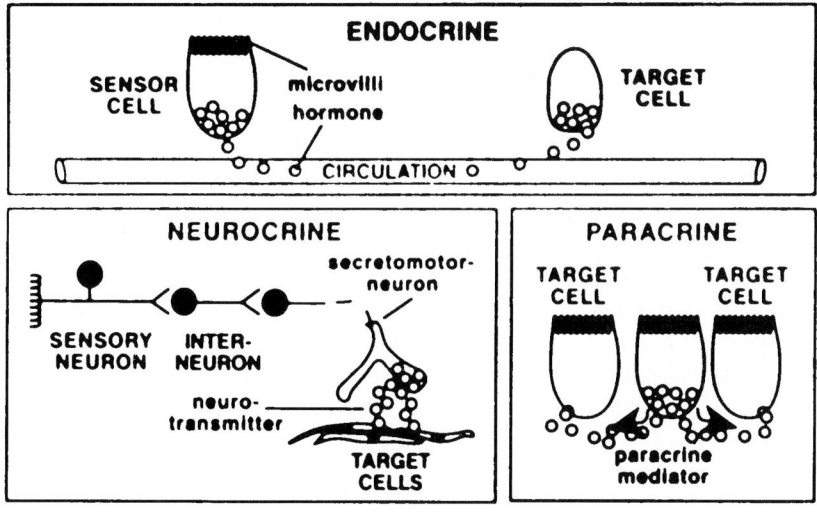

way, the multiplicity of mucosal-specific cells adds a layer of complexity and control to the presence of multiple hormones present in the mucosa. Finally, the ENS, with its many neuronal connections to mucosal cells, integrates the stimuli controlling GI hormone release. Both preganglionic parasympathetic cholinergic nerves and postganglionic fibers, mediated by neurocrine peptides, are important regulators of the GI response to feeding. In addition, chemosensory neurons detect intraluminal events and regulate mucosal function by intrinsic mucosal reflexes.

Some peptide hormones are important mitogens for the cells of the intestinal tract. Gastrin stimulates the growth of gastric oxyntic gland mucosa. Glucagonlike peptides 1 and 2 are produced in gut endocrine cells. These peptides are released by nutrient ingestion, and regulate cell proliferation and differentiation in the intestine in addition to their role in energy disposal. Insulinlike growth factor-I is also produced by gut mucosal cells, and is a potent trophic factor for intestinal mucosa. Glucagonlike peptide-1 (GLP-1) and GLP-2 also have antiapoptotic activity, thereby enhancing their effect on mucosal growth.

INTEGRATED RESPONSE TO A MEAL

The integrated response of the GI tract to a meal represents a coordinated series of events that includes the regulation of food intake, stimuli-evoked responses in anticipation of the meal, ingestion and transfer of the meal to the stomach, digestion and absorption of the meal, and the elimination of waste products of the meal, bringing into play all of the individual regulatory controls reviewed earlier.

Regulation of Food Intake

The GI tract is involved in the earliest part of feeding, beginning with the control of nutrient ingestion. Peptide hormones and other neurotransmitters in the gut have been implicated in the short-term regulation of energy intake. Olfactory and visual signals, along with mood and degree of physical activity, can regulate intake via hypothalamic and brain stem centers. Taste buds in the tongue can affect energy intake during a meal. Gut hormones that have been suggested as regulators of food intake include insulin, glucagon, CCK, and GRP. Neurotransmitters possibly involved include serotonin, dopamine, epinephrine, opiates, and γ-butyric acid. There is considerable evidence to support the role of CCK and GRP as satiety factors, both of them neurally released. Insulin probably acts as a stimulant of the hunger drive. Recently, two other hormonal systems that affect the hypothalamus have been related to production of satiety, the leptin-NPY system, and ghrelin. The abundance of potential satiety agents makes it appear likely that the gut signals, important in the short-term control of energy intake, are multiple and perhaps additive.

The molecular basis for the signal from fat stores that influence food intake was discovered to be leptin, a hormone arising from adipose tissue. The phenotype of leptin deficiency in *ob/ob* mice and in human congenital leptin deficiency is very similar, including early-onset obesity, increased food intake, hypometabolism, hyperinsulinemia, and defective function of the hypothalamo-pituitary-thyroidal axis. Replacement of leptin in deficient humans has dramatic effects on intake of food, but none on the basal metabolic rate, even in the face of weight loss. There are also important interactions between leptin and several hypothalamic systems, especially NPY, a stimulant of food intake that acts on the ventromedial and paraventricular hypothalamic nuclei. Deletion of the NPY gene partially reverses the phenotype in *ob/ob* mice, confirming the balance between the actions of leptin and NPY. Although no monogenic disorders of NPY overexpression have been reported in humans, leptin receptor deficiency also presents with severe hyperphagia and weight gain. In addition, mild growth retardation and altered insulinlike growth factor-I secretion in these children suggests that the leptin receptor may interact with other hormonal systems.

The melanocortin-4 receptor is also involved in the response to leptin. Mutations in the agouti mouse model generate an endogenous peptide antagonist to the melanocortin-4 receptor, and mutations in the receptor itself represent the most commonly observed monogenic disorder presenting with extreme obesity. The ligands for the melanocortin-4 receptor include peptides derived from the prohormone proopiomelanocortin by the action of prohormone convertase 1. The major peptide that results is α-melanocyte-stimulating hormone. Prohormone proopiomelanocortin and α-melanocyte-stimulating hormone are clearly linked to the leptin-NPY system in animals, and mutation of prohormone proopiomelanocortin and especially of the converting enzyme prohormone convertase 1 are associated with cases of inherited obesity in humans. Other hypothalamic hormones that may play a role in the complex regulation of food intake include glucagonlike peptide I, 5-hydroxytryptamine, catecholamines, and orexins.

Hypothalamic regulation of food intake seems to exert its control over the long term, as it is modified in response to signals from energy stores. Signals from the gut work over a shorter time and modify intake of specific meals. CCK from the duodenum appears to signal the hypothalamus via vagal afferent fibers, and also induces the release of leptin from gastric chief cells. Another peptide that is released from the stomach is ghrelin, so named because of its action on the hypothalamus as a growth hormone–releasing peptide. Plasma ghrelin is increased by fasting and decreased by feeding, and levels are low in patients with obesity. Levels increase after caloric restriction, but not so much after gastric-bypass surgery, suggesting that ghrelin may be in part responsible for the inability to decrease caloric restriction long term, but may help to explain the reduced appetite seen in some patients after gastric-bypass surgery.

Two nonhormonal gut peptides, enterostatin (the amino-terminal peptide of colipase) and apolipoprotein A-IV, have also been implicated as physiologically relevant satiety factors. The regulation of food intake clearly involves many systems, and more are likely to be discovered in the future.

Stimuli-Evoked Responses

The anticipatory responses to a meal are mediated by the CNS. Visual, olfactory, and auditory senses as well as the presence of food in the mouth can activate secretory responses from the salivary glands, stomach, and pancreas, and can initiate relaxation in the stomach, contraction of the gallbladder, and relaxation of the sphincter of Oddi. These actions prepare the GI tract to initiate digestion when the meal arrives. This preparation is important because digestive products of foodstuffs (e.g., amino acids, free fatty acids) are important stimuli in creating the maximum responses necessary to digest and absorb a meal. Thus, these nutrient products must be produced early in the meal. This cephalic phase of the meal is mediated through various brain centers, but the efferent signals all reach the gut through the vagus nerve. Once the meal enters the GI tract, the ENS becomes activated and works in concert with the CNS. For example, distention of the esophagus and/or stomach causes a contractile response mediated entirely by the ENS.

The most documented anticipatory CNS-mediated response is the cephalic phase of gastric secretion. Sensory input from the eye, nose, ear, and mouth send afferent signals to the dorsal vagal complex in the midbrain, where they are integrated and transmitted to GI organs by vagal efferent nerves. In the stomach, the response is to produce acid and pepsin. Acetylcholine release from the vagus stimulates pepsinogen release into the lumen of the stomach. In the distal stomach, the vagal efferent nerves activate the ENS to produce GRP to release gastrin, stimulating acid and pepsinogen production. Thus, when food enters the stomach, some of the protein is rapidly converted to oligopeptides by the action of pepsin, produced from pepsinogen and activated in the presence of low pH. These oligopeptides stimulate the release of more gastrin to perpetuate the digestive process. In this process, as well as in other anticipatory responses, appetizing meals stimulate more response than bland or unappetizing meals. Thus, the higher centers of the CNS are important in regulating the initial response of the GI tract.

Although these anticipatory responses are clearly present at each meal, it is not certain to what degree they are essential for the assimilation of nutrients. For example, the stomach can be removed and digestion and absorption can proceed fairly completely. Anticipatory responses to a meal may be more important in determining the amount of food eaten at a meal than the absorption of nutrients. The loss of anticipatory relaxation of the proximal stomach

allows only small volumes to be consumed at one time, and maintenance of sufficient food intake to maintain weight becomes difficult. Although this deficit can be overcome by cognitive training, the response to a meal is impaired. Impairment in the senses of sight, taste, and/or smell affects the cognitive drive that creates the desire to eat.

Mouth

Chewing and salivary secretion form the food into a round and smooth portion that can be swallowed. The mouth serves as the receptacle for these two functions: secretion and motility. Secretion into the oral cavity originates from the salivary glands and consists of fluid, electrolytes, and proteins. The structure and function of salivary glands, composed of acini that secrete their products through ducts, are analogous to the pancreas. Chloride (Cl) enters the lumen of the salivary gland through Cl channels, and Na enters paracellularly to maintain electroneutrality. In the ducts, the fluid is modified as Na and Cl leave the lumen; some Na is exchanged for K and some Cl is exchanged for bicarbonate (HCO_3^-), producing a final salivary secretion rich in HCO_3^-. Stimulation of the parasympathetic nerves is the major factor in regulating salivary secretion by direct acinar and duct cell innervation and by altering the blood supply. However, vasoactive peptides are also released to regulate blood flow. Sympathetic nerve input also stimulates secretion, but to a much lesser extent.

Proteins present in salivary secretions are important during the initial stages of nutrient assimilation. The influence of salivary amylase on starch digestion in the mouth and esophagus is small because of the short residence time of food in the mouth. However, in the stomach the attachment of amylase to its substrate protects the enzyme from inactivation at the slightly acid environment (pH of 5 to 6) of the stomach when it is buffered by food. Thus, the enzyme achieves a significant initial hydrolysis of dietary starch while still in the stomach. In addition, a non–bile salt-dependent triglyceride lipase is produced by Ebner glands at the base of the tongue. Although the oral production is relatively small, the gastric mucosa produces more of this lipase. As is the case with salivary amylase, the digestion of triglycerides because of this lingual/gastric lipase occurs primarily in the gastric lumen. The best dietary substrates for this enzyme are triglycerides that contain medium-chain fatty acids. The salivary glands also secrete haptocorrin (also known as R protein), a carrier protein that protects vitamin B_{12} from acid-peptic digestion in the stomach. Most of the other salivary proteins function largely to enhance lubrication, provide antibacterial action, and enhance mucosal integrity.

The motility functions of the oral cavity are coordinated with the upper esophageal sphincter to propel the food bolus into the esophagus. This action requires the coordination of extrinsic muscles to modify the shape of the pharyngeal cavity and to close the airways, and of intrinsic muscles to propel the bolus caudally. These two groups work in succession so that food does not reflux into the nose or larynx. These muscular units work in reverse order during the act of vomiting, again with the purpose of preventing the luminal contents from entering the airways.

Esophagus

The esophagus carries the food bolus from the mouth to the proximal stomach. Relaxation of the upper esophageal sphincter occurs immediately after swallowing, along with increased pharyngeal pressure. These pressure changes move the bolus into the esophagus. The esophagus is the first gut organ in which the phenomenon of peristalsis is encountered. Peristalsis along the length of the esophagus (primary peristalsis) is enhanced by distention in the esophagus produced by the food bolus (secondary peristalsis). The coordinated caudal movement of contraction and relaxation waves moves the food bolus along the length of the esophagus. The act of swallowing initiates both pharyngeal and esophageal peristalsis and relaxation of the lower esophageal sphincter, allowing the swallowed bolus to enter the proximal stomach. Immediately after a swallow, the lower esophageal sphincter pressure also decreases to that of the stomach, and remains low until the swallow is completed. At the end of the swallow, the lower esophageal sphincter contracts, stripping the end of the esophagus of any remaining food contents. The most important neurotransmitters for the motility pattern in the esophagus are acetylcholine (contraction) and VIP/NO (relaxation). Although the esophagus is often depicted as an open tube, the walls of the esophagus are actually approximated to each other during fasting conditions and in areas not distended by a food bolus during feeding. Thus, the bolus cannot travel down the esophagus in the absence of peristalsis. Surprisingly, gravity is not a significant factor in the function of the esophagus.

Stomach

Although the oral cavity initiates some changes in the food bolus, it is not until residence in the stomach that the physical and chemical characteristics of the meal are altered. The food bolus enters the stomach as large particles after chewing action in the mouth. In the stomach, the food is mixed and ground with secreted fluid and enzymes and converted to a suspension of particles small enough to pass the pylorus into the duodenum. In addition, fats are converted into an emulsion by mixing action, and small amounts of fatty acids and monoglycerides are formed. Protein and starch digestion also proceeds to create monomeric and oligomeric nutrients that can act further in the duodenum to potentiate the intestinal response to a meal. The two major components responsible for these overall actions of the stomach are motility and acid/peptic secretion.

The anticipatory cephalic phase and distention of the stomach by a meal both lead to receptive relaxation of the proximal stomach, thus accommodating the meal without increasing gastric pressure. Vagal afferent fibers in the gastric wall respond to changes in tension in the muscular coat of the stomach. These responses are processed in the dorsal vagal nucleus in the medulla, and create vagal efferent responses that not only relax the proximal stomach, but also increase gastrin, acid, and pepsinogen secretion; initiate antral and gallbladder contraction; relax the sphincter of Oddi; and stimulate pancreatic secretion. These vagovagal reflexes are important in the coordinated function of the organs of the upper GI tract (stomach, duodenum, gallbladder, and pancreas), and are part of the reason that these organs are considered as a cluster unit. The likely neural mediators of these reflexes are VIP and NO. Although the functions of the four upper GI organs are being considered separately, it is important to realize that these functions do not proceed in isolation, but are part of a carefully programmed response involving the entire cluster unit.

Antral (distal stomach) contractions are initiated by distention of the stomach. The propulsion, grinding, and retropulsion action in the distal stomach serves to grind the meal into small pieces and to mix it with gastric secretions rich in acid and pepsin. The food bolus is ground until the particle size becomes less than 2 mm so it can pass through the pylorus during the propulsive component. Peristalsis in the stomach is slow at a frequency of approximately three cycles per minute, mediated in large part by vagal and intrinsic gastric wall cholinergic neurons.

Gastric emptying is a closely regulated phenomenon and is modulated by factors other than particle size. The fastest rate of gastric emptying occurs with isotonic solutions. Most solid meals produce hypertonic solutions, and most liquids are either hypotonic or hypertonic. Thus, most meals will not be emptied at the fastest possible rate. The rate of gastric emptying after a meal is normally approximately 2 mL/min. At this rate, the digestive and absorptive functions of the upper small intestine are not overwhelmed. Other inhibitory mechanisms affecting the rate of gastric emptying involve H+ ion concentration and caloric load delivered to the duodenum.

Another major function of the stomach is to produce secretions rich in hydrogen and pepsinogen. The parietal and chief cells are most responsible for the products entering the gastric lumen after a meal (Table 70.3). Postprandially, the volume of gastric secretion increases and the ion concentration changes, almost entirely the result of parietal cell secretion. Non–parietal cell secretion from mucous and chief cells contributes HCO_3^--rich fluid in the fasting state. After a meal, hydrogen is exchanged for Na^+, and Cl^- replaces HCO_3^- secretion. Most of these secretory changes occur during the gastric phase of acid secretion, which occurs maximally about 60 to 90 minutes after ingestion of food.

TABLE 70.3. GASTRIC CELL SECRETORY PRODUCTS AND FUNCTION

CELL TYPE	PRODUCT	FUNCTION
Surface cells	Mucus	Lubrication
Neck cells	Bicarbonate	Protection
	Trefoil peptides	
Parietal cells	H^+	Protein digestion
	Intrinsic factor	Binding of cobalamin (vitamin B_{12})
Chief cells	Pepsinogen	Protein digestion
	Gastric lipase	Triglyceride digestion
Endocrine cells	Gastrin	Regulation of acid secretion
	Histamine	
	Somatostatin	

The mechanism of enhanced parietal cell secretion involves four different cell types: parietal cells, enterochromaffinlike (ECL) cells, somatostatin (D) cells, and gastrin (G) cells. These cells are distributed in two different anatomic portions of the stomach; the parietal, ECL, and fundic D cells in the fundus, and the antral D cell and G cells in the antrum. It is mainly the interaction of gastrin, somatostatin, and other transmitters that affects the production of histamine from the ECL cells that, in turn, determines the rate of gastric acid secretion. Gastrin is released from the G cells in response to a meal by multiple mechanisms; acetylcholine and GRP acting through vagal and intrinsic nerves release gastrin during the cephalic and gastric phases of secretion, and luminal amino acids released by pepsin also stimulate gastrin release during the gastric phase. Gastrin acts in an endocrine fashion by binding to CCK-B receptors on the ECL cell, causing histamine release by exocytosis. Somewhat later, synthesis of histidine decarboxylase is activated, causing additional histamine production. Finally, gastrin stimulates ECL cell growth. As a result of these three effects, ECL cell histamine production is increased and drives parietal cell activation and secretion. Gastrin accounts for about 70% of the stimulated histamine release, the remainder being driven by acetylcholine via muscarinic receptors, by epinephrine via adrenergic receptors, and by gastrin directly via CCK-B receptors. These multiple neural transmitters and peptides are involved in the regulation of acid secretion, working as endocrine and paracrine hormones.

Gastric acid secretion is further regulated by feedback inhibition, mediated largely by somatostatin released from specialized endocrine (D) cells in the antrum and fundus. The fundic D cells are probably more important than antral D cells in regulating histamine production from ECL cells. Different conditions mediate the release of somatostatin from D cells in these two locations. Calcitonin gene-related peptide, secretin, and VIP all seem to stimulate release of somatostatin from fundic D cells. The second arm of the feedback loop occurs in antral D cells. When the pH in the antral lumen falls below 3.0, somatostatin is released from antral D cells, inhibiting gastrin release from G cells by paracrine mechanisms. Moreover, luminal acid directly decreases gastrin release from G cells. This example of the regulation of gastric acid secretion after a meal is provided as one of the best-known examples of the intricate and complex coordination of GI function, using elements of the CNS, ENS, and GI hormones.

Gastric parietal cells also produce intrinsic factor, a carrier protein necessary for ileal absorption of vitamin B_{12}. Vitamin B_{12} fits into a hydrophobic pit of the intrinsic factor protein, forming the intrinsic factor-vitamin B_{12} complex that is the obligatory ligand for receptor-mediated absorption in the terminal ileum.

Duodenum

The duodenum is at the center of another elaborately coordinated regulatory process, integrating the functions of gastric emptying, bile formation, gallbladder and duodenal motility, and pancreatic and biliary secretion. For this reason, the concept of the duodenal cluster unit has been developed. This concept is also embryologically cogent. Each of the organs of the duodenal cluster unit (stomach, duodenum, liver, common bile duct, gallbladder, and pancreas) are derived from closely related structures at an early stage of fetal development. The liver, gallbladder, common bile duct, and ventral pancreas bud off together from the antimesenteric side of the duodenum, whereas the dorsal pancreatic bud develops from the mesenteric surface. The ventral pancreas then rotates to join the dorsal pancreas. It is not surprising, therefore, that sensors in the duodenum can regulate function in the other organs of the cluster unit.

The duodenum acts as both a simple mixing chamber and a regulatory center by containing cells and nerve endings that sense nutrient content, pH, and osmolarity. The major hormones involved in regulating the duodenal cluster unit are CCK and secretin, although their effects are not exclusive. Moreover, the GI hormones that act in the duodenal cluster unit may act via an endocrine mechanism (through the blood stream) or via paracrine mechanisms (locally within the intestinal mucosa). An acid pH leads to release of secretin and activation of extrinsic and intrinsic nerves to increase pancreatic and biliary secretion of water and HCO_3^- e. The presence of digestive products of nutrients (amino acids, fatty acids, monosaccharides) leads to release of CCK and activation of extrinsic and intrinsic nerves, which inhibit gastric emptying and acid secretion, stimulate gallbladder contraction, stimulate pancreatic enzyme secretion, and initiate the small bowel motility pattern of the fed state.

Gastric acid secretion can be inhibited by the neural or hormonal systems originating in the duodenum (Table 70.4). This process is distinguished from inhibition by antral somatostatin in that the regulation of gastric acid secretion by duodenal acid, hyperosmolarity, and fatty

TABLE 70.4. REGULATION OF GASTRIC ACID SECRETION

REGION	STIMULUS	MEDIATION	INHIBITS GASTRIN Release	DIRECTLY INHIBITS ACID Secretion
Oxyntic gland area Antrum	Acid (pH <3.0) Yes	Somatostatin	Yes	Yes Secretin Yes
Duodenum	Acid Hyperosmotic solutions	Nervous reflex Unidentified Enterogasterone	No No	Yes Yes
Duodenum and jejunum	Fatty acids (candidates include GLP-1, GLP-2, PGE$_2$)	GIP Unidentified Enterogasterone	Yes No	Yes Yes

GLP, glucagonlike peptide; PGE$_2$, prostaglandin E$_2$.

acids also leads to inhibition of gastric emptying. In this way the duodenal mucosa is doubly protected from an excessive influx of acid. GIP, formerly called gastric inhibitory polypeptide, released by the duodenum, inhibits gastric acid secretion and stimulates insulin release from pancreatic β cells.

The release of CCK from duodenal CCK cells after a meal is of crucial importance for meal digestion. CCK acts as a hormone to stimulate pancreatic secretion and to increase antral, pyloric, and duodenal contractions. Moreover, CCK acting as a neurocrine peptide stimulates vagal afferent fibers that form part of the vagal efferent outflow after a meal, with subsequent effects on proximal gastric relaxation, increased acid output, gut motility, and pancreatic secretion. In fact, most of the effects of CCK after a meal may be effected through its role as a neurocrine peptide. CCK is important in regulation of the biliary system and its components. The peptide stimulates gallbladder contraction and relaxes the sphincter of Oddi, allowing concentrated bile to enter the duodenum. This action is mediated by both the hormonal and the neurocrine functions of CCK. Fatty acids in the duodenal lumen release CCK, which in turn acts humorally on CCK-A receptors in the gallbladder. Moreover, in response to sensory afferent nerves activated by CCK, vagal efferent nerves mediated by acetylcholine contract the gallbladder, and vagal afferent nerves releasing VIP/NO relax the sphincter of Oddi.

There is a complex system regulating the release of CCK from endocrine I (CCK-secreting) cells in the duodenum. Luminal nutrients, especially protein and amino acids and free fatty acids, initiate the signal. Protein in particular is involved in stimulating the release of three peptides that in turn release CCK: monitor peptide produced in pancreatic acinar cells, diazepam-binding inhibitor from porcine intestine, and CCK-releasing peptide produced in rat duodenal mucosal cells. Pancreatic phospholipase A2 from pancreatic juice also may act as a secretin-releasing peptide. Release of both peptides is mediated by parasympathetic (vagal) efferent nerves. Between meals these peptides are degraded by luminal trypsin that is

highly concentrated. Thus, little CCK secretion occurs during fasting. However, as large quantities of protein enter the gut after a meal, the amount overwhelms luminal trypsin activity, and most of the putative regulatory peptides escape degradation. In this way the ingestion of protein regulates the release of CCK, which, in turn, stimulates the release of proteolytic enzymes from the pancreas, in conjunction with vagal efferent stimulation. Another important role of the duodenal cluster unit is to neutralize the gastric acid delivered to the proximal duodenum and maintain a constant intraluminal pH. There are multiple organs involved in this regulation, including the duodenal mucosa, biliary system, and pancreas. The meal itself provides buffers, mostly in the form of peptides and fatty acids. Most of the neutralization comes from HCO$_3^-$ secreted from the pancreas, biliary ducts, and duodenal mucosa. Secretin mediates the biliary and pancreatic response, whereas the ENS mediates the mucosal response. The major mucosal sensor is the endocrine secretin (S) cell, which is activated to release secretin when the luminal pH falls below 4.5. A low intraluminal pH stimulates duodenal HCO$_3^-$ secretion via both central and enteric nerves, by local prostaglandin production, and by hormones. Mechanisms invoked can be cyclic adenosine monophosphate mediated (dopamine agonists, enteropeptide [EP$_3$] receptor agonists, VIP), cyclic guanosine monophosphate mediated (guanylin, uroguanylin), calcium mediated (muscarinic M$_3$ agonists, CCK$_A$ agonists), or inhibition by neurotransmitters (α$_2$-adrenoceptor agonists, NPY receptor agonists, NO).

A final important role for the duodenum is to produce and maintain isotonicity of luminal contents, thereby avoiding large shifts of fluid across the semipermeable membrane of the gut. This function is one performed by the duodenal mucosa alone, without other organs in the cluster unit. Most meals are either hypertonic or hypotonic. Thus, the duodenum must either add or absorb fluid and electrolytes. Remarkably, this adjustment is made within the duodenum. Under normal circumstances, however, the maximum rate of gastric emptying is about 2 mL/min, so the proximal duodenum is not presented with larger volumes than it can accommodate for isotonic adjustment.

Thus, passage through the duodenum changes the physical properties of the meal because of the contributions of the organs in the duodenal cluster unit. Large amounts of pancreatic hydrolases and bile salts are added, digesting nearly all ingested macromolecules (except dietary fiber) to oligomers or monomers solubilized in a form compatible with absorption. Intestinal fluid leaving the duodenum is more isosmotic, and the pH is made more neutral.

Biliary System

Bile salts are crucial for solubilization and absorption of lipid soluble nutrients. Bile salts are synthesized and secreted by the liver, conjugated to either taurine or glycine to improve solubility, stored and concentrated in the gallbladder, and delivered to the duodenal lumen in response to a meal. Between meals the gallbladder stores and concentrates the bile salts that are extracted by the liver from the blood. There are two major factors that regulate the supply of bile salts after a meal. First, contraction of the gallbladder and relaxation of the sphincter of Oddi release the gallbladder contents into the upper duodenum. This provides the first and immediate load of bile salts to enhance digestion by pancreatic lipase and fatty acid/monoglyceride and cholesterol solubilization. Second, bile salts subsequently move down the small intestine to the ileum, where they are absorbed by a receptor-mediated mechanism and returned to the liver via the bloodstream. The enterohepatic circulation (reabsorption in the ileum, uptake by the liver, and secretion back into the intestine) preserves bile salts and diminishes the need for new synthesis in the 1 to 2 hours after a meal. The entire body pool of bile salts (~3 to 4 g) is recirculated two to four times after each meal, providing 6 to 16 g of bile salts to the upper duodenum during the first hours after a meal. With a total luminal volume from diet and secretions of 2 to 3 L after each meal, this provides a large margin of safety for maintaining a luminal concentration above the critical micellar concentration of 2 to 4 mM needed for lipid solubilization and activation of pancreatic lipase.

Pancreas

There are three phases of pancreatic secretion after a meal: cephalic, gastric, and intestinal (Table 70.5). These phases have been described in an attempt to classify the multitude of events that occur postprandially. As seen in the other organs described earlier, pancreatic secretion is mediated by neural (vagal) efferent responses and by gut hormones. In humans, the cephalic phase of secretion is largely if not exclusively mediated by the vagus nerve. In this phase and in the gastric phase, the pancreas secretes mostly water and HCO_3^-. Pancreatic polypeptide, located in specific pancreatic polypeptide cells in the pancreatic islets, acts as a negative feedback mechanism for the vagally stimulated portion of pancreatic secretion. Pancreatic polypeptide is released in response to vagal efferent stimulation and inhibits the vagal efferent effect on the pancreas.

In the intestinal phase, pancreatic enzymes are added to the large volume of fluid secreted. As noted earlier, products of proteolysis and lipolysis stimulate the CCK (endocrine I) cells to release CCK, which acts humorally on the pancreatic acinar cells to produce enzymes. At the same time, H^+ ions stimulate the S cell to release secretin, which acts humorally on the pancreatic duct cells to secrete a HCO_3^--rich fluid necessary to neutralize gastric acid and allow pancreatic enzymes to be effective. In addition, enteropancreatic reflexes within the ENS, sensitive to distention, osmolarity, and various nutrients, stimulate pancreatic enzyme secretion mediated by acetylcholine, GRP, and VIP. Most of the hydrolases secreted by the pancreas are proteases and are secreted in an inactive precursor form to prevent digestion within the pancreas (Table 70.6). Trypsinogen accounts for 40% of the pancreatic protein secreted. In the intestinal lumen, trypsinogen is activated to trypsin by the enzyme enterokinase, produced by duodenal enterocytes. Trypsin, in turn, converts trypsinogen and all of the other proenzymes to their active form, and the intraluminal phase of intestinal digestion is initiated.

Pancreatic insulin secretion in response to a meal is enhanced by the release of GIP from the GIP cell, a mucosal endocrine cell. Although GIP was first recognized for its ability to inhibit gastric acid secretion, it was

TABLE 70.5. PHASES OF PANCREATIC SECRETION AFTER A MEAL

PHASES	PANCREATIC RESPONSE (%)	STIMULANTS	MEDIATORS
Cephalic	25	Sight, smell, taste, eating	Vagal innervation
Gastric	10	Distention	Vagal-cholinergic pathways
Intestinal	50–75	Amino acids	Cholecystokinin, secretin
		Fatty acids	Enteropancreatic reflexes
		Calcium and hydrogen ions	Other hormones (?)
		Distention	

From Johnson LR, Alpers DH, Jacobson ED et al., eds. Physiology of the Gastrointestinal Tract, vol 1. 3rd ed. New York: Raven Press, 1994.

TABLE 70.6. INTESTINAL BRUSH-BORDER MEMBRANE HYDROLASE ACTIVITY IN NORMAL HUMAN BIOPSY SPECIMENS

HYDROLASE	APPROXIMATE ACTIVITY (UNITS/g PROTEIN)
Glucoamylase	250
Sucrase	100
α-Dextrinase	100
Lactase	45

later found that the major function of this peptide is to mediate meal-stimulated insulin release from the pancreas. This observation led to changing the name of GIP from gastric inhibitory polypeptide to glucose insulinotropic polypeptide. Intraluminal glucose stimulates GIP release, which acts humorally to augment the glucose-mediated release of insulin from β cells in pancreatic islets. This action of GIP helps to maintain blood glucose levels within a reasonable range after a meal and provides another example of the redundancy that is characteristic of the regulation of GI function after a meal.

NUTRIENT ABSORPTION

Fluid and Electrolytes

The GI tract absorbs large volumes of fluid each day. Approximately 9 L of water are delivered to the upper small intestine daily from dietary intake (2000 mL), saliva (1500 mL), gastric secretions (2500 mL), bile (500 mL), pancreatic secretions (1500 mL), and small intestinal secretions (1000 mL). Ninety-eight percent of the daily fluid load is absorbed, whereas only 100 to 200 mL/day is excreted in stool; approximately 85% (7.5 L) of water is absorbed in the jejunum and ileum and 13% (1.4 L) in the colon.

Water is absorbed passively throughout the intestine and is regulated primarily by active electrolyte absorption. Specific features of epithelial cells throughout the intestine are important in regulating fluid and electrolyte absorption. First, the apical (luminal) membrane contains specific electrolyte transporters and channels. Second, the basolateral (serosal) membrane contains an NA pump that provides the drive for electrolyte absorption. Third, intestinal epithelial cells are linked to each other by tight junctions that are located close to the apical surface. The permeability of the intestinal epithelium depends on the number of tight junctions. The permeability of these intercellular junctions to solute, ion, and water movement decreases distally through the intestine. Therefore the jejunum is more permeable or "leaky" than the ileum, which is more leaky than the cecum, which is more leaky than the rest of the colon.

Fluid and electrolytes are absorbed from the intestinal lumen directly through (transcellular pathway) or between (paracellular pathway) epithelial cells. Passive transport

does not require energy and can occur transcellularly or paracellularly. The lipid content of the epithelial cell membrane prevents passive diffusion of charged electrolytes. Specialized proteins present in the apical membrane form channels or pores, which permit electrolyte transport. Passive transport through membrane channels is regulated by concentration and electrochemical gradients across the membrane. Ion channels are usually specific for certain ions and can be opened or closed by cellular messages. In the open state, more than 1 million ions can pass through per second, but no ions pass when the channel is closed. Passive transport can also occur via carriers, which are proteins located in the cell membrane. Carriers are specific for certain solutes or ions and facilitate their passive movement along a concentration or electrochemical gradient across the cell membrane. Carrier-mediated transport is much slower than movement through channels.

Active transport requires energy and permits the movement of a solute or ion against a concentration or electrochemical gradient. Active transport only occurs transcellularly and is mediated by a "pump" that moves ions in and out of the cell. The most important epithelial cell pump is the Na pump (also known as Na/K-ATPase) and moves three Na ions across the basolateral membrane in exchange for two K ions (Fig. 70.10). Therefore, the Na pump makes the intracellular Na concentration low and the intracellular potential difference negative compared with the extracellular environment.

Secondary active transport represents transport that combines both passive and active processes. For example, the negative intracellular voltage of epithelial cells enhances cation entry and anion exit from the cell. Thus, ions may move passively against their concentration gradients because of the electrical potential difference across the cell generated by the active Na pump. The use of oral rehydration therapy in patients with severe diarrhea, such as those with cholera or short bowel syndrome, takes advantage of secondary active transport and the Na-glucose cotransporter in small intestinal epithelium (see Fig. 70.10). This transporter, present in the apical membrane, binds both Na and glucose. Glucose is transported across the cell membrane into the cell against its concentration gradient because of the low Na concentration and the negative potential difference present in the cell. As glucose accumulates in the cell, it moves along its concentration gradient across the basolateral membrane via a specific transport carrier. Similar Na cotransport mechanisms also facilitate absorption of amino acids, vitamins, and bile salts. The Na pump also drives passive absorptive or secretory transport of hydrogen, Cl, K, and HCO_3^- (see Fig. 70.10). Transport regulation can occur at the channel, carrier, or pump levels.

Water is absorbed passively throughout the GI tract and follows the absorption of electrolytes and other osmotically active nutrients. As noted earlier, water moves

Apical   **Basolateral**

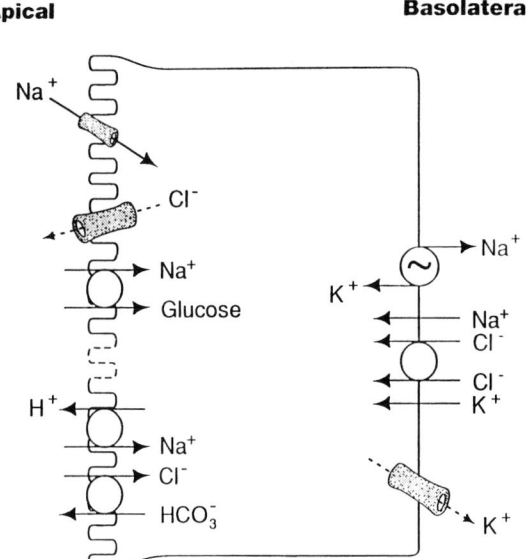

Figure 70.10. Electrolyte and solute absorption. Sodium can travel from the intestinal lumen into the epithelial cell by (1) an ion channel (apical side **top**), (2) the sodium (Na^+)-glucose cotransporter (apical side **middle**), or (3) an Na^+-hydrogen (H) exchanger (apical side **bottom**). The release of H creates a favorable gradient for bicarbonate (HCO_3) exit, which facilitates chloride (Cl) entry via the Cl/HCO_3 exchanger. The Na/potassium (K)/Cl cotransporter in the basolateral membrane also increases Cl uptake. Electrogenic Cl secretion occurs via a Cl channel on the apical membrane. Intracellular glucose accumulation favors glucose transport across the basolateral membrane via a specific carrier protein. The Na pump (Na/K-adenosine triphosphatase [ATPase]) provides the energy for these processes by generating low intracellular Na concentrations and a transmembrane electrochemical gradient. (From Sleisinger MH, Fordtran JS, Scharschmidt BF et al., eds. Gastrointestinal Disease. 5th ed. Philadelphia: WB Saunders, 1993:954–76, with permission.)

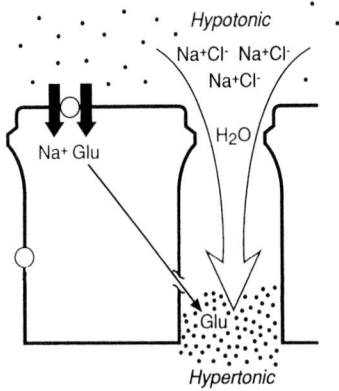

Figure 70.11. Electrolyte and water absorption in the jejunum. The sodium (Na)-glucose cotransporter present in the small intestinal binds both sodium and glucose and transports them across the epithelial cell membrane. As glucose accumulates in the cell, it moves along its concentration gradient across the basolateral membrane via a specific transport carrier. Water is absorbed passively by both transcellular and paracellular routes in response to an increase in osmolarity of the intracellular and subepithelial spaces. The Na-nutrient cotransporter shown in this figure and the electroneutral Na chloride (NaCl) exchange transporter are responsible for most water absorption. Water absorbed between epithelial cells can increase the absorption of solutes present in water by "solvent drag."

both transcellularly and paracellularly in response to an increase in osmolarity of the intracellular and subepithelial spaces. Na absorption is the most important factor in regulating water absorption. The Na-nutrient cotransporter and electroneutral NaCl exchange transporter are responsible for most water absorption. Furthermore, water absorbed between epithelial cells can increase the absorption of solutes present in water, a process known as solvent drag (Fig. 70.11). Movement of both Na and water in response to an osmotic gradient is much greater in the jejunum than in the ileum because of the increased leakiness of the junctions between epithelial cells in the jejunum compared with those in the ileum. In the jejunum, Na is primarily absorbed by uptake via the Na-nutrient cotransporter and solvent drag. Therefore, ingestion of fluids or a meal with a low Na content increases the osmolality in the upper small intestine and causes net secretion of water and Na into the lumen. Patients with a jejunostomy and less than 100 cm of jejunum have difficulty maintaining fluid and electrolyte balance; thus, longer lengths of small intestine are often required for optimal fluid and electrolyte absorption. Balance studies

performed after liquid ingestion in patients with a very short bowel ending in a jejunostomy show that drinking solutions with Na concentrations less than 90 mmol/L leads to net Na and water losses, whereas drinking a solution with at least 90 mmol/L causes net Na and fluid absorption. Although most water is absorbed in the small intestine, approximately 1 to 1.5 L enters the colon each day. Ninety-five percent of the fluid that enters the colon is absorbed. Moreover, the colon has the capacity to absorb up to approximately 5 L of fluid per day.

Lipid

Approximately 100 g of fat, equivalent to approximately 40% of total energy intake, is consumed daily in an adult Western diet. The majority (95%) of fat intake consists of long-chain triglycerides (LCTs), whereas the remainder includes cell membrane phospholipids, cholesterol, other sterols, and fat-soluble vitamins. In addition, a large quantity of endogenous lipids (~60 g) are delivered into the intestinal lumen daily from bile (containing ~30 g of bile salts, 10 to 15 g of phospholipids, and 1 to 2 g of cholesterol), desquamated intestinal cells (containing ~5 g of membrane lipids), and dead bacteria (containing ~10 g of membrane lipids). The upper limit of normal fecal fat output while consuming a 100-g-fat diet is approximately 7 g/day. Therefore, at least 95% of fat delivered to the intestine is usually absorbed. Most dietary fat is absorbed before the fat contained in a meal reaches the ileum. However, even when no dietary fat is ingested, a small amount of fat can still be detected in stool because of the contribution from endogenous sources.

Assimilation of dietary fat provides a good general index of intestinal absorptive function because it involves most of the components involved in digestive and absorptive processes. Triglycerides are particularly difficult to digest and absorb because they are insoluble in water. Therefore, absorption requires: (a) the breakdown of ingested fat into an emulsion, which enhances contact between lipolytic enzymes and triglycerides; (b) enzymatic hydrolysis of triglycerides; (c) water-soluble micelle formation, which permits transport across the unstirred water layer to intestinal epithelial cells; (d) uptake of fatty acids by epithelial cells; (e) repackaging of fatty acids into water-soluble chylomicrons within the epithelial cell; and (f) secretion of chylomicrons into the systemic circulation by lymphatic vessels.

The stomach is important in initiating fat digestion. Approximately 20% of ingested triglycerides are hydrolyzed in the stomach by gastric lipase, which is produced by chief cells, functions in an acid environment, and is resistant to denaturation by pepsin. In addition, gastric muscle contractions, gastric acidity, and pepsin mash food particles and release dietary lipids from their protein interactions, generating an emulsion of small particles that is delivered into the duodenum.

In the duodenum, the emulsion particles are further stabilized by the addition of bile salts and phospholipids secreted by the gallbladder. The presence of gastric acid in the duodenum stimulates secretin release from duodenal mucosa. Secretin enters the portal circulation and stimulates the pancreas to secrete HCO_3^-, which raises the intraluminal pH to greater than 6. The presence of fatty acids and amino acids in the duodenum stimulates CCK release from duodenal mucosa, which then enters the portal circulation and stimulates the pancreas to secrete lipase, colipase, and other digestive enzymes, and stimulates gallbladder contraction and bile flow into the duodenum. Lipase and colipase are secreted by the pancreas in a 1:1 molar ratio and act at the surface of the emulsion particles to hydrolyze triglycerides to monoglycerides and fatty acids. The near-neutral pH of the duodenum maximizes lipase and colipase activity; pancreatic lipase is not functional in an acidic environment. Colipase is a critical cofactor for lipolysis by acting as a link between pancreatic lipase and triglycerides. In fact, pancreatic lipase is unable to gain access to triglycerides within the emulsion without colipase because of interference from bile salts and phospholipids coating the emulsion particles. Although pancreatic lipase is responsible for the majority of intestinal triglyceride lipolysis, the pancreas also secretes bile salt-activated lipase, which hydrolyzes ester linkages in cholesterol, phospholipids, and fat-soluble vitamins. Fat digestion by gastric and pancreatic lipases is very effective, and most ingested triglycerides are hydrolyzed within the first 100 cm of jejunum.

Fatty acids, monoglycerides, and other lipids interact with bile salts to form water-soluble mixed micelles. Bile

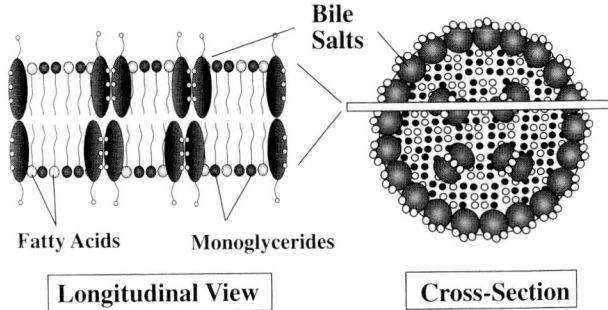

Figure 70.12. Structure of a mixed lipid–bile salt micelle. The products of lipolysis are solubilized in the interior of the particle. The bile sale molecules orient with their hydroxyl groups *(black circles)* facing the aqueous phase or when they are in the interior of the micelle, facing each other. Fatty acids and monoglycerides orient in the micelle with their polar head groups in contact with the aqueous phase and their hydrocarbon tails in the interior of the micelle. (From Chang EB, Sitrin MD, Black DD, eds. Gastrointestinal, Hepatobiliary, and Nutritional Physiology. Philadelphia: Lippincott-Raven, 1996:147, with permission.)

salts contain both water-soluble and lipid-soluble portions, allowing them to surround the digested lipid products; their hydrophobic side pointing toward the interior and the hydrophilic side toward the exterior. Thus, bile salts make fatty acids, monoglycerides, cholesterol, and other intraluminal lipids soluble in water by "hiding" these lipid products inside of mixed micelles (Fig. 70.12). Although bile salts secreted in bile are diluted by luminal fluid, the intraduodenal concentration (10 to 20 mmol/L) is still well above the critical micellar concentration (2 to 3 mmol/L). The products of triglyceride digestion by pancreatic lipase can also coalesce to form vesicles. Lipid within these vesicles is usually transferred to micelles but can also transport lipid directly to the mucosa. It is believed that the formation of vesicles permits absorption of more than half of ingested triglycerides when bile salts are absent, such as in patients with severe cholestasis. However, vitamins D, E, and K are particularly insoluble and require micelle formation for adequate absorption.

Mixed micelles must pass through a 40-µm-deep unstirred water layer located at the surface of intestinal epithelium to deliver their contents to the apical portion of the enterocytes. The quantitative diffusion of fatty acids through the unstirred water layer is enhanced more than 100-fold when fatty acids are carried within micelles rather than as monomeric fatty acids. Fatty acid and lipid uptake across the epithelial brush-border membrane occurs by passive diffusion, facilitated diffusion, and active transport. Members of the ATP-binding cassette transporter superfamily have been identified in the human small intestine that may transport fatty acids, monoglycerides, and cholesterol across the enterocyte apical membrane. Defects in the *ABCG5* and *ABCG8* genes are associated with the rare autosomal-recessive disorder, sitosterolemia.

After fatty acids and lipolytic products enter the intestinal epithelial cell, they are bound to cytosolic fatty acid binding proteins. These binding proteins are found predominantly in villus cells in the jejunum; their expression declines progressively down the GI tract. Fatty acid binding proteins are important for intracellular trafficking by directing fatty acids from the cell membrane to the smooth endoplasmic reticulum for triglyceride synthesis. Furthermore, this intracellular fatty acid transport system enhances fatty acid uptake by maintaining a fatty acid concentration gradient and prevents potentially toxic interactions between fatty acids and intracellular organelles.

Fatty acids and monoglycerides present in smooth endoplasmic reticulum are used to produce triglycerides and phospholipids. Triglyceride, phospholipid, cholesterol, and fat-soluble vitamins are joined by apolipoproteins, made in the rough endoplasmic reticulum, to form chylomicrons, which consist of a core of triglyceride, cholesterol esters, fat-soluble vitamins, and other lipids and a surface of phospholipids, free cholesterol, and apolipoproteins (apolipoproteins B-48, A-IV, and A-I) (Fig. 70.13). These nascent chylomicrons are transferred to the Golgi apparatus and are incorporated into secretory vesicles, which fuse with the basolateral membrane of the epithelial cells and are released by exocytosis into the extracellular space. These chylomicrons move through the lamina propria into the villous core, which contains a network of capillaries and a single lymph lacteal. Chylomicrons cannot enter the bloodstream directly because they are too large to pass through the fenestrations between capillary endothelial cells. Fat absorption stimulates lacteal distention, which produces gaps between endothelial cells and facilitates chylomicron uptake by the lymphatic system and ultimate delivery into the systemic circulation. Newly formed circulating chylomicrons interact with other circulating lipoproteins and exchange components, thereby acquiring additional apolipoproteins, including apolipoproteins C-II and E, that serve important functions in chylomicron metabolism.

Medium-chain triglycerides (MCTs) contain fatty acids with a chain length of six to 12 carbon atoms. A normal diet usually does not contain appreciable amounts of MCTs, but specialized diets for patients who have fat malabsorption or require a low-LCT diet may include supplementation with MCT oil or MCT-enriched liquid formulas. Absorption of MCTs differs markedly from that of LCTs. MCTs are hydrolyzed more rapidly by lipases than are LCTs, do not require bile salts for absorption because MCTs are water soluble, and can be absorbed as an intact triglyceride. Once inside the intestinal epithelial cell, MCTs and medium-chain monoglycerides are rapidly hydrolyzed to medium-chain fatty acids by specific cellular lipases. Medium-chain fatty acids do not bind to fatty acid binding proteins, are not re-esterified to triglycerides, and are not packaged in chylomicrons. After leaving the enterocyte, medium-chain fatty acids enter the portal system, where they become bound to albumin and are transported to the liver.

Carbohydrate

A typical Western diet contains 200 to 300 g/day of carbohydrate (45% of total energy intake), which includes starch derived from cereals and plants (amylose, amylopectin); sugars derived from fruits and vegetables (glucose, fructose, sucrose), milk (lactose), and refined processed foods (sucrose, fructose, oligosaccharides, polysaccharides); and fiber derived from plant wall polysaccharides and lignin. Starch consists of long chains of glucose molecules joined together by α-1,4 linear linkages (amylose) or by both α-1,4 linear and α-1,6 branched linkages (amylopectin) (Fig. 70.14). Ingested sugars consist of monosaccharides (glucose, fructose) and disaccharides (sucrose containing glucose linked with fructose, lactose containing glucose linked with galactose). Approximately

Figure 70.13. Chylomicrons are fat droplets that are coated with a monolayer of phospholipid and cholesterol. Dispersed in the monolayer are apoproteins (Apo) A-1, apoA-IV, and Apo B and probably also some Apo C-11 and Apo C-111. These proteins help direct the tissue uptake and catabolism of the chylomicrons. In the circulation, chylomicrons also acquire additional apoproteins. Although triglyceride is the major lipid carried in chylomicrons, they are also carriers of cholesterol, fat-soluble vitamins, and small amounts of many other trace lipophilic molecules. (From Patton JS, Hoffman AF. Lipid Digestion. Undergraduate Teaching Project, Unit 19. Bethesda, MD: American Gastroenterological Association, 1986, with permission.)

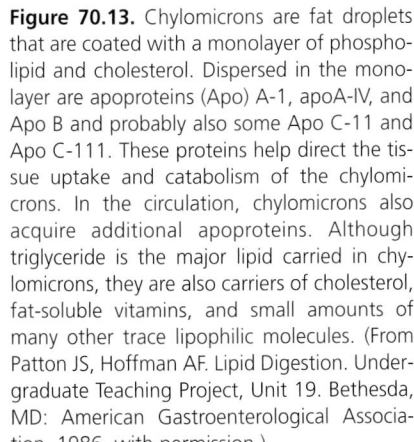

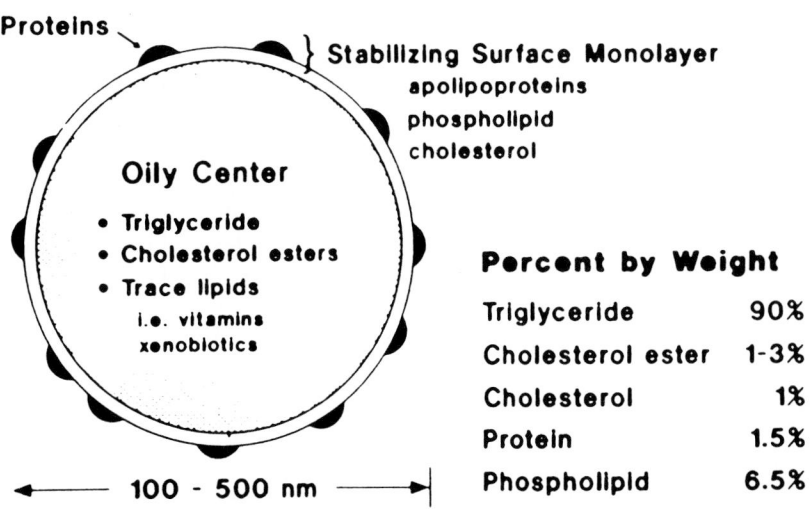

Proteins

Stabilizing Surface Monolayer
apolipoproteins
phospholipid
cholesterol

Oily Center
- Triglyceride
- Cholesterol esters
- Trace lipids
  i.e. vitamins
  xenobiotics

← 100 - 500 nm →

Percent by Weight	
Triglyceride	90%
Cholesterol ester	1-3%
Cholesterol	1%
Protein	1.5%
Phospholipid	6.5%

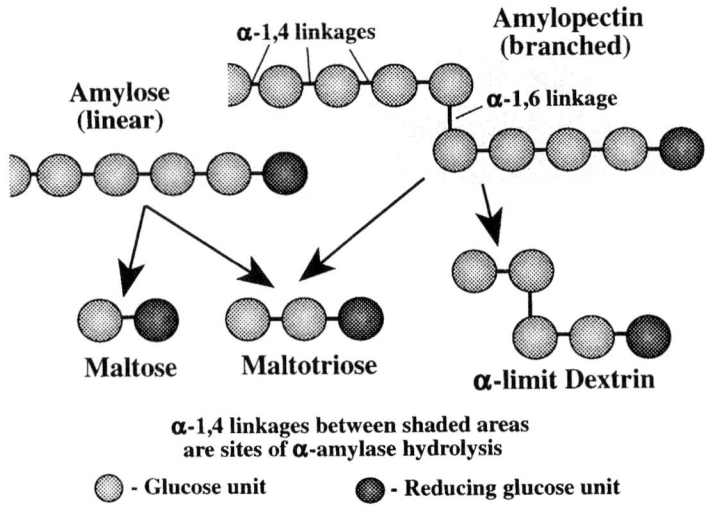

Figure 70.14. Starch (amylose and amylopectin) digestion by pancreatic amylase produces maltose, maltotriose, and α-limit dextrans. (From Chang EB, Sitrin MD, Black DD, eds. Gastrointestinal, Hepatobiliary, and Nutritional Physiology. Philadelphia: Lippincott-Raven, 1996:122, with permission.)

10 to 20 g of dietary fiber are ingested daily in an average Western diet, consisting mostly of celluloses and hemicelluloses, but also pectin, gums, and lignin. Cellulose consists of glucose molecules joined together by β-1,4 linear linkages, whereas hemicellulose consists of pentose and hexose monomers joined together by both β-1,4 linear and branched linkages. Most dietary carbohydrates are completely digested and absorbed in the jejunum. However, dietary fiber cannot be digested in the small intestine because the β-1,4 bond is resistant to amylase.

Amylase secreted by the salivary glands and pancreas cleaves the α-1,4 bond but not the α-1,6 bonds of starch, generating linear oligosaccharides, branched α limit dextrins, maltotriose, and maltose (see Fig. 70.14). Pancreatic amylase is responsible for most starch digestion. The contribution from salivary amylase is not clear and depends on the duration and amount of contact between salivary amylase and ingested starches. Presumably, slow and careful chewing would increase starch digestion by salivary amylase. Furthermore, the physical interaction between salivary amylase and its substrate provides some protection from acid denaturation after ingested carbohydrates and amylase enter the stomach.

Brush-border membrane hydrolases, glucoamylase (maltase), sucrase-α dextrinase (sucrase-isomaltase), and lactose-phlorizin hydrolase (lactase) are required to completely hydrolyze dietary disaccharides and the products of amylase starch digestion before their complete absorption can occur. Glucoamylase cleaves α-1,4 bonds releasing one glucose molecule at a time from oligosaccharides containing up to nine residues. Sucrase-α dextrinase represents two enzyme subunits with distinct properties. Sucrase hydrolyzes sucrose disaccharides to glucose and fructose and short-chain α-1,4–linked oligosaccharides to glucose. α-Dextrinase also hydrolyzes short-chain α-1, 4–linked oligosaccharides to glucose and can also hydrolyze α-1,6–linked α limit dextrins. Lactase hydrolyzes lactose to glucose and galactose. Digestion of disaccharides,

trisaccharides, and oligosaccharides at the surface brush-border membrane usually exceeds the capacity of monosaccharide enterocyte transport. However, hydrolysis of lactose is the rate-limiting step for absorption because lactase activity is lower than all other brush-border hydrolases, even in persons who have complete lactase activity (Table 70.6).

The brush-border membrane hydrolases are glycoproteins produced by enterocytes. These hydrolases are secreted from the cell and inserted into the brush-border membrane; the hydrophobic end attaches to the membrane, whereas the oligosaccharidase component projects into the lumen. Brush-border hydrolases are only expressed in villous enterocytes, predominantly in the duodenum and jejunum with decreased expression distally. Enzyme expression and activity is regulated by transcriptional, translational, and posttranslational processes, which are modified by dietary intake, pancreatic enzyme activity, trophic factors, and GI diseases.

Transport proteins, known as glucose transporters, present in the apical and basolateral cell membranes facilitate monosaccharide absorption (Fig. 70.15). These transporters are expressed only in villous cells. Glucose and galactose absorption occur principally by an Na-monosaccharide cotransporter, $SGLT_1$, that delivers two Na molecules for every monosaccharide across the cell membrane. GLUT-5 facilitates Na-independent fructose absorption, but fructose is not as well absorbed as glucose. Glucose and fructose exit the enterocyte through the basolateral membrane into the portal circulation via the Na-independent GLUT-2 transporter.

Starches and dietary fiber not absorbed in the small intestine enter the colon, where colonic bacteria can metabolize these carbohydrates to short-chain fatty acids (SCFAs) (acetate, propionate, and butyrate), carbon dioxide, and hydrogen. Absorption of SCFAs appears to occur via the monocarboxylate transporter, MCT1, allowing the colon to salvage a considerable amount of energy that

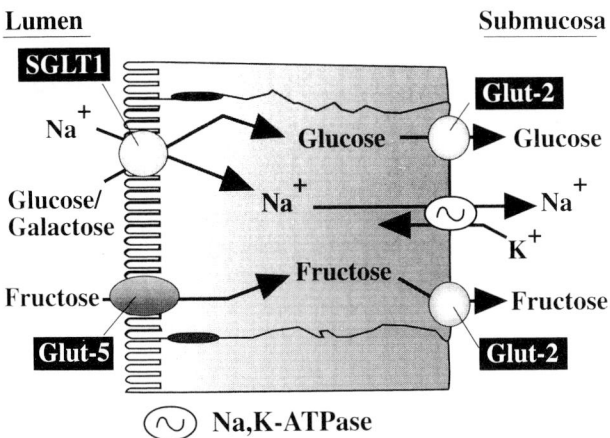

Lumen   **Submucosa**

Figure 70.15. Monosaccharide absorption by the enterocyte occurs by active and passive processes. Glucose and galactose are absorbed by a sodium (Na)-dependent glucose/galactose transporter (SGLT$_1$), driven by an Na$^+$ gradient generated by Na$^+$/potassium (K$^+$)/adenosine triphosphatase (ATPase) at the basolateral membrane of the enterocyte. Fructose is absorbed by facilitated diffusion using a transporter called GLUT-5. All monosaccharides exit the enterocyte by facilitated diffusion via a carrier protein called GLUT-2. (From Chang EB, Sitrin MD, Black DD, eds. Gastrointestinal, Hepatobiliary, and Nutritional Physiology. Philadelphia: Lippincott-Raven, 1996:125, with permission.)

would otherwise have been lost in stool. Butyrate is a preferred large intestine fuel and provides approximately 70% of daily colonic fuel requirements, propionate may have important effects on hepatic metabolism, and acetate provides an important systemic fuel. Furthermore, SCFA absorption enhances colonic Na and water absorption.

Protein

Approximately 70 to 100 g of protein, representing approximately 15% of total energy intake, is ingested daily as part of a typical Western diet. Additional proteins are presented to the GI tract from salivary, gastric, biliary, pancreatic, and intestinal secretions (~35 g/day), desquamated intestinal cells (~30 g/day), and plasma protein (~2 g/day). Normally, more than 95% of the total protein load delivered to the gut is absorbed.

Protein digestion begins in the stomach, where a family of proteolytic enzymes (pepsins) hydrolyzes peptide bonds. Pepsins are generated from pepsinogens, which are inactive proenzymes produced mostly by chief cells. When exposed to the acidic environment of the stomach, pepsinogen undergoes a conformational change with loss of a terminal peptide to its active pepsin form. Pepsin is active at low pH and is inactivated in an alkaline environment. The stomach is not essential for protein digestion, and patients with atrophic gastritis and even a total gastrectomy can absorb protein normally. However, the release of amino acids in the stomach triggers part of the initial GI response to a meal: gastric acid secretion, CCK secretion, gastrin secretion, and gastric emptying.

A significant amount of protein digestion occurs in the duodenum; 60% of protein is digested by the time it reaches the proximal jejunum. Several proteases (Table 70.7), in the form of inactive proenzymes, are secreted into the duodenal lumen by the pancreas. Enterokinase, a brush-border enzyme that is released into the lumen by bile acids, cleaves the N-terminal peptide from trypsinogen to form trypsin. Trypsin activates additional trypsinogen molecules as well as the other pancreatic proenzymes. Pancreatic proteases act as either endopeptidases (trypsin, chymotrypsin, and elastase) or exopeptidases (carboxypeptidase A and B). Endopeptidases and exopeptidases work efficiently in concert to degrade protein into smaller subunits. However, proline-containing peptides are resistant to cleavage by pancreatic proteases. After pancreatic hydrolysis of proteins is completed, approximately 70% of amino nitrogen is present as oligopeptides containing 2 to 6 amino acids and 30% is present as free amino acids.

The mucosal brush-border membrane contains approximately 20 peptidases that cleave specific amino acids present in dipeptides, tripeptides, and oligopeptides, thereby generating free amino acids, dipeptides, and tripeptides. These peptidases are produced by enterocytes, released at the cell surface, and anchored to the cell membrane with the active site projecting into the lumen. Most brush-border peptidases are aminopeptidases, which sequentially cleave the N-terminal amino acid from oligopeptides. Several specific peptidases are able to hydrolyze proline-containing peptides, thus compensating for the inability of pancreatic proteases to cleave the proline-amino acid bond.

Amino acids, dipeptides, and tripeptides generated by intraluminal and brush-border protein hydrolysis are transported across the enterocyte apical cell membrane by specific transport mechanisms. Amino acid transport is facilitated by several transport systems (Table 70.8). Some amino acids can use many different carriers because of overlapping specificity between systems. Amino acid transport in

TABLE 70.7. PANCREATIC PROTEASES

PROTEASE	FUNCTION
Endopeptidases	
Trypsin	Cleaves internal bonds at lysine or arginine residues and cleaves other pancreatic proenzymes
Chymotrypsin	Cleaves bonds at aromatic or neutral amino acid residues
Elastase	Cleaves bonds at aliphatic amino acid residues
Exopeptidases	
Carboxypeptidase A	Cleaves aromatic amino acids from carboxy terminal end of protein and peptides
Carboxypeptidase B	Cleaves arginine or lysine from carboxy terminal end of proteins and peptides

TABLE 70.8. BRUSH-BORDER MEMBRANE AMINO ACID TRANSPORT SYSTEMS

TRANSPORT SYSTEM	AMINO ACIDS	SODIUM DEPENDENT	DISTRIBUTION
Neutral amino acids			
N	Neutral amino acids	Yes	Hepatocytes, muscle
B^0	Neutral amino acids	Yes	All epithelial
PHE	Phenylalanine, methionine	Yes	Intestine
IMINO	Proline, hydroxyproline	Yes	Intestine
β	β-Alanine, taurine	Yes	Kidney, brain
L	Branched chain and aromatics	No	Hepatocytes, choroid plexus
Acidic amino acids			
X^-_{GA}	Glutamate, aspartate	Yes	Gut, brain, liver
Basic			
B^{0+}	Neutral and basic amino acids	Yes	Gut, kidney
Y^+L	Neutral and basic amino acids	Yes	All epithelial
$b^{0,+}$	Neutral and basic amino acids	No	All epithelial
Di/tri-peptide			
hPept1	Dipeptides and tripeptides	Yes	Gut, kidney
hPept2	Dipeptides and tripeptides	Yes	Kidney

most systems is coupled to Na uptake (Na dependent). However, amino acid uptake can also occur by Na-independent processes by facilitated or passive diffusion. Dipeptides and tripeptides are absorbed intact by intestinal epithelia by a sodium-independent process that involves hydrogen-peptide cotransport along a hydrogen gradient. The human dipeptide/tripeptide transporters belong to the proton-dependent oligopeptide transporter family, and include hPepT1, expressed only in the intestine, and hPepT2, expressed in both kidney and intestine. Peptide transport represents an important mechanism for amino acid absorption; in the jejunum, most amino acids are absorbed faster as peptides than as free amino acids.

Enterocyte absorption of digested dietary and intestinal proteins generates intracellular amino acids, dipeptides, and tripeptides. Peptides present in the enterocyte are hydrolyzed to individual amino acids by several cytosolic peptidases. In fact, dipeptidases and tripeptidases are much more abundant inside the cell than in the brush-border membrane. Intracellular amino acids are transported out of the enterocyte through the basolateral membrane by active transport, facilitated diffusion, and simple diffusion. During meals, most amino acid transport out of the cell occurs by facilitated or simple diffusion because of the large amino acid concentration gradient across the cell membrane. Several amino acid transport systems have been identified. Passive diffusion and the L-facilitated carrier system are principally involved in amino acid exit from the enterocyte, whereas the active Na^+-dependent A and ASC systems and the Na^+-independent asc, b^0, and y^+ systems are principally involved in amino acid uptake.

Absorbed amino acids can have several fates: some provide fuel for the small intestine itself (particularly glutamate and glutamine) and some are used for protein synthesis, whereas most are transported into the portal circulation for metabolism in the liver or for subsequent delivery to peripheral tissues via the bloodstream. Despite

the presence of intracellular peptidases, approximately 10% of portal blood amino nitrogen is in the form of peptides that have escaped intracellular hydrolysis. After a meal, villous cells receive their amino acid requirements from absorption of luminal proteins. In contrast, crypt cells receive most of their amino acids from the bloodstream, as do villous cells during postabsorptive conditions.

Minerals

Mineral absorption involves three general events: (a) intraluminal events that transform ingested minerals into absorbable forms, (b) mucosal events that govern mineral uptake by intestinal epithelium, and (c) postmucosal events that regulate the mineral transport into the mesenteric and portal circulation for subsequent delivery to the liver and peripheral tissues. Although some general comments regarding intestinal mineral absorption will be made in this section, the specific absorptive processes for each mineral are reviewed in depth in Chapters 8 through 18.

Minerals ingested in the diet are frequently bound to proteins within a matrix of organic molecules. Therefore, mechanical separation by mastication and dispersion, and digestion by pancreatic enzymes, are needed to convert ingested minerals into forms necessary for effective absorption. Unlike other nutrients, intestinal absorption of some minerals is regulated by body stores to prevent excessive uptake and toxicity. Furthermore, the absorption of one mineral can decrease the absorption of another. For example, there are absorptive interactions between calcium and magnesium and between iron, zinc, and copper. These interactions can be used therapeutically; oral zinc supplementation inhibits copper absorption in patients with Wilson disease, who have excessive tissue copper loads.

Mineral absorption can be complicated because some minerals are released into the lumen as charged ions whereas others are a component of an organic complex.

For example, iron is ingested as a component of heme (animal sources) and nonheme (animal and plant sources) iron compounds (see Chapter 12). Dietary nonheme iron is usually present in the ferric (Fe^{3+}) form, which is soluble in the acid pH of the stomach but insoluble at pH above 3. Other dietary compounds and intestinal secretions can either enhance iron absorption by making iron more soluble (by forming unstable chelates or reducing iron to the more soluble ferrous [Fe^{2+}] form) or decrease iron absorption by making iron less soluble (by precipitating iron or forming stable chelates). Heme iron is soluble at the alkaline pH of the small intestine and is more efficiently absorbed than nonheme iron. Iron is predominantly absorbed in the duodenum, whereas other minerals are predominantly absorbed throughout the small intestine.

Vitamins

Water-soluble vitamins (thiamin, riboflavin, niacin, pyridoxine, biotin, pantothenate, folate, cobalamin, and ascorbic acid) are usually present in foods as part of a coenzyme system and are often associated with proteins. This complex arrangement must be digested to a simpler form before the vitamins can be transported across the apical epithelial cell membrane. Vitamins are usually present in the diet in low concentrations and require active carrier systems for adequate absorption. However, water-soluble vitamins are also absorbed by passive diffusion. Therefore, oral vitamin supplementation with large doses can often overcome defects in normal vitamin transport by achieving high intraluminal concentrations. All water-soluble vitamins are absorbed primarily in the upper small intestine with the exception of vitamin B_{12}, which is absorbed principally in the terminal ileum. The specific mechanisms involved in the absorption of each water-soluble vitamin are reviewed in Chapters 23 through 31.

Absorption of fat-soluble vitamins (vitamins A, D, E, and K) requires bile salts for solubilization within micelles, which enhance their delivery through the unstirred water layer to the enterocyte apical membrane. Therefore, the absence of bile salts can seriously impair fat-soluble vitamin absorption, particularly the highly insoluble vitamins D and K. Vitamin K is unique in that body stores reflect absorption of both vitamin K_1 (phylloquinone) ingested in the diet and vitamin K_2 (menaquinone) produced by intestinal bacteria. Vitamin K of bacterial origin comes predominantly from vitamin K synthesized by small intestinal bacteria or colonic bacteria that refluxed into the small intestine because absorption by the colon is limited. Once inside the enterocyte, fat-soluble vitamins become incorporated within the core of chylomicrons for transport into intestinal lymphatics. Most ingested fat-soluble vitamins are absorbed in the proximal small intestine, although often less than 50% of total dietary intake is absorbed. The specific mechanisms involved in the absorption of each fat-soluble vitamin are reviewed in Chapters 19 through 22.

INTESTINAL MICROFLORA

The human GI tract contains approximately 10^{14} bacteria consisting of more than 500 different species. Bacteria become progressively more abundant down the GI tract; the colon has more than 100-fold more species and 100,000-fold more organisms than any other intestinal area (Table 70.9). These organisms serve important metabolic and defense functions. The mitotic index and cell turnover rate are lower, and intestinal transit times are prolonged in animals without intestinal flora. Moreover, anaerobic bacteria in the colon produce SCFAs, especially butyric acid, a preferred substrate for the colonocyte. Nonetheless, in the absence of colonic flora, animals have healthy colonic mucosa.

The mouth contains mostly anaerobic bacteria. However, the distribution of the oral flora is not uniform and bacterial composition and density vary with location. The most densely populated areas are the gingival crevices. Poor oral hygiene and immunologic variations permit overgrowth of subgingival organisms, leading to gingivitis. Most of the bacteria that enter the stomach are killed by the acid environment. However, some species, such as *Lactobacillus*, *Streptococcus viridans*, *Staphylococcus*, *Peptostreptococcus*, *Neisseria*, and the yeast *Candida*, are found in the stomach because they are more acid-resistant than other organisms. *Helicobacter pylori*, an important cause of gastritis and ulcer disease, may be the only organism to truly colonize the stomach. The duodenum and proximal small bowel (jejunum) also contain few microorganisms, consisting mostly of aerobes and facultative anaerobes. In the ileum, there is a marked increase in bacteria number increase as well as a shift from aerobic to anaerobic organisms. In the colon, the number of microorganisms increases 100,000-fold, consisting almost entirely of strict anaerobes such as *Bacteroides*, anaerobic *Lactobacilli*, and *Clostridia*. The ileocecal valve represents a physical barrier between the small and large intestine. Resection of the ileocecal valve permits translocation of bacteria flora from the colon to the remaining ileum, where the bacterial population becomes similar to that of the colon.

The interaction between enteric microflora and the host is complex. The presence of enteric organisms enhances

TABLE 70.9. INTESTINAL MICROFLORA

	AEROBES/ FACULTATIVE ANAEROBES[a]	ANAEROBES	TOTAL BACTERIA
Stomach	$0-10^3$	0	$0-10^3$
Jejunum	$0-10^4$	0	$0-10^4$
Ileum	10^2-10^5	10^3-10^7	10^5-10^8
Colon	10^2-10^9	10^9-10^{12}	$10^{10}-10^{12}$

[a]Values are per milliliter or gram of contents.

From Silk DBA, Grimble GK, Rees RG. Proc Nutr Soc 1985;44:63.

the defense against pathogenic bacteria by stimulating antibody production, increasing cell-mediated immunity, and preventing the overgrowth of more pathogenic organisms. The mucosal barrier is a combined physical/chemical complex function composed in part of mucus secretion, mucin glycoproteins, trefoil peptides, and surfactant phospholipids. It forms a separation of luminal contents from the mucosa and creates a framework for host-bacterial interactions. The innate immune system of the GI tract provides another set of defense mechanisms against pathogenic bacteria and parasites. Pattern recognition receptors (also called Toll-like receptors) are present in some epithelial cells, and are more broadly expressed in macrophages and other immune cells. These receptors sense the presence of various bacterial macromolecules and initiate a nonspecific inflammatory response. Endogenous antimicrobial peptides, known as defensins, are produced by Paneth cells at the base of intestinal crypts and offer a broad spectrum of antimicrobial activity. Goblet cells also produce small cysteine-rich proteins, which have antihelminthic activity. Normal flora effectively compete for intraluminal fuels and adhere better to the intestinal wall, preventing pathogenic bacteria from establishing residence. The importance of this defense mechanism is illustrated by germ-free animals that cannot survive exposure to hostile microbes.

Intestinal bacteria also have important metabolic and nutritional functions, including hydrolysis of cholesterol esters, androgen, estrogen, and bile salts; use of carbohydrate, lipid, and protein; and consumption (vitamin B_{12} and folate) and production (biotin, folate, and vitamin K) of vitamins. All compounds that enter the alimentary tract by ingestion or intestinal secretion are potential substrates for bacterial metabolism (Table 70.10).

IMMUNE SYSTEM

The alimentary tract houses a major portion of the body's immune system and is directed toward defending the host against bacterial, viral, parasitic, and food antigens that are constantly present in the intestinal lumen. The intestinal immune system consists of two arms, the innate immune system and the adaptive immune system. Components of the innate immune system include Paneth cells and goblet cells that secrete various defensive peptides, macrophages, and myelomonocytic cells. This arm of the immune system is more primitive and orchestrates defensive and inflammatory responses triggered by the presence of various bacteria-derived macromolecules. The adaptive immune system regulates antigen-specific immune responses and consists of the following components: (a) T lymphocytes, (b) B lymphocytes, (c) natural killer cells, (d) myelomonocytic cells (monocytes, neutrophils, eosinophils, and basophils), (e) cytokines, (f) antibodies (IgG, IgM and secretory IgA) and (g) gut-associated lymphoid tissue (GALT).

TABLE 70.10. BIOCHEMICAL REACTIONS BY INTESTINAL BACTERIA

REACTION	REPRESENTATIVE SUBSTRATE
Hydrolysis	
Glucuronides	Estradiol-3-glucuronide
Glycosides	Cycasin
Sulfamates	Cyclamate, amygdalin
Amides	Methotrexate
Esters	Acetyldigoxin
Nitrates	Pentaerythritol trinitrate
Dehydroxylation	
C-Hydroxy groups	Bile acids
N-Hydroxyl groups	N-Hydroxyfluorenylacetamide
Decarboxylation	Amino acids
D-Demethylation	Biochanin A
Deamination	Amino acids
Dehydrogenase	Cholesterol, bile acids
Dehalogenation	DDT
Reduction	
Nitro groups	*P*-Nitrobenzoic acid
Double bonds	Unsaturated fatty acids
Azo groups	Food dyes
Aldehydes	Benzaldehydes
Alcohols	Benzyl alcohols
N-Oxides	4-Nitroquinoline-1-oxide
Nitrosamine formation	Dimethylnitrosamine
Aromatization	Quinic acid
Acetylation	Histamine
Esterification	Galic acid

From Kim YS, Erickson RH. Gastroenterology 1985;88:1071–3.

The secretion of the dimeric Ig, IgA, is an important GI tract protective mechanism. Secretory IgA, the predominant intestinal Ig, is produced by B lymphocytes in the lamina propria. Secretory IgA binds dietary antigens, thereby preventing their absorption, and can bind to pathogenic microorganisms, thereby preventing epithelial cell adherence and intestinal colonization.

GALT contains anatomically organized and nonorganized compartments within the submucosa, lamina propria, and epithelium to provide specialized host defense functions (Fig. 70.16). An important component of GALT is organized follicle-associated epithelium, which contains M cells that overlie Peyer patches. M cells provide a selective site for sampling intraluminal antigens by permitting the transport of large molecules and microorganisms. These antigens come into contact with lymphocytes and macrophages located within an indented space below the M cell before entering Peyer patches. A Peyer patch consists of a collection of lymphoid follicles that release lymphocytes after antigen processing. These lymphocytes migrate to mesenteric lymph nodes, the systemic circulation, and back to specific mucosal sites, where they provide protective immunity from the offending antigen. In addition, GALT contains a nonorganized distribution of intraepithelial T lymphocytes, lamina propria immune cells (T and B lymphocytes, plasma cells, and macrophages), and mucosal and submucosal mast cells.

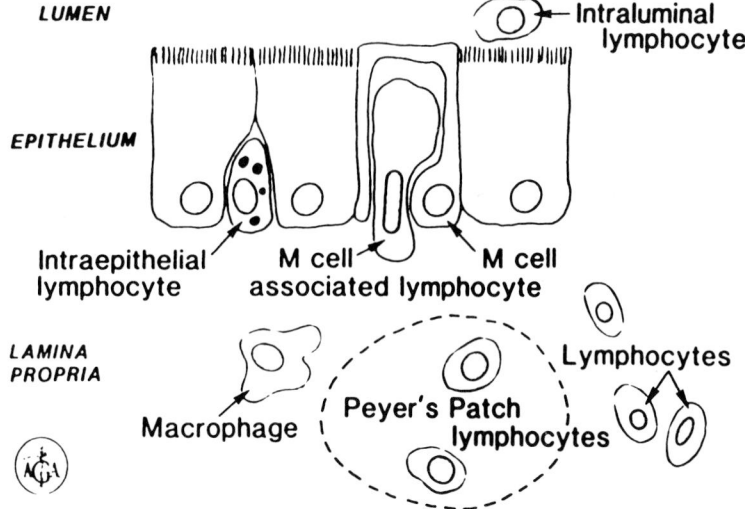

Figure 70.16. Gut-associated lymphoid tissue (GALT) including intraepithelial lymphocytes, M cells, and M cell associated lymphocytes overlying the lymphoid follicles of a Peyer patch. In addition, lymphocytes and macrophages are present within the lamina propria. (From Ernst PB, Befus AD, Bienenstock J. Immunol Today 1985;6:50, with permission.)

A specialized form of macrophage is the dendritic cell, bone marrow–derived antigen-presenting cells that probably play an important role in maintaining the balance between tolerance and active immunity. The two major functions of dendritic cells are the acquisition of antigen and the stimulation of lymphocytes. The population of these cells in the mucosa is dynamic, and they respond differently to various microorganisms. They sense the microbial environment by expressing pattern recognition receptors, including Toll-like receptors that recognize bacterial cell wall components. Dendritic cells are involved in the production of mucosal tolerance in mice, and are altered in human inflammatory bowel disease. The highly plastic dendritic cell provides an important link between the host and the establishment of commensal bacterial flora and the response to pathogens.

REFERENCES

1. Podalsky DK. Am J Physiol 1993;264:G179–86.
2. Neutra MR, Forstner JF. Gastrointestinal mucus: synthesis, secretion, and function. In: Johnson LR, ed. Physiology of the Gastrointestinal Tract, vol 1. 2nd ed. New York: Raven Press, 1987.
3. Gordon JI. Cell Biol 1989;108:1187.
4. Rubin DC. Small intestine: anatomy and structural anomalies. In: Yamada T, Alpers DH, Kaplowitz N et al., eds. Textbook of Gastroenterology. 4th ed. Philadelphia: Lippincott Williams & Wilkins, 2003:1466–85.
5. Cohn SM, Birnbaum EH. Colon: anatomy and structural anomalies. In: Yamada T, Alpers DH, Kaplowitz N et al., eds. Textbook of Gastroenterology. 4th ed. Philadelphia: Lippincott Williams & Wilkins, 2003:1685–98.
6. Granger DN, Richardson PDI, Kvietys PR et al. Gastroenterology 1980;78:837–63.
7. Chou CC. Fed Proc 1983;42:1658.
8. Geboes K, Geboes KP, Maleux G. Best Pract Res Clin Gastroenterol 2001;15:1–14.
9. Crissinger KD, Granger DN. Gastrointestinal blood flow. In: Yamada T, Alpers DH, Kaplowitz N et al., eds. Textbook of Gastroenterology. 4th ed. Philadelphia: Lippincott Williams & Wilkins, 2003:498–520.
10. Johnson LR, Alpers DH, Jacobson ED et al., eds. Physiology of the Gastrointestinal Tract, vol 1. 3rd ed. New York: Raven Press, 1994.
11. Furness JB, Clerc N, Vogalis F et al. The enteric nervous system and its extrinsic connections. In: Yamada T, Alpers DH, Kaplowitz N et al., eds. Textbook of Gastroenterology. 4th ed. Philadelphia: Lippincott Williams & Wilkins, 2003:12–34.
12. Hasler WL. Motility of the small intestine and colon. In: Yamada T, Alpers DH, Kaplowitz N et al., eds. Textbook of Gastroenterology. 4th ed. Philadelphia: Lippincott Williams & Wilkins, 2003:220–47.
13. Miller LJ. Gastrointestinal hormones and receptors. In: Yamada T, Alpers DH, Kaplowitz N et al., eds. Textbook of Gastroenterology. 4th ed. Philadelphia: Lippincott Williams & Wilkins, 2003:48–76
14. Walsh JH, Mayer EA. Gastrointestinal hormones. In: Sleisenger MH, Fordtran JS, Scharschmidt BF et al., eds. Gastrointestinal Disease. 5th ed. Philadelphia: WB Saunders, 1993:18–44.
15. Drucker DJ. Mol Endocrinol 2003;17:161–71.
16. Howarth GS. J Nutr 2003;133:2109–12.
17. Pandol SJ, ed. Gastrointestinal system, section 6. In: West JB, ed. Physiological Basis of Medical Practice. 12th ed. Baltimore: Williams & Wilkins, 1991:606–722.
18. Raybould HE, Pandol SJ, Yee H. The integrated responses of the gastrointestinal tract and liver to a meal. In: Yamada T, Alpers DH, Kaplowitz N, eds. Textbook of Gastroenterology. 4th ed. Philadelphia: Lippincott Williams & Wilkins, 2003:2–11.
19. Johnson LR, ed. Essentials of Medical Physiology. Part V: Gastrointestinal Physiology. New York: Raven Press, 1992:449–530.
20. Sachs G, Prinz C. News Physiol Sci 1996;11:57–62.
21. Chey WY, Chang T. Pancreatology 2001;1:320–35.
22. Flemstrom G, Isenberg JI. News Physiol Sci 2001;16:23–8.
23. O'Rahilly S, Sadaf Farooqi I, Yeo GSH et al. Endocrinology 2003;144:3757–64.
24. Druce M, Bloom SR. Curr Opin Clin Nutr Metab Care 2003;6:361–7.
25. Pico C, Oliver P, Sanchez J et al. Br J Nutr 2003;90:735–41.
26. Anonymous. Nutr Rev 2003;61:101–4.
27. Anderson JM, Van Itallie CM. Am J Physiol 1995;269:G467–76.
28. Horisberger J-D, Canessa C, Rossier BC. Cell Physiol Biochem 1993;3:283–94.
29. Semenza N, Kessler M, Schmidt U et al. Ann NY Acad Sci 1985;456:83–96.

30. Ghisan FK. Pediatr Clin North Am 1988;35:35–51.

31. Spiller RC, Jones BJM, Silk DBA. Gut 1987;28:681–7.

32. Debognie JC, Phillips SF. Gastroenterology 1978;74:698–703.

33. Levitt M. Gastroenterology 1983;85:769–70.

34. Hopfer U. Membrane transport mechanisms for hexoses and amino acids in the small intestine. In: Johnson LR, ed. Physiology of the Gastrointestinal Tract. New York: Raven, 1987:1499–526.

35. Fine KD, Santa Ana CA, Porter JL et al. Gastroenterology 1993;105:1117–25.

36. Mueckler M, Caruso C, Baldwin SA et al. Science 1985;229:941.

37. Hunziker W, Spiess M, Semenza G et al. Cell 1986;46:227–34.

38. Pappenheimer Jr, Reiss KZ. J Membr Biol 1987;100:123–36.

39. Ruppin H, Bar-Meir S, Soergel KH et al. Gastroenterology 1980;78:1500–7.

40. Erickson RH, Kim YS. Annu Rev Med 1990;41:133–9.

41. Kim YS, Erickson RH. Gastroenterology 1985;88:1071–3.

42. Silk DBA, Grimble GK, Rees RG. Proc Nutr Soc 1985;44:63.

43. Tobey N, Heizer W, Yeh R et al. Gastroenterology 1985;88:913.

44. Carey MC, Hernell. Semin Gastrointest Dis 1992;3:189–208.

45. Lowe ME. Gastroenterology 1994;107:1524–36.

46. Staggers, JE, Hernell O, Stafford RJ et al. Biochemistry 1990;29:2028–40.

47. Hernell O, Staggers JE, Carey MC. Biochemistry 1990;29:2041–56.

48. Chang EB, Sitrin MD, Black DD eds. Gastrointestinal, Hepatobiliary, and Nutritional Physiology. Philadelphia: Lippincott-Raven, 1996:91–210.

49. Sleisenger MH, Fordtran JS, Scharschmidt BF et al., eds. Gastrointestinal Disease. 5th ed. Philadelphia: WB Saunders, 1993:954–76.

50. Hyde R, Taylor PM, Hundal HS. Biochem J 2003;373:1–18.

51. Castagna M, Shayakul C, Trott D et al. J Exp Biol 1997;200:269–86.

52. Nielsen CU, Brodin B. Curr Drug Targets 2003;4:373–88.

53. Enerson BE, Drewes LR. J Pharm Sci 2003;92:1531–44.

54. Schmitz G, Kaminski WE. Curr Atheroscler Rep 2002;4:243–51.

55. Goldin BR, Lichtenstein AH, Gorbach SL. Nutritional and metabolic roles of intestinal flora. In: Shils ME, Olson JA, Shike M, eds. Modern Nutrition in Health and Disease. 8th ed. Philadelphia: Lea & Febiger, 1994:569–82.

56. Toskes P, Donaldson RM. Enteric bacterial flora. In: Sleisenger MH, Fordtran JS, Scharschmidt BF et al., eds. Gastrointestinal Disease. 5th ed. Philadelphia: WB Saunders, 1993:1106–18.

57. Bourlioux P, Koletzko B, Guarner F et al. Am J Clin Nutr 2003;78:675–83.

58. Brandtzaeg P, Sollid L, Thrane P et al. Gut 1988;29:1116.

59. Perdue MH, Bienenstock J. Curr Opin Gastroenterol 1991;7:421.

60. Cooper M. N Engl J Med 1987;317:1452.

61. Stagg AJ, Hart AL, Knight SC et al. Gut 2003;52:1522–9.

62. Sanderson IR. Mol Immunol 2003;40:393.

63. He W, Wang ML, Jiang HQ et al. Gastroenterology 2003;125:1388.

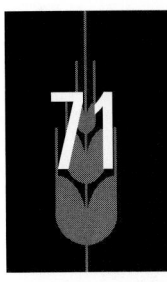

ASSESSMENT OF MALABSORPTION[1]

DARLENE G. KELLY

MEDICAL HISTORY 1443
DIET HISTORY 1444
FAMILY HISTORY 1444
PHYSICAL EXAMINATION .1444
LABORATORY STUDIES 1444
    Initial Testing 1445
    Tests of Mucosal Dysfunction 1446
    Tests of Luminal Dysfunction 1447
SUMMARY 1450

The term malabsorption is used broadly to include intraluminal processes that primarily involve maldigestion, dysfunction at the mucosal level that alters transport or absorption per se, and postabsorptive handling of nutrients. From a nutritional point of view, the end result of malabsorption caused by maldigestion tends to be more specific in that only one or a few nutrients may be affected, whereas mucosal disease usually involves generalized malabsorption. Maldigestion and malabsorption are the results of numerous disorders, and the history often gives a clue that may help to distinguish the actual cause (Table 71.1).

Malabsorption may be implicated in the patient who presents not only with growth failure or weight loss, but also with delayed sexual maturation, bloating, and flatulence. Gastrointestinal symptoms may range from frequent passage of large volumes of watery diarrhea and flatulence, usually associated with carbohydrate maldigestion, to steatorrhea consisting of less frequent bulky, oily, foul-smelling stool, more commonly seen with fat maldigestion or malabsorption. However, it is not uncommon for gastrointestinal symptoms to be absent or minimal. Other signs and symptoms that can result from malabsorption include fatigue, malaise, edema, easy bruising, bleeding, muscle weakness, hyporeflexia, bone pain, pathologic fractures, altered taste sensation, poor wound healing, cramps, paresthesias, tetany, and numbness. Although these features are not specific to malabsorption and none is pathognomonic

of intestinal dysfunction, malabsorption should be included in the differential diagnostic considerations when they are present. A careful history and physical examination should be used to guide an efficient laboratory evaluation of malabsorption (Table 71.2).

MEDICAL HISTORY

A history of childhood growth failure or diarrhea in an adult may suggest the presence of a chronic or latent process such as Crohn's disease or celiac disease. Previous surgical procedures, especially gastric and intestinal resections, may be important in the pathogenesis of malabsorption. Gastric surgery often alters the ability to take in sufficient calories, to regulate stomach emptying and/or small bowel transit, or to absorb specific nutrients such as iron and calcium. Intestinal resection even when restricted can selectively alter nutrient absorption (i.e., vitamin B_{12} and bile salts with ileal resection), and when extensive can cause generalized malabsorption because of decreased mucosal surface area. Bacterial overgrowth of the small bowel may be the consequence of surgical resections as a result of decreased gastric acid production, creation of a blind loop, or abdominal irradiation. Prior abdominal or pelvic radiation therapy can contribute to significant nutritional compromise as a result of radiation enteritis and dysmotility from desmoplastic reactions of the serosal surface of the bowel (Fig. 71.1) or fibrotic changes in the muscularis.

Associated nongastrointestinal symptoms often help to determine the diagnosis of malabsorption syndromes. Chronic iron deficiency anemia or osteopenia can be the sole symptom in individuals who have celiac disease (see Chapter 77). Rheumatologic symptoms, including Raynaud phenomenon and arthralgias, may be suggestive of scleroderma, inflammatory bowel disease, or Whipple's disease. All of these disease states can cause significant malabsorption. Mesenteric ischemia, presenting as postprandial pain, may be seen in patients who have extensive vascular disease. The presence of endocrine diseases, such as hyperthyroidism, diabetes mellitus, and hypoparathyroidism, can suggest that malabsorption may be a result of these disorders. Pulmonary disease in children with steatorrhea may point to a diagnosis of cystic fibrosis.

Medication history often explains malabsorption of certain nutrients. For example, cholestyramine binds bile

---

[1]**Abbreviations: Co,** cobalt; **Ig,** immunoglobulin; **INR,** international normalized ratio; **MCV,** mean corpuscular volume; **RDW,** red cell distribution width; **SeHCAT,** homocholic acid taurine; **tTG,** tissue transglutaminase.

TABLE 71.1. MALABSORPTION/MALDIGESTION DIAGNOSES IN THE UNITED STATES

Most common
Crohn's disease
Celiac disease/sprue
Lactase deficiency
Short bowel syndrome
Radiation enteritis
Pancreatic insufficiency
Cholestatic diseases
Small bowel bacterial overgrowth
Radiation enteritis
Iatrogenic (medication related)
Hyperthyroidism
Infectious diarrheas
Postgastrectomy malabsorption
Less common
Acquired immunodeficiency syndrome–associated
malabsorption
Factitious diarrhea
Amyloidosis
Cystic fibrosis
Protein-losing enteropathy
Eosinophilic gastroenteritis
Whipple's disease
Tropical sprue
Scleroderma
Sarcoidosis
Eosinophilic gastroenteritis
Mesenteric vascular insufficiency
Other disaccharidase deficiencies
Rare
Common variable immunodeficiency syndrome
Cronkhite-Canada syndrome
Lymphangiectasia
Genetic malabsorption syndromes
Amino acid transport deficits
Abetalipoproteinemia
Acrodermatitis enteropathica
Systemic mastocytosis

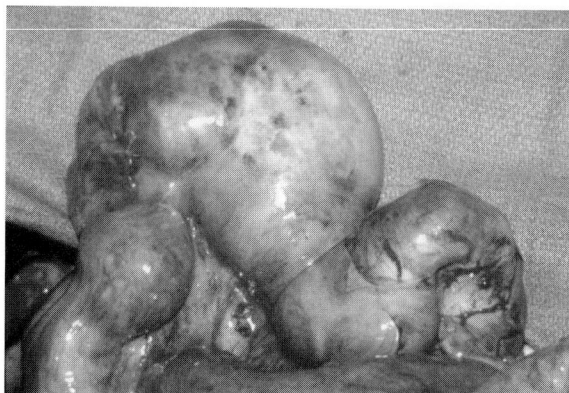

Figure 71.1. Desmoplastic reaction of small bowel observed at operation. This reaction results in the formation of a "casing" that entraps multiple loops of small intestine, inhibiting normal bowel transit. As a result of altered motility, small intestinal bacterial overgrowth syndrome commonly occurs, as well as pseudoobstruction of the small intestine. These changes are occasionally seen as a result of recent radiation therapy, particularly whole-abdominal irradiation used in ovarian cancer. (Intraoperative photograph Courtesy of Karl Podratz, M.D.)

salts, decreasing solubilization of fat and fat-soluble vitamins. Similarly, a history of alcohol abuse may contribute to chronic liver disease or pancreatic insufficiency, both of which may cause fat malabsorption. Other social factors, including homosexual practices or intravenous drug abuse that predispose people to human immunodeficiency virus and *Giardia lamblia* infection, may provide clues to causes of malabsorption.

DIET HISTORY

Although diet histories are often inaccurate, especially when taken by the inexperienced, they should not be omitted because they may be helpful in detecting one of the common reasons for growth failure and weight loss, namely inadequate intake. This may result from anorexia related to the underlying disease or to psychosocial issues, such as depression, stress, or eating disorders. Additionally, various other factors lead to poor intake. Often, pain curtails food intake. Occasionally, one learns that health professionals and well-meaning acquaintances have instituted programs that unnecessarily restrict the diet. A careful history of dietary practices that reveals a poor intake may prevent an uncomfortable, expensive, and time-consuming evaluation of presumed malabsorption.

FAMILY HISTORY

Several malabsorptive disorders can be characterized by a positive family history, including inflammatory bowel diseases, celiac disease, and lactase deficiency. Lack of a positive family history, however, does not exclude these diagnoses. A history in family members of various nongastrointestinal disease states often associated with malabsorption may be helpful in arriving at an ultimate diagnosis.

PHYSICAL EXAMINATION

In severe or prolonged malabsorption, wasting of muscle mass (particularly noticed in the temporal, buccal, and gluteal regions) and of subcutaneous fat stores is common. When there is marked hypoalbuminemia, peripheral edema or even anasarca can be found. On abdominal examination, distension, visible peristalsis, and borborygmi are sometimes present. Abdominal tenderness is not usually present except in inflammatory conditions. Other stigmata of malnutrition, which are discussed elsewhere (see Chapter 38), may be suggestive of specific nutrient deficiencies.

LABORATORY STUDIES

Laboratory tests used to diagnose malabsorptive disorders can be broadly divided into categories. The initial tests are typically those considered to be screening tests, primarily

TABLE 71.2. SYMPTOMS AND LABORATORY EVALUATION OF NUTRIENT MALABSORPTION

MALABSORBED NUTRIENT	CLINICAL MANIFESTATIONS	LABORATORY TESTS
Fat	Pale, bulky greasy malodorous stool; diarrhea without distention or gas	Fecal fat
Protein	Edema, muscle atrophy	Fecal nitrogen, albumin, α-1-antitrypsin
Carbohydrate	Watery diarrhea, flatus, borborygmi, abdominal distension	Breath H_2 excretion
Vitamin B_{12}	Macrocytic anemia, fatigue, neurologic sequelae	Hemoglobin, MCV, Schilling test, serum B_{12}
Folic acid	Macrocytic anemia	Hemoglobin, MCV, serum and red blood cell folate
B-complex vitamins	Angular cheilosis, painless glossitis, acrodermatitis	Vitamin blood levels
Iron	Microcytic anemia, fatigue, painful glossitis', koilonychia	Hemoglobin, MCV, serum ferritin, serum iron, iron-binding capacity
Magnesium	Paresthesias, tetany	Serum magnesium, 24 hr urinary magnesium
Calcium and vitamin D	Paresthesias, tetany, bone pain or fractures, positive Chvostek/Trousseau signs, muscle cramps	Serum calcium and phosphate, plasma vitamin D, serum alkaline phosphatase, serum parathyroid hormone
Vitamin A	Night blindness, follicular hyperkeratosis	Retinal esters
Vitamin E	Decreased deep tendon reflexes	Serum tocopherol
Vitamin K	Easy bruising, hemorrhage	Prothrombin time/international normalized ratio (INR)
Fluid, electrolytes	Tachycardia, hyperpnea, dry mouth	Electrolyte panel, creatinine, blood urea nitrogen
Bile salts	Watery diarrhea	

MCV, mean corpuscular volume.
Adapted from Newcomer AD. Physiologic and diagnostic approach to diarrheal diseases. In: Winawer, SJ, Almy TP, eds. Management of Gastrointestinal Diseases. New York: Gower Medical, 1992:12.1–12.18, with permission.

general hematology (complete blood count) and chemistry studies. This initial battery of tests may be helpful in directing subsequent assessment. A second group of tests is diagnostic or suggestive of generalized mucosal failure. The next series of studies is used to determine specific dysfunction of luminal digestion or specialized absorption mechanisms. Based on knowledge of absorption, it should be possible to systematically direct an efficient and focused laboratory workup. The choice and order of laboratory tests, however, is not universally agreed on and may be modified by availability and expertise at any given institution. Finally, it must be remembered that reference ranges for any laboratory test result are laboratory specific, so test results must be interpreted in light of the normal values for the specific laboratory used.

Initial Testing

The complete blood count, particularly hemoglobin or hematocrit, mean corpuscular volume, and red cell distribution width (RDW), in conjunction with a peripheral blood smear, may be used to suggest the presence of iron deficiency (microcytosis and hypochromasia), macrocytosis related to vitamin B_{12} or folate deficiency, or possibly a combination of these suggested by an elevated RDW. Iron deficiency is most commonly encountered in blood loss, but can occur from malabsorption, especially after gastric resection and occasionally as the sole manifestation of

celiac disease. Vitamin B_{12} malabsorption occurs after gastric resection, distal ileal resection, bacterial overgrowth, and extensive ileal Crohn's disease and in cases of prolonged pancreatic insufficiency. Folate deficiency is found in proximal mucosal disease, such as celiac disease or tropical sprue. By contrast, elevated folate levels are often encountered in intestinal bacterial overgrowth syndrome as a result of microbial synthesis of the vitamin. Based on the findings of the blood count and smear, follow-up tests may be indicated, including measurement of ferritin (1), red blood cell and serum folate, or vitamin B_{12} levels. A Schilling test can then be used to determine whether the vitamin B_{12} deficiency is the result of inadequate production of intrinsic factor, small bowel bacterial overgrowth and preferential use of the vitamin by the bacteria, pancreatic insufficiency causing failure of cleavage of the vitamin from R protein by trypsin, or ileal disease (Table 71.3). In this test, a fasting patient is given a dose of oral cobalt-58 ([58]Co)-tagged vitamin B_{12} and a dose of [57]Co-tagged vitamin B_{12} bound to intrinsic factor. This is followed in 1 hour by a nonradioactive flushing dose of parenteral vitamin B_{12}. Then a 24-hour urine collection is completed, and the radioactivity in the urine is measured using a scintillation counter. In pernicious anemia, less than 5% of the [58]Co-tagged vitamin B_{12}, but more than 10% of the [57]Co-tagged vitamin B_{12} dose bound to intrinsic factor, is excreted. If both labels are found in low quantities in the urine, the etiology is malabsorption. The test

TABLE 71.3. DIAGNOSIS OF VITAMIN B$_{12}$ DEFICIENCY WITH THE SCHILLING TEST

CAUSE OF DEFICIENCY	FREE B$_{12}$	B$_{12}$ WITH INTRINSIC FACTOR	+ ANTIBIOTICS	+ PANCREATIC ENZYMES
Normal	Normal	—	—	—
Pernicious anemia (lack of intrinsic factor)	Abnormal	Corrected	—	—
Bacterial overgrowth	Abnormal	Abnormal	Corrected	—
Pancreatic insufficiency	Abnormal	Abnormal	Abnormal	Corrected
Ileal disease or resection	Abnormal	Abnormal	Abnormal	Abnormal

From Raimondo M, DiMagno EP. Pract Gastroenterol 1996;20:54–9, with permission of Churchill Livingstone.

can be repeated after a course of antibiotics intended to treat small bowel bacterial overgrowth. If this corrects uptake of the vitamin, bacterial overgrowth is the cause of a low serum vitamin B$_{12}$ level. A final step can be performed when pancreatic insufficiency is suspected of being the cause of low levels of vitamin B$_{12}$. This involves giving oral pancreatic enzymes in conjunction with the test dose of radiolabeled vitamin B$_{12}$. The Schilling test requires normal renal function and a complete 24-hour urine collection for valid measurements. Additionally, it requires that the patient receive radioactivity, and the completion of all phases of the test can be quite cumbersome. These factors have caused some laboratories to discontinue its use in lieu of using a combination of serum vitamin B$_{12}$ and measurement of serum intrinsic factor blocking antibodies with or without measurement of serum methylmalonic acid (a metabolite of vitamin B$_{12}$) and gastrin levels. This battery of tests does not distinguish causes of vitamin B$_{12}$ deficiency other than pernicious anemia.

Serum albumin is commonly regarded as helpful in assessing malabsorption and nutritional status, but it must be remembered that albumin levels are also affected by a variety of disorders, including sepsis, trauma, liver disease, cancer, and inflammation (2). Hypoalbuminemia in gastrointestinal disease is frequently indicative of protein-losing gastroenteropathy rather than of malabsorption (3). It is unusual for hypoproteinemia to be present at the initial diagnosis of malabsorption based on mucosal disease or pancreatic insufficiency. In pancreatic insufficiency, low lipase levels causing steatorrhea and wasting markedly antedate (by 5 years on average) clinically significant decreased protease production and resulting protein maldigestion (4). Albumin levels are useful, however, in interpreting levels of minerals, because many minerals, notably calcium, magnesium, selenium, and zinc, are albumin-bound, and low levels are to be expected in hypoalbuminemic patients.

Although a common cause of a decreased serum calcium level is a low albumin level, a clinically significant decrease in the calcium level may also occur as a result of decreased calcium absorption. This may be the result of poor absorption of vitamin D or of luminal binding of calcium with unabsorbed fats to form unabsorbable soaps. A serum 25 hydroxy-cholecalciferol level is helpful in determining whether a low calcium level (in the setting of a

normal albumin) is based on malabsorption of fat-soluble vitamins and vitamin D deficiency (see Chapter 20). Hypomagnesemia is commonly found after distal small bowel and colonic resection and in short bowel syndrome, as well as occasionally in Crohn's disease and celiac disease. Decreased serum zinc levels are most commonly observed in patients with enterocutaneous fistula, in which losses of zinc are high (see Chapter 13).

An increased prothrombin time/international normalized ratio (INR) resulting from vitamin K deficiency, frequently found in conjunction with evidence of vitamin D deficiency, is suggestive of fat malabsorption that is often accompanied by fat-soluble vitamin malabsorption. Decreased levels of vitamin A and E may be found in this setting as well.

Tests of Mucosal Dysfunction

Gut mucosal failure resulting in weight loss, diarrhea, and generalized nutritional deficiencies may occur in such disorders as celiac disease, Crohn's disease, Whipple's disease, radiation enteritis, mesenteric ischemia, and intestinal resection. Although various mechanisms are involved in these disorders, the overall result tends to be generalized nutritional deficiencies.

The serum carotene level is frequently used as a screening tool for mucosal failure. However, the test is quite insensitive, and apart from mucosal disease and fat malabsorption, low concentrations can be found in patients with poor dietary intake of carotene and with liver disease. Normal levels of carotene may help exclude severe mucosal disease as a cause of malabsorption.

The traditional D-xylose test is also used to noninvasively screen for malabsorption and to distinguish mucosal from intraluminal disease. For this test, a 25-g dose of D-xylose is given orally, and urine is collected for 5 hours. Urinary excretion of less than 4 g D-xylose in 5 hours is found in more than 90% of patients with celiac disease, whereas a small percentage of those with pancreatic dysfunction and no mucosal disease have decreased excretion (5). Negative results can occur in mucosal disease limited to the distal small bowel or with mild proximal disease. False-positive results are found in myxedema, vomiting, and ascites; after gastric surgery when rapid transit decreases absorption; in bacterial overgrowth syndrome;

and during treatment with aspirin, neomycin, glipizide, and indomethacin. Incomplete urine collections and renal insufficiency also cause false-positive results. In this case, serum levels obtained either 1 or 2 hours after the test dose or a 5-hour breath test (6) can be done to help circumvent these problems. A newer approach to improving the accuracy of D-xylose serum testing uses intravenous and oral doses of D-xylose in two separate tests and measures serum concentrations at baseline and at intervals up to 3 hours after the dose (7). Although this technique increased sensitivity to 90% and specificity to 95%, compared to 71% and 100% respectively for the standard 1-hour D-xylose test, it does increase the complexity of the test markedly. The application of this test awaits further testing.

In general, the gold-standard diagnostic tests are structural studies for mucosal disorders. In the case of short bowel syndrome, the history of resection, details of residual small bowel length, and anatomy (proximal versus distal) provide sufficient evidence to determine whether the malabsorption is consistent with the degree of resection. When details of resection are unavailable, x-ray studies of the small intestine may be helpful in confirming the length of remaining small bowel (Fig. 71.2). In cases of Crohn's

disease or ischemia, the radiologic studies are helpful in determining the diagnosis as well as the extent of disease. Enteroclysis is currently considered the gold standard for assessment of small bowel mucosal disease. Infusion of barium via an enteric tube avoids or delays flocculation of barium, allows better distension of the lumen, and provides a better assessment of the folds of Kerkring to provide a more accurate diagnosis (8). On the horizon is computerized tomography enterography, which may eventually replace other radiological studies by providing high-resolution three-dimensional detail. Specialized radiological examinations, such as angiography or Doppler ultrasonography for the diagnosis of mesenteric insufficiency and lymphangiography for the identification of intestinal lymphangiectasia, are essential for the establishment of some diagnoses. A recent application of radiologic techniques predicting celiac disease found that increased gallbladder volume, free fluid in the abdominal cavity, and enlarged mesenteric lymph nodes using ultrasound techniques had specificities of 96 to 97% (9).

Another structural test that is often helpful in diagnosing suspected mucosal disease is the small bowel biopsy (Fig. 71.3). The biopsy can be diagnostic in diseases such as amyloidosis, mastocytosis, and Whipple's disease (Fig. 71.4). In other diseases, including bacterial overgrowth, celiac disease, and radiation enteritis, the findings are suggestive but not diagnostic. The importance of establishing an accurate diagnosis in celiac disease, in addition to correcting the resulting malabsorption, is related to the risk for malignant complications (discussed in Chapter 77) and to the fact that the diet is complicated and somewhat unpalatable. For the diagnosis to be based solely on biopsy results, the classical mucosal changes of absence of villi, elongation of crypts, and lymphocytic infiltration of the

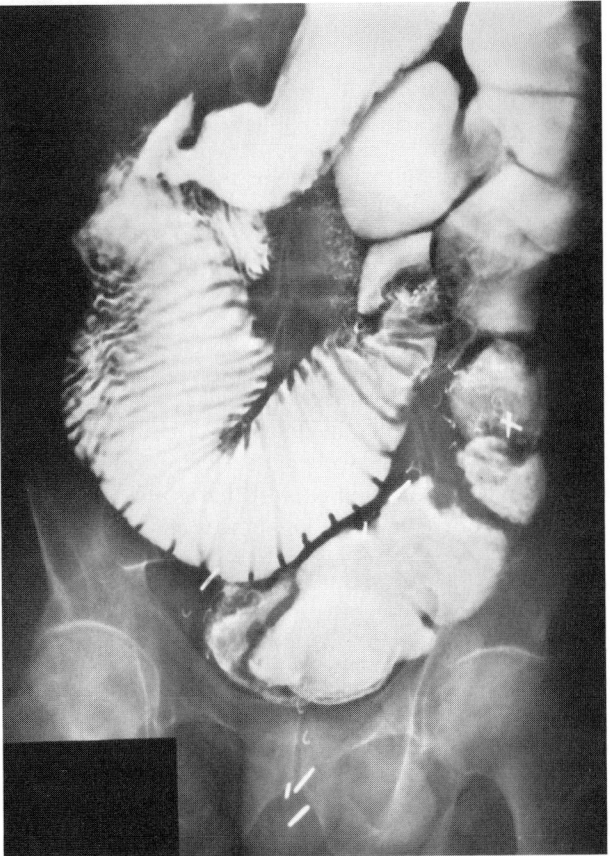

Figure 71.2. Short bowel syndrome. A small bowel follow-through x-ray study demonstrates the approximate residual length of this very short bowel, as well as the marked dilatation of the residual duodenum and jejunum. The jejunum is anastomosed to the distal colon.

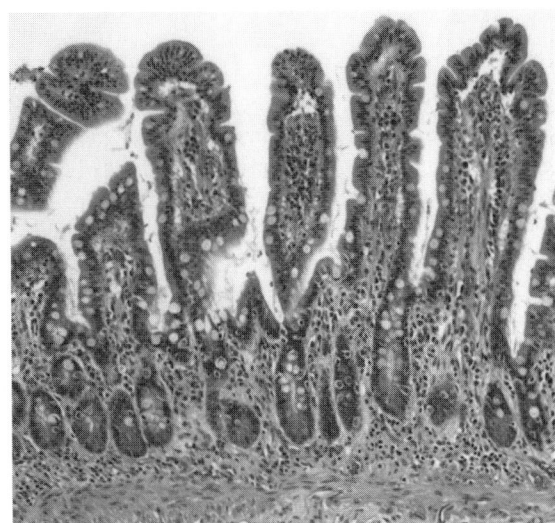

Figure 71.3. Normal small bowel biopsy. This shows normal villi and crypts of the jejunum (Hematoxylin and eosin). (Courtesy of Lawrence Burgart, M.D.)

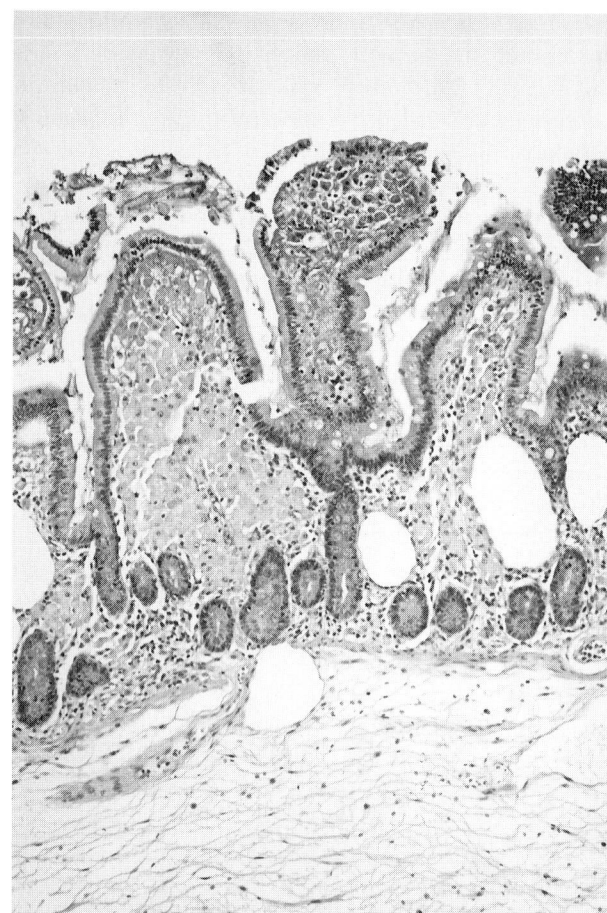

Figure 71.4. Whipple's disease, small bowel section. The lamina propria contains numerous macrophages with abundant eosinophilic cytoplasm, resulting in thickened and mildly blunted villi. Whereas *Mycobacterium avium intracellulare* infection could show similar changes, special stains for mycobacteria were negative, and polymerase chain reaction was positive for Whipple bacilli *(Tropheryma whippelii)*. The dilated lymphatic spaces are also characteristic of Whipple's disease (Hematoxylin and eosin). (Courtesy of K.P. Batts, M.D.)

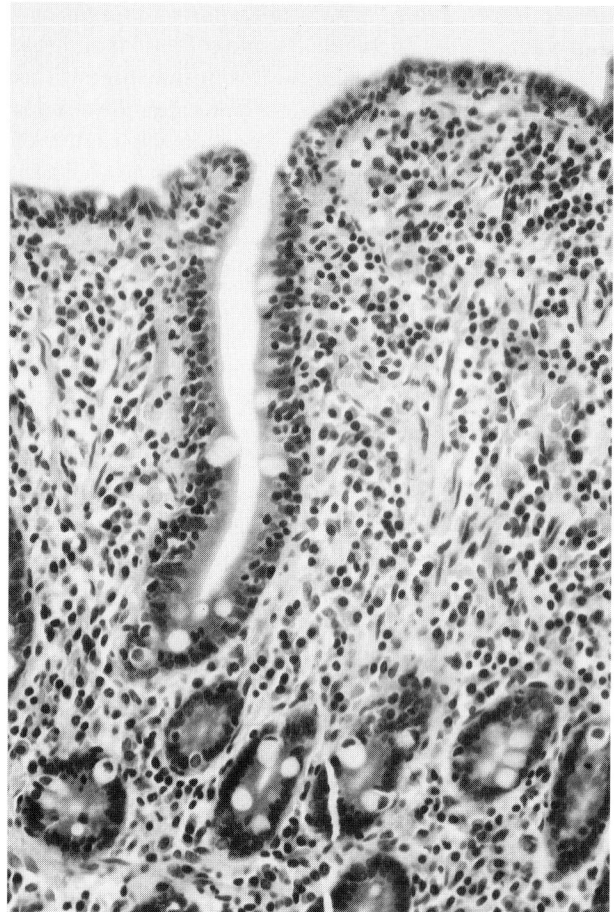

Figure 71.5. Celiac disease, small bowel biopsy. The total villous atrophy, crypt hyperplasia, and relatively squat, cuboidal surface epithelium are all features indicative of mucosal injury. The prominent intraepithelial lymphocytosis and the similar inflammatory infiltrate in the lamina propria are suggestive of celiac disease (Hematoxylin and eosin). (Courtesy of K.P. Batts, M.D.)

epithelium and lamina propria must be shown (Fig. 71.5), with subsequent resolution during 6 to 12 months of a strict gluten-free diet. This is most important in children, in whom infectious gastroenteritis can mimic celiac disease. However, the biopsy results can be confirmed with noninvasive antibody-specific immunoassays. The use of these assays must be undertaken with the awareness that immunoglobulin (Ig) A deficiency is ten to 15 times more common in celiac disease, so IgA-specific assays are less likely to give a diagnosis in cases of IgA deficiency. Within the last decade, tissue transglutaminase (tTG) has been identified as the enzyme responsible for deamidating the structure of the gliadin chain of gluten to allow binding of the antigenic segment of the molecule to the gene responsible for celiac disease (10). Antibodies to tTG have been reported to be 85 to 100% sensitive and 76 to 100% specific for diagnosing active, untreated celiac disease (11).

Use of human recombinant IgG tTG antibody assays may increase sensitivity for diagnosing celiac disease in those who have IgA deficiency. IgA endomysial antibody immunofluorescence also has excellent sensitivity and specificity, but this is a more expensive test that is also more time-consuming. Some investigations have found a combination of tTG and endomysial assays to increase sensitivity and specificity somewhat (12). However, other studies have reported that tTG identified celiac disease in a subset of patients who were negative for endomysial antibodies (13). IgA antigliadin is less sensitive (reportedly as low as 31%) and specific (reportedly as low as 58%) (14). An unequivocal response to a strict gluten-free diet also provides supporting evidence to confirm the diagnosis of celiac disease.

Although mechanisms of fat absorption involve both luminal and mucosal steps, tests indicating the presence of excess fat in stool can be extremely helpful in diagnosing mucosal dysfunction because fat malabsorption is a feature of most mucosal diseases. Microscopic examination of a single sample of feces using Sudan red stain is favored by some as a key screening test (15). However, it is only reliable when there is moderate or severe steatorrhea. The gold standard test for fat malabsorption remains the 48- or 72-hour quantitative fecal fat determination. This test is done by giving a 100-g-fat diet for 1 to 2 days before starting and continuing throughout the collection period. It is critical that accurate records are made of fat intake because fat absorption is proportional to intake. Patients then collect all stool excreted during the specified collection period. The stool is homogenized and dried, then subjected to nuclear magnetic resonance testing. Using the estimated fat intake, a coefficient of fat absorption can be calculated using this formula:

$$\frac{(\text{Dietary fat intake} - \text{Fecal fat excreted}) \times 100}{\text{Dietary fat intake}}$$

$$= \text{Coefficient of fat absorption}$$

Although normal fecal fat levels are quoted as up to 7% of intake, it has been shown that with cathartic-induced diarrhea in healthy subjects, up to 14% of fat intake can appear in stool as a result of rapid gut transit (16). Although fecal fat quantitation is fraught with problems of incomplete collection and unpopularity among patients and laboratory personnel, it not only offers a coefficient of fat absorption, but also gives data concerning the amount of stool excreted and the amount of water in the stool. These advantages of the fecal fat determination make it a superior test to triolein breath tests and Sudan staining (17).

Bile acid malabsorption can be a cause of chronic diarrhea and ultimately of malabsorption of fat and fat-soluble vitamins if the bile acid pool becomes depleted. This can be determined using the selenium-75 homo-cholic acid taurine (SeHCAT) test (18). This test uses an oral dose of a radiolabeled synthetic bile acid followed by gamma camera scan after 7 days to determine retention of the tracer dose. Investigators found this test to be helpful in those with no other obvious cause for their diarrhea.

Tests of Luminal Dysfunction

Bacterial overgrowth syndrome results from surgical creation of blind loops, radiation-induced alterations of normal gut transit, and as a result of achlorhydria from gastric atrophy, gastrectomy or prolonged treatment with acid inhibitors. The effect of bacterial overgrowth on nutritional status is related to bacterial deconjugation of bile salts, use of vitamin B_{12} by the bacteria, and mucosal damage causing disaccharidase destruction, protein-losing enteropathy, altered intestinal transport, and secretion of water and electrolytes (Fig. 71.6). The results are malabsorption of fats, fat-soluble vitamins, vitamin B_{12}, and carbohydrates (19). The medical history, constellation of symptoms, and results of screening blood tests may be highly suggestive of this diagnosis and should prompt one to order a small bowel aspirate for quantitative aerobic and anaerobic cultures. Cultures of duodenal and jejunal aspirates yield bacterial numbers exceeding the normal level of 10^5 colony-forming units per milliliter, but specific pathogenic organisms are usually not identified. Alternatively, noninvasive tests have been developed for bacterial overgrowth, with the ^{14}C-xylose breath test offering specificity and sensitivity similar to that of cultures, albeit at the expense of exposure to low doses of radionuclide (20). A subsequent barium x-ray study often identifies the cause of bacterial overgrowth. Effective treatment with antibiotics, usually on a cyclic basis, confirms this diagnosis as the cause of malabsorption.

Giardia lamblia infestation results in weight loss in up to 65% of cases. If stool examination results for ova and parasites have been negative, examination of a duodenal aspirate or of a biopsy can be helpful in making this diagnosis (21).

In acquired immunodeficiency syndrome particularly, infectious causes of malabsorption are quite common. However, the newer combination therapies have greatly reduced the frequency of severe malabsorption in this disease. Stool and jejunal fluid cultures and examinations for ova and parasites, as well as jejunal and colonic mucosal cultures and histology, are helpful in identifying the organisms involved (22).

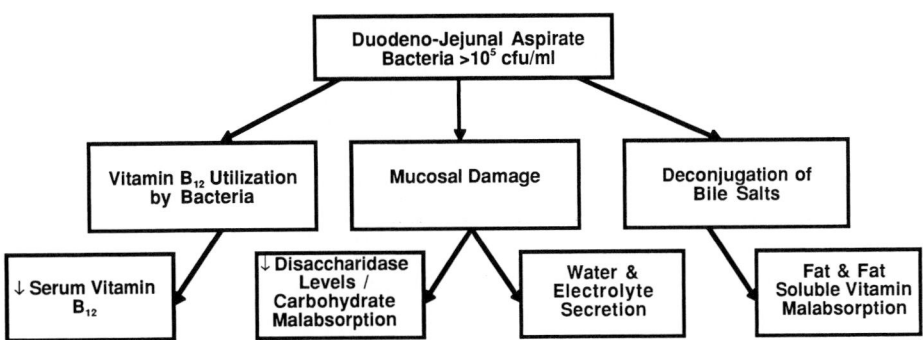

Figure 71.6. The pathogenesis of malabsorption in bacterial overgrowth syndrome.

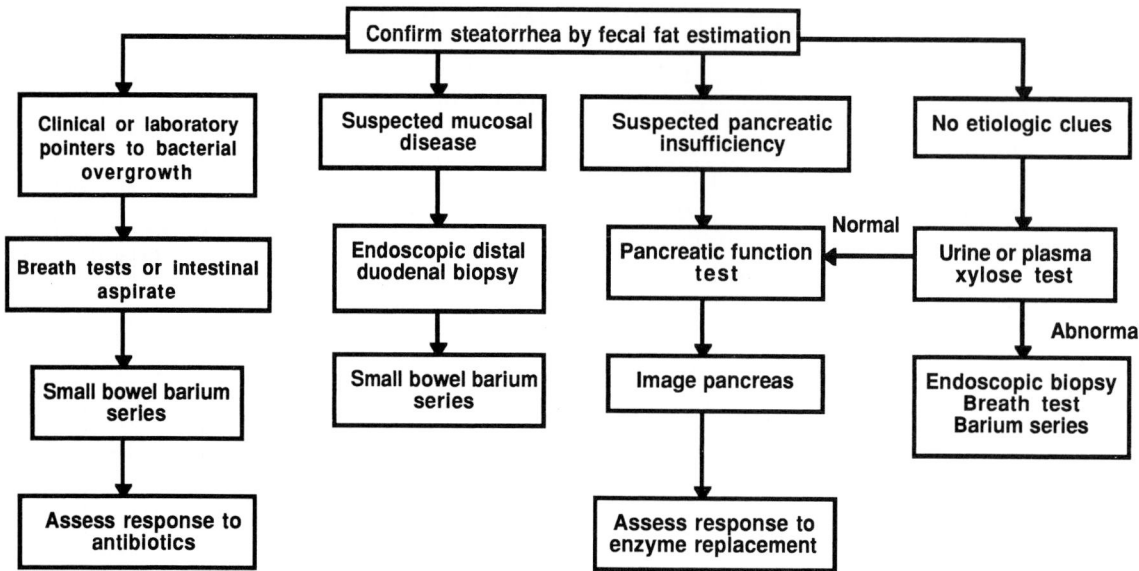

Figure 71.7. An algorithm for the evaluation of steatorrhea. (Modified from Riley SA, Turnberg LA. Maldigestion and malabsorption. In: Sleisenger MH, Fordtran JS, Scharschmidt BF et al., eds. Gastrointestinal Disease Pathophysiology/Diagnosis/Management. Philadelphia: WB Saunders, 1993:1009–27, with permission.)

Pancreatic insufficiency is manifest years after chronic pancreatic fibrosis occurs, owing to the large reserve of pancreatic enzymes. Steatorrhea does not occur until lipase levels are less than 10% of normal (23). The tests that are considered the gold standard for diagnosis are those that directly measure stimulated pancreatic exocrine function (Fig. 71.7). These tests use intravenous cholecystokinin and/or secretin and a duodenal tube to collect pancreatic juice for measurement of lipase and trypsin and/or bicarbonate. This test is highly sensitive and specific (96 and 93%, respectively) but is invasive, costly (~$900 as of 2004), and of limited availability (21). Tubeless assays such as the fecal chymotrypsin, bentiromide, and pancreolauryl test results tend to be abnormal when intestinal malabsorption is present. In the initial diagnosis of chronic pancreatitis, a simple plain film of the abdomen is an inexpensive way of identifying the calcification of the organ that is pathognomonic for the disease. In many patients, a very high level of fecal fat and the presence of pancreatic calcification are highly suggestive of pancreatic insufficiency, and a successful trial of adequate enzyme replacement may be sufficient for diagnosis in such cases. However, pancreatic malignancy can also present with pancreatic insufficiency, so ultrasound, computerized tomography, or endoscopic retrograde cholangiopancreatography may be necessary to exclude the diagnosis in some cases.

Isolated disaccharidase deficiency presents with watery diarrhea, distension, and flatulence (see Chapter 74). For patients who have symptoms clearly associated with milk ingestion, especially those in whom ethnic origin and family history are consistent, a trial of lactose withdrawal and relapse with rechallenge may be all that is needed for a diagnosis of lactase deficiency. In those for whom symptoms

are more subtle and less clearly associated with specific foods, hydrogen breath tests performed with various disaccharides often will clarify the diagnosis of disaccharidase deficiency.

SUMMARY

The general approach to the evaluation of weight loss and malabsorption should include a carefully obtained history, particularly including a diet history, and a physical examination. Laboratory investigations should be tailored to the individual patient based on this information, as well as on an understanding of the physiology and pathophysiology of intestinal absorption. There is no universal agreement among experts in gastroenterology on a protocol for diagnosing malabsorption; this in part is the result of differences in the availability of specialized tests and in laboratory expertise at individual clinical settings. New tests are introduced on a regular basis, and these must be evaluated for diagnostic value, safety, and cost.

REFERENCES

1. Fairbanks VF. Hosp Pract 1991;26:15–24.
2. McMahon MM, Bistrian BR. Dis Mon 1990;36:375–415.
3. Riley SA, Turnberg LA. Maldigestion and malabsorption. In: Sleisenger MH, Fordtran JS, Scharschmidt BF et al., eds. Gastrointestinal Disease Pathophysiology/Diagnosis/Management. Philadelphia: WB Saunders, 1993:1009–27.
4. DiMagno E, Malagelada J-R, Go V. Ann NY Acad Sci 1975;252:200–7.
5. Craig RM, Atkinson AJ. Gastroenterology 1988;106:615–23.
6. Casellas F, Malagelada J-R. Dig Dis Sci 1994;39:2320–6.
7. Ehrenpreiss ED, Salvino M, Craig RM. J Clin Gastroenterol 2001;33:36–40.

8. Herlinger H. Radiologe 1993;33:335–42.

9. Fraquelli M, Colli A, Colucci A et al. Arch Intern Med 2004;164:169–74.

10. Mowat AM. Lancet 2003;361:1290–2.

11. Johnston SD, McMillan SA, Tham JSA et al. Eur J Gastroenterol Hepatol 2003;15:1001–4.

12. Bilboa JR, Vitoria JC, Ortiz L et al. Autoimmunity 2002;35:255–9.

13. Tesei N, Sugai E, Vazquez H et al. Aliment Pharmacol Ther 2003;17:1415–23.

14. Tursi A, Brandimarte G, Giorgetti GM. J Clin Gastroenterol 2003;36:219–21.

15. Roberts IM. Compr Ther 1994;20:10–5.

16. Fine KD, Fordtran JS. Gastroenterology 1992;102:2163–4.

17. Newcomer AD. Physiologic and diagnostic approach to diarrheal diseases. In: Winawer SJ, Almy TP, eds. Management of Gastrointestinal Diseases. New York: Gower Medical, 1992:12.1–12.18.

18. Wildt S, Rasmussen SN, Madsen JL et al. Scand J Gastroenterol 2003;38:826–30.

19. Toskes PP. Adv Intern Med 1993;38:387–407.

20. Saltzman JR, Russell RM. Compr Ther 1994;20:523–30.

21. Hill DR. *Giardia lamblia.* In: Mandell GL, Douglas JRG, Bennett JE, eds. Principles and Practice of Infectious Disease. 3rd ed. New York: Churchill Livingstone, 1990:2110–5.

22. Friedman SL. Gastrointestinal manifestations of the acquired immunodeficiency syndrome. In: Sleisenger MH, Fordtran JS, Scharschmidt BF et al., eds. Gastrointestinal Disease Pathophysiology/Diagnosis/Management. Philadelphia: WB Saunders, 1993:239–67.

SELECTED READINGS

Högenauer C, Hammer HF. Maldigestion and malabsorption. In: Feldman M, Friedman LS, Sleisinger MH, eds. Sleisinger and Fordtran's Gastrointestinal and Liver Disease Pathophysiology/Diagnosis/Management. 7th ed. Philadelphia: WB Saunders, 2002:1755–82.

Kelly DG. Small intestine and its disorders. In: Shearman D, Finlayson N, Carter D et al. eds. Diseases of the Gastrointestinal Tract and Liver. 3rd ed. Edinburgh: Churchill Livingstone, 1997:13.1–13.41.

Raimondo M, DiMagno EP. Chronic pancreatitis: selective use of diagnostic laboratory procedures. Pract Gastroenterol 1996;20:54–9.

Singh VV, Toskes PP. Small bowel bacterial overgrowth: presentation, diagnosis, and treatment. Curr Gastroenterol Rep 2003;5:365–72.

Thomas PD, Forbes A, Green J et al. Guidelines for the investigations of chronic diarrhoea. Gut 2003;52[Suppl 5]:1–15.

Wallach J. Interpretation of Diagnostic Tests. 7th ed. Philadelphia: Lippincott Williams & Wilkins, 2000.

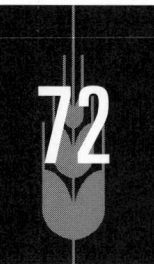

72 NUTRITION AND DENTAL MEDICINE[1]

DOMINICK P. DePAOLA, RIVA TOUGER-DECKER, DIANE RIGASSIO-RADLER, AND MARY P. FAINE

CELLULAR AND STRUCTURAL CHARACTERISTICS
    OF THE ORAL TISSUES 1152
ROLE OF NUTRITION IN CRANIOFACIAL AND ORAL
    TISSUE DEVELOPMENT .1155
NUTRITION AND DENTAL CARIES 1157
    Role of Carbohydrates In Dental Caries 1158
    Factors Affecting Cariogenicity 1161
    Measuring the Cariogenic Potential of Human
        Food 1162
    Root Caries 1162
    Early Childhood Caries 1163
FLUORIDE 1163
    Mechanisms of Action 1164
    Water Fluoridation 1164
    Dietary Supplementation 1165
    Dental Fluorosis 1165
EFFECT OF NUTRITION ON ORAL SOFT TISSUES 1166
NUTRIENT DEFICIENCIES .1166
NUTRIENT EXCESSES 1167
PERIODONTAL DISEASE 1168
ALVEOLAR BONE HEALTH, OSTEOPOROSIS, AND
    DENTATE STATUS 1169
DENTATE STATUS 1169
FOOD-RELATED INJURY 1171
FAILURE TO THRIVE IN CHILDREN 1171
ORAL SURGERY 1171
ORAL INFECTIONS AND IMMUNE DEFICIENCY
    DISEASES 1172
ORAL AND PHARYNGEAL CANCERS 1172
EFFECTS OF SALIVA ON ORAL HEALTH AND
    NUTRITION 1172
DISORDERS OF GASTROESOPHAGEAL REFLUX AND
    BULIMIA 1173
THE AGING PATIENT 1174
DIABETES AND ORAL HEALTH 1174
ORAL MALODORS AND DIET 1175

CELLULAR AND STRUCTURAL CHARACTERISTICS OF THE ORAL TISSUES

Distinctive characteristics of oral tissues may render them particularly sensitive to nutritional extremes. For example, the inability of enamel to remodel and the high cellular turnover rate of oral mucosa, the rates of alveolar bone growth, and the production of saliva, make oral tissues a unique indicator of physiologic perturbations.

In the same vein, nutrition and oral health and disease transcend the relationship between fermentable carbohydrates and dental caries. The oral cavity is the site of chronic disease such as caries, periodontal disease, acquired immunodeficiency syndrome (AIDS), nutritional anemias, herpes, salivary gland disorders, osteoporosis, and cancer, congenital anomalies such as cleft lip and palate, and environmentally induced birth defects such as fetal alcohol syndrome, that could relate to nutritional status. In fact, cleft lip and palate are highly prevalent birth defects that have a complex genetic and environmental etiology linked to maternal nutrient status, folate in particular.

The linkages between oral disease and systemic health are becoming clarified and scientifically validated on a frequent basis with some startling and profound observations. Within the past decade, clear linkages have been established between periodontal disease and cardiovascular disease, diabetes, pulmonary disease, stroke, and adverse pregnancy outcomes. For example, the infectious nature of the oral diseases has been demonstrated to increase the risk of cardiac disease (1), as well as increasing the risk of giving birth to a low-birth-weight infant (2). Because the inherent nature of the infectious oral diseases dictates that the host have an adequately functioning immune and cellular repair system and there are unequivocal data linking nutrient intake and these host defense mechanisms, the relationships among oral health, systemic health, and nutrition require the careful attention of physicians, dentists, nurses, and virtually all health care providers.

To appreciate these complex relationships better, it is vital to understand the structure and function of the craniofacial-oral-dental complex. Teeth are specialized structures necessary for the initial processing of food, and they are composed of three mineralized tissues, enamel, dentin, and cementum, which encase the highly vascular dental pulp or "nerve." These relationships can be seen in the schematic cross

[1]**Abbreviations: ADA,** American Dental Association; **AIDS,** acquired immunodeficiency syndrome; **APF,** acidulated phosphate fluoride; **DMFS,** decayed-missing-filled surfaces; **DMFT,** decayed-missing-filled teeth; **GI,** gastrointestinal; **HIV,** human immunodeficiency virus; **NHANES,** National Health and Nutrition Examination Survey; **NIDCR,** National Institute of Dental and Craniofacial Research.

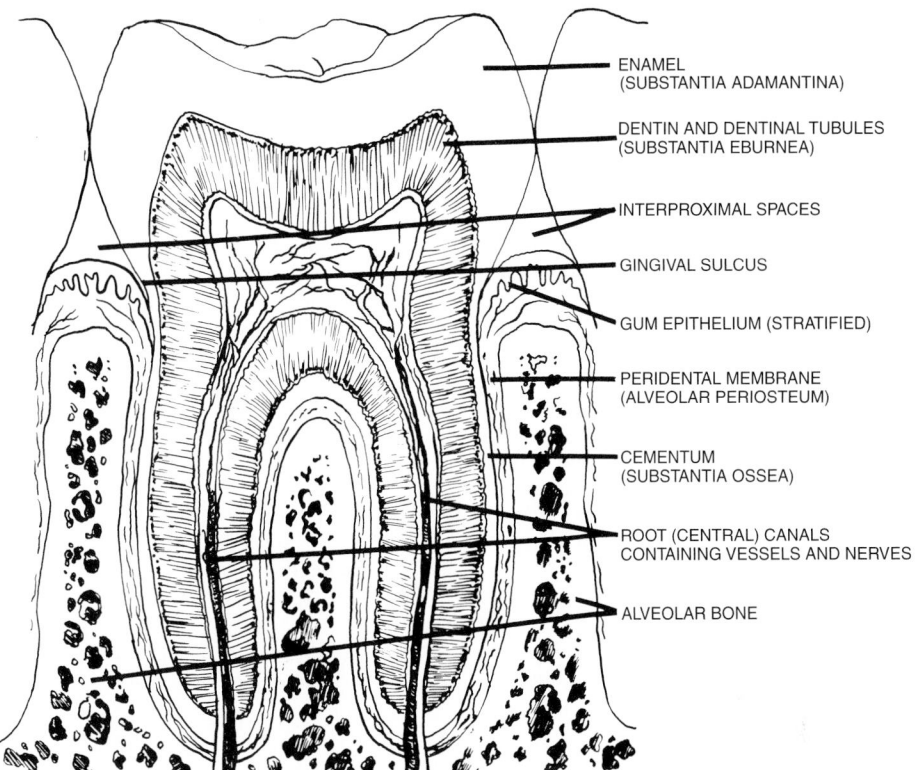

ENAMEL
(SUBSTANTIA ADAMANTINA)

DENTIN AND DENTINAL TUBULES
(SUBSTANTIA EBURNEA)

INTERPROXIMAL SPACES

GINGIVAL SULCUS

GUM EPITHELIUM (STRATIFIED)

PERIDENTAL MEMBRANE
(ALVEOLAR PERIOSTEUM)

CEMENTUM
(SUBSTANTIA OSSEA)

ROOT (CENTRAL) CANALS
CONTAINING VESSELS AND NERVES

ALVEOLAR BONE

Figure 72.1. Schematic illustration of teeth in contact with the alveolar bone.

section of a tooth in Figure 72.1. The teeth are retained in their bony sockets by means of a fibrous structure termed the periodontal membrane or ligament. Influences that affect the integrity of this structure and bone surrounding the socket result in periodontal disease that may progress sufficiently to cause loosening and loss of the teeth (3).

Each tooth develops from a tooth bud or germ located in the jaws. The bud consists of an epithelial component that arises as an invagination from the surface and produces enamel. The mesenchymal component consists of the dental papilla, which produces the tooth pulp and dentin, and the dental follicle, which produces the cementum and periodontal ligament once the tooth has formed. Table 72.1 details the chronology of the human dentition. The primary teeth begin forming about 6 weeks in utero when cells in the primitive oral cavity differentiate to form the dental lamina, which is the site of tooth bud development. The formation of the crown of the tooth begins with the secretion of a dentin matrix containing collagen fibrils. Mineral ions then enter the matrix to form small crystals on or between the collagen fibrils. Enamel formation begins as soon as the first dentin layer has been laid down. This mineralization process constitutes the maturation of enamel and continues after all the matrix is formed. As can be seen in Table 72.1, the mineralization process begins as early as 4 months in utero and continues into late adolescence. After the tooth erupts into the oral cavity, it continues to incorporate minerals (including fluoride) into its structure from saliva, food, and drinking fluids (4).

The life history of a tooth may be divided into three main eras: (a) the period during which its crown is forming and mineralizing in the jaw, (b) the period of maturation when the tooth is erupting into the oral cavity and its root or roots are forming, and (c) the maintenance period while it is functioning in the oral cavity (4). During the preeruptive period, the developing enamel and dentin are subject to nutritional deficiencies or imbalances in the same manner as any other developing tissues. Indeed, nutrient deficiencies can affect either the secretory or the maturation stage of enamel formation. Following eruption into the oral cavity, the enamel is bathed in saliva and is exposed to oral microorganisms and their byproducts as well as food, so nutritional deficiencies or excesses and dietary habits may affect teeth in a totally different or more local manner (4).

At least three striking differences exist between the mineralized tissues of teeth and other tissues of the body. First, enamel contains no capillary or lymphatic vessels to act as transport systems; however, the intimate relationships between the organic and the inorganic components of enamel suggest that pathways in the enamel exist for diffusion of ions and small molecules from saliva, and possibly from blood. Although the dentin likewise contains no vascular elements, it is more readily permeable to the passage of extracellular fluids from the blood, by reason of the dentinal tubules that traverse the dentin. The interchange between elements in the enamel takes place through the bathing of its external surface with saliva. In contrast, the

TABLE 72.1. CHRONOLOGY OF DEVELOPMENT OF THE HUMAN DENTITION

TOOTH	HARD TISSUE FORMATION BEGINS	AMOUNT OF ENAMEL FORMED AT BIRTH	ENAMEL COMPLETED	ERUPTION	ROOT COMPLETED
Primary dentition					
Maxillary					
Central incisor	4 mo in utero	Five sixths	1½ mo	7½ mo	1½ y
Lateral incisor	4½ mo in utero	Two thirds	2½ mo	9 mo	2 y
Cuspid	5 mo in utero	One third	9 mo	18 mo	3¼ y
First molar	5 mo in utero	Cusps united	6 mo	14 mo	2½ y
Second molar	6 mo in utero	Cusp tips still isolated	11 mo	24 mo	3 y
Mandibular					
Central incisor	4½ mo in utero	Three fifths	2½ mo	6 mo	1½ y
Lateral incisor	4½ mo in utero	Three fifths	3 mo	7 mo	1½ y
Cuspid	5 mo in utero	One third	9 mo	16 mo	3¼ y
First molar	5 mo in utero	Cusps united	5½ mo	12 mo	2¼ y
Second molar	6 mo in utero	Cusp tips still isolated	10 mo	20 mo	3 y
Permanent dentition					
Maxillary					
Central incisor	3–4 mo	—	4–5 y	7–8 y	10 y
Lateral incisor	10–12 mo	—	4–5 y	8–9 y	11 y
Cuspid	4–5 mo	—	6–7 y	11–12 y	13–15 y
First bicuspid	1½–1¾ y	—	5–6 y	10–11 y	12–13 y
Second bicuspid	2–2¼ y	—	6–7 y	10–12 y	12–14 y
First molar	At birth	Sometimes a trace	2½–3 y	6–7 y	9–10 y
Second molar	2½–3 y	—	7–8 y	12–13 y	14–16 y
Mandibular					
Central incisor	3–4 mo	—	4–5 y	6–7 y	9 y
Lateral incisor	3–4 mo	—	4–5 y	7–8 y	10 y
Cuspid	4–5 mo	—	6–7 y	9–10 y	12–14 y
First bicuspid	1¾–2 y	—	5–6 y	10–12 y	12–13 y
Second bicuspid	2¼–2½ y	—	6–7 y	11–12 y	13–14 y
First molar	At birth	Sometimes a trace	2½–3 y	6–7 y	9–10 y
Second molar	2½–3 y	—	7–8 y	11–13 y	14–5 y

interchange in the dentin occurs by the movement of ions present in the blood supply to the pulp or periodontal membrane (3). Second, owing to the absence of cells, mineralized dental tissues do not have a microscopically or chemically detectable ability to repair improperly formed or mineralized areas, and the tooth does not have the ability to repair itself after a portion has been destroyed by tooth decay or mechanical injury. An exception is the remineralization of slightly demineralized, superficial areas of the enamel where the organic matrix and surface integrity are still intact, commonly referred to as "white spots." In addition, secondary dentin is formed by the odontoblasts, which persist throughout life on the pulpal surface of the dentin, in response to chemical stimuli from an advancing carious lesion in an effort to wall off the noxious influence. Lack of ability to repair dental tissues is in direct contrast to bone, with its continual turnover and ability to remodel (3). Third, unlike other tissues, the mineralized tissues of teeth undergo a partial change of environment. When the tooth begins to emerge into the oral cavity, the vascular supply to the enamel organ is severed, and the enamel surface comes in contact with a complex mixture of saliva, microorganisms, food debris, and epithelial remnants. Thus, instead of a pure systemic environment, the erupted tooth has, in addition, an oral or external environment. As a consequence, the enamel and cementum surfaces on which carious lesions are initiated by microbial action are largely outside the influences of humoral immune systems, so immune relationships with the caries process are primarily limited to those in saliva (3).

The development and maintenance of the soft tissues and bone that support the teeth are also subject to nutrient defects. The periodontium, as seen in Figure 72.1, comprises the gingiva, the periodontal ligament (peridental membrane), which joins the root cementum to the alveolar bone, the root cementum, which is a specialized, mineralized tissue similar to bone that covers the root of the tooth, and the alveolar bone, which forms and supports the sockets of the teeth. The alveolar bone grows in response to dental eruption, is modified by dental changes, and resorbs when teeth are lost. The finite space between the tooth and the gingiva, known as the gingival sulcus, is lined by a nonkeratinized epithelium. In addition, dental plaque, one of the primary agents responsible for the initiation of both dental caries and gingivitis, contains a high concentration of bacteria, which, in the gingival sulcus, are juxtaposed with a "naked" epithelium. Thus, bacteria and their byproducts or antigens can permeate the gingival epithelium and precipitate a classic inflammatory response that denotes periodontal disease. In fact, an intact immune system, which is highly dependent on nutrient status, is vital to maintain periodontal health. The diversity of hard and soft tissues that comprise the oral structures and the distinctive nutritional needs of each contribute to the uniqueness of the mouth as an external reflection of past and present nutritional problems (5, 6).

ROLE OF NUTRITION IN CRANIOFACIAL AND ORAL TISSUE DEVELOPMENT

Many severe and even moderate nutrient deficits can result in defects in tooth development. The most commonly studied nutrients and conditions that have affected tooth integrity, enamel solubility, and salivary flow and composition in animal models include protein-calorie malnutrition, ascorbic acid, vitamin A, vitamin D, calcium and phosphorus, iron, zinc, and fluoride. Only protein-calorie malnutrition, deficiencies of vitamin A, ascorbic acid, vitamin D, and iodine, and fluoride excess have been demonstrated to affect human dentition (Table 72.2).

Enamel hypoplastic defects and hypomineralization have been the hallmarks of undernutrition or overnutrition during tooth development (7, 8). Vitamin A deficiency has been implicated as a critical factor in tooth health because it frequently accompanies protein-calorie malnutrition and is known to affect epithelial tissue development, tooth morphogenesis, and odontoblast differentiation (9). Protracted vitamin A deficiency during tooth development results in atrophy of the enamel organ, metaplasia of the ameloblasts, and defective apposition and calcification of dentin (6). The interference with calcification is manifested clinically by enamel hypoplasia (10). Additionally, vitamin A excess, when present during the first trimester of pregnancy, can result in severe craniofacial and oral clefts and limb defects (11).

Vitamin D, calcium, and phosphorus deficiencies all result in significant effects on tooth development and resistance to the caries challenge. Vitamin D deficiency appears to exert its metabolic effect through lowering plasma calcium levels; it has been difficult to localize vitamin D metabolites in target tooth and bone cells (12). Leaver demonstrated that extreme calcium and phosphorus deficiencies may result in hypomineralization of developing teeth (13). The deficit must be severe enough to

TABLE 72.2. EFFECTS OF NUTRIENT DEFICIENCIES ON TOOTH DEVELOPMENT

NUTRIENT	EFFECT ON TISSUE	EFFECT ON CARIES	HUMAN DATA
Protein-calorie malnutrition	Tooth eruption delayed Tooth size Enamel solubility decreased Salivary gland dysfunction	Yes	Yes
Vitamin A	Decreased epithelial tissue development Tooth morphogenesis dysfunction Decreased odontoblast differentiation Increased enamel hypoplasia	Yes	Yes
Vitamin D/ calcium/phosphorus	Lowered plasma calcium Hypomineralization (hypoplastic defects) Tooth integrity compromised Delayed eruption patterns	Yes	Yes
Ascorbic acid	Dental pulpal alterations Odontoblastic degeneration Aberrant dentin	No	No
Fluoride	Stability of enamel crystal (enamel formation) Inhibition of demineralization Stimulation of remineralization Mottled enamel (excess) Inhibition of bacterial growth	Yes	Yes
Iodine	Delayed tooth eruption Altered growth patterns Malocclusion	No	Yes
Iron	Slow growth Tooth integrity Salivary gland dysfunction	Yes	No

reduce plasma levels of calcium and phosphorus. This finding suggests that this mechanism in the human population is unlikely, because of the highly effective homeostatic mechanisms that mobilize calcium from the skeleton to maintain normal plasma calcium levels. Bawden postulated that vitamin D hypovitaminosis may be more important in considering hypomineralization resulting from inadequate calcium transport into developing dental tissues (14). Vitamin D deficiency has also been shown to affect tooth structure and to delay eruption patterns of teeth (15).

In childhood vitamin D deficiency, teeth are characterized microscopically by a widened layer of predentin, by the presence of interglobular dentin, and by interference with enamel formation (hypoplastic defects) (16). Young children with rickets have delayed eruption of the deciduous teeth, and the sequence of eruption is altered (6). The permanent incisors, cuspids, and first molars are usually affected because their development coincides with the age at which rickets is most common (6). Vitamin D–resistant rickets results in more frequent and severe tooth defects relative to primary rickets, including large pulps with developmental "exposures" of the pulp.

Vitamin C deficiency has also been demonstrated to affect tooth development and eruption. Deciduous and permanent teeth of scorbutic infants contain minute pulpal hemorrhages attributable to vitamin C deficiency. In older vitamin C–deficient children, the dental pulp undergoes hyperemia, edema, necrosis, and aberrant calcification, whereas the dentin shows odontoblastic degeneration and irregular formation (17). The relation of vitamin C deficiency to dental caries is poorly defined, however. Indeed, although it is likely that the primary mechanism of vitamin C deficiency–induced tooth, gingival, and bone disease is mediated through the disruption of collagen biosyntheses, no study has clearly demonstrated the relationship between scurvy and dental caries (18). In areas where goiter is endemic, children born to mothers with severe iodine deficiency are characterized by marked mental and physical growth retardation. Eruption of the primary and secondary teeth is often greatly delayed and precluded. Malocclusion is relatively common because of the altered patterns of craniofacial growth and development (6).

Perhaps the most intriguing and important data on nutritional status during development and oral disease come from observations on malnutrition and dental caries. Several studies have demonstrated that tooth eruption is delayed, tooth integrity is compromised (especially enamel surface solubility), and dental caries is increased in chronically malnourished animals and children (19, 20). Studies in Lima, Peru demonstrated significant delays in tooth eruption and exfoliation in three groups of malnourished children; such delays were associated with and appeared to be the direct cause of a significant temporal delay in caries development in the primary teeth (21). These data support previous studies on malnourished children in India and Guatemala (22, 23).

The development of teeth and salivary glands is intimately associated with the nutrient supply. Teeth subjected to nutritional insult during critical stages of development show a diminished ability to withstand caries and thus are at a higher risk. In many studies, impaired salivary function has accompanied the morphologic changes in teeth, which may be a primary factor in the subsequent increase in caries susceptibility (24). These data also explain the positive association between socioeconomic status and the prevalence of dental caries in deciduous but not permanent teeth (20). Nutritional injuries early in life may affect tooth formation and may result in increased caries susceptibility, whereas chronic malnutrition is associated with delayed tooth emergence and a shift of the curve for caries prevalence versus age (20). Thus, in understanding any cross-sectional survey on caries prevalence, the nutritional history must be taken into account.

On a broader scale, 7% of babies born in the United States each year have some mental or physical defect evident at birth or later (25). Prominent among these defects are structural, functional, or biochemical abnormalities involving the craniofacial complex. The most common of these malformations are cleft lip and cleft palate, affecting one in 600 white infants, with the incidence higher among Asians, Native Americans, and Inuit and lower among blacks (25, 34). One in 1600 babies born alive suffers from craniofacial anomalies other than cleft lip or palate, including jaw deformities, defects in ossification, malformed or missing teeth, facial asymmetries, and defects that are a component of other syndromes, such as fetal alcohol syndrome (25). Fetal alcohol syndrome consists primarily of small size for gestational age, dysmorphism (especially of the face and eyes, heart, joints, and internal genitalia), and mental deficiency. Of particular interest are the facial aberrant growth patterns, which include a low nasal bridge, short palpebral fissures, indistinct philtrum of the lip, thin upper lip, short nose, small midface, epicanthic folds, and small head circumference (26).

In addition, certain other craniofacial oral-dental disorders such as craniosynostosis, hemifacial microsomia, anodontia, amelogenesis imperfecta, dentinogenesis imperfecta, osteogenesis imperfecta, chondrodystrophies, and juvenile periodontitis represent major challenges to human oral health (27). Neural tube defects, among the most common birth defects with a rate of occurrence of 1 to 2 in 1000 births and linked to folate deficiency, range in severity and can result in incomplete formation of cranial bones (28). Many of these malformations and disorders have a genetic basis or an environmental cause. Certain nutrients given in excess, especially early in pregnancy (e.g., retinoic acid, and other lipophilic molecules such as vitamins K and E) are known to induce craniofacial oral-dental malformations. As stated previously, therapeutic doses of 13-*cis*-retinoic acid administered to treat cystic acne have resulted in significant craniofacial oral-dental malformations when the agent is taken during the first trimester of pregnancy. The molecular mechanisms during these genetic-environmental interactions are not precisely known but are believed to interface with developmental processes by reducing the number of cells required for normal morphogenesis of the head, face, jaws, skeleton, and neural tube, among others (28).

Most investigators believe that craniofacial malformations have a multifactorial basis, in which particular genes alter the ability of the developing fetus to adapt to environmental factors (25). Indeed, evidence from studies of identical twins clearly establishes the role of environmental and genetic factors in cases of isolated cleft lip or cleft palate (25).

The regulatory genes and gene products functioning as transcriptional factors for the bronchial arches that give rise to the midface and lower face are being discovered, and their interaction with nutrients (e.g., retinoic acid via its specific receptors) has been found to be critical to craniofacial oral-dental morphogenesis (29). A superfamily of genes is now considered to interact with nutrients during early stages of craniofacial development in the mammalian embryo (i.e., at about 19 to 26 days of gestation in the human embryo). Endogenous retinoic acid appears to function as a developmental organizer during limb development and limb regeneration. Excess exogenous retinoic acid produces significant craniofacial malformations associated with clefting, dental development, hemifacial microsomia, spina bifida, eye defects, and limb morphogenesis (30). What the function of endogenous retinoic acid is in craniofacial development and how excess levels of retinoic acid may produce congenital malformations are two central questions in this area (28, 31) (see also the discussion on differentiation and morphogenesis). A striking illustration of the need to understand the effects of nutrition on birth defects is the recent datum that demonstrated that folate supplements provided around the time of conception significantly reduced the recurrence of neural tube defects among high-risk persons in the United Kingdom (32). Similar data are being established relating folic acid or multivitamins in congenital craniofacial malformations such as cleft lip and/or cleft palate (28, 33). Although the data remain equivocal, Hayes reviewed the evidence relating folate to cleft lip and palate formation and provided a succinct summary in Table 72.3.

NUTRITION AND DENTAL CARIES

Dental caries is one of the most frequently occurring preventable infectious diseases of the oral cavity and is a major cause of tooth loss in children and adults in the United States. As the most common pediatric chronic disease, it occurs five to eight times more often than asthma, the second most common chronic pediatric disease (34). However, approximately 80% of the caries incidence in children and adolescents can be found in about 25% of the population (34). According to data from the third National

TABLE 72.3. POSSIBLE EFFECTS OF FOLIC ACID ON ORAL CLEFT DEVELOPMENT

Insufficient folic acid intake may be related to cleft origin
Clefts have been seen in children of women taking folate antagonists during pregnancy
Folic acid supplementation periconceptionally results in reduction of neural tube defects that may be related to oral clefts
Neural tube defects and oral clefts are both considered midline defects and occur together more often than by chance
Folic acid protects against cleft development

From Hayes CA. Nutrition in the growth and development of oral structures: a closer look. In: Palmer CA, ed. Diet and Nutrition in Oral Health. Englewood Cliffs, NJ: Prentice-Hall, 2002:167–81, with permission.

Health and Nutrition Examination Survey (NHANES III), about 25% of the adult population has untreated dental caries, and most cases occur in persons of lower income and in ethnically diverse populations (Fig. 72.2). More than one third of adults have treated dental caries, that is, cavities that were filled (35).

Caries can also occur in the primary teeth. As shown in Figure 72.3, in young children aged 5 to 9 years, more than 40% had caries in their primary teeth. Data in Figure 72.2 demonstrate that most caries in the primary teeth occurred in Mexican-American children, followed by

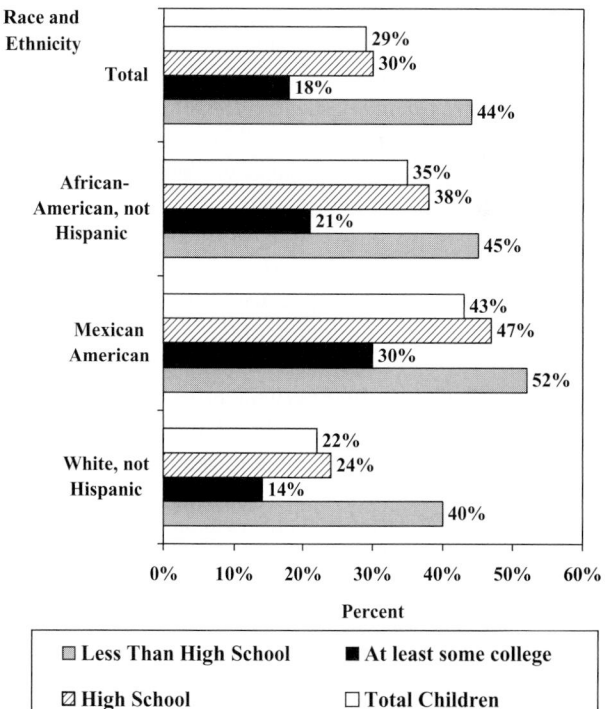

*Educational attainment of family reference person

Figure 72.2. Percentage of US children and adolescents who are caries free by age and ethnicity. (From National Center for Health Statistics. Plan and Operation of the Third National Health and Nutrition Examination Survey 1988–94. Series 1, no. 322. Hyattsville, MD: National Center for Health Statistics, 1994; DHHS Publ. no. [PHS] 94–1308.).

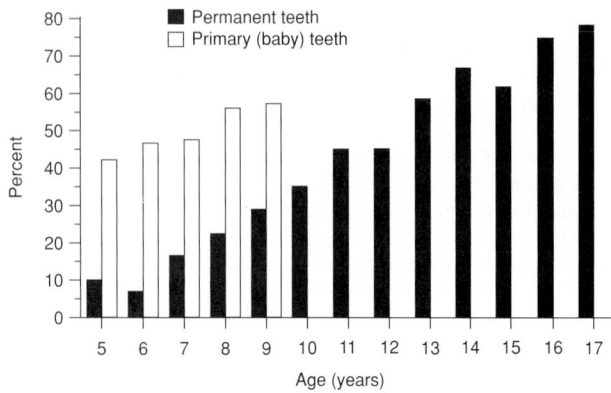

Figure 72.3. Caries in primary and permanent dentition. (From Oral Health. Preventing Cavities, Gum Disease, and Oral Cancer, at a Glance 2004, http://www.cdc.gov/nccdphp/org_oh.htm.)

African-American, non-Hispanic children. The US Surgeon General has labeled children's tooth decay as America's silent epidemic because it represents the nation's number 1 unmet health need (34).

Since the mid-1970s, the incidence of dental caries has declined, mainly because of preventive measures such as fluoride and dental sealants (36, 37). However, as stated earlier, dental caries is still the most common childhood infectious disease (34, 38). Dietary intake may contribute to dental caries (see the next section, on the cause of dental caries); additionally, preserving the integrity of dentition may be essential to overall nutritional status because untreated dental decay may lead to pain, eventual tooth loss with subsequent masticatory dysfunction, and compromised dietary intake.

The extent of dental decay in a population may be measured by DMFS (decayed-missing-filled surfaces), representing the sum of the number of permanent tooth surfaces (out of a possible 128 surfaces on 32 teeth) that are decayed, missing, or filled (39). According to NHANES III, conducted between 1988 and 1991, among US children aged 5 to 17 years old who were examined, more than half (54.7%) had a caries-free permanent dentition; however, the mean DMFS was 2.5 (40). In comparison, in the 1979 to 1980 survey conducted by the National Institute of Dental Research (NIDR) survey, 37% of school children examined had no caries in their permanent teeth, and the mean DMFS was 4.77. However, dental decay increases with age, so by 15 years of age, about two thirds of US teens had experienced caries in their permanent dentition (see Fig. 72.3). Cavitation occurs most frequently on the occlusal or chewing surface of the tooth. Decay on the smooth surfaces of teeth has declined since 1980; and interproximal (between teeth) caries has nearly been eradicated in the younger age groups.

Caries was also common in the primary teeth based on NHANES III data. Although more than 60% of those children younger than 9 years of age had a caries-free deciduous dentition, the average number of decayed or filled primary tooth surfaces was 3.1 (40). Mexican-American children had the highest mean number of decayed-filled primary tooth surfaces (4.8). About 31% of children aged 6 to 8 years had untreated decay in their primary or permanent teeth (41). The prevalence of unfilled tooth surfaces was greater among low-income, Mexican-American, and non-Hispanic black children and teens.

Based on data collected in the NHANES III survey, 93.8% of dentate adults have treated or nontreated coronal caries. The average number of decayed and filled coronal tooth surfaces for adults aged 25 to 34 years was 16.5, and it climbed to 73.1 in adults 65 to 74.9 years of age (42).

The rate of edentulousness also continues to decline. In the 1988 to 1991 survey, 26% of adults 65 to 69 years of age were edentulous as compared with 32% of adults in the 1985 to 1986 NIDR adult survey (34, 35). Many adults have had fluoride exposure part of their lives; as a result, teeth are being retained longer.

Although historically it was thought that dental caries was irreversible, caries is really a dynamic process that has three phases: (a) demineralization (loss of mineral when plaque pH falls to less than 5.5), (b) equilibrium, and (c) remineralization (occurs when plaque pH rises above the critical level to neutral or alkaline levels) of tooth enamel. In the early stage of tooth decay, often resulting from frequent fermentable carbohydrate exposure and poor oral hygiene, incipient lesions may develop rapidly. During periods when no bacterial fermentation is occurring, calcium, phosphorus, and fluoride that have been released from the tooth enamel can be redeposited in the enamel to remineralize the tooth. A clinical cavity (caries) is the final stage in the disease process. The average time for progression of incipient caries to a carious lesion in children is about 18 ± 6 months.

Role of Carbohydrates in Dental Caries

Dental caries is a multifactorial oral infectious disease. Fermentable carbohydrates are only one component in the etiology, along with the oral environment and dental plaque (Fig. 72.4). Fluoridated water and oral hygiene practices can have a dramatic impact on caries risk. Tooth erosion, which impairs tooth integrity, is not an infectious disease, but the resultant defects increase risk of caries. Presence and adequacy of saliva, immune status, and lifestyle behaviors affect caries risk.

In addition to fluoride, primary factors influencing this balance are nutrition and diet. Nutrition has a systemic effect, whereas diet has a local effect. For example, systemically, malnutrition has a negative impact on the volume, antibacterial properties, and physiochemical properties of saliva. In addition, as detailed earlier in this chapter, nutrition during development can affect the integrity of the tooth and salivary glands and the ability of the tooth to withstand bacterial challenge. Systemic diseases and medications affecting the integrity of the oral cavity and or salivary

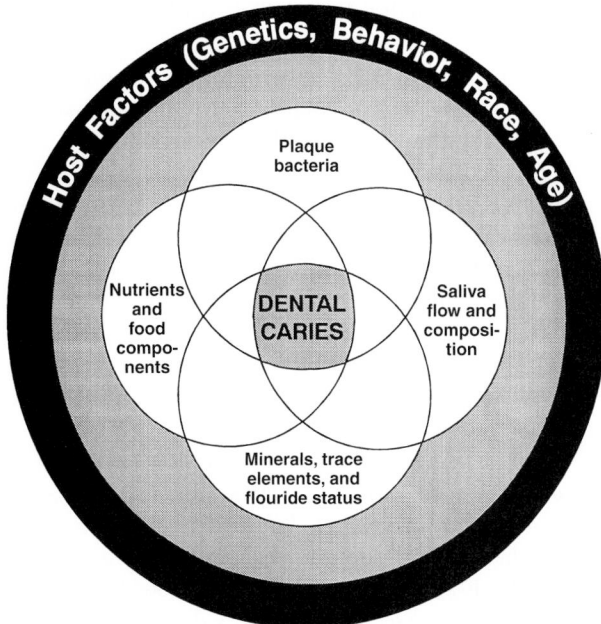

Figure 72.4. Major factors that interact in the dental caries process. (Adapted from Navia JM. Am J Clin Nutr 1994;59:719S–27S, with permission.)

flow can also have a potent impact on nutritional well-being as well as caries risk.

Locally, dietary sources of fermentable carbohydrates are metabolized to acids by plaque bacteria, thus causing a drop in pH. Fermentable carbohydrates are carbohydrates (sugars and starch) that begin digestion in the oral cavity with salivary amylase. The low pH favors the growth of *mutans* streptococci (primary bacteria in the development of caries). In contrast, a diet with plenty of calcium-rich cheese eaten around mealtime favors remineralization.

Sugars are fermentable carbohydrates. Sugars are found in the diet either as intrinsic, which are those found naturally in foods such as fruits, honey, and dairy products, or extrinsic, which are sugars added to foods during processing (43). Examples of added sugars include white or brown sugar, honey, molasses, maple, malt, corn syrup or high-fructose corn syrup, fructose, and dextrose (44). Other disaccharides, in particular trehalose and isomaltose, have a lesser cariogenic risk than sucrose. Starches are subsequently digested by salivary amylase to oligosaccharides, which may be fermented by the oral microflora. According to Lingstrom and associates, only the gelatinized starches are susceptible to breakdown by salivary amylase into maltose, maltotriose, and dextrins (45).

Epidemiologic surveys, animal experiments, and early controlled human studies have all linked sugars to the development of dental caries. Sreebny showed that the average, decayed-missing-filled teeth (DMFT) index in 12-year-old children in 47 countries was highly correlated with the grams of sugar available per capita on a daily basis (46). Populations with low sugar intakes had low caries

scores; children who had high sugar consumption developed high rates of caries. In contrast, studies from the later part of the twentieth century and the 2001 Caries Consensus Conference reported that diet could only explain a relatively small percentage of caries risk because of the introduction and widespread use of fluoride toothpastes (47–49). Konig and Navia (50) provided four inherent limitations in quantifying the relationship between dietary sources of sugars and dental caries: (a) variability in sugar consumption patterns that alters duration of exposure of the teeth to the sugars; (b) the lack of specificity provided by diet recalls or food diaries, which only approximate a self-reported intake of actual sugars and eating patterns; (c) the finding that sugar intake patterns can be calculated annually, but caries formation can take several years; and (d) other factors, including fluoride, calcium, and phosphorus in the diet, along with oral hygiene habits and education level, all of which influence caries risk (50).

Results of the 2001 National Institutes of Health Consensus Development Conference on Caries at which 69 studies on diet and caries published between 1980 and 2000 were reviewed showed that only two found a strong diet-caries relationship, 16 showed a moderate relationship, and 18 showed a weak relationship (49). The authors did not differentiate between sugars consumed as sucrose and other monosaccharides and disaccharides; these authors concluded that diets that promote coronal caries also promote root caries. The authors emphasized that the reviewed studies differ from sugar-caries studies published in the decades before fluoride. Although the papers reviewed indicated a decline in caries risk in relation to sugar intake, they attributed the relative drop to fluoride use. The evidence for the diet-caries relationship is clear in their conclusion that "sugar consumption is likely to be a more powerful indicator for risk of caries infection in persons that don't have regular exposure to fluoride" (49).

As the per capita consumption of sucrose increased in England and the United States in the last 100 years, the prevalence of caries rose. Since the later part of the twentieth century, sugar intake by adults and children has increased considerably; per capita consumption of added sugars increased 23% from 1970 to 1999 (43, 51). Added sugars intake increased in the period from 1989 to 1991 to the period from 1994 to 1996, an increase from 13.2 to 15.8% of total energy intake (52). In 2000, the most frequently reported source of added sugars in the US diet was from nondiet soft drinks, accounting for up to one third of the intake of sugars (53, 54).

In rodents, monkeys, and humans, the presence of sucrose in the mouth increases the volume and rate of plaque formation. Sucrose has a unique role in permitting bacteria to colonize on the teeth. When high concentrations of sucrose are present, *Streptococcus mutans* is able to produce extracellular polysaccharides, glucans, which form an organic matrix on the tooth. These insoluble, sticky polymers permit bacterial colonies to adhere to the tooth. In addition to glucans, *S. mutans* produces intracellular polysaccharides, primarily fructans, from sucrose that are stored and used in glycolysis when dietary carbohydrates are unavailable.

The critical concentration of carbohydrate in a food that will cause human caries is unknown; however, foods with 15% sugars by weight are considered high-sugar foods. In animals, caries scores increase as the sugar content increases (55). The Hopewood House Study showed that children eating diets containing complex carbohydrates but few refined sugars had low caries increments (56). In a longitudinal study of school children in England where the fluoride level in the drinking water was low, the relationship of sugar intake to caries increment was examined; the highest significant correlation was between grams of sugar eaten daily and caries experience (57).

The other monosaccharides and disaccharides—glucose, fructose, maltose, and lactose—found in fruits, dairy products, and processed foods are also readily used by oral microorganisms. These sugars diffuse rapidly through dental plaque to become available for bacterial fermentation. Within a few minutes of ingestion, fructose and glucose cause falls in plaque pH similar to sucrose; thus, they are considered as cariogenic as sucrose.

When eaten with meals, citrus fresh fruits are of low cariogenic potential. This is attributed to the high water content and the presence of citric acid, which stimulates saliva secretion. Fresh fruits vary in sucrose content from 10 to 15% by weight in apples, bananas, and some grapes, 7 to 8% in citrus fruits, to 2% in berries, cherries, and pears. Foods of high acid content may prevent bacterial fermentation but cause enamel erosion.

Sugars in solution have been considered less harmful to teeth than solid sweets because beverages clear the mouth quickly. In the 1940s, however, Stephan showed that a 10% glucose rinse lowered the plaque pH to less than 5.5 (58). The total amount of sugars in carbonated beverages, fruit drinks, and fruit juices is about 10%, and sport drinks contain about 4.4% total sugars. Based on sugar content, acidity, and changes in plaque pH after rinsing with these beverages, all of them appear to have similar cariogenic potential (59). Analysis of dental data from 1971 to 1974 (NHANES I) showed that frequent between meal intake of sweetened beverages was associated with increased caries (60). Teenagers and young adults who used sugar-sweetened soft drinks three or more times between meals on a daily basis increased their odds of having a high DMFT score by 179%. Since that time, food manufacturers have replaced some of the sucrose in beverages with high-fructose corn syrup, saccharin, or aspartame. Whether beverages formulated with high-fructose corn syrup are less cariogenic is unknown. Substitution of sport drinks or ion drinks for carbonated beverages or fruit drinks was associated with decalcification of Japanese children's teeth (61). Most of these drinks have a pH lower than 4. Slowly drinking sugar-sweetened tea or coffee can

also lead to enamel dissolution. The use of sugar-based liquid oral medication may affect the oral health of chronically sick children. English children taking long-term liquid oral medicine had significantly more caries of deciduous anterior teeth than their siblings (62).

Sugar alcohols notably seen in sugar-free gums and beverages can have a positive impact on caries risk. Examples include sorbitol, xyitol, mannitol, erythritol, and isomalt. Sugar-free gums with these polyols serve to stimulate saliva, thereby speeding clearance of fermentable carbohydrates from the oral cavity and serving as an oral buffer. Chewing sugar-free gum following meals and snacks when brushing is not possible is a reasonable caries risk-reduction measure.

Xylitol, a five-carbon sugar alcohol, has been used in Canada, Asia, and Europe to replace sucrose in candies, gum, and medicines much longer than in the United States, where it is approved for use in special dietary products by the Food and Drug Administration. Ingestion of solutions of xylitol does not cause a drop in plaque pH because oral bacteria lack the enzymes to ferment xylitol to organic acids. A 2-year clinical trial in Finland showed that young adults using foods sweetened solely with xylitol developed no new caries, whereas groups assigned to fructose and sucrose developed caries (63). Xylitol also appears to have an antimicrobial affect, causing increased buffer activity with a subsequent rise in pH and enhancing remineralization (64). A major deterrent to widespread use of xylitol in the United States has been its high cost. It is used in some sugarless gums and candies but not typically as the sole sweetner, most often in combination with sorbitol and mannitol.

Saccharin, found in beverages, dietetic foods, dentifrices, and as a table sweetener for diabetics, inhibits tooth decay in rats. Low caries scores and low recoveries of *S. mutans* resulted when rats were challenged with a cariogenic diet supplemented with saccharin (65). The effects of saccharin on human oral bacteria have not been reported. Aspartame does not support the growth of *S. mutans*, acid production in the mouth, or plaque formation. Frequent rinsing with aspartame was no more cariogenic in rats than distilled water (66). Because soft drinks are a popular cariogenic snack, the use of aspartame in these beverages is safer for teeth.

Frequent use of chewing gum sweetened with xylitol or xylitol/sorbitol mixtures causes significant reductions in dental plaque as well as plaque and saliva levels of *S. mutans* (67, 68). Gum chewing stimulates salivary flow and pushes saliva into the interproximal area, where salivary buffers can neutralize bacterial acids. Chewing also removes food particles from plaque and the soft tissues. The net result is that the stimulation of salivary flow caused by the physical act of chewing, coupled with the helpful effects of a noncaloric sweetener, can be beneficial to dental health by "neutralizing" the plaque bacteria's acid response to fermentable carbohydrate-containing foods.

The effect of starch-containing foods on teeth is dependent on the form, whether the starch is raw or cooked, and on whether sucrose is present. Because starch is a large molecule, it cannot diffuse through dental plaque. When cereal grains are refined in the production of breads or crackers and are cooked, however, they are more easily hydrolyzed by salivary and plaque amylases. Fermentation of the resulting sugar, maltose, yields acids that demineralize enamel rapidly. Mixtures of starches and sugars in ready-to-eat breakfast cereals, bread, pastries, and many convenience foods are often retained longer in the interproximal plaque than high-sugar foods. This may make heated sugar-starch combinations more cariogenic than sugar alone (69, 70). Foods previously thought to be of low cariogenicity, such as breads, muffins, crackers, and chips, are no longer considered safe for teeth especially when they are eaten between meals, because of their retentive properties and their ability to act as substrate for plaque microbial fermentation.

Factors Affecting Cariogenicity

Sugar and starches are not the only factors that determine the cariogenic potential of a food. Frequency of intake, clearance time from the oral cavity, nutrient composition, acid content and position of a food in the meal are also important.

In rats, the intervals between eating snacks and meals have a profound effect on the number of S. mutans bacteria in plaque and the number of cavities formed. Little caries develops in rats fed a cariogenic diet two or three times a day. As the frequency of sugar and starch exposures increases, the caries risk increases. The more often fermentable carbohydrates are consumed, the more often plaque pH will fall to acidic levels; given that pH drops can last as long as 30 minutes after each "insult," the risk of demineralization rises considerably the more often one eats.

The sequence of eating foods in a meal affects the magnitude of a drop in plaque pH. If a piece of aged cheese is eaten following an acidogenic food such as canned pears in syrup, the plaque pH will rise above the danger zone immediately (71). The pH drop in response to sugared coffee will be rapid but will rise if followed by an unsweetened food. If sugared coffee is drunk at the end of a meal, however, a prolonged drop in plaque pH will occur. By placing acidogenic items between other foods, the risk of demineralization is lessened.

Clearance time of foods and fluids from the oral cavity likewise affects caries risk. Clearance time is based on several factors inherent in the individual person as well as the food or fluid. Beverages clear rapidly from the oral cavity. In contrast, clearance time of solids varies, depending on their retentiveness in the mouth. Stickiness is not synonymous with retentiveness; marshmallows or jellies are sticky; however, their retentive properties are low, so they

are cleared from the mouth more quickly than refined starches such as cookies, cakes, and chips. The quantity of glucose in the oral cavity is greater initially with "sticky" foods such as marshmallows and jellies but is cleared more rapidly than the glucose produced by refined grains, which first requires breakdown of the starches by salivary amylase. Kashket and colleagues demonstrated these principles; his research explores the salivary clearance rates of high-starch and high-sugar foods (72, 73).

Nutrient composition and acidity of the foods and fluids also affect caries risk. Food components can have two protective effects on tooth enamel. Some foods decrease the solubility of enamel (demineralization), and other foods stimulate salivary secretion or remineralization of tooth enamel. Substances that make the enamel less soluble include fluoride in tea, an unidentified factor in cocoa, phytate, oxalate, and proteins in milk. The impact of cheese is discussed later. Pairing of high-acid food or cariogenic foods with calcium-rich dairy products that are more alkaline provides a dietary buffering system, reducing the cariogenic risk of the combined foods because a low-pH food is paired with a high-pH food. Another example is combining refined starch and sugar-containing cereals with milk, a high-pH food, to attenuate the cariogenic risk of the meal.

Cheese seems to prevent demineralization and to promote remineralization (74). Some speculation exists that a protective pH rise factor is present, but it has yet to be identified. More than 21 aged cheeses have been identified that do not cause the plaque pH to fall (75). The protective properties of these cheeses are attributed to their texture, which increase salivary secretion rate, and their protein, calcium, and phosphorus, content which neutralizes plaque acids. The data of cheese and dental caries have recently been reviewed by DePaola and Kashket (76).

Although sugar-containing foods that are acidic such as sports drinks, fruit juices, and fruits can serve as fermentable carbohydrates, acidic foods, by nature of their low pH, can also increase caries risk. Any food or beverage with a pH lower than 5.5 (the critical pH for dissolution of enamel) increases risk of tooth erosion. However, the level of risk of erosion of such products depends on the availability of food buffers eaten with the acidic food and the buffer systems in the oral cavity. In healthy persons with an adequate quantity and quality of saliva and good oral hygiene practices, acidic foods or fluids are not a significant risk factor when they are consumed as part of a healthy diet. However, vitamin C in hard candy or chewable form will cause a drop in pH because of the citric acid in the product (77). Product labels should be read cautiously to look for sources of sugar as well as acids that can increase the erosive potential of the saliva. Patients typically consume vitamin C candies or chewables when they have a cold and may be concurrently taking cold medicines that can reduce salivary flow. The combined impact of increased acid and reduced saliva increases risk of tooth erosion.

Saliva and protective components in foods modify the effect of fermentable carbohydrates on the teeth (78). The importance of saliva in caries prevention is perhaps best demonstrated by the rampant caries that develop in xerostomic patients. Saliva flow is stimulated by mastication of foods, by citric acid in fruits, and by sugars. The composition of saliva is also influenced by dietary components.

Four protective mechanisms of saliva are important in preventing caries. First, saliva prevents the aggregation of bacteria on the tooth's surface and speeds the clearance of food particles and sugars from the mouth. A second mechanism is the buffering action of proteins, bicarbonates, and phosphates in saliva that dilute and neutralize plaque acids. Third, immunoglobulins present in saliva protect the teeth by depressing bacterial activity. Finally, the presence of calcium, phosphate, and fluoride ions in saliva promotes the remineralization of tooth enamel.

In summary, the relationships between diet and dental caries is dynamic; fluoride is the primary public health preventive measure to prevent dental caries. Diet is the primary public health measure from a nutrition perspective, with a focus on seven key dietary recommendations (79):

1. Combine a balanced diet with good oral hygiene, to maximize oral and systemic health and to reduce risk of caries.
2. Combine foods to reduce risk of caries, including dairy products with fermentable carbohydrates and other sugars at meals rather than between meals; drink sweetened and acidic beverages with meals rather than between meals.
3. Chew sugarless gums (particularly those with sugar alcohols) and eat dairy products such as cheese after consumption of fermentable carbohydrates.
4. Chew sugarless gums between meals.
5. Drink, rather than sip, sweetened or acidic beverages.
6. Moderate eating frequency of fermentable carbohydrates to reduce repeated exposures to acids, sugars, and other fermentable carbohydrates.
7. Avoid giving an infant or child a bottle of milk, juice, or other acidic or sugar-containing beverage while the child is in bed.

Measuring the Cariogenic Potential of Human Food

The measurement of plaque acidogenicity is recognized as a valid indirect technique for determining the cariogenic potential of foods in humans. The results of three indirect types of tests (79), when taken together on a variety of commonly consumed foods, reveal that the foods with high cariogenic potential are those high in fermentable carbohydrate content, that are eaten frequently, and that adhere to the teeth (80). Tests also demonstrated that the following foods cause the pH at interproximal sites to fall to less than pH 5.5, a finding implying that, if they are ingested frequently, the risk of caries will substantially increase: dried fruits, breads, cereals, cookies, snack crackers, and potato chips (81). Generally, the more processing a food undergoes, the greater its cariogenicity. Foods that are noncariogenic (do not drop the plaque pH to <5.5) include some vegetables, meats, fish, aged cheeses, and nuts. These tests are useful predictors of cariogenicity, but additional factors will determine whether caries actually develops. These factors include the following: host susceptibility, virulence of the oral bacteria, how frequently a food is eaten, the sequence in which foods are eaten in a meal, and the interaction between foods eaten concurrently.

In addition to the continuing concern regarding food cariogenicity and caries prevalence and experience in the physiologically normal population, two other specific groups have been targeted as high-risk groups, primarily because of eating and social behavioral patterns. These two groups are the infant/toddler at risk of early childhood caries and the elderly, at risk of developing root surface caries.

Root Caries

Dietary factors are important in the initiation and progression of root caries. When gingival tissues recede, the root surfaces of teeth are exposed to the oral environment. Because roots lack the protective enamel layer, they are highly susceptible to dental caries. Root caries lesions are primarily a disease of older adults. In the NHANES III survey, root surface lesions were found in 54% of men and in 41% of women 65 to 74 years of age. The mean number of decayed and filled root surfaces for 65 to 74 year olds was 2.2 (82). About 60% of the lesions had been restored. Older adults at greatest risk of developing root caries include persons with coronal caries, gingival recession, low saliva flow, low fluoride exposure, and frequent intake of fermentable carbohydrates.

High levels of S. mutans are found in adults with root caries (83). Examination of ancient skulls and dentition of members of primitive societies revealed that root caries was more common than coronal caries. Because these groups consumed starches but not refined sugars, complex carbohydrates are implicated in the development of root caries. Adults who have periodontitis or have had periodontal surgery resulting in exposed root surfaces frequently develop root caries if their intake of fermentable carbohydrates is high (84). A high sugar intake is positively associated with root caries, and a high cheese intake is negatively associated with root caries (85, 86). In a cross-sectional study of healthy, free-living elderly persons, a high daily intake of liquid-solid and sticky, slow-dissolving fermentable foods such as ice cream, gelatin, hard candies, and antacids was positively correlated with root caries (87).

In a 2-year longitudinal study of elderly Bostonians, subjects in the highest quintile for root caries had significantly higher intakes of sweetened liquids, solid fermentable carbohydrates, and starches than subjects who were free of root caries (88). Adults who were free of root caries ate 50% more cheese and 25% more milk than persons with caries. Because root caries develop more rapidly than coronal caries, preventive measures are critical. Nutrition counseling, home oral care, and fluoride therapy should be provided to older adults with gingival recession. Thus, the dietary origin of root caries seems to be similar to that of coronal caries.

Early Childhood Caries

Severe tooth decay in infants and toddlers is a preventable disease associated with inappropriate feeding practices. Early childhood caries, often referred to as nursing caries or baby bottle tooth decay, occurs between 1 and 3 years of age, develops rapidly, and can cause severe dental pain and infection. The prevalence of early childhood caries in the United States is estimated to be between 1 and 12%. However, much higher prevalence rates have been reported among Hispanic, Southeast Asian, inner-city, and Native American/Alaska Native children (>50%) (89).

Children with nursing caries are at greater risk of developing additional caries in the primary and permanent teeth than children who are caries free (90). Initially, the smooth surfaces of the four primary maxillary incisor teeth are involved, and later, decalcification of the maxillary and mandibular molars and canines occurs (91). The tongue protects the lower anterior four incisors. First, white spot lesions develop on the gingival third of the maxillary front teeth; this stage often goes undetected by parents. Within 6 months, these lesions may progress to a dull white band of demineralization rapidly developing along the gum line of the upper incisors. If the disease advances further, a brown or black collar encircles the necks of the teeth. The four maxillary incisors may be completely destroyed, so only brownish root stumps remain. When nursing caries progresses to the development of abscesses, the abscesses may affect the underlying developing permanent dentition. Restoration of severe caries is expensive and emotionally traumatic for parents and children. The young child must often be treated using general anesthesia. Loss of incisors alters the arch dimension, affects appearance and speech, and may have a psychologic impact on the child.

Early childhood caries results from the interaction of pathogenic oral microorganisms, fermentable carbohydrates, and susceptible teeth. S. mutans is not part of the indigenous flora of the oral cavity at birth. When the deciduous teeth erupt at about 6 months of age, bacterial colonies begin to form in the mouth. S. mutans is believed to be transmitted to infants by caregivers. If mothers have high levels of S. mutans, their infants are at greater risk of having elevated levels of these cariogenic organisms in their plaque (92). Early malnutrition may increase a tooth's susceptibility to caries.

Early decay of the primary dentition may result from use of a nursing bottle at naptime and/or bedtime that contains milk, fruit juice, or another sweetened solution. When a child habitually falls asleep with a bottle in his or her mouth, sweetened liquids pool around the teeth and leads to demineralization of the enamel. The same pattern of dental decay may result from ad libitum breast-feeding (93). Breast-fed infants with rampant decay have reportedly been allowed to sleep with the mother and remain on the breast for long periods of time. During sleep, the protective action of saliva is greatly reduced by diminished flow rates. Severity of the disease is linked to the number of decay-causing bacteria present in the oral cavity, the number of feedings per day, and duration of bottle or breast-feeding.

To prevent early childhood caries, education must occur before a child's primary teeth erupt. All caregivers—parents, grandparents, and day-care workers—must be counseled about the recommended feeding practices with the baby bottle. Nap or nighttime bottle feeding in bed should be discouraged. If a bedtime bottle is offered, the only safe liquid is water. Parents should be encouraged to offer juices from a cup after 6 months of age. Allowing breast-fed infants to sleep with the nipple in the mouth during the night should be avoided after the first primary tooth begins to erupt. Infants should be removed from the breast when they fall asleep. Children should be weaned from the bottle by 12 months of age. One-to-one counseling with caretakers of infants and community-wide education programs have been successful in reducing baby bottle tooth decay among southwestern Native American children (94). The American Academy of Pediatric Dentistry recommends that infants visit a dentist within 6 months after the first tooth erupts in the mouth.

FLUORIDE

The decline in coronal caries in industrialized countries in the past 50 years is attributed primarily to the widespread use of fluorides. This mineral is universally present in nature; trace amounts are found in soils, water, plants, and foodstuffs. Currently, the primary sources of fluoride for humans are community water supplies, foods, beverages, dentifrices, and other dental products. The ionic fluoride ingested in water has a systemic effect before tooth eruption and a topical effect after eruption. Dietary fluoride supplements are prescribed for children when fluoride is lacking in the water supply. Professionally applied topical applications of fluoride in higher concentrations are used to protect erupted teeth and are not swallowed. The preventive benefits of fluoride depend on the concentration of fluoride used, whether it is given systematically or topically, and the type of agent used, whether in water, tablet, drops, a rinse, or a gel. The caries-preventive properties of systemic and topical fluoride are additive. Fluoride is more effective in the prevention of smooth surface caries than occlusal caries.

Mechanisms of Action

Although the cariostatic properties of fluoride are widely recognized, the mechanisms of action of fluoride in the oral environment are not fully understood. At least three mechanisms are recognized (95). First, fluoride ions replace some of the hydroxyl groups of the hydroxyapatite in developing teeth to form fluoridated hydroxyapatite. This increases the stability of the enamel crystals because fluoridated hydroxyapatite is less soluble to organic acids than hydroxyapatite. Fluoride uptake by calcified tissues is extremely high (90%) in infancy but decreases with age. Second, low concentrations of fluoride in the saliva can decrease the rate of demineralization and enhance remineralization of early carious lesions. When enamel is partially demineralized by organic acids, calcium, phosphate, and fluoride from the tooth can diffuse back into the surface layers of enamel and accelerate recrystallization. Third, fluoride has direct effects on the acidogenic plaque bacteria. In higher concentrations, fluoride inhibits growth of S. *mutans* found in dental plaque, and in low concentrations inhibit bacterial enzymes, thus reducing acid production from catabolism of fermentable carbohydrates.

Water Fluoridation

Fluoridation of community water supplies is the most effective method of providing fluoride to large populations. Through extensive epidemiologic studies of communities with naturally fluoridated water in the United States in the 1930s, the protective properties of fluoride in the prevention of dental caries were fully recognized (96). In 21 US cities, an inverse relationship was shown between caries prevalence in children and the fluoride content of the drinking at an optimal range (Fig. 72.5).

In 1945, Grand Rapids, Michigan, became the first city in the world to fluoridate their drinking water. Between 1950 and 1980, clinical studies conducted in 20 countries showed that adding fluoride to community water supplies resulted in a 40 to 50% caries reduction in primary teeth and a 50 to 60% reduction in dental caries in permanent teeth (97). Comparisons of caries in US children who had always lived in optimally fluoridated communities with children never exposed to fluoridated drinking water revealed 25% lower DMFS scores in the fluoridated group (98). The decline in caries prevalence among children living in communities with nonfluoridated water is attributed to intake of foods and beverages processed with fluoridated water, the use of fluoride-containing dentrifices, and the use of topical fluorides in the dental office and at home. Adults also experience benefits from the consumption of fluoridated water. The prevalence of coronal and root caries seems to be 20 to 30% lower in adults living in optimally fluoridated communities than in adults residing in cities with lower levels of fluoride in the water supply (99).

According to the US Public Health Service, the desirable fluoride concentration for dental caries prevention is about one part per million (0.7–1.2 ppm, based on climactic temperature). By 1990, 42 of the 50 largest cities in the United States had fluoridated their water supplies. In 1992, in the United States, approximately 144 million people, or 62% of the population on public water supplies, drink water with 0.7 ppm or higher levels of fluoride. This includes 9 million people who drink water with natural fluoride at optimal levels. Continuous exposure to fluoride is desirable. In communities where water fluoridation has been interrupted or eliminated, a significant increase in dental caries has been observed (100). In fact, the US Centers for Disease Control and Prevention have identified water fluoridation as one of the nations top ten disease-prevention efforts ever developed.

Water fluoridation is the most cost-effective method of preventing tooth decay in the United States. The current average cost for delivering fluoride in the drinking water is less than a dollar per person per year. Even though scientists, health professionals, and the courts generally agree that community water fluoridation is safe, effective, economical, and legally valid, some members of the public remain confused about fluoride's safety. Opponents to fluoridation have attempted to link it to AIDS, Alzheimer disease, and cancer, but they have provided no scientific evidence to support their claims. More than 50 epidemiologic studies have demonstrated no association between water fluoride and the risk of cancer. In addition, animal studies have failed to establish a relationship between fluoride and cancer (95).

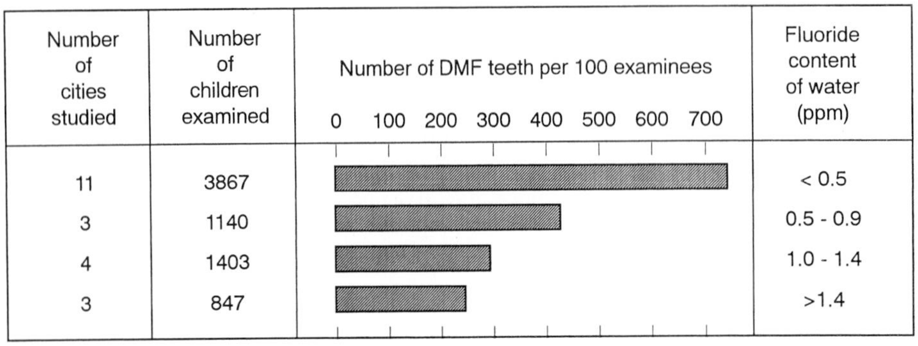

Number of cities studied	Number of children examined	Number of DMF teeth per 100 examinees	Fluoride content of water (ppm)
11	3867		< 0.5
3	1140		0.5 - 0.9
4	1403		1.0 - 1.4
3	847		>1.4

Figure 72.5. The relationship between caries prevalence and fluoride content of drinking water in 21 cities. (From Newbrun E. Fluorides and Dental Caries. 3rd ed. Springfield, IL: Charles C Thomas 1986, with permission.)

TABLE 72.4. SUPPLEMENTAL FLUORIDE DOSAGE SCHEDULE (mg/dª) ACCORDING TO FLUORIDE CONCENTRATION OF DRINKING WATER

CONCENTRATION OF FLUORIDE IN DRINKING WATER (ppm)

AGE	<0.3	0.3–0.6	>0.6
6 mo–2 y	0.25 mg	0	0
3–6 y	0.50 mg	0.25 mg	0
6–16 y	1.00 mg	0.50 mg	0

ppm, parts permission.
ª2.2 mg sodium fluoride contain 1 mg fluoride.

From ADA Council on Access, Prevention, and Interpersonal Relations. J Am Dent Assoc 1995;126:19S, with permission.

Dietary Supplementation

Children living in cities and rural areas with suboptimal water fluoridation can receive the caries-preventive benefits of fluoride by taking a prescribed fluoride supplement. When children are given fluoride drops or tablets daily from 6 months of age through the early teenage years, a low prevalence of caries is found. The level of dietary supplementation is determined by the age of the child and the concentration of fluoride in the water supply. Well water should be tested for fluoride concentration by the local authorities. Table 72.4 presents the recommended levels of daily fluoride supplementation as approved by the American Dental Association (ADA) Council on Scientific Affairs and the American Academy of Pediatrics. No fluoride supplementation is recommended in areas where the drinking water contains 0.6 ppm fluoride or greater. For those consuming water with less than 0.30 ppm fluoride, 1 mg of fluoride is not recommended until the age of 6 years. The upper limit of fluoride intake appears to be 0.05 mg/kg of body weight. Future dosage schedules may be based on body weight rather than age.

Liquid fluoride supplements (drops) are recommended for infants and young children. A list of accepted fluoride supplements is published regularly by the ADA Council on Scientific Affairs (101). Fluoride-vitamin supplements are not recommended by the ADA because, when vitamins are discontinued, the use of fluorides may cease. Few healthy, full-term, formula-fed infants require a vitamin-mineral supplement. The fluoride present when commercial formula is diluted with fluoridated water is 95 to 100% available. If infant formula is prepared with nonfluoridated water, however, fluoride drops should be prescribed. The fluoride concentration of breast milk and cow's milk is very low (0.1 ppm).

For older children, fluoride tablets are available in the following doses: 0.25 mg F, 0.5 mg F, or 1 mg F. Tablets are formulated with neutral sodium fluoride or acidulated phosphate fluoride (APF). The caries-preventive effects of neutral fluoride tablets are similar to those of APF tablets. Chewable fluoride tablets seem to have topical as well as systemic benefits.

Other countries have incorporated fluoride into the food supply by fluoridating salt, milk, flour, or sugar. If community water fluoridation is impractical, these foods appear to be possible vehicles for fluoride. Unfortunately, individual intake of these foods varies widely, so formulating a dosage regimen is difficult.

Primary tooth development begins before birth; therefore, the efficacy of prenatal fluoride supplementation is of interest. During pregnancy, fluoride diffuses across the placental barrier and is incorporated into fetal bones and teeth. The concentration of fluoride in fetal blood appears to be about 25% of that of maternal blood (102). Although prenatal supplements are considered safe for the mother and fetus, the benefits of supplementation in reducing caries are unproven. Dental caries rates of children whose mothers received fluoride supplements during pregnancy were not significantly different at 3 and 5 years of age than in children whose mothers did not receive prenatal fluoride supplements (103). Both groups lived in cities lacking fluoridation of the water supply.

Dental Fluorosis

Fluorosis is characterized by white opaque flecks, white or brown staining, or, in severe cases, pitting of the tooth enamel. Because the crowns of all permanent teeth form between birth and 14 years of age, the effects of excess systemic fluoride are limited to this age group. The most critical time for developing fluorosis appears to be the first or second year of life, when maturation of upper anterior permanent teeth enamel occurs and the daily fluoride ingestion is greater than 2 ppm (104). Fewer than 2% of school children in the 1986 to 1987 NIDR survey had moderate to severe fluorosis (105). An increase in the prevalence of mild or very mild dental fluorosis is observed more often in fluoridated than nonfluoridated communities (Fig. 72.6). This is primarily a cosmetic problem and does not increase the teeth's susceptibility to caries.

Exposure to multiple sources of fluoride increases a child's risk of developing fluorosis (106, 107). More than two thirds of fluorosis cases can be explained by inappropriate use of fluoride supplements and use of more than the recommended amount of toothpaste (106). If a child is receiving optimal amounts of fluoride from dietary sources or fluoridated water and swallows large amounts of dentifrice, fluorosis can occur. Nearly all US toothpastes contain fluoride, which is readily absorbed when ingested. Toothpaste is generally swallowed rather than expectorated by children younger than 6 years of age. Therefore, parents should dispense a pea-sized amount of toothpaste for young children, to prevent excess intake of fluoride.

Substantial amounts of fluoride can be introduced into the infant's diet through food processing. In the 1970s, it was discovered that infant formulas contained variable and often

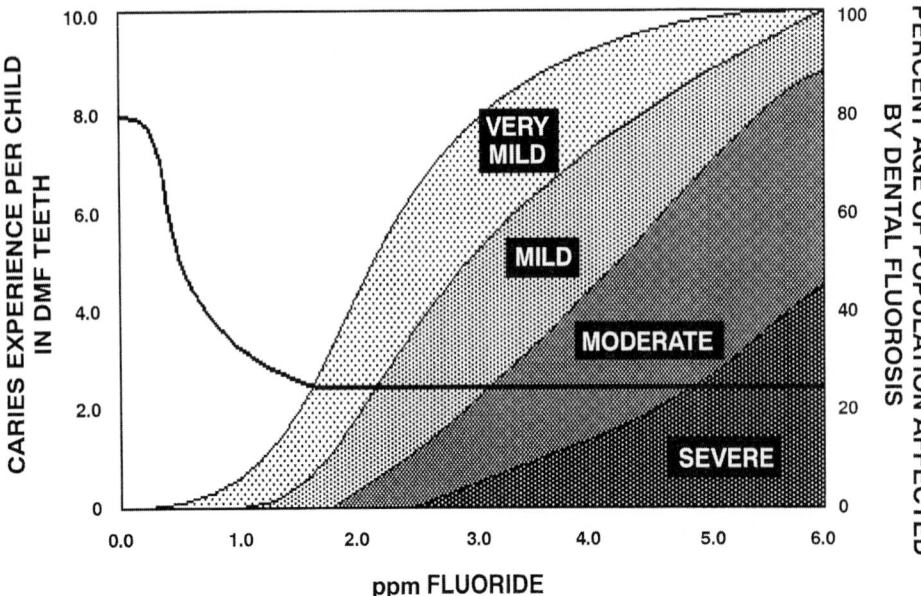

Figure 72.6. Prevalence of dental caries and dental fluorosis in relation to fluoride in drinking water. (From US Department of Health and Human Services, Public Health Service. Review of Fluoride Benefits and Risks, Report of the Ad Hoc Subcommittee on Fluoride of the Committee to Coordinate Environmental Health and Related Programs. Washington, DC: US Government Printing Office, 1991.)

high levels of fluoride. To reduce the risk of infants' receiving too much fluoride, beginning in 1979, infant formula manufacturers voluntarily reduced the amount of fluoride in formulas. Soy-based formulas appear to have higher fluoride levels than milk-based formulas because the soy products contain components that bind fluoride. Ready-to-feed infant fruit juices, tea, fish, dried seafood products, and chicken products can contain high levels of fluoride. Continued monitoring of the fluoride content of a "market basket" of infant and toddler foods in the United States is needed to ensure that fluoride intake remains within safe limits.

EFFECT OF NUTRITION ON ORAL SOFT TISSUES

The integrity of the teeth, oral mucosa, and tongue may be compromised by nutrient deficiencies and excesses, local oral diseases, and oral manifestations of systemic diseases, as discussed in subsequent sections of this chapter. Clinicians must be adept at combining physical examination factors with a comprehensive diet and nutrition history as well as medical and medication history to determine possible causes of oral lesions and other alterations in the integrity of the oral mucosa or tongue. Although it is not the primary role of nondentist practitioners to diagnose oral diseases, it is incumbent on these professionals to screen for and detect abnormal conditions and to refer patients appropriately to dentists for comprehensive care.

Oral screening for nutritional deficits and excesses can be easily done by dietetic, medical, nursing, and other health professionals (108, 109). An intraoral and extraoral screen should identify existing or potential problems with one or more of the following:

1. Oral manifestations of a nutritional disorder.
2. Oral manifestations of a systemic disease that affects diet and nutritional status such as diabetes.

3. Local oral conditions interfering with ingestion, mastication, swallowing ability, taste, and saliva.
4. Dietary influences on the oral cavity and their contributions to oral diseases (109, 110).

Once any or all of these finding are determined, the professional should consult with and refer patients to general dentists or appropriate dental specialists for diagnosis and care as well as provide appropriate diet intervention and nutritional care.

NUTRIENT DEFICIENCIES

The oral mucosa is particularly susceptible to physiologic or anatomic changes resulting from nutritional deficit or toxicity. Because the turnover rate of oral mucosal cells is relatively rapid (gingival sulcular epithelial cells have a turnover rate of 3 to 7 days), sufficient nutrients must be available at the appropriate times and in the correct concentration for DNA replication, protein synthesis, and cell and tissue maturation to occur. The oral epithelium acts as an effective barrier against the invasion of toxic substances, particularly antigens derived from oral microbes, into the underlying collagenous connective tissue. Inadequate nutrition can cause the oral epithelia to either break down or to be compromised, thus increasing the tissue's susceptibility to infectious disease.

For these reasons, the oral cavity is one of the first regions of the body to exhibit clinical signs of nutrient deficits and malnutrition. Virtually every classic nutrition deficiency or toxicity, including scurvy, beriberi, and pellagra, has signs and symptoms in the oral cavity and surrounding structures. The lips, tongue, oral mucosa, and gingiva may all reflect nutritional aberrations long before signs are apparent elsewhere in the body (Table 72.5).

TABLE 72.5. NUTRITION RISK FACTORS TO CONSIDER IN PHYSICAL EXAMINATION

BODY AREA	NUTRITION RISK SYMPTOMS	NUTRITION IMPLICATIONS
Hair	Dull, shedding, easily pluckable	Generalized protein calorie malnutrition
Face	a. Malar pigmentation (dark skin over cheeks and under eyes) Bitemporal wasting	Niacin, B vitamins, malnutrition
	b. Nasolabial seborrhea	Niacin, riboflavin, vitamin B_6
	c. Edematous	Protein deficiency
	d. Moon face	Corticosteroid impact
	e. Lack of color	Inadequate iron, undernutrition
Eyes	Pale eye membranes	Inadequate iron
	Bitot spots, conjunctival xerosis, keratomalacia, corneal xerosis	Inadequate vitamin A
Lips	Cheilosis (red/swelling)	Inadequate niacin, riboflavin
	Angular fissures	Inadequate niacin, vitamin B_6, riboflavin, iron
Gingiva	Spongy, bleeding, abnormal redness	Inadequate vitamin C
Tongue	a. Glossitis (red, raw, fissured)	Inadequate folate, niacin, riboflavin, iron, vitamins B_6 and B_{12}
	b. Pale, atrophic, smooth/slick (filiform papillary atrophy)	Inadequate iron, vitamin B_{12}, niacin, folate
	c. Magenta color	Inadequate riboflavin
Nails	Spoon shaped, brittle, ridged	Inadequate iron
Back muscles	Bony prominences along shoulder girdle Tendons prominent to palpation	Malnutrition

From Touger-Decker R. Clinical and laboratory assessment of nutrition status. Dent Clin North Am 2003:47:259–78, with permission.

Nutritionally induced oral changes may include anatomic lesions, color changes, functional changes (e.g., burning mouth and tongue), textural changes, and inflammation of the lips, oral mucosa, corners of the mouth, tongue, and gingiva (111).

For example, the dorsum of the tongue may undergo changes in size or color, and taste changes may result from atrophy or hypertrophy of tongue papillae. Long-standing nutrient deficiencies may lead to atrophy of the papillae and denudation of the dorsum. A bright red, painful tongue and swelling of the oral mucosa may be early symptoms of pernicious anemia resulting from a lack of vitamin B_{12}. Inflammation, a burning sensation, and tenderness of the tongue or palate may be caused by a deficiency of vitamin B complex, protein, or iron. Burning mouth syndrome has been associated with vitamin B complex deficiencies (112), and vitamin B complex supplementation resolved the symptoms in 85% of subjects. A bright red, inflamed mucosa, from a vitamin B complex deficiency, may be seen in persons with long-term alcoholism. The mucosa may become pale in iron-, folic acid–, or vitamin B_{12}–induced anemias. Atrophy of the filiform papillae of the tongue (glossitis) is a sign of malnutrition usually resulting from multiple nutritional deficiencies. A highly significant positive correlation shown between papillae health and plasma vitamin E status provides some indication that vitamin E may be a marker nutrient for papillary health (113).

In ascorbic acid deficiency, the classic oral signs of scurvy are first seen in the oral cavity and include red swollen interdental papillae that bleed readily and inflamed and swollen marginal and attached gingiva. Although no longer a public health problem, ascorbic acid deficiency may occur most likely secondary to increased losses combined with dietary deficiency. No scientifically sound evidence supports a direct relationship between periodontal disease and ascorbic acid status in any population other than smokers, and even there the evidence is weak. Consumption of ascorbic acid in excess of recommended allowances has not been shown to be associated with increased periodontal health (114).

No clinical sign is of significance by itself, however, because several etiologic factors usually contribute to a differential diagnosis. For example, inflammation or cracking of the lips may be be caused by allergies, licking of the lips, or drooling, as well as by nutritional aberrations. Angular cheilosis can result not only from vitamin deficiencies, but also when overclosure of the jaw in denture wearers allows the skin folds at the corners of the mouth to provide a moist area for bacterial or fungal infections to develop. Table 72.6 provides a functional oral assessment tool that can be used as a broad clinical examination guide for nondentist health providers.

NUTRIENT EXCESSES

Nutrient excesses can also affect the oral cavity. Vitamin A toxicity can impair the proper development of the oral mucosal epithelium and can result in a variety oral changes including delayed wound healing (115). Clinical effects reported in a patient taking 200,000 IU/day of vitamin A for more than 6 months included gingival erosions

TABLE 72.6. FUNCTIONAL ORAL NUTRITION RISK EVALUATION[a]

STRUCTURE	PATIENT-FOCUSED EXAMINATION	MANAGEMENT
Lips	Dryness; sensation; cracking or fissuring, swelling; history of blisters or ulcers	Alter diet texture and consistency
Gingiva and oral mucosa	Soreness/pain; bleeding spontaneously, change in appearance; swelling, growths, discharge; bad taste; halitosis	Alter diet texture, temperature, and consistency
	Red or white patches/lesions	Screen for oral cancer, nutrient deficiencies
	Erosion/ulceration; focal pigmentation; erythema	
Teeth	Toothache/pain; looseness and mobility; dental prosthesis (removable or fixed);edentulism	Adjust diet, consistency; evaluate caries risk; consider altered taste/smell
Tongue	Soreness/pain; burning; rough patches; dryness; cracking or fissuring; growths; changes in taste; ulcers	Screen for systematic disease, nutrient deficiencies; alter diet texture
Temporomandibular joint	Difficulty or painful opening; grinding sounds on joint opening/chewing with limited range or pain; weakness of chewing muscles	Change diet consistency, food "hardness"; limit "chewy" foods
Salivary glands	Mucosal dryness; too little or too much saliva; drooling; change in color, consistency, difficulty swallowing dry food, altered taste, dry eyes; gland pain or swelling	Increase fluids; evaluate for dysgeusia, dysphagia; limit spices, "hard" foods; review changes in prescriptions; evaluate zinc status
Neck	Tender/swollen lymph nodes, other swellings	Medical consultation
Skin	Change in appearances; rashes, sores, lumps, itching	Medical consultation

[a] For each section, ask about patient complaints, duration of symptoms, and any changes in appearance, size, acuity, frequency, and pain.

From Touger-Decker R, Sirois D. Approaches to oral nutrition health risk assessment. In: Touger-Decker R, Sirois DA, Mobley CC, eds. Nutrition and Oral Medicine. Totowa, NJ: Humana Press, 2005, with permission.

and ulcerations, bleeding, swelling, loss of keratinization, and color changes in the oral cavity, along with desquamation of the lips and dry mouth. Two months after withdrawal of the supplementation, all clinical manifestations had disappeared (116).

Rebound scurvy is a condition in which scurvy develops as an adaptation result of fast withdrawal after chronic high intake levels of vitamin C in animals (117). Its existence in human populations has been questioned (118), but some supportive evidence exists (119), which has been reported clinically in patients who abruptly terminated a habit of megadosing on vitamin C. The resulting scurvy is again, first manifested in the oral cavity and diagnosed by the dental professional.

PERIODONTAL DISEASE

Periodontal disease is a general term describing bacterial infection of either the gingiva (that part of the oral mucosa that covers the root and the apical portion of the crown) or both the gingiva and the attachment apparatus (ligamentous attachment of the tooth to the surrounding alveolar bone). If the infection is confined to the gingival unit, the resulting disease is called gingivitis. If the infection involves the destruction of tissue attaching tooth to bone, the disease is termed periodontitis. The two diseases are not a continuum of the same process, but are in fact two separate diseases, each associated with different plaque flora. The cause of gingivitis is relatively simple,

whereas the etiology of periodontitis is extremely complex. Although bacterial plaque is the major etiologic agent in both conditions, other local and systemic factors, many unidentified, play a large role as well.

Most forms of periodontitis result in a slow loss of attachment of the tooth from the surrounding alveolar bone. Although most persons have some degree of mild periodontal disease, severe periodontal destruction is confined to approximately 24% of the adult population (35).

Select disease states increase risk of periodontal disease. Such conditions include diabetes mellitus (types 1 and 2), osteoporosis (discussed in detail in the next section), and smoking. Menopause and pregnancy are also associated with periodontal disease, with the association most likely not nutritional but hormonal. Increasing relationships between periodontal disease and systemic health are emerging with its association with adverse pregnancy outcomes and cardiovascular disease, among other chronic disease links.

The reaction of the periodontal tissues to microbial antigens and byproducts is a classic chronic inflammatory-immune response like that observed in infectious diseases in general. Optimal functioning of the host's cellular and humoral immune system and phagocytic system and the integrity of the oral mucosa (particularly the gingival sulcular epithelium) are important to the maintenance of periodontal health and the prevention of periodontal disease.

Several animal and human studies have demonstrated a positive correlation between nutrient deficits of ascorbic acid, iron, folate, and zinc and the increased permeability or diminished integrity of the gingival sulcular epithelium (an important host defense mechanism) (120–122). Zinc deficiency in rats resulted in parakeratotic and hyperplastic buccal epithelium resulting from decreased keratinolytic enzyme activity (123). Dietary vitamin E supplementation was shown to accelerate gingival wound healing in albino rats and to decrease alveolar bone loss in rice rats (124, 125).

The area of nutrition/diet and periodontal disease has been fraught with limited scientific evidence and many claims for curative roles of nutrients. Clearly, relationships exist between periodontal disease and wound healing, nutrition status, and immune response, and relationships also exist between periodontal disease and individual nutrients (food and supplement forms) and select host defense and health variables. Deficiencies of select nutrients may compromise the systemic response to inflammation and infection and may alter nutrient needs (126, 127). Although limited research has demonstrated that persons who smoke and consume a diet low in vitamin C had significantly higher levels of periodontal disease, there are no recommendations for smokers to take supplemental doses of vitamin C for prevention or treatment of periodontal disease (126).

Nutrient deficiencies can compromise the associated inflammatory response and wound healing, given the direct influence of nutritional well-being on the synthesis and release of cytokines and their action (127). Malnutrition can cause adverse alterations in the volume, antibacterial, and physiochemical properties of saliva. Supplemental intake of any nutrients beyond the dietary reference intakes is not recommended for the prevention or treatment of periodontal disease. Boyd and Madden have recently summarized the nutrient effects on the periodontium in Table 72.7 (128).

ALVEOLAR BONE HEALTH, OSTEOPOROSIS, AND DENTATE STATUS

One of the more dramatic clinical signs of severe periodontal disease is resorption of alveolar bone, which ultimately results in tooth loss. The literature has long speculated that calcium deficiency is a major etiologic factor in periodontitis, and that periodontal disease may be a harbinger of systemic metabolic bone disorders (129, 130), which would then lead to tooth loss. Given that currently one in two women and one in eight men over the age of 65 years have osteoporosis and the predictions of the 2004 Surgeon General's report on bone health and osteoporosis, which states that by the year 2020 one in two US adults over the age of 50 years will have or be at high risk of developing osteoporosis, the relationship of this disease with periodontal disease deserves attention (131).

The alveolar process (crest of the maxilla and mandible) is composed primarily of trabecular bone. Histologically, it

is the same type of bone found in the distal radius, neck of the femur, and vertebrae. When negative calcium balance occurs in the body, calcium is more easily mobilized from skeletal sites consisting of trabecular rather than cortical bone. Thus, the alveolar bone provides a potential labile source of calcium available to meet other tissue needs. Because the alveolar process is thought to undergo resorption before other bones, change detected in the alveolar process may be used for early diagnosis of osteoporosis. In women, a high correlation has been shown between dental bone mass and total bone mass. Women with low bone density have fewer teeth. Women with severe residual ridge resorption have osteopenia on the iliac crest, and those with severe postmenopausal osteoporosis are three times more likely to be edentulous than physiologically normal control subjects (132).

Longitudinal studies and NHANES III data (133–135) have demonstrated significant relationships among tooth loss, periodontal disease, low calcium intake, and osteoporosis in older men and women who are at increased risk of both osteoporosis and periodontal disease. Dietrich found that higher serum $25(OH)D_3$ levels are associated with decreased loss of tooth attachment in adults more than 50 years old (136). Payne and associates examined changes in alveolar bone height in postmenopausal women with and without osteoporosis over 24 months (137). The relationship between alveolar bone loss and bone mineral density was significant. Women with osteoporosis lost significantly more alveolar bone than those without the condition. According to Krall, "the available evidence supports the hypothesis that poor systemic bone status contributes to tooth loss and periodontal disease but is not conclusive" (138).

DENTATE STATUS

Resorption of the alveolar process is a widespread problem among patients with dentures. Remodeling of the alveolar bone occurs in response to occlusal forces associated with chewing. With the loss of teeth, the alveolar bone is no longer required for tooth support; as a consequence, bone resorption is accelerated, and bone height is diminished. Bone loss is greatest during the first 6 months following tooth extractions. The reduction in residual ridge height is more pronounced in women than in men, and resorption is greater in the mandible than in the maxilla. Severe mandibular resorption makes it difficult to construct a mandibular denture with good stability and retention. Bone resorption and loss are common denominators of both periodontal disease and osteoporosis, and a low calcium intake may compound bone loss in denture wearers (139). Calcium supplementation for new denture wearers may help to maintain calcium balance and may slow the rate of alveolar resorption. In a study of postmenopausal women, researchers described an association between calcium and vitamin D supplementation and reduced risk of

TABLE 72.7. NUTRIENT EFFECTS ON THE PERIODONTIUM

NUTRIENT	FUNCTIONAL CHANGES RESULTING FROM INADEQUATE INTAKE	GROUPS AT RISK OF INADEQUATE INTAKE	FOOD SOURCES OF NUTRIENT
Protein	Compromised antibacterial properties of saliva Impaired acute-phase response to infection ↓Neutrophil function Lag period in the initiation of wound healing ↓Collagen synthesis	Persons with poorly controlled diabetes Patients with advanced cancer Patients with advanced AIDS Patients fasting ≥4 d or those with chronic poor nutrient intakes	Meat Dairy Legumes
Vitamin A	↓Production of γ-interferon ↓Collagen synthesis ↓Epithelialization ↓Incidence of infection	Patients with cystic fibrosis Patients with advanced AIDS Persons with GI conditions with malabsorption Persons taking weight-loss medication: orlistat	Fortified dairy foods Dark green leafy vegetables Meat and dairy
B-complex Vitamins	Inability to produce adequate energy ↓Protein synthesis, including DNA and RNA Breakdown of the mucosal barrier to pathogens	Persons with HIV infection Elderly vegans (vitamin B$_{12}$) Postgastrectomy patients Patients taking medications: H$_2$ blockers, phenytoin, methrotrexate	Enriched breads and cereals Green leafy vegetables Meat and dairy
Vitamin C	↓Neutrophil function Breakdown of the mucosal barrier to pathogens ↓Collagen synthesis	Smokers Substance abusers Elderly persons Persons with chronic disease People who avoid fruits and vegetables	Citrus fruits Dark green leafy vegetables Potatoes Cantaloupe
Vitamin D	Impaired absorption of calcium	Elderly women in northern latitudes those with little sun exposure	Fortified milk Eggs Liver
Vitamin E	↓Overall immune response ↓Antibody production	Persons with GI conditions with malabsorption Patients with advanced AIDS	Nuts and seeds Polyunsaturated oils Whole grains
Vitamin K	↓Bone density and possibly bone strength	Persons receiving anticoagulant therapy	Green leafy vegetables Liver
Boron	Impaired wound healing Possible association with bone calcification		Legumes Fruits, especially dried Vegetables
Calcium	Inadequate formation of peak bone mass Accelerated bone loss postmenopausally Osteoporosis Possible association with tooth loss	Young women Postmenopausal women	Milk and milk products Tofu processed with calcium Legumes
Copper	↓Tensile strength of collagen ↑Bone fragility ↓Proliferation neutrophils	Persons with an increased intake of antacids Persons taking megadoses of iron/zinc Alcohol abusers Patients with cystic fibrosis Patients with short bowel syndrome Postgastric bypass patients Persons taking medications: dexamethasone, penicillamine	Poultry Nuts Legumes Cereals Dried fruit Shellfish Chocolate Organ meats
Iron	↓Neutrophil phagocytic activity ↓Proliferation lymphocytes	Young children Women of childbearing age	Meat Eggs Legumes Dried fruit
Magnesium	More rapid development of ostenopenia	Persons with chronic alcoholism Medications: diuretics Elderly persons Postmenopausal women Persons with diabetes	Green leafy vegetables Whole grains Nuts
Zinc	↑Susceptibility to infection ↓Protein synthesis, including DNA and RNA	Elderly persons? Persons with alcoholism	Meats Whole grains

AIDS, acquired immunodeficiency syndrome; GI, gastrointestinal; HIV human immunodeficiency virus.

Adapted from Boyd LD, Madden TE. Nutrition and the periodontium. In: Palmer CA, ed. Diet and Nutrition in Oral Health. Englewood Cliffs, NJ: Prentice-Hall 2003:202–12, with permission.

tooth loss; those who experienced tooth loss were significantly more likely to experience systemic bone loss (140). Problems associated with small sample sizes, varying definitions of periodontal disease and osteoporosis, and the lack of prospective data have been cited as reasons for inconclusive results; longitudinal studies are advocated (139, 141). Positive calcium balance may be especially important along with adequate nutrition status to help preserve the integrity of the residual ridges of edentulous postmenopausal women.

Although an intact dentition is not absolutely essential to maintain nutritional health, loss of teeth or of the supporting periodontium can affect food selection and subsequent nutritional status. Periodontal disease, with its associated tissue soreness, pain, tooth sensitivity, bone resorption, and tooth mobility, can lead to a preference for soft foods of low nutritional value and the avoidance of foods requiring chewing. The same may be true of persons with severe dental caries and those with dentures.

Missing teeth, the absence of natural posterior occluding tooth surfaces, or ill-fitting dentures may impair biting and chewing and resultant dietary intake, often manifesting in a diet with less vegetable and fiber intake and more cholesterol, fat, and calories than in people with more teeth (142–147). Oral pain and discomfort may also influence daily activities, which, in turn, may affect dietary intake and quality of life (148). Edentulousness has also been associated with GI disorders (149), and among the frail elderly, poor oral health is associated with the involuntary weight loss resulting from protein-calorie malnutrition (150).

Dentures can also affect taste and swallowing ability, especially if they are maxillary (upper) dentures. The denture covers the hard and soft palate, where some taste buds are located, and thus can blunt normal taste sensitivity. A maxillary denture can also impede swallowing. When the hard palate is covered, it is difficult for the tongue to determine the location of food in the mouth, form a bolus, and swallow, which may contribute to dysphagia.

The dentally impaired can maintain good dietary intake and adequate nutrition status by making appropriate food selections and adapting gradually to new dentures. Persons receiving new dentures should be counseled on choosing foods that are easy to masticate, eating slowly, chewing longer, cooking foods longer, and cutting large, hard foods into bite-sized pieces.

FOOD-RELATED INJURY

Thermal or mechanical injury can result from drinking hot beverages, chewing ice cubes, or puncturing oral tissues, resulting in tooth or mouth pain. This, in turn, may alter a person's food selection behavior. Fortunately, the oral tissues have a more rapid tissue turnover rate than other body tissues, possibly as an adaptation to just such insults. As a result, tissue repair is fairly rapid and should not

cause long-term dietary problems. Tooth sensitivity is often associated with gingival recession, which is common in middle-aged and older adults. Other causes of sensitivity can include toothbrush abrasion, caries, and the side effects of periodontal treatment. Tooth sensitivity sometimes can be corrected by the use of over-the-counter desensitizing products.

FAILURE TO THRIVE IN CHILDREN

Oral conditions are often overlooked as contributing factors to eating problems or failure to thrive in children. Sore teeth and gums may lead a child to avoid chewing or eating. The foods they will or can eat may not provide adequate calories or nutritional value to meet their growth needs (151). If caregivers are not alerted to look for oral problems, or if the children may not be receiving regular dental care, the oral implications of the problem may be missed.

ORAL SURGERY

The degree of oral impairment and its impact on diet and nutrition status in oral surgery patients are usually conditions of the extent and location of the surgery and the nutritional well-being of the patient before surgery. In general oral surgical situations, food consumption is impaired for a relatively short period, and the risk of nutritional deficiency is low except in those already at nutritional risk. A soft or liquid diet may be recommended. In patients undergoing dental implant surgery, the number and location of implants will dictate the extent of oral impairment. Implants placed in the anterior (or front) teeth will affect biting ability for a short time, whereas implants placed in the back teeth will affect chewing ability. In both instances, the extent of impact is typically limited to 7 to 10 days. When teeth are extracted in preparation for dentures and the patient is rendered edentulous, a graduated diet must be provided. During the initial 1 to 3 days, the diet should be limited to soups, liquids, ice cream, yogurts, puddings, and mashed potatoes. Gradually, soft, nonirritating foods such as cooked fruits and vegetables, pastas, and meats/fish/poultry with gravies and sauces can be introduced. A similar diet regimen is used for patients who have teeth extracted and immediate dentures placed.

For the patient who has a wired jaw, however, eating may be impaired for long periods, and specific dietary guidelines are needed to attain and maintain nutritional status. Depending on the nature of the condition that led to the wired jaw, energy needs may also be increased. Severe trauma resulting in a fractured jaw and wiring increases energy needs considerably. Diets for patients with wired jaws are based on three main principles: all foods must be blenderized, strained, and able to go through a straw. Table foods can be blenderized and liquefied using soups and other fluids and strained to go through a straw. High-protein, high-calorie meal replacement formulas such as Instant Breakfast may be needed to meet energy and protein needs. Dietary fiber needs may be met by preparing vegetables and cereals in an appropriate form for consumption. Vitamin-mineral supplements may be needed to meet micronutrient needs. It is essential that diet suggestions be provided that will allow the patient to meet his or her caloric needs via liquid food sources alone (152).

ORAL INFECTIONS AND IMMUNE DEFICIENCY DISEASES

Oral infections such as herpes simplex and oral candidiasis can result in painful oral lesions that impair the desire and ability to eat. Usually, palliative oral care and appropriate food choices (bland, temperate, easily masticated) can effectively help to maintain nutritional status. However, when these conditions are long standing, such as in human immunodeficiency virus (HIV) infection and AIDS, nutritional status can be undermined, thus contributing to further virulence of the disease.

People living with HIV infection may have oral lesions manifesting from the disease process (Kaposi sarcoma or major aphthous ulcers), pathogens causing infections (candidiasis or herpes simplex), oral infectious diseases (dental caries or periodontal disease), or side effects of many of the medications used to treat HIV (xerostomia, oral ulceration, dysguesia, apathy toward oral hygiene and eating) (153–156). The occurrence of many of these lesions can be drastically curtailed or their severity reduced by the use of prophylactic regimens.

Because the oral cavity is the beginning of the GI tract, ulcerations in the mouth as a result of the systemic GI disease may be evident and may even precede GI symptoms (157, 158). Pyostomatitis vegetans is a rare eruption of the oral mucosa that is characterized by small yellow pustules and is considered a marker for inflammatory bowel disease. In one study, oral zinc supplementation caused a regression of the pyostomatitis vegetans, a finding leading to the conclusion that this oral lesion may be caused by zinc deficiency secondary to malabsorption (159).

Adequate nutrition in people living with Crohn's disease is often difficult even when the oral cavity is healthy, because these persons usually need to avoid certain foods as a result of maldigestion, and they are at increased risk of micronutrient deficiencies because of malabsorption (160). Attention to the nutrition needs of these patients is essential, to reduce the risk of further compromise resulting from oral lesions.

ORAL AND PHARYNGEAL CANCERS

Diet has been shown to play a role in oral and pharyngeal cancer risk as well as prevention. Consumption of charcoal-grilled and salt-preserved foods has been implicated as having a possible role in risk of oral and pharyngeal cancers. In contrast, increased consumption of fruits and vegetables may have a protective effect (161–164). However, increased consumption of alcohol and cigarette smoking have been shown to reduce the protective effect (163). Diets rich in fruits and vegetables are inversely associated with oral and pharyngeal cancer risk, particularly in respect to foods rich in β-carotene, potassium, vitamins B_6 and C, and folate (165). Antioxidant nutrients including vitamins C and E, β-carotene, and flavinoids have been suggested as protective dietary components against oral cavity cancers (161, 166). The protective effect of fruit-rich diets has been shown across population subgroups in Italy, the United States, and Japan. However, although nutritional epidemiology studies globally have demonstrated protective effects of fruits and vegetables for oral and pharyngeal cancer, the micronutrient impact has been based on food not supplemental sources. Clinical trials and longitudinal studies are needed to support the protective effects found in these epidemiologic studies.

In laboratory and animal studies, both β-carotene and vitamin E can inhibit oral carcinogenesis and cause clinical regression of oral leukoplakia (167), which is a precursor to oral cancer. However, methodologic difficulties have resulted in less definitive results in humans to date (168, 169).

Radiation therapy may adversely affect nutrition and oral health status and may cause xerostomia, loss of taste, increased risk of fungal infections, mucositis and its attendant pain, and/or osteoradionecrosis (161). If not treated before irradiation, chronic pulpal and periodontal infections can become acute because of radiation-associated changes and can lead to osteoradionecrosis. These lesions are extremely painful and difficult to treat and can impair systemic nutrition for months.

Some of the same oral lesions associated with HIV infections are also seen in patients with cancer who are undergoing chemotherapy. The antimetabolic activity of these drugs often induces mucositis, rendering the tissues more susceptible to physical trauma from sharp tooth edges and hard bits of food. Ulceration, secondary infection, and painful stomatitis may result. Generally, the more intense the cytotoxic therapy, the more common the oral complications. Through the use of proper prophylactic therapy before chemotherapy, many lesions can be prevented or minimized, with the result of fewer problems in ingesting required nutrients (170, 171). For detailed discussion of radiation therapy, see Chapter 83.

EFFECTS OF SALIVA ON ORAL HEALTH AND NUTRITION

Saliva is a primary factor in both the function and maintenance of the oral cavity. In addition to saliva's importance in speech and deglutition, certain antimicrobial and nonantimicrobial systems in saliva protect both the hard and soft tissues of the mouth. Cessation or severe decrease of salivary flow from such causes as surgical removal of salivary glands, radiation therapy, uncontrolled diabetes mellitus, or Sjögren's syndrome can lead to microbial infection of the oral cavity, rampant caries, and loss of taste acuity, as well as an inability to lubricate, masticate, and swallow food (172–174). All these conditions have a profound effect on selection of ingestion of foods and thus on systemic nutrition. In fact, significant deficiencies of fiber, vitamin B_6, iron, calcium, and zinc were found in xerostomic older adults (175). Additionally, comfort in wearing dentures depends on lubrication of the soft tissues by saliva; patients with oral dryness have poor retention of their dentures and may develop ulcerations at denture borders, thus making mastication difficult and painful and possibly affecting dietary intake and nutrition status.

It was once believed that the aging process brought with it a "natural" reduction of salivary flow, but, in fact, salivary flow in healthy persons does not decrease with age (176). Nearly 50% of elderly people take medications that diminish salivary flow, however, so although salivary flow is decreased, it generally still does not interfere with either deglutition or the maintenance of hard and soft tissues (177). Nonetheless, these patients often feel as if their mouths are dry, and they frequently use hard candies or gum to stimulate salivary flow throughout the day. Because most of the candies and gum used contain fermentable carbohydrates, the constant exposure may result in rampant caries and altered food intake because of discomfort or loss of integrity of the dentition. Patients taking xerostomia-producing drugs should be counseled about side effects and should be advised to use candies and gums containing relatively nonfermentable sugar alcohols such as sorbitol, mannitol, or xylitol. The use of artificial saliva, although not a panacea, may be beneficial to some of these patients. To prevent rampant caries in such persons, aggressive home care emphasizing effective oral hygiene and daily fluoride application is usually recommended (178).

Many classes of drugs can cause xerostomia. Patients taking drugs that are anticholinergic (e.g., antihistamines, tricyclic antidepressants, and antipsychotics) medications, as well as α-adrenergic receptor blockers (narcotics, antianxiety and hyponotic agents, antiemetics and selective serotonin reuptake inhibitor antidepressants) are prone to xerostomia. In persons experiencing such side effects, aggressive oral hygiene, topical fluoride, and use of sugar-free gums and candies, along with frequent water consumption, can help to reduce caries risk.

DISORDERS OF GASTROESOPHAGEAL REFLUX AND BULIMIA

Both gastric reflux and self-induced vomiting, such as observed in eating disorders, commonly lead to irritation of oral tissues and destruction of dental enamel (179). The extent of oral tissue damage depends on the frequency of

the purging and the cariogenicity of the diet. Because they are often the first health-care providers to see these patients, dentists may make an early diagnosis of eating disorders. Some symptoms that may cause these patients to seek dental treatment are sensitivity to hot and cold temperatures or to air or dental pain, as well as concern about the appearance of their teeth.

Enamel erosion is primarily caused by chronic regurgitation of the acidic contents of the stomach. Erosion may also result from frequent intake of fruit juices high in citric acid, sucking on chewable vitamin C tablets, disulfiram (Antabuse) therapy for alcoholism, or exposure to industrial acids. Contact and thermal hypersensitivity occurs when the dentin is exposed. The acidic oral environment causes irritation of the oral mucosa including the gingiva, palate, and pharynx.

The most obvious clinical symptom of bulimia nervosa is loss of tooth enamel (permylosis) and dentin on the lingual and incisal surfaces of anterior teeth and occlusal surfaces of posterior teeth. Perioral stomatitis, along with swollen salivary, parotid, and submandibular glands, can occur as a result of hypersalivation. The degree of gland swelling is typically relative to the frequency of vomiting. Redness of the throat and calluses on the knuckles may also be additional signs of bulimia. Erosion of the lingual (tongue) side surfaces of the teeth, particularly the anterior (front) teeth, can occur but may take months to develop; thermal sensitivity to foods and fluids may also occur.

With repeated vomiting, esophageal tears may develop. The lips may become cracked, and fissures may develop at the corners of the mouth. When compared with physiologically normal adults, low resting salivary flow rates have been found in patients with eating disorders that may result in xerostomia (180). The dental caries profile and periodontal status of patients with bulimia nervosa are similar to those of healthy young adults without eating disorders (181). Low levels of dental caries, dental plaque, and gingival recession have been reported; however, high intakes of fermentable carbohydrates during binges may cause caries.

Dental treatment must be coordinated with the primary health care provider. Definitive restorative treatment cannot occur until the vomiting behavior is under control. Temporary restorations are placed on eroded tooth surfaces to prevent further loss of enamel and to prevent hypersensitivity. The patient is encouraged to practice meticulous oral hygiene. Patients are cautioned against brushing immediately after vomiting, to prevent further erosion of dental enamel. Instead, a sodium bicarbonate or magnesium hydroxide rinse is recommended to neutralize acid in the mouth. Neutral pH sodium fluoride rinses (0.5%) or the home application of stannous fluoride gels (0.4%) in custom trays will prevent dental erosion and will enhance remineralization of teeth (182). Patients should be counseled to limit fruit juices with high citric acid content and to avoid sticky, sweet foods between meals. Foods of low cariogenicity—nuts, seeds, cheese and vegetables—are desirable snacks. If dry mouth is a problem, chewing paraffin wax, sugarless chewing gum, or sugar-free lemon drops may be used to stimulate saliva flow.

THE AGING PATIENT

In the past three decades, the population of persons aged 65 years and older has increased considerably. In 2003, this group accounted for approximately 12% of the US population and represented close to 36 million people (183). In the 1900s, the numbers of elderly persons increased approximately from a population of 3 million to 35 million at the beginning of the twenty-first century. The population of those 85 years old and older increased from just over 100,000 at the turn of the twentieth century to 4.2 million 100 years later in 2000, with a projected increase to 21 million by 2050, according to the US Census Bureau. The aging process involves a host of changes that can affect and be affected by oral health. Older patients frequently have one or more chronic diseases and/or other problems that can affect their oral health and/or dental treatment (109); the bidirectional relationship often cited between nutrition and oral health is particularly evident in the elderly. Tooth loss, partial and complete edentulism, and ill-fitting dentures all influence diet quality and often appetite. Poor oral health can be a contributing factor in the development of involuntary weight loss in the elderly (184). Because today's elderly persons tend to retain more of their natural teeth, new patterns of oral diseases, including root and coronal decay, are becoming more common. Oral manifestations of chronic diseases, xerostomia, side effects of polypharmacy on the oral cavity, osteoporosis, menopause, and eating problems associated with denture placement are examples of the scope of dental nutrition problems faced by the elderly (185). Tooth loss, edentulism, and removable prostheses can all negatively affect eating habits and can create long-term changes that are not easily reversed. Possible consequences include altered masticatory function, compromised sense of taste, and subjective complaints of indigestion (186, 187). The term "oral invalids" has been coined in reference to denture wearers (188). Research has documented that denture wearers have about one fifth the chewing ability of their dentate counterparts (140) and take more drugs (including laxatives and antireflux agents) for GI disorders (187).

The hypogeusia observed in some elderly persons is possibly associated with specific disorders leading to taste loss, rather than a normal component of the aging process (180). Xerostomia is a common sequela of multiple drug use and often results in root caries. Nearly 50% of those aged 75 years and older take two or more medications daily (191), and one third to one half of older adults may experience xerostomia (192). With between 68% of 65 to 69 year olds and 51% of those more than 80 years old at least partially dentate, dental caries remains a potential problem. Root caries affects more than 60% of dentate persons, and the caries rate increases with age (193). Periodontal disease is also a problem for older adults; approximately one third show evidence of severe periodontitis (193). Oral cancer is also more common with age, almost tripling between the group aged 55 to 64 years and those aged 85 years old or older. Tooth loss, pain, malpositioning, loss of vertical dimension, joint dysfunction, and dental prostheses can all impair mastication. In addition, social interactions surrounding eating and subsequent nutrition can be impaired by mobile or fractured teeth and by the condition and/or retention of dental prostheses (191).

Because elderly persons are at particular risk of nutritional and oral problems, all health professionals are encouraged to broaden the scope of their routine screening beyond their own discipline. To accomplish this, the Nutrition Screening Initiative (a collaborative project of the American Academy of Family Physicians, the American Dietetic Association, and the National Council on the Aging) has developed simple screening questionnaires based on the major contributors to nutrition risk, to be used by health professionals to screen the elderly (194). Screening forms are provided for medical problems, drug interactions, psychosocial factors, nutrition, and oral health. When these forms are used consistently, all health care providers, including dietetic and dental professionals, will be able to screen for a variety of factors contributing to nutrition risk and to refer to the appropriate provider for further care.

DIABETES AND ORAL HEALTH

Oral implications of uncontrolled diabetes mellitus may include, but are not limited to, increased risk and incidence of infection, poor wound healing, increased incidence and severity of caries, candidiasis, periodontal disease, xerostomia, alterations in taste, and burning mouth or tongue (195). The oral manifestations in such patients are most likely related to the results of polyuria, altered response to infection, microvascular changes, and, possibly, salivary hyperglycemia (increased glucose in saliva). Caries risk may be related to the inherent increased risk of infection, salivary hyperglycemia, and xerostomia. Candidiasis, often presenting on the tongue, is a fungal infection often associated with hyperglycemia (196). Denture stomatitis, angular cheilitis, and thrush are often associated with candidal infection (196). Periodontal disease has been referred to as the "sixth complication of diabetes mellitus" (197). Persons with diabetes are at greater risk of developing periodontal disease, and the severity of the disease is relative to the duration of diagnosis of diabetes. Altered taste may result from altered salivary chemistry (from diabetes out of control), xerostomia, burning mouth or tongue, and/or candidiasis. All potential causes should be explored to determine whether the patient has any other underlying disorder.

Careful evaluation and monitoring of glycemic control are critical in determining the risk assessment for progression to the oral complications of diabetes. Persons with type 1 or type 2 diabetes who complain of dry mouth, burning tongue, or altered taste, as well as those presenting with candidiasis, should be evaluated for their diabetes control. Appropriate intervention includes management of diabetes and of oral health in such patients.

With proper management techniques, oral health can be maintained despite the diabetes. A regimen of controlled diet, conscientious and effective oral hygiene, and topical fluoride, when indicated, can maintain oral health integrity throughout life (195, 198).

ORAL MALODORS AND DIET

Halitosis or malodorous breath is a common problem that has been extensively studied for many years. A number of reviews concluded that the primary source of malodorous breath was the release of volatile sulfur-containing gases that originate in the oral cavity (199, 200). The putative causes of the malodor range from oral infections, such as gingivitis and periodontitis, to sinusitis, Zenker diverticula, and prolonged fasting (201). Significant data, however, support the notion that gases produced by the gut microflora can also be a source of breath malodor (202). Suarez and associates conducted an interesting study investigating the mouth versus gut origin of malodorous gases using the sulfur-containing gases of garlic as probes (203). The findings of these investigators demonstrated that breath odor after garlic ingestion originates from the mouth initially and, subsequently, from the gut.

In reviewing these data, Hasler (204) concluded that by using differential means of collecting air samples from the mouth and pulmonary alveoli, Suarez and colleagues were able to show that most gases seemed to be generated from only oral sources, for example, methanethiol and allyl mercaptan. However, allyl methyl sulfide was not metabolized by gut mucosal and hepatic tissues and thus was exhaled for prolonged periods after ingestion of garlic. This study has important ramifications because it illustrates that aggressive oral hygiene, including tongue brushing, will not alleviate some sources of breath malodors. Interestingly, Paster recently studied the microbial profile of persons with breath malodors following ingestion of a variety of potentially noxious substance and concluded that specific oral microbiota may be responsible for some of these malodors (205). Hasler speculated that the findings of Suarez and colleagues raise the question whether a dietary supplement could be developed to assist gut metabolism of substances, like allyl methyl sulfide, so garlic lovers could enjoy their meals similar to the manner in which supplemental lactose enables milk-intolerant persons to tolerate dairy products (204). Similarly, the

finding of Paster suggest that specific microbial targets could assist in thwarting the malodor derived from oral origins.

REFERENCES

1. Genco RJ, Trevisan M, Wu T et al. JAMA 2001;285:40–1.
2. Madianos PN, Bobetsis GA, Kinane D. J Clin Periodontol 2002;29[Suppl 3]:22–30.
3. Shaw JH, Sweeney EA. Nutrition in relation to dental medicine. In: Shils ME, Young VR, eds. Modern Nutrition in Health and Disease. 7th ed. Philadelphia: Lea & Febiger, 1988:1070–1.
4. US Department of Health and Human Services. Surgeon General's Report on Nutrition and Health: Dental Diseases. Publ. no. 88–50210. Washington, DC: US Government Printing Office, 1988:345–80.
5. Palmer CA, DePaola D. Nutrition as the foundation of general and oral health. In: Palmer CA, ed. Diet and Nutrition in Oral Health. Englewood Cliffs, NJ: Prentice-Hall, 2003:1–12.
6. Dreizen S. Pediatrician 1989;16:139–46.
7. Sweeney EA, Saffir AJ, deLeon R. Am J Clin Nutr 1971;4:29–31.
8. Sawyer DR, Kwoku AL. J Dent Child 1985;54:141–5.
9. Punysingh JT, Hoffman S, Harris SS et al. J Oral Pathol 1984;13:40–57.
10. Boyle PE. J Dent Res 1933;13:139–50.
11. Slavkin H. J Am Dent Assoc 1996;127:681–2.
12. Kim YS, Stumpf WA, Clark SA et al. J Dent Res 1983;62:58–9.
13. Leaver AG. Clin Orthop 1971;8:90–107.
14. Bawden JW. Anat Rec 1989;24:226–33.
15. Mellanby M. Br Dent J 1923;44:1031–41.
16. Wolf JJ. Am J Dis Child 1935;49:905–11.
17. Boyle PE. J Dent Res 1934;14:172.
18. Schiltz JR, Rosenbloom J, Levinson GE. J Embryol Exp Morphol 1977;37:49–57.
19. Alvarez JO, Eguren JC, Caleda J et al. J Dent Res 1990;69:1564–6.
20. Alvarez JO, Navia JM. Am J Clin Nutr 1989;49:417–26.
21. Alvarez JO, Lewis CA, Saman C et al. Am J Clin Nutr 1988;48:368–72.
22. Rami-Reddy V, Vijayalakshmi PB, Chandrasekhar-Reddy BK. Odont Pediatr 1986;7:1–5.
23. Delgado H, Habicht JP, Yarbrough C et al. Am J Clin Nutr 1975;38:216–24.
24. Menaker L, Navia JM. J Dent Res 1973;52:688–91.
25. National Institute of Dental Research. Mineralized tissues, craniofacial development, dentofacial malrelations and trauma. In: Broadening the Scope: Long-Range Research Plan for the Nineties. NIH Publ. no. 90–1188. Washington, DC: US Government Printing Office, 1990.
26. Iber FL. Nutr Today 1990;15:5.
27. Slavkin HC. Cleft Palate J 1990;27:101–9.
28. Slavkin HC. J Am Dent Assoc 1997;128:1308–13.
29. Akam M. Cell 1989;57:347–9.
30. Lammer EJ, Chen DT, Hoar RM et al. N Engl J Med 1985;313:837–41.
31. Slavkin HC. Personal communication, 1992.
32. MRC Vitamin Study Research Group. Lancet 1991;338:131–7.
33. Tolarova M, Harris J. Teratology 1995;51:71–8.
34. US Department of Health and Human Services, National Institute of Dental and Craniofacial Research, National Institutes of Health. Oral Health in America: A Report of the Surgeon

General. Rockville, MD: US Department of Health and Human Services, 2000.

35. National Institute of Dental Research. Oral Health of United States Adults: The National Survey of Oral Health in US Employed Adults and Seniors 1985–1986. NIH Publ. no. (PHS) 87–2868, Washington, DC: US Government Printing Office, 1987.

36. NIH Consensus Statement. (2001). Diagnosis and Management of Dental Caries Throughout Life. Retrieved November 9, 2002, from http://consensus.nih.gov/cons/115/115_intro.htm

37. Peterson PE. The World Oral Health Report. Geneva: World Health Organization, 2003.

38. US Department of Health and Human Services. Oral Health. In Healthy People 2010: Understanding and Improving Health. 2nd ed, vol 2. Washington, DC: U.S. Government Printing Office, 2000.

39. WHO Oral Health Country/Area Profile Programme.Caries Prevelance: DMFT and DMFS. Retrieved November 9, 2002, from http://www.whocollab.od.mah.se/expl/orhdmft.html

40. Kaste LM, Selwitz RJ, Oldakowski JA et al. J Dent Res 1996;75:631–41.

41. Gift HC, Drury TF, Nowjack–Raymer RE. J Public Health Dent 1996;56:84–91.

42. Winn DM, Brunelle JA, Selwitz RH et al. J Dent Res 1996;75:684–95.

43. Johnson RK, Frary C. J Nutr 2001;131:2766S–71S.

44. Mobley C, Dodds MW. Top Nutr 1998;7:1–18.

45. Lingstrom P, van Houte J, Kashket S. Crit Rev Oral Biol Med 2000;11:366–80.

46. Sreebny LM. Worl Rev Nutr Diet 1982;40:19–65.

47. Cleaton-Jones P, Richardson BD, Sinwel R et al. Caries Res 1984;18:472–7.

48. Persson LA, Stecksen-Blicks C, Holm AK. Commun Dent Oral Epidemiol 1984;12:390–7.

49. Burt BA, Pai S. J Dent Educ 2001;65:1017–24.

50. Konig KG, Navia JM. Am J Clin Nutr 1995;62:275S–83S.

51. Kantor KS. A Dietary Assessment of the US Food Supply: Comparing per Capita Food Consumption with Food Gguide Pyramid Serving Recommendations. Food and Rural Economics Division, Economics Research Service. US Department of Agriculture, Agricultural Economic Report no. 772. Washington DC: US Government Printing Office, 1998.

52. Krebs-Smith SM. J Nutr 2001;131:527S–35S.

53. Murphy S, Johnson R. Am J Clin Nutr 2003;78:815S–26S.

54. Guthrie JF, Morton JF. J Am Diet Assoc 2000;100:43–51.

55. Ishii T, Konig KG, Muhlemann HR. Helv Odontol Acta 1968;12:41–7.

56. Harris R. J Dent Res 1963;42:1387–99.

57. Rugg-Gunn AJ, Hackett AF, Appleton DR. Caries Res 1987;21:464–78.

58. Stephan RJ. J Am Dent Res 1940;27:718–23.

59. Birkhed D. Caries Res 1984;18:120–7.

60. Ismail Al, Burt BA, Eklund SA. J Am Dent Assoc 1984;109:241–5.

61. Motokawa W, Braham R, Ishii K et al. Quintessence Int 1990;21:983–7.

62. Maguire A, Rugg-Gunn AJ, Butler TJ. Caries Res 1996;30:16–21.

63. Scheinen A, Makinen KK. Acta Odontol Scand 1975;34:179–216.

64. MachiulskieneV, Nyvad B, Baelum V. Commun Dent Oral Epidemiol 2001;29:278–88.

65. Tanzer JM, Slee AM. J Am Dent Assoc 1983;106:331–3.

66. Lout RK, Messer LB, Soberay A et al. Caries Res 1988;22:237–41.

67. Hildebrandt GH, Sparks BS. J Am Diet Assoc 2000;131:909–16.

68. Scheinen A, Makinen KK, Larmas M. Acta Odontol Scand 1975;39:269–78.

69. Mundorff SA, Featherstone JDB, Bibby BC et al. Caries Res 1990;24:344–55.

70. Pollard MA, Imfeld T, Higham SM et al. Caries Res 1996;30:132–7.

71. Rugg–Gunn AJ, Edgar WM, Jenkins GN. J Dent Res 1981;60:867–72.

72. Kashket S, van Houte J, Lopez LR et al. J Dent Res 1991;70:1314–9.

73. Kashket S, Zhang J, van Houte J. J Dent Res 1996;75:1885–91.

74. Silva MF, Jenkins GN, Burgess RC et al. Caries Res 1986;20:263–9.

75. Jensen ME, Harlander SK, Schachtele CF et al. Evaluation of the acidogenic and antacid properties of cheeses by telemetric recording of dental plaque. In: Hefferen JJ, Koehler HM, Osborn JC, eds. Food, Nutrition and Dental Health. Park Forest South, IL: Pathotox ,1984.

76. DePaola DP, Kashket S. Nutr Rev 2002;60:97–103.

77. Moynihan P. Annex 6: The Scientific Basis for Diet, Nutrition and the Prevention of Dental Diseases. Background paper for the Joint FAO/WHO Expert Consultation on Diet, Nutrition and the Prevention of Chronic Diseases. Geneva: Food and Agriculture Organization/World Health Organization, 2002, Last accessed November 11, 2002. http://www.who.int/hpr/nutrition/CommentsExpertConsultationReportOrgs/Associated CountryWomenoftheWorld.pdf.

78. Lagerlof F, Oliveby A. Adv Dent Res 1994;8:229–38.

79. Touger-Decker R, van Loveren C. Am J Clin Nutr 2003;78 [Suppl]:881S–92S.

80. DePaola, DP. J Dent Res 1986;65:1540–3.

81. Schachtele CF, Harlander SK. J Can Dent Assoc 1984;50:213–9.

82. Winn DV, Brunelle JH, Selwitz RH et al. J Dent Res 1996;75:642–51.

83. van Houte J, Jordan R, Laraway R et al. J Dent Res 1990;69:1463–8.

84. Ravald N, Hemp SE, Birkhed D. J Clin Periodontol 1986;13:758–67.

85. Papas AS, Joshi A, Belanger AJ et al. Am J Clin Nutr 1995;61:417S–22S.

86. Papas AS, Joshi A, Palmer CA et al. Am J Clin Nutr 1995;61:423S–9S.

87. Papas AS, Palmer CA, McGandy R et al. Gerodontics 1987;3:30–7.

88. Papas AS, Palmer CA, Rounds MC et al. Ann NY Acad Sci 1989;561:124–42.

89. Billings RJ. J Public Health Dent 1996;56:37.

90. O'Sullivan DV, Tinanoff N. J Dent Res 1993;72:1577–8.

91. Ripa LW. Pediatr Dent 1988;10:268–82.

92. Berkowitz R. J Public Health Dent 1996;56:51–4.

93. Gardner DE, Norwood JR, Eisenson JE. J Dent Child 1977;44:186–91.

94. Bruerd B, Jone C. Public Health Rep 1995;111:63–5.

95. US Department of Health and Human Services, Public Health Service: Review of Fluoride Benefits and Risks. Report of the Ad Hoc Subcommittee on Fluoride of the Committee to Coordinate Environmental Health and Related Programs. Washington, DC: US Government Printing Office, 1991.

96. Dean HT. Epidemiological studies in the United States. In: Moulton FR, ed. Dental Caries and Fluoride. Washington, DC: American Association for Advancement of Science, 1946.

97. Murray JJ, Rugg-Gunn AJ. Fluorides and Dental Caries. 2nd ed. Bristol, UK: John Wright & Sons, 1982.

98. Brunelle JA. Carlos JP. J Dent Res 1990;69:723–7.

99. Newbrun E. J Public Health Dent 1989;49:279–89.

100. Centers for Disease Control and Prevention. MMWR Morb Mortal Wkly Rep 1992;41:372–81.

101. American Dental Association. ADA Guide to Dental Therapeutics. Chicago: American Dental Association, 1998.

102. Kula K, Wei SHY. Fluoride supplements and dietary sources of fluoride. In: Wei SHY, ed. Clinical Uses of Fluoride. Philadelphia: Lea & Febiger, 1985.

103. Leverett DH, Vaughn BW, Adair SM et al. J Public Health Dent 1993;53:205(abst).

104. Ismail Al, Messer JG. J Public Health Dent 1996;56:22–7.

105. Brunelle JA. J Dent Res 1989;68:995.

106. Levy SM, Kahout FJ, Firitsy MC et al. J Am Dent Assoc 1995; 126:1625–32.

107. Pendry DG. J Am Dent Assoc 1995;126:1617–24

108. Mackle T, Touger-Decker R, O'Sullivan Maillet J et al. J Am Diet Assoc 2004;103;1632–8.

109. Touger-Decker R, Mobley C. J Am Diet Assoc 2003;103: 615–625.

110. Touger-Decker R. Dent Clin North Am 2003 47:259–78.

111. Dreizen S. Pediatrician 1989;16:139–46.

112. Lamey, PJ, Allam BF. Br Dent J 1986;160:81–3.

113. Drinks P, Langer E, Voeks S et al. J Am Coll Nutr 1993;12:1, 14–20.

114. Woolfe SN, Hume WR, Kenney EP. J West Soc Periodontol Abstr 1980;28:44–56.

115. Hathcock J, Hattan DC, Jenkins M et al. Am J Clin Nutr 1990; 52:183–202.

116. DeMenezes AC, Costa IM, El–Guindy MM. J Periodontol 1984;55:474–6.

117. Tsao CS, Leung PY. J Nutr 1988;118:895–900.

118. Gerster H, Moser V. Nutr Res 1988;8:1327–32.

119. Omaye ST, Skala JH, Jacob RA. Am J Clin Nutr 1988;48: 379–81.

120. Genco, RJ, Wilson ME, DeNardin E. Periodontal complications and neutrophil abnormalities. In: Genco R, Goldman H, Cohen DW,eds. Contemporary Periodontitis. St. Louis: CV Mosby, 1990.

121. Vogel RI, Lamster IB, Wechsler SA et al. J Periodontol 1986; 57:472–9.

122. Alvares O, Siegel I. J Oral Pathol 1981;10:40–8.

123. Hsu DJ, Daniel JC, Gerson SJ. Arch Oral Biol 1991;36:10, 759–63.

124. Kim JE, Shklar G. J Periodontol 1983;54:305–8.

125. Cohen ME, Meyer DM. Arch Oral Biol 1993;38:7, 601–6.

126. Nishida M, Grossi SG, Dunford RG et al. J Periodontol 2000; 71:1215–23.

127. Enwonwu CO. Am J Clin Nutr1995;61[Suppl]:430S–6S.

128. Boyd LD, Madden TE. Nutrition and the periodontium. In: Palmer CA, ed. Diet and Nutrition in Oral Health. Englewood Cliffs, NJ: Prentice-Hall, 2003:202–12.

129. Whalen J, Krook L. Nutrition 1996;12:53–4.

130. Kribbs PJ. J Prosthet Dent 1990;63:86–9.

131. US Department of Health and Human Services. Bone Health and Osteoporosis: A Report of the Surgeon General. Rockville, MD: Office of the Surgeon General, Last accessed December 16, 2004. http://www.surgeongeneral.gov/library/bonehealth/content.html.

132. Jeffcoat MK, Chesnut C. J Am Dent Assoc 1993;124:49–56.

133. Krall E, Wehler C, Garcia RI et al. Am J Med 2001:111: 452–6.

134. Nishida M, Grossi SG, Dunford RG et al. J Periodontol 2000; 71:1057–66.

135. Yoshihara A, Seida Y, Hanada N et al. J Clin Periodontol 2004; 21:680–4.

136. Dietrich T. Am J Clin Nutr 2004;80:108–13.

137. Payne JB, Reinhardt RA, Nummikoski PV et al. Osteoporosis Int 1999;10:34–40.

138. Krall E. Osteoporosis. In: Touger-Decker R, Sirois DA, Mobley CC, eds. Nutrition and Oral Medicine. Totowa, NJ: Humana Press, 2005:261–70.

139. Wactawski-Wende J. Ann Periodontol 2001:6:197–208.

140. Krall EA, Wehler C, Garcia RI et al. Am J Med 2001:111: 452–6.

141. Chesnut CHR. Ann Periodontol 2001;6:193–6.

142. Marshall TA, Warren, JJ, Hand, JS et al. J Am Dent Assoc 2002; 133:1369–79.

143. Mojon P, Budtz-Jorgensen E, Rapin CH. Age Ageing 1999;28: 463–8.

144. Moynihan PJ, Butler TJ, Thomason JM et al. J Dent 2000;28: 557–63.

145. Nowjack-Raymer RE, Sheiham A. J Dent Res 2003;82:123–6.

146. Papas AS, Palmer CA, Rounds MC et al. Spec Care Dent 1998;18:17–25.

147. Sahyoun NR, Lin CL, Krall E. J Am Diet Assoc 2003;103:61–6.

148. Allen F. Health Qual Life Outcomes 2003;1:40.

149. Sheiham A, Steele JG, Marcenes W et al. Br Dent J 2002;192: 703–6.

150. Ritchie CS, Joshipura K et al. J Gerontol A Biol Sci Med Sci 2000:55:M366–71.

151. McKinney L, Palmer C, Dwyer JT, Garcia R. Top Clin Nutr 1991;6:70–5.

152. Patten JA. Compend Contin Educ Dent 1995;16:200–14.

153. Kademani, D, Glick M. Quintessence Int 1998;29:523–34.

154. Narani N, Epstein JB. J Clin Periodontol 2001;28:137–45.

155. Sifri R, Diaz VAJ, Gordon L et al. J Am Board Fam Pract 1998;11:434–44.

156. Sirois DA. Mt Sinai J Med 1998;65:322–32.

157. Das KM. Dig Dis Sci 1999;44:1–13.

158. Siegel MA, Jacobsen JJ, Braun RJ. Diseases of the gastrointestinal tract. In: Greenberg MS, Glick M, eds. Burket's Oral Medicine Diagnosis and Treatment. 10th ed. Hamilton, Ontario, Canada: BC Decker 2003:389–406.

159. Ficarra G, Cicchi P, Armorosi A et al. Oral Surg Oral Med Oral Pathol 1993;75:220–4.

160. Griffiths AM. Inflammatory bowel disease. In: Shils ME, Olson JA, Shike M et al., eds. Modern Nutrition in Health and Disease. 9th ed. Philadelphia: Williams & Wilkins, 1999:1141–9.

161. Morse DE. Oral and pharyngeal cancer. In: Touger-Decker R, Sirois DA, Mobley CC, eds. Nutrition and Oral Medicine. Totowa, NJ: Humana Press, 2005:205–22.

162. Franceschi S, Favero A, Conti E et al. Br J Cancer 1999;80: 614–20.

163. Tavani A, Gallus S, La Vecchia C et al. Eur J Cancer Prev 2001; 10:191–5.

164. DeStefani E, Ronco A, Mendilaharsu M et al. Oral Oncol 1999;34:222–6.

165. Negri E, Franceschi S, Bosetti C et al. Int J Cancer 2000;86: 122–7.

166. Petridou E, Zavras A, Lefatzis D et al. Cancer 2002;94:2981–8.

167. Benner S, Winn R, Lippman S et al. J Natl Cancer Inst 1993;85: 44–7.

168. Garewal H. Am J Clin Nutr 1995;62[Suppl]:1410S–16S.

169. Garewal H, Meyskens F, Friedman S et al. Prev Med 1993;22: 701–11.

170. Toth BB, Martin JW, Flemming RJ. Clin Periodontol 1990;17: 508–15.

171. Dwyer J, Efstathion A, Palmer C, Papas A. Nutr Rev 1991;49: 11:332–7.

172. Bardow A, Nyvad B, Nauntofte B. Arch Oral Biol 2001;46: 413–23.

173. Grisius MM, Fox PC. Salivary gland diseases. In Greenberg MS, Glick M, eds. Burket's Oral Medicine Diagnosis and Treatment. 10th ed. Hamilton, Ontario, Canada: BC Decker, 2003:235–70.

174. Mobley C, Saunders MJ. J Am Diet Assoc 1997;97[Suppl 2]:S123–6.

175. Rhodus NL, Brown J. J Am Diet Assoc 1990;90:1688–92.

176. Heft MW, Baum BJ. J Dent Res 1984;63:1182–5.

177. Beck JD, Hunt RJ. J Dent Educ 1985;49:407–25.

178. Diaz–Arnold AM, Marek CA. J Prosthet Dent 2002;88: 337–43.

179. Schroeder PL, Filler SJ, Ramirez B et al. Ann Intern Med 1995;122:11:809–10.

180. Tylenda AA, Robert MW, Elin RJ. J Am Dent Assoc 1991;122: 37–41.

181. Roberts MW, Li SH. J Am Dent Assoc 1987;115:407–10.

182. Gross KBW, Brough KM, Randolph PM. J Dent Child 1986;53:378–81.

183. He W, Sengupta M, Velkoff VA et al. 65+ in the United States: 2004. Current population reports, special studies; P23. Washington, DC: US Government Printing Office.

184. Mojon P, Budtz-Jørgensen E, Rapin C. Age Ageing 1999;28: 463–8.

185. Dolan TA, Atchison KA. J Dent Educ 1993;57:876–85.

186. Sheiham A, Steele J. Public Health Nutr 2001;4:797–803.

187. Brodeur JM, Laurin D, Vallee R et al. J Prosthet Dent 1993;70: 468–73.

188. Slagter AP, Olthoff LW, Bosman F et al. J Prosthet Dent 1992; 68:299–307.

189. Moynihan P, Bradbury J. Nutrition 2001;17:177–8.

190. Bartoshuk LM. Chemical sensation: taste. In: Pollack R, Kravitz R, eds. Nutrition in Oral Health and Disease. Philadelphia: Lea & Febiger, 1985.

191. Berkey D, Berg R, Ettinger R et al. J Am Dent Assoc 1996;127: 321–32.

192. Atkinson JC, Fox PC. Clin Geriatr Med 1992;8:499–511.

193. US Public Health Service, National Institute of Dental Research. Oral Health of United States Adults: National Findings. NIH Publ. no. (PHS) 88–1593, series 10, no. 165. Washington, DC: US Government Printing Office, 1988.

194. Nutrition Screening Initiative. Nutrition Screening Manual for Professionals Caring for Older Americans. Washington, DC, (Nutrition Screening Initiative, 2626 Pennsylvania Avenue NW, Suite 301, Washington, DC 20037).

195. Touger-Decker R, Sirois D. Dental care of the person with diabetes. In: Powers MA ed. Handbook of Diabetes Nutrition Management. 2nd ed. Rockville, MD: Aspen, 1996.

196. Samarananayake LP. Host factors and oral candidosis. In: Samarananayake LP, MacFarlane TW, eds. Oral Candidosis. London: Wright, 1990:66–103.

197. Loe H. Diabetes Care 1993;16:329–34.

198. Holdren RS, Patton LL. Diabetes Spectrum 1993;6:11–7.

199. Tonzetich J. J Periodontol 1977;48;13–29.

200. Greenstein RB, Goldberg S, Marky-Cohen S et al. J Periodontol 1997;68;1176–81.

201. Bollen CM, Rompen EH, Demanez JP. Rev Med Liege 1999: 54;32–6.

202. Levitt MD, Gibson GR, Christl SU. Gas metabolism in the large intestine. In: Gibson GR, Macfarlane GT, eds. Human Colonic Bacteria: Role in Nutrition, Physiology and Diesease. Boca Raton, FL: CRC Press, 1995:131–54.

203. Suarez F, Springfield J, Furne J et al. Am J Physiol 1999;276: G425–30.

204. Hasler WJ. Gastroenterology 1999;117:1248–9.

205. Paster B. Personal communication, 2004.

SELECTED READINGS

Bowen WH, Tabak L. Cariology for the Nineties. Rochester, NY: University of Rochester Press, 1993.

DePaola DP, Mobley C, Tougher-Decker R. Nutrition and oral medicine. In: Berdanier CD, ed. CRC Handbook of Nutrition and Food. Boca Raton, FL: CRC Press, 2002:1113–34.

DePaola DP, Schachtele CP. Diet and oral disease. In: Stipanuk MH, ed. Biochemical and Physiological Aspects of Human Nutrition. Philadelphia: WB Saunders, 2000:866–81.

Enwonwu CO. Cellular and molecular effects of malnutrition and their relevance to periodontal diseases. J Clin Periodontol 1994;21:643–57.

Enwonwu CO, Phillips RS, Falkier WA. Nutrition and oral infectious disease: state of the science. Compend Contin Educ Dent 2002;23: 431–46.

Harris NO, Garcia-Godoy F. Primary Preventative Dentistry. Norwalk, CT: Appleton & Lange, 1999.

Palmer CA, ed. Diet and Nutrition in Oral Health. Englewood Cliffs, NJ: Prentice-Hall, 2003.

Tougher-Decker R, Sirois DA, Mobley CC, eds. Nutrition and Oral Medicine. Totowa, NJ: Humana Press, 2005.

Whitford GM. Flouride. In: Stipanuk MH, ed. Biochemical and Physiological Aspects of Human Nutrition. Philadelphia: WB Saunders, 2000:810–24.

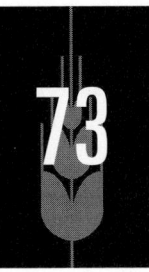

73 THE ESOPHAGUS AND STOMACH[1]
WILLIAM F. STENSON

MOUTH, PHARYNX, AND ESOPHAGUS 1179
GASTRIC MOTILITY 1179
   Gastric Motility after a Meal 1179
   Gastric Motility during Fasting 1180
   Gastric Emptying 1181
   Disorders of Gastric Emptying 1181
GASTRIC SECRETION AND DIGESTION 1182
   Acid Secretion 1182
   Protein and Fat Digestion 1184
   Intrinsic Factor 1184
DIET IN GASTROESOPHAGEAL DISEASES 1184
   Gastroesophageal Reflux Disease 1184
   Peptic Ulcer Disease .1185
NUTRITION AND GASTRIC SURGERY 1185
   Surgery and Gastric Emptying 1185
   Dumping Syndrome .1186
   Iron and Calcium 1187

MOUTH, PHARYNX, AND ESOPHAGUS

The digestive process is initiated by placing food in the mouth (see also Chapter 70). Chewing and salivary secretion result in formation of a food bolus, a rounded, lubricated mass suitable for swallowing (Fig. 73.1). Movement of the bolus from the mouth to the pharynx initiates the process of swallowing. The presence of the bolus in the pharynx activates glossopharyngeal and vagal fibers connected to the swallowing center in the brainstem (1). The swallowing center coordinates initiation of swallowing, opening of the upper esophageal sphincter, peristalsis in the upper esophagus, and momentary cessation of breathing. The presence of food in the mouth also activates neural pathways that result in salivary secretion, gastric acid secretion, pancreatic secretion, contraction of the gallbladder, and relaxation of the sphincter of Oddi. Thus, although the mouth and pharynx have little direct role in digestion and absorption of nutrients, neurally mediated events initiated by the presence of food in the mouth and pharynx are important in coordinating the initial phases of

the integrated response of the entire gastrointestinal (GI) tract to a meal.

Human saliva contains two digestive enzymes, salivary amylase and lingual lipase. Lingual lipase has a limited role in digestion of dietary triglycerides; however, salivary amylase plays an important role in digestion of dietary starches. Although salivary amylase is secreted with the saliva into the mouth, little starch digestion occurs in the mouth because of the limited time of interaction of food with saliva there. Most of the enzymatic activity of salivary amylase occurs in the stomach, where there is a much longer time for it to interact with dietary starch. After leaving the pharynx, the food bolus passes through the upper esophageal sphincter to enter the esophagus (2, 3). In the resting state, both the upper esophageal sphincter and the lower esophageal sphincter (LES) are closed. After initiation of a swallow, pressure in the pharynx increases, and the upper esophageal sphincter relaxes. This combination of events pushes the food bolus from the pharynx into the upper esophagus. Then the upper sphincter closes, and a peristaltic wave pushes the bolus through the esophagus. The LES relaxes after initiation of the swallow and contracts again after the bolus passes through it.

GASTRIC MOTILITY

Gastric Motility after a Meal

After a meal, the stomach relaxes, and its volume increases to accommodate the ingested food (see also Chapter 70). In addition to this reservoir function, the stomach also grinds food into smaller particles through the action of the antral musculature. Finally, the stomach releases the gastric contents into the duodenum in a regulated fashion. The net effects of the motor activity of the stomach are to prepare food for digestion and absorption in the intestine by reducing it to small particles and to present these particles to the intestine at a rate that facilitates digestion and absorption by allowing maximal mixing with pancreatic and biliary secretions and maximal contact time with the small intestinal mucosa (4).

Motility is markedly different in the proximal and distal parts of the stomach (5). The proximal stomach, which includes the fundus and the upper part of the body, relaxes as it is filled with food. This relaxation increases gastric volume without increasing intragastric pressure. Relaxation of

[1]**Abbreviations: GERD,** gastroesophageal reflux disease; **GI,** gastrointestinal; **LES,** lower esophageal sphincter; **MMC,** migrating motor complex.

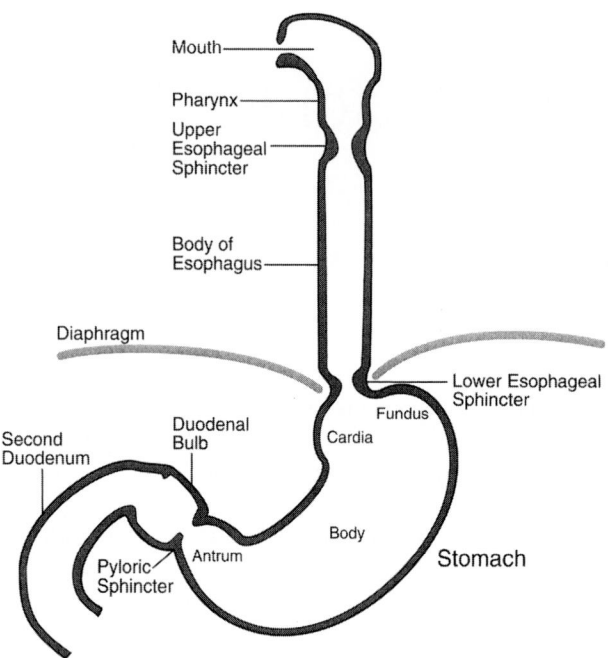

Figure 73.1. Anatomy of the human upper gastrointestinal tract.

the proximal stomach in response to a meal includes both receptive relaxation and gastric accommodation (5, 6). *Receptive relaxation* is a reduction in proximal gastric tone in response to swallowing; it is mediated by neural pathways and occurs within 10 seconds of swallowing. In contrast, *gastric accommodation* is the reflex relaxation of the proximal stomach in response to gastric distention; this process is mediated by vagovagal reflexes. The vagal afferents are activated by the effects of gastric distention on pressure receptors in the gastric wall. The afferent messages are processed in the brain in the dorsal vagal complex of the medulla. This processing, in turn, initiates vagal efferent activity, which elicits effects in the stomach and other portions of the GI tract. In the stomach, the vagal efferent activity causes muscle relaxation in the proximal stomach (gastric accommodation) and muscle contraction in the antrum; it also induces secretion of gastric acid, pepsinogen, and gastrin. Vagal efferent activity induced by gastric distention also causes increased enzyme secretion in the pancreas, contraction of the gallbladder, and relaxation of the sphincter of Oddi.

The period of relaxation in the proximal stomach after a meal is followed by a period of contraction, which increases intragastric pressure. The proximal stomach produces slow, sustained tonic contractions to push the contents of the meal into the distal stomach. The intragastric pressure created by the tonic contraction of the proximal stomach increases the rate of gastric emptying, especially the emptying of liquids. Contraction of the proximal stomach is regulated by neural and hormonal input; among the hormones that influence this process are cholecystokinin, motilin, and gastrin.

The distal stomach includes the lower part of the body and the antrum. In contrast to the tonic contractions of the proximal stomach, the contractions of the distal stomach are phasic. (In *tonic contractions*, the muscle contracts over a long period; in *phasic contractions*, rhythmic contraction and relaxation occur.) Tonic contractions of the proximal stomach influence the rate of gastric emptying, whereas phasic contractions of the distal stomach grind food into small particles. Phasic motor activity in the distal stomach migrates as a ring contraction, increasing in amplitude as it approaches the pylorus; these contractions can generate intragastric pressures as high as 100 mm Hg. Phasic contractions originate in an area of spontaneously depolarizing muscle in the proximal body termed the gastric pacemaker; depolarization travels in a wavelike manner from the pacemaker through the distal body and the antrum. The pattern of phasic antral contractions seen in the fed state begins 5 to 10 minutes after the ingestion of a meal and persists as long as food remains in the stomach. Fluoroscopic studies demonstrate that antral contractions first propel ingested material distally toward the pylorus. The pylorus is closed tightly enough that larger food particles cannot pass. The ingested material is then directed back from the distal antrum into the more proximal stomach, and the process is repeated (7). This to-and-fro action mixes and grinds solid food.

The pylorus is a sphincter that sits at the junction of the antrum and the duodenal bulb. It regulates the flow of intraluminal contents from the stomach into the duodenum (8). The rate of gastric emptying is determined by the pressure generated in the proximal stomach and by the size of the pyloric opening; the higher the pressure and the larger the opening, the faster the rate of emptying. During feeding, the pylorus acts as a sieve that impairs the emptying of particles greater than 1 mm in diameter (9). If the stomach is presented with a meal that is a mixture of small (<1 mm) and large (>2 mm) particles, the pylorus passes the smaller ones and retains the larger ones. Antral grinding of the larger particles reduces them to a size that can pass through the pylorus.

Gastric Motility during Fasting

In addition to the motor activity seen in the stomach in response to a meal, there is also activity in the fasting state. The migrating motor complex (MMC) clears the stomach and small intestine of undigested food particles and other particulate debris (10). The MMC has three phases of activity that repeat at periods of 90 to 100 minutes. Phase I, which occupies 40 to 60% of the cycle, is a period of little phasic motor activity. Phase II, which lasts 20 to 30% of the cycle length, is a period of irregular contractions of various amplitudes. Phase III lasts 5 to 10 minutes and is marked by high-pressure, propagative waves accompanied by pyloric relaxation. These waves clear undigested food particles from the stomach. Phase III is mediated by cyclic release of motilin from duodenal mucosal cells.

Gastric Emptying

Liquids and solids each empty from the stomach at different rates, and these rates are regulated by different mechanisms (5, 11). Liquids, such as water or isotonic saline, empty rapidly from the stomach. The volume emptied into the duodenum is a constant fraction of the volume of liquid in the stomach. Thus, the initial rate of emptying of a 400-mL bolus of water is twice that of a 200-mL bolus; half the volume of a bolus of water empties from the stomach in about 10 to 15 minutes (12). The rate of emptying of liquids from the stomach is determined by the tonic contractions of the proximal stomach but is also influenced by the degree of pyloric resistance and the capacity of the duodenum to receive a volume of fluid.

When nutrients such as glucose are present in a liquid meal, the rate of gastric emptying is slowed in response to feedback from the small intestine (13). Neural reflexes from the small intestine modulate contraction of the muscles of the proximal stomach and thus affect intragastric pressure and the rate of gastric emptying. The rate of emptying of a liquid from the stomach is influenced by its caloric concentration, osmolality, fat content, and pH. Liquids of high caloric density empty more slowly than those with fewer calories per unit volume. The emptying of nutrients occurs at a rate that delivers approximately 200 kcal/hour into the intestine. Carbohydrates and amino acids modulate intestinal nutrient delivery through their effects on small intestine osmolality. Nutritional liquids of high osmolality empty more slowly than those of low osmolality. A bolus of 300 mL of 0.1 M glucose empties from the stomach three times as fast as a bolus of 300 mL of 0.3 M glucose (14). The effects of fats on gastric emptying are complex. Liquid fats empty from the stomach more slowly than aqueous liquids. Fats bind to solid food particles and float on the surface of aqueous gastric secretions, and this feature slows their emptying from the stomach. The rate of liquid emptying from the stomach is also influenced by pH; acid solutions empty more slowly than neutral solutions. This reflex prevents acid solutions from entering the duodenum at a rate high enough to lower the pH of the duodenal contents and thus diminish the activity of pancreatic enzymes. Slowing the release of acid solutions from the stomach provides more time for neutralization by bicarbonate in biliary and pancreatic secretions.

Digestible solids empty from the stomach at a slower rate than liquids. Food particles need to be reduced in diameter to a maximum of 1 to 2 mm to allow passage through the pylorus (15). Small particles have a higher surface volume ratio than large particles, and this makes more of their contents accessible to the action of digestive enzymes in the intestine. Digestible solids empty after an initial lag phase that persists for up to an hour after the end of a meal. During the lag phase, extensive mixing and grinding of solid food occur, but little or no solid material exits the stomach. The smaller the food particles are, the shorter the lag phase is. After this initial grinding period, the particles empty at a linear rate that is independent of the volume remaining in the stomach. Food particles larger than 2 mm in diameter that cannot be further reduced in size are emptied from the stomach by active contraction during phase III of the MMC. These strong contractions also clear foreign bodies from the stomach. In adults, coins as large as a quarter are cleared through the pylorus by the MMC.

Disorders of Gastric Emptying

Most disturbances of gastric motor activity delay gastric emptying (16). Gastroparesis is a chronic motility disorder of the stomach characterized by delayed gastric emptying in the absence of mechanical obstruction. In gastroparesis, accommodation is impaired; the stomach fails to distend in response to a meal and fails to shrink in response to emptying. Peristaltic contractions are weak, resulting in a failure to break down food particles and emulsify fats. Emptying of liquids is normal, but emptying of solids is delayed. Partially digested food may be retained in the stomach to form a bezoar. The symptoms associated with delayed gastric emptying are nausea, vomiting, early satiety (feeling full after eating a small portion of a normal meal), weight loss, and abdominal distention. Delayed gastric emptying can result in vomiting of recognizable food particles many hours after ingestion of a meal. Delayed gastric emptying caused by disorders of gastric motility may be difficult to distinguish from that caused by gastric outlet obstruction by ulcer, scarring, or tumor; the two conditions cause the same set of symptoms.

Delayed gastric emptying is seen in a variety of conditions. Certain drugs can delay gastric emptying; among these are opiates, tricyclic antidepressants, phenothiazines, and calcium channel blockers. Alcohol, tobacco, and marijuana can also delay gastric emptying. Delayed gastric emptying is seen in anorexia nervosa. Malnutrition itself can delay gastric emptying; treatment of patients with anorexia nervosa with dietary supplements to induce weight gain improves gastric emptying. Radiation therapy to the upper abdomen can result in delayed gastric emptying within months or many years.

The most common cause of clinically significant delayed gastric emptying is diabetic gastroparesis (17–19). This is especially common in insulin-dependent diabetes of long standing and is often associated with peripheral or autonomic neuropathy. At least 25% of insulin-requiring diabetics who have had their disease for 10 years, will have delayed emptying of liquids and/or solids (20). For some patients with long-standing insulin-dependent diabetes, gastroparesis is a major cause of morbidity; severe upper abdominal discomfort, frequent vomiting, and substantial weight loss are common. The pathogenesis of the delay in gastric emptying in diabetes is not well understood, but evidence indicates that it results primarily from neuropathy of the autonomic nervous system, with vagal neuropathy being the dominant abnormality (21). Reduced vagal input to the distal stomach results in reduced antral contractions. Pyloric dysfunction also occurs in diabetes and results in increased pyloric resistance and impairment of emptying. Evaluation of diabetic gastroparesis is difficult, and most patients are treated on the basis of suggestive symptoms in an appropriate clinical setting. Delayed gastric emptying may be suspected from retained gastric contents after a fast for a radiologic upper GI examination or endoscopy.

A radionuclide gastric-emptying study is the most sensitive clinical test. Solid-phase radionuclide tracers are normally used, because delayed emptying for either liquids or solids may be detected by this method. Radionuclide emptying studies have a broad range of normal values, and the results need to be carefully standardized. The correlation between symptoms and radionuclide studies is not good; some asymptomatic patients have markedly abnormal radionuclide studies, and some patients with severe symptoms have relatively normal studies.

The first approach to symptomatic relief in diabetic gastroparesis is better control of blood glucose concentrations; hyperglycemia itself is thought to have adverse effects on gastric motor function. Other approaches include removing offending medications, increasing the liquid content of the diet, and reducing dietary fat. Over the past few years, several drugs that stimulate GI motility have become available. Although some of these prokinetic agents are effective in diabetic gastroparesis, their efficacy is variable and tends to diminish over time. Metoclopramide has dopamine-antagonist and cholinergic-enhancing effects (22). The cholinergic effects increase the amplitude and frequency of antral contractions and relax the pylorus. Thus, metoclopramide produces an effect that mimics phase III of the MMC. The central dopamine antagonism of metoclopramide can cause side effects that mimic Parkinson disease. The prokinetic effect of metoclopramide on the stomach is diminished after about 4 weeks of therapy. Cisapride accelerates emptying of both liquids and solids by enhancing the coordination of gastric and duodenal motor events (23). Like metoclopramide, cisapride produces a phase III–like effect through acetylcholine release. The prokinetic effects of cisapride are more sustained than those of metoclopramide but still diminish after 6 months. In contrast to metoclopramide, which activates motility primarily in the stomach and proximal small intestine, cisapride activates motility in the entire GI tract from esophagus to colon; as a consequence, diarrhea is its major side effect. Cisapride is only available to approved physicians through limited-access protocols. Injection of botulinum toxin into the pyloric sphincter has been beneficial in diabetic gastroparesis in preliminary studies (24–26).

Accelerated gastric emptying occurs most commonly in patients who have had gastric surgery for peptic ulcer disease. This topic is discussed later in the section Nutrition and Gastric Surgery.

GASTRIC SECRETION AND DIGESTION

The major organ for digestion and absorption of nutrients is the small intestine (see also Chapter 70). The stomach primarily prepares ingested food for digestion and absorption in the small intestine by grinding it into smaller particles and regulating its flow into the small intestine for optimal digestion and absorption. Although the intestine is the major digestive organ, appreciable digestion of carbohydrates, protein, and fats occurs in the stomach (27). Moreover, the stomach is the source of intrinsic factor, a protein required for absorption of vitamin B_{12} in the ileum. Although the stomach facilitates digestion of macronutrients, its contribution to digestion is not absolutely required. Patients who have undergone total gastrectomy can maintain normal nutritional status on a regular diet despite the absence of the stomach. The only exception to this is the requirement for administration of parenteral vitamin B_{12} to compensate for the malabsorption of dietary vitamin B_{12} as a result of the absence of intrinsic factor. In patients with gastrectomies, the major morbidity is not the absence of the stomach as a digestive organ but, rather, the absence of the stomach as a food reservoir and regulator of the flow of ingested food into the small intestine.

Digestive events in the stomach are tied to the functional capacity of the different populations of cells forming the gastric epithelial lining. The gastric lining consists of thick folds, each of which contains microscopic gastric pits (28). Four or five gastric glands drain into each of these pits. The mucosa of the body and fundus of the stomach contains oxyntic glands (Fig. 73.2). (The term oxyntic gland comes from the oxyntic, or parietal, cell, which is a prominent component of these glands.) Oxyntic glands are lined by parietal cells that secrete gastric acid and intrinsic factor and by chief cells that secrete pepsinogen and gastric lipase. In contrast, the pyloric glands that form the mucosa of the antrum contain almost no parietal cells or chief cells but, rather, contain mucus-secreting cells and G cells, which produce the hormone gastrin.

Acid Secretion

The physiologic function most closely associated with the stomach is the production of gastric acid (27). The physiologic stimulus for gastric acid production is food. Although gastric acid is produced in response to a meal, it plays a relatively minor role in digestion. Patients treated with drugs that inhibit gastric acid secretion by blocking the parietal cell proton pump do not have clinically significant problems with maldigestion or malabsorption. Nonetheless, gastric acid does play some role in digestion.

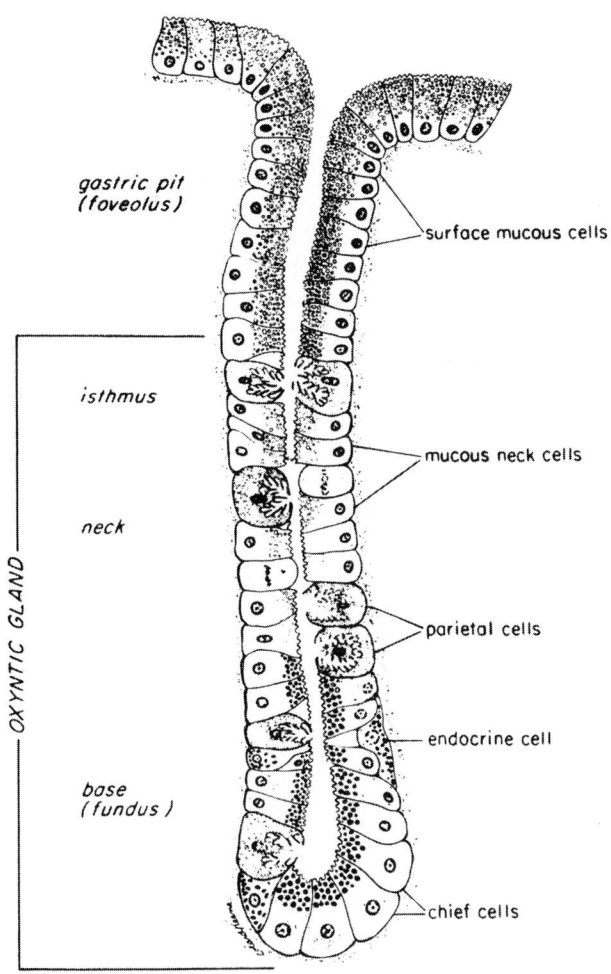

Figure 73.2. Gastric gland from the body of a mammalian stomach. (From Ito S, Winchester RJ. J Cell Biol 1963;16:541–78, with permission.)

gastric pit (foveolus)

surface mucous cells

OXYNTIC GLAND

isthmus

mucous neck cells

neck

parietal cells

endocrine cell

base (fundus)

chief cells

Conversion of pepsinogen to pepsin requires an acid pH that can only be achieved by gastric acid secretion. Moreover, pepsins, which break down proteins into peptides, have pH optima in the acid range. Gastric lipase cleaves triglycerides to yield free fatty acids. The pH optimum for gastric lipase is between 4 and 5.5; this enzyme is much less active at the neutral pH seen in the absence of gastric acid secretion. However, neither pepsin nor gastric lipase is required for digestion of food. The functional reserves of pancreatic peptidases and pancreatic lipase are large enough to make up for the loss of the contribution of pepsins and gastric lipase to digestion. Gastric acid secretion is important in the absorption of iron, particularly nonheme iron. Ferric salts are insoluble at neutral or slightly acid pH, whereas ferrous salts are much more soluble in this pH range (29). In acidic solutions (pH <4), ferric salts dissolve and can be reduced to ferrous salts, which remain in solution at the neutral pH found in the duodenum where they are absorbed.

Gastric acid is secreted constantly, but the rate of secretion is increased with meals. During fasting, gastric acid is secreted at about 15% of its maximal rate. The food-stimulated increase in gastric acid secretion occurs in three phases: cephalic, gastric, and intestinal (27). The cephalic phase refers to the stimulation of gastric acid secretion by the smell, taste, or even thought of food. Gastric acid secretion induced by chewing or swallowing food is also part of the cephalic phase. The cephalic phase is mediated primarily by the vagus nerve; vagotomy abolishes this phase of gastric acid secretion. When food enters the stomach, gastric acid secretion is stimulated. One mechanism for the gastric phase of acid secretion is distention of the stomach by food, which activates stretch receptors in the gastric wall and thus initiates gastric acid secretion mediated by a vagovagal reflex. A second mechanism is activation of chemoreceptors by amino acids and peptides formed by partial digestion of dietary proteins by pepsins. The entry of partially digested food into the small intestine initiates the intestinal phase of acid secretion. This process is mediated by distention of the small intestine and by the presence of proteins and the products of protein digestion in the partially digested food. In contrast to the cephalic and gastric phases of gastric secretion, the intestinal phase is not mediated by vagal reflexes; the intestinal phase remains intact even after vagotomy.

Gastric acid secretion increases at the start of a meal; within 1 hour after the end of the meal, the rate of acid secretion reaches a peak that is near the maximal capacity of the stomach to secrete acid. Within 2 to 3 hours after a meal, gastric acid production is reduced by the presence of acid and the products of digestion in the stomach and intestine. Although the rate of acid secretion peaks within the first hour after a meal, the total amount of acid in the stomach rises for an additional 1 to 2 hours.

The presence of acid in the gastric antrum shuts down gastrin release and thus reduces acid secretion. The presence of acid, fat, or hyperosmotic solutions in the duodenum inhibits gastric acid secretion. The inhibition of acid secretion by duodenal contents is at least partially humoral, because it persists after vagotomy. Certain hormones including somatostatin, secretin, and cholecystokinin have been suggested as possible mediators of the inhibition of gastric acid secretion by duodenal contents.

Gastric acid secretion by parietal cells is regulated by acetylcholine, gastrin, and histamine (30). Parietal cells have specific receptors for each of these ligands. Acetylcholine is a neurotransmitter produced by the vagus and other parasympathetic nerves. Gastrin is a peptide hormone produced by G cells in the gastric antrum. Gastrin secretion is stimulated by specific nutrients in the gastric lumen that include amino acids and small peptides but not glucose or fat. Gastrin release is also stimulated by a high pH in the gastric lumen. Histamine is secreted by mucosal mast cells and enterochromaffin-like cells. Drugs that suppress the hydrogen/potassium adenosine triphosphatase in gastric parietal cells are called proton pump inhibitors, and they strongly decrease acid secretion. Another class of drugs that block the binding of histamine to its receptor on parietal cells (H_2-receptor antagonists) are also potent inhibitors of gastric acid secretion.

Protein and Fat Digestion

In the stomach, dietary proteins are cleaved into smaller peptides by the action of pepsins, proteases that are maximally active at low pH (pH 1.5–2.5) and are inactivated by neutral or alkaline conditions (31). Pepsinogens, the inactive precursors of pepsins, are secreted by chief cells and are autocatalytically cleaved to form pepsins under acidic conditions (pH <6). Secretion of pepsinogens by chief cells, like secretion of gastric acid by parietal cells, occurs in response to the ingestion of food. Gastrin and acetylcholine are important mediators of pepsinogen secretion in response to a meal. Chief cells store pepsinogen in apical granules; stimulation by gastrin or acetylcholine results in the exocytosis of these granules. Parallel stimulation of parietal cells provides the acid environment required for cleavage of pepsinogens to form pepsins. Protein digestion by pepsins, which cleave only 10 to 15% of the peptide bonds in dietary proteins, yields a mixture of peptides with relatively few free amino acids. Peptides generated by pepsin digestion of dietary proteins act as signals for secretion of gastrin by G cells in the antral mucosa. These peptides are further hydrolyzed to amino acids by the action of pancreatic peptidases in the intestine. The stomach contributes to fat digestion both by emulsifying dietary fats to prepare them for digestion by lipases in the intestine and by lipolysis of ingested fats by gastric lipase (32). Emulsification of dietary fats is initiated in the stomach by body heat, which liquefies most dietary fat, and by the grinding action of the antrum, which promotes the interaction of dietary lecithin with dietary triglyceride droplets. Gastric lipase, like pepsinogens, is secreted by chief cells in the oxyntic mucosa; its secretion is regulated by the same mechanisms that regulate secretion of pepsinogens. Gastric lipase differs from pancreatic lipase in several important respects. It has a pH optimum of 4 to 5.5, as opposed to the neutral pH optimum of pancreatic lipase. Moreover, gastric lipase acts preferentially on the 3-position long-chain fatty acid esterified on triglyceride. Thus, the major products of gastric lipase action on triglycerides are free fatty acids and diglycerides. Moreover, gastric lipase is activated by bile salts, whereas pancreatic lipase is not. Under normal circumstances, gastric lipase accounts for the digestion of 20 to 30% of total dietary fats, with pancreatic lipase accounting for most of the rest. When pancreatic lipase is present in decreased amounts, as in patients with pancreatitis or surgical resections of the pancreas, gastric lipase can account for a considerably larger percentage of lipid digestion. Gastric lipase is also important in lipid digestion in neonates, because pancreatic lipase secretion is quite limited during the first weeks of life.

Intrinsic Factor

Intrinsic factor is secreted from parietal cells in response to stimulation by gastrin and acetylcholine (33). Dietary vitamin B_{12} (cobalamin) can be absorbed in the ileum only when it is complexed with intrinsic factor (see Chapter 29). Other luminal porteins can also bind cobalamin; in the acidic environment of the stomach, cobalamin preferentially binds to R protein, which is secreted in saliva, rather than intrinsic factor. In the duodenum and jejunum, salivary R protein is degraded by pancreatic proteases, and cobalamin is released. In the neutral pH of the small intestine, cobalamin preferentially binds to intrinsic factor. The intrinsic factor–cobalamin complex is then bound to a specific ileal receptor and absorbed. Even though the stomach secretes intrinsic factor in excess, a partial gastrectomy (especially one that involves resection of a significant portion of the body) may result in substantial loss of intrinsic factor secretory capacity, with clinically significant effects on cobalamin absorption. In the complete absence of intrinsic factor secretion (e.g., after total gastrectomy), dietary cobalamin is not absorbed. The very large stores of cobalamin in the liver prevent development of the clinical manifestations of cobalamin deficiency for 3 to 6 years after gastrectomy. In addition to total or partial gastrectomy, the other common cause of intrinsic factor deficiency is pernicious anemia, a disease that typically affects elderly white persons. It is characterized by atrophy of the oxyntic mucosa with resultant loss of gastric acid and intrinsic factor secretion. Over a period of years, the absence of intrinsic factor leads to clinical cobalamin deficiency. Patients with pernicious anemia and those with total gastrectomy should receive parenteral cobalamin once a month. Although parenteral cobalamin is the conventional therapy for those with pernicious anemia or gastrectomy, oral cobalamin, if given in high enough doses, is also effective (34). In patients with partial gastrectomies, the risk of cobalamin deficiency is great enough that either the serum cobalamin level should be monitored carefully or the patient should be given prophylactic vitamin B_{12} therapy. Pernicious anemia is associated with a two- or three-fold increase in the risk of gastric cancer.

DIET IN GASTROESOPHAGEAL DISEASES

Gastroesophageal Reflux Disease

Gastroesophageal reflux disease (GERD) consists of irritation and inflammation of the esophagus in response to reflux of gastric acid into the esophagus (35). In physiologically normal persons, reflux of gastric contents into the esophagus is largely blocked by the LES at the junction of the esophagus and stomach. The LES is normally closed except during swallowing. Despite the presence of the LES, some reflux of gastric contents into the esophagus occurs in physiologically normal persons. This reflux elicits esophageal contractions that push the refluxed gastric contents back into the stomach. GERD occurs when reflux of gastric contents into the esophagus occurs with excessive frequency or in excessive volume or if the refluxed gastric contents fail to elicit esophageal contractions to push them back into the stomach. When too much gastric acid is in contact with the esophageal mucosa for too long a time, the person may experience heartburn. In milder cases of GERD, the patient experiences heartburn, but the esophageal mucosa remains endoscopically and histologically normal. In more severe cases, the refluxed gastric contents cause the esophageal mucosa to become inflamed and ulcerated. Healing of these esophageal ulcers can result in stricturing of the esophagus and thus difficulty in swallowing. Among the factors that contribute to GERD are an excessive volume of acidic contents in the stomach, looseness of the LES, and motility disorders in the esophagus that impair its ability to generate a coordinated contraction in response to reflux of gastric contents. The amount of acid refluxed, the severity of heartburn, and the damage to the epithelium do not always correlate. Sometimes, severe heartburn is seen in the absence of mucosal injury, or severe injury is seen in patients with minimal heartburn.

GERD is treated with drugs, physical measures, and diet. The drugs used to treat GERD are those that decrease gastric acid secretion (H_2-receptor antagonists and proton pump inhibitors), those that neutralize gastric acid (antacids), and those that enhance gastric emptying (metoclopramide and cisapride). One physical measure used to treat GERD is elevation of the head of the bed, to keep gastric acid in the stomach and out of the esophagus during sleep.

Diet affects GERD in several ways. If the esophageal mucosa is damaged and sensory pain fibers are exposed or sensitized, acidic foods such as orange juice or tomato juice may elicit pain on swallowing. The more important impact of diet on GERD involves the effects of food on LES pressure and gastric acid secretion, which depend on both the kinds of food consumed and the timing of their ingestion. The amount of gastric acid in the stomach reaches a maximum 2 to 3 hours after a meal. When a person is in the upright position, gravity keeps gastric acid in the lower portions of the stomach; however, reclining allows gastric acid to enter the upper part of the stomach, where it can more easily reflux into the esophagus. Patients with GERD frequently complain that their symptoms worsen if they lie down after eating. Thus, patients with GERD should be told not to eat within 3 hours before going to bed. Alcohol, chocolate, and fatty foods have been implicated in relaxing the LES and inducing GERD. In physiologically normal persons, coffee tightens the LES; however, in patients with GERD, it does not. Furthermore, coffee and alcohol both increase gastric acid secretion. Thus, a bad combination of events for a patient with GERD is a large, fatty meal eaten late in the evening and accompanied by alcohol, coffee, and chocolate.

Peptic Ulcer Disease

Peptic ulcer disease includes both gastric and duodenal ulcers (36). For many years, gastric acid secretion was thought to playa major role in the pathogenesis of peptic ulcer disease; however, more recent studies identified *Helicobacter pylori* as a causal agent for many, if not most, cases of peptic ulcer disease. Aspirin and other nonsteroidal antiinflammatory drugs play a part in the causation of many other cases of peptic ulcer disease. Although gastric acid is not the primary cause in the majority of cases of peptic ulcer disease, it does play a causal role when it is secreted at extremely high rates, as is seen in Zollinger-Ellison syndrome.

Although gastric acid is not a primary cause of most cases of peptic ulcer disease, inhibition of gastric acid secretion is therapeutic. Both H_2-receptor antagonists, which inhibit gastric acid secretion by blocking the histamine receptor on parietal cells, and proton pump inhibitors, which inhibit the parietal cell pump that secretes hydrogen ions into the gastric lumen, are therapeutic in peptic ulcer disease. Although these drugs that profoundly inhibit gastric acid secretion are therapeutic in peptic ulcer disease, evidence indicates that dietary manipulations that modulate gastric acid secretion are therapeutic.

Many patients with ulcers remark that certain foods, particularly spicy foods, cause them epigastric discomfort, but no evidence indicates that these foods cause peptic ulcer disease. Moreover, no causal role in peptic ulcer disease has been demonstrated even for foods known to be potent inducers of gastric acid secretion, such as milk, alcohol, and coffee. Just as no evidence exists for a causal role for diet in peptic ulcer disease, no evidence demonstrates that diet influences the rate of ulcer healing. Many patients with ulcers have been told to avoid alcohol, coffee, and other potent secretagogs, yet no evidence indicates that these dietary factors, at least when taken in moderate quantities, retard ulcer healing. Theoretic reasons exist to limit the consumption of alcohol, in particular, in patients with peptic ulcer disease. Beer and wine, even in modest amounts, induce near-maximal gastric acid secretion without providing any significant buffering capacity. Some interest has been shown in the potential role of dietary fiber in peptic ulcer disease; some studies suggest that the incidence of recurrence of peptic ulcer disease is higher in patients on low-fiber diets than in those on high-fiber diets (37).

NUTRITION AND GASTRIC SURGERY

Surgery and Gastric Emptying

The markedly improved medical therapy for peptic ulcer disease in recent years resulted in a profound decrease in surgery for this disease. Two commonly performed surgical procedures for peptic ulcer disease are truncal vagotomy with pyloroplasty and truncal vagotomy with antrectomy (for discussion of gastric surgery for cancer, see Chapter 83, and for obesity, see Chapter 64). Truncal vagotomy involves cutting the main trunks of the vagus nerve on each side of the distal esophagus. Vagotomy is part of the surgical treatment of peptic ulcer disease because it eliminates the neural components of the stimulation of gastric acid secretion. However, truncal vagotomy also eliminates neural input to the antral musculature and thus reduces antral contractions and delays emptying of solids from the stomach. Truncal vagotomy also impairs relaxation of the pylorus, which further impairs gastric emptying. To compensate for these effects, truncal vagotomy is often accompanied by pyloroplasty, which is a surgical revision of the pylorus that makes it incapable of acting as a barrier to the emptying of gastric contents. Vagotomy with pyloroplasty results in accelerated emptying of liquids, whereas the emptying of solids is frequently slowed (38).

Vagotomy with antrectomy is a more aggressive surgical procedure for peptic ulcer disease. Antrectomy is the resection of the antrum and pylorus; resection of the antrum removes the gastrin-secreting portion of the stomach and thus eliminates the gastrin-dependent component of the stimulation of gastric acid secretion. There are two operations for attaching the gastric remnant to the intestine after antrectomy (Fig. 73.3). In the Billroth I operation,

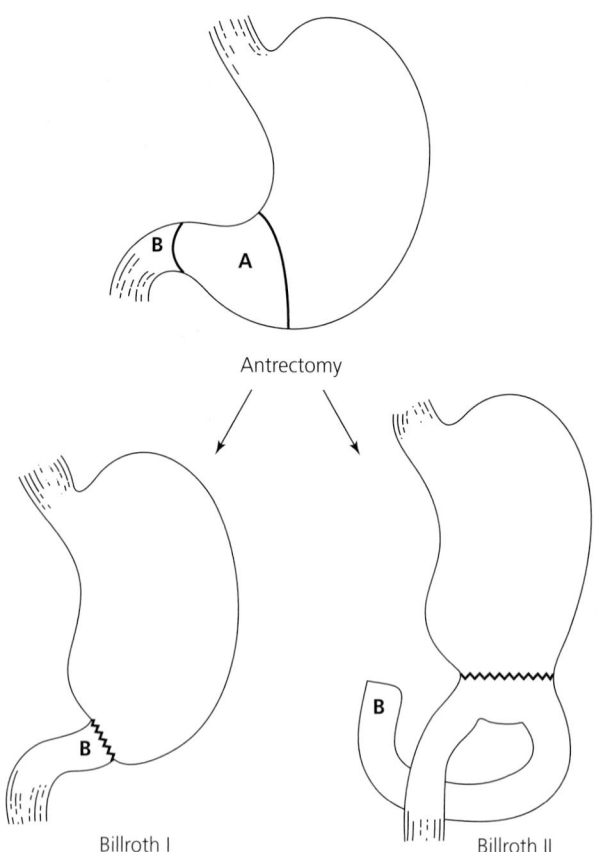

Antrectomy

Billroth I   Billroth II

Figure 73.3. Billroth I and Billroth II procedures. *A,* antrum; *B,* duodenal bulb.

the gastric remnant is anastomosed to the duodenal bulb, and the flow of gastric contents is directly into the bulb. In the Billroth II operation, the gastric remnant is anastomosed to the jejenum, and the proximal side of the duodenum is closed; in this procedure, gastric contents bypass the duodenum and proximal jejunum. Vagotomy with antrectomy results in rapid and unregulated entry of gastric contents into the intestine; it also allows solid food particles to enter the intestine without having been reduced in size by antral grinding. With antrectomy, the intestine sees the sudden entry of a large volume of liquids and unground solids after a meal, rather than the slow, regulated presentation of liquids and finely ground particles seen with an intact stomach. The larger the gastric resection is, the more severe the problems with rapid entry into the intestine will be.

The highly selective vagotomy, or proximal gastric vagotomy, is a surgical procedure for peptic ulcer disease that is designed to reduce gastric acid secretion without interfering with antral motility. In a standard truncal vagotomy, the vagal input to gastric secretion and to antral contraction is lost. Truncal vagotomy also eliminates vagal innervation of the gallbladder, pancreas, and small intestine. In highly selective vagotomy, the vagal branches going to the body of the stomach are cut, whereas the branches going to the antrum are not. This results in decreased acid secretion without impaired antral motility, thus eliminating the need for pyloroplasty and the associated rapid gastric emptying (39). This procedure also spares the vagal innervation of the gallbladder, pancreas, and small intestine.

Dumping Syndrome

Vagotomy with pyloroplasty results in rapid entry of liquids into the intestine, whereas vagotomy plus antrectomy results in rapid entry of both solids and liquids. When nutrients empty from the stomach and enter the intestine in a rapid and unregulated fashion, the digestive and absorptive capacity of the intestine can be overwhelmed. The symptom complex induced by accelerated gastric emptying is termed the dumping syndrome (38). Diarrhea, abdominal pain, and the symptoms associated with hypoglycemia (diaphoresis, palpitations, weakness) are prominent components of the dumping syndrome. In response to rapid entry of a hypertonic meal into the intestine, water enters the intestinal lumen through the intestinal wall in an attempt to make the intestinal contents isosmotic. The sudden influx of the meal and water into the proximal intestine stretches the intestinal wall and causes abdominal distention and pain. Diarrhea results from the inability of the intestine to deal with the sudden load of volume and osmoles. This early phase of the dumping syndrome may also be marked by systemic symptoms, including weakness, tachycardia, and palpitations, thought to result from the sudden fluid shifts from the intravascular space into the intestine with the release of vasoactive substances (bradykinin, serotonin, substance P). There is also a late phase of the dumping syndrome, which is related to hypoglycemia. Rapid gastric emptying results in rapid glucose absorption from the intestine and an abrupt increase in insulin secretion. Not infrequently, insulin is secreted in excess of the amounts required to handle the glucose load. When carbohydrate absorption abruptly ceases and circulating insulin remains high, the patient can have a transient episode of hypoglycemia. In the dumping syndrome, diarrhea and abdominal pain occur 30 to 60 minutes after the meal, and the symptoms of hypoglycemia occur later. Some of the symptoms (weakness and palpitations) associated with hypoglycemia in the late phase of the dumping syndrome are similar to those seen with fluid shifts in the early phase. Dietary management usually controls the symptoms of the dumping syndrome. The core of dietary management is to avoid the sudden entry of large volumes into the proximal intestine. This is achieved by eating frequent small meals and by avoiding the intake of liquids with meals. Meals should be low in osmolality, and simple sugars should be avoided.

Iron and Calcium

Absorption of iron and calcium is frequently impaired after gastric ulcer surgery. Iron deficiency anemia is common in patients with vagotomy and antrectomy. Several contributing factors are recognized. Frequently, total food intake is slightly decreased, especially in patients with antrectomy. There is also decreased digestion of iron-containing foods, particularly meats. Diminished acid secretion results in a higher gastric pH, which impairs the solubility of ferric ions and diminishes their conversion to the more easily absorbed ferrous ions (29). Moreover, the duodenum is an important site for iron absorption, and gastric surgery either bypasses the duodenum (Billroth II) or causes ingested materials to pass through the duodenum rapidly (Billroth I). When all these factors are combined with the marginal iron intake prevalent in society, the result is iron deficiency anemia.

Osteomalacia is also common after surgery for peptic ulcer disease (40). Osteomalacia is marked by low serum calcium, low urinary calcium, elevated alkaline phosphatase, and elevated parathyroid hormone levels and widened osteoid seams in the bones. The clinical outcome of this process is a fracture rate that is two to three times that of the general population (41). The mechanism for osteomalacia after gastric ulcer surgery is not fully defined. In physiologically normal persons, the duodenum is an important site for calcium absorption, and the rapid transit through the duodenum seen after gastric ulcer surgery may contribute to calcium malabsorption. However, it is not clear that calcium malabsorption per se is a major feature in the pathogenesis of osteomalacia.

REFERENCES

1. Diamant NE. Physiology of the esophagus. In: Sleisenger MH, Fordtran JS, eds. Gastrointestinal Disease. 5th ed. Philadelphia: WB Saunders, 1993:319–30.
2. Biancani P, Behar JB. Motility: esophageal motor function. In: Yamada T, ed. Textbook of Gastroenterology. 2nd ed. Philadelphia: JB Lippincott, 1995:159–81.
3. Conklin JL, Christensen J. Motor functions of the pharynx and esophagus. In: Johnson, LR, ed. Physiology of the Gastrointestinal Tract. 3rd ed. New York: Raven Press, 1994:903–29.
4. Jansson G. Acta Physiol Scand Suppl 1969;326:1–42.
5. Mayer EA. The physiology of gastric storage and emptying. In: Johnson LR, ed. Physiology of the Gastrointestinal Tract. 3rd ed. New York: Raven Press, 1994:929–76.
6. Hasler WL. The physiology of gastric motility and gastric emptying. In: Yamada T, ed. Textbook of Gastroenterology. 2nd ed. Philadelphia: JB Lippincott, 1995:181–v206.
7. Cannon WB. Am J Physiol 1898;1:359–370.
8. Schulze-Delrieu K, Wall JP. Am J Physiol 1983;245:G257–64.
9. Meyer JH, Thompson JB, Cohen MB et al. Gastroenterology 1979;76:804–13.
10. Rees WDW, Malagelada JR, Miller LJ et al. Dig Dis Sci 1982;27:321–9.
11. Read NW, Houghton LA. Gastoenterol Clin North Am 1989;18:359–73.
12. McHugh PR, Moran TH. Am J Physiol 1979;236:G254–60.
13. Huntj N, Stubbs DF. J Physiol (Lond) 1975;245:209–25.
14. Lin HC, Doty JE, Reedy TJ et al. Am J Physiol 1989;256:G404–11.
15. Mayer EA, Thompson JB, Jehn D. Gastroenterology 1984;87:1264–71.
16. Lin HC, Hasler WL. Disorders of gastric emptying. In: Yamada T, ed. Textbook of Gastroenterology. 2nd ed. Philadelphia: JB Lippincott, 1995:1318–46.
17. Feldman M, Schiller LR. Ann Intern Med 1983;98:378–84.
18. Jones KL, Russo A, Berry MK et al. Am J Med 2002;113:449–55.
19. Talley NJ. Am J Gastroenterol 2003;98:264–71.
20. Keshavarzian A, Iber FL, Vaetch J. Am J Gastroenterol 1987;82:29–35.
21. Feldman M, Corbett DB, Ramsey EJ. Gastroenterology 1979;77:12–7.
22. Schulze-Delrieu K. Gastroenterology 1979;77:768–79.
23. McCallum RW. Am J Gastroenterol 1991;86:135–49.
24. Lacy BE, Zayal EN, Crowell MD et al. Am J Gastroenteroal 2002,97:1548–52.
25. Ezzeddine D, Jit R, Katz N et al. Gastrointest Endosc 2002;55:920–3.
26. Miller LS, Szych GA, Kantor SB et al. Am J Gastroenterol 2002;97:1653–60.
27. DelValle J, Lucey MR, Yamada T. Gastric secretion. In: Yamada T, ed. Textbook of Gastroenterology. 2nd ed. Philadelphia: JB Lippincott, 1995:295–325.
28. Ito S, Winchester RJ. J Cell Biol 1963;16:541–78.
29. Conrad ME. Factors Affecting Iron Absorption. New York: Academic Press, 1970:87–115.
30. Hersey SJ, Sachs G. Physiol Rev 1995;75:155–90.
31. Hersey SJ. Gastric secretion of pepsins. In: Johnson LR, ed. Physiology of the Gastrointestinal Tract. 3rd ed. New York: Raven Press, 1994:1227.
32. Hamosh M. Gastric and lingual lipases. In: Johnson LR, ed. Physiology of the Gastrointestinal Tract. 3rd ed. New York: Raven Press, 1994:1239–54.

33. Seetharam B. Gastrointestinal absorption and transport of cobalamin. In: Johnson LR, ed. Physiology of the Gastrointestinal Tract. 3rd ed. New York: Raven Press, 1994:1997–2026.

34. Kuzminski AM, Giacco EJD, Allen RH et al. Blood 1998;92:1191.

35. Kahrilas PJ, Hogan J. Gastroesophageal reflux disease. In: Sieisenger MH, Fordtran JS, eds, Gastrointestinal Disease. 5th ed. Philadelphia: WB Saunders, 1993:378–400.

36. Soll AH. Gastric, duodenal, and stress ulcer. In: Sleisenger MH, Fordtran JS, eds. Gastrointestinal Disease. 5th ed. Philadelphia: WB Saunders, 1993:580–678.

37. Rydning A, Berstad A. Scand J Gastroenterol 1986;21:1–5.

38. Meyer JH. Chronic morbidity after ulcer surgery. In: Sleisenger MH, Fordtran JS, eds. Gastrointestinal Disease. 5th ed. Philadelphia: WB Saunders, 1993:731–92.

39. Lavigne ME, Wiley ZD, Martin P. Am J Surg 1979;138:644–51.

40. Klein KB, Orwoll ES, Lieberman DA. Gastroenterology 1987;92:608–16.

41. Nilsson BE, Westlin NE. Acta Chir Scand 1971;137:533–4.

SELECTED READINGS

Conklin JL, Christensen J. Motor functions of the pharynx and esophagus. In: Johnson LR, ed. Physiology of the Gastrointestinal Tract. 3rd ed. New York: Raven Press, 1994:903–29.

Hersey SJ, Sachs G. Physiol Rev 1995;75:155–90.

Mayer EA. The physiology of gastric storage and emptying. In: Johnson LR, ed. Physiology of the Gastrointestinal Tract. 3rd ed. New York: Raven Press, 1994:929–76.

Parkman HP, Fisher RS. Disorders of gastric emptying. In: Yamada T, ed. Textbook of Gastroenterology. 3rd ed. Philadelphia: Lippincott Williams & Wilkins, 2003:1292–320.

Quigley EMM. Gastric motor and sensory function and motor disorders of the stomach. In: Feldman M, Friedman LS, Sleisenger MH, eds. Gastrointestinal and Liver Disease. 7th ed. Philadelphia: WB Saunders, 2002:691–714.

Rege RV, Jones DB. Current role of surgery in peptic ulcer disease. In: Feldman M, Friedman LS, Sleisenger MH, eds. Gastrointestinal and Liver Disease. 7th ed. Philadelphia: WB Saunders, 2002:797–809.

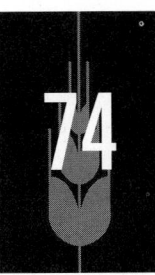

74 INTESTINAL DISACCHARIDASE DEPLETIONS[1]

STEVEN R. HERTZLER, YEONSOO KIM, RUBINA KHAN, MICHELLE ASP, AND DENNIS SAVAIANO

DEVELOPMENT OF THE BRUSH BORDER
  DIGESTIVE ENZYMES 1189
LACTASE-PHLORIZIN HYDROLASE 1189
  Location and Functions 1189
  Types of Hypolactasia and Lactase
    Nonpersistence 1190
  Clinical Assessment of Lactase Activity 1192
  Lactose Maldigestion and Symptoms
    of Lactose Intolerance 1193
  Dietary Approaches for Overcoming
    Lactose Intolerance 1193
  Gene Therapy for Lactose Intolerance 1196
SUCRASE-ISOMALTASE AND
  MALTASE-GLUCOAMYLASE 1196
TREHALASE 1197
SUMMARY 1198

The goals of the following chapter include (a) to review the physiology of the dissacharidases in the human intestinal tract, (b) to highlight the clinical consequences associated with reduced activity of these enzymes, and (c) to describe the dietary approaches for management of these conditions, with special reference to hypolactasia.

Disaccharides are a significant source of carbohydrates in the diet. The primary disaccharides include sucrose (O-α-D-glucopyranosyl-(1→2)-β-fructofuranoside), lactose (O-β-D-galactopyranosyl-(1→4)-β-glucopyranose), maltose (O-α-D-glucopyranosyl-(1→4)-α-glucopyranose), and trehalose (O-α-D-glucopyranosyl-(1→1)-α-glucopyranose). Lactose is the primary carbohydrate in human milk, which contains approximately 7% lactose by weight, among the highest of all mammalian milks (Table 74.1). Sucrose, lactose, and maltose comprise approximately 30%, 6%, and 1 to 2%, respectively, of the total carbohydrate in the diet (1). The majority of the maltose present in the intestine is derived from starch digestion, with only small amounts contributed from grains and fermented beverages. The only significant dietary sources of trehalose are mushrooms and other fungi.

---

[1] **Abbreviations: LNP,** lactase nonpersistence; **LPH,** lactase-phlorizin hydrolase; **PNG,** pyridoxine 5'-β-D-glucoside; **RER,** rough endoplasmic reticulum; **SI,** sucrase-isomaltase.

Because the small intestine is normally impermeable to disaccharides, the activity of intestinal disaccharidases is required for absorption of their component monosaccharides (2). In humans and other mammals, four enzymes or enzyme complexes for disaccharide digestion are known: sucrase-isomaltase (SI), lactase-phlorizin hydrolase (LPH or lactase), maltase-glucoamylase, and trehalase (3). In contrast to the other enzymes that hydrolyze α-glucosidic bonds, lactase hydrolyzes β-glucosidic bonds. Low levels of any of these enzymes in the intestinal mucosa result in carbohydrate malabsorption that may also be associated with clinical symptoms such as diarrhea, abdominal pain, and flatulence.

DEVELOPMENT OF THE BRUSH BORDER DIGESTIVE ENZYMES

The carbohydrate-digesting enzymes produced by the small intestine are anchored in the brush border. The disaccharidases present include sucrase, lactase, glucoamylase, isomaltase, and trehalase. Table 74.2 shows the substrates and products of each disaccharidase (4). SI activity at 34 weeks of gestation reaches 70% of the adult level and rises to the adult level at birth (5). Glucoamylase and trehalase activities are detected at 13 weeks of gestation (6). Lactase activity develops later in gestation. The lactase activity is only 30% that of a full-term infant at 34 weeks of gestation and is still just 70% of the full-term level by 35 to 38 weeks (5).

The activity of disaccharidases in the brush border is recognized as the rate-limiting step in disaccharide digestion (7). Thus, congenital or acquired enzyme deficiencies cause poor absorption of disaccharides. In addition, losses of disaccharidase activity can occur secondary to damage to the intestinal mucosa by certain diseases (e.g, alcoholism, celiac disease), infections, medications, surgery, or radiation exposure (8).

LACTASE-PHLORIZIN HYDROLASE

Location and Functions

The highest activity of LPH in humans is found in the jejunum, approximately 50 to 200 cm distal to the ligament of Treitz; the activity of LPH is 25% lower at Treitz ligament and is minimal in the ileum (9). The gene for

TABLE 74.1. LACTOSE CONTENT OF SELECTED DAIRY FOODS

FOOD	TYPICAL SERVING SIZE	LACTOSE CONTENT PER SERVING (g)
Whole milk	245 g (1 cup)	11
2% reduced-fat milk	245 g (1 cup)	9–13
Nonfat milk	245 g (1 cup)	12–14
Lactose-reduced milk		
70% lactose-reduced	245 g (1 cup)	3–4
100% lactose-reduced	245 g (1 cup)	0–1
Low-fat yogurt	245 g (1 cup)	11–15
Cheese		
Blue, parmesan	56.7 g (2 oz)	1–2
Camembert	56.7 g (2 oz)	0–1
Cheddar, gouda	56.7 g (2 oz)	1–2
Cottage cheese	210 g (1 cup)	7–8
Ice cream: 10% fat	133 g (1 cup)	9–10
Ice cream: 16% fat	148 g (1 cup)	9–10
Ice milk	132 g (1 cup)	9–10

Adapted from Moore BJ. Dairy foods: are they politically correct? Nutr Today 2003;38:82–90, with permission.

LPH is located on chromosome 2, and it directs the synthesis of a pre-pro form of LPH in the enterocytes. The pre-pro LPH is processed intracellularly (and possibly by pancreatic proteases) into the mature form that is anchored in the cell membrane at the brush border. The human enzyme has two catalytic sites, both on the luminal side of the enterocyte cell membrane. These active sites, β-galactosidase (EC 3.2.1.23) and phlorizin hydrolase (EC 3.2.1.62), comprise Glu1749 in domain IV and Glu1273 in domain III, respectively (10). The β-galactosidase portion is able to hydrolyze lactose, cellobiose, *o*-nitro-phenyl-β-glucopyranoside, and *o*-nitro-phenyl-β-galactopyranoside (10). Phlorizin hydrolase is able to hydrolyze phlorizin, β-glycopyranosyl-ceramides, and *m*-nitro-phenyl-β-glucopyranoside (10).

Beyond its well-recognized role in lactose digestion, evidence indicates that LPH could be involved in the hydrolysis of other nutritionally important β-glucosides. For example, although the glycosylated forms of isoflavones and flavonoids occur in nature, only the aglycone forms can be absorbed from the intestine. It was previously assumed that the colonic microflora was mainly responsible for this deconjugation. However, two studies (11, 12) have since demonstrated that the lactase catalytic site of LPH is able to hydrolyze glycosylated isoflavones and flavonoids and to make them available for absorption in the small intestine. Similarly, the hydrolysis of a β-glucosidic linkage is necessary to release pyridoxine from pyridoxine 5'-β-D-glucoside (PNG), an important step in increasing the bioavailability of this form of vitamin B_6 that provides roughly 15% of the total vitamin B_6 in a mixed diet (13). Mackey and colleagues (13) reported that LPH purified from rat small intestinal mucosa possesses the capability to hydrolyze PNG in vitro. Future studies are needed to determine whether the bioavailability of isoflavones and PNG could be compromised in those persons who have experienced the loss of small intestinal lactase activity.

Types of Hypolactasia and Lactase Nonpersistence

Full-term infants, regardless of racial or ethnic background, generally possess high levels of lactase activity. Congenital lactase deficiency is the rare condition in which lactase is absent at birth. Even in Finland, where the condition is most common, only 42 cases were reported from 1966 to 1998 (14). In these infants, lactase activity in jejunal biopsy specimens is reduced to 0 to 10 IU/g protein, and severe diarrhea results from unabsorbed lactose (14). Treatment with a lactose-free formula eliminates the diarrhea and promotes normal growth and development. The congenital lactase deficiency just described is a separate clinical entity from congenital lactose intolerance. Congenital lactose intolerance is a rare and serious disease with vomiting, failure to thrive, dehydration, disacchariduria including lactosuria,

TABLE 74.2. ROLE OF BRUSH BORDER ENZYMES IN DIGESTION OF DISACCHARIDES AND STARCH

ENZYME	ENZYMATIC ACTIVITY	SUBSTRATE	PRODUCTS
Lactase	β-(1-4) Galactosidase	Lactose	Glucose, Galactose
Sucrase	α-(1-4) Glucosidase Hydrolysis of the α-1, β-2 glucose-fructose bond in sucrose	Sucrose, maltose, maltotriose, α-limit dextrins with terminal α 1-4 links	Glucose, fructose, malto-oligosaccharides with terminal α 1-6 linkages
Glucoamylase	α-(1-4) Glucosidase	Maltose, maltotriose, malto-oligosaccharide	Glucose, malto-oligosaccharide with terminal α 1-6 linkage
Isomaltase	α-(1-6) Glucosidase	Maltose, isomaltose, α-limit dextrins (malto-oligosaccharide with terminal α 1-6 links)	Glucose, malto-oligosaccharides
Trehalase	α- and β-Glucosidase (tested on renal trehalase)	Trehalose	Glucose

renal tubular acidosis, aminoaciduria, liver damage, and cataracts as possible clinical sequelae (15–18). The cause of this disorder is not lactase deficiency, but rather the gastric absorption of intact lactose (16). Although this condition can be fatal in early infancy if it is not recognized, a milk-free diet leads to rapid recovery, and often patients may be able to tolerate a normal diet (with milk) after 6 months of age (15).

The loss of intestinal lactase activity (hypolactasia) is either congenital or acquired, and lactase is the only digestive enzyme for which greatly reduced activity in adulthood is common. Acquired hypolactasia is subdefined as primary or secondary. Primary hypolactasia (also referred to as lactase nonpersistence, LNP) is a geneticallyprogrammed, irreversible loss of the majority (90–95%) of intestinal lactase activity that occurs sometime after weaning, probably between 3 and 5 years of age (19, 20). The genetic trait for LNP affects approximately 75% of the world's population (Table 74.3), with the exception that most Northern Europeans and a few pastoral tribes in African and the Middle East maintain high lactase levels throughout life (21). Because this loss of lactase is actually the normal pattern in mammalian physiology (humans are the only known mammalian species to have a subpopulation that retains lactase activity) and is not pathogenic, the use of the term lactase deficiency to describe the primary loss of lactase is incorrect. Finally, the terms LNP and lactose intolerance should not be used interchangeably. The former term simply describes the loss of lactase activity, whereas the latter pertains to the development of clinical symptoms resulting from lactose maldigestion. This relationship is discussed in more detail later in this chapter.

Two major competing hypotheses have been offered to explain the pattern of LNP distribution in the world's population. The first, the geographic hypothesis, was proposed by Simoons in 1978 (22). According to this hypothesis, a mutation for lactose persistence occurred several thousand years ago, before the origins of dairying. In those geographic regions where dairy farming was practiced, persons with the mutation coding for lactose digestion had improved tolerance to milk and gained a selective advantage over their counterparts, especially when they were living under marginal nutritional conditions.

More recently, the malaria hypothesis was proposed by Anderson and Vullo (23). These authors suggested that malaria selected for LNP. Noting that LNP is common in geographic areas of world that are endemic for malaria, the authors posited that the genetic tendency for LNP would cause lactose maldigestion and intolerance symptoms leading to a corresponding decline in milk intake in affected persons. Because milk products are excellent sources of riboflavin, it was further proposed that many of these persons may have had marginal riboflavin deficiency. A state of marginal riboflavin deficiency that could be tolerated by the person and yet still lead to localized flavin deficiency in the erythrocytes is theorized to inhibit the multiplication of malaria parasites and thus to reduce mortality from malaria. Although this hypothesis is interesting, a study conducted in northern Sardinia showed no differences in the prevalence of LNP in villages with a past history of low, intermediate, or high malaria morbidity and mortality (24). A further commentary on this study (25) pointed out that, in contrast to the data on LNP, the frequencies of glucose-6-phosphate dehydrogenase deficiency and β-thalassemia trait (two disorders that are known to be selected for by malaria) were strikingly higher in the areas with a high past malarial endemicity versus the area with low malarial endemicity. Thus, the limited evidence presented so far does not support the malaria hypothesis.

In persons with LNP, lactase activity in the jejunal enterocytes is found in a mosaic-type pattern, meaning that some jejunal enterocytes produce high levels of lactase, whereas others, even those sharing the same villus, do not produce lactase (26, 27). Thus, rather than a uniform reduction in lactase production among all enterocytes, persons with LNP may have a patchy distribution of lactase-producing enterocytes that are low in number relative to the nonlactase–producing enterocytes. However, in lactase-persistent persons, all enterocytes may produce lactase.

Many studies have been conducted to evaluate the molecular basis for LNP. It is known that LNP is an autosomal recessive trait and that the gene for human LPH is located on chromosome 2q21 (28). Initial studies suggested that alterations in the posttranslational modifications of LPH were responsible for the low lactase activity in hypolactasia (29, 30). Rossi and colleagues (26) found that intestinal biopsies of hypolactasic persons in southern Italy had substantial levels of lactose mRNA. Thus, it was thought that hypolatasic persons do synthesize the lactase protein, but posttranslational modifications cause it to be

TABLE 74.3. PREVELANCE OF LACTASE NONPERSISTENCE IN VARIOUS ETHNIC GROUPS

GROUP	PREVALENCE (%)
Northern European	2–7
White (United States)	6–22
Central European	9–23
Indian (Indian subcontinent)	
Northern	20–30
Southern	60–70
Hispanic	50–80
Ashkenazi Jewish	60–80
African-American	60–80
Black African	70–95
Native American	80–100
Asian	85–100

Adapted from Srinivasan R, Minocha A. When to suspect lactose intolerance: symptomatic, ethnic, and laboratory clues. Postgrad Med 1998;104:109–23, with permission, copyright 1998 The McGraw-Hill Companies; data also from Sahi T. Genetics and epidemiology of adult-type hypolactasia. Scand J Gastroenterol 1994;29[Suppl 202]:7–20.

either malfolded and enzymatically inactive or result in its intracellular degradation (31). Sebastio and associates (32) studied persons with the hypolactasic phenotype and the lactase-persistent phenotype. These investigators noted no clear difference in the lactase mRNA levels in the intestinal biopsies of persons with either phenotype. The authors concluded that expression of lactase is controlled at the posttranscriptional level.

Despite this evidence, the current opinion is that lactase regulation is primarily at the level of transcription. Numerous studies (33–35) demonstrated the importance of the presence of an adequate lactase mRNA level to have expression of LPH activity. Krasinski and associates (36) found that LPH mRNA levels in rats were abundant before weaning, but these levels declined two- to fourfold during weaning. The LPH activity observed in the rats corresponded with the protein and mRNA levels at the different life stages. Thus, transcriptional mechanisms were thought to be responsible for regulation of lactase biosynthesis. Escher and colleagues (37) studied lactase-specific activity and lactase mRNA levels in Asian, black, and white patients. These investigators observed that lactase activity always corresponded with the lactase mRNA levels, a finding thereby suggesting that transcriptional regulation is responsible for variable lactase activity. Further, studies of the porcine LPH gene have identified a sequence CE-LPH1 in the promoter region that binds a *trans*-acting nuclear factor NF-LPH1. High levels of NF-LPH1 were found in enterocytes of newborn pigs that had high lactase activity, whereas the levels were lower in adult pigs that had low lactase activity. The investigators suggested that the nuclear factor NF-LPH1 could be implicated in the lowering of lactase activity at weaning and could provide an explanation for the molecular regulation of hypolactasia (38). Subsequent studies showed that other nuclear factors may also interact with the CE-LPH1 promoter region (39).

The molecular basis for regulation of lactase activity in LNP is still being actively studied. Although it is widely accepted that transcriptional control is the primary mechanism (28), the contribution of posttranslational events in regulating the activity cannot be ignored (40).

Secondary acquired hypolactasia is caused by enterocyte damage resulting from disease, medication, surgery, or radiation (41). Table 74.4 lists some of the causes of secondary hypolactasia. In one study of malnourished patients, lactase was reduced to a greater degree than other disaccharidases and was the last of the disaccharidases to recover (42). A possible explanation is that the quantity of lactase is only about 50% as high as that of the other disaccharidases, even in lactase-persistent persons (43). A key issue in the management of secondary hypolactasia is the need for, and the severity of, lactose restriction in the diet. Although removing lactose-containing dairy foods may improve clinical tolerance, it also may deprive a malnourished patient of the nutritional value of these foods. Later in this chapter, several strategies are presented for the incorporation of dairy foods into the diet while reducing the possibility of lactose intolerance. Secondary hypolactasia can be reversed once the underlying problem has been resolved, but the process is slow and can take 6 months or longer (41).

Clinical Assessment of Lactase Activity

Lactase activity is assessed by either direct or indirect methods. The direct measurement of the lactase activity obtained by a small intestinal mucosal biopsy or intestinal perfusion is the most accurate, but these methods are invasive and carry the potential risk of complications, such as intestinal bleeding (44). Thus, direct methods are rarely performed clinically.

Indirect methods for assessing the digestion of a dose of lactose include breath tests (hydrogen, $^{13}CO_2$, $^{14}CO_2$), blood tests (glucose and galactose), urine tests (galactose, lactose/lactulose ratio), fecal tests (pH, reducing substances), and intolerance symptoms. Of these methods, the breath hydrogen test is currently the most widely used. This test operates on the principle that lactose that

TABLE 74.4. POTENTIAL CAUSES OF SECONDARY HYPOLACTASIA

DISEASES		
SMALL BOWEL	MULTISYSTEM	IATROGENIC
Human immunodeficiency virus enteropathy	Carcinoid syndrome	Chemotherapy
Regional enteritis (e.g., Crohn disease)	Cystic fibrosis	Radiation enteritis
Sprue (celiac and tropical)	Diabetic gastropathy	Surgical resection of intestine
Whipple disease (intestinal lipodystrophy)	Protein-energy malnutrition	Medications
Ascaris lumbricoides infection	Zollinger-Ellison syndrome	Colchicine (antigout)
Blind loop syndrome	Alcoholism	Neomycin (antibiotic)
Giardiasis	Iron deficiency	Kanamycin (antibiotic)
Infectious diarrhea		Aminosalicylic acid (antibiotic)
Short gut		

From Savaiano D, Hertzler S, Jackson KA et al. Nutrient considerations in lactose intolerance. In: Coulston AM, Rock CL, Monsen ER, eds. Nutrition in the Prevention and Treatment of Disease. San Diego: Academic Press, 2001:563–75, with permission.

escapes digestion in the small intestine will be fermented by the colonic bacteria, resulting in the generation of hydrogen gas (the only known source of molecular hydrogen in the body). A portion of this hydrogen gas diffuses from the colonic lumen into the blood and is ultimately excreted via the pulmonary route. This method has excellent sensitivity and specificity, but careful attention to the test protocol is required. For an excellent review of these diagnostic methods and protocols, see the article by Arola (44).

Lactose Maldigestion and Symptoms of Lactose Intolerance

The well-documented high prevalence of LNP in much of the world's population has unfortunately misled many to believe that lactose intolerance is equally common. However, a large body of evidence now exists demonstrating that symptoms of lactose intolerance in response to physiologic amounts of lactose (8–16 fl oz of milk) affect only a small fraction of lactose maldigesters (45). An example is a study by Carroccio and associates (46). In this study, 323 Sicilians (72 children aged 5–16 years, 141 adults aged 17–64 years, and 110 elderly adults aged 65–85 years) underwent breath hydrogen testing with a 25-g lactose dose (1 g/kg for children) to determine lactose digestion status and were queried for the presence of lactose intolerance in the ensuing 24-hour period. Of the 323 persons studied, 117 (36%) were classified as lactose maldigesters. Just 13 of the lactose maldigesters were also lactose intolerant, which was only 4% of the total study group (11% of the lactose maldigesters).

Another concern is that many persons may self-diagnose lactose intolerance when they may not be lactose maldigesters. Two studies by Suarez and associates and another by Johnson and colleagues (47–49) demonstrated that about 30 to 33% of subjects who claim to have lactose intolerance (even severe) are, in fact, lactose digesters. Of the 49 subjects in the study by Carroccio and colleagues (46) who had self-reported milk intolerance at entry into the study, just five were both lactose maldigesters and lactose intolerant. It is likely that some persons who self-diagnose themselves with lactose intolerance may have an underlying bowel disorder that is masquerading as lactose intolerance. These findings strongly indicate that diagnosing lactose intolerance solely on the basis of reported symptoms following milk ingestion is unreliable. Objective tests of lactose maldigestion or evaluations of symptoms in a double-masked, placebo-controlled study are necessary (50).

Symptoms of lactose intolerance are primarily gastrointestinal and include flatulence, cramping, abdominal pain, nausea, distention, bloating, and diarrhea (51). The causes of lactose intolerance symptoms have not been fully elucidated, but they appear to be related to the ability of the colonic microflora to process undigested lactose (52). Differences in the types of bacteria and/or their metabolic activities affect how lactose is fermented. Investigators have proposed that a dominance of lactic acid bacteria in the colon would improve the fermentation of lactose into short-chain fatty acids and other products that are easily absorbed from the colon (53). Thus, the potential for osmotic diarrhea resulting from unfermented lactose would diminish. Further, lactic acid bacteria may also reduce intestinal gas production either directly or indirectly. First, lactic acid bacteria are able to ferment lactose without producing hydrogen (54). Second, the pH-lowering effect of lactic acid may inhibit bacteria that are major hydrogen producers (e.g., clostridia, *Escherichia coli*) (55, 56). Given that hydrogen gas can account for 50% or more of total colonic gas during active fermentation (57), reducing hydrogen production could appreciably lower the volume of gas produced and could therefore reduce flatulence symptoms. However, other studies suggest that subjective symptoms may result from a person's increased sensitivity to a normal amount of gas versus an increase in the absolute volume of gas (58, 59).

It is common for many lactose-maldigesting persons to avoid lactose completely in the belief that any amount of lactose will cause intolerance symptoms. However, the relationship between lactose maldigestion and the development of lactose intolerance is complex. The symptom response is influenced by several physiologic and psychosocial factors. Multiple strategies for overcoming lactose intolerance symptoms are available and are reviewed in the following section.

Dietary Approaches for Overcoming Lactose Intolerance

An overview of dietary strategies for managing lactose intolerance is given in Table 74.5.

Dose of Lactose

Historically, a 50-g lactose challenge (equivalent to 1 L of milk) has been used in lactose tolerance testing. Between 80 and 100% of lactose maldigesters will experience intolerance symptoms when such an unphysiologic amount of lactose is fed on an empty stomach (19). However, the symptom responses to a typical serving of milk (e.g., 8 fl oz of milk [240 mL] containing 12 g lactose) are typically much lower and are often absent in lactose maldigesters. Residual lactase activity may help to explain tolerance to smaller lactose loads. Bond and Levitt (60), using an intestinal intubation technique, demonstrated that lactose maldigesters may absorb anywhere from 42 to 75% of a 12.5-g lactose dose. The combination of the relatively small amount of lactose and residual lactase activity usually results in negligible symptom responses at lactose doses of 12 g or less. Some studies (61–63) identified a

TABLE 74.5. DIETARY STRATEGIES FOR LACTOSE INTOLERANCE

FACTORS AFFECTING LACTOSE DIGESTION	DIETARY STRATEGY	INVESTIGATORS, YEAR (REFERENCE)
Dose of lactose	Consume a cup of milk or less at a time, containing up to 12 g lactose.	Suarez et al., 1995 (47) Hertzler and Savaiano, 1996 (69) Suarez et al., 1997 (48)
Intestinal transit	Consume milk with other foods, rather than alone, to slow the intestinal transit of lactose.	Solomons et al., 1985 (72) Martini and Savaiano, 1988 (73) Dehkordi et al., 1995 (74)
Yogurts	Consume yogurts containing active bacterial cultures. A serving, or even two, should be well tolerated. Lactose in yogurts is better digested than the lactose in milks. Pasteurized yogurts do not improve lactose digestion; however, these products, when consumed, produce few if any symptoms.	Kolars et al., 1984 (84) Gilliland and Kim, 1984 (88) Savaiano et al., 1984 (85) Shermak et al., 1995 (92) Savaiano et al., 1984 (85) Kolars et al., 1984 (84) Gilliland and Kim, 1984 (88)
Digestive aids	Over-the-counter lactase supplements (pills, capsules, and drops) may be used when large doses of lactose (>12 g) are consumed at once. Lactose-hydrolyzed milks also are well tolerated.	Moskovitz et al., 1987 (124) Lin et al., 1993 (121) Ramirez et al., 1994 (119) Nielsen et al., 1984 (126) Biller et al., 1987 (108) Rosado et al., 1989 (116) Brand and Holt, 1991 (112)
Colon adaptation	Consume lactose-containing foods daily to increase the colon bacteria's ability to metabolize undigested lactose.	Perman et al., 1981 (55) Johnson et al., 1993 (132) Hertzler and Savaiano, 1996 (69) Pribila et al., 2000 (133)

Adapted from Savaiano D, Hertzler S, Jackson KA et al. Nutrient considerations in lactose intolerance. In: Coulston AM, Rock CL, Monsen ER, eds. Nutrition in the Prevention and Treatment of Disease. San Diego: Academic Press, 2001:563–75, with permission.

few persons who may be sensitive to as little as 3 to 5 g lactose. However, one of these studies (61) did not have appropriate masking of treatment identities, whereas another study, this time double-masked (62), found that only three of 59 lactose maldigesters had a positive symptom response to 3 g lactose, a number that was not different from the 0-g lactose placebo. Further, a double-masked study by Suarez and colleagues (47) found that even subjects who claimed to be severely lactose intolerant did not report more symptoms when 8 fl oz/day of regular versus 100% lactose-hydrolyzed milk was fed for 7 days. Hertzler and associates (64), using breath hydrogen analysis, determined that a 2-g lactose dose was completely absorbed, whereas some evidence indicated lactose maldigestion (without symptoms) at a 6-g dose. Good tolerance to doses of lactose up to 7 g was confirmed in another study as well (65).

Larger, but still physiologic, loads of lactose (e.g., 15–25 g) generally cause symptoms in about 50% of lactose maldigesters (66). In general, 12 g lactose or greater can cause abdominal pain in some lactose maldigesters, whereas significant increases in flatulence symptoms may not be present until the lactose dose reaches 20 g (64, 67). However, if a total of approximately 25 g lactose is consumed as two separate doses of 12 g each at breakfast and dinner, symptoms are minimal (48). Lactose maldigesters may be able to tolerate even a large amount of lactose (34 g or more) on a daily basis if the total dose is subdivided into smaller doses (i.e., 12 g or less) throughout the day (68, 69).

Gastrointestinal Transit Effects

Gastrointestinal transit time is negatively correlated with peak breath hydrogen and intolerance symptoms in lactose maldigesters (70, 71). Delaying gastrointestinal transit may enhance lactose digestion by increasing the time in which residual lactase is able to hydrolyze lactose. Greater digestion of lactose in the small intestine will decrease the amount of lactose reaching the colon, thus decreasing the osmotic load as well as reducing hydrogen production by colonic bacteria. In addition, slower fermentation of lactose in the colon may allow for more efficient disposal of fermentation gases and thereby reduce the potential for symptoms.

The most successful approach for slowing the transit of lactose to the colon is for milk to be consumed with meals. Consuming lactose-containing foods as part of a meal has been shown to increase the time to peak breath hydrogen, to decrease overall hydrogen production, and to decrease symptoms of intolerance in lactose maldigesters (72–74). Other gastrointestinal transit-related factors that have been studied include altering the energy content, viscosity, temperature, and fat content of milk. Increasing the energy content or viscosity of milk does not improve lactose digestion or tolerance, although increasing the energy content may slow gastric emptying somewhat (75, 76). A study of lactose solutions (50 g) at 2 to 3°C (cold), 20 to 21°C (room temperature), and 55 to 58°C (hot) detected no effect of temperature on lactose digestion or overall gastrointestinal symptoms, although the cold solution was associated with somewhat greater abdominal pain and less flatulence than the other solutions (77). With regard to fat content, an initial study by Leichter (78) reported improved lactose tolerance to whole milk versus skim milk. However, the report made no mention of randomization in this study, nor was a statistical evaluation of intolerance symptoms performed. Subsequent studies found no significant effects of whole versus skim milk on lactose digestion (74) or tolerance (79, 80).

Cocoa has been studied for its ability to increase tolerance to lactose. One mechanism by which cocoa may exert its effect is by slowing the rate of gastric emptying. Chocolate milk has been shown in two studies to decrease breath hydrogen and symptoms of intolerance compared with plain milk (74, 81), but masking treatment identities is difficult in these types of studies, and differences in taste and appearance cannot be excluded as possible confounding variables. Milk chocolate was also studied for its ability to increase tolerance to lactose in persons with self-described lactose intolerance (82). No differences in gastrointestinal symptoms or stool frequency and consistency were found when subjects consumed 100-g chocolate samples containing either 12 or 2 g lactose. The results of this study provide additional support for the theory that chocolate may improve lactose digestion; however, objective evidence (i.e., breath hydrogen testing) was not obtained.

Microbe-Containing Dairy Foods

The lactose in yogurt with live cultures is digested better than lactose in milk, and it is well tolerated by those who are lactose intolerant (83–88). During manufacturing, most commercial yogurts are enriched to 6% lactose before fermentation because of the addition of milk solids. However, as the numbers of lactic acid bacteria (*Lactobacillus delbrueckii* subsp. *bulgaricus* and *Streptococcus salivarius* subsp. *thermophilus*) increase to approximately 100 million cells/mL, 20 to 30% of the lactose is used, resulting in a lactose concentration of 4% in the final product (89), a concentration that is similar to that of milk. During fermentation, the β-galactosidase activity of the yogurt increases. Because of the buffering of gastric acid by yogurt's calcium and phosphorus, substantial numbers of live cells may enter the duodenum (90). After entry into the duodenum, the intact bacterial cells interact with bile acids and cause disruption of the cell membrane and access of lactose to the β-galactosidase. This process is termed autodigestion and is limited to the amount of

lactose normally present in yogurt (85, 91). Although the inherent β-galactosidase activity of yogurt is an important determinant of lactose digestion, it is not the only consideration. Yogurts with widely differing β-galactosidase activities (87), and even pasteurized yogurt, all tend to improve tolerance, even if lactose maldigestion increases somewhat (86, 88, 92). Thus, factors such as physical form, gelling, or the energy density of yogurt may be important as well. Most commercial "frozen yogurts," however, are an exception to this rule. Because these products are typically pasteurized after culturing, β-galactosidase activity is reduced to zero, and the breath hydrogen and symptom responses are similar to those of ice milk or ice cream (93).

Kefir is a fermented dairy beverage that, compared with yogurt, contains a more diverse array of microorganisms, typically including a yeast, in its starter culture. One study demonstrated that kefir possesses β-galactosidase activity equal to or higher than that of yogurt and that it improves both lactose digestion and lactose intolerance symptoms (94). Thus, kefir represents a potential alternative to yogurt for lactose-intolerant persons.

Unlike fermented dairy beverages, unfermented acidophilus milks are made by the addition of *Lactobacillus acidophilus* cells to cold milk, with no multiplication of the organism unless the storage temperature exceeds 40°F (5°C) (95). Various strains of *L. acidophilus* exist, with the NCFM strain the most extensively studied and used in commercial products. Most studies that have evaluated the effect of acidophilus milk on lactose digestion and tolerance have reported no improvement (85, 96–99). One potential explanation for these findings is that many commercial products do not have sufficient *L. acidophilus* cell counts. Some studies reporting a positive effect of acidophilus milk on lactose digestion used cell counts that are much higher than what is available commercially (100, 101). Another possibility is that the strains of *L. acidophilus* used are not sensitive to bile acids in the intestine (95). Thus, bile acids will not disrupt the bacterial cell membrane in the intestinal lumen, thereby preventing exposure of lactose to bacterial β-galactosidase. In support of this concept is a study in which the feeding of a milk containing sonicated *L. acidophilus* cells improved lactose digestion compared with the same milk that had unsonicated cells (96). Subsequent research has focused on developing unfermented milks with different types of bacteria that have high β-galactosidase activity (102) or with strains of *L. acidophilus* having different degrees of bile acid sensitivity or lactose uptake (103).

Lactose-Hydrolyzed Milk and Lactase Enzyme Supplements

Lactose-intolerant persons now have several methods available for improving lactose digestion from dairy products. The level of intact lactose in milk can be greatly reduced or eliminated by the incubation of regular milk with lactases derived from yeasts (e.g, *Kluyveromyces lactis*) or other fungi (e.g., *Aspergillus oryzae, A. niger*). In addition, tablets or capsules containing lactase can be taken with lactose-containing meals. Use of these enzymes and milks treated with them has been affirmed as Generally Recognized as Safe by the US Food and Drug Administration (104). The most commonly available products currently are milks treated to achieve 70 or 100% lactose hydrolysis (105,106) and caplets containing different concentrations of lactase (106). New products are appearing regularly on the grocery shelves.

Lactose digestion and lactose intolerance symptoms are improved by lactose-hydrolyzed milk (50–100% lactose hydrolysis) (98, 107–118). The same is generally true for lactase supplements containing doses of lactase in the range of 3000 to 6000 FCC units (up to 9000 FCC units may be required for doses of lactose exceeding 20 g) (119–124). In addition, one study demonstrated that hydrolysis of 80% of the lactose in a commercial meal-replacement supplement significantly reduced breath hydrogen excretion and also tended to decrease lactose intolerance symptoms (125). Although lactose-hydrolyzed milks and lactase supplements are generally effective for improving lactose digestion, these products are rarely necessary for lactose maldigesters, unless large amounts of lactose are going to be consumed, or if the lactose will be consumed in the absence of other foods, as could be the case with a lactose-containing meal replacement. Another consideration is the increased financial expense associated with lactase supplements or lactose-hydrolyzed milk versus regular milk (47). Finally, the added sweetness caused by hydrolysis of lactose to glucose and galactose could either increase (126) or decrease (118) its acceptability.

Colonic Adaptation to Malabsorbed Lactose

The loss of lactase in LNP is permanent. Several studies demonstrated that the ingestion of 50 g lactose or more per day for periods of 1 to 14 months has no impact on jejunal lactase activity as measured by intestinal biopsies (127–129). Despite this finding, milk-feeding programs in school children in Ethiopia, India, and China (each having a high prevalence of lactose maldigesters) showed that tolerance to lactose improves greatly within about 4 weeks of the initiation of milk consumption (129–131). In addition, Johnson and colleagues (132) reported that 77% of lactose-intolerant African-Americans could tolerate 12 g or more lactose when lactose was increased gradually and fed daily over a period of 6 to 12 weeks. The postulated mechanism for this improved tolerance is colonic bacterial adaptation to malabsorbed lactose.

Thus far, good evidence exists for human colonic bacterial adaptation to lactose. Hertzler and Savaiano (69) fed 20 lactose maldigesters either lactose or dextrose for 10 days in a randomized crossover study. The dose of each carbohydrate was gradually increased from 0.6 to 1.0 g/kg/day over the course of the feeding period. The lactose feeding period dramatically decreased the breath hydrogen response to a 0.35-g/kg lactose challenge. In addition, fecal β-galactosidase activity increased three-fold, and flatulence symptoms in response to the lactose challenge were decreased by 50%. A similar decrease in breath hydrogen excretion was reported in a study of African-American adolescent girls who were fed a dairy-rich diet containing approximately 33 g lactose/day for 21 days (133). Finally, Briet and associates (134) reported colonic adaptation to a dose of 34 g lactose/day for 13 days and a corresponding drop in lactose intolerance symptoms in response to a 50-g lactose challenge. However, it was noted in this study that a control group of subjects fed sucrose for the same length of time also showed a decrease in the symptom response to the lactose challenge, even though no evidence of metabolic adaptation was seen in that group. Studies are currently under way in our laboratory to define the minimum dose of milk required to induce metabolic adaptation and the kinetics of that adaptation.

Gene Therapy for Lactose Intolerance

During and colleagues (135) explored the possibility of using gene therapy as a potential cure for LNP. An adeno-associated virus vector containing the lactase gene (AAVlac) was administered via an orogastric tube to hypolactasic rats. An adeno-associated virus with the luciferase (AAVluc) gene and phosphate-buffered saline served as controls. The adeno-associated virus vector was chosen because it is a defective, helper-dependent virus and because it is nonpathogenic in humans and other species. Following a single administration of AAVlac, four of four rats tested were positive for lacZ mRNA within 3 days, whereas none of the rats that received AAVluc or phosphate-buffered saline were positive. An acute lactose challenge was given on day 7 after administration, and an elevation of plasma glucose from 114±4 to 130±3 mg/dL in 30 minutes was observed in the rats that received AAVlac. The control rats had a flat glucose curve. The positive blood glucose response to a lactose challenge and the positive lacZ mRNA persisted at 4 and 6 months, respectively, after the vector administration. Many questions regarding gene therapy for lactose intolerance remain unanswered. No human studies have been conducted to date, but the concept is intriguing.

SUCRASE-ISOMALTASE AND MALTASE-GLUCOAMYLASE

SI is an integral enzyme in the small intestinal brush border that contains a sucrase (EC 3.2.1.48) domain for the hydrolysis of the α-1,2-glucose to fructose bond in sucrose and an isomaltase (EC 3.2.1.10) domain for hydrolyzing maltose and α-1,6-linked limit dextrins (4).

The activity of SI is distributed along the entire length of the small intestine. The highest activity is found in the jejunum, with 20 to 30% less activity found either proximal to the ligament of Treitz or in the distal ileum (9). The function of SI considerably overlaps with the maltase-glucoamylase complex (EC 3.2.1.3 and EC 3.2.1.20) that primarily hydrolyzes maltose. In fact, approximately 80% of the maltase activity is accounted for by SI and only 20% by maltase-glucoamylase (4). The activity of maltase-glucoamylase progressively increases to its maximal level in the distal ileum (9).

The gene encoding human SI has been localized to the long arm of chromosome 3 (136, 137). In the rough endoplasmic reticulum (RER), SI is synthesized as a long polypeptide chain carrying two similar but not identical active sites (pro-SI) (4). The pro-SI is inserted into the RER via its N-terminal region. In the RER, the peptide elongates and is glycosylated with mannose residues at asparagines sites. The glycoprotein then migrates to the Golgi complex, where mannose residues are cleaved, and glycosylation with N-acetyl galactosamine and sialic acid occurs. After this glycosylation, the pro-SI is inserted into the enterocyte membrane, with the sucrase domain protruding farthest out into the lumen. Pro-SI is then rapidly processed by trypsin, yielding the two subunits of sucrase and isomaltase.

The regulation of SI expression involves factors at the level of transcription, translation, glycosylation, and processing by luminal proteases. Several descriptions of various derangements of the intracellular processing and transport of pro-SI that can lead to deficient enzyme activity have been published (138–141). In addition, some evidence has been presented that sucrase, more than other intestinal disaccharidases, may be inducible to some degree by dietary sucrose in animals and in healthy human adults with normal sucrase activity (4, 142, 143). However, neither sucrose nor fructose increases sucrase activity in patients with SI deficiency (4).

Much less is known about SI deficiency compared with hypolactasia, but the research base is currently growing. Although reports exist of acquired or adult-onset SI deficiency (144–146), the congenital type of SI deficiency is most common. In congenital SI deficiency, there is always a nearly complete absence of sucrase activity, whereas isomaltase activity can vary from the existence of only traces of activity to a nearly normal level (4). Congenital SI deficiency is transmitted via autosomal recessive inheritance, and it appears that only a few population groups have significant numbers of people with this disorder. Estimates of the prevalence of congenital SI deficiency (4) in different populations are as follows: Native Greenlanders (2–10%), Native Alaskans (3%), Canadian native peoples (3.6–7.1%), Danes (<0.1%), and white North Americans (≤0.2%). Investigators have proposed that the reason that SI deficiency is high only in Arctic regions is because the diet in these areas has been composed mainly of animal products

for centuries. Thus, patients with sucrose malabsorption who ate animal foods would have no intolerance symptoms, and their chances of survival would be just as great as if normal sucrase activity was present (147).

Dietary therapy for SI deficiency consists of sucrose restriction. It is not usually necessary to make the diet starch free, except in infants or in older children who do not respond to a sucrose-free diet (4). In glucoamylase deficiency, however, elimination of dietary starch appears to be more important and has successfully resolved carbohydrate malabsorption symptoms in children diagnosed with this condition (148). In some reported cases of congenital glucoamylase deficiency in infants and children, patients have had coexisting lactase and sucrase deficiencies as well, necessitating more comprehensive diet therapy (149, 150).

An additional dietary management strategy for SI deficiency involves the use of enzyme supplement therapy. Sacrosidase is a liquid product prepared from the yeast *Saccharomyces cerevisae* that containing approximately 9000 IU/mL of sucrase activity. Although sacrosidase promotes sucrose hydrolysis, it is unlike the human enzyme in that it does not have isomaltase activity. However, this product reduces the breath hydrogen response to a sucrose challenge and decreases sucrose intolerance symptoms such as diarrhea, flatulence, abdominal pain, and bloating (151, 152).

TREHALASE

Trehalase (trehalose 1-glucohydrolase; EC 3.2.1.28) is a disaccharidase that hydrolyses trehalose to two molecules of glucose (153). The enzyme is present in the brush border membrane of small intestine and proximal convoluted tubules of the kidney (154). The highest activity of this enzyme is observed in the proximal part of the jejunum (3). As with SI deficiency, trehalase deficiency is rare outside of Arctic populations. Gudmand-Høyer and colleagues found that trehalose activity was low in 14 of 29 Greenlanders (153). Trehalose maldigestion resulting from trehalase deficiency causes symptoms similar to that of lactose maldigestion (155). However, young mushrooms are the only significant contributors of trehalose in the present-day diet, perhaps contributing as much as 6 g trehalose in a 150-g serving (155). Thus, trehalose ingestion from foods is not likely to exceed 20 g/day, and, according to a study conducted by Oku and Nakamura, this amount is insufficient to cause diarrhea or abdominal symptoms (156).

Trehalase is the only disaccharidase present in the human plasma (154). The significance of plasma trehalase is yet undefined, but trehalase activity in plasma may be associated with glucose metabolism. In one study, high plasma trehalase activity in an individual was associated with greater likelihood of developing diabetes (154). Serum trehalase activity has been found to be low in patients with rheumatoid arthritis, a finding suggesting that processes leading to inflammation could affect the enzyme activity (157).

In summary, intestinal trehalase deficiency is rare, and because dietary trehalose intake is also low, this disorder has very little clinical or nutritional significance. The physiologic importance of high or low plasma trehalase levels is still unclear.

SUMMARY

Unexplained gastrointestinal symptoms such as flatulence, abdominal pain, and diarrhea can often be traced to low levels of intestinal disaccharidase activity. However, hypolactasia is the only disaccharidase depletion that affects significant numbers of people worldwide. Fortunately, many dietary approaches are available for the management of the disaccharidase depletions covered in this chapter.

REFERENCES

1. Johnson LR. Gastrointestinal Physiology. 6th ed. St. Louis, MO: Mosby, 2001.
2. Southgate DAT. Am J Clin Nutr 1995;62[Suppl]:203S–11S.
3. Gudmand-Høyer E, Skovberg H. Scand J Gastroenterol 1996;31[Suppl 2]:111–21.
4. Treem WR. J Pediatr Gastroenterol Nutr 1995;21:1–14.
5. Kien CL, Heitlinger LA, Li BU et al. Semin Perinatol 1989;13:78–87.
6. Tso P, Crissinger K. Overview of digestion and absorption. In: Stipanauk MH, ed. Biochemical and Physiological Aspects of Human Nutrition. Philadelphia: WB Saunders, 2000:75–90.
7. Bayless TM, Christopher NL. Am J Clin Nutr 1969;22:181–90.
8. Srinivasan R, Minocha A. Postgrad Med 1998;104:10923.
9. Skovbjerg H. Clin Chim Acta 1981;112:205–12.
10. Zecca L, Mesonero JE, Stutz A et al. FEBS Lett 1998;435:225–8.
11. Day AJ, Cañada FJ, Diaz JC et al. FEBS Lett 2000;468:166–70.
12. Wilkinson AP, Gee JM, Dupont S et al. Xenobiotica 2003;33:255–64.
13. Mackey AD, Henderson GN, Gregory JF. J Biol Chem 2002;277:26858–64.
14. Järvelä I, Enattah NS, Kokkonen J et al. . Am J Hum Genet 1998;63:1078–85.
15. Hoskova A, Sabacky J, Mrskos A et al. Arch Dis Child 1980;55:304–16.
16. Berg NO, Dahlqvist A, Lindberg T et al. Acta Paediatr Scand 1969;58:525–7.
17. Hirashima Y, Shinozuka S, Ieiri T et al. Eur J Pediatr 1979;130:41–5.
18. Russo G, Mollica F, Mazzone D et al. Acta Paediatr Scand 1974;63:457–60.
19. Newcomer AD, McGill DB. Clin Nutr 1984;3:53–8.
20. Gilat T, Russo S, Gelman-Malachi E et al. Gastroenterology 1972;62:1125–7.
21. Sahi T. Scand J Gastroenterol 1994;29:7–20.
22. Simoons FJ. Dig Dis 1978;23:963–80.
23. Anderson B, Vullo C. Gut 1994;35:1487–9.
24. Meloni T, Colombo C, Ruggiu G et al. Ital J Gastroenterol Hepatol 1998;30:490–3.
25. Auricchio S. Ital J Gastroenterol Hepatol 1998;30:494–5.
26. Rossi M, Maiuri L, Fusco MI et al. Gastroenterology 1997;112:1506–14.
27. Maiuri L, Rossi M, Raia V et al. . Gastroenterology 1994;107:54–60.
28. Grand RJ, Montgomery RK, Chitkara DK et al. Gut 2003;52:617–9.
29. Witte J, Lloyd M, Lorenzsonn V et al. J Clin Invest 1990;86:1338–42.
30. Lorenzsonn V, Lloyd M, Olen WA. Gastroenterology 1993;105:51–9.
31. Naim HY. Histol Histopathol 2001;16:553–61.
32. Sebastio G, Villa M, Sartorio R et al. Am J Hum Genet 1989;45:489–97.
33. Montgomery RK, Büller HA, Rings EHHM et al. FASEB J 1991;5:2824–32.
34. Lloyd M, Mevissen G, Fischer M et al. J Clin Invest 1992;89:524–9.
35. Fajardo O, Naim HY, Lacey SW. Gastroenterology 1994;106:1233–41.
36. Krasinski SD, Estrada G, Yeh KY et al. Am J Physiol 1994;267:G584–94.
37. Escher JC, Koning ND, van Engen CGJ et al. J Clin Invest 1992;89:480–83.
38. Troelsen JT, Olsen J, Norén O et al. J Biol Chem 1992;267:20407–11.
39. Troelsen JT, Mitchelmore C, Spodsberg N et al. Biochem J 1997;322:833–8.
40. Naim HY, Lentze MJ. J Biol Chem 1992;267:25494–504.
41. Scrimshaw NS, Murray EB. Am J Clin Nutr 1988;48:1083–1159.
42. Khambadkone MR, Jain MK, Ganapathy S. Indian Pediatr 1994;31:1351–5.
43. Gray G. Gastroenterology 1993;105:931.
44. Arola H. Scand J Gastroenterol 1994;29[Suppl 202]:26–35.
45. McBean LD, Miller GD. J Am Diet Assoc 1998;98:671–6.
46. Carroccio A, Montalto G, Cavera G et al. J Am Coll Nutr 1998;17:631–6.
47. Suarez FL, Savaiano DA, Levitt MD. N Engl J Med 1995;333:1–4.
48. Suarez FL, Savaiano DA, Arbisi P, Levitt MD. Am J Clin Nutr 1997;65:1502–6.
49. Johnson AO, Semenya JG, Buchowski MS et al. Am J Clin Nutr 1993;57:399–401.
50. Suarez F, Levitt M. Gut 1997;41:715–6.
51. Srinivasan R, Minocha A. Postgrad Med 1998;104:109–123.
52. Vonk RJ, Priebe MG, Koetse HA et al. Eur J Clin Invest 2003;33:70–5.
53. Hill MJ. Bacterial adaptation to lactase deficiency. In: Delmont J, ed. Milk Intolerances and Rejection. Basel: Karger, 1983:22–6.
54. Ballongue J. Bifidobacteria and probiotic action. In: Selminen S, vonWright A, eds. Lactic Acid Bacteria. New York: Marcel Dekker, 1993:369–71.
55. Perman J, Modler S, Olson AC. J Clin Invest 1981;67:643–50.
56. Vogelsang H, Ferenci P, Frotz S et al. Gut 1988;29:21–6.
57. Tomlin J, Lowis C, Read NW. Gut 1991;32:665–9.
58. Hammer HF, Petritsch W, Pristautz H et al. Wien Klin Wochenschr 1996;108:175–9.
59. Levitt MD, Furne J, Olsson S. Ann Intern Med 1996;124:422–4.
60. Bond JH, Levitt MD. Gastroenterology 1976;70:1058–62.
61. Bedine MS, Bayless TM. Gastroenterology 1973;65:735–43.
62. Newcomer AD, McGill DB, Thomas PJ et al. Gastroenterology 1978;74:44–6.

63. Gudmand-Høyer E, Simony K. Dig Dis 1977;22:177–81.
64. Hertzler SR, Huynh B-C, Savaiano DA. J Am Diet Assoc 1996;96:243–6.
65. Vesa TH, Korpela RA, Sahi T. Am J Clin Nutr 1996;64:197–201.
66. Savaiano DA, Levitt MD. J Dairy Sci 1987;70:397–406.
67. Gremse DA, Greer AS, Vacik J et al. Clin Pediatr 2003;42:341–5.
68. Suarez FL, Adshead J, Furne JK et al. Am J Clin Nutr 1998;68:1118–22.
69. Hertzler SR, Savaiano DA. Am J Clin Nutr 1996;64:232–6.
70. Ladas S, Papanikos J, Arapakis G. Gut 1982;23:968–73.
71. Labayen I, Forga L, Gonzalez A et al. Aliment Pharmacol Ther 2001;15:543–9.
72. Solomons NW, Guerrero A-M, Torun B. Am J Clin Nutr 1985;41:199–208.
73. Martini MC, Savaiano DA. Am J Clin Nutr 1988;47:57–60.
74. Dehkordi N, Rao DR, Warren AP et al. J Am Diet Assoc 1995;95:484–6.
75. Vesa TH, Marteau PR, Briet FB et al. J Nutr 1997;127:2316–20.
76. Vesa TH, Marteau PR, Briet FB et al. Am J Clin Nutr 1997;66:123–6.
77. Peuhkuri K, Vapaatalo H, Nevala R et al. Scand J Clin Invest 2000;60:75–80.
78. Leichter JL. Am J Clin Nutr 1973;26:393–6.
79. Cavalli-Sforza LT, Strata A. Hum Nutr Clin Nutr 1986;40C:19–30.
80. Vesa TH, Lember M, Korpela R. Eur J Clin Nutr 1997;51:633–6.
81. Lee CM, Hardy CM. Am J Clin Nutr 1989;49:840–4.
82. Jarvinen RMK, Loukaskorpi M, Uusitupa MIJ. Eur J Clin Nutr 2003;57:701–5.
83. Gallagher CR, Molleson AL, Caldwell JH. J Am Diet Assoc 1974;65:418–9.
84. Kolars JC, Levitt MD, Aouji M et al. N Engl J Med 1984;310:1–3.
85. Savaiano DA, AbouElAnouar A, Smith DE et al. Am J Clin Nutr 1984;40:1219–23.
86. Lerebours E, Ndam CND, Lavoine A et al. Am J Clin Nutr 1989;49:823–7.
87. Martini MC, Lerebours EC, Lin W-J et al. Am J Clin Nutr 1991;54:1041–6.
88. Gilliland SE, Kim HS. J Dairy Sci 1984;67:1–6.
89. Răsic J, Kurmans JA. The nutritional-physiological value of yogurt. In: Yogurt: Scientific Grounds, Technology, Manufacture, and Preparations. Copenhagen: Technical Dairy Publishing House, 1978:99–137.
90. Martini MC, Bollweg GL, Levitt MD et al. Am J Clin Nutr 1987;45:432–6.
91. Martini MC, Kukielka D, Savaiano DA. Am J Clin Nutr 1991;53:1253–8.
92. Shermak MA, Saavedra JM, Jackson TL et al. Am J Clin Nutr 1995;62:1003–6.
93. Martini MC, Smith DE, Savaiano DA. Am J Clin Nutr 1987;46:36–40.
94. Hertzler SR, Clancy SM. J Am Diet Assoc 2003;103:582–7.
95. Newcomer AD, Park HS, O'Brien PC. Am J Clin Nutr 1983;38:257–63.
96. Mc Donough FE, Hitchins AD, Wong NP. Am J Clin Nutr 1987;45:570–4.
97. Lin M-Y, Savaiano DA, Harlander S. J Dairy Sci 1991;74:87–95.
98. Onwulata CI, Rao DR, Vankineni P. Am J Clin Nutr 1989;49:1233–7.
99. Saltzman JR, Russell RM, Golner B et al. Am J Clin Nutr 1999;69:140–6.
100. Montes RG, Bayless TM, Saavedra JM et al. J Dairy Sci 1995;78:1657–64.
101. Kim HS, Gilliland SE. J Dairy Sci 1983;66:959–66.
102. Jiang T, Mustapha A, Savaiano DA. J Dairy Sci 1996;79:750–7.
103. Mustapha A, Jiang T, Savaiano DA. J Dairy Sci 1997;80:1537–45.
104. US Food and Drug Administration. Available at:http://www.cfsan.fda.gov/~dms/opa–enzy.html. Accessed November 25, 2003.
105. Land O Lakes. Dairy Ease nutritional information. Available at:http://www.dairyease.com/benefits/nutritional_whole.html. Accessed November 25, 2003.
106. Lactaid. Lactaid products. Available at:http://www.lactaid.com. Accessed November 25, 2003.
107. Rosado JL, Morales M, Pasquetti A et al. Rev Invest Clin 1988;40:141–7.
108. Biller JA, King S, Rosenthal A et al. J Pediatr 1987;111:91–4.
109. Payne-Bose D, Welsh JD, Gearhart HL et al. Am J Clin Nutr 1977;30:695–7.
110. Payne DL, Welsh JD, Manion CV. Am J Clin Nutr 1981;34:2711–5.
111. Pedersen ER, Jensen BH, Jensen HJ. Scand J Gastroenterol 1982;17:861–4.
112. Brand JC, Holt S. Am J Clin Nutr 1991;54:148–51.
113. Turner SJ, Daly T, Hourigan JA et al. Am J Clin Nutr 1976;29:739–44.
114. Paige DM, Bayless TM, Mellits ED et al. J Agric Food Chem 1979;27:677–80.
115. Cheng AHR, Brunser O, Espinoza J et al. Am J Clin Nutr 1979;32:1989–93.
116. Rosado JL, Morales M, Pasquetti A. JPEN J Parenter Enteral Nutr 1989;13:157–61.
117. Nagy L, Mozsik G, Garamszegi M et al. Acta Med Hung 1983;40:239–45.
118. Reasoner J, Maculan TP, Rand AG et al. Am J Clin Nutr 1981;34:54–60.
119. Ramirez FC, Lee K, Graham DY. Am J Gastroenterol 1994;89:566–70.
120. Gao K-P, Mitsui T, Fujiki K et al. Nagoya J Med Sci 2002;65:21–8.
121. Lin M-Y, DiPalma JA, Martini MC et al. Dig Dis Sci 1993;38:2022–7.
122. Sanders SW, Tolman KG, Reitberg DP. Clin Pharm 1992;11:533–8.
123. DiPalma JA, Collins MS. J Clin Gastroenterol 1989;11:290–3.
124. Moskovitz M, Curtis C, Gavaler J. Am J Gastroenterol 1987;82:632–5.
125. Suarez FL, Zumarraga LM, Furne JK et al. J Am Diet Assoc 2001;101:1447–52.
126. Nielsen OH, Schiotz PO, Rasmussen SN et al. J Pediatr Gastroenterol Nutr 1984;3:219–23.
127. Gilat F, Russo S, Gelman-Malachi E et al. Gastroenterology 1972;62:1125–7.
128. Keusch GT, Troncale FJ, Thavaramara B et al. Am J Clin Nutr 1969;22:638–41.
129. Reddy V, Pershad J. Am J Clin Nutr 1972;25:114–9.
130. Habte D, Sterky G, Hjalmarsson B. Acta Paediatr Scand 1973;62:649–54.
131. Greenfield H. Nutr Today 2003;38:77–81.
132. Johnson AO, Semenya JG, Buchowski MS et al. Am J Clin Nutr 1993;58:879–81.
133. Pribila BA, Hertzler SR, Martin BR et al. J Am Diet Assoc 2000;100:524–28.
134. Briet F, Pochart P, Marteau P et al. Gut 1997;41:632–5.
135. During MJ, Xu R, Young D et al. Nat Med 1998;4:1131–5.

136. West LF, Davis MB, Green FR et al. Ann Hum Genet 1988;52:57–61.

137. Green F, Edwards Y, Hauri HP et al. Gene 1987;57:101–10.

138. Lloyd ML, Olsen WA. N Engl J Med 1987;316:438–42.

139. Jacob R, Zimmer K-P, Schmitz J et al. J Clin Invest 2000;106:281–7.

140. Ouwendijk J, Moolenaar CEC, Peters WJ et al. J Clin Invest 1996;97:633–41.

141. Moolenaar CEC, Ouwendijk J, Wittpoth M et al. J Cell Sci 1997;110:557–67.

142. Rosensweig NS, Herman RH. J Clin Invest 1968;47:2253–62.

143. Schmitz J, Odievre M, Rey J. Gastroenterology 1972;62:389–92.

144. Muldoon C, Maguire P, Gleeson F. Am J Gastroenterol 1999;94:2298–9.

145. Ringrose RE, Preiser H, Welsh JD. Dig Dis Sci 1980;25:384–7.

146. Cooper BT, Scott J, Hopkins J et al. Dig Dis Sci 1983;28:473–7.

147. Gudmand-Høyer E, Fenger HJ, Kern-Hansen P et al. Scand J Gastroenterol 1987;22:24–8.

148. Lebenthal E, Khin-Maung U, Zheng BY et al. J Pediatr 1994;124:541–6.

149. Nichols BL, Avery SE, Karnsakul W et al. J Pediatr Gastroenterol Nutr 2002;35:573–9.

150. Karsakul W, Luginbuehl U, Hahn D et al. J Pediatr Gastroenterol Nutr 2002;35:551–6.

151. Treem WR, McAdams L, Stanford L et al. J Pediatr Gastroenterol Nutr 1999;28:137–42.

152. Treem WR, Ahsan N, Sullivan B et al. Gastroenterology 1993;105:1061–68.

153. Gudmand-Høyer E, Fenger HJ, Skovbjerg H et al. Scand J Gastroenterol 1988;23:775–8.

154. Eze, LC. Biochem Genet 1989;27:487–95.

155. Arola H, Koivula T, Karvonen AL et al. Scand J Gastroenterol 1999;34:898–903.

156. Oku T, Nakamura S. Eur J Clin Nutr 2000;54:783–8.

157. Yoshida K, Mizukawa H, Haruki E. Clin Chim Acta 1993;215:123–4.

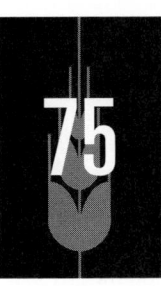

75   SHORT BOWEL SYNDROME[1]

KHURSHEED N. JEEJEEBHOY

DEFINITION 1201
ETIOLOGY 1201
PATHOPHYSIOLOGIC CONSIDERATIONS 1201
   Stomach 1201
   Small Bowel 1202
   Unique Functions of the Ileum 1202
   Colon 1202
   Effect of Loss of Intestinal and Colonic Function
      on the Absorption of Fluid and Electrolytes . . .1202
   Effect of Intestinal Resection on Nutrient
      Absorption 1202
ADAPTATION OF THE INTESTINE 1203
   Effect of Excluding Food from the Bowel Lumen .1203
   Factors Influencing Bowel Atrophy 1203
   Hormonal Factors Influencing Intestinal
      Adaptation 1203
   Does Bowel Rest Induce Gut Atrophy in
      Humans? 1204
SPECIFIC ASPECTS OF MANAGEMENT 1204
   Control of Gastric Hypersecretion and Motility . .1204
   Jejunal Resection with Intact Ileum and Colon . .1204
   Ileal Resection of Less Than 100 cm with
      Colon Largely Intact .1204
   Ileal Resection Between 100 and 200 cm with
      Colon Largely Intact .1204
   Resection in Excess of 200 cm of Small Bowel
      and Partial Colectomy 1204
   Resection Leaving Less Than 60 cm Small
      Bowel or Only Duodenum: Massive Bowel
      Resection 1204
GENERAL MANAGEMENT CONSIDERATIONS 1204
   Control of Diarrhea 1204
   Intravenous Fluids 1204
   Maintenance of Fluid and Electrolyte Balance
      Orally 1204
   Maintenance of Energy Balance 1205
   Carbohydrate Versus Fat Feeding 1205
   Micronutrient Supplements 1206
   Parenteral Supplementation and Nutrition 1206

COMPLICATIONS 1207
   Gastric Hypersecretion and Peptic Ulceration . . .1207
   Cholelithiasis 1207
   Renal Stones 1207
   ᴅ-Lactic Acidosis 1207
PHARMACOLOGIC APPROACHES TO PROMOTE
   ABSORPTION 1207
   Somatostatin Analog 1207
   Growth Hormone 1207
   Glucagonlike Peptide-2 1207

DEFINITION

The short bowel syndrome is caused by reduction in the area of functioning intestine resulting in an inability to maintain fluid and electrolyte balance and/or meet macronutrient and micronutrient requirements.

ETIOLOGY

The causes of short bowel syndrome are given in Table 75.1. Most cases of short bowel syndrome result from massive intestinal resection of the distal small bowel with a variable degree of colonic resection. Loss of both ileum and colon causes the most severe degrees of malabsorption.

PATHOPHYSIOLOGIC CONSIDERATIONS

To understand and treat this condition, it is necessary to understand normal function and how it is altered by the short bowel syndrome.

Stomach

The rate of gastric emptying regulates the progress of the meal through the small bowel. Gastric emptying is rapid and exponential for liquids and is slow and regulated by particle size for solids. Furthermore, intestinal contents entering the distal intestine inhibit gastric emptying (1).

Gastric hypersecretion occurs after small bowel resection and reduces nutrient absorption by inactivating pancreatic enzymes. Gastric motility is enhanced by small bowel resection (2). Although proximal resection does not increase the rate of intestinal transit, ileal resection significantly

---

[1] **Abbreviations: GLP**, glucagonlike peptide; **HPN**, home parenteral nutrition; **NPO**, nil per os; **ORS**, oral rehydration solution; **SCFA**, short-chain fatty acid; **TPN**, total parenteral nutrition.

TABLE 75.1. CAUSES OF SHORT BOWEL SYNDROME

Intestinal resection
    Ileal resection
    Ileocolic resection
    End jejunostomy
Mucosal disease
    Celiac disease
    Whipple disease
    Lymphoma
    Ulcerative jejunoileitis
    Abetalipoproteinemia
Small bowel disease
    Radiation injury and chemotherapy
    Inflammatory bowel disease
    Neoplasms
    Autoimmune disease
    Infection (e.g., human immunodeficiency virus)
Gut bypass
    Intestinal fistulas
    Surgical bypass

accelerates intestinal transit (3). In this situation, the colon aids in slowing intestinal transit, so in patients with a short bowel without a colon, a marker fed by mouth was completely excreted in a few hours (4).

Small Bowel

Small bowel motility is three times slower in the ileum than in the jejunum (5). In addition, the ileocecal valve may slow transit, especially when the ileum has been resected (6). The adult small bowel receives about 5 to 6 L/day of endogenous secretions and 2 to 3 L/day of exogenous fluids. Most of this volume is reabsorbed in the small bowel. The amount reabsorbed in the small intestine depends on the nature of the meal (7). With a low-osmotic meal, usually low in soluble carbohydrates (meat and salad meal), most of the fluid is absorbed in the jejunum, whereas with a meal high in osmolarity and soluble carbohydrates, such as lactose (milk and doughnut meal), less is absorbed proximally and more flows distally. In addition, the absorptive processes are different in the jejunum as compared with the ileum. In general, water absorption is a passive process resulting from the active transport of nutrients and electrolytes. The transport of sodium creates an electrochemical gradient and also drives the uptake of carbohydrates and amino acids across the intestinal mucosa. In the ileum, sodium chloride absorption is neutral. However, the net absorption depends not only on these processes but also on the extent of backdiffusion of the transported material back into the intestinal lumen through "leaky" intercellular junctions. In the jejunum, these junctions are very leaky, and thus jejunal contents are always isotonic. Fluid absorption in this region of the bowel is very inefficient when compared with the ileum. Investigators have estimated that the efficiency of water absorption is 44 and 70% of the ingested load in the jejunum and ileum, respectively. For sodium, the corresponding estimates are

13 and 72% (7). Hence the ileum is important in the conservation of fluid and electrolytes.

Unique Functions of the Ileum

The ileum uniquely absorbs vitamin B_{12} and bile salts. Bile salts are essential for the efficient absorption of fats and fat-soluble vitamins. Normally, the intestinal concentration of bile salts required for fat absorption cannot be met by synthesis alone but is attained by ileal resorption and recycling into the intestine. With ileal resection, the loss of bile salts increases, resulting in the depletion of the bile salt pool and causing fat malabsorption. In addition, loss of bile salts into the colon reduces the ability of the colon to reabsorb salt and water. In the colon, bile salts are also dehydroxylated to deoxy bile salts, which induce colonic water secretion. Both the foregoing factors enhance diarrhea.

Colon

The colon has the slowest transit time, varying between 24 and 150 hours. The intercellular junctions are the tightest in this part of the bowel, and the efficiency of water and salt absorption in the colon exceeds 90% (8). Carbohydrate not absorbed in the small bowel is fermented in the colon to short-chain fatty acids (SCFAs), which, in turn, have two important actions. First, SCFAs enhance salt and water absorption (9). Second, the energy content of malabsorbed carbohydrates is salvaged by being absorbed as SCFAs. Our observations suggest that in patients with short bowel syndrome, this salvage may be greater than in physiologically normal persons (10). Thus, the colon becomes an important organ for fluid and electrolyte conservation and for the salvage of malabsorbed energy substrates in patients with a short bowel.

Effect of Loss of Intestinal and Colonic Function on the Absorption of Fluid and Electrolytes

The effect of intestinal resection depends on the extent and site of resection. Proximal resection results in no bowel disturbance because the ileum and colon absorb the increased fluid and electrolyte load efficiently. The remaining ileum continues to absorb bile salts, and thus little reaches the colon to impede salt and water reabsorption. In contrast, when the ileum is resected, the colon receives a much larger load of fluid and electrolytes and also receives bile salts that reduce its ability to absorb salt and water and result in diarrhea. In addition to the ileum, if the colon is also resected, the ability to maintain fluid and electrolyte homeostasis is severely impaired (11).

Effect of Intestinal Resection on Nutrient Absorption:

Absorption of nutrients occurs throughout the small bowel, and the removal of the jejunum alone results in the ileum taking over most of the lost function. In this situation, no malabsorption occurs (12). In contrast, even a loss of a 100 cm of ileum causes steatorrhea (13). The degree of malabsorption increases with the length of resection, and the variety of nutrients malabsorbed increases (14, 15). Balance studies of energy absorption have shown that the absorption of fat and carbohydrate were equally reduced to between 50 and 75% of intake (16). However, nitrogen absorption was reduced to a lesser extent than that of carbohydrate and fat. Nitrogen absorption was 81% of intake. In patients with a short bowel, Ladefoged and colleagues (15) found that the degrees of calcium, magnesium, zinc, and phosphorus absorption were reduced but did not correlate with the remaining length of bowel. These investigators recommended that parenteral supplementation be mandatory in these patients. Our studies showed similar reduction in absorption, but only half our patients required parenteral replacement. The data taken as a whole suggest that it is easier to meet needs for energy and nitrogen by increasing oral intake than it is to meet the needs for electrolytes and divalent ions. A review of the literature before the availability of parenteral nutrition shows that resections up to 33% result in no malnutrition, and those up to 50% can be tolerated without special aids, but patients who undergo resections in excess of 75% require nutritional support to avoid severe malnutrition (17).

ADAPTATION OF THE INTESTINE

Following resection, the remaining small bowel hypertrophies and increases absorptive function (18, 19). This process enhances the ability of the remaining bowel to recover the lost function and is thus an important compensatory process. The factors that influence this adaptation are complex and are discussed later, as are the effects of total parenteral nutrition (TPN).

Eating exposes the gastrointestinal tract to unique stimuli that do not occur when the gastrointestinal tract is kept constantly empty, a process called bowel rest. The advent of TPN resulted in the ability to rest the bowel for short or long periods without causing malnutrition, a situation that had not been possible previously. This process nourished the body but excluded the gut from the nutrient and hormonal stimuli that occur during ingestion of an oral diet. The advent of defined formula diets without residue and diets composed of monomers such as glucose instead of polymeric starch modified the stimuli received by the gut when exposed to a normal diet. Moreover, because nutrients are absorbed progressively along the length of the bowel, the jejunum is exposed to a higher concentration of nutrients than the ileum. Resection of the proximal bowel causes the ileum to receive more nutrients. Conversely, resection of the ileum does not alter the jejunal nutrient load but may reduce stimuli from hormones released by the ileum.

Effect of Excluding Food from the Bowel Lumen

Hypoplasia of the mucosa is the most obvious change in experimental animals when food is excluded from the lumen. At the same time, body composition can be simultaneously maintained by the use of TPN (20).

In growing or neonatal animals, TPN and bowel rest maintained normal body growth but resulted in reduced bowel length and in gastric and pancreatic hypoplasia (21–23). Despite the occurrence of mucosal hypoplasia, the development of disaccharidase enzymes proceeded, glucose transport was accelerated, and mucosal levels of these enzymes increased in neonatal animals receiving TPN (22, 23). Hypoplasia occurred mainly in the proximal small bowel and was less evident distally (24). In addition, TPN and bowel rest increased intestinal permeability (25) and altered the response to endotoxin (26). These dramatic effects of withdrawing food by mouth and giving TPN in animals are not as pronounced in humans. A month of TPN does not cause atrophy; only after several months of being nil per os (NPO) does villus atrophy occur in humans (27).

The nature of the feedings influences the degree of hypoplasia. Refined liquid feedings cause relative hypoplasia as compared with a solid diet (21).

Factors Influencing Bowel Atrophy

In general, it appears that the decreased digestive and absorptive activities of the mucosa during bowel rest are the major reasons for hypoplasia. This concept is supported by the finding that simply increasing the tonicity of the bowel contents results in an increase of the mucosal mass (28). Absorption of amino acids causes a nonspecific increase of mucosal function and mass (29). Finally, disaccharide hydrolysis followed by absorption stimulates mucosal growth to a greater extent than equivalent monosaccharide absorption (30).

SCFAs produced by fermentation in the colon were shown to prevent or reduce mucosal atrophy in animals receiving TPN and bowel rest, even when these substances were given parenterally (31). Dietary fiber is the main source of colonic fermentable substrate for SCFA production. Therefore, fiber in the diet aids in the maintenance of mucosal mass. For the same reasons, defined formula diets are not quite as good as a solid diet in this regard. Glutamine is a nutrient for the bowel mucosa, and the supplementation of TPN with glutamine preserves gastric and colonic mass in TPN-fed animals but does not preserve small bowel mucosal height (32).

Hormonal Factors Influencing Intestinal Adaptation

Glucagonlike peptides 1 and 2 (GLP-1 and GLP-2) are produced by the gut endocrine cells and have a profound effect on intestinal function. Preliminary data suggest that GLP-2 can improve intestinal absorption in patients with a short bowel (33).

Does Bowel Rest Induce Gut Atrophy in Humans?

In the rat, bowel rest with TPN causes atrophy in days (34), but in humans, even after 21 days of bowel rest with TPN, no change occurs in gut hormone production after a meal (35), nor is any histologic atrophy evident (27). In a study of children, bowel rest caused atrophy only when prolonged beyond 9 months (27). However, the size of the microvilli is reduced, and brush border enzyme activity falls (36).

In summary, animal data suggest that when the bowel is not used, it atrophies. Mucosal atrophy results from a combination of the lack of functional stimulation and the absence of hormonal, biliary, and pancreatic secretion. The only convincing trophic factors are GLP-1 and 2, SCFAs and their precoursor, dietary fiber, and glutamine. In addition, some evidence suggests a role for vitamin A, zinc, and glutathione as weaker trophic factors (37).

SPECIFIC ASPECTS OF MANAGEMENT

Control of Gastric Hypersecretion and Motility

Reducing acid secretion improves absorption in patients with a short bowel (38). Furthermore, hypersecretion can cause nausea, reflux, and hemorrhage from severe esophageal ulceration; these effects are prevented by proton pump inhibitors (39).

Jejunal Resection with Intact Ileum and Colon

Patients in this category can be fed orally immediately and rarely have any problems.

Ileal Resection of Less than 100 cm with Colon Largely Intact

Patients in this category have so-called bile salt–induced diarrhea, and they are best helped by the administration of 4 g of cholestyramine one to three times a day to bind bile salts. Bile salts are absorbed by the ileum and are recycled. After ileal resection, bile salts remain unabsorbed and enter the colon, where they cause water secretion and diarrhea. Vitamin B_{12} absorption is also impaired in some patients.

Ileal Resection between 100 and 200 cm with Colon Largely Intact

These patients have little difficulty in maintaining nutrition with an oral diet, but they have almost complete malabsorption of bile salts. In consequence, they have a deficiency of bile salts in the intestinal lumen because bile salt synthesis alone without recycling of bile salts through the ileum is unable to maintain an adequate concentration in the intestinal lumen. These patients have colonic water secretion resulting from entry of bile salt into the colon as well as malabsorption of fatty acid caused by a low concentration of bile salts in the intestinal lumen. Malabsorbed fatty acids entering the colon increase water secretion. For such patients, fat restriction is mandatory. In patients with a larger resection, the bile salt pool is depleted, and cholestyramine alone is no longer able to prevent diarrhea. Parenteral vitamin B_{12} replacement is required.

Resection in Excess of 200 cm of Small Bowel and Partial Colectomy

Patients in this group require the graduated adaptation program indicated later, in the discussion of general management considerations.

Resection Leaving Less than 60 cm Small Bowel or Only Duodenum: Massive Bowel Resection

Patients in this category need HPN indefinitely. However, many patients even in this category may show a surprising degree of adaptation. They may require less parenteral nutrition and may benefit from orally absorbed nutrients. In these patients, parenteral nutrition can be reduced when weight gain is excessive, and cautious reduction of HPN does not cause electrolyte imbalance and dehydration.

GENERAL MANAGEMENT CONSIDERATIONS

Control of Diarrhea

Diarrhea results from a combination of increased secretions, increased motility, and osmotic stimulation of water secretion caused by malabsorption of luminal contents. Initially, keeping the patient NPO to reduce any osmotically driven water secretion controls diarrhea. Gastric hypersecretion can be controlled by the continuous infusion of appropriate doses of proton pump inhibitors. In addition, loperamide can be used to slow gastric and intestinal transit. If loperamide does not work, then codeine or phenoxylate may be tried.

Intravenous Fluids

In the immediate postoperative period, all patients require intravenous fluids and electrolytes to replace losses. Sodium and potassium chloride as well as magnesium are the most important ions to be replaced, and plasma levels of these ions should be monitored frequently. Fluid is infused according to measured losses to maintain an adequate urine output of between 1 and 2 L/day. The infusion is tapered as oral intake is increased as long as a desired urine output is maintained.

Maintenance of Fluid and Electrolyte Balance Orally

The next consideration is to determine the nature of oral feedings. In patients who have more than 100 cm of remaining jejunum, refeeding should be progressive, with

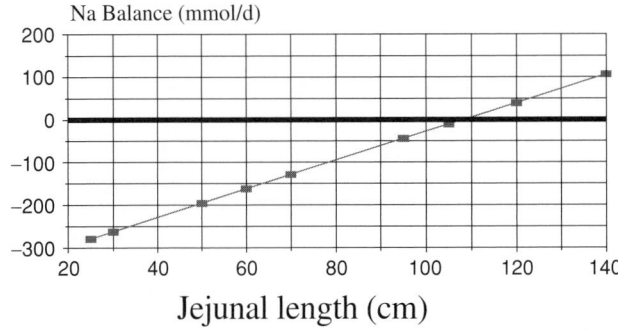

Figure 75.1. Jejunal efflux or absorption of sodium (Na) in relation to length of remaining small bowel. The *dark solid line* is the demarcation at which sodium secretion changes to absorption. (From Nightingale JMD, Lennard-Jones JE, Walker ER et al. Lancet 1990;336:765–8, with permission.)

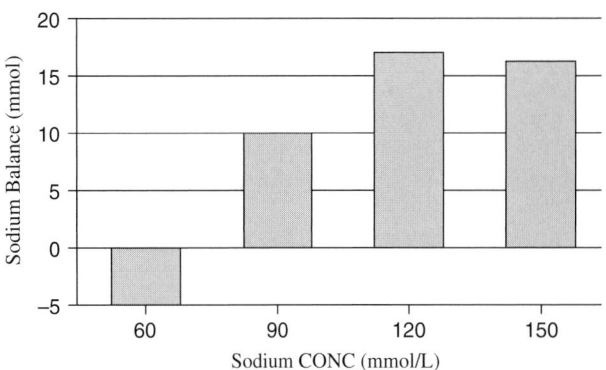

Figure 75.3. Effect of increasing the sodium content of oral rehydration solution on fluid absorption. (From Lennard-Jones JE. Clin Ther 1990;12[SupplA]:129–38, with permission.)

a view ultimately to feeding a normal oral diet. In patients with less than 100 cm of jejunum as the only small bowel remaining, dietary intake and fluids cause increased fluid loss (40) (Fig. 75.1). By contrast, in patients who have little small bowel left, the initial target should be small-volume isotonic feedings containing oral rehydration solution (ORS; Fig. 75.2). Investigators have shown that fluid absorption improves with increasing sodium concentration (Fig. 75.3). In addition to providing sufficient sodium to absorb fluids, it is necessary to ingest 10 to 15 g of sodium chloride as tablets with meals to aid the absorption of dietary carbohydrate. Such a regimen avoids osmotic stimulation of secretion and yet stimulates the bowel to absorb, thus promoting adaptation.

Maintenance of Energy Balance

The absorption of energy is better preserved than that of fluid and electrolytes and becomes limiting when the bowel is very short (Fig. 75.4). Comparison of Figures 75.1 to 75.4 shows that fluid and electrolyte losses become limiting when 100 cm of jejunum remains, whereas energy absorption becomes limiting when jejunal length is less than 60 to 70 cm. Hyperphagia is the key to meeting

energy requirements. In a group of patients with a short bowel, we found that the absorption of carbohydrate and fat energy was about 60% of intake (Fig. 75.5), whereas protein absorption was about 80% (16). Our unpublished data in patients receiving HPN suggest that body weight equilibrates at an absorbed energy intake at about 32 kcal/kg/day. In a 60-kg physiologically normal person, about 1800 kcal/day will be sufficient to maintain weight. If absorption is about 60% of intake, it will be necessary to increase oral energy intake to 3000 to 4000 kcal/day to absorb about 1800 kcal/day.

Progressive feeding should be attempted, as shown in Figures 75.6 and 75.7. The diet should be lactose free because lactase levels in such patients are reduced.

Carbohydrate Versus Fat Feeding

The ability of the colon to salvage malabsorbed carbohydrate can be used to improve nutrition in patients with a short bowel who have a colon. In these patients, hyperphagia with complex carbohydrates can result in the salvage of as much as a 1000 additional kilocalories (41). In

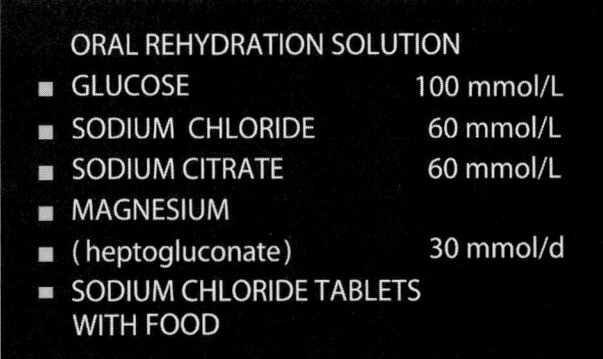

Figure 75.2. Composition of oral rehydration solution.

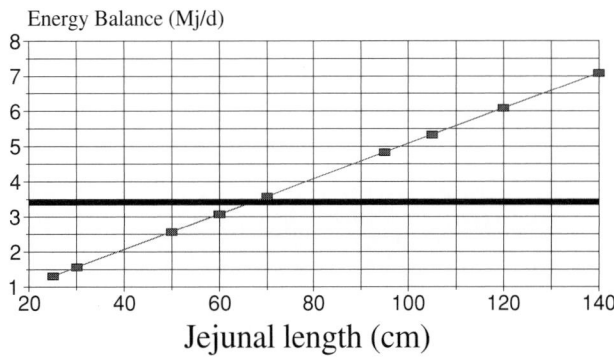

Figure 75.4. The relationship of energy absorption to length of remaining small bowel. The *dark solid line* shows the level at which energy absorption will meet the requirements of an average adult. (From Nightingale JMD, Lennard-Jones JE, Walker ER et al. Lancet 1990;336:765–8, with permission.)

	FAT	CARBO-HYDRATE	PROTEIN	TOTAL ABSORPTION
DIET	871 ± 97	608 ± 56	396 ± 36	1875 ± 174
STOOL	405 ± 73	239 ± 42	76 ± 15	719 ± 108
ABSORPTION (%)	54 ± 4	61 ± 7	81 ± 5	62 ± 3

*THERE WAS NO CHANGE IN ABSORPTION IN ANY OF THE PARA-METERS MEASURED OVER THE 10-DAY STUDY PERIOD.

Figure 75.5. Absolute and percentage of dietary absorption of protein, carbohydrates, and fats in patients with a very short bowel.

contrast, in patients with a jejunostomy and no colon, a high-fat diet was as well absorbed as carbohydrate (42), and did not result in additional loss of divalent ions. Because of its palatability and high energy density, a high-fat diet is more readily consumed. Fat restriction has been advocated, especially in patients with a remaining colon, because malabsorbed long-chain fatty acids can cause colonic water secretion and may bind divalent ions such as magnesium and calcium (43). However, in two cross-over studies of patients with a short bowel with variable lengths of remaining colon, we showed that a high-fat diet was comparable to a high-carbohydrate diet in regard to total fluid, energy, nitrogen, sodium, potassium, and divalent ion absorption (16, 44). We therefore recommend a low-lactose diet containing high calories from both fat and carbohydrate and a high nitrogen intake in most patients with a short bowel. The objective is to promote hyperphagia by making the diet palatable and acceptable. In adults who require about 30 kcal/kg/day, we aim to increase intake gradually to about 60 kcal/kg/day to provide sufficient absorbed calories despite malabsorption. The rationale for this approach is discussed by Woolf and associates (44).

Micronutrient Supplements

A summary of supplements (see details in Part II, Sections B and C) is given in Figure 75.8. Vitamin B_{12} absorption should be measured, and if it is subnormal, injections of 200 to 500 μg/month should be started. Supplements of potassium, magnesium, and zinc are given while one is monitoring serum levels. In particular, potassium as

- BOWEL ADAPAPTION REQUIRES CONSTANT ADJUSTMENT OF THE REGIMEN.
- AVOID HIGH FIBER NUTRIENT POOR FOODS.
- ADD SALT TO DIET TO MAKE IT "ISOTONIC."
- RESTRICT HYPO- AND HYPERTONIC FLUIDS.
- SIP LIQUIDS

Figure 75.6. The objectives of promoting oral intake in patients with a short bowel.

- ENCOURAGE "HYPERPHAGIA" TO COMPENSATE FOR MALABSORPTION.
- AVOID SOLUBLE CARBOHYDRATES — SUGAR AND LACTOSE.
- INCREASE BOTH FAT AND COMPLEX CARBOHYDRATE INTAKE.
- FAT SLOWS TRANSIT.
- FAT ALLOWS INTAKE OF MORE ENERGY FOR THE SAME VOLUME.
- CARBOHYDRATE IS ABSORBED BY THE COLON AS SHORT - CHAIN FATTY ACIDS.
- FAT MAY CAUSE WATER SECRETION IN COLON.
- UNABSORBED CARBOHYDRATE AND EXCESS SCFA CAN ALSO CAUSE OSMOTIC DIARRHEA.

Figure 75.7. Energy intake and the effects of dietary fat and carbohydrate. SCFA, short-chain fatty acid.

gluconate may be added to a concentration of 12 mmol/L in the ORS. In addition, we have found that magnesium heptogluconate is especially useful as a supplement to correct hypomagnesemia without causing diarrhea. It is possible to add 30 mmol of magnesium per liter of ORS and sipped over the day.

Parenteral Supplementation and Nutrition

In patients with less than 100 cm of remaining jejunum and in those with a combined small bowel and colon resection, parenterally infused fluids and electrolytes, especially magnesium, markedly improve the quality of life and in some cases are lifesaving. This infusion is started in such patients within a few days of the resection, and initially, 32 kcal/kg of a mixed-energy substrate and 1 g/kg amino acids are infused, with sodium 150 to 200 mM, potassium 60 to 100 mM, calcium 9 to 11 mM, magnesium 7 to 15 mM, and zinc 70 to 100 μmol/day. Among trace elements, zinc is the most important because we have found large losses in patients with a high endogenous output of intestinal fluids (45). Oral feedings are simultaneously started, and attempts are made to reduce parenteral feeding as oral feedings are increased.

- Zinc and selenium losses high
- Zinc gluconate 100 mg/d
- Selenium   60-100 g/d
- Malabsorption of fat-soluble vitamins
- Vitamin A 10,000 IU/d
- 1,25 OH Vitamin D 0.25-0.5 g/d
- Vitamin E 1200 IU/d
- Calcium gluconate   1500 mg/d
- Severe osteoporosis
- Pamidronate 30 mg IV/ every 3 months

Figure 75.8. Micronutrient supplementation in patients with a short bowel.

It will become apparent whether a patient needs parenteral feeding on a long-term basis. If that is the case, then the patient should be started on a program of home parenteral nutrition (HPN). We have found that as the bowel adapts over months and even years, the patient requires less parenteral feeding, and ultimately about 30% of our patients initially requiring HPN can be weaned off HPN by using up to 2 L of ORS, a high-calorie diet, and supplements of potassium, magnesium, calcium, fat-soluble vitamins, and zinc. These patients are monitored regularly until their weight is stable and they are in electrolyte balance. Hypomagnesemia is a particularly serious problem in these patients. Ingestion of magnesium salts orally enhances diarrhea, and therefore it often becomes difficult to use magnesium supplements orally. I have successfully used magnesium heptogluconate for this purpose. This preparation is available as a palatable liquid that is added to the Gastrolyte supplement in quantities of 30 mM/day. If this approach is not successful, then magnesium sulfate is infused through an indwelling catheter in doses of 12 mM one to three times a week to supplement the oral intake.

Vitamin supplementation needs comment. These patients can absorb water-soluble vitamins but have difficulty absorbing fat-soluble vitamins. They require large doses of vitamin A, D, and E to maintain normal levels. In addition, pills often pass out whole in these patients; hence liquid preparations have to be used. I recommend the measurement of these vitamin levels and supplementation with aqueous preparations of vitamin A and E (Aqasol A and E) and 1,25 dihydroxy-vitamin D in doses that normalize the plasma levels. Normalization may not be possible with oral vitamins in some patients, especially vitamin E levels. In others, an oral diet with intravenous fluid and electrolytes becomes necessary, and in the remainder, full parenteral nutrition is given (parenteral nutrition is discussed in Chapter 99).

COMPLICATIONS

Gastric Hypersecretion and Peptic Ulceration

Gastric hypersecretion occurs immediately after intestinal resection and tends to be transient. However, in some patients, peptic ulceration may occur. Treatment with histamine (H_2)-blockers (46) and, more recently, proton pump inhibitors (47) has been successful.

Cholelithiasis

As mentioned earlier, after ileal resection the bile salt concentration in bile falls. The reduction of the concentration of chenodeoxycholate in the bile increases cholesterol secretion (48). The combination of reduced bile salts and increased cholesterol makes the bile lithogenic (49). Intestinal resection may also increase the formation of pigment stones (50).

Renal Stones

Hyperoxaluria occurs in patients with short bowel syndrome as a result of increased absorption of oxalate by the colon (51), which is enhanced by bile salts entering the colon (52). Hyperoxalauria is associated with renal stone formation, and the propensity to form stones is reduced by supplementation with citrate and the use of thiazide diuretics (53). Prevention involves taking a low-oxalate diet, cholestyramine to bind bile salts, and citrate supplementation sufficient to normalize urinary citrate levels.

D-Lactic Acidosis

In some patients with a short bowel, episodic slurred speech, ataxia, and altered affect occur (54). The cause of this syndrome in which the patient appears "drunk" to relatives is fermentation of malabsorbed carbohydrate in the colon to D-lactate and absorption of this metabolite (55). Low soluble carbohydrate intake and antibiotics have been used to treat these episodes (56).

PHARMACOLOGIC APPROACHES TO PROMOTE ABSORPTION

Somatostatin Analog

Long-acting somatostatin analog has become available and can be given subcutaneously in doses of 50 to 100 µg before meals. All studies have shown a reduction in the volume of output and an increase in sodium or chloride absorption (57–59). However, the reduction did not seem to be sufficient to avoid parenteral nutrition in patients who required it (59). With the availability of long-acting octreotide (Sandostatin LAR), it is now possible to give octreotide as a single monthly dose of between 5 and 10 mg.

Growth Hormone

In an uncontrolled study, a combination of growth hormone, oral glutamine, and a high-carbohydrate, low-fat diet allowed 57% of patients previously receiving HPN to stop this therapy (60); However, this finding was not confirmed by two randomized controlled trials (61, 62), but it was supported by a third trial using low-dose growth hormone (63).

Glucagonlike Peptide-2

In eight patients with short bowel syndrome and an end jejunostomy who had very low levels of GLP-2, the twice-daily administration of 400 µg of GLP-2 improved energy absorption, reduced stool weight, and increased body weight (64). This hormone is rapidly hydrolyzed after injection by dipeptidyl peptidase, and an analog with alanine substituted by glycine resistant to this hydrolysis is now available. Clinical trials are now in progress to determine whether this analog can significantly improve absorption and nutrition in patients with short bowel syndrome.

REFERENCES

1. Malagelada J-R. Gastric, pancreatic and biliary response to a meal. In: Johnson JR, ed. Physiology of the Gastrointestinal Tract. New York: Raven Press, 1981.
2. Nylander G. Acta Chir Scand 1967;133:131–8.
3. Reynell PC, Spray GH. Gastroenterology 1956;31:361–8.
4. Woolf GM, Miller C, Kurian R et al. Gastroenterology 1983;84:823–8.
5. Summers RW, Kent TH, Osborne JW. Gastroenterology 1970;59:731–9.
6. Ricotta J, Zuidema GD, Gadacz TR et al. Surg Gynecol Obstet 1981;152:310–4.
7. Fordtran JS, Locklear TW. Am J Dig Dis 1966;11:503–21.
8. Powell DW. Intestinal water and electrolyte transport. In: Johnson LR, ed. Physiology of the Gastrointestinal Tract. 2nd ed. New York: Raven Press, 1987.
9. Binder HJ, Mehta P. Gastroenterology 1989;96:989–96.
10. Royall D, Wolever TMS, Jeejeebhoy KN. Am J Gastroenterol 1990;85:1307–12.
11. Cummings JH, James WPT, Wiggins HS. Lancet 1973;1:344–7.
12. Booth CC, Aldis D, Read AE. Gut 1961;2:168–74.
13. Hoffman AF, Poley JR. Gastroenterology 1972;62:918–34.
14. Hylander E, Ladefoged K, Jarnum S. Scand J Gastroenterol 1980;15:853–8.
15. Ladefoged K, Nicolaidou P, Jarnum S. Am J Clin Nutr 1980;33:2137–44.
16. Woolf GM, Miller C, Kurian R et al. Dig Dis Sci 1987;32:8–15.
17. Haymond HE. Surg Gynecol Obstet 1953;61:693–705.
18. Flint JM. Johns Hopkins Med J 1912;23:127–44.
19. Althausen TL, Doig RK, Uyeyama K et al. Gastroenterology 1950;16:126–39.
20. Lo CW, Walker WA. Nutr Rev 1989;47:193–8.
21. Goldstein RM, Hebiguchi T, Luk G et al. J Pediatr Surg 1985;20:785–91.
22. Shulman RJ. Gastroenterology 1988;95:85–92.
23. Gall DG, Chung M, O'Laughlin EV et al. Biol Neonate 1987;51:286–96.
24. Morgan W, Yardley J, Luk G et al, Dudgeon D. Pediatr Surg 1987;22:541–5.
25. Purandare S, Offenbartl K, Westrom B et al. Scand J Gastroenterol 1989;24:678–82.
26. Fong YM, Marano MA, Barber A et al. Ann Surg 1989;210:449–56.
27. Jeejeebhoy KN. Am J Clin Nutr 2001;74:160–3.
28. Weser E, Babbitt J, Vandeventer A. Dig Dis Sci 1985;30:675–81.
29. Levine GM. Gastroenterology 1986;91:49–55.
30. Weser E, Babbit J, Vandeventer A. Gastroenterology 1986;91:521–7.
31. Koruda MJ, Rolandelli RH, Bliss DZ et al. Am J Clin Nutr 1990;51:685–9.
32. Grant JP, Snyder PJ. J Surg Res 1988;44:506–13.
33. Drucker DJ. Gut 2002;50:428–35.
34. Hughes CA, Prince A, Dowling RH. Clin Sci 1980;59:329–36.
35. Greenberg GR, Wolman SL, Cristofides ND et al. Gastroenterology 1981;80:988–93.
36. Guedon C, Schmitz J, Lerebours E et al. Gastroenterology 1986;90:373–8.
37. Ziegler TR, Evans ME, Fernandez-Estývariz C et al. Annu Rev Nutr 2003;23:229–61.
38. Cortot A, Fleming CR, Malagelada JR. N Engl J Med 1979;300:79–80.
39. Tang S-J, Jose M, Nieto JM et al. J Clin Gastroenterol 2002;34:62–3.
40. Nightingale JMD, Lennard-Jones JE, Walker ER et al. Lancet 1990;336:765–8.
41. Nordgaard I, Hansen BS, Mortensen PB. Lancet 1994;343:373–6.
42. McIntyre PB, Fitchew M, Lennard-Jones JE. Gastroenterology 1986;91:25–33.
43. Ovesen L, Chu R, Howard L. Am J Clin Nutr 1983;38:823–8.
44. Woolf GM, Miller C, Kurian R et al. Dig Dis Sci 1987;32:8–15.
45. Wolman SL, Anderson GH, Marliss EB et al. Gastroenterology 1979;76:458–67.
46. Murphy JP Jr, King DR, Dubois A. N Engl J Med 1979;300:80–1.
47. Tang SJ, Nieto JM, Jensen DM et al. J Clin Gastroenterol 2002;34:62–3.
48. Farkkila MA. Surgery 1988;104:18–25.
49. Pitt HA, King W 3rd, Mann LL et al. Am J Surg 1983;145:106–12.
50. Pitt HA, Lewinski MA, Muller EL et al. Surgery 1984;96:154–62.
51. Dobbins JW, Binder HJ. N Engl J Med 1977;296:298–301.
52. Chadwick VS, Gaginella TS, Carlson GL et al. J Lab Clin Med 1979;94:661–74.
53. Pak CYC, Peterson R, Sakhaee K et al. Am J Med 1985;79:284–8.
54. Traube M, Bock JL, Boyer JL. Ann Intern Med 1983;98:171–3.
55. Satoh T, Narisawa K, Konno T et al. Eur J Pediatr 1982;138:324–6.
56. Ramakrishnan T, Stokes P. JPEN J Parenter Enteral Nutr 1985;9:361–3.
57. Dharmsathaphorn K, Gorelick FS, Sherwin RS et al. J Clin Gastroenterol 1982;4:521–4.
58. Ladefoged K, Christensen KC, Hegnhoj J et al. Gut 1989;30:943–9.
59. O'Keefe SJD, Peterson ME, Fleming R. JPEN J Parenter Enteral Nutr 1994;18:26–34.
60. Byrne TA, Persinger RL, Young LS et al. JPEN J Parenter Enteral Nutr 1995;222:243–55.
61. Scolapio JS, Camilleri M, Fleming CR et al. Gastroenterology 1997;113:1074–81.
62. Jeppesen PB, Szkudlarek J, Hoy CE et al. Scand J Gastroenterol 2001;36:48–54.
63. Seguy D, Vahedi K, Kapel N et al. Gastroenterology 2003;124:293–302.
64. Jeppesen PB, Hartmann B, Thulesen J et al. Gastroenterology 2001;120:806–15.

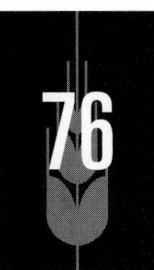

INFLAMMATORY BOWEL DISEASE¹

ANNE M. GRIFFITHS

DIET AND THE PATHOGENESIS
    OF INFLAMMATORY BOWEL DISEASE 1209
        Pathogenesis of Inflammatory Bowel
            Disease: Current Concepts 1209
        The Role of Diet 1210
INTESTINAL EFFECTS OF INFLAMMATORY
    BOWEL DISEASE 1210
        Fat Absorption 1210
        Enteric Losses 1211
        Digestion and Absorption of Specific Nutrients . .1211
        Drug-Nutrient Interactions 1211
NUTRITIONAL CONSEQUENCES
    OF INFLAMMATORY BOWEL DISEASE 1211
        Malnutrition 1211
        Growth Impairment 1212
        Specific Nutrient Deficiencies 1213
NUTRITION IN THE MANAGEMENT
    OF INFLAMMATORY BOWEL DISEASE 1213
        General Dietary Measures 1214
INTENSIVE NUTRITIONAL SUPPORT
    IN INFLAMMATORY BOWEL DISEASE 1214
        Adjunctive Nutritional Therapy 1214
        Primary Nutritional Therapy of Active Disease . . .1215
        Long-Term Nutritional Support 1216

Inflammatory bowel disease (IBD) encompasses at least two forms of chronic intestinal inflammation: Crohn's disease (CD) and ulcerative colitis (UC) (1). The two conditions are currently defined empirically on the basis of clinical, radiologic, endoscopic, and histologic features. Debate continues regarding whether these two major forms of IBD represent different manifestations of the same disease or distinct disorders with some pathogenetic and clinical similarities. The latter contention is favored by genetic and immunologic data. The natural history of IBD is variable. The observed spectrum of disease severity and nutritional impact is wide, in part related to the site, nature, and extent of intestinal involvement.

---

¹**Abbreviations: CD,** Crohn's disease; **ECCDS,** European Collaborative Crohn's Disease Study; **IBD,** inflammatory bowel disease; **IGF-I,** insulin growth factor-I; **PUFA,** polyunsaturated fatty acid; **REE,** resting energy expenditure; **TPN,** total parenteral nutrition; **UC,** ulcerative colitis.

CD is a panenteric transmural inflammatory process with focal microscopic inflammation identifiable throughout the gastrointestinal tract. The anatomic distribution of macroscopic disease varies, but includes the terminal ileum more frequently than any other site. Initial patterns of localization include terminal ileal disease only (25–35% of patients), involvement of the terminal ileum and colon (35–45%), isolated colonic disease (15–25%), and, least commonly, proximal or diffuse small intestinal inflammation (5–10%). After intestinal resection, CD almost invariably recrudesces in a new site, most commonly proximal to the anastomosis. Wherever it occurs, macroscopic disease is characteristically segmental with spared areas (skip lesions).

The inflammation in UC is confined to the colonic mucosa, and hence is curable by colectomy. Inflammation universally includes the rectum, but extends proximally to varying degrees in a continuous fashion. Patients are typically classified as having proctitis, rectosigmoiditis, left-sided colitis, or extensive or pancolitis, depending on the length of diseased colon.

Many nutritional issues are important in the care of patients with IBD. Many patients think that their problem is caused by or requires a special diet. This chapter reviews the question of the role of diet in the pathogenesis of IBD, discusses the problems of malnutrition and specific nutritional deficiencies and their management, and examines the use of nutritional therapies in the primary modulation of intestinal inflammation. Separate consideration of CD and UC is warranted because of differences both in the impact of disease on nutritional state and in the responsiveness of acute disease to nutritional therapies.

DIET AND THE PATHOGENESIS OF INFLAMMATORY BOWEL DISEASE

Pathogenesis of Inflammatory Bowel Disease: Current Concepts

The increased concordance for IBD, particularly CD, in monozygotic versus dizygotic twins has provided strong evidence that genetic factors are important in its pathogenesis. The landmark identification of NOD2/CARD15 as a CD susceptibility gene represented the first time a gene in any complex disorder had been first localized through linkage studies in families with multiple affected members (2) and then positionally cloned (3). NOD2/CARD15 encodes an intracellular receptor involved in the innate immune system that regulates the immediate response to microbial pathogens (4). Hence, the recognition of NOD2/CARD15 polymorphisms in roughly one third of patients with both familial and sporadic CD (3) clearly links genetic susceptibility and enteric bacteria, two factors long hypothesized as important in the etiopathogenesis of IBD (1).

As expected for a complex genetic trait, however, NOD2/CARD15 polymorphisms are neither necessary nor sufficient for CD to develop, and are not involved in susceptibility to UC. Several other loci are recognized to contain genes determining IBD susceptibility and influencing its phenotypic expression (5). Moreover, environmental factors clearly play a role, as evidenced by the incomplete concordance in monozygotic twins, the increasing incidence of CD in recent decades, and the changing incidence of IBD in migrant populations (e.g., increased UC in Asian persons after emigration to England) (6).

The fundamental question regarding the pathogenesis of IBD has been framed as follows: Does the chronic, recurring inflammatory activity reflect an appropriate response to a persistently abnormal stimulus (e.g., a persistent causative agent in the intestinal lumen) or an abnormally prolonged response to a normal stimulus (i.e., aberrant regulation of the immune response) (1)? Although the search for a specific pathogen, in CD particularly, continues, the most widely accepted working hypothesis is that IBD represents a dysregulated immune response to intraluminal antigens, conceivably dietary, but more likely common enteric bacteria (1). An enormous antigenic load is regularly presented through the lumen of the gastrointestinal tract, but regulatory mechanisms normally prevent the immune and inflammatory responses from proceeding to cause tissue injury. The intestinal inflammation of IBD may be viewed as an exaggeration of the physiologic inflammatory response always present in the normal lamina propria of the intestine and colon. Predisposing genes such as NOD2/CARD15 and its mutant protein must interact with exogenous or endogenous triggers and modifying factors to result in a chronic inflammatory process in which tissue injury is mediated by the immune system (1).

The Role of Diet

No specific dietary toxin or antigen has been determined. The rarity of IBD has limited traditional epidemiologic methods of determining causation to case control studies, which have failed to provide a meaningful lead to the pathogenesis of CD and UC. Persson and colleagues reviewed studies examining the reported preillness intake of refined sugar, cereals, fiber, and milk products in patients with CD or UC compared with controls (7). An increased intake of refined sugar before the development of symptomatic CD has been fairly consistently reported, suggesting perhaps a modulating role, but the methodologic weaknesses of the study design must be recognized (7). The association may represent a behavioral adaptation to rather than a cause of disease. Many IBD patients have circulating antibodies to milk protein, but it is likely that this is also a secondary phenomenon; the inflamed intestine is abnormally permeable, permitting entry of intact dietary proteins, to which an appropriate immune response is then mounted (8).

Nutritional factors modulating the risk of IBD development have been examined. Breast-fed infants may have a reduced risk of developing CD (6). Although not truly dietary, a clear dichotomy between UC and CD is indicated by the opposing effect of cigarette smoking on the two disorders (6). Smoking decreases and cessation of smoking increases the risk of developing UC, whereas smokers are at an increased risk of developing CD. Some investigators suggest that smoking may be a determinant of the type of IBD that develops in predisposed subjects. Finally, in a correlation study from Japan, the increasing incidence of CD in the racially homogeneous population was shown to parallel increasing daily intake of animal protein, total fat, and animal fat, especially n-6 polyunsaturated fatty acids (PUFAs) relative to n-3 PUFAs (9). These trends indicating Westernization of the diet in Japan were determined from sequential population surveys of dietary habits. n-3 PUFAs found in marine oils have an antiinflammatory effect through modulation of proinflammatory cytokine synthesis (10). One placebo-controlled study using enteric-coated fish oil capsules designed for ileal release showed a substantial reduction in clinical relapse rate among patients with CD in clinical remission, with persistence of elevated erythrocyte sedimentation rate (11), but these observations have not been replicated. Prior studies with pharmacologic amounts of eicosapentanoic acid, but without a coating to facilitate release in the distal intestine, showed no or minimal clinical benefit in UC and CD.

INTESTINAL EFFECTS OF INFLAMMATORY BOWEL DISEASE

The impact of IBD on the gastrointestinal tract and on its digestive and absorptive functions varies depending on the site(s), nature, and extent of intestinal inflammation.

Fat Absorption

Digestion and absorption of fat are unaffected by UC. In CD involving the ileum, the processes of fat digestion and absorption may be altered either by loss of gut surface area because of inflammation or by depletion of the circulating bile salt pool because of bile acid malabsorption in the diseased ileum or deconjugation by bacteria. However, studies in 1973 and 1986 confirmed that significant impairment of fat absorption occurs only when the extent of inflammatory involvement is massive, when the absorptive surface has been reduced by extensive small intestinal resection, or conceivably when there is bacterial overgrowth secondary to luminal stenosis and incomplete bowel obstruction (12, 13). Fillipson and colleagues studied fecal excretion in CD patients before intestinal resection and found predominantly mild steatorrhea in 24% of patients with ileal disease, 26% of those with ileocolonic involvement, and 17% of those with Crohn colitis. After resection of the ileum and ileocecal valve, fecal fat excretion was elevated in 48% of patients (12). The frequency and severity of steatorrhea correlated with the extent of the ileal resection, and was infrequent and mild with resections of less than 30 cm.

Enteric Losses

More prevalent and significant than fat malabsorption is enteric leakage of protein, blood, minerals, electrolytes, and trace elements from the bowel during periods of active inflammation in both UC and CD. Patients with CD, even when clinically asymptomatic, frequently have laboratory evidence of protein-losing enteropathy and consequent hypoalbuminemia (14).

Digestion and Absorption of Specific Nutrients

Specific digestive or absorptive defects may occur in CD, but these also are not universal (12, 13). Vitamin B_{12} malabsorption is the most common because its site of absorption corresponds to the area most often inflamed. The prevalence of vitamin B_{12} malabsorption correlates with the extent of distal ileal disease, and following surgery, with the length of distal ileum resected. Vitamin B_{12} malabsorption has been reported in 21% of patients with less than 30 cm of terminal ileum involved, in 48% of those with 30 to 60 cm affected, and in 71% of patients with 60 to 90 cm resected (12). Other digestive or absorptive defects are uncommon, presumably reflecting the reserve of the gut and the large surface area that is usually relatively uninflamed. Lactase deficiency and lactose intolerance may coexist with IBD but are in general no more common that would be expected in an age- and ethnically matched control population (15).

Drug-Nutrient Interactions

Certain drugs used in the management of IBD contribute to selected nutrient malabsorption. For example, sulfasalazine reduces folate absorption. Although supplementation to prevent overt deficiency does not seem routinely necessary, there may be a benefit to folic acid administration in modifying the dysplasia risk associated with longstanding UC (16). Calcium metabolism is disturbed by corticosteroid treatment, which causes decreased absorption and increased urinary excretion.

NUTRITIONAL CONSEQUENCES OF INFLAMMATORY BOWEL DISEASE

Malnutrition

Weight loss and emaciation are the most prevalent nutritional disturbances in IBD (17, 18). Twenty to 75% of adult patients experience weight loss with exacerbations, the incidence and magnitude of the loss varying with disease severity. At the time of first diagnosis, approximately 85% of pediatric patients with CD and 65% of pediatric patients with UC have lost weight.

Etiology of Malnutrition

As summarized in Table 76.1, multiple factors contribute to malnutrition. However, reduced intake rather than excessive loss or increased need is the major cause of the weight loss. Abdominal cramps and diarrhea are aggravated by eating, hence the patient consumes less. Disease-related anorexia may be profound; cytokines produced by the inflamed bowel are likely responsible. Tumor necrosis factor-α produced by inflammatory cells has been shown to produce anorexia in rats with experimental colitis (19).

Intestinal malabsorption may be a factor leading to energy imbalance, but is seldom the major cause, as discussed above. Increased energy expenditure associated with active inflammation has been suggested as a further mechanism accounting for the frequency of malnutrition. In general, resting energy expenditure (REE) does not differ from normal in patients with inactive disease but can exceed predicted rates in the presence of fever and sepsis (20). Furthermore, in comparison with comparably malnourished patients with anorexia nervosa, a lack of compensatory reduction in REE has been described (21). Reduction in REE is a normal biologic response for conserving energy. Production of inflammatory mediators

TABLE 76.1. ETIOLOGIC FACTORS CAUSING MALNUTRITION IN INFLAMMATORY BOWEL DISEASE

Decreased nutrient intake
  Disease-related anorexia
  Iatrogenic factors (unjustified dietary restrictions)
Malabsorption
  Diminished absorptive surface (disease, fistulae, resection)
  Bacterial overgrowth
  Bile salt deficiency
Increased gut losses
  Protein-losing enteropathy
  Electrolytes, minerals, trace metals (diarrhea and fistulae)
  Bleeding
Increased requirements
  Sepsis, fever
  Increased cell turnover

may explain the lack of REE adaptation in patients with CD and may further augment the ongoing malnutrition.

Growth Impairment

Inflammatory disease occurring during early adolescence is likely to have a major impact on nutritional status and growth because of the very rapid accumulation of lean body mass that normally occurs at this time. Further, boys are more vulnerable to disturbances in growth than are girls because their growth spurt comes at a later stage of normal pubertal development and is ultimately longer and greater. Growth impairment is much less common in UC than in CD, at least in part because the more subtle intestinal symptoms in CD often go unrecognized and the inflammatory disease therefore goes untreated for longer periods of time.

Prevalence of Growth Impairment in Crohn's Disease

Several studies published within the past decade have characterized the growth of children with CD treated in the 1980s and into the 1990s (22–27). These studies are important as a benchmark of outcomes with traditional therapy. It is to be hoped that our improved understanding of the pathogenesis of growth impairment together with the greater efficacy of immunomodulatory and emerging biologic therapies in treating intestinal inflammation may lead to enhanced growth of young patients diagnosed in the current decade.

Height velocity is the most sensitive parameter by which to recognize impaired growth. As summarized in Table 76.2, the percentage of patients with CD whose growth is affected varies with the definition of growth impairment and with the nature of the population under study (tertiary referral center versus population-based) (22–27). It has nevertheless been consistently observed that impairment of linear growth is common before diagnosis of CD as well as during the subsequent years, and that final adult height has often been compromised

(22–27). In contrast, linear growth is seldom impaired at the time of diagnosis of UC; even in follow-up, linear growth is usually maintained unless long-term daily corticosteroid therapy is inappropriately used.

In caring for children with IBD, it is important to obtain preillness height measurements so that the impact of the chronic intestinal inflammation can be fully appreciated. The greater the height deficit at diagnosis, the greater is the need for catch-up growth.

Pathophysiology of Growth Impairment

As summarized in Table 76.3, several interrelated factors contribute to growth impairment in children with CD. Chronic undernutrition has long been implicated and remains an important and remediable cause of growth retardation (28). However, a simple nutritional hypothesis fails to explain all of the observations related to growth patterns among children with IBD. Within the past decade, the direct growth-inhibiting effects of proinflammatory cytokines released from the inflamed intestine increasingly have been recognized and are now the focus of very intriguing research (29, 30).

Insulinlike growth factor-I (IGF-I), produced by the liver in response to growth hormone stimulation, normally mediates growth hormone effects on the growth plate of bones. An association between impaired growth in CD and low IGF-I levels is well recognized (31). Malnutrition, cytokines, and chronic daily corticosteroid therapy may all suppress IGF-I production. The relative contributions of malnutrition and inflammation to linear growth delay have been explored recently by Ballinger and colleagues using a rat model of trinitrobenzesulfonic acid colitis (29). Two control groups were used: healthy free-feeding controls with free access to food, and a pair-fed group composed of healthy animals with daily food intake restricted to match that of colitic rats (29). Plasma IGF-I concentrations reflected linear growth. In the colitic rats, IGF-I levels were reduced to 35% of control values. Comparison with the healthy but undernourished pair-fed rats suggested

TABLE 76.2. PREVALENCE OF LINEAR GROWTH IMPAIRMENT IN PEDIATRIC CROHN'S DISEASE

STUDY (REFERENCE)	TIME OF ASSESSMENT	PATIENTS STUDIED	DEFINITION OF LINEAR GROWTH IMPAIRMENT	PERCENTAGE WITH GROWTH IMPAIRMENT
Kanof et al. (27)	At diagnosis	Prepubertal (Tanner I or II) patients (n = 50)	Decrease in height velocity	88
Kirschner (22)	At diagnosis	—	Decrease in height percentile >1 SD	36
Griffiths et al. (23)	During follow-up	Prepubertal (Tanner I or II) patients (n = 100)	Height velocity ≤2 SD for age for ≥2 years	49
Hildebrand et al. (24)	Before diagnosis or during follow-up	Population-based cohort of 46 children	Height velocity ≤2 SD for age for 1 year	65
Markowitz et al. (25)	At maturity	38 children in tertiary care setting	Failure to reach predicted adult height	37

SD, standard deviations.

TABLE 76.3. FACTORS CONTRIBUTING TO GROWTH ABNORMALITIES IN CHILDREN WITH CROHN'S DISEASE

FACTOR	REASON
Suboptimal intake	Fear of worsening gastrointestinal symptoms, anorexia
Stool losses	Mucosal damage or resection leading to protein-losing enteropathy, steatorrhea
Increased nutritional needs	Fever, chronic deficits
Corticosteroid treatment	Inhibition of insulinlike growth factor-I
Disease activity	Direct role of circulating inflammatory cytokines in linear growth inhibition

TABLE 76.4. RELATIVE FREQUENCIES OF SUBOPTIMAL MICRONUTRIENT LEVELS IN INFLAMMATORY BOWEL DISEASE[a]

	CROHN'S DISEASE	ULCERATIVE COLITIS
Vitamin B$_{12}$	++	−
Iron	++	+++
Folate	+++	++
Magnesium	+	−
Vitamin D	++	−
Vitamin E	+	+
Vitamin A	+	+
β-Carotene	+	+
Vitamin K	+	−
Vitamin C	+	+
Zinc	++	++
Copper	+	
Selenium	+	+

[a]Clinical manifestations are uncommon except with iron and folate.

From Gassull MA, Stange E. Nutrition and diet in inflammatory bowel disease. In: Satsangi J, Sutherland LR, eds. Inflammatory Bowel Diseases. London: Churchill Livingstone, 2003:461–74, with permission.

that malnutrition accounted for 53% of the total depression of IGF-I in colitic rats, with the remaining 47% attributable to inflammation (29). These results support earlier data from interleukin-6 transgenic mice that also showed cytokine-mediated reduction in IGF-I production by the liver, demonstrating a mechanism by which chronic inflammation leads to stunting directly and separately from undernutrition (30).

From the foregoing discussion, it is clear that enhancement of linear growth is best achieved through both control of intestinal inflammation (but without chronic corticosteroid therapy) and assurance of adequate nutrition (32).

Specific Nutrient Deficiencies

As with protein-calorie malnutrition, deficiencies of vitamins, minerals, and trace elements may result from either inadequate intake or increased losses. The majority of studies of micronutrition have focused on adults; reported frequencies pertain predominantly to CD (33). Observations based on small numbers of patients may not be generalizable. It is difficult to obtain an accurate and meaningful representation of the prevalence of specific deficiencies, but an appreciation of their relative frequencies, as summarized in Table 76.4, is useful.

Water-Soluble Vitamins

Of the water-soluble vitamins, folic acid and vitamin B$_{12}$ deficiencies are relatively commonly encountered; others are extremely rare.

Fat-Soluble Vitamins

Vitamin D deficiency is the most commonly reported fat-soluble vitamin deficiency (34). However, although osteomalacia may be encountered in CD, especially after ileal resection, a more prevalent problem seems to be osteopenia and osteoporosis related to a direct effect of inflammatory disease on bone deposition (35).

Minerals and Trace Elements

Iron deficiency is common, and is related to gut losses and inadequate intake (36). The ability to absorb iron is usually preserved. A low serum ferritin level is the most reliable indicator of reduced iron stores. Anemia in IBD is frequently caused by the chronic disease impact rather than iron deficiency. Of other minerals and trace elements, zinc has received considerable attention (37). As discussed in Chapter 13, low intake and diarrheal losses put patients at risk of zinc depletion. Nevertheless, the true frequency of deficiency and its role in growth retardation are highly controversial because of inaccuracies in the measurement of total body zinc. Low serum levels of zinc reflect more the degree of hypoproteinemia than the depletion of body stores. Avoidance of milk products and the effects of corticosteroids on calcium absorption and excretion predispose to calcium deficiency; documented hypocalcemia, however, is usually caused by hypoalbuminemia.

NUTRITION IN THE MANAGEMENT OF INFLAMMATORY BOWEL DISEASE

Nutritional support is a vital component of the management of patients with IBD. The macronutrient deficiency that is frequently encountered can lead to alterations in cellular immunity with an increased risk of infection, prolonged cellular renewal of inflamed tissues and delayed wound healing, diminished skeletal muscle function, and, in children, growth retardation. Undernutrition and its associated complications may therefore become as debilitating as the underlying IBD. Management goals must include correction and prevention of nutritional deficits as well as control of symptoms. Nutritional assessment techniques are discussed in Chapters 49 to 54. Table 76.5 correlates with the above discussion of nutritional problems encountered in

TABLE 76.5. RECOMMENDED NUTRITIONAL ASSESSMENT OF PATIENTS WITH INFLAMMATORY BOWEL DISEASE

Subject assessment
  Detailed history
  Complete physical examination, pubertal staging[a]
  Diet evaluation (3-day diary)
Anthropometry
  Height, weight
  Growth velocity[a]
  Height for age percent,[a] weight for height percent
  Midarm circumference
  Triceps skinfold thickness
Laboratory data
  Complete blood count, red-cell morphology
  Serum albumin level
  Folic acid and vitamin B_{12} levels
  Serum iron level, total iron-binding capacity, ferritin level
  Calcium, magnesium, alkaline phosphatase levels
  Bone age[a]
Additional tests if growth failure or significant malnutrition
  is present
  Vitamin A, D, and E levels
  Prothrombin time, partial prothrombin time
  Zinc level
  Phosphorus level

[a]In pediatric populations.

IBD and summarizes the evaluation that should be considered the essential minimum for patient care.

General Dietary Measures

For the majority of ambulatory patients, the most important advice is to consume a diet liberal in protein and with calories sufficient to maintain or restore weight, or to support growth in children and adolescents. Consumption of 35 to 40 kcal/kg ideal body weight per day and 1 to 1.5 g/kg ideal body weight of protein per day will meet the protein and energy requirements of most adult patients with active IBD. For children, recommendations should be made according to height, age, and need for catch-up growth. Liquid dietary supplements may help motivated patients to achieve these goals, although in young patients these will often simply displace ingested calories from regular food without increasing total caloric intake (38).

The merits and necessity of dietary restrictions need to be critically examined. Controlled studies have not supported a role for a low-residue diet, nor for a high-fiber, low-refined-sugar diet in the maintenance of remission in IBD (39, 40). One group of investigators has suggested that the exclusion of specific foods on the basis of individual clinical intolerance improves the short-term clinical course of CD (41). A major problem with dietary modifications, however, is that they frequently result in a less appetizing diet, which discourages optimal caloric intake. Imposition of dietary restrictions can result in a major source of conflict between children with IBD and their parents. Except in specific circumstances (e.g., a low-residue diet to reduce obstructive symptoms in the setting

of small intestinal stricture), a full diet for age is most appropriate.

INTENSIVE NUTRITIONAL SUPPORT IN INFLAMMATORY BOWEL DISEASE

There are three broad indications for undertaking intensive nutritional support in patients with IBD. The first indication is as adjunctive therapy to correct or avoid malnutrition and in children to facilitate growth. The second is as primary therapy of active intestinal inflammation in CD, but not in UC. The third includes the small proportion of CD patients who may require long-term nutritional support because of extensive intestinal resections and consequent short bowel syndrome. Nutritional therapy in these contexts may be provided by enteral nutrition using formulated food or via parenteral nutrition using a centrally placed intravenous catheter. Enteral nutrition has come to constitute the preferred and more frequent approach by virtue of its lower complication rates and its easier and less costly administration. Circumstances favoring long-term total parenteral nutrition (TPN) are limited to the patient with a very short gut.

Adjunctive Nutritional Therapy

Adjunct to Drug Treatment

Intensive nutritional support improves the nutritional status of the anorectic or malnourished patient with CD or UC. In the setting of acute severe colitis, provision of TPN prevents further decline of body protein and improves respiratory and peripheral muscle function (42). Postoperative respiratory complications were reduced among patients who ultimately require colectomy (42). These data argue for the early use of parenteral nutrition in conjunction with pharmacologic therapy, but do not justify delaying colectomy to improve the nutritional state in the malnourished patient with fulminant disease in whom medical therapy is clearly failing.

Preoperative Nutritional Support

Adjunctive nutritional therapy has frequently been advocated before planned surgery in CD and UC to decrease postoperative morbidity. The rationale is based on observations that protein-calorie malnutrition impairs wound healing and diminishes immunocompetence, thereby increasing the risk of infection. Collins and colleagues found that provision of calories with amino acids resulted in a lower complication rate postoperatively than the provision of either amino acids alone or standard intravenous solutions (43). Clinically important benefits are observed only among patients with severe malnutrition (44).

Nutritional Treatment of Growth Impairment

When chronic nutritional insufficiency was recognized to be a significant factor in growth delay associated with CD, several reports documented restoration of growth after consistent provision of adequate nutrition either enterally or parenterally (17, 28, 45–47). The most commonly used approach involves nocturnal nasogastric infusion of formulated food (45–47). Such intensive nutritional support rather than simple dietary counseling to increase caloric intake is required when growth is retarded (17). The success of supplementary enteral nutrition in many young patients with poor weight gain and impaired linear growth cannot be denied. Unfortunately, others with persistent chronically active inflammatory disease have remained stunted despite provision of adequate calories, providing clinical evidence of the direct role of chronic inflammation in linear growth inhibition. The timely use of effective immunomodulatory drugs and the availability of more efficacious biologic therapies promise to improve the clinical course and ultimate stature attained by this subset of children with previously refractory CD.

Primary Nutritional Therapy of Active Disease

Enteral Nutrition in Crohn's Disease

Liquid diet therapy is an effective alternative to pharmacologic therapy of active CD. Although not popular as primary therapy in North America, enteral nutrition is regarded as first-line therapy for pediatric patients in centers in the United Kingdom (31) and is commonly used in other parts of Europe and Canada.

Evidence-Based Therapeutic Indications: Active Disease. The potential role of exclusive enteral nutrition as primary therapy of active CD was discovered fortuitously. Patients given elemental formulas preoperatively experienced an improvement not only in their nutritional status as intended, but also in the inflammatory activity of their disease (48). These observations of primary therapeutic efficacy were first confirmed in the small controlled trial conducted by O'Morain and colleagues (49). Adult patients achieved clinical remission by drinking an elemental (amino-acid–based) formula as often as with conventional corticosteroids (49). However, in the subsequent and much larger European Collaborative Crohn's Disease Study (ECCDS), randomized trials of enteral nutrition versus corticosteroid and sulfasalazine therapy, the drug therapy proved superior to semielemental formulas containing oligopeptides as the protein source (50, 51).

The controversy surrounding seemingly divergent outcomes has fueled several metaanalyses, each of which has concluded that there is a treatment benefit to corticosteroids in comparison with enteral nutrition (52–54). Analyzing results of eight trials on an intention-to-treat basis, the pooled odds ratio for the likelihood of clinical remission with liquid diet therapy versus corticosteroids is 0.35 (95% confidence intervals, 0.23-0.53) (52). Furthermore, poor compliance, although contributory, does not constitute the major explanation for the lower response rates to enteral nutrition, as is evident from secondary metaanalysis excluding dropouts for apparent intolerance (52).

No controlled trials of enteral nutrition versus placebo or less effective drugs in active CD have been conducted. However, comparison of observed response rates to exclusive liquid diet therapy (53–82%) with usual placebo response rates (18–42%) in the controlled clinical trial setting suggests that enteral nutrition is of therapeutic benefit, when tolerated, even if efficacy does not equal that of corticosteroid treatment (52–54). Moreover, a reduction in gastrointestinal protein loss, a decrease in intestinal permeability, and a reduction in fecal excretion of indium-labeled leucocytes have each been shown, suggesting a direct effect on intestinal inflammation (55). Open trials in children have documented endoscopic healing and decreased mucosal cytokine production after exclusive enteral nutrition (56), which are intriguing observations, particularly in contrast with the common lack of mucosal healing despite an apparent clinical response to corticosteroid therapy.

Factors Influencing Efficacy: Anatomic Localization of Inflammation. The results of the ECCDS did not confirm a relationship between the sites of intestinal inflammation and the outcome, but the numbers of patients with isolated colonic disease were small even in these trials (50, 51). The lack of site-specific data concerning rates of induction of clinical remission in other trials precludes prospective appraisal of the relationship between anatomic localization of CD and responsiveness to exclusive enteral nutrition. Anecdotes often suggest that Crohn colitis is less amenable to treatment with enteral nutrition, but in a comparative trial of two liquid diets, two thirds of patients had disease confined to the colon, and excellent clinical response rates of 67 and 73% to elemental and polymeric formulas, respectively, were nevertheless observed (57).

Formula Composition. Both decreased antigenicity related to the use of amino-acid–based formulas and low total fat content and/or low ratio of n-6 to n-3 PUFAs have been hypothesized to facilitate reduction of intestinal inflammation. To test these theories, several clinical trials have compared the efficacy of elemental versus nonelemental formulas of varying protein and fat composition. Existing data combined in metaanalysis do not support an advantage to elemental (amino-acid–based) feedings compared with more palatable polymeric formulations (52, 58). The importance of fat composition to efficacy is less clear, but the treatment benefit, if any, achieved by reduction in the content of total fat or n-6 PUFAs is small (58).

Bowel Rest. When used in the treatment of active CD, enteral nutrition is generally combined with avoidance of oral intake. The necessity, however, of complete avoidance of other food is challenged by the results of a randomized controlled trial of adjunctive nutritional support (59). Partial parenteral nutrition plus an ad libitum oral diet proved as effective in inducing clinical remission as either elemental liquid diets administered by nasogastric tube or TPN and complete bowel rest among patients hospitalized because of continuing activity of their disease despite high-dose steroid therapy (59).

Age/Disease Duration. It has been suggested by some that enteral nutrition is more efficacious as primary therapy of active CD in children in comparison with adults (60). Several small trials of enteral nutrition in children were reported to have extremely high success (60), but caution is always required in drawing firm conclusions from very small studies (61). The Canadian Pediatric Collaborative Trial of enteral nutrition versus corticosteroids (62) used an oligopeptide-containing liquid diet very similar in composition to that used among adults in the ECCDS (51). These two trials included 78 children and 107 adults, respectively. It seems likely that the higher remission rate overall with enteral nutrition in the pediatric study (75%) versus the adult study (53%) reflects differences in the nature of the patients randomized rather than an inherent difference in the responsiveness of childhood CD. Pediatric patients were stratified before randomization according to duration of disease (newly diagnosed versus disease in relapse). The subgroup of children with disease in relapse and of longer duration had a rate of clinical response to enteral nutrition very similar to that of adult patients (51, 62). It is possible that recent-onset CD is particularly amenable to healing through the use of enteral nutrition.

If not inherently more efficacious, enteral nutrition did seem to be more feasible among children, who become adept at swallowing Silastic nasogastric feeding catheters. Formula can be infused nocturnally in the home setting and not interfere with normal activities. There is enough evidence of the short-term efficacy of enteral nutrition in active disease to support presentation as an alternate primary treatment for young patients, particularly those with predominantly small intestinal disease, for whom corticosteroids are being considered.

Evidence-Based Therapeutic Indications: Maintenance of Remission. Maintenance of clinical and ideally histologic remission, whether induced pharmacologically, nutritionally, or surgically, is the major challenge of CD management. In most studies of enteral nutrition, 60 to 70% of patients experience a relapse within 12 months of resuming a normal diet (57). Chronic intermittent bowel rest with nocturnal infusion of an elemental diet 1 month out of 4 has been recommended as a means of sustaining remission (47). The beneficial effects on disease activity and growth of such cyclic enteral nutrition were confirmed in a pediatric randomized controlled trial versus alternate-day prednisone (63). During an 18-month period of follow-up, the difference between the percentage of patients remaining in continuous remission with alternate-day prednisone (47%) and with cyclic enteral nutrition (67%) was not statistically significant, but linear growth was significantly better among patients randomized to receive

the nutritional therapy (63). Continuation of nocturnal nasogastric feeding four to five times weekly as a supplement to an unrestricted ad libitum daytime diet was also associated with prolonged disease quiescence and improved growth in a historical cohort study (46). In the long term, allowing normal food at times when family and friends are eating is particularly important in achieving compliance. If long-term therapy either in a cyclic exclusive or a continuous supplementary fashion is contemplated, insertion of a gastrostomy tube may make administration easier (64).

Mechanism of Action. The mode of action of enteral nutrition as primary treatment of active CD remains conjectural (65). Hypotheses, which have been largely discarded, include simply overall nutritional repletion or elimination of dietary antigen uptake. Diminution of intestinal synthesis of inflammatory mediators via reduction of dietary fat remains a possible factor (58), as does alteration in intestinal microbial flora, a possibility that has yet to be explored, but that fits with current understanding of CD pathogenesis (1, 3, 4).

Parenteral Nutrition: Efficacy

Studies of TPN as primary treatment of active CD have been summarized in detail by Greenberg (18). In contrast with studies of enteral nutrition in active disease, there are numerous retrospective reports, but few prospective, randomized, controlled trials of TPN. From retrospective series among CD patients, one can expect an in-hospital remission rate of 64% after 14 to 21 days of treatment, with isolated colonic CD responding less often than disease involving the small intestine alone or the small intestine plus colon (18). Two small prospective-controlled trials suggest that TPN combined with bowel rest is of no primary therapeutic efficacy in the management of patients with acute UC or of those with acute Crohn's colitis, although it will improve their nutritional status (66, 67). Only two randomized studies have compared TPN with exclusive enteral nutrition in the treatment of active disease; remission rates with either modality were comparable (59, 68). No evidence suggests that TPN is superior to enteral nutrition in the treatment of acute inflammation. Indeed, enteral provision of nutrients may optimize the repair of inflamed mucosa. TPN administration in animals kept nil per os is associated with subtotal villous atrophy of the intestine, and this physical alteration of the mucosal barrier has been shown to promote translocation of bacteria normally confined to the gastrointestinal tract (69). Permeability, in contrast, normalizes with enteral nutrition such that access to factors that putatively may perpetuate intestinal inflammation is reduced (55).

Long-Term Nutritional Support

Fortunately, only a few patients with CD have inadequate gastrointestinal reserve for the maintenance of a normal nutritional state on standard oral or enteral diets. Nevertheless, patients with CD are often the largest single group of adults in home TPN programs (70). The usual clinical setting involves persistent active inflammation after multiple small bowel resections. Either the remaining small bowel is incapable of sufficient nutrient absorption to sustain nutritional homeostasis (short bowel syndrome) or resection of the colon and ileum results in substantial losses of isotonic fluid, electrolytes, minerals, and trace elements, but with relatively normal macronutrient absorption (end-jejunostomy syndrome). Both these circumstances may require permanent home parenteral nutrition for the provision of complete nutritional support, or alternatively, to facilitate fluid and electrolyte balance. These situations should become less common with the advent of more effective biologic therapies and with more conservative approaches to surgery, that is, surgery for complications of disease only, limited resections of only the most severely diseased bowel, and use of stricturoplasty to preserve absorptive surface area.

REFERENCES

1. Podolsky DK. N Engl J Med 1991;325:928–35, 1008–14.
2. Hugot J-P, Laurent-Puig P, Gower-Rousseau C et al. Nature 2001;411:599–603.
3. Hugot J-P, Chamaillard M, Zouali H et al. Nature 2001;411:599–603.
4. Philpott DJ, Viala J. Best Pract Res Clin Gastroenterol 2004;18:447–9.
5. Bonen DK, Cho JH. Gastroenterology 2003;124:521–36.
6. Calkins BM, Mendeloff AI. Epidemiol Rev 1986;8:60–91.
7. Persson P-G, Alhbom A, Hellers G. Scand J Gastroenterol 1987;22:385–9.
8. Lochs H, Genser D, Bühner S. Role of nutrition in IBD. In: Tytgat GNJ, Bartelsman JFWM, van Deventer SJH, eds. Inflammatory Bowel Diseases. New York: Kluwer Academic, 1995.
9. Shoda R, Matsueda K, Yamato S et al. Am J Clin Nutr 1996;63:741–5.
10. Blok WL, Katan MB, van der Meer JWM. J Nutr 1996;126:1515–33.
11. Belluzzi A, Brignola C, Campieri M et al. N Engl J Med 1996;334:1557–60.
12. Filipsson S, Hulten L, Lindstedt G. Scand J Gastroenterol 1978;13:529–36.
13. Dyer NH, Dawson AM. Br J Surg 1973;60:134–40.
14. Griffiths AM, Drobnies A, Soldin SJ et al. J Pediatr Gastroenterol Nutr 1986;5:907.
15. Kirschner BS, Defavaro MV, Jensen W. Gastroenterology 1981;81:829–32.
16. Lashner BA et al. Gastroenterology 1997;112:29–32.
17. Seidman E, LeLeiko N, Ament M et al. J Pediatr Gastroenterol Nutr 1991;12:424–38.
18. Greenberg GR. Semin Gastrointest Dis 1993;4:69–86.
19. Murch SH. Inflammatory mediators and suppression of growth in paediatric chronic IBD. In: Tytgat GNJ, Bartelsman JFWM, van Deventer SJH, eds. Inflammatory Bowel Diseases. New York: Kluwer Academic, 1995.
20. Chan ATH, Fleming CR, O'Fallon WM et al. Gastroenterology 1986;91:75–8.
21. Ascue M, Rashid M, Griffiths A et al. Gut 1997;41:203–8.
22. Kirschner BS. Acta Paediatr Scand Suppl 1990;366:98–104.
23. Griffiths AM, Nguyen P, Smith C et al. Gut 1993;34:939–43.
24. Hildebrand H, Karlberg J, Kristiansson B. J Pediatr Gastroenterol Nutr 1994;18:165–73.
25. Markowitz J, Grancher K, Rosa J et al. J Pediatr Gastroenterol Nutr 1993;16:373–80.
26. Motil KJ, Grand RJ, Davis-Kraft L et al. Gastroenterology 1993;105:681–91.
27. Kanof ME, Lake AM, Bayless TM. Gastroenterology 1988;95:1423–7.
28. Kelts DG, Grand RJ, Shen G et al. Gastroenterology 1979;76:720–7.
29. Ballinger A, Azooz O, El-Haj Y et al. Gut 2000;46:1–6.
30. DeBenedetti F, Alonzi T, Moretta A et al. J Clin Invest 1997;99:643–50.
31. Kirschner BS, Sutton MM. Gastroenterology 1986;91:830–6.
32. Walker-Smith JA. Arch Dis Child 1996;75:351–4.
33. Harries AD, Heatley RV. Postgrad Med J 1983;59:690–7.
34. Driscoll RH, Meredith SC, Sitrin M et al. Gastroenterology 1982;83:1252–8.
35. Bjarnson I, Macpherson A, Mackintosh C et al. Gut 1997;40:228–33.
36. Bartels U, Strandberg Pedersen N, Jarnum S. Scand J Gastroenterol 1978;13:649–56.
37. Hendricks KM, Walker WA. Nutr Rev 1988;46:40–6.
38. Harries AD, Danis V, Heatley RV et al. Lancet 1983;1:887–90.
39. Levenstein S, Prantera C, Luzi C et al. Gut 1985;26:989–93.
40. Ritchie JK, Wadsworth J, Lennard-Jones JE et al. BMJ 1987;295:517–20.
41. Riordan AM, Hunter JO, Cowan RE. Lancet 1993;343:1131–4.
42. Christie PM, Hill GL. Gastroenterology 1990;99:730–6.
43. Collins JP, Oxby CB, Hill GL. Lancet 1978;1:788–91.
44. The Veterans Affairs TPN Cooperative Study Group. N Engl J Med 1991;325:525–32.
45. Aiges H, Markowitz J, Rosa J, et al Gastroenterology 1999;97:905–10.
46. Wilschanski M, Sherman P, Pencharz P et al. Gut 1996;38:543–8.
47. Belli DC, Seidman E, Bouthillier L et al. Gastroenterology 1988;94:603–10.
48. Vointk AJ, Echave V, Feller JH et al. Arch Surg 1973;107:329–33.
49. O'Morain C, Segal AW, Levi AJ. BMJ 1984;288:1859–2862.
50. Lochs H, Steinhardt HJ, Klaus-Ventz B et al. Gastroenterology 1991;101:881–8.
51. Malchow H, Steinhardt HJ, Lorenz-Meyer H et al. Scand J Gastroenterol 1990;25:235–44.
52. Griffiths AM, Ohlsson A, Sherman P et al. Gastroenterology 1995;108:1056–67.
53. Fernandez-Banares F, Cabre E, Esteve-Comas M et al. JPEN J Parenter Enteral Nutr 1995;19:356–62.
54. Messori G, Trallori G, D'Albasio G et al. Scand J Gastroenterol 1996;31:267–72.
55. Teahon K, Smethurst P, Pearson M et al. Gastroenterology 1991;101:84–7.
56. Fell JME, Paintin M, Arnoud-Battandier F et al. J Pediatr Gastroenterol Nutr 1997;24:474.
57. Rigaud D, Cosnes J, Le Quintrec Y et al. Gut 1991;32:1492–7.
58. Zachos M, Tondeur M, Griffiths AM. Cochrane Rev 2001;3:1–24.
59. Greenberg GR, Fleming CR, Jeejeebhoy KN et al. Gut 1988;29:1309–15.
60. Heuschkel RB, Menache CC, Megerian JT et al. J Pediatr Gastroenterol Nutr 2000;31:8–15.

61. Griffiths AM. J Pediatr Gastroenterol Nutr 2000;31:3–5.
62. Seidman E, Griffiths AM, Jones A et al. Gastroenterology 1993;104:778A.
63. Seidman E, Jones A, Issenman R et al. J Pediatr Gastroenterol Nutr 1996;23:344.
64. Israel DM, Hassall E. Am J Gastroeterol 1995;90:1084–8.
65. Fernandez-Banares F, Cabre E, Gonzalez-Huix F et al. Gut 1994;35:S55–9.
66. Dickinson RJ, Ashton RM, Axon ATR. Gastroenterology 1980;79:1199–204.
67. McIntyre PB, Powell-Tuck J, Wood SR et al. Gut 1986;27:481–4.
68. Alun Jones V. Dig Dis Sci 1987;32:1009–75.
69. Feldman FJ, Dowling RH, McNaughton J et al. Gastroenterology 1976;5:712–9.
70. Richards DM, Irving MH. Gut 1997;40:218–22.

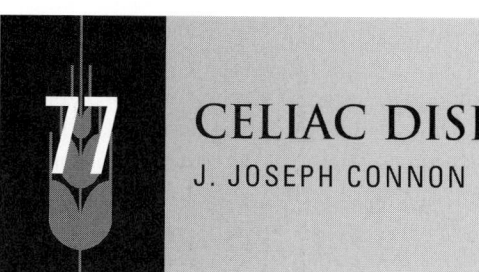

CELIAC DISEASE[1]

J. JOSEPH CONNON

HISTORICAL BACKGROUND 1219
PREVALENCE 1219
PATHOLOGY 1219
GENETICS 1220
PATHOGENESIS 1220
CLINICAL MANIFESTATIONS 1221
    Diarrhea 1221
    Weight Loss 1222
    Malaise 1222
    Monodeficiency Syndromes 1222
    Associated Diseases 1222
INVESTIGATIONS 1222
    Hematology 1222
    Biochemistry 1223
    Radiology 1223
    Antigliadin and Antiendomysial Antibodies 1223
    Intestinal Biopsy 1223
MANAGEMENT 1223
TREATMENT FAILURE 1224

HISTORICAL BACKGROUND

Celiac disease had its roots both literally and metaphorically, when primitive humans switched from the hunter-gatherer mode to a more settled agricultural experience. This occurred about 10,000 BC and involved the cultivation of cereals such as wheat, barley, oats, and rye from their wild grass precursors, such as emmer and einkorn. An illness resembling celiac disease was described as early as the first century AD by Aretaeus of Cappadocia (1). In the nineteenth century, Dr. Samuel Gee provided an excellent clinical description and recommended dietary treatment of a diarrheal illness that he termed "the celiac affection" (2). However, determination of the cause and dietary therapy of celiac disease awaited the observations of W. R. Dicke, a Dutch pediatrician, who noted improvement followed by deterioration of his patients with celiac disease as bread was first withdrawn and then reintroduced into their diet during and after the Second World War (3). Further progress in understanding the disease

was facilitated by development of peroral intestinal biopsy devices by Shiner (4) and Crosby and Kugler (5) that confirmed Paulley's observation of intestinal mucosal flattening in surgically obtained specimens (6).

PREVALENCE

Celiac disease has worldwide distribution, but it has significant variations in clinical prevalence, ranging from 1:300 in Ireland (7) to 1:10,000 in the United States (8). Serologic testing for antiendomysial or antitransglutaminase antibodies resulted in an upward revision of figures, ranging from 2.5:1000 in Denmark (9) to 7.7:1000 in Switzerland (10). It is extremely rare in Black, Chinese, and Japanese persons, but it has been described in India (11). Celiac disease is more common in women, especially during the reproductive years, but this may be an artifact related to increased case finding. The prevalence of celiac disease is higher in adults than in children, and most such adults have no history of childhood symptoms. Peak prevalence in women occurs between 35 and 44 years of age (12). In Scotland, the incidence of childhood celiac disease appears to have fallen since 1976, perhaps because of changes in weaning practice (13), involving later introduction of cereal products to the infant diet. Significant variances in the incidence of celiac disease between Danish and Swedish infants have also been related to differences in the age of introduction of gluten to the diet. An increased prevalence of celiac disease in diabetic patients has been reported from Sweden and Italy (14, 15).

PATHOLOGY

The normal small bowel mucosa is thrown up in a series of concertina-like folds called the valvulae conniventes. Microscopically, the absorptive surface of the mucosa is configured as millions of villi covered by columnar epithelial cells, whereas the secretory mucosa primarily consists of the crypts of Lieberkühn. In advanced celiac disease, the valvulae are thinner and more widely spaced than normal, and scalloping of their free margins has been described at endoscopy (16, 17). Mucosal nodularity, especially in the duodenal bulb, has been noted. The microscopic changes are usually diffuse rather than focal and diminish in severity caudally. Changes range in severity

---

[1]**Abbreviations: HLA,** human leukocyte antigen; **Ig,** immunoglobulin.

from intraepithelial infiltration by CD8 lymphocytes to complete loss of villi, crypt hyperplasia, and infiltration of the lamina propria by plasma cells, CD4 lymphocytes, neutrophils, eosinophils, and mast cells (18). The remaining absorptive cells are cuboidal and vacuolated. Occasionally, changes are patchy (19).

The progression of celiac disease was graded pathologically by Marsh as follows: stage I, increased intraepithelial lymphocytes; stage II, crypt hyperplasia; and stage III, villous atrophy (20).

The effects of gluten extend beyond the small intestine. A lymphoplasmacytoid reaction responsive to gluten has been demonstrated in the rectal mucosa of patients with celiac disease (21). Changes similar to those of celiac disease have been described in other local and systemic disorders that affect the intestinal mucosa. These include lymphoma, giardiasis, tropical sprue, bacterial overgrowth, viral gastroenteritis, cow's milk protein intolerance, and graft-versus-host disease (22).

Dietary exclusion of gluten usually results in restoration of a more normal mucosal appearance within 2 to 3 months. In children, complete recovery may occur, but the presence of some residual villous blunting and lymphocytic infiltration is the rule (23). If rechallenge with gluten is believed necessary to confirm the diagnosis, 10 g/day gluten should be added to the diet for up to 2 months, followed by rebiopsy. Some patients are unable to tolerate gluten for more than a few days because of nausea, bloating, and diarrhea. Occasionally, gluten challenge fails to cause typical histologic changes in patients, who have a relapse years later (24). In one study, smaller amounts of gluten (0.1 g/kg/day) caused a relapse in patients who were challenged, a finding suggesting that less than 10 g daily may be a sufficient challenge, especially in patients who experience symptoms after a larger dose. The presence of normal mucosa, even on a normal diet, does not preclude the eventual development of celiac disease (latent celiac disease) (25).

Because some gluten-sensitized people may have a normal mucosa, even in the presence of antigluten antibodies, and others with advanced jejunal mucosal atrophy may be asymptomatic, Marsh emphasized the need to reconsider traditional definitions of celiac disease (26). He proposed that gluten sensitivity be regarded as a state of heightened T- and B-cell–based immunologic responsiveness to gluten proteins in persons with DQW2 alleles (see later).

GENETICS

Strong evidence indicates an inherited predisposition to celiac disease (27), which occurs up to 100 times more frequently in first-degree relatives of patients with the disease than in the general population. About half of these relatives are asymptomatic. Identical twin studies have shown a disease concordance of 70% (28). Both human leukocyte antigen (HLA) and non-HLA genes have been linked with

celiac disease. In aggregate, the contribution of the non-HLA genes is greater (29), but no specific gene has been identified, although a clustering on chromosome 5 appears to occur (30). Genes coding for HLA molecules are part of the major histocompatibility complex on chromosome 6. The molecules encoded by HLA class I and II genes are required for presentation of gliadin to T-cell receptors of CD4 lymphocytes. More than 95% of patients with celiac disease have the genotype (HLA alleles DQA1* 0501/DQB1* 0201) (31), which encodes for a specific cell-surface glycoprotein molecule, the DQ2 α, β heterodimer. This DQ2 molecule, which is present in most patients with celiac disease, has an affinity for certain gluten epitopes, especially those that have been deamidated. Antigen-presenting cells in the lamina propria that have DQ2 on their cell surface can present the gluten epitope to the α/β T-cell receptor on CD4 T lymphocytes; the result is the development of an immune or inflammatory reaction culminating in the pathologic findings associated with celiac disease. The remaining 5% of patients have HLA DQA103 and HLA DQB1* 0302 alleles that code for DQ8 (32).

Intriguing genetic associations have been found between patients with celiac disease and homozygotes and heterozygotes for the *HFE* gene, which determines hereditary hemochromatosis. Investigators have suggested that those patients carrying the *HFE* gene may be protected from malabsorption of iron (33).

PATHOGENESIS

Gluten is a protein component of wheats, oats, barley, and rye. Alcohol extraction of gluten produces a soluble fraction containing prolamines and an insoluble fraction, the glutenins. Both are toxic to the intestinal mucosa of patients with celiac disease. Prolamines are so called because of their high content of proline and glutamine. Nontoxic cereals such as rice, oats, and corn have a low prolamine content. Wheat prolamines can be subfractionated into α, β, γ, and ω gliadins, all of which are harmful to susceptible intestinal mucosa (34).

Normally, a state of oral tolerance exists for gluten. In persons who do not have celiac disease, the peptide products of gluten digestion by pancreatic and brush border enzymes traverse the apical membrane into the enterocyte, where they are further processed by hydrolases to nonimmunogenic products. A tiny fraction of undigested gluten enters the lamina propria through tight junctions and generates oral tolerance. Intercellular tight junctions are composed of vertically and horizontally intersecting fibers, and if these are damaged, increased intestinal permeability results. The mucosal permeability of patients with celiac disease to macromolecules is significantly increased (35).

Increased expression of zonulin, a peptide capable of loosening tight junctions, has been found in celiac intestinal mucosa (36). However, it remains unclear whether enhanced access of gluten to the lamina propria is a primary phenomenon that plays an initiating role in the onset of celiac disease or is simply a consequence of gluten-induced intestinal damage.

A 33-amino acid peptide fragment of gliadin (33-mer) has been found that resists both peptic and brush border digestion. This peptide has a strong affinity for transglutaminase and contains three epitopes that can activate T cells in patients with celiac disease. On theoretic grounds, endopeptidases could be constructed that could detoxify gluten peptides such as 33-mer in the intestinal lumen, thus potentially precluding the need for a gluten-free diet (37).

The causal relationship between dietary gluten and mucosal changes in susceptible patients is unquestioned. However, many questions remain regarding the mechanism by which gluten exerts its harmful effects. Initially, investigators suggested that incomplete brush border hydrolysis of gluten as a consequence of enzyme deficiency led to formation of toxic products (38), but the inability to demonstrate abnormally low mucosal peptidase or carbohydrase activity following treatment with a gluten-free diet rendered this hypothesis untenable (39).

Various antibodies directed against both dietary antigens and self-antigens have been found in serum and intestinal secretions of celiac patients (40–42). Antigliadin immunoglobulin A (IgA) antibodies are found in up to 90% of patients with untreated celiac disease, and their titer gradually diminishes on gluten withdrawal (43). Other food-related antibodies such as antiovalbumin and anticasein have been described. It appears likely that antibody production is related to the increased paracellular intestinal permeability found in celiac disease.

IgA antibodies directed against specific tissue components have also been identified. These include antireticulin (44), antijejunal (45), and antiendomysial antibodies (46), which can be detected by immunofluorescence technique in both human and animal tissues. These antibodies likely recognize a common antigen (47). The endomysium is a delicate connective tissue layer surrounding intestinal smooth muscle, and antiendomysial antibodies have been found in more than 95% of patients with celiac disease (48, 49). The specificity of both antiendomysial and antigliadin antibodies is 90%. Antiendomysial antibody titers decrease after institution of a gluten-free diet. Tissue transglutaminase is the target of antiendomysial antibodies (50).

The peptide-binding groove of antigen-presenting cells in patients with the DQ2 allele has a higher than expected affinity for gluten peptides. Based on the peptide-binding motif of DQ2, one would expect a binding preference for negatively charged peptides (51), whereas gluten proteins contain few negatively charged residues. However, tissue transglutaminase can generate negatively charged peptides within gluten by deamidating glutamine to the more negatively charged glutamic acid (52). T cells derived from celiac mucosa have been shown preferentially to recognize

deamidated gluten peptides. Finally, transglutaminase expression is significantly elevated in celiac disease.

There is widespread agreement that interaction between CD4 cells and prolamin peptides bound to a celiac-associated HLA-DQ molecule is important in bringing about the pathologic changes associated with celiac disease. Class II HLA molecules bind peptide fragments and present them after further intracellular processing on the cell surface, where they may interact with immunologically competent cells and cause crypt cell hyperplasia and villous atrophy (53). Translocation of gliadin has been shown in intraenterocyte vacuoles positive for HLA-DR antigens in patients with untreated celiac disease (54).

Kagnoff and associates noted significant structural amino acid homology between a gliadin fragment and a nonstructural component, E1B, of type 12 adenovirus and suggested that adenovirus infection of susceptible subjects induces gluten sensitization through the process of molecular mimicry (55). Although this and other groups (56) found a significant increase in the prevalence of antiadenovirus 12 antibodies in patients with untreated celiac disease, other investigators have failed to confirm this finding (57, 58).

CLINICAL MANIFESTATIONS

The presentation of celiac disease is highly variable, ranging from mild, nonspecific features through monodeficiency states to a full-blown classic panmalabsorption syndrome (59). In adults, the classic form of the disease is now the least common presentation, and several authors have emphasized the need to consider celiac disease in patients with features resembling irritable bowel disease occurring in association with another trigger finding such as anemia, weight loss, or a monodeficiency state (60, 61). Moreover, many of these patients with atypical presentations do not have gastrointestinal symptoms.

Diarrhea

Diarrhea is found in 70% of patients (62). It is usually intermittent, occurs three to four times daily, and is of a mushy consistency. Patients with celiac disease often have crampy abdominal pain that, in association with diarrhea and bloating secondary to fermentation of lactose and other maldigested compounds, may simulate the irritable bowel syndrome (63). In a few patients, the diarrhea is more severe, and stools have the classic malabsorptive features of large volume, frothiness, offensive odor, greasy appearance, and a tendency to float. This last quality results from the increased gaseous content of the feces, rather than their fat concentration.

Most childhood cases classically present up to 24 months of age after weaning with a cereal-containing diet. Diarrhea is associated with failure to grow, abdominal distention, anemia, vomiting, and edema.

Weight Loss

Some weight loss is usual, but the amount is highly variable, depending as much on associated anorexia as on malabsorption. Patients with villous atrophy confined to the proximal small intestine may lose no weight.

Malaise

A loss of general well-being is found in 80% of patients but is often so insidious in onset that it is only recognized retrospectively, after institution of a gluten-free diet.

Monodeficiency Syndromes

Isolated monomalabsorption of substances absorbed from the duodenum and proximal and midjejunum is well recognized (64). These include iron, vitamins D and K, calcium, magnesium, and folic acid (12, 65, 66). A combination of iron and folate deficiency is not unusual. Bone mineral density is reduced in association with increased bone turnover and increased secretion of parathormone. The abnormal bone density may respond only partially to treatment with a gluten-free diet (67, 68). The increased metabolic demands of pregnancy may unmask marginal absorption, especially of iron and folate.

Associated Diseases

The clinical features of celiac disease may sometimes be overshadowed by the more dramatic manifestations of associated diseases, thus delaying diagnosis. Many of these diseases have an autoimmune basis. They include dermatitis herpetiformis (69), intestinal lymphoma (70), diabetes (71), thyroid disease (72), IgA deficiency (73), neurologic problems including cerebellar atrophy (74, 75), inflammatory bowel disease (76), and sclerosing cholangitis (77). Celiac disease is found in 3 to 8% of patients with insulin-requiring diabetes (78). Malabsorption of glucose can cause difficulties in diabetes control.

The possibility of celiac disease should also be considered in unexplained transaminasemia (79) and hyperamylasemia (80). The latter results from binding of amylase to serum proteins and responds to gluten exclusion. Other diseases linked with celiac disease include psychiatric disorders, farmer's lung, autoimmune thrombocytopenia, anemia, and Berger's disease, but the evidence for these associations is not conclusive (81).

Dermatitis Herpetiformis

Dermatitis herpetiformis causes pruritic, vesicular, and papular lesions with an erythematous background, primarily on the extensor surfaces of the limbs. The lesions demonstrate granular deposition of IgA at the junction of the dermis and epidermis (82). Although intestinal symptoms are uncommon, virtually all patients with the granular pattern of IgA deposition show patchy mucosal changes identical to those of celiac disease. Linear deposition of IgA is not associated with celiac disease. Both the cutaneous and mucosal abnormalities respond to a gluten-free diet, and in some patients, dapsone therapy can be withdrawn (83, 84).

Malignancy

Certain malignant disorders have been associated with celiac disease, notably small intestinal lymphoma. The relative risk of lymphoma is unclear because of the very wide range of reported incidence figures. One multicenter case-control investigation found a sixfold increase in the risk of lymphoma (85). Celiac-associated lymphoma is generally agreed to be of T-cell origin, although it has been described as malignant histiocytosis (86). Although investigators have suggested that the mucosal atrophy associated with this lymphoma is secondary to the lymphoma rather than vice versa (87), many are reluctant to accept that the malignant features of lymphoma may be delayed for many years and that gluten exclusion would restore a normal mucosal appearance in intestinal lymphoma. Moreover, antigliadin antibodies have been noted in patients who develop lymphoma in the course of celiac disease, whereas these antibodies are absent in patients who present with lymphoma without a prior history of celiac disease (88).

Various presentations have been noted including diarrhea, intestinal obstruction, intestinal perforation, weight loss, abdominal pain, intestinal bleeding, fever, and finger clubbing. IgA levels may increase. Enteropathy-associated T-cell lymphoma may be very difficult to diagnose (89). If routine investigations, including small bowel radiography and abdominal computed tomography, are negative and the clinical picture is suspicious, a laparotomy with full-thickness biopsies should be done. Local resection is rarely possible, and response to systemic chemotherapy is poor.

Other cancers also occur with increased frequency in celiac disease, including esophageal and pharyngeal cancer, as well as small intestinal adenocarcinoma (90). A reduced incidence of small bowel lymphoma has been reported in patients adhering to a gluten-free diet (91, 92).

INVESTIGATIONS

The purpose of investigations in patients with suspected celiac disease is twofold. First, they confirm that the clinical features are indeed the result of celiac disease. Second, they enable one to search for evidence of nutritional deficiencies, complications such as lymphoma, and the presence of frequently associated diseases.

Hematology

Anemia is present in 40 to 80% of patients (93, 94). Unexplained iron or folate deficiency anemia rather than florid malabsorption is increasingly responsible for raising the suspicion of celiac disease (95). The simultaneous deficiency of both iron and folate produces a dimorphic blood picture, giving rise to an increased red cell distribution width. Hyposplenism is common in celiac disease and produces Howell-Jolly bodies (96). Folate deficiency may cause a slightly low serum vitamin B_{12} level that responds to folate replacement. Rarely, mucosal atrophy extending to the terminal ileum or bacterial overgrowth secondary to celiac-associated intestinal stasis may produce vitamin B_{12} deficiency (97). Fecal occult blood tests are positive in 41% of patients with celiac disease who have normal upper and lower gastrointestinal tracts (98). The cause is uncertain but may be related to small bowel ulceration, and it may contribute to iron deficiency.

Biochemistry

Biochemical abnormalities in celiac disease essentially reflect both the extent and the duration of malabsorption and range from none to multiple changes involving fluids, minerals, proteins, fat, and gut hormones. The stool fat content is usually increased in patients with celiac disease and diarrhea, but it may be normal in those presenting in a monosymptomatic fashion with iron, folate, or vitamin D deficiency (99). Steatorrhea tends to be less marked in celiac disease than in chronic pancreatitis, and stool fat concentration is also relatively lower because of greater fluid losses in the celiac stool. The importance of stool fat measurement has diminished with increasing use of endoscopic small bowel biopsy.

D-Xylose is an inert sugar absorbed in the upper small intestine. Serum or urinary levels following oral administration provide a measure of jejunal absorptive capacity, but the reliability of the test is influenced by variations in gastric emptying, age, and renal function (100). Selective mucosal absorption has been tested with probes of different molecular size for both diagnosis and follow-up of celiac disease. These molecules include mannitol, lactulose, and lactobiose. In patients with celiac disease, larger molecules are selectively absorbed, probably via paracellular routes, and transcellular absorption of smaller molecules diminishes as a result of villous atrophy (101). Although high sensitivity and negative predictive values have been claimed for tests of differential urinary excretion, they have not yet gained wide acceptance. Transaminase levels are frequently elevated in adult patients and normalize following treatment with a gluten-free diet (102, 103).

Radiology

The primary role of radiology of the small bowel is exclusion of other diseases such as Crohn disease, jejunal diverticulosis, strictures, or lymphoma, and barium studies are not routinely required. In celiac disease, the radiologic appearance is often normal, but one may see dilatation of the lumen and thickening of mucosal folds.

Antigliadin and Antiendomysial Antibodies

Increasing recognition of the subtle and atypical modes of presentation of celiac disease has underscored the importance of noninvasive screening tests. Both IgG and IgA antigliadin antibodies are present in untreated celiac disease, but they lack sufficient diagnostic sensitivity and specificity. IgG antigliadin antibodies are more sensitive, whereas IgA antibodies are more specific (104). IgG antigliadin antibodies are valuable in serologic testing of patients with IgA deficiency, and IgA antibody testing is useful in children less than 2 years of age, in whom antiendomysial antibody testing is insensitive (105). Antiendomysial antibodies, which are detected by binding to a variety of smooth muscle basement membranes including monkey esophagus and human umbilical cord (106), have a sensitivity and specificity of close to 100%. This results in a predictive accuracy of 100%, even with prevalence rates as low as 0.2% (107–109). Titers of both antigliadin antibodies and antiendomysial antibodies fall rapidly in patients on a gluten-free diet.

Antiendomysial antibodies are directed against tissue transglutaminase. They can be measured by the enzyme-linked immunosorbent assay technique and have sensitivities and specificities of up to 98 and 100%, respectively. The test is less subject to observer error than endomysial antibody testing and is much easier to automate. A few patients with celiac disease are negative on endomysial antibody testing and positive on anti-transglutaminase testing and vice versa.

The role of serologic testing remains controversial. It will likely become a valuable screening test but will not supplant intestinal biopsy as a diagnostic test. The positive predictive values of antiendomysial and antitransglutaminase antibody testing are sufficiently high for use as a population screening tool.

The desirability of mass screening is unclear. Proponents argue that it will reduce the burden of disease by preventing complications related to celiac disease, whereas others are concerned about feasibility and quality of life issues related to putting large numbers of entirely asymptomatic patients on life-long gluten-free diets.

Intestinal Biopsy

Endoscopic biopsy of the second or third portion of the duodenum has replaced use of the Crosby or Watson capsule. Although these latter devices provide larger biopsy specimens, frustration with the technical difficulties associated with them compared with the ease of obtaining multiple, albeit smaller, endoscopic samples led to a marked decline in their use. An immediate diagnosis of villous atrophy can be made by dissecting-microscopic examination of the biopsy material. Gastric antral histologic changes have been reported in patients with celiac disease.

Endoscopy may reveal macroscopic changes in some patients. These include thinning, wider separation, and scalloping of the margins of the valvulae conniventes (7, 8). En face, the mucosa may have a mosaic appearance that is enhanced when it is partially covered with blood following biopsy. Diagnostic sensitivity and specificity of about 90% have been reported. Marked duodenal nodularity is found in some patients.

The appearance of celiac disease on biopsy specimens is nonspecific, and definitive diagnosis requires repeat biopsy to demonstrate histologic improvement on a gluten-free diet and reversion to abnormality after gluten challenge. In adults, the last step is frequently omitted.

MANAGEMENT

The underlying genetic defect in celiac disease is, of course, not curable, but the condition is unique in that its phenotypic expression is usually reversible by dietary exclusion of gluten. The importance of a life-long gluten-free diet cannot be overemphasized. The ubiquity of gluten as a food additive and pill excipient mandates an effective relationship among the patient, the physician, and the dietitian. Patients should carefully examine food labels for possible presence of gluten and should be familiar with the recommendations of authoritative bodies such as the American Dietetic Association's National Center for Nutrition (hotline: 1-800-366-1655) and the Celiac Sprue Association (www.csaceliacs.org).

Dietary avoidance of gluten is central to the management of celiac disease. Most patients notice a significant symptomatic improvement within days. Changes in mucosal histology take longer. A reduction in intraepithelial lymphocyte infiltration occurs within a few weeks (110), but recovery of the normal villous appearance usually takes 2 to 3 months. Some patients never fully recover, even though they feel well. The diet of patients with demonstrated deficiencies should be supplemented initially with appropriate vitamins and minerals, but long-term supplementation is unnecessary.

Wheat, barley, rye, and oats are the main sources of gluten, and foodstuffs derived from these products have been traditionally excluded. Oats contain less gluten than other cereals, and one Finnish study showed no adverse nutritional or mucosal effects from a daily intake of 50 g of oats (111). Adherence to a strict gluten-free diet may be difficult because cereal products are present in a variety of prepared foods, but deliberate noncompliance is a much larger problem. Dietary surveys show that 30% of patients admit to taking gluten and remaining asymptomatic (112, 113). However, in some patients, ingestion of even small amounts of gluten results in bloating and diarrhea. Attainment of expected adult stature may be compromised by gluten intake during childhood and adolescence (114). The desirability of adhering to a gluten-free diet is heightened by a study demonstrating a reduction in the malignancy rates of compliant patients (73). See Appendix Table A-36-a-f for details of a gluten-free diet and associated precautions.

Significant differences exist internationally in the constituents of a gluten-free diet. In Canada, the diet must not contain any wheat, barley, rye, oats, or triticale, whereas in many European countries, levels ranging from 5 to 50 μg/day gliadin are acceptable. The Celiac Sprue Association USA, in addition to recommending complete exclusion of gluten-containing cereals, also advises avoiding buckwheat and any foods using cereal mash in their manufacture. These include distilled alcoholic beverages and white vinegar, which contain no detectable gliadins. Beer contains 3 μg/L prolamin and probably should be avoided. In vitro studies have shown that gliadin-deficient wheat is less toxic to enterocytes, thus revealing potential approaches to dietary treatment (115).

TREATMENT FAILURE

Most patients show a rapid clinical response to the institution of a gluten-free diet, often within a week or so. Histologic improvement is a longer, more drawn-out process, sometimes requiring 2 years for restoration to normal. Some patients, however, fail to respond to the diet either from the beginning of treatment or after a variable period of improvement (116). The most important and frequent reason for a poor response is continuation of gluten in the diet, either deliberately or inadvertently. If this possibility is excluded, virtually every cause of chronic diarrhea, such as inflammatory bowel disease, bacterial overgrowth, giardiasis, and chronic pancreatitis, must be considered before one concludes that refractory celiac disease is present (117).

Refractory celiac disease is rare and is a diagnosis of exclusion. Somewhat arbitrarily, a failure of response to treatment after a 6-month period of gluten exclusion is required before one makes the diagnosis.

A growing sense exists that most patients with refractory disease have occult or cryptic lymphoma, classified as enteropathy-associated T-cell lymphoma (118, 119). A phenotypically abnormal, monoclonal population of intraepithelial lymphocytes has been described in 75% of patients with refractory sprue. These patients have a particularly poor response to treatment.

Therapy is based on anecdoctal reports in a small number of patients using a variety of approaches including total parenteral nutrition, corticosteroids (120), azathioprine (121, 122), infliximab(123), and cyclosporine (124, 125).

REFERENCES

1. Hude C. Aretaeus: Corpus Medicorum Graecorum II. 2nd ed. Berlin: Academy of Sciences, 1958.
2. Gee SJ. St. Bartholomews Hosp Res 1888;24:17–20.
3. Dicke WK. Coeliakie. PhD thesis. University of Utrecht, Utrecht, the Netherlands, 1950.

4. Shiner M. Lancet 1956;1:85.

5. Crosby WH, Kugler HW. Am J Dig Dis 1957;2:236–41.

6. Paulley JW. Proc R Soc Med 1949;42:241.

7. Mylotte M, Egan-Mitchell B, McCarthy CF et al. BMJ 1973; 1:703–5.

8. Talley NJ, Valdovinos M.Peteson TM et al. Am J Gastroenterol 1994;89;843–6.

9. Weile I, Grodzindky E, Skogh T et al. FAPMIS 2001;109: 745–50.

10 Rutz R, Ritzler E, Fierz W et al. Swiss Med Wkly 2002;132: 43–7.

11. Misra RC, Kasthuri D, Chuttani HK. BMJ 1966;2:1230–2.

12. Logan RAF, Rifkind EA, Busuttil A et al. Gastroenterology 1986;90:334–42.

13. Ascher H, Krantz I, Kristiansson B. Arch Dis Child 1991;66:608–11.

14. Sigurs N, Johansson C, Elfstrand PO et al. Acta Paediatr 1993; 82:748–51.

15. Sategna-Guidetti C, Grosso S, Pulitano R et al. Dig Dis Sci 1994;39:1633–7.

16. Jabbari M, Wild G, Goreski CA et al. Gastroenterology 1988; 95:1518–22.

17. Brocchi E, Corazza G, Treggiari EA et al. N Engl J Med 1988; 319:741–4.

18. Rubin CE, Brandborg LL, Phelps PC et al. Gastroenterology 1960;38:28–49.

19. Scott BB, Losowsky MS. Gut 1976;17:984–92.

20. Marsh MN. Gastroenterology 1992;102:330–54.

21. Ensarim A, Marsh MN, Loft DE et al. Gut 1993;34:1225–9.

22. Cooke WT, Holmes, GKT. Celiac Disease. New York: Churchill Livingstone, 1984.

23. Rubin CE, Eidelman S, Weinstein WM. Gastroenterology 1970;58:409–13.

24. Kuitunen P, Savilahti E, Verkasalo M. Acta Paediatr Scand 1986;75:340–2.

25. Mäki M, Holm K, Koskimies S et al. Arch Dis Child 1990; 65:1137–41.

26. Marsh MN. Q J Med 1995;85:913.

27. Mylotte M, Egan-Mitchell B, Fottrell PF et al. Q J Med 1974; 43:359–69.

28. Polanco I, Biemond I, van Leeuwen A et al. In: McConnell RD, ed. Genetics of Celiac Disease: Proceedings of an International Symposium. Lancaster, UK: MTP Press, 1981.

29. Molberg O, McAdam SN, Sollid LM. J Pediatr Gastroenterol Nutr 2000;30:232–40.

30. Greco L. Am J Hum Genet 1998;62:669–75.

31. Sollid L, Thorsby E. Gastroenterology 1993;105:910–22.

32. Tosi R, Vismara D, Tanigaki N et al. Clin Immunopathol 1983; 28:395–404.

33. Butterworth JR, Cooper BT, Rosenberb MC et al. Gastroenterology 2002;123:444–9.

34. Ciclitira PJ, Evans DJ, Fagg NLK et al. Clin Sci 1984;66:357–64.

35. Cobden I, Dickinson RJ, Rothwell J et al. BMJ 1978;2:1060.

36. Fasano A, Not T, Wang W et al. Lancet 2000;355:1518–9.

37. Shan L, Molberg O. Parrot I et al. Science 2002;297:2275–9.

38. Frazer AC, Fletcher RF, Ross CA. Lancet 1959;2:252–5.

39. Davidson AGF, Bridges MA. Clin Chim Acta 1987;163:1–40.

40. Kenrick KG, Walker-Smith JA. Gut 1970;11:635–40.

41. Ferguson A. Carswell F. BMJ 1972;1:75–7.

42. O'Mahony S, Arranz E, Barton JR et al. Gut 1991;32:29–35.

43. Kelly CP, Feighery CF, Weir DG. Gastroenterology 1988;94: A221.

44. Mäki M, Hallstrom O, Vesikari T et al. J Pediatr 1984;105: 901–5.

45. Kárpáti S, Török E, Kosnaii J. Invest Dermatol 1986;87:703–6.

46. Volta U, Molinaro N, Fusconi M et al. Dig Dis Sci 1991;36: 752–6.

47. Kárpáti S, Meurer M, Burgin-Wolff A et al. Gut 1992;191–3.

48. Chorzelski TP, Suley J, Tchorzewska H et al. Ann NY Acad Sci 1983;420:325–34.

49. Kumar V, Lerner A, Valeski JE et al. Immunol Invest 1989; 18:533–44.

50. Dieterich W et al. Nat Med 1997;3:797–801.

51. Johannsen BH, Vardal F, Eriksen JA et al. Int Immunol 1996;8:177–82.

52. Van de Wal Y, Kooy Y, van Veelen P et al. J Immunol 1998; 161:1585–8.

53. Lundin KEA, Sollid LM, Qvigstad E et al. J Immunol 1990; 145:136–9.

54. Ciclitira PJ, Harms E. Gut 1995;36:703–9.

55. Kagnoff MF, Austin RK, Hubert JJ et al. J Exp Med 1984; 160:1544–57.

56. Lahdaaho ML, Parkkonen P, Reunala T et al. Clin Immunol Immunopathol 1993;69:300–5.

57. Howdle PD, Blair Zajdel ME, Smart CJ et al. Scand J Gastroenterol 1989;24:282–6.

58. Mahon J, Blair GE, Wood GM. Gut 1991;32:1114–6.

59. Mann JG, Brown WR, Kern F. Am J Med 1970;48:375–6.

60. Rifkind EA, Busuttil A, Ferguson A. BMJ 1980;281:1637.

61. Swinson CM, Levi AJ. BMJ 1980;281:1258–60.

62. Dawson AM. Neth J Med 1987;31:256–62.

63. Hasler WL. Gastroenterology 2002;122:2086–7.

64. Rossi E. Eur J Pediatr 1982;138:4–5.

65. Weir DG, Hourihane DOB. Gut 1974;15:450–7.

66. Mora S, Bareta G, Beccio S et al. J Pediatr 2001;139:516–21.

67. Gonzalez D, Mazure R, Mautalen C et al. Bone 1995;16:231–4.

68. Cecchetti L, Tarozzi C, Corra O et al. Gastroenterology 1995; 109:122–8.

69. Marks J, Shuster S, Watson AJ. Lancet 1966;2:1280–2.

70. Holmes GKT, Stokes PL, Sorahan TM et al. Gut 1976;17: 612–9.

71. Walker-Smith JA. Arch Dis Child 1975;50:668.

72. Midhagen G, Jarnerot G, Kraaz W. Scand J Gastroenterol 1988; 23:1000–4.

73. Mawhinney H, Tomkin GH. Lancet 1971;2:121–4.

74. Finelli PF, McEntee WJ, Ambler M et al. Neurology 1980;30: 245–9.

75. Hadjivassiliou M, Grinewald RA, Davies-Jones GA. J Neurol Neurosurg Psychiatry 2002;72:560–3.

76. Shah A, Mayberry JF, Williams G et al. Q J Med 1990;74:283–8.

77. Hay JE, Wiesner RH, Shorter RG et al. Ann Intern Med 1988;109:713–7.

78. Hansen D, Bennedbaek FN, Hansen LK et al. Acta Paediatr 2001;90:1238–43.

79. Kaukinen K, Halme L, Collin P et al. Gastroenterology 2002; 122:881–8.

80. Rabsztyn A, Green PH, Berti I et al. Am J Gastroenterol 2001; 96:1096–1100.

81. Mulder CJ, Tytgat GN. Neth J Med 1987;31:286–9.

82. Lawley TJ, Strober W, Yaoita H et al. J Invest Dermatol 1980; 74:9.

83. Weinstein WM, Brow JR, Parker F et al. Gastroenterology 1971;60:362–9.

84. Fry L, Seah PP, Riches DJ et al. Lancet 1973;1:288–91.

85. Askiing J, Linet M, Gridley G et al Gastroenterology 2002; 123:1428–35.

86. Isaacson PG, O'Connor NT, Spencer J et al. Lancet 1985;2: 688–91.

87. Wright DH, Jones DB, Clark H et al. Lancet 1991;337:1373–4.

88. O'Farrelly C, Feighery C, O'Briain DS et al. BMJ 1986;293: 908–10.

89. Isaacson PG. Celiac Disease: malignant lymphoma. In: Jewell DP, Ireland A, eds. Topics in Gastroenterology, vol 14. Boston: Blackwell Scientific Publications, 1986.

90. Swinson CM, Slavin G, Coles EC et al. Lancet 1983;1:111–5.

91. Holmes GKT, Prior P, Lane MR et al. Gut 1989;30:333–8.

92. Corrao G, Corazza GR, Bagnardi M et al. Lancet 2001;358: 356–61.

93. Hoffbrand AV. Clin Gastroenterol 1974;3:71–89.

94. Corazza GR, Valentini RA, Andreani ML. Scand J Gastroenterol 1995;30:153–6.

95. Logan RAF, Tucker G, Rifkind EA. BMJ 1983;286:95–7.

96. Ferguson A, Hutton MM, Maxwell JD et al. Lancet 1970;1: 163–4.

97. Dickey W. Eur J Gastroenterol Hepatol 2002;14:425–7.

98. Fine KD. N Engl J Med 1996;334:1190–1201.

99. McGuigan JE, Volwiler W. Gastroenterology 1964;47:636–41.

100. Craig RM, Atkinson AJ Jr. Gastroenterology 1988;95:223–31.

101. Juby LD, Rothwell J, Axon AT. Gastroenterology 1989;96:79–85.

102. Dickey W, McMillan SA, Collins JS et al. J Clin Gastroenterol 1995;20:290–2.

103. Bardella MT, Fraquelli M, Quatrini M et al. Hepatology 1995; 22:833–6.

104. Burgin-Wolff A, Berger R, Gaze H et al. Eur J Pediatr 1989;148:496–502.

105. Farrell RJ, Kelly CP. N Engl J Med 2002;346:180–88.

106. Ladinser B, Rossipal E, Bittschieler K. Gut 1994;35:776–8.

107. Hallström O. Gut 1989;30:1225–32.

108. Ferenci P, Granditsch G, Penner E. Am J Gastroenterol 1995; 90:394–8.

109. Corrao G, Corazza GR, Andreani ML. Gut 1994;35:771–5.

110. Yardley JH, Bayless TM, Norton JH et al. N Engl J Med 1962;267:1173–9.

111. Janatuinen EK, Pikkarainen PH, Kemppainen TA. N Engl J Med 1995;333:1033–7.

112. Kumar PJ, Clark ML, Dawson AM. Q J Med 1985;57:803.

113. Bardella MT, Molteni N, Prampolini L. Arch Dis Child 1994; 70:211–3.

114. Colaco J, Egan-Mitchell B, Stevens FM et al. Arch Dis Child 1987;62:706–8.

115. Frisono M, Corazza GR, Lafiandra D. Gut 1995;36:375–8.

116. Trier J, Falchuk Z, Carey M et al. Gastroenterology 1978;75: 307–16.

117. Ryan BM, Kelleher D. Gastroenterology 2000;119:243–51.

118. Carbonel F, Grollet-Bioul L, Brouet J et al. Blood 1998;92: 3879–86.

119. Cellier C, Delabesse E, Helmer C et al. Lancet 2000; 356 (9225):203–8.

120. Peters T, Jones P, Jenkins W et al. Clin Sci Mol Med 1978; 55:293–300.

121. Vaidya A, Bolanos J, Berkelhammer C. Am J Gastroenterol 1999;94:1967–8.

122. Maurino E, Niveloni S, Chernavsky A et al. Am J Gastroenterol. 2002;97:2592–602.

123. Gillett HR, Arnott ID, McIntyre M et al. Gastroenterology 2002;122:800–5.

124. Bernstein E, Whitington P. Gastroenterology 1988;95:199–204.

125. Longstreth GF. Ann Intern Med 1993;119:1014–6.

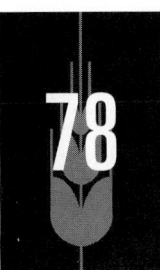

78 NUTRITION IN PANCREATIC DISORDERS[1]
MASSIMO RAIMONDO AND JAMES S. SCOLAPIO

ACUTE PANCREATITIS 1227
   Clinical Presentation .1227
   Clinical Assessment and Prediction of Need
      for Specialized Nutritional Treatment 1227
   Imaging and Serum Tests 1228
   Nutrition Treatment 1228
CHRONIC PANCREATITIS 1230
   Etiology and Epidemiology 1230
   Clinical Presentation .1231
   Nutrition Assessment .1231
   Nutrition Management 1232
   Pancreatic Enzyme Replacement 1232
   Pain Management 1233
   Patient Monitoring 1233
PANCREATIC CANCER 1233
SUMMARY 1233

The exocrine pancreas controls digestion of nutrients. Deranged pancreatic function during inflammatory and neoplastic conditions may lead to temporary or permanent nutritional imbalances. Acute pancreatitis, in the moderate and severe forms of the disease, is complicated by prolonged hospitalization with organ failure that may preclude patients from eating. Chronic pancreatitis and pancreatic cancer are characterized by significant reduction in secretion of pancreatic enzymes leading to malabsorption. In the former, atrophy and fibrosis of the acinar cells are responsible for the malabsorption, whereas in the latter, obstruction of the pancreatic duct by the tumor precludes pancreatic enzymes from entering the duodenum. This chapter deals with principal clinical features of these diseases, with particular emphasis on assessments of the nutritional deficits, oral, parenteral, or enteral nutrition (EN) in acute pancreatitis, and pancreatic enzymes and diet in chronic pancreatitis and pancreatic cancer. Refer to Chapter 70 for a discussion of the role of the pancreas in normal digestion.

---

[1]**Abbreviations: APACHE,** Acute Physiology and Chronic Health Evaluation; **CCK,** cholecystokinin; **EN,** enteral nutrition; **H₂,** histamine; **PPI,** proton-pump inhibitor; **REE,** resting energy expenditure; **SIRS,** systemic inflammatory response syndrome; **TPN,** total parenteral nutrition.

ACUTE PANCREATITIS

Clinical Presentation

Alcohol abuse and biliary lithiasis account for acute pancreatitis in 75 to 85% of patients. In addition to these common causes of acute pancreatitis, other factors have been implicated in the pathogenesis of the disorder, such as metabolic, traumatic, operative, infectious, and pharmacologic causes. Patients with acute pancreatitis typically present with acute abdominal pain localized in the upper quadrants and elevation of amylase and lipase in the serum.

The clinical spectrum of acute pancreatitis ranges in severity from a mild form with edematous inflammation (interstitial pancreatitis), which usually resolves in a few days, to a fulminate process, which can progress to necrotizing pancreatitis resulting from inflammation and tissue necrosis following intrapancreatic and extrapancreatic spreading of active pancreatic enzymes. In acute pancreatitis, the cause of toxicity and complications is extravasation of enzymes into the pararenal spaces, lesser sac, and peritoneal cavity and into the circulation by absorption through retroperitoneal venous and lymphatic vessels. The extravasation of enzymes into the abdominal cavities produces a "burn," resulting in loss of protein and fluid. This third-space loss and escape of enzymes into the circulation cause hypovolemia and hypotension. In addition to circulatory collapse, this process also leads to release of chemokines, thought to be key mediators in the human systemic inflammatory response syndrome (SIRS) (1). Further, escape of pancreatic enzymes and other pancreatic secretions into the pancreas and peripancreatic areas causes pancreatic and peripancreatic necrosis. Lipase most likely is the enzyme responsible for the initiation of necrosis by digesting pancreatic and peripancreatic fat.

Clinical Assessment and Prediction of Need for Specialized Nutritional Treatment

Mild acute interstitial pancreatitis is characterized by abdominal pain, nausea, vomiting, anorexia, and low or no mortality (<2%). Although local complications such as third-space losses leading to hypovolemia and systemic complications such as respiratory or renal failure may occur in interstitial pancreatitis, these complications are uncommon, and resolution of symptoms and recovery occur in several days. In these patients, simple supportive medical treatment suffices, and EN or parenteral nutrition is rarely needed. However, in severe necrotizing pancreatitis, characterized by end-organ failure, the mortality rate may approximate 30% if the necrotic tissue is infected (2). Patients with this disorder need nutrition support as soon as severe pancreatitis is recognized because a prolonged, complicated clinical course is extremely likely.

Clinical Predictors of Severity

Severity of acute pancreatitis is the major predictor of the outcome of an attack of pancreatitis, and it determines the type of treatment patients will receive. A particular concern is how to recognize patients with developing pancreatic necrosis who are predisposed to systemic complications such as SIRS or lung failure. Numerous predictors of severity have been proposed; many of them carry the name of the principal investigator who devised them. Among them are the criteria of Ranson (3), the first criteria proposed. In addition, Bank and associates (4), Agarwal and Pitchumoni (5), and Corfield and associates (6) suggested criteria. All these criteria have the disadvantage that they require 48 hours to measure at least some of the components of the criteria. Ranson's criteria (Table 78.1) use age and laboratory measurements at admission and further clinical and laboratory measurements at 48 hours; patients with up to two signs have 0% mortality, those with three to five signs have a mortality of 10 to 20%, and those with six signs or more have a mortality greater than 50%. Patients with three or more signs have a high risk of developing pancreatic necrosis and systemic complications. The other named criteria are simpler and in general rely on the development of cardiac, pulmonary, renal, metabolic, hematologic, and neurologic complications within the first 48 hours; the presence of at least one complication identifies patients who have a high risk of complications and death.

The Acute Physiology and Chronic Health Evaluation (APACHE-II) score is a system based on laboratory testing and vital signs. The advantage of the APACHE score is

TABLE 78.1. RANSON'S CRITERIA OF SEVERITY OF PANCREATITIS

At admission
  Age >55 y
  White blood cell count >16,000/mm^3
  Glucose >200 mg/dL
  Lactate dehydrogenase >350 IU/L
  Aspartate aminotransferase >250 U/L
During initial 48 h
  Hematocrit decrease of >10 points
  Blood urea nitrogen increase of >5 mg/dL
  Calcium <8 mg/dL
  Arterial oxygen tension <60 mm Hg
  Base deficit >4 mEq/L
  Fluid sequestration >6 L

that it can be used repeatedly and at any time during the course of an attack and that it is in common use. Scores lower than 9 predict survival, but scores higher than 13 predict a high probability of death (7–12). Unfortunately, in a study by Lankisch and associates, the APACHE-II score on admission to the hospital did not provide a reliable diagnosis of necrotizing pancreatitis, and it showed different rates of overestimation or underestimation of clinical status (13).

Imaging and Serum Tests

Of the imaging and laboratory tests, computed tomography is currently considered the best to assess the severity of acute pancreatitis. Originally, the scoring system of Balthazar and Ranson and their colleagues (14, 15) was used (grades A to E: A, normal pancreas; B, focal or diffuse enlargement; C to –E, pancreatic enlargement, C with mild peripancreatic inflammation, D with fluid in the anterior pararenal space, and E with fluid collections in more than one area). The prognosis for grades A and B is excellent. For grade C, the rate of pancreatic necrosis and infection approximates 10%, but for grades D and E, the rate of infection is 50%, and mortality may reach 15%. Currently, the most accurate test is bolus contrast-enhanced computed tomography when severe pancreatitis is suspected. This technique clearly differentiates interstitial from necrotizing pancreatitis.

Elevations in serum amylase and lipase concentrations are used in the diagnosis of pancreatitis. Among the numerous other biochemical markers (C-reactive protein, α_2-macroglobulin, phopholipase A_2 activity, and urinary trypsinogen activating peptide), no single parameter has yet achieved widespread clinical acceptance and use.

The severity of acute pancreatitis is independent of the elevation in serum amylase or lipase level on admission. Patients with only a slight increase can also have or develop severe acute pancreatitis. This is especially true for patients with alcohol-induced acute pancreatitis whose amylase levels are lower than in other etiologic groups (16). No enzyme assay has a predictive role in determining the severity or etiology of acute pancreatitis. Once the diagnosis of acute pancreatitis is established, daily measurements of amylase and lipase have no value in assessing the clinical progress of the patient or ultimate prognosis (17).

Nutrition Treatment

Mild Acute Pancreatitis

Most patients who experience mild pancreatitis are treated for several days with supportive care including pain control, intravenous fluids, and nothing by mouth. Most patients eat within 5 to 7 days and do not require specialized nutrition support. When to begin oral feedings, what to feed, and how often to feed are questions that occur with every patient with acute pancreatitis.

Unfortunately, answers to these questions are not based on scientific data obtained in patients with acute pancreatitis. Instead, the principles of refeeding are based on physiologic studies in healthy persons to determine the effects of nutrients on pancreatic enzyme secretion and personal anecdotal experience. The criteria we use to initiate oral feedings are as follows: absence of abdominal pain and tenderness, reduction of amylase levels near to normal levels, and absence of complications.

We begin feeding patients by giving 100 to 300 mL of liquids containing no calories every 4 hours for the first 24 hours. Clear liquid diets have no fat and therefore present less risk of pancreatic stimulation as initial feeding. If this diet is tolerated, oral feeding is advanced to giving the same volume of liquids containing low-fat nutrients. Subsequently, if patients continue to do well, feedings are changed gradually over 3 to 4 days to soft and finally solid foods. All the diets contain greater than 50% carbohydrate calories, and the total caloric content is gradually increased from 160 to 640 kcal per meal.

These recommendations are based on studies in healthy persons that found that the rate of pancreatic enzymes secretion was related to the nutrient composition of meals (18) and the rate of the delivery of kilocalories to the duodenum (19). Secretion of pancreatic enzymes decreased as more carbohydrate fraction was ingested, particularly when carbohydrates were 50% or more of the total caloric content of the diet. In another study, when nutrients were infused into the duodenum, pancreatic enzymes secretion was directly related to the rate of kilocalories infused: fewer pancreatic enzymes were secreted at rates of 40 kcal/hour compared with 90 or 160 kcal/hour (19).

Moderate to Severe Acute Pancreatitis

On admission to the hospital, all patients presenting with acute pancreatitis are allowed nothing by mouth. In addition, in moderate to severe attacks of pancreatitis, gastric contents may be aspirated from the stomach through a nasogastric tube in presence of ileus or to minimize nausea and vomiting. Although resting energy expenditure (REE) in patients with uncomplicated acute pancreatitis (measured by indirect calorimetry) is no greater than in comparable healthy persons, 82% of patients with sepsis are hypermetabolic ($120\pm12\%$ of predicted value) (20). Indeed, patients with pancreatitis exhibit some of the same metabolic, cardiovascular, and hemodynamic features observed in sepsis. In addition, if pseudocysts, abscesses, or fistulas develop, a protracted course with increased metabolic needs should be anticipated; it is in this setting that nutritional complications are most likely to arise.

Considerable progress has been made in the management of moderate to severe acute pancreatitis. The paradigm in severe acute pancreatitis seems to have shifted toward the use of more enterally based nutritional approaches. Several lines of evidence suggest that EN can influence the clinical course of acute pancreatitis. In fact, several randomized clinical studies in both mild and severe forms of pancreatitis have been published. McClave and colleagues published the results of a randomized trial evaluating the effects of EN versus total parenteral nutrition (TPN) in mild acute pancreatitis (21). The overall group of patients had alcoholic acute pancreatitis or recurrent pancreatitis in addition to chronic pancreatitis. In this study, EN was better and cheaper than TPN. In the same year, Kalfarentzos and associates reported their results of a randomized trial of EN versus TPN in severe acute pancreatitis. Most of the patients of this study were women with biliary pancreatitis. In this study, EN was well tolerated and was associated with fewer septic and overall complications. Furthermore, EN was three times less expensive than TPN (22). In another randomized controlled trial of EN versus TPN in patients with severe biliary pancreatitis, Windsor and colleagues observed a significant reduction of the incidence of SIRS in the EN-treated group (23). However, Powell and colleagues showed that early EN compared with no nutrition did not affect the overall outcome, had no effect on markers of SIRS, and presumably had an adverse effect on intestinal barrier function (24). Most recently, Abou-Assi and coworkers reported their experience with a randomized comparative study of early hypocaloric EN versus TPN in acute pancreatitis. They studied 53 patients, 26 in the EN group and 27 in the TPN group. Most of their patients had biliary pancreatitis. They observed that the EN group had fewer treatment-related complications; patients required less nutritional support (6.7 versus 10.8 days); the cost saving with EN was $2362 per patient. On average, EN support in the study was able to deliver 54% of the estimated nutritional requirements (25). These studies used jejunal feedings as the enteral route, whereas the type of feeding was a semielemental formula. The results of these studies must be interpreted with caution, however, because the theoretic benefits of EN over TPN have not yet translated into improved outcomes in patients with severe acute pancreatitis. What is clearly demonstrated in these trials is that EN is feasible, practical, and cheaper than TPN. A major advantage of the intestinal route is the elimination of the complications of parenteral nutrition. Among the complications of parenteral nutrition is catheter sepsis, the incidence of which is reported to be 2.1% even if the catheter is managed appropriately (26). Other complications of parenteral nutrition include metabolic abnormalities and the less frequent catheter sepsis, pneumothorax, vein thrombosis, thrombophlebitis, and catheter embolism. TPN maintains "pancreatic rest" better than jejunal elemental feedings. The further down the upper gastrointestinal tract an elemental diet is infused, the less stimulation of pancreatic exocrine secretion will occur, because the normal cephalic, gastric, and intestinal (more potent) phases of pancreatic stimulation are bypassed.

Other advantages of the EN over TPN include the maintenance of intestinal integrity and the gut mucosal barrier, which may decrease the risk of bacterial translocation and subsequent septic complications of acute pancreatitis, and lower cost resulting from elimination of complications related to TPN.

Complications of Pancreatitis

Pancreatic pseudocysts complicate patients with severe acute pancreatitis. Chronic unremitting pain worsened by meals is one of the most common symptoms. No controlled studies have evaluated different forms of nutritional support in patients with pseudocysts (EN, TPN, nothing by mouth). Anecdotal evidence suggests that most TPN-treated patients have clinical and radiographic regression of their pseudocysts. However, the increased risk of catheter-related and metabolic complications suggests that this therapy should be limited to patients who are unable to sustain EN. Endoscopic, radiologic, and surgical approaches are sometimes used to decompress large symptomatic pancreatic pseudocysts.

Because of inhibition of pancreatic activity, which reduces exocrine secretion and further prevents the release and activation of enzymes, octreotide has been suggested as a specific treatment in patients with pseudocysts. Unfortunately, the results of clinical investigations using somatostatin or its analog are controversial, because these trials have low statistical power.

CHRONIC PANCREATITIS

Etiology and Epidemiology

The etiology of chronic pancreatitis includes alcohol in 70% of the cases in Western societies, and it is idiopathic in approximately 20% of cases. Since the mid-1990s, much has been learned about the role of genetic mutations in chronic pancreatitis. Up to 37% of patients with idiopathic chronic pancreatitis have been found to have mutations in the cystic fibrosis gene (CFTR) (27, 28). Mutations in the cationic trypsinogen gene (PRSS1) were identified to cause hereditary pancreatitis in 1996 by Whitcomb and colleagues (29). Hereditary pancreatitis is an autosomal dominant disorder characterized by recurrent attacks of acute pancreatitis starting in childhood or adolescence, with frequent progression to chronic pancreatitis. Witt and associates reported an association of mutations in the serine protease inhibitor, SPINK 1 (PSTI), in 23% of patients with idiopathic chronic pancreatitis (30). Other causes of chronic pancreatitis include tropical (nutritional) pancreatitis, hyperparathyroidism with associated hypercalcemia, hypertrigyceridemia, and obstruction of the pancreatic duct. Regarding tropical or nutritional pancreatitis, the etiology is not clearly understood. Malnutrition and deficiency of certain micronutrients such as zinc, copper, and selenium may cause antioxidant deficiency and

unopposed free radical injury resulting in chronic pancreatitis (31). Tropical pancreatitis is seen in geographic areas within 30 degrees latitude of the equator. Populations with tropical pancreatitis have been studied for genetic mutations, and no association has been found with cystic fibrosis or cationic trypsinogen gene mutations. However, 44% of these persons have been found to carry SPINK 1 mutations, a finding suggesting a genetic predisposition (32).

Of the various causes of chronic pancreatitis, alcohol ingestion is associated with poorest dietary intake and the worst nutritional deficiencies. Both experimental and epidemiologic studies indicate that the risk of alcohol-induced pancreatitis is higher in people consuming a high-fat, high-protein diet (33). The effects of alcohol with a high-protein, high-fat diet appear to be additive. Genetic as well as environmental factors may explain this observation because many patients with chronic alcoholism develop chronic pancreatitis without evidence of a high-fat diet. Moreover, only a few people who drink alcohol develop pancreatic disease, a finding suggesting other genetic and environmental influences in the development of chronic pancreatitis.

The prevalence of chronic pancreatitis in autopsy studies ranges between 0.04 and 5% (34). Clinical studies suggest large differences in prevalence in different parts of the world. A study from Copenhagen in 1978 reported an incidence of 8.2 cases per 100,000 persons (35).

Pathophysiology

Chronic pancreatitis is a progressive inflammatory disease in which irreversible morphologic damage and loss of organ function are accompanied by organ fibrosis. The mechanism resulting in fibrosis is not known. Fibrosis may result from a deregulation of the normal repair process following tissue injury (36). One of the mediators of fibrotic reactions during regeneration in many tissues is transforming growth factor-β (37). This growth factor stimulates the deposition of extracellular matrix, which most likely results in pancreatic gland damage. With progressive pancreatic damage, a decrease in digestive enzyme release from the exocrine pancreatic gland results in nutrient malabsorption. The acinar cells of the pancreas secrete digestive enzymes. The ductal epithelial cells secrete bicarbonate, and the islet cells secrete insulin and other hormones. Approximately 80% of the pancreas gland is made of acinar cells. The proteolytic enzymes, which include trypsinogen, chymotrypsinogen, procarboxypeptidase, and proaminopeptidase, are secreted in the proenzyme form. Enterokinase, an enzyme produced by the duodenal mucosa, converts trypsinogen to trypsin, which then activates the other proteolytic enzymes. The other enzymes, lipase (fat digestion), amylase (carbohydrate digestion), and ribonuclease, are secreted in their active form and therefore do not require activation by trypsin.

Bicarbonate originates from the intralobular and small interlobular ducts of the pancreas. The most potent stimulant of pancreatic enzyme and bicarbonate secretion is secretin. The duodenal pH and duodenal products of fat in the diet influence secretin release. Cholecystokinin (CCK) is the other major gut hormone that controls pancreatic secretion. The hydrolytic products of digestion, including protein and fat, stimulate release of CCK. CCK release occurs within 10 to 30 minutes of eating a protein or fat meal. By stimulation of vagal cholinergic afferent nerves originating in the duodenal mucosa, the pancreatic acinar cells are then stimulated to release the digestive enzymes mentioned earlier. Activated pancreatic enzymes then inhibit the release of CCK and exocrine pancreas secretion. This negative feedback mechanism may have clinical significance in chronic pancreatitis because large doses of exogenous pancreatic enzymes may reduce pancreatic stimulation and may lessen abdominal pain in subgroups of patients with chronic pancreatitis.

Malabsorption does not occur until pancreatic enzyme secretion is reduced to less than 10% of normal (38). Therefore, steatorrhea occurs late in the course of chronic pancreatitis. Lipase secretion decreases earlier than the secretion of proteolytic enzymes. For this reason, fat malabsorption is diagnosed earlier than that of protein. Along with the reduction in enzyme secretion, bicarbonate secretion is also reduced, resulting in a duodenal pH of less than 4. Low duodenal pH inactivates pancreatic enzymes and precipitates bile acids. As a result of intestinal malabsorption, weight loss is one of the presenting features of chronic pancreatitis.

Clinical Presentation

The most common presenting symptom of chronic pancreatitis is abdominal pain. The pain is usually described as a dull, epigastric pain with radiation to the middle back. This pain is usually intermittent and is aggravated by food intake. The mechanism of pain in chronic pancreatitis is unclear. Many patients with presumed chronic pancreatitis have drug-dependent personalities, and it may be very difficult to determine the true cause of a patient's pain. Weight loss is also a common feature of chronic pancreatitis. Weight loss occurs because of malabsorption and a patient's fear of eating; hence daily caloric intake is significantly reduced. The weight loss is usually gradual. Rapid weight loss would suggest another diagnosis such as pancreatic cancer. Steatorrhea occurs when exocrine secretion of pancreatic enzymes is insufficient to maintain normal absorption of dietary fat. The patient may note a change in stool characteristics including oil droplets and stools that float and have a bad odor. Fat-soluble vitamin deficiency (vitamins A, D, E, K) may occur with associated signs and symptoms. Other clinical features of chronic pancreatitis may include symptoms of diabetes mellitus, this is, polyuria and polydipsia. Jaundice may also occur because of common bile duct compression by the inflamed pancreas. Occasionally, a ruptured pancreatic duct may present with ascites and pleural effusions. Early satiety may result from extrinsic compression of the stomach or duodenum by a pancreatic pseudocyst.

Nutrition Assessment

Nutrition assessment begins with taking a history specifically related to the pattern of weight loss and the quantity and quality of a patient's diet. Questions should be asked related to bowel function, including diarrhea and signs to suggest malabsorption such as oil droplets and visualization of undigested food particles in the stool. In addition, patients should be asked whether they have postprandial abdominal pain that is limiting the amount and type of food they consume. If postprandial pain is not limiting their caloric intake, patients should be specifically asked why they think their food intake has been reduced. Patients are usually very insightful regarding the cause. Patients should be referred to a dietitian for appropriate estimation of the type and amount of daily food intake. Often, a written food diary is helpful. Given that alcohol abuse is the leading cause of chronic pancreatitis, an estimation of the amount of alcohol consumption is important. Alcohol is also known as the "empty calorie" (i.e., 7 kcal/kg without protein or vitamins). The relative risk of chronic pancreatitis increases linearly as a function of the amount of alcohol consumed. The amount of alcohol required appears to have no threshold. In most studies, the time between heavy alcohol consumption and chronic pancreatitis is 18 years (39). The duration of alcohol consumption required to produce chronic pancreatitis is shorter than that required to produce cirrhosis of the liver. Patients rarely have both alcohol-induced liver disease and pancreatitis.

The physical examination should begin with accurate height and weight measurements. The body mass index of a patient can be calculated as follows: kg (weight)/m^2 (height). Signs of peripheral edema and ascites should be noted because these conditions will artificially increase a patient's weight. Poor dentition, loss of subcutaneous fat, and loss of temporal muscle mass are other signs of weight loss and inadequate nutrition. Laboratory tests including serum electrolytes, albumin, prothrombin time (vitamin K dependent), and a 72-hour fecal fat determination are also important in the nutritional assessment of a patient. Serum levels of vitamin B$_{12}$ and fat-soluble vitamins should also be checked.

Vitamin B$_{12}$ can bind two carrier proteins in the digestive tract, haptocorrin (R binder) and intrinsic factor, but only its binding to intrinsic factor allows its absorption. The cobalamin-R-protein complex is split by pancreatic enzymes in the duodenum, where cobalamin is bound to intrinsic factor. Malabsorption of vitamin B$_{12}$ is observed in about 30% of adult patients with exocrine pancreatic insufficiency.

Regarding the nutrition ranking of the patient, we use the subjective global assessment score to evaluate the nutritional status of each patient (40). Minimal reduction of food intake with less than 5% loss in body weight is scored A. Evidence of reduced food intake with 5 to 10% weight loss and little evidence of body wasting is scored B. Reduced food intake with greater than 10% weight loss and loss of subcutaneous fat and muscle is scored C. A patient with a score of C is considered severely malnourished, and nutrition support (i.e., oral supplements, tube feeding, or parenteral nutrition) should be considered.

Nutrition Management

Nutritional management begins with an estimation of the caloric requirements of the patient. Caloric needs can be calculated using the Harris-Benedict equation or by indirect calorimetry. Energy requirements using the Harris-Benedict equation can be calculated as follows:

$$^{HB}REE = 66.5 + (13.75 \times W) + (5.0 \times H) - 6.75 \times A \text{ (for men)}$$

$$^{HB}REE = 665.1 + (9.56 \times W) + (1.85 \times H) - (4.676 \times A) \text{ (for women)}$$

where ^{HB}REE = Harris-Benedict REE, W = weight (kg), H = height (cm), and A = age (years). Although energy requirements may be increased by 15 to 30% of what is expected based on the Harris-Benedict equation, excess overfeeding should be avoided (20). Ideally, the patient should be maintained in positive nitrogen balance by feeding total calories based on the Harris-Benedict equation plus 20%, which is approximately 25 to 30 kcal/kg/day. Dietary management begins with total abstinence from alcohol. Prognosis after abstinence from alcohol is controversial. Trapnell reported that 75% of his patients with chronic alcoholic pancreatitis experienced pain relief when they stopped drinking (41). Marks and colleagues found that symptoms did not progress as rapidly once a patient discontinued alcohol consumption (42). Other investigators have found progression of symptoms despite abstinence from alcohol. Despite the controversy, total abstinence should be recommended. Protein should supply approximately 1.0 to 1.5 g/kg/day, lipids should comprise approximately 30% of the total calories, and 40 to 60% of the nutrient mixture should be carbohydrate. Hyperglycemia may occur, and insulin may be required to maintain a serum glucose concentration of less than 200 mg/dL. Glycemia greater than 200 mg/dL results in a greater risk of infection (43). A low-fat diet, with fat making up less than 30% of total calories, should be given to selected patients to minimize steatorrhea. Semielemental diets (e.g., Peptamen) containing fat in the form of medium-chain triglycerides are reported to cause less stimulation of pancreatic exocrine secretion and diarrhea compared with standard formulas of long-chain triglycerides (44–46). Serum triglycerides levels should be maintained at less than 400 mg/dL.

Replacement of combined antioxidants (selenium, methionine, vitamins A, C, and E) has been shown to reduce pancreatic inflammation and pain in patients with both acute and chronic pancreatitis (47–52). Small studies have suggested that daily antioxidants should include 600 μg of organic selenium, 9000 IU of vitamin A, 500 mg of vitamin C, 270 IU of vitamin E, and 2 g of methionine. Antioxidants can be administered in parenteral nutrition as well. In patients given EN, a multivitamin or the oral preparation Selenium ACE (Wassen International, Leatherhead, UK) can be given orally or via feeding tube.

Pancreatic Enzyme Replacement

Treatment of exocrine insufficiency relies on pancreatic enzyme replacement (53). Ingestion of exogenous pancreatic enzymes in sufficient quantities can correct protein malabsorption and can improve steatorrhea. Exogenous preparations vary in the amount of porcine lipase per tablet from 4500 to 20,000 USP. The minimal required dose of lipase is 28,000 IU per meal. Commercially available preparations containing 4500 USP units of lipase would require approximately eight tablets with each meal. Pancreatic lipase is more fragile to an acid environment than is trypsin. Low gastric and duodenal pH (pH<4) will inactivate lipase. Therefore, commercial products of porcine lipase rarely abolish steatorrhea because the ingested lipase is inactivated within the intestinal lumen by acid and proteases. Timing of pill intake in relation to the meal is crucial. We typically recommend one tablet to be taken with the first bite, one tablet with the last bite, and the remaining tablets (particularly in case of non–enteric-coated preparations) taken during the meal. Weight maintenance, symptomatic improvement of diarrhea, and a decrease in 72-hour fecal fat excretion are the goals of therapy. If steatorrhea persists, the addition of a histamine (H_2) antagonist or proton-pump inhibitor (PPI) may be of benefit. If correction with an H_2 antagonist or PPI fails, gastric intubation studies should be performed to adjust the dose of the H_2 blocker or PPI to a pH higher than 4.

Enteric-coated preparations may be also effective (i.e., Creon). Enteric coating is effective only if pancreatic enzymes are delivered to the upper small intestine with ingested food, to allow adequate mixing of the lipolytic activity with each meal. Reduction of steatorrhea using the enteric-coated preparation Pancrease does not appear to be superior to nonenteric preparations (54). Microencapsulated preparations containing large amounts of lipase (75,000–225,000 USP/day) have been withdrawn from the market because of reports of colonic strictures in children with cystic fibrosis (55). Suzuki and colleagues published results showing correction of steatorrhea in dogs using bacterial lipase and a high-fat, high-calorie diet (56, 57). Raimondo and DiMagno reported that, in vitro, lipolytic activity of bacterial lipase (isolated from the bacteria *Burkholderia plantarii*) survives better than porcine lipase in human gastric and duodenal juice in presence of physiologic postprandial concentration of bile acids (58). Clinical studies to confirm the in vitro activity of the bacterial lipase for the correction of steatorrhea in pancreatic exocrine insufficiency are under way.

Pain Management

Appropriate management of a patient's postprandial abdominal pain is also important in the nutritional management of patients with chronic pancreatitis. Abdominal pain is the primary reason that patients require hospitalization. The presumed causes of pain are increased pancreatic duct pressure, entrapment of nerves, and pancreatic ischemia. Several studies in patients with pain from chronic pancreatitis have reported increased intraductal pressure compared with healthy persons (59). Patients with a dilated pancreatic duct have been reported to have improved pain scores following surgical decompression. Pain also appears to decrease spontaneously in advanced phases of chronic pancreatitis as the inflammatory process is replaced by fibrosis. Exogenous administration of pancreatic enzymes may also reduce pain associated with chronic pancreatitis. Three controlled studies reported pain relief in 73% of patients treated with non–enteric-coated pancreatic enzymes (60–62). Two other studies showed that oral administration of pancreatic enzymes did not significantly relieve abdominal pain compared with placebo (63, 64). A metaanalysis of pancreatic enzyme supplementation to reduce pain in patients with chronic pancreatitis failed to show a beneficial effect (65).

Oral analgesics are often necessary to treat a patient's pain. Nonsteroidal antiinflammatory medications may be useful in some cases. If these medications are not helpful, narcotics may be needed. Referral to a specialized pain clinic is very important in our opinion, given the high degree of narcotic dependency in this patient population. Dosing 30 to 60 minutes before mealtime may also be helpful in reducing a patient's postprandial abdominal pain. For patients in whom medications fail, celiac plexus block using steroids may be helpful. However, the effect is usually short-lived, lasting approximately 6 months or less, and repeat treatment is usually required (66). For patients with pain despite analgesia and celiac plexus block, an endoscopic or surgical approach should be considered. Appropriate candidates for each method will depend on the pancreatic duct characteristics on imaging studies.

Patient Monitoring

The goals of nutrition therapy in patients with chronic pancreatitis are to maintain weight, to ensure a proper supply of vitamins and minerals, to minimize stool fat loss, and to maintain adequate control of the patient's abdominal pain. Patients should weigh themselves once weekly and should report any significant weight loss to their health care provider. Patients should also work closely with a dietitian to monitor caloric intake. If a patient has inadequate caloric intake, oral supplements or enteral feeding may be necessary. Monitoring the effect of pancreatic enzyme replacement on the steatorrhea by a 72-hour fecal fat collection should be documented. Monitoring the patient's abdominal pain is also necessary because as postprandial abdominal pain increases, the patient's oral intake will decrease, resulting in weight loss. Serum levels of fat-soluble vitamins and of vitamin B_{12} should be evaluated biannually.

PANCREATIC CANCER

In pancreatic cancer, at least a component of weight loss is due to increased REE likely related to the production of proinflammatory cytokines (67). The administration of a nutritional supplement containing fish oil to patients with pancreatic cancer has been shown to induce an increase in weight, an increase in fasting insulin concentration, a decrease in REE and a normalization of the metabolic cost of feeding and substrate utilization. It has been shown previously that fish oil lowers the production of proinflammatory cytokines in cancer patients (68). Fish oil–enriched nutritional supplement may be beneficial in reversing weight loss in cachectic patients with cancer by modulating the metabolic response to feeding, thus explaining the improved response to nutritional support (69).

In addition, a common error in patients with pancreatic cancer is to not recognize that malabsorption is an important cause of weight loss. About 75 to 80% of pancreatic adenocarcinomas, the type of 90% of pancreatic cancers, arise in the head of the pancreas and are associated with obstruction of the pancreatic duct and severe exocrine pancreatic insufficiency. Furthermore, some patients who undergo the standard radical pancreaticoduodenectomy require enzyme replacement therapy, and their treatment should be optimized with aggressive pancreatic enzyme replacement. These patients should receive pancreatin as described for the treatment of chronic pancreatitis. In our experience, steatorrhea and creatorrhea can be appreciably improved. For full discussion of nutrition in pancreatic cancer, see Chapter 83.

SUMMARY

During the initial stages of acute pancreatitis, eliminate oral intake and maintain hydration with intravenous fluids. EN with placement of a nasojejunal tube (by radiologic or endoscopic guidance) is needed if recovery takes longer than several days. Replace the jejunal feedings by the parenteral route if paralytic ileus ensues and if prolonged nutritional support is necessary because of the presence of complications (abscesses or pseudocysts). Oral intake is started when clinical findings suggest a resolution of inflammation.

During early chronic pancreatitis in patients with abdominal pain but no steatorrhea, a diet low in fat, low in protein, and high in carbohydrate is indicated. Preliminary data suggest that during the late stage of the disease, a diet containing high fat, low protein, and moderate carbohydrate along with sufficient amount of lipolytic activity (bacterial or porcine lipase) is capable of improving steatorrhea by increasing the coefficient of fat absorption (57). TPN is indicated for complications of chronic pancreatitis (e.g., severe exacerbation, ascites, symptomatic pseudocyst) or in patients following pancreatic surgery for pain control. Most patients with pancreatic cancer have malabsorption and require appropriate treatment with pancreatic enzymes.

REFERENCES

1. Rau B, Baumgart K, Kruger CM et al. Intensive Care Med 2003;29:622–9.
2. Roscher R, Beger HG. Bacterial infection of pancreatic necrosis. In: Beger HG, Bèuchler M, eds. Acute Pancreatitis: Research and Clinical Management. Berlin: Springer-Verlag, 1987:314–7.
3. Ranson JH, Rifkind KM, Roses DF et al. Surg Gynecol Obstet 1974;139:69–81.
4. Bank S, Wise L, Gersten M. Am J Gastroenterol 1983;78:637–40.
5. Agarwal N, Pitchumoni CS. Pancreas 1986;1:69–73.
6. Corfield AP, Cooper MJ, Williamson RC et al. Lancet 1985;2:403–7.
7. Demmy TL, Burch JM, Feliciano DV et al. Am J Surg 1988;156:492–6.
8. Larvin M, McMahon MJ. Lancet 1989;2:201–5.
9. Wilson C, Heath DI, Imrie CW. Br J Surg 1990;77:1260–4.
10. Stanten R, Frey CF. Arch Surg 1990;125:1269–74.
11. Larvin M, Chalmers AG, Robinson PJ et al. Br J Surg 1989;76:465–71.
12. Karimgani I, Porter KA, Langevin RE et al. Gastroenterology 1992;103:1636–40.
13. Lankisch PG, Warnecke B, Bruns D et al. Pancreas 2002;24:217–22.
14. Balthazar EJ, Ranson JH, Naidich DP et al. Radiology 1985;156:767–72.
15. Balthazar EJ, Robinson DL, Megibow AJ et al. Radiology 1990;174:331–6.
16. Lankisch PG, Burchard-Reckert S, Lehnick D. Gut 1999;44:542–4.
17. Yadav D, Agarwal N, Pitchumoni CS. Am J Gastroenterol 2002;97:1309–18.
18. Boivin M, Lanspa SJ, Zinsmeister AR et al. Gastroenterology 1990;99:1763–71.
19. Holtmann G, Kelly DG, DiMagno EP. Gut 1996;38:920–4.
20. Dickerson RN, Vehe KL, Mullen JL et al. Crit Care Med 1991;19:484–90.
21. McClave SA, Greene LM, Snider HL et al. JPEN J Parenter Enteral Nutr 1997;21:14–20.
22. Kalfarentzos F, Kehagias J, Mead N et al. Br J Surg 1997;84:1665–9.
23. Windsor AC, Kanwar S, Li AG et al. Gut 1998;42:431–5.
24. Powell JJ, Murchison JT, Fearon KC et al. Br J Surg 2000;87:1375–81.
25. Abou-Assi S, Craig K, O'Keefe SJ. Am J Gastroenterol 2002;97:2255–62.
26. Grant JP, James S, Grabowski V et al. Ann Surg 1984;200:627–31.
27. Sharer N, Schwarz M, Malone G et al. N Engl J Med 1998;339:645–52.
28. Cohn JA, Friedman KJ, Noone PG et al. N Engl J Med 1998;339:653–8.
29. Whitcomb DC, Gorry MC, Preston RA et al. Nat Genet 1996;14:141–5.
30. Witt H, Luck W, Hennies HC et al. Nat Genet 2000;25:213–6.
31. Pitchumoni CS. Clin Gastroenterol 1984;13:941–59.
32. Durno C, Corey M, Zielenski J et al. Gastroenterology 2002;123:1857–64.
33. Levy P, Mathurin P, Roqueplo A et al. Pancreas 1995;10:231–8.
34. Skyhoj Olsen T. Acta Pathol Microbiol Scand 1978;86:361.
35. Copenhagen Pancreatitis Study Scand J Gastroenterol 1981;16:305–12.
36. Rodemann HP, Binder A, Burger A et al. Kidney Int Suppl 1996;54:S32–6.
37. Roberts AB, Heine UI, Flanders KC et al. Ann NY Acad Sci 1990;580:225–32.
38. DiMagno EP, Go VL, Summerskill WH. N Engl J Med 1973;288:813–5.
39. Almela P, Aparisi L, Grau F et al. Rev Esp Enferm Dig 1997;89:741–6, 747–52.
40. Detsky AS, McLaughlin JR, Baker JP et al. JPEN J Parenter Enteral Nutr 1987;11:8–13.
41. Trapnell JE. Br J Surg 1979;66:471–5.
42. Marks IN, Girdwood AH, Bank S et al. S Afr Med J 1980;57:640–3.
43. Alexiewicz JM, Kumar D, Smogorzewski M et al. Ann Intern Med 1995;123:919–24.
44. Keith RG. Surg Gynecol Obstet 1980;151:337–43.
45. Vison N, Hecketsweiler P, Butel J et al. Gut 1978;19:194–8.
46. Shea JC, Bishop MD, Parker EM et al. Pancreatology 2003;3:36–40.
47. Braganza JM, Jeffrey IJ, Foster J et al. Pancreas 1987;2:489–94.
48. Braganza JM, Thomas A, Robinson A. Int J Pancreatol 1988;3:209–16.
49. Uden S, Bilton D, Nathan L et al. Aliment Pharmacol Ther 1990;4:357–71.
50. DeWaele B, Vierendeels T, Willems G. Clin Nutr 1992;11:83.
51. Mathew P, Wyllie R, Van Lente F et al. Am J Gastroenterol 1996;91:1558–62.
52. Van Gossum A, Closset P, Noel E et al. Dig Dis Sci 1996;41:1225–31.
53. Layer P, Keller J. Pancreas 2003;26:1–7.
54. Layer P, Go VL, DiMagno EP. Am J Physiol 1986;251:G475–80.
55. Taylor CJ. Lancet 1994;343:615–6.
56. Suzuki A, Mizumoto A, Rerknimitr R et al. Gastroenterology 1999;116:431–7.
57. Suzuki A, Mizumoto A, Sarr MG et al. Gastroenterology 1997;112:2048–55.
58. Raimondo M, DiMagno EP. Gastroenterology 1994;107:231–5.
59. Ebbehoj N, Borly L, Bulow J et al. Scand J Gastroenterol 1990;25:1046–51.
60. Isaksson G, Ihse I. Dig Dis Sci 1983;28:97–102.
61. Ramo OJ, Puolakkainen PA, Seppala K et al. Scand J Gastroenterol 1989;24:688–92.
62. Slaff J, Jacobson D, Tillman CR et al. Gastroenterology 1984;87:44–52.
63. Halgreen H, Pedersen NT, Worning H. Scand J Gastroenterol 1986;21:104–8.
64. Mossner J, Secknus R, Meyer J et al. Digestion 1992;53:54–66.
65. Brown A, Hughes M, Tenner S et al. Am J Gastroenterol 1997;92:2032–5.
66. Pap A, Nauss LA, DiMagno EP. Pancreas 1990;5:725–9.
67. Falconer JS, Fearon KC, Plester CE et al. Ann Surg 1994;219:325–31.
68. Barber MD, Ross JA, Voss AC et al. Br J Cancer 1999;81:80–6.
69. Barber MD, McMillan DC, Preston T et al. Clin Sci (Lond) 2000;98:389–99.

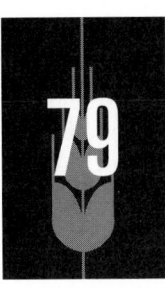

79 NUTRITION IN LIVER DISORDERS AND THE ROLE OF ALCOHOL[1]

CHARLES S. LIEBER

ROLE OF THE LIVER IN MAINTAINING NORMAL
   NUTRITION 1235
     Bile Salts 1235
     Intermediary Metabolism 1236
NUTRITIONAL CONSEQUENCES OF LIVER INJURY ...1236
     Acute Liver Injury 1236
     Chronic Liver Injury 1237
     Dietary Intake 1237
     Maldigestion and Malabsorption 1237
     Metabolic Changes 1237
NUTRITIONAL THERAPY OF LIVER DISORDERS 1237
     Protein and Amino Acids: Treatment and
       Prevention of Hepatic Encephalopathy 1237
     Choline, Methionine, and
       S-Adenosyl-ʟ-Methionine 1238
     Carbohydrates 1241
     Lipids, Fatty Liver, Hyperlipidemia,
       and Ketoacidosis 1242
     Nonalcoholic Fatty Liver and Steatohepatitis 1244
     Vitamins 1245
EFFECT OF NUTRITION ON THE LIVER 1245
NUTRITIONAL VALUE OF ALCOHOLIC BEVERAGES ...1246
NUTRITIONAL STATUS OF PATIENTS WITH
   ALCOHOLISM 1247
EFFECTS OF ETHANOL ON DIGESTION AND
   ABSORPTION 1248
     Gastrointestinal Tract 1248
     Bile Salts 1249
     Pancreatitis and Pancreatic Insufficiency 1249
     Alterations of Nutrient Metabolism 1249
EFFECT OF ETHANOL ON THE METABOLISM
   OF URIC ACID 1253
EFFECTS OF DIETARY FACTORS ON ETHANOL
   METABOLISM 1253

ALCOHOL, NUTRITION, AND ORGAN DAMAGE
   IN PATIENTS WITH ALCOHOLISM 1254
     Liver 1254
     Stroke 1254
     Heart 1255
     Blood and Bone Marrow 1255
SUMMARY OF NUTRITIONAL THERAPY
   IN ALCOHOLISM 1255

The interactions among liver function, nutrition, and exogenous factors such as medications and other potential toxins, predominantly alcohol, are complex. The functional integrity of the liver is essential for the proper use of nutrients. This chapter first delineates the liver's role in nutritional status. Next, the nutritional complications of liver dysfunction and corrective approaches are assessed. Nutritional factors that may themselves result in liver injury are discussed, and the role of alcoholism as a prominent example of the actions of toxins is reviewed. More detailed information, including additional older literature references, can be found elsewhere (1, 2).

ROLE OF THE LIVER IN MAINTAINING NORMAL NUTRITION

Bile Salts

Bile salts are synthesized in the liver from cholesterol, are secreted in bile, and are mixed with the intestinal contents in response to a meal. In the intestine, bile salts are active in the intraluminal phase of fat assimilation, its principal action being that of a detergent. Triglycerides enter the duodenum in the form of an emulsion. The surface of this emulsion is covered by a relatively polar layer of phospholipids and proteins that must be removed by bile salts before lipolysis via pancreatic lipase can proceed.

The products of lipolysis form mixed micelles with bile salts promote the intestinal uptake of long-chain fatty acids. In contrast, the absorption of short- and medium-chain fatty acids proceeds in the absence of bile (3). Following uptake of fatty acids, bile salts are conserved by being recycled through an enterohepatic circulation. Bile salts, especially cholic acid, a conjugate of trihydroxy bile acid, are reabsorbed from the distal small bowel by an

[1] **Abbreviations: ADH,** alcohol dehydrogenase; **BCAA,** branched-chain amino acids; **CoA,** coenzyme A; **DLPC,** dilinoleophosphatidylcholine; **HDL,** high-density lipoprotein; **LDL,** low-density lipoprotein; **MEOS,** microsomal ethanol oxidizing system; **NAD,** nicotinamide adenine dinucleotide (-H reduced); **NAFL,** nonalcoholic fatty liver; **NAFLD,** nonalcoholic fatty liver disease; **NASH,** nonalcoholic steatohepatitis; **PC,** phosphatidylcholine; **PPC,** polyenylphosphatidylcholine; **SAMe,** S-adenosly-ʟ-methionine; **VLDL,** very-low-density lipoprotein.

active, sodium-dependent process. Dihydroxy bile salts are absorbed by passive diffusion from the proximal small bowel. The liver extracts these reabsorbed bile salts from the portal vein blood and returns them to the biliary tree. Hepatic synthesis of bile salts replenishes the fraction of the bile salt pool that escapes reabsorption and is excreted in the feces.

Intermediary Metabolism

The liver plays a fundamental role in intermediary metabolism. Only highlights are covered here, to allow an overall view for the understanding of the nutritional complications of liver injury.

Carbohydrates

The liver regulates the synthesis, storage, and breakdown of glycogen, a polymeric form of glucose. Large amounts of glycogen can be stored within the hepatocyte without major effects on the intracellular osmotic pressure. Glycogen is formed when the intake of glucose (or other gluconeogenic fuels) exceeds energy requirements; glycogen is broken down when intake lags behind energy needs. The principal enzymes controlling glycogenesis and glycogenolysis are glycogen synthase and phosphorylase, respectively. A reciprocal relationship exists between these two enzymes. Stimulation of glycogen synthetase is usually accompanied by inhibition of phosphorylase, and vice versa. Factors that control these enzymes include intracellular levels of glucose-6-phosphate and hormones such as epinephrine, glucagon, and insulin. Epinephrine and glucagon raise blood glucose levels by activating phosphorylase whereas insulin lowers blood glucose, in part by stimulating glycogen synthetase.

Hepatocytes also possess enzymes that enable them to synthesize glucose from various precursors such as amino acids, pyruvate, and lactate (gluconeogenesis). It is well established that hypoglycemia promotes this process. The link between hypoglycemia and gluconeogenesis is probably mediated by the secretion of cortisol from the adrenal medulla. Cortisol secretion is under pituitary control (adrenocorticotropic hormone) and mobilizes glycogenic amino acids from various tissues.

Fat

The liver is a major site of fatty acid breakdown and triglyceride synthesis. The breakdown of fatty acids provides an alternative source of energy when glucose is unavailable, as during fasting or starvation. Triglycerides in adipose tissue are hydrolyzed to release fatty acids. Bound to albumin in the blood, the released fatty acids are rapidly removed by the hepatocyte and are transported into the mitochondria by a carnitine-mediated process. Within the mitochondria, numerous enzymes degrade the fatty acid molecule to acetyl coenzyme A

(CoA) fragments, a sequence known as β-oxidation. In turn, acetyl CoA can enter the citric acid cycle and generate adenosine triphosphate by oxidative phosphorylation. Triglyceride synthesis occurs when carbohydrate intake exceeds energy requirements; under such conditions, glucose may overwhelm the glycogen reservoir, and the acetyl CoA generated by glycolysis is not needed for oxidative phosphorylation. During such times of nutrient abundance, acetyl CoA is converted to fatty acids, and ultimately, triglycerides, which are transported to the adipose tissues as part of the very-low-density lipoproteins (VLDLs).

Proteins

The liver plays a central role in the synthesis and degradation of protein. Plasma proteins, including albumin, coagulation factors, transferrin, and ceruloplasmin, constitute about one half of the protein synthesized in the liver. These export proteins are synthesized on the rough endoplasmic reticulum. Protein synthesis by the liver is influenced by the nutritional state, as well as by hormones and alcohol. Insulin and steroids stimulate the synthesis of hepatic proteins, whereas glucagon inhibits synthesis and promotes their degradation.

As reviewed elsewhere (4), the effect of ethanol per se on overall protein metabolism, measured as nitrogen balance, is nitrogen sparing when ethanol is given as additional calories, but it causes increased urinary urea when given as an isocaloric substitute for carbohydrate. Ethanol interferes with amino acid absorption in the gut; given in single doses, it causes impaired hepatic amino acid uptake, decreased gluconeogenesis, decreased leucine oxidation, increased serum branched-chain amino acids (BCAAs), and impaired synthesis of lipoproteins, albumin (5), and fibrinogen. Given over time, ethanol impairs protein secretion from the liver, probably related to alterations in microtubles and retention of proteins in enlarged hepatocytes (6).

NUTRITIONAL CONSEQUENCES OF LIVER INJURY

Acute Liver Injury

Regardless of cause, acute liver injury is often associated with anorexia, nausea, and vomiting. When the liver injury is the result of alcohol, these symptoms may be exacerbated by concomitant alcoholic gastritis. Thus, acute liver injury is likely to decrease the oral intake of food, but if the illness is short-lived, nutritional consequences are minimal. Both alcoholic and nonalcoholic acute liver injury may cause fasting hypoglycemia. This has been attributed to depleted liver glycogen reserves and a block in gluconeogenesis form amino acids (see the discussion of carbohydrates later, in the section on nutritional therapy of liver disorders).

Chronic Liver Injury

Nutritional complications are frequent when liver functions become impaired in chronic liver injury, particularly cirrhosis. Regardless of origin, cirrhosis is likely to cause patients to have abnormal anthropometric measurements (i.e., muscle wasting) and to be anergic to common antigens on skin testing (7). Circulating levels of both fat- and water-soluble vitamins are low in a high percentage of patients with alcoholic cirrhosis. Low serum levels of fat-soluble vitamins (rather than the water-soluble variety) are more characteristic of nonalcoholic cirrhosis (8). These nutritional deficiencies arise as a result of inadequate dietary intake, maldigestion, malabsorption, and/or defective metabolism.

Dietary Intake

Inadequate intake of protein is common, especially among patients with alcoholism and cirrhosis. Indeed, if a patient with alcoholism continues to drink, protein intake may be low, and the bulk of dietary calories may be derived from carbohydrates and alcohol. Calories derived from alcohol are, in a sense, "empty" because alcoholic beverages are devoid of proteins, minerals, vitamins, and significant amounts of carbohydrate. Furthermore, their actual caloric contribution has been shown to be less than that of an equivalent amount of carbohydrates, as discussed later in the section on the nutritional value of alcoholic beverages. Changes in mental status that result from hepatic encephalopathy may also contribute to the poor intake of patients with advanced liver disease. Hepatic coma, in turn, is likely to result in hospitalization, which may exacerbate nutritional deficiencies in these patients. Malnutrition in hospitalized patients arises as a result of both diagnostic (radiologic or endoscopic procedures) and therapeutic (e.g., variceal sclerotherapy) interventions.

Maldigestion and Malabsorption

Decreases in bile salt secretion and pool size have been demonstrated in patients with cirrhosis (9). In light of the role of bile salts in fat digestion (see the discussion of bile salts), a contraction of the bile salt pool results, as expected, in impaired micelle formation and leads to abnormalities of fat absorption, especially in patients with underlying pancreatic insufficiency. Steatorrhea, in turn, causes deficiencies in fat-soluble vitamins with corresponding clinical manifestations (see later).

Metabolic Changes

Defects in protein metabolism in patients with chronic liver failure include decreased hepatic synthesis of export proteins (see earlier), decreased urea synthesis, and decreased metabolism of aromatic amino acids. Decreased synthesis of plasma proteins may lead to hypoalbuminemia and may exacerbate the formation of ascites in patients with portal hypertension. Depressed levels of coagulation factors may predispose these patients to the risk of gastrointestinal hemorrhage. The failure to detoxify ammonia and the abnormal amino acid profile of patients with cirrhosis may, in part, increase the likelihood of hepatic encephalopathy. Despite the abnormalities in intermediary metabolism, overall nitrogen balance can be maintained at positive levels by amounts of dietary protein similar to those in persons who do not have cirrhosis (35–50 g/day).

Glucose tolerance is frequently abnormal in the cirrhotic patient and has been linked to insulin resistance (see later). Furthermore, because glycogen stores are often depleted in the cirrhotic liver, fatty acid oxidation appears to supplant glucose as a source of fuel during fasting.

Abnormalities of water- and fat-soluble vitamins are common in patients with cirrhosis. In addition to inadequate intake and decreased uptake, vitamin metabolism per se may be deranged in chronic liver injury, as reviewed elsewhere (10). Defects have been described in the phosphorylation of thiamin by patients with alcoholic cirrhosis, in the synthesis of retinol-binding protein, in the degradation of pyridoxal-5'-phosphate, and in the conversion of vitamin D to its active form. Hepatic vitamin A levels are depressed by both heavy alcohol consumption and drug use (11, 12). It is conceivable that part of the hepatic depletion may result from mobilization inasmuch as hepatic lipoprotein secretion is increased by long-term alcohol consumption (13). Induced hepatic microsomes may enhance the degradation of both retinol and retinoic acid (14–16). As a result of these derangements, vitamin repletion strategies require modification in patients with liver failure, as discussed in the following section.

NUTRITIONAL THERAPY OF LIVER DISORDERS

Protein and Amino Acids: Treatment and Prevention of Hepatic Encephalopathy

To the extent that patients with liver injury, either acute or chronic, are in negative nitrogen balance, it has been assumed that liver regeneration will be delayed and muscle wasting will be accelerated. However, when feeding protein or administering amino acids, one must be aware of the precarious balance between the need to restore protein intake and the potential risk of precipitating hepatic encephalopathy. Often only a small margin of safety exists in this respect. The amount of dietary protein that can be tolerated will vary considerably. At times, only minimal amounts of protein can be ingested without altering the patient's mental state. Under such circumstances, the breakdown of remaining protein stores can be minimized by the provision of calories in the form of fats and carbohydrates.

In acute liver injury, much work has focused on the role of protein or amino acid supplementation on the outcome of alcoholic hepatitis. Both enteral and parenteral routes have been employed in these investigations. In general, studies in patients with acute hepatitis have demonstrated that hepatic encephalopathy can usually be avoided by judicious titration of dietary protein, that relatively little dietary protein can be associated with positive nitrogen balance, and that symptomatic as well as biochemical improvement (if not prognosis) can be expected (17). However, temporary reduction of dietary protein to less than required levels may be necessary to overcome episodes of acute liver failure.

Positive nitrogen balance can be attained in patients with chronic liver injury (cirrhosis) with daily amounts of dietary protein (0.74 g/kg) similar to that required by physiologically normal persons (18). Conflicting results have been obtained regarding the extent to which the source of the dietary protein (animal or vegetable) affects overall nitrogen balance (19).

Attempts have been made to normalize the plasma amino acid pattern found in patients with cirrhosis. The ratio of the BCAAs isoleucine, leucine, valine, and lysine to aromatic amino acids (phenylalanine, tryptophan, and tyrosine) is abnormally low in these patients, especially those who are malnourished. Investigators hoped that correction of the abnormal amino acid profile in patients with cirrhosis would be beneficial in the treatment of hepatic encephalopathy. To this end, mixtures with high ratios of BCAAs to aromatic amino acids were administered, and the source of protein has been varied (e.g., using vegetable-derived protein relatively lacking in aromatic amino acids). A potential benefit seemed plausible in light of the false neurotransmitter hypothesis of Fischer and Baldessarini (20). In this scheme, the entry of aromatic amino acids into the brain is favored by low plasma levels of BCAAs. In the brain, sympathomimetic amines are generated from these aromatic amino acids, especially phenylalanine, the presence of which hinders neuronal transmission by competitive interactions with bona fide neurotransmitters at the receptor level. Initial human studies involving infusion of BCAA-enriched amino acid mixtures were encouraging, but these early clinical trials were not fully controlled or randomized (21). Using tighter designs, most subsequent studies failed to confirm the efficacy of intravenous or orally administered enriched mixtures in treating acute hepatic encephalopathy, and most of the evidence does not support the routine clinical use of these mixtures in acute encephalopathy (22). However, it remains possible that a subset of protein-intolerant patients with chronic encephalopathy (and better liver function) may benefit from BCAAs (23).

Some success has been achieved in treating hepatic encephalopathy using protein derived from vegetable sources. However, improvement in encephalopathy did not correlate with changes in the plasma amino acid profile. As a result, investigators have suggested that the beneficial effects of vegetable protein are mediated by fiber content rather than by amino acid composition per se (24). Fiber may increase the elimination of nitrogenous waste, but the high fiber content of these diets is poorly tolerated.

Dietary restrictions of amino acids or protein are important in certain inherited liver abnormalities, including disorders of the urea cycle and hypertyrosinemia (see Chapter 58).

Choline, Methionine, and *S*-Adenosyl-ʟ-Methionine

For several decades, protein, methionine, and choline deficiencies have been implicated in the pathogenesis of liver injury. In growing rats, deficiencies in dietary protein and lipotropic factors (choline and methionine) can produce a fatty liver (25), and investigators have reported that ethanol increases choline requirements in the rat (26), possibly by enhancing choline oxidation (27). Primates, however, are far less susceptible to protein and lipotrope deficiency than are rodents (28). Clinically, choline treatment of patients suffering from alcoholic liver injury was found to be ineffective in the presence of continued alcohol abuse (29). Human liver contains very little choline oxidase activity, and this may explain the species differences with regard to choline deficiency. In humans, choline deficiency (and thus a need for choline supplementation) has been documented in only very limited circumstances of extremely restricted diets (30). Moreover, in baboons fed ethanol, fatty liver as well as fibrosis (including cirrhosis) developed (31, 32) (Fig. 79.1), with striking ultrastructural changes (33), despite an amount of choline given at twice the dose recommended for the baboon. Nevertheless, because the possibility existed that massive choline supplementation could have a favorable effect on the process, this was the subject of an experimental study in baboons. These animals were given either normal or choline-supplemented diets (fivefold the recommended amount) with or without ethanol. Choline supplementation failed to prevent alcohol-induced steatosis and fibrosis. All parameters remained normal in the eight baboons fed the regular control diet. However, in the choline-supplemented controls, serum bilirubin, aspartate aminotransferase , and glutamate dehydrogenase activities increased moderately, and serum albumin decreased. Occasional fat droplets appeared in hepatocytes with mitochondrial changes (enlargement and alterations of the cristae) and an abundance of "myelin" figures in the cytoplasm, findings indicating that the choline excess had exerted moderate hepatotoxicity (34). We concluded that massive choline supplementation does not prevent alcoholic liver injury but, in fact, may be hepatotoxic.

Liberal supplementation with methionine (31) also failed to prevent alcohol-induced liver injury, including cirrhosis, from developing in baboons. In human patients as well, methionine supplementation was contemplated for the treatment of liver diseases, especially alcoholic disorders, but some difficulties have been encountered. Indeed, excess methionine was shown to have some adverse effects (35). Furthermore, whereas circulating methionine levels are normal in some patients with alcoholic liver disease, in others, elevated levels were reported

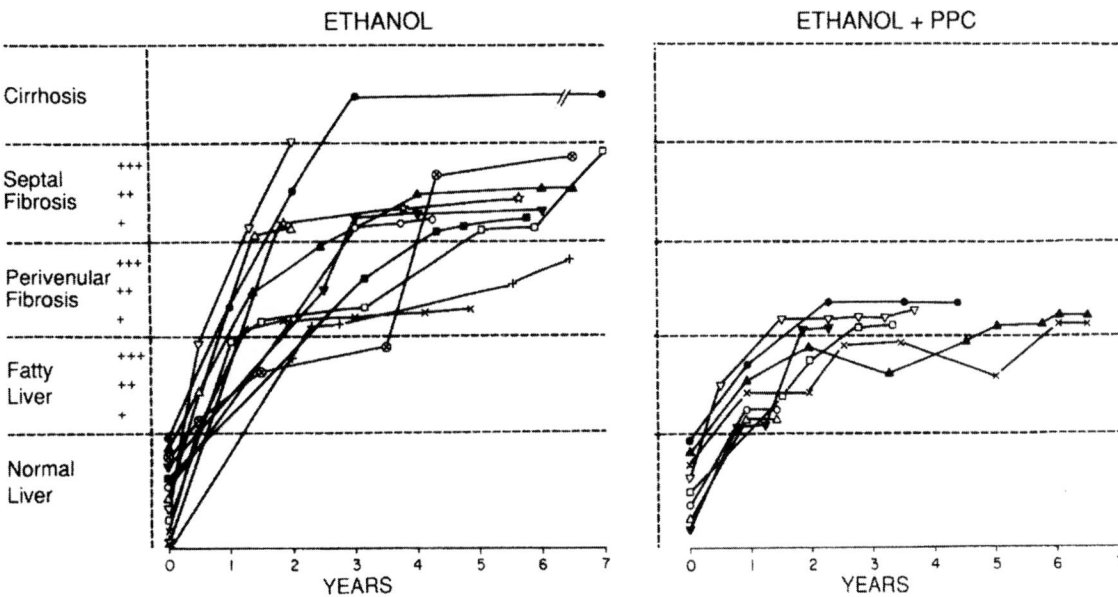

Figure 79.1. Sequential development of alcoholic liver injury in baboons fed ethanol with an adequate diet **(left)** and prevention of septal fibrosis and cirrhosis by supplementation with polyenylphosphatidylcholine (PPC) **(right)**. Liver morphology in animals pair fed control diets (with or without PPC) remained normal (not shown). Whereas no cirrhosis or septal fibrosis developed in the animals fed alcohol with PPC, in the aggregate, 67 baboons fed ethanol with adequate diets (usually for 5 years) in this (32), as well as other (29, 40, 277) studies, cirrhosis developed in 14, and septal fibrosis was observed in an additional 14 animals, an incidence comparable to that observed in patients with alcoholism. (Data from Lieber CS, Robins SJ, Li J et al. Phosphatidylcholine protects against fibrosis and cirrhosis in the baboon. Gastroenterology 1994;106:152–9.)

(36). Moreover, a delay in the clearance of plasma methionine was observed after its systemic administration to patients with liver damage or after an oral load (37). Because about half of the methionine is metabolized by the liver, the foregoing observations suggested impaired hepatic metabolism of this amino acid in patients with alcoholic liver disease. Indeed, Martin-Duce and colleagues (38) reported decreases of S-adenosyl-L-methionine (SAMe) synthetase activities in cirrhotic liver. Long-term alcohol consumption was found to be associated with enhanced methionine utilization and depletion (39). As a consequence, one could anticipate SAMe depletion as well as its decreased availability. Therefore, the baboon model of alcohol-induced liver injury was used to verify the latter hypothesis and to explore the possibility that SAMe repletion could oppose some of the adverse effects of alcohol on the liver (40). This study revealed that, in the baboon, long-term ethanol consumption is indeed associated with a significant depletion of hepatic SAMe, and SAMe supplementation attenuates ethanol-induced liver injury. The significant hepatic SAMe depletion in primates after long-term ethanol consumption (40) results, in part, from increased utilization of reduced glutathione (GSH) secondary to enhanced free radical and acetaldehyde generation by the induced microsomal ethanol oxidizing system (MEOS) (Fig. 79.2), as well as by GSH leakage (41). Under these conditions, increased GSH turnover may ensue, as evidenced by a rise in α-amino-n-butyric acid (see Fig. 79.2; 79.3). However, the production of SAMe may become rate limiting, especially because the activity

of the corresponding synthetase is decreased in cirrhosis (38). As a consequence of this enzymic defect, SAMe depletion ensues, and methionine supplementation may be ineffective in alcoholic liver disease, whereas SAMe can correct the defect.

Potentially, SAMe depletion may have numerous adverse effects. SAMe is the principal methylating agent in various vital transmethylation reactions including those involved in nucleic acid and protein synthesis. Investigators have demonstrated that methylation is also important to cell membrane function (42), with a role of phospholipid methylation in membrane fluidity and the transport of metabolites and transmission of signals across membranes. Thus, decreased SAMe, by being detrimental for methyl-transferase activity, may promote the membrane injury that has been documented in alcohol-induced liver damage (43). Not only is SAMe the methyl donor in almost all transmethylation reactions, but also it plays a key role in the synthesis of polyamines and provides one of the sources of cysteine needed for glutathione production. Alcohol-induced depletion of glutathione has been shown to be particularly striking in primates (40, 44). Thus, replenishment of methionine (in its activated form SAMe) may be particularly indicated in primates subjected to an alcoholic insult.

Replenishment of the hepatocyte with SAMe is feasible through ingestion of the compound; it has been shown that blood levels of SAMe are increased after oral administration in humans (45). Although investigators have claimed that the liver does not take up SAMe from the bloodstream (46), other results have indicated uptake of SAMe by isolated

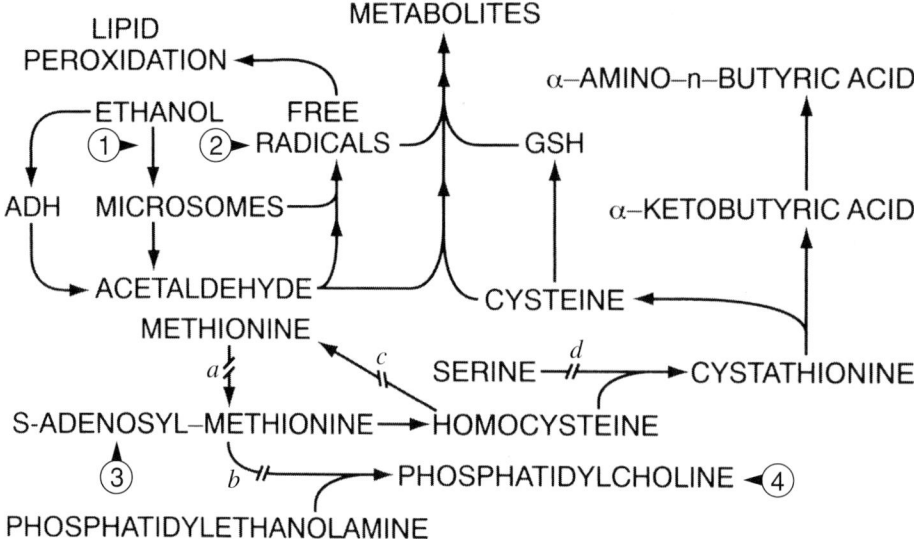

Figure 79.2. Lipid peroxidation and other consequences of alcoholic liver disease and/or increased free radical generation and acetaldehyde production by ethanol-induced microsomes, with sites of possible therapeutic interventions. Metabolic blocks caused by liver disease (a,b), folate (c), vitamin B$_{12}$ (c), or vitamin B$_6$ (d) deficiencies are illustrated, with corresponding depletions in S–adenosylmethionine, phosphatidylcholine, and glutathione (GSH). New therapeutic approaches include (1) downregulation of microsomal enzyme induction, especially of CYP2E1, (2) decrease of free radicals with antioxidants, and replenishment of S–adenosylmethionine (3) and of phosphatidylcholine (4). ADH, alcohol dehydrogenase. (From Lieber CS. Alcoholic liver disease: new insights in pathogenesis lead to new treatments. J Hepatol 2000;32:113–28, with permission.)

hepatocytes, as reviewed elsewhere (47). Results in baboons (40) also clearly indicated hepatic uptake of exogenous SAMe. Furthermore, in these baboons, the ethanol-induced hepatic SAMe depletion was partially corrected with oral SAMe administration. Because the SAMe transport system does not appear to be saturated under physiologic conditions, it is likely that SAMe levels in biologic compartments regulate, at least in part, the rate of transport

across membranes. Indeed, hepatic levels of SAMe are increased with increasing extracellular levels (48), and the intracellular concentrations reached are greater than or close to the Michaelis-Menten constant for SAMe of both phospholipid methyltransferase (49, 50) and catechol-O-methyltransferase (51). Furthermore, the effective utilization of SAMe for both transmethylation and transsulfuration has been demonstrated in vivo (52).

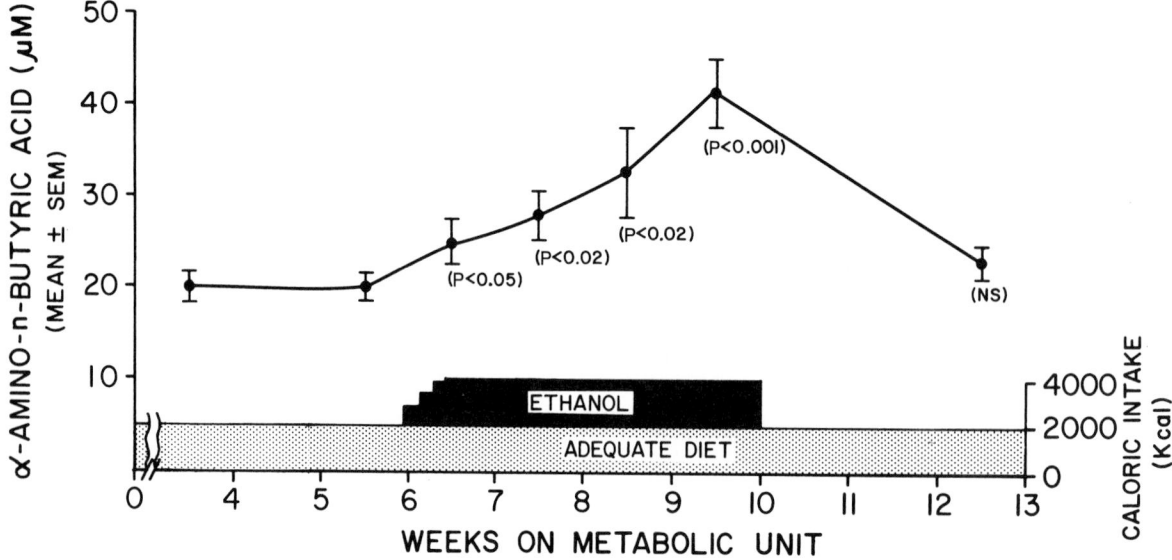

Figure 79.3. Effect of ethanol consumption on plasma α-amino-n-butyric acid (mean ± SEM). Consumption of ethanol (4 g/kg/day) in addition to an adequate diet in three human volunteers resulted in a doubling of plasma α-amino-n-butyric acid after 2 to 4 weeks that was reversed after cessation of drinking. (From Shaw S, Lieber CS. Plasma amino acid abnormalities in the alcoholic: respective role of alcohol, nutrition and liver injury. Gastroenterology 1978;74:677–82, with permission.)

Thus, the therapeutic use of SAMe is a good example of the beneficial effect by replenishment of a naturally occurring molecule that has been depleted by liver disease. The exact role of SAMe in the treatment of liver disorders was clarified in part by studies showing that this molecule is beneficial for intrahepatic cholestasis, as reviewed in detail by Osman and associates (53). Treatment with a stable salt of SAMe resulted in both improvement of standard liver function tests and reduction in symptoms such as itching. It has also been successfully used in severe cholestasis of pregnancy, in which it has the advantage of few, if any, untoward effects. Recurrent intrahepatic cholestasis and severe jaundice caused by androgens or estrogens are also conditions in which treatment with SAMe appears to be helpful, perhaps because of changes in membrane phospholipid composition. Experimentally, SAMe prevented total parenteral nutrition–induced cholestasis in the rat (54). Potentially beneficial clinical effects of SAMe include enhanced bile salt conjugation with taurine in patients with liver cirrhosis (55). Other observations indicated that administration of exogenous SAMe prevents the glutathione depletion observed in the liver of patients affected by liver disease (56). Loguercio and colleagues (57) also measured glutathionine and cysteine concentrations in erythrocytes of patients with alcoholism with and without liver cirrhosis. Glutathione levels were decreased, whereas those of cysteine were increased in all patients. Parenteral treatment with SAMe corrected the erythrocyte thiol alterations. Furthermore, in patients given SAMe, long-term treatment doubled the plasma concentration of the secondary sulfur-containing amino acids cystine and taurine, which were on average low normal at baseline, without any change in the concentration of methionine, neutral amino acids, and polyamines.

Therapeutic success was also achieved in a long-term randomized, placebo-controlled, double-blind, multicenter trial of SAMe in patients with alcoholic liver cirrhosis (58). One hundred twenty-three patients with Child class A, B, or C cirrhosis were studied for 2 years. When the Child C patients were excluded, the overall mortality or liver transplantation rate was significantly lower in the treated group (12% versus 29%, $p = .025$). An additional positive feature of this investigation was the confirmation of a virtually total lack of side effects of SAMe.

More recently, SAMe was also found to be beneficial in the treatment of acute (59) and chronic (60) viral hepatitis. The role of SAMe in the treatment of alcoholic liver disease was reviewed in two international symposia (40, 61, 62).

Lack of methionine may also result from a deficit in methylation of homocysteine to methionine (see Fig. 79.2), mainly by the folate- and vitamin B_{12}–dependent enzyme methionine synthetase. Because in most patients with alcoholism the folate status is disturbed (attributable to multiple mechanisms, including an inadequate diet), elevated plasma homocysteine levels in these patients could have been anticipated and were indeed noted in a group of such

patients (63). Because hyperhomocysteinemia has been associated with premature vascular disease (64), the increased plasma homocysteine in patients with alcoholism could contribute to the enhanced incidence of stroke found in these patients. Furthermore, the SAMe-dependent methylation of specific DNA cytosine bases to form 5-methylcytosine may block gene expression, and abnormalities in DNA methylation contribute to the loss of the normal controls on protooncogene expression (65). In fact, a methyl-deficient diet has been linked to early stages of colorectal neoplasia (66). These observations illustrate the need to correct underlying malnutrition in the patient with alcoholism, malnutrition that may exist irrespective of the patient's social and medical situation (67). Nutritional support was successful in decreasing nutrition-associated complications in patients with alcoholic liver disease (68). The rationale for the various modalities of nutritional intervention has also been reviewed (69). It is now clear that mere overall nutritional repletion may not suffice, and "supernutrients" may be needed, such as SAMe and possibly polyunsaturated phospholipids (see later). Indeed, many essential nutrients, including methionine, must first be activated in the liver or in other tissues before they can exert their key functions. This activating process, however, is altered by liver disease. A case in point is methionine that has to be converted to SAMe before it can act as the main cellular methyl donor (see Fig. 79.2). Such an activated nutrient that is lacking because of the defective activation in liver diseases and thus must be provided exogenously has been defined as a supernutrient.

Carbohydrates

Patients with cirrhosis are prone to develop diabetes. As already noted, insulin resistance appears to account for this abnormality. In patients with portal hypertension complicated by portosystemic shunting, an alteration in the metabolism of insulin may contribute to this resistance. Insulin resistance caused by alcohol has been demonstrated in healthy subjects and in elderly men (70) using the insulin clamp technique whereby glucose utilization is measured during glucose infusions at steady blood glucose and insulin levels (71). Depleted body stores of potassium and elevated levels of growth hormone are probably additional significant factors (72). As in other patients with diabetes, nutritional management plays an important role in therapy. Specifically, provision of calories in the form of complex carbohydrates is effective in reducing insulin requirements. Increasing the intake of complex carbohydrate may also be advantageous in terms of hepatic encephalopathy because the nonabsorbable fiber found in such foods lowers colonic pH. Indeed, the efficacy of lactulose, one of the mainstays in the treatment of hepatic encephalopathy, has been related to these same effects.

Patients with inherited disorders of hepatic carbohydrate metabolism may also benefit from dietary manipulation (see Chapter 58). This heterogenous group of disorders, which includes galactosemia, glycogen storage disease, and fructose intolerance, can be traced to specific enzymatic deficiencies. These defects impair the orderly flow of substrates along pathways involved in anaerobic glycolysis. The accumulation of these substrates in various organs, especially the liver and muscle, results in organ injury and, frequently, hypoglycemia. Galactosemia can be successfully controlled by strict dietary exclusion of milk products containing galactose. Likewise, fruits, vegetables, and sucrose must be eliminated from the diet of children who are fructose intolerant. At least in type I glycogen storage disease (von Gierke disease), biochemical improvement can be expected when hypoglycemia is prevented with frequent feedings of glucose-rich formulas.

The clinical problems of carbohydrate metabolism include hyperglycemia, which is frequent, but rarely severe or life-threatening, and hypoglycemia, which is infrequent, mostly occurring in conjunction with fasting or prolonged poor food intake or with disaccharide (mostly lactose) malabsorption or after acute alcohol intoxication, when it can be lethal if overlooked and untreated.

In the fed state, when liver glycogen is abundant, glycogenolysis supports blood glucose levels. In the fasting state, the following pathways that can support blood glucose are interfered with by concomitant metabolism of alcohol: glycogenesis from amino acids as well as formation of glucose from glycerol, lactate, and galactose (73). Increase in reduced nicotinamide adenine dinucleotide (NADH) from hepatic metabolism of alcohol (Fig. 79.4) is

partly responsible for these metabolic changes. Changes in enzyme activities relevant to various metabolic steps of gluconeogenesis (74) and lipogenesis (75) have also been described. Clinically, hypoglycemia must be suspected when an alcohol drinker exhibits altered mental status (even in the fed state, especially in children). Provision of glucose, usually intravenously, is simple and effective.

Lipids, Fatty Liver, Hyperlipidemia, and Ketoacidosis

Alcohol ingestion is associated with fatty infiltration of the liver, hyperlipidemia, and ketosis, each of which is largely explained by the effects of alcohol on the metabolism of lipids (69).

Fat accumulation in the liver is also strikingly affected by the amount and type of dietary triglycerides (see later). With alcohol, the more dietary triglycerides that are present in the diet, the more fat accumulates in the liver (Fig. 79.5), at least down to a level of 10% of total energy. At lower levels, fat accumulates even when dietary fat is extremely low, probably because of stimulation of lipogenesis.

Fatty liver contains triglycerides with fatty acids derived from dietary sources, when available, but of endogenously synthesized ones when dietary fatty acids are sparse (76). High-fat diets increase the amount of fat that accumulates. Low-fat diets, high-protein diets, and even hypocaloric diets will lessen the amount of fat that accumulates because of alcohol, but they will not completely prevent fatty liver. Dietary fat composed of triglycerides of medium chain

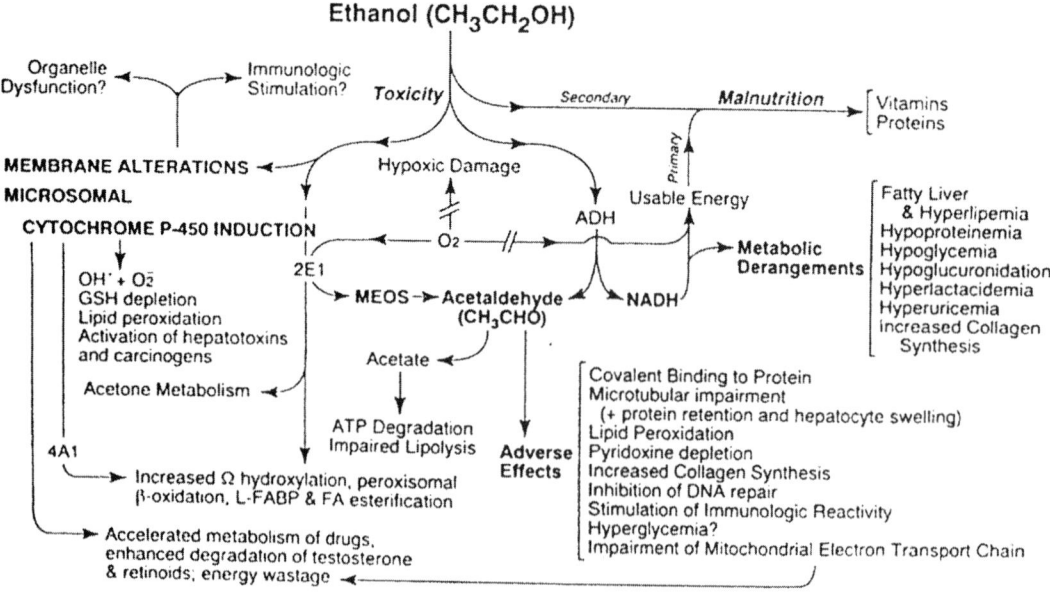

Figure 79.4. Hepatic, nutritional, and metabolic abnormalities after ethanol abuse. Malnutrition, whether primary or secondary, can be differentiated from metabolic changes or direct toxicity, resulting partly from alcohol dehydrogenase (ADH)-mediated redox changes, or effects secondary to microsomal induction or acetaldehyde production. ATP, adenosine triphosphate; FA, fatty acid; MEOS, microsomal ethanol oxidizing system; NADH, reduced nicotinamide adenine dinucleotide. (From Lieber CS. Alcoholic liver disease: new insights in pathogenesis leads to new treatments. J Hepatol 2000;32:113–28, with permission.)

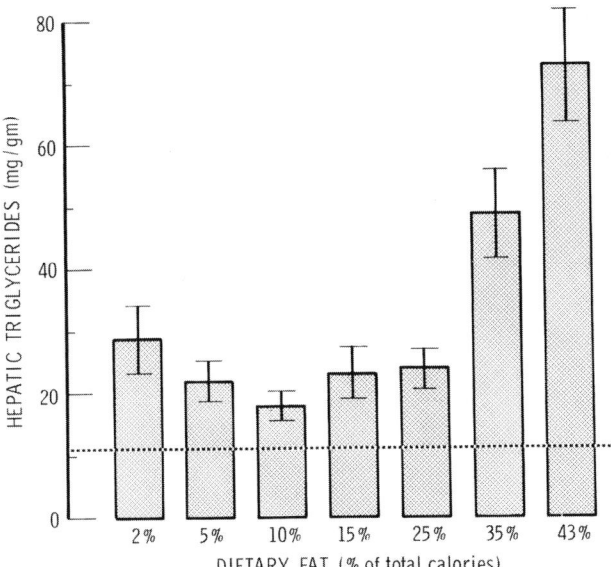

Figure 79.5. Effect of varying amounts of dietary fat on hepatic triglycerides. These were measured in seven groups of rats given ethanol (36% of calories) and a diet with normal protein (18% of calories). Average hepatic triglyceride concentration in the control animals is indicated by the *dotted line*. (From Lieber CS, DeCarli LM. Quantitative relationship between the amount of dietary fat and the severity of the alcoholic fatty liver. Am J Clin Nutr 1970;23:474–8, with permission.)

length causes less hepatic fat accumulation than fat containing triglycerides of long-chain fatty acids (77, 78). The increase in the NADH/NAD ratio consequent to the oxidation of alcohol to acetaldehyde by alcohol dehydrogenase (ADH) reduces the NAD availability for fatty acid oxidation by the citric acid cycle and thereby depresses fatty acid oxidation. Furthermore, because of structural damage to mitochondria, oxidation of two carbon fragments from all sources is inhibited. Fatty acid elongation by mitochondria is stimulated, probably by the increased NADH/NAD ratio. Glycerolipid synthesis is increased as a result of the greater availability of fatty acids, the conversion of dihydroxyacetone phosphate to glycerol-3-phosphate favored by the increased NADH/NAD ratio, and possibly the increased capacity of lipid-synthesizing systems. Indeed, activity both of the rate-limiting enzyme, phosphatidate phosphohydrolase, which removes phosphorus from phosphatidic acid to form diacylglycerol, and of diacylglycerol acyl transferase, which catalyzes the formation of triglycerides, is increased.

Human consumption of ethanol consistently results in hyperlipidemia; its extent is modified by associated dietary and pathologic conditions. The major increase occurs in serum triglycerides with some cholesterol elevation; the involved lipoproteins are VLDLs and chylomicrons, formed by the intestine. High-density lipoproteins (HDLs) are also increased by ethanol. Alcoholic hyperlipemia is usually classified as type IV according to the International Classification of Hyperlipidemias and Hyperlipoproteinemias because it is composed mostly of VLDLs, but it may be

classified as type V when chylomicrons are also present. About 6% of patients with alcoholism have type II hyperlipidemia, with hypercholesterolemia resulting from increased low-density lipoproteins (LDLs). Alcohol-induced hyperlipemia may change rapidly in composition because of more rapid clearing of triglycerides than of cholesterol and phospholipids. When alcohol is administered for several weeks at a dose of 300 g/day, the initial increase in triglycerides gradually abates (79). This change may result from liver damage or increased lipoprotein lipase activity. Hyperlipemia is usually absent with severe liver injury (e.g., cirrhosis), and hypolipemia may be present (13).

Some patients have exceptionally striking hyperlipemia during alcohol ingestion. This most likely represents an underlying genetic defect in lipid metabolism aggravated by the effects of alcohol, such as hyperchylomicronemia (type I) resulting from decreased postheparin lipoprotein lipase activity (80), carbohydrate sensitive hyperlipidemia, diabetes, obesity, or pancreatitis.

Moderate alcohol intake is associated with an increase in the fasting levels of a species of HDL cholesterol (HDL$_3$) whose significance regarding risk for heart disease, unlike that for HDL$_2$, has not been fully established. In one study, men who drank red wine (46g/kg/d of ethanol) tended to have elevated serum apolipoprotein A1 levels (81). Alcohol withdrawal led to a rapid decrease in both apolipoprotein A1 and HDL$_3$ (82). Therefore, it is not clear whether any decreased risk of coronary heart disease associated with moderate alcohol intake can be explained by increased levels of HDL resulting from alcohol. HDL$_2$ increases with more substantial alcohol intake, but such a high level of intake is not cardioprotective and may even be deleterious (83).

Other possible mechanisms for a coronary protective effect of ethanol have been suggested. Modest ethanol intake is associated with enhanced fibrinolysis via its effect on the plasma concentration of plasminogen activator (84). Furthermore, platelet aggregation is decreased by an acetaldehyde-mediated increase in prostacyclins (85) and by congeners in wine (86). Because apparent protection has been noted in people taking only one drink per week (87) or per month (88), factors other than alcoholic beverages are at play, such as lifestyle, that contribute to the coronary-protective effect observed in modest drinkers.

Alcohol intake is often accompanied by ketosis (89), with minimal or absent acidosis. The blood glucose level is usually normal (90). The extent of ketosis will be underestimated unless care is taken to measure β-hydroxybutyrate in addition to acetoacetate, more common with diabetic ketosis. Abstinence from alcohol and a return to normal diet are usually the only required treatments. Fluid and electrolytes may be given. Insulin is usually not required.

Dietary phospholipids have also striking effects on liver structure and function. Indeed, in primates, long-term ethanol consumption results in a decrease of liver phospholipids and of phosphatidylcholine (PC); both can be corrected by PC supplementation (32). The total phospholipid content of the mitochondrial membranes is decreased, with a significant reduction in the levels of PC (33) and associated striking morphologic changes with a corresponding functional counterpart, namely, diminished mitochondrial oxidation mainly from decreased cytochrome oxidase activity (33). The latter appears to result from alterations in the phospholipid composition of the mitochondrial membranes. Indeed, in vitro cytochrome oxidase activity could be restored with phospholipids extracted from normal mitochondria or synthetic ones, with PC the most active species (33).

The mechanism whereby long-term ethanol consumption alters phospholipids has not been clarified but may be related, at least in part, to decreased phospholipid methyltransferase activity described in cirrhotic livers (38). That this is not simply secondary to cirrhosis, but may in fact be a primary defect related to alcohol, is suggested by the observation that the enzyme activity is already decreased before cirrhosis develops (32). Another mechanism whereby ethanol may affect phospholipids is via formation of phosphatidylethanol, with a possible impact on signal transduction, as shown in isolated rat hepatocytes (91). A third mechanism is increased lipid peroxidation, as reflected by increased F_2 isoprostanes (92), which could explain the associated decrease of arachidonic acid in phospholipids (33).

In patients with alcoholism, reduction in phospholipid methyltransferase activity together with the decreased activity of SAMe synthetase (see earlier) may promote the membrane injury that was documented experimentally in alcohol-induced liver damage (43). The question then arose whether such deficiency could be attenuated, at least in part, by bypassing the enzyme defects through phospholipid supplementation. This was tested by feeding baboons alcohol in a diet supplemented with polyunsaturated lecithin. Administration of phospholipid preparations rich in polyunsaturated polyenylphosphatidylcholines (PPCs) (40) or virtually pure PPCs (32) (see Fig. 79.1) was found, in the nonhuman primate, to prevent alcohol-induced fibrosis and cirrhosis completely.

Whereas some discussion still exists about the relative contributions of hepatocytes and stellate cells in the production of collagen in the liver, stellate cells are "activated" after long-term alcohol consumption and appear to play a major role (93, 94). Normal stellate cells, when isolated and cultured on plastic surfaces, undergo spontaneous transformation into myofibroblast-like cells, thereby mimicking in vitro the "activation" that prevails in vivo after long-term alcohol consumption (95). These cells in culture produce collagen (95). When acetaldehyde is added to these cells, they respond with a further increase in collagen accumulation (95), with enhanced mRNA for collagen (96). Other aldehydes (e.g., malonaldehyde) are produced from lipid peroxidation, and they may also stimulate collagen production. Acetaldehyde stimulates collagen synthesis in cultured myofibroblasts as well (97), and a similar effect was observed with lactate. These cells were shown to proliferate in the perivenular zones of the liver after long-term alcohol consumption (98); they are similar to "activated" stellate cells, although they can be differentiated by ultrastructural and cytochemical characteristics (99). The normal liver contains a negligible number of "activated" stellate cells, whereas after long-term alcohol consumption, most stellate cells (>80%) are transformed. The protection afforded by PC against fibrosis (see Fig. 79.1) was associated with a lesser transformation of stellate cells to transitional cells in vivo (48% versus 81%). Thus, to the extent that the transformation of stellate cells in alcohol-fed animals was responsible for the fibrosis, the lesser transformation after PC may be one of the reasons for the decreased fibrosis.

Fibrosis and the associated collagen accumulation do not result simply from enhanced collagen production, but rather from an imbalance between collagen production and breakdown. Breakdown was assessed in cultured rat stellate cells by measuring collagenase activity with different phospholipids, including various species of PC. Under those conditions, a mixture of PCs affected the breakdown, but not the synthesis of collagen (100). The PC preparation used contained 18:2-18:2 PC (DLPC), 16:0-18:2 PC and other minor PC species. We found that pure DLPC stimulates collagenase activity in vitro. Increased collagenase activity can be expected to oppose collagen accumulation and the development of fibrosis by promoting the breakdown of collagen. Collagenase activity is generally increased during the early stage of liver injury (101). Indeed, fibrosis coincides with the stage at which collagen breakdown slackens and stops keeping pace with increased production (102). Therefore, these findings suggest that studies of collagenase activity associated with hepatic injury may be relevant to the elucidation of the pathogenesis of liver fibrosis and its treatment and prevention.

PC were used before empirically and mostly in open-label studies in nonalcoholic liver diseases: beneficial histologic effects were reported in the recovery from kwashiorkor (103), in patients with cirrhosis who were positive for the hepatitis B surface antigen (104), and in patients with chronic active hepatitis in terms of inflammatory parameters (105). In addition, PC attenuated experimental nonalcoholic hepatic fibrosis and accelerated its regression (106). PC was also used for the treatment of alcoholic hepatitis (105). Clinical trials for the prevention or treatment of alcoholic hepatic fibrosis or cirrhosis were recently completed. Investigators noted a marked attenuation of alcohol consumption, which resulted in a striking decrease of fibrosis progression (107), but in a subgroup of patients who continued to drink, some beneficial effects of PPC were observed (108).

Nonalcoholic Fatty Liver and Steatohepatitis

In our aging and overfed population, obesity and diabetes are common and frequently associated with nonalcoholic fatty liver disease (NAFLD), which comprises nonalcoholic fatty liver (NAFL) and nonalcoholic steatohepatitis (NASH). Whereas NAFL is usually benign, NASH is recognized as a precursor to "cryptogenic" cirrhosis (109). NAFLD and NASH combined are now the most common liver diseases in the United States (110). No therapy for NASH has been demonstrated to be clearly effective (111–114). However, because in a large segment of these patients either obesity or diabetes plays a crucial pathogenic role, see Chapters 64 and 65 for the best possible management of obesity and diabetes. Furthermore, the pathology of the liver in alcoholic steatosis and alcoholic steatohepatitis is remarkably similar to that of NAFLD, including NASH, a finding suggesting some common pathogenic mechanism. Studies carried out since the 1980s of possible mechanisms revealed one common link, namely, the induction of cytochrome P4502E1 with the associated oxidative stress (115). In fact, managing diabetes, obesity, and oxidative stress is the cornerstone of treatment and prevention of NASH (116).

Vitamins

Fat-Soluble Vitamins

Poor dietary intake and changes in bile salt metabolism and pancreatic function increase the likelihood of fat-soluble vitamin deficiency in patients with both alcoholic and nonalcoholic cirrhosis.

Vitamin A. The diet of the patient with nonalcoholic cirrhosis should start with a daily supplement of 5,000 to 15,000 IU of vitamin A. In patients with alcoholic cirrhosis, caution must be exercised in this respect because microsomal induction may increase the toxicity of this vitamin (11, 117) (see later), and ethanol potentiates liver damage caused by excessive vitamin A (118). Although β-carotene, the precursor of vitamin A, is less toxic than vitamin A itself, studies in nonhuman primates have shown that its toxic effects are also enhanced by alcohol (119). Furthermore, β-carotene increases the risk of pulmonary cancer in smokers (120), an effect related to an interaction between β-carotene and alcohol (121, 122). Thus, vitamin A or β-carotene supplementation must be used cautiously in patients with alcoholism.

Vitamin D. Supplementation of the diet with this vitamin may fail to halt the progression of osteoporosis and osteopenia. However, there appears to be no hazard in recommending ingestion of additional 25-OH D_3 (100–300 nmol or 40–120 μg/day) when patients complain of bone pain or demonstrate pathologic fractures (123).

Vitamin E. In children with biliary atresia and cholestasis, vitamin E deficiency may be associated with numerous neurologic alterations. Although these children may benefit from supplementation, repletion of vitamin E stores in adults with liver injury is of no proven clinical efficacy. Actually, in patients with liver disease of various causes, hepatic vitamin E concentrations were rather

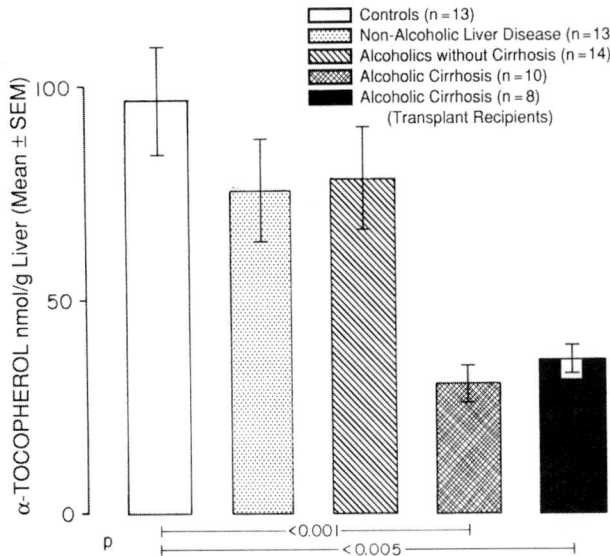

Figure 79.6. Effects of various liver diseases on total hepatic tocopherol levels. Only the cirrhotic groups had significantly lower α-tocopherol levels. (From Leo MA, Rosman A, Lieber CS. Differential depletion of carotenoids and tocopherol in liver disease. Hepatology 1993; 17:977–86, with permission.)

normal except in the presence of cirrhosis, alcoholic or nonalcoholic (Fig. 79.6).

Vitamin K. Deficiency of this vitamin leads to easy bruisability and, at times, to overt bleeding from esophageal varices or hemorrhoids. When the prothrombin time is lengthened, parenteral supplementation of vitamin K (10 mg/day for 3 days) will serve to discriminate between vitamin K deficiency or malabsorption and failure of the liver to synthesize normal coagulation factors. After parenteral vitamin K administration, an abnormal prothrombin time will be corrected in the former setting, but not in the latter.

Water-Soluble Vitamins and Trace Minerals

Deficiencies of water-soluble vitamins (folic acid, thiamin, and pyridoxine) are most likely to occur in the malnourished patient with alcoholism and advanced liver injury.

Patients with Wilson disease or those with chronic cholestasis (e.g., primary biliary cirrhosis) have excessive copper accumulation in the liver (124). Although chelation of copper by penicillamine is highly effective, it is also advantageous to reduce the intake of foods rich in this mineral such as chocolate, shellfish, and liver. Zinc deficiency also occurs in patients with alcoholism and liver injury.

EFFECT OF NUTRITION ON THE LIVER

Protein deficiency (kwashiorkor) is associated with the development of a fatty liver, at least in children (125). Other studies indicated that severe malnutrition can also lead to liver injury in adults (126). However, other factors, including hepatotoxins (e.g., aflatoxin) and parasites (schistosomiasis), prevalent in war-ravaged or developing countries, may have obscured the relationship between liver injury and poor nutrition in these reports.

Because malnutrition is also common in patients with alcoholism, these early findings were used to bolster the argument that malnutrition, rather than alcohol consumption per se, could explain the pathogenesis of alcohol-induced liver injury. Since the 1980s, however, a more balanced view has evolved. Based on studies in rodents, nonhuman primates, and humans, it is now established that alcohol can cause liver damage in the absence of dietary deficiencies, as reviewed by Lieber and DeCarli (127). Epidemiologic data also support this revised concept: a close correlation exists between per capita alcohol consumption and the likelihood of cirrhosis (128). Moreover, no relationship has been documented between nutritional status and the severity of alcohol-induced liver injury as defined histologically (129). The foregoing notwithstanding, it is now becoming clear that nutrition and the toxic effects of alcohol are often intertwined at the biochemical level. For example, by inducing microsomal cytochromes, long-term ethanol consumption is known to result in energy wastage and to promote the breakdown of nutrients, including retinol (16, 122, 130). A detailed discussion of the specific interaction of alcohol with diet, nutrition, and liver function is provided in the following sections.

NUTRITIONAL VALUE OF ALCOHOLIC BEVERAGES

The interactions between nutrition and alcoholism occur at many levels and are complex. Alcoholic beverages provide calories but almost no other useful constituents (131). Ethanol-containing beverages alter appetite and affect the level of food intake and utilization. They displace required nutrients from the diet. Ethanol and nutrients have multiple interactions at almost every level of the gastrointestinal tract. Ethanol alters the storage, mobilization, activation, and metabolism of nutrients and is toxic to many tissues. Alcoholism remains one of the major causes of nutritional deficiency in the United States; alcohol-related illness poses an enormous medical burden and often calls for complex nutritional therapy. Nutritional therapy is frequently a balance between maximizing recovery and avoiding iatrogenic complications.

Alcoholic beverages contain water, ethanol, variable amounts of carbohydrate, and little else of nutritive value. The carbohydrate content varies greatly: whiskey, cognac, and vodka have none, red and dry white wines have 2 to 10 g/L, beer and dry sherry have 30 g/L, and sweetened white and port wines have as much as 120 g/L (132). The protein and vitamin content of these beverages is extremely low except for beer. Even if one used beer as a nutrient source, 1 L would be necessary daily for nicotinic acid requirement, 15 to 20 L for protein, and 25 L for thiamin. Iron content may be appreciable, especially in wine

(132). The amounts of iron, lead, or cobalt may reach harmful levels. The significance of congener content is mostly obscure (131).

Americans consume on average 4.5% of total calories as ethanol (133), and adult drinkers consume more than 10%. Heavy drinkers may derive more than half their daily calories from ethanol. Combustion of ethanol in a bomb calorimeter yields 7.1 kcal/g; however, its biologic value is probably less. Lowered body weight in alcohol drinkers compared with nondrinkers is especially clear in women (134). When study subjects were given additional calories as alcohol under metabolic ward conditions, they did not gain weight (135, 136), and isocaloric substitution of ethanol for carbohydrate, as 50% of total calories (in a balanced diet) under metabolic ward conditions, resulted in a decline in body weight (Fig. 79.7).

Evidence indicates that ethanol increases the metabolic rate, and this finding would explain, at least in part, ethanol's reduced biologic energy value. Indeed, ethanol increases oxygen consumption in physiologically normal subjects, and it does so to a greater degree in patients with alcoholism (137). Substitution of ethanol for carbohydrates increased metabolic rate and diet-induced thermogenesis in humans and rodents (138). Resting energy expenditure (139) also increased in humans (138). Only a small portion of the energy waste in rats could be attributed to brown fat thermogenesis (140). Investigators theorized that energy waste during ethanol consumption may occur via oxidation without phosphorylation by the MEOS (136). The MEOS is inducible by long-term ethanol consumption, which aggravates energy waste (141, 142). The MEOS is not solely responsible for energy wastage from ethanol. Even when the MEOS is induced, much of the ethanol is metabolized by ADH to acetaldehyde, and much of the energy from ethanol is produced by the oxidation of acetaldehyde to carbon dioxide and water. Acetaldehyde may contribute

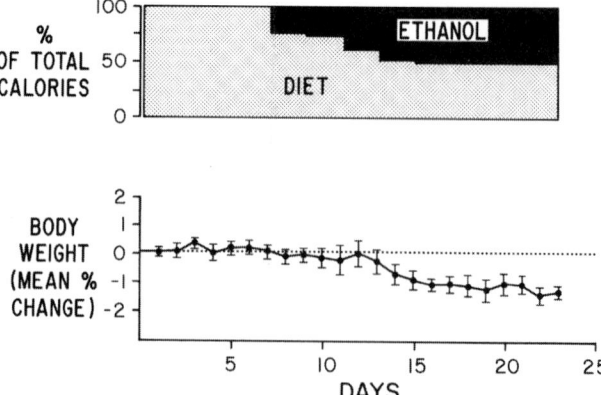

Figure 79.7. Effect of the isocaloric substitution of carbohydrate by ethanol on body weight. Substitution of ethanol up to 50% of total calories resulted in body weight loss. (From Pirola RC, Lieber CS. The energy cost of the metabolism of drugs, including ethanol. Pharmacology 1972;7:185–96, with permission.)

to energy wastage by promoting catecholamine release and by impairing various mitochondrial shuttles and mitochondrial oxidative phosphorylation. Acetate, the next product in the oxidation of ethanol, is also associated with several energy-consuming features. It increases myocardial contractility, coronary blood flow, and cardiac output. Hepatic damage, secondary to ethanol, decreases energy utilization, particularly from fat (142). Indeed, investigators observed that the damage is greater when alcohol consumption is associated with a diet rich in fat (76, 143, 144). The damage comprises striking alternations of the liver mitochondria, demonstrated by electron microscopy, both in humans (145) and in rats (146), and this probably explains why alcohol's effect on body weight is striking only in association with a diet containing substantial amounts of fat (Fig. 79.8).

In any event, impairment of the activities of the respiratory chain or the citric acid cycle, or both, may explain the decreases in oxygen uptake and in carbon dioxide production from citric acid cycle intermediates and fatty acids, as well as the increase in ketone body production, found, for instance, in mitochondria from ethanol-fed rats (147). Evidence for increased ketone production was also obtained in vivo, in experimental animals as well as in humans, in studies carried out under metabolic ward conditions (89). Thus, not only does ethanol, when present, become a preferred fuel and displace other fuels, such as fats (77, 148, 149), carbohydrates, and proteins (149), but also it impairs the

energy utilization derived from the oxidation of these other fuels, particularly fat, most likely because of the mitochondrial impairment associated with alcohol abuse.

NUTRITIONAL STATUS OF PATIENTS WITH ALCOHOLISM

Alcoholism can undermine nutritional status. Investigators estimated that 20,000 patients with alcoholism were suffering major illnesses resulting from malnutrition in the United States each year, accounting for 7.5 million days of hospitalization (150). Patients with alcoholism hospitalized for medical complications of this condition have the most severe malnutrition. They have inadequate dietary protein (151), with signs of protein malnutrition (150, 152), and anthropomorphic measurements indicative of impaired nutrition: muscle mass estimated by the creatinine-height index is reduced (152, 153), and triceps skin folds are thin (152–154). Continued drinking results in weight loss, whereas abstinence results in weight gain in patients with and without liver disease (154).

Many patients who drink to excess are either not malnourished or are less malnourished than the group hospitalized for medical problems. In one study, women drinking one or more drinks per day weighed on average 2.3 kg less than nondrinkers, and they and their male counterparts continued a more stable weight over the next 10 years than the nondrinkers, whose weight rose (155).

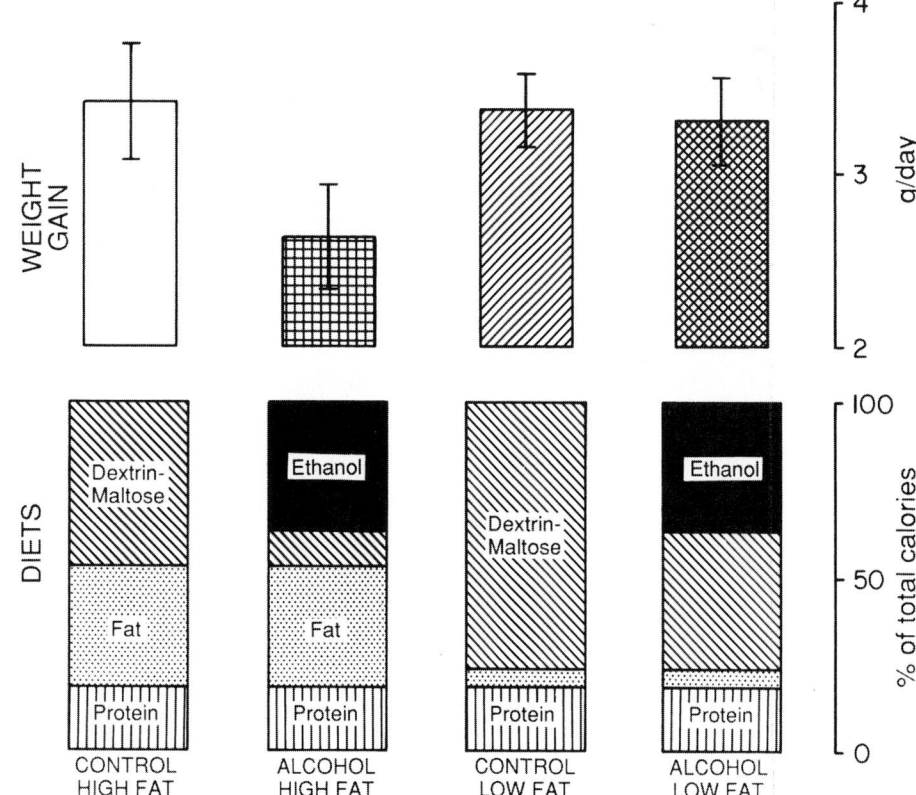

Figure 79.8. Effects of ethanol and/or dietary fat on body weight gain in rats. The ethanol-induced deficit in weight gain was not observed in the presence of a very-low-fat diet (5% of energy). (From Lieber CS. Perspectives: do alcohol calories count? Am J Clin Nutr 1991; 54: 976–82, with permission.)

Other surveys, however, found that alcohol consumption, especially when accompanied by high fat intake and sedentary behavior (156), favors truncal obesity, particularly in women (157). Those with moderate alcohol intake (158), even those admitted to a hospital for alcohol rehabilitation rather than for medical problems (159), often hardly differ nutritionally from controls (matched for socioeconomic status and health history), except women have a lower level of thiamin excretion than control patients following a thiamin load test (159).

The wide range in nutritional status of the alcoholic population reflects, in part, differences in what they eat. Moderate alcohol intake, accounting for 16% of total calories (alcohol included), is associated with slightly increased total energy intake (160). Perhaps because of the energy considerations already discussed, this group with higher total caloric intake has no weight gain despite physical activity levels comparable to those of the non–alcohol-consuming population. These levels of alcohol intake, and even slightly higher levels (23%) (161), are associated with a substitution of alcohol for carbohydrate in the diet. In those persons consuming more than 30% of total calories as alcohol, significant decreases in protein and fat intake also occur, and their intake of vitamins A and C and thiamin may descend to less than the recommended daily allowances (160). Calcium, iron, and fiber intake are also lowered (161).

The mechanisms underlying the altered pattern of food intake are not exactly known. Suppression of appetite has been postulated (162), but it has not been much studied. Depressed consciousness during inebriation, hangover, and gastroduodenitis resulting from ethanol partly explain the decreased food intake.

EFFECTS OF ETHANOL ON DIGESTION AND ABSORPTION

Alcohol consumption is associated with motility changes in the gastrointestinal tract, including diarrhea (163), that affect the digestion and absorption of nutrients. Ethanol's effects may be direct or indirect, acute or chronic. One of the most striking changes, intestinal malabsorption secondary to folic acid deficiency, is not a direct effect of ethanol, but rather results from diminished folic acid intake and utilization accompanying alcoholism.

Gastrointestinal Tract

Patients with cirrhosis of the liver resulting from alcohol consumption have edema, interstromal fat infiltration and fibrosis of the parotid glands, decreased basal and citric acid–stimulated salivary flow, and lower salivary concentrations of sodium, bicarbonate, and proteins (164). Changes in esophageal peristalsis and lower esophageal sphincter pressure follow no consistent patterns (165–167), and they usually do not lead to clinically significant dysphagia. However, the changes in saliva and esophageal motility and the direct

effect of ethanol may be important in causing esophagitis and strictures, which are common in patients with alcoholism and interfere dramatically with food intake.

Alcohol consumption is a cause of acute gastritis and duodenitis (168). These areas of the gut are exposed to the highest concentrations of ethanol for the longest times. Damage to the gastric mucosal "barrier" is important in making the mucosa more susceptible to acid and hyperosmolarity. Damage is probably the result of a combination of diminished gastric mucus production, altered mucosal blood flow, inhibition of active transport, increased permeability from mast cell release of histamine and leukotriene C_4, cell membrane disruption, hyperosmolarity, changes in prostaglandin and cyclic adenosine monophosphate content of mucosa, and lipoperoxidative mechanisms. Erosive gastritis occurs, as does nonerosive hemorrhagic gastritis consisting of subepithelial hemorrhage of the foveolar region with surrounding edema (169). The effects of ethanol on gastric emptying of meals are concentration dependent; higher concentrations cause more consistent delays of passage of solid contents (170) while enhancing movement of liquid contents (171).

In the jejunum, ethanol decreases type I (impeding) waves, whereas in the ileum it increases type III (propulsive) activity. Decreases in villus height (172) and disaccharide activity (173) of mucosal biopsy specimens have been found in patients with alcoholism who have associated lactose intolerance, especially in African-American patients with cirrhosis (173) (Fig. 79.9). The possibility of lactase deficiency must be considered in dietary treatment. Monosaccharide absorption is variably affected by

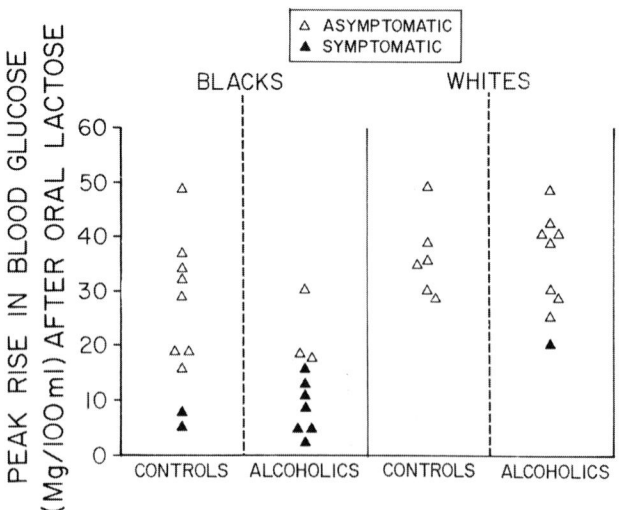

Figure 79.9. Effect of lactase deficiency on the rise in serum glucose after oral lactose administration. Blood glucose rose the least in subjects with the most severe lactase deficiency, namely, black patients with alcoholism. A good correlation was noted between symptoms and the lack of rise in glucose. (From Perlow W, Baraona E, Lieber CS. Symptomatic intestinal disaccharidase deficiency in patients with alcoholism. Gastroenterology 1977;72:680–4, with permission.)

ethanol; glucose is absorbed less well in rabbits after acute ethanol exposure (174), but long-term ethanol exposure enhances galactose absorption in rats (175) and glucose absorption in humans (176).

Acute depression of amino acid absorption can readily be demonstrated with high concentrations of ethanol (0.5–3.0%) in experimental models of ethanol exposure, using short segments of gut perfused in vivo or gut sacs bathed in vitro.

Bile Salts

Steatorrhea, when it occurs in patients with alcoholism, is mostly the result of folic acid deficiency (see later), but luminal bile salt deficiency may be a contributory factor. Intraluminal bile salts are decreased by short-term ethanol administration (177). In rodents, long-term ethanol administration delays the half-time excretion of cholic and chenodeoxycholic acids by decreasing the daily excretion and expanding the pool size slightly (178). Patients with alcoholic cirrhosis may have bile low in deoxycholic acid, possibly because of impaired conversion of cholate to deoxycholate by bacteria (179). Thus, decreased cholic acid synthesis, decreased bile acid pool size (180), low concentrations of bile salts in intestinal juice, and bacterial deconjugation of bile salts by altered intestinal flora all promote steatorrhea in cirrhosis. Pigmented gallstones are more frequent in patients with cirrhosis (181).

Pancreatitis and Pancreatic Insufficiency

See Chapter 78.

Alterations of Nutrient Metabolism

Water-Soluble Vitamins

Patients with alcoholism tend to have clinical or laboratory signs of water-soluble vitamin insufficiency correlated with the increasing amount of alcohol intake and a corresponding decrease in vitamin intake. This is true for thiamin, riboflavin, pyridoxine, folic acid, and ascorbic acid, but it has not been demonstrated for vitamin B_{12}. Alcohol's effects on absorption, activation, and storage must also be considered.

Folic Acid. Folic acid absorption is usually increased by partial starvation. Folate concentrations are less elevated in rats when alcohol is consumed (182). Investigators have not clearly shown, however, that either protein deficiency or alcohol consumption (183) decreases folate absorption in vivo. Thus, it is still unsettled what aspects of malnutrition adversely affect folate absorption and under which clinical circumstances alcohol may interfere with folate absorption. The fact remains, however, intestinal absorption is decreased in drinking and abstaining patients with alcoholism. The mechanism is presumably histologic and/or metabolic alcohol damage to the intestinal mucosal cells.

Alcohol accelerates the production of megaloblastic anemia in patients with depleted folate stores (184), and it suppresses the hematologic response to folic acid in folic acid–depleted patients (185).

The clinical approach to folate deficiency without anemia is straightforward. A diet providing adequate folate, perhaps with additional folate, will replete stores in a matter of weeks. If malabsorption persists after this period, evaluation for causes other than folate deficiency should be instituted. When the patient is anemic, the diagnostic evaluation is more complex (184). In addition to folate deficiency, the direct effect of alcohol on the bone marrow, liver disease, hypersplenism, bleeding, iron deficiency, infection, and the use of anticonvulsants are all commonly encountered and will exert separate and combined influences on the hematologic picture. In well-nourished patients with alcoholism, folic acid deficiency is a rare cause of anemia (186), and a search for folic acid deficiency (serum or red cell folate levels) as an explanation for anemia is unwarranted unless some of the morphologic features of the deficiency are present (e.g., macroovalocytes, hypersegmentation of polymorphonuclear leukocytes, megaloblastosis of the bone marrow).

Vitamin B_{12}. Patients with alcoholism do not commonly develop vitamin B_{12} deficiency. Their serum levels are usually normal even when they are deficient in folate, whether they have cirrhosis or not (182). This is probably the result of large body stores of vitamin B_{12} and reserve capacity for absorption.

Vitamin C. The vitamin C status of hospitalized patients with alcoholism is lower than that of nonalcoholic patients as measured by serum ascorbic acid, peripheral leukocyte ascorbic acid, or urinary ascorbic acid after an oral challenge (187). In one study, in addition to a lower mean ascorbic acid level, some 25% of patients with cirrhosis had serum ascorbic acid levels lower than the range of healthy controls (187). Ascorbic acid status is low in patients with alcoholism with and without liver disease. Daily supplementation with 175 to 500 mg of ascorbic acid may be necessary for weeks or months to restore plasma and urinary ascorbate to normal levels (187).

Fat-Soluble Vitamins

Vitamin A and β-Carotene. The interaction of alcoholism and vitamin A involves the intake and possibly the absorption of the vitamin and its metabolism; evidence indicates that alcohol may modulate the role of vitamin A in hepatotoxicity and carcinogenesis (188).

Persons in the United States who take 24% of total calories as alcohol ingest only 75% of the recommended dietary allowance for vitamin A (161). Probably those with intense alcoholism (i.e., persons consuming 50% or more of daily calories as alcohol) consume even less vitamin A.

Alcohol consumption is associated with raised blood β-carotene levels in both men (189) and women (190).

Lower blood β-carotene levels in drinkers in population studies may result from the lowering effect of concomitant smoking (191). Chronic alcoholic pancreatic insufficiency may substantially reduce vitamin A absorption, and the mean plasma vitamin A is lower in these patients than in physiologically normal controls, a finding correlating with the severity of steatorrhea (192). In one study, despite the lack of clinical signs of vitamin A deficiency, low blood β-carotene levels were found in 98% of patients with chronic alcoholism (150 g alcohol/day for 5 to 25 years) who were admitted to a hospital (193).

The effect of short-term consumption of alcohol on vitamin A blood levels has been variously reported as unchanged in humans (194) or increased as lipoprotein-bound retinol in rats (14). Feeding of baboons with alcohol raised their blood β-carotene concentrations (119). Serum and liver levels of carotenoids and retinoids were measured in patients with liver diseases of alcoholic and nonalcoholic origin, in normal livers of transplant donors, and in sera of physiologically normal control subjects (195). Total retinoids were decreased in the livers of patients with alcoholism and in nonalcoholic patients with liver disease, and decreases were more profound as alcoholic liver disease progressed to cirrhosis. Impaired conversion of ingested carotenes to hepatic retinoids during alcohol consumption may partially explain the decreased liver retinoid content, especially at advanced stages of alcoholic liver disease when plasma β-carotene is not much raised by carotene feeding (119, 189). The effect of long-term alcohol consumption on hepatic vitamin A in experimental animals has been profound and is consistent with observations in humans: hepatic vitamin A stores are diminished whether dietary vitamin A is low, normal, or high. Rodents fed alcohol (5 g/kg/day) had a 20% decrease in the liver (196). Higher intakes of alcohol (36% of calories or ~14 g/kg/day) decreased hepatic vitamin A by 60% in 4 to 6 weeks and by 72% in 7 to 9 weeks, without changes in serum vitamin A or retinol binding protein. In another study (197), five times the usual amount of vitamin A was given, and that still did not prevent hepatic depletion induced by alcohol. When baboons were fed 50% of calories as alcohol, a 60% decrease in hepatic vitamin A occurred after 4 months and a 95% decrease after 24 to 84 months (197). In another study, hepatic vitamin A levels showed a progressive decrease with increasing severity of lesions (including cirrhosis) in human patients (Fig. 79.10) (11). Enhancement of hepatic vitamin A degradation by alcohol consumption is one likely explanation for the drop in vitamin content. Vitamin A degradation by metabolism of retinoic acid to 4-hydroxy and 4-oxoretinoic acid and other polar metabolites is catalyzed by microsomal enzymes induced by ethanol consumption, but these enzymes are not active enough to deplete vitamin A stores. A more likely candidate responsible for depleting hepatic vitamin A is a microsomal pathway for oxidation of retinol to polar metabolites (15), also inducible

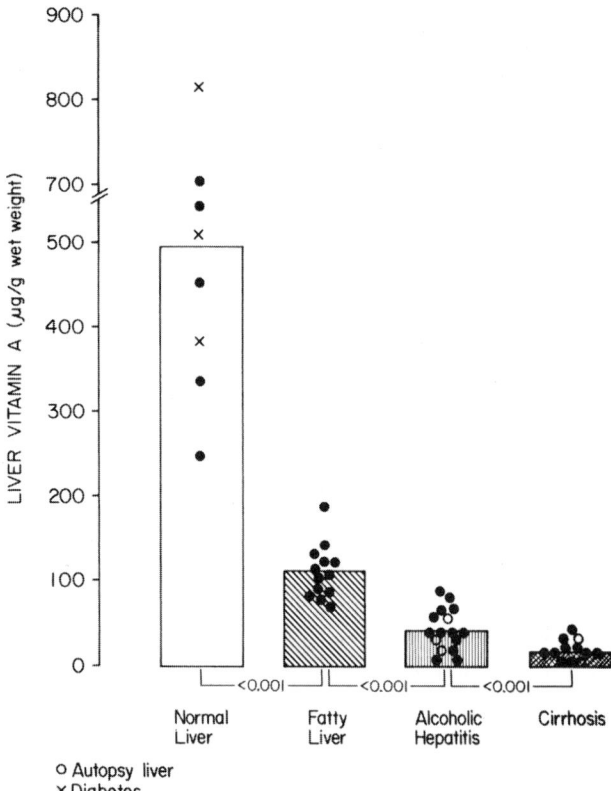

Figure 79.10. Hepatic vitamin A levels in subjects with normal livers and various stages of alcoholic liver injury. To convert vitamin A values to micromoles per gram, multiply by 0.003491. Numbers below the graph denote *p* values. (From Leo MA, Lieber CS. Hepatic vitamin A depletion in alcoholic liver injury. N Engl J Med 1982;307:597–601, with permission.)

by alcohol consumption (198). In addition, alcohol promotes vitamin A mobilization from the liver (198).

An important clinical consequence of low tissue vitamin A concentration is night blindness. Abnormal dark adaption occurs in 15% of patients with alcoholism without cirrhosis and in 50% of those with cirrhosis (199). One hepatic lesion resulting from diminished vitamin A includes the presence of multivesicular lysosomes and is potentiated by concomitant alcohol intake (200). Hepatotoxicity from increased vitamin A includes fibrosis (11, 200), which is potentiated by concomitant alcohol consumption (201). The squamous metaplasia of rodent trachea resulting from vitamin A depletion is also enhanced by ethanol (202). Ethanol increases vitamin A levels in lung and esophagus (203). The role of alcohol in increasing vitamin A content of some tissues while having the opposite effect in others, speeding or altering the conversion of vitamin A to metabolites, probably has important consequences for the hepatotoxicity, fibrosis, and squamous metaplasia described earlier. Alcohol-mediated alterations of vitamin A status could be relevant to the association of low vitamin A levels with malignant diseases: mean levels of vitamin A were lower in both smokers and drinkers with oropharyngeal squamous cancer than in control patients (203).

Several factors complicate vitamin A therapy in the setting of alcoholism: assessment of tissue stores of vitamin A is difficult, vitamin A in high doses is toxic, even usual doses of vitamin A are potentially toxic with continued intake of alcohol (or other microsome-inducing drugs), and monitoring vitamin A hepatotoxicity is difficult in the presence of continued alcohol intake. Replacement with β-carotene was considered less hazardous, but, in association with continued alcohol intake, it also shows evidence of hepatotoxicity (119, 204). Vitamin A replacement must therefore be modest for patients who cannot be ensured an alcohol- and drug-free environment. Replacement of vitamin A should be considered for patients who are confirmed as vitamin deficient and in whom abstinence from alcohol can be ensured. Night blindness (or abnormal dark adaptation) with low serum vitamin A (<30 μg/dL or <1 μmol/L) may be considered evidence of deficiency. Vitamin A given at 2000 μg/day for several weeks should provide an adequate trial. Especially in the presence of night blindness, patients with a low serum zinc level (<80 μg/dL) should be treated with doses of 600 mg/day zinc sulfate. Considering the interrelationship of vitamin A and zinc metabolism, zinc therapy may also be tried when vitamin A therapy fails to correct night blindness. Documented fat malabsorption should prompt parenteral replacement of vitamin A.

β-Carotene, the precursor of vitamin A, is less toxic than vitamin A, but its deleterious effects are also enhanced by alcohol. Indeed, β-carotene increases the risk of pulmonary cancer in smokers (120). As discussed before, this effect is related to a concomitant consumption of alcohol (121, 122). Thus, vitamin A or β-carotene supplementation must be used cautiously in patients with alcoholism.

Vitamin D. Patients with alcoholism have abnormalities of calcium, phosphorus, and vitamin D homeostasis. They have decreases in bone density and bone mass (205), increased susceptibility to fractures (206), and increased osteonecrosis (207). Low blood calcium, phosphorus, and magnesium and low, normal, or high vitamin D_3 levels have been reported, consistent with disturbed calcium metabolism (205).

In patients with alcoholic liver disease, vitamin D deficiency probably derives from too little vitamin D substrate, which results from poor dietary intake, malabsorption caused by cholestasis or pancreatic insufficiency, and insufficient sunlight. The status of 25-hydroxylation appears adequate even in advanced liver disease (205). These patients have a lower concentration of vitamin D binding globulin, a protein synthesized in the liver (208), but because of the excess of binding sites, its decrease is an unlikely cause of 25-OH vitamin D_3 deficiency. Although blood levels of 25-OH vitamin D_3 and 1,25-OH vitamin D_3 may be normal or even elevated in patients with alcoholism, the stores of

vitamin D_3 are often depleted, severely so in nutritionally depleted patients with alcoholism (205). Insufficient intake of calcium and phosphorus or decreased calcium absorption in the presence of normal or increased 1,25-OH vitamin D_3 (and parathormone) may accelerate bone loss in patients with alcoholism.

The diagnosis of osteopenia in liver disease may require bone densitometry because other clinical parameters of liver disease correlate poorly with osteopenia (209). Moreover, levels of free 25-OH vitamin D_3 may be normal in liver disease when total levels are low (210). Bone disease in patients with liver disease should be treated by increasing intake of vitamin D_3, by ultraviolet light therapy, and by correction of fat malabsorption to keep plasma calcium and phosphorus concentrations normal. Of course, abstinence from alcohol is important.

Vitamin K. Vitamin K deficiency in alcoholism may arise when fat absorption is interrupted by pancreatic insufficiency, biliary obstruction, or intestinal mucosal abnormality secondary to folic acid deficiency. Dietary vitamin K inadequacy is not a likely cause of clinical deficiency unless patients have concomitant sterilization of the colon, a reliable source of the vitamin. Alcohol-induced hepatocyte injury interferes with use of available vitamin K, with a consequent drop in blood levels of clotting factors II, VII, IX, and X, whose syntheses depend on this vitamin. Vitamin K serves as a cofactor for the microsomal carboxylase that affects posttranslational modification of these proteins, namely, the conversion of glutamic acid (Glu) residues to γ-carboxyglutamic acid (Gla) residues, a process that is necessary for function. Abnormally high levels of inactive factor II (prothrombin) are found in the plasma in the presence of cirrhosis or vitamin K deficiency (211).

Vitamin E and Selenium. Vitamin E and selenium serve protective roles as antioxidants and interact physiologically (212). Vitamin E is a powerful antioxidant that prevents peroxidation of cellular and subcellular membrane phospholipids. Selenium is also involved in antioxidant functions and is a component of red blood cell glutathione peroxidase. Vitamin E and selenium function synergistically: vitamin E reduces selenium requirement, prevents its loss from the body, and maintains it in an active form; selenium spares vitamin E and reduces the requirement for the vitamin (213).

Vitamin E deficiency is not a recognized complication of alcoholism, although patients with chronic alcoholic pancreatitis have a lower ratio of vitamin E to total plasma lipid (192). Vitamin E deficiency occurs in adults with diverse causes of fat malabsorption (212) and primary biliary cirrhosis (214) with clinical manifestations, including decreased erythrocyte survival and neurologic disturbances (e.g., areflexia, gait disturbance, decreased proprioception and vibratory sensation, ophthalmoplegia). When rodents were fed ethanol repeatedly, their hepatic vitamin E levels, measured as α-tocopherol, were low (215); this was accompanied by increased hepatic lipid peroxidation when alcohol was combined with a low–vitamin E diet (216). The mechanism of hepatic vitamin E depletion by ethanol is probably enhanced oxidation of α-tocopherol to α-tocopherol quinone in liver microsomes (217). Alcohol-induced liver injury may be mediated, in part, by stress on cellular antioxidant mechanisms interrelated with vitamin E and selenium. Considering the findings in humans with fat malabsorption or severe cholestasis, and the evidence of vitamin E depletion by long-term alcohol feeding of experimental animals, it would seem that great potential for vitamin E deficiency exists in patients with chronic alcoholism who may combine low vitamin E intake with steatorrhea from chronic pancreatitis or prolonged cholestasis. However, as already mentioned (see Fig. 79.6), in a study of patients with liver disease, including those with alcoholism, hepatic vitamin E concentrations were normal, except in patients with cirrhosis. In any event, vitamin E supplementation in patients with chronic decompensated alcoholic cirrhosis for a year achieved significant elevations of serum vitamin E (217).

Selenium metabolism is of great theoretic interest to hepatologists in view of the proposed lipoperoxidative mechanism of drug- and alcohol-induced liver injury (203). Serum selenium levels have been reported to be low in alcoholism, especially in the presence of liver disease, but this may be a consequence of liver injury (203), because nonalcoholic patients with liver disease also have low selenium levels. Alcohol intake was not found to influence selenium excretion in the urine (218).

Water, Minerals, and Electrolytes

Salt and Water Retention. Patients with alcoholism and chronic liver disease often have disorders of water and electrolyte balance. Retention of sodium and water is clinically apparent as weight gain, peripheral edema, ascites, and pleural effusions. Patients may have respiratory difficulties and umbilical herniation as further complications. Not only is sodium retained avidly, but also a water load cannot be excreted normally. Low body potassium levels may result from vomiting, diarrhea, hyperaldosteronism, and muscle wasting; potassium depletion may contribute to the appearance of renal vein ammonia and may worsen hepatic encephalopathy (219).

The pathogenesis of fluid retention and ascites is complex. At the hepatic level, portal hypertension, hypoalbuminemia, and alteration of lymph flow are important factors for ascites formation (220). Endocrine accompaniments and other phenomena suggest that the body is reacting to a diminished "effective circulating volume" (total blood volume is normal or elevated, but a disproportionately large fraction is sequestered in the splanchnic region) (221).

Patients with cirrhosis and fluid overload may require urgent relief, as when ascites and pleural effusion cause respiratory difficulties or when imminent rupture of an umbilical hernia may result in lethal peritonitis. Dietary management combines sodium and water restriction in selected cases of deficient water excretion. It is difficult to provide a palatable diet on a long-term basis with less than 0.5 to 1 g of sodium and 1500 to 2000 mL of total fluid daily, the amount recommended.

Magnesium. Neuromuscular excitability in acute alcohol withdrawal resembles that seen in magnesium deficiency. Investigators found that acute doses of ethanol caused magnesium loss in the urine (222). Patients with alcoholism have low blood magnesium and low body-exchangeable magnesium levels; symptoms in these patients resemble those in patients with magnesium deficiency of other causes. Hospitalized patients with alcoholism with normal serum total magnesium levels have significantly lower serum ionized magnesium (223). Magnesium replacement should be given to symptomatic patients with low serum magnesium, anorectic patients with low serum magnesium, and hypocalcemic patients with alcoholism who do not respond to calcium replacement. Most patients with alcoholism will replete body stores of magnesium readily from normal dietary sources.

Iron. In patients with alcoholism either deficiency or excess of iron may occur. These patients may be iron deficient as a result of the several gastrointestinal lesions to which they are prone and that may bleed. Iron therapy should be restricted to patients with clearly diagnosed cases of deficiency.

Iron overload of the liver was described in Bantus who consumed alcoholic beverages prepared in iron containers that thereby contributed a large amount of elemental iron to their diet. However, in most patients with alcoholism, the iron content of the liver is normal or only modestly elevated, although one may see stainable iron in reticuloendothelial cells, possibly because of bouts of hemolysis. The clinician should have little difficulty in distinguishing the hepatic iron increases of alcoholic liver disease from the much higher amounts characteristic of genetic hemochromatosis, using a measure of absolute iron content per gram of liver with upward adjustments for age (224, 225). Of great potential significance is the contribution hepatic iron may make to liver damage via its role in lipid peroxidation (226) in conjunction with the effects of alcohol. Its possible role in promoting fibrogenesis (227) is also of great potential significance.

Alcoholism has been reported to result in qualitative changes in transferrin, the serum transport protein for iron: a higher fraction of molecules bears a reduced sialic acid content (228). This provides a useful test for long-term alcohol consumption (229).

Zinc. Patients with alcoholic cirrhosis have low plasma zinc (230), low liver zinc (231), and an increase in urinary zinc levels (232). The low zinc status in patients with chronic alcoholism and cirrhosis is thought to result from decreased intake and decreased absorption as well as increased urinary excretion. Many persons in the United

States have a diet that is marginal in zinc (233). Some instances of night blindness not fully responsive to vitamin A replacement have responded to zinc. It is possible that the hypogonadism of some patients with alcoholism may involve perturbations of vitamin A and zinc interactions. Currently, the therapeutic use of zinc in alcoholism is restricted to the treatment of night blindness not responsive to vitamin A.

Copper and Other Trace Metals. Hepatic copper content is increased in advanced alcoholic cirrhosis (234). Nickel levels are consistently high in alcoholic liver disease; manganese and chromium are unchanged (234). Intracellular shifts in trace metals have been described on acute administration of alcohol (235). The clinical significance of trace metal changes is obscure, except for the cardiotoxicity ascribed to alcoholic beverages with high cobalt content.

EFFECT OF ETHANOL ON THE METABOLISM OF URIC ACID

It is an ancient observation that drinking alcoholic beverages is associated with precipitation of acute gouty attacks. An important mechanism of alcoholic hyperuricemia is decreased urinary excretion of uric acid secondary to elevated serum lactate. This is illustrated in data from a representative patient (Fig. 79.11) (236). Lactate is produced in the liver from pyruvate by the action of NADH generated in the metabolism of ethanol by ADH (see Fig. 79.4). Depending on the metabolic state of the liver, NADH generation either enhances hepatic lactate production or prevents the liver from using lactate originating in peripheral tissues, especially lactate produced from muscle activity during alcohol withdrawal. The renal mechanism neither depends on pH of the urine (236) nor is abolished by probenecid (237); it remains unexplained. Alcohol-associated ketosis or starvation may also exacerbate the hyperuricemia.

The purine content (guanosine) of some beers may also be a contributing factor for hyperuricemia and gout in patients with alcoholism (238). Patients with gout should refrain from significant alcohol intake, especially of purine-containing beers. The hyperuricemia encountered in the recent drinker should be observed during several days to a week of abstinence, which will allow alcoholic hyperuricemia to recede; thus, a costly workup for other causes of hyperuricemia may be avoided.

EFFECTS OF DIETARY FACTORS ON ETHANOL METABOLISM

Alcohol is metabolized to acetaldehyde by cytosolic ADH and the MEOS. As discussed before, MEOS, but not ADH, is inducible by long-term alcohol consumption. Furthermore, MEOS activity in the liver showed greater induction when given with a normal rather than a low-fat diet in rats (239), and the induction of P4502E1, the

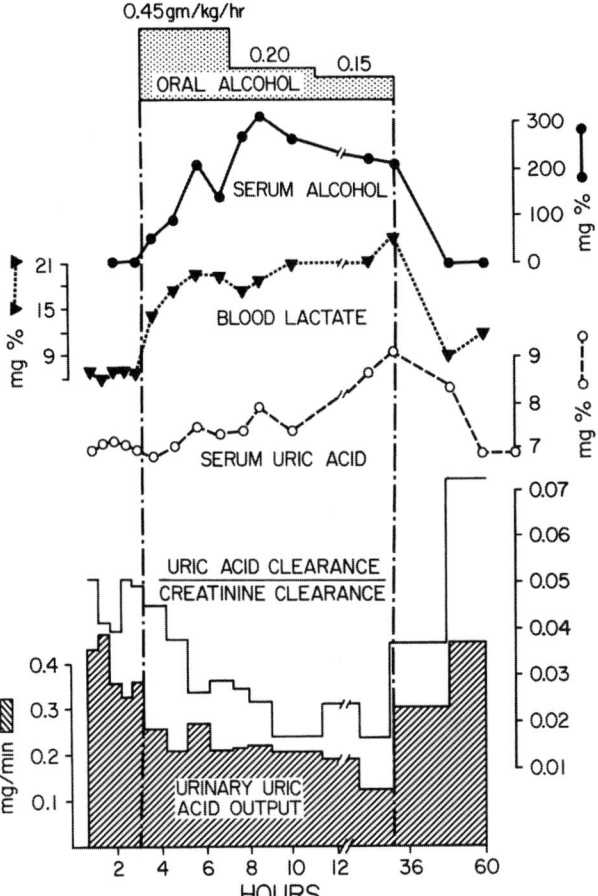

Figure 79.11. Blood and urine studies in a representative subject given alcohol orally. The rise in serum uric acid concentration was accompanied by a rise in blood lactate and by a decrease in urinary uric acid output. The creatinine clearance remained unchanged, and the ratio of uric acid clearance to creatinine clearance paralleled primary uric acid output. (Data from Lieber CS, Jones DP, Losowsky MS et al. Interrelation of uric acid and ethanol metabolism in man. J Clin Invest 1962;41:1863–70.)

cytochrome P450 specific for ethanol metabolism, was highest with low-carbohydrate diets (240). Low-protein diets reduced hepatic ADH and lower ethanol oxidation rates in rats (241) and in humans (242). Prolonged fasting also decreased ethanol oxidation rates, as shown in isolated rat liver cells. A mechanism for lowered metabolism of ethanol during fasting is the lack of available metabolites to shuttle into the mitochondria the reducing equivalents generated by ethanol oxidation in the cytosol (243). For a given alcohol intake, malnourished patients with alcoholism may develop higher blood alcohol levels and may sustain them longer than normally nourished persons, with possible deleterious consequences.

An additional isozyme of ADH, σ-ADH, was discovered in the stomach (244) and contributes to the metabolism of ethanol before it reaches the portal circulation and the liver, so-called first-pass metabolism of ethanol. This ADH isozyme has been characterized and its gene has been cloned (245). It is absent or decreased in Asians, and this feature is associated with a lower metabolism of alcohol (246). In addition, women younger than 50 years of age have a smaller first-pass metabolism of ethanol than do men (247). The reason is lesser class III ADH activity (248). This feature may contribute to the greater vulnerability of women to the effects of ethanol, especially after long-term alcohol abuse, which decreases gastric ADH activity and the first-pass metabolism of ethanol, thereby increasing blood levels even further (69, 248).

Gastric ADH is also inhibited by the histamine (H_2)-receptor antagonists taken orally as well as by other drugs, such as aspirin, as reviewed elsewhere (249, 250).

ALCOHOL, NUTRITION, AND ORGAN DAMAGE IN PATIENTS WITH ALCOHOLISM

Liver

Malnutrition contributes to the development of alcoholic fatty liver: fatty liver is present in protein deficiency, particularly in children with kwashiorkor. A highly visible "skid row" subset of patients with alcoholism with fatty liver is also malnourished. Furthermore, rodents subjected to diets deficient in lipotropes (see earlier) readily develop fatty livers. However, our current understanding is that alcohol per se, given in sufficient quantities, can cause fatty liver in humans and animals despite the presence of an otherwise adequate diet (251). The lipid and protein composition of the diet has modulating effects on the amount and types of fat that accumulate in the liver. As already discussed (see Fig. 79.5), reduction of dietary fat to 10% of total calories (but not lower) greatly lessens, but does not completely eliminate, hepatic fat accumulation. Furthermore, provision of higher than usually recommended dietary protein (25% of total calories) will not eliminate hepatic fat accumulation. The amount of fat accumulating in the ethanol-induced fatty liver is but one parameter of damage and must be considered along with organelle dysfunction and metabolic imbalances.

Alcoholic cirrhosis has been directly linked to the overall ethanol consumption by its drop in the United States during the Prohibition Era and in Europe during World War II, when alcoholic beverages were rationed (252). The studies of Lelbach (253) also showed the direct influence of intensity of alcohol consumption (g/kg/day × years) on the incidence of chronic liver disease in patients admitted to alcohol rehabilitation spas in Europe. Neither the beverage source of ethanol nor concomitant malnutrition was noted to have an influence. These findings were confirmed in France (254), and the direct effect of ethanol in causing hepatic fibrosis and cirrhosis was demonstrated in the baboon model of hepatic injury (31).

The direct hepatotoxic effect of ethanol has also been shown histologically (by light and electron microscopy) and biochemically in patients both with and without alcoholism

regardless of dietary variation in fat, protein, vitamins, and lipotropes (135, 145, 255).

The role of nutrition in the recovery from alcoholic liver injury was studied by clinicians before the pathogenesis of the injury was fully understood. Patek and colleagues (256) demonstrated the efficacy of a normal-protein, normal-fat, vitamin-enriched diet in the treatment of cirrhosis as measured by clinical response. Erenoglu and associates (257), extending previous work, treated cirrhotic patients with 198 mL of absolute ethanol daily and an adequate diet; these investigators found no adverse effects and a possible benefit from high dietary protein. As already discussed, the aggregate evidence indicates that acute liver damage consistently occurs if sufficient alcohol is consumed and is not preventable by a nutritious diet. Safe levels of intake probably exist. Chronic liver injury from alcohol appears to be dose and time related but with no indication that dietary manipulation will act preventively. Patients with precursor lesions of cirrhosis, such as perivenular fibrosis (258), require special attention. By and large, the treatment approach is still mainly abstinence or very low consumption, but this level of alcohol intake is lower than that which many patients with alcoholism consume spontaneously, in view of the lack of control that most patients with alcoholism have in limiting their alcohol intake. Efforts to define populations with varying degrees of susceptibility to ethanol-induced liver disease on the basis of genetics or viral exposure have not yet been convincing; however, girls and women are more susceptible than boys and men (247, 248). We cannot advise a different approach for any group, but ongoing studies revealed a remarkable effectiveness for the Brief Intervention Technique to reduce excessive alcohol consumption to a moderate level (107, 259).

Stroke

The incidence of stroke is strongly associated with advancing age, black race, obesity, and hypertension. Moderate to heavy alcohol consumption, more than 45 g/day, has been identified as an independent predictor of stroke after accounting for the increased risk resulting from hypertension and cigarette smoking (260). A review of most of the English language literature concluded that moderate alcohol intake, less than 60 g/day, has a complex association with ischemic stroke in white populations: very low levels are possibly protective and higher levels are definitely deleterious, with little, if any, association in Japanese populations. By contrast, moderate drinking increases hemorrhagic stroke (intracerebral and subarachoid hemorrhage) in diverse populations (261). Alcohol consumption may contribute to stroke by raising blood pressure to hypertensive levels as shown by most (262, 263), but not all (264), studies. Sodium intake and phosphorus intake were also positively identified as nutrient predictors of hypertension (262). Some authors have detected an immediacy of alcohol intake just before stroke, although others have not.

Heart

The acute effects of even small amounts of hard liquor (several ounces) include measureable myocardial depression (265), dose-dependent impairment of left ventricular emptying at rest (266), and electrophysiologic effects such as slight delay in atrial conduction and shortening of both the atrioventricular conduction time and the effective ventricular myocardial refractory period (267). These effects usually are not clinically apparent in people with normal hearts, especially because the impaired left ventricular emptying disappears with exercise (266). Patients with angina pectoris, even with congestive heart failure, have responses in left ventricular performance similar to those seen in controls at blood alcohol levels of 100 mg/dL (268). Patients with myocardial ischemia may experience an unfavorable distribution of coronary blood flow away from ischemic areas (269). Thus, the result of alcohol intake is not always predictable because it depends on the relative influence of alcohol on peripheral vasodilatation, coronary blood flow, direct myocardial depression, electrophysiologic changes, and the extent of underlying cardiac reserve (270). Patients with chronic alcoholism or heart disease (270) and even physiologically normal nonalcoholic subjects may develop atrial arrhythmias after substantial acute alcohol ingestion (271).

Long-term alcohol consumption may result in heart disease by its association with hypertension, as discussed earlier in relation to stroke, or by its association with severe thiamin deficiency in the beriberi heart syndrome. Alcohol intake is associated with elevations of serum homocysteine, as discussed earlier in relation to folic acid. Elevation of serum homocysteine has been linked to premature vascular disease. The relevance of alcohol-induced changes in serum HDL cholesterol to the appearance of heart disease is not established. As reviewed before, the question whether alcohol per se reduces coronary artery disease and cardiac death rate is still a matter of debate.

A fairly characteristic syndrome known as alcoholic cardiomyopathy has been described in a subset of patients with alcoholism and heart disease. It is a congestive cardiomyopathy seen typically in men aged 30 to 55 years who have been drinking 30 to 50% of calories as alcohol for 10 to 15 years (270). Arrhythmias are frequent. Coronary artery disease, hypertension, valvular abnormalities, and congenital heart disease must be excluded before the diagnosis of this disorder is made. Treatment with rest, diuretics, and abstention from alcohol may yield dramatic improvement (268), but many times it does not.

Blood and Bone Marrow

In addition to the anemias caused by blood loss and folic acid deficiency already discussed, alcohol has direct or at least unexplained effects on the blood elements. Alcohol consumption is associated with vacuolization of erythroid precursors, which is not prevented by adequate diet and

pharmacologic doses of folic acid (272). Alcohol intake also causes granulocytopenia, probably mediated by nutritional inadequacy (272), thrombocytopenia, and impairment of platelet function (273, 274), which are partly attributed to direct effects because they are not mediated by folic acid or other identifiable nutritional deficiencies.

SUMMARY OF NUTRITIONAL THERAPY IN ALCOHOLISM

Nutritional therapy in alcoholism is directed at the prevention of illnesses resulting from alcoholism, the treatment of documented or presumed deficiencies, and the management of complications of alcoholism. Persons consuming more than 30% of total calories as alcohol have a high probability of ingesting less than the recommended daily amounts of carbohydrate, protein, fat, vitamins A, C, and B (especially thiamin), and minerals such as calcium and iron. It is sensible to recommend a complete diet comparable to that of persons who do not have alcoholism to forestall deficiency syndromes, but some organ damage from direct toxicity of alcohol (e.g., alcoholic liver disease) cannot thereby be prevented. It may be beneficial to correct specific deficiencies in S-adenosylmethionine and PC illustrated in Figure 79.2. Downregulation of CYP2E1 induction may thereby also be achieved (275). One may also contemplate the use of antioxidants (to oppose the oxidative stress) and antifibrotic agents (276).

The management of observed deficiencies of protein and calories is straightforward in the absence of organ damage. The treatment of gross malnutrition of protein in severe acute and chronic liver disease is discussed earlier. Nervous system damage from thiamin lack is serious and treatable with a great margin of safety; therefore, thiamin deficiency should be presumed if not definitely disproved. Parenteral therapy with 50 mg/day of thiamin should be given until similar doses can be taken by mouth. Riboflavin and pyridoxine should be routinely given at the dosages usually contained in standard multivitamin preparations. Adequate folic acid replacement can be accomplished with the usual hospital diet. Additional replacement is optional unless deficiency is severe. Vitamin A replacement should be given only for well-documented deficiency and to patients whose abstinence from alcohol is ensured (see the earlier discussion of hepatotoxicity of hypervitaminosis A, especially when combined with alcohol). Vitamin A at doses of 2000 to 3000 µg/day may then be given. Zinc replacement should be administered for night blindness unresponsive to vitamin A replacement. Magnesium replacement is recommended for symptomatic patients with low serum magnesium levels. Iron deficiency that has been clearly diagnosed may be corrected orally. Wernicke-Korsakoff syndrome requires at least 50 mg/day of thiamin (parenterally if necessary) for prolonged periods. Beriberi heart failure responds quickly to thiamin. Peripheral nerve damage will necessitate months or years of vitamin B therapy. Acute pancreatitis may require withholding oral feeding for prolonged periods, during which time venous alimentation must be given. Chronic pancreatic exocrine insufficiency is treated by dietary manipulation (often decreases in fat) with oral pancreatic enzymes at mealtime. In patients with severe liver disease, such as advanced cirrhosis, one major challenge in the nutritional therapy of alcoholism is to achieve nutritional replenishment without secondary exacerbation of encephalopathy.

Acknowledgments
Original studies were supported, in part, by National Institutes of Health grant AA11115, the Department of Veterans Affairs, the Kingsbridge Research Foundation, and the Chrisptopher D. Smithers Foundation. I am grateful to Ms. Y. Rodriguez for the skillful typing of this chapter.

REFERENCES

1. Feinman L, Lieber CS. Nutrition and diet in alcoholism. In: Shils ME, Olson JA, Shike M et al, eds. Modern Nutrition in Health and Disease. 9th ed. Baltimore: Williams & Wilkins, 1998: 1523–42.
2. Lieber CS. Nutrition in liver disorders. In: Shils ME, Olson JA, Shike M et al, eds. Modern Nutrition in Health and Disease. 9th ed. Baltimore: Williams & Wilkins, 1998:1177–89.
3. Westergaard H, Dietschy JM. J Clin Invest 1976;58:97–108.
4. Adibi SA, Baraona E, Lieber CS. Effects of ethanol on amino acid and protein metabolism. In: Lieber CS, ed. Medical and Nutritional Complications of Alcoholism: Mechanisms and Management. New York: Plenum, 1992:127–63.
5. Preedy VR, Siddig T, Why H et al. Alcohol Alcohol 1994;29:141–7.
6. Baraona E, Leo M, Borowsky SA et al. Science 1975;190:794–5.
7. McCullough AJ, Mullen KD, Smanik EJ et al. Gastroenterol Clin North Am 1989;18:619–43.
8. Mezey E. Liver and biliary system. In: Paige DM, ed. Clinical Nutrition. 2nd ed. St. Louis: CV Mosby, 1988;186–97.
9. Vlahcevic ZR, Buhac I, Farar JT et al. Gastroenterology 1971;60:491–8.
10. Feinman L, Lieber CS. Nutrition: medical problems of alcoholism. In: Lieber CS, ed. Medical and Nutritional Complications of Alcoholism: Mechanisms and Management. New York: Plenum, 1992:515–30.
11. Leo MA, Lieber CS. N Engl J Med 1982;307:597–601.
12. Leo MA, Lowe N, Lieber CS. Am J Clin Nutr 1984;40:1131–6.
13. Borowsky SA, Perlow W, Baraona E et al. Dig Dis Sci 1980;25:22–7.
14. Sato M, Lieber CS. Arch Biochem Biophys 1982;213:557–64.
15. Leo MA, Lieber CS. J Biol Chem 1985;260:5228–31.
16. Leo MA, Lowe N, Lieber CS. J Nutr 1987;117:70–6.
17. Simon D, Galambos JT. J Hepatol 1988;7:200–7.
18. Gabuzda GJ, Shear L. Am J Clin Nutr 1970;23:479–84.
19. Shaw S, Rubin KP, Lieber CS. Dig Dis Sci 1983;28:585–9.
20. Fischer JE, Baldessarini RJ. Lancet 1971;2:75–80.
21. Fischer JE, Yoshimura N, Aguirre A et al. Am J Surg 1974;127:40–7.
22. Vilstrup H, Gluud C, Hardt F et al. J Hepatol 1990;10:291–6.
23. Horst D, Grace ND, Conn HO et al. Hepatology 1984;4:279–87.
24. Weber FL, Minco D, Fresard KM et al. Gastroenterology 1985;89: 538–44.
25. Best CH, Hartroft WS, Lucas CC et al. BMJ 1949;2:1001–6.
26. Klatskin G, Hrehl WA, Conn HO. J Exp Med 1954;100:605–14.
27. Thompson JA, Reitz RC. Ann NY Acad Sci 1976;273:194–204.
28. Hoffbauer FW, Zaki FG. Arch Pathol 1965;79:364–9.
29. Lieber CS, Teschke R, Hasumura Y et al. Fed Proc 1975;34:2060–74.
30. Chawla RK, Wolf DC, Kutner MH et al. Gastroenterology 1989;97:1514–20.
31. Lieber CS, DeCarli LM. J Med Primatol 1974;3:153–63.
32. Lieber CS, Robins SJ, Li J et al. Gastroenterology 1994;106:152–9.
33. Arai M, Leo MA, Nakano M et al. Hepatology 1984;4:165–4.
34. Lieber CS, Leo MA, Mak KM et al. Hepatology 1985;5:561–72.
35. Finkelstein JD, Martin JJ. J Biol Chem 1986;261:1582–7.
36. Montanari A, Simoni I, Vallisa D et al. Hepatology 1988;8:1034–9.
37. Horowitz JH, Rypins EB, Henderson JM et al. Gastroenterology 1981;81:668–75.
38. Martin–Duce AM, Ortiz P, Cabrero C et al. Hepatology 1988;8:65–8.
39. Finkelstein JD, Cello JP, Kyle WE. Biochem Biophy Res Commun 1974;61:525–31.
40. Lieber CS, Casini A, DeCarli LM et al. Hepatology 1990;11:165–72.
41. Speisky H, MacDonald A, Giles G et al. Biochem J 1985;225:565–72.
42. Hirata F, Axelrod J. Science 1980;209:1082–90.
43. Yamada S, Mak KM, Lieber CS. Gastroenterology 1985;88:1799–806.
44. Shaw S, Jayatilleke E, Ross WA et al. J Lab Clin Med 1981;98:417–25.
45. Bombardieri G, Pappalardo G, Bernardi L et al. Int J Clin Pharmacol Therapy Toxicol 1983;21:186–8.
46. Hoffman DR, Marion DW, Cornatzer WE et al. J Biol Chem 1980;22:10822–7.
47. Lieber CS. Am J Clin Nutr 2002;76:1183S–7S.
48. Engstrom MA, Benevenga NJ. J Nutr 1987;117:1820–6.
49. Zappia V, Galletti P, Porcelli M. FEBS Lett 1978;90:331–5.
50. Audubert F, Vance D. J Biol Chem 1983;258:10695–701.
51. Quiram DR, Winshilboum RM. J Neurochem 1976;27:1197–203.
52. Giulidori P. Stramentinoli G. Anal Biochem 1984;137:217–20.
53. Osman E, Owen JS, Burroughs AK. Aliment Pharmacol Ther 1993;7:21–8.
54. Belli DC, Fournier LA, Lepage G et al. J Hepatol 1994;21:18–23.
55. Angelico M, Gandin C, Nistri A et al. Scand J Clin Invest 1994;54:459–64.
56. Vendemiale G, Altomare E, Trizio T et al. Scand J Gastroenterol 1989;24:407–15.
57. Loguercio C, Nardi G, Argenzio F et al. Alcohol Alcohol 1994;29:597–604.
58. Mato JM, Cámara J, Fernández de Paz J et al. J Hepatol 1999;30:1081–9.
59. Bao-en W. Clin Drug Invest 2001;21:765–73.
60. Bao-en W. Clin Drug Invest 2001;21:685–94.
61. Lieber CS. Alcohol 2002;27:173–7.
62. Lieber CS, Packer L. Am J Clin Nutr 2002;76:1148S–50S.
63. Hultberg B, Berglund M, Andersson A et al. Alcohol Clin Exp Res 1993;17:687–9.
64. Stampfer MJ, Malinow MR, Willett WC et al. JAMA 1992;268:877–81.
65. Holliday R. Science 1987;283:163–70.

66. Giovannucci E, Stampfer MJ, Colditz GA et al. J Natl Cancer Inst 1993;85:875–84.
67. Koehn V, Burnand B, Niquille M et al. JPEN J Parenter Enteral Nutr 1993;17:35–40.
68. Hirsch S, Bunout D, de la Maza P et al. JPEN J Parenter Enteral Nutr 1993;17:119–24.
69. Lieber CS. Alcohol Clin Exp Res 2000;24:417–8.
70. Boden G, Chen X, Desantis R et al. Diabetes 1993;42:28–34.
71. Yki–Järvinen H, Nikkilä EA. Metabolism 1985;61:941–5.
72. Collins JR, Lacy WW, Stiel JN et al. Arch Intern Med 1970;126:608–14.
73. Krebs HA, Hems FR, Stibbs M. Biochem J 1969;112:117–24.
74. Duruibe V, Tejwani GA. Mol Pharmacol 1981;20:621.
75. Guthrie GD, Myers KJ, Gesser EJ et al. Alcohol Clin Exp Res 1990;14:17–22.
76. Lieber CS, Spritz N, DeCarli LM. J Clin Invest 1966;45:51–62.
77. Lieber CS, Lefevre A, Spritz N et al. J Clin Invest 1967;46:1451–60.
78. Nanji AA, Yang EK, Fogt F et al. J Pharmacol Exp Ther 1996;277:1694–700.
79. Lieber CS, Jones DP, Mendelson J et al. Trans Assoc Am Physicians 1963;76:289–300.
80. Losowsky MS, Jones DP, Davidson CS et al. Am J Med 1963;35:794–803.
81. Simonetti P, Brusamolino A, Pellegrini N et al. Alcohol Clin Exp Res 1995;19:517–22.
82. Lamisse F, Schellenberg F, Bouyou E et al. Alcohol Alcohol 1994;29:25–30.
83. Lieber CS. N Engl J Med 1984;310:846–8.
84. Ridker PM, Vaughan DE, Stampfer MJ et al. JAMA 1994;272:929–33.
85. Guivernau M, Baraona E, Lieber CS. J Pharmacol Exp Ther 1987;240:59–64.
86. Renaud S, de Lorgeril M. Lancet 1992;339:1523–6.
87. Boffetta P, Garfinkel L. Epidemiology 1990;1:342–8.
88. Gronbaek M, Deis A, Sorensen TI et al. BMJ 1995;310:1165–9.
89. Lefevre A, Adler H, Lieber CS. J Clin Invest 1970;49:1775–82.
90. McGhee A, Henderson JM, Millikan WJ Jr et al. Ann Surg 1983;197:288–93.
91. Hoek JB, Thomas AP, Rooney TA et al. FASEB J 1992;6:2386–96.
92. Lieber CS, Leo MA, Aleynik SI et al. Alcohol Clin Exp Res 1997;21:375–9.
93. Mak KM, Leo MA, Lieber CS. Gastroenterology 1984;87:188–200.
94. Mak KM, Lieber CS. Hepatology 1988;8:1027–37.
95. Moshage H, Casini A, Lieber CS. Hepatology 1990;12:511–8.
96. Casini A, Cunningham M, Rojkind M et al. Hepatology 1991;13:758–65.
97. Savolainen E–R, Goldberg B, Leo MA et al. Alcoholism Clin Exp Res 1984;8:384–9.
98. Nakano M, Lieber CS. Am J Pathol 1982;106:145–55.
99. Takase S, Leo MA, Nouchi T et al. J Hepatol 1988;6:267–76.
100. Li J, Kim CI, Leo MA et al. Hepatology 1992;15:373–81.
101. Maruyama K, Feinman L, Okazaki I et al. Biochim Biophys Acta 1981;658:14–31.
102. Maruyama K, Feinman L, Fainako M et al. Life Sci 1982;30:1379–84.
103. Alliet J, Comlan G, Goudier D. Quest Med 1976;29:85–104.
104. Fassati P, Horejsi J, Passati M et al. Casopis Lekaru Ceskych 1981;10:56–60.
105. Bird GLA, Panos MZ, Polson MZ et al. Z Gastroenterol 1991;29:21–4.
106. Ma X, Zhao J, Lieber CS. J Hepatol 1996;24:604–13.
107. Lieber CS, Weiss DG, Groszmann R et al. I. Alcohol Clin Exp Res 2003;27:1757–64.
108. Lieber CS, Weiss DG, Groszmann R et al. Alcohol Clin Exp Res 2003;27:1765–72.
109. James FW, Day CP. J Hepatol 1998;29:495–501.
110. Yu AS, Keeffe EB. Rev Gastroenterol Disord 2002;2:11–19.
111. Lee RG, Keeffe EB. Non-alcoholic fatty liver: causes and complications. In: Bircher J, Benhamou JP, McIntyre M et al, eds. Textbook of Clinical Hepatology. 2nd ed. Oxford: Oxford University Press, 1999:1251–7.
112. Matteoni CA, Younossi ZM, Gramich T et al. Gastroenterology 1999;116:1413–1419.
113. Kumar KS, Malet PF. Mayo Clin Proc 2000;75:733–9.
114. Fong DG, Nehra V, Lindor KD et al. Hepatology 2000;32:3–10.
115. Lieber CS. Hepatol Res 2004;28:1–11.
116. Oneta CM, Dufour JF. Swiss Med Wkly 2002;132:493–505.
117. Leo MA, Sato M, Lieber CS. Gastroenterology 1983;84:562–72.
118. Leo MA, Kim C, Lieber CS. Nutr Rev 1988;46:32.
119. Leo MA, Kim CI, Lowe N et al. Hepatology 1992;15:883–91.
120. Alpha-Tocopherol Beta-Carotene Cancer Prevention Study Group. N Engl J Med 1994;330:1029–35.
121. Leo MA, Lieber CS. N Engl J Med 1994;331:612.
122. Albanese D, Heinonen OP, Taylor PR et al. J Natl Cancer Inst 1996;88:1560–71.
123. Long RG, Meinhard E, Skinner RK et al. Gut 1978;19:85–90.
124. Gibbs K, Walshe JM. Clin Sci 1971;41:189–202.
125. Cook GC, Hutt MS. BMJ 1967;3:454–7.
126. Ramalingaswami V. Nature 1964;201:546–51.
127. Lieber CS, DeCarli LM. J Hepatol 1991;12:394–401.
128. Conn HO, Atterbury CE. Cirrhosis. In: Schiff L, Schiff ER, eds. Diseases of the Liver. Philadelphia: JB Lippincott, 1987:725–864.
129. Pequingot G, Chabert C, Eydoux H et al. Rev Alcohol 1974;20:191–202.
130. Sato M, Lieber CS. J Nutr 1982;12:1188–96.
131. Feinman L, Lieber CS. Alcohol Clin Exp Res 1988;12:2–6.
132. Pekkanen L, Forsander O. Nutr Bull 1977;4:91–102.
133. Scheig R. Am J Clin Nutr 1970;23:467–73.
134. Williamson DF, Forman MR, Binkin NJ et al. Am J Public Health 1987;77:1324–30.
135. Lieber CS, Jones DP, DeCarli LM. J Clin Invest 1965;44:1009–21.
136. Pirola RC, Lieber CS. Pharmacology 1972;7:185–96.
137. Tremolieres J, Carre L. Rev Alcoolisme 1961;7:202–27.
138. Stock MJ, Stuart JA. Nutr Metabol 1974;17:297–305.
139. Klesges RC, Mealer CZ, Kesges LM. Am J Clin Nutr 1994;59:805–9.
140. Rothwell NJ, Stock MJ. Metabolism 1984;33:768–71.
141. Pirola RC, Lieber CS. J Nutr 1975;105:1544–8.
142. Lieber CS. Am J Clin Nutr 1991;54:976–82.
143. Lieber CS, Spritz N. J Clin Invest 1966;45:1400–11.
144. Lieber CS, DeCarli LM. Am J Clin Nutr 1970;23:474–8.
145. Lane BP, Lieber CS. Am J Pathol 1966;49:593–603.
146. Iseri OA, Lieber CS, Gottlieb LS. Am J Pathol 1966;48:535–55.
147. Cederbaum AI, Lieber CS, Rubin E. Arch Biochem Biophys 1976;176:525–38.
148. Lieber CS, Schmid R. J Clin Invest 1961;40:394–9.
149. Shelmet JJ, Reichard GA, Skutches CL et al. Nutr Today 1971;6:2–9.
151. Patek AJ Jr, Toth IG, Saunders MG et al. Arch Intern Med 1975;135:1053–7.
152. Mendenhall C, Bongiovanni G, Goldberg S et al. JPEN J Parenter Enteral Nutr 1985;9:590–6.

153. Morgan MY. Acta Chir Scand 1981;507:81–90.

154. Simko V, Connell AM, Banks B. Am J Clin Nutr 1982;3: 197–203.

155. Liu S, Serdula MK, Williamson DF et al. Am J Epidemiol 1994; 140:912–20.

156. Armellini F, Zamboni M, Frigo L et al. Eur J Clin Nutr 1993; 47:52–60.

157. Tremblay A, Buemann B, Theriault G et al. Eur J Clin Nutr 1995;49:824–31.

158. Bebb HT, Houser HB, Witschi JC et al. Am J Clin Nutr 1971; 24:1042–52.

159. Neville JN, Eagles JA, Samson G et al. Am J Clin Nutr 1968;21: 1329–40.

160. Gruchow HW, Sobociaski KA, Barboriak JJ et al. Am J Clin Nutr 1985;42:289–95.

161. Hillers VN, Massey LK. Am J Clin Nutr 1985;41:356–62.

162. Westerfeld WW, Schulman MP. JAMA 1959;170:197–203.

163. Keshavarzian A, Saverymuttu SH, Tai PC et al. Gastroenterology 1985;88:1041–9.

164. Dutta SK, Dukehart M, Narang A et al. Gastroenterology 1989; 96:510–8.

165. Winship DH, Caflisch CR, Zboralske FF et al. Gastroenterology 1968;55:173–8.

166. Silver LS, Worner TM, Korsten MA. Am J Gastroenterol 1986; 81:423–7.

167. Keshavarzian A, Iber F, Ferguson Y. Gastroenterology 1987;92: 651–7.

168. Gottfried EB, Korsten MA, Lieber CS. Am J Gastroenterol 1978;70:587–92.

169. Laine L, Weinstein WM. Gastroenterology 1988;94:1254–62.

170. Barboriak JJ, Meade RC. Am J Clin Nutr 1970;23:1151–3.

171. Jian R, Cortot A, Ducrot F et al. Dig Dis Sci 1986;31:604–14.

172. Hermos JA, Adams WH, Liu YK et al. Ann Intern Med 1972; 76:957–65.

173. Perlow W, Baraona E, Lieber CS. Gastroenterology 1977;72: 680–4.

174. Thomson AB. Dig Dis Sci 1984;29:267–74.

175. Mazzanti R, Debnam ES, Jenkins WJ. Gut 1987;28:56–60.

176. Green PH, Tall AR. Am J Med 1979;67:1066–76.

177. Marin GA, Ward NL, Fischer R. Am J Dig Dis 1973;18:825–33.

178. Lefevre A, DeCarli LM, Lieber CS. J Lipid Res 1972;13:48–55.

179. Knodell RG, Kinsey M, Boedeker EC et al. Gastroenterology 1976;71:196–201.

180. Vlahcevic ZR, Juttijudata P, Bell CC et al. Gastroenterology 1972;62:1174–83.

181. Nicholas P, Rinaudo PA, Conn HO. Gastroenterology 1972; 63: 112–21.

182. Racusen LC, Krawitt EL. Am J Dig Dis 1977;22:915–20.

183. Lindenbaum J, Lieber CS. Effects of ethanol on the blood, bone marrow and small intestine of man. In: Roach MK, McIsaac WM, Cleaven PJ, eds. Biological Aspects of Alcohol, vol 3. Austin, TX: University of Texas Press, 1971:27–45.

184. Lindenbaum J, Lieber CS. Alcohol and the hematologic system. In: Lieber CS, ed. Medical Disorders of Alcoholism: Pathogenesis and Treatment, vol 22. Philadelphia: WB Saunders, 1982:313–62.

185. Sullivan LW, Herbert V. J Clin Invest 1964;43:2048–62.

186. Eichner ER, Buchanan B, Smith JW et al. Am J Med Sci 1972; 273:35–42.

187. Bonjour JP. Int J Vitam Nutr Res 1979;49:434–41.

188. Leo MA, Lieber CS. Am J Clin Nutr 1999;69:1071–85.

189. Ahmed S, Leo MA, Lieber CS. Am J Clin Nutr 1994;60:430–6.

190. Forman MR, Beecher GR, Lanza E et al. Am J Clin Nutr 1995;62:131–5.

191. Rimm E, Colditz G. Ann NY Acad Sci 1993;686:323–33.

192. Marotta F, Labadarios D, Frazer L et al. Dig Dis Sci 1994;39: 993–8.

193. Althausen TL, Uyeyama K, Loran MR. Gastroenterology 1960; 38:942–5.

194. Russell RM, Giovetti A, Garrett M et al. Gastroenterology 1979;77:A36.

195. Leo MA, Rosman A, Lieber CS. Hepatology 1993;17:977–86.

196. Nadkarni GD, Deshpande UR, Pahuja DN. Experientia 1979; 35:1059–60.

197. Sato M, Lieber CS. J Nutr 1981;111:2015–23.

198. Leo MA, Kim C, Lieber CS. Alcohol Clin Exp Res 1986;10: 487–92.

199. Bonjour JP. Int J Vitam Nutr Res 1981;51:4166–77.

200. Leo MA, Lieber CS. Hepatology 1983;3:1–11.

201. Leo MA, Arai M, Sato M et al. Gastroenterology 1982;82: 194–205.

202. Mak KM, Leo MA, Lieber CS. Trans Assoc Am Physicians 1984;98:210–21.

203. Lieber CS. Alcohol and the liver. In: Arai IM, Frenkel MS, Wilson JHP, eds. Liver Annual VI. Amsterdam: Excerpta Medica 1987:163–240.

204. Leo MA, Lieber CS. N Engl J Med 1994;331:612.

205. Gascon-Barré M. J Am Coll Nutr 1985;4:565–74.

206. Nilsson BE. Acta Chir Scand 1970;136:383–4.

207. Solomon L. J Bone Joint Surg Br 1973;55:246–61.

208. Long RG. Vitamin D in chronic liver disease. In: Bianchi L, Gerok W, Landmann L et al, eds. Liver in Metabolic Diseases. Boston,:MTP Press, 1983:421–7.

209. Bonkovsky HL, Hawkins M, Steinberg K et al. Hepatology 1990;12:273–80.

210. Bikle DD, Halloran BP, Gee E et al. J Clin Invest 1986;78: 748–52.

211. Blanchard R, Furie BC, Jorgensen M et al. N Engl J Med 1981; 305:242–8.

212. Bieri JG, Corash L, Hubbard VS. N Engl J Med 1983;308: 1063–71.

213. Martin DW Jr. Fat-soluble vitamins. In: Martin DW Jr, Mayes PA, Rodwill VW et al, eds. Harper's Review of Biochemistry, 20th ed. Los Altos, CA: Lange Medical Publications, 1985: 118–27.

214. Knight RE, Bourne AJ, Newton M et al. Gastroenterology 1986;91:209–11.

215. Bjorneboe GE, Bjorneboe A, Hagen BF et al. Biochim Biophys Acta 1987;918:236–41.

216. Kawase T, Kato S, Lieber CS. Hepatology 1989;10:815–21.

217. de la Maza MP, Petermann M, Bunout D et al. J Am Col Nutr 1995;14:192–6.

218. Rodriguez Rodriguez EM, Sanz Alaejob MT, Diaz Romero C. Eur J Clin Chem Clin Biochem 1995;33:127–33.

219. Shear L, Gabuzda GJ. Am J Clin Nutr 1970;23:614–8.

220. Summerskill WH, Barnardo DE, Baldus WP. Am J Clin Nutr 1970;23:499–507.

221. Epstein FH. N Engl J Med 1982;307:1577–8.

222. McCollister R, Prasad AS, Doe RP et al. J Lab Clin Med 1958; 52:928–32.

223. Wu C, Kenny MA. Clin Chem 1996;42:625–9.

224. Bassett ML, Halliday JW, Powell LW. Hepatology 1986;6:24–9.

225. Olynyk J, Hall P, Sallie R et al. Hepatology 1990;12:26–30.

226. Bacon BR, Britton RS. Hepatology 1990;11:127–37.

227. Chojkier M, Houglum K, Solis-Herruzo J et al. J Biol Chem 1989;264:16957–62.

228. Stibler H, Sydow O, Borg S. Pharmacol Biochem Behav 1980;13[Suppl 1]:47–51.

229. Behrens UJ, Worner TM, Braly LF et al. Alcohol Clin Exp Res 1988;12:427–32.
230. Vallee BL, Wacker WEC, Bartholomay AF et al. N Engl J Med 1956;225:403–8.
231. Vallee BL, Wacker WEC, Bartholomay AF et al. N Engl J Med 1957;257:1055–65.
232. Sullivan JF. Gastroenterology 1962;42:439–42.
233. Sandstead HH. Am J Clin Nutr 1973;26:1251–60.
234. Volini F, de la Huerga J, Kent G et al. Trace metal studies in liver disease using atomic absorption spectroscopy. In: Sunderman FW, Sunderman FW Jr, eds. Laboratory Diagnosis of Liver Disease. St. Louis: W.H. Green, 1968:199–206.
235. Szutowski MM, Lipska M, Bandolet JP. Pol J Pharmacol Pharm 1976;28:397–401.
236. Lieber CS, Jones DP, Losowsky MS et al. J Clin Invest 1962;41:1863–70.
237. MacLachlan MJ, Rodnan GP. Am J Med 1967;42:38–57.
238. Gibson T, Rodgers AV, Simmonds HA et al. Br J Rheumatol 1984;23:203–9.
239. Lieber CS, Lasker JM, DeCarli LM et al. J Pharmacol Exp Ther 1988;247:791–5.
240. Lieber CS. Alcohol Clin Exp Res 1999;23:991–1007.
241. Bode CH, Goebell H, Stahler M. Gesampte Exp Med 1970;152:111–24.
242. Bode CH, Buchwald B, Goebell H. German Med Mon 1971;1:149–51.
243. Meijer AJ, van Woerkom GM, Willianmson JR et al. Biochem J 1975;150:205–9.
244. Hernandez–Munoz R, Caballeria J, Baraona E et al. Alcohol Clin Exp Res 1990;14:946–50.
245. Yokoyama H, Baraona E, Lieber CS. Genomics 1996;31:243–5.
246. Dohmen K, Baraona E, Ishibashi H et al. Alcohol Clin Exp Res 1996;20:1569–76.
247. Frezza M, Di Padova C, Pozzato G et al. N Engl J Med 1990;322:95–9.
248. Baraona E, Abittan CS, Dohmen K et al. Alcohol Clin Exp Res 2001;25:502–507.
249. Gentry RT, Baraona E, Amir I et al. Life Sci 1999;65:2505–12.
250. Lieber CS. Molecular basis and metabolic consequences of ethanol metabolism. In: Heather N, Peters TJ, Stockwell T, eds. Handbook of Alcohol and Alcohol-Related Problems, London: John Wiley & Sons, 2001:75–102.
251. Lieber CS, Leo MA. Alcohol and the liver. In: Lieber CS, ed. Medical and Nutritional Complications of Alcoholism: Mechanisms and Management. New York: Plenum, 1992:185–239.
252. Lederman S. Alcohol, alcoholisme, alcoholisation: Paris, Institut national d'études demographiques, travaux, et documents. Cahier No. 41. Paris: Presses Universitaires de France, 1964.
253. Lelbach WK. Acta Hepatosplenol (Stuttgart) 1967;14:9–39.
254. Tuyns AJ, Esteban J, Pequignot G. Br J Addict 1984;79:389–93.
255. Lieber CS, Rubin E. Am J Med 1968;44:200–6.
256. Patek AJ, Post J, Ratnoff OB. JAMA 1948;138:543–9.
257. Erenoglu E, Edreira JG, Patek AJ Jr. Ann Intern Med 1964;60:814–23.
258. Worner TM, Lieber CS. JAMA 1985;254:627–30.
259. Fleming MF, Mundt MP, French MT et al. Alcohol Clin Exp Res 2002;26:36–43.
260. Gill JS, Zezulka V, Shipley MJ et al. N Engl J Med 1986;315:1041–6.
261. Camargo CA Jr. Stroke 1989;20:1611–26.
262. Gruchow HW, Sobovinski KA, Barboriak JJ. JAMA 1985;15:1567–70.
263. Witteman JC, Willett WC, Stampfer MJ et al. Am J Cardiol 1990;65:633–7.
264. Coates RA, Corey PN, Ashley MJ et al. Prev Med 1985;14:1–14.
265. Lang RM, Borow K, Neuman A et al. Ann Intern Med 1985;102:742–7.
266. Kelbaek H. Prog Cardiovasc Dis 1990;32:347–64.
267. Gould L, Reddy R, Becker W et al. J Electrocardiology 1978;11:219–26.
268. Kupari M. Eur Heart J 1984;5:412–8.
269. Friedman HS, Neal C, Dowd A et al. Am J Cardiol 1981;47:61–7.
270. Segel LD, Klausner SC, Gnadt JT et al. Med Clin North Am 1984;68:147–61.
271. Thornton JR. Lancet 1984;2:1013–5.
272. Lindenbaum J, Lieber CS. N Engl J Med 1969;281:333–8.
273. Haut MJ, Cowan DH. Am J Med 1974;56:22–33.
274. Lindenbaum J, Hargrove RL. Ann Intern Med 1968;68:526–32.
275. Aleynik MK, Leo MA, Alcohol Clin Exp Res 1999;23:96–100.
276. Lieber CS. Annu Rev Nutr 2000;20:395–430.
277. Popper H, Lieber CS. Am J Pathol 1980;98:695–716.
278. Shaw S, Lieber CS. Gastroenterology 1978;74:677–82.
279. Lieber CS. J Hepatol 2000;32:113–28.

80 MOLECULAR BASIS OF CARCINOGENESIS[1]
DANA RATHKOPF AND GARY K. SCHWARTZ

A MOLECULAR MODEL FOR CARCINOGENESIS 1260
ONCOGENES 1260
TUMOR SUPPRESSOR GENES 1261
MISMATCH REPAIR GENES AND MICROSATELLITE
    INSTABILITY 1261
DNA METHYLATION 1262
MULTISTEP MODEL OF CARCINOGENESIS 1263
CELL CYCLE 1263
CONCLUSION AND FUTURE DIRECTIONS 1265

A MOLECULAR MODEL FOR CARCINOGENESIS

The hypothesis governing the current model of molecular carcinogenesis is that cancer results from the accumulation of genetic abnormalities. The fundamental gene families controlling this process are called oncogenes and tumor suppressor genes. Alterations to these gene families can occur through mutation, deletion, or insertion of the DNA base sequence. In addition, epigenetic modulation through DNA methylation affecting gene expression without actual alteration of the DNA base sequence can also result in abnormal cellular behavior. Whether these disruptions of genetic expression are caused by acquired environmental factors (chemicals, radiation, dietary factors, viruses), inherited factors (familial genetics), or sporadic events, the end result is an alteration in the cell cycle leading to uncontrolled cellular growth and carcinogenesis.

ONCOGENES

Oncogenes are normal genes that can be activated to stimulate uncontrolled cellular proliferation. Insight into this class of genes can be traced back to 1911, when it was established that extracts from avian sarcomas could induce sarcoma in otherwise healthy birds (1). Years later, the avian sarcoma extract was identified as the Rous sarcoma virus (named after the article's original author). By studying the genomic material of the virus, it was realized that certain normal genes could be converted by viruses into cancer-causing genes called *oncogenes*. The Rous sarcoma virus was found to contain the *src* oncogene, which contributes to carcinogenesis by encoding for a protein that disrupts the cytoskeleton (2).

In 1982, with the isolation of the c-*myc* oncogene in Burkitt lymphoma (c-*myc* is the cellular homolog to the avian leukemia virus oncogene *VMYC*), the concept of viral oncogenesis was expanded to include human malignancies. Cytogenetic analysis of Burkitt lymphoma demonstrated constitutive rearrangement of the c-*myc* oncogene resulting in uncontrolled cellular replication (1).

It has since been established that normal cell genes (*protooncogenes*) responsible for cell growth and differentiation can undergo DNA alteration via point mutation, translocation, or amplification, resulting in inappropriate cellular function and subsequent tumor formation. When activated, these previously normal cells, or protooncogenes, are referred to as oncogenes. Only one of the two alleles in a given gene needs to be affected to trigger malignant transformation, and the activated oncogenic form is therefore dominant over the protooncogene. In addition, the oncoprotein is frequently biochemically more active than the normal gene product. Only the tumor tissue containing the activated oncogene is affected; the remaining healthy cells retain the normal protooncogene and gene product (3). Examples of frequently encountered oncogenes, mechanism of activation, functional properties, and associated cancers are listed in Table 80.1.

Oncogenes implicated in the development of colorectal cancer include c-*myc*, c-*erbB2*, and *ras*. The *ras* oncogene is mutated in up to 50% of large polyps and sporadic colorectal cancers (2). More than 95% of pancreatic cancers exhibit a K-*ras* mutation suggesting a causative relationship between the *ras* mutation and pancreatic malignancy (4).

Located on chromosome 12, the *ras* oncogene is activated by a point mutation at any of three particular codons (12, 13, or 61), and the result is an amino acid substitution. Normally, Ras is a guanine nucleotide binding protein that is located on the inner surface of the cell membrane. In its activated state, the Ras protein binds to guanosine triphosphate (GTP) and plays a role in transducing biologic signals from the cell surface to the cell nucleus through secondary

---

[1]**Abbreviations: APC,** adenomatous polyposis coli; **CDK,** cyclin-dependent kinase; **CDKI,** cyclin-dependent kinase inhibitor; **DCC,** deleted in colorectal carcinoma; **GDP,** guanosine diphosphate; **GTP,** guanosine triphosphate; **INK4,** inhibitor of cyclin-dependent kinase 4; **KIP,** kinase inhibitor protein; **MMR,** mismatch repair; **MSI-H,** high-frequency microsatellite instability; **MSI-L,** low-frequency microsatellite instability; **MSS,** microsatellite stable.

TABLE 80.1. ONCOGENES

ONCOGENE	FUNCTIONAL PROPERTIES	ASSOCIATED TUMORS
bcr-abl	Chimeric nonreceptor tyrosine kinase	Acute lymphocytic leukemia, chronic myelogenous leukemia
b-Cat	Transcriptional coactivator	Melanoma, colorectal cancer
bcl-2	Antiapoptosis	B-cell lymphoma, colorectal cancer
cdk4	cyclin-dependent kinase	sarcoma
erb-B1	Growth factor receptor	Squamous cell carcinoma, glioblastoma, astrocytoma
erb-B2/neu	Growth factor receptor	Breast, gastric, ovarian cancer
gli	Transcription factor	Sarcoma, glioma
met	receptor tyrosine kinase	Carcinomas; sarcomas of lung, breast, cervix
mdm-2	p53 binding protein	Gastric sarcomas
myc family (c-, l-, n-)	transcription factor	c-: Burkitt lymphoma. Small cell lung carcinoma, acute T-cell lymphoma
		l-: small cell lung carcinoma
		n-: neuroblastoma, small cell lung carcinoma
plm-RARa	Chimeric transcription factor	Acute promyelocytic leukemia
ras family (H-, K-, N-)	p21 GTPase	H-: bladder cancer
		K-: pancreatic cancer, colorectal cancer, lung adenocarcinoma, endometrial cancer
		N-: myeloid leukemia
ret	Receptor tyrosine kinase	Thyroid cancer (papillary, medullary), sarcoma
smo	Transmembrane signaling	Basal cell skin cancer
trk	Receptor tyrosine kinase	Thyroid carcinoma, colorectal carcinoma
ttg	Transcription factor	T-cell acute lymphocytic leukemia
w2a-pbx1	Chimeric transcription factor	Pre–B-cell acute lymphocytic leukemia

messengers called mitogen-activated protein kinases, and the process ultimately results in cell division. This signal is autoregulated by hydrolysis of GTP to guanosine diphosphate (GDP), thereby turning the signal cascade "off" and leaving the Ras protein in its neutral GDP-bound state. The mutated, oncogenic form of the Ras protein lacks the ability to autoregulate signal transduction and as a result is continuously "on," thus allowing for uncontrolled cellular proliferation and carcinogenesis (5).

TUMOR SUPPRESSOR GENES

The concept of an "antioncogene," later termed a *tumor suppressor gene*, was first described by Knudson in 1971, when he described the "two-hit" hypothesis to demonstrate the epidemiology of retinoblastoma in children (2). To transform a normal cell into a malignant cell, two discrete "hits" or molecular events need to occur so both alleles of a tumor suppressor gene will be mutated. The first "hit" can be either inherited, as in the case of hereditary retinoblastoma in which patients have a germ-line mutation in one of the *rb-1* alleles, or spontaneous. Whether the first mutation is inherited or spontaneous, the tumor suppressor gene remains functional in the heterozygous state until a second "hit" occurs, at which time the gene is rendered incapacitated, and uncontrolled cellular proliferation occurs. As shown in Table 80.2, various cancer types have been associated with a loss of tumor suppressor gene function.

In fact, many of the inherited cancer syndromes involve tumor suppressor gene mutations. For example, the

development of certain breast cancers, brain cancers, leukemias, and sarcomas in patients with the Li-Fraumeni syndrome has been associated with a *p53* gene defect, and hereditary neurofibromatosis has been linked to a mutation in the *nf-1* gene (1). Because both alleles of a given tumor suppressor gene need to be mutated to result in loss of function, familial syndromes often exhibit variable penetrance. Affected family members tend to inherit one mutated gene and one normal gene, thus exposing them to an increased predisposition to cancer. If the normal allele becomes mutated as well, then the tumor suppressor gene loses its protective function, and uncontrolled growth and, ultimately, cancer can occur. As a result, not all family members actually develop cancer, and this is likely because they are able to maintain one intact normal allele, which preserves the functionality of the gene. Unfortunately, family members who do develop disease often do so at a younger age than the general population because the inherited germ-line mutation predisposes them to cancer by necessitating only one spontaneous mutation to lead to loss of gene function and subsequent carcinogenesis.

MISMATCH REPAIR GENES AND MICROSATELLITE INSTABILITY

Mismatch repair (MMR) genes are responsible for correcting errors of DNA replication. Defects in MMR genes allow small tandem sequences of nucleotide bases called *microsatellites* to be repeated, resulting in genomic instability. In

TABLE 80.2. TUMOR SUPPRESSOR GENES

TUMOR SUPPRESSOR GENE	SYNDROME	FUNCTION	ASSOCIATED TUMORS
P53	Li-Fraumeni syndrome	Cell-cycle regulation, apoptosis	Brain tumors, sarcoma, leukemia, breast cancer
RB1	Familial retinoblastoma	Cell-cycle regulation	Retinoblastoma, osteogenic sarcoma
WT1	Wilms tumor	Transcriptional regulation	Pediatric kidney cancer, hepatoblastoma
NF1	Neurofibromatosis, type 1	Catalysis of ras inactivation	Neurofibroma, sarcoma, glioma
APC	Familial adenomatous polyposis	Signaling through adhesion molecules to nucleus	Colorectal cancer
DCC	Deleted in colorectal carcinoma	Transmembrane receptor involved in axonal guidance via netrins	Colorectal cancer
BRCA1/BRCA2	Familial breast cancer	Repair of DNA double-strand breaks	Breast and ovarian cancer
MSH2/MLH1	Hereditary nonpolyposis colorectal cancer, types 1 and 2	DNA mismatch repair	Colorectal cancer
VHL	von Hippel-Lindau syndrome	Regulation of transcription elongation/ubiquitination of known substrates (HIF-1α)	Kidney cancer (clear cell), hemangioblastoma, pheochromocytoma
DPC4 (SMAD4)	Deleted in pancreatic cancer 4	Regulation of signal transduction	Pancreatic cancer, colorectal cancer

1997, the National Cancer Institute proposed a panel of five validated reference markers for detecting microsatellite instability. Tumors expressing two or more of these markers were defined as having high-frequency microsatellite instability (MSI-H), one marker was low frequency (MSI-L), and no markers indicated microsatellite stable (MSS). Because of the small number of reference markers, no distinction was made between MSI-L and MSS tumors (6).

MSI-H tumors are responsible for approximately 15% of colorectal cancers. These tumors have been associated with distinct clinical and pathologic features including proximal location, poor differentiation, mucinous cell type, and peritumoral lymphocytic infiltration (7). Although MSI-H colorectal tumors appear to have a better overall prognosis when adjusted for stage, a study by Ribic and colleagues demonstrated that MSI-L and MSS tumors benefit more from fluorouracil-based adjuvant chemotherapy (8).

MMR genes are frequently mutated in hereditary nonpolyposis colorectal cancer syndrome resulting in MSI-H. Affected persons can develop accelerated tumorigenesis because they lack the ability to correct errors that occur during DNA replication. More than 400 MMR gene mutations have been identified, with approximately 50% affecting MLH1, 40% MSH2, 10% MSH6, and 5% PMS2 (9). The risk of colon cancer is as high as 85% in persons with MMR genetic mutations, and other organs can be affected as well, including the uterus, ovary, hepatobiliary system, genitourinary system, pancreas, and small intestine (2).

MMR genes can also be affected by epigenetic processes that are not associated with hereditary germ-line abnormalities but still result in tumors exhibiting MSI-H. An example of this is hypermethylation of the promoter sequence of MLH1 and is discussed later (7).

DNA METHYLATION

DNA methylation is an epigenetic process that is increasingly implicated in the development of carcinogenesis. Enzyme-induced methylation of the DNA structure can occur without alteration in the base pair sequence. This can result in either direct inhibition of gene expression or indirect alteration of the gene product by increasing the likelihood of a mutational event. Both wide areas of hypomethylation along the genome and localized areas of hypermethylation within the gene promoter regions have been associated with altered patterns of oncogene and tumor suppressor gene expression (10). These epigenetic events may alter the behavior of the cell and may ultimately contribute to malignant transformation.

Promoter regions are areas where DNA transcription into RNA begins. These regions frequently contain stretches of DNA called CpG islands. CpG islands are clusters of dinucleotide base pairs in which cytosine precedes guanine. These cytosine-guanine dinucleotide base pairs are capable of being methylated by the methyl donor S-adenosyl-methionine and the enzyme DNA methyltransferase, which catalyzes the addition of a methyl group to the cytosine ring. In cancer, CpG islands in the promoter region tend to be hypermethylated. This results in epigenetic silencing of transcription and can functionally inactivate one or both copies of a given gene (11). Examples of epigenetic hypermethylation in tumor suppressor genes include the MMR gene *MLH1* and colorectal cancer, the *VHL* gene and renal cancer, the *RB* gene and retinoblastoma, and the *APC* gene and colorectal cancer (10).

MULTISTEP MODEL OF CARCINOGENESIS

Accumulations of specific alterations in oncogenes and tumor suppressor genes resulting in tumorigenesis have been well described by Fearon and Vogelstein's multistep model of colon cancer carcinogenesis (12). In this model, sporadic colon cancer results from the accumulation of multiple somatic mutations involving activation of oncogenes and inactivation of tumor suppressor genes. Each subsequent genetic event allows for a selective growth advantage for the affected colon cell. The cumulative effect of these genetic events ultimately leads to the development of sporadic colon cancer. This model can be extrapolated to fit a multitude of different cancer types.

In the Vogelstein model of colorectal carcinogenesis, genetic alterations of oncogenes (e.g. *ras*) and tumor suppressor genes (e.g. *APC, DCC, p53*) drive the process of colorectal tumorigenesis forward from a normal epithelial cell, to an adenoma of increasing malignant potential, and ultimately to invasive carcinoma (Fig. 80.1). This process of malignant transformation involves somatic mutations of at least four or five genes in a given cell. It is the accumulation of these genetic alterations, not the sequence, that ultimately determines the abnormal behavior of the cell and contributes to carcinogenesis (3).

Mutation of the adenomatous polyposis coli (*APC*) tumor suppressor gene appears to be one of the initial steps toward colorectal carcinogenesis. The *APC* gene is thought to play a role in cell signal transduction and growth through the modulation of the β-catenin protein, and loss of this function likely results in patients' developing hyperproliferative epithelium. Because this mutation often occurs early in the process of tumorigenesis, the *APC* gene is referred to as the "gatekeeper" gene (2).

Familial adenomatous polyposis is the result of a single germ-line mutation of the *APC* gene on chromosome 5q and is frequently transmitted through autosomal dominance. Familial adenomatous polyposis can also arise as a de novo mutation of the *APC* gene in up to one third of affected persons (2). Whether inherited or sporadic, hundreds to thousands of colonic polyps develop in persons with familial adenomatous polyposis. Although the rate of multistep malignant transformation is low, the large number of polyps essentially ensures the development of colorectal cancer at a young age, and as a result, prophylactic colectomy is frequently performed.

Subsequent epigenetic and genetic events such as DNA hypomethylation and mutation of the ras oncogene on chromosome 12p contribute to clonal expansion of preexisting small adenomas and ultimately result in larger, more dysplastic tumors (3). In addition, up to 70% of colorectal carcinomas and 50% of advanced adenomas have an abnormality of the deleted in colorectal carcinoma (*DCC*) tumor suppressor gene on chromosome 18q. The *DCC* gene was first identified in 1989 and is thought possibly to play a role in colon cancer carcinogenesis through disruption of cell-cell or cell-matrix interactions (13).

Loss of the *p53* tumor suppressor gene on chromosome 17p tends to occur late in the process of tumorigenesis and triggers the transformation from a late adenoma to an invasive carcinoma. Normally, *p53* plays a role in G_1 cell-cycle arrest and facilitates DNA repair or induction of apoptosis. As many as 75% of sporadic colorectal tumors exhibit *p53* inactivation, and this is associated with a worse prognosis as measured by overall survival time (2).

The transition from normal colonic mucosa to adenocarcinoma is therefore a genetic and epigenetic phenomenon that occurs gradually over time. In some instances, the development from normal colonic mucosa to adenoma can take 5 to 20 years, and then progression from adenoma to carcinoma can take an additional 5 to 15 years. This gradual development of disease offers a significant opportunity for early detection and prevention (14).

CELL CYCLE

Cancer arises from an imbalance between regulatory mechanisms in a normal cell. The cell cycle is a complex cellular mechanism. The activation of cell-cycle checkpoints, in the setting of DNA damage, induces cell-cycle arrest, which provides the cell sufficient time to repair damaged DNA. Defects in cell-cycle regulation result in uncontrolled cellular proliferation, the accumulation of abnormal DNA, and subsequent malignant transformation. Thus, the cell cycle serves to protect genetic fidelity. As a result, the cell cycle is a fundamental component of carcinogenesis, and a basic understanding of its molecular underpinnings will likely help to elucidate means of cancer prevention and even future cancer therapy.

The four phases of the cell cycle are G_1, S (DNA synthesis), G_2, and M (mitosis) (Fig. 80.2). Each transition point (from G_1 to S or G_2 to M) is tightly regulated to prevent

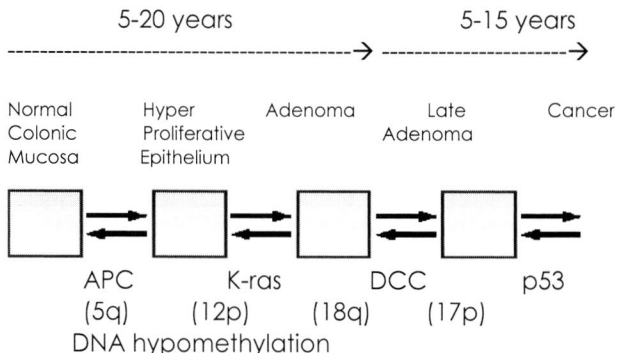

Figure 80.1. Colorectal tumorigenesis. Colorectal tumorigenesis proceeds through a series of genetic events involving oncogenes (*ras*) and tumor suppressor genes (*APC, DCC, p53*).

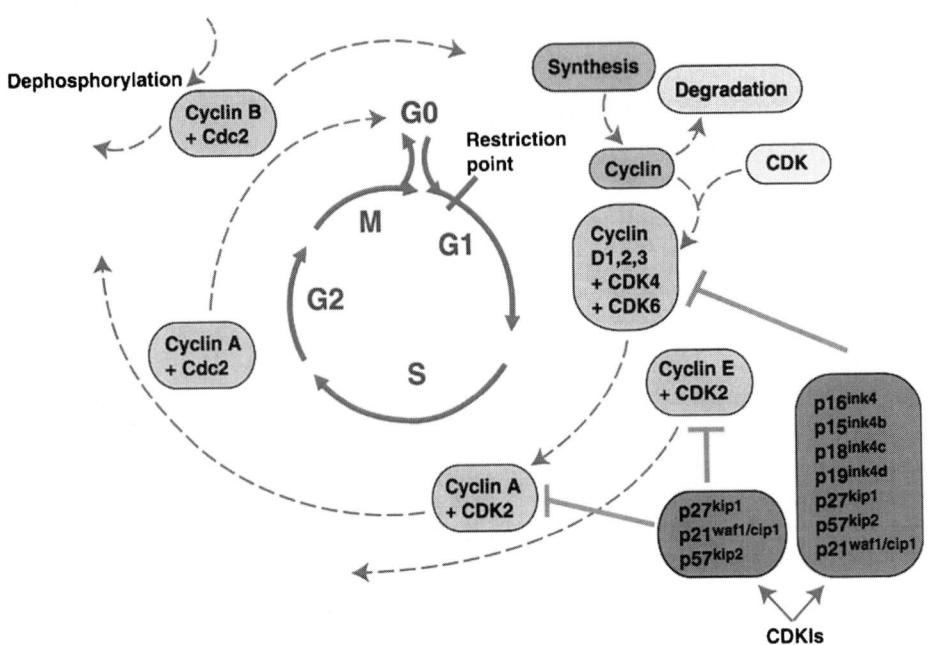

Figure 80.2. Cellcycle regulation. The cell cycle consists of four phases: G_1, S (DNA synthesis), G_2, and M (mitosis). G_0 is the where the cell performs routine functions such as cell growth. Progression through the cell cycle is regulated by cyclins, cyclin-dependent kinases (CDKs), and cyclin-dependent kinase inhibitors (CDKIs). (From Shah MA, Schwartz GK. Cell cycle modulation: an emerging target for cancer therapy. Horizons Cancer Ther 2003; 4:3–21, with permission.)

premature exit with damaged or incompletely repaired DNA repair. The biology of the cell cycle involves a complex array of interdependent mechanisms. Progression of a cell through the cell cycle is driven by cyclin-dependent kinases (CDKs). When these CDKs are complexed with positive regulatory proteins called cyclins, cells progress within the cell cycle from a period of relative quiescence (G_0) through to cell growth and proliferation.

At least nine structurally related CDKs have been identified (CDK1–CDK9), and even more cyclins have been discovered (cyclins A–T). These complexes are activated via phosphorylation by CDK-activating kinase (15). The pattern of expression of each CDK/cyclin complex determines the relative position of a given cell within the cell cycle. For example, cyclin D isoforms (cyclin D1–D3) interact with CDK2, CDK4, and CDK6 to move the cell through G_1, cyclin E/CDK2 is active at the G_1/S interface, cyclin A/CDK1 is important in G_2, and cyclin B/CDK1 is necessary for mitosis to occur (16). Overexpression of these cyclins results in unregulated cell growth and allows for an early step in malignant transformation.

CDK inhibitors (CDKIs) are negative regulators of the CDKs and prevent the cell from entering into consecutive phases of the cell cycle. The INK4 (inhibitor of CDK4) class of CDKIs binds and inhibits cyclin D–associated kinases and prevents progression through G_1. Similarly, the KIP (kinase inhibitor protein) group of CDKIs affects cyclin E and cyclin A when complexed with CDK2 by negatively regulating progression from G_1 through S (17).

Loss of expression of an INK4 or KIP family member results in the inability to inhibit a CDK, thus inducing unregulated cell growth in a normal cell and resulting in accumulation of abnormal DNA and malignant transfor-

mation. For example, *p16* is an INK4 gene that is particularly sensitive to epigenetic silencing by hypermethylation of its promoter region, and this results in inhibition of transcription and loss of gene expression. When this occurs, uncontrolled proliferation can result. Accordingly, loss of *p16* function has been associated with a multitude of malignancies including melanoma and lung, breast, and colorectal tumors (10).

Checkpoints are integral to cell-cycle function. For example, the S-phase checkpoint slows progression of the cell while undergoing DNA synthesis and is sometimes referred to as the replication checkpoint. When DNA damage occurs, a complicated pathway of ATM/ATR kinase activation, Chk1/Chk2 phosphorylation, and Cdc25 inhibitory phosphorylation can result in cyclin B/CDK1 inactivation, which halts late G_2 phase progression and ultimately prevents mitosis (16).

Tumor suppressor genes and oncogenes via signal transduction pathways also regulate cell-cycle entry and exit. In malignant transformation, these checkpoints are compromised, and as a result, carcinogenesis and uncontrolled cellular proliferation occurs. The retinoblastoma gene product (pRb) is an example of a tumor suppressor gene product that helps to regulate the cell cycle. In its active state, pRb is hypophosphorylated and forms an inhibitory complex with a transcription factor known as E2F, which prevents the G_1-S transition (Fig. 80.3). When pRb is phosphorylated, E2F is released, allowing for transcriptional activation of integral S-phase proteins such as thymidylate synthase and dihydrofolate reductase and thus permitting DNA synthesis and progression through the cell cycle (17).

P53 is another tumor suppressor gene that contributes to cell-cycle regulation. *P53* expression is activated by

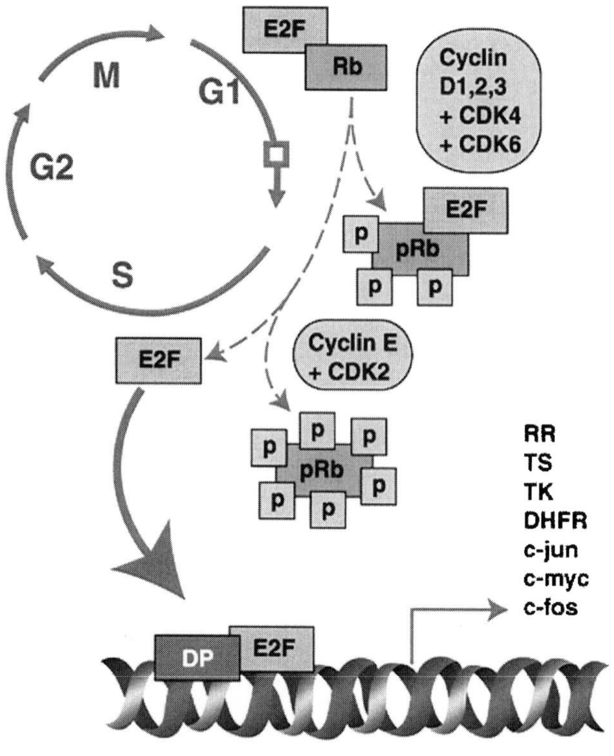

DNA damage. P53 then serves as a transcription factor that results in the induction of p21. P21 is a KIP that binds to and inhibits the activation of the cyclin A or the cyclin E/CDK2 complex and results in cell-cycle arrest at the G_1–S interphase (17). Thus, normal cells that acquire mutations in tumor suppressor genes such as p53 or pRb are able to undergo unregulated cell-cycle growth, with accumulation of abnormal DNA and eventual malignant transformation.

Figure 80.3. *Rb* and the G_1–S transition. The retinoblastoma gene product (pRb) is hypophosphorylated in the active state and complexes with a group of transcription factors collectively known as E2F. Cyclin-dependent kinase (CDK)–mediated phosphorylation inactivates RB and releases E2F, allowing for transcriptional activation of integral S-phase proteins such as ribonucleotide reductase (RR), thymidylate synthase (TS), thymidine kinase (TK), dihydrofolate reductase (DHFR), c-jun, c-myc, and c-fos. (From Shah MA, Schwartz GK. Cell cycle modulation: an emerging target for cancer therapy. Horizons Cancer Ther 2003; 4:3–21, with permission.)

CONCLUSION AND FUTURE DIRECTIONS

In this chapter, we attempt to illustrate key steps in the molecular basis of carcinogenesis that leads to malignant transformation. An understanding of these processes has significant clinical implications. The identification of specific genetic events that result in neoplasia provides the ability to screen and identify family members who are at high risk of developing hereditary malignancies. In high-risk family members, the results of these screening tests can be used to recommend surgical interventions with removal of organs (i.e., prophylactic colectomy, mastectomy, or oophorectomy) that are especially susceptible to malignant transformation.

Even more exciting is the development of nonsurgical approaches to prevent malignant transformation. An understanding of the cell cycle and of the mechanisms by which malignant transformation is initiated and maintained has and will continue to result in promising new therapeutic approaches. In numerous current examples, changes in the cell-cycle machinery associated with the process of carcinogenesis are being used as potential targets for chemoprevention and early intervention.

Recently, APC deletions have been associated with overexpression of enzymes that cause a decrease in acetylation of histones on DNA, believed to be an early step in carcinogenesis. Oral inhibitors of these enzymes are now undergoing clinical development and provide a new means for cancer prevention in populations at high risk of developing cancer. The association of cyclooxygenase-2 with Barrett esophagus and the rapid increase in adenocarcinoma of the gastroesophageal junction point to the use of oral cyclooxygenase-2 inhibitors in cancer prevention. The use of this class of drugs has already proven successful in cancer prevention in persons with familial adenomatous polyposis who are at high risk of colon cancer (18).

In addition, recent advances in the understanding of the cell cycle have led to the development of a class of drugs that target the motors of the cell cycle, the CDKs. Small-molecule CDKIs are currently in clinical development. This promising class of drugs is being studied both alone and in combination with standard chemotherapeutic agents in an effort to reintroduce cell-cycle arrest and reverse cell-cycle–mediated drug resistance. Thus, a detailed understanding of the molecular basis of carcinogenesis provides the platform from which new and exciting targeted therapies can be developed with the ultimate goal of noninvasive cancer prevention and early intervention.

REFERENCES

1. Savage PD. In Shils ME, Olson JA et al., eds. Modern Nutrition in Health and Disease. 9th ed. Philadelphia: Lippincott Williams & Wilkins, 1998:1235–42.
2. Calvert PM, Frucht H. Ann Intern Med 2002;137:603–12.
3. Ringer DP, Schipper LE. In: Lenhard RE, Osteen RT, Gansler T, eds. The American Cancer Society's Clinical Oncology. Atlanta, GA: American Cancer Society, 2001.
4. Scharovsky OG, Rozados VR, Gervasoni SI et al. J Biomed Sci 2000;7:292–8.
5. Goodsell DS. Oncologist 1999;4:263–4.
6. Boland CR, Thibodeau SN, Hamilton SR et al. Cancer Res 1998;58:5248–57.
7. de la Chapelle A. N Engl J Med 2003;349:209–10.
8. Ribic CM, Sargent DJ, Moore MJ et al. N Engl J Med 2003;349:247–57.
9. Peltomaki P. J Clin Oncol 2003;21:1174–9.
10. Shahjehan WA, Laird PW, DeMeester TR. Ann Surg 2001;234:10–20.
11. Herman JG, Baylin SB. N Engl J Med 2003;349:2042–54.

12. Fearon ER. Vogelstein B. Cell 1990;61:759–67.
13. Mehlen P, Fearon ER. J Clin Oncol 2004;22:3420–8.
14. Alberts DS. Cancer J 2002;8:208–21.
15. Kaldis P, Russo AA, Chou HS et al. Mol Biol Cell 1998;9:2545–60.
16. Shah MA, Schwartz GK. Horizons Cancer Ther 2003;4:3–21.
17. Shah MA, Schwartz GK. Clin Cancer Res 2001;7:2168–81.
18. Janne PA, Mayer RJ. N Engl J Med 2000;342:1960–6.
19. King MW. SciLinks 2001, modified 6/25/04. http://web.indstate.edu
20. Kuznetsova AV, Meller J, Schnell PO et al. Proc Natl Acad Sci USA 2003;100:2706–11.

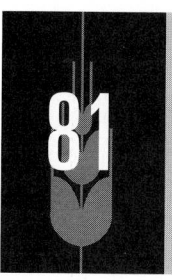

EPIDEMIOLOGY OF DIET AND CANCER RISK[1]

WALTER C. WILLETT AND EDWARD GIOVANNUCCI

CANCER AS A PUBLIC HEALTH PROBLEM 1267
EPIDEMIOLOGIC INVESTIGATION OF DIET
    AND CANCER RELATIONSHIPS 1268
CURRENT STATE OF KNOWLEDGE OF SPECIFIC
    ASPECTS OF DIET 1269
      Energy Balance, Growth Rates, and Body Size . . .1269
      Macronutrients .1270
      Food Groups .1272
      Dietary Fiber and Cancer Risk 1273
      Alcoholic Beverages 1274
      Vitamin and Mineral Supplements 1274
SUMMARY 1275

CANCER AS A PUBLIC HEALTH PROBLEM

Following cardiovascular disease, cancer is the second leading cause of death in most affluent countries and also contributes importantly to mortality rates among adults in developing countries (1, 2). At current rates in the United States, about one in three women and slightly less than one in two men will be diagnosed with cancer during their lifetime (3). Although overall cancer rates among adults vary only modestly around the world, the types of cancers are dramatically different (1, 2). In most affluent countries, cancers of the lung, colon, breast, and prostate contribute most to incidence and mortality. In poorer regions and in the Far East, cancers of the stomach, liver, oral cavity, esophagus, and uterine cervix are most important. However, cancer incidence rates are highly dynamic; populations that move from countries with low rates of specific cancers to areas with high rates, or the reverse, almost invariably achieve the rates characteristic of the new homeland (4–6). The time required to attain the new rate can vary, however, from several decades in the case of colon cancer to about three generations for breast cancer (6–9). Although genetics influences the development of cancer, the striking changes in cancer rates within countries demonstrate the importance of noninherited factors.

The dramatic variations in cancer rates around the world and changes over time imply that these malignancies

are potentially avoidable if we could identify and then avoid the causal factors. For a few cancers, the primary causes are well known, such as smoking in the case of lung cancer, but for most others the etiologic factors are less well established. However, dietary and nutritional factors are likely to account for many of these variations in cancer rates, as suggested by observations that national rates of specific cancers are strongly correlated with aspects of diet such as per capita consumption of fat (10). In addition, numerous studies in animals clearly demonstrate that dietary manipulations influence tumorigenesis.

Many steps in the pathogenesis of cancer have been identified in which dietary factors could plausibly act either to increase or to decrease the probability that a clinical cancer will develop. For example, carcinogens in food that can directly damage DNA are discussed in Chapter 82, and other dietary factors may block the endogenous synthesis of carcinogens or induce enzymes involved in the activation or deactivation of exogenous carcinogenic substances (11). Oxidative damage to DNA is likely to be an important cause of mutations and can potentially be enhanced by some dietary factors, such as polyunsaturated fats and iron, or reduced by dietary antioxidants or nutrients that are cofactors for antioxidant enzymes, such as selenium or copper (12). Inadequate intake of dietary factors needed for DNA synthesis, repair, and methylation, such as folate, could also influence mutation rates or gene expression. The rate of cell division will influence whether DNA lesions are replicated and is thus likely to influence the probability of cancer (12). Thus, energy balance and growth rates, which can be influenced by a variety of essential nutrients, could affect cancer rates. Dietary factors can influence endogenous hormone levels, including estrogens and various growth factors, which can influence cell cycling and, thus, potentially cancer incidence. Estrogenic substances found in some plant foods can also interact with estrogen receptors and thus could either mimic or block the effects of endogenous estrogens (11). Many other aspects of diet can alter cell proliferation or differentiation either by direct hormonal effects, such as by vitamins A or D, or indirectly by influencing inflammatory or irritative processes, such as specific fatty acids that are precursors of prostaglandins or that inhibit their synthesis. Many other examples can be given by which dietary factors could plausibly influence the development of cancer (11, 12).

---

[1]**Abbreviation: IGF,** insulinlike growth factor.

EPIDEMIOLOGIC INVESTIGATION OF DIET AND CANCER RELATIONSHIPS

The strong suggestions from international comparisons, animal studies, and mechanistic investigations that various aspects of diet could importantly influence the risk of cancer raise two critical sets of questions: Which dietary factors are actually important determinants of human cancer? What is the nature of the dose-response and temporal relationships? The nature of the dose-response relationships is particularly important because in large amounts a substance could be carcinogenic to humans, but no important risk would be imparted within the range of actual intake. Alternatively, another factor could be critical for protection against cancer, but all persons in a population may already be consuming sufficient amounts to receive the maximal benefit. In either case, no potential exists for reduction in cancer rates by altering current intakes. The important factors to identify are those for which at least some part of the population is either consuming a toxic level or is not eating a sufficient amount for optimal health. Because carcinogenesis is a multistage process that typically takes decades, the temporal relationship is also critical to identify.

Various epidemiologic approaches can be used to investigate the relationships between diet and human cancer (Table 81.1). Relationships between diet and cancer incidence in epidemiologic studies can be evaluated by collecting data on dietary intake, by using biochemical indicators of dietary factors, or by measuring body size and composition. Food frequency questionnaires have been used to assess diet in most epidemiologic studies because they provide information on usual diet over an extended period, they are efficient for use in large populations, and they are sufficiently valid based on comparisons with more detailed assessments of diet and biochemical indicators (13). Biochemical indicators of diet can be useful in some situations, but for many dietary factors of interest, such as total fat, fiber, and sodium, no useful indicators exist. DNA specimens have been collected from participants in many studies and allow for the examination of gene-diet interactions. Until recently, most information on diet and cancer was obtained from case-control studies. However, large ongoing prospective cohort studies of diet and cancer in various countries are now generating data that are transforming our epidemiologic understanding of nutrition and cancer. Epidemiologic investigations should be viewed as complementary to animal studies, in vitro investigations, studies in humans of diet on intermediate end points, such as hormone levels, DNA damage, or precancerous lesions, and randomized trials with cancer as the

TABLE 81.1. TYPES OF STUDIES THAT ADDRESS EFFECT OF DIET ON HUMAN CANCER

STUDY	METHODS	POTENTIAL LIMITATIONS
Descriptive	Comparison of cancer rates in populations having different diets by assessing average intake of specific nutrients and determining cancer incidence or mortality	Diet is only one of many variables that distinguish different populations. Gathering even crude data on average nutrient intake is difficult. These studies are probably best used to generate hypotheses.
Case-control	Comparison of earlier diets reported by patients with a particular type of cancer with diets reported by matched controls without cancer	Selection bias can occur if controls do not accurately represent the population from which cases arose. Recall bias results when patients systematically differ from controls in ability to recall diets; memory of dietary habits can be faulty among patients and controls[a]; in studies of rapidly fatal cancers, researchers must often rely on recall of proxy respondents such as spouses.
Cohort (prospective or follow-up)	Comparison of incidence of cancer in people whose diets and other potentially relevant traits are determined before follow-up begins	Selection bias and recall bias should not occur, but cohort studies must enroll thousands or even tens of thousands of people and monitor their health for many years before statistical power can be achieved.
Interventional	Comparison of incidence of cancer in two groups randomized to specific interventions or sometimes to no interventions	Compliance with substantial dietary changes is difficult for many people. Subjects cannot be easily blinded to their status. Optimal dosages (e.g., of supplemental nutrients) and dose-response relationships can be difficult to ascertain. Duration of intervention required is generally unknown but may be decades.

[a] In case-control and cohort studies of the effect of vitamins, measurements of vitamins in blood are sometimes substituted for dietary recall questionnaires; however, this strategy is not universally applicable. For example, retinol levels in blood do not accurately reflect intake of vitamin A, for example, whereas β-carotene blood levels are a good index of dietary intake. Blood levels must be interpreted with caution in case-control studies because cancer can change the level of a vitamin in the plasma.
From Willett WC. Adv Oncol 1995;11:3–8, with permission from Cliggott Publishing Co.

outcome. Although conditions can be controlled to a much greater degree in laboratory studies than in free-living human populations, the relevance of findings to humans will always be uncertain, particularly in regard to dose-response and temporal relationships. Ultimately, our knowledge is best based on a synthesis of epidemiologic, metabolic, animal, clinical, and mechanistic studies.

CURRENT STATE OF KNOWLEDGE OF SPECIFIC ASPECTS OF DIET

Diet is a complex composite of various nutrients and non-nutritive food constituents, and many types of human cancer exist, each with its own pathogenic mechanisms; thus, the combinations of specific dietary factors and cancer are almost limitless. This brief overview focuses primarily on the major cancers of affluent populations and aspects of diet for which strong hypotheses and substantial epidemiologic data exist. Several aspects of diet for which preventive roles have been hypothesized are discussed in further detail in Chapter 82.

Energy Balance, Growth Rates, and Body Size

Studies by Tannenbaum and Silverstone (14, 15) during the first half of the twentieth century indicated that energy restriction could profoundly reduce the development of mammary tumors in animals. This finding has been consistently replicated in a wide variety of mammary tumor models and for many other tumors (16–20). For example, restriction in energy intake by approximately 30% can reduce mammary tumors by as much as 90% (21). The possibility that this relationship, which is consistent and strong in animal studies, could also apply to humans received relatively little attention until recently.

In evaluating the effect of energy restriction on cancer rates in humans, it may be tempting to examine the association between energy intake and incidence of cancer. However, such an approach is likely to be misleading because, in free-living populations, variation in energy intake is determined largely by energy expenditure in the form of physical activity (22). Thus, for example, energy intake is inversely associated with risk of coronary heart disease, as a result of the protective effect of exercise against this disease (13). The most sensitive indicators of the balance between energy intake and expenditure are growth rates and body size, which can be measured well in epidemiologic investigations, although they also reflect genetic and other nonnutritional factors. Adult height can thus provide an indirect indicator of preadult nutrition, and adult weight gain and obesity reflect positive energy balance later in life. In populations that were traditionally short, such as the Japanese, rapid gains in height during the last several decades (23) have corresponded with increases in breast and colon cancer rates. Further support for an important role of growth rates comes from epidemiologic studies of

age at menarche. An early menarche is a well-established risk factor for breast cancer. In past decades, the difference in the age of menarche in China, approximately 17 years (24), compared with 12 and 13 years of age in the United States (25), contributed importantly to differences in breast cancer rates between these populations, although the trend is toward earlier age of menarche in China (26). Body mass index, height, and weight have consistently been strong determinants or correlates of age at menstruation (27–29), but the composition of diet appears to have little effect, if any. Collectively, these studies provide strong evidence, consistent with animal experiments, that rapid growth rates before puberty play an important role in determining future risk of breast and probably other cancers. Whether the epidemiologic findings are caused only by restriction of energy intake in relation to requirements for maximal growth, or whether the limitation of other nutrients, such as essential amino acids, may also play a role cannot be determined from available data.

A positive energy balance during adult life and the resultant accumulation of body fat also contribute importantly to several human cancers. The best-established relationships are with cancers of the colon, kidney, pancreas, esophagus (adenocarcinoma), endometrium, and gallbladder (30–37). The relation between body fat and breast cancer is more complex. Before menopause, women with greater body fat have reduced risks of breast cancer (38, 39), and after menopause a positive, but weak, association with adiposity is seen. These findings are probably the result of anovulatory menstrual cycles in fatter women before menopause (40), which should reduce risk, and the synthesis of endogenous estrogen by adipose tissue in postmenopausal women (41), which is presumed to increase the risk of breast cancer. The relationship between body size and prostate cancer has not been consistent; most studies have not indicated an appreciable association with incidence of prostate cancer, although some studies have suggested that overweight men may have higher mortality from prostate cancer (42). One study showed that obesity in adolescence may reduce the risk of prostate cancer, and younger men or those with a positive family history of prostate cancer may be at reduced risk if they are obese (43).

The association between obesity and cancer risk may be explained in part by alterations in the metabolism and levels of hormones, including sex steroids, insulin, and insulinlike growth factors (IGFs), which influence cell proliferation, differentiation and apoptosis. In animal models, reductions in IGF-I mediate at least part of the effect of energy reduction (44). Insulin is known to be a powerful modulator of bioavailable IGF-I (45). In human studies, increasing evidence indicates that high circulating levels of IGF-I and insulin are associated with an increased risk of some cancers that occur in affluent populations, particularly colon cancer (45, 46). In fact, indirect evidence (47) suggests that factors related to energy balance and dietary patterns that increase insulin and IGF-I exposure throughout the life span could largely account for the approximately one third of cancers in men in affluent countries that are believed to be influenced by nutrition (48). The avoidance of weight gain in adulthood appears to be an important factor for the prevention of some cancers, although a benefit of intended weight loss in reducing risk has not been well studied in humans. However, one prospective study found that women who experienced intentional weight loss episodes of 20 or more pounds had a reduced risk of cancer, particularly breast cancer (49).

Macronutrients

Fat

In the landmark 1982 National Academy of Sciences review of diet, nutrition, and cancer (50), reduction in fat intake to 30% of calories was the primary recommendation; this objective was echoed in subsequent dietary recommendations as well (51, 52). Two lines of evidence stimulated interest in dietary fat as a cause of cancer. First, a vast literature indicated that diets high in fat could promote tumor growth in animal models (reviewed elsewhere) (20, 50, 53–57). However, the influence of fat in animal models has not been definitely established to be independent of the effect of energy intake (20, 21, 56–58). Second, a possible relation of dietary fat intake to cancer incidence was also hypothesized because the large international differences in rates of cancers of the breast, colon, prostate, and endometrium are strongly correlated with apparent per capita animal fat consumption (10, 59–61).

Fat and Breast Cancer. Although a major rationale for the dietary fat hypothesis was the international correlation between fat consumption and national breast cancer mortality (10), other evidence has not been as supportive. For example, in a study of 65 Chinese counties (62), in which per capita fat intake varied from 6 to 25% of energy, only a weak positive association was seen between fat intake and breast cancer mortality. Notably, five counties consumed approximately 25% of energy from fat, yet this population experienced rates of breast cancer far lower than those of US women with similar fat intake (63). Breast cancer incidence rates increased substantially in the United States during the twentieth century, as did estimates of per capita fat consumption based on food disappearance data. However, surveys based on reports of individual actual intake, rather than food disappearance, indicated that consumption of energy from fat, either as absolute intake or as a percentage of energy, actually declined in the 1970s and 1980s (64, 65), a time during which breast cancer incidence increased (66). Numerous case-control studies have investigated the effect of dietary fat on breast cancer risk. In the largest study so far (67), animal fat and total fat intake were not associated with breast cancer. The results from 12 smaller case-control studies were summarized in a metaanalysis by Howe and associates (68), which included 4312 cases and 5978 controls. The pooled relative risk was 1.35 (p <.0001) for a 100-g increase in daily total fat intake, although the risk was somewhat stronger for postmenopausal women (relative risk, 1.48; p <.001). This magnitude of association, however, could potentially be compatible with biases caused by recall of diet or the selection of controls in case-control studies (69).

A substantial body of data from cohort studies is now available to assess prospectively the relation between dietary fat intake and breast cancer in developed countries. In a pooled analysis of prospective studies that included 4980 incident cases of breast cancer (70), no overall association was seen for total fat intake over the range of 20 to 45% of energy from fat. A similar lack of association was seen among postmenopausal women only and for specific types of fat. Only among the small number of women consuming less than 15% of energy from fat was a significant association seen, but this was in the opposite than expected direction; breast cancer risk was elevated twofold in this group. An update of the pooled analysis with 7329 cases continued to support the lack of association with total fat intake (71). In the Nurses' Health Study, analyses were conducted with 14 years of follow-up (2956 cases) and with up to four assessments of fat intake, which improved the measurement of long-term intake; no indication of an increased risk associated with high fat intake was detected (72). Thus, the prospective studies that have included mostly postmenopausal women provided strong evidence against an association with dietary fat. However, a study conducted among 90,655 premenopausal women age 26 to 46 years at baseline found a statistically significant positive association between animal fat, mainly from red meat and high-fat dairy sources, and risk of premenopausal breast cancer (73). No association was seen with vegetable fat intake. The possibility that diet later in life may have less influence on postmenopausal breast cancer, whereas diet earlier in life may affect premenopausal breast cancer, requires confirmation. Some of the inconsistencies in fat and breast cancer risk may be resolved when results from a large, ongoing intervention trial of a low fat diet in women, the Women's Health Initiative, is completed (74). However, the diet pattern also includes increased intakes of fruits, vegetables, and grains, which will complicate interpretation of results. In addition, because women were postmenopausal at randomization, and they were up to 75 years old, effects at younger ages cannot be addressed.

Although total fat intake has been unrelated to breast cancer risk in prospective epidemiologic studies, some evidence suggests that the type of fat may be important. In animal mammary tumor models, the tumor-promoting effect of fat intake was observed primarily for polyunsaturated fats when fed in the presence of high-fat diets containing approximately 45% of energy (75, 76). However, in a metaanalysis of case-control studies (68), increased risk of breast cancer was somewhat greater for saturated fats (relative risk, 1.46) and monounsaturated fats (relative risk, 1.41) than for polyunsaturated fats (relative risk, 1.25). In the Nurses' Health Study, an inverse association between monounsaturated fat and breast cancer was present (63), although only a weak nonsignificant association was found in a pooling study of eight cohort studies (71). Rates of breast cancer are relatively low in southern European countries, which have high average intakes of monounsaturated fats because of the use of olive oil as the primary fat source. In case-control studies in Spain and Greece, women who used more olive oil had reduced risks of breast cancer (77, 78). Furthermore, olive oil was shown to be protective relative to other sources of fats in some animal studies (57). Specific oils may be rich in bioactive compounds (e.g., tocopherols) that could be protective.

Fat and Colon Cancer. In comparisons among countries, rates of colon cancer are strongly correlated with national per capita disappearance of animal fat and meat, with correlation coefficients ranging between 0.8 and 0.9 (10, 61). These epidemiologic investigations and animal studies led to the hypothesis that dietary fat increases excretion of bile acids, which can be converted to colonic carcinogens or promoters (79). However, more recent evidence from many studies that higher body weight increases risk and higher levels of physical activity reduce risk of colon cancer (80) indicates that at least part of the high rates in affluent countries previously attributed to fat intake are probably the result of sedentary lifestyle and excess energy intakes.

With some exceptions (81–84), case-control studies have generally shown an association between risk of colon cancer and intake of fat (85–92) or red meat (93–98). However, in many of these studies, a positive association between total energy intake and risk of colon cancer has also been observed (85–89, 91, 92). A metaanalysis by Howe of 13 case-control studies found a statistically significant association between total energy intake and colon cancer, but saturated, monounsaturated, and polyunsaturated fats were not associated with colon cancer independently of total energy intake (99).

The relation between dietary fat and colon cancer was examined in several large prospective studies. These also failed to confirm a positive association with total energy intake in case-control studies (100–104), a finding suggesting that results from the case-control studies were distorted by reporting bias. Although excessive energy intake relative to requirements (i.e., obesity) is likely to increase risk, total energy intake is likely to reflect physical activity, a protective factor (80). Most of the studies did not support an association between fat intake and colon cancer risk independent of energy intake. One exception was the Nurses' Health Study, which showed about a twofold higher risk of colon cancer among women in the highest compared with those in the lowest quintile of animal fat

intake (100). However, in a multivariate analysis of these data, which included red meat and animal fat intakes in the same model, red meat intake remained significantly predictive of the risk of colon cancer, whereas the association with animal fat was eliminated (see the later discussion on meat intake).

Fat and Prostate Cancer. Associations between fat intake and prostate cancer risk were seen in many case-control studies (105–115), but sometimes only in subgroups. In a large case-control study of various ethnic groups within the United States (116), consistent associations with prostate cancer risk were seen for saturated fat, but not with other types of fat. However, whether the association between fat and prostate cancer is independent of total energy intake was generally not considered in case-control studies.

The association between fat intake and prostate cancer risk has been assessed in only a few cohort studies. In a cohort of 8000 Japanese men living in Hawaii, no association was seen between intake of total or unsaturated fat and prostate cancer risk (117). However, diet was assessed with a single 24-hour recall in this study, so the lack of association may not be informative, because measurement error would be expected to be substantial. In a study of 14,000 Seventh-Day Adventist men living in California, a positive association between the percentage of calories from animal fat and prostate cancer risk was seen, but this was not statistically significant (118). In the Health Professionals Follow-up Study of 51,000 men, a positive association was seen with intake of red meat, total fat, and animal fat, an association largely limited to aggressive prostate cancers (119, 120). No association was seen with vegetable fats. In another cohort from Hawaii, increased risks of prostate cancer were seen with consumption of beef and animal fat (121).

A somewhat puzzling observation is that high intake or blood level of α-linolenic acid, a fatty acid comprising only about 1% of total energy intake, was associated with an increased risk of prostate cancer (especially advanced cancers) in two distinct prospective studies (119, 122, 123), as well as in five case-control studies in diverse populations: Uruguay (124), Spain (125), Norway (126), China (127), and the United States (128). However, other studies did not support this association (129–133). It is critical to determine whether this association is causal, because this fatty acid is beneficial in regard to cardiovascular disease (134, 135). Although further data are desirable, the evidence from international correlations, case-control studies, and cohort studies is reasonably consistent in support of an association between consumption of fat-containing animal products and prostate cancer incidence, particularly advanced prostate cancer.

Fat and Other Cancers. Rates of other cancers that are common in affluent countries, including those of the endometrium and ovary, are, of course, also correlated with fat intake internationally. Although these correlations were studied in a small number of case-control investigations, consistent associations with fat intake were not seen (136–145). In a prospective study among Iowa women (146), no evidence of relation between fat intake and risk of endometrial cancer was observed. Positive associations have been hypothesized between fat intake and risks of skin cancer (147) and lung cancer(148, 149), but relevant data in humans are nonsupportive (150, 151).

Summary of Fat and Cancer. As the findings from large prospective studies emerged, support for a major relationship between fat intake and breast cancer risk weakened considerably. For colon cancer, the associations seen with animal fat internationally were supported in numerous case-control and cohort studies. However, more recent evidence suggested that this association could be explained by factors in red meat other than simply its fat content. Further, the importance of energy balance on colon cancer risk indicates that international correlations probably overstate the contribution of dietary composition to differences in colon cancer incidence. The available evidence most strongly supports an association between animal fat consumption and risk of aggressive or advanced prostate cancer. As with colon cancer, however, the possibility remains that other factors in foods containing animal fat contribute to risk.

Carbohydrates

Coincident with the strong emphasis on lowering dietary fat over the past several decades, the tendency has been for greater consumption of grains (152, 153). Although the mechanisms linking obesity to increased cancer risk are unknown, diets high in refined carbohydrates are known to exacerbate many of the metabolic effects of obesity, including hypertriglyceridemia, hyperglycemia, and hyperinsulinemia (154–156). Fasting plasma insulin concentrations, in turn, are inversely correlated with IGF-binding protein-1 and thus an increase in bioactive IGF-I (45). In a group of case-control studies from Italy, diets high in glycemic load were related to a higher risk of colorectal (157), ovarian (158), and endometrial (159) cancers and were weakly related to breast cancer risk (160). In cohort studies, null associations for glycemic load index were observed for breast cancer (161, 162), but positive associations were seen for pancreatic (163), uterine (164), and colorectal cancer (165). For colon cancer, many studies in diverse populations found that sugar, sucrose, and the major sources of starch were associated with increased risk (45). Although much work is still needed, enough data exist to suggest that abnormal glucose and insulin metabolism, especially in obese, sedentary persons, is important to consider in carcinogenesis.

Protein

Epidemiologic studies have not found a clear association between a high protein intake, at least in adulthood, and the risk of cancer. It is conceivable that an abundance of essential amino acids could complement the influence of high energy intakes in enhancing growth rates, which is a risk factor for cancer (see earlier). In most studies in adults, no evidence indicated deleterious effects of some of the major sources of protein, including fish, poultry, and plant sources. Red meat and dairy products, the other major protein sources, are discussed in the following section.

Food Groups

Meat

Red meat intake has been associated with risk of several cancers, most notably of the colon, rectum, and prostate. Findings for red meat and colon cancer have been mixed, although in a metaanalysis of 13 prospective studies, a 12 to 17% increase in risk with each 100-g increment of red meat intake (slightly more than 3 oz) and a 49% increased risk for each 25-g increment of processed meats (about one slice) were observed (166). These findings were largely confirmed in another metaanalysis (167). A positive association between red meat and processed meat intake and colon cancer risk has been observed in many, although not all, case-control studies (168), even though meat-related variables, method of assessment, and country of study have been quite diverse. To clarify the relationship between meat and prostate cancer, future studies need to examine components of red meat more closely. For example, mutagenic N-nitroso (NOC) compounds, formed endogenously from nitrogenous residues from red meat (169), and NOC precursors in processed meats (170), could explain the risks associated with processed meats. In an intervention study, heme iron (abundant in red meat), but not ferrous iron, stimulated endogenous NOC production in healthy volunteers (171).

In a review of red meat and prostate cancer, 15 of 21 studies found more than 30% increased risks associated with higher red meat intakes; six of these were statistically significant (172). Six of eight prospective studies found at least a 40% increased risk; three of these were statistically significant. Whether the association is the result of the fat content or of other components of meat remains unclear. The evidence regarding meat for other cancers is less consistent. In a large pooled analysis of eight cohort studies, no association was observed among red meat intake, total meat intake, and breast cancer risk (173). Other cancers, including bladder, pancreas, and kidney cancers, may also be associated with meat constituents, but not all studies are consistent (174).

Dairy Products

In the United States, dairy products are the major source of dietary calcium and vitamin D and an important source of protein, saturated fat, and minerals. Besides these components, which have been hypothesized to influence cancer risk, dairy products also contain other hypothetically protective (175) and adverse (176) components. Epidemiologic studies of dairy products and colorectal (177) and breast cancer risk (173) have been inconsistent and mostly null, but some studies suggest a possible lower risk of these cancers with higher intakes of low-fat dairy products (178, 179). For colorectal cancer, the benefit seems largely from calcium and possibly vitamin D (see later). In contrast, dairy products have been associated in some studies with increased risk of prostate cancer (180), and one study showed high-fat dairy products to be associated with an increased risk of premenopausal breast cancer (73). In one review (180), seven of 14 case-control studies and five of nine cohort studies reported a statistically significant higher risk of prostate cancer among men who consumed higher intakes of milk or dairy products. Men with higher intakes have had approximately a twofold increase in risk of total or advanced prostate cancer. The underlying mechanism has not been established, although the effect of calcium on lowering $1,25(OH)_2$ vitamin D has been proposed (180).

Fruits and Vegetables

Fruits and vegetables have received much interest because they contain numerous substances with potential anticarcinogenic activity. Results from more than 250 epidemiologic studies of fruits and vegetables and cancer were summarized in several large reviews (174, 181, 182), which concluded that diets high in fruits and vegetables were consistently associated with lower risk of some, but not all, cancers. Most of these studies were case-control studies. However, more recent null or weak findings on fruits and vegetables and cancer from large prospective cohort studies raised doubt about the strength of the association between fruits and vegetables and cancer risk. For example, prospective studies of stomach cancer and colon or colorectal cancer demonstrated weaker associations for fruits and vegetables than did case-control studies, as reviewed in the literature (174, 183). An intervention study that included higher intakes of whole grains, fruits, and vegetables on recurrence of colorectal adenomas did not find a reduction in risk (184). A large pooled analysis of eight prospective cohort studies found negligible associations between fruits and vegetables and breast cancer (185). These findings from more rigorous studies indicated that plant foods probably play a smaller direct role in cancer prevention than previously thought.

Several factors may account for the apparently divergent results from the earlier case-control studies and the more recent prospective and intervention studies. First, in some of the case-control studies, recall or selection biases may have occurred. Second, some risk factors for specific cancers have emerged relatively recently (e.g., tobacco, obesity, physical inactivity for colon cancer), and these factors were not controlled for in many of the previous analyses. Third, the strength of the results may have been exaggerated in some of the previous reports because several subgroupings of fruits and vegetables (e.g., citrus fruits) may have been considered, but only significant findings were emphasized in the reports. Finally, the source of the potentially protective agents may have changed; for example, in many previous studies, the main source of folate was fruits and vegetables; in the United States, however, multivitamins and fortified foods are the most common sources associated with higher intakes. A final point is that some types of fruits and vegetables may have potential deleterious effects. For example, potatoes and some fruit juices, which have a high glycemic index and increase insulin secretion, comprise the majority of total fruit and vegetable consumption in the United States (186).

Although a strong global protective role for total fruits and vegetables on total cancer risk now appears unlikely, fruits and vegetables contain varying levels of potentially protective compounds for specific cancer sites. Combining fruits and vegetables in analyses may obscure potentially strong protective effects of certain phytochemical or botanical subgroups on some cancer sites. From an epidemiologic perspective, some of the promising leads include tomato or lycopene-containing foods and prostate cancer (187), cruciferous vegetables and several cancer sites including prostate, bladder, and lung (174), allium vegetables and stomach cancer (188), folate-rich fruits and vegetables and colon cancer, and citrus fruits and lung cancer (189). Fruits and vegetables contain a myriad of biologically active chemicals, including both recognized nutrients and many more nonnutritive constituents, that could potentially play a role in protection against cancer (11). The identification of the specific protective constituents, or combination of constituents, is a daunting task and may never be completely possible. Further details on the types and amounts of fruits and vegetables that appear to be particularly protective could provide additional practical dietary guidance.

Dietary Fiber and Cancer Risk

Interest in dietary fiber is largely the result of Dr. Denis Burkitt's observation of low rates of colon cancer in areas of Africa where fiber consumption and stool bulk were high (190). Although fiber was originally seen simply as providing bulk to dilute potential carcinogens and to speed their transit through the colon, other hypotheses have suggested that fiber may act by binding carcinogenic substances (191), altering the colonic flora (192–195), reducing the pH (196), or serving as the substrate for the generation of short-chain fatty acids that are the preferred substrate for colonic epithelial cells (197).

A 1992 metaanalysis of case-control studies appeared to support the fiber hypothesis (198), but a later reanalysis of these data, considering study heterogeneity and limited to studies with validated diet assessment instruments, was less supportive (199). Prospective cohort studies of dietary fiber and colon cancer risk, mostly conducted since the mid-1990s, generally have not supported an association (100, 103, 200–202). In contrast, more recently published results from a large European study involving ten countries found a 25% lower risk of colon cancer associated with higher fiber intakes compared with low intakes (203). However, other potentially responsible factors were not included in the analysis (e.g., physical activity, smoking, or other nutrients in high fiber diets such as folate); thus, it is difficult to isolate fiber as the responsible factor. Intervention trials of wheat bran fiber (204), isphaghula husk (psyllium fiber) (205), and a high-fiber/low-fat diet (184) failed to reduce the risk of recurrent adenomatous polyps. In fact, psyllium fiber appeared to increase risk (205), a finding suggesting that purified forms of a single fiber source may give unexpected results.

Higher intake of fiber has also been hypothesized to reduce risk of breast cancer by interrupting the enterohepatic circulation of estrogens (206). However, in prospective studies, little or no relationship was observed between fiber intake and risk of breast cancer (63, 207–209).

Alcoholic Beverages

High consumption of alcohol, particularly in combination with cigarette smoking, is a well-established cause of cancer of the oral cavity, larynx, esophagus, and liver (210). Substantial evidence from case-control and cohort studies indicated that amounts as low as one or two drinks per day increase risk of breast cancer (211–213). In addition, moderate alcohol consumption also appears to be associated with risk of cancers of the colon and rectum (214). In the upper gastrointestinal tract, the carcinogenic effects of alcohol could result from direct contact, and, in the liver, this could result from toxicity during catabolism of alcohol. However, in the large bowel and breast tissue, the mechanisms remain unclear. Nonetheless, an intriguing potential mechanism may involve the well-established antifolate effects of alcohol (215). Evidence from animal and human studies shows that "methyl-poor" diets (high-alcohol–low-methionine low-folate) are associated with three- to fourfold increases in the risk of both colorectal adenomas and cancer compared with "methyl-rich" diets (low-alcohol, high-methionine, high-folate diets) (216). These results are quite consistent in men, and less so in women, possibly because of their lower alcohol intake. This mechanism may extend to other cancer sites (217–222), although the studies are not as consistent, and further work is needed.

Vitamin and Mineral Supplements

Calcium

Calcium has been inversely related to the risk of colorectal cancer (177) and adenomas (223) but positively associated with risk of other cancers, including prostate cancer (180). Although previous epidemiologic studies suggested a weak relationship, if any, with colorectal cancer risk

(224), more recent prospective studies showed a more consistent inverse association between calcium intake and colorectal and colon cancer risk (178, 225). A role of calcium was also supported by randomized intervention trials with recurrent colorectal adenomas as the outcome (205, 223). The optimal dose and form of calcium that may be most protective are not known, but prospective studies suggested that benefits may plateau at 1000 mg/day or less (178, 225). Some data suggest an increased risk of prostate cancer with higher calcium intake (180), particularly higher than 1500 mg/day and for advanced (metastatic) prostate cancer (226). Few studies on calcium and breast cancer have been reported. One hospital-based case-control study reported a statistically significant lower risk (20%) of breast cancer with high versus low calcium intakes (227), whereas results in three other studies were not significant (227–230). A prospective study reported a significant inverse association between calcium and breast cancer, but only in premenopausal women (179).

Vitamin D

Vitamin D (see also Chapter 20) has been of interest based on ecologic studies that found that populations with greater exposure to ultraviolet light had lower risks of breast (231), colon (232), and prostate cancer (233). Although some epidemiologic studies support a role of sunlight, dietary vitamin D, and circulating vitamin D metabolites in reducing risk of these cancers, the data are mixed, and these relationships require clarification (177). Data for a biologic mechanism involving the effects of vitamin D in proliferation and differentiation are strong (234), so a potential role of vitamin D deserves more careful study in plasma- or serum-based studies.

Folate

Folate is important for DNA methylation, repair, and synthesis (235–238). Epidemiologic studies have linked low folate intake with a higher risk of several cancers, most notably colorectal (216), breast (218), and possibly cervical cancer (218). Long-term use of folic acid–containing multivitamin supplements is associated with a 20 to 70% reduction in risk of colon cancer (239–242). Isolated studies in other cancers, including esophageal cancer (243) and leukemia (244), also suggest that inadequate folate intake or metabolism may contribute to carcinogenesis in other sites. Supporting a role of folate is that genotypes for *MTHFR*, an enzyme known to be involved in folate metabolism, predict risk of colon cancer dependent on folate intake or status (216, 245). As discussed earlier, folate requirements may be higher in alcohol drinkers.

Vitamins C and E

Oxidant byproducts from normal metabolism, from smoking, or from chronic inflammation damage DNA, protein, and lipids; DNA repair enzymes efficiently repair damage, but antioxidant defenses are imperfect (12). Antioxidants may reduce the risk of cancer by neutralizing reactive oxygen species or free radicals that can damage DNA. Vitamin C is the major water-soluble antioxidant , and α-tocopherol is the major lipid-soluble, membrane-localized antioxidant in humans. However, epidemiologic studies did not consistently support roles for vitamins C and E on cancer risk (174), and chemoprevention trials of stomach cancer in high-risk populations did not conclusively support a benefit from vitamin C supplements (246), although several antioxidant nutrients were associated with regression of gastric dysplasia (247). In the Alpha-Tocopherol Beta-Carotene (ATBC) trial, no association between supplemental α-tocopherol and lung cancer was found, but a 34% lower incidence of prostate cancer among the population of heavy smokers was noted (248). Subsequent prospective analyses of vitamin E supplements (usually as α-tocopherol) or levels in patients with prostate cancer supported a possible role limited to smokers, but not in nonsmokers (249, 250). In several studies, long-term use of vitamin E supplements was related to a lower risk of bladder cancer (251, 252).

Selenium

Selenium functions through selenoproteins, including selenium-dependent glutathione peroxidases that defend against oxidative stress. The selenium content of food varies depending on the selenium content of soil where plants are grown or animals are raised. Because content can vary more than tenfold, nutrient databases for selenium are unreliable. Most epidemiologic evidence on the anticarcinogenic role of selenium stems from biomarker and intervention studies. Selenium was strongly associated with reduced prostate cancer risk in one trial of selenium supplementation and skin cancer (253), as well as in two nested case-control studies of toenail and serum selenium biomarkers (254, 255). The SELECT trial, an ongoing supplement trial funded by the National Cancer Institute, is comparing supplemental selenium, vitamin E, and a combination with placebo on primary prevention of prostate cancer.

SUMMARY

Evidence from both animal and epidemiologic studies indicates that throughout life, excessive energy intake in relation to requirements increases the risk of human cancer. Rapid growth rate in childhood leading to greater adult height increases the risk of breast, colon, prostate, and other cancers, and accumulation of body fat in adulthood is related to cancers of the colon, kidney, pancreas, esophagus (adenocarcinoma), and endometrium, as well as postmenopausal breast cancer. Evidence suggests that the percentage of energy from fat in the diet is not a major cause of cancers of the breast or colon. Higher intake of meat and dairy products has been associated with greater

risk of prostate cancer, which may be related to a specific component of fat. In addition, consumption of red and processed meat may be associated with risk of colon cancer. Based on prospective studies, a diet high in fruits and vegetables and fiber may not be as protective against cancer as initially indicated by case-control studies. Nonetheless, some micronutrients and phytochemicals may offer some benefits against some specific cancers. Excessive consumption of alcohol increases risks of upper gastrointestinal tract cancer, and even moderate intake appears to increase the risk of cancers of the breast and large bowel. Although many details remain to be learned, evidence is strong that remaining physically active and lean throughout life, consuming an abundance of fruits and vegetables, and avoiding high intakes of red meat, foods high in animal fat, highly processed carbohydrates, and excessive alcohol will substantially reduce the risk of human cancer.

REFERENCES

1. Parkin DM. Cancer Surv 1994;19–20:519–61.
2. Parkin DM, Muir CS, Whelan SL et al, eds. Cancer Incidence in Five Continents, vol 6. No. 120. Lyon, France: International Agency for Research on Cancer Scientific Publications, 1992.
3. American Cancer Society. Cancer Facts and Figures 2003. Atlanta, GA: American Cancer Society, 2003.
4. Haenszel W, Kurihara M. J Natl Cancer Inst 1968;40:43–68.
5. Buell P. J Natl Cancer Inst 1973;51:1479–83.
6. Shimizu H, Ross RK, Bernstein L et al. Br J Cancer 1991;63:963–6.
7. Thomas DB, Karagas MR. Cancer Res 1987;47:5771–6.
8. Kolonel LN, Hankin JH, Lee J et al. Br J Cancer 1981;44:332–9.
9. Ziegler RG, Hoover RN, Pike MC et al. J Natl Cancer Inst 1993;85:1819–27.
10. Armstrong B, Doll R. Int J Cancer 1975;15:617–31.
11. Steinmetz KA, Potter JD. Cancer Causes Control 1991;2:427–42.
12. Ames BN, Gold LS, Willett WC. Proc Natl Acad Sci USA 1995;92:5258–65.
13. Willett WC. Nutritional Epidemiology. 2nd ed. New York: Oxford University Press, 1998.
14. Tannenbaum A. Cancer Res 1942;2:468–75.
15. Tannenbaum A, Silverstone H. Adv Cancer Res 1953;1:451–501.
16. Ross MH, Bras G. J Natl Cancer Inst 1971;47:1095–113.
17. Weindruch R, Walford RL. Science 1982;215:1415–8.
18. Birt DF. J Nutr 1995;125[Suppl]:1673S–6S.
19. Birt DF, Kris ES, Choe M et al. Cancer Res 1992;52[Suppl]:2035S–9S.
20. Birt DF. Adv Exp Med Biol 1986;206:69–83.
21. Boissonneault GA, Elson CE, Pariza MW. J Natl Cancer Inst 1986;76:335–8.
22. Willett WC, Stampfer MJ. Am J Epidemiol 1986;124:17–27.
23. Micozzi MS. Horm Res 1993;39[Suppl 3]:49–58.
24. Chen J, Campbell TC, Junyao L et al. Diet, Life-Style, and Mortality in China: A Study of the Characteristics of 65 Chinese Counties. Oxford: Oxford University Press, 1990.
25. Wyshak G, Frisch RE. N Engl J Med 1982;306:1033–5.
26. Wang D, Murphy M. J Biosoc Sci 2002;34:349–61.
27. Moisan J, Meyer F, Gingras S. Cancer Causes Control 1990;1:149–54.

28. Maclure M, Travis LB, Willett WC et al. Am J Clin Nutr 1991; 54:649–56.

29. Merzenich H, Boeing H, Wahrendorf J. Am J Epidemiol 1993; 138:217–24.

30. Austin H, Austin JM, Jr., Partridge EE et al. Cancer Res 1991; 51:568–72.

31. Goodman MT, Nomura AMY, Kolonel LN et al. In: Rao RS, Deo MA, Sanghvi LD, eds. Proceedings of the International Cancer Congress, New Delhi, India. Bologna, Italy: Monduzzi Editore, 1994:2325–8.

32. Parazzini F, La Vecchia C, Bocciolone L et al. Gynecol Oncol 1991;41:1–16.

33. Tornberg SA, Carstensen JM. Br J Cancer 1994;69:358–61.

34. Garfinkel L. Cancer 1986;58[Suppl]:1826–9.

35. Martinez ME, Giovannucci E, Spiegelman D et al. Am J Epidemiol 1996;143:S73.

36. Giovannucci E, Ascherio A, Rimm EB et al. Ann Intern Med 1995;122:327–34.

37. Calle EE, Rodriguez C, Walker–Thurmond K et al. N Engl J Med 2003;348:1625–38.

38. Tretli S. Int J Cancer 1989;44:23–30.

39. London SJ, Colditz GA, Stampfer MJ et al. JAMA 1989;262: 2853–8.

40. Rich-Edwards JW, Goldman MB, Willett WC et al. Am J Obstet Gynecol 1994;171:171–7.

41. Hankinson SE, Willett WC, Manson JE et al. J Natl Cancer Inst 1995;87:1297–302.

42. Nomura AM. Epidemiol Rev 2001;23:126–31.

43. Giovannucci E, Rimm EB, Liu Y et al. J Natl Cancer Inst 2003;95:1240–4.

44. Kari FW, Dunn SE, French JE et al. J Nutr Health Aging 1999; 3:92–101.

45. Giovannucci E. J Nutr 2001;131:3109S–20S.

46. Pollak M. Eur J Cancer 2000;36:1224–8.

47. Giovannucci E, Rimm EB, Liu Y et al. Int J Epidemiol 2004; 33:217–25.

48. Doll R, Peto R. J Natl Cancer Inst 1981;66:1191–308.

49. Parker ED, Folsom AR. Int J Obes Relat Metab Disord 2003; 27:1447–52.

50. Committee on Diet Nutrition and Cancer, Assembly of Life Sciences, National Research Council. Diet, Nutrition, and Cancer. Washington, DC: National Academy Press, 1982.

51. Committee on Diet and Health, National Research Council. Recommended Dietary Allowances. 10th ed. Washington, DC: National Academy Press, 1989.

52. Food and Nutrition Board, Institute of Medicine. Recommended Dietary Allowances. 10th rev ed. Washington, DC: National Academy Press, 1989.

53. Albanes D. Cancer Res 1987;47:1987–92.

54. Sonnenschein E, Glickman L, Goldschmidt M et al. Am J Epidemiol 1991;133:694–703.

55. Appleton BS, Landers RE. Adv Exp Med Biol 1986;206: 99–104.

56. Freedman LS, Clifford C, Messina M. Cancer Res 1990;50: 5710–9.

57. Welsch CW. Cancer Res 1992;52[Suppl 7]:2040S–8S.

58. Ip C. In: Mettlin CJ, Aoki K, eds. Recent Progress in Research on Nutrition and Cancer: Proceedings of a Workshop Sponsored by the International Union against Cancer, Nagoya, Japan, November 1–3, 1989. New York: Wiley-Liss, 1990: 107–17.

59. Carroll MD, Abraham S, Dresser CM. Dietary Intake Source Data: United States, 1976–1980, series 11. Hyattsville, MD: National Center for Health Statistics, 1983.

60. Prentice RL, Sheppard L. Cancer Causes Control 1990;1: 81–97.

61. Rose DP, Boyar AP, Wynder EL. Cancer 1986;58:2263–71.

62. Marshall JR, Qu Y, Chen J et al. Eur J Cancer 1992;28A: 1720–7.

63. Willett WC, Hunter DJ, Stampfer MJ et al. JAMA 1992;268: 2037–44.

64. Stephen AM, Wald NJ. Am J Clin Nutr 1990;52:457–69.

65. McDowell MA, Briefel RR, Alaimo K et al. Energy and Macronutrient Intakes of Persons Ages 2 Months and over in the United States: Third National Health and Nutrition Examination Survey, Phase I: 1988–1991. DHHS Publication No. (PHS) 95–1250. Hyattsville, MD: National Center for Health Statistics, Centers for Disease Control, Public Health Service, US Department of Health and Human Services, 1994.

66. American Cancer Society. 1994. Cancer Facts and Figures. Atlanta, GA: American Cancer Society, 1994.

67. Graham S, Marshall J, Mettlin C et al. Am J Epidemiol 1982; 116:68–75.

68. Howe GR, Hirohata T, Hislop TG et al. J Natl Cancer Inst 1990;82:561–9.

69. Giovannucci E, Stampfer MJ, Colditz GA et al. Am J Epidemiol 1993;137:502–11.

70. Hunter DJ, Spiegelman D, Adami HO et al. N Engl J Med 1996;334:356–61.

71. Smith-Warner SA, Spiegelman D, Adami HO et al. Int J Cancer 2001;92:767–74.

72. Holmes MD, Hunter DJ, Colditz GA et al. JAMA 1999;281:914–20.

73. Cho E, Spiegelman D, Hunter DJ et al. J Natl Cancer Inst 2003;95:1079–85.

74. Rossouw JE, Finnegan LP, Harlan WR et al. J Am Med Womens Assoc 1995;50:50–5.

75. Hopkins GJ, Carroll KK. J Natl Cancer Inst 1979;62:1009–12.

76. Hopkins GJ, Kennedy TG, Carroll KK. J Natl Cancer Inst 1981;66:517–22.

77. Martin-Moreno JM, Willett WC, Gorgojo L et al. Int J Cancer 1994;58:774–80.

78. Trichopoulou A, Katsouyanni K, Stuver S et al. J Natl Cancer Inst 1995;87:110–6.

79. Giovannucci E, Stampfer MJ, Colditz GA et al. J Natl Cancer Inst 1992;84:91–8.

80. Giovannucci E. Gastroenterol Clin North Am 2002;31:925–43.

81. Macquart-Moulin G, Riboli E, Cornee J et al. Int J Cancer 1986;38:183–91.

82. Berta JL, Coste T, Rautureau J et al. Gastroenterol Clin Biol 1985;9:348–53.

83. Tuyns AJ, Haelterman M, Kaaks R. Nutr Cancer 1987;10: 181–96.

84. Meyer F, White E. Am J Epidemiol 1993;138:225–36.

85. Jain M, Cook GM, Davis FG et al. Int J Cancer 1980;26: 757–68.

86. Potter JD, McMichael AJ. J Natl Cancer Inst 1986;76:557–69.

87. Lyon JL, Mahoney AW, West DW et al. J Natl Cancer Inst 1987;78:853–61.

88. Graham S, Marshall J, Haughey B et al. Am J Epidemiol 1988; 128:490–503.

89. Bristol JB, Emmett PM, Heaton KW et al. BMJ 1985; 291:1467–70.

90. Kune GA, Kune S, Watson LF. Nutr Cancer 1987;9:5–56.

91. West DW, Slattery ML, Robison LM et al. Am J Epidemiol 1989;130:883–94.

92. Peters RK, Pike MC, Garabrandt D et al. Cancer Causes Control 1992;3:457–73.

93. Manousos O, Day NE, Trichopoulos D et al. Int J Cancer 1983; 32:1–5.
94. La Vecchia C, Negri E, Decarli A et al. Int J Cancer 1988; 41:492–8.
95. Miller AB, Howe GR, Jain M et al. Int J Cancer 1983; 32:155–61.
96. Young TB, Wolf DA. Int J Cancer 1988;42:167–75.
97. Benito E, Obrador A, Stiggelbout A et al. Int J Cancer 1990; 45:69–76.
98. Lee HP, Gourley L, Duffy SW et al. Int J Cancer 1989; 43:1007–16.
99. Howe GR. Advances in the biology and therapy of colorectal cancer. Paper presented at the MD Anderson thirty-seventh annual clinical conference, MD Anderson Cancer Center, Houston, TX, 1993.
100. Willett WC, Stampfer MJ, Colditz GA et al. N Engl J Med 1990;323:1664–72.
101. Goldbohm RA, van den Brandt PA, van't Veer P et al. Cancer Res 1994;54:718–23.
102. Bostick RM, Potter JD, Kushi LH et al. Cancer Causes Control 1994;5:38–52.
103. Giovannucci E, Rimm EB, Stampfer MJ et al. Cancer Res 1994;54:2390–7.
104. Thun MJ, Calle EE, Namboodiri MM et al. J Natl Cancer Inst 1992;84:1491–500.
105. Talamini R, La Vecchia C, Decarli A et al. Br J Cancer 1986; 53:817–21.
106. Rotkin ID. Cancer Treat Rep 1977;61:173–80.
107. Mishina T, Watanabe H, Araki H et al. Prostate 1985;6:423–36.
108. Talamini R, Franceschi S, La Vecchia C et al. Nutr Cancer 1992;18:277–86.
109. Schuman LM, Mandel JS, Radke A et al. In: Magnus K, ed. Trends in Cancer Incidence: Causes and Practical Implications. Washington, DC: Hemisphere Publishing, 1982:345–54.
110. Graham S, Haughey B, Marshall J et al. J Natl Cancer Inst 1983;70:687–92.
111. Ross RK, Shimizu H, Paganini-Hill A et al. J Natl Cancer Inst 1987;78:869–74.
112. West DW, Slattery ML, Robison LM et al. Cancer Causes Control 1991;2:85–94.
113. Kolonel LN, Yoshizawa CN, Hankin JH. Am J Epidemiol 1988; 127:999–1012.
114. Heshmat MY, Kaul L, Kovi J et al. Prostate 1985;6:7–17.
115. Kolonel LN. Cancer Causes Control 1996;7:83–94.
116. Whittemore AS, Kolonel LN, Wu AH et al. J Natl Cancer Inst 1995;87:652–61.
117. Severson RK, Nomura AMY, Grove JS et al. Cancer Res 1989; 49:1857–60.
118. Mills PK, Beeson WL, Phillips RL et al. Cancer 1989; 64:598–604.
119. Giovannucci E, Rimm EB, Colditz GA et al. J Natl Cancer Inst 1993;85:1571–79.
120. Michaud DS, Augustsson K, Rimm EB et al. Cancer Causes Control 2001;12:557–67.
121. Le Marchand L, Kolonel LN, Wilkens LR et al. Epidemiology 1994;5:276–82.
122. Gann PH, Hennekens CH, Sacks FM et al. J Natl Cancer Inst 1994;86:281–6.
123. Leitzmann MF, Stampfer MJ, Michaud DS et al. Am J Clin Nutr 2004;80:204–16.
124. De Stefani E, Deneo-Pellegrini H, Boffetta P et al. Cancer Epidemiol Biomarkers Prev 2000;9:335–8.
125. Ramon JM, Bou R, Romea S et al. Cancer Causes Control 2000;11:679–85.
126. Harvei S, Bjerve KS, Tretli S et al. Int J Cancer 1997;71: 545–51.
127. Yang YJ, Lee SH, Hong SJ et al. Clin Biochem 1999;32:405–9.
128. Newcomer LM, King IB, Wicklund KG et al. Prostate 2001; 47:262–8.
129. Andersson S-O, Wolk A, Bergström R et al. Int J Cancer 1996; 68:716–22.
130. Schuurman AG, van den Brandt PA, Dorant E et al. Cancer 1999;86:1019–27.
131. Meyer F, Bairati I, Fradet Y et al. Nutr Cancer 1997;29:120–6.
132. Bairati I, Meyer F, Fradet Y et al. J Urol 1998;159:1271–5.
133. Freeman VL, Meydani M, Yong S et al. J Urol 2000; 164: 2168–72.
134. Ascherio A, Rimm EB, Giovannucci EL et al. BMJ 1996; 313:84–90.
135. Colditz GA. Cancer Causes Control 2000;11:677–8.
136. Cramer DW, Welch WR, Hutchison GB et al. Obstet Gynecol 1984;63:833–8.
137. La Vecchia C, Decarli A, Negri E et al. J Natl Cancer Inst 1987;79:663–9.
138. Shu XO, Gao YT, Yuan JM et al. Br J Cancer 1989;59:92–6.
139. Byers T, Marshall J, Graham S et al. J Natl Cancer Inst 1983;71: 681–6.
140. Slattery ML, Schuman KL, West DW et al. Am J Epidemiol 1989;130:497–502.
141. Risch HA, Jain M, Marrett LD et al. J Natl Cancer Inst 1994;86:1409–15.
142. Levi F, Franceschi S, Negri E et al. Cancer 1993;71:3575–81.
143. Barbone F, Austin H, Partridge EE. Am J Epidemiol 1993; 137:393–403.
144. Potischman N, Swanson CA, Brinton LA et al. Cancer Causes Control 1993;4:239–50.
145. Shu XO, Zheng W, Potischamn N et al. Am J Epidemiol 1993; 137:155–65.
146. Zheng W, Kushi LH, Potter JD et al. Am J Epidemiol 1995; 142:388–94.
147. Black HS, Herd JA, Goldberg LH et al. N Engl J Med 1994; 330:1272–5.
148. Hankin JH, Zhao LP, Wilkens LR et al. Cancer Causes Control 1992;3:17–23.
149. Alavanja MC, Brown CC, Swanson C et al. J Natl Cancer Inst 1993;85:1906–16.
150. van Dam RM, Huang ZP, Giovannucci E et al. Am J Clin Nutr 2000;71:135–41.
151. Smith–Warner SA, Ritz J, Hunter DJ et al. Cancer Epidemiol Biomarkers Prev 2002;11:987–92.
152. Chanmugam P, Guthrie JF, Cecilio F et al. J Am Diet Assoc 2003;103:867–72.
153. Popkin BM, Siega-Riz AM, Haines PS. N Engl J Med 1996; 335:716–20.
154. Wolever TMS, Jenkins DJA. Am J Clin Nutr 1986;43:167–72.
155. Miller JC. Am J Clin Nutr 1994;59:747S–52S.
156. Pereira MA, Jacobs DR Jr, Pins JJ et al. Am J Clin Nutr 2002; 75:848–55.
157. Franceschi S, Dal Maso L, Augustin L et al. Ann Oncol 2001; 12:173–8.
158. Augustin LS, Polesel J, Bosetti C et al. Ann Oncol 2003;14: 78–84.
159. Augustin LS, Gallus S, Bosetti C et al. Int J Cancer 2003;105: 404–7.
160. Augustin LSA, Dal Maso L, Vecchia CL et al. Ann Oncol 2001; 12:1533–8.
161. Terry PD, Jain M, Miller AB et al. J Natl Cancer Inst 2003;95: 914–6.

162. Jonas CR, McCullough ML, Teras LR et al. Cancer Epidemiol Biomarkers Prev 2003;12:573–7.

163. Michaud DS, Liu S, Giovannucci E et al. J Natl Cancer Inst 2002;94:1293–300.

164. Folsom AR, Demissie Z, Harnack L. Nutr Cancer 3002; 46:119–24.

165. Higginbotham S, Zhang ZF, Lee IM et al. J Natl Cancer Inst 2004;96:229–33.

166. Sandhu MS, White IR, McPherson K. Cancer Epidemiol Biomarkers Prev 2001;10:439–46.

167. Norat T, Lukanova A, Ferrari P et al. Int J Cancer 2002; 98:241–56.

168. Kushi L, Giovannucci E. Am J Med 2002;113:63S–70S.

169. Bingham SA, Hughes R, Cross AJ. J Nutr 2002;132:3522S–5S.

170. Mirvish SS, Haorah J, Zhou L et al. J Nutr 2002;132:3526S–9S.

171. Cross AJ, Pollock JR, Bingham SA. Cancer Res 2003;63: 2358–60.

172. Kolonel LN. Epidemiol Rev 2001;23:72–81.

173. Missmer SA, Smith-Warner SA, Spiegelman D et al. Int J Epidemiol 2002;31:78–85.

174. World Cancer Research Fund, American Institute for Cancer Research. Food, Nutrition and the Prevention of Cancer: A Global Perspective. Washington, DC: American Institute for Cancer Research, 1997.

175. Parodi PW. J Nutr 1997;127:1055–60.

176. Outwater JL, Nicholson A, Barnard N. Med Hypotheses 1997; 48:453–61.

177. Platz EA, Giovannucci E. 1999. In: Heber D, Blackburn GL, Go VL, eds. Nutritional Oncology. San Diego: Academic Press, 1999:223–52.

178. Wu K, Willett WC, Fuchs CS et al. J Natl Cancer Inst 2002; 94:437–46.

179. Shin MH, Holmes MD, Hankinson SE et al. J Natl Cancer Inst 2002;94:1301–10.

180. Chan JM, Stampfer MJ, Ma J et al. Am J Clin Nutr 2001; 74:549–54.

181. Block G, Patterson B, Subar A. Nutr Cancer 1992;18:1–29.

182. Steinmetz KA, Potter JD. Cancer Causes Control 1991; 2:325–57.

183. Terry P, Terry JB, Wolk A. J Intern Med 2001;250:280–90.

184. Schatzkin A, Lanza E, Corle D et al. N Engl J Med 2000; 342:1149–55.

185. Smith-Warner SA, Spiegelman D, Yaun SS et al. JAMA 2001; 285:769–76.

186. Krebs-Smith SM, Kantor LS. J Nutr 2001;131:487S–501S.

187. Giovannucci E. J Natl Cancer Inst 1999;91:317–31.

188. Milner JA. J Nutr 2001;131:1027S–31S.

189. Smith-Warner SA, Spiegelman D, Yaun SS et al. Int J Cancer 2003;107:1001–11.

190. Burkitt DP. Cancer 1971;28:3–13.

191. Story JA, Kritchevsky D. Am J Clin Nutr 1978;31[Suppl]: 199S–202S.

192. Reddy BS, Mastromarino A, Wynder EL. Cancer Res 1975;35: 3403–6.

193. Reddy BS. Fed Proc 1971;30:1772.

194. Reddy BS, Weisburger JH, Wynder EL. J Nutr 1975;105: 878–84.

195. Klurfeld DM. Cancer Res 1992;52[Suppl]:2055S–9S.

196. Cummings JH. Lancet 1983;1:1206–9.

197. Stephen AM, Cummings JH. Nature 1980;284:283–4.

198. Howe GR, Benito E, Castelleto R et al. J Natl Cancer Inst 1992;84:1887–96.

199. Friedenreich CM, Brant RF, Riboli E. Epidemiology 1994; 5:66–79.

200. Steinmetz KA, Kushi LH, Bostick RM et al. Am J Epidemiol 1994;139:1–15.

201. Fuchs CS, Colditz GA, Stampfer MJ et al. N Engl J Med 1999; 340:169–76.

202. Heilbrun LK, Nomura A, Hankin JH et al. Lancet 1985;1:925.

203. Bingham SA, Day NE, Luben R et al. Lancet 2003;361: 1496–501.

204. Alberts DS, Martinez ME, Roe DJ et al. N Engl J Med 2000; 342:1156–62.

205. Bonithon-Kopp C, Kronborg O, Giacosa A et al. Lancet 2000;356:1300–6.

206. Gorbach SL, Goldin BR. Prev Med 1987;16:525–31.

207. Rohan TE, Howe GR, Friedenreich CM et al. Cancer Causes Control 1993;4:29–37.

208. Verhoeven DTH, Assen N, Goldbohm RA et al. Am J Epidemiol 1996;143[Suppl]:37S.

209. Terry P, Jain M, Miller AB et al. Cancer Epidemiol Biomarkers Prev 2002;11:1507–8.

210. International Agency for Research on Cancer. IARC Mongr Eval Carcinog Risks Hum 1988;44:194–207.

211. Longnecker MP, Newcomb PA, Mittendorf R et al. J Natl Cancer Inst 1995;87:923–9.

212. Longnecker MP. Cancer Causes Control 1994;5:73–82.

213. Smith-Warner SA, Spiegelman D, Yaun S-S et al. JAMA 1998;279:535–40.

214. Potter JD. Cancer Causes Control 1996;7:127–46.

215. Hillman RS, Steinberg SE. Annu Rev Med 1982;33:345–54.

216. Giovannucci E. J Nutr 2002;132:2350S–5S.

217. Zhang SM, Willett WC, Selhub J et al. J Natl Cancer Inst 2003; 95:373–80.

218. Eichholzer M, Luthy J, Moser U et al. Swiss Med Wkly 2001; 131:539–49.

219. Feigelson HS, Jonas CR, Robertson AS et al. Cancer Epidemiol Biomarkers Prev 2003;12:161–4.

220. Rohan TE, Jain MG, Howe GR et al. J Natl Cancer Inst 2000;92:266–9.

221. Zhang S, Hunter DJ, Hankinson SE et al. JAMA 1999;281: 1632–7.

222. Sellers TA, Kushi LH, Cerhan JR et al. Epidemiology 2001;12: 420–8.

223. Baron JA, Beach M, Mandel JS et al. N Engl J Med 1999; 340:101–7.

224. Martinez ME, Willett WC. Cancer Epidemiol Biomarkers Prev 1998;7:163–8.

225. McCullough ML, Robertson AS, Rodriguez C et al. Cancer Causes Control 2003;14:1–12.

226. Giovannucci E, Rimm EB, Wolk A et al. Cancer Res 1998;58: 442–7.

227. Negri E, La Vecchia C, Franceschi S et al. Int J Cancer 1996; 65:140–4.

228. Katsouyanni K, Willett W, Trichopoulos D et al. Cancer 1988; 61:181–5.

229. Potischman N, Swanson CA, Coates RJ et al. Int J Cancer 1999; 82:315–21.

230. Levi F, Pasche C, Lucchini F et al. Int J Cancer 2001;91:260–3.

231. Garland FC, Garland CF, Gorham ED et al. Prev Med 1990; 19:614–22.

232. Garland CF, Garland FC. Int J Epidemiol 1980;9:227–31.

233. Hanchette CL, Schwartz GG. Cancer 1992;70:2861–9.

234. Lamprecht SA, Lipkin M. Ann NY Acad Sci 2001;952:73–87.

235. Duthie SJ, Narayanan S, Blum S et al. Nutr Cancer 2000; 37:245–51.

236. Duthie SJ. Br Med Bull 1999;55:578–92.

237. Wickramasinghe SN, Fida S. Blood 1994;83:1656–61.

238. Blount BC, Mack MM, Wehr CM et al. Proc Natl Acad Sci USA 1997;94:3290–5.
239. White E, Shannon JS, Patterson RE. Cancer Epidemiol Biomarkers Prev 1997;6:769–74.
240. Jacobs EJ, Connell CJ, Patel AV et al. Cancer Causes Control 2001;12:927–34.
241. Giovannucci E, Rimm EB, Ascherio A et al. J Natl Cancer Inst 1995;87:265–73.
242. Giovannucci E, Stampfer MJ, Colditz GA et al. Ann Intern Med 1998;129:517–24.
243. Prasad MP, Krishna TP, Pasricha S et al. Nutr Cancer 1992; 18:85–93.
244. Thompson JR, Gerald PF, Willoughby ML et al. Lancet 2001;358:1935–40.
245. Chen J, Giovannucci E, Kelsey K et al. Cancer Res 1996;56: 4862–4.
246. Blot WJ, Li JY, Taylor PR et al. J Natl Cancer Inst 1993;85:1483–92.
247. Correa P, Fontham ET, Bravo JC et al. J Natl Cancer Inst 2000; 92:1881–8.
248. Anonymous. N Engl J Med 1994;330:1029–35.
249. Gann PH, Ma J, Giovannucci E et al. Cancer Res 1999;59: 1225–30.
250. Chan JM, Stampfer MJ, Ma J et al. Cancer Epidemiol Biomarkers Prev 1999;8:893–9.
251. Michaud DS, Spiegelman D, Clinton SK et al. Am J Epidemiol 2002;152:1145–53.
252. Jacobs EJ, Henion AK, Briggs PJ et al. Am J Epidemiol 2002; 156:1002–10.
253. Clark LC, Combs GF, Jr., Turnbull BW et al. JAMA 1996;276: 1957–63.
254. Yoshizawa K, Willett WC, Morris SJ et al. J Natl Cancer Inst 1998;90:1219–24.
255. Nomura AMY, Lee J, Stemmermann GN et al. Cancer Epidemiol Biomarkers Prev 2000;9:883–7.

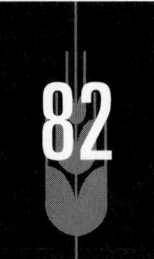

CHEMOPREVENTION OF CANCER[1]

MICHAEL B. SPORN

CARCINOGENESIS AND CANCER 1281
CHEMOPREVENTION BASED ON MECHANISM 1282
PHARMACOLOGY OF CHEMOPREVENTION 1283
   Nuclear Receptor Ligands 1283
   Antiinflammatory Agents 1285
   Chromatin Modifiers 1286
IMPORTANCE OF ANIMAL EXPERIMENTS 1286
EDUCATIONAL AND SOCIETAL ISSUES 1287
CLINICAL APPLICATIONS .1288

The data shown in Tables 82.1 and 82.2, for deaths from cancer at common epithelial target sites in 1971 and in 2004, provide a striking commentary on the continuing magnitude of the cancer problem. They clearly emphasize that conventional chemotherapy of advanced invasive and metastatic disease has failed to effect major reductions in the mortality rates for the common forms of epithelial malignancy, such as carcinoma of the lung, colon, breast, prostate, ovary, and pancreas (1, 2). These unfortunate statistics clearly indicate that new approaches to the control of cancer are critically needed. Although great advances have been made in basic scientific knowledge relating to cancer, as well as in the clinical treatment and cure of some malignancies (such as testicular cancer, as well as certain leukemias and lymphomas), the fact remains that the National Cancer Institute's stated goal (promulgated at the start of the War on Cancer in the 1970s) of a 50% reduction in overall cancer mortality by the year 2000 has not been met (3).

Indeed, death rates from some of the common cancers continue to increase. This is particularly striking with respect to the dramatic increase during the past 30 years in the number of lung cancer deaths in women, which can be attributed in large part to an increased use of tobacco by women. However, there have also been striking increases in the number of deaths in women of both pancreatic and ovarian cancer, as well as deaths in men of prostate cancer,

for which there is no obvious dietary or other environmental cause.

It is therefore essential that we now reevaluate some of our basic assumptions about the nature of cancer and how we approach the problem of treatment or prevention of this disease. These assumptions dictate current practice and have resulted in the present undesirable outcome for many cancer patients. Most importantly, we need to begin to adopt a more intensive and imaginative approach to the prevention of cancer. At present, both basic and clinical research on cancer are driven by an obsessive quest for the elusive goal of cure of advanced disease (cancer research suffers from the mythology of a magic bullet), an approach that is often unrealistic because of the genetic heterogeneity and extent of the tumor burden characteristic of late-stage malignancy. Given the genotypic and phenotypic heterogeneity of advanced malignant lesions as they occur in individual patients, one wonders just exactly what are the unique and specific molecular and cellular targets for the putative cure.

Thus, a lesion that is anatomically defined in reality will contain many different types of cells, each with its own phenotype and genotype (4–6). Indeed, the postulation of a mutator phenotype in cancer (7, 8) suggests that individual cancer cells can contain thousands of mutations, which may be the result of alteration of the very genes that are designed to maintain stability of the genome itself. As a consequence, the idea that we will eventually treat invasive cancer with some sort of single gene therapy seems pathetically naive. Which gene in which cell shall we fix? A more realistic approach would be to suppress mutation in the first place, or if this cannot be done, then to suppress the phenotypic appearance of the genetic transformation that drives the carcinogenic process.

The overall topic of chemoprevention, which is a pharmacologic approach to intervention with the goal of arresting or reversing the process of carcinogenesis, is discussed in this chapter. In the original article in which my colleagues and I coined the term chemoprevention (9), we indicated that, in contrast to the cytotoxic approach of chemotherapy of invasive cancer, in which a deliberate attempt is made to kill cancer cells by blocking key metabolic pathways, in chemoprevention an attempt is made during the period of preneoplasia to arrest or reverse premalignant cells during their progression to invasive malignancy, using physiologic

---

[1]**Abbreviations: COX-2,** inducible cyclooxygenase; **ER,** estrogen receptors; **iNOS,** inducible nitric oxide synthase; **NF-κB,** nuclear factor-κB; **PPARγ,** peroxisome proliferator-activated receptor γ; **RAR,** retinoic acid receptors; **RXR,** retinoid X receptors; **SERM,** selective estrogen receptor modulator; **VDR,** vitamin D receptor.

TABLE 82.1. TOTAL CANCER DEATHS IN MEN IN THE UNITED STATES[a]

SITE	1971	2004
Lung	53,000	92,000
Colorectal	22,000	28,000
Prostate	17,000	30,000
Pancreas	10,000	15,000

[a] Data have not been adjusted for age or population; the latter has increased by approximately 40% during the past 30 years.

Data from American Cancer Society. Estimated Cancer Deaths and New Cases by Sex and Site: 1971 Cancer Facts and Figures. New York: American Cancer Society, 1970, and from Jemal A, Tirwari RC, Murray T et al. CA Cancer J Clin 2004;54:8–29.

mechanisms that are not cytotoxic. There is a good reason to believe that such mechanisms are normally operative in people during the period of preneoplasia (10), but that they are relatively ineffective if the exposure to carcinogens or cocarcinogens is excessive. A nutritional, physiologic, or pharmacologic enhancement of these protective mechanisms is thus required if we are to achieve the goal of prevention of invasive cancer. The eventual success of this approach will depend on the development of new synthetic drugs. However, because specific chemicals that have chemopreventive activity are also ingested as nutrients in the diet, nutritional approaches also fall under the overall rubric of chemoprevention. In this chapter, an overview of the process of carcinogenesis is first presented, because an understanding of carcinogenesis is the fundamental basis for the development of effective chemoprevention, and then strategies and agents that can be used to prevent cancer both in animals and in a clinical setting are discussed.

CARCINOGENESIS AND CANCER (see also chapter 80)

In several reviews that my colleagues and I have written, we have suggested that the very name cancer, a term widely used by clinicians, laboratory scientists, and laypersons alike to describe the phenomenon of malignancy, is indeed a misnomer. The disease in reality is a process, namely, carcinogenesis, rather than a state, as implied by the term cancer.

TABLE 82.2. TOTAL CANCER DEATHS IN WOMEN IN THE UNITED STATES[a]

SITE	1971	2004
Lung	11,000	69,000
Colorectal	24,000	28,000
Breast	31,000	40,000
Pancreas	8,000	16,000
Ovary	10,000	16,000

[a] Data have not been adjusted for age or population; the latter has increased by approximately 40% during the past 30 years.

Data from American Cancer Society. Estimated Cancer Deaths and New Cases by Sex and Site: 1971 Cancer Facts and Figures. New York: American Cancer Society, 1970, and from Jemal A, Tirwari RC, Murray T et al. Ca Cancer J Clin 2004;54:8–29.

As has been noted elsewhere (11), the actual disease is an evolving molecular and cellular process, not a static circumstance, the onset of which can be dated to the time when a pathologist can finally see malignant cells invading through a basement membrane on a slide. Classic terminology, which originated more than a century ago, ignores the importance of the critical dimension of time in the development of epithelial carcinogenesis; by now, we know that there is a latency period, often 20 years or more, between the initiation of carcinogenesis and the onset of the terminal, invasive, and metastatic phase of the disease (12). Classic pathology and clinical oncology have dealt with cancer in the three dimensions of space (the size and location of lesions); to understand the process of carcinogenesis, which is the reality of the disease, we must now add the dimension of time (11).

A more realistic and modern view would be to consider the process of carcinogenesis as a four-dimensional process of dysregulation of gene function (this may be caused by mutation, deletion, amplification, or translocation, or even by some other mechanism). As a consequence of this genetic dysfunctionality, a series of events starts with clonal expansion and clonal heterogeneity of initiated and promoted cells, then proceeds to local tissue invasion, and finally terminates in metastasis of tumor cells, which usually is the cause of death of malignancy. At the present rate of discovery of oncogenes and suppressor genes (13), it is conceivable that hundreds of genes will eventually be implicated in the process of dysregulation that finally leads to the invasive or metastatic phenotype; in any individual patient with metastatic carcinoma, this is manifested by a wide array of genotypes and phenotypes within the population of tumor cells in that patient (7, 8).

It is thus important to develop a kinetic perspective of the entire process of carcinogenesis, particularly the kinetics of the development of the early lesions of the disease. It must be emphasized that there is only a stochastic probability, not an unqualified certainty, that an early stage will progress to a later one. Indeed, the natural history of many forms of epithelial carcinogenesis indicates that many, if not most, early lesions disappear spontaneously (3, 10, 11). Because these early lesions often disappear, it has been erroneously concluded in the past that they are not relevant to cancer. Indeed it is widely believed by many physicians that the patient with an early, noninvasive lesion does not have cancer. This is clearly a fallacious interpretation. To the extent that everyone is subject to mutation, either endogenous or exogenous, everyone is part of the carcinogenic process. Given the ubiquitous nature of both natural and synthetic carcinogenic substances in our environment, it is doubtful whether the genome of any man or woman has sustained no damage over the course of that person's lifetime. In this regard, a major development since the mid-1980s has been the finding and validation that DNA damage and mutation arise from endogenous products of cellular metabolism, particularly reactive oxygen and reactive nitrogen species (14–20). Thus, carcinogenesis is an endemic disease process, driven in large part by mutagenic agents derived from our own metabolism, and essentially no one is entirely healthy from a genomic perspective. Everyone is at risk, and indeed, although progression from early to late lesions may be stochastic, at the present time an epidemiologist can accurately predict that at least one in five persons in the entire population of the United States will eventually die of end-stage malignancy if the current death rates continue (2, 21).

There are several other logical fallacies that have resulted from the failure to understand the chronic nature of the process of carcinogenesis. The worst fallacy is the widespread notion that people are healthy until they have cancer, as if one could accurately set a date on which the cancer truly began. The date that a woman can first feel a lump in her breast or that this lump can be detected on a mammogram is totally irrelevant to the understanding of the pathogenesis of invasive breast cancer. Carcinogenesis begins with the earliest damage to any regulatory gene that is relevant to the disease process, even though it may be many years before the phenotypic manifestations of this damage are apparent. Corollary fallacies are the notions that it is unethical to treat healthy people with a preventive agent and that one must wait until a diagnosis of "cancer" is made before it is ethically justified to treat that patient with a "cancer drug" (11).

There is tremendous disparity in the manner in which the oncology medical community, as compared with the cardiovascular medical community, approaches this entire problem of the detection and management of early disease. Thus, the oncology community lags far behind the cardiovascular community in recognizing the importance of early precursor lesions as antecedents of clinically symptomatic disease. In cardiovascular medicine, there has been a major emphasis on the natural history of the disease process, and coupled with this, there has been the use of intensive chemoprevention to arrest or reverse the pathogenesis of cardiovascular disease. The process of atherogenesis has been exhaustively studied, and no one any longer doubts the relationship between precursor lesions, such as fatty streaking of arteries or the development of arterial plaques, and the life-threatening clinical outcomes, myocardial infarction and stroke. In any person, there is no certainty that individual arterial lesions will progress, but this uncertainty is not used as an argument against pharmacologic intervention designed to prevent further progression. Thus, during atherogenesis, just as in carcinogenesis, progression of lesions is stochastic, but a different approach to management of early cardiovascular lesions is in widespread clinical use. Accordingly, synthetic drugs that are cholesterol-lowering, antihypertensive, and antiplatelet agents are widely prescribed for chemoprevention of cardiovascular disease, with the knowledge that some recipients will not benefit and some will even experience undesirable side effects. However, the benefit-versus-risk analysis has clearly been favorable for active intervention, and an acceptance of the concept of chemoprevention has prevailed (21).

Why has there been such a lag in acceptance of the relevance of early lesions to the progression of carcinogenesis? I have suggested elsewhere (11) that in the past the primary reason may have been the perception that nothing could be done about such lesions: the clinician, lacking any means of prevention and aware that the lesion might even disappear spontaneously, has not wished to alarm the patient with a diagnosis of cancer; similarly, the patient has not wished to confront the possibility of having a potentially lethal disease when there was no means of prevention. It is important to emphasize that this situation has changed, and that now, with the development of effective agents for the chemoprevention of cancer, the earliest possible detection and definition of precursor lesions has become increasingly necessary. Moreover, with new and better markers of progression, we now are able to give patients a more realistic assessment of their risk of proceeding to invasive carcinoma, and of the possibility of halting this progression by the use of a chemopreventive agent. The outlook for the patient with an early lesion is much brighter than it was 10 years ago. This is particularly true for women with precursor lesions in the breast, which are estrogen receptor–positive, because dramatic advances have been made in the use of chemopreventive agents for preventing progression of such lesions, as will be discussed later (22–24).

CHEMOPREVENTION BASED ON MECHANISM

Successful implementation of chemoprevention depends on a mechanistic understanding of carcinogenesis at the molecular, cellular, and tissue levels (see Chapter 80). If one considers carcinogenesis as a disease of aberrant differentiation, which is almost axiomatic at the present time (see the classic reviews of Pierce [25] and Mintz [26] and their colleagues), then one must consider the potential role that the 2000 to 3000 proteins that regulate gene transcription may play in this process (27), because differentiation is ultimately determined by the expression of specific genes. In addition to gene mutation, there is strong evidence that dysfunctional epigenetic control, such as aberrant methylation of DNA or acetylation of histones, is also associated with carcinogenesis (28–30). Likewise, in addition to the transcription factors themselves, defects in the complex signal transduction cascades that regulate the activity of these regulators can also contribute to the carcinogenic process.

Carcinogenesis, however, is more than the result of having too many cells; it is the result of too many aggressive, invasive cells that are in the wrong place at the wrong time and often are dysfunctional. Although molecular lesions in genes that regulate the cell cycle might enhance carcinogenesis, the tumorigenic process also affects the normal relationships between epithelial cells and their underlying stromal cells (31–33). Carcinogenesis can therefore be redefined as a disease of tissue, which involves multiple cell types. The end result (invasive and metastatic carcinoma) is the final stage of many dysfunctional steps at both the cellular and tissue level. This complex process will probably require many pharmacologic agents to prevent end-stage disease. At present, it seems unlikely that a single "magic bullet" will ever be found that can either prevent carcinoma at multiple organ sites or treat metastatic malignancy resulting from a wide range of primary tumor sites. It is much more likely that eventually practical chemoprevention regimens will rely on the use of multiple pharmacologic agents (21).

PHARMACOLOGY OF CHEMOPREVENTION

The most rational approach to chemoprevention is to design and test new agents that act on specific molecular and cellular targets. In addition, it is essential that the efficacy and safety of new agents are validated in experimental models before clinical trials are begun. Although epidemiologic studies can provide valuable leads for development of chemopreventive agents, they need to be confirmed with experimental data in cell culture and animals before clinical trials.

Empiric approaches to chemoprevention, based solely on epidemiologic data that merely correlate dietary patterns and risk of developing cancer, are fraught with danger, as was dramatically seen in the clinical failure of the trials with β-carotene to prevent cancer at common sites, such as the lung, prostate, and colon (34–36). The selection of β-carotene for these trials was based largely on data indicating that consumption of high amounts of fruits and vegetables was associated with a reduced risk of cancer, and there were almost no data in experimental animals to support the suggestion that β-carotene itself prevented cancer at the above sites. In particular, there was essentially no experimental basis for implicating β-carotene as the most important single agent (in diets containing high amounts of fruits and vegetables) that might be responsible for a potential chemopreventive effect of such diets.

Fortunately, many new agents are now available to target molecular and cellular processes known to be important in carcinogenesis; these agents also prevent cancer in experimental animals (21, 37, 38). Some of these agents are now discussed.

Nuclear Receptor Ligands

Members of the nuclear receptor superfamily are transcription factors that selectively regulate cell differentiation and proliferation in specific organs, many of which are important sites for carcinogenesis (39). Thus, their ligands represent agents ideal for chemoprevention. Nuclear receptors involved in carcinogenesis and targeted for chemoprevention include the two estrogen receptors (ER-α and ER-β), the androgen receptor, the three retinoic acid receptors (RAR-α, β, and γ), the three retinoid X receptors (RXR-α, β, and γ), the vitamin D receptor (VDR), and peroxisome proliferator-activated receptor γ (PPARγ) (Table 82.3).

Transcriptional activity of these receptors is controlled by the binding of specific ligands, which activate transcription in one cellular context and repress transcription in another. Although this phenomenon of contextual action was puzzling when originally discovered, it is now understood in terms of the selective recruitment and displacement of other proteins, which are transcriptional coactivators and corepressors, that interact with the transcription factors themselves (40, 41). Thus, tamoxifen should no longer be viewed as an estrogen antagonist; it is a selective estrogen receptor modulator (SERM) that can be antiestrogenic in one organ, such as the breast, and proestrogenic in others, such as bone and the uterus (40). The antiestrogenic activity of tamoxifen in the breast is desirable for chemoprevention because estrogen enhances the growth of almost all breast cancer cells during the early stages of carcinogenesis; in contrast, stimulation of uterine epithelium by tamoxifen can potentially cause endometrial carcinoma (22, 42). Raloxifene thus represents a major improvement (Table 82.3) over tamoxifen because it is not uterotrophic but still is strongly antiestrogenic in the breast (23, 24, 43). For chronic administration of a SERM for breast cancer prevention, it is also important that it be proestrogenic in bone to avoid osteoporosis that results from estrogen deprivation, and raloxifene again fulfills this criterion (23, 24).

The SERM concept and its extension to other members of the nuclear receptor superfamily that are also selective modulators, for example, selective PPAR-γ modulators (44), has great importance for the entire field of chemoprevention because a single modulator drug that can have the total spectrum of desired actions (both agonistic and antagonistic) in different organs of the body is now within reach (41). Although this goal has not yet been achieved, the development of newer SERMs, such as raloxifene and arzoxifene (which are antiestrogenic in breast and uterus and proestrogenic in bone), indicates that it will be possible to achieve further benefits of SERMs while eliminating some of the undesirable actions of older agents (42).

Chemopreventive benefits of SERMs may not be limited to actions in the breast; the recent identification of ER-α and ER-β in the prostate suggests that they could provide a useful target for prevention of prostate cancer (45). Indeed, prevention of prostate cancer in a rat model with tamoxifen (which binds to both ER-α and ER-β) was shown several years ago (46). Likewise, estrogen receptors in the colon also have the potential to modulate carcinogenesis in that organ (47). However, up to the present, clinical efficacy of SERMs for cancer prevention has been shown only in the breast, for tamoxifen (22) and raloxifene (23, 24).

TABLE 82.3. EXAMPLES OF CHEMOPREVENTIVE AGENTS WITH DEFINED MOLECULAR TARGETS

TYPE OF AGENT	STRUCTURE	MOLECULAR TARGET	REFERENCES
Ligands for nuclear receptors			
Raloxifene (selective estrogen receptor modulator)		Estrogen receptors	23, 24, 43
Bexarotene (rexinoid)		Retinoid X receptors	49, 50, 52
Rosiglitazone		Peroxisome proliferator-activated receptor γ	39, 48
Calcitriol		Vitamin D receptor	53
Antiinflammatory agents			
Celecoxib		Cyclooxygenase	66–68
Curcumin		Nuclear factor-κB	71

TABLE 82.3. EXAMPLES OF CHEMOPREVENTIVE AGENTS WITH DEFINED MOLECULAR TARGETS (Continued)

TYPE OF AGENT	STRUCTURE	MOLECULAR TARGET	REFERENCES
Chromatin modifiers			
Suberoylanilide hydroxamic acid		Histone deacetylase	29, 81
5-Aza-2′-deoxycytidine		DNA (demethylating agent)	81, 82

The importance of PPARγ as a target for chemoprevention is underscored by the widespread clinical use of their ligands, the thiazolidinediones (such as rosiglitazone, Table 82.3) for chronic treatment of type II diabetes. There is major current interest in the use of PPAR-γ ligands for chemoprevention of cancer (44, 48), and a side benefit of their use in diabetes therapy might be the prevention of cancer. Such data remain to be obtained.

Rexinoids, which are ligands that are selective for binding to any or all of the three RXRs, are another group of highly promising chemopreventive agents. As RXRs form functional heterodimers with many other nuclear receptors, including the RARs, VDR, and PPAR-γ, the rexinoids have the unique ability to modulate the actions of many other transcription factors (49). They have already proven useful as single agents in animal models for preventing both ER-positive (50) and ER-negative (51) breast cancer. Prevention of ER-negative cancers is a particularly important achievement because these malignancies generally have a poor prognosis. Moreover, although RXRs are not known to interact directly with ERs, the combination of the rexinoid LGD 1069 and tamoxifen has unusual potency not only in preventing but also in treating breast cancer in rats (50, 52).

The synthetic analogs of vitamin D (deltanoids), many of which have potent differentiative and antiproliferative activities (53), are yet another set of promising ligands for chemoprevention. Numerous epidemiologic studies indicate an inverse association between vitamin D intake and human cancer risk, especially in the colon (54), and new laboratory findings show that the VDR can protect the colon from the carcinogenic effects of bile acids (55). However, ingestion of increased amounts of natural forms of vitamin D is dangerous because of the resultant increase in blood calcium levels (hypercalcemia). The development of new synthetic deltanoids, which are strongly antiproliferative but have a much lesser propensity to cause hypercalcemia, has been a major advance (53). The VDR is a classic transcription factor and has been shown to interact functionally with Smad3, a component of the signal transduction pathway for the regulatory cytokine transforming growth factor-β (56).

Thus, in summary, ligands for the nuclear receptor superfamily display complex interactions: they control gene expression directly, and they interact with a much larger set of regulatory pathways (27, 57) through cross-talk with signal transduction cascades. With progress in the synthesis of new deltanoids that are almost totally noncalcemic, it seems that VDR ligands will be increasingly important. Abundant data show that they are highly active for prevention in animal models (53), but clinical proof is yet to come. Observations that were originally made in nutritional studies thus have had major impact on the development of new pharmacologic agents for cancer prevention.

Antiinflammatory Agents

The concept that inflammation and carcinogenesis are related phenomena has been the subject of many studies that have attempted to link these two processes in a mechanistic fashion (58–60). The enzymes that mediate the constitutive synthesis of nitric oxide and prostaglandins from arginine and arachidonate, respectively, have relatively little significance for either inflammation or carcinogenesis. In contrast, inducible nitric oxide synthase (iNOS) and inducible cyclooxygenase-2 (COX-2) both have critical roles in the response of tissues to injury or infectious agents. These inducible enzymes are essential components of the inflammatory process, the ultimate repair of injury, and carcinogenesis (61–64). Although physiologic activity of iNOS and COX-2 may provide a definite benefit to the organism, aberrant or excessive expression of either iNOS or COX-2 has been implicated in the pathogenesis of cancer. There has been particularly strong interest in the connection between inflammation and cancer in the area of colorectal cancer, in which inflammatory bowel disease is thought to play a strong etiologic role (65).

This entire topic has recently taken on a new importance as antiinflammatory agents that inhibit the formation of prostaglandins have been shown to be useful in chemoprevention (Table 82.3). Nonsteroidal antiinflammatory agents, and especially the newer selective inhibitors of COX-2 such as celecoxib, inhibit colon carcinogenesis in experimental animals (66) and have been shown to cause a significant reduction of colorectal polyps in human subjects (67). Mechanistically, these studies are particularly interesting because the beneficial effects of these agents seem to be mediated by their effects on stromal cells of the intestine, especially their ability to suppress angiogenesis, which is part of the stromal reaction (reviewed in reference 68).

In addition to COX-2, the enzyme iNOS provides another target for the use of antiinflammatory agents in chemoprevention. The evidence for a significant role of iNOS in carcinogenesis is increasing as new studies indicate that elevation of iNOS may contribute to the pathogenesis of human colon, brain, breast, and gynecologic cancer (15, 19). It is clear that the product of iNOS, namely nitric oxide, is a potent mutagen (14), and that nitric oxide or its metabolites can also activate COX-2 (69).

Beyond the use of agents that act directly as inhibitors of the enzymatic activity of COX-2 or iNOS, or as inhibitors of the induction of these enzymes, the transcription factor nuclear factor-κB (NF-κB), which regulates the activities of many genes involved in the inflammatory process, provides an excellent target for the development of new chemopreventive agents (70). For example, several natural products that have both antiinflammatory and anticarcinogenic activity, such as curcumin, resveratrol, and caffeic acid phenethylester, block either the activation or the transcriptional activity of NF-κB (71). The development of new inhibitors for NF-κB is being widely pursued for many therapeutic indications beyond cancer (for example, inflammatory bowel disease or neurodegenerative disease) and illustrates the diverse applications of studies of regulation of gene transcription in modern pharmacology. However, suppression of NF-κB activity is not without risk, because it can increase susceptibility to infections such as tuberculosis.

Chromatin Modifiers

A new area of research that has started to impact on chemoprevention is the study of chromatin modifiers. These can alter the activities of many other agents that are ligands either for transcription factors or for other proteins that modulate the activities of transcription factors. Chromatin structure can be modified with drugs that either increase the acetylation of histones (histone deacetylase inhibitors) or demethylate cytosine residues in DNA, and thereby increase the ability of transcription factors to stimulate gene expression (28, 29). The two classes of agents are interactive (72), and members of both classes have been used successfully for chemoprevention in experimental animals (Table 82.3). Mechanistically, chromatin modifiers interact with ligands for the nuclear receptor superfamily, as can be seen in the ability of trichostatin A (a histone deacetylase inhibitor) or 5-aza-2′-deoxycytidine (a DNA demethylating agent) to enhance the ability of all-*trans*-retinoic acid either to differentiate human leukemia cells (73) or to suppress the proliferation of human breast cancer cells (74). The practical use of many chromatin modifiers has been limited so far by their toxicity, but the development of less toxic new agents such as suberoylanilide hydroxamic acid (29) indicates that this problem can be solved.

IMPORTANCE OF ANIMAL EXPERIMENTS

Demonstrating the efficacy of chemopreventive agents in appropriate animal models is essential before the agents can enter into clinical trials. As noted earlier, failure to observe this caveat with β-carotene has had unfortunate consequences in the past. I do not wish to imply that epidemiologic studies cannot provide important leads for further clinical studies of chemopreventive agents; I am only suggesting that such information be reinforced with laboratory data before extremely expensive and time-consuming clinical trials are begun. Fortunately, excellent rodent models of breast, prostate, lung, and colon cancer exist. The recent development of transgenic mice for carcinogenesis studies has been a major advance and now offers the possibility of studying the prevention of ER-negative breast cancer (51), an addition to the well-established rat models for ER-positive breast cancer. Furthermore, significant new transgenic models of pancreatic cancer also are being developed (75, 76).

Although transgenic models of carcinogenesis have become widely used, in many respects models that use chemical carcinogens still are extensively useful. This is particularly true if one wishes to study classes of preventive agents that are selective for modulating the initiation, promotion, or progression phases of carcinogenesis because one can easily control the timing of the carcinogenic insult as well as the dosimetry of the carcinogenic damage. Thus, agents that scavenge electrophiles that damage DNA (e.g., ascorbic acid or α-tocopherol) or agents that induce phase 2 enzymes that protect against such damage e.g., the potent inducer from broccoli, sulforaphane (77), are most readily studied in an experimental design of the sort shown in Figure 82.1, in which the chemopreventive agent is given just before and during the time of the administration of the carcinogen. Conversely, agents that affect promotion and progression (as opposed to initiation) by altering cell

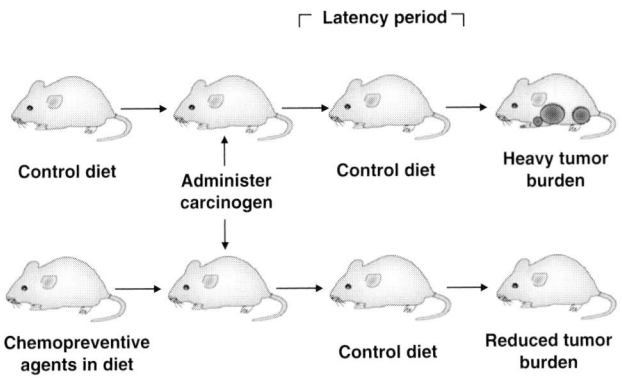

Figure 82.1. Study design for effects on initiation.

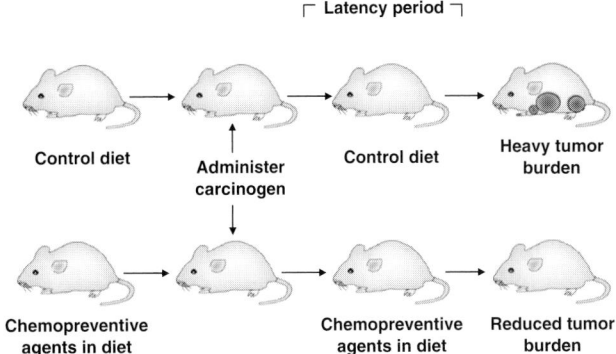

Figure 82.3. Study design for effects on both initiation and promotion/progression.

differentiation and DNA synthesis can be evaluated in a study design as shown in Figure 82.2, in which treatment with the preventive agent is not started until after carcinogen administration has been completed (during the latency period). The ultimate ideal chemopreventive regimen would be one that both blocked initiation and suppressed promotion and progression, and a design of the sort shown in Figure 82.3 would allow such an evaluation to be made. Because in the real world of human carcinogenesis, continuing mutagenic DNA damage during the latency period undoubtedly drives the carcinogenic process (7, 8, 17, 20), it is important to consider the use of such experimental designs. Thus, although in the classic mouse skin model of carcinogenesis initiation and promotion/progression can be neatly separated, in actual practice in many human situations such distinctions may not exist.

Figure 82.4 clearly shows the sophistry of suggesting that chemopreventive agents only "delay" the onset of cancer but do not "prevent" it. Most chemoprevention experiments in experimental animals are performed in groups of animals that either have been treated with a massive dose of carcinogen or have a genetic defect that results in the majority of the control animals developing malignant tumors in a short time period. This use of animals with overwhelming carcinogenic burden is not a particularly valid model of human carcinogenesis, but rather is a reflection of the

practical and economic considerations that enable an investigator to evaluate a preventive agent in a reasonable time at a reasonable cost.

Because one can easily evaluate a preventive agent with a relatively small number of animals when the controls have 100% tumor incidence within a short latency period, this is a preferred method for laboratory studies. However, in humans the latency period for carcinogenesis is long; it can be 10 to 20 years, or even more at many sites (12). Moreover, the incidence of invasive cancer is fortunately low in the total human population. Most heavy smokers do not develop invasive lung cancer, although all probably have genetic lesions and cellular abnormalities in their bronchial epithelium. Therefore, when very high doses of carcinogen are used in chemopreventive studies, it may seem that a preventive agent is only delaying the onset of cancer. However, when more relevant low doses of carcinogen are used, one can show suppression of the onset of cancer over very long periods, even the lifetime of an animal in some cases (shown schematically in Fig. 82.4). The important concept to emphasize is that an effective chemopreventive agent can extend the latency period for onset of cancer, often more than doubling this parameter so that an animal may never develop a visibly invasive carcinoma. Chemopreventive agents that double the latency period for human carcinogenesis would have an immense impact on useful, high-quality life for millions of people (78). The development of effective antimutagenic agents will be particularly important for this entire problem of extending latency.

EDUCATIONAL AND SOCIETAL ISSUES

There are many aspects of the chemoprevention issue that go well beyond the scientific ones that have been discussed in this chapter, and these deal largely with the public and professional acceptance of the entire concept of the use of drugs to prevent cancer and the willingness of the pharmaceutical industry to participate in the manufacture and distribution of such drugs as well as to promote their use. These are practical issues of major importance to the field, and are not discussed here. However, the reader is referred

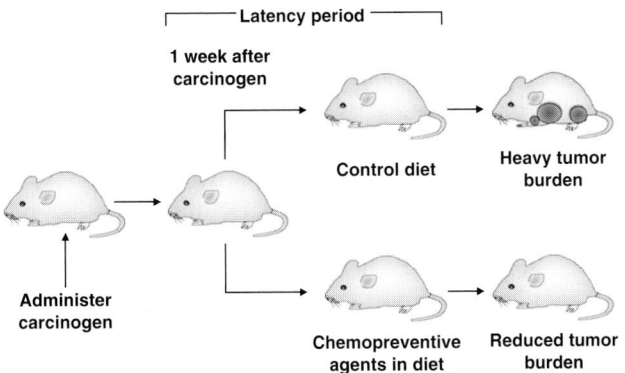

Figure 82.2. Study design for effects on promotion/progression.

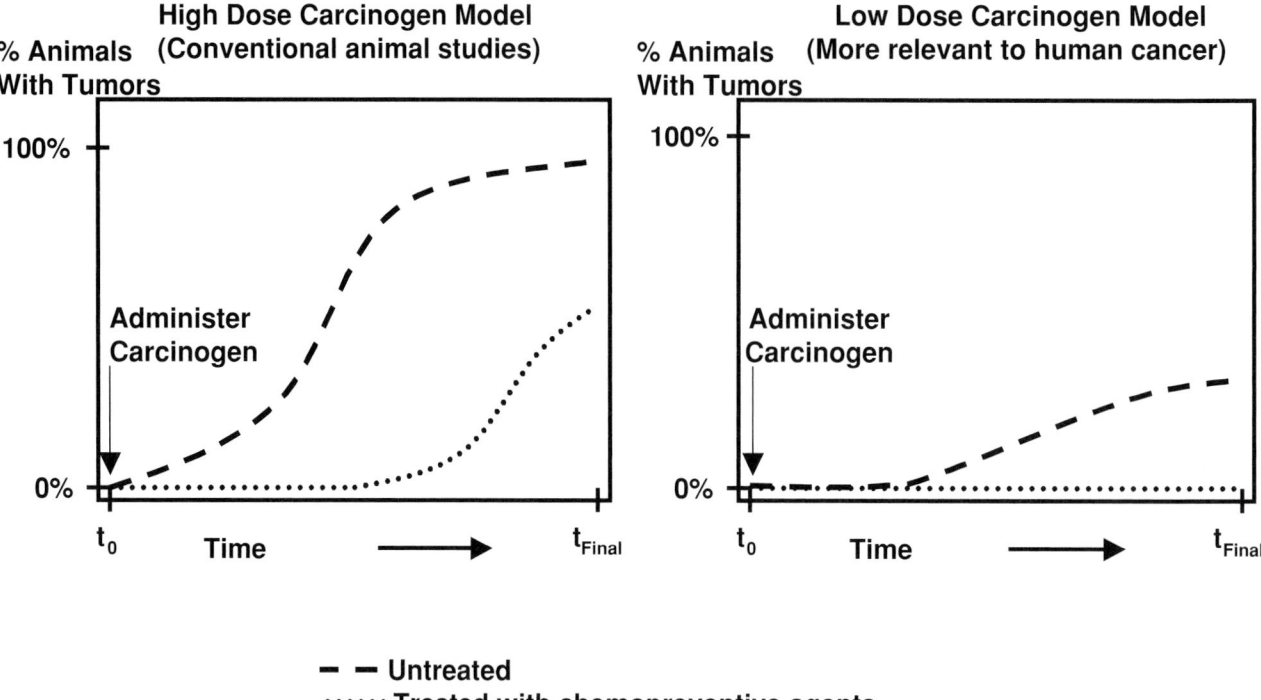

Figure 82.4. Chemopreventive agents can extend the latency period of carcinogenesis. If the dose of carcinogen is low enough, lifetime protection can result with the use of a preventive agent.

to a published report of a special Working Group of the American Association for Cancer Research for a detailed discussion of these matters (79).

CLINICAL APPLICATIONS

By now, there are dozens of ongoing clinical trials of various chemopreventive agents in the cancer field. The dramatic success of both tamoxifen (22) and raloxifene (23, 24) in preventing estrogen receptor–positive breast cancer in postmenopausal women has given tremendous impetus to this area of clinical cancer research. For an extensive review and discussion, the reader is referred to the overview of this topic that Lippman and I wrote (80).

Acknowledgment
I thank Megan Padgett for expert assistance in preparation of this review.

REFERENCES

1. American Cancer Society. Estimated Cancer Deaths and New Cases by Sex and Site: 1971 Cancer Facts and Figures. New York: American Cancer Society, 1970.
2. Jemal A, Tirwari RC, Murray T et al. CA Cancer J Clin 2004; 54:8–29.
3. Sporn MB. Lancet 1996;347:1377–81.
4. Fidler IJ, Kripke ML. Science 1977;197:893–5.
5. Poste G, Greig R. Invasion Metastasis 1982;2:137–76.
6. Heppner GH. Cancer Res 1984;44:2259–65.
7. Loeb LA, Loeb KR, Anderson JP. Proc Natl Acad Sci USA 2003; 100:776–81.
8. Loeb LA. Cancer Res 2001;61:3230–9.
9. Sporn MB, Dunlop NM, Newton DL et al. Fed Proc 1976;35: 1332–8.
10. Sporn MB. Cancer Res 1976;36:2699–702.
11. Sporn MB. Cancer Res 1991;51:6215–8.
12. O'Shaughnessy JA, Kelloff GJ, Gordon GB et al. Clin Cancer Res 2002;8:314–46.
13. Hanahan D, Weinberg RA. Cell 2000;100:57–70.
14. Tamir S, Tannenbaum SR. Biochim Biophys Acta 1996;1288: F31–6.
15. Ambs S, Merriam WG, Bennett WP et al. Cancer Res 1998;58: 334–41.
16. Ames BN. Mutat Res 1989;214:41–6.
17. Marnett LJ. Carcinogenesis 2000;21:361–70.
18. Feig DI, Reid TM, Loeb LA. Cancer Res 1994;54:1890S–4S.
19. Hussain SP, Hofseth LJ, Harris CC. Nat Rev Cancer 2003;3: 276–85.
20. Sharma RA, Farmer PB. Clin Cancer Res 2004;10:4901–12.
21. Sporn MB, Suh N. Nat Rev Cancer 2002,2:537–43.
22. Fisher B, Costantino JP, Wickerham DL et al. J Natl Cancer Inst 1998;90:1371–88.
23. Cauley JA, Norton L, Lippman ME et al. Breast Cancer Res Treat 2001;65:125–34.
24. Cummings SR, Eckert S, Krueger KA et al. JAMA 1999;281: 2189–97.
25. Pierce GB, Shikes R, Fink LM. Cancer: A Problem of Developmental Biology. Englewood Cliffs, NJ: Prentice-Hall, 1978.

26. Mintz B, Fleischman RA. Adv Cancer Res 1981;34:211–78.

27. Brivanlou AH, Darnell JE Jr. Science 2002;298:813–8.

28. Baylin SB, Herman JG, Graff JR et al. Adv Cancer Res 1998;72: 141–96.

29. Marks P, Rifkind RA, Richon VM et al. Nat Rev Cancer 2001;1: 194–202.

30. Robertson KD, Jones PA. Carcinogenesis 2000;21:461–7.

31. Bissell MJ, Radisky D. Nat Rev Cancer 2001;1:46–54.

32. Clark WH Jr. Acta Oncol 1995;31:2–21.

33. Liotta LA, Kohn EC. Nature 2001;411:375–9.

34. Hennekens CH, Buring JE, Manson JE et al. N Engl J Med 1996;334:1145–9.

35. Alpha-Tocopherol, Beta Carotene Cancer Prevention Study Group. N Engl J Med 1994;330:1029–35.

36. Omenn GS, Goodman GE, Thornquist MD et al. N Engl J Med 1996;334:1150–5.

37. Kelloff GJ. Adv Cancer Res 1999;78:188–334.

38. Sporn MB, Suh N. Carcinogenesis 2000;21:525–30.

39. Mangelsdorf DJ, Thummel C, Beato M et al. Cell 1995;83:835–9.

40. Katzenellenbogen BS, Katzenellenbogen JA. Science 2002;295: 2380.

41. Smith CL, O'Malley BW. Endocr Rev 2004;25:45–71.

42. Sporn MB. Clin Cancer Res 2004;10:5313–5.

43. Anzano MA, Peer CW, Smith JM et al. J Natl Cancer Inst 1996; 99:123–5.

44. Sporn MB, Suh N, Mangelsdorf DJ. Trends Mol Med 2001;7: 395–400.

45. Horvath LG, Henshall SM, Lee CS et al. Cancer Res 2001;61: 5331–5.

46. Lucia MS, Anzano MA, Slayter MV et al. Cancer Res 1995;55: 5621–7.

47. Campbell-Thompson M, Lynch IJ, Bhardwaj B. Cancer Res 2001;61:632–40.

48. Kopelovich L, Fay JR, Glazer RI et al. Mol Cancer Ther 2002; 1:357–63.

49. Chawla A, Repa JJ, Evans RM et al. Science 2001;294:1866–70.

50. Bischoff ED, Gottardis MM, Moon TE et al. Cancer Res 1998; 58:479–84.

51. Wu K, Kim HT, Rodriquez JL et al. Cancer Epidemiol Biomarkers Prev 2002;11:467–74.

52. Gottardis MM, Bischoff ED, Shirley MA et al. Cancer Res 1996; 56:5566–70.

53. Guyton KZ, Kensler TW, Posner GH. Annu Rev Pharmacol Toxicol 2001;41:421–42.

54. Martinez ME, Willett NS. Cancer Epidemiol Biomarkers Prev 1998;7:163–8.

55. Makishima M, Lu TT, Xie W et al. Science 2002;296:1313–6.

56. Yanagisawa J, Yanagi Y, Masuhiro Y et al. Science 1999;283: 1317–21.

57. Misteli T. Science 2001;291:843–7.

58. Sporn MB, Roberts AB. J Clin Invest 1986;78:329–32.

59. Ohshima H, Bartsch H. Mutat Res 1994;305:253–64.

60. Coussens LM, Werb Z. Nature 2002;420;860–7.

61. Moncada S, Palmer RMJ, Higgs EA. Pharmacol Rev 1991;43: 109–41.

62. Nathan CF, Xie QW. Cell 1994;78:915–8.

63. Salvemini D, Seibert K, Masferrer JL et al. J Clin Invest 1994; 93:1940–7.

64. Nathan C. Nature 2002;420;846–52.

65. Itzkowitz SH, Yio X. Am J Physiol 2004;287:G7–17.

66. Reddy BS, Hirose Y, Lubet R et al. Cancer Res 2000;60:293–7.

67. Steinbach G, Lynch PM, Phillips RK et al. N Engl J Med 2000; 342:1946–52.

68. Gupta RA, DuBois RN. Nat Rev Cancer 2001;1:11–21.

69. Landino LM, Crews BC, Timmons MD et al. Proc Natl Acad Sci USA 1996;93:15069–74.

70. Yamamoto Y, Gaynor RB. J Clin Invest 2001;107:135–42.

71. Bharti AC, Aggarwal BB. Biochem Pharmacol 2002;64:883–8.

72. Cameron EE, Bachman KE, Myohanen S et al. Nat Genet 1999; 21:103–7.

73. Ferrara FF, Fazi F, Bianchini A et al. Cancer Res 2001;61:2–7.

74. Widschwendter M, Berger J, Hermann M et al. J Natl Cancer Inst 2000;92:826–32.

75. Aguirre AJ, Bardeesy N, Sinha M et al. Genes Dev 2003;17: 3112–26.

76. Hingorani SR, Petricoin EF III, Maitra A et al. Cancer Cell 2003;4:437–50.

77. Talalay P, Dinkova-Kostova AT, Holtzclaw WD. Adv Enzyme Regul 2003;43:121–34.

78. Lippman SM, Hong WK. Clin Cancer Res 2002;8:305–13.

79. Chemoprevention Working Group. Cancer Res 1999;59:4743–58.

80. Sporn MB, Lippman SM. Chemoprevention of cancer. In: Kufe DW, Pollock RE, Weichselbaum RR et al., eds. Cancer Medicine. 6th ed. Hamilton, Ontario, Canada: BC Decker, 2003:413–22.

81. Kopelovich L, Crowell JA, Fay JR. J Natl Cancer Inst 2003; 95:1747–57.

82. Lantry LE, Zhang Z, Crist KA et al. Carcinogenesis 1999;20: 343–6.

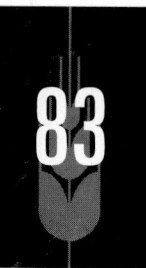

83 NUTRITION SUPPORT OF THE PATIENT WITH CANCER[1]

MARK SCHATTNER AND MOSHE SHIKE

TRENDS AND IMPACT OF CANCER 1290
PREVALENCE OF MALNUTRITION IN PATIENTS
    WITH CANCER 1291
SIGNIFICANCE OF MALNUTRITION IN PATIENTS
    WITH CANCER 1291
CAUSES OF MALNUTRITION 1292
    Alterations of Metabolism 1292
    Impaired Caloric Intake, Maldigestion,
        and Malabsorption 1295
NUTRITIONAL THERAPIES 1297
    Oral Dietary Therapy 1297
    Enteral Nutrition 1298
    Total Parenteral Nutrition 1299
    Pharmacotherapy 1300
EFFECT OF NUTRITION SUPPORT ON TUMOR
    GROWTH 1303
NUTRITIONAL MANAGEMENT OF PATIENTS
    WITH SPECIFIC CANCERS 1303
    Cancer of the Head and Neck 1304
    Cancer of the Esophagus 1304
    Cancer of the Stomach 1305
    Cancer of the Pancreas 1305
    Cancer of the Colon and Rectum 1306
    Gynecologic Cancers 1306
    Patients Undergoing Bone Marrow
        Transplantation 1306
    During Palliative Care 1307
SUMMARY 1308

More than 1.3 million new cases of invasive cancer were diagnosed in the United States in 2003 (1). Eighty percent of these patients suffered from weight loss and malnutrition during the course of their illness (2). This has a significant negative impact. In patients with cancer, malnutrition is associated with longer hospitalization (3), reduced responses

to and increased complications from anticancer therapies (4, 5), increased cost (5), worse quality of life and performance status (6), and decreased survival (7, 8). The pathogenesis of malnutrition in patients with cancer is multifactorial (9). Therapies include oral diets, enteral nutrition, parenteral nutrition, drugs, and specific nutrients. Correct application of these therapies requires understanding their indications, limitations, and efficacy.

TRENDS AND IMPACT OF CANCER

Cancer is a major public health issue, with an incidence of more than 1.3 million cases per year in the United States (excluding skin cancer) (Table 83.1). Forty three percent of men and 39% of women will be diagnosed with cancer during their lifetime (1). Lung, breast, and colorectal cancers account for more than one half of all new cancers in women, whereas lung, prostate, and colorectal cancers comprise 55% of all incident cancers among men (1). These four cancers cause more than half of the 556,500 cancer-related deaths each year. In the United States, cancer causes 23% of all deaths, making it second only to heart disease (29.6% of all deaths) as a cause of mortality (1).

From 1992 to 1999, overall cancer death rates declined by 1.5% per year in men and 0.6% per year in women (1). However, because of the growing population and the continuing decline in mortality from cardiovascular disease, the absolute number of deaths from cancer in the United States continues to increase. This increase is predominantly the result of more deaths from lung cancer (1).

Within the United States, variability in the incidence of cancer and in its associated mortality among various populations is significant. The incidence and mortality rates for African-Americans are the highest of any group and are approximately 10% higher than in whites (1). The reason for the poorer survival rate is, in part, that for most common cancers, African-Americans are more likely to be diagnosed with regional or metastatic disease, rather than localized disease, which can be more effectively treated. A portion of the survival difference persists even when comparing whites and African-Americans with the same stage of disease, a finding suggesting that comorbidities or access to health care may play a role (1). Recent data show that when whites and African-Americans receive equal-quality health care, these differences disappear (10).

---

[1]**Abbreviations: CRF,** corticotropin-releasing factor; **EPA,** eicosapentaenoic acid; **GI,** gastrointestinal; **IFN-γ,** interferon-γ; **IL,** interleukin; **LMF,** lipid-mobilizing factor; **α-MSH,** α-melanocyte–stimulating hormone; **NPY,** neuropeptide Y; **PD,** pancreaticodoudenectomy; **PEG,** percutaneous endoscopic gastrostomy; **PEJ,** percutaneous endoscopic jejunostomy; **TNM,** tumor, node, metastasis (conforms to American Joint Committee on Cancer standards); **TNF-α,** tumor necrosis factor-α; **TPN,** total parenteral nutrition.

TABLE 83.1. INCIDENCE AND MORTALITY OF VARIOUS CANCERS IN THE UNITED STATES IN 2003

SITE	INCIDENCE	MORTALITY
Lung	171,900	157,200
Colon, rectum	147,500	57,100
Pancreas, gallbladder, bile duct, liver	54,800	47,900
Breast	212,600	40,200
Prostate	220,900	28,900
Ovary, uterus, cervix, vulva	83,700	26,800
Lymphoma	61,000	24,700
Leukemia	30,600	21,900
Esophagus	19,900	13,000
Stomach	22,400	12,100
Oral cavity, pharynx, larynx	37,200	11,000

Data from Jemal A, Taylor M, Samules A et al. CA Cancer J Clin 2003;53:5–26.

Cancer has an enormous economic impact. In the United States, medical expenditures directed toward cancer treatment account for 5% of all medical expenditures and 10% of Medicare spending (11). The direct cost of caring for patients with cancer is more than 40 billion dollars annually (12).

PREVALENCE OF MALNUTRITION IN PATIENTS WITH CANCER

The prevalence of malnutrition among patients with cancer depends on the tumor type and stage, the organs involved, and the anticancer therapy. Concurrent nonmalignant conditions such as diabetes and intestinal diseases can be important contributing factors. Determining the true prevalence of malnutrition can be difficult because it depends on the sensitivity and specificity of the parameters used for nutritional assessment and because of the lack of universal agreement on the validity of these parameters. Most studies use weight loss as the primary measure, and involuntary weight loss of more than 10% is generally agreed to be a sign of significant malnutrition and a cause for concern.

The prevalence of weight loss during the 6 months preceding the diagnosis of cancer was reported from a multicenter cooperative study of patients with 12 types of cancer (8). The lowest frequency (31–40%) and severity of weight loss were found in patients with sarcomas, breast cancer, and hematologic cancers. An intermediate frequency of weight loss was found in patients with colon, prostate, and lung cancers (54–64%). Patients with cancer of the pancreas and stomach had the highest frequency (>80%) and severity of weight loss. Approximately 35% of the patients with lung cancer lost more than 5% of their body weight. This finding underscores that even if the tumor does not involve the gastrointestinal (GI) tract directly, significant weight loss can occur because of systemic and metabolic derangements and loss of appetite. A review conducted by the American College of Surgeons of

more than 5000 patients with esophageal cancer showed that 57% of patients presented with weight loss (13). Malnutrition is also common among patients with cancer of the head and neck. A study of 108 patients with laryngeal cancer found that 30% presented with weight loss (14). Even when head and neck cancer is detected at an early stage (T1 or T2, N0), 26% of patients present with a weight loss of more than 5% of their body weight (15). A well-designed study using the prognostic Nutritional Index found that 54% of women with gynecologic cancer were malnourished at presentation (16).

Among patients receiving medical treatment for a variety of cancers, 40% were found to be malnourished (2, 17). Among surgical patients in a Veterans Administration hospital, 39% of those undergoing a major operation for cancer were malnourished, as judged by either a nutrition risk index or a combination of weight loss and low serum proteins (18). In a study from Memorial Sloan-Kettering Cancer Center in New York, most patients with pancreatic cancer undergoing curative resection were malnourished, as determined by weight loss (19). Malnutrition is not limited to the hospitalized patient. In a study of more than 600 ambulatory patients with cancer, loss of at least 5% of body weight was seen in 59% of the patients (20).

Children with cancer are at high risk of malnutrition and subsequent growth retardation. In a study of children with a variety of malignancies who were receiving treatment at a pediatric oncology day-hospital, up to 26% were found to be undernourished (21). In a cohort of 1019 children presenting with acute lymphoblastic leukemia, a threefold increase in the incidence of malnutrition was detected as compared with reference data of healthy children (22).

SIGNIFICANCE OF MALNUTRITION IN PATIENTS WITH CANCER

The impact of malnutrition on the patient with cancer was demonstrated in a report by Warren in 1932 (23). Based on data from autopsies, the conclusion was that cachexia was the leading cause of death in a group of 400 patients with various cancers. More recent studies confirmed the significant impact of malnutrition on the quality of life and prognosis of the patient with cancer. In a multicenter cooperative study of patients receiving chemotherapy (8), those who presented with weight loss at the time of diagnosis had decreased performance status and survival when compared with those without weight loss. When data from four randomized trials involving 152 patients with GI cancer receiving chemotherapy were examined, weight loss was found to be an independent predictor of a decrease in survival, response to therapy, and quality of life (24). Malnourished patients are also at increased risk of severe chemotherapy-induced hematologic toxicities such as neutropenic fever or severe thrombocytopenia (25). In a study of patients with limited, inoperable lung cancer, weight loss was a major predictive factor for survival (17).

The negative impact of malnutrition was also demonstrated in surgical patients with malignant and benign diseases. Malnourished patients undergoing a major operation were at greater risk of postoperative morbidity and mortality than were well-nourished patients (18, 26). Furthermore, weight loss was found to be a better predictor of mortality than even tumor, node, metastasis (TNM) staging among patients with recurrent cancers of the head and neck (27).

These studies do not establish a clear causal relationship between malnutrition and poor outcome. It is reasonable to suppose that a poor nutritional state is an independent prognostic factor for poor outcome, but malnutrition may merely indicate a more serious type and stage of illness, rather than independently causing a poor outcome. A few studies have attempted to isolate the effect of malnutrition from the direct effects of the disease (8, 24, 27). Without a clear demonstration that reversal of malnutrition independently improves outcome, it is difficult to establish it as an independent factor in the course of the disease. However, one must appreciate that in a particular patient, various ill effects result from malnutrition and may improve with specialized nutrition support.

CAUSES OF MALNUTRITION

The origin of weight loss and malnutrition in patients with cancer is multifactorial. Impaired food intake and absorption resulting from tumor or treatment effects and widespread alterations in metabolism induced by the tumor lead to the profound malnutrition that accompanies malignancy. In considering nutrition therapy, these alterations have to be kept in mind. The provision of nutrients may not be adequate to reverse malnutrition in the patient with cancer because it only bypasses the supply aspect and does not address the inefficient utilization secondary to metabolic derangements.

Alterations of Metabolism

Cancer induces widespread cellular and metabolic alterations that affect carbohydrates, protein, lipids, mineral, vitamins, and hormones. A complex picture is emerging from the understanding of the role of cytokines and various other mediators that are induced by cancer. The overall effect is that of a wasteful and inefficient metabolic state that contributes to weight loss and malnutrition.

Currently, enteral or parenteral nutrition support can overcome impaired nutrient intake, digestion, and absorption in almost every patient; however, the efficacy of these therapies is limited by the persistent alterations in metabolism that lead to inefficient utilization of the delivered energy and nutrients. Improved understanding of the effects of cancer on the cytokines, neuropeptides, and other mediators outlined later holds the promise of improving the outcome of nutrition support among patients with cancer.

Energy Expenditure

The hypothesis that increased energy expenditure leads to weight loss experienced by patients with cancer was supported by initial studies (28, 29). However, later observations showed that the effect of cancer on energy expenditure is variable and complex. A study of 173 patients with various types of GI cancer showed that 36% were hypometabolic, 22% were hypermetabolic, and 42% had normal resting energy expenditure (30). These findings were not explained by differences in tumor burden, nutritional status, or duration of disease. Tumor type, however, was predictive; patients with gastric, pancreatic, and biliary cancer were the most hypermetabolic. In a study of 104 patients with gastric or colon cancer and 47 patients with non–small cell lung cancer, indirect calorimetry detected an increase in resting energy expenditure in the patients with lung cancer but not in those with gastric or colon cancer (31). This same study showed that the resting energy expenditure returned to normal after curative resection of lung cancer, a finding indicating that the increase in energy expenditure was tumor driven. Among patients with hematologic malignancies, the effect on energy expenditure is also variable and is best predicted by tumor type. In general, patients with leukemia are more likely than patients with lymphoma to experience increased energy expenditure (32). The exact contribution of the increase in energy expenditure to weight loss in patients with cancer cannot be quantified at the present time; however, in some patients, such as those with small cell lung cancer, it may be substantial.

Carbohydrate Metabolism

Glucose intolerance has been frequently noted in patients with cancer (33, 34). Contributors to glucose intolerance and hyperglycemia include increased endogenous glucose production, increased resistance to both exogenous and endogenous insulin, and perhaps inadequate insulin release. There may be other nonspecific factors such as weight loss, bed rest, and sepsis that cause similar changes in other diseases (35). The alterations in glucose metabolism seen in patients with cancer are in sharp contrast to the compensatory alterations seen in patients with uncomplicated starvation. In simple starvation, weight loss is associated with a reduction in glucose turnover, whereas in patients with cancer, weight loss is accompanied by increased glucose turnover (36). Rates of glucose and urea turnover and glucose oxidation have been determined in normal volunteers, in a group of patients with early GI (i.e., colon) cancer, and in those with advanced GI (i.e., esophagus, stomach, and pancreas) cancer (37). Basal rates of glucose turnover were similar in the normal and early cancer groups but were significantly higher in the advanced cancer group. The glucose oxidation rate increased progressively in proportion to tumor burden (23.9% for controls, 32.8% for early tumors, and 43.0% for advanced tumors).

After curative resection in the early tumor groups, glucose use decreased significantly (37). In those with early and advanced GI cancer, glucose infusion only partially suppressed glucose production by 76 and 69%, respectively, whereas in normal volunteers, glucose production was almost completely suppressed (94%) (37). This phenomenon contributes to the difficulty in achieving weight gain in patients with active cancer even when adequate calories are supplied.

An increase in wasteful metabolic cycles such as the Cori cycle contributes to altered glucose metabolism in patients with cancer. In the Cori cycle, lactate formed by glucose oxidation in muscle and red blood cells is transported to the kidney and liver, where it is reconverted to glucose. There is a net loss of four high-energy phosphate bonds for each passage though the Cori cycle. If anaerobic glycolysis by tumor cells with the release of lactate is substantial, then a large amount of energy would be wasted in this futile cycle. Initial studies noted increased Cori cycle activity in patients with metastatic disease and weight loss but not in patients with cancer and stable weight (38). More recent data show that an increase in the Cori cycle has only a minor role in alterations of glucose metabolism (39); however, other futile cycles have been identified.

Protein Metabolism

In simple starvation, protein catabolism slowly decreases to preserve lean body mass. This adaptive process is frequently lost in patients with cancer and weight loss. The rates of whole-body protein turnover and the synthetic and the catabolic rates of muscle protein increase with advancing stage of disease and degree of weight loss (40, 41).

The increased protein turnover has been shown to result from increased hepatic protein synthesis, increased muscle protein degradation, and impaired protein synthesis (42, 43). These derangements are not reversed by the administration of parenteral nutrition (44), thereby limiting the efficacy of total parenteral nutrition (TPN) in malnourished patients with active malignancies. Organ imaging in a small sample size of patients with cancer cachexia indicated that liver size is generally spared, presumably as the result of transfer of nitrogen to the liver (45). Patients with cancer and significant weight loss have decreased lean body muscle mass, although the percentage of nonmuscle lean body mass (i.e., visceral protein) rises markedly (46).

At least three distinct pathways are involved in the increased proteolysis seen in patients with cancer. One pathway is lysosomal energy-dependent proteolysis, another involves calcium-dependent proteases, and the third is the ubiquitin-proteasome dependent pathway (47). The ubiquitin-associated pathway is the predominant mechanism of muscle protein loss in cancer (48). In this pathway, polyubiquitin chains are attached to proteins that are then recognized and degraded by a proteasome complex. This pathway is regulated, in part, by proteolysis-inducing factor,

a 24-kDa glycoprotein produced by tumors (49) (see later). Effective treatment of the underlying cancer has been shown to reverse ubiquitin-dependent proteolysis of skeletal muscle (50). In a murine model of colon cancer within 11 days of eradication of tumors with cystemustine, rates of ubiquitin-dependent proteolysis decreased below basal levels observed in healthy control mice (50). Better understanding of this process holds the promise of improving therapy to attenuate the loss of protein seen in patients with cancer (51). Already, agents such as pentoxifylline (52), torbafylline (53), and eicosapentaenoic acid (EPA) (54) have been shown to attenuate muscle loss via downregulation of the ubiquitin-proteasome pathway in animal models of cancer cachexia.

Lipid Metabolism

Depletion of adipose tissue and lipid stores is commonly seen in patients with cancer who have lost weight. Anorexia and impaired nutrient intake contribute to this loss of fat; however, an imbalance between lipogenesis and lipolysis has been suggested (7). Decreased lipogenesis has not been well described. However, several causes of increased lipolysis have been proposed, including decreased food intake, stress response to illness with adrenal medullary stimulation and increased circulating catecholamine levels, insulin resistance, and release of lipolytic factors produced by the tumor itself or by myeloid tissue cells (55). One such factor has been well characterized (56). Lipid-mobilizing factor (LMF), a 24-kDa glycoprotein produced by tumors, has been shown to stimulate increased lipid mobilization from adipocytes (57) (see later).

Mediators of Altered Metabolism

Various mediators including glycoproteins, proinflammatory cytokines, and neuropeptides have been implicated in the widespread metabolic derangements described earlier.

Glycoproteins. Recently, two glycoproteins, proteolysis-inducing factor and LMF, have been found to be important mediators of the cachexia seen in a wide variety of cancers, particularly pancreatic cancer, but also ovarian, lung, colorectal, and breast cancer (58).

Proteolysis-Inducing Factor. Proteolysis-inducing factor, a 24-kDa glycoprotein, is produced by human tumors, and its expression directly correlates with the severity of weight loss experienced by patients with cancer (59). In animal models, infusion of proteolysis-inducing factor leads to loss of body weight and skeletal muscle along with increased expression of key components of the adenosine triphosphate-ubiquitin–dependent proteolytic pathway (60). This finding suggests that the primary effect of proteolysis-inducing factor is increased proteolysis and cachexia by upregulation of the ubiquitin-proteasome dependent pathway of proteolysis (49). However, proteolysis-inducing factor has several other actions that may also result in cancer cachexia. For example, it increases expression of proinflammatory cytokines, including interleukin-6 (IL-6), which are independently associated with cancer cachexia (61). In addition, it induces shedding of syndecans (a group of transmembrane proteoglycans), and this results in impaired wound repair and increased metastasis (61). One of the mechanisms by which EPA affects cancer cachexia is via downregulation of proteolysis-inducing factor and subsequent decrease in the ubiquitin-proteasome dependent pathway of proteolysis (54).

Lipid Mobilizing Factor. LMF, a glycoprotein produced by a variety of tumors, leads to increased lipolysis and glucose oxidation (62). LMF has recently been shown to be identical to the plasma protein zinc-α_2-glycoprotein (63). It is thought to act through binding of β-adrenergic receptors and subsequent upregulation of mitochondrial uncoupling proteins (64, 65). Animal studies demonstrated that LMF causes loss of body weight (specifically a loss of body fat) independent of caloric food intake (66). The activity of LMF in the urine and serum of patients with cancer has been shown to correlate with the degree of weight loss (67) and tumor burden (68). In addition to its effect on lipid metabolism, preliminary evidence indicates that LMF may protect tumor cells from free radical toxicity and may therefore make tumors less responsive to certain chemotherapeutic agents that induce oxidative damage (69).

Proinflammatory Cytokines. Proinflammatory cytokines are protein molecules synthesized and released by peripheral lymphocytes and monocytes as well as by neurons and glial cells within the central nervous system. Production and release of a specific cytokine is often regulated by levels of other cytokines (i.e., a cytokine cascade); therefore, the metabolic effect of a single cytokine is often difficult to distinguish from the effect of others.

Tumor Necrosis Factor-α. Tumor necrosis factor-α (TNF-α) was first isolated in 1975 (70) and was found to be involved in cancer mediated cachexia in a rabbit model in 1985 (71). Since that time, data from animal studies confirmed that TNF-α is a significant mediator of cachexia (72, 73). In one study (73), infusion of TNF-α in rats produced weight loss, net nitrogen loss, and skeletal muscle catabolism. Blockade of TNF-α with neutralizing antibodies has been shown to increase food intake and fat mass in tumor-bearing mice (74). Similarly, knockout mice lacking a TNF receptor experience less protein degradation when they are implanted with a tumor (75). Data from human studies are less consistent. Infusion of TNF-α into physiologically normal subjects for 4 weeks did not modify resting energy expenditure, body weight, serum TNF-α, or common laboratory nutritional markers (76). No significant elevations of serum TNF-α were found in patients with solid tumors without sepsis (77). In contrast, TNF-α levels can be very high in the serum of patients with leukemias (78, 79), and these levels become undetectable levels in patients with complete remission (79). Similarly, recent data show that transcription of TNF-α mRNA is increased in patients with pancreatic cancer and falls after tumor resection (80).

Failure to observe elevated serum TNF-α levels does not necessarily signify that TNF-α is not involved in cancer-induced cachexia. Increased production of TNF-α by peripheral mononuclear blood cells was found in patients with pancreatic cancer, although serum TNF-α was not present (77). Additionally, increased soluble TNF-α has been detected in hypermetabolic patients with lung cancer (81). These data suggest that local activity at the production site, without first circulating through the blood, may be important in the development of the hypercatabolic state.

Interleukin-6. IL-6 is involved in many processes including inflammation, response to infection, hematopiesis, and liver and neuronal regeneration (82). Its role in cancer-induced cachexia has been well established in animal models (83, 84). Levels of IL-6 correlate with degree of cachexia and fall with tumor resection. Furthermore, blockade of the effects of IL-6 with monoclonal antibodies (83) or by gene knockout (85) suppressed the development of cancer cachexia in a murine model.

Studies in humans have shown higher IL-6 levels in patients with cancer than in healthy persons. Lymph node involvement and overtly metastatic disease are associated with further elevation of serum IL-6 levels (86, 87). Elevated serum IL-6 has been related to weight loss in patients with a variety of cancers, including those with cancer of the lung (81, 88), prostate (89), and colon (90). In patients with esophageal cancer, the degree of weight loss, tumor size, and tumor invasion correlate with IL-6 levels (91). In a small study of 11 patients with human immunodeficiency virus infection and lymphoma, blockade of IL-6 with a monoclonal antibody led to a clear improvement of cachexia (92). The rise in IL-6 levels seen in patients with cancer-induced cachexia is not always related to an acute-phase response and may be seen independently (77).

Interleukin-1. Expression of IL-1 is upregulated in tumor-bearing mice and correlates with clinical manifestations of cancer, including cachexia (93). Infusion of IL-1 in animals leads to anorexia, weight loss, loss of peripheral proteins stores, and alterations in glucose metabolism similar to those seen in human patients with cancer-induced cachexia (73, 94). Selective blockade of the IL-1 receptor decreases tumor-induced cachexia without decreasing tumor burden, a finding suggesting direct involvement of IL-1 in cancer cachexia.

Studies in humans have been less consistent. Levels of IL-1 have been shown to be elevated in some (95), but not all, cancers (96). However, a study in patients with pancreatic cancer showed that a genetic polymorphism of the IL-1 gene is associated with increased IL-1 production, a greater acute-phase response, and significantly shorter survival (97).

Interferon-γ. Interferon-γ (IFN-γ) is often sited as a mediator of cancer cachexia. It has been shown to play a prominent role in some animal models of cancer cachexia

(98, 99), and treatment with monoclonal antibodies directed against IFN-γ can prevent or reverse the wasting seen in these models (100). However, data in human studies are inconsistent; some studies show increased IFN-γ levels in patients with cancer (101), whereas others show decreased levels (102).

Neuropeptides. The central nervous system is one of the most important targets (either directly or via second messengers) of the cytokines outlined earlier. The primary effect of these cytokines is seen in the hypothalamus, where they affect mediators of energy balance such as neuropeptide Y (NPY), corticotropin-releasing factor (CRF), and melanocortins.

Neuropeptide Y. NPY is a 36-amino acid orexigenic (appetite-stimulating) neuropeptide found in the hypothalamus (103). Increased NPY levels in the hypothalamus stimulate feeding and decrease energy expenditure (104). Normally, NPY levels rise in the setting of starvation or increased metabolic demand to restore energy balance (105). However, this homeostatic mechanism is lost in cancer cachexia. In animal models of cancer cachexia, hypothalamic levels of NPY are inappropriately low, and the orexigenic effects of NPY infused into the hypothalamus are markedly diminished (106, 107). IL-1 is one of the key mediators of this phenomenon. Infusion of IL-1 specifically reduces NPY in the hypothalamus (108), and high-levels of NPY can counteract the anorexic effects of IL-1 (105). Data from human studies are very limited; however, in one study of 73 patients with cancer cachexia, circulating NPY levels were found to be significantly lower than in a control population (109).

Corticotropin-Releasing Factor. CRF is a 41-amino acid peptide primarily made in the hypothalamus. Increased levels of CRF lead to anorexia, lipolysis, and weight loss in part via an inhibition of the effects of NPY (110, 111). CRF also interacts with IL-1. IL-1 stimulates CRF production, and blockade of CRF with anti-CRF antibodies attenuates the cachetic effects of IL-1 (112). In a rat model of sarcoma, inappropriately high levels of CRF were detected in tumor-bearing animals with anorexia (113).

Melanocortins. Melanocortins such as α-melanocyte–stimulating hormone (α-MSH) bind to the type 4 melanocortin receptor (MC4-R) in the hypothalamus and inhibit appetite. Animal models have demonstrated that blockade of this binding will attenuate weight loss in tumor-bearing animals (114). The mechanism by which tumors lead to increased α-MSH activity is unclear; however, the proinflammatory cytokines reviewed in this section likely play a role (115).

Impaired Caloric Intake, Maldigestion, and Malabsorption

Impaired caloric intake is the most significant cause of malnutrition among patients with cancer (7, 116). Changes in taste and appetite, learned food aversions, depression, and disturbances of the GI tract frequently prevent ingestion of adequate calories by patients with cancer. In a prospective study (117), approximately one half of the most common and most distressing symptoms in patients with advanced cancers were GI symptoms, including early satiety (71%), taste change (60%), and anorexia (56%). GI symptoms are also very prevalent early in the course of the disease in patients who are otherwise functional. Grosvenor and colleagues reported on 254 patients with varied malignancies and favorable performance status (ECOG level 0–2) and found symptoms of abdominal fullness, taste change, and constipation in more than 40% (118).

Changes of Taste and Appetite

The proinflammatory cytokines and neuropeptides outlined earlier contribute to diminished appetite among patients with cancer. Unpleasant alterations of taste and smell compound this anorexia and further limit caloric intake. An early study noted that 25 of 50 patients with metastatic carcinoma from various primary sites stated that food did not taste good (119). This change was associated with an elevated taste threshold for sweetness (i.e., food tasted less sweet) and a lowered taste threshold for bitterness (119). Subsequent articles challenged the concept of a consistent pattern of altered taste (120, 121), and others found no abnormalities (122, 123).

Treatment-related alterations in taste are very common and have been reviewed (124). Chemotherapeutic agents including cisplatin, carboplatin, cyclophosphamide, doxorubicin, 5-fluorouracil, levamisole, and methotrexate have been linked to adverse changes in taste (125). These changes may persist for months after completion of therapy (125, 126). Radiation therapy, especially to the head and neck, is also associated with significant changes in taste, some of which may never recover (127, 128). Finally, almost one half of all patients undergoing resection of a gastric or esophageal cancer were found to suffer a postoperative taste deficit that could last for up to 1 year (129).

When cancer- and treatment-related changes in taste of foods cause rejection of nutritious foods, they contribute to anorexia and decreased intake. Hospitalized patients with cancer may have a further reduction in oral intake because of limitations of meal delivery systems. In a traditional meal delivery system, meal trays are delivered three times a day. If patients are absent from the hospital room or if their symptoms are particularly severe at the time of meal delivery, they may miss an entire meal. Innovative programs of a "room service" style of meal delivery in which a patient can obtain a meal delivered at any time have been shown to increase meal consumption and patient satisfaction (130, 131). Studies to determine whether this type of program also leads to improved caloric intake are currently under way.

Learned Food Aversions

Patients who receive chemotherapy or radiation therapy for cancer may develop aversions to dietary items that were consumed at the time of treatment (132, 133). In a classic study by Bernstein and colleagues (134), children who were given emetogenic chemotherapy were tested for a learned food aversion. The test group was offered an unusual flavor of ice cream shortly before chemotherapy administration, whereas controls were given ice cream, but not this flavor. When tested later for aversions to the unusually flavored ice cream, controls chose it three times more frequently than did the experimental group. Similar findings have been reported in adults (135). The risk of developing a learned food aversion is directly related to the emetogenic potential of the therapy. Nausea is the only treatment-related side effect associated with learned food aversions (136).

The mechanism of learned food aversions experienced by patients with cancer has not been well described. However, it is most likely similar to other conditioned food preferences and aversions, which are discussed in Chapter 45, with reference to neural pathways.

Several management strategies can be effective in prevention of learned food aversions. One such strategy involves the use of an alternative target (e.g., an odor) for aversion formation to prevent aversion to a dietary item. In a study of 209 patients undergoing chemotherapy or radiation therapy, exposure to an alternative or "scapegoat" stimulus before treatment resulted in a significant reduction in development of aversions to dietary items (137). Hypnosis (138) has also been shown to be effective in the management of learned food aversions. Finally, newer antiemetic medications have greatly reduced the nausea and vomiting associated with anticancer therapy, including anticipatory nausea and vomiting, and therefore should greatly decrease the risk of developing a learned food aversion (139).

Depression

Major depression develops in approximately 25% of patients with cancer (140). The mechanism is likely a combination of the cognitive stressors of being diagnosed with a malignancy and neurohumoral changes induced by the tumor (141). Regardless of the mechanism, depression is associated with impaired oral intake and malnutrition among patients with cancer (142–144). Evaluation for and treatment of depression should be incorporated in the management of patients with cancer and malnutrition.

Disturbances of the Gastrointestinal Tract

Localized effects of various neoplasms or complications from treatment may lead to nutritional problems caused by the direct effects on the GI tract. Intestinal obstruction, dysmotility, malabsorption, and primary cancers of the intestine can all lead to significant malnutrition.

Intestinal Obstruction. The most common direct effect of alimentary tract neoplasms on nutritional status relates to partial or complete obstruction at one or more sites. Approximately 15% of surgical hospital admissions for acute abdominal pain are associated with intestinal obstruction (145). Malignancy is the second most common cause of obstruction, accounting for 26% of all cases in adults (146). Esophageal, gastric, colonic, and pancreatic cancers frequently lead to direct mechanical obstruction by the primary tumor. However, peritoneal seeding by any tumor may lead to intestinal dysfunction without frank mechanical obstruction. This is especially common in gynecologic malignancies. Up to 42% of patients with ovarian cancer will develop intestinal obstruction during the course of their illness (147). Acute obstruction almost always leads to immediate medical attention. However, neoplasms may obstruct more slowly and progressively, causing an ongoing decrease in food intake and weight loss. Many patients wait until one or more of their symptoms and signs (anorexia, dysphagia, weight loss, weakness, nausea, vomiting, pain, or diarrhea) cause them to seek medical care. In addition, recurrent bouts of obstruction are very common and occur in most patients who experience a bowel obstruction caused by cancer (148). Options for the management of malignant bowel obstruction have been recently reviewed (149).

Intestinal Dysmotility. Altered intestinal motility in patients with cancer may have many causes (150). Tumors can induce an immune-mediated destruction of components of the enteric nerve plexus resulting in a paraneoplastic syndrome of gastroparesis and intestinal pseudoobstruction (151–153). Tumor resections are often associated with prolonged postoperative ileus (154). Radiation therapy can cause acute and chronic alteration in GI motility. Finally, chemotherapeutic agents (155) and other medications (especially narcotics) that are frequently used by patients with cancer have adverse effects on GI motility. Any significant disruption of intestinal motility can impair caloric intake, and the severity of dysmotility is directly related to the degree of malnutrition (156).

Malabsorption. Although malabsorption will not directly limit caloric intake, it will greatly reduce the utilization of ingested nutrients and can result in malnutrition. Patients with cancer may experience malabsorption for a variety of reasons. Investigators initially suggested that malignant tumors external to the GI tract induced abnormal intestinal mucosa with resultant malabsorption (157). Later studies showed similar changes (abnormal mucosal structure, epithelial cell loss, and decreased xylose absorption) in the intestinal mucosa of patients with severe malnutrition but without cancer, a finding suggesting that the changes are caused by malnutrition in addition to direct effect of the tumor (158). Anticancer treatments such as chemotherapy, radiation therapy, and surgery can directly induce malabsorption. In a recent review of patients with TPN dependence resulting from radiation enteritis, malabsorption was the primary cause for intestinal failure in approximately 10% of the cases (159). Diarrhea induced by 5-fluorouracil is associated with malabsorption as measured by impaired D-xylose absorption (160). Finally, even a limited bowel resection such as that done to create an ileal neobladder in patients with bladder cancer is associated with a decrease in D-xylose absorption (161).

Small bowel bacterial overgrowth may also contribute to malabsorption in patients with cancer. Typically, this occurs in the setting of anatomic abnormalities such as strictures, surgically created blind loops, loss of the ileocecal valve (allowing bacteria to migrate from the colon into the small bowel), fistulas, or loss of the protective barrier provided by gastric acid (as seen following total gastrectomy). Anaerobic bacteria can then colonize the small intestine, where they deconjugate bile salts, metabolize nutrients, and damage enterocytes leading to maldigestion and malabsorption. In some series, evidence of bacterial overgrowth can be detected in up to 90% of patients following gastrectomy when measured using a glucose breath test (162).

Exocrine pancreatic insufficiency is commonly encountered after pancreatic resections and can result in maldigestion and malabsorption (163). Many of these patients have recurrent disease and associated cachexia. However, even those who are cured of their cancer may have chronic pancreatic insufficiency. In one series, 16 of 17 long-term survivors (median follow-up, 32 months) had evidence of exocrine pancreatic insufficiency after removal of pancreatic tumors (164). Even among patients who are able to regain weight after pancreatic resection, 36% show significant pancreatic insufficiency as measured by fecal chymotrypsin levels (165). Other malignant conditions such as lymphoma (166) and gastric cancer (167) have also been associated with pancreatic insufficiency. Rarely, radiation therapy can induce pancreatic insufficiency (168).

Fistulas resulting in bypass of a significant portion of bowel can result in malabsorption. The degree of malabsorption depends on the site and extent of the bypass. Severe malabsorption occurs with fistulas between stomach and large bowel (gastrocolic), between small bowel and large bowel (enterocolic), between small bowel and small bowel (enteroenteric), and from small bowel to skin (enterocutaneous). Fistulas may result from direct tumor invasion or from therapy such as surgery or radiation. Up to 85% of fistulas occur in the postoperative setting, most commonly after a cancer operation (169). Cancer, chemotherapy, and radiation all reduce the likelihood of spontaneous closure (169). Nutritional management of patients with a fistula must be individualized and must address ongoing losses of fluid and nutrients from the fistula (170).

Malabsorption caused by protein-losing enteropathy is associated with a variety of malignancies including gastric cancer (171), lymphoma (172), and melanoma (173). It is also a rare complication of chemotherapy and radiation therapy (174). Pathologically, it is characterized by infiltration of the lamina propria of the small intestine with tumor cells, with subsequent obstruction and dilation of the lymphatics within the intestinal villi. Clinically, this manifests as hypoalbuminemia, hypoglobulinemia, and lymphopenia, which may reverse with treatment of the underlying condition.

Malignancies of the Small Bowel. Primary malignancies of the small bowel are uncommon and account for fewer than 2% of all GI tract cancers (175). They may be associated with pain, bleeding, weight loss, and partial obstruction. Diarrhea and steatorrhea are especially common with lymphomas of the small intestine. Diagnosis is often delayed. In one large series, mean time from presentation to diagnosis was 7 months (176). Several diseases are associated with malabsorption and an increased risk of small bowel cancer. Celiac sprue, with its associated villous atrophy and inflammation, is linked to increased rates of several malignancies, including intestinal lymphomas and adenocarcinomas (177) (see Chapter 77). Immunoproliferative small intestinal disease (also know as α-heavy chain disease and Mediterranean lymphoma), an endemic disease in the parts of the Mediterranean basin and North Africa, presents with chronic diarrhea and malabsorption and can progress to frank lymphoma (178). Crohn's disease is associated with increased rates of small bowel adenocarcinoma (179).

NUTRITIONAL THERAPIES

Four types of nutritional therapies are used: oral dietary therapy, enteral nutrition, parenteral nutrition, and pharmacotherapy aimed at improving appetite and food intake. Depending on the patient's condition, nutritional support in the patient with cancer has two distinct objectives: (a) provision of nutrition during anticancer therapies to counteract their nutritionally related side effects and to improve outcome following these therapies and (b) support in patients with long-term or permanent severe impairment of the GI tract. In these patients, nutritional support may be required indefinitely. Results of numerous clinical trials support the use of specialized nutritional support only in limited situations during anticancer therapies. In the group with prolonged GI failure, nutrition support may be a lifesaving therapy because patients could die of adverse effects of starvation without specialized nutrition support.

Oral Dietary Therapy

Patients who are able to eat but who have impairment of the GI tract or special metabolic requirements may benefit from specialized oral dietary therapy (180). Often, this may obviate the need for more costly and complex interventions such as parenteral nutrition. In oral dietary therapy, the regular diet is modified based on the pathophysiologic changes induced by the underlying disorder, with the goal of providing optimal nutrition. For example, patients who have had a gastrectomy should be placed on a diet composed of small, frequent meals containing foods high in calories. Simple carbohydrates and insoluble fiber should be limited. This will limit symptoms of dumping syndrome, which is frequently encountered after gastrectomy (see later). Patients with cancer of the head and neck and resulting dysphagia should be evaluated by a therapist specializing in swallowing. Often, the dysphagia is not complete, and foods of certain consistencies may be safely ingested. For example, following partial glossectomy, puddings and pureed foods can often be safely swallowed, whereas thin liquids are associated with an increased frequency of aspiration. Once it has been determined what consistency of foods a patient can safely swallow, a dietitian can develop a meal plan that will provide adequate nutrition.

When the main problem is inadequate food consumption, various commercial oral supplements can be used, but usually for only short periods because of taste fatigue. Some preparations provide complete nutrition, whereas others are intended to supplement deficits of specific nutrients (see Chapter 98). Problems common in patients with cancer such as partial small bowel obstruction, chronic radiation enteritis, and short bowel syndrome may all be amenable to dietary therapies. In partial small bowel obstruction or motility dysfunction, a diet composed of frequent, small, calorically dense meals with minimal amounts of fiber is indicated. Patients with radiation enteritis should receive a low-fiber and lactose-free diet. Dietary management of patients with short bowel syndrome includes frequent small meals, limitation of fiber, lactose, and simple sugars, taking liquids separately from meals, and supplementation of calcium and zinc orally, as well as magnesium and vitamin B_{12} (see Chapter 75).

Bye and colleagues (181) conducted a prospective, randomized trial of a low-fat, low-lactose diet in 143 patients undergoing radiation therapy. The intervention group had significantly less diarrhea. Diarrhea in the control group correlated with increased fatigue and decreased physical function. The authors concluded that dietary intervention during radiotherapy reduced the severity of diarrhea, influenced the patients' ability to cope with diarrhea, and gave these patients more control over their situation.

The successful implementation of prescribed diets depends to a large extent on a dietitian's converting the prescribed diet to a meal plan and working with the patient to implement it. In a prospective, randomized study of 57 patients undergoing chemotherapy for ovarian, breast, or lung cancer, those who received intensive dietary counseling had improved long-term food intake (182). Similar data have been demonstrated in patients with cancer undergoing surgery (183) and radiotherapy (183, 184), as well as in patients with acute leukemia undergoing induction chemotherapy (185). Although dietary counseling improves caloric intake in patients with active cancer, it may not be sufficient to improve tolerance of chemotherapy, the degree

of toxicity experienced by patients, the frequency of treatment delays, response rates, quality of life, or survival (186, 187).

Enteral Nutrition

Enteral nutrition is a critical therapy for the prevention and treatment of malnutrition associated with cancer (see Chapter 98). Placement of feeding tubes into the stomach or small intestine can overcome some of the most common causes of impaired food intake in patients with cancer. For example, enteral nutrition can provide optimal nutrition to patients with obstructions or defects in the oropharynx, esophagus, stomach, or duodenum. It can also allow patients with a limited absorptive capacity (e.g., short bowel syndrome, radiation enteritis,) to be fed by continuous infusions over 8 to 16 hours a day.

Indications

Although routine use of enteral nutrition may improve laboratory parameters of protein kinetics in patients with cancer (188), no evidence supports the routine use of enteral nutrition in well-nourished patients with cancer undergoing chemotherapy (189) or surgery (190–192). Data from randomized trials examining the efficacy of enteral nutrition given as an adjuvant therapy in patients receiving chemotherapy for a variety of cancers failed to demonstrate a clear benefit in terms of survival or response to treatment (193–197). The validity of the conclusions of these studies, however, is limited by their small size and poor design. Similar difficulties plague the studies examining the role of standard enteral nutrition in the perioperative period (198–200). Although data on early (postoperative day 1) enteral feeding following resection of an upper GI tract tumor showed improved protein metabolism, no evidence indicates that this translates into improved clinical outcome (201). In a prospective randomized study of early enteral feeding in 195 patients after resection of upper GI malignancy, no benefit was noted (202). Complication rates, mortality, and length of hospital stay were not affected by early postoperative enteral feedings (202). Therefore, routine use of enteral nutrition support in patients receiving chemotherapy or undergoing operations for cancer cannot be justified.

In patients undergoing chemoradiation therapy to the head or neck, mucositis that impairs oral intake is almost universal (203). Therefore, routine use of enteral nutrition even among those who are well nourished at the initiation of therapy has been shown to prevent episodes of dehydration and treatment interruptions effectively (204–206) (see the later discussion of nutrition support in patients with cancer of the head and neck). In all other instances, the decision to initiate enteral nutrition must be individualized. In general, enteral nutrition is indicated in any malnourished patient with a functional GI tract who is unable to ingest sufficient nutrients orally as long as enteral access can safely be achieved. Enteral nutrition is preferred over parenteral nutrition (207, 208) because it is more physiologic, simpler, safer (209), and less costly (210).

Enteral Access and Formula

A detailed discussion of access for enteral feeding and of commercially available formulas is presented in Chapter 98. Formulas have been developed for patients with diabetes mellitus, renal insufficiency, pulmonary insufficiency, and hepatic encephalopathy. The efficacy of these formulas has been described (211). Formulas designed to modulate the immune response have been developed and suggested to offer a specific benefit to the patient with cancer. Various nutrients including arginine, glutamine, ω-3 fatty acids, and polyribonucleotides (RNA) have been shown to alter immune response (7). In 1990, Cerra demonstrated that an enteral formula supplemented with these nutrients could alter the outcome of in vitro tests of immune response (212). This finding prompted several clinical trials to evaluate the effect of these formulas on patients with cancer and other diseases. To date, at least 15 prospective, randomized studies evaluating the effect of these formulas on patients with cancer have been performed. Although some studies have shown a decrease in infectious complications (213–215), none have shown a statistically significant survival benefit (216, 217). A metaanalysis of six randomized trials of standard enteral nutrition versus immune-modulating enteral nutrition in patients with cancer yielded similar conclusions (218). This analysis included 487 patients with GI cancer and demonstrated that supplementation with an immune-modulating formula was associated with an approximately 50% reduction in infectious complications and a decreased length of stay; however, no effect on survival was noted.

Home Enteral Nutrition

Home enteral nutrition allows many patients to receive outpatient treatment. In addition, dysphagia caused by cancer or anticancer therapies may persist after eradication of the underlying malignancy. In this setting, home enteral nutrition is often necessary and may be required for prolonged periods. Each year, Medicare pays for home enteral nutrition for approximately 73,000 patients at a cost of over 137 million dollars (219). Cancer, the most common indication for home enteral nutrition, accounts for over 40% of patients (220). Outcome in these patients is dependent on the underlying cancer; however, many of these patients do well. A review of 3931 patients in the North American Registry showed that 30% of patients with cancer were able to resume oral intake and discontinue enteral feeding during the first year, and 36% were alive after 1 year (219). Home enteral nutrition is safe, with a hospitalization rate for complications related to home enteral nutrition of less than 0.4 per patient per year

(219, 221). Quality of life has not been well studied in patients with cancer who are receiving home enteral nutrition. A French study reported on 30 patients with head and neck or esophageal cancer maintained on home enteral nutrition for 28 days (222). These investigators found the tube feedings to be physically well tolerated and associated with an improvement in a global health status/quality-of-life scaled score.

Even in patients who have been dependent on enteral nutrition for more than 1 year, a significant percentage (24% in our series) may be able to resume enough oral intake to obviate the need for further enteral nutrition (221). This finding indicates the need for repeated evaluations to determine whether improvements in swallowing allow the discontinuation of enteral nutrition. For those patients who have a permanent dependence on enteral nutrition support, complete nutrition can be safely provided indefinitely.

Total Parenteral Nutrition

TPN is an effective method for delivery of nutrients directly into the blood and thus overcomes major causes of cancer cachexia, including decreased food intake and dysfunction of the GI tract. Survival for more than 20 years in patients nourished exclusively by TPN clearly demonstrates the lifesaving role of this method of nutritional support. Initially, it seemed logical that TPN would be an effective adjuvant therapy for most patients with cancer undergoing radiation therapy, surgery, or chemotherapy because of the accompanying cachexia and inability to eat adequately. In addition, TPN may have a stimulatory effect on tumor cell-cycle kinetics (223, 224). It was hoped that this effect would induce improved tumor response to cell-cycle–specific chemotherapy. However, proof of such benefits remains elusive. Randomized studies have shown that TPN benefits only a select subgroup of patients with cancer during anticancer therapy.

Total Parenteral Nutrition During Cancer Therapy

In patients receiving chemotherapy with or without radiation, TPN can lead to improvements of several nutritional parameters. Both body weight and body fat increase (225). Deficits of specific vitamins, minerals, and trace elements can be corrected, and hydration status can be improved (225, 226). TPN, however, does not alter many of the metabolic derangements encountered in the patient with cancer. Increased glucose oxidation and turnover persist (227), as do muscle proteolysis (228, 229) and increased lipolysis (230). Finally, TPN is does not stop the overall losses of body nitrogen (231). The relevant issue for the clinician is the effect of TPN on the morbidity and mortality associated with cancer therapy and whether TPN can allow more intense anticancer therapy as was initially hoped. Numerous randomized trials have examined these issues. Studies of patients undergoing chemotherapy for carcinoma of the ovary (232), lung (233, 234), colon (235), testes (236), lymphoma (237), and other tumors (238) have been conducted. However, the patients in these studies were largely unselected. Many were not malnourished, and others had adequate oral intake with intact GI function, thus making intravenous nutrition unnecessary and futile. Numerous metaanalyses concluded that nondiscriminatory use of TPN in patients undergoing chemotherapy offers no improvement in mortality, response to chemotherapy, or reduction in treatment-associated complications (239–241). This conclusion was echoed in a joint consensus statement from the National Institutes of Health, the American Society for Parenteral and Enteral Nutrition, and the American Society for Clinical Nutrition (242). The improvement in nutritional parameters afforded by TPN in patients receiving chemotherapy is not necessarily translated into improved clinical outcome. Thus, the routine use of TPN in these patients is not indicated. In some circumstances, however, nutritional support with parenteral nutrition should be considered. These include prevention of the effects of starvation in a patient unable to tolerate oral or enteral feedings for a prolonged period (usually >7–10 days), maximization of performance status in a malnourished patient before chemotherapy or surgery, and use in patients undergoing bone marrow transplantation (see later) (243).

A few randomized studies have examined the use of TPN in patients receiving radiotherapy to the abdomen and pelvis (244–247). Theses studies did not show any clear benefit from the routine administration of TPN.

The role of TPN in the perioperative period has been extensively studied (248–255). In an early study by Mueller and associates (253), a 10-day course of preoperative TPN was associated with nutritional improvement and significant reduction in major postoperative complications and mortality. These impressive results were not confirmed in subsequent studies. At Memorial Sloan-Kettering Cancer Center, a prospective study of 117 patients undergoing curative resection for pancreatic cancer who were randomized to receive TPN or intravenous fluids in the postoperative period showed no benefit from routine use of postoperative TPN (254). The group receiving TPN had a significant increase in postoperative infectious complications. The largest prospective randomized trial investigating the role of TPN in the perioperative setting was the Veterans Administration Cooperative Study (248). In this study, 395 patients with cancer and benign disease were randomized to receive 7 to 15 days preoperative and 3 days postoperative TPN or oral feeding plus intravenous fluids. TPN did not improve morbidity or 90-day mortality. However, subgroup analysis showed that severely malnourished patients had fewer infectious complications when they received TPN. The authors concluded that the routine administration of perioperative TPN should be limited to patients who are severely malnourished unless other specific indications exist. These data and others provided the basis for the joint consensus statement from

the National Institutes of Health, the American Society for Parenteral and Enteral Nutrition, and the American Society for Clinical Nutrition (242) regarding the use of perioperative TPN that states the following: (a) a course of 7 to 10 days of preoperative TPN in a malnourished patient with GI cancer results in a 10% reduction in postoperative complications; (b) routine use of postoperative TPN in malnourished surgical patients who did not receive preoperative TPN results in a 10% *increase* in complications; and (c) if by postoperative day 5 to 10, a patient is unable to tolerate oral or enteral feedings, then TPN is indicated to prevent the adverse effects of starvation. This panel, however, cautioned that in the majority of studies looking at perioperative TPN, the amount and type of parenteral nutrition given were not optimal, and often patients were given excess calories. Therefore, the results may differ with the provision of relatively hypocaloric formulas (242).

Home Total Parenteral Nutrition

Long-term TPN in the home can be a lifesaving treatment in an appropriately selected group of patients. It is clear that patients with cancer who have had severe GI injury, such as massive intestinal resection or severe radiation enteritis, and in whom the cancer has been cured or is well controlled, benefit from long-term TPN at home (256). Survival rates and TPN-related complications in such patients are comparable to those seen in patients with benign diseases (Crohn's disease, intestinal necrosis) who require home TPN. Among patients with widely metastatic disease and poor prognosis, home TPN offers very limited benefit (257). Median survival is only 4 months (258). Recently developed techniques for placing feeding tubes make it possible to hydrate and feed patients enterally, even in the presence of GI obstruction (259), and thus obviate the need for home TPN in patients with upper GI tract dysfunction. In terminally ill patients, TPN should be avoided. The concern that such patients should not be "starved to death" is not a justification for TPN. A noncontrolled study of terminally ill patients with cancer who were hospitalized at a long-term care facility suggested that these patients did not experience hunger or thirst, and in those patients who experienced such symptoms, small amounts of food alleviated the symptoms (260). In such patients, the utilization of TPN either in the home or at health care facilities cannot be justified.

Pharmacotherapy

Agents that will reverse the wasting seen in advanced cancers have long been sought to complement or replace the provision of nutrients via the oral, enteral or parenteral route. Hormones, appetite stimulants, and, most recently, cytokine antagonists have been examined (261, 262) (Table 83.2).

TABLE 83.2. DRUGS WITH POTENTIAL NUTRITIONAL IMPACT

CLASS OF AGENT	EXAMPLE	EFFICACY	ADVERSE EFFECTS
Hormones	Insulin, growth hormone	Attenuation of tumor-induced weight loss, *no* improvement in quality of life or survival	Hypoglycemia, hypokalemia
	Ghrelin	Increased appetite and caloric intake	Promotion of tumor growth
	Melatonin	Less weight loss and improved survival in uncontrolled studies	Headache, insomnia (rare)
Appetite stimulants	Anabolic steroids (norandrolone propionate)	Transient appetite improvement, weight gain (primarily fluid)	Negative nitrogen balance, calcium loss, hyperglycemia, immunosuppression
	Megestrol acetate	Improved appetite, attenuated weight loss, improved quality of life	Hyperglycemia, fluid retention, adrenal insufficiency, deep venous thrombosis
	Dronabinol	Improved appetite, weight gain	Dizziness, confusion, ataxia
	Cyproheptadine	Improved appetite	Blurred vision, dry mouth, nausea
	Hydrazine sulfate	Increased caloric intake in some studies	Rare hepatorenal failure
Cytokine inhibitors	Monoclonal antibodies (anti-TNF) Suramin	Improved caloric intake, preservation of protein stores in animal models	Clinical trials lacking
	Thalidomide	Weight gain and increased lean body mass	Somnolence, headache
	Pentoxifylline	Inhibition of TNF-α, no significant weight gain	Dizziness, headache, dyspepsia, nausea
	Eicosapentaenoic acid	Attenuation of weight loss, improved appetite, in uncontrolled studies	Fishy aftertaste, loose stools, nausea
Drugs to relieve symptoms	Antiemetics	Control of chemotherapy-induced nausea, possible prevention of learned food aversions	Somnolence, diarrhea
	Antidepressants	Improved anorexia, possible weight gain	Headache, insomnia

TNF, tumor necrosis factor.

Hormones

Studies of growth hormone (263–265), insulin-like growth factor-I alone (165), or insulin-like growth factor-I with insulin (266) in cancer-bearing rodent models showed significant attenuation of tumor-induced weight loss. In clinical trials, these agents provided modest gain in weight but no other benefits and no improvement in quality of life (267).

Ghrelin, a potent orexigenic peptide hormone produced by the stomach, has been shown to increase appetite and caloric intake in physiologically normal persons (268) and in animal models of cancer cachexia (269). Therefore, it was hoped that this could be an effective treatment for cancer-induced cachexia; however, its use will likely be limited by its promotion of cellular proliferation and invasion of certain types of cancer (270).

Melatonin, the major product of the pineal gland, has been reported to have a variety of anticancer and anticachectic effects (271), possibly mediated by inhibition of TNF production (272, 273). It is available in an oral preparation and has been suggested as a possible therapy for cachexia. In a prospective randomized study of 100 patients with untreatable solid tumors, those who received melatonin (20 mg/day orally) had less weight loss than those who received just supportive care (273). In a follow-up study

performed by the same researchers, 1440 patients with advanced, untreatable cancer were randomized to supportive care or supportive care plus melatonin 20 mg/day. The investigators found significantly less cachexia and significantly greater 1-year survival among patients treated with melatonin (271). These studies were not placebo controlled, and further study is needed before the routine use of melatonin can be recommended.

Appetite Stimulants

Anabolic steroids have no proven efficacy in treating cancer cachexia. In a murine model, administration of norandrolone propionate resulted in weight gain, but this was largely the result of fluid retention (274). In human trials, steroids such as dexamethasone produced transient improvement of nutritional parameters and appetite, but continued use is associated with negative nitrogen balance, net calcium loss, glucose intolerance, and immunosuppression (267). Megestrol acetate and medroxyprogesterone acetate are progestational agents that have been shown to improve appetite and ameliorate weight loss in numerous, but not all, studies of patients with cancer and cachexia (267, 275). Doses in these studies ranged from 160 to 1280 mg/day, and maximal weight gain was generally seen within

8 weeks. The change in weight is largely the result of increased adipose tissue and edema (276). Nevertheless, improvement in quality of life has consistently been demonstrated in several large prospective studies in patients with cancer cachexia treated with megestrol acetate (277–279). It is generally well tolerated and has fewer side effects than dexamethasone (280), but it can exacerbate underlying diabetes mellitus and rarely leads to adrenal suppression (281). It may also be associated with a small increase in the risk of deep venous thrombosis (282). The mechanism of action is not well defined; however, preliminary data indicate that its effect is mediated, in part, via alterations in IL-6 levels (283, 284). A large prospective study directly compared a progestational agent (megestrol acetate), a corticosteroid (dexamethasone), and an anabolic corticosteroid (fluoxymesterone) for the treatment of cancer anorexia/cachexia (285). The results showed that fluoxymesterone was less effective and more toxic than either megestrol acetate or dexamethasone. Megestrol acetate and dexamethasone had similar appetite-stimulating efficacy but differed in toxicity; dexamethasone caused more corticosteroid-type toxicity, whereas megestrol acetate had a higher rate of deep venous thrombosis.

Dronabinol, a marijuana derivative, improved appetite and caused weight gain in small studies (267). A recent large randomized trial of 469 patients with advanced cancer and cachexia compared dronabinol with megestrol acetate (286). A greater percentage of megestrol acetate– treated patients reported appetite improvement and weight gain compared with dronabinol-treated patients. Combination therapy with both agents was not superior to treatment with megestrol acetate alone. Adverse effects include dizziness, ataxia, and confusion. The mechanism of action of dronabinol is not known, but discovery of two cannabinoid receptors, CB1 and CB2, in neuronal and immune cells may lead to better understanding and use of dronabinol in the therapy of cancer (287). US Food and Drug Administration approval is currently limited to treatment of nausea and vomiting during chemotherapy and for cachexia in patients with human immunodeficiency virus infection.

Cyproheptadine is a potent antihistamine and serotonin antagonist that competes with histamine for H_1-receptor sites on effector cells in the GI tract, blood vessels, and respiratory tract. It has been shown to increase appetite among patients with anorexia nervosa (288) and wasting resulting from tuberculosis (289). In a prospective, randomized, placebo-controlled trial involving 295 patients with advanced cancer, cyproheptadine, at a dose of 8 mg orally three times a day, resulted in a small, subjective improvement in appetite but could not prevent weight loss (290). However, in patients with diarrhea and weight loss resulting from the carcinoid syndrome, cyproheptadine can result in significant weight gain (291). The cause is most likely a direct blockade of the excess serotonin and histamine produced by the tumor.

Hydrazine sulfate inhibits gluconeogenesis and has been studied as an adjuvant therapy for cancer for several decades. A prospective, placebo-controlled trial of hydrazine sulfate in 65 patients with advanced non–small cell lung cancer showed that hydrazine sulfate, at a dose of 60 mg orally three times a day, was associated with significantly greater caloric intake and serum albumin maintenance (292). However, several subsequent larger studies failed to show any benefit (293–295). Therefore, hydrazine sulfate cannot be recommend for the treatment of cancer cachexia outside of research protocols.

Cytokine Inhibitors

Inhibitors of cytokines involved in cancer cachexia and anorexia have the potential to be potent agents in the treatment of malnutrition in cancer. Monoclonal antibodies against TNF lead to improved food intake and diminished loss of protein and fat in murine models of cancer cachexia (296). Similar data are available for anti–IL-6 (297, 298) and anti–IFN-γ (299). Suramin, a direct IL-6 receptor antagonist, decreased several key parameters of cachexia in tumor-bearing mice (300). A study from Japan of a novel inhibitor of IL-1 and TNF-α showed that direct injection of the drug into tumor did not alter tumor growth but did result in attenuation of loss of body weight and epididymal fat in tumor-bearing mice (301).

Human studies using the anticytokine approach are more limited. Thalidomide has been shown to inhibit TNF-α and to have various other antineoplastic effects (302). It also has demonstrated utility in the prevention of weight loss associated with acquired immunodeficiency syndrome and tuberculosis (303, 304). Taken together, these data make thalidomide a potentially useful agent for cancer cachexia. A recent small, open-label study in patients with cachexia resulting from advanced esophageal cancer demonstrated that a 2-week course of thalidomide was associated with a gain of weight and lean body mass (305). Larger studies are currently under way.

Pentoxifylline is an orally available methylxanthine derivative used in the treatment of peripheral vascular disease. It has been shown to inhibit production of TNF-α in patients with cancer (306). However, a prospective, randomized, double-blind, placebo-controlled trial involving 70 patients with advanced cancer cachexia did not show any improvement in appetite or weight gain (307).

EPA is an α-3 ω fatty acid found in high concentrations in fish oils. Laboratory and clinical studies have shown that EPA has several potential anticachetic effects, including (a) attenuation of protein degradation induced by proteolysis-inducing factor (308), (b) prevention of excess hepatic protein turnover (309), (c) inhibition of IL-6 production (310, 311), and (d) inhibition of tumor-derived LMF (312). Trials examining the clinical efficacy of EPA supplements in the management of cancer cachexia have yielded mixed results. EPA, given at a dose of 6g/day orally for 12 weeks, was able to prevent further weight loss among 26 patients with advanced pancreatic cancer who were losing weight at enrollment (313). A study of 20 patients with advanced pancreatic cancer who were prescribed two cans of a nutritional supplement containing 310 kcal, 16.1 g protein, and 1.09 g EPA per can were able to gain weight, improve appetite, and enhance performance status (314). However, this study did not include a comparison control group. In contrast, a recent prospective, double-blind, placebo controlled trial of a 2-week course of fish oil supplements in 60 patients with cancer cachexia failed to show any benefit in terms of improvement in appetite, tiredness, nausea, well-being, caloric intake, nutritional status, or functional status (315).

Drugs to Relieve Symptoms

The use of medications to relieve cancer or treatment-related symptoms that impair oral intake is an important adjuvant to nutritional support in these patients. For example, optimal antiemetic therapy can now adequately control acute and delayed emesis in 70 to 90% of patients (316). Despite this finding, the incidence of chemotherapy-induced nausea and emesis is underestimated by oncologists and nurses (317). This highlights the importance of a careful history and review of systems when completing a nutritional evaluation of a patient with cancer. Many patients with cancer assume that nausea and vomiting are normal during treatment and do not report it as a problem unless they are specifically asked.

Antidepressant medications should be considered when evaluating a patient with cancer and malnutrition. Depression occurs in 25 to 45% of patients with cancer and can lead to loss of appetite and weight loss (140, 318). Pharmacotherapy for depression using selective serotonin reuptake inhibitors or tricyclic antidepressants is effective in patients with cancer (318). Methylphenidate, a stimulant, has also been shown to be effective for the treatment of cancer-related depression (319). Although the relief of depression may improve appetite, in patients without cancer, selective serotonin reuptake inhibitors and tricyclic antidepressants are associated with weight gain that is independent of the response of the underlying depression (320). Pilot studies suggest that these drugs may also produce weight gain in patients with cancer (321). As for methylphenidate, it is associated with anorexia in patients without cancer; however, in patients with cancer-related depression and anorexia, its use is associated with relief of anorexia (322). Therefore, methylphenidate can be used to treat depression in patients with cancer who have depression and malnutrition.

EFFECT OF NUTRITION SUPPORT ON TUMOR GROWTH

Data from animal studies have led to a concern that nutrition support may enhance tumor growth (323, 324). Investigators have suggested that provision of energy and essential nutrients, as well as the influence of hormones and growth factors that are stimulated in response to nutrition support, may promote tumor growth. Such a finding has not been conclusively demonstrated in humans; however, studies are limited by small sample sizes and difficulty in measurements of tumor growth in vivo (7, 325).

Attempts to modulate tumor growth via nutritional manipulation have had mixed results. The initial approach used TPN to stimulate tumor growth and thereby synchronize a greater percentage of the malignant cells into S phase. It was hoped that the cytotoxic effects of a cell-cycle–specific chemotherapeutic agent such as doxorubicin (Adriamycin) would then be enhanced (326, 327). Limited studies in humans have confirmed that TPN may stimulate a greater percentage of tumor cells to enter S phase (328). However, clinical utility of such a strategy in terms of improved response rates or survival has not been demonstrated. Tumors preferentially use glucose as an energy source. Therefore, attempts to impair tumor growth by altering the source of calories and providing a greater percentage of calories from lipids have been conducted. These have been largely unsuccessful, and no significant effect on tumor growth has been demonstrated (329, 330). A novel approach using parenteral nutrition that has been deprived of methionine combined with 5-flourouracil has been shown to improve response rates and survival in an animal model (331). In a small human study, methionine-depleted TPN enhanced the cytotoxic effects of 5-flourouracil in patients with gastric cancer (332).

Parenteral or enteral supplementation of glutamine has also been investigated as a means to alter tumor growth. The metabolic roles and clinical significance of glutamine and its precursors are discussed in detail in Chapter 35. In 1994, Fahr and colleagues reported that a 3-week course of glutamine supplementation led to a 40% reduction in tumor growth in a rat model (333). This inhibition of tumor growth was accompanied by increased activity of host natural killer T lymphocytes, a finding suggesting that the decrease in tumor growth was the result of greater immune-mediated destruction of malignant cells. Similar results have been demonstrated in other tumor models (334, 335). However, data supporting the clinical utility of glutamine supplementation to slow cancer growth in humans are lacking (336, 337).

NUTRITIONAL MANAGEMENT OF PATIENTS WITH SPECIFIC CANCERS

Reversal of the undesirable clinical, metabolic, and nutritional changes secondary to progressive systemic and localized effects of cancer depends primarily on complete disease eradication or major palliation. As with all chronic wasting diseases, one cannot not and should not expect to induce significant improvement in the nutritional state in a short time. Generally, urgent antineoplastic treatment should not be postponed until nutritional rehabilitation is achieved. In such a situation, vitamin and mineral deficiencies, blood loss, and electrolyte and fluid imbalances can usually be corrected rapidly. Nutritional therapy should be incorporated in the overall treatment program as early as possible.

When surgery, radiation, and chemotherapy are indicated for a malnourished patient, efforts to improve nutritional and metabolic status using specialized nutritional support via the oral, enteral, or parenteral route may help to decrease morbidity and mortality and improve quality of life. The efficacy of such intervention in patients with specific tumors is discussed in the following sections.

Cancer of the Head and Neck

This group includes patients with cancer of the pharynx, larynx, salivary glands, and oral or nasal cavity. The annual incidence is approximately 45,000 in the United States (1). Patients with cancer of the head and neck often develop malnutrition because of the location of the tumor and its effect on swallowing. Thus, the cardinal impact of these cancers is a lack of adequate nutrients. This is compounded by the finding that many patients also have a history of alcohol and tobacco use that predisposes them to malnutrition. Investigators have estimated that up to 57% of patients with cancer of the head and neck have significant weight loss before beginning treatment (338). Therapies used to treat the tumor, including surgery, radiation, and chemotherapy, also adversely affect nutritional status. Most patients experience acute toxicity related to treatment. In a review of 158 patients with squamous cell carcinoma of the head and neck who were treated with definitive radiation or chemoradiation therapy, at 1 month, significant treatment induced mucositis, and dysphagia developed in 76 and 87%, respectively (339). These effects led to an additional 10% loss of body weight resulting from treatment (340). Silent aspiration may be detected in more than 50% of patients treated for head and neck cancer (341). These adverse effects on oral intake may become chronic and may persist even after the tumor has been treated. Approximately 10% of all survivors of head and neck cancer will be permanently dependent on enteral nutrition via a percutaneous endoscopic gastrostomy (PEG) (342). In an analysis from Memorial Sloan-Kettering, head and neck cancer accounted for 72% of all patients requiring long-term (>1 year) enteral nutrition in the home (221).

In the majority of patients, the GI tract beyond the oropharynx is intact, and therefore enteral nutrition is appropriate. PEG placement before initiation of radiotherapy has been shown to prevent weight loss, treatment interruption, and hospitalization for dehydration (204–206). For malnourished patients undergoing tumor resection, a course of 7 to 10 days of preoperative enteral nutrition support is associated with a 10% reduction in morbidity (343) and improved quality of life (344). Factors shown to predict the need for perioperative enteral support include recent heavy alcohol use, tongue base involvement and surgery, pharyngectomy, composite resection, reconstruction with a myocutaneous flap, radiation therapy, tumor size, and moderately–to poorly differentiated histology (345). In patients with inoperable cancer, enteral nutrition during palliative radiation successfully maintained nutritional status, as measured by serum proteins and anthropometric data, and allowed more patients to return to their regular activities than those patients receiving only oral nutrition (346). Most patients with head and neck cancer will regain their ability to eat and can have the PEG tube removed. However, a few have prolonged dependence on enteral feeding. In these patients, complete enteral nutrition can be safely provided via a PEG tube or low-profile gastrostomy device indefinitely, with few complications (221, 347).

Cancer of the Esophagus

Since the mid-1970s, the incidence of adenocarcinoma of the esophagus has increased in the United States and other Western countries, whereas the incidence of esophageal squamous cell carcinoma has remained largely unchanged (348). Approximately 14,000 new cases of esophageal squamous cell and adenocarcinoma were diagnosed in the United States in 2003 (1). Dyphagia is almost universal in patients with cancer of the esophagus and is associated with an average weight loss of 10 kg at presentation (349). Approximately 80% of patients with esophageal cancer will present with or develop malnutrition (350). Treatment for esophageal cancer includes resection, chemotherapy, and radiation therapy. Frequently, these modalities are combined. Recent analysis of several large prospective trials involving 1116 patients showed that use of chemoradiation therapy followed by surgery improves survival (351). All these therapies may impair oral intake and compound malnutrition. Radiation therapy can cause esophagitis and strictures, whereas chemotherapy can lead to odynophagia from esophagitis and mucositis (352). Esophagectomy requires bilateral vagotomy, and delayed gastric emptying is often seen even after pyloroplasty (353). The anastomotic leaks and strictures that occur prevent oral intake (354), and dilation is required in up to 53% of patients (353). Although all these complications from the tumor or the therapies prevent oral intake, the remaining GI tract is usually functional. Therefore, enteral nutrition via a gastrotomy or jejunostomy is an effective method of nutritional support. In a prospective study of patients with esophageal cancer who were undergoing chemoradiation, enteral nutrition effectively prevented weight loss during therapy (355).

PEG tubes can be placed in more than 97% of patients with esophageal cancer, with a procedure-related mortality of less than 1%, and these tubes do not prevent future esophagectomy and gastric pull-up (356). When compared with parenteral nutrition, perioperative enteral nutrition is associated with fewer complications and less production of endotoxin and proinflammatory cytokines following esophagectomy (357, 358). Placement of direct percutaneous endoscopic jejunostomy (PEJ) tubes is useful in the management of complications following esophagectomy. In a report from Memorial Sloan-Kettering (359) of 25 patients with complications after esophagectomy that prevented oral intake and led to dependence on TPN, direct PEJ tubes were successfully placed in 84%. No major procedure-related complications occurred. Minor complications were seen 19% of patients. All patients were able to be weaned off TPN in an average of 3 days. In this setting, PEJ placement greatly facilitated discharge from the hospital by alleviating the need for home parenteral nutrition.

Cancer of the Stomach

Although the rate of gastric cancer continues to decline worldwide, it remains one of the most common causes of cancer-related mortality (360, 361). Despite advances in limited endoscopic resections for early gastric cancer, total or subtotal gastrectomy remains the cornerstone of treatment (360). Following total or subtotal gastrectomy, patients may complain of early satiety and may be unable to ingest adequate nutrients to prevent weight loss (362). Loss of the gastric reservoir may also lead to dumping syndrome, characterized by postprandial diaphoresis, tachycardia, faintness, diarrhea, and cramping. Usually, these signs and symptoms occur within 15 to 30 minutes following ingestion of a meal (early dumping). Another set of symptoms that often occur in conjunction with those just mentioned, but usually 1.5 to 2 hours after eating (late dumping), is characterized by sweating, tachycardia, and faintness; confusion may also occur. This set of symptoms and signs is related to catecholamine discharge mediated by a heightened insulin response and hypoglycemia resulting from rapid entry of the meal into the upper small bowel (363). This syndrome may be intense enough to discourage food consumption (364). When dietary management with an antidumping diet (365) (small, frequent meals, high protein, low simple carbohydrates, low insoluable fiber) and pharmacotherapy with octreotide (366) cannot adequately control symptoms, slow, continuous enteral feeding through a direct PEJ tube can provide complete nutrition (367).

Interest has also been renewed in the use of a jejunal pouch during surgical reconstruction after gastrectomy to minimize the adverse effects of the dumping syndrome. The Hunt-Lawrence-Rodino pouch (368) uses a loop of jejunum to create a reservoir for digestion and absorption and has been suggested to have a pseudopyloric function that slows the release of ingested food from the pouch into the small intestine and therefore minimizes the dumping syndrome (369). A recent study compared patients who underwent standard total gastrectomy with those who underwent gastrectomy with pouch creation and found that the patients with the pouch had a better nutritional status (as measured by the prognostic nutritional index) at

1 and 3 months and greater preservation of their body weight at 1 year (369).

In addition to the dumping syndrome and its associated impairment of oral intake, nutritional status following gastrectomy may be further affected by fat malabsorption resulting from bacterial overgrowth and impaired timing of pancreatic enzyme release (370). Clinical trials of supplements of pancreatic enzymes have had mixed results (371, 372). However, in a patient with steatorrhea, a therapeutic trial of pancreatic enzymes and antibiotics is reasonable. Deficiencies of iron, calcium, and fat-soluble vitamins may also develop. Treatment is with oral administration of iron plus ascorbic acid and with supplements containing both water-soluble and fat-soluble vitamins. Loss of gastric acidity, intrinsic factor, and R protein inhibits cobalamin availability and absorption from food; therefore, parenteral supplementation is required.

Cancer of the Pancreas

In the United States, the incidence of pancreatic cancer has been relatively stable since the mid-1970s, with an annual incidence of approximately 30,000 (1). Prognosis remains very poor; therefore, mortality rates almost mimic incidence rates. Pancreatic cancer is often associated with presenting complaints of abdominal pain, anorexia, nausea, vomiting, and weight loss. In a prospective study of patients with unresectable pancreatic cancer, all patients had experienced weight loss by the time of presentation, with a median loss of 14% of preillness weight (373). Weight loss is progressive, and by the time of last followup, patients had lost approximately one fourth of their pre-illness weight. Obstruction of the pancreatic duct may cause deficiency of digestive enzymes, whereas bile insufficiency may result from tumor obstruction of the ampulla of Vater or the common bile duct behind the pancreatic head. Maldigestion and malabsorption will occur and exacerbate the weight loss (374).

Most patients have unresectable cancer at presentation or disease recurrence within a year after surgery. These patients often suffer from partial or complete gastric outlet obstruction, intestinal dysmotility from intraabdominal metastasis, and pancreatic exocrine insufficiency. Oral dietary therapy with frequent, small, calorically dense meals and sufficient pancreatic enzyme supplements should be recommended. However, these measures often fail to improve the nutritional status. In patients who are candidates for antineoplastic therapy, a continuous infusion of enteral feeding formula though an endoscopically placed jejunostomy can provide significant numbers of calories (375).

For patients who are thought to have resectable disease (~20% of all patients), surgery offers the only chance of cure. The resection of most pancreatic cancers requires pancreaticodoudenectomy (PD). In the standard operative procedure, the distal half of the stomach is removed, the pancreas is transected (usually at the neck but varying amounts and rarely the entire gland may be removed), and the entire duodenum and a few centimeters of jejunum distal to the ligament of Treitz are resected. The long-term nutritional effects of PD have been studied. McLeod and colleagues of Toronto examined the nutritional status of 25 patients who were alive and free of disease more than 6 months after undergoing PD (376). In general, these patients were well nourished (as measured by a subjective global assessment, anthropometrics, and weight); however, ten patients developed diabetes mellitus, and five developed steatorrhea. The authors concluded that the nutritional status of those who remain free of malignancy following PD can be excellent. Long-term follow-up (median, 4.6 years) of a similar group confirmed these findings (377). A modification of the standard PD in which the stomach and pylorus are not disrupted does not seem to offer any long-term nutritional benefit (378).

Cancer of the Colon and Rectum

Although largely preventable, colon cancer remains the second most common cause of cancer-related mortality in the United States (1). Patients with colon cancer usually present with little or no weight loss. Surgical therapy involves removal the segment of colon containing the tumor. More extensive resections (usually total proctocolectomy) are performed in patients with underlying ulcerative colitis or hereditary colon cancer syndromes. Adjuvant chemotherapy is currently indicated for patients with stage III (node-positive disease) and advanced stage II disease (379). First-line therapy is a 5-fluorouracil–based regimen that can result in transient diarrhea but rarely creates nutritional problems.

Resection of the right colon with the ileocecal valve and a portion of the terminal ileum may be associated with watery diarrhea resulting from (a) loss of the braking effect of the ileocecal valve, (b) entry of increased amounts of bile salts into the colon with stimulation of water excretion into the colonic lumen (choleretic diarrhea), and (c) impaired water and sodium absorption caused by some loss of surface area in the colon (380). Cholestyramine binds bile salts and often markedly attenuates the diarrhea (381). Typically, a sufficient length of distal ileum remains to absorb adequate vitamin B_{12}. Resections of the left side of the colon or the rectum rarely have a significant impact on nutritional status. Usually, patients with colon cancer maintain a good nutritional status and do not require specialized nutrition support.

Gynecologic Cancers

In 2003, 83,700 women were diagnosed in the United States with new gynecologic cancers, and 26,800 died of these diseases (1). Response rates to chemotherapy have doubled from 40 to 80%, and the median survival has tripled since the 1980s (382). However, most patients still die of their disease. Gynecologic malignances and their multimodal therapies may be associated with severe malnutrition. Although some nutritional problems occur in patients with cervical and endometrial cancer, these problems are most commonly seen in those with ovarian cancer, particularly in advanced stages, when intraabdominal metastases severely impair GI function. A study of 67 consecutive patients hospitalized with gynecologic cancers at the University of Texas found that 54% of the women were malnourished, as determined by the prognostic nutritional index (16).

Up to 42% of patients with ovarian cancer will develop intestinal obstruction during the course of their illness (383). Frequently, women are alert and functional and have no other organ system dysfunction when bowel obstruction develops (382). Optimum management of these patients is not well defined. Surgery can be considered but is associated with a perioperative mortality of up to 32% and a reobstruction rate of 50% even in select populations (384). The alternative for these women is placement of a gastrostomy tube (PEG) for drainage and palliative care. Drainage PEG tubes can be successfully placed in 89% of patients, with a low (4%) complication rate (385). Placement of these tubes eliminates nausea and vomiting, but the problem of malnutrition remains. Although many of these women will quickly die as a result of progression of their disease, some have a good performance status and quality of life and without intervention will die of dehydration and malnutrition rather than progression of disease.

Few data exist on the use of TPN in patients with bowel obstruction resulting from carcinomatosis from a primary gynecologic malignancy. A study from Memorial Sloan-Kettering Cancer Center examined 21 patients with malignant bowel obstruction from ovarian cancer. All patients had a drainage PEG and received intravenous chemotherapy. Eleven patients also received TPN support. Those patients who were given TPN had significantly longer survival (386). The use of home TPN in patients with an active tumor and GI failure should be individualized. In general, this approach does not improve survival or quality of life (387). However, in a subgroup of patients who have a Karnofsky performance status of 50 or better at the time of GI failure, TPN is associated with improved nutritional status and quality of life (388). In our registry of patients receiving home parenteral nutrition, we have approximately 70 patients with a gynecologic malignancy and GI failure. Their survival on home TPN is quite variable but mostly less than 1 year. Approximately 25% of patients survive for longer than 6 months.

Patients Undergoing Bone Marrow Transplantation

Bone marrow transplantation involves eradication of the patient's own bone marrow with high doses of cytotoxic chemotherapy and radiation. Once this process of cytoreduction is complete, the patient receives the transplant, which is designed to repopulate the bone marrow with healthy, nonmalignant cells. The patient may receive a transplant of his or her own cells (an autologous transplant) or may be given cells from a donor (an allogeneic transplant). Approximately 50,000 transplants are performed around the world each year; two thirds are autologous and the remainder are allogeneic (389). Current indications include leukemia, lymphoma, multiple myeloma, aplastic anemia, congential immunodeficiencies, and some solid tumors.

Among patients undergoing allogeneic bone marrow transplantation, severe GI toxicity from cytoreduction is almost universal. Severe mucositis causes odynophagia, whereas infectious gastroenteritis or graft-versus-host disease (a condition in which the transplanted cells lead to immune-mediated destruction of host tissues, including the mucosa of the digestive tract) may lead to severe nausea, vomiting, and diarrhea. The difficulty in maintaining adequate caloric intake during the transplant led to the study of routine use of TPN. In 1987, Weisdorf and associates reported a prospective randomized study of routine use of TPN in 137 well-nourished patients undergoing bone marrow transplantation (390). Patients were randomized to either TPN or hydration with a 5% dextrose solution containing electrolytes, minerals, trace elements, and vitamins beginning during their cytoreduction and continuing for 4 weeks after the transplant. During a median follow-up period of 2 years, overall survival, time to relapse, and disease-free survival were significantly improved in the TPN group. However, 40 of 66 control patients did receive TPN when nutritional compromise was detected. The authors concluded that the routine use of TPN was indicated for patients undergoing bone marrow transplantation.

The GI toxicity associated with bone marrow transplantation has limited the study of enteral nutrition support in these patients. However, if tolerated, the enteral route is preferred because it is more physiologic and may help to maintain the integrity of the digestive tract. In addition, prolonged use of TPN may delay the resumption of adequate oral intake and may predispose to metabolic and infectious complications (391). In a study comparing TPN with an individualized enteral feeding program (dietary counseling, high-protein snacks, and/or tube feeding), patients randomized to TPN experienced more frequent hyperglycemia and central venous catheter complications but less frequent hypomagnesemia than those receiving the enteral feeding program (392). No significant differences were noted in the time to engraftment, length of stay, or survival. The authors concluded that TPN should be reserved for patients undergoing bone marrow transplantation who demonstrate intolerance to enteral feeding. Poor tolerance of enteral feeding may be improved with direct delivery of nutrients to the jejunum. A pilot study of 15 patients undergoing allogeneic bone marrow transplantation demonstrated that enteral feeding via a nasojejunal tube could be safely administered and were well tolerated (393). Larger prospective randomized trials of enteral versus parenteral nutrition support during bone marrow transplantation will need to be conducted before routine use of enteral nutrition can be recommended (394).

Role of Glutamine Supplementation

Because of issues of chemical stability, glutamine is not routinely included in parenteral nutrition. Data from animal studies suggested that parenteral or enteral supplementation of glutamine may ameliorate the GI toxicity caused by radiation or chemotherapy (395). This finding led to interest in the use of glutamine during bone marrow transplantation. Several studies have been reported, with mixed results (396). In a prospective, double-blind, randomized trial of 45 patients undergoing allogeneic bone marrow transplantation, those who received glutamine-supplemented parenteral nutrition had fewer infectious complications and shortened length of stay compared with patients receiving standard parenteral nutrition (397). Other studies were not able demonstrate similar benefits (398, 399). Therefore, the efficacy of glutamine supplementation requires stronger data before routine use can be advocated.

During Palliative Care

Before the advent of enteral and parenteral nutrition, the inability to receive nutrients through oral intake inevitably led to wasting and death. Therefore, in most patients, the natural history of cancer led to death because of dehydration and starvation (400). In patients with potentially curable or stable disease, nutritional support is an important and often critical part of the overall treatment plan. Conversely, the efficacy of nutritional support in the terminally ill patient is very limited. For patients with cancer that is no longer responsive to therapy and whose performance status has deteriorated to a point that they can no longer care for themselves (Karnofsky performance status <50), dietary therapy, enteral nutrition, or parenteral nutrition will not improve survival or quality of life and should therefore be avoided (401, 402). In general, cachexia, anorexia, or dehydration in the terminal phase is not uncomfortable (401). In these patients, dietary restrictions (i.e., low-salt diets) should be discontinued, and patients should be instructed to eat and drink as desired. For patients who are distressed by their anorexia, megestrol acetate can offer some improvement in quality of life (see earlier). If symptoms of thirst, dry mouth, or mucositis develop, these patients can often be successfully palliated with sips of fluid, ice chips, glycerine swabs, nonalcoholic mouthwashes, or viscous lidocaine. Medications should also be reviewed, and, if possible, any drugs with anticholinergic effects should be discontinued in patients with xerostomia.

It is often difficult for patients and families to understand why nutrition support is not being recommended. The reason is that, for most treatments (operations, chemotherapy, radiation therapy), the patient's knowledge and experience may be very limited, and thus the physician's recommendations usually form the basis for the patient's decisions. This is not the case with nutrition. People understand the role of nutrition in sustaining life, and it is often difficult for a lay person to understand why parenteral nutrition may not be indicated. This is exemplified by a study form the University of Michigan, which showed that 90% of women undergoing treatment for gynecologic cancer could envision a time when they would refuse ventilatory support, but only 37% could foresee a time when they would refuse artificial nutrition (403). In the terminally ill cancer patient, it is the physician's responsibility to explain thoroughly the reasons for withholding TPN. The importance of this step was demonstrated in a study of 197 patients with terminal cancer (404). In this report, although 58% of patients said that they understood artificial nutrition and 78% had received some sort of artificial nutrition in the past, their knowledge was poor. On average, patients were able to answer only 24% of questions correctly. However, increased patient knowledge about the efficacy of artificial nutrition was associated with a decreased desire to use artificial nutrition.

Among patients with terminal cancer, the basis for the recommendations for both initiation and withdrawal of an ongoing therapy should be the same. As stated in the President's Commission for the Study of Ethical Problems in Medicine and Biomedical and Behavioral Research, "A justification that is adequate for not commencing a treatment is also sufficient for ceasing it. Moreover, establishing a higher requirement for cessation might unjustifiably discourage vigorous initial attempts to treat seriously ill patients that sometimes succeed" (405).

At Memorial Sloan-Kettering Cancer Center, TPN is used infrequently in patients with cancer who do not receive any further anticancer therapy. TPN is used under these conditions only when it is judged that this approach will enhance the quality of life of a patient who is not at imminent risk of dying in spite of widely metastatic disease. When one considers the chance of improving the patient's quality of life, the burden of TPN administration and monitoring and the risk of complications have to be considered.

SUMMARY

Cancer is frequently associated with significant degrees of malnutrition caused by numerous mechanisms. The development of parenteral and enteral nutrition now allows virtually any patient to be fed; however, the efficacy of these therapies remains limited by alterations in host metabolism. Currently, *routine* use of specialized nutrition support among patients with an active malignancy is limited to select populations such as those undergoing radiation to the head and neck and those undergoing allogeneic bone marrow transplants. All other prescriptions for nutritional support must be done on a case-by-case basis. As antineoplastic therapies and understanding of cancer-induced cachexia improve, specialized nutrition support may become a more effective adjuvant during anticancer therapy. In patients who are cured of their malignancy but who have been left with GI tract failure as a result of treatment (i.e., chronic radiation enteritis), long-term specialized nutrition support is efficacious and often lifesaving.

REFERENCES

1. Jemal A, Taylor M, Samules A et al. CA Cancer J Clin 2003;53: 5–26.
2. Ollenschlager G, Veill B, Thomas W et al. Cancer Res 1991; 121:249–59.
3. Naber T, Schermer T, de Bree A et al. Am J Clin Nutr 1997;66: 1232–9.
4. Andreyev HJ, Norman AR, Oates J et al. Eur J Cancer 1998;34: 503–9.
5. Reilly J, Hull S, Albert N et al. JPEN J Parenter Enteral Nutr 1998;12:371–6.
6. O'Gorman P, McMillan DC, McArdle CS. Nutr Cancer 1998; 32:76–80.
7. Nitenberg G, Raynard B. Crit Rev Oncol Hematol 2000;34: 137–68.
8. Dewys WD, Begg C, Lavin PT et al. Am J Med 1980;69:491–7.
9. Shike M. Hematol Oncol Clin North Am 1996;10:221–34.
10. Bach PB, Schrag D, Brawley OW et al. JAMA 2002;287:2106–13.
11. Hodgson TA, Cohen AJ. Health Care Financ Rev 1999;21: 119–64.
12. Brown ML, Riley GF, Schussler N et al. Med Care 2002;40 [Suppl 4]:104–17.
13. Daly JM, Fry WA, Little AG et al. J Am Coll Surg 2000;190: 562–72.
14. Miziara ID, Cahali MB, Murakami MS et al. Rev Laryngol Otol Rhinol 1998;119:101–4.
15. Collins MM, Wight RG, Middlesbrough UK. Ann R Coll Surg Engl 1999;81:376–81.
16. Santoso JT, Canada T, Latson B et al. Obstet Gynecol 2000;95: 844–6.
17. Lanzotti VJ, Thomas DR, Boyle LE. Cancer 1977;39:303.
18. Veterans Affairs Total Parenteral Nutrition Cooperative Study. N Engl J Med 1991;325:525.
19. Brennan MF, Pisters PWT, Posner M et al. Ann Surg 1994;220: 436.
20. Tchekmedyian NS. Oncology 1995;9:79–84.
21. Schiavetti A, Fornari C, Bonci E et al. Nutr Cancer 2002;44: 153–5.
22. Reilly JJ, Weir J, McColl JH et al. J Pediatr Gastroenterol Nutr 1999;29:194–7.
23. Warren RS, Starnes HF, Gabrilove JL et al. Arch Surg 1987; 122:1936.
24. Persson C, Gilmelius B. Anticancer Res 2002;22:3661–8.
25. Alexandre J, Gross-Goupil M, Falissard B et al. Ann Oncol 2003;14:36–41.
26. Dempsey DT, Mullen JL, Buzby GP. Am J Clin Nutr 1985; 47[Suppl 2]:352.
27. Nguyen TV, Yueh B. Cancer 2002;95:553–62.
28. Nixon DW, Kutner M, Heymsfield S et al. Metabolism 1988;37: 1059–64.
29. Falconer JS, Fearon KC, Plester CE et al. Ann Surg 1994;219: 325–31.
30. Dempsey DT, Feurer ID, Knox LS et al. Cancer 1984;53: 1265–73.
31. Fredrix EW, Soeters PB, Wouters EF et al. Cancer Res 1991;51:6138–41.

32. Humberstone DA, Shaw JH. Cancer 1988;62:1619–24.

33. Kern KA, Norton JA. JPEN J Parenter Enteral Nutr 1988;12: 286–98.

34. Yoshikawa T, Noguchi Y, Doi C et al. Nutrition 2001;17:590–3.

35. Sauerwein HP, Romijn JA. Clin Nutr 2001;20:2–8.

36. Holroyde CP, Reichard GA. Cancer Treat Rep 1981;65[Suppl 5]: 55–9.

37. Shaw JH, Wolfe RR. Surgery 1987;101:181–91.

38. Holroyde CP, Gabuzda TG, Putnam RC et al. Cancer Res 1975;35:3710–4.

39. Cersosimo E, Pisters PW, Pesola G et al. Surgery 1991;109: 459–67.

40. Eden E, Ekman L, Bennegard K et al. Metabolism 1984;33: 1020–7.

41. Smith KL, Tisdale MJ. Br J Cancer 1993;68:314–8.

42. Pisters PW, Pearlstone DB. Crit Rev Clin Lab Sci 1993;30: 223–72.

43. Lundholm K, Bennegard K, Eden E et al. Cancer Res 1982;42: 4807–11.

44. Norton JA, Stein TP, Brennan MF. Ann Surg 1981;194:123–8.

45. Heymsfield SB, McManus CB. Cancer 1985;55[Suppl]:238–49.

46. Cohn SH, Gartenhaus W, Sawitsky A et al. Metabolism 1981; 30:222–9.

47. Tiao G, Fagan JM, Samuels N et al. J Clin Invest 1994;94:2255–64.

48. Hasselgren PO, Wray C, Mammen J. Biochem Biophys Res Commun 2002;290:1–10.

49. Lorite MJ, Smith HJ, Arnold JA et al. Br J Cancer 2001;85: 297–302.

50. Tilignac T, Temparis S, Combaret L et al. Cancer Res 2002;62: 7133.

51. Attaix D, Aurousseau E, Combaret L et al. Reprod Nutr Dev 1998;38:153–65.

52. Combaret L, Ralliere C, Taillandier D et al. Mol Biol Rep 1999; 1–2:95–101.

53. Combaret L, Tilignac T, Claustre A et al. Biochem J 2002;361: 185–92.

54. Whitehouse AS, Smith HJ, Drake JL et al. Cancer Res 2001;61: 3604–9.

55. Klein S, Wolfe RR. J Clin Invest 1990;86:1403–8.

56. Todorov PT, McDevitt TM, Meyer DJ et al. Cancer Res 1998; 58:2353–8.

57. Hirai K, Hussey HJ, Barber MD et al. 1998;58:2359–65.

58. Tisdale MJ. Support Care Cancer 2003;11:73–8.

59. Cabal-Manzano R, Bhargava P, Torres-Duarte A et al. Br J Cancer 2001;84:1599–601.

60. Lorite MJ, Thompson MG, Drake JL et al. 1998;78:850–6.

61. Watchorn TM, Waddell I, Ross JA. Am J Physiol 2002;282: E763–9.

62. Russell ST, Tisdale MJ. Br J Cancer 2002;87:580–4.

63. Sanders PM, Tisdale MJ. Cancer Lett 2004;212:71–81.

64. Russell ST, Hirai K, Tisdale MJ. Br J Cancer 2002;86:424–8.

65. Bing C, Russell ST, Beckett EE et al. Br J Cancer 2002;86: 612–8.

66. Russell ST, Zimmerman TP, Domin BA et al. Biochim Biophys Acta 2004;1636:59–68.

67. Groundwater P, Beck SA, Barton C et al. Br J Cancer 1990;62: 816–21.

68. Beck SA, Groundwater P, Barton C et al. Br J Cancer 1990;62: 822–5.

69. Sanders PM, Tisdale MJ. Br J Cancer 2004;90:1274–8.

70. Carswell EA, Old LJ, Kassel RL et al. Proc Natl Acad Sci USA 1975;72:3666–70.

71. Beutler B, Greenwald D, Hulmes JD et al. Nature 1985;316: 552–4.

72. Oliff A, Defeo-Jones D, Boyer M et al. Cell 1987;50:555–63.

73. Ling PR, Schwartz JH, Bistrian BR. Am J Physiol 1997;272: E333–9.

74. Gelin J, Moldawer LL, Lonnroth C et al. Cancer Res 1991;51: 415–21.

75. Llovera M, Garcia-Martinez C, Lopez-Soriano J et al. Mol Cell Endocrinol 1998;142:183–9.

76. Hardin TC, Koeller JM, Kuhn JG et al. JPEN J Parenter Enteral Nutr 1993;17:541–5.

77. Falconer JS, Fearon KC, Plester CE et al. Ann Surg 1994; 219:325–31.

78. Adami F, Guarini A, Pini M et al. Eur J Cancer 1994;30A: 1259–63.

79. Saarinen UM, Koskelo EK, Teppo AM et al. Cancer Res 1990; 50:592–5.

80. Ariapart P, Bergstedt-Lindqvist S, van Harmelen V et al. Pancreatology 2002;2:491–4.

81. Staal-van den Brekel AJ, Dentener MA et al. J Clin Oncol 1995; 13:2600–5.

82. Heinrich PC, Behrmann I, Haan S et al. Biochem J 2003; 374:1–20.

83. Strassmann G, Fong M, Kenney JS et al. J Clin Invest 1992;89: 1681–4.

84. Barton BE, Murphy TF. Cytokine 2001;16:251–7.

85. Cahlin C, Korner A, Axelsson H et al. Cancer Res 2000;60: 5488–93.

86. Mantovani G, Maccio A, Mura L et al. J Mol Med 2000;78: 554–61.

87. Dosquet C, Schaetz A, Faucher C et al. Eur J Cancer 1994; 30A:162–7.

88. Scott HR, McMillan DC, Crilly A et al. Br J Cancer 1996;73: 1560–2.

89. Pfitzenmaier J, Vessella R, Higano CS et al. Cancer 2003; 97:1211–6.

90. Fordy C, Glover C, Henderson DC et al. Br J Surg 1999;86: 639–44.

91. Oka M, Yamamoto K, Takahashi M et al. Cancer Res 1996;56: 2776–80.

92. Emilie D, Wijdenes J, Gisselbrecht C et al. Blood 1994;84: 2472–9.

93. Nakatani S, Iwagaki H, Okabayashi T et al. Res Commun Mol Pathol Pharmacol 1998;102:241–9.

94. Fong Y, Moldawer LL, Marano M. Am J Physiol 1989;256: R659–65.

95. Ikemoto S, Sugimura K, Yoshida N et al. Anticancer Res 2000; 20:317–21.

96. Moradi MM, Carson LF, Weinberg B et al. Cancer 1993; 72:2433–40.

97. Barber MD, Powell JJ, Lynch SF et al. Br J Cancer 2000;83: 1443–7.

98. Matthys P, Dijkmans R, Proost P et al. Int J Cancer 1991;49: 77–82.

99. Langstein HN, Doherty GM, Fraker DL et al. Cancer Res 1991;51:2302–6.

100. Matthys P, Heremans H, Opdenakker G et al. Eur J Cancer 1991;27:182–7.

101. Aleman MR, Santolaria F, Batista N et al. Cytokine 2002;19: 21–6.

102. Shibata M, Nezu T, Kanou H et al. J Clin Gastroenterol 2002; 34:416–20.

103. Tatemoto K. Proc Natl Acad Sci USA 1982;79:5485–9.

104. Stanley BG. Neuropeptide Y in multiple hypothalamic sites controls eating behavior, endocrine, and autonomic systems for body energy balance. In: Colmers WF, Wahlestedt C, eds. The

Biology of Neuropeptide Y and Related Peptides. Totowa, NJ: Humana Press, 1993:457–509.

105. Inui A. Cancer Res 1999;59:4493–501.

106. Chance WT, Balasubramaniam A, Dayal R et al. Life Sci 1994; 54:1869–74.

107. Chance WT, Balasubramaniam A, Thompson H et al. J Peptides 1996;17:797–801.

108. Gayle D, Ilyin SE, Plata-Salaman CR. Brain Res Bull 1997; 44:311–7.

109. Jatoi A, Loprinzi CL, Sloan JA et al. Cancer 2001;92:629–33.

110. Heinrichs SC, Menzaghi F, Koob GF. Vitam Horm 1998;54: 51–66.

111. Schwartz MW, Dallman MF, Woods SC. Am J Physiol 1995; 269:R949–57.

112. Uehara A, Sekiya C, Takasugi Y et al. Am J Physiol 1989; 257:R613–7.

113. McCarthy HD, McKibbin PE, Perkins AV et al. Am J Physiol 1993;264:E638–43.

114. Wisse BE, Frayo RS, Schwartz MW et al. Endocrinology 2001; 142:3292–301.

115. Wisse BE, Schwartz MW, Cummings DE. Ann NY Acad Sci 2003;994:275–81.

116. Ollenschlaeger G, Konkol K, Wickramanayake PD et al. Am J Clin Nutr 1989;50:454–9.

117. Komurcu S, Nelson KA, Walsh D, Ford RB et al. Am J Hosp Palliat Care 2002;19:351–5.

118. Grosvenor M, Bulcavage L, Chlebowski RT. Cancer 1989;63: 330–4.

119. DeWys WD, Walters K. Cancer 1975;36:1888–96.

120. Williams LR, Cohen MH. Am J Clin Nutr 1978;31:122–5.

121. Carson JA, Gormican A. J Am Diet Assoc 1977;70:361–5.

122. Kamath S, Booth P, Lad TE et al. Cancer 1983;52:386–9.

123. Trant AS, Serin J, Douglass HO. Am J Clin Nutr 1982;36: 45–58.

124. Comeau TB, Epstein JB, Migas C. Support Care Cancer 2001; 9:575–80.

125. Wickham RS, Rehwaldt M, Kefer C et al. Oncol Nurs Forum 1999;26:697–706.

126. Epstein JB, Phillips N, Parry J et al. Bone Marrow Transplant 2002;30:785–92.

127. Fernando IN, Patel T, Billingham L et al. Clin Oncol 1995; 7:173–8.

128. Saito T, Miyake M, Kawamori J et al. Radiat Med 2002;20: 257–60.

129. Harris AM, Griffin SM. J Surg Oncol 2003;82:147–50.

130. Pietersma P, Follett-Bick S, Wilkinson B et al. Support Care Cancer 2003;11:611–4.

131. McLymont V, Cox S, Stell F. J Nurs Care Qual 2003;18:27–37.

132. Mattes RD, Curran WJ Jr, Alavi J et al. Cancer 1992;70:192–200.

133. Scalera G. Nutr Neurosci 2002;5:159–88.

134. Bernstein IL, Webster MM, Bernstein ID. Cancer 1982;50: 2961–3.

135. Jacobsen PB, Bovbjerg DH, Schwartz MD et al. Behav Res Ther 1993;31:739–48.

136. Schwartz MD, Jacobsen PB, Bovbjerg DH. Physiol Behav 1996;59:659–63.

137. Mattes RD. Nutr Cancer 1994;21:13–24.

138. Levitan AA. Psychiatr Med 1992;10:119–31.

139. Schnell FM. Oncologist 2003;8:187–98.

140. Valente SM, Saunders JM, Cohen MZ. Cancer Pract 1994;2: 65–71.

141. Raison CL, Miller AH. Biol Psychiatry 2003;54:283–94.

142. Christensen L, Somers S. J Am Coll Nutr 1994;13:597–600.

143. Padilla GV. Surg Clin North Am 1986;66:1121–35.

144. Westin T, Jansson A, Zenckert C et al. Arch Otolaryngol Head Neck Surg 1988;114:1449–53.

145. Irvin TT. Br J Surg 1989;76:1121–5.

146. McEntee G, Pender D, Mulvin D et al. Br J Surg 1987;74: 976–80.

147. Randall TC, Rubin SC. Oncology 2000;14:1159–63.

148. Miller G, Boman J, Shrier I et al. Can J Surg 2000;43:353–8.

149. Potluri V, Zhukovsky DS. Curr Pain Headache Rep 2003;7: 270–8.

150. DiBaise JK, Quigley EM. Dig Dis Sci 1998;43:1369–401.

151. De Giorgio R, Bovara M, Barbara G et al. Gastroenterology 2003;125:70–9.

152. Pardi DS, Miller SM, Miller DL et al. Am J Gastroenterol 2002;97:1828–33.

153. Moskovitz DN, Robb KV. Can J Gastroenterol 2002;16:171–4.

154. Miedema BW, Johnson JO. Lancet Oncol 2003;4:365–72.

155. Sninsky CA. Gastroenterology 1987;92:472–8.

156. Husebye E, Hauer-Jensen M, Kjorstad K et al. Dig Dis Sci 1994;39:2341–9.

157. Creamer, B. BMJ 1964;5422:1435–6.

158. Barry RE. Gut 1974;15:562–70.

159. Scolapio JS, Ukleja A, Burnes JU et al. Am J Gastroenterol 2002;97:662–6.

160. Daniele B, Secondulfo M, De Vivo R. J Clin Gastroenterol 2001;32:228–30.

161. Hara S, Miyake H, Okada H et al. Int J Urol 2002;9:628–31.

162. Iivonen MK, Ahola TO, Matikainen MJ. Scand J Gastroenterol 1998;33:63–70.

163. Ghaneh P, Neoptolemos JP. Ann NY Acad Sci 1999;880:308–18.

164. Lemaire E, O'Toole D, Sauvanet A et al. Br J Surg 2000;87: 434–8.

165. Ong HS, Ng EH, Heng G et al. Aust NZ J Surg 2000;70: 199–203.

166. Bernardeau M, Auroux J, Cavicchi M et al. Pancreatology 2002; 2:427–30.

167. Friess H, Bohm J, Muller MW et al. Am J Gastroenterol 1996; 91:341–7.

168. Dookeran KA, Thompson MM, Allum WH. Eur J Surg Oncol 1993;19:95–6.

169. Falconi M, Pederzoli P. Gut 2001;49[Suppl 4]:2–10.

170. Makhdoom ZA, Komar MJ, Still CD. J Clin Gastroenterol 2000;31:195–204.

171. Mak KL, Hui PK, Chan WY et al. Arch Pathol Lab Med 1996; 120:78–80.

172. Padilla F, Hall WH, Boyd CM et al. South Med J 1975;68: 354–7.

173. Raymond AR, Rorat E, Goldstein D et al. Am J Gastroenterol 1984;79:689–92.

174. Rao SS, Dundas S, Holdsworth CD. Dig Dis Sci 1987;32: 939–42.

175. Gill SS, Heuman DM, Mihas AA. J Clin Gastroenterol 2001;33: 267–82.

176. O'Riordan BG, Vilor M, Herrera L. Dig Dis Sci 1996;14: 245–57.

177. Green PH, Fleischauer AT, Bhagat G et al. Am J Med 2003; 115:191–5.

178. Fine KD, Stone MJ. Am J Gastroenterol 1999;94:1139–52.

179. Christodoulou D, Skopelitou AS, Katsanos KH. Eur J Gastroenterol Hepatol 2002;14:805–10.

180. Potter J, Langhorne P, Roberts M. BMJ 1998;317:495–501.

181. Bye A, Ose T, Jaasa S. Acta Obstet Gynecol Scand 1995; 74:147.

182. Ovensen L, Allingstrup L, Hannibal J et al. J Clin Oncol 1993; 11:2043.

183. Dawson ER, Morley SE, Robertson AG et al. Nutr Cancer 2001;41:70–4.
184. Macia E, Moran J, Santos J et al. J. Nutrition 1991;7:205.
185. Ollenschlager G, Thomas W, Konkol K et al. Eur J Clin Invest 1992;22:546.
186. Evans WK, Nixon DW, Daly JM et al. J Clin Oncol 1987;5:113–24.
187. Ovesen L, Allingstrup L, Hannibal J et al. J Clin Oncol 1993;11:2043–9.
188. Harrison LE, Hochwald SN, Heslin MJ et al. JPEN J Parenter Enteral Nutr 1997;21:202–7.
189. Lipman TO. Hematol Oncol Clin North Am 1991;5:91–102.
190. Smith RC, Hartemink RJ, Hollinshead JW et al. Br J Surg 1985;72:458–61.
191. Heslin MJ, Latkany L, Leung D et al. Ann Surg 1997;226:567–77.
192. Page RD, Oo AY, Russell GN et al. Eur J Cardiothorac Surg 2002;22:666–72.
193. Strong RM, Condon SC, Solinger MR et al. JPEN J Parenter Enteral Nutr 1992;16:59.
194. Evens WK, Nixon DW, Daly JM. J Clin Oncol 1987;5:113.
195. Elkort RJ, Baker FL, Vitale JJ et al. JPEN J Parenter Enteral Nutr 1981;5:385.
196. Bozzetti F. JPEN J Parenter Enteral Nutr 1989;4:406.
197. Bounous G, Gentile JM, Hugon J. Can J Surg 1971;14:312.
198. Smith RC, Hartemink RJ, Hollinshead JW et al. Br J Surg 1985;72:458.
199. Ryan JA, Page CP, Babcock L. Am Surg 1981;47:393.
200. Flynn MB, Leightty FF. Am J Surg 1987;154:359.
201. Hochwald SN, Harrison LE, Heslin MJ et al. Am J Surg 1997;174:325.
202. Heslin MJ, Latkany L, Leung D et al. Ann Surg 1997;226:577.
203. Vissink A, Jansma J, Spijkervet FK et al. Crit Rev Oral Biol Med 2003;14:199–212.
204. Lee JH, Machtay M, Unger L et al. Arch Otolaryngol Head Neck Surg 1998;124:871–5.
205. Scolapio JS, Spangler PR, Romano MM et al. J Clin Gastroenterol 2001;33:215–7.
206. Raykher A, Schattner M, Friedman A et al. Proceedings of the 26th Congress of the European Society of Parenteral and Enteral Nutrition, Lisbon, 2004.
207. Bozzetti F, Gavazzi C, Mariani L et al. World J Surg 1999;23:577–83.
208. Nitenberg G, Raynard B. Crit Rev Oncol Hematol 2000;34:137–68.
209. Braunschweig CL, Levy P, Sheean PM et al. Am J Clin Nutr 2001;74:534–42.
210. Tchekmedyian NS. Semin Oncol 1998;25:62–9.
211. Matarese LE. Gastrintest Endosc Clin North Am 1998;8:593–609.
212. Cerra FB, Lehman S, Konstantinides N et al. Nutrition 1990;6:84–7.
213. Daly JM, Lieberman MD, Goldfine J. et al. Surgery 1992;112:56–67.
214. Braga M, Gianotti L, Radaelli G et al. Arch Surg 1999;134:428–33.
215. Braga M, Gianotti L, Vignali A et al. Surgery 2002;132:805–14.
216. Calder PC. BMJ 2003;327:117–8.
217. McCowen KC, Bistrian BR. Am J Clin Nutr 2003;77:764–70.
218. Heys SD, Walker LG, Smith I et al. Ann Surg 1999;229:467–77.
219. Howard L, Patton L, Scheib et al. Gastrointest Endosc Clin North Am 1998;8:705–22.
220. Howard L, Ament C, Fleming CR et al. Gastroenterology 1995;109:355–65.
221. Schattner M, Barrera R, Nygard S et al. Nutr Clin Pract 2001;16:292–5.
222. Roberge C, Massoud C, Poiree B et al. Br J Cancer 2000;8292:263–9.
223. Baron PL, Lawrence W, Chan WM et al. Arch Surg 1986;121:1282.
224. Bozzetti F, Gavazzi C, Cozzaglio L et al. Tumori 1999;85:163–6.
225. Shike M, Russel DM, Detsky A et al. Ann Intern Med 1984;101:303.
226. Lowry SF, Smith JC, Brennan MF. Am J Clin Nutr 1981;34:1853.
227. Shaw JH, Humberstone DM, Wolfe RR. Ann Surg 1988;207:283.
228. Jeevanandam M, Horowitz GS, Lowry SF et al. Lancet 1984;1:1423.
229. Sharp JW, Roncagli T. Cancer Pract 1993;1:119.
230. Shaw JH, Wolfe RR. Ann Surg 1987;205:368.
231. Nixon DW, Moffitt S, Lawson DH et al. Cancer Treat Rep 1981;65[Suppl 5]:121.
232. Abu-Rustum NR, Barakat RR, Venkatraman E et al. Gynecol Oncol 1997;64:493.
233. Serrou B, Cupissol D, Plagne R et al. Cancer Treat Rep 1981;65[Suppl 5]:151.
234. Valdivieso M, Bodner GP, Benjamin RS et al. Cancer Treat Rep 1981;65[Suppl 5]:154.
235. Nixon DW, Moffitt S, Lawson DH et al. Cancer Treat Rep 1981;65[Suppl 5]:121.
236. Samuels Ml, Selig DE, Ogden S et al. Cancer Treat Rep 1981;65:615.
237. Daly JM, Reynolds J, Thom A et al. Ann Surg 1988;208:512.
238. Fletcher JP, Little JM. Surgery 1986;100:21.
239. American College of Physicians. Ann Intern Med 1989;110:734.
240. Klein S, Simes J, Blackburn GL. Cancer 1986;58:1378.
241. McGeer AJ, Detsky AS, O'Rourke K. Nutrition 1990;6:233.
242. Klein S, Kinney J, Jeejeebhoy MB et al. Am J Clin Nutr 1997;66:683.
243. Weisdorf SA, Lysne J, Wind D et al. Transplantation 1987;43:833.
244. Ghavimi F, Shils ME, Scott BF et al. J Pediatr 1982;4:530.
245. Kinsella TJ, Malcom A, Bothe A et al. Int J Radiat Oncol Biol Phys 1981;7:543.
246. Klein S, Koretz RL. Nutr Clin Pract 1994;9:91.
247. Van Eys J, Copeland EM, Cangier A et al. Med Pediatr Oncol 1980;8:63.
248. Veterans Affairs Total Parenteral Nutrition Cooperative Study Group. N Engl J Med 1991;325:525.
249. Detsky AS, Baker JP, O'Rourke K et al. Ann Intern Med 1989;107:195.
250. Fan ST, Lo M, Lai ECS et al. N Engl J Med 1994;331:1547.
251. Hotler AR, Fischer JE. J Surg Res 1977;23:31.
252. Hotler AR, Rosen HM, Fischer JE. Acta Chir Scand 1976;86[Suppl]:466.
253. Mueller JM, Brenner U, Dienst C et al. Lancet 1982;1:68.
254. Brennan MF, Pisters PWT, Posner M et al. Ann Surg 1994;220:436.
255. Bozzetti F, Gavazzi C, Miceli R et al. JPEN J Parenter Enteral Nutr 2000;24:7–14.
256. Howard L, Ament M, Fleming R et al. Gastroenterology 1995;109:355.
257. Sharp JW, Roncagli T. Cancer Pract 1993;1:119.
258. Bozzetti F, Cozzaglio L, Biganzoli E et al. Clin Nutr 2002;21:281–8.
259. Schattner M. J Clin Gastroenterol 2003;36:297–302.
260. McCann RM, Hall WJ, Groth-Junker A. JAMA 1994;272:1263.
261. Argiles JM, Moore–Carrasco R, Busquets S et al. Drug Discov Today 2003;8:838–44.

262. Mantovani G, Maccio A, Madeddu C et al. Expert Rev Anti-cancer Ther 2003;3:381–92.

263. Wolf RF, Ng B, Weksler B et al. Ann Surg Oncol 1994;1:314–20.

264. Bartlett DL, Stein TP, Torosian MH. Surgery 1995;117:260.

265. Ng EH, Rock CS, Lazarus DD et al. Am J Physiol 1992;262: R426.

266. Tomas FM, Chandler CS, Coyle P et al. Biochem J 1994;301: 769.

267. Ottery FD, Walsh D, Strwford A. Semin Oncol 1998;25[Suppl 6]:35.

268. Wren AM, Seal LJ, Cohen MA et al. J Clin Endocrinol Metab 2001;86:5992.

269. Hanada T, Toshinai K, Kajimura N et al. Biochem Biophys Res Commun 2003;301:275–9.

270. Duxbury MS, Waseem T, Ito H et al. Biochem Biophys Res Commun 2003;309:464–8.

271. Lissoni P. Support Care Cancer 2002;10:110–6.

272. Kotler DP. Ann Intern Med 2000;133:622–34.

273. Lissoni P, Paolorossi F, Tancini G et al. Eur J Cancer 1996;32A: 1340–3.

274. Lyden E, Cvetkovska E, Westin T. Metabolism 1995;44:445.

275. Tomiska M, Tomiskova M, Salajka F et al. Neoplasma 2003;50: 227–33.

276. Strang P. Anticancer Res 1997;17:657.

277. Beller E, Tattersall M, Lumley T et al. Ann Oncol 1997;8:277.

278. Skarlos DV, Fountzilas G, Pavlidis N et al. Acta Oncol 1993;32: 37.

279. De Conno F, Martini C, Zecca E et al. Eur J Cancer 1998;34: 1705–9.

280. Loprinzi CL, Kugler JW, Sloan JA et al. J Clin Oncol 1999;17: 3299–306.

281. Meacham LR, Mazewski C, Krawiecki N. J Pediatr Hematol Oncol 2003;25:414–7.

282. Rowland KM Jr, Loprinzi CL, Shaw EG et al. J Clin Oncol 1996;14:135–41.

283. Mantovani G, Maccio A, Lai P et al. Crit Rev Oncol 1998;9: 99–106.

284. Yeh S, Wu SY, Levine DM et al. J Nutr Health Aging 2000;4: 246–51.

285. Loprinzi CL, Kugler JW, Sloan JA et al. J Clin Oncol 1999;17: 3299–306.

286. Jatoi A, Windschitl HE, Loprinzi CL et al. J Clin Oncol 2002; 20:567–73.

287. Walsh D, Nelson KA, Mahmoud FA. Support Care Cancer 2003;11:137–43.

288. Goldberg SC, Halmi KA, Eckert ED et al. Br J Psychiatry 1979; 134:67–70.

289. Rahman KM. Med J Malaysia 1975;29:270–4.

290. Kardinal CG, Loprinzi CL, Schaid DJ et al. Cancer 1990;65: 2657–62.

291. Moertel CG, Kvols LK, Rubin J. Cancer 1991;67:33–6.

292. Chlebowski RT, Bulcavage L, Grosvenor M et al. J Clin Oncol 1990;8:9–15.

293. Loprinzi CL, Goldberg RM, Su JQ et al. J Clin Oncol 1994;12: 1126–9.

294. Loprinzi CL, Kuross SA, O'Fallon JR et al. J Clin Oncol 1994; 12:1121–5.

295. Kosty MP, Fleishman SB, Herndon JE et al. J Clin Oncol 1994; 12:1113–20.

296. Sherry BA, Gelin J, Fong Y et al. FASEB J 1989;3:1956.

297. Fujimoto-Ouchi K, Tamura S, Mori K et al. Int J Cancer 1995; 61:522.

298. Gelin J, Moldawer LL, Lonnroth C et al. Cancer Res 1991;51: 415.

299. Matthys P, Dijkmans R, Proost P et al. Int J Cancer 1991;49:77.

300. Strassmann G, Kambayashi T. Cytokines Mol Ther 1995;1:107.

301. Yamamoto N, Kawamura I, Nishigaki F et al. Anticancer Res 1998;18:139.

302. Fanelli M, Sarmiento R, Gattuso D et al. Expert Opin Invest Drugs 2003;12:1211–25.

303. Haslett PA, Semin Oncol 1998;2[Suppl 6]:53.

304. Klausner JD, Makonkawkeyoon S, Akarasewi P et al. J Acquir Immune Defic Syndr Hum Retrovirol 1996;11:247–57.

305. Khan ZH, Simpson EJ, Cole AT et al. Aliment Pharmacol Ther 2003;17:677–82.

306. Dezube BJ, Sherman ML, Fridovich-Keil JL et al. Cancer Immunol Immunother 1993;36:57–60.

307. Goldberg RM, Loprinzi CL, Mailliard JA et al. J Clin Oncol 1995;13:2856–9.

308. Whitehouse AS, Tisdale MJ. Br J Cancer 2003;89:1116–22.

309. Barber MD, Preston T, McMillan DC et al. Clin Sci (Lond) 2003;106:359–64.

310. Wigmore SJ, Fearon KC, Maingay JP et al. Clin Sci (Colch) 1997;92:215–21.

311. Barber MD, Fearon KC, Tisdale MJ et al. Nutr Cancer 2001; 40:118–24.

312. Price SA; Tisdale MJ. Cancer Res 1998;58:4827–31.

313. Wigmore SJ, Barber MD, Ross JA et al. Nutr Cancer 2000;36: 177–84.

314. Barber MD, Ross JA, Voss AC et al. Br J Cancer 1999;81: 80–6.

315. Bruera E, Strasser F, Palmer JL et al. J Clin Oncol 2003;21: 129–34.

316. Licitra L, Spinazze S, Roila F. Crit Rev Oncol Hematol 2002; 43:93–101.

317. Grunberg SM, Deuson RR, Mavros P et al. Cancer 2004;100: 2261–8.

318. Fisch M. J Natl Cancer Inst Monogr 2004;32:105–11.

319. Homsi J, Nelson KA, Sarhill N et al. Am J Hosp Palliat Care 2001;18:403–7.

320. Kulkarni SK, Kaur G 2001;37:559–571.

321. Theobald DE, Kirsh KL, Holtsclaw E et al. J Pain Symptom Manage 2002;23:442–7.

322. Fernandez F, Adams F. Head Neck Surg 1986;8:296–300.

323. Grossie VB Jr, Nishioka K, Chang TH et al. JPEN J Parenter Enteral Nutr 1989;13:590–5.

324. Istfan NW, Wan JM, Bistrian BR. JPEN J Parenter Enteral Nutr 1992;16[Suppl]:76S–82S.

325. Bozzetti F, Gavazzi C, Mariani L et al. World J Surg 1999;23: 577–83.

326. Torosian MH, Mullen JL, Miller EE et al. Surgery 1983;94: 291–9.

327. Torosian MH, Tsou KC, Daly JM et al. Cancer 1984;53: 1409–15.

328. Frank JL, Lawrence W Jr, Banks WL Jr et al. Cancer 1992;69: 1858–64.

329. Hak LJ, Raasch RH, Hammer VB et al. JPEN J Parenter Enteral Nutr 1984;8:657–9.

330. Mares-Perlman JA, Francis AM, Shrago E. Am J Clin Nutr 1988;48:50–6.

331. Xiao HB, Cao WX, Yin HR et al. World J Gastroenterol 2001;7: 698–701.

332. Goseki N, Yamazaki S, Shimojyu K et al. Jpn J Cancer Res 1995;86:484–9.

333. Fahr MJ, Kornbluth J, Blossom S et al. JPEN J Parenter Enteral Nutr 1994;18:471–6.

334. Kaufmann Y, Kornbluth J, Feng Z et al. JPEN J Parenter Enteral Nutr 2003;27:411–8.

335. Shewchuk LD, Baracos VE, Field CJ. J Nutr 1997;127:158–66.
336. Medina MA. J Nutr 2001;131[Suppl]:2539S–42S.
337. Bozzetti F, Biganzoli L, Gavazzi C et al. Nutrition 1997;13:748–51.
338. Lees J. Eur J Cancer Care 1999;8:133–6.
339. Mekhail TM, Adelstein DJ, Rybicki LA et al. Cancer 2001;91:1785–90.
340. Newman LA, Vieira F, Schwiezer V et al. Arch Otolaryngol Head Neck Surg 1998;124:589–92.
341. Smith CH, Logemann JA, Colangelo LA et al. Dysphagia 1999;14:1–7.
342. Machtay M, Rosenthal DI, Hershock D et al. J Clin Oncol 2002;20:3964–71.
343. Bertrand PC, Piquet MA, Bordier I et al. Curr Opin Nutr Metab Care 2002;4:435–40.
344. Van Bokhorst–de Van der Schuer MA, Langendoen SI et al. Clin Nutr 2000;19:437–44.
345. Schweinfurth JM, Boger GN, Feustel PJ. Head Neck 2001;23:376–82.
346. Daly JM, Hearne B, Dunaj J et al. Am J Surg 1984;148:514–20.
347. Shike M, Berner YN, Gerdes H et al. Otolaryngol Head Neck Surg 1989;101:549–54.
348. Lukanich JM. Semin Thorac Cardiovasc Surg 2003;15:158–66.
349. Goodwin WJ, Byers PM. Med Clin North Am 1993;77:597–610.
350. Riccardi D, Allen K. Cancer Control 1999;6:64–72.
351. Urschel JD, Vasan H. Am J Surg 2003;185:538–43.
352. Herskovic A, Martz K, Al-Sassaf M et al. N Engl J Med 1992;326:1592–8.
353. Finley FJ, Lamy A, Clifton J et al. Am J Surg 1995;169:471–5.
354. Lerut T, Coosemans W, Decker G et al. Dig Surg 2002;19:92–8.
355. Bozzetti F, Cozzaglio L, Gavazzi C et al. Tumori 1998;84:681–6.
356. Stockeld D, Fagerberg J, Granstrom L et al. Eur J Surg 2001;167:839–44.
357. Baigrie RJ, Devitt PG, Watkin DS. Aust NZ J Surg 1996;66:668–70.
358. Takagi K, Yamamori H, Toyoda Y et al. Nutrition 2000;16:355–60.
359. Bueno JT, Schattner MA, Barrera R et al. Gastrointest Endosc 2003;57:536–40.
360. Hohenberger P, Gretschel S. Lancet 2003;362:305–15.
361. Wainess RM, Dimick JB, Upchurch GR et al. J Gastrointest Surg 2003;7:879–83.
362. Bae JM, Park JW, Yang HK et al. World J Surg 1998;22:254–60.
363. Gebhard B, Holst JJ, Biegelmayer C et al. Dig Dis Sci 2001;46:1915–23.
364. Vander Kleij FGH, Vecht J, Lamers et al. Scand J Gastroenterol 1996;31:1162–6.
365. Hasler WL. Curr Treat Options Gastroenterol 2002;5:139–145.
366. Vecht J, Lamers CB, Masclee AA. Clin Endocrinol (Oxf) 1999;51:619–24.
367. Shike M, Schroy P, Ritchie MA et al. Gastrointest Endosc 1987;33:372–4.
368. Herfarth CH, Stern J, Buhl K. Z Gastroenterol 1988;26:397–403.
369. Nozoe T, Anai H, Sugimachi K. Am J Surg 2001;181:274–8.
370. Bragelmann R, Armbrecht U, Rosemeyer D et al. Scand J Gastroenterol Suppl 1996;218:26–33.
371. Armbrecht U, Lundell L, Stockbrugger RW. Aliment Pharmacol Ther 1988;2:493–500.
372. Bragelmann R, Armbrecht U, Rosemeyer D et al. Eur J Gastroenterol Hepatol 1999;11:231–7.
373. Wigmore S, Plester C, Richardson R et al. Br J Cancer 1997;75:106–9.
374. Gupta R, Ihmaidat H. Eur J Surg Oncol 2003;29:634–43.
375. Shike M, Latkany L, Gerdes H et al. Gastrointest Endosc 1996;44:536–40.
376. McLeod RS, Taylor BR, O'Connor BI et al. Am J Surg 1995;169:179–85.
377. Royall D, Jeejeebhoy KN, O'Connor B et al. J Am Coll Nutr 1996;15:73–8.
378. Melvin WS, Buekers KS, Muscarella P et al. J Gastrointest Surg 1998;2:72–8.
379. Merkel S, Wein A, Gunther K, Papadopoulos T et al. Cancer 2001;92:1435–43.
380. Arrambide KA, Santa Ana CA, Schiller LR et al. Dig Dis Sci 1989;34:193–201.
381. Jacobsen O, Hojgaard L, Hylander Moller E et al. BMJ 1985;290:1315–8.
382. Rubin S. Gynecol Oncol 1999;75:311–2.
383. Randall TC, Rubin SC. Oncology 2000;14:1159–63.
384. Feuer DJ, Broadley KE, Shepherd JH et al. Gynecol Oncol 1999;75:313–22.
385. Herman LL, Hoskins WJ, Shike M. Gastrointest Edosc 1992;38:314–8.
386. Abu-Rustum NR, Barakat RR, Venkatraman E et al. Gynecol Oncol 1997;64:493–5.
387. Ripamonti C, Twycross R, Baines M et al. Support Care Cancer 2001;9:223–33.
388. Cozzaglio L, Balsola F, Costentino F et al. JPEN J Parenter Enteral Nutr 1997;21:339–42.
389. Goldman JM, Horowitz MM. Int J Hematol 2002;76[Suppl 1]:393–7.
390. Weisdorf SA, Lysne J, Wind D et al. Transplantation 1987;43:833–8.
391. Charuhas PM, Fosberg KL, Bruemmer B et al. JPEN J Parenter Enteral Nutr 1997;21:157–61.
392. Szeluga DJ, Stuart RK, Brookmeyer R et al. Cancer Res 1987;47:3309–16.
393. Sefcick A, Anderton D, Byrne JL et al. Bone Marrow Transplant 2001;28:1135–9.
394. Raynard B, Nitenberg G, Gory-Delabaere G et al. Br J Cancer 2003;89[Suppl 1]:101S–6S.
395. Klimberg VS, Souba WW, Dolson DJ et al. Cancer 1990;66:62–8.
396. Ziegler TR. Br J Nutr 2002;87[Suppl 1]:S9–S15.
397. Ziegler TR, Young LS, Benfell K et al. Ann Intern Med 1992;116:821–8.
398. Schloerb PR, Amare M. JPEN J Parenter Enteral Nutr 1993;17:407–13.
399. Schloerb PR, Skikne BS. JPEN J Parenter Enteral Nutr 1999;23:117–22.
400. Warren S. Am J Med Sci 1932;184:610.
401. Bachmann P, Marti-Massoud C, Blanc-Vincent MP et al. Br J Cancer 2003;89[Suppl 1]:107S–10S.
402. Torelli GF, Campos AC, Meguid MM. Nutrition 1999;15:665–7.
403. Brown D, Roberts JA, Elkins TE et al. Gynecol Oncol 1994;55:355.
404. Chiu TY, Hu WY, Chuang RB et al. J Pain Symptom Manage 2004;27:206–14.
405. President's Commission for the Study of Ethical Problems in Medicine and Behavior Research. Deciding to Forego Life Sustaining Treatment: A Report on the Ethical, Medical, and Legal Issues in Treatment Decisions. Washington, DC: US Government Printing Office, 1983;3:61.

84 BONE BIOLOGY IN HEALTH AND DISEASE[1]

ROBERT P. HEANEY

BONE COMPOSITION AND STRUCTURE 1314
   Bone Mineral 1314
   Protein Matrix 1314
   Noncollagenous Matrix Proteins 1315
BONE CELLS AND THEIR FUNCTIONS 1315
BONE ARCHITECTURE 1316
BONE DEVELOPMENT 1317
REVISION OF BONY MATERIAL 1317
BONE FUNCTIONS 1318
   Mechanical Functions 1318
   Homeostatic Functions 1319
NUTRIENTS IMPORTANT TO SKELETAL INTEGRITY . . .1320
   Calcium and Phosphorus 1320
   Vitamin D 1320
   Vitamin K 1321
   Micronutrients 1321
SKELETAL DISORDERS AND THEIR
   NUTRITIONAL CORRELATES 1321
   Osteoporosis 1321
   Rickets and Osteomalacia 1321
   Paget Disease of Bone 1322
   Parathyroid Dysfunction 1322
   Osteogenesis Imperfecta 1322
   Bony Manifestations of Diseases of
      Nonskeletal Systems 1322
   Aluminum and Bone 1322
SKELETAL MANIFESTATIONS OF SYSTEMIC
   NUTRIENT DEFICIENCIES 1323
   Protein-Calorie Malnutrition 1323
   Magnesium Deficiency 1323
INVESTIGATION OF NUTRIENT EFFECTS
   ON THE SKELETON .1323
   Change in Bone Mass 1323
   The Remodeling Transient 1324
   Bone Histomorphometry 1324
   Biochemical Markers of Bone Remodeling 1324

---

[1]**Abbreviations: Al,** aluminum; **BMD,** bone mineral density; **[Ca2+],** concentration of calcium ions; **CT,** calcitonin; **DXA,** dual-energy x-ray absorptiometry; **OI,** osteogenesis imperfecta; **PTH,** parathyroid hormone.

BONE COMPOSITION AND STRUCTURE

Bone is a tissue in which cells make up only 2 to 5% of the volume, and nonliving material, 95 to 98%. It is the nonliving material that gives the bone its mechanical properties of hardness, stiffness, and resiliency. This nonliving material consists of a mineral-encrusted protein matrix (also called osteoid), with the mineral comprising about half the volume and the matrix the other half. Unlike in other connective tissues, virtually no free water is present in the bony material itself. Embedded in this solid material are cells, called osteocytes, residing in lacunae in the matrix and communicating with one another through an extensive network of long cellular processes lying in channels called canaliculi, which ramify throughout the bone. As a consequence of this arrangement, virtually no volume of normal bone is more than a few micrometers from a living cell. Furthermore, even in the dense bone of the shafts of long bones, an extensive network of vascular channels exists, so the most remote osteocyte is typically no more than 90 μm away from a capillary.

Bone Mineral

The mineral of bone is a carbonate-rich, imperfect hydroxyapatite with variable stoichiometry. Calcium comprises 37 to 40%, phosphate 50 to 58%, and carbonate 2 to 8% of this mineral. These values vary somewhat from species to species, and the carbonate component is particularly sensitive to systemic acid-base status (decreasing in acidosis and increasing in alkalosis). In addition, bone mineral contains small amounts of sodium, potassium, magnesium, citrate, and other ions present in the extracellular fluid at the time the mineral was deposited, adsorbed onto the crystal surfaces, and trapped there as the water in the recently deposited matrix is displaced by the growing mineral crystals.

Protein Matrix

The protein matrix of bone, as for tendons, ligaments, and dermis, consists predominantly of collagen, which comprises about 90% of the organic matrix. For bone, the collagen is type I. Collagen is a long, fibrous protein, coiled as a triple helix. For the molecules of the protein to coil tightly, no side chains can project from the peptide backbone on the side facing inward. Hence every third amino acid in the body of the collagen molecule is glycine. Projecting outward, however, are the side chains of various amino acids, such as lysine, which allow the posttranslational formation of tight, covalent bonds between collagen fibers. This cross-linking helps to prevent fibers from sliding along one another when bone is stressed along the axis of the fibers.

Noncollagenous Matrix Proteins

Noncollagenous proteins make up about 10% of the organic matrix of bone (1). These proteins include a family of proteins in which glutamic acid residues are carboxylated in the γ position, called gla-proteins, the best studied of which is osteocalcin (or bone gla-protein [BGP]), which comprises about 1.5% of the matrix proteins. Other proteins include osteonectin, fibronectin, matrix gla-protein, osteopontin, and bone sialoprotein. The functions of these many constituents are not entirely clear. Some doubtless serve as chemoattractants for osteoclasts or as points of osteoclast attachment while others stimulate osteoblasts to lay down new bone. Because of these properties of the matrix proteins, bone seems to contain some of the chemical signals for its own remodeling (see later).

The shape and three-dimensional structure of bone are determined by its protein matrix. A bone that has been completely demineralized in the laboratory (by soaking in ethylenediaminetetraacetic or other acid) looks entirely normal, and when sectioned, stained, and examined under a microscope, it reveals all the fine structure of bone. In fact, prior demineralization has been the traditional first step in studying bone histologically (because mineralized bone tends to damage the microtome knives used by histologists to make their sections).

BONE CELLS AND THEIR FUNCTIONS

The four principal bone cells are lining cells, osteoblasts, osteoclasts, and osteocytes. They are responsible both for maintaining the mechanical properties of bone and for mediating the calcium homeostatic function of bone.

Lining cells are flat, fibrocytelike cells covering free surfaces of bone. They are probably derived from, or closely related to, the osteoblast cell line. They form a membrane that completely covers free bone surfaces and insulates them from the cells and hormones in the general circulation.

Osteoblasts are derived from marrow stromal cells; they are the cells that lay down bone, first by synthesizing, depositing, and orienting the fibrous proteins of the matrix and then by initiating changes that render the matrix capable of mineralization. Osteoblasts lay this matrix down between and beneath themselves on a preexisting bone surface, thereby pushing themselves backward as they add new bone.

Bone matrix, when freshly deposited, consists of about half protein and half water, and is not immediately mineralizable, just as the similar collagen-based structures, tendon and ligament, do not normally calcify. So the osteoblast still has more work to do after forming and depositing the matrix. The details of the process are not completely clear, but they involve secretion of proteins by the osteoblast into the matrix that it had previously laid down. These somehow help to create a three-dimensional configuration that attracts calcium and phosphate ions and arranges them in the apatite crystal habitus. Osteoblasts also secrete an enzyme called alkaline phosphatase that hydrolyzes organic phosphate compounds in the vicinity. These phosphate components would otherwise function as mineralization inhibitors. Finally, as mineral is deposited, it displaces the water of the original matrix. The apatite crystals that form are spindle shaped and are oriented parallel to and between the collagen fibers.

Osteoclasts are derived from the monocyte-macrophage line of cells, are usually multinucleated, and are the cells that resorb bone. They do this first by attaching firmly to a microscopic bony surface and then by walling off a small region of that surface. The attachment involves linkage between proteins called integins in the cell membrane of the osteoclast with proteins in the bone matrix, such as osteopontin, that exhibit a particular amino acid sequence (RGD, i.e., arginine-glycine-asparagine). Once firmly attached, osteoclasts secrete acid and proteolytic enzymes into this confined space. These dissolve the mineral and digest the matrix. The osteoclasts then release the breakdown products into the extracellular fluid around the resorption site, whence they are carried away by the circulating blood. After working for a short period of time (measured in days), the osteoclasts undergo programmed cell death (apoptosis), leaving their excavation to be refilled by osteoblasts.

The calcium and phosphorus released into the bloodstream will usually be used to mineralize remodeling sites elsewhere in the skeleton that are currently in their formation phase. The protein fragments are metabolized or excreted. Some of the amino acids released in collagen degradation reenter the body's amino acid pool and can be reused for protein synthesis elsewhere. However, those that have undergone posttranslational modification (e.g., proline to hydroxyproline and the amino acids involved in collagen cross-linking) cannot be reutilized. For this reason, bone remodeling requires a continuing supply of fresh dietary protein.

Osteocytes are osteoblasts that have stopped matrix synthesis and have become embedded in bone as other bone-forming cells around them continue to add new layers of matrix. Osteocytes are responsible for monitoring the amount of strain (bending) that occurs in their domains when bone is mechanically loaded and for reporting that information to lining cells on nearby anatomic bone surfaces, which may then initiate local bone remodeling projects. The full extent of their function is not known, but

TABLE 84.1. HUMORAL FACTORS ACTING ON BONE CELLS

OSTEOBLASTS	OSTEOCLASTS
Parathyroid hormone	Calcitonin
1,25(OH)$_2$ vitamin D	Bisphosphonate drugs
Glucocorticoids	Interleukin-1
Insulinlike growth factors (IGFs)	Colony-stimulating factor-1 (CSF-1)
Transforming growth factor-β (TGF-β)	Transforming growth factor-α (TGF-α)
Interleukin-6	Transforming growth factor-β (TGF-β)
Parathyroid hormone–related peptide (PTHrP)	Gallium nitrate
Osteoprotegerin	

it is clear that bone with dead osteocytes (from whatever cause) is excessively fragile.

The activity of these bone cells is influenced by a large number of both systemic and local hormonal agents. Additionally, the cells influence the activity of one another. Table 84.1 lists a few of the many agents influencing osteoblasts and osteoclasts. This is a rapidly developing field of investigation, and much is still to be learned. The osteoblasts, or cells of the osteoblast lineage, occupy a central position, not just in forming bone, but also in processing systemic signals to the bone remodeling apparatus (see the later section on revision of bony material). Thus, although parathyroid hormone (PTH) is responsible for stimulating bone resorption, no PTH receptors are present on the osteoclast. Rather, they are found on osteoblasts (and related cells) that, in response to PTH binding, release or express on their surfaces agents that stimulate osteoclast activity. By contrast, the osteoclasts do possess calcitonin (CT) receptors and are thus able to respond very rapidly to the antiresorptive stimulus provided by CT.

BONE ARCHITECTURE

Bone consists of a dense outer shell, or cortex, and an internal, chambered system of interconnected plates, rods, and spicules called cancellous or trabecular bone (Fig. 84.1). In the shafts of the long bones, the cortical component predominates, creating a hollow tube, whereas nearer the joints, the cortex becomes thinner and the interior is made up of an extensive latticework of cancellous bone. Bones such as the vertebrae, pelvis, sternum, and shoulder blades possess a thin outer rind of cortex and a more or less even distribution of cancellous bone on the inside. The internal, three-dimensional architecture of cancellous bone is arranged along the lines of force a particular bone experiences and hence provides maximum structural strength with minimum material.

The proportions both of mineral and matrix and of calcium and phosphorus are essentially identical in cortical and cancellous bone. The issue has been sometimes confused in the literature because of the difficulty of removing adherent

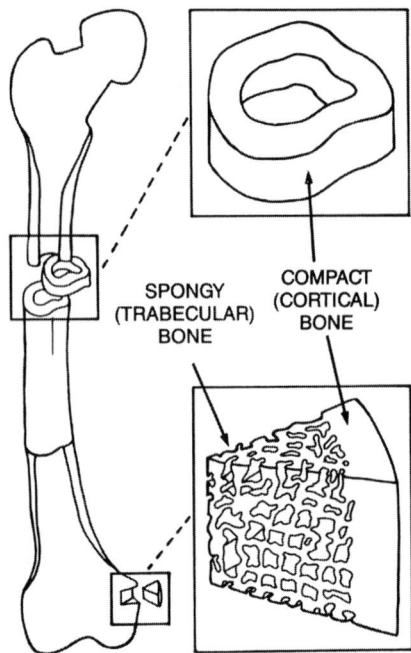

Figure 84.1. Gross and microarchitecture of a typical long bone. (Copyright Robert P. Heaney, 1996.)

marrow elements from cancellous bone samples prior to analysis. Fundamentally, however, bone is bone. On the other hand, cancellous bone turns over (remodels) much more rapidly than cortical bone. This is partly because of the much greater surface area of cancellous bone. (Remodeling always proceeds from a microanatomic bone surface burrowing into the bony material. See the later section on revision of bony material.) It is also partly the result of the generally greater contact with hemopoietic marrow in cancellous bone. In fact, the partition between bone with and bone without red marrow is probably more important than the partition between cortical and trabecular bone.

The end segments of bones are called epiphyses (Fig. 84.2). The shafts of long bones are called diaphyses, and

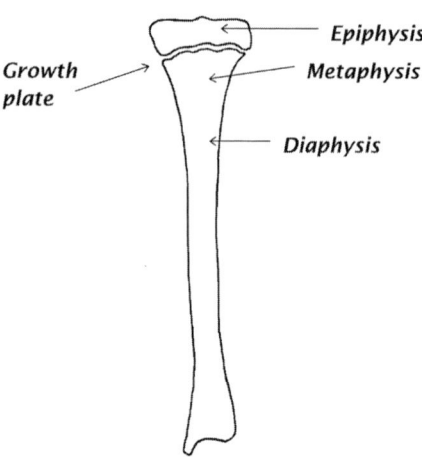

Figure 84.2. Principal regions of a growing long bone. (Copyright Robert P. Heaney, 1996.)

the flared portion of the shaft merging with the region of the growth plate is called a metaphysis. The lining cells on the outside of the bone form a tough sheet or membrane, called the periosteum, while the cells on the inside surfaces of both cortical and trabecular bone are called the endosteum.

The spaces between the trabecular plates and spicules are filled with bone marrow. Early in life, much of that marrow is hemopoietic, but later the blood-producing marrow is confined to the bones of the trunk, and the peripheral skeletal marrow spaces are filled mostly with fat.

In dense cortical bone, remodeling over the years produces a series of internal structures called osteons or haversian systems, in which concentric cylindric layers of bone are laid down along the course of a capillary. These are produced by the usual remodeling process (see later, in the section on revision of bony material). First, a tubular hole is created in the bone by osteoclastic resorption; then, it is filled in by successive waves of osteoblasts moving from the outside inward.

At their ends, where bones meet one another in a joint, the bony surface is covered with a layer of cartilage, rather than with periosteum. In health, this cartilage is highly hydrated and is lubricated by synovial fluid held there by a tough connective tissue sac called the joint capsule. This arrangement ensures that the bones move on one another smoothly.

BONE DEVELOPMENT

In utero, most bones are formed first as cartilage models, which are gradually replaced by bone. In this process, blood vessels invade the cartilage, calcification ensues, and the calcified cartilage is then removed by osteoclasts and replaced by bone laid down by osteoblasts. In infancy and childhood, bone growth and development follow a similar pattern. However, to accommodate growth, most bones possess one or more plates of cartilage perpendicular to the main axis of growth, separating, for example, the bone at the ends of a long bone from the bone of the shaft. This structure, called a growth plate (see Fig. 84.2), consists of rapidly proliferating cartilage cells that, as they multiply, push the ends of the bones away from the shafts. Blood vessels invade these columns of proliferating cartilage cells from the shaft side and initiate calcification of the cartilage and bony replacement in a process similar to what occurs in utero. Meanwhile, the ends of the bone are being pushed still further away, so there continues to be an anatomic and temporal sequence consisting of growth plate, proliferating cartilage, calcifying cartilage, and bony replacement, progressing down the metaphysis from the epiphyses toward the diaphysis.

Growth stops when the ossification process catches up with the formation of new cartilage at the growth plate and bony bridges develop across the growth plate, thus firmly anchoring the ends to the shaft of the bone. This closure process is initiated by the high levels of estrogen produced at puberty in both girls and boys. During the time when growth in length is occurring, the process of modeling (see later) shapes the outsides of the bones to keep them in proper proportion with the growth in length. At midshaft, this typically involves periosteal new bone formation and endosteal resorption, while at the metaphysis, periosteal resorption and endosteal formation occur.

REVISION OF BONY MATERIAL

Although the intercellular bony material, which makes up 95 to 98% of the volume of bone, is nonliving, nevertheless it is capable of being revised and replaced, just as are soft tissues, whose cellular constituents are turning over constantly and invisibly. In bone, the revision process occurs at discrete locations and is readily visualizable microscopically. The process normally follows a stereotyped sequence of activation first, then resorption, then reversal, and finally formation. This sequence is shown diagrammatically in Figure 84.3.

In the activation step, lining cells on a bone surface retract, exposing the bony substance directly to the circulating blood. Mineralized bone serves as a chemoattractant for osteoclast precursors, which migrate to the exposed site, coalesce, attach to bone as osteoclasts, and begin to erode into the bone. After removing a suitable volume of bone, osteoclasts undergo apoptosis and disappear from the scene. A reversal phase follows. Then osteoblasts move in and begin to replace the bone removed from the cavity. They orient the collagen fibers in parallel arrays, layer by layer, often alternating direction of the fibers every few micrometers. In this way, they build what is termed lamellar bone, which is similar in a sense to plywood (in which the grain of the wood runs in different directions in different layers). In the adult, osteoblasts advance at a rate of about 0.5 μm/day, and mineralization lags about 10 days behind the advancing matrix deposition.

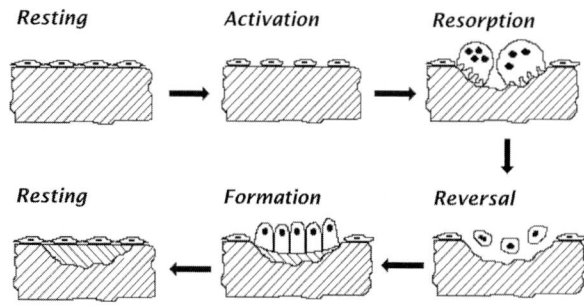

Figure 84.3. Schematic diagram of some of the major bone cells, indicating their role in the bone remodeling sequence. In the resting state, the bone surface is covered by lining cells. These retract at activated sites. Multinucleated osteoclasts move in and excavate a cavity. Then, after reversal, columnar osteoblasts deposit new bone matrix. Finally, the resting state is reestablished. (Copyright Robert P. Heaney, 1996.)

Some of the osteoblasts, as already noted, stay behind in cavities within the bone and become osteocytes.

When this revision process is finished at a particular site, the remaining surface osteoblasts become quiescent, flatten out, and turn into lining cells, effectively sealing the new bone surface until, at some later time, a new remodeling project is initiated locally. In healthy adults, this sequence, from start to finish, takes about 3 months at any given site. The resorptive phase takes about 2 to 3 weeks, and formation takes 2 to 3 months. The process is faster in infants and small children and is slower in elderly persons.

The process just described is technically called remodeling. One of its principal purposes is to replace damaged volumes of bone with fresh new material. During growth, however, and indeed at any time when the shape of the bone is being revised, the resorptive and formative processes occur, not at the same site, but in different parts of the bone. For example, the small shafts of the long bones of a child enlarge to adult size by osteoblastic formation on the periosteal surface and by corresponding osteoclastic resorption on the endosteal surface. This process is technically called modeling and is similar to remodeling in most respects, except the new bone is laid down at a location different from the site of resorption.

One of the ways in which this revision process can be readily visualized is by the administration of carefully timed doses of a fluorescent compound such as one of the tetracycline antibiotics. The molecules of these markers bind to mineralizing bone sites and are trapped as the site is buried by layers of new bone. The markers become readily visible when undecalcified bone biopsy specimens are viewed microscopically under ultraviolet illumination (Fig. 84.4).

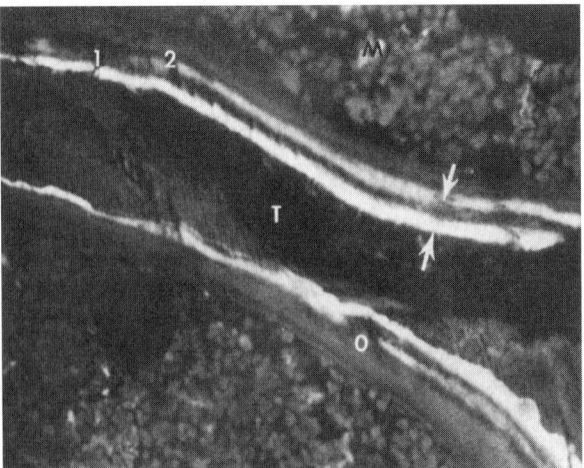

Figure 84.4. Section through trabecular bone obtained from the iliac crest. M, marrow; T, trabecular bone; *1* and *2*, first and second tetracycline labels. The distance between the *arrows* represents the amount of bone deposited during the time between administration of the two tetracycline labels.

BONE FUNCTIONS

Bone serves two distinct functions: the provision of mechanical rigidity and stiffness to our bodies; and the provision of a homeostatic buffer, particularly to help our bodies maintain a constant level of calcium in the circulating body fluids and to provide a reserve supply of phosphorus. The mechanical function is necessary so that we can resist gravity and move about on dry land. (Strictly speaking, a rigid skeleton would not be necessary in a fully buoyant medium such as water. For example, some originally bony fish, such as the sturgeon, have lost nearly all of their skeleton over the millennia of evolution. Still they function mechanically perfectly well.) The homeostatic function is the older of the two, from the standpoint of evolution, and is in a sense the more fundamental, because the body will sacrifice the structural function before it will risk losing the homeostatic one. In other words, the body will weaken the bone structurally to maintain the calcium levels of the blood and extracellular fluid.

Mechanical Functions

In the mechanical function of bone, nature strikes a balance between a skeleton so massive that it would resist most forces, but be too heavy to carry around, and one so flimsy that, although adequate to meet calcium homeostatic needs, it would be too fragile to sustain the mechanical forces of exertion or of minor injuries. Bone finds the middle ground by adjusting its mass using a classic negative feedback loop so it bends under routine use by about 0.05 to 0.10% in compression or tension and by 0.1 to 0.20% in shear (Fig. 84.5). This bending set point is a major determinant of bone size during growth and bone density during adult remodeling.

In the operation of this control loop, the osteocytes detect the amount of bending (or strain) in a local region of bone and send signals to nearby cells of the remodeling apparatus, which mediate the balance between resorption and formation. The result is that, when bone is loaded locally so heavily that its strain is greater than the reference amount (as with an increase in strenuous exercise), the processes of modeling and remodeling work to increase local bone density. When bone is loaded less heavily, so that its strains are less than this reference amount, remodeling removes more bone than it replaces, thereby lightening the structure and making it less stiff. For example, the bones in the dominant arm tend to be denser than those of the nondominant side, and the bones of athletes denser than those of nonathletes. This effect on bone mass is illustrated in Figure 84.6, which shows how this difference in bone mass between the dominant and nondominant arms is exaggerated in world-class racquet sports players, relative to nonathletes.

The strength of a bony structure is proportional to approximately the square of the bony density. This relationship makes bone strength sensitive to relatively small

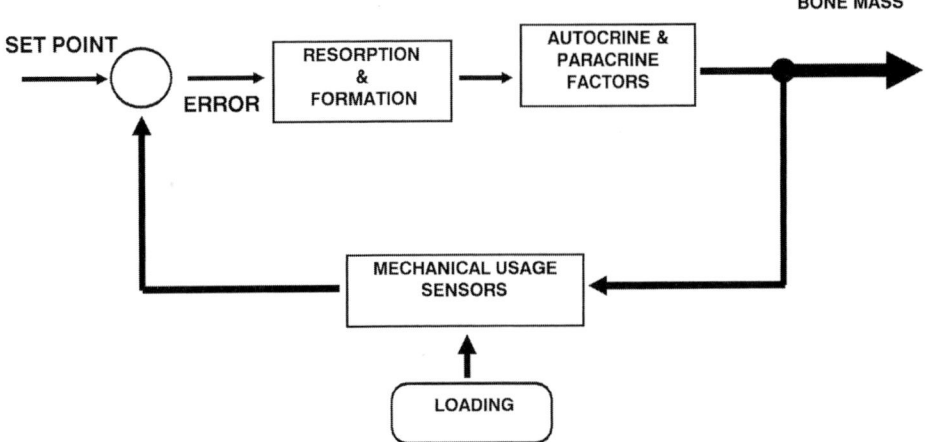

Figure 84.5. Feedback loop regulating bone mass. Mechanical sensors detect the amount of bending occurring under loading, compare that with the reference level, or set point, and if the two differ, send signals to the remodeling apparatus, either to initiate remodeling or to adjust the balance between resorption and formation. (Copyright Robert P. Heaney, 1990.)

changes in density and helps to explain why fracture risk doubles at bone density values only 10 to 15% lower than normal.

It is important to grasp the meaning of this doubling of fracture risk. If an average person's risk of fracture is, for example, one chance in 100 in any given year, doubling of risk means simply that the risk is now two chances in 100. The average person will not perceive any difference, because the typical person will not actually experience fracture (i.e., 98 out of 100 will be fracture free). Nevertheless, at a population level, the group of all persons experiencing this decline in bone mass will have twice as many fractures overall, and health care costs or demands on the health care system will rise accordingly.

Homeostatic Functions

The bone remodeling process also mediates the homeostatic function of bone. Whereas the pattern of strain under

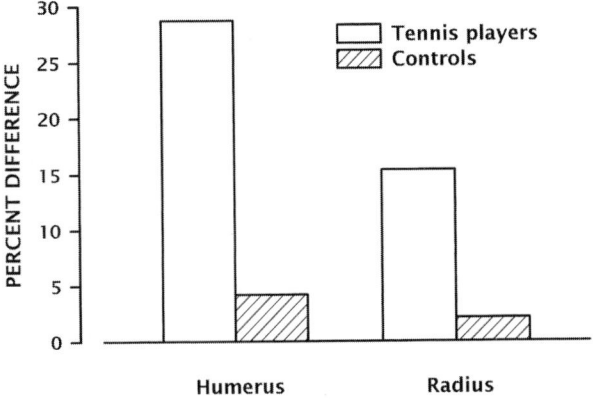

Figure 84.6. Difference in humeral and radial bone mass between dominant and nondominant arms of world-class tennis players and nonathletic controls. Even in the controls, the greater use of the dominant arm results in more bone on that side. This difference is greatly amplified in the tennis players. (Data from Kannus P, Haapasalo H, Sievanen H et al.) The site-specific effects of long-term unilateral activity on bone mineral density and content. Bone 1994;15:279–84; (Copyright Robert P. Heaney, 1996.)

loading is the major determinant of *where* bone remodeling occurs, PTH is the principal determinant of *how much* remodeling is occurring and how readily bone cells in any given locus respond to local stimuli to initiate a remodeling project. PTH secretion is directly responsive to the body's need for calcium. However, calcium is never simply removed from bone. Instead, whole volumes of bone are removed, and their calcium is then scavenged to meet the body's needs.

As noted earlier, resorption precedes formation. This produces local asynchrony of mineral movement: remodeling at any given site first makes its calcium and phosphorus available to the body (as mineral is removed during resorption). The same site later creates a demand for calcium and phosphorus as the mineralizing site extracts mineral from the blood flowing past it. Averaged over the whole skeleton, these processes are about equal at any given time: new remodeling sites are releasing as much calcium as the older sites are depositing. However, this local asynchrony also means that, when remodeling activity is increased, resorption changes first, and more calcium is released from bone than previously initiated remodeling sites need. This makes an additional supply of calcium temporarily available to the body. Conversely, when remodeling is acutely suppressed, resorption drops immediately while previously initiated formation continues, and thus the skeleton is able to soak up a temporary excess of calcium from the blood. Modulation of remodeling in this way by the hormones PTH and CT is a major part of the basis of the regulation of blood calcium levels by the skeleton.

Two examples with nutritional relevance illustrate how this system operates. During the absorption of large quantities of calcium from milk in infant feeding, CT is secreted to suppress osteoclastic resorptive activity, thereby reducing release of calcium from bone. This allows the demands of rapidly mineralizing bone to be met by absorbed calcium from the milk, and at the same time it prevents the absorbed calcium from causing a dangerous increase in the concentration of calcium ions ($[Ca^{2+}]$) in the blood. Later, during the postabsorptive phase, CT levels drop and PTH rises to stimulate resorption again. This action sustains the blood $[Ca^{2+}]$ calcium at normal levels in the presence of steady mineral demands of bone formation and wide swings in calcium input from the intestine.

Another example is found during antler formation in deer. Because the skeletal remodeling cycle lasts several weeks at any given site, the asynchrony between calcium availability in resorption and calcium demand in formation is capable of prolonged support of unbalanced calcium needs. Each spring, the demands of the growing antler exceed the calcium available from the late winter foliage that makes up the deer's diet. So a burst of PTH-mediated remodeling occurs throughout the skeleton at the time antler mineralization begins. This creates a temporary surplus of calcium from the resorptive phase of skeletal remodeling, which is used to mineralize the bone of the rapidly forming antler. Later, when the new bony remodeling sites throughout the skeleton enter their own formation phase and now have a net demand for calcium, they are filled in with calcium made available from the then calcium-rich summer grasses and foliage.

NUTRIENTS IMPORTANT TO SKELETAL INTEGRITY

Total nutritional status influences bone cell function just as it does the function of other tissues. However, cellular malnutrition affects mainly bone currently being remodeled, whereas the strength of bony structures at any given time is dependent, not so much on current cell function, as on the mass of bony material accumulated by bone cellular activity over many years. For that reason, acute nutritional stresses or deficiencies rarely produce overt skeletal symptoms in adults, even when they severely compromise bone cell function. Children and growing animals show effects more promptly, both because they have less skeletal capital in their bone banks and because they are revising it much more rapidly. Nevertheless, a few nutrients, when deficient, are more likely than others to produce skeletal manifestations. These include calcium, phosphorus, vitamin D, vitamin K, and certain of the trace minerals.

Calcium and Phosphorus

In addition to buffering absorptive oscillations in blood calcium levels, bone serves as a nutrient reserve for both calcium and phosphorus. This reserve is to the calcium (and phosphorus) functions of the body as body fat is to energy metabolism. Unlike most nutrient reserves, however, this one (bone) has acquired a distinct function in its own right, that is, mechanical and structural support. In other words, we walk around on our calcium reserve. It follows that any influence, nutritional or otherwise, that alters the size of the calcium reserve will alter bone strength.

Bone is a very rich source of calcium: Total skeletal calcium averages 1100 to 1500 g, and each cubic centimeter of bone contains more calcium than the entire circulating blood volume in an adult. Thus, in comparison with other nutrients, the calcium reserve is huge. Although low-calcium diets usually deplete the bony reserves, they do so slowly. Thus, whereas the *population-level* risk of fracture rises immediately, it will take many years for bone strength to be sufficiently reduced to lead to a perceptible increase in an *individual person's* risk of fracture (see earlier). The slow expression of the effect of calcium deficiency led many nutritional scientists in the past to the erroneous conclusion that calcium was not important for adult bone strength. Nevertheless, a nutritional deficiency that develops over 30 years is just as much a deficiency as one that develops over 30 days.

Low intakes of calcium and phosphorus can both limit bone acquisition during growth and cause bone loss after maturity. Calcium intake operates most directly through modulation of remodeling, as described earlier. In the antler example previously cited, if summer foliage were not calcium rich, each cycle of antler formation would deplete the skeleton, bony replacement would fail to occur, and bone mass would fall progressively over the animal's adult life. Because human calcium requirements rise with age (3), and because calcium intakes tend to fall in elderly persons, precisely such depletion occurs in most human populations as they age.

Inadequate phosphorus availability also affects bone, but in a different way. The osteoblast environment is one of continuous mineralization, with the matrix extracting phosphate (as well as calcium) from the fluid bathing the bone-forming cells. Although calcium makes up about 40% of the bone mineral, phosphate (PO_4^{3-}) accounts for nearly 60%. Thus, phosphorus is fully as important for bone building as is calcium. Rapid growth is not possible without a high blood phosphate level, a fact that explains the substantially higher blood phosphate values in children. When phosphate levels in the blood entering bone are low, mineralization extracts as much phosphate as it can from the fluid around the osteoblast. In so doing, it creates a local environment severely depleted of phosphate. However, osteoblasts, like all cells, need phosphate for their own metabolism. The result is serious interference with osteoblast function: matrix deposition is slowed, and osteoblast initiation of mineralization is reduced even more. These abnormalities produce the typical histologic pattern in bone of rickets and osteomalacia (see later).

Vitamin D

Vitamin D has many bony effects, such as facilitating the development of osteoclast precursors at an activated remodeling locus and augmenting osteoclast response to resorptive stimuli. The vitamin also stimulates synthesis and release of osteocalcin by osteoblasts (see earlier).

However, its major importance for bone is to facilitate absorption of calcium (and to some extent phosphorus) from the diet. Severe vitamin D deficiency causes rickets and osteomalacia (see later). Milder shortages of the vitamin reduce calcium availability to the body and produce a situation of calcium deficiency, resulting in osteoporosis. Because of the traditional (if simplistic) identification of vitamin D *deficiency* with rickets and osteomalacia, it has been customary to refer to less extreme degrees of vitamin D shortage as *insufficiency*. This distinction is no longer useful. All degrees of vitamin D inadequacy that produce disease should be termed *deficiency* (see also Chapter 20).

Vitamin K

Vitamin K functions in the γ-carboxylation of the glutamic acid residues of three bone gla-proteins (see also Chapter 22), the best studied of which is osteocalcin. Vitamin K deficiency results both in undercarboxylation of osteocalcin and in reduced osteocalcin synthesis. The net effect of these changes on bone strength or integrity is not certain. However, low vitamin K status is associated in epidemiologic studies with low bone mass, increased hip fracture risk, and increased cardiovascular mortality (4).

Micronutrients

Vitamin C and certain trace minerals (notably copper, zinc, and manganese) are important cofactors for the synthesis or cross-linking of matrix proteins. Copper and vitamin C are perhaps the best studied in this regard. Copper is the cofactor for lysyl oxidase, the enzyme responsible for cross-linking collagen fibrils. Interference with cross-linking results in structurally weak bone. Ascorbic acid is also a required cofactor for the cross-linking of collagen fibrils, and in its absence bone strength is impaired. In the presence of deficiencies of these micronutrients during growth, severe bone abnormalities can result. These abnormalities include stunting of growth, deformity of bones, and epiphyseal dysplasia. Whether adults can develop sufficient deficiencies of these nutrients to interfere significantly with bone integrity remains unknown.

SKELETAL DISORDERS AND THEIR NUTRITIONAL CORRELATES

Osteoporosis

Osteoporosis is a multifactorial condition of the skeleton in which skeletal strength is reduced sufficiently so that fractures occur on minor trauma (see also Chapter 86). Generally, osteoporosis exhibits reduced bone mass (i.e., both matrix and mineral) as well as various microstructural disturbances of bony architecture (5). A simple decrease in quantity of bone is sometimes called osteopenia (literally, "shortage of bone"). By current World Health Organization standards, bone mass is measured by x-ray absorptiometry as an areal density, termed bone mineral density (BMD). Osteopenia is characterized by a BMD value at hip or spine between −1 and −2.5 standard deviations below the young adult normal mean. BMD values more than 2.5 standard deviations below young adult normal are now called osteoporosis, whether or not a fracture is present. BMD is, unfortunately, a poor way to represent bone structural strength, because it explicitly eliminates the important influence of bone size. A larger bone with a lower density is usually stronger—less likely to fracture—than a smaller, denser bone.

A common feature of most cases of osteoporosis is elevated bone remodeling, particularly in postmenopausal women (6). Remodeling activity, although designed to repair weakened bone, actually makes it temporarily weaker during the remodeling process, and when remodeling is in excess of mechanical need, it causes only weakness. Estrogen deficiency, low calcium intake, and vitamin D deficiency all contribute to a harmful postmenopausal rise in bone remodeling.

Lack of exercise and alcohol abuse also contribute to the development of this disorder. Given diets typical of the elderly persons in Europe and North America, it can be estimated that inadequate calcium intake is responsible for one third to two thirds of osteoporotic fractures. (For this reason, the US Food and Drug Administration allows an osteoporosis health claim on the labels of certain calcium-rich foods.)

Rickets and Osteomalacia

Rickets is a disorder of the growth apparatus of bone (see earlier) in which the growth cartilage fails to mature and mineralize normally (7). Growth is stunted, and various deformities about the growth plates occur. Osteomalacia is the corresponding disorder in adults in which the newly deposited bone matrix fails to mineralize adequately. New matrix formation is slowed in both conditions, but mineralization is retarded even more; thus, unmineralized matrix accumulates on microscopic bone surfaces. For this reason, the proportion of mineral to matrix drops. In severe cases, unmineralized bone may constitute so large a proportion of the skeleton that individual bones lose their stiffness and become severely deformed (bowed legs and misshapen pelves).

The stereotypical forms of rickets and osteomalacia are those associated with vitamin D deficiency. The principal pathogenesis of these common forms follows from insufficient intestinal absorption of calcium and phosphorus from the diet. In attempting to keep blood calcium levels close to normal levels, the body raises PTH secretion. Because one of the effects of PTH is to increase renal clearance of phosphate, this adaptive response drives the already reduced blood phosphate concentrations down to levels such that severe phosphate deficiency develops, first locally in the vicinity of the osteoblasts and chondrocytes and then in other tissues as well (producing, e.g., muscle weakness, tenderness, and pain).

Rickets and osteomalacia also develop for reasons other than vitamin D deficiency, including fluoride toxicity and cadmium poisoning, as well as in association with certain rare vascular malignant diseases. The toxins or some products of tumor metabolism interfere with normal osteoblast function or, alternatively, lower the renal phosphorus threshold. Typical of the latter mechanism is a group of heritable abnormalities of renal phosphate transport, the most common of which is X-linked hypophosphatemia (8). These conditions have in common the inability to maintain the blood phosphate levels required for growth. Such forms of rickets produce their bony effects solely because of severe hypophosphatemia. This group of disorders in the past was called vitamin D–resistant rickets. These disorders do not respond to usual doses of vitamin D (hence their name). Therapy is directed at elevating serum phosphate levels.

Paget Disease of Bone

Paget disease is a local, but often multifocal disorder of the bone remodeling process, and it is of uncertain etiology. Resorption proceeds erratically, with formation filling in with new bone behind it. Bone architecture and even external bone shape are disordered. During the early resorptive phase, the bone is excessively fragile and may fracture readily. The high level of bone remodeling is usually accompanied by high levels of remodeling markers (see later), particularly serum alkaline phosphatase. When the process involves the skull, bony growths may constrict the cranial nerve passages and may lead to, for example, deafness. No nutritional correlates of this disorder are known.

Parathyroid Dysfunction

Because PTH is the principal determinant of the amount of remodeling activity in the skeleton, one could expect significant skeletal manifestations of parathyroid functional disorders. The reality, however, is complicated. Patients with hypoparathyroidism have reduced remodeling, slightly greater than average bone mass, and probably fewer fractures. By contrast, patients with severe, longstanding hyperparathyroidism may have reduced bone mass, subperiosteal bone loss, widespread, very active bone remodeling, and even cysts in bone filled with osteoclastlike cells. Such cases are extremely rare today, and generally patients with primary hyperparathyroidism have no abnormalities of the skeleton detectable by ordinary x-ray studies. Untreated mild primary hyperparathyroidism is now known to result in increased fracture risk, not for reasons of decreased bone mass, but because of increased PTH-mediated bone remodeling. When PTH hypersecretion is pulsatile, and the peaks are short-lived, PTH is actually trophic for bone and can produce quite large increases in spine bone density. For that reason, PTH 1-34 is now an approved therapy for osteoporosis.

Osteogenesis Imperfecta

Osteogenesis imperfecta (OI) is a group of heritable disorders in which one of several mutations may occur in the genes encoding for the collagen molecules that comprise the bulk of bone matrix (9). Patients with OI have fragile skeletons with reduced bone mass. In one of the common forms of OI, long bones typically have narrow shafts as well as reduced mass. Patients with OI commonly suffer many fractures throughout life, often starting in utero. When some other amino acid replaces glycine in the collagen molecule, the triple helix will not coil properly, collagen synthesis is reduced, and the matrix is abnormal. The severity of the defect depends on the position of the substitution in the chain of the collagen molecule. Fractures heal normally. Other collagen-based connective tissues are also affected in certain forms of the disease, including dentin, ligaments and tendons, and sclerae. Despite the manifest abnormality of the bone matrix, the reason for the reduction in bone mass is unclear.

Bony Manifestations of Diseases of Nonskeletal Systems

Patients with chronic liver disease, but especially with biliary cirrhosis, commonly have a bone disease that is basically osteoporosis (10). Patients who are to undergo liver transplantation often have severe osteoporosis, attributable to a combination of the underlying disease, the immobilization that inevitably accompanies the severe disability of these very sick patients, and the treatments they have received.

Patients with end-stage renal disease often have a complex bone disease consisting of a varying mixture of osteosclerosis, osteomalacia, and hyperparathyroid bone disease (11). Exact expression of these varied abnormalities depends on the medical regimens the patients receive, specifically the way in which these regimens manage calcium, phosphorus, and vitamin D metabolism for the patient.

Patients with a variety of disorders of the small intestine, but especially those with gluten-sensitive enteropathy, malabsorb fat-soluble vitamins and hypersecrete calcium and magnesium into the digestive juices. As a result, these patients are commonly deficient in vitamin D, calcium, and magnesium. They often have severe osteoporosis and may have osteomalacia as well.

Patients who have had organ transplants commonly have osteoporosis (12), in part because they present for organ transplantation with already reduced bone mass and in part because the immunosuppressive therapy used to sustain the transplant itself causes bone loss.

Aluminum and Bone

Aluminum (Al) is not strictly speaking a nutrient, but it is extremely common in the environment, is a major component of antacids, and is widely used as cookware. Only a small fraction of ingested Al is absorbed, and in healthy persons, absorbed Al is promptly excreted in the urine. However, in patients with severely compromised renal function, particularly in those treated with large doses of Al-containing antacids to block phosphorus absorption, Al accumulates at the mineralizing sites of the bone remodeling process. It was thought at one time to be responsible for the unique bony pathologic features of end-stage renal disease, but it is now considered only a minor contributor to renal osteopathy. Experimentally, Al has shown an ability to increase trabecular bone density in animals, particularly in combination with fluoride. The ultimate significance of this finding remains uncertain.

SKELETAL MANIFESTATIONS OF SYSTEMIC NUTRIENT DEFICIENCIES

Protein-Calorie Malnutrition

As noted earlier, the cells of bone are as dependent on total nutrition as are other cells, and bone suffers in starvation just as do other tissues. However, bone strength is not immediately affected in acute malnutrition, especially in adults. The bony effects of protein-calorie malnutrition are most obvious in two situations: one is during growth, when both growth rates and bone mass accumulation are retarded by malnutrition; and the other is in the repair of fractures, especially in elderly persons. Protein-calorie malnutrition is common among old elderly persons, and when they break a bone, such as the hip, serious complications and even death may ensue. Protein supplementation has been shown to reduce these complications substantially, and it is an important and necessary component of the treatment of most patients with hip fractures (13). The reason for the trophic effect of protein on bone is partly that dietary protein helps to sustain normal insulinlike growth factor I concentrations, needed for bone growth and repair (14), and partly that, as already discussed, bone formation requires fresh dietary protein.

Magnesium Deficiency

Magnesium deficiency occurs in severe intestinal malabsorption (e.g., gluten-sensitive enteropathy, fistulas, or ileal resection, especially with high-fat diets) or with urinary losses from renal tubular defects. Initially, magnesium deficiency impairs bony responsiveness to PTH and thus leads to hypocalcemia despite a rising PTH level. As deficiency progresses, parathyroid response falters, and PTH secretion falls. The hypocalcemia of magnesium deficiency is thus the result of impairment of the calcium regulatory system and is unresponsive to calcium supplementation (15) (see also Chapter 9). Less severe degrees of magnesium deficiency in these same syndromes are associated with reduced bone mass, also unresponsive to

calcium supplementation. In addition to other needed treatments (e.g., calcium), magnesium supplements are necessary in these patients.

INVESTIGATION OF NUTRIENT EFFECTS ON THE SKELETON

As already noted, the effects of nutrient deficiencies on the skeleton express themselves slowly in adults. For this same reason, nutrient effects on the skeleton of any kind are difficult to detect and easy to misinterpret.

Change in Bone Mass

As noted earlier, bone is a composite of mineral and matrix, and bone mass refers to the quantity of such bone present in the whole organism (or in a particular body region). Technically, changes in bone mass itself cannot be measured in vivo, because no way of detecting the organic component of the composite is known. However, in conditions of health, and in fact in most bone diseases, the proportion of mineral and matrix is about the same (50:50, by volume). In addition, quite good methods are available for measuring bone mineral. Mineral content can be measured either for the whole skeleton or for various regions of interest by x-ray absorptiometric methods (see later). *Change* in bone mass is measured either by classic metabolic balance methods or by serial absorptiometry.

The classic nutritional approach to nutrient status is the measurement of a metabolic balance, in this case calcium (or phosphorus) balance. Because more than 99% of body calcium is in the skeleton, total body calcium balance reflects predominantly bone balance. Moreover, because calcium is essentially never removed from or added to preformed bone tissue (rather, units of tissue itself are removed or added), it follows that body calcium balance is a direct measure of bone tissue balance. The balance method is theoretically the ideal way of assessing change in bone mass, but it is expensive, and balance studies are difficult to perform accurately. The principal source of this difficulty, for poorly absorbed nutrients such as calcium, is that most of the ingested calcium ends up in the feces. Accurate timing of fecal excretion is nearly impossible. Moreover, the lag time between ingestion and fecal excretion averages several days in healthy adults, and failure to take that lag time into account leads to serious misinterpretation of calcium balance results (16). Colored dye markers demarcating treatment periods are not adequate safeguards. Rather, continuous intake markers (e.g., polyethylene glycol [PEG 4000]) are required, and fecal output must be adjusted both for its polyethylene glycol content and for the time lag.

A newer approach, and one ideally suited to measurement of the quantity of bone present, is the direct measurement of bone mineral (17), either in a specific region or in the skeleton as a whole, by the technique of dual-energy x-ray absorptiometry (DXA). A tightly collimated beam of x-rays is passed back and forth across the body (or one of its regions), and absorption of its photons is measured by a detector on the side opposite the x-ray source. Absorption is a function of the amount of mineral present in the path of the beam. This method measures, for example, spine mineral content in as little as 2 to 5 minutes and has a reproducibility on the order of 1 to 2% in healthy young adults.

Because total body calcium in an adult is in the range of 900 to 1500 g, and because change in bone mass (in other words, positive or negative calcium balance) is rarely more than ±100 mg/day (and usually much less), it follows that closely spaced, repeat measurements by DXA will produce results within the reproducibility error of the method. For that reason, measurements in persons must usually be separated by 12 to 24 months. (Less time will not allow for measurable change to occur.) Thus, although DXA permits rapid and accurate measurement of bone *mass*, it is not very sensitive to the sorts of *change in mass* that have physiologic or nutritional significance.

The Remodeling Transient

Any intervention, nutritional or otherwise, that alters bone remodeling activity will produce a transient change (18) in calcium balance (or bone mass), which results from the asynchrony of the remodeling cycle (see earlier). Because of the temporal separation of resorption and formation at each remodeling site, suppression of remodeling will produce a prompt but temporary increase in bone mass (Fig. 84.7). If this follows, for example, the administration of supplemental calcium, phosphorus, or vitamin D, the retention

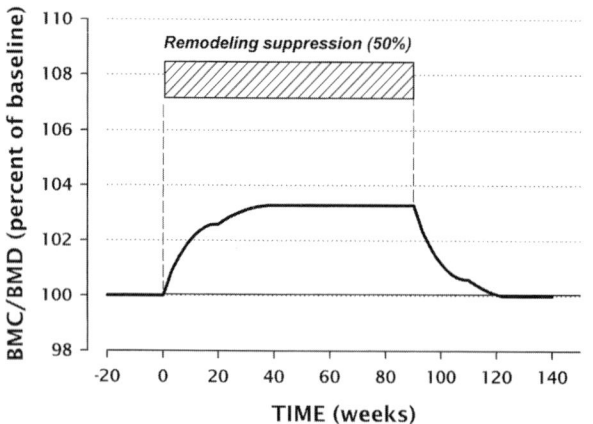

Figure 84.7. Positive bone remodeling transient in a healthy person who is not calcium deficient, in response first to a large increase in calcium intake (sufficient to suppress remodeling by 50%) and then to its later withdrawal. The vertical axis is bone mass (i.e., either bone mineral content [BMC] or bone mineral density [BMD]), expressed as a percentage of the baseline value. The initial rise in bone mass does not continue past one remodeling cycle (40 weeks in this illustration), and the bone gained by remodeling suppression is lost once again when remodeling returns to its previous level. (Copyright Robert P. Heaney, 1996.)

of bone mineral should not be interpreted to mean that the patient has a preexisting deficiency. (Such a deficiency may be present, of course, but positive balance will occur whether or not deficiency is present, simply because, initially, the resorptive component of remodeling is reduced more than the formative component.) Because the remodeling cycle lasts at least 3 months in healthy young adults, bone mass and calcium balance continue to change under the influence of this asynchronous remodeling for at least that long. The process may actually take a year or more in elderly persons for formation and resorption once again to come into equilibrium. Response to nutritional interventions can be interpreted only *after* the transient is complete. If, at that time, balance is more positive (or bone mass by DXA is still increasing), only then can one safely conclude that the subjects needed more of the nutrient than they had previously been receiving.

Bone Histomorphometry

The term histomorphometry means the measurement of shapes on histologic specimens of bone (19). As noted earlier, many substances attach to bone crystals as they are forming and then become trapped as more bone is laid down on top of them. Some of those substances, like the tetracycline antibiotics, fluoresce brilliantly when they are illuminated by ultraviolet light. Histomorphometry takes advantage of that property by giving patients paired, timed doses of tetracycline several days before obtaining a bone biopsy (typically from the iliac crest). Specimens are sectioned on special microtomes without first removing the mineral and are then examined with an ultraviolet microscope. Figure 84.4 presents a typical photomicrograph from such a labeled biopsy. Because the distance between fluorescent lines can be measured with a calibrated eyepiece or by shape-sensing software, and because the times of administration are known, one can derive a direct and reasonably precise estimate of the rate at which the remodeling cells are working and how active the remodeling process may be. Among other histologic features, measurements are made not only of the distance between labels but also of the extent of bone surface covered with a label. This method is very useful for studying bone biology and disease, but it has limited applicability to the study of nutritional problems affecting bone.

Biochemical Markers of Bone Remodeling

In the synthesis of bone collagen, the ends of the collagen molecules are clipped off as the triple helix is assembled, the proline molecules in the peptide chain are converted to hydroxyproline, and cross-links are developed between the side chains of adjacent collagen fibrils, involving particularly lysine and hydroxylysine protruding from the backbone of the peptide chain. Additionally, both alkaline phosphatase and the noncollagenous proteins are secreted into the matrix; in this process, some of these substances

TABLE 84.2. BIOCHEMICAL MARKERS OF BONE REMODELING

FORMATION	RESORPTION
Serum alkaline phosphatase	Urine hydroxyproline
Bone specific	Urine pyridinium cross-links
Total	Pyridinoline
Serum osteocalcin	Deoxypyridinoline
Serum procollagen type I	Peptide cross-links
propeptide	Urine amino terminal cross-
Carboxyterminal (P1CP)	links (NTx)
	Urine carboxyterminal cross-
Amino terminal (P1NP)	links (CTx)
	Serum carboxyterminal cross-
	links (CTx)

leak into the bloodstream, where they can be measured. Later, when bone is broken down, the hydroxyproline residues and the cross-links, because they cannot be recycled, are metabolized or excreted. All these activities leave residues or produce effects that can be measured in serum or urine. Collectively, these circulating or excreted substances are called biochemical biomarkers of bone remodeling (20). They reflect in a general way the level of bone remodeling activity. Table 84.2 summarizes the principal markers currently in use, together with the component of remodeling they are thought to reflect most directly. In this connection, when remodeling activity changes, ultimately both resorption and formation generally change, almost always in the same direction, and often to very nearly the same extent. Under steady-state conditions, therefore, a marker for either formation or resorption may be used as an index of remodeling activity.

Although measurements of bone biomarkers can be a relatively inexpensive way of assessing bone remodeling activity under differing nutritional conditions, they are at most only semiquantitative. In other words, a 50% drop in a resorption marker does not mean a 50% reduction in the amount of bone resorbed. In addition, the markers exhibit important discrepancies among themselves. For example, serum alkaline phosphatase is high in nutritional rickets despite a generally low level of new bone apposition, and $1,25(OH)_2$ vitamin D elevates serum osteocalcin apparently without altering actual bone-forming activity (21).

The effects of nutritional deficiencies on the relationship between marker level and the process it reflects have not been studied. Nevertheless, to the extent that a nutritional deficiency alters bone remodeling, one can expect to find corresponding changes in remodeling marker levels. Thus, the accelerated bone loss of the aged that results from calcium deficiency is associated with elevated excretion of deoxypyridinoline and hydroxyproline. Calcium supplementation both stops or slows the bone loss and reduces urinary excretion of these resorption markers.

REFERENCES

1. Gokhale JA, Robey PG, Boskey AL. The biochemistry of bone. In: Marcus R, Feldman D, Kelsey J, eds. Osteoporosis, Vol 1. 2nd ed. San Diego: Academic Press, 2001:107–88.
2. Kannus P, Haapasalo H, Sievanen H et al. Bone 1994;15:279–84.
3. NIH Consensus Conference. JAMA 1994;272:1942–8.
4. Vermeer C. Vitamin K and bone health. In: Burckhardt P, Dawson-Hughes B, Heaney RP, eds. Nutritional Aspects of Osteoporosis, 2nd ed. San Diego: Elsevier Academic Press, 2004:79–92.
5. Marcus R, Majumder S. The nature of osteoporosis. In: Marcus R, Feldman D, Kelsey J, eds. Osteoporosis, Vol 2. 2nd ed. San Diego: Academic Press, 2001:3–17.
6. Heaney RP. Bone 2003;33:457–65.
7. Pettifor JM. Nutritional and drug-induced rickets and osteomalacia. In: Favus MJ, ed. Primer on the Metabolic Bone Diseases and Disorders of Mineral Metabolism. 5th ed. Washington, DC: American Society for Bone and Mineral Research, 2003: 399–407.
8. Glorieux FH. Hypophosphatemic vitamin D resistant rickets. In: Favus MJ, ed. Primer on the Metabolic Bone Diseases and Disorders of Mineral Metabolism. 5th ed. Washington, DC: American Society for Bone and Mineral Research, 2003:414–7.
9. Shapiro JR. Osteogenesis imperfecta and other defects of bone development as occasional causes of adult osteoporosis. In: Marcus R, Feldman D, Kelsey J, eds. Osteoporosis, Vol 2. 2nd ed. San Diego: Academic Press, 2001:271–301.
10. Herlong HF, Recker RR, Maddrey WC. Gastroenterology 1982;83:103–8.
11. Goodman WG, Coburn JW, Ramirez JA et al. Renal osteodystrophy in adults and children. In: Favus MJ, ed. Primer on the Metabolic Bone Diseases and Disorders of Mineral Metabolism. 5th ed. Washington, DC: American Society for Bone and Mineral Research, 2003:430–47.
12. Epstein S. J Bone Miner Res 1996;11:1–7.
13. Delmi M, Rapin C-H, Bengoa J-M et al. Lancet 1990;335: 1013–6.
14. Wüster C, Rosen C. Growth hormone, insulin-like growth factors: potential applications and limitations in the management of osteoporosis. In: Marcus R, Feldman D, Kelsey J, eds. Osteoporosis, Vol 2. 2nd ed. San Diego: Academic Press, 2001: 747–67.
15. Rude RK. Magnesium depletion and hypermagnesemia. In: Favus MJ, ed. Primer on the Metabolic Bone Diseases and Disorders of Mineral Metabolism. 5th ed. Washington, DC: American Society for Bone and Mineral Research, 2003:292–5.
16. Heaney RP. Bone Miner 1986;1:99–114.
17. Faulkner KG. Clinical use of bone densitometry. In: Marcus R, Feldman D, Kelsey J, eds. Osteoporosis, Vol 2. 2nd ed. San Diego: Academic Press, 2001:433–58.
18. Heaney RP. J Bone Miner Res 1994;9:1515–23.
19. Recker RR, Barger-Lux MJ. Transilial bone biopsy. In: Bilezikian JP, Raisz L, Rodan GA, eds. Principles of Bone Biology. 2nd ed. San Diego: Academic Press, 2002:1595–664.
20. Garnero P, Delmas PD. Biochemical markers of bone turnover in osteoporosis. In: Marcus R, Feldman D, Kelsey J, eds. Osteoporosis, Vol 2. 2nd ed. San Diego: Academic Press, 2001: 459–77.
21. Feldman D, Malloy PJ, Gross C. Vitamin D: biology, action, and clinical implications. In: Marcus R, Feldman D, Kelsey J, eds. Osteoporosis, Vol 1. 2nd ed. San Diego: Academic Press, 2001: 257–303.

NUTRITION AND DIET IN RHEUMATIC DISEASES[1]

SARAH L. MORGAN AND JOSEPH E. BAGGOTT

DEFINITION OF RHEUMATIC DISEASES 1326
GENERAL NUTRITIONAL ASPECTS OF ARTHRITIS 1326
   Strategies to Improve Nutritional Status 1326
   Drug-Nutrient Interactions 1327
GOUT 1327
   Definition 1327
   Mechanisms of Hyperuricemia 1327
   Metabolic Profile 1328
   Dietary Therapy 1328
OSTEOARTHRITIS 1329
   Definition 1329
   Nutrient Intakes and Nutritional Status 1329
   Relationship between Obesity and Osteoarthritis 1329
   Vitamin D 1330
   Glucosamine and Chondroitin Sulfate as Therapy 1330
RHEUMATOID ARTHRITIS .1330
   Definition 1330
   Mechanisms Affecting Nutritional Status 1330
   Nutrient Intakes and Vitamin Levels 1330
   Nutritional Status 1331
   Body Composition of Patients 1331
   Diet Therapy 1332
ω-3 FATTY ACIDS AS THERAPY FOR ARTHRITIS 1335
ANTIOXIDANTS AND ARTHRITIS 1335
METHOTREXATE AND FOLATE: AN EXAMPLE
   OF A PREVENTABLE DRUG-NUTRIENT
   INTERACTION 1335
SUMMARY 1336

DEFINITION OF RHEUMATIC DISEASES

"Rheumatic diseases are characterized by inflammation (redness and/or heat, swelling, and pain) and loss of function of one or more connecting or supporting structures of the body. Rheumatic diseases typically affect joints, tendons, ligaments, bones, and muscles producing symptoms such as pain, swelling, and stiffness. Some rheumatic diseases involve internal organs" (1). Some examples of rheumatic diseases are infectious arthritis, osteoarthritis, psoriatic arthritis, rheumatoid arthritis, fibromyalgia, systemic lupus erythematosus, gout, polymyositis, bursitis, and tendinitis. The best estimates are that arthritis and other rheumatic diseases affected 70 million adults in the United States in 2001 (2, 3). If arthritis prevalence rates remain stable, the number of persons with arthritis could double by 2030 (4). This chapter discusses the nutritional correlates and therapies of gout, osteoarthritis, and rheumatoid arthritis.

GENERAL NUTRITIONAL ASPECTS OF ARTHRITIS

The nutritional aspects of rheumatic diseases are evaluated from several perspectives including (a) the nutritional status of patients with arthritis, (b) the effects of drug therapies on nutrients and nutritional status (drug-nutrient interactions), (c) the involvement of nutrients in disease or drug mechanisms, and (d) the evaluation of diet therapy and supplements used as treatments.

In 1981, a link between nutrition and arthritis was only beginning to be accepted (5). In 1981, the Arthritis Foundation, in *The Truth about Diet and Arthritis*, stated: "the possible relationship between diet and arthritis has been thoroughly and scientifically studied. The simple proven fact is no food has anything to do with causing arthritis and no food is effective in treating or 'curing' it" (6). Twenty years later, their brochure, *Diet and Your Arthritis*, stated, "Research has shown several connections between food, nutritional supplements (vitamins, minerals and ω-3 fatty acids) and certain forms of arthritis or related conditions, such as gout, osteoporosis, osteoarthritis, rheumatoid arthritis, and reactive arthritis" (7). The use of nutritional therapies for arthritis is increasing (8–13).

Strategies to Improve Nutritional Status

Strategies exist to help patients in the preparation of food (14). Many different adaptive tools are available to aid in the preparation and consumption of adequate diets including cookbook holders, door knob extenders, extended drinking straws, over-the-sink cutting boards, jar lid openers, rolling trivets, nonskid pads, easy-grip utensils, pan holders, and handles for milk cartons. For example, Figure 85.1A shows proper posture when preparing foods, Figure 85.1B shows the use of a rolling cutting board to minimize lifting, and Figure 85.1C shows an

---

[1]**Abbreviations: AA,** arachidonic acid; **BMI,** body mass index; **Ig,** immunoglobulin; **RDA,** recommended dietary allowance; **TNF,** tumor necrosis factor.

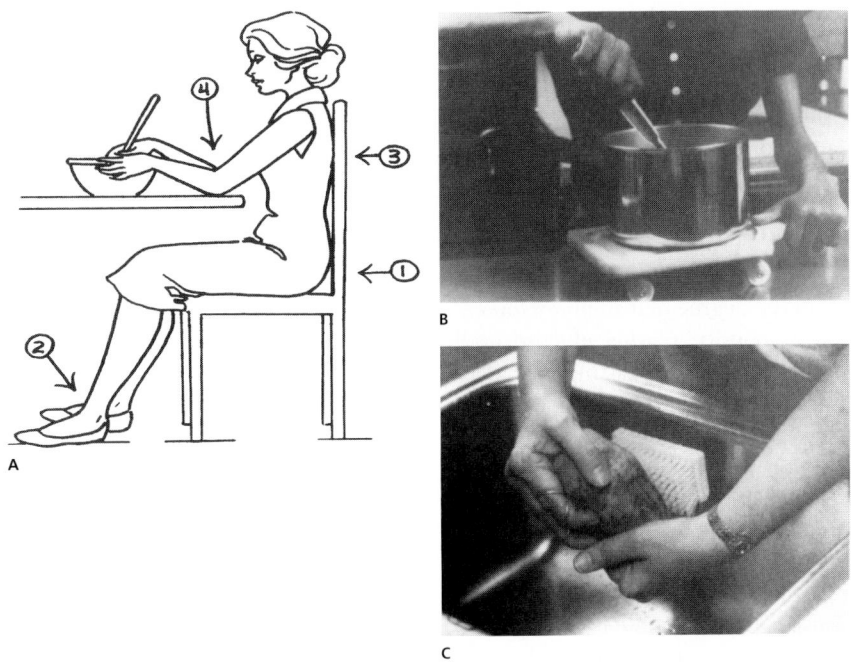

Figure 85.1. A. Correct posture for food preparation. **B.** The use of a rolling cutting board to minimize lifting. **C.** The attachment of a vegetable brush with suction cups to the sink for scrubbing vegetables. (From University of Alabama Research Foundation. The Essential Arthritis Cookbook. Mankato, MN: Appletree Press, 1999:45, 47, 61, with permission.)

energy-saving technique of attaching a brush with suction cups to the sink for scrubbing fresh vegetables.

Drug-Nutrient Interactions

Drugs used to treat arthritis interact with and affect the need for a wide variety of nutrients. Examples of some common drug-nutrient interactions include iron deficiency caused by gastrointestinal bleeding from aspirin or nonsteroidal antiinflammatory drug use and altered folate status after treatment with the antifolate, methotrexate, in patients with rheumatoid arthritis. Table 85.1 outlines other possible drug-nutrient interactions.

TABLE 85.1. ARTHRITIS DRUG-NUTRIENT INTERACTIONS

DRUG	AFFECTED NUTRIENT STATUS
Aspirin	↓ Folate, ↓iron, ↓vitamin C
Salicylate	↓ Folate
Nonsteroidal antiinflammatory drugs	↓Iron, ↓folate
Sulfasalazine	↓Folate
Methotrexate	↓Folate
Corticosteroids	↓Calcium, ↓vitamin D, ↓potassium, ↓zinc, ↓vitamin C, ↓magnesium, ↓folate, ↓selenium
Tetracycline	↓Calcium, ↓magnesium, ↓iron,
Colchicine	↓Vitamin B₁₂, ↓sodium, ↓potassium,
D-Penicillamine	↓Vitamin B₆, ↓magnesium, ↓zinc, ↓copper

Data from references 14 and 144 to 146.

GOUT

Definition

"Gout is a crystalline arthritis that results from deposits of uric acid in joints. The crystals cause inflammation, swelling, and pain in the affected joint, especially the big toe (podagra)" (1). The clinical spectrum of gout can range from an acute arthritis to accumulation of uric acid crystalline deposits, called tophi, or uric acid urolithiasis and, less frequently, renal failure (gout nephropathy) (15).

Mechanisms of Hyperuricemia

Uric acid is the end product of purine catabolism in humans. At most, dietary purines can contribute one third of the uric acid of the blood uric acid level (16). Patients with gout who consumed a purine-free diet had little change in plasma uric acid levels compared with uric acid levels after a regular diet (17). Hyperuricemia is defined as a serum uric acid level greater than 7.0 mg/dL in men and greater than than 6.0 mg/dL in women, and it is a common feature in all types of gout. Overt manifestations of gout are more likely when the serum urate level is greater than 9.0 mg/dL and urinary uric acid excretion is greater than 800 mg/day (18).

The basic mechanisms of hyperuricemia are overproduction (~10% of patients) and underexcretion (~90% of patients) of uric acid. Overproduction, for example, could result from myeloproliferative disorders, malignant diseases, and hemolytic anemias. Metabolic errors that cause increased purine and urate production include hypoxanthine-guanine phosphoribosyltransferase deficiency, phosphoribosylpyrophosphate synthetase overactivity, and glucose-6-phosphatase deficiency (19). Impaired urate clearance may result from renal failure, dehydration, diabetic ketoacidosis, ethanol intake, diuretics, low-dose aspirin, and the use of ethambutol, pyrazinamide, levodopa, methoxyflurane, and cyclosporine (19).

Strong correlations exist between insulin resistance and serum uric acid levels and between renal uric acid clearance impairment and the degree of insulin resistance (20, 21). The presence of obesity, plasma glucose and insulin response to a 75-g glucose load, fasting uric acid concentration, insulin-mediated glucose disposal, and urinary uric acid clearance were measured in 36 healthy persons who were not diabetic and who had no history of gout (21). A significant correlation was noted between the degree of insulin resistance and the serum uric acid concentration. Urinary uric acid clearance was also inversely related to the degree of insulin resistance. In an additional study, serum uric levels and a timed urinary uric acid collection were evaluated in 568 physiologically normal Italian men (20). Elevated serum uric acid levels were related to increased resorption of sodium in the kidney proximal tubule versus the distal tubule. This finding suggested that insulin resistance produces increased sodium resorption along with elevated serum uric acid levels.

Metabolic Profile

The prevalence of gout appears to be rising in the United States (22). Gout is much more frequent in men than in women and is most common in persons aged 40 to 60 years (15, 23). Using the Rochester Epidemiology Project computerized medical record system, cases of acute gout were abstracted in 1977 to 1978 and 1995 to 1996 (22). More than a twofold increase in primary gout occurred between the two time periods, and this was not related to thiazide diuretic therapy. The authors speculated that increasing prevalence of the underlying metabolic risk factor, insulin resistance, could play a role. The classic profile of a patient with gout is an obese, hypertensive, middle-aged man who drinks alcohol (15). Using data from the Tecumseh Community Health Study, a significant correlation was seen between serum uric acid levels and body weight (24). The metabolic profile of syndrome X, which includes hyperlipidemia, obesity, diabetes mellitus, and hypertension (see also Chapter 62), is frequent in patients with gout (25), and patients with hyperuricemia have more insulin resistance and dyslipidemia than patients with normouricemia (26).

Dietary Therapy

Pharmacologic therapy with allopurinol, which decreases oxidation of purines to uric acid, and uricosuric agents, such as probenecid and sulfinpyrazone, has changed the therapy of gout. Dietary therapies can be considered to have additive benefits to pharmacologic therapy, although they rarely lower serum urate levels by greater than 1 mg/dL, even with severe purine restriction (15, 17, 27, 28). However, the dietary management of gout is still useful, particularly during a gouty flare. Conventional therapies include the following recommendations (see later for updated recommendations):

1. Maintain a healthy body weight because weight loss in overweight patients has been shown to decrease plasma urate levels (29, 30).
2. Undertake gradual weight loss because fasting and rapid weight loss can increase urate levels (31).
3. Follow a diet low in fat, saturated fat, and cholesterol because patients with gout often have hyperlipidemia.
4. Consume alcohol in moderation or not at all because alcohol increases blood uric acid levels by mechanisms including (a) alcohol-induced lactic acidemia and lactate competition for urate excretion by the kidney, (b) stimulation of purine biosynthesis, and (c) the high purine content of beer (16).
5. Consume liberal amounts of fluid daily (2–3 quarts/day) to prevent the formation of uric acid kidney stones.
6. Consume moderate amounts of protein and foods low in purine content to prevent excessive uric acid production.

Foods with the highest purine content include kidney, liver, and other organ meats and certain seafoods. Foods that are moderate in purine content include muscle meats, whole-grain breads and cereals, poultry, dried beans and peas, asparagus, spinach, and mushrooms. Foods low in purine content that can be eaten in unlimited amounts are vegetables (except for those in the moderate-purine category), fruits, milk, cheese, eggs, non–whole-grain breads, sugar, and nuts.

More recent trials have caused a rethinking of these guidelines. After 16 weeks of a 1600-kcal diet consisting of 40% complex carbohydrates, 30% monounsaturated and polyunsaturated fat, and 30% protein, 13 white men with recent gouty attacks had significantly lower serum uric acid, total cholesterol, and triglyceride levels. The diet resulted in a mean weight loss of 7.7 kg and a significantly lowered incidence of acute gouty attacks (32). The authors suggested that the lower insulin resistance resulted in increased renal urate clearance (21, 32, 33). A similar reduction in serum urate levels was found using a stepwise reduction from 1500 to 1200, 1200 to 1000, and finally 1000 to 800 kcal/day over 12 weeks in 27 overweight persons (31). In another study, 15 overweight persons with gout received a low-purine, alcohol-free diet for 1 week and then a low-carbohydrate, weight-reduction diet until the desired weight was achieved (29). These persons then received a low-purine diet for a week. An average 8-kg weight loss was achieved, along with a significant decrease in plasma uric acid levels. Increased renal uric acid clearance was associated with a lower serum uric acid level. Therefore, the new goals for gout management include a major emphasis on diet therapy to reduce insulin resistance and to produce weight loss in overweight patients.

OSTEOARTHRITIS

Definition

"Osteoarthritis is a common type of arthritis affecting an estimated 21 million adults in the United States. Osteoarthritis primarily affects cartilage, which is the tissue that cushions the ends of bones within the joint. In osteoarthritis, the cartilage begins to fray and may entirely wear away. Osteoarthritis can cause joint pain and stiffness. Disability results most often when the disease affects the spine and the weight-bearing joints (the knees and hips)" (1).

Nutrient Intakes and Nutritional Status

A series of 12 patients with osteoarthritis was evaluated with diet history questionnaires. More than 50% of the patients consumed diets with less than 67% of the recommended dietary allowances (RDAs) for iron, zinc, vitamin E, folate, and vitamin B_6 (34). Eighty-two older ambulatory patients were assessed by a registered dietitian using a food-frequency questionnaire and a weight history (35). Eighty percent had a body mass index (BMI) of greater than or equal to 27, and the average weight gain since early adulthood was 59 lb (~27 kg). Dietary assessment revealed that dietary intakes were not optimal in the grain and dairy groups. Dietary intakes in 77 patients who were participating in a multidisciplinary program for the management of osteoarthritis were evaluated (36). Seventy-nine percent of the patients were obese as determined by BMI, and the degree of obesity was related to the pain of arthritis. Using a 24-hour dietary recall and a food-frequency questionnaire, dietary intakes of vitamin D, folate, pyridoxine, and zinc were less than 80% of the RDA (see Appendix Table A-2-b). In another study, patients with osteoarthritis averaged 15 lb (6.8 kg) overweight, whereas patients with rheumatoid arthritis averaged 10 lb (4.5 kg) underweight (37).

In a study of patients with rheumatoid arthritis and osteoarthritis who were undergoing joint surgery, the patients with osteoarthritis had a higher average BMI than did the patients with rheumatoid arthritis (27.7 versus 21.6) and a higher upper arm muscle circumference as an indicator of somatic muscle protein (38). Osteoarthritis at weight-bearing joints such as the knees and hips is increased in obese persons; however, osteoarthritis of non–weight-bearing joints is also increased in obese persons, a finding suggesting alterations in cartilage and bone metabolism at these sites (39–44). Because many of these studies are cross-sectional, it can logically be asked whether the obesity may be caused by a more sedentary lifestyle after the development of arthritis. However, being overweight at age 37 years increased the risk of developing osteoarthritis in people in their 70s (45).

Relationship between Obesity and Osteoarthritis

Many nutritional factors favor the progression of osteoarthritis, including obesity (46, 47). The relationship of obesity and metabolic factors associated with obesity with osteoarthritis is controversial. Whether magnified weight forces across a joint (three to six times the body weight is exerted against the knee during walking) or metabolic factors such as insulin resistance increase the risk of osteoarthritis is not clear (48). Oliveria and colleagues (49) evaluated 134 matched case-control pairs of women and found that osteoarthritis of the hand, hip, and knee was positively related to body weight, even after controlling for estrogen use, smoking, height, and health care use. The Chingford Study (50) assessed blood pressure, blood glucose, serum cholesterol, triglycerides, and uric acid levels and weight-bearing knee radiographs in 1003 women. The investigators found radiographic evidence of knee osteoarthritis in 118 women. For unilateral knee osteoarthritis, elevated blood glucose and moderately elevated serum cholesterol levels were significantly related to radiographic evidence of osteoarthritis. For bilateral knee osteoarthritis, the associations with hypertension and elevated cholesterol were significant. In contrast, the Baltimore Longitudinal Study of Aging (51) evaluated physical and metabolic findings in white persons (464 men and 275 women more than 40 years old) including knee radiographs, blood pressure, fasting lipid levels, a 2-hour glucose tolerance test, and anthropometric measurements. No metabolic factors were found to be related to osteoarthritis, even after adjusting for age and obesity. Given the relationship of osteoarthritis with non–weight-bearing sites, it is likely that both weight-bearing status and metabolic factors play a role.

Data from the Framingham Osteoarthritis Study (52) suggest that a weight loss of 5 kg will reduce the risk of development of knee osteoarthritis over the subsequent 10 years by 50%. Persons who underwent gastric bypass operations, with a mean weight loss of 46 kg, experienced less joint pain in the knees and the hips after the operation (53). Messier and associates (54) evaluated 24 community-dwelling adults who were more than 60 years of age and who had a BMI greater than 28, knee pain, radiographic evidence of knee osteoarthritis, and self-reported disability. The study subjects participated in either a program of exercise and diet or an exercise-alone program. The exercise program consisted of weight training and walking, and the dietary intervention included counseling by nutritionists as well as a cognitive-behavioral modification program designed to produce a weight loss of 15 lb (6.7 kg) over 6 months. At 6 months, the investigators noted a mean loss of 19 lb (8.6 kg) in the exercise and diet group versus a mean loss of 4 lb pounds (1.8 kg) in the exercise-alone group. Both groups reported significant improvements in self-reported disability and knee pain intensity and frequency as well as modest improvements in knee strength. However, no statistical differences in knee pain scores or in self-reported measurements of physical function were reported between the two groups. The authors concluded that weight loss in patients with knee arthritis could lead to improvements in pain, disability, and performance. Toda and colleagues (55) demonstrated that changes in body fat and increasing exercise, but not decreasing body weight, were responsible for improving symptoms of osteoarthritis in persons receiving a low-calorie diet, mazindol, and nonsteroidal antiinflammatory drugs. In conclusion, it is likely that weight reduction will lessen osteoarthritis pain and disability.

Vitamin D

Participants in the Framingham Heart Study had two knee radiographs, assessments of vitamin D dietary intake by a food-frequency questionnaire, and measurement of serum 25-hydroxyvitamin D levels. Persons with low dietary intakes of vitamin D and low 25-hydroxyvitamin D levels (<30 ng/mL) were more likely to have progression of established osteoarthritis, but these factors did not affect the risk for development of osteoarthritis. The authors hypothesized that low vitamin D status hinders the response of bone to cartilage damage occurring in osteoarthritis (56).

The Study for Osteoporotic Fractures Research Group found that the development of hip joint space narrowing was increased in persons in the middle and lowest tertile of serum 25-hydroxyvitamin D levels compared with the highest tertile (57). Elderly women with low serum 25-hydroxyvitamin D levels were three times more likely to develop hip joint space narrowing than women with levels in the highest tertile. The authors postulated that the relationship of vitamin D levels with osteoarthritis could be through their effect on bone and cartilage metabolism (46). These observations merit further prospective evaluations.

Glucosamine and Chondroitin Sulfate as Therapy

The use of nutraceuticals as therapy has increased since the mid-1990s (8–13). Numerous trials have evaluated both glucosamine and chondroitin sulfate in osteoarthritis therapy. Glucosamine occurs in hyaluronic acid, which is a glycosaminoglycan in synovial fluid, and chondroitin sulfate is a glycosaminoglycan found in cartilage, tendons, and ligaments. A metaanalysis of glucosamine and chondroitin sulfate for the treatment of osteoarthritis evaluated 15 clinical trials and concluded that both compounds had moderate to large treatment effects on symptoms. However, problems with the quality of the studies and a publication bias from drug company support likely overestimated the treatment

effects (58). Additionally, a metaanalysis of injected hyaluronic acid for the treatment of knee osteoarthritis concluded that this subtance had little or no efficacy (59). Presumably, one reason for using glucosamine and chondroitin sulfate supplements would be to increase hyaluronic acid biosynthesis. Investigators have suggested that, until more placebo-controlled, double-blind trials can be completed, caution be used with these agents (60). A large National Institutes of Health trial is currently under way.

RHEUMATOID ARTHRITIS

Definition

"Rheumatoid arthritis is an inflammatory disease of the synovium or lining of the joint, and results in pain, stiffness, swelling, joint damage, and loss of function of the joints. Inflammation most often affects joints of the hands and feet and tends to be symmetrical. This symmetry helps distinguish rheumatoid arthritis from other forms of the disease. About 1% of the US population, (about 2.1 million people) have rheumatoid arthritis" (1). Published reports noted that patients with rheumatoid arthritis had excess deaths, deterioration of radiographs, and reduced functional status, despite disease-modifying antirheumatic drug treatment (61–64).

Mechanisms Affecting Nutritional Status

Rheumatoid arthritis can affect nutritional status through several mechanisms (65–67) (Table 85.2). Joint swelling and tenderness can impair food preparation, involvement of the temporomandibular joint can impair chewing, and general joint involvement can impair self-feeding. In addition, patients may have xerostomia that can impair food intake. Many of the pharmacologic therapies used to treat rheumatoid arthritis also have side effects that further inhibit food intake, such as nausea with methotrexate or proteolysis with corticosteroid therapy (68, 69). Moreover, the catabolic and inflammatory aspects of the disease affect nutritional status.

Nutrient Intakes and Vitamin Levels

In 1996, Kremer (70) found that patients with rheumatoid arthritis ingest diets that are too high in total fat, too low in fiber, and deficient in micronutrients. Forty-one patients with active rheumatoid arthritis were evaluated with 3-day dietary records. In this study population, the diets were deficient in pyridoxine, zinc, magnesium, folate, and copper when compared with the RDAs and the typical American diet. Kremer suggested that patients with rheumatoid arthritis should be routinely prescribed a multiple vitamin with trace minerals.

Morgan and associates (67, 71) evaluated the nutrient intake of methotrexate-treated adults with rheumatoid arthritis by using dietary recalls and circulating vitamin

TABLE 85.2. ADVERSE EFFECTS OF RHEUMATOID ARTHRITIS ON NUTRITIONAL STATUS

Increased nutrient requirements
Increased metabolism and nitrogen losses increase protein requirements.
Inflammation increases micronutrient requirements (i.e., antioxidant vitamins).

Diminished intake
Articular disease diminishes the ability to self-feed, shop, and prepare foods.
Morning stiffness may decrease morning appetite.
Temporomandibular joint disease may impair the ability to chew.
Depression from chronic disease may impair food intake.
Sjögren syndrome and xerostomia may impair food intake.

Diminished absorption
Abnormalities of the small bowel, liver, and pancreas may decrease absorption of nutrients.
Drug therapy such as salicylazosulfpyridine may inhibit nutrient absorption.

Inadequate utilization
Drugs therapy such as methotrexate, salicylazosulfapyridine, and nonsteroidal antiinflammatory drugs may inhibit enzymes of intermediary metabolism.
Vitamin B_{12} deficiency can reduce folate uptake and retention by the cells.

Increased excretion
Urinary excretion of nutrients may be increased in the catabolic state of active disease and by some drug treatments such as prednisone.
Chronic blood loss from nonsteroidal antiinflammatory agents may increase the need for hematopoietic precursors (e.g., iron).

From Morgan SL, Hine RJ, Vaughn WH et al. Arthritis Care Res 1993;6:4–10, with permission. Arthritis Care and Research © 1993, Wiley.

levels. In the first study, 32 patients, aged 28 to 75 years, with a mean disease duration of 12 years, were evaluated (67). Intakes of pyridoxine, calcium, magnesium, and zinc were less than 33% of the 1989 RDA values. Thirty percent of the patients had a deficient plasma folate level, and 23% had a deficient erythrocyte folate level before starting methotrexate therapy. In a subsequent study, 79 patients were followed for 1 year after starting methotrexate therapy (71). A total of five 24-hour dietary recalls were taken. Analyses of vitamin A, thiamin, riboflavin, pyridoxine, plasma and erythrocyte folate, vitamin B_{12}, vitamin C, vitamin E, and total carotenoid intakes were performed. The mean age of the study population was 53 years, and the mean disease duration was 9 years. The patients consumed less than 67% of the reference dietary intake for folate, vitamin B_{12}, vitamin E, calcium, iron, magnesium, copper, and zinc. Before the start of methotrexate therapy, 47% of patients had deficient plasma folate levels, and 11% had deficient erythrocyte folate levels.

Nutritional Status

Helliwell and colleagues (72) evaluated 50 patients with rheumatoid arthritis and 50 normal control subjects using anthropometric and biochemical measurements including serum albumin, transferrin, retinol-binding protein, thyroxine-binding prealbumin, zinc, and folic acid levels. Patients were classified as being malnourished if they had a reduction in one anthropometric measurement with two or more biochemical abnormalities. The upper arm muscle circumference was reduced in 14% of patients, and most of the biochemical measures were low in the patients. Thirteen of 50 patients met the criteria for malnutrition, versus none of the controls (72).

Collins and associates (73) studied 38 hospitalized patients with rheumatoid arthritis. A likelihood of malnutrition index was calculated that included serum folate and vitamin C levels, triceps skinfold or BMI calculation, arm muscle area corrected for bone area, total lymphocyte count, serum albumin, and hematocrit. Twenty-seven of 38 patients had a high likelihood of malnutrition index.

Mody and colleagues (74) assessed the nutritional status of 220 patients with rheumatoid arthritis by using triceps skinfold, upper arm muscle circumference, BMI, percentage of ideal body weight, and serum albumin measurements. Forty-five of 220 patients (20%) had a low value in one or more anthropometric measurement, and six patients (3%) had a low albumin level. This subcategory of malnourished patients had more severe functional disabilities. Obesity, defined as a BMI greater than 30, was also found in 10% of this population. In contrast, Kalla and associates (75) compared 65 patients with rheumatoid arthritis with 71 matched controls by using anthropometric measurements and serum protein levels. Lean body mass was estimated by anthropometric measures and was similar in the controls and in the patients. Corticosteroid therapy did not have an effect on anthropometric measurements.

Hernandez-Beriain and associates (76) evaluated 75 outpatients with rheumatoid arthritis who had variable functional class, radiologic stage, seropositivity status, presence of extraarticular disease, and disease duration. Nutritional status was evaluated by measurements of weight, height, midupper arm circumference, and triceps skinfold and by calculation of midarm muscle area and midarm fat area. Lean body mass, as evaluated by midupper arm circumference, was lower in patients with a lower rheumatoid arthritis functional class. In 24% of the patients, measurements were lower than the tenth percentile, and in 14% of patients they were lower than the fifth percentile. The authors concluded that patients with a poorer functional class, with more severe radiographic disease, or with extraarticular disease had worse nutritional status and loss of lean body mass than did patients with less severe disease.

Body Composition of Patients

Comorbidities of rheumatoid arthritis include weight loss and loss of lean body mass, termed rheumatoid cachexia, which is the end product of the hypermetabolism associated with this disease (77–80). Sir James Paget first described rheumatoid cachexia in 1873 (81).

Several studies have documented significant clinical wasting in patients with rheumatoid arthritis. Munro and Capell (82) evaluated BMI, upper arm fat mass (an estimate of body fat mass), and upper arm muscle area (an estimate of body somatic muscle mass) by anthropometric measurements. Greater than half the patients with rheumatoid arthritis had values in the lowest tenth percentile for upper arm muscle area, a finding reflecting a loss in somatic muscle stores and the catabolic nature of the disease. In addition, female patients had a correlation between low fat mass and elevated erythrocyte sedimentation rates and C-reactive protein levels. The wasted patients were also more disabled in their ability to perform activities of daily living, as assessed by the Health Assessment Questionnaire.

Roubenoff and colleagues (77) investigated body composition in patients with rheumatoid arthritis and correlated rheumatoid cachexia with cytokine levels. In a group of 24 patients, 67% were cachectic, and their lean body mass was inversely associated with numbers of swollen joints. This finding suggested that protein catabolism and gluconeogenesis may be required to maintain a high level of disease activity. Chronic caloric deficits were apparently not a cause of lower lean body mass. Elevated tumor necrosis factor-α (TNF-α) levels were found in three of five patients with flaring joints. TNF-α levels were not elevated in patients with less active disease. A later study evaluated the relationship between cytokine production and body composition in 23 adult patients whose disease was considered by their rheumatologists to be under good control, without changes in medication dosage over the past 3 months (83). Patients were compared with 23 healthy adults matched for age, sex, race, and weight. Lean body mass was 13% lower in those with rheumatoid arthritis than in matched controls, a finding indicating a loss of approximately one third of mobilizable muscle cell mass. This finding was surprising in patients who were considered to have minimal disease. Cytokine production from peripheral blood mononuclear cells was also increased in these patients, and higher interleukin-1β and TNF-α production was associated with increased resting energy expenditure. Several strategies have been used to try to alter the detrimental effects of chronic stress of rheumatoid arthritis on body composition (84, 85). Progressive resistance exercise has been shown to increase strength, but it is not accompanied by changes in body composition (84, 85). Rall and associates (86) showed that treatment with methotrexate normalized leucine kinetics, probably as a result of a reduction in protein catabolism.

Morgan and colleagues (71) measured BMI in 79 patients who were starting methotrexate for rheumatoid arthritis. Sixty percent of the patients had a BMI lower than 25, 10% of patients were moderately underweight (BMI, 18–20.9), and 4% were severely underweight (BMI, <18). Forty percent of patients were overweight;

with 30% having grade I obesity (BMI, 25–29.9), 9% having grade II obesity (BMI, 30–40) and 1% had grade III obesity (BMI, >40). Roubenoff and colleagues (87) found that the low physical activity levels of women with rheumatoid arthritis result in lower total energy expenditures. Although patients with rheumatoid arthritis are at risk for cachexia, poor food choices and inactivity make them also at risk for obesity (88, 89).

Diet Therapy

Effect of Foods on Rheumatic Symptoms

In 1943, 31 patients with arthritis were evaluated to determine their dietary history for the year before the onset of rheumatoid arthritis (90). Although their dietary intakes were not substantially different from the dietary intakes of a cross-section of families in the North Atlantic United States, more than two thirds of patients had diets deficient in calcium, thiamin, and riboflavin, and approximately 50% had a low intake of vitamin C. In general, it has not been possible to identify any nutrient intake differences in patients who develop rheumatoid arthritis.

More recent surveys have looked at the effect of diet on rheumatic symptoms (91, 92). In a study of 742 patients with rheumatoid arthritis, juvenile rheumatoid arthritis, ankylosing spondylitis, psoriatic arthropathy, primary fibromyalgia, and osteoarthritis, one third of patients with rheumatoid arthritis reported a worsening of symptoms with specific foods (91). Forty-three percent of patients with juvenile rheumatoid arthritis reported an exacerbation of symptoms with specific foods. The foods most frequently cited were meat, wine, alcohol, coffee, sweets, sugar, chocolate, apples, and citrus fruits.

Specific Diets as Therapy

Panush and colleagues (93) conducted a double-blind, placebo-controlled trial of diet therapy for patients with active rheumatoid arthritis who met American College of Rheumatology criteria. The experimental diet was modeled after the "Dong Diet" (94, 95) and was free of additives, preservatives, fruit, red meat, herbs, and dairy products. The placebo diet also excluded items from some major food groups so it mimicked the experimental diet. Clinical evaluations occurred at entry and termination of the 10-week trial, and compliance with both diets was greater than 95%. No differences were seen between the experimental diet and the placebo diet in patients' global assessment of disease, examiners' assessment of disease, duration of morning stiffness, 50-foot walking time, grip strength, numbers of tender or swollen joints, and erythrocyte sedimentation rates. The authors described two patients who improved markedly on the experimental diet and who elected to continue the experimental diet after the termination of the protocol.

Fifty patients with rheumatoid arthritis according to the 1987 American College of Rheumatology criteria were followed in a 24-week double-blind, randomized trial of a well-balanced diet versus a diet low in saturated fat, high in polyunsaturated fat, and with "hypoallergenic" foods (96). The caloric content of the experimental diet was set to facilitate weight loss and to achieve the patient's ideal body weight. The investigators noted a significant reduction in the number of tender joints and erythrocyte sedimentation rate between the experimental diet and the balanced diet. No other measures of disease activity were significantly different. No difference was observed between the study groups in the number of patients experiencing a 20 or 50% improvement in disease. Weight loss during the protocol may have had a beneficial effect on disease activity. These studies reinforce the conclusion no specific therapeutic diet exists for rheumatoid arthritis.

Food Allergy

That allergic responses to food may be related to rheumatoid arthritis disease activity is a relatively old idea. In the early 1900s, many reports of arthritis caused by specific foods appeared (5, 97–104). Van der Laar and colleagues (105) reported circumstantial evidence for a relationship between rheumatoid arthritis and food allergy, as shown in Table 85.3. The human gut contains immunologically active cells in the Peyer patches (105–109). Mechanisms that may alter the handling of food antigens include atrophic gastritis, increased intestinal permeability, and alteration in gut flora.

Thirty-five patients, who reported food-related gastrointestinal symptoms, were evaluated to determine whether a relationship existed between joint swelling or arthralgias and the presence of immune complexes in the serum (110). The number of patients with circulating immune complexes was higher in patients with arthralgias than in those patients without arthralgias, and levels of complexes were higher in the patients with arthralgias. The authors used this evidence to support the idea that food-related gastrointestinal symptoms may involve

TABLE 85.3. CIRCUMSTANTIAL EVIDENCE FOR A RELATION AMONG RHEUMATOID ARTHRITIS, FOOD, AND ALLERGY

I	Food intolerances in individual patients suffering RA
II	Food-induced symptoms in other arthritides
III	Modulation of the immune response by nutritional components
IV	Different antigen handling by the gut in RA
V	Presence of increased IgE and of rheumatoid factor activity of IgE in RA
VI	Frequent occurrence of eosinophilia in RA
VII	Mast cell infiltration of the inflamed synovial membrane in RA

IgE, immunoglobulin E; RA, rheumatoid arthritis.

From van de Laar MAFJ, van der Korst JK. Semin Arthritis Rheum 1991;21:12–23, with permission from Elsevier.

immunologic or allergic mechanisms. However, the success of elemental diets, which do not contain antigenic proteins, has been variable (111, 112).

In a study of 704 patients, 28% believed in an association between a specific food and their disease activity (92). The foods that were thought to have an unfavorable effect on their arthritis included preservatives, beef, pork, food additives, milk, and sugar. Patients with a history of allergy, a history of drug allergy, or a family history of allergy were more likely to report an association between foods and disease activity.

Panush and associates (113) described a patient with inflammatory arthritis that worsened with milk intake. She was fasted for several days, then was given an elemental diet for 33 days, and finally was given blinded food challenges. Placebo foods such as lettuce and carrots caused no exacerbations in joint symptoms. Four blinded milk challenges caused increases in morning stiffness and swollen and joints. Immune studies suggested delayed and cutaneous hyperreactivity to milk. An additional case study documented a patient whose rheumatoid arthritis was worsened by intake of milk and cheese (114).

In conclusion, it is likely that food allergy plays some role in rheumatoid arthritis in a small percentage of patients; however, in the majority, it is not likely a major factor. If patients indicate that they have an arthritis flare associated with a food, a prudent course of action would be to avoid the offending food. Referral to a registered or licensed dietitian can be beneficial to make sure that the diet is nutritionally adequate.

Fasting and Vegetarian Diets

The use of fasting and vegetarian diets has been extensively reviewed (5, 98) (see also Chapters 48 and 103). Preliminary reports of improvements in disease activity with fasting led to speculation on the relationship of rheumatoid arthritis with dietary antigens, because fasting would lower the antigen stimulus to the gut mucosa.

In 1979, Sköldstam and colleagues (115) studied patients with rheumatoid arthritis who were randomized to a control diet or to a 10-day fast, followed by a lactovegetarian diet. The fasting patients received 800 kcal/day from fruit and vegetable juices. These patients were purged with castor oil and received five water enemas on the first day of the fast. After fasting, the patients began a lactovegetarian diet for 1 week and then were discharged with instructions to follow the diet for an additional 9 weeks. Yogurt was allowed, but other dairy products were discouraged. Ten patients served as controls and consumed a more typical diet. When compared with the control group, five of 15 patients had a 10% decrease in erythrocyte sedimentation rate and a five-point or more decrease in the Ritchie articular index of joint tenderness. However, only one of 14 in the diet group had persistent improvement after 9 weeks of the vegetarian diet. The fasting patients lost an average of 3.5 kg during the fasting period, and this could itself have altered disease activity.

In an additional study by the same group (116), 20 patients were followed for several months on the ordinary diet and then, after fasting, began a vegan diet. They were inpatients for 4 weeks and were fasted initially for about 10 days. The vegan diet also did not include refined sugar, corn flour, salt, strong spices, preservatives, alcoholic beverages, tea, and coffee. At the end of the trial, the patients improved in their pain perception; however, they had no significant changes in grip strength, tender joint counts, and an index of joint tenderness compared with the control period. The authors concluded that the benefit of the diet was only in subjective assessments, but the underlying disease was not suppressed.

Kjeldsen-Kragh and associates (117) completed a randomized, single-blinded controlled trial of patients who stayed at a health farm for 4 weeks. After an initial 10-day subtotal fast, the patients were changed to a gluten-free vegan diet for 3.5 months and then a lactovegetarian diet for the remainder of the trial. A control group stayed at a convalescent home and ate a general diet. Compared with the control group, at 1 month, the diet group had a significant improvement in the number of tender joints, the Ritchie articular index, the number of swollen joints, the pain score, the duration of morning stiffness, grip strength, erythrocyte sedimentation rate, C-reactive protein level, and the health assessment questionnaire score. The patients in the convalescent home had a decrease only in the pain score. At 13 months, a persistent improvement was noted in the diet group compared with the control group in most of the indices. The radiographic score deteriorated slightly in both groups at the end of the trial. Although food allergy was suspected, the authors stated that it probably did not explain the results. These investigators speculated that changes in fatty acids in the diet or weight loss could have affected disease activity.

Numerous subanalyses were completed on the subjects undergoing the foregoing, single-blind protocol. The nutritional status of the patients on the fast and vegetarian diet compared with the control group was studied over 13 months (118). The BMI and triceps skinfold significantly decreased in the diet group versus the control group; however, the upper arm muscle area was not different. No significant differences were reported in serum albumin, hemoglobin, ferritin, zinc, and copper levels between the two groups, findings suggesting that the fasting and vegetarian diet had only a minor effect on nutritional status. Platelet counts, white blood cell counts, total immunoglobulin (Ig) G, IgM rheumatoid factor, and complement factors C3 and C4 were significantly lower in the diet group after 1 month (119). At 1 year, only white blood cell count, IgM rheumatoid factor, and C3 and C4 were significantly different. The diet group was classified as diet responders and diet nonresponders based on subjective improvement in joint disease activity. The responders had

greater decreases in platelet count, C3, and C4 than the nonresponders. Stool samples were also analyzed for bacterial fatty acid profiles (120). Fecal flora changed markedly when the patients changed from the omnivorous diet to the vegan diet and differed markedly between patients with high and low response. The authors speculated that changes in gut flora could be beneficial to disease activity by reducing intestinal inflammation and reducing absorption of bacterial and dietary antigens.

Differences in psychologic factors between the subjects who volunteered for the trial and other patients without rheumatoid arthritis not in the trial and between diet responders and nonresponders were evaluated (121). The study patients had a stronger belief in their ability to influence their health status and a lower belief that chance affects their health. The study patients also had a greater belief in the efficacy of alternative forms of treatment. When the diet group was classified as responders and nonresponders, responders had a significantly lower belief in the effectiveness of traditional medical care than nonresponders. This finding suggested that patients with specific psychologic characteristics were selected for the clinical trial and that the expectations concerning the efficacy of alternative therapies could have contributed to the effect of the vegetarian diet.

A 2-year follow-up of the study patients found that all the diet responders and half of the diet nonresponders were still following a modified diet (121). No food item was identified that worsened joint disease. A significant difference was also noted in the pain score, the duration of morning stiffness, the number of tender joints, the Ritchie articular index, and the number of swollen joints between diet responders and the control patients. This finding suggests that some subgroup of patients with rheumatoid arthritis can benefit from a vegetarian diet, and the effects of the diet can be sustained.

In a more recent study, Nenonen and associates (122) randomized 43 patients to a control diet or a diet that was an uncooked vegan diet, rich in lactobacilli. One half of the dietary group experienced nausea or diarrhea during the dietary intervention and stopped the diet prematurely. The Health Assessment Questionnaire score, the duration of morning stiffness and pain at rest and with movement, the Ritchie articular index, and C-reactive protein levels were not different between the control and diet groups at 2 months. However, a composite disease activity score that measured subjective changes in arthritis was significantly improved in the dietary intervention group compared with the control group. The bacterial fatty acid profile of stool in groups with and without improvement was evaluated (123). A significant difference was seen in fecal flora between patients with improvement and those with little improvement after 1 month of the diet. The authors speculated that changes in fecal flora are related to changes in disease activity.

Finally, McDougall and colleagues (124) reported on a 4-week, very-low-fat (10% of total calories) vegan diet intervention in free-living patients with rheumatoid arthritis.

Before starting the diet and 4 weeks afterward, these patients were evaluated by a rheumatologist who was blinded to the study design. The investigators noted a significant loss in body weight in these patients, but erythrocyte sedimentation rate, C-reactive protein, and rheumatoid factor levels did not change. The joint tenderness score, the joint swelling score, and the severity of morning stiffness decreased significantly, but no significant change in duration of morning stiffness was reported. The patients who had the largest degree of improvement had the most active disease at the beginning of the study, and those with long-standing disease showed little improvement. The authors concluded that a vegan diet could improve patients' symptoms and speculated that changes in intestinal permeability to antigens and levels of food and bacterial antigens could be mechanisms.

In conclusion, fasting and a vegetarian type of diet may have beneficial effects in a subset of patients, although the evaluation of these studies is hampered by the lack of placebo-controlled, double-blind designs. Food allergy may be related to disease activity in these patients. Fasting is obviously not a long-term therapeutic approach to the management of rheumatoid arthritis.

ω-3 FATTY ACIDS AS THERAPY FOR ARTHRITIS

Perhaps the first suggestion that the composition of dietary fat could affect inflammation was the observation that Native Greenlanders have a low prevalence of asthma, psoriasis, and rheumatoid arthritis when compared with Europeans (125). The Native Greenlanders' daily intake of the fish oil containing the ω-3 series of fats, mainly eicosapentaenoic and docosahexenoic acids (see Chapter 5), was about 8 g versus only 0.2 g in Europeans. The finding that the ω-3 series fatty acid can replace the ω-6 series fatty acids (i.e., linoleic acid and arachidonic acid [AA]) in cell membrane phospholipid (and thus alter function) and can interfere with AA metabolism to inflammatory eicosanoids (126) undoubtedly stimulated the clinical trials of fish oil fatty acids in the treatment of rheumatoid arthritis. A supplement mixture of both eicosapentaenoic and docosahexenoic acids was used, generally in the range of 2 to 5 g and 1 to 3 g/day, respectively. Reviews of well-controlled studies (70, 127) concluded that this regimen generally lowered the duration of morning stiffness and physician and patient global assessment of disease, with some reduction in the number of swollen joints. Based on low cost, low toxicity, and the possibility for lowering the dose of potentially toxic drugs, it is now the consensus that fish oil supplements should be a part of standard therapy in rheumatoid arthritis (128, 129).

The mechanism of action of fish oil fatty acid has been reviewed (126). In general, these ω-3 fatty acids compete with and block formation of inflammatory prostaglandins, prostacyclins, thromboxanes, and leukotrienes produced from fatty acids of the ω-6 series (see also Chapter 5). Metabolism of ω-3 fatty acid to the foregoing compounds is slower, and the resulting prostaglandins, thromboxanes, and prostacyclins with three double bonds or leukotrienes with five double bonds are less inflammatory and bioactive. Even moderate fish oil supplementation will alter membrane phospholipids composition, mainly by replacing AA, whereas high-dose fish oil supplements will alter both membrane composition and neutrophil function (130). In addition, studies have shown that fish oil supplements suppress the production of the proinflammatory interleukin 1-β (129). More recent studies using human osteoarthritic cartilage show that ω-3, but not ω-6, fatty acids suppress mRNA production of both cyclooxygenase and lipoxygenase enzymes, a finding suggesting that these fatty acids may act at the level of protein synthesis as well as interfering with existing amounts of enzyme (131).

ANTIOXIDANTS AND ARTHRITIS

Without question, activated immunologic cells directly produce reactive oxygen species, including superoxide free radical, hydrogen peroxide, and hypochlorous acid (132, 133) (see also Chapter 44). In addition, joint tissue itself is probably damaged by reactive oxygen species generated by the ischemia and reperfusion process (134). Proposed in this process is a mechanically induced temporary occlusion of capillary beds (ischemia) that depletes adenosine triphosphate levels and as a result increases purine base levels. During reperfusion, purine bases are oxidized, oxygen is used by xanthine oxidase, and uric acid and the superoxide free radical are formed.

A broader question remains: Is antioxidant therapy of benefit to patients with rheumatoid arthritis and osteoarthritis? Many patients with rheumatoid arthritis have low vitamin C nutriture; however, no reports indicate that supplemental vitamin C alters the clinical course of the disease (126). Although the guinea pig model of osteoarthritis benefits from supplemental ascorbic acid, no study in humans appears to be available to confirm this finding (46, 135). Conversely, it is possible that adequate vitamin C nutrition reduces the risk of osteoarthritis (136).

Vitamin E has the potential of interfering with AA metabolism and therefore should have antiinflammatory properties (136). Again, few reports of only moderate beneficial effects of vitamin E therapy for rheumatoid arthritis and osteoarthritis exist (46). In conclusion, it is likely that patients with arthritis suffer from overproduction of reactive oxygen species rather than underprotection by antioxidant nutrients (137, 138).

METHOTREXATE AND FOLATE: AN EXAMPLE OF A PREVENTABLE DRUG-NUTRIENT INTERACTION

Methotrexate therapy is widely viewed as the current standard in the treatment of rheumatoid arthritis. Evidence exists that low-dose methotrexate blocks purine nucleotide

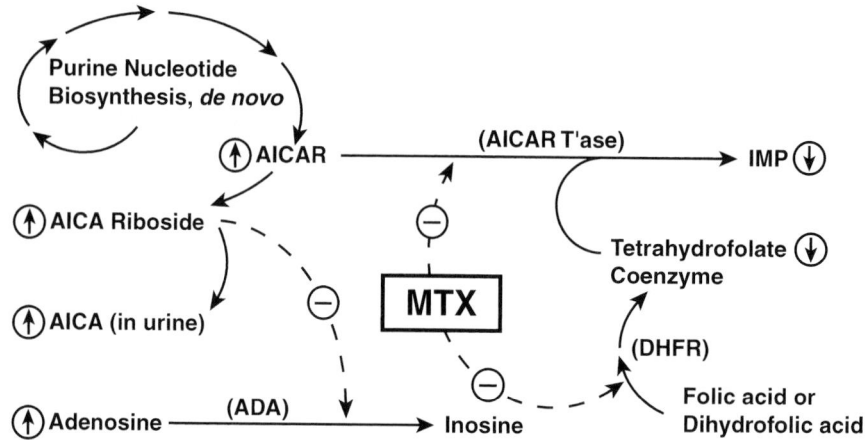

Figure 85.2. Proposed mechanism of action of low-dose methotrexate (MTX) therapy for rheumatoid arthritis. ADA, adenosine deaminase; AICA, aminoimidazolecarboxamide; AICAR, AICA ribotide; AICAR T'ase, AICAR transformylase; DHFR, dihydrofolate reductase; IMP, inosine monophosphate. (*Dotted lines with negative signs in circles* indicate enzyme inhibition; *circles with arrows* indicate increased or decreased in vivo levels.)

biosynthesis at a folate-dependent step catalyzed by aminoimidazolecarboxamide ribotide transformylase, and that this produces immunosuppression via adenosine accumulation (139, 140) (Fig. 85.2). Because methotrexate is a general antifolate, the the drug has the potential to produce a functional deficiency of folate. Indeed, Morgan and associates (141, 142) found that certain methotrexate toxicities such as cytopenias resemble those found in uncomplicated folate deficiency, whereas others such as liver toxicity probably are the toxic effect of methotrexate. Because methotrexate toxicity, even in the presence of efficacy, is a major reason for discontinuing the drug, compelling reasons exist to ameliorate these side effects.

Several studies demonstrated that folic acid supplementation of methotrexate-treated patients with rheumatoid arthritis lowers drug toxicity while preserving efficacy (141, 142). The mechanism is not known; however, it is possible that the folic acid supplement replenishes folate coenzyme levels in organs susceptible to methotrexate-induced folate deficiency (i.e., enterocyte, liver), whereas it has little effect on methotrexate cytotoxicity in immunologic cells. It is now routinely recommended that patients with rheumatoid arthritis receiving methotrexate also be supplemented with folic acid (143).

SUMMARY

Reduced capacity for food preparation and poor intake result in poor nutritional status for some patients. In recent decades, both overweight and underweight patients have appeared. For the overweight patient, it is especially important to lose weight and normalize insulin sensitivity, which will probably alleviate some symptoms of gout and osteoarthritis and possibly of rheumatoid arthritis.

The hypermetabolic state of rheumatoid arthritis leads to loss of lean body mass. The removal of specific foods from the diet and fasting followed by a vegetarian diet may

help a small subset of patients with rheumatoid arthritis. Specific diets and glucosamine and chondroitin sulfate supplements remain unproven therapies for the treatment of rheumatoid or osteoarthritis. Conversely, ω-3 fatty acid supplements have some benefit in the treatment of rheumatoid arthritis. Although oxidative stress is associated with arthritis, antioxidant therapy is not a proven treatment. An example of a preventable adverse drug-nutrient interaction is the use of folic acid supplements to prevent methotrexate toxicity in patients with rheumatoid arthritis.

Acknowledgment

The clerical support of Ms. Jackie Rainey is gratefully acknowledged.

REFERENCES

1. National Institute of Arthritis and Musculoskeletal and Skin Diseases. *www.niams.nih.gov/hi/topics/arthritis/artrheu.htm.* Bethesda, MD: National Institutes of Medicine, 2002.
2. Centers for Disease Control and Prevention. MMWR Morb Mortal Wkly Rep 2001;50:120–5.
3. Centers for Disease Control and Prevention. MMWR Morb Mortal Wkly Rep 2002;51:948–50.
4. Centers for Disease Control and Prevention. MMWR Morb Mortal Wkly Rep 2003;52:489–91.
5. Henderson C, Panush R. Rheum Dis Clin North Am 1999;25: 937–65.
6. Arthritis Foundation. Atlanta, GA: Arthritis Foundation, 1981.
7. Arthritis Foundation. Atlanta, GA: Arthritis Foundation, 2003.
8. Taibi DM, Bourguigon C. Fam Comm Health 2003;26: 41–52.
9. Fautrel B, Adam V, St-Pierre Y et al. J Rheumatol 2002;29: 2435–41.
10. Panush RS. J Rheumatol 2002;29:656–8.
11. Kaboli PJ, Doebbeling BN, Saag KG et al. Arthritis Rheum 2001;45:398–403.
12. Ramsey SD, Spencer AC, Topolski TD et al. Arthritis Rheum 2001;45:222–7.
13. Rao JK, Mihaliak K, Kroenke K et al. Ann Intern Med 1999; 131: 409–16.

14. Arthritis Center and Department of Nutrition Sciences at the University of Alabama at Birmingham. The Essential Arthritis Cookbook. Mankato, MN: Appletree Press, 1999.
15. Boulware DW, Becker MA, Edwards NL. Gout and crystal induced synovitis. In: Koopman WJ, Boulware DW, Heudebert GR, eds. Clinical Primer of Rheumatology. Philadelphia: Lippincott Williams & Wilkins, 2003:262–77.
16. Fam AG. J Rheumatol 2002;29:1350–54.
17. Porcelli B, Vannoni D, Leoncini R et al. In: Sahota A, Taylor M, eds. Purine and Pyrimidine Metabolism in Man VIII. New York: Plenum Press, 1995:47–52.
18. Gutman A. Postgrad Med 1972;51:61–6.
19. Becker MA, Roessier BJ. Hyperuricemia and gout. In: Scriver CR, Beaudet AL, Sly WS, Valle D, eds. The Metabolic and Molecular Bases of Inherited Disease. 7th ed. New York: McGraw-Hill, 1995:1655–77.
20. Cappuccio FP, Strazzullo P, Farinaro E et al. JAMA 1993;270: 354–9.
21. Facchini F, Chen Y-D, Hollenbeck C et al. JAMA 1991;266: 3008–11.
22. Arromdee E, Michet C, Crowson C et al. J Rheumatol 2002;29: 2403–6.
23. Yeomans A. Nurse Pract 1991;16:18–26.
24. Myers AR, Epstein FH, Dodge HJ et al. Am J Med 1968;45: 520–8.
25. Nakamura T, Tsutani H, Ueda T. Jpn J Clin Med 1996;54: 3248–5.
26. Zavvroni I, Mazza S. J Intern Med 1993;234:25–30.
27. Emerson BT. N Engl J Med 1996;334:445–51.
28. Yu T-F. Am J Med 1974;56:676–85.
29. Nicholls A, Scott JT. Lancet 1972;2:1223–4.
30. Emerson BT. Adv Exp Med Biol 1974;41:429–33.
31. Yamashita S, Matsuzawa Y, Tokunaga K et al. Int J Obes 1986; 10: 255–64.
32. Dessein P, Shipton E, Stanwix A et al. Ann Rheum Dis 2000;59: 539–43.
33. Snaith M. Lancet 2001;358:525.
34. Kowsari B, Finnie S, Carter R et al. J Am Diet Assoc 1983;82: 657–59.
35. White-O'Connor B, Sobal J, Muncie J, H.L. J Am Diet Assoc 1989;378–82.
36. White-O'Connor B, Sobal J. Clin Ther 1986;9:30–43.
37. Eising L. J Bone Joint Surg 1963;45:69–81.
38. Haugen M, Homme K, Reigstad A et al. Arthritis Care Res 1999;12:26–32.
39. Bray GA. Endocrinol Metab Clin North Am 1996;25:907–19.
40. Hartz AJ, Fischer ME, Bril G et al. J Chronic Dis 1986;39: 311–19.
41. van Saase J, Vandenbroucke JP, van Romunde L et al. J Rheumatol 1988;15:1152–8.
42. Leach RE, Baumgard S, Broom J. Clin Orthop 1973;93:271–3.
43. Watson M. Rheum Rehab 1976;15:264–9.
44. Acheson RM, Collart AB. Ann Rheum Dis 1975;34:379–87.
45. Felson D, Anderson JJ, Naimark A et al. Ann Intern Med 1988; 109:18–24.
46. McAlindon T, Felson D. Ann Rheum Dis 1997;56:397–402.
47. Felson D, Zhang Y. Arthritis Rheum 1998;41:1343–55.
48. Felson D. Ann Rheum Dis 1996;55:668–70.
49. Oliveria SA, Felson D, Cirillo PA et al. Epidemiology 1999;10: 161–6.
50. Hart DJ, Doyle DV, Spector TD. J Rheumatol 1995;22: 1118–23.
51. Martin K, Lethbridge-Cejku, Muller DC et al. J Rheumatol 1997;24:702–7.
52. Felson D, Zhang Y, Anthony JM et al. Ann Intern Med 1992; 116:535–9.
53. McGoey BV, Deitel M, Saplys R et al. J Bone Joint Surg Br 1990;72:322.
54. Messier SP, Loeser RF, Mitchell MN et al. J Am Geriatr Soc 2000;48:1062–72.
55. Toda Y, Toda T, Takemura S et al. J Rheumatol 1998;25:2181–6.
56. McAlindon T, Felson D, Zhang Y et al. Ann Intern Med 1996; 125:353–59.
57. Lane N, Gore R, Cummings S et al. Arthritis Rheum 1999;42: 854–60.
58. McAlindon T, LaValley M, Gulin J et al. JAMA 2000;283: 1469–75.
59. Lo G, LaValley M, McAlindon T et al. JAMA 2003;290:3115–21.
60. Callaghan J, Buckwalter J, Schenck R. Clin Orthop 2000;381: 88–90.
61. Chehata JC, Hassell AB, Clarke SA et al. Rheumatology 2001; 40:447–52.
62. Riise T, Jacobsen BK, Gran JT et al. Clin Rheumatol 2001;20: 123–7.
63. Wong J, Ramey D, Singh G. Arthritis Rheum 2001;44:2746–9.
64. Gordon P, West J, Jones H et al. J Rheumatol 2001;28:2409–15.
65. Martin R. Proc Nutr Soc 1998;57:231–4.
66. Touger-Decker R. J Am Diet Assoc 1988;88:327–31.
67. Morgan SL, Hine RJ, Vaughn WH et al. Arthritis Care Res 1993;6:4–10.
68. Heimburger DC, Weinsier RL. Therapeutic diets. In: Shanahan J, ed. Handbook of Clinical Nutrition. 3rd ed. St. Louis: CV Mosby, 1997:235–66.
69. Roubenoff R, Roubenoff RA, Ward LM et al. Am J Clin Nutr 1990;52:1113–7.
70. Kremer J, Bigaouette J. J Rheumatol 1996;23:229–4.
71. Morgan SL, Anderson AM, Hood SM et al. Arthritis Care Res 1997;10:9–17.
72. Helliwell M, Coombes E, Moody B et al. Ann Rheum Dis 1984; 43:386–90.
73. Collins R, Dunn T, Harrell W et al. Clin Rheumatol 1987; 6:391–8.
74. Mody GM, Brown GM, Meyers OL et al. S Afr Med J 1989;76: 255–7.
75. Kalla AA, Brown GM, Meyers OL. S Afr Med J 1992;82:411–4.
76. Hernandez-Beriain J, Segura-Garcia C, Rodriguez-Lozano B et al. Scand J Rheumatol 1996;25:383–7.
77. Roubenoff R, Roubenoff RA, Cannon JG et al. J Clin Invest 1994;93:2379–86.
78. Walsmith J, Roubenoff R. Int J Cardiol 2002;85:89–99.
79. Rall L, Walsmith J, Snydman L et al. Arthritis Rheum 2002;46: 2574–7.
80. Zoico E, Roubenoff R. Nutr 2002;60:39–51.
81. Paget J. Lancet 1873;2:727–9.
82. Munro R, Capell H. Ann Rheum Dis 1997;56:326–9.
83. Roubenoff R. J. Nutr 1997;127:1014S–6S.
84. Rall LC, Roubenoff R. Arthritis Care Res 1996;9:151–6.
85. Rall L, Roubenoff R, Cannon JG et al. Med Sci Sports Exerc 1996;28:1356–65.
86. Rall LC, Rosen CJ, Dolnikowski G et al. Arthritis Rheum 1996;39:1115–24.
87. Roubenoff R, Walsmith J, Lundgren N et al. Am J Clin Nutr 2002;76:774–9.
88. Ahluwalia IB, Mack KA, Murphy W et al. MMWR CDC Surveill Summ 2003;52:1–80.
89. Haffner S, Taegtmeyer H. Circulation 2003;108:1541–5.
90. Bayles TB, Richardson H, Hall FC. N Engl J Med 1943;229: 319–24.

91. Haugen M, Kjeldsen-Kragh J, Nordvåg B et al. Clin Rheumatol 1991;10:401–7.
92. Tanner SB, Callahan LF, Panush R et al. Arthritis Care Res 1990;3:189–95.
93. Panush R, Carter R, Katz P et al. Arthritis Rheum 1983;26:462–71.
94. Dong CH, Banks J. The Arthritic's Cookbook. New York: Thomas Y. Crowell, 1973.
95. Dong CH, Banks J. New Hope for the Arthritic. New York: Thomas Y. Crowell, 1975.
96. Sarzi-Puttini P, Comi D, Boccassini L et al. Scand J Rheumatol 2000;29:302–7.
97. Panush R. Rheum Dis Clin North Am 1991;17:259–72.
98. Panush R. In: Koopman WJ, ed. Arthritis and Allied Conditions: A Textbook of Rheumatology. 14th ed. Philadelphia: Lippincott Williams & Wilkins, 2001:965–86.
99. Lewin P, Taub SJ. JAMA 1936;106:2144.
100. Hench BS, Bauer W, Dawson MH et al. Ann Intern Med 1940;13:1838–90.
101. Hench BS, Bauer W, Boland E et al. Ann Intern Med 1941;15:1002–1108.
102. Marquardt JL, Snyderman R, Oppenheim JJ. Cell Immunol 1973;9:263–272.
103. Epstein S. Ann Allergy 1969;26:343–439.
104. Pottenger RT. Ann Intern Med 1928;12:323–33.
105. van de Laar M, van der Korst J. Semin Arthritis Rheum 1991;21:12–23.
106. Cunningham-Rundles C. Rheum Dis Clin North Am 1991;17:287–307.
107. Inman RD. Rheum Dis Clin North Am 1991;17:309–21.
108. Sköldstam L, Magnusson KE. Rheum Dis Clin North Am 1991;17:363–71.
109. Delafuente J. Rheum Dis Clin North Am 1991;17:203–12.
110. Bengtsson U, Hanson L, Ahlstedt S. Clin Exp Allergy 1996;26:1387–94.
111. Kavanagh R, Workman E, Nash P et al. Br J Rheumatol 1995;34:270–3.
112. Holst-Jensen SE, Pfeiffer-Jensen M, Monsrud M et al. Scand J Rheumatol 1998;27:329–36.
113. Panush RS, Stroud RM, Webster EM. Arthritis Rheum 1986;29:220–6.
114. Parke AL, Hughes G. BMJ 1981;282:2027–9.
115. Sköldstam L, Larsson L, Lindström F. Scand J Rheumatol 1979;8:249–55.
116. Sköldstam L. Scand J Rheumatol 1986;15:219–23.
117. Kjeldsen-Kragh J, Borchgrevink C, Laerum E et al. Lancet 1991;338:899–902.
118. Haugen M, Kjeldsen-Kragh J, Skakkebek N et al. Clin Rheumatol 1993;12:62–9.
119. Kjeldsen-Kragh J, Mellbye O, Haugen M et al. Scand J Rheumatol 1995;24:85–93.
120. Peltonen R, Kjeldsen-Kragh J, Haugen M et al. Br J Rheumatol 1994;33:638–43.
121. Kjeldsen-Kragh J, Haugen M, Forre O et al. Br J Rheumatol 1994;33:569–75.
122. Nenonen M, Helve T, Rauma A-L et al. Br J Rheumatol 1998;37:274–81.
123. Peltonen R, Nenonen M, Helve T et al. Br J Rheumatol 1997;36.
124. McDougall J, Bruce B, Spiller G et al. J Altern Complement Med 2002;8:71–5.
125. Horrobin DF. Med Hypotheses 1987;22:421–8.
126. Adam O. Eur J Clin Nutr 1995;49:703–17.
127. James MJ, Cleland L. Sem Arthritis Rheum 1997;27:85–97.
128. Cleland L, James M. J Rheumatol 2000;2:2305–7.
129. Kremer J. Am J Clin Nutr 2000;71:349S–51S.
130. Healy D, Wallace F, Miles E et al. Lipids 2000;35:763–8.
131. Curtis C, Rees S, Cramp J et al. Proc Nutr Soc 2002;61:381–9.
132. Aruoma O. Food Chem Toxicol 1994;32:671–83.
133. Halliwell B. FASEB J 1987;1:358–64.
134. Winyard P, Blake D. Adv Pharmacol 1997;38:403–21.
135. Sowers MF, Lachance L. Rheum Dis Clin North Am 1999;25:315–32.
136. Darlington L, Stone T. Br J Nutr 2001;85:251–69.
137. Cimen M, Cimen Ö, Kacmaz H et al. Clin Rheumatol 2000;19:275–77.
138. Gambhir J, Lali P, Jain A. Clin Biochem 1997;30:351–55.
139. Baggott JE, Morgan SL, Ha TS et al. Clin Exp Rheum 1993;11:101–5.
140. Baggott JE, Morgan SL, Sams WM et al. Arch Dermatol 1999;135:813–7.
141. Morgan SL, Baggott JE, Vaughn WH et al. Arthritis Rheum 1990;33:9–18.
142. Morgan SL, Baggott JE, Vaughn WH et al. Ann Intern Med 1994;121:833–41.
143. Morgan SL, Baggott JE, Alarcon G. Biodrugs 1997;8:164–75.
144. Roe D. Diet and Drug Interactions. Ithaca, NY: Van Nostrand Reinhold, 1989.
145. Roe D. Drug-Induced Nutritional Deficiencies. 2nd ed. Ithaca, NY: AVI Publishing, 1985.
146. Pelton R, LaValle JB, Hawkins EB et al. Drug-Induced Nutrient Depletion Handbook. Hudson, OH: Lexi-Comp, 2000:416–26.

SELECTED READINGS

Kremer J. n-3 fatty acid supplements in rheumatoid arthritis. Am J Clin Nutr 2000;71:349S–51S.

Morgan SL, Baggott JE, Vaughn WH et al. Supplementation with folic acid during methotrexate therapy of rheumatoid arthritis: results from a double-blind, placebo-controlled trial. Ann Intern Med 1994;121:833–41.

National Institute of Arthritis and Musculoskeletal and Skin Diseases.

www.niams.nih.gov/hi/topics/arthritis/artrheu.htm. Bethesda, MD: National Institutes of Health, 2002.

Panush RS. Diets, other complementary and alternative therapies, and the rheumatic diseases. In: Koopman WJ, ed. Arthritis and Allied Conditions: A Textbook of Rheumatology. 14th ed. Philadelphia: Lippincott Williams & Wilkins, 2001:965–86.

86 OSTEOPOROSIS[1]

BESS DAWSON-HUGHES

BONE DENSITY ASSESSMENT 1339
EPIDEMIOLOGY OF OSTEOPOROSIS 1340
   Patterns of Peak Bone Density and Bone Loss . . .1340
   Epidemiology of Fractures 1341
   Falls 1342
NUTRITIONAL DETERMINANTS OF BONE
  DENSITY AND FRACTURE RISK 1342
   Calcium 1342
   Vitamin D 1343
   Phosphorus 1344
   Protein 1344
   Vitamin A 1346
   Vitamin K 1346
   Sodium 1346
   Caffeine 1347
   Alcohol 1347
   Fluoride 1347
   Trace Minerals 1347
OTHER RISK FACTORS FOR OSTEOPOROTIC
  FRACTURE 1348
   Body Weight and Body Composition 1348
   Smoking 1348
   Physical Activity 1348
   Heredity 1348
   Glucocorticoid Medications 1348
PREVENTION OF OSTEOPOROSIS 1349
THERAPIES FOR OSTEOPOROSIS 1349
   Estrogen 1349
   Bisphosphonates 1349
   Calcitonin 1349
   Raloxifene 1349
   Parathyroid Hormone (1-34) 1350

One and a half million osteoporotic fractures of the spine, hip, wrist, and other sites occur each year, primarily in postmenopausal white women. The number of osteoporosis cases among men and nonwhite persons, however, is expected to increase substantially over the next several decades as life expectancy increases and the world population expands. In the United States, direct medical costs of fractures among the population age 45 and older totaled nearly $14 billion in 1995 (1). Treatment of men accounted for approximately $3 billion, or 20% of the total amount. In addition, fractures of the hip and spine often contribute to disability, dependence, and increased risk of death.

Osteoporosis is characterized by low bone mass, microarchitectural deterioration, compromised bone strength, and an increased risk of fracture. For a discussion of normal bone development, metabolism, and composition, see Chapter 84.

Osteoporotic bone tissue is characterized by demineralized, disconnected trabeculae and thinning of the outer cortical surfaces (Fig 86.1) (2). The etiology and symptoms of osteoporosis and its link to menopause were first described by Albright and colleagues in 1941 (3). Several causes were known or suspected at that time, including immobilization, diet, and metabolic diseases. In subsequent years, the list of risk factors has grown, and it is now recognized that bone mass throughout the life span and the risk of osteoporotic fracture are determined by heredity and by a large number of environmental factors. Diet remains of critical interest in this multifactorial disease because it is one of the few determinants that can be modified safely.

BONE DENSITY ASSESSMENT

Much of our knowledge of the influence of nutrition and other factors on bone status and fracture risk has been gained since the introduction of precise, noninvasive methods of measuring bone mineral density (BMD). Widely used methods for both clinical diagnosis and research purposes include single x-ray absorptiometry, which is appropriate for measuring sites without much overlying fat and muscle tissue (e.g., wrist and heel), and dual x-ray absorptiometry (DXA) for sites such as the hip, spine, and whole body, where thicker layers of soft tissue surround the bone. Bone density is proportional to the amount of energy that is absorbed as it passes from an energy source located on one side of the bone to a detector on the opposite side. Low-radiation x-ray absorptiometry has largely

---

[1] **Abbreviations: AI,** adequate intake; **BMD,** bone mineral density; **CI,** confidence interval; **DXA,** dual x-ray absorptiometry; **FDA,** US Food and Drug Administration; **FNB,** Food and Nutrition Board; **PTH,** parathyroid hormone; **RDA,** recommended dietary allowance; **RE,** retinol equivalents.

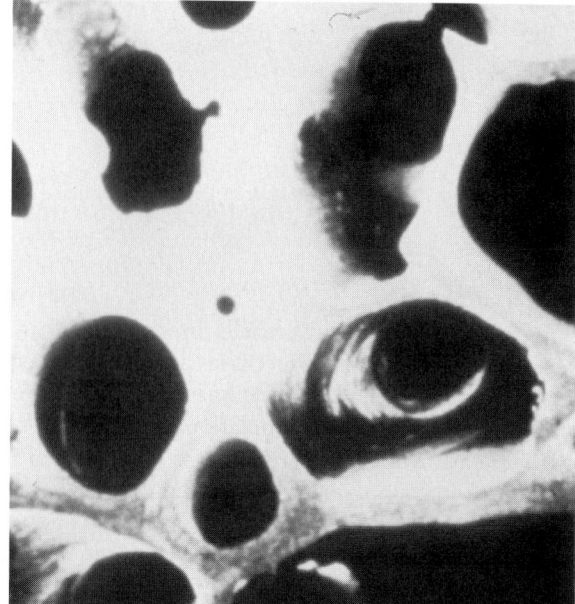

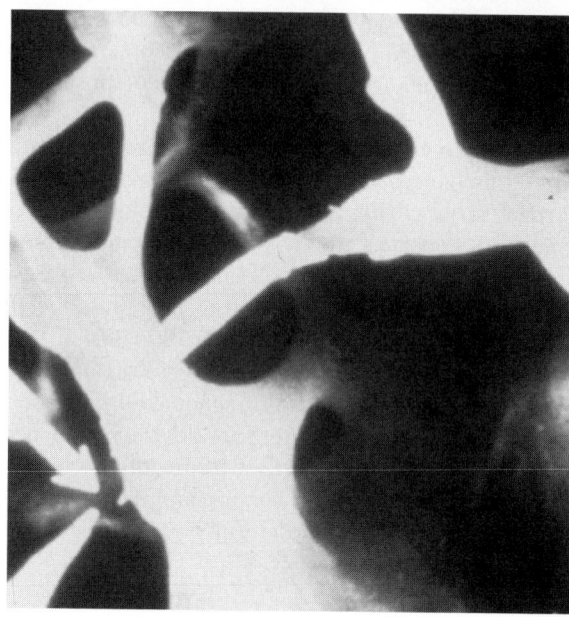

Figure 86.1. Electron micrographs of iliac crest biopsies illustrating normal bone **(A)** and osteoporotic bone **(B)**. Normal bone consists of a series of plates interconnected by thick rods. The osteoporotic bone has few plates, and several rods are fractured or disconnected. (From Dempster DW, Shane E, Horbert W et al. J Bone Miner Res 1986;1:15–21, with permission of the American Society for Bone and Mineral Research.)

replaced the older technologies that used a photon energy source.

Quantitative computed tomography and quantitative ultrasound are two alternative research techniques for assessing bone status. Quantitative computed tomography is primarily used to selectively assess trabecular bone, which is metabolically more active than cortical bone. Quantitative ultrasound measures the attenuation and velocity of sound waves as they pass through bone and other tissues. These measures are thought to assess qualitative factors such as bone architecture and elasticity in addition to bone mineral mass. Advantages of ultrasound are the lack of radiation exposure and the compact size of ultrasound units, which allows bone status measurements in field settings. A disadvantage is that the measurements are not as precise (reproducible) as DXA measurements.

EPIDEMIOLOGY OF OSTEOPOROSIS

The descriptive epidemiology of osteoporosis depends to some extent on the method used to define the disorder. Fractures resulting from moderate trauma (e.g., a fall from standing height or less) are the most important clinical outcome of osteoporosis. The incidence of fractures at the hip and spine increases sharply in the fourth decade of life, and continues to increase exponentially with age in men and women. At age 50, a white woman has a 30% chance of fracture. Osteoporosis can also be defined solely in terms of BMD, regardless of whether an individual has suffered a fracture. There is a continuous inverse relationship between BMD and risk of fracture (4) as shown in Figure 86.2. The fracture rate for a given decrease in BMD is greater in older than in younger persons (left panel), which indicates that qualitative properties of bone that are not measured by BMD are important in determining fracture risk.

Overall, the likelihood of fracture increases 1.5- to 2.5-fold for each standard deviation decrease in bone density. The World Health Organization criteria for the definition of osteoporosis are based on this relationship: BMD that is not more than 1 standard deviation below a young same-sex mean reference value is considered normal, osteopenia (low bone mass) is defined as BMD between 1 and 2.5 standard deviations below the reference value, and osteoporosis is defined as BMD 2.5 standard deviations or more below the reference value. Using these criteria and considering the United States population age 50 years and older, 20% of white women and 5% of black women have osteoporosis and 52% of white women and 35% of black women have osteopenia or low bone mass (5). Seven percent of white men and 3% of black men have osteoporosis, and 35% of white men and 19% of black men have osteopenia.

Patterns of Peak Bone Density and Bone Loss

BMD in the older adult is influenced by the peak bone mass achieved in young adulthood and the rate of bone loss in later years. The patterns of peak BMD, rates of bone loss, and fracture incidence vary with sex, age, ethnic group, and possibly skeletal site. Women, on average, have lower BMDs than men. This sex difference becomes evident in adolescence and is enhanced in later adulthood by several years of rapid bone loss surrounding menopause. Blacks tend to have higher BMDs than whites and Asians, and this difference is first apparent in early childhood (6).

Growth in childhood is accompanied by an increase in bone mass. Bone mass accumulates rapidly during the

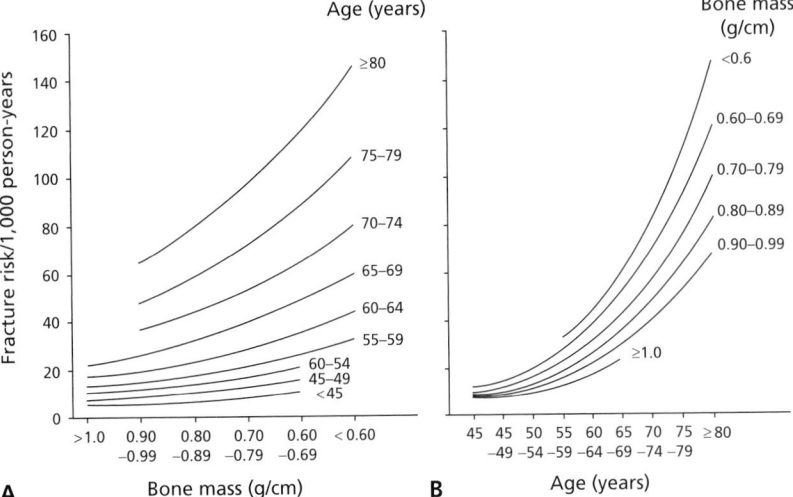

Figure 86.2. Relationships between bone mass of the radius, age, and rate of all nonvertebral fractures in women. For a given age, the risk of fracture increases with progressively decreasing bone mass **(A)**. The relationship between fracture risk and age is stronger, however, as seen by the steeper rise in risk with advancing age at a given level of bone mass **(B)**. (From Hui SL, Slemenda CW, Johnston CC Jr. J Clin Invest 1988; 81:1804–9, with permission.)

growth spurt that normally occurs between the ages of 11 and 14 years in girls and 13 to 17 years in boys. After the growth spurt, bone continues to increase in density but at a slower rate until peak bone mass is achieved sometime in young adulthood, about the same time that the bones cease to grow in length and the epiphyses close (7). Small increments in bone mass may continue until the late 20s or 30s.

Bone loss in young adults is believed to be minimal, and the age of onset may vary by skeletal site (8). Longitudinal studies of women indicate that bone loss at the hip and radius occurs before menopause, but the rate is not greater than 1% per year. Within the first 1 to 5 years after the onset of menopause, the rate of bone loss is two to six times premenopausal levels, but it gradually returns to about 1% annually by the tenth year after menopause. In older women, bone loss continues at a rate of approximately 1% annually into advanced ages (9, 10). An apparent increase in lumbar spine density with age has been reported in elderly women and men, but this is attributed to coexisting osteoarthritis or calcification of soft tissue in the spine scan field, which interferes with DXA bone density measurements.

The higher average bone mass seen in men beginning at puberty is maintained throughout the life span, and it is not clear at what age bone loss begins in men. Cross-sectional studies indicate that decreases in bone density at various skeletal sites among men more than 50 years old are similar in magnitude to the declines seen in women more than 10 years after menopause (11, 12). These findings have been confirmed in several longitudinal studies in men, in which rates of bone loss from the hip (10) and radius (13) were approximately 1%/year.

Epidemiology of Fractures

The incidence of fractures peaks in childhood and then declines until age 40, when rates begin to increase again. Most fractures among children and young adults result

from severe trauma and are not highly dependent on bone density, but after age 40, an increasing proportion of fractures results from mild or moderate trauma. The incidence of fractures most closely associated with osteoporosis in men and women residing in Rochester County, Minnesota, a predominantly white population (14), is shown in Figure 86.3.

Radius

The incidence of fractures of the forearm or distal radius (Colles fracture) increases after age 40 and tends to level off by age 55 in men and age 65 in women. The ratio of forearm fracture in women and men varies from 2:1 at age 35 to more than 8:1 after age 80 (15).

Femur

Beginning at age 40, the rate of hip fracture doubles about every 6 or 7 years in men and women in the United States, and this exponential increase continues among the very

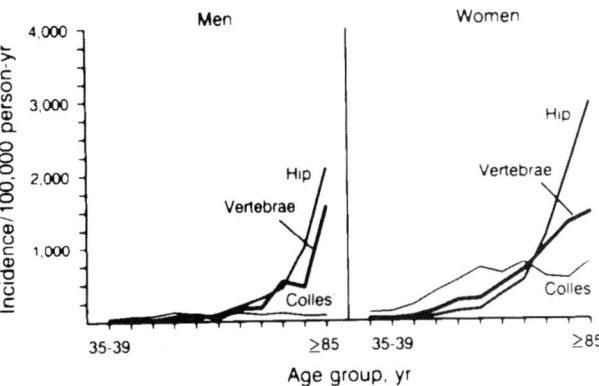

Figure 86.3. Age-specific incidence rates of hip, vertebral, and Colles fracture in Rochester, Minnesota men and women. (From Cooper C, Melton LJ III. Trends Endocrinol Metab 1992;314:224–9, with permission.)

old (16). The incidence of hip fractures in white Americans is shown in Figure 86.3 (14). The risk of hip fracture by age 85 is 11.2% for white women, 4.1% for white men, 3.6% for black women, and 2.0% for black men in the United States (17). Men and women of Asian descent living in the United States also have a reduced risk of hip fracture, comparable with that in blacks. Of all osteoporotic fractures, those at the hip are associated with the highest risk of death and disability.

Spine

A vertebral compression facture is typically diagnosed when the height of the vertebra decreases by 20% or more. As a result, the normally cube-shaped vertebra frequently becomes concave or wedge shaped. A consequence of anterior wedging of multiple vertebrae is kyphosis, or the curved spine known as a dowager's hump. Vertebral fractures are more than three times more common in women than in men in the United States (15). There is considerable geographic variation in the prevalence of this type of fracture. Estimates of the prevalence of vertebral fractures in the population older than 65 years vary from less than 3% in Finland to more than 20% in the United Sates (18). Because vertebral fractures can be asymptomatic or easily misdiagnosed, rates of vertebral compression fracture estimated by radiographic evaluations are much higher than those obtained from hospital admissions and clinical presentation.

Other Sites

Osteoporotic fractures at sites other than the radius, spine, or hip account for approximately half of all fractures among women age 65 years and more. Pelvic fracture resulting from moderate trauma in women in Rochester, Minnesota, increased from 17/100,000 person-years at ages 35 to 54 to 446/100,000 more than age 85 (19). In men, the rate reached 64/100,000 by age 85. Fractures of the humerus display a similar gender-specific pattern, increasing from 120/100,000 at ages 50 to 69 to 317/100,000 at more than age 70 in women, and from 27 to 51/100,000 in men (20). In contrast, fractures of the ankle, ribs, patella, and hands do not seem to follow the age- or sex-specific incidence patterns of other osteoporotic fractures (16).

Falls

More than 90% of fractures among elderly people are caused by falls. Factors associated with an elevated risk of falling include use of sedatives, diminished muscle strength, gait and balance difficulties, arthritis, poor vision, Parkinson disease, and disabilities of the lower extremities (21, 22). The chance of falling increases as more risk factors are present. In addition to bone density, biomechanical and individual characteristics influence the likelihood of fracture because of a fall. Hip fractures occur more frequently after a fall to the side (23), whereas Colles fractures are more often associated with forward falls. The height of the fall is directly related to the force of impact and risk of fracture, but persons with a high body mass index are less likely to sustain a fracture (23). Most falls occur after tripping or slipping on environmental hazards (21), a finding that implies that nonmedical interventions can significantly reduce the number of falls and fractures.

NUTRITIONAL DETERMINANTS OF BONE DENSITY AND FRACTURE RISK

Many nutritional factors have been examined for associations with osteoporosis and bone mass. Calcium, phosphorus, trace minerals, and protein are components of bone tissue. Vitamin D regulates calcium balance, and other nutrients influence calcium absorption and excretion. Thus, dietary intakes of these nutrients may affect bone mass, although the strength of associations may be expected to vary according to developmental phase, menopausal status, and habitual intake by the subjects studied.

Calcium

Calcium Intake and Bone Mass in Childhood

Bone mass during childhood and adolescence can be increased by increasing calcium intake to the 1997 Food and Nutrition Board (FNB) adequate intake (AI) values of 1300 mg (32.5 mmol)/day for ages 9 through 18 years and 1000 mg (25 mmol) for ages 19 through 50 years, for both men and women (see Appendix Tables II A-2-a-2 and A-2-b-1). A 3-year, randomized, double-blind, placebo-controlled trial was conducted in twins ages 6 to 14 years, during which the usual daily calcium intake (22.5 mmol, or 900 mg) of one of each pair was supplemented with 17.5 mmol (700 mg)/day (24). In prepubertal twins, the child taking the calcium supplement gained a total of 3 to 5% more bone mass at the radius and spine than his or her sibling, but there was no clear benefit of supplementation among older children. In another randomized study of calcium supplementation in girls, mean age 11.9 years, a daily calcium intake of 32.8 mmol (1314 mg) was associated with 2.6% higher bone densities at the spine and whole-body bone density at the end of 2 years (25). A daily calcium intake of 30 mmol achieved with dairy foods instead of supplements was associated with larger gains in BMD at the spine and whole body in 9- to 13-year-old girls than in a control group (26). Intakes of phosphorus, vitamin D, and protein were also increased, and it is not certain whether calcium or a combination of nutrients was responsible for the gains in bone mass. The benefit to bone mass of 18 months of added calcium in prepubertal children disappeared when supplementation was halted (27), suggesting that adequate calcium intake may need to be maintained throughout childhood and adolescence to have a meaningful impact on peak bone mass. Gains in peak bone mass may afford some protection against fracture in later life.

Calcium Intake and Bone Loss in Adult Women

Increased calcium intake causes about a 10 to 15% reduction in the bone remodeling rate in adult women, as measured by serum and urine biochemical markers of bone turnover. Calcium does not impede the refilling of open remodeling space, however, and the refilling that occurs over 12 to 18 months is usually accompanied by a 1 to 3% increase in BMD. The higher BMD is usually maintained as long as the calcium intake remains constant.

Premenopausal Intake. Prospective studies indicate that increasing calcium intake may reduce the rate of bone loss in premenopausal women. Spinal bone loss was significantly lower in a group of women who used dairy foods to raise calcium intake from 22.5 to 37.5 mmol (900–1500 mg) daily (28). A similar level of calcium intake (37 mmol) attained through supplementation slowed bone loss from the humerus but not the radius or ulna (29). The effect of calcium on bone density at other skeletal sites such as the hip in young women is unknown.

Postmenopausal Intake. The responsiveness of bone to nutritional intervention is blunted in the first few years of menopause, as decreasing endogenous estrogen levels create a new set point of bone metabolism. A 2-year controlled study of women ages 46 to 55 years found that daily supplements of 25 or 50 mmol (1 or 2 g) retarded spinal bone loss only within the first year (30). Calcium had no benefit on metacarpal bone minerals. Limited responses to added calcium were also observed in early menopausal women with low usual calcium intakes, less than 16.2 mmol, or 650 mg (31). In contrast, a 3-year study of early menopausal women found that calcium reduced bone loss from the femoral neck, and the effect of supplementation was sustained during the second and third years (32). Calcium supplementation also slowed the loss of total body calcium in that study.

Controlled trials of calcium supplementation in later postmenopausal women confirm earlier studies that demonstrated a reduction in bone loss (31, 33). Several also suggest that the benefits can be maintained over an extended period. In a 4-year study in which total calcium intake was increased to 42.5 mmol/day (1700 mg), a reduction in total body bone loss became apparent after the first year but bone loss continued at a slower rate throughout all remaining years of the study (34). Other factors have emerged in addition to menopausal age that may modify the effect of calcium intake on bone loss. The level of usual calcium intake affected the degree to which a supplement containing 500 mg (12.5 mmol) elemental calcium retarded bone loss among late menopausal women participating in a randomized, placebo-controlled study

(31). The largest reductions in bone loss from the spine, hip, and radius were observed in women with usual daily calcium intakes lower than 10 mmol (400 mg), and the benefit of increased calcium intake on weight-bearing sites such as the hip seems to be enhanced in women who also have high levels of physical activity (35, 33).

Calcium Intake and Bone Loss in Men

To date, there are few longitudinal studies of calcium supplementation in men. A placebo-controlled study in men ages 30 to 87 found that added calcium did not reduce bone loss at the spine over 3 years (13). These men habitually consumed a high level of calcium, more than 27.4 mmol (1100 mg)/day, and the treatment group received an additional 25 mmol/day. In contrast, supplementation with 12.5 mmol (500 mg) of calcium, together with 17.5 µg (700 IU)/day of vitamin D, reduced rates of bone loss from the spine, hip, and total body in men with a usual mean calcium intake of 17.5 mmol (700 mg)/day (36). These findings suggest that there is a threshold of calcium intake above which more calcium has no measurable effect, or that vitamin D is a critical component of the intervention. In this trial, which included women as well as men (36), discontinuation of the supplemental calcium and vitamin D was associated with an increase in the remodeling rate and loss of the bone density gains over the next 2 years (37). This study underscores the importance of consistency in meeting the calcium intake requirement.

Calcium Intake and Fracture Rates

Evidence for the effect of supplemental calcium on fracture rates comes largely from small studies with BMD change as their primary end points (34, 38, 39). Calcium supplementation reduced the rate of all fractures in a 4-year study of postmenopausal women, but the total number of fractures was very small (34). In an 18-month trial, the rate of vertebral compression fractures was about 32% lower in the treatment group than in a placebo group, but again the number of fractures was small and the difference was not statistically significant (38). In the largest of these intervention studies, calcium lowered the risk of fracture in postmenopausal women who had a pre-existing vertebral fracture but not in women with no prior vertebral fracture (39). The true impact of calcium on fracture rates needs better definition.

Vitamin D

Vitamin D is obtained from the diet in the forms of ergocalciferol (vitamin D_2) and cholecalciferol (vitamin D_3) as well as from cutaneous synthesis after exposure to sunlight. It is hydroxylated to 25-hydroxyvitamin D (25(OH)D, or calcidiol) in the liver and then to the active metabolite, 1,25-dihydroxyvitamin D (1,25(OH)$_2$D, or calcitriol), in the kidney. 1,25(OH)$_2$D stimulates the active transport of calcium across the intestine and is necessary for maintenance of healthy bone. Plasma level of 25(OH)D is the best clinical indicator of vitamin D status, and it reflects both dietary and endogenous contributions. Sunlight exposure seems to have a stronger influence on the 25(OH)D level than diet at vitamin D intake levels typically consumed in the United States; however, diet takes on increased importance in wintertime at high latitudes in healthy adults and throughout the year in persons who have limited sun exposure or a diminished ability to synthesize the vitamin. In the United States, elderly people ingest an average of about 5.0 μg (200 IU)/day.

The concentrations of parathyroid hormone (PTH), 25(OH)D, and 1,25(OH)$_2$D vary with season. In the northern hemisphere, PTH is higher and levels of 25(OH)D and 1,25(OH)$_2$D are lower in winter than in summer. The most striking seasonal variability is seen in persons with dietary vitamin D intake lower than 5 μg, or 200 IU (40). Rates of bone loss also have been reported to vary by season, with more rapid loss during the period in which PTH is elevated and vitamin D levels are low (41).

The role of vitamin D insufficiency in osteoporosis is increasingly recognized. Increasing intake of vitamin D can increase intestinal calcium absorption (42), lower circulating levels of PTH (36), and reduce rates of bone loss (43, 41). Supplemental vitamin D also lowers the risk of falling (44). Evidence also indicates that supplementation with vitamin D can lower fracture risk. Annual intramuscular injections of vitamin D$_2$ given to institutionalized and free-living elderly persons in Finland reduced the number of fractures (45). Injections overcame the problems of poor intestinal absorption and noncompliance. Randomized trials of oral vitamin D$_3$ with fractures as an outcome are summarized in Table 86.1. Note that in several of these trials, calcium was given along with the vitamin D (36, 46–48). A large controlled trial of 20 μg vitamin D$_3$ and calcium supplementation in elderly institutionalized French women showed a substantial reduction in risk of fracture (46). With supplementation, a significant 26% reduction in the occurrence of hip fractures and other nonvertebral fractures was noted. The same supplement regimen had a similar impact on hip fracture risk in a second population of institutionalized elderly French women (47). In healthy men and women age 65 years and older, supplementation with 17.5 μg (700 IU) of vitamin D$_3$ and 12.5 mmol (500 mg)/day of calcium lowered the risk of nonvertebral fracture by 50% over 3 years (36).

Two large studies have examined the impact of vitamin D$_3$ alone on fractures. Supplementation of a large group of community-dwelling elderly men and women in the United Kingdom with 2500 μg (100,000 IU) of vitamin D$_3$ orally every 4 months (equivalent to 833 IU/day) lowered the risk of any first fracture by 30% (49). In contrast, supplementation with 10 μg (400 IU)/day of vitamin D$_3$ had no effect on hip or other fractures in elderly Dutch men and women (50). Other low-dose vitamin D intervention trials have had similar negative results (48, 51). From

these trials, it seems that a dose of vitamin D of 17.5 to 20 μg (700 to 800 IU)/day is needed to significantly suppress PTH levels and lower fracture rates in elderly people and that an adequate intake of calcium is also important.

The 1997 FNB AI values for vitamin D were increased to 10 μg for men and women ages 51 through 70 years and to 15 μg for men and women ages 71 years old and older (52). Evidence suggests that the 25(OH)D level needed to minimize fracture risk is not lower than 80 nmol/L and that an intake of 800 to 1000 IU/day of vitamin D$_3$ is needed to bring the group mean value to this level. An even higher intake of vitamin D$_2$ would be needed to reach the level of 80 nmol/L (53).

Phosphorus

An increase in serum phosphorus concentration arising from high dietary phosphorus intake stimulates PTH secretion, which in turn suppresses 1,25(OH)$_2$D production and intestinal calcium absorption. As a consequence, excess phosphorus intake may be a concern. Increased phosphorus has an opposing effect on calcium lost through the urine, and this action may adequately offset the adverse effects on calcium absorption and bone metabolism in healthy adults. The phosphorus-calcium ratio may be more important than the level of phosphorus alone. A diet high in phosphorus (55 mmol or 1700 mg/day) and low in calcium (10 mmol/day) produced an increase in PTH secretion (54). If extended over a long period, it is suspected that this common dietary pattern could lead to unfavorable bone balance, but this has not been demonstrated.

Prolonged dietary phosphorus deficiency can deplete the serum level and result in enhanced resorption of this mineral from bone. For a portion of the elderly population, phosphorus deficiency is a concern. Low serum phosphorus levels can result from malnutrition, excessive use of phosphorus-binding antacids, and intestinal malabsorption. The phosphorus content of calcium triphosphate supplements may have contributed to some degree to the reduction in fracture rate in the French studies of vitamin D and calcium interventions (55, 47). The 1997 FNB recommended dietary allowance (RDA) for phosphorus in men and women older than 19 years (700 mg/day) is lower than the 1989 RDA of 1200 mg at 19 to 24 years and 800 mg thereafter (see Appendix Tables II A-2-a-2 and A-2-b-2).

Protein

Excess dietary protein has been proposed as a contributor to osteoporosis risk because of its calciuric effect. Over a wide range of protein intakes, an increase in dietary protein of 1 g results in the loss of an additional 1 mg of calcium in the urine. This effect results from the acid load imparted by dietary protein. More recently, however, protein has been shown to increase circulating levels of

TABLE 86.1. SUMMARY OF RANDOMIZED TRIALS OF ORAL VITAMIN D₃ SUPPLEMENTATION

INVESTIGATORS	DESCRIPTION OF SUBJECTS	STUDY LENGTH	DOSE OF VITAMIN D_3 (μg/d)	PUBLISHED SERUM 25(OH)D VALUES ON TREATMENT (nmol/L)	STANDARDIZED[a] SERUM 25(OH)D VALUES ON TREATMENT (nmol/L)	EFFECT ON SERUM PTH (%)	PREVENTATIVE EFFECT ON NONVERTEBRAL FRACTURE (HIP AND OTHERS)
Chapuy et al., 1994 (46)	3,270 women, institutionalized, mean age 84 y	3 y	20[b]	100	71	−47	+
Chapuy et al., 2002 (47)	583 women, institutionalized, mean age 85.2 y		20[b]	100	71	−33	Trend[c]
Dawson-Hughes et al., 1997 (36)	213 women and 176 men, free-living, mean age 71 y	3 y	17.5[b]	112	99	F, −33 M, −23	+
Trivedi et al., 2003 (49)	649 women and 2,037 men, free-living, mean age 75 y	5 y	20.5[d]	74	—	—	+
Lips et al., 1996 (50)	1,916 women and 662 men, 60% institutionalized, mean age 80 y	3.5 y	10	54	54	−6	NS
Meyer et al., 2002 (48)	858 women and 286 men, institutionalized, mean age 53 y	2 y	10[b,e]	64	—	—	NS
Komulainen et al., 1998 (51)	232 women, free-living, mean age 53 y	5 y	7.5	—	—	—	NS

PTH, parathyroid hormone; NS, not significant.

[a]Serum 25(OH)D values standardized to DiaSorin equivalent values (i.e., high-performance liquid chromatography followed by a competitive protein-binding assay), based on a cross-calibration study (122).

[b]Subjects also given supplemental calcium.

[c]Hip fracture risk ratio = 1.69 (95% confidence interval, 0.96–3.00), $p = .07$.

[d]Supplement given as a 2,500-μg (100,000-IU) tablet every 4 months.

[e]Vitamin D given as cod liver oil.

insulinlike growth factor-I, a bone growth factor (56, 57). The impact of dietary protein on calcium absorption remains an open question. Several recent studies have examined the effects of increasing protein intakes from food sources on indices of bone turnover and bone loss. One observed a decrease in deoxypyridinoline, a marker of bone resorption (56), and the other reported no change in indices of bone turnover (57). Finally, in patients with recent hip fractures, protein supplementation for 6 months significantly lowered the rate of bone loss from the hip over a 1-year period (58).

The composition of the diet may influence the impact of dietary protein on the skeleton. For instance, the impact of dietary protein on rates of bone loss seems to be more favorable among subjects with higher rather than lower calcium intakes (37). It can also be anticipated that the overall acid-base balance of the diet will influence the impact of dietary protein on bone. A high intake of alkaline foods such as fruits and vegetables may mitigate the calciuric effect of protein and promote a net positive impact of protein on the skeleton. The studies cited earlier have tested protein intakes up to about 1.6 g/kg/day. The impact of higher protein intakes on the skeleton has not been defined, but may be negative because of the increased calciuria.

Vitamin A

Vitamin A is ingested as preformed vitamin A (retinol and retinyl esters) from animal foods and as the precursor, β-carotene, from carrots, green plants, and some fruits. Carotene is cleaved to retinol in the intestine and retinol is transported by chylomicrons to the liver, where it is stored mainly as retinyl palmitate. Vitamin A and its precursors are measured in retinol equivalents (RE) and in international units, and 3 μg RE equals 10 IU. Vitamin A is present in plasma as retinol, bound to a specific retinol-binding protein. Increasing carotene intake does not increase plasma retinol levels because its absorption and transformation into vitamin A are controlled. Recommended intakes go as high as 1667 RE (5000 IU)/day, but the FNB recently recommended 700 RE for women and 900 RE for men as AIs (59).

Bone has nuclear receptors for vitamins A and D. The receptors of both vitamins bind to target genes as heterodimers. In rats, 1,25(OH)$_2$D activates the vitamin D receptor, retinoid X receptor complex (60). This interaction has also been demonstrated recently in humans (61). In this study, administration of retinyl palmitate decreased the plasma calcium increase in response to oral administration of 1,25(OH)$_2$D.

Vitamin A deficiency is characterized by night blindness, retarded growth, and immune deficiencies, and vitamin A excess or toxicity causes accelerated bone resorption, hypercalcemia, and fractures (62). The impact of mild to moderately increased intakes of vitamin A on BMD and fracture rates has been examined in several observational studies. Higher retinol intakes have been associated with greater rates of bone loss (63, 64) and higher rates of hip fracture (65). One recent study linked higher serum retinol levels with increased fracture incidence (66). Small, short-term intervention studies have not detected any effect of vitamin A on biochemical markers of bone turnover (67). More data are needed to better define the boundary between adequate and excessive intakes of vitamin A and the possible impact of vitamin D status on that boundary.

Vitamin K

Vitamin K is a fat-soluble vitamin that may influence rates of bone loss. Vitamin K refers to a family of compounds consisting of phylloquinone (vitamin K$_1$), present in green leafy vegetables and other plants, and a series of menaquinones (vitamin K$_2$) that are present in liver, meats, and foods prepared by fermentation, such as cheeses. The AI of vitamin K is set at 120 μg/day for men and 90 μg/day for women (59).

Vitamin K is a cofactor for the formation of γ-carboxyglutamyl residues in the bone proteins osteocalcin, matrix γ-carboxyglutamyl protein, and protein S. Osteocalcin is produced by the osteoblast, and this 49-amino acid protein confers mineral-binding properties to the bone matrix protein, osteoid (68). Some of the osteocalcin present in serum is undercarboxylated, and a high proportion of undercarboxylated osteocalcin reflects nutritional deficiency of vitamin K. Matrix γ-carboxyglutamyl protein is present in bone and cartilage, where it is bound to both the organic and mineral components. Protein S, a cofactor for the anticoagulant activities of protein C, is also present in bone. Deficiency of each of these vitamin K-dependent proteins has been associated with osteopenia.

Low dietary phylloquinone intake (69, 70) and a high ratio of undercarboxylated-to-total osteocalcin (71) have been associated with increased risk of hip fracture in women, whereas associations with change in BMD have been equivocal. One prospective intervention trial using a pharmacologic menaquinone-4 dose of 45 mg/day found that it reduced bone loss in postmenopausal women (72). Additional trials testing nutritional replacement levels of vitamin K are needed to define the impact of this vitamin on age-related bone loss. Finally, long-term use of the vitamin K antagonist, warfarin, may be expected to promote bone loss, but this has not been a consistent finding.

Sodium

Sodium causes an increase in renal calcium excretion. At the high levels of sodium intake typical in the United States, more than 90% of ingested sodium is excreted, and urinary sodium is thus a reliable estimate of dietary intake. For each 500-mg increment in sodium excretion (or sodium intake), there is approximately a 10-mg increase in the amount of calcium lost in urine. Because on average only 25% of ingested calcium is absorbed, calcium intake must be increased 40 mg to compensate for a 500-mg increment in sodium intake. The impact of sodium intake on the rate of bone loss was evaluated in postmenopausal women (73). Over a wide range of sodium excretion (1 to 6 g/day), there was an increasingly negative change in total hip BMD with higher levels of urinary sodium but no association with change in BMD at the femoral neck or the spine. In that population, optimal intakes to minimize bone loss were estimated at approximately 25 mmol (1000 mg)/day of calcium and no more than 87 mmol (2000 mg)/day of sodium.

Caffeine

Caffeine ingestion causes a short-term (within 1 to 3 hours) increase in urinary calcium excretion, but controlled studies have failed to document sustained effects of caffeine on urinary or fecal calcium excretion (74, 75). Such a temporary increase may be expected to have a minor effect on net calcium balance. However, among older persons with low calcium intakes, the effect may possibly take on relatively greater importance as the body fails to adequately compensate for the additional calcium loss. A study of postmenopausal women found that coffee intake of two or more cups per day was associated with reduced BMD in those who did not drink milk on a daily basis (76). Bone loss was more rapid in a subgroup of postmenopausal women with calcium intakes lower than the RDA of 800 mg/day and caffeine intakes of more than two cups of brewed coffee per day (75). Coffee consumption has also been associated with an increased risk of hip fracture (77) in elderly women.

Alcohol

Chronic alcoholism and osteoporosis commonly occur simultaneously in men (78). Ethanol directly affects bone tissue by suppressing bone formation. Its use is also associated with multiple nutritional deficiencies, hepatic damage, and hypogonadism, all of which have deleterious effects on bone metabolism. Moderate or social use, on the other hand, seems to have the opposite effect on BMD and bone loss. Several population studies have reported that moderate alcohol use is associated with higher mean bone density levels (79) and reduced rates of bone loss (80). Alcohol stimulates the conversion of androstenedione to estrone, an estrogenic compound with bone-preserving properties. A potential reduction in fracture risk among alcohol users arising from a modest increase in bone density may be offset by an increased likelihood of falling, however.

Fluoride

Fluoride stimulates osteoblast activity and can replace hydroxyl ions in the hydroxyapatite structure of bone. This substitution results in bone with increased crystalline size but decreased elasticity and quality. Thus, although the compression strength of fluoride-enriched bone is greater, the tensile quality may decline. An association between increased bone density on radiographs and naturally occurring high fluoride in drinking water, at concentrations between 0.21 and 0.30 mmol (4 to 5.8 mg)/L, was observed in an early study (81). In contrast, fluoridated drinking water that supplies 0.05 to 0.16 mmol (1 to 3 mg)/day has neither beneficial nor deleterious effects on bone density (82) or hip fracture rates (83).

When used in high doses as a therapeutic agent for osteoporosis, fluoride increases spinal bone density, but the effect on fracture incidence is less clear. No protection against vertebral fractures was found in two trials of 3.9 mmol (75 mg) fluoride, and there was a suggestion that nonvertebral fractures may have increased during fluoride therapy (84, 85). More recently, a lower dose of slow-release sodium fluoride (1.3 mmol or 25 mg/day) administered cyclically increased bone density of the spine and hip and decreased the rate of vertebral fracture (86).

Trace Minerals

Increasing boron intake may result in a decrease in urinary excretion of calcium, phosphorus, and magnesium and a simultaneous increase in serum estradiol level (87). Such findings suggest that boron may play a role in maintaining calcium balance. Although the mechanism is unknown, it is postulated that boron is necessary for formation of certain steroid hormones or hydroxylation of 25(OH)D. More information is needed on usual dietary intakes and boron requirements before its importance in the development of osteoporosis can be fully understood.

Strontium has been proposed as an agent for improving BMD. It has similarities to calcium and has long been used as a marker for assessing calcium absorption. In two studies in Europe, strontium ranelate in doses of 1 to 2 g/day for 2 years increased BMD by 2 to 3% relative to placebo in postmenopausal women (88, 89). The nature of its effect on bone is unknown, but its similarity to calcium suggests that it is likely involved in the mineralization process.

Bone tissue contains approximately half of the body stores of magnesium. In animals, dietary magnesium restriction is associated with increased bone resorption and decreased formation. When magnesium depletion is induced in humans, decreased PTH secretion, hypocalcemia, hypocalciuria, and a positive calcium balance result. Reports of altered levels of magnesium in bone of osteoporotic and control subjects have not been substantiated.

Manganese, zinc, and copper are cofactors for enzymes essential to bone tissue. The effect of these three trace minerals on bone loss at the spine, alone or in combination with calcium, was evaluated in a 2-year trial of postmenopausal women (90). Spine BMD in the group supplemented with a combination of 25 mol (1 g) calcium, 0.09 mmol (5 mg) manganese, 0.04 mmol (2.5 mg) copper, and 0.23 mmol (15 mg) zinc showed no decline compared with that in the control group, which lost an average of 3.5% of bone mass. The role of these trace minerals in maintaining bone mass has not yet been established.

OTHER RISK FACTORS FOR OSTEOPOROTIC FRACTURE

Body Weight and Body Composition

Bone loss that occurs during prolonged immobilization and weightlessness in space flight demonstrates the importance of gravitational force in preserving bone density. Body weight is directly correlated with bone density, and higher weight protects against fracture (91). Apart from the contribution of total weight to bone mass, the two major components of body weight, fat-free mass (primarily muscle) and fat tissue, may influence bone through other mechanisms. Fat tissue is a source of endogenous estrogen. In postmenopausal women, this source takes on increased importance as gonadal hormone production declines. Muscle size is influenced by some of the same factors that stimulate bone formation, such as physical activity, insulin, growth hormones, and androgens. There is no agreement on whether the fat (92) or fat-free (93) component of body weight is more important in building and preserving bone density. However, excess body fat is strongly associated with an increased risk of numerous chronic diseases. Voluntary weight loss has been associated with bone loss, with BMD changes of about 1 to 2% occurring with a 10% reduction in weight. This association is present in men and women, and seems to be stronger in postmenopausal than in premenopausal women. Increased aerobic exercise during weight loss may mitigate bone loss (94). Involuntary weight loss is frequently accompanied by rapid bone loss because the underlying cause of the weight loss often has an independent adverse effect on bone.

Smoking

Cigarette smokers often possess characteristics associated with low bone density independently of their exposure to tobacco. These include lower body weight, greater consumption of caffeine and alcohol, and, in women, earlier menopause. After controlling for some or all of these factors, women who smoke still have lower bone density and more rapid rates of bone loss than nonsmokers (95, 96). The effect of smoking is thought to be related, in part, to alterations in estrogen metabolism. Smoking increases the hepatic conversion of estradiol into biologically inactive metabolites at the expense of active hormones estrone and estriol (97). Although one population study of hip fracture in elderly women reported that smoking reduced the benefit of hormone replacement therapy (98), another found no difference in bone loss rates between smokers who did use supplemental estrogen and those who did not (96).

Smoking is associated with lower BMD, increased rate of bone loss, and higher fracture risk in men as well (99). It is not known whether smoking affects circulating androgen levels or has other direct effects on bone tissue.

Physical Activity

Part of the decrease in bone density that accompanies aging may be the result of declining physical activity levels in later life. Vigorous, high-impact activity in young men and premenopausal women results in modest increases in bone mass. Evidence suggests that initiating an exercise regime in older, previously sedentary persons will increase bone density or slow bone loss. It is not known whether any one type of activity is best for maintaining bone health. Stabilization of bone mass has been demonstrated with resistive (100), weight-bearing aerobic (101), and high-impact loading exercises (102). In postmenopausal women, aerobic exercise for 20 minutes, three to seven times per week, in conjunction with muscle-strengthening exercise is recommended to help stabilize bone density. Strength and balance exercises also improve muscle function and reduce falls and thereby are expected to reduce risk of fracture (103).

Heredity

Like many anthropometric traits, bone density displays a family resemblance. Heritability accounts for about 80% of the variance in peak bone mass (104) and for a much smaller and not clearly defined proportion of the variance in rates of bone loss in adults. Numerous studies involving genome-wide mapping of quantitative trait loci linked to discrete traits for bone strength such as bone size, cortical thickness, and trabecular architecture and population-based association studies for candidate genes involved in bone metabolic pathways are underway.

The vitamin D receptor was the first genetic marker to be associated with bone density and rates of bone loss in several different populations (105, 106). Interactions of vitamin D receptor alleles with calcium intake illustrate an environmental-hereditary interaction (107, 108). Women with the low-bone density genotype exhibit more-rapid bone loss when their usual calcium intake is very low (107) and lack a compensatory increase in calcium absorption in response to a reduction in dietary calcium (108). Genes coding for low density lipoprotein receptor-related protein 5 are now known to be responsible for the familial high bone mass and juvenile-onset osteoporosis-pseudoganglioma syndromes (109, 110). Many other candidate genes are under investigation, including receptors of hormones such as estrogen and PTH, of growth factors such as insulinlike growth factor-I, of bone collagen such as collagen type I, $\propto$1.

Glucocorticoid Medications

Glucocorticoids are a class of drugs used to treat a range of chronic inflammatory diseases such as rheumatoid arthritis, inflammatory bowel diseases, asthma, and systemic lupus, and to suppress the rejection of transplanted organs. Adverse effects associated with their use include decreased intestinal absorption and increased urinary excretion of calcium, reduced gonadal hormone levels, inhibition of osteoblast function, and increased bone resorption; each of these mechanisms can result in accelerated bone loss and increased risk of fracture. Osteoporosis occurs in more than half of patients who receive long-term glucocorticoid treatment. It is estimated that 4 million cases of osteoporosis in the United States, or 20% of the total number, are attributable to corticosteroid use (111).

PREVENTION OF OSTEOPOROSIS

Recommendations to help prevent osteoporosis derive from knowledge of the modifiable risk factors described earlier. As this knowledge increases and becomes more refined, recommendations for prevention will change accordingly. Currently, a healthy diet involving adequate intakes of calcium, vitamin D, protein, and vitamin K, as defined by the National Academy of Sciences, is recommended. As data accumulate, one can anticipate that the amount of vitamin D recommended will increase. Avoiding excess intakes of phosphorus, vitamin A, protein, sodium, caffeine, and alcohol is also important. Weight-bearing and muscle-strengthening exercises for 30 to 40 minutes/day reduce bone loss and lower the risk of falling. Finally, avoiding smoking is very important for bone health.

THERAPIES FOR OSTEOPOROSIS

Diet modification and a healthy lifestyle are not sufficient treatment for established osteoporosis, although they are important components of therapy. For patients with osteoporosis, a growing number of treatments are available. These medications are described briefly later.

Estrogen

Estrogen receptors have been identified in normal human osteoblast-like bone cells in vitro, providing a means by which estrogen can directly influence bone turnover (112). Estrogen enhances calcium absorption through its trophic effect on $1,25(OH)_2D$ and perhaps also directly. When administered to postmenopausal women, estrogen lowers the bone remodeling rate and retards bone loss (113).

Women who have not had a hysterectomy who use estrogen also require progestin to protect the uterine lining. Estrogen alone is used in women who have had their uterus removed. Estrogen is approved by the US Food and Drug Administration (FDA) for treatment of vasomotor symptoms and for the prevention of osteoporosis. The Women's Health Initiative found that the combination of estrogen and medroxy-progesterone (hormone therapy) lowered risk of hip fracture by 34% (hazard ratio, 0.66 [95% confidence interval (CI), 0.45 to 0.98]) in a study

of more than 16,000 postmenopausal women ages 50 to 79 years (114). In the same study, however, hormone therapy significantly increased the risks of myocardial infarction, stroke, invasive breast cancer, pulmonary emboli, and deep vein phlebitis (114). Because of these risks, the FDA advises that hormone therapy should be used in the lowest possible dose for the shortest duration, and when hormone therapy is being considered for treatment of osteoporosis alone, nonestrogen treatments should be considered first.

Bisphosphonates

Bisphosphonates are structural analogues of pyrophosphate. Their metabolic actions include inhibition of hydroxyapatite formation and inhibition of bone resorption through a direct dose-related effect on osteoclasts. Two amino-bisphosphonates, alendronate and risedronate, have been approved by the FDA for the prevention and treatment of osteoporosis.

Alendronate given for 3 years to postmenopausal women with osteoporosis increases bone density and lowers vertebral, nonvertebral, and hip fractures by about 50% (115). Risedronate also significantly lowers fracture rates at these sites in postmenopausal women. In clinical trials, these drugs were tolerated as well as placebo. Clinical experience indicates, however, that some patients experience upper gastrointestinal symptoms. These drugs must be taken after a prolonged fast with 8 ounces of water at least 30 minutes before eating or drinking, and patients should remain upright (sitting or standing) during this interval.

Calcitonin

Calcitonin, a small peptide hormone produced by the C cells of the thyroid gland, is secreted in response to increased serum calcium concentrations. Its primary function is to inhibit bone resorption. Women with osteoporosis have an attenuated calcitonin response to a calcium challenge.

Salmon calcitonin is a more potent inhibitor of bone resorption than is human calcitonin. A controlled clinical trial in more than 1200 osteoporotic late-menopausal women revealed that nasal calcitonin in a dose of 200 IU/day lowered the vertebral fracture rates by 21% (risk reduction, 0.79 [95% CI, 0.62 to 1.0]) (116). There is currently no evidence that calcitonin lowers fracture risk at other skeletal sites.

Raloxifene

Raloxifene is a selective estrogen receptor modulator that is FDA approved for the prevention and treatment of osteoporosis. Raloxifene lowers the bone remodeling rate like other antiresorptive drugs described earlier. In controlled clinical trials, raloxifene lowers the risk of vertebral fracture by 40% (risk reduction, 0.6 [95% CI, 0.50 to 0.70]) (117). Currently, there is no evidence that it significantly reduces nonvertebral fracture rates. Raloxifene increases the risk of deep vein phlebitis to a degree similar to that of estrogen. It also increases hot flashes by about 6% over placebo. Raloxifene seems to decrease the risk of estrogen-receptor–positive breast cancer (118). Its effects on the cardiovascular system have not yet been defined.

Parathyroid Hormone (1-34)

PTH (1-34), or teriparatide, is the first anabolic agent to be FDA approved for the treatment of osteoporosis. When administered subcutaneously in a dose of 20 μg/day, PTH (1-34) increased spinal BMD by 9% and femoral neck BMD by 3% over 18 months in osteoporotic older women (119). It also lowered the risk of vertebral fractures by 65% (risk reduction, 0.35 [95% CI, 0.22 to 0.55]) and nonvertebral fractures by 56% (risk reduction, 0.46 [95% CI, 0.25 to 0.88]) in the same population (119). PTH (1-34) is generally well tolerated, although a few patients experience leg cramps and dizziness. The drug is not approved for use extending beyond 2 years. PTH (1-34) caused osteosarcoma in rats (treated with high doses for extended periods); therefore, patients at increased risk for osteosarcoma (e.g., patients with Paget disease, prior radiation therapy, prior skeletal malignancy, bone metastases, and hypercalcemia) should not receive this therapy.

The combination of PTH (1-34) and alendronate did not have the anticipated additive positive effect on BMD in postmenopausal women (120, 121). The optimal approach to using sequential and combination therapies requires further definition.

REFERENCES

1. Ray NF, Chan JK, Thamer M et al. J Bone Miner Res 1997; 12:24–35.
2. Dempster DW, Shane E, Horbert W et al. J Bone Miner Res 1986;1:15–21.
3. Albright F, Smith PH, Richardson AM. JAMA 1941;116: 2465–74.
4. Hui SL, Slemenda CW, Johnston CC Jr. J Clin Invest 1988; 81:1804–9.
5. America's Bone Health: The State of Osteoporosis and Low Bone Mass. Washington, DC: National Osteoporosis Foundation, 2002:55.
6. Bell NH, Shary J, Stevens J et al. J Bone Miner Res 1991;6: 719–23.
7. Theintz G, Buchs B, Rizzoli R et al. J Clin Endocrinol Metab 1992;75:1060–5.
8. Sowers MR, Galuska DA. Epidemiol Rev 1993;15:374–98.
9. Ensrud KE, Palermo L, Black DM et al. J Bone Miner Res 1995;10:1778–87.
10. Jones G, Nguyen T, Sambrook P et al. BMJ 1994;309:691–5.
11. Glynn NW, Meilahn EN, Charron M et al. J Bone Miner Res 1995;10:1769–77.
12. Hannan MT, Felson DT, Anderson JJ. J Bone Miner Res 1992; 7:547–53.
13. Orwoll ES, Oviatt SK, McClung MR et al. Ann Intern Med 1990;112:29–34.
14. Cooper C, Melton LJ III. Trends Endocrinol Metab 1992;314: 224–9.
15. Cooper C, Atkinson EJ, O'Fallon WM et al. J Bone Miner Res 1992;7:221–7.
16. Nevitt MC. Rheum Dis Clin North Am 1994;20:535–59.
17. Barrett JA, Baron JA, Karagas MR et al. J Clin Epidemiol 1999; 52:243–9.
18. Kanis JA, McCloskey EV. Bone 1992;13[Suppl 10]:1S–10S.
19. Melton LJ III, Sampson JM, Morrey BF et al. Clin Orthop 1981;155:43–7.
20. Rose SH, Melton LJ III, Morrey BF et al. Clin Orthop 1982; 168:24–30.
21. Tinetti ME, Speechley M, Ginter SF. N Engl J Med 1988;319: 1701–7.
22. Grisso JA, Kelsey JL, Strom BL et al. N Engl J Med 1991; 324:1326–31.
23. Greenspan SL, Myers ER, Maitland LA et al. JAMA 1994; 271:128–33.
24. Johnston CC Jr, Miller JZ, Slemenda CW et al. N Engl J Med 1992;327:82–7.
25. Lloyd T, Andon MB, Rollings N et al. JAMA 1993;270:841–4.
26. Chan GM, Hoffman K, McMurry M. J Pediatr 1995;126:551–6.
27. Lee WT, Leung SS, Leung DM et al. Am J Clin Nutr 1996; 64:71–7.
28. Baran D, Sorensen A, Grimes J et al. J Clin Endocrinol Metab 1990;70:264–70.
29. Smith EL, Gilligan C, Smith PE et al. Am J Clin Nutr 1989;50: 833–42.
30. Elders PJ, Netelenbos JC, Lips P et al. J Clin Endocrinol Metab 1991;73:533–40.
31. Dawson-Hughes B, Dallal GE, Krall EA et al. N Engl J Med 1990;323:878–83.
32. Aloia JF, Vaswani A, Yeh JK et al. Ann Intern Med 1994; 120:97–103.
33. Lau EM, Woo J, Leung PC et al. Osteoporos Int 1992;2: 168–73.
34. Reid IR, Ames RW, Evans MC et al. Am J Med 1995;98:331–5.
35. Prince R, Devine A, Dick I et al. J Bone Miner Res 1995; 10:1068–75.
36. Dawson-Hughes B, Harris SS, Krall EA et al. N Engl J Med 1997;337:670–6.
37. Dawson-Hughes B, Harris SS, Krall EA et al. Am J Clin Nutr 2000;72:745–50.
38. Chevalley T, Rizzoli R, Nydegger V et al. Osteoporos Int 1994; 4:245–52.
39. Recker RR, Hinders S, Davies KM et al. J Bone Miner Res 1996;11:1961–6.
40. Krall EA, Sahyoun N, Tannenbaum S et al. N Engl J Med 1989; 321:1777–83.
41. Dawson-Hughes B, Dallal GE, Krall EA et al. Ann Intern Med 1991;115:505–12.
42. Heaney RP, Dowell MS, Hale CA et al. J Am Coll Nutr 2003; 22:142.
43. Ooms ME, Lips P, Roos JC et al. J Bone Miner Res 1995; 10:1177–84.
44. Bischoff HA, Stahelin HB, Dick W et al. J Bone Miner Res 2003;18:343–51.
45. Heikinheimo RJ, Inkovaara JA, Harju EJ et al. Calcif Tissue Int 1992;51:105–10.
46. Chapuy MC, Arlot ME, Delmas PD et al. BMJ 1994;308:1081–2.
47. Chapuy MC, Pamphile R, Paris E et al. Osteoporos Int 2002; 13:257–64.
48. Meyer HE, Smedshaug GB, Kvaavik E et al. J Bone Miner Res 2002;17:709–15.

49. Trivedi DP, Doll R, Khaw KT. BMJ 2003;326:469.

50. Lips P, Graafmans WC, Ooms ME et al. Ann Intern Med 1996; 124:400–6.

51. Komulainen MH, Kroger H, Tuppurainen MT et al. Maturitas 1998;31:45–54.

52. Food and Nutrition Board, Institute of Medicine. Dietary Reference Intakes for Calcium, Phosphorus, Magnesium, Vitamin D, and Fluoride. Washington, DC: National Academy Press, 1997:250–287.

53. Trang HM, Cole DE, Rubin LA et al. Am J Clin Nutr 1998; 68:854–8.

54. Calvo MS, Kumar R, Heath H. J Clin Endocrinol Metab 1990; 70:1334–40.

55. Chapuy MC, Arlot ME, Duboeuf F et al. N Engl J Med 1992; 327:1637–42.

56. Arjmandi BH, Khalil DA, Smith BJ et al. J Clin Endocrinol Metab 2003;88:1048–54.

57. Roughead ZK, Johnson LK, Lykken GI et al. J Nutr 2003; 133:1020–6.

58. Schurch MA, Rizzoli R, Slosman D et al. Ann Intern Med 1998;128:801–9.

59. Food and Nutrition Board, Institute of Medicine Food. Dietary Reference Intakes for Vitamin A, Vitamin K, Arsenic, Boron, Chromium, Copper, Iodine, Iron, Manganese, Molybdenum, Silicon, Vanadium, and Zinc: A Report of the Panel on Micronutrients. Washington, DC: National Academy Press, 2001:65–126.

60. Haussler MR, Haussler CA, Jurutka PW et al. J Endocrinol 1997;154[Suppl 73]:57S–73S.

61. Johansson S, Melhus H. J Bone Miner Res 2001;16:1899–1905.

62. Frame B, Jackson CE, Reynolds WA et al. Ann Intern Med 1974;80:44–8.

63. Freudenheim JL, Johnson NE, Smith EL. Am J Clin Nutr 1986;44:863–76.

64. Promislow JH, Goodman-Gruen D, Slymen DJ et al. J Bone Miner Res 2002;17:1349–58.

65. Feskanich D, Singh V, Willett WC et al. JAMA 2002;287:47–54.

66. Michaelsson K, Lithell H, Vessby B et al. N Engl J Med 2003; 348:287–94.

67. Kawahara TN, Krueger DC, Engelke JA et al. J Nutr 2002; 132:1169–72.

68. Furie BC, Furie B. Thromb Haemost 1997;78:595–8.

69. Feskanich D, Weber P, Willett WC et al. Am J Clin Nutr 1999; 69:74–9.

70. Booth SL, Tucker KL, Chen H et al. Am J Clin Nutr 2000; 71:1201–8.

71. Luukinen H, Kakonen SM, Pettersson K et al. J Bone Miner Res 2000;15:2473–8.

72. Shiraki M, Shiraki Y, Aoki C et al. J Bone Miner Res 2000; 15:515–21.

73. Devine A, Criddle RA, Dick IM et al. Am J Clin Nutr 1995; 62:740–5.

74. Barger-Lux MJ, Heaney RP, Stegman MR. Am J Clin Nutr 1990;52:722–5.

75. Harris SS, Dawson-Hughes B. Am J Clin Nutr 1994;60:573–8.

76. Barrett-Connor E, Chang JC, Edelstein SL. JAMA 1994;271: 280–3.

77. Kiel DP, Felson DT, Hannan MT et al. Am J Epidemiol 1990; 132:675–84.

78. Kelepouris N, Harper KD, Gannon F et al. Ann Intern Med 1995;123:452–60.

79. Felson DT, Zhang Y, Hannan MT et al. Am J Epidemiol 1995; 142:485–92.

80. Hansen MA, Overgaard K, Riis BJ et al. Osteoporos Int 1991; 1:95–102.

81. Bernstein DS, Sadowsky N, Hegsted DM et al. JAMA 1966; 198:499–504.

82. Cauley JA, Murphy PA, Riley TJ et al. J Bone Miner Res 1995; 10:1076–86.

83. Suarez-Almazor ME, Flowerdew G, Saunders LD et al. Am J Public Health 1993;83:689–93.

84. Riggs BL, Hodgson SF, O'Fallon WM et al. N Engl J Med 1990;322:802–9.

85. Kleerekoper M, Peterson EL, Nelson DA et al. Osteoporos Int 1991;1:155–61.

86. Pak CY, Sakhaee K, Adams-Huet B et al. Ann Intern Med 1995; 123:401–8.

87. Nielsen FH, Hunt CD, Mullen LM et al. FASEB J 1987; 1:394–7.

88. Meunier PJ, Slosman DO, Delmas PD et al. J Clin Endocrinol Metab 2002;87:2060–6.

89. Reginster JY, Deroisy R, Dougados M et al. Osteoporos Int 2002;13:925–31.

90. Strause L, Saltman P, Smith KT et al. J Nutr 1994;124:1060–4.

91. Cummings SR, Nevitt MC, Browner WS et al. N Engl J Med 1995;332:767–73.

92. Reid IR, Legge M, Stapleton JP et al. J Clin Endocrinol Metab 1995;80:1764–8.

93. Aloia JF, Vaswani A, Ma R et al. Am J Clin Nutr 1995;61: 1110–4.

94. Ryan AS, Nicklas BJ, Dennis KE. J Appl Physiol 1998;84: 1305–10.

95. Krall EA, Dawson-Hughes B. J Bone Miner Res 1991;6: 1323–9.

96. The Postmenopausal Estrogen/Progestin Interventions (PEPI) Trial Investigators. JAMA 1996;276:1389–96.

97. Michnovicz JJ, Hershcopf RJ, Naganuma H et al. N Engl J Med 1986;315:1305–9.

98. Kiel DP, Baron JA, Anderson JJ et al. Ann Intern Med 1992; 116:716–21.

99. Slemenda CW, Christian JC, Reed T et al. Ann Intern Med 1992;117:286–91.

100. Kelley GA, Kelley KS, Tran ZV. Am J Phys Med Rehabil 2001; 80:65–77.

101. Kohrt WM, Snead DB, Slatopolsky E et al. J Bone Miner Res 1995;10:1303–11.

102. Snow CM, Shaw JM, Winters KM et al. J Gerontol 2000;55: M489–91.

103. Campbell AJ, Robertson MC, Gardner MM et al. BMJ 1997; 315:1065–9.

104. Eisman JA. Endocr Rev 1999;20:788–804.

105. Morrison NA, Qi JC, Tokita A et al. Nature 1994;367:284–7.

106. Riggs BL, Nguyen TV, Melton LJ III et al. J Bone Miner Res 1995;10:991–6.

107. Krall EA, Parry P, Lichter JB et al. J Bone Miner Res 1995;10: 978–84.

108. Dawson-Hughes B, Harris SS, Finneran S. J Clin Endocrinol Metab 1995;80:3657–61.

109. Johnson ML, Gong G, Kimberling W et al. Am J Hum Genet 1997;60:1326–32.

110. Boyden LM, Mao J, Belsky J et al. N Engl J Med 2002;346: 1513–21.

111. American College of Rheumatology. Arthritis Rheum 1996;39: 1791–801.

112. Eriksen EF, Colvard DS, Berg NJ et al. Science 1988;241: 84–6.

113. Cauley JA, Robbins J, Chen Z et al. JAMA 2003;290:1729–38.

114. Writing Group for the Women's Health Initiative Investigators. JAMA 2002;288:321–33.

115. Cranney A, Wells G, Willan A et al. Endocr Rev 2002;23: 508–16.

116. Chesnut CH III, Silverman S, Andriano K et al. Am J Med 2000;109:267–76.

117. Cranney A, Tugwell P, Zytaruk N et al. Endocr Rev 2002; 23:524–8.

118. Cauley JA, Norton L, Lippman ME et al. Br Cancer Res Treat 2001;65:125–34.

119. Neer RM, Arnaud CD, Zanchetta JR et al. N Engl J Med 2001; 344:1434–41.

120. Black DM, Greenspan SL, Ensrud KE et al. N Engl J Med 2003;349:1207–15.

121. Finkelstein JS, Hayes A, Hunzelman JL et al. N Engl J Med 2003;349:1216–26.

122. Lips P, Chapuy MC, Dawson-Hughes B et al. Osteoporos Int 1999;9:394–7.

87 | BEHAVIORAL DISORDERS AFFECTING FOOD INTAKE: EATING DISORDERS AND OTHER PSYCHIATRIC CONDITIONS[1]

JANELLE W. COUGHLIN AND ANGELA S. GUARDA

OVERVIEW OF EATING DISORDERS 1353
   Anorexia Nervosa 1353
   Bulimia Nervosa 1353
   Eating Disorder Not Otherwise Specified 1354
EPIDEMIOLOGY 1354
ETIOLOGY: RISK AND SUSCEPTIBILITY FACTORS 1354
   Genetics 1354
   Personality 1355
   Developmental Factors 1355
   Sociocultural Factors 1355
CONSEQUENCES AND COMPLICATIONS 1356
   Social and Developmental Complications 1356
   Psychologic Complications 1356
   Physical Complications and Signs 1356
TREATMENT 1357
   Evidence-Based Treatment 1357
   Role of the Nutritionist 1358
   Prognosis and Outcomes 1359
OTHER PSYCHIATRIC CONDITIONS AFFECTING
   FOOD INTAKE 1359
   Mood Disorders 1359
   Schizophrenia 1359
   Substance Use Disorders 1360
   Psychotropic Medications 1360

Eating disorders are driven behavioral disorders resulting in significant functional impairment and, in extreme cases, death. Although they occur along a spectrum, so diagnostic boundaries are often blurred, the fourth edition of the *Diagnostic and Statistical Manual of Mental Disorders* (1) distinguishes three major categories of eating disorders: anorexia nervosa (AN), bulimia nervosa (BN), and eating disorder not otherwise specified (EDNOS). Binge-eating disorder (BED) is often accompanied by obesity and is subsumed under the EDNOS category. BED is currently under consideration as a distinct eating disorder and has become the focus of significant clinical and scientific attention.

Unlike BED, AN and BN are perhaps better thought of as "dieting disorders" (2). Both are characterized by an overvalued fear of fatness that drives a set of disturbed behaviors, including restricting food intake, binge eating, excessive exercise, self-induced vomiting, and abuse of laxatives, diuretics, and diet pills. Engagement in these behaviors, coupled with the physiologic consequences of starvation and/or the binge-purge-restrict cycle, sustains and heightens food preoccupation and body image disturbance. This chapter reviews the diagnosis, epidemiology, etiology, complications, and treatment of eating disorders. Although obesity is often the consequence of repetitive overeating and/or binge eating, it is primarily a medical condition and is addressed in a chapter reserved solely for this topic. The chapter concludes with a summary of other psychiatric conditions and frequently prescribed psychotropic medications that may affect food intake.

OVERVIEW OF EATING DISORDERS

Anorexia Nervosa

AN is a syndrome of self-starvation characterized by weight loss to a level below 85% of expected body weight. Weight loss is accompanied by fear of fatness and, in girls and women, amenorrhea or the absence of three or more consecutive menstrual cycles. AN is further subdivided into a restricting (AN-R) or a binge-eating/purging (AN-P) subtype. Individuals with AN-R restrict food intake and often excessively exercise and fidget in the service of weight loss but do not binge or engage in purging behaviors. By contrast, AN-P includes regular binge-eating and/or purging behaviors (e.g., self-induced vomiting and abuse of laxatives, diuretics, and enemas).

Bulimia Nervosa

BN is a dieting disorder characterized by episodes of binge eating followed by compensatory behaviors aimed at preventing weight gain. Binge eating is defined as consumption of an amount of food definitely larger than most people would eat in a similar period, under similar circumstances, and is associated with a sense of loss of control over eating. Typical binge foods are high-fat, high-calorie, "forbidden" foods, and amounts consumed are 1000 to 2000 calories or more per binge (3). Between binges, bulimic individuals

---

[1]**Abbreviations: AN,** anorexia nervosa; **BED,** binge-eating disorder; **BMI,** body mass index; **BN,** bulimia nervosa; **CBT,** cognitive-behavioral treatment; **EDNOS,** eating disorder not otherwise specified; **IPT,** interpersonal psychotherapy.

typically restrict intake and only consume "safe," low-calorie, low-fat foods. Other compensatory behaviors following a binge can include purging, by vomiting, abuse of laxatives or diuretics, or excessive exercise. As in AN, dieting and preoccupation with thinness develop into a consuming passion difficult to interrupt. The distinction between AN-P and BN is primarily one of weight; that is, individuals who binge and purge but are below 85% of ideal body weight and are amenorrheic are given the diagnosis of AN-P, whereas those who are less underweight, or more commonly of normal weight or overweight, are given the diagnosis of BN. The two subtypes of BN are purging (BN-P) and nonpurging (BN-NP). Individuals with BN-NP do not self-induce vomiting or abuse laxatives or diuretics; rather, episodes of binge eating alternate with fasting or excessive exercise.

Eating Disorder Not Otherwise Specified

EDNOS is a heterogeneous diagnostic category. It includes partial-syndrome cases of AN and BN, BED, and atypical eating disorders. For partial-syndrome AN or BN, the diagnosis of EDNOS does not imply minor clinical significance. Indeed, these cases may be associated with morbidity equal to or greater than full-syndrome cases of AN or BN (4). An example would be an individual whose baseline weight was obese and who developed intense fear of fatness and extreme dieting behaviors, rapidly losing more than 40% of his or her body weight yet failing to meet the underweight criterion for AN or the binge frequency criterion for BN.

BED is defined as regular binge eating, twice a week or more, associated with a subjective sense of loss of control over eating but lacking the compensatory behaviors typical of BN. BED differs from BN in several additional ways. Individuals with BN tend to restrict their food choices and calorie intake when not bingeing yet are more impulsive and consume more calories during binges than do individuals with BED. Patients with BED overeat more consistently throughout the day than do patients with BN (5) and are more likely to be overweight or obese.

Examples of atypical eating disorders include globus hystericus, or fear of swallowing, resulting in severe weight loss and functional impairment, and psychogenic vomiting syndromes. In some cases, these may be factitious disorders, conditions in which the behavior persists in part because the sick role has become rewarding to the affected individual.

EPIDEMIOLOGY

Epidemiologic data on eating disorders is limited for several reasons. Both AN and BN have relatively low prevalence in the general population. Furthermore, most patients are ambivalent about seeking treatment and minimize their symptoms. A minority of cases reaches clinical attention, so research on clinical samples inevitably underestimates the true incidence of these psychiatric conditions (6).

The prevalence of AN among young women is approximately 0.3%, with girls and women ten times more likely to develop AN than boys and men (6). The age- and sex-adjusted incidence in the general population is approximately eight cases per 100,000 population per year. Across the life span, AN is most likely to have its onset among girls and women ages 15 to 19 years, who comprise an estimated 40% of documented new cases. In one epidemiologic sample, incidence rates in this age group increased steadily from 1935 to 1989 (7). It is unclear how much this increase reflects better detection and increased care seeking as awareness of the diagnosis among both clinicians and the general public has increased.

Incidence rates of BN are consistently higher than those reported for AN across studies, approximating 12 cases per 100,000 population per year (6). These are likely to be underestimates because of the more secretive nature of this disorder and because affected individuals lack the starved habitus that makes AN easier to detect. The higher incidence and prevalence of BN are also partly explained by research suggesting that as many as 40% of patients with AN progress to BN over time as a result of the challenges of maintaining a low body weight through primarily restrictive behaviors (8). In comparison with AN, the age of onset in BN is later, with 20- to 24-year-old women being at greatest risk. Prevalence rates for BN are 1% for girls and women and 0.1% for boys and men, the same gender distribution found in AN (6).

EDNOS is a phenomenologically heterogeneous group, and epidemiologic information on it is scant at best, although the prevalence of partial-syndrome eating disorders is at least twice that of full-syndrome eating disorders (9). Only three population studies of the prevalence of BED have been completed, and these reveal a prevalence rate of 2 to 3%, a more equal female-to-male distribution (approximately 2:1), and a later age of onset than that of AN or BN of 30 to 50 years (10). Rates of BED are much higher, on the order of approximately 25%, in clinical samples of obese individuals seeking weight-loss treatment (11).

ETIOLOGY: RISK AND SUSCEPTIBILITY FACTORS

Although knowledge of the pathogenesis of eating disorders remains limited, it is clear that the etiology of these conditions is multifactorial and in most cases includes the interaction of both genetic and environmental predisposing factors. These interactions and how they contribute to risk remain largely unexplored and are believed to vary significantly among individuals.

Genetics

Family, twin, and molecular studies suggest that eating disorders are genetically influenced. Cross-transmission of AN, BN, and EDNOS within families suggests a shared familial liability (12). Prevalence of eating disorders in relatives of eating-disordered probands is seven to 12 times that of controls, and monozygotic twins have significantly higher concordance rates of AN and BN than their dizygotic counterparts (13); however, eating disorders do not necessarily breed true (i.e., relatives of probands with AN have increased rates of AN or BN, not increased rates of AN specifically). Twin studies have found heritability estimates of 58 to 76% for AN, 54 to 76% for BN, 38 to 61% for BED, and 32 to 72% for attitudes commonly associated with eating disorders (e.g., body dissatisfaction and weight preoccupation) (13, 14). Attempts to identify biologic markers for AN and BN have led some researchers to investigate polymorphisms in serotonin- and dopamine-related genes. Other studies have targeted leptin and estrogen receptors, genes involved in weight regulation, feeding, and energy expenditure (15). Although promising, research on these biologic markers has produced inconsistent findings and therefore awaits further investigation.

Personality

Research has identified several personality traits associated with eating disorders including elevated harm avoidance (15), neurotic personality features, and low self-esteem (16). Perfectionism, conscientiousness, persistence, and obsessive qualities are often discriminating features of AN, whereas elevated impulsivity, novelty seeking, negative emotionality, stress reactivity, and personality traits associated with antisocial, borderline, histrionic, and narcissistic personality disorders are more commonly associated with BN (15, 17). Family studies have found increased levels of some of these traits in first-degree relatives of individuals with eating disorders, a finding suggesting that the heritability of AN and BN may be related in part to the heritability of these personality characteristics (17).

Developmental Factors

Eating disorders are significantly more prevalent in menstruating girls and women than in prepubertal girls, a finding implicating a role for ovarian hormones and sexual development in the activation of disordered eating (18). Perception of being overweight prepubertally (19) and early-onset menarche (20) have emerged as specific aspects of puberty that may increase eating disorder vulnerability. Early-maturing girls have higher adiposity before menarche, are more dissatisfied with their bodies, and are more likely to engage in weight-loss efforts than girls who go through puberty on time or later in life (20). Environmental changes associated with the transition to college, including high levels of stress, performance and achievement demands, and role and identity changes, are factors significantly related to disordered eating (21) and may make this developmental milestone one that places late adolescents at risk of developing eating disorders. Past trauma, namely, childhood sexual abuse, may heighten the risk of

developing eating disorders; however, early sexual abuse has been associated with other psychiatric conditions, thus making it difficult to determine whether a direct link between eating disorders and childhood sexual abuse exists or whether early sexual abuse and mental health are more broadly linked (22).

Sociocultural Factors

The sociocultural model of eating disorders posits that eating disorders and body image disturbances are the result of pervasive societal pressures on girls and women to be thin. According to this model, messages idealizing thinness are transmitted to members of society through the mass media, peers, and families. Although this model explains why eating disorders are more common in Western cultures that value thinness, only a small minority of the population develops eating disorders; therefore, sociocultural factors alone are not a sufficient explanation for the development of an eating disorder. However, pressures to be thin starting around the age of puberty may trigger the onset of dieting behavior in otherwise vulnerable individuals.

Mass Media

Slender female models and images (e.g., cartoons, computer graphics) saturate the mass media of Western culture. Internalization, or acceptance, of these societal standards of thinness may lead to low self-esteem, negative affect, dieting, and/or eating disorders in girls and women (23). Experimental studies have consistently shown that girls and women exposed to media images of thinness experience greater body dissatisfaction in comparison with those exposed to heavier or neutral images (24). The negative effect of these images is heightened when girls and women viewing slender images have already internalized thin beauty ideals or have high baseline levels of body image disturbance.

Peers

Pressure to be thin from peers (25) and past history of weight-related teasing (26) may impact body dissatisfaction among girls and women and may increase the risk of disordered eating behaviors; however, at least one study reported that weight-related teasing does not predict body dissatisfaction in adolescent girls (27). Because most studies of teasing are retrospective, they are also affected by recall bias, which may be stronger in individuals with body dissatisfaction who are at risk of eating disorders. Similarly, although members of adolescent female cliques often have comparable levels of body image disturbance, it is unclear whether body image is directly influenced by peers or whether adolescents simply seek homogeneous peer groups. Among college sorority sisters, bingeing and purging behaviors are passed from one individual to another, much like the spreading of a disease (a contagion effect), a finding suggesting a direct social influence of peers on disordered eating (28).

Family

Parents are the most dominant sociocultural factor affecting young children, and parents' direct comments about their child's weight, particularly comments of mothers, have been identified as the most consistent factor associated with children's concerns and behaviors related to weight and shape (29, 30). Familial dynamics are also important predisposing factors in eating disorders. Girls who eat alone, who have parents who are not married, (31) or who perceive their family communication, parental caring, and parental expectations as low (32) are at increased risk of disordered eating. Indeed, investigators have suggested that low perceived social support from the family, coupled with low self-esteem, high body concern, and use of escape-avoidance coping, places women at high risk of developing eating disorders (33).

CONSEQUENCES AND COMPLICATIONS

Social and Developmental Complications

Eating is a highly social activity, and eating disorders inevitably impair interpersonal function. Affected individuals become socially isolated in an attempt to hide or avoid confrontation regarding their food choices or amounts eaten and spend increasing time engaged in eating rituals and exercise routines that take precedence over age-appropriate social engagements. Formation of intimate relationships and sexual function are often impaired by starvation's effect on libido and heightened body image concerns. Because they primarily affect young women and girls, AN and BN often result in the interruption of normal developmental tasks including separation-individuation from parents, identity formation, and the development of meaningful peer relationships.

Psychologic Complications

Individuals with eating disorders describe a consuming and constant preoccupation with food and weight that occupies much of their waking time and worsens with starvation. Furthermore, starvation results in a syndrome characterized by low mood, apathy, anhedonia, and decreased concentration and energy that is indistinguishable from major depression but reverses within days or weeks of refeeding (34). Besides starvation-related increases in obsessional preoccupation with food and weight and depressive symptoms, family studies have confirmed increased rates of affective disorders, alcohol abuse, and anxiety disorders in first-degree relatives of individuals with AN and BN (17). This finding suggests that comorbid psychiatric conditions are common and may complicate the treatment

course unless they are addressed in parallel with the eating disorder. Finally, demoralization and loss of self-esteem often accompany patients' attempts to control their behaviors and the realization that these behaviors have impaired their functioning.

Physical Complications and Signs

Physical complications arise as a consequence of starvation and/or purging behaviors. The diagnostic group at highest risk is therefore AN-P, underweight starved patients who employ purging techniques in the service of weight loss. Besides complications of the eating disorder itself, treatment and refeeding are associated with potential medical risks.

Starvation-Related Complications

Malnutrition and starvation in AN are associated with numerous physical signs and symptoms. Patients often appear emaciated, with muscle wasting and weakness on examination, and may develop lanugo, the growth of fine, diffuse body hair. Physiologic responses to self-starvation are aimed at conserving energy and include bradycardia, hypotension, hypothermia, and interruption of the hypothalamic-pituitary-ovarian axis. Estrogen, follicle-stimulating hormone, and luteinizing hormone revert to prepubertal levels, as a result of disturbances in gonadotropin-releasing hormone pulsatility, resulting in amenorrhea and infertility. In prepubertal patients, normal secondary sexual characteristics, such as breast development and height, may be halted by malnutrition (35). Patients frequently complain of cold intolerance, fatigue, and gastrointestinal symptoms, including bloating, early satiety, and constipation. Starvation also results in delayed gastric emptying, delayed gastrointestinal transit times, and constipation (36). Anemia is common, and pancytopenia and bone marrow suppression can occur in severely malnourished patients (37). Osteoporosis is a largely irreversible consequence of AN, occurring relatively early in the course of the disorder; most affected girls and women develop significant decreases in bone density within a year of onset, and osteoporosis can also be a complication for boys and men with AN (38). Osteoporosis results in elevated fracture risk, and patients with chronic AN are at risk of debilitating hip fractures and spinal compression fractures. Unlike in menopausal osteoporosis, little evidence suggests a protective role for estrogen in preventing bone loss, and weight restoration is the only intervention known to stop bone mineral loss (39).

Purging-Related Complications

Patients who vomit may present with visible bilateral parotid and salivary gland hypertrophy and with the Russell sign, calluses on the dorsum of the hand resulting from reflexive biting during manual stimulation of the gag reflex to induce vomiting. Dental caries and enamel erosion of the lingual surface of the teeth are also common. Recurrent vomiting can lead to esophagitis and reflux, and some patients ruminate or chew and spit food as part of their disorder (40). Ipecac abuse is especially dangerous because its active ingredient, emetine, is cardiotoxic and has a long half-life, accumulating in cardiac muscle and increasing the risk of life-threatening cardiomyopathy.

Laxative abusers often use large quantities of laxatives daily and may develop laxative dependence and constipation. Besides acute dehydration and presyncopal or syncopal symptoms, chronic laxative and diuretic abuse can lead to renal damage and nephrocalcinosis. Both vomiting and laxative abuse can result in electrolyte and acid-base imbalances as well as dehydration. The most common serious electrolyte imbalance is hypokalemia, which increases the risk of potentially lethal cardiac arrhythmias.

Refeeding Syndrome

Refeeding syndrome is the term used to describe the constellation of severe metabolic abnormalities that may arise in AN as a result of rapid weight restoration (41). These complications are more likely to occur with parenteral and enteral refeeding than with oral refeeding but are risks in any severely malnourished patient. In severely starved patients with a body mass index (BMI, measured as weight in kilograms divided by the square of the height in meters) of 14 or lower, refeeding should be initiated gradually, starting with 1200 to 1500 cal/day and advancing to 3500 cal/day in increments no larger than 500 calories every 2 to 3 days (42). The initial diet should be low in salt, lactose, and fat to minimize malabsorption and edema. Severe hypophosphatemia, a serious potential complication of refeeding, results from the intracellular shift of serum phosphate needed for the regeneration of adenosine triphosphate, 2,3-diphosphoglycerate, and glycerol-3-phosphate involved in cellular anabolic processes. Hypophosphatemia is associated with cardiac and neuromuscular dysfunction and with hematologic red and white blood cell dysfunction. Intracellular shifts in potassium and magnesium leading to low serum levels of these two electrolytes contribute to an increased risk of cardiac arrhythmia, as well as to gastrointestinal and neuromuscular complications. Rapid extracellular fluid expansion resulting in peripheral edema is common in malnourished patients during early refeeding, and in extreme cases, congestive heart failure is a risk. Abrupt cessation of laxative or diuretic abuse and vomiting behavior can contribute to fluid retention. Patients who purge using these techniques tend to have chronically elevated aldosterone levels from metabolic alkalosis induced by volume depletion, which may take several weeks to normalize (43). Finally, severely underweight patients are at risk of Wernicke encephalopathy related to thiamin deficiency. Thiamin supplementation intramuscularly or intravenously before refeeding in severely starved patients is recommended (44).

TREATMENT

AN and BN are behavioral disorders and, like addictions, once established, tend to take on a life of their own. Although certain stressors and risk factors are associated with their onset, disordered eating patterns eventually sustain themselves. Initial treatment goals include normalizing eating patterns and restoring weight in underweight patients. Starvation perpetuates a preoccupation with food (34), and weight restoration is well established as necessary, if not sufficient, for recovery from AN (45). Similarly, in BN, repeated engagement in the restrict-binge-purge cycle exacerbates symptomatic preoccupations with weight and shape and the drive to diet. Psychotherapy aimed at elucidating underlying individual vulnerabilities to these disorders may provide a meaningful narrative to patients to help them understand the development of their disorder, but it is unlikely to bring about behavioral change. Primarily insight-oriented approaches are therefore best reserved for a later stage in treatment once eating behavior has been normalized.

Patients with AN or BN tend to be ambivalent about treatment because they experience their dieting behaviors as rewarding and do not want to stop them. Successful treatment can be seen as requiring a cognitive shift or conversion, from viewing dieting as a solution to seeing it as the primary impairment to healthy function. Treating clinicians often find themselves in a battle of wills with patients who deny or minimize the severity of their problems. Motivating patients with AN or BN to change their behavior requires significant role induction and the building of a strong therapeutic alliance between clinician and patient. The clinician is faced with the task of repeatedly confronting the patient about the self-destructive consequences of his or her behavior in the presence of the patient's resistance to change.

Evidence-Based Treatment

To date, the most comprehensive guidelines for the treatment of eating disorders are the American Psychiatric Association's practice guidelines (45) and the clinical guidelines of the National Institute for Clinical Excellence (46). Decisions about the appropriate setting for treatment and the introduction of pharmacotherapy should be made by professionals familiar with these guidelines who are able to assess psychiatric, behavioral, and medical factors associated with eating disorders. Treatment often requires collaboration and close communication within a multidisciplinary team, which may include psychiatrists, general practitioners, psychologists, social workers, professional counselors, nutritionists, nurses, and/or occupational therapists.

Outpatient Treatment

Randomized clinical trials provide strong empirical evidence in support of cognitive-behavioral treatment (CBT) of eating disorders, particularly for BN and BED (46). CBT involves several components: (a) normalization of eating behavior, (b) self-monitoring and maintaining of food records, (c) correcting cognitive distortions that sustain disordered eating habits, and (d) relapse-prevention techniques. Interpersonal psychotherapy (IPT), a treatment that focuses on maladaptive interpersonal patterns and relationships, is an effective alternative to CBT for treatment of both BN and BED; however, IPT is typically of longer duration and has fewer studies supporting its efficacy in comparison with CBT.

In contrast to BN and BED, a paucity of controlled research addresses the outpatient treatment of AN. One exception is adolescent AN of short duration. This subset of patients has been found to respond best to outpatient family therapy that instructs parents to take control of their child's food intake (47). Family therapy is equally effective whether the patient is treated separately from his or her parents or conjointly as a family, although parent training and separated family therapy techniques are easier to learn and disseminate among clinicians than conjoint family therapy (48, 49). In the case of adult AN, evidence-based trials of outpatient interventions are scant and are plagued by methodologic problems such as high dropout rates. Furthermore, most outpatient trials have been ineffective at achieving weight restoration in this population. A double-blind controlled trial of CBT for relapse prevention in AN, however, suggests that once weight is restored in an inpatient setting, follow-up outpatient CBT is more effective than nutritional counseling in preventing relapse at 1-year follow-up (50).

Inpatient Treatment and Partial Hospitalization

The presence of comorbid psychiatric problems, a dangerously low BMI, metabolic complications or abnormalities, suicidality, pregnancy, type 1 diabetes, and self-injurious behaviors often warrant inpatient hospitalization in patients with eating disorders (45). Most patients admitted to inpatient specialty units for eating disorders have AN, because uncomplicated BN is usually treatable in an outpatient setting. Only those patients with BN who are treatment resistant or who have serious medical or psychiatric comorbidity are likely to be admitted as inpatients. Although few randomized clinical trials exist, naturalistic studies have yielded certain conclusions about the efficacy of acute inpatient treatment for AN. Behavioral units are well established in achieving rapid weight restoration in severely underweight patients on the order of 2 to 4 lb/week (~1–2 kg/week) (42, 45). The less structured partial-hospital setting can also be effective for weight restoration; however, rates of weight gain are slower, averaging 0.5 to 2 lb/week, and some patients may not be treatable in this setting because of compliance problems. Partial-hospital treatment can also be useful when applied in a stepdown sequence as a transitional level of care between inpatient and weekly outpatient treatment. In this model, inpatient treatment is used to block eating disorder behaviors and to establish healthy eating patterns, and patients are then given increasing levels of independence over eating as they make the transition to a less restrictive setting.

Medications

The role of pharmacotherapy in the treatment of eating disorders is limited. Most randomized controlled trials are of short duration, and many lack adequate follow-up data. Although several agents have been found useful, especially for the treatment of BN and BED, no agent to date has been conclusively shown to assist patients with AN to gain weight outside the setting of a structured inpatient behavioral refeeding program. One small randomized, controlled study suggested that fluoxetine may be helpful in preventing relapse in weight-restored patients who had AN (51), and some preliminary open-label and uncontrolled studies suggest that the atypical antipsychotics, olanzapine in particular, may hold promise in acutely underweight patients with AN.

In the case of BN, several controlled studies have found that antidepressants are helpful in decreasing urges to binge and purge, although their effect is usually smaller than that of CBT. The best studied antidepressant in BN is fluoxetine, which, at high doses of 60 to 80 mg/day, was found superior to placebo in decreasing bulimic behaviors (52). Lower doses are ineffective, however, and few patients achieve abstinence with medication alone. Importantly, it appears that the antibulimic effect of fluoxetine is independent of its antidepressant effects.

In the case of BED, the most promising data are from a recent controlled trial of the anticonvulsant topiramate, which was effective in decreasing binges and in significantly decreasing weight in patients with BED (53). This agent, however, is poorly tolerated and has frequent, uncomfortable side effects including paresthesias and mental confusion as well as a risk of metabolic acidosis and oligohydrosis.

Role of the Nutritionist

In the case of both AN and BN, education about normal eating should include instruction on scheduling three regular meals a day, eating normal portion sizes, expanding food repertoire, which is often very narrow, and avoiding diet foods. Patients should be encouraged to consume all foods in moderation and in normal combinations and to avoid fat-free or sugar-free diet products. An exception to the latter may be the case for patients with BED or BN who are overweight. These patients are likely to benefit from additional guidance on eating fewer high-calorie, high-fat foods, introducing more fruits, vegetables, and whole-grain unprocessed foods, and engaging in a regular exercise program as well as decreasing sedentary activities, such as watching television. Vegetarianism that develops after the onset of dieting behavior is common in both AN and BN and should be discouraged because it is often used to disguise dieting. Careful questioning usually reveals that preferred vegetarian foods are limited to those low in calories.

Instruction in the diabetic exchange system as a method of estimating portion sizes is easily adapted to the treatment of eating disorders, and this system is useful in teaching portion sizes without focus on calorie counting. Patients with BN or BED should be instructed to eat approximately 2000 cal/day with an initial goal of weight maintenance. Although most patients with BN are dissatisfied with their body shape and want to lose weight, it is important to stress that interrupting bulimic behavior and weight maintenance are the initial goals of treatment. Restricting intake in the service of weight loss is likely to exacerbate bingeing behavior unless the bulimia is in remission for 6 months or more. In the case of BED, many clinicians believe that behavioral weight-loss management strategies can exacerbate bingeing unless they are introduced after a normal eating pattern is established. Data on very-low-calorie diets and behavioral weight-loss strategies in BED are currently mixed, although some studies suggest that the combination of CBT and behavioral weight-loss strategies may prove effective when instituted in a complementary fashion.

Patients with AN who need to gain weight should be instructed to consume the same normal, healthy, 2000-cal diet plus three high-calorie liquid supplements between meals, totaling an additional 1000 to 1500 cal/day to gain weight. These supplements should be thought of as "prescribed medication." On a diet of 3000 to 3500 cal/day, patients should be able to gain 1 to 4 lb/week. While on a weight-gain diet, patients should stop all exercise, or they will be unlikely to gain weight. For severely underweight persons with a BMI of 14.5 or lower, calories may need to be titrated more slowly to minimize the risk of refeeding edema (see the earlier section on refeeding complications). Compulsive weighing should be discouraged, and patients should be instructed to limit weighing to weekly sessions with a nutritionist or their therapist. The treating clinician should instruct patients on how to keep a food log and should review food diaries weekly because self-monitoring is one of the most effective tools in achieving behavioral change. The outpatient treatment of eating disorders often requires a multidisciplinary approach and may initially involve weekly meetings with a nutritionist, an eating disorder therapist, and a physician. Excellent communication among clinicians is essential to this team approach, and clinicians need to be alert to the potential for "splitting" in the service of the eating disorder. This occurs when patients distort the recommendations of one clinician in their report to another member of the team.

Prognosis and Outcomes

Outcomes studies of AN and BN suggest that approximately 50% of patients with eating disorders recover fully,

25 to 30% improve significantly, and 15 to 20% continue to have unrelenting eating disorders following treatment, with mortality rates ranging from 1 to 13% in AN and 0 to 3% in BN (54, 55). Naturalistic studies reveal that the risk of relapse in these disorders is substantial, and recovery is characterized by a fluctuating course with frequent readmissions and exacerbations (56). Less is known about the long-term outcomes of BED treatment; however, the disorder appears to be unstable, waxing and waning with and without treatment and responding well to placebo and wait-list conditions (57).

OTHER PSYCHIATRIC CONDITIONS AFFECTING FOOD INTAKE

Mood Disorders

Although significant changes in body weight are commonly associated with eating disorders, it is not uncommon for individuals who are clinically depressed to lose or gain weight. Major depression is characterized by depressed mood and diminished interest in pleasurable activities accompanied by changes in sleep patterns, difficulty concentrating, loss of libido, lack of energy, feelings of worthlessness or guilt, thoughts of death or suicide, and a disturbance in appetite (1). Children who are depressed often present as irritable, instead of sad and tearful, and may fail to gain weight as expected.

In contrast to eating disorders, changes in appetite that occur during depressive episodes are not driven by fear of fatness and obsession with dieting and food. Rather, depressed individuals frequently report that they have lost interest in eating and tend to identify their weight loss as a problem. These individuals are less likely to become distressed over the thought or reality of resuming normal eating and may even express a desire to do so. Furthermore, their eating pattern does not reflect the restriction of fats, sweets, and high-calorie foods that is typical of AN. Rather, they just eat less and describe losing a taste for food. Not all depressed individuals report decreased appetite, however; some display a marked increase in appetite and cravings and note that they find themselves coping with sadness by overeating and indulging in high-calorie foods. Besides depression, adjustment disorders in response to acute stressors and grief reactions can also be characterized by transient anorexia or loss of appetite accompanied by weight loss.

Schizophrenia

Schizophrenia is a psychotic disorder in which delusions, hallucinations, disorganized speech and behaviors, and affective flattening are often present (1). Individuals frequently become paranoid in response to delusional thoughts, which are erroneous, often bizarre, perceptions of reality that are strongly held, even in the presence of clear contradictory evidence. Although the content of delusions may include a variety of themes, they sometimes involve food or eating. An example of a delusion involving food or eating includes a person's belief that his or her food is contaminated or that he or she is being watched while eating. Such paranoid thinking often results in refusal to eat and, in turn, significant weight loss. Psychiatric management, which includes antipsychotic medication, supportive psychotherapy, and family-based interventions, is commonly recommended for individuals exhibiting delusional and other psychotic symptoms. Cessation of delusional thinking is often necessary for behaviors, such as eating and self-care, to improve.

Substance Use Disorders

Substance use disorders can also affect weight and eating. The effect of different substances on food intake varies depending on substance class and level of use. Substance dependence is characterized by tolerance, withdrawal, extensive and persistent use, functional impairment, and continued use in the presence of physical and psychologic consequences (1). Substance abuse lacks the tolerance and withdrawal that characterize substance dependence but includes significant adverse and harmful substance-related consequences. Substance intoxication is a more reversible psychologic and behavioral reaction to a substance and does not necessarily imply frequent and persistent use.

Marijuana use is associated with increased appetite and food intake, and symptoms of cannabis withdrawal include increased irritability, depression, and decreased food intake (58). Alcoholism is associated with abnormal consummatory behaviors and susceptibility to overweight, obesity, and eating disorders (59). Patients with severe alcoholism may eat sporadically and obtain most of their caloric intake from alcohol, resulting in nutritional deficiencies, including risk of Wernicke-Korsakoff syndrome from inadequate thiamin intake (see Chapter 23). Whereas obesity is prevalent among individuals with a history of significant alcohol consumption, overweight is uncommon in the advanced stages of alcoholism, during which multiple, often irreversible, organ dysfunction is accompanied by severe illness, weight loss, and malnutrition. Cocaine and other amphetamines stimulate the central nervous system and usually decrease appetite and food intake, resulting in weight loss, which can be severe at times. Occasionally, individuals with an eating disorder may abuse these substances preferentially to lose weight.

Drug-induced disturbances in food intake are unlikely to be reversed without significant changes in substance use. Treatment of substance-induced effects on appetite is therefore secondary to treatment of substance dependence, abuse, and intoxication.

Psychotropic Medications

Many psychopharmacologic agents used in the treatment of psychiatric disorders have effects on appetite and food intake (60). Regularly weighing patients who are taking psychotropic medications is crucial to the recognition of weight-related side effects early in treatment. If these problems arise, switching to a different agent that is weight neutral or lowering the dose can be helpful interventions and will increase patient compliance with medication. Several antidepressants, mood stabilizers, and antipsychotics are associated with weight gain and increased appetite, whereas stimulant drugs used in the treatment of attention deficit hyperactivity disorder tend to reduce appetite and may result in weight loss.

Among the antidepressants, the older tricyclic drugs, especially amitriptyline and imipramine, as well as the newer agent mirtazapine, are associated with the largest weight gains. The monoamine oxidase inhibitors, phenelzine and tranylcypromine, are less likely to be associated with weight changes but require adherence to a strict low-tyramine diet to avoid the risk of a hypertensive crisis. For this reason, the latter agents are poor choices in patients unlikely to follow a prescribed diet. The two most frequently used mood stabilizers, lithium and valproate, can both result in weight gain. Lithium can also cause fluid retention and edema in some patients. In contrast, the newer mood stabilizer, topiramate, has been associated with significant weight loss and appetite suppression, with average weight loss of 3 to 10 kg ($\sim$7–22 lb) over several weeks.

Several antipsychotic agents are associated with weight gain. Of the conventional neuroleptics, chlorpromazine and thioridazine have the highest rates of weight gain. Although the newer atypical neuroleptics, clozapine, olanzapine, and quietapine, have a more favorable side effect profile in other respects compared with conventional agents, they often result in significant weight gain and may affect glucose metabolism, resulting in new-onset type 2 diabetes mellitus.

Psychostimulant drugs used in the treatment of attention deficit hyperactivity disorder, including dextroamphetamine, pemoline, and methylphenidate, decrease appetite and often result in weight loss. These drugs may occasionally present a problem because they can suppress growth. Therefore, all children treated with psychostimulants should be regularly monitored using developmental growth charts and periodic weight and height measurements.

REFERENCES

1. American Psychiatric Association. Diagnostic and Statistical Manual of Eating Disorders. 4th ed. Washington, DC: American Psychiatric Association, 2000:583–95.
2. Beumont PJV, Touyz SW. Eur Child Adolesc Psychiatry 2003;12 [Suppl]:120S–4S.
3. Fairburn CG, Harrison PJ. Lancet 2003;361:407–16.
4. Watson TL, Andersen AE. Acta Psyhiatr Scand 2003;108:175–82.
5. Walsh BT, Boudreau G. Int J Eat Disord 2003;34[Suppl]: 30S–8S.
6. Hoek HW, van Hoeken D. Int J Eat Disord 2003;34:383–96.
7. Lucas AR, Crowson CS, O'Fallon WM et al. Int J Eat Disord 1999;148:397–405.

8. Eckert ED, Halmi KA, Marchi P et al. Psychol Med 1995;25: 143–56.

9. Shisslak CM., Crago M., Estes LS. Int J Eat Disord 1995;18: 209–19.

10. Dingemans AE, Bruna MJ, van Furth EF. Int J Obes 2003;26: 299–307.

11. Yanovski SZ. Int J Eat Disorders 2003;34[Suppl]:117S–20S.

12. Strober M, Freeman R, Lampert C et al. Am J Psychiatry 2000; 157:393–401.

13. Klump KL, Kaye WH, Strober M. Psychiatr Clin North Am 2001;24:215–25.

14. Bulik CM, Sullivan, PF, Kendler KS. Int J Eat Disord 2003; 33:293–8.

15. Klien DA, Walsh BT. Int J Psychiatry 2003;15:205–16.

16. Cervera S, Lahortiga F, Martinez-Gonzalez MA et al. Int J Eat Disord 2003;33:271–80.

17. Lilenfeld LR, Kaye WH, Greeno, CG et al. Arch Gen Psychiatry 1998;55:603–10.

18. Klump KL, McGue M, Iacono WG. Int J Eat Disord 2003;33: 287–92.

19. Ackard DM, Peterson CB. Int J Eat Disord 2001;29:187–94.

20. Striegel-Moore RH, McMahon RP, Biro FM et al. Int J Eat Disord 2001;30:421–33.

21. Rosen JC, Compas BE, Tacy B. Int J Eat Disord 2001;29:280–8.

22. Everill JT, Waller G. Int J Eat Disord 1995;53:1–11.

23. Thompson JK, Stice E. Curr Directions Psychol Sci 2001;10: 181–3.

24. Groesz LM, Levine MP, Murnen SK. Int J Eat Disord 2002;31: 1–16.

25. Stice E, Maxfield J, Wells T. Int J Eat Disord 2003;34:108–17.

26. Lunner K, Werthem EH, Thompson JK et al. Int J Eat Disord 2000;28:430–5.

27. Stice E, Whitenton K. Dev Psychol 2002;38:669–78.

28. Crandall CS. J Pers Soc Psychol 1988;55:588–98.

29. Thelen MH, Cormier JF. Behav Ther 1995;26:85–99.

30. Smolak L, Levine MP, Schermer F. Int J Eat Disord 1999;25: 263–71.

31. Martinez-Gonzalez MA, Gual P, Lahortiga F et al. Pediatrics 2003;111:315–20.

32. Neumark-Sztainer D, Story M, Hannan PJ et al. Int J Eat Disord 2000;28:249–58.

33. Ghaderi A. Eat Behav 2003;3:387–96.

34. Keys A, Brozek J, Henschel A et al. The Biology of Human Starvation, vols 1 and 2. Minneapolis: University of Minnesota Press, 1950.

35. Russell GF. J Psychiatr Res 1985;19:363–9.

36. Hadley SJ, Walsh BT. Curr Drug Targets CNS Neurol Disord 2003;2:1–9.

37. Devuyst O, Lambert M, Rodhain J et al., QJM 1993;86:791–9.

38. Bachrach LK, Guido D, Katzman DK et al. Pediatrics 1990;86:440.

39. Mehler PS. Int J Eat Disord. 2003;33:113–26.

40. Guarda AS, Coughlin JW, Cummings M et al. Eat Behav 2004;5: 231–9.

41. Solomon SM, Kirby, DF. JPEN J Parenter Enteral Nutr 1990; 14:90–7.

42. Guarda AS, Heinberg LJ. Inpatient and partial hospital approaches to the treatment of eating disorders. In: Thompson JK, ed. Handbook of Eating Disorders and Obesity. New York: John Wiley and Sons, 2003:297–322.

43. Schulte M, Mehler P. Metabolic abnormalities in eating disorders. In: Mehler PS, Andersen AE, eds. Eating Disorders: A Guide to Medical Care and Complications. Baltimore: Johns Hopkins University Press, 1999:76–86.

44. Winston AP, Jamieson CP, Madira W et al. Int J Eat Disord 2000; 28:451–4.

45. American Psychiatric Association. Am J Psychiatry 2000;157 [Suppl]:1S–39S.

46. National Institute for Clinical Excellence. Eating Disorders: Core Interventions in the Treatment and Management of Anorexia Nervosa, Bulimia Nervosa and Related Eating Disorders. Clinical guideline 9. London: National Collaborating Center for Mental Health, 2004:1–35.

47. Eisler I, Dare C, Russell GFM et al. Arch Gen Psychiatry 1997: 54:1025–30.

48. Eisler I, Dare C, Hodes M et al. J Child Psychiatry Psychol 2000; 41:727–36.

49. Lock J, Le Grange D, Agras WS et al. Treatment Manual for Anorexia Nervosa: A Family-Based Approach. New York: Guilford Press, 2001.

50. Pike KM, Walsh BT, Vitousek K et al. Am J Psychiatry 2003:160: 2046–9.

51. Kaye WH, Nagata T, Weltzin TE et al. Biol Psychiatry 2001;49: 644–52.

52. Romano S, Halmi K, Sarkar NP et al. Am J Psychiatry 2002;159: 96–102.

53. McElroy SL, Arnold LM, Shapira NA et al. Am J Psychiatry 2003;160:255–61.

54. Agras WS, Brandt HA, Bulik CM et al. Int J Eat Disord 2004;35: 509–21.

55. Keel PK, Mitchell J E. Am J Psychiatry 1997;154:313–21.

56. Strober, M., Freeman, R., Morrell W. Int J Eat Disord 1997;22: 339–60.

57. Stunkard AJ, Allison KC. Int J Eat Disord 2003;34[Suppl]: 107S–16S.

58. Haney M. J Clin Pharmacol 2002;42[Suppl]:34S–40S.

59. Thiele T, Navarro M, Sparta DR et al. Neuropeptides 2003;37: 321–37.

60. Vanina Y, Podolskaya A, Sedky K et al. Psychiatr Serv 2002;53: 842–7.

SELECTED READINGS

American Dietetic Association. Nutrition intervention in the treatment of anorexia nervosa, bulimia nervosa, and eating disorders not otherwise specified (EDNOS). J Am Diet Assoc 2001;101:810–9.

American Psychiatric Association Work Group on Eating Disorders. Practice guidelines for the treatment of patients with eating disorders (revision). Am J Psychiatry 2000;157[Suppl 1]:1–39.

Keys A, Brozek J, Henschel A et al. The Biology of Human Starvation, vols 1 and 2. Minneapolis: University of Minnesota Press, 1950.

88 NUTRITIONAL DISORDERS OF THE NERVOUS SYSTEM[1]

GUSTAVO C. ROMÁN

NUTRITION AND COGNITIVE FUNCTION 1363
MICRONUTRIENT DEFICIENCIES AND
  COGNITIVE FUNCTION 1363
    Iodine Deficiency Disorders 1364
    Cognitive Effects of Iron Deficiency 1365
    Cognitive Effects of Zinc Deficiency 1366
NUTRITIONAL NEUROPATHIES AND
  MYELONEUROPATHIES 1366
    Cuban Epidemic Neuropathy 1366
NEUROLOGIC DISORDERS ASSOCIATED WITH
  SPECIFIC VITAMINS 1367
    Vitamin A 1367
    Vitamin B₁ (Thiamin) and Beriberi 1368
    Vitamin B₂ (Riboflavin) 1371
    Niacin Deficiency (Pellagra) 1371
    Vitamin B₆ (Pyridoxine) 1371
    Vitamin B₁₂ (Cobalamin) 1372
    Folic Acid 1374
    Pantothenic Acid (Vitamin B₅) 1375
    Vitamin E (α-tocopherol) 1375
    Vitamin D 1376
DIETARY AND VITAMIN TREATMENT
  IN NEUROLOGY 1376
    Migraine 1376
    Stroke 1376
    Orthostatic Hypotension 1376
    Hepatic Encephalopathy 1376
    Idiopathic Intracranial Hypertension 1378
    Childhood Epilepsy 1378

[1]**Abbreviations: ALA,** α-linolenic acid; **ATP,** adenosine triphosphate; **CNS,** central nervous system; **CoA,** coenzyme A; **CSF,** cerebrospinal fluid; **GABA,** γ-aminobutyric acid; **HIV,** human immunodeficiency virus; **IDD,** iodine deficiency disorder; **IF,** intrinsic factor; **IQ,** intelligence quotient; **5MH₄F,** 5-methyltetrahydrofolate; **MMA,** methylmalonic acid; **MS,** multiple sclerosis; **NAD,** nicotinamide adenine dinucleotide; **NADP,** nicotinamide adenine dinucleotide phosphate; **NADPH,** reduced nicotinamide adenine dinucleotide phosphate; **1,25(OH)₂D,** 1,25-dihydroxyvitamin D; **POW,** prisoner of war; **SAM,** S-adenosylmethionine; **SCD,** subacute combined degeneration; **T₃,** triiodothyronine; **T₄,** thyroxine; **Tc,** transcobalamin; **TPN,** total parenteral nutrition; **WKS,** Wernicke-Korsakoff syndrome.

Brain function is unavoidably dependent on a constant dietary supply of appropriate nutrients. Regrettably, large segments of the world population have limited access to basic foodstuffs. Despite increases in agricultural production, hunger remains a widespread worldwide problem as a result of poverty, war, population displacement, and social unrest. Hunger creates a vicious cycle of poor health, lack of energy, and mental impairment that reduces people's ability to work, thereby increasing poverty. According to the United Nations' Food and Agriculture Organization, in 2004, some 852 million people worldwide were malnourished (1). This represents more than 35% of tropical Africa's population, about 25% of the people in India, and 5 to 20% of Latin America and Caribbean populations. Of them, 150 million children worldwide are underweight, and 182 million are physically and cognitively stunted. Moreover, protein-energy malnutrition contributes to 5 million child deaths per year.

Less recognized, however, are the effects of malnutrition on the nervous system. These may range from isolated involvement of the peripheral nervous system that produces blindness, deafness, paralysis, or sensory deficits to complex lesions of the spinal cord and central nervous system (CNS) that lead to mental retardation, cognitive dysfunction, and gait limitations. Nutritional deficiencies affecting the nervous system are not restricted, however, to developing nations. Selected groups in the developed world also suffer from the neurologic consequences of nutritional deficiencies as a result of meager diets. Populations at risk include the poor, the homeless, people addicted to alcohol and substance abusers, some patients with chronic psychiatric conditions, and demented elderly persons. Also affected are persons with peculiar dietary habits such as strict vegans or those suffering from eating disorders such as bulimia and anorexia nervosa, as well as patients with impaired absorption of nutrients from intestinal malabsorption syndromes. A rampant form of malnutrition peculiar to developed nations is obesity, frequently accompanied by a metabolic syndrome, hypertension, and diabetes that may present with secondary neurologic manifestations as a result of stroke, obstructive sleep apnea, and peripheral neuropathy.

NUTRITION AND COGNITIVE FUNCTION

A constant dietary supply of appropriate nutrients including glucose, amino acids, fatty acids, vitamins, and minerals is required for normal brain function (2). Food is also needed to maintain the integrity of brain membranes and the production of neurotransmitters (3). Although the brain represents only 2% of the body mass, it consumes 20% of the energy provided by the diet and 20% of the oxygen inhaled. Children consume twice more glucose than adults do, and the newborn brain requires 60% of the energy provided by the diet. Therefore, the effects of prolonged hypoglycemia can be devastating for newborns and children, given that the brain is totally dependent on dietary glucose, and glycogen reserves are limited. In the elderly, decreased cognitive performance occurs with relatively mild hypoglycemia (4).

The brain requires a dietary supply of amino acids to synthesize neurotransmitters and proteins. The quality of dietary proteins influences brain protein formation. Tryptophan, a precursor of serotonin (5-hydroxytryptamine)—the neurotransmitter involved in appetite and satiety, sleep, blood pressure, pain sensitivity, and mood—is particularly important because 5-hydroxytryptamine cannot cross the blood-brain barrier. Metabolically active brain sites such as hippocampus, basal ganglia, and hypothalamus are particularly sensitive to the effects of malnutrition, loss of energy, and amino acid supply.

Studies in experimental animals and in humans have demonstrated the importance of appropriate nutrition during crucial—and relatively brief—periods of brain growth (5–9). Neurons and glia are formed and begin migration by 22 weeks of gestation, and by late pregnancy marked axonal and neural proliferation result in substantial brain growth. Brain weight at birth is about 350 g, increasing during the first year of life to about 1100 g or 70% of the adult brain weight. In 1969, Winick and Rosso (10, 11) demonstrated that early malnutrition stunts brain growth and development. Children dying of severe malnutrition during pregnancy and from marasmic malnutrition in early life had smaller head circumferences, decreased brain weight, and lower brain content of total protein, DNA and RNA compared with normal controls. Early malnutrition also affects processes involved in brain maturation such as neurogenesis, neuronal and glial migration, number of synapses, and degree of myelination.

These changes are largely irreversible and cause permanent cognitive deficiencies (4, 8, 12, 13). The extent of the cognitive and neurologic damage depends on factors such as severity and duration of the nutritional deficiency, the stage of brain development, and associated diseases such as diarrhea from *Giardia lamblia* (14) and other causes, as well as familial, social, cultural, and economic factors. Nonetheless, substantial evidence indicates that reduced breast-feeding, low birth weight, iron and iodine deficiency, and protein-energy malnutrition are associated

with long-term deficits in psychomotor brain function (9). Follow-up studies of perinatal malnutrition have shown, 15 and 20 years later, residual deficits in brain size, cognition, and psychosocial achievements (4, 8). Ivanovic and Leiva and their colleagues (15, 16) demonstrated, among high school students in Chile, residual effects of early malnutrition manifested by smaller head circumferences and brain volumes determined by magnetic resonance imaging. Lower intelligence quotient (IQ) and more severe learning difficulties resulted in worse school performance, higher school desertion, and lower enrollment in higher education institutions in those with history of early malnutrition, compared with classmates from a common socioeconomic background who had a normal nutritional history.

Similar, although less severe, problems also occur in premature and low-birth-weight infants (17). In clinical trials comparing breast milk with preterm formula alone or as a supplement to maternal milk, in preterm infants weighing less than 1200 g, children fed banked breast milk took longer to reach 2000 g than those fed a high-protein preterm formula. Lucas and colleagues (18) found that IQs, short-term memory, and attention at 8 years of age were better in children fed maternal milk than in controls, even after adjustment for maternal education and social class. Interestingly, breast milk lowers low-density lipoprotein cholesterol and C-reactive protein, findings indicating decreased risk of atherosclerosis late in life (19).

Maternal milk contains a number of factors, particularly lipids, that promote brain maturation in periods of rapid growth. The brain is 60% structural lipid and depends on dietary lipids. Lack of both linoleic acid and α-linolenic acid (ALA) is incompatible with life. Of major dietary importance are ω-3 fatty acids of the ALA family (2). Arachidonic acid and docosahexaenoic acid are large contributors to nonmyelin membranes and must be provided by the diet. Differentiation and functioning of cultured brain cells, oligodendrocytes, and astrocytes require ALA and ω-3 fatty acids. Brain and visual development are affected by diets with insufficient amounts of essential fatty acids, such as those found in soy oil–based formula products (17).

In adults, decreased dietary levels of ω-3 fatty acids (particularly from fish consumption) increase the risk of depression (20), in particular postpartum depression, Alzheimer disease (21), and vascular dementia (22). An appropriate dietary provision of ω-3 fatty acids during aging may prevent abnormal phospholipid metabolism, thus ensuring membrane maintenance and brain function (23).

MICRONUTRIENT DEFICIENCIES AND COGNITIVE FUNCTION

From the public health viewpoint, iodine is the most important micronutrient for the prevention of brain disorders causing lower intellectual functioning, psychomotor delay, and mental retardation (24). Universal salt iodization may solve the worldwide problem of iodine deficiency disorders (IDDs). The World Health Organization considers that 50 million people have some degree of mental impairment caused by IDDs (25, 26).

Also of major public health importance is the deficiency of other micronutrients capable of affecting the nervous system; these include deficiencies of iron, zinc, and selenium, as well as vitamin B_{12}, folate, and vitamin A. The magnitude of these problems is staggering (24): for instance, 2 billion people—more than 30% of the world's population—suffer from iron deficiency anemia, most often in developing countries in association with malaria and hookworm infections.

Iodine Deficiency Disorders

IDDs occur in areas of the earth where iodine was leached from the soil by the effects of rain, glaciations, and flooding waters. These areas typically include flood plains and mountainous regions such as the Alps, the Balkans, the Andes, the Himalayas, and the New Guinea Highlands (27). The neurologic importance of IDDs resides in the definite risk of fetal brain damage resulting in thyroid hormone deficiency during critical periods of brain development, both in utero and in the early postpartum period (26, 28, 29).

In areas with moderate iodine deficiency (I ingestion = 20–49 μg/day), clinically euthyroid children and adults often have abnormalities of psychomotor and intellectual development including lower IQ, slower visual-motor performances, loss of fine motor skill, deficits in perceptual and neuromotor abilities, apathy, and low developmental quotients (28, 29). A metaanalysis of 19 studies from eight countries included 2676 subjects ranging in age from 2 to 30 years living in iodine-deficient regions. Iodine deficiency resulted in a mean loss of 13.5 IQ points at global population level; that is, 82% of children with normal iodine intake scored better than iodine-deficient children (30). Loss of intellectual capacity and deafness from IDDs constitute public health problems with major impact on socioeconomic development.

Endemic Cretinism and Other Forms of Iodine Deficiency Disorders

Endemic cretinism is a congenital disorder of the CNS manifested by deaf-mutism, mental retardation, spastic diplegia, squint, and signs of bulbar damage (31). Partial manifestations include isolated deafness or deaf-mutism and mental retardation without pyramidal tract signs. In some endemic places (New Guinea, Thailand, Indonesia, the Andes), the usual signs of childhood myxedema— coarse puffy skin, macroglossia, umbilical hernia, short stature, and skeletal disproportion—occur rarely, whereas these signs predominate in other endemic areas (China, Congo). Therefore, two forms of the syndrome of endemic cretinism are recognized: neurologic and myxedematous.

Endemic cretinism is different from congenital hypothyroidism, which occurs in one in 3500 newborns (32). Congenital hypothyroidism results from deficient thyroid function in the fetus and the newborn, resulting from endocrine factors unrelated to dietary iodine deficiency.

Halpern and colleagues (33) studied the neurologic features associated with both types of endemic cretinism in 104 persons with myxedematous cretinism from China and in 35 persons from central Java, Indonesia, who had the predominantly neurologic form. Both types of endemic cretinism had a similar pattern of neurologic involvement with mental retardation, proximal pyramidal and extrapyramidal signs, squint, deafness, primitive reflexes, and typical gait with laxity and deformities of joints. Those with serious hypothyroidism had calcification of basal ganglia on cerebral computed tomography. Therefore, both forms of endemic cretinism represent the most severe degree of brain damage from in utero maternal and fetal hypothyroidism, resulting from dietary iodine deficiency. The myxedematous type is explained by continuing postnatal thyroid hormone deficiency with impaired growth, skeletal retardation, and sexual immaturity. Thiocyanate toxicity from cassava consumption plays a role in myxedematous endemic cretinism. The combined effect of iodine and selenium deficiency is also relevant.

Thiocyanate Toxicity. Numerous staple foods in the tropics contain large amounts of cyanogenic glycosides. These include cassava (*Manihot esculenta* Crantz: *yuca* in Spanish, *manioc* in French), yam, sweet potato, corn, millet (*Sorghum* sp.), bamboo shoots, and beans such as *Phaseolus vulgaris* (34). Tobacco smoke (*Nicotiana tabacum*) also contains considerable amounts of cyanide (150–300 μg per cigarette). Hydrolysis of plant glycosides releases cyanide as hydrocyanic acid. Acute intoxication occurs by rapid cyanide absorption through the gastrointestinal tract or the lungs. Detoxification is mainly to thiocyanate in a reaction mediated by a sulfur-transferase (rhodanase) converting thiosulfate into thiocyanate and sulfite. The sulfur-containing essential amino acids, cystine, cysteine, and methionine, provide the sulfur for these detoxification reactions. Also important is vitamin B_{12} with conversion of hydroxocobalamin to cyanocobalamin.

Thiocyanate from cassava is goitrogenic (35); it inhibits thyroid peroxidase and prevents the incorporation of iodine into thyroglobulin (36). Thiocyanate may also form thiourea. These mechanisms explain the damaging neurologic effects of cyanide, diets poor in sulfur-containing amino acids, and low dietary iodine intake.

Selenium. In 1990, Vanderpas and associates (37) found combined iodine and selenium deficiency associated with cretinism in northern Zaire (Congo). Selenium is present in high concentrations in the normal thyroid (28), in glutathione peroxidase and superoxide dismutase, the enzymes for detoxification of toxic derivatives of oxygen. It is also present in deiodinase, the enzyme for peripheral conversion of thyroxine (T_4) to triiodothyronine (T_3).

Selenium deficiency decreases T_4 catabolism and allows excessive production of peroxide (H_2O_2) with thyroid cell destruction, fibrosis, and thyroid failure (28).

Pathogenesis of Brain Lesions Induced by Iodine Deficiency

Thyroid hormones affect neuronal differentiation, migration, neural networking, and synaptogenesis (28, 29), through binding of T_3 to nuclear receptors regulating gene expression in different brain regions. Thyroid hormone receptors are present in the human fetus by 8 weeks of gestation and increase about tenfold between 10 and 18 weeks of gestation. Kester and associates (38) found that T_3 is required by the human cerebral cortex before midgestation. T_4 from the mother is the only source and correlates with deiodinase activity in the cortex. For these reasons, even moderately low T_4 maternal levels may be damaging to the fetus. Haddow and colleagues (39) found in mothers with increased thyroid-stimulating hormone during the second trimester of pregnancy, that the strongest predictor of infant mental development was the mothers' free T_4 levels at 12 weeks of gestation. Furthermore, low levels of free T_4 at both 12 and 32 weeks of gestation resulted in worse infant cognitive outcome.

Recently, Lavado-Autric and colleagues (40) and Ausó and associates (41) produced in the rat an experimental model of transient maternal hypothyroxinemia—low T_4 but normal T_3—demonstrating that transient and mild thyroid function deficits in the mother during early gestation produced permanent abnormalities in cortical cytoarchitecture, with presence of heterotopic neuronal migration in hippocampus and somatosensory cortex. Migration of cortical neurons along the scaffolding provided by radial glia is regulated by the *reelin-dab* signaling system. Reelin is an extracellular protein secreted by Cajal-Retzius neurons that binds to membrane receptors on migrating neurons, phosphorylating the disabled homolog 1 (Dab1) to guide cells to their destination. Hypothyroidism reduces reelin expression and enhances Dab1 expression and could explain these migratory abnormalities (32, 43).

Treatment and Prevention

The results of salt iodination programs in Switzerland offer important evidence of their beneficial effects at population levels (44). Before 1922, the prevalence of cretinism in some Swiss Cantons was 0.5%, and 100% of the schoolchildren had goiter; 30% of young men were unfit for military service because of large goiters. Salt iodination began in 1922 at low levels; by 1930, no cases of cretinism occurred, and goiter disappeared rapidly among schoolchildren. Some Cantons that allowed salt iodination only in 1952 lagged behind in these achievements. The incidence of isolated deafness, mental deficiency, and short stature also decreased after implementation of salt iodination.

In 1966, Pharoah and colleagues (45) demonstrated, in a case-controlled trial in the Jimi Valley of New Guinea, the effects of iodine in the prevention of congenital cretinism. Each alternate family received intramuscular injections of iodine in oil, whereas controls received saline injections. Of the women who received placebo, 534 children were born, and 26 of these children had endemic cretinism, whereas among 498 children of treated women, seven children had endemic cretinism, but six of these women were already pregnant when they received iodine injections. In 1994, Cao and colleagues (46) studied an area of severe iodine deficiency in Xinjiang, China. Oral iodine was provided to 689 children from birth to 3 years of age and to 295 women at each trimester of pregnancy. Neurologic abnormalities occurred in 2% of children born to mothers treated early versus 9% among those treated in the third trimester. Microcephaly decreased from 27% in the untreated group to 11% in the treated children, and developmental quotients at 2 years of age also increased. Treatment in the third trimester of pregnancy or after delivery did not improve neurologic status, but head growth and developmental quotients improved slightly. Treatment during the first trimester improved neurologic outcome. In conclusion, based on these and other controlled clinical trials, treatment with iodized oil or iodized salt before or during early pregnancy prevents endemic cretinism and brain damage (47). Provision of iodized salt is the most cost-effective strategy.

Cognitive Effects of Iron Deficiency

Iron is an essential cofactor for numerous proteins involved in neuronal function. Both iron deficiency anemia and excessive iron accumulation in the brain are associated with neurologic disturbances. The brain has limited access to plasma iron because of the blood-brain barrier (48). Apathy and poverty of movement have been observed in iron-deficient children. A review by Grantham-McGregor and Ani (49) showed that anemic children usually have poor cognition and lower school achievement than nonanemic children. With treatment, most but not all of them tend to improve; however, school achievement generally remains lower in those with prior iron deficiency anemia than in nonanemic controls. Lozoff and Brittenham (50) showed that severe and chronic iron deficiency in infancy continues to cause developmental and behavioral delay more than 10 years after iron treatment. Iron deficiency causes lower cognitive, motor, attentional, and developmental scores, including failure to respond to test stimuli, short attention span, unhappiness, increased fearfulness, withdrawal, and increased body tension. In adults, anemia limits maximal physical performance, endurance, and spontaneous activity.

With aging, there is accumulation of iron-containing molecules in the brain, particularly in Alzheimer and Parkinson diseases, perhaps caused by enhanced generation of reactive oxygen species and higher neuronal vulnerability. Iron accumulation also occurs in congenital aceruloplasminemia,

Friedreich ataxia, Hallervorden-Spatz disease, neuroferritinopathy, neurodegeneration with brain iron accumulation, and in restless legs syndrome (48).

Cognitive Effects of Zinc Deficiency

Dietary zinc deficiency is a common nutritional disorder around the world (24). Zinc treatment of deficient children improves growth, immunity, and motor development in infants and toddlers. Zinc deprivation during periods of rapid growth impairs brain and sexual development. There are few studies in children on the cognitive, motor, and behavioral changes associated with zinc deficiency and supplementation (51).

NUTRITIONAL NEUROPATHIES AND MYELONEUROPATHIES

The polyneuropathies observed in association with alcoholism are usually considered nutritional, although a specific vitamin cannot be identified as causal. Alcohol may play a secondary neurotoxic role, but it also displaces food in the diet, increases the metabolic demands for B-group vitamins, and decreases absorption of thiamin, folic acid, and liposoluble vitamins because of impaired pancreatic function. Symptoms vary from weakness, dysesthesias, and pain to the asymptomatic patient with absent ankle reflexes. Sensory and motor deficits predominate distally and symmetrically in the legs; the face and trunk are not involved. Sensitivity to pressure palsies is often present. On neuropathologic examination, the nutritional neuropathies show predominantly sensory axonal degeneration.

It appears pointless to incriminate one particular factor as the cause of a polyneuropathy appearing in conditions of severe dietary restriction, alcoholism, or widespread malabsorption. Nevertheless, B-group vitamin deficiencies have long been thought to be the main cause of nutritional disorders, particularly when associated to alcoholism.

Neurologic signs occur relatively late during malnutrition. Symptoms appear when a combination of factors finally leads to a deficiency of essential nutrients that is severe enough to injure the nervous system, or when protective nutrients—such as sulfur-containing amino acids and antioxidant carotenoids such as lycopene—become unavailable. The most sensitive elements are highly active metabolic neurons, such as dorsal root ganglia, large myelinated distal axons, bipolar retinal neurons, cochlear neurons. These are the first ones to suffer damage and to manifest the earliest symptoms. Axons require active transport mechanisms to maintain the integrity of neurotubules and to secure axonal flow. Neurotransmitter precursors, glycoproteins, lipids, and amino acids are transported from the soma to the distal axon at rates of 200 to 410 mm/day. There is also a retrograde transport system. Nutritional deficiencies and toxic products disrupt adenosine triphosphate (ATP) production, and axonal flow begins to fail in the typical "dying-back neuropathy" pattern. The distal ends of the longest and largest axons are the first ones to display pathologic changes; the clinical consequences are the stocking-and-glove distribution of sensory and motor symptoms.

In addition to alcoholism, nutritional neuropathies are also observed with dietary restriction (vegans and food faddists), with malabsorption (sprue, pernicious anemia, gastrointestinal tract resections, bariatric surgery), antivitamins (isoniazid), excessive use of pyridoxine, and prolonged inadequate parenteral therapy. A nutritional origin has also been postulated in tropical neuropathies and myeloneuropathies (52, 53). These include the following: Strachan's Jamaican neuropathy (1888), characterized by sensory symptoms of feet and hands, ataxic gait, absent knee reflexes, and decreased sight and hearing; and Mádan's Cuban retrobulbar optic neuropathy (1898), considered to be identical to tobacco-alcohol amblyopia in nondrinking malnourished patients (54). Nutritional neuropathies and myeloneuropathies were common among prisoners of war (POWs) interned in Japanese prison camps in tropical and subtropical regions, mainly in the Far East, during World War II (55). A similar condition was Peraita's Spanish Civil War neuropathy (1939). More recently, in 1993 to 1994, an epidemic of nutritional neuropathy in Cuba affected more than 50,000 people and constituted one of the worst nutritional neurologic epidemics of the last century. This phenomenon emphasizes the pervasiveness and importance of nutrition as a cause of neurologic problems.

Cuban Epidemic Neuropathy

The epidemic of neuropathy in Cuba (54, 56–60) began as an outbreak of optic neuropathy; however, other nutritional syndromes affecting peripheral nerves and spinal cord (Table 88.1) were also observed.

TABLE 88.1. CLINICAL SYNDROMES OBSERVED DURING THE EPIDEMIC OF NUTRITIONAL NEUROPATHY IN CUBA AND POSSIBLE CAUSES

CLINICAL MANIFESTATIONS	POSSIBLE CAUSE
Optic neuropathy	
Decreased visual acuity	Folate-vitamin B_{12} deficiency +
Cecocentral scotoma	methanol
Dyschromatopsia	Cyanide (tobacco)
Dorsolateral myelopathy	
Proprioceptive loss	Vitamin B_{12} deficiency
Pyramidal tract weakness	
Sensorineural deafness	
High-frequency (4–8 kHz) loss	Folate-vitamin B_{12} deficiency
Peripheral neuropathy	
Stocking-glove sensory loss	Thiamin deficiency
Arreflexia	
Burning feet	Niacin, pantothenic acid, thiamin, pyridoxine deficiencies
Myeloneuropathy	Multivitamin deficiency including vitamin E

Epidemiology

A total of 50,862 patients were diagnosed and treated in the island during the epidemic for an incidence rate of 462/100,000, with balanced rates for predominantly optic forms (242/100,000) and peripheral forms (219/100,000). Few cases occurred in children, adolescents, and the elderly. Most cases (87%) occurred between the ages of 25 and 64 years. Optic forms predominated in men aged 45 to 64 years and peripheral forms in women aged 25 to 44 years. The geographic west-to-east pattern of decreasing incidence showed the highest rates in the tobacco-growing province of Pinar del Rio. Risk factors included irregular diet, weight loss, cigar smoking, alcohol, and excessive sugar consumption (60).

Clinical Manifestations

Neurologic symptoms were preceded by weight loss, anorexia, chronic fatigue, lack of energy, irritability, sleep disturbances, and difficulties with concentration and memory.

Optic Neuropathy. Patients complained of blurred vision, photophobia, decreased visual acuity, and loss of color vision for red and green. Examination showed central and cecocentral scotomata, loss of axons in the maculopapillary bundle, and temporal disc pallor in advanced cases (57). One third of patients also presented cheilosis, glossitis, dermatitis, peripheral neuropathy, or funicular spinal cord involvement, and 20% had hearing loss. Vision improved with parenteral B-group vitamins and folic acid treatment.

Dorsolateral Myelopathy. Patients had leg weakness, difficulty walking, increased urinary frequency, impotence in males, brisk knee reflexes, crossed-adductor responses, contrasting with decreased ankle reflexes, but spasticity and Babinski signs were usually absent. Proximal motor weakness was present in one third of these cases, with loss of position sense in the feet, positive Romberg sign, and sensory ataxia in severe cases. Vitamin B_{12} deficiency was probably responsible for most of these cases that resembled subacute combined degeneration (SCD).

Sensorineural Deafness. Patients had high-pitch tinnitus and bilateral and symmetric high-frequency (4–8 kHz) hearing loss. No associated vestibular symptoms was reported. Hearing loss has been associated with folate-cobalamin deficiency in the elderly.

Peripheral Neuropathy. Symptoms included painful dysesthesias of the soles and palms, "burning feet," numbness, cramps, paresthesias, and sensitivity of nerves to pressure, but with minimal motor involvement. Objective signs were often mild and included loss or decreased perception of vibration, light touch, and pinprick distally in the limbs in a glove-and-stocking pattern. Achilles tendon reflexes were decreased or absent. Motor nerve conduction velocities were normal, and sensory nerve potential

amplitudes were decreased only in severe cases. Some patients presented hot skin and excessive sweating or coldness and hyperhydrosis of hands and feet. Sural nerve biopsies in 34 patients (58) showed an axonal neuropathy with predominant loss of myelinated large-caliber fibers and a less important loss of small-caliber fibers.

Myeloneuropathy. Patients had a combination of peripheral distal sensory polyneuropathy and funicular spinal cord involvement, manifested by spastic-ataxic gait, sphincter disturbances, brisk knee reflexes, and absent ankle reflexes.

Etiology and Treatment

Cuban neuropathies were due to nutritional deficiencies produced by poor diets resulting from political and economic problems (60, 61). Deficit of B vitamins, mainly vitamin B_{12}, compounded by lack of essential sulfur-containing amino acids and carotenoids such as lycopene in the diet, appears to have been the immediate cause. From a number of toxic agents investigated, only cigar smoking and alcohol were contributory. Treatment with parenteral B-group vitamins and provision of multivitamins to the Cuban population controlled the outbreak.

NEUROLOGIC DISORDERS ASSOCIATED WITH SPECIFIC VITAMINS

Vitamin A

Vitamin A Deficiency

The causes of vitamin A deficiency include defective dietary intake of preformed vitamin A (retinyl esters) of animal origin, or of fruits and vegetables containing provitamin A carotenoids, or from altered intestinal absorption such as in intestinal parasitic infections (giardiasis, ascaridiasis, and strongyloidiasis), or more rarely with abetalipoproteinemia or after biliopancreatic bypass surgery. Raw soybeans contain the enzyme *lipoxidase*, which oxidizes and destroys carotene.

The main manifestations of vitamin A deficiency occur in the eye (62–64), where it is needed for the synthesis of RNA and glycoproteins in cornea and conjunctiva. Retinal is the essential chromophore that combines with both rod and cone opsins to form rhodopsin for phototransduction. Clinical manifestations of vitamin A deficiency include night blindness, conjunctival xerosis, Bitot spots, and corneal xerosis that may lead to corneal ulceration and keratomalacia (62, 64). Vitamin A deficiency also affects metabolic and immune functions, thus worsening morbidity and mortality in children (62, 65). Vitamin A attenuates the severity of diarrhea and measles (66).

Vitamin A Intoxication

Excessive intake of vitamin A produces increased intracranial pressure, with irritability, anorexia, confusion, headache, vomiting, lethargy, malaise, abdominal pain, hepatomegaly, and myalgias. Funduscopic examination reveals papilledema, consistent with pseudotumor cerebri in the absence of focal neurologic signs. In addition to pharmaceutical preparations, vitamin-A–rich foods include polar bear liver and halibut liver.

Excessive vitamin A intake (>10,000 IU/day) increases the risk of cleft palate, harelip, macroglossia, eye abnormalities, and hydrocephalus. Retinoids are vitamin A derivatives used in dermatology. Isotretinoin (Accutane) has substantial teratogenic effects estimated at 15 to 45% of exposures in utero, mainly in the first trimester of pregnancy; risks persist up to 1 month after discontinuation of the drug (67). Malformations involve the face, the ears, the CNS, and the heart; there is also a 20 to 30% rate of spontaneous abortion.

Vitamin B₁ (Thiamin) and Beriberi

The main manifestations of deficiency are a sensorimotor axonal peripheral neuropathy (dry beriberi) and a cardiac form (shoshin beriberi) also called wet beriberi because of edema secondary to congestive heart failure. Beriberi was a major cause of morbidity and mortality in populations depending on polished rice for their staple diet (China, Japan, Indonesia, the Philippines), but it also occurred among poorly nourished children and adults in the Indian subcontinent, the Far East, Africa, and tropical South America. In the 1950s, with universal enrichment of rice, grains, and flour products with thiamin, significant control of beriberi was achieved around the world (see Chapter 23).

Beriberi continues to occur, mainly in alcoholic patients, malnourished elderly persons, and, more rarely, in pregnant women as a result of due to hyperemesis gravidarum. In the tropics, beriberi occurs under conditions of low thiamin intake, carbohydrate-rich diets, and high energy expenditure. Thiamin is not stored in the body, and signs of thiamin depletion occur in just 18 days with a thiamin-deficient diet (68) or with total parenteral nutrition (TPN). In 1997, a nationwide shortage of multivitamins for TPN led to reports of lactic acidosis from thiamin deficiency (69). Intractable heart failure is another common manifestation of undiagnosed beriberi.

Pathogenesis

Thiamin is required for energy production in all metabolically active tissues and is found in high concentrations in skeletal muscle, heart, liver, kidneys, and brain. Thiamin serves as coenzyme for the mitochondrial pyruvate dehydrogenase enzyme complex (pyruvate dehydrogenase and α-ketoglutarate dehydrogenase) and for transketolase.

Pyruvate Dehydrogenase. Thiamin is critical for mitochondrial energy production from glycolysis, that is, the sequence of cytosol reactions that convert glucose into pyruvate; this is followed by the oxidative decarboxylation of pyruvate to form acetyl coenzyme A (CoA) in the mito-

chondrial matrix. As a cofactor for the mitochondrial pyruvate dehydrogenase enzyme complex, thiamin is at a crucial link point between glycolysis and the citric acid cycle—the final common pathway for the oxidation of fuel molecules such as amino acids, fatty acids, and carbohydrates, resulting in electron transfers and production of ATP. Not surprisingly, intravenous glucose infusion in patients with thiamin deficiency may consume all thiamin reserves and may precipitate a coma as a result of acute Wernicke encephalopathy.

α-Ketoglutarate Dehydrogenase. This enzyme catalyzes the oxidative decarboxylation of α-ketoglutarate to form succinyl CoA in Krebs cycle. As a result, in beriberi the levels of pyruvate and α-ketoglutarate in the blood are higher than normal, especially after ingestion of glucose.

Transketolase. This enzyme transfers two-carbon units from one sugar to another in the pentose phosphate pathway, using reduced nicotinamide adenine dinucleotide phosphate (NADPH) as the hydrogen and electron donor in reduction reactions. The transketolase activity in red cells is low in thiamin deficiency; this is the most accurate diagnostic test for beriberi.

Independent of its function in carbohydrate metabolism, thiamin is also active in neurons, axonal membranes and axonal transport, and in sodium gating in neuronal membranes. In addition, loss of α-ketoglutarate dehydrogenase activity may account for alterations of several neurotransmitters, including γ-aminobutyric acid (GABA), glutamate, and aspartate during thiamin deficiency (68).

Clinical Manifestations of Thiamin Deficiency and Beriberi

The major manifestations of thiamin deficiency involve the cardiovascular system (shoshin or wet beriberi), the peripheral nervous system (dry beriberi or beriberi neuropathy), and the CNS (Wernicke-Korsakoff syndrome [WKS]).

Alcoholic Ketoacidosis. Beriberi may present as alcoholic ketoacidosis, characterized by increased levels of lactate from the anaerobic glycolysis of pyruvate as a result of the blockage of the oxidative decarboxylation of pyruvate. Unexplained lactic acidosis from thiamin deficiency may also occur in patients in intensive care settings with serious systemic diseases, liver failure, hemodialysis, severe vomiting, gastric malignancy, intestinal obstruction, pyloric stenosis, severe gastritis, after gastrectomy, or receiving TPN with insufficient thiamin (69).

Cardiac Beriberi (Shoshin). The typical presentation in patients with alcoholism is high-output cardiac failure with tachycardia and wide pulse pressure. Cardiomegaly, pedal edema, and pulmonary edema are common. Cardiac beriberi may present in Western hospitals with intractable cardiac failure, collapsed peripheral circulation, lactic acidosis, and shock (70). With intravenous thiamin, cardiac failure responds dramatically, with massive diuresis, correction of acidosis, reduction in pulmonary-capillary wedge pressure, and hemodynamic normalization. In tropical areas, cardiac beriberi may occur in children less than 6 months of age, born to malnourished mothers with signs of neuropathy or pedal edema. The child becomes restless, with rapid pulse, abdominal edema, and cardiogenic shock that responds only to thiamin.

Cardiac beriberi may occur in healthy young adults in the tropics following strenuous exercise. An outbreak at a military garrison in Colombia (71) was characterized clinically by progressive loss of endurance, pedal edema, feet dysesthesias, frequent foot-drop, acute congestive heart failure, pulmonary edema, and elevated mortality. The shoshin beriberi resulting from thiamin deficiency was confirmed by typical lesions in the heart. The enormous energy expenditure of soldiers training in the humid tropical conditions, the reduced intake of thiamin, the carbohydrate-rich diet, and the possible presence of fish thiaminase in the diet probably contributed to this outbreak (71). Urgent treatment must be initiated based on clinical suspicion alone. The recommended dose of thiamin in alcoholic ketoacidosis or cardiac shoshin beriberi is 100 mg intravenously, followed by 100 mg intramuscularly daily for 5 days.

Beriberi Neuropathy. Beriberi produces a distal symmetric sensorimotor peripheral neuropathy (72, 73). Despite the name "dry beriberi," signs of polyneuropathy usually coexist with pedal edema resulting from shoshin. Acute quadriplegia with brisk reflexes in shoshin beriberi may result from central-pontine myelinolysis (72, 74). The theory that vagal neuropathy in beriberi caused cardiac failure is outdated. Cardiac failure in beriberi results from mitochondrial energy failure and is rapidly reversible by thiamin.

Beriberi neuropathy begins slowly with tingling of the toes, painful "burning feet," or coldness and inability to get the feet warm. Cruickshank (55) collected notes on 400 cases of beriberi he treated at the Changi prison camp in Singapore. He wrote:

> Men complained of numbness, tingling or pins-and-needles in fingertips and toes, sometimes spreading to involve the whole body, but sometimes just around the mouth or the umbilicus, or on the side of the thighs. Men complained of "not feeling the floor," which forced them to walk unsteadily. All had dulled sensations in hands and feet as if they were constantly wearing gloves and socks. Aching, stiffness, and tightness or cramps in the calves after a day of labor and a tendency to drag the feet were also prominent. But the most common manifestation of thiamin deficiency in these men was the swelling of the feet, present in 317 of the first 400 patients. This was accompanied by breathlessness, lassitude and weakness in half of the cases, and by a fast heart rate and cardiac palpitations in a small fraction.

Calf tenderness and sharp stabbing pains in the feet when walking are typical. Decreased sweating or hyperhidrosis of the feet, redness, dryness and atrophy of the skin, and distal hair loss are suggestive of autonomic involvement. Foot-drop presents with "steppage" gait, often resulting from sensitivity to compression of the lateral peroneal nerve at the head of the fibula. Children often have aphonia from paralysis of the recurrent laryngeal nerves. There is global arreflexia and loss of all sensory modalities in a typical stocking distribution, with late involvement of the hands. About 80% of patients with WKS have coexistent beriberi neuropathy.

Recently, Koike and associates (75) confirmed that postgastrectomy neuropathy is clinically and pathologically identical to beriberi with similar erythrocyte transketolase activity, thiamin levels, and nerve biopsies. Motor- and sensory-nerve conduction velocities were normal, but compound muscle and sensory action potentials were reduced. Sural nerve biopsies showed axonal degeneration with predominant loss of large myelinated fibers; however, both small myelinated and nonmyelinated fibers were slightly decreased. Subperineurial edema was present in most cases. About 46% of teased fibers showed axonal degeneration, and 5% had segmental demyelination and remyelination. Beriberi follows a progressive pattern, with impairment of both superficial and deep sensation and motor weakness. The recommended dose of thiamin in beriberi neuropathy is 100 mg intravenously, followed by 100 mg intramuscularly daily for 5 days, and permanent oral maintenance. Moreover, beriberi neuropathy and shoshin beriberi often coexist. In the presence of edema, there is a risk of sudden cardiac death, and the treatment with intravenous thiamin must be initiated immediately.

Wernicke-Korsakoff Syndrome. The two components of WKS are Wernicke encephalopathy and Korsakoff amnesic-confabulatory psychosis with polyneuropathy (76). There is an apparent genetic predisposition to WKS (77). Fibroblasts from patients with WKS showed decreased binding of transketolase to thiamin diphosphate than in control cell lines. Transketolase deficiency persisted despite excess thiamin, a finding indicating genetic rather than dietary abnormalities. Transketolase in fibroblasts from patients with WKS was catalytically defective (78).

Wernicke Encephalopathy. This disorder is characterized by acute onset of nystagmus, abducens and conjugate gaze palsies, gait ataxia, and mental confusion from lesions of nuclei at the level of third and fourth ventricle and in the periaqueductal gray. The disease may begin with ataxia, followed by nystagmus and confusion. The typical ocular abnormalities are horizontal and vertical nystagmus, bilateral lateral rectus palsy, and weakness of conjugate gaze. Internuclear ophthalmoplegia is common, and patients with advanced cases may exhibit complete ophthalmoplegia. Ataxia is severe, with wide-based stance and slow, hesitant, short-stepped gait; tandem walking may be impossible. Intention tremor is absent. Drowsiness, confusion, apathy, and loss of attention and memory occur in the acute stage. Ocular signs and confusion respond rapidly to intravenous thiamin, but the ataxia and memory deficits may fail to improve.

Neuropathologic findings in Wernicke encephalopathy include symmetric lesions of the periventricular regions of the thalamus and hypothalamus and characteristic involvement of the mammillary bodies. Lesions affect periaqueductal gray, dorsal motor nuclei of the vagus, vestibular nuclei, and superior cerebellar vermis. Histology of these lesions shows necrosis, neuronal loss, tissue edema, vacuolization, small foci of hemorrhages, prominence of capillaries, and endothelial proliferation. Purkinje cells and other layers of the cerebellar cortex are affected, particularly in the superior vermis, with late astrocytic and microglial proliferation.

Treatment of Wernicke encephalopathy is a neurologic emergency because of the risk of death from brainstem involvement, or chronic dementia from Korsakoff syndrome. Oral glucose load or intravenous glucose infusions must be avoided in patients with history of alcoholism, in whom deficit of thiamin is likely. Thiamin must be administered on clinical suspicion alone. The recommended dose of thiamin for Wernicke encephalopathy is 100 mg intravenously, followed by 100 mg intramuscularly daily for 5 days. Maintenance oral doses of thiamin and B-complex vitamins should be continued indefinitely in alcoholic patients.

Korsakoff Syndrome. This syndrome is considered a chronic phase of Wernicke encephalopathy. Usually, patients are completely amnesic of events that occurred during the acute phase of the illness. The memory loss affects both new learning (anterograde amnesia) and past memories (retrograde amnesia). The most severe deficits are those of learning and storage of new information. Patients also exhibit executive dysfunction, loss of spatial organization, and problems with visual and verbal abstractions. Korsakoff syndrome is associated not only with memory impairment but also with executive dysfunction and global deficits (79) indicative of impairment of frontal lobe connections. Interruption of the hippocampo-mammillothalamic tract at several levels (mammillary bodies and dorsal medial and anterior thalamic nuclei) explains the severe amnesia. Other behavioral and cognitive deficits result from interruption of prefrontal corticosubcortical circuits that underlie executive function and attention. Confabulation is typical of Korsakoff syndrome, particularly during the confusional early phase. Even with timely thiamin treatment, only about 20% of patients recover from the memory deficits. Donepezil, a cholinesterase inhibitor, has been used in patients with chronic Korsakoff syndrome with some positive results.

Cerebellar Ataxia. Alcoholic cerebellar degeneration is similar to the ataxia of thiamin deficiency. There is loss of Purkinje cells in anterior and superior cerebellar vermis manifested by abnormalities of gait, station, and truncal ataxia. The Nigerian epidemic seasonal ataxia, observed after ingestion of the African silkworm *Anaphe venata*, is probably the result of a heat-resistant thiaminase that induces thiamin deficiency (80).

Nutritional Amblyopia. Nutritional amblyopia is also known as tobacco-alcohol amblyopia, deficiency amblyopia, nutritional optic neuropathy, and tropical amblyopia (Mádan, 1898). The pathologic lesion appears to be confined to the maculopapillary bundle resulting in central or cecocentral scotomata, loss of color vision, and pallor of the temporal side of the optic disc. Nutritional amblyopia was also observed among POWs in the Far East between 1942 and 1945 (55, 72, 81–87). Cruickshank (55) described camp blindness, as follows:

> On examination there was lowered visual acuity of one or both eyes with difficulty in reading. Central or paracentral scotomata just above or below the point of fixation were constant findings. They varied in size but were usually larger for red than for black or white. Ophthalmoscopy in the early stages usually revealed a normal fundus. In patients with symptoms of long duration, pallor of the temporal side of the disc developed, frequently corresponding with the maculopapillary bundle.

The specific deficit responsible for nutritional amblyopia has not been established. A combination of deficits of thiamin, vitamin B_{12}, folate and perhaps riboflavin has been invoked. In patients with Cuban optic neuropathy, Sadun (88, 89) postulated an acquired mitochondrial energy failure of macular neurons resulting from a combination of dietary deficiency of folic acid and ingestion of low doses of methanol, manifested by elevation of formate in serum and cerebrospinal fluid (CSF). Retinal mitochondria can be impaired genetically (Leber hereditary optic neuropathy), by nutritional deficit of folate and vitamin B_{12}, or by toxic factors (methanol, ethambutol, or cyanide). These metabolic optic neuropathies are characterized by bilaterally symmetric visual impairment with loss of central visual acuity, dyschromatopsia, cecocentral visual field defects, temporal optic disc atrophy, and specific loss of the nerve fiber layer in the maculopapillary bundle. The resulting mitochondrial derangement would lead to ATP depletion that compromises axonal transport.

Burning Feet. According to Bruyn and Poser (90), "burning feet" were first described in 1826 by J. Grierson, a British medical officer in the Indian Army. This complex symptom was also commonly found in POW camps in tropical regions, where it was called "the happy feet," probably because pain kept patients walking at night. More recently, the condition known as burning feet is a symptom of patients with distal sensory neuropathy from human immunodeficiency virus (HIV) infection (91). Cruickshank (92), who studied 500 cases of burning feet, described the following symptoms appearing among POWs about 3 months after imprisonment:

> The suffering men were unable to sleep because of the severe burning pain in the soles of the feet. The earliest sign was a dull throbbing in the balls of the feet appearing in the evening at the end of the work day. The pains were always worst at night, keeping the patient awake. The patients became worn out from pain and loss of sleep; rapid loss of weight occurred and the appetite often became poor. Tightly gripping

and massaging the feet gave some relief and men adopted a characteristic attitude in bed, sitting forward, cross-legged, gripping their feet. On examination the patient's face wears an expression of chronic distress with dark shadows under the eyes. The constant pain and the loss of sleep produce an exhausted, red-eyed, irritable patient. Some are almost tearful from the pain. The only abnormal findings in the feet were hyperaesthesia to pin prick and light touch in the majority and excessive sweating in some of the severe cases, sensory deficits in a stocking and glove distribution, and depressed or absent ankle reflexes, without severe paresis.

In Cruickshank's experience, thiamin and riboflavin deficiencies were not a likely cause of burning feet among POWs. He used nicotinic acid (niacin) with good results in 68% of 500 cases, but pellagra or niacin deficiency alone is not a probable cause of this syndrome. Pantothenic acid was useful in some patients, and experimental deficiency of pantothenic acid in pigs produces dorsal myelopathy and sensory neuropathy. Folic acid deficiency per se has been associated with cases of myelopathy and sensory neuropathy in humans. The treatment of burning feet remains symptomatic.

Patients with HIV infection and burning feet show a dying-back axonal degeneration of long axons in distal regions, loss of unmyelinated fibers, and variable degree of macrophage infiltration in peripheral nerves and dorsal root ganglia. Skin biopsies (81) show reduction in nerve fiber density, increased frequency of varicosities, and fragmentation of cutaneous nerve fibers.

Vitamin B$_2$ (Riboflavin)

Riboflavin Deficiency

Ariboflavinosis is associated with nonspecific signs such as angular cheilosis, glossitis (beefy-red tongue), scaling dermatitis, normochromic normocytic anemia, and superficial interstitial keratitis. Recommended treatment is with vitamin B complex that usually contains a mixture of riboflavin, thiamin, niacin, folic acid, vitamin B$_{12}$, pantothenic acid, and biotin. In the presence of a deficiency syndrome with interstitial keratitis, vitamin A is also recommended.

Niacin Deficiency (Pellagra)

Since the 1600s, pellagra (Ital. *pelle*, skin + *agra*, rough) was epidemic in Mediterranean Europe and north Africa. In the southeastern United States from 1910 until 1935, the incidence reached 170,000 cases/year. Pellagra continues to occur among patients with alcoholism, malabsorption syndromes, and chronic diseases and in malnourished populations that consume corn (maize) as staple food. Niacin, as nicotinamide, is an essential component of NAD and NADP, two coenzymes crucial in oxidation-reduction reactions. Nicotinic acid is used for the treatment of hyperlipidemia, particularly in type 2 diabetes (93).

Humans obtain niacin from the diet or from tryptophan. Dietary leucine, found in millet in Asia and Africa, blocks the conversion from tryptophan to niacin. The traditional Central and South American treatment of corn with alkaline lime before baking the tortillas increases niacin content. Pellagra may occur in carcinoid syndrome as a result of conversion of tryptophan to serotonin by the tumor, as well as in Hartnup disease, caused by defective intestinal absorption of several amino acids.

The three Ds—dermatitis, diarrhea, and dementia—characterize the clinical manifestations of pellagra. The dermatitis typically occurs in areas exposed to sunlight, including the neck (Casal's collar, 1762). The dermatitis of acute pellagra begins as an erythema that resembles sunburn with slow tanning and exacerbation by sunlight. Oral scalding, burning sensations of the tongue, glossitis, anorexia, abdominal pain, and recurrent bouts of diarrhea also occur. The dementia is preceded by insomnia, fatigue, nervousness, irritability, and depression. Suicide by drowning was said to be a common occurrence. The cognitive deficits include confusion, mental dullness, apathy, and memory impairment. Typical neuropathologic lesions of pellagra affect Betz cells in the motor cortex, smaller pyramidal cortical neurons, large neurons of basal ganglia and motor cranial nuclei, dentate nucleus, and anterior horn cells. Affected neurons appear swollen, rounded, with eccentric nuclei and loss of Nissl particles. Some alcoholic patients have similar brain lesions in the absence of overt pellagra. Pellagra neuropathy is indistinguishable from beriberi neuropathy, but it fails to respond to niacin treatment alone, and B-complex vitamin treatment is recommended.

Diagnosis and Treatment

No definitive laboratory test exists for pellagra. The diagnosis is supported by low levels of serum niacin, tryptophan, NAD, and NADP. A combined excretion of *N*-methylnicotinamide and pyridone of less than 1.5 mg/24 hours indicates severe niacin deficiency. Treatment is with niacin (nicotinic acid) or with nicotinamide, which does not cause the flushing caused by niacin. The adult dose for acute pellagra is nicotinamide, 100 mg orally every 6 hours for several days or until resolution of major acute symptoms, followed by oral administration of 50 mg every 8 to 12 hours until all skin lesions heal. In severe cases with neurologic involvement, 1 g three to four times daily should be provided, initially by the parenteral route. The dose for children is 10 to 50 mg orally every 6 hours until resolution of the symptoms and signs of pellagra. Therapy should also include other B vitamins, zinc, and magnesium, as well as a diet rich in calories. Some data support the use of niacin in HIV-infected patients because HIV induces niacin depletion.

Vitamin B$_6$ (Pyridoxine)

Vitamin B$_6$ exists in three natural forms: pyridoxol, pyridoxal, and pyridoxamine. Ingested pyridoxol is phosphorylated and then oxidized to pyridoxal phosphate, an important coenzyme in the metabolism of amino acids, including the conversion of α-ketoglutarate to glutamate and of glutamate to GABA. Vitamin B_6 deficiency may cause niacin deficiency as a result of impaired tryptophan metabolism. Increased homocysteine responds to pyridoxine, vitamin B_{12}, or folate, depending on the type of depletion.

Vitamin B_6 Deficiency

Pyridoxine is found in virtually all foods, thus making dietary deficiency unlikely, although increased requirements occur with pregnancy and lactation, estrogen use, hyperthyroidism, high-protein diets, and in the elderly. Faulty preparation may destroy pyridoxine in baby formula, resulting in infantile seizures. Infants of mothers deficient in vitamin B_6 may also suffer neonatal seizures. The latter two mechanism of seizure causation are different from pyridoxine dependency, a rare autosomal recessive disorder causing intractable seizures in neonates and infants.

The clinical manifestations of pyridoxine deficiency resulting from use of the antagonist desoxypyridoxine include seborrheic dermatitis, angular cheilosis, glossitis, peripheral neuropathy, and convulsions. Pyridoxine deficiency is common in patients with alcoholism because of displacement of pyridoxal phosphate by acetaldehyde. Isoniazid and penicillamine combine with pyridoxal phosphate to inactivate it. Long-term treatment of tuberculosis with isoniazid may result in a distal, symmetric neuropathy that may progress to sensory ataxia and limb weakness. Pathologic examination reveals axonal degeneration and regeneration of both myelinated and unmyelinated fibers. Isoniazid acetylation by N-acetyltransferase is a genetically determined polymorphism; the acetylated drug is more easily excreted by the kidney. In Western populations, half are slow acetylators, with an increased risk of developing neuropathy (and hepatotoxicity) with standard doses. Isoniazid neuropathy is reversible by discontinuation of the drug or vitamin B_6 supplementation. Acute isoniazid overdose is characterized by the clinical triad of repetitive seizures that are unresponsive to anticonvulsants, metabolic acidosis with a high anion gap, and coma. The recommended therapy for isoniazid intoxication is pyridoxine. Prevention of neuropathy in patients taking isoniazid is with oral pyridoxine, 50 to 100 mg/day for the duration of the isoniazid treatment.

Vitamin B_6 Intoxication

Megadoses of pyridoxine greater than 200 mg/day have been associated with sensory neuropathy and severe ataxia, but without weakness (94). In experimental animals (95), histologic examination revealed widespread neuronal degeneration in the dorsal root ganglia and gasserian ganglia, as well as degeneration of sensory nerve fibers in peripheral nerves, the dorsal columns of the spinal cord,

and the descending spinal tract of the trigeminal nerve. The mechanism of action of megadoses of pyridoxine producing toxic, peripheral sensory neuronopathy remains unclear. The treatment is symptomatic.

Vitamin B_{12} (Cobalamin)

Vitamin B_{12} Absorption

Cobalamin absorption is quite complex and involves at least five separate cobalamin-binding molecules, receptors, and transporters (96). In the stomach, cobalamin is bound to haptocorrin and then to intrinsic factor (IF) produced by gastric parietal cells. The IF-cobalamin complex passes into distal ileum, where it binds to high-affinity IF receptors on ileal epithelial cells, to be absorbed in the distal small intestine. Cobalamin is then released for subsequent binding to transcobalamin II (TcII). The TcII-cobalamin complex is transported across the cell to be released into the circulation. All cells in the body have surface receptors for TcII-cobalamin complex. However, 90% of the cobalamin in plasma is protein bound to TcI and TcIII, probably as storage forms.

Vitamin B_{12} deficiency

Diverse factors may cause cobalamin deficiency, including absent dietary supply (vegans), antibodies against IF (pernicious anemia), gastrectomy, gastritis involving parietal cells in gastric fundus, malabsorption syndromes (tropical sprue), surgical resection or bypass of distal ileum, competition for vitamin B_{12} (by bacterial proliferation in the intestine in the blind-loop syndrome or by intestinal parasitism with the fish tapeworm *Diphyllobotrium latum*), and rare genetic enzyme deficiencies (methylmalonic aciduria).

Repeated inhalation of nitrous oxide in anesthesia or as a recreational drug produces cobalamin deficiency (97). Nitrous oxide interacts with vitamin B_{12} resulting in selective inhibition of methionine synthase, a key enzyme in methionine and folate metabolism; this results in alteration of one-carbon donors and methyl-group transfer reactions that are critical for purine, thymidylate, and DNA syntheses.

It is becoming increasingly recognized that elderly persons are prone to vitamin B_{12} deficiency (98). About 10 to 15% of elderly persons have cobalamin levels lower than 150 pmol/L, and almost half (43%) have serum elevations of sensitive markers such as homocysteine or methylmalonic acid (MMA). Atrophic gastritis occurs in 20 to 50% of the elderly and results in gastric achlorhydria and low pepsinogen secretion that prevent the release of cobalamin protein complexes from the food and cause alkalinization of the small intestine and bacterial overgrowth, decreasing the bioavailability of cobalamin. Drugs such as proton pump inhibitors or H_2 receptor antagonists inhibit cobalamin absorption. There are rare cases of familial deficiency of TcI/haptocorrin (99); however, plasma holotranscobalamin is not an early marker of cobalamin deficiency (100).

Epidemiology. Pernicious anemia is common throughout the world (101, 102), especially in persons of European or African descent. Dietary deficiency of vitamin B_{12} from vegetarianism is increasing, particularly in Asia, North America, and Europe, and causing hyperhomocysteinemia, which raises the risk for vascular disease. Breast-fed infants of vitamin B_{12}-deficient vegan mothers are at risk of severe developmental abnormalities, growth failure, anemia, lower academic performance, attentional deficits, and delinquent behavior (24, 101, 102). Dietary vitamin B_{12} deficiency is a severe problem in the Indian subcontinent, Mexico, Central and South America, and some African countries (101).

Pathogenesis. Cobalamin deficiency impairs conversion of L-methylmalonyl CoA to succinyl CoA resulting in increase MMA, and *methylations*, such as the synthesis of methionine, an important component for the synthesis of S-adenoyslmethionine (SAM). The provision of activated methyl groups by SAM is the end result of the activated methyl cycle, important in the synthesis of neurotransmitters such as norepinephrine and glutamate, as well as in myelin synthesis.

Methionine can be regenerated by the transfer to homocysteine of a methyl group from methyltetrahydrofolate (MTH_4F). This reaction is catalyzed by homocysteine methyltransferase, a crucial methylcobalamin-dependent reaction. Cobalamin deficit results in increased homocysteine levels.

Neurologic Manifestations of Vitamin B_{12} Deficiency

Manifestations of vitamin B_{12} deficiency (Table 88.2) are mediated by the foregoing metabolic alterations and by abnormal production of cytokines (tumor necrosis factor-α, interleukin-6) and deficit of epidermal growth factor, a neurotrophic factor (103). Signs of neurologic involvement may occur before development of megaloblastic anemia and, rarely, with normal serum levels of vitamin B_{12}. More sensitive indicators of neural damage are increases in serum MMA and homocysteine. The spinal cord, brain, optic nerves, and peripheral nerves may be affected by vitamin B_{12} deficiency.

Subacute Combined Degeneration. The typical spinal cord lesions of vitamin B_{12} deficiency are the degeneration of posterior and lateral columns causing SCD, manifested by a triad of sensory ataxia, spasticity, and leg weakness (104). Symptoms begin with paresthesias, tingling, and pins-and-needles sensations in the feet and then in the hands; Lhermitte sign may be present. These symptoms are constant and evolve toward unsteadiness of gait from pyramidal weakness and loss of proprioception and postural sense, as well as Romberg sign. As the disease progresses, stiffness and weakness of the legs develop,

TABLE 88.2. NEUROLOGIC LESIONS AND MANIFESTATIONS OF VITAMIN B_{12} (Cobalamin) Deficiency

Subacute combined degeneration
  Lesion of myelin in lateral and dorsal columns with typical honeycomb appearance
  Clinical triad: sensory ataxia, spasticity, and leg weakness
Optic neuropathy
  Loss of macular ganglion cells and axons of maculopapillary bundle
  Clinical signs: poor visual acuity, cecocentral scotomata, dyschromatopsia
Peripheral neuropathy
  Axonal sensory neuropathy
  Stockings-and-gloves sensory loss, arreflexia
Neuropsychiatric symptoms
  Cerebral myelin involvement
  Confusional episodes, maniac depressive mood, cognitive decline, dementia
Less common symptoms
  Vocal cord paralysis
  Taste and smell changes
  Tinnitus and hearing loss
  Tabetic-type pains
  Gaze limitations
  Cerebellar signs

with brisk knee reflexes, crossed-adductor responses, and Babinski sign. In a large series of patients with pernicious anemia (104), common symptoms included loss of cutaneous sensation, weakness, urinary or fecal incontinence, and orthostatic hypotension. About one in four patients had no evidence of anemia. The final stage in untreated cases is an ataxic paraplegia, with spasticity and contractures; flaccid paraplegia may occur in some patients with severe peripheral nerve involvement. Response to treatment was inversely related to duration and severity of the neurologic symptoms and the anemia before diagnosis.

Early pathologic changes involve separation of myelin lamellae, vacuolization, and axonal damage with minimal gliosis, involving first the dorsal columns of the cervical and upper thoracic cord. Late lesions are scattered irregularly in posterior and lateral funiculi and disclose a typical honey-comb appearance. Vacuolar myelopathy, pathologicly identical to SCD, occurs in patients with acquired immunodeficiency syndrome (105). Based on a postulated abnormality of cobalamin-dependent transmethylation leading to reductions of SAM (106), a clinical trial with L-methionine was completed; unfortunately, the results were negative (107).

Optic Neuropathy. Visual symptoms resulting from involvement of the optic nerves occur commonly in pernicious anemia. Clinically, patients have loss of visual acuity and color vision and cecocentral scotomata, similar to those of other nutritional optic neuropathies, described earlier. At autopsy, spongy degeneration of the optic nerves is usually found. In a model of dietary vitamin B_{12}

deficiency in monkeys (108), neuropathologic examination revealed loss of ganglion cells in the macula with early involvement of the maculopapillary bundles, extending to the retrobulbar portion of the optic nerves. CNS changes in the monkeys occurred after 33 to 45 months of deficiency, similar to the time required to produce vitamin B_{12} deficiency in humans.

Peripheral Neuropathy. A mild form of sensory peripheral neuropathy probably occurs in vitamin B_{12} deficiency, with a typical stocking-and-glove distribution, but most of the sensory symptoms result from dorsal column involvement. A review of clinical electrophysiologic studies in SCD (109) showed posterior column dysfunction and damage to the central motor pathway. A few patients had axonal neuropathy and, more rarely, demyelinating neuropathy. Motor evoked potentials and median somatosensory evoked potentials became normal with cobalamin treatment, but tibial somatosensory evoked potentials remained abnormal in most patients.

Other Forms of Presentation. Unusual forms of presentation of vitamin B_{12} deficiency (110) include cranial neuropathies with hoarseness from vocal cord paralysis, disturbances of taste and smell, tinnitus, nocturnal tabetic-type pains, upward or lateral gaze limitation, cerebellar dysfunction, and movement disorders occurring in addition to more typical manifestations of SCD.

Neuropsychiatric Symptoms. Mental symptoms are frequent in pernicious anemia and range from confusional episodes and maniac behavior to depression and progressive cognitive decline of memory, orientation, and mentation leading to dementia. Cerebral white matter lesions typical of vitamin B_{12} deficiency are the probable neuropathologic substrate. Neuropsychiatric symptoms have been correlated with reduced CSF levels of SAM (111).

Diagnosis and Treatment

The diagnosis of vitamin B_{12} deficiency from pernicious anemia is usually made in the presence of positive anti-IF antibodies, low levels of vitamin B_{12}, and increased levels of MMA and homocysteine. Macrocytic anemia and neutrophil polysegmentation may not be present.

The neurologic complications of vitamin B_{12} deficiency usually respond to intramuscular injections of 1000 μg of vitamin B_{12} daily for 5 days to replenish the stores, followed by monthly injections of 500 to 1000 μg indefinitely. A sublingual form of vitamin B_{12} is also available. For preventive treatment, oral preparations of vitamin B_{12} appear to be adequate.

Folic Acid

After intestinal absorption, mainly 5-methyltetrahydrofolate ($5MTH_4F$) enters the circulation; folate reserves are limited, and deficits may occur after a few months of negative balance. Tetrahydrofolates act as acceptors of one-carbon fragments for the synthesis of purines, methionine, and deoxythymidine monophosphate for the synthesis of DNA. Decreased absorption is present in patients with alcoholism and in malabsorption, as well as with ingestion of phenytoin and oral contraceptives. There are increased requirements for folic acid in pregnancy and lactation, in infants and adolescents, and in patients with active hematopoiesis and cancer.

Neurologic Manifestations of Folate Deficiency

Folate deficiency produces megaloblastic anemia identical to that of vitamin B_{12} deficiency, but isolated folic acid deficiency rarely produces SCD and peripheral neuropathy. Folic acid deficiency may produce isolated increase of homocysteine.

Recently, Ramaekers and Blau (112) described a neurologic syndrome called idiopathic cerebral folate deficiency in children with low CSF levels of $5MTH_4F$ but with normal folate metabolism outside the nervous system. Onset is at about 4 months of age, with restlessness, irritability, and altered sleep, followed by psychomotor retardation, cerebellar ataxia, spastic paraplegia, dyskinesias, and visual and hearing loss; one third of the children have seizures. Periventricular demyelination and cerebral atrophy are seen. The syndrome is caused by nonfunctional CSF receptor-mediated folate receptor protein 1 (FR1). Cases usually responded to oral folate supplementation. Secondary forms of cerbral folate deficiency include long-term use of antifolate and anticonvulsant drugs, Rett syndrome, Aicardi-Goutieres syndrome, 3-phosphoglycerate dehydrogenase deficiency, dihydropteridine reductase deficiency, aromatic amino acid decarboxylase deficiency, and Kearns-Sayre syndrome.

Congenital errors of folate metabolism include (113) methylenetetrahydrofolate reductase deficiency, characterized by mental retardation, seizures, schizophrenia, or vascular disease, without hematologic abnormalities. This is the most common congenital error of folate metabolism. Laboratory tests show low folate in serum, red blood cells, and CSF, associated with homocystinuria. Methionine synthase deficiency causes megaloblastic anemia associated with mental retardation. Glutamate formiminotransferase-cyclodeaminase deficiency presents with severe mental retardation. Rarely, dihydrofolate reductase deficiency presents with folate-responsive neonatal megaloblastic anemia.

Neural Tube Defects and Folate. One of the most common malformations of the CNS is spina bifida, resulting from fusion failure of the caudal neural tube. Up to 70% of the cases of spina bifida cases can be prevented by maternal folic acid supplementation (114). Other causes include chromosome abnormalities, single gene disorders, and teratogenic exposure. The mechanism of protection is unknown, but it may include genes that regulate folate transport and metabolism. Maternal risk factors also include low dietary intake of iron, magnesium, and niacin

(115), as well as maternal use of some antiepileptic drugs (116).

Homocysteine in Stroke and Dementia. Vitamin B_{12}, vitamin B_6, and folic acid are key enzymes in the metabolism of methionine and limit production of homocysteine, a sulfur-containing amino acid. Increased serum homocysteine levels are associated with increased risk of stroke, cerebrovascular and cardiovascular disease, cognitive decline, and dementia (117). In the population-based Framingham cohort (118), elevated homocysteine levels were a risk factor for Alzheimer disease and vascular dementia. Garcia and Zanibbi (119) found that increased levels of homocysteine over 2.3 years correlated with changes in executive function.

Hyperhomocysteinemia acts in vitro as an agonist on the glutamate-binding site of the N-methyl-D-aspartate receptor, with resulting excess intracellular influx of calcium and production of reactive oxygen species. Hyperhomocysteinemia is an independent risk factor for cardiovascular disease and stroke (120), thus increasing platelet aggregation. At the endothelial level, homocysteine induces atherogenesis by increasing oxidative damage and promoting oxidation of low-density lipoproteins. The Rotterdam Scan Study (121) found an association among elevated homocysteine levels, silent brain infarcts, and white matter lesions.

Homocysteine levels can be lowered by supplementation with vitamin B_{12}, vitamin B_6, and folic acid. Recently, folic acid fortification of grain products was implemented in numerous countries to prevent neural tube defects, in particular spina bifida; however, prevention of stroke and myocardial infarction could also be expected. In patients with increased homocysteine despite folate intake, intramuscular cyanocobalamin injections, 1000 μg/month, should be initiated. The damaging effects of homocysteine on the endothelium can also be reduced by consumption of antioxidants, such as those in vitamin C, vitamin E, lycopenes, and selenium.

Genetic susceptibility to folate deficiency occurs in subjects with gene mutations of the enzyme 5,10-methylenetetrahydrofolate reductase (MH_4FR). A common gene mutation (C677T) results in decreased activity of this enzyme (122) and increased homocysteine levels. The effects are probably worsened by low folate and riboflavin levels; this mutation may increase the risk of depression in the elderly as a result of the dysfunction of methylation metabolic pathways critical to the synthesis of SAM, norepinephrine, and serotonin (122).

Pantothenic Acid

Pantothenate is bound to CoA, a critical component of carbohydrate and fatty acid metabolism, and it acts against apoptosis and cell damage by quenching oxygen free radicals. Recently, the Hallervorden-Spatz syndrome was linked with the gene *PANK2* on chromosome 20, which encodes pantothenate kinase, an essential step for the synthesis of CoA from pantothenate (123), thus causing abnormalities of fatty acid synthesis and energy metabolism and increased concentration of cysteine-iron deposits in basal ganglia. Hallervorden-Spatz syndrome is characterized pathologically by iron deposits and axonal spheroids in basal ganglia.

Vitamin E (α-Tocopherol)

This liposoluble vitamin was initially identified as an indispensable nutrient for fertility in animals; however, α-tocopherol is also a potent antioxidant that prevents cell membrane injury from lipid peroxidation. Tocopherol is absorbed into chylomicrons in the small intestine and is transported bound to α-tocopherol transfer protein.

Vitamin E deficiency occurs with poor diets, malabsorption (124), short bowel and blind loop syndromes (125), cystic fibrosis (126), celiac disease, and chronic cholestatic liver disease, as well as in abetalipoproteinemia and in isolated genetic defects of the α-tocopherol transfer protein. The Italian form of ataxia with vitamin E deficiency (127) is a rare autosomal recessive disorder caused by mutations in the α-tocopherol transfer protein gene on chromosome 8q13. Affected patients have a progressive spinocerebellar syndrome and low plasma levels of vitamin E (127). Vitamin E deficiency has also been described in patients with tropical myeloneuropathies, probably associated to dietary deficiency and tropical malabsorption (128).

There is a rare syndrome of isolated vitamin E deficiency with neurologic manifestations with onset in childhood, without fat malabsorption (129). Symptoms include tremor, gait ataxia, tremulous, dysarthric speech, loss of proprioception and vibratory sensation, and global arreflexia. Cerebellar deficits include dysmetria, slowed finger movements, and postural tremor. The gait is wide based, with prominent lordosis and genu recurvatum with pseudodystonic extension of the knees and inversion of the feet. Ophthalmoplegia, retinitis pigmentosa, dysarthria, generalized muscle weakness, and extensor plantar responses are present in some cases. The symptoms progress from hyporeflexia, ataxia, limitations in upward gaze, and strabismus to long-tract defects, weakness, and visual field constriction. Patients with severe, prolonged deficiency may develop complete blindness, dementia, and cardiac arrhythmias (130).

On neuropathology, vitamin E deficiency shows a large-fiber axonal sensory neuropathy, with damage to dorsal root ganglia, along with a spinocerebellar disorder with typical axonal spheroids, that is, swollen and dystrophic axons that involve posterior funiculi and Clarke columns. Sensory-nerve conduction velocities may be absent, with low amplitude of sensory nerve action potentials.

Treatment must be tailored to the underlying cause of vitamin E deficiency and may include oral or parenteral vitamin E supplementation. Even in genetic cases, vitamin E therapy allowed neurologic stabilization in most patients, although a few have developed spasticity and retinitis pigmentosa (130). The more advanced the deficits, the more limited the response to therapy will be. Therefore, early treatment, periodic neurologic and ophthalmologic examinations, and determinations of serum vitamin E levels are essential in patients at risk of vitamin E deficiency.

Vitamin E is currently recommended in the treatment of dementia of Alzheimer disease (131), based on its antioxidant properties; however, mixed results have been obtained from clinical trials. Likewise, despite a number of trials, no convincing evidence of a protective effect of vitamin E in cardiovascular disease or stroke has been reported (132).

Vitamin D

In humans, vitamin D produced by exposure to sunlight is metabolized in the liver and then in the kidney to 1,25-dihydroxyvitamin D (1,25(OH)$_2$D). Vitamin D receptors are present in the intestine and bone, as well as in the brain, heart, stomach, pancreas, activated T and B lymphocytes, skin, and gonads (133). 1,25(OH)$_2$D is one of the most potent inhibitors of cell proliferation in both normal and hyperproliferative cells, inducing them to mature (134). Vitamin D is a natural immunoregulator with anti-inflammatory action. Vitamin D regulates T-helper cell (Th1) and dendritic cell function while inducing regulatory T-cell function (133, 134). Low vitamin D status has been implicated in the etiology of autoimmune diseases (134), such as multiple sclerosis (MS).

MS occurs with lower prevalence in equatorial regions of the world that have significantly higher exposure to sunlight; Nordic countries with fewer days of sunlight have a much higher prevalence of MS. Munger and colleagues (135) studied the dietary intake of vitamin D in relation to MS incidence in two cohorts in the United States, representing more than 187,000 women (The Nurses' Health Study I and II) followed from 1980 to 2000 and 1991 to 2001. Higher dietary intakes of vitamin D from supplements were inversely associated with risk of MS (risk ratio, 0.59; 95% confidence interval = 0.38–0.91; p for trend = .006).

Furthermore, in experimental allergic encephalomyelitis, an experimental model of MS, the active metabolite 1,25-(OH)$_2$D prevented and reduced disease activity by modulating dendritic cell and T-cell function and regulating macrophages (136).

In summary, although controlled clinical trials have not been completed, exposure to sunlight (137, 138) and vitamin D supplementation may be considered for patients with MS and in persons at risk. The recommended oral dose of vitamin D in supplements is[1] 400 IU/day (10 µg/day). Supplemental vitamin D intake is mostly from multivitamins and usually also includes vitamins A, C, and E, folic acid, and the B-group vitamins.

DIETARY AND VITAMIN TREATMENT IN NEUROLOGY

Numerous neurologic conditions, ranging from migraine, stroke, and hepatic encephalopathy to rare metabolic disturbances, respond to dietary treatment or to specific vitamins.

Migraine

The most common dietary recommendations in neurology are given to patients with migraine; advice includes avoidance of hypoglycemia, nitrates, monosodium glutamate, and biogenic amines, in particular tyramine and phenylethylamine. Despite the value of these recommendations in daily practice, a few clinical trials (139) showed no conclusive relation between biogenic amines in red wine and wine intolerance, tyramine on migraine, or phenylethylamine in chocolate and headache attacks in persons with headache. Riboflavin supplementation helps to prevent recurrence of migraine.

Stroke

Dietary advice for prevention of stroke and for poststroke treatment (140), as well as for patients with cardiovascular disease, includes recommendations to decrease intake of saturated animal fats and sodium to control hypertension, hyperlipidemia, and body mass index. The DASH diet (Dietary Approaches to Stop Hypertension) recommends lowering the dietary intake to 150, 100, or 50 mmol/day of sodium, according to the severity of hypertension and to increase consumption of fruits, juices, and vegetables (141).

Orthostatic Hypotension

To increase the circulating volume, patients with orthostatic hypotension are advised to increase their sodium intake to 150 to 250 mEq/day of sodium (10 to 20 g of salt) and to raise their oral fluid intake to 20 oz/day, along with high potassium supplementation when they are taking fludrocortisone.

Hepatic Encephalopathy

The term *hepatic encephalopathy* refers to the neuropsychiatric manifestations of patients with liver disease, in particular alcoholic or posthepatitis cirrhosis, and following portosystemic shunts (most commonly, transjugular intrahepatic portosystemic shunt) that alter the normal urea cycle. Manifestations range from cognitive slowing, asterixis, and drowsiness to coma, with typical triphasic slow waves in the electroencephalogram. The pathogenesis probably involves increased levels of ammonia, false neurotransmitters, activation of inhibitory GABA-benzodiazepine neurotransmission, alterations of ATP-dependent sodium/potassium channels, zinc deficiency, and excess manganese in the brain.

Although traditionally a low-protein diet is advised, recent studies showed that diets with normal protein content can be administered safely during episodes of hepatic encephalopathy resulting from cirrhosis (142). A systematic review of randomized trials found insufficient evidence regarding the benefice of using nonabsorbable disaccharides such as lactulose (β-galactosidofructose) or lactitol (β-galactosidosorbitol) to increase intestinal removal of ammonia and related products (142). There are also mixed results with the use of zinc, a cofactor of enzymes in the

TABLE 88.3. INBORN ERRORS OF METABOLISM WITH NEUROLOGIC MANIFESTATIONS THAT RESPOND TO NUTRITIONAL TREATMENT

CONDITION	MAIN CLINICAL FEATURES	TREATMENT
Neuropathies		
Abetalipoproteinemia	Diarrhea, steatorrhea, ataxia, retinitis pigmentosa	Vitamins A, E, K
Refsum disease	Cerebellar ataxia, retinitis pigmentosa, CSF protein, peroxisomal disorder	Phytanic acid, dietary restriction
Mitochondrial diseases	MELAS, MERFF, Leigh, NARP, sensory ataxia	CoQ$_{10}$ creatine, L-carnitine, vitamins C, B$_1$, B$_2$, K
Myopathies		
McArdle disease (GSD V)	Myophosphorilase deficiency, exercise intolerance, myopathy, rhabdomyolysis	Branched-chain amino acids, high-protein diet, vitamin B$_6$, carbohydrate load before exercise
Cori-Forbes disease (GSD III)	Debrancher enzyme deficiency, hypoglycemia	Normoglycemia
Pompe disease (GSD IIa)	Acid maltase deficiency, myopathy, cardiomyopathy	High-protein diet
Tarui disease (GSD VII)	Muscle phosphofructokinase deficiency, exercise intolerance, myopathy, rhabdomyolysis, hemolysis	Carbohydrate load before exercise
Glucose transporter defect	Hypoglycemia, low CSF glucose, neonatal seizures, ataxia, microcephaly, ataxia, retardation	Carbohydrate loading, thioatic acid
Carnitine disorders	Myopathy, rhabdomyolysis, hypoglycemia	High carbohydrate, low-fat diet, no fasting, vitamins B$_2$, A, E, K
Very-long-chain acyl-CoA dehydrogenase deficiency	Myopathy, rhabdomyolysis, hypoglycemia, cardiomegaly	Medium-chain triglycerides[a], vitamins A, E, K
Smith-Lemil-Opitz disease	Elevated 7-dehydrocholesterol, microcephaly, retardation	High-cholesterol diet
Mitochondrial myopathies	Leigh-type pyruvate dehydrogenase	Ketogenic diet
	Benign pyruvate dehydrogenase complex	Ketogenic diet, thiamin, lipoic acid, CoQ$_{10}$ creatine, vitamins C, B$_2$, K
Inborn Vitamin Disorders		
Pyridoxine (B$_6$) deficiency	Neonatal seizures	Pyridoxine (B$_6$)
Biotin deficiency	Biotin-dependent carboxilases, organic aciduria, seizures, hypotonia, retardation, skin rash, alopecia	Biotin
Biopterin deficiency	Developmental delay, seizures, hypotonia	Tetrahydrobiopterin, 5OH-tryptophan, L-dopa
Cobalamin deficiency	Methylmalonic academia, homocysteinemia	Cobalamin
	Megaloblastic anemia, seizures, myelopathy, retardation	Protein restriction, carnitine, betaine
Aminoacidopathies		
Hartnup disease	Neutral amino aciduria, ataxia, behavioral changes	Tryptophan
Maple syrup disease	Branched chain amino acid (leucine, isoleucine, valine) aciduria, vomiting, spasticity	Dietary restriction, vitamin B
Phenylketonuria	Phenylalanine, spasticity, retardation	Dietary restriction
Homocystinuria	Homocysteine, lens subluxation, stroke, seizures, retardation	Dietary restriction, pyridoxine, (vitamin B$_6$), betaine
Propionic acidemia	Hypotonia, seizures, acidosis	Protein restriction, carnitine
Isovaleric acidemia	Vomiting, ketosis, acidosis	Protein restriction, glycine, carnitine
Glutaric academia type I	Macrocephaly, spasticity, dystonia	Tryptophan restriction, lysine restriction, carnitine, vitamin B$_2$

CoA, coenzyme A; CoQ, coenzyme Q; CSF, cerebrospinal fluid; GSD, glycogen storage disease; MELAS, mitochondrial encephalomyopathy lactic acidosis and strokelike episodes; MERFF, myoclonus epilepsy with ragged-red fibers; NARP, neuropathy, ataxia and retinitis pigmentosa.
[a]Medium-chain triglyceride treatment is formally contraindicated in patients with medium-chain acyl-CoA dehydrogenase deficiency.

urea cycle. In contrast, the use of L-ornithine-L-aspartate (143), a substrate for conversion of ammonia to urea and glutamine, has shown positive results in controlled clinical trials, by reducing blood ammonia levels and improving mental function in patients with advanced hepatic encephalopathy.

Idiopathic Intracranial Hypertension

This syndrome is characterized by headache, papilledema, and absence of focal neurologic signs. It may result from thrombosis of venous sinuses and from a number of endocrine conditions. The two most common nutritional causes are obesity and hypervitaminosis A. Weight reduction, either by diet or by bariatric surgery, is effective in controlling the symptoms. A low-salt diet and fluid restriction help to alleviate the edema.

Childhood Epilepsy

The ketogenic diet has been used for more than 80 years for treatment of childhood epilepsy, in particular for refractory cases such as the Lennox-Gastaut syndrome (144, 145). It is important to maintain ketosis avoiding calorie and fluid restrictions (145). The ketogenic acid is also used in neonatal seizures resulting from glucose transporter deficiency and in some mitochondrial disorders (benign pyruvate dehydrogenase complex deficiency).

Numerous other single- or multiple-nutrient approaches are used in patients with several inborn errors of metabolism with neurologic manifestations, including carbohydrate metabolism disorders, fatty acid metabolism disorders, mitochondrial disorders, phytanic acid accumulation (Refsum disease), and abetalipoproteinemia. These conditions are summarized in Table 88.3.

REFERENCES

1. Food and Agriculture Organization. The State of Food Insecurity in the World 2004. Rome: Food and Agriculture Organization of the United Nations, 2004. www.fao.org
2. Bourre J-M. Rev Neurol 2004;160:762–92.
3. Hernández-Rodríguez J, Manjarrez-Gutiérrez G. Nutr Rev 2001;59:49S–57S.
4. Benton D. Nutr Rev 2001;59:20S–1S.
5. Stoch MB, Smythe PM. Arch Dis Child 1963;68:546–52.
6. Stoch MB, Smythe PM. S Afr Med J 1967;41:1027–30.
7. Dobbing J. Am J Dis Child 1970;120:411–5.
8. Morgane P, Austin-Lafrance R, Bronzino J et al. Neurosci Biobehab Rev 1993;17:91–128.
9. Grantham-McGregor SM, Walker SP, Chang S. Proc Nutr Soc 2000;59:47–54.
10. Winick M, Rosso P. Pediatr Res 1969;3:181–4.
11. Winick M, Rosso P. J Pediatr 1969;74:774–8.
12. Stoch MB, Smythe PM. Arch Dis Child 1976;51:327–36.
13. Stoch MB, Smythe PM, Moodie A et al. Dev Med Child Neurol 1982;24:419–36.
14. Berkman DS, Lescano AG, Gilman RH et al. Lancet 2002;359:564–71.
15. Ivanovic D, Leiva B, Pérez H et al. Nutrition 2000;16:1056–63.
16. Leiva B, Inzunza N, Pérez H et al. Arch Latinoamer Nutr 2001;51:64–71.
17. Gordon N. Brain Dev 1997;19:165–70.
18. Lucas A, Morley R, Cole TJ et al. Lancet 1992;339:261–4.
19. Singhal A, Cole TJ, Fewtrell M et al. Obstet Gynecol Surv 2005;60:19–21.
20. Freeman MP. Ann Clin Psychiatry 2000;12:159–65.
21. Standridge JB. Am J Geriatr Pharmacother 2004;2:119–32.
22. Appel LJ. Am Fam Physician 2004;70:34–5.
23. Bourre J. Nutr Health Aging 2004;8:163–74.
24. Black MM. J Nutr 2003;133:3927S–31S.
25. World Health Organization/Unicef/ICCIDD. Indicators for Assessing Iodine Deficiency Disorders and Their Control through Salt Iodization. (WHO/NUT/94.6). Geneva: World Health Organization, 1994:1–55.
26. World Health Organization. Iodine. In: Trace Elements in Human Nutrition and Health. Geneva: World Health Organization, 1996:49–71.
27. Delange F, Bürgi H, Chen ZP et al. Thyroid 2002;12:915–24.
28. Hetzel BS. J Nutr 2000;130:493S–5S.
29. Delange F. Postgrad Med J 2001;77:217–20.
30. Bleichrodt N, Born MP. A metaanalysis of research on iodine and its relationship to cognitive development. In: Stanbury JB, ed. The Damaged Brain of Iodine Deficiency. New York: Cognizant Communication, 1994:195–200.
31. Hornabrook RW. Endemic cretinism. In: Hornabrook RW, ed. Topics in Tropical Neurology. Philadelphia: FA Davis, 1975:91–108.
32. Gillam MP, Kopp P. Curr Opin Pediatr 2001;13:358–63.
33. Halpern JP, Boyages SC, Maberly GF et al. Brain 1991;114:825–41.
34. Conn EC. Acta Horticult 1994;375:31–43.
35. Delange F, Ekpechi LO, Rosling H. Acta Horticult 1994;375:289–93.
36. Chandra AAK, Mukhopaadhyay S, Lahari D et al. Indian J Med Res 2004;119:180–5.
37. Vanderpas JB, Contempre B, Duale NL et al. Am J Clin Nutr 1990;52:1087–93.
38. Kester MHA, Martinez de Mena R, Obregon MJ et al. J Clin Endocrinol Metab 2004;89:3117–28.
39. Haddow JE, Palomaki GE, Allan WC et al. N Engl J Med 1999;341:549–55.
40. Lavado-Autric R, Ausó E, García-Velasco JV et al. J Clin Invest 2003;111:1073–82.
41. Ausó E, Lavado-Autric R, Cuevas E et al. Endocrinology 2004;145:403–7.
42. Zoeller RT. J Clin Invest 2003;111:954–57.
43. Forrest D. Endocrinology 2004;145:4034–6.
44. Burgi H, Supersaxo Z, Selz B. Acta Endocrinol (Copen) 1990;123:577–90.
45. Pharoah POD, Buttfield IH, Hetzel BS. Lancet 1971;1:308–10.
46. Cao X-Y, Jiang X-M, Dou Z-H et al. N Engl J Med 1994;331:1739–4.
47. Delange F. Bull WHO 1996;74:101–8.
48. Zecca L, Youdim MBH, Riederer P et al. Nat Rev Neurosci 2004;5:863–73.
49. Grantham-McGregor S, Ani C. J Nutr 2001;131:649S–66S.
50. Lozoff B, Brittenham GM. Hematol Oncol Clin North Am 1987;1:449–64.
51. Salgueiro MJ, Weill R, Zubillaga M et al. Biol Trace Elem Res 2004;99:49–69.
52. Román GC. Baillieres Clin Neurol 1995;5:469–76.
53. Román GC. Curr Opin Neurol 1998;11:539–45.

54. Ordunez-Garcia PO, Nieto FJ, Espinosa-Brito AD et al. Am J Public Health 1996;86:738–43.

55. Cruickshank BK. Effects of malnutrition on the central nervous system and the nerves. In: Vinken PJ, Bruyn GW, eds. Handbook of Clinical Neurology, vol. 28. Amsterdam: Elsevier, 1976.

56. Román GC. J Neurol Sci 1994;127:11–28.

57. Sadun AA, Martone JF, Reyes L et al. JAMA 1994;271:663–4.

58. Borrajero I, Perez JL, Dominguez C et al. J Neurol Sci 1994;127:68–76.

59. Thomas PK, Plant GT, Baxter P et al. J Neurol 1995;242: 629–38.

60. Cuba Neuropathy Field Investigation Team. N Engl J Med 1995;333:1176–82.

61. Román GC. Neurology 1994;44:1784–6.

62. Diniz A da S, Pacheco Santos LM. J Pediatr (Rio J) 2000;76 [Suppl]:311S–22S.

63. Biesalski HK, Nohr D. J Nutr 2004;134[Suppl]:3453S–7S.

64. Smith J, Steinemann TL. Int Ophthalmol Clin 2000;40:83–91.

65. Beaton GH, Martorell R, L'Abbé KA et al. Bol Sanit Panam 1994;117:506–18.

66. D'Souza RM, D'Souza R. J Trop Pediatr 2002;48:323–7.

67. Collins MD, Mao GE. Annu Rev Pharmacol Toxicol 1999;39: 399–430.

68. Singleton CK, Martin PR. Curr Mol Med 2001;1:197–207.

69. Silverman B, Franklin GM, Bolin R et al. MMWR Morb Mortal Wkly Rep 1997;46:523–8.

70. Smith SW. J Emerg Med 1998;16:587–91.

71. Martínez M, Román GC, de la Hoz F et al. Biomedica (Colombia) 1996;16:41–51.

72. Spillane JD. Nutritional Disorders of the Nervous System. Edinburgh: E & S Livingstone, 1947.

73. Cruickshank EK. Proc Nutr Soc 1046;5:121–7.

74. Aguiar AC, Costa VM, Ragazzo PC et al. Arq Neuropsiquiatr 2004;62:733–6.

75. Koike H, Iijima M, Mori K et al. Nutrition 2004;20:961–6.

76. Victor M, Adams RD, Collins GH. The Wernicke-Korsakoff Syndrome: A Clinical and Pathological Study of 245 Patients, 82 with Post-Mortem Examinations. Philadelphia: FA Davis, 1971.

77. Blass JP, Gibson GE. N Engl J Med 1977;297:1367–70.

78. Jung EH, Sheu KF, Blass JP. J Neurol Sci 1993;114:123–7.

79. Brokate B, Hildebrandt H, Eling P et al. Neuropsychology 2003;17:420–8.

80. Adamolekun B, McCandless DW, Butterworth RF. Metab Brain Dis 1997;12:251–8.

81. Fisher CM. Can Serv Med J 1955;11:157–99.

82. Denny-Brown D. Medicine (Baltimore) 1947;26:41–113.

83. Wilkinson PB, King A. Lancet 1944;1:528–31.

84. Spillane JD, Scott GI. Lancet 1945;2:261–4.

85. Clarke CA, Sneddon IB. Lancet 1946;1:734–7.

86. Hobbs HE, Forbes FA. Lancet 1946;2:149–53.

87. Smith DA. Brain 1946;69:209–22.

88. Sadun A. Trans Am Ophthalmol Soc 1998;96:881–923.

89. Sadun A. Semin Ophthalmol 2002;17:29–32.

90. Bruyn GW, Poser CM. The History of Tropical and Neurological Nutritional Disorders. Canton, MA: Science History Publications, 2000:144.

91. Pardo CA, McArthur JC, Griffin JW. J Peripher Nerv Syst 2001; 6:21–7.

92. Cruickshank EK. Lancet 1946;2:369–71.

93. Grundy SM, Vega GL, McGovern ME et al. Arch Intern Med 2002;162:1568–76.

94. Schaumburg H, Kaplan J, Windebank A et al. N Engl J Med 1983;309:445–8.

95. Krinke G, Schaumburg HH, Spencer PS et al. Neurotoxicology 1981;2:13–24.

96. Russell-Jones GJ, Alpers DH. Pharm Biotechnol 1999;12: 493–520.

97. Ahn SC, Brown AW. Arch Phys Med Rehabil 2005;86: 150–3.

98. Wolters M, Strohle A, Hahn A. Prev Med 2004;39:1256–66.

99. Carmel R. Clin Chem 2003;49:1367–74.

100. van Asselt DZ, Thomas CM, Segers MF et al. Ann Clin Biochem 2003;40:65–9.

101. Stabler SP, Allen RH. Annu Rev Nutr 2004;24:299–326.

102. Rogers LM, Boy E, Miller JW et al. Am J Clin Nutr 2003;77: 433–40.

103. Scalabrino G, Buccellato FR, Veber D et al. Clin Chem Lab Med 2003;41:1435–7.

104. Healton EB, Savage DG, Brust JC et al. Medicine (Baltimore) 1991;70:229–45.

105. Petito CK, Navia BA, Cho ES et al. N Engl J Med 1985;312: 874–9.

106. Di Rocco A, Bottiglieri T, Werner P et al. Neurology 2002;58: 730–5.

107. Di Rocco A, Werner P, Bottiglieri T et al. Neurology 2004;63: 1270–5.

108. Chester EM, Agamanolis DP, Harris JW et al. Acta Neurol Scand 1980;61:9–26.

109. Hemmer B, Glocker FX, Schumacher M et al. J Neurol Neurosurg Psychiatry 1998;65:822–7.

110. Ahn TB, Cho JW, Jeon BS. Eur J Neurol 2004;11:339–41.

111. Bottiglieri T, Hyland K. Acta Neurol Scand Suppl 1994;154: 19–26.

112. Ramaekers VT, Blau N. Dev Med Child Neurol 2004;46: 843–51.

113. Zittoun J. Baillieres Clin Haematol 1995;8:603–16.

114. Mitchell LE, Adzick NS, Melchionne J et al. Lancet 2004;364: 1885–95.

115. Groenen PM, van Rooij IA, Peer PG et al. J Nutr 2004;134: 1516–22.

116. Frey L, Hauser WA. Epilepsia 2003;44[Suppl]:4–13.

117. Garcia A, Zanibbi K. Can Med Assoc J 2004;171:897–904.

118. Seshadri S, Beiser A, Selhub J et al. N Engl J Med 2002;346: 476–83.

119. Garcia A, Haron Y, Evans L et al. J Am Geriatr Soc 2004;52: 66–71.

120. Homocysteine Studies Collaboration. JAMA 2002;288:2015–22.

121. Vermeer SE, Van Dijk EJ, Koudstaal PJ et al. Ann Neurol 2002;51:285–9.

122. Almeida OP, Flicker L, Lautenschlager NT et al. Neurobiol Aging 2005;26:251–7.

123. Gordon N. Eur J Paediatr Neurol 2002;6:243–7.

124. Harding AE, Muller DPR, Thomas PK et al. Ann Neurol 1982;12:419–24.

125. Brin MF, Fetell MR, Green PH. Neurology 1985;35:338–42.

126. Sitrin MD, Lieberman F, Jensen WE et al. Ann Intern Med 1987;107:51–4.

127. Mariotti C, Gellera C, Rimoldi M et al. Neurol Sci 2004;25: 130–7.

128. Tranchant D, Darracq R, Ticolat R. Presse Med 1986 ;15: 1729–30.

129. Jackson CE, Amato AA, Barohn RJ. Muscle Nerve 1996;19: 1161–5.

130. Tanyel MC, Mancano LD. Am Fam Physician 1997;55: 197–201.

131. Berman K, Brodaty H. CNS Drugs 2004;18:807–25.

132. Jialal I, Devaraj S. J Nutr 2005;135:348–53.

133. Holick MF. J Cell Biochem 2003;88:296–307.

134. Cantorna MT, Mahon BD. Exp Biol Med 2004;229:1136–42.

135. Munger KL, Zhang SM, O'Reilly E et al. Neurology 2004;62: 60–5.

136. VanAmerongen BM, Dijkstra CD, Lips P et al. Eur J Clin Nutr 2004;58:1095–109.

137. Dumas M, Jauberteau-Marchan MO. Med Hypotheses 2000;55:517–20.

138. McMichael AJ, Hall AJ. Neuroepidemiology 2001;20:165–7.

139. Jansen SC, van Dusseldorp M, Bottema KC et al. Ann Allergy Asthma Immunol 2003;91:233–40.

140. Schwamm LH, Pancioli A, Acker JE et al. Stroke 2005;36: 690–703.

141. Ard JD, Coffman CJ, Lin PH et al. Am J Hypertens 2004;17: 1156–62.

142. Shawcross D, Jalan R. Lancet 2005;365:431–3.

143. Kircheis G, Wettstein M, Dahl S et al. Metab Brain Dis 2002; 17:453–62.

144. Freeman JM, Kelly MT, Freeman JB. The Epilepsy Diet Treatment: An Introduction to the Ketogenic Diet. New York: Demo Publications, 1994.

145. Vaisleib II, Buchhalter JR, Zupanc ML. Pediatr Neurol 2004; 31:198–202.

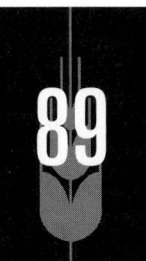

89 THE HYPERCATABOLIC STATE[1]
STEPHEN F. LOWRY AND J. MARTIN PEREZ

METABOLIC RESPONSES TO INJURY AND DISEASE . . .1381
    Energy Expenditure .1382
    Protein Metabolism .1384
    Glucose Metabolism 1386
    Lipid Metabolism 1387
MEDIATORS OF THE HYPERCATABOLIC RESPONSE . . .1389
    Neuroimmunoendocrine Response 1389
    Cytokines 1391
SYSTEMIC AND ORGAN REACTIONS 1393
    Gastrointestinal Tract 1393
    Cachexia 1393
GENERAL NUTRITION AND ANABOLIC SUPPORT 1394
    Macronutrients 1394
    Anabolic Therapy 1394
    Micronutrients 1395
NUTRITIONAL SUPPORT IN ORGAN FAILURE 1395
    Lung 1395
    Kidney 1395
    Liver 1396
    Heart 1396

The hypercatabolic state is induced by endogenous production of a variety of mediators in response to diverse stimuli including trauma, sepsis, and specific advanced diseases. This state is characterized by progressive severe loss of body protein, alterations in carbohydrate metabolism, increased oxidation of lipids, and increased extracellular volume that may result in organ failure and that, at present, may be ameliorated to some extent by nutritional support but can be reversed only by major palliation or cure of the underlying disease process. The metabolic response, however, also serves the purpose of healing and resolution of inflammation. The hypercatabolic state is characterized by

hypermetabolism and implies a disruption of normal metabolic homeostasis. Since the pioneering work of Cuthbertson (1) in 1945, much research has focused on mechanisms underlying this often-dramatic host metabolic response to injury or disease, as well as the means of modifying such responses via direct nutritional intervention or modulation of the inflammatory milieu. This chapter describes the hypermetabolic state, the neuroimmunoendocrine and cytokine mediators of this response, the metabolic consequences of prolonged net hypermetabolism to the host, and, briefly, how this condition influences aspects of nutrient use. The clinical features of this response, in general, are qualitatively similar, regardless of the nature of the insult. However, the catabolic response to cancer and immunocompromised states, such as human immunodeficiency virus (HIV), are distinct and are reviewed separately.

METABOLIC RESPONSES TO INJURY AND DISEASE

The temporal sequence of postinjury metabolic events is well known from the careful evaluation by many investigators. Cuthbertson (1) initially established the basis for understanding the biologic response to injury. He found that urinary excretion of nitrogen, potassium, and phosphorus was markedly increased in patients with long bone fractures. The relative concentrations of these excreted nutrients were similar to those of muscles, and he concluded that muscle was the source of these losses. These and subsequent isotopic dilution studies by Moore and colleagues (2) characterized the ebb and flow phases of the postinjury response. The early ebb phase occurs immediately after insult and is characterized by hemodynamic instability with decreased cardiac output and oxygen consumption, low core temperature, and elevated glucagon, catecholamine, and free fatty acid levels. This phase typically lasts from 12 to 24 hours and is modified to some degree by the extent and adequacy of fluid resuscitation.

The subsequent flow phase is fundamentally a metabolic response that alters energy and protein use to preserve critical organ function and repair damaged tissue. Total body oxygen consumption, metabolic rate, and amino acid efflux from peripheral muscle stores all increase, counterregulatory hormone concentrations are elevated, glucose metabolism is altered, and lactate production, urinary nitrogen

[1]**Abbreviations: ACTH,** adrenocorticotropic hormone; **AIDS,** acquired immunodeficiency syndrome; **ATP,** adenosine triphosphate; **CNS,** central nervous system; **GH,** growth hormone; **HALS,** HIV-associated lipodystrophy syndrome; **HIV,** human immunodeficiency virus; **HPA,** hypothalamic-pituitary-adrenal axis; **IFN-γ,** interferon-γ; **IGF,** insulinlike growth factor; **IL,** interleukin; **POMC,** propiomelanocortin; **REE,** resting energy expenditure; **IL-1ra,** interleukin-1 receptor antagonist; **T₃,** triiodothyronine; **T₄,** thyroxine; **TNF,** tumor necrosis factor; **UPPS,** ubiquitin-proteosome proteolytic system.

TABLE 89.1. METABOLIC ALTERATIONS FOLLOWING INJURY

EBB PHASE	FLOW PHASE
Increased blood glucose	Normal/slightly increased blood glucose
Increased circulating free fatty acids	Normal/slightly increased free fatty acids
Decreased insulin	Normal/increased insulin
Increased catecholamines	Increased catecholamines
Decreased cardiac output	Increased cardiac output
Decreased oxygen consumption	Increased oxygen consumption
Decreased core temperature	Elevated core temperature

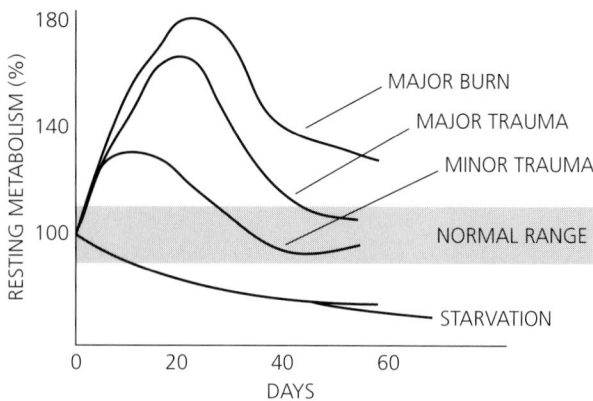

Figure 89.1. Effect of injury on metabolic rate. (Adapted from Wilmore DW. The Metabolic Management of the Critically Ill. New York: Plenum Medical Book, 1977, with permission.)

losses, and tissue protein catabolism all increase (3) (Table 89.1). This metabolic response has evolved to enhance survival in times of stress and provides a mechanism to resolve the consequences of tissue injury and inflammation. The mobilization of energy from stored adipose tissue and amino acids from lean muscle essentially serve as building blocks for acute-phase reactants and tissue renewal. With the resolution of the inciting event, a period of recuperative anabolism ensues in which metabolic homeostasis is reestablished in concert with replenishment of fat and muscle stores. The discussion later focuses on the flow phase response and the endogenous mediators that regulate this response.

Energy Expenditure

Injury and Sepsis

During the postinsult flow phase, increased energy expenditure by the body occurs, as well as an increased metabolic rate. Total body oxygen consumption increases in concert with increased oxidation of fuel sources (carbohydrates, amino acids, and lipids). To some extent, the elevation of the metabolic rate correlates with the cause and/or the severity of the initial injury. Energy expenditure may increase minimally with mild injury (4), 15 to 25% after long bone fractures (1), and as much as double with burn injury over more than 40% of total body surface (5) (Fig. 89.1). The physiologic consequences of the flow phase insult serve as the basis for modern critical care medicine in which key features such as support of adequate cardiac hemodynamics, optimized ventilation strategies, fluid administration, monitoring of organ function, and nutrition are supported in the critically ill patient.

The increased metabolic rate requires mobilizing the body's nutrient stores to provide substrates for the increased energy demand. The body's stores of carbohydrates, primarily glycogen, are quickly depleted in the first 24 hours after injury. Thereafter, fat and protein serve as the main energy sources. In the hypermetabolic state there is an obligatory net protein loss that partly serves to provide substrates for gluconeogenesis and amino acids for increased synthesis of acute-phase proteins. Nitrogen is used as a

surrogate marker of protein loss because of the fixed relation between the two substances (e.g., protein in grams/6.25 = nitrogen in grams). After an inciting event, an increase in urinary nitrogen excretion occurs that is generally related to the magnitude of the injury and the adequacy of insult resolution. The nitrogen loss is primarily in the form of urea, but other contributing losses are in the form of creatinine, ammonia, uric acid, and amino acids excreted in urine. Skeletal muscle represents the majority of protein-containing tissues, and the net protein loss characteristic of the catabolic response results in loss of lean muscle mass.

Stored triglycerides are also mobilized and oxidized to provide substrates for the hypermetabolic state but are unable to prevent protein catabolism. During this state, there is also a marked increase in the counterregulatory hormones: glucocorticoids, catecholamines, and glucagon mediated in large part by the central nervous system (CNS) and at the level of individual tissues. These hormones promote a variety of metabolic effects, as discussed later. Also important in the response to injury are the cytokines, which have effects that are mediated by both endocrine and paracrine mechanisms. These acute alterations in metabolic and hormonal responses serve to maintain tissue functions (Fig 89.2).

Cancer

In contrast to the hypermetabolic state universally seen after trauma, hypermetabolism is not an invariable finding in patients with cancer (see also Chapter 83). Because patients in the advanced stages of cancer often become cachectic, it was hypothesized that this weight loss was the result of increased energy expenditure and net negative energy balance. Studies do not confirm this hypothesis but indicate a variable metabolic response to cancer; some investigators report a hypermetabolic response, whereas others observe no change or a hypometabolic response (6–8) (Fig. 89.3). One study failed to demonstrate a correlation between resting energy expenditure (REE)

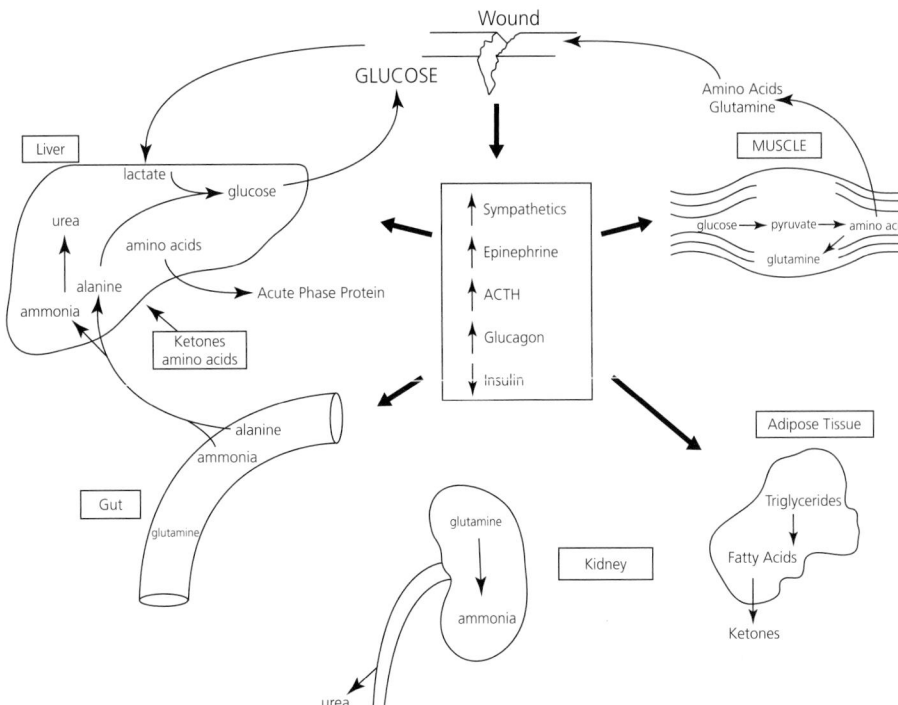

Figure 89.2. Neuroendocrine and metabolic consequences of injury. ACTH, adrenocorticotropic hormone.

and weight loss or tumor burden (9). Other studies demonstrated no significant difference in REE in with gastric or patients with colon cancer who were losing weight or were at a stable weight (7).

Numerous studies show that the variations in REE seen in patients with cancer may be influenced by tumor histology (10–13). One study found that patients with nonsmall cell lung cancer had an elevated REE, whereas patients with gastric or colorectal cancer did not. Another

study demonstrated a hypermetabolic state in patients with gastric cancer, whereas patients with esophageal or colorectal cancers were evenly distributed in their metabolic response, and patients with pancreatic or hepatobiliary neoplasms were mostly hypometabolic (12). In contrast, a study of cachectic patients with advanced pancreatic cancer demonstrated an increase in REE (13). The elevated REE observed in certain patients with cancer may be a phenomenon resulting, in part, from tumor-related metabolism in addition to the host response. Elevated adrenergic activity and sensitivity has been demonstrated in tumor-bearing animals and patients with cancer (14). The increased adrenergic activity and sensitivity may result in part from systemic inflammation, stress response to starvation, cancer-related anemia, decreased stroke volume, and an increased heart rate. These changes may be seen as compensatory in nature to systemic inflammation of cancer and poor nutrition. Limited studies have demonstrated the possible role of β-blockers to effectively reduce β-adrenergic mediated lipolysis and decrease cardiovascular energy-related expenditure. β-Blockade has been demonstrated to lower resting metabolism in patients with cancer (15). Thus, the metabolic response to tumor burden varies and may depend in part on tumor type and/or their endogenous mediators involved in the tumor-host interaction.

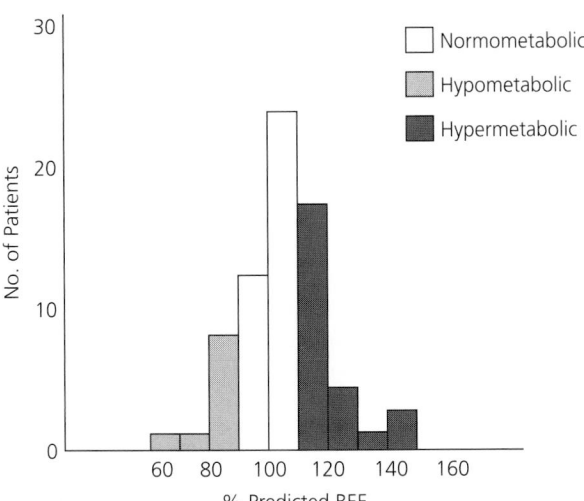

Figure 89.3. Preoperative resting energy expenditure (REE) in patients with cancer. (Adapted from Luketich JD, Mullen JL, Fuerer ID et al. Ablation of abnormal energy expenditure by curative tumor resection. Arch Surg 1990;125:337–41, with permission.)

Acquired Immunodeficiency Syndrome

Another patient population in which a hypermetabolic response is often observed is those with HIV infection.

Several studies suggest that the REE is elevated in patients with early HIV infection and increases further with subsequent acquired immunodeficiency syndrome (AIDS) (16–19). This REE increase may occur in an asymptomatic patient with normal CD4 lymphocyte counts (20). Certain secondary infections may cause even further elevations in the REE, although it appears that even latent HIV infection can cause an increase in REE above basal levels. Other studies have indicated that a small percentage of AIDS patients without secondary infection may, in fact be, hypometabolic and demonstrate a metabolic response similar to that seen in starvation (17). This response has been strongly associated with oral candidiasis or odynophagia, which suggests that poor food intake may impose a starvation metabolic response in addition to the hypermetabolic response (21). Additionally, one study found that in HIV-positive subjects, REE was unchanged in comparison with controls (22). These apparent inconsistencies may be explained by methodologic differences in these studies in accounting for differences in body composition, which in turn may impact the accuracy of REE determinations. REE determinations typically are based on healthy populations, thus making accurate determinations difficult when body compositional changes are present. Furthermore, the use of highly active antiretroviral therapy may render previously developed equations inaccurate for determining REE in HIV disease states.

Thus, the hypermetabolic response in the host can be initiated by a variety of initial insults, including trauma, burns, infection (including HIV), and cancer. The increased energy expenditure results in an alteration of fuel metabolism, leading to a breakdown of protein and fat and alterations in glucose metabolism to provide the necessary substrates for these increased energy demands.

Protein Metabolism

Injury and Sepsis

Protein represents a large reserve of body fuel. In response to the increased energy demands after injury, skeletal muscle stores are mobilized. This leads to increased amino acid efflux from peripheral stores and increased urinary nitrogen excretion. The extent of urinary nitrogen loss correlates with the severity of the injury. The result is a net negative nitrogen balance as protein catabolism exceeds protein synthesis. This acceleration of protein catabolism generally parallels the increase in oxygen consumption and represents a constant fraction of total oxidation after injury (4). If allowed to proceed unabated, the net protein catabolism leads to loss of lean muscle mass and in turn may contribute to organ dysfunction or failure (23).

The mechanism of muscle catabolism during sepsis involves increased protein breakdown in a similar fashion to injury, especially myofibrillar protein, as well as reduced

protein synthesis and inhibition of amino acid uptake by muscle (24–26). In animal models, important mediators of this catabolism during sepsis include glucocorticoids as well as certain cytokines, particularly tumor necrosis factor (TNF) and interleukin-1 (IL-1) (27). The current understanding of cytokine function in muscle homeostasis, including muscle catabolism, anabolism, and links between other intermediaries in metabolism, remains incomplete. Cytokines appear to have a bidirectional effect on muscle during inflammation with myocytes capable of producing cytokines; expressing cytokine receptors, adhesion molecules, and costimultory molecules; and influencing the course of inflammation itself (28).

Cytokines that affect muscle homeostasis can be produced by the myocyte or by nonmyocyte cells (i.e., macrophages), either locally at the site of injury or from a distance. Cytokines, therefore, can exert their effects in an endocrine, autocrine, or paracrine manner depending on the nature of the injury and the particular cytokine (29). The principal sources of extrinsic cytokine production appear to be neutrophils and macrophages resident in muscle (30). Intrinsic muscle cytokines include IL-1β, IL-6, IL-8, and transforming growth factor β. Granulocyte macrophage-colony stimulating factor production by myoblasts appears to be induced by exposure to IL-1α, IL-1β, and TNF-α (31).

The relevance of cytokines in pathologic conditions such as injury and sepsis remains incompletely characterized despite extensive studies searching for putative mediators in muscle protein breakdown. The body of literature does indicate a complex network including but not limited to TNF-α, IL-1β, IL-6, gp130 proteins, interferons, and growth/differentiation factor-8 involved in the regulation of muscle protein homeostasis. Individual cytokine contributions to the overall milieu remain difficult to elucidate. Certainly, data exist that would argue against the hypothesis that cytokines alone are responsible for all of the metabolic changes seen in injury and infection. First, cytokine levels have not been found to be uniformly elevated in all injured patients. Second, the effects of intravenously administered cytokines appear to be temporally limited. Third, some evidence exists that cytokines do not appear to have a direct effect on muscle protein breakdown (32).

The intracellular mechanisms involved in muscle protein breakdown in sepsis and injury are not clearly defined; however, animal studies indicate that sepsis induces a nonlysosomal, energy-dependent proteolysis (33). This involves activation of the ubiquitin-proteasome-dependent pathway that increases mRNAs encoding ubiquitin and proteasomes in muscle. In this pathway, proteins destined for degradation are ligated to the polypeptide ubiquitin and then degraded by a protease that acts on ubiquinated proteins (34–36). The ubiquitination of proteins destined to undergo proteolysis by the proteasome is regulated by ubiquitin ligases as well as other enzymes. Recent studies have demonstrated E2(14k) and E3α, ubiquitin ligases, to be involved in increased breakdown of proteins in atrophying muscle (37). Other studies indicated that the mRNA for ubiquitin increases during glucocorticoid excess and acidosis, and may occur in septic states (36, 38). In rats, endotoxemia can induce increased ubiquitin mRNA, IL-6, TNF-α, and net release of 3-methylhistidine, a marker of protein breakdown (39). Studies have also demonstrated that the ubiquitin-proteasome system does not break down the complexes of proteins contained in actomyosin or myofibrils, which constitute the bulk of muscle protein (35, 40). Therefore, additional proteases such as caspase-3 may release constituent proteins of actomyosin before ubiquitin-proteasome system activation (41). It is likely that the ubiquitin pathway is important in proteolysis in sepsis and in other catabolic conditions, but further studies are needed to delineate the mechanisms leading to ubiquitin-proteasome system activation.

The increased amino acid efflux from peripheral stores after injury provides a substrate for enhanced hepatic gluconeogenesis and acute-phase protein synthesis. It also allows synthesis of new protein tissue in wounds and proliferation of cellular components involved in the inflammatory response. There is increased splanchnic uptake of glucogenic amino acids, particularly alanine and glutamine. This increase in uptake in burn patients corresponds with the quantity and distribution of peripheral tissue amino acid release (42). The enhanced splanchnic uptake is achieved by increased glutamine uptake in the gut enterocytes, whereas alanine is released by the gastrointestinal tract in increasing amounts during stress (43).

During the postinjury response, alanine and glutamine are also preferentially released from muscle stores. Although these amino acids make up approximately 6% of protein in muscle stores, they constitute 60 to 80% of the free amino acids released in response to insult (44, 45). This effect may be influenced by glucocorticoid activity; in a study using a canine model, both acute and chronic glucocorticoid excess increased glutamine and alanine release (46). Glutamine availability may become limited during catabolic illness, and mortality in critically ill patients has been associated with low glutamine levels (47, 48). Glutamine supplementation in some studies has improved immune function and reduced intestinal permeability (49). Glutamine supplementation has been demonstrated to preserve skeletal muscle and improve nitrogen balance (50). Given that glutamine is a precursor to glutathione, it has been demonstrated that supplementation results in a higher antioxidant capacity mediated in part by glutamine (51). A recent metaanalysis of 14 randomized trials comparing the use of glutamine supplementation in surgical and critically ill patients showed that glutamine supplementation may be associated in critically ill patients with a reduction in complication and mortality rates; the greatest benefit was seen with high-dose parenteral glutamine (see Chapter 35) (52).

Despite net peripheral proteolysis, liver mass is usually preserved during injury, often with an increase in total liver protein, RNA, and DNA (53). Preservation of liver mass occurs with sustained or increased hepatic capacity for gluconeogenesis and synthesis of acute-phase proteins (54).

In summary, skeletal protein catabolism may serve three main purposes. First, it provides amino acids that can serve as a substrate for protein synthesis by the wound or liver. Second, the released amino acids can be converted to glucose by the liver as an energy source during the hypermetabolic response. Third, it provides a source of glutamine to be used as a fuel source by the gut and possibly by other tissues involved in the metabolic response to stress.

Cancer

Patients with cancer and significant weight loss may have protein kinetics similar to those seen in traumatized or infected patients. Whole-body protein turnover rates are increased, in some patients, with increases in protein synthesis as well as catabolism (55–57). However, there are conflicting reports in the literature regarding difference in whole-body protein turnover between patients with cancer and controls. Attempts have been made to correlate the increase in protein turnover rates with changes in REE or weight loss. Isotope infusion studies suggest a significant increase in whole-body protein catabolism in patients with cancer and cachexia compared with non-cachectic patients with cancer or patients with benign disease (59). However, although the protein turnover rate is increased in other studies, it does not appear to correlate with energy expenditure or weight loss in most patients with cancer (7).

AIDS

In contrast with other patient populations, those infected with HIV in general show an elevated REE with decreased protein synthesis and catabolism in the absence of secondary infection (60). Preliminary data indicate that protein catabolism and a negative nitrogen balance occur when an AIDS patient becomes secondarily infected (19). The loss of lean body mass is a common finding in patients with HIV infection and predicts morbidity and mortality (61–63). Multiple factors are implicated in the loss of lean body mass, including reduced nutritional intake, nutrient malabsorption, elevated REE, and altered lipid, carbohydrate, and protein metabolism (64–68). Asymptomatic HIV-infected patients do not appear to have significant lean body mass losses as compared with HIV-infected adults with secondary infections (69, 70). Protein turnover appears to be increased in HIV-infected patients when compared with healthy controls; however, net protein balance appears to be positive in asymptomatic HIV-infected patients (65, 66). This is in contrast to HIV-infected children, in whom growth failure secondary to low rates of lean tissue deposition is common (73). Moreover, growth failure in HIV-infected children appears to be a significant factor in a poor prognosis (71–73). In a study comparing children with HIV infection and age-matched children without HIV infection with regard to whole-body and splanchnic protein kinetics and synthesis of acute-phase proteins, children with HIV infection but without secondary infection have reduced protein balance because of an inability to downregulate protein catabolism along with increased levels of synthesis of acute-phase reactants (73).

Glucose Metabolism

Injury and Sepsis

Hyperglycemia is a common response to septic or traumatic injury. It results from both increased hepatic gluconeogenesis and decreased glucose uptake by insulin-dependent tissues. In the ebb phase, insulin levels are depressed, but they become normal to elevated during the flow phase, although remaining depressed in relation to the degree of hyperglycemia. The persistent hyperglycemia suggests injury-induced insulin resistance (3). In addition, studies using hepatic vein cannulations in thermally injured patients show increased uptake of gluconeogenic amino acids by the splanchnic tissues (42). These amino acids are then used for gluconeogenesis, resulting in increased splanchnic production of glucose and further contributing to the hyperglycemic state.

Altered glucose metabolism in response to stress results in decreased skeletal muscle uptake of glucose and decreased glucose incorporation into fatty acids by adipocytes (74). The decreased uptake by skeletal muscle is the result of peripheral insulin resistance, which may be mediated in part by excess cortisol and catecholamines (75, 76). Recent evidence also indicates that TNF-α induces insulin resistance (77). In these stressed patients, hyperglycemia fails to suppress hepatic gluconeogenesis or glycogenolysis; administration of a dextrose infusion suppresses gluconeogenesis less effectively in septic or trauma patients than in healthy volunteers (78, 79). Amino acid infusions are also unable to inhibit gluconeogenesis in trauma patients (80). This alteration in glucose metabolism maintains glucose availability to noninsulin-dependent tissues such as the CNS, kidneys, wound tissue, and hematologic cells, which are vital for survival.

During the stress response, another source of glucose results from the change to anaerobic glycolysis in skeletal muscle and hypoxic tissue (i.e., the wound) producing increased amounts of lactate. Lactate can be converted into glucose in the liver via the Cori cycle, which is increased in both burn and trauma patients (81, 82). In burn patients, lactate is the most important gluconeogenic substrate (83). The resultant lacticacidemia may be mediated in part by both catecholamines and cytokines (84, 85). In critically ill patients, elevated lactate levels may reflect impaired tissue oxygenation; however, elevated lactate levels may persist despite evidence of adequate tissue oxygenation. The

higher lactate levels in this circumstance reflect excess production of pyruvate as a consequence of accelerated glycolysis stemming from increased glucose uptake and glycogen breakdown rather than tissue hypoxia (86).

The efficiency of glucose oxidation is altered by injury (87) and in postoperative (88) and burn patients (89), further contributing to the hyperglycemic state. Maximum glucose oxidative capacity appears to be inversely related to the severity of the injury. The decrease in oxidation may be the result of reduced activity of intracellular enzymatic metabolic pathways, such as pyruvate dehydrogenase (90).

Cancer

Glucose intolerance has long been observed in association with malignancy, and as early as 1919 was proposed as a means to distinguish patients who were more likely to have gastric carcinoma than peptic ulcer disease (91). Since that initial report, many investigators have confirmed glucose intolerance in diverse cancer populations with advanced disease (92–94). Glucose intolerance results from increased resistance to both exogenous and endogenous insulin (95). The mechanism underlying this insulin resistance is not well defined, but because monocyte insulin receptors from patients with cancer are normal, a postreceptor defect has been postulated (96). However, this effect may not be cancer induced per se but may be related to the effects of cancer, such as weight loss, because glucose intolerance also occurs in response to weight loss attributable to calorie deprivation in benign disease (97) as well as response to sepsis (98, 99).

Numerous reports have noted increased endogenous glucose production in patients with cancer (91, 92, 100, 101), with an observed increase in glucose turnover rate affected by tumor stage (102, 103), histology (93, 101), and type. In a study comparing patients with early (limited to gut wall) and advanced gastrointestinal malignancies (esophagus, stomach, and pancreas), rates of glucose turnover were significantly higher in patients with advanced lesions (102). Similar findings were observed in patients with advanced colon cancer (103), indicating that increased glucose turnover is consistent with an advanced stage. Other studies make it evident that tumor histology also affects glucose turnover rates. Studies in sarcoma (101) and leukemic patients (93) indicate a glucose turnover rate two to three times that seen in normal volunteers (93). In contrast, patients with lymphoma had a glucose turnover rate similar to that of normal volunteers (93). Other studies indicate that the increased glucose turnover is related specifically to the cancer. The increase in glucose turnover rate is significantly higher in patients with cancer and weight loss than in the cancer-free population with comparable weight loss (97). Another study demonstrated that patients with cancer and progressive weight loss had markedly elevated rates of glucose turnover, whereas weight-stable patients with cancer had glucose turnover rates similar to those in normal volunteers (99). These findings contrast with the decreased glucose turnover rates in patients with weight loss attributable to uncomplicated starvation (104).

Regulation of hepatic glucose production is altered in patients with cancer. Although infusion of glucose in normal subjects suppresses hepatic gluconeogenesis, glucose infusion reduces glucose production by only 70% in patients with early or advanced gastric cancer (102). In sarcoma or leukemic patients, hepatic glucose production was decreased by less than one third (93, 101).

Increased gluconeogenesis via the Cori cycle represents a substantial proportion of the observed increase in glucose turnover rate in patients with cancer. During this cycle, lactate released from anaerobic glycolysis in peripheral tissue is recycled to glucose in the liver in an energy-requiring reaction. Increased Cori cycle activity occurs in patients with cancer, particularly those with weight loss (99). The increase in Cori cycle activity seems to be a specific response to the neoplasm and not directly related to weight loss. The source of the lactate molecules remains a matter of debate. Tumor cells may be one source of lactate production (105). Other studies indicate that the tumor itself may exert distal effects on the host carbohydrate metabolism; the rates of glucose uptake and lactate release from forearm tissue of patients with cancer were significantly higher than those in tissue from physiologically normal subjects (97, 106). Taken together, it seems probable that increased glycolysis in both the tumor and host tissues contributes to the increased lactate production. The Warburg effect describes the phenomenon of dramatically increased contribution by glycolytic adenosine triphosphate (ATP) turnover to total ATP production under aerobic conditions (107). The net effect is the perception that a high glycolytic rate is typical of malignant cells. In fact, fluorodeoxyglucose positron emission tomography has become an effective cancer detection technique, largely based on the assumption that cancer tissues have a higher rate of glucose uptake than normal tissues (108). Recent studies, however, have challenged the perception that the Warburg effect explains fully the altered glucose metabolism seen in malignant cells. A recent analysis of studies that use a comprehensive energy analysis, accounting for all sources of ATP production and precise oxygen consumption measurements, has yielded a mean value of total ATP production of 20% for normal cells and 17% for malignant cells (109). These limited data do not support the long-held conviction of aerobic glycolytic cancer metabolism.

Increased glucose oxidation is also observed in patients with cancer and weight loss (99, 110, 111). The increase in oxidation rate is not proportional to the increased glucose availability, which implies a loss of efficiency in the oxidation process (97, 102). The effects of alteration in carbohydrate metabolism incurred by patients with cancer on energy balance and use are difficult to quantitate but are likely to influence whole-body kinetics and, to some extent, development of cancer cachexia.

Acquired Immunodeficiency Syndrome

Although there are only a few studies on carbohydrate metabolism in HIV-infected patients, hyperglycemia does not appear to be a prevalent finding in patients who are HIV positive. Evidence indicates that abnormal glucose metabolism in patients with AIDS may be related to pentamidine toxicity. Moreover, HIV infection has been reported to cause islet β-cell dysfunction, leading to insulin-dependent diabetes mellitus in the absence of islet cell or insulin antibodies (112). Abnormalities of glucose homeostasis (insulin resistance) and related metabolic abnormalities such as hypertriglyceridemia, low high-density lipoprotein levels, or development of an atherogenic profile are frequently associated with body composition changes in HIV-infected patients receiving antiretroviral therapy (113–115). Before the era of antiviral therapy, the observed hyperglycemia of HIV disease was thought to be a direct effect of HIV infection. Among HIV-infected patients with lipodystrophy, fasting glucose levels are most often normal, but impaired glucose tolerance is a common result with standard oral glucose tolerance testing (116). HIV-associated lipodystrophy syndrome (HALS) has been described as the centrifugal loss of fat with centripetal fat reorganization (i.e., loss of subcutaneous fat in the face and buttocks, and a fat loss from the extremities with an increase of visceral abdominal fat). A variant of HALS has also been described with a predominance of fat pad accumulation in the neck region, in the mammae, or by subcutaneous lipomatosis. HALS has been associated with insulin resistance (117). A 50% reduction in insulin sensitivity was documented in HIV-infected patients with lipodystrophy as compared with HIV-infected patients who had not experienced fat redistribution (118). Duration and modality of antiretroviral therapy appear to contribute to insulin resistance (119). The mechanism of insulin resistance in patients with HALS is not fully understood; however, in vitro study demonstrates inhibited insulin-responsive facilitative glucose transporter (GLUT 4) (120). Additional defects in insulin secretion likely also contribute to the overall metabolic alterations seen in HALS.

Lipid Metabolism

Injury and Sepsis

Lipid is a major source of fuel for the body, representing 80% of the body's energy reserves. In response to stress, lipid mobilization and use can potentially preserve proteins. Immediately after insult, enhanced lipolysis mediated by sympathetic stimulation of adipose tissue occurs, as well as activation of lipase by norepinephrine and glucagon (121). Leptin, a hormone that stimulates fatty acid oxidation and is expressed by adipocytes, is related to cytokines in that it is considered a stress-related hormone. Leptin suppresses adrenal synthetic activity and may be responsible for the functional adrenal insufficiency seen in sepsis (122, 123). Insulin, insulinlike growth factor-I (IGF-I), thyroid hormones, somatotropin release-inhibiting factor glucocorticoids, and β-adrenergic agonists are known to enhance leptin production. Leptin levels correlate with early sepsis, and survivors appear to have higher plasma levels than controls (124). However, leptin levels are not elevated in patients with sepsis of longer duration and do not predict outcome (125). The overall net result of these hormones and cytokines is an increase in free fatty acids and glycerol concentration in the circulation.

Several studies have indicated that there may be a preference for oxidation of fat as a source of energy in septic or trauma patients (126). In the nonstressed condition, the normal respiratory quotient is approximately 0.85 (127). In the injured patient, the respiratory quotient is lower, indicating increased lipid oxidation (5). A decreased respiratory quotient is also seen in patients with worsening sepsis, and isotopic studies have corroborated increased fat oxidation in these patients (128, 129). Other studies have demonstrated that with increased severity of sepsis, oxidation and clearance of lipids from the bloodstream decrease, a finding suggesting poor use and that may account for the feeding-resistant protein wasting with preservation of fat stores seen in critical illness (130). Overall, the increased amount of free fatty acids serves as a fuel source for tissues except red blood cells and the CNS.

Cancer

A large body of evidence indicates that most of the weight loss seen in cancer cachexia is the result of depletion of body fat (103, 131, 132). Fat is stored mainly as triglycerides in adipocytes, which is hydrolyzed to glycerol and free fatty acid. This is accomplished by the action of specific lipases that are regulated by hormones that may stimulate (e.g., catecholamines) or inhibit (e.g., insulin) lipolysis. The turnover rates of glycerol and free fatty acids have been used in studies as a measurement of lipolysis. The effect that cancer has on the lipolysis rate is unclear. Whole-body lipolytic rates in patients with cancer have been reported to be both increased and normal (133, 135). In a study using stable isotopes, the turnover rate of glycerol and free fatty acids in weight-stable and weight-losing patients with cancer was compared with that seen in healthy volunteers. No significant differences were noted in weight-stable patients and normal volunteers, but investigators reported a significant increase in the rate of glycerol and free fatty acid release in the weight-losing patients with cancer (134, 135). However, in a similar study using cachectic patients without cancer as a control group for weight loss, the rate of lipolysis was similar in cachectic patients with and without cancer (136). Thus the increased weight loss itself may account for the increased lipolysis.

The role of leptin in mediating cachexia in patients with cancer is poorly understood. However, the systemic inflammatory response is associated with increased substrate use and increased energy expenditure in patients with cancer and chronic disease (137), and is in part mediated by the actions of IL-6. Leptin and IL-6 share the common receptor gp130 (138). Additionally, IL-6 and leptin share structural and functional similarities with similar patterns of secretion during injury (139). Despite these intriguing data, few studies have examined the relationship between leptin levels and cancer. The few studies to date have focused on weight-losing patients with cancer rather than on longitudinal studies of the relationship between leptin, cancer disease progression, appetite, and changes in REE in weight-stable patients.

In their discussion of lipolysis in patients with cancer of the esophagus, Klein and Wolfe propose four possible mechanisms for increased lipolysis in patients with cancer: (a) increased lipolytic rates caused by decreased food intake and malnutrition; (b) increased lipolysis when expressed per kilogram of body weight caused by body fat loss and an increased percentage of body weight as lean body mass; (c) stimulation of lipolysis caused by the stress response with adrenal medullary stimulation, increased circulating catecholamines, and insulin resistance; and (d) the release of lipolytic factors produced by the tumor or by myeloid tissue cells (140).

An increased rate of fat oxidation has been reported in many patient populations with cancer (97, 110, 133). A study of patients with colorectal or gastric cancer found that patients with cancer and weight loss oxidized fat more rapidly than patients with cancer and no weight loss or patients with benign disease and weight loss (111). Therefore, as with stressed patients, it appears that the body responds to the tumor-bearing state with a preference for fat oxidation.

Human Immunodeficiency Virus Infection

In contrast to injury and sepsis, adipose tissue is often conserved in patients with AIDS at the expense of body cell mass (141). Various direct and indirect lipid metabolic changes have been described in HIV-infected patients with lipodystrophy, to include insulin resistance, hypertriglyceridemia, and low high-density lipoprotein levels (142). These metabolic changes are often accompanied by body compositional changes as described in the HALS syndrome, which is the predominant lipid disorder seen in HIV (see the discussion under glucose metabolism, HIV). The role of protease inhibitors in lipodystrophy associated with HIV remains largely uncharacterized; however, recent studies indicate impaired differentiation of preadipocytes, apoptosis of subcutaneous adipocytes, and reduced mRNA levels of key transcription factors involved in adipogenesis, such as sterol regulatory element-binding protein 1c and peroxisome-proliferator-activated receptor γ (143–145).

Grunfeld and Feingold, in their review of metabolic disturbances in HIV, described decreased triglyceride clearance attributable to decrease lipoprotein lipase activity, with a resultant marked triglyceridemia (19). Hepatic synthesis of fatty acids increases (146), and the levels of circulating free fatty acids are elevated (147). There appears to be no correlation between the alterations in triglyceride metabolism and wasting in AIDS (19, 147).

MEDIATORS OF THE HYPERCATABOLIC RESPONSE

A characteristic postinjury neuroendocrine response occurs, with an increase in catecholamines and glucocorticoids. However, despite extensive investigation of the hormonal milieu and response to injury and stress, hormone increases with normal subjects have not been able to reproduce the amount of protein catabolism seen in severe injury. This indicates that hormonal changes alone cannot account for all the metabolic consequences of severe stress and injury. Therefore, increased attention to other possible mediators of hypercatabolic stress mechanisms has largely focused on the role of immunopeptide regulation of host metabolic response to injury. These endogenous mediators of postinjury hypermetabolism, including the humoral mediators of the neuroendocrine system, the autonomic nervous systems, and the cytokines, can integrate and transfer information from the injury site to affect a response beneficial to the host. The next section focuses on the role of these mediators in the postinjury response.

Another recent hypothesis attempts to correlate the amount of protein catabolism observed in the hypermetabolic state with the cellular hydration state (148). The cell swelling theory argues that cellular volume is the key signal for the metabolic orientation of the cell metabolism: cellular swelling leads to anabolism, whereas cellular shrinkage promotes catabolism (149). A recent study of sequential changes in intracellular water, total body protein, total body potassium, and intracellular potassium in critically ill patients with blunt trauma or sepsis demonstrated that the loss of protein and potassium is accompanied by progressive cellular dehydration (150). Cellular dehydration is influenced by many factors, including altered nutrition, hormones, cytokines, and oxygen radicals. Although it proposes an interesting mechanism for the proteolysis observed in critically ill patients, this hypothesis remains to be substantiated in clinical trials.

Neuroimmunoendocrine Response

The neuroendocrine and immune systems are interrelated by sharing, in common, chemical mediators (hormones, cytokines, steroids, neuropeptides, and neurotransmitters) and their associated receptors. These shared chemical mediators and receptors in turn allow for an integrated molecular response of the neuroimmunoendocrine system to stress, inflammation, and infection. Sensory afferent and postganglionic sympathetic neurons also influence inflammation by secreting proinflammatory or antiinflammatory neuropeptides, such as substance P and somatostatin, into the site of inflammation.

Early studies by Hume and Egdahl established the importance of an intact CNS in mediating the early response to injury (151). Their original studies demonstrated that sectioning the peripheral nerve, cervical spinal cord, or medulla oblongata in dogs could block the increase in adrenocorticoid steroids after a burn injury. Other clinical studies show lower adrenocorticotropic hormone (ACTH) or growth hormone (GH) release in response to minor tissue injury (herniorrhaphy) in patients receiving spinal anesthesia than in those receiving general anesthesia (152). The CNS also appears to be instrumental in the hypermetabolic response to injury. One study demonstrated that administration of inert gas anesthesia to hypermetabolic burn patients lowered their core temperatures and metabolic rates (153). A study of patients with head injuries who were in barbiturate coma established that metabolic rate and nitrogen excretion were reduced to basal levels with administration of the barbiturate (154).

Afferent signals from the site of injury, baroreceptors sensing hypovolemia, and infection can elicit hypothalamic mechanisms to stimulate the anterior pituitary to secrete prolactin, ACTH, antidiuretic hormone, and GH (44). ACTH release stimulates an increase in adrenal glucocorticoid secretion. Evidence of increased ACTH secretion has been observed after elective operations, extensive trauma (155–157), thermal injury (158, 159), and infection (160, 161). Circulating levels of GH are markedly increased immediately after injury and tend to decrease to normal levels within 24 to 48 hours. However, in protracted critical illness the dominant profile of endocrine response is that of suppression of anterior pituitary hormone secretion. Cortisol appears unaffected and remains high; this effect is potentially mediated by endothelin (162, 163).

Thyroid-stimulating hormone levels do not appear to be greatly affected by injury. However, a characteristic pattern of normal thyroxine (T_4), elevated triiodothyronine receptor (rT_3), and depressed triiodothyronine (T_3) during prolonged periods of stress is related in part to calorie deficiency (164, 165) and to response to an inflammatory stimulus (166). In patients with this euthyroid sick syndrome, proposed mechanisms include impaired responsiveness of the thyroid to thyroid-stimulating hormone, reduced serum binding of thyroid hormones, and reduced peripheral conversion of T_4 to T_3. Glucocorticoids inhibit the enzymatic conversion of T_4 to T_3. Cytokines appear not to inhibit this glucocorticoid-mediated inhibition of the conversion of T_4 to T_3 (167).

Catecholamines

The catecholamines, specifically epinephrine and norepinephrine, are rapidly produced in response to a variety of insults. Elevated levels are most pronounced during the early postinjury period (48 hours) and decrease during recovery (168, 169). Postinjury levels of catecholamines correlate to some extent with the severity of initial injury (169). Mild injury may elicit a moderate increase in catecholamines, whereas more severe injuries may be associated with a prolonged increase in urinary or circulating levels of catecholamines (3).

The net metabolic influence of catecholamines is to increase energy expenditure, hepatic glycogenolysis, glycolysis, and lipolysis with resultant increase in free fatty acid concentration. Paradoxically, catecholamine excess acutely decreases the efflux of amino acids from peripheral tissue while increasing lactate release from skeletal muscle. This was confirmed by studies in which epinephrine infusion into healthy subjects resulted in increased energy expenditure, hyperglycemia, lactic acidosis, and decreased amino acid efflux (5, 170, 171). Although the precise effect of adrenergic stimulation on protein kinetics is controversial, studies indicate that β stimulation promotes gluconeogenesis and may limit skeletal muscle nitrogen loss, whereas α-adrenergic stimulation leads to protein catabolism (172, 173). A recent study of β-blockade in pediatric patients with severe burns demonstrated attenuation of hypermetabolism and reversal of muscle-protein catabolism. Propranolol, in this study, was thought to increase the intracellular recycling of free amino acids, resulting in reincorporation into bound protein (174). β-Blockade, however, has not been associated with improved survival and has the potential of converting intermediate-thickness burn wounds to full-thickness if hypoperfusion results. Taken together, these studies indicate appreciable catecholamine influence on extreme changes in protein metabolism seen in severe stress and injury.

Cortisol

Glucocorticoid excess promotes negative nitrogen balance (170) but shows little influence on overall energy expenditure (171). The lines of evidence indicating the role of glucocorticoids in the catabolism of muscle tissues are (a) glucocorticoids levels are increased in a number of conditions characterized by muscle atrophy; (b) in humans or experimental animals, treatment with glucocorticoids induces a catabolic response in skeletal muscle; (c) in vitro, cultured muscle cells treated with glucocorticoids show a net protein loss; (d) muscle wasting can be inhibited by adrenalectomy or by treating animals with a glucocorticoid receptor antagonist (175). Cortisol effects a slight increase in free fatty acid concentration, promotes hepatic gluconeogenesis, and increases peripheral tissue amino acid efflux. In normal subjects, cortisol infusion alone produced the same net sustained nitrogen loss as that produced by combined cortisol, epinephrine, norepinephrine, and glucagon infusion (170). In addition, short-term cortisol infusion in high physiologic concentrations in healthy subjects increased plasma amino

acid concentration, particularly the branched-chain amino acids (leucine, isoleucine, and valine) (176, 177). Glucocorticoids mediate muscle catabolic activity in part via the ubiquitin-proteasome pathway and calcium-dependent protein degradation (178). During sepsis and other catabolic conditions, glutamine use increases with increased glutamine synthetase expression and activity in skeletal muscle and lung. Overall, glutamine levels are reduced in muscle during critical illness and are proposed to be an important mechanism of stimulated muscle breakdown and inhibited protein synthesis (179, 180). Glucocorticoids appear to regulate the expression and activity of glutamine synthetase in skeletal muscle, thus possibly playing a role in glutamine-mediated muscle breakdown (181, 182).

Insulin

Insulin levels are initially decreased during the ebb phase after injury, but are mildly to markedly increase during the early flow phase. Hyperglycemia and hyperinsulinemia are characteristic of the early stress response. As stated earlier, the body becomes resistant to insulin in such tissues as adipocytes and skeletal myocytes (75, 183). The splanchnic tissues also display a relative resistance to insulin, manifested by continued hepatic gluconeogenesis despite elevated glucose levels (183, 184). Insulin resistance may be mediated in part by cortisol (76) as well as by catecholamines (75). The role of the characteristic hyperinsulinemia observed after injury remains unclear because critical organs, including the CNS, hematogenous cells, wounds, and the kidney, incorporate glucose in an insulin-independent manner. Nevertheless, continuous infusion of glucose and insulin resulted in decreased urine urea nitrogen excretion as well as decreased amino acid efflux and decreased 3-methylhistidine excretion (a marker of protein catabolism) (185); therefore, the increase in insulin may serve to decrease protein catabolism during the flow phase. Hyperglycemia and glucose intolerance have long been recognized features of various types of critical illness and injury states including burns (186, 187), myocardial infarction (188), and surgery (189). Recent studies examining the relationship between insulin, blood glucose, and clinical outcomes in critically ill patients have reported decreased infectious complications (190), improved skin grafting success in burn patients, and a reduction in morbidity and mortality in patients subjected to an intensive insulin regimen (191). These results have for the first time demontrated a clinical benefit from insulin therapy; however, the question remains whether the derived benefit is the result of the effects of lowered blood glucose, insulin action independent of lowered blood glucose, or both.

Glucagon

Circulating glucagon levels increase during the hypermetabolic postinjury phase and correlate roughly with the severity of injury (155, 192, 193). Glucagon appears to exert little independent influence on peripheral tissue metabolism (194), but is a potent stimulant of the hepatic cyclic adenosine monophosphate system, facilitating hepatic uptake of amino acids (195) and gluconeogenesis (196). Glucagon is also influenced by the autonomic nervous system (197).

Cytokines

Proinflammatory Cytokine Peptides

Proinflammatory cytokine peptides were originally studied for their effect on immunologic homeostasis in several areas, but they also exert potent activity toward regulation of hemodynamic and metabolic responses (198). During early postinjury or infectious conditions, the initial cytokine response to such insults likely mediates beneficial protective signaling of the immune system. Nevertheless, excessive acute production of some cytokines, such as TNF, may promote septic shock. Prolonged production of tissue cytokines sustains some metabolic effects of the hypercatabolic state.

Diverse cell types of both myeloid and nonmyeloid origin produce the proinflammatory cytokine peptides. These proteins may function by autocrine (acting on the same cell), paracrine (acting on cells in the immediate area), or systemic mechanisms of action. They produce local tissue responses by cell-to-cell interaction at very low concentrations, but also may exert systemic effects in higher concentrations. Although many cytokines are now well characterized, those showing the more prominent proinflammatory activities, including TNF-α, IL-1, IL-6, and interferon-γ (IFN-γ), have been more widely studied from a metabolic perspective (Table 89.2).

Tumor Nectrosis Factor

TNF is a 17-kDa protein primarily secreted from monocytes and macrophages. Although originally isolated as a soluble factor that produced cachexia during infection and (as implied by the name) in vivo necrosis of some solid tumors (199), this cytokine has been implicated as the initiating signal for a variety of cellular and metabolic events seen in critically ill patients. TNF administration to healthy subjects elicits a systemic response resembling that observed during septicemia (200), including increased stress hormone release, temperature elevation, and increased acute-phase protein synthesis (201). The systemic effects of bacterial liposaccharide (endotoxin) are replicated, if not largely mediated, by TNF (201). Indeed endotoxin infusion induces a rapid increase in circulating TNF levels, and blocking TNF with antibodies in animal models alleviates many of the toxic effects of endotoxin (202, 203). TNF may circulate predominately as a complex with its soluble receptors, making detection of the bioactive ligand more difficult. Increased levels of these soluble TNF receptors are seen in response to diverse inflammatory stimuli, including sepsis, cancer, and AIDS (77). Nevertheless, elevated TNF levels are detected in many disease states, including bacterial infection, infected thermal injury, tumor-bearing states, sepsis, and AIDS (74, 204). The metabolic effects of TNF and perhaps also the other proinflammatory cytokines seem to promote redistribution of body protein and lipid stores (200). The result is a net loss of peripheral tissue protein with a concomitant increase in hepatic uptake. Alterations in fat metabolism elicited by TNF resemble the changes seen in infection. They include promotion of cellular lipolysis and hepatic lipogenesis with decreased free fatty acid synthesis and decreased clearance of extracellular lipids (202, 205–207). Increased TNF-α levels have been demonstrated in obesity-induced insulin resistance, a finding suggesting a role for TNF-α in mediating insulin resistance. Soluble TNF receptors have also been demonstrated to neutralize unbound TNF and inhibit the development of TNF-α-induced insulin resistance and adipogenesis (208).

Interleukin-1

IL-1 is produced by macrophages/monocytes, neutrophils, lymphocytes, and keratinocytes (198). Its production is

TABLE 89.2. MAJOR CYTOKINES INVOLVED IN HYPERMETABOLIC RESPONSE

CYTOKINE	CELL SOURCE	METABOLIC EFFECTS
Tumor necrosis factor-α	Monocytes/macrophages, lymphocytes, Kupffer cells, glial cells, endothelial cells, natural killer cells, mast cells	Decrease free fatty acid synthesis Increased lipolysis Increased peripheral amino acid loss Increased hepatic amino acid uptake Fever
Interleukin-1	Monocytes/macrophages, neutrophils, lymphocytes, keratinocytes, Kupffer cells	Increased adrenocorticotropic hormone Increased hepatic acute-phase protein synthesis Fever
Interleukin-6	Monocytes/macrophages, keratinocytes, endothelial cells, fibroblasts, T cells, epithelial cells	Increased acute-phase protein synthesis Fever
Interferon-γ	Lymphocytes, pulmonary macrophages	Increased monocyte respiratory burst

From Matarese G, La Cava A. The intricate interface between immune system and metabolism. Trends Immunol 2004;25:195–6, with permission.

stimulated by TNF and endotoxin, and like TNF, it may represent an early cytokine response to injury. Once released, it exerts multiple immunologic and metabolic effects, including stimulation of ACTH (209), induction of fever, hepatic acute-phase protein synthesis, and alteration of energy metabolism (198). IL-1 also induces anorexia and inhibition of fatty acid synthesis and adipocyte differentiation (210, 211). Like TNF activity, IL-1 activity is regulated by shedding of soluble receptors, as well as by unique, naturally occurring receptor antagonist (IL-1ra) (212). IL-1ra binds to the IL-1 receptor without an agonist influence. IL-1ra-deficient mice exhibit growth retardation, resistance to high-fat-diet-induced obesity, and reduced activity of lipoprotein lipase, and have low insulin levels (211). In humans, IL-1ra is upregulated in serum of obese persons and correlates with insulin resistance (213).

Interleukin-6

IL-6 is the most frequently detected cytokine in patients with acute infection (214), injury, and tumor-bearing states (215) and after elective surgical procedures (216). The biologic actions of this protein include regulation of acute-phase protein synthesis after injury (217, 218) and differentiation of lymphocytes (219). It also induces fever via prostaglandin production (220). In one study, administration of IL-6 to humans induced modest changes in the kinetics of glucose and protein (221). IL-6 is produced in large part by adipose tissue, and circulating levels correlate with body mass index, insulin sensitivity, and glucose tolerance.

Interferon-γ

IFN-γ is secreted from lymphocytes and macrophages and exerts antiviral effects as well as protection against bacteria, fungi, and parasites. It enhances TNF production in response to endotoxin (222) and increases the cytotoxicity of monocytes, possibly by increasing their respiratory burst activity (223). A direct role for IFN-γ in directing altered metabolic processes has not been defined in humans, although its administration does induce cachexia and loss of protein and lipid stores in animals (224).

Antiinflammatory Cytokines

Regulation of the various cytokines produced in response to injury or disease is complex and involves counterregulation by antiinflammatory cytokines such as IL-10, which downregulates secretion of proinflammatory cytokines (i.e., TNF and IL-1) as well as suppressing macrophage and T-cell functions. Counterregulatory mechanisms likely are important in maintaining a counterbalance to unopposed systemic inflammation and hypercatabolism and may play a role in restoration of metabolic homeostasis and anabolism.

Neuroendocrine Response and Cytokines

The response to injury, infection, and ischemia/reperfusion is associated with concurrent activation of the hypothalamic-pituitary-adrenal axis (HPA). Recent work suggests that organ systems express and respond to a large number of common regulatory and counterregulatory molecules, such as cytokines, neuropeptides, neurotransmitters, and steroids, which provide an integrated and bidirectional molecular response to stressors. The end result is an integration of the nervous, endocrine, and immune systems to these perturbations (225–228). Cytokines, including IL-1, IL-6, TNF, and leukemia inhibitory factor, appear to mediate the complex HPA axis response to stress or inflammation (229). Cytokines may function like classic endocrine secretagogues acting locally or may impact a distant target (230). During stress, cytokines stimulate pituitary corticotroph propiomelanocortin (POMC) gene expression and ACTH secretion in the hypothalamus and pituitary (228–231). The gp130 cytokine family, consisting of leukemia inhibitory factor, IL-6, IL-11, ciliary neurotrophic factor, and oncostatin M, participates in ACTH regulation and mediates the immunoneuroendocrine interface (232, 233). Through intracellular signaling systems such as cyclic adenosine monophosphate and the JAK/STAT/SOCS pathway and in synergy with POMC inducers and corticotropin-releasing hormone, cytokines mediate cell proliferation, mature ACTH secretion, and impart negative feedback to the HPA axis (225).

Glucocorticoid secretion, mediated by ACTH and indirectly through cytokines, is a potent antiinflammatory mechanism. The α-glucocorticoid receptor binds the steroid hormone, translocates to the nucleus, and binds to the glucocorticoid-responsive elements (234). Some glucocorticoid-responsive elements downregulate the transcription of other genes (e.g., most cytokines) and prevent transcription initiated by transcriptional factors such as nuclear factor-κB (235). Glucocorticoids can inhibit production of TNF or IL-6 (218, 236, 237), and in the case of TNF, the mechanism appears to include altering transcription of the mRNA (238). Cortisol infusion attenuates the endogenous TNF response to endotoxin administration (218, 219). Catecholamine infusion also inhibits endotoxin-induced TNF production while simultaneously increasing release of IL-10 (239). Proinflammatory cytokines such as TNF and IL-1 initiate a cascade of inflammatory responses by activating nuclear factor-κB, which, in turn, stimulates proinflammatory genes. Glucocorticoids bound to glucocorticoid receptor interact with nuclear factor-κB in the nucleus and alter its ability to promote transcription of cytokine-responsive genes (240). These two opposing regulatory systems are coupled to maintain the homeostatic balance of the inflammatory response. Glucocorticoids, in turn, antagonize the actions of growth hormone and the sex steroids on adipose tissue (lipolysis) and muscle/bone anabolism (241). Chronic activation of the system would lead to a decrease in lean body mass through the loss of muscle and bone and suppression of osteoblastic activity (235).

Hence, the neuroimmunoendocrine milieu elicited by injury, infection, or other hypermetabolic conditions may serve to alter cytokine mediator activities in a complex manner. It remains to be determined to what extent these parallel signaling pathways direct the human metabolic response.

SYSTEMIC AND ORGAN REACTIONS

Gastrointestinal Tract

The gastrointestinal tract provides important nutrient absorptive and metabolic functions and recently has emerged as an immunologically important organ. Since the late 1960s, parenteral nutritional provided a lifesaving therapy to patients with hypercatabolic disorders (242). Total parenteral nutrition administration provides fluids, macronutrients, and micronutrients in sufficient quantity to meet nutritional needs and prevents progressive starvation-induced malnutrition, and in turn changed the outcome of patients who would have otherwise died (243). However, subsequent studies have demonstrated that enteral processing of nutrients affects the metabolic response to septic insults and improved host defenses. In a study of randomized severely burned children receiving a standard enteral or a protein-supplemented diet, those receiving high-protein diets had fewer septic complications and a lower mortality (244). In vitro evidence also demonrated that in a rat model of *Escherichia coli* peritonitis, enteral support lowered mortality (245). More recent studies have focused on intestinal permeability after injury and translocation of intraluminal bacteria to mesenteric lymph nodes and to the systemic circulation (246–248). These studies suggest that maintenance of intestinal barrier function is required to reduce permeability to intraluminal organisms. Total parenteral nutrition and bowel rest, on the other hand, are associated with an exaggerated response to injury (249). The gut mucosa normally provides a barrier to foreign material such as bacteria, their products, and other ingested particles. Enteral feeding is essential to maintain the integrity of the mucosal barrier (250, 251). In animal studies, bowel rest and parenteral nutrition produce increased translocation of bacteria to intestinal lymphoid tissue (252). Whether bacterial translocation is an important source of systemic bacteremia and sepsis during disease states in humans is a matter of debate; however, it may be that stimulation of splanchnic immune cells by foreign antigens that have crossed the mucosal barrier influences systemic immunologic and metabolic processes during disease states. Cytokines secreted by splanchnic cells or lymphocytes or macrophages influence both the immune and the hemodynamic responses to injury as well as the metabolic response (253, 254). In this way, the intestine may partially regulate the immune response to injury or disease.

Cachexia

The primary manifestation of the metabolic derangements associated with cancer is the syndrome of cachexia. Cancer cachexia is a profound change in metabolic processes principally characterized by muscle loss and alterations in fat and carbohydrate metabolism as a direct result of tumor mediators or indirectly by the host response to the tumor itself. Clinically, cachexia is variably associated with degrees of anorexia, changes in taste perception, early satiety, pain, oral and gastrointestinal dysfunction, psychologic factors, weakness, and weight loss (255). In a retrospective case control study of patients with cachexia, the degree of wasting was found to be an important prognostic factor, with progressive weight loss correlating with mortality (256). Various metabolic changes in nutrient processing have been documented in cachexia to include relative glucose intolerance, insulin resistance with increased rates of glucose production, and recycling via lactate. Lipogenesis appears altered in cancer cachexia, but lipolysis rates are not significantly increased (257, 258). Other metabolic changes include decreased concentration or responsiveness to thyroid hormone, growth hormone, and testosterone; increased cachexia-related presence or activity of glucagon, cortisol, proinflammatory cytokines, and eicosanoids, and a proteolysis-inducing glycoprotein of tumor origin have also been demonstrated. Cachexia is also found in other disease states such as advanced cardiopulmonary disease, rheumatoid arthritis, and chronic infection.

In terms of individual cytokines, TNF, IL-1, IL-6, interferon-γ, and ciliary neurotrophic factor have been implicated in cachexia. Although difficult to detect in the blood of patients with cancer, TNF appears to lead to anorexia, weight loss, an acute-phase protein response, protein and fat breakdown, increased levels of cortisol and glucagon, reduced insulin levels, insulin resistance, anemia, fever, and elevated energy expenditure in animals (259–261) and humans (262–265). TNF has been demonstrated to be elevated in peripheral blood monocytes from patients with advanced pancreatic cancer (266). In contradistinction, it is rare to detect elevated TNF levels in patients with cancer, antibodies to TNF in animal models of cachexia do not appear to affect weight loss (267), and the pattern of weight loss seen in cancer cachexia appears to differ from the weight loss seen in experimental animals given TNF (268).

IL-6 administration produces weight loss in human subjects and is produced by some cancer cell lines (269, 270). IL-6 levels are elevated in some patients with cancer cachexia (271, 272); antibodies to IL-6 suppress the development of cachexia to some degree in animal models (273). In patients with AIDS-related lymphoma, administration of IL-6 produced weight gain and stabilized levels of the acute-phase reactant C-reactive protein (274). Despite similar IL-6 levels, experimental tumor clones produce different patterns of weight loss, a finding suggesting that IL-6 alone cannot fully explain tumor cachexia (275). Ciliary neurotrophic factor, a member of the IL-6 superfamily, produces weight loss, protein degradation, fever, and an acute-phase protein response in animals (276, 277).

Various animal experiments examining the role of IFN-γ have demonstrated greater cachexia in mice injected with TNF-α CHO (Chinese hamster ovary)–stable transfectants as compared with native tumor alone and attenuation of the IFN response with antibodies to IFN in animal cachexia models (278, 279). Tumor-derived proteolysis-inducing factor is glycoprotein of tumor origin that consists of a short polypeptide chain that is highly glycosylated. This factor was originally described in tumor-bearing mice with MAC-16 (mouse adenocarcinoma colon-16) adenocarcinoma. Purified factor, when given to animals or applied to muscle cells in vivo, induces an intense protein catabolism (280–282). A similar tumor-derived proteolytic factor has been described in a broad spectrum of human malignancies to include pancreatic, breast, lung, ovary, melanoma, and the gastrointestinal tract. The presence of the factor is typically found in patients with active weight loss. Further studies will demonstrate the contributing role of tumor-derived proteolysis-inducing factor in mediating cancer cachexia.

Ubiquitin-proteosome proteolytic system (UPPS), in addition to the lysosomal and mitochondrial proteolysis systems, appears to be a significant contributor to muscle loss in cachexia. UPPS may be expressed in a subset of patients who develop cancer cachexia as the dominant mechanism of muscle loss. Most cytosolic and nuclear proteins are long-lived and are hydrolyzed by the ubiquitin-proteasome system. Protein hydrolysis by UPPS is generally characterized by a multienzymatic process driven by ATP. Several features of the UPPS pathway allow for tight regulation and avoidance of nonspecific protein degradation, isolation of the proteolytic sites within the proteosome, allowing only unfolded proteins passage into the proteasome, and the need for ATP hydrolysis all serve as regulatory points in the process of protein degradation and minimize nonspecific protein degradation that could disturb the tight balance of protein degradation and formation within the cell. In cancer cachexia, animal and human studies indicate a role for the UPPS in mediating loss of muscle mass. However, muscle proteolysis appears to be mediated only in part by the UPPS system. Injection of hepatoma cells into the peritoneal cavity of rats induced weight and muscle mass to fall below levels of controls even though tumor accounted for less than 3% of body weight. The muscle loss was thought to be the result of activation of ATP-dependant proteolysis. Increased levels of ubiquitin-conjugated proteins and associated mRNAs for ubiquitin and proteasome subunits were detected in

muscle (283). Bossola and colleagues reported increased ubiquitin mRNA levels in muscle biopsies of patients with gastric cancer (284). Further studies are needed to determine the role of the ubiquitin-proteasome proteolytic pathway in mediating cancer cachexia, including the identification of signaling events that regulate activity, the role of intracellular signaling systems, and the interaction with immune mediators and cells.

Various mediators are involved in the abnormal metabolism seen in cancer cachexia, and it has become increasingly apparent that individual mediators do not work alone in vivo and that a complex network of cytokines in combination with other factors are involved in the pathogenesis of cachexia.

GENERAL NUTRITION AND ANABOLIC SUPPORT

Macronutrients

Treatment of patients who are hypermetabolic for extended periods should in all likelihood include nutrient supplementation. Nutritional management of stress patients is reviewed in Chapter 91 and is only briefly mentioned here.

The fundamental objectives of nutrition support of the hypermetabolic patient are to provide sufficient nonprotein energy sources and sufficient protein substrate to alleviate or at least minimize catabolism of endogenous energy and protein sources. Enteral and parenteral nutrition support in depleted patients often demonstrably improve nitrogen balance during the catabolic phase of injury (285). Enteral nutrient provision is clearly the preferred route of feeding in the presence of a functional intestinal tract. Recent studies indicate some possible benefit to enteral feedings in selected patient populations (286–288).

There is also evidence to suggest that some nutrients may become conditionally essential during catabolic illness. Among these is the amino acid glutamine (see Chapter 35), which is a major component of the tissue free amino acid pool and appears to be rapidly depleted in periods of stress. It is also essential for nucleotide and glutathione synthesis, as well as for gluconeogenesis. Other studies suggest that other amino acids, such as arginine, may also be limiting to the maintenance of lymphocyte function and wound healing (289, 290).

Anabolic Therapy

Although nutritional supplementation may improve body nitrogen and calorie balance during hypermetabolic states, progressive depletion of structure protein still continues. Consequently, additional means of adjuvant anabolic therapy, such as insulin, IGF-I, anabolic steroids, or GH, have been investigated in an effort to decrease muscle protein loss in hypermetabolic patients. Administration of GH or IGF-I increases skeletal muscle amino acid uptake and muscle mRNA synthesis during full nutritional support (291, 292).

IGF-I infusion in healthy humans also increases peripheral glucose disposal, reduces lipolysis, and decreases total branched-chain amino acid levels, a finding suggesting a protein anabolic effect (293, 294). Insulin administration also reduces protein loss in burn and trauma patients, resulting in decreased urinary urea excretion and reduced protein breakdown rates (295, 296). Studies using a combination of GH and insulin in patients with cancer indicate that this combination of therapy may lead to whole-body nitrogen retention and skeletal muscle sparing (297). GH affects nitrogen balance positively by exerting an anabolic effect on proteins (298). In clinical trials, the effect of GH also seems to depend on the severity of injury. In patients under mild to moderate stress, GH does promote improved nitrogen balance with an anabolic effect on protein synthesis. However, severely stressed patients (those losing >1.5 g/kg/day protein), exogenous GH is not demonstrably effective as an anabolic agent (299). Although most studies show anabolic effects of GH treatment of patients with mild to moderate catabolism, improved clinical outcome has been difficult to document in most hypermetabolic patient populations. A study of ventilator-dependent critically ill patients does suggest that prolonged GH treatment may promote pulmonary function in this group (300). In contradistinction, a study of high-dose recombinant human growth hormone in critically ill patients (cardiac surgery, abdominal surgery, multiple trauma, or acute respiratory failure) demonstrated an increase in mortality, hospital and intensive care unit length of stay, and duration of mechanical ventilation as compared with controls (301). The increased morbidity and mortality demontrated in this study secondary to multiple organ failure, septic shock, and uncontrolled infection could be the result of the effects of human growth hormone on the immune system (277). Further studies are needed to characterize the effects of human growth hormone on immune function.

Severe burn injury is characterized by marked catabolism with impaired wound healing and impaired musculoskeletal function. Human growth hormone administration in severe burn injury has been demonstrated to decrease postburn catabolism, maintain body mass, and increase the rate of burn wound healing (302–304). Human growth hormone administration, however, may exacerbate insulin resistance and result in significant hyperglycemia. Oxandrolone, a testosterone analog, has been used in burn patients to restore lean body mass in the postburn recovery period (305).

Micronutrients

The major intracellular elements, potassium, magnesium, and phosphate, follow patterns of nitrogen loss in response to acute infection (306). The liver sequesters zinc as well as iron, with a decrease in circulating plasma levels. This may represent a host survival mechanism during infection

by making zinc and iron unavailable to the replicating bacteria. Increases in serum iron concentration during infection may impair the host resistance to infection. Zinc is essential for wound healing; thus, adequate levels must be maintained in the stressed individual to ensure healing. Ceruloplasmin synthesis is increased by the liver concomitant increase in copper levels. Catabolic destruction or urinary loss of many vitamins, most notably vitamin A occurs, and this may contribute to morbidity and mortality in some infections. Vitamins and trace elements should be components of all parenteral and enteral formulas (see Chapters 98 and 99). Levels of these additives should be monitored periodically during long-term parenteral administration (307).

NUTRITIONAL SUPPORT IN ORGAN FAILURE

The hypermetabolic patient who has a response to therapeutic interventions will proceed to an anabolic stage of recovery, and eventually to positive nitrogen balance. However, some patients continue to be hypermetabolic and may develop multiorgan system failure. The pathogenesis of organ system failure remains to be completely clarified, but it is multifactorial. With the onset of multiorgan system failure, nutritional requirements may be modified.

Lung

Respiratory insufficiency may be the end result of protein-energy malnutrition, leading to a decrease in muscle mass of respiratory muscles as well as disturbances in respiratory drive (308) (see also Chapter 93). The net result is increased CO_2 retention and difficulty in oxygenation. This process may be exacerbated by vasoactive factors released during infection that increase pulmonary vascular permeability with an ensuing ventilatory mismatch. It is hypothesized that increased CO_2 production from the carbohydrate provided in supplemental nutrition increases CO_2 retention. Therefore an increased proportion of calories from lipid might be used in these patients.

Kidney

The etiology of acute renal failure in the injured or septic patient is multifactorial and can include shock, nephrotoxic drugs, glomerulonephritis, and urinary tract obstruction (see also Chapter 94). The multiple metabolic consequences of renal failure include fluid and electrolyte abnormalities as well as alterations in protein, carbohydrate, lipid, trace element, and vitamin metabolism (309), with decreased clearance of phosphate, potassium, and magnesium and elevated concentrations as the result of impaired glomerular filtration. Acidosis develops from decreased excretion of acid and increased tissue catabolism. Uremia ensues because of increased protein breakdown and decreased urea clearance. When renal tubular disorder is present (e.g., as the result of nephrotoxic drugs), renal loss of minerals may occur. Dialysis is initiated to minimize these metabolic disturbances. Traditionally, patients with acute renal failure have been treated with low-protein nutritional support to decrease urea production. However, there are no data to indicate that a low-protein diet intake can decrease loss of renal function or improve recovery of renal function in acute renal failure (286). Therefore, protein should not be restricted; nutritive sufficient amounts should be given, with increased metabolites and waste products treated with appropriate dialysis. The protein requirements in dialysis patients are higher than normal because of increased catabolism in these patients and loss of nutrients in the dialysate (286). Data suggest that hypercatabolic patients with acute renal failure require 1.25 to 1.5 g/kg/day of protein, with higher requirements for patients receiving dialysis. Close regulation of magnesium, potassium, and phosphate is also necessary in patients with renal failure.

Liver

Hepatic dysfunction in the critically ill patient ranges from mild abnormalities in liver function to fulminant liver failure with severe jaundice and wasting. Nutritional requirements in such patients depend on the primary disease process underlying the liver dysfunction (see also Chapter 79). Infectious processes that affect the liver itself, such as hepatitis, localized abscesses, and pylephlebitis, may result in liver dysfunction. Altered amino acid metabolism is a key feature of liver disease with low levels of circulating branched chain amino acids (leucine, isoleucine, and valine) and elevated levels of circulating aromatic amino acids (phenylalanine, tyrosine, tryptophan, and methionine). In the presence of acute encephalopathy, the protein load should be decreased, and parenterally administered amino acids are generally better tolerated than those administered enterally (310). Some have advocated use of solutions high in branched-chain amino acids, with no aromatic amino acids, but the benefit of such solutions is controversial (182). Zinc deficiency may be supplemented empirically as there is evidence suggesting supplementation with improved amino acid metabolism and clinical grade of encephalopathy (311).

Occasionally, hypoglycemia may occur in end-stage liver failure. More often, minor elevations in liver function tests occur during the course of intravenous feeding. This generally resolves after cessation of parenteral feeding and, in the absence of drastically altered liver function or associated inflammatory processes, is of minimal consequence to the acute recovery process.

Heart

The goals of nutrition in patients with chronic congestive heart failure include reduction of cardiac workload, maintenance of dry weight, and achieving optimal nutritional status within the constraints of limited fluid volume and restricted sodium intake (see Chapter 69). Close monitoring of sodium and fluid status with avoidance of sodium depletion is especially important in elderly patients on strict sodium diets.

REFERENCES

1. Cuthbertson D. Br Med Bull 1945;3:96–102.
2. Moore F. Metabolic Care of the Surgical Patient. Philadelphia: WB Saunders, 1959.
3. Lowry SF. Host metabolic response to injury. In: Gallin JI, Fauci AS, eds. Advances in Host Defense Mechanisms, vol 6. New York: Raven Press, 1986:169–90.
4. Duke JH, Jorgensen SB, Broell JR et al. Surgery 1970;68:168–74.
5. Wilmore D, Long JM, Mason AD et al. Ann Surg 1974;180:653–69.
6. Bozzetti F, Pagnoni A, Del Vecchio M. Surg Gynecol Obstet 1980;150:229–34.
7. Fearon KCH, Hansell DT, Preston T et al. Cancer Res 1988;48:2590–5.
8. Knox CS, Crosby LO, Feuer IB et al. Ann Surg 1983;197:152–62.
9. Knox L, Crosby LO, Feurer ID et al. Clin Res 1980;38:620A(abst).
10. Fredrix EW, Soeters PB, Wouters EFM et al. Cancer Res 1991;51:6138–41.
11. Fredrix EW, Wouters EFM, Soeters PB et al. Cancer 1991;68:1612–21.
12. Dempsey DT, Feurer ID, Knox LS et al. Cancer 1984;53:1265–73.
13. Falconer JS, Fearon KCH, Plester CE et al. Ann Surg 1994;219:325–31.
14. Drott C, Persson H, Lundholm K et al. Clin Physiol 1989;9:427–39.
15. Hyltander A, Kornell U, Lundholm K et al. Eur J Clin Invest 1993;23:46–52
16. Hommes MJ, Romijn JA, Godfried MH et al. Metabolism 1990;39:1186–90.
17. Melchior JC, Salmon D, Rigaud D et al. Am J Clin Nutr 1991;53:437–41.
18. Melchior JC, Raguin G, Rigaud D et al. Abstracts of the Seventh International Conference on AIDS. Florence, Italy, June 16–21, 1991;1:293(abst).
19. Grunfeld C, Feingold KR. N Engl J Med 1992;327:329–37.
20. Hommes MJT, Romijn JA, Endert E et al. Am J Clin Nutr 1991;54:311–5.
21. Centers for Disease Control. MMWR Morb Mortal Wkly Rep 1987;36[Suppl 1]:1S–15S.
22. Suttmann U, Ockenga J, Hoogestraat L et al. Metabolism 1993;42:1173–9.
23. Lowry SF. Nutritional support of the trauma patient. In: Shires GT, ed. Principles of Trauma Care, vol 3. New York: McGraw-Hill, 1985:592–608.
24. Hasselgren PO, James JH, Benson DW et al. Metab Clin Exp 1989;38:634–40.
25. Hummel RP, Hasselgren PO, James JH et al. Metab Clin Exp 1988;37:1120–7.
26. Hasselgren PO, James JH, Fischer JE. Ann Surg 1986;203:360–5.
27. Zamir O, Hasselgren PO, Higashiguchi T et al. Mediat Inflam 1992;1:247–50.
28. Nagaraju K. Acta Physiol Scand 2001;171:215–23.
29. Curfs JH, Meis JF, Hoogkamp-Korstanje JA. Clin Microbiol Rev 1997;10:742–80.

30. Cannon JC. J Gerontol A Biol Sci Med Sci 1995;50A:120–3.
31. Nagaraju K, Ruben N, Merritt G et al. Clin Exp Immunol 1998;113:407–14.
32. Hill AG. World J Surg 2000;24:624–9.
33. Tiao G, Fagan JM, Samuels N et al. J Clin Invest 1994;94: 2255–64.
34. Hersko A, Ciechanover A. Annu Rev Biochem 1992;61:761–807.
35. Mitch WE, Goldberg AL. N Engl J Med 1996;335:1897–905.
36. Price SR. Int J Biochem Cell Biol 2003;35:617–28.
37. Solomon V, Baracos V, Sarraf P et al. Proc Natl Acad Sci USA 1998;13:12602–7.
38. Price SR, England BK, Bailey JL et al. Am J Physiol 1994:267: C955–60.
39. Chai J, Wu Y, Sheng Z. Crit Care Med 2003;31:1802–7.
40. Lecker SH, Solomon V, Mitch WE et al. J Nutr 1999;129: 227S–37S.
41. Du J, Wang X, Miereles C et al. J Clin Invest 2004;113:115–23.
42. Wilmore DW, Goodwin CW, Aulick LH et al. Ann Surg 1980; 192:491–504.
43. Souba WW, Wilmore DW. Surgery 1983;94:342–50.
44. Bessey PQ. Metabolic response to critical illness. In: Wilmore DS, ed. Care of the Surgical Patient. New York: Scientific American, 1994:3–31.
45. Shou J. Glutamine. In: Zaloga GP, ed. Nutrition in Critical Care. Philadelphia: Mosby, 1994:123–41.
46. Muhlbacher F, Kapadia CR, Colpoys MF et al. Am J Physiol 1974;247:E75–E83.
47. Planas M, Schwartz S, Arbos MA et al. JPEN J Parenter Enteral Nutr 1993;17:299–300.
48. Oudemans-Van Straaten HM, Bosman RJ, Trekes M et al. Intensive Care Med 2001;27:84–90.
49. Ogle CK, Ogle JD, Mao JX et al. JPEN J Parenter Enteral Nutr 1994;18:128–33.
50. Hammarqvist F, Wernerman J, Ali R et al. Ann Surg 1989; 209:455–66.
51. Amores-Sanchez M, Medina M. Mol Genet Metab 1999;67: 100–5.
52. Novak F, Heyland DK, Avenell A et al. Crit Care Med 2002; 30:2022–9.
53. Kinney JM, Elwyn DH. Annu Rev Nutr 1983;3:433–66.
54. Wannemacher RW Jr, Pekarek RS, Thompson WL et al. Endocrinology 1975;96:651–61.
55. Carmichael MJ, Clague MD, Kier MJ et al. Br J Surg 1980; 67:736–9.
56. Eden E, Ekman L, Lindmark L et al. Metabolism 1984;33: 1020–7.
57. Heber D, Chlebowski RT, Ishibashi DE et al. Cancer Res 1982; 42:4815–9.
58. Dworzak F, Ferrari P, Gavazzi C et al. Cancer 1998;82:42–8.
59. Shaw JHF, Humberstone DA, Douglas RG et al. Surgery 1991; 109:37–50.
60. Stein TP, Nutinsky C, Condoluci D et al. Metabolism 1990; 39:876–81.
61. Kotler DP, Wang J, Pierson RN. Am J Clin Nutr 1985;42: 1255–65.
62. Kotler DP, Tierney AR, Wang J et al. Am J Clin Nutr 1989; 50:444–7.
63. Oliver CJ, Rose A, Blagojevic N et al. Total body protein status of males infected with the human immunodeficiency virus. In: Ellis KJ, Eastman JD, eds. Human Body Composition: In Vivo Methods, Models, and Assessment. New York: Plenum Press, 1993:197–200.
64. Melchior JC, Salmon D, Rigaud D et al. Am J Clin Nutr 1991; 53:437–41.

65. Grunfeld C, Pang M, Doerrler W et al. J Clin Endocrinol Metab 1992;74:1045–52.
66. Hellerstein MC, Grunfeld C, Wu K et al. J Clin Endocrinol Metab 1993;76:559–65.
67. Selberg O, Suttman U, Melzer A et al. Metabolism 1995; 44:1159–65.
68. Yarasheski KE, Zachwieja JJ, Gischler J et al. Am J Physiol 1998;275:E577–83.
69. Yaresheski KE, Zachwieja JJ, Gischler J et al. Am J Physiol 1998;275:E577–83.
70. Macallan DC, McNurlan MA, Milne E et al. Am J Clin Nutr 1995;61:818–26.
71. Abrams EJ, Matheson PB, Thomas PA et al. Pediatrics 1995; 96:451–8.
72. Tovo PA, de Martino M, Gabiano C et al. Lancet 1992;339: 1249–53.
73. Jahoor F, Abramson S, Heird WC. Am J Clin Nutr 2003; 78:182–9.
74. Fong Y, Lowry SF. Metabolic consequences of critical illness. In: Barie PS, Shires GT, eds. Surgical Intensive Care, vol 1. Boston: Little, Brown, 1993:893–905.
75. Deibert DC, DeFronzo RA. J Clin Invest 1980;65:717–21.
76. Diethelm AG. Ann Surg 1977;185:251–63.
77. Tracey KJ, Cerami A. Annu Rev Cell Biol 1993;9:317–43.
78. Nelson KM, Long CL, Bailey R et al. Metabolism 1992;41: 68–75.
79. Shaw JHF, Januskiewicz J, Horsborough R. Circ Shock 1985; 16:77–8.
80. Long CL, Nelson KM, Geiger JW et al. J Trauma 1996; 40:335–41.
81. Wolfe RR, Herndon DN, Jahoor F et al. Am J Physiol 1977; 232:415–8.
82. Wolfe RR, Herndon DN, Jahoor F et al. N Engl J Med 1987; 317:403–8.
83. Warren RS, Starnes HF, Gabrilove JL et al. Arch Surg 1987; 122:1396–400.
84. Bearn AG, Billing B, Sherlock S. J Physiol London 1951; 115:430.
85. Shaw JHF, Wolfe RR. Ann Surg 1989;209:63–72.
86. Wolfe RR, Martini WZ. World J Surg 2000;24:639–47.
87. Clowes GHA, O'Donnell TF, Blackburn GF et al. Surg Clin North Am 1976;56:1169–84.
88. Wolfe RR, O'Donnell TF Jr, Stone MD et al. Metabolism 1980; 29:892–900.
89. Burke JF, Wolfe RR, Mullany CJ et al. Ann Surg 1979;190: 274–85.
90. Vary TC, Siegal JH, Wakatani T et al. Am J Physiol 1986; 13:634–40.
91. Rohdenberg GL, Bernhard A, Krehbiel O. JAMA 1919;72: 1528–9.
92. Holroyde CP, Skutches CL, Boden G et al. Cancer Res 1984; 44:5910–3.
93. Humberstone DA, Shaw JHF. Cancer 1988;207:283–9.
94. Lundholm K, Edstrom S, Karlberg I et al. Cancer 1982;50: 1142–50.
95. Lawson DH, Richmond A, Nixon DW et al. Annu Rev Nutr 1982;2:277–301.
96. Douglas RG, Shaw JHF. Br J Surg 1990;77:246–54.
97. Eden E, Edstrom S, Bennegard K et al. Cancer Res 1984;44: 1717–24.
98. Cheblowski RT, Heber D. Surg Clin North Am 1986;66: 957–68.
99. Holroyde CP, Gabuzda TG, Putnam RC et al. Cancer Res 1975; 35:3710–4.

100. Waterhouse C. Cancer 1974;33:66–71.
101. Shaw JHF, Humberstone DM, Wolfe RR. Ann Surg 1988;207: 283–9.
102. Shaw JHF, Wolfe RR. Surgery 1987;101:181–91.
103. Kokal WA, McCullough A, Wright PO et al. Ann Surg 1983; 198:146–50.
104. Holyrode CP, Reichard GA. Cancer Treat Rep 1981;65 [Suppl]:55–9.
105. Warburg O. The Metabolism of Tumours. New York: Richard F Smith, 1930.
106. Burt ME, Brennan MF. Semin Oncol 1984;11:127–35.
107. Warburg O. Science 1956;123:309–14.
108. Yonekura Y, Benua RS, Brill AB et al. J Nucl Med 1982;23: 1133–7.
109. Zu XL, Guppy M. Biochem Biophys Res Commun 2004;313: 459–65.
110. Holyrode CP, Meyers RN, Smirk RD et al. Cancer Res 1977; 37:3109–14.
111. Hansell DT, Davies JWL, Burns HJG. Ann Surg 1986;203: 240–5.
112. Vendrell J, Nubiola A, Goday A et al. Lancet 1987;2:1212.
113. Hadigan C, Meigs JB, Corcoran C et al. Clin Infect Dis 2001; 32:130–9.
114. Carr A, Samaras K, Burton S et al. AIDS 1998;12:F51–8.
115. Vigoroux C, Charakhanian S, Salhi Y et al. Diabetes Metab 1999;25:225–32.
116. Hadigan C, Meigs JB, Corcoran C et al. Clin Infect Dis 2001; 32:130–9.
117. Carr A, Samaras K, Burton S et al. AIDS 1998;12:F51–8.
118. Andersen O, Haugaard SB, Andersen UB et al. Metabolism 2003;52:1343–53.
119. Carr A, Samaras K, Thorisdottir A et al. Lancet 1999;353: 2093–9.
120. Murata H, Hruz PW, Mueckler M. J Biol Chem 2000;275: 20251–4.
121. Wolfe RR, Bagby GJ. Lipid metabolism in shock. In: Altura BM, Lefer AM, Schumer W et al, eds. Handbook of Shock and Trauma. New York: Raven, 1983:199–219.
122. Bornstein SR, Uhlmann K, Haidan A et al. Diabetes 1997;46: 1235–8.
123. Aygen B, Inan M, Doganay M et al. Exp Clin Endcrinol Diabetes 1997;105:182–6.
124. Bornstein SR, Licinio J, Tauchnitz R et al. J Clin Endocrinol Metab 1998;83:3063–70.
125. Carlson GL, Saeed M, Little RA et al. Am J Physiol 1999; 276:E658–62.
126. Askanazi J, Carpentier YA, Elwyn DH et al. Ann Surg 1980; 191:40–6.
127. Wolfe RR, Allsop JR, Burke JF. Metabolism 1979;28:210–20.
128. Nanni G, Siegel JH, Coleman B et al. J Trauma 1984;24:14–30.
129. Stoner HB, Little RA, Frayn RN et al. Br J Surg 1983;70:32–5.
130. Tissot S, Normand S, Khalfallah Y et al. Am J Physiol 1995;269: E753–8.
131. Lundholm K. Surg Clin North Am 1986;66:1023–4.
132. Cohn S, Gartenhaus W, Sawitsky A et al. Metabolism 1980;30: 222–9.
133. Legaspi A, Jeevanandam M, Starnes HF et al. Metabolism 1987;36:958–63.
134. Shaw JHF, Wolfe RR. Ann Surg 1987;205:368–76.
135. Eden E, Edstrom S, Bennegard K et al. Surgery 1985;97: 176–84.
136. Klein S, Wolfe RR. J Clin Invest 1990;86:1403–8.
137. Fearon KC, Barber MD, Falconer JS et al. World J Surg 1999; 23:584–8.
138. Stone M, Osamura RY. Pituitary 2001;4:15–23.
139. Wallace AM, Sattar N, McMillan DC. Clin Cancer Res 4:2977–9.
140. Klein S, Wolfe RR. J Clin Invest 1990;86:1403–8.
141. Kotler DP, Tierney AR, Wang J et al. Am J Clin Nutr 1989;50: 444–7.
142. Carr A, Samaras K, Thorisdottir A et al. Lancet 1999;353: 2093–9.
143. Dowell P, Flexner C, Kwiterovich PO et al. J Biol Chem 2000; 275:41325–32.
144. Domingo P, Matias-Guiu X, Pujol RM et al. AIDS 1999; 13:2261–7.
145. Bastard JP, Caron M, Vidal H et al. Lancet 2002;359:1026–31.
146. Hellerstein MK, Grunfeld C, Wu K et al. J Clin Endocrinol Metab 1993;76:559–65.
147. Grunfeld C, Kotler DP, Hamadeh R et al. Am J Med 1989; 86:27–31.
148. Haussinger D, Roth E, Lang F et al. Lancet 1993;341:1330–2.
149. Ritz P, Salle A, Simard G et al. Eur J Clin Nutr 2003;57:S2–5.
150. Finn PJ, Plank LD, Clark MA et al. Lancet 1996;347:654–6.
151. Hume DM, Egdahl RH. Ann Surg 1959;150:697–712.
152. Newsome HH, Rose JC. J Clin Endocrinol Metab 1971; 33:481–7.
153. Taylor JW, Hander EW, Skreen R et al. J Surg Res 1976; 20:313–20.
154. Dempsey DT, Guenter P, Mullen JL et al. Surg Gynecol Obstet 1985;160:128–34.
155. Meguid MM, Brennan MF, Aoki TT et al. Arch Surg 1974; 109:776–83.
156. Hume DM, Bell CC, Bartter F. Surgery 1962;52:174–87.
157. Carey LC, Cloutier CT, Lowery BD. Ann Surg 1971;174: 451–60.
158. Popp MB, Srivastava LS, Knowles HC et al. Surg Gynecol Obstet 1977;145:517–24.
159. Wise L, Margraf HW, Ballinger WF. Arch Surg 1972;105:213–20.
160. Marchuk JB, Finely RJ, Graces AC et al. J Surg Res 1977; 23:177–82.
161. Beisel WR. Am J Clin Nutr 1977;30:1236–47.
162. Van den Berghe G, de Zegher F, Bouillon R. J Clin Endocrinol Metab 1998;83:1827–34.
163. Vermes I, Bieshuizen A, Hampsink RM et al. J Clin Endocrinol Metab 1995;80:1238–42.
164. O'Brien JT, Bybee DE, Burman BD et al. Metabolism 1980; 29:721–7.
165. Richmand DA, Molitch MD, O'Donnell TF. Metabolism 1980; 29:936–42.
166. Van der Poll T, Van Zee KJ, Endert E et al. J Clin Endocrinol Metab 1995;80:1341–6.
167. Davies PH, Sheppard MC, Franklyn JA. Mol Cell Endocrinol 1997;129:191–8.
168. Jaattela A, Alho A, Avikainen V et al. Br J Surg 1975;62:177–81.
169. Davies CL, Newman RJ, Molyneux SG et al. J Trauma 1984;24: 99–105.
170. Gelfand RA, Matthews DE, Bier DM et al. J Clin Invest 1984;74:2238–48.
171. Fong Y, Albert JD, Tracey KJ et al. J Trauma 1991;31:1467–76.
172. Kraenzlin ME, Keller U, Keller A et al. J Clin Invest 1989;84: 388–93.
173. Shaw JHF, Holdaway CM, Humberston DA. Surgery 1988;103: 520–5.
174. Herndon DN, Hart DW, Wolf SE et al. N Engl J Med 2001; 345:1223–9.
175. Hasselgren P. Curr Opin Clin Nutr Metab Care 1999;2:201–5.
176. Shamoon HP, Soma V, Sherwin RS. J Clin Endocrinol Metab 1980;50:495–501.

177. Simmons PS, Miles JM, Gerich JE et al. J Clin Invest 1984; 73:412–20.

178. Wang L, Luo GJ, Wang JJ et al. Shock 1998;10:298–306.

179. MacLennan PA, Brown RA, Rennie MJ. FEBS Lett 1987;215: 187–91.

180. MacLennan PA, Smith K, Weryk B et al. FEBS Lett 1988;237: 133–6.

181. Abcouwer SF, Bode BP, Souba WW. J Surg Res 1995;59:59–65.

182. Lukaszewicz GC, Souba WW, Abcouwer SF. Shock 1997;7: 332–8.

183. Porte D Jr, Robertson RP. Fed Proc 1973;32:1792–6.

184. Flaim KE, Hutson SM, Lloyd CE et al. Am J Physiol 1985;249: E447–53.

185. Inculet RI, Finley RI, Duff JH et al. Surgery 1986;99:752–8.

186. Yu CC, Hua HA, Tong C. Burns 1989;15:145–6.

187. Wolfe RR, Herndon DN, Jahoor F et al. N Engl J Med 1987; 317:403–8.

188. Ellenberg M, Osserman KE, Pollack H. Diabetes 1952;1:16.

189. Ross H, Johnston IDA, Wellborn TA et al. Lancet 1966;2:563.

190. Gore DC, Chinkes D, Heggers J et al. J Trauma 2001;51:540.

191. Van den Berghe G, Wouters P, Weeks F et al. N Engl J Med 2001;19:1359–67.

192. Alberti KGMM, Batsone GF, Foster KJ et al. JPEN J Parenter Enteral Nutr 1980;4:141–6.

193. Wolfe BM, Culebras JM, Aoki TT et al. Surgery 1979;86: 248–56.

194. Pozefsky T, Tancredi RG, Moxley RT et al. Diabetes 1976;25: 128–35.

195. Warren RS, Donner DB, Starnes HF et al. Proc Natl Acad Sci USA 1987;84:8619–22.

196. Felig P, Wahren J, Hendler R. J Clin Invest 1976;58:761–5.

197. Iversen J. J Clin Invest 1973;52:2102–16.

198. Fong Y, Lowry SF. Cytokines and the cellular response to injury and infection. In: Harken AH, Wilmore DW, eds. Care of the Surgical Patient. New York: Scientific American, 1996:1–21.

199. Carswell EA, Old LJ, Kassel RL et al. Proc Natl Acad Sci USA 1975;72:3666–70.

200. Van der Poll RJA, Endert E Romijn JA et al. Am J Physiol 1991; 261:E457–65.

201. Michie HR, Spriggs DR, Manogue KR et al. Surgery 1988; 1004:280–6.

202. Fong Y, Lowry SF. Clin Immunol Immunopathol 1990;55: 157–70.

203. Van Zee KJ, Kohno T, Fischer E et al. Proc Natl Acad Sci USA 1992;89:4845–9.

204. Lahdevirta J. Maury CPJ, Teppo AM et al. Am J Med 1988; 85:289–91.

205. Beutler B, Mahoney J, Le Trang N et al. J Exp Med 1985; 161;984–5.

206. Feingold KR, Grunfeld C. J Clin Invest 1987;80:184–90.

207. Zechner R, Newman TC, Sherry B et al. Mol Cell Biol 1988; 8:2394–401.

208. Fruhbeck G, Gomez-Ambrosi J, Muruzabal FJ et al. Am J Physiol Endocrinol Metab 2001;280:E827–47.

209. Tracey KJ, Lowry SF. Adv Surg 1990;23:21–56.

210. Haddad JJ, Saade NE, Safieh-Garabedian B et al. J Neuroimmunol 2002;133:1–19.

211. Matsuki T, Horai R, Sudo K et al. J Exp Med 2003;198:877–88.

212. Fischer E, Van Zee KJ, Marano MA et al. Blood 1992;79: 2196–200.

213. Juge-Aubry CE, Somm E, Guisti V et al. Diabetes 2003;52: 1104–10.

214. Helfgott DC, Tatter SB, Santhanam U et al. J Immunol 1989; 142:948–53.

215. Gelin J, Moldawer LL, Lonroth C et al. Biochem Biophys Res Commun 1988;157:575–9.

216. Shenkin A, Fraser WD, Series J et al. Lymphokine Res 1989;8: 123–7.

217. Ritchie DG, Fuller GM. Ann NY Acad Sci 1983;408:490–502.

218. Castell JV, Gomez-Lechon MJ, David M et al. FEBS Lett 1989;242:237–9.

219. Garman RD, Jacobs KA, Clark SC et al. Proc Natl Acad Sci USA 1987;84:7629–33.

220. Helfgott DC, Fong Y, Moldawer LL et al. Clin Res 1989; 37:564A.

221. Stouthard JM, Romijn JA, Van der Poll T et al. Am J Physiol 1995;268:E813–9.

222. Luedke CE, Cerami A. J Clin Invest 1990;86:1234–40.

223. Nathan CF, Murray HW, Weibe ME et al. J Exp Med 1983;158: 670–89.

224. Matthys P, Duksman R, Proost P et al. Int J Cancer 1991;49: 77–82.

225. Chesnokova V, Melmed S. Endocrinology 2002;143:1571–4.

226. Wilder RL. Annu Rev Immunol 1995;13:307–38.

227. Besedovsky H, Del Ray A. Endocr Rev 1996;18:206–28.

228. Turnbull AV, Rivier CL. Physiol Rev 1999;79:1–71.

229. Tsigos C, Papanicolaou DA, Defensor R et al. Neuroendocrinology 1997;66:54–62.

230. Reichlin S. Recent Prog Horm Res 1999;54:133–81.

231. Chrousos G. Ann NY Acad Sci 1998;851:311–35.

232. Auernhammer CJ, Melmed S. Endocr Rev 2000;21:313–45.

233. Arzt E. J Clin Invest 2001;108:1729–33.

234. Annane D, Cavaillon JM. Shock 2003;20:197–207.

235. Scheinman RI, Gualberto A, Jewell CM et al. Mol Cell Biol 1995;15:943–53.

236. Ray A, LaForge KS, Sehgal PB. Mol Cell Biol 1990;10: 5736–46.

237. Zuckerman SH, Shellhaas J, Butler LD. Eur J Immunol 1989; 19:301–5.

238. Han J, Thompson P, Beutler B. J Exp Med 1990;172:391–4.

239. Van der Poll T, Coyle SM, Barbosa K et al. J Clin Invest 1996; 97:713–9.

240. Webster JC, Oakley RH, Jewell CM et al. Proc Natl Acad Sci USA 2001;98:6865–70.

241. Chrousos GP. In J Obes Relat Metabl Disord 2000;24[Suppl 2]; S50–5.

242. Dudrick SJ, Wilmore DW, Vars HM et al. Ann Surg 1969;70: 974–84.

243. Kudsk KA. Am J Surg 2002;183:390–8.

244. Alexander JW, Macmillan BG, Stinnett JD et al. Ann Surg 1980; 192:505–17.

245. Kudsk, KA, Stone JM, Carpenter G et al. J Trauma 1983;23: 605–9.

246. Ziegler TR, Smith RJ, O'Dwyer ST et al. Arch Surg 1988;123: 1313–9.

247. Deitch EA. J Trauma 1990;30:S184–9.

248. Deitch EA, Winteton J, Ma L et al. Ann Surg 1987;205:681–92.

249. Fong Y, Marano MA, Barber A et al. Ann Surg 1989;210: 449–57.

250. Robin CN, Williamson MB, Chir M. N Engl J Med 1978;298: 1393–402.

251. Streilen JW, Stein-Streilen J, Head J. Regional specialization in antigen presentation. In: Phillips SM, Escobar MR, eds. The Reticuloendothelial System, vol 9. New York: Plenum, 1986: 37–94.

252. Alverdy JC, Aoys E, Moss GS. Surgery 1988;104:185–90.

253. Fong Y, Lowry SF, Cerami A. JPEN J Parenter Enteral Nutr 1988;12:72S–7S.

254. Fong Y, Moldawer LL, Marano M et al. J Immunol 1989;142: 2321–4.

255. McDonald N, Easson AM, Mazurak VC et al. J Am Coll Surg 2003;197:143–61.

256. Kotler DP. J Nutr 1992;122:723–7.

257. Jeevanandam M, Horowitz GD, Lowry SF et al. Metabolism 1986;35:304.

258. Vlassara H, Spiegel RJ, San Doval D et al. Horm Metab Res 1986;18:698.

259. Tracey KJ, Wei HE, Manogue KR et al. J Exp Med 1988; 167:1211.

260. Mahony SM, Tisdale MJ. Br J Cancer 1988;58:345.

261. Moldawer, LL, Andersson C, Gelin J et al. Am J Physiol 1988; 254:G450.

262. Starnes HF, Warren RS, Jeevanandam M et al. J Clin Invest 1988;82:1321.

263. Warren RS, Starnes HF, Gabrilove JL et al. Arch Surg 1987; 122:1396.

264. Selby P, Hobbs S, Viner C et al. Br J Cancer 1987;56:803.

265. Michie HR, Spriggs DR, Manogue KR et al. Surgery 1988; 10:280.

266. Falconer JS, Fearson KH, Plester CE et al. Ann Surg 1994;219: 325.

267. Smith BK, Kluger MJ. Am J Physiol 1993;265:R615.

268. Mahoney SM, Beck SA, Tisdale MJ. Br J Cancer 1988;57:385.

269. Wigmore, SJ, Ross JA, Fearon KH et al. Br J Surg 1994;81: 1814.

270. Stouthard JL, Goey H, deVries EE et al. Br J Cancer 1996;73: 789.

271. Fearon KH, McMillan DC, Preston T et al. Ann Surg 1991;213: 26.

272. Scott, HR, McMillan DC, Crilly A et al. Br J Cancer 1996;73: 1560.

273. Strassman G, Fong M, Kenney JS et al. J Clin Invest 1992;89: 1681.

274. Emilie D, Wijdenes J, Gisselbreck C et al. Blood 1994;84:2472.

275. Soda K, Kawakami, M, Kashii A et al. Int J Cancer 1995;62:332.

276. Henderson JT, Seniuk NA, Richardson PM et al. J Clin Invest 1994;93:2632.

277. Espat NJ, Auffenberg T, Rosenberg JJ et al. Am J Physiol 1996; 271:R185.

278. Matthys P, Dijkmans R, Proost P et al. Int J Cancer 1991;49:77.

279. Langstein HN, Doherty GM, Fraker DL et al. Cancer Res 1991;51:2302.

280. Cariuk P, Lorite MJ, Todorov PT et al. Br J Cancer 1997;76: 606–13.

281. Lorite MJ, Thompson MG, Drake JL et al. Br J Cancer 1998; 78:850–6.

282. Todorov PT, Field WN, Tisdale MJ. Br J Cancer 1999;80:1734–7.

283. Baracos VE, DeVivo C, Hoyle DH et al. Am J Physiol 1995; 268:E996–E1006.

284. Bossola M, Muscaritoli M, Costelli P et al. Ann Surg 2003; 237:382–9.

285. Shenkin A, Neuhauser M, Bergstrom J et al. Am J Clin Nutr 1980;33:2119–27.

286. Moore FA, Moore EE, Jones TN et al. J Trauma 1989;29: 916–23.

287. Moore FA, Feliciano DV, Andrassy RJ et al. Ann Surg 1992; 216:171–83.

288. Kudsk KA, Croce MA, Fabian TC et al. Ann Surg 1992;215: 503–13.

289. Efron D, Kirk SJ, Regan MC et al. Surgery 1991;110:327–34.

290. Barbul A, Lazarou S, Efron DT et al. Surgery 1990;108:331–7.

291. Thompson WA, Coylse SM, Lazarus D et al. Surg Forum 1991; 42:23–5.

292. Fong Y, Rosenbaum M, Tracey KJ et al. Proc Natl Acad Sci USA 1989;86:3371–4.

293. Boulware SD, Tamborlane W, Sherwin R. Am J Physiol 1992; 262:130–3.

294. Clemmons DR, Smith-Banks A, Celniker AC et al. J Clin Endocrinol Metab 1992;75:1192–7.

295. Hinton P, Allison SP, Littlejohn S et al. Lancet 1971;1:767–9.

296. Woolfson AMJ, Heatley RV, Allison SP. N Engl J Med 1979; 300:14–7.

297. Wolf RF, Pearlstone DB, Newman E et al. Ann Surg 1992;216: 280–8.

298. Ziegler TR, Gatzen C, Wilmore DW. Annu Rev Med 1994;45: 459–80.

299. Koea JB, Breier BH, Douglas RJ et al. Br J Surg 1996;83: 196–202.

300. Knox JB, Wilmore DW, Demling RH et al. Am J Surg 1996; 171:576–80.

301. Takala, J, Ruokonen E, Webster NR et al. N Engl J Med 1999; 341:785–92.

302. Gatzen C, Schettinger MR, Kimbrough TD et al. Surgery 1992; 112:181–5.

303. Jorgensen P, Oxlund H. Wound Rep Reg 1996;40:40–7.

304. Knox J, Demling R, Wilmore D et al. J Trauma 1995;39: 526–31.

305. Demling R, DeSanti L. J Trauma 1997;43:47–52.

306. Beisel WR, Sawyer WD, Ryll ED et al. Ann Intern Med 1967; 67:744–79.

307. August D, Teitelbaum D, Albina J et al. JPEN J Parenter Enteral Nutr 2002;26:32SA.

308. Arora NS, Rochester DF. Am Rev Respir Dis 1982;126:5–8.

309. Suleiman MY, Zaloga GP. Renal failure. In: Zaloga G, ed. Nutrition in Critical Care. St. Louis: Mosby, 1993:661–84.

310. Rombeau Jl, Rolandelli RH, Wilmore DW et al. Nutritional support. In: Harken AH, Wilmore DW, eds. Care of the Surgical Patient. New York: Scientific American, 1994:3–35.

311. Marchesini G, Fabbri A, Bianchi G et al. Hepatology 1996;23: 1084–92.

90 NUTRITION AND INFECTION[1]

RICHARD D. SEMBA

HISTORICAL OVERVIEW 1401
GENERAL PRINCIPLES 1402
MALNUTRITION AND SPECIFIC INFECTIOUS
    DISEASES 1403
    Measles 1403
    Malaria 1404
    Diarrheal Disease 1404
    Acute Respiratory Infections 1405
    Hookworm Infection 1405
    Human Immunodeficiency Virus Infection 1405
    Tuberculosis 1407
NUTRITIONAL INTERACTIONS 1408
    Vitamin A 1408
    Zinc 1408
    Iron 1409
    Other Nutrients 1409
PREVENTION 1409

The duration and severity of many infectious diseases are related to host immunity and nutritional status. Lack of specific nutrients may lead to dysregulated or ineffective immune response and higher morbidity and mortality. Over the last three decades, a large series of clinical trials has demonstrated that vitamin A and zinc play an important role in reducing the morbidity and mortality of specific infectious diseases. The effect of micronutrients on immune function and resistance to infection appears to be specific for both the micronutrient and the particular pathogen.

HISTORICAL OVERVIEW

A temporal relationship among famine, starvation, and subsequent outbreaks of epidemic disease has long been recognized (1, 2). The relationship between less obvious malnutrition and infection was largely characterized in the twentieth century. In the early twentieth century, the idea of certain "substances," "accessory food factors," or "vita-

mines" that are essential for health emerged (3–5), and there was a rapid growth of knowledge regarding vitamins and deficiency diseases in the period following 1912 (6). Outbreaks of infections were observed among animals subjected to certain experimental diets (7–10). An increased susceptibility to infections was especially common in animals that were deficient in vitamin A, and soon vitamin A became known as the "antiinfective" vitamin (11). Carl Bloch, a pediatrician in Copenhagen, clearly attributed an increased susceptibility to infection and mortality in infants and young children to the lack of vitamin A, and he advocated the use of milk, cream, and butter for children to reduce their infections (12). In 1932 in London, Joseph Ellison discovered that vitamin A supplementation reduced the mortality of children with measles (13, 14). From 1920 through 1940, vitamin A underwent considerable evaluation in at least 30 therapeutic trials for different infectious diseases (15). Public health efforts became focused on the eradication of vitamin A deficiency because of its known association with reduced resistance to infection. By the early 1940s, it was generally accepted that vitamin A was important in maintaining mucosal immunity against infections (16). Concerns about ensuring an adequate vitamin A intake were reflected in the widespread use of cod liver oil for children, institution of milk programs in schools, and the fortification of milk with vitamin A.

In the 1930s, investigators showed that zinc was essential for the growth of animals (17, 18), and adults were noted to have low zinc levels in China (19, 20). In the 1960s, a syndrome described as human zinc deficiency and consisting of dwarfism, delayed sexual maturation, and iron deficiency anemia was found in young men who practiced geophagia and had low dietary intakes of zinc (21). Growth and sexual maturation occurred with zinc supplementation, a finding demonstrating that zinc was a limiting essential nutrient (22, 23). In the 1970s, acrodermatitis enteropathica, a syndrome characterized by dermatitis, diarrhea, and depressed immunity, was linked to zinc deficiency (24–27). The recommended dietary allowance for zinc was not established by the National Research Council until 1974, which belies the relatively recent recognition of zinc as an essential nutrient. In the late 1980s and 1990s, zinc supplementation was evaluated as therapy for diarrheal disease, pneumonia, malaria, and

[1]**Abbreviations: AIDS,** acquired immunodeficiency syndrome; **HIV,** human immunodeficiency; **IFN,** interferon; **IL,** interleukin; **MHC,** major histocompatibility complex; **NF-κB,** nuclear factor-κB; **TNF,** tumor necrosis factor.

child growth and development (28). Zinc was recommended as therapy for infections such as diarrhea and dysentery as early as the nineteenth century (29).

The study of nutrition and infection was facilitated by developments in immunology, such as the description of humoral antibodies, serologic tests for the diagnosis of infectious diseases, and assays for measurements of immunologic protection (30). By the late 1930s and early 1940s, it became generally accepted that some dietary deficiencies could increase the risk of infectious diseases (16, 31, 32). With fortification of foods, improvement in diet, and a general increase in the standard of living, many micronutrient deficiencies declined as public health problems in developed countries. Important observations were made in developing countries that linked malnutrition with infections and high mortality. In 1933, Cicely Williams described kwashiorkor among young children in west Africa who were rapidly weaned onto a diet of maize (33). In the 1950s, Donald McLaren observed that keratomalacia was more common among the Oriya people compared with the Kui people in the Khond Hills of Orissa, India, despite a relatively similar rice-based diet among both groups (34). The Kui people had a custom in which it was expected that couples would abstain from sexual intercourse until at least the child was able to walk, whereas the Oriyas did not have this custom and resumed intercourse within a month or two of delivery. Among the Oriyas, closely spaced pregnancies and early weaning increased the risk of keratomalacia among their infants, in a pattern analogous to the situation of kwashiorkor.

In 1968, a World Health Organization expert committee reviewed the interactions between nutrition and infection and published a comprehensive monograph, *Interactions of Nutrition and Infection* (35). The authors concluded:

> Infections are likely to have more serious consequences among persons with clinical or subclinical malnutrition, and infectious diseases have the capacity to turn borderline nutritional deficiencies into severe malnutrition. In this way, malnutrition and infection can be mutually aggravating and produce more serious consequences for the patient than would be expected from a summation of the independent effects of the two.

This work provided the important foundation for research on nutrition and infection that has followed to the present, much of which has taken place in developing countries where micronutrient deficiencies are more prevalent (36).

GENERAL PRINCIPLES

Infection with a pathogen usually triggers a series of responses; these vary depending on the infectious agent. Response to bacterial infection commences with the release of microbial products such as lipopolysaccharides and peptidoglycans from bacterial cell walls, bacterial DNA, and exotoxins; viral infections start with the release of viral double-stranded RNA and viral glycoproteins.

Depending on the type of pathogen and its ability to evade the immune response, the location of the infection, host immune status, and other factors, there may be a localized response with influx of polymorphonuclear leukocytes, macrophages, and natural killer cells. Polymorphonuclear cells release inflammatory mediators from granules, including reactive oxygen intermediates such as hydroxyl radicals, hydrogen peroxide, reactive nitrogen, and superoxide anion, and antimicrobial enzymes such as lysozyme, proteases, collagenases, and phospholipases. Macrophages may phagocytize antigens and express cytokines such as interleukin (IL)-1 that attract T lymphocytes to the site of inflammation (see also Chapter 43). The complement system may be activated. If the pathogen is not contained, these localized events may amplify and lead to a larger systemic condition, the acute-phase response, which is characterized by fever, somnolence, anorexia, and cachexia and is accompanied by metabolic alterations such as loss of muscle and negative nitrogen balance, fat catabolism, and impaired gluconeogenesis. The acute-phase response can also be triggered by other factors, including trauma, burns, surgery, tissue infarction, exposure to chemicals or radiation, and advanced cancer.

During the acute-phase response, changes occur in many plasma proteins, or acute-phase proteins, which have been defined as proteins whose plasma concentrations increase (positive acute-phase proteins) or decrease (negative acute-phase proteins) by at least one fourth during inflammatory disorders (37, 38). C-reactive protein, (38), α-1-acid glycoprotein (39), and serum amyloid A (40) are among the best characterized positive acute-phase proteins. The liver is the main site of synthesis of most acute-phase proteins. C-reactive protein, α-1-acid glycoprotein, and serum amyloid A are components of the innate immune response. C-reactive protein binds to phosphocholine and phospholipid constituents of damaged cells, activates complement, and induces inflammatory cytokines (38). Serum amyloid A can induce enzymes that are important in the repair process following tissue damage and also serves as a chemoattractant for immune effector cells (40). α-1-Acid glycoprotein has been described as having immunomodulatory properties such as inhibition of polymorphonuclear cell activation and modulation of cytokine secretion (39). Other positive acute-phase proteins include ferritin, haptoglobin, and ceruloplasmin, and negative acute-phase proteins include albumin and transthyretin.

Cytokines play an important role in the acute-phase response as inducers of acute-phase proteins and hormones, as modulators of inflammation, and as activators and inhibitors of central nervous system functions related to appetite and metabolism (41). Cytokines that have been implicated in the anorexia that occurs during infection include IL-1β, IL-6, and tumor necrosis factor-α (TNF-α) (41). IL-1β and TNF-α are produced primarily by macrophages and can be triggered by stimuli such as bacterial wall products, lipopolysaccharide, viruses, parasites, and microbial superantigens. IL-6 is produced by monocytes, T lymphocytes, endothelial cells, and fibroblasts and is a major stimulator of the production of acute-phase proteins in the liver. These cytokines may have a direct effect on hypothalamic neurons involved in appetite, and other neural mediators, such as serotonin, corticotropin-releasing factor, and β-melanocyte stimulating hormone, and decreases in dopamine and neuropeptide Y. There may be increased cytokines in the circulation as well as the brain that modulate appetite during the acute-phase response (42).

MALNUTRITION AND SPECIFIC INFECTIOUS DISEASES

The impact of malnutrition on the severity of infection has been investigated most extensively in children with measles, diarrheal disease, respiratory infections, and malaria and in children and adults with tuberculosis and human immunodeficiency virus (HIV) infection. In general, the severity of morbidity and mortality during different infections is worse among persons with malnutrition. Malnutrition has been estimated to account for about one half of the mortality that occurs with among children in developing countries (Fig. 90.1) (43). This mortality occurs in the presence of major infectious diseases and is widely considered to be related to alterations in immunity that are associated with malnutrition.

Measles

Measles is estimated to account for 1 million deaths and a great deal of morbidity among the 30 million cases of measles per year, most of which occur in developing countries (44) where malnutrition is more prevalent. Deaths from measles are largely the result of an increased suscep-

tibility to secondary bacterial and viral infections, and the underlying mechanism includes immune suppression related to malnutrition, especially vitamin A deficiency (45). Complications may occur in 10 to 30% of cases and include pneumonia, diarrhea, malnutrition, otitis media, mouth ulcers, corneal epithelial keratitis, corneal ulceration, and blindness (see also Chapters 19 and 38).

Measles virus is an enveloped RNA virus in the genus *Morbillivirus* of the family Paramyxoviridae. There is one known serotype and eight clades (A–H) of measles. Measles is spread when a susceptible person inhales aerolized droplets containing measles virus. Viral replication occurs initially in macrophages in the lymphoid tissue of the nasopharynx, respiratory mucosa, and lungs (46). The measles virus enters human cells via a cell-surface receptor known as signaling lymphocyte activation molecule (SLAM, or CDw 150) (47). Viremia allows measles virus to spread to multiple organs, including the skin, liver, and conjunctiva, and a prodrome of fever, cough, and conjunctivitis occurs approximately 14 days after infection. Antibody responses against measles virus proteins are detectable at the onset of the rash. Infants are protected against measles virus infection by passively acquired maternal antibody to measles. T-cell–driven cellular immune responses, including activation of CD4$^+$ and CD8$^+$ lymphocytes, occur during measles (46). Delayed-type hypersensitivity skin test responses and in vitro proliferation of lymphocytes to viral antigens are often minimal or absent in measles infection (46). The immune response to measles is thought to be consistent with T-helper type 2–like immune responses in which antibody responses predominate and are driven by IL-4, IL-6, and IL-10. Immune suppression often accompanies measles infection and increases the susceptibility to secondary infections.

Malnutrition is an important determinant of the severity of measles (48–52). In the classic, early investigation of a measles outbreak in the Faroe Islands by Peter Panum and August Manicus in 1846, the most severe diarrheal disease and highest mortality were described among those patients with greatest poverty and poor diet (53). Malnourished children have more severe disease and higher mortality (51, 52), and mortality is greater among children who develop prolonged diarrhea (50). More persistent measles infection and viral shedding have been reported in malnourished children (48). A close synergism exists between measles and vitamin A deficiency, because children with measles who are vitamin A deficient have a much higher risk of xerophthalmia, corneal ulceration, keratomalacia, and subsequent blindness (54).

Vitamin A supplementation reduces the morbidity and mortality of measles among preschool children (13, 55–58). Vitamin A supplementation appears to reduce the infectious complications associated with measles immune suppression, such as pneumonia and diarrheal disease, and these effects have been associated with modulation of immune responses by vitamin A (59, 60).

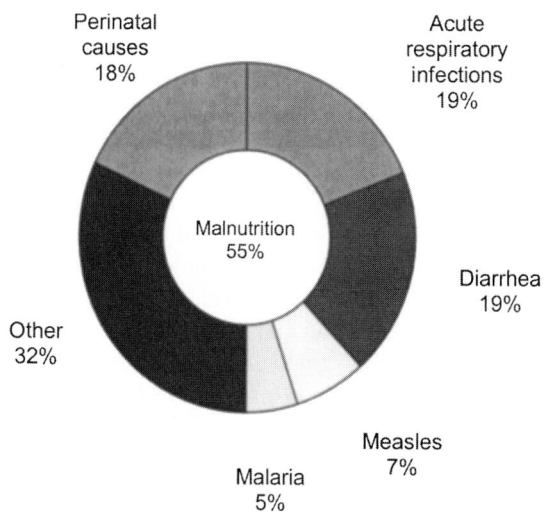

Figure 90.1. Malnutrition and child mortality.

Zinc supplementation does not appear to have an effect on morbidity among children with measles that is accompanied by pneumonia (61).

Malaria

Malaria, a parasitic infection with protozoan organisms of the genus *Plasmodium*, causes an estimated 1 to 3 million deaths worldwide each year (62). Of the four malaria species that infect humans (*P. falciparum*, *P. vivax*, *P. malariae*, and *P. ovale*), the most serious morbidity and mortality are caused by *P. falciparum*, and nearly 90% of all cases and fatalities occur in sub-Saharan Africa (63). Malarial infection begins when a female mosquito takes a blood meal and releases sporozoites from the salivary bland into the circulating blood of the host. Sporozoites then enter hepatocytes, and in the preerythrocytic cycle, sporozoites grow and develop in the liver into thousands of merozoites. The hepatocytes then release merozoites, which invade erythrocytes. In the asexual erythrocytic cycle, merozoites develop into schizonts, and erythrocytes rupture, releasing more merozoites that can invade erythrocytes. In the sexual stage, some merozoites develop into gametocytes that are taken up in a blood meal by a mosquito, and within the mosquito, these gametocytes develop in microgametes and macrogametes.

Natural history studies suggest that the severity of malaria may be related to nutritional status. Although some studies in the older literature have reported that malnutrition is protective against malaria, comprehensive reviews show that persons with better nutritional status have less severe malaria and a lower risk of death (63, 64). Nutritional indicators of poor vitamin A status have been associated with malaria (65–67). A randomized, placebo-controlled clinical trial was conducted in Papua New Guinea to examine the effects of vitamin A supplementation, 60 mg retinol equivalents every 3 months, on malarial morbidity in preschool children (68). Children between 6 and 60 months of age were randomly allocated to receive vitamin A or placebo every 3 months. A weekly morbidity surveillance and clinic-based surveillance were established for monitoring acute malaria, and children were followed for 1 year. Vitamin A significantly reduced the incidence of malaria attacks by about 20 to 50% for all except those with extremely high levels of parasitemia. Similarly, vitamin A supplementation reduced clinic-based malaria attacks, which consisted of self-solicited visits to the clinic by mothers who thought that their children should be seen because of fever. Vitamin A supplementation had little impact in children less than 12 months of age and the greatest effect among children aged 13 to 36 months.

Two clinical trials showed that zinc supplementation reduces the morbidity of malaria (69, 70). In The Gambia, 110 children were randomized to receive 70 mg zinc or placebo twice weekly for 1.24 years. Zinc supplementation was associated with a 30% reduction in the incidence of clinical malaria episodes (69). In Papua New Guinea, 274 preschool children, aged 6 to 60 months, received 10 mg zinc or placebo/day for 46 weeks. Zinc supplementation resulted in a 38% reduction in malaria morbidity, in which the outcome was a health center visit with elevated *P. falciparum* parasitemia and a fever (70). A clinical trial from Burkina Faso in which children were supplemented with 12.5 mg zinc or placebo/day for 6 months did not show an effect of zinc supplementation on clinical malaria episodes (71). However, the method to assess malaria episodes was based on daily visits and temperature monitoring of the children 6 days/week for detection of malaria episodes rather than self-report to the health center because of a fever. Thus, the trial in Burkina Faso was designed to detect early manifestations of a malaria episode and less severe morbidity and cannot be compared directly with the trials in The Gambia and Papua New Guinea. In addition, an unusually high proportion (86%) of all fevers found in the children (894 of 1041 fever episodes) in Burkina Faso were attributed to malaria (71). The impact of zinc supplementation on more severe malaria episodes (69, 70) is likely to be of greater programmatic relevance. Zinc supplementation did not appear to reduce the morbidity of malaria (reduction of fever or parasitemia) when it was given as adjunct therapy with chloroquine to children, aged 6 months to 5 years, who presented with an attack of acute uncomplicated falciparum malaria (72).

Diarrheal Disease

Diarrheal diseases cause an estimated 3.5 million deaths/year, mostly among those less than 2 years of age (73). The main causes of diarrheal diseases among children in developing countries are rotavirus, *Escherichia coli*, and *Shigella*, *Vibrio cholerae*, *Salmonella*, and *Entamoeba histolytica*. The epidemiology, clinical features, immunology, and pathogenesis of diarrhea may differ according to characteristics of the pathogen, such as production of toxins, tissue invasion, fluid and electrolyte loss, and location of infection. Diarrhea is generally defined as the condition in which three or more liquid stools are passed in a 24-hour period (73). In developing countries, community-based studies suggest that children less than 5 years of age have a median incidence of 2.6 diarrheal episodes/year (73). In general, host defenses in the gut include gastric acidity, the presence of normal microflora, gut motility, mucus production, integrity of microvilli, local secretion of antibody, and cell-mediated immunity, and micronutrient malnutrition may impair some of these host defenses. Malnourished infants and children are at higher risk of more severe disease and higher mortality from diarrhea (74, 75), and an increased incidence of diarrhea is found among children with evidence of depressed immunity (76).

Clinical vitamin A deficiency is associated with diarrheal disease in children (77–82). Vitamin A supplementation or fortification has been shown to reduce the morbidity and mortality of diarrheal diseases among preschool children in clinical trials conducted in developing countries over the last 2 decades (83). Trials were conducted in Indonesia, India, Ghana, and other developing countries (84–90). The severity of diarrheal disease was reduced by vitamin A supplementation in a clinical trial in Brazil (91). The reduction in diarrheal disease mortality appears to account for most of the reduction in overall mortality when vitamin A is given through fortification or supplementation on a community level (92). One of the mechanisms by which vitamin A may improve clinical outcomes in diarrheal disease is through restoration of gut integrity (93). Urinary losses of vitamin A during diarrhea may be substantial in some children (94), and persistent diarrhea may reduce the bioavailability of vitamin A (95). Vitamin A supplementation (60 mg retinol equivalents) reduces morbidity in children with acute shigellosis (96), but the effects of vitamin A supplementation on other specific diarrheal pathogens have not been completely clarified.

Recent randomized controlled trials in developing countries showed that zinc supplementation can reduce the incidence of diarrhea by about 18% (97). Zinc supplementation also reduces the incidence of pneumonia, because a pooled analysis showed a reduction of mortality of 41% (95% confidence interval, 17–59%) (98). When used as therapy for acute or persistent diarrhea, zinc supplementation reduced the duration of diarrhea (97). One trial showed that zinc supplementation reduced mortality among small-for-gestational age term infants by 68% when given from 1 to 9 months of age (99), and further clinical trials are in progress to determine whether zinc supplementation reduces infant and young child mortality (97).

Acute Respiratory Infections

Acute respiratory infections are a major cause of morbidity and mortality among infants and children in developing countries, and these infections account for an estimated 4 million deaths per year (100). Malnutrition is a major determinant of morbidity and mortality during acute respiratory infections in children (101). The main causes of acute lower respiratory infections in children are respiratory syncytial virus, adenovirus, parainfluenza virus, influenza virus, *Streptococcus pneumoniae*, and *Haemophilus influenzae* (102). The nonspecific immune defenses of the respiratory tract consist of cilia in the tracheobronchial tree, mucus secretion by goblet cells, and phagocytic activity by alveolar macrophages (102). Acute respiratory infections in children have been associated with poor weight gain and stunting (102).

Controlled clinical trials showed that zinc supplementation reduced the incidence of pneumonia among children (103–108). A pooled analysis of four randomized trials showed that zinc supplementation decreased the incidence of pneumonia by 41% (28). Among infants and young children, zinc supplementation reduced the morbidity of severe acute lower respiratory infection (109, 110). Vitamin A supplementation has shown little to no effect on reducing the incidence or severity of acute respiratory infections among preschool children (92), but it does reduce the morbidity of acute respiratory infections associated with measles infection (83).

Hookworm Infection

About one fourth of the world's population is infected with hookworm (111). Hookworm infection is a major cause of iron deficiency. Two species of hookworm, *Ancyclostoma duodenale* and *Necator americanus*, account for a great deal of human morbidity and mortality. Hookworm is usually spread from person-to-person through contamination of soil and vegetation with feces that contain hookworm eggs. In the soil, the eggs develop into larvae that can penetrate human skin on contact. The infective larvae may leave a pruritic, papulovesicular eruption on the skin, so-called "ground itch." The hookworm larvae migrate through the skin to the alveoli of the lungs, where they may be coughed up and ingested. The hookworms attach to the intestinal mucosa and cause chronic blood loss and depletion of iron stores (111). Hookworms elicit antibody and cellular immune responses in humans, but limited evidence suggests that these immune responses give any protection against infection (112). Hookworm infection is associated with growth retardation among infants and children, iron deficiency and impaired mental development in school children, and fatigue and decreased work capacity among adults (113). Poor hygiene is the major risk factor for hookworm infection, and hookworm infection, in turn, increases the risk of iron and other micronutrient deficiencies.

Pioneering studies conducted in the early part of the twentieth century in the United States showed that deworming of heavily infected school children improved hemoglobin concentrations and increased growth (114, 115). Hookworm infection was associated with poor mental development (116, 117), and treatment for hookworm in infected children improved performance on mental development tests compared with infected children who were not treated (118). These studies were conducted at a time when hookworm infection was common in the southern part of the United States (119). More recent studies in developing countries showed that treatment of school children for hookworm infection was associated with improved iron status (120) and better growth (121), and a combination of hookworm treatment and iron supplementation was associated with improved cognitive performance (122) and growth (123).

Human Immunodeficiency Virus Infection

An estimated 39.4 million persons are infected with HIV worldwide (124). HIV infection causes a progressive decline in immunity that can lead to the acquired immunodeficiency syndrome (AIDS). HIV-1 is spread person-to-person by three major routes: sexual contact, mother-to-child transmission, and through transmission by blood products such as shared needles and syringes. Wasting syndrome, characterized by unintentional loss of more than 10% body weight, was common among HIV-infected adults in industrialized countries before the advent of highly active antiretroviral therapy around 1995. Wasting syndrome is still highly prevalent among HIV-infected adults in sub-Saharan Africa, south Asia, and southeast Asia in situations with limited access to highly active antiretroviral therapy.

Poor nutrition may play an important role in disease progression in HIV-infected persons (125). During HIV infection, nutritional intake may be affected by anorexia, central nervous system disease, dysphagia, and odynophagia (painful swallowing) (126). Esophageal candidiasis is not infrequent during HIV infection and usually causes dysphagia and odynophagia. Decreased food intake may occur even in asymptomatic HIV-infected adults and has been associated with significant weight loss (127). Fairly high proportions of HIV-infected individuals do not consume at least the recommended dietary allowance for some B-complex vitamins, vitamin E, and zinc (128, 129), and it has been suggested that the recommended dietary allowances should be higher for persons with HIV infection (130). Diarrhea and malabsorption of fats, carbohydrates, and vitamin B_{12} appear to be common in all stages of HIV infection. Cryptosporidia, microsporidia, cytomegalovirus, and *Mycobacterium avium-intracellulare* are major causes of diarrhea in patients with AIDS, and many pathogens are resistant to treatment and lead to severe weight loss and death (131). Fat malabsorption may be common during HIV infection and can reduce the absorption of fat-soluble vitamins, such as vitamins A and E.

Jejunal and duodenal villous atrophy with or without crypt hyperplasia occurs in all stages of HIV disease (132). Increased intestinal permeability may occur in about one fourth of asymptomatic HIV-infected adults and may increase with HIV disease progression (133). Physiologic studies of human duodenal biopsies showed that HIV-infected patients with diarrhea have epithelial barrier defects, a finding suggesting that a passive leak of ions, substrates, and water could contribute to diarrhea during HIV infection (134). With the advent of highly active antiretroviral therapy in the mid-1990s in developed countries, many of the more severe nutritional problems associated with HIV infection declined in prevalence. However, most persons with HIV infection live in developing countries and have more limited access to high active antiretroviral therapy.

A fairly high prevalence of micronutrient deficiencies has been reported in many HIV-infected risk groups (125). Vitamin A deficiency is common among HIV-infected pregnant women (135, 136) and children (137) in developing countries. A few studies suggested that serum vitamin C concentrations are lower among HIV-infected adults compared with healthy controls (138). A high proportion of HIV-infected adults appear to have low levels of vitamin B_6 (139, 140), vitamin B_{12} (141), and folate (142). Iron deficiency is common among HIV-infected pregnant women (143), female injection drug users (144), and children (145, 146). Low blood zinc concentrations have been described in HIV-infected adults (139, 147). Low serum or plasma levels of selenium consistent with deficiency have been reported in HIV-infected adults (148).

Nutrients can be involved in the pathogenesis of HIV infection through their roles as antioxidants and in immune function. Antioxidant nutrients such as the carotenoids, tocopherols, vitamin C, and selenium have been implicated in the pathogenesis of HIV infection through their interactions with reactive oxygen intermediates and nuclear factor-κB (NF-κB), a transcriptional promotor of proteins that are involved in the inflammatory and acute-phase responses. NF-κB is involved in the transcription of HIV-1. Thus, antioxidants may potentially be involved in the pathogenesis of HIV infection by their effects on reactive oxygen intermediates and interactions of reactive oxygen species with NF-κB, with subsequent upregulation of HIV expression. Vitamin A plays a central role in the growth and function of T and B cells, antibody responses, and maintenance of mucosal epithelium, including that of the respiratory, gastrointestinal, and genitourinary tracts (149). Zinc plays an important role in the growth, development, and function of neutrophils, macrophages, natural killer cells, and T and B lymphocytes (150).

Longitudinal studies suggested that certain micronutrient deficiencies are associated with increased morbidity and mortality during HIV infection. Low plasma or serum vitamin A levels are associated with accelerated HIV progression (151), increased mortality (152), and, in children, growth failure (153). High serum vitamin E levels were associated with a lower risk of progression to AIDS (154). The risk of progression to AIDS may be higher in those with vitamin B_{12} deficiency (155). Low serum zinc levels are associated with reduced secretory function of the thymus (156) and HIV disease progression (151, 157). Low serum or plasma selenium concentrations are associated with an increased risk of progression to AIDS and higher mortality (158–160).

Several large clinical trials of micronutrient supplementation for HIV-infected adults have been conducted. A trial in Tanzania showed that multivitamin supplementation slowed progression to AIDS when this therapy was given to HIV-infected pregnant women through pregnancy and during lactation (161), and it also reduced fetal deaths and low birth weight (162). Vitamin A and β-carotene supplementation reduced preterm delivery among pregnant women in Durban, South Africa (163), and daily vitamin A supplementation alone for pregnant women reduced the proportion of infants with low birth weight and increased their hemoglobin concentrations in Malawi (164). A reduction in oxidative stress and an apparent decrease in viral load were noted in a clinical trial of vitamins E (800 mg/day) and C (1 g/day) in HIV-infected adults in Toronto (165). A recent clinical trial in Uganda showed that periodic high-dose vitamin A supplementation reduced the mortality of HIV-infected preschool children by 46% (137).

Tuberculosis

Tuberculosis is an infection caused by *Mycobacterium tuberculosis* or related organisms such as *M. bovis*. *M. tuberculosis*, a slowly growing acid-fast-staining bacillus, is the most common cause of tuberculosis in humans. The spectrum of disease ranges from asymptomatic latent tuberculous infection to disseminated disease. The most common form of tuberculosis is latent infection. Active tuberculosis, the form of disease that disrupts normal host physiology to produce symptoms, is generally classified as pulmonary or extrapulmonary disease. Pulmonary disease, the most common form of active tuberculosis, accounts for about 80% of cases, and clinical manifestations include chronic cough and sometimes hemoptysis, dyspnea, and chest pain. Other constitutional symptoms include fevers, night sweats, and weight loss. Extrapulmonary disease accounts for about 20% of active tuberculosis cases, and the most common extrapulmonary sites are the lymph nodes (most often the cervical lymph nodes), pleura, kidneys, meninges, and bone or joints.

Tuberculosis is usually transmitted from person to person via the aerial route, and most persons who are infected do not develop clinical disease. About 5% of those infected may develop clinical manifestations such as pulmonary or miliary disease, and disease may occur at the time of primary infection or years later. Once infected, a person has about a 10% lifetime risk of developing active tuberculosis. Malnutrition increases the risk of developing clinical disease. In the absence of effective chemotherapy, tuberculosis is characterized by wasting and high mortality. The association of poor nutrition with tuberculosis is evident in older terms for tuberculosis such as the Greek term *aphthisis* or "to waste away," and "consumption."

Worldwide, tuberculosis is the leading infectious cause of death, accounting for 2 million deaths annually (166). About one third of the world's population, or 1.8 billion persons, are infected with *M. tuberculosis*, and this group represents an enormous pool of persons at risk of development of future disease. In sub-Saharan Africa, the Indian subcontinent, and southeast Asia, half or more of adults have latent tuberculosis infection. Each year, between 7 and 8 million people throughout the world develop active tuberculosis, and most cases occur in sub-Saharan Africa and Asia. Tuberculosis is responsible for about one fourth of all preventable deaths in developing

countries, and many of these deaths are associated with underlying HIV infection. The annual risk of infection, a marker of *M. tuberculosis* transmission, is estimated at 1 to 2% per year. Similarly for active tuberculosis, the annual global incidence increased from 62 cases/100,000 population in the 1980s to 75 cases/100,000 population in the 1990s (167).

M. tuberculosis is transmitted through the airborne route from infectious cases to susceptible contacts. An infected person will cough and produce an aerosol of tiny droplet particles that contain live *M. tuberculosis*. When these particles are inhaled by a susceptible contact, they impact deep in the lung parenchyma in the alveoli. The initial interaction between the host immune system and *M. tuberculosis* occurs in the alveoli, where pulmonary macrophages engulf, process, and present mycobacterial antigens in conjunction with major histocompatibility complex (MHC) class II molecules. When the complex of mycobacterial antigen and MHC molecule is recognized by antigen-specific CD4 lymphocytes, the CD4 lymphocytes release interferon-γ (IFN-γ) and IL-2. The IFN-γ serves to activate macrophages and enhance their ability to contain mycobacteria. This response is regulated, in part, by IL-12, which induces differentiation of Th-1 cells and augments the release of IFN-γ from the T lymphocytes (168). The activated macrophages release a number of cytokines including TNF-α (169), IL-1 (170), and IL-6 (171) that are responsible for the recruitment of cells to the site of infection, formation of granuloma, and development of the delayed-type hypersensitivity response. This process is downregulated by effects of monocyte-derived transforming growth factor-β and IL-10 on CD4 lymphocytes (172, 173). Within this network of cytokines, TNF-α appears to play a more central role in the pathogenesis of tuberculosis. TNF-α is essential for granuloma formation (174) and activates macrophage clearance of the organism. Further, proteins and polysaccharides of *M. tuberculosis* stimulate mononuclear phagocytes to express TNF-α as well as other cytokines (175). Overexpression of TNF-α also appears to be responsible for many of the systemic signs and morbidity of tuberculosis, such as fever, night sweats, and cachexia.

Malnutrition is well known among adults with tuberculosis (176, 177). In Tanzania, 77% of male patients and 58% of female patients with smear-positive pulmonary tuberculosis had a body mass index of less than 18.5 on admission (178). In general, adults gained weight during 6 months of treatment with chemotherapy, but weight was lost after treatment had finished. The length of stay in the hospital was the primary determinant of weight gain in patients receiving chemotherapy, a finding suggesting that nutritional intake in the hospital was better than could be achieved at home. Progressive nutritional recovery generally occurs during tuberculosis chemotherapy; however, serum albumin levels and mean arm muscle circumference have been reported as subnormal after 12 months, a finding suggesting that body protein reserves may not be fully recovered during treatment (179). Altered amino acid metabolism may contribute to wasting in tuberculosis (180). Body composition studies suggest that body cell mass is relatively depleted in adults with tuberculosis and HIV infection (181, 182).

Experimental animal studies showed that protein-calorie malnutrition has a marked effect on resistance to tuberculosis (183). Restoration of a full protein diet could reverse the fatal course of tuberculosis in malnourished mice. T-cell subset alterations were described in malnourished cattle infected with *M. bovis* (184). In a guinea pig model, animals on a protein-restricted diet were vaccinated with *M. bovis* bacille Calmette-Guérin vaccine and then infected via the respiratory route with virulent *M. tuberculosis*. Protein deficiency was associated with loss of tuberculin skin sensitivity, reduced lymphocyte proliferation responses to mycobacterial antigens, decreased IL-2 production, and reduced $CD2^+$ lymphocytes in the thymus and peripheral blood (185, 186).

Multiple micronutrient deficiencies are common during tuberculosis (187). Cod liver oil, a rich source of vitamin A, was a main treatment for tuberculosis in the era before antibiotics (15). Animal studies suggest that vitamin A improves immune responses to tuberculosis and enhances survival (188, 189). Although the association between malnutrition and tuberculosis is well known, few controlled clinical trials have been conducted to investigate whether improved nutrition will reduce the risk of developing active disease or will improve the clinical outcome of tuberculosis. In Harlem, New York City, a trial was conducted in the 1940s to determine whether a vitamin and mineral supplement could reduce the incidence of tuberculosis in families with an active case of tuberculosis. One hundred ninety-four families received either a vitamin and mineral supplement or no supplement. The attack rate of tuberculosis was 0.16/100 person-years in families taking the vitamins and minerals and 0.91/100 person-years among families in the control group (190).

NUTRITIONAL INTERACTIONS

Vitamin A

Vitamin A plays an essential role in both innate and adaptive immunity (191). Vitamin A deficiency is associated with loss of cilia in the respiratory tract, loss of microvilli in the gastointestinal tract, loss of mucin and goblet cells in the respiratory, gastrointestinal, and genitourinary tracts, squamous metaplasia with abnormal keratinization in the respiratory tract, alterations in antigen-specific secretory immunoglobulin A concentrations, impairment of alveolar monocyte/macrophage function, and decreased integrity of the gut. Vitamin A is necessary for the function of natural killer cells (192) and neutrophils (193), and altered T-cell subsets have been described during vitamin A deficiency (194). Vitamin A deficiency may influence T-lymphocyte-related immunocompetence through modulation of numbers or distribution of T cells, changes in phenotype, alterations in cytokine production, or decreased expression or function of cell-surface molecules involved in T-cell signaling (191). Vitamin A deficiency impairs the growth, activation, and function of B lymphocytes. The hallmark of vitamin A deficiency is an impaired capacity to generate an antibody response to T-cell–dependent antigens (195, 196), including tetanus toxoid (197) and diphtheria antigens in humans (198), and T-cell–independent type 2 antigens such as pneumococcal polysaccharide (199). These findings suggest that vitamin A deficiency may compromise immunity to many types of infections in which the main immune defense depends on antibody responses. Clinical trials showed that vitamin A supplementation reduces morbidity and mortality from measles, diarrheal disease, and HIV infection in children, decreases pregnancy-related mortality (200), and reduces the morbidity of *P. falciparum* malaria (Table 90.1).

Zinc

Zinc plays a role in both innate and adaptive immunity. Zinc deficiency impairs the function of neutrophils (201) and natural killer cells (202) and the chemotactic responses of monocyte/macrophages (150). In preschool children, zinc supplementation was associated with an increase in delayed-type hypersensitivity skin responses to multiple antigens (203). Another trial among low-birth-weight infants showed that zinc supplementation had no effect on delayed-type hypersensitivity skin responses to phytohemagglutinin (204). The investigators noted that phytohemagglutinin is a strong antigen, and the test may have been insensitive to detect more subtle differences in immunity. Another study that used a multiple antigen skin

TABLE 90.1. SOME NOTABLE TRIALS OF VITAMIN A AND INFECTIOUS DISEASES

LOCATION	DATE	SUBJECTS	OBSERVATION	REFERENCE
London[a]	1932	Children	Reduced measles mortality	13
Indonesia	1986	Children	Reduced diarrheal disease mortality	84
South Africa	1990	Children	Reduced measles mortality	56
Papua New Guinea	1999	Children	Reduced malaria morbidity	68
Nepal	1999	Women	Reduced pregnancy-related mortality	200
Uganda	2005	Children	Reduced mortality during HIV/AIDS	137

HIV/AIDS, human immunodeficiency virus/acquired immunodeficiency syndrome.
[a]Vitamin A in the form of cod liver oil.

test to seven antigens (tetanus, diphtheria, tuberculin, *Candida, Trichophyton,* and *Proteus*) showed that zinc supplementation reduced anergy by skin testing (205). The numbers of circulating CD4$^+$ and CD8$^+$ lymphocytes decrease during zinc deficiency (150, 205). Numbers of circulating CD8$^+$ CD73$^+$ T cells, which are mostly precursors for cytotoxic T lymphocytes, are reduced during zinc deficiency (206). A decrease in CD8$^+$ CD73$^+$ T cells could possibly increase the susceptibility of zinc-deficient persons to viral, parasitic, and bacterial infections (206). Zinc deficiency plays a role in thymic atrophy and may modulate maturation of T lymphocytes (150, 207). Zinc deficiency is associated with impaired antibody responses to T-cell–dependent and T-cell–independent antigens (150). In experimental human zinc deficiency, peripheral blood mononuclear cells showed a decrease in IFN-γ and IL-2 production, but no change in IL-4, IL-6, and IL-10 production, a finding suggesting a possible depression of Th-1–like responses during zinc deficiency (208). Clinical trials showed that zinc supplementation reduces the duration of diarrhea (209, 210) and the incidence of diarrhea and pneumonia, and it may reduce infant mortality (Table 90.2).

Iron

In contrast to vitamin A deficiency and zinc deficiency, less is known about the role of iron in human immunity and infection, and many of the available data are inconsistent (211). Iron deficiency appears to affect neutrophil function (211, 212), impair natural killer cell function, and reduce delayed-type hypersensitivity skin testing (211, 213). It is not clear whether iron deficiency affects lymphocyte proliferation responses to mitogens or the composition of T-cell subsets in peripheral blood, because results from various studies have been inconsistent (211, 214). Iron deficiency does not appear to impair antibody responses following immunization in children (211, 215). Few solid data from observational studies show that iron deficiency increases the morbidity and mortality of infectious diseases (214), and it appears to be fairly clear that increased infectious disease morbidity is not part of the syndrome of iron deficiency (213). Oral iron supplementation has not been associated with a reduction in the morbidity of infectious diseases (214), and a recent systematic review of 28 controlled clinical trials showed that iron

supplementation has no apparent effect on the incidence of infectious diseases, including malaria, except for a slightly increased risk of diarrhea (214). Although it has been speculated that iron supplementation may worsen HIV infection because of prooxidant effects and upregulation of HIV expression through NF-κB, little evidence from interventional studies currently indicates that iron supplementation has a detrimental effect on clinical outcome in HIV infection (216).

Other Nutrients

Selenium is an important component of the antioxidant defense system because it is contained in selenoproteins such as gluthione peroxidase (217). Coxsackie B3 virus can mutate in selenium-deficient mice (218), a finding suggesting the potential for viral mutation in populations in which selenium deficiency is endemic. Fatty acids play a role in immune function through modulation of inflammatory mediators and inflammatory cells (219). Carotenoids are lipophilic antioxidants (220), and their role in infectious diseases has not been well characterized.

PREVENTION

The causes of malnutrition are complex and involve food, society, health, and caring practices. The theoretic framework for the causes of malnutrition used by UNICEF classifies the causes as immediate (individual level), underlying (household or family level), and basic (societal level) (Fig. 90.2) (221). A malnourished child has reduced immunity to infection and can have more severe and frequent episodes of illness. Illnesses such as diarrheal disease can reduce appetite, increase malabsorption of nutrients, and hasten losses of nutrients and thus further perpetuate a cycle of malnutrition and infection. On the level of the household, problems may exist with food security, that is, access to safe food of sufficient quality and quantity to ensure adequate health for all family members. The quality and quantity of food should meet the requirements for protein, energy, and micronutrients. Access to food can depend on financial, social, and physical access to food. Given the close relationship between malnutrition and infection, factors that affect hygiene on the household level, such as clean water and sanitation, will have an effect on malnutrition. Inadequate maternal and child

TABLE 90.2. SOME NOTABLE TRIALS OF ZINC SUPPLEMENTATION AND INFECTIOUS DISEASES

LOCATION	DATE	SUBJECTS	OBSERVATION	REFERENCE
India	1988	Infants	Reduced duration of diarrhea	209
The Gambia	1993	Children	Reduced malaria morbidity	69
India	1995	Infants	Reduced risk continued diarrhea	210
Vietnam	1996	Children	Reduced incidence diarrhea, pneumonia	103
Papua New Guinea	2000	Children	Reduced malaria morbidity	70
India	2001	Infants	Reduced mortality	99

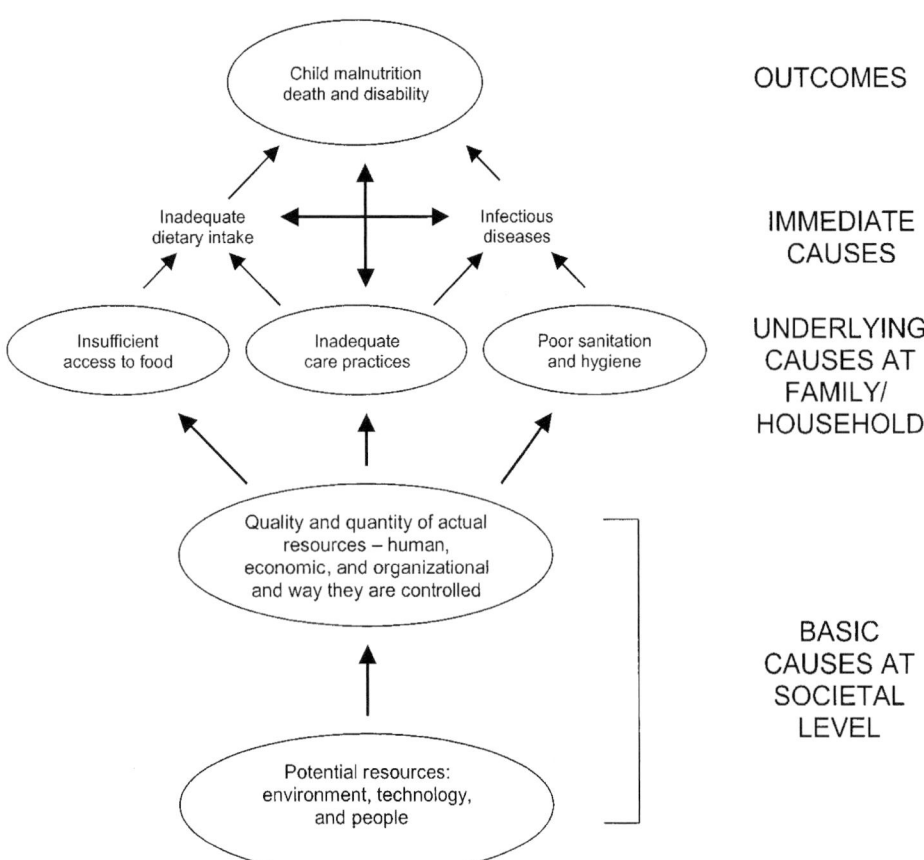

Figure 90.2. UNICEF conceptual framework of child malnutrition.

care practices are also an underlying household cause of malnutrition. Lack of or early cessation of breast-feeding, the lack of safe, high-quality complementary foods, withholding of food and liquids to a child with diarrhea, inadequate practices of food sharing at the table, poor knowledge of personal hygiene, and lack of immunizations are some specific examples of practices at the household level that are underlying causes of malnutrition (221). On the societal level, low status of women, inadequate health services, lack of jobs, and poverty are causes that underlie malnutrition.

The theoretic framework of UNICEF for the causes of malnutrition suggests multiple levels for interventions to reduce morbidity and mortality from infectious diseases. It also suggests that such strategies range from improved roads and sanitation, maternal education, and immunizations to food fortification and micronutrient supplementation.

REFERENCES

1. Sigerist HE. Bull Hist Med 1941;9:81–100.
2. Villermé LR. Des epidémies sous les rapportes de l'hygiène publique, de la statistique médicale et de l'économie politique. Paris, 1833.
3. Grijns G. Geneeskundig Tijdschrift Nederl Indië 1901;41:3.
4. Hopkins FG. Analyst 1906;31:385–404.
5. Funk C. J State Med 1912;20:341–68.
6. Carpenter KJ. J Nutr 2003;133:3023–32.
7. Osborne TB, Mendel LB. Feeding Experiments with Isolated Food-Substances. Publ. no. 156. Washington, DC: Carnegie Institute of Washington, 1911.
8. Osborne TB, Mendel LB. J Biol Chem 1913;15:311–26.
9. Mellanby E. Lancet 1926;1:515–9.
10. Sherman HC, Burtis MP. Proc Soc Exp Biol Med 1928;25:649–50.
11. Green HN, Mellanby E. BMJ 1928;2:691–6.
12. Bloch CE. Am J Dis Child 1924;27:139–48.
13. Ellison JB. BMJ 1932;2:708–11.
14. Semba RD. Nutrition 2003;19:390–4.
15. Semba RD. J Nutr 1999;129:783–91.
16. Heilbron IM, Jones WE, Bacharach AL. Vitam Horm 1944;2:155–13.
17. Todd WR, Elvehjem CA, Hart EB. Am J Physiol 1934;107:146–56.
18. Stirn FE, Elvehjem CA, Hart EB. J Biol Chem 1935;109:347–59.
19. Eggleton WGE. Biochem J 1939;33:403–6.
20. Eggleton WGE. Chin J Physiol 1940;15:33–44.
21. Prasad AS, Halsted JA, Nadimi M. Am J Med 1961;31:532–46.
22. Prasad AS, Miale A, Farid Z et al. J Lab Clin Med 1963;61:537–49.
23. Sandstead HH, Prasad AS, Schulert AR et al. Am J Clin Nutr 1967;20:422–42.
24. Barnes PM, Moynahan EJ. Proc R Soc Med 1973;66:327–9.
25. Julius R, Schulkind M, Sprinkle T et al. J Pediatr 1973;83:1007–11.
26. Endre L, Katona Z, Gyurkovits K. Lancet 1975;1:1196.
27. Oleske JM, Westphal ML, Shore S et al. Am J Dis Child 1979;133:915–8.
28. Bhutta ZA, Black RE, Brown KH et al. J Pediatr 1999;135:689–97.

29. Trousseau A, Pidoux H. Traité de thérapeutique et de matière médicale. 4th ed. Paris: Béchet Jeune, 1851.

30. Silverstein AM. A History of Immunology. San Diego: Academic Press, 1989.

31. Robertson EC. Medicine 1934;13:123–206.

32. Clausen SW. Physiol Rev 1934;14:309–50.

33. Williams CD. Arch Dis Child 1933;8:423–33.

34. McLaren DS. J Trop Pediatr 1956;2:135–40.

35. Scrimshaw NS, Taylor CE, Gordon JE. Interactions of Nutrition and Infection. Geneva: World Health Organization, 1968.

36. Semba RD, Bloem MW, eds. Nutrition and Health in Developing Countries. Totowa, NJ: Humana Press, 2001.

37. Gitlin JD, Colten HR. Molecular biology of the acute phase plasma proteins. In: Pick E, Landy M, eds. Lymphokines, vol 14. San Diego: Academic Press, 1987:123–53.

38. Gabay C, Kushner I. N Engl J Med 1999;340:448–54.

39. Fournier T, Medjoubi-N N, Porquet D. Biochim Biophys Acta 2000;1482:157–71.

40. Uhlar CM, Whitehead AS. Eur J Biochem 1999;265:501–23.

41. Langhans W. Nutrition 2000;16:996–1005.

42. Plata-Salamán CR. Int J Obes 2001;25[Suppl 5]:48S–52S.

43. Pelletier DG, Frongillo EA, Habicht JP. Am J Public Health 1993;83:1130–3.

44. World Health Organization. Wkly Epidemiol Rec 1998;50:389–96.

45. Perry RT, Halsey NA. J Infect Dis 2004;189[Suppl 1];4S–16S.

46. Griffin DE. Curr Top Microbiol Immunol 1995;191:117–34.

47. Tatsuo H, Ono N, Tanaka K et al. Nature 2000;406:893–7.

48. Dossetor J, Whittle HC, Greenwood BM. BMJ 1977;1:1633–5.

49. Chen LC, Rahman M, Sarder AM. Int J Epidemiol 1980;9:25–33.

50. Koster FT, Curlin GC, Aziz KM et al. Bull WHO 1981;59:901–8.

51. Smedman L, Lindeberg A, Jeppsson O et al. Ann Trop Paediatr 1983;3:169–76.

52. Alwar AJE. East Afr Med J 1992;69:415–8.

53. Manicus A. Ugeskrift Laeger 1847;6:189–210.

54. Semba RD, Bloem MW. Surv Ophthalmol 2004;49:243–55

55. Barclay AJG, Foster A, Sommer A. BMJ 1987;294:294–6.

56. Hussey GD, Klein M. N Engl J Med 1990;323:160–4.

57. Coutsoudis A, Broughton M, Coovadia HM. Am J Clin Nutr 1991;54:890–5.

58. Ogaro FO, Orinda VA, Onyango FE et al. Trop Geogr Med 1993;45:283–6.

59. Coutsoudis A, Kiepiela P, Coovadia HM et al. Pediatr Infect Dis J 1992;11:203–9.

60. Benn CS, Balde A, George E et al. Lancet 2002;359:1313–4.

61. Mahalanabis D, Chowdhury A, Jana S et al. Am J Clin Nutr 2002;76:604–7.

62. Phillips RS. Clin Microbiol Rev 2001;14:208–26.

63. Shankar AH. Malaria. In: Semba RD, Bloem MW, eds. Nutrition and Health in Developing Countries. Totowa, NJ: Humana Press, 2001:177–207.

64. Caulfield LE, Richard SA, Black RE. Am J Trop Med Hyg 2004;71[Suppl 2]:55–63.

65. Stürchler D, Tanner M, Hanck A et al. Acta Trop 1987;44:213–27.

66. Galan P, Samba C, Luzeau R et al. Int J Vit Nutr Res 1990;60:224–8.

67. Friis H, Mwaniki D, Omondi B et al. Am J Clin Nutr 1997;66:665–71.

68. Shankar AH, Genton B, Semba RD et al. Lancet 1999;354:203–9.

69. Bates CJ, Evans PH, Dardenne M et al. Br J Nutr 1993;69:243–55.

70. Shankar AH, Genton B, Baisor M et al. Am J Trop Med Hyg 2000;62:663–9.

71. Müller O, Becher H, van Zweeden AB et al. BMJ 2001;322:1–6.

72. Zinc Against Plasmodium Study Group. Am J Clin Nutr 2002;76:805–12.

73. Lanata CF, Black RE. Diarrheal diseases. In: Semba RD, Bloem MW, eds. Nutrition and Health in Developing Countries. Totowa, NJ: Humana Press: 2001:93–129.

74. Chen LC, Huq E, Huffman SL. Am J Epidemiol 1981;114:284–92.

75. Black RE, Brown KH, Becker S. Am J Clin Nutr 1984;39:87–94.

76. Baqui AH, Black RE, Sack RB et al. Am J Epidemiol 1993;137:355–65.

77. McLaren DS, Shirajian E, Tchalian M et al. Am J Clin Nutr 1965;17:117–30.

78. Doesschate JT. Causes of blindness in and around Surabaja, East Java, Indonesia. Doctoral thesis. University of Jakarta, Jakarta, Indonesia, 1968.

79. Sommer A. Nutritional Blindness: Xerophthalmia and Keratomalacia. New York: Oxford University Press, 1982.

80. Cohen N, Rahman H, Sprague J et al. World Health Stat Q 1985;38:317–30.

81. Khatry SK, West KP Jr, Katz J et al. Arch Ophthalmol 1995;113:425–9.

82. Schaumberg DA, O'Connor J, Semba RD. Eur J Clin Nutr 1996;50:761–4.

83. Beaton GH, Martorell R, L'Abbe KA et al. Effectiveness of Vitamin A Supplementation in the Control of Young Child Morbidity and Mortality in Developing Countries. ACC/SCN State-of-the-Art Nutrition Policy Discussion paper no. 13. New York: United Nations, 1993.

84. Sommer A, Tarwotjo I, Djunaedi E et al. Lancet 1986;1:1169–73.

85. Vijayaraghavan K, Radhaiah G, Prakasam BS et al. Lancet 1990;336:1342–5.

86. Rahmathullah L, Underwood BA, Thulasiraj RD et al. N Engl J Med 1990;323:929–35.

87. West KP Jr, Pokhrel RP, Katz J et al. Lancet 1991;338:67–71.

88. Kothari G. J Trop Pediatr 1991;37:141.

89. Daulaire NMP, Starbuck ES, Houston RM et al. BMJ 1992;304:207–10.

90. Ghana VAST Study Team. Lancet 1993;342:7–12.

91. Barreto ML, Santos LMP, Assis AMO et al. Lancet 1994;344:228–31.

92. Vitamin A and Pneumonia Working Group. Bull WHO 1995;73:609–19.

93. Filteau SM, Rollins NC, Coutsoudis A et al. J Pediatr Gastroenterol Nutr 2001;32:464–70.

94. Mitra AK, Alvarez JO, Guay–Woodford L et al. Am J Clin Nutr 1998;68:1095–103.

95. Kelly P, Musuku J, Kafwenbe E et al. Aliment Pharmacol Ther 2001;15:973–9.

96. Hossain S, Biswas R, Kabir I et al. BMJ 1998;316:422–6.

97. Black RE. J Nutr 2003;133:1485S–9S.

98. Zinc Investigators' Collaborative Group. J Pediatr 1999;135:689–97.

99. Sazawal S, Black RE, Menon VP et al. Pediatrics 2001;108:1280–6.

100. Kirkwood BR, Gove S, Rogers S et al. Bull WHO 1995;73:793–8.

101. Victora CG, Kirkwood BR, Ashworth A et al. Am J Clin Nutr 1999;70:309–20.

102. Lanata C, Black RE. Acute lower-respiratory infections. In: Semba RD, Bloem MW, eds. Nutrition and Health in Developing Countries. Totowa, NJ: Humana Press, 2001: 131–62.

103. Ninh NX, Thissen JP, Collette L et al. Am J Clin Nutr 1996;63:514–9.

104. Sazawal S, Black RE, Bhan MK et al. Am J Clin Nutr 1997;66:413–8.

105. Sazawal S, Black RE, Jalla S et al. Pediatrics 1998;102:1–5.

106. Meeks-Gardner J, Witter MM, Ramdath DD. Eur J Clin Nutr 1998;52:34–9.

107. Penny ME, Peerson JM, Marin RM. J Pediatr 1999;135:208–17.

108. Bhandari N, Bahl R, Taneja S. BMJ 2002;324:1358–60.

109. Mahalanabis D, Lahiri M, Paul D et al. Am J Clin Nutr 2004;79:430–6.

110. Brooks WA, Yunus M, Santosham M, et al. Lancet 2004;363:1683–8.

111. Pawlowski ZS, Schad GA, Stott GJ. Hookworm Infection and Anemia: Approaches to Prevention and Control. Geneva: World Health Organization, 1991.

112. Loukas A, Prociv P. Clin Microbiol Rev 2001;14:689–703.

113. Hotez PJ, Brooker S, Bethony JM et al. N Engl J Med 2004;351:799–807.

114. Smillie WG, Augustine DL. Am J Dis Child 1926;31:151–68.

115. Smillie WG, Augustine DL. South Med J 1926;19:19–28.

116. Smillie WG, Spencer CR. J Educ Psychol 1926;17:314–21.

117. Waite JH, Neilson IL. JAMA 1919;73:1877–9.

118. Strong EK. Effects of Hookworm Disease on the Mental and Physical Development of Children. Rockefeller Foundation International Health Commission publ. no. 3. New York: Rockefeller Foundation, 1916.

119. Semba RD. Nutrition: epidemiology and public health overview. In: Ward JW, Warren C, eds. A Safer and Healthier America: The Advancement of Public Health in the 20th Century. New York: Oxford University Press, 2005.

120. Stoltzfus RJ, Albonico M, Chwaya HM et al. Am J Clin Nutr 1998;68:179–86.

121. Stephenson LS, Latham MC, Kurz KM et al. Am J Trop Med Hyg 1989;41:78–87.

122. Boivin MJ, Giordani B. J Pediatr Psychol 1993;18:249–64.

123. Dossa RA, Ategbo EA, de Koning FL et al. Eur J Clin Nutr 2001;55:223–8.

124. UNAIDS. AIDS Epidemic Update. December 2004.

125. Semba RD, Tang AM. Br J Nutr 1999;81:181–9.

126. Castetbon K, Kadio A, Bondurand A et al. Eur J Clin Nutr 1997;51:81–6.

127. McCorkindale C, Dybevik K, Coulston AM et al. J Am Diet Assoc 1990;90:1236–41.

128. Tang AM, Graham NMH, Kirby AJ et al. Am J Epidemiol 1993;138:937–51.

129. Baum M, Cassetti L, Bonvehi P et al. Nutrition 1994;10:16–20.

130. Baum MK, Shor-Posner G, Bonvehi P et al. Ann NY Acad Sci 1992;669:165–73.

131. Sharpstone D, Gazzard B. Lancet 1996;348:379–83.

132. Kotler DP, Gaetz HP, Lange M et al. Ann Intern Med 1984;101:421–8.

133. Keating J, Bjarnason I, Somasundaram S et al. Gut 1995;37:623–9.

134. Stockmann M, Fromm M, Schmitz H et al. AIDS 1998;12:43–51.

135. Semba RD, Miotti PG, Chiphangwi JD et al. Lancet 1994;343:1593–7.

136. Phuapradit W, Chaturachinda K, Taneepanichskul S et al. Obstet Gynecol 1996;87:564–7.

137. Semba RD, Ndugwa C, Perry RT et al. Nutrition 2005 (in press).

138. Tang AM, Smit E. Vitamins C and E, and HIV infection. In: Friis H, ed. Micronutrients and HIV Infection. Boca Raton, FL: CRC Press, 2000:111–33.

139. Beach RS, Mantero-Atienza E, Shor-Posner G et al. AIDS 1992;6:701–8.

140. Tang AM, Graham NMH, Chandra RK et al. J Nutr 1997;127:345–51.

141. Paltiel O, Falutz J, Veilleux M et al. Am J Hematol 1995;49:318–22.

142. Boudes P, Zittoun J, Sobel A. Lancet 1990;335:1401–2.

143. Semba RD, Kumwenda N, Hoover DR et al. Eur J Clin Nutr 2000;54:872–7.

144. Semba RD, Shah N, Strathdee SA et al. J Acquir Immune Defic Syndr Hum Retrovirol 2002;29:142–4.

145. Mueller BU, Tannenbaum S, Pizzo PA. J Pediatr Hematol Oncol 1996;18:266–71.

146. Totin D, Ndugwa C, Mmiro F et al. J Nutr 2002;132:423–9.

147. Koch J, Neal EA, Schlott MJ et al. Nutrition 1996;12:515–8.

148. Mantero-Atienza E, Sotomayor MG, Shor-Posner G et al. Nutr Res 1991;11:1237–50.

149. Semba RD. Nutr Rev 1998;56[Suppl 2]:38S–48S.

150. Shankar AH, Prasad AS. Am J Clin Nutr 1998;68[Suppl 2]:447S–63S.

151. Baum MK, Shor-Posner G, Lu Y et al. AIDS 1995;9:1051–6.

152. Semba RD, Graham NMH, Caiaffa WT et al. Arch Intern Med 1993;153:2149–54.

153. Semba RD, Miotti P, Chiphangwi JD et al. J Acquir Immune Defic Syndr Hum Retrovirol 1997;14:219–22.

154. Tang AM, Graham NMH, Semba RD et al. AIDS 1997:11:613–20.

155. Tang AM, Graham NM, Chandra RK et al. J Nutr 1997;127:345–51.

156. Falutz J, Tsoukas C, Gold P. JAMA 1988;259:2850–1.

157. Graham NMH, Sorensen D, Odaka N et al. J Acquir Immune Defic Syndr Hum Retrovirol 1991;4:976–80.

158. Baum MK, Shor-Posner G, Lai S et al. J Acquir Immune Defic Syndr Hum Retrovirol 1997;15:370–4.

159. Campa A, Shor-Posner G, Indacochea F et al. J Acquir Immune Defic Syndr Hum Retrovirol 1999;20:508–13.

160. Kupka R, Msamanga GI, Spiegelman D et al. J Nutr 2004;134:2556–60.

161. Fawzi WW, Msamanga GI, Spiegelman D et al N Engl J Med 2004;351:23–32.

162. Fawzi WW, Msamanga GI, Spiegelman D et al. Lancet 1998;351:1477–82.

163. Coutsoudis A, Pillay K, Spooner E et al. AIDS 1999;13:1517–24.

164. Kumwenda N, Miotti PG, Taha TE et al. Clin Inf Dis 2002;35:618–24.

165. Allard JP, Aghdassi E, Chau J et al. AIDS 1998;12:1653–9.

166. Frieden TR, Sterling TR, Munsiff SS et al. Lancet 2003;362:887–99.

167. Raviglione MC, Snider DE, Kochi A. JAMA 1995;273:220–6.

168. Toossi Z. Infect Agents Dis 1996;5:98–107.

169. Takashima T, Ueta C, Tsuyuguchi I et al. Infect Immun 1990;58:3286–92.

170. Wallis RS, Vjecha M, Amir-Tahmasseb M et al. J Infect Dis 1993;167:43–8.

171. Ogawa T, Uchida H, Kusumoto Y et al. Infect Immun 1991;59:3021–5.

172. Hirsch CS, Hussain R, Toossi Z et al. Proc Natl Acad Sci USA 1996;93:3193–8.

173. Toossi Z, Gogate P, Shiratsuchi H et al. J Immunol 1995;54:465–73.

174. Kindler V, Sappino AP, Grau GE et al. Cell 1989;56:731–40.

175. Valone SE, Rich EA, Wallis RS et al. Infect Immun 1988;56:3313–5.

176. Nkhoma WA, Harries AD, Reeve PA et al. East Afr Med J 1987; 64:643–7.

177. Harries AD, Nkhoma WA, Thompson PJ et al. Eur J Clin Nutr 1988;42:445–50.

178. Kennedy N, Ramsay A, Uiso L et al. Trans R Soc Trop Med Hyg 1996;90:162–6.

179. Onwubalili JK. Eur J Clin Nutr 1988;42:363–6.

180. Macallan DC, McNurlan MA, Kurpad AV et al. Clin Sci 1998; 94:321–31.

181. Paton NI, Castello–Branco LR, Jenning G et al. J Acquir Immune Defic Syndr Hum Retrovirol 1999;20:265–71.

182. Shah S, Whalen C, Kotler DP et al. J Nutr 2001;131:2843–7.

183. Chan J, Tian Y, Tanaka KE et al. Proc Natl Acad Sci USA 1996; 93:14857–61.

184. Doherty ML, Monaghan ML, Bassett HF et al. Vet Immunol Immunopathol 1996;49:307–20.

185. Bartow RA, McMurray DN. Infect Immun 1990;58:1843–7.

186. McMurray DN, Bartow RA. J Nutr 1992;122:738–43.

187. Van Lettow M, Fawzi WW, Semba RD. Nutr Rev 2003;61:81–90.

188. Solotorovsky M, Squibb RL, Wogan GN et al. Am Rev Respir Dis 1961; 84:226–35.

189. Ferraro F, Mattei M, Colizzi V. Z Erkrank Atm Org 1988;171: 45–9.

190. Downes J. Milbank Mem Fund Q 1950;28:127–59.

191. Semba RD. Vitamin A. In: Hughes DA, Bendich A, Darlington LG, eds. Dietary Enhancement of Human Immune Function. Totowa, NJ: Humana Press, 2003.

192. Zhao Z, Murasko DM, Ross AC. Nat Immun 1994;13:29–41.

193. Twining SS, Schulte DP, Wilson PM et al. J Nutr 1996;127: 558–65.

194. Semba RD, Muhilal, Ward BJ et al. Lancet 1993;341:5–8.

195. Wiedermann U, Hanson LA, Kahu H et al. Immunology 1993; 80:581–6.

196. Smith SM, Hayes CE. Proc Natl Acad Sci USA 1987;84: 5878–82.

197. Semba RD, Muhilal, Scott AL et al. J Nutr 1992;122:101–7.

198. Rahman MM, Mahalanabis D, Hossain S et al. J Nutr 1999;129:2192–5.

199. Pasatiempo AMG, Bowman TA, Taylor CE et al. Am J Clin Nutr 1989;49:501–10.

200. West KP Jr, Katz J, Khatry SK et al. BMJ 1999;318:570–5.

201. Briggs WA, Pedersen MM, Mahajan SK et al. Kidney Int 1982; 21:827–32.

202. Allen JI, Perri RT, McClain CJ et al. J Lab Clin Med 1983;102: 577–89.

203. Sempertegui F, Estrella B, Correa E et al. Eur J Clin Nutr 1996;50:42–6.

204. Lira PIC, Ashworth A, Morris SS. Am J Clin Nutr 1998;68 [Suppl]:418S–24S.

205. Sazawal S, Jalla S, Mazumder S et al. Indian Pediatr 1997;34: 589–97.

206. Beck FWJ, Kaplan J, Fine N et al. J Lab Clin Med 1997;130: 147–56.

207. Ibs KH, Rink L. J Nutr 2003;133:1452S–6S.

208. Prasad AS. J Infect Dis 2000;182[Suppl 1]:62S–8S.

209. Sachdev HPS, Mittal NK, Mittal SK et al. J Pediatr Gastroenterol Nutr 1998;7:877–8.

210. Sazawal S, Black RE, Bhan MK, et al. N Engl J Med 1995;333: 839–44.

211. Kuvibidila S, Baliga BS: Role of iron in immunity and infection. In: Calder PC, Field CJ, Gill HS, eds. Nutrition and Immune Function. Oxon, UK: CAB International, 2002:209–228.

212. Murakawa H, Bland CE, Willis WT et al. Blood 1987;69: 1464–8.

213. Farthing MJG. Acta Paediatr Scand Suppl 1989;361:44–52.

214. Gera T, Sachdev HPS. BMJ 2002;325:1142–51.

215. Bagchi K, Mohanram M, Reddy V. BMJ 1980;280:1249–51.

216. Clark TD, Semba RD. Med Hypotheses 2001;57:476–9.

217. McKenzie R, Arthur JR, Miller SM et al. Selenium and the immune system. In: Calder PC, Gill HS, eds. Nutrition and Immune Function. Wallingford, UK: CAB International, 2002: 229–50.

218. Beck MA, Shi Q, Morris et al. Nat Med 1995;1:433–6.

219. Calder PC, Field CJ. Fatty acids, inflammation and immunity. In: Calder PC, Field CJ, Gill HS, eds. Nutrition and Immune Function, Oxon,UK: CAB International, 2002:57–92.

220. Hughes DA. Carotenoids. In: Hughes DA, Darlington LG, Bendich A, eds. Diet and Human Immune Function. Totowa, NJ: Humana Press, 2004:165–83.

221. UNICEF. The State of the World's Children 1998. New York: Oxford University Press, 1998.

SELECTED READINGS

Hughes DA, Darlington LG, Bendich A, eds. Diet and Human Immune Function. Totowa, NJ: Humana Press, 2004.

Keusch GT. The history of nutrition: Malnutrition, infection and immunity. J Nutr 2003;133:336S–40S.

McLaren DS, Frigg M. Sight and Life Manual on Vitamin A Deficiency Disorders (VADD). 2nd ed. Basel: Task Force Sight and Life, 2001.

Pelletier DL, Frongillo EA. Changes in child survival are strongly associated with changes in malnutrition in developing countries. J Nutr 2003;133:107–19.

Semba RD, Bloem MW, eds. Nutrition and Health in Developing Countries. Totowa, NJ: Humana Press, 2001.

Walker CF, Black RE. Zinc and the risk for infectious disease. Annu Rev Nutr 2004;24:255–75.

91

NUTRITION IN THE CARE OF THE PATIENT WITH SURGERY, TRAUMA, AND SEPSIS[1]

KENNETH A. KUDSK AND GORDON S. SACKS

HISTORY OF NUTRITION SUPPORT 1415
IDENTIFICATION OF THE AT-RISK SURGICAL PATIENT .1415
    Trauma Patients 1415
    General Surgical Patients 1417
PHYSIOLOGIC RESPONSE TO SURGERY AND INJURY .1418
    Intermediary Metabolism Changes: Protein 1419
    Fat 1419
    Glucose 1420
    Cytokine Mediators of Metabolic Responses 1420
NUTRITIONAL REQUIREMENTS 1420
    Estimating Total Caloric Requirements 1420
    Glucose Requirements 1421
    Protein Requirements 1421
    Fat Requirements 1422
    Vitamin Requirements 1422
    Trace Element Requirements 1423
ROUTES OF NUTRITION SUPPORT 1424
    Enteral Route 1424
    Perioperative Nutrition Support 1424
ROLE OF GUT IN HOST DEFENSE 1424
TYPES OF NUTRIENT DIET 1425
    Enteral Diet 1425
    Parenteral Diet 1428
MONITORING NUTRITION SUPPORT THERAPY 1431
ANABOLIC AGENTS 1431
    Human Growth Hormone 1431
    Insulinlike Growth Factor-I 1432
    Oxandrolone 1433

Nutrition plays an important and integral role in the preoperative and postoperative preparation of patients undergoing major general surgical procedures and in the support of severely injured patients. In general, when applied to select populations of patients undergoing major general surgical procedures, nutrition support has been shown to reduce the complications of major wound complications such as wound dehiscence and anastomotic leak. When nutrition support is provided enterally, an added benefit in the reduction of septic complications has been well documented. In trauma patients with severe injuries, the use of postinjury enteral support has been shown to reduce the risk of septic complications in particular. Nutrition does not play a key role in the treatment of sepsis per se, but rather in the prevention of sepsis following anastomotic and wound dehiscence or the development of pneumonia or intraabdominal abscesses. The role of nutrition in the treatment of septic complications is not well defined, but it is clear that it reduces the subsequent development of complications. The key issues are the appropriate use of the technique and, in particular, choice of the appropriate patient population for this complicated, sophisticated therapy. Specialized forms of nutrition support have the potential for causing injury as well as providing benefit. When these therapies are used in patients who are not at risk of wound or septic complications, only the complications of therapy are seen. However, when the therapy is applied to patients who have an increased risk of wound failure or septic complications, nutrition appears to reduce these complications.

The field of nutrition support constitutes specialized delivery of nutrients to patients unable to take adequate oral intake. Nutrition support is delivered either intravenously through centrally placed catheters with infusion of concentrated formulas containing macronutrients and micronutrients or enterally via tubes placed either into the stomach or small bowel to bypass postoperative gastric atony or small

[1] **Abbreviations: AAG,** α_1-acid glycoprotein; **ADH,** antidiuretic hormone; **ALB,** albumin; **APACHE,** Acute Physiology and Chronic Health Evaluation; **ARDS,** acute respiratory distress syndrome; **ATI,** abdominal trauma index; **BCAA,** branched-chain amino acids; **BEE,** basal energy expenditure; **CRP,** C-reactive protein; **DH,** delayed hypersensitivity; **FDA,** US Food and Drug Administration; **GCS,** Glasgow Coma Scale; **GH,** growth hormone; **hGH,** human growth hormone; **ICU,** intensive care unit; **Ig,** immunoglobulin; **IGF-I,** insulinlike growth factor-I; **IGFBP-3,** insulinlike growth factor binding protein-3; **IL,** interleukin; **ISS,** injury severity score; **IVLE,** intravenous lipid emulsion; **LCFA,** long-chain fatty acids; **LCT,** long-chain triglycerides; **MAdCAM-1,** mucosal addressin cellular adhesion molecule; **MCFA,** medium-chain fatty acid; **MCT,** medium-chain triglycerides; **NCJ,** needle catheter jejunostomy; **PN,** parenteral nutrition; **PINI,** Prognostic Inflammatory and

Nutritional Index; **PNI,** Prognostic Nutritional Index; **PUFA,** polyunsaturated fatty acid; **RDA,** recommended dietary allowance; **rGH,** recombinant growth hormone; **RQ,** respiratory quotient; **$t_{1/2}$,** half-life; **TFN,** transferrin; **TNF,** tumor necrosis factor; **TPN,** total parenteral nutrition; **TSF,** triceps skinfold thickness.

bowel ileus in the preoperative and postoperative periods. Although techniques for intragastric feeding have been available for hundreds of years, parenteral nutrition (PN) is a relatively new, highly technical field, which rapidly advanced during the 1970s. The goals of nutrition support are to prevent further deterioration of nutritional status, to replenish host defenses and lean tissue, to improve clinical outcome, and to support adjunctive therapies, which would otherwise be impossible in a catabolic, malnourished patient.

Many patients could not survive their illness without specialized nutrition support. Patients with total or near-total intestinal loss as a result of infarction or following multiple resections, malnourished patients with chronic inflammatory mucosal disease that interferes with normal absorption, or patients with fistulas that preclude ingestion of adequate oral nutrition are specific examples. Definite indications for many patients are less clear, particularly when no preexisting malnutrition exists and they are likely to resume adequate oral intake within a relatively short period. However, evidence indicates that preemptive nutritional therapy reduces the risk of subsequent complications in some patient populations. Active work is currently pursuing the identification of those specific patient populations who will benefit. This is important because complex specialized nutritional therapy carries the potential of risk as well as of benefit. Despite somewhat meager evidence for use of nutrition support in some patients, however, this therapy is prescribed because of the well-established relationship between severe malnutrition and morbidity and mortality, the high rate of protein malnutrition in hospitalized patients, the recognition that prolonged starvation further impairs nutritional vigor and reduces the ability to heal, and generalization of well-designed clinical trials demonstrating benefit in at-risk patient populations. Although nutrition support carries its own risks and benefits, risks are minimized and benefits magnified when experienced professionals deliver this complex technical therapy to appropriate patient populations.

HISTORY OF NUTRITION SUPPORT

Contemporary nutrition therapy can be traced back to the 1700s, when Hunter (1) administered intragastric feeding with an eelskin-covered whalebone. Small-bore feeding tubes appeared in the early 1950s to administer blenderized foods. In the early 1900s, intravenous fat, carbohydrate, protein, and alcohol infusions were attempted, but extensive dilution (needed to avoid venous thrombosis) frequently caused congestive heart failure and fluid overload. After the introduction of the subclavian catheter (2), Dudrick and colleagues (3) successfully administered hypertonic solutions into the central circulation, where these solutions were rapidly diluted by the blood flow. The technique provided adequate macronutrients and micronutrients to support nutritional needs. Early experience led to

identification of severe, potentially fatal complications including severe hyperglycemia, the refeeding syndrome, and trace metal deficiencies. Early advocates noted that patients who would otherwise have died, particularly those with fistulas, survived with therapy, underwent successful surgical procedures, and left the hospital alive (4).

In the late 1970s, research interest in the use of the gastrointestinal tract for nutrient administration was renewed. Early experimental work demonstrated increased susceptibility to infections when the gut was not fed (5, 6). These findings were later confirmed in studies of trauma patients and were reconfirmed in other surgical populations (7–11). Since then, the bias has swung toward delivery of nutrients via the gastrointestinal tract when feasible, to avoid immunologic and metabolic complications associated with PN.

Current work focuses on the pharmacologic effect of specialized nutrients administered either parenterally or enterally in support of specific immunologic and healing properties. These specialized nutrients can help—or hurt—depending on the individual patient's condition. Researchers are defining specific patient populations, designing specialized formulas that may be patient-population specific, and developing new techniques to administer these agents.

IDENTIFICATION OF THE AT-RISK SURGICAL PATIENT

Identification of the at-risk surgical patient is limited by the tools available. Several scoring systems quantify the risk of post injury complications, particularly septic complications in severely injured patients sustaining blunt or penetrating trauma. These systems have successfully allowed stratification by risk in nutritional studies. In multiple trials, enteral nutrition support, using formulas with or without specialty pharmacologic nutrients, improves outcome by reducing septic complications compared with fasted or parenterally fed patients (7–12). Nutritionally, trauma patients are not traditionally considered "at risk" because most are young and well nourished, although alcohol and drug abuse is not uncommon. General surgical patients, those with preexisting nutritional deficits, have been more difficult to stratify because scoring systems are not readily applied. Several general principles exist. Preoperative albumin (ALB) is the single best indicator of postoperative complications and mortality following general surgery (13). Unfortunately, ALB levels may reflect liver disease, fluid resuscitation, or inflammation, rather than nutritional status. However, nutritional risk is still possible using parameters such as weight loss and serum protein levels.

Trauma Patients

Specific nutritional therapy improves clinical outcome in trauma patients with critical injuries. In most studies, the

Injury Severity Score (ISS) (14), Abdominal Trauma Index (ATI) (15), or a combination of the two has been used to stratify patients according to complication risk. The ISS scores the three most severely injured body regions of six: head and neck, musculoskeletal, soft tissue, abdominal, thoracic, and head. The ISS correlates best with mortality, but also with morbidity. In randomized prospective studies, patients with an ISS greater than 18 to 20 have improved outcome with early enteral feeding compared with PN or fasting.

The ISS, however, underestimates risk from severe injuries isolated to one body area. The ATI is effective in identification of patients with serious intraabdominal injures who are at risk of subsequent infectious complications (Table 91.1) (15). Each intraabdominal organ carries its own risk factor (see Table 91.1) that, when multiplied

TABLE 91.1 CALCULATED RISK OF SEPSIS BY THE ABDOMINAL TRAUMA INDEX[a]

ORGAN INJURED	RISK FACTOR	SCORING	ORGAN INJURED	RISK FACTOR	SCORING
HIGH RISK			**LOW RISK**		
Pancreas	(5)	1. Tangential 2. Through-and-through (duct intact) 3. Major débridement or distal duct injury 4. Proximal duct injury 5. Pancreaticoduodenectomy	Kidney	(2)	1. Nonbleeding 2. Minor débridement or suturing 3. Major débridement 4. Pedicle or major calyceal 5. Nephrectomy
Large intestine	(5)	1. Serosal 2. Single wall 3. ≤25% wall 4. >25% wall 5. Colon wall and blood supply	Ureter	(2)	1. Contusion 2. Laceration 3. Minor débridement 4. Segmental resection 5. Reconstruction
Major vascular	(5)	1. ≤25% wall 2. >25% wall 3. Complete transection 4. Interposition grafting or bypass 5. Ligation	Bladder	(1)	1. Single wall 2. Through-and-through 3. Débridement 4. Wedge resection 5. Reconstruction
MODERATE-HIGH RISK					
Duodenum	(4)	1. Single wall 2. ≤25% wall 3. >25% wall 4. Duodenal wall and blood supply 5. Pancreaticoduodenectomy	Extrahepatic biliary	(1)	1. Contusion 2. Cholescystectomy 3. ≤25% wall 4. >25% wall 5. Biliary enteric reconstruction
Liver	(4)	1. Nonbleeding peripheral 2. Bleeding, central, or minor débridement 3. Major débridement or hepatic artery ligation 4. Lobectomy 5. Lobectomy with caval repair or extensive bilobar débridement	Bone	(1)	1. Periosteum 2. Cortex 3. Through-and-through 4. Intraarticular 5. Major bone loss
MODERATE RISK					
Stomach	(3)	1. Single wall 2. Through-and-through 3. Minor débridement 4. Wedge resection 5. >35% resection	Small bowel	(1)	1. Single wall 2. Through-and-though 3. ≤25% wall 4. >25% wall 5. Wall and blood supply or >5 injuries
Spleen	(3)	1. Nonbleeding 2. Cautery or hemostatic agent 3. Minor débridement or suturing 4. Partial resection 5. Splenectomy	Minor vascular	(1)	1. Nonbleeding small hematoma 2. Nonbleeding large hematoma 3. Suturing 4. Ligation of isolated vessels 5. Ligation of named vessels

[a]The abdominal trauma index is calculated by multiplying the risk of sepsis (column 2) by the severity of injury (column 3) for each individual organ injured and summing the individual scores for all injuries.

Adapted from references 8 and 15 and reprinted from Kudsk K, Brown R. In: Moore EE, Feliciano DV, Mattox KI eds. Trauma. 4th ed. New York: McGraw-Hill, 2000, with permission.

by the magnitude of that organ's injury, correlates with likelihood of sepsis from that injury. Injuries to the pancreas, colon, major vascular structures, duodenum, and liver pose the highest risk. The ATI can be rapidly calculated during celiotomy by summing the risk factors of each individual organ injury. Patients with an ATI greater than 20 to 25 are at greatest risk of subsequent septic complications. However, even with ATI values less than 20, the simultaneous presence of serious extraabdominal injuries such as severe pulmonary contusion, multiple rib fractures, closed head injury with a Glasgow Coma Scale score (GCS) of 6, spinal cord injury, major soft tissue injuries requiring repeated surgical therapy, or multiple lower extremity fractures identify the high-risk patient population. Most of these patients have an ISS greater than 20. With an ATI greater than 20 to 25 or an ISS of more than 18 to 20, early enteral nutrition is tolerated in most patients, and it improves clinical outcome by maintaining host defenses and reducing septic complications to shorten the hospital stay (9, 12).

General Surgical Patients

Nutritional status is a continuum ranging from the well-nourished patient to the cachexic patient. Severely malnourished patients are most likely to develop wound dehiscence, infections, anastomotic leaks, and other complications. Several techniques of nutritional assessment can estimate the place of a patient on this nutritional spectrum.

The simplest, most effective screening technique involves an adequate history and physical examination with identification of unintentional weight loss. A strong correlation exists between deterioration in protein states and postoperative complications after gastrointestinal surgery (16). Unintentional weight loss of greater than 10% over the past 6 months or more than 20% in the presence of increased metabolic requirements indicates nutritional risk. Two calculations are commonly used (17):

$$\% \text{ body weight loss} = \frac{\text{usual weight} - \text{current weight}}{\text{usual weight}} \times 100$$

or

$$\% \text{ usual body weight} = \frac{\text{current body weight}}{\text{usual body weight}} \times 100$$

Other symptoms such as abdominal pain, chronic diarrhea, anorexia, or lethargy usually accompany these clinical changes in weight. Anthropometric measurements with weight and height have compared patients with population norms, but an indepth medical history is usually adequate. Skinfold thickness to determine fat mass, urinary collection to assess a creatinine-height index, and other specific techniques such as delayed cutaneous hypersensitivity to a battery of antigens are no longer common practice (18–20). Assessments of immunologic status with total peripheral lymphocyte count or lymphocyte transformation are not specific for nutritional deficiencies and are confounded by severe injury.

Laboratory tests may confirm preexisting malnutrition. Protein-calorie malnutrition decreases ALB synthesis, but simultaneous decreases in protein degradation can maintain adequate serum levels. This is seen in marasmus when both protein and calorie intake are severely restricted, such as in patients with esophageal obstruction. Lowered levels of constitutive transport proteins such as ALB ($[t_{1/2}]$ = 21 days), transferrin (TFN; $t_{1/2}$ = 8 days), or thyroxin-binding prealbumin ($t_{1/2}$ = 2–3 days) may reflect the degree of malnutrition (21). However, inflammatory conditions (e.g., trauma, diverticulitis, sepsis, peritonitis) increase serum interleukin-6 (IL-6), which stimulates the acute-phase protein response (22). This response stimulates C-reactive protein (CRP) and α_1-acid glycoprotein (AAG) production while inhibiting constitutive protein production. Therefore, initial serum protein assessment should include CRP along with ALB or prealbumin to determine the influence of inflammation. Low ALB or prealbumin concentrations with a low CRP more likely indicate preexisting malnutrition; elevated CRP with depressed ALB and prealbumin may reflect inflammation, protein-calorie malnutrition, or both.

Combinations of these parameters have been used in predictive models to quantify the risk of postoperative complications. The Prognostic Nutritional Index (PNI) (23) correlates with the incidence of complications as follows:

$$\text{PNI } (\%) = 158 - 16.6 \, (\text{ALB}) - 0.78 \, (\text{TSF}) - 0.20 \, (\text{TFN}) - 5.8 \, (\text{DH})$$

where PNI is the percentage of risk of complication, ALB is serum ALB in g/dL, TSF is the triceps skinfold thickness in mm, TFN is the serum TFN in mg/dL, and DH is delayed hypersensitivity reactive to one of three recall antigens. With DH, 0 is nonreactive, 1 represents less than 5 mm of induration, and 2 represents more than 5 mm of induration. Because DH is no longer commonly used, an alternative uses a lymphocyte score of 0 to 2 where 0 means fewer than 1000 total lymphocytes/mm^3, 1 signifies 1000 to 2000/mm^3, and 2 represents more than 2000/mm^3. The equation is most affected by ALB and is susceptible to nonnutritional factors that reduce ALB, such as inflammation, preexisting liver disease, and edema. The PNI predicts the complication rate better than ALB alone (24).

The Prognostic Inflammatory and Nutritional Index (PINI) (25) correlates recovery with a ratio of acute-phase protein levels to constitutive protein levels as follows:

$$\text{PINI} = \frac{\text{CRP} \times \text{AAG}}{\text{PA} \times \text{ALB}}$$

CRP, AAG, and prealbumin are measured in mg/dL, whereas ALB is measured in g/dL. The result correlates well with outcome. Because the AAG elevation and ALB depression are prolonged and are slow to recover, CRP and prealbumin responses reflect patient recovery. However, sensitivity and specificity are lost when AAG and ALB are not included in the PINI.

The subjective global assessment (26, 27) evaluates nutritional status by examining changes in organ function, changes in body composition, the disease process, and the restriction of nutrient intake. Interobserver variability is good in its predictive value. It is more valuable than anthropometric measurements (which also correlate with a degree of malnutrition), which suffers from significant interobserver variability and influences of hydration state and age.

Although no current standard exists to determine nutritional status, a complete history and physical examination, determination of body weight changes, and the use of selected serum tests can identify patients at risk of nutrition-related complications. Preoperative protein levels and the degree of stress are complementary factors in risk assessment.

Some of the most stressful gastrointestinal operations are esophagectomy and pancreatic procedures. Complications increase as preoperative ALB levels drop in elective surgery on these organs (Fig. 91.1) (28). Patients undergoing esophagectomy with ALB levels lower than 3.5 g/dL, or pancreatic or gastric operations with an ALB level lower than

3.25 g/dL, have a significantly increased risk of major postoperative complications that increases as ALB levels drop. Further work will determine whether additional markers improve the ability to predict complications when correlated with the degree of surgical stress. This will allow improved stratification for preoperative intervention studies.

PHYSIOLOGIC RESPONSE TO SURGERY AND INJURY

The body produces a characteristic response to any injury such as trauma, elective surgery, or inflammation (29–32). The less the insult, the more blunted and short-lived the response will be, whereas the greater the injury, the more prolonged and severe the response will be, particularly if complications ensue. The response increases metabolic rate, glucocorticoid and catecholamine secretion, proinflammatory cytokine production, and water retention. Water retention and lower urinary output result from augmented vasopressin and mineralocorticoid secretion as well as from increases in interstitial edema caused by increased permeability. Uncomplicated postoperative recovery results in diuresis of this fluid on the third to the fourth postoperative day as the endocrine response abates. Hyperglycemia results from catecholamine suppression of insulin secretion by the pancreas (the central effect) and inhibited uptake of glucose by peripheral tissues in response to circulating insulin levels (the peripheral effect).

It is believed that each response provides a specific benefit such as salt and water retention to maintain blood volume, increased hepatic glucose production to provide adequate fuel, and mobilization of amino acids for gluconeogenesis, hepatic protein production, fibroblast proliferation, and immunologic upregulation. The changes accelerate catabolism of protein, especially muscle protein. Catecholamines stimulate hepatic glycogenolysis and gluconeogenesis. Cortisol stimulates glycogenolysis, gluconeogenesis, and muscle proteolysis and potentiates effects of catecholamines in the liver.

Other hormones are secreted in response to injury. Arginine vasopressin (formerly known as antidiuretic hormone [ADH]), increases water absorption and stimulates hepatic glycogenolysis and gluconeogenesis. Glucagon levels increase to augment glycolysis, lipolysis, and gluconeogenesis. Insulinlike growth factor-I (IGF-I) and growth hormone (GH) are depressed, and this induces an imbalance in regulatory hormones leading to reduced anabolic hormone and accelerated lean tissue loss. In addition, concomitant immobilization produces significant decreases in muscle mass because exercise is a fundamental determinant of muscle mass. Even without injury, protein loss resulting from complete immobilization continues for approximately 3 weeks even with adequate nutrition (33).

The stress response differs from starvation without injury (34, 35). Starvation reduces energy expenditure and increases lipogenesis and ketone body production. It does

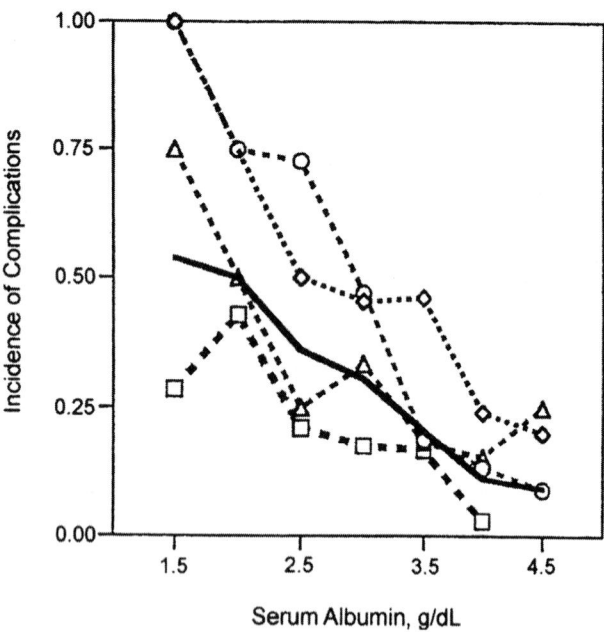

Figure 91.1. Complications increase as albumin levels drop in surgical populations (*solid line*). Complication rates, however, vary by surgical procedure. Patients undergoing esophageal (*squares connected by dots*) and pancreatic (*circles connected by dots*) procedures have developed complications at a higher rate at the same albumin level compared with patients undergoing gastric (*triangles connected by dashed lines*) or colon (*squares connected by dashed lines*) procedures. (From Kudsk KA, Tolley EA, DeWitt C et al. Preoperative albumin and surgical site identifies surgical risk of major post-operative complications. JPEN Parenter Enteral Nutr 203;27:1–9, with permission from the American Society for Parenteral and Enteral Nutrition [ASPEN]. ASPEN does not endorse the use of this material of any form other than its entirety.)

not generate an acute-phase protein response. Stress increases energy expenditure, accelerates hepatic protein production, stimulates the acute-phase protein response, and accelerates proteolysis with no ketone body production. Fatty acids, ketone bodies, and glycerol are the primary energy substrates in starvation meeting 95% of entry needs. In stress, amino acids are a more important source of glucose production through hepatic gluconeogenesis. Protein provides 15 to 20% of energy, whereas fat provides 80 to 85%.

Intermediary Metabolism Changes: Protein

Injury increases protein synthesis and catabolism resulting from immobilization, the hormonal milieu, the cytokine response, and starvation (36, 37). Loss of muscle mass increases in relation to the severity of injury. Muscle loss is characterized by increased 3-methyl-histidine excretion derived from the metabolism of muscle fiber actin and myosin (38). The intracellular branched-chain amino acid (BCAA) concentrations rise while nonessential amino acids decrease. The metabolic processes have been studied and reviewed in detail (39–41). In severe stress, glutamine and alanine account for more than 70% of the amino acids released by proteolysis and intramuscular metabolism, although they constitute only 10% of the muscle composition. Skeletal muscle metabolizes the BCAAs valine, isoleucine, and leucine, whereas other amino acids are released into the systemic amino acid pool (Fig. 91.2).

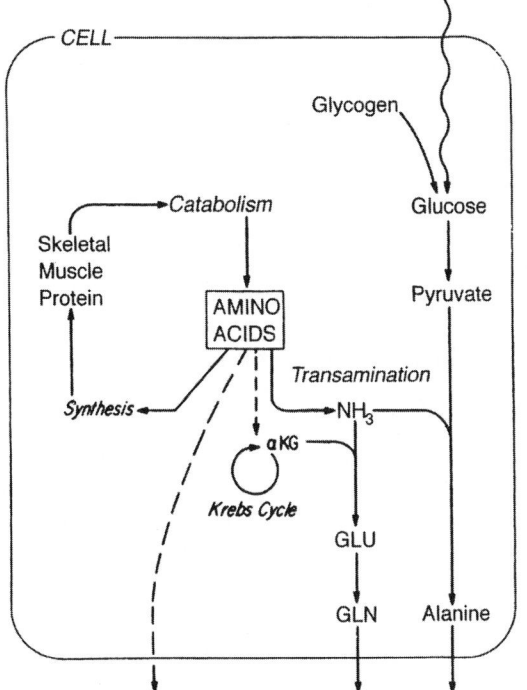

Figure 91.2. Major biochemical reactions that lead to synthesis of glutamine (GLN) and alanine in skeletal muscle. GLU, glucose; αKG, α-ketoglutarate.

As BCAAs are deaminated and the carbon chains metabolized in the Krebs cycle, the waste nitrogen is disposed of in two methods. Nitrogen is transaminated onto pyruvate, which results from intracellular glucose metabolism. This produces alanine, which is released to be cleared and deaminated by the liver. The nitrogen is excreted as urea, and the residual pyruvate is converted by the liver into glucose. This results in no net gluconeogenesis. The second process to eliminate nitrogen is through transamination of α-ketoglutarate, which is produced in the Kreb cycle. α-Ketoglutarate is capable of accepting two nitrogen moieties sequentially to produce glutamic acid and subsequently glutamine after the second nitrogen is added.

Glutamine is the most abundant amino acid in the cytosol in health, but intracellular levels drop during stress and sepsis despite increases in production because it is rapidly transported from the cell. Circulating glutamine provides fuel for enterocytes and for immunologic cells, especially T lymphocytes. Within the gut-associated lymphoid tissue and other splanchnic tissue, glutamine is converted to ammonia and alanine. These products, together with ornithine and citrulline, which are produced within the gastrointestinal tract, are cleared by the liver. Ornithine and citrulline are constituents of the urea acid cycle for urea production. The kidney is also capable of producing glucose in small quantities through glutamine metabolism.

Muscle protein catabolism increases more than synthesis during stress, but net increases in hepatic gluconeogenesis and protein production occur (42, 43). Hepatic protein production is affected by IL-6, which is found in higher concentration in the portal vein than the systemic circulation (44). IL-6 directly effects liver protein production by blunting production of the constitutive proteins, ALB and prealbumin, and by stimulating production of the acute-phase proteins, CRP and AAG.

Fat

Fat is the primary fuel source to support metabolic needs following injury. Lipolysis is enhanced through the increased glucagon, cortisol, epinephrine, and possibly GH (45). This occurs despite increased levels of plasma insulin induced by hyperglycemia. The importance of fat is obvious through a depressed respiratory quotient (RQ) found in septic patients (46). The RQ ratio reflects the ratio of carbon oxide production to oxygen consumption ranging from approximately 0.6 to 0.7 in starvation (almost pure fat metabolism) to 1.0 when metabolism is completely glucose driven. During stress, the RQ ranges between 0.8 and 0.85. As patient recovery ensues, the RQ ratio increases toward 1.0.

Fat administration during illness can affect various aspects of metabolism. Although mammals produce only saturated fat (i.e., no double bonds), various types of polyunsaturated fatty acids (PUFAs) exist in nonmammalian fat.

For example, vegetable oil is primarily ω-6 fatty acids (unsaturated at the sixth double bond from the methylated end of the molecule), whereas fish oil or canola oil consists primarily of ω-3 fatty acids (an unsaturated double bond at the third position). These issues are not crucial while these fatty acids are incorporated into membranes of cells during health, but they become important during stress, when increased intracellular calcium activates phospholipase A_2 to release the fatty acids from the cell wall. ω-6 Fatty acids are incorporated into cell walls as arachadonic acid, whereas ω-3 fatty acids are not. As arachadonic acid is released and metabolized in stress, cyclooxygenase produces the prostanoid prostaglandin E_2, a vasodilator, and lipoxygenase produces the leukotrienes B_4 and 5-hydroxy-6,8,11,14-eicosatetranoic acid (47, 48). These immunosuppressive prostaglandins and leukotrienes of the 2 and 4 series decrease T-cell function and inhibit migration of cytotoxic cells (48). The leukotrienes themselves are important proinflammatory chemoattractants. When intracellular enzymes produce prostaglandins from ω-3 fatty acids in the cell wall, the products are prostaglandins and leukotrienes of the 3 and 5 series, which are less immunosuppressive and proinflammatory than their ω-6 counterparts. These issues are important in the immune-enhancing diets. Within 5 days of administration of ω-3 fatty acids, significant increases in concentrations in cell membranes are measurable (47).

Glucose

The hyperglycemia following injury occurs for several reasons. As indicated earlier, epinephrine blunts the excretion of insulin in response to hyperglycemia (the central effect) whereas cortisol blunts the ability of cells to transport circulating insulin into the cell (the peripheral effect). In addition, hepatic gluconeogenesis accelerates despite hyperglycemia. This gluconeogenesis is not blunted by glucose administration (43). Increased production of alanine and glutamine by muscle and lactate by hypoxic tissues provides substrate for hepatic glucose production. Lactate production is dramatically increased in hypoxic or hypotensive patients, whereas alanine production increases by as much as 40% following severe injury (37).

Glucose oxidation becomes less efficient after severe injury (49). This is only partially explained by the onset of insulin resistance (50). The hyperglycemia may be protective in some circumstances because experimental models have demonstrated reduction in mortality and increases in blood pressure with hyperglycemia (51, 52). However, more recent work studying glucose control with insulin infusions in patients in intensive care units (ICUs) demonstrated a reduction in mortality with exogenous insulin control of hyperglycemia (53). The primary effect was seen in cardiac patients; it still is unproven whether these results are generalizable to general surgical, general medical, or trauma patients.

Cytokine Mediators of Metabolic Responses

Many mediators are released by injured tissue or by the inflammatory response of immunologic defenses following injury during sepsis. The release of these mediators is influenced by the severity of injury: significant after severe trauma but minimally increased following surgical procedures such as inguinal hernia repair or laparoscopic cholecystectomy. These mediators affect both the immunologic response and metabolism. Exogenous administration of tumor necrosis factor (TNF) produces tachycardia, fever, an increase in oxygen consumption, and other signs of stress and sepsis (54). Its peak response is short-lived, but TNF affects the subsequent release of other inflammatory mediators. IL-1 affects proteolysis (together with TNF) and carbohydrate metabolism (55). IL-1β stimulates adrenocorticotropic hormone release and increases proteolysis through effects on insulin and glycogen. TNF-α, IL-1β, and IL-2 inhibit lipoprotein lipase and reduce lipid uptake by peripheral tissues (56). IL-2 also inhibits α-adrenergic stimulation of hormone-sensitive lipases to stimulate lipolysis. IL-6 is important in prostaglandin production, the acute-phase protein response, B-cell proliferation, and immunoglobulin synthesis (57). It is released by numerous tissues, with higher concentrations in the portal than the systemic circulation. IL-6 is a primary stimulant for hepatic acute-phase protein production of CRP and AAG in levels proportion to the IL-6 levels. These acute-phase proteins serve numerous functions including augmented clearance from the blood of nuclear material from necrotic cells, enhancement of phagocytosis, and chemoattraction in the nonspecific immune response. Other acute-phase proteins include α_1-antitrypsin, heparin cofactor II, plasminogen activator inhibitor, fibrinogen, von Willebrand factor, the complement proteins C2, C3, C5, and C9, and various metal-binding proteins such as ceruloplasm, magnesium superoxide dismutase, hemopexin, and haptoglobin (58). Each serves various functions in response to the cytokine polypeptide signals produced after injury, bacteremia, or endotoxin.

NUTRITIONAL REQUIREMENTS

Estimating Total Caloric Requirements

With either enteral feeding or PN, the nutrient prescription should meet the metabolic demands of the patient. Overfeeding should be avoided because it increases oxygen consumption, generates hepatic lipogenesis, produces immunosuppression (secondary to hyperglycemia or lipid deposition), and increases carbon dioxide production.

The most common way to determine basal energy expenditure (BEE) is by the Harris-Benedict formula:

In males: BEE = 66 + (13.8 × W) + (5 × H) − (6.8 × A)

In females: BEE = 665 + (9.6 × W) + (1.8 × H) − (4.7 × A)

where W is the weight in kg, H is height in cm, and A is age in years. Traditionally, these values were multiplied by stress and activity factors to account for metabolic effects of injury or sepsis. Recent use of indirect calorimetry, however, shows that these stress and activity factors often result in overfeeding (59, 60). Most critically ill general surgical patients rarely exceed the calculated BEE by more than 20%.

In indirect calorimetry, metabolic carts measure expired carbon dioxide and oxygen consumption via expired gas to determine the overall resting energy expenditure via the Weir equation. The measurements under controlled conditions approximate the Harris-Benedict equation within 5 to 10%, a finding demonstrating that large stress factors are inappropriate and unnecessary. An RQ ratio analyzes the substrate being used by the patient because each fuel has a characteristic RQ during metabolism (carbohydrate RQ = 1.0; protein RQ = 0.8; fat RQ = 0.7). Because lipogenesis has an RQ value of approximately 8, a calculated RQ greater than 1 is diagnostic of overfeeding.

Unfortunately, the drawbacks to indirect calorimetry are significant (61). Small percentage errors in measurement of either the inspired or expired oxygen consumption in patients administered a high oxygen concentration may produce a 100% error in calculation. These mismeasurements can occur from chest tube losses or leaks around a tracheostomy. Therefore, the patients who could benefit most from these measurements—those most critically ill requiring significant ventilator support—are those patients most likely to have tainted values. The technique is labor intensive and requires committed personnel using defined protocols. Because most hypermetabolic patients rarely have increases greater than 15% above their calculated BEE, provision of 25 to 30 kcal/kg/day allows 90% of the patients to reach energy requirements, with overfeeding occurring in only 10 to 20% of patients (59). Thus, these values should be used with the calculated BEE to feed routine postoperative or trauma patients. Total requirements are met by administering a combination of fat (10 kcal/g intravenously or 9.1 kcal/g enterally), carbohydrate (4.0 kcal/g enterally and 3.4 kcal/g hydrated glucose), and protein (4 kcal/g).

A modest caloric intake may yield better clinical outcomes in some critically ill patients. Patients in medical ICUs who are receiving between approximately 9 and 18 kcal/kg/day via enteral feedings and/or PN are more likely to achieve spontaneous ventilation before ICU discharge and to be alive at hospital discharge than are those patients receiving the most calories (i.e., 18–28 kcal/kg/day) (62). A modest caloric intake is also associated with a higher likelihood of achieving spontaneous ventilation before ICU discharge when compared with those patients with the lowest caloric intake (0–9 kcal/kg/day). Apparently, a specific range for caloric intake may exist for which calories exceeding or failing to meet this intake can have a negative impact on patient outcome. Trauma studies have demonstrated that patients undergoing enteral nutrition who are receiving only 40% of goal nutrient intake still exhibit significantly fewer infectious complications compared patients undergoing PN who are receiving more than half of the goal calories ordered (9). Whether it is the result of preventing the metabolic complications from excessive overfeeding or some other unknown mechanism, the provision of less than 100% of calculated energy needs can have a beneficial effect in critically ill patients.

Emerging evidence suggests that obesity is an independent risk factor for ICU death (63, 64). To prevent further delivery of excess calories that create a positive caloric balance, the concept of "permissive underfeeding" has been used in the management of obese patients requiring PN in the postoperative period. Provision of a hypocaloric, high-protein regimen promotes utilization of endogenous fat stores for energy needs in stressed obese patients while maintaining lean tissue mass. One study showed that a hypocaloric, high-protein PN formulation administered to obese patients produced an average weight loss of 2.3 kg/week over 48 days. Positive nitrogen balances or nitrogen equilibrium was demonstrated in all patients, as well as complete healing of wound dehiscence, abscesses, and closure of fistulas (65). Typical hypocaloric PN formulations provide 14 kcal/kg/day of actual body weight as nonprotein calories and 1.2 g/kg/day as protein (66).

Glucose Requirements

Hepatic gluconeogenesis produces hyperglycemia as glucose production increases from 2 to 2.5 mg/kg/minute under normal conditions to 4 to 5 mg/kg/minute in severely stressed patients (67). Intravenous infusions of glucose aggravate this hyperglycemia as a result of central and peripheral insulin resistance. The maximal rate of glucose oxidation is 5 mg/kg/minute (7.2 g/kg per day), which is easily exceeded (68, 69). In a 70-kg patient, 2 L of a 25% dextrose solution contains 500 g of glucose, which reaches this maximal level. Traditional recommendations were to maintain blood glucose values to less than 200 mg/dL because of the immunosuppressive effects on neutrophils, but more recent data suggest that even tighter control (80–120 mg/dL) with insulin improves clinical outcome (53). Mortality dropped in a large group of patients in ICUs (primarily cardiac surgical patients). It was unclear whether insulin had the primary effect on the cardiac response or was secondary to other effects because general surgical patients in that study (including patients with trauma, vascular, and other intraabdominal procedures) showed no significant improvement with the aggressive insulin treatment. Further work is necessary, but current recommendations are that glucose should be maintained at much less than 200 mg/dL via insulin whenever possible.

Protein Requirements

Protein (or amino acids) should be administered at 1.2 to 1.5 g/kg/day to patients without renal dysfunction. If blood

TABLE 91.2. GENERAL GUIDELINES FOR PROTEIN REQUIREMENTS BASED ON STRESS OR CHANGES IN ORGAN DYSFUNCTION

CLINICAL SITUATION	RECOMMENDED PROTEIN INTAKES
Maintenance	1 g/kg/d actual BW
Stress or repletion	1.3–2 g/kg/d actual BW
Renal failure/predialysis	0.8–1 g/kg/d dry BW
Renal failure/hemodialysis	1.2–1.5 g/kg/d dry BW
Renal failure/peritoneal/CVVHD	1.5–2 g/kg/d dry BW
Burn injury	2–2.5 g/kg/d dry BW
Hepatic failure	0.6–1.2 g/kg/d dry BW
Liver transplant	1–1.5 g/kg/d dry BW
Bone marrow transplant	1.5–2 g/kg/d dry BW

BW, body weight; CVVHD, continuous venovenous hemodialysis.

urea nitrogen increases to more than 100 mg/dL, protein should be decreased to 1.0 to 1.3 g/kg/day. With the use of hemodialysis or renal supportive techniques such as continuous arterial venous hemodialysis or continuous venovenous hemodialysis, protein requirements actually increase to 1.5 to 2 g/kg/day, to account for protein losses across the dialysis membranes. Burn patients typically require 2 to 2.5 g/kg/day because of excessive urinary losses and wound losses. General guidelines for protein needs based on clinical condition and organ dysfunction are summarized in Table 91.2.

Fat Requirements

Glucose should provide approximately 50 to 60% of total caloric requirements (~80% of nonprotein calories). The current recommendation is that the balance of nonprotein calories should be administered as fat at a dose of 1 to 1.5 g/kg/day in critically ill patients with triglyceride levels lower than 300 mg/dL. Hyperlipidemia with serum triglyceride levels higher than 500 mg/dL mandates withholding lipid administration. The maximum recommended dose of intravenous lipid is 2.5 g/kg/day in the adult, but this should rarely be used (70). Fat calories can be increased to 50% of nutrient requirements in select patients with severe hyperglycemia or high carbon dioxide production, but with the potential complication of hyperlipidemia, cholestasis, immunosuppression, and increased infection (71). In general, patients with suspected overfeeding with increased carbon dioxide production should be treated by reduction in total calories (72).

Vitamin Requirements

In April 2000, the US Food and Drug Administration (FDA) amended the requirements for marketing of an "effective" adult parenteral multivitamin formulation and recommended changing the 12-vitamin formulation that had been available in the United States since 1979 (73). Changes mandated by the FDA to parenteral multivitamin formulations include higher dosages of vitamins B_1 (thiamin), vitamin B_6 (pyridoxine), vitamin C (ascorbic acid), and folic acid, as well as the addition of vitamin K (phylloquinone). See Table 91.3 for a comparison of the vitamin content of old and new parenteral multivitamin formulations. These modifications are based on the recommendations of a 1985 workshop sponsored jointly by the American Medical Association's Division of Personal and Public Health Policy and the FDA's Division of Metabolic and Endocrine Drug Products. Practitioners and researchers have suggested that vitamin requirements may be greater in seriously ill patients requiring enteral nutrition or PN (74). In addition, higher dosages of particular vitamins, such as vitamin C or vitamin E, may play a critical role in antioxidant defense.

TABLE 91.3. OLD VERSUS NEW FOOD AND DRUG ADMINISTRATION RECOMMENDATIONS FOR ADULT PARENTERAL MULTIVITAMIN FORMULATIONS

VITAMIN	OLD RECOMMENDATIONS[a]	NEW RECOMMENDATIONS[b]
Vitamin A	3,300 International Units (1 mg retinol)	3,300 International Units (1 mg retinol)
Vitamin D_2	200 International Units (5 μg cholecalciferol)	200 International Units (5 μg cholecalciferol)
Vitamin E	10 mg (α-tocopherol)	10 mg (α-tocopherol)
Vitamin K	as needed	150 μg
Thiamin (B_1)	3 mg	6 mg
Riboflavin (B_2)	3.6 mg	3.6 mg
Pyridoxine (B_6)	4 mg	6 mg
Niacin	40 mg	40 mg
Pantothenate	15 mg	15 mg
Biotin	60 μg	60 μg
Folate	400 μg	600 μg
Cyanocobalamin (B_{12})	5 μg	5 μg
Ascorbic acid (C)	100 mg	200 mg

[a]Data from American Medical Association Department of Foods and Nutrition. JPEN J Parenter Enteral Nutr 1979;3:258–62.
[b]Data from Department of Health and Human Services, Food and Drug Administration. Fed Reg 2000;65:64607–19.

Supplemental vitamin E has shown benefit in patients undergoing surgical treatment of abdominal aortic aneurysm (75). Patients receiving oral vitamin E, 600 IU (400 mg of RRR-α-tocopherol or α-tocopherol equivalents)/day for 8 days preoperatively, demonstrated reduced evidence of ischemia-reperfusion tissue injury on muscle biopsies. Patients undergoing the same surgical procedure who were not receiving supplemental vitamin E displayed muscle biopsy findings consistent with tissue perfusion injury. Because of their antioxidant properties, supplemental dosages of vitamins C and E have been studied for their impact on pulmonary complications and organ failure in critically ill surgical patients. In this study, 595 trauma patients or patients requiring emergency surgery were randomly assigned to a control group receiving standard care with no antioxidant therapy or a treatment group receiving α-tocopherol, 1000 IU every 8 hours orally and ascorbic acid 1000 mg every 8 hours intravenously, for the duration of the ICU stay or for 28 days (76). Although no difference in pulmonary morbidity (i.e., pneumonia, acute respiratory distress syndrome [ARDS]) was detected, multiple-organ dysfunction syndrome was significantly less likely to occur in the antioxidant-supplemented group versus the control group. The total incidence of multiple-organ dysfunction syndrome in both groups was only 4% (26/595); thus, the potential for benefit of antioxidant supplementation was quite limited.

Plasma concentrations of vitamins C and E have been shown to be reduced in seriously ill patients with ARDS compared with healthy volunteers (77). Standard intake of parenteral multivitamins in PN failed to maintain plasma concentrations of vitamin E and vitamin C in patients with ARDS over a 6-day study period. In addition, serum concentrations of malondialdehyde continued to rise in the patients with ARDS compared with the healthy controls. Excessive production of the lipid peroxidation product malondialdehyde has been previously reported in acutely ill patients with ARDS, a finding suggesting that these patients may require higher dosages of specific vitamins to maintain antioxidant defense mechanisms. Although these data suggest that low plasma vitamin concentrations may have important functional consequences, changes in blood vitamin concentrations may not necessarily reflect a deficiency state.

The effect of the acute-phase response on fluid distribution and on measured vitamin concentrations has been documented in patients undergoing uncomplicated orthopedic surgical procedures (78). Decreased plasma concentrations of vitamin A, vitamin E, and pyridoxal-5′-phosphate in addition to concentrations of leukocyte vitamin C were accompanied by an equally significant increase in plasma CRP concentrations over a 7-day period. Vitamin concentrations returned to baseline with resolution in the acute-phase response, and self-correction of decreased vitamin measurements mirrored the changes in CRP concentrations. Thus, reduction in vitamin concentrations should be

interpreted with care during the acute-phase response, and supplementation of vitamins may not be indicated. Supplemental vitamins may be indicated only when low vitamin concentrations persist during the absence of an acute-phase response.

Acute injury or illness has been associated with progressive vitamin deficiencies during convalescence. Children with thermal injuries covering 40% or more of the total body surface area have been deficient in vitamin D up to 7 years following the burn injury (79). Low concentrations of circulating 25-hydroxy-vitamin D also correlated with bone mineral density Z-scores, a finding suggesting that vitamin D depletion after a burn injury could be a contributing factor to postburn bone loss. New evidence suggests that a defect in the skin production of cholecalciferol, vitamin D_3, is responsible for low serum concentrations of vitamin D (80). A fivefold reduction was observed in the conversion of 7-dehydrocholesterol to previtamin D_3 in burn scar skin compared with unburned control skin. Implications of these data are that survivors of a large burn injury should be assessed for hypovitaminosis D, bone disease, and other consequences of vitamin D deficiency. At a minimum, burn victims should receive a daily multivitamin with 200 to 400 IU/day of vitamin D on discharge from the hospital.

Trace Element Requirements

The Nutrition Advisory Group of the American Medical Association recommended that trace elements be added to PN formulations daily. Standard trace element solutions contain selenium, chromium, zinc, copper, and manganese. These minerals play essential roles in numerous metabolic pathways, and biochemical and functional alterations may develop in the presence of severe deficiency states. Significant reductions in plasma selenium have been associated with higher rates of ventilator-associated pneumonia, organ failure, and mortality in critically ill patients (81). Interventional studies have evaluated the effect of selenium replacement on outcome in patients in ICUs who have systemic inflammatory response syndrome. A small, randomized, prospective study demonstrated that a regimen of 9 days of intravenous selenium replacement (dose range, 155–535 μg/day) reduced the requirements for hemodialysis and significantly lowered Acute Physiology and Chronic Health Evaluation (APACHE) III scores compared with control patients receiving only 35 μg of selenium/day (82). High urinary and cutaneous losses of selenium, zinc, and copper have been documented in burn and trauma patients (83). Supplementation of these three trace elements has improved immune response in severely burned patients. The total number of infectious episodes was reduced in patients supplemented with trace elements compared with controls receiving standard doses of trace elements. Specifically, pulmonary infections were significantly lower as a result of trace element supplementation and the length of ICU stay was shorter in the supplemented group when normalized for burned surface area (83).

ROUTES OF NUTRITION SUPPORT

In general, the enteral route is preferable to PN in patients in whom access to and function of gastrointestinal tract allow enteral delivery of nutrients. Many patients previously fed intravenously are capable of tolerating enteral feeding. Although gastroparesis follows intraabdominal surgery or occurs during critical illness and after injury, access directly into the small intestine allows nutrition to be provided in quantities adequate to meet nutrient needs. Experimentally, PN decreases brush border hydrolase activity, probably increases mucosal permeability, results in atrophy of villous height, and generates inhibitory affects on gut mucosal immunity (84–88). Each of these factors is beneficially affected by enteral feeding.

Enteral Route

Substantial clinical data support the use of enteral nutrition. Many of these studies were performed in trauma patients (7–9, 11, 12) in whom small bowel cannulation during celiotomy allowed randomization to early enteral feeding versus PN or no specialized nutrition. Almost uniformly, studies showed significant reductions in pneumonia and intraabdominal abscesses (in those at risk of intraabdominal abscesses). In particular, patients with an ATI of 20 or greater or an ISS of 18 to 20 or greater—the patients most at risk of infectious complications—were most likely to benefit (9). In patients with isolated closed head injury, gastroparesis resolves usually within 3 to 4 days unless patients are kept in a barbiturate coma. Following severe head injury, enteral feeding should be instituted as gastroparesis resolves because earlier feeding via small bowel tubes placed endoscopically provides no additional benefit (89). If gastroparesis persists, a tube should be advanced blindly, endoscopically, or via fluoroscopy into the distal duodenum or the proximal small intestine for enteral feeding.

Similar results were found in studies of general surgical patients. In numerous trials, early enteral nutrition improved postoperative infections, immunologic parameters, and gastrointestinal tract function (10, 90–92). However, no benefit of early enteral feeding was reported in studies primarily enrolling well-nourished patients undergoing major surgical procedures, in whom an uncomplicated postoperative course is usual (93, 94). However, studies recruiting significant numbers of patients with preexisting malnutrition showed improved outcome with enteral feeding and PN (91, 92, 95, 96). Early postoperative nutrition should be instituted to preclude further loss in lean body mass, with nutrients delivered via the gastrointestinal tract rather than parenterally when possible. Enteral feeding and PN have been studied in inflammatory bowel disease (97, 98), following transplantation (99, 100), and in patients with mild to moderate pancreatitis (101, 102). Uniformly, reports have supported beneficial effects with the use of enteral feeding rather than PN when clinically tolerated.

Perioperative Nutrition Support

Multiple studies have evaluated preoperative and postoperative nutrition support, although they have provided conflicting results. A critical issue in the interpretation of these data is patient selection because many studies recruited patients who were not at risk of nutrition-related complications. Particularly when a PN arm of a trial was included, the results often demonstrated an increase in septic complications with PN in patients who could otherwise have had uncomplicated courses. The classic example is the Veterans Affairs Cooperative study (95), which randomized preoperative surgical patients to PN for 7 to 15 days preoperatively or to a control group with free access to a diet. The amount of PN administered in that study exceeded current recommendations, and this may have aggravated the negative effects. Overall, the trend was toward a reduction in healing complications (wound dehiscence, anastomotic dehiscence, fistula formation) in the parenterally fed group, but a significantly increased rate of infectious complications, particularly pneumonia. After stratification by the degree of preexisting malnutrition, severely malnourished patients clearly benefited from PN, with a significant reduction in healing complications and no increase (and some decrease) in infectious complications. In trials of perioperative nutrition, almost all trials with negative results or a negative effect of nutrition recruited mostly well-nourished patients (93–95). However, trials that included large numbers of malnourished patients demonstrated significant benefit with perioperative nutrition (91, 92, 95). One can conclude that well-nourished patients—identified after a careful nutritional history and physical examination—are unlikely to benefit preoperatively from either PN or enteral feeding. If, however, patients have preexisting nutritional deficits, data support the use of early nutrition support in the preoperative and/or postoperative periods.

One exception to this observation exists. Well-nourished patients undergoing elective colorectal procedures randomized to receive 7 days of an oral diet supplemented with arginine, ω-3 fatty acids, and nucleotides had significant improvement in their postoperative recovery with dietary pretreatment (103). This observation of preoperative feeding in well-nourished patients hold significant promise, but its generalizability to a wide range of surgical patients is as yet unclear and untested.

ROLE OF GUT IN HOST DEFENSE

The general consensus is that nutrients should be administered via the gastrointestinal tract rather than parenterally whenever possible. This consensus resulted from numerous randomized prospective clinical trials in trauma patients and general surgical patients (7–12, 89–92). Significant experimental work has documented alterations in gastrointestinal histology as well as in mucosal immunity when the gastrointestinal tract remains unfed.

Experimentally, changes in the height of the villi occur very rapidly in animal models (85). These changes also occur within humans, but not to the same extent as in rodents (104). Injury, hemorrhagic shock, ischemia, and sepsis alter gut permeability to macromolecules as well as to bacteria (86, 105). Gut permeability does increase in trauma patients, but permeability returns to normal quite quickly and has not been linked clinically to a pathologic condition (106, 107). Recently, products released from the gastrointestinal tract into the thoracic duct have been implicated as a factor in the development of multiple-organ dysfunction in animal models of shock in ischemia reperfusion (108, 109). The substance believed to be responsible has not yet been identified. It is also unclear whether starvation of the gut potentiates the release of this factor in animal models.

The gut, however, plays a pivotal role in mucosal immunity. Bacteria are normally kept in check and with combination of peristalsis, competing bacterial populations, mucin, immunoglobulin A (IgA), and other factors. Experimentally, the lack of enteral feeding results in a significant reduction in T and B cells within the lamina propria, Peyer patches, and intraepithelial space (110). This reduction in cell numbers is associated with a reduction in the IgA-stimulating cytokines IL-4 and IL-10 in direct proportion to the decrease in IgA levels within the intestinal lumina (111). Peyer patches are the entry site for the $\alpha_4\beta_7$/L-selectin–positive T and B cells, which are destined for the mucosal immune system (112, 113). These molecules interact with mucosal addressin cellular adhesion molecule-1 (MAdCAM-1) on the high endothelial venules of the Peyer patches. MAdCAM-1 expression is decreased experimentally when the gastrointestinal tract is not fed (114). After cells normally enter the Peyer patches, where they are sensitized to antigens absorbed from the intestinal lumen and processed by the dendritic cells in this location, they are distributed back to the gastrointestinal tract as well as to extraintestinal sites such as the lung, genitourinary tract, and lactating mammary gland (115). With the reduction in MAdCAM-1, fewer cells are processed and distributed throughout the body. Just as IgA levels dropped within the intestinal tract, they also are reduced within the respiratory tract of parenterally fed mice. This results in a loss in respiratory defenses against bacteria and viruses in immunized animals (116, 117). Memory is not lost because the reinstitution of enteral feeding leads to rapid resumption of these immune defenses to protect the intestine and the respiratory tract. The result of enteral feeding is maintenance of immunity with both antiviral and antibacterial defenses in the respiratory tract, reduction in bacterial translocation within the gastrointestinal tract, and maintenance of normal intestinal architecture as defenses against bacterial invasion.

Systemic and intraperitoneal protection is also affected by the route of nutrient administration. Enteral feeding reduces the lethality of intraperitoneal bacteria compared with animals that are parenterally fed isonitrogenous and isocaloric diets. These early studies were confirmed by Lin and coworkers, who demonstrated that enteral feeding in rats results in increased intraperitoneal levels of TNF and the inhibition of bacterial proliferation (118). This resulted in a blunted systemic TNF response to intraperitoneal sepsis. This finding was confirmed by Fong and colleagues (119) in human subjects. When parenterally fed individuals were administered intravenous endotoxin, TNF responses were augmented in parenterally fed individuals compared with those fed enterally. As a result of these multiple facets, enteral feeding remains the preferred method for delivery of nutrients.

TYPES OF NUTRIENT DIET

Enteral Diet (see also chapter 98)

Gastroparesis complicates the course of most trauma patients with severe injuries and of most critically ill patients. This condition precludes early intragastric feeding. One important exception is burned patients, who develop less gastroparesis when they are tube fed within 8 to 12 hours of admission (120). When gastroparesis occurs, enteral access obtained beyond the ligament of Treitz allows enteral feeding using a multitude of formulas that vary in concentration, fiber, content, electrolyte load, and complexity of macronutrients. Even when nutrients are infused directly into the intestine, chemically defined diets are usually not necessary (121). These formulas are usually reserved for patients with mucosal disease or significant gastrointestinal intolerance. In most critically ill or postsurgical patients, administration of an isotonic diet containing soluble fiber limits diarrhea, which usually is secondary to antibiotics, bacterial overgrowth, *Clostridium difficile* infection, gastric motility agents, or sorbitol-rich elixirs rather than the enteral formula (122–124). In general, isotonic diets containing 1 kcal/mL and are usually well tolerated and can be administered through nasojejunal tubes, 5- and 7-French needle catheter jejunostomies (NCJs), or size 14, 16, or 18 catheters. Diets should be started only in hemodynamically stable patients, usually at a rate of 15 to 25 mL/hour, and advanced every 12 to 24 hours as tolerated with direct small bowel feedings. Intragastric feedings are started at a faster rate, usually 50 mL/hour, to test for gastroparesis. If residuals are not elevated (>200–250 mL 4 hours after institution of feeding), diets can be advanced more rapidly to goal rate. For the most part, any complex enteral formula is acceptable for intragastric feedings.

Specific Substrates

Clinical evidence indicates that specific substrates may be beneficial in certain critically ill or critically injured patients. The nutrients glutamine, arginine, ω-3 fatty acids, and nucleotides have been combined in various formulas commonly referred to as immune-enhancing diets. Production of glutamine, the most abundant amino acid in the body, is increased during stress and sepsis. However, both serum levels and intracellular levels drop as this particular amino acid becomes conditionally essential during times of high metabolic rate. It serves as substrate for the gastrointestinal enterocyte, rapidly proliferating cells, and T lymphocytes. Both enteral feedings and PN supplemented with glutamine have been shown to be effective (12, 125, 126). Unfortunately, glutamine is difficult to solubilize, and with heat and sterilization it degrades into ammonia and pyroglutamate, two toxic products. Its use has been limited with intravenous feeding, but it is used in several commercial enteral products. Arginine is a precursor of nitric oxide, nitrites, and nitrates and promotes proliferation of T cells after stimulation. It plays a role in cellular immunity and fibroblast proliferation and serves as a secretagogue for GH, prolactin, glucogon, and insulin production (127). (See Chapters 35 and 36 for additional information on these two amino acids).

PUFAs contain double bonds at various positions. Mammals do not make unsaturated fatty acids, and these substances are largely obtained from the diet. ω-6 Fatty acids are obtained from vegetable oils, whereas ω-3 fatty acids are found in high concentrations in fish oil and canola oil (rapeseed oil). Humans cannot synthesize these PUFAs, but can rapidly incorporate them into cell membranes, where during stress or sepsis, they are released and are subsequently metabolized into end products. ω-6 Fatty acids are incorporated into the cell membrane as arachadonic acid and are subsequently metabolized with phospholipases producing prostaglandin E_2, thromboxane A_2, and leukotriene B_4 of the 2 and 4 series. Prostanoids and leukotriene are immunosuppressive and proinflammatory. They inhibit killer cell activity, impair antibody formation, and blunt cell-mediated immunity. ω-3 PUFAs are metabolized to prostanoids of the 3 and 5 series including prostaglandin PGI_3, thromboxane A_3, and leukotriene B_5 via the lipoxygenase pathway. These end products are neither immunosuppressive nor proinflammatory. Nucleotides provide RNA for various functions including cell proliferation, DNA and RNA synthesis, and immunocyte function.

The use of these formulas has been studied in certain populations. In particular, trauma patients with severe injuries were shown in several clinical trials to benefit significantly from the early use of these diets when such diets were administered enterally (12, 128). No benefit was found when these diets were used in well-nourished elective general surgical patients unlikely to have postoperative complications (93, 94), with the exception of two studies that preoperatively loaded the patients with 1 L of these diets before colorectal surgery (96). Under those circumstances, patients who were otherwise not malnourished appeared to benefit. In studies of patients who underwent upper gastrointestinal resection for malignancies (91, 92), as well as trauma patients, these immune-enhancing diets reduced infectious complications, hospital stay, and total complications.

More recently, however, their use in frankly septic patients has been questioned, and although the issue is still controversial, investigators have speculated that arginine may be deleterious in patients who are septic. Fortunately, most patients who are extremely septic do not tolerate enteral feeding, and, given these data, clinicians should be circumspect in administering it to frankly septic patients (129). In one study, the increase in mortality was limited to elderly men who were septic with pneumonia (130). More recent data demonstrate that this finding may be more generalizable to a wider range of septic patients (131).

The reason for this increase in mortality may reside in cellular responses to sepsis as opposed to trauma. Trauma patients have a clear increase in cellular arginase, which leads to rapid metabolism of arginine (132). In these conditions, supplemental arginine may be beneficial in normalizing serum levels. In frank sepsis, however, more arginine has metabolized to nitric oxide because arginase levels are depressed. Investigators have speculated that this increase in nitric oxide may be the origin of increased mortality resulting from increased vasodilatation through this end product.

In summary, these specialty-supplemented diets appear to benefit severely malnourished patients undergoing elective surgical procedures and trauma patients with severe injuries. Their use in frankly septic patients may not be appropriate, however.

Access for Enteral Feeding

Most enteral feeding is delivered through small-bore tubes introduced into the stomach. This method is the most common in medical and surgical ICUs, particularly when surgical access has not been obtained or celiotomy has not been performed. Small-bore tubes (versus large nasogastric tubes) reduce the incidence of complications from reflux, pressure, and necrosis in the nasal alae or irritation resulting in ulcers or strictures. The stylet of the tubes allows easy passage, but the position must be confirmed by either aspiration of gastric juice or radiographic confirmation to eliminate the inadvertent infusion of nutrients into the pulmonary tree. Simple air insufflation will not distinguish between a tube placed in the left lower lobe and that located within the stomach; additional confirmation is necessary. Unfortunately, these tubes are frequently dislodged and provide potential for reflux and aspiration with intragastric feeding. Thus, with intragastric feeding, the head of the patient's bed should be kept elevated at least 30 to 35 degrees because the gastroesophageal junction is the most dependent area of the stomach in supine patients.

In patients in whom residuals are high and intragastric feeding is not tolerated, as evidenced by recurrent aspiration or reflux of tube feedings back into throat, tube access must be obtained distally. If celiotomy is not indicated, small-bore tubes can be advanced either blindly (success rates of 95%) or via fluoroscopy or endoscopy. Although no strong evidence indicates that advancement of the tube out of the stomach will preclude gastric aspiration, the studies have often just placed the tube into the proximal duodenum and have not simultaneously decompressed the stomach to preclude aspiration with gastric juices. Intuitively, advancement of the tube into the fourth portion of the duodenum or ideally into the small intestine seems advantageous in the protection against subsequent aspiration because the administration of direct small bowel feedings rarely refluxes back into the stomach. Intragastric feeding is not recommended in patients who are severely neurologically impaired and have free esophageal reflux or who have recurrent pneumonia secondary to reflux. A major drawback to nasojejunal or oral jejunal tubes is that they are frequently dislodged and serve as a temporary measure at best.

If celiotomy is necessary, the surgeon should consider obtaining access as part of the preoperative and intraoperative plan. In patients in whom recurrent aspiration pneumonia or severe gastroesophageal reflux is an issue, or in whom gastroparesis is expected, direct small bowel access can be obtained with large-bore tubes (14-, 16-, or 18-French tubes) or with 5- and 7-French NCJs or transgastric jejunostomies. NCJs are useful and can be expected to function for 3 to 4 weeks as long as they are cared for properly. Medications should not be administered via the NCJs because elixirs coagulate tube feedings and lead to early loss. NCJs do not require the use of chemically defined diets and usually tolerate commercially prepared, fiber-containing diets without problems. The advantages of the 14-, 16-, or 18-French tubes, however, is that if they become dislodged or clog, they can be removed and replaced with a tube of similar diameter. They also tolerate administration of medications better as long as the tubes are irrigated with 20 to 30 mL of water before and after their administration. Needle catheters cannot be replaced once they cease to function. Important points in the creation of any jejunostomy are as follows:

1. A tube should be located far enough distal to the ligament of Treitz in an area of the intestine with long enough mesentery so if the patient develops distention, the small intestine attachment point is not pulled off the anterior abdominal wall.
2. A Witzel tunnel should be performed around all tubes so the tube at no point is in contact with the direct peritoneal cavity, to preclude dislodgment into the peritoneal cavity.
3. A jejunostomy should be sutured to the anterior abdominal wall for approximately 4 cm, to preclude volvulus at the attachment point.
4. The jejunostomy should be sutured to the abdominal wall at the lateral edge of the rectus sheath or more laterally, to reduce the incidence of small bowel herniation over the jejunostomy site.
5. The external portion of the catheter should be kept short, to minimize inadvertent dislodgment of the tube by confused patients.

Tube feedings can be administered into the small intestine as soon as the patient becomes hemodynamically stable and is no longer receiving vasopressors required for hemodynamic stability. Resuscitation should be complete, with evidence of splanchnic perfusion (usually reflected in adequate urinary output). Isotonic solutions are preferable to hypertonic solutions to minimize the chance of diarrhea. In addition, fiber supplementation is advantageous because the soluble fiber is metabolized by bacteria to produce short-chain fatty acids (acetoacetate, butyrate, propionate) that are substrates for colonocyte metabolism and allow them to preserve their function of water absorption. Formulas with medium-chain triglycerides (MCTs) may be better tolerated than those with long-chain triglycerides (LCTs) because MCTs are more easily digested. However, some LCTs must be simultaneously administered because MCTs have no essential fatty acids. Abdominal distention, emesis, diarrhea, tube dislodgment, and electrolyte abnormalities are the most common complications associated with enteral delivery of nutrients. Aspiration is most likely with intragastric feeding and can be minimized by administration of prokinetic agents as necessary, elevation of the head of the bed to at least 30 degrees, frequent checking of residuals, and discontinuation of feedings if residuals are high or if evidence shows reflux from the stomach into the esophagus. Advancement of the tube beyond the ligament of Treitz may allow successful feeding if residuals are high.

Possible Complications

Diarrhea usually is a result of sorbitol and elixirs used to administer medications, antibiotic usage with bacterial overgrowth, *Clostridium difficile* infection, or failure to discontinue gastric motility agents after recovery of normal gastric emptying has occurred. In addition, magnesium-containing antacids may cause diarrhea. In patients with diarrhea, *Clostridium difficile* toxin should be checked; diets converted to a fiber containing isotonic diet, and all enterally administered medications discontinued. In addition, the need for antibiotic therapy should be reviewed, and such treatment should be discontinued as necessary.

Tube dislodgment is prevented primarily through vigilant nursing care during movement or turning of the patient. With surgically placed small-bore feeding tubes, the external portion should be kept short and well fixed with a suture at the skin level.

Electrolyte abnormalities are not uncommon with enteral feeding as well as with PN. The refeeding syndrome with subsequent hypokalemia, hypophosphatemia, or hypomagnesaemia is not uncommon in malnourished patients who are administered enteral feeding, and patients with this syndrome warrant supplementation with these specific electrolytes. In addition, most enteral products only have 30 to 40 mEq of sodium, so hyponatremia can occur, if patients have multiple intravenous fluids (particularly piggybacks) in 5% dextrose in water. Hypernatremia can occur when concentrated formulas are used. Approximately 1 mL of water should be administered for each calorie to maintain hydration.

Other rare complications include small bowel necrosis or pneumatosis intestinalis. Although the origin of this disorder is unknown, it has been associated with small bowel feedings in patients who are receiving pressors, are hemodynamically unstable, or are underresuscitated. Intragastric feedings are safe in these circumstances because small intestinal intolerance occurs with gastroparesis, which protects the small intestine. High gastric residuals will occur in patients whose intestine is not ready to be fed. Thus, enteral feedings can safely be administered in burn patients, even those receiving pressors. If residuals remain low, it is a sign that small bowel tolerance is adequate, and patients can advance rapidly to their goal rate.

Parenteral Diet (see also chapter 99)

Glucose

The monohydrated form of glucose is used in PN formulations to provide carbohydrate and to meet increased energy requirements. Recent notable attention has been given to glucose metabolism in surgical patients with injury, trauma, or sepsis. One study showed a dramatic reduction in mortality and infectious complications with an aggressive insulin protocol, maintaining serum glucose concentrations in a range of 80 to 120 mg/dL (53). Although these results appear promising, the effect was primarily in cardiac surgical patients, and it did not have an impact on patients undergoing trauma-related, vascular, transplant, or general surgical procedures. Although the results are encouraging, they need to be duplicated in more general ICU patient populations before intensive insulin regimens are adopted as standard medical practice.

Amino Acids

In the routine surgical patient receiving PN, certain standard amino acid solutions appear to be comparable in nutrient value. Some specialty parenteral formulas for stress, sepsis, hepatic failure, or renal failure have been commercially available, but results in these circumstances have been unclear, and current practices recommend the use of standard amino acid formulas in these patient populations. Several patient populations have been studied with the use of supplemental glutamine. Glutamine is not contained in commercially available amino acid products in the United States because of its limited stability in solution and its breakdown to potentially dangerous metabolic byproducts, pyroglutamic acid and ammonia. For safe administration of glutamine in the United States, cold sterilization and filtration processes are used to ensure the purity and stability of the intravenous form prepared from nonsterile glutamine powder. In several clinical trials, glutamine supplementation was shown to have a beneficial effect on lymphocytes (133, 134), and it reduces the incidence of clinical infections in bone marrow transplant recipients (135). These results have not been duplicated in patients with solid organ malignancies. Studies in critically ill patients have been limited, but they seem to demonstrate reductions in hospital stay and improved survival. Experimentally, glutamine supplementation appeared to improve proximal duodenal mucosal thickness, thus preventing total PN (TPN)-induced mucosal atrophy.

Intravenous Lipid Emulsions

In the United States, all intravenous lipid emulsions (IVLEs) available for parenteral administration are composed of fatty acids derived from soybean oil or soybean-safflower oil combinations. These vegetable oils are long-chain fatty acids (LCFAs) and deliver the essential fatty acids, linoleic acid (ω-6) and α-linolenic acid (ω-3). Linoleic acid is the major fatty acid component of IVLEs, ranging from 44 to 65%, with α-linolenic acid present in much smaller concentrations of 4 to 11%. Alterations in immune function have been associated with large infusions of IVLEs over short periods. These effects are primarily the result of end products of ω-6 fatty acid metabolism that are proinflammatory and immunosuppressive. When infusions of IVLEs exceed 0.12 g/kg/hour, there appears to be a greater tendency for impairment of neutrophil or monocyte/macrophage function (136). Impairment of cellular immunity by IVLEs has been inconsistent, and no studies have documented significant changes in humoral immunity with infusions of IVLEs.

Adverse pulmonary hemodynamics, including hypoxemia and deterioration in gas exchange, can occur with high rates of IVLEs. Elevations of mean pulmonary artery pressure and pulmonary venous admixture and a decline in the ratio of arterial oxygen tension to fractional inspired oxygen were noted with IVLE infusion rates greater than 0.12 g/kg/hour in patients with ARDS with (137) and without sepsis (138, 139). Trauma patients not receiving any IVLEs with PN during the first 10 days of hospitalization experienced almost a 2-week reduction in mechanical ventilator days compared with patients randomized to receive PN with IVLE. Unfortunately, these beneficial effects on pulmonary function cannot be attributed solely to any deleterious effects of IVLEs; the reason may be that the lipid-free PN group also received fewer calories than the group receiving PN in combination with IVLE (140).

In an attempt to circumvent the problems with LCFA-based IVLEs, investigators assessed alternative lipid sources such as MCTs. MCTs possess several metabolic advantages over LCFAs. MCTs are cleared more rapidly from the serum, are independent of carnitine for transport into mitochondria, and are less likely to be deposited in the liver or adipose tissue. Experiments were performed with MCTs in mechanically ventilated patients, and MCTs appear to be tolerated, although they may increase oxygen consumption. Pure MCT formulations do not provide the essential fatty acids, linoleic acid and α-linolenic acid; thus, they must always be combined with LCFAs. Medium-chain fatty acids (MCFAs) are also ketogenic, so they must be used with extreme caution in diabetic patients and are contraindicated in patients with ketosis or acidosis.

Researchers developed combination products incorporating both MCFAs and LCFAs into lipid emulsion products to take advantage of the benefits of MCFAs and to minimize any adverse effects. Combination products exist in two forms: physical mixtures of MCFAs and LCFAs or structured triglycerides. Structured triglycerides are formulated by hydrolysis and reesterification of MCFAs and LCFAs on the same glycerol backbone. As a result, essential fatty acid components are supplied and MCFAs are rapidly cleared from the bloodstream with both fatty acid groups residing on same glycerol molecule. Structured triglyceride products have resulted in a more positive nitrogen balance, significant weight gain, and enhanced lipid clearance in catabolic patients when compared with physical mixtures of MCFAs and LCFAs (141). Despite these encouraging results, combination IVLE products are not currently marketed in the United States for use in clinical practice.

Electrolytes

In response to surgery and injury, fluid and electrolyte imbalances often occur, and adjustments are required in the PN formulations to maintain homeostasis.

Sodium. Sodium is principally an extracellular cation with no established recommended dietary allowance (RDA) for healthy persons. Its inclusion in the PN formulation is based on clinical need. The sodium concentration is usually chosen to reflect 0.45% saline; therefore, 80 mEq/L of sodium is added to the PN formulation. Certain disease states can cause fluid overload, which is manifested as hypervolemic hyponatremia, such as worsening edema with congestive heart failure, cirrhosis, or nephrotic syndrome. This hyponatremia is the result of excess total body sodium in the presence of an even greater excess in total body water. In this case, severe sodium restriction is often required, and it is not uncommon for sodium to be withheld from the PN formulation.

A less common cause of hyponatremia in critically ill patients is the syndrome of inappropriate ADH secretion. Insults to the central nervous system such as head injury, meningitis, and subarachnoid hemorrhage are associated with this clinical phenomenon. Pharmacologic agents, including carbamazepine, chlorpropamide, tricyclic antidepressants, clonidine, and cyclophosphamide, may also be responsible for this electrolyte alteration. The diagnosis of syndrome of inappropriate ADH secretion is determined by a combination of low serum sodium (in the absence of fluid overload), a decrease in serum osmolality, an elevated urine osmolality relative to serum osmolality, and a urine sodium concentration greater than 40 mEq/L. Because of the effect of ADH on the kidney, water is absorbed without sodium, so urine sodium and tonicity are high relative to serum. The appropriate therapy is water restriction; thus, all free water should be eliminated from the PN formulation.

Conversely, patients with large nasogastric fluid losses, high ileostomy or pancreatic fistula outputs, or major small bowel losses often require substantial quantities of sodium per day. If these sodium and fluid losses are not replaced, the patient can become hypernatremic. Generally, if serum sodium is greater than 150 mEq/L, no more than 40 mEq/day of sodium should be added to the PN formulation. Patients' medication records should also be reviewed for "hidden" sources of sodium, such as ALB, medications in 0.9% saline, and sodium-containing antibiotics (i.e., Timentin). Other medications can cause dehydration as a result of volume depletion from excessive diarrhea, such as lactulose therapy in patients with hepatic encephalopathy.

Potassium. Potassium is principally an intracellular cation with no established RDI; thus, its inclusion in PN is dictated by clinical need. If patients' renal functions are normal, generally 40 mEq/L of potassium is sufficient to maintain homeostasis. Potassium requirements can be greatly influenced by acid-base status. During metabolic acidosis (pH <7.2), an excess of hydrogen ions is present in the circulation, and potassium exchanges its intracellular position for hydrogen ions in an attempt to abate the transfer, thus causing hyperkalemia. Conversely, hypokalemia results during metabolic alkalosis.

Renal insufficiency (creatinine clearance <30 mL/min) is also associated with impaired potassium clearance and hyperkalemia. In general, hyperkalemia in acute renal failure warrants potassium removal from the nutrient solution. Once levels have decreased to 4.0 mEq/L, potassium should be added in modest doses (e.g., 10 mEq/L). Many medications are associated with alterations in serum potassium concentrations. For example, the risk of developing hyperkalemia is increased in the presence of potassium-sparing medications such as angiotensin-converting enzyme inhibitors, spironolactone, triamterene, and amiloride. Heparin is an aldosterone antagonist that causes sodium wasting and potassium retention. Both therapeutic doses of heparin and low-dose heparin have been reported to cause this abnormality, especially in patients with diabetes and chronic renal dysfunction. Trimethoprim is a component of the combination product trimethoprim-sulfamethoxazole used frequently for gram-negative systemic infections. It is a weak diuretic with potassium-sparing activities. Reduction of potassium in the PN formulation is warranted when patients are receiving these medications, even when renal function is normal.

Pharmacotherapeutic agents associated with hypokalemia include potassium-wasting medications, such as amphotericin B, aminoglycosides, antipseudomonal penicillins (i.e., ticarcillin), loop and thiazide diuretics, glucocorticoids, insulin, and inhaled β-agonists (i.e., albuterol). If serum potassium concentrations exceed 5.1 mEq/L, no more than 20 mEq/day of potassium should be included in the PN formulation.

Calcium. Calcium is always administered as the gluconate salt in PN because it is more stable and less likely to precipitate with inorganic phosphorus salts. Up to 98% of total body calcium is in bone and can be readily mobilized in times of need under the influence of parathyroid hormone. The parenteral RDA for calcium is approximately 10 mEq or 200 mg/day. Certain patients, such as those with severe short bowel syndrome and those requiring massive blood transfusions, may require substantially greater quantities of calcium, and such increases in the PN admixture should be accomplished gradually. Dosage increases of 5 mEq/day for acute care are reasonable, and simultaneous monitoring of serum phosphorus is recommended during such times. Calcium is highly protein bound (especially to ALB). The following formula may be used to adjust serum calcium concentrations for low ALB concentrations: corrected calcium = [(4 − ALB) × 0.8] + measured calcium. Low amounts of calcium may be required for patients with hyperphosphatemia, metastatic cancer, or hyperparathyroidism. Usually, 10 mEq/day is a sufficient amount to add to the PN formulation.

Magnesium. Magnesium is closely linked to calcium metabolism where it is necessary for parathyroid hormone secretion. The parenteral RDA for magnesium is approximately 10 mEq or 120 mg/day. Patients with short bowel syndrome, alchoholism, and thermal injury often require larger doses to achieve magnesium homeostasis and can be advanced incrementally by 50% of the parenteral RDA as with calcium. Medications associated with magnesium wasting include amphotericin B, aminoglycosides, cyclosporine, cisplatin, loop and thiazide diuretics, and piperacillin. Dysrhythmias, hypocalcemia (an unusual problem in trauma patients), and irritability are avoided with magnesium monitoring and appropriate treatment. Intravenous magnesium replacement therapy is usually necessary in patients with moderate to severe magnesium deficiency resulting from poor absorption of oral magnesium salts. Magnesium has a renal tubular threshold similar to that of glucose, so rapid administration over a short time

TABLE 91.4. GRADUATED DOSING SCHEME FOR MAGNESIUM REPLACEMENT THERAPY

SERUM MAGNESIUM CONCENTRATION (mg/dL)[a]	MAGNESIUM DOSE/INFUSION PERIOD[b]
1.5–1.8	0.5 mEq/kg/12 h
1.1–1.4	1 mEq/kg/24 h
≤1	1.5 mEq/kg/24 h

[a]Normal magnesium concentration (1.7–2.3 mg/dL).
[b]Use 50% of recommended doses when creatinine clearance <30 mL/min.

will invariably result in high urinary losses. A weight-based dosing regimen for magnesium deficiency has been developed in which intravenous doses are infused slowly over 12 to 24 hours to facilitate better retention (Table 91.4). Magnesium status should also be considered when evaluating a hypokalemic patient because magnesium is an important cofactor for the sodium-potassium/adenosine triphosphatase pump. Magnesium replacement therapy should be considered for low-normal serum magnesium concentrations in the presence of hypokalemia because magnesium is an intracellular cation, and serum concentrations may not accurately reflect intracellular status. Generally, 12 mEq/L is appropriate to add to the TPN; if the patient has renal dysfunction, then add 4 mEq/L. Hypermagnesemia usually occurs in association with renal dysfunction or failure. Magnesium should be removed from the PN of these patients until the serum concentration returns to the normal range.

Phosphorus. The role of phosphorus in physiologic processes is diverse, and it influences multiple organ systems including respiration, myocardial function, platelet, red and white blood cell function. The parenteral RDA of phosphorus is approximately 30 mmol or 1000 mg/day. If phosphorus is omitted from PN formulations in the presence of normal renal function, potentially life-threatening hypophosphatemia can occur within a week of PN therapy. Hypophosphatemia is a common metabolic complication of critically ill patients receiving nutrition support, reported to occur in approximately 30% of patients receiving PN. Several patient populations are at a greater risk of developing phosphorus deficiency, such as patients with a history of alcohol abuse, poor nutritional status before injury, or long-term use of antacids or sucralfate. Drug-induced hypophosphatemia results from intracellular shift of phosphorus into the cell or urinary wasting. Medications associated with hypophosphatemia include antacids, sucralfate, diuretics, theophylline, and insulin. Generally, 30 mmol/day of phosphorus should be added to the PN formulation. Treatment of hypophosphatemia is dictated by the severity of the condition, and intravenous replacement doses are most frequently used. In patients requiring both potassium and phosphate, potassium phosphate (usually 15–22.5 mmol/L) can be added to the PN formulation. A graduated dosing scheme for replacement of

TABLE 91.5. GRADUATED DOSING SCHEME FOR PHOSPHORUS REPLACEMENT THERAPY[a]

SERUM PHOSPHORUS CONCENTRATION (mg/dL)	PHOSPHORUS DOSE/INFUSION PERIOD[b]
2.3–3	0.16 mmol/kg/4 h
1.6–2.2	0.32 mmol/kg/4–6 h
≤1.5	0.64 mmol/kg/8 h

[a]Normal phosphorus serum concentration (2.5–4.5 mg/dL).
[b]Use 50% of the recommended dose when creatinine clearance <30 mL/min.

phosphorus in patients receiving specialized nutrition support (i.e., PN, enteral nutrition, or both) has been developed and is based on the serum phosphorus concentration of the patient (Table 91.5).

Hyperphosphatemia is much less prevalent than hypophosphatemia in surgical patients and usually is associated with renal compromise. Medications associated with increased serum phosphorus concentrations include IVLEs and Fleet enemas in the presence of renal dysfunction. If a patient has renal dysfunction, then 3 to 5 mmol/L of phosphorus added to a PN formulation is appropriate because the excretion of phosphorus will be reduced.

The use of chloride and acetate salts in PN should be based on the acid-base status of the patient. For example, in cases of metabolic alkalosis, only chloride salts of either sodium or potassium should be used. Conversely, in cases of acidemia, the emphasis should be placed on acetate salts of either sodium or potassium. Under no circumstances should salts such as calcium chloride or sodium bicarbonate be used in a PN formulation, because these can result in the formation of insoluble precipitates that can be deposited in the pulmonary vasculature and can cause fatal respiratory failure.

MONITORING NUTRITION SUPPORT THERAPY

Fluid status should be evaluated on a daily basis in critically ill patients. The PN formulation should be concentrated and reduced in sodium content when patients suddenly gain 1 to 2 kg over a 24-hour period. Laboratory measurements for glucose, sodium, potassium, acid-base status, and renal function should be performed each day, whereas measurements for calcium, phosphorus, and magnesium should be performed at least three times a week. Triglyceride concentrations, liver function tests, complete blood count with differential, prothrombin time, and thromboplastin time should be assessed weekly during the acute phase of injury in this patient population.

A nitrogen balance can be calculated after a 24-hour urine collection for volume and urea nitrogen to determine the severity of catabolism (142). Nitrogen balance is defined as the difference between nitrogen intake and nitrogen excretion. Patients who have spinal cord or severe head injuries will remain in negative nitrogen balance even when a dose of protein of 2 g/kg/day is given

because of disuse atrophy. Nitrogen equilibrium, or a zero nitrogen balance, is acceptable in a stressed, previously healthy, young surgical patient.

Serum protein concentrations can be used as a measure of nutritional status because an increase in these certain protein concentrations can reflect protein anabolism. Serum ALB concentration is the most commonly used protein for assessing nutritional status. However, it is a poor marker for nutritional status in critically ill patients because of rapid falls in response to stress or injury resulting from redistribution from the intravascular space to the interstitial space and because of its long half-life (~21 days). Other serum proteins, such as prealbumin and TFN, are more sensitive to nutrition support administration because of their shorter half-lives of 2 and 7 days, respectively. Assessment of CRP in combination with these short-term serum proteins should be considered. CRP is recognized as a positive acute-phase protein, and its synthesis is increased during inflammation and stress. If CRP is elevated and the serum prealbumin concentration has suddenly decreased, this may indicate the presence of an underlying inflammatory condition rather than a deterioration in nutritional status. However, combined low prealbumin and CRP concentrations may reflect inadequate provision of calories or protein. These basic principles can be used to assist the clinician in making the appropriate adjustments in a patient's nutrition regimen.

ANABOLIC AGENTS

Because toxicities are associated with excessive administration of specialized nutrition support, anabolic agents as adjunctive therapy with PN or enteral nutrition to enhance recovery have been considered. Some data support the administration of GH, IGF-I, or anabolic steroids to critically ill patients. Much of the research in critically ill patients has been performed in patients with thermal and other injuries.

Human Growth Hormone

A decreased mortality rate has been reported in patients receiving human GH (hGH) compared with control patients (11 versus 37%, $p < .03$) (143). Pediatric burn patients receiving 0.2 mg/kg/day of hGH versus placebo demonstrated a significant decrease in donor-site healing times at first harvest (9.1±0.4 versus 7.4±0.6, $p < .05$, respectively) and second harvest (9.0±0.7 versus 5.7±0.3, $p < .05$, respectively). Length of hospital stay (divided by percentage of total body surface area) was also shortened by the use of recombinant GH (rGH), with 0.80±0.10 days divided by the percentage of total body surface area in the placebo group versus 0.52±0.04 days divided by the percentage of total body surface area burn in the treatment group ($p < .05$) (144).

The encouraging results observed with rGH was tempered by the FDA in 1997 when it released a drug warning reporting a significantly higher mortality rate in critically ill patients receiving hGH. The FDA warning was in response to two parallel studies conducted in Finland and elsewhere in Europe. A multicenter, double-blind, randomized, placebo-controlled trial was performed involving a total of 532 patients in ICUs (247 Finnish patients and 285 other European patients) (145).The patient population consisted of four separate groups: cardiac surgery, abdominal surgery, multiple trauma, and acute respiratory failure. Patients received either a daily dose of 0.10 ± 0.02 mg/kg of hGH or placebo until they were discharged from the ICU or for a maximum of 21 days. The patients who received hGH exhibited a higher mortality compared with those who did not receive the drug ($p < .001$). The Finnish study mortality rate was 39% in the hGH group and 20% in the placebo group compared with the other European study, in which 44% died in the hGH group versus 18% in the placebo group. The relative risk of death for patients receiving hGH was 1.9 (95% confidence interval, 1.3–2.9) in the Finnish study and 2.4 (95% confidence interval, 1.6–3.5) in the other European study. Increased mortality persisted even after the data were analyzed accounting for diagnostic group, APACHE II score, and age. The primary causes of death in both treatment groups were multiple-organ failure, uncontrolled infection, and septic shock. Most of the deaths in the non-Finnish European study occurred in the first 10 days of treatment, whereas 50% of deaths in the Finnish study occurred during the first 10 days of treatment, and the remainder occurred more than 3 weeks after enrollment.

Factors responsible for the increased mortality are unclear. Takala and associates (145) theorized that hGH caused a modulation in immune function. hGH has been reported to augment or inhibit the production of reactive oxygen species and proinflammatory cytokines as well as to reduce or increase the susceptibility to endotoxin or bacterial challenge in animals. Thus, depending on the underlying clinical condition, hGH could be either beneficial or detrimental in a catabolic patient. Major differences between the populations could also account for differences in mortality. In the study by Takala and colleagues (145), the average age was 60 years, and approximately 95% of patients had respiratory failure. Fewer than 10% were trauma patients. Earlier trials with hGH were conducted in younger patients with primarily trauma, burn, and surgical diagnoses. One investigator proposed that the increased mortality in the study by Takala and colleagues (145) may have resulted from negative hypermetabolic and proinflammatory effects of hGH in the study populations (146).

Other investigators have suggested that growth signals transmitted to damaged cells may trigger cell death in some tissues. Administration of hGH is known to increase IGF-I concentrations, and both serum GH and IGF-I concentrations have been associated with increased myocyte apoptosis in patients with acromegalic cardiomyopathy

(147). Apoptotic signals could be triggered by stimulation of the GH and IGF-I receptor pathways in compromised cells that results in cellular death and, ultimately, organ failure.

Impaired glycemic control induced by hGH could have increased infectious complications. Increased blood glucose concentrations are a common adverse effect of hGH, and this effect has been observed in patients receiving hGH. The cause of hyperglycemia has been attributed to defective nonoxidative glucose disposal, an increase in splanchnic glucose release, and increased peripheral resistance (148). Tightly controlled glucose concentrations have been reported to decrease morbidity and mortality in critically ill patients (53). In addition, insulin resistance induced by hGH could deprive cells of glucose, thereby leading to an energy deficit.

GH causes an initial energy deficit directly by increasing cellular metabolic rate and indirectly by increasing plasma catecholamine concentrations, which, in turn, increase energy demand. Patients with an activated systemic inflammatory response have no worsening energy deficit or further increased metabolic rate. The possibility of sudden energy deficit in the septic, traumatized, and thermally injured patient is decreased because the systemic inflammatory response has been activated. Because patients did not have systemic inflammation as a component of their disease process in the study by Takala and associates (145), increased mortality could have been the result of an energy deficit induced by hGH. Despite the mechanism, hGH should not be used in the critically ill patient. Although thermally injured or trauma patients may be an exception, research with growth factors in critical care has been redirected from hGH to anabolic steroids. Oxandrolone and other anabolic steroids have become the more popular agents of research because of positive findings and fewer adverse effects.

Insulinlike Growth Factor-I

As with GH, administration of IGF-I in the critical care population has been investigated as a means to diminish or block the catabolic process, especially in the trauma and thermally injured patient. Kudsk and associates (149) studied the effects of IGF-I and aggressive PN on CD4/CD8 ratios in head-injured patients. Fourteen patients admitted with a GCS of 4 to 10 were randomized to receive a continuous infusion of recombinant IGF-I (0.01 mg/kg/hour) or saline. Both groups received PN, which provided a total protein intake of 2 g/kg/day and a maximum nonprotein caloric delivery of 40 kcal/kg/day. IGF-I administration increased CD4/CD8 ratios and elevated IGF-I levels.

The effect of IGF-I and aggressive nutrition support on the catabolic state and clinical outcome of head-injured patients has been investigated. Patients were randomized to receive a continuous infusion of IGF-I (0.1 mg/kg/hour) beginning within 72 hours of injury and continuing for

14 days. Nutrition support was delivered at a goal of 1.25 times the measured energy expenditure. PN was used until bowel sounds returned and gastric residual volumes were less than 700 mL in 24 hours. Patients treated with IGF-I demonstrated weight gain despite a significantly higher measured energy expenditure and lower calorie intake ($p = .02$), decreased nitrogen excretion, and improved nitrogen balances. Improvements in GCS scores were also noted in those patients receiving IGF-I (150).

Administration of IGF-I has also been studied in thermally injured patients. Ten adult patients were consecutively studied after receiving saline (pretreatment), IGF-I, and IGF-binding protein-3 (IGFBP-3) for 5 days. An escalating dosing scheme delivered 1, 2, and 4 mg/day. IGF and IGFBP-3 concentrations increased as expected, and no glucose abnormalities developed. No clinical outcome data were collected in this study (151).

Oxandrolone

Nutrition support and the administration of anabolic steroids have long been investigated in the surgical and trauma patient for the preservation of lean body mass. Early studies investigating the use of nandrolone and stanozolol reported improvements in nitrogen balance as a result of decreases in nitrogen excretion. Clinical outcome data were not included (152–154). Gervasio and colleagues (155) investigated oxandrolone administration in multiple-trauma patients. In a prospective, double-blind, placebo-controlled study, 60 trauma patients were randomized to receive oxandrolone, 10 mg twice daily (n = 30), or placebo (n = 30) for a maximum of 28 days or until discharge if earlier. Enteral nutrition was initiated within 48 hours of admission. Measurement of total urinary nitrogen at baseline showed both groups to be highly catabolic (oxandrolone 17.2±4.9, placebo 19.1±10.8 g/day; not significant). On days 7 and 10, urinary nitrogen increased in both groups, but no significant differences were noted between the groups. Nitrogen balance was negative throughout the study. No significant difference in serum prealbumin concentrations over time was detected between the oxandrolone group and the placebo group. Hospital length of stay (oxandrolone 30.8±17.9, placebo 27.0±25.7 days), ICU stay (oxandrolone 17.1±7.8, placebo 15.5±9.7 days), and frequency of pneumonia or sepsis (oxandrolone 48, placebo 43 episodes) did not differ significantly between groups. The investigators concluded that oxandrolone did not have any beneficial effect on nutritional or clinical outcomes during the first 28 days after multiple trauma. Thus, more clinical research with IGF-I and anabolic steroids is needed in trauma patients.

REFERENCES

1. Hunter JA. Trans Soc Improve Med Chir Know 1793;1:182–6.
2. Aubaniac R. Semin Hop Paris 1952;28:3445–7.
3. Dudrick SJ, Wilmore DW, Vars HM et al. Surgery 1968;64:134–6.
4. Rhoads JE, Dudrich SJ. In: Rombeau JL, eds. Clinical Nutrition: Parenteral Nutrition. 2nd ed. Philadelphia: WB Saunders 1993:1–10.
5. Kudsk KA, Carpenter G, Petersen S et al. J Surg Res 1981;31:105–10.
6. Kudsk, KA, Stone JM, Carpenter G et al. J Trauma 1983;23:605–9.
7. Moore EE, Jones TN. J Trauma 1986;26:874–9.
8. Moore FA, Moore EE, Jones TN et al. J Trauma 1989;29:916–23.
9. Kudsk KA, Croce MA, Fabian TC et al. Ann Surg 1992;215:503–11.
10. Beier-Holgersen R, Boesby S. Gut 1996;39:833–5.
11. Moore FA, Feliciano DV, Andrassy RJ et al. Ann Surg 1992;216:172–83.
12. Kudsk KA, Minard G, Croce MA. Ann Surg 1996;224:531–40.
13. Khuri SF, Daley J, Henderson W et al. J Am Coll Surg 1997;185:315–27.
14. Baker SP, O'Neill B. J Trauma 1976;16:822–85.
15. Borlase BC, Moore EE, Moore FA. J Trauma 1990;30:1340–4.
16. Winsor JA, Hill GL. Ann Surg 1988;208:209–14.
17. Blackburn GL, Bistrian BR, Maini BS et al. JPEN J Parenter Enteral Nutr 1977;1:11–22.
18. Forbes GF, Bruining GJ. Am J Clin Nutr 1976;29:1359–63.
19. Hall JC, O'Quigley J, Giles GR et al. Am J Clin Nutr 1980;33:1846–51.
20. Jeejeebhoy KN. In: Rombeau JL, Caldwell MD eds. Clinical Nutrition: Enteral and Parenteral Feeding. Philadelphia: WB Saunders, 1990;118–226.
21. Kudsk KA, Jacobs DO. In: Norton JA, Bollinger RR, Chang AE et al., eds. Surgery: Scientific Basis and Current Practice. New York, Springer, 2000:123–50.
22. Kudsk KA, Minard G, Wojtysiak SL et al. Surgery 1994;116:516–23.
23. Buzby GP, Mullen JL, Mathews DC et al. Am J Surg 1980;139:160–7.
24. Kyle UG, Pirlich M, Schuetz T et al. JPEN J Parenter Enteral Nutr 2004;28:99–104.
25. Ingenbleek Y, Carpentier YA. Int J Vitam Nutr Res 1984;55:91–101.
26. Detsky AS, McLaughlin JR, Baker JP et al. JPEN J Parenter Enteral Nutr 1987;11:8–13.
27. Enia G, Sicuso C, Alati G et al. Nephrol Dial Transplant 1993;8:1094–8.
28. Kudsk KA, Tolley EA, DeWitt RC et al. JPEN J Parenter Enteral Nutr 2003;271–9.
29. Hershey SD, Moore EE, Jones TN. In: Maull KI ed. Advances in Trauma. Chicago: Year Book, 1986.
30. Moore FD. Ann Surg 1953;137:289–315.
31. Gann DS, Foster AH. In: Schwartz SI, eds. Principles of Surgery. 6th ed. New York: McGraw-Hill, 1994.
32. Cuthbertson DP. JPEN J Parenter Enteral Nutr 1979;3:108–29.
33. Deitrick JE, Whedon GD, Shorr E. Am J Med 1948;4:3–13.
34. Cerra FB. In: Mattox KL, Feliciano DV, Moore EE, eds. Trauma. 3rd ed. Stamford, CT: Appleton & Lange, 1996:1155–76.
35. Shaw-Delanty SN, Elwyn DH, Askanazi J et al. Clin Nutr 1990;9:305–10.
36. Shaw JHF, Wolfe RR. Ann Surg 1989;207:63–72.
37. Shaw JHF, Klein S, Wolfe RR. Surgery 1985;97:557–68.
38. Threlfall CJ, Maxwell AR, Stoner HB. J Trauma 1984;24:516–23.
39. Wilmore DW, Smith RJ, O'Dwyer ST et al. Surgery 1988;104:917–23.

40. Souba WW. Annu Rev Nutr 1991;11:285–308.

41. Windmueller HG, Spaeth AE. J Biol Chem 1974;249:5070–9.

42. Van Gool J, Boers W, Ladiges NCJ. Biochem J 1984;220: 125–32.

43. Long CL, Kinney JM, Geiger JW. Metabolism 1976;25: 193–201.

44. Ohzato H, Yoshizaki, K, Nishimoto N et al. Surgery 1992;111: 201–9.

45. Stoner HB, Frayn KN, Barton RN et al. Clin Sci 1979;56: 563–73.

46. Nanni G, Siegel JH, Coleman B et al. J Trauma 1984;24:14–30.

47. Kenler AS, Swails WS, Driscoll DF et al. Ann Surg 1996;223: 316–33.

48. Gurr MI. Prog Lipid Res 1983;22:257–87.

49. Wolfe R, O'Donnell T, Stone M et al. Metabolism 1980;29: 892–900.

50. Stremple JF, Thomas H, Sakach V et al. Surgery 1976;80:4–13.

51. McNamara JJ, Molot MD, Dunn RA et al. Ann Surg 1972;176: 247–50.

52. Frayn KN. Br Med Bull 1985;41:232–9.

53. van den Berghe G, Wouters P, Weekers F et al. N Engl J Med 2001;345:1359–67.

54. Tracey KJ, Beutler B, Lowry S et al. Science 1986;234:470–4.

55. Besedovsky H, Del Rey A, Sorkin E et al. Science 1986;233: 652–4.

56. Gagner M, Shizgal HM, Forse RA. Surgery 1986;100:298–305.

57. Kudsk K, Brown R. In: Moore EE, Feliciano DV, Mattox KI eds. Trauma. 4th ed. New York: McGraw-Hill, 2000:1369–405.

58. Pannen BHJ, Robotham JL. New Horizons 1995;3:183–97.

59. Hunter DC, Jaksik T, Lewis D et al. Br J Surg 1988;75:875–8.

60. Hwang T-L, Hwang S-L, Chen M-F. J Trauma 1993;34:247–51.

61. Campbell SM, Kudsk KA. JPEN J Parenter Enteral Nutr 1988; 12:610–2.

62. Krishnan JA, Parce PB, Martinez A et al. Chest 2003;124: 297–305.

63. Goulenok C, Monchi M, Chicke J–D et al. Chest 2004;125: 1441–5.

64. Bercault N, Boulain T, Kuteifan K et al. Crit Care Med 2004; 32:998–1003.

65. Dickerson RN, Rosato EF, Mullen JL. Am J Clin Nutr 1986; 44:747–55.

66. Choban PS, Burge J, Scales D et al. Am J Clin Nutr 1997; 66:546–50.

67. Long CL, Schaffel N, Geiger JW et al. JPEN J Parenter Enteral Nutr 1979;3:452–6.

68. Wolfe R, Allsop J, Burke J. Metabolism 1979;28:210–20.

69. Wolfe RR, Shaw JHF. Am J Physiol 1985;248:E236–43.

70. Pelham LD. Am J Hosp Pharm 1981;38:198–208.

71. Allardyce DB. Surg Gynecol Obstet 1982;154:641–7.

72. Talpers SS, Romberger DJ, Dunce SB et al. Chest 1992;102: 551–5.

73. Department of Health and Human Services, Food and Drug Administration. Fed Reg 2000;65:64607–19.

74. DeBiasse MA, Wilmore DW. New Horizons 1994;2:122–30.

75. Novelli GP, Adembri C, Gandini E et al. Am J Surg 1997;173: 206–9.

76. Nathens AB, Neff MJ, Jurkovich GJ et al. Ann Surg 2002;236: 814–22.

77. Metnitz PGH, Bartens C, Fischer M et al. Intensive Care Med 1999;25:180–5.

78. Louw JA, Werbeck A, Louw ME et al. Crit Care Med 1992;20: 934–41.

79. Klein GL, Langman CB, Herndon DN. J Trauma 2002;52: 346–50.

80. Klein GL, Chen TC, Holick MF et al. Lancet 2004;363:291–2.

81. Forceville X. Intensive Care Med 2001;27:16–8.

82. Angstwurm MWA, Schottdorf J, Schopohl J et al. Crit Care Med 1999;27:1807–13.

83. Berger MM, Spertini FS, Shenkin A et al. Am J Clin Nutr 1998; 68:365–71.

84. Johnson LR, Copeland EM, Dudrick SJ et al. Gastroenterology 1975;68:1177–83.

85. Levine GM, Derin JJ, Steiger E et al. Gastroenterology 1974; 67:975–82.

86. Purandare S, Offenbartl K, Westrom B et al. Scand J Gastroenterol 1989; 24:678–82.

87. Kudsk KA. Am J Surg 2002;183:370–98.

88. Genton L, Kudsk KA. Am J Surg 2003;186:253–8.

89. Minard G, Kudsk KA, Melton S et al. JPEN J Parenter Enteral Nutr 2000;24:145–9.

90. Fan St, Lo CM, Lai EC et al. N Engl J Med 1994;331:1547–52.

91. Daly JM, Liebernab MD, Goldfine J et al. Surgery 1992;112: 56–67.

92. Daly JM, Weintraub FN, Shou J et al. Ann Surg 1995;221: 327–38.

93. Brennan MF, Pisters PWT, Posner M et al. Ann Surg 1994; 220:436–44.

94. Heslin MJ, Latkany L, Leung D et al. Ann Surg 1997;226: 567–77.

95. Veteran Affairs Total Parenteral Nutrition Cooperative Study Group. N Engl J Med 1991;325:525–32.

96. Braga M, Gianotti L, Nespoli L et al. Arch Surg 2002;137: 174–80.

97. Ginzalez-Huix F, Fernandez-Banares F, Esteve-Comas M et al. Am J Gastroenterol 1993;88:227–32.

98. Gonzalez-Huix F, de Leon R, Fernandez-Banares F et al. Gut 1993;34:778–2.

99. Wicks C, Somasundaram S, Bjarnason I et al. Lancet 1994;344: 837–40.

100. Hasse JM, Blue LS, Liepa GU et al. JPEN J Parenter Enteral Nutr 1995;19:437–43.

101. McClave SA, Greene LM, Snider HL et al. JPEN J Parenter Enteral Nutr 1997;21:14–20.

102. Windsor AC, Kanwar S, Li AG et al. Gut 1998;42:431–5.

103. Gianotti L, Braga M, Nespoli L et al. Gastroenterology 2002; 122:1763–70.

104. van der Hulst RRWJ, von Meyenfeldt MF, van Kreel BK et al. Lancet 1993;341:1363–5.

105. Deitch EA. Perspect Crit Care 1988;1:1–13.

106. Janu P, Li J, Minard G et al. Surg Forum 1996;47:7–9.

107. Moore FA, Moore EE, Poggetti R et al. J Trauma 1991;31: 629–36.

108. Deitch EA, Shi HP, Lu Q et al. Crit Care Med 2004;32:533–8.

109. Adams CA Jr, Hauser CJ, Adams JM et al. Shock 2002;18: 513–7.

110. Li J, Gocinski B, Henken B et al. J Trauma 1995;39:44.

111. Wu Y, Kudsk KA, DeWitt RC et al. Ann Surg 1999;229:662–8.

112. Fukatsu K, Zarzaur B, Johnson C et al. Surg Forum 2000;51: 211–4.

113. Ikeda S, Kudsk KA, Fukatsu K et al. Ann Surg 2003;237: 677–85.

114. Zarzaur BL, Fukatsu K, Johnson CJ et al. Surg Forum 2001;52: 194–6.

115. Svanborn C. In: Ogra PL, Lamm ME, McGhee JR, eds. Handbook of Mucosal Immunology. San Diego: Academic Press, 1974.

116. Kudsk KA, Li J, Renegar KB. Ann Surg 1996;223:629.

117. King BK, Kudsk KA, Li J et al. Ann Surg 1999;229:272–8.

118. Lin M-T, Saito H, Fukushima R et al. Ann Surg 1996;223: 84–93.
119. Fong Y, Marano MA, Barber E et al. Ann Surg 1989;210: 449–56.
120. McDonald WS, Sharp CW Jr, Deitch EA. Ann Surg 1991;213: 177–83.
121. Collier P, Kudsk KA, Glezer J et al. Nutr Clin Pract 1994;9: 101–3.
122. Edes TE, Walk BE, Austin JL. Am J Med 1990;88:91–3.
123. Eisenberg PG. Nutr Clin Pract 1993;8:119–23.
124. Guenter PA, Settle RG, Permutter S et al. JPEN J Parenter Enteral Nutr 1991;15:277–80.
125. Houdijk APJ, Rijnsburger ER, Jansen J et al. Lancet 1998; 352: 772–6.
126. Griffiths RD, Jones C, Palmer TE. Nutrition 1997;13:295–302.
127. Kirk SJ, Barbul A. JPEN J Parenter Enteral Nutr 1990;14: 226S–9S.
128. Moore FA, Moore EE, Kudsk KA et al. J Trauma 1994;37: 607–15.
129. Heyland DK, Novak F, Drover J et al. JAMA 2001;286:944–53.
130. Dent D, Heyland DK, Levy H et al. Crit Care Med 1995;30: A17.
131. Bertolini G, Iapchino G, Radrizzani D et al. Intensive Care Med 2003;29:834–40.
132. Ochoa JB, Makarenkova V, Bansal V. Nutr Clin Pract 2004;19: 216–25.
133. Chang W-K, Yang KD, Shaio M-F. Clin Immunol 1999;93: 294–301.
134. Wilmore DW, Shabert JK. Nutrition 1998;14:618–26.
135. Ziegler TR, Young LS, Benfell K et al. Ann Intern Med 1992; 116:821–8.
136. Klein S, Miles JM. JPEN J Parenter Enteral Nutr 1994;18: 396–7.
137. Smirniotis V, Kostopanagiotou G, Vassiliou J et al. Intensive Care Med 1998;24:1029–33.
138. Hwang TL, Huang SL, Chen MF. Chest 1990;97:934–8.
139. Venus B, Smith RA, Patel C et al. Chest 1989;95:1278–81.
140. Battistella FD, Widergren JT, Anderson JT et al. J Trauma 1997;43:52–60.
141. Kruimel JW, Naber TH, van der Vliet JA et al. JPEN J Parenter Enteral Nutr 2001;25:237–44.
142. Miller SJ. Hosp Pharm 1990;25:61–5, 70.
143. Knox J, Demling R, Wilmore D et al. J Trauma 1995;39:526–32.
144. Herndon DN, Barrow RE, Kunkel KR et al. Ann Surg 1990; 212:424–73.
145. Takala J, Ruokonen E, Webster NR et al. N Engl J Med 1999; 341:785–92.
146. Demling R. N Engl J Med 1999;341:837–9.
147. O'Connor R. Adv Biochem Eng Biotechnol 1998;62:137–66.
148. Jeevanandam M, Holaday NJ, Peterson SR. Metabolism 1996; 45:450–6.
149. Kudsk KA, Mowatt-Larssen C, Bukar J et al. Arch Surg 1994; 129:66–70.
150. Hatton J, Rapp RP, Kudsk KA et al. J Neurosurg 1997;86: 779–86.
151. Debroy MA, Wolf SE, Zhang XJ et al. J Trauma 1999;47: 904–10.
152. Hausmann DF, Nutz V, Rommelsheim K et al. JPEN J Parenter Enteral Nutr 1990;14:111–4.
153. Mosebach KO, Hausmann DF, Caspari R et al. Acta Endocrinol Suppl 1985;271:60–9.
154. Hansell DT, Davies JW, Shenkin A et al. JPEN J Parenter Enteral Nutr 1989;13:349–58.
155. Gervasio JM, Dickerson RN, Swearingen J et al. Pharmacotherapy 2000;20:1328–31.

92 NUTRITIONAL ASPECTS OF HEMATOLOGIC DISEASES[1,2]

CHRISTOPHER R. CHITAMBAR AND AŚOK C. ANTONY

GENERAL CONCEPTS 1436
ANEMIA AND ITS CLINICAL CONSEQUENCES 1436
IRON 1437
   Physiology 1437
   Absorption and Availability of Dietary Iron 1438
   Prevalence of Iron Deficiency 1440
   Signs and Symptoms in Iron Deficiency Anemia .1441
   Diagnosis of Iron Deficiency 1442
   Differential Diagnosis .1442
   Iron Deficiency in Pregnancy 1443
   Infants, Children, and Adolescents 1443
   Iron Fortification and Treatment 1443
   Functional Iron Deficiency with the Use
      of Recombinant Erythropoietin 1444
COBALAMIN AND FOLATE 1444
   Nutritional Aspects of Cobalamin and Folate
      Deficiency 1444
   Intracellular Metabolism and Cobalamin-Folate
      Interrelationships 1447
   Consequences of Folate and Cobalamin
      Deficiency in Proliferating Cells 1447
   Neurologic Dysfunction with Cobalamin
      Deficiency 1447
   Signs and Symptoms in Cobalamin Deficiency . .1448
   Laboratory Data 1449
   Diagnosis of Cobalamin Deficiency 1451
   Nutritional Cobalamin Deficiency 1451
   Pathogenesis of Folate Deficiency 1454
   Folate-Responsive Neural Tube Defects
      and Neurocristopathies 1455
   Therapy for Cobalamin and Folate Deficiency . . .1457
   Hematologic Response to Cobalamin or Folate . .1457
   Masked Megaloblastosis 1457
   Routine Supplementation of Cobalamin
      and Folate 1457

LESS COMMON NUTRITIONAL DEFICIENCIES
   AFFECTING THE BLOOD 1458
      Ascorbic Acid (Vitamin C) 1458
      Pyridoxine 1458
      Protein-Energy (Kwashiorkor) 1458
      Vitamin E 1458
      Riboflavin 1458
      Copper 1458

GENERAL CONCEPTS

The formation of blood cells (hematopoiesis) is sited in the bone marrow cavity (medulla) of virtually all bones in the newborn, but in adults, active blood formation is confined to the central skeleton (skull, vertebral column, ribs, and pelvis) and the upper ends of the humerus and femur. All hematopoietic cells arise from a very small population of self-renewing stem cells that can be detected only with monoclonal antibodies directed against unique antigens present on these cells. Stem cells, under the influence of a range of growth factors, give rise to red blood cells, white blood cells including polymorphonuclear neutrophils, eosinophils, basophils, monocytes, lymphocytes, and platelets.

The nutritional requirements for hematopoiesis are no different from those of any other tissue. However, turnover of blood cells is normally greater than that of other tissues in the body, and availability of three nutrients can become limiting: iron, cobalamin (vitamin B_{12}), and pteroylglutamic acid (folic acid or folate). Iron is required as the oxygen carrier in the hemoglobin molecule in erythrocytes, and cobalamin and folate are essential in the synthesis of three of the four nucleotides of DNA required for the doubling of the DNA content of the cell before mitosis. Lack of other nutrients only rarely causes anemia; these include vitamin A, vitamin B_6, riboflavin, ascorbic acid, vitamin E, and copper.

ANEMIA AND ITS CLINICAL CONSEQUENCES

Impairment of normal red cell production results in a fall in the hemoglobin concentration, red cell count, and packed cell volume to less than the levels shown in Table 92.1.

[1]We are honored to update Professor I. Chanarin's ninth edition chapter and have retained some of his original text and color photographs.
[2]Abbreviations: **CoA**, coenzyme A; **DRI**, dietary reference intake; **MCV**, mean corpuscular volume; **MMA**, methylmalonic acid; **NHANES**, National Health and Nutrition Examination Survey; **NTD**, neural tube defect; **RDA**, recommended dietary allowance; **rHuEpo**, recombinant human erythropoietin; **sTfR**, serum soluble transferrin receptor.

TABLE 92.1. VALUES IN A BLOOD COUNT BELOW WHICH ANEMIA IS PRESENT[a]

	WOMEN	MEN
Red cell count (10⁶/mm³)	4.0	4.5
Hemoglobin (g/dL)	12	13.5
Hematocrit Packed cell volume (%)	36	41

[a]Data for men and women (18–50 y) of all races in the United States.

Persons living at an altitude of 4000 feet or more have higher blood values. The fall in blood values, in turn, leads to a reduction in the oxygen-carrying capacity of the blood and impairment of oxygen delivery to tissues. The effects of anemia are the result not only of impaired oxygen delivery but also of the compensatory mechanisms that develop.

The compensatory mechanisms are of three kinds. An increase in the level of 2,3-diphosphoglycerate in anemic red blood cells leads to increased binding of this compound to deoxyhemoglobin and so reduces its affinity for oxygen. As a result, a greater proportion of the oxygen on hemoglobin can be released to tissues. A second adjustment to anemia is speeding circulation of blood by increasing cardiac output; this becomes clinically obvious when the hemoglobin concentration falls to less than 7 g/dL. Finally, the decline in oxygenation of the kidneys results in increased production of the erythropoietic hormone, erythropoietin, which leads to increased blood production and extension of hematopoiesis into fatty bone marrow. In chronic anemia, these compensatory mechanisms allow the patient to continue relatively normal activity, so the severity of anemia often appears out of keeping with the paucity of symptoms.

Most patients with significant anemia are fatigued and tire easily after exertion. They are pale, most evident on inspection of mucous membranes. Palpitations (awareness of the heart beat), tinnitus (ringing or whistling noise in the ears or head), headache, irritability, dizziness, and weakness may be present. Patients are short of breath and have a rapid heart beat and pulse and visible arterial pulsation. They often have systolic heart murmurs on cardiac auscultation that disappear when the anemia has been corrected. In older people, cardiac pain (angina) and cardiac failure may develop, the latter characterized by swelling of the feet, enlarged liver, and pulmonary edema.

Soreness of the mouth and tongue is often present in iron, cobalamin, or folate deficiencies. In the latter two deficiencies, impaired squamous cell renewal in mouth and tongue can be blamed, and a high iron requirement may also explain these findings in iron deficiency. Cracks may appear at the angles of the mouth, termed *angular stomatitis* (Fig. 92.1). Other findings in particular deficiencies are dealt with later in this chapter.

IRON

Iron is essential for cell viability and cell proliferation; it is an essential component of proteins involved in energy metabolism (mitochondria, electron transport, and the citric acid cycle), respiration (hemoglobin and myoglobin), and DNA synthesis (ribonucleotide reductase). Because the major requirement for iron in the body is for hemoglobin production, most of the iron in the body is present in red blood cells. Blood loss from the gastrointestinal tract and menstrual blood loss in women are major causes of iron deficiency in adults. Gastrointestinal malabsorption of iron and increased requirements for iron during growth and pregnancy that are not met by dietary intake are additional causes of iron deficiency. Hookworm infestation of the gut is a common cause of iron deficiency in many parts of the world and may coexist with dietary deficiency. The depletion of body iron stores blunts erythropoiesis and results in anemia, the most common clinical manifestation of iron deficiency. The discussion in this section focuses primarily on factors producing negative iron balance and the resultant hematologic consequences. Basic aspects of iron metabolism are dealt with in Chapter 12.

Physiology

In the body, iron is present in hemoglobin (1600–2400 mg in an adult), myoglobin (300 mg), and various heme and nonheme enzymes (150 mg), including cytochromes necessary for oxidative reactions producing energy. Ferritin and hemosiderin in the liver, spleen, and bone marrow are the primary sites for iron storage. The relative distribution of iron in the body based on body weight is summarized in Table 92.2 (1–3).

Whereas men have some 500 to 1000 mg of storage iron and older men have even more, iron stores in women seldom reach 500 mg. Indeed, when iron requirements are high, as in growing children, in menstruating women, and in pregnancy, iron stores are usually absent or low. The initial phase in the development of iron deficiency is a progressive

TABLE 92.2. NORMAL DISTRIBUTION OF IRON-CONTAINING COMPOUNDS IN MEN AND WOMEN (MILLIGRAMS PER KILOGRAM OF BODY WEIGHT)

COMPOUND	MEN	WOMEN
Storage		
Ferritin	9	4
Hemosiderin	4	1
Transport protein		
Transferrin	<1	<1
Functional compounds		
Hemoglobin	31	31
Myoglobin	4	4
Respiratory enzymes	2	2
Total	50	42

Data from references 1 to 3.

decrease in body iron stores that can be recognized as a diminution and, eventually, an absence of stainable iron in the bone marrow or liver. In otherwise healthy persons, serum ferritin levels are a good marker of body iron stores, and these levels decrease in parallel with the decrease in iron stores. Anemia eventually ensues when the amount of iron available from body stores and gastrointestinal absorption is insufficient to meet the requirements for hemoglobin production; the anemia worsens as iron deficiency becomes more severe.

In adults, approximately 22 mg of iron is turned over each day: 20 to 21 mg iron is recovered and recycled from senescent red cells removed from the circulation at the end of their life span, whereas only about 1 mg/day in men and 2 mg/day in women will enter the body from absorption of dietary iron. The latter values constitute iron requirements and arise from iron lost as a result of desquamation of epithelial cells and by iron lost in menstruation. Substantial amounts of additional iron are required during pregnancy and during growth in childhood. Iron losses have been assessed as follows: In men, iron losses have been measured at 0.9 mg/24 hours or 14 μg/kg/24 hours (4). Extrapolation of data from men indicates a basal iron loss of 0.8 mg/24 hours for a 55-kg woman. Median menstrual blood loss in healthy women is between 25 and 30 mL per cycle. Averaged over the entire menstrual cycle, the daily iron loss is 0.5 mg/24 hours. One fourth of women lose more than 0.8 mg/24 hours, 10% more than 1.3 mg/24 hours, and 5% more than 1.6 mg/24 hours. When basal iron losses are added, the daily iron requirement in 5% of women exceeds 2.4 mg/24 hours. Oral contraceptives reduce menstrual loss by about half, whereas intrauterine devices double the loss.

Pregnant women require iron to replace basal iron losses (220 mg iron during pregnancy going to term), to expand their red cell mass (500 mg), and to provide iron for the placenta and developing fetus. The full-term fetus has about 290 mg of iron, and placenta has about 25 mg. Thus, the total additional iron requirement in pregnancy is about 1000 mg. The increased requirement for iron starts in the second trimester; the daily iron requirement increases from 0.8 mg in the first trimester to 4.4 mg in the second and to 6.3 mg daily in the third trimester. In the latter two

thirds of pregnancy, iron needs cannot be met by dietary iron alone, and unless at least 500 mg of iron is available as iron stores present before pregnancy, iron supplements need to be given during pregnancy. Further iron loss results from bleeding during delivery. During pregnancy, iron loss from menstruation ceases, and during the puerperium, reduction of the red cell mass makes the iron in these surplus red cells available. Following delivery, several months elapse before menstruation is restored in a lactating woman. However, a daily loss of 0.3 mg in breast milk occurs, and hence the mean iron requirement during 6 months of lactation is 1.1 mg/day.

A normal newborn has about 75 mg iron/kg, of which two thirds is in hemoglobin. The physiologic decrease in red cell mass in the first 2 months of life returns some iron to stores. Absorption of dietary iron becomes significant only at 4 to 6 months of life, when initial iron stores have become considerably depleted. Premature (low-birth-weight) infants have much reduced iron stores and need dietary iron at a much earlier age than full-term infants. In childhood, additional iron is required for the expanding red cell mass and for growth.

Requirements are shown in Table 92.3 for the Food and Agriculture Organization and World Health Organization (4) and in Table 92.4 for the 1989 US recommended dietary allowances (RDA) (3). More recent dietary reference intakes (DRIs) for iron are also listed in Table 92.5 (5) for comparison.

Absorption and Availability of Dietary Iron

Dietary Sources of Iron

Iron in food is present in high-molecular-weight species, the digestion of which is important for the release and absorption of iron. Iron is available as heme iron and nonheme (inorganic) iron. The latter may be present as the ferrous (reduced, Fe[II]) or ferric (oxidized, Fe[III]) form. The duodenum is the primary site of both heme and nonheme iron absorption in the gut.

Heme iron (iron porphyrin) is present in the hemoglobin and myoglobin of animal foods and is highly bioavailable. After being split from globin, iron porphyrin is trans-

TABLE 92.3. IRON REQUIREMENTS FOR INFANTS AND CHILDREN

AGE (y)	MEAN BODY WEIGHT (kg)	GROWTH REQUIREMENT (mg/24 h)	BASAL LOSSES (mg/24 h)	TOTAL REQUIREMENT (mg/24 h)
0.25–1	3	0.56	0.21	0.77
1–2	11	0.24	0.25	0.49
2–6	16	0.22	0.34	0.55
6–12	29	0.38	0.55	0.94
12–16 males	53	0.66	0.80	1.45
12–16 females	51	0.35	0.79	1.62[a]

[a] Allowing for menstrual loss of 0.47 mg/24 h.

From Food and Agriculture Organization/World Health Organization. FAO/WHO Requirements of Vitamin A, Iron, Folate and Vitamin B$_{12}$. FAO Food and Nutrition Series no. 23. Rome: Food and Agriculture Organization, 1988:1–107, with permission.

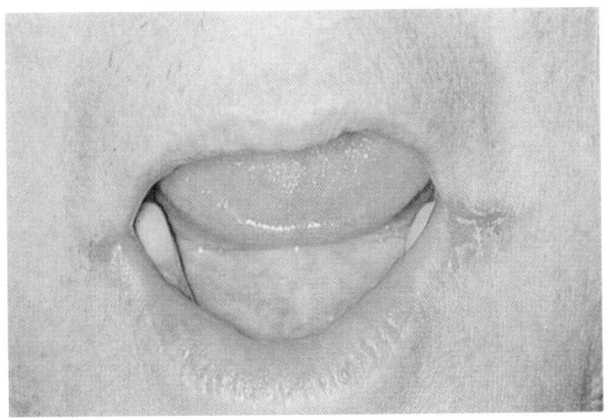

Figure 92.1. Angular stomatitis and a smooth, shiny tongue in iron deficiency anemia.

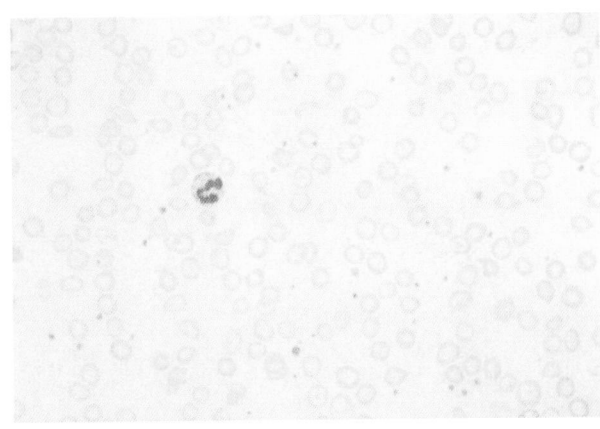

Figure 92.2. Peripheral blood film from a patient with severe iron deficiency anemia.

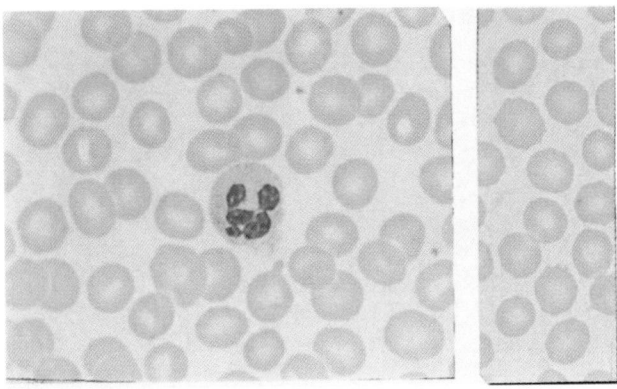

Figure 92.3. Early macrocytic anemia. The red blood cells are large, compared with those in the strip on the right, which is a normal blood film.

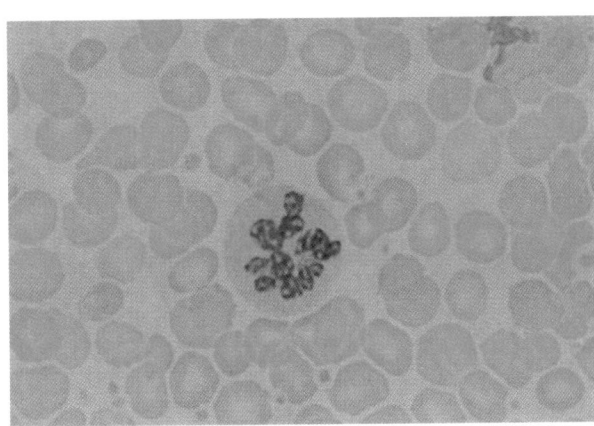

Figure 92.4. Blood film from a patient with cobalamin deficiency showing a striking hypersegmented neutrophil polymorphonuclear leukocyte. The red blood cells show variation in size (anisocytosis) and are generally larger than normal (macrocytosis).

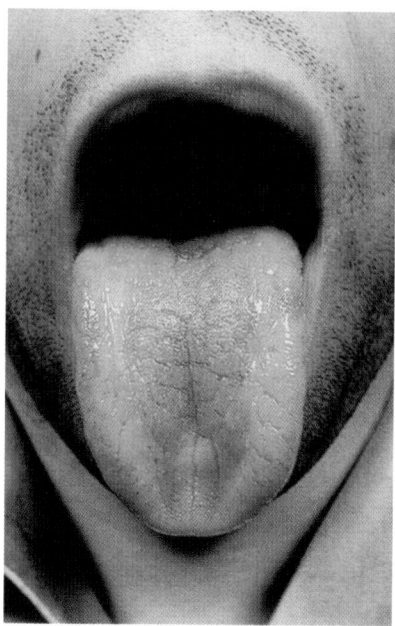

Figure 92.5. Red, "beefy" tongue in a 23-year-old man with cobalamin deficiency. For 1 year, he complained that spicy food and, in particular, whiskey, produced a painful mouth and tongue.

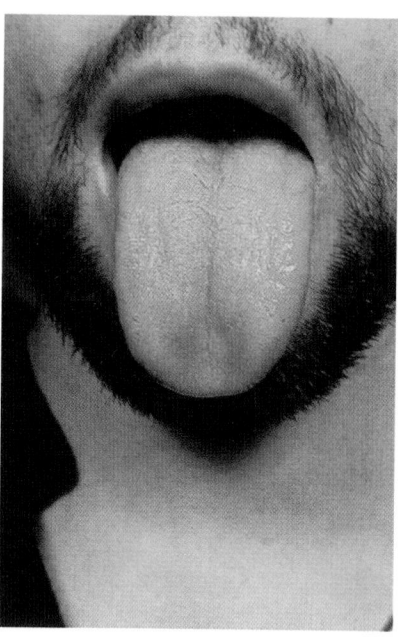

Figure 92.6. Same patient as in Figure 92.5 about 2 weeks after the start of cobalamin treatment. The tongue is normal in appearance, and the unpleasant symptoms related to whiskey had disappeared.

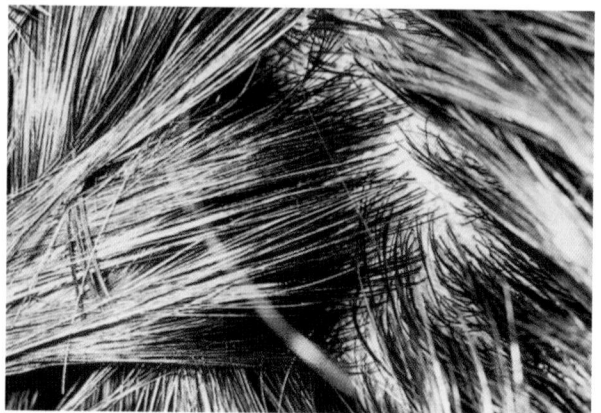

Figure 92.7. Scalp hair of a 19-year-old Indian with nutritional cobalamin deficiency and severe megaloblastic anemia. On presentation, his hair was a dingy gray. This photograph was taken about 2 months after the start of oral cobalamin, 5 μg/day. Cobalamin restored the normal pigment to the hair, which now grew jet black.

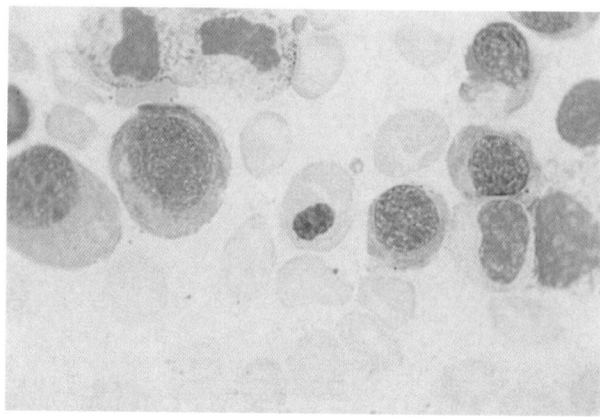

Figure 92.8. Bone marrow film from a patient with severe megaloblastic anemia. The cells with finely stippled nuclei and gray cytoplasm are red cell precursors called megaloblasts.

TABLE 92.4. RECOMMENDED DIETARY ALLOWANCE (RDA) FOR IRON IN THE UNITED STATES IN 1989 AND THE PROPORTION OF US POPULATION HAVING DIETS MEETING 100% OF THE RDA FOR IRON FROM 1994 TO 1996[a]

SEX AND AGE (y)	RDA (mg/d)	PROPORTION OF US POPULATION MEETING 100% OF THE 1989 RDA FOR IRON (%)
Both sexes		
<1	6–10	87.9[b]
1–2	10	43.9
3–5	10	61.7
Females		
6–11	10	60.9
12–19	15	27.7
20–29	15	25.9
30–39	15	26.6
40–49	15	22.1
50–59	10	55.2
60–69	10	59.3
≥70	10	59.2
Males		
6–11	10	79.8
12–19	12	83.1
20–29	10	86.9
30–39	10	88.9
40–49	10	85.9
50–59	10	83.8
60–69	10	85.5
≥70	10	78.5

[a]Recommendations to prevent and control iron deficiency in the United States.

[b]Excludes breast-fed infants.

From Centers for Disease Control and Prevention. MMWR Morb Mortal Wkly Rep 1998;47:1–29.

ported across the brush border membrane to the interior of the enterocyte. Within the cell, iron is split from the tetrapyrrol portion of heme and may exit the enterocyte to the circulation through a pathway similar to that of nonheme iron. Heme provides 10 to 15% of food iron in a mixed diet. Twenty to 30% of heme iron is absorbed independent of the overall composition of the diet and, in persons ingesting a diet of high meat content, heme iron may provide one fourth of the iron requirements.

Nonheme iron is present in cereals, pulses (seeds of leguminous plants), fruits, vegetables, and dairy products. It provides 85 to 90% of dietary iron in a mixed diet and is the only source of iron in a largely vegetarian diet.

Factors Influencing Iron Absorption

The mixture of foods in a diet contains factors that either promote or inhibit iron absorption, and thus the amount of iron absorbed may vary considerably. Absorption of food iron is inhibited by phytates, polyphenols (6, 7) including tannins present in tea, certain proteins, and certain dietary fibers. Inhibitors act by strongly binding ionic iron. Phytates are

salts of inositol hexaphosphates, and about 90% arise from dietary cereals. Even small amounts of phytates have a strong inhibitory effect on iron absorption. Bran has a high phytate content, as does high-extraction-rate flour. Fiber-rich foods have abundant phytates. A high dietary iron content does not counteract the inhibitory effect of fiber. Polyphenols are widely present in plants and some bind iron, particularly those in tea, coffee, and cocoa. They are also present in vegetables such as spinach and in some herbs and spices. Calcium as a salt or in milk and cheese interferes with both heme and nonheme iron absorption (8).

Absorption of food iron is enhanced by the presence of meat, poultry, seafood, and ascorbic acid. Ascorbic acid, as such or derived from fruit and vegetables, is a potent enhancer of iron absorption, probably by reducing ferric to ferrous iron. Apart from their effect as a reducing agent, iron-ascorbate complexes are absorbed as such. Recent studies indicate that ferric iron is first reduced to ferrous iron by the action of a reductase and is transported across the luminal surface of the enterocyte by the divalent metal transporter DMT-1 (9). Other weak organic acids such as

TABLE 92.5. RECOMMENDED DIETARY REFERENCE INTAKE FOR IRON BY LIFE STAGE GROUP

LIFE STAGE GROUP	RDA (mg/d)	SELECTED FOOD SOURCES AND SPECIAL CONSIDERATIONS
Both sexes		Special food sources:
7–12 mo	11	Fruits, vegetables, and fortified
1–3 y	7	bread and grain products
4–8 y	10	such as cereal (nonheme iron sources), meat, and poultry (heme iron sources)
Females		Special considerations:
9–13 y	8	Nonheme iron absorption is
14–18 y	15	lower for those consuming
19–50 y	18	vegetarian diets than for
51–70 y	8	those eating nonvegetarian
>70 y	8	diets. Therefore, it has been
Pregnancy		suggested that the iron
14–18 y	27	requirement for those
19–50 y	27	consuming a vegetarian diet
Lactation		is approximately twofold
14–18 y	10	greater than for those
19–50 y	9	consuming a nonvegetarian diet.
		Recommended intake
		assumes 75% of iron is from
		heme iron sources.
Males		
9–13 y	8	
14–18 y	11	
19–70 y	8	
>70 y	8	

RDA, recommended dietary allowance.

From Food and Nutrition Board, Institute of Medicine. Dietary Reference Intakes for Vitamin A, Vitamin K, Arsenic, Boron, Chromium, Copper, Iodine, Iron, Manganese, Molybdenum, Nickel, Silicon, Vanadium, and Zinc. Washington, DC: National Academy Press, 2001:18–9, with permission.

citric acid may also enhance absorption of nonheme iron. It is not clear why meat, fish, and other seafood enhance the absorption of nonheme iron.

Apart from the composition of the diet, the amount of iron absorbed is affected by the subject's iron status. Substantial iron stores decrease iron absorption, particularly of nonheme iron, and conversely, iron deficiency is accompanied by an increase in iron absorption to a maximum of 4 mg/24 hours. This, however, is still short of the daily iron requirement in the latter months of pregnancy.

Total Dietary Iron Intake

Daily iron intake per capita in 137 countries ranged from 14.4 to 20.2 mg (4). Animal produce was a major contributor of iron in only 23 of these countries. This iron intake should be enough to meet a requirement of 1 to 2 mg/day, but it often does not do so because of the low availability of the iron in these diets. A comparison of the diet and iron status of 50 vegetarians and 50 matched subjects on mixed diets showed that the vegetarians consumed 16.8 mg iron/ day compared with 14.6 mg in persons ingesting a mixed diet, but those on a mixed diet had larger iron stores. Serum ferritin levels in vegetarians were 36.6 ng/mL, compared with 105.4 ng/mL in those on a mixed diet (10).

Diets provide iron of low, intermediate, or high bioavailability (4). The data refer to iron absorption by persons with no iron stores but with normal iron transport. A diet low in iron bioavailability (iron absorption ~5%) is a monotonous diet of cereals, roots, and/or tubers and negligible amounts of meat, fish, or foods likely to contain ascorbate. These foods often contain inhibitors to iron absorption present in maize, beans, whole wheat flour, and sorghum and are largely consumed in lower socioeconomic groups in developing countries. Diets consisting largely of cereals may allow only 1 to 2% of the iron to be absorbed. This diet does not meet the needs of menstruating or pregnant women but may suffice under other circumstances.

Diets of intermediate iron bioavailability (iron absorption ~10%) consist mainly of cereals, roots, and/or tubers, some food supplying ascorbate, and minimal food of animal origin. A low-bioavailability diet can be changed into one of intermediate bioavailability by increased intake of meat, fish, or ascorbate. A high-bioavailability diet can be changed to one of intermediate iron availability by simultaneous consumption of tea or coffee, which contains inhibitors to iron absorption. This diet may meet the needs of some menstruating women but not the needs of pregnant women.

A diet high in iron bioavailability (iron absorption ~15%) is a mixed diet with good quantities of meat, poultry, fish, and foods of high ascorbate content. It is typical of the diet in industrialized countries. It is adequate for menstruating women but without substantial iron stores will not meet the needs in many pregnancies.

Human breast milk contains about 0.5 mg iron/L. The bioavailability is high; 50% of this iron is absorbed. This contrasts with cow's milk formulas or unfortified cow's milk, in which only 10 to 20% of the iron is available for absorption. Cow's milk formulas are usually fortified with iron to supply 6 to 12 mg/L. Breast milk supplies sufficient iron to full-term infants to meet their needs for the first 4 to 5 months of life. Weaning foods often consist of cereals with iron of low bioavailability. Thus, many cereals have iron and ascorbate added, and they are a major source of iron in the first 1 to 2 years of life.

Prevalence of Iron Deficiency

Iron deficiency is a significant public health issue. It is estimated that at least 700 million persons worldwide have overt iron deficiency anemia. Major factors contributing to widespread iron deficiency include diets low in available iron, demands for iron that cannot be met during pregnancy and growth, menorrhagia in women of childbearing age, and gastrointestinal blood loss. Causes of gastrointestinal blood loss include gastric ulcer disease, gastric irritation resulting from long-term use of nonsteroidal antiinflammatory medication (including aspirin) or steroids, gastroesophageal hiatal hernia, colonic diverticulosis, malformations of blood vessels involving the gastrointestinal mucosa (angiodysplasia), malignancy, and, in certain parts of the world, hookworm infestation (*Ancylostoma duodenale* or *Necator americanus*). Urinary iron losses leading to iron deficiency may occur in conditions associated with intravascular hemolysis such as paroxysmal nocturnal hemoglobinuria and red cell fragmentation from prosthetic heart valves. Malabsorption of iron may occur following surgical resection of the stomach (total or partial gastrectomy), surgery that results in bypassing the duodenum, gastric achlorhydria, sprue, or inflammatory gastrointestinal conditions (enteritis).

With regard to dietary causes, in African countries, millet, sorghum, or maize is the staple food, and in many parts of Asia, it is rice. Anemia is present in 36% of the population in developing countries and in about 8% of the population of developed countries. It is the most prevalent nutritional deficiency in the world. The prevalence of iron deficiency and iron deficiency anemia in the United States, based on data from the National Health and Nutrition Examination Survey (NHANES) of 1999 to 2000 and from NHANES III (1988–1994), is shown in Tables 92.6 and 92.7 (11).

A mixed diet is expected to supply enough iron in persons with a normal iron requirement. Observations made in persons who are largely vegetarian underscores the finding that purely nutritional factors are of great importance. A study of megaloblastic anemia in a community of strict lifelong vegetarians generally taking cow's milk as the only form of animal food showed that two thirds (53 women and 38 men) of 138 persons had overt iron deficiency.

TABLE 92.6. PREVALENCE OF IRON DEFICIENCY: UNITED STATES NATIONAL HEALTH AND NUTRITION EXAMINATION SURVEYS, 1988 TO 1994 AND 1999 TO 2000[a]

SEX/AGE GROUP (y)	1988–1994 %	1988–1994 (95% CI)	1999–2000 %	1999–2000 (95% CI)
Both sexes				
1–2	9	(6–11)	7	(3–11)
3–5	3	(2–4)	5	(2–7)
6–11	2	(1–3)	4	(1–7)
Males				
12–15	1	(0.1–2)	5	(2–8)
16–69	1	(0.6–1)	2	(1–3)
≥70	4	(2–)	3	(2–7)
Females (nonpregnant)				
12–49	11	(10–12)	12	(10–14)
12–15	9	(6–12)	9	(5–12)
16–19	11	(7–14)	16	(10–22)
20–49	11	(10–13)	12	(10–16)
White, non-Hispanic	8	(7–9)	10	(7–13)
African-American, non-Hispanic	15	(13–17)	19	(14–24)
Mexican-American	19	(17–21)	22	(17–27)
50–69	5	(4–7)	9	(5–12)
≥70	7	(5–8)	6	(4–9)

CI, confidence interval.

[a] All racial/ethnic groups except where noted.

Adapted from Centers for Disease Control and Prevention. MMWR Morb Mortal Wkly Rep 2002;51:897–9.

Stainable iron stores in bone marrow were absent in 70%. No abnormal blood loss occurred (12).

Signs and Symptoms in Iron Deficiency Anemia

In early stages of iron deficiency, persons can be entirely asymptomatic, and the discovery of iron deficiency anemia may be made only as a result of a routine blood count. In other instances, especially in athletes, iron deficiency may result in symptoms of decreased endurance without the presence of anemia. Eventually, however, patients with iron deficiency will develop symptoms secondary to anemia. Depending on the severity of anemia, these symptoms

TABLE 92.7. PREVALENCE OF IRON DEFICIENCY ANEMIA IN SELECTED POPULATIONS: UNITED STATES NATIONAL HEALTH AND NUTRITION EXAMINATION SURVEYS, 1988 TO 1994 AND 1999 TO 2000

SEX/AGE GROUP (y)	1988–1994 %	1999–2000 %
Both sexes		
1–2	3	2
Females (nonpregnant)		
12–19	2	2
20–49	5	4
50–69	2	3
≥70	2	1

Adapted from Centers for Disease Control and Prevention. MMWR Morb Mortal Wkly Rep 2002;51:897–9.

include fatigue, lightheadedness, and dyspnea on exertion. Severely anemic patients may display clinical symptoms of heart failure. Whereas these symptoms may be caused by anemia regardless of its origin, additional clinical findings may be attributable to iron deficiency directly. These include difficulty in swallowing and a sensation of a lump in the throat. Some patients have a sore mouth and tongue, which may be aggravated by hot drinks or spicy food. Angular stomatitis and possibly reversible gastric atrophy may occur.

Pica (eating of materials such as ice, clay, paper, or dirt) may be seen, particularly in children. Obsessive eating of ice (pagophagia) may be specific to iron deficiency and disappears within 1 to 2 weeks of iron treatment. Eating of ice was noted in 8.1% of 553 African-American women with iron deficiency in pregnancy (13). Patients with iron deficiency may complain of a sensation of pins and needles (paresthesia) in the hands and feet.

Examination of iron-deficient persons reveals pallor of the conjunctiva and skin, pale blue sclera, and nails that break easily and may be misshapen and even spoon shaped (koilonychia). The heart and pulse rate may be rapid, and in severely anemic patients of long standing, the spleen may be enlarged, with the edge palpable under the left costal margin. Radiography may show a web in the esophagus (postcricoid web) and atrophic gastritis. Less well established are observations indicating impaired work performance and muscle function, possibly resulting from an effect of iron lack on enzymes.

Cell-mediated (T-lymphocyte) immunity and neutrophil killing of phagocytosed bacteria may be impaired in iron-deficient patients (14). Neutrophils ingest and kill organisms by the production of active oxygen species, a process referred to as the oxidative burst. Because generation of the oxidative burst requires the activity of iron-containing enzymes, including reduced nicotinamide-adenine dinucleotide phosphate oxidase and cytochrome B, iron deficiency may lead to a decrease in the magnitude of this bactericidal function in neutrophils. Conversely, because microorganisms require iron for their growth, iron deficiency may provide protection against infection by limiting iron availability to pathogenic organisms. Indeed, iron treatment, particularly with parenteral iron, has been reported to precipitate latent infection such as pyelonephritis and activate latent malaria (presumably by providing iron to microorganisms) (14).

In children, impaired mental development was found when hemoglobin levels were lower than 10 g/dL at 5 years of age (15). This impairment was manifested in lower scores in mental and motor function that returned to normal when tests were repeated after iron therapy. Iron-deficient children showed reduced attention and poor learning performance. The iron content of parts of the brain is comparable to that of liver and continues to increase until the third decade of life. Iron uptake in the central nervous system is mediated by a transferrin system comparable to that in the bone marrow. In pregnancy, iron deficiency is accompanied by increased maternal morbidity including premature labor and low-birth-weight infants (16).

Patients with iron deficiency anemia may have additional clinical complaints that are not the result of anemia per se but are related to the cause of iron deficiency. For example, the presence of tarry or bright red stools would suggest iron loss from gastrointestinal bleeding, whereas the presence of dark (Coca Cola–colored) urine would suggest urinary iron loss from genitourinary bleeding or intravascular hemolysis.

Diagnosis of Iron Deficiency

The diagnosis of iron deficiency is established by measuring the hemoglobin and hematocrit and the levels of iron, transferrin, and ferritin in the blood. With the development of negative iron balance, the serum ferritin (reflective of iron stores) decreases to less than the normal level (<11 μg/L), followed by a decrease in serum iron to less than the normal range of 11 to 28 μM (65–165 μg/dL in women); the serum iron binding capacity rises to greater than the normal range of 47 to 70 μM (260–420 μg/dL), whereas transferrin saturation falls to less than the normal range of 15 to 45%. Eventually, transferrin levels increase to greater than normal. An early indicator of iron deficiency is an increase in the red cell protoporphyrin level to more than the normal value of 30 μg/dL; however, this test is not routinely performed in clinical practice. With the development of iron deficiency, erythropoiesis is affected, and hemoglobin production diminishes, leading to anemia and the development of constitutional symptoms. In clinical practice, the presence of iron deficiency is usually suspected when the blood count shows a reduction in hemoglobin and hematocrit levels and a decrease in the mean corpuscular volume (MCV) of circulating red blood cells to less than 80 fL (femtoliters). These smaller red blood cells (referred to as microcytes) contain less hemoglobin than normal red cells, so the mean corpuscular hemoglobin is also reduced to less than 27 pg (picograms) per red cell. Although the development of microcytic and hypochromic red cells is characteristic of iron deficiency anemia, the decrease in hemoglobin generally precedes the appearance of microcytosis. Hence, in early iron deficiency anemia, the red cells are normocytic and normochromic. With severe iron deficiency anemia, red cell morphology may be significantly altered, with red cells appearing as thin rings with bizarre shapes (Fig. 92.2).

Although the diagnosis of iron deficiency as the cause of anemia can usually be established by blood tests and a review of the peripheral blood smear, in certain conditions (e.g., chronic inflammation), measurements of serum iron, transferrin, and serum iron binding capacity may not be reliable indicators of iron deficiency. In these situations, an analysis of the bone marrow to demonstrate the absence of stainable iron in the marrow has long been considered the standard for establishing iron deficiency.

More recently, investigators have shown that soluble transferrin receptor levels in the circulation are increased in iron deficiency. Hence, measurement of serum soluble transferrin receptor (sTfR) level and calculation of the ratio of sTfR to log ferritin (i.e., logarithmic transformation of the serum ferritin level) are of value in estimating body iron stores when serum iron and transferrin levels are not reliable and analysis of the marrow is not feasible. The ratio of sTfR to log ferritin is increased in iron deficiency. A present obstacle to the routine use of sTfR measurements for determining iron deficiency appears to be the lack of standardization among available assays (17). Hence, this assay has not yet found its place in routine clinical practice.

Iron deficiency anemia is not associated with changes in white blood cell number. However, an increase in the platelet count is often seen.

Differential Diagnosis

Whereas microcytic hypochromic anemia is the hallmark finding of iron deficiency anemia, small red blood cells (microcytes) may be seen in a few other conditions that should be differentiated from iron deficiency to avoid inappropriate diagnostic testing and treatment. The MCV that is reported from analysis of the complete blood count on an automated counter represents a mean of the population of red blood cells being examined. Therefore, the automated complete blood count report should always be coupled with an examination of the peripheral blood smear by light microscopy to confirm the changes in red cell morphology. The red blood cells are larger in the newborn than in adults; however, cells that are substantially smaller than adult red blood cells soon replace these cells. Not until the midteens does the mean MCV reach adult levels. The diagnosis of iron deficiency in children requires confirmation by serum iron and serum ferritin levels.

Because thalassemic syndromes produce a decrease in globin synthesis, they are characterized by small red cells. Mild to moderate microcytic hypochromic anemia occurs in thalassemia trait. However, unlike iron deficiency, in which the red cell count is decreased, in thalassemia trait the red cell count is elevated, often exceeding 5.5 to 6 million/μL. This latter finding is a useful clue to the presence of thalassemia trait but requires confirmation by hemoglobin electrophoresis. In uncomplicated thalassemia trait, serum iron and ferritin levels are normal, and the hemoglobin A_2 level in red cells is raised in β-thalassemia trait. An important caveat in measuring hemoglobin A_2 levels by hemoglobin electrophoresis to establish a diagnosis of β-thalassemia trait is that coexisting iron deficiency will block the elevation of hemoglobin A_2. Hence, iron deficiency, if suspected, should be treated before one measures hemoglobin A_2.

Anemia of chronic disease may resemble iron deficiency; both are characterized by small red blood cells and a low serum iron level. However, the serum iron binding capacity is normal or low in the anemia of chronic disorders, whereas in iron deficiency it is raised. Because ferritin is an acute-phase reactant, its levels may be elevated in the anemia of chronic disease. Because sTfR concentration is not elevated in chronic disease (in contrast to ferritin), the use of the sTfR:log ferritin ratio to discriminate between iron deficiency anemia and anemia of chronic disease has been suggested. In a study of 129 consecutive anemic patients, an sTfR:log ferritin ratio of less than 1 was seen in anemia caused by inflammation or chronic disease, whereas a value of more than 4 was seen in iron deficiency anemia (18). However, whereas the sTfR:log ferritin ratio has diagnostic value, its routine use awaits standardization of the sTfR assay. Distinguishing iron deficiency from anemia of chronic disease may therefore still require direct examination of the marrow for iron stores. Measurement of markers of inflammation such as C-reactive protein may also be useful in establishing the presence of inflammation as a cause of anemia (17). Copper deficiency may be accompanied by microcytic anemia that is unresponsive to iron therapy.

Nutritional deficiency, as a factor in producing iron deficiency, may be suspected from a careful assessment of the diet. A diet likely to be deficient in available iron is a strictly vegetarian one from which foods of animal origin are excluded. At the same time, exclusion of blood loss is essential. A good clinical history often provides a clue to gastric or gut problems, medication with aspirin or nonsteroidal analgesics, and menstrual blood loss. Fecal blood loss is often intermittent, and repeated tests for occult blood loss are needed. Where hookworm is endemic, the stool should be analyzed for the presence of hookworm ova.

Iron Deficiency in Pregnancy

Pregnancy is accompanied by important changes in plasma and red cell volume that affect the hemoglobin concentration. The plasma volume expands by about 1000 mL, and the red cell volume by about 300 mL. The greater expansion of plasma volume results in dilution of red cells. The mean hemoglobin falls from 13.5 g/dL in nonpregnant women to 12.5 and 12.0 g/dL at 15 and 30 weeks of pregnancy, respectively. Thereafter, some hemoconcentration occurs, with a rise in hemoglobin to a mean of 12.8 g/dL at 38 weeks. At 30 weeks' gestation, hemoglobin in iron-replete women ranges from 10.0 to 14.5 g/dL. At the same time, physiologic changes are noted in the size of the red cells. These cells increase in size from a mean of 85 to 89 fL, but in some women the increase can reach 20 fL, so the MCV is 105 fL. This is not influenced by folate supplements but is diminished or absent if the woman also has iron deficiency and/or β-thalassemia trait.

An extra 1000 mg of iron is required in the second and third trimester to meet the needs of a normal pregnancy. This has to be set against the total body iron present in a woman of 2500 mg with a normal iron absorption of 1 to 2 mg/day, increasing to 4 mg/day in the third trimester. It is unusual for sufficient iron stores to be present to meet such demands, and this amount is more than can be absorbed from a good diet. Serum iron and ferritin levels both fall steadily throughout pregnancy. In a study of more than 2000 women who were not given any iron during pregnancy, not only did the hemoglobin level remain low to term, but even 1 year after childbirth, the mean hemoglobin of the group was still less than the level present in the first blood sample taken in early pregnancy (19). Iron deficiency in pregnancy is the result of increased demands for iron that cannot be met from stores and diet. It is coupled with poor nutrition insofar as a poor iron intake prevents formation of adequate iron stores and fails to provide sufficient iron to meet immediate needs.

The diagnosis of iron deficiency in pregnancy is the same as in other situations. It is found in about one third or more of pregnant women who do not receive an iron supplement from early pregnancy. A hemoglobin level lower than 10 g/dL is low. Since the mid-1970s, a combined iron and folic acid tablet has been given in pregnancy in most developed countries and has proved so successful in removing anemia as a significant problem in pregnancy that a generation of midwives and obstetricians in practice in affluent societies has seen little anemia in antenatal practice, and many of these practitioners advocate treatment only when anemia is diagnosed. It may be that better diet and the widespread use of oral contraceptives have improved the iron status of women, but these measures are unlikely to have changed the balance so greatly that women now have sufficient iron in pregnancy. A recent study comparing iron and placebo in pregnancy in Dublin showed the expected fall in hemoglobin in the placebo group; the mean hemoglobin level at term in the supplemented group was 13.6 g/dL, compared with 11.9 g/dL in the placebo group (20).

Some resistance to iron medication in pregnancy also exists because of the side effects experienced, including abdominal cramps and constipation. Because these symptoms are related to the dose of iron ingested, decreasing the amount of iron can minimize them. Whereas most physicians prescribe 200 to 300 mg/day ferrous sulfate or its equivalent, as little as 30 mg ferrous sulfate once daily is fully adequate (21).

Infants, Children, and Adolescents

In utero iron stores are built up in the fetus in the last few weeks of pregnancy. Premature birth curtails transfer of iron from mother to child, and premature infants need iron supplements at an earlier age than full-term infants. Thereafter, rapid growth with expansion of the red cell mass increases iron needs, and if diet fails to supply enough iron, iron deficiency appears.

Iron Fortification and Treatment

In populations whose dietary iron content may be inadequate, food has been fortified with iron as a strategy to enhance its intake. However, this approach has been challenging because metallic iron remains insoluble and is not bioavailable, whereas soluble iron compounds tend to render food such as bread unpalatable. The addition of iron to individual foods such as cereals has been more successful, and iron is widely added to prepared infant foods. At present, 2.7 mg iron is added to 100 g flour in the United States.

Iron deficiency anemia is treated with iron salts; three preparations are available: ferrous sulfate, ferrous gluconate and ferrous fumarate. Ferrous sulfate is the least expensive and most frequently prescribed. A 325-mg tablet of ferrous sulfate (which contains 65 mg of elemental iron) administered three times a day effectively delivers the amount of iron needed to achieve an optimal hematologic response. The frequency of side effects from these different iron preparations appears to be similar, and, when administered in doses containing equivalent amounts of elemental iron, all three are equally efficacious in the treatment of iron deficiency. Another oral preparation of iron, a polysaccharide-iron complex (Niferex), apparently has fewer side effects than ferrous sulfate, but it is more expensive. However, a randomized, comparative study suggested that iron in this complex is not absorbed as well as ferrous sulfate (22).

In an attempt to decrease some of the side effects associated with oral iron administration, prolonged-release or enteric-coated iron tablets have also been marketed. However, because iron is absorbed in the duodenum, such iron preparations may dissolve slowly and transit beyond the duodenum, thus failing to deliver iron to the appropriate site of absorption.

Iron is maximally absorbed when iron tablets are ingested apart from meals (on an empty stomach); however, this is often associated with symptoms such as nausea, heartburn, abdominal cramping, diarrhea, or constipation. These symptoms often deter patients from taking iron tablets over the long period required to replete iron stores. Gastrointestinal symptoms are related to the dose of iron ingested and can be reduced by decreasing the dose. Moreover, because these symptoms improve as tolerance to iron salts develops, it is reasonable to start treatment with a lower dose of iron salts and then increase it gradually. Iron taken with meals or close to meals is absorbed 40 to 50% less than iron taken on an empty stomach, but it is better tolerated and hence is more likely to be acceptable to patients. These strategies to decrease the gastrointestinal side effects of oral iron are important in ensuring patient compliance with treatment. In addition, iron absorption is increased in the presence of ascorbate (as in orange juice) and meat and is decreased in the presence of tea, milk, and cereals. A response to iron therapy is evidenced by a clinical benefit characterized by a rise in hemoglobin level of about 1 g/dL/week. Patients with iron deficiency anemia require treatment with iron for at least 6 months to replete iron stores.

Whereas iron deficiency is effectively treated with oral iron compounds, in certain clinical situations the repletion of iron stores requires the parenteral administration of soluble iron preparations. These conditions include impaired gastrointestinal iron absorption, inflammatory bowel conditions, inability to tolerate oral iron or noncompliance with oral iron compounds, chronic gastrointestinal blood loss resulting in iron deficiency that cannot be overcome by oral iron administration, and patients with renal failure who are undergoing hemodialysis and who cannot achieve a positive iron balance with oral therapy alone. Parenteral iron compounds include iron-dextran complex (Imferon), ferric sodium gluconate (Ferrlecit), and iron sucrose. All three compounds may be administered intravenously. Although iron-dextran may also be administered intramuscularly, the intravenous administration produces much less patient discomfort than intramuscular administration and is recommended. Until recently, in the United States, iron-dextran was the only parenteral compound available, and its intravenous administration is associated with the risk of anaphylactic and delayed reactions. Ferric sodium gluconate and iron sucrose were recently approved, have much better safety profiles, and are therefore preferable to iron-dextran.

Functional Iron Deficiency with the Use of Recombinant Erythropoietin

Recombinant human erythropoietin (rHuEpo) is used to increase erythropoiesis in anemic patients with renal failure and other disorders, including cancer. In these conditions, body iron stores are adequate or may even be increased. However, iron cannot be adequately mobilized to meet the increased requirement for erythropoiesis when patients are treated with rHuEpo, a situation referred to as functional iron deficiency. Optimal erythroid response to rHuEpo therefore requires the concurrent administration of oral or intravenous iron compounds (23).

COBALAMIN AND FOLATE

Nutritional Aspects of Cobalamin and Folate Deficiency

Bone marrow progenitors and precursor cells are highly dependent on cobalamin (vitamin B_{12}) and folate for DNA synthesis. Folate is critically important to the integrity and developmental program of neural tube and neural crest cells during uterine development. Postnatally, however, folate deficiency manifests primarily as hematologic abnormalities. Because adequate cobalamin is required for normal functioning of intracellular folate-mediated reactions, cobalamin deficiency leads to a functional intracellular folate deficiency state that is characterized by similar hematologic findings (see Chapters 28 and 29). However, because cobalamin is independently required for maintenance of the nervous system, cobalamin deficiency gives rise to a unique spectrum of neurologic abnormalities.

Nutritional deficiency of cobalamin and folate can lead to megaloblastic changes in hematopoietic cells that have a common biochemical feature involving a defect in DNA synthesis, with lesser alterations in RNA and protein synthesis, leading to a state of unbalanced cell growth and impaired cell division. Morphologically, megaloblastic cells exhibit an arrested nuclear maturation with relatively normal cytoplasmic maturation in all proliferating cells. The peripheral blood picture is characteristic and reflective of megaloblastic hematopoiesis within the bone marrow.

Cobalamin

Cobalamin is a pink, water-soluble vitamin. The main part of the molecule is similar in structure to heme but with cobalt replacing iron in the center of the pyrrole ring. In humans, nutritional cobalamin deficiency occurs in vegetarians and in infants of mothers with cobalamin deficiency and in those with inability to absorb or use this vitamin normally (see Chapter 29).

Nutrition. Cobalamin is produced in nature only by cobalamin-producing microorganisms, and humans receive cobalamin solely from the diet. Herbivores obtain their dietary quota of cobalamin from plants contaminated with cobalamin-producing bacteria that grow in roots and nodules of legumes. Exogenous contamination of plants by manure used in fertilization may also be another source of cobalamin, so in theory, organically grown leafy vegetables (e.g., cabbage, cauliflower, broccoli, lettuce, spinach) may have higher cobalamin contents than those exposed to nonorganic (chemical) fertilizers. Moreover, insecticides could render such vegetables free of minute insects that could otherwise be inadvertently consumed and be a contributory source of cobalamin. In the human large bowel, numerous bacteria can produce cobalamin, but this site is too distal for physiologic cobalamin absorption, which occurs in the terminal ileum. However, the human small intestine also often harbors a considerable microflora, and this is even more extensive in apparently healthy persons from South India, in whom at least two groups of organisms in the small bowel (*Pseudomonas* and *Klebsiella* spp) may synthesize significant amounts of the vitamin (24). Lower animals can also receive cobalamin by eating insects and other animals and via coprophagy.

Animal protein is the major dietary cobalamin source for nonvegetarians. Meats from parenchymal organs are richest in cobalamin (>10 μg cobalamin/100 g wet weight); fish and animal muscle, milk products, and egg yolk have 1 to 10 μg/100 g wet weight (see Appendix Table A-23-a for a detailed list of vitamin B$_{12}$ in food). An average nonvegetarian Western diet contains 5 to 7 μg/ day of cobalamin, which adequately sustains normal cobalamin equilibrium. Daily food intake in men taking a mixed diet containing 70 g protein and 2400 kcal supplied 5.2 μg

cobalamin, and a diet with 53 g protein and 1400 kcal in women had 5.6 μg cobalamin (25). The daily intake ranged from 0.4 to 85.5 μg, heavily influenced by consumption of liver or other rich sources. A vegetarian diet supplies between 0.25 and 0.5 μg cobalamin/day, derived from bacterial activity in the food, from water, and from animal products such as milk. Unambiguous evidence now indicates that most vegetarians do not receive adequate dietary cobalamin (discussed later in this chapter), and diets supplying 0.5 μg cobalamin or less daily are associated with a high proportion of cobalamin deficiency. The RDA in men and nonpregnant women is 2.4 μg; in pregnant women, 2.6 μg; in lactating women, 2.8 μg; and in children 9 to 18 years, between 1.5 and 2 μg (26).

Cobalamin is exceptionally well stored in tissues in its coenzyme forms. Of the total body content of 2 to 5 mg in adults, approximately 1 mg is in the liver. An obligatory loss of 0.1%/day (1.3 μg) occurs regardless of total body cobalamin content. With a daily requirement of 1.0 μg, such cobalamin stores should suffice for 2500 days or more. It takes approximately 3 to 4 years to deplete cobalamin stores when dietary cobalamin is abruptly malabsorbed because this interferes with the otherwise very efficient enterohepatic circulation, which accounts for turnover of 5 to 10 μg/day of cobalamin (27). Cobalamin is stable and resists high-temperature cooking processes, but it can readily be converted to inactive analogs by ascorbic acid and is destroyed in very alkaline conditions (pH >12).

Absorption. Cobalamin in food is usually in coenzyme form [5′-deoxyadenosyl cobalamin and methylcobalamin] bound to its respective enzymes and nonspecifically bound to proteins. In the stomach, peptic digestion at low pH is a prerequisite for cobalamin release from food protein, and persons who have hypochlorhydria or achlorhydria (as a result of use of proton pump inhibitors or gastrectomy) can have inadequate release of protein-bound cobalamin. After release by proteolysis, cobalamin preferentially binds to a high-affinity cobalamin-binding protein (known as R-protein) in the stomach. However, release to the gastric cobalamin-binding protein, intrinsic factor, is effected only after the R-protein is degraded by pancreatic proteases. Intrinsic factor also binds cobalamin that is recirculated via the bile, and intrinsic factor–cobalamin complexes are then absorbed in the terminal ileum through interaction with specific intrinsic factor–cobalamin receptors (now called cubulin).

The amount of cobalamin that is absorbed from a single dose or meal is limited, probably because of saturation of cubulin binding sites in the small gut. This amount is about 1.0 to 1.5 μg (28). A second dose of cobalamin given 4 to 6 hours after the first is absorbed normally, so if three adequate meals are taken daily in a mixed diet, up to 4.5 μg of cobalamin can be absorbed.

After a 3- to 5-hour delay, intestinally absorbed cobalamin that is transferred to transcobalamin II within enterocytes appears in the portal blood and is then rapidly cleared from the circulation by binding to transcobalamin II receptors on cells (27). The internalized cobalamin is then reduced and converted to 5′deoxyadenosyl-cobalamin and methyl-cobalamin coenzyme forms.

Cobalamin in large doses can also passively diffuse through buccal, gastric, and jejunal mucosa, so less than 1% of a large dose of oral cobalamin (~1 mg) appears in the circulation within minutes. This property is used to advantage in some persons with cobalamin malabsorption in lieu of parenteral replacement (27).

Mitochondrial methylmalonyl-coenzyme A (CoA) mutase in the presence of 5′deoxyadenosyl-cobalamin converts methylmalonyl-CoA to succinyl-CoA, thereby converting the products of propionate metabolism (i.e., methylmalonyl-CoA) into easily metabolized products. Cytoplasmic methyl-cobalamin functions as a coenzyme for methionine synthase, which catalyzes the transfer of methyl groups from methyl-cobalamin to homocysteine to form methionine (29–31). In this process, methyl-cobalamin is converted to Cob(I)alamin. The methyl group of 5-methyl-tetrahydrofolate is donated to Cob(I)alamin, thus regenerating methyl-cobalamin; 5-methyl-tetrahydrofolate is thus converted to tetrahydrofolate. Folates and cobalamin are thus required together for normal one-carbon metabolism. Once methionine is formed, it can become adenylated to S-adenosyl-methionine and then donate its methyl group in a critical series of biologic methylation reactions involving more than 80 proteins, phospholipids, neurotransmitters, RNA, and DNA (see Chapters 28, 29, and 32).

Renal conservation of cobalamin is mediated through a large, 550-kDa membrane protein called megalin that is found in renal proximal epithelial cells and that functions as a multiligand receptor for a variety of macromolecules (32, 33).

Folates

Folates are a group of labile compounds required for transfer of single-carbon units in various biochemical pathways including synthesis of three of the four nucleotides of DNA. They are discussed in Chapter 28.

Nutrition. Folates are synthesized by microorganisms and plants and are found as reduced and polyglutamated forms throughout nature. Particularly rich sources include green leafy vegetables (spinach, lettuce, broccoli, beans), fruits (bananas, melons, lemons), yeast, mushrooms, and animal protein (liver, kidney) (28); (see Appendix Table A-23-a for a detailed list of folate content of foods). The RDA of folate is as follows: men and nonpregnant women, 400 μg; pregnant women, 600 μg; lactating women, 500 μg; children 9 to 18 years, between 300 and 400 μg (26). Whereas a balanced Western diet contains adequate amounts of folate, the net dietary intake of folate in many developing countries is often insufficient to sustain folate balance (28). Folates are highly susceptible to breakdown during cooking for more than 15 minutes; cultural and ethnic cooking practices involve prolonged boiling of lentils in spices for more than 30 minutes in large volumes of water (34), and such dishes are regular accompaniments for most meals among Indians. Frying foods in an open pan results in loss of 50 to 95% of folate. Moreover, in many cultures, it is not common to eat fresh raw or stir-fried vegetables or salads that are rich in folate. Food additives such as nitrites can oxidize folates and reduce folate bioavailability, whereas reducing agents such as ascorbate have a protective effect (35).

Absorption, Enterohepatic Circulation, Cellular Uptake, Retention, and Excretion. Most dietary folates are bioavailable (with some exceptions such as cabbage, lettuce, orange). Dietary folates, which are in the form of pteroyl*poly*glutamates, must be hydrolyzed to pteroyl*mono*glutamate by an enzyme present in the brush border membranes of small intestinal cells before transport into jejunum via membrane-associated reduced-folate carriers (28). Dietary folate deficiency leads to marked upregulation in intestinal folate uptake and reduced-folate carriers and in the activity of pteroylpolyglutamate hydrolase (36), findings suggesting physiologic adaptation. Ingested human milk, which contains specific high-affinity folate-binding proteins (37), also facilitates the nutritional bioavailability of ingested folate in neonates (38), but the precise mechanism is unclear (39).

Studies with tritium-labeled folates showed almost complete absorption of reduced folate monoglutamates and approximately 80% absorption of folic acid. Precise data on the absorption of reduced folate polyglutamates are not available, but absorption is estimated to be approximately 70% (25).

Passive diffusion of orally administered folic acid is probably the primary mechanism of intestinal mucosal folate absorption at high pharmacologic concentrations (28), with peak folate levels in plasma achieved within 1 to 2 hours. Whereas such folic acid enters the portal blood unchanged, food folate is reduced and methylated within the enterocyte to 5-methyl-tetrahydrofolate before release into plasma.

Substantial enterohepatic circulation of up to 90 μg of folate and ingestion of dietary folate contribute to maintain the normal serum folate level. Up to 95% of folates are cleared from plasma within 3 minutes by tissues by two distinct components that are involved in cellular folate transport: reduced-folate carriers, which constitute a low-affinity but high-capacity system; and folate receptors, which have a high affinity but relatively lower capacity for transporting physiologic serum 5-methyl-tetrahydrofolate (37, 40). Passive diffusion can also occur at pharmacologic parenteral concentrations. Folate deficiency can upregulate the transport pathways and, in the case of folate receptors, at the transcriptional, posttranscriptional, and translational levels (41).

Polyglutamation of folate is the major factor for intracellular retention (42), but folate turnover and/or catabolism can be accelerated intracellularly by the activity of heavy-chain ferritin (43), which limits the amount of newly imported (unbound) folate monoglutamates before they can function as cofactors with intracellular enzymes. Following glomerular filtration, luminal folate is captured by folate receptors in the brush border membranes of proximal renal tubular cells (44) and is transported back to the blood via transport across basolateral membranes.

Intracellular Metabolism and Cobalamin-Folate Interrelationships

Folic acid is not a biologically active form of folate; when given therapeutically, it requires reduction to tetrahydrofolate. Physiologically, however, 5-methytetrahydrofolate is what is transported into cells. Both these folate forms can be converted to tetrahydrofolate, and after acquisition of polyglutamyl tails, these forms are retained within cells and are optimum substrates for the various enzymes involved in folate-mediated reactions involving the transfer of one-carbon units (e.g., methyl-, formyl-, methylene, among others). These reactions, which are critical for purine and pyrimidine synthesis, are broadly categorized under the descriptive term one-carbon metabolism. Tetrahydrofolate can be converted to 10-formyl-tetrahydrofolate (used in de novo biosynthesis of purines) and 5,10-methylene-tetrahydrofolate (for synthesis of thymidylate). Furthermore, these forms can be interconverted via intermediates. A key form of folate is 5,10-methylene-tetrahydrofolate, which can be used in either the *thymidylate cycle* via thymidylate synthase for thymidine and DNA synthesis or the *methylation cycle* after its conversion to 5-methyl-tetrahydrofolate, which, via methionine synthase, leads to formation of methionine and tetrahydrofolate (see Chapter 28).

Consequences of Folate and Cobalamin Deficiency in Proliferating Cells

In either cobalamin or folate deficiency, a net decrease in 5,10-methylene-tetrahydrofolate interrupts the reaction mediated by thymidylate synthase, which converts deoxyuridine monophosphate to deoxythymidine monophosphate. The excess deoxyuridine monophosphate is then phosphorylated to deoxyuridine triphosphate and is incorporated into DNA. However, this faulty incorporation (in lieu of deoxythymidine triphosphate) is immediately recognized by an editorial enzyme and is excised. When this faulty incorporation and excision cycle is repeated multiple times, it leads to DNA fragmentation and to perturbation of the cell cycle giving rise to megaloblastosis.

All proliferating cells exhibit megaloblastosis, including epithelial cells lining the gastrointestinal tract (buccal mucosa, tongue, small intestine), cervix, vagina, and uterus (28). However, megaloblastic changes are most striking in the blood and bone marrow. Ineffective hematopoiesis extends into the long bones, and the bone marrow aspirate exhibits trilineal hypercellularity involving erythroid, myeloid, and megakaryocyte lines.

The earliest manifestation of megaloblastosis is an increase in MCV with macroovalocytes (≤14 μm). Because these cells have adequate hemoglobin, the central pallor, which normally occupies about one third of the cell, is decreased (Fig. 92.3).

As anemia becomes more severe, poikilocytosis and anisocytosis become evident. Nuclear hypersegmentation of DNA in polymorphonuclear neutrophils strongly suggests megaloblastosis when associated with macroovalocytosis; normally, fewer than 5% of polymorphonuclear neutrophils have more than five lobes, and no cells have more than six lobes in the peripheral blood (Fig. 92.4).

Megaloblastosis in rapidly proliferating cells of the gastrointestinal tract leads to a variable degree of morphologic changes and atrophy of the epithelial cells of the luminal lining. This leads to functional defects, which include a failure in secretion of intrinsic factor and malabsorption of cobalamin and folate in certain subsets of patients. Thus, a vicious cycle whereby megaloblastosis begets more megaloblastosis is established that can be interrupted only by specific therapy with cobalamin or folate.

The hematologic manifestations of folate deficiency include pancytopenia with megaloblastic marrow with cardiopulmonary symptoms and signs of anemia, as well as gastrointestinal (megaloblastosis with or without malabsorption), dermatologic (skin pigmentation), and genital (megaloblastosis of cervical epithelium) manifestations, infertility (sterility), and psychiatric conditions (Table 92.8). Most of these manifestations are noted during the history and physical examination. When cases of neuropathy accompanying folate deficiency are encountered, the possibility of alcoholism with thiamin deficiency must be considered. In any case, every patient with neuropathy, myelopathy, or psychiatric manifestations associated with megaloblastosis must be investigated in detail to rule out cobalamin deficiency.

Neurologic Dysfunction with Cobalamin Deficiency

Because megaloblastosis resulting from either folate or cobalamin deficiency leads to a functional folate coenzyme deficiency, the morphologic manifestations of both deficiencies are indistinguishable (see Table 92.8). However, only cobalamin deficiency results in a patchy demyelination process, which is expressed clinically as cerebral abnormalities and subacute combined degeneration of the spinal cord (28). The demyelinating process involves patchy swelling of the myelin sheath followed by its breakdown (demyelination), leading to axonal degeneration with foci that eventually coalesce with secondary degeneration of long tracts. Lesions begin in the dorsal columns of the thoracic segments of the spinal cord and then spread *contiguously* to involve

TABLE 92.8. MEGALOBLASTIC SEQUELAE OF FOLATE AND COBALAMIN DEFICIENCY AND SEVERAL CLINICAL MANIFESTATIONS ARE THE SAME[a] (BUT THE NEUROLOGIC SPECTRUM OF DYSFUNCTION WITH COBALAMIN DEFICIENCY IS DISTINCT)

Hematologic	Pancytopenia with megaloblastic marrow
Cardiopulmonary	Congestive heart failure
Gastrointestinal	Beefy-red tongue and added stigmata of broad-spectrum malabsorption in folate deficiency[b]
Dermatologic	Melanin pigmentation and premature graying
Genital	Cervical/uterine dysplasia
Reproductive	Infertility/sterility
Psychiatric	Depressed affect/cognitive dysfunction
Neuropsychiatric[c]	Unique to cobalamin deficiency with cerebral, myelopathic, or peripheral neuropathic disturbances including optic and autonomic nerve dysfunction

[a] Inadequate hemoglobinization (from inadequate iron stores and/or globin synthesis) will mask the expected erythroid megaloblastic morphology in the bone marrow and peripheral smear, and only specific therapy (e.g., iron) will unmask classic megaloblastic manifestations. Megaloblastic leukopoiesis will be unchanged, and hypersegmented polymorphonuclear leukocytes should be visible on the smear.
[b] If folate deficiency is uncorrected for more than 2 to 3 years, cobalamin deficiency will supervene.
[c] Dorsal tract involvement is earliest manifestation in more than 70% patients with cobalamin deficiency. Neuropsychiatric manifestations are unassociated with megaloblastosis in up to 30% patients.
Adapted from Antony AC. Megaloblastic anemias. In: Hoffman R, Benz EJ Jr, Shattil SJ et al., eds. Hematology: Basic Principles and Practice. 4th ed. New York: Churchill Livingstone, 2005:519–56.

corticospinal, spinothalamic, and spinocerebellar tracts. Degeneration of the dorsal root ganglia, of the celiac ganglia, and of the Meissner and Auerbach plexus also occurs.

A greater awareness of cobalamin deficiency coupled with use of sensitive metabolite diagnostic tests, the widespread use of supplementary folates taken by humans, including fortification of food with folate, and the routine fortification of foods of livestock (chickens, pigs, cows) can be expected to blunt hematologic presentations leading to pure neuropsychiatric disease.

Paresthesias and ataxia are commonly the first symptoms, and diminished vibratory sensation and proprioception in the lower extremities are common objective early signs. Although multiple neurologic syndromes are often seen in the same patient, the spectrum of objective signs could include loss of fine/coarse touch, decreased or increased deep tendon reflexes with spasticity or muscle weakness, urinary or fecal incontinence, orthostatic hypotension, amaurosis, dementia, psychosis, and mood disturbances (45). Although neurologic deficits are generally mild in most cases, the severity is proportionate to the duration of symptoms before diagnosis. The demonstration of cognitive improvement after treatment with cobalamin in 11 of 18 geriatric subjects with low cobalamin levels and quantitative cognitive dysfunction and the

observation of a limited window of opportunity for effective intervention also highlight the importance of early diagnosis for this population (46).

Signs and Symptoms in Cobalamin Deficiency

Vast numbers of persons who have nutritional cobalamin deficiency and a low serum cobalamin level as a result are apparently well, with no clinical problems. Thus, among a community of 15,000 Hindu Indians, largely vegetarian, of whom 54% had low serum cobalamin levels, only ten patients per year with cobalamin-deficient megaloblastic anemia were seen in one local hospital (21). Most are just in balance, with low cobalamin stores and low cobalamin intake. However, what has been previously been termed a subclinical state of cobalamin deficiency—in which disease manifestations are cryptic based on traditional physical diagnosis—needs to be revisited in the light of far more sophisticated questionnaires, instruments, and other methods used to test brain function. Carmel and collaborators opened this Pandora's box in the cobalamin field by asking: Does mild subclinical cobalamin deficiency affect the adult nervous system? These investigators have consistently found, in one half or more of their patients with metabolically defined, mild, preclinical cobalamin deficiency (47–49), clear-cut abnormalities in electroencephalographic, evoked potential, and P300 event-related potentials (the last are electric signals from the brain found when the subject performs various cognitive tasks and are established electrophysiologic markers of cognitive ability). Of major significance, in most cases these abnormalities were reversed with cobalamin therapy, a finding supporting a causal relationship. This is a more significant issue in cobalamin-deficient children (discussed later). Thus, these studies, using more sensitive tests with metabolites coupled with sophisticated neurophysiologic testing instruments, forced the conclusion that such persons do indeed have both metabolic and clinical evidence of deficiency.

From the classic clinical presentation standpoint, patients may come to notice because macrocytosis has been found in a blood count. Such patients may have few complaints, although almost invariably, they feel better after cobalamin therapy. In a series of 95 Asian Indians (52 women and 43 men, age range, 13–80 years) with nutritional megaloblastic anemia seen over 14 years (21), complaints included tiredness (33%), shortness of breath (25%), loss of appetite (23%), weight loss (22%), generalized aches (19%) generally resulting from calcium and vitamin D deficiency, vomiting (19%), paresthesia (11%), change in skin pigmentation (8%), sore mouth (7%), diarrhea (6%), headache (5%), and infertility (5%). In 6%, macrocytosis in a blood count was the first indication of clinical cobalamin deficiency. All these patients had a megaloblastic bone marrow, and all had low serum cobalamin levels.

Examination showed pallor, a beefy red tongue in some patients (Fig. 92.5) that responded well to specific therapy (Fig. 92.6), and yellowish sclera in 13%. Indian patients may show increased pigmentation about the nails, and one patient with severe anemia showed splenomegaly. This 19-year-old male patient also had lost hair pigmentation and had gray hair; hair grown after the start of oral cobalamin therapy was jet black (Fig. 92.7).

Neuropathy, if present, may manifest as symmetric tingling sensations in fingers and/or toes. Patients may have spastic movements, stiffness, and weakness. Difficulty with micturition includes hesitancy, a poor urinary stream, and even retention. Constipation and postural hypotension may be caused by an effect on the autonomic nervous system. Irritability, memory disturbance, mild depression, and even hallucinations may occur. Visual impairment is uncommon. Loss of vibration sense, appreciation of passive movement, and a positive Romberg sign may be present. There may be exaggerated reflexes and an extensor plantar response, but other patients have flaccid paralysis. Muscles may be wasted. Abnormal nerve conduction is found on electrophysiologic testing in 25% of patients.

In severe anemia, patients have a fast pulse rate and low blood pressure. A soft systolic murmur may be present. Patients with severe anemia may be in cardiac failure with distended neck veins, swollen ankles, and cardiac enlargement.

Laboratory Data

Highly sensitive metabolite tests are now routinely available for clinical diagnosis of cobalamin and folate deficiency (Table 92.9). Total homocysteine can be measured in either plasma (50) or serum (51). In general, plasma levels are slightly lower. The normal value for serum total homocysteine is 5.1 to 13.9 μM and serum methylmalonic acid (MMA) is 73 to 271 nM, and in general, the higher the values, the more severe the clinical abnormalities (50). The earliest clinically evaluable manifestations of negative cobalamin balance are increased serum MMA and total homocysteine levels (52–55), which occur when the total cobalamin in serum is still normal. Likewise, metabolic evidence of folate deficiency (i.e., increased total homocysteine) is often found when serum folates are still in the low-normal range. With continued negative cobalamin or folate balance, serum cobalamin and folate levels decrease. Only later does one note morphologic expression of perturbed DNA in polymorphonuclear neutrophils, macroovalocytosis, and anemia (see Table 92.9). The combined use of serum total homocysteine and MMA can distinguish between cobalamin and folate deficiency because most patients with folate deficiency have normal MMA levels (53–55).

Although both total homocysteine and MMA are elevated in patients with dehydration and renal failure, propionic acid derived from anerobic fecal bacterial

TABLE 92.9. STEPWISE APPROACH TO DIAGNOSIS OF COBALAMIN AND FOLATE DEFICIENCY

Megaloblastic anemia OR neurologic-psychiatric manifestations consistent with cobalamin deficiency
PLUS
Test results[a] on serum cobalamin and serum folate

COBALAMIN[b] (pg/mL)	FOLATE[c] (ng/mL)	PROVISIONAL DIAGNOSIS	PROCEED WITH METABOLITES?
>300	>4	Cobalamin/folate deficiency is unlikely	No
<200	>4	*Consistent* with cobalamin deficiency	No
200–300	>4	*Rule out* cobalamin deficiency	Yes
>300	<2	*Consistent* with folate deficiency	No
<200	<2	*Consistent* with (1) combined cobalamin plus folate deficiency or (2) isolated folate deficiency	Yes
>300	2–4	*Consistent* with (1) folate deficiency or (2) an anemia unrelated to vitamin deficiency	Yes

Test Results on metabolites: serum methylmalonic acid and total homocysteine[d]

METHYLMALONIC ACID (normal = 70–270 nM)	TOTAL HOMOCYSTEINE (normal = 5–14 μM)	DIAGNOSIS
Increased	Increased	Cobalamin deficiency is confirmed; folate deficiency still possible
Normal	Increased	Folate deficiency is likely; <5% may have cobalamin deficiency
Normal	Normal	Cobalamin and folate deficiency is excluded

[a] Cost for each of these tests in Indiana in 2003: serum cobalamin, $25; serum folate, $20 plus markup costs for venipuncture, $12, and costs for registered nurse visit, $35).
[b] Serum cobalamin levels: abnormally low, less than 200 pg/mL; clinically relevant low-normal range, 200 to 300 pg/mL.
[c] Serum folate levels: abnormally low, less than 2 ng/mL; clinically relevant low-normal range, 2 to 4 ng/mL.
[d] The costs in Indiana in 2003 for testing serum methylmalonic acid is $45 and for testing total homocysteine is $34. Any frozen-over sample from serum folate/cobalamin determination can be subjected to metabolite tests.
Adapted from Antony AC. Megaloblastic anemias. In: Hoffman R, Benz EJ Jr, Shattil SJ et al., eds. Hematology: Basic Principles and Practice. 4th ed. New York: Churchill Livingstone, 2005:519–56.

metabolism can also contribute substantially to methylmalonate production (56). In this setting, the gut flora contribution to MMA can be reduced by treatment with metronidazole.

More than 10% of subjects with normal serum cobalamin levels, such as elderly persons in the Framingham population (57), many elderly European persons (58), children on macrobiotic diets (59), alcoholic patients with folate deficiency (60), and even patients with thyroid disease can have a raised serum MMA. Moreover, one third of sera from pregnant women had raised levels of MMA irrespective of the serum cobalamin level (61). Conversely, measurement of MMA levels in 548 elderly subjects in the Framingham study showed raised levels in 82 (15%) (57). Basal levels of MMA are usually less than 500 nM, and in renal failure the value rarely increases to more than 1,000 nM (51, 62). Because of variables related to age and mild renal dysfunction that can falsely elevate these metabolites (a not uncommon finding in elderly persons), proof of metabolic deficiency *especially in the presence of normal serum vitamin levels* requires demonstration of a reduction in metabolite levels with vitamin supplementation (63).

Homocysteine is a continuous (progressive) risk factor for occlusive vascular disease (i.e., higher levels predict higher risk) that is modifiable and likely causal. Therefore, the lower the level is, the better (see Chapters 28 and 34).

Serum Cobalamin Levels

For the most part, serum cobalamin is an established biochemical indicator of cobalamin deficiency in patients with hematologic or neurologic abnormalities consistent with cobalamin deficiency (see Table 92.9). The serum cobalamin is less than 300 pg/mL in 99% of patients with clinical hematologic or neurologic manifestations of cobalamin deficiency (52, 55). Conversely, a cobalamin level of greater than 300 pg/mL predicts folate deficiency or another hematologic disease (see Table 92.9). However, if the serum folate levels are borderline normal and the patient has megaloblastic anemia with cobalamin levels higher than 300 pg/mL, metabolite tests or a therapeutic trial may be necessary to rule out underlying folate deficiency (see Table 92.9).

Serum Folate Levels

When combined with a clinical picture of megaloblastic anemia and additional results of cobalamin levels, the serum folate is the cheapest and most useful initial biochemical test to diagnose folate deficiency (see Table 92.9) (64). However, a low serum folate level alone should never dictate therapy, and it is important to consider the clinical picture, peripheral smear, and bone marrow morphology and to rule out underlying cobalamin deficiency. Serum folate level is highly sensitive to folate intake, and a single (hospital) meal can normalize it in a patient with true folate deficiency. Although red blood cell folates correlate well with tissue (hepatic) folate stores, the current red blood cell folate tests are too unreliable for routine clinical use.

Diagnostic Approach and Important Caveats in the Use of Serum Tests

Based on the lower costs of serum cobalamin and folate testing compared with serum MMA and total homocysteine testing, it is recommended (see Table 92.9) first to use the cheaper tests that will assist in diagnosis of the majority of obvious cases of cobalamin and folate deficiency (64, 65). Clinicians should also restrict use of serum MMA and total homocysteine testing to the following patients: (a) those with borderline cobalamin and folate levels; (b) those with existing conditions known to perturb folate and cobalamin tests leading to difficulties in the interpretation of test results; (c) when both cobalamin and folate levels are low, in which a high MMA value is useful in confirming cobalamin deficiency (rather than attributing the condition to folate deficiency alone); and (d) those with clearly low serum levels but in whom an alternative explanation exists for the syndrome that led to obtaining a serum cobalamin level (e.g., a diabetic or alcoholic patient with peripheral neuropathy, or an alcoholic patient with a high MCV and a low serum cobalamin level without anemia). Here, serum metabolites can assist in the diagnosis of vitamin deficiency.

Diagnostic algorithms consistently stress the value of clinical data to improve the pretest probability of serum cobalamin and serum folate tests, which, by themselves, have inherent limitations in sensitivity and specificity (28, 66). So, without detailed clinical information, the combined results of serum cobalamin, serum folate, and serum metabolite (total homocysteine and MMA) tests are not sufficiently unambiguous to diagnose and distinguish cobalamin deficiency from combined cobalamin-*plus*-folate deficiency accurately. In combined cobalamin-*plus*-folate deficiency, both vitamins would be needed to restore baseline values, particularly of homocysteine (63). In the context of diagnosing a subclinical deficiency of cobalamin (or folate) based on increased serum MMA and/or total homocysteine *despite* normal serum cobalamin (or folate) levels, positive attribution can be confidently made only after the *demonstrated* reversal of laboratory values following treatment with cobalamin (and/or folate) (63, 66–68). This is similar in principle to that used to confirm clinically significant nutrient deficiency (28, 69).

Other Tests

Neither the existing tests using red cell folates nor the newer holo-transcobalamin II or urine MMA tests have been clinically validated as being superior to the serum tests discussed earlier in the many patient groups at risk; these tests require further evaluation to define their proper niche in the clinical diagnostic algorithm for cobalamin deficiency (28, 70). Moreover, it remains to be shown from more than one laboratory that these measures can replace existing tests in the diagnosis of early vitamin deficiency. Finally, the deoxyuridine suppression test that is performed on megaloblastic cells is not widely available for routine clinical use.

Bone Marrow

The blood changes are caused by abnormal blood formation in the bone marrow, and these changes, termed *megaloblastic*, are easily recognized with properly fixed and stained marrow preparations (Fig. 92.8). When the blood count, blood film, and clinical picture all strongly suggest megaloblastic anemia, bone marrow examination can be omitted. In fact, because of the widespread availability of sensitive metabolite tests, most clinicians rely on a detailed history, physical examination, and these laboratory test results to make a provisional diagnosis and then verify that therapy restores the clinical abnormalities to normal. This approach avoids the discomfort associated with a bone marrow test altogether in most cases.

Cobalamin Absorption Tests

Other than nutritional cobalamin deficiency, all the conditions producing cobalamin deficiency share a failure in the intestinal absorption of cobalamin. The usual cobalamin absorption test, such as the Schilling test, involves giving the patient an injection of 1000 μg of cobalamin. This constitutes complete treatment and means that the chance of obtaining positive evidence for the diagnosis of nutritional cobalamin deficiency, by demonstrating a response to 5 μg cobalamin once daily by mouth, is lost. If the absorption of cobalamin is normal and the patient responds hematologically following the injection of cobalamin, then the likely diagnosis remains nutritional cobalamin deficiency, provided the patient is a long-standing vegetarian or "near-vegetarian," as discussed in the section on nutritional cobalamin deficiency. If the patient has malabsorption of cobalamin, the most likely diagnosis is pernicious anemia (absent cobalamin-binding intrinsic factor resulting from autoimmune destruction of gastric parietal cells) or another disorder producing cobalamin deficiency. Such disorders include sequelae of gastric surgery, abnormal small gut flora resulting from blind intestinal loops, strictures, diverticula, gut resections, and Crohn's disease. Disorders of the wall of the small gut producing cobalamin malabsorption include gluten sensitivity, tropical sprue, sequelae of ileal bypass or resection, radiation damage, and drugs including alcohol. Five of 95 patients with nutritional cobalamin deficiency were found to have transient cobalamin malabsorption that disappeared after a few months of cobalamin therapy (21), and one third had steatorrhea and xylose malabsorption. These latter findings also disappeared with cobalamin therapy.

Diagnosis of Cobalamin Deficiency

Diagnosis of nutritional cobalamin deficiency depends on establishing cobalamin deficiency in a person whose diet largely lacks all sources of cobalamin and in excluding other causes of cobalamin malabsorption such as in pernicious anemia, small intestinal bacterial overgrowth, and intestinal resection. As indicated earlier, consumption of milk and occasional eggs and cheese will not supply enough cobalamin. Finding antibodies to intrinsic factor makes it likely that the diagnosis is pernicious anemia. Anti–intrinsic factor antibodies are found in the serum of approximately 60% of patients with pernicious anemia and in the gastric juice of 75%; approximately 90% of patients with pernicious anemia have anti–intrinsic factor antibodies in either serum or gastric juice (27). Similar intrinsic factor antibodies are quite rare in the general population; anti–intrinsic factor antibodies are thus highly specific and confirmatory for pernicious anemia. In the study of Indian vegetarians, 95 patients had nutritional cobalamin deficiency, but another 20 had pernicious anemia, and only four had folate-deficient megaloblastic anemia, associated with excess alcohol in two and pregnancy in the other two (21).

Nutritional Cobalamin Deficiency

Vegetarian diets can be classified as being lactovegetarian, ovovegetarian, lactoovovegetarian, or vegan, respectively, if they include dairy products, eggs, both dairy products and eggs, or no animal products at all (59). Vegan diets contain a very low cobalamin content warranting routine cobalamin supplementation. This was recognized as early as 1955 when Wokes and colleagues (71) systematically compared a group of American, Dutch, and British vegans and identified many with significantly lower cobalamin levels than nonvegetarians; a few vegans even had mild symptoms. Within the next year, however, Dhopeshwarkar and associates (72) called attention to the observation that asymptomatic Indian lactovegetarians (who comprise a majority of the population in India) had distinctly lower serum cobalamin levels than nonvegetarians. This finding was confirmed over the years by several studies in various populations from different geographic regions in India (73–76). Quantitatively, nearly one half of asymptomatic lactovegetarians had significantly lower serum levels of cobalamin from low dietary intake of cobalamin when compared with nonvegetarians (76). Until 2003, however, it was unclear whether these persons could be classified as definitely clinically cobalamin deficient. It was nevertheless recognized that because vegetarianism has been in effect over several millennia in India, much of this population was at risk of low cobalamin status throughout life. The superimposition of additional conditions that perturb either cobalamin absorption (gastrectomy, proton-pump inhibitors, medical disease, or surgical resection or bypass of the ileum) or cobalamin metabolism (nitrous oxide exposure) can easily tip such persons into frank cobalamin deficiency. Thus, cobalamin deficiency has been noted among vegetarians in India (59) and among Indian vegetarians living in the United Kingdom (21, 77).

However, an important study from the West (78) documented that asymptomatic lactoovovegetarians and lactovegetarians with low cobalamin levels have an increased blood total homocysteine and MMA consistent with biochemical evidence of cobalamin deficiency (with or without folate deficiency). Although ultimate proof of deficiency must be based on complete normalization of abnormal test results following specific vitamin replacement (69), a high likelihood exists that these data reflect a true cobalamin deficiency, given the low cobalamin content of vegetarian diets.

So what is the significance of, and how are we to interpret, low cobalamin levels in nonvegetarians in developing countries? Not every nonvegetarian in the developing world has a diet similar to that of a nonvegetarian in developed countries (71). The reason is very simple: muscle meats (cattle, goats, sheep, fowl, fish) are expensive, and only persons in the upper economic strata (a minority) and less frequently those in the middle and lower income bracket can afford this luxury with any regularity. Even when available, portions are small: for example, an average steak in the United States could easily be extended into a meal for six to eight persons when made into a stew or curry. So apart from voluntary vegetarianism, even professed nonvegetarians in developing countries have a cobalamin status that is marginally better than lactoovovegetarians, and only daily meat eaters have a cobalamin status comparable to that of nonvegetarians in the West.

Thus, there are two closely related groups whose diets are quite similar and who exhibit clinical and biochemical evidence of dietary cobalamin deficiency: (a) voluntary vegetarians who base their dietary preferences on religious or philosophical grounds (they comprise a majority of the Indian population) and (b) poverty-imposed near-vegetarians who also live in developing countries worldwide and who consume meager quantities of meat infrequently. In fact, these poverty-imposed near-vegetarians have a cobalamin status that is only marginally better than that of lactoovovegetarians (59). This can explain why recent studies in vegetarians and nonvegetarians in India reported increased metabolites consistent with cobalamin deficiency (79).

Infants born of cobalamin-depleted vegetarian mothers living under extremely low socioeconomic conditions in the developing world are also at risk of cobalamin deficiency because prolonged breast-feeding over the first 2 years is not an uncommon practice. These infants, who otherwise have a background of adequate general nutrition, exhibit apathy, megaloblastic anemia, skin pigmentation, involuntary movements, and developmental regression that is rapidly corrected by cobalamin. Almost all such infants develop normally for the first 4 months of life. Thereafter, they decline and are usually seen clinically between 6 and 14 months of age. The infants become irritable and lethargic, decline solid food, and are weak. They stop smiling, do not support their heads, and do not turn over. They have marked hypotonia and some choreoathetoid movements of upper limbs or constant wringing of hands. Their eyes do not fix or follow objects. They may even be in a coma. Some have abnormal pigment on the back of their hands and about the nails. One sees developmental delay, anemia (sometimes very severe), and usually enlarged liver and spleen. The blood is macrocytic, and the bone marrow is megaloblastic. The serum cobalamin level is low, as is that of the mother. Response to cobalamin is excellent, and provided the delay in diagnosis has not been too long, recovery is complete and rapid (59).

Similar cases have been described in the West among infants breast-fed by long-standing vegetarians in whom low maternal serum and breast milk cobalamin concentrations—which closely correlate with cobalamin insufficiency in the infant (80–82)—can lead to impaired psychomotor functioning well into youth and later adolescence (83).

The results from a longitudinal cohort study on the importance of cobalamin during the early years of life were most enlightening. This study related to the effects of a cobalamin-deficient macrobiotic diet consisting of cereals (primarily unpolished rice), a variety of pulses and vegetables, and small amounts of seaweed, fermented foods, nuts, seeds, fruit with occasional servings of fish, but no meat and dairy products. By 1989, Dagnelie and associates reported that infants given a macrobiotic diet had cobalamin deficiency (84). These investigators then identified that infants of a macrobiotic cohort at a mean age of 15 months had markedly impaired cobalamin status and impaired psychomotor functioning compared with control infants (85). Following dietary advice, most families then switched these children to a lactovegetarian, lactoovovegetarian, and even an omnivorous diet on average after their sixth birthdays. However, on subsequent follow up, one fifth of these children had continued impaired cobalamin status despite a dietary change (86). The issue here is likely related to insufficient replenishment of cobalamin stores solely by a diet that is only somewhat richer in cobalamin than previously. So cobalamin-deficient vegetarians need immediately to focus on completely replenishing stores with a cobalamin supplement before relying on dietary modifications to maintain adequate cobalamin nutritional status. Next, these investigators determined whether cognitive functioning was affected in their cohort of adolescents between the ages of 10 and 16 years who had a history of compromised cobalamin status. These were the same children who had been switched to a lactovegetarian or omnivorous diet usually by their sixth birthdays; they were compared with a control group of children who were omnivorous since birth. The data were dramatic in that control subjects performed better on most psychologic tests (83). Significantly, a relation between test score and cobalamin deficiency was observed for a test measuring fluid intelligence, and this was more pronounced within the subgroup of those with the poorest cobalamin intake earlier in childhood. The most important associations were between cobalamin status and performance on tests that measured fluid intelligence, spatial ability, and short-term memory (83). Among these parameters, fluid intelligence is particularly important because it involves the use of faculties related to reasoning, the capacity to solve complex problems, abstract thinking ability, and the ability to learn. Because this intelligence is critical to functioning as independent adults, a compromise in cobalamin during childhood (age < 6 years) has potential long-term consequences well into adulthood.

Reports on nutritional macrocytic anemia have identified cobalamin deficiency as the basis for anemia in up to 50% of cases of children aged 6 months to 12 years in India (87). Moreover, studies of anemic children (age 3 months–3 years) in an urban Indian slum revealed that one fifth had cobalamin deficiency (88); it is likely that the use of metabolite testing would have detected many more asymptomatic cobalamin-deficient children because only anemic children were studied. In analogy to the tip of the iceberg, these studies along with the rich literature on the low cobalamin status of adult vegetarians suggest with a fairly high degree of certainty that low cobalamin status may be widespread among children in India.

Parallel results from the Western hemisphere come from studies of Guatemalan school children (89). Before looking at these results, however, we need to step back and look at an earlier study of the general cobalamin status of Guatemalan mothers and their infants (90). In that study, cobalamin deficiency was highly prevalent in these lactating women and was associated with depletion of the vitamin in their infants (90). This finding, too, is reminiscent of results in macrobiotic women and their infants. So it is not surprising that now, when Guatemalan children are studied, they also continue to have low cobalamin status through either dietary insufficiency alone or combined with as yet uncharacterized gastrointestinal malabsorption (89). The risk of lower cognitive and neuromotor performance is real among these children (91). Here, too, reasoning, short-term memory, and perception were poorer in the low-cobalamin group than in the adequate-cobalamin group (92). This study is instructive in that Guatemalan children represent the category of poverty-imposed near-vegetarianism that is prevalent throughout the developing world. Therefore, collectively, this work on the adverse consequences of cobalamin deficiency in children fed a vegetarian diet and those with poverty-imposed near-vegetarianism has significant implications for millions of children worldwide.

The findings that clear-cut biochemical evidence of perturbed cobalamin metabolism exists in vegetarians (78) and that hyperhomocysteinemia is a risk factor for occlu-

sive vascular diseases (93), some neural tube defects (NTDs) (94), congenital heart defects (95), dementia, and Alzheimer disease (96) suggest that vegetarians should be routinely taking relatively inexpensive (generic) cobalamin-containing supplements (59) (Table 92.10).

Poverty afflicts approximately one third of the Indian Subcontinent (97), and a World Bank report (98) on the crisis of malnutrition in India highlighted the finding that one half of all children less than 4 years are malnourished, 30% of all newborns are underweight, and 60% of all women are anemic. So any discussion of vegetarianism and cobalamin deficiency in developing countries immediately raises the question whether folate deficiency—which consistently accompanies poverty and malnutrition—has become an uncommon cause of megaloblastic anemia. Although some studies suggest that this is the case (88, 99), nagging questions remain about whether such patients had combined cobalamin-*plus*-folate-deficiency (69). This question is unanswered because testing using metabolites before and after cobalamin replacement has not been carried out in these populations (59).

Undiagnosed pernicious anemia is common among free-living elderly persons in the United States (>60 years of age) who have only minimal clinical manifestations of

---

TABLE 92.10. INDICATIONS FOR PROPHYLAXIS WITH COBALAMIN OR FOLATE

Prophylaxis with cobalamin
    Infants of mothers with pernicious anemia[a]
    Infants on specialized diets[a]
    Vegetarians and poverty-imposed near-vegetarians[a]
    Patients after total gastrectomy[b]
Prophylaxis with folic acid[c]
    All women contemplating pregnancy (≥400 μg/d)[d]
    Pregnant and lactating women, premature infants
    Mothers at risk for delivery of infants with neural tube defects[e,f]
    Hemolytic anemias/hyperproliferative hematologic states
    Patients with rheumatoid arthritis or psoriasis receiving therapy with methotrexate[g]

[a] For vegetarians, prophylaxis with cobalamin 5- to 10-μg tablets/day orally should suffice. In food-cobalamin malabsorption secondary to inability to cleave food cobalamin by acid and pepsin, replacement therapy should be with tablets of more than 100 μg/day orally. In all other conditions involving any abnormality of cobalamin absorption, cobalamin tablets of 1000 μg/day should be administered orally to ensure that cobalamin transport via passive diffusion across the intestine is sufficient to meet daily needs.
[b] Consider late development of cobalamin deficiency and iron malabsorption (prophylaxis with oral cobalamin and iron).
[c] Ensure that the patient does not have cobalamin deficiency before initiating long-term folate prophylaxis.
[d] For prevention of first occurrence of neural tube defect.
[e] Previous delivery of a child with neural tube defects (anencephaly, spina bifida, meningocele) gives a tenfold greater risk for subsequent delivery of infant with neural tube defects.
[f] Folic acid (4 mg/day) administered *periconceptionally and throughout the first trimester.*
[g] To reduce toxicity of the antifolate.
Adapted from Antony AC. Megaloblastic anemias. In: Hoffman R, Benz EJ Jr, Shattil SJ et al., eds. Hematology: Basic Principles and Practice. 4th ed. New York: Churchill Livingstone, 2005:519–56.

cobalamin deficiency; that is, 1.9% of a survey population had unrecognized and untreated pernicious anemia (100). The prevalence was 2.7% in women and 1.4% in men, but 4.3% of the African-American women and 4.0% of the white women had pernicious anemia. It is significant that this study *did not* include elderly patients with cobalamin deficiency caused by other disorders or the still unknown number of younger people with unrecognized pernicious anemia and other causes of cobalamin deficiency (100). If these findings can be extrapolated, approximately 800,000 elderly people in the United States have undiagnosed and untreated pernicious anemia!

Already as a result of food fortification with folic acid (discussed later), hyperhomocysteinemia in the United States is most frequently the result of cobalamin deficiency, especially among elderly persons (57, 101–103), who need *more than* 100 μg/day oral cobalamin to normalize elevated metabolites (104). Nearly one half (40–50%) of the elderly persons with subclinical cobalamin deficiency have food-cobalamin malabsorption, and a few have pernicious anemia; the cause among the remaining 50 to 60% cases of subclinical cobalamin deficiency is not known but is suspected to be nutritional insufficiency of cobalamin.

Pathogenesis of Folate Deficiency

Folate deficiency is usually recognized in the course of certain clinical presentations that predispose to negative folate balance and subsequent deficiency. It is instructive therefore to conceptualize cellular folate deficiency as arising from etiologic categories of *decreased supply* (reduced intake/absorption/ transport/utilization) or *increased requirement* (metabolic consumption/destruction/excretion). However, in the same patient, more than one mechanism may result in net folate deficiency. The precise contribution of one mechanism over the other is often not obvious. Specific tests to define each mechanism are not routinely available for clinical use.

Nutritional Causes of Folate Deficiency

The body stores of folate are adequate for only approximately 4 months (28). Folate stores are probably depleted much earlier in persons who are chronically in negative folate balance or who have additional conditions that can "tip" them into true folate deficiency. The incidence of folate deficiency in the setting of general malnutrition in developing countries is very high and is invariably a problem of multiple vitamin deficiencies when associated with protein-calorie malnutrition (~38,000 children die *every day* of hunger and starvation-related illness) (105). Decreased availability of folate-rich foods (in winter, after natural disasters, or during the wet season in central Africa), poverty, various cultural and ethnic diets (consisting of maize, rice, or well-cooked beans and vegetables), and cooking techniques that destroy food folate, coupled

with the anorexia that accompanies chronic illnesses, are just a few of the reasons for rapid development of folate deficiency (27, 28, 106, 107).

The rapidly proliferating tissues in children have an absolute requirement for exogenously supplied folate. Although human or cow's milk is barely adequate to maintain folate balance in breast-fed infants, superimposition of associated illnesses that lead to anorexia or folate malabsorption readily shifts these infants into negative folate balance. Infants fed powdered milk formulas, goat's milk (only 6 μg/L folate), or milk that has been boiled (>50% of folate may be destroyed) are at high risk in this regard, as are those on restricted formulas for phenylketonuria and maple syrup urine disease. In Western countries, food faddism, alcoholism, and slimming diets usually lead to decreased folate intake in young to middle-aged persons (28). Although fortification of food with folic acid has markedly reduced folate deficiency in the West, edentulous, infirm, or neglected elderly persons who are too ill to prepare their meals, as well as psychiatric patients, are still at risk of nutritional folate deficiency (28).

Growth

Poor dietary folate intake, particularly when the folate requirement is increased (e.g., in children with sickle cell anemia and with the increased requirement for normal growth), can delay growth and the onset of menstruation in girls. This was shown dramatically in Nigeria, where folate therapy in women who were more than 20 years old was followed by growth spurts and the onset of normal menses (25).

Pregnancy

The increased folate requirement in pregnancy arises from its role in increasing the mother's red cell mass, formation of the placenta, growth of the uterus and the fetus, and, finally, providing folate to be transferred to the fetus. Folate requirement increases throughout pregnancy and is maximal near term.

At the same time, urinary loss of folate in increased in pregnancy because of a lower renal threshold. Folate in the urine in pregnancy averages 14 μg/day, versus 4.2 μg/day in nonpregnant women and 3.5 μg/day in the puerperium. In some women, the urinary loss in pregnancy exceeds 50 μg/day (25). The extent of folate catabolism in pregnancy needs to be quantified (108). The increased folate requirement, which has been assessed at 100 μg/day (25), has to be met from the diet and from whatever folate stores are available.

Overall, iron deficiency is the major cause of anemia in pregnancy, and folate deficiency comes next. Except for malnutrition in children, pregnancy with poor folate intake is the most common cause of megaloblastic anemia in the world. The frequency of significant folate deficiency is related to the efforts made in its detection. Overt megaloblastic anemia is easily recognized, but more often it is concealed by the accompanying iron deficiency; however, hypersegmented polymorphonuclear neutrophils are seen in the blood smear.

The RDA for folate in pregnancy in the United States is 600 μg/day (109). Treatment of megaloblastic anemia in pregnancy is 5 mg folic acid given once or twice daily and continued for 4 weeks after delivery.

Pregnancy and lactation are associated with significantly higher folate requirements (>600 μg/day) for growth of the fetus, placenta, breast, and other maternal tissues. This demand for folate must be met by adequate dietary intake. Maternal-to-fetal folate transfer though the placenta is mediated by placental folate receptors (110, 111) that function in concert with dietary folate to effect continued unidirectional transplacental folate transport (40) to the developing fetus. Folate deficiency in the pregnant mother will lead to decreased placental weight and premature, low-birth-weight infants (112, 113).

The incidence of megaloblastic bone marrow in the United States, Canada, and the United Kingdom during late pregnancy has been reported to be approximately 25%, but in South India it was reported to be as high as 55% (28); these figures for the United States and Canada presumably changed following the advent of the food folate fortification program. Folate deficiency is eight times as high in twin pregnancies. Multiparity (multiple frequent pregnancies with a prolonged state of negative folate balance) and hyperemesis gravidarum commonly lead to folate deficiency. Because the anemia of pregnancy is most frequently caused by iron deficiency, combined iron and folate deficiency (dimorphic anemia) is the more frequent clinical presentation. Increased utilization of folates in newborns leads to a drop in folate levels by approximately 6 weeks. This drop is exaggerated in premature infants, who because of feeding difficulties, infection, or hemolytic disease often develop pure folate deficiency (28).

Lactation

Most patients with megaloblastic anemia in pregnancy are diagnosed in the puerperium. With delivery, folate requirements decline, and undiagnosed megaloblastosis will remit with dietary folate. This must be the case with the majority of women who have megaloblastic bone marrow at this time and who never come to clinical notice in the usual course of events. In some women, however, dietary folate is insufficient, and lactation poses a persistent increase in folate requirement. Human milk after the second month of lactation contains 25 μg/L of folate; with secretion of 700 mL, this involves a loss of about 20 μg/day of folate. Milk contains an avid folate-binding protein (114), and small doses of folate given to the mother appear in the milk without any measurable rise in the maternal serum level (25). In developing countries, megaloblastic

anemia is more often diagnosed 2 to 18 months after birth than during pregnancy (25). The RDA during lactation is 500 μg/day of folate (109). Treatment of megaloblastic anemia found during lactation is 5 mg of oral folic acid once daily. See the DRIs for folate and cobalamin in Appendix Table A-2-e.

Folate and Alcohol

A strong association exists among excessive alcohol consumption, folate deficiency, and megaloblastic anemia, and not infrequently, alcohol abuse turns out to be the explanation for an otherwise puzzling case of anemia. Alcohol has a direct toxic effect on hematopoietic cells in the bone marrow and perhaps on cells in the peripheral blood as well; it promotes excessive iron absorption, and patients who substitute alcohol for food can develop nutritional folate deficiency. The direct toxic effect is most obvious in persons with a high alcohol intake and is best seen in the bone marrow, where megaloblastosis, vacuolation of red and white cell precursors, and ringed sideroblasts (i.e., red cell precursors with iron granules forming a ring around the nucleus) are noted. These changes disappear within 10 days of alcohol withdrawal.

The peripheral blood in alcoholic patients may show a mixture of hypochromic and normochromic red cells, called a dimorphic blood picture, or just macrocytosis present in more than 80% of alcoholic patients who ingest more than 80 g ethanol daily. The first diagnosis in a patient with a normal hemoglobin level and large red blood cells is alcohol abuse. Indeed, routine health screens carried out on the employees of a large US insurance company showed that almost all the employees with large red blood cells and a normal hemoglobin level were taking excessive amounts of alcohol. The changes in the peripheral blood, although resulting from a direct toxic effect of alcohol on the bone marrow, take up to 100 days to disappear, related more to the survival of red cells in the circulation than to events in the marrow.

Folate deficiency occurs in one third of alcoholic patients because of a tendency to substitute alcohol for food. These persons give a history of not taking an adequate meal during the day. This deficiency is seen in spirit drinkers rather than beer drinkers, because beer is a good source of folate (28).

Folate-Responsive Neural Tube Defects and Neurocristopathies

NTDs are the most common major congenital malformations of the central nervous system. They arise from disturbances in neurulation that involve incomplete closure of neural tissues leading to major midline defects; this process leads to a spectrum of birth defects including anencephaly (in which most of the brain and skull are absent), encephalocele (in which the brain protrudes through a defect in the skull), and spina bifida (in which the spinal canal is not closed). The neural tube, which starts out as a tiny ribbon of tissue, normally folds inward to form a tube by the twenty-eighth day after conception. Because NTDs originate in the first month of pregnancy (before many women know they are pregnant), it is critical for a woman to have enough folic acid in her system before conception (periconceptionally) to ensure availability for the embryo. Because embryonic neural tube and neural crest cells have critical bursts of proliferative activity (with occasional doubling times as fast as 5 hours!), folate deficiency of these cells leads to megaloblastosis and cell death and profoundly affects neural tube cell and neural crest cell-mediated midline closure during embryogenesis (115). When folate is plentiful, normal functioning of folate receptors is critical for the prevention of NTDs (116–118). The more severe defects are incompatible with life, and the more severe forms of spina bifida lead to very serious handicaps, with paralysis of legs and the bladder.

Women with a prior history of giving birth to a baby with an NTD have a tenfold higher risk of having a second and subsequent baby with an NTD. For such women, periconceptional folic acid in high doses (4 mg/day) can decrease the recurrence of NTDs by 72% (119). Moreover, periconceptional folate supplementation (800 µg/day) can also reduce the first time occurrence of NTD by close to 75% (120). This finding was confirmed in a massive study from China (121). Other studies also suggest that that periconceptional folate deficiency also leads to oral clefts, conotruncal heart defects, and urinary tract abnormalities and limb reduction defects (122–129), which can be prevented by periconceptional folate supplementation.

Studies in the West demonstrated that women cannot obtain enough folic acid by eating a "balanced Western diet" (130). Only those who received folic acid supplements or who had folate-fortified foods improved their folate status. Because 50% of pregnancies in the United States are unplanned and compliance with taking folic supplements to prevent NTDs is only at approximately 50%, by January 1998, the fortification of foods (rice, flour, pasta, macaroni, breads, cake at 140 µg folic acid/100 g food) was enacted into US law. This level was chosen to ensure that women of childbearing age would have an increase in folic acid intake of 100 µg/day (~25% of the RDA).

As a consequence, the prevalence of folate deficiency (based on a plasma folate <3 ng/mL) was reduced in the United States after food fortification from approximately 20% to approximately 1% (131), and independent studies confirmed a near doubling of serum folate after food fortification from 12 to 20 ng/L (132). In addition, the birth prevalence of NTDs has decreased by 19% in the United States (133); this finding may represent an underestimate based on the methodology used to obtain these data (134). Likewise, in Ontario, Canada, the prevalence of open

NTDs decreased from 1.13 per 1000 pregnancies before food fortification to 0.58 per 1000 pregnancies thereafter (135). Nevertheless, questions remain about the effectiveness of the folic acid fortification program for women in the 15- to 35-year age group in preventing NTDs. Because of an incomplete knowledge base among some women (136, 137), there is continued concern that this group is still not obtaining an adequate amount of dietary folate. This is the basis for recommendations to continue to educate women to take folate supplements at 400 µg/day (beyond what they are already receiving through food folate fortification).

In many developing countries such as India, it sometimes appears that anyone and everyone even remotely related to the newly married couple—and sometimes the whole village—plans the first pregnancy! Such an event represents an excellent window of opportunity to institute good nutritional practices for the mother and future baby. Among such cultures, in which pregnancies are carefully planned, it appears that folate supplementation in the form of daily consumption of folic acid tablets is considered best (138). Moreover, in places where food production and distribution are strictly local, the fortification of food at any federal- or state-supervised central production facility will not reach the masses. This is the case in India, where approximately three fourths of the population lives in villages and small towns. However, when popular brand-name foods advertise that their products are fortified with folic acid, this could reach a wider population. This approach is widely employed in the United States (e.g., for orange juice) and could be popularized in developing countries, where similar products are avidly sought out as frequently as Coca Cola.

One of the serious shortcomings of existing public health policy lies in the lack of translation of scientific information (from randomized controlled trials) to developing countries that constitute the bulk of the world's population. In fact, currently, no formal program exists in most developing countries for prevention of NTDs using periconceptional folic acid. Nevertheless, bright points of lights are shown by efforts in smaller countries. For example, the Malaysian government has distributed informative pamphlets emphasizing the importance of folic acid in the prevention of NTDs in primary health care centers; this information is similar to that found on the US March of Dimes Web site. However, nagging questions remain about the actual compliance with such recommendations among the population of women at risk, as well as questions regarding any outcomes on the actual reduction of NTDs since these educational initiatives were begun. Within this context, it is evident that the methods employed to teach the educated minority in many developing countries will need to be quite different from those used to teach the less educated. Even here, however, no information exists on the best method to reach these groups of women from the behavioral research standpoint.

These are major challenges for nutritionists and public health policy makers in the immediate future.

Therapy for Cobalamin and Folate Deficiency

Routinely, treatment with full doses of parenteral cobalamin (1 mg/day) and oral folate (folic acid) (1–5 mg) before knowledge of the type of vitamin deficiency is established should be reserved for the severely ill patient. An appropriate regimen for conditions in which cobalamin replenishment will rapidly correct cellular cobalamin deficiency but will not correct the underlying problem that led to the deficiency (e.g., pernicious anemia) is 1 mg of intramuscular cobalamin/day (week 1), 1 mg twice weekly (week 2), 1 mg/week for 4 weeks, and then 1 mg/month for life (~15% or 150 μg will be retained 48 hours after each 1 mg cobalamin injection).

Large doses of cobalamin can be given by mouth; even in pernicious anemia, about 1% is absorbed by passive diffusion. This supplement must be taken daily to achieve an adequate intake of at least 1 μg/day. A randomized study clearly demonstrated equivalence between 2 mg cobalamin tablets daily and traditional parenteral treatment for patients with relatively replete cobalamin stores (139). Therefore, this is an alternative for patients who refuse monthly parenteral therapy or who prefer daily oral therapy or in those with disorders of hemostasis. Cobalamin tablets, 1 to 2 mg/day, can also be recommended for patients with cobalamin malabsorption (27, 28, 140). However, it is imperative that the physician ensure that (a) the patient's depleted cobalamin stores are rapidly repleted by parenteral cobalamin *before* switching to oral cobalamin in the long term, and (b) the patient is compliant and demonstrates adequate cobalamin levels and resolution of hematologic and neurologic abnormalities on follow-up.

For nutritional cobalamin deficiency (e.g., in vegetarians) when the entire circuitry in cobalamin absorption is intact, oral cobalamin of 5 to 10 μg (found in conventional multivitamin tablets in the United States) taken for a lifetime of vegetarianism will suffice, but again, only after replenishing exhausted cobalamin stores with higher doses. If there is malabsorption of food-bound cobalamin, then it has been demonstrated that for elderly persons, higher doses of cobalamin of more than 100 μg/day will be required (104).

Oral folate (folic acid) at doses of 1 to 5 mg/day results in adequate absorption (even when intestinal malabsorption of physiologic food folate is present). Therapy should be continued until complete hematologic recovery is documented. If the underlying cause leading to folate deficiency is not corrected, folate may be continued.

Hematologic Response to Cobalamin or Folate

The response to treatment provides further evidence for the diagnosis of cobalamin or folate deficiency, provided the response is optimal. In cobalamin deficiency, an injec-

tion of cobalamin is followed by a most gratifying clinical response with a remarkable feeling of well-being within 1 to 2 days and a dramatic return of appetite.

A rise occurs in reticulocytes (young red blood cells), which reach a peak 5 to 7 days after the start of treatment, and a rise is also seen in hemoglobin and red cells, which exceed 3 million/μL by the third week.

Masked Megaloblastosis

The term masked megaloblastosis is reserved for conditions in which true cobalamin or folate deficiency with anemia is not accompanied by classic findings of megaloblastosis in the peripheral blood and bone marrow. This occurs when patients have a coexisting condition that neutralizes the tendency to generate megaloblastic cells (usually involving reduction in red blood cell hemoglobinization, as in iron deficiency or thalassemia). So if patients have a second blood disorder that produces small red cells (e.g., thalassemia trait or iron deficiency), the MCV may be normal. In this case, the blood film will nevertheless be abnormal, with bizarre red cell fragments and features of dimorphic anemia with large and small cells. Cobalamin or folate therapy restores the smaller red cells that characterize thalassemia trait.

Because strict lifelong vegetarians have a high incidence of overt iron deficiency (≤70% [21]), the manifestations of megaloblastic anemia resulting from accompanying cobalamin and or folate deficiency will be significantly masked. Indeed, appropriate replacement with cobalamin or folate will elicit a maximal therapeutic benefit only when iron deficiency is corrected. Conversely, if combined iron and cobalamin deficiency (total gastrectomy) or iron and folate deficiency (pregnancy) is treated with iron alone, megaloblastosis will be unmasked.

Routine Supplementation of Cobalamin and Folate

Routine *periconceptional* supplementation of folate for (a) physiologically normal women (120, 121) and (b) in higher doses for women at risk for delivery of babies with NTDs (119) provides effective prophylaxis against the development of NTDs (see Table 92.10). Supplementation with folate throughout pregnancy also helps to to prevent premature delivery of low-birth-weight infants (28, 112, 113), and routine supplementation for premature infants and lactating mothers is also recommended.

In addition to hematologic diseases leading to increased folate requirements (e.g., autoimmune hemolytic anemia, β-thalassemia), folic acid supplements appear to reduce the toxicity of methotrexate in rheumatoid arthritis and psoriasis (141–143).

Chronic hyperhomocysteinemia is now established as a major risk factor in occlusive vascular diseases (144–146). These conditions include myocardial infarctions from coronary atherosclerosis (147), extracranial carotid artery stenosis (148, 149), and stroke (150), vascular disease in end-stage renal failure (151, 152), thromboangitis obliterans, aortic atherosclerosis (153), venous thromboembolism (147, 154, 155), and placental abruption or infarction (156), some NTDs (94), and congenital heart defects (95), as well as dementia and Alzheimer disease (96). There also appears to be gathering evidence that low folate status can predispose to carcinogenesis.When presented with these findings, one would have expected this to lead to widespread use of vitamin supplements. However, this is not the case. Longitudinal studies on Seventh-Day Adventists in the West revealed widespread apathy toward taking supplements (157) among these groups. More surprising are cross-sectional studies of Asian Indian physicians living in the United States who are vegetarians with a high incidence of hyperhomocysteinemia attributed to vegetarianism. This finding highlights the difficulty in convincing even highly educated at-risk populations to take cobalamin supplements routinely (158, 159). This situation, coupled with the even greater challenge to teach less well-educated vegetarians in developing countries about the value of taking vitamin supplements and then to implement a program to ensure the consumption of such supplements, is the next frontier in preventive medicine for nutritionists.

LESS COMMON NUTRITIONAL DEFICIENCIES AFFECTING THE BLOOD

Ascorbic Acid (Vitamin C)

Ascorbic acid and folate are both heat-labile, water-soluble vitamins, and they occur in the same kind of foods. A diet deficient in one is likely to be deficient in the other. Ascorbate in food protects folate from oxidative destruction. Many patients with clinical scurvy have megaloblastic hematopoiesis or even frank megaloblastic anemia. Most of these patients respond only to ascorbate, but some may respond to folate. The relationship is likely to be a nutritional deficiency of both these substances in the same person. No good evidence indicates a biochemical relationship other than the protective effect of ascorbate as a reducing agent preventing oxidation of labile tetrahydrofolate analogs, which occurs in an in vitro situation.

Pyridoxine

Pyridoxine-responsive anemias are not uncommon and are associated with pyridoxine antagonists such as cycloserine and pyrazinamide used to treat tuberculosis and with a group of anemias called sideroblastic anemias in which iron accumulates in erythroblasts as a ring around the nucleus. The accumulation of iron granules linked to mitochondria accompanies a failure of hemoglobin formation, so the cytoplasm of the erythroblast is pale and, if this cell matures, will give rise to an iron-deficient red blood cell. Apart from pyridoxine antagonists, sideroblastic anemia occurs as preleukemic refractory anemia in older people and as sex-linked hereditary anemia in male patients. Folate deficiency is common, so a megaloblastic overlay is present.

All these disorders are suspected by examination of the stained blood film, which shows a mixture of iron-deficient (hypochromic) and normochromic red blood cells, also called a dimorphic blood picture. A dimorphic blood film is also present after a blood transfusion to an iron-deficient patient or after iron treatment in iron deficiency. The pyridoxine responsiveness is not the result of nutritional deficiency but rather reflects a biochemical problem with pyridoxine metabolism, and high doses of pyridoxine in excess of 100 mg/day are needed for a response. Folate-deficient patients respond to folate in small doses.

Protein-Energy (Kwashiorkor)

Children with protein malnutrition as recorded in developing countries almost invariably have other problems, including infection and lack of other nutrients. Anemia is common and may be normocytic and normochromic. Hemoglobin levels may be less than 8 g/dL, and the blood film may show anisocytosis. Some patients show evidence of scurvy, and slow hematologic responses follow repletion with protein. Bone marrows are often megaloblastic, and low blood folate levels are not infrequent. In some patients, megaloblastosis resulting from folate deficiency becomes evident only after protein repletion has been started.

Vitamin E

α-Tocopherol serves as an antioxidant. Deficiency of vitamin E is rare but does occur in premature infants at about 4 to 6 weeks of age. These patients have anemia that does not respond to iron and is recognizable from the appearance of the blood film, which shows contracted red blood cells and polychromasia. Polychromatic red cells are new red cells or reticulocytes; when increased under these circumstances, they indicate a response to increased red blood cell destruction (hemolytic anemia), presumably from loss of the protective effect of vitamin E. The hemolytic anemia is accompanied by a raised platelet count and edema of the dorsum of the feet and pretibial area. These symptoms and signs disappear with vitamin E treatment.

Riboflavin

Experimental deficiency in volunteers was accompanied by anemia affecting only the red blood cells. Clinically, anemia resulting from riboflavin deficiency is rare and is said to accompany alcohol abuse when a smooth, cherry-red tongue is a feature.

Copper

Copper deficiency has been described in malnourished children and in patients receiving parenteral nutrition containing inadequate copper. Copper is required in certain enzymes; it is carried in plasma bound to a protein termed *ceruloplasmin*. The level is low in copper deficiency. Anemia and neutropenia rarely occur in copper deficiency and are said to be similar to those in iron deficiency but unresponsive to iron (see Chapters 14 and 38).

REFERENCES

1. Bothwell T, Charlton R, Cook J et al. Iron metabolism in man. Blackwell Scientific Publications, 1979.
2. Bothwell T, Charlton R. Iron deficiency in women. Washington, DC: The Nutrition Foundation, 1981.
3. Centers for Disease Control and Prevention. MMWR Morb Mortal Wkly Rep 1998;47:1–29.
4. Food and Agriculture Organization/World Health Organization. FAO/WHO Requirements of Vitamin A, Iron, Folate and Vitamin B₁₂. FAO Food and Nutrition Series no. 23. Rome: Food and Agriculture Organization, 1988:1–107.
5. Food and Nutrition Board, Institute of Medicine. Dietary Reference Intakes for Vitamin A, Vitamin K, Arsenic, Boron, Chromium, Copper, Iodine, Iron, Manganese, Molybdenum, Nickel, Silicon, Vanadium, and Zinc. Washington, DC: National Academy Press, 2001:18–9.
6. Gillooly M, Torrance JD, Bothwell TH et al. Am J Clin Nutr 1984;40:522–7.
7. Gillooly M, Bothwell TH, Charlton RW et al. Br J Nutr 1984;51:37–46.
8. Hallberg L, Rossander-Hulten L, Brune M et al. Eur J Clin Nutr 1992;46:317–27.
9. Miret S, Simpson RJ, McKie AT. Annu Rev Nutr 2003;23:283–301.
10. Alexander D, Ball MJ, Mann J. Eur J Clin Nutr 1994;48:538–46.
11. Centers for Disease Control and Prevention. MMWR Morb Mortal Wkly Rep 2002;51:897–9.
12. Chanarin I, Rothman D. BMJ 1971;2:81–4.
13. Edwards CH, Johnson AA, Knight EM et al. J Nutr 1994;124:954S–62S.
14. Brock J. Iron in infection, immunity, inflammation, and neoplasia. In: Brock JH, Halliday JW, Pippard MJ, Powell LW eds. Iron Metabolism in Health and Disease. Philadephia: WB Saunders, 1994:353–89.
15. Lozoff B, Jimenez E, Wolf AW. N Engl J Med 1991;325:687–94.
16. Lieberman E, Ryan KJ, Monson RR et al. Am J Obstet Gynecol 1988;159:107–14.
17. Cook JD, Flowers CH, Skikne BS. Blood 2003;101:3359–64.
18. Punnonen K, Irjala K, Rajamaki A. Blood 1997;89:1052–7.
19. Magee H, Milligan E. BMJ 1951;4743:1307–10.
20. Barton DP, Joy MT, Lappin TR et al. Am J Obstet Gynecol 1994;170:896–901.
21. Chanarin I, Malkowska V, O'Hea AM et al. Lancet 1985;2:1168–72.
22. Tinawi M, Martin KJ, Bastani B. Nephron 1996;74:291–4.
23. Cazzola M, Mercuriali F, Brugnara C. Blood 1997;89:4248–67.
24. Albert MJ, Mathan VI, Baker SJ. Nature 1980;283:781–2.
25. Chanarin I. The Megaloblastic Anemias. Oxford: Blackwell Scientific Publications, 1979.
26. Food and Nutrition Board, Institute of Medicine. Dietary Reference Intakes for Thiamin, Riboflavin, Niacin, Vitamin B₆, Folate, Vitamin B₁₂, Pantothenic Acid, Biotin, and Choline. Washington, DC: National Academy Press, 1998:306–56.
27. Antony AC. Megaloblastic anemias. In: Hoffman R, Benz EJ Jr, Shattil SJ et al., eds. Hematology: Basic Principles and Practice. New York: Churchill Livingstone, 1991:392–422.
28. Antony AC. Megaloblastic anemias. In: Hoffman R, Benz EJ Jr, Shattil SJ et al., eds. Hematology: Basic Principles and Practice. 4th ed. New York: Churchill Livingstone, 2005:519–56.
29. Banerjee RV, Matthews RG. FASEB J 1990;4:1450–9.
30. Kolhouse JF, Utley C, Stabler SP et al. J Biol Chem 1991;266:23010–5.
31. Chen Z, Chakraborty S, Banerjee R. J Biol Chem 1995;270:19246–9.
32. Moestrup SK, Verroust PJ. Annu Rev Nutr 2001;21:407–28.
33. Moestrup SK, Birn H, Fischer PB et al. Proc Natl Acad Sci USA 1996;93:8612–7.
34. Herbert V. Am J Clin Nutr 1987;46:387–402.
35. Hoppner K, Lampi B. Int J Vitam Nutr Res 1992;62:244–7.
36. Said HM, Chatterjee N, Haq RU et al. Am J Physiol 2000;279:C1889–95.
37. Antony AC. Blood 1992;79:2807–20.
38. Olivares M, Hertrampf E, Llaguno S et al. Bol Oficina Sanit Panam 1989;106:185–92.
39. Sirotnak FM, Tolner B. Annu Rev Nutr 1999;19:91–122.
40. Antony AC. Annu Rev Nutr 1996;16:501–21.
41. Antony AC, Tang Y-S, Khan R et al. J Clin Invest 2004;113:285–301.
42. Shane B. Vitam Horm 1989;45:263–335.
43. Suh JR, Herbig AK, Stover PJ. Annu Rev Nutr 2001;21:255–82.
44. McMartin KE, Morshed KM, Hazen-Martin DJ et al. Am J Physiol 1992;263:F841–8.
45. Healton EB, Savage DG, Brust JC et al. Medicine (Baltimore) 1991;70:229–45.
46. Martin DC, Francis J, Protetch J et al. J Am Geriatr Soc 1992;40:168–72.
47. Karnaze DS, Carmel R. Arch Neurol 1990;47:1008–12.
48. Carmel R, Gott PS, Waters CH et al. Eur J Haematol 1995;54:245–53.
49. Gott PS, DeGiorgio CM, Schreiber SS et al. J Clin Neurophysiol 1997;14:447(abst).
50. Rasmussen K, Moller J, Lyngbak M et al. Clin Chem 1996;42:630–6.
51. Stabler SP, Lindenbaum J, Allen RH. J Nutr 1996;126:1266S–72S.
52. Stabler SP, Allen RH, Savage DG et al. Blood 1990;76:871–81.
53. Stabler SP, Marcell PD, Podell ER et al. J Clin Invest 1988;81:466–74.
54. Allen RH, Stabler SP, Savage DG et al. Am J Hematol 1990;34:90–8.
55. Lindenbaum J, Savage DG, Stabler SP et al. Am J Hematol 1990;34:99–107.
56. Bain MD, Jones M, Borriello SP et al. Lancet 1988;1:1078–9.
57. Lindenbaum J, Rosenberg IH, Wilson PW et al. Am J Clin Nutr 1994;60:2–11.
58. Joosten E, van den Berg A, Riezler R et al. Am J Clin Nutr 1993;58:468–76 [erratum appears in Am J Clin Nutr 1994;60: 147].
59. Antony AC. Am J Clin Nutr 2003;78:3–6.
60. Savage DG, Lindenbaum J, Stabler SP et al. Am J Med 1994;96:239–46.
61. Metz J, McGrath K, Bennett M et al. Am J Hematol 1995;48:251–5.
62. Stabler SP. J Am Geriatr Soc 1995;43:1290–7.
63. Naurath HJ, Joosten E, Riezler R et al. Lancet 1995;346:85–9.
64. Antony AC. Pernicious anemia and other megaloblastic anemias. In: Rakel RE, ed. Conn's Current Therapy:1996. Philadelphia: WB Saunders, 1996:350–3.

65. Savage DG, Lindenbaum J. Folate-cobalamin interactions. In: Bailey LB, ed. Folate in Health and Disease. New York: Marcel Dekker, 1995:237–85.

66. Savage D, Lindenbaum J, S Stabler et al. Am J Med 1994;96: 239–46.

67. Pennypacker LC, Allen RH, Kelly JP et al. J Am Geriatr Soc 1992;40:1197–204.

68. Allen RH, Stabler SP, Savage DG et al. Am J Hematol 1990;34: 90–8.

69. Antony AC. Am J Clin Nutr 2001;74:157–9.

70. Carmel R. Clin Chem 2002;48:407–9.

71. Wokes F, Badenoch J, Sinclair HM. Am J Clin Nutr 1955;3: 375–82.

72. Dhopeshwarkar GA, Trivedi JC, Kulkarni BS et al. Br J Nutr 1956;10:105–10.

73. Banerjee DK, Chatterjea JB. BMJ 1960;2:992–4.

74. Mehta BM, Rege DV, Satoskar RS. Am J Clin Nutr 1964;15: 77–84.

75. Jathar VS, Patrawalla SP, Doongaji DR et al. Br J Psychiatry 1970;117:699–704.

76. Jathar VS, Inamdar-Deshmukh AB, Rege DV et al. Acta Haematol 1975;53:90–7.

77. Britt RP, Harper C, Spray GH. Q J Med 1971;40:499–520.

78. Herrmann W, Schorr H, Obeid R et al. Am J Clin Nutr 2003; 78:131–6.

79. Refsum H, Yajnik CS, Gadkari M et al. Am J Clin Nutr 2001; 74:233–41.

80. Bjorke Monsen AL, Ueland PM, Vollset SE et al. Pediatrics 2001;108:624–30.

81. Specker BL, Miller D, Norman EJ et al. Am J Clin Nutr 1988; 47:89–92.

82. Specker BL, Black A, Allen L et al. Am J Clin Nutr 1990;52: 1073–6.

83. Louwman MW, van Dusseldorp M, van de Vijver FJ et al. Am J Clin Nutr 2000;72:762–9.

84. Dagnelie PC, van Staveren WA, Vergote FJ et al. Am J Clin Nutr 1989;50:818–24.

85. Dagnelie PC, van Staveren WA. Am J Clin Nutr 1994;59: 1187S–96S.

86. van Dusseldorp M, Schneede J, Refsum H et al. Am J Clin Nutr 1999;69:664–71.

87. Saraya AK, Singla PN, Ramachandran K et al. Am J Clin Nutr 1970;23:1378–84.

88. Gomber S, Kumar S, Rusia U et al. Ind J Med Res 1998;107: 269–73.

89. Rogers LM, Boy E, Miller JW et al. Am J Clin Nutr 2003;77: 433–40.

90. Casterline JE, Allen LH, Ruel MT. J Nutr 1997;127:1966–72.

91. Allen LH, Penland JG, Boy E et al. FASEB J 1999;13:A544(abst).

92. Penland J, Allen L, Boy E et al. L. FASEB J 2000;14: A561(abst).

93. Refsum H, Ueland PM, Nygard O et al. Annu Rev Med 1998; 49:31–62.

94. van der Put NM, Steegers-Theunissen RP, Frosst P et al. Lancet 1995;346:1070–1.

95. Rosenquist TH, Ratashak SA, Selhub J. Proc Natl Acad Sci USA 1996;93:15227–32.

96. Seshadri S, Beiser A, Selhub J et al. N Engl J Med 2002;346: 476–83.

97. Nath I, Reddy KS, Dinshaw KA et al. Lancet 1998;351: 1265–75.

98. Measham A, Chatterjee M. The Crisis of Malnutrition in India: New World Bank Report addresses Food Program Shortcomings. http://wbln1018.worldbank.org/sar/sa.nsf/

2991b676f98842f0852567d7005d2cba/9c8acc61f27739468525 686b0056d709?OpenDocument. World Bank Group, 1999. Accessed on April 14, 2003.

99. Sarode R, Garewal G, Marwaha N et al. Trop Geogr Med 1989; 41:331–6.

100. Carmel R. Arch Intern Med 1996;156:1097–100.

101. Pennypacker LC, Allen RH, Kelly JP et al. J Am Geriatr Soc 1992;40:1197–204.

102. Johnson MA, Hawthorne NA, Brackett WR et al. Am J Clin Nutr 2003;77:211–20.

103. Stabler SP, Allen RH, Fried LP et al. Am J Clin Nutr 1999;70: 911–9.

104. Rajan S, Wallace JI, Brodkin KI et al. J Am Geriatr Soc 2002;50: 1789–95.

105. Grant J. The State of the World's Children: 1988. Oxford: Oxford University Press, 1988.

106. Mukiibi JM, Paul B, Mandisodza A. Central Afr J Med 1989;35: 310–3.

107. Duff EM, Cooper ES. Am J Public Health 1994;84:473–6.

108. McPartlin J, Halligan A, Scott JM et al. Lancet 1993;341: 148–9.

109. Food and Nutrition Board, Institute of Medicine. Dietary Reference Intakes for Thiamin, Riboflavin, Niacin, Vitamin B_6, Folate, Vitamin B_{12}, Pantothenic Acid, Biotin, and Choline. Washington, DC: National Academy Press, 1998:196–305.

110. Antony AC, Utley C, Van Horne KC et al. J Biol Chem 1981; 256:9684–92.

111. Verma RS, Gullapalli S, Antony AC. J Biol Chem 1992;267: 4119–27.

112. Baumslag N, Edelstein T, Metz J. BMJ 1970;1:16–7.

113. Iyengar L, Rajalakshmi K. Am J Obstet Gynecol 1975;122: 332–6.

114. Antony AC, Utley CS, Marcell PD et al. J Biol Chem 1982;257: 10081–9.

115. Antony AC, Hansen DK. Teratology 2000;62:42–50.

116. Piedrahita JA, Oetama B, Bennett GD et al. Nat Genet 1999; 23:228–32.

117. Hansen DK, Streck RD, Antony AC. Birth Defects Res Part A 2003;67:475–87.

118. Rothenberg SP, da Costa MP, Sequeira JM et al. N Engl J Med 2004;350:134–42.

119. MRC Vitamin Study Research Group. Lancet 1991;338:131–7.

120. Czeizel AE, Dudas I. N Engl J Med 1992;327:1832–5.

121. Berry RJ, Li Z, Erickson JD et al. N Engl J Med 1999;341: 1485–90.

122. Czeizel AE, Toth M, Rockenbauer M. Teratology 1996;53: 345–51.

123. Tolarova M, Harris J. Teratology 1995;51:71–8.

124. Shaw GM, Lammer EJ, Wasserman CR et al. Lancet 1995;346: 393–6.

125. Werler MM, Hayes C, Louik C et al. Am J Epidemiol 1999;150: 675–82.

126. Shaw GM, O'Malley CD, Wasserman CR et al. Am J Med Genet 1995;59:536–45.

127. Czeizel AE. Am J Med Genet 1996;62:179–83.

128. Botto LD, Khoury MJ, Mulinare J et al. Pediatrics 1996;98: 911–7.

129. Yang Q, Khoury MJ, Olney RS et al. Epidemiology 1997;8: 157–61.

130. Cuskelly GJ, McNulty H, Scott JM. Lancet 1996;347:657–9.

131. Jacques PF, Selhub J, Bostom AG et al. N Engl J Med 1999; 340:1449–54.

132. Lawrence JM, Chiu V, Petitti DB. N Engl J Med 2000;343:970; author reply 972.

133. Honein MA, Paulozzi LJ, Mathews TJ et al. JAMA 2001;285: 2981–6 [erratum appears in JAMA 2001;286:2236].
134. Mills JL, England L. JAMA 2001;285:3022–3.
135. Ray JG, Meier C, Vermeulen MJ et al. Lancet 2002;360:2047–8.
136. Anonymous. MMWR Morb Mortal Wkly Rep 1999;48:325–7.
137. Feldkamp M, Friedrichs M, Marti K. Am J Med Genet 2002; 107:67–9.
138. Botto LD, Moore CA, Khoury MJ et al. N Engl J Med 1999; 341:1509–19.
139. Kuzminski AM, Del Giacco EJ, Allen RH et al. Blood 1998;92: 1191–8.
140. Lederle FA. JAMA 1991;265:94–5.
141. Leung CF, Lao TT, Chang AM. Eur J Obstet Gynecol Reprod Biol 1989;33:209–13.
142. Morgan SL, Baggott JE, Vaughn WH et al. Arthritis Rheum 1990;33:9–18.
143. Duhra P. J Am Acad Dermatol 1993;28:466–9.
144. Selhub J. Annu Rev Nutr 1999;19:217–46.
145. Boers GH. Thromb Haemost 1997;78:520–2.
146. Selhub J, D'Angelo A. Thromb Haemost 1997;78:527–31.
147. Nygard O, Nordrehaug JE, Refsum H et al. N Engl J Med 1997;337:230–6.
148. Selhub J, Jacques PF, Bostom AG et al. N Engl J Med 1995; 332:286–91.
149. Aronow WS, Ahn C, Schoenfeld MR. Am J Cardiol 1997;79: 1432–3.
150. Perry IJ, Refsum H, Morris RW et al. Lancet 1995;346: 1395–8.
151. Dennis VW, Robinson K. Kidney Int Suppl 1996;57:11S–7S.
152. Robinson K, Gupta A, Dennis V et al. Circulation 1996;94: 2743–8.
153. Konecky N, Malinow MR, Tunick PA et al. Am Heart J 1997; 133:534–40.
154. Graham IM, Daly LE, Refsum HM et al. JAMA 1997;277: 1775–81.
155. D'Angelo A, Selhub J. Blood 1997;90:1–11.
156. Goddijn-Wessel TA, Wouters MG, van de Molen EF et al. Eur J Obstet Gynecol Reprod Biol 1996;66:23–9.
157. Armstrong BK, Davis RE, Nicol DJ et al. Am J Clin Nutr 1974; 27:712–8.
158. Hokin BD, Butler T. Am J Clin Nutr 1999;70:576S–8S.
159. Carmel R, Mallidi PV, Vinarskiy S et al. Am J Hematol 2002;70: 107–14.

93 NUTRITION, RESPIRATORY FUNCTION, AND DISEASE[1,2]

BRUCE SUCKLING, MARGARET M. JOHNSON, AND ROBERT CHIN, JR.

STRUCTURE AND FUNCTION OF THE RESPIRATORY
   SYSTEM 1462
     Control of Breathing .1462
     Respiratory Muscles .1462
     Lung Parenchyma 1463
     Pulmonary Physiology 1463
COMMON PULMONARY PATHOPHYSIOLOGY 1464
EFFECTS OF MALNUTRITION ON DEVELOPMENT,
   STRUCTURE, AND FUNCTION OF THE
   RESPIRATORY SYSTEM 1465
     Development 1465
     Respiratory Muscles .1465
     Ventilatory Drive 1465
     Host Defenses 1465
PROTOTYPICAL LUNG DISEASES: RELATION
   TO NUTRITIONAL STATUS 1465
     Critical Illness and Acute Respiratory Failure 1465
     Obstructive Lung Disease 1467
     Asthma 1470
     Lung Cancer 1470
     Cystic Fibrosis 1471
     Lung Transplantation 1471
     Other Clinical Considerations 1472

Cellular respiration is essential for the functioning of all tissues. Food substrate is converted to usable energy by the formation of high-energy phosphate bonds. Oxygen (O_2) fuels this process, and carbon dioxide (CO_2) is produced as a byproduct. The respiratory system supplies the necessary O_2 and eliminates the CO_2 produced. Adequate nutrition is essential for development, growth, and function of the respiratory system. This chapter summarizes the normal structure and function of the respiratory system, the changes encountered with common diseases, and the impact of nutritional status on the epidemiology and pathophysiology of pulmonary disease.

STRUCTURE AND FUNCTION OF THE RESPIRATORY SYSTEM

Control of Breathing

Afferent signals arising from pontomedullary portion of the brainstem control resting rhythmic breathing patterns. Voluntary and involuntary input from higher cerebral centers can override these rhythmic impulses and alter respiratory patterns as needed to meet the changing metabolic demands of the organism. Peripheral and central chemoreceptors, which sense changes in partial pressure of arterial O_2 (PaO_2) and of CO_2 ($PaCO_2$), as well as pH, alter central respiratory output to match peripheral ventilatory demands to maintain pH and respirable gas levels within a narrow, physiologic range.

Respiratory Muscles

Inspiration is achieved when a negative intrathoracic pressure is generated by the active contraction of the inspiratory muscles, leading to expansion of the thoracic cage. The negative intrathoracic pressure generated creates a pressure gradient between the mouth, and the distal air spaces, the alveoli. Moving down this pressure gradient, air fills the lungs until the alveoli and atmospheric pressure equilibrate. Relaxation of the inspiratory muscles returns the thoracic cage to its resting position, thus reversing the pressure gradient and leading to exhalation.

The diaphragm, the primary muscle of respiration, is dome shaped at rest. With contraction, it flattens and descends, increasing both the vertical and anterior-posterior dimensions of the thoracic cage. Although the diaphragm contracts rhythmically throughout life, it does not have intrinsic automaticity properties like cardiac muscle and, thus, can fatigue when demand exceeds supply. Fatigue (1) is a reversible inability of a muscle to generate a prior

---

[1]**Editors' Note:** Chapter 1β by John Kinney traces the development of knowledge on the relationships of food, work, and heat, topics that relate to this chapter.

[2]**Abbreviations: ARDS,** acute respiratory distress syndrome; **BMI,** body mass index; **CF,** cystic fibrosis; **CO_2,** carbon dioxide; **COPD,** chronic obstructive pulmonary disease; **FEV_1,** forced expiratory volume in 1 second; **FVC,** forced vital capacity; **IBW,** ideal body weight; **MEP** and **MIP,** maximum pressures attainable with expiration and inspiration, respectively; **O_2,** oxygen; **$PaCO_2$,** partial pressure of carbon dioxide in the arterial blood; **PaO_2,** partial pressure of oxygen in the arterial blood; **Pdi/Pdmax,** ratio of diaphragmatic pressure generation to peak pressure; **REE,** resting energy expenditure; **RR,** respiratory rate; **Ti/Ttot,** ratio of inspiratory time to the total respiratory cycle; **TTdi,** tension time index; **V_A,** minute alveolar ventilation; **V_E,** minute ventilation; **V_{O_2},** oxygen consumption; **V_T,** tidal volume.

attainable force. Weakness is the chronic inability to attain adequate force. Both fatigue and weakness may cause inadequate ventilation. Bellemare and Grassino defined the product of the ratio of inspiratory time to the total respiratory cycle (Ti/Ttot) and the ratio of diaphragmatic pressure generation to peak pressure (Pdi/Pdmax) as the tension time index (TTdi) (2):

$$TTdi = Pdi/Pdimax \div Ti/Ttot$$

A TTdi greater than 0.15 is associated with electromyographic changes of diaphragm fatigue (3). Any mechanism that increases Pdi/Pdimax and or Ti/Ttot induces fatigue. If malnutrition leads to a reduced attainable peak pressure, the pressure required to generate a breath represents a greater percentage of the new, but reduced, peak pressure and subsequently an increased TTdi. Adaptive mechanisms can lead to the generation of a lower peak pressure for each breath that, consequently, results in lower tidal volume (VT), assuming constant lung mechanics. Because minute ventilation (VE) is the product of respiratory rate (RR) and VT, RR must increase to maintain the same VE. Increased RR increases Ti/Ttot, again leading to respiratory muscle fatigue.

Diseases directly affecting the respiratory muscles are uncommon, but the respiratory muscles are an important compensatory mechanism in lung disease. If the respiratory muscles can respond to increased bulk airflow demands, function can be maintained. However, in increased demand states such as exercise, or in the presence of muscle dysfunction from malnutrition, the compensatory mechanisms are overwhelmed, leading to diminished functional capabilities.

Lung Parenchyma

The lungs are composed of the conducting airways, the alveoli, and the capillary beds, which form the gas exchanging units, the supporting interstitial structures, the pulmonary vasculature, and immune effector cells.

Tracheobronchial Tree (Conducting Airways)

The conducting airways are a series of progressively, dichotomously branching tubular structures extending from the trachea. The trachea and proximal main airways, the bronchi, offer structural support to the airways but do not participate in gas exchange. Gas exchange occurs at the level of the distal respiratory bronchioles and the alveoli. The tracheobronchial tree is lined with ciliated columnar bronchial epithelial cells and submucosal glands that humidify, warm, and filter the inspired air and contribute to the bronchial mucus layer (4). In response to chronic irritation, as from tobacco smoke, these glands increase their output and size narrowing the airway lumen.

Smooth muscle, innervated by the parasympathetic and the nonandrenergic, noncholinergic nervous pathways,

lines the tracheobronchial tree. Muscle contraction imparts rigidity to the airways and reduces the caliber of the airway lumen. Airway edema, inflammation, and excessive mucus also contribute to luminal narrowing (4), which effects the bulk flow of gas. Airflow is inversely related to airway resistance, which, in turn, is inversely related to the fourth power of the radius of the tracheobronchial tree as defined by Poiseuille's law ($V = P$ pi $r^4/8nl$ where V = flow, P = driving pressure, r = radius, n = viscosity and l = length).

Terminal Respiratory Units

The terminal respiratory unit, consisting of respiratory bronchioles, alveolar ducts, and alveoli, is the gas-exchanging unit. Gas exchange occurs at the alveolar-capillary membrane, which consists of the alveolar epithelium and capillary endothelium, their basement membranes, the contiguous interstitial space, and the surfactant lining (4). Surfactant is a complex phospholipid and protein mixture, produced by type II pneumocytes, that reduces the surface tension of the alveolus and thereby decreases its tendency to collapse at low lung volumes.

Pulmonary Physiology

The ultimate purpose of the respiratory system is to transfer O_2 from the inspired air to the bloodstream and CO_2 from the bloodstream to the exhaled air. The respiratory and cardiac systems work in conjunction to provide a continuous supply of oxygenated blood to the peripheral tissues. After circulating in the periphery where O_2 is extracted, blood is returned to the right side of the heart and is pumped through the pulmonary arteries to the pulmonary capillaries. At the alveolar-capillary interface, O_2 diffuses down a concentration gradient from the O_2-rich alveolar gas to the pulmonary capillary blood. Most of the transferred O_2 binds to hemoglobin in the red blood cells; a small percentage is dissolved in the plasma. Simultaneously, CO_2 diffuses down a concentration gradient from the capillary blood to the alveolus.

Inspired, O_2-enriched gas must be continuously replenished at the alveolar level. As described, inspired gas travels through the airways down a negative pressure gradient generated by diaphragm contraction. Approximately 30% of each inspired breath remains in the conducting airways and thus does not participate in gas exchange. The volume of air remaining in the conducting airways is called the anatomic dead space. A small fraction of each inspired breath reaches alveoli that are not perfused and thereby do not allow gas transfer. This volume of gas is physiologic dead space. The sum of the anatomic and physiologic dead space is the total dead space. Effective minute alveolar ventilation (VA) is the difference between the total VE and dead space ventilation (Table 93.1).

Efficient gas exchange is contingent on the delivery of gas to perfused alveoli. Inadequate gas flow causes perfused

TABLE 93.1. DEFINITION OF RESPIRATORY PHYSIOLOGY TERMS AND ABBREVIATIONS

TERM	DEFINITION
Tidal volume (V_T)	Volume of gas moved during a single respiration
Minute ventilation (V_E)	Amount of air moved in and out of the lungs in 1 minute; V_E = V_T * respiratory rate (RR) per minute
Dead-space ventilation	Amount of inspired gas that does not participate in gas exchange; ventilation of nonperfused alveoli
V_D/V_T	Fraction of each tidal volume that is dead space
Alveolar minute ventilation (V_A)	Amount of inspired air able to participate in gas exchange; alveolar ventilation is the difference between total minute ventilation and dead-space ventilation
Forced vital capacity (FVC)	Volume of gas that can be forcibly exhaled after a maximal inhalation
Forced expiratory volume in 1 second (FEV_1)	Volume of gas expired in the first second of a forced expiration
Stroke volume (SV)	Amount of blood pumped by the heart in a single beat
Cardiac output (CO)	Volume of blood pumped by the heart in one minute; (HR * SV)
Pao_2	Partial pressure of oxygen in the arterial blood
$Paco_2$	Partial pressure of carbon dioxide in the arterial blood
Vo_2	Oxygen consumption (mL/min)
Vco_2	Carbon dioxide production (mL/min)
Compliance	Change in volume per unit change of pressure
Respiratory quotient (RQ)	Molecules of oxygen used/molecule of carbon dioxide produced
Mixed venous blood	Deoxygenated blood returned to the heart; samples for measurements are obtained from a catheter in the pulmonary artery

alveoli not to be ventilated. Deoxygenated blood from these areas mixes with O_2-rich blood from normal areas, reducing total O_2 content of the postcapillary blood. The complete absence of ventilation to perfused alveoli is called shunt.

Efficient gas exchange also requires adequate capillary blood flow to match gas delivery. Supplying inspired air to nonperfused alveoli increases physiologic dead space, thereby decreasing the effective V_T. This is commonly seen in emphysema as a result of capillary bed obliteration from air space enlargement and in acute respiratory distress syndrome (ARDS) as a result of thrombotic occlusion of the precapillary vessel.

Increased V_E initially can compensate for mismatching between gas and blood flow. Ultimately, however, if metabolic demands exceed these compensatory mechanisms, gas exchange abnormalities will develop.

Additional Respiratory System Functions

In addition to gas exchange functions, the lung acts as a "filter" for the blood and also has extensive metabolic functions. The lung synthesizes surfactant and other substances including histamine and arachidonic acid. The effects of nutrition on these functions are largely unknown.

COMMON PULMONARY PATHOPHYSIOLOGY

Various diseases can affect the respiratory system and ultimately compromise gas exchange. Bulk gas flow can be diminished by airway obstruction or restriction as a result of decreased respiratory system compliance (see Table 93.1). In obstructive disease, the airway lumen is narrowed, creating increased resistance to flow. Prototypical obstructive diseases include asthma, emphysema, and chronic bronchitis. In airway obstruction, the resistance to flow increases the work required to deliver adequate V_A to match perfusion. Arterial hypoxemia results when gas flow fails to match perfusion. CO_2 excretion is initially maintained by the increased V_A, but ultimately it may fail to meet demand, leading to an increase in partial pressure of CO_2, hypercarbic respiratory failure, and arterial acidemia.

Decreased compliance of the respiratory system leads to restrictive disease. The loss of compliance can be result from abnormalities in the lung parenchyma, respiratory muscles, or chest wall. Pulmonary fibrosis, the prototypical restrictive disease, is characterized by a loss of compliance of the lung parenchyma as a result of interstitial fibrosis. Other diseases, such as pneumonia and pulmonary edema, decrease the lung compliance by filling the alveolar spaces. Decreased compliance increases the work required to maintain adequate bulk gas flow. In addition, these processes also result in the loss of functioning alveolar-capillary units, thus worsening ventilation-perfusion mismatching and resulting in hypoxemia. Compensation again occurs, usually with an increased RR, but the V_T may fall because of the increased work required to inflate noncompliant lungs. With disease progression or with increased metabolic demands, CO_2 elimination decreases, $Paco_2$ rises, and hypercapnic hypoxemic respiratory failure ensues.

Pulmonary function tests measure exhaled gas volumes and flow rates. The forced vital capacity (FVC), the volume of gas that can be forcibly exhaled after a maximal inhalation, reflects total lung volume. The forced expiratory volume in 1 second (FEV_1) measures the volume of gas that is forcibly exhaled in the first second of exhalation. In restrictive lung diseases, the FVC and FEV_1 are reduced proportionally. In obstructive diseases, the FEV_1

is reduced out of proportion to the FVC, resulting in a decreased FEV_1/FVC ratio, the hallmark of airflow obstruction. Abnormalities in the maximum pressures attainable with inspiration and expiration (MIP and MEP, respectively) can identify abnormal respiratory muscle function. Arterial blood gas determinations, which measure the arterial pH, $PaCO_2$, and PaO_2, can evaluate the efficiency of gas exchange. Other tests, including timed walk tests or cardiopulmonary exercise tests, can more comprehensively assess the interaction of the respiratory and cardiac systems with the peripheral muscles. These tests allow one to measure the impact of various nutritional interventions on lung function.

EFFECTS OF MALNUTRITION ON DEVELOPMENT, STRUCTURE, AND FUNCTION OF THE RESPIRATORY SYSTEM

Development

Both animal and human investigations demonstrate that inadequate nutrition during fetal development can adversely alter organ development. In animal models, fetal malnutrition can result in pulmonary hypoplasia (5, 6). Inadequate protein during development diminishes collagen and elastin synthesis and causes pathologic changes similar to those in emphysema (7). The timing of nutrition insults affects their manifestations. Animal models demonstrate that early malnutrition leads to small but normally proportioned animals, whereas later insults result in lung size disproportionately small for body size (8). In humans, a direct correlation exists between low birth weight and subsequent decreases in pulmonary function (9, 10).

Respiratory Muscles

Diaphragm weight correlates with body weight in animal models and both healthy and emphysematous humans (11–13). Poorly nourished patients have diminished maximal respiratory muscle strength as measured by MIP and MEP (13). The extent of muscle strength loss exceeds the loss of muscle mass, a finding suggesting coexistent myopathy of the remaining muscle (13).

The diaphragm is composed of both type I and type II fibers, and malnutrition affects these fibers differently. In grossly underfed rats, the cross-sectional area of both types of fibers is greatly reduced, but the fast-twitch fibers are quantitatively more affected (14). Others investigators have confirmed greater fast-twitch muscle atrophy in both general malnutrition and protein deficiency specifically (15, 16). Interestingly, Sieck and associates demonstrated greater resistance to fatigue in an in vitro nerve-diaphragm muscle strip preparation from nutritionally depleted animals. Similar to previous findings, these preparations showed a selectively greater decrease in type II fibers. It was hypothesized that the relative greater atrophy of the more fatigable type II

fibers accounted for the overall increase in fatigue resistance (17). These observations suggest that malnutrition should clinically diminish peak pressure generation but have a more limited impact on endurance.

Ventilatory Drive

The impact of nutrition on respiratory drive is incompletely understood. Caloric and nutrient restrictions decrease the hypoxic respiratory drive in normal subjects (18, 19). Ryan and associates described a patient with severe anorexia nervosa (46% of ideal body weight [IBW]), who developed both low V_E and mouth occlusion pressure in response to hypercapnea that reversed on refeeding (20). Mouth occlusion pressure reflects the output of the respiratory center, a finding suggesting that malnutrition affects both central respiratory control and muscle strength.

Host Defenses

Malnutrition increases general susceptibility to infections, but it specifically alters pulmonary defense mechanisms. Infant rats deprived of adequate protein calories develop reduced T-lymphocyte–dependent alveolar macrophage function (21). Animal models of severe malnourishment have also demonstrated decreased alveolar macrophage counts (22) and phagocytosis and microbial killing (23). In patients with tracheostomies, nutritional status inversely correlates with lower respiratory tract bacterial colonization (24).

Lower respiratory tract infections are a significant source of morbidity and mortality in patients with chronic obstructive pulmonary disease (COPD). Malnourished patients are predisposed to pulmonary infections because of inadequate clearance of respiratory secretions resulting from ineffective cough from muscle weakness and a greater propensity for alveolar collapse (atelectasis).

PROTOTYPICAL LUNG DISEASES: RELATION TO NUTRITIONAL STATUS

Critical Illness and Acute Respiratory Failure

Critically ill patients typically have multisystem organ failure, commonly including the respiratory system. Respiratory dysfunction is most often the result of ARDS, which is a syndrome characterized by diffuse radiographic infiltrates and hypoxemic respiratory failure in the setting of a severe systemic critical illness or isolated pulmonary disease. In this section, we review nutritional supplementation in the critically ill patient, with specific attention to ARDS.

Nutrition in Critical Illness: Metabolic Requirements

The nutritional milieu of critical illness is characterized by hypermetabolism, protein catabolism, including muscle proteolysis, insulin resistance leading to impaired glucose utilization, and hyperglycemia. Nutritional support focuses on providing the appropriate amount and composition of nutrients to counter these abnormalities. Because of the inherent complications of both underfeeding and overfeeding, proper estimation of caloric requirements is an essential but challenging task. Energy requirements can be estimated using standard population-based regression formulas, such as the Harris-Benedict equation (25). However, predictive formulas were derived from physiologically normal subjects at rest and do not address the stress and hypercatabolism of critical illness. "Correction stress factors," ranging from 1.2 to 1.5 times the calculated resting energy expenditure (REE),have been developed (26) to account for the increase demands associated with critical illness, but their correlation with indirect calorimetery measurements is suboptimal (27, 28).

O_2 consumption (Vo_2), which can be used as an estimate of caloric needs, can be calculated by the Fick equation $Vo_2 = CO \div (Cao_2 - Cvo_2)$ where CO is the cardiac output, and Cao_2 and Cvo_2 are the O_2 content of arterial and mixed venous blood, respectively. This approach requires invasive monitoring with a pulmonary artery catheter, the need for a relatively stable patient, the inherent inaccuracy of using multiple measurements each with their own standard errors to calculate a final product, and the intermittent timing of the measurements.

Alternatively, Vo_2 can be assessed with a metabolic cart that measures exhaled gases directly. This technique is not universally available, and it requires expensive equipment, technical expertise, and a stable fraction of inspired O_2. Despite these limitations, this technique offers the advantage of continuous measurements rather than intermittent snapshots of one's caloric needs.

The Vo_2 (mL/min) obtained by either the Fick equation or by the gas exchange method is converted to kilocalories/day by using the caloric value of O_2 (4.69–5.05 kcal/L of O_2 consumed) or by using the modified Weir equation if Vco_2 (CO_2 production) is also known (26).

Substrate Supplementation: Implications for Ventilatory Requirements

Patients with acute respiratory failure typically are in a hypercatabolic state and rely, in part, on proteolysis of protein stores to meet their immediate metabolic needs. Gluconeogenesis from amino acids supplies glucose-dependent tissues such as the brain, red blood cells, and healing wounds if glucose supplies are limited (29). Nutritional interventions may spare consumption of endogenous protein. In normal fasting patients, inhibition of glucose neosynthesis with protein sparing can be accomplished by administration of 100 g/day of glucose. By contrast, injured or septic patients require up to 600 g/day (30). Intravenous fat emulsions can also spare protein if they are administered with a minimum of 500 kcal/day of carbohydrate (31). Exogenous protein

supplementation also can replace endogenous protein stores to limit proteolysis (31).

The appropriate mix of carbohydrate, fat, and protein calories must be individualized. Carbohydrates produce more CO_2 during oxidation than fat or protein. For every molecule of glucose completely oxidized, six molecules of CO_2 are produced, giving a respiratory quotient of 1 (see Table 93.1), whereas the oxidation of fat and protein produces less CO_2, with a respiratory quotient of 0.7 and 0.8, respectively. To maintain a normal partial pressure of arterial CO_2 in the presence of increased CO_2 production, V_A must be increased by increasing either RR or V_T. In the presence of underlying lung disease, the ability to increase V_A is limited.

Timing and Route of Nutritional Support

Malnutrition at the onset of critical illness is associated with poor outcomes (32, 33). This association and the inherent perception that feeding is beneficial led to the assumption that nutritional supplementation is indicated in critical illness. Admittedly, no confirmatory data to endorse this contention, but it is highly unlikely that a study withholding nutritional support could or will be performed.

Enteral Feeding and Pulmonary Issues. Enteral feeding is most commonly accomplished through a nasogastric tube or nasoduodenal tube. Potential mechanical risks are associated with enteric feeding tubes, including misplacement in the tracheobronchial tree or pleural space, and thus radiographic confirmation of proper placement is mandatory before initiation of feeding. Theoretically, enteral feeding into the duodenum rather than the stomach reduces the risk of aspiration by bypassing illness-induced delayed gastric emptying and by the use of the pylorous as a barrier to regurgitation. Studies comparing the effect of gastric and duodenal feedings on aspiration are challenging to perform because of difficulties confirming clinically relevant aspiration, and currently available data are conflicting (34, 35). Maintaining patients in a semirecumbent position, rather than supine, appears to decrease the risk of pulmonary aspiration (36).

Parenteral Nutrition and Pulmonary Issues. Parenteral nutrition is delivered through a central or peripheral vein. Central vein infusions allow for the delivery of more concentrated solutions and thus minimize obligate fluid requirements. In patients with ARDS, limited fluid intake may improve outcomes (37).

Access for parenteral nutrition is obtained through percutaneous catheterization of a central vein. Catheter-related thrombosis and infection may complicate catheter use. The addition of 6000 U/day of heparin to the parenteral nutrition formula limits the risk of thrombosis (38). The use of chlorhexidine skin preparation (39) and full-body drapes at the time of catheter insertion (40), restricting catheter use exclusively to alimentation (41), and minimizing line disruption all decrease infectious complications.

Infusions of lipid emulsions have been shown to decrease diffusing capacity and O_2 saturation (42). These alterations are the result of mismatching of ventilation and perfusion induced by the lipids, but their clinical relevance is unknown.

Acute Respiratory Distress Syndrome/Acute Lung Injury

The role of specific nutritional support in ARDS has been studied. Patients with ARDS have lower levels of dietary antioxidants including vitamin E, vitamin C, retinol, and β-carotene than healthy controls (43). Decreased plasma concentrations of tocopherol and vitamin E and elevated lipoperoxides indicative of oxidative damage are commonly seen in patients with ARDS (44), findings prompting speculation that antioxidant supplementation may be beneficial. However, a randomized prospective trial examining the efficacy of supplementation with α-tocopherol and vitamin C showed no change in pulmonary mortality or the development of ARDS. However, the intervention group did have significantly lower incidence of multisystem organ failure, shorter intensive care unit stays, and fewer days of mechanical ventilation (45).

The specific dietary lipid alters the profile of eicosanoids produced by inflammatory cells, and this finding may have clinical relevance. Linoleic acid, an n-6 fatty acid, is converted to arachidonic acid, which is the precursor of many proinflammatory prostaglandins and leukotrienes (46). Alternatively, linolenic acid, an n-3 fatty acid, is converted into eicosapentanoic acid, which produces eicosanoids with much less inflammatory potential (46).

Gadek and colleagues prospectively assessed the effects of enteral feedings enriched with eicosapentaenoic acid (and fish oil), γ-linolenic acid, and antioxidants in 98 patients with ARDS. Compared with controls, the treatment group had more ventilator-free and intensive care unit–free days, earlier improvements in oxygenation, less new organ failure development, and a nonsignificant trend toward decreased mortality (16% versus 25%; $p = .31$) (47).

Production of O_2 free radicals is thought to contribute to acute lung injury, and micronutrient supplementation may offer protective effects. In rats, a deficiency of selenium, an essential cofactor of the antioxidant enzyme glutathione peroxidase, increases susceptibility to lung injury induced by exposure to high O_2 concentrations (48, 49). Although most enteral feeding formulas contain recommended levels of micronutrient, it remains speculative whether additional supplementation is beneficial.

Chronic Lung Diseases

Chronic lung disease is generally classified as obstructive or restrictive, based on the primary physiologic abnormality, as discussed earlier. Obstructive lung diseases include asthma, chronic bronichitis, emphysema, cystic fibrosis (CF), and bronchiectasis. Emphysema and chronic bronchitis are overwhelmingly most commonly the result of tobacco abuse and are collectively labeled COPD.

Restrictive diseases include infiltrative or fibrotic diseases of the lung paranchyma as well as extrapulmonary processes such as muscular weakness, thoracic cage abnormalities, and neurologic diseases that result in similar physiologic impairments. Restrictive diseases are characterized by a loss of compliance of the pulmonary system and increased work of breathing.

Investigations of the interrelationships between nutrition and chronic pulmonary disease have focused on COPD, asthma, and CF. However, it is likely that results from these populations could be extrapolated to others.

Obstructive Lung Disease

COPD causes substantial and increasing morbidity and mortality in the United States and worldwide. Currently, 16 million patients have been diagnosed with COPD, and double that many may have impaired lung function not yet diagnosed (50). Emphysema is thought to be caused by an imbalance of proteases and antiproteases resulting in destruction of the elastin and collagen matrix supporting the lung architecture. Neutrophils, which migrate into the lung in response to tobacco smoke exposure, release elastase and other proteases. Oxidants inhaled from tobacco smoke and released from activated inflammatory cells recruited into the airways impair endogenous antiproteases and contribute to the development of emphysema.

Several naturally occurring antioxidants are present in the lower respiratory tract to counter inhaled oxidants. The extent to which dietary supplementation with antioxidants may protect against tobacco or other environmentally induced pulmonary damage is not established. Concerns exist about deleterious effects of β-carotene supplementation (see later, in the section on lung cancer). A rat model of emphysema induced by elastase has shown reversibility of pathologic changes with all-*trans*-retinoic acid. Attempts to duplicate these results in humans are ongoing (51).

Only 15 to 50% of chronic smokers develop clinically relevant COPD, and the amount of tobacco exposure does not fully account for disease development. Therefore, it is hypothesized that one's diet may serve either a predisposing or protective role in COPD development. Supporting this hypothesis is the observation of pathologic changes similar to emphysema in patients with anorexia nervosa (52).

Dietary antioxidants intake and pulmonary function are inversely related (53–56). Serum levels of β-carotene and retinol correlated with maintenance of ventilatory function in the β-Carotene and Retinol Efficacy Trial (57). These findings mirrored those of an earlier trial (58). However, baseline data from participants in the Atherosclerosis Risk in Communities study failed to demonstrate this relationship (59).

Because the type of ingested dietary fat may affect systemic inflammation, the Atherosclerosis Risk in Communities study investigated the relationship between dietary intake of n-3 fatty acids and the subsequent development of COPD in 8960 current or former smokers. There was a quantity-dependent inverse relationship between the two after controlling for the intensity of tobacco use (60). Sharp and associates and Schwartz and Weiss demonstrated similar results in 6346 and 2526 subjects, respectively (55, 61).

Mechanisms of Malnutrition

Malnutrition affects up to 60% of patients with COPD (62–64), and it is associated with poor outcomes (65–67). Persons who are less than 90% of IBW have greater 5-year mortality after correction for the severity of lung disease (62). In a cohort of 4088 patients, 5-year survival was 24% in those with a body mass index (BMI) lower than 20 and 59% for those with a BMI greater than 30 (Fig. 93.1) (65). Data suggest that inadequate nutrition may be a reversible risk factor for deleterious outcomes in COPD, and improvement in nutritional status has been linked with improvements in survival (68), but it remains uncertain whether dietary interventions can enhance clinical outcomes.

Malnutrition and weight loss in association with advanced lung disease are recognized as the pulmonary cachexia syndrome. Inadequate intake resulting from hyperinflation-induced early satiety and chronic systemic inflammation primarily contribute to pulmonary cachexia (69). Patients with COPD are generally hypermetabolic. Measured REE exceeds the predicted REE by the Harris-Benedict equation in patients with COPD with and without weight loss (13, 70, 71). The increased work of breathing and greater energy expenditure for respiratory muscle activity account for the bulk of the increase in REE. Additionally, diet-induced thermogenesis and the O_2 cost associated with eating limit the ability to consume adequate calories to effect weight gain.

Investigations examining the adequacy of caloric intake are challenging. Most rely on patient food recall that is inherently inaccurate (72). Commonly, intake is adequate to meet energy requirements at rest but insufficient for metabolic demands of activity or for intercurrent illness (68, 72, 73). Schols and associates found that although patients with COPD with and without weight loss had similar REEs, those with weight loss had an inadequate dietary intake in relation to their energy expenditure (74). Baarends and colleagues noted higher total free-living energy expenditure in eight patients with stable COPD who were admitted to pulmonary rehabilitation as compared with matched controls. REE was similar between the two groups, a finding supporting that hypothesis of a higher metabolic demand for physical activity in patients with COPD as compared with controls (75).

COPD is characterized by an enhanced inflammatory state primarily resulting from chronic airway inflammation and circulating inflammatory mediators that may contribute to malnutrition (76). Skeletal muscle loss has been correlated with circulating levels of inflammatory mediators in patients with stable COPD, a finding suggesting that weight loss and loss of fat-free mass are associated with the host's amplified inflammatory state (69). Additionally, tumor necrosis factor-α, a cytokine that can induce cachexia, is elevated in weight losing patients with COPD even in the absence of an acute infection (77).

The recognized association of nutritional depletion and COPD prompted investigators to examine whether low body mass is a risk factor for the subsequent development of COPD. An observational retrospective study of 650 subjects demonstrated an increased relative risk of developing COPD in men in the lowest BMI tertile relative to the highest tertile after controlling for other pertinent factors (78). These data suggest that early nutritional interventions may prevent or delay disease development.

Nutritional Supplementation

Despite the correlation of poor nutritional status with worsened outcome and the theoretic benefit of improved nutritional status, it remains challenging to demonstrate improved clinical outcomes with nutritional support.

Numerous investigators have prospectively studied the effects of prolonged (>2 weeks) nutritional supplementation on patients with COPD (Table 93.2). Most of these studies are small, thus limiting their conclusions. Although the heterogeneity in study design limits the utility of meta-analysis, a recent review of the available data suggests no significant benefit in lung function, anthropometric measures, or exercise capacity in patients with stable COPD (79).

The ideal study design to assess the value of nutritional supplementation is debatable. Less than IBW is commonly used as a marker of inadequate nutrition and changes in respiratory muscle function as the outcome assessed, but this approach has limitations. Although related to prognosis (62), body weight below IBW is only one marker of inadequate nutritional status. Change in respiratory muscle function may be a suboptimal outcome measure because it does

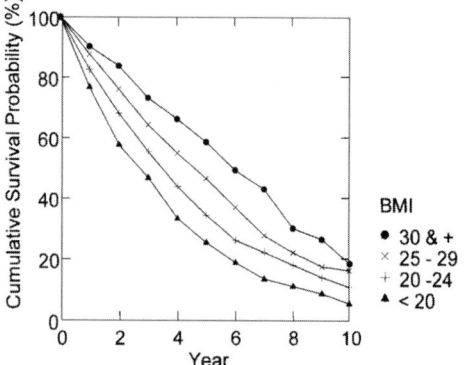

Figure 93.1. Prognostic influence of body mass index in patients with chronic obstructive pulmonary disease. (From Chailleux E. *Chest* 2003; 123:1463, with permission.)

TABLE 93.2. RANDOMIZED CONTROLLED TRIALS EVALUATING NUTRITIONAL SUPPORT IN CHRONIC OBSTRUCTIVE PULMONARY DISEASE

AUTHOR, Y	NO.	DURATION (WK)	WEIGHT GAIN?	OTHER OUTCOMES
Wilson, 1986	6	3	Yes	Improved MIP
Lewis, 1987	10	8	No	No change in MIP
Knowles, 1988	25	8	No	No change in MIP
Efthimiou, 1988	7	12	Yes	Improved MIP
Otte, 1989	28	13	Yes	No change in pulmonary function
Fuenzalida, 1990	9	21	Yes	Improved immune response
Whittaker, 1990	6	2.3	Yes	MIP improved
Rogers, 1992	15	4	Yes	Improved MIP
Schols, 1995	135	8	Yes	Improved MIP
Creutzberg, 2003	64	8	Yes	Improved MIP, handgrip strength, peak workload, symptoms
Cai, 2003	60	3	Yes	Increased FEV$_1$

FEV$_1$, forced expiratory volume in 1 second; MIP, maximum inspiratory pressure.

not strongly correlate with prognosis, lacks functional significance, and is affected by forces other than nutrition. The learning effects of many functional tests, such as timed walk tests, limit their usefulness as outcome measurements.

Recognizing individual variability, tailoring dietary interventions based on specific needs is likely to result in the most appropriate interventions. Slinde and colleagues demonstrated significant anthropometric and functional improvements with a 1-year individualized dietary intervention in patients undergoing rehabilitation (80). To understand better the heterogeneous response seen in studies of nutritional supplementation, Creutzberg and associates identified advanced age, anorexia, and an elevated systemic inflammatory response as characteristics of persons unable to achieve weight gain (81).

Anabolic Steroid/Growth Hormone Administration

Administration of supplemental growth hormone and anabolic steroids has been studied as adjuvant therapy to improve nutritional status in patients with COPD. Various investigators have shown improvements in nitrogen balance (82), body weight, lean body mass (83, 84), and maximum inspiratory pressures with growth hormone use (85). Rudman and associates supplemented the diet of healthy elderly men with growth hormone to test the hypothesis that declining growth hormone levels contribute to the decrease in lean body mass and an increase in fatty tissue with aging (86). The treatment group had a significant increase in lean body mass and a decrease in adipose tissue mass compared with controls (86). In a similar trial, Burdet and colleagues demonstrated an increase in lean body mass with growth hormone but no effect on inspiratory or peripheral muscle strength (84). The use of exogenous growth hormone may allow protein synthesis while minimizing the thermogenic effect of nutritional replacement by reducing the total number of calories needed for anabolism. Schols and colleagues compared the effects of nutritional supplementation with or without

anabolic steroids with placebo in patients with COPD enrolled in a rehabilitation program. Nutritional support in combination with anabolic steroids increased fat-free body mass and MIP in subjects who were depleted at baseline (87). In 23 malnourished patients with COPD who had reduced respiratory muscle strength, synthetically derived testosterone improved BMI, weight, and lean body mass but did not affect exercise capacity (88). In two similarly designed studies, supplementation with growth hormone increased lean body mass but did not improve functional capabilities (83, 84). Recognizing that body weight is an independent predictor of survival, supplements that increase weight should improve outcomes, but data validating this assumption are lacking.

Nutrient Composition and Administration

As described earlier, the oxidation of carbohydrates produces more CO_2 for each mole of O_2 consumed than fats. Therefore, it has been suggested that a high-fat diet would be superior to a high-carbohydrate diet in patients with limited ventilatory reserve. Angelillo and associates randomized COPD patients with hypercarbia to a high-carbohydrate (74% carbohydrate calories) or a low-carbohydrate (28% carbohydrate calories) diet (89). The low-carbohydrate diet resulted in lower CO_2 production and arterial $Paco_2$ and higher Pao_2. Kwan and Mir documented similar findings in patients fed a low-carbohydrate diet (90).

The impact of dietary composition on exercise performance is unclear. Brown and colleagues showed a reduction in 12-minute walk distance after a large-carbohydrate meal in patients with COPD (91). In normal subjects, however, altering dietary fat and carbohydrate proportions did not change exercise gas exchange or mean VE (92).

Electrolyte deficiencies including hypokalemia, hypocalcemia, and hypophosphatemia can also adversely affect respiratory muscle function (see Chapters 8, 9, and 10). Diaphragmatic contractility improves after phosphorus replacement in hypophosphatemic patients with acute respiratory failure (93). This observation is particularly relevant to patients with COPD who require mechanical ventilation because intracellular shifts of phosphorus follow correction of respiratory acidosis with ventilatory support. The clinical manifestations of hypophosphatemia result from intracellular phosphorus depletion resulting from chronic hypophosphatemia. Aubier and colleagues also reported that acute lowering of the serum calcium can also reduce maximum diaphragmatic contractility (93). Restoring normal intracellular concentrations of these ions may improve respiratory muscle strength.

Despite the paucity of proven beneficial effects of nutritional supplementation in malnourished patients with COPD, it is recommended that interventions be undertaken to restore or maintain a normal BMI. Such supplementation should be instituted in conjunction with a regular exercise program and routine reassessment of the patient's progress and nutritional status.

Asthma

Prostanoids released from inflammatory cells contribute greatly to the pathophysiologic changes of asthma, and dietary fat composition may alter prostanoid production. Epidemiologic studies from the 1960s and 1970s demonstrated a low incidence of asthma in populations whose diets were rich in fish oil, which contains eicosapentaenoic acid (94), a finding leading to clinical investigations of this acid in asthma. Although supplementation can effect in vitro changes in inflammatory cells, the effects on clinical markers of disease vary (95, 96). A review of randomized trials failed to substantiate a therapeutic role for either dietary or supplemental eicosapentaenoic acid (97).

Vitamin C has been hypothesized to be beneficial in the treatment of atopic asthma, but a metaanalysis by Bielory and Gandhi examining this question failed to demonstrate efficacy conclusively (98). Both inhaled and intravenous magnesium supplements have been suggested to augment standard β-agonist therapy in acute asthma. The efficacy of magnesium therapy has been more fully established in pediatric populations than in adults (99–102).

Antioxidant supplementation has been suggested as a means to modulate effects of airway injury in patients with asthma who are exposed to ozone and other air pollutants. Children with asthma in Mexico City were randomized to receive either a combined vitamin E and C supplement or placebo. Supplementation attenuated the decrement in small airway function in those children with moderate to severe disease (103).

Lung Cancer

Lung cancer is the leading cause of cancer deaths. Most cases are attributable to tobacco abuse, with a direct relationship between the dose and duration of smoking and disease incidence. However, only approximately 10 to 20%

of heavy smokers develop lung cancer, a finding suggesting a role for either genetic or environmental predispositions.

Retinol, Carotenoids, and α-Tocopherol

Epidemiologic studies suggested that reduced intake and serum levels of carotenoids or retinoids correlated with increased incidence of lung cancer. The National Cancer Institute in Milan prospectively examined the use of retinoids in the prevention of secondary tumors in patients with lung cancer (104). Patients with localized disease were randomized to retinyl palmitate treatment or to a control group. A greater disease-free interval and fewer new malignancies related to tobacco use were seen in the treatment group, but there was no improvement in overall survival. Subsequently, the Alpha-Tocopherol, Beta-Carotene Cancer Prevention Group randomized 29,133 male smokers to α-tocopherol, β-carotene, both agents, or placebo (105). Supplementation with α-tocopherol or β-carotene did not decrease the incidence of lung cancer. However, total mortality was 8% higher in those participants who received β-carotene than in those who did not, primarily from an increase in mortality from lung cancer and ischemic heart disease. In the β-Carotene and Retinol Efficacy Trial, former smokers, current smokers, and asbestos workers were randomized to receive β-carotene and vitamin A or placebo. The intervention group had a 1.28 greater relative risk for lung cancer development (106). These troubling results raised still unresolved concerns regarding prooncogenic effects of β-carotene and prompted early termination of the trial.

Alternatively, the Physicians Health Study randomized 22,000 male physicians to β-carotene (50 mg) supplementation or placebo every other day for an average of 12 years. No difference in the rates of overall malignancy or any specific type of malignancy was seen (107). Finally, 1024 asbestos workers were studied in South Africa in a nonblinded fashion, with a comparison made between supplemental β-carotene (30 mg) and retinol (25,000 IU). The incidence of malignant mesothelioma was significantly lower in the retinol group compared with the β-carotene group but overall lung cancer incidence was the same (108). Currently, neither β-carotene nor α-tocopherol supplementation can be recommended for lung cancer chemoprevention.

Fruits and Vegetables

Diets rich in fruits and vegetables may decrease the incidence of lung cancer. More than ten studies have demonstrated an inverse relationship between fruit and vegetable intake and the incidence of lung malignancy irrespective of tobacco history (109–111). Special attention has been paid to intake of carrots in particular. Consumption of five or more carrots a week in women was associated with a decreased risk of lung cancer (112, 113).

Dietary Fat

Epidemiologic data in the 1980s serendipitously uncovered a potential relationship between dietary intake of saturated fat and lung cancer (114). Subsequent case-control studies demonstrated a positive association between saturated fat intake and lung cancer incidence (115–118) and attributable mortality. In a multicountry study including more than 12,000 participants, lung cancer mortality correlated with saturated fat consumption (119).

Cystic Fibrosis

CF is an autosomal recessive disorder characterized by impaired chloride transport in various organs. Clinical manifestations include broncheictasis, recurrent respiratory infections, and pancreatic dysfunction resulting in fat-soluble vitamin deficiency. Malnutrition is exceedingly common in CF, and inadequate weight gain is often the dominant finding in children at presentation. Nutritional status has been directly correlated with mortality and morbidity (120), and maintenance of adequate nutrition is a vital goal of therapy (see Chapter 69).

Numerous factors lead to malnutrition in CF. Malabsorption resulting from pancreatic dysfunction is the major contributing factor. Moreover, similar to patients with COPD, REE is 25 to 80% greater in patients with CF (121), primarily because of the increased work of breathing (122).

Abnormal cellular mitochondrial function also contributes to increased Vo_2 (123). Although the mechanism is incompletely delineated, it is likely that the CF gene abnormalities alter cellular aerobic respiration.

Because of chronic infection, circulating inflammatory cytokines, catecholamines, and cortisol are elevated in CF, and increased REE has been correlated with elevated levels of circulating catecholamines and tumor necrosis factor-α (124). Antimicrobial treatment of pulmonary infections can reduce REE and promote weight gain (122), but the chronicity and recurrence of infection make it difficult to achieve sustained improvements.

Nutritional assessment should be undertaken at the time of the diagnosis and periodically thereafter to ensure adequate nutrient intake. It is generally recommended that a patient with CF consume 120 to 150% of the recommended caloric intake of age- and sex-matched controls (125).

Pancreatic insufficiency decreases the absorption of fat-soluble nutrients such as β-carotene and vitamins K, A, D, and E. β-Carotene deficiency is common in patients with CF, and supplementation is recommended (126). Vitamin K deficiency typically occurs only in conjunction with antibiotic use, and thus supplementation is recommended at those times (127).

Up to 50% of patients have vitamin A deficiency, leading to visual defects in up to 18% (128). Low vitamin A levels correlate with poor lung function and offer prognostic value (129). Serum measurements of vitamin A or retinol-binding protein should be obtained when the patient is in a noninfected state because levels vary widely in the presence of with inflammation.

Osteoporosis is a persistent problem in CF that is frequently accompanied by vitamin D deficiency. Malabsorption, inadequate exposure to sunlight, and poor hepatic function all contribute to this deficiency. Supplementation of both calcium and vitamin D is recommended to ensure bone health.

Vitamin E is highly fat-soluble and correlates well with fat malabsorption. Severely deficient states are characterized by hemolytic anemia, neuromuscular degeneration, and cognitive deficits. Annual assessment of vitamin E levels and supplementation, when deficient, are recommended.

Iron and zinc deficiency are common in CF. Iron supplements are indicated in the presence of iron deficiency anemia. Zinc supplementation has been advocated in children who have failed to meet developmental landmarks appropriately (125).

Despite advances in our understanding of the genetic defect of CF, treatment is still largely supportive. A high-calorie, high-protein diet with supplemental pancreatic enzymes and multivitamins is generally recommended. Supplementation with n-3 fatty acids may be beneficial, but confirmatory research is necessary (130, 131). Aggressive nutritional intervention, even using enteral feedings when indicated, may aid in weight maintenance and improve lung function (132).

Lung Transplantation

Lung transplantation is a therapeutic option for patients with end-stage lung disease resulting from a variety of illnesses. Malnutrition and obesity are commonly recognized problems both before and after lung transplantation, and they have a direct impact on a patient's clinical course.

Malnutrition is encountered in up to 60% of patients seeking evaluation for lung transplantation (133). A BMI less than 17 kg/m^2 is associated with an increased risk of mortality (134). It is unclear whether improving malnutrition perioperatively improves outcomes, and interventions to do so have met with various degrees of success (135, 136). Delaying lung transplantation to improve nutritional status may adversely affect the outcome (137).

Lung transplantation may reverse malnutrition. In 37 patients followed after lung transplantation, total weight and fat-free mass increased 16.6 and 14.0%, respectively, in the first year after the transplant (138). Greater weight gain following transplantation is associated with improved survival (139).

Pretransplant obesity has also been recognized as a powerful predictor of mortality (134, 140), but whether obesity alone should preclude lung transplantation is undetermined. Weight reduction may improve function sufficiently in some patients to delay or obviate the need for transplantation (141).

Other Clinical Considerations

Compromised nutritional status may exacerbate or be worsened by respiratory illness. For example, protein malnutrition causing hypoalbuminemia alters the threshold for transudation of fluid into the lung parenchyma and pleural space and results in pulmonary edema and pleural effusions.

Specific respiratory diseases impose particular nutritional demands. Patients with malignant disease metastatic to the pleura may drain large amounts of protein into the pleural space. Repeated thoracentesis to drain this fluid results in severe protein wasting. Patients with chylothorax caused by disruption of the thoracic duct may lose massive amounts of protein, fat, and electrolytes into the pleural space. Parenteral alimentation or oral medium-chain triglycerides are often beneficial in replacing the lost nutrients.

Systemic corticosteroids, which are used in a variety of pulmonary diseases, have numerous potential deleterious side effects including fluid retention and weight gain, with resultant increases in work of breathing. In animal models, steroids are associated increased atrophy of type II fibers in the diaphragm (142). In 64 nutritionally depleted patients with COPD, the beneficial effects of nutritional supplementation were attenuated in those receiving systemic steroids (143). Dietary suppressants, including aminorex and fenfluramine (Redux), have been associated with the development of pulmonary hypertension (144).

Although this chapter focuses on the adverse respiratory effects of malnutrition and low body weight, obesity also profoundly affects respiratory function. Excessive weight on the chest and elevation of the hemidiaphragm because of increased abdominal pressure may cause restrictive ventilatory impairment. In extreme cases, these mechanical changes interact with abnormalities of the respiratory center (decreased sensitivity to hypoxemia and hypercarbia) and culminate in the obesity-hypoventilation syndrome. Moreover, increased body weight is a major risk factor for obstructive sleep apnea, which may lead to the development of pulmonary hypertension. Weight loss is the primary treatment for both these conditions.

REFERENCES

1. Roussos C, Macklem PT. N Engl J Med 1982;307:786–97.
2. Bellemare F, Grassino A. J Appl Physiol 1982;53:1190–5.
3. Bellemare F, Grassino A. J Appl Physiol 1983;55:8–15.
4. Murray JF. The Normal Lung: The Basis for Diagnosis and Treatment of Pulmonary Disease. 2nd ed. Philadelphia: WB Saunders, 1986.
5. Lechner AJ, Winston DC, Bauman JE. J Appl Physiol 1986;60:1610–4.
6. Fariday EE. J Appl Physiol 1975;39:535–40.
7. Kalenga M, Eeckhout Y. Pediatr Res 1989;26:125–7.
8. Shaheen S, Barker DJ. Thorax 1994;49:533–6.
9. Chan KN, Noble-Jamieson CM, Elliman A et al. Arch Dis Child 1989;64:1284–93.
10. Barker DJ, Godfrey KM, Fall C et al. BMJ 1991;303:671–5.
11. Rochester DF, Pradel-Guena M. J Appl Physiol 1973;34:68–74.
12. Goldberg AL, Odessey R. Am J Physiol 1972;223:1384–91.
13. Sherman MS, Lang DM, Matityahu A. Chest 1993;103:1038–44.
14. Lewis MI, Sieck GC, Fournier M et al. J Appl Physiol 1986;60:596–603.
15. Goldspink G, Ward PS. J Physiol (Lond) 1979;296:453–69.
16. Oldfors A, Mair WG, Sourander P. J Neurol Sci 1983;59:291–302.
17. Sieck GC, Lewis MI, Blanco CE. J Appl Physiol 1989;66:2196–205.
18. Doekel RC Jr, Zwillich CW, Scoggin CH et al. N Engl J Med 1976;295:358–61.
19. Baier H, Somani P. Chest 1984;85:222–5.
20. Ryan CF, Whittaker JS, Road JD. Chest 1992;102:1286–8.
21. Martin TR, Altman LC, Alvares OF. Am Rev Respir Dis 1983;128:1013–9.
22. Moriguchi S, Sone S, Kishino Y. J Nutr 1983;113:40–6.
23. Shennib H, Chiu RC, Mulder DS et al. Surg Gynecol Obstet 1984;158:535–40.
24. Niederman MS, Merrill WW, Ferranti RD et al. Ann Intern Med 1984;100:795–800.
25. Harris JA, Benedict FG. Standard Basal Metabolism Constants for Physiologists and Clinicians: A Biometric Study of Basal Metabolism in Man. Philadelphia: JB Lippincott, 1919:223.
26. Damask MC, Schwarz Y, Weissman C. Crit Care Clin 1987;3:71–96.
27. Weissman C, Kemper M, Askanazi J et al. Anesthesiology 1986;64:673–9.
28. Liggett SB, Renfro AD. Chest 1990;98:682–6.
29. Wilmore DW. J Am Coll Nutr 1983;2:3–13.
30. Elwyn DH, Kinney JM, Jeevanandam M et al. Ann Surg 1979;190:117–27.
31. Edens NK, Gil KM, Elwyn DH. Clin Chest Med 1986;7:3–17.
32. Giner M, Laviano A, Meguid MM et al. Nutrition 1996;12:23–9.
33. Heys SD, Walker LG, Smith I et al. Ann Surg 1999;229:467–77.
34. Zaloga GP. Chest 1991;100:1643–6.
35. Strong RM, Condon SC, Solinger MR et al. JPEN J Parenter Enteral Nutr 1992;16:59–63.
36. Torres A, Serra-Batlles J, Ros E et al. Ann Intern Med 1992;116:540–3.
37. Humphrey H, Hall J, Sznajder I et al. Chest 1990;97:1176–80.
38. Imperial J, Bistrian BR, Bothe A Jr et al. J Am Coll Nutr 1983;2:63–73.
39. Chaiyakunapruk N, Veenstra DL, Lipsky BA et al. Ann Intern Med 2002;136:792–801.
40. Hu KK, Lipsky BA, Veenstra DL et al. Am J Infect Control 2004;32:142–6.
41. Kruse JA, Shah NJ. Nutr Clin Pract 1993;8:163–70.
42. Hageman JR, Hunt CE. Clin Chest Med 1986;7:69–77.
43. Metnitz PG, Bartens C, Fischer M et al. Intensive Care Med 1999;25:180–5.
44. Richard C, Lemonnier F, Thibault M et al. Crit Care Med 1990;18:4–9.
45. Nathens AB, Neff MJ, Jurkovich GJ et al. Ann Surg 2002;236:814–22.
46. Zaloga GP. Nutrition and prevention of systemic infection. In: Taylor RW, Shoemaker WC, eds. Critical Care State of the Art. Fullerton, CA: Society of Critical Care Medicine, 1991:31–80.
47. Gadek JE, DeMichele SJ, Karlstad MD et al. Crit Care Med 1999;27:1409–20.

48. Coursin DB, Cihla HP. Thorax 1996;51:479–83.

49. Kim HY, Picciano MF, Wallig MA. J Nutr 1992;122:1760–7.

50. National Heart, Lung, and Blood Institute, US Department of Health and Human Services. Chronic Obstructive Pulmonary Disease. Bethesda, MD: National Institutes of Health, 2003.

51. Massaro GD, Massaro D. Nat Med 1997;3:675–7.

52. Chan IH, Birmingham CL, Mayo JR. In: 89th Scientific Assembly and Annual Meeting of the Radiological Society of North America, 2003.

53. Britton JR, Pavord ID, Richards KA et al. Am J Respir Crit Care Med 1995;151:1383–7.

54. Strachan DP, Cox BD, Erzinclioglu SW et al. Thorax 1991; 46:624–9.

55. Schwartz J, Weiss ST. Am J Clin Nutr 1994;59:110–4.

56. Schwartz J, Weiss ST. Am J Epidemiol 1990;132:67–76.

57. Chuwers P, Barnhart S, Blanc P et al. Am J Respir Crit Care Med 1997;155:1066–71.

58. Morabia A, Menkes MJ, Comstock GW et al. Am J Epidemiol 1990;132:77–82.

59. Shahar E, Folsom AR, Melnick SL et al. Am J Respir Crit Care Med 1994;150:978–82.

60. Shahar E, Folsom AR, Melnick SL et al. N Engl J Med 1994; 331:228–33.

61. Sharp DS, Rodriguez BL, Shahar E et al. Am J Respir Crit Care Med 1994;150:983–7.

62. Wilson DO, Rogers RM, Wright EC et al. Am Rev Respir Dis 1989;139:1435–8.

63. Sahebjami H, Doers JT, Render ML et al. Am J Med 1993;94: 469–74.

64. Schols AM, Soeters PB, Dingemans AM et al. Am Rev Respir Dis 1993;147:1151–6.

65. Chailleux E, Laaban JP, Veale D. Chest 2003;123:1460–6.

66. Gray-Donald K, Gibbons L, Shapiro SH et al. Am J Respir Crit Care Med 1996;153:961–6.

67. Thomas DR. Clin Geriatr Med 2002;18:835–9.

68. Schols AM, Slangen J, Volovics L et al. Am J Respir Crit Care Med 1998;157:1791–7.

69. Eid AA, Ionescu AA, Nixon LS et al. Am J Respir Crit Care Med 2001;164:1414–8.

70. Goldstein SA, Thomashow BM, Kvetan V et al. Am Rev Respir Dis 1988;138:636–44.

71. Donahoe M, Rogers RM, Wilson DO et al. Am Rev Respir Dis 1989;140:385–91.

72. Ryan CF, Road JD, Buckley PA et al. Chest 1993;103:1038–44.

73. Wilson DO, Rogers RM, Sanders MH et al. Am Rev Respir Dis 1986;134:672–7.

74. Schols AM, Soeters PB, Mostert R et al. Am Rev Respir Dis 1991;143:1248–52.

75. Baarends EM, Schols AM, Pannemans DL et al. Am J Respir Crit Care Med 1997;155:549–54.

76. Vernooy JH, Kucukaycan M, Jacobs JA et al. Am J Respir Crit Care Med 2002;166:1218–24.

77. Di Francia M, Barbier D, Mege JL et al. Am J Respir Crit Care Med 1994;150:1453–5.

78. Harik-Khan RI, Fleg JL, Wise RA. Chest 2002;121:370–6.

79. Ferreira I, Brooks D, Lacasse Y et al. Chest 2001;119:353–63.

80. Slinde F, Gronberg AM, Engstrom CR et al. Respir Med 2002;96:330–6.

81. Creutzberg EC, Schols AM, Weling-Scheepers CA et al. Am J Respir Crit Care Med 2000;161:745–52.

82. Suchner U, Rothkopf MM, Stanislaus G et al. Arch Intern Med 1990;150:1225–30.

83. Casaburi R, Porszasz J, Burns MR et al. Am J Respir Crit Care Med 1997;155:1541–51.

84. Burdet L, de Muralt B, Schutz Y et al. Am J Respir Crit Care Med 1997;156:1800–6.

85. Pape GS, Friedman M, Underwood LE et al. Chest 1991;99: 1495–500.

86. Rudman D, Fellor AG, Angraj HS. N Engl J Med 1991;323:1–6.

87. Schols AM, Soeters PB, Mostert R et al. Am J Respir Crit Care Med 1995;152:1268–74.

88. Ferreira IM, Verreschi IT, Nery LE et al. Chest 1998;114:19–28.

89. Angelillo VA, Bedi S, Durfee D et al. Ann Intern Med 1985;103: 883–5.

90. Kwan R, Mir MA. Am J Med 1987;82:751–8.

91. Brown SE, Nagendran RC, McHugh JW et al. Am Rev Respir Dis 1985;132:960–2.

92. Sue CY, Chung MM, Grosvenor M et al. Am Rev Respir Dis 1989;139:1430–4.

93. Aubier M, Murciano D, Lecocguic Y et al. N Engl J Med 1985; 313:420–4.

94. Horrobin DF. Med Hypotheses 1987;22:421–8.

95. Arm JP, Horton CE, Spur BW et al. Am Rev Respir Dis 1989; 139:1395–400.

96. Thien FC, Mencia-Huerta JM, Lee TH. Am Rev Respir Dis 1993;147:1138–43.

97. Woods RK, Thien FC, Abramson MJ. Cochrane Database Syst Rev 2002:CD001283.

98. Bielory L, Gandhi R. Ann Allergy 1994;73:89–100.

99. Ciarallo L, Sauer AH, Shannon MW. J Pediatr 1996;129:809–14.

100. McLean RM. Am J Med 1994;96:63–76.

101. Silverman RA, Osborn H, Runge J et al. Chest 2002;122: 489–97.

102. Hughes R, Goldkorn A, Masoli M et al. Lancet 2003;361: 2114–7.

103. Romieu I, Sienra-Monge JJ, Ramirez-Aguilar M et al. Am J Respir Crit Care Med 2002;166:703–9.

104. Pastorino U, Infante M, Maioli M et al. J Clin Oncol 1993;11: 1216–22.

105. Alpha-Tocopherol, Beta-Carotene Cancer Prevention Study Group. N Engl J Med 1994;330:1029–35.

106. Omenn GS, Goodman GE, Thornquist MD et al. N Engl J Med 1996;334:1150–5.

107. Hennekens CH, Buring JE, Manson JE et al. N Engl J Med 1996;334:1145–9.

108. de Klerk NH, Musk AW, Ambrosini GL et al. Int J Cancer 1998;75:362–7.

109. Brennan P, Fortes C, Butler J et al. Cancer Causes Control 2000;11:49–58.

110. Jansen MC, Bueno-de-Mesquita HB, Rasanen L et al. Int J Cancer 2001;92:913–8.

111. Voorrips LE, Goldbohm RA, Verhoeven DT et al. Cancer Causes Control 2000;11:101–5.

112. Speizer FE, Colditz GA, Hunter DJ et al. Cancer Causes Control 1999;10:475–82.

113. Rachtan J. Acta Oncol 2002;41:389–94.

114. Byers TE, Graham S, Haughey BP et al. Am J Epidemiol 1987; 125:351–63.

115. Hinds MW, Kolonel LN, Lee J et al. Am J Clin Nutr 1983;37: 192–3.

116. Jain M, Burch JD, Howe GR et al. Int J Cancer 1990;45: 287–93.

117. Stefani ED, Boffetta P, Deneo-Pellegrini H et al. Nutr Cancer 1999;34:100–10.

118. Shekelle RB, Rossof AH, Stamler J. Am J Epidemiol 1991;134: 480–4; discussion 543–8.

119. Mulder I, Jansen MC, Smit HA et al. Int J Cancer 2000;88: 665–71.

120. Corey M, McLaughlin FJ, Williams M et al. J Clin Epidemiol 1988;41:583–91.

121. Pencharz P, Hill R, Archibald E et al. J Pediatr Gastroenterol Nutr 1984;3[Suppl 1]:147S–53S.

122. Bell SC, Saunders MJ, Elborn JS et al. Thorax 1996;51:126–31.

123. Feigal RJ, Shapiro BL. Nature 1979;278:276–7.

124. Elborn JS, Cordon SM, Western PJ et al. Clin Sci (Lond) 1993;85:563–8.

125. Borowitz D, Baker RD, Stallings V. J Pediatr Gastroenterol Nutr 2002;35:246–59.

126. Renner S, Rath R, Rust P et al. Thorax 2001;56:48–52.

127. Beker LT, Ahrens RA, Fink RJ et al. J Pediatr Gastroenterol Nutr 1997;24:512–7.

128. Rayner RJ, Tyrrell JC, Hiller EJ et al. Arch Dis Child 1989;64:1151–6.

129. Duggan C, Colin AA, Agil A et al. Am J Clin Nutr 1996;64:635–9.

130. De Vizia B, Raia V, Spano C et al. JPEN J Parenter Enteral Nutr 2003;27:52–7.

131. Beckles WN, Elliott TM. Cochrane Database Sys Rev 2002;CD002201.

132. Steinkamp G, von der Hardt H. J Pediatr 1994;124:244–7.

133. Calanas-Continente AJ, Cervero Pluvins C, Munoz Gomariz E et al. Nutr Hosp 2002;17:197–203.

134. Madill J, Gutierrez C, Grossman J et al. J Heart Lung Transplant 2001;20:288–96.

135. Forli L, Bjortuft O, Vatn M et al. Ann Nutr Metab 2001;45:159–68.

136. Forli L, Pedersen JI, Bjortuft O et al. Respiration 2001;68:51–7.

137. Snell GI, Bennetts K, Bartolo J et al. J Heart Lung Transplant 1998;17:1097–103.

138. Kyle UG, Nicod L, Romand JA et al. Transplantation 2003;75:821–8.

139. Singer LG, Brazelton TR, Doyle RL et al. J Heart Lung Transplant 2003;22:894–902.

140. Kanasky WF Jr, Anton SD, Rodrigue JR et al. Chest 2002;121:401–6.

141. Forsythe J, Cooley K, Greaver B. Prog Transplant 2000;10:234–8.

142. Lewis MI, Monn SA, Sieck GC. J Appl Physiol 1992;72:293–301.

143. Creutzberg EC, Wouters EF, Mostert R et al. Nutrition 2003;19:120–7.

144. Abenhaim L, Moride Y, Brenot F et al. N Engl J Med 1996;335:609–16.

94 NUTRITION, DIET, AND THE KIDNEY[1]

JOEL D. KOPPLE

KIDNEY FUNCTION 1475
INTERRELATIONSHIPS BETWEEN NUTRIENTS
   AND KIDNEY FUNCTION 1476
     Effects of Malnutrition on the Kidney 1476
     Effects of Protein and Amino Acid Intake
       on Renal Function 1477
EFFECT OF NUTRITIONAL INTAKE ON THE RATE
   OF PROGRESSION OF RENAL FAILURE 1477
     Mechanisms of Progression 1477
     Experimental Evidence in Chronic Renal Failure .1478
     Human Studies in Chronic Renal Failure 1479
NUTRITIONAL ALTERATIONS IN THE NEPHROTIC
   SYNDROME 1482
NUTRITIONAL AND METABOLIC CONSEQUENCES
   OF CHRONIC RENAL FAILURE 1482
     Clinical, Nutritional, and Metabolic Disorders . . .1482
     Wasting Syndrome and Protein-Energy
       Malnutrition 1484
     Inflammation in Chronic Renal Failure and in
       Patients Undergoing Maintenance Dialysis . . .1485
     Why Are Protein-Energy Malnutrition and
       Inflammation of Great Concern to
       Nephrologists? 1485
DIETARY MANAGEMENT OF CHRONIC RENAL
   DISEASE AND CHRONIC RENAL FAILURE 1486
     General Principles 1486
     Urea Nitrogen Appearance and the Ratio of
       Serum Urea Nitrogen to Serum Creatinine . . .1489
     Dietary Prescription .1490
     Prioritizing Dietary Goals 1499
NUTRITIONAL THERAPY IN ACUTE RENAL FAILURE . .1499
     General Principles 1499
     Peripheral Parenteral Nutrition 1504
     Supplemental Parenteral Nutrition 1505
     Amino Acids that May Predispose to Acute
       Renal Failure 1505

KIDNEY FUNCTION

The kidney has three primary functions: excretory, endocrine, and metabolic. All three functions may be impaired in renal disease and may affect the patient's nutritional status and management. When injury, necrosis, and scarring of the renal parenchyma cause a loss of renal function, the quantity of the substances that are filtered by the kidney falls. However, many aspects of renal function undergo adaptive changes that preserve homeostasis and minimize the derangements in plasma and tissue concentrations of substances that normally are excreted by the kidney. Prominent among these adaptions are nephron hypertrophy and an increase in blood flow and glomerular filtration rate (GFR) in those nephrons that are still functional. Chronic kidney disease (CKD) has recently been classified into five stages, as shown in Table 94.1 (1).

Water and many organic compounds and minerals accumulate in renal failure (2). Low-protein diets (LPDs) reduce accumulation of many of these substances. Eventually, renal failure may become so severe that the aforementioned adaptive mechanisms are no longer adequate to maintain homeostasis, even with special dietary therapy that restricts the intake of fluid, electrolytes, and protein. The accumulation of these compounds, the endocrine and metabolic disturbances, and the clinical signs and symptoms that result from renal failure are referred to as uremia. If this condition is not treated by maintenance hemodialysis (MHD), chronic peritoneal dialysis (CPD), or renal transplantation, clinical deterioration and death will eventually supervene.

Excretion and regulation of body water, minerals, and organic compounds are clearly the most important functions of the kidney. Without renal excretory function, patients rarely live longer than 4 to 5 weeks and often less

---

[1] **Abbreviations: ACEI**, angiotensin-converting enzyme inhibitor; **ARB**, angiotensin receptor blocker; **BMI**, body mass index; **CKD**, chronic kidney disease; **CPD**, chronic peritoneal dialysis; **CRF**, chronic renal failure; **CAVH**, continuous arteriovenous hemofiltration; **CAVHD**, with concurrent hemodialysis; **CVVH**, continuous venovenous hemofiltration; **CVVHD, CVVH** with concurrent

hemodialysis using low dialysate flow rates; **DRI**, dietary reference intake; **ESRD**, end-stage renal disease; **GFR**, glomerular filtration rate; **HDL**, high-density lipoprotein; **IDL**, intermediate-density lipoprotein; **IGF**, insulinlike growth factor; **LDL**, low-density lipoprotein; **LPD**, low-protein diet; **MD**, maintenance dialysis; **MDRD**, Modification of Diet in Renal Disease; **MHD**, maintenance hemodialysis; **PEM**, protein-energy malnutrition; **rhIGF-I**, recombinant human insulinlike growth factor-I; **SUN**, serum urea nitrogen; **TLC**, Therapeutic Lifestyle Changes; **TPN**, total parenteral nutrition; **UNA**, urea nitrogen appearance; **VLDL**, very-low-density lipoprotein.

TABLE 94.1. NATIONAL KIDNEY FOUNDATION DOQI STAGES OF CHRONIC KIDNEY DISEASE[a]

STAGE	DESCRIPTION	GFR (mL/min/1.73m²)
1	Kidney damage with normal normal or increased GFR	≥90
2	Kidney damage with mild decreased GFR	60–89
3	Moderate decreased GFR	30–59
4	Severe decreased GFR	15–29
5	Kidney failure	<15 (or receiving dialysis) therapy

[a]Chronic kidney disease is defined as kidney damage or a glomerular filtration rate (GFR) <60 mL/min/1.72m² for 3 months. Kidney damage is defined as pathologic abnormalities or markers of damage, including abnormalities in blood or urine tests or imaging studies.

From National Kidney Foundation. Am J Kidney Dis 2000;35[Suppl]:6, with permission.

than 10 days, particularly if they are hypercatabolic. In contrast, anephric patients can be kept alive for years with intermittent MHD or CPD, even though many of the endocrine and metabolic disorders that occur with a failing kidney are not completely corrected.

The kidney elaborates certain hormones that have diverse metabolic effects, including 1,25-dihydroxycholecalciferol, erythropoietin, renin, and kallikreins; these have been reviewed elsewhere (3–6). Vitamin D_3 (cholecalciferol is hydroxylated in the liver to form 25-hydroxycholecalciferol. This compound is then converted in the kidney to 1,25-dihydroxycholecalciferol (1,25-dihydroxyvitamin D), the most potent natural form of vitamin D (see Chapter 20). In renal failure, impaired synthesis of 1,25-dihydroxyvitamin D contributes to a vitamin D–deficient state associated with impaired intestinal calcium absorption, hyperparathyroidism, resistance to the actions of parathyroid hormone on bone, and the development of renal osteodystrophy.

Erythropoietin stimulates erythropoeisis in bone marrow (6, 7), and the anemia of chronic renal failure (CRF) is primarily caused by impaired erythropoiesis resulting from reduced erythropoietin production in the diseased kidneys. Compounds that accumulate in renal failure may also suppress erythropoiesis, and mild hemolysis often contributes to the anemia. Recombinant DNA-synthesized human erythropoietin is commonly used to increase the blood hemoglobin levels of patients with advanced CRF and those undergoing maintenance dialysis (MD) (8).

Renin stimulates the conversion of angiotensinogen to angiotensin I, which, in turn, is converted to angiotensin II by angiotensin-converting enzyme. Angiotensin II is a potent vasoconstrictive agent that raises blood pressure and also may stimulate collagen formation and cell proliferation in the kidney and probably other tissues. Renal renin secretion is stimulated by renal ischemia (e.g., in renal artery stenosis) and sometimes by other renal diseases; increased plasma renin levels can cause hypertension. Renal disease, and particularly renal failure, also may engender hypertension by other mechanisms, including the retention of sodium chloride and water.

INTERRELATIONSHIPS BETWEEN NUTRIENTS AND KIDNEY FUNCTION

Kidney function both regulates and is influenced by the body's pools and concentrations of water, minerals, and many other nutrients and their metabolites. (See Chapter 8 for a discussion of electrolytes, water, and acid-base balance and their regulating factors. Individual nutrients are discussed in relevant chapters.)

Effects of Malnutrition on the Kidney

Malnutrition can have important but usually reversible effects on renal function. In humans, malnutrition decreases the GFR (9, 10), as well as the capacity to concentrate and acidify urine (9–12). If nutritional intake improves, these functions may normalize. GFR falls reversibly in obese subjects placed on weight-reduction diets that contain no protein or calories but that provide water, vitamins, and small quantities of minerals. This phenomenon is partly the result of a reduction in extracellular body water, circulating blood volume, and renal blood flow. Increased salt and water intake rapidly reverses this condition. The low or absent protein intake also contributes to the lower renal blood flow and GFR (9, 10). LPDs in rats cause almost a 35% reduction in GFR, increased resistance in the arterioles leading into (afferent) and out of (efferent) the glomerulus, a 25% reduction in the glomerular capillary plasma flow, and almost a 50% decrease in the glomerular capillary ultrafiltration coefficient (13). A reduction in insulinlike growth factor I (IGF-I) levels may contribute to these changes (14, 15).

Malnourished individuals often have lower specific gravity in random urine specimens and therefore increased daily urine volumes. Impaired concentrating ability probably contributes to the nocturia that may occur in malnutrition. The inability of the malnourished patient to concentrate urine normally appears to result from the low protein intake and consequent low rate of urea synthesis (11). Urea is critical for normal urinary concentration. Some of the urea filtered by the glomerulus is reabsorbed in the renal tubule. The urea accumulates in the interstitium of the renal medulla where, when the collecting duct aquaporin receptors are expressed, urea and other chemicals attract water from the lumen of the distal tubule and collecting duct by osmotic pressure. The loss of water from the lumen of the distal tubule and collecting duct by osmotic pressure increases the concentration of urine. When less urea accumulates in the renal medulla, the ability to attract water from collecting duct and, hence, the urinary concentrating ability are diminished. The capacity to dilute urine is normal in malnutrition.

Malnourished subjects are more likely to develop acidosis after an acid load (12). Urinary phosphate and ammonia are primary carriers of acid in the urine. Hydrogen ion secretion into the lumen of the distal nephron lowers the pH of tubular fluid and converts HPO_4^{2-} to $H_2PO_4^-$ and stimulates ammonia production and the conversion of ammonia to NH_4^+. In individuals who have a low phosphorus intake, the phosphate filtered in the kidney is largely reabsorbed; this response conserves body phosphate pools; less phosphorus is excreted in the urine, however, and this reduces the capacity of the kidney to excrete acid. Infusion of phosphate increases urinary excretion of titratable acid in malnourished patients (12). Renal production and excretion of ammonium are also reduced in malnutrition, both under basal conditions and after an acid load (12).

During prolonged starvation, the kidney may account for up to 45% of endogenous glucose production, although part of the rise in the renal contribution to total glucose synthesis is the result of a fall in total body glucose production (16). In extended starvation, net renal extraction of lactate, pyruvate, amino acids, and glycerol also occurs (15). The carbon skeleton in these compounds is virtually completely converted into glucose. During prolonged starvation, free fatty acids and β-hydroxybutyrate are also extracted by the kidney, and acetoacetate is released (16).

Acute starvation and other conditions associated with increased catabolism of nucleic acids, purines, and amino acids, such as may occur with chemotherapy of leukemia and certain other tumors, can cause a marked increase in uric acid production. Hyperuricemia can lead to deposition of uric acid sludge in the kidney and lower urinary tract and may cause acute renal failure. Treatment consists of allopurinol, which inhibits the synthesis of uric acid, maintenance of good hydration and a large urine flow, and alkalinization of the urine, because the solubility of uric acid increases markedly in alkaline solutions (17).

Effects of Protein and Amino Acid Intake on Renal Function

Protein intake appears to engender both an immediate and a more long-term increase in renal blood flow and GFR in humans. A transient increase in renal blood flow and GFR of about 20 to 28% occurs about 2 hours after ingestion of a protein or amino acid load and generally lasts about 1 hour (18, 19). Renal blood flow and GFR increase transiently and more quickly following an intravenous infusion of a mixture of essential and nonessential amino acids (20) or a 30-minute infusion of arginine hydrochloride (21).

EFFECT OF NUTRITIONAL INTAKE ON THE RATE OF PROGRESSION OF RENAL FAILURE

Mechanisms of Progression

Physicians have known for many decades that patients with chronic renal disease who have sustained a substantial loss of GFR often continue to lose renal function inexorably until they develop terminal renal failure (22–31). Although the rate of progression of renal failure varies greatly among patients, in many individuals the decline in kidney function is linear (22–24). The percentage of patients with renal insufficiency who will progress to renal failure is not known, but it seems likely that most patients who sustain a loss of GFR of 50% or greater will show continued progression of renal failure. Renal failure may progress because of continued activity of the underlying renal disease or because of the superimposition of other diseases that may contribute to renal injury such as hypertension, adverse effects of nephrotoxic medications (antibiotics or radiocontrast material), obstruction, kidney infection, hypercalcemia, or hyperuricemia. However, it is not rare for progression to continue even after the initial cause of the renal disease seems to have disappeared and when superimposed illnesses are not present (26–29). For example, progression of renal failure may continue in patients who have relief of urinary tract obstruction, control of hypertension, discontinuance of nephrotoxic drugs, or partial recovery from acute renal failure.

Studies of animal and in vitro models of chronic renal disease or renal failure have led to the following observations. There is a rather common set of physiologic and biochemical responses to chronic loss of renal function that is, to a large degree, independent of the underlying type of kidney disease. When the loss of functioning nephrons becomes sufficient to cause renal insufficiency, the remaining individual functioning nephrons generally undergo an increase in the glomerular plasma flow and GFR and an enlargement in size of both the glomeruli and the tubules (i.e., nephron hypertrophy) (30, 31). The capillary blood flow of the remaining glomeruli increases, as does the blood pressure gradient across the capillary wall (31, 32). In addition, the chemical and electrical as well as pore size barriers to the movement of plasma proteins across the glomerulus and into the renal tubule are impaired (33, 34). Migration of leukocytes and monocytes, platelet aggregation, collagen deposition, cellular proliferation, and other inflammatory and scarifying changes may occur to a greater or lesser degree and may cause progressive renal damage. Many of these changes, some of which could be considered adaptive physiologic responses, are believed to promote further renal injury and lead to progressive renal failure.

Current thinking regarding potential causes of progressive renal failure is summarized in Table 92.2. Most of these processes have been investigated only in animal models, and it is inferred that they may play a role in human renal disease. It is pertinent that many of these mechanisms appear to be susceptible to amelioration or reversal by nutritional therapy. For example, protein-restricted diets have been shown to reduce renal blood flow, GFR, and proteinuria in human patients with renal disease (21). ▪

TABLE 94.2. POTENTIAL CAUSES AND MECHANISMS OF PROGRESSION OF RENAL FAILURE[a]

Continued activity of the underlying renal disease
  Systemic hypertension[b]
  High-protein diet[b]
  High-phosphorus diet[b]
  High-total-fat or high-cholesterol diet[b]
  High calcium-phosphorus product in sera[b]
  Vitamin D overdose (causing hypercalcemia)[b]
  High serum oxalate levels (can be enhanced by high ascorbic acid intake)[b]
  Proteinuria[b]
  Angiotensin II[b]
  Aldosterone[b]
  Hyperuricemia
  Acidemia
  Inflammatory response in kidney with release of cytokines and monokines
  Platelet aggregation in kidney
  Increased mesangial matrix production
  Deposition of other proteins in glomerulus
  Lipoprotein and lipid deposition in glomerulus
  Release of growth factors in kidney
  Glomerular and tubular hypertrophy
  Intraglomerular capillary pressure and capillary blood flow
  Intraglomerular transcapillary hydraulic pressure
  Increased generation of reactive oxygen metabolites in remaining functional nephrons
  Calcium phosphate or calcium oxalate deposition in the kidney
  Nephrotoxic medicines (e.g., radiocontrast material, aminoglycoside antibiotics)
  Enhanced renal tubular generation of ammonia leading to complement activation
  Lead, cadmium toxicity

[a]For many of these factors, evidence that they may cause progressive renal failure is derived from animal models or in vitro systems.
[b]These causes of progressive renal failure may act through one or more of the mechanisms listed in the lower half of this table.

Experimental Evidence in Chronic Renal Failure

Dietary protein restriction has been used for many decades to minimize uremic toxicity (35). In the first half of the twentieth century, research studies in rats indicated that LPDs can retard progression of renal failure (36–38). However, the results were inconsistent (38). In the 1970s and 1980s, studies in rats and humans indicated that diets low in protein and phosphorus or low or high in certain fats retarded the rate of progression of renal failure caused by a variety of renal diseases (39–47). Moreover, administration of prostaglandins may affect the progression of CKD in animals (48–50).

Proteins

In experimental animals with renal disease, a high-protein diet stimulated an increase in GFR, glomerular capillary blood flow, blood pressure gradients across the glomerular capillary wall, and enlargement of individual nephrons, whereas an LPD blunted or prevented this response (31). Moreover, normal rats with renal injury who were fed a high-protein diet developed renal failure, and when such animals were fed an LPD, the progression of renal failure was retarded or arrested (37, 38, 42). It has been hypothesized that a high protein intake, by increasing both glomerular capillary blood flow and transcapillary glomerular hydraulic pressure, causes progressive renal injury to the basement membrane (filtering wall) of the glomerulus (32, 51, 52).

High-protein diets may also promote renal insufficiency by other mechanisms. These include the following: (a) induction of nephron hypertrophy with activation of growth factors that stimulate cell hypertrophy, proliferation, and scarring in the glomerulus; (b) enhanced oxidation rates in the nephron with increased generation of reactive oxygen species (53); (c) an acid load that stimulates renal ammonium production and activation of complement (54); (d) increased generation of urea, which itself may cause hypertrophy of segments of the renal tubule (55); and (e) generation of angiotensin II, aldosterone, and other hormones (56, 57). An LPD retards or stops progressive renal damage by preventing or reducing these phenomena. Transforming growth factor-β plays a central role in scarring of the diseased kidney (58). This growth factor acts on many other mediators that promote renal fibrosis and protein matrix accumulation (59). The degree to which these processes can be modified or slowed by modifications of nutrient intake is not clear. Most of these mechanisms of progression of kidney disease have been studied only in animals, and it is inferred that they are operative in humans. Diets providing soya protein, a vegetable protein, as compared with casein, an animal protein, may more effectively retard the progression of kidney failure in rats with remnant kidneys (60) and in human patients with chronic renal disease (see later).

Diabetic rats with moderate hyperglycemia develop renal hypertrophy and increased hemodynamics (61), and similar abnormalities appear to occur in the intact kidney of humans with diabetes mellitus. Early during the course of diabetes mellitus, patients develop increased renal blood flow, increased GFR, and large kidneys (62). Ultimately, in a large proportion of these patients, glomerulosclerosis occurs and renal failure supervenes (63, 64). In the early stages of diabetes, strict glucose control may reverse these phenomena.

Phosphorus and Calcium

As previously indicated, a low phosphorus intake independent of protein intake appears to retard progression of renal failure (39, 65, 66). One theory of the mechanism of action of the low phosphorus intake is that it decreases the deposition of calcium phosphate in kidney tissue, which may cause further renal damage (65–68). Indeed, in renal tissue obtained by biopsy or autopsy, direct correlation exists between the calcium content and the serum creatinine concentration (67). In general, the calcium concentration of renal tissue is increased more in diseased kidneys with greater renal histopathologic changes.

Lipids and Lipoproteins

Many animal studies suggest a pathogenic role for dietary fat intake and hyperlipoproteinemia. Rats, rabbits, and guinea pigs fed a high-cholesterol diet develop hypercholesterolemia and progressive glomerulosclerosis and renal failure (44, 69, 70). The lipid composition of renal cortical tissue is altered, and both mesangial cellularity and matrix formation increase (69). Glomerular capillary pressure rises, even though systemic blood pressure is not very elevated. The cholesterol-induced renal injury is much greater when cholesterol-supplemented rats have underlying renal diseases. Mesangial cells and monocytes have receptors for certain lipoproteins (71). Monocytes may ingest low-density lipoprotein (LDL) cholesterol and other lipoproteins, which may initiate a series of biochemical and physiologic processes that promote tissue injury. Drugs that lower serum lipoprotein levels may ameliorate glomerular injury in rats (72).

In addition to a number of growth factors, many other compounds may affect renal physiology and the progression of renal failure (2, 6). These include various eicosanoids, angiotensin, and probably aldosterone. The essential fatty acid linoleic acid can be metabolized in the kidney to several families of eicosanoids, including prostaglandins. Prostaglandins have far-reaching effects on the blood flow and blood pressure inside the glomerulus, the propensity for platelets to clot in the glomerulus, and the inflammatory process. Eicosanoids may have antagonistic effects; some increase glomerular blood flow and pressure and may impair platelet clotting, whereas others do the opposite and may also stimulate an inflammatory response. In renal insufficiency, elaboration of certain eicosanoids and other cytokines is increased in the kidney (47, 73), and these substances appear to play an important role in the complex adaptive processes undergone by the nephron as kidney function deteriorates (74, 75). In various rat models of chronic renal disease, feeding or infusions of linoleic acid, vasodilatory prostaglandins or injections of thromboxane or leukotriene B_4 may retard progression of renal failure (48–50, 76, 77). In rats with Heymann nephritis, dietary protein itself reduces eicosanoid synthesis (78). Hence the beneficial effects of dietary protein restriction may be partly caused by its effects on eicosanoid production. Angiotensin II causes vasoconstriction, alters glomerular permeability to serum proteins, and may stimulate mesangial cell proliferation and aldosterone secretion (5).

Medications

Although the foregoing studies in animals indicate an important role for dietary restriction of protein and phosphorus and reduction or increase of certain dietary fats to control progressive renal failure, there is evidence that certain medicines may substitute for or possibly add to the benefits of nutrient restriction. Angiotensin-converting enzyme inhibitors (ACEIs) (medications that decrease blood pressure by inhibiting the enzyme that catalyzes the conversion of angiotensin I to angiotensin II) and angiotensin receptor blockers (ARBs) also lower glomerular capillary blood flow and blood pressure gradients across the glomerular capillary wall in rats with renal insufficiency (5, 79). These agents decrease high blood pressure and retard progressive renal failure in animals and humans, particularly but not only in diabetic patients (80–84). ACEIs and ARBs reduce urinary protein excretion in patients with kidney disease and reduce or abolish microalbuminuria in diabetic and nondiabetic patients (86, 87). Evidence is accumulating that aldosterone receptor blockers inhibit activation of a number of cytokines that promote renal fibrosis and collagen matrix formation (88). This medication also reduces proteinuria in patients with renal disease (89). Studies of whether aldosterone receptor blockers inhibit progression of renal disease in humans are clearly needed. Antihypertensive medications also slow CKD by reducing blood pressure.

Medications that bind phosphorus in the intestinal tract enhance the effectiveness of dietary phosphorus restriction in reducing the progression of renal failure in animals (39, 66). These drugs are of particular value as an adjunct to dietary phosphorus restriction, because it is difficult to lower dietary phosphorus intake to necessary levels without making diets highly restrictive, unpalatable, and difficult for adherence.

Human Studies in Chronic Renal Failure

To what extent are the animal data applicable to patients? From the mid-1970s to the present, many but not all dietary studies in humans with renal insufficiency indicated that a low intake of dietary protein and phosphorus will retard the rate of progression of renal failure (90–101). Some evidence indicates that a low protein or phosphorus intake may each act separately to slow progressive renal failure (65). The earlier studies of this question in humans suffered from one or more major defects in experimental design. Later studies, in general, were better designed. Diet studies generally evaluated low-protein, low-phosphorus diets that provide about 0.40 to 0.60 g protein/kg body weight/day or a very-LPD containing about 0.28 g/kg/day (e.g., ~16–25 g protein/day). This latter diet was supplemented with ten to 20 g/day of the nine essential amino acids or of mixtures of several essential amino acids and ketoacid or hydroxyacid analogs of the other essential amino acids (90, 92–95, 97, 100). These diets were compared with either a more liberal diet containing approximately 1.0 g or more of protein/kg/day and more phosphorus or with an ad libitum diet.

The ketoacid or hydroxyacid analog is structurally identical to its corresponding essential amino acid, except that the amino (NH_2) group attached to the second (α) carbon of the amino acid is replaced with a keto group or a hydroxy group, respectively. The ketoacid and hydroxyacid analogs can be transaminated in the body to the respective amino acids, although some of the analogs are degraded rather than transaminated. Because the ketoacids and hydroxyacids lack the nitrogen-containing amino group on the α carbon, these compounds provide the patient with a lesser nitrogen load. As they are degraded in the body, they should engender fewer waste products that normally accumulate in renal failure. Ketoacid analogs of the branched-chain amino acids, especially of leucine, may be somewhat more likely to promote protein anabolism, possibly by decreasing protein degradation (102, 103).

The largest and most intensive examination of whether low-protein, low-phosphorus diets retard the rate of progression of renal disease was the Modification of Diet in Renal Disease (MDRD) Study, funded by the National Institutes of Health (100, 101). This project investigated, in an intention-to-treat analysis, the effects of three levels of dietary protein and phosphorus intakes and two blood pressure management goals on the progression of chronic renal disease. A total of 840 adults with various types of renal disease, but excluding diabetes mellitus, was divided into two study groups according to GFR.

In Study A, 585 patients with a GFR, measured by ^{131}I-iothalamate clearances, of 25 to 55 mL/1.73 m^2/minute were examined. Patients were randomly assigned to either a usual-protein, usual-phosphorus diet (1.3 g/kg standard body weight/day of protein and 16–20 mg/kg/day of phosphorus) or to a low-protein, low-phosphorus diet (0.58 g/kg/day of protein and 5–10 mg/kg/day of phosphorus) and also to either a moderate or strict blood pressure goal: mean arterial blood pressure 107 mm Hg (113 mm Hg for those ≥61 years of age) or 92 mm Hg (98 mm Hg for those ≤61 years of age). Study B included 255 patients with a baseline GFR of 13 to 24 mL/1.73 m^2/minute. Patients were randomly assigned to the low-protein, low-phosphorus diet or to the very-low-protein, very-low-phosphorus diet (0.28 g/kg/day of protein and 4–9 mg/kg/day of phosphorus) with a ketoacid-amino acid supplement (0.28 g/kg/day). They were also randomly assigned to either the moderate or strict blood pressure control groups, as in Study A. The adherence to the dietary protein prescription in the different diet groups was good (100).

Among participants in Study A, those prescribed the LPD had significantly faster declines in GFR during the first 4 months than those assigned to the usual-protein diet. Thereafter, the rate of decline of the GFR in the low-protein, low-phosphorus group was significantly slower than in the group fed the usual-protein, usual-phosphorus diet.

Over the course of the entire treatment period, there was no difference in the overall rate of progression of renal failure in the two diet groups. However, it is likely that the initial greater fall in GFR in the patients prescribed the LPD may reflect a hemodynamic response to the reduction in protein intake rather than a greater rate of progression of the parenchymal renal disease. This response may in fact be beneficial, reflecting a reduction of intrarenal hyperfiltration and intrarenal hypertension. If this explanation is correct, and it is not proven that it is correct, the subsequently slower rate of progression of disease after the first 4 months of dietary treatment is consistent with a beneficial effect of this intervention on the renal disease. In Study B, the very-LPD group had a marginally slower decline of GFR than the LPD group; the average rate of decline did not differ significantly between the two groups ($p = .066$).

In the MDRD study, the very-low-protein, ketoacid/amino acid–supplemented diet was not compared with the usual protein intake. Moreover, it is possible that the lack of significant effect of the LPD on the progression of renal failure may reflect the rather short mean duration of treatment in the MDRD study, 2.2 years. Indeed, if the trend toward slower progression of renal failure in the LPD groups that was present at the termination of the MDRD study had persisted during a longer follow-up period, a statistically significantly slower progression would have been observed with the 0.60 g/kg protein diet in Study A and the very-low-protein, ketoacid-amino acid–supplemented diet in Study B. Several other characteristics of the patient population and study design of the MDRD may have led to the lack of a statistically significant difference in progression of renal failure between the diet groups (104).

It is also reported that vegetarian LPDs providing soy protein may retard progression of CRF more effectively than diets of similar protein content that contain animal protein (60, 105, 106). The mechanisms of such an effect is not known, but it may be related to the total content and different composition of fats in the vegetarian diet. This latter diet is reported to improve the serum lipid profile in patients with chronic renal disease and the nephrotic syndrome (106, 107).

Four published metaanalyses have evaluated several clinical trials of the effects of LPDs on the rate of progression of kidney failure. In general the LPDs were also low in phosphorus. These metaanalyses each evaluated a somewhat different series of clinical trials, only some of which included the MDRD Study (108–111). Three of the metaanalyses used, as the key outcome, the onset of end-stage renal disease (ESRD) as determined by the patient with CRF starting treatment with MHD or CPD or receiving a kidney transplant (108, 109, 111). These metaanalyses reported statistically significant reductions in the relative risk of a patient with CRF assigned to the LPDs reaching this end point to 0.54, about 0.67, and 0.61, respectively. One metaanalysis used the rate of decrease in GFR as the key outcome (110). This latter study described a slowing in the progression of renal failure of only 6%, which, although statistically significant, was of questionable clinical significance.

The discrepancy between these two sets of findings may be explained in part by the fact that ingestion of LPDs leads to a reduction in the generation of metabolic products of protein and amino acids, and some of these metabolic products are toxic. Indeed, patients ingesting LPDs are reported to be started on MHD or CPD at lower GFRs than persons eating higher protein intakes. These metaanalyses also examined clinical trials that used an intention-to-treat type of analysis, whereby the data from individuals assigned to a given dietary intake were included in the results whether or not these persons adhered to the dietary prescription or even were available for follow-up testing.

One metaanalysis analyzed the results of five prospective clinical trials of the effects of such diets on progression of renal failure in patients with insulin-dependent diabetes mellitus (109). This analysis indicated that LPDs also retard disease progression in these patients. However, the results were much less definitive because much smaller numbers of patients were analyzed; in two of the trials, there was no randomized, concurrent control group, and the key end points were less definitive.

In a secondary analysis of Study B in which the decrease in GFR was correlated with the actual quantity of protein ingested, there was no effect of ingesting the LPD versus the very-LPD supplemented with ketoacids-amino acids on the progression of renal failure (101). However, in Study A, when the data from the two groups were combined and then analyzed, there was a significant inverse relationship between the protein intake actually ingested, as determined from the urea nitrogen appearance (UNA) (see later), and the rate of decline in GFR (101). The actual dietary protein intake associated with the lowest rate of decline in GFR was about 0.62 g/kg/day.

A recent 12-year follow-up analysis was conducted in the Study A MDRD patients concerning the hazard ratio, adjusted for baseline characteristics, of incurring ESRD or a combination of either ESRD or all-cause mortality (112). ESRD was defined as commencing MD therapy or receiving a kidney transplant. This study indicated that during the first 6 years after the onset of the dietary protein prescription, there was a statistically significant adjusted lower hazard ratio of incurring ESRD, or the combination of either ESRD or mortality, in those assigned to the 0.60 g protein/kg/day diet versus those assigned to the 1.3-g protein/kg/day diet (112). This difference tended to reverse itself in the second 6-year period of follow-up.

In Study B patients, those assigned to the ketoacid-supplemented diet had a significantly greater hazard ratio, adjusted for baseline factors, for death after they developed ESRD during the 12 years after assignment to their diet prescription (113). These data are particularly intriguing because patients were monitored only, on average, for the first 2.2 years of follow-up and were then referred back to their usual physicians. Moreover, with few exceptions, ketoacid mixtures were not available in the United States, except for those persons participating in the MDRD Study during the time they were assigned to this diet. Thus, it would have been very difficult for the Study B patients to continue taking ketoacids after the MDRD Study ended.

The Nurses' Health Study compared spontaneous protein intakes of individual women with different levels of GFR, determined from their serum creatinine concentrations (114). Women (n = 1624), ages 42 to 68 years, had their protein intake measured in 1990 and again in 1994 using a semiquantitative food-frequency questionnaire. Those women with mildly reduced baseline estimated GFR levels that were greater than 55 mL/minute/1.73 m^2 but less than 80 mL/minute/1.73 m^2 showed a fall in GFR of -1.69 mL/minute/1.73 m^2/10-g increase in protein intake. However, after adjustment for measurement of error, the change in estimated GFR was -7.72 mL/minute/1.73 m^2/10-g increase in protein intake. This association was of borderline statistical significance. A high intake of nondairy animal protein with mild renal insufficiency was associated with a significantly greater fall in estimated GFR (-1.21 mL/minute/1.73 m^2/10-g increase in nondairy animal protein intakes. A recent retrospective study in renal transplant recipients indicated that those recipients who spontaneously ingested higher-protein diets experienced greater losses of GFR (115).

Taken together, the post hoc analysis of the MDRD Study data, the results of the approximately 12 years of follow-up to the MDRD Study, the Nurses Health Study, the study in renal transplant recipients, and the four metaanalyses all point to the probability that LPDs will retard the rate of progression of renal failure in patients with CKD. Moreover, because these LPDs often engender sufficiently lower uremic toxicity for a given level of reduced renal function, patients fed these diets may be able to avoid MHD or CPD therapy at GFR levels that would require patients ingesting higher protein intakes to commence such therapy.

An interesting question is whether diets may promote or retard the development of renal failure in persons with no underlying renal disease. At the present time, there are no clear answers to this question. Another unresolved issue is whether LPDs will retard progression of renal failure in patients receiving ACEIs and/or ARBs. Because dietary protein restriction exerts many of the same hemodynamic and other physiologic effects on the kidney as do ACEIs and ARBs (51, 52, 85), it is possible that the renal-protective effects of LPDs, when combined with ACEIs and ARBs, are replicative, rather than additive. In one rather small study, 62 patients with type 2 diabetes mellitus were randomly assigned to an LPD (0.60 g protein/kg/day) or a more usual-protein diet (116); most of the patients were receiving ACEIs. In this 4-year trial, the LPD group experienced a 10% incidence of death or ESRD as compared with 27% in the patients eating the usual-protein diet ($p < .042$). There was no difference in the rate of decline in GFR in the two groups (116).

Because proteinuria is associated with greater progression of renal failure and increased risk of cardiovascular disease, and because ACEIs and ARBs, even in combination, may reduce proteinuria but do not eradicate it, there may be a role for LPDs at least in persistently proteinuric patients. More research in this area is clearly needed.

NUTRITIONAL ALTERATIONS IN THE NEPHROTIC SYNDROME

The nephrotic syndrome is a kidney disorder characterized by losses of large quantities of protein in the urine (≥3.0 g/day), low serum albumin concentrations, high serum levels of cholesterol and other fats, and accumulation of excess body water to form edema (117). This condition is caused by diseases that affect the glomerulus and increase glomerular permeability to protein. Because patients with the nephrotic syndrome have large urinary protein losses and their appetite is frequently poor, they often develop protein malnutrition and debility. Certain vitamins and most trace elements are protein bound in plasma, and these patients are therefore also at risk of developing deficiencies of these nutrients when these proteins are lost in the urine. Excessive urinary iron, copper, and vitamin D losses and vitamin D deficiency have been reported in patients with the nephrotic syndrome (117, 118). Malnutrition may occur in nephrotic patients even when they do not have advanced kidney failure. For a given type of renal disease, heavy proteinuria is associated with more rapid progression of renal failure, possibly because of the incorporation of proteins into the glomerular mesangium which may cause sclerosis or inflammatory responses (119). Many growth factors and other bioactive substances are also bound to proteins that are filtered by the leaky glomerulus in patients with the nephrotic syndrome. It is postulated that some of these bioactive compounds may promote progressive renal damage (120).

As indicated earlier, protein-restricted diets, ACEIs, ARBs, and aldosterone receptor antagonists may each reduce renal losses of protein (121–124). Using these medications to reduce proteinuria while maintaining a sufficiently high protein intake to increase both albumin and total body protein mass may be desirable.

NUTRITIONAL AND METABOLIC CONSEQUENCES OF CHRONIC RENAL FAILURE

CRF causes pervasive nutritional and metabolic disorders that may affect virtually every organ system. These abnormalities are reviewed briefly.

Clinical, Nutritional, and Metabolic Disorders

Advanced CRF is a complex disorder caused by a marked reduction in the excretory, endocrine, and metabolic

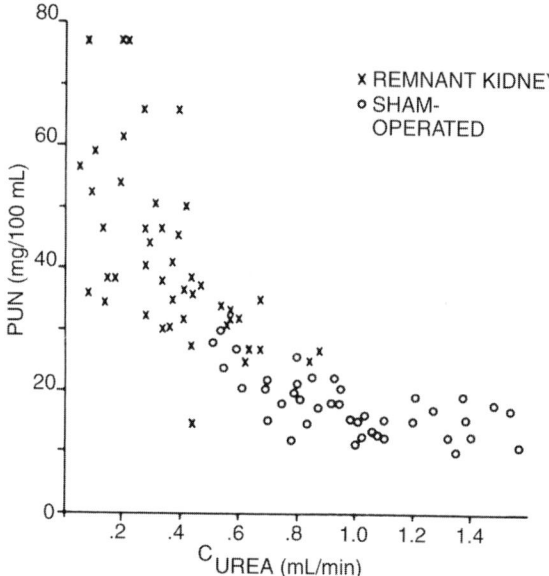

Figure 94.1. Relationship between the plasma urea nitrogen (PUN) and the glomerular filtration rate as indicated by urea clearance in Sprague-Dawley rats with chronic renal insufficiency and sham-operated controls. Chronic renal failure was produced by ligation of two thirds to three fourths of the arterial supply to the left kidney and contralateral nephrectomy. (From Kopple JD. Nutrition and the kidney. In: Alfin-Slater RB, Kritchevsky D, eds. Human Nutrition: A Comprehensive Treatise, vol 4. New York: Plenum Publishing, 1979:409–57, with permission.)

functions of the kidney. Patients with CRF eventually develop uremia, which refers to the accumulation of nitrogenous metabolites in the blood in combination with the clinical signs and symptoms of advanced renal failure. Most of these compounds are products of amino acid and protein metabolism. Quantitatively, the most prominent are urea, creatinine, other guanidine compounds, and uric acid (Fig. 94.1). It is generally believed that some of these compounds are toxic in high concentrations.

The many signs and symptoms of uremia include weakness, a feeling of ill health, insomnia, fatigue, loss of appetite, nausea, vomiting, weight loss, diarrhea, itching, muscle cramps, hiccups, twitching or jerking of the extremities, fasciculations, tremors, emotional irritability, and decreased mental concentration and comprehension. A characteristic fetid breath is often present.

Altered serum concentrations of other electrolytes and acidosis can occur and can have profound and life-threatening effects on the physiologic processes and metabolism of the body (see Fig. 94.1). Abnormalities in water and electrolyte balance and acidosis are caused by impaired ability of the failing kidney to regulate, by excretion, the content of water, salts, and acids in the body. The sodium and water disturbances associated with renal failure can lead to congestive heart failure and hypertension or, if excessive sodium depletion occurs, reduction in extracellular fluid volume and a fall in blood pressure. When renal failure is not end stage or nearly so, most of these clinical and metabolic disorders can be ameliorated or prevented with dietary therapy. Untreated uremia can lead to lethargy, loss of consciousness, coma, convulsions, and death.

Advanced CRF causes pervasive alterations in the absorption, excretion, or metabolism of many nutrients. These disorders include the following: accumulation of chemical products of protein metabolism (2); a decreased ability of the kidney either to excrete a large sodium load or to conserve sodium rigorously when dietary sodium is restricted (125); impaired renal ability to excrete water, potassium, calcium, magnesium, phosphorus, trace elements, acids, and other compounds; a tendency to retain phosphorus (126–128); decreased intestinal absorption of calcium (127) and possibly iron (128); and a high risk of developing certain vitamin deficiencies, particularly vitamin B_6, vitamin C, folic acid, and the most potent known form of vitamin D, 1,25-dihydroxycholecalciferol (127, 129). The patient with CRF is also likely to accumulate certain potentially toxic chemicals, such as aluminum, that normally are ingested in small amounts and excreted in the urine (128).

Uremia is also a polyendocrinopathy, and many of the metabolic and clinical manifestations of uremia are caused by the endocrine disorders. Many hormone concentrations are elevated in renal failure, particularly those of the peptide hormones, because of the impaired ability of the kidney to degrade peptides. These elevated peptide hormones include parathyroid hormone, leptin, glucagon, insulin, growth hormone, prolactin, luteinizing hormone, often follicle-stimulating hormone, and gastrin (127, 130–138). Increased secretion of some hormones, such as parathyroid hormone and insulin, may contribute to elevated plasma levels. CRF patients have altered thyroid hormone levels that are similar to the euthyroid sick syndrome, but hypothyroidism is not common (139). Of the hormones elaborated by the kidney, plasma erythropoietin and 1,25-dihydroxycholecalciferol are reduced (58, 127), and plasma renin activity may be increased, normal, or decreased.

Serum IGF-I levels are usually normal in renal failure, but there is resistance to the activity of IGF-I (140, 141). There is increased sensitivity to the actions of glucagon, which is reversed by hemodialysis, although hyperglucagonemia persists (131). Resistance to the peripheral action of insulin occurs (142). These effects on insulin and glucagon contribute to the mild glucose intolerance usually present in nondiabetic patients with CRF (132). Impaired actions of hormones in uremia may result from circulating inhibitors in serum, downregulation of receptor number, or postreceptor defects in the signal transduction system. Cytosolic calcium participates in certain cell-signaling systems. Elevated basal cytosolic calcium, induced by hyperparathyroidism, appears to be one of the postreceptor signal transduction disorders induced by CRF (143).

Most of the products of metabolism that accumulate in renal failure do so as the result of decreased excretion. The ability of the failing kidney to synthesize or metabolize many compounds, including amino acids, is also impaired. In chronic renal insufficiency, the kidney displays reduced catabolism of glutamine, impaired synthesis of alanine, and decreased conversion of glycine to serine and citralline to urea (144, 145). Serum and tissue taurine levels are often low.

Quantitatively, the most important end product of nitrogen metabolism is urea (146). In a clinically stable patient with CRF who eats at least 40 g of protein/day, the net quantity of urea produced each day contains an amount of nitrogen equal to about 80 to 90% of the daily nitrogen intake. Guanidines are the next most abundant end product of nitrogen metabolism. Guanidine compounds include creatinine, creatine, and guanidinosuccinic acid (2, 146). The "middle molecules" are a class of compounds that are midway in size between the small, readily dialyzable substances that accumulate in renal failure and small proteins. Most middle molecules are considered to have molecular weights of approximately 300 to 2500 and contain amino acids. Some middle molecule compounds are increased in uremic sera (2, 146). Despite decades of study, the compounds that cause uremic toxicity are not well defined. Probably, many compounds contribute to uremic toxicity. Prime suspects for uremic toxins include urea, guanidine compounds, phenolic acids, middle molecules, proinflammatory cytokines (see later), and some of the hormones elevated in uremic plasma, especially parathyroid hormone and possibly glucagon (2, 131, 143, 146–148).

Altered gastrointestinal function may affect nitrogen metabolism in patients with CRF. The gastrointestinal tract metabolizes urea, uric acid, creatinine, and choline and synthesizes or releases from larger molecules dimethylamine, trimethylamine, ammonia, sarcosine, methylamine, and methylguanidine (146). The gut metabolism or synthesis of many of these compounds is increased in CRF, possibly because of the rise in the quantity of intestinal bacterial flora (149).

Some of the metabolic alterations in uremia are adaptive homeostatic responses that offer both benefits and disadvantages to the patient (147). Hyperparathyroidism is an example. As the kidneys fail, impaired excretion of phosphorus leads to phosphorus retention. Concomitantly, the diseased and scarred renal parenchyma is less able to convert 25-hydroxycholecalciferol to the most potent metabolite of vitamin D, 1,25-dihydroxycholecalciferol, a powerful suppressor of parathyroid hormone secretion (127). Low plasma concentrations of 1,25-dihydroxycholecalciferol lead to an increase in parathyroid hormone secretion. In addition, deficiency of 1,25-dihydroxycholecalciferol both impairs intestinal calcium absorption and causes resistance to the actions of parathyroid hormone in bone. These alterations also promote hypocalcemia and contribute to the development of hyperparathyroidism.

Elevated serum parathyroid hormone reduces renal tubular reabsorption of phosphorus (enhancing urine phosphorus excretion), lowers serum phosphorus, promotes renal synthesis of 1,25-dihydroxycholecalciferol, mobilizes calcium from bone, and increases intestinal calcium absorption, although intestinal calcium absorption usually remains low or, in mild renal insufficiency, normal. The benefits derived from these homeostatic actions are that more normal concentrations of plasma phosphorus and calcium are maintained in patients with mild to more advanced renal insuffiency. The trade-off is the development of hyperparathyroidism (147, 148). Parathyroid hormone has been implicated as a pervasive uremic toxin that adversely affects many organs and tissues and contributes to the uremic syndrome (148).

Anemia, which usually is primarily the result of impaired erythropoiesis caused by deficiency of erythropoietin, can be treated effectively with this hormone (8). To reduce the risks and the high costs of therapy, usually sufficient erythropoietin is given to raise the hematocrit only to about 33 to 35%. Large doses of iron, usually given intravenously to maintain serum total iron binding saturation at around 40%, will often decrease the dosage needed of erythropoietin (150). When kidney failure is a complication of an underlying systemic disease, such as diabetes mellitus, hypertension, or lupus erythematosus, other manifestations of these underlying diseases may also adversely affect the patient and may be progressive. All these problems do not seriously affect every patient, and many patients with CRF or who are undergoing dialysis lead full and productive lives.

With the institution of dietary therapy or treatment with MHD or CPD, blood levels of many metabolic products that accumulate in uremic plasma decrease, and the patient may experience clinical improvement. MHD or CPD enables patients to live for many years with essentially no renal function. Despite such improvement, however, many clinical and metabolic disorders may persist or even progress. These include the following: (a) oxidative and carbonyl stress; (b) an inflammatory state; (c) a type IV hyperlipidemia and other disorders of lipid metabolism (151, 152); (d) a high incidence of cardiovascular, cerebrovascular, and peripheral vascular disease (153); (e) osteodystrophy with disordered bone architecture, osteoporosis, or osteomalacia (aluminum toxicity often contributes to the osteomalacia) (127, 154); (f) anemia (6–8); (g) impaired immune function and decreased resistance to infection; (h) mildly impaired peripheral and central nervous system function; (i) muscle weakness and atrophy; (j) frequent occurrence of viral hepatitis (155); (k) sexual impotence and infertility; (l) generalized wasting and malnutrition (156–164); (m) a general feeling of ill health or emotional depression; and (n) poor rehabilitation (165). Most of these complications can be aggravated by poor nutritional intake or improved with good nutrition.

The foregoing considerations indicate that the intestinal absorption, excretion, and/or metabolism of virtually every nutrient may be altered in CRF. In addition, the decreased intake of food and excessive intake of certain minerals, such as phosphorus, sodium, or potassium, may alter clinical or nutritional status. Moreover, medicinal therapy may

adversely affect nutrient metabolism in renal failure. For example, anticonvulsant medications may cause deficiencies of vitamin D and folic acid; hydralazine, isoniazid, and other medications may cause vitamin B_6 deficiency (166). Part of the challenge of dietary therapy for such patients is to provide for the altered requirements and tolerance of many nutrients that occur in CRF.

Wasting Syndrome and Protein-Energy Malnutrition

Patients with CRF, and particularly in those undergoing MHD or CPD, frequently show evidence of wasting or protein-energy malnutrition (PEM). The phrase, protein wasting syndrome, is preferable because not all causes of PEM are the result of inadequate nutrient intake (156–164, 167). The changes are summarized in Table 94.3. The plasma amino acid pattern, which is pathognomonic for renal failure, also has similarities to that found in malnutrition. The findings of malnutrition are sometimes observed in nondialyzed patients with CRF, but they are more prevalent in patients undergoing MHD or CPD. Not every dialysis-treated patient has evidence of these

TABLE 94.3. EVIDENCE FOR PROTEIN-ENERGY MALNUTRITION IN PATIENTS WITH ADVANCED CHRONIC RENAL FAILURE

ANTHROPOMETRY, BODY COMPOSITION, AND ISOTOPE DILUTION STUDIES[a]	BIOCHEMISTRY[a]
Decreased	Decreased
Body weight	Serum
Height (children)	Total protein
Growth (children)	Albumin
Body fat (skinfold thickness)	Transferrin
Fat-free solids	Prealbumin
Intracellular water	C3
Muscle mass (midarm muscle	C3 Activator
circumference)	Cholinesterase
Total body potassium	Plasma
(nondialyzed patients)	Leucine
Total body nitrogen (patients on	Isoleucine
chronic peritoneal dialysis)	Total tryptophan
	Valine
	Tyrosine
Total albumin mass, synthesis,	
and catabolism	
Valine pools (nondialyzed	Valine:glycine ratio
patients)	Essential:nonessential
	ratio
	Muscle
	Alkali soluble protein
	RNA:DNA ratio
	Valine
	Tyrosine
	Normal to Increased
	Plasma
	glycine

[a]Patients with chronic renal failure may have normal values for these parameters, but statistical comparisons indicate that the levels are often abnormal in these persons.

disorders; however, virtually every survey of patients undergoing MD indicates that, as a group, these patients show evidence of malnutrition (156–164, 167). Malnutrition is only mild to moderate in most malnourished patients undergoing chronic dialysis. About 6 to 8% of dialysis-treated patients have severe wasting. In addition to PEM, patients with CRF are at higher risk for malnutrition of iron, zinc, and certain vitamins, including vitamin B_6, vitamin C, folic acid, 1,25-dihydroxycholecalciferol, and possibly carnitine (168–173).

There are many causes of wasting or PEM in CRF (157). First, dietary intake is often inadequate, particularly for energy requirements (156, 161, 174, 175). The low dietary intake is mainly the result of anorexia. This is caused by uremic toxicity, a CRF-related inflammatory state, the anorexigenic effects of acute or chronic superimposed illnesses, and emotional depression. Associated illnesses may also impair the patient's physical ability to procure, ingest, or digest foods or to receive or utilize tube feeding. In addition, the dietary prescription in renal failure, which is low in protein and other nutrients and which may be difficult to prepare or unpalatable, can lead to low nutrient intakes.

Second, the superimposed illnesses frequently found in patients with CRF often induce a catabolic state (176–178). Third, the dialysis procedure itself may induce wasting. Hemodialysis and peritoneal dialysis remove free amino acids, peptides, or bound amino acids (179–182), water-soluble vitamins (129), proteins (with peritoneal dialysis and, rarely, with hemodialysis) (180, 183), glucose (during hemodialysis with glucose-free dialysate) (184), and probably other bioactive compounds. Hemodialysis also increases net protein breakdown, especially by activating the complement cascade system and inducing release of catabolic cytokines (see later) (185, 186). Fourth, excessive accumulation of acid in blood (acidemia) may engender protein catabolism (187). Fifth, patients with CRF sustain blood losses. Because blood is a rich source of protein, these losses may contribute to protein depletion. The blood losses are caused by frequent blood drawing for laboratory testing, the common occurrence of occult gastrointestinal bleeding, and sequestration of blood in the hemodialyzer and blood tubing (188).

Other possible but not well-established causes of wasting include the following: (a) altered endocrine activity, particularly resistance to insulin (142) and IGF-I (140, 141), hyperglucagonemia (131), hyperparathyroidism (127, 143, 147, 148), and deficiency of 1,25-dihydroxycholecalciferol (127); (b) endogenous uremic toxins; (c) exogenous uremic toxins, such as aluminum; and (d) loss of metabolic functions of the kidney. Because the kidney is a metabolic organ that synthesizes or degrades many biologically valuable compounds, including amino acids (144, 145), the loss of these activities in kidney failure could possibly disrupt the body's metabolism and promote wasting.

Inflammation in Chronic Renal Failure and in Patients Undergoing Maintenance Dialysis

Patients with CRF and those undergoing MD frequently show evidence of inflammation. This evidence includes increased serum levels of such acute-phase proteins as C-reactive protein, and serum amyloid A, and ceruloplasmin. Serum levels of negative acute-phase proteins, including albumin, transferrin, transthyretin (prealbumin), and cholesterol-carrying lipoproteins may decrease not only as a result of PEM but also as a direct result of inflammation (175, 189–193). Most surveys suggest that serum C-reactive protein levels are increased in about 30 to 50% of US and European MHD-treated patients and are perhaps lower in Asian MHD-treated patients (193). Serum proinflammatory cytokines, including tumor necrosis factor-α, interleukin-1, and interleukin-6, are commonly elevated in patients with advanced CRF (193–197). In patients with advanced CRF and those undergoing MD, there is also an accumulation in serum of compounds that cause oxidant or carbonyl stress (193, 198, 199). Oxidant stress refers to cellular injury caused by exposure of the cell to compounds that oxidize chemicals in the cell (198). Carbonyl stress refers to cellular injury caused by carbon containing compounds that react with compounds in the cell (199). Homocysteine is such a carbonyl-reactive compound that is increased in serum in patients with CRF and those undergoing MD and that, when elevated, exerts a number of adverse effects on the vascular endothelium (200–204).

Causes of inflammation in patients with CKD include comorbid illnesses, CRF per se, (which itself leads to an increase in serum levels of a number of oxidants, reactive carbonyl compounds, and proinflammatory cytokines), oxidant and carbonyl stress, chronic low-grade infection such as is caused by *Chlamydia*, and reaction to the vascular access prostheses necessary to perform hemodialysis, the hemodialyzer itself, the peritoneal dialysis catheter (for CPD) and (for MHD or CPD) dialyzer tubing, or impure dialysate (190–192, 205).

Why Are Protein-Energy Malnutrition and Inflammation of Great Concern to Nephrologists?

The reason for the current high interest in PEM and inflammation is that measures of either of these two conditions are epidemiologically linked to increased risk of morbidity and mortality in patients undergoing MD (19). Markers of inflammation have been particularly linked to atherosclerosis and cardiovascular morbidity and mortality (191–193, 205). Moreover, laboratory research indicates that certain acute-phase proteins, oxidants, reactive carbonyl compounds, and proinflammatory cytokines can be directly toxic to the endothelium. These compounds may cause inflammation, cellular proliferation, and increased matrix deposition in the endothelium with the formation of inflamed atherosclerotic plaques, which are likely to rupture and increase the likelihood of myocardial infarction or stroke.

The increased risk of morbidity and mortality in MD-treated patients with PEM and/or inflammation is of particular importance because the adjusted mortality rate for MD-treated patients in the United States is very high, approximately 24% per year (178). Hence, in a population that is already at high risk for morbidity and mortality, the identification of clinical characteristics that demonstrate the presence of a subgroup of these individuals who are at even greater risk for these adverse outcomes is a cause for alarm. At the same time, it is a potential opportunity to develop interventions that may improve such poor prognoses.

There is an overlap between the manifestations of PEM and inflammation. Thus, both PEM and inflammation display reduced serum levels of such negative acute-phase proteins as albumin, transferrin, transthyretin, and cholesterol-carrying lipoproteins (189, 192, 195, 205). The lowest serum levels of these proteins are generally found with inflammation rather than PEM. Inflammation may cause PEM by inducing anorexia—for example, tumor necrosis factor-α and interleukin-6 are anorexigens—and also by engendering a hypercatabolic state (192, 195, 206, 207). Whether PEM may predispose to inflammation, for example by increasing the risk of infection or enhancing the inflammatory response to other stimuli, is not certain.

The relative contributions of PEM and inflammation to the high morbidity and mortality of CRF patients are controversial, especially because the syndrome of PEM shares many clinical manifestations with inflammation. Because inflammatory processes may cause endothelial injury and/or predispose to atherosclerosis and vascular thrombosis, it is easy to perceive why there would be a causal connection between inflammation and morbidity and mortality from vascular disease.

These considerations have led some investigators to question whether PEM by itself is hazardous or whether it is only an important risk factor for morbidity and mortality when it occurs in association with inflammation (208). Intuitively, it seems that a nutrient intake that is inadequate to maintain a healthy quantity of body protein mass or that does not provide adequate energy must eventually place the patient at risk for increased morbidity and mortality. We suspect that PEM may, among its other adverse consequences, predispose to inflammation and vascular disease. This is a question that demands further investigation. PEM and inflammation occur together so commonly in patients with ESRD that some investigators have described them as components of a single syndrome referred to as the malnutrition-inflammation complex syndrome (209).

Some researchers have recently pointed out that relationships between traditional risk factors and mortality are markedly altered or even reversed in patients undergoing MD as compared with the public at large. These altered relationships, referred to as risk factor reversal, paradoxic risk factors, or reverse epidemiology have been observed

for body mass index (BMI) or weight for a given height, predialysis serum total cholesterol, LDL-cholesterol and predialysis creatinine, serum urea nitrogen (SUN), UNA (net urea production; see later), blood pressure, magnitude of acidosis, and possibly serum homocysteine and parathyroid hormone levels (210–219).

Although several explanations have been advanced to explain these phenomena, the most likely mechanism is related to the malnutrition inflammation complex syndrome (210, 212, 216, 217). MD-treated patients who eat inadequately, who have major comorbid conditions, or who have evidence of systemic inflammation are more likely to have low BMI and low serum cholesterol and homocysteine and also to be at greater risk of mortality. Individuals who are healthier are more likely to have a greater appetite and to have a higher body weight, a greater protein intake, and, hence, a higher UNA and greater metabolic acid production and metabolic acidosis. Serum total cholesterol, LDL cholesterol, and homocysteine tend to be higher in healthy people who have greater food intakes. Because of their greater muscle mass and appetite, these persons tend to have higher predialysis serum creatinine and urea concentrations. They are less likely to suffer from cardiac pump failure and to have low blood pressures. Moreover, because they are healthier, they are more likely to live longer.

Survival bias may also account for some of the paradoxic risk factors, that is, those persons with increased levels of the normal risk factor. These explanations cannot completely account for the reverse epidemiology in MD-treated patients because it turns out that markedly obese persons (those with BMI of ≥45 kg/m²) have greater unadjusted 2-year mortality rates than those patients who are overweight or mildly obese (213, 220). Clearly, further research is indicated in this area.

DIETARY MANAGEMENT OF CHRONIC RENAL DISEASE AND CHRONIC RENAL FAILURE

A recommended plan for nutrient intake is given in Table 94.4 for patients with CRF who are not undergoing dialysis therapy as well as for patients undergoing MHD or CPD. The following text explains this approach to the dietary management of these patients.

General Principles

The widespread metabolic and nutritional disorders, frequent occurrence of PEM, high incidence of cardiovascular, cerebrovascular, and peripheral vascular disease, and the possibility that diet may retard the progression of renal failure indicate that nutritional management is a critical aspect of the treatment of CRF. The four goals of dietary therapy are (a) to maintain good nutritional status, (b) to prevent or to minimize uremic toxicity and the metabolic derangements of renal failure, (c) to reduce risk factors for cardiac

TABLE 94.4. RECOMMENDED NUTRIENT INTAKE FOR NONDIALYZED PATIENTS WITH CHRONIC RENAL FAILURE AND PATIENTS UNDERGOING MAINTENANCE HEMODIALYSIS OR CHRONIC PERITONEAL DIALYSIS

	CHRONIC RENAL FAILURE[a]	MAINTENANCE HEMODIALYSIS OR CHRONIC PERITONEAL DIALYSIS[b]
Protein	Low-protein diet: 0.60–0.75 g/kg/d ≥0.35 g/kg/d of high biologic value protein	Hemodialysis[b] 1.1–1.2 g/kg/d ≥50% high biologic value protein CPD 1.2–1.3 g/kg/d ≥50% high biologic value protein. CPD patients may be given up to 1.5 g/kg/d
Energy[c]	≥35 kcal/kg/d unless the patient's relative body weight is >120% or the patient gains unwanted weight	
Fat (% of total energy intake)[d,e]	30–40	30–40
Polyunsaturated: saturated fatty acid ratio[e]	1.0:1.0	1.0:1.0
Carbohydrate[f]	Rest of nonprotein calories	
Total fiber intake[e]	20–25 g	20–25 g
Minerals	Range of Intake	
Sodium	1,000–3,000 mg/d[g]	750–1,000 mg/d[g]
Potassium	40–70 mEq/d	40–70 mEq/d
Phosphorus	5–10 mg/kg/d[b,j,k]	8–17 mg/kg/d[b,k]
Calcium	1,400–1,600 mg/d[i]	1,400–1,600 mg/d[i]
Magnesium	200–300 mg/d	200–300 mg/d
Iron	≥10–18 mg/d[j]	See text
Zinc	15 mg/d	15 mg/d
Water	≤3,000 mL/d as tolerated[g]	usually 750–1,500 mL/d[g]
Vitamins	Diets to be Supplemented with These Quantities	
Thiamin	1.5 mg/d	1.5 mg/d
Riboflavin	1.8 mg/d	1.8 mg/d
Pantothenic acid	5 mg/d	5 mg/d
Niacin	20 mg/d	20 mg/d
Pyridoxine HCl	l5 mg/d	5–10 mg/d
Vitamin B_{12}	3 μg/d	3 μg/d
Vitamin C	60 mg/d	60 mg/d
Folic acid	1–10 mg/d	1–10 mg/d[l]
Vitamin A	No addition	No addition
Vitamin D	See text	See text
Vitamin E	15 IU/d	15 IU/d
Vitamin K	None[k]	None[k]

CPD, chronic peritoneal dialysis.

[a] GFR >4–5 mL/1.73 m^2/min and ~75 mL/1.73 m^2 or lower (see text).

[b] Protein intake for hemodialysis-treated patients generally should be at or near 1.2 g/kg/d; for CPD-treated patients who are not malnourished, it should be ~1.2 to 1.3 g/kg/d.

[c] This includes energy intake from dialysate in the CPD-treated patients.

[d] Refers to percentage of total energy intake (diet plus dialysate); if triglyceride levels are markedly elevated, the percentage of fat in the diet may be increased to ~40% of total calories; otherwise, 30% of total calories is preferable.

[e] These dietary recommendations are considered less crucial than the others, unless hypercholesterolemia is present (see text).

[f] Should be primarily complex carbohydrates, if tolerated by the patient.

[g] Can be higher in CPD-treated patients or in those nondialyzed patients with chronic renal failure and hemodialysis-treated patients who have greater urinary losses.

[h] Phosphate binders (especially sevelemer hydrochloride) are often needed as well.

[i] Dietary intake usually must be supplemented to provide these levels.

[j] 10 mg/d for males and nonmenstruating females; ≥18 mg/d for menstruating females; may be increased with erythropoietin therapy.

[k] Vitamin K supplements may be needed for patients who are not eating and who are receiving antibiotics.

[l] Doses to be determined by serum homocysteine levels and the response to previous folate supplements.

and vascular disease, and (d) to retard or to stop the rate of progression of renal failure.

Adherence to specialized diets is difficult and stressful for most patients and their families. Generally, it requires patients to undergo a major change in their behavior patterns and to forsake many of their traditional sources of daily pleasure. The patient must procure special foods, prepare special recipes, usually forgo or severely limit intake of many favorite foods, and often eat foods that are not desirable. Demands are made on the time, effort, and emotional support system of the family or close associates. Therefore, it is incumbent on the physician not to prescribe radical changes in dietary intake without a clear indication that such changes may be beneficial to the patient. To ensure successful dietary therapy,

TABLE 94.5. RECOMMENDED MEASURES FOR MONITORING NUTRITIONAL STATUS OF MAINTENANCE DIALYSIS PATIENTS

CATEGORY	MEASURE	MINIMUM FREQUENCY OF MEASUREMENT
I. Measurements that should be performed routinely in all patients	Predialysis or stabilized serum albumin	Monthly
	% of usual postdialysis (MHD) or postdrain (CPD) body weight	Monthly
	% of standard (NHANES II) body weight	Every 4 mo
	Subjective global assessment	Every 6 mo
	Dietary interview and/or diary	Every 6 mo
	nPNA	Monthly MHD; every 3–4 mo CPD
II. Measures that can be useful to confirm or extend the data obtained from the measures in category I	Predialysis or stabilized serum prealbumin	As needed
	Skinfold thickness	As needed
	Midarm muscle area, circumference, or diameter	As needed
	Dual-energy x-ray absorptiometry	As needed
III. Clinically useful Measures that, if low may suggest the need for the need for a more rigorous examination of protein-energy nutritional status	Predialysis or stabilized serum,	
	Creatinine	As needed
	Urea nitrogen	As needed
	Cholesterol	
	Creatinine index	As needed

CPD, chronic peritoneal dialysis; MHD, maintenance hemodialysis; nPNA, net protein equivalent of total nitrogen appearance.

From National Kidney Foundation DOQI clinical practice guidelines for nutrition in chronic renal failure. Am J Kidney Dis 2000;35[Suppl 2]:1S–140S, with permission.

patients with renal failure must undergo extensive training in the principles of nutritional therapy and the design and preparation of diets, and they need continuous encouragement regarding dietary adherence. When nutritional intake is not carefully monitored, patients tend to adhere poorly to dietary prescriptions. They may eat too little of certain nutrients rather than too much.

A team approach to dietary management may improve adherence to the special diet. The team should include the physician, dietitian, close family members, nursing staff, and, where available, psychiatrists or social workers. Diet plans should be designed specifically for the individual tastes of the patient. A problem-oriented approach to dietary compliance can be very effective (193). At each visit, the physician should monitor dietary intake and should discuss the results with the patient. The physician must strongly support the dietitian's efforts to train and counsel the patient and to obtain dietary compliance. The patient's family and close associates can provide moral support to the patient and assist with acquisition and preparation of foods. To promote adherence to the diet, the entire medical team should assume an energetic, positive, and sympathetic approach. Research indicates that the foregoing techniques can enable many patients to attain acceptable levels of dietary compliance (221).

Patients with advanced renal failure are at particular risk for inadequate energy intake. Because the prescribed diets are often marginally low in some nutrients, such as protein, and high in others, such as energy fuels, and malnutrition is not infrequent, it is important to evaluate the adequacy of the diet and the patient's nutritional status periodically. Such evaluation should include assessment of protein-energy nutritional status, mineral and bone metabolism, parathyroid status, and bone densitometry, risk factors for cardiovascular disease (e.g., serum lipid panel, homocysteine, and C-reactive protein levels, and urine albumin excretion including the presence of microalbuminuria. The National Kidney Foundation KDOQI Clinical Practice Guidelines for Nutrition in Chronic Renal Failure recommendations for evaluation of nutritional status in patients undergoing MD are shown in Table 94.5.

The dietitian is often best qualified to perform anthropometry. To maintain good dietary compliance and to monitor fluid and electrolyte disorders and clinical and nutritional status, it is often preferable for the physician and dietitian to see the patient with stage 3 to 5 CKD monthly. Patients with slowly progressive mild or moderate renal insufficiency, under some circumstances, may see the physician and dietitian less frequently.

Recent cross-sectional studies indicate that dietary protein and energy intake begin to fall and that protein-energy nutritional status begins to deteriorate when the GFR decreases to roughly one half normal (~50–55 mL/minute) (223). The decline in nutritional status is gradual and usually mild to moderate until the GFR falls rather severely, to less than 10 mL/minute, and when the patient is commencing MD therapy (156, 174, 223, 224). Although nutritional status may improve during the first few months of dialysis therapy (225), the protein-energy nutritional status at the onset of chronic dialysis treatment appears to be a good predictor of both nutritional status 2 to 3 years later and of longevity (156, 226). Hence, particular effort should be made to prevent malnutrition when the patient approaches the time when dialysis should be instituted and during the first few weeks of chronic dialysis therapy. Such effort should be directed toward maintaining good nutritional intake during this period, rapidly instituting therapy for supervening illnesses, and maintaining good nutritional intake during such illnesses.

Urea Nitrogen Appearance and the Ratio of Serum Urea Nitrogen to Serum Creatinine

The control of protein intake is pivotal to the nutritional management of patients with acute renal failure or CRF. Hence, one must accurately monitor nitrogen intake. Fortunately, this is possible for most patients. Those who are in nitrogen balance should have a total nitrogen output equal to nitrogen intake minus about 0.5 g nitrogen/day for unmeasured losses from growth of skin, hair, and nails and from sweat, respiration, flatus, and blood drawing (227). For clinical purposes, a slightly positive or negative balance does not substantially alter the use of the nitrogen output to estimate intake. If patients are in very positive or negative balance, such as from pregnancy or severe infection, nitrogen output may not reflect intake. However, it is usually readily apparent to the clinician whether the patient is in very positive or negative balance and whether the nitrogen output will reflect intake.

The measurement of total nitrogen output is too laborious and expensive to be widely applied for clinical uses. However, because urea is the major nitrogenous product of protein and amino acid degradation, the UNA can be used to estimate total nitrogen output and hence nitrogen intake (228–230). UNA refers to the amount of urea that appears or accumulates in body fluids and all outputs, such as urine, dialysate, and fistula drainage. The term UNA is used rather than urea production or generation because some urea is degraded in the gastrointestinal tract; the ammonia released from urea is largely transported to the liver and converted back to urea (231, 232). Thus, the enterohepatic urea cycle has little effect on urea or total nitrogen economy, and this cycle can be ignored without compromising the ability of the UNA to estimate total nitrogen output or intake accurately. Moreover, the recycling of urea cannot be measured without costly and time-consuming isotope studies.

UNA is calculated as follows:

Equation 1:

$$\text{UNA (g/day)} = \text{urinary urea nitrogen (g/day)}$$
$$+ \text{ dialysate urea nitrogen (g/day)}$$
$$+ \text{ change in body urea nitrogen (g/day)}$$

Equation 2:

$$\text{Change in body urea nitrogen (g/day)} =$$
$$(\text{SUN}_f - \text{SUN}_i, \text{g/L/day}) \times \text{BW}_i (\text{kg}) \times (0.60 \text{ L/kg})$$
$$+ (\text{BW}_f - \text{BW}_i, \text{kg/day}) \times \text{SUN}_f (\text{g/L}) \times (1.0 \text{ L/kg})$$

where i and f are the initial and final values for the period of measurement, SUN is serum urea nitrogen (grams per liter), BW is body weight (kilograms), 0.60 is an estimate of the fraction of body weight that is water, and 1.0 is the fractional distribution of urea in the weight that is gained or lost (i.e., 100%).

The estimated proportion of body weight that is water may be increased in patients who are edematous or lean and decreased in persons who are obese or very young. Changes in body weight during the 1- to 3-day period of measurement of UNA are assumed to be entirely the result of changes in body water. In patients undergoing hemodialysis, the urea concentration in dialysate is low and difficult to measure accurately, and UNA can be calculated during the interdialytic interval and then normalized to 24 hours. Because many patients undergoing dialysis have little or no urinary excretion, the equation for calculating their UNA during the interdialytic interval often can be simplified to Equation 2.

In our metabolic studies, the relationship between UNA and total nitrogen appearance (output) in chronically uremic patients not undergoing dialysis is as follows (230):

Equation 3:

$$\text{Total nitrogen appearance (g/day)} = 1.19 \text{ UNA (g/day)} + 1.27$$

If the patient is more or less in neutral nitrogen balance, the UNA also will correlate closely with nitrogen intake. Equation 4 describes our observed relationships between UNA and dietary nitrogen intake in clinically stable nondialyzed chronically uremic patients who are in neutral protein balance.

Equation 4:

$$\text{Dietary nitrogen intake (g/day)} = 1.20 \text{ UNA (g/day)} + 1.74$$

Multiplication of Equation 3 by 6.25 will convert total nitrogen output to net protein degradation (g/day), that is, the difference between the absolute rates of protein degradation and protein synthesis in the study. Multiplication of Equation 4 by 6.25 will convert dietary nitrogen intake to dietary protein intake (grams/day). When both nitrogen intake and UNA are known, nitrogen balance can be estimated from the difference between nitrogen intake and nitrogen output estimated from the UNA. If the patient is markedly anabolic, such as from pregnancy, particularly in its later stages, Equation 4 will underestimate nitrogen intake. For patients who have large protein losses, such as from nephrotic syndrome or peritoneal dialysis, or who are acidemic and have sufficient kidney function to excrete large quantities of ammonium, Equations 3 and 4 will underestimate both nitrogen output and nitrogen intake. In most circumstances, however, these conditions are not present, and the UNA provides a powerful tool for monitoring nitrogen output and intake or estimating balance. Maroni and associates and other researchers have described similar techniques for monitoring these parameters (228, 229).

The relationships among the UNA, total nitrogen appearance, and dietary nitrogen intake in patients undergoing continuous ambulatory peritoneal dialysis are shown in Equations 5 and 6 (230). Other researchers have described rather similar equations (233). Because protein losses in peritoneal dialysate are variable, in some equations an independent term is added for the daily nitrogen losses from protein in peritoneal dialysate. As indicated previously, multiplication of these terms by 6.25 can convert the equations to net protein output (grams/day) or, in clinically stable patients who are in approximately neutral protein balance, to dietary protein intake (grams/day).

Equation 5:

$$\text{Total nitrogen appearance (g/day)} = 0.94 \text{ UNA} + 5.54$$

Equation 6:

$$\text{Dietary nitrogen intake (g/day)} = 0.97 \text{ UNA} + 6.80$$

The UNA (also called Gu) can be calculated in hemodialysis-treated patients by urea kinetic modeling (228, 234). This technique essentially involves the predialysis and postdialysis SUN and body weight, the urea clearance characteristics of the dialysis, and the blood flow, dialysate flow, and duration of the dialysis therapy. The relationships among UNA, net protein degradation, and dietary protein intake in MHD-treated patients have been described in other studies (230, 234). Net protein degradation in dialysis-treated patients, normalized to body weight, is usually referred to as protein catabolic rate (nPCR) or our preferred term: protein equivalent of total nitrogen appearance (nPNA) (235). A critique of the precision and reproducibility of these calculations is presented elsewhere (230, 234). The nPCR or nPNA often reported refers to net total body protein degradation, which underestimates total protein intake (compare Equations 3 and 4 with Equations 5 and 6).

The ratio of SUN to serum creatinine also correlates closely with dietary protein or amino acid intake in chronically uremic patients who are not undergoing dialysis treatment. This relationship can be used to estimate the recent daily intake of such patients. Although this ratio is not as precise as the UNA and is influenced by certain clinical factors (236), it is easy and inexpensive to measure.

Dietary Prescription

For purposes of nutritional prescription, the body weights in this chapter refer to the standard (normal) body weights from data from the National Health and Nutrition Examination Survey (237). Exception are persons who are obese (e.g., >115% of standard body weight) and those who are very underweight (e.g., <90% of standard body weight). For these patients, their adjusted actual body weight (designated aBW in the next equation) may be used for the body weight term (238). The adjusted actual body weight appears to be gaining in popularity but has not yet been validated by experimental data. The adjusted actual body weight, modified from the American Dietetic Association report (238), is calculated as follows:

$$\text{Adjusted aBW} = \text{standard (normal) BW} \\ + ([\text{edema-free aBW} - \text{standard} \\ \text{(normal) BW}] \times 0.25)$$

Protein Intake

When the Glomerular Filtration Rate Is Higher than 70 mL/1.73 m²/Minute. Virtually no data exist concerning the optimal dietary protein and phosphorus intakes for patients with chronic renal disease and mild impairment in renal function. At present, we do not routinely restrict protein for patients with a GFR higher than 70 mL/1.73 m²/minute, except perhaps to 0.80 to 1.0 g/kg body weight/day, unless renal function is clearly declining. In the latter case, the patient is treated as indicated in the next paragraph.

When the Glomerular Filtration Rate is 25 to 70 mL/1.73 m²/Minute. The studies, including the meta-analyses (see earlier), indicating that low-protein, low-phosphorus diets may retard the need for chronic dialysis, dialysis, or renal transplantation must be qualified because it is not yet certain that these diets will be effective in patients receiving ACEIs and/or ARBs. This should be explained to the patient, but it is emphasized that regardless of whether or not protein is restricted, many other aspects of dietary therapy cannot be ignored. If the patient agrees to dietary therapy, a diet is offered providing 0.60 g protein/kg/day, of which at least 35 g/kg/day is protein of high biologic value, to ensure a sufficient intake of the essential amino acids. This quantity of protein should maintain neutral or positive nitrogen balance (229, 230, 239, 240), and for many patients, it should not be excessively burdensome. If this diet is too difficult to adhere to or if the patient cannot maintain an adequate energy intake on this diet, the protein intake may be increased up to 0.75 g/kg/day.

When the Glomerular Filtration Rate is Lower than 25 mL/1.73m²/Minute Without Dialysis. At this level of renal failure, the potential advantages to using a low-protein, low-phosphorus diet become more compelling. First, at this degree of renal insufficiency, potentially toxic products of nitrogen metabolism begin to accumulate in larger quantities. The LPD generates fewer potentially toxic nitrogenous metabolites. Second, because the LPD generally contains less phosphorus and potassium, the intake of these minerals can be reduced more readily with this diet (see later sections on recommended phosphorus and potassium intakes). Third, some patients with chronic renal insufficiency eat too little protein, rather than too much. Specific training and encouragement to follow a prescribed diet may increase the likelihood that the patient will not ingest too little protein. Patients should be prescribed a protein intake as described in the previous paragraph (see Table 94.4).

Because of the lack of evidence from the MDRD Study that the ketoacid-amino acid–supplemented very-LPDs retard the rate of progression of renal failure and because such diets may not be safe (see earlier) (113), they are not recommended. Moreover, the ketoacid-essential amino acid supplements are not currently available in the United States. There is insufficient research experience to evaluate the potential for essential amino acid–supplemented very-LPDs to retard progression or their safety, and these diets are therefore not currently recommended.

When the Glomerular Filtration Rate Falls Below About 5 mL/1.73m²/Minute. No evidence indicates that patients fare as well with low-nitrogen diets as with regular dialysis and higher protein intakes. Because patients with these low GFR levels may be at high risk of malnutrition and long-term sequelae of uremic toxicity (156, 174, 223, 224), it is recommended that MD treatment or renal transplantation be inaugurated at this time. If patients with a higher GFR (≤20 mL/minute) cannot maintain a sufficiently high energy intake to maintain their body weight and there is no other identifiable cause for weight loss, chronic dialysis therapy should be considered at these higher levels of renal function (241). This is especially important because evidence of PEM at the commencement of MD therapy is a predictor of higher mortality.

Nephrotic Syndrome. Evidence indicates that a rather LPD (e.g., 0.80 g protein/kg/day) may slow progression of renal failure, cause a decrease in urine protein excretion, and maintain or actually slightly increase serum albumin levels (122, 123, 242). This has led to recommendations for a reduction in dietary protein prescription for nephrotic patients. A vegetarian, soy-based, LPD also decreases proteinuria and serum lipid levels in nephrotic patients (105–107). Until more information is available, it is recommended that patients with the nephrotic syndrome be prescribed a diet containing about 0.70 g protein/kg/day and an additional 1.0 g/day of high biologic value protein for each gram of urinary protein lost each day above 5.0 g/day. ACEIs and ARBs reduce proteinuria (121), lower blood pressure, retard progression of renal failure, and may protect against atherosclerotic disease and therefore should be given preference in the treatment of hypertension in these patients (81–84). LPDs, when added to ACEIs and ARBs, may further reduce proteinuria. *Aldosterone receptor antagonists may also reduce proteinuria (89), but serum potassium must be carefully monitored with ACEIs, ARBs, and aldosterone receptor antagonists because these three classes of drugs may each reduce urinary potassium excretion and cause dangerous hyperkalemia.* Patients with the nephrotic syndrome should be given multivitamins, including vitamin D supplements, and must be monitored for depletion of protein and protein-bound nutrients including vitamin D analogs and trace elements.

Maintenance Dialysis Therapy. Although few studies of dietary protein requirements have been conducted in patients undergoing MHD (243, 244), it seems clear that these patients have greater protein needs because of the removal of amino acids and peptides by dialysis procedures (179–181) and probably because of such other metabolic disorders as inflammation, activation of complement, and other catabolic stimuli of hemodialysis (186, 242). Based on available evidence from nitrogen balance studies and clinical monitoring of outpatients, the National Kidney Foundation KDOQI Clinical Practice Guidelines recommend that MHD-treated patients receive 1.1 to 1.2 g protein/kg/day (see Table 94.4) (241). CPD-treated patients lose each day into dialysate about 9 g protein, a small amount of peptides, and about 2.5 to 4.0 g/day of amino acids and are also subjected to inflammatory and other metabolic stimuli (181, 183). Based on nitrogen balance studies, the National Kidney Foundation KDOQI guidelines recommend that CPD-treated patients should be prescribed 1.2 to 1.3 g protein/kg/day (241, 245). Patients undergoing CPD who are protein depleted may be prescribed up to

1.5 g protein/kg/day (216). At least 50% of the daily protein intake of all patients undergoing MD should be of high biologic value.

Some physicians suggest that patients undergoing MHD or CPD may maintain their body protein mass with lower dietary protein intakes (e.g., ~0.9 g protein/kg/day). The foregoing recommendations, although based on relatively small numbers of studies, are designed to maintain good protein nutrition for most (i.e., ~97%) of patients undergoing MD. This reasoning is consistent with the deliberations used by the World Health Organization to determine the recommended dietary protein intakes for physiologically normal adults (246). Hence, although some patients may maintain good protein nutrition with lower daily protein intakes, there is no demonstrated method for identifying which patients can maintain nitrogen balance on these lower-protein diets. Because of the high incidence of protein malnutrition in these patients (155–164, 167, 193), we suggest that the higher protein intakes recommended in this chapter should be prescribed.

Energy

Studies in nondialyzed patients with CRF and those undergoing MHD indicate that energy expenditure is normal or nearly normal when patients are lying in bed, sitting, following ingestion of a standard meal, and during defined exercise (247–249). Nitrogen balance studies in nondialyzed patients with stage 4 and 5 CKD who are ingesting diets providing 0.55 to 0.60 g protein/kg/day and 15, 25, 35, or 45 kcal/kg/day indicate that the energy intake necessary to ensure neutral or positive nitrogen balance is approximately 35 kcal/kg/day (247). Similar findings were obtained in nitrogen balance studies of MHD-treated patients who were ingesting 1.1 g protein per kg/day and 25, 35, or 45 kcal/kg/day (250). However, virtually every survey of energy intake in nondialyzed patients with stage 4 or 5 CKD and in those undergoing MHD or CPD indicates that, on average, the dietary intake is lower than this level and usually substantially less than 30 kcal/kg daily (251–255). In nondialyzed patients with CRF and in those undergoing MHD, the finding that decreased body fat is one of the more prominent alterations in nutritional status supports the contention that these patients require more energy than they usually ingest (251, 253–255). In contrast, CPD-treated patients not uncommonly gain fat, probably because of the additional energy intake from glucose absorbed from the dialysate in the peritoneal cavity.

The National Kidney Foundation KDOQI Guidelines recommend that patients less than 60 years old who are undergoing MHD and CPD should ingest at least 35 kcal/kg/day, and those who are 60 years or older should ingest 30 kcal/kg/day (241). The same energy intakes, adjusted for age, are recommended for patients with GFR levels lower than 50 kcal/kg/day. Patients who are obese with an edema-free body weight greater than 120% of desirable body weight may be treated with lower caloric intakes. Some patients, particularly those with mild renal insufficiency and young or middle-aged women, may become obese on this energy intake or may refuse to ingest the recommended calories out of fear of obesity. These patients may require a lower energy prescription.

Many commercially available high-calorie foodstuffs are low in protein, phosphorus, sodium, and potassium. A nephrology dietitian can recommend these foodstuffs as well as other low-protein, high-calorie foods that can be prepared easily at home.

Lipids and Obesity

Patients with stage 4 and 5 CKD and patients undergoing MHD and CPD have a high incidence of increased serum triglyceride levels, intermediate-density lipoprotein (IDL), very LDL (VLDL), and serum lipoprotein (a); serum high-density lipoprotein (HDL) cholesterol is often low in patients with CRF and MHD (151, 256–260). Patients undergoing CPD often have higher serum total cholesterol, triglycerides, LDL cholesterol, and apolipoprotein B levels than do MHD-treated patients (261, 262). Qualitative changes in the apolipoprotein concentrations also occur; among these is an increase in small dense LDL (263).

A major metabolic abnormality in CRF and in MD-treated patients is a decreased rate of catabolism of triglyceride-rich lipoproteins. This reduced catabolic rate leads to increased quanatius of apolipoprotein B–containing triglyceride-rich lipoproteins in IDL and VLDL and reduced concentrations of HDL. The key alteration in the apolipoprotein levels appears to be a decreased ratio of apoprotein A-1 to apoprotein C-III (264).

In addition, because diets for patients with CKD are usually restricted in protein, sodium, potassium, and water, it may be difficult to provide sufficient energy without resorting to a large intake of purified sugars that may increase triglyceride production. Activities of plasma and hepatic lipoprotein lipase and lecithin cholesterol acyltransferase are decreased (265). Moreover, impaired actions of carnitine may sometimes be present (266, 267).

Patients with the nephrotic syndrome usually have hypertriglyceridemia with increased serum total cholesterol and LDL cholesterol. LDL, IDL, VLDL, and lipoprotein (a) are increased (268), and serum HDL tends to be low. Serum phospholipids and apoproteins B, C-II, C-III, and E are increased, whereas apoproteins A-I and A-II are normal (269). Elevated serum cholesterol is caused by increased hepatic synthesis of lipoproteins and cholesterol and reduction in LDL receptor activity that plays an important role in the clearance of IDLs. These changes are stimulated by urinary albumin losses. Decreased activity of lipoprotein lipase contributes to the elevated serum triglyceride levels. Plasma cholesterol ester transfer protein is elevated, and catabolism of LDL apolipoprotein is decreased, at least by the more typical receptor pathway.

Renal transplant recipients may have type IIb hyperlipidemia with high serum total cholesterol and LDL cholesterol. LDL and IDL lipoproteins are increased. Type II-a and type IV hyperlipidemia also is often present after kidney transplantation, particularly if renal failure persists (270–272). Medical therapy (glucocorticoids, cyclosporine, sirolimus, tacrolimus, diuretics, antihypertensives), renal failure, fasting hyperinsulinemia, and obesity, which occurs frequently after renal transplantation, all may add to the high incidence of serum lipid disorders in renal transplant recipients.

Because these lipid and apolipoprotein abnormalities may contribute to the high incidence of atherosclerosis and cardiovascular disease in patients with CRF, those undergoing MD, and those receiving renal transplants, attention has been directed toward reducing serum cholesterol and triglycerides and increasing HDL cholesterol. At present, we recommend a dietary plan based on the National Cholesterol Education Program Therapeutic Lifestyle Changes (TLC) diet for patients with CRF, those undergoing MHD and CPD, patients with the nephrotic syndrome, and renal transplant recipients, especially if their serum LDL levels are greater than 100 mg/dL. Because these patients are all at high risk of cardiovascular, cerebrovascular and peripheral vascular disease, we prefer to set a target LDL cholesterol value of 70 mg/dL.

The TLC diet provides the following (273): no more than 25 to 35% of total calories from fat, polyunsaturated fatty acids providing up to 10% of total calories, monounsaturated fatty acids providing up to 20% of total calories, saturated fatty acids providing less than 7% of total calories, and a cholesterol content of 200 mg/day or lower. Carbohydrate intake should be 50 to 60% of total calories and derived predominantly from foods rich in complex carbohydrates. Fiber intake should be 20 to 30 g/day (273). We treat hypertriglyceridemia by further dietary modification or pharmacologically when serum triglyceride levels are approximately 400 mg/dL or greater. The patient's energy intake should be monitored with this diet to ensure that it does not fall, but patients are encouraged to control calorie intake to avoid becoming substantially overweight or frankly obese (i.e., BMI >28 kg/m^2).

The most potent LDL-cholesterol lowering therapy is hydroxymethyl glutarate coenzyme A treatment (i.e., statins) (274). These medications often lower LDL cholesterol by as much as 35%, and some statins increase serum HDL cholesterol by about 2 to 4 mg/dL. Statins also appear to protect the vasculature by their antiinflammatory properties. Although several serious adverse effects may be caused by statins, including altered liver function tests and potentially severe myopathy, this class of drugs is generally so well tolerated that these agents have become the treatment of choice for many nephrologists. However, a recent randomized prospective controlled study in diabetic MHD-treated patients failed to show any benefit in adverse cardiovascular events or survival from statin therapy (275).

Several investigators have reported that serum triglycerides may decrease if hypertriglyceridemic patients who are undergoing dialysis take L-carnitine, a compound that is often low in their plasma and possibly muscle (see later) (276, 277). However, other investigators have not confirmed this effect (278, 279). Fibric acids (e.g., gemfibrozil) also lower serum triglyceride levels in uremic patients, but owing to the altered pharmacokinetics of this drug in renal failure, the risk of developing myopathy or other toxicities is high (280). ω-3 Fatty acids, such as eicosapentaenoic acid and docosahexaenoic acid, which are found in fish oil, lower serum triglyceride and total cholesterol levels as well as phospholipids and may be tried (281). Fish oil also decreases platelet aggregation and exerts antiinflammatory effects (281). Some evidence suggests that ω-3 fatty acids or fish oil may retard the progression of CRF, particularly when it is caused by immunoglobulin A nephropathy (282). Ingestion of activated charcoal may lower serum cholesterol and triglycerides in chronically uremic rats (283).

If serum triglyceride levels are substantially elevated, serum carnitine should be measured. If serum carnitine is low, 0.5 to 1.0 g/day orally may be given to nondialyzed patients with CRF and to patients undergoing MD. Alternatively, patients undergoing hemodialysis may be given L-carnitine, 1.5 g orally or intravenously, at the end of each dialysis. Fish oil supplements may be tried for severe hypertriglyceridemia (284).

No established treatment exists for the low serum concentrations of HDL in uremic patients, although a small amount of alcohol (e.g., one glass of red wine/day) and exercise may increase levels (249). Torcetrapib, a potent inhibitor of cholesteryl ester transfer protein, that increases serum HDL cholesterol is currently undergoing clinical trials (285). As indicated earlier, whereas it is uncommon for hemodialysis-treated patients to gain substantial amounts of body fat, patients undergoing CPD commonly gain excessive body fat probably because of the additional 400 to 700 kcal they receive from the glucose absorbed from dialysate.

Virtually no long-term data are available on the effects of dietary fat and carbohydrate intake, obesity, or changing serum lipid levels on the clinical course of patients with specific renal diseases, the nephrotic syndrome, renal failure, or renal transplantation. The recommendations given here are largely derived from data obtained from populations without renal disease, from the recognition that patients with renal disease or renal failure have a high incidence of abnormal serum lipid and lipoprotein levels and atherosclerotic vascular disease, and from studies in animals with renal disease that indicate that high lipid intakes or elevated lipoprotein levels may accelerate the rate of progression of renal failure, as previously discussed.

Carnitine

L-Carnitine is an essential nutrient that is both synthesized in the body and ingested. Carnitine facilitates the transfer of long-chain (>10 carbon) fatty acids into mitochondria and probably other cellular structures (286). Because fatty acids are the major fuel source for skeletal and myocardial muscle at rest and during mild to moderate exercise, this process is considered necessary for normal skeletal muscle and myocardial function (see Chapter 33).

Patients with stage 4 and 5 CKD have normal serum free carnitine and increased acylcarnitines (fatty acid-carnitine compounds) (278, 279). In MHD-treated patients, particularly those undergoing MHD for at least 1 year, serum free carnitine is low, acylcarnitines are increased, and, for those receiving MHD for at least 3 to 4 years, skeletal muscle free carnitine is also reduced (287, 288). The cause of low serum and skeletal muscle carnitine is probably primarily the loss from dialysis, but reduced synthesis and possibly decreased dietary intake of carnitine may contribute to these low levels (278, 279). It has been suggested that the actions of carnitine actions may be impaired in CRF, possibly because of interference by the increased concentrations of acylcarnitines.

Clinical studies in patients with CRF suggest that carnitine may improve physical exercise capacity, reduce dialysis-related symptoms including skeletal muscle cramps and hypotension, improve overall sense of well-being, increase blood hemoglobin levels, reduce cardiac arrhythmias and improve cardiac function, increase protein balance, and possibly reduce inflammation (289–298). Some studies indicate that carnitine will lower serum triglyceride levels, whereas other studies have not confirmed this (278, 279). Many nephrologists are unconvinced by this foregoing research, in part because of the suboptimal experimental design of many of these studies, given that many of the reported benefits are not easy to quantify and clinical trials of carnitine therapy often given conflictory results. L-Carnitine appears to be a safe drug.

Until more definitive information is available, we consider using L-carnitine for patients who satisfy both the following criteria: (a) disabling or very bothersome skeletal muscle weakness or cardiomyopathy, skeletal muscle cramps or hypotension during hemodialysis treatment, severe malaise, or anemia refractory to erythropoietin therapy for no apparent reason; and (b) when the foregoing disorders do not respond to standard treatments. The patient is given a 3- to 6-month trial of L-carnitine (9 months for refractory anemia). If the symptoms do not improve by the end of the treatment period, carnitine therapy is discontinued. L-Carnitine may be administered orally, intravenously, or into dialysate. Oral L-carnitine is less expensive, but intestinal absorption is somewhat unpredictable in nonuremic persons and has not been examined well in patients with CRF. The optimal dose of carnitine is not defined. Carnitine may be infused intravenously, 10 to 20 mg/kg, at the end of each hemodialysis, three times weekly, or given orally about 0.50 g/day (289, 292).

Carbohydrates

The patient should be encouraged to eat complex rather than purified carbohydrates to reduce triglyceride synthesis and, when pertinent, to improve glucose tolerance.

Fiber

Studies in the physiologically normal population suggest that high dietary fiber intake may reduce the incidence of constipation, irritable bowel syndrome, diverticulitis, and neoplasia of the colon (294). Fiber may improve glucose tolerance in diabetic patients including those with CRF (295). Soluble fiber, which is soluble in the intestinal lumen but is not absorbed, includes pectins, certain gums, and psyllium. Supplemental soluble dietary fiber may also reduce plasma total cholesterol and LDL cholesterol levels in hypercholesterolemic men (296) and may decrease serum fasting triglycerides in hypertriglyceridemic patients with diabetes mellitus (297). A high dietary fiber intake also may reduce the SUN by decreasing colonic bacterial ammonia generation and enhancing fecal nitrogen excretion (298). High fiber intakes may promote fecal losses of trace elements. Foods high in fiber are often high in potassium, phosphorus, and low-quality protein. Thus, caution must be exercised when prescribing high-fiber diets to patients with renal failure. Because patients with renal failure may benefit from fiber intake, we currently encourage them to eat 20 to 25 g/day of total fiber.

Phosphorus

In patients with CRF, a high dietary phosphorus intake can lead to a high plasma phosphorus and calcium phosphorus product with increased risk of calcium phosphate deposition in soft tissues including arteries (127). Moreover, hyperphosphatemia, by lowering serum calcium, provides a strong stimulus to the development of hyperparathyroidism, a serious complication of CRF that is associated with increased morbidity and mortality. As previously discussed, both animal and human studies suggest the possibility that a low phosphorus intake may reduce the progression of CRF (39, 65, 67).

The optimal dietary phosphorus intake for patients with moderate CKD (stages 3 and 4) has not been well established. One approach is to maintain dietary phosphorus intake at about 1000 to 1200 mg/day. For both nondialyzed and dialyzed patients, the morning fasting serum phosphorus concentrations should always be maintained at or above 2.7 mg/dL and no higher than 4.6 mg/dL (1). Because a rough correlation exists between the protein and phosphorus content of the diet, it is easier to restrict phosphorus if protein intake is reduced.

The National Kidney Foundation KDOQI Clinical Practice Guidelines for Bone Metabolism and Disease in Chronic Kidney Disease recommends for patients with stage 5 CKD (GFR <15 mL/1.73 m²/minute or who are receiving MHD) that serum phosphorus be maintained between 3.5 and 5.5 mg/dL (1). This so often requires a low phosphorus intake of around 800 to 1000 mg/day, particularly when the serum phosphorus levels are greater than 4.6 mg/dL at stages 3 and 4 CKD and greater than 5.5 mg/dL in those with kidney failure (stage 5). Dietary phosphorus intake should also be restricted to 800 to 1000 mg/day when the plasma levels of intact pH are greater than these target ranges (see later).

Serum phosphorus levels should be monitored monthly following the initiation of dietary phosphorus restriction to ensure that serum phosphorus remains within the normal range. In stage 5 CKD, this level of dietary phosphorus restriction often does not maintain serum phosphorus levels within normal limits. Hence, phosphate binders, which bind phosphate in the intestinal tract rendering it unavailable for absorption, are also used.

Traditionally, the two most commonly used phosphate binders have been aluminum carbonate and aluminum hydroxide. Usually, two to four 500-mg capsules taken three to four times/day are generally needed. Greater doses may be used if necessary. As a result of evidence that aluminum-induced osteomalacia, anemia, and possibly dementia can be caused by aluminum phosphate binders, such binders are generally used as a last resort (299, 300).

Several alkaline calcium salts will also bind phosphate. These include calcium carbonate, calcium acetate, and calcium citrate. Calcium acetate may be slightly more potent than calcium carbonate at binding phosphate in the intestinal tract, whereas calcium citrate appears to be the least effective binder (301–304). Calcium acetate may be more likely to induce gastrointestinal discomfort (304). Patients should not ingest calcium citrate if they are also taking aluminum binders because the citrate anion may complex with aluminum and enhance its intestinal absorption (301).

The calcium salts are taken in divided doses with meals and should not be given unless the serum phosphorus level is normal or nearly normal, to avoid precipitation of calcium phosphate in soft tissues. Thus, hyperphosphatemic patients may be treated with other binders of phosphate until serum phosphorus falls to normal, or near normal, and at that time, they may be changed to calcium carbonate or calcium acetate. Calcium binder doses should not provide more than about 1500 mg of elemental calcium/day (total calcium intake from diet plus binders, 200 mg/day), to prevent excessive accumulation of calcium in soft tissues (1). Calcium comprises 40% of calcium carbonate, 25% of calcium acetate, 21% of calcium citrate, and 9% of calcium gluconate.

Two other noncalcium-, nonaluminum-, and nonmagnesium-containing phosphate binders are currently available. These are sevelamer HCl (305, 306) and lanthanum carbonate (307, 308). Sevelamer HCl is often given in doses of two to six 800 mg capsules three or four times/day with meals. This drug is generally well tolerated, although some patients develop discomfort or nausea and can become acidotic because of the large hydrochloride content of this preparation. Lanthanum carbonate appears to be roughly as effective as sevelamer HCl and the calcium salts as a phosphate binder. Small quantities of lanthanum accumulate in plasma of MD-treated patients with daily doses; it has not been shown that these are harmful to the patient. If such patients remain hyperphosphatemic (serum phosphorus >5.5 mg/dL), these latter phosphate binders may need to be given in combination with calcium binders.

Phosphate binders, in general, bind only up to 300 to 400 mg phosphorus/day, even when given in maximum doses. Thus, the use of phosphate binders does not substitute for the need to restrict dietary phosphorus. For patients with stage 3 or 4 CRF (i.e., a GFR between 30 and 60 mL/1.73 m²/minute) or with a higher GFR and progressive loss of renal function, 7 to 12 mg phosphorus/kg/day may be prescribed with the 0.55- to 0.60-g protein/kg/day diet. Even this level of reduction in phosphorus intake is difficult for many patients to accept, and lower phosphorus intakes make the diet too restrictive for virtually all patients.

Calcium, Vitamin D, and Parathyroid Hormone

Patients with CRF, including those undergoing MD therapy, usually have an increased dietary calcium requirement because they have both vitamin D deficiency and resistance to the actions of vitamin D. These disorders, which lead to impaired intestinal calcium absorption, are compounded by the low calcium content of diets for uremic patients. A 40-g protein, low-phosphorus diet, for example, generally provides only about 300 to 400 mg of calcium daily. Dietary calcium intake is low because many foods that are high in calcium are high in phosphorus, such as dairy products, and are therefore restricted for CRF patients.

Nondialyzed patients with stage 5 CKD usually require 1200 to 1600 mg/day of calcium for neutral or positive calcium balance unless they are receiving supplemental 1,25-dihydroxycholecalciferol (calcitriol) or another vitamin D sterol (309). The current recommendation is to provide a total daily calcium intake (diet plus supplement) of 1400 to 1600 mg/day. Thus, LPDs need to be supplemented with approximately 1000 to 1400 mg of elemental calcium daily. Supplemental calcium should not be initiated unless the serum phosphorus concentration is normal (e.g., 2.5–~5.5 mg/dL) to prevent calcium phosphate deposition in soft tissues. In addition, frequent monitoring of serum calcium is important because hypercalcemia may develop, particularly if serum phosphorus should fall to low-normal or low levels. This is especially likely to occur if the patient also has hyperparathyroidism, a common complication of CRF (127). Patients undergoing MHD or peritoneal dialysis may require 1.0 g/day of supplemental oral calcium even though there is net calcium uptake from dialysate. The supplemental calcium should be taken in two or three divided doses each day. An

easy way to provide supplemental calcium is with the use of a calcium binder of phosphorus.

The DOQI Guidelines on Bone Metabolism and Disease in Chronic Renal Failure make the following recommendations (1): For patients with stage 3 and 4 CKD, serum levels of calcium, corrected for any change in albumin levels should be maintained within the normal range for the laboratory used. For stage 5 CKD, serum levels of corrected total calcium should be maintained within the normal range for the laboratory used, but preferably toward the lower end of normal (8.4–9.5 mg/dL). As indicated earlier, total elemental calcium intake for the diet and calcium-based phosphate binders should not exceed 2000 mg/day. The serum calcium-phosphorus product should be maintained at less than 55 mg²/dL². This should be attained primarily by controlling serum levels of phosphorus within the target range, as indicated earlier. If the serum total corrected calcium is below the lower limit for the laboratory used (<8.4 mg/dL), the patient should receive ingest more calcium to increase serum calcium levels if there are clinical signs of hypocalcemia or if the plasma intact parathyroid hormone level is above the target range for CKD. Corrected serum albumin may be calculated as follows (1):

$$\text{Corrected serum calcium (mg/dL)} = \text{total serum calcium (mg/dL)} + 0.0704 \times [34 - \text{serum albumin (g/L)}]$$

A simpler equation, which is about as accurate, is as follows:

$$\text{Corrected total calcium (mg/dL)} = \text{total calcium (mg/dL)} + 0.8 \times [4 - \text{serum albumin (g/dL)}]$$

As indicated earlier, treatment with vitamin D analogs will decrease the daily calcium requirement by enhancing intestinal calcium absorption. To reduce the total daily calcium load to the dialysis-treated patient who is taking calcium binders of phosphate, the calcium content of dialysate is often reduced. Currently, this is somewhat more effective with daily CPD than with thrice weekly MHD. Generally, the dialysate calcium concentration in patients undergoing MHD or CPD should be 2.5 mEq/L.

Secondary hyperparathyroidism can be treated in patients with CRF by vitamin D analogs. In patients with stage 5 CKD, serum intact parathyroid hormone should be maintained within a target range of 150 to 300 pg/mL.

If the serum level of 25-hydroxyvitamin D is less than 30 ng/mL supplementation with vitamin D₂ (ergocalciferol) should be initiated. For patients with stage 5 CRF, therapy with an active vitamin D sterol (calcitriol, alphacalcidol, paricalcitol, or doxercalciferol) should be provided if the plasma levels of parathyroid hormone are greater than 300 pg/mL (1).

A recent retrospective study in about 60,000 patients undergoing MHD indicated that the treatment of these with the vitamin D analog paricalcitrol is associated with a lower mortality rate than patients receiving 1,25(OH)₂ vitamin D. A recent addition to therapeutic treatment of secondary hyper-parathyroidism in patients with stage 4 and 5 CKD is the use of a drug (cinacalcet) that increases the sensitivity of the calcium receptor in the parathyroid gland allowing lower levels of serum calcium to suppress parathyroid hormone secretion. This agent appears to increase the ability to suppress hyperparathyroidism in patients with CRF who are hyperparathyroid and whose serum calcium and phosphorus levels and serum calcium-phosphorus product are at or above the acceptable range. Serum calcium can be corrected for hypoalbuminemia by the equation noted earlier.

A syndrome called aplastic or hypoplastic bone disease has been described in patients undergoing chronic dialysis (127). It is characterized by relatively low serum parathyroid hormone concentrations, decreased bone osteoblasts, and marked reduction in bone turnover. The syndrome can be caused by aluminum toxicity, but it also occurs in the absence of such toxicity (127, 314, 315). It has been postulated that treatment with large doses of calcium binders of phosphate or vitamin D with consequent suppression of parathyroid hormone is a cause of this disorder (127, 314, 316).

Magnesium

In CRF, there is net absorption of approximately 50% of ingested magnesium from the intestinal tract (314). The absorbed magnesium is excreted primarily by the kidney. Hence, in renal failure, hypermagnesemia may occur (317). Because the restricted diets of uremic patients are low in magnesium (usually ~100–300 mg/day for a 40-g protein diet), their serum magnesium levels are usually normal or only slightly elevated unless these patients take substances that are high in magnesium content, such as magnesium-containing antacids and laxatives (309, 317). Nondialyzed chronically uremic patients require about 200 mg/day of magnesium to maintain neutral balance (309). The optimal dietary magnesium allowance for the patient undergoing chronic dialysis has not been well defined. It is influenced by the level of magnesium in the dialysate; at current dialysate magnesium concentrations, the optimal magnesium allowance is probably about 200 to 250 mg/day.

Sodium and Water

Sodium is freely filterable by the glomerulus. In the normal kidney, the renal tubules reabsorb well over 99% of the filtered sodium. As renal insufficiency progresses, both the GFR and fractional tubular reabsorption of sodium fall progressively. Thus, many patients with renal failure are able to maintain sodium balance with a normal salt intake. Normally, only about 1 to 3 mEq/day of sodium are excreted in the feces, and in the nonsweating person, only a few milliequivalents/day of sodium are lost through the skin. Despite an adaptive reduction in the renal tubular reabsorption of sodium when ESRD supervenes, patients may be unable to excrete the quantity of sodium ingested, and they may develop edema, hypertension, or congestive heart failure. This syndrome is particularly likely to occur when the GFR is less than 4 to 10 mL/minute. When renal insufficiency is complicated by congestive heart failure, the nephrotic syndrome, or advanced liver disease, the propensity for sodium retention is increased. With decreased ability to excrete sodium, restriction of sodium and water intake and the use of diuretic medications may be necessary. In renal failure, hypertension often is more easily controlled with sodium restriction and may be accentuated with increased sodium intake probably because of expansion of the extracellular fluid volume (318).

In addition, nondialyzed patients with CRF often have an inability to conserve sodium normally (125, 126). A low sodium intake may not be sufficient to replace urinary and extrarenal sodium losses, and the patient may develop sodium depletion, a decrease in extracellular fluid volume, blood volume, and renal blood flow, and a further reduction in GFR. Volume depletion may be difficult to recognize. An unexplained weight loss or a decrease in blood pressure may be a sign of this condition. Nondialyzed patients with CRF who do not have evidence of fluid overload, hypertension, or heart failure may be cautiously given a greater sodium intake to determine whether their GFR can be improved slightly by extracellular volume expansion.

In general, when sodium balance is well controlled, thirst will regulate water balance adequately. However, when the GFR falls to less than 2 to 5 mL/minute, there is a particular risk of overhydration. In diabetic patients, hyperglycemia may also increase thirst and enhance positive water balance. For patients with far-advanced renal failure whose total body water is at the desired level (as indicated by normal or near-normal blood pressure, absence of edema, and normal serum sodium), urine volume may be a good guide to water intake. The daily water intake should equal the urine output plus approximately 500 mL to replace insensible losses.

In most nondialyzed patients with advanced renal failure, a daily intake of 1000 to 3000 mg (40–130 mEq) of sodium and 1500 to 3000 mL of fluid will maintain sodium and water balance. However, the requirement for sodium and water varies markedly, and each patient must be managed individually. Patients undergoing MHD or CPD usually become oliguric or anuric after several weeks to 1 or 2 years of treatment. For hemodialysis-treated patients, sodium and total fluid intake generally should be restricted to 1000 to 1500 mg/day and 750 to 1500 mL/day, respectively. Patients undergoing CPD usually tolerate a greater sodium and water intake because salt and water can be easily removed each day by using hypertonic dialysate, which increases the flow of water from the body into the peritoneal cavity, where it can be drained. Maintaining a large dietary sodium and water intake allows the quantity of fluid removed from the CPD-treated patient and, hence, the daily dialysate volume to be increased. This increase may be advantageous because the daily clearance of small molecules with CPD is directly related to the volume of dialysate outflow. In nondialyzed chronically uremic patients or in those undergoing MD who are not anuric and who gain excessive sodium or water despite attempts at dietary restriction, a potent loop diuretic, such as furosemide or bumetanide, may be tried to increase urinary sodium and water excretion.

Potassium

Normally, the kidney provides the major route for potassium excretion. In renal failure, potassium retention may occur and may lead quickly to fatal hyperkalemia. Two factors act to mitigate this process in renal failure. First, as long as urine output remains at approximately 1000 mL/day or greater, tubular secretion of potassium in the remaining functioning nephrons tends to be increased, and therefore the renal potassium clearance does not fall as markedly as the GFR. Second, fecal excretion of potassium is increased owing to enhanced large intestinal secretion (239). Thus, patients with CRF usually do not become hyperkalemic except in the following circumstances: (a) excessive intake of potassium; (b) acidosis, oliguria, or hypoaldosteronism (e.g., secondary to decreased renin secretion by the diseased kidney or renal tubular resistance to the actions of aldosterone); or (c) catabolic stress. Patients with stage 4 or 5 CKD (GFR <29 mL/minute) including those undergoing MHD, in general, should receive no more than 70 mEq of potassium/day. Some patients, particularly those with less advanced CRF, may tolerate higher potassium intakes; they may be identified by liberalizing their dietary potassium and carefully monitoring serum potassium levels. As emphasized earlier, the common use of ACEIs, ARBs, and/or aldosterone receptor blockers increases the risk of hyperkalemia by reducing the secretion or action of aldosterone. Even persons with normal kidney function may need to restrict their potassium intake if they take these medications and develop hyperkalemia.

Trace Elements

Several factors tend either to increase or decrease the body burden of certain trace elements in patients with renal failure (319–321). Many trace elements are excreted primarily in the urine, and they may accumulate with renal failure (320, 322). Elements such as iron, zinc, and copper, which are protein bound, may be lost in excessive quantities when there are large urinary protein losses, such as in the nephrotic syndrome (322). Occupational exposure or pica may increase the burden of some trace elements. The effect of the altered dietary intake of the uremic patient on body pools of trace elements is unknown (321). Because many trace elements bind avidly to serum proteins, when present even in small quantities in dialysate, they may be taken up into blood and cause toxicity. It is therefore recommended that, as a routine practice, dialysate should be purified of trace elements before use.

In certain circumstances, therapeutic doses of trace elements may be administered through dialysis, as has been done for zinc (323). Assessment of the trace element pools in patient with renal failure is difficult because the serum binding protein concentrations or affinities for trace elements may be altered, and red cell levels of trace elements may not reflect concentrations in other tissues.

Dietary requirements for trace elements have not been well defined in uremic patients (see Table 94.4). Trace element supplementation should be undertaken with caution because impaired urinary excretion of trace elements increases the risk of overdosage. Oral iron supplements are often given to patients who are iron deficient or, as a routine treatment, for patients who have a propensity to develop iron deficiency (e.g., those who frequently have marginal or low serum iron, reduced percentage of saturation of the iron binding capacity, or decreased ferritin levels). Iron requirements increase when erythropoietin therapy is started and hemoglobin synthesis rises. Ferrous sulfate, 300 mg up to three times/day, one half hour after meals, may be used. Some patients develop anorexia, nausea, constipation, or abdominal pain with ferrous sulfate and may tolerate other iron compounds better, such as ferrous fumarate, gluconate, or lactate. Patients who are intolerant to oral iron supplements or in whom oral iron therapy does not maintain adequate serum iron levels may be treated with intramuscular or, more usually, intravenous iron. Intravenous iron is commonly needed in MD-treated patients who are receiving treatment with erythropoietin (324, 325).

The zinc content of most tissues is normal in renal failure (321), although usually serum and hair zinc may be low and red cell zinc is increased (320, 323, 326, 327). In nondialyzed chronically uremic patients, the fractional urinary excretion of zinc is increased; however, because the GFR is reduced, total urinary excretion of zinc may be normal or reduced (319). Fecal zinc is increased (326), and a dietary zinc intake greater than the dietary reference intakes (DRIs) (328) may be necessary to maintain normal body zinc pools. Further studies are needed to confirm this. Some reports indicate that dysgeusia, poor food intake, and impaired sexual function, which are common problems of uremic patients, may be improved by giving patients zinc supplements (323, 326, 329, 330). However, other studies have not confirmed this (283).

As previously indicated, in nondialyzed chronically uremic patients and in those receiving MD, increased body burden of aluminum has been implicated as a cause of a progressive dementia syndrome (particularly in hemodialysis-treated patients), osteomalacia, weakness of the muscles of the proximal limbs, and anemia (127, 299, 300, 314, 315). Although contamination of dialysate with aluminum previously was the major source of aluminum toxicity in many dialysis centers, current methods of water treatment have removed virtually all aluminum from dialysate. At present, ingestion of aluminum binders of phosphate is probably the major cause of the excess body burden of aluminum (299, 300). Consequently, many nephrologists now use aluminum binders sparingly if at all, and they rely more on low-phosphorus diets and nonaluminum phosphate binders (see earlier) to control serum phosphorus levels (301–304). Aluminum toxicity may be treated by reduction of aluminum intake and by intravenous infusions of desferrioxamine, a chelator of aluminum (330). This chelator can be removed from the body by hemodialysis or peritoneal dialysis. Because deferrioxamine may predispose to serious infections, nephrologists tend to use this medication infrequently.

Vitamins

Patients with more advanced CKD (i.e., stages 3–5) are prone to deficiencies of water-soluble vitamins unless supplements are given (129). Vitamin deficiencies occur for the following reasons: First, vitamin intake is often low because of anorexia and poor food intake and also because many foods that are high in water-soluble vitamins are often restricted owing to the elevated potassium content. The typical diet for nondialyzed patients with CRF and for patients undergoing MD is frequently less than the DRIs for certain water-soluble vitamins (332) (see Appendix Table A-2-e for these data). Second, the metabolism of certain water-soluble vitamins tends to be altered in CRF (333, 334). Third, many medications interfere with the intestinal absorption, metabolism, or actions of vitamins (166, 185). Fourth, dialysis treatment removes water-soluble vitamins.

Vitamin B_6, vitamin C, and folic acid are the water-soluble vitamins most likely to be deficient in nondialyzed patients with CRF and in those undergoing MHD. Vitamin B_{12} deficiency is uncommon in CRF because the daily requirement is small (2 μg/day for nonpregnant, nonlactating adults) (332), the body can store relatively large quantities of this vitamin, and vitamin B_{12} is protein bound in plasma and hence is poorly dialyzed.

Some studies have suggested that many patients undergoing MHD may subsist for months with no vitamin supplementation and without developing deficiencies of water-soluble vitamins (335). However, these latter studies have not demonstrated that, without vitamin supplements, a small but substantial proportion of patients will not develop water-soluble vitamin deficiencies, particularly after 1 or more years of dialysis treatment. Because water-soluble vitamin deficiencies are caused by several different mechanisms in these patients, because vitamin deficiency may develop gradually, after months or years of dialysis treatment, and because water-soluble vitamin supplements are safe, it would seem prudent to continue to use them routinely.

Daily supplements for most vitamins are not well defined in renal failure (129). Evidence indicates that, in addition to vitamin intake from foods, the daily supplements of vitamins indicated in Table 94.4 will prevent or correct vitamin deficiency: pyridoxine hydrochloride, 5 mg in nondialyzed patients and 10 mg in those undergoing MHD or peritoneal dialysis (336); folic acid, 1 mg; and the DRIs for normal individuals for the other water-soluble vitamins (332). Patients with renal failure probably require less than 1.0 mg/day of folic acid; however, because this vitamin is safe and some evidence suggests that there may be competitive interference with its actions (333, 337), it may be advisable to prescribe this dose of folic acid until more definitive studies of the requirements are conducted. A supplement of only 60 mg/day of vitamin C is advised because ascorbic acid can be metabolized to oxalate. Large doses of ascorbic acid have been associated with increased plasma oxalate levels in patients with renal failure (338, 339). Oxalate is highly insoluble, and there is concern that high plasma oxalate concentrations may lead to precipitation in soft tissues. Moreover, in the nondialyzed patient with chronic renal insufficiency, it is possible that oxalate deposition in the kidney may cause further impairment in renal function.

Because serum retinol binding protein and vitamin A are elevated in uremia (340), the routine use of supplemental vitamin A is not recommended, particularly because even relatively small doses of vitamin A (i.e., 7500–15,000 IU/day) may cause bone toxicity (341). Additional vitamins E and K are probably not necessary. However, patients who receive antibiotics for extended periods and who do not ingest foods containing vitamin K may need vitamin K supplements (342).

Treatment with calcitriol is described earlier. Calcitriol increases intestinal calcium and phosphorus absorption, raises serum calcium, lowers serum parathyroid hormone, decreases serum alkaline phosphatase activity, reduces bone resorption, decreases endosteal fibrosis, and often improves osteomalacia (127). Therapy with calcitriol or other active vitamin D sterols is indicated for hyperparathyroidism, osteitis fibrosa, mixed osteomalacia, and severe hypocalcemia. Some patients with stage 5 CKD and vitamin D deficiency develop myopathy, primarily of the proximal limb muscles, and may present with severe weakness. Strength may improve with vitamin D therapy. Calcitriol has many immunologic effects in vitro (343, 344); whether treatment of patients with renal failure with this substance improves their immune function is not known. Children with stage 3 to 5 CKD require vitamin D analogs to promote growth.

Treatment of nondialyzed patients with stage 3 to 5 CKD with calcitriol usually is started at 0.25 to 0.50 μg/day. The serum calcium must be monitored carefully, and if it is low and does not rise by at least 0.5 mg/dL with any particular dosage, the dose may be increased by 0.25 to 0.50 μg/day every 4 to 6 weeks. Hypercalcemia is treated by temporary withdrawal of calcitriol. Ultimately, the best criterion for effective treatment with 1,25-dihydroxycholecalciferol is improvement in bone anatomy as determined by bone histology, radiographs, and densitometry. Improvement in muscle function or abolition of severe hypocalcemia also may indicate appropriate dosage of calcitriol. With time, the requirements for 1,25-dihydroxycholecalciferol and the tolerance for this vitamin may decrease, and the maintenance dosage may have to be reduced. This change may occur after there has been sufficient bone healing so the skeleton no longer serves as a sink for calcium and phosphorus.

Calcitriol should not be started unless serum calcium is not elevated (8.4–9.5 mg/dL), serum phosphorus is not more than slightly increased, and the calcium-phosphorus product is less than 55 mg^2/dL^2. Indications for other vitamin D sterols are described earlier. As indicated previously, serum calcium and phosphorus should be monitored during therapy to ensure that the concentrations are normal. In renal failure, many of the beneficial effects of 1,25-dihydroxycholecalciferol (calcitriol) can be reproduced by administration of other vitamin D sterols, often with less risk of hypercalcemia (see earlier).

Acidosis

Metabolic acidosis occurs frequently in nondialyzed patients with CRF because the ability of the kidney to excrete acidic metabolites is impaired. In the earlier stages of CRF, metabolic acidosis can also be caused by excessive renal losses of bicarbonate. The rate of acid production is probably normal or below normal in stable chronically uremic patients. Acidosis is reported to cause bone reabsorption, increased net protein degradation (345–347), and symptoms of lethargy and weakness.

Ingestion of low-nitrogen diets may prevent or reduce the severity of the acidosis by decreasing the endogenous generation of acidic products of protein metabolism. Alkali supplements are usually effective for preventing or treating the acidosis of CRF. Calcium carbonate, 5 g/day, may correct mild acidosis and reduce intestinal phosphate absorption, but care must be taken to prevent soft tissue calcification. For more severe acidosis, sodium bicarbonate or citrate may be administered orally or intravenously. If the nondialyzed chronically uremic patient is not oliguric and is not likely to develop edema, sodium is usually readily excreted when it is administered as sodium bicarbonate or citrate.

Alkali therapy should probably be initiated if the arterial pH is less than 7.37. The National Kidney Foundation DOQI Guidelines recommend that the serum bicarbonate be maintained at 22 mEq/L (124) or greater. It is my personal view that the serum bicarbonate is preferably maintained at normal concentrations (24–25 mEq/L). Before alkali therapy is implemented, it must be ascertained that the low serum bicarbonate is not a compensatory response to chronic respiratory alkalosis. If acidosis is severe and is not controlled by the foregoing measures, hemodialysis or peritoneal dialysis may be employed.

Prioritizing Dietary Goals

The number and magnitude of dietary modifications for CRF patients are so great that if they are all presented to the patient at one time, demoralization and noncompliance are likely to occur. Hence, we often list goals for dietary treatment according to priority. Control of sodium, potassium, protein, phosphorus, energy, calcium, and magnesium intake generally is emphasized. Conversely, unless the patient has a lipid disorder that carries a high risk of atherosclerotic disease, recommendations concerning the types and amounts of carbohydrates and fats ingested are usually given lower priorities. Moreover, a high dietary fiber intake is given a lower priority.

NUTRITIONAL THERAPY IN ACUTE RENAL FAILURE

Acute renal failure is characterized by a sudden reduction or cessation in GFR. The most common causes of acute renal failure include shock, severe infection, trauma, medications, obstruction, and certain types of glomerulonephritis. In most instances, if the patients survive the underlying diseases, they will recover from the acute renal failure. With acute renal failure, they are likely to develop fluid and electrolyte disorders, uremic toxicity, and wasting. These disorders are particularly prone to develop when the patient is both oliguric and hypercatabolic, common complications of acute renal failure.

Patients with acute renal failure, and particularly those with underlying catabolic illnesses, frequently undergo metabolic changes that promote degradation of protein and amino acids and consumption of fuel substrates. Energy expenditure is often increased (348). In vitro studies with rat muscle tissue indicate that protein degradation is enhanced and protein synthesis is reduced (349, 350). In addition, hepatic gluconeogenesis is increased. If the liver from these animals is perfused or incubated with amino acids, the elevated hepatic glucose and urea production will be further enhanced (351). The metabolic changes promoting catabolism are frequently severe in patients with acute renal failure, thus causing them to be among the sickest and most metabolically deranged patients in the hospital. As a result of these metabolic derangements, these patients are often unable to use protein, amino acids, and energy substrates efficiently. Hence, it may be difficult to maintain and to improve the nutritional status of these patients by enteral or parenteral nutrition (352–354).

General Principles

Because available data concerning optimal nutritional therapy for patients with acute renal failure are both limited and conflicting, it is not possible to justify strongly any treatment plan for such patients. The following therapeutic approach is based on analysis of the literature and personal experience.

Fluid and mineral balance should be carefully monitored in patients with acute renal failure to prevent overhydration or electrolyte disorders. Water intake, in general, should equal output from urine and all other measured sources (e.g., nasogastric aspirate, fistula drainage) plus 400 mL/day. This regimen takes into account the contributions of endogenous water production from metabolism and the insensible water losses (from respiration, skin losses) to water balance. In general, if the patient is catabolic, weight should be allowed to decrease by 0.2 to 0.5 kg/day to avoid excessive accumulation of fluid. Sodium, potassium, phosphorus, and magnesium intake should be restricted to prevent accumulation of these minerals. Energy and, if feasible, protein intake should satisfy the patient's nutritional requirements, which may exceed normal. By controlling the water and electrolyte intake and lowering the UNA, one may be able to reduce the need for dialysis treatments.

The patient's desirable nutrient intake will depend on the nutritional status, catabolic rate, residual GFR, and the clinical indications for initiating dialysis therapy. For example, in a patient who is wasted, one may be more inclined to give a surfeit of nutrients and to provide dialysis as needed. A patient with acute renal failure who has a high residual GFR also may receive larger quantities of nutrients, because there is less risk of developing fluid and electrolyte disorders or accumulating potentially toxic metabolites. Conversely, for a patient who has little or no urine flow and who is not very catabolic or uremic, the intake of small quantities of water, minerals, and amino acids may reduce the need for dialysis; this approach may be particularly beneficial if it is anticipated that the patient will not tolerate dialysis well. Similarly, a patient who is starting to recover from acute renal failure may be given this latter treatment to avoid dialysis for a few days until renal function becomes adequate. In these latter patients, high-calorie diets providing small amounts of essential amino acids or ketoacids with little or no protein may be used for short periods.

Whenever feasible, patients with acute renal failure should receive oral nutrition. If the patient will not eat adequately, the use of liquid formula diets, elemental diets, and tube or enterostomy feeding should be considered. Often parenteral nutrition is the only technique that will provide adequate nutrient intake (Table 94.6).

Specific Nutrient Intakes

Protein and Amino Acid Intake. The quantity of nitrogen and the composition of the amino acid formulations that are administered enterally or parenterally to patients with acute renal failure are the subject of controversy. Numerous studies of the effectiveness of various formulations were performed in the 1970s and early 1980s (355–361).

These data suggest that high-calorie solutions providing about 21 g/day of essential amino acids may be used more effectively than isocaloric preparations containing larger quantities of essential and nonessential amino acids (e.g., 40–70 g/day) provided in a ratio of essential to nonessential amino acids of 1.0:1.0 (354). The essential amino acids solutions seem to reduce the UNA and total nitrogen output more than the essential and nonessential amino acids. Consequently, nitrogen balance seems to be no more negative with the former preparations, but the accumulation of nitrogenous metabolites is less. Studies in clinically stable patients with CRF also indicate that diets providing small amounts of essential amino acids as the sole nitrogen source maintain nitrogen balance more effectively than diets providing similar quantities of protein (361). The data from rat studies are also inconclusive (362–365).

These conflicting observations are probably the result of the following factors: (a) the clinical course of patients with acute renal failure is so complex and variable that it would be necessary to study large numbers of patients to show statistically significant benefits of nutritional therapy, if it exists; (b) many of these studies were retrospective or not randomly controlled; this fact may have led to unintentional biases in the results; (c) the optimal composition of nutrients in the total parenteral nutrition (TPN) solutions has not been defined, and the use of suboptimal formulations of nutrients may reduce the clinical benefits of nutritional therapy; and (d) catabolic patients with acute renal failure may need both good nutrition and metabolic intervention to suppress catabolic processes and to promote anabolism; providing nutrients without metabolic intervention may not have a beneficial effect on nutritional status or clinical outcome, particularly in the first days after the onset of acute renal failure.

It is pertinent that the prospective studies of parenteral nutrition in patients with acute renal failure compared different regimens of nutritional therapy; that is, infusion of high-calorie solutions containing amino acids versus isocaloric infusions without amino acids and administration of isocaloric solutions with essential amino acids as compared with essential and nonessential amino acids (352, 353, 357, 360). No prospective, randomized study has compared the clinical course of patients receiving nutritional therapy with that of patients receiving no nutritional support.

Our current policy for amino acid or protein intake in patients with acute renal failure is as follows (see Table 94.6). Patients may be prescribed a low enteral or intravenous nitrogen intake if there is a low UNA (i.e., ≤4–5 g N/day), if they have no evidence of severe protein malnutrition, if one anticipates that the patient will recover renal function within the next 1 or 2 weeks, and if there is an indication to avoid dialysis therapy (354). Under these conditions, we may prescribe 0.3 to 0.5 g/kg/day of primarily high-quality protein or essential amino acids, preferably with arginine. We do not give more than 0.4 g/kg/day of essential amino acids as the sole nitrogen source because larger quantities of the nine essential amino acids may cause serious amino acid imbalances (354, 366). Diets providing

TABLE 94.6. TYPICAL COMPOSITION OF SOLUTIONS FOR TOTAL PARENTERAL NUTRITION IN PATIENTS WITH ACUTE RENAL FAILURE[a]

		DAILY QUANTITY OR CONCENTRATION TO BE INFUSED
Volume	Liters	1.0
Essential and nonessential free crystalline amino acids (4.25–5.0%)[b] or	g/L	42.5–50
Essential amino acids (5%)[b]	g/L	12.5–25
Dextrose (D-glucose)[c]	g/L	350
Lipid emulsion[c]	10 or 20%	50 or 100 g/500 mL
Energy (approx.)[c]	kcal/L	1,140
Electrolytes[d]		
Sodium[e]	mmol/L	40–50
Chloride[e]	mmol/L	25–35
Potassium	mmol/d	≥35
Acetate	mmol/d	35–40
Calcium	mmol/d	5
Phosphorus	mmol/d	8
Magnesium	mmol/d	4
Iron	mmol/d	2
Trace elements		See text
Vitamins		
Vitamin A[f]		See text
Vitamin D		See text
Vitamin K[g]	mg/wk	7.5
Vitamin E[b]	IU/d	10
Niacin	mg/d	20
Thiamin HCl (B$_1$)	mg/d	2
Riboflavin (B$_2$)	mg/d	2
Pantothenic acid (B$_3$)	mg/d	10
Pyridoxine HCl (B$_6$)	mg/d	10
Ascorbic acid (C)	mg/d	60
Biotin	μg/d	100
Folic acid	mg/d	2
Vitamin B$_{12}$	μg/d	3

[a]These nutrients are present in each bottle containing 500 mL of 8.5–10% crystalline amino acids or 250–500 mL of 5% essential amino acids and 500 mL of 70% dextrose. The vitamins and trace elements are an exception because they are added to only one bottle per day. The patient's fluid status and serum electrolytes and glucose must be monitored closely. The composition and volume of the infusate may need to be changed if the patient is very uremic, acidotic, or volume overloaded, if the serum electrolyte concentrations are not normal or if they are changing, or if dialysis therapy is not readily available or is particularly hazardous to the patient (see text).

[b]For patients who are more catabolic (e.g., urea nitrogen appearance ≥5 g/d), who are undergoing regular dialysis treatments (particularly for ≥2 wk), or who are wasted, essential and nonessential amino acids may be infused: ~1.0–1.2 g/kg/d for hemodialysis-treated patients and 1.2–1.3 g/kg/d for patients receiving intermittent or chronic peritoneal dialysis (see text). For patients who are less wasted, are less catabolic, are not undergoing regular dialysis therapy, and will not be receiving total parenteral nutrition for more than 2 or 3 wk, 0.30–0.50 g/kg/d of the nine essential amino acids (preferably with arginine) may be infused. Patients undergoing continuous venovenous hemofiltration (CVVH) or CVVH with concurrent hemodialysis using low dialysate flow rates may be given up to 1.5–2.5 g/kg/d of essential and nonessential amino acids depending on their clinical and metabolic status. See text for discussion of the formulations of amino acids. Only solutions of crystalline amino acids should be used.

[c]To attain an energy intake of 30–40 kcal/kg/d, 70% dextrose is added as necessary (see text). Lower energy intakes may be used in very obese patients. For the higher levels of energy intake (i.e., 35–40 kcal/kg/d), additional 70% dextrose may be added to the solutions. To balance the sources of calories and to prevent essential fatty acid deficiency, lipid emulsions may be used. For patients who are septic or at high risk for sepsis, about 10–20% of calories or less may be given as lipids. For more stable patients, 20–30% of calories may be given as lipids. The lipid emulsions probably should be infused over at least 12 hours, if not 24 hours, to reduce the hyperlipidemia that occurs with intravenous infusion of lipid emulsions (see text). The lipid emulsions may be infused in a separate line or mixed with the amino acid and dextrose solutions and infused soon after mixing (see text). A 20% lipid emulsion may be used to reduce the water load. The approximate calorie values are as follows: dextrose monohydrate, 3.4 kcal/g; amino acids, 3.5 kcal/g; lipid emulsions 10%, 1.1 kcal/mL; 20%, 2.0 kcal/mL.

[d]When one is adding electrolytes, the amounts intrinsically present in the amino acid solution should be taken into account.

[e]Refers to the final concentrations of electrolytes after any additional 70% dextrose or other solutions have been added.

[f]Vitamin A probably should be avoided unless total parenteral nutrition is continued for more than several days (see text).

[g]Should be given orally or parenterally and not in the total parenteral nutrition solution because of antagonisms.

[h]May need to be increased with use of lipid emulsions.

0.10 to 0.30 g/kg/day of miscellaneous protein and 10 to 20 g/day of essential amino acids or ketoacids may also be used in patients who can eat. These regimens should minimize the rate of accumulation of nitrogenous metabolites and, unless the patient is severely catabolic, will usually maintain neutral or only mildly negative nitrogen balance. Hence, the need for dialysis therapy may be minimized or avoided. If the patient has substantial residual renal function (e.g., GFR of 5–10 mL/minute) and is not very catabolic, we may treat the individual as a nondialyzed patient with CRF. The patient would receive 0.55 to 0.60 g protein or amino acids/kg desirable body weight/day.

For patients who are more catabolic and have a higher UNA (>5 g N/day), are severely wasted, or are undergoing regular dialysis therapy and either have or are anticipated to have acute renal failure for more than 2 weeks, we are inclined to prescribe a higher protein or amino acid intake, up to 1.0 to 1.2 g/kg body weight/day. If tolerated, 1.2 g protein or amino acids/kg/day is preferable. In comparison with small quantities of essential amino acids, these larger nitrogen intakes may improve nitrogen balance, particularly after the first 1 or 2 weeks of dialysis treatments. However, the UNA almost invariably rises, and the increased azotemia and, in those patients receiving TPN, the larger volumes of fluid necessary to provide this amount of amino acids may increase the need for dialysis.

If acute renal failure persists for more than 2 to 3 weeks, patients undergoing regular dialysis are treated as MD-treated patients, with about 1.0 to 1.2 g/kg/day of protein or amino acids for hemodialysis-treated patients or 1.2 to 1.5 g/kg/day for patients undergoing peritoneal dialysis.

Other Maneuvers to Improve Protein Balance and Clinical Outcome

Continuous arteriovenous hemofiltration (CAVH), CAVH with concurrent hemodialysis (CAVHD), continuous venovenous hemofiltration (CVVH), and CVVH with concurrent hemodialysis using low dialysate flow rates (CVVHD) are used increasingly for the management of very ill patients with acute renal failure or other causes of fluid or nitrogen intolerance (e.g., severe liver or congestive heart failure). With CAVH, catheters are placed into a large artery and vein, such as the femoral artery and vein (367). The blood flows through a small filtering apparatus where some of the plasma water is filtered; the remaining blood is returned to the vein. CVVH and CVVHD are often preferred to CAVH or CAVHD because these procedures reduce the risks of complications caused by arterial catheter placement.

The following are among the advantages to this treatment (for simplicity, CVVH or CVVHD will also refer to CAVH without or with dialysis): (a) large quantities of water, electrolytes, and metabolic products may be removed each day; (b) because the rate of removal of water and electrolytes is slow, CVVH or CVVHD is less likely to cause or worsen hypotension or induce other adverse physiologic changes (e.g., cardiac arrhythmias); and (c) the high daily clearances of water and small molecules, including metabolic waste products, allow one more safely to administer large amounts of amino acids and other nutrients to the patient. Physicians frequently combine parenteral nutrition therapy with CVVH/CVVHD to provide intravenous nutrition and, at the same time, to control the water and salt balance and remove the metabolic products that accumulate in renal failure.

When CVVH/CVVHD is not used, patients with acute renal failure who receive parenteral nutrition may require treatment with a hemodialyzer as often as every day rather than three times weekly, which is the usual treatment for clinically stable patients receiving MHD. With CVVH, and particularly CVVHD, standard hemodialysis treatments are usually needed less frequently and often can be avoided altogether. Indeed, CVVH/CVVHD often allows patients with acute renal failure to receive the magnitude of infused nutrients that are normally given to hypercatabolic, critically ill patients who do not have fluid, electrolyte, or nitrogen intolerance (i.e., patients who do not have renal, liver, or heart failure). For patients receiving CVVHD, we often prescribe 1.5 to 2.5 g/kg/day of mixtures of essential and nonessential amino acids intravenously or similar amounts of protein given enterally. Amino acid losses with CVVH/CVVHD are generally about 4 to 7 g/day and are slightly higher when patients are receiving amino acid infusions as compared with when they are not (368, 369).

Nutritional Dialysis. Some investigators have proposed adding amino acids and additional glucose to the dialysate of patients undergoing CAPD or MHD (370, 371). The nutrients diffuse into the body during dialysis. At present, these techniques may provide supplemental nutrition but cannot be used for total nutritional support.

Because the metabolic status of patients with acute renal failure often facilitates the catabolism of protein, amino acids, and other energy substrates (349–354, 360), there may be advantages to administering agents that promote anabolic processes or reduce catabolic pathways. As mentioned previously, the nitrogen intake appears to be used more efficiently if a greater proportion of the administered amino acids is essential (352, 354, 361). This hypothesis has not yet been tested clinically. In addition, studies in catabolic patients without renal failure suggest that intravenous infusions in which a large proportion of the amino acids are composed of branched-chain amino acids (i.e., isoleucine, leucine, and valine) may have a specific anabolic effect (372, 373). Not all studies confirm these findings. Ketoacid analogs of the branched-chain amino acids have also been shown to promote anabolism both when studied in in vitro preparations and when given to nonuremic persons who are not hypercatabolic (102, 103).

The intravenous infusion of the salt complex of α-ketoglutarate and ornithine in postoperative patients receiving TPN is reported to reduce UNA and to increase nitrogen balance (374). Severely stressed patients without renal failure display a rapid fall in intracellular muscle glutamine (375). Administration of glutamine improves protein balance in these patients (375, 376). Arginine also may increase nitrogen balance (377).

Anabolic steroidal compounds, many of which are androgenic and resemble testosterone, have been used in patients with acute renal failure (378, 379). These agents can reduce UNA and increase nitrogen balance; they also have been reported to decrease the need for dialysis treatments. In vitro studies of skeletal muscle from rats with acute renal failure indicate that insulin may increase synthesis and reduce degradation of protein (350). Studies in catabolic patients who do not have renal failure indicate that insulin may decrease the UNA (380, 381). Recombinant DNA-synthesized human growth hormone has been used to improve nitrogen balance in postoperative, acutely stressed patients without renal failure, and the results have been encouraging (382, 383). This hormone has also improved nitrogen balance in stable, malnourished patients undergoing MHD (384). However, patients who are acutely stressed from infection or physical trauma or who receive low quantities of nutrients sometimes become refractory to growth hormone, possibly because of downregulation of growth hormone receptors with reduced ability to express IGF-I (385). Moreover, in very ill patients in intensive care units, the use of growth hormone has been associated with increased mortality rates (386). Therefore, for the present, growth hormone should not be given to such patients.

These findings could be construed to suggest that there may be benefits of recombinant human IGF-I (rhIGF-I) therapy over growth hormone treatment for hypercatabolic patients with acute renal failure. Indeed, studies in rats with ischemic- or toxin-induced acute renal failure indicated that rhIGF-I may enhance recovery of renal function (387, 388). However, a 1999 study suggested that rhIGF-I therapy does not enhance the rate of recovery of renal function, reduce the need for dialysis treatment, or improve survival in sick patients in intensive care units who have acute renal failure (389). Because IGF-I appears to stimulate growth of dedifferentiated cells, neither growth hormone nor rhIGF-I should be given to patients with active malignancy.

Several other growth factors (i.e., epidermal growth factor [390], hepatocyte growth factor [391]), hormones (thyroxin [392], atrial natriuretic peptide [393]), and adenine nucleotides (394) are reported to enhance recovery of renal function in experimental animals or in preliminary studies in humans. None of these agents have yet been shown to improve renal function in well-controlled clinical trials in humans with acute renal failure.

Energy. Several lines of evidence suggest that patients with acute renal failure may benefit from a high energy intake. Because patients with acute renal failure are frequently in negative energy and nitrogen balance (348, 352, 353, 360), some investigators contend that a greater energy intake may reduce protein wasting. Moreover, unlike nonuremic acutely ill patients who may receive large quantities of amino acids, patients with acute renal failure are usually given relatively small amounts of amino acids because of their excretory impairment. It is possible, although not proven, that higher energy intakes may improve the use of low nitrogen intakes. In two studies of patients with acute renal failure who were not randomized for energy intake, those who died were found to have a

higher energy expenditure and more negative energy balance (348) or lower energy intake (348, 352) than those who survived. As a result of these findings, we usually administer about 30 to 40 kcal/kg standard (normal) weight/day (see Table 94.6) (237, 395), except in patients who are obese (e.g., >125% standard body weight) or very underweight.

The higher intakes (i.e., 40 kcal/kg/day) are used for patients who have a higher UNA, who are severely ill, and who are less obese. For example, if nitrogen balance, estimated from the difference between the patient's nitrogen intake and the nitrogen output calculated from the UNA, is negative, we try to provide an energy intake close to 40 kcal/day. Alternatively, the patient's energy needs may be estimated by multiplying the Harris-Benedict equation (396) or the newer World Health Organization equations (397) for calculating the daily energy requirements of physiologically normal persons by a stress factor to adjust for the patient's illness (398, 399) and by 1.25. This latter term (1.25) is included to provide a surfeit of energy to promote anabolism or to diminish the rate of catabolism of the patient; the value of this term has not been clearly demonstrated. Energy expenditure, measured by indirect calorimetry, can also be multiplied by 1.25 to estimate the daily energy requirement.

These energy intakes are higher than currently recommended for severely stressed patients without renal failure. However, because nitrogen intolerance limits the amount of amino acids or protein that can be given to the patient with renal failure and higher energy intakes tend to reduce nitrogen losses, the patient with renal failure may benefit from a larger energy load. Unfortunately, prospective studies to test this hypothesis are not available.

Larger energy intakes are not used because there appears to be little nutritional advantage to administering more calories to catabolic patients. Indeed, because high energy intakes generate more carbon dioxide from the infused carbohydrate and fat, they can promote hypercapnia if pulmonary function is impaired (400). Carbon dioxide retention is particularly likely to occur with very high carbohydrate loads. In addition, high energy intakes may cause obesity and fatty liver (401), and they may increase the water load to the patient.

Because most patients with acute renal failure do not tolerate large water intakes, glucose is usually administered in a 70% solution. The glucose and amino acid solutions are mixed, so the amino acids and energy are provided simultaneously (see Table 94.6). Patients receiving TPN for more than 5 days should receive lipid emulsions. Patients require about 25 g/day of a lipid emulsion to prevent essential fatty acid deficiency. Some investigators have recommended giving up 30 to 40% calories as lipid emulsions to provide sufficient fatty acids to organs that normally use lipids as their main energy source and to more closely approximate normal US dietary intake. However, some researchers have reported that infusions of large amounts of fat emulsions, such as 50 g over 8 to 12 hours, may impair the function of the reticuloendothelial system (402); these researchers have questioned whether infusion of lipid emulsions could lower host resistance. A prudent approach may be to infuse lipid emulsions over at least 12 hours, if not 24 hours, to prevent marked increases in plasma lipids. For patients who are septic or at high risk of severe sepsis, probably no more than 10 to 20% of total calories should be provided from fat. For patients who are not septic and not at high risk of infection, about 20 to 30% of calories may be given as lipid emulsions.

Intravenous lipid emulsions are available in 10% (1.1 kcal/mL) and 20% (2.0 kcal/mL) solutions. Traditionally, lipid emulsions have been infused separately from the glucose and amino acid mixtures. With careful attention to aseptic control, the lipid emulsions may be mixed with glucose and amino acids; the mixtures should be infused shortly after preparation (403).

Minerals. A mineral prescription for parenteral nutrition in acute renal failure is shown in Table 94.6. Any recommended intake of minerals is tentative and must be adjusted according to the clinical status of the patient. If the serum concentration of an electrolyte is increased, it may be advisable to reduce the quantity infused or to not administer it at the onset of parenteral nutrition. The patient must be monitored closely, because the hormonal and metabolic changes that often occur with initiation of parenteral nutrition may cause the serum electrolytes to fall rapidly. This occurrence is particularly likely for serum potassium and phosphorus. Conversely, a low concentration of a mineral may indicate a need for greater than usual intake of that element. Again, metabolic changes and the impaired GFR can lead to a rapid rise in the serum concentrations during repletion.

Trace elements are probably not necessary in parenteral nutrition solutions given to catabolic patients with acute renal failure unless this is the sole source of nutritional support for at least 2 to 3 weeks. The nutritional requirements for trace elements have not been established for uremic patients receiving TPN.

Vitamins. The vitamin requirements have not been well defined for patients with acute renal failure. Tentative recommendations for vitamin intake for patients receiving parenteral nutrition are shown in Table 94.6. Much of the recommended intake is based on information obtained from studies in chronically uremic patients, physiologically normal persons, or nonuremic acutely ill patients. Vitamin A is probably best avoided for the first several days of nutritional support, because in CRF serum vitamin A levels are elevated, and small doses of vitamin A have been reported to cause toxicity to chronically uremic patients (340, 341). After the first several days of nutritional therapy, a dose of vitamin A that is between one half and the complete DRIs (328) for normal individuals may be given daily.

Vitamin D is fat soluble, and vitamin stores should not become depleted during the few days to weeks that most patients with acute renal failure receive parenteral nutrition. However, the turnover of its active analog, 1,25-dihydroxycholecalciferol, is much faster. Hence, this analog may be needed in patients with acute renal failure (344).

Although vitamin K is fat soluble, vitamin K deficiency has been reported in nonuremic patients who are not eating and are receiving antibiotics (342). Vitamin K therefore should be given routinely to patients receiving parenteral nutrition (see Table 94.6). Ten milligrams/day of pyridoxine hydrochloride (8.2 mg/day of pyridoxine) is recommended because studies in clinically stable or sick patients undergoing MHD indicate that this quantity may be necessary to prevent or to correct vitamin B_6 deficiency (336). Patients should probably not receive more than 60 mg of ascorbic acid/day because of the risk of increased oxalate production (338, 339).

The nutrient intake of patients with acute renal failure must be carefully reevaluated each day and sometimes more frequently. This reevaluation is particularly important because these patients may undergo rapid changes in their clinical and metabolic condition.

Peripheral Parenteral Nutrition

Parenteral nutrition through a peripheral vein avoids the risks of inserting a catheter into the inferior vena cava. Because the osmolality of the infusate must be restricted to reduce the risk of thrombophlebitis, it is necessary to use a larger volume of fluid and/or a lower intake of nutrients. Both approaches may have undesirable consequences for patients with acute renal failure. It has been argued that the financial cost of TPN administered through a peripheral vein is about the same as or greater than the cost of administration through a central vein because of the large quantities of isotonic lipid emulsions used to provide the energy needs when peripheral veins are used.

Peripheral partial parenteral nutrition may be advantageous for patients with acute renal failure who are able to ingest or be tube fed a part of their daily nutritional requirements. The peripheral infusions may enable these patients to receive adequate nutrition without resorting to TPN through a large flow vein. In these patients, it is often most practical to infuse an 8.5 to 10% amino acid solution or a 20% lipid emulsion into a peripheral vein and to administer as much as possible of the other essential nutrients, including carbohydrates, through the enteral tract.

The peripheral vascular access used for hemodialysis can also be used for parenteral nutrition. Because there is a high blood flow through the vascular access used for hemodialysis, hypertonic solutions can be used, and the water load to the patient can be reduced. This technique probably increases the risk of infection or thrombosis in the vascular access, however, and it should not be used in patients who will need a hemodialysis access for extended periods.

Supplemental Parenteral Nutrition

Infusion of amino acids and glucose and/or lipids may be given as a nutritional supplement to patients with acute renal failure or CRF who eat poorly. Supplemental amino acids, glucose, and/or lipids can be infused conveniently during the hemodialysis procedure. Because most patients in need of nutritional supplements have decreased intake of both amino acids and energy, I infuse 40 to 42 g of essential and nonessential amino acids and 200 g of D-glucose (150 g of D-glucose if the hemodialysate contains glucose). This preparation is infused throughout the hemodialysis procedure at a constant rate into the blood leaving the dialyzer. Such a technique minimizes the normal fall in amino acid and glucose pools that occurs as a result of dialysis of these nutrients. Most of the infused glucose and amino acids are retained; the amino acid losses into dialysate increase by only about 4 to 5 g (181). Lipid infusions have been substituted for some of the infused glucose but are more expensive and possibly pose some risk of reducing host resistance to infection (402). Patients who have low serum phosphorus or potassium concentrations at the onset of dialysis treatment may require supplements of these electrolytes during the amino acid and glucose supplementation. To prevent reactive hypoglycemia, the infusion should not be stopped until the end of hemodialysis, and the patient should eat a carbohydrate source 20 to 30 minutes before the end of the infusion.

Whether intravenous supplements with amino acids, glucose, and/or lipids thrice weekly for about 3 to 4 hours during hemodialysis are beneficial to MHD-treated patients who eat poorly is controversial. Two 1994 retrospective analyses suggested that in malnourished patients undergoing MHD, intradialytic parenteral nutrition may reduce the mortality rate (404, 405). One study indicated that this benefit was observed only when the serum albumin was 3.3 g/dL or lower (405). Intradialytic parenteral nutrition should be used only in patients who cannot increase their intake of foods or take oral supplements. The intravenous supplements should be continued only if nutritional or clinical assessment indicates that these nourishments are beneficial.

Amino Acids that May Predispose to Acute Renal Failure

Several studies in rats suggested that amino acid or protein intake may increase the susceptibility to and severity of acute renal failure caused by ischemia or aminoglycoside nephrotoxicity (406–409). Although some studies demonstrated this effect with large doses of intravenous amino acids or dietary protein (406–409), the quantities of amino acids and protein that may be prescribed for patients can also predispose to renal failure in animal studies (407, 408). D-Serine, DL-ethionine, and L-lysine appear to be particularly nephrotoxic (407, 409). It is not known whether amino acid or protein intake will predispose to renal failure in humans. If either one does, then patients who receive nephrotoxic medications or who are at high risk of renal ischemia could benefit from low amino acid or protein intakes for transient periods. Conversely, in vitro studies also indicated that some amino acids, particularly L-glycine and L-alanine, may protect renal tubular cells from ischemic or nephrotoxic injury (410). Clearly, more research is needed in this area.

REFERENCES

1. National Kidney Foundation. Am J Kidney Dis 2003;42[Suppl 3]:1S–201S.
2. Lindholm B, Heimbürger O, Stenvinkel P et al. Uremic toxicity. In: Kopple JD, Massry SG, eds. Nutritional Management of Renal Disease. Philadelphia: Lippincott Williams & Wilkins, 2003:63–98.
3. Takeda M, Endou H. Renal cell metabolism. In: Massry SG, Glassock RJ, eds. Massry and Glassock's Textbook of Nephrology. 4th ed, vol 1. Philadelphia: Lippincott Williams & Wilkins, 2001:110–21.
4. Hausmann MJ, Rabkin R, Dahl DC. Role of kidney in hormone metabolism. In: Massry SG, Glassock RJ, eds. Massry and Glassock's Textbook of Nephrology. 4th ed, vol 1. Philadelphia: Lippincott Williams & Wilkins, 2001:141–50.
5. Don BR, Schambelan M, Lo JC. Endocrine hypertension: effects of hormones on renal function. In: Greenspan FS, Gardner DG, eds. Basic and Clinical Endocrinology. 7th ed. New York: McGraw-Hill, 2004:414–38.
6. Hausmann MJ, Rabkin R. Kidney and endocrine system. In: Massry SG, Glassock RJ, eds. Massry and Glassock's Textbook of Nephrology. 4th ed, vol 1. Philadelphia: Lippincott Williams & Wilkins, 2001:139–230.
7. Kokko KE, Montero A, Lakkis FG et al. Hormones and the kidney. In: Schrier RW, ed. Diseases of the Kidney. 7th ed, vol 1. Philadelphia: Lippincott Williams & Wilkins, 2001:265–313.
8. Eschbach JW, Kelly MR, Haley R et al. N Engl J Med 1989; 321:158–62.
9. Klahr S. Effect of malnutrition and of changes in protein intake on renal function. In: Kopple JD, Massry SG, eds. Nutritional Management of Renal Disease. 2nd ed. Philadelphia: Lippincott Williams & Wilkins, 2004:213–21.
10. Klahr S, Tripathy K. Arch Intern Med 1966;118:322–5.
11. Klahr S, Tripathy K, Garcia FT et al. Am J Med 1967;43:84–96.
12. Klahr S, Tripathy K, Lotero H. Am J Med 1970;48:325–31.
13. Ichikawa I, Purkerson, ML, Klahr S et al. J Clin Invest 1980;65: 982–8.
14. Hirschberg R, Kopple JD, Blantz RC et al. J Clin Invest 1991; 87:1200–6.
15. Hirschberg, R, Kopple JD. J Am Soc Nephrol 1991;1:1034–40.
16. Owen OE, Felig P, Morgan AP. J Clin Invest 1969;48:574–83.
17. Gutman AB, Yu T-F. Am J Med 1968;45:756–79.
18. Bosch JP, Lew S, Glabman S et al. Am J Med 1986;81:809–15.
19. Smoyer WE, Brouhard BH, Rassin DK et al. J Lab Clin Med 1991;118:166–75.
20. Castellino P, Hunt W, DeFronzo RA. Kidney Int Suppl 1987;32:15S–20S.
21. Hirschberg R, Kopple JD. Kidney Int 1987;32:382–7.
22. Mitch WE, Walser M, Buffington GA et al. Lancet 1976;2: 1326–8.
23. Rutherford WE, Blondin J, Miller JP et al. Kidney Int 1977;11: 62–70.

24. Barsotti G, Guiducci A, Ciardella F et al. Nephron 1981;27: 13–117.
25. Cotran R. Kidney Int 1982;21:528.
26. McCormack LJ, Beland JE, Schnekloth RE et al. Am J Pathol 1958;34:1011–22.
27. Kleinknecht C, Grunfeld J-P, Gomez PC et al. Kidney Int 1973; 4:390–400.
28. Rodriguez-Iturbe B, Garcia, R, Rubio L et al. Clin Nephrol 1976;5:198–206.
29. Torres VE, Velosa JA, Holley KE et al. Ann Intern Med 1980; 92:776–84.
30. Deen WM, Maddox DA, Robertson CR et al. Am J Physiol 1974;227:556–62.
31. Hostetter TH, Olson JL, Rennke HG et al. Am J Physiol 1981; 241:F85–93.
32. Hostetter TH, Troy JL, Brenner BM. Kidney Int 1981;19: 410–5.
33. Olson JL, Hostetter TH, Rennke HG et al. In: Proceedings of the American Society of Nephrology. Thorofare, NJ: Charles B. Slack, 1979:87A.
34. Olson JL, Hostetter TH, Rennke HG et al. Kidney Int 1982;22: 112–26.
35. Kopple JD, Shinaberger JH, Coburn JW et al. Am J Clin. Nutr 1968;21:508–15.
36. Blatherwick NR, Medlar EM. Arch Intern Med 1937;59: 572–96.
37. Farr LE, Smadel JE. J Exp Med 1939;70:615–27.
38. Addis T. Glomerular nephritis. In: Diagnosis and Treatment. New York: Macmillan, 1948.
39. Ibels LS, Alfrey AC, Haut L et al. N Engl J Med 1978;298: 122–6.
40. Karlinsky ML, Haut LL, Buddington B et al. Kidney Int 1980; 17:293–302.
41. Haut LL, Alfrey AC, Guggenheim S et al. Kidney Int 1980;17: 722–31.
42. Kirsch R, Frith L, Black E et al. Nature 1968;217:578–9.
43. Kenner CH, Evan AP, Blomgren P et al. Kidney Int 1985;27: 739–50.
44. French SW, Yamanaka W, Ostwald R. Arch Pathol 1967;83: 204–10.
45. Hurd ER, Johnston JM, Okita JR et al. J Clin Invest 1981;67: 476–85.
46. Rothschild MA, Oratz M, Evans CD et al. Albumin synthesis. In: Rosemoer M, Oratz M, Rothschild A, eds. Albumin Structure, Function and Uses. New York: Pergamon Press, 1977: 227–55.
47. Barcelli UO, Weiss M, Pollack VE. J Lab Clin Med 1982;100: 786–97.
48. Zurier RB, Damjanov O, Sayadoff DM et al. Arthritis Rheum 1977;20:1449–56.
49. Kelley VE, Winkelstein A, Izui S. Lab Invest 1979;41:531–7.
50. McLeish KR, Gohara AF, Cunning WT III. J Lab Clin Med 1980;96:470–9.
51. Brenner BM, Meyer TW, Hostetter TH. N Engl J Med 1982;307:652–9.
52. Meyer TW, Lawrence WE, Brenner BM. Kidney Int 1983;24 [Suppl 16]:243S–7S.
53. Schrier RW, Harris DCH, Chan L et al. Am J Kidney Dis 1988; 12:243–9.
54. Nath KA, Hostetter MK, Hostetter TH. J Clin Invest 1985; 76:667–75.
55. Bouby N, Bachmann S, Bichet D et al. Am J Physiol 1990;258: F973–9.
56. Paller MS, Hostetter TH. Am J Physiol 1986;251:F34–9.
57. Williams M, Young JB, Rosa RM et al. J Clin Invest 1986;78: 1687–93.
58. Wang S, Hirschberg R. J Biol Chem 2004;279:23200–6.
59. Wang S, Wilkes MC, Leof EB et al. FASEB J 2005;19:1–11.
60. Walls J, Williams SJ. Contr Nephrol 1988;60:179–87.
61. Mauer SM, Steffes MW, Azar S et al. Kidney Int 1989;35: 48–59.
62. Mogensen CE. Diabetes 1976;25:872–9.
63. Mogensen CE, Steffes MW, Deckert T et al. Diabetologia 1981;21:89–93.
64. Mogensen CE, Christensen CK, Vittinghus E. Diabetes 1983; 32[Suppl 2]:64–78.
65. Barsotti G, Giannoni A, Morelli E et al. Clin Nephrol 1984;21: 4–59.
66. Lumlertgul D, Burke TJ, Gillum OM et al. Kidney Int 1986; 29:658–66.
67. Gimenez LF, Solez K, Walker GW. Kidney Int 1987;31:93–9.
68. Harris DCH, Hammond WS, Burke TJ et al. Kidney Int 1987; 31:41–6.
69. Kasiske BL, O'Donnell MP, Schmitz PG et al. Kidney Int 1990;37:880–91.
70. Wellmann K, Wolk BW. Lab Invest 1970;22:144–5.
71. Keane WF, O'Donnell MP, Kasiske BL et al. J Am Soc Nephrol 1990;1:69S–74S.
72. Kasiske BL, O'Donnell MP, Cleary MP et al. Kidney Int 1988; 33:667–72.
73. Susuki S, Shapiro R, Mulrow PJ et al. Prostaglandins Med 4: 377–82.
74. Knecht A, Fine LG, Kleinman KS et al. Am J Physiol 1991;261: F292–9.
75. Komers R, Meyer TW, Anderson S. Pathophysiology and nephron adaptation in chronic renal failure. In: Schrier RW, ed. Diseases of the Kidney. 7th ed, vol 3. Philadelphia: Lippincott Williams & Wilkins, 2001:2689–718.
76. Rahman MA, Nakazawa M, Emancipator SN et al. Kidney Int 1986;29:343(abst).
77. Badr KF, Brenner BM, Wasserman M et al. Kidney Int 1986; 29:328(abst).
78. Don BR, Blake S, Hutchison FN et al. Am J Physiol 1989;256: F711–8.
79. Anderson S, Meyer TW, Rennke HG et al. J Clin Invest 1985; 76:612–9.
80. Tolins JP, Raij L. Hypertension 1990;16:452–61.
81. Ruggenenti P, Perna A, Benini R et al. J Am Soc Nephrol 1999; 10:997–1006.
82. Brenner BM, Cooper ME, de Zeeuw D et al. N Engl J Med 2001;345:861–9.
83. Lewis EJ, Hunsicker LG, Clarke WR et al. N Engl J Med 2001; 345:851–60.
84. Ruggenenti P, Perna A, Gherardi G et al. J Kidney Dis 2000;35: 1155–65.
85. Hostetter TH, Rosenberg ME. J Am Soc Nephrol 1990;1: 55S–8S.
86. Lewis EJ, Hunsicker LG, Bain RP et al. N Engl J Med 1993; 329:1456-62.
87. Viberti G, Mogensen CE, Groop LC et al. JAMA 1994;271: 275–9.
88. Blasi ER, Rocha R, Rudolph AE et al. Kidney Int 2003;63: 1791–800.
90. Walser M. Clin. Nephrol 1976;3:180–6.
91. Maschio G, Oldrizzi L, Tessitore N et al. Kidney Int 1982;22: 371–6.
92. Alvestrand A, Ahlberg M, Bergstrom J. Kidney Int Suppl 1983; 24:268S–72S.

93. Barsotti G, Morelli E, Giannoni A et al. Kidney Int Suppl 1983; 24:278S–84S.
94. Gretz N, Korb E, Strauch M. Kidney Int Suppl 1983;24: 263S–7S.
95. Mitch WE, Walser M, Steinman TI et al. N Engl J Med 1984; 311:623–9.
96. Rosman JB, Meijer S, Sluiter WJ et al. Lancet 1984;2:1291–5.
97. Walser J, LaFrance ND, Ward L et al. Kidney Int 1987;32:123–8.
98. Ihle BU, Becker GJ, Whitworth JA et al. N Engl J Med 1989; 321:1773–7.
99. Zeller J, Whittaker E, Sullivan L et al. N Engl J Med 1991;324: 78–84.
100. Klahr S, Levey AS, Beck GJ et al. N Engl J Med 1994;330: 877–84.
101. Levey AS, Adler S, Caggiula AW et al. Am J Kidney Dis 1996; 27:652–63.
102. Mitch WE, Walser M, Sapir DG. J Clin Invest 1981;67:553–62.
103. Tischler ME, Desautels M, Goldberg AL. J Biol Chem 1982; 257:1613–21.
104. Kopple JD. Nutritional management of nondialyzed patients with chronic renal failure. In: Kopple JD, Massry SG, eds. Nutritional Management of Renal Disease. 2nd ed. Philadelphia: Lippincott Williams & Wilkins, 2004:379–414.
105. Williams AJ, Baker F, Walls J. Nephron 1987;46:83–90.
106. D'Amico G, Gentile MG, Manna G et al. Lancet 1992;339: 1131–4.
107. D'Amico G, Remuzzi G, Maschio G et al. Clin Nephrol 1991; 35:237–42.
108. Fouque D, Laville M, Boissel JP et al. BMJ 1992;304:216–20.
109. Pedrini MT, Levey AS, Lau J et al. Ann Intern Med 1996;124: 627–32.
110. Kasiske BL, Lakatua JD, Ma JZ et al. Am J Kidney Dis 1998;31: 954–61.
111. Fouque D, Wang P, Laville M et al. Nephrol Dial Transplant 2000;12:1986–92.
112. Levey AS, Greene T, Sarnak MJ et al. J Am Soc Nephrol 2003; 15:586A.
113. Levey AS, Greene T, Sarnak MJ et al. J Am Soc Nephrol 2003; 15:586A.
114. Knight EL, Stampfer MJ, Hankinson SE et al. Ann Intern Med 2003;138:460–7.
115. Bernardi A, Biasia F, Pati T et al. Am J Kidney Dis 2003;41: 146S–5S.
116. Hansen HP, Tauber-Lassen E, Jensen BR et al. Kidney Int 2002;62:220–8.
117. Schnaper HW, Robson AM. Nephrotic syndrome: minimal change disease, focal glomerulosclerosis, and related disorders. In: Schrier RW, ed. Diseases of the Kidney. 7th ed, vol 2. Philadelphia: Lippincott Williams & Wilkins, 2001:1773–831.
118. Don BR, Kaysen GA. Nutritional management of nephrotic syndrome. In: Kopple JD, Massry SG, eds. Nutritional Management of Renal Disease. 2nd ed. Philadelphia: Lippincott Williams & Wilkins, 2004:415–32.
119. Ibels LS, Gyory AZ. Medicine (Baltimore) 1994;73:79.
120. Hirschberg R, Wange S. Curr Opin Nephrol Hypertens 2005; 14:43–52.
121. Taguma Y, Kitamoto Y, Futaki G et al. N Engl J Med 1985;313: 1617–20.
122. Kaysen GA, Gambertoglio J, Jimenez I et al. Kidney Int 1986; 29:572–7.
123. Zeller KR, Raskin P, Rosenstock J et al. Kidney Int 1986;29: 209.
124. Kaysen GA, Davies RW. J Am Soc Nephrol 1990;1:75S–9S.
125. Gonick HC, Maxwell MH, Rubini ME et al. Nephron 1966;3: 37–52.
126. Falkenhain M, Hartman J, Hebert LA. Nutritional management of water, sodium, potassium, chloride and magnesium in renal disease and renal failure. In: Kopple JD, Massry SG, eds. Nutritional Management of Renal Disease. 2nd ed. Philadelphia: Lippincott Williams & Wilkins, 2004:287–98.
127. Moe SM. Calcium, phosphorus, and vitamin D metabolism in renal disease and chronic renal failure. In: Kopple JD, Massry SG, eds. Nutritional Management of Renal Disease. 2nd ed. Philadelphia: Lippincott Williams & Wilkins, 2004:261–85.
128. Vanholder R, Cornelis R, Dhondt A et al. Trace element metabolism in renal disease and renal failure. In: Kopple JD, Massry SG, eds. Nutritional Management of Renal Disease. 2nd ed. Philadelphia: Lippincott Williams & Wilkins, 2004:299–313.
129. Chazot C, Kopple JD. Vitamin metabolism and requirements in renal disease and renal failure. In: Kopple JD, Massry SG, eds. Nutritional Management of Renal Disease. 2nd ed. Philadelphia: Lippincott Williams & Wilkins, 2004:315–56.
130. Rabkin R, Simon NM, Steiner S et al. N Engl J Med 1970;282: 182–7.
131. Sherwin RS, Bastl C, Finkelstein FO et al. J Clin Invest 1976; 57:722–31.
132. Vajda FJE, Martin TJ, Melick RA. Endocrinology 1969;84:162–4.
133. Cuttelod S, Lemarchand-Beraud T, Magnenat P et al. Metabolism 1974;23:101–13.
134. Davidson WD, Moore TC, Shippey W et al. Gastroenterology 1974;66:522–5.
135. Samaan N, Freeman RM. Metabolism 1970;19:102–13.
136. Nagel TC, Frenkel N, Bell RH et al. J Clin Endocrinol Metab 1973;36:428–32.
137. Lim VS, Fang, VS. Am J Med 1975;58:655–62.
138. Tourkantonis A, Spiliopoulos A, Pharmakioltis A et al. Nephron 1981;27:271–2.
139. Hershman JM, Krugman LG, Kopple JD et al. Metabolism 1979;27:755–9.
140. Fouque D, Peng SC, Kopple JD. Kidney Int 1995;47:876–83.
141. Ding H, Gao X-L, Hirschberg R et al. J Clin Invest 1996;97: 1064–75.
142. McCaleb ML, Wish JB, Lockwood DH. Endocrinol Res 1985;11:113–25.
143. Fadda GZ, Hajjar SM, Perna AF et al. J Clin Invest 1991;87: 255–61.
144. Kopple JD, Fukuda S. Am J Clin Nutr 1980;33:1363–72.
145. Tizianello A, De Ferrari G, Garibotto B et al. J Clin Invest 1980;65:1162–73.
146. Kopple JD. Products of nitrogen metabolism and their toxicity. In: Massry SG, Glassock RJ, eds. Massry and Glassock's Textbook of Nephrology. 4th ed, vol 2. Philadelphia: Lippincott Williams & Wilkins, 2001:1262–78.
147. Bricker NS. N Engl J Med 1972;286:1093–9.
148. Massry SG, Smogorzewski M. Semin Nephrol 1994;14:219–31.
149. Simenoff ML, Burke JF, Saukkonen JJ et al. Lancet 1976;2: 818–21.
150. Taylor JE, Peat N, Porter C et al. Nephrol Dial Transplant 1996;11:1079–83.
151. Krol E, Rutkowski B, Wroblewska M et al. Miner Electrolyte Metab 1996;22:13–5.
152. Attmann PO, Alaupovic P. Nephron 1991;57:401–10.
153. Lindner A, Charra B, Sherrard D et al. N Engl J Med 1974; 290:697–701.
154. Malluche HH, Faugere MC. Kidney Int 1990;38:193–211.
155. Briggs WA, Lazarus JM, Birtch AG et al. Arch Intern Med 1973;132:21–8.
156. Kopple JD. Nutrition in renal failure: causes of catabolism and wasting in acute or chronic renal failure. In: Robinson RR, ed.

Nephrology, vol 2. Proceedings of the IXth International Congress of Nephrology. New York: Springer-Verlag, 1984: 1498–515.

157. Cianciaruso B, Brunori G, Kopple JD et al. Am J Kidney Dis 1995;26:475–86.

158. Canada-USA Peritoneal Dialysis Study Group. J Am Soc Nephrol 1996;7:198–207.

159. Woodrow G, Oldroyd B, Turney JH et al. Nephrol Dial Transplant 1996;11:1613–8.

160. Palop L, Martinez JA. Am J Clin Nutr 1997;66:498S–503S.

161. Dwyer JT, Cunniff PJ, Maroni BJ et al. J Renal Nutr 1998;8: 11–20.

162. Aparicio M, Cano N, Chauveau P et al. Nephrol Dial Transplant 1999;14:1679–86.

163. Chung SH, Na MH, Lee SH et al. Perit Dial Int 1999;19: 517S–22S.

164. Williams AJ, McArley A. J Ren Nutr 1999;9:157–62.

165. Carlson DM, Duncan DA, Naessens JM et al. Mayo Clin Proc 1984;59:769–75.

166. Hirschberg R. Drug-nutrient interactions in renal failure. In: Kopple JD, Massry SG, eds. Nutritional Management of Renal Disease. 2nd ed. Philadelphia: Lippincott Williams & Wilkins, 2004:593–603.

167. Lowrie EG, Lew NL. Am J Kidney Dis 1990;15:458.

168. Delano BG, Manis JG, Manis T. Nephron 1977;19:26.

169. Lawson DH, Bodd K, King PC et al. Clin Sci 1971;41:345–51.

170. Mahajan SK Prasad AS, Lambujon J et al. Am J Clin Nutr 1980; 33:1517–21.

171. Kopple JD, Mercurio K, Blumenkrantz MJ et al. Kidney Int 1981;19:694–704.

172. Sprenger KBG, Bundschu D, Lewis K et al. Kidney Int Suppl 1983;24:315S–8S.

173. Bellinghieri G Savica V, Mallamace A et al. Am J Clin Nutr 1983;38:523–31.

174. Kopple JD, Berg R, Houser H et al. Kidney Int Suppl 1989;36: 184S–94S.

175. Mehrotra R, Kopple JD. Causes of protein-energy malnutrition in chronic renal failure. In: Kopple JD, Massry SG, eds. Nutritional Management of Renal Disease. 2nd ed. Philadelphia: Lippincott Williams & Wilkins, 2004:167–82.

176. Grodstein GP, Blumenkrantz MJ, Kopple JD. Am J Clin Nutr 1980;33:1411–6.

177. Keane WF, Collins AJ. Am J Kidney Dis 1994;24:1010–8.

178. US Renal Data System. Am J Kidney Dis 2005;45[Suppl 1]: 1S–280S.

179. Wolfson M, Jones MR, Kopple JD. Kidney Int 1982;21:500–6.

180. Ikizler TA, Flakoll PJ, Parker RA et al. Kidney Int 1994; 46:830–7.

181. Kopple JD Blumenkrantz MJ, Jones MR et al. Am J Clin Nutr 1982;36:395–402.

182. Chazot C, Shahmir E, Matias B et al. Kidney Int 1997;52: 1663–70.

183. Blumenkrantz MJ, Gahl GM, Kopple JD et al. Kidney Int 1981;19:593–602.

184. Wathen RL Keshaviah P, Hommeyer P et al. Am J Clin Nutr 1978;31:1870–5.

185. Gutierrez A, Alvestrand A, Wahren J et al. Kidney Int 1990;38: 487–94.

186. Gutierrez A, Bergström J, Alvestrand A. Clin Nephrol 1992; 38:20.

187. Mehrotra R, Kopple JD, Wolfson M. Kidney Int Suppl 2003;88: 13S–25S.

188. Linton AL, Clark WF, Driedger AA et al. Nephron 1977;19: 95–8.

189. Kopple JD. Dietary Considerations in patients with chronic renal failure, acute renal failure, and transplantation. In: Schrier RW ed. Diseases of the Kidney. 7th ed. Philadelphia: Lippincott Williams & Wilkins, 2001:3085–3138.

190. Kalantar-Zadeh K, Ikizler TA, Block G et al. Am J Kidney Dis 2003;43:864–81.

191. Zimmerman J, Herrlinger S, Pruy A et al. Kidney Int 1999;55: 648–58.

192. Stenvinkel P, Yuen, JY. Role of inflammation in malnutrition and atherosclerosis in chronic renal failure. In: Kopple JD, Massry SG, eds. Nutritional Management of Renal Disease. 2nd ed. Philadelphia: Lippincott Williams & Wilkins, 2004:199–212.

193. Kalantar-Zadeh K, Stenvinkel P, Pillon L et al. Adv Ren Replace Ther 2003;10:155–9.

194. Pereira BJG, Shapiro L, King AJ et al. Kidney Int 1994;45:890–6.

195. Bologa RM, Levine DM, Parker TS et al. Am J Kidney Dis 1998;32:107–14.

196. Witko-Sarsat V, Friedlander M, Khoa TN et al. J Immunol 1998;161:2524–32.

197. Mezzano D, Pais EO, Aranda E et al. Kidney Int 2001;60: 1844–50.

198. Horl WH. Oxidant stress. In: Kopple JD, Massry SG, eds. Nutritional Management of Renal Disease. 2nd ed. Philadelphia: Lippincott Williams & Wilkins, 2004:99–110.

199. Miyata T, Kurokawa K. Carbonyl stress in uremia. In: Kopple JD, Massry SG, eds. Nutritional Management of Renal Disease. 2nd ed. Philadelphia: Lippincott Williams & Wilkins, 2004:111–5.

200. Bachmann J, Tepel M, Raidt H et al. J Am Soc Nephrol 1995;6: 121–5.

201. Robinson K, Gupta A, Dennis V et al. Circulation 1996;94: 2743–8.

202. Kalantar-Zadeh K, Block G, Humphreys MH et al. J Am Soc Nephrol 2004;15:442–53.

203. Welch GN, Loscalzo J. N Engl J Med 1998;338:1042–50.

204. Kopple JD. Am Soc Artificial Int Organs J 1997;43:246–50.

205. Kalantar-Zadeh K, Kopple JD. Nutritional management of patients undergoing maintenance hemodialysis. In: Kopple JD, Massry SG, eds. Nutritional Management of Renal Disease. 2nd ed. Philadelphia: Lippincott Williams & Wilkins, 2004:433–56.

206. Garcia-Martinez C, Llovera M, Agell N et al. Biochem Biophys Res Commun 1994;201:682–6.

207. Sarraf P, Frederich RC, Turner EM et al. J Exp Med 1997;185: 171–5.

208. Stenvinkel P, Heimburger O, Lindholm B et al. Nephrol Dial Transplant 2000;15:953–60.

209. Kalantar-Zadeh K, Kopple JD. Am J Kidney Dis 2001;38: 1343–50.

210. Kopple JD, Zhu X, Lew NL et al. Kidney Int 1999;56:1136–48.

211. Port FK, Ashby VB, Dhingra RK et al. J Am Soc Nephrol 2002; 13:1061–6.

212. Kalantar-Zadeh K, Block G, Humphreys MH et al. Kidney Int 2003;63:793–808.

213. Liu Y, Coresh J, Eustace JA et al. JAMA 2004;291:451–9.

214. Kalantar-Zadeh K, Block G, Humphreys MH et al. J Am Soc Nephrol 2004;15:442–53.

215. Kalantar-Zadeh K, Kopple JD, Humphreys MH et al. Nephrol Dial Transplant 2004;19:1507–19.

216. Johansen KL, Young B, Kaysen GA et al. Am J Clin Nutr 2004; 80:324–32.

217. Leavey SF, McCullough K, Hecking E et al. Nephrol Dial Transplant 2001;16:2386–94.

218. Kalantar-Zadeh K, Kilpatrick RD, McAllister CJ et al. (submitted).

219. Kalantar-Zadeh K, Kilpatrick RD, McAllister CJ et al. J Am Soc Nephrol 2004;15:126A.
220. Kopple JD. Am J Clin Nutr 2005 (in press).
221. Burrowes JD, Cockram DB. Achieving patient adherence to diet therapy. In: Kopple JD, Massry SG, eds. Nutritional Management of Renal Disease. 2nd ed. Philadelphia: Lippincott Williams & Wilkins, 2004:629–39.
222. Haynes RB. Strategies for improving compliance: A methodologic analysis and review. In: Sacket DL, Haynes RB, eds. Compliance with Therapeutic Regimens. Baltimore: Johns Hopkins University Press, 1976:69–82.
223. Kopple JD, Greene T, Chumlea WC et al. Kidney Int 2000;57:1688–703.
224. Ikizler TA, Greene JH, Wingard RL et al. J Am Soc Nephrol 1995;6:1386–91.
225. Mehrotra R, Berman N, Alistwani A et al. Am J Kidney Dis 2002;40:133–42.
226. Salusky I, Fine RN, Nelson P et al. In: Proceedings of the American Society of Nephrology 15th Annual Meeting, December 1982:66A(abst).
227. Calloway DH, Odell ACF, Margen S. J Nutr 1971;101:775–86.
228. Sargent JA, Gotch FA. J Am Diet Assoc 1979;75:547–51.
229. Maroni BJ, Steinman TI, Mitch WE. Kidney Int 1985;27:58–65.
230. Kopple JD, Gao X-L, Qing DP-Y. Kidney Int 1997;52:486–94.
231. Varcoe R, Halliday D, Carson ER et al. Clin Sci Mol Med 1975;43:379–90.
232. Walser M. J Clin Invest 1974;53:1385–92.
233. Bergström J, Fürst P, Alvestrand A et al. Kidney Int 1993;44:1048–57.
234. Blake P, Daugirdas J. Quantification and prescription: General principles. In: Jacobs C, Kjellstrand CM, Koch KM et al., eds. Replacement of Renal Function by Dialysis. 4th rev. ed. Dordrecht: Kluwer Academic Publishers, 1996:619–56.
235. Kopple JD, Jones MR, Keshaviah PR et al. Am J Kidney Dis 1995;26:963–81.
236. Kopple JD, Coburn JW. JAMA 1974;227:41–4.
237. Frisancho AR. Am J Clin Nutr 1984;40:808.
238. American Dietetic Association. Manual of Clinical Dietetics. Chicago: American Dietetic Association, 1988:Appendix 48, 623.
239. Kopple JD, Coburn JW. Medicine (Baltimore) 1973;52:583–95.
240. Kopple JD. Treatment with low protein and amino acid diets in chronic renal failure. In: Barcelo R, Bergeron M, Carriere S et al., eds. Proceedings of the VIIIth International Congress of Nephrology. Basel: S. Karger, 1978:497–507.
241. National Kidney Foundation. Am J Kidney Dis 2000;35[Suppl 2]:1S–140S.
242. Kaysen GA, Al-Bander H. Am J Nephrol 1990;10:36.
243. Borah MF, Schoenfeld PY, Gotch FA et al. Kidney Int 1978;14:491–500.
244. Kopple JD, Shinaberger JH, Coburn JW et al. Trans Am Soc Artif Intern Organs 1969;15:302–8.
245. Blumenkrantz MJ, Kopple JD, Moran JK et al. Kidney Int 1982;21:849–61.
246. World Health Organization. Energy and Protein Requirements. Report of a Joint FAO/WHO/UNU Expert Consultation. Technical Report Series no. 724. Geneva: World Health Organization, 1985:1–206.
247. Kopple JD, Monteon FJ, Shaib JK. Kidney Int 1986;29:734–42.
248. Monteon FJ, Laidlaw SA, Shaib JK et al. Kidney Int 1986;30:741–7.
249. Schwickardi M, Lange H. In: Abstract of the VIIth International Congress on Nutrition and Metabolism in Renal Disease, Stockholm, May 29–Jun 1, 1994:51.
250. Slomowitz LA, Monteon FJ, Grosvenor M et al. Kidney Int 1989;35:704–11.
251. Wolfson M, Strong CJ, Minturn D et al. Am J Clin Nutr 1984;39:547–55.
252. Marckmann P. Clin Nephrol 1988;29:75–8.
253. Kopple JD. Kidney Int 1978;14:340–8.
254. Kluthe R, Luttgen FM, Capetianu T et al. Am J Clin Nutr 1978;31:1812–20.
255. Blumenkrantz MJ, Kopple JD, Gutman RA et al. Am J Clin Nutr 1980;33:1567–85.
256. Appel G. Kidney Int 1991;39:169–83.
257. Attman PO. Nephrol Dial Transplant 1993;8:294.
258. Cocchi R, Viglino G, Cancarini G et al. Miner Electrolyte Metab 1996;22:22–5.
259. Wanner C, Bartens W, Nauck M et al. Miner Electrolyte Metab 1996;22:26–30.
260. Wanner C. Lipid metabolism in renal disease and renal failure. In: Kopple JD, Massry SG, eds. Nutritional Management of Renal Disease. 2nd ed. Philadelphia: Lippincott Williams & Wilkins, 2004:35–62.
261. Roncari DAK, Breckenridge WC, Khanna R et al. Perit Dial Bull 1988;1:136–41.
262. Boeschoten EW, Zuyderhoudt FMJ, Krediet RT et al. Perit Dial Bull 1988;19:8–13.
263. Deighan CJ, Caslake MJ, McConnell M et al. Am J Kidney Dis 2000;35:852–62.
264. Samuelsson O, Attmann PO, Knight-Gibson C et al. Nephrol Dial Transplant 1991;9:1580–5.
265. Chan MK, Varghese Z, Moorhead JF. Kidney Int 1981;19:625–37.
266. Ciman M, Rizzoli V, Moracchiello M et al. Am J Clin Nutr 1980;33:1489–92.
267. Bellinghieri G, Savica V, Mallamace A et al. Am J Clin Nutr 1983;38:523–31.
268. Wanner C, Rader D, Bartens W et al. Ann Intern Med 1993;119:263–9.
269. Joven J, Villabona C, Vilella E et al. N Engl J Med 1990;323:579–84.
270. Ibels LS, Alfrey AC, Weil R III. Am J Med 1978;64:634.
271. Nelson J, Beauregard H, Gelinas M et al. Transplant Proc 1988;20:1264–70.
272. Dimëny E, Fellstrom B, Larsson E et al. Transplant Proc 1992;24:366.
273. National Cholesterol Education Program (NCEP) Expert Panel on Detection, Evaluation, and Treatment of High Blood Cholesterol in Adults (Adult Treatment Panel III). JAMA 2001;285:2486–97.
274. Thomas ME, Harris KPG, Ramaswamy C et al. Kidney Int 1993;44:1124–9.
275. Wanner C. Presentation at the 37th Annual Meeting of the American Society of Nephrology. October 27–November 1, 2004.
276. Ciman M, Rizzoli V, Moracchiello M et al. Am J Clin Nutr 1980;33:1489–92.
277. Bellinghieri G, Savica V, Mallamace A et al. Am J Clin Nutr 1983;38:523–31.
278. Guarnieri G, Toigo G, Crapesi L et al. Kidney Int Suppl 1987;32:116S–27S.
279. Wanner C, Horl WH. Nephron 1988;50:89.
280. Pierides AM, Alvarez-Ude F, Kerr DNS et al. Lancet 1979;2:1279–82.
281. Leaf A, Weber PC. N Engl J Med 1988;318:549.
282. Donadio JV Jr, Bergstralh EJ, Offord KP et al. N Engl J Med 1994;331:1194–9.

283. Manis T, Deutsch J, Feinstein EI et al. Am J Clin Nutr 1980;33: 1485–8.

284. Hamazaki T, Nakazawa R, Tateno S et al. Kidney Int 1984;26: 1–84.

285. Brousseau ME, Schaefer EJ, Wolfe ML et al. N Engl J Med 2004;350:1491–4.

286. Bremer J. Physiol Rev 1983;63:1420.

287. Vacha GM, Corsi M, Giorcelli G et al. Curr Ther Res 1985;37: 505.

288. Hiatt WR, Koziol BJ, Shapiro JI et al. Kidney Int 1992;41: 1613–9.

289. Golper TA, Wolfson M, Ahmad S et al. Kidney Int 1990;38: 904–11.

290. Ahmad S, Robertson HT, Gloper TA et al. Kidney Int 1990;38: 912–8.

291. van Es A, Henny FC, Kooistra MP et al. Contrib Nephrol 1992; 98:28–35.

292. Golper TA, Ahmad S. Semin Dial 1992;5:94–8.

293. Labonia WD. Am J Kidney Dis 1995;26:757–64.

294. Symposium on Role Dietary Fiber in Health. Am J Clin Nutr 1978;31:1S–291S.

295. Parillo M, Riccardi G, Pacioni D et al. Diabetes Care 1985;8: 620.

296. Anderson JW, Zettwoch N, Feldman T et al. Arch Intern Med 1988;148:292.

297. Anderson JW, Chen WL. Am J Clin Nutr 1979;32:346.

298. Rampton DS, Cohen SL, Crammond VDeB et al. Clin Nephrol 1984;21:159–63.

299. Cannata JB, Briggs JD, Junor BJR. BMJ 1983;286:1937–8.

300. Sedman AB, Miller NL, Warady BA et al. Kidney Int 1984;26: 201–4.

301. Nolan CR, Califano JR, Butzin CA. Kidney Int 1990;38:937–41.

302. Schaefer K, Scheer J, Asmus G et al. Nephrol Dial Transplant 1991;6:170–5.

303. Mai ML, Emmett M, Sheikh MS et al. Kidney Int 1989;36: 690–5.

304. Pflanz S, Henderson IS, McElduff N et al. Nephrol Dial Transplant 1994;9:1121.

305. Chertow GM, Burke SK, Raggi P. Kidney Int 2002;62:245–52.

306. Chertow GM. J Am Soc Nephrol 2003;14:310S–4S.

307. Al-Baaj F, Speake M, Hutchison AJ. Nephrol Dial Transplant 2005 (in press).

308. Lacour B, Lucas A, Auchere D et al. Kidney Int 2005;67: 1062–9.

309. Kopple JD, Coburn JW. Medicine (Baltimore) 1973;52: 597–607.

310. Teng M, Wolf M, Lowrie E et al. N Engl J Med 2003;349: 446–56.

311. Lindberg JS, Culleton B, Won G et al. J Am Soc Nephrol 2005; 16:800–7.

312. Moe SM, Chertow GM, Coburn JW et al. Kidney Int 2005;67: 760–71.

313. Colloton M, Shatzen E, Miller G et al. Kidney Int 2005;67: 467–76.

314. Sherrard DJ, Hercz G, Pei Y et al. Kidney Int 1993;43:436–42.

315. Faugere MC, Malluche HH. Kidney Int 1986;30:717–22.

316. Hercz G, Pei Y, Greenwood C et al. Kidney Int 1993;44:860–6.

317. Randall RE Jr, Cohen MD, Spray CC Jr et al. Ann Intern Med 1964;61:73–8.

318. Koomans HA, Roos JC, Boer P et al. Hypertension 1982;4:190–7.

319. Lawson DH, Boddy K, King PC et al. Clin Sci 1971;41:345–51.

320. Chen SM. J Formosan Med Assoc 1990;89:220.

321. Rudolph H, Alfrey AC, Smythe WR. Trans Am Soc Artif Intern Organs 1973;19:456–65.

322. Cartwright GE, Gubler CJ, Wintrobe MM. J Clin Invest 1964; 33:685.

323. Sprenger KBG, Bundschu D, Lewis K et al. Kidney Int Suppl 1983;24:315S–8S.

324. Taylor JE, Peat N, Porter C et al. Nephrol Dial Transplant 1996; 11:1079–83.

325. Ahsan N. J Am Soc Nephrol 1998;9:664–8.

326. Mahajan SK, Bowersox EM, Rye DL et al. Kidney Int Suppl 1989;27:269S–73S.

327. Mansouri K, Halsted JA, Gombos EA. Arch Intern Med 1970; 125:88–93.

328. Food and Nutrition Board, Institute of Medicine. Dietary Reference Intakes for Vitamin A, Vitamin K, Arsenic, Boron, Chromium, Copper, Iodine, Iron, Manganese, Molybdenum, Nickel, Silicon, Vanadium, and Zinc. Washington, DC: National Academy Press, 2002.

329. Mahajan SK, Abraham J, Hessburg T et al. Kidney Int Suppl 1983;24:310S–4S.

330. Antoniou LD, Shalhoub RJ, Sudhakar T et al. Lancet 1977;2: 895–8.

331. Rodger RS, Sheldon WL, Watson MJ et al. Nephrol Dial Transplant 1989;4:888.

332. Food and Nutrition Board, Institute of Medicine. Dietary Reference Intakes for Thiamin, Riboflavin, Niacin, Vitamin B$_6$, Folate, Vitamin B$_{12}$, Panthothenic Acid, Biotin, and Choline. Washington, DC: National Academy Press, 1999.

333. Jennette JC, Goldman ID. J Lab Clin Med 1975;86:834–43.

334. Spannuth CL Jr, Warnock LG, Wagner C et al. J Lab Clin Med 1977;90:32–7.

335. Descombes E, Hanck AB, Fellay G. Kidney Int 1993;43: 1319–28.

336. Kopple JD, Mercurio K, Blumenkrantz MJ et al. Kidney Int 1981;19:94–104.

337. Kopple JD, Swendseid ME. Kidney Int Suppl 1975;7:79S–84S.

338. Balcke P, Schmidt P, Zazgornik J et al. Ann Intern Med 1984; 101:344–5.

339. Pru C, Eaton J, Kjellstrand C. Nephron 1985;39:112–6.

340. Smith FR, Goodman DS. J Clin Invest 1971;50:2426–36.

341. Yatzidis H, Digenis P et al. BMJ 1975;2:352–3.

342. Udall JA. JAMA 1965;194:127.

343. Kopple JD, Massry, S.G. Am J Nephrol 1988;8:437–48.

344. Reichel H, Koeffler HP, Norman AW. N Engl J Med 1989;320: 980–91.

345. May RC, Kelly RA, Mitch WE. J Clin Invest 1987;79:1099–103.

346. Reaich D, Channon SM, Scrimgeour CM et al. Am J Physiol 1992;263:E735–9.

347. Mehrotra R, Kopple JD, Wolfson M. Kidney Int Suppl 2003;88: 13S–25S.

348. Mault JR, Bartlett RH, Dechert RE et al. Trans Am Soc Artif Intern Organs 1983;29:390–4.

349. Flugel-Link RM, Salusky IB, Jones MR et al. Am J Physiol 1983;244:E615–23.

350. Clark AS, Mitch WE. J Clin Invest 1983;72:836–45.

351. Frohlich J, Scholmerich J, Hoppe-Seyler G et al. Eur J Clin Invest 1974;4:453–8.

352. Feinstein EI, Blumenkrantz MJ, Healy H et al. Medicine (Baltimore) 1981;60:124–37.

353. Feinstein EI, Kopple JD, Silberman H. Kidney Int Suppl 1983;26:319S–23S.

354. Kopple JD. JPEN J Parenter Enteral Nutr 1996;20:3–12.

355. Abel RM, Abbott WM, Beck CH Jr et al. Am J Surg 1974;128: 317–23.

356. Abel RM, Shih VE, Abbott WM et al. Ann Surg 1974;180: 350–5.

357. Abel RM, Beck CH Jr, Abbott WM et al. N Engl J Med 1973; 288:695–9.

358. Baek SM, Makabali GG, Bryan-Brown CW et al. Surg Gynecol Obstet 1975;141:405–8.

359. McMurray SD, Luft FC, Maxwell DR et al. Arch Intern Med 1978;138:950–5.

360. Leonard CD, Luke RG, Siegel RR. Urology 1975;6:154–7.

361. Kopple JD, Swendseid ME. Am J Clin Nutr 1974;27:806–12.

362. Toback FG. Kidney Int 1977;12:193–8.

363. Toback FG, Teegarden DE, Havener LJ. Kidney Int 1979;15: 542–7.

364. Toback FG, Dodd RC, Maier, ER et al. Clin Res 1979;27: 432A(abst).

365. Oken DE, Sprinkel FM, Kirschbaum BB et al. Kidney Int 1980;17:14–23.

366. Nakasaki H, Katayama T, Yokoyama S et al. JPEN J Parenter Enteral Nutr 1993;17:86–90.

367. Mehta RL. Semin Nephrol 1994;14:64–82.

368. Davenport A, Roberts NB. Crit Care Med 1989;17:1010.

369. Davies SP, Reaveley DA, Brown EA et al. Crit Care Med 1991; 19:1510–5.

370. Feinstein EI, Collins JF, Blumenkrantz MJ et al. Prog Artif Organs 1984;1:421–6.

371. Kopple JD, Bernard D, Messana J et al. Kidney Int 1995;47: 1148–57.

372. Cerra FB, Upson D, Angelico R et al. Surgery 1982;92: 192–200.

373. Daly M, Mihranian MH, Kehoe JI et al. Surgery 1983;94: 151–9.

374. Leander U, Fürst P, Vesterberg K et al. Clin Nutr 19854:43–51.

375. Hammarqvist F, Wernerman J, Ruston A et al. Ann Surg 1989;209:455–61.

376. Stehle P, Zander J, Mertes N et al. Lancet 1989;1:231–3.

377. Daly JM, Reynolds J, Thom A et al. Ann Surg 1988;208:512–23.

378. McCracken BH, Parsons FM. Lancet 1958;2:885–6.

379. Gjorup S, Thaysen JH. Acta Med Scand 1960;167:27–238.

380. Hinton P, Allison SP, Littlejohn S et al. Lancet 19711:767–9.

381. Woolfson AMJ, Healtley RV, Allison SP. N Engl J Med 1979;300:14–7.

382. Ponting GA, Halliday D, Teale JD et al. Lancet 1988;1:438–40.

383. Wilmore DW. N Engl J Med 1991;325:695.

384. Kopple JD, Brunori G, Leiserowitz M et al. Nephrol Dial Transplant 2005 (in press).

385. Dahn MS, Lange P, Jacobs LA. Arch Surg 1988;123:1409.

386. Takala J, Ruokonen E, Webster NR et al. N Engl J Med 1999; 341:785–92.

387. Miller SB, Martin DR, Kissane J et al. Proc Natl Acad Sci USA 1992;89:11876–80.

388. Ding H, Kopple JD, Cohen A et al. J Clin Invest 1993;91: 2281–7.

389. Hirschberg R, Kopple JD, Lipsett P et al. Kidney Int 1999;55: 2423–32.

390. Humes HD, Cieslinski DA, Coimbra TM et al. J Clin Invest 1989;84:1757–61.

391. Miller SB, Martin Dr, Kissane J et al. Am J Physiol 1994;266: F129–34.

392. Siegel NJ, Gaudio KM, Katz LA et al. Kidney Int 1984;25:906–11.

393. Rahman SN, Kim GE, Mathew AS et al. Kidney Int 1994;45: 1731–8.

394. Siegel NJ, Glazier WB, Chaudry IH et al. Kidney Int 1980;17: 338–49.

395. Kopple JD, Jones MR, Keshaviah PR et al. Am J Kidney Dis 1995;26:963–81.

396. Harris JA, Benedict FG. A biometric study of basal metabolism. In: Man. Publ. no. 279. Washington, DC: Carnegie Institute, 1919.

397. Garrel DR, Jobin N, de Jonge LHM. Nutr Clin Pract 1996;11: 99–103.

398. Wilmore DW. The metabolic management of the critically ill. In: The Metabolic Management of the Critically Ill. New York: Plenum Press, 1977:314.

399. Kopple JD. Nutritional management of acute renal failure. In: Kopple JD, Massry SG, eds. Nutritional Management of Renal Disease. 2nd ed. Philadelphia: Lippincott Williams & Wilkins, 2004:549–72.

400. Askanazi J, Elwyn DH, Silverberg BS et al. Surgery 1980;87: 596–8.

401. Jeejeebhoy KN, Langer B, Tsallas G et al. Gastroenterology 1976;71:943–53.

402. Seidner DL, Mascioli EA, Istfan NW et al. JPEN J Parenter Enteral Nutr 1989;13:614–9.

403. Driscoll DF, Baptista BJ Bistrian BR et al. Am J Hosp Pharm 1986;43:416–9.

404. Capelli JP et al. Am J Kidney Dis 1994;23:808.

405. Chertow GM et al. Am J Kidney Dis 1994;24:912.

406. Zager RA, Johannes G, Tuttle SE et al. J Lab Clin Med 1983; 101:130–40.

407. Zager RA, Venkatachalam MA. Kidney Int 1983;24:620–5.

408. Malis CD, Racusen C, Solez K et al. J Lab Clin Med 1984;103: 660–76.

409. Andrews PM, Bates SB. Kidney Int Suppl 1987;32:76S–80S.

410. Weinberg JM. Semin Nephrol 1990;10:491–500.

95 FOOD ALLERGIES AND INTOLERANCES[1]

STEVE L. TAYLOR AND SUSAN L. HEFLE

DEFINITION AND CLASSIFICATION 1512
IMMUNOGLOBULIN E–MEDIATED FOOD ALLERGIES .1513
    Mechanism 1513
    Symptoms 1514
    Sources 1515
    Food Allergens 1516
    Prevalence 1516
    Persistence 1516
    Prevention 1516
    Diagnosis 1517
    Management 1518
    Minimal Eliciting Dose (Threshold) 1519
    Detection of Residues of Allergenic Foods 1520
    Effects of Processing on Allergenicity 1520
    Allergenicity of Foods Produced through
       Agricultural Biotechnology 1520
DELAYED HYPERSENSITIVITY REACTIONS 1521
CELIAC DISEASE 1521
    Mechanism 1521
    Symptoms and Sequelae 1521
    Sources 1521
    Causative Factor 1521
    Prevalence and Persistence 1522
    Management and Minimal Eliciting Dose 1522
    Detection 1522
FOOD INTOLERANCES 1522
LACTOSE INTOLERANCE 1522
    Sources, Properties, and Occurrence in Foods . . .1523
    Prevalence 1523
    Minimal Eliciting Dose and Management 1523
FAVISM 1523
SULFITE-INDUCED ASTHMA 1524
    Sources, Properties, and Occurrence in Foods . . .1524
    Prevalence and Severity 1524
    Management 1524
ALLERGYLIKE INTOXICATIONS
    (HISTAMINE POISONING) 1525
    Symptoms and Features 1525

Diagnosis and Treatment 1525
Sources and Formation 1526
Toxicology 1526
Preventive Measures .1527
CONCLUSIONS 1527

Centuries ago, the Roman philosopher Lucretius stated, "What is food to one is bitter poison to another." Food allergies and related illnesses can be collectively referred to as "individualistic adverse reactions to foods." These illnesses affect certain persons within the population, but not others. Although these individualistic adverse reactions to foods are often grouped together under the general heading of food allergy, in fact, a variety of different types of illnesses are involved. Several different types of individualistic adverse reactions to foods occur, having different symptoms, severity, prevalence, and causative factors, although this fact is not recognized by some physicians and many consumers. When properly diagnosed by medical professionals, food allergies and related diseases can be successfully treated and symptoms can be avoided by following specific avoidance diets. Nutritional advice is often desirable in the construction of safe and effective avoidance diets.

However, consumers sometimes do not seek medical attention for these conditions, relying instead on self-diagnosis or parental diagnosis of the conditions experienced by infants and young children. Consumers perceive that food allergies are quite common (1), whereas, in fact, many self-diagnosed cases of food allergy incorrectly associate foods with a particular malady or ascribe various mild forms of postprandial eating discomfort to this category of illness. As a result, some consumers mistakenly attempt to avoid certain foods. Although the result of such needless avoidance diets is harmless in many cases, nutritional problems can occur, especially when attempts are made to avoid many foods.

DEFINITION AND CLASSIFICATION

Most consumers and some physicians improperly classify any abnormal response to ingestion of food as a food allergy. In fact, several different types of individualistic

[1] **Abbreviations: DBPCFC,** double-blind, placebo-controlled food challenge; **G6PDH,** glucose-6-phosphate dehydrogenase; **Ig,** immunoglobulin; **OAS,** oral allergy syndrome; **RAST,** radioallergosorbent test; **SPT,** skin-prick test.

TABLE 95.1. CLASSIFICATION OF INDIVIDUALISTIC ADVERSE REACTIONS TO FOODS

True food allergies
  Antibody-mediated food allergies
    Immunoglobulin E–mediated food allergies (peanut, cows' milk, etc.) including oral allergy syndrome
    Exercise-associated food allergies
  Cell-mediated food allergies
    Celiac disease
    Food protein–induced enterocolitis
    Food protein–induced enteropathy
    Food protein–induced proctitis
    Other types of delayed hypersensitivity
  Either antibody-mediated and/or cell-mediated
    Allergic eosinophilic gastroenteritis
    Allergic eosinophilic esophagitis
Food intolerances
  Anaphylactoid reactions
  Metabolic food disorders
    Lactose intolerance
    Favism
  Idiosyncratic reactions
    Sulfite-induced asthma

adverse reactions are known to occur, and only certain types of reactions can be correctly classified as true food allergies.

A classification scheme for the different types of individualistic adverse reactions to foods or food sensitivities that occur in association with food ingestion is provided in Table 95.1. Two major groups of food sensitivity are known: true food allergies and food intolerances (2). Although true food allergies involve abnormal immunologic mechanisms, food intolerances do not. The differences between immunologic food allergies and nonimmunologic food intolerances are significant for the affected person. Food intolerances can usually be managed by limiting the amount of the food or food ingredient that is eaten; total avoidance is usually not necessary for food intolerances. In contrast, total avoidance of the offending food is typically necessary with true food allergies. In addition, allergylike intoxications can occur with certain foods (3). Although this form of food poisoning is sometimes clinically confused with food allergy, it is distinctly different because all consumers would be potentially susceptible.

Food allergies are abnormal immunologic responses to a particular food or food component, usually a naturally occurring protein (4, 5). Immediate hypersensitivity reactions and delayed hypersensitivity reactions are well-documented types of immunologic responses that can occur in certain persons on ingestion of specific foods. Immediate hypersensitivity reactions are immunoglobulin E (IgE)-mediated reactions, and symptoms ensue within minutes of the ingestion of the offending food. Delayed hypersensitivity reactions are cell-mediated reactions, and symptoms develop 48 to 72 hours after ingestion of the offending food. The role of cell-mediated reactions in food

allergies is far less well established, with the exception of celiac disease, the only type of delayed hypersensitivity discussed in this chapter.

In contrast, food intolerances do not involve abnormal responses of the immune system (6). Three mechanistically distinct forms of food intolerances are recognized: anaphylactoid reactions, metabolic food disorders, and idiosyncratic reactions.

As the name implies, allergylike intoxications are often confused with true food allergies because the symptoms are identical (3). Histamine poisoning is the primary example of an allergylike intoxication.

IMMUNOGLOBULIN E–MEDIATED FOOD ALLERGIES

IgE-mediated food allergies are arguably the most important class of food sensitivities. Although the number of affected persons is relatively small, the reactions in some persons in this group can be life-threatening, especially if a significant quantity of the offending food is inadvertently ingested. In addition, the degree of tolerance for the offending food is small, making the implementation of safe and effective avoidance diets more difficult.

Mechanism

IgE-mediated or immediate hypersensitivity reactions are associated with the rapid onset of symptoms, usually within minutes to a few hours, after the ingestion of the offending food. Immediate hypersensitivity reactions are mediated by an allergen-specific IgE antibody, as depicted in Figure 95.1 (4). Food allergens are typically naturally occurring proteins in foods (7). In IgE-mediated food allergies, exposure to the allergen stimulates the production of allergen-specific IgE antibodies by plasma cells in susceptible persons (6). The allergen-specific IgE attaches itself to the surface of mast cells in various tissues and basophils in the blood. This process is known as sensitization.

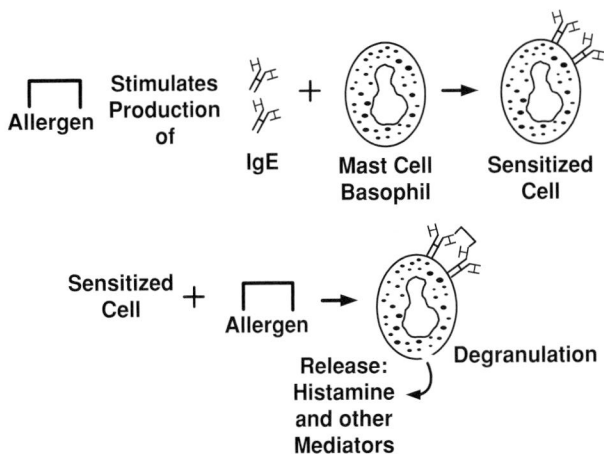

Figure 95.1. Mechanism of immunoglobulin E–mediated food allergy.

During the sensitization phase, the susceptible person will form allergen-specific IgE antibodies on exposure to a specific food protein. However, even among susceptible persons, exposure to food proteins does not usually result in the formation of IgE antibodies. In physiologically normal persons, exposure to a food protein in the gastrointestinal tract results in oral tolerance through either the formation of protein-specific IgG, IgM, or IgA antibodies or no immunologic response whatsoever (clonal anergy) (8, 9). Heredity and other physiologic factors are important in predisposing persons to the development of IgE-mediated allergies, including food allergies (10). Monozygotic and dizygotic twins demonstrate that genetics is an extremely important parameter and that identical twins may even inherit the likelihood of responding to the same allergenic food, e.g., peanuts (11, 12). Approximately 65% of patients with clinically documented allergy have first-degree relatives with allergic disease (10). Conditions that increase the permeability of the small intestinal mucosa to proteins, such as viral gastroenteritis, premature birth, and cystic fibrosis, also seem to increase the risk of development of food allergy.

Although the sensitization process is symptomless, the affected person is now primed for an allergic reaction. On subsequent exposure to the allergenic food, the allergen cross-links IgE molecules on the surface of the mast cell or basophil membrane, causing these cells to release various mediators of the allergic reaction into the bloodstream and tissues. Dozens of physiologically active mediators of the allergic reaction have been identified (4). Histamine is one of the most important mediators of the immediate hypersensitivity reaction and can elicit inflammation, pruritus, and contraction of the smooth muscles in the blood vessels, gastrointestinal tract, and respiratory tract (6). Other important mediators include various leukotrienes and prostaglandins (6). The released mediators interact with receptors in various tissues, eliciting a wide range of physiologic responses. Because the mediators are released into the bloodstream, systemic reactions involving multiple tissues and organs can ensue.

Allergies to pollens, mold spores, animal danders, dust mites, certain drugs (e.g., penicillin), and bee venom also occur through this same IgE-mediated mechanism. Susceptible persons may form allergen-specific IgE to one or several substances, including food allergens. Occupational food allergies are also known to occur, in which persons are affected by contact with or inhalation of the offending food rather than by its ingestion (13).

Symptoms

Numerous symptoms can be associated with IgE-mediated food allergies, ranging from mild and annoying to severe and life-threatening (Table 95.2) (2). Only a few of these symptoms will be apparent in each allergic person. The nature of the symptoms and their severity depend on several factors,

including the person, the amount of the offending food ingested, the tissue receptors that are affected, and the length of time since the last previous exposure.

As noted in Table 95.2, the symptoms of IgE-mediated reactions can involve the gastrointestinal tract, skin, or respiratory tract. Gastrointestinal and cutaneous symptoms are among the more common manifestations of IgE-mediated food allergies. Although respiratory symptoms are much less commonly encountered in food-allergic reactions, persons with respiratory manifestations of their food allergies may be more likely to experience severe and life-threatening reactions (14). Mild respiratory symptoms (rhinitis, rhinoconjunctivitis) are much more likely to be encountered with exposure to environmental allergens such as pollens or animal danders that are airborne and inhaled directly into the respiratory tract. Although these mild respiratory symptoms are mostly annoying, those few food-allergic persons who experience serious respiratory manifestations (asthma, laryngeal edema) in association with the inadvertent ingestion of the offending food are most likely to be at risk for life-threatening episodes (14).

Among the many symptoms involved in IgE-mediated food allergies, anaphylactic shock is the most severe manifestation. Anaphylactic shock can involve multiple organ systems (gastrointestinal, respiratory, cutaneous, and cardiovascular) and numerous symptoms. Death can ensue from severe hypotension coupled with respiratory and cardiovascular complications. Comparatively few persons are susceptible to suffering such severe reactions to food ingestion. The severity of an allergic reaction is dependent on the degree of sensitivity of the person and the amount of the offending food that is ingested (2). The inadvertent ingestion of allergenic foods has resulted in deaths (14–16). Anaphylactic shock is a common cause of these fatalities. Deaths have occurred with most of the common allergenic

TABLE 95.2. SYMPTOMS ASSOCIATED WITH IMMUNOGLOBULIN E–MEDIATED FOOD ALLERGY

Gastrointestinal	Nausea
	Vomiting
	Diarrhea
	Abdominal cramping
	Oral allergy syndrome
Cutaneous	Urticaria
	Dermatitis or eczema
	Angioedema
	Pruritus
Respiratory	Rhinitis
	Rhinoconjunctivitis
	Asthma
	Laryngeal edema
	Heiner syndrome
Generalized	Anaphylactic shock

For additional information, see Sampson HA. J Allergy Clin Immunol 2004;113:805–19.

foods (all of the "big eight" except wheat), although peanuts, tree nuts, and crustacean shellfish seem to be more frequently implicated in severe food allergies than some of the other commonly allergenic foods. The prevalence of severe allergic reactions to foods is rather uncertain. Although the number of deaths occurring from IgE-mediated food allergies is not recorded in most countries, approximately 100 deaths are thought to occur in the United States each year (16, 17).

Although severe and potentially fatal allergic reactions such as anaphylactic shock are obviously a focus of much concern, it is important to note that mild symptoms are much more likely to occur with IgE-mediated food allergies than are severe ones. Perhaps the most common and possibly the most mild form of IgE-mediated food allergy is the so-called oral allergy syndrome (OAS) (18). OAS symptoms are confined to the oropharyngeal area and include pruritus, urticaria, and angioedema. OAS is most frequently associated with the ingestion of various fresh fruits and vegetables (18). OAS is an IgE-mediated reaction to specific proteins present in fresh fruits and vegetables, although fresh fruits and vegetables contain comparatively low quantities of protein (18). These fruit and vegetable allergens are apparently quite susceptible to digestive proteases in the gastrointestinal tract (19), thus systemic reactions to these foods are rarely encountered. These fruit and vegetable allergens are also apparently heat-labile (19), because the heat-processed versions of these foods typically are not involved in initiation of OAS. With OAS, affected persons are initially sensitized to one or more pollens in the environment, such as birch and mugwort pollens, that cross-react with related proteins found in the fresh fruits and vegetables (19, 20). With OAS, sensitization to the pollen increases the likelihood of sensitization to specific foods.

Exercise-induced food allergies are a subset of the immediate hypersensitivity reactions to foods. In these cases, exercise must be done coincident with ingestion of the food for symptoms to occur (21). Exercise-induced food allergies have been associated with numerous foods including shellfish, wheat, celery, and peach. The symptoms of exercise-induced food allergies are individualistic, variable, and similar to those involved in other food allergies. Exercise-induced allergies can also exist without any role for food intake (21). The mechanism of this illness is not well understood, although the involvement of IgE antibodies is apparent.

Sources

The Food and Agriculture Organization of the United Nations has established that peanuts, soybeans, fish, crustacean shellfish, milk, eggs, tree nuts, and wheat are the most common allergenic foods on a worldwide basis (22). As many as 90% of all IgE-mediated food allergies may be caused by these eight foods or food groups, sometimes referred to as the "big eight". The big eight actually involves many more than eight foods because several food groups are included. Fish refers to all species of finfish, although some species of fish, such as cod and salmon, are more commonly allergenic than others (23, 24). Shrimp, prawns, crab, lobster, and crayfish are included in the category of Crustacea; most persons with crustacean allergy are sensitive to all species of Crustacea (25). Egg-allergic persons are allergic to the eggs of all avian species (26). Furthermore, both egg white and egg yolk contain allergens (27), although egg white is considered to be the more potent sensitizing fraction. Milk-allergic persons are primarily sensitized to cows' milk, but typically also are reactive to the milk of other species, including goats and sheep (28). The commonly allergenic tree nuts include almonds, walnuts, pecans, cashews, Brazil nuts, macadamias, pistachios, hazelnuts (filberts), hickory nuts, chestnuts, and pine nuts (pinyon nuts) (2). Coconuts, kola nuts, and shea nuts, although considered to be tree nuts, are rarely allergenic.

Cross-reactions do not inevitably occur with closely related foods. Although there are several hundred species of edible legumes, peanuts and soybeans account for most legume-related food allergies. However, several of the other legumes, including lentils, beans, and garbanzo beans (chickpeas), have occasionally caused serious allergic reactions (29, 30).

Although the eight most commonly allergenic foods and food groups account for more than 90% of all IgE-mediated food allergies on a global basis, over 160 other foods have been documented in the medical literature on one or more occasions to elicit food allergies (31). Any food that contains protein has the potential to elicit allergic sensitization on a more infrequent basis. Generally, foods that are major sources of protein and that are frequently consumed in the diet are most likely to cause allergic reactions. However, certain foods that are considered to be good sources of protein, such as beef, pork, chicken, and turkey, are rarely allergenic (31).

Although the Food and Agriculture Organization list of the eight most commonly allergenic foods or food groups is reasonably well accepted, various regulatory jurisdictions have established their own lists of commonly allergenic foods. These lists are used for food labeling regulations in these areas. The lists reflect the fact that unique cultural dietary patterns may affect the comparative prevalence of specific allergenic foods. For example, lists in Canada, the European Union, and Australia/New Zealand include sesame seed, a common allergenic food among certain Asian and Middle Eastern cultures (32). By contrast, sesame seed allergy seems to be comparatively uncommon in the United States. Buckwheat is included on the list of commonly allergenic foods in Japan and Korea and seems to be a commonly allergenic food in those countries, probably because of frequent exposure to saba noodles (33). Mustard is on the list of commonly allergenic foods in the European Union, although the prevalence of mustard allergy is not very well established; mustard allergy has principally been reported in France and Spain for unexplained reasons (34).

Among the large group of 160 less commonly allergenic foods (31), several foods or food groups are noteworthy because they are known to elicit severe reactions in some affected persons. These foods or food groups include the molluscan shellfish (35), cottonseed meal or protein (36), sesame seed (32), sunflower seed (37), poppy seed (38), buckwheat (33), and celery (39).

Food Allergens

Virtually all of the allergens in foods are naturally occurring proteins (7). However, foods contain millions of proteins and only a very small percentage are known to be allergens. Allergenicity does not appear to be an inherent property of proteins, although all proteins are certainly capable of provoking immune reactions under selected circumstances of exposure. Some of the commonly allergenic foods, including peanuts, eggs, milk, and soybeans, contain multiple allergens (7). Other commonly allergenic foods appear to contain only a single major allergen, including cod, shrimp, and Brazil nuts (7). Major allergens are generally defined as proteins for which 50% or more of the allergic patients studied have specific IgE (7). Plant food allergens tend to fall into certain functional categories, such as some of the pathogenesis-related proteins or certain classes of storage proteins (40). For example, the 2S albumins, storage proteins rich in sulfur-containing amino acids, are major allergens in Brazil nuts, sesame seeds, walnuts, sunflower seeds, and mustard (41). Similarly, several pan-allergens seem to exist in allergenic animal species, such as parvalbumin in fish (42) and tropomyosin in crustacean shellfish (43).

Prevalence

Allergic diseases affect a significant portion of the general population, estimated at 10 to 25% (4). The prevalence of IgE-mediated food allergies in the United States can be estimated at 3.5 to 4.0% of the overall population. This estimate is based on surveys indicating the prevalence of shrimp, peanut, tree nut, and fish allergies as 1.9, 0.6, 0.5, and 0.4% of the overall population (44, 45). IgE-mediated food allergies are more common among infants and young children than among adults; the prevalence in children under the age of 3 years is in the range of 5 to 8% (46, 47). Although food allergies develop most commonly in early childhood, food allergies can develop later in life. For example, Crustacea are among the most common allergenic foods among adults (25, 45), but that particular food allergy is rarely seen among young children, probably because of their infrequent ingestion of Crustacea.

The prevalence of IgE-mediated food allergies to specific foods has been evaluated primarily on the basis of random digit-dial telephone surveys (44, 45). For certain types of food allergies, including immediate hypersensitivity reactions associated with noteworthy symptomology, these telephone surveys are arguably reasonably accurate. However, clinical confirmation of these estimates has not been obtained. As noted previously, there is general agreement that eight foods or food groups comprise the most IgE-mediated food allergies (22). This knowledge is based primarily on comparative prevalence studies conducted in allergy clinics with groups of allergic patients, such as estimates of the comparative prevalence of various food allergies in a group of pediatric patients with atopic dermatitis, which showed that milk, eggs, peanuts, soybeans, and wheat were the most common allergenic foods for this particular group (48).

Fewer studies have attempted to determine the prevalence of specific food allergies among the general population. The prevalence of adverse reactions to foods as confirmed by double-blind, placebo-controlled food challenge (DBPCFC) during the first 3 years of life among 480 consecutively born infants in a community in Colorado was 8% (46). Of these children, 25 (5.2%) were suspected to be allergic to cows' milk, but DBPCFC confirmed a sensitivity to cows' milk in only 11 (2.3%) of these infants (46). In a prospective study of 1749 newborns born in a single hospital in Denmark during 1985, 39 (2.2%) were found to have adverse reactions to cows' milk (49). Similarly, Jakobsson and Lindberg (50) followed up a cohort of 1079 Swedish newborns and found that 1.9% developed a sensitivity to cows' milk. A prevalence rate of 2.8% was observed in challenge studies conducted on a group of Dutch infants (51). The overall prevalence of food allergies among a birth cohort in Australia was estimated at about 8.5%, although some of these young children likely had multiple food allergies (52). The prevalence of specific food allergies was 3.2% for egg, 2.0% for milk, 1.9% for peanut, and 0.42% for sesame seed (52).

Persistence

Many young children outgrow their food allergies in early childhood within a few months to several years after the onset of the hypersensitivity (6). As many as 80 to 87% of food-allergic children are able to tolerate the offending food by 3 years of age (53). Allergies to certain foods, such as cows' milk (54), are more commonly outgrown than are allergies to certain other foods, such as peanuts (55). The mechanisms involved in the loss of sensitivity to specific foods are not precisely known, but the development of immunologic tolerance is definitely involved (9).

Prevention

The prevention of allergic sensitization and the development of IgE-mediated food allergies in infants requires early identification of high-risk infants. IgE-mediated food allergies are most likely to develop in high-risk infants, those infants born to parents with histories of allergic disease of any type (e.g., pollens, mold spores, animal danders, bee venoms, food). Several strategies have been advocated for the prevention of allergic sensitization in high-risk infants, although agreement on the optimal approach has certainly not been achieved. Among the strategies are exclusion of commonly allergenic foods such as cows' milk, eggs, and peanuts from the infant diet, breast-feeding for an extended period, possible use of a hypoallergenic infant formula, and the exclusion of commonly allergenic foods from the diet of the nursing mother (56, 57). Maternal dietary restriction during pregnancy (excluding commonly allergenic foods such as peanuts) did not prevent the development of food allergy in infants in several studies (56, 57), which suggests that sensitization does not occur in utero. However, the avoidance of peanuts during pregnancy has been advocated by some clinicians (58). Breast-feeding for extended periods of time delays but may not prevent the development of IgE-mediated food allergies (59). However, the observation has been made that infants can on occasion be sensitized to allergenic foods through exposure to the allergens in breast milk (60, 61). Apparently, certain allergenic food proteins are resistant to digestion, are absorbed at least to a small extent from the small intestine, and are secreted in breast milk, leading to sensitization. Maternal dietary avoidance of certain commonly allergenic foods, such as peanuts, during the lactation period is advocated because it will help to prevent sensitization through breast milk. However, the elimination of certain other commonly allergenic foods, such as milk and eggs, is not recommended for nursing mothers because these foods are usually considered to be too important nutritionally. Emerging evidence indicates that the use of probiotics during lactation may also help to lessen the likelihood of allergic sensitization (62). Hypoallergenic infant formula can also prevent the development of food allergies in high-risk infants (63), although these formulas are more often used to prevent reactions after sensitization has already occurred. In particular, the use of partial whey hydrolysate formula has been advocated for this purpose because this partial hydrolysate is more likely to prevent sensitization than is a formula based on whole milk (64). The partial hydrolysate whey formula is also more palatable to the infant. High-risk infants may still develop food allergies once solid foods are introduced into the diet (59).

Diagnosis

The diagnosis of food allergies and related illnesses can be approached in various ways. Self or parental diagnosis is a common practice, but is often unreliable (65). Without expert medical assistance, persons often identify food as a causative factor when it is not, or else they identify the wrong food or too many foods. Misdiagnosis obviously leads to unnecessary avoidance diets. These avoidance diets can be nutritionally harmful in some circumstances, especially in infants and young children. Thus, obtaining a competent diagnosis is essential to proper management of the condition.

The first step is to confirm the role of one or more specific foods as causative factors in the illness. Careful history-taking will often lead to the development of a relatively short list of suspected foods, especially in cases of immediate hypersensitivity, in which the rapid onset of symptoms after ingestion of the food allows easier identification of the culprit food. If the number of foods suspected is confined to one or a limited number, and especially if the symptoms are very noteworthy, a food diary may be kept. This diary should record all foods consumed and any symptoms that occur coincident with ingestion of those foods. This will aid the physician in determining whether an adverse reaction is occurring after the ingestion of a particular food.

Once a particular food is suspected as the cause of the adverse reaction, confirmation should be sought. This can be approached rather simply by elimination of the food from the diet to see whether symptoms disappear (particularly in the case of symptoms that tend to be long-lasting, such as atopic dermatitis or eczema). If the adverse reaction is not especially severe, the food can be reintroduced to the diet to determine whether symptoms reappear. However, the most reliable diagnostic procedure is the DBPCFC (66). The DBPCFC will unequivocally link ingestion of a specific food to elicitation of a specific set of symptoms. The DBPCFC should not be used when there is a history of life-threatening anaphylaxis to a suspected food (66). The DBPCFC is particularly useful when the role of a specific food or foods in a reaction is nebulous. Open challenges or single-blind challenges alternatively may be used in some situations.

Confirmation of an IgE-mediated food allergy requires additional diagnostic effort. The skin-prick test (SPT) or the radioallergosorbent test (RAST) and similar immunoassays are the most common procedures used to confirm the existence of an IgE-mediated mechanism (64, 67). The simplest procedure is the SPT (65, 68), which involves the application of a small amount of food extract to the skin, usually on the inside of the forearm or on the back. The site is pricked with a needle to allow the extract (antigen) to enter. A wheal-and-flare developing at the site demonstrates that IgE in the skin has reacted with some protein in the extract. The RAST method is an in vitro test that can be performed using a sample of the patient's blood serum (66, 69). The serum is reacted with an allergen bound to some solid matrix. The degree of binding of allergen-specific IgE in the serum to the solid-phase allergen is assessed with radiolabeled antihuman IgE. Although the results of the RAST are considered to be equally as reliable as the SPT, these tests are considerably more expensive. However, this may be the test of choice for patients with extreme sensitivities because SPTs may be hazardous in such patients (67, 70). The RAST method has become highly standardized. For some foods, RAST scores in specific commercial systems have been correlated with the results of DBPCFC, negating the need to perform the DBPCFC in all cases (71).

Management

Treatment or management of IgE-mediated food allergies can be approached in two different ways. Allergic reactions can be treated to resolve the symptoms. However, preferably, the avoidance of the allergenic food(s) will prevent the occurrence of allergic reactions.

Pharmacologic approaches are available for the treatment of the symptoms that occur during an allergic reaction (72). Antihistamines are useful for the treatment of most mild to moderate allergic reactions and function by blocking histamine receptors in the tissues. Epinephrine or adrenaline is a much more powerful drug that has the ability to resolve severe anaphylactic reactions in many cases. Those patients with a history of life-threatening reactions to foods are advised to carry an epinephrine-filled syringe with them at all times (73).

The major means of treatment for true food allergies is their prevention through implementation of a specific avoidance diet (74). Once the offending food(s) has been identified through diagnostic procedures as described earlier, the patient must avoid the food or foods to prevent reactions. For example, if allergic to peanuts, simply avoid peanuts in all forms. Considerable responsibility is placed on these persons; they must acquire considerable knowledge of food composition. Dietitians can be helpful in teaching clients to interpret food labels to detect ingredients made from the offending food. The passage of the Food Allergen Labeling and Consumer Protection Act of 2004 in the United States will simplify recognition of ingredients that must be avoided. The Act requires the use of common or usual names so casein and whey will be identified as originating from milk and semolina will be identified as originating from wheat on ingredient statements. Compliance with such avoidance diets is enhanced if the number of foods eliminated is kept to a minimum. Thus, accurate diagnosis is an important initial step.

Only a few hypoallergenic foods are available for use by such patients. In the case of infants with cows' milk allergy, several alternative formulas can be fed. Soybean-based infant formula works well in many cases (75), although some infants will develop soybean allergy as a result of that exposure (76). Casein hydrolysate formula can also be used successfully in the majority of cases (77). This formula is based on extensively hydrolyzed casein. Although casein is a common cows' milk allergen (7), the hydrolysis of the casein to a mixture of very small peptides and amino acids eliminates the allergenicity. Still, there have been a few exceptional case reports of allergic reactions to casein hydrolysates (78, 79).

In the construction of safe and effective avoidance diets, questions often arise regarding the need to avoid ingredients derived from commonly allergenic sources. Ingredients derived from the commonly allergenic foods will also be allergenic if they contain protein residues from the source material. Examples of ingredients derived from commonly allergenic sources include edible oils, protein hydrolysates, lecithin, flavors, gelatin, lactose, starch, soy sauce, and isinglass.

Edible oils can be derived from commonly allergenic sources such as peanuts and soybeans, or from other well-described allergenic foods such as sunflower seeds and sesame seeds. The processing of edible oils removes virtually all of the protein from the source material when hot solvent extraction is used. Refined, bleached, and deodorized oils from peanuts, soybeans, and sunflower seed have been documented to be safe for ingestion by persons allergic to the source material through use of clinical challenge trials (80). However, some oils from other sources, such as sesame seed and tree nuts, may receive less processing and contain allergenic residues (81, 82). Cold-pressed oils may also contain allergenic residues (83).

Protein hydrolysates are frequently derived from commonly allergenic sources such as soybean, wheat, milk, and peanuts. Several different hydrolytic processes can be used in their manufacturing, including acid hydrolysis and enzymatic hydrolysis. The degree of hydrolysis of the protein hydrolysate products varies according to the functional use, source, and method of hydrolysis. If the proteins are only partially hydrolyzed, they are likely to retain their allergenicity (6). If they are extensively hydrolyzed, they may be safe for most persons allergic to the source material (6). However, as already noted, extensively hydrolyzed casein in hypoallergenic infant formula can occasionally trigger allergic reactions in exquisitely sensitive cows' milk-allergic infants (78, 79). However, infant formulas based on partial whey hydrolysates were even more likely to elicit allergic reactions in cows' milk-allergic infants (84).

Several sources exist commercially for lecithin, including both soybean and egg, although soybean is by far the more common source. Commercial soy lecithin contains trace residues of soy proteins. Commercial soy lecithin contains soy protein residues, including IgE-binding proteins (85, 86). However, the levels of soy allergens in soy lecithin may be insufficient to elicit allergic reactions in most soybean-allergic persons, and many soybean-allergic persons do not avoid lecithin.

Although flavorings, especially natural flavoring, can occasionally be derived from allergenic sources, most flavoring formulations do not contain protein, especially protein derived from allergenic sources. However, some flavor formulations do contain components that are derived from allergenic sources (87). Allergic reactions have occurred to flavors, but only on rare occasions (88, 89).

Beef and pork are the most common sources of gelatin used in foods. Beef and pork gelatin are generally not considered to be allergenic when ingested. However, gelatin can also be derived from fish. Recently, a clinical trial documented that fish gelatin derived from codfish skins would not provoke allergic reactions in cod-allergic persons at levels up to 3.61 g of cumulative intake (90). Thus, although fish gelatin is actually protein from an allergenic source, the gelatin derived from collagen may not be allergenic. Reports of allergic reactions to fish gelatin among fish-allergic persons have not been documented (91). However, fish collagen may be an allergen for at least some fish-allergic persons (92), although that finding does not necessarily indicate that fish gelatin is allergenic.

Lactose is derived from cows' milk. Commercially, lactose contains residual milk protein from the whey fraction. However, no well-documented reports exist for allergic reactions to lactose used as a food ingredient among milk-allergic persons (93).

Starch used as a food ingredient is most frequently derived from corn, and corn is not a particularly common source of food allergies (31). Occasionally, starch may be derived from wheat. No evidence exists for IgE-mediated allergic reactions to wheat starch (91), although wheat starch is documented to contain wheat protein residues (94).

Many types of soy sauce are available in the marketplace. Two general types of soy sauce are available in the US marketplace. One form is naturally fermented using wheat and soybeans as fermentation substrates. The other form is simply a mixture of extensively hydrolyzed soybean protein, salt, caramel coloring, and water. The naturally fermented type of soy sauce has vastly reduced IgE-binding activity but does retain some IgE-binding activity (95). The second type of soy sauce does not have residual IgE-binding activity. Although naturally fermented soy sauce retains some IgE-binding activity, the risk posed to soy- and wheat-allergic persons is uncertain. Documented cases of allergic reactions to soy sauce do not exist (91).

Isinglass is also a fish collagen-based ingredient. Isinglass is used commercially to remove fine particulates from various beverages such as beers, ales, wines, and champagnes. Isinglass is derived from the swim bladders of several species of tropical fish. No reports exist of allergic reactions to isinglass. Residual levels of isinglass in the beverages would be predicted to be extraordinarily low.

In the construction of safe and effective avoidance diets, questions also often arise regarding the potential allergenicity of closely related foods. Cross-reactions occur between closely related foods in the case of certain food groups but not others, so it does not seem to be possible to offer uniform advice on this particular aspect. As noted earlier, cross-reactions are known to occur among the various crustacean species (shrimp, crab, lobster, and crawfish) (25), different species of avian eggs (26), and cows' milk and goats' milk (27). In contrast, patients allergic to one or more species of fish can sometimes consume other fish species without adverse reactions (96), although parvalbumin appears to be a panallergen present in all species of fish (97). Thus, the patterns of fish allergy seem to be variable from one person to another (96), but the matter deserves more clinical study. In addition, some peanut-allergic persons are allergic to other legumes such as soybeans (98), but this is not a common occurrence (99). Clinical hypersensitivity to one legume, such as peanuts or soybeans, does not warrant exclusion of the entire legume family from the diet unless allergy to each individual legume is confirmed by clinical challenge trials (99). As noted earlier, cross-reactions are not inevitable among related species and the legume family is a good example of this.

In addition to cross-reactions among related foods, cross-reactions are also known to occur between certain types of pollens and foods, especially with OAS. Examples include ragweed pollen and melons, mugwort pollen and celery, mugwort pollen and hazelnuts, and birch pollen and various foods including carrots, apples, hazelnuts, and potatoes (100). Cross-reactions are also known to occur between allergies to natural rubber latex and certain foods such as bananas, chestnuts, and avocados (101).

Minimal Eliciting Dose (Threshold)

Many persons with IgE-mediated food allergies are exquisitely sensitive to the offending food (102). This low threshold for the offending food also complicates the construction of a safe and effective avoidance diet. The low eliciting dose results from the interaction of a rather small amount of allergen with IgE antibodies on the surfaces of mast cells and basophils, which triggers the release of large quantities of biologically active mediators. Hence, exposure to a small dose of the allergen can elicit a clinically significant reaction. With these persons, adverse reactions occur after exposure to trace amounts of the offending food, which may arise through various processing or preparation errors (103). Food processing errors can include the failure to adequately clean shared equipment, the use of rework (a common practice in certain segments of the industry involving the incorporation of leftover or misformulated quantities of a food product into subsequent batches of related products with identical or related formulations), and the inadvertent addition of an ingredient that is not supposed to be in the formulation (88, 104–105). However, with packaged foods, the majority of food ingredients are declared on the ingredient statement on the label. Additionally, many food processors have begun to add precautionary labeling to food products, including terms such as "made on shared equipment with peanuts" or "may contain peanuts." This sort of labeling alerts allergic consumers to the possible presence of hazardous residues of allergenic foods in the product.

Restaurants and other food service facilities are often a bigger challenge for food-allergic consumers. The existence of unlabeled foods in restaurant or other food service settings is a major challenge for the implementation of effective avoidance diets. Many adverse reactions have occurred in such settings (14, 15). Additionally, errors can occur in food preparation, including the use of shared cooking/serving equipment or surfaces and mistakes or substitutions in following recipes (103).

For practical purposes, complete avoidance of the offending food must be emphasized to the allergic person. However, minimal eliciting or threshold doses do exist below which allergic persons will not experience adverse reactions. In one of the first experiments documenting this concept, Hourihane and colleagues (106) evaluated the threshold doses in a group of peanut-allergic persons who were challenged with low but varying doses of peanuts. In this group of 12 persons, the most sensitive person began to experience subjective symptoms when exposed to 100 μg of peanut protein and to experience mild, objective symptoms when exposed to 2 mg of peanut protein (106). However, four other peanut-allergic persons in this same study with equally impressive histories of serious allergic reactions to peanuts had no reaction when exposed to the highest dose used in the trial, 50 mg of peanut protein (106). Thus, the threshold dose for peanuts was shown to be low and variable among peanut-allergic persons. Surprisingly, some peanut-allergic persons with histories of severe reactions were able to tolerate 50 mg or more of peanuts. Since that initial clinical research, additional studies have documented that the minimal eliciting doses for peanuts, milk, and eggs are likely in the low milligram range for the most sensitive persons but that considerable individual variability exists (102, 107–109). In addition, the possibility exists that the threshold doses vary from one allergenic food to another. Modeling may be an approach to estimation of a safe dose for allergic persons using the data acquired from existing challenge trials (110). Some uncertainty exists because the existing challenge data were acquired using several different clinical protocols, but consensus has been achieved on the development of a consensus clinical protocol for low-dose challenge studies (111).

Detection of Residues of Allergenic Foods

Food allergies are being increasingly recognized as sources of illness. The wider recognition of food allergies extends to regulatory agencies. One of the fastest growing areas of recalls of packaged foods in the United States is the undeclared presence of allergenic foods (89). Considerable improvements have recently been made in the ability to detect reliably the presence of residues of allergenic foods contaminating other foods (112, 113). The ability to detect the presence of undeclared allergens in foods has provided the food industry with the tools necessary to ensure that their manufacturing practices are adequate to eliminate such occurrences and regulatory agencies with the

tools necessary for enforcement of labeling provisions on packaged foods. Enzyme-linked immunosorbent assays with detection limits in the low parts per million (mg/kg) range are available for the detection of residues of peanuts, eggs, cows' milk, almonds, gluten (wheat, rye, barley), walnuts, pecan, shrimp, and hazelnuts (see references 114 and 115 as examples).

Effects of Processing on Allergenicity

Most food processing operations have little effect on the allergenicity of most foods. Allergenic food proteins tend to be remarkably stable to food processing conditions (19). Most allergenic food proteins are quite heat-stable; typical heat processing conditions do not alter the allergenicity of the resulting products (19). Several exceptions do exist. For example, the allergens in some fruits and vegetables are heat sensitive (116). In addition, the allergens present in some species of fish may be destroyed by canning processes, although other heating processes do not seem to affect these allergens (117). Additionally, food allergens tend to be resistant to proteolysis, allowing these proteins to survive digestive processes and arrive in the intestine in immunologically active form (19, 118). Thus, food allergens may survive, in whole or in part, the acid and enzymatic hydrolysis methods used to prepare protein hydrolysates (19). The difficulty encountered in sufficiently hydrolyzing casein to make hypoallergenic infant formula has already been described.

Allergenicity of Foods Produced through Agricultural Biotechnology

The development of genetically engineered foods through biotechnology is an area of some concern with respect to food allergies. Genetically engineered foods will contain one to several novel proteins. Because most food allergens are proteins, the potential exists for the transfer of allergens in the genetic modification of foods. However, only a few of the many thousands of proteins in nature are allergens, so this possibility is somewhat limited by chance alone. An approach has been developed for the evaluation of the potential allergenicity of genetically engineered foods (119, 120). This strategy takes into account the source of the genetic material, the possible amino acid sequence homology with known allergens, the immunoreactivity of the novel protein, and the digestive stability of the protein. Obviously, the opportunity for transfer of an allergen is greatest when the genetic material is obtained from a known allergenic source. Only one case of the transfer of an allergen through genetic modification has been documented thus far. The development of a genetically engineered soybean variety with improved levels of methionine was achieved through the transfer of a high-methionine protein from Brazil nuts, but this particular Brazil nut protein was subsequently identified as the major Brazil nut allergen and commercial interest in this transgenic variety of soybeans was dropped (121). Currently marketed genetically engineered crops contain rather low levels of the novel proteins and present virtually no risk of eliciting allergic sensitization or reactions (120).

DELAYED HYPERSENSITIVITY REACTIONS

Delayed hypersensitivity reactions are associated with symptoms that appear 6 to 24 or more hours after the ingestion of the offending food. This reaction develops slowly, often reaching its peak at 48 or more hours after the ingestion of the offending food. The inflammatory responses associated with delayed hypersensitivity reactions also subside slowly. Delayed hypersensitivity reactions involve the stimulation of sensitized tissue-bound lymphocytes, T cells, which release cytokines and lymphokines, producing a localized inflammatory response (4). With food-induced, delayed hypersensitivity reactions, the symptoms are likely confined primarily to the gastrointestinal tract. Recently, several gastrointestinal maladies primarily affecting infants have been identified as immune-mediated reactions (4). IgE may play a role in some of these conditions, although IgE may not be the sole factor involved. T cells and other immune effector cells may also be involved. For the purposes of this chapter, celiac disease is discussed as the primary example of delayed hypersensitivity reactions associated with foods; it is perhaps the best-studied example, although the mechanism of this illness remains somewhat unclear.

CELIAC DISEASE

Celiac disease, also known as celiac sprue, nontropical sprue, and gluten-sensitive enteropathy, is a malabsorption syndrome occurring in sensitive persons on the consumption of wheat, rye, barley, triticale, spelt, and kamut (5). Celiac disease serves as a good example of delayed hypersensitivity reactions associated with foods. Celiac disease has been extensively studied, although it is not yet thoroughly understood. The cause-and-effect relationship between celiac disease and ingestion of certain foods is very well established.

Mechanism

Celiac disease is associated with a cell-mediated, localized inflammatory reaction in the intestinal tract (5, 122). The inflammatory reaction results in a so-called flat lesion in the gut. The cell-mediated immunologic reaction in the gut is characterized by this villous atrophy along with crypt hyperplasia, lymphoid infiltration of the epithelium, edema of the lamina propria, and impaired absorptive function of the epithelium including increased fluid secretion and enhanced permeability (123). The absorptive epithelium of the small intestine becomes damaged by this inflammatory process. This results in a decreased number of the epithelial cells that are critical to digestion and absorption. The mucosal enzymes necessary for digestion and absorption are also altered in the damaged cells. Thus, the absorptive cells are functionally compromised. This mucosal damage leads to nutrient malabsorption (6). It seems as though a defect in mucosal processing of gliadin in celiac patients provokes the generation of toxic peptides that contribute to the abnormal immunologic response and the subsequent inflammatory reaction (124).

Symptoms and Sequelae

The inflammatory process occurring in celiac disease results in a severe malabsorption syndrome characterized by diarrhea, bloating, weight loss, anemia, bone pain, chronic fatigue, weakness, various nutritional deficiencies, muscle cramps, and, in children, failure to thrive (123, 125). Although the risk of death is quite low (126), untreated celiac disease is associated with considerable discomfort in many celiac sufferers. Persons suffering from celiac disease for long periods are also at increased risk for development of T-cell lymphomas (123, 127). Celiac patients also are more likely than others to have various other diseases, especially diseases of an autoimmune nature (125). Examples would include dermatitis herpetiformis, thyroid diseases, Addison disease, pernicious anemia, autoimmune thrombocytopenia, sarcoidosis, insulin-dependent diabetes mellitus, IgA nephropathy, and Down syndrome (125).

Sources

Celiac disease is associated with the ingestion of wheat, rye, barley, and triticale (22, 128). Although oats were once thought to be a causative factor in celiac disease, the role of oats has now been discounted (129). However, oats are often contaminated with wheat in commerce, so caution may still be necessary with respect to the ingestion of oats by celiac sufferers (6). Spelt and kamut, which are basically varieties of wheat, are also thought to trigger celiac disease in susceptible persons (6).

Causative Factor

The prolamin fractions of wheat, rye, and barley are implicated in the causation of celiac disease. Because the prolamin fraction of wheat is known as gluten, celiac disease is sometimes referred to as gluten-sensitive enteropathy. In wheat, the gliadin or alcohol-soluble fraction is the component of the gluten fraction that is involved in the elicitation of celiac disease (124, 130). Because the prolamins are the major storage proteins in these grains, all varieties of wheat, rye, and barley are considered hazardous for celiac sufferers. The level of these proteins in wheat, rye, and barley is rather high.

Prevalence and Persistence

The prevalence of celiac disease remains a subject of intense scrutiny. The diagnosis of celiac disease can on occasion be rather difficult. Celiac disease appears to be latent or subclinical in some persons, with symptoms only appearing occasionally (131, 132). The prevalence of celiac disease seems highest in certain European populations and in Australia (125, 133), although this may relate to more thorough diagnostic approaches. Celiac disease may occur in as many as one in every 250 people in some European groups (125). In the United States, the prevalence of celiac disease is generally perceived to be much lower. However, improved diagnosis has led to an increased estimate of prevalence in the United States of one in every 133 people (134), although many of these persons would have latent celiac disease. Considerable variability is observed in the prevalence of celiac disease among various European populations (125, 133, 135).

Celiac disease is a lifelong condition. Although celiac disease may occur in a latent phase in some affected persons, oral tolerance for gluten proteins does not seem to occur.

Management and Minimal Eliciting Dose

Like IgE-mediated food allergies, celiac disease is treated by implementation of an avoidance diet (136). Those with celiac disease attempt to avoid all sources of wheat, rye, barley, and related grains, including a wide variety of common food ingredients derived from these grains (136). The need to avoid ingredients that do not contain protein from the implicated grains is somewhat debatable but is widely practiced (6). Most of these persons also avoid oats, but that is likely wise considering the frequent contamination of oats with wheat from shared farms, harvesting equipment, and storage facilities (6). Although evidence is scant, two varieties of wheat spelt and kamut, are likely to trigger celiac disease in susceptible persons (6).

Gluten-free foods are available commercially. The definition of gluten-free in most countries is below 200 ppm gluten. Canada has the most stringent definition, having adopted a limit of 20 ppm for gluten-free foods. Other countries are considering adoption of this limit. The United States has no definition for gluten-free.

The minimal eliciting dose for wheat, rye, barley, and related grains among celiac sufferers is unknown. Many persons with celiac disease go to great lengths to avoid all sources of wheat, rye, barley, and triticale. Although this has not been conclusively proven, a few isolated studies have concluded that levels of 10 mg/day of gliadin will be tolerated by most patients with celiac disease (137).

Detection

An enzyme-linked immunosorbent assay has been developed for the detection of gluten and related proteins from wheat, rye, and barley (138). Current enzyme-linked immunosorbent assay kits on the market allow the detection of gluten at levels of 10 ppm or greater. Such assays are used to ensure that gluten-free products are properly labeled.

FOOD INTOLERANCES

As noted earlier, food intolerances are the other major category of food-associated adverse reactions that affect only certain persons in the population. Food intolerances include all of those individualistic adverse reactions to foods in which the immune system is not directly involved in the pathogenesis of the illness. The major categories include anaphylactoid reactions, metabolic food disorders, and idiosyncratic reactions.

Anaphylactoid reactions are associated with the release of histamine and other mediators of allergic disease from mast cells without the intervention of IgE (6). Some foods may contain substances that destabilize mast cells membranes, causing the spontaneous release of histamine. However, no such substances have ever been identified in foods, so the existence of this particular category of food intolerance remains controversial. Therefore, anaphylactoid reactions will not be discussed in further detail here.

Metabolic food disorders result from a genetically inherited defect in the ability to metabolize a food component or a genetically inherited sensitivity to a food component that affects some critical metabolic process. The premier examples of metabolic food disorders are lactose intolerance and favism. Lactose intolerance results from an inherited deficiency of the enzyme β-galactosidase in the intestinal mucosa (139). In favism, an inherited deficiency in the enzyme glucose-6-phosphate dehydrogenase (G6PDH) in the erythrocytes results in a heightened sensitivity to several naturally occurring oxidant compounds found in fava beans (140).

Idiosyncratic reactions are adverse reactions to foods that occur through unknown mechanisms (6). Obviously, a wide variety of mechanisms could theoretically be involved in these idiosyncratic reactions, and a range of symptoms could occur. However, the role of foods in many of these reactions has not been well established. Sulfite-induced asthma is discussed as an example because the cause-and-effect relationship has been well established in this case. The role of specific foods or food ingredients in most idiosyncratic reactions remains to be clearly established.

LACTOSE INTOLERANCE

Lactose intolerance is a metabolic food disorder associated with a deficiency of the enzyme β-galactosidase or lactase in the intestinal mucosa (139). As a result, lactose, the primary sugar in milk and milk products, cannot be metabolized into its component monosaccharides, galactose and glucose. In contrast to the monosaccharides, the undigested lactose cannot be absorbed across the small intestinal mucosa. The undigested lactose thus passes into the colon, where resident bacteria metabolize the lactose into CO_2, H_2, and H_2O. The characteristic symptoms of lactose intolerance are bloating, flatulence, abdominal cramping, and frothy diarrhea (6, 139).

Sources, Properties, and Occurrence in Foods

Lactose is the principal sugar in milk and milk products. Lactose is a disaccharide, 4'-(β-D-galacto-pyranoside)-D-glucopyranose. This disaccharide is quite unique and is found exclusively in milk and milk products. Lactose is present in appreciable amounts in many dairy products, such as milk, ice cream, cottage cheese, and yogurt. Hard cheeses contain only small amounts of lactose. The usual treatment for lactose intolerance is the avoidance of dairy products containing lactose. Persons with lactose intolerance seem to tolerate yogurt and acidophilus milk better than other dairy products even though these products contain appreciable amounts of lactose (141, 142). Apparently, these fermented products have inherent lactase activity that is partially able to survive digestive processes and assist with the metabolism of lactose in the small intestine (139).

Prevalence

Lactose intolerance affects a large number of people on a worldwide basis. It occurs with high frequency among black Americans, Native Americans, Hispanics, Asians, Jews, and Arabs, affecting as many as 60 to 90% of persons in such groups (143). The prevalence among white North Americans is about 6 to 12% (144). β-Galactosidase levels are high in virtually all infants at birth (139). However, after infancy, people in the ethnic groups mentioned earlier lose 90% of intestinal β-galactosidase activity (145, 146). This normal pattern of loss of β-galactosidase activity is transmitted by a recessive gene and should be considered a normal physiologic event (139). The levels of β-galactosidase found in infants persist into adulthood in a few ethnic populations such as white populations, presumably as an adaptation to the widespread historical use of dairy products in these cultures (139). β-Galactosidase persistence is inherited as an autosomal dominant characteristic (147). Although genuine lactose intolerance affects many persons on a worldwide basis, 15 to 30% of self-diagnosed, lactose-intolerant persons in the United States have satisfactory levels of β-galactosidase and thus should not display the symptoms of lactose intolerance on the ingestion of dairy products (148).

Minimal Eliciting Dose and Management

In contrast to IgE-mediated food allergies, lactose-intolerant persons can tolerate some amount of lactose in their diets (2). In the majority of lactose-intolerant persons, symptoms after the consumption of 12 g of lactose, an amount equivalent to 1 cup of milk, are trivial (148). The frequency and severity of symptoms increase as the lactose dose exceeds 12 g (147, 149). Lactose-intolerant persons do have some variability in their individual tolerances for lactose (139). Lactose ingested with a meal containing high amounts of solids or fat is better tolerated than a similar amount of lactose in fluid milk (139). As noted previously, lactose in yogurt and acidophilus milk is better tolerated than lactose from other dairy products (141, 142). Most adults consume less than 25 g/day of lactose, whereas infants commonly consume greater than 50 g/day (139). On a body weight basis, infants ingest significantly greater amounts of lactose than adults.

Lactose intolerance is not a severe illness. The symptoms are confined to the gastrointestinal tract and are usually rather mild (6). Symptom severity can vary from one person to another depending on β-galactosidase activity, gastrointestinal transit time, lactose load, and colonic fermentation (139, 146). The symptoms of lactose intolerance can be avoided by the implementation of a dairy product avoidance diet (6). However, because dairy products provide 75% of the calcium intake in US diets, the implementation of dairy product avoidance diets from childhood can place persons at increased risk of postmenopausal osteoporosis (139). The emergence of lactose-hydrolyzed dairy products onto the marketplace in recent years provides lactose-intolerant persons with another means of controlling their reactions.

Overall, the risk posed by lactose to lactose-intolerant persons is much less than the risk posed by allergenic foods to persons with IgE-mediated food allergies. Although lactose intolerance may affect a larger number of persons, the symptoms are in general much more mild, and the tolerance for lactose in the diet equates to fewer problems in the implementation of a safe and effective avoidance diet.

FAVISM

Favism results from an intolerance to the consumption of fava beans or the inhalation of pollen from the *Vicia faba* plant. Sensitive persons suffer from acute hemolytic anemia on exposure (140). The characteristic symptoms of favism include pallor, fatigue, dyspnea, nausea, abdominal and/or back pain, fever, and chills. Rarely, hemoglobinuria, jaundice, and renal failure will occur. The onset time is quite rapid, usually occurring in 5 to 24 hours after ingestion. Recovery is prompt and spontaneous assuming no further exposure. Favism occurs most frequently in areas where the plant grows and the crop is harvested and sold in local markets. Favism is most prevalent when the *Vicia faba* plant is in bloom, causing elevated levels of airborne pollen, and also when the beans are available in the market.

Persons susceptible to favism are those with an inherited deficiency of erythrocyte G6PDH (140). G6PDH is a critical enzyme in erythrocytes, where it is essential for maintaining adequate levels of the reduced form of glutathione and nicotinamide adenine dinucleotide phosphate; glutathione and nicotinamide adenine dinucleotide phosphate prevent oxidative damage to the cells. Thus, the red blood cells of persons with G6PDH deficiency are more susceptible to oxidative damage. Fava beans contain several naturally occurring oxidants, including vicine and convicine, which are able to damage the erythrocytes of G6PDH-deficient persons. G6PDH deficiency is the most common inherited enzymatic defect in human beings on a worldwide basis, affecting 100 million people (140). G6PDH deficiency occurs with the highest frequency among Sephardic Jewish communities in Israel, Sardinians, Cypriot Greeks, American blacks, and certain African populations. The trait is virtually nonexistent in northern European nations, North American Indians, and Eskimos. Favism occurs primarily in the Mediterranean area, the Middle East, China, and Bulgaria, where the genetic trait is fairly prevalent and where fava beans are frequently consumed. The diagnosis of G6PDH deficiency is made through an assay for enzymatic activity of G6PDH in isolated red blood cells. Obviously, susceptible persons can avoid favism by avoiding the ingestion of fava beans and/or the inhalation of the plant pollen.

SULFITE-INDUCED ASTHMA

Sulfite sensitivity is an idiosyncratic reaction of undefined mechanism associated with the ingestion of sulfites in foods and medications (150). Although scattered reports exist of other manifestations of sulfite sensitivity including anaphylaxis (150, 151), asthma is the only symptom that has been clearly linked to sulfite ingestion in multiple subjects as the result of carefully controlled clinical challenge studies (150, 152).

Sources, Properties, and Occurrence in Foods

Sulfites are used as food additives in a variety of foods (153). Sulfites exist in several forms: sulfur dioxide, sodium metabisulfite, potassium metabisulfite, sodium bisulfite, potassium bisulfite, and sodium sulfite, although all of these ingredients have similar chemistries in foods depending on pH (153). Sulfites can also occur naturally in foods, especially fermented foods, as the result of formation by yeast (153). The residual levels of sulfites in foods range from less than 10 ppm in many food products to greater than 2000 ppm in certain dried fruits (153). Naturally occurring levels of sulfites are typically quite low. Sulfites are added to foods for a variety of purposes, including the control of enzymatic and nonenzymatic browning (e.g., potatoes), the prevention of undesirable bacterial growth (e.g., corn wet milling and wine making), the conditioning of dough (e.g., some frozen dough products), the prevention of oxidation, and the bleaching of selected products (e.g., maraschino cherries and hominy). When added to foods, the fate of sulfites is

complex (153). In acidic foods, sulfites can be released from foods into the surrounding atmosphere as SO_2 gas. Sulfites can also react with numerous food components, including carbohydrates, proteins, and others. These reactions can be either reversible or irreversible depending on the nature of the reaction. Very little free, unbound sulfite remains in most sulfited foods, with a few exceptions such as lettuce (154).

Prevalence and Severity

Although asthma is the most prominent symptom involved in sulfite sensitivity, only a few patients with asthma are sulfite sensitive (155). Challenge studies indicate that patients with severe or steroid-dependent asthma are primarily at risk (155). Patients with severe or steroid-dependent asthma make up only about 20% of the overall asthmatic population. However, only about 5% of these patients with severe asthma are sulfite sensitive (155). Extrapolating from these challenge study results, perhaps 150,000 patients with sulfite-sensitive asthma exist in the US population.

Despite the small size of the at-risk population, sulfites are capable of causing severe reactions in sensitive persons. The provocation of asthma can be life-threatening in some situations. Deaths have occurred from the ingestion of sulfites by patients with sulfite-sensitive asthma (150, 156), although the number of deaths is rather small. Anaphylaxis seems to be another rare but severe manifestation of sulfite sensitivity (151). However, only a few such cases have been described in the medical literature.

Management

Patients with sulfite-sensitive asthma must avoid the ingestion of sulfites in their diets (153). Fortunately, the presence of sulfites must be declared on the ingredient labels of packaged foods when residual levels exceed 10 ppm (2). In addition, sulfite use is banned from many fresh food products such as lettuce, in which high residual levels were associated with provocation of particularly severe reactions (157). However, patients with sulfite-sensitive asthma can tolerate the ingestion of small quantities of sulfites (152, 155). Challenge results support the hypothesis that patients with sulfite-sensitive asthma are more tolerant of sulfites in foods than they are of inorganic sulfites in capsules or other common challenge vehicles (150, 157). Apparently, the reaction of sulfites with food components removes some of the sulfite in foods from having the capability to trigger asthmatic reactions in sensitive persons (157). The tolerance for sulfited foods seems to vary with the nature of the food, suggesting that the form of bound sulfite is likely an important issue (157). Because of the release of SO_2 vapor from acidic beverages, patients with sulfite-sensitive asthma may be more sensitive to sulfited beverages than to other forms of sulfite in foods (157, 158). Patients with sulfite-sensitive asthma also seems to be more sensitive to residues of unbound sulfites in foods such as lettuce (157) than they are to sulfited foods that contain bound sulfites, such as shrimp and potatoes (157).

Overall, sulfites pose a considerable risk to patients with sulfite-sensitive asthma. Although the size of the affected population is comparatively quite small, the reactions can be severe and life-threatening. Patients with sulfite-sensitive asthma can tolerate some sulfite in their diets, but the thresholds are low in some persons. Patients with sulfite-sensitive asthma must follow avoidance diets that exclude most significant sources of sulfite from their diets.

ALLERGYLIKE INTOXICATIONS (HISTAMINE POISONING)

Histamine poisoning is the most commonly encountered allergylike intoxication (3). Outbreaks of histamine intoxication are often referred to as scombroid fish poisoning, and occur with some frequency in the United States, Europe, Japan, and other countries.

Symptoms and Features

As noted earlier, histamine is one of the primary mediators released from mast cells in IgE-mediated food allergies. Thus, similar symptoms occur in histamine intoxication and IgE-mediated food allergy. As with IgE-mediated food allergies, the symptoms can be variable and are not particularly definitive, although the illness is typically rather mild (159). Gastrointestinal symptoms such as nausea, vomiting, diarrhea, and abdominal cramps are common. Tingling, itching, and burning sensations often occur in the mouth. Cutaneous symptoms including flushing, urticaria, and angioedema, and other itchy rashes appear as well. Hypotension is a common manifestation. Other common symptoms include headache and palpitations. Although the list of possible symptoms is long, most patients suffer only a few of these symptoms. In the study of a large series of outbreaks in the United Kingdom, the most common symptoms were rash, diarrhea, flushing and sweating, and headache (160). Such symptoms are not particularly definitive, which leads to frequent misdiagnosis of histamine intoxication. Although histamine intoxication is usually rather mild, serious cardiac and respiratory complications can occur on rare occasions, especially in persons with preexisting cardiac and respiratory complications (3, 161).

Symptoms of histamine poisoning typically appear within minutes to a few hours after ingestion of the offending food (3). Histamine intoxication is a self-limited illness, and symptoms usually subside within a few hours, even without treatment. However, when untreated, symptoms can persist for as long as 24 to 48 hours (3). The dose of exposure and/or the susceptibility of the affected person may affect symptom duration. Effective treatment (see later) leads to a prompt resolution of the symptoms.

Diagnosis and Treatment

The diagnosis of histamine poisoning is often contingent on associating the ingestion of one of the more commonly implicated foods with the rapid onset of symptoms typical of histamine intoxication (3). A beneficial response of the patient to antihistamines would further strengthen the diagnosis (3). The diagnosis of histamine intoxication can be confirmed only by analysis of the suspect food with the detection of unusually high levels of histamine (3). Samples of the incriminated food should be sought immediately whenever histamine intoxication is suspected. The accepted procedure for the analysis of histamine in the incriminated food involves extraction, clean-up, and fluorometric analysis (162). In cases in which food samples are not available, the confirmation of the diagnosis of histamine intoxication is probably impossible. Vomitus and/or stomach contents could be analyzed for histamine, but baseline data on histamine levels in these materials are not readily available (3). Analysis for histamine in the blood or histamine metabolites in the urine could be attempted. The rapid metabolism of histamine would be expected to complicate blood analysis. Urine analysis for histamine and its metabolites has not been attempted to our knowledge (3).

Because of the similarities in symptoms and the beneficial effects of antihistamines, histamine poisoning is often misdiagnosed as an allergic reaction to food. However, histamine intoxications can be readily distinguished from IgE-mediated food allergies (3). With histamine intoxication, the patient typically has no prior history of allergic reactions to the implicated food or perhaps does not even have any sort of allergic history. By contrast, the patient usually is well aware of existing IgE-mediated food allergies. In addition, SPTs with commercial extracts of the food will be negative if no IgE-mediated allergy exists in the patient. However, if an extract is made of the actual incriminated food, the SPT can be positive because of the presence of histamine in the extract (3). In many situations, the presence of symptoms in dining companions offers another clue. With histamine intoxication, the attack rates in group outbreaks are often 50 to 100%. Meanwhile, with IgE-mediated food allergies, it would be rare to encounter two persons sharing the same meal who would experience the same food allergy. Finally, histamine intoxication can be distinguished from IgE-mediated food allergy by analysis of the incriminated food and detection of abnormally high levels of histamine.

Antihistamines are the most effective treatment for histamine intoxication. Both H_1 and H_2 antagonists are effective (163, 164). Even without treatment, the symptoms of histamine intoxication will usually subside within a few hours (3). However, treatment with antihistamines will shorten the duration of the illness and lessen the discomfort experienced by the patient.

Sources and Formation

The most common cause of histamine poisoning is certain types of spoiled fish (3). This illness is sometimes referred to as scombroid fish poisoning because of its frequent association with fish from the families *Scomberesocidae* and *Scombridae*, such as tuna, skipjack, mackerel, and bonito. Scombroid fish poisoning is a bit of a misnomer, however, because certain types of nonscombroid fish are also commonly involved, including mahi-mahi, bluefish, jack mackerel, sardines, yellowtail, anchovies, and herring. In the United States, mahi-mahi has become one of the most frequent offending foods in cases of histamine intoxication (3). These species of fish do not elicit histamine poisoning unless they contain elevated levels of histamine; the Food and Drug Administration considers 50 mg of histamine per 100 g of fish to be hazardous for tuna based on the investigation of numerous outbreaks (165).

Outbreaks of histamine poisoning from cheese occur with far less frequency than outbreaks involving fish (3). Swiss cheese has been implicated in several outbreaks of histamine intoxication in the United States. (3, 166). Typically, the histamine contents of cheeses are quite low.

Histamine may be a cause of wine intolerance (167), although few clinical studies have been conducted to confirm this possibility. In a challenge study with 125 mL of red wine containing 50 μg of histamine, 22 of 28 patients experienced a significant increase in plasma histamine within 30 minutes, along with some symptoms consistent with histamine intoxication (167).

Histamine formation in foods is associated with the growth of bacteria possessing the enzyme histidine decarboxylase, which is able to convert the amino acid histidine into histamine. Few bacterial species are capable of the prolific histamine formation necessary to develop hazardous levels in food products. In fish, *Morganella morganii* and *Klebsiella pneumoniae* are two species with such capabilities (3, 168). When fish such as tuna with high levels of free histidine in their edible tissues are contaminated with such histamine-producing bacteria (and most are not), the bacteria can convert large amounts of histidine to histamine in a relatively short period of time when the fish are held at elevated temperatures. Such fish will not necessarily appear to be spoiled, although they contain hazardous levels of histamine.

In cheese, certain species of lactobacilli are probably responsible for histamine formation. Histamine formation is a rather unusual trait among lactobacilli (3). Several factors may contribute to histamine formation in cheese, including higher ripening temperatures, excessive proteolysis, high pH, and low salt concentrations (169). The Swiss cheese-making process is especially conducive to histamine formation, and the levels of histamine in Swiss cheese appear to be dependent primarily on the number of histamine-producing bacteria in the raw milk supply (169).

Toxicology

Histamine is much less potent when taken orally than it is when released or administered intravenously (170). Humans can tolerate milligram levels of histamine orally without untoward effects (171). The lack of toxicity of orally administered histamine is not particularly surprising because humans have several enzymes in the intestinal mucosa, diamine oxidase and histamine-N-methyltransferase, that are capable of detoxifying histamine (170).

In fact, the role of histamine in scombroid fish poisoning has been questioned (172, 173). There was no correlation observed between the dose of histamine and the likelihood of an adverse reaction when human subjects consumed mackerel samples that had been implicated in outbreaks of scombroid fish poisoning (172, 173). However, the antihistamine chlorpheniramine abolished the adverse effects observed in some persons with specific samples of spoiled mackerel (173). Thus, Ijomah and colleagues (173) postulated that spoiled fish contain an as-yet-unidentified substance that induces the release of endogenous histamine from mast cells, and that scombroid fish poisoning is the result of the release of endogenous histamine rather than the ingestion of exogenous histamine. Thus, histamine poisoning could possibly be an anaphylactoid reaction as described earlier. In contrast, Morrow and colleagues (174) asserted that exogenous histamine was the likely causative agent in scombroid fish poisoning because high levels of histamine and one of its metabolites, N-methylhistamine, were found in the urine of three persons experiencing scombroid fish poisoning from marlin. They were unable to find elevated urinary levels of the prostaglandin D_2 metabolite, $9\alpha,11\beta$-dihydroxy-15-oxo-2,3,18,19-tetranorprost-5-ene-1,20-dioic acid, suggesting that mast cell degranulation had not occurred (174). The use of tryptase as a measure of mast cell degranulation would have been preferable, but to our knowledge that has never been tried.

Some individual variability is likely in susceptibility to histamine poisoning (3). Considerable variability was observed in individual susceptibility to ingestion of mackerel fillets that had been implicated in a scombroid fish poisoning outbreak (172). Some persons are likely compromised in their ability to detoxify and excrete histamine (3). Several drugs, including isoniazid, can inhibit the detoxification of histamine and are likely to potentiate the toxicity of histamine. Isoniazid has been implicated as a contributing factor in several outbreaks of histamine poisoning (175, 176). Alternatively, persons taking antihistamines for various reasons may be protected to some extent from the effects of histamine (3).

Preventive Measures

Although the role of exogenous histamine remains somewhat controversial, the bulk of the scientific evidence suggests that histamine plays some central role in scombroid fish poisoning. The key to the prevention of histamine intoxication is to prevent spoilage and histamine formation (3). Although efforts have focused on preventing the formation of histamine, the histamine-releasing factor, if present, must also be formed during spoilage because freshly caught and/or properly refrigerated/frozen fish do not cause illness (3). Holding fish at temperatures below 5°C after catching them prevents histamine formation (170). Good hygienic practices may also be important in the control of histamine formation (170). Most histamine-producing bacteria in fish are enteric bacteria, so human handling of the fish after catching may be the source of contamination. Good hygienic practices during distribution, storage, handling, processing, and preparation could prevent contamination of the fish. With cheese, histamine formation can be controlled by reducing the number of histamine-producing bacteria in the raw milk (169). Thus, the risk should be quite small in any cheese made from pasteurized milk (3).

CONCLUSIONS

Food allergies and other individualistic adverse reactions to foods affect only a small percentage of the population. However, the reactions can be very severe and even life-threatening in some cases of IgE-mediated food allergy and sulfite-induced asthma. The primary management strategies for these illnesses are the avoidance of the offending food or food ingredient. However, the avoidance of a specific food or food ingredient can be a daunting daily task, and complete success is unlikely.

IgE-mediated food allergies are well understood and relatively easy to diagnose. Management can be quite difficult. The prevalence of IgE-mediated food allergies appears to be increasing in the United States, and awareness of the consequences of IgE-mediated food allergies is increasing around the world. Much research progress has been made in recent years in the identification and characterization of the allergenic proteins in foods, methods for the detection of allergenic residues in foods, and food industry practices for controlling allergenic residues. However, many unresolved issues remain, such as clear establishment of minimal eliciting doses, allowing the development of safe and effective regulatory guidelines; the allergenicity of food ingredients derived from allergenic sources; the prediction of the allergenicity of novel proteins contained in genetically engineered foods; methods for preventing allergic sensitization in infants; and improved treatment modalities for those with food allergies, especially severe food allergies.

The role of delayed hypersensitivity reactions in food allergies is much less clear. Certainly, celiac disease may be more common than previously appreciated. In addition, severe consequences such as an increased prevalence of lymphoma may accompany celiac disease. A better understanding of the role of other foods in delayed hypersensitivity reactions would be helpful in the treatment of affected persons.

The role of certain food ingredients in food intolerances such as lactose intolerance and sulfite-induced asthma is well established. However, the food intolerances and the role of foods or food additives in these illnesses is much less clear. Here, research should be focused on establishment of clear cause-and-effect relationships.

Histamine poisoning can be confused diagnostically with food allergy. However, histamine poisoning can be readily distinguished in many circumstances by the presence of multiple cases among persons sharing the same meal. Histamine poisoning is not an individualistic adverse reaction to food. Unlike true food allergies, histamine poisoning can be controlled by limiting bacterial histamine formation in foods.

REFERENCES

1. Sloan AE, Powers ME. J Allergy Clin Immunol 1986;78:127–33.
2. Taylor SL, Hefle SL. Food Technology 2001;55:68–83.
3. Taylor SL, Hefle SL. Allergylike intoxications from foods. In: Frieri M, Kettelhut B, eds. Food Hypersensitivity and Adverse Reactions—A Practical Guide for Diagnosis and Management. New York: Marcel Dekker, 1999:141–53.
4. Sampson HA. J Allergy Clin Immunol 2004;113:805–19.
5. Murray J. Gluten-sensitive enteropathy. In: Metcalfe DD, Sampson HA, Simon RA, eds. Food Allergy—Adverse Reactions to Foods and Food Additives. 3rd ed. Malden, MA: Blackwell Science, 2003:242–61.
6. Taylor SL, Hefle SL. Allergic reactions and food intolerances. In: Kotsonis FN, Mackey MA, eds. Nutritional Toxicology. 2nd ed. New York: Taylor and Francis, 2002:93–121.
7. Bush, RK, Hefle SL. Crit Rev Food Sci Nutr 1996;36S:119–63.
8. Sicherer SH, Sampson HA. Clin Exp Allergy 1999;29:507–12.
9. Holt PG, Bjorksten B. Development of immunological tolerance to food antigens. In: Metcalfe DD, Sampson HA, Simon RA, eds. Food Allergy—Adverse Reactions to Foods and Food Additives. 3rd ed. Malden, MA: Blackwell Science, 2003:81–90.
10. Chandra RK. Food allergy: Setting the theme. In: Chandra RK, ed. Food Allergy. St. John's, Newfoundland: Nutrition Research Education Foundation, 1987:3–5.
11. Lack G, Fox DES, Golding J. J Allergy Clin Immunol 1999;103:S95.
12. Sicherer SH, Furlong TJ, Maes HH et al. J Allergy Clin Immunol 2000;106:53–6.
13. Aresery M, Cartier A, Wild L et al. Occupational reactions to food antigens. In: Metcalfe DD, Sampson HA, Simon RA, eds. Food Allergy—Adverse Reactions to Foods and Food Additives. 3rd ed. Malden, MA: Blackwell Science, 2003:270–95.
14. Sampson HA, Mendelson L, Rosen J. N Engl J Med 1992;327:380–4.
15. Yunginger JW, Sweeney KG, Sturner WQ et al. JAMA 1988;260:1450–2.

16. Bock SA, Munoz-Furlong A, Sampson HA. J Allergy Clin Immunol 2001;107:191–3.

17. Miller R, Ghatek A, Rothman P et al. J Allergy Clin Immunol 2000;105:S349.

18. Pastorello E, Ortolani C. Oral allergy syndrome. In: Metcalfe DD, Sampson HA, Simon RA, eds. Food Allergy—Adverse Reactions to Foods and Food Additives. 3rd ed. Malden, MA: Blackwell Science, 2003:169–82.

19. Taylor SL, Lehrer SB. Crit Rev Food Sci Nutr 1996;36:S91–S118.

20. Calkhoven PG, Aalbers M, Koshte VL et al. Allergy 1987;42:382–90.

21. O'Connor ME, Schocket AL. Exercise- and pressure-induced syndromes. In: Metcalfe DD, Sampson HA, Simon RA, eds. Food Allergy—Adverse Reactions to Foods and Food Additives. 3rd ed. Malden, MA: Blackwell Science, 2003:262–9.

22. Food and Agriculture Organization. Report of the FAO Technical Consultation on Food Allergies, Rome, November 13–14. Food and Agricultural Organization of the United Nations, 1995.

23. Bernhisel-Broadbent J, Scanlon SM, Sampson HA. J Allergy Clin Immunol 1992;89:730–7.

24. Hansen TK, Bindslev-Jensen C. Allergy 1992;47:610–7.

25. O'Neill CE, Lehrer SB. Food Technology 1995;49:103–16.

26. Langeland T. Allergy 1983;39:399–412.

27. Anet J, Back JF, Baker RS et al. Int Arch Allergy Immunol 1985;77:364–71.

28. Dean TP, Adler BR, Ruge F et al. Clin Exp Allergy 1993;23:205–10.

29. Martin JA, Compaired JA, de la Hoz B et al. Allergy 1992;47:185–7.

30. Kalogeromitros D, Armenaka M, Galatas I et al. Ann Allergy Asthma Immunol 1996;77:480–2.

31. Hefle SL, Nordlee JA, Taylor SL. Crit Rev Food Sci Nutr 1996;36S:69–89.

32. Taylor SL, Hefle SL, Soylemez G et al. Food Allergy Intolerance 2002;3:115–22.

33. Imai T, Akasawa A, Iikura Y. Int Arch Allergy Immunol 2001;124:312–4.

34. Rance F, Dutau G, Abbal M. Allergy 2000;55:496–500.

35. Taylor SL. Molluscan shellfish allergens. In: Villalba A, Reguera B, Romalde JL et al, eds: Molluscan Shellfish Safety, Proceedings of the 4th International Conference on Molluscan Shellfish Safety. Vilanova de Arousa, Spain: Consellaria de Pesce e Asuntos Maritmos, 2003:595–605.

36. Atkins FM, Wilson M, Bock SA. J Allergy Clin Immunol 1988;82:242–50.

37. Noyes J H, Boyd GK, Settipane GA. J Allergy Clin Immunol 1979;63:242–4.

38. Kalyoncu AF, Stalenheim G. Allergy 1993;48:295.

39. Ballmer-Weber B, Besler M, Hoffmann-Sommergruber K et al. Internet Symptoms Food Allergens 2000;2:145–67.

40. Breiteneder H, Ebner C. J Allergy Clin Immunol 2000;106:27–36.

41. Pastorello EA, Pravettoni V, Calamari M et al. Allergy 2002;57 [Suppl 72]:106–10.

42. Bugajska-Schretter A, Elfman L, Fuchs T. J Allergy Clin Immunol 1998;101:67–74.

43. Reese G, Ayuso R, Lehrer SB. Int Arch Allergy Immunol 1999;119:247–58.

44. Sicherer SH, Munoz-Furlong A, Sampson HA. J Allergy Clin Immunol 2004;114:159–65.

45. Sicherer SH, Munoz-Furlong A, Sampson HA, Sicherer SH. J Allergy Clin Immunol 2004;113:S100.

46. Bock SA. Pediatrics 1987;79:683–8.

47. Sampson HA. Curr Opin Immunol 1990;2:542–7.

48. Sampson HA, McCaskill CC. J Pediatr 1985;107:669–75.

49. Host A, Halken S. Allergy 1990;45:587–96.

50. Jakobbson I, Lindberg T. Acta Pediatr Scand 1979;68:853–9.

51. Schrander JJP, van den Bogart JPH, Forget PP et al. Eur J Pediatr 1993;152:640–4.

52. Hill DJ, Hosking CS, Zhie CY et al. Environ Toxicol Pathol 1997;4:101–10.

53. Bock SA. J Allergy Clin Immunol 1982;69:173–7.

54. Hill DJ, Hosking CS. Nutr Res 1992;12:109–21.

55. Bock SA, Atkins FM. J Allergy Clin Immunol 1989;83:900–4.

56. Wood RA. Natural history and prevention of food hypersensitivity. In: Metcalfe DD, Sampson HA, Simon RA, eds. Food Allergy—Adverse Reactions to Foods and Food Additives. 3rd ed. Malden, MA: Blackwell Scientific, 2003:425–37.

57. Zeiger RS, Heller S, Mellon MH et al. J Allergy Clin Immunol 1989;84:72–89.

58. Warner JO, Jones CA, Kilburn SA et al. Pediatr Allergy Immunol 2000;13S:6–8.

59. Zeiger RS, Heller S. J Allergy Clin Immunol 1995;95:1179–90.

60. Van Asperen PP, Kemp AS, Mellis CM. Arch Dis Child 1983;58:253–6.

61. Gerrard JW. Ann Allergy 1979;42:69–72.

62. Kirjavainen PV, Apostolou E, Salminen SJ et al. Allergy 1999;54:909–15.

63. Businco L, Dreborg S, Einarsson R et al. Pediatr Allergy Immunol 1993;4:101–11.

64. Vandenplas Y, Hauser B, Van den Borre C et al. Eur J Pediatr 1995;154:488–94.

65. Bock SA, Lee WY, Remigio LK et al. J Allergy Clin Immunol 1978;62:327–34.

66. Bock SA, Sampson HA, Atkins FM et al. J Allergy Clin Immunol 1988;82:986–97.

67. Van Arsdel PP, Larson EB. Ann Intern Med 1989;110:304–12.

68. Dreborg S. Allergy Proc 1991;12:251–4.

69. Yunginger JW, Ahlstedt S, Eggleston PA et al. J Allergy Clin Immunol 2000;105:1077–84.

70. Metcalfe DD. Nutr Rev 1984;42:92–7.

71. Sampson HA, Ho DG. J Allergy Clin Immunol 1997;100:444–51.

72. Furukawa CT. Nondietary management of food allergy. In: Chiaramonte LT, Schneider AT, Lifshitz F, eds. Food Allergy—A Practical Approach to Diagnosis and Management. New York: Marcel Dekker, 1988:365–75.

73. Atkins FM. Nutr Rev 1983;41:229–34.

74. Taylor SL, Bush RK, Busse WW. N Engl Reg Allergy Proc 1986;7:527–32.

75. Cordle CT. J Nutr 2004;134:1213S–9S.

76. Zeiger RS, Sampson HA, Bock SA et al. J Pediatr 1999;134:614–22.

77. Hill DJ, Hosking CS. The management and prevention of food allergy. In: Frieri M, Kettelhut B, eds. Food Hypersensitivity and Adverse Reactions—A Practical Guide to Diagnosis and Management. New York: Marcel Dekker, 1999:423–47.

78. Saylor JD, Bahna SL. J Pediatr 1991;118:71–4.

79. Rosenthal E, Schlesinger Y, Birnbaum Y et al. Acta Paediatr Scand 1991;80:958–60.

80. Hefle SL, Taylor SL. Food Technology 1999;53:62–70.

81. Teuber SS, Brown RL, Haapanen LAD. J Allergy Clin Immunol 1997;99:502–7.

82. Kanny G, de Hauteclocque C, Moneret-Vautrin DA. Allergy 1996;51:952–7.

83. Hoffman DR, Collins-Williams C. J Allergy Clin Immunol 1994;93:801–2.

84. Businco L, Cantani A, Longhi M et al. Ann Allergy 1989;62:
    333–5.
85. Muller U, Weber W, Hoffmann A et al. Z Lebensm Unter
    Forsch 1998;207:341–51.
86. Gu X, Beardslee T, Zeece M et al. Int Arch Allergy Immunol
    2001;126:218–25.
87. Taylor SL, Dormedy ES. Adv Food Nutr Res 1998;42:1–44.
88. Gern JE, Yang E, Evrard HM et al. N Engl J Med 1991;324:
    976–9.
89. McKenna C, Klontz KC. Ann Allergy Asthma Immunol 1997;
    79:234–6.
90. Hansen TK, Poulsen LK, Stahl Skov P et al. Food Chem Toxi-
    col 2004;42:2037–44.
91. Taylor SL, Hefle SL. Can J Allergy 2000;5:106–10.
92. Hamada Y, Nagashima Y, Shiomi K. Biosci Biotechnol Biochem
    2001;65:285–91.
93. Taylor SL, Hefle SL. Curr Allergy Clin Immunol 2001;14:12–8.
94. Lardizabal AL, Niemann LM, Hefle SL. J Allergy Clin
    Immunol 2004;113:S99.
95. Herian AM, Taylor SL, Bush RK. J Food Sci 1993;58:385–8.
96. Bernhisel-Broadbent J, Scanlon SM, Sampson HA. J Allergy
    Clin Immunol 1992;89:730–7.
97. Hansen TK, Bindslev-Jensen C, Skov PS et al. Ann Allergy
    Asthma Immunol 1997;78:187–94.
98. Herian AM, Taylor SL, Bush RK. Int Arch Allergy Appl
    Immunol 1990;92:193–8.
99. Bernhisel-Broadbent J, Sampson HA. J Allergy Clin Immunol
    1989;83:435–40.
100. Vieths S, Scheurer S, Ballmer-Weber B. Ann N Y Acad Sci
     2002;964:47–68.
101. Blanco C, Carrillo T, Castillo R et al. Ann Allergy 1994;73:309–14.
102. Taylor SL, Hefle SL, Bindslev-Jensen C et al. J Allergy Clin
     Immunol 2002;109:24–30.
103. Taylor SL, Nordlee JA, Rupnow JH. Food allergies and sensi-
     tivities. In: Taylor SL, Scanlan RA, eds. Food Toxicology—A
     Perspective on the Relative Risks. New York: Marcel Dekker,
     1989:255–95.
104. Yunginger JW, Gauerke MB, Jones RT et al. J Food Prot 1983;
     46:625–8.
105. Laoprasert N, Wallen ND, Jones RT et al. J Food Prot 1998;
     61:1522–4.
106. Hourihane JO'B, Kilburn SA, Nordlee JA et al. J Allergy Clin
     Immunol 1997;100:596–600.
107. Wensing M, Penninks AH, Hefle SL et al. J Allergy Clin
     Immunol 2002;110:915–20.
108. Morisset M, Moneret-Vautrin DA, Kanny G et al. Clin Exp
     Allergy 2003;33:1046–51.
109. Osterballe M, Bindslev-Jensen C. J Allergy Clin Immunol 2003;
     112:196–201.
110. Bindslev-Jensen C, Briggs D, Osterballe M. Allergy 2002;57:
     741–6.
111. Taylor SL, Hefle SL, Bindslev-Jensen C et al. Clin Exp Allergy
     2004;34:689–95.
112. Taylor SL, Nordlee JA. Food Technology 1996;50:231–4, 238.
113. Poms R, Klein CL, Anklam E. Food Addit Contam
     2004;21:1–31.
114. Hefle SL, Jeanniton E, Taylor SL. J Food Prot 2001;64:1812–6.
115. Hlywka JJ, Hefle SL, Taylor SL. J Food Prot 2000;63:252–7.
116. Jankiewicz A, Baltes W, Bogl K et al. J Sci Food Agric 1997;75:
     357–70.
117. Bernhisel-Broadbent J, Strause D, Sampson HA. J Allergy Clin
     Immunol 1992;90:622–9.
118. Astwood JD, Leach JN, Fuchs RL. Nat Biotechnol 1996;14:
     1269–73.
119. Metcalfe DD, Astwood JD, Townsend R et al. Crit Rev Food
     Sci Nutr 1996;36S:165–86.
120. Taylor SL, Hefle SL. J Allergy Clin Immunol 2001;107:765–71.
121. Nordlee J, Taylor SL, Townsend JA et al. N Engl J Med 1996;
     334:688–92.
122. Strober W. J Allergy Clin Immunol 1986;78:202–11.
123. Marsh MN. Gastroenterology 1992;102:330–54.
124. Cornell HJ. Amino Acids 1996;10:1–19.
125. Troncone R, Greco L, Auricchio S. Pediatr Clin North Am
     1996;43:355–73.
126. Logan RFA, Rifkind EA, Turner ID et al. Gastroenterology
     1989;97:265–71.
127. O'Mahoney S, Ferguson A. Gluten-sensitive enteropathy (celiac
     disease). In: Metcalfe DD, Sampson HA, Simon RA, eds. Food
     Allergy—Adverse Reactions to Foods and Food Additives.
     Boston: Blackwell Scientific, 1991:186–98.
128. Anand BS, Piris J, Truelove SC. Q J Med 1978;47:101–10.
129. Janatuinen EK, Pikkarainen PH, Kemppainen TA et al. N Engl
     J Med 1995;333:1033–7.
130. Wieser H. Acta Pediatr Suppl 1996;412:3–9.
131. Duggan JM. Med J Aust 1997;166:312–5.
132. Troncone R. Acta Pediatr 1995;34:1252–7.
133. Logan RFA. Descriptive epidemiology of celiac disease. In:
     Branski D, Rozen P, Kagnoff MF, eds. Gluten-Sensitive
     Enteropathy: Frontiers in Gastrointestinal Research, vol 19.
     Basel: Karger, 1992:1–14.
134. Fasano A, Berti I, Gerarduzzi T et al. Arch Intern Med 2003;
     163:286–92.
135. George EK., Mearin ML, van der Velde EA et al. Pediatr Res
     1995;37:213–8.
136. Hartsook EI. Cereal Foods World 1984;29:157–8.
137. Hekkens WTJM, van Twist de Graaf M. Nahrung 1990;34:483–7.
138. Skerritt JH, Hill AS. 1991. J Assoc Off Anal Chem 1991;74:
     257–64.
139. Suarez FL, Savaiano DA. Food Technology 1997;51:74–6.
140. Mager J, Chevion M, Glaser G. Favism. In: Liener IE, ed.
     Toxic Constituents of Plant Foodstuffs. 2nd ed. New York:
     Academic Press, 1980:265–94.
141. Gallagher CR, Molleson AL, Caldwell JH. Cult Dairy Prod J
     12977;10:22–4.
142. Kolars JC, Levitt MD, Aouji M et al. N Engl J Med 1984;310:
     1–3.
143. Kocian J. Int J Biochem 1988;20:1–5.
144. Sandine WE, Daly M. J Food Prot 1979;42:435–7.
145. Gilat T, Russo S, Gelman-Malachi E et al. Gastroenterology
     1972;62:1125–7.
146. Scrimshaw NS, Murray EB. Am J Clin Nutr 1988;48:1083–159.
147. Johnson AO, Semenya JG, Buchowski MS. Am J Clin Nutr
     1993;57:399–401.
148. Suarez FL, Savaiano DA, Levitt MD. N Engl J Med 1995;
     333:1–4.
149. Reasoner J, Maculan TP, Rand AG et al. Am J Clin Nutr 1981;
     34:54–60.
150. Bush RK, Taylor SL, Hefle SL. Adverse reactions to food and
     drug additives. In: Adkinson ND, Yunginger JW, Busse WW
     et al, eds. Middleton's Allergy Principles and Practices. 6th ed.
     Mosby: St. Louis, 2003:1645–63.
151. Prenner BM, Stevens JJ. Ann Allergy 1976;37:180–2.
152. Stevenson DD, Simon RA. J Allergy Clin Immunol 1981;68:
     26–32.
153. Taylor SL, Higley NA, Bush RK. Adv Food Res 1986;30:1–76.
154. Martin LB, Nordlee JA, Taylor SL. J Food Prot 1986;49:126–9.
155. Bush RK, Taylor SL, Holden K et al. Am J Med 1986;81:
     816–21.

156. Yang WH, Purchase ECR, Rivington RN. J Allergy Clin Immunol 1986;78:443–9.

157. Taylor SL, Bush RK, Selner JC et al. J Allergy Clin Immunol 1988;81:1159–67.

158. Delohery J, Simmul R, Castle WD et al. Am Rev Respir Dis 1984;130:1027–32.

159. Taylor SL, Stratton JE, Nordlee JA. Clin Toxicol 1989;27:225–40.

160. Bartholomew BA, Berry PR, Rodhouse JC et al. Epidemiol Infect 1987;99:775–82.

161. Borysiewicz L, Krikler D. Br Med J 1981;282:1434.

162. Anonymous. Histamine in seafood—Fluorometric method. In: Helrich K, ed. Official Methods of Analysis of the Association of Analytical Chemists. 15th ed. Arlington, VA: Association of Official Analytical Chemists, 1990:876–7.

163. Dickinson G. Ann Emerg Med 1982;11:487–9.

164. Blakesley ML. Ann Emerg Med 1983;12:104–6.

165. Food and Drug Administration. Decomposition and histamine—Raw, frozen tuna and mahi-mahi; canned tuna; and related species. Compliance Policy Guide 7108.24, 1995:3.

166. Taylor SL, Keefe TJ, Windham ES et al. J Food Prot 1982;45:455–7.

167. Wantke F, Gotz M, Jarisch R. N Engl Reg Allergy Proc 1994;15:27–32.

168. Halasz A, Barath A, Simon-Sarkadi L et al. Trends Food Sci Technol 1994;5:42–9.

169. Sumner SS, Roche F, Taylor SL. J Dairy Sci 1990;73:3050–8.

170. Taylor SL. Crit Rev Toxicol 1986;17:91–128.

171. Weiss S, Robb GP, Ellis LB. Arch Intern Med 1932;49:360–2.

172. Clifford MN, Walker R, Ijomah P et al. Food Addit Contam 1991;8:641–52.

173. Ijomah P, Clifford MN, Walker R et al. Food Addit Contam 1991;8:531–42.

174. Morrow JD, Margolies GR, Rowland J et al. N Engl J Med 1991;324:716–20.

175. Uragoda CG, Kottegoda SR. Tubercle 1977;58:83–9.

176. Senanayake N, Vyravanathan S. Toxicon 1981;19:184–5.

96 NUTRITION IN THE OLDER PERSON[1]

JOHN E. MORLEY

INDICATORS OF DECLINE AND MORTALITY 1531
 Causes of Weight Loss and Its Management 1532
 Effect of Anorexia and Weight Loss Factors 1534
METABOLIC AND NUTRITION-RELATED DISEASES
 IN OLDER PERSONS 1536
 Insulin Resistance Syndrome 1536
 Diabetes Mellitus 1536
 Vitamin Deficiency 1536
CONCLUSION 1537

"... for wasting which represents old age (sarcopenia) and wasting that is secondary to fever (cachexia) and wasting which is called doalgashi (starvation)"

... Maimonides (1135–1204)

Human life expectancy was 18 years in the Bronze Age. This rose to 33 years in England during the Middle Ages, 35.5 years in the eighteenth century, and 40.9 years in the nineteenth century. In the United States, life expectancy increased from 49.2 years at the beginning of the twentieth century to 79 years at the end of the century. At the beginning of the twentieth century, 4% of the US population was more than 65 years of age, and this number had grown to 12.8% by the end of the century. The longest-lived persons in the world live in Japan, and Italy has the largest population over 65 years of age. Women live longer than men. The United States, despite having the largest health care budget, fails to be in the top ten for life expectancy from birth or for life expectancy over the age of 65 years. Eight of ten countries with the longest life expectancy consume 1% or more of their calories from fish (1).

INDICATORS OF DECLINE AND MORTALITY

Although much of the nutrition focus in younger and middle-aged persons is on obesity, in older persons the major problem is weight loss. The best indicator of mortality in community-dwelling (2–4), hospitalized (5), or institutionalized (6) elderly persons is weight loss. Low total calorie intake is associated with increased mortality (7). Low dietary

---

[1] **Abbreviations: AIDS,** acquired immunodeficiency syndrome; **CCK,** cholecystokinin; **CNAQ,** Council of Nutrition Appetite Questionnaire; **NASH,** nonalcoholic steatohepatitis.

intake, low body mass index, decreased arm muscle area, and low serum albumin are associated with hip fracture (8). When weight loss is reversed in older, institutionalized persons, survival is improved (9). Weight loss, even when intentional, increases the propensity to fracture a hip (10). Weight loss is associated with an increased propensity for an older person to be institutionalized (11).

Since the pioneering work of Reuben Andres, numerous studies have shown that, with aging, the body mass index associated with the lowest mortality has increased (12). When body mass index is plotted against mortality, the data are best fitted by a quadratic (U-shaped) curve, rather than by a simple regression (13). Thus, being underweight (body mass index <21) and being overweight are predictors of increased mortality and functional decline in older persons.

With aging, there is an increase in waist-to-hip ratio (14). This was more marked in persons who smoke cigarettes (15). Two studies in persons aged 55 to 69 years have shown that this increase in central adiposity is associated with an increase in coronary artery disease mortality and total mortality (16, 17).

Both low serum albumin and low cholesterol are strong predictors of death in older persons (18–21). To a large extent, the reason is that albumin and cholesterol levels decline not only in association with protein-energy intake, but also in response to increasing levels of circulating cytokines, such as tumor necrosis factor-α or interleukin-1 (22). A serum albumin level lower than 30 g/L is strongly associated with subsequent mortality.

Food intake decreases over the life span. In the third National Health and Nutrition Examination Survey, there was a linear decrease in food intake in male subjects from a peak ingestion aged 16 to 19 years of 3097 to 1776 kcal in men more than 80 years of age (23). By the sixth decade, calorie intake had reduced by 32%, and in those more than 80 years by 39%. In women, caloric intake decreased by 14% in those in their 60s and 22% in those more than 80 years of age. Numerous longitudinal studies have confirmed this decline in caloric intake with aging (24, 25). These calories have consistently shown that a fall in fat intake predominately accounts for the decline in total calories.

In older persons, fat is a key to survival. Fat acts as a storage organ for calories in times of famine. In the

United States, it has been shown that the most hospitalized elderly patients receive inadequate calories to maintain their weight and to ingest adequate vitamins and minerals (26). This makes weight loss the true skeleton in the hospital closet! Fat also acts as a protective organ, thus decreasing the propensity to hip fracture. Subcutaneous fat is important for the maintenance of thermoregulation. Finally, fat is a highly metabolic tissue, releasing a variety of peptides such as leptin, adiponectin, and cytokines.

Protein-energy undernutrition has a variety of deleterious effects in older persons. These include pressure ulcers, infections, hip fracture, cognitive abnormalities, anemia, muscle weakness, fatigue, edema, and mortality. In addition, protein-energy undernutrition tends to worsen the negative age-related changes that occur in the immune system, such as delayed hypersensitivity, thymic involution, decreased mitogen lymphocyte proliferation, decreased interleukin-2, and decreased response to immunization. In addition, protein-energy malnutrition can produce a marked decrease in the numbers of helper/inducer (CD_4^+) T cells (27). This change has been associated with unusual infections in older persons.

Overall metabolic rate declines with aging (Fig. 96.1). The reasons are a marked decrease in physical activity and a smaller decline in resting metabolic rate (28). The decrease in resting metabolic rate is predominantly the result of the decline in lean body mass that occurs with aging. Thus, the decline in resting metabolic rate with aging is minimal when corrected for lean body mass. A small decline in resting metabolic rate also occurs with aging because of a decline in the body's ability to generate energy, such as from the decline in sodium-potassium/adenosine triphosphatase activity (29). A delayed or decreased thermic effect of feeding occurs with aging. This appears to be predominantly related to the delay in the rate of gastric emptying that occurs with large caloric loads (>500 kcal) in older persons.

Causes of Weight Loss and Its Management

The four major causes of weight loss in older persons are anorexia, sarcopenia, cachexia, and dehydration.

Anorexia of Aging

Physiologic Anorexia. With aging, a physiologic anorexia occurs as delineated earlier in the chapter. This is predominantly in response to the decline in activity over the life span. The causes of this physiologic anorexia include social isolation, alterations in taste and smell, changes in gastrointestinal function leading to early satiation, and, in men, a decline in testosterone resulting in elevated leptin levels (Fig. 96.2) (30).

In social situations, older persons eat more than when they eat alone (31). Suda and colleagues (32) showed that nutritional risk could be significantly decreased by having the person delivering the Meals-on-Wheels sit with the older person while he or she ate a meal. Enhancing the environment in the dining room in a nursing home leads to weight gain (33). Multiple changes in taste and smell with aging decrease one's enjoyment of food. The use of food enhancers, such as monosodium glutamate, leads to an increased weight gain (34). Poor dentition is associated with a decline in food intake (35).

When food enters the fundus of the stomach, it causes the release of nitric oxide, with consequent relaxation of the smooth muscle and fundal dilation. This is called adaptive relaxation. With aging, there is a decrease in the release of nitric oxide. This leads to a decrease in fundal compliance and thus allows smaller volumes of food to be contained in the fundus (36). The faster egress of food from the fundus to the antrum causes antral stretch to occur sooner, and the result is earlier satiation. This early satiation is seen with large meals (>500 calories) and is associated with a slowing of gastric emptying (37).

When food reaches the duodenum, the satiating hormone, cholecystokinin (CCK) is released. Older persons have an increase in basal circulating CCK levels and a

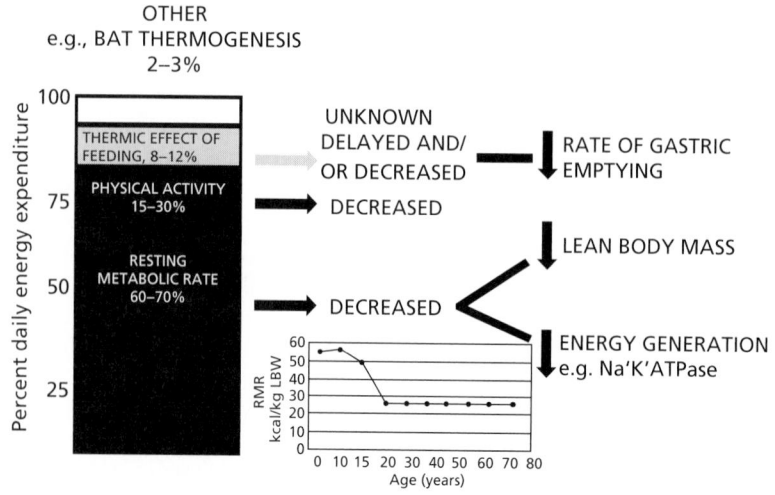

Figure 96.1. Changes in metabolic rate with age. BAT, brown adipose tissue; LBW, lean body weight; RMR, resting metabolic rate. (Adapted from Morley JE et al. Pharm Biochem Behav 1995;50:369–73, with permission.)

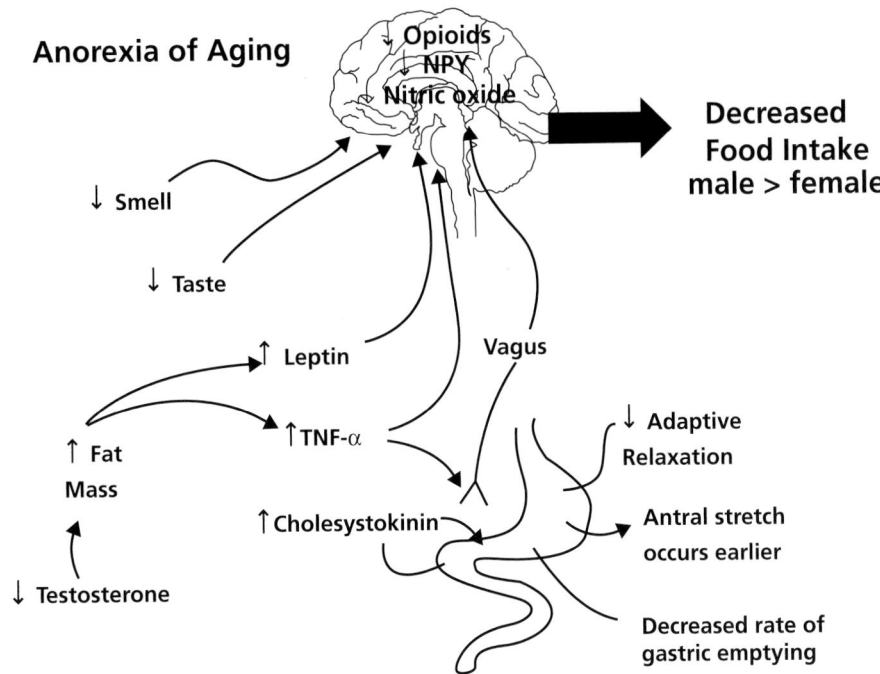

Figure 96.2. The causes of the physiologic anorexia of aging. TNF-α, tumor necrosis factor-α. (From Wilson MMG, Morley JE. J Appl Physiol 2003;95:1728–36, with permission.)

marked increase in CCK levels in response to a lipid meal (38). The reasons are a decline in clearance of CCK with aging and the fact that this hormone is a more effective satiating agent in older persons (39). For these reasons, CCK plays an important role in the decline in fat intake with aging.

Ghrelin is a peptide hormone released from the fundus of the stomach. This hormone increases food intake and growth hormone release and improves memory. Ghrelin levels appear to decline slightly with aging, a finding suggesting a role in the physiologic anorexia of aging and the age-related decline in growth hormone secretion.

Testosterone levels decline with aging in men (40). This decline in testosterone in men is associated with an increase in leptin levels (41). Leptin is a hormone produced from adipose tissue that is anorectic and is associated with an increase in metabolic rate. Testosterone treatment in older men leads to a decrease in leptin levels (42). Thus, it is reasonable to postulate that the decline in testosterone coupled with the increase in leptin is responsible for the increased anorexia seen in older men compared with older women.

Pathologic Anorexia. Besides the physiologic anorexia of aging, there is also a pathologic anorexia of aging. The causes of weight loss in the elderly are conveniently remembered by the mnemonic MEALS-ON-WHEELS (Table 96.1). The major factor responsible for weight loss in community-dwelling and institutionalized elderly persons is depression. Numerous medications can produce anorexia; in the presence of the polypharmacy often seen with older persons, medications are an important cause of anorexia (Table 96.2). Another important cause of weight loss is therapeutic diets. In older persons, the use of therapeutic diets, such as diabetic, low-cholesterol, and low-salt diets, is questionable, and such diets are no longer recommended in institutions (43). Cancers account for

TABLE 96.1. PATHOLOGIC CAUSES OF WEIGHT LOSS IN OLDER PERSONS: THE MEALS-ON-WHEELS MNEMONIC

*M*edications (e.g., digoxin, theophylline, cimetidine)
*E*motional (e.g., depression)
*A*lcoholism, elder abuse, anorexia tardive
*L*ate life paranoia
*S*wallowing problems
*O*ral factors
*N*osocomial infections (e.g., tuberculosis)
*W*andering and other dementia-related factors
*H*yperthyroidism, *H*ypercalcemia, *H*ypoadrenalism
*E*nteral problems (e.g., gluten enteropathy)
*E*ating problems
*L*ow-salt, low-cholesterol and other therapeutic diets
*S*tones (cholecystitis)

TABLE 96.2. CLASSES OF MEDICATIONS THAT CAUSE ANOREXIA AND/OR WEIGHT LOSS IN OLDER PERSONS

Antidepressants (selective serotonin reuptake inhibitors)
Sympathomimetics
Antiarrythmics
Antihypertensives
Opiates
Antibiotics
Antineoplastics
Antiepileptics
H₂ antagonists
Xanthines
Digitalis

approximately 10% of the weight loss seen in older persons, whereas depression is responsible for 30%.

Effect of Anorexia and Weight Loss Factors

Sarcopenia

Sarcopenia is the excessive loss of muscle, with the maintenance of fat mass. It is strongly correlated with a decline in function and death in older persons (44). It occurs in about 10% of persons more than 65 years old. Obese persons who lose muscle mass, that is, obese sarcopenic or "fat frail" persons, have particularly poor outcomes.

The causes of sarcopenia are multifactorial. They include a decline in testosterone and insulinlike growth factor-I an increase in proinflammatory cytokines, a decrease in physical activity, peripheral vascular disease, and a decline in food intake. Diminished intake of creatine, which has a specific role in muscle function, may be particularly important. A decrease in the number of nerve end plates innervating muscle also plays a role in the pathogenesis of sarcopenia. The decline in testosterone not only leads to a decrease in muscle protein synthesis but also leads to reduced production of satellite precursor cells, which are essential for the repair of muscle (45).

Cachexia

Cachexia is the excessive loss of lean body mass together with a loss of body fat associated with disease processes (46). Cachexia can coexist with adequate calorie intake. The major factor responsible for cachexia appears to be excess cytokine, such as interleukin-1, interleukin-6, and tumor necrosis factor-α release. Cytokines decrease protein synthesis in muscle through activation of nuclear factor-κ β, and by enhancing the action of the ubiquitin-proteasome system, they induce proteolysis. This leads to an increase in amino acids available for the liver to produce C-reactive protein and other acute-phase proteins. Cytokines also produce insulin resistance. They decrease the activity of lipoprotein lipase in the liver and thus produce lipolysis and a decline in gastrointestinal motility. Cytokines are anorectic and induce sickness behavior.

Many diseases are associated with cachexia. These include cancer, rheumatoid arthritis, congestive heart failure (cardiac cachexia), renal failure, acquired immunodeficiency syndrome (AIDS) and other infections, and chronic obstructive pulmonary disease. With the exception of AIDS, all these conditions occur more commonly in older persons, and even the prevalence of AIDS is increasing in the elderly.

Dehydration

With aging, the perception of thirst is decreased. The reason is a decline in the μ opioid drinking drive (47). This decreased thirst drive makes older persons highly vulnerable

to developing dehydration when they have fevers, are exposed to high environmental temperatures, are given diuretics, have other causes of excessive urination such as diabetes, or develop diarrhea.

It is commonly considered that a ratio of blood urea nitrogen to creatinine greater than 20:1 is indicative of dehydration. However, in older persons, this can occur because of gastrointestinal bleeding, congestive heart failure, and renal failure. In some older persons with heart disease, mild degrees of dehydration are often necessary to prevent symptomatic heart failure. An elevated sodium level is a better indicator of dehydration in older persons. Diagnosis of dehydration in an older person depends on measuring or calculating serum osmolality (see Chapter 8). Failure to do this has been shown to miscategorize large numbers of older persons as dehydrated when they are not suffering from dehydration.

Although the equivalent of eight glasses of fluid a day is recommended for older persons, drinking four to six glasses a day has been shown to be sufficient to prevent dehydration (48).

Management

Weights need to be measured regularly in older persons. A loss of 5% or more of weight requires aggressive intervention. Changes in appetite that will lead to weight loss in older persons can be recognized by the answers to the mini-Council of Nutrition Appetite Questionnaire (CNAQ, pronounced snack) (Table 96.3). The MiniNutritional Assessment is a validated clinical tool, which does not require laboratory measurements, for determining nutritional risk in older persons (Table 96.4) (49). The DETERMINE questionnaire has been shown to have inadequate sensitivity and specificity to be useful in recognizing nutritional risk in older persons. All older persons who are losing weight should be screened for cognitive problems by using either the MiniMental Status Examination (50) or the St. Louis University Mental Status Examination (51).

It is important to ascertain that an older person losing weight has adequate help with shopping, meal preparation, and feeding. In nursing homes, it can take more than 30 minutes to feed a demented patient adequately (52). Liquid calorie supplements, when used, should be given between meals, at least 1 hour before the meal (53). The Cochrane Collaboration metaanalysis showed that calorie supplements in older persons produce a small increase in weight and decrease mortality (54).

Tube feeding, either nasogastric or gastrointestinal, clearly can be lifesaving in some persons who cannot swallow. However, most older persons who receive tubes have mild degrees of dysphagia and aspiration for which the indication of tube feeding is questionable. Many of these patients were first placed on diets of altered consistency in an attempt to prevent aspiration. These diets rarely work and are unpalatable, leading to continued weight loss.

TABLE 96.3. APPETITE QUESTIONNAIRE TO PREDICT WEIGHT LOSS IN OLDER PERSONS: THE MINI-COUNCIL OF NUTRITION APPETITE QUESTIONNAIRE (CNAQ)[a]

1. My appetite is
   A. very poor
   B. poor
   C. average
   D. good
   E. very good

2. When I eat
   A. I feel full after eating only a few mouthfuls
   B. I feel full after eating about a third of a meal
   C. I feel full after eating over half a meal
   D. I feel full after eating most of the meal
   E. I hardly ever feel full

3. Food tastes
   A. very bad
   B. bad
   C. average
   D. good
   E. very good

4. Normally I eat
   A. less than one meal a day
   B. one meal a day
   C. two meals a day
   D. three meals a day
   E. more than three meals a day

[a]Instructions: Complete the questionnaire by circling the correct answers and then tally the results based on the following numeric scale: A = 1, B = 2, C = 3, D = 4, E = 5.
Scoring: If the mini-CNAQ is less than 14, there is a significant risk of weight loss.

No evidence indicates that demented persons with weight loss have better outcomes when they are tube fed. Overall, it would appear that in the United States, there is an excessive use of tube feeding. Given the poor outcomes in older tube-fed patients, this would appear to be an ethically unsound approach (see also Chapter 101). Peripheral parenteral nutrition may have a role in some older patients in hospitals who are not eating adequate calories.

Because of the poor appetite in older persons, orexigenics are becoming more used. A metaanalysis showed that megestrol acetate increases food intake, produces weight gain, and enhances quality of life (55). Megestrol acetate, a glucorticoid progestational agent, has been shown to produce weight gain in older nursing home residents (56, 57). Its glucocorticoid effects decrease the activity of the hypothalamic-pituitary-adrenal axis; very occasionally, adrenal insufficiency may occur during withdrawal of the drug. Like other glococorticoids, megestrol acetate decreases testosterone levels. Finally, megestrol acetate produces a small increase in the incidence of deep vein thrombosis. However, the incidence is less than that seen with antipsychotics.

Dronabinol, a synthetic cannabis agent, increases appetite in older persons. It has not been shown to increase weight gain significantly in this population (58). It also calms agitated behavior, decreases pain, and is antinauseatic. For these reasons, it has been suggested to be an excellent drug to treat persons at the end of life. The antiserotonergic agent, cyproheptadine, does not appear to be an effective orexigenic agent in older persons. Oxoglutarate has been successfully used as an orexigenic agent in Europe.

Anabolic agents include the testosteronelike steroids and growth hormone. Growth hormone has been shown to reverse weight loss, increase lean body mass, and improve functional status in malnourished older persons (59, 60). Testosterone appears to be better than growth hormone at reversing the decline in strength that occurs with sarcopenia (61). Nandrolone has been successfully used to treat sarcopenia and malnutrition. The oral anabolic agents appear to be less effective than the parenteral anabolics, perhaps because of the first-pass liver effect of the oral anabolic drugs.

Overall, many treatable causes of weight loss exist in older persons. Because of the poor outcomes associated with weight loss, it is important in older persons that weight loss be aggressively managed.

TABLE 96.4. MININUTRITIONAL ASSESSMENT[a]

A. Has food intake declined over the past 3 months as a result of loss of appetite, digestive problems, or chewing or swallowing difficulties?
   0 = severe loss of appetite
   1 = moderate loss of appetite
   2 = no loss of appetite

B. Weight loss during last 3 months
   0 = weight loss >3 kg (6.6 lb)
   1 = does not know
   2 = weight loss between 1 and 3 kg (2.2 and 6.6 lb)
   3 = no weight loss

C. Mobility
   0 = bed or chair bound
   1 = able to get out of bed/chair but does not go out
   2 = goes out

D. Has suffered psychologic stress or acute disease in the past 3 months
   0 = yes
   2 = no

E. Neuropsychologic problems
   0 = severe dementia or depression
   1 = mild dementia
   2 = no psychologic problems

F. Body mass index (BMI) (weight in kg)/(height in m)^2
   0 = BMI <19
   1 = BMI 19–21
   2 = BMI 21–<23
   3 = BMI ≥23

[a]Screening Score (subtotal max. 14 points):
12 points or greater: normal, no need for further assessment.
11 points or below: possible malnutrition, continue assessment.

Adapted from Rubenstein LZ, Harker JO, Salva A et al. Screening for undernutrition in geriatric practice: Developing the short-form Mini-Nutritional Assessment (MNA-SF). J Gerontol Med Sci 2001;57A:M366–72, with permission.

TABLE 96.5. COMPARISON OF THE TYPES OF DIABETES MELLITUS

	DIABETIC TYPES		
	TYPE 1	TYPE 1 1/2	TYPE 2
Age	Young	Old	Middle-Aged
Body habitus	Thin	Thin or mild visceral obesity	Obese
Coma	Ketoacidotic	Mixed/lactic acidosis	Hyperosmolar
Glucose-induced insulin release	Very low	Low	Increased but insufficient to overcome insulin resistance
Insulin-mediated glucose disposal	Normal	Mild or decreased	Markedly decreased
Fasting hepatic glucose output	Increased	Normal	Increased

From Morley JE. J Gerontol Med Sci 2000;55A:M255–6, with permission.

METABOLIC AND NUTRITION-RELATED DISEASES IN OLDER PERSONS

Insulin Resistance Syndrome

Since the mid-1990s, there has been increased recognition of the importance of insulin resistance in middle-aged and older adults (62). Insulin resistance is a syndrome that is particularly associated with the presence of visceral obesity. Insulin resistance leads to hyperinsulinemia, hypertension, diabetes mellitus, hyperuricemia, clotting abnormalities, hypertriglyceridemia, myosteatosis (fat infiltration in muscle), nonalcoholic steatohepatitis, and cognitive abnormalities. It has been suggested that the insulin resistance syndrome can lead to Alzheimer disease. The reason is that insulin and amyloid β protein are degraded by the same enzyme, insulin-degrading enzyme, in the brain. High insulin levels will, therefore, slow the degradation of amyloid β protein. Amyloid β protein is associated with the senile plaques, cognitive abnormalities, and free radical damage that occur in Alzheimer disease.

Diabetes Mellitus

Many persons with diabetes mellitus who are more than 70 years old are thin, not obese (63). Although they have some degree of insulin resistance, they also have a decline in insulin production. This type of diabetes in the older person has been characterized as type 1½ (Table 96.5). Older persons should be screened for diabetes mellitus every 2 years. Both a fasting glucose concentration and a postprandial glucose level should be obtained.

Diabetes mellitus represents a major cause of functional decline in older persons. Persons with diabetes also have problems with mobility and are more likely to have injurious falls. Diabetes is associated with an increased rate of hip fracture. Depression is a major factor in hospitalization of older patients with diabetes and is associated with increased mortality. Diabetes mellitus is associated with pain that can lead to functional impairment, poor sleep, and decreased quality of life. Approximately 10% of older persons with diabetes mellitus are zinc deficient (64). This deficiency is associated with poor healing of vascular ulcers. Pressure ulcers occur more commonly in older persons with diabetes mellitus.

Vitamin Deficiency

Vitamin deficiency occurs commonly in older persons (Table 96.6). Although very few older persons present with frank vitamin deficiency, vitamin deficiency is commonly

TABLE 96.6. PREVALENCE OF VITAMIN DEFICIENCIES IN OLDER PERSONS

VITAMIN	INDEPENDENT	HOSPITALIZED	NURSING HOME
Vitamin A	1%	?	?
B$_1$ (thiamin)	13–43%	40%	2–5%
B$_2$ (riboflavin)	3–42%	12%	1–34%
B$_6$ (Pyridoxine)	5–56%	19%	21–93%
Folate	2.5–34%	24%	4–24%
Vitamin B$_{12}$ (cyanocobalamin)	4–43%	?	4–29%
Vitamin C (ascorbic acid)	?	?	0–5%
Vitamin D[a]	2–5%	22%	35%

?, unknown.
[a] Based on measured levels as intake interacts with sunlight.

TABLE 96.7. STUDIES ON EFFECTS OF VITAMIN ADMINISTRATION IN OLDER SUBJECTS

AUTHOR AND DATE (REFERENCE)	TREATMENT	OUTCOME
Cognition		
Eastley, 2000 (65)	Vitamin B_{12}	Improvement in mild cognitive impairment patients on verbal fluency test
Hassing, 1999 (66)	Folic acid	Improvement in impairment of word recall and object recall
Deijen, 1992 (67)	Vitamin B_6	Improvement in long–term memory
Smidt, 1991 (68)	Thiamin	Improvement in cognitive function
Wilkinson, 1997 (69)	Thiamin	Improved cognition
Immune function		
Buzina–Suboticanec, 1998 (70)	Multivitamin	Improvement in delayed cutaneous hypersensitivity
Chandra, 1992 (71)	Vitamin-trace element supplement	Increased natural killer cells, proliferation of white cells following mitogen exposure, increase interleukin-2 production, and decreased infections
Pike and Chandra, 1995 (72)	Vitamin-trace element supplement	Increase in CD57 and no decrease in CD4 T cells compared with placebo
Bogden, 1994 (73)	Vitamin-trace element supplement	Improved delayed cutaneous hypersensitivity
Chavance, 1993 (74)	Multivitamin	No difference in infections
Biochemical		
Mann, 1987 (75)	Multivitamin	Increase in vitamins C, B_2, B_{12}, and folate, but no effect on vitamins A and E
Kauwell, 2000 (76)	Folate	415 mg/d of folate, but not 200 mg/d reduced serum homocysteine levels
van der Wielen, 1995 (77)	Fortified fruit juice	Decreased serum homocysteine and increased body weight
Hip fracture		
Chapuy, 1994 (78)	Vitamin D and calcium	Decreased hip fracture and decreased mortality rate

associated with cognitive dysfunction and immune alterations that respond to vitamin replacement (Table 96.7).

Folate and vitamin B_{12} deficiency are associated with elevated levels of homocysteine, which are associated with cognitive decline, hip fracture, and atherosclerotic disease. Besides deficiency of folate and vitamin B_{12}, renal failure and hypothyroidism are associated with elevated homocysteine levels in the elderly.

In a longitudinal study vitamin D levels were found to decline even in healthy older persons living in New Mexico. Vitamin D deficiency is very common among older persons as a result of one or more of the following: decreased synthesis of cholecalciferol, excessive use of sunblock, decreased sun exposure by clothing or by being housebound, or impaired renal or hepatic synthesis of vitamin D metabolites (see Chapter 20). Replacement of vitamin D and calcium decreases the rate of hip fracture in the elderly. Older persons with vitamin D deficiency have decreased strength and more falls and functional impairment.

CONCLUSION

Numerous alterations in nutrition occur with aging. Weight loss, rather than obesity, is the major problem. Diabetes mellitus and insulin resistance syndrome are important conditions involving nutrition in older persons. The role of nutrition in cognitive dysfunction has become

an important area of research. Vitamin D deficiency plays a key role in hip fracture, loss of muscular strength, and functional impairment. Changes in the metabolism of other vitamins are mainly associated with cognitive dysfunction and impaired immune function.

REFERENCES

1. Morley JE. J Am Geriatr Soc 1991;39:836–8.
2. Pamuk ER, Williamson DF, Madans J et al. Am J Epidemiol 1992;136:686–97.
3. de Groot CP, Enzi G, Matthys C et al. J Nutr Health Aging 2002; 6:4–8.
4. Losonczy KG, Harris TB, Cornoni–Huntley J et al. Am J Epidemiol 1995;141:312–21.
5. Liu L, Bopp MM, Roberson PK et al. J Gerontol Med Sci 2002;57A:M741–6.
6. Morley JE, Silver AJ. Ann Intern Med 1995;123:850–9.
7. Morley JE, Thomas DR. Nutrition 1999;15:499–503.
8. Morley JE. Am J Clin Nutr 1997;66:760–73.
9. Yamashita BD, Sullivan DH, Morley JE et al. J Nutr Health Aging 2002;6:275–81.
10. Ensrud KE, Ewing SK, Stone KL et al. J Am Geriatr Soc 2003; 51:1740–7.
11. Payette H, Coulombe C, Boutier V et al. J Gerontol Med Sci 1999;54A:M440–5.
12. Andres R, Elahi D, Tobin JD et al. Ann Intern Med 1985; 103:1030–3.
13. Build Study 1979. Chicago: Society of Actuaries and Association of Life Insurance Medical Directors of America, 1980.

14. Shimokata H, Tobin JD, Muller DC et al. J Gerontol 1989;44:M66–73.
15. Shimokata H, Muller DC, Andres R. JAMA 1989;262:1185–6.
16. Prineas RJ, Folsom AR, Kaye SA. Ann Epidemiol 1993;3:35–41.
17. Folsom AR, Kaye SA, Sellers TA et al. JAMA 1993;269:483–7.
18. Agarwal N, Acevedo F, Leighton LS et al. Am J Clin Nutr 1988;48:1173–8.
19. Hermann FR, Safran C, Levkoff SE et al. Arch Intern Med 1992;152:125–30.
20. Brescianini S, Maggi S, Farchi G et al, ILSA Group. J Am Geriatr Soc 2003;51:991–6.
21. Foody JM, Wang Y, Kiefe CI et al. J Am Geriatr Soc 2003;51:930–6.
22. Baez–Franceschi D, Morley JE. Z Gerontol Geriatr 1999;32 [Suppl 1]:I12–9.
23. Anonymous. MMWR Morb Mortal Wkly Rep 1994;43:116–25.
24. Koehler KM. Nutr Rev 1994;8:S34–7.
25. Sjogren A, Osterberg T, Steen B. Age Ageing 1994;23:108–12.
26. Sullivan DH, Sun S, Walls RC. JAMA 1999;281:2013–9.
27. Kaiser FE, Morley JE. J Am Geriatr Soc 1994;42:1291–4.
28. Wilson MM, Morley JE. J Appl Physiol 2003;95:1728–36.
29. Simat BM, Morley JE, From AH et al. Am J Clin Nutr 1984;40:339–45.
30. Morley JE, Silver AJ. Neurobiol Aging 1988;9:9–16.
31. de Castro JM. J Gerontol Med Sci 2002;57:M368–77.
32. Suda Y, Marske CE, Flaherty JH et al. J Nutr Health Aging 2001;5:118–23.
33. Mathey MF, Vanneste VG, de Graaf C et al. Prev Med 2001;32:416–23.
34. Mathey MF, Siebelink E, de Graaf C et al. J Gerontol Med Sci 2001;56A:M200–5.
35. Ritchie CS, Joshipura K, Silliman RA et al. J Gerontol Med Sci 2000;55A:M366–71.
36. Chapman IM, MacIntosh CG, Morley JE et al. Biogerontology 2002;3:67–71.
37. Clarkston WK, Pantano MM, Morley JE et al. Am J Physiol 1997;272:R243–8.
38. MacIntosh CG, Horowitz M, Verhagen MA et al. Am J Gastroenterol 2001;96:997–1007.
39. MacIntosh CG, Morley JE, Wishart J et al. J Clin Endocrinol Metab 2001;86:5830–7.
40. Morley JE, Perry HM III. J Steroid Biochem Molecul Biol 2003;85:367–73.
41. Baumgartner RN, Ross RR, Waters DL et al. Obes Res 1999;7:141–9.
42. Sih R, Morley JE, Kaiser FE et al. J Clin Endocrinol Metab 1997;82:1661–7.
43. Tariq SH, Karcic E, Thomas DR et al. J Am Diet Assoc 2001;101:1463–6.
44. Morley JE, Baumgartner RN, Roubenoff R et al. J Lab Clin Med. 2001;137:231–43.
45. Bhasin S, Taylor WE, Singh R et al. J Gerontol Med Sci 2003;58A:M1103–10.
46. Kotler DP. Ann Intern Med 2000;133:622–34.
47. Silver AJ, Morley JE. J Am Geriatr Soc 1992;40:556–60.
48. Lindeman RD, Romero LJ, Liang HC et al. J Gerontol Med Sci 2000;55A:M361–5.
49. Guigoz Y, Lauque S, Vellas BJ. Clin Geriatr Med 2002;18:737–57.
50. Tombaugh TN, McIntyre NJ. J Am Geriatr Soc 1992;40:922–35.
51. Banks WA, Morley JE. J Gerontol Med Sci 2003;58A:314–21.
52. Simmons SF, Babineau S, Garcia E et al. J Gerontol Med Sci 2002;57A:M665–71.
53. Wilson MM, Purushothaman R, Morley JE. Am J Clin Nutr 2002;75:944–7.
54. Milne AC, Potter J, Avenell A. Cochrane Database of Systematic Reviews 2004:4.
55. Pascual Lopez A, Roque I, Figuls M et al. J Pain Sympt Mgt 2004;27:360–9.
56. Yeh SS, Hafner A, Chang CK et al. J Am Geriatr Soc 2004;52:1708–12.
57. Karcic E, Philpot C, Morley JE. J Nutr Health Aging 2002;6:191–200.
58. Morley JE. Clin Geriatr Med 2002;18:853–66.
59. Chu LW, Lam KS, Tam SC et al. J Clin Endocrinol Metab 2001;86:1913–20.
60. Kaiser FE, Silver AJ, Morley JE. J Am Geriatr Soc 1991;39:235–40.
61. Bhasin S. J Gerontol Med Sci 2003;58A:1002–8.
62. Morley JE. J Gerontol Med Sci 2004;59A:139–42.
63. Morley JE. J Gerontol Med Sci 2000;55A:M255–6.
64. Niewoehner CB, Allen JI, Boosalis M et al. Am J Med 1986;81:63–8.
65. Eastley R, Wilcock GK, Bucks RS. Int J Geriatr Psychiatry 2000;15:226–33.
66. Hassing L, Wahlin A, Winblad B et al. Biol Psychiatry 1999;45:1472–80.
67. Deijen JB, van der Beek EJ, Orlebeke JF et al. Psychopharmacology 1992;109:489–96.
68. Schmidt IJ, Cremin FM, Grivetti LE et al. J Gerontol 1991;46:M16–22.
69. Wilkinson TJ, Hanger HC, Elmslie J et al. Am J Clin Nutr 1997;66:925–8.
70. Buzina–Suboticanec K, Buzina R, Stavljenic A et al. Int J Vit Nutr Res 1998;68:133–41.
71. Chandra RK. Lancet 1992;340:1124–7.
72. Pike J, Chandra RK. Int J Vit Nutr Res 1995;65:117–21.
73. Bogden JD, Bendich A, Kemp FW et al. Am J Clin Nutr 1994;60:437–47.
74. Chavance M, Herbeth B, Lemoine A et al. Int J Vit Nutr Res 1993;63:11–6.
75. Mann BA, Garry PJ, Hunt WC et al. J Am Geriatr Soc 1987;35:302–6.
76. Kauwell GPA, Lippert Bl, Wilsky CE et al. J Nutr 2000;130:1584–90.
77. van der Wielen RP, van Heereveld HA, de Groot CP et al. Eur J Clin Nutr 1995;49:665–74.
78. Chapuy MC, Arlot ME, Delmes PD et al. BMJ 1994;308:1081–2.

97 DRUG-NUTRIENT INTERACTIONS

LINGTAK-NEANDER CHAN

INCIDENCE 1540
DEFINITION AND CLASSIFICATION 1540
    Classification 1540
HOST AND DRUG OR NUTRIENT FACTORS 1541
MECHANISM 1541
    Ex Vivo Bioinactivations 1541
    Effect of Meal Intake on Drug and Nutrient
        Absorption 1542
    Alteration of Gastrointestinal Motility 1543
    Gastric Acid Secretion Effect 1543
    Modulation of Presystemic Clearance 1544
    Disease States, Diet, and Genetics on
        Enzymatic Metabolism and Drug Responses . .1546
    Interactions Involving
        Alteration of Physiologic Functions 1547
SPECIFIC DRUG INTERACTIONS 1547
    Interactions Associated with Tyramine
        Intake: The "Cheese Effect" 1547
    Interactions with the Anticoagulant
        Warfarin 1548
    Interactions Associated with Dietary
        Supplements 1549
CLINICAL APPROACH TO MANAGEMENT 1549
OTHER FACTORS ALTERING THE DISPOSITION OF
    DRUGS AND NUTRIENTS 1551
    SUMMARY 1551

That disease states and therapies may precipitate malnutrition (1–3) has long been recognized. In the earlier days, drug-nutrient interactions (sometimes referred to as drug-food interactions) were limited to determine whether meal intake would impair drug absorption. Case studies and review articles focused primarily on the influence of food on the bioavailability of drug. Later on, some researchers and clinicians observed that enteral feeding could also affect the pharmacokinetics of drugs (4, 5). More carefully

---

[1]**Abbreviations: ATP,** adenosine triphosphate; **AUC,** area under the concentration time curve; **CYP,** cytochrome P450; **GI,** gastrointestinal; **INR,** international normalized ratio; **MAO,** monoamine oxidase; **P-gp,** P-glycoprotein; t_{max}, time to reach maximal serum or plasma concentration; **TPGS,** D-α-tocopheryl-polyethylene-glycol-1000 succinate or water-soluble vitamin E.

designed studies in specific patient populations, such as patients with head trauma and surgical patients, were then conducted.

With the improved knowledge in physiology and molecular biology, the help of modern technology such as gene cloning and computerized diagnostic imaging studies, and the birth of such medical specialties as critical care medicine, nutrition support, transplant, and geriatrics, clinicians are now managing much sicker patients who would not have survived before. Often, patients who present with severe acute illnesses also have multiple underlying chronic diseases, such as hypertension, hyperlipidemia, obesity, chronic infections (e.g., acquired immunodeficiency syndrome), which require long-term nutritional and pharmacotherapeutic intervention. The practice of polypharmacy (i.e., using multiple drugs to manage different disease states) further increases patients' risk of drug-nutrient interactions. For example, the use of combination drug regimens to prevent allograft rejection, opportunistic infections, and other intervention-induced complications, such as hyperlipidemia, weight gain, and metabolic bone diseases, has already put transplant recipients at risk of drug-nutrient interactions (6). In the process of treating these patients, more complicated issues on drug delivery and nutrition support may continue to surface. Inevitably, managing drug-nutrient interaction has become a major challenge most clinicians are facing today.

Failure to identify and properly manage drug-nutrient interactions can lead to very serious consequences. In the case of treating an infection, for instance, some drug-nutrient interactions can result in reduced absorption of certain oral antibiotics and may lead to suboptimal antibiotic concentrations at the site of infection (7, 8). This predisposes the patient to treatment failure. In patients who have underlying comprised immune function (e.g., elderly patients, patient undergoing chemotherapy, transplant recipients), failure to clear the infectious organisms effectively may prolong treatment course or length of hospital stay or may even contribute to morbidity. In this regard, drug-nutrient interaction also becomes a burden on health care costs. In some disease states, the impacts of unrecognized and unmanaged drug-nutrient interactions may take years to surface. Metabolic bone disease secondary to vitamin D deficiency in transplant recipients or in patients with epilepsy usually takes months to years to progress (9–13). Without proper monitoring of minerals and vitamins levels and early interventions, accelerated bone loss or even bone fracture can result.

Until recently, drug-nutrient interactions were not clearly defined and characterized in the medical and scientific literatures (14). Properly designed studies on the epidemiology of drug-nutrient interactions do not exist in the medical and scientific literature. As a result, standardized management approaches and consensus toward specific drug-nutrient interactions are lacking. The aims of this chapter are to (a) define and classify drug-nutrient interactions based on their mechanism of interactions, (b) characterize drug-nutrient interactions based on the information from the literature, and (c) provide an overview on the general management approaches.

INCIDENCE

Because drug-nutrient interaction cannot occur without the concurrent use of drugs, patients who take medications to manage their chronic diseases are more likely to experience significant drug-nutrient interactions than are relatively healthy persons. The Sloan Survey showed that more than 80% of the survey responders in the United States would be taking at least one medication (prescription drugs, over-the-counter drugs, dietary supplements) and more than 25% would be taking more than five medications in a given week (15). These figures imply that the overall likelihood of identifying potential drug-nutrient interaction in most patients is high. Geriatric patients are particularly at risk because more than 30% of all the prescription drugs are taken by this population. Together with an altered ratio of body fat to muscle as a result of aging and reduced physiologic reserves, it can be expected that elderly patients are more likely to experience adverse events from drug-nutrient interactions. Other patient populations who have increased risks of suffering from adverse events associated with drug-nutrient interactions include patients with multiple medical disorders and critically ill patients (Table 97.1).

TABLE 97.1. PATIENT POPULATIONS WITH SIGNIFICANTLY HIGHER RISK OF EXPERIENCING ADVERSE EVENTS FROM DRUG-NUTRIENT INTERACTIONS

Patients with acquired immunodeficiency syndrome
Patients with cancer
Elderly patients
Malnourished patients
Patients with gastrointestinal tract dysfunctions or surgery
  (e.g., gastric bypass surgery, Crohn disease)
Patients receiving enteral nutrition
Pregnant women
Transplant recipients

DEFINITION AND CLASSIFICATION

Drug-nutrient interaction is defined as an *alteration* of *pharmacokinetics* or *pharmacodynamics* of a drug or nutritional element or a *compromise* in *nutritional status* as a result of the addition of a drug (14). Pharmacokinetics refers to the quantitative description of drug disposition, which include absorption, distribution, metabolism, and excretion of the compound. Pharmacokinetic parameters such as half-life, bioavailability, time to reach maximal concentration (t_{max}), and area–under–the–concentration time curve (AUC) are often used to provide quantitative comparisons. Half-life refers to the time it takes for the drug concentration (usually in the plasma) to reduce by one half. It is commonly used to reflect the rate of removal or clearance of the drug from the body. Bioavailability refers to the fraction of the drug administered becomes available in the body. By definition, intravenous administration provides 100% bioavailability. Oral administration, in many cases, produces lower bioavailability because of incomplete absorption or loss of the active component from presystemic effect. Oral bioavailability is usually the most significant parameter affected by drug-nutrient interactions, although the rate of absorption, metabolic clearance, and tissue distribution of compounds may also be altered. The parameter t_{max} is used to estimate the rate of absorption. Age, underlying medical conditions, types of diet consumed, surgical interventions to the gastrointestinal (GI) tract (e.g., Roux-en-Y gastric bypass surgery), and concurrent medications can all affect t_{max}. The parameter AUC is used to reflect the overall exposure of a drug by the patient. It is affected by oral bioavailability, clearance, and in some cases the rate of absorption also.

Pharmacodynamics refers to the clinical or physiologic effects of the drug. For example, coadministration of folic acid to a patient taking the antiepileptic agent phenytoin may lead to a reduction in serum phenytoin concentration (pharmacokinetic effect). If the reduction in phenytoin concentration is clinically significant, the patient may experience increased frequency or duration of seizure activities (pharmacodynamic effect).

The four types of drug-nutrient interactions are categorized based on the nature and the mechanisms of the interactions (14). Each type is briefly described in the following paragraphs, and the terms *object agent* and *precipitant agent* are used. An object agent refers to the drug or the nutritional element that is affected by the interaction. A precipitant agent refers to the drug or the nutritional element that causes the interaction.

Classification

Type I : Ex vivo bioinactivations, which refer to the interaction between the drug and the nutritional element or formulation through biochemical or physical reactions. Some of the examples of this type of interaction involve hydrolysis, oxidation, neutralization, precipitation, and complexation. These reactions usually take place when the interacting agents are in direct physical contact and occur usually before the nutrients or drugs enter the body. In other words, these interactions usually occur in the delivery device.

Type II : Interactions affecting absorption, which affect drugs and nutrients delivered only by mouth or via enteral delivery devices. These interactions cause either an increase or decrease of oral bioavailability of the object agent. The precipitant agents may modify the function of an *enzyme (type A interaction)* or a *transport mechanism (type B interaction)* that is responsible for the biotransformation or transport of the object agent before reaching systemic circulation. In some cases, *complexation, binding, and/or other deactivating processes* occur in the GI tract (*type C interaction*) and impair the object agent from being absorbed.

Type III : Interactions affecting systemic or physiologic disposition, which occur after the drug or the nutritional element has been absorbed from the GI tract and entered the systemic circulation. The mechanisms involve changing the cellular or tissue distribution, systemic transport, or penetration to specific organ or tissues of the object compound. In some cases, the interaction between the precipitant agent and the object agent may involve changing the function of other cofactors (e.g., clotting factors) or hormones.

Type IV : Interactions affecting the elimination or clearance of drugs or nutrients, which may involve the modulation, antagonism, or impairment of renal or enterohepatic elimination.

HOST AND DRUG OR NUTRIENT FACTORS

The two factors that play the most significant role in the occurrence of drug-nutrient interactions are the host and the drug (or nutrient) itself (Fig. 97.1). The host factor refers to the individual's response to a drug or nutrient. Age, sex, body size, body composition, lifestyle, underlying diseases and medical conditions, and genetics can affect the response (see Table 97.1). For example, elderly patients are more like to experience adverse events as a result of drug-nutrient interaction because reserved physiologic functions are reduced with age (16). Investigators have also observed that nutritional malnourishment and obesity both exaggerate a patient's response to drugs and nutrients (17–19). Patients with multiple chronic diseases are also more likely to experience adverse events. Genetics can be an important factor in determining the appropriate dose and clinical response to a particular drug of nutrient. Genetic polymorphism of the methylenetetrahydrofolate reductase gene (*MTHFR*) may affect the amount of pyridoxine, cobalamin, folic acid, and riboflavin requirement

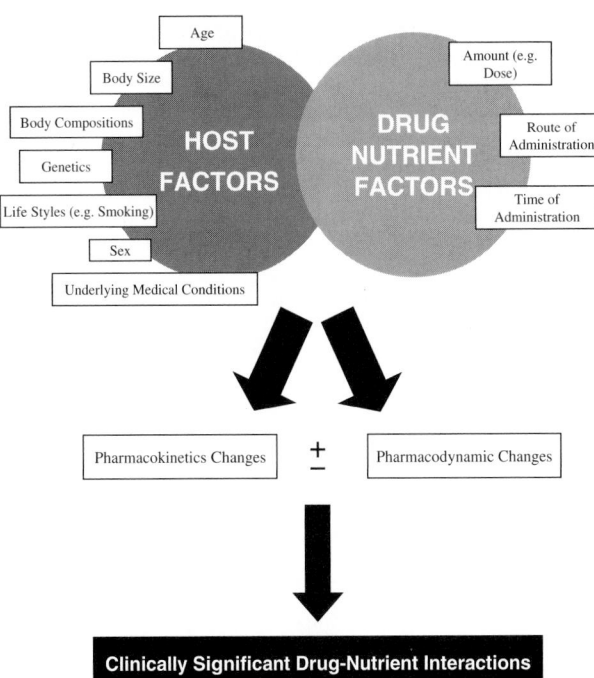

Figure 97.1. Factors contributing to drug-nutrient interactions. Not all pharmacokinetic or pharmacodynamic changes may lead to clinically significant interactions.

(20–22). It is possible that polymorphism in some cases may protect the patient from experiencing clinically significant drug-nutrient interactions.

The drug or nutrient factor is always affected by the amount, time, and route of administration. For instance, type II drug-nutrient interaction occurs exclusively when both the nutrient and the drug are administered orally or via the enteral route, and it can essentially be eliminated by administration via the intravenous route. Many type IIc interactions (complexation in the GI tract) can be avoided by simply spacing out the administration time. Type I interactions are far more common with drugs and nutrients administered intravenously. The potential for drug-nutrient interactions increases exponentially with addition of every drug or dietary supplement (23).

MECHANISM

Ex Vivo Bioinactivations

Before reaching the GI tract or the venous blood (as in the case of intravenous administration), drugs and nutrients are sometimes mixed in the delivery system. This practice is especially common in managing patients requiring enteral and parenteral nutritional support. Physicobiochemical reactions may occur ex vivo between drugs and nutrients in a delivery vehicle or tubings, in which the active ingredients can be deactivated before being absorbed. The physical changes as the result of the interaction, often described as incompatibility, are sometimes visible on inspection. This is especially the case for intravenous products, because most

TABLE 97.2. SUGGESTED APPROACHES TO MINIMIZE TYPE I DRUG-NUTRIENT INTERACTION

- Do not mix drugs directly with feeding formulas (enteral or parenteral).
- Hold enteral feeding before administering drugs through an enteral feeding tube; holding time varies from a few minutes to preferably 2 hours for drug such as phenytoin.
- Flush the feeding tube with water before and after drug administration.
- Use preformulated oral solutions, elixirs, or suspensions instead of crushing tablets when administering drugs through enteral feeding tubes, to increase dose accuracy and to minimize clogging.
- For parenteral agents, always consult with pharmacists or references to determine the compatibility of these agents.
- Do not rely on visual inspection to determine compatibility among intravenously administered products; use published references.
- Consider monitoring drugs levels for drugs with narrow therapeutic indices.

of the parenteral products are in a clear solution form. Precipitation from calcium and phosphate salts is a classic example of physical incompatibility resulting in the formation of the insoluble particles. However, some of the precipitants formed may be too small to be visible by naked eyes, making the visual inspection method unreliable to determine the presence of an interaction (24). Intravenous lipids products, conversely, are formulated as opaque emulsions (oil mixed in water). Therefore, physical incompatibility cannot be determined by visual inspection. As a general rule, practitioners should not rely on visual inspection to determine the presence of type I interactions (Table 97.2).

Effect of Meal Intake on Drug and Nutrient Absorption

Concurrent meal intake and drug administration can influence oral absorption of drug and nutrients, and this situation is an example of type II interactions. The overall impact may include changing the rate of absorption, changing the magnitude of absorption, or both. The mechanisms affecting drug or nutrient absorption with concurrent meal intake usually involve one or more of the following factors: (a) altering gastric acid and gastrin secretion, (b) altering GI transit time, (c) changing dissolution of drugs in solid dosage forms, (d) binding or complexation of micronutrient or macronutrient with food contents, and (e) changing bile flow (25–27).

Meal intake generally stimulates gastric and intestinal secretions (28, 29). Increased secretions in the GI tract theoretically improve dissolution of drugs from their solid dosage form and facilitate absorption. In addition, meals with higher fat content stimulate the release of bile salts, which favors the intestinal uptake of highly lipophilic compounds or compounds that require bile salts for optimal absorption (30). Furthermore, high-fat meals promote the

release of cholecystokinin, which slows GI motility and increases the contact time between the drug molecules and the intestinal epithelial tissues (31). All these factors combined tend to favor a more complete absorption of many drugs and nutrients. For example, the oral bioavailability of albendazole and griseofulvin is dramatically increased when taken with a fatty meal (32, 33). However, the potential physicochemical interactions, the potential binding affinity between the individual drug and food contents, the dose of the drug administered, and the composition of the meals make drug absorption in the presence of food rather erratic and unpredictable. Therefore, concurrent food intake actually contributes to the variation in the magnitude of the drug and nutrient interaction observed (26). For instance, the data on how food affects the oral bioavailability of verapamil, a calcium channel blocker commonly used in the treatment of hypertension, are very inconsistent. Some studies showed a small reduction of verapamil oral bioavailability caused by concurrent food intake, and a similar number of studies failed to show any clinically relevant change in verapamil bioavailability and pharmacodynamic changes. The AUCs of verapamil observed were similar with or without food. The only consistent finding among the studies was that food slowed down the rate of verapamil absorption (34–37). Therefore, it appears that verapamil can be taken without regard to food, as long as it is on a consistent basis.

Many practitioners do not recognize the difference between "delayed" absorption versus "decreased" absorption. Delayed absorption of a drug by food does not necessarily lead to reduced absorption. In many cases, food may impair the rate of drug absorption, as measured by the time required to reach the highest serum drug concentration (or t_{max}) without affecting the total amount absorbed as measured by AUC. Delayed absorption of drugs caused by food may be explained by the highly variable physiologic response to feeding among individual persons, as well as the inconsistency in food contents consumed between meals. Drugs such as famciclovir, methotrexate, verapamil, levetiracetam, levodopa have delayed absorption in the presence of food as measured by increased t_{max}; however, the total amount absorbed is comparable with or without food as quantified by the AUCs (38–44). In these cases, food can delay the onset of the drug action; however, the efficacy should not be affected. Despite a detectable difference in the pharmacokinetic parameter, these drug-nutrient interactions may not be considered clinically significant. On the contrary, if food intake causes a significant reduction in the AUC of a drug, it implies that the overall amount absorbed is *reduced*. This kind of interaction is more clinically significant, and pharmacodynamic changes may be detected. In this case, patients should receive specific instructions on taking the drug with regard to meal intake. More importantly, patient's compliance should be emphasized and monitored to warrant stable and consistent drug

TABLE 97.3. DRUGS THAT ARE RECOMMENDED TO TAKE WITH FOOD TO MAXIMIZE ABSORPTION

Albendazole	Ketoconazole
Amiodarone	Lithium
Atazanavir	Lopinavir
Atovaquone	Lovastatin
Cefuroxime	Mefloquine
Erythromycin ethylsuccinate	Nelfinavir
Ganciclovir	Rifapentine
Griseofulvin	Ritonavir
Hydralazine	Saquinavir
Itraconazole (capsule only)	

Data from references 27 and 129.

responses and to prevent undesired effects or therapeutic misadventures.

The presence of food causes distention of the stomach and stimulates the autonomic nervous system to alter GI tone (45, 46). Together with the endocrinologic changes induced by the food contents (e.g., releases of insulin, cholecystokinin, gastrin), splanchnic blood flow is also increased (47–49). Increased blood delivery to the liver through the hepatic portal vein can augment presystemic metabolism (i.e., deactivation of the drug before reaching the systemic circulation). However, because the metabolism of most drugs depends primarily on the host's intrinsic clearance (i.e., the amount and the availability of the drug metabolizing enzymes) but not hepatic blood flow, food-induced augmentation of splanchnic and hepatic blood flow rarely causes clinically significant drug-nutrient interactions. The exception is ethanol, a compound with high extraction ratio whose metabolism appears to be highly affected by hepatic blood flow. Concurrent food intake with 530 kcal increased the presystemic metabolism of ethanol metabolism by up to 49%, with men showing more dramatic increase than women (50). Hepatic blood flow can be estimated by the use of intravenous indocyanine green (51). Tables 97.3 and 97.4 summarize the commonly prescribed medications that are recommended to be taken with food or on an empty stomach,

TABLE 97.4. DRUGS THAT SHOULD NOT BE TAKEN WITH FOOD TO ALLOW OPTIMAL ABSORPTION

Ampicillin[a]	Isoniazid[a]
Captopril[b]	Norfloxacin[c]
Ciprofloxacin[c]	Ofloxacin[c]
Didanosin[a,c]	Rifampin[b]
Dicloxacillin[a]	Tetracycline[c]
Doxycycline[c]	Voriconazole[b]
Indinavir[d]	Zafirlukast[b]

[a] Acid liability; food intake may deactivate the drug.
[b] Mechanism unknown.
[c] Chelation and/or binding with food content or divalent and trivalent cations (e.g., calcium magnesium).
[d] Food may deactivate the drug through precipitation.

Data from references 27, 130, and 131.

respectively. In summary, whether a drug should be taken with food or on an empty stomach depends mostly on the characteristics of the drug. When in doubt, it is recommended to consult the primary literature. Drugs with decreased oral absorption in the presence of food should be taken on an empty stomach. Drugs with delayed but not decreased absorption in the presence of food may be taken without regard to meal intake.

Alteration of Gastrointestinal Motility

Gastric emptying and intestinal transit time may alter the rate and magnitude of drug or nutrient absorption from the GI tract. Upper GI tone is initially increased by meal. Continued food consumption leads to the release of inhibitory neuroendocrines and peptides such as secretin, glucagon-like peptides, and cholecystokinin that inhibit gastric emptying and eventually cause satiety (52–56). Decreased GI motility increases the contact time for the drug or nutrient with the GI epithelial tissue, thus potentially allows more complete absorption of the drug molecules or nutrients into the portal vein.

The autonomic nervous system affects both GI tone and secretions in the GI tract. Increased GI secretion provides a complementary effect on absorption and the digestive process (57, 58). Vagal stimulation increases upper GI contraction and decreases pyloric sphincter contractions. As a result, gastric emptying is promoted, and the time required for the drug or nutrient to reach the small intestine is shortened. Decreased gastric emptying time may reduce drug absorption owing to less complete dissolution (for solid dosage forms). Conversely, drug and nutrient absorption may be increased by the coadministration of opioid derivatives, which slows GI motility, or drugs with anticholinergic effect (e.g., sedating antihistamines, phenothiazines, tricyclic antidepressants) that blocks the vagus nerve. However, anticholinergic effect may also decrease the secretion in the intestine and affect nutrient absorption. Overall speaking, significantly decreased GI tone may precipitate toxicities as a result of more complete absorption, whereas elevated GI motility may increase the risk of therapeutic failure.

Gastric Acid Secretion Effect

Some nutrients require gastric acid to maximize their absorption from the GI tract. Dietary cobalamin (vitamin B_{12}), for example, is highly bound to the protein content in food. It requires gastric acid and pepsin to be liberated from the dietary protein so it can bind to the host vitamin carrier, salivary R-protein. This cobalamin-R-protein complex can then be hydrolyzed by the pancreatic enzyme in the duodenum to produce free cobalamin, which can subsequently bind to the intrinsic factor to in the jejunum for adequate absorption in the terminal ileum (59, 60). Acid reducing agents such as proton-pump inhibitors and type 2 histamine receptor (H_2) antagonists have been reported to cause cobalamin malabsorption leading to megaloblastic anemia (61–63).

Modulation of Presystemic Clearance

Presystemic clearance, previously known as first-pass metabolism, refers to the metabolism of orally ingested compounds before reaching the systemic circulation (e.g., via the portal vein into the liver for metabolism). This process is usually catabolic, which decreases the amount of active compounds available for systemic circulation. However, it can also provide metabolic activation of compounds, as in the case of prodrugs. The extent of presystemic clearance may affect the potency and efficacy of a particular drug or nutrient. Research has clearly demonstrated that both the intestine and the liver account for the majority of the presystemic metabolism in humans (64, 65). The stomach does play a minor role. Class III alcohol dehydrogenase, for example, is present in the gastric mucosa and is responsible for the activation of some biogenic amines, steroids, and, to a minor extent, degradation of the ingested alcohol derivatives (66).

A significantly higher content of drug metabolizing enzyme, represented by cytochrome P450 (CYP)3A4, is present in the intestinal epithelial tissues. CYP3A4 plays a pivotal role in regulating the oral bioavailability of a large number of drugs and perhaps, nutrients. Functional alteration of CYP3A4 either through induction or inhibition can have a profound impact on the amount of drugs or nutrients absorbed. As a result, the potency of drugs or nutrients can be affected. In addition, the rate of how substrates are presented to these intestinal enzymes seems to be regulated by transport proteins. Whereas most of the intestinal transporters facilitate the absorption of drugs or nutrients, some transporters efflux molecules already absorbed in the cytoplasm of the enterocyte back into the intestinal lumen, thus decreasing the bioavailability of certain compounds. This efflux system appears to minimize xenobiotic exposure by the host. It is believed that these efflux pumps regulate the rate of drugs being presented to the cytoplasmic enzymes and prevent the saturation of these enzymes. P-glycoprotein (P-gp) is the representative of this type of efflux system. P-gp belongs to the family of adenosine triphosphate (ATP)-binding cassette (ABC) transporters. This transporter uses ATP and mobilizes solutes against concentration gradient. It is well established that intestinal P-gp and CYP3A4 combined are the most important factor that regulate oral bioavailability of most drugs. It is thought that P-gp regulates the rate of substrates presented to CYP3A4 to provide a more stable and consistent rate of presystemic metabolism (67–69). For instance, cyclosporine is a known substrate for both CYP3A4 and P-gp. After oral administration, absorption of cyclosporine across the epithelium in the small intestine is limited by P-gp efflux and prehepatic CYP3A4 metabolism. P-gp, located mostly on the apical side of the enterocytes,

regulates how fast and how much cyclosporine can reach the CYP3A4 enzymes, which are present in the endoplasmic reticulum of the enterocytes. The efflux mechanism of P-gp will transport some of the already absorbed cyclosporine molecules from the cytosol of the enterocytes back into the intestinal lumen. This action provides CYP3A4 enzymes repeated opportunities to metabolize the drug when it again enters the enterocyte. Cyclosporine absorption and pharmacodynamics are affected by disrupting the harmony of this coupled transport-metabolic system with the use of nutrients (e.g., water-soluble vitamin E, grapefruit juice) or herbal supplement (e.g., St. John's wort).

Modulation of Enzymes in the Gastrointestinal Tract (Type IIA Interactions)

Induction or inhibition of the enzyme in the gut by nutrients may lead to a significant change in oral bioavailability of drugs or vice versa. Some food products and dietary supplements are known to affect intestinal CYP3A4 activity and change the pharmacokinetic profiles of the object drugs. Grapefruit juice is a classic example of a selective intestinal CYP3A4 inhibitor. Grapefruit juice causes a type IIA interaction with certain prescription drugs by deactivating and destroying intestinal CYP3A4 enzymes. It has been reported that the overall exposure of some object drugs can be increased by more than fivefold when taken with grapefruit juice (70, 71). Dose reduction of the object drugs or avoidance of the juice, especially in patients taking drugs with narrow therapeutic window, is necessary to prevent serious adverse events such as seizures and renal failure (Table 97.5). Strong evidence implied that 6′,7′-dihydroxybergamottin, a furanocoumarin-derivative in the juice, is primarily responsible for enzymatic inhibition. The onset of this interaction is immediate. A significant increase in the absorption of the object drugs can be detected with the first glass of grapefruit juice consumed. The magnitude of the enzymatic inhibition increases with repeated grapefruit juice consumption. Because the mechanism of inhibition involves degradation of the CYP3A4 enzymes, this interaction cannot be avoided by spacing out the administration time of the object drugs and grapefruit juice (72). On the discontinuation of grapefruit juice, increased absorption of the object drugs is expected to continue for 3 to 5 more days. The most significant interactions occur when patients consume the frozen concentrates instead of the freshly squeezed juice. No evidence suggests that eating grapefruit in moderation results in detectable inhibition of CYP3A4 enzymes.

St. John's wort, an herbal supplement widely available over the counter, also causes type IIA drug-nutrient interactions. St. John's wort is a very potent *inducer* of CYP3A4 (73, 74). As a result, the oral bioavailability and overall exposure (measured by AUC) of many prescription drugs can be reduced resulting in therapeutic failure. Because the mechanism of this drug-nutrient interaction involves

TABLE 97.5. DRUGS WITH INCREASED ORAL ABSORPTION WHEN TAKEN WITH GRAPEFRUIT JUICE AND POSSIBLE ASSOCIATED ADVERSE REACTIONS

Albendazole[a, b, c]	Nimodipine[j]
Amiodarone[d]	Nicardipine[j]
Artemether[e]	Nislodipine[j]
Atorvastatin[f]	Nitrendipine[j]
Buspirone[g, h]	Praziquantel[b, c]
Carbamazepine[i]	Saquinavir[b]
Carvedilol[e, j]	Scopolamine[i]
Cyclosporine[c, k, l, m]	Sertraline[i]
Diazepam[i]	Sidenafil[b, j, p, q]
Ethinylestradiol	Simvastatin[f]
Erythromycin[b, g, n]	Tacrolimus[g, k]
Felodipine[j]	Triazolam[c, i]
Midazolam[i, o]	Verapamil[d, e, g]
Nifedipine[j, p]	

[a] Elevation of liver function tests
[b] Gastrointestinal discomforts
[c] Central nervous system symptoms
[d] Heart block
[e] Bradycardia
[f] Rhabdomyolysis
[g] Cardiovascular symptoms
[h] Dystonic reactions
[i] Drowsiness, prolonged sedations
[j] Hypotension
[k] Acute renal failure
[l] Headache
[m] Seizure
[n] QT prolongation, torsades de pointes
[o] Respiratory depression
[p] Myocardial infarction
[q] Priapism

upregulation of the *CYP3A4* gene, CYP3A4 activity remains elevated for weeks after discontinuation of St. John's wort (75). Close monitoring of the object drug over a lengthy period is necessary to minimize the risk of treatment failure.

Significantly decreased drug concentrations or loss of therapeutic potency associated with St. John's wort use has been reported with alprazolam, cyclosporine, digoxin, fex-ofenadine HCl, imatinib, indinavir, irinotecan, methadone, oral contraceptives, simvastatin, tacrolimus, and verapamil (76–87). St. John's wort caused an average of 50% reduction of AUC with most of the interacting drugs studied. Acute allograft rejection was reported in a patient who received a heart transplant as a result of this interaction. It is likely that the efficacy and safety of many more drugs can be affected by St. John's wort. Since many drugs currently in use are metabolized by CYP3A4.

Modulation of Transporters in the Gastrointestinal Tract (Type IIB Interactions)

Water-soluble vitamin E (also known as D-α-tocopheryl-polyethylene-glycol-1000 succinate, or TPGS) is the classic example showing how interactions can take place through the inhibition of intestinal P-gp (type IIB interaction) by a nutrient. Coadministration of TPGS to liver transplant recipients and healthy volunteers increased cyclosproine

oral bioavailability for up to 80% (6). P-gp inhibition by TPGS was confirmed using in vitro models (88, 89). TPGS at 400 IU twice daily also increased AUC of digoxin in healthy volunteers, although no significant pharmacodynamic changes (e.g., bradycardia, atrioventricular block) were observed (90). The lack of adverse cardiovascular effect can be explained by the age of the study sample (young healthy subjects). This drug-nutrient interaction is highly clinically significant as vitamin E is widely available commercially and is believed to be a safe nutritional supplement. Lack of proper monitoring in patients receiving TPGS and P-gp substrates with narrow therapeutic index may lead to serious adverse reactions resulting in injury or death. This interaction appears to occur with TPGS only. Other vitamin E formulations, such as α-tocopherol acetate capsules, have so far failed to demonstrate any clinically significant drug-nutrient interactions with P-gp substrates (90). It is likely that the surfactant polyethylene glycol 1000 added the liquid vitamin E formulation is responsible for the drug-nutrient interaction (89). The addition of a surfactant to the vitamin E formulation is supposed to increase the solubility of vitamin E and enhance its absorption, even in the absence of adequate bile flow. Conversely, St. John's wort, in addition to being a CYP3A4 inducer, is also a P-gp inducer (91). Patients taking St. John's wort showed significantly lower serum concentrations drugs that are P-gp substrates such as digoxin, cyclosporine, and indinavir (76).

Binding and Chelation Interactions in the Gastrointestinal Tract (Type IIC Interactions)

The fact that enteral nutrition can impair drug absorption has been documented for decades. Although enteral feeding is the preferred method of providing nutrition support and also allows easy access for administering drugs to patients who are unable to swallow, therapeutic failure has been extensively documented in the literature when specific drugs were administered directly into the enteral feeding system. Some data suggest that the protein component of the enteral formulas may bind to drug molecules and thus decrease their bioavailability. Binding between formulas and drugs has been suggested in the cases of warfarin and phenytoin (14). Other examples of type IIC drug-nutrient interaction include chelation between divalent and trivalent cations with drugs. Tetracyclines and fluoroquininones are believed to interact with food and enteral formulas through this mechanism (27).

A well-recognized type II drug-nutrient interaction is that between feeding formulas and the antiepileptic agent phenytoin. This interaction was first reported by Bauer in 1982 in a series of neurosurgical patients. Phenytoin initiated at standard doses failed to achieve therapeutic concentrations in patients receiving continuous nasogastric feeding. However, the average phenytoin concentration was increased by fourfold once the feeding was discontinued.

Similarly, in patients who had been previously stabilized on phenytoin, initiation of continuous tube feedings resulted in more than 70% reduction of mean serum phenytoin concentration. The finding was consistent when the investigator recruited five healthy volunteers to take a single oral dose of phenytoin suspension alone and then consume a nasogastric tube feeding preparation orally at a rate of 100 mL/hour, in whom phenytoin serum concentrations were 71.6% lower with concurrent tube feeding (4). To date, more than 30 articles have been published as case reports or clinical studies involving this interaction with variable results. A recent systematic review on this topic revealed that 25 reports supported the presence of this interaction with only four studies refuting the interaction (92). As much as 80% reduction of phenytoin concentration was reported in at least one study. All four negative studies used healthy volunteers as study subjects instead of patients; continuous enteral feeding method was used in only one of these four studies, whereas interrupted feeding approach was used in the other three studies. It can therefore be concluded that this interaction exists in patients receiving continuous enteral feeding and will result in decreased phenytoin absorption from the GI tract. Nevertheless, the exact mechanism of the interaction remains unknown, with at least five mechanisms proposed by various investigators. Overall, the pattern and the nature of this interaction are similar to a type IIC drug-nutrient interaction, although adsorption of phenytoin to the feeding tube causing drug loss has also been proposed. Close and frequent monitoring of serum phenytoin concentration (e.g., twice to three times a week) is highly recommended in patients receiving continuous enteral feeding.

Disease States, Diet, and Genetics on Enzymatic Metabolism and Drug Responses

Biotransformation or metabolism of drugs and nutrients takes place essentially in most organ systems of the human body. Drug metabolizing enzymes such as CYP2E1 and alcohol dehydrogenase are found in the brain, CYP3A4 is found abundantly in the enterocytes of the small intestine, whereas CYP1A and other phase II metabolic enzymes can be found in the pulmonary alveolar cells. Nevertheless, the high and sustained amount of blood flow and the abundance of metabolizing enzymes make the liver the powerhouse for xenobiotic metabolism. As drugs and nutrients are metabolized, they usually first undergo phase I metabolism, which results in the opening up of the functional groups through oxidation, reduction, hydroxylation, and so forth. This process usually increases the activity of the compound to allow further reactions to take place. The second phase (i.e., phase II reaction) is a synthetic process involving conjugation of the compound with endogenous

molecules such as glucuronic acid, sulfate, glutathione, glycine, and acetate, resulting in a more hydrophilic compound that favors its excretion into bile or urine. Some compounds do not have to go through phase I metabolism before undergoing phase II metabolism. Lorazepam, for example, undergoes phase II metabolism (glucuronidation) by uridine diphosphate glucuronosyltransfersae (UGT) 2B7 without any phase I reaction involved. The kidney eliminates the resultant conjugated, inactive metabolite. Similarly, some compounds can be eliminated from the body unchanged with going through any biotransformation at all.

The enzyme system responsible for the metabolism of most nutrients and drugs is the CYP enzyme superfamily, primarily located in the endoplasmic reticulum of the hepatocytes and enterocytes. Starvation, change in diet, genetics, and some coexisting disease states may affect CYP enzyme activities (93, 94). For example, administration of parenteral nutrition appeared to decrease CYP1A, CYP2C, and activities but increase CYP2E1 activity (95–97). Vegetarian diet may have a direct impact on drug metabolism. The activity of CYP1A enzyme seems to be suppressed in Asian vegetarians but unaffected in white vegetarians (98–100). It is possible that the reduced CYP activity was related to an overall reduction in the intake of protein calories. Charcoal-rich food induces CYP1A enzyme in humans. Induction of CYP enzymes usually increases the risk of therapeutic failure, because the metabolic clearance of the drugs will be augmented. On the contrary, inhibition or suppression of CYP enzymatic activities increases the risk of drug-related toxicity.

Sex differences in pharmacokinetics and pharmacodynamics exist, probably related to the intrinsic enzymatic expressions and activities (101). Additionally, some CYP enzymes exhibit genetic polymorphism. CYP2C19 poor metabolizers are found in up to 20% of Chinese, Korean, and Japanese subjects, as supposed to less than 5% in white subjects (102–104). It appears that patients who are poor metabolizers of CYP2C19, identified as carriers of the *CYP2C19*2* or *CYP2C19*3* gene, are more susceptible to proton-pump inhibitor-induced vitamin B$_{12}$ malabsorption (63). Mutation of the *CYP27B1* gene, which is responsible for the final activating step for the biologically active form of vitamin D, is associated with type I vitamin D–dependent rickets (105). Examples of other polymorphic genes that are closely linked to altered nutritional responses include apolipoprotein E (*APOE*), 5,10-methylenetetrahydrofolate reductase (*MTHFR*), and peroxisome proliferator-activated receptor-γ2 (*PPARγ2*) (106, 107).

The direct effect of nutrients on human CYP activity has not been extensively investigated. Data from other species suggest that vitamins can modulate the activity of various CYP enzymes and dietary changes (93, 94) (Table 97.6).

TABLE 97.6. DIETARY FACTORS THAT MODULATE CYTOCHROME P ACTIVITY

DIETARY FACTORS	SPECIES	TISSUE	CYP ACTIVITY
Caloric restriction	Rat	Liver	↑ CYP3A4
Charcoal-rich food	Human	Liver	↑ CYP1A1, 1A2
Corn oil supplementation	Rat	Liver	↑ CYP2B1, 2E1, 3A4
Garlic oil + fish oil	Rat	Liver	↑ CYP1A1, 2E1 3A1
Iron deficiency	Rat	Intestine	↓ total CYP
MCT oil supplementation	Rat	Liver	↑ CYP1A2
Parenteral nutrition	Human	Hepatocytes	↑ CYP2E1
		Liver	↓ CYP1A
Protein deficiency	Human	Whole body	↓ CYP1A2
Protein supplementation	Human	Whole body	↑ CYP1A2
Starvation	Rat	Liver	↓ CYP1A, 2C11
			↑ CYP2B, 2E1, 3A
Thiamin deficiency	Rat	Liver	↑ CYP2E1
Vitamin A deficiency	Rat	Liver	↓ CYP2C11
Vitamin A supplementation	Rat	Skin	↓ CYP1A
		Liver	↑ CYP2A, 3A, ↓ 2C
Vitamin C deficiency	Guinea pig	Liver	↓ CYP1A2
Vitamin E supplementation	Rat	Liver	↑ CYP2C11

CYP, Cytochrome P450; MCT, medium-chain triglyceride.

Data from references 82, 83, and 138.

Interactions Involving Alteration of Physiologic Functions

The mechanism of many drug-nutrient interactions involves the direct interference of the pharmacologic actions of the drug or the physiologic and biologic functions of the nutrients. In some cases, a drug was designed to antagonize the physiologic function of a nutrient. Increased or inconsistent intake of that particular nutrient would alter the pharmacologic effect of the drug. A classic example is the interaction between warfarin and vitamin K (108). Sometimes, a drug can decrease the catabolism of certain nutritional elements that are responsible for the biosynthesis of hormones, neurotransmitters, and other biologically active peptides. As the result, the patient may experience a heightened biologic response secondary to the drug-nutrient interaction. The combination of tyramine-rich food and monoamine oxidase (MAO) inhibitor is a well-recognized example (109).

In some cases, a drug and a nutrient compete for the same intracellular transport mechanism or metabolic pathway. Over time, such drug-nutrient interaction can result in an exaggerated response because of increased accumulation of the object compound or clinical deficiency of the object compound because of inadequate intracellular uptake. The interaction between carnitine and valproic acid may fit this description. Although the exact mechanism is not certain, valproic acid is known to cause idiopathic hyperammonemia without the presence of hepatitis. The presentation is often accompanied by carnitine deficiency. Research suggests that valproic acid interferes with carnitine uptake through multiple pathways that include competition for the carnitine transporter in the tissues,

alteration of β-oxidation by valproic acid leading to impaired carnitine metabolic recycling, and inhibition of intramitochondrial β-oxidation enzymes (110). Regardless of the mechanism, most cases of valproic acid–induced carnitine deficiency can easily be treated with carnitine supplementation.

SPECIFIC DRUG INTERACTIONS

Interactions Associated with Tyramine Intake: The "Cheese Effect"

Tyramine is structurally similarly to dopamine. It is a trace amine with sympathomimetic activities and is formed by the decarboxylation of tyrosine aromatic L-amino acid decarboxylase. Depending on the diet, food intake can be a significant source of tyramine for some people (111). In addition, fermented food and protein-rich foods that have begun to spoil also contain other biogenic amines (e.g., 2-phenylethylamine) with sympathomimetic activities (112). Tyramine is inactivated primarily by the enzymes MAOs. Drugs demonstrating inhibitory effect on MAO can decrease the catabolism of tyramine. This drug-nutrient interaction may lead to an exaggerated catecholamine response by the patient that can range from headache, hallucination, and vomiting to hypertensive emergencies and death (113, 114). Patients who are taking medications that can inhibit MAO should receive specific nutritional counseling and monitoring.

Food rich in tyramine should be minimized or avoided (Table 97.7). Fortunately, with improved food processing technology and sanitation in food manufacturing and storage, contamination of food products by other biogenic

TABLE 97.7. FOOD PRODUCTS THAT ARE LIKELY TO CONTAIN HIGHER AMOUNT OF TYRAMINE

Aged and fermented products (e.g., sauerkraut, fermented soy products)
Anchovies
Avocado
Beans (especially fava beans and broad beans)
Brewer's yeast
Cheese (except cream cheese and cottage cheese)
Chocolates
Cream from pasteurized milk
Hydrolyzed protein extracts
Liquid and powdered protein supplements
Meat extracts
Processed meat products (e.g., sausages, pate, liver products)
Raspberries
Sour cream
Yogurt (especially homemade)

amines has significantly decreased. Together with the much-accepted use of the newer generations of antidepressants such as the selective serotonin reuptake inhibitors (e.g., fluoxetine, paroxetine, sertraline) over the older, first-generation nonselective MAO inhibitors (e.g., phenelzine and tranylcypromine), the risk of drug-nutrient interactions related to the "cheese" effect is becoming less common. Drugs with known MAO inhibitory effect are summarized in Table 97.8.

Interactions with the Anticoagulant Warfarin

Warfarin is the most widely prescribed anticoagulant in the world. It is used in the management of many disease states and medical conditions requiring chronic anticoagulation, including thromboembolic events (e.g., pulmonary embolism, ischemic stroke, deep vein thrombosis), for acquired hypercoagulatory disorders, and for preventing

TABLE 97.8. DRUGS THAT HAVE SHOWN INHIBITORY EFFECTS ON MONOAMINE OXIDASES AND ARE LIKELY TO CAUSE CLINICALLY SIGNIFICANT DRUG-NUTRIENT INTERACTION WITH DIET CONTAINING LARGE AMOUNT OF TYRAMINE

DRUG	MOST COMMON CLINICAL USE
Furazolidone	Parasite infections (giardiasis)
Isocarboxazid	Depression
Linezolid	Bacterial infection (especially Gram-positive bacteria)
Phenelzine	Depression
Selegiline[a]	Parkinson disease, usually used in combination with levodopa/carbidopa
Tranylcypromine	Depression
Kava[b]	Dietary supplement

[a]Inhibits primarily type B monoamine oxidase (MAO-B). Magnitude of interaction with tyramine should be less profound than the nonselective MAO inhibitors such as the antidepressants.
[b]High suspicion although clinical significance not known.

Data from references 135 to 137.

clot formation after the insertion of vascular mechanical devices (e.g., mechanical heart valves, inferior vena cava filters, arterial stents). Warfarin competes with vitamin K at its binding sites and thus inhibits the synthesis of vitamin K–dependent clotting factors II, VII, IX, and X, and coagulation inhibitors proteins C and S (115).

Administration of high doses of vitamin K can reverse the anticoagulation effect of warfarin. Although the most significant interactions with warfarin are usually through drug-drug interactions that inhibit warfarin metabolism (e.g., with CYP2C9 inhibitors such as fluconazole, amiodarone, sulfonamide antibiotics), inconsistent dietary intake of vitamin K may possibly alter the pharmacodynamic effect of warfarin as well. However, formal investigations on the effect of dietary vitamin K on patients' responses to warfarin therapy are very limited. Most of data have been published only as case reports with very few prospective trials (116–118). Among the prospective studies, only one has a crossover design to compare the effect of low (mean intake 26 μg/day) versus high (mean intake 591 μg/day) vitamin K intake within the same cohorts. Although a statistically significant change in the international normalized ratio (INR) was detected (INR increased from 2.6 ± 0.5 to 3.3 ± 0.9 in 7 days with vitamin K–depleted diet and decreased from 3.1 ± 0.8 to 2.8 ± 0.6 in 4 days with vitamin K–enriched diet), the clinical significance of the change was questionable (119). Estimation of dietary vitamin K intake in other studies is confounded by the use of self-administered questionnaire or retrospective dietary recall. It appears that in the absence of other triggering factors such as drug-drug interactions or acute illnesses that could alter clotting factor synthesis, a more dramatic change in the dietary content of vitamin K is needed to precipitate a measurable change in the pharmacodynamic effect of warfarin. One study reported that an average increase in dietary vitamin K intake by 100 μg for a 4-day period only caused a reduction of INR by 0.2 (120).

It is likely that the physical health of the patient, age, and the genotype of CYP2C9, which is the most important enzyme responsible for metabolism of warfarin, provide a more significant contribution to the interpatient variability of warfarin dose requirement, whereas variation in dietary vitamin K intake contributes to minor intrapatient variation. Nevertheless, sufficient clinical reports exist to raise the concern regarding the possible drug-nutrient interaction between inconsistent dietary vitamin K intake and warfarin. To minimize this potential drug-nutrient interaction, instead of advising patients to avoid food products rich in vitamin K, the more practical approach is to instruct them to have a relatively constant and stable intake of vitamin K. Dietary sources of vitamin K come from not only green vegetables, but also from certain plant oils and prepared foods containing these plant oils, such as baked foods, margarines, and salad dressings. When an interaction between warfarin and vitamin K intake from dietary source is suspected, clinicians should carefully review with the patients not only the intake of green vegetables, but also the type of oil used in the food preparation.

Interactions Associated with Dietary Supplements

One of the emerging issues in drug-nutrient interaction is the interaction between dietary supplements and prescription drugs. Dietary supplements such as herbs, natural products, and homeopathic products are widely available in grocery stores and convenient markets. In the United States, dietary supplements are defined as "..a product (other than tobacco) intended to supplement the diet that bears or contains one or more of the following dietary ingredients: a vitamin, mineral, herbs or other botanicals, amino acids, a dietary substance used by man to supplement the diet by increasing the total dietary intake; or a concentrate, metabolite, constituent, extract, or combination of any ingredient described above; and intended for ingestion in the form of a capsule, powder, softgel, or gelcap, and not represented as a conventional food or as sole item of a meal or diet." These products are regulated under the Dietary Supplement Health and Education Act. Under this act and the current regulations, dietary supplements do not have to undergo the same rigorous testing for safety and efficacy before being marketed, as in the case for prescription drugs and other medical devices. In addition, the US Food and Drug Administration does not monitor the manufacturing practices of the companies marketing these products and leaves the manufacturer responsible for data supporting any product claims in the labeling (121). As a result, the risks and potential adverse effects of many of these dietary supplements have not been formally investigated.

Recently, increasing numbers of reports in the medical and scientific literature indicate that clinically significant drug-nutrient interactions can be precipitated by the concurrent use of dietary supplements. Table 97.9 includes a list of the most commonly used dietary supplements used by the public in the United States (15). St. John's wort has the most extensive drug-nutrient interaction profile among these supplements. The mechanism of St. John's

TABLE 97.9. TOP TEN MOST COMMONLY USED DIETARY SUPPLEMENTS IN NORTH AMERICA.

1. Ginseng
2. Ginkgo
3. Garlic
4. Glucosamine
5. St. John's wort
6. Echinacea
7. Lecithin
8. Chondroitin
9. Creatine
10. Saw palmetto

wort-drug interactions is not limited to induction of CYP3A4 and P-gp, as previously described. St. John's wort can also interfere with the pharmacodynamic effects of many psychotropic drugs such as tricyclic antidepressants and selective serotonin reuptake inhibitors. Symptoms consistent with serotonin syndrome, characterized by severe mental status changes, tremor, autonomic instability, myalgias, and motor restlessness, have been reported in numerous cases of the combination of the psychotropic drugs with St. John's wort (74, 122). Table 97.10 includes examples of the reported or highly suspected drug-nutrient interactions associated with other dietary supplements.

CLINICAL APPROACH TO MANAGEMENT

Essentially all clinically significant drug-nutrient interactions can be prevented or properly managed without causing adverse events to the patients. To prevent significant drug-nutrient interactions effectively, clinicians must first increase their awareness to identify important drug-nutrient interactions. Special attentions should to be paid to the more susceptible patient populations. Obtaining complete and accurate medical, dietary, and drug histories is essential to the identification of potential drug-nutrient interactions. Clinicians should specifically ask whether the patient consumes certain food products such as grapefruit juice or dietary supplements on a regular basis. Many patients perceive dietary supplement use as a way to maintain good health and do not recognize their potential to

TABLE 97.10. EXAMPLES OF REPORTED DRUG-NUTRIENT INTERACTIONS ASSOCIATED WITH DIETARY SUPPLEMENT USE THAT MAY HAVE CLINICAL SIGNIFICANCE

DIETARY SUPPLEMENT (PRECIPITING AGENT)	OBJECT DRUG AFFECTED	POTENTIAL RISKS
Coenzyme Q	Warfarin	Decreased efficacy of warfarin
Dong quai	Warfarin	Potentiation of anticoagulation
Folic acid	Phenytoin	Decreased phenytoin absorption
Garlic supplement	Protease inhibitors	Decreased efficacy of protease inhibitors
Ginseng	Oral hypoglycemics	Increased hypoglycemic effect
Kava	Benzodiazepines	Increased sedation
Vitamin E	Aspirin	Additive antithrombotic effect
Vitamin E	Warfarin	Increased risk of bleeding

Data from references 76, and 132 to 134.

affect drug therapy. Therefore, the use of supplements and of other dietary products tends be underreported in medical and drug histories (123). Without complete documentation, possible drug-nutrient interactions can be missed.

Once documentation is complete, clinicians can then determine whether potential drug-nutrient interactions are present. Not all drug-nutrient interactions are clinically significant. The presence of a potential drug-nutrient interaction combination per se does not warrant a clinically significant event necessitating an intervention. Many hypothetic drug-nutrient interactions do not have clinical significance in most patients because of adequate physiologic compensations (especially in younger patients), relatively limited magnitude of the interactions leading to insignificant pharmacodynamic changes, the highly variable nature of human diet and food contents, or a combination of these factors. Clinicians should use good judgment and focus on the relevant interactions. Generally speaking, special attentions should be paid to patients who receive both drugs and feeding via enteral feeding tubes or those require specialized nutrition support (see Table 97.2; Table 97.11). Drugs known to be affected by type I and type II interactions should be identified. Proper monitoring parameters such as plasma drug concentrations or nutrient concentrations should be followed if necessary. Attention should also be paid to drugs with narrow therapeutic indices, because altered absorption or metabolism can lead to treatment failure or toxicities. Drugs or nutrients that can modulate the activities of metabolic enzymes or transporters are more likely to cause clinically significant

TABLE 97.11. PRACTICE GUIDELINES REGARDING DRUG-NUTRIENT INTERACTIONS AS RECOMMENDED BY THE AMERICAN SOCIETY FOR PARENTERAL AND ENTERAL NUTRITION

1. Medication profiles of patients receiving specialized nutrition support should be reviewed for potential effects on nutrition and metabolic status.
2. Medications coadministered with enteral nutrition should be reviewed periodically for potential incompatibilities.
3. When medications are administered via an enteral feeding tube, the tube should be flushed before and after each medication is administered.
4. Liquid medication formulations should be used, when available, for administration via enteral feeding tubes.
5. Patients receiving enteral nutrition who develop diarrhea should be evaluated for antibiotic-associated causes, including colitis caused by *Clostridium difficile.*
6. Coadministration or admixture of medications known to be incompatible with parenteral nutrition should be prevented.
7. In the absence of reliable information concerning compatibility of a specific drug with a specialized nutrition support formula, the medication should be administered separately from the specialized nutrition support.
8. Each parenteral nutrition formulation compounded should be inspected for signs of gross particulate contamination, discoloration, particulate formation, and phase separation at the time of compounding and before administration.

TABLE 97.12 APPROACHES TO AN IDENTIFIED DRUG-NUTRIENT INTERACTION WITH KNOWN CLINICAL SIGNIFICANCE.

1. Make no changes to the existing regimens; continue to monitor patients for signs and symptoms of possible complications associated with the interaction (e.g., monitoring plasma concentrations of drugs or nutrients, or other related laboratory tests).
2. Make immediate changes to the current regimens.
   a. Substitute the offending agent with an alternative agent not known to cause similar interactions. Sometime, drugs in the same therapeutic class may not have the same drug-nutrient interaction profile.
   b. Make necessary dose adjustment to the object drug.
   c. Supplement the loss or deficient nutrient.
   d. Change the route of administration for the object drug.

interactions. Some drug-nutrient interactions may take a long time before any symptom can be detected. Phenytoin-induced folate deficiency and vitamin D deficiency associated with corticosteroid use, for instance, may take months to years before the patient shows symptoms associated with metabolic bone diseases. It is therefore important that the monitoring effort be continued over a prolonged period, so any possible signs associated with the drug-nutrient interactions can be detected at the earliest possible time. If in doubt, monitor and follow the relevant clinical or laboratory parameters and consult with your center's clinical pharmacist or other experts in managing the relevant adverse drug reactions.

If an established drug-nutrient interaction is identified in a patient, the clinician's approach may include (a) changing the management approach immediately or (b) making no changes to the existing regimen and continuing followup (Table 97.12). Clinicians should weigh the risks versus benefits before any intervention is made. In some cases, the risks of changing the therapeutic regimen outweigh the benefits because of the lack of efficacy for the alternative agents. Sometimes, no established alternative approach is available. The most sensible option therefore is to continue to monitor for therapeutic effects or toxicities.

If a change to the existing therapeutic regimen is preferred, clinicians may choose to use alternative agents to the interacting agents, adjust the dose of the object agent, supplement the object agent to replace the deficiency, or use a combination of these methods. In some cases, an alternative drug in the same therapeutic class can be used because a drug-nutrient interaction does not always apply to the entire drug class. Class IIC interaction applies to ciprofloxacin and ofloxacin; however, food does not reduce the bioavailability of other fluoroquinolone antibiotics such as levofloxacin. Levofloxacin may be a better choice for patients receiving continuous enteral feeding in whom intermittent bolus feedings cannot be tolerated (Table 97.13). In some cases, changing the route of administration may prevent or minimize the interaction. Knowing

TABLE 97.13. USING THE QUINOLONE CLASS ANTIBIOTICS AS AN EXAMPLE TO ILLUSTRATE THAT NOT ALL DRUGS IN THE SAME CLASS HAVE THE SAME DRUG-NUTRIENT INTERACTION PROFILE

TOTAL AMOUNT ABSORBED REDUCED BY CONCURRENT FOOD INTAKE	TOTAL AMOUNT ABSORBED NOT REDUCED BY CONCURRENT FOOD INTAKE
Ciprofloxacin	Gatifloxacin
Norfloxacin	Gemifloxacin
Ofloxacin	Levofloxacin
	Moxifloxacin

the mechanism of the drug-nutrient interaction would be extremely helpful to decide what approach may be more practical or preferable. Unfortunately, because of the lack of systematic investigations, as previously mentioned, the exact mechanisms for most clinically significant drug-nutrient interactions have not been established. Clinicians must therefore exercise good clinical judgment before deciding on any intervention. Consulting the literature, even if based solely on anecdotal reports, may still be useful because such case reports provide the experience of how others managed that specific interaction and the subsequent outcome. The goal of managing clinical significant drug-nutrient interactions is to avoid therapeutic misadventures without sacrificing the intended treatment goals and outcomes.

OTHER FACTORS ALTERING THE DISPOSITION OF DRUGS AND NUTRIENTS

Many other factors besides the presence of a drug-nutrient interaction can alter the disposition of drugs or nutrients. Sometimes, malabsorption of a drug may be related to the positioning of the enteral feeding tube. Altered absorption and metabolism of digoxin, ciprofloxacin, phenytoin, and tacrolimus have been reported when these agents are administered via a jejunostomy tube (124–127). The change in drug absorption in these examples is associated with the pharmacokinetic characteristics of the drugs and is precipitated by the technical aspect of enteral nutrition and drug delivery. It is likely that the pharmacokinetic profiles of many drugs are different between gastric and small bowel administration. However, these changes are not directly associated with drug-nutrient interactions.

Occasionally, the use of certain drugs may affect GI tract function and may lead to a loss of bodily electrolytes and fluid. This can be contributed to either by the active ingredient of the drug or by the excipients in the formulation. For instance, sorbitol is used in some oral liquid formulations as a solvent and a taste-masking agent (128). Patients may experience diarrhea from an excessive amount of sorbitol, which, in turn, can lead to malabsorptive disorders. In this case, nutrient or drug malabsorption is not related to a drug-nutrient interaction, but to an

adverse reaction to a drug or a product instead. Changing product formulations may sometimes alleviate the symptoms. Clinicians should carefully evaluate each patient's history, clinical course, complaints, and therapy, to determine properly whether a drug-nutrient interaction contributes to the patient's presentation.

SUMMARY

Advanced technology and improved understanding in science and medicine have allowed clinicians to manage patients with diseases of increased complexity and severity. Inevitably, clinicians are also facing the challenge of encountering more complicated therapeutic regimens that will more likely precipitate drug-nutrient interactions. Most drug-nutrient interactions can be prevented or properly managed with careful and thorough review and assessment of patient's history and treatment regimens. Failure to do so may lead to very serious adverse consequences. These may include drug toxicities, osteoporosis, arrhythmias, atherosclerosis, thromboembolic events, excessive bleeding, endocrine disorders, end organ damage, or even death. These complications not only contribute to morbidity or mortality, but they also increase the economic burden on our health care system.

Clinicians must be vigilant for drug-nutrient interactions, especially those with clinically significant consequences. Elderly patients and patients who are critically ill, malnourished, or receiving multiple concurrent medications have significantly increased risks of suffering adverse events related to drug-nutrient interactions. Epidemiologic data are desperately needed to help clinicians better identify the clinically important drug-nutrient interactions. Such data will allow clinicians to pay further medical attentions to the patient populations who are at risk of these serious interactions. Overall, the mechanism of most drug-nutrient interactions requires further investigations so specific and effective management approaches can be studied and compared. Once these comparative data become available, a scientific and clinically useful ranking system on the likelihood and severity of drug-nutrient interactions can be developed, which should allow even more accurate and effective identification and management of important drug-nutrient interactions. Until such a system is established and validated, clinicians must continue to rely on clinical case reports, basic concepts of pharmacokinetics and pharmacodynamics, and reasonable extrapolation from in vitro data, and they must exercise good clinical judgment in approaching drug-nutrient interactions in practice.

REFERENCES

1. Jolliffe N, Most RM. Vitam Horm 1943;1:49–107.
2. Biehl JP, Vilter RW. JAMA 1954;156:1549–52.
3. Biehl JP, Vilter RW. Proc Soc Exp Biol Med 1954;85:389–92.
4. Bauer LA. Neurology 1982;32:570–2.

5. Ozuna J, Friel P. J Neurosurg Nurs 1984;16:289–91.

6. Chan L-N. J Parenter Enteral Nutr. 2001;25:132–41.

7. Neuvonen PJ. Drugs 1976;11:45–54.

8. Radandt JM, Marchbanks CR, Dudley MN. Clin Infect Dis 1992;14:272–84.

9. Offermann G, Pinto V, Kruse R. Epilepsia 1979;20:3–15.

10. Farhat G, Yamout B, Mikati MA et al. Neurology 2002;58: 1348–53.

11. Mikati M, Wakim RH, Fayad M. J Med Liban 2003;51:71–3.

12. Drezner MK. Epilepsy Behav 2004;5[Suppl 2]:41S–7S.

13. Fitzpatrick LA. Epilepsy Behav 2004;5[Suppl 2]:3S–15S.

14. Chan L-N. Curr Opin Clin Nutr Metab Care 2002;5:327–32.

15. Kaufman DW, Kelly JP, Rosenberg L et al JAMA 2002;287: 337–44.

16. Noble RE. Metabolism 2003;52[Suppl 2]:27–30.

17. Cheymol G. Clin Pharmacokinet 2000;39:215–31.

18. Murry DJ, Riva L, Poplack DG. Int J Cancer Suppl 1998;11: 48–51.

19. Krishnaswamy K. Clin Pharmacokinet 1989;17[Suppl 1]:68–88.

20. Varela-Moreiras G. Biomed Pharmacother 2001;55:448–53.

21. Bailey LB, Gregory JF III. J Nutr 1999;129:919–22.

22. Carmel R, Green R, Rosenblatt DS et al. Hematology (Am Soc Hematol Educ Program) 2003;62–81.

23. Hansten PD. Sci Med 1998; Jan/Feb:16–25.

24. Mirtallo JM. J Infus Nurs 2004;27:19–24.

25. Fleisher D, Li C, Zhou Y. Clin Pharmacokinet 1999;36:233–54.

26. Singh BN. Clin Pharmacokinet 1999;37:213–55.

27. Schmidt LE, Dalhoff K. Drugs 2002;62:1481–502.

28. Pedrazzoni M, Ciotti G, Davoli L et al. J Endocrinol Invest 1989;12:409–12.

29. Borovicka J, Schwizer W, Mettraux C et al. Am J Physiol 1997; 273:G374–80.

30. Costarelli V, Sanders TA. Br J Nutr 2001;86:471–7.

31. Konturek JW, Thor P, Maczka M et al. Scand J Gastroenterol 1994;29:583–90.

32. Ogunbona FA, Smith IF, Olawoye OS. J Pharm Pharmacol 1985;37:283–4.

33. Lange H, Eggers R, Bircher J. Eur J Clin Pharmacol 1988;34: 315–7.

34. Conway EL, Phillips PA, Drummer OH et al. J Pharm Sci 1990;79:228–31.

35. Hoon TJ, McCollam PL, Beckman KJ et al. Am J Cardiol 1992;70:1072–6.

36. Hashiguchi M, Ogata H, Maeda A et al. J Clin Pharmacol 1996; 36:1022–8.

37. Waldman SA, Morganroth J. J Clin Pharmacol 1995;35:163–9.

38. Gill KS, Wood MJ. Clin Pharmacokinet 1996;31:1–8.

39. Oguey D, Kolliker F, Gerber NJ et al. Arthritis Rheum 1992;35: 611–4.

40. Kozloski GD, DeVito JM, Kisicki JC et al. Arthritis Rheum 1992;35:761–4.

41. Hamilton RA, Kremer JM. J Rheumatol 1995;22:630–2.

42. Dupuis LL, Koren G, Silverman ED et al. J Rheumatol 1995; 22:1570–3.

43. Patsalos PN. Clin Pharmacokinet 2004;43:707–24.

44. Crevoisier C, Zerr P, Calvi-Gries F et al. Eur J Pharm Biopharm 2003;55:71–6.

45. Wiley J, Tatum D, Keinath R et al. Gastroenterology 1988;94: 1144–9.

46. Kaneko H, Sakakibara M, Mitsuma T et al. Am J Gastroenterol 1995;90:603–9.

47. Brundin T, Wahren J. Am J Physiol 1991;260:E232–7.

48. Dauzat M, Lafortune M, Patriquin H et al. Eur J Appl Physiol Occup Physiol 1994;68:373–80.

49. Szinnai C, Mottet C, Gutzwiller JP et al. Scand J Gastroenterol 2001;36:540–4.

50. Ramchandani VA, Kwo PY, Li T-K. J Clin Pharmacol 2001;41: 1345–50.

51. Gao L, Ramzan I, Baker AB. Anaesth Intensive Care 2000;28: 375–85.

52. Peikin SR. Gastroenterol Clin North Am 1989;18:757–75.

53. Greiff JM, Rowbotham D. Clin Pharmacokinet 1994;27: 447–61.

54. Schirra J, Katschinski M, Weidmann C et al. J Clin Invest 1996; 97:92–103.

55. Levanon D, Zhang M, Orr WC et al. Am J Physiol 1998;274: G430–4.

56. Chey WY, Chang TM. J Gastroenterol 2003;38:1025–35.

57. Rezek M, Novin D. J Nutr 1976;106:812–20.

58. Moran TH, Ladenheim EE, Schwartz GJ. Int J Obes Relat Metab Disord 2001;25[Suppl 5]:S39–S41.

59. Herzlich B, Herbert V. Am J Gastroenterol 1986;81:678–80.

60. Neal G. Gut 1990;31:59–63.

61. Howden CW. J Clin Gastroenterol 2000;30:29–33.

62. Ruscin JM, Page RL II, Valuck RJ. Ann Pharmacother 2002;36: 812–6.

63. Sagar M, Janczewska I, Ljungdahl A et al. Aliment Pharmacol Ther 1999;13:453–8.

64. Hall SD, Thummel KE, Watkins PB. Drug Metab Dispos 1999; 27;161–6.

65. Ito K, Kusuhara H, Sugiyama Y. Pharm Res 1999;16:225–31.

66. Lee SL, Wang MF, Lee AI et al. FEBS Lett 2003;544:143–7.

67. Wacher VJ, Salphati L, Benet LZ. Adv Drug Deliv Rev 2001;46: 89–102.

68. Benet LZ, Cummins CL. Adv Drug Deliv Rev 2001;50[Suppl 1]:S3–S11.

69. Benet LZ, Cummins CL, Wu CY. Int J Pharm 2004;277:3–9.

70. Dresser GK, Spence JD, Bailey DG. Clin Pharmacokinet 2000; 38:41–57.

71. Huang SM, Hall SD, Watkins P et al. Clin Pharmacol Ther 2004;75:1–12.

72. Lown KS, Bailey DG, Fontana RJ et al. J Clin Invest 1997;99: 2545–53.

73. Zhou S, Gao Y, Jiang W et al. Drug Metab Rev 2003;35:35–98.

74. Henderson L, Yue QY, Bergquist C et al. Br J Clin Pharmacol 2002;54:349–56.

75. Mannel M. Drug Saf 2004;27:773–97.

76. Mucksavage JJ, Chan L-N. Dietary supplement interactions with medications. In: Boullata JI, Armenti VT, Malone M, eds. Handbook of Drug-Nutrient Interactions. Totawa, NJ: Humana Press, 2004:217–33.

77. Mai I, Bauer S, Perloff ES et al. Clin Pharmacol Ther 2004; 76:330–40.

78. Bauer S, Stormer E, Johne A et al. Br J Clin Pharmacol 2003; 55:203–11.

79. Frye RF, Fitzgerald SM, Lagattuta TF, et al. Clin Pharmacol Ther 2004;76:323–9.

80. Smith P. Pharmacotherapy 2004;24:1508–14.

81. Mueller SC, Uehleke B, Woehling H et al. Clin Pharmacol Ther 2004;75:546–57.

82. Tannergren C, Engman H, Knutson L et al. Clin Pharmacol Ther 2004;75:298–309.

83. Morimoto T, Kotegawa T, Tsutsumi K et al. J Clin Pharmacol 2004;44:95–101.

84. Hebert MF, Park JM, Chen YL et al. J Clin Pharmacol 2004;44: 89–94.

85. Hall SD, Wang Z, Huang SM et al. Clin Pharmacol Ther 2003; 74:525–35.

86. Pfrunder A, Schiesser M, Gerber S et al. Br J Clin Pharmacol 2003;56:683–90.
87. Markowitz JS, Donovan JL, DeVane CL et al. JAMA 2003; 290:1500–4.
88. Dintaman JM, Silverman JA. Pharm Res 1999;16:1550–6.
89. Johnson BM, Charman WN, Porter CJ. AAPS Pharm Sci 2002;4:E40.
90. Chan L, Humma LM, Schriever CA et al. Clin Pharmacol Ther 2004;75:P95.
91. Hennessy M, Kelleher D, Spiers JP et al. Br J Clin Pharmacol 2002;53:75–82.
92. Au Yeung SC, Ensom MH. Ann Pharmacother 2000;34:896–905.
93. Guengerich FR. Am J Clin Nutr 1995; 61:651S–8S.
94. Ioannides C. Xenobiotica 1999;29:109–54.
95. Cashman JR, Lattard V, Lin J. Drug Metab Dispos 2004;32:222–9.
96. Dickerson RN, Charland SL. Pharmacotherapy 2002;22:1084–90.
97. Earl-Salotti GI, Charland SL. JPEN J Parenter Enteral Nutr 1994;18:458–65.
98. Muclow JC, Caraher MT, Henderson DB et al. Br J Clin Pharmacol 1979;7:416–7.
99. Wilmana PF, Brodie MJ, Muclow JC et al. Br J Clin Pharmacol 1979;8:523–8.
100. Brodie MJ, Boobis AR, Toverud EL et al. Br J Clin Pharmacol 1980;9:523–5.
101. Gandhi M, Aweeka F, Greenblatt RM, et al. Annu Rev Pharmacol Toxicol 2004;44:499–523.
102. Evans WE, McLeod HL. N Engl J Med 2003;348:538–49.
103. Mizutani T. Drug Metab Rev 2003;35:99–106.
104. Evans WE, Relling MV. Nature 2004;429:464–8.
105. Nebert DW, Russell DW. Lancet 2002; 360:1155–62.
106. Paoloni-Giacobino A, Grimble R, Pichard C. Clin Nutr 2003;22 429–35.
107. Loktionov A. J Nutr Biochem 2003;14:426–51.
108. Booth SL, Centurelli MA. Nutr Rev 1999;57:288–96.
109. Volz HP, Gleiter CH. Drugs Aging 1998;13:341–55.
110. Tein I. J Inherit Metab Dis 2003;26:147–69.
111. Youdim MB, Weinstock M. Neurotoxicology 2004;25:243–50.
112. Suzzi G, Gardini F. Int J Food Microbiol 2003;88:41–54.
113. Brown C, Taniguchi G, Yip K. J Clin Pharmacol 1989;29:529–32.
114. Yamada M, Yasuhara H. Neurotoxicology 2004;25:215–21.
115. Wittkowsky AK. Semin Vasc Med 2003;3:221–30.
116. Karlson B, Leijd B, Hellstrom K. Acta Med Scand 1986;220:347–50.
117. Pedersen FM, Hamberg O, Hess K et al. J Intern Med 1991;229:517–20.
118. Lubetsky A, Dekel-Stern E, Chetrit A et al. Thromb Haemost 1999;81:396–9.
119. Franco V, Polanczyk CA, Clausell N et al Am J Med 2004;116:651–6.
120. Khan T, Wynne H, Wood P et al. Br J Haematol 2004;124:348–54.
121. Dietary Supplement Health and Education Act (DSHEA), Public Law 103-417, 25 October 1994; codified at 42USC 287C–11.
122. Mills E, Montori VM, Wu P et al. BMJ 2004;329:27–30.
123. Hensrud DD, Engle DD, Scheitel SM. Mayo Clin Proc 1999;74:443–7.
124. Ehrenpreis ED, Guerriero S, Nogueras JJ et al. Ann Pharmacother 1994;28:1239–40.
125. Healy DP, Brodbeck MC, Clendening CE. Antimicrob Agents Chemother 1996;40:6–10.
126. Rodman DP, Stevenson TL, Ray TR. Pharmacotherapy 1995;15:801–5.
127. Hasegawa T, Nara K, Kimura T et al. Pediatr Transplant 2001;5:204–9.
128. Madigan SM, Courtney DE, Macauley D. Clin Nutr 2002;21:531–2.
129. Orrick JJ, Steinhart CR. Ann Pharmacother 2004;38:1664–74.
130. Burman WJ, Gallicano K, Peloquin C. Clin Pharmacokinet 2001;40:327–41.
131. Purkins L, Wood N, Kleinermans D, et al. Br J Clin Pharmacol 2003;56[Suppl 1]:17–23.
132. De Smet PAGM. N Engl J Med 2002;347:2046–56.
133. Anonymous. J Am Coll Surg 2002;194:251.
134. Heck AM, DeWitt BA, Lukes AL. Am J Health Syst Pharm 2000;57:1221–7.
135. Livingston MG, Livingston HM. Drug Saf 1996;14:219–27.
136. Volz HP, Gleiter CH. Drugs Aging 1998;13:341–55.
137. Antal EJ, Hendershot PE, Batts DH et al. J Clin Pharmacol 2001;41:552–62.
138. Chen H-W, Tsai C-W, Yang J-J, et al. Br J Nutr 2003;89:189–200.

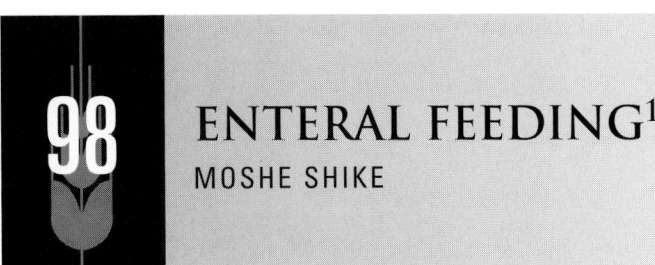

98 ENTERAL FEEDING[1]

MOSHE SHIKE

HISTORY 1554
FEEDING TUBES 1555
   Nasogastric and Nasoenteral Tubes 1555
   Gastrostomy and Jejunostomy Tubes 1555
ENTERAL FEEDING FORMULAS 1556
   Definitions 1556
   Classification 1556
   Composition 1557
NUTRIENT ABSORPTION AND UTILIZATION 1560
   Protein 1560
   Carbohydrates 1561
   Fat 1561
   Vitamins and Trace Elements 1561
   Fiber 1562
INDICATIONS AND CONTRAINDICATIONS 1562
   Specific Indications 1562
METHODS OF INFUSION .1563
COMPLICATIONS 1563
ENTERAL FEEDING IN VARIOUS
   MEDICAL CONDITIONS 1564
HOME ENTERAL NUTRITION 1564
DRUGS IN ENTERAL FEEDING 1564

Enteral feeding is a method of provision of nutrients into the gastrointestinal (GI) tract through a tube. This method is used for nutritional support in patients who cannot ingest or digest sufficient amounts of food but have adequate intestinal functional capacity. Enteral feeding is now widely used in many different clinical disorders.

HISTORY

The history of enteral feeding has been reviewed by Randall (1) and more recently by Harkness (2). The practice of placing nutrients into the GI tract not through the mouth originated in ancient times with the Egyptians, who used nutrient enemas for preservation of general health. Ancient

Greek physicians used enemas containing wine, whey, milk, and barley broth for the treatment of diarrhea. In the nineteenth century, European physicians administered nutrient enemas that included beef extracts, milk, and whiskey. Rectal feeding was widely used until the beginning of the twentieth century, when Einhorn pointed out its limitations (3). In 1598, a Venetian physician, Capivacceus, was the first to use a hollow tube attached to an animal's bladder for feeding into the esophagus. The use of a small silver tube passed from the nose to the esophagus was reported in 1617 for feeding patients suffering from tetanus. A major development in provision of nutrition through tubes occurred at the end of the eighteenth century, when John Hunter used a nasogastric tube made from eel skin to feed a patient with neurogenic dysphagia. The use of nasogastric tubes became widespread in the nineteenth century.

The concept of early postoperative enteral feeding was introduced by Andresen in 1918, when he started jejunal feeding in a patient following a gastrojejunostomy (4). Jejunal feeding gained popularity because of the realization that although gastric emptying may be impaired postoperatively, small bowel peristalsis is preserved. In 1959, Barron reported on postoperative enteral feeding in a few hundred patients (5). He used juices and foods broken into fine mixtures and also GI secretions collected from drainage from biliary, pancreatic, gastric, and intestinal fistulas. These substances were infused via polyethylene tubes passed through the nose.

Specialized enteral feeding formulas appeared in the 1930s with the introduction of casein hydrolysate for enteral and parenteral feeding. Subsequently, other proteins and crystalline amino acids were used in combination with various amounts of carbohydrates, fats, minerals, and vitamins. A commercial enteral feeding formula, Nutramigen, was introduced in 1942. Major progress in utilization of chemically defined formulas was achieved in studies that were sponsored by the National Aeronautics and Space Administration (6). These studies demonstrated that physiologically normal volunteers could be maintained during a 6-month period, in a normal nutritional and physical state while being fed solely with chemically defined formulas. Based on these observations, Randall and colleagues conducted a series of studies using commercial chemically defined diets (1) and demonstrated the

---

[1] **Abbreviations: AAA,** aromatic amino acid; **BCAA,** branched-chain amino acid; **EAA,** essential amino acid; **GI,** gastrointestinal; **HEN,** home enteral nutrition; **LCT,** long-chain triglyceride; **MCT,** medium-chain triglyceride; **PEG,** percutaneous endoscopic gastrostomy; **PEJ,** percutaneous endoscopic jejunostomy.

usefulness of these diets in patients with a variety of GI diseases.

Enteral feeding is clearly a major advance in the ability to provide nutrients to patients with various illnesses and thus potentially to affect morbidity, mortality and quality of life. However, this method may not always result in benefits to patients who are unable to eat. This issue has been raised particularly regarding patients with dementia (7).

FEEDING TUBES

Enteral feeding requires infusion of formulas through a tube into the upper GI tract. Feeding tubes can be divided into two categories: those entering the GI tract through the nose (nasogastric or nasoenteral tubes) and those entering through the abdominal wall (gastrostomies, jejunostomies). The type of access for enteral feeding depends on the state of the upper GI tract, the anticipated length of feeding, and the expertise of the local professionals. Generally, feedings for periods less than 4 weeks can be provided through nasal tubes, whereas feedings for longer periods require more permanent tubes (gastrostomies and jejunostomies).

Nasogastric and Nasoenteral Tubes

Various types of nasogastric and nasoenteral tubes are available commercially. Most are made of silicone or polyvinyl. Tubes used in adults vary in length between 30 and 43 inches with diameters from 8 to 14 French. The shorter tubes are used for nasogastric feeding and the longer for nasoenteral feeding. The thinner tubes are softer, tend to clog, and are more difficult to use. The tips of some tubes are weighed with tungsten or silicone to facilitate passage through the GI tract. The tubes come with a stylet, which facilitates insertion through the nose and into the GI tract. Nasogastric tubes are usually used for short-term enteral feeding, mostly in the hospital. The tubes are placed at the bedside by health professionals, and verification of the location of the tip of the tube in the stomach or the small intestines is required. This can be done by a radiograph of the abdomen. Listening for airflow over the upper abdomen can provide misleading information (8) and can lead to serious complications. Procedures using color, pH, and quantity of aspirated fluid are also inadequate to determine the location of the feeding tube tip.

Nasoenteral tubes should be used whenever a risk of aspiration exists or when gastric motility is impaired. Advancement of such tubes from the stomach into the small bowel may be facilitated by administration of prokinetic drugs (9). Placement of tubes in the duodenum or jejunum can also be facilitated by endoscopic or radiographic techniques (10), with a success rate of 85 to 95%. Contraindications to placement of nasogastric tubes include obstruction of the upper GI tract, severe reflux, cranial or facial trauma, gastric dysmotility, and aspiration risk. Nasoenteral tubes can be used in patients with reflux, gastric dysmotility, or aspiration risk.

Complications related to nasogastric and nasoenteral tubes can be divided into two categories: those resulting from the the tube insertion and those arising from feeding. Insertion-related complications include trauma and bleeding from the nose and upper GI tract, perforation, misplacement of the tube into the respiratory tract, aspiration pneumonia, and vomiting as a result of pharyngeal irritation. Postinsertion complications include tube migration, aspiration of infused formula, erosion of the GI tract mucosa, and ear and nose infections.

Malfunction of nasogastric and nasoenteral tubes occurs commonly because of clogging with formulas or medications, kinking, or bursting (secondary to forceful injection of solutions). These complications can be avoided with appropriate care of the tube (e.g., thorough cleansing after each feeding). Complication rates of feeding tubes vary, depending on the experience of the professional inserting the tube and on the care of the tube after it is placed. These rates vary between 7.6 and 19% (11, 12). Comprehensive reviews of nasogastric and nasoenteral feeding tubes, techniques, complications, and recommendations for practice have been published (10, 12).

Gastrostomy and Jejunostomy Tubes

For long-term enteral feeding (>4 weeks), gastrostomy or jejunostomy tubes are advantageous for the following reasons: (a) they have a larger diameter (15 to 28 French) and thus do not tend to clog; the wider tubes also allow for a quicker and easier administration of formulas and medications; (b) the risk of aspiration is considerably decreased because the tubes are fixed in the stomach or intestines and do not migrate into the esophagus, as may happen with nasogastric tubes; and (c) they are more convenient and aesthetically acceptable.

The advantages of feeding patients who have had acute strokes through an endoscopically placed gastrostomy tube over a nasogastric tube were documented in a randomized study demonstrating that use of the former was associated with more optimal provision of nutrients, a better nutritional state, and less mortality (13). However, other studies failed to demonstrate advantages related to aspiration, although percutaneous endoscopic gastrostomy (PEG) feeding was found to be more convenient (14).

The various methods of placement of gastrostomy and jejunostomy tubes have been reviewed (14). Gastrostomy and jejunostomy tubes can be placed surgically, Endoscopically, or radiologically by fluoroscopy, sonography, or tomography (15). The surgical method requires a minor operation, but it has a complication rate of 2.5 to 16% and a mortality rate of 1 to 6% (16–18). A less invasive surgical approach involves use of a laporoscope for access into the abdomen (19, 20). No definite randomized studies have compared endoscopic and surgical gastrostomy tube placement. However, the general consensus is that the endoscopic approach is preferable over the two surgical approaches (21). Radiologic techniques are also commonly used for placement of percutaneous gastrostomies and percutaneous jejunostomy tubes (22).

PEG, first reported in 1980, is the most commonly used method for placement of a gastrostomy tubes. The technical aspects of the procedure have been reported (14, 23, 24). In patients with gastric resection and in those with increased risk for aspiration (gastroparesis, severe reflux, neurologic disorders), percutaneous endoscopic jejunostomy (PEJ) tubes are preferable. (25). Adequate randomized studies comparing gastric and small bowel feedings have not been performed. Existing data suggest that feeding into the small bowel, particularly in severely ill patients, has the advantages of lessened gastroesophageal reflux, increased nutrient delivery, and a lower rate of pneumonia in mechanically ventilated patients.

Placement of PEG and PEJ is associated with a morbidity rate of 5 to 15% and a mortality rate of 0.3 to 1% (14, 23–25). Complications include wound infections and, rarely, severe infections such as fasciitis and peritonitis. Leakage at the tube site tends to occur in patients receiving steroids or chemotherapy. These medications should be avoided as much as possible during the first 7 days following placement of a PEG. Bleeding, interposition of abdominal organs (liver, small bowel, colon) between the stomach and the abdominal wall with intestinal perforation, and liver laceration are rare complications (12). In the long term, PEG and PEJ tubes function well with few complications (12, 14, 24, 25). They usually last approximately 2 years and require replacement when signs of tube deterioration appear. Active patients who are receiving long-term enteral feeding can benefit from a skin-level button gastrostomy or jejunostomy (26), which is less obtrusive and more convenient compared with the tubes.

ENTERAL FEEDING FORMULAS

Definitions

More than 100 commercial formulas are available for enteral feeding. The composition of different products varies greatly, with some intended for general nutrition and others designed for specific metabolic or clinical conditions. Enteral feeding formulas have been classified according to various criteria. The names given to different classes of formulas have not always been consistent and often overlap, thus leading to lack of clarity and confusion. The general term medical foods has been used since 1989 by the US Food and Drug Administration to define enteral nutrition products (27): "Medical foods (MF) are distinguished from other foods for special dietary purposes or foods which make health claims (e.g., fiber in relation to cancer) by the requirement that they (MF) be used under medical supervision." In general, to be considered a medical food, a product must, at a minimum, meet the following criteria: (a) the product is a food for oral or tube feeding, and (b) the product is labeled for the dietary management of a medical disorder, disease, or condition.

The definitions and regulatory aspects of enteral feeding products have been summarized by Talbot (28). Defined-formula diets was suggested as a general term to indicate that the ingredients (including nutrients processed from foods and/or relatively purified compounds, simple or complex) are prepared commercially by designated procedures so their composition is established fairly well, although not necessarily with chemical precision (29). The term elemental has been used mostly to indicate formulas containing predigested protein.

Classification

The following is a classification based on practical considerations according to clinical indications:

1. Polymeric formulas: These contain macronutrients in the form of isolates of intact protein, triglycerides, and carbohydrate polymers. They can be used orally or through a tube and provide complete nutrition. They also contain vitamins, minerals, trace elements, and, in some cases, fiber. These are the most commonly used formulas for enteral feeding.

2. Monomeric formulas: These usually contain proteins as peptides and/or amino acids, fat as long-chain triglycerides (LCTs) or a mixture of LCTs and medium-chain triglycerides (MCTs), and carbohydrates as partially hydrolyzed starch maltodextrins and glucose oligosaccharides. They also contain vitamins, minerals, and trace elements. These formulas are often used for patients with impaired digestion or absorption; however, it is questionable whether they are more advantageous than polymeric formulas.

3. Blenderized foods: These are natural foods, semiliquified in a blender, that can be used for the provision of nutrition by the oral route or through a tube. Currently, these foods are rarely used.

4. Formulas for specific metabolic needs: These are intended for patients who have unique metabolic requirements: inborn errors of metabolism, renal failure, diabetes, and other illnesses presenting specific needs.

5. Immune-enhancing formulas: These formulas contain specific nutrients thought to improve the immune response. In spite of extensive research, no clear evidence of clinical advantages exist, although some studies identified specific patients in whom these formulas offer benefits.

6. Modular formulas: These are single nutritional components that can be given by themselves or mixed with other enteral products to provide formulas that meet

special nutritional or metabolic needs (i.e., increased calories, protein, and minerals).

7. Hydration solutions: These provide minerals, water, and small amounts of carbohydrates.

Composition

Polymeric Formulas

Many different polymeric commercial formulas are available. Protein constitutes 12 to 20% of total calories, carbohydrates 40 to 60%, and fats 30 to 40%. In the standard formulas, the ratio of nitrogen to nonprotein calories is about 1 g/150 kcal. In the high-nitrogen formulas, this ratio can be as high as 1 g/75 kcal. An extensive review of protein, peptides, and amino acids in enteral nutrition has been published (30). Polymeric formulas contain whole proteins: casein, lactalbumin, whey, egg white, or a combination of these. Carbohydrates are usually glucose polymers in the form of starch and its hydrolysates. Fats are of vegetable origin, such as corn oil, safflower oil, or sunflower oil.

Vitamins, minerals, and essential trace elements are present in adequate quantities so a daily intake of 1500 to 2000 kcal provides the necessary maintenance requirements of these nutrients both for adults (31) and children (32). The amounts of minerals such as sodium and potassium vary considerably among the various formulas, thus allowing a choice when restriction of the intake of specific minerals is necessary.

Polymeric formulas are lactose and gluten free. The osmolality varies between 300 and 650 mOsm/kg. Some polymeric formulas contain fiber in the form of complex nondigestable or partially digestable carbohydrates. The amounts of fiber range between 6 and 14 g/1000 kcal. The caloric density is between 1 and 2 kcal/mL. The high-caloric formulas allow provision of large amounts of calories in a smaller volume. Administration of these formulas requires close follow-up because they can be associated with dehydration and severe serum electrolytes abnormalities. The ranges of the nutrient contents of polymeric formulas are listed in Table 98.1.

Monomeric Formulas

The main feature of monomeric formulas is that they require less digestion than regular foods or polymeric formulas. Protein is in the form of peptides and free amino acids and is derived from hydrolysis of casein, whey, and other proteins. The net absorption of dipeptides and tripeptides, and the amino acids generated from their digestion is faster and more efficient than the absorption of equivalent amounts of free amino acids (33).

Carbohydrates are in the form of partially hydrolyzed starch (maltodextrins and glucose oligosaccharides). Fat is usually a mixture of MCTs and LCTs of plant origin and provides only 1 to 5% of the calories. Protein contributes 12 to 20% of the total calories. The caloric density of monomeric formulas varies between 1 and 1.5 kcal/mL. These formulas contain sufficient minerals, trace elements, and vitamins; 2000 kcal will usually provide the daily requirements of these nutrients. Monomeric formulas are lactose free and do not contain fiber. The partially digested macronutrients contribute to the higher osmolality in comparison with that of polymeric formulas. The osmolality of monomeric formulas ranges between 270 and 650 mOsm/kg.

Based on physiologic considerations, these formulas are suitable for patients with impaired digestion, such as those with pancreatic insufficiency or short bowel syndrome. Clinical trials to demonstrate such an advantage, however, have not been adequate.

When the osmolality of enteral formulas is greater than 300 mOsm/kg, the formulas tend to induce shift of free water into the intestinal lumen and can thus induce rapid transit and diarrhea. The osmolality of monomeric formulas is usually higher than that of the polymeric formulas with the same caloric density.

Natural Foods

Blenderized natural foods are available commercially or can be prepared by the patient. The commercial blenderized food formulas are prepared from milk, beef, fruits, vegetables, and fiber; hence their nutrient content is not determined precisely, and their nutritional completeness is not ensured. Commercial blenderized food products are usually more expensive than polymeric formulas. Patients who use enteral feeding in the home can prepare blenderized foods from regular foods in the household. If this practice is used, the nutritional adequacy of the blenderized foods must be ensured, particularly if patients are receiving long-term therapy.

Formulas for Specific Metabolic Needs

These formulas are mostly complete nutritional products in which specific nutrients are added or removed to meet special metabolic requirements. Specific metabolic formulas can be divided into two categories. The first category includes formulas designed for use in patients with inherited metabolic disorders. These formulas are low in or devoid of specific nutrients, such as phenylalanine or other amino acids, that cannot be properly metabolized because of enzymatic defects or deficiencies (see Chapters 58 and 59). The second category includes formulas designed for use in patients with specific medical conditions, such as liver failure, renal failure, or critical illness with multiple organ failure. Formulas in this category are designed to lessen the metabolic burden on the failing organs.

High Branched-Chain Amino Acid Formulas. These formulas contain about 40 to 50% of the amino acids as leucine, isoleucine, and valine. The concentration of the aromatic amino acids (AAAs) tryptophan, tyrosine, and phenylalanine is low. Formulas high in

TABLE 98.1. RANGES OF NUTRIENT CONTENT OF ENTERAL FEEDING PRODUCTS

NUTRIENTS	BLENDERIZED FOODS OR MILK-BASE FORMULAS: COMPLETE	POLYMERIC FORMULAS: COMPLETE	POLYMERIC FORMULAS WITH FIBER: COMPLETE	MONOMERIC FORMULAS	DISEASE-SPECIFIC FORMULATIONS
kcal/mL	0.7–1.0	0.5–2.0	1.0–1.2	1.0–1.33	1.0–2.0
Protein g/L					
Intact	42.0–84.0	17.5–83.7	39.7–53.0	0	30.0–83.0
Hydrolyzed	0	0	0	31.5–58.1	0
Amino acids	0	0	0	20.6–38.2	19.4–69.7
Carbohydrate g/L	82.8–192.0	68.0–250.0	123.0–162.0	127.0–226.3	93.7–365.6
Fat g/L	20.0–42.8	17.5–106.0	35.0–46.0	1.45–52.0	7.4–96.0
MCT:LCT ratio	NA	20:80–73:27[a]	NA	40:60–70:30[a]	25:75–70:30[a]
Fiber g/L	4.24	NA	5.9–14.4	NA	NA
Osmolality	300–450	120–710	303–480	270–650	320–910
Volume to meet 100% RDA	—	750–2000	1250–1800	1500–2250	947–3000
Nonprotein calorie:N ratio	131:1	75:1–167:1	116:1–148:1	125:1–284:1	NA
Vitamin A (IU)	3332–9000	1250–10,000	3300–5000	2500–5000	735–6700[a]
Vitamin D (IU)	266.8–800.0	100.0–560.0	267.0–420.0	140.0–280.0	84.5–423.0[a]
Vitamin E (IU)	24–42	15–75	21–64	15–40	10–60[a]
Vitamin K (μg)	66.8–80.0	38.0–320.0	48.0–160.0	22.3–160.0	35.0–160.0[a]
Vitamin C (mg)	60.0–120.0	56.0–317.0	120.0–254.0	33.3–200.0	30.0–317[a]
Thiamin (mg)	1.48–2.12	0.75–4.0	1.2–3.22	0.83–2.00	0.69–3.17[a]
Riboflavin (mg)	1.68–4.76	0.85–4.8	1.36–3.64	0.94–2.4	0.7–3.59[a]
Niacin (mg)	16.0–28.0	10.0–56.0	16.0–42.4	11.1–28.0	8.82–42.0[a]
Vitamin B$_6$ (mg)	2.0–2.8	1.0–8.0	1.6–4.24	1.11–4.0	1.07–8.61[a]
Folate (μg)	266.8–560.0	200.0–1,080.0	270.0–540.0	210.0–540.0	47.6–1056.0[a]
Pantothenic acid (mg)	6.68–14.0	5.0–28.0	8.0–21.2	5.00–14.0	2.62–21.1[a]
Vitamin B$_{12}$ (μg)	4.8–12.0	3.0–16.0	4.8–12.7	2.0–8.0	2.94–12.7[a]
Biotin (μg)	49.2–440.0	150.0–800.0	240.0–400.0	100.0–400.0	142.5–634.0[a]
Sodium (mg)	760–1320	350–1184	500–930	460–1000	235–1310[a]
Potassium (mg)	1400–3640	600–2500	1250–1800	782–1661	882–1902[a]
Chloride (mg)	1132–3600	500–2000	1000–1440	819–2501	677–1691[a]
Calcium (mg)	668–2320	250–1400	667–910	451–800	491–1284[a]
Phosphorus (mg)	868–2000	250–1400	667–850	499–700	491–1056[a]
Magnesium (mg)	240–560	100–680	267–340	200–400	192–423[a]
Iron (mg)	12.0–25.2	4.5–24.0	12.0–15.0	9.0–13.3	8.82–19.0[a]
Iodine (μg)	100.0–212.0	37.5–200.0	100.0–127.0	74.7–101.3	73.5–158.4[a]
Copper (mg)	1.32–2.8	0.5–3.0	1.3–1.7	1.0–1.6	0.96–2.11[a]
Zinc (mg)	12.0–21.2	3.75–30.0	12.0–20.0	8.33–15.0	7.35–23.8[a]
Manganese (mg)	0.16–4.0	1.0–5.4	1.77–3.8	0.94–3.33	1.23–5.3[a]

LCT, long-chain triglyceride; MCT, medium-chain triglyceride. NA. Not available; RDA, recommended dietary allowance.
[a] Information available only on some of the formulas.

branched-chain amino acids (BCAAs) have been designed for use in two conditions: (a) hepatic failure and encephalopathy and (b) severe illness and stress with multiple organs failure, such as sepsis and major injury. Patients with hepatic encephalopathy tend to have decreased levels of BCAAs and increased levels of AAAs in blood and in cerebrospinal fluid. The AAAs act as false neurotransmitters in the central nervous system and can contribute to hepatic encephalopathy (34). Formulas high in BCAAs and low in AAAs were designed to improve hepatic encephalopathy. Most randomized studies examining the use of high-BCAA formulas in patients with hepatic encephalopathy showed no benefit (35), whereas some showed decreased morbidity and

mortality (35, 36) (see Chapter 79). A comprehensive review has been published (35).

Major acute illnesses associated with severe metabolic stress, such as sepsis, severe trauma, and burns, are associated with accelerated muscle catabolism (see Chapters 89 and 91). Because BCAAs are used extensively by muscles, formulas high in BCAAs have been proposed to be beneficial for muscle preservation in severely ill and catabolic patients. Results of clinical trials have been inconclusive, and a comprehensive review found no specific benefit from BCAAs in these patients (37).

Formulas High in Essential Amino Acids. These formulas are designed for patients with renal failure, many of whom may have trauma and/or sepsis (see Chapter 94).

The failing kidneys have a reduced capacity for clearance of various metabolites. Serum levels of some nonessential amino acids are elevated, and those of essential amino acids (EAAs: leucine, isoleucine, and valine) are decreased. The objectives of nutritional support in patients with renal failure are to provide optimal nutrition and at the same time to minimize the load of metabolites presented for handling by the compromised kidneys. The latter objective is particularly important in patients with seriously impaired renal function in whom an effort is made to avoid dialysis. Renal formulas contain EAAs, histidine, small amounts of fat, and electrolytes. They do not contain vitamins or trace elements, which must be supplemented as needed. The low content of electrolytes allows flexibility because electrolytes can be added as needed. Most of the clinical studies on the role of highEAA feeding regimens have been performed with parenteral nutrition, and although some metabolic benefits have been noted, a clear clinical advantage has not been documented (38). The few studies in which enteral nutrition was examined suggest that administration of EAAs is associated with improved nitrogen balance and an attenuation of the rise in blood urea nitrogen (39).

High-Fat/Low-Carbohydrate Formulas for Pulmonary Insufficiency. In these formulas, the fat content is increased to approximately 50% of total calories, with a corresponding decrease in carbohydrate content. Although calories of any source increase oxygen consumption and carbon dioxide production and thus present an added burden to the failing lungs, carbohydrate metabolism requires more oxygen and produces more carbon dioxide compared with fat, hence the concept that replacing carbohydrates by fat presents a lighter burden on the respiratory system. In most patients, the difference is not clinically significant; however, in those with borderline pulmonary function (40, 41), the difference may be important (see Chapter 93).

Immune-Modulating Formulas. Specific nutrients can influence the immune response (see Chapter 43). Experimental studies, mostly in animals, suggest that nutrients that are nonessential, such as certain ω-3 fatty acids (42, 43), RNA (42, 44), arginine (45), and glutamine may exert beneficial effects on the immune response and defense against infections. Arginine, a nonessential amino acid, is a precursor of nitrous oxide (see Chapter 2), which may not be adequately produced in the critically ill patient. Arginine affects immune function and stimulates a variety of hormones. ω-3 Fatty acids have many essential metabolic effects mediated mostly by their impact on prostaglandin production. Enhanced production of ω-3–derived prostaglandins (as opposed to those derived from ω-6) decreases the severity of the inflammatory response and improves immunity (see Chapter 43).

The potential benefits of immune formulas were examined in numerous randomized trials in patients after major surgery, trauma, multiple organ failure, and burn injury.

Some studies demonstrated that postoperative administration of immune-enhancing enteral feeding resulted in better immunologic and metabolic outcomes, with a decrease in infectious and wound complications and a decrease in postoperative hospitalization. Other investigators did not find such benefits. Comparison and interpretation of clinical studies of immune-modulating formulas are hindered by heterogenety of patients (trauma, postsurgical status, burns, multiorgan failure, different study designs, different outcome measures, and different products used). An early metaanalysis of 11 studies (1009 patients) found a decrease in major infectious complications and in hospital stay; however, a nonsignificant trend toward increased morality was reported (46). Another metaanalysis of studies in 1482 critically ill patients found no excess mortality and a significant reduction in infections, duration of mechanical ventilation, and hospital stay (47). The most recent meta-analysis included 22 randomized studies with 2419 patients, with a variety of conditions (postsurgical status, critical illness, burn injury, and trauma). The study included subgroup analysis and found that immune-modulating nutrition was associated with a significantly lower infection rate in surgical patients but not in the critically ill, who were found to have a trend toward higher mortality (48). These analyses suggest a possible benefical effect in surgical patients with a decrease in infectious complications and hospital stay. No such benefits were evident in critically ill patients, in whom a trend toward increased mortality was noted. A comprehensive review of immunonutrition has been published (49).

Formulas for Diabetes. Diet is important in the strategy for metabolic control and reduction of complications in patients with diabetes (see Chapter 65). Enteral formulas have been designed to normalize blood glucose and lipid concentrations by decreasing carbohydrates, increasing fat (particularly monounsaturated fat), and adding fiber. Numerous products are available. The one used in most studies was Glucerna. It contains a reduced amount of carbohydrates (~35% of total calories) in the form of maltodextrins, fructose, and soy polysaccharides designed to prevent rapid glucose absorption and rise in the blood glucose concentration. Lipids provide about 50% of the calories, with monounsaturated fatty acids accounting for 70% of these calories. In 1500 kcal, the formula provides the daily requirements of minerals, vitamins, and trace elements and about 20 g of fiber. When compared with other enteral formulas, Glucerna was shown to result in a significantly attenuated rise in the blood glucose concentration in patients with type 1 (50) and type 2 (51) diabetes, as well as in those with stress-induced hyperglycemia (52). A reduction in serum lipids was also noted (53). Although the impact of feeding the disease-specific formula on long-term clinical complications has not been evaluated, the better metabolic control suggests that such an advantage may well be expected. A review of studies of diabetic formulas supported the concept of their advantages (54).

Modular Formulas

Modular formulas provide each of the macronutrients or micronutrients singly and can be used to prepare specialized formulas or to augment regular enteral or oral feeding. Protein modular products are powders that have to be mixed with water before their administration. Carbohydrates are available in the form of glucose polymers and fat as triglycerides of long-chain polyunsaturated or medium-chain fatty acids. These nutrients can be added when extra calories or proteins are required. They are particularly useful when the patient cannot receive the required amount of a macronutrient by increasing the amount of the enteral formula because of limited tolerance to other components in the formulas. The use of these nutrients to modify commercial products or to prepare a special formula is limited by the difficulty they present in their administration. Fat requires an emulsifier to keep it dispersed with other enteral products. Glucose polymers added to enteral formulas can increase the osmolality and can induce diarrhea. Protein powder is difficult to mix and tends to clump, thereby creating mechanical difficulties when it is mixed with other formulas.

When requirements increase for certain micronutrients, those available for oral intake and parenteral use can also be used for enteral feeding; thus, in patients needing additional potassium, an oral potassium solution can be added to regular enteral feedings to increase potassium intake. Caution must be exercised, however, when adding nutrients to enteral formulas to prevent precipitation, which can decrease absorption. Thus, phosphate added to enteral feedings may cause precipitation of calcium, which can clog small-diameter tubes and may not be absorbed in the intestines. Such problems can be avoided by administering additives separately from the feeding formula, unless advance testing has been adequate.

Hydration Solutions

Hydration solutions have been designed mostly to provide fluid and minerals to children and adults with acute diarrhea to prevent dehydration. The solutions contain sodium and glucose. Osmolarity varies between 224 and 311 mmol/L (55). Glucose facilitates sodium absorption in the small bowel. Hydration solutions have been used successfully in developing countries during epidemics of infectious diarrhea to treat or to prevent dehydration (55). These solutions can be taken orally or administered through tubes to patients with excessive fluid and mineral requirements.

NUTRIENT ABSORPTION AND UTILIZATION

Protein

Protein is digested in the proximal intestinal tract and is absorbed in the form of dipeptides, tripeptides, or as single amino acids (see Chapter 70). In enteral formulas with intact protein, the process of protein digestion and absorption is not different from that of regular foods. In some formulas, protein is provided in the form of small peptides or amino acids. Based on physiologic considerations, these may be particularly useful when digestion is impaired or inadequate.

In subjects with physiologically normal GI tracts, studies designed to determine whether low-molecular-weight hydrolysates (dipeptides to pentapeptides) were better absorbed than intact proteins or free amino acids yielded conflicting results; some showed better absorption (56, 57), and others showed no difference (58).

In undernourished patients with no malabsorption who were fed by a jejunal tube, nitrogen absorption was as effective from a formula with intact protein (Isocal) as from an isocaloric isonitrogenous formula containing protein hydrolysates (Criticare HN) (59). Jones and colleagues showed that only small absorptive differences existed between a formula containing free amino acids and an intact protein diet infused by tube over 24 hours in a randomized study in 70 malnourished patients (60). With similar nitrogen and caloric intakes, nutritional parameters were about the same, but the intact protein formula was associated with a better nitrogen balance.

The same issues were addressed in patients with compromised digestive and absorptive capacity. A crossover study in seven patients with the short bowel syndrome examined the absorption from a defined-formula diet with whole protein, one with protein hydrolysates, and three solid diets (61). The diets varied in fat, fiber, and carbohydrates. The investigators concluded that a liquid diet containing peptides, oligosaccharides, and MCTs is not more beneficial than a polymeric diet in patients with short bowel syndrome. A randomized study in patients who received enteral feeding following GI operations found no significant difference in tolerance of polymeric formulas compared with that of elemental formulas (62).

Enteral formulas differ not only in their sources and amounts of amino acids, but also in their content of carbohydrates, fats, and other nutrients. This point should be considered in the evaluation of results of comparative studies because these variables are essentially uncontrolled in most studies. Furthermore, in most of the comparative studies, the amino acid composition of the free amino acid formulas was different from that of the protein hydrolysate or intact protein formulas. Thus, no clear, consistent clinical data support the use of formulas in which the protein is in the form of hydrolysates or free amino acids.

The comparative value of enteral and parenteral fed amino acid mixtures regarding protein accretion was investigated in healthy dogs using a multilabeled leucine tracer. The authors concluded that enteral feeding was superior to total parenteral nutrition (63).

Glutamine

Glutamine is a nonessential amino acid (see Chapter 35). It is the most abundant free amino acid in the body. It is synthesized mostly in muscle and is used as the primary fuel in the small intestines. Glutamine has become increasingly recognized as important for maintenance of healthy intestinal mucosa and for protection from injury induced by chemotherapy, radiation, or other factors (64). In addition, glutamine is important in maintenance of acid-based equilibrium through the generation of ammonia. Glutamine is unstable in aqueous solutions and spontaneously breaks down to ammonia and pyroglutamic acid; thus, inclusion of glutamine in nutritional formulas poses a manufacturing problem.

In catabolic states, release of glutamine from muscle and its utilization by the GI mucosa increase (65, 66). This process may result in loss of muscle tissue. When catabolism is prolonged, glutamine synthesis and release from muscle decrease and may be inadequate to meet the requirements, especially of the GI mucosa. Thus, glutamine consequently has been proposed as an essential nutrient in catabolic patients (67). In some studies, glutamine was shown to improve the morphology, immune response, and barrier function of the GI mucosa, particularly in the absence of oral intake (68). Animal studies suggested that these effects result in less bacterial translocation and sepsis. However, such an impact appears to be less significant in humans (see Chapter 35).

Proteins in enteral formulas contain glutamine. Determination of the glutamine content is difficult because it requires hydrolysis of the protein with heat and acid, a process that also results in conversion of glutamine to glutamate. Formulas with intact protein contain glutamine in quantities less than 14% of the total amino acids. However, formulas are available with added free glutamine (Vivonex, Alitraq). For reviews of clinical studies with glutamine, see Chapter 35.

Carbohydrates

Starches in enteral formulas are present in various polymer lengths. The osmolality of a formula is influenced to a major extent by the sources and amounts of glucose, sucrose, and the shorter-chain glucose units and, to a lesser extent, by free amino acids and electrolyte concentrations.

In the patient with normal GI function, starch hydrolysis is rapid. Most of the glucose is absorbed in the proximal small bowel. In patients with severe pancreatic insufficiency, oligosaccharides may be useful because they can be hydrolyzed in the intestinal brush border enzymes and do not require pancreatic enzymes.

Rapid infusion into the stomach or jejunum of large volumes of high-osmolality formulas should be avoided in patients with esophagectomy, gastrectomy, intestinal dysfunction, and vagatomy because these formulas can induce rapid transit, abdominal discomfort, and diarrhea.

Hyperosmolar nonketotic coma can occur with high-carbohydrate feedings; coma is most likely to develop in the diabetic patient who is infected and dehydrated. Excess carbohydrate calories in enteral feeding can result in hypercarbia in patients with respiratory insufficiency.

Fat

The fat content of enteral formulas varies from less than 2 to 45% of the total calories. Lipids, mostly in the form of corn oil or soy oil, contain large amounts of polyunsaturated fatty acids; some contain lecithin (as an emulsifier), and others have MCTs in small or large proportions. The rationale for adding MCTs is based on the concept that they are easily hydrolyzed and absorbed via portal blood rather than the lymphatics (69). MCTs are ketogenic, and they should be avoided in patients with diabetes, ketosis, or acidosis (69). The relatively large amounts of polyunsaturated fat in most formulas provide more than an adequate amount of essential fatty acids, the need for which is approximately 3 to 4.5% of the total calories (see Chapter 5). Some enteral formulas contain part of the fat in the form of fish oil, which has a high content of ω-3 fatty acids.

The efficiency of fat absorption depends on the rate of infusion, the concentration of the nutrient, and the digestive and absorptive capacities of the GI tract (see Chapter 70). Patients with exocrine pancreatic insufficiency with no measurable pancreatic lipase activity may absorb more than 50% of dietary fat through digestion by lingual and gastric lipases (70). Nevertheless, administration of pancreatic extracts is useful in patients with pancreatic insufficiency.

Patients with the short bowel syndrome have been reported to absorb 54% of the fat from a diet containing 46% of the calories as fat (71). Dietary fat did not have an adverse effect on absorption of magnesium, calcium, and zinc. This finding dispels the notion that patients with the short bowel syndrome must be on a low-fat diet and has an important implication regarding the use of enteral feeding in such patients. A high-fat enteral feeding formula administered through a continuous drip can provide a large amount of calories and thus can ensure absorption of adequate calories in spite of malabsorption. A study compared the effectiveness of five different levels of fat (10–50% of nonprotein calories) in enteral feedings given to guinea pigs with 30% total-body-surface full-thickness burn injury (72). Fat content between 5 and 15% of nonprotein calories was deemed most optimal. These findings may have significant implications for enteral feeding in patients with burn injury.

Vitamins and Trace Elements

Most enteral formulas are designed to provide the required daily amounts of vitamins and trace elements with an intake of 1500 to 2000 kcal. Patients maintained on enteral feeding for periods exceeding 6 months were shown to have normal or high blood levels of various vitamins (31). The stability of vitamins in commercial enteral feeding formulas has been determined only to a limited extent. Specific data regarding absorption of vitamins from enteral formulas are lacking. However, the adequate or high levels of vitamins in the blood of patients who received long-term enteral feeding (31) suggest that both stability and absorption are adequate.

Most enteral formulas contain sufficient amounts of trace elements, including iron, zinc, copper, and iodine, so intake of 1500 to 2000 kcal/day provides adequate maintenance amounts of these nutrients. Zinc and other micronutrient deficiencies, however, can occur when the caloric intake from enteral feeding is low or when GI losses of zinc persistently exceed intake, as can happen in patients with active Crohn disease or malabsorption (73). In such conditions, supplementation with specific trace elements may be required.

Fiber

Fiber is an important component of the diet and has beneficial metabolic and physiologic effects (see Chapter 4). The amounts recommended by Pilch of dietary fiber for healthy persons in the United States are 10 to 13 g/1000 kcal (74). The adequate intake of the new dietary reference intakes for fiber are based on a slightly higher level of 14 g/1000 kcal (see Chapter 4 and Appendix Table A-2-d-3). The fiber content of various enteral formulas has been published (75). Polymeric formulas are manufactured with fiber from different sources including soy and oat, among others. Soy polysaccharide is a tasteless and odorless material that physically can be added easily to enteral formulas. Only about 6% of soy polysaccharide is water soluble. It improves lipid metabolism and control of diabetes. The amounts of soy polysaccharide in enteral formulas vary between 2.5 and 5.9 g/250 mL (75). Pectin and gum are poor fibers for enteral formulas because of high viscosity. However, partially hydrolyzed guar gum is water soluble, has low viscosity, and can be easily added to enteral formulas (76). Some enteral feedings contain a combination of fibers: oat, pectin, gum arabic, and hydrolyzed gums, providing both soluble and insoluble fibers. Fiber derived from oats may have a cholesterol-lowering effect, whereas most insoluble fibers, such as cellulose and hemicellulose, act mostly as laxatives and stool bulking agents. If a formula without fiber is used, fiber can be administered separately in other forms, such as natural bran or Metamucil. In spite of physiologic considerations pointing to GI function and metabolic benefits of dietary fiber, results of studies on its role in enteral feeding have been inconsistent, although most studies have been poorly designed.

In a study of healthy young male subjects, the effects of adding 0, 30, or 60 g/day of soy fiber to a formula (Ensure) were compared. The results showed that fiber increased fecal weight and frequency of bowel movements. All dosages of fiber resulted in decreased transit time in the GI tract (77).

The effects on bowel function of a fiber-containing enteral formula (Enrich, 12.8 g fiber/1000 kcal) were compared in a crossover randomized study with the effects of a formula without fiber (Ensure) (78). Feeding the no-fiber formula was associated with increased laxative use and resultant diarrhea.

The addition of soluble fiber to enteral feeding was found to decrease diarrhea in elderly patients (79) and in severly ill, mechanically ventilated septic patients (80). However, no such effect was noted in surgical patients (81). Fiber in enteral formulas was reported in a randomized study to reduce the rate of postoperative infections following major abdominal surgery (82). Fiber in enteral feedings also improved healing of experimental colonic anastomosis in rats (83).

The effects of fiber in enteral formulas on absorption of minerals and vitamins have been examined. The addition of 120 g/day of soy polysaccharides to an elemental formula reduced the absorption of magnesium, zinc, and phosphorus, but it did not affect potassium and calcium absorption. The balance for all five minerals was positive (84). In another study, the effect of adding 20, 30, and 40 g of soy polysaccharides was studied. Forty grams of fiber caused a negative balance for copper and iron, whereas zinc, calcium, and magnesium were in a positive balance (85). The inclusion of soy polysaccharide in enteral formulas does not appear to result in significant malabsorption and deficiency of minerals and trace elements in the short term. The effects in patients maintained on long-term enteral feeding as the primary or sole diet are unclear, however. Appropriate monitoring of these nutrients is prudent. The addition of fiber to enteral feeding in diabetic patients may improve glycemic control. Specialized formulas low in carbohydrates and high in monounsaturated fat with added fiber have been specifically formulated for diabetic patients (52).

INDICATIONS AND CONTRAINDICATIONS

Enteral feeding is indicated in patients who cannot ingest adequate amounts of food but who have adequate GI function to allow digestion and absorption of enteral formulas delivered into the GI tract through tubes. The choice of appropriate feeding formulas and the method of administration, based on sound pathophysiologic considerations of the GI tract, are essential to maximize the digestion and absorption of enteral feeding in the compromised GI tract.

Specific Indications

Specific indications for enteral feeding are as follows:

1. Severe dysphagia from obstruction or dysfunction of the oropharynx or esophagus.
2. Coma or delirious state.
3. Persistent anorexia.

4. Nausea or vomiting. Patients who suffer from nausea and vomiting arising from a gastric disorder (gastroparesis, gastritis, gastric outlet obstruction) can be safely fed into the jejunum. If these symptoms are the result of intestinal obstruction, however, enteral feeding is contraindicated.

5. Fistulas of the distal small bowel or colon.

6. Severe malabsorption secondary to decreased absorption capacity of the GI tract, such as a short bowel or inflammatory disease. In these conditions, a pump-controlled slow drip of enteral formula can maximize utilization of the limited absorption capacity, which may be overwhelmed by the large volume of food and fluids delivered to the intestines from oral or bolus feeding.

7. Recurrent aspiration. In this condition, formulas should be delivered through a jejunostomy (25).

8. Diseases or disorders that require administration of specific formulas that cannot be taken orally for prolonged periods (see Chapters 58 and 59).

9. Increased nutritional requirements that cannot be met by oral intake. This indication applies mostly to patients with burn injury, who have high nutritional requirements.

10. Growth induction in children with Crohn disease and other diseases (see Chapter 76). The indications for enteral feeding in specific clinical conditions are reviewed in the chapters dealing with these conditions.

The use of tube feeding in patients with advanced cognitive disorders including dementia is controversial. Observations and some expert opinion indicate that enteral feeding may provide no benefit to elderly patients with advanced dementia and may be associated with increased risks and discomfort (86, 87). Considering the lack of convincing evidence and the natural inclination of families and health care professionals "not to starve the patient," decisions regarding enteral feeding in patients with dementia should be made on individual basis after careful consideration of the patient's status and documented wishes, and in consultation with the patient's family (see Chapter 101).

Enteral feeding is contraindicated in patients with complete intestinal obstruction, paralytic ileus, severe pseudointestinal obstruction, severe diarrhea, or extreme malabsorption. In patients with a proximal intestinal fistula, enteral feeding can be attempted only if the tip of the feeding tube is distal to the fistula.

METHODS OF INFUSION

Enteral feedings can be administered either by bolus (24) or by continuous drip (25). When possible, the bolus method is preferable because it takes less time, gives the patient more freedom, and is easier to use. It does not require pump control. The feeding bolus can be given by administering up to 750 mL over 5 to 10 minutes with a syringe or a gravity-driven drip from a bag. The outflow of the bolus from the stomach into the duodenum is regulated by the pyloric sphincter. Thus, a bolus containing one third of the daily volume can be well tolerated (24). When the tip of the feeding tube is in the duodenum or the jejunum, the formula must be delivered in a continuous drip (preferably pump controlled) to avoid intestinal distention and dumping. Feeding into the small bowel usually can be tolerated at a rate as high as 150 mL/hour.

The bolus in gastric feeding must be administered with the patient sitting or reclining at 45 degrees to prevent aspiration. When feeding into the stomach, iso-osmolar and hyperosmolar formulas can be used because the pylorus regulates the volume passed into the duodenum. When feeding into the small bowel, iso-osmolar formulas are usually preferable to avoid high osmolarity–induced secretion of free water from the intestinal wall into the lumen that can cause abdominal distention and diarrhea.

COMPLICATIONS

Enteral feeding can be a safe and effective nutritional support method. Its safety depends on (a) the choice of the appropriate formula and infusion method, (b) delivery of the formula into the appropriate part of the GI tract, and (c) the clinical and metabolic evaluation of the patient before and during enteral feeding.

The most severe complication of enteral feeding is aspiration. Numerous factors may predispose a patient to aspiration: location of the tip of the feeding tube in the esophagous or upper stomach, impaired gastric emptying, decreased lower esophageal sphincter pressure, large volume of feeding, patient's position during feeding, and various medications that decrease GI peristalsis. The risk of aspiration can be reduced by appropriate positioning of the feeding tube, elevating the patient's upper body to 45 degrees, and avoiding enteral feeding when contraindicated. The placement of a gastrotomy tube per se does not affect the lower esophageal pressure. However, gastric distention caused by a rapid delivery of intragastric bulous of enteral feeding can induce relaxation of the sphincter (88). The incidence of aspiration depends on how vigorously it is looked for and on the type of patient. In a prospective study, the incidence of aspiration was 2.4 per 1000 enteral feeding days (89). Little morbidity and no mortality resulted from aspiration. However, other studies reported aspiration rates between 17 and 32% in patients receiving gastric feeding (90, 91).

Several methods have been used to detect aspiration of enteral feeding. These include adding blue dyes to the formula and testing for glucose levels in upper respiratory secretions (92). Rigorous studies have not been conducted to assess the validity and safety of these tests. One evaluation of these methods concluded that they should be abandoned because the glucose method is insensitive, whereas the blue dye added to formulas may be severely toxic and can cause mitochondrial dysfunction and death (93). Determination of residual volume in the stomach during enteral feeding is widely used to assess tolerance to feeding and aspiration risk, but this practice has not been assessed adequately. Postpyloric feeding may reduce aspiration risk, as was shown by a randomized study using radioisotopic methods (94).

Bacterial contamination of enteral feeding formulas can occur because the formulas are an ideal growth medium for bacteria. Occasional case reports of sepsis associated with feeding of contaminated enteral feedings have been published.

Nonspecific symptoms of abdominal cramps, distention, and bloating can occur and are usually caused by too rapid an infusion or by an underlying intestinal disorder. Defining diarrhea and determining its causes in patients receiving enteral feeding may be difficult, and the method of reporting may significantly alter the incidence of this complication (95). An important cause of diarrhea during enteral feeding is concomitant administration of medications, particularly antibiotics and magnesium-containing products. In some reports, as many as half of the patients receiving enteral feeding who were also receiving antibiotics developed diarrhea, with antibiotics and magnesium acting synergistically (96). Studies in healthy volunteers demonstrated that significant colonic secretion of water sodium and chloride occurs during enteral feeding (97). This may contribute to diarrhea, especially in patients with compromised intestinal function.

Constipation occurs commonly in patients receiving long-term enteral feedings. This condition may be alleviated by administering formulas with insoluble fiber or giving fiber separately from the feedings.

The frequency and severity of metabolic abnormalities in patients receiving enteral feeding depend mostly on the general medical condition of the patient. Thus, patients with renal failure are at risk of developing increased azotemia, hyperkalemia, hypermagnesemia, and hyperphosphatemia, whereas the diabetic patient is at risk of hyperglycemia. These potential complications are not inherent to enteral feeding and can be avoided by careful monitoring of the patient. Dehydration is a potential complication in patients given formulas with high calorie and nitrogen content. Patients receiving such products must be monitored closely to prevent dehydration and metabolic complications.

Case reports have noted intestinal necrosis associated with jejunal feeding. This complication occurred in critically ill patients with sepsis hypotension and multiple organs failure (98), although it is not clear that the feeding per se was the cause of the complication.

ENTERAL FEEDING IN VARIOUS MEDICAL CONDITIONS

The role of enteral feeding in specific medical conditions is presented in the following chapters: inherited metabolic diseases, Chapters 58 and 59; inflammatory bowel diseases, Chapter 76; pancreatic disorders, Chapter 78; cancer, Chapter 83; and surgery and trauma, Chapter 91.

HOME ENTERAL NUTRITION

Home enteral nutrition (HEN) is increasingly used to provide nutrients and fluids outside the hospital. The main indications are for neurologic and malignant diseases. The National Registry of home total parenteral nutrition and HEN reported the clinical data on 3931 patients (99). The two most common diagnoses of patients receiving HEN were cancer, which accounted for 42%, and swallowing disorders, 30%. The latter group included mostly patients with strokes. The therapy was safe in the home. Complications of HEN that require hospitalization occurred at an annual rate of 0.4 and 0.3% in the patients with cancer and in those with swallowing disorders, respectively. The 1-year survival was 30% for patients with cancer and 55% for those with neurologic disorders. Thirty percent of the patients with cancer and 15% of the neurologic patients were able to resume full oral nutrition. In patients with cancer of the head and neck whose tumors are successfully treated, HEN has been used for periods exceeding 10 years and has provided good nutrition and rehabilitation and good quality of life (100). Regular medical follow-up is essential to ensure appropriate functioning of the feeding tube and optimization of the nutrition regimen.

DRUGS IN ENTERAL FEEDING

The absorption, activity, toxicity, and disposal of medications may be altered by the site in the GI tract into which they are delivered (101). Therefore, each drug administered through a feeding tube must be evaluated for potential changes in absorption and activity. The rate-limiting step to oral drug absorption is dissolution (102). The crushing of tablets and preparation of slurries often used for administration through a tube modify this process and can alter the drug kinetics and activity (103). The crushing of tablets may result in quicker absorption and higher maximal concentration in the blood, with an increase in dose-related toxicity (104). Faster absorption may also result in enhanced clearance and reduced duration of effect. Depending on gastric emptying times, the increased or decreased exposure to gastric acid can also significantly alter the amount of drug available for intestinal absorption. For example, digoxin taken orally is partially degraded by stomach acid. Mixing drugs with enteral formula may result in decline in drug activity (105). Thus, phenytoin was found to bind to enteral formulas, with a resulting decrease in concentrations in the blood when the drug was administered with enteral feeding (106). Therefore, larger doses are required when the drug is administered with a formula.

Postpyloric administration may have a major impact on drug activity (107) by skipping the acid milieu of the stomach and the regulated passage through the pylorus. Drugs are absorbed more quickly when they are un-ionized. Gastric acidity enhances drug un-ionization and absorption. Skipping the stomach, as in jejunal feeding, will thus render the drug less absorbable in the intestinal tract. Drugs such as ketocanazole will be poorly absorbed when delivered directly in the less acid millieu of the intestines.

Little research has been done to document drug activities when drugs are administered with enteral feeding. Nevertheless, guidelines regarding specific drugs have been published, based mostly on physiologic considerations rather than actual clinical observations (108). When administering drugs through tubes, it is advisable to do it separately from the feeding formula and to monitor the patient carefully with regard to the drug effect, toxicity, and plasma levels when feasible.

Acknowledgments

I am grateful to Lianne Latkany, M.S., R.D., and Silvia Herszkopf, M.S., R.D., for helpful comments on the manuscript.

REFERENCES

1. Randall HT. JPEN J Parenter Enteral Nutr 1984;8:113–6.
2. Harkness L. J Am Diet Assoc 2002;102:399–404.
3. Einhorn M. Med Rec 1910;78:98–101.
4. Andresen AFR. Ann Surg 1918;67:565–6.
5. Barron J. Surg Clin North Am 1959;39:1481–91.
6. Winitz M, Seedman, DA, Graff J. Am J Clin Nutr 1970;23:525–45.
7. Finucane TE, Christmas C, Travis K. JAMA 1999;282:1365–70.
8. Metheny N. Nurs Res 1990;39:262–7.
9. Kirby DF, Delegge MH, Fleming CR. Gastroenterology 1995;108:1282–301.
10. Waitzberg DL, Plopper C, Terra RM. World J Surg 2000;24:1468–76.
11. Benya R, Langer S, Mobrahan S. JPEN J Parenter Enteral Nutr 1990;14:108–9.
12. McClave SA, Chang W-K. Gastrointest Endosc 2003;58:739–51.
13. Norton B, Homer-Ward M, Donnelly MT et al. BMJ 1996;312:13–6.
14. Vanek VW. Nutr Clin Pract 2003;18:50–74.
15. Ho SG, Marchinkow LO, Legiehn GM et al. Clin Radiol 2001;56:902–10.
16. Shellito M. Ann Surg 1985;201:763–7.
17. Gallagher MW, Tyson KRT, Ashcraft KW. Surgery 1973;74:536–9.
18. Holder TM, Leape LL, Ashcraft KW. N Engl J Med 1972;286:1345–7.
19. Tomicic JT, Luks Fi, Shalon L et al. Eur J Pediatr Surg 2002;12:107–10.
20. Collins JB, Georgeson KE, Vicente Y. J Pediatr Surg 1995;32:1065–71.
21. Campos AC, Marchesini JB. Curr Opin Clin Nutr Metab Care 1999;2:265–9.
22. Ho CS, Young EY. AJR Am J Roentgenol 1992;158:251–7.
23. Ponsky JL, Gauderer MWL, Stellato TA. Arch Surg 1983;118:913–4.
24. Shike M, Berner YN, Gerdes H. Otolaryngol Head Neck Surg 1989;101:549–54.
25. Shike M, Latkany L, Gerdes H. Gastrointest Endosc 1996;44:536–40.
26. Shike M, Wallach C, Gerdes H. JPEN J Parenter Enteral Nutr 1989;13:648–50.
27. US Food and Drug Administration (FDA). Compliance Program Guidance Manual. Program No. 7321.002. Washington, DC: FDA, 1989–1991.
28. Talbot JM. Guidelines for the Scientific Review of Enteral Food Products for Medicinal Purposes. Bethesda, MD: Life Sciences Research Office, Federation of American Societies for Experimental Biology, 1990.
29. Shils ME, ed. Introduction. In: Proceedings of Conference: Defined-Formula Diets for Medical Purposes. Chicago: American Medical Association, 1977.
30. Young RU, YU Y-M, Borgonha S. Nestle Nutrition Workshop Series. Clinical and Performance Program. Basel: S. Karger, 2000;3:1–23.
31. Berner Y, Morse R, Frank O et al. JPEN J Parenter Enteral Nutr 1989;13:525–8.
32. Johnson TE, Janes SJ, MacDonald A et al. Arch Dis Child 2002;86:411–5.
33. Grimble GK, Silk DBA. Nutr Clin Pract 1990;5:227–30.
34. Fischer JE, Yoshimura N, Aquirre A et al. Am J Surg 1974;127:40–7.
35. Mascarenhas R, Mobrahan S. Nutr Rev 2004;62:33–8.
36. Butterworth RF. J. Hepatol 2000;32:171–80.
37. Klein S, Kinney J, Jeejeebhoy K et al. JPEN J Parenter Enteral Nutr 1997;21:133–56.
38. Feinstein EI, Kopple JD, Silberman H. Kidney Int 1983;26:5319–23.
39. Kopple JD. JPEN J Parenter Enteral Nutr 1996;20:3–12.
40. Kwan R, Mir MA. Am J Med 1987;82:751–8.
41. Weissman C, Askanazi J, Rosenbaum SH et al. Ann Intern Med 1983;98:41–4.
42. Schloerb PR. JPEN J Parenter Enteral Nutr 2000;25:3S–6S.
43. Alexander JW, Saito H, Trocki O et al. Ann Surg 1986;204:1–8.
44. Kulkarni AD, Fanslow WC, Drath DB et al. Arch Surg 1986;121:169–72.
45. Kirk SJ, Barbul A. JPEN J Parenter Enteral Nutr 1990;14:226S–9S.
46. Heys SD, Walker LG, Smith I et al. Ann Surg 1999;229:467–77.
47. Beale RJ, Bryg DJ, Bihari DJ. Crit Care Med 1999;27:2799–2805.
48. Zaloga G, Mizock B, Ochoa J et al. Syllabus of the Annual Meeting of the American Society for Parenteral and Enteral Nutrition (ASPEN). Silver Spring, MD: ASPEN, 2003;229–36.
49. McCowen KC, Bristian BR. Am J Clin Nutr 2003;77:764–70.
50. Peters AL, Davidson MB. JPEN J Parenter Enteral Nutr 1992;16:69–74.
51. Sanz A, Albero R, Playan J. JPEN J Parenter Enteral Nutr 1994;18:31S.
52. Grahm TW, Harrington TR, Isaac RM. Clin Res 1989;37:138A.
53. Abbruzzese B. FASEB J 1993;7:A847.
54. Coulston AM. Clin Nutr 1998;17:46–56.
55. World Health Organization (WHO). WHO Expert Consultation on Oral Hydration: A New Reduced Osmolarity Formulation. WWW.who.int/child/adolescent-health/New-Publication/News/statment.htm. Accessed June, 2003.
56. Grimble GK, Keohane PP, Higgins BE et al. Clin Sci 1986;71:65–9.

57. Silk DBA, Grimble GK. Nutrition 1992;8:1–12.
58. Moriarty KJ, Hegarty JE, Fairclough PD et al. Gut 1985;26: 694–9.
59. Heymsfield SB, Bleier J, Whitmire L et al. Am J Clin Nutr 1984;39:243–50.
60. Jones BJM, Lees R, Andrews J et al. Gut 1983;24:78–84.
61. McIntyre PB, Fitchew M, Lennard-Jones JE. Gastroenterology 1986;91:25–33.
62. Ford EG, Hull SF, Jennings LM et al. J Am Clin Nutr 1992;11: 11–6.
63. Yu YM, Young VR, Tompkins RG et al. JPEN J Parenter Enteral Nutr 1995;19:209–15.
64. Souba WW, Herskowitz K, Salloum RM. JPEN J Parenter Enteral Nutr 1990;14:45S–50S.
65. Souba WW, Smith RJ, Wilmore DW. JPEN J Parenter Enteral Nutr 1985;9:608–17.
66. Stehle P, Zander J, Merters N et al. Lancet 1989;1:231–3.
67. Smith FR. JPEN J Parenter Enteral Nutr 1990;14:40S–4S.
68. Buchman A: Am J Clin Nutr 2001;74:25–32.
69. Bach AC, Babayan VK. Am J Clin Nutr 1982;36:950–62.
70. Abrams CK, Hamosh M, Dutta SK et al. Gastroenterology 1987;92:125–9.
71. Woolf GM, Miller C, Kurian R et al. Dig Dis Sci 1987;32:8–15.
72. Mochizuki H, Trocki O, Dominioni L et al. JPEN J Parenter Enteral Nutr 1984;8:638–46.
73. Sturniolo GC, Molokhia MM, Shields RR et al. Gut 1980;21: 387–91.
74. Pilch SM, ed. Physiological Effects and Healthy Consequences of Dietary Fiber. Washington, DC: US Food and Drug Administration, Federation of American Societies of Experimental Biology, 1987.
75. Fredstrom SB, Baglien KS, Lampe JW et al. JPEN J Parenter Enteral Nutr 1991;15:450–3.
76. Slavin JL, Greenberg NA. Nutrition 2003;19:549–52.
77. Slavin JL, Nelson NL, McNamara EA et al. JPEN J Parenter Enteral Nutr 1985;9:317–21.
78. Shankardass K, Chuchmach S, Chelswick K et al. JPEN J Parenter Enteral Nutr 1990;14:508–12.
79. Nakao M, Ogura Y, Satake S et al. Nutrition 2002;18:35–9.
80. Spapen H, Dilteor M, Van Malderen C et al. Clin Nutr 2001;20:301–5.
81. Khalil L, Ho KH, Png D et al. Singapore Med J 1998;39:156–9.
82. Rayes N, Seehofer D, Muller AR. Z Gastroenterol 2002;40: 867–76.
83. Demetriades H, Botsios D, Kazantzidou D. Eur Surg Res 1999;31:57–63.
84. Heymsfield SB, Roongspisuthipong C, Evert M et al. JPEN J Parenter Enteral Nutr 1988;12:265–73.
85. Taper LJ, Milam RS, McCallister MS et al. Am J Clin Nutr 1988;48:305–11.
86. Finucane TE, Christmas C, Travis K. JAMA 1999;282:1365–70.
87. Gillick MR. N Engl J Med 2000;342:206–10.
88. Coben RM, Weintraub A, DiMarino AJ et al. Gastroenterology 1994;106:13–8.
89. Mullan H, Roubenoff RA, Roubenoff RJ. JPEN J Parenter Enteral Nutr 1992;16:160–4.
90. Strong RM, Condon SC, Salinger MR et al. JPEN J Parenter Enteral Nutr 1992;16:59–63.
91. Montecalvo MA, Steger KA, Farber HW et al. Crit Care Med 1992;20:1377–87.
92. Maloney JP, Ryan TA. JPEN J Parenter Enteral Nutr 2002;26:S34–S42.
93. McClave SA, DeMeo MT, DeLegge MH et al. JPEN J Parenter Enteral Nutr 2002;26:S80–S5.
94. Heyland DK, Drover J, MacDonald S. Crit Care Med 2001;29: 1495–1501.
95. Bliss DZ, Guenter PA, Settle RG. Am J Clin Nutr 1992;55: 753–9.
96. Silk DBA. Clin Nutr 1987;6:61–74.
97. Bowling TE, Raimundo AH, Grimble GK et al. Lancet 1993;342:1266–88.
98. Schunn CD, Daly JM. J Am Coll Surg 1995;180:410–6.
99. Howard L, Ament M, Fleming CR et al. Gastroenterology 1995;109:355–65.
100. Shike M, Schattner M. Unpublished data.
101. Gilbar PJ, Kam FS. Aust J Hosp Pharm 1997;27:214–20.
102. Gibaldi M. In: Prescott LF, Nimmo WS. eds. Drug Absorption: Proceedings of the Edinburgh International Conference. Aukland, NZ: ADIS Press, 1979:1–5.
103. Marshall D, Souther J. Health Syst Pharm 1996;1:12–20.
104. Cleary JD, Evans PC, Hikal AH et al. Am J Health Syst Pharm 1999;56:1529–34.
105. Wright DH, Pietz SL, Konstantinodes FN. JPEN J Parenter Enteral Nutr 2000;24:42–8.
106. Au Yeung SC, Ensom MH. Ann Pharmacother 2000;34:896–905.
107. Beckwith MC, Feddema SS, Barton RG et al. Hosp Pharm 2004;39:225–37.
108. Feinberg M, Rosen G. Consult Pharm 1993;8:975–83.

99 PARENTERAL NUTRITION[1]

REX O. BROWN AND GAYLE MINARD

NOMENCLATURE 1568
INDICATIONS 1568
VENOUS ACCESS: PERIPHERAL AND CENTRAL 1569
DELIVERY SYSTEMS 1570
PARENTERAL COMPONENTS AND REQUIREMENTS . .1571
   General Requirements .1571
   Water 1571
   Carbohydrates 1572
   Lipids 1574
   Amino Acids 1578
   Minerals 1580
   Vitamins 1585
COMPLICATIONS OF ORGAN FUNCTION 1588
   Hepatic Dysfunction .1588
   Gallstones 1589
   Metabolic Bone Disease 1589
COMPATIBILITY OF DRUGS WITH PARENTERAL
   NUTRITION SOLUTIONS 1591
HOME PARENTERAL NUTRITION 1591
   Patient Numbers and Categories 1592
   Patient Outcome 1592
   Quality of Life and Support Needs 1592
   Cost-Effectiveness 1593
SMALL BOWEL TRANSPLANTATION 1593
EFFECTS OF TROPHIC AGENTS 1593

The history of parenteral nutrition (PN) has recently been summarized in great detail by Vinnars and Wilmore (1). One could argue that the first event that eventually led to

[1] **Abbreviations: AIDS,** acquired immunodeficiency syndrome;
AMA, American Medical Association; **apoE,** apolipoprotein E; **ASPEN,** American Society for Parenteral and Enteral Nutrition; **BCAA,** branched-chain amino acid; **Cr^{3+},** chromium; **EFA,** essential fatty acid; **FDA,** Food and Drug Administration; **FFA,** free fatty acid; **GSHPx,** glutathione peroxidase; **HDL,** high-density lipoprotein; **HIV,** human immunodeficiency virus; **HPN,** home parenteral nutrition; **ICV,** ileocecal valve; **JI,** jejunum and ileum; **LBW,** low birth-weight; **LCT,** long-chain triglyceride; **LDL,** low-density lipoprotein; **LPL,** lipoprotein lipase; **LpX,** lipoprotein X; **MCT,** medium-chain triglyceride; **Mn^{2+},** manganese; **PICC,** peripherally inserted central catheters; **PL,** phospholipid; **PN,** parenteral nutrition; **PPN,** peripheral parenteral nutrition; **PVC,** polyvinyl chloride; **REE,** resting energy expenditure; **RES,** reticuloendothelial system; **RQ,** respiratory quotient; **TG,** triglyceride; **TNA,** total nutrient admixture; **TPN,** total parenteral nutrition.

the parenteral route being used medically was the discovery of the blood circulation by Harvey in 1628. That event was followed by efforts to introduce fluid, salt, and food directly into the bloodstream of a dog by Sir Christopher Wren in 1658 (1). Latta actually treated patients with cholera successfully by administering parenteral salt and water in 1831. Other milestones in the development of PN were the realization of the importance of glucose in human metabolism by Bernard in 1859 and the discovery of essential amino acids by Rose (1). Subsequently this led to intravenous administration of glucose by Beidle and Krauts in 1896, intravenous administration of intravenous protein as fibrinogen hydrolysate by Elman in 1937, and the development of the first intravenous fat emulsion (Lipomul) in the United States in 1960 (1). The scientific groundwork resulting in successful PN was laid in the third to fifth decades of the twentieth century with developments in the ability to provide pyrogen-free fluids as a result of Seibert's work and of the recognition of the metabolic and nutritional changes and needs associated with disease (1).

Peripheral PN (PPN) using 5 or 10% glucose, protein hydrolysates, intravenous fat (Lipomul), electrolytes, and multivitamins was used from 1955 to 1965 by various clinicians for limited periods. Serious side effects led to withdrawal of intravenous Lipomul from the United States market in the early 1960s. This created a serious problem requiring that glucose be given either in large, relatively isotonic volumes for peripheral vein infusion or else in hyperosmolar form requiring infusion into a major vein. Although central catheters threaded into veins had been used as early as 1944, they were uncommon. A safe and effective intravenous lipid preparation (Intralipid) had been developed by Wretlind in 1961 (2) and approved for use in most European countries by 1963; it was not approved for use in Canada or in the United States until 1977. Intralipid availability in Europe in the early 1960s led to increased use of PN through peripheral veins.

Widespread interest and increased use of PN occurred after publication of reports by Dudrick and colleagues (3). Using percutaneous central catheters to deliver nutrient solutions with glucose as the source of nonprotein calories, these investigators demonstrated convincingly that PN as the sole source of nutrients resulted in good growth in malnourished infants and positive nitrogen balance and nutritional and clinical improvement in malnourished adults over periods of many weeks.

After the early reports of successful use of central PN, its use expanded rapidly in the clinical practice of nutrition support. Many institutions that used PN frequently developed multidisciplinary nutrition support teams. The American Society for Parenteral and Enteral Nutrition (ASPEN) was formed in 1978, and one of its goals was to promote the safe and efficacious use of specialized nutrition support (PN and enteral nutrition). The first set of clinical guidelines for the use of specialized nutrition support were published by ASPEN in 1993 (4). A revision of these guidelines that provided a markedly increased depth and scope of nutrition support practice was published in 2002 (5). A National Advisory Group of ASPEN published a report on safe practices for PN formulations in 1998 (6). A revision of these guidelines was published in late 2004 (6a). The American Gastroenterological Association issued a medical position statement on PN in 2001 (7).

The major physiologic difference between parenteral and enteral nutrients is the direct entry of parenteral solutions into the systemic circulation, bypassing the alimentary tract and the first circulatory pass through the liver, as happens with enteral nutrients. Other problems related to the parenteral route involve venous access, sterile and stable solutions, technique of administration, and nutritional adequacy.

NOMENCLATURE

Various descriptive terms have been applied to the procedure used in supplying nutrition support. The term hyperalimentation entered the clinical nutritional lexicon in various ways to indicate the need for large amounts of calories and certain other nutrients. Co Tui and colleagues used the term in 1944 and 1945 when describing large amounts of casein hydrolysate and carbohydrates given postoperatively by tube to patients who had undergone gastrectomy (8) and orally or by tube to patients with peptic ulcer (9). The term was reintroduced by the University of Pennsylvania group (3) to describe techniques for supplying total nutritional support by the intravenous route. Hyperalimentation became widely used in the context of high caloric formulation, and the term was often shortened to hyperal. Because it was applied also to tube feeding, intravenous hyperalimentation and enteral hyperalimentation appeared in the literature.

Both historically and etymologically, the term hyperalimentation has implied needing and providing amounts of nutrients that exceed normal requirements (particularly for energy and amino acids). It is now clear that used in this way, the term has a potentially misleading connotation because provision of excess energy and certain nutrients is often undesirable. For this reason, the term is no longer used. It was replaced by the designation total parenteral nutrition (TPN) and more recently by the general designation of PN.

INDICATIONS

The primary objective of PN is maintaining or improving the nutritional and metabolic status of patients who, for a critical period of time, cannot be adequately nourished by oral or tube feeding (Table 99.1). The value and use of this treatment method in the management of patients with specific clinical problems are discussed in relevant chapters in this book and in the ASPEN Guidelines for the Use of Parenteral and Enteral Nutrition in Adult and Pediatric Patients (5). Normal nutritional requirements for adults and children are cited, as well as specific recommendations for nutrition support throughout the life cycle and diseases frequently encountered in these two populations. Other publications outline indications for the use of PN in various disease states and clinical conditions (7, 10, 11).

The decision to undertake PN requires weighing various factors and considering the patient's diagnosis and prognosis as discussed in the relevant chapters. It is not a defensible substitute for oral or tube feeding when adequate provision by either of these methods is feasible.

The conditions for PN listed in Table 99.1 are generally accepted indications. However, its use in a variety of other conditions is often controversial because of the paucity of appropriate studies that give statistically valid data supporting or negating the value of PN. Initially it was thought that PN might be primary therapy for many diseases, but it is clearly adjunctive treatment in most cases. For instance, a metaanalysis of PN in critically ill patients demonstrated that PN did not affect mortality in this population, but does decrease complication rates, especially in undernourished patients (12). Some of the data that reflect negatively on PN have more to do with overfeeding than harm actually caused by the PN itself. Jeejeebhoy recently

TABLE 99.1. CLINICAL STATES LIKELY TO BENEFIT FROM PARENTERAL NUTRITION

CLINICAL STATE	EXAMPLES
Motility disorders	Ileus (postoperative or disease related)
	Severe intestinal pseudoobstruction
	Intractable vomiting
	Diffuse peritonitis
Mechanical intestinal obstruction not immediately remediable by surgery	Partial or complete small bowel obstruction
Perioperative state with profound undernutrition in which enteral nutrition is not feasible	Obstructing esophageal or gastrointestinal tumor
Hypermetabolic critically ill patient in whom enteral nutrition is not feasible	Persistent ileus
Very LBW premature infant in whom enteral feeding is inappropriate	Immature gastrointestinal tract, gastrointestinal atresia
Intestinal ischemia/sloughing	Toxic epidermal necrolysis

reviewed the merits of PN in patients who meet the criteria for its use (13).

VENOUS ACCESS: PERIPHERAL AND CENTRAL

The advantage of infusing nutrient solution directly into a peripheral vein (PPN) is that it does not require the insertion and maintenance of a central venous catheter. In an attempt to minimize peripheral vein damage, 10 or 20% isotonic lipid emulsion as the main caloric source is substituted for the hypertonic glucose solutions used in central PN. For example, a typical 3-L preparation composed of 2% amino acids, 3% lipid, and 6% dextrose provides 9.6 g of nitrogen and 1512 nonprotein calories, with an osmolality of 574 mosm/L. This osmolality is much less than a typical central PN solution of 20% dextrose, 5% amino acids, and 2% lipid, which has an osmolality of 1566. PPN requires that the patient has adequate venous access, because even the lower osmolality can be very irritating to the vein. Frequent (48- to 72-hour) catheter changes are recommended to prevent thrombophlebitis. Some institutions use low-dose heparin infusion and/or corticosteroids to try to prevent phlebitis, however, these strategies have no proven efficacy and are not without risk. In addition, the use of PPN necessitates significant fluid administration to provide adequate calories, particularly in the patient with high caloric requirements. PPN may be useful for the patient who needs nutritional support for a short period of time and who has adequate peripheral veins, however, because of these limitations, many clinicians do not routinely prescribe this treatment.

Providing sufficient energy by the central route without providing a large percentage as lipid necessitates infusing hypertonic glucose solutions. Consequently, the catheter tip must be in a vessel with high blood flow causing rapid dilution; this minimizes the occurrence of phlebitis and thrombosis. Numerous routes for such vascular access have been used; the most common are subclavian, jugular, and femoral veins, although reports of the use of azygous vein, facial vein, and other unusual sites have been reported. Central catheters placed via the subclavian vein are reported to have a lower bacterial colonization rate when compared with internal jugular or femoral vein approaches (14). Arteriovenous fistulas of the internal type have been prepared, usually with a bovine graft, and external fistulas also have been used; some of the early patients discharged home on PN had one such fistula. Other vascular approaches have been adopted when the usual vessels were not patent or were otherwise unavailable.

Peripherally inserted central catheters (PICC lines) are used for intermediate to long-term PN. If these types of catheters are used for PN, the tip of the catheter must be positioned in a central vein such as the superior or inferior vena cava. Kearns and colleagues (15) have reported a significantly higher incidence of thrombosis and infection and decreased catheter survival when the tip of a PICC resided in the axillosubclavian-innominate vein compared with use of the superior vena cava. Cowl and colleagues (16) reported a higher rate of thrombosis and difficulty in placement when PICCs were compared with standard subclavian/internal jugular approaches.

Several reviews on the prevention of catheter complications have been published (17, 18). In an effort to reduce the incidence of infection, tunneled central catheters were introduced in 1973. Not only are they associated with a lower risk of infection, but also they can remain in place and functional for long periods of time. These are usually placed surgically within the subclavian or jugular vein, with the tip in the superior vena cava. The extravascular portion of the catheter is tunneled before being brought out through the skin. The catheter is often anchored at the skin exit with a Dacron cuff, which eliminates the need for sutures in the skin and also acts as a barrier to bacteria. In another method, chambers of silicone or other elastomers, termed ports, are implanted subcutaneously. The chamber is connected by a catheter, usually placed into the subclavian vein with its tip in the superior vena cava (19). Nutrient solution is infused into the chamber via special needles inserted through the skin.

Insertion and use of an indwelling central venous catheter pose various risks to the patient, including pneumothorax, hemothorax, thrombosis, infection, vascular or nerve injury, hypersensitivity reactions, and microbial contamination. Reported complication rates range from 0.3 to 12%, and vary according to definition of complications, physician expertise, preparation used, frequency of manipulation of the catheter, and other factors (20). Thrombogenicity varies with the catheter material; the earlier and stiffer polyvinyl and polyethylene catheters were associated with more thrombus formation than silicone or polyurethane catheters. Multilumen catheters have increased in use, and they provide additional access for infusing medications and blood and for blood sampling without interfering with PN administration. There are conflicting reports about the frequency of catheter-related sepsis (21, 22). Placement site is related to infection rates; e.g., femoral and jugular sites tend to have higher rates than the subclavian site (22). Similarly, catheter tunneling (e.g., jugular) reduces the incidence of line sepsis (23) and also reduces other problems such as dislodgment.

The use of antibiotic-coated catheters has been associated with a decrease in line colonization and infection. The first coated catheters on the market were coated externally with chlorhexidine and silver sulfadiazine. Maki and colleagues demonstrated a statistically significant reduction in colonization and bloodstream infection from 24.1 and 4.6% down to 13.5 and 1%, respectively, when compared with noncoated catheters (24). Raad and colleagues performed a similar study using catheters bonded internally and externally with minocycline and rifampin (25). They showed a reduction in colonization and bloodstream infection from 26 and 8% down to 5 and 0%, respectively.

Darouiche and colleagues subsequently compared both catheters and showed that catheters impregnated with minocycline and rifampin were associated with a 7.9% colonization and 0.3% infection rate compared with 22.8 and 3.4% for catheters impregnated with chlorhexidine and silver sulfadiazine (26). These catheters are more expensive, but are probably worthwhile if long-term use is anticipated. It remains to be seen whether use of these catheters will lead to increased antibiotic resistance. Currently, the use of antimicrobial-impregnated and heparin-bonded central catheters appears to be justified (17, 27, 28).

All types of complications, not just infectious, have also been shown to be less frequent when experienced personnel (preferably members of a nutrition support team) exercise necessary precautions, including using an aseptic technique in catheter insertion and maintenance, checking proper placement by radiographic study before use, and adequately caring for the insertion site. In 2002 the US Centers for Disease Control and Prevention published comprehensive guidelines for the prevention of intravascular catheter-related infection (29).

The use of ultrasound may facilitate central line placement. It reduces the number of failed insertion attempts, particularly in the hands of inexperienced personnel, but it does not seem to significantly decrease insertion time.

In general, a diagnosis of line sepsis should be seriously considered when the patient has spiking fever, elevated white blood cell count, and/or shaking chills. With onset of fever, sources of infection should be sought, and blood cultures should be drawn from both the catheter and a peripheral vein. Appropriate antibiotic treatment should be instituted as indicated.

When microbial colonization is suspected in a percutaneously placed catheter (positive blood cultures without another source), the catheter should be changed over a wire using the Seldinger technique (30, 31). The tip and/or subcutaneous portion of the removed catheter should be cultured. Most catheters removed on suspicion of sepsis are found to be sterile. Alternatively, an endoluminal brush can be inserted in the catheter to remove biofilm for culture. If an endoluminal brush is used to sample the catheter, the acridine orange leukocyte cytospin test may be useful for detecting infected catheters in situ (32). If the insertion site of a central venous catheter appears infected, or if the catheter that was exchanged over a wire has more than 15 colony-forming units when cultured, a new line should be inserted at a new site. More permanent central access (tunneled catheters or ports) may sometimes be treated with infusion of antibiotics, but frequently need replacement.

Experience indicates that with good technique in both catheter placement and solution preparation and with proper maintenance, indwelling catheters of the percutaneous or tunneled type may remain safely in place for months and years without infection or disruption (33, 34).

Several comprehensive reports have been published regarding the catheter-related sepsis rate in patients who have long-term catheters for intravenous access. Buchman and colleagues reported on 527 patients receiving home PN (HPN) who were followed up for a median time of 206 days (range, 7 to 6344 days) (35). Eighty-one percent of the adults and 3% of the children were never infected. The number of adults who were infection free in this retrospective review is higher than in most reports addressing this topic. Thirty-six patients were infection free for more than 10 years. The catheter-related sepsis rate was 0.37 per patient-year for all patients and 0.51 per patient-year for children. Patients with catheters for more than 10 years had a catheter-related sepsis rate of 0.28 per patient-year. Risk factors for sepsis are Crohn disease, presence of jejunostomy, smoking, and central vein thrombosis (36).

DELIVERY SYSTEMS

Nutrient solutions for PN are now delivered exclusively from plastic bags via electronic pumps. Central PN solutions are generally delivered using peristaltic pumps of various types. These have become increasingly sophisticated, automated, and expensive. They ensure even flow rates, overcome the increased resistance of filters of small porosity (especially with continued use), minimize the likelihood of clotting at the catheter tip, and reduce the need for frequent nursing surveillance. Most of them have an air-in-line alarm system that prevents the occurrence of air embolism.

The use of pliable plastic bags of various sizes eliminates the danger of breakage, simplifies transportation and storage, and reduces storage space requirements before and after filling compared with use of glass or formed-plastic bottles. The usual water solutions of nutrient formulations do not extract measurable amounts of phthalate plasticizer used in the manufacture of polyvinyl chloride (PVC) bags; however, albumin, lipids, and blood take up the plasticizer (36). The amount of plasticizer eluted from PVC administration sets by lipid emulsions is relatively small compared with that from the bags. Plasticizer-free ethylene vinyl acetate tubing and bags have essentially replaced products using PVC. Another elastomer contains the plasticizer trioctyl trimellitate, which is not extracted by lipid. These are useful with certain lipid formulas. The manufacturers of Intralipid (Fresenius Kabi AB) have recently converted all of their products from glass to plastic bags. These products are available in 50-, 100-, 250-, 500-, and 1000-mL plastic containers. The plastic bags are made of polypropylene and are latex free and void of di-(2-ethylhexyl)-phthalate.

Dual-chambered plastic bags that allow admixture of macronutrients immediately before infusion of PN are available. These are very convenient for HPN, especially for patients who receive intravenous lipids on a regular basis. Dual-chambered bags are manufactured either empty or with the macronutrients in them (i.e., dextrose in one chamber and amino acids in the other chamber). When lipid is used, the dextrose, amino acids, and electrolytes are added to the bottom chamber of the empty bag and the desired intravenous lipid dose to the upper chamber. Before administration, the plastic divider is removed and the admixture with lipid is prepared. This increases stability because the total nutrient admixture (TNA) is not prepared until just before infusion.

Filters continue to be recommended during administration of PN formulations (37). The importance of this practice became apparent after two deaths reported from improper admixing of calcium and phosphorus into a TNA (38). In general, filters will remove or reduce the infusion of particulate matter, air, and microorganisms into the patient. Particulates are found in large-volume injectables. Particulates have been found to clog pulmonary capillaries and actually cause pulmonary embolus when they exceed 5 μm (microns). Potentially, they could also deposit in other soft tissues such as the brain, spleen, renal medulla, and lung. For those centers that use PPN, in-line filters have been reported to decrease the incidence of phlebitis (39). The two filters used commonly during administration of PN formulations are 0.22- and 1.2-μm (micron) filters. The 0.22-μm (micron) filter is effective at removing microorganisms, particulates, and air. A 0.22-μm (micron) filter with a nylon membrane that has been positively charged has the ability to remove pyrogen (e.g., gram-negative endotoxin) by electromagnetic forces (6). TNAs should be filtered with 1.2-μm (micron) filters because the lipid particles in a stable emulsion are between 0.1 and 1 μm (micron) in size. Although lipid particles could be forced through a 0.22-μm (micron) filter, it would destabilize the emulsion. The 1.2-μm (micron) filter will remove organisms such as *Candida albicans* because they are large particles in the range of 3 to 6 μm (microns).

Patients who receive HPN will have several bags of PN stored in a home refrigerator to enhance compatibility before administration. These patients should be taught to remove the PN formulation 2 to 3 hours before administration so the product is closer to room temperature during infusion.

Insulin adsorption varies appreciably depending on the binding characteristics of the nutrients present, the type of plastic in the delivery system, the presence of filters, and the concentration of insulin added (40). When insulin is added to PN formulations for diabetic patients, the dosage must be closely monitored until properly adjusted (40, 41). An in vitro study simulating the clinical setting showed that 90% of regular insulin added to admixtures with and without lipid was available after infusion through tubing (42).

Because of adherence and loss of vitamins A and E (particularly the former) when PN formulations are infused slowly to very-low-birth-weight (LBW) infants, a delivery system using minimal tubing and more rapid infusion has been recommended.

PARENTERAL COMPONENTS AND REQUIREMENTS

General Requirements

The weight of a relatively unstressed middle-aged patient with restricted activity, who has no fever or other hypermetabolic condition, should be maintained in an acceptable range by approximately 30 kcal (7.2 kJ)/kg body weight/day. A ratio of grams of nitrogen to kilocalories (N:kcal) of approximately 1:130 to 150 (1:31 to 36 N/kJ) is an appropriate formula for such a patient (43). Malnourished non-hypercatabolic adults can achieve a positive nitrogen balance on a caloric intake of approximately 1.3 times resting energy expenditure (REE) while receiving PN supplying 1.13 g of amino acids/kg (180 mg N/kg)/day (44). When twice this amount of amino acids was given, nitrogen retention was better; such patients appear to behave like growing children in this respect. More calories are required for weight gain, depending on the weight gain desired. Shaw and colleagues developed a graphic presentation of the effects of nitrogen and energy intakes on nitrogen and fat balance in depleted patients (45). The amount of additional protein needed is usually proportionally higher than that of energy; for example, for adult patients acutely stressed by trauma, burns, or infection, the N:kcal ratio is generally increased (1:100) with such patients receiving as much as 30 to 35 total kcal/kg or occasionally more. The goals for infants and children are reviewed in Chapter 51.

All essential and sufficient nonessential amino acids should be provided in amounts needed to sustain adequate protein synthesis and intermediary metabolism. Essential fatty acids (EFAs) should be supplied regularly. Electrolyte, trace element, and vitamin intakes should meet individual requirements. No matter how adequate the formula is in other respects, a deficiency of any essential nutrient may lead to negative nitrogen balance. A single deficiency of potassium, sodium, phosphate, or nitrogen impaired or abolished retention of other elements (46), and zinc depletion also caused negative nitrogen balance.

Water

The fluid component must meet individual requirements as determined by evaluation of the clinical and laboratory data. Consideration of the close interrelationships of water, electrolytes, hormonal factors, and organ function are very important when prescribing a PN formulation. Proper management of fluid and electrolytes is an essential aspect of nutrition support. In addition to clinical factors that could cause excessive retention or loss, consideration must be given to fluid intake with medications and "keep-vein-open" infusions, as well as changes in insensible water loss. Meticulous recording of fluid intake and output is necessary. Assessment of volume status by hemodynamic monitoring may be required in some critically ill patients.

Standard PN admixtures can be administered to the patient with increased fluid needs, especially when extrarenal losses are involved, with a supplemental intravenous solution to meet needs in the acute care setting. In the home setting, the extra fluid requirements can be added to the PN admixture in one plastic bag or can be given separately. For the patient who is fluid overloaded, the PN prescription should be made as concentrated as possible to minimize intake.

Expansion of extracellular fluid is common in hospitalized patients with malnutrition, and this increases body weight and decreases serum albumin concentrations. Starker and colleagues described different patterns of change in body weight and serum albumin concentrations in various clinical situations during the first week of PN (47).

Carbohydrates

Glucose is the commonly used carbohydrate for caloric contribution in PN and is usually the major source of energy. Parenteral glucose is in the form of the monohydrate, with 1 g providing approximately 3.4 kcal. It is readily available in various concentrations in liquid form, is relatively inexpensive, and is rapidly metabolized by most patients. Using primarily glucose to meet large energy needs within a tolerable fluid volume requires an extremely hypertonic solution (Table 99.2).

A solution containing 3% glycerol, amino acids (3%), and electrolytes (Procalamine, B Braun) is available for use in PPN. The glycerol is a good energy source in traumatized patients when it is given with 10% lipid. Compared with glucose, glycerol required only about half the amount of insulin to maintain the glycemia of diabetics in the range of 150 to 200 mg/dL (48).

Glucose Metabolism and Hormonal Changes

Infusion of intravenous glucose into humans results in an increase in insulin secretion, resulting in increased insulin serum concentrations. In stable patients, this adaptive response is often adequate for maintaining normal or near-normal serum concentrations of glucose. Abrupt cessation of PN can result in rebound hypoglycemia in some patients because the secretion of insulin is not blunted

immediately with the withdrawal of the PN infusion. Therefore, clinical practice dictates that intravenous dextrose (usually 5 or 10%) be administered after withdrawal of PN to prevent hypoglycemia. Adaptation to increasing loads of parenteral glucose and other nutrients decreased as the duration of infusion was shortened in test subjects, who were relatively stable adults being prepared for or already receiving HPN (49). Glucose and various hormone concentrations were measured in the course of 24-, 17-, and 12-hour infusions of the same PN formulas and volumes and during the postinfusion period. Tapering the 24- and 17-hour infusions resulted in a decrease in serum glucose concentrations to fasting levels in less than 30 minutes, together with a decline in insulin. No significant changes in glucagon, cortisol, or growth hormone were noted. With the 12-hour infusion, one of the five patients developed marked hyperglycemia, hyperinsulinemia, hyperglucagonemia, and increased growth hormone and cortisol concentrations; the elevated hormone concentrations persisted into and beyond the tapering period (49). Because such patients are not uncommon, tolerance to glucose must be checked before large amounts are infused in cyclic fashion. Other studies in adults found that abrupt termination of PN was rarely associated with significant hypoglycemia or its symptoms (50). The literature on the effects of abrupt termination in young children is contradictory, but symptoms (when they occurred) were mild (51), perhaps because the children remained in bed for a time after termination. Sudden increases or decreases in glucose infusion can be averted by the use of infusion pumps that can gradually increase infusion of the admixture and taper it automatically, without changing the pump settings.

Altered Substrate Metabolism in Hypercatabolic Patients

Glucose metabolism in patients with trauma, injury, burns, and sepsis or advanced cancer that induces weight loss differs markedly from that of physiologically normal persons. The reasonably stable patient can oxidize infused glucose to carbon dioxide (CO_2) efficiently up to approximately 14 mg/kg/minute, whereas the critically ill patient has only about half that capacity: 5 mg/kg/minute in burned patients and 6 to 7 mg/kg/minute in postoperative patients. Infusion above the limiting rate results in conversion of glucose to fat, with an increase in energy expenditure and an increase above 1 in the respiratory quotient (RQ). Conversion of excess glucose to fat is energy dependent; after oxidation of the resultant fat, the derived energy (as adenosine triphosphate sources) is 30% of that theoretically obtained by direct oxidation of the converted glucose. Other potentially detrimental effects of providing glucose in excess exist. Wolfe and colleagues (52) have calculated that at an infusion rate of 9 mg/kg/minute into the stressed patient, 206 g/day of triglyceride were synthesized in the liver. Only a

TABLE 99.2. OSMOLALITIES AND ENERGY VALUES OF INTRAVENOUS DEXTROSE PREPARATIONS

PERCENTAGE (%)	OSMOLALITY (mOsm/kg H$_2$O)	kcal/L
5	278	170
10	523	340
15	896	510
20	1,250	680
25	1,410	850
30	1,569	1,020
70[a]	3,660	2,330

[a] Used in preparation of parenteral nutrition only.

small fraction of newly synthesized fat would have to remain in the liver for fatty liver to develop (52). Other undesirable effects of excess glucose relate to the risk of hyperglycemia and glycosuria, with resultant water sodium and other minerals losses.

Elwyn and colleagues demonstrated that malnourished persons had no increase in REE with increasing glucose intake in amounts below those needed for energy equilibrium; however, with excess glucose, REE increased by 1 kcal for each 5 kcal of intake in association with fat deposition and increase in RQ above 1 (53). In contrast, the injured and/or septic patient given a large amount of glucose with lipid-free PN showed major increases in both resting CO_2 production and O_2 consumption; however, the nonprotein RQ remained below 1 (54). This finding is compatible with other evidence indicating that some fat oxidation persists despite a glucose intake that normally abolishes fat oxidation (52).

Differences in energy expenditure were apparent when surgical patients receiving a high-glucose PN formula were compared with those receiving a relatively isocaloric glucose-fat formulation with 60% of nonnitrogen calories as fat. Although the mean doses of energy were similar between groups, the actual administration of PN was not controlled and both groups were overfed by today's standards (44 and 46 kcal/kg/day). The group receiving all nonprotein calories as glucose demonstrated a 21% increase in REE from baseline, and the mean RQ exceeded 1. The group receiving the mixture of glucose and fat demonstrated only a 7% increase in REE from baseline, and the RQ was less than 1 in all cases (55).

As would be expected from the absence of lipids and their phospholipids (PLs), PN solutions with glucose as the major nonnitrogen energy source have been associated with low serum cholesterol and triglyceride concentrations (see later). A 26% increase occurred in the fractional catabolic rate of low-density lipoprotein (LDL) with an associated reduction of plasma cholesterol levels through changes in both LDL and high-density lipoprotein (HDL) (56).

Control of Serum Glucose Concentrations During Hyperglycemia

Throughout the history of PN, control of hyperglycemia has been an important component of the management of patients receiving this intervention. The administration of PN with a substantial component of dextrose contributes to hyperglycemia; however, it is usually this administration with the combination of an acute disease state (trauma, burns, sepsis), a chronic disease condition (diabetes mellitus), and/or concomitant pharmacotherapy (corticosteroids, protease inhibitors) that often results in moderate to severe hyperglycemia. Critically ill patients are particularly at risk for stress-induced hyperglycemia (57). In fact, sustained endotoxemia in the rat model resulted in the

downregulation of early steps in the insulin-signaling cascade through reduction in insulin receptors (58). Osmotic dehydration from uncontrolled hyperglycemia has long been recognized as a complication of PN. Other risks of uncontrolled hyperglycemia include postoperative nosocomial infections in patients with diabetes mellitus (59), impairment of superoxide production from neutrophils (60), and exacerbation of hypercatabolism in thermal injury (61). After intervention with regular insulin to control hyperglycemia in thermally injured children, the body cell mass and bone mass were better preserved when compared with a similar group without the aggressive regular insulin dosing (62).

A major clinical trial addressing hyperglycemia in critically ill patients was published by Van den Berghe and colleagues (63) in which 1548 patients hospitalized in an intensive care unit were randomized to intensive insulin therapy or standard insulin treatment. All patients were receiving parenteral or enteral nutrition during the study. The intensive insulin therapy group received regular insulin as a continuous infusion to maintain serum glucose concentrations in the normal range of 80 to 110 mg/dL (4.4–6.1 mmol/L). The standard insulin treatment group received regular insulin as a continuous infusion when the serum glucose concentration exceeded 215 mg/dL. The goal in this group was to maintain the serum glucose concentrations between 180 and 200 mg/dL (10–11.1 mmol/L).

The results from this major study demonstrated decreased mortality in the group receiving intensive insulin therapy. Several other improvements in hospital morbidity were realized in the group receiving intensive insulin therapy for patients residing in an intensive care unit for more than 5 days: decreased length of intensive care unit stay, decreased time receiving ventilatory support, decreased prevalence of acute renal failure, and decreased bacteremia (63).

It is still unclear whether the benefit realized by patients receiving aggressive insulin therapy results from the control of hyperglycemia or the administration of the anabolic agent insulin itself. Both Finney and colleagues (64) and Van den Berghe and colleagues (65) have subsequently published data that suggest that the improvements in mortality and clinical outcome result from the control of hyperglycemia and not necessarily the administration of insulin. Lazar and colleagues (66) showed that diabetic patients undergoing coronary artery bypass graft surgery had better clinical outcomes when their postoperative serum glucose concentrations were controlled with glucose, insulin, and potassium therapy. Jeschke and colleagues (67) demonstrated that the administration of regular insulin to a group of thermally injured children resulted in a downregulation of proinflammatory cytokines and an upregulation of the antiinflammatory cascade when compared with a similar group who did not receive regular insulin but did have a similar state of glycemia. It is likely that both control of hyperglycemia and administration of insulin have beneficial effects in the intensive care unit patient.

Some practitioners are advocating the use of hypocaloric PN for all patients who require this method of nutrition support when hospitalized in the intensive care unit (68, 69). This has also been termed permissive underfeeding and would theoretically avoid some of the problems of hyperglycemia by using a lower-calorie dose. Prospective, randomized clinical trials are needed in this area of nutrition support.

Ventilatory Response to Glucose

When malnourished persons were given glucose infusion in amounts exceeding the REE, with resultant lipogenesis, minute ventilation at rest increased by about 32%; it increased appreciably more in hypermetabolic patients who had an elevated resting ventilation before PN (70). In patients with decreased sensitivity to CO_2 with compromised lung function or with hyperventilation, the added ventilatory stimulus of high-glucose PN may aggravate preexisting pulmonary dysfunction.

Lipids

Composition

Lipid emulsions consist of tiny droplets (≤ 0.5 µm [micron]) with triglyceride as the core and cholesterol derived from egg yolk phosphatides surrounded by a solubilizing and stabilizing surface layer of the emulsifying PLs. A few intravenous lipid preparations are available as 10, 20, and 30% concentrations that serve as a source of calories and EFAs (Table 99.3).

The cholesterol content per liter of Intralipid is appreciably higher than that of Liposyn II and III, presumably because of the phosphatide used. Per kilocalorie, the 20% emulsion has only half and the 30% only one third as much cholesterol as the 10% preparation. The increase in serum cholesterol concentration after a single infusion of lipid emulsion is transient and usually reverts to near preinfusion concentrations within 4 to 6 hours. As noted later, however, more frequent use of lipid infusions is associated with elevated plasma PL and free cholesterol levels. Long-term PN often results in low serum concentrations of cholesterol; in fact, PN was once investigated for its cholesterol-lowering effects in hyperlipidemic patients.

Addition of glycerin (glycerol) makes the emulsion isotonic. It is also a carbohydrate source. The isotonicity and tolerance of the endothelium of small vessels for the intravenous lipid preparation permit peripheral vein infusion of a large number of calories. In the United States, the 30% intravenous lipid emulsion can only be used as part of a TNA; in Europe, it can be directly infused into patients (71).

As noted in Table 99.3, Intralipid and Liposyn III contain more linolenic acid (C18:3,n-3) than Liposyn II because of soybean oil, whereas Liposyn II has more linoleic acid (C18:2,n-6) because of incorporation of safflower oil. The nutritional role of these EFAs and their metabolism and requirements are discussed in Chapter 5 and elsewhere in this book. EFA deficiency can be prevented in adults receiving PN by providing a minimum of 4% of total calories as linoleic acid via intravenous fat emulsion (72). Requirements for infants and children are noted later in this discussion and reviewed in Chapter 51. Newer lipid formulations under clinical study are reviewed later.

Metabolism

After infusion of intravenous fat emulsions into humans, lipoprotein lipase acts on the triglyceride portion of this product, converting it into free fatty acids (FFAs). The FFAs can enter the mitochondria via carnitine to be oxidized directly for energy, stored in adipose tissue, or transported to the liver via albumin to be synthesized into complex lipids. Although the particle sizes of lipid emulsions

TABLE 99.3. COMPARISON OF PARENTERAL LIPID EMULSION PRODUCTS

	INTRALIPID[a]	INTRALIPID	INTRALIPID	LIPOSYN III[a]	LIPOSYN III	LIPOSYN II[b]	LIPOSYN II
Total fat (%)	10	20	30	10	20	10	20
kcal/mL	1.1	2	3	1.1	2	1.1	2
Glycerin (%)	2.25	2.25	1.7	2.5	2.5	2.5	2.5
Egg phospholipid (%)	1.2	1.2	1.2	1.2	1.2	1.2	1.2
Linoleic acid (%)	50	50	50	54.5	54.5	65.8	65.8
Linolenic acid (%)	9	9	9	8.3	8.3	4.2	4.2
Oleic acid (%)	26	26	26	22.4	22.4	17.7	17.7
Palmitic acid (%)	10	10	10	10.5	10.5	8.8	8.8
Cholesterol (mg/dL)	250–300	250–300	250–300	19–21	19–21	13–22	13–22
Phosphorus (mg/dL)	150–200	150–200	150–200	267–500	267–500	267–500	267–500
α-Tocopherol (mg/dL)	8–12	16–24	24–36	8–12	16–24		
Osmolality (mOsm/L)	300	300	300	284–292	284–292	260–280	260–280
pH	8	8	8	8.3	8.3	8.3	8.3
Vitamin K (µg[micrograms]/L)	308	608				132	270

[a] Intralipid and Liposyn III are made from soybean oil.
[b] Liposyn II is made from one half soybean oil and one half safflower oil.

are within the range of those of chylomicrons, significant differences exist between the two types of particles (73). In emulsions, PLs are in excess; some serve as surface emulsifiers of the triglycerides (TGs) and the rest is present as liposomes (74). The latter take up from the circulation free cholesterol, various lipoproteins, in particular apolipoprotein E (apoE), and albumin (75) to yield the abnormal lipoprotein X (LpX) (76).

On short-term ultracentrifugation in saline, two thirds of the PLs separate from TGs in 10% Intralipid, whereas only one third separated in the 20% emulsion. The former would contribute four times the amount of liposomal LpX of the 20% emulsion when expressed per gram of TG. The significance of this difference is illustrated by a study in which 1.75 g/kg/day of long-chain TGs was infused into postoperative patients as one of two 10% emulsions with PL:TG ratios of either 0.12 or 0.06. Over an infusion period of 5 days, plasma PL, free cholesterol, and apoE levels increased progressively only when the PL:TG ratio was 0.12. FFAs and TGs remained constant with all formulations (77).

The LpX concentration is appreciably higher in the plasma of patients receiving 10% Intralipid than in those receiving 20% Intralipid, presumably because of the higher PL content per kilocalorie infused in the 10% preparation. The half-life of LpX appears to be 2 to 4 days, with small amounts still present 7 days after termination of the lipid infusion (78). Excess PL induces alterations of plasma lipids even in a few days; use of lipid emulsions with a PL:TG weight ratio of 0.06 is preferable (i.e., 20 or 30%).

Tolerance

When the concentration of lipid increases to the level at which binding sites on lipoprotein lipase (LPL) are saturated, a maximum elimination capacity has been reached. In physiologically normal adults, this maximum rate is about 3.8 g of fat/kg/24 hours, which corresponds to about 35 kcal/kg/24 hours. It increases in starvation (~50%) and even more in trauma (79).

Daily infusion of fat emulsion over 1 week or more is associated with increased tolerance, as indicated by decreased preinfusion serum TGs. Serum FFAs are cleared more rapidly with simultaneously administered carbohydrate. The clearance rate from plasma is not equivalent to the oxidative rate of lipid.

Llop and colleagues (80) studied intravenous lipid tolerance in 260 patients requiring PN in a multicenter clinical trial. All patients had preinfusion serum TG of less than 265 mg/dL (<3 mmol). The patients were given Intralipid at a dose of 0.83 ± 0.37 g/kg/day (mean ± SD) and were studied for 7 days or until PN was discontinued (if <7 days). Of the 260 patients, 68 (26.2%) developed hypertriglyceridemia [greater than 265 mg/dL (>3 mmol)] during the infusion of intravenous lipid. Using odds ratios, the following clinical factors were found to be major associations with the development of hypertriglyceridemia: serum glucose concentration greater than 200 mg/dL (10 mmol/L), dose of intravenous lipid greater than 1.5 g/kg/day, corticosteroid (prednisone) administration greater than 0.5 mg/kg/day, or the presence of pancreatitis, renal failure, or sepsis (80). This clinical trial is helpful in identifying patients who are at most risk for developing hypertriglyceridemia during PN with lipid emulsion.

Effect of Lipid Infusion with Parenteral Nutrition

When lipid (supplying one third of the calories) is infused for approximately 8 hours, together with a glucose-based PN formula given over 24 hours, fat oxidation is approximately 6 kcal/kg/minute; it decreases to about 3 kcal/kg/minute after cessation of lipid. A PN formula with glucose and no lipid is associated with a fat oxidation rate of about 2 kcal/kg/minute, decreasing to approximately 0 by the end of 24 hours (81).

Hypermetabolic patients with sepsis and/or trauma in the basal state have increased rates of lipolysis, as indicated by higher glycerol flux and fat oxidation than in physiologically normal persons (e.g., 5.3 versus 2.2 μmol(micromoles)/kg/minute and 2 versus 1 mg/kg/minute, respectively) (82). In patients with sepsis who were given PN with lipid, most of the fat oxidized was from endogenous fat stores rather than from infused cleared lipid (82).

Nonnitrogen Caloric Sources and Nitrogen Retention

Solid evidence exists for the nitrogen-sparing effect of carbohydrate (including glycerol), with and without amino acids. In the absence of amino acids, fat seems not to spare nitrogen beyond its glycerol content released on hydrolysis and its metabolism as a carbohydrate precursor. At low energy intakes, the effects of carbohydrate on nitrogen balance are much greater than those of fat. Increasing amounts of carbohydrate from 0 up to about 100 to 150 g intake (400 to 600 kcal) increase nitrogen balance by approximately 7.5 mg of N per added kcal (1.8 mg N/kJ). This effect is not shared by fat. Above this amount, however, the effect of added carbohydrate on increased nitrogen balance is only about 1.5 mg N per added kilocalorie; this effect is thought to be shared by fat (83). A review of nitrogen balance studies in patients with various inflammatory diseases, however, indicated that fat and carbohydrate were comparable in promoting nitrogen balance (84), presumably after the minimum of 100 g glucose had been met (83).

Total Nutrient Admixture

Use of intravenous lipid emulsions has increased as their cost has decreased and their clinical efficacy has been appreciated. They have been infused by piggybacking the tubing from the separate emulsion container into the tubing from the water-based PN solution. Admixtures of amino acids, dextrose, minerals, vitamins, and a fat emulsion are also used frequently; these are designated TNAs.

Stability and Safety Factor. The admixture system is potentially unstable. The relevant properties of the phosphatide emulsifiers and various factors influencing stability of the fat emulsions in the presence of various additives in the admixture have been reviewed (85). The cumulative effects on aggregation of various cations of different charges can be predicted from an equation defining the critical aggregation number at and above which neutralization of anionic surface groups results in lipid particle aggregation.

Driscoll and colleagues found that iron dextran was the most disruptive component of TNAs (86). They studied the effects of many additives, including amino acids, lipids, dextrose, and monovalent, divalent, and trivalent ions. TNAs were assessed for stability by particle-size analysis, done by light obscuration and dynamic light-scattering methods. Based on these results, using more sophisticated analysis, addition of any dose of iron dextran to a TNA is discouraged.

Microbial Growth. Less microbial growth over 24 hours occurs in TNAs than in intravenous lipid emulsions per se. This finding led the Centers for Disease Control of the United States Public Health Service to recommend a 12-hour maximal infusion time for intravenous lipid emulsions not in TNAs. The major advantages and disadvantages of the TNA system are listed in Table 99.4.

Catheter Occlusion

Various investigators have reported blockage of catheters in patients receiving TNA for periods of 37 to 206 days, with deposition of a soft, creamy material on the internal catheter surface (87). Such material obtained after filtration of a specific TNA formulation stored for 7 days at 4°C in four different commercial EVA bags averaged 99.4% fat and less than 0.5% mineral salts (87). Of concern was finding plasticizer particles (means of 2890 to 16,204 from different bags) with a size range of 1.4 to 43.8 μm (microns) that had been flushed out of the bags with saline before adding the TNA solution. Sterile 70% ethanol has been used successfully by some investigators to unclog catheters that were occluded with fat from a TNA (88). In fact, if urokinase is unsuccessful, ethanol should be used to attempt to clear the catheter, especially in patients who have been receiving TNAs.

Complications of Lipid Infusions

Because the ability to metabolize these emulsions is related directly to infant maturity, the risk of lipid accumulation in blood and its sequelae is greatest in the premature infant, the small-for-age gestational LBW infant, and the nutritionally depleted older child.

TABLE 99.4. ADVANTAGES AND DISADVANTAGES OF THE TOTAL NUTRIENT ADMIXTURE SYSTEM

Advantages	Decreased nursing personnel time and subsequent cost savings because of simplified administration
	Increased compliance in home patients because of ease of administration
	Decreased training time for home patients requiring daily lipid emulsion
	Potential decrease in rate of extrinsic contamination because of fewer manipulations of intravenous delivery system by nursing personnel
	Less likelihood of lipid toxicity by increased dilution and duration of lipid infusion
	Decreased pharmacy preparation time
Disadvantages	Supports growth of a variety of microorganisms significantly better than dextrose/amino acid formulations, but less than emulsions per se
	Undesired effects (i.e., oiling out) when base solution ratios and/or additives exceed the amounts tested under stipulated controlled conditions
	Inability to filter TNA with a 0.22-μm (micron) bacterial-retention filter
	Inability to use total membrane sampling of TNA systems for a pharmacy quality assurance sterility testing program
	Unknown consequences of long-term administration of larger particle size (>4 μm [microns]) in TNA system

TNA, total nutrient admixture.

Possible Altered Pulmonary Function. Lipid accumulation in the hepatic reticuloendothelial system (RES) with the likelihood of depressed immune responses and its competition with bilirubin and other substances for albumin binding have been described. Cases have been reported, primarily in young children, of bleeding dyscrasia in association with high plasma lipid concentrations and platelets engorged with lipid. Reports of altered pulmonary function during acute hyperlipidemia have varied; whereas decreased pulmonary diffusion capacity has been noted by some, other investigators have found no change in lung dynamics, but rather have found decreased arterial oxygenation. Still others have not found oxygen impairment in neonates with hyperlipidemia (79) or in healthy men. Patients with acute respiratory distress syndrome who received 500 mL of 20% intravenous lipid emulsion over 8 hours (maximum rate suggested in package inserts) demonstrated a significant decrease in PaO_2/FiO_2 and mean pulmonary arterial pressure and a significant increase in pulmonary vascular resistance and pulmonary venous admixture (89). Intravenous lipid emulsions should be administered cautiously to patients with acute respiratory distress syndrome, and at lower doses and infused over longer periods of time than those noted earlier by Venus and colleagues (89). While recognizing the toxic potential of lipid infusions in infants, biochemical evidence of EFA deficiency occurred in more than half of premature infants at 7 days of age (90).

Various fat emulsions given intravenously are known to elicit lipid particles and deposition of a ceroid pigment in the RES of the bone marrow, lymph nodes, and spleen, and the Kupffer cells and hepatocytes of the livers of adults, children, and laboratory animals. To date, no deleterious effect of these histologic changes on hepatic function has been noted.

Effects of Immunity. The increased uptake of long-chain lipids by the RES in patients with hepatosplenomegaly and decreased clearance of lipids have led to concern about possible depression of immune responses with such infusions and increased susceptibility to infection. Mice injected with streptococci demonstrated higher mortality rates and incidence of bacteremia and decreased neutrophil chemotaxis when Intralipid was given. In healthy and in burned guinea pigs, intravenous long-chain triglyceride (LCT) infusion at 75% or more of total nonprotein calories resulted in RES overload and an altered pattern of intravenously administered pseudomonas (91).

Using clearance of sulfur colloid technetium-99 as a marker of RES function, 3 days of administration of long-chain intravenous fat emulsion resulted in significant impairment in humans receiving PN at a dose of 0.13 g/kg/hour for 10 hours daily. It took 3 days of lipid administration for this measurement of immunologic impairment to occur (92). A follow-up study demonstrated little change from baseline in the clearance of sulfur colloid technetium-99 when a lipid emulsion containing both LCTs and medium-chain triglycerides (MCTs) was used (93).

Various immune functions were studied in malnourished patients with cancer who were maintained on either a glucose PN formula or one with both glucose and lipid; depressed cell-mediated immunity was noted before starting PN, and no alteration in these parameters was observed with fat infusion (94). In a randomized trial, preoperative PN patients who received 50% of their caloric intake as lipids experienced more major complications and deaths than control subjects receiving lipid-free PN (95). A metaanalysis of randomized studies showed that patients with cancer who were receiving chemotherapy and PN had a fourfold greater risk of significant infection than control subjects who did not receive PN (96). Metaanalysis of the same data by another group revealed that the infection rate for patients receiving PN who did not receive intravenous lipids did not differ from that of the control subjects, and those receiving lipids one to three times per week had a risk of infection 2.3 times that of controls ($p < .02$), whereas those given lipids daily had 6.3 times the risk ($p < .01$) (97). Freeman and colleagues (98) analyzed risk factors associated with bacteremia because of coagulase-negative staphylococci in neonatal intensive care units; this organism was the most common blood culture isolate in this situation. Infants with this type

of bacteremia were 5.8 times as likely as control subjects to have received intravenous lipid emulsion before the onset of bacteremia; because lipid infusions were common, 56.6% of all cases of nosocomial infections were attributed to lipid administration. Although such data are suggestive, whether intravenous lipid is immunosuppressive in humans and whether it leads to increased infection remain unresolved.

Conversely, Lenssen and colleagues (99) studied 512 patients who underwent either autologous or allogeneic bone marrow transplantation. All patients received PN in the postoperative period, so that oral feeding and PN provided 1.5 times basal energy expenditure. Patients were then stratified by several clinical factors and randomized to either a low dose or a standard dose of intravenous lipid. The low dose was 6 to 8% of total parenteral calories from intravenous lipids, and the standard dose was 25 to 30% of total parenteral calories from intravenous lipids. No significant differences in the incidence in bacteremia and fungemia were noted between the two groups of lipid doses. There was still no significant difference between groups when the observation period was extended to 60 days after transplantation. These data strongly suggest that moderate doses of intravenous lipids have no appreciable effect on infection in this immunocompromised patient population.

Newer Intravenous Lipids

MCTs derived from coconut oil, mixed LCTs and MCTs, short-chain fatty acids, and n-3 fatty acids are all under current study as lipid fuels in PN.

Medium-Chain Triglyceride/Long-Chain Triglyceride Mixtures. MCTs may have a role when they are given orally or enterally by tube in the management of malabsorptive disorders (see Chapter 75). Experimental laboratory animal studies have indicated that MCT is cleared and oxidized more rapidly than LCT and is equivalent in providing energy and supporting protein synthesis. MCT (with octanoic acid as the main fatty acid) has been tested experimentally in laboratory animals as physical mixtures of MCT and LCT and as chemically structured TGs. The latter has fatty acids of various chain lengths (short, medium, or long) esterified on the same glycerol backbone; the amounts of the different fatty acids depend on the starting proportions of the types of fatty acids in their preparation.

Mixtures of MCT and LCT (as soybean oil) in equal amounts have been given intravenously to patients (100). Clinical investigations have been conducted in the United States with 75/25 physical mixtures of MCT and LCT (93). Long-term studies were conducted in Belgium in patients with inflammatory bowel disease with 20% LCT or a 20% MCT/LCT mixture (equal amounts), with glucose providing an equal proportion of energy; each emulsion was infused for 3 months, followed by the other in random order (74). Abnormal liver function test results did not develop in any of the patients receiving an MCT/LCT mixture; abnormal liver function test results developed in three of eight patients receiving LCT and regressed to normal when LCT was replaced by an MCT/LCT mixture. Medium-chain fatty acids released in high amounts during MCT/LCT infusion were oxidized in greater proportions than long-chain fatty acids and produced more ketone bodies. LCT infusion led to a significant increase in the LDL:HDL cholesteryl ester ratio, whereas MCT/LCT infusion did not; LCT infusion caused an imbalance in the fatty acid pattern of erythrocyte PLs, which was corrected by MCT/LCT infusion (74). Results similar to the above were reported in a study of HPN patients randomized to a structured lipid of MCT/LCT or LCT (101).

Ultrasonic comparison of liver size and gray-scale value (which relates to liver density and incorporation of fat and connective tissue) was done before and after patients were given PN with either 10% Intralipid or a 10% mixture of MCT and LCT in equal amounts; no changes were noted in either parameter with the MCT/LCT infusion, whereas both increased significantly with LCT (102). Although the rates and amounts of MCT infused in these and other studies appear to be safe, infusion of octanoate as the salt or as MCT in various laboratory species at higher doses can produce lactic acidosis and encephalopathy.

Structured TG (40:60, MCT:LCT by weight) emulsions have been shown to be well tolerated at 1 g/kg/day by postoperative patients in short-term studies (5 to 7 days) when compared with 20% Intralipid (103). One-day repeated crossover studies comparing this structured TG preparation with 20% Intralipid at 1 and 1.5 g/kg/day indicated similar tolerance in postoperative patients, and the former was associated with greater whole-body fat oxidation (104). It has been suggested that such structured TGs may be less toxic and less likely to promote acidosis. One reason given for favoring MCT over LCT has been the belief that unlike long-chain fatty acid transport, carnitine is not required for medium-chain fatty acid transport into the mitochondria. Measurements of the concentrations of the various plasma carnitine fractions in healthy subjects before and during infusion of glucose or amino acids, LCT, and 1:1 MCT-LCT revealed significant differences in the carnitine fractions between the LCT and MCT-LCT infusions; such data support the hypothesis that medium-chain fatty acid metabolism involves carnitine in some manner and suggest the need for more study of these interactions. Intravenous lipid emulsions with olive oil have also been investigated in pediatric patients receiving PN (105).

n-3 Fatty Acids. Important physiologic differences among the prostanoids and leukotrienes, derived from linoleic and linolenic acids, have directed attention to the possible advantages of including n-3 fatty acids and/or dihomo-γ-linolenic acid as TGs or PLs in intravenous fat emulsions to allow conversion to their eicosanoids. Eicosanoid synthesis must be carefully regulated to pro-

vide their various mediators in appropriate quantities in response to appropriate stimuli while avoiding harmful excesses of these potent compounds.

Mashima and colleagues (106) developed and originally tested in rats an intravenous lipid emulsion containing purified fish oil (1.5%) that supplied eicosapentanoic acid, docosahexanoic acid, and soybean oil (8.5%). It was reportedly well tolerated by patients for up to 6 weeks and raised their low eicosapentanoic acid and docosahexanoic acid serum concentrations to normal.

Twenty postoperative trauma patients who received isonitrogenous and isocaloric PN were randomized to either soybean oil 1 g/kg/day or a combination of soybean oil 0.85 g/kg/day and fish oil 0.15 g/kg/day as part of the PN formula (107). After 5 days of PN administration, patients receiving intravenous lipid emulsion with fish oil demonstrated a 2.5-fold increase in eicosapentanoic acid, a 1.5-fold increase in leukotriene B_5, and a 7-fold increase in leukotriene C_5. In the group receiving the soybean oil fat emulsion, eicosapentanoic acid and leukotriene B_5 remained unchanged, whereas leukotriene C_5 doubled (107). Such data demonstrate the potential usefulness of modified lipids in elevating concentrations of desired eicosanoids and leukotrienes.

Furukawa and colleagues (108) demonstrated a decrease in interleukin-6 when eicosapentanoic acid was given with PN that had 20% of total calories added as soybean oil lipid emulsion when compared with this PN formulation without eicosapentanoic acid. In this study, the eicosapentanoic acid was given orally or via feeding tube, not intravenously (108).

Short-Chain Fatty Acids. Supplementation of PN solutions with short-chain fatty acids prevents PN–associated mucosal atrophy and facilitates morphologic adaptation to small bowel resection in rats. Rats with 80% small bowel resection had better ileal glucose absorption and higher expression of glucose transporter 2 messenger RNA, glucose transporter 1, and sodium, potassium/adenosine triphosphatase RNA when receiving a glucose-lipid PN formulation with sodium acetate, propionate, and butyrate than with non–short-chain fatty acids PN (109).

Lipids as Pharmacologic Vehicles. Some drugs are now marketed in intravenous lipid emulsions. One example is propofol, originally marketed for induction of anesthesia, but used more often for sedation in the critical care setting. It is prepared by the manufacturer in 10% fat emulsion, and some patients who needed large doses of propofol receive more than 1000 kcal/day from fat (110). In addition, several lipid formulations of amphotericin B have been marketed in the United States; however, the caloric contribution of lipid formulations of amphotericin B is negligible.

Amino Acids

Intravenous amino acid solutions have evolved from the original hydrolysates of casein or blood fibrin to formulations of crystalline L-amino acids of different compositions and varying concentrations based in part on the amino acid composition of high-quality dietary proteins. Formulations of crystalline L-amino acids have been developed for specific clinical problems, with varying claims for superiority over more general formulas for use in renal and hepatic failure, in trauma, and for growth of infants (111). Commercial formulations differ between and within manufacturers in amino acid composition and concentrations, depending on clinical purpose; in addition, they may have added electrolytes and/or glucose. Concentrated standard amino acids in a 15 and 20% solution are now available for patients who are fluid overloaded and require PN. Many pharmacies that use automated compounders will stock one strength (usually 15 or 20%) of standard amino acids to make all PN formulations using this component.

The eight amino acids essential for physiologically normal adults are present in all formulas, as are histidine and arginine, which are needed for young children. Glycine, alanine, and proline are present in moderately high concentrations in the general adult formulations as sources of nonessential amino nitrogen. The ratio by weight of essential to total amino acids in the pediatric and standard adult solutions varies between 0.41 and 0.54; higher ratios are present in formulas designed for patients with renal or hepatic failure.

Calculating the Energy Contribution of Amino Acids

Should the amino acids in PN be included in the total energy calculations of the formulation? The basic issue is whether the amino acids avoid oxidation by being incorporated in significant amounts of newly synthesized protein, being lost as such in urine or through the gut, or else being diverted into carbohydrate stores. In fact, the amounts of new protein laid down in successfully renourishing a child or an adult are a small proportion of the amino acid equivalent given (e.g., 3 to 4 g protein/day of 60 to 90 g of protein equivalent given to adults). Although the energy cost of protein synthesis from amino acids is high, this is a small factor in terms of daily synthesis, even in growing, malnourished, and hypercatabolic persons. Finally, accumulation of stored glucose (as glycogen) derived from gluconeogenesis from amino acids is limited, and the amino acids are mostly metabolized if hyperglycemia is minimized. It is our opinion that the energy contributed by the amino acids in the PN formulation should be included in the total calculation.

Achieving nitrogen equilibrium or positive nitrogen balance requires sufficient essential amino acids and sufficient nonessential amino nitrogen, adequate nonnitrogen energy, and other nutrients (such as potassium and phosphorus) essential for nitrogen use.

Branched-Chain Amino Acids

Leucine, isoleucine, and valine make up the branched-chain amino acids (BCAAs). These essential amino acids are taken up by muscle for metabolism. Do injured and/or septic patients need more BCAAs than are usually present in general PN formulations? Claims have been contradictory concerning beneficial effects (e.g., improved nitrogen balance with higher BCAA levels than the 19 to 25% in standard US amino acid formulations). There continue to be studies suggesting benefit in mortality in septic patients using these products (112). An expert panel concluded: "In clinical studies, while some positive results in parameters of nitrogen metabolism have been noted using BCAA-enriched solutions in the most severely ill patients, little or no major effect on outcome has yet been demonstrated" (113). Additional negative studies have been published (114). In the hepatic failure patient with hepatic encephalopathy who requires PN, BCAA-enriched amino acid formulations should be considered for those patients who are intolerant to both a dose of protein of 1 g/kg/day and traditional pharmacotherapy such as lactulose (115, 116).

Taurine

Considered a nonessential amino acid for humans, taurine is of nutritional interest with respect to PN because its plasma, platelet, and urine levels are depressed in children and adults maintained on long-term PN. No other substantial evidence for deficiency has been forthcoming. In fact, the low levels in adult and pediatric patients receiving long-term PN did not appear to be correlated with any index of visual function. Because of limited ability of LBW infants to synthesize taurine, the low levels of its precursor cysteine in PN solutions, and the reduced capacity to reabsorb taurine, this amino acid is added to some pediatric formulas.

Arginine

Arginine is a semiessential amino acid during the stress of trauma or major surgery. It has been suggested that supplementation with arginine will enhance immune function in this patient population. Arginine is also a secretagogue of growth hormone. Another potential benefit of arginine supplementation is through enhancement of nitric oxide synthesis, which can provide vasodilation, resulting in improved blood flow and oxygen delivery to tissues. One concern with arginine administration has been its effects on nitric oxide synthesis in patients with ongoing severe sepsis or septic shock. Until more data are available, withholding supplemental arginine in these clinical conditions of hemodynamic instability appears to be prudent, even though some positive data in the animal model exist (117).

Glutamic Acid and Glutamine

The central role of glutamic acid and glutamine in metabolism is reviewed in Chapters 2 and 35. Although glutamic acid was present in the early parenteral protein hydrolysates, it was omitted from the free amino acid formulations because it is synthesized in the body and glutamine synthetase catalyzes its reaction with ammonia to form glutamine. Interest in the clinical importance of glutamine has increased in recent years, partly because of its role as an energy and nitrogen source in rapidly dividing cells (e.g., intestine and stimulated lymphocytes) and partly because under conditions that include hypercatabolic disease states, glutamine concentrations can decrease markedly.

The issues for PN concern proof of stability in solutions, safety, and evidence of the efficacy of glutamine in improving nitrogen balance, muscle protein kinetics, and clinical outcome when added to standard formulas given to hypercatabolic patients. Concern about the stability of glutamine stored with PN components was alleviated; glutamine was stable for 22 days at 40°C when dissolved in sterile water and added to various PN solutions at concentrations of 1 and 1.5% with cold sterilization using two membrane filters (118). Infusing 20 to 57 g (136 to 390 mmol) of glutamine in PN solutions for more than 5 days did not significantly change serum ammonia and glutamate concentrations.

In an increasing number of clinical studies in stressed patients, L-glutamine has been given intravenously in PN solutions as such (119, 120), as the dipeptide L-alanyl-L-glutamine (120–122), or as its α-keto precursors, α-ketoglutarate or ornithine α-ketoglytarate. In these studies, glutamine in its various forms was provided in daily amounts ranging from approximately 0.19 to 0.57 g/kg of body weight (119). Given to postoperative patients in short 3- to 5-day studies, glutamine decreased the negative nitrogen balance noted in the control subjects, increased intramuscular free glutamine concentration (121), and maintained skeletal muscle ribosome concentrations. Morlion and colleagues (123) demonstrated not only improved nitrogen balance and improved lymphocyte recovery, but also a shortened postoperative length of stay in patients receiving glutamine supplementation of PN after major abdominal surgery. After bone marrow transplantation, glutamine significantly decreased the negative nitrogen balance of the subjects during post-transplantation days 7 to 11; over 3 weeks, glutamine infusion increased plasma glutamine without increasing plasma glutamate or changing the ammonia concentration gradient between the groups. Fewer patients given glutamine developed clinical infection and microbial colonization, and their hospital stay was shortened (119). These results have not been reproduced to date. Villus height was maintained and intestinal permeability was lower in patients receiving PN plus glycyl L-glutamine than in patients receiving PN alone (124). As noted earlier, glutamine in a protocol with growth hormone enhanced absorption. Tremel and colleagues (122) have demonstrated that glutamine-supplemented PN prevents intestinal atrophy and permeability when compared with standard PN in critically ill patients. A comprehensive review of glutamine supplementation during PN suggests a decrease in infectious complications and hospital length of stay (125). Critically ill patients may actually benefit with a significantly better mortality when compared with those receiving standard PN (126, 127).

Issues remain to be resolved concerning the reported beneficial effects of glutamine in hypercatabolic patients. How much glutamine is necessary and safe for optimal results? On the basis of their work and that of others, Furst and colleagues suggest that in routine postoperative patients, about 13 g (89 mmol) of glutamine daily meets the intestinal mucosal need for cell replication plus increased need for cell replication plus increased muscle needs, whereas severely injured or stressed patients may need 27 to 40 g (187 to 237 mmol)/day (128).

Short-Chain Peptide Use

Adibi has summarized the advantages of using short-chain peptides in place of free amino acids in PN solutions: (a) increased usable nitrogen sources in more concentrated form (minimizing fluid volume), (b) decreased osmolality with its advantage for PPN, and (c) perhaps most important, the increased solubility as dipeptides of poorly soluble amino acids or the increased stability of unstable free forms (129). How well used are small peptides given intravenously? Adibi summarized his studies in baboons, in which a series of free amino acids and their dipeptides as the relevant nitrogen sources were infused, and his studies of glutamine in peptide form (129). In a 1-week crossover study and in 4-week studies comparing free amino acids and dipeptides, no significant differences were noted with respect to nitrogen balance; plasma and muscle amino acid concentrations; urinary losses; plasma concentration of insulin, glucose, and lipids; and other parameters (130).

Minerals

Sodium, potassium, calcium, magnesium, phosphate, and chloride are essential nutrients. Because a significant proportion of patients receiving or needing PN have malabsorption of the alimentary tract or impaired renal reabsorption or both, often associated with large fluid ionic losses, a continuing concern in the care of such patients is the adequacy of fluid and electrolyte balance (131).

The basic daily needs of patients with reasonably normal cardiovascular, intestinal, renal, hormonal, and hydration status are 50 to 60 mEq (mmol) of sodium, 40 mEq (mmol) of chloride and bicarbonate (including those associated with amino acids as acetate), and 40 to 60 mEq (mmol) of potassium. Excessive losses from the intestine or kidney and abnormal retention require appropriate changes, with suitable monitoring as needed.

Calcium, Phosphorus, and Magnesium

Calcium and phosphorus (as inorganic phosphate) are needed in relatively large amounts by infants; however, when both are present in relatively large concentrations, solubility in the PN solution becomes a problem. It has been recommended that glycerophosphate or glucose phosphate be given together with calcium gluconate or calcium glycerophosphate as more soluble forms of these nutrients. Reference curves have been developed to estimate calcium and phosphate compatibility in commonly used neonatal PN solutions (132). The electrolyte needs of infants and children per kilogram per day are given in Chapter 51. Recommended pediatric concentrations of calcium, phosphorus, and magnesium per liter of PN solution are given by Greene and colleagues (133). Adults require between 10 and 25 mEq of calcium/day via PN.

Negative calcium balance related to hypercalciuria may occur in adults receiving PN, especially during the infusion period of cyclic PN; supplementation with either sodium or potassium acetate (replacing equimolar amounts of NaCl or KCl) resulted in major decreases in urinary calcium in patients receiving 24-hour and cyclic PN, primarily because of increased renal tubular reabsorption with reduced excretion to near-infusion levels (134). Reports are contradictory concerning whether urinary calcium excretion with 12-hour cyclic PN is greater than that with continuous 24-hour infusion (134). Although this may not be a significant issue for the short-term patient, it may be important for those on prolonged PN because chronic negative calcium balance would result in skeletal calcium loss.

Six patients receiving long-term PN (mean of 18.7 years) demonstrated a significantly decreased bone mass when compared with physiologically normal volunteers (135). The patients had higher serum parathyroid hormone concentrations compared with physiologically normal persons, but had an abnormally low response to sodium acetate infusions, which suggested that they had secondary hyperparathyroidism (135).

Hypophosphatemia has multiple causes; however, in PN patients it is often associated with sudden infusion of glucose, the metabolism of which stimulates transfer of phosphate from plasma to cells (see Chapter 10). Hypophosphatemia was treated during provision of PN by using a graduated dosing scheme based on the serum phosphorus concentration in patients with normal renal function (136). For serum phosphorus concentrations below 1.5 mg/dL, 0.64 mmol/kg was given over 8 hours; doses of 0.32 mmol/kg over 4 to 6 hours and 0.16 mmol/kg over 4 hours were given for serum phosphorus concentrations of 1.6 to 2.2 mg/dL and 2.3 to 3.0 mg/dL, respectively (136). Recently, we have noted that the low dose for mild hypophosphatemia is not as effective as when the study was conducted. There are some data supporting more aggressive replacement of phosphorus in patients with moderate to severe hypophosphatemia (137).

The importance of magnesium and magnesium balance is being appreciated more, especially in the critical care setting, where serum magnesium concentrations are being assessed with increased frequency and risk factors for magnesium depletion are now well recognized (see Chapter 11). Although the serum magnesium concentration does not always accurately reflect magnesium status, a low concentration usually indicates magnesium deficiency. Doses for management of moderate to severe deficiency in various clinical situations for various age groups are given in Chapter 11 and elsewhere (138). Hypermagnesemia may occur with fluctuating or progressively deteriorating renal function or decreasing intestinal or renal magnesium loss; periodic monitoring of serum magnesium is necessary.

Trace Elements

Acceptable direct evidence indicates that iron, iodide, zinc, copper, chromium (Cr^{3+}), and selenium are essential human nutrients. Manganese (Mn^{2+}) has been found essential for all experimental species studied, but clear evidence for Mn^{2+} deficiency in human beings is lacking. A single well-documented case of molybdenum deficiency was noted in a patient receiving long-term PN. (The biochemical and physiologic roles of these trace elements and the effects of their depletion in humans and other species are reviewed in Chapters 12 through 18.)

Several generalizations about essential trace elements are in order. The cationic trace elements (iron, zinc, copper, Cr^{3+}, and Mn^{2+}) in their salt forms are highly regulated and tend to be absorbed in small amounts from food by the normal intestine. When in excess in the body, all these elements may be toxic. Giving them intravenously risks excessive retention because intestinal controls are bypassed. Iron particularly is poorly excreted in the urine after PN or blood infusion. Copper, Mn^{2+}, and (to a much smaller extent) molybdate are excreted through the bile into the intestinal tract, hence continued administration of the usual amounts of copper and Mn^{2+} in the presence of excretory liver dysfunction imposes a risk (see later). In contrast, all the anionic forms of trace elements (iodide, selenite, or molybdate) are well absorbed and excreted in the urine; again, excess imposes a risk of toxicity. Many trace elements are present as contaminants in PN components and so contribute variably to the input.

Iron. The intravenous requirement for the term infant is estimated to be about 100 μg(micrograms)/kg/day; the premature infant probably needs double that amount intravenously. Older children need 1 to 2 mg/day. Nonmenstruating women and men whose condition is stable need about 1 mg, and menstruating women need double that amount per day. Iron loss through frequent venipuncture for various tests may be estimated on the basis of 1 mg of iron lost for every 1 mL of packed red cells removed (see Chapter 12).

When evidence indicates iron depletion, iron may be given intravenously as dilute iron dextran solution in varying amounts after ensuring that the patient has no hypersensitivity to a test dose. Other parenteral iron products include iron sucrose and sodium ferric gluconate. Because neither of the latter two products has been tested in PN formulations, they should be administered separately from the PN formulation. As noted earlier, addition of iron dextran and other iron salts disrupts TNA stability.

Patients who receive chronic PN without iron and eat very little invariably become iron deficient over time. Iron should be added to the PN solution (preferably a dextrose/amino acid PN) to either prevent or treat iron deficiency in this situation. This can be accomplished by adding small daily doses of iron dextran to the PN solution (e.g., 1 to 2 mg/day) or by giving regular doses of therapeutic iron dextran via PN (e.g., 25 to 50 mg/day for 2 to 4 weeks). Patients who have a duodenum and proximal jejunum and eat a normal diet during chronic PN usually absorb enough iron to prevent deficiency. These patients may not need supplemental iron via PN. Regular measurement of hemoglobin, serum iron concentration, mean corpuscular volume, and serum ferritin concentration helps in assessing iron stores. During acute stress such as infections, measuring serum iron and ferritin concentrations may not be helpful in the diagnosis of iron deficiency because serum iron concentration decreases while serum ferritin concentration increases.

Iodide. Serum iodide often remains normal in infants and adults with no added iodide in PN. During 4 or more years of observation in adult patients receiving long-term PN at home without added iodide, the various parameters of thyroid function have remained within normal limits. This is explained by iodide contamination of various mineral additives, by efficient absorption in the upper gastrointestinal tract of iodides from any ingested diet, and by the use of iodide-containing topical antimicrobial solutions. However, Centers for Disease Control and Prevention guidelines support the use of chlorhexidine solution for site care dressings of central catheters. This would remove the iodine intake through the skin using previously recommended solutions with this trace element. For the occasional previously depleted adult patient with malabsorption who may have a low serum iodide concentration, 1 μg (microgram)/kg/day appears adequate during the repletion period. The same amount has been recommended for infants to avoid any risk of deficiency or toxicity.

After the recommendation of an expert committee of the Nutrition Advisory Group of the American Medical Association (AMA) to the Food and Drug Administration (FDA) in 1979 (139), commercial intravenous solutions of zinc, copper, Mn^{2+}, and Cr^{3+} became available, ending a period in which such solutions were available only to physicians and pharmacists who personally prepared them. We have modified the 1979 suggested intakes on the basis of newer information in Table 99.5. Some data relevant to PN are reviewed briefly later. The 2002 ASPEN guidelines have suggested marked decreases in both copper and Mn^{2+} during administration of PN (5).

Zinc. Pediatric dosages of zinc have been more precisely defined by Greene and colleagues (133) (see Table 99.5). The original recommendations of the AMA committee (139) for stable and for hypermetabolic patients are deemed reasonable. As in adults, severe diarrhea secondary to infectious disease and the short bowel syndrome in children are associated with increased zinc losses and increased need. The guidelines in the appropriate footnote for zinc in Table 99.5 are helpful in estimating intestinal losses (140). Periodic checks of serum concentrations in such circumstances are essential. Zinc contamination of PN additives is variable depending on the specific sources. As a result, total zinc in the formulation may be as high as 0.3 to 0.4 mg/L (141).

Copper. The pediatric copper dose recommendations in Table 99.5 are the same as the AMA recommendations (139). The work of Shike and colleagues showed that unlike zinc, increased stool volume is not associated with a major increase in copper excretion, and urinary losses tend to be low; thus, copper accumulates in the body when infused in amounts exceeding those needed for maintenance (142). On the basis of these and other findings, it is suggested that the range for copper be lowered to 0.3 to 0.5 mg/day for stable patients, hence the upper limit of the recommendation

TABLE 99.5. RECOMMENDED PARENTERAL DOSES FOR TRACE ELEMENTS

TRACE ELEMENT[a]	PRETERM (μg[MICROGRAMS]/ kg/d)	TERM (μg[MICROGRAMS]/ kg/d)	CHILDREN (μg[MICROGRAMS]/ kg/d)	STABLE ADULT (μg[MICROGRAMS]/d)	ADULT WITH GASTROINTESTINAL LOSSES (μg[MICROGRAMS]/d)
Zinc	400	100–250	50	2,500–4,000[b]	Add[c]
Copper	20	20	20	300–500	500
Chromium	0.2	0.2	0.2	10–15	20
Manganese	1	1	1	60–100	—
Selenium	2	2	2	40–80	—
Molybdenum	0.25	0.25	0.25	0	—

[a]Conversion factors: zinc 1 μg(microgram) = 0.0153 μmol(micromoles); copper 1 μg(microgram) = 0.0157 μmol; chromium 1 μg(microgram) = 0.0192 μmol(micromoles); manganese 1 μg(microgram) = 0.0182 μmol(micromoles); selenium 1 μg(microgram) = 0.0127 μmol(micromoles).
[b]Add additional 2,000 μg(micrograms)/day to hypermetabolic patients.
[c]Add 12 mg/L of small bowel losses and 17 mg/kg of stool or ileostomy losses.

in Table 99.5 is at the lower limit of the AMA recommendation. Caution in copper administration in obstructive jaundice is emphasized because the major excretory route is through bile. It should be noted that copper deficiency has occurred during PN administration when it was removed secondary to cholestasis (143).

Manganese. The Mn^{2+} content in PN components (144) and the blood concentrations found in PN patients given varying amounts of Mn^{2+} (145) suggested an appreciable reduction in the AMA recommendations. The current pediatric recommendations of 1 μg(microgram)/kg/day with a total of 50 μg(micrograms)/day for older children in Table 99.5 are below the AMA recommendation of 2 to 10 μg(micrograms)/kg/day.

Mn^{2+} contamination of various PN additives produced in the United States may result in an adult receiving 8 to 22 μg(micrograms)/day (144). HPN patients receiving 60 to 120 μg(micrograms)/day (~1.5 to 3 μg(micrograms)/kg/day) of added Mn^{2+} had normal serum concentrations (145). As suggested earlier, it appears wise to provide only 60 to 100 μg(micrograms)/day to adults (see Table 99.5) (145), rather than the 150 to 180 μg(micrograms)/day of the AMA recommendations.

The potential for excessive retention escalates when cholestasis is present (which interferes with Mn^{2+} elimination from the body) and there is continued provision of the amount of Mn^{2+} listed in Table 99.5 in PN. Even with normal liver function, higher dosages in infants and children (146, 147) and in several adults (148–152) on long-term PN resulted in high blood concentrations associated with high signal intensity in Tl-weighted imaging in the basal ganglia (146–150, 153). Concentrations of plasma (154) or whole blood (146) Mn^{2+} in children showed a significant positive correlation with bilirubin levels. Reducing or omitting supplementary Mn^{2+} resulted in major decreases in blood Mn^{2+} over periods varying from weeks to months (146–148) in children and adults, and the high-intensity signal on magnetic resonance brain imaging disappeared in one adult (155) and in a child (147) and was markedly reduced in another adult (148). The amounts of Mn^{2+} given to patients in whom high blood concentrations and imaging changes developed (146–148, 155) were appreciably greater than those in either the AMA recommendations or Table 99.5.

The exact relation of Mn^{2+} to the high-intensity signal in the basal ganglia is uncertain. Some investigators postulate deposition of a paramagnetic metal (i.e., Mn^{2+}) (146, 155); others suggest that the disappearance with cessation of Mn^{2+} infusion is more likely to be related to Mn^{2+}-induced reversible changes in the ultrastructural membrane composition (156). Also uncertain is the possible role of high concentrations of blood Mn^{2+} per se as one of the many factors in PN that can lead to hepatotoxicity (146).

Neurologic signs were present in one adult on long-term PN containing 1 to 2 mg/day of Mn^{2+}; these improved, and serum and urinary Mn^{2+} concentration decreased when

Mn^{2+} was omitted from PN. Nine months later the patient died of a massive gastrointestinal hemorrhage secondary to her cancer. At autopsy, the Mn^{2+} content of the caudate nucleus and centrum ovale was two to three times that found in some patients not receiving PN (157). In another study, complete withdrawal of Mn^{2+} resulted in a decrease in serum concentrations and brain deposition of Mn^{2+} (149).

Chromium. As noted in the 1979 AMA report, quantitative data on Cr^{3+} requirements were lacking at that time, and the qualitative suggestions were based on estimates from balance data on healthy persons (139). The current situation is not appreciably clearer, largely because of the difficulty of measuring plasma Cr^{3+} concentrations (normally very low), lack of information on tissue levels of this ion, and lack of controlled studies on very low Cr^{3+} intake.

The relatively few cases of well-documented symptomatic Cr^{3+} depletion have occurred in long-term adult PN patients receiving little or no supplementary Cr^{3+}. It has been associated with sudden occurrence of glucose intolerance, glycosuria, weight loss, and neurologic symptoms, especially peripheral neuropathy. Development of symptoms appeared to be related to prolonged glucose infusions and intestinal fluid losses—both of which increase Cr^{3+} need. The patients responded well to Cr^{3+}, often 250 μg(micrograms) Cr^{3+} infused daily for weeks (158). Cr^{3+} toxicity has not been observed, even with doses greater than 250 μg(micrograms)/day.

A pediatric formula containing 4 μg(micrograms) of Cr^{3+} as a contaminant, given over 16 months, did not produce signs or symptoms suggesting Cr^{3+} deficiency (159). Children aged 1.3 to 14 years who were receiving Cr^{3+} during long-term PN at 0.15 ± 0.09 μg(microgram)/kg/day had higher serum Cr^{3+} concentrations than control subjects (2.1 ± 1.2 versus 0.10 ± 0.03 μg(micrograms)/L). Supplementation was discontinued for 1 year (during which time the Cr^{3+} intake was estimated to be 0.05 ± 0.01 μg(microgram)/kg/day), at which time the serum Cr^{3+} concentration was 0.5 ± 0.3 μg(microgram)/L, and no signs of deficiency were observed (160). It was suggested that the parenteral Cr^{3+} pediatric intake should be lowered to 0.05 μg(microgram)/kg/day and that current values of Cr^{3+} as contaminants may be sufficient for adults. A period of 1 year of reduced Cr^{3+} intake after a period of high intake without signs or symptoms may not be an adequate test of need in long-term patients. We believe that for children and adults on long-term PN, the recommendations given in Table 99.5 are still valid pending further studies. However, for periods of 1 year or less, the recommendations of Moukarzel and colleagues (160) may be tried with adequate precautions.

Selenium. Recommendations for selenium were not made in the 1979 AMA report. That year saw the first reports in English relating selenium deficiency to Keshan disease in China (see Chapter 16) and the report of Van Rijn and colleagues of a case of selenium deficiency in a patient receiving PN (161). Considerable clinical and biochemical information has accrued since then, including selenium deficiency in patients receiving PN, with some deaths associated with cardiomyopathy and reports of muscle tenderness and weakness.

Low plasma concentrations of selenium less than 10 μg (micrograms)/mL or less than 0.13 μmol(micromoles)/L may be present without symptoms. Cohen and colleagues followed up five patients on HPN without added selenium for an average of 18.6 months (162). Selenium-dependent glutathione peroxidase (GSHPx) in plasma reached very low levels less than 15% of normal values, 0.32 units/mL) in approximately 1 year; GSHPx in red cells reached that level (24 units/g hemoglobin) in 1 to 2 years. At the time plasma GSHPx was at this concentration, plasma selenium was 0.19 ± 0.07 pmol/mL. There was no evidence of either cardiac or skeletal muscle dysfunction in this study (162). After infusion of 400 μg(micrograms) of selenium as selenite, plasma GSHPx increased within 6 hours; that in red cells did not reach normal concentrations until 3 to 4 months later, similar to the time required for new red cells to appear (162).

Selenious acid (as selenite salts) is available for intravenous use. Use of 40 to 60 μg(micrograms)/day in PN usually maintains normal plasma concentrations during short-term PN. Patients requiring long-term PN or HPN usually require 100 to 120 μg(micrograms)/day to maintain normal serum concentrations of selenium. Administration of 100 μg(micrograms)/day in the infusate will increase low concentrations in previously depleted patients receiving PN into a control range (161).

Selenoprotein P concentrations in plasma (measured by radioimmunoassay) correlate well with extracellular GSHPx and selenium as markers for selenium status in deficient patients on long-term PN.

Molybdenum. A single documented case of molybdenum deficiency was reported in a patient with Crohn disease receiving long-term PN; clinical and biochemical abnormalities were reversed by daily supplementation with 300 μg(micrograms) of ammonium molybdate (163). Tissue levels of molybdenum and balance data were not obtained, nor were molybdenum-dependent enzyme activities measured. Two patients with active Crohn disease and malabsorption had ileostomy losses of 560 and 300 to 350 μg(micrograms)/day of this ion.

In view of a time lapse of at least 6 months from the initiation of PN to development of symptoms in the single reported patient, the lack of simple biochemical criteria as diagnostic clues, and the reportedly high molybdenum content of PN solutions, it is recommended that molybdenum not be added at present to PN infusions in adults and that it be withheld in children unless they are to receive long-term PN.

Multitrace Element Additives. The most commonly used commercially available trace element combination products, which contain four to five individual metals, are listed in Tables 99.6. A combination product containing six

TABLE 99.6. TRACE ELEMENT COMBINATION PRODUCTS FOR ADULTS, PEDIATRIC PATIENTS, AND NEONATES

	ZINC (μg[MICROGRAMS])	COPPER (μg[MICROGRAMS])	CHROMIUM (μg[MICROGRAMS])	MANGANESE[a] (μg[MICROGRAMS])	SELENIUM (μg[MICROGRAMS])
Adult					
Four-element product (per 3 mL)	3,000	1,200	12	300	—
Four-element product concentrate (per 1 mL)	5,000	1,000	10	500	—
Five-element product (per 3 mL)	3,000	1,200	12	300	60
Five-element product concentrate (per 1 mL)	5,000	1,000	10	500	60
Neonates					
Four-element product (per 1 mL)	1,500	100	0.85	25	—
Pediatrics					
Four-element product (per 1 mL)	1,000	100	1	25	—
Five-element product (per 1 mL)	1,000	100	1	25	15

[a]Daily dose of manganese exceeds the dose suggested in Table 99.5.

trace elements (molybdenum plus zinc, copper, Mn^{2+}, Cr^{3+}, and selenium) and one containing seven trace elements (iodine plus the six mentioned earlier) are also commercially available.

Use of multiple trace elements in a fixed formula poses the risk of excessive dosage of one or more of the constituents to patients receiving the formula long-term and who have metabolic abnormalities that require restriction or omission. Furthermore, evidence reviewed in this chapter and recommendations in Table 99.6 suggest that routine needs for some trace elements are appreciably lower than those recommended in the AMA-FDA report (139). A combination of individual trace elements or a decreased volume of a given multitrace element formulation may be necessary when restriction of one or more of the latter is indicated.

Potential Toxicity of Other Trace Elements. The issue of toxicity of parenterally administered lead, cadmium, mercury, and aluminum present as contaminants merits consideration because they bypass the normal barriers of the gastrointestinal tract.

Aluminum. Aluminum is of special concern because its toxicity was well delineated in patients with renal disease who were treated with aluminum-containing phosphate-binding antacids and/or who received aluminum-contaminated water in hemodialysis. Neurologic changes include apraxic motor abnormalities involving speech, myoclonus, seizures, and dementia. Also seen is an osteomalacia refractory to therapy with vitamin D analogs, calcium, or phosphate; bone pain; pathologic fractures; aluminum deposition on bone osteoid front; and a microcytic anemia without evidence of iron deficiency (164).

Reports of serious metabolic bone disease in a group of patients receiving HPN for 6 to 72 months were followed by the discovery that the casein hydrolysate used as the source of amino acids contained relatively large amounts of aluminum (2313 ± 149 μg(micrograms)/L) (165). Aluminum concentrations in plasma, urine, and bone were markedly elevated in all patients studied, and the bone morphology was that of osteomalacia, ranging from mild to severe. Intense periarticular and lower extremity pain in long bones and weight-bearing joints developed within 5 months in five of the initial 11 patients despite improvement in their overall nutritional state. Patients with impaired renal clearance are at increased risk. As noted later, use of casein hydrolysate at this institution was discontinued, and the patients' bone status improved.

Although free amino acid solutions have much smaller amounts of aluminum (e.g., 26 ± 20 μg(micrograms)/L of 10% solution), other PN ingredients may have significant amounts and may contribute to the total burden. Premature infants are at increased risk because of their poor renal clearance. Widely varying concentrations of aluminum have been found in the same component from different manufacturers or in different salts of the same mineral; careful

selection can reduce aluminum contamination from 288 μg(micrograms)/L of PN solution to 10.9 μg(micrograms)/L (166). There is evidence from a study conducted in Cambridge in the United Kingdom that preterm infants given PN for a median period of 9.5 days (range, 5 to 15) with a solution providing 45 μg(micrograms)/kg/day of aluminum had dose-related reduced developmental attainment at the postterm age of 18 months, compared with a control group given a solution containing 4 to 5 μg(micrograms)/kg/day of aluminum (167).

A joint working group on standards for aluminum content of PN solutions supported the FDA proposal to set an upper limit of 25 μg(micrograms) Al/L (0.93 μmol(micromoles)/L) in large-volume parenteral solutions (e.g., amino acids, lipids, dextrose), small-volume parenteral solutions (e.g., calcium, potassium, sodium, magnesium salts), and pharmacy bulk packages. This is mandated to ensure that the aluminum load from PN formulations is less than 5 μg (micrograms)/kg/day. PN formulations delivering aluminum loads of 15 to 30 μg(micrograms)/kg/day should be considered unsafe, and those greater than 30 μg(micrograms)/kg/day are considered toxic. It also recommended that salts of calcium, phosphate, and magnesium trace element and multivitamin solutions state the amount of aluminum on their label and that pharmacists and physicians be educated about the risk of aluminum (168). Despite the recommendations of its advisory panel in 1986, the FDA finally established the date of July 26, 2004, as the implementation date for labeling compliance.

Vitamins

Formulations

The original parenteral multivitamin formulations in the United States were based on those proposed in 1975 by the Nutrition Advisory Group of the AMA for intravenous vitamin formulations (169). The adult formulation was approved by the FDA in 1979 and was designated here as the AMA-FDA adult formula. In 1984, its recommended pediatric formula was approved, and these guidelines were published in 1988. In 1985, an FDA/AMA-sponsored workshop proposed several changes for parenteral formulations of vitamins. See Table 99.7 for comparisons between the 1975 and 1985 workshop recommendations. The new guidelines were published in the Federal Register in 2000. The major change was to include vitamin K (150 μg (micrograms)) in the adult formulation for the first time. The daily adequate intake for vitamin K via the gastrointestinal tract in health is 90 μg(micrograms) for women and 120 μg(micrograms) for men; however, vitamin K is known to be synthesized by bacteria in the gastrointestinal tract. The parenteral dose of vitamin K likely mimics closely what the normal subject would require via the gastrointestinal tract in health. This dose is much lower than previously suggested parenteral doses of vitamin K during PN (5 to 10 mg/week or 1 mg/day).

TABLE 99.7. COMPOSITION OF PARENTERAL MULTIVITAMINS FOR ADULTS (AMOUNT/D)

VITAMIN	AMA-FDA 1975 WORKSHOP	AMA-FDA 1985 WORKSHOP	MVI-12[a]	MVI-ADULT[a] INFUVITE ADULT[b]
A (μg[micrograms]) [IU]	1,000 [3,300]	1,000 [3,300]	1,000 [3,300]	1,000 [3,300]
D_2 (μg) [IU]	5 [200]	5 [200]	5 [200]	5 [200]
E (mg) [IU]	10 [10]	10 [10]	10 [10]	10 [10]
K (μg[micrograms])	0	150	0	150
Thiamin (mg)	3	6	3	6
Riboflavin (mg)	3.6	3.6	3.6	3.6
Pyridoxine (mg)	4	6	4	6
Niacin (mg)	40	40	40	40
Pantothenate (mg)	15	15	15	15
Biotin (μg[micrograms])	60	60	60	60
Folate (μg[micrograms])	400	600	400	600
Cobalamin (μg[micrograms])	5	5	5	5
Ascorbate (mg)	100	200	100	200

[a]Manufactured by Mayne Pharmaceuticals.
[b]Manufactured by Baxter.

Stability. Some adsorption and/or destruction of individual vitamins may occur through contact with plastic containers and tubes and in passage through filters, exposure to light and heat, and interactions with other substances present in solutions. Factors affecting the solubility and stability of vitamins in various pharmaceutical preparations have been reviewed (170).

Appreciable amounts of retinol appear to be lost from solution by a combination of adsorption and photodegradation when the flow through tubing is slow. This is particularly true with the increased light intensity used in neonatal nurseries. With exposure to bright sunlight, 100% of retinol in PN solutions can be lost in 3 hours. Use of polyolefin tubing rather than polyvinyl tubing reduces vitamin A loss. Little loss of vitamin D occurs in plastic delivery systems. DL-α-tocopherol is stable in sunlight, but 50% of vitamin K can be lost from PN solutions in 3 hours. Riboflavin and pyridoxine are also unstable when exposed to direct sunlight for a matter of hours. Thiamin, folate, riboflavin, and pyridoxine are stable under fluorescent light.

Addition of the multivitamin solution to other PN constituents presents the possibility of some loss of specific vitamins. Thiamin is split and loses biologic activity in the presence of sulfite compounds that are components of amino acid solutions in the United States; hence, multivitamin solutions should not be added directly to undiluted amino acid solutions, but rather to the ultimate solution shortly before infusion into the patient. Ascorbic acid is progressively lost in the presence of copper ion (Cu^{2+}) and oxygen.

Adult Needs

The issue of vitamin needs for the sick and injured has long been of concern. Varying amounts of vitamins have been administered to postoperative and other patients who are receiving PN, with differing intervals between the times of vitamin infusion and those of blood sampling; blood levels have been the usual criteria, although some investigators have used enzymatic methods. Few investigators have completely surveyed all 13 vitamins. Much of the published data obtained in seriously ill adult patients is based on information gathered from a few weeks to a few months, the critical time range for most patients. These data indicate a relatively narrow range of requirements for certain of these nutrients, and adequate blood levels or related enzyme activities may be attained in hypercatabolic patients with daily infusion dosages for some that are appreciably below the old MVI (multiple vitamin infusion) concentrate formula and in some cases, below, at, or not far above the AMA-FDA adult dosages (171).

A survey of 290 medical inpatients revealed a 57% incidence of vitamin D deficiency using a serum concentration of 25-OH vitamin D as the marker (172). Twenty-two percent of this population was considered severely deficient. Low vitamin D intake, winter season, and housebound status were independent predictors of vitamin D status.

A dietary workshop on folic acid, vitamin B_{12}, and choline was published recently (173). The importance of folic acid administration in preventing neural tubular defects was reemphasized, as well as the utility of using the enzymes homocysteine and methylmalonic acid for the diagnosis of folic acid deficiency and vitamin B_{12} deficiency in macrocytic anemia (173). Choline status was not addressed in the detail given to folate and vitamin B_{12}.

There is evidence that serum choline concentrations are depressed in patients who receive long-term PN (174). Impairment of the transsulfuration pathway of methionine to choline appears to be a possible mechanism for this disorder. In a small pilot study, choline supplementation for HPN patients demonstrated significant improvement in a test measuring verbal and visual memory when compared with HPN patients not receiving choline (174). Compher and colleagues (175) have suggested an association between vitamin B_{12} deficiency and choline deficiency.

The adequacy of the original adult AMA-FDA formulation was tested in 16 adults with severe malabsorption or intestinal obstruction who had been receiving HPN for 1 to 9 years. These patients were studied serially over many months on this formulation (MVI-12) (176). Blood was sampled at least 36 hours after the preceding infusion of vitamins was terminated. Mean values for plasma vitamin A were near or above the upper limit of reference values, in part because five subjects had renal insufficiency; the high values were associated with elevated retinol-binding protein levels. Thiamin, pyridoxine, niacin, biotin, riboflavin, vitamin B_{12}, and folate levels were within the reference ranges for all patients; pantothenate levels tended to be within or above the reference ranges; and thiamin tended to be toward the lower half of the reference range, as did vitamin E levels. In addition to the label amount of 10 mg/dL α-tocopherol acetate, additional vitamin E was given as a constituent of the intravenous lipid. The low plasma lipid levels of these patients tended to decrease circulating vitamin E concentrations. A few subjects had ascorbic acid values persistently below 0.3 mg/dL, which may have been caused by loss of this vitamin during storage for 30 hours. Concentrations of 25-OH vitamin D and 1,25(OH)2 vitamin D in eight persons over 430 to 588 days on MVI-12 were within the reference range, as were parathormone levels. Prothrombin times were normal, with 5 mg of vitamin K oxide added once per week (176).

In another study, the plasma vitamin E concentrations measured in patients over 28 to 250 days on this formulation increased from 2.1 ± 4.6 to 16.5 ± 4.6 μmol(micromoles)/L (mean ± SD) (177). In a study using some of the same patients as in the study by Shils and colleagues (176) on HPN, the same multivitamins, and twice the volume of Intralipid, plasma α-tocopherol levels of 17.5 ± 6.6 μmol (micromoles) in seven patients were not statistically different from values in controls (178). When a different source of vitamin E was given to patients on long-term HPN, the average plasma α-tocopherol concentration was 11.14 μmol(micromoles)/L (normal, 18.11 μmol (micromoles)/L) and there were significantly higher breath pentane levels (a measure of lipid peroxidation) as in controls (179).

The amounts of vitamin E present in Intralipid as α-tocopherol are given in Table 99.3 together with concentrations of other isomers. (See Chapter 21 for a discussion of vitamin E isomer activities.) In addition, as noted in this table, lipid emulsions contain appreciable amounts of vitamin K, with roughly twice as much in those containing soybean oil only. Consequently, with regular lipid infusions, separate vitamin K infusions may be reduced or eliminated.

A major function of vitamin D is improved efficiency of absorption of calcium and phosphate by the small intes-tine. PN bypasses this route, so why is this vitamin included in parenteral solutions? Calcitriol, as the active form of vitamin D, plays an intimate role with parathyroid hormone in bone turnover; the vitamin also plays a role in cellular differentiation (see Chapter 20). Whether the current parenteral dosage recommendations are higher than necessary for these functions remains to be demonstrated.

Pediatric Needs

Greene and colleagues summarized research on vitamin concentrations in term-gestation infants and children and problems related to the needs of preterm and underweight newborn infants (180). They concluded that the vitamin dosages suggested for children in the 1975 AMA report were adequate for continued use in term infants and children up to 11 years of age. This formulation is commercially available as MVI-Pediatric and Infuvite Pediatric (Table 99.8). Use of this formulation for underweight infants was found to increase blood tocopherol to a high level; the manufacturer and the FDA then recommended that the daily dose be reduced successively to 65% and then to one third of a vial for infants weighing less than 1000 g. Further problems have surfaced in providing this formulation to very LBW infants, including large losses of retinol through the delivery sets and elevated riboflavin and vitamin B_6 plasma concentrations (180). Greene and colleagues recommended a revised formulation for the very LBW infant (133) (see Table 99.8); currently, this is not in production.

Thiamin Deficiency

There continue to be reports of severe thiamin deficiency in adult patients receiving PN. This occurs despite (a) the availability and safety of its parenteral preparation in multivitamin or individual form, (b) widespread knowledge of

TABLE 99.8. COMPOSITION OF PARENTERAL MULTIVITAMINS FOR CHILDREN[a]

VITAMIN	VERY LOW BIRTH WEIGHT (/kg)	TERM TO 11 Y OF AGE (/d)
A (μg[micrograms]) [IU]	500 [1,670]	700 [2,300]
D_2 (μg[micrograms]) [IU]	4 [160]	10 [400]
E (mg) [IU]	2.8 [2.8]	7 [7]
K (μg[micrograms])	80	200
Thiamin (mg)	0.35	1.2
Riboflavin (mg)	0.15	1.4
Pyridoxine (mg)	0.18	1
Niacin (mg)	6.8	17
Pantothenate (mg)	2	5
Biotin (μg[micrograms])	6	20
Folate (μg[micrograms])	56	140
Cobalamin (μg[micrograms])	0.3	1
Ascorbate (mg)	25	80

[a]These doses of parenteral vitamins can be delivered by either MVI-Pediatric (Mayne Pharmaceuticals) or Infuvite Pediatric (Baxter).

its increased need with use of high-glucose formulas, (c) its known instability in contact with the sulfite in amino acids, necessitating minimum storage at room temperature before use, and (d) the fairly rapid onset (1 to 2 months) of life-threatening metabolic changes characteristic of its deficiency. Unfortunately, the problem was complicated by periodic production difficulties with intravenous multivitamin preparations in the United States, resulting in nationwide shortages in the 1990s (181). In published reports in a period of 3 years, 15 cases have been described with four deaths (182, 183); several patients had severe lactic acidosis and peripheral neuropathy and/or ataxia.

COMPLICATIONS OF ORGAN FUNCTION

Complications related to vascular access, catheter-related sepsis, concentration problems resulting from formula composition, and underlying diseases were discussed earlier. They can be prevented or minimized by having responsibility vested in experienced physicians, nurses, dietitians, and pharmacists working as a team that closely supervises their inpatients and outpatients. Disorders related directly to PN, including liver dysfunction, gallstones, and decreased bone mass, will be addressed in this section.

Hepatic Dysfunction

Fatty liver (steatosis), intrahepatic cholestasis, and portal inflammation can occur, particularly in children, but also in adults (184, 185). It can progress to portal tract fibrosis and infiltration, liver failure, and death.

Children

Since the first description of PN-associated cholestasis and early cirrhosis in 1971 in a premature infant (186), a large and continuing literature has confirmed PN as a contributing risk factor for hepatobiliary dysfunction of varying degree and incidence. Reviews of the biochemical, clinical, and histopathologic changes in adults and children have emphasized the multifactorial nature of the problem (184, 185). In children, the degree of prematurity, infection, inability to consume food orally, extent of intestinal dysfunction, number of surgical procedures, duration of PN, and long-term administration of excessive calories are risk factors (184, 185). Immaturity of the hepatic excretory function and the enterohepatic circulation, particularly in the neonate, is one reason for development of cholestasis. Cholestasis has been reported in various series to occur in 7.4 to 42.1% of infants, with wide variations among differing populations, criteria, hospital practices, and clinical conditions (187).

Intravenous lipid emulsions with their endogenous content of phytosterols from vegetable oils were addressed as a potential cause of cholestatic liver disease in a preliminary study of children (188). Five of 29 patients who were receiving PN and had severe cholestatic liver disease had significantly increased concentrations of campesterol, stigmasterol, sitosterol, and isofucosterol (all phytosterols); they also had elevated concentrations of cholestanol and sitostanol (a phytostanol). The 24 patients receiving PN who did not have severe cholestatic disease had normal or slightly elevated phytosterol levels. Thrombocytopenia, a common complication in patients with hereditary phytasterolemia, was clearly evident in the five patients with severe cholestatic liver disease. The dose of intravenous fat emulsion was substantially higher in the five patients with liver disease than in the other 24 patients (188). The possible relationship of high blood Mn^{2+} levels to the development of cholestasis was mentioned earlier (146).

Adults

In adults, preexisting liver and other diseases, sepsis, preexisting malnutrition, extent of bowel resection and/or damage (such as from radiation), excess nonprotein calories, little or no oral intake, and duration on PN are also associated risk factors. Increases may occur in serum transaminase, alkaline phosphatase, γ-glutamyl-transferase, and less frequently, bilirubin as indicators of hepatic dysfunction.

Adult patients receiving long-term PN (median, 18 months) who were given relative excesses of carbohydrate, fat, and amino acids showed abnormal hepatic function and cholestatic changes. When the amounts of these macronutrients were reduced, jaundice was reversed and liver function test results and histologic features improved (189). Other investigators noted increasing steatosis with administration of excess calories as carbohydrate or lipid or both (190). Forty-three patients who received PN were randomized to receive either glucose as the sole nonprotein calorie source or a combination of glucose and fat. The dose of nonprotein energy used in this study was moderate compared with that in many of the previous studies. Although the patients were not dramatically overfed (1.5 times calculated basal energy expenditure), alkaline phosphatase and γ-glutamyl-transferase increased significantly in both groups. Aspartate aminotransferase, alanine aminotransferase, and direct bilirubin increased more in the group receiving only glucose as nonprotein calories. It appears that liver enzyme laboratory test results are affected by administration of PN, even when used in moderate doses and when part of the energy dose is given as intravenous lipid emulsion (191).

Data from various studies strongly suggest that patients with little or no remaining small intestine are at increased risk of developing serious hepatic dysfunction with fibrotic changes; the rapidity of development and the severity of the disease vary among series. Unlike in children, actual liver failure in adults is uncommon.

Amelioration or Prevention

A variety of agents have been tested on patients receiving PN who have developed evidence of associated significant hepatic dysfunction and who require continued PN. Currently studies are being conducted with Sincalide (cholecystokinin octapeptide) and tauroursodeoxycholic acid (a hydrophilic bile acid) in neonates. Giving a mixture of MCT and LCT to PN patients as the intravenous lipid source did not cause a change in liver size or grayscale value, whereas LCT infusion increased both (129). On the grounds that metronidazole could depress formation by intestinal bacteria of potentially damaging bile acids, this drug has been tested in patients receiving PN and has been reported by some to reduce abnormalities in liver enzymes compared with untreated control subjects (192, 193). Other antibiotics such as neomycin, gentamycin, and polymyxin B are also being evaluated. It is theorized that the use of enteral antibiotics reduces the bacterial load of the gut, which in turn decreases the amount of lipopolysaccharide that crosses into the portal circulation. Ursodeoxycholic acid, an epimer of chenodeoxycholic acid, has been given with benefit to adults (194) and children (195) on long-term PN who developed cholestatic liver disease. Jaundice and enzyme abnormalities regressed, and their clinical condition improved. Discontinuance of the ursodeoxycholic acid resulted in an increase in liver enzymes, which again regressed when this drug was readministered. Ursodeoxycholic acid given intravenously for 3 weeks to newborn piglets on PN was effective in reducing cholestasis by normalizing bile flow, bile acid secretion, and the bilirubin content of liver and serum; bile composition remained abnormal (196). Cholecystokinin in synthetic form was given intravenously twice daily from onset of PN for at least 14 days to 26 neonates on PN in a case-matched study; its use was associated with a significant trend toward lower serum direct bilirubin levels (197). Cholestyramine, choline, and lecithin have been reported to decrease hepatic steatosis (198). Phenobarbital and rifampin have also been reported to help reduce cholestasis, although results are very inconsistent. Studies are also ongoing with s-adenosyl methionine (an amino acid) because deficiencies have been associated with cholestasis.

Using a mouse model, Tazuke and colleagues (199) demonstrated an upregulation of multidrug resistance 1 genes and a downregulation of multidrug resistance 2 genes associated with the administration of PN. These aberrations were not seen when mice received normal saline as a control. This was a short-term study, so it was not able to measure hepatic injury; however, it does present new information that may help understand the mechanism of PN-associated liver dysfunction seen in some patients (199).

Gallstones

Sludge in the gallbladder has been observed repeatedly as a PN- and bowel rest–associated risk factor; this situation can progress to gallstone formation as the duration of PN increases. Patients who receive long-term PN maintenance because of resection or disease of the terminal ileum usually malabsorb bile salts. Thus, the bile salt pool decreases, and lower levels of bile salts are present in the gallbladder. This situation in turn increases the tendency of cholesterol to precipitate in the bile forming the nidus of gallstones. There is also an increase in unconjugated bilirubin and calcium, which are present in the stones that form from the accumulated sludge in the gallbladder (200). Impaired gallbladder contraction is important. Ultrasonography indicated development of biliary sludge within 12 days of starting PN in 14 of 23 patients. By 6 weeks, all had sludge, with six developing stones and three requiring surgery. The sludge disappeared 4 weeks after instituting oral feeding (201). Stasis and resulting sludge were prevented in the PN prairie dog model given daily injections of cholecystokinin (202). When chenodeoxycholate was given intravenously to a group of prairie dogs on PN for about 40 days, they did not develop gallstone or calcium bilirubinate crystals; the controls on only TPN had gallstones (5 of 6) or crystals (6 of 6) (203).

Gallstones are a significant problem in adults, but even more so in children on PN. For example, nine of 29 children receiving PN developed cholelithiasis; 64% of these with ileal disorders or resections developed stones (204); six of 13 children with less than 38 cm of small bowel remaining required a cholecystectomy (205). Some physicians recommend routine cholecystectomy whenever total or subtotal resection of the terminal ileum is performed (206). Emergency cholecystectomy in PN patients may not be a benign procedure; for example, in a study from 1984, the operative morbidity was 54% and hospital mortality was 11% in 35 patients (23 adult, 12 children) with PN-associated gallbladder disease (207). Most investigators now, however, quote a mortality rate of less than 5% (208).

These potential problems have led to the following suggestions for management of such patients at risk: nutrition should be provided enterally whenever possible in an effort to decrease biliary stasis, liver function studies should be checked periodically, ultrasound should be used liberally when a cholestatic picture is evident if gallstones are detected, elective cholecystectomy should be considered, and if laparotomy is to be done for any reason, cholecystectomy should be considered at that time.

Metabolic Bone Disease

Metabolic bone disease is usually a long-term complication of PN administration; however, it is prevalent in several disease states such as short bowel syndrome, inflammatory bowel disease, and cancer (209, 210). Patients with these disease states make up a substantial portion of patients receiving HPN, so metabolic bone disease is a multifactorial disorder. Administration of corticosteroids has also been associated with metabolic bone disease because these drugs increase bone resorption and impair osteoblastic activity (209). Pironi and colleagues (211) have done work addressing the prevalence of metabolic bone disease in adult patients receiving long-term PN in Europe. Of 165 patients, 84% had T-scores via dual-energy x-ray absorptiometry that were decreased by more than 1 standard deviation from normal, which meets criteria for osteopenia. Forty-one percent of these patients had T-scores that were decreased by more than 2.5 standard deviations from normal, meeting criteria for osteoporosis (211). Calcium, phosphorus, magnesium, and sodium balance all may be factors in the development of metabolic bone disease, as well as vitamins D and K intake. High doses of protein, especially when given via cyclic PN, increase urinary excretion of calcium, potentially contributing to the development of metabolic bone disease.

Rickets has been described in infants receiving PN. The causative factor appeared to be a need for more calcium and phosphate in the small fluid volume required by the neonate, rather than more vitamin D.

Reference has been made earlier to the effects of aluminum contamination on bone (164). When contaminated casein hydrolysate was replaced by crystalline amino acids, increased bone formation occurred with reduced osteoid area, decreased amounts of aluminum at the bone surface, and in plasma, and reduced calcium excretion.

The histomorphologic features of bone were examined in relation to formula composition in patients receiving long-term HPN who were not subsisting on aluminum-contaminated casein hydrolysate. In a prospective study in Toronto by Shike and colleagues, bone biopsies of HPN patients initially showed a hyperkinetic pattern, possibly resulting from initial malnutrition; at 6 to 73 months on HPN, the histologic features changed, with 12 of 16 patients having some degree of osteomalacia (212). In this study, 500 IU of vitamin D2 were given every other day; all other vitamins were supplied except biotin. Because seven of these patients were hypercalcemic and six had elevated 25(OH) vitamin D concentrations, further studies were performed on 11 patients before and after withdrawal of vitamin D2 (and, by necessity, the accompanying vitamin A) for 6 months (212). Six of ten patients had less osteoid and increased tetracycline uptake with the vitamin modification, but there was continuing evidence of a high turnover rate. In the three symptomatic patients, bone pain subsided, fractures healed, and urinary loss of calcium and phosphate was decreased. It was recommended that vitamin D solutions not be added to PN solutions of home patients (213). The mechanism of the postulated adverse role of this vitamin was not delineated. Others have noted improvement in HPN patients with respect to bone fractures and pain after withdrawal of vitamin D from the PN formulations (214). Withdrawal of vitamin D for 4.5 ± 0.2 years from 9 HPN patients with low parathyroid hormone and calcitriol concentrations was associated

with normalization of these values and some increase in lumbar spine bone mineral; there was no decrease in the mean concentration of calcidiol (214).

In a study in New York City of 12 HPN patients given crystalline amino acids (with the exception of two who had been transferred from casein hydrolysate 6 years earlier), the average daily vitamin D intake over the years had been 284 IU replaced 3 to 10 months earlier by 200 IU daily (215). Histomorphometry with tetracycline labeling revealed osteopenia, subnormal osteoid volume, and normal trabecular osteoid seam width; the calcification rate was normal. Of the seven women, four were in the 66- to 77-year range, and at least one had been a heavy cigarette smoker for many years. Six patients had minor bone complaints associated with osteoarthritis or postmenopausal osteoporosis (215). Serum calcium, parathyroid hormone, and calcitriol values were normal. The reasons for the marked difference in the histologic features of bone between the Toronto and New York studies are not apparent, but there were some formula differences. The PN formulas in the New York study had appreciably fewer fat calories, proportionately more glucose calories, and a different vitamin formulation, including biotin.

A longitudinal study of bone with regional densitometry and bone biopsy was performed in 14 patients on long-term PN who had either never been on protein hydrolysate or had not been for at least 7 years (216). Most subjects had osteopenia with heterogeneity in bone status, complaints of bone pain, and some documented fractures while on HPN; all 11 women were amenorrheic. In the follow-up period (27 ± 14 months), some patients had improved bone mass, some had no change, and others lost bone. Serum calcium, which had been low at baseline in six patients, normalized in most; parathyroid hormone was high in five; calcitriol was normal.

It has been suggested that PN patients lose a significant amount of bone mass early as a result of hypocalcemia that then stabilizes. Amenorrhea and/or smoking are also factors. The conclusion is that osteopenia is characteristic of long-term PN patients but that present PN formulations do not necessarily cause deterioration of bone health and may benefit some (216).

Pironi and colleagues (217) reported impaired bone formation in patients who were on PN for more than 1 year. Poor bone formation was positively correlated with low serum osteocalcin concentrations in this population. An inadequate vitamin K intake (and presumably low osteocalcin concentrations) has been associated with hip fractures in women (218).

Substantial data now demonstrate that parenteral phosphorus administration via PN in home nutrition patients decreases hypercalciuria (219, 220). It is likely that phosphorus induces this favorable response by increasing renal tubular calcium absorption (219).

Home PN patients should have calcium, phosphorus, and magnesium concentrations monitored regularly. Sufficient acetate should be administered to buffer titratable acids generated by the patient. Vitamin K should be provided daily either as a component of the parenteral vitamin product or as a separate component if it is not contained in the vitamin constituent.

COMPATIBILITY OF DRUGS WITH PARENTERAL NUTRITION SOLUTIONS

The frequency of drug interventions for coexistent illnesses or complications of PN requires ensuring that administering a drug as part of the PN solution or in conjunction with that solution will not produce incompatibility or an adverse reaction. Significant information on this issue has been summarized (221–223). Table 99.9 contains compatibility information for PN solutions and many commonly used drugs. Both dextrose/amino acid PN solutions and TNAs are listed in this table. Drugs that can or should be administered as continuous infusions and that are compatible with PN solutions are ideal additives, especially in the critical care setting, where fluid intake often must be regulated. Not all combinations of drugs and different PN solutions have been studied. In addition, some drugs are compatible

TABLE 99.9. COMPATIBILITIES OF SELECTED DRUGS WITH PARENTERAL NUTRITION SOLUTIONS

Dextrose/Amino Acids	
Compatible with	Albumin
	Folic acid
	Regular human insulin
	Phytonadione
	Cimetidine
	Heparin
	Iron dextran
	Ranitidine
	Famotidine
	HCl
	Metoclopramide
	Thiamin
Total nutrient admixtures	
Compatible with	Albumin
	Heparin
	Phytonadione
	Cimetidine
	Regular human insulin
	Ranitidine
	Famotidine
	Metoclopramide
	Thiamin
Dextrose/amino acids	
Incompatible with	Amphotericin B
	Phenytoin
	Ampicillin
	Metronidazole
Total nutrient admixtures	
Incompatible with	Amphotericin B
	Methyldopa
	HCl
	Phenytoin
	Iron dextran

TABLE 99.10. DRUGS INCOMPATIBLE WITH PARENTERAL NUTRITION SOLUTIONS WITH SIMULATED Y-SITE ADMINISTRATION

Acyclovir
Amphotericin B
Cefazolin
Ciprofloxacin
Cisplatin
Cyclosporine
Cytarabine
Doxorubicin
Fluorouracil
Furosemide
Ganciclovir
Methotrexate
Metoclopramide
Midazolam
Minocycline
Mitoxantrone
Potassium phosphate
Promethazine
Sodium bicarbonate

in traditional dextrose/amino acid PN solutions but not in TNAs (e.g., iron dextran). Still other drugs are compatible in PN solutions because they are diluted in a large volume of fluid and are incompatible when given during Y-site administration with the same PN solution. This problem undoubtedly occurs because the drug concentration is high when coinfused with PN through the same tubing. Trissel and colleagues (222) found that 82 of 102 drugs were compatible during Y-site administration with PN solutions; the 20 incompatible drugs are listed in Table 99.10.

HOME PARENTERAL NUTRITION

Since the first patients were discharged from the hospital to home on PN in 1969 and the early 1970s, in the United States and Canada (224), HPN as primary outpatient nutritional support has mushroomed. An HPN registry for the United States and Canada was established at the New York Academy of Medicine during the years 1978 to 1983 to collect and compile the data being accrued by an increasing number of medical centers that discharged patients on HPN. Data were distributed regularly to participants and interested parties. In 1984, this registry became a joint effort of the Oley Foundation and the American Society for Enteral and Parenteral Nutrition, originally designated the OASIS Registry and, more recently, the North American Home Parenteral and Enteral Nutrition Patient Registry (HPEN Registry) produced by the Oley Foundation. Today it is very difficult to assess the actual number of patients receiving HPN, but Delegge has estimated that 40,000 patients receive this therapy currently (225). Issues related to suitability, training, formulations, and home support have been extensively identified, and standards on organization, patient selection, and management have been developed (5).

Patient Numbers and Categories

Because Medicare in the United States is the largest single payer for HPN, its data provide useful information on national use, growth, and costs (226). In 1992, an estimated 10,035 Medicare beneficiaries were on HPN of the total Medicare enrollment of nearly 35 million, or 288 per million, at an expenditure of $156 million. Based on the figures for patients in the HPEN Registry in 1992, with 25% covered by Medicare, it was estimated that 40,000 patients used HPN therapy in that year (226). As mentioned earlier, 40,000 patients receiving HPN is still considered the closest estimate (225).

Of the 5481 HPN patients entering the registry during their first year on therapy between 1985 and 1992, the ten top specific diagnoses in percentages were neoplasm, 40.4; Crohn disease, 10.8; ischemic bowel, 6.2; motility disorders, 5.7; acquired immunodeficiency syndrome (AIDS), 5.5; congenital bowel disease, 3.3; chronic pancreatitis, 3; radiation enteritis, 2.7; chronic obstruction, 2.3; and cystic fibrosis, 1 (226).

Patient Outcome

Detailed data have been published for 11 diagnoses concerning survival, likelihood of rehabilitation to full and to partial function, and frequency of HPN and non-HPN complications (226). Annual survival rates of those with gastrointestinal diseases were 87% or better, with a 50 to 73% likelihood of complete rehabilitation in 1 year except for those with radiation enteritis or obstruction with chronic adhesions. In the three most common gastrointestinal diseases (Crohn disease, ischemic bowel disease, and motility disorders), survival rate more than 1 year for patients 18 years or less was about 95%; for those 35 to 55, 90%; and for those 65 and older, about 70%. Howard and colleagues (227) have estimated that between 25 and 33% of all patients receiving home nutrition support are more than 65 years of age. Their outcomes are reasonable, so age should not be considered a barrier for offering these means of support. Younger patients were more likely to resume full oral nutrition and have more complete rehabilitation, but they had more septic admissions. The registry to 1992 lists 66 patients with these three gastrointestinal diseases plus radiation enteritis who have survived 15 to 20 years on HPN. Only about 30% of patients with cancer who were receiving HPN were alive at 6 months, and 20% at 1 year (226). The mortality of patients with AIDS at 1 year was 90%; decreased use of HPN has likely occurred in human immunodeficiency virus (HIV)-infected patients as the effectiveness of newer medications surfaced.

Egger and colleagues (228) support the use of body weight gain or maintenance along with a subjective global assessment of the patient to document efficacy of HPN. They reported that patients were often underweight with depressed skinfold measurements; however, visceral protein concentrations were normal.

The frequency of HPN-related complications was similar in all diagnostic groups: one to two rehospitalizations per year, one half because of sepsis (226). Complications associated with HPN accounted for only 5% of deaths. If earlier experience continues to hold true, a minority of patients account for a majority of rehospitalizations. Howard and colleagues (229) have recently reviewed the management of complications of HPN.

One of the more dramatic successes of HPN is the much better outcome of the newborn with abnormalities of the gastrointestinal tract requiring extensive intestinal resection. In a Los Angeles HPN program for the years 1977 to 1984, 13 children were left with less than 38 cm of remaining jejunum and ileum (JI) beginning in the first month of life; of these, 69% survived, compared with 23% previously (203). Five of these had HPN discontinued after 4 to 32 months and had normal growth and development, whereas two remained on partial HPN after 9 and 55 months, and two required PN after 66 and 68 months; these four children have grown normally. Of those with 15 to 38 cm without an ileocecal valve (ICV) and those with less than 15 cm with and without an ICV, 70% survived; three of the ten discontinued HPN. Ultimate survival with normal growth and without HPN is now possible with as little as 11 cm residual JI and an intact ICV and as little as 25 cm JI without an ICV (203).

The course of 87 children with major resections managed from 1970 to 1988 in a Paris hospital have been analyzed. HPN was introduced in 1980. Fourteen of the 16 deaths occurred before 1980. Of those with less than 40 cm of JI who were born before 1980, 42% survived. Of those born after 1980, 94% in this category survived. The presence of an ICV did not significantly affect survival. The average time needed for adequate bowel adaptation was 27.3 months for those with less than 40 cm and 14 months for those with 40 to 80 cm (204).

Quality of Life and Support Needs

HPN presents various stresses to the patient and family members (230), including the sudden need to cope with the technical aspects, time demands, and safety issues of HPN after hospital discharge; management of handicaps resulting from primary and secondary illness and their treatments; concerns about meeting costs; patient dependency; and excessive dependence on others. A smooth transition to home care requires (a) adequate predischarge assessment and training of the patient and family in HPN management and (b) close support by the healthcare team via telephone contact and follow-up at home or in the physician's office to ensure that the patient's condition remains satisfactory. Dietary intake and other factors at home may require modification of the PN formulation from that deemed satisfactory in the hospital setting.

Data are available from a survey of 178 randomly selected families with a member on HPN for an average of

4.6 years, with 116 follow-up questionnaires (231). Patient and caregiver mean family scores for quality of life, self-esteem, life satisfaction, family cohesion, and quality of patient-caregiver relationship were similar to published norms for other healthy populations and other groups of chronically ill patients. HPN family adaptability and coping scores were higher. There were problems associated with financial strain and mild depression in patients related to increasing duration of PN and being barred from work (although able to) because of their disability classification.

Cost-Effectiveness

Estimates of the cost of HPN vary from $75,000 to $150,000 per patient-year (232). Many factors enter into the total cost of maintaining a patient on HPN; such charges vary considerably, depending in part on the method used in their estimations and on differences in the perspectives chosen for the analyses, particularly the matter of estimating benefits gained and/or the effectiveness gained. Goel has discussed these issues and has reviewed the pertinent literature relating to hospital PN and to HPN (233). Daily costs of HPN were estimated to be 60 to 70% lower than those of hospital PN. Goel has also summarized factors involved in cost-effectiveness analysis, the variability in determining precise costs, and the inclusion of effectiveness as measured by quality-adjusted life-year—a composite measure of life expectancy and morbidity.

A cost-effectiveness analysis of HPN in a cohort of 72 patients from 1970 to 1982 in Toronto was compared with the alternative costs that would have accrued from intermittent hospital care, including PN on each admission for the same patients not receiving HPN. It was concluded that HPN was cost-effective (234). In commenting on his study (234) and others, Detsky said, "Home parenteral nutrition is indeed a mature technology that almost certainly provides considerable survival benefit and reasonable quality of life. The estimated incremental cost-effectiveness ratio for this technology would even be better when delivered to patients without disseminated cancer or advanced HIV infection."

SMALL BOWEL TRANSPLANTATION

Successful small bowel transplantation was demonstrated to be technically feasible in laboratory animals in the late 1950s. Until the late 1980s, attempts were unsuccessful in patients because the immunosuppressive drugs available in that period could not prevent rejection of the transplanted intestine (235). With the availability of cyclosporine and tacrolimus, single successful transplants of isolated bowel were reported from Kiev and Paris (235), and a successful combined liver-small bowel transplantation was performed in London, Ontario (236). Today, tacrolimus is used almost exclusively for intestinal transplants (237). Three types of intestinal allografts are now being performed. For example,

between May 1990 and February 1995, the University of Pittsburgh's transplantation group performed 71 small bowel transplantations in 67 patients: 23 received an isolated intestine, 32 a combined intestine and liver, and 23 a multivisceral transplant (238).

A series of reviews summarizes techniques, problems, advances, and results (237–239). In an early review, survival and graft function were 58% and 50% at 18 months, respectively (238). Others have reported a survival of 69% (isolated intestine), 66% (intestinal/liver transplant), and 63% (multivisceral grafts) since 1995 (239). Successful small bowel grafts can absorb oral nutrients, including fat, despite denervation and disruption of lymphatics at the time of surgery. Therefore feeding jejunostomies are usually placed during the transplant, and enteral nutrition is usually begun by postoperative day 7 (237). This has allowed complete weaning from PN in a mean of 1 month according to most reports (237, 239). Within the International Intestinal Transplant Registry, 77% of patients undergoing intestinal transplantation have been completely weaned from PN, 14% require partial PN, and 9% still require complete PN (6% lost their graft, 3% still have the graft) (239).

The review of the International Intestinal Transplant Registry concludes: "to become the standard treatment for intestinal failure, transplantation must offer greater safety, lower costs, and a better quality of life than PN." Although progress has been made, "further refinements are needed before bowel transplantation becomes a routine surgical procedure" (240). Intestinal transplantation to date has been considered and performed in the context of serious hepatobiliary disease or loss of venous access, both secondary to PN complications (237–239).

EFFECTS OF TROPHIC AGENTS

Standard PN solutions cannot adequately support patients whose catabolic state is so advanced that they cannot develop a net positive peripheral uptake of amino acids despite adequate provision of energy and known essential nutrients (241). Strategies that have been adopted to try to improve this situation have included (a) having the patient perform regular exercise; (b) providing increased amounts of such nutrients such as arginine, BCAAs, n-3 polyunsaturated fatty acids, or glutamine; (c) blocking the signals of interleukins, which initiate responses to inflammation; (d) providing hormones and related growth factors that appear to enhance protein retention, such as recombinant human growth hormone, insulinlike growth factor-I, the β-adrenergic agonist clenbuterol, and low-dose bradykinin; and (e) a combination of the above.

There have been a large number of small clinical trials measuring the efficacy of human growth hormone or insulinlike growth factor-I. A multicenter study that was being conducted in Europe in critically ill patients was discontinued prematurely because the mortality rate was twice as high in the group receiving human growth hormone when compared with a placebo group (242). One hypothesis about this profound difference was the prevalence of hyperglycemia that almost universally occurs with administration of this hormone in critically ill patients.

The concept of using trophic agents with a modified diet was applied in an open study to selected patients with short bowel syndrome requiring HPN in an effort to increase hyperplasia and hypertrophy. Some 47 long-term patients who had no cancer, diabetes, dysmotility, inflammatory obstructive symptoms, or active inflammatory bowel disease were hospitalized on a regimen of diet (60% carbohydrate, 20% fat, and 20% protein), glutamine (0.6 g/kg/day) orally, and recombinant growth hormone (0.14 mg/kg/day) parenterally for 26 days (243). They were discharged on 30 g glutamine/day and the diet. After 4 weeks, 27 of the subjects were off PN, 14 were on reduced PN, and six were continued on PN. After 5 months to 5 years, 19 patients (40%) were off PN, an equal number were on reduced PN, and nine (20%) were on their original PN formula (243).

A study of eight long-term HPN patients compared the effects on bowel function of a similar triple regimen with those of placebo in a randomized, double-blind, crossover format (244). Although the treated patients had modest improvements in sodium and potassium absorption and in gastric emptying delay, there were no consistent improvements in small bowel morphology, stool losses, or macronutrient absorption. The two studies (243, 244) differed with respect to duration, degree of bowel resection, hospital stay and supervision, and route of medication administration. Two follow-up studies have not been able to produce the results observed in the initial study (245, 246). The three studies with negative results have studied very small patient populations with short bowel syndrome, enhancing the chance for a type 2 error.

A small clinical trial has demonstrated improvement in the Crohn's Disease Activity Index Score after human growth hormone administration in patients with this disease. It took 4 months of hormone administration before a significant difference in the above score was appreciated (247). This study suggests that a longer period of drug administration with growth hormone is needed before clinical and statistically significant results are observed. The potential role of glucagonlike peptide 2 is addressed in Chapter 75 on short bowel syndrome.

REFERENCES

1. Vinnars E, Wilmore D. JPEN J Parenter Enteral Nutr 2003;27: 225–31.
2. Schuberth O, Wretlind A. Acta Chir Scand 1961;278[Suppl]:1–21.
3. Dudrick S, Wilmore DW, Vars HM et al. Surgery 1968;64:134–42.
4. Anonymous. JPEN J Parenter Enteral Nutr 1993;17: 1SA–26SA.
5. Anonymous. JPEN J Parenter Enteral Nutr 2002;26:1SA–138SA.
6. Anonymous. JPEN J Parenter Enteral Nutr 1998;22:49–66.
6a. Anonymous. JPEN J Parenter Enteral Nutr 2004;28: S39–S70.
7. Anonymous. Gastroenterology 2001;121:966–9.
8. Co Tui, Wright AM, Mulholland JH et al. Ann Surg 1944;120: 99–122.
9. Co Tui, Wright AM, Mulholland JH et al. Gastroenterology 1945;5:5–17.
10. Anonymous. Nutr Clin Pract 2002;17:384–91.
11. Klein S, Kinney J, Jeejeebhoy K et al. Am J Clin Nutr 1997;66: 683–706.
12. Heyland DK, MacDonald S, Leefe L et al. JAMA 1998;280: 2013–9.
13. Jeejeebhoy KN. Am J Clin Nutr 2001;74:160–3.
14. Norwood S, Wilkins HE, Vallina VL et al. Crit Care Med 2000; 28:1376–82.
15. Kearns PJ, Coleman S, Wehner JH. JPEN J Parenter Enteral Nutr 1996;20:20–4.
16. Cowl CT, Weinstock JV, Al-Jurf A et al. Clin Nutr 2000;19: 237–43.
17. McGee DC, Gould MK. N Engl J Med 2003;348:1123.
18. Polderman KH, Girbes AR. Intensive Care Med 2002;28: 18–28.
19. Fonkalsrud EW, Berquist W, Burke M et al. Am J Surg 1982; 143:209–11.
20. Mansfield PE, Hohn DC, Fornage BD et al. N Engl J Med 1994;331:1735–8.
21. Clark-Christoff N, Watters VA, Sparks W et al. JPEN J Parenter Enteral Nutr 1992;16:403–7.
22. Kemp L, Burge J, Choban P et al. JPEN J Parenter Enteral Nutr 1994;18:71–4.
23. Timsit JF, Sebille V, Farkas JC et al. JAMA 1996;276:1416–20.
24. Maki DG, Stolz SM, Wheeler S et al. Ann Intern Med 1997; 127:257–66.
25. Raad I, Darouiche R, Dupuis J et al. Ann Intern Med 1997;127: 267–74.
26. Darouiche RO, Raad II, Heard SO et al. N Engl J Med 1999; 340:1–8.
27. Marin MG, Lee JC, Skurnick JH. Crit Care Med 2000;28: 3332–8.
28. Mermel LA. Ann Intern Med 2000;132:391–402.
29. Anonymous. MMWR Morb Mortal Wkly Rep 2002;51:1–26.
30. Shils ME. Am J Clin Nutr 1975;28:1429–35.
31. Newsome HH, Armstrong CW, Mayhall GC et al. JPEN J Parenter Enteral Nutr 1984;8:560–2.
32. Kite P, Dobbins BM, Wilcox MH et al. Lancet 1999;354: 1504–7.
33. Press OW, Ramsey PG, Larson EB et al. Medicine (Baltimore) 1984;63:189–200.
34. Peterson FB, Clift RA, Hickman RO et al. JPEN J Parenter Enteral Nutr 1986;10:58–62.
35. Buchman AL, Moukarzel A, Goodman B et al. JPEN J Parenter Enteral Nutr 1994;18:297–302.
36. O'Keefe SJ, Burnes JU, Thompson RL. JPEN J Parenter Enteral Nutr 1994;18:256–63.
37. Allwood MC. Int J Pharm 1986;29:233–6.
38. Bethune K, Dip PG, Allwood M et al. Nutrition 2001;17:403–8.
39. Hill SE, Heldman S, Goo ED et al. JPEN J Parenter Enteral Nutr 1996;20:81–7.
40. Alcutt A, Lort D, McCollum N. Br J Surg 1983;70:111.
41. Seres DS. Nutr Clin Pract 1990;5:111–7.
42. McMahon M, Manji N, Driscoll DF et al. JPEN J Parenter Enteral Nutr 1989;13:545–53.
43. Marcuard SP, Dunham B, Hobbs A et al. JPEN J Parenter Enteral Nutr 1990;14:262–4.
44. Smith RC, Burkinshaw L, Hill GL. Gastroenterology 1982;82: 445–52.

45. Shaw SN, Elwyn DH, Askanazi J et al. Am J Clin Nutr 1983; 37:930–40.
46. Rudman E, Millikan WJ, Richardson TJ et al. J Clin Invest 1975;55:94–104.
47. Starker PM, LaSala PA, Forse A et al. JPEN J Parenter Enteral Nutr 1985;9:300–2.
48. Lev-Ram A, Johnson J, Hwang DL et al. JPEN J Parenter Enteral Nutr 1987;11:271–4.
49. Byrne WJ, Lippe BM, Strobel CT et al. Gastroenterology 1981; 80:947–56.
50. Krzywda A, Andris DA, Whipple JK et al. JPEN J Parenter Enteral Nutr 1993;17:64–7.
51. Bendorf K, Friesen CA, Roberts CC. JPEN J Parenter Enteral Nutr 1996;20:120–2.
52. Wolfe R, ODonnell TF, Stone MD et al. Metabolism 1980;29: 892–900.
53. Elwyn DH, Gump FE, Munroe HN et al. Am J Clin Nutr 1979;32:1597–611.
54. Askanazi J, Carpentier YA, Elwyn DH et al. Ann Surg 1980;191: 40–6.
55. MacFie J, Halmfield JH, King RF et al. JPEN J Parenter Enteral Nutr 1983;7:1–5.
56. Chait A, Foster D, Miller DG et al. Proc Soc Exp Biol Med 1981;168:97–104.
57. McCowen KC, Malhotra A, Bistrian BR. Crit Care Clin 2001;17:107–24.
58. McCowen KC, Ling PR, Ciccarone A et al. Crit Care Med 2001;29:839–46.
59. Pomposelli JJ, Baxter JJ, Babineau TJ et al. JPEN J Parenter Enteral Nutr 1998;22:77–81.
60. Perner A, Nielsen SE, Rask-Madsen J. Intensive Care Med 2003;29:642–5.
61. Gore DC, Chinkes DL, Hart DW et al. Crit Care Med 2002;30: 2438–42.
62. Thomas SJ, Morimoto K, Herndon DN et al. Surgery 2002;132: 341–7.
63. Van den Berghe G, Wouters P, Weekers F et al. N Engl J Med 2001;345:1359–67.
64. Finney SJ, Zekveld C, Elia A et al. JAMA 2003;290:2041–7.
65. Van den Berghe G, Wouters PJ, Bouillon R et al. Crit Care Med 2003;31:359–66.
66. Lazar HL, Chipkin SR, Fitzgerald CA et al. Circulation 2004; 109:1497–502.
67. Jeschke MG, Klein D, Herndon DN. Ann Surg 2004;239: 553–60.
68. McCowen KC, Friel C, Sternberg J et al. Crit Care Med 2000; 28:3606–11.
69. Patino JF, de Pimiento SE, Vergara A et al. World J Surg 1999; 23:553–9.
70. Askanazi J, Rosenbaum SH, Hyman AI et al. JAMA 1980;243: 1444–7.
71. Kalfarentzos F, Kokkinis K, Leukaditi K et al. Clin Nutr 1998; 17:31–4.
72. Barr LH, Dunn GD, Brennan ME. Surgery 1981;193:304–11.
73. Kemin Q, Maysoon A, Seo T et al. JPEN J Parenter Enteral Nutr 2003;27:58–64.
74. Carpentier YA. Clin Nutr 1989;8:115–25.
75. Mendez AJ, He LJ, Huang HS et al. Lipids 1988;23:961–7.
76. Griffin E, Breckenridge C, Kuksis A et al. J Clin Invest 1979;64: 1703–12.
77. Roulet M, Wiesel PH, Filet M et al. JPEN J Parenter Enteral Nutr 1993;17:107–12.
78. Rigaud D, Serog P, Legrand A et al. JPEN J Parenter Enteral Nutr 1984;8:529–34.
79. Adamkin DH, Gelke KN, Andrews BE. JPEN J Parenter Enteral Nutr 1984;8:563–7.
80. Llop J, Sabin P, Garau M et al. Clin Nutr 2003;22:577–83.
81. Elwyn DH, Kinney JM, Gump FE et al. Metabolism 1980;29: 125–32.
82. Goodenough RD, Wolfe RR. JPEN J Parenter Enteral Nutr 1984;8:357–60.
83. Elwyn DH. Repletion of the malnourished patient. In: Blackburn GL, Grant JP, Young VR et al., eds. Amino Acids: Metabolism and Medical Application. Boston: John Wright/PSG, 1983: 359–75.
84. Jeejeebhoy KN. Lipid emulsions. In: Fischer JE, ed. Total Parenteral Nutrition. 2nd ed. Boston: Little, Brown, 1991:410–3.
85. Driscoll DF. JPEN J Parenter Enteral Nutr 2003;27:433–8.
86. Driscoll DF, Bhargava HN, Li L et al. Am J Hosp Pharm 1995;52:623–34.
87. Rubin M, Bilik R, Aserin A et al. JPEN J Parenter Enteral Nutr 1989;13:641–3.
88. Holcombe BJ, Forloines-Lynn S, Garmhausen LW. J Intrav Nurs 1992;15:36–41.
89. Venus B, Smith RA, Patel C et al. Chest 1989;95:1278–81.
90. Gutcher GR, Farrell PM. Am J Clin Nutr 1991;54:1024–8.
91. Sobrado J, Moldawer L, Pomposelli JJ et al. Am J Clin Nutr 1985;42:855–63.
92. Seidner DL, Mascioli EA, Istfan NW et al. JPEN J Parenter Enteral Nutr 1987;13:614–9.
93. Jensen GL, Mascioli EA, Seidner DL et al. JPEN J Parenter Enteral Nutr 1990;14:467–71.
94. Ota DM, Jessup JM, Babcock GE et al. JPEN J Parenter Enteral Nutr 1985;9:23–7.
95. Muller JM, Keller HW, Brenner U et al. World J Surg 1986;10: 53–63.
96. American College of Physicians. Ann Intern Med 1989;110: 734–6.
97. Desai TK, Kinzie J. JPEN J Parenter Enteral Nutr 1990;14: 75(abst).
98. Freeman J, Goldmann DA, Smith NE et al. N Engl J Med 1990;323:301–8(letter).
99. Lenssen P, Bruemmer BA, Bowden RA et al. Am J Clin Nutr 1998;67:927–33.
100. Nijveldt RJ, Tan AM, Prins HA et al. Clin Nutr 1998;17:23–9.
101. Rubin M, Moser A, Vaserberg N et al. Nutrition 2000;16: 95–100.
102. Baldermann H, Wicklmayr M, Rett K et al. JPEN J Parenter Enteral Nutr 1991;15:601–3.
103. Sandstrom R, Hyltander A, Krner V et al. JPEN J Parenter Enteral Nutr 1993;17:153–7.
104. Sandstrom R, Hyltander A, Krner V et al. JPEN J Parenter Enteral Nutr 1995;19:381–6.
105. Goulet O, de Potter S, Antebi H et al. Am J Clin Nutr 1999;70: 338–45.
106. Mashima Y, Tashiro T, Yamamori H et al. Advances in Polyunsaturated Fatty Acid Research. New York: Elsevier Science, 1993:239–40.
107. Morlion BJ, Torwesten E, Lessire H et al. Metabolism 1996;45: 1208–13.
108. Furukawa K, Tashiro T, Yamamori H et al. Ann Surg 1999;229: 255–61.
109. Tappenden KA, Thomson ABR, Wild GE et al. Gastroenterology 1997;112:792–802.
110. Lowrey TS, Dulap AW, Brown RO, et al. Nutr Clin Pract 1996; 11:147–9.
111. Kearns LR, Phillips MC, Ness-Abramof R et al. Nutr Clin Pract 2001;16:219–25.

112. Garcia-de-Lorenzo A, Oritz-Leyba C, Planas M et al. Crit Care Med 1997;25:418–24.

113. Brennan MF, Cerra F, Daly JM et al. JPEN J Parenter Enteral Nutr 1986;10:446–52.

114. Von Meyenfeldt MF, Soeters PB, Vente JP et al. Br J Surg 1990;77:924–9.

115. Anonymous. JPEN J Parenter Enteral Nutr 2002;26[Suppl]: 65SA–8SA

116. Patton KM, Aranda-Michel J. Nutr Clin Pract 2002;17:332–40.

117. Yeh CL, Yeh SL, Lin MT et al. Nutrition 2002;18:631–5.

118. Hornsby-Lewis L, Shike M, Brown P et al. JPEN J Parenter Enteral Nutr 1994;18:266–7.

119. Ziegler TR, Young LS, Benfell K et al. Ann Intern Med 1992; 116:821–8.

120. Schloerb PR, Amare M. JPEN J Parenter Enteral Nutr 1993; 17:407–13.

121. Stehle P, Zander J, Merten N et al. Lancet 1989;1:231–3.

122. Tremel H, Kienle B, Sacha L et al. Gastroenterology 1994;107: 1595–601.

123. Morlion BJ, Stehle P, Wachtler P et al. Ann Surg 1998;227: 302–8.

124. van der Hulst R, van Kreel BK, von Meyenfeldt MF et al. Lancet 1993;341:363–5.

125. Novak F, Heyland DK, Avenell A et al. Crit Care Med 2002;30: 2022–9.

126. Griffiths RD, Allen KD, Andrews FJ et al. Nutrition 2002;18: 546–52.

127. Goeters C, Wenn A, Mertes N et al. Crit Care Med 202;30: 2032–7.

128. Furst P, Albers S, Stehle P. JPEN J Parenter Enteral Nutr 1990;14[Suppl]:118S–24S.

129. Adibi SA. Metab Clin Exp 1987;36:1001–11.

130. Vazquez IA, Paleos GA, Steinhardt HJ et al. Am J Clin Nutr 1986;44:24–32.

131. Maroulis J, Kalfarentzos F. Clin Nutr 2000;19:295–304.

132. Dunham B, Marcuard S, Khazanie PG et al. JPEN J Parenter Enteral Nutr 1991;15:608–11.

133. Greene HL, Hambidge M, Schanler R et al. Am J Clin Nutr 1988;48:1324–42.

134. Berkelhammer CH, Wood RJ, Sitrin MD. Am J Clin Nutr 1988; 48:1482–9.

135. Goodman WG, Misra S, Veldhuis JD et al. Am J Clin Nutr 2000; 71:560–8.

136. Clark CL, Sacks GS, Dickerson RN et al. Crit Care Med 1995; 23:1504–11.

137. Charon T, Bernard F, Skrobik Y et al. Intensive Care Med 2003;29:1273–8.

138. Sacks GS, Brown RO, Dickerson RN et al. Nutrition 1997;13: 303–8.

139. Shils ME, Burke AW, Greene HL et al. JAMA 1979;241: 2051–4.

140. Wolman SL, Anderson GH, Marliss EB et al. Gastroenterology 1979;76:458–67.

141. Solomons NW, Layden TJ, Rosenberg IH et al. Gastroenterology 1976;70:1022–5.

142. Shike M, Roulet M, Kurian R et al. Gastroenterology 1981;81: 290–7.

143. Spiegel JE, Willenbucher RF. JPEN J Parenter Enteral Nutr 1999;23:169–72.

144. Kurkus J, Alcock NW, Shils ME. JPEN J Parenter Enteral Nutr 1984;8:254–7.

145. Shike M, Ritchie ME, Shils ME. Clin Res 1986;34:804A(abst).

146. Fell JME, Reynolds AP, Meadows N et al. Lancet1996;347: 1218–21.

147. Ono J, Harada K, Kodaka R et al. JPEN J Parenter Enteral Nutr 1995;19:310–2.

148. Ejima A, Imanura T, Nakamura S et al. Lancet 1992;339:426 (letter).

149. Bertinet DB, Tinivella M, Balzola FA et al. JPEN J Parenter Enteral Nutr 2000;24:223–7.

150. Reimund JM, Dietemann JL, Warter JM et al. Clin Nutr 2000; 19:343–8.

151. Takagi Y, Okada A, Sando K et al. Am J Clin Nutr 2002; 75:112–8.

152. Siepler JK, Nishikawa RA, Diamantidis T et al. Nutr Clin Pract 2003;18:370–3.

153. Reynolds N, Blumsohn A, Baxter JP et al. Clin Nutr 1998;17: 227–30.

154. Hambidge KM, Sokol RJ, Fidanze SJ et al. JPEN J Parenter Enteral Nutr 1989;13:168–71.

155. Mirowitz SA, Westrich TJ, Hirsch JD. Radiology 1991;181: 117–20.

156. Mirowitz SA, Westrich TJ. Radiology 1992;185:535–6.

157. Alves G, Thiebot J, Tracqui A et al. JPEN J Parenter Enteral Nutr 1997;21:41–5.

158. Verhage AH, Cheong WK, Jeejeebhoy K. JPEN J Parenter Enteral Nutr 1996;20:123–7.

159. Kien CL, Veillon C, Patterson KY et al. JPEN J Parenter Enteral Nutr 1986;10:662–4.

160. Moukarzel AA, Song MK, Buchman AL et al. Lancet 1992;339: 385–8.

161. Van Rijn AM, Thompson CD, McKenzie JM, et al. Am J Clin Nutr 1979;43:2076–85.

162. Cohen HJ, Brown MR, Hamilton D et al. Am J Clin Nutr 1989; 49:132–9.

163. Abumrad NN, Schneider AJ, Steel D et al. Am J Clin Nutr 1981;34:2551–9.

164. Klein GA. Am J Clin Nutr 1995;61:449–56.

165. Klein GL, Alfrey AC, Miller NL et al. Am J Clin Nutr 1982;35: 1425–9.

166. Wu WW, Kaplan LA, Horn J et al. JPEN J Parenter Enteral Nutr 1986;10:591–5.

167. Bishop NJ, Morley R, Day JP et al. N Engl J Med 1997;336: 1557–61.

168. Klein GL, Alfrey AA, Shike M et al. Am J Clin Nutr 1991;53: 399–402.

169. Vanamee P, Shils ME, Burke AW et al. JPEN J Parenter Enteral Nutr 1979;3:258–62.

170. De Ritter EJ. Pharm Sci 1982;71:1073–96.

171. Kirkemo AK, Burt ME, Brennan M. Am J Clin Nutr 1982;35: 1003–9.

172. Thomas MK, Lloyd-Jones DM, Thadhani RI et al. N Engl J Med 1998;338:777–83.

173. Anonymous. Nutrition 1999;15:92–6.

174. Buckman AL, Sohel M, Brown M et al. JPEN J Parenter Enteral Nutr 2000;25:30–5.

175. Compher CW, Kinosian BP, Stoner NE et al. JPEN J Parenter Enteral Nutr 2002;26:57–62.

176. Shils ME, Baker H, Frank O. JPEN J Parenter Enteral Nutr 1985;9:179–88.

177. Chen F, Boyce HW, Tripiett L. JPEN J Parenter Enteral Nutr 1983;7:462–4.

178. Steephen AC, Traber MG, Ito Y et al. JPEN J Parenter Enteral Nutr 1991;15:647–52.

179. Lemoyne M, Gossum AV, Kurian R et al. Am J Clin Nutr 1988; 48:1310–5.

180. Greene HL, Smith R, Pollack P et al. J Am Coll Nutr 1991; 10:281–8.

181. Centers for Disease Control and Prevention. MMWR Morb Mortal Wkly Rep 1997;46:523–8.

182. Centers for Disease Control and Prevention. MMWR Morb Mortal Wkly Rep 1989;38:43–6.

183. Zak J, Burns D, Lingenfelser T et al. JPEN J Parenter Enteral Nutr 1991;15:200–1.

184. Buchman A. JPEN J Parenter Enteral Nutr 2002;26[Suppl]: S43–8.

185. Guglielmi FW, Penco JM, Gentile A et al. Clin Nutr 2001; 20[Suppl]:51–5.

186. Peden Y, Witzleben C, Shelton M et al. J Pediatr 1971;78: 180(letter).

187. Bell RL, Ferry GD, Smith EO et al. JPEN J Parenter Enteral Nutr 1986;10:356–9.

188. Clayton PT, Bowron A, Mills KA et al. Gastroenterology 1993; 105:1806–13.

189. Messing B, Colombel JF, Heresbach D et al. Nutrition 1992;8: 30–6.

190. Wagner WH, Lowry AC, Silberman H. Am J Gastroenterol 1983;78:199–202.

191. Buchmiller CE, Kleiman-Wexler RL, Ephgrave KS et al. JPEN J Parenter Enteral Nutr 1993;17:301–6.

192. Payne-James JJ, Silk DB. Dig Dis Sci 1991;9:10–24.

193. Lambert JP, Thomas SM. JPEN J Parenter Enteral Nutr 1985; 9:501–3.

194. Lindor KD, Burnes J. Gastroenterology 1991;101:250–3.

195. Spagnuolo MM, Iorio R, Vegnente A et al. Gastroenterology 1996;111:716–9.

196. Duerksen DR, van Aerde JE, Gramlich L et al. Gastroenterology 1996;111:111–17.

197. Teitelbaum DH, Han-Marker T, Drongowski RA et al. JPEN J Parenter Enteral Nutr 1997;21:100–3.

198. Buchman AL, Dubin M, Venden D et al. Gastroenterology 1992;102:1363–70.

199. Tazuke Y, Kiristioglu I, Heidelberger KP et al. JPEN J Parenter Enteral Nutr 2004;28:1–6.

200. Muller EL, Grace FA, Pitt HA. J Surg Res 1986;40:55–62.

201. Messing B, Bories C, Kustlinger F et al. Gastroenterology 1983; 84:1012–9.

202. Dory JE, Pitt HA, Porter-Fink V et al. Ann Surg 1985;201:76–80.

203. Broughton G, Fitzgibbons RJ, Geiss RW et al. JPEN J Parenter Enteral Nutr 1996;20:187–93.

204. Roslyn JJ, Berquist WE, Pitt HA et al. Pediatrics 1983;71: 784–9.

205. Dorney SF, Ament ME, Berquist WE et al. J Pediatr 1985;107: 521–5.

206. Goulet ON, Revillion Y, Jan D et al. J Pediatr 1991;119:18–23.

207. Roslyn JJ, Pitt HA, Mann LL. Am J Surg 1984;148:58–63.

208. Miltenburg DM, Schaffer R III, Breslin T et al. Pediatrics 2000;105:1250–3.

209. Seidner DL. JPEN J Parenter Enteral Nutr 2002;26[Suppl]: S37–S42.

210. Buchman AL, Moukarzel A. Clin Nutr 2000;19:217–31.

211. Pironi L, Morselli AM, Pertkiewicz M et al. Clin Nutr 2002;21: 289–96.

212. Shike M, Harrison JE, Sturtridge WC et al. Ann Intern Med 1980;92:343–50.

213. Shike M, Sturtridge WC, Tam CS et al. Ann Intern Med 1981; 95:560–8.

214. Verhage AH, Cheong WI, Allard JP et al. JPEN J Parenter Enteral Nutr 1995;19:431–6.

215. Shike M, Shils ME, Heller A et al. Am J Clin Nutr 1986;44: 89–98.

216. Saitta JC, Ou SM, Sherrard DJ et al. JPEN J Parenter Enteral Nutr 1993;17:214–9.

217. Pironi L, Zolezzi C, Ruggeri E et al. Nutrition 2000;16:272–7.

218. Feskanich D, Weber, P, Willett WC et al. Am J Clin Nutr 1999; 69:74–9.

219. Wood RJ, Sitrin MD, Rosenberg IH. Am J Clin Nutr 1988;48: 632–6.

220. Berkelhammer C, Wood RJ, Sitrin MD. JPEN J Parenter Enteral Nutr 1998;22:142–6.

221. Mirtallo JM. Parenteral formulas. In: Rombeau JL, Rolandelli RH, eds. Parenteral Nutrition. 3rd ed. Philadelphia: WB Saunders, 2001:118–39.

222. Trissel LA, Gilbert DL, Martinez JF et al. Am J Health Syst Pharm 1997;54:1295–300.

223. Trissel LA, Gilbert DL, Martinez JF et al. JPEN J Parenter Enteral Nutr 1999;23:67–74.

224. Shils ME, Wright WL, Turnbull A et al. N Engl J Med 1970; 283:341–4.

225. Delegge MH. JPEN J Parenter Enteral Nutr 2002;26[Suppl]: S60–2.

226. Howard L, Ament M, Fleming CR et al. Gastroenterology 1995;109:355–65.

227. Howard L, Malone M. Am J Clin Nutr 1997;66:1364–70.

228. Egger NG, Carlson GL, Shaffer JL. Nutrition 1999;15:1–6.

229. Howard L, Ashley C. Gastroenterology 2003;124:1651–61.

230. Gulledge AD, Srp F, Sharp JW et al. Nutr Clin Pract 1987;2: 183–94.

231. Smith CE. JPEN J Parenter Enteral Nutr 1993;17:501–6.

232. Howard L, Heaphey L, Fleming CR et al. JPEN J Parenter Enteral Nutr 1991;15:384–93.

233. Goel V. Program in Technology and Health Care. Washington, DC: Georgetown University School of Medicine, 1989:41–51.

234. Detsky AS, McLaughlin JR, Abrams HB et al. JPEN J Parenter Enteral Nutr 1986;10:49–57.

235. Wood RF, Ingraham-Clark CL. Br Med J 1992;304:1453–4.

236. Grant D, Wall W, Mimeault R et al. Lancet 1990;335:181–4.

237. Janson DD. Nutr Clin Pract 2002;17:361–4.

238. Lee RG, Nakamura K, Tsamandas AC et al. Gastroenterology 1996;110:1820–34.

239. Iyer KR. JPEN J Parenter Enteral Nutr 2002;26[Suppl]: S49–S54.

240. Grant D, International Intestinal Transplant Registry. Lancet 1996;347:1801–3.

241. Wilmore DW. N Engl J Med 1991;325:695–702.

242. Takala J, Ruokonen E, Webster NR et al. N Engl J Med 1999; 341:785–92.

243. Byrne TA, Persinger RL, Young LS et al. Ann Surg 1995;222: 243–55.

244. Scolapio JS, Camilleri M, Fleming CR et al. Gastroenterology 1997;113:1074–81.

245. Scolapio JS. JPEN J Parenter Enteral Nutr 1999;23:309–13.

246. Szkudlarek J, Jeppesen PB, Mortensen PB. Gut 2000;47: 199–205.

247. Slonim AE, Bulone L, Damore MB et al. N Engl J Med 2000; 342:1633–7.

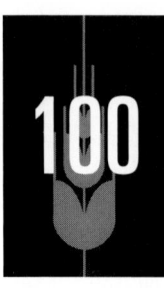

100 CHRONIC DISEASE MANAGEMENT: THE TEAM APPROACH[1]

MAURICE E. SHILS, ABBY S. BLOCH, AND PATRICIA BROWN

EXTENT AND COSTS OF CHRONIC DISEASES 1599
ADEQUACY OF MEDICAL CARE 1599
   Inadequate Adherence to Quality Guidelines . . .1599
   Problems in Adherence to Prescriptions
      and Directives 1600
   Increasing Difficulties in Meeting Health
      Care Costs 1600
CHANGING RELATIONS OF PHYSICIANS
   TO PATIENTS 1600
   Hospitalists 1600
   Increasing Nonphysician Clinical Professionals . .1601
CHANGING ATTITUDES IN PHYSICIAN-PATIENT
   RELATIONS 1601
   The Chronic Care Model 1602
   Involvement of Nonphysician Professionals 1602
   Recent Appraisals of Quality Care by
      Professional Societies 1605
NEED FOR ADDITIONAL SUPPORT PROGRAMS 1605
   Community Support 1605
   Improved Communication and
      Information Systems 1605
   Demonstration and Evaluation Projects 1605
   Medical School Changes 1605
   Professional Societies .1606
   Federal Agencies 1606
   Lay Workers 1606

It may appear somewhat strange to a potential reader checking titles in this book to find another chapter title concerned with chronic disease and to note that this chapter is in a section concerned with systems of nutrition support. Nevertheless, there are at least two related major reasons for this chapter and its placement: first, the increasing close relationships of various chronic diseases with nutrition, and second, increasing recognition that multiprofessional team interactions may well improve prevention and management of these diseases. As authors, our interest in clinical teams stems from our close interaction as physician, dietitian, and

nurse members of a hospital clinical nutrition team concerned with the education and management of seriously ill patients who required long-term nutrition support.

We present five brief statements from the literature that delineate the areas of concern better than does the list of section titles.

"We have observed a growing sense of dissatisfaction among both patients and professionals with programs that are not relevant, and, an increased awareness of the need to develop programs that are adequate to deal with the complexities of living with a chronic illness such as diabetes." Funnell, Anderson, Arnold et al., 1991 (1).

"Shifting from the acute-care/compliance-focused paradigm to an empowerment/collaborative approach requires a new vision of diabetes education and a new definition and enactment of the roles of educators and patients." Anderson and Funnell, 2002 (2).

"A more clinical argument against the focus on patient safety is that medical injuries do not cause as many deaths as errors of omission . . . Our health care system fails with embarrassing frequency to provide medical interventions known to benefit patients. These failures are not the fault of physicians alone, they reflect poor coordination among all parties including patients." Lee, 2002 (3).

"In a population increasingly afflicted by chronic conditions, the health care system is poorly organized to provide care to those with such conditions." Committee on the Quality of Health Care in America, 2001 (4).

"As its ultimate goal, the chronic care model envisions an informed, activated patient interacting with a prepared, proactive team, resulting in high-quality, satisfying encounters and improved outcomes." Bodenheimer, Wagner, and Grumbach, 2002 (5).

The second and final report of the Committee on the Quality of Health Care in America of the Institute of Medicine (IOM), National Academies of Science is concerned with issues about the health care delivered to US residents and how the system can be improved (4). After reviewing various quality problems, the report lists four key aspects that help explain the problems: "The growing complexity of science and technology, *the increase in chronic conditions* [emphasis ours], a poorly organized delivery system, and constraints of exploiting the revolution in information technology" (4). The same Executive Summary states: "To initiate the process of change, the committee believes the

---

[1] **Abbreviations: ADA,** American Dietetic Association; **CV,** cardiovascular; **HMO,** health maintenance organization; **IOM,** Institute of Medicine; **MNT,** medical nutrition therapy; **NHANES,** National Health and Nutrition Examination Survey.

health care system must focus greater attention on the developments of care processes for the common conditions that affect many people. A limited number of such conditions, about 15 to 25, account for the majority of health care services . . . nearly all of these conditions are chronic . . . Care of the chronically ill needs to be a collaborative, multidisciplinary process. Effective methods of communication, both among caregivers and between caregivers and patients, are critical to providing high quality care" (4).

EXTENT AND COSTS OF CHRONIC DISEASES

This IOM report defines a chronic condition as "an illness that lasts longer than 3 weeks and that is not self-limiting" (4). It cites a 1996 Robert Wood Johnson Foundation report noting that chronic conditions affected about 100 million US residents, the number could grow to 134 million by 2020, disabling chronic conditions affect all age groups, and about two thirds of those with such conditions were less than 65 years of age. In 1990, the direct medical cost for such conditions was $425 billion, nearly 70% of all personal health care expenditures. Lost productivity resulting from premature death or inability to work added another $234 billion.

As pointed out in a joint scientific statement of the American Cancer Society, the American Diabetes Association, and the American Heart Association, cardiovascular (CV) diseases, cancer, and diabetes accounted for nearly two of every three deaths in the United States, about 1.5 million people in 2001 (6). The number of prevalent cases in the United States estimated in 2001 was 64,400,000 of CV diseases; 9,600,000 of cancer; and 18,200,000 of diabetes.

In a prospective study of more than 900,000 US adults, who were free of cancer in 1982, there were 57,145 deaths from cancer during 16 years of follow-up (7). In those with a body mass index of 40 or more in 1982, the death rates from all cancers were 52% higher for men and 62% higher for women than in those of normal weight. It was estimated that the current patterns of overweight and obesity could account for 14 and 20%, respectively, of all deaths from cancer in men and women.

Excess body weight is also an independent risk factor for stroke. The percentage of patients hospitalized for ischemic stroke increased from 16 to 30% with an increase of 3 kg/m^2 in body mass index (8).

From 1990 to 2001, the prevalence of diabetes increased by 61%. This increase, primarily in type 2 diabetes, which accounts for 90 to 95% of all diagnosed cases, was attributed to major increases in body weight occurring in the United States during that period (9).

Among adults at least 20 years of age in data from the 1999–2002 National Health and Nutrition Examination Survey, 65.1% were overweight or obese, and among children aged 6 through 19 years, in 1999 to 2002, 31.0% were at risk of overweight or were overweight, whereas 16.0%

were obese (10, 11). The ominous clinical significance of these statistics is reflected in reports of the occurrence of type 2 diabetes in children (12), the finding of high blood pressure in overweight and obese children (13), and the prevalence of the metabolic syndrome among obese children and adolescents (12).

A recent report estimated the level and the change in health care spending between 1997 (evaluating 34,459 persons) and 2000 (evaluating 25,096 persons) for noninstitutionalized persons (14). The report noted that 15 medical conditions accounted for between 43 and 61% of inflation-adjusted growth of the $199 billion in these 13 years. Most of this growth was for care of people with chronic diseases, with the greatest increases for CV disease, pulmonary conditions, mental disorders, cancer, and hypertension. The rise in treated disease prevalence was a key factor accounting for the rise in spending. There was a 59% spending increase for mental disorders, a 60% increase for stroke and cerebral ischemia, a 42% increase for pulmonary disorders, a 50% increase for arthritis, and a 19% increase for hypertension. For some of these diseases, a rise in the costs per treated case accounted for most of the growth in spending; this was particularly the case for CV disease (69%) and hypertension (60%). Population growth accounted for about 19 to 35% of the increase in spending for the top 15 medical conditions.

ADEQUACY OF MEDICAL CARE

The 2001 IOM report lists poorly organized delivery systems of patient care as one of the key aspects of problems of medical care (4).

Inadequate Adherence to Quality Guidelines

A major study by McGlynn, Asch, Adams, and coworkers evaluated the quality of care for a broad spectrum of medical conditions by obtaining information directly from patients and from their medical records over a recent 2-year period in 12 metropolitan areas across the United States (15). National guidelines and other proposed indicators of quality for all phases of screening, diagnoses, treatment, and follow-up were used to assess potential problems with overuse or underuse of key processes. The proportion of recommended acute care actually provided was 53.5%, whereas the recommended care for chronic conditions actually provided was 56.1%. The specific percentages (with 95% confidence limits) of recommended care actually received for various chronic disease states were as follows: coronary artery disease, 68.0 (64.2–71.8); hypertension, 64.7 (62.6–66.7); CV disease, 59.1 (49.7–68.4); asthma, 53.8 (50.0–57.0); hyperlipidemia, 48.6 (44.1–53.2); diabetes mellitus, 45.4 (42.7–48.3); and atrial fibrillation, 24.7 (18.4–30.9).

In the 1999–2000 NHANES cross-sectional surveys of persons previously diagnosed with diabetes mellitus, only 7.3% (confidence interval, 2.8–11.9%) of these adults attained the recommended goals for glycosylated hemoglobin, blood pressure, and total cholesterol (16). As a result of poor clinical management, it was estimated that men in the United States who have this disease at age 40 years will lose almost 12 years of life and 19.6 quality-adjusted life years. Women of this age will lose 14.3 life years and 22 quality-adjusted life years (17).

Ades estimates that the percentage of eligible patients who participate in formal programs of cardiac rehabilitation varies from 10 to 47% (18). After he reviewed the deficiencies of care of chronically ill patients, Ades listed the components of cardiac rehabilitation and associated goals in a table covering almost a full page of small type. He noted management issues including those for hyperlipidemias, hypertension, diabetes, psychologic aspects, weight reduction, cessation of smoking, physical activity, diet or other counseling, and training. Missing in the author's plan is a clear statement of how health professionals other than the primary physician could or should be involved, particularly in a setting in which some such patients would require long-term and complex management.

In a 2-year period in which 2804 persons sustained a study-defined bone fracture (of whom 80.7% were women), only 8.4% had bone density measurements, and of these, only 42.4% had pharmacologic treatment during those years (19). Approximately 95.5% of men in the study were not evaluated or treated in accordance with guideline recommendations.

In persons with atrial fibrillation who are at risk of ischemic stroke, data indicate that only approximately one third to slightly more than one half of those actually receive warfarin therapy that can reduce risk substantially; elderly patients are the least likely to be treated (20). For additional reports of underuse of both screening for chronic disease and their available treatments, Table A-1 in reference 4 summarizes the data of more than 70 surveys published between 1993 and 1998.

Problems in Adherence to Prescriptions and Directives

For those patients who initiate medications for one or more chronic diseases, long-term adherence is frequently problematic. Elderly patients in a study in New Jersey had the proportion of days with statin ingestion at 79% in the first 3 months of treatment, 56% in the second 3-month period, and 42% after 120 months; only one patient in four maintained an 80% rate of medication use after 5 years (21). The 2-year adherence rates to this class of drugs were 40.1% among those with recent acute coronary syndrome (22,379 patients started), 36.1% among those with chronic coronary artery disease (36,106 patients started), and 25.4% among those taking the drugs for primary prevention (85,020 patients started) (22).

In an accompanying editorial, Applegate discussed the problem of poor adherence to physician recommendations

and some of the causes. He noted that other studies revealed similar adherence problems for prescribed medications and procedures in the management of hyperlipidemias, hypertension, and heart failure (23).

An interesting statistic concerning physician-patient relations is the finding that only one third of those patients who underuse statins because of cost ever discussed this issue with their physicians in advance; many never discussed this issue at all (24).

Patient Health Literacy

Nearly one half of adults in the United States have trouble interpreting medical information, according to two recent reports (25, 26). Consent forms, prescription drug directives, and oral instructions are considered overly complex or poorly communicated. These problems have resulted in errors, mistakes in prescription ingestion, failed appointments, health problems, inflated costs, and extra work for professionals. The Agency for Healthcare Research and Quality report that reviewed the literature on the health impacts of low reading and comprehension skills linked these issues to higher rates of hospitalization, greater use of emergency services, and a decreased likelihood of having had tests for cancer in women. Patients with better reading skills tended to use more preventive services (25).

The IOM report called for integrating health literacy into the curricula from elementary schools through medical school. It noted that some medical schools offer specific health literacy training for better patient communication (26).

Increasing Difficulties in Meeting Health Care Costs

Peter Bendetti compared health care insurance status changes in the United States between 1993 and 2003. The number of uninsured people increased from 39.7 million to 45 million in these 10 years. Between 2000 and 2003, nearly 4 million workers lost employee-sponsored insurance, whereas those employed now share health care costs that are increasing faster than their income. He concluded that the problems of uninsurance, uncompensated care, high cost, poor quality, and limited access remain (27).

CHANGING RELATIONS OF PHYSICIANS TO PATIENTS

Over the past 30 or so years, the time spent by physicians in hospitals caring for their private patients has decreased from an estimated 40% to about 10% (28).

Hospitalists

In recent years, hospitals, medical groups, and health maintenance organizations (HMOs) with no associated house staff have employed physicians, termed "hospitalists," who care for their hospitalized patients; on discharge, the patients return to the care of their original physicians (28, 29). The estimated number of hospitalists has increased to approximately 8000, with further growth projected (28).

A decrease in ambulatory care for patients with chronic disease is reflected in the progressive decline (~50%) in medical school graduates matching for the family practice specialty between 1997 and 2002 (30).

Increased hospitalist time in patient care has been associated with reduced duration of length of patient stay in hospitals. This leads us to ask: For the patient with a newly diagnosed chronic disease, who on discharge will have care transferred to his or her busy personal physician on an outpatient basis, how much in-hospital training has occurred to improve understanding and self-involvement in care? Has the shortened hospital stay reduced the opportunity for important self-care training for patients with chronic disease? One would also be interested in knowing whether Medicare or insurance companies that may save money by the shortened stays are using the savings for outpatient education.

Increasing Nonphysician Clinical Professionals

As noted by Aiken, the ratio of physicians to nonphysician health care workers in 1900 was approximately one in three; in the early 1980s, the ratio was one in 16, with a continuing rise in the denominator (31). Trends in outpatient care provided by physicians and nonphysician clinicians between 1987 and 1997 indicate a rise from 30.6 to 36.1% in visits to the nonphysicians; the trend also indicates an increase in those who visit both (32).

One of the issues raised by Druss and colleagues in their survey (32) of this issue (but that they do not answer) is this: How much of the involvement by the nonphysician clinicians is cooperative and how much is competitive? Of the ten different nonphysician health care workers listed (physician assistants, nurses, chiropractors, physical or nonoccupational therapists, psychologist, optometrists, podiatrists, social workers, midwives, and "others"), few would appear to be truly competitive. In addition, the number of multidisciplinary teams working together is relatively small. Notably missing from their list of nonphysician health care professionals are clinical dietitians/nutritionists.

In the editorial discussing this paper by Druss and colleagues, Aiken emphasizes the increased services to outpatients and particularly the consolidations of such services in large organizations employing nonphysicians in health care disciplines in response to increasing pressure for cost containment. Additional factors have been the shift in illness from acute to chronic conditions and the increasing emphasis on prevention. Dr. Aiken closes her editorial by expressing the hope that the report by Druss and associates "will help change the nature of the discussion about the interdisciplinary workforce, shifting the focus from competing interests of physicians and other health care professionals, a problem that is unnecessarily exaggerated, to the core areas of health care in which physicians and other clinicians who work together can promote their mutual interests and those of their patients" (31).

CHANGING ATTITUDES IN PHYSICIAN-PATIENT RELATIONS

From the early 1980s, and probably earlier, physicians and public health educators have recognized the need for new approaches in the care of those with chronic diseases. In this chapter, we concentrate on more recent documents that effectively state the problems and suggest reasonable solutions.

The titles of two papers, 9 years apart, by health professionals at the Michigan Diabetes Research and Training Center and University of Michigan Medical Center, summarize important aspects of the wake-up call. The 1991 paper is entitled *Empowerment: An Idea Whose Time Has Come in Diabetes Education* (1), and the 2000 paper is *Compliance and Adherence Are Dysfunctional Concepts in Diabetes Care* (2).

Taking the idea of empowerment of the patient from others in philosophy, psychology, and health education, Funnell and coauthors defined the term as "an interactive process of cultivating the power in others through the sharing of knowledge, expertise and resources" (1). These authors pointed out that patients with chronic diseases often have other serious problems (family issues, socioeconomic problems, and comorbid conditions) that are obstacles to overall health care management. When they also have nonphysician expert support, "the patients are no longer just consumers of our services but active partners in the provision of their diabetic care." These authors outlined a patient empowerment education program and developed a multipoint table of differences between the traditional medical model and the "empowering" person-centered model. The traditional model, for example, is one in which the "goal is compliance with recommendations" and "a lack of compliance is viewed as a failure of patients and provider." In contrast, the empowering person-centered model has the following view: "the goal is to enable patients to make informed choices. Behavioral strategies are used to help patients change behaviors of their choosing. A lack of goal achievement is viewed as feedback and is used to modify goals and strategies."

The title of the 2000 commentary of Anderson and Funnell quoted earlier (2) is based on the concept that the empowering approach results in a new degree of expertise and understanding on the part of the patient together with a collaborative relation with the physician. The result is that the terms *compliance* and *adherence* do not properly indicate the desired relationships.

The Chronic Care Model

Wagner and associates developed a model for primary care of chronic disease patients at the Group Health Cooperative of Puget Sound, Washington in cooperation with the Group Health's McColl Institute for Health Care Innovation (33, 34).

The six components of this model, as noted by Wagner and coauthors (5), are as follows: (a) community resources such as hospitals, senior centers, or home care agencies that provide patients with education classes, exercise facilities, and case managers; (b) health care organizations, including provider organizations, insurers, and other forms of reimbursement essential for care; (c) self-management support taught to the patient and family members that helps them to acquire the skills, confidence, tools, and information necessary to manage their illnesses (e.g., diet, exercise, self-management, social support); (d) delivery system design including necessary practice teams, each with a clear division of labor; these nonphysician personnel (who may be trained by the provider or elsewhere) who support patient self-management arrange routine periodic examination, ensure appropriate follow-up, and have planned visits; (e) evidence-based clinical practice guidelines to provide the standards for optimal chronic care; physicians leading education sessions for practice teams reinforce these standards; (f) clinical information systems, with computerized information in the form of reminders to the patients and care teams, feedback to physicians on patient data and registries for planning individual patient care, recording test data, or plans for such, and charts to be printed for each visit.

This paper also reviews the aspects of the chronic care programs adopted by four ongoing organizations in the United States: one a network of private practices, one of 700 community health centers, and two integrated delivery systems (5). These authors reviewed research evidence from 39 studies of various chronic diseases; 32 of these indicated that interventions that had chronic care models improved outcome measures for diabetic patients. Eighteen of 27 studies concerned with congestive heart failure, asthma, and diabetes demonstrated reduced health care costs or decreased use of health care services. Nevertheless, the authors point out that such programs are negatively affected as hospitals renounce capitations in favor of per diem payment as readmissions decrease or as success also decreases emergency room visits and income. The authors point out that the business aspect for chronic care would be better if Medicare paid for chronic care start-up costs including necessary clinical information services, reimbursed involved nonphysician personnel, and increased rates for provider organizations with superior performance.

Patient Self-Management and Collaborative Care

A noteworthy review of this area is that of Bodenheimer and colleagues (35). Two of their tables are reproduced here, one that compares traditional with collaborative care in chronic illness (Table 100.1) and another that compares traditional patient education with self-management education (Table 100.2).

This report provides the Web sites for the Michigan Diabetes Training Center (36), the Health Inequalities, London (37), and the Stanford Patient Education Research Center (38); these are organizations involved in training for such programs.

Involvement of Nonphysician Professionals

The types and numbers of nonprofessional members of a management team will vary depending on the needs of patients with a specific disease. However, a common need

TABLE 100.1. COMPARISON OF TRADITIONAL AND COLLABORATIVE CARE IN CHRONIC ILLNESS

ISSUE	TRADITIONAL CARE	COLLABORATIVE CARE
What is the relationship between the patient and health professionals?	Professionals are the experts who tell patients what to do. Patients are passive.	Shared expertise shared with active patients. Professionals are experts about the disease, and patients are experts about their lives.
Who is the principal caregiver and problem solver? Who is responsible for outcomes?	The professional	The patient and professional are the principal caregivers; they share responsibility for solving problems and for outcomes.
What is the goal?	Compliance with instructions. Noncompliance is a personal deficit of the patient.	The patient sets goals, and the professional helps the patient make informed choices. Lack of goal achievement is a problem to be solved by modifying strategies.
How is behavior changed?	External motivation	Internal motivation. Patients gain understanding and confidence to accomplish new behaviors.
How are problems identified?	By the professional (e.g., changing unhealthy behaviors)	By the patient (e.g., pain or inability to function); and by the professional
How are problems solved?	Professional solve problems for the patient.	Professionals teach problem-solving skills and help the patient in solving problems.

TABLE 100.2. COMPARISON OF TRADITIONAL PATIENT EDUCATION AND SELF-MANAGEMENT EDUCATION

ISSUE	TRADITIONAL PATIENT EDUCATION	SELF-MANAGEMENT EDUCATION
What is taught?	Information and technical skills about the disease	Skills on how to act on problems
How are problems formulated?	Problems reflect inadequate control of the disease.	The patient identifies problems he or she experiences that may or may not be related to the disease.
What is the relation of education to the disease?	Education is disease specific and teaches information and technical skills related to the disease.	Education provides problem-solving skills that are relevant to the consequences of chronic conditions in general.
What is the theory underlying the education?	Disease-specific knowledge creates behavior change, which, in turn, produces better clinical outcomes.	Greater patient confidence in his or her capacity to make life-improving changes (self-efficacy) yields better clinical outcomes.
What is the goal?	Compliance with the behavior changes taught to the patient to improve clinical outcomes	Increased self-efficacy to improve clinical outcomes
Who is the educator?	A health professional	A health professional, peer leader, or other patients, often in group settings

From Bodenheimer T, Lorig K, Holman H et al. JAMA 2002;288:2469–75, with permission. Copyright 2002, American Medical Association. All rights reserved.

for the success of a team is recognition by the patient, close family members, and key team members that concern for the patient is a priority of all. Equally important are the composition, quality, and close interaction of the multifaceted education team with the patient (39).

Among the active health organizations with chronic care models, we were particularly impressed by the description of the Kaiser Permanente Northern California Plan (40). Chronic disease management there is divided into three levels depending on the degree of care needed, whereas the number of nonphysician professionals concerned depends on the level of education and management needed. Not only are nurses, dietitians, health educators, pharmacists, and therapists available—some who may work extensively with patients having poorly controlled conditions for a 6- to 15-month period—but also medical social workers are involved as needed. Case managers, who attend training programs, update seminars, and peer group meetings, are mentored with specialist physicians.

In a review of the published literature in English between 1997 and 2002 from a number of countries, Newman, Steed, and Mulligan summarized the individual studies by intervention groups, duration, and types of professionals involved in self-management interventions with adults who had diabetes, asthma, rheumatoid arthritis, or osteoarthritis (41).

Another recent paper that went further back in searching Medline and Health Star reports (1964–1999) found 71 self-management education trials (42). Although the authors found the trials to vary substantially and suboptimally in methodology and in conducting and reporting results, they found that diabetic patients in such programs demonstrated reductions in glycosylated hemoglobin and systolic blood pressure.

In a description of two other health care organizations with important components of the chronic care model,

Grumbach and Bodenheimer discussed the issue of team composition and size (43). They reviewed the five concepts developed by various students of team building and noted that these are incorporated in the systems of these two health care groups. Inherent in all is the combining of the key elements with the use of specific measurable objectives to achieve successful patient outcomes. These authors stressed that the teams of physicians and nonphysician professionals that have greater cohesiveness are associated with better clinical outcomes. This paper and its references are recommended for those interested in learning more about multiprofessional team operations.

Roles of the Advance Practice Nurse

In reviewing the organization of medical management groups involved in multidisciplinary care of patients, the role of the advance practice nurse is prominent. Since the first nurse practitioners started work in 1965, the number exceeded 62,000 by the year 2000. Edward Salsberg, director of the Center for Workforce Studies at the American Association of Medical Colleges in Washington, is quoted: "Nurse practitioners are very quickly becoming a real cornerstone of the delivery system" (44).

The nursing profession has an efficient program permitting experienced nurses to obtain an advanced degree with further experience and new clinical skills under expert supervision. The title of advance practice nurse has officially been adopted by a number of key nursing organizations as the single definition for both the clinical nurse specialist and the nurse practitioner. The scope of practice of these two categories is determined by individual states through their licensing under Nurse Practice Acts. The Federal Balanced Budget Act of 1997 extended Medicare coverage for their professional services. The educational opportunities continue to advance. For example, it is reported that the

School of Nursing at Columbia University in New York is expected to introduce a 4-year "degree of nursing practice" program in 2005 (44).

Both clinical teams analyzed by Grumbach and Bodenheimer have a registered nurse who is the advice nurse who answers patient questions and performs triage on patients who telephone or come to the physician's office (43). Another nurse is the team coleader working with the physician coleader to solve day-to-day problems, thus ensuring that clinical systems are functioning well and interacting with team members as indicated. The authors quoted Wagner to the effect "that nurses' training makes them better than physicians at following chronic care management protocols" and "that they may also have better education and communication skills than do physicians" (45). These authors also noted two metaanalyses providing evidence that nurse practitioners delivered care of equivalent quality to that provided by primary care physicians, but with the caveat that the numbers of clinicians were small, and long-term outcomes of patients with chronic illnesses or complex situations were examined by only a few of the reports (46, 47).

The Diabetes Self-Management Education Report lists a nurse as a key member of the instructional team and notes that nurses have been used most often as instructors (48).

Roles of the Dietitian/Nutritionist

Clinical dietitians in hospital practice obviously play an important role in patient management as advisors on diet and nutrition based on their evaluation of patients' needs in acute situations. In the hospital outpatient setting, dietitians either follow patients after discharge or on physician's referral for variable periods from another clinic. In such settings, continuing multidisciplinary interactions with long-term patients with physicians and nurses is not usual except in some circumstances where there has been early specialization, such as pediatrics, hemodialysis, or home care in which skilled nonphysician professionals supervise parenteral and enteral feeding. Broader specialization developed in the 1980s and is reflected in the increasing number of specialty practice groups in the American Dietetic Association (ADA).

According to the year 2002 membership data of the ADA, some 34% (nearly 24,200 members) were hospital-based clinical dietitians concerned with inpatient issues; 11.6% (about 8000 members) were clinical dietitians involved with outpatients (clinics or ambulatory care). Only 1.7% of clinical dietitian members were employed by HMOs or other physician practice groups; this low number is undoubtedly the result of the past and present history of inability to obtain reasonable payment from patient insurance or Medicare for dietitian service programs.

Dietitians in Chronic Disease Research. The importance of nutrition and of the roles of dietitians in the prevention and management of different types of diabetes mellitus is well summarized in a number of papers (49–51). The joint statements of key clinical societies and others concerned with chronic diseases are reviewed in the earlier part of this chapter (6, 65); these statements call for the increased role of dietitians in managed care. The American Diabetes Association has designated dietitians as well as nurses as essential professionals in teaching and management of diabetes (48). Examples of successful dietitian collaborative research exist in management of hypertension (52) and in cholesterol control (53–55).

Dietitians as Medicare/Medicaid Providers. The Medicare, Medicaid, and State Children's Health Insurance Program Benefits Improvement and Protection Act of 2000 has allowed registered dietitians and qualified nutrition professionals enrolled as Medicare providers to receive reimbursement for medical nutrition therapy (MNT) provided to Medicare Part B beneficiaries with diabetes and kidney disease since the beginning of 2002 (56).

In February 2004, the Center for Medicare and Medicaid Services announced to their state directors the three major disease management models that could qualify under Medicaid for matching funds. As discussed by Pritchett, one of these is disease management as an individual provider, through contract with a disease-management provider (57). This author proceeded to discuss the chronic care model discussed earlier and noted the similarities of E. H. Wagner's presentations with the ADA's Nutrition Care Process and Model (58).

In 2004, Congress passed Medicare reform legislation as the Voluntary Chronic Care Improvement under Traditional Fee-for-Service that will allow some beneficiaries to receive medical nutrition therapy beginning in January 2006 as a phase 1 program to test and evaluate chronic care improvement programs. For those organizations demonstrating competence and success over 3 years, phase 2 will begin enrolling beneficiaries nationwide (59, 60).

It remains to be seen how effective these proposed reforms will be in meeting the goals of the chronic care model. We hope that dietitians will be fully involved in the development of these reforms.

Medical Nutrition Therapy Protocols. Such protocols have been developed and published through the ADA together with MNT protocols for other chronic diseases that can be adopted and implemented in outpatient, home health, and long-term care (61).

Increased Educational and Practice Opportunities. The introduction of managed care systems related to the chronic care model into various patient care sites as recommended by Holman (62) will certainly require clinical dietitians. We suggest this important multidisciplinary role be assigned to a separate unit of the existing hospital clinical dietary staff that will have an academic affiliation in the clinical department responsible for such clinical and educational activities. The opportunities for long-term multidisciplinary interactions involving administration, student, and resident teaching and patient education and communication call for broader basic and clinical knowledge and practical experience in long-term care and prevention of chronic diseases.

In her review of educational and practice opportunities open to nurses, Annalyn Skipper made a significant point relevant to dietitians: "Dietetics is rapidly moving to an intervention-oriented outcome-focused discipline. To demonstrate the value of advanced practice in dietetics, it will be important to focus on what the advanced practice dietitian can do rather than what the advanced practice dietitian knows. To be successful advanced-level practitioners, dietitians will need to identify skills of value to patients and health care organizations and become proficient in performing these skills" (63).

On this same issue, Delehanty and Nathan, after reviewing the role of dietitians in long-term diabetes research and care, concluded: "The evidence suggests that dietetic professionals have an increasingly important role in the early initiation of MNT . . . and in establishing the long-term relationships required to shape behavior and sustain the lifestyle habits that translate into increasingly significant health benefits and cost savings over time" (49).

In a paper discussing the practice-doctorate program in place since 2003 at her institution, Touger-Decker mentioned prior conferences and reports within the ADA concerning such advance training (64). The Doctorate in Clinical Nutrition is Web-based at the University of Medicine and Dentistry of New Jersey, and the program is described in detail on its Web site (65).

Recent Appraisals of Quality Care by Professional Societies

In 2004, the American Cancer Society, the American Diabetes Association, and the American Heart Association issued a joint report reviewing strategies for the prevention and early detection of cancer and CV diseases as the beginning of a new collaboration among the three organizations; this report was published in each of the major journals of these organizations (6). The report notes that the annual physical examination has little empiric evidence of its value. It calls for "age- and gender-appropriate" models for periodic health maintenance visits by "fairly reimbursed" clinicians for encounter-based visits and notes the importance of detailed family histories and of preventive care.

The American Diabetes Association, the North American Association for the Study of Obesity, and the American Society for Clinical Nutrition also issued a statement in 2004 emphasizing overweight and obesity as important risk factors for type 2 diabetes and the need for lifestyle modifications designed to reduce energy intake and increase physical activity (66). Specific recommendations are made for achieving weight loss by decreased caloric intake and for a progressive program of physical activity.

Changes in office practices are proposed that include close follow-up with attention to behavioral change, self-monitoring, and frequent patient-provider contact. The program should include the enlistment of health care professionals (e.g., nurse, medical assistants, and dietitians).

NEED FOR ADDITIONAL SUPPORT PROGRAMS

The numerous issues concerning chronic illnesses from childhood to old age dictate that societal as well as professional and patient interactions must also change to have a fully effective system emphasizing prevention as well as disease management.

Community Support

Health programs in preschool and schools through high school and college involving local and state boards of education together with parents and medical societies should emphasize health programs and early detection of risk factors. Relevant school boards should have public health representatives to help guide the necessary activities with more involvement of nurses, dietitians, and physical exercise experts for relevant ages. Increasingly, the family unit should be the focus of education and health supervision.

Improved Communication and Information Systems

The need for improved and widespread use of technology for organized care management processes has been emphasized in the IOM report (4) and in a recent survey of the current availability of such technology (67).

Demonstration and Evaluation Projects

Citing the report by Donaldson and Mohr (68), the IOM Report (4) provided examples of types of projects that could be supported by a major Health Care Innovative Fund (e.g., $1 billion over 3–5 years) that should be created by Congress to finance such proposals designed to implement changes (4).

Medical School Changes

Holman reviewed what he considers to be the current inadequacies of clinical education in medical schools and house-staff education and outlined the changes that will broaden the knowledge of physicians in working with patients and nonphysicians professionals (62). He cited as an example the recent academic medical centers initiatives, oriented primarily to residents, that is supported by the Robert Wood Johnson Foundation. He pointed out the lack of training programs for medical students and called for the creation of ambulatory care programs practicing the chronic care model; these should be the sites of student and faculty learning with the ability to design and evaluate new forms of practice and education. Students interested in primary or specialty medicine should be assigned to supervise longitudinal care of patients with chronic diseases.

Medical school clinical teaching departments, divisions, and sections do not recognize clinical nutrition as a teaching or practice title unless added to an existing subspecialty title. This situation is in large part the result of the lack of a generally recognized nutrition subspecialty board and an examination for licensing in that discipline, although nutrition as an examination topic occurs frequently in a number of other subspecialty examinations. Furthermore, such medical school organization and practice systems nowadays make it difficult for someone with an advanced degree in nutrition science (Ph.D. or Sc.D.) who also has an M.D. to make a reasonable salary as a medical school clinician without board certification in a recognized subspecialty.

The recognition of the importance of nutrition issues in medicine appears to be increasing, especially among younger physicians, but our impression is that this is usually not related to any significant increase in formal nutrition education in many medical schools; rather, it stems from their exposure to nutrition-related clinical situations and to the medical literature that they read. The addition of the term *nutrition* to the existing titles of gastroenterology, endocrinology, or metabolic sections does not automatically imply that the clinical section has an M.D. with extensive nutrition background and the clinical experience to interact with medical students and house staff, dietitians, nurses, or sick patients.

It appears to us that an added point to Holman's review (62) would be increased medical school faculty attention to having in their inpatient and ambulatory care programs someone with an Sc.D. or Ph.D. degree as well as an M.D. degree with significant basic and clinical training and experience in clinical nutrition to act as a team-member.

Professional Societies

The complexity and importance of the needs mentioned earlier should stimulate various medical, nursing, and dietetic organizations to review their programs through their national and regional branches. The need to influence school boards and parent groups to modify or establish nutrition and health activities during and after school has been mentioned. Collaborative practical and educational activities with essential nonphysician professionals should be established on a continuing basis. Whatever physician practice group is involved, a family-based approach seems desirable.

Federal Agencies

Evidence indicates that the US Department of Agriculture has initiated grants to individual school boards to increase availability of vegetables and fruits in school food programs. The Centers for Disease Control and Prevention has also supported increased physical activity programs in certain schools. The very large multicommunity health center organization mentioned earlier is assisted with funds from the Federal Bureau of Primary Health Care and other federal and state agencies.

Lay Workers

As noted by E. H. Wagner (69), community health workers or health aides can bridge the gap of language and cultural differences between middle class health professionals and socioeconomically, ethnically, and culturally different patient populations. Lay volunteers who have experienced certain illnesses have been shown to be effective in self-management programs, where they have been used for patients with arthritis (70) and for other chronic diseases (71).

REFERENCES

1. Funnell MM, Anderson RM, Arnold MS et al. Diabetes Educ 1991;17:37–41.
2. Anderson RM, Funnell MM. Diabetes Educ 2000;26:97–603.
3. Lee TH. N Engl J Med 2002;347:1965–7.
4. Committee on Quality Health in America, Institute of Medicine. Crossing the Quality Chasm: A New Health System for the 21st Century. Washington, DC: National Academy Press, 2001.
5. Bodenheimer T, Wagner EH, Grumbach K. JAMA 2002;288: 1909–14.
6. Eyre H, Kahn R, Robertson RM et al. Circulation 2004;109: 3244–55.
7. Calle EF, Rodriquez C, Walker-Thurmond K et al. N Engl J Med 2003;348:1625–38.
8. Rodriquez BC, D'Agostino R, Abbott RD et al. Stroke 2002;33: 230–6.
9. Mokad AH, Ford ES, Bonham B et al. Diabetes Care 2000;23: 1278–83.
10. Dietz WH. N Engl J Med 2004;350:855–7.
11. Hedley AA, Ogden CL, Johnson CG et al. J AMA 2004;291: 2847–50.
12. Weiss R, Dziura J, Burgert TS et al. N Engl J Med 2004;350: 2362–74.
13. Ingelfinger JR. N Engl J Med 2004;350:2123–6.
14. Thorpe KE, Florence CS, Joski P. Health Affairs 2004;Web exclusive:W4–437.
15. McGlynn EA, Asch SM, Adams J et al. N Engl J Med 2003;348: 2635–45.
16. Saydah SH, Fradkin J, Couie CC. J Am Diet Assoc 2004;291: 335–42.
17. Venrat Narayan KM, Boyle JP, Thompson TJ et al. JAMA 2003; 290:1884–90.
18. Ades PA. N Engl J Med 2001;345:892–902.
19. Feinstein A, Elmer PJ, Orwoll E et al. Arch Intern Med 2003; 163:2165–72.
20. Waldo AL. JAMA 2003;290:1093–5.
21. Benner JS, Glynn RJ, Mogun H et al. JAMA 2002;288: 455–61.
22. Jackevicius CA, Mandani M, Tu JV. JAMA 2002;288:462.
23. Applegate WB. JAMA 2002;288:495–7.
24. Piette JD, Heisler M, Wagner TH. Arch Intern Med 2004;164: 1749–55.
25. (AHRQ) Agency for Healthcare Research and Quality. Literacy and Health Outcomes. http://www.ahrq.gov/clinic/epcsums/ litsum.htm.

26. Institute of Medicine. Health Literacy, a Prescription to End Confusion. http://www.edu.report.asp?id=19723.
27. Bendetti PP. JAMA 2004;292:2000–6.
28. Wachter RM. N Engl J Med 2004;350:935–6.
29. Hoff TH, Whitcomb MF, Williams K et al. Arch Intern Med 2001;161:851–8.
30. Whitcomb MF, Cohen JJ. N Engl J Med 2004;351:710–2.
31. Aiken LH. N Engl J Med 2003;348:164–6.
32. Druss BG, Marcus SC, Olfson M et al. N Engl J Med 2003;348: 130–7.
33. Wagner EH, Austin BT, von Korff M et al. Milbank Q 1996;74: 511–44.
34. Katon W, von Korff M, Lin E et al. JAMA 1995;273:1026–31.
35. Bodenheimer T, Lorig K, Holman H et al. JAMA 2002;288: 2469–75.
36. http://www.med.umich.edu/mdrtc.
37. http://www.doh.uk/healthinequalities.
38. http://www.stanford.edu/group/perc.
39. Messing C, Boucher J, Cypress M et al. Diabetes Care 2004;27 [Suppl 1]:143–50.
40. Bodenheimer T, Wagner EH, Grumbach K. JAMA 2002;288: 1775–9.
41. Newman S, Steed L, Mulligan K. Lancet 2004;364:1523–37.
42. Warsi A, Wang PS, La Valley MP et al. Arch Intern Med 2004; 164:1641–9.
43. Grumbach K, Bodenheimer T. JAMA 2004;291:1246–51.
44. Blackman A. The Journal report: Personal health. Wall Street Journal (online), Oct 11, 2004.
45. Wagner EH. BMJ 2000;320:569–72.
46. Brown SA, Grimes DA. Nurse Res 1995;44:332–9.
47. Horrocks S, Anderson E, Salisbury C. BMJ 2002;324:819–23.
48. Diabetes Self-Management Education Report. Diabetes Care 2002;25:2165–71.
49. Delehanty LM, Nathan DJ. Am Diet Assoc 2004;104:1846–56.
50. Wylie-Rosett J, Delehanty L. J Am Diet Assoc 2002;102:1065–8.
51. Lemon CC, Lacey K, Lohse B et al. J Am Diet Assoc 2004;104: 1805–15.
52. Windhauser MM, Ernst DB, Karanja NM et al. J Am Diet Assoc 1999;8[Suppl]:S90–95.
53. Shaffer J, Wexler LF. Arch Intern Med 1995;155:2330–5.
54. Delehanty LM, Sonnenberg LM, Hayden D et al. J Am Diet Assoc 2001;101:1012–23.
55. Delehanty LM, Hayden D, Aminuman A et al. Ann Behav Med 2002;24:269–79.
56. Hodorowicz MA. Nutr Clin Pract 2003;18:48–9.
57. Pritchett E. J Am Diet Assoc 2004;104:1345–8.
58. Lacey K, Pritchett E. J Am Diet Assoc 2003;103:1061–72.
59. Hager MH. J Am Diet Assoc 2004;104:890–1.
60. Smith R. J Am Diet Assoc 2004;104:734–5.
61. American Dietetic Association. Medical Nutrition Therapy Protocols http://www.eatright.org.
62. Holman H. JAMA 2004;292:1057–9.
63. Skipper AJ. J Am Diet Assoc 2004;104:1007–12.
64. Touger-Decker R. J Am Diet Assoc 2004;104:1456–8.
65. http://shrp.umdnj.edu/nutr/.
66. Klein S, Sheard NF, Pi-Sunyer X et al. Am J Clin Nutr 2004;80: 257–63.
67. Casalino L, Gillies RR, Shortell SM et al. JAMA 2003;289: 434–42.
68. Donaldson MS, Mohr JJ. Exploring Innovation and Quality Improvement in Healthcare Microsystems: Across-Case Analyses. Washington, DC: National Academy Press, 2000.
69. Wagner EH. BMJ 2000;320:569–72.
70. Lorig KR, Mazonson PD, Holman HR. Arthritis Rheum 1993; 6:439–46.
71. Lorig KR, Sobel DS, Stewart AL et al. Med Care 1999;37:5–14.

NUTRITION AND MEDICAL ETHICS: THE INTERPLAY OF MEDICAL DECISIONS, PATIENTS' RIGHTS, AND THE JUDICIAL SYSTEM[1]

MAURICE E. SHILS

NUTRITION SUPPORT AS AN ETHICAL ISSUE 1608
   Prevention and Management of
      Undernutrition 1608
   Prevention and Management of Chronic
      Diseases 1609
CHANGING VIEWS ABOUT MEDICAL ETHICS 1609
   Hippocratic Tradition 1609
   "Principalism" 1609
   Alternative Ethical Approaches 1610
ISSUES CONCERNING NUTRITION SUPPORT OF
   THE COMPETENT PATIENT 1610
   The Bouvia Case 1610
   Patient-Physician Interaction and Decision
      Making 1610
   Recommendation of the President's
      Commission 1611
   Resolving Differences Between Patient
      and Physician 1612
   Patient Self-Determination Act 1613
   Patient Decision-Making and Its
      Consequences 1614
NUTRITION SUPPORT OF THE INCOMPETENT
   PATIENT 1614
   The Vegetative State 1615
   The Minimally Conscious State 1618
   Advanced Dementia .1618
   Advance Care Directives 1618
   Palliataive Care; Hospice 1619
   Attitude Changes in the Care of Ill Children 1619
   Physiologic Responses to Food-Water
      Restriction 1619

Nutrition has progressively been recognized as an important aspect of individual and public health through its contributions in preservation of health throughout the life cycle and in the prevention and management of various diseases. Ethical issues enter into the provision of nutrition by physicians and other health professionals when needed in health maintenance and in the management of those who will benefit by its inclusion in their care. Much attention has been given in recent years to the ethical and legal aspects of providing, withholding, and discontinuing nutrition and fluids to patients with advanced or incurable diseases, especially for those unable to make critical decisions by themselves.

NUTRITION SUPPORT AS AN ETHICAL ISSUE

Without clinical craftsmanship, the physician-humanist is without authenticity. Incompetence is inhumane because it betrays the trust the patient places in the physician's capacity to help and not harm.

Edmund D. Pellegrino, M.D. (1)

A more clinical argument against the focus on patient safety is that medical injuries do not cause as many deaths as errors of omission.... Our health care system fails with embarrassing frequency to provide medical interventions known to benefit patients. These failures are not the fault of physicians alone, they reflect poor coordination among all parties, including patients.

Thomas H. Lee, M.D. (2)

Prevention and Management of Undernutrition

Physicians have increasingly become more sensitive to the need for remedial action in disease-related undernutrition resulting from inadequate intake or poor utilization of calories and essential nutrients. It is recognized that the undernutrition accompanying a disease may be secondary to disease-related metabolic changes and may respond only with palliation or cure of the basic problem; however, one cannot say with certainty that provision of improved nutrition support will always be futile (3, 4); hence, the effort of such support is worthwhile for a trial period.

It is also a fact that physicians may overlook the presence of serious undernutrition in their patients or may delay initiation of nutrition support in the expectation that the underlying problem will soon be controlled and the patient will resume eating, a hope often delayed. At intervals over many years, reports of the prevalence of hospital-based malnutrition resurface with their notations of increased mortality. An ethical issue arises when the risks of serious undernutrition are ignored or there is inadequate treatment of a potentially curable condition.

---

[1]**AMA,** American Medical Association; **CHD,** coronary heart disease; **PVS,** persistent vegetative state.

Prevention and Management of Chronic Diseases

The important role of diet and nutrition in the management of a number of chronic diseases is now well established. What is also apparent is a significant failure to adhere to and follow-up such recommendations for preventive and therapeutic care by physicians (see Chapter 100) (5, 6).

In contrast to those earlier beliefs that coronary heart disease (CHD) occurs in about half of those who have modifiable traditional cardiovascular risk factors such as smoking, diabetes mellitus, hypertension, and hypercholesterolemia (7), more recent observations indicate that the prevalence of at least one of these risk factors is associated with the development of clinically significant CHD in 80 to 90% and in 95% of those with a fatal CHD event (8–10). In contrast, those men in age groups 18 to 39 years and 40 to 59 years who had none of the risk factors had death rates from CHD and cardiovascular disease of 0.8 to 0.15% and 0.23 to 0.29%, respectively (11). It is also clear that treatment of such risk factors decreases the incidence of CHD (10). In addition to the risk factors cited earlier for CHD, we must consider obesity with those metabolic and biochemical factors that jointly constitute the metabolic syndrome (12) (see Chapters 62 to 65.) Of even greater significance in terms of potential gains through prevention is accruing evidence that risk factors can be detected with some certainty at earlier ages, for example, risk factors for cardiac disease appearing in adolescents (13) (see Chapter 52) and detection of abnormal blood pressure in overweight and obese children (13, 14). These are signals to institute healthful lifestyle changes. In controlling such risks, dietary and nutrition changes must be considered in addition to increased physical activities.

What has previously been viewed as an issue of personal behavior (e.g., obesity) or as a simple relationship (I prescribe and you take) between physician and patient now needs to be viewed in a different light as a very large and growing public health problem. The high incidence of failure of physicians to evaluate and treat potential or actual chronic disease adequately (see Chapter 100) and the failure of a large percentage of patients to continue therapies must be viewed as societal, professional, and personal ethical problems. Similarly, state departments of education and their local school boards must move away from the common attitude that they have no ethical responsibility to students, parents, and the community for instituting adequate health and nutrition education, proper diets, and physical education.

CHANGING VIEWS ABOUT MEDICAL ETHICS

Clinical ethics deals with situations in which there are strong reasons both for and against a course of action. Decisions often are difficult because ethical guidelines conflict and people of integrity and good will may disagree over what to do.

Bernard Lo, M.D. (15)

Hippocratic Tradition

The moral principles to which medical professionals are exposed during their training and in their professional organizations have a long history. The Hippocratic tradition of some 2500 years developed from interactions of ancient Greek philosophic schools and medicine with modifications of Stoic attitudes to duty and virtue. These were further modified by the views of Galen, with subsequent religious Christian input to remove pagan influences (16). Ethical precepts from the Hippocratic tradition include beneficence and malfeasance (the obligation to promote the patient's welfare while balancing benefits and harm), duty, compassion, and confidentiality as well as prohibitions on abortion and euthanasia. The tradition combined precepts on gentlemanly conduct, education, and practical judgment including a good physician-patient relationship. These would lead physicians toward right and good decisions for their patients in situations of moral choice. Inherent in this system of medical practice and ethics was the authoritarian role of the physician; this long era has been termed one of the paternalism (17) or the quiescent period (18).

"Principalism"

The traditional Hippocratic system of professional ethics was increasingly questioned in the United States in the mid-1960s in conjunction with many professional and societal changes that included depersonalization and fragmentation in many physician-patient relationships and challenges to governmental authority with the rise in the civil rights, antiwar, feminist, and consumer rights movements in an increasingly multiethnic pluralistic democratic society. As physician-patient relationships came under increasing scrutiny with claims for more patient rights, series of principles of medical ethics were advanced (designated by some as "principalism"). These were effectively set out by Beauchamp and Childress in the first edition of *Principles of Biomedical Ethics* (19) and its successors. Its first two principles (nonmaleficence and beneficence) were similar to those in the Hippocratic ethic; the third concept, patient *autonomy*, contravened paternalism, whereas the fourth, *justice* (an area of diverse views often involving elements of fairness and entitlement for individuals), was completely at odds with the old tradition.

The term *autonomy* signifies the right of the competent person to make choices freely about medical care and denotes the obligation of the health care provider to communicate effectively with the patient and to solicit those decisions. As detailed by Beauchamp and Childress, autonomous actions require that definitions be available including criteria so someone could give or refuse informed consent and make other decisions. Furthermore, the principle of respect for autonomy must be evaluated in given situations in competition with the other principles (19). Widespread acceptance of principalism in the United States was circumscribed to a period of about

20 years from the mid-1960s, as other ethical concepts became more prominent.

Alternative Ethical Approaches

Advocacy has increased in the past decade for alternative ethical approaches that place more emphasis on the value of a more personal decision-making interaction of physician and patient (20–24). Alternative ethical approaches include casuistry (analysis of a specific case in relation to a system of principles and cross-cultural narrative) and virtue ethics. These gained advocacy with the increasing cost of new medical techniques and drugs and changes in medical practice; such as the institution of diagnosis-related groups (DRGs) in 1983 and, more recently, the widespread movement toward managed-care systems owned or directed by for-profit insurance corporations and nonprofit organizations vying competitively. These raised serious concerns, divided physician loyalties, and imposed limitations on medical care (22).

In addition to secular ethical positions, some bioethicists have formulated their positions on the basis of particular religious traditions (25, 26) and some attempt to construct a basis for secular ethics for those "who do not share a contentful moral vision" (27).

ISSUES CONCERNING NUTRITION SUPPORT OF THE COMPETENT PATIENT

Many of the ethical and legal issues concerning medical practice and patient-physician relations are associated with provision of nutrition and hydration. Before the practical application of artificial feeding techniques, the inability to maintain adequate nutrition by mouth meant progressive body wasting until death. Except for deaths occurring very rapidly from violence, trauma, or acute overwhelming infections, the more usual direct causes of death in those with more chronic illness were dehydration and anorexia or obstruction leading to starvation. Under these circumstances, there was little that a physician could do to restore health while maintaining a good nutritional state. The situation began to change significantly in the nineteenth century as effective therapies, initially surgical treatments and then vaccinations and later advances in diagnosis and other treatments, enhanced the societal importance of, and regard for, the physician.

Concerning oversight of medical care in general, the prevailing judicial position in the past was that of "compelling state interest" such as preservation of life, prevention of suicide, and certification of physician education. This legal position in conjunction with the paternalistic role of the physician eventually led to contentious legal issues.

The patient's right to refuse medical treatment was not established until 1891, in a case in which the US Supreme Court upheld the right of a personal injury plaintiff to refuse a medical examination (28). This decision established the general rights of individuals to make choices regarding bodily examination and treatment under the principle that common law guards the right of every individual to the possession and control of his or her own person on the basis of the doctrine of informed consent.

In the past, the issue of provision of nutrition and fluids caused the most controversy among adult patients, their surrogates, physicians, hospital administrators, state courts, and eventually the US Supreme Court. The right of competent individuals to decide for themselves whether or not to receive medical therapy (autonomy) was not automatically granted. Withholding or withdrawal of artificial nutrition and hydration became a contentious issue because some physicians, ethicists, theologians, and "right-to-life" groups considered such acts assisted suicide or euthanasia (and hence likely to involve criminal penalties) or cessations of "ordinary" medical procedures.

The Bouvia Case

This case posed the right of a competent patient to starve to death.

Elizabeth Bouvia, a quadriplegic patient in her mid-20s, was hospitalized in California with severe cerebral palsy and arthritic pain requiring morphine injection. While able to ingest food orally with assistance, she asked that such feeding be stopped. The hospital refused to accede to her wishes, and a lower court ruling in 1984 supported the hospital (29). When her condition deteriorated to the point that feeding by nasogastric tube was necessary, the Appellate Court ruled in 1986 that her refusal of treatment was not a form of suicide, thus rejecting the arguments of hospital officials that removing the tube would make them a party to suicide (30). With the additional support given later by the US Supreme Court decision in the Cruzan case (see later), the right of an irreversibly ill, but competent patient to refuse artificial feeding is unlikely to be seriously challenged again.

Bouvia's condition was classified as a state of severe and permanent paralysis, which may acutely or progressively result in a "permanent locked-in state." This was first described as a medical condition in 1966 by Cranford as irreversible loss of motor function with preservation of normal consciousness, possible long-term survival of years or even decades, and physical and psychologic suffering of a degree that may become extreme because of the patient's awareness of the condition (31).

Patient-Physician Interactions and Decision Making

In an incisive essay, Pellegrino stated "that a more sensitive and compelling guide to the care of the sick is to be found in the fact of illness as a human experience rather than in the assigned role of the profession. Without supplanting traditional professional ethics, the intrinsic dehumanizing nature of illness imposes additional obligations of greater sensitivity" (32). Persons with "illness as an acute event or as a chronic accompaniment of life are deprived in varying degrees of those things which distinguish humanity from other forms of existence." These include loss of freedom of action, freedom to make choices, and freedom from the power of others as well as threats to personal self-image. These disabilities "must be the infrangible base for the obligations of physicians and all others who profess to heal. . ., these obligations constitute the substance of professional medical ethics,. . . Its rooting in the existential situation is more authentic and more human . . . than the traditional one in the self declared duties of the profession . . . The professional can make a valid claim for technical authority but this no longer extends to moral authority . . . The patient has the human right to his own moral agency if he or she wishes to exercise it. The physician has the moral obligation to ascertain the degree to which the patient wishes to exercise his moral prerogatives and to provide the fullest exposition which will enable the privilege to be exercised" (32).

The principle of respect for autonomy of the competent patient may result in tension between a patient or the parent of a minor and the physician when the patient's decision seems inappropriate. What appears legally to be a clear-cut situation, that is, the rights of a competent patient, may be a complex and difficult situation for all concerned with the welfare of the individual person. The old Spanish proverb quoted elsewhere in this context is apt: "The appearance of the bull changes as one leaves the grandstand and enters the ring" (33). The patient's viewpoint may reflect a lucid and rational decision or an undisclosed or undiagnosed problem such as depression, other mental difficulty, side effect of medication (34), an unspoken complicating social problem, strong opposing family influence, misunderstanding of the physician's intentions, or the patient's failure to know, comprehend, or accept the severity or irreversibility of the disease.

Disagreement may occur, for example, when the patient wishes parenteral or enteral feeding stopped and the physician believes that continued feeding is in the patient's best interest. An even more difficult situation arises when economic or related pressures raise questions about stopping parenteral feeding in an intestinally obstructed patient with cancer in whom all therapy has failed but who is still competent and ambulatory, and for whom such continued support at home could conceivably extend life for months.

Recommendations of the President's Commission

Several recommendations on this issue were considered by the President's Commission for the Study of Ethical Problems in Medicine and Biomedical and Behavioral Research reported in 1983 (35). It held that "health care professionals serve patients best by maintaining a presumption in favor of sustaining life while recognizing that competent patients are entitled to choose to forgo any treatments, including those that sustain life" and "the voluntary choice of a competent and informed patient should determine whether or not life-sustaining therapy will be undertaken, while healthcare institutions and professionals should try to enhance patients' abilities to make decisions on their own behalf and to promote understanding of the available options."

In such situations, members of the hospital nutritional support team, who are often and intimately involved in a major aspect of the patient's care, may be helpful in affording insight into the patient's status and expressed position. The physician's discussion of the medical situation with patient and family, the basis for the medical recommendations, the therapeutic alternatives with their probabilities of success, and the offer of a second opinion are all essential to the decision-making process.

This commission also examined the role of traditional moral distinctions as they relate to decisions about medical care and whether they are acceptable or unacceptable. It noted that from the viewpoint of most competent patients, decisions about alternative available courses of treatment are made on the basis of factors that include benefits in terms of extension of life, the nature and quality of that life, the degree of suffering involved, and the various costs to themselves and to others (35). It noted that other criteria have been used in judging the acceptability or unacceptability of life-and-death decisions and stated:

These bases are traditionally presented in the form of opposing categories. Although the categories causing death—by acting versus by omitting the act; withholding versus withdrawing treatment; the intended versus the unintended but foreseeable consequences of a choice; and ordinary versus extraordinary treatment—do reflect factors that can be important in assessing the moral and legal acceptability of decisions to forego life sustaining treatment, they are inherently unclear. Worse, their invocation is often so mechanical that it neither illuminates an actual case nor provides an ethically persuasive argument.

Several of the Commission's conclusions about such distinctions are relevant to the issue of nutrition and hydration and have, in fact, had a significant influence on the attitudes of physicians and the courts. For example:

The distinction between acting and omitting to act provides a useful rule-of-thumb by separating cases that probably deserve more scrutiny from those that are likely not to need it. Nonetheless, the mere difference between acts and omissions—which is often hard to draw in any case—never by itself determines what is morally acceptable. Rather, the acceptability of particular actions or omissions turns on other morally significant considerations, such as the balance of harms and benefits likely to be achieved, the duties owed by others to a dying person, the risks imposed on others in acting or refraining, and the certainty of outcome.... A justification that is adequate for not commencing a treatment is also sufficient for ceasing it. Moreover, erecting a higher requirement for cessation might unjustifiably discourage vigorous initial attempts to treat seriously ill patients that sometimes succeed (35).

Although these principles are sound, their implementation in actual medical situations may be contentious. They often involve end-of-life decisions in which differences arise among patient, family members, and physicians in the absence of advance directives.

The guidelines of the Hastings Center also expressed concern that the terms *ordinary* and *extraordinary*

> *obscure ethically important questions rather than helping to resolve them. Prevalence of a treatment or its degree of technological complexity is sometimes used to make the distinction between 'ordinary' and 'extraordinary.' We reject the distinction. No treatment is intrinsically 'ordinary' or 'extraordinary.' All treatments that impose undue burdens on the patient without overriding benefits or that simply provide no benefits may justifiably be withheld or withdrawn. While traditional definitions of 'extraordinary' hinged on this comparison of benefits and burdens, the term has become so confusing that it is no longer useful (36).*

Resolving Differences Between Patient and Physician

When all the stated precautions and efforts have been honored in decision making but the choice of the competent and informed patient is contrary to the judgment of the physician, where does this leave the physician? Cranford stated: "The physician too has a set of values to which he owes allegiance. He has a double obligation, to protect those of the patient and to be faithful to his own" (31). To deal humanely with the conflicts that must occasionally arise, "the physician must know enough about his own beliefs to decide when he can compromise, when he cannot, and when he must give the patient the opportunity to transfer his care to another physician whose values more closely coincide," as Pellegrino stated (32).

In this situation, the President's Commission took the position that "health care professionals or institutions may decline to provide a particular option because that choice would violate their conscience or professional judgment, though in doing so they may not abandon a patient" (35). In that instance, responsibility for the care of the patient must be transferred to another physician who accepts the patient's decision and acts accordingly. Abandonment means leaving the patient without care, a serious and punishable infraction of both the legal and ethical obligations of the physician. There has been a recent emphasis on nonabandonment "as an open-ended commitment over time" (37) of the physician to the patient (37, 38), for example, accepting competent patient decisions on demanding or stopping artificial feeding. Objection has been raised to the apparent elevation of nonabandonment to a principle rather than considering it one of the essential derivatives of medical ethics (39).

When the patient's request is opposed by the hospital administration, the solutions open to the hospital are to yield to staff pressure on behalf of the patient, to transfer the patient to another hospital willing to accept the patient, or to yield to a court order when it supports the patient. Often in the past and continuing to some degree today, it has been the reluctance of the hospital administration to discontinue tube feeding or some other life support—usually because of fear of civil or criminal penalties or on religious grounds—that has led to legal actions by patients or family members.

Religious and Spiritual Views

Patients, family members, surrogates, and physicians may hold religious and spiritual beliefs that influence their decisions on medical treatments and end-of-life issues. There is increasing diversity of such beliefs in the population of the United States and in many other countries; in addition, there are variations of personal belief in mainstream religions. The need for medical decisions in periods of crisis may awaken or increase religious and spiritual concerns that may lead to questions about treatment, hesitancy in decisions, or actual objections (40). A group of 13 professionals, mostly physicians, in various programs in medical ethics, has considered the importance of physicians' attention to such patient and family concerns to ensure that the best care is provided and the patient and family are given a respectful hearing with discussion in a effort to gain an understanding of the physician's views on prognosis and treatment (40). This approach does not require the physician's agreement with the patient or modification of his or her medical views. As with the other *JAMA* "Perspectives on Care" mentioned elsewhere in this chapter, these authors consider this issue through case histories and physician-patient discussions together with pertinent literature reviews.

The physician and hospital must each make their positions clear to patients and surrogates concerning such end-of-life issues so, if necessary, alternatives can be found without rancor and undue distress. It is equally important that physicians, nurses, and other members of the health care team "be skilled in the two essential aspects of good clinical care of dying patients—technical issues in the compassionate withdrawal of life-prolonging therapy and counseling and emotional support for patients, families, and staff during this process" (41).

Distinguishing Patient Refusal from Requests

Physicians may differentiate between the competent patient's refusal of a recommended treatment and the request for a nonrecommended treatment (42). Refusals must be honored even when the physician knows that death will result. In contrast, a physician may believe that there is no moral or legal obligation to honor a request for treatment that the physician firmly believes will have an undesirable effect or result in death. This is a matter of judgment focusing on the issue of treatments deemed useless or futile by the physicians or hospital.

Denial of Treatment as Medically Futile

Statements such as those made by the President's Commission (35) and the chief counsel for the American Medical Association (AMA) (43) supporting the physician's right to deny futile treatments have been under increasing scrutiny and criticism as being too simplistic. This area has considerable relevance to artificial nutrition, especially by the intravenous route, because of its expense, increased risk of infection, and evidence of little or no benefit in advanced disease, particularly in patients with cancer who are unresponsive to disease-specific therapy.

Justifications for physician refusal of futile interventions for the competent patient include (a) the specific intervention proposed has no physiologic rationale, (b) the intervention has already been tried and failed to achieve any apparent benefit, (c) maximal treatment for the underlying advanced disease is a failure, and (d) the intervention will not help achieve the goal of care, is burdensome, and may worsen the quality of life (15).

With respect to nutrition, how valid are these justifications? Item (a) earlier is obviously questionable or incorrect in the case of intravenous feeding, because it does provide essential nutrition and hydration; (b) would not hold if nutrition has not previously been given; arguments (c) and (d) may hold true. However the challenge to statement (d) rests on the answer to the question: whose goal or value is most valid—the physician's or the patient's? If the patient wishes to continue the requested treatment—even for a limited period—to achieve his or her goal (e.g., survival for additional months to see an only child married or the first grandchild born), what is the justification for saying "nay"?

Even if the likelihood of success, in the opinion of the physician, is very small, how can one know if a particular patient will or will not respond? Furthermore, can the patient be certain that the physician is fully conversant with the medical literature on this point, or has not misinterpreted the situation, or that other physicians in the same hospital or elsewhere will be in agreement? Uncertainty and changes of therapeutic options in medicine are hardly uncommon (44, 45).

The basis of physician opinion may be that the prospective benefit for the patient does not justify the required resources. However, futility is not to be confused with resource allocation (which requires well-tested clinical data plus administrative and societal decisions for acceptability), even though they do share a common purpose (46, 47). A continuum of conditions and situations extends from those that are obviously futile, to those that produce an effect but are deemed by the physician to be of no net benefit, to those in which the physician is believed to be in error by other physicians or by the patient. In the case of the incompetent patient, the same issues about futile treatments arise in the physician-surrogate relationship.

This issue has resulted in a large number of papers, letters, editorials, and conferences in the medical and bioethics literature (43–49), to the point where the question has been posed: "Is futility a futile concept?" based on the argument that its proponents have not paid sufficient attention to the problematic nature of the data supporting the use of their definitions (49).

It is not surprising that strongly held differences of opinion may arise between and among physicians, patients, families, and surrogates about treatment that arguably is futile. Collaborative procedures have been advocated or instituted to help solve such problems and settle such differences constructively, short of the courts (50, 51).

Patient Self-Determination Act

As a result of the recommendation of the President's Commission and other similar suggestions, federal legislation (the Patient Self-Determination Act of 1990) was enacted and became law on December 1, 1991 (52). This law applies to hospitals, nursing homes, hospices, health care maintenance organizations, and health care companies receiving Medicare and Medicaid funds. At the time of admission, enrollment, or on initiating home care, these groups are required to inform patients about their legal rights in that specific state and assist them in making decisions concerning their medical care and formulating advance directives. Such a directive must be in the patient's medical record, indicating whether life support has been rejected. This federal law, as well as most state laws and court decisions on this subject, also allow hospitals and nursing homes to express their administrative positions on these subjects to the patient before or at admission. One goal of the statute is to encourage (but not require) adults to complete advance directives in the form of treatment directives, a proxy appointment, or both while they are competent. Another goal is to influence both health care givers and institutions to honor advance directives.

As a result of the majority decision of the US Supreme Court on the Cruzan case (see later) and the Patient Self-Determination Act, advance directives must be based on the legal requirement of individual states. Thus, standards in the United States have been established in varying degrees for truth in prognosis (53), informed consent, and advance care directives.

In the approximately 15 years of the existence of advance care directives, numerous surveys and studies have commented on what has become a complicated and variable matter. It has been noted that most patients do not execute directives in part because physicians frequently fail to discuss this issue (43) or because patients fail to see the notices about directives when they are distributed on admission (54). Even when such directives are executed, only about 39% of patients in one study wished to have the directives observed strictly by the physician (55). In addition, significant numbers of directives are either ignored or overridden by the physician; sometimes more treatment is given than requested and sometimes less (43, 56).

Attitudes toward executing directives, especially by older persons, are significantly influenced by a number of factors including dependence on family decisions, educational and economic status, religious views, ethnic backgrounds, and national origins. For example, Korean-Americans and Mexican-Americans were more likely to hold a family-centered model of medical decision making, rather than the patient autonomy model favored by most African-American and European-American respondents (57). Most Navajo informants considered advance care planning a dangerous violation of their traditional values (58). To develop the understanding of and respect for cultural differences that will help to avoid inappropriately paternalistic judgments, physicians do well to seek assistance from family members and others who are knowledgeable in this area (59).

Patient Decision-Making and Its Consequences

The processes of decision making concerning medical intervention, life support of the seriously ill, and the issue of quality of life and its expected duration have been ongoing. Earlier, studies used measures of physiologic competence (e.g., organ function or metabolic indices), economic or environmental factors, or overall individual performance to ascertain whether any of these factors are improved by specific therapies. More recently, efforts have been spent obtaining information on the relative importance patients assign to the value of their lives and how it may be influenced by their therapies (60, 61). The subjective health values and ratings of 1438 seriously ill but competent patients with at least one of nine diseases with a projected overall mortality rate of 50% were compared with similar ratings obtained from the patients' surrogates and their physicians. The health values of the patients varied greatly from one to another, but the individual patient showed excellent test-retest reliability. Patients' preferences for living at current health levels compared with living in excellent health correlated strongly with their preferences for care that extended life even though it was at the expense of pain and discomfort (62).

In a more recent study of 226 persons 60 or more years of age, all of whom had limited life expectancy because of cancer, congestive heart failure, or advanced lung disease, acceptance of projected treatments depended on its results. If either severe functional impairment or cognitive impairment were likely, 74.4 and 88.8%, respectively, would object to treatment as compared with almost all who chose treatment when the outcome was reasonable survival rather than death (63). In an accompanying editorial, the difficulties with advance directives were emphasized both in the failure of adherence to them, once drawn, and particularly by the difficulty faced by healthy persons who have to make a judgment for the future with no certainty (64).

In addition to the cultural differences noted earlier are important differences in the responses of elderly persons about the use of living wills and desire for life-sustaining treatments between those who have chosen to forgo life-sustaining treatments and those who have not indicated such a preference. Persons with living wills were less likely

to change their expressed wishes (14%) over a 2-year period than those without (41%) (65). During the study period, those patients who had been hospitalized, had an accident, became more immobile or depressed, or had less social support showed appreciable change in the stability of choice and now wanted increased treatment. Such data indicate the need for periodic review of preferences for life-sustaining treatments.

Consequences of Having No Advance Directive or an Inadequate One

A suitable advance directive (for a given state) communicates the individual's wishes about future treatment to physician, hospital, and immediate family. It also safeguards against the wishes of dissident family members. It is equally important, in those states that require it, that the wishes be stated clearly also to the surrogate. The unfortunate consequences of failure in these respects are discussed in selected cases reviewed in the next section.

Even though an advance directive may exist, problems may occur for a number of reasons, in large part because of inadequate communication among patients, their doctors, and their families. Hanson and associates looked at this issue by interviewing family members of 461 elderly persons who had died recently of one of a variety of chronic diseases (lung, heart, cancer, and liver) (66). Approximately half of the deaths occurred in the hospital, one fourth in nursing homes, and the others at home. Respondents reported that in 23% of the cases, neither patient nor family members participated in discussions about treatment decisions; a living will made no difference. Eight percent felt that more should have been done to prolong life, whereas 18% believed that more should have been done to increase comfort. In response to open-ended questions about satisfactory aspects of care, nearly all comments about hospice were positive, whereas only 69%, 58%, and 51% of comments were positive about hospital care, physician services, and nursing homes, respectively. Forty-four percent of respondents indicated a need for better communication by physicians.

NUTRITION SUPPORT OF THE INCOMPETENT PATIENT

The major medical, ethical, and legal issues relating to nutrition support have involved incompetent patients. More than 30 separate state court decisions on this issue between 1983 and 1995 have been summarized (67). Cantor reviewed in detail in 2001 the complex "legal framework that provides options for preserving a modicum of dignity in the dying process" in the years since the Quinlan case (68).

There are many causes of incompetence, ranging from severe memory loss without physical disability in various types of dementia progressing to loss of cognitive ability eventually requiring hand or tube feeding, acute traumatic or nontraumatic brain injury from stroke, cardiorespiratory arrest, or metabolic or developmental disorders. Until physicians have had sufficient time to develop a firm diagnosis and prognosis of the individual patient who is unable to take sufficient food and fluid by mouth, nutrition and hydration are indicated.

Traditionally, the right of the state to preserve the life of the incompetent patient has been manifest in the requirement for a court-appointed guardian or surrogate to act on behalf of the adult patient. In the case of minors, courts have almost always affirmed the authority of the parents or (if needed) a surrogate to make decisions.

The Vegetative State

The Multi-Society Task Force on the persistent vegetative state (PVS) defined this condition as a "clinical condition of complete unawareness of the self and the environment accompanied by sleep-wake cycles with partial preservation of hypothalamic and brain stem autonomic functions" (69). Seven diagnostic criteria were given. Facial and reflex movements, groans, and cries may occur, and small amounts of food placed in the mouth may be swallowed (31, 69). Clinical observation, the results of positron emission tomographic studies and neuropathologic examination support the belief that these patients are unaware and insensate and lack the cerebral cortical capacity to be conscious of pain (70). In its 1994 report, the Task Force referred to estimates of PVS in the United States of 10,000 to 25,000 adults and 4000 to 10,000 children (67).

Guidelines were also developed by a multidisciplinary working group convened by the Royal College of Physicians (71). This group preferred the following definition: "vegetative state: to describe the condition which may be transient with recovery/or which might persist to death." The term *continuing vegetative state* was applied when the condition persisted for more than 4 weeks and recovery from coma became unlikely. A "permanent" state exists "when the diagnosis of irreversibility can be established with a high degree of clinical certainty." The working group accepted the US Multi-Society Task Force on PVS suggestion for use of the term *permanent* for adults and children with traumatic injury of 12 months' duration, and 3 months' duration for those with nontraumatic injuries.

In the study of 257 patients, the cumulative mortality rate at 3 years was 70%, and at 5 years, 84% (72). Survival beyond 10 years was unusual, but some patients lived for 30 years (20, 61). Progressive spasticity and bed rest lead to muscle atrophy and limb, hand, and foot contraction. The term *permanent vegetative state* is prognostic, because the outcome cannot be known with absolute accuracy. It may be used after the time lapses noted, which strongly indicate that recovery is very unlikely.

The Multi-Society Task Force noted that relatively few patients of the 754 in PVS had verified recovery of consciousness after 12 months following traumatic injury, or more than 3 months after a nontraumatic injury; the few who recovered were left with severe disability (70). Jennet reviewed in detail prognosis for recovery and survival of many of the same and other reports (73). The need for competent and persistent serial evaluation of all vegetative patients and the use of additional evaluation techniques have been emphasized (73–75).

Most survivors of cardiac arrest are comatose after resuscitation, and meaningful neurologic recovery occurs in a small proportion of cases. Because treatment can be lengthy, expensive, and difficult for family and staff, Booth and associates evaluated the precision and accuracy of various clinical signs in predicting poor outcome in postcardiac arrest coma. Absent corneal reflexes, absent papillary responses, absent withdrawal response to pain and no motor response, all at 24 hours, plus no motor response at 72 hours, were found to strongly predict death or poor neurologic outcome. When the summary likelihood ratios were at the 95% confidence interval, the probability of a poor outcome was 97% (76).

The impact of PVS on the patient's family and friends is one of distress and helplessness. Psychologic consequences of seeing the loved one remain unresponsive with increasing atrophy and contractures as weeks and months pass are exacerbated by developing monetary and social problems. Many such cases have led to multiple court decisions that have focused the attention of the public, other courts, and medical societies on biomedical and ethical issues related to the requests for withdrawal of life-sustaining treatments including withdrawal of artificial nutrition and hydration (68). Some instructive cases with important court decisions affecting adults are summarized in the following sections.

The Quinlan Case

The case of Karen Ann Quinlan was a landmark effort to discontinue life support.

She was a young woman in New Jersey who was in PVS on a respirator. The state's Supreme Court, on a reversal of a lower court decision, made medical legal history in 1976 when, at the request of the parents and despite the opposition of the patient's physician and hospital, it ruled that the father should be Karen's legal guardian, and as he wished, the respirator was discontinued (77). When this was done, the patient was able to breathe spontaneously, and she survived for 9 years on tube feeding until she died from overwhelming infection. Withdrawal of tube feeding was not considered an option by the parents. This position reflected a view then widely held, namely, that food and hydration were not in the category of a special life-support system but rather a humanitarian action necessary for the comfort of the patient.

The Barber-Nejde Case

Another troubling judicial issue was the legal liability of physicians when nutrition was withheld from an incompetent patient who was not terminally ill and who, while competent, had not clearly indicated in writing or verbally to a reliable witness a desire not to be artificially fed when terminally or incurably ill.

This concern is illustrated by the case of Clarence Herbert, who had suffered respiratory arrest in association with routine intestinal surgery (78). Following resuscitation, he remained comatose over the following several days. On the advice of physicians that prognosis for recovery was poor and, with consent of family, use of the respirator was stopped. The patient then breathed spontaneously but without change in his comatose state. Two days later, again after consultation with the family, the attending physicians ordered removal of the nasogastric tube, intravenous nutrition, and air mist. The patient died 6 days later. He had not previously executed a format directive under the California Natural Death Act, nor had he written anything concerning his wishes in such circumstances; however, he had stated to his wife that he did not want to be kept alive by machine or "become another Karen Ann Quinlan."

A nurse reported the actions of the physicians to local authorities, who then filed criminal charges for murder against both attending physicians, Drs. Barber and Nejde. Despite a municipal court magistrate ruling that death had resulted from brain damage secondary to anoxia and that the conduct of the physicians was not "unlawful," the district attorney appealed the case to Los Angeles Superior Court. The murder charge was reinstated by a judge who decided that there was no legal justification for the physicians' action. When the physicians appealed to the California Court of Appeals, that court dismissed the criminal charges in October 1983.

The Conroy Case

Another important case, occurring at the same time, further delineated the complex medicolegal issues and varied court decisions that arise when the status of an incurably ill patient is presented to different jurists.

Claire Conroy was an 84-year-old woman severely ill with advanced atherosclerosis, diabetes, and organic brain syndrome. A nephew filed a petition to authorize removal of the nasogastric feeding tube from the patient, although there was no clear evidence of what the patient would have desired. A trial judge authorized removal of the feeding tube but not cessation of any voluntary or assisted oral feeding. The decision was appealed by the nursing home and, pending the hearing, tube feeding was continued until the patient's death. Despite Conroy's death, the New Jersey Appellate Court heard the appeal and reversed the earlier trial judge's decision (79). It held that (a) she was neither comatose nor terminally ill, (b) the feeding tube
was not a particularly invasive treatment as was the respirator in the Quinlan case, and (c) if the nasogastric tube had been removed in accordance with the trial judge's decision, Mrs. Conroy would have died not as a result of her condition but from a "new and independent condition: dehydration and starvation and that this would constitute murder (euthanasia)." The case was then appealed to the New Jersey Supreme Court that sanctioned withdrawal of artificial nutrition and hydration in this type of case but with a time constraint of expected survival of 1 year or less (80).

In his review of the case, Emanuel noted that the court laid down three standards for terminating such care and stipulated that one of them be satisfied before treatment could be stopped (81). The court designated the first a "subjective standard," which permits termination of treatment when an incompetent patient left clear indication, such as a living will, that he or she would have refused that treatment. It called the second a "pure objective standard," which permits termination of life-sustaining treatment for patients if the burden of the care outweighs the benefits, although they have not left indication of their preferences about life-sustaining care; for example, administering life-sustaining care would be inhumane because it would perpetuate severe pain. Others label this the "best interests standard," wherein the patient's surrogate objectively evaluates the benefits and risks of a treatment and decides which most benefits the patient. The court, acting as surrogate, accepted this standard. The third standard, called by the court a "limited objective standard," is a combination of the first two and permits termination of care if there is some evidence (e.g., remarks made during a conversation) or opinion of the surrogate that the patient would not want the treatment and if the burden and pain of continued life outweigh the benefits; this is similar to the substituted judgment standard.

The judicial ambivalence is further demonstrated in the decision of the same New Jersey Supreme Court in the later Nancy Jobes case (82). Family members took this case to court when the nursing home refused to discontinue tube feedings of Mrs. Jobes who was in PVS. Instead of adopting its previous "Conroy" criteria, the court returned to the "substituted judgment" of the Quinlan case.

Emanuel and Emanuel briefly reviewed the judicial and legislative history and endorsement of decision making for incompetent patients by proxy or surrogate and their ethical justification (83). They summarized objections to proxy making on the grounds that "proxy decision makers cannot divine or implement the incompetent patient's wishes regarding the termination of life sustaining care." Alternative solutions were suggested, with recognition that each has limitations. While agreeing with the array of concerns about proxy decision making, Lynn, in an accompanying editorial, took the position that "a morally justifiably and pragmatic policy for decision making for incompetent adults, at this point, will have to rely heavily on appointed and family proxies, with a morally defensible and practical plan" (84) that provides options similar to those suggested by the Coordinating Council on Life Sustaining Medical Treatment Decision-Making by the Courts (85).

American Medical Association Statement of 1986

In the midst of these and other pertinent judicial decisions, the AMA, through its Council on Ethical and Judicial Affairs, issued in 1984 (and in revised form in 1986) statements on withholding or withdrawing life-prolonging medical treatment. The 1986 statement consists of four short paragraphs that include the following, which also relate to food and fluids (86):

In the absence of the patient's choice or an authorized proxy, the physician must act in the best interest of the patient. … For humane reasons, with informed consent, a physician may do what is medically necessary to alleviate severe pain, or cease or omit treatment to permit a terminally ill patient whose death is imminent to die. Even if death is not imminent but a patient's coma is beyond doubt irreversible and there are adequate safeguards to confirm the accuracy of the diagnosis and with the concurrence of those with responsibility for the care of the patient, it is not unethical to discontinue all means of life prolonging medical treatment. Life prolonging medical treatment includes medication and artificially or technologically supplied respiration, nutrition, or hydration.

The change in physician attitudes resulting from the continuing widespread interest and discussion of these issues is evidenced by significant differences between the 1984 and 1986 statements. For example, the first version refers only to terminally ill patients, whereas the later one includes those in irreversible coma; the 1984 version did not define "life prolonging medical treatment," whereas in 1986, these are specifically designated and include nutrition or hydration.

The Cruzan Case

This case was the first to involve the US Supreme Court on the issue of discontinuance of tube feeding an incompetent patient. Like the Quinlan case, it aroused widespread public and professional interest and resulted in a decision with far-reaching implications.

In January 1983, at the age of 25 years, Nancy Cruzan suffered irreversible brain damage following an automobile accident and was then supported in the hospital by tube feeding. In 1986, her parents requested discontinuance of the feedings but had to resort to legal action at the insistence of the Missouri state hospital administration. In July 1988, a trial court ruled that tube feeding could be withheld; however, on appeal, the Missouri Supreme Court, by a four to three decision, reversed the trial court on the grounds that no reliable evidence was presented indicating that Cruzan would have refused artificial feeding (87).

On June 25, 1990, the US Supreme Court affirmed the state court's reversal by a vote of five to four (88). Three of the four dissenting justices stated that incompetent as well as competent patients had the constitutional right to be free of unwanted medical treatment, and the fourth stated that the Constitution required that the best interest of the patient be followed. Six of the nine justices explicitly found no distinction between fluids and nutrition delivered artificially and other medical treatments; none of the other three found a constitutionally relevant distinction (88, 89).

The words of one of these judges, Sandra Day O'Connor, are instructive: "The liberty guaranteed [by the Fourteenth Amendment] must protect, if it protects anything, an individual's deeply personal decision to reject medical treatment, including the artificial delivery of food and water" (90).

Six months later, nearly 8 years after the parents' first request, a judge in Missouri Circuit Court, in a brief order, authorized the parents as coguardians "to cause the removal of nutrition and hydration from our ward, Nancy Beth Cruzan" (91). This was done, and Cruzan died 12 days later.

Evidence of the impact of the Supreme Court's decision was the rapid collapse of the medical, institutional, surrogate, and legal opposition in Missouri to discontinuing Cruzan's feedings and the speed with which many states enacted health proxy legislation (92). Major problems still remained, however, because of the variability in important judicial positions and requirements among state judges and laws.

The Schiavo Case

This long-term case of PVS illustrates the interplay of family dissent, politics, and religious beliefs.

In 1993, Terri Schiavo at age 27 developed acute potassium deficiency while on a severe weight-reducing regimen that lead to transient cardiac arrest, coma, PVS, and tube feeding. With no advance directive, her husband made efforts in Florida courts to have the tube withdrawn but was successfully opposed by her parents. On October 15, 2003, however, a District Court of Appeals judge ordered the tube removed, whereupon the parents appealed to Governor Jeb Bush, and the state legislature quickly passed a law ordering the tube replaced. The feedings were resumed, and another guardian was appointed. On the grounds that the legislation was unconstitutional, Mr. Schiavo appealed to the Circuit Court and on April 6, 2004, a presiding judge ruled in his favor. The governor's office then filed an appeal to the Florida Supreme Court. "In late September 2004 this court ruled unanimously that the Governor violated "a cornerstone of American Democracy in overriding a court decision" (93a). Another Governor's appeal was rejected by the US Supreme Court; other appeals by the Schindler family were followed by court rejections. A Florida court judge again ordered the feeding tube removed and this was done on March 18, 2005. Two days later on March 20, the U.S. House and Senate passed a special bill that was then signed by President Bush that allowed the Schindlers to appeal to various federal courts. These and state courts, in turn, rejected their appeals. Mrs. Schiavo died on March 31, 2005 (93b).

In addition to PVS and the "locked-in syndrome" described in the Bouvia case, other types of severe incapacity continue to raise ethical, family, and legal questions, in part, because of the need for artificial feeding to sustain the patient.

The Minimally Conscious State

This is a fairly recently defined condition in which the patient has some evidence of cognition, some sporadic intelligible speech, and indications of understanding by "yes" or "no" communication or eye movements; nevertheless, the patient is totally dependent and requires tube feeding (94–96). This category includes patients who have regained some consciousness following severe head injury with an initially comatose period.

As would be expected, court cases have been filed for such patients who left no advance directives and have been receiving tube feeding. In the case of Nelson (97) and of Wrenland (98), wives and children requested feeding tube removal, but other family members opposed this request. Despite persistent efforts, the eventual outcome was denial of the request by the courts.

Advanced Dementia

Dementia is also in the category of disabling neurologic conditions with the potential for prolonged survival and the resulting issue of life-sustaining medical treatment. Dementia includes Alzheimer disease, multiinfarcts of the brain, other vascular dementias with variable cognitive deficits (31, 34), the variants of Creutzfeldt-Jakob disease, and dementias associated with parkinsonism and progressive supranuclear palsy (99). These disorders are characterized by gradual onset of progressive neurologic deterioration occurring over years to decades, with the time to prognostic certainty usually months to a year or more.

PVS is the ultimate and terminal form of dementia as the result of complete loss of neocortical function (31, 69). An estimated 4 million patients in the United States have various stages of dementia, of which 1.3 to 1.9 million have Alzheimer disease (34). Increasing proportions of patients are surviving to the advanced states in which they are unable to eat orally and swallow normally.

As occurred with the cases with the minimally conscious state, a woman with advanced Alzheimer disease who was receiving tube feeding, without an advance directive, had her case appealed by her sister and guardian so feeding could be discontinued; the appeal was denied in 1997 by a Wisconsin court (100). In the same year, the

Supreme Court agreed that a "best interests" judgment by a guardian was allowable only for patients with PVS; other patients had to have an advance directive or other clear evidence of their wishes (100, 101). Some courts in other states have on occasion disagreed with this view.

Mitchell and colleagues recently reviewed use of tube feedings in those residents of national Medicare- and Medicaid-certified nursing homes who had advanced cognitive impairments; the assessments were made within 60 days of April 1, 1999 (102). Thirty-four percent (98) of such patients were being tube fed. Interestingly, these investigators made no mention of the 66% of such patients without feeding tubes; however, the inability of such patients to eat orally and to swallow suggests that the patients died with minimum nutrition support. The closing comments in this review include the statement: "Comprehensive implementation of advance care planning is likely to reduce the use of feeding tubes." In a further study, Mitchell and associates found that most patients with advanced dementia in the Medicare- and Medicaid-licensed nursing homes that were studied do not die within 6 months and do not receive the comprehensive palliative care that they deserve under the current hospice eligibility requirements (103).

Advance Care Directives

It is apparent from the few cases described in this chapter, and documented more fully in Cantor (68), that the failure to have an adequate advance directive by an initially competent patient (now incompetent) will lead to an outcome that neither the patient nor close family members originally wanted. As noted by Cantor (65) and by Gillick (90), there are states (e.g., New York, Michigan, Wisconsin) where the advance directive is insufficient if the surrogate—absent a family member with the advance directive—has no proof of such a directive.

Under both common law and constitutional law, a competent individual has the right, with few exceptions, either to consent to or to refuse any medical treatment that is offered even though rejection of treatment may result in death. Despite the importance of this issue and the existence of the Patient Self-Determination Act of 1990 and relevant state laws, few adults have written directives. Gillick cites a figure of 15 to 20% (90). After reviewing more than 100 research papers on this subject, Miles and colleagues concluded that "advance treatment preferences have been difficult to form, communicate, and implement" (104).

A major responsibility rests on every physician or other health professional who is in a position to advise patients and every lawyer who assists in preparing a will to discuss the importance of an advance directive—be it a living will type or power of attorney in a form suitable for the relevant state. In those states where a proxy or surrogate is likely, that specific person should be specifically included.

The periodic publication in the *JAMA* in recent years of a series of papers termed "Perspectives on Care at the Close of Life" produced and edited at the University of California at San Francisco provides information and insight through interviews with varieties of patients, their families, physicians, and other health care providers on issues of decision making and care, together with relevant research-oriented documentation.

Palliative Care; Hospice

In the quarter-century since the founding of hospice care in England, this system has expanded greatly in the United States and elsewhere. Hospice exists as independent nonprofit, hospital-based, or private programs with care available at home or in nursing homes. Such care is designed for patients with a life-limiting illness or injury who understand their prognosis, make advanced plans, and designate a surrogate decision maker. Entry to hospice has traditionally meant that aggressive efforts at cure or palliation in acute care hospitals are replaced by pain control, symptom management, social and psychologic support, and dignity-concerned approaches for the patient and family. The amount of time in hospice depends on care needs (105, 106). The Medical Hospice Benefits provision created by Congress in 1982 provides a per diem reimbursement for care of those patients likely to have life expectancy no longer than 6 months in whom the goal is palliation. In her "Perspective on Care at the Close of Life," Lynn discusses such a case from the viewpoints of the patient and his or her family, the guidelines of the national hospice organization, and the available options (105). Morrison and Meier reviewed protocols for communicating with patients about topics in palliative care and approaches to management and care coordination at various stages of serious chronic illnesses (107). In their discussion, they mention the National Comprehensive Cancer Network for patients with advanced incurable cancer and the National Consensus Project for Quality Palliative Care, a collaborative effort of five national palliative care organizations.

Recently, some hospice-type programs have added therapeutic management for patients with advanced acquired immunodeficiency syndrome (108), and some of these programs include aggressive disease treatments through some hospitals and insurance companies (104, 110). Indicative of the influence of the hospice programs is the enrollment rise from 246,000 patients in 1992 to 885,000 in 2002 (110).

Attitude Changes in the Care of Ill Children

In contrast to issues concerning incompetent adults, forgoing medically provided nutrition and hydration in children has until relatively recently received much less discussion and legal review. In a review of the status of this issue in 1995, Nelson and associates noted that pediatri-

cians were more likely than internists to continue artificial nutrition and hydration in PVS against parental desires, even though other life support systems had been discontinued (111). These authors listed three major medical categories of children for whom it was considered ethically permissible to forgo such nutrition and hydration: neurologic devastation, such as PVS from severe brain injury or anencephaly; irreversible total intestinal failure, such as total bowel necrosis or neural dysplasia; and proximate death (days or weeks) in conditions such as advanced, unresponsive cancer. The issue of total intestinal failure is discussed in light of the possibility of a successful bowel transplant and the presence of other serious disease in recipient and donor. Various judicial decisions concerned with cessation of artificial feeding (in most of which the courts upheld the desire by the parents for termination) were reviewed, as well as federal statutory law and state laws (111).

A recent review entitled "Pediatric Palliative Care" documented very significant changes in such concerns with emphasis on the need for extension of designated palliative care teams in all health care facilities that serve life-threatened children (112). The authors pointed out that in contrast to adults, particularly those who are elderly or suffering from long illnesses in which death is often acceptable or even welcome, "a child's death remains emotionally difficult, unnatural, and unexpected for families and health care providers alike." These investigators noted that, as the result of advances in medical science and technology, there is much longer survival of children with rare disorders and complex medical conditions; this presents special problems in care and in prognosis because of certain medical problems in which premature death is likely or expected. The concept of palliative care in children encompasses efforts at curing and healing combined with the areas of hospice philosophy of attention to social, psychologic, and spiritual needs of the child and family and ameliorating pain and suffering extended widely to home, hospital, and school (112). The review documented an extensive literature including a guide to children's palliative care service by the Royal College of Pediatrics and Child Health in 1997, on pediatric palliative care from the National Academies Press in 2001 and 2003, and support for this concept by the American Academy of Pediatrics in 2000. In contrast to the limited coverage noted by Nelson and associates in 1995 (105, 111), the authors' list of conditions appropriate for palliative care includes multiple diseases of various causes.

Physiologic Responses to Food-Water Restriction

Young, healthy, active persons in negative water balance develop thirst, dry mouth, and headache, followed by fatigue; cognitive impairment occurs as dehydration progresses and becomes severe with abnormal electrolytes, rising blood urea, and hemoconcentration. Renal failure ensues unless water is available. In healthy elderly people, in contrast, reduced thirst may occur with water deprivation (113).

Those involved in palliative care of terminally ill patients have reported frequently that the conscious competent patient with an advancing severe illness unresponsive to therapy and in little or no pain becomes progressively weaker, with decreasing communication, increasing anorexia, decreased desire for fluids, and progressive apathy. In such patients with little intake of fluids, signs and symptoms of dehydration appear: dryness of skin and mouth, decreased urinary output, and occasional thirst. Nausea, vomiting, and cramps are reportedly rare in this situation, and the dehydrated patient rarely needs oral pharyngeal suction; this is in contrast to the hydrated patient (31, 113–120). Obtundation usually progresses to a peaceful death.

There are significant numbers of reports (summarized in 119) that many terminally ill patients have relatively few of the changes in blood and urine chemistry that indicate clinical dehydration and that thirst is usually absent. In a brief report about terminally ill patients, no differences were noted in biochemical parameters and state of consciousness in those given intravenous fluids and those given only oral fluids (120). In their detailed study of 32 competent terminally ill cancer patients, McCann and colleagues concluded that "food and fluid administered beyond the specific requests of patients may play a minimal role in providing comfort to terminally ill patients"; 97% either did not experience hunger at all or only initially, 66% either did not experience thirst or only initially, and the rest were comfortable with mouth care and sips of water (121).

The relationships among symptoms, laboratory evidence of dehydration, and medications were studied in 82 patients dying of cancer in a hospice; none were given artificial fluid therapy, and the time from entry into the study to death ranged from 1 to 5 days (median, 2 days). Fifty percent had normal serum osmolalities below the upper limit of normal and a urea concentration below 11.0 mmol/L, which was not considered evidence of dehydration. The others had evidence of dehydration. There was no statistically significant relationship between hydration status and the symptoms of dry mouth and thirst noted by about 85% of those able to respond clearly to questions. Almost all the latter patients were receiving medications known to cause dry mouth and/or had other causes for this condition such as mouth breathing, candidiasis, and past treatment with chemotherapeutic agents and radiotherapy (122).

Management of symptoms that may arise when artificial nutrition and hydration are withheld or withdrawn is outlined in Table 101.1.

When palliative care becomes unacceptable for some patients because of pain or other symptoms and other factors, competent patients may request help hastening death for a variety of reasons. Some may voluntarily stop eating and drinking or may request terminal sedation

TABLE 101.1. MANAGEMENT OF SYMPTOMS THAT OCCASIONALLY COMPLICATE WITHDRAWAL OF ARTIFICIAL NUTRITION AND HYDRATION

SYMPTOM	MANAGEMENT
Thirst (rare)	Sips of fluids (patients commonly take much less than required for physiologic volume replacement)
Dry mouth (common)	Glycerine swabs, ice chips, sips of fluid; review of medication list for any that cause dry mouth
Dry mouth (if aggravated by glycerine or lemon swabs)	Artificial saliva, petroleum jelly, lip balm
Mouth debris or poor hygiene	Nonalcoholic mouthwashes, dilute hydrogen peroxide
Oral inflammation	Diphenhydramine liquid, viscous lidocaine; antimonilial therapy
Pain, restlessness (rare)	Morphine or benzodiazepines in titrated doses
Nausea (rare)	Antiemetic drugs

From Brody H, Campbell ML, Faber-Langendoen K et al. N Engl J Med 1997;336:652–7, with permission.

(118, 123). In a report from various Oregon hospice units concerning 102 competent patients who died as a consequence of voluntarily stopping food and fluids, 85% died within 2 weeks, and most died with little or no suffering, generally peacefully during this period, with a "good" death (118). Such reports put into question the use of tube and orally administered fluids to the dying patient. The common use of intravenous isotonic glucose—with or without electrolytes or vitamin additives—in this situation also seems less defensible because this prevents ketosis and inhibits some dehydration, thereby overcoming such contributions to comfort and prolonging the dying process.

In the management of such patients with the stated goal of comfort, one must also consider some of the undesirable effects of tube feeding, whether via nasal or gastrostomy tube. These include increased agitation, accidental or self-extubation often requiring restraints, and aspiration pneumonia (124, 125); in addition, leakage, diarrhea, or impaction may occur. As Cranford has stated, "to a large extent limiting nutrition and hydration is more a medical than a moral issue" (31).

REFERENCES

Note: The references to judicial decisions follow the form generally used in legal writing. Following the case name, the first number refers to the volume of the reporter series for the decisional court; the reported series follows as an abbreviation, then the number of the first page of the printed judicial decision, and finally the year of the decision. For example, *Smith v Jones*, 261 F2d448 (1990) can be found in vol. 261 of the second series of the *Federal Reporter* beginning on page 448. Published court decisions are generally available to the public through state, county, or city bar association libraries or law school libraries. West Publishing Company and Mead Data Services also provide case text databases on a fee-for-service basis to libraries and law firms.

1. Pellegrino ED. JAMA 1974;227:1288–94.
2. Lee TH. N Engl J Med 2002;347:1965–7.
3. Pennington CR. Nutrition 1996;12:56–7.
4. Akner G, Cederholm T. Am J Clin Nutr 2001;74:6–24.
5. Institute of Medicine. Crossing the Quality Chasm: A New Health System for the 21st Century. Washington, DC: National Academy Press, 2001.
6. McGlynn EA, Asch SM, Adams J et al. N Engl J Med 2003;348:2635–45.
7. Braunwald EN. N Engl J Med 1997;337;1360–9.
8. Greenland P, Knoll MD, Stamler J et al. JAMA 2003;290:891–7.
9. Khot NW, Khot MB, Bajzer CT et al. JAMA 2003;290:898–904.
10. Canto JG, Iskandrian AE. JAMA 2003;290:947–9[Editorial].
11. Stamler J., Stamler R, Neaton JD et al. JAMA 1999;282;2012–8.
12. Bray GA, Champagne CM. J Am Diet Assoc 2004;104:86–9.
13. Weiss R, Dzivra J, Burger TS et al. N Engl J Med 2004;350:2362–74.
14. Ingelfinger JR. N Engl J Med 2004;350:2123–6.
15. Lo B. Resolving Ethical Dilemmas: A Guide for Clinicians. Baltimore: Williams & Wilkins, 1995.
16. Conrad LI, Neve M, Nutton V et al. The Western Medical Tradition: 800 BC–1800 AD. New York: Cambridge University Press, 1995:1.
17. Siegler M. Mayo Clin Proc 1993;68:461–7.
18. Pellegrino ED. JAMA 1993;269:1158–62.
19. Beauchamp TL, Childress JF. Principles of Biomedical Ethics. New York: Oxford University Press, 1979.
20. Mahowald MD. Clin Geriatr Med 1994;10:403–18.
21. Wolf SM. Am J Law Med 1994;20:395–487.
22. Pellegrino ED. JAMA 1994;271:1668–70.
23. Beauchamp TL, Childress JF. Principles of Biomedical Ethics. 5th ed. New York: Oxford University Press, 2001.
24. Jones AH. Lancet 1997;349:1243–6.
25. Pellegrino ED, Thomasma DC. The Christian Virtues in Medical Practice. Washington, DC: Georgetown University Press, 1996.
26. Freedman F. Duty and Healing: Foundation of a Jewish Bioethics. Available at http://www.mcgill.ca/CTRG/bfreed/.
27. Engelhardt HT Jr. The Foundations of Bioethics. 2nd ed. New York: Oxford University Press, 1996.
28. *Union Pacific Ry v Botsford,* 141 US 250, 251 (1891).
29. *Bouvia v county of Riverside,* 159780 Riverside Co. CA. Sup. Ct. 1984.
30. *Bouvia v Superior Court (Glenchur),* 179 cal. App. 3d 1127 1986;225 cal. Rpts. 297.
31. Cranford RD. Law Med Health Care 1991;19:13–22.
32. Pellegrino ED. NY State J Med 1977;77:1456–62.
33. Nevins M. Am Coll Physicians Observer 1986;Mar:13–6.
34. Howe EG, Gordon DS, Valentin M. Law Med Health Care 1991;19:27–33.
35. President's Commission for the Study of Ethical Problems in Medicine and Biomedical and Behavioral Research. Deciding to Forego Life-Sustaining Treatment. A Report on the Ethical, Medical, and Legal Issues in Treatment Decisions. Washington, DC: United States Government Printing Office, 1983.
36. Hastings Center. Guidelines on the Termination of Life Sustaining Treatment and the Care of the Dying. Briarcliff Manor, NY: Hastings Center, 1987:50.
37. Quill TE, Cassel CK. Ann Intern Med 1995;122:368–74.
38. Cimino JE. Top Clin Nutr 1993;9:29–34.
39. Pellegrino ED. Ann Intern Med 1995;122:377–8.
40. Lo B, Ruston D, Kates LW et al. JAMA 2002;287:749–54
41. Brody H, Campbell ML, Faber-Langendoen K et al. N Engl J Med 197;336:652–7.
42. Gert B, Bernat JL, Mogulnicki RP. Hastings Cent Rep 1994;24:13–5.
43. Orentlicher D. JAMA 1992;267:2101–4.
44. Tiemstra JD. J Clin Ethics 1995;6:163–5.
45. Logan RL, Scott PJ. Lancet 1996;347:595–8.
46. Veach RM, Spicer CM. Am J Law Med 1992;18:15–56.
47. Gatter RA Jr, Moskop JC. J Med Philos 1995;20:191–205.
48. Schneiderman LJ, Jecker NS. Doctors, Patients, and Futile Treatment, Baltimore: Johns Hopkins University Press, 1995.
49. Brody AB, Halevy A. J Med Philos 1995;20:123–44.
50. Spielman BJ. Law Med Ethics 1995;23:136–42.
51. American Medical Association Committee on Ethical and Judicial Affairs. JAMA 1999;281:937–41.
52. Patient Self-Determination Act, sections 4206 and 4751 of the Omnibus Budget Reconciliation Act of 1960;P.L. 101–508 Nov 5, 1990.
53. Annas GJ. N Engl J Med 1994;330:223–5.
54. Cugliari AM, Miller T, Sokal J. Arch Intern Med 1995;155:1893–8.
55. Sehyal A, Gallbraith A, Chesney M et al. JAMA 1992;267:59–63.
56. Danis M, Southerland LI, Barrett JM et al. N Engl J Med 1991;324:882–8.
57. Blackhall LJ, Murphy ST, Frank G et al. JAMA 1955;274:820–5.
58. Carrese JA, Rhodes LA. JAMA 1995;274:826–9.
59. Gostin LO. JAMA 1995;274:844–5.
60. Guyatt GH, Feeny DH, Patrick DL. Ann Intern Med 1993;118:622–9.
61. Gill TM, Feinstein AR. JAMA 1994;272:619–26.
62. Tsevat J, Cook EF, Green ML et al. Ann Intern Med 1995;122:514–20.
63. Fried TR, Bradley EH, Towle VR et al. N Engl J Med 2002;346:1061–6.
64. Meier DE, Morrison RS. N Engl J Med 2002;346:1087–9.
65. Danis M, Garrett J, Harris R et al. Ann Intern Med 1994;120:567–73.
66. Hanson LC, Danis M, Garett J. J Am Geriatr Soc 1997;45:1339–44.
67. American Medical Association Council on Ethical and Judicial Affairs. Code of Medical Ethics: Current Opinions with Annotations, 1996–1997 ed. Chicago: American Medical Association, 1996;275:41–51.
68. Cantor NL. J Law Med Ethics 2001;29:182–96.
69. Multi-Society Task Force on PVS. N Engl J Med 1994;330:1499–508.
70. Multi-Society Task Force on PVS. N Engl J Med 1994;330:1572–9.
71. Royal College of Physicians Working Group. J R Coll Physicians Lond 1996;30:119–21.
72. Ashwell S, Cranford R. N Engl J Med 1995;333:130[Correction].
73. Jennet B. The Vegetative State: Medical Facts, Ethical and Legal Dilemmas. Cambridge: Cambridge University Press 2002.
74. Cranford R. BMJ 1996;313:5–6[Editorial].
75. Zeman A. Lancet 1997;350:795–9.
76. Booth CM, Boone RH, Tomlinson G et al. JAMA 2004:291:870–79.
77. *In re Quinlan* 70 NJ 10, 355 A2d;647, 1976.
78. Myers DW. Arch Intern Med 1985;145:125–7.
79. *Matter of Claire Conroy* 453, 464 A 2d 303 (NJ App. 1983).
80. *Matter of Claire Conroy* rev'd cf also 98 NJ 321, 486A 2d 1209 (1985).

81. Emanuel EJ. Lancet 1988;1:170–1.
82. Emanuel EJ. Lancet 1988;1:106–7.
83. Emanuel EJ, Emanuel LL. JAMA 1992;267:2067–71.
84. Lynn J. JAMA 1992;267:2082–4.
85. Coordinating Council on Life-Sustaining Medical Treatment Decision-Making by the Courts. Guidelines for State Court Decision-Making in Authorizing or Withholding Life Sustaining Medical Treatment. Williamsburg, VA: National Center for State Courts, 1991.
86. American Medical Association Council on Ethical and Judicial Affairs. Withholding or Withdrawing Life Prolonging Medical Treatment. Chicago: American Medical Association, 1986.
87. *Cruzan v Harmson* 760 SW 2d 408 (MO 1988).
88. *Cruzan v Missouri Department of Health* 760 sw 2d 408 aff 110 S. Ct. 2841 (1990).
89. Annas GJ. Law Med Health Care 1991;19:32–9.
90. Gillick MR. N Engl J Med 2004;350:7–8.
91. *Cruzan v Mouton Estate* No CV 384–9P (Circ. Ct Jasper Co, filed Dec. 14, 1990) (Teel).
92. King PA. Law Med Health Care 1991;325:511–2.
93. Associated Press. Winston-Salem J April 7, 2004:A14.
93a. Washington Post. Quoted in Winston-Salem J September 24, 2004.
93b. Associated Press. Winston-Salem J April 1, 2005:p.1.
94. Multi-Society Task Force on PVS. N Engl J Med 1994;330:23–4, 142.
95. Giacino J, Ashwal S, Childs N et al. Neurology 2002;58:349–53.
96. Boly M, Faymonville ME. Peigneux P et al. Arch Neurol 2004;61:233–8.
97. Nelson L, Cranford RE, Martin M et al. Contemp Health Law Policy 1999;15:427–53.
98. Lo B, Dornbrand L, Wolf L et al. N Engl J Med 2002;346:1489–93.
99. Case Records of the Massachusetts General Hospital. Case 26–1997. N Engl J Med 1997;337:549–56.
100. Multi-Society Task Force on PVS. N Engl J Med 1994;330:143.
101. Shapiro RS. In re Edna MF. Theor Med 1999;20:45–54.
102. Mitchell LS, Teno JM, Roy J et al. JAMA 2003;290:73–80.
103. Mitchell LS, Kiley DK, Hamel MB et al. JAMA 2004;291:2734–40.
104. Miles SH, Koepp R, Weber EP. Arch Intern Med 1996;156:1062–8.
105. Lynn J. JAMA 2001;285:925–32.
106. Chochinov HM. JAMA 2002;287;2253–60.
107. Morrison RS, Meier DE. N Engl J Med 2004;350:2582–90.
108. Selwyn PA, Forstein M, JAMA 2003;290:806–14.
109. Petersen A. Wall Street J May 20, 2004:D5.
110. National Hospice and Palliative Care Org (www.nhpco.org).
111. Nelson LJ, Rushton CH, Cranford RE et al. J Law Med Ethics 1995;23:33–46.
112. Himelstein BP, Hilden JM, Boldt AM et al. N Engl J Med 2004;350:1752–62.
113. Phillips P, Rolls BJ, Ledingham GG Jr et al. N Engl J Med 1984;311:753–9.
114. Zerwekh JV. Nursing 1983;83:47–51.
115. Printz LA. Geriatrics 1988;43:84–8.
116. Schmitz P. Law Med Health Care 1991;19;19:23–6.
117. Dunlop R J, Ellershaw JE, Baines MJ. J Med Ethics 1995;21:141–3.
118. Ganzini L, Goy ER, Miller LL et al. N Engl J Med 2003;349;359–65.
119. Fletcher JC, Spencer EM. Lancet 1995;345:271–2.
120. Waller A, Adunski A, Hershkowitz J. Lancet 1991;337:745.
121. McCann RM, Hall WJ, Groth-Juncker A. JAMA 1994;272:1263–6.
122. Ellershaw JE, Sutcliffe JM, Saunders CM. J Pain Symptom Manage 1995;10:192–7.
123. Quill TE, Lo B, Brock DW. 1997:278:2099–104.
124. Giocon JO, Silverstone FA, Graner LM et al. Arch Intern Med 1988;148:429–3.
125. Quill TE. Arch Intern Med 1989;149:1937–41.

SELECTED READINGS

Beauchamp TL, Childress JF. Principles of Biomedical Ethics. 5th ed. New York: Oxford University Press, 2001.

Lo B. Resolving Ethical Dilemmas: A Guide for Clinicians. 2nd ed. Philadelphia: Lippincott Williams & Wilkins, 2000.

Pellegrino E, Mazzarella P, Corsi P, eds. Transcultural Dimensions in Medical Ethics. Frederick, MD: University Publishing, 1992.

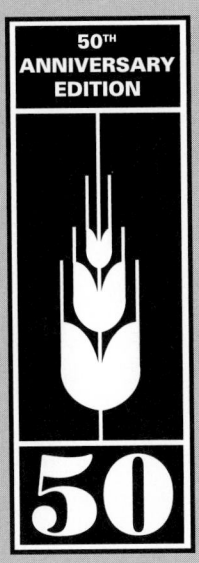

50TH
ANNIVERSARY
EDITION

50

PART VI

DIET AND NUTRITION IN HEALTH OF POPULATIONS

102 FOUNDATIONS OF A HEALTHY DIET[1]
WALTER C. WILLETT AND MEIR J. STAMPFER

QUANTITY VERSUS QUALITY OF DIET 1626
DOES DIETARY GUIDANCE NEED TO BE
   INDIVIDUALIZED? 1626
SPECIFIC CONSIDERATIONS IN FORMULATING
   A HEALTHY DIET 1627
   Dietary Fat and Specific Fatty Acids 1627
   Carbohydrates 1628
   Protein 1629
   Vegetables and Fruits 1629
   Calcium and Dairy Products 1630
   Salt and Processed Meats 1630
   Alcohol 1630
   Vitamin Supplements 1630
  SUMMARY 1631
REPRESENTATION OF AN OVERALL HEALTHY
   DIET AND VALIDATION 1632
   Guidelines and Pyramids 1632
   Indices..............................1633
CONCLUSIONS 1633

Nutritional science has provided a wealth of data ranging from detailed molecular descriptions of nutrients and their actions to epidemiologic findings from large prospective studies and controlled randomized studies on selected population groups. Integrating this vast literature into a description of a healthy diet is a challenging but yet essential step to provide the public and those responsible for food programs with the best information regarding their food choices. Efforts to develop descriptions of a healthy diet include the *US Dietary Guidelines for Americans* (1), a synthesis by the Institute of Medicine (2), and recommendations of the World Health Organization (3). Because information on diet and health is accruing rapidly, these syntheses of dietary information require frequent updating, which is recognized by the requirement that the *US Dietary Guidelines* be reviewed every 5 years. In this chapter, considerations for developing the definition of a healthy diet are discussed, and some of the main issues are

reviewed briefly, recognizing that they are addressed in detail elsewhere in this text. Finally, several alternative representations of a healthy diet are described.

Until recently, a primary focus of human nutrition was the prevention of nutrient deficiency, and achieving the recommended dietary allowance (RDAs) (4) for essential nutrients was the central objective. This approach led to the development of the seven food groups during World War II and later the "basic four" (meat, dairy, grains, and fruits and vegetables) as the definition of a healthy diet to be conveyed to the public (5). This effort successfully eliminated clinically evident nutrient deficiencies from the United States and Europe. In the last several decades, the definition of a healthy diet has been expanded to include the optimization of long-term health. An underlying motivation for this expansion in scope was epidemiologic evidence that coronary heart disease (CHD) and cancer had become the major causes of death in Western countries. Thus, considerations regarding a healthy diet have come to include macronutrient composition, qualitative aspects of macronutrients such as the glycemic index, food constituents not considered to be nutrients such as fiber and carotenoids, and possible benefits of essential nutrients at intakes higher than those known to prevent deficiency.

In describing a healthy diet, an immediate issue is whether this should be expressed as foods or as nutrients. Using foods is attractive because this provides an easy form of communication that is recognizable by all. Although this is in principle desirable, those attempting to describe an optimal diet only in terms of foods find this challenging. The main reason is that the same foods can be made in many ways. For example, a cracker can be made with lard, partially hydrogenated vegetable oil, or nonhydrogenated corn oil, and vegetables served at a restaurant can be prepared in butter, margarine of unknown composition, or olive oil. The implications for health vary greatly. This issue is becoming increasingly important as the proportion of the food supply that is already processed or is eaten away from home increases. Most groups that have grappled with these issues have developed guidelines that are hybrids using a combination of food and nutrient criteria. For example, many written guidelines include both a quantitative description of fat intake and suggestions about servings of fruits and vegetables. However, when

---

[1]**Abbreviations: CHD,** coronary heart disease; **HDL,** high-density lipoprotein; **HEI,** Healthy Eating Index; **HIV,** human immunodeficiency virus; **LDL,** low-density lipoprotein; **RDA,** recommended dietary allowance.

translating dietary guidance into graphic form (e.g., a food guide pyramid), this is often done by only using foods, an approach that may fail to convey key information.

QUANTITY VERSUS QUALITY OF DIET

Excessive body fat resulting from an imbalance between energy intake and expenditure is the most important nutritional problem in developed countries and is rapidly becoming a global epidemic; a definition of a healthy diet that fails to address this problem would be deficient. Some well-intended guidelines are highly prescriptive in terms of energy intake or servings per day of each food group. A fundamental problem is that even the healthiest combination of foods consumed in slight excess, by only a percentage or two, over an extended period will lead to overweight. Even with the best of methods, our assessments of intake are not sufficiently precise to measure these fine differences, and our assessments of energy expenditure are at least as imperfect. This problem is further compounded by the highly imprecise estimation of quantities of foods by individual persons, and even by differences in definitions of serving sizes among branches of government (e.g., the US Food and Drug Administration and the US Department of Agriculture). For these reasons, attempts to address overweight by detailed definitions of energy intake in dietary guidelines will not be successful. Weight itself, however, is well measured and represents a sensitive indicator of the long-term balance between energy intake and expenditure. For this reason, a definition of a healthy diet needs to be closely linked with the importance of maintaining a healthy weight and the need to make adjustments in intake or physical activity if an imbalance exists. Whether the qualitative aspects of diet may help to facilitate weight control is discussed later.

DOES DIETARY GUIDANCE NEED TO BE INDIVIDUALIZED?

For many years, nutritionists have recognized that individual persons differ in their response to nutrient intakes; for example, in the response of serum cholesterol to dietary cholesterol (6) or of blood pressure to sodium intake (7). In extreme cases of inborn genetic defects, for example, phenylketonuria, standard diets can be lethal. The elucidation of the human genome and rapid identification of polymorphisms in almost all genes is creating new opportunities to individualize dietary guidance. For example, a homozygous polymorphism in the methylenetetrahydrofolate reductase (MTHFR) gene, present in about 10% of the population, increases the amount of dietary folic acid needed to minimize blood levels of homocysteine (8). Does this mean that special dietary guidance needs to be given to those persons? Although we could now easily screen for MTHFR polymorphisms and give these persons different dietary advice, this is still probably not a logical

strategy. First, other functionally important polymorphisms in genes related to folic acid requirements will probably be discovered. Second, having different dietary advice for folic acid for different persons would create considerable complexity within populations and even within families. Because these variations probably exist for almost every nutrient, the possible combinations are almost infinite and would mean that each person would have a unique dietary recommendation. An alternative is to define healthy diets that would be sufficiently high in folic acid to meet the needs of this subset of the population. This has been the general approach in setting RDAs whereby a margin of error has been added above average requirements to include individual variations in nutrient needs. This is an appropriate approach when variation in requirements is known to exist and we have no practical way of identifying individual persons with different requirements or the reason for these differences, and it will often still be a reasonable strategy even though we have the potential to identify individual differences in requirements.

The ability to identify individual persons with different requirements will allow more detailed studies to be sure that their needs are being met. In addition, for some carefully selected genetic variants, different dietary approaches may be appropriate (e.g., phenylketonuria, as mentioned earlier). It also may well be that diets to reduce blood cholesterol levels eventually will be prescribed based on genetic information.

Genetic variation is only one of several factors that can influence nutritional requirements, and it may not even be the most important. Age and pregnancy have long been recognized as factors to be considered, and requirements are often specific for certain age groups and for pregnant women. However, as Hegsted pointed out (9), if requirements are expressed in terms of dietary quality (e.g., as nutrient densities), many of the differences in requirements will diminish. One fundamentally important influence on the response to diet is the underlying degree of insulin resistance. This was described by Jeppesen and colleagues (10, 11), who noted that the adverse effects of high carbohydrate intake on metabolic markers of the insulin resistance syndrome were strongly correlated with baseline insulin resistance. This relation has been confirmed in population studies showing a much stronger relation between the dietary glycemic load and blood triglyceride levels (12) and risk of CHD (13) among persons with a greater body mass index, a major determinant of insulin resistance. The implication is that a person who is lean and active can better tolerate a high-carbohydrate diet than someone who is less active and overweight. This finding also has important implications on a population basis because of strong evidence that most Asian groups have a higher prevalence of insulin resistance for genetic reasons compared with European populations (14). Neel (15) had earlier described this as the "thrifty gene." Until recently, these populations were generally highly active and lean and thus protected from the adverse effects of this genetic predisposition. However, with the reductions in activity and gains in body weight that typically accompany a modern lifestyle, the ability to tolerate a diet high in refined carbohydrates diminishes. Still, this does not necessarily require different dietary recommendations if diets with low amounts of refined carbohydrate, even if not as critical, would also be desirable for other populations.

SPECIFIC CONSIDERATIONS IN FORMULATING A HEALTHY DIET

Traditionally, animal experiments and small human metabolic studies formed the basis of dietary recommendations. Inevitably, the study of chronic disease in humans has required epidemiologic approaches. Until recently, these largely consisted of international comparisons and case-control studies, which examined dietary factors retrospectively in relation to cancer and other diseases. Now, large prospective studies of many thousands of persons are providing data based on both biochemical indicators of diet and dietary questionnaires that have been rigorously validated (16). Ideally, each potential relationship between diet and a health outcome would be evaluated in a randomized trial, but this is often not feasible because of practical constraints. The best available evidence will be based on a synthesis of epidemiologic, metabolic, animal, and mechanistic studies. Major aspects of diet are discussed briefly here.

Dietary Fat and Specific Fatty Acids

Until recently, reviews on diet and health consistently recommended reducing total fat intake, usually to 30% of energy or less (17, 18), to decrease CHD and cancer. The classic diet-heart hypothesis rested heavily on observations that total serum cholesterol levels predict CHD risk; serum cholesterol has thus functioned as a surrogate marker of risk in hundreds of metabolic studies. These studies, summarized as equations by Keys (19) and Hegsted (20), indicated that, compared with carbohydrates, saturated fats and dietary cholesterol increase, and polyunsaturated fat decreases, serum cholesterol, whereas monounsaturated fat has no influence. These widely used equations, although valid for total cholesterol, have become less relevant with the recognition that the high-density lipoprotein (HDL) cholesterol fraction is strongly and inversely related to CHD risk and that the ratio of total cholesterol to HDL is a better predictor (21–24).

Substitution of carbohydrate for saturated fat (the basis of the American Heart Association diets) tends to reduce HDL as well as total and low-density lipoprotein (LDL) cholesterol; thus, the ratio does not change appreciably (25). In contrast, substituting monounsaturated fat for saturated fat reduces LDL without affecting HDL, thus providing an improved ratio (25). In addition, monounsaturated fats, compared with carbohydrate, reduce blood sugar

and triglycerides in persons with adult-onset diabetes (26). Although different saturated fats vary in their influence on LDL levels, this usually does not have practical importance because intakes of the various saturated fats are strongly correlated with each other, and no good evidence indicates that stearic acid is a lesser risk factor for CHD than other saturated fatty acids (27).

Uncertainty About Optimal Polyunsaturated Fat Intake

The earlier metabolic studies predicting total serum cholesterol (19, 20) suggested that polyunsaturated fat intake should be maximized, and the American Heart Association recommended intakes of up to 10% of energy (compared with US averages of about 3% in the 1950s and 6% at present). Concerns have arisen from animal studies in which ω-6 polyunsaturated fat (typically as corn oil) has promoted tumor growth (28), and the possibility that high intakes of ω-6 relative to ω-3 fatty acids could promote coronary thrombosis. However, as described later, available evidence from human studies has not supported these concerns at levels of ω-6 fatty acid intakes lower than 10% of calories.

Dietary Fat and Incidence of Coronary Heart Disease

In Keys' pioneering ecologic study of diets and CHD in seven countries (29, 30), total fat intake had little association with population rates of CHD; indeed, the lowest rate was in Crete, which had the highest fat intake because of the large consumption of olive oil. Saturated fat intake, however, was positively related to CHD. In contrast to international comparisons, little relationship has been seen with saturated fat intake in prospective studies of individuals (16, 31, 32). Some studies, however, tend to support a modest association between dietary cholesterol and CHD risk (33), and inverse associations have been seen with polyunsaturated fat (31, 32). Similarly, dietary intervention trials have generally shown little effect on CHD incidence when carbohydrate replaces saturated fat, but replacing saturated fat with polyunsaturated fat has reduced the incidence of CHD (34–37). At intakes within the dietary range, the benefits of ω-3 fatty acids appear to be primarily in prevention of fatal arrhythmias that can complicate CHD, rather than in prevention of infarction (38–40). The amount of ω-3 fatty acids needed to prevent arrhythmia is remarkably small—on the order of 1 g/day or less (40), and fish consumption twice a week appears to provide most of the potential reduction of sudden death (41).

Trans Fatty Acids

Trans fatty acids are formed by the partial hydrogenation of liquid vegetable oils in the production of margarine and vegetable shortening, and they can account for as much as 40% of these products. *Trans* fatty acids increase LDL and decrease HDL (42–47), raise the proportion of small, dense and atherogenic LDL particles (48), raise lipoprotein (a) (46, 49), and increase inflammatory markers that have been related to CHD risk (50, 51). In the most detailed prospective study, *trans* fatty acid intake was strongly associated with risk of CHD (32), and, as predicted by metabolic studies, this association was stronger than for saturated fat. The association between *trans* fatty acid intake (52) and risk of CHD has been confirmed in other prospective studies. The Food and Drug Administration has announced that food labeling will be required to include the *trans* fat content as of 2006.

Relation between Dietary Fat and Risk of Type 2 Diabetes. The relation between dietary fat and risk of type 2 diabetes appears to be similar to that for CHD (53). The overall percentage of fat does not appear to be related to risk. However, polyunsaturated fat is inversely associated with risk, consistent with its effect on insulin resistance, and *trans* fat has been positively associated with risk (53), consistent with evidence of its effects on inflammatory markers noted earlier. Consumption of red meat, particularly processed red meat, has been associated with greater risk (54).

Dietary Fat and Cancer. One justification for low-fat diets has been the belief that these would reduce the incidence of cancers of the breast, colon and rectum, and prostate (17, 55). The primary evidence has been that countries with low fat intake (also the less affluent areas) have had low rates of these cancers (55, 56). These correlations have been primarily with animal fat and meat intake, rather than with vegetable fat consumption.

The hypothesis that fat intake increases breast cancer risk has been supported by most animal models (57, 58), although no association was seen in a large study that did not use an inducing agent (59). Moreover, much of the effect of dietary fat in the animal studies appears to be the result of an increase in total energy intake, and energy restriction profoundly decreases disease incidence (28, 57, 59). Data from many large prospective studies, including approximately 8000 cases in more than 300,000 women, have been published (60). In none of these studies was the risk of breast cancer significantly elevated among those with the highest fat intake, and the summary relative risk for the highest versus lowest category of dietary fat composition was 1.03 (60). In the largest study (61), no reduction in risk was seen even below 20% of energy from fat. Thus, over the range of fat intake consumed by middle-aged women in these studies, which included the present dietary recommendations, dietary total fat did not appear to increase breast cancer risk. Recently, higher intake of animal fat, particularly from dairy products, during the premenopausal years was associated with a greater risk of breast cancer. Vegetable fat was not associated with risk of breast cancer in this study, a finding suggesting that some

components of animal foods rather than fat per se may increase risk (62).

Associations between animal fat consumption and colon cancer incidence have been seen in some (63–65), although not all (66), studies, whereas little relation has been seen with vegetable fat. However, the associations between red meat consumption, particularly processed meats, and colon cancer have been even stronger than the association of fat in some analyses (64, 65). These data suggest that relationships with red meat are the result of components other than fat, such as heat-induced carcinogens (67) or the high content of readily available iron (68). Like rates of breast and colon cancer, prostate cancer rates are much higher in affluent compared with poor and Eastern countries (56). More detailed epidemiologic studies are few, but associations with animal fat or red meat consumption have been suggested in some prospective studies (69, 70). A positive association has been seen between intake of α-linolenic acid, primarily attributable to consumption of fat from red meat (71).

Overweight is an important cause of morbidity and mortality, and short-term studies have suggested that reducing the fat content of the diet induces weight loss (72). However, in randomized studies lasting a year or longer, reductions in fat to 20 to 25% of energy had minimal effects on overall long-term body weight (73).

Summary. Little evidence indicates that dietary fat per se is associated with risk of CHD. Metabolic and epidemiologic data are consistent in suggesting that intake of partially hydrogenated vegetable fats should be minimized. Metabolic studies, epidemiologic studies, and randomized trials support a reduction in saturated fats, but these data suggest that the benefits will be small if carbohydrate rather than unsaturated fat replaces the saturated fat. Definitive data are not available on the optimal intake of polyunsaturated and monounsaturated fats, but the metabolic data as well as the experience of Southern European populations suggest that consuming a substantial proportion of energy as monounsaturated fat would be desirable.

Available evidence also suggests that total fat reduction would have little effect on breast cancer risk, although reducing red meat intake may well decrease the incidence of colon cancer and possibly prostate cancer.

Carbohydrates

As protein varies only modestly across a wide range of human diets, higher carbohydrate consumption is, in practice, the reciprocal of a low-fat diet. For reasons discussed under the topic of fat, a high-carbohydrate diet can have adverse metabolic consequences. In particular, such diets are associated with an increase in triglycerides and a reduction in HDL cholesterol (24), and these adverse responses are aggravated in the context of insulin resistance (10, 74).

Complex Carbohydrates

The traditional distinction between simple and complex carbohydrates is not useful in dietary recommendations, because some forms of complex carbohydrates, such as starch in potatoes, are very rapidly metabolized to glucose. Instead, emphasis is better placed on whole-grain and other less refined complex carbohydrates as opposed to the highly refined products and sugar generally consumed in the United States. Adverse consequences of highly refined grains appear to result both from the rapid digestion and absorption of these foods, as well as from the loss of fiber and micronutrients in the milling process. The glycemic response after carbohydrate intake, which has been characterized by the glycemic index, is greater with highly refined foods as compared with less refined, whole grains (75). The greater glycemic response resulting from highly refined carbohydrates is accompanied by increased plasma insulin levels and augments the other adverse metabolic changes caused by carbohydrate consumption noted earlier to a greater degree than with less refined foods (12). Higher intakes of refined starches and sugar, particularly when associated with low fiber intake, appear to increase the risk of non–insulin-dependent diabetes (76, 77) and possibly the risk of CHD (13). In contrast, higher intake of fiber from grain products has consistently been associated with lower risks of CHD and diabetes (53, 78). Whether these benefits are mediated by only fiber per se or in part by the accompanying micronutrients is not clear, but for practical reasons this distinction is not essential.

Anticipated reductions in colon cancer risk by diets high in grain fiber diets have not been supported in most prospective studies (79, 80). However, reduced constipation and a lower risk of colonic diverticular disease (81) are clear benefits of such diets.

The importance of micronutrients in the prevention of many chronic conditions has reemphasized the problem of "empty calories" associated with diets high in sugar and highly refined carbohydrates. In the standard milling of white flour, as much as 60 to 90% of vitamins B_6 and E, folate, and other nutrients are lost (82); this may be nutritionally critical for persons with otherwise marginal intakes. Thiamin, riboflavin, folate, and niacin are currently replaced by fortification, but other nutrients remain substantially reduced.

Protein

Average protein consumption in the United States substantially exceeds conventional requirements (17), and adequate intake can be maintained on most reasonable diets. Optimal protein intake has been widely debated, and high intakes are advocated in many popular diets, but long-term data are limited. Substituting protein for carbohydrate improves blood lipids and has been associated with lower risk of CHD (83).

Protein Sources

The specific sources of dietary protein do have important implications for long-term health, probably more related to the other constituents of these foods than to the protein per se. As noted earlier, fish consumption is related to lower risk of sudden cardiac death, probably due to its content of ω-3 fatty acids. In addition, regular consumption of nuts has been related to a lower risk of CHD in multiple studies (84) and type 2 diabetes (85), likely because of their high content of unsaturated fatty acids and possibly also their high content of micronutrients and other phytochemicals. Soy products are high in polyunsaturated fatty acids and would presumably be beneficial with regard to CHD risk, but little direct evidence is available, and the same applies to other legumes. Poultry fat is relatively unsaturated compared with that of red meat, which is the primary contributor to saturated fat intake in the US diet. Not surprisingly, the dietary ratio of red meat to chicken plus fish has been positively related to risk of CHD (27). As noted earlier, consumption of red meat, particularly processed meats, has also been related to risks of several cancers and type 2 diabetes. This extensive body of evidence supports the replacement of red meat with a combination of nuts, fish, poultry, and legumes as protein sources for overall long-term health.

Vegetables and Fruits

Advice to eat a generous amount of vegetables and fruits (17) has been largely justified by anticipated reductions in cancer and cardiovascular disease. However, more recent cohort studies have tended to show much weaker—or no—relation between overall fruit and vegetable consumption and risks of common cancers (86). The possibility remains for a small overall benefit or benefits only of specific fruits or vegetables against specific cancers. For example, considerable evidence suggests that lycopene, mainly from tomato products, reduces the risk of prostate cancer, but overall consumption of fruits is unrelated to risk (87).

In contrast to the data for cancer, the epidemiologic evidence quite consistently supports a benefit of higher intake of fruit and vegetable consumption for the prevention of cardiovascular disease (78, 88). Evidence that elevated blood homocysteine is an independent risk factor for CHD and cerebrovascular disease (89, 90), and that levels can be reduced by increasing folic acid intake (91), suggests one mechanism. High intake of vegetables reduces blood pressure (92); the active factor remains unclear, but potassium is a likely contributor (93).

Other benefits of higher fruit and vegetable intake are likely to include lower risk of neural tube defects, the most common severe birth defect (94), as a result of higher folic acid intake. Intake of the carotenoids lutein and zeaxanthin, which are high in green leafy vegetables, has been inversely related to the risk of cataracts (95, 96).

Calcium and Dairy Products

Recommendations to maintain adequate calcium intake (17) and to consume large amounts of dairy products on a daily basis (97) derive primarily from the importance of calcium in maintaining bone strength. Calcium supplements in conjunction with vitamin D have reduced fracture incidence in some studies (98), but benefits of calcium cannot be distinguished from those of vitamin D. Uncertainty remains regarding the optimal calcium intake. Intakes of 1200 mg/day or higher are recommended for those older than 50 years in the United States (99), whereas a more recent review in the United Kingdom concluded that 700 mg/day was adequate (100). Many populations have low fracture rates, despite minimal dairy product consumption and low overall calcium intake by adults (101). Several large prospective studies have directly addressed the relation of dairy product consumption to fracture incidence; higher consumption of calcium or dairy products as an adult has consistently not been associated with lower fracture incidence (102, 103). At best, the benefits of high calcium intake are minor compared with those from regular physical activity (104, 105) or additional vitamin D (102).

Inverse associations have been reported between calcium intake and blood pressure in some studies (106), but in a review of trials of supplementation, little overall effect was seen (107). Low calcium intake and low dairy product consumption are associated with a modestly elevated risk of colon cancer (108), but most benefits appear to be achieved with calcium intake of about 800 mg/day. Evidence from a randomized trial that calcium supplementation modestly reduces colon adenoma recurrence adds important evidence of causality to the epidemiologic studies (109).

Although recommended calcium intakes can be achieved by a high consumption of greens and certain other vegetables, greatly increased intakes would be required for most women to achieve currently recommended levels by diet without regular use of milk and other dairy products. Calcium supplements are an inexpensive form of calcium without accompanying calories or saturated fat. Thus, dairy product consumption can be considered an optional rather than a necessary dietary component. Enthusiasm regarding high dairy consumption should also be tempered by the suggestion in many studies that this is associated with increased risks of advanced or fatal prostate cancer (110, 111). Whether an increased risk is the result of the calcium, endogenous hormones, or other factors in milk remains unclear.

Salt and Processed Meats

Reduction of salt (sodium chloride) intake from an average of approximately 8 to 10 g/day to less than 6 g/day will, on average, decrease blood pressure to a small degree. In a comprehensive review, Law and associates (112) concluded that a 3 g/day reduction would reduce the incidence of stroke by 22% and of CHD by 16%. Although the decrease in risk of cardiovascular disease achieved by reducing salt consumption is modest for most persons, the overall number of deaths potentially avoided is large, thereby supporting policies to reduce salt consumption, particularly in processed foods and by institutions.

In many case-control studies, the consumption of salty and pickled foods has been associated with stomach cancer (70). However, because this cancer is relatively rare in the United States, further benefit from reducing salt intake would be small.

Alcohol

Many adverse influences of heavy alcohol consumption are well recognized, but moderate consumption has both beneficial and harmful effects, thus greatly complicating decisions for individual persons. Overwhelming epidemiologic data indicate that moderate consumption (one to two drinks/day) reduces the risk of myocardial infarction (113, 114) by approximately 30 to 40%. Although this effect has been hypothesized to be the result of antioxidants in red wine, similar protective effects for equivalent amounts of alcohol have been seen for all types of alcoholic beverages (115, 116). Conversely, modest positive associations with risk of breast cancer incidence have been observed in more than 30 studies (117) for similar levels of alcohol intake, possibly because alcohol appears to increase endogenous estrogen levels (118, 119). The overall effect of alcohol, as represented by total mortality, appears beneficial for up to about two drinks/day in men (120). Overall, a similar relation with total mortality is seen among women, but no net benefit was observed among those at low risk of CHD because of younger age or lack of coronary risk factors (121). Several studies suggest that the adverse effects of alcohol on cancer risk may be mitigated by adequate intake of folate.

Vitamin Supplements

The role of vitamin supplements and food fortification has been debated on both a philosophic basis and a scientific level. Some nutritionists have believed as a matter of principle that nutritional needs should be met by diet alone. Often this is not possible, however, for example, when iodine levels are low in the soil, and iodine fortification has been a great public health advance. In addition, a large percentage of the US population appears to have suboptimal blood levels of vitamin D, largely because of limited solar exposure at northern latitudes during the winter. In addition, low incomes and limited access can be serious barriers to optimal food intakes; to achieve the recommended 400 μg/day of folic acid by diet alone can be expensive. Many of these shortcomings can be remedied efficiently and effectively by some combination of fortification and supplementation.

Only recently have data become available that address the effects of vitamin supplements against the background of actual diets in the United States, which appear far from ideal (122). The most firmly established benefit is that folic acid supplements in the amounts contained in multiple vitamins can reduce the risks of neural tube defects by approximately 70% (123). This is probably an indicator of more widespread consequences of suboptimal folate intakes, because inverse associations have also been seen with colonic neoplasias (124); low folate intake, along with suboptimal vitamin B_6, is likely to contribute to elevated blood homocysteine levels and risk of cardiovascular disease (90, 125). Since 1998, grain products in the United States have been fortified with folic acid; the extent to which this has reduced the value in taking supplemental folic acid is unclear, but some US residents still have intakes lower than the RDA of 400 µg/day (126).

Many elderly persons have suboptimal vitamin B_{12} status, mainly because of a loss of stomach acid, which is needed to liberate vitamin B_{12} from food sources. In contrast, vitamin B_{12} in supplements or from food sources is readily absorbed without stomach acid.

The majority of the US population appears to have suboptimal blood levels of vitamin D, as assessed by the relation to bone density (127). Over nearly the entire range of vitamin D levels in blood, higher levels are directly related to bone density, a finding suggesting that most US residents do not have optimal vitamin D status. Because natural sources of vitamin D are few (mainly fish), and recommendations to increase sun exposure would lead to elevations in skin cancer, increases in supplementation and fortification are the only good options. The current RDA of 400 µg/day is probably far too low to achieve optimal levels, and intakes of at least several times this amount are probably desirable (128).

In a randomized trial conducted in a region of China with low consumption of fruits and vegetables, a supplement containing β-carotene, vitamin E, and selenium reduced incidence of stomach cancer (129). In a recent study conducted among Tanzanian women infected with human immunodeficiency virus (HIV), a multiple vitamin containing B vitamins, vitamin E, and vitamin C reduced progression of the disease and HIV-related mortality (130). Whether these benefits would be seen in the background of dietary intakes in the United States is not clear.

Any recommendation for use of nutritional supplements should carefully consider possible adverse effects. One of the few adverse effects of vitamin supplement use at the RDA level appears to be an increase in risk of hip fractures resulting from vitamin A, when it is consumed as 5000 IU/day in the form of retinol. Higher intake of preformed vitamin A (retinol) has been associated with excess risk of hip fracture in prospective studies (131, 132), and elevated risks were seen for both use of multiple vitamins and specific supplements of vitamin A. In addition, serum retinol levels have been associated with future risk of fractures (133). These effects may result from competition at the vitamin D receptor (134), which may not have occurred if vitamin D levels were adequate. The amount of retinol in most multiple vitamins has been reduced.

Current evidence, although far from complete, suggests that supplements of folate and possibly other vitamins, at the RDA level contained in most nonprescription multivitamin preparations, may have substantial benefits for at least an important subgroup of the US population, perhaps characterized in part by increased requirements or by suboptimal diets. Intakes of folate as well as other micronutrients appear marginal for many US residents (122, 135), and the risks of using multivitamins appear minimal; given that the cost of supplements is low (especially compared with the cost of fresh fruits and vegetables), the use of a daily multiple vitamin appears rational for most of the US population.

SUMMARY

Any description of a healthy diet must be made with the recognition that information is currently incomplete and conclusions are subject to change with new data. Most of the major diseases contributing to morbidity and mortality in the United States develop over many decades, and large-scale nutritional epidemiologic studies were only begun in the early 1980s; thus, a full picture of the relation between diet and disease will require additional decades of careful investigation. Nevertheless, in combining available metabolic, clinical, and epidemiologic evidence, several general conclusions that are unlikely to change substantially can be drawn.

1. Staying lean and active throughout life will have major health benefits. Because most members of developed countries work at sedentary jobs, weight control will usually require conscious daily physical activity as well as some effort to avoid overconsumption of calories.
2. Dietary fats should be primarily in the form of nonhydrogenated plant oils. Butter and lard and fat from red meat should be used sparingly, if at all, and *trans* fatty acids from partially hydrogenated vegetable oils should be minimized.
3. Grains should be consumed primarily in a minimally refined, high-fiber form, and intakes of refined starches and simple sugars should be low.
4. Vegetables and fruits should be consumed in abundance (five servings/day is minimal) and should include green leafy and orange vegetables daily.
5. Red meat should be consumed only occasionally and in low amounts, if at all; nuts, legumes, poultry, and fish in moderation are healthy alternatives.
6. The optimal consumption of dairy products and calcium intake is not known, but dairy products should be considered as optional. High consumption of milk (e.g., more than two servings/day) is not likely to be beneficial for middle-aged and older adults, and it may increase

risk of prostate cancer. Adequate calcium intake may be particularly important for growing children, adolescents, and lactating women; supplements should be considered if dietary sources are low.

7. For most people, taking a daily RDA-level multiple vitamin containing folic acid provides a sensible nutritional safety net. Because menstrual losses of iron may not be adequately replaced by iron intake on the low-energy diets of women in a sedentary society, it is sensible for most premenopausal women to use a multiple vitamin that also contains iron.

8. Salt intake should be kept low.

REPRESENTATION OF AN OVERALL HEALTHY DIET AND VALIDATION

To inform the public and provide guidance for food programs and services, many summary representations of a healthy diet have been developed. The approaches include written guidelines, graphic displays, and dietary indices or scores.

Guidelines and Pyramids

Examples of dietary guidelines include the *Dietary Guidelines for Americans* (1), which are updated every 5 years, the Population Nutrient Intake Goals created by the World Health Organization (3), and those developed by the professional organizations such the American Heart Association and American Cancer Society (Table 102.1). These have usually been created by committees of experts, ideally using the best available evidence. However, in reality, consistency with earlier versions of the same guideline and with other guidelines is often given high priority, even when the other guidelines were based on little evidence. Thus, these processes are inherently slow to evolve and may lag behind available evidence considerably.

Graphic depictions of a healthy diet have often been used to convey information to the public in a way that is intended to be more friendly and effective. Examples of this include the US Food Guide Pyramid (136), a figure meant to be based on the *Dietary Guidelines for Americans*, and the Healthy Eating Pyramid developed at Harvard School of Public Health (137) (Fig. 102.1). Many other countries

TABLE 102.1 EXAMPLES OF DIETARY GUIDELINES

FACTOR	US DIETARY GUIDELINES[a]	WORLD HEALTH ORGANIZATION DIETARY GOALS[b]	AMERICAN HEART ASSOCIATION EATING PLAN FOR HEALTHY AMERICANS[c]	AMERICAN CANCER SOCIETY GUIDELINES ON NUTRITION AND PHYSICAL ACTIVITY[d]
Weight control	BMI <25	BMI <25	Adjust calories to maintain healthy weight	Maintain healthful weight throughout life. Strive for BMI <25
Fat	<30% E	15–30% E	<30% E, <10% polyunsaturated, <15% monounsaturated	
Protein	2–3 servings/d	10–15% E		Emphasize plant sources
Carbohydrates	6–11 servings/d (whole grains, cereal, bread)	55–75% E	6+ or more servings grains, starchy vegetables	Choose whole grains
Fruits and vegetables	5+ servings/d	400 g/d	5+ servings/d	5+ servings per day
Dairy	2–3 servings/d		2–4 servings/d	
Alcohol	0–1 serving/d, women		0–1 serving/d, women	0–1 serving/day, women
	0–2 servings/d, men		0–2 servings/d, men	0–2 serving/day, men
Sugar, sweets		Free sugars <10% of E		
Physical activity	30 min most days	30 min most days	30 min/d	30–45 minutes 5+ times/week
Other	Take salt in moderate amounts		<2,400 mg sodium, 300 mg cholesterol/d	Limit red meat

BMI, body mass index; E, energy.
[a]Data from US Department of Agriculture, US Department of Health and Human Services. Nutrition and Your Health: Dietary Guidelines for Americans. 5th ed. Washington, DC: US Government Printing Office, 2000.
[b]Data from World Health Organization (WHO), Food and Agriculture Organization (FAO). Diet, Nutrition and the Prevention of Chronic Diseases: Report of a Joint WHO/FAO Expert
Consultation. Report no. 916. Geneva: World Health Organization, 2003.
[c]Data from Krauss RM, Eckel RH, Howard B et al. Stroke 2000;31:2751–66.
[d]Data from Byers T, Nestle M, McTiernan A et al. CA Cancer J Clin 2002;52:92–119.

USDA Food Guide Pyramid

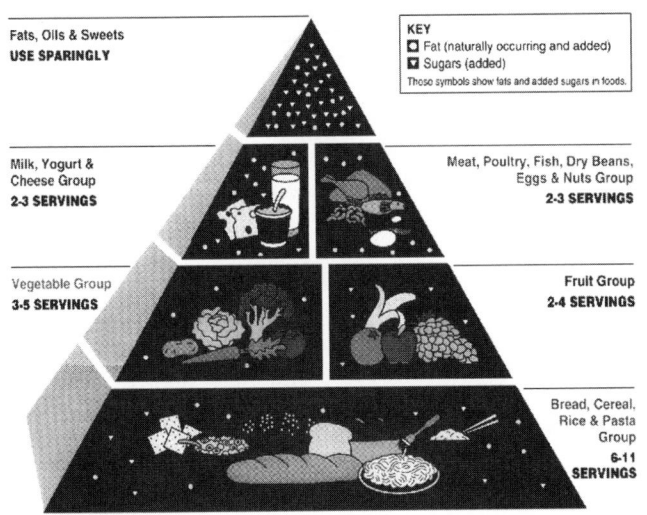

Healthy Eating Pyramid

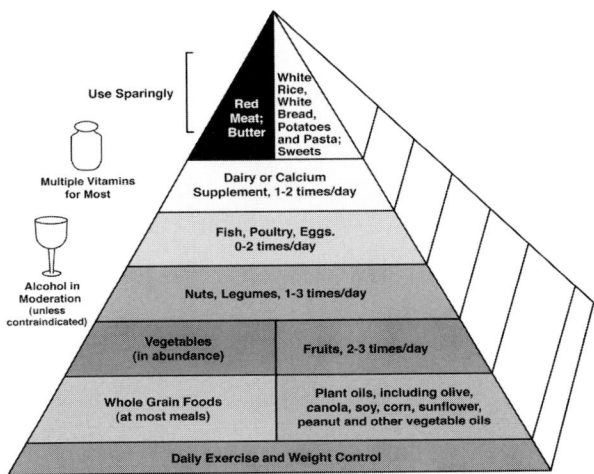

Figure 102.1. Examples of graphic representations of a healthy diet: the US Department of Agriculture Food Guide Pyramid and the Healthy Eating Pyramid. (Food Guide Pyramid from US Department of Agriculture. The Food Guide Pyramid. Home and Garden Bulletin no. 252. Washington, DC: US Government Printing Office, 1992; Healthy Eating Pyramid from Willett WC. Eat, Drink and Be Healthy: The Harvard Medical School Guide to Healthy Eating. New York: Simon & Schuster, 2001, with permission.)

and organizations have developed similar graphics, and there is no consensus on the ideal shape or method of conveying information. Condensing the massive literature on diet and health into a simple figure is challenging, and it requires that only the most important information be addressed. Whether these figures should represent volume, energy, or frequency of consumption is also unclear.

Indices

Dietary indices or scores have been created to represent a healthy diet. These are usually based on a priori information from many sources, and they have been used to assess diets of individuals or food programs (Table 102.2). One example is the Healthy Eating Index (HEI) (138), which

TABLE 102.2 PRESENTATION OF A HEALTHY DIET BY INDICES

HEALTHY EATING INDEX[a]	REVISED HEALTHY EATING INDEX[b]	CORONARY HEART DISEASE DIETARY INDEX[c]	MEDITERRANEAN DIET SCORE[d]
Grains (servings/d)	Vegetables (servings/d)	Low *trans* fat	Vegetables (g/d)
Vegetables (servings/d)	Fruits (servings/d)	High ratio of polyunsaturated to saturated fat	Legumes (g/d)
Fruits (servings/d)	Nuts and soy protein (servings/d)	High cereal fiber	Fruits and nuts (g/d)
Milk (servings/d)	Ratio of white to red meat	High marine ω-3 fatty acids	Cereals (g/d)
Meat (servings/d)	Cereal fiber (g/d)	High folate	Fish (g/d)
Total fat (% E)	*Trans* fat (% E)	Low glycemic load	Red meat, poultry (g/d)
Saturated fat (% E)	Ratio of polyunsaturated fat to saturated fat		Dairy products (g/d)
Cholesterol mg/d	Duration of multivitamin use		Alcohol
Sodium (mg/d)	Alcohol (servings/d)		Ratio of monounsaturated to saturated fat
Variety Each item scored 0–10, Total Score range, 0–100	Each item scored 1–10, except multivitamin use 2.5–7.5. Score range 2.5–87.5	Each item scored 1–5 (quintiles) Score range 6–30	Each item scored 0–1 by adherence. For items 1–5, at or above median intake scores 1. For items 6–9, at or above median intake scores 0. Score range, 0–9

E, energy.
[a]Data from US Department of Agriculture. The Healthy Eating Index. Washington, DC: US Department of Agriculture, 1995.
[b]Data from McCullough ML, Feskanich D, Stampfer MJ et al. Am J Clin Nutr 2002;76:1261–71.
[c]Data from Stampfer MJ, Hu FB, Manson JE et al. N Engl J Med 2000;343:16–22.
[d]Data from Trichopoulou A, Costacou T, Bamia C et al. N Engl J Med 2003;348:2599–608.

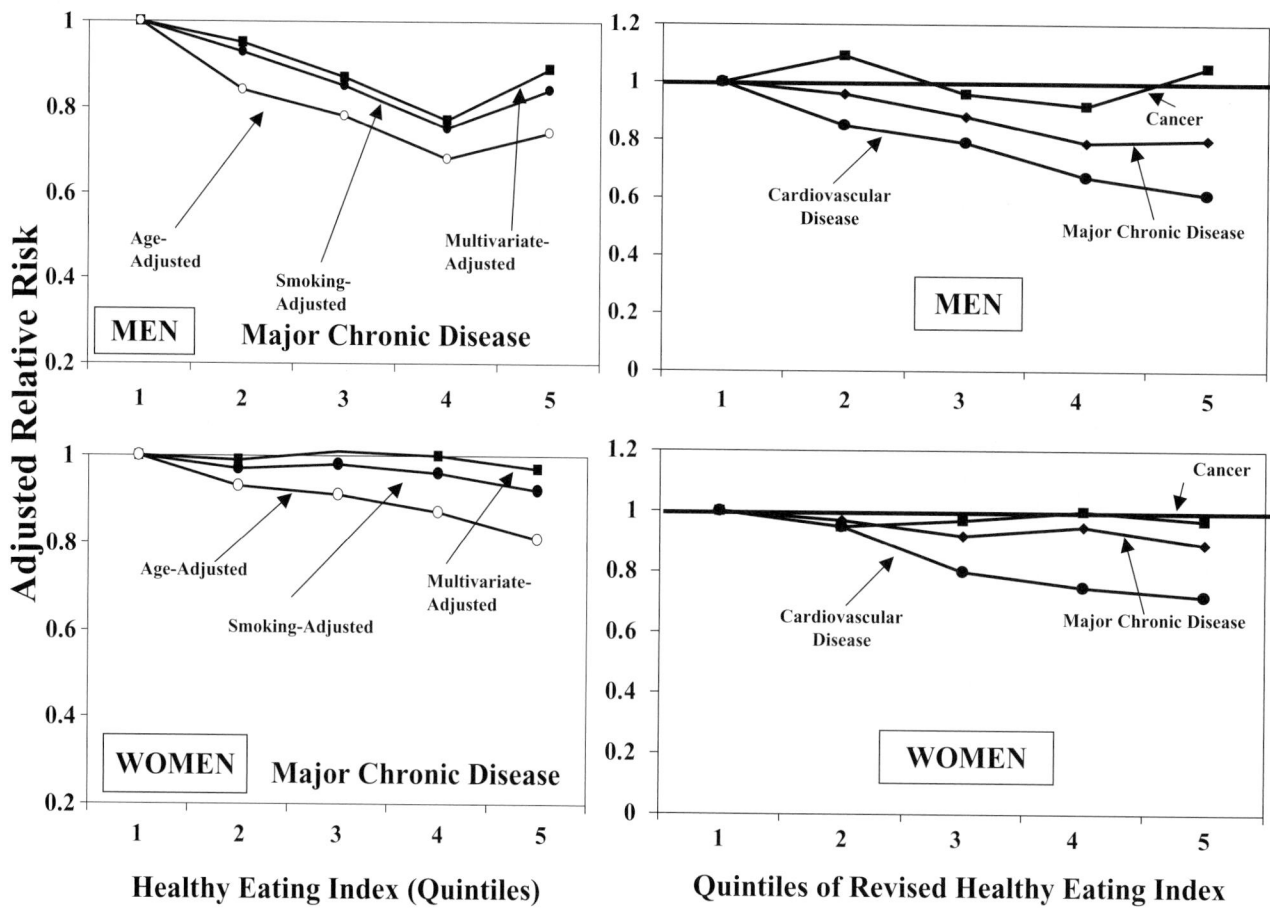

Figure 102.2. Relation of the Healthy Eating Index score to the risk of major chronic disease. All data for the Revised Healthy Eating Index are multivariate-adjusted. (Data from references 142 to 144.)

was designed to be a quantitative measure of adherence to the *Dietary Guidelines for Americans* and the Food Guide Pyramid. Conceptually, this index has been an important advance because it provides a method for determining the degree to which federal food programs are consistent with the guidelines. Other indices include those designed to summarize the important dietary factors in predicting risk of CHD (139) and the Mediterranean diet (140). An alternative approach to creating a dietary score is to use stepwise regression or other multivariate techniques to create a prediction score based on a health outcome in a specific population. This has been used to develop a prediction score for colon cancer (141).

Validation of Dietary Indices

The value of any dietary index or score will depend on whether greater adherence is related to better health. If the index emphasizes irrelevant aspects of diet or fails to make important distinctions, its usefulness will be impaired. A direct assessment of the validity of an index is to determine whether individual persons with higher scores have better long-term health outcomes, taking into account other risk factors. As an example, the HEI has been widely used to

evaluate individual diets and food programs, but until recently the validity of the index had not been examined. To address this issue, McCullough and colleagues, in parallel studies of 67,272 women and 38,622 men, examined whether higher scores on the HEI predicted future risk of major chronic disease, defined as any cancer, myocardial infarction, stroke, or death excluding those resulting from trauma (142, 143). Although clear inverse relations were seen in age-adjusted analyses, after accounting for smoking, physical activity, and other risk factors, persons with the highest HEI scores did not fare appreciably better than those with low scores (Fig. 102.2), a finding indicating that the overall index had little value. A revised HEI, reflecting modified guidelines that took into account the type of fat, form of carbohydrate, and sources of protein did significantly predict lower rates of major chronic disease, especially cardiovascular disease, in both men and women (144). Notably, the 2005 *Dietary Guidelines* were modified substantially to emphasize the distinctions among types of fat and forms of carbohydrate, although sources of protein were not differentiated (145). In evaluations of other indices, a five-variable dietary score developed by Stampfer strongly predicted lower risk of CHD (146) (Fig. 102.3). When combined with not smoking, regular physical activity,

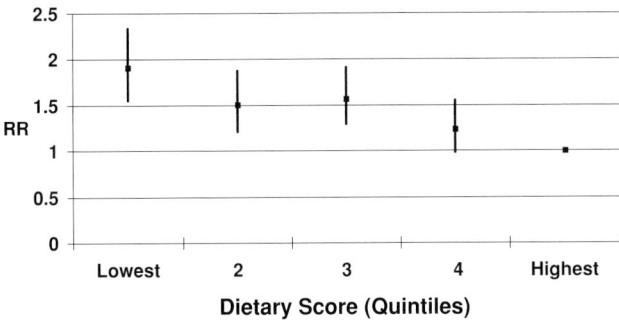

Figure 102.3. Multivariate relative risk of coronary heart disease for dietary score. The score is based on intake of *trans* fat, polyunsaturated-to-saturated fat ratio, long-chain ω-3 fatty acids, cereal fiber, and glycemic load. (Data from Stampfer MJ, Hu FB, Manson JE et al. N Engl J Med 2000;343:16–22.)

avoidance of overweight, and moderate alcohol consumption, these findings indicated that more than 80% of CHD is avoidable by diet and lifestyle changes. In another analysis, the Mediterranean dietary index predicted overall lower cardiovascular, cancer, and total mortality in a Greek population (147).

CONCLUSIONS

Because rates of cardiovascular disease and most cancers have been low in specific populations, we have long recognized that these conditions are not inevitable, and dietary factors have been suspected as being important. A convergence of metabolic, clinical, and epidemiologic evidence has identified specific aspects of diet that contribute to the cause or prevention of these diseases. When combined, these dietary factors can have a major impact. Dietary guidelines and indices should be subjected to empiric validation because widely used guidelines have not always proven useful. Future research should add further refinement to our understanding of an optimal diet, especially regarding the effects of dietary choices during childhood and early adult life on long-term health.

REFERENCES

1. US Department of Agriculture and of Health and Human Services. Nutrition and Your Health: Dietary Guidelines for Americans. 5th ed. Washington, DC: US Government Printing Office, 2000.
2. Food and Nutrition Board, Institute of Medicine. Dietary Reference Intakes for Energy, Carbohydrate, Fiber, Fat, Fatty Acids, Cholesterol, Protein, and Amino Acids (Macronutrients). Washington, DC: National Academy of Sciences, 2002.
3. World Health Organization (WHO)/Food and Agriculture Organization (FAO). Diet, Nutrition and the Prevention of Chronic Diseases. Report of a joint WHO/FAO expert consultation. Report no. 916. Geneva: World Health Organization, 2003.
4. Food and Nutrition Board, Institute of Medicine. Recommended Dietary Allowances. 10th rev ed. Washington, DC: National Academy of Sciences, 1989.
5. Hayes O, Trulson MF, Stare FJ. J Am Diet Assoc 1955;31:1103–7.
6. Katan MB, Beynen AC, de Vries JH et al. Am J Epidemiol 1986;123:221–34.
7. Beeks E, Kessels AG, Kroon AA et al. J Hypertens 2004;22:1243–9.
8. Bailey LB, Gregory JF 3rd. J Nutr 1999;129:919–22.
9. Hegsted DM. Clin Nutr 1985;4:159–63.
10. Jeppesen J, Chen YDI, Zhou MY et al. Am J Clin Nutr 1995;61:787–91.
11. Jeppesen J, Chen YD, Zhou MY et al. Am J Clin Nutr 1995;62:1201–5.
12. Liu S, Manson JE, Stampfer MJ et al. Am J Clin Nutr 2001;73:560–6.
13. Liu S, Willett WC, Stampfer MJ et al. Am J Clin Nutr 2000;71:1455–61.
14. Dickinson S, Claggier S, Faramus E et al. J Nutr 2002;132:2574–9.
15. Neel J. Am J Hum Genet 1962;14:353–62.
16. Willett WC. Nutritional Epidemiology. 2nd ed. New York: Oxford University Press, 1998.
17. US Department of Agriculture, US Department of Health and Human Services. Nutrition and Your Health: Dietary Guidelines for Americans, 4th ed. Home and Garden Bulletin no. 232. Washington, DC: US Government Printing Office, 1995.
18. US Department of Health and Human Services. The Surgeon General's Report on Nutrition and Health. DHHS publication (PHS) no. 50210. Washington, DC: US Government Printing Office, 1988.
19. Keys A. Am J Clin Nutr 1984;40:351–9.
20. Hegsted DM. Am J Clin Nutr 1986;44:299–305.
21. Castelli WP, Abbott RD, McNamara PM. Circulation 1983;67:730–4.
22. Ginsberg HN, Barr SL, Gilbert A et al. N Engl J Med 1990;322:574–9.
23. Mensink RP, Katan MB. Lancet 1987;1:122–5.
24. Mensink RP, Katan MB. Arterioscler Thromb Vasc Biol 1992;12:911–9.
25. Mensink RP, Zock PL, Kester AD et al. Am J Clin Nutr 2003;77:1146–55.
26. Garg A, Grundy SM, Koffler M. Diabetes Care 1992;15:1572–80.
27. Hu FB, Stampfer MJ, Manson JE et al. Am J Clin Nutr 1999;70:1001–8.
28. Welsch CW. Cancer Res 1992;52[Suppl 7]:2040S–8S.
29. Keys A. Seven Countries: A Multivariate Analysis of Death and Coronary Heart Disease. Cambridge, MA: Harvard University Press, 1980.
30. Verschuren WM, Jacobs DR, Bloemberg BP et al. JAMA 1995;274:131–6.
31. Shekelle RB, Shryock AM, Paul O et al. N Engl J Med 1981;304:65–70.
32. Hu F, Stampfer MJ, Manson JE et al. N Engl J Med 1997;337:1491–9.
33. Shekelle RB, Stamler J. Lancet 1989;1:1177–9.
34. Multiple Risk Factor Intervention Trial Research Group. JAMA 1982;248:1465–77.
35. Stamler J, Wentworth D, Neaton JD. JAMA 1986;256:2823–8.
36. Frantz IDJ, Dawson EA, Ashman PL et al. Arteriosclerosis 1989;9:129–35.
37. Sacks F. J Cardiovasc Risk 1994;1:3–8.
38. de Lorgeril M, Renaud S, Mamelle N et al. Lancet 1994;343:1454–9.
39. Leaf A. Prostaglandins Leukot Essent Fatty Acids 1995;52:197–8.

40. GISSI Prevention Investigators. Lancet 1999;354:447–55.

41. Albert CM, Hennekens CH, O'Donnell CJ et al. JAMA 1998;279:23–8.

42. Booyens J, Louwrens CC. Med Hypoth 1986;21:387–408.

43. Mensink RPM, Katan MB. N Engl J Med 1990;323:439–45.

44. Zock PL, Katan MB. J Lipid Res 1992;33:399–410.

45. Judd JT, Clevidence BA, Muesing RA et al. Am J Clin Nutr 1994;59:861–8.

46. Nestel P, Noakes M, Belling Bea. J Lipid Res 1992;33:1029–36.

47. Sundram K, Ismail A, Hayes KC et al. J Nutr 1997;127:514S–20S.

48. Lichtenstein AH, Ausman LM, Jalbert SM et al. N Engl J Med 1999;340:1933–40.

49. Mensink RP, Zock PL, Katan MB et al. J Lipid Res 1992;33:1493–501.

50. Mozaffarian D, Pischon T, Hankinson SE et al. Am J Clin Nutr 2004;79:606–12.

51. Baer DJ, Judd JT, Clevidence BA et al. Am J Clin Nutr 2004;79:969–73.

52. Ascherio A, Katan MB, Zock PL et al. N Engl J Med 1999;340:1994–8.

53. Hu FB, van Dam RM, Liu S. Diabetologia 2001;44:805–17.

54. van Dam RM, Willett WC, Rimm EB et al. Diabetes Care 2002;25:417–24.

55. Prentice RL, Sheppard L. Cancer Causes Control 1990;1:81–97.

56. Armstrong B, Doll R. Int J Cancer 1975;15:617–31.

57. Ip C. Quantitative assessment of fat and calorie as risk factors in mammary carcinogenesis in an experimental model. In: Mettlin CJ, Aoki K, eds. Recent Progress in Research on Nutrition and Cancer: Proceedings of a Workshop Sponsored by the International Union Against Cancer, held in Nagoya, Japan, November 1–3, 1989. New York: Wiley-Liss, 1990:107–17.

58. Freedman LS, Clifford C, Messina M. Cancer Res 1990;50:5710–9.

59. Appleton BS, Landers RE. Adv Exp Med Biol 1986;206:99–104.

60. Smith-Warner SA, Spiegelman D, Adami HO et al. Int J Cancer 2001;92:767–74.

61. Holmes MD, Hunter DJ, Colditz GA et al. JAMA 1999;281:914–20.

62. Cho E, Spiegelman D, Hunter DJ et al. J Natl Cancer Inst 2003;95:1079–85.

63. Whittemore AS, Wu-Williams AH, Lee M et al. J Natl Cancer Inst 1990;82:915–26.

64. Willett WC, Stampfer MJ, Colditz GA et al. N Engl J Med 1990;323:1664–72.

65. Giovannucci E, Rimm EB, Ascherio A et al. J Natl Cancer Inst 1995;87:265–73.

66. Phillips RL, Snowdon DA. Cancer Res 1983;43[Suppl]:2403S–8S.

67. Gerhardsson de Verdier M, Hagman U, Peters RK et al. Int J Cancer 1991;49:520–5.

68. Babbs CF. Free Radic Biol Med 1990;8:191–200.

69. Kolonel LN. Cancer Causes Control 1996;7:83–94.

70. World Cancer Research Fund (WCRF)/American Institute for Cancer Research (AICR). Food, Nutrition and the Prevention of Cancer: A Global Perspective. Washington, DC: American Institute for Cancer Research, 1997.

71. Giovannucci E, Rimm EB, Stampfer MJ et al. Cancer Res 1994;54:2390–7.

72. Bray GA, Popkin BM. Am J Clin Nutr 1998;68:1157–73.

73. Willett WC, Leibel RL. Am J Med 2002;113[Suppl 9B]:47S–59S.

74. Jeppesen J, Hollenbeck CB, Zhou MY et al. Arterioscler Thromb Vasc Biol 1995;15:320–4.

75. Jenkins DJ, Wolever TM, Taylor RH et al. Am J Clin Nutr 1981;34:362–6.

76. Salmeron J, Manson JE, Stampfer MJ et al. JAMA 1997;277:472–7.

77. Salmeron J, Ascherio A, Rimm EB et al. Diabetes Care 1997;20:545–50.

78. Hu FB, Willett WC. JAMA 2002;288:2569–78.

79. Fuchs CS, Colditz GA, Stampfer MJ et al. N Engl J Med 1999;340:169–76.

80. Terry P, Giovannucci E, Michels KB et al. J Natl Cancer Inst 2001;93:525–33.

81. Aldoori WH, Giovannucci EL, Rockett HR et al. J Nutr 1998;128:714–9.

82. Schroeder HA. Am J Clin Nutr 1971;24:562–73.

83. Hu FB, Stampfer MJ, Manson JE et al. Am J Clin Nutr 1999;70:221–7.

84. Hu FB, Stampfer MJ. Curr Atheroscler Rep 1999;1:204–9.

85. Jiang R, Manson JE, Stampfer MJ et al. JAMA 2002;288:2554–60.

86. Michels KB, Giovannucci E, Joshipura KJ et al. IARC Sci Publ 2002;156:139–40.

87. Giovannucci E. J Natl Cancer Inst 1999;91:317–31.

88. Joshipura KJ, Hu FB, Manson JE et al. Ann Intern Med 2001;134:1106–14.

89. Stampfer MJ, Malinow MR, Willett WC et al. JAMA 1992;268:877–81.

90. Selhub J, Jacques PF, Bostom AG et al. N Engl J Med 1995;332:286–91.

91. Tucker KL, Olson B, Bakun P et al. Am J Clin Nutr 2004;79:805–11.

92. Sacks FM, Svetkey LP, Vollmer WM et al. N Engl J Med 2001;344:3–10.

93. Sacks FM, Willett WC, Smith A et al. Hypertension 1998;31:131–8.

94. Werler MM, Shapiro S, Mitchell AA. JAMA 1993;269:1257–61.

95. Chasan-Taber L, Willett WC, Seddon JM et al. Am J Clin Nutr 1999;70:509–16.

96. Brown L, Rimm EB, Seddon JM et al. Am J Clin Nutr 1999;70:517–24.

97. Welsh S, Davis C, Shaw A. Nutr Today 1992;27:12–23.

98. Chapuy MC, Arlof ME, Duboeuf F et al. N Engl J Med 1992;327:1637–42.

99. Food and Nutrition Board Institute of Medicine. Dietary Reference Intakes for Calcium, Phosphorus, Magnesium, Vitamin D, and Fluoride. Washington D.C., National Academy Press, 1997. http://www.nos.org.uk/infosheets.calcium.pdf

100. Report of the Panel on Dietary Reference Values of the Committee on Medical Aspects of Food Policy. London Her Majesty's Stationery office 1991 (Table 15).

101. Nordin BEC. Clin Orthop 1966;45:17–20.

102. Feskanich D, Willett WC, Colditz GA. Am J Clin Nutr 2003;77:504–11.

103. Michaelsson K, Melhus H, Bellocco R et al. Bone 2003;32:694–703.

104. Feskanich D, Willett W, Colditz G. JAMA 2002;288:2300–6.

105. Wickham CAC, Walsh K, Cooper C et al. BMJ 1989;299:889–92.

106. McCarron DA, Morris CD, Henry HJ et al. Science 1984;224:1392–8.

107. Cutler JA, Brittain E. Am J Hypertens 1990;3:137S–146S.

108. Cho E, Smith-Warner S, Spiegelman D et al. J Natl Cancer Inst 2004;96:1015–22.

109. Baron JA, Beach M, Mandel JS et al. N Engl J Med 1999;340:101–7.

110. Giovannucci E, Rimm EB, Wolk A et al. Cancer Res 1998; 58:442–7.
111. Giovannucci E. Nutritional and environmental epidemiology of prostate cancer. In: Kantoff PW, Carroll PR, D'Amico AV, eds. Prostate Cancer: Principles and Practice. Philadelphia: Lippincott Williams & Wilkins, 2002:117–39.
112. Law MR, Frost CD, Wald NJ. BMJ 1991;302:819–24.
113. Klatsky AL, Armstrong MA, Friedman GD. Am J Cardiol 1990; 66:1237–42.
114. Rimm EB, Giovannucci EL, Willett WC et al. Lancet 1991; 338:464–8.
115. Hines LM, Rimm EB. Postgrad Med J 2001;77:747–52.
116. Mukamal KJ, Conigrave KM, Mittleman MA et al. N Engl J Med 2003;348:109–18.
117. Smith-Warner SA, Spiegelman D, Yaun S-S et al. JAMA 1998; 279:535–40.
118. Reichman ME, Judd JT, Longcope C et al. J Natl Cancer Inst 1993;85:722–7.
119. Hankinson SE, Willett WC, Manson JE et al. J Natl Cancer Inst 1995;87:1297–302.
120. Boffetta P, Garfinkel L. Epidemiology 1990;1:342–8.
121. Fuchs CS, Stampfer MJ, Colditz GA et al. N Engl J Med 1995; 332:1245–50.
122. Block G, Abrams B. Ann NY Acad Sci 1993;678:244–54.
123. MRC Vitamin Study Research Group. Lancet 1991;338: 131–7.
124. Giovannucci E. J Nutr 2002;132:2350S–5S.
125. Rimm EB, Willett WC, Hu FB et al. JAMA 1998;279: 359–64.
126. Choumenkovitch SF, Selhub J, Wilson PWF et al. J Nutr 2002; 132:2792–8.
127. Bischoff-Ferrari HA, Dietrich T, Orav EJ et al. Am J Med 2004;116:634–9.
128. Holick MF. Am J Clin Nutr 2004;79:362–71.
129. Blot WJ, Li JY, Taylor PR et al. J Natl Cancer Inst 1993;85: 1483–92.
130. Fawzi WW, Msamanga GI, Spiegelman D et al. N Engl J Med 2004;351:23–32.
131. Feskanich D, Singh V, Willett WC et al. JAMA 2002;287:47–54.
132. Melhus H, Michaelsson K, Kindmark A et al. Ann Intern Med 1998;129:770–8.
133. Michaelsson K, Lithell H, Vessby B et al. N Engl J Med 2003;348:287–94.
134. Johansson S, Melhus H. J Bone Miner Res 2001;16: 1899–905.
135. Block G, Patterson B, Subar A. Nutr Cancer 1992;18:1–29.
136. US Department of Agriculture. The Food Guide Pyramid. Home and Garden Bulletin no. 252. Washington, DC: US Government Printing Office, 1992:1–30.
137. Willett WC. Eat, Drink, and Be Healthy: The Harvard Medical School Guide to Healthy Eating. New York: Simon & Schuster, 2001.
138. Kennedy ET, Ohls J, Carlson S et al. J Am Diet Assoc 1995; 95:1103–8.
139. Stampfer MJ, Hu FB, Manson JE et al. N Engl J Med 2000; 343:16–22.
140. Trichopoulou A, Lagiou P, Kuper H et al. Cancer Epidemiol Biomarkers Prev 2000;9:869–73.
141. McCullough ML, Robertson AS, Rodriguez C et al. Cancer Causes Control 2003;14:1–12.
142. McCullough ML, Feskanich D, Stampfer MJ et al. Am J Clin Nutr 2000;72:1214–22.
143. McCullough ML, Feskanich D, Rimm EB et al. Am J Clin Nutr 2000;72:1223–31.
144. McCullough ML, Feskanich D, Stampfer MJ et al. Am J Clin Nutr 2002;76:1261–71.
145. US Department of Agriculture, US Department of Health and Human Services. Nutrition and Your Health: Dietary Guidelines for Americans. 6th ed. Home and Garden Bulletin no. 232. Washington, DC: US Government Printing Office, 2005. http://www.health.gov/dietaryguidelines/dga2005/document/
146. Stampfer MJ, Hu FB, Manson JE et al. N Engl J Med 2000; 343:16–22.
147. Trichopoulou A, Costacou T, Bamia C et al. N Engl J Med 2003;348:2599–608.

SELECTED READINGS

McCullough ML, Feskanich D, Stampfer MJ et al. Diet quality and major chronic disease risk in men and women: Moving toward improved dietary guidance. Am J Clin Nutr 2002;76:1261–71.

Stampfer MJ, Hu FB, Manson JE et al. Primary prevention of coronary heart disease in women through diet and lifestyle. N Engl J Med 2000;343:16–22.

Trichopoulou A, Costacou T, Bamia C et al. Adherence to a Mediterranean diet and survival in a Greek population. N Engl J Med 2003; 348:2599–608.

US Department of Agriculture, US Department of Health and Human Services. Nutrition and Your Health: Dietary Guidelines for Americans. 6th ed. Washington, DC: US Government Printing Office, 2005.

Willett WC. Eat, Drink and Be Healthy: The Harvard Medical School Guide to Healthy Eating. New York: Simon & Schuster, 2001.

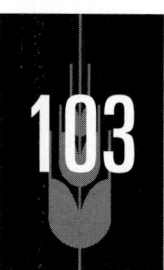

103 NUTRITIONAL IMPLICATIONS OF VEGETARIAN DIETS[1]
PATRICIA K. JOHNSTON AND JOAN SABATÉ

OVERVIEW 1638
   Historical Context 1638
   Definitions and Rationale for Vegetarian
      Dietary Practices 1638
   Trends in Vegetarian Dietary
      Practices 1639
DIETARY INTAKE AND NUTRITIONAL STATUS
   OF VEGETARIANS 1639
   Dietary Intake 1640
   Nutrient Status 1641
VEGETARIAN DIETS IN CHRONIC DISEASE
   PREVENTION 1644
   Coronary Heart Disease 1644
   Hypertension 1645
   Diabetes 1645
   Cancer 1645
   Osteoporosis 1646
VEGETARIAN DIETS IN THE LIFE CYCLE 1646
   Pregnancy and Lactation 1647
   Infancy and Childhood 1647
   Adolescence 1648
   Adulthood and Elderly Persons 1648
   Women's Issues 1648
VEGETARIAN DIETS IN CHRONIC DISEASE
   MANAGEMENT 1649
   Coronary Heart Disease 1649
   Hypertension 1649
   Diabetes 1649
   Renal Disease 1650
   Rheumatoid Arthritis 1650
DIETARY GUIDELINES FOR A HEALTHY
   VEGETARIAN LIFESTYLE 1650
   Dietary Recommendations 1650
   Food Guides 1650
   Nutrition Counseling 1651
CONCLUSION 1652

---

[1]**Abbreviations: ALA,** α-linolenic acid; **BMI,** body mass index; **CHD,** coronary heart disease; **DHA,** docosahexaenoic acid; **LA,** linoleic acid; **LOV,** lactoovovegetarian.

1638

OVERVIEW

Historical Context

For centuries, vegetarian diets have been used in different parts of the world for various reasons. Even in ancient times, some advocated such diets for a variety of health-related, religious, or ethical reasons. Although Pythagoras is considered the founder of the vegetarian movement and advocates included other ancient Greeks, Hebrew writings documented the practice of vegetarian diets even from Old Testament Bible times. Eastern religions, including Buddhism, Zainism, and Hinduism, also promote vegetarian diets and continue to urge preservation of animal life; vegetarians are found among their adherents.

In the eighteenth century, Benjamin Franklin was perhaps the most famous of the scientists, physicians, and philosophers who supported vegetarian diets. The vegetarian movement expanded considerably in the nineteenth century with the formation of societies, establishment of health care facilities, publication of books, and opening of restaurants, all promoting vegetarian diets. The twentieth century witnessed a further expansion of interest and knowledge. Details of the history of vegetarian dietary practices have been reviewed (1, 2).

Definitions and Rationale for Vegetarian Dietary Practices

The term *vegetarian* encompasses a wide range of dietary practices with potentially differing implications for health. It is not uncommon for persons who call themselves vegetarians to consume meat. It was reported that 20% of vegetarians said they ate meat at least once a month (3). Consumption of fish or poultry is even more common.

The varied dietary practices considered to be vegetarian result in differing nutritional intakes and necessitate that health professionals ascertain what actually is eaten rather than depend on what persons call themselves. Unfortunately, there is no consistent definition for vegetarian in the various scientific studies, although researchers may classify subjects on reported dietary intake rather than on what the subjects call themselves or their diets.

Cereal grains, fruits, vegetables, legumes, nuts, and seeds form the basis of vegetarian diets, with varying amounts of dairy products and eggs. The types of animal products included frequently are used to identify the kind of vegetarian diet. Lactoovovegetarians (LOVs), sometimes called ovolactovegetarians, and lactovegetarians are the largest subgroups. Both exclude meat, poultry, fish, and other seafood, but they may consume dairy products, and in the case of the LOVs, also eggs.

Persons who exclude all animal products may be called strict, total, or pure vegetarians. However, these descriptors are also sometimes used, albeit inaccurately, to mean simply exclusion of flesh foods. The term *vegan* is explicitly used to define persons who do not consume any animal products. Some vegans also refrain from using honey and animal products such as leather or wool.

Macrobiotic diets are often classified as vegetarian, although they may include fish. The macrobiotic diets of today are an outgrowth of a ten-step approach to eating that culminated in a diet composed almost exclusively of brown rice. The use of such a restrictive diet resulted in severe nutritional deficiencies and has since been modified. Although it still emphasizes brown rice and other whole grains, it also includes sea vegetables, legumes, and root vegetables. Standard macrobiotic diet recommendations include 40 to 60% whole grains, 20 to 30% vegetables, 5 to 10% beans and sea vegetables. Fruits, white meat fish, seeds, and nuts may be consumed occasionally. Meat, poultry, eggs, dairy products, as well as refined sugars, honey, artificial sweeteners, and genetically modified foods, are generally avoided (4).

Occasionally, one encounters a fruitarian, a person who consumes only raw foods. The fruitarian diet consists of fruits (including those vegetables botanically classified as such), nuts, and seeds. A raw food diet, also called "living food diet," includes uncooked, fermented, or sprouted plant foods and the juice made from sprouts.

Thus, a broad spectrum of dietary practices may be classified as vegetarian. The reasons for adopting a vegetarian lifestyle are also varied. Historically, vegetarian diets were associated with certain religious practices. Currently, however, health appears to be the primary reason for adopting a vegetarian diet (3). Government and other health-related organizations recommend a plant-based diet (5–7). Other reasons encompass ecologic and environmental issues relating to the large differences in resources necessary to support animal- and plant-based diets. Another common reason relates to ethical concerns about the treatment of animals and may extend to the use of animals for clothing or research. In many cases, however, multiple reasons underlie vegetarian dietary practices.

Trends in Vegetarian Dietary Practices

A 1994 survey reported that some 12.4 million people in the United States call themselves vegetarians (8). This represented approximately 7% of the population and a near doubling in the number of reported vegetarians over an 8-year period. Analysis of the respondents' answers to

TABLE 103.1. MAIN THEMES OF ARTICLES ON VEGETARIAN NUTRITION PUBLISHED IN BIOMEDICAL LITERATURE BETWEEN 1966 AND 1995

DECADE	1966–1975	1976–1985	1986–1995	P^a
Nutrition adequacy issues	48%	37%	24%	.001
Preventive and therapeutic applications	24%	38%	40%	.196
Other themes	28%	25%	36%	—

^{a} Chi-square test for linear trends.

Adapted from Sabaté J, Duk A, Lee CL. Am J Clin Nutr 1999;70[Suppl]:601S–19S.

the survey questions showed that approximately 1% of the population were true vegetarians (those who do not eat meat, fish, or fowl). However, the same poll administered in the year 2000 concluded that 2.5% of the population can be considered vegetarian (9).

The growing vegetarian population necessitates that health professionals be informed about the potential benefits and risks associated with these dietary practices. Position papers and scientific reviews have been published, as well as the proceedings from four international congresses addressing this topic (10–16). In addition, two books on vegetarian diets address most of the important topics related to the nutritional status of vegetarians and provide useful summaries of the literature as well as dietary suggestions for different conditions (8, 17).

Professional interest in vegetarian nutrition is at an all-time high. This is only partly explained by the increasing number of vegetarians. The number of scientific publications on vegetarian diets is also growing. Sabaté and colleagues (18) documented publication trends in the biomedical literature of articles related to vegetarian nutrition using a bibliographic database (18). The rate of publication of vegetarian articles increased steadily both in nutrition journals and in other journals. The main focus of vegetarian nutrition research has also changed over time (Table 103.1). Although the major theme before the 1980s focused primarily on the nutritional adequacy of vegetarian diets, 40% of all vegetarian nutrition articles published in the decade 1986 to 1995 emphasized preventive and therapeutic applications of vegetarian diets, mainly with respect to chronic diseases (18).

DIETARY INTAKE AND NUTRITIONAL STATUS OF VEGETARIANS

Many and varied ways exist to meet nutrient needs, and the adequacy of a diet depends not on what it is called but on the foods that are included in it. A vegetarian diet need not be deficient in nutrients; however, the more foods eliminated from any diet, the greater the risk of deficiency.

Most vegetarians ingest an adequate diet; however, those following restrictive dietary patterns may not ingest all the required nutrients in adequate amounts. Inadequate diets engender significant concern, especially when they are consumed by pregnant and lactating women, infants, children, and the elderly. As the understanding of both beneficial and problematic aspects of vegetarian dietary practices increases, attention can better be focused on those issues of greatest consequence for preventing disease and promoting health. Thus, our attention here is addressed to those questions that are most frequently raised.

Dietary Intake

To answer the question "What do vegetarians in the United States eat?" nutrient and food consumption patterns of self-defined vegetarians and nonvegetarians were compared in a representative sample of the US population (19). The dietary patterns of vegetarians were generally considered healthier than those of nonvegetarians, even for vegetarians who may consume some fish, poultry, or red meat. Diets of vegetarians tended to be lower in total fat, saturated fat, and cholesterol, and higher in fiber, than the diets of nonvegetarians. Vegetarians tended to consume more grains, legumes, vegetables, fruit, and wine than nonvegetarians. Other studies also reported that, among vegetarians, intakes of soy and nutrients such as folate, vitamin C, vitamin E, and magnesium are higher than among nonvegetarians, but intakes of retinol, vitamin B_{12}, vitamin D, calcium, and zinc are lower (20–23).

Much attention is currently focused on the benefits of dietary antioxidants. It is not surprising that vegetarians, in view of their diet, are reported to have higher blood levels of β-carotene, vitamin C, and vitamin E, all nutrients thought to play important roles in the prevention of chronic disease (24). Mineral element antioxidant intakes are variable in vegetarian and other diets. Vegetarian diets usually provide more copper than in most mixed diets. Although the intake of zinc may be similar, its bioavailability is generally lower in the context of a vegetarian diet. The amount of selenium is variable, based on soil content (25). This section highlights specific nutrient intakes and adequacy when various vegetarian diets are practiced. In addition to the nutrients mentioned here, others including iodine and riboflavin have been identified as being inadequate in more restrictive vegetarian diets (26).

Energy Intake and Weight Status

Some, but not all, investigators report that vegetarians weigh less than nonvegetarians, with the difference being least among the LOVs and greatest among the vegans. The lower weight among vegetarians is consistent with the lower intake of calories that is often reported. The energy-yielding nutrients protein and fat are generally consumed in somewhat greater amounts by nonvegetarians, whereas larger amounts of carbohydrates are consumed by vegetarians (27). The result of this difference is that vegetarians tend to have a lower energy intake and lower body

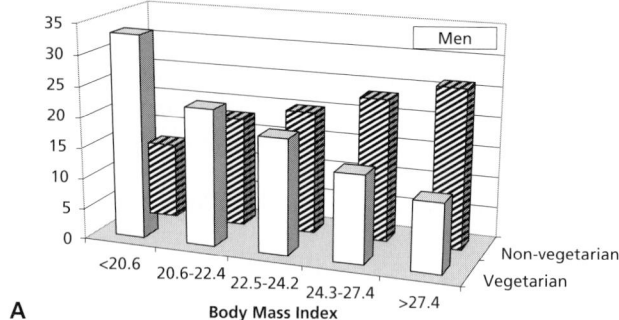

A

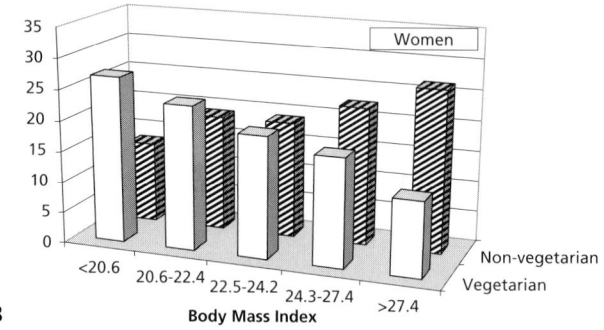

B

Figure 103.1. Distribution in categories of body mass index (BMI) of vegetarians and nonvegetarians of the Adventist Health Study cohort. For both men **(A)** and women **(B)**, a striking inverse relationship exists between BMI and vegetarian status. (From Sabaté J, ed. Vegetarian Nutrition. Boca Raton, FL: CRC Press, 2001:97, with permission.)

mass index (BMI) than do omnivores (21, 28, 29). Thus, they may be closer to desirable weight and they may more closely approximate dietary recommendations for the distribution of macronutrients than do omnivores. As illustrated in Figure 103.1, vegetarians may also demonstrate more desirable weight patterns than omnivores (30).

Various other reasons have been suggested for the weight difference between vegetarians and nonvegetarians. In addition to the higher intake of carbohydrates in vegetarians, which may be less efficiently converted to body fat, they include perhaps greater control of food intake, possibly greater physical activity, and greater intake of fiber, which may enhance satiation (31).

Although overweight is a frequent concern in the general population, maintaining adequate weight through appropriate caloric intake may be a concern to some vegetarians. Those at risk include children, adolescents, the elderly, and those who include no added oils or fat in the diet.

Vegetarian Diets and Weight Loss

The general understanding that vegetarian diets are associated with lower weight status may be the rationale for some people, girls and women especially, to adopt such a diet, in the hope of weight loss. There is the view, however, that among similarly health-conscious vegetarians and nonvegetarians, relative weight and weight loss efforts are quite similar (32). Vegetarian dietary practices have been found among patients with anorexia nervosa, although most were not vegetarians before the anorexia (see also Chapter 87). The risk of extreme eating behaviors and disorders may be more likely among adolescent vegetarians (33). However, it has been suggested that vegetarian diets are used as a convenient and socially acceptable way to reduce caloric intake (34). A study of eating behavior found that vegetarian women had lower dietary restraint scores, indicating that they were not motivated by weight loss to adopt the vegetarian diet (35). Thus, it is inappropriate to conclude that vegetarians are more prone to eating disorders than the general population.

Nutrient Status

Protein

One of the most frequent questions regarding the nutritional adequacy of vegetarian diets relates to attaining adequate protein, yet little supporting evidence exists for such concerns with usual dietary intake in healthy vegetarians. However, the inadequate energy intake in some vegetarians may compromise protein status as well. Moreover, because of the lower digestibility of plant proteins, the protein requirement of vegans may be higher than those of nonvegetarians (36).

The nutritional quality of plant proteins may be underestimated in studies of animals, because animals have greater protein needs per body weight than humans. More relevant human data confirm the adequacy of plant proteins to meet the needs of both adults and children. Foods of plant origin are often said to lack certain indispensable amino acids and thus to provide protein of lesser quality than that in foods of animal origin. Although a certain plant food may be low in a specific amino acid, it is inaccurate to say that it is incomplete when consumed in the context of a diet. A single plant food, if fed as the only protein source, may prove inadequate. However, this is likely to occur only in a research setting. Appropriate mixtures of plant foods provide protein of equivalent quality to that in animal foods, and such mixtures are commonly consumed.

Two amino acids are of particular interest in vegetarian diets: lysine, the limiting amino acid in cereal grains, and methionine, the limiting amino acid in legumes. Lysine occurs in significant amounts in the intracellular spaces of the skeletal musculature, where it is deposited after a protein-rich meal (37). Subsequently, it is available to buffer a low-lysine amino acid mixture resulting from consumption of a meal deficient in this amino acid. Methionine is of interest because it is the limiting amino acid in soy and other legumes, which are often a major source of protein in vegetarian diets. Soy protein isolates have been used successfully in refeeding children recovering from malnutrition; they provide a protein quality comparable to that of milk. Soy protein isolates may be used as the sole source of protein for adults and children; however, modest supplementation with methionine may be appropriate for

soy-based infant formulas, although the amount needed is lower than predicted from studies in rats (37).

Protein complementation occurs when a food low in a particular amino acid is combined with a food containing an adequate amount of that amino acid. Animal studies have influenced our attitudes toward combining complementary proteins within one meal. In these studies, an amino acid otherwise absent from the diet was added several hours later. Such a delay in providing a supplementary amino acid to rapidly growing rats and pigs affected the overall utilization of the other proteins in the meal. However, similar effects were not seen in human adults when the plant protein was distributed among several meals. The supplementary effect was somewhat lower in young children when the complementary proteins were fed at intervals longer than 6 hours; however, this is a longer between-meal period than is usual in young children, and their usual meals are not entirely devoid of an amino acid, as in the case of laboratory studies (37). It therefore can be concluded that combinations of plant foods consumed throughout the day provide adequate amino acids for nitrogen retention and use.

Plant proteins in their natural form are, in general, less digestible than animal protein sources. Well-processed soy isolates, however, are as digestible as egg protein (37). Processing methods may have beneficial or detrimental effects on the nutritional quality of plant proteins. Consuming a broad variety of foods prepared in many different ways ensures an adequate intake of amino acids from plant proteins.

Vegetarians, in general, consume less total protein and even less animal protein than omnivores; however, studies have consistently shown that they more than meet the recommended dietary allowances, and the recommendation for 10% of calories as protein. In addition, they more than meet the needs for the indispensable amino acids. Current evidence suggests that a lower intake of animal protein may be beneficial and may lower urinary calcium excretion and slow the progression of renal disease. In addition, compared with sources of animal protein, sources of plant protein contribute less total fat, saturated fat, and cholesterol and more carbohydrate and fiber. In more restrictive diets, in which variety or energy intake is limited, greater attention must be given to providing an adequate protein intake, especially in pregnant women, infants, growing children, and the elderly.

Iron

Nonheme iron from plant foods is less available than heme iron, and plant foods contain a variety of substances known to reduce iron availability; thus, the iron status of vegetarians is often questioned. However, plant foods also contain other substances that enhance iron uptake, and well-planned vegetarian diets often contain more iron than omnivorous diets.

Some studies suggest that long-term LOVs, even with a higher fiber intake, maintain iron status no different from that of omnivores (38). Other studies, however, indicate that vegetarians may have reduced iron stores, even though iron deficiency anemia as determined by hemoglobin levels is no more prevalent than among omnivores (39). Although no significant difference in iron intake was noted, a study found significantly lower hemoglobin levels in vegetarian children than in omnivorous children in England (40). The authors suggested that dietary advice was needed to ensure an optimal absorption of iron. Poor iron status was independently associated with vegetarianism in a study of British young people (41). Another study found lower serum ferritin levels in both male and female vegetarians than in omnivorous controls, although the vegetarians consumed significantly more iron (42). Although lower iron stores increase the risk of iron deficiency, the optimal level of tissue iron storage continues to be debated, particularly in view of evidence of an association between elevated iron stores and reduced insulin sensitivity (43), as well as coronary heart disease (CHD) (44).

The high levels of iron in well-planned vegetarian diets combined with the frequent intake of fruits and vegetables rich in vitamin C (ascorbate) appear to protect against iron deficiency (45), which is more likely to be encountered among those on restrictive vegetarian diets such as macrobiotic diets. Iron deficiency is also more prevalent in developing countries where dietary choices are limited and there is a greater reliance on unleavened and unrefined cereal products (38).

Folate

Intake and blood levels of folate are often higher in vegetarians than in omnivores because of the greater use of fruits and vegetables in vegetarian diets. This was found to be the case for pregnant vegetarians as well (46). Elevated folate is of concern in persons whose vitamin B_{12} intake is low because folate may delay the appearance of megaloblastic anemia and thus mask a developing vitamin B_{12} deficiency, with its potentially irreversible neurologic effects (47).

Vitamin B_{12}

Vitamin B_{12} is of particular interest because the usual dietary sources of this vitamin are animal products. Relevant metabolic indicators suggest that persons who include only plant foods in their diet, such as vegans and others who consume only raw foods, are at increased risk of deficiency (48–50), unless care is taken to include a reliable source of vitamin B_{12}. In contrast, however, some are of the view that a vegetarian diet only partly explains the metabolic signs of vitamin B_{12} deficiency (51). Vitamin B_{12} deficiency can result in serious and irreversible neurologic and neuropsychiatric abnormalities. These potentially significant consequences necessitate giving attention to this vitamin in any discussion of vegetarian diets.

In addition, inactive analogs of this vitamin occur in foods and are found in the body. However, they are not differentiated in the usual microbiologic assays used to assess either vitamin B_{12} status or its content in foods, which are likely overestimated unless a method specific for cobalamin, the active form, is used (52).

Plants do not synthesize or store vitamin B_{12}. The ultimate source of this vitamin is microbial synthesis. Vitamin B_{12} occurs in plants only if they are contaminated by bacteria producing it (52). Such contamination is more likely where strict sanitary procedures are not followed in handling food, and vitamin B_{12} from soil or other sources of microbial contamination may be a reasonable explanation for the limited vitamin B_{12} deficiency occurring among vegan populations in developing countries. Animals either ingest the vitamin or absorb what is produced by bacteria in their intestines, thus becoming a source of vitamin B_{12} for those who consume animal products.

As noted, the microbiologic assays often used to assess vitamin B_{12} content determine the inactive vitamin B_{12} analogs, as well as cobalamin, the active form of the vitamin. Labels on many food products give values for the nonactive analogs, rather than for cobalamin. This is misleading and causes confusion for the consumer. Assays specific for cobalamin indicate that many food products commonly *thought to* be sources of vitamin B_{12} in actuality contain mostly inactive analogs (52); these include spirulina, tempeh, other fermented foods, and most sea algae. Investigators suggested that persons relying on spirulina as a source of vitamin B_{12} could develop a deficiency more rapidly because some of the analogs contained in it block vitamin B_{12} metabolism (52).

Serum vitamin B_{12} levels in vegans are generally lower than those in omnivores, with intermediate levels found in LOVs. Persons adopting a vegan diet showed a more rapid reduction in serum vitamin B_{12} than anticipated, and those using vitamin B_{12} supplements or foods fortified with vitamin B_{12} had higher mean serum vitamin B_{12} levels over time (53). Similarly, serum vitamin B_{12} levels declined over a 2-year period in six of nine subjects adhering to a "living food diet" (54).

It is remarkable that so few reported cases of vitamin B_{12} deficiency exist even among vegans. Observations, however, suggest that suboptimal vitamin B_{12} status may occur well before the deficiency is discovered. Reasons for the low incidence of vitamin B_{12} deficiency include the very small requirement, relatively large stores, and a very efficient enterohepatic circulation that recovers most of the vitamin B_{12} that is excreted in the bile. Intestinal bacteria produce vitamin B_{12}; however, most of this occurs below the ileal site for vitamin B_{12} absorption, and the vitamin B_{12} produced is excreted in the feces (52). Some evidence indicates that small amounts are produced in the small intestine, although it is unclear how much of this is the active form (52). Some vegans may consume the vitamin in foods eaten outside their homes.

Limited evidence indicates that some seaweeds may contribute active vitamin B_{12}, presumably from contamination with plankton. Vegans consuming *Chlorella* or Nori seaweed had serum vitamin B_{12} concentrations twice as high as those not consuming these seaweeds (54). In another study, increased consumption of seaweeds by a mother led to normalization of urinary methylmalonic acid in her breast-fed infant (55). In contrast, ample consumption of seaweed by vitamin B_{12}–deficient infants did not improve their abnormal hematologic indices, and there was no relationship between algae consumption by macrobiotic adults and their vitamin B_{12} status (56, 57). Reliable sources of vitamin B_{12} must be ensured to prevent deficiency in persons who consume no animal foods.

Calcium and Vitamin D

Adequate calcium and vitamin D intakes are important to ensure optimal bone status over the lifetime. Evidence suggests that calcium also may be important in regulating blood pressure and preventing colon cancer. Milk and dairy products supply 70% of calcium in US diets, and questions regarding calcium adequacy are often expressed when the intake of these foods is limited, as in vegan diets.

Calcium intake among LOVs appears to be similar to that of omnivores, whereas intake in vegans is less. The long-term impact of this lower intake of calcium on bone health is not yet known, although some evidence suggests that concern is warranted (58). In addition to the lower intake of calcium, vegans also consume less vitamin D. The low consumption of vitamin D may be further exacerbated in some cases by limited exposure to sunlight. Low vitamin D concentrations and secondary hyperparathyroidism were documented during the winter in vegans living at northern latitudes (59). Vitamin D deficiency was also documented in British Asian vegetarians and is a frequent concern regarding macrobiotic diets in children (60, 61). Dietary intake of vitamin D was significantly lower in both vegan and lactovegetarians compared with omnivores during the winter in Finland (62), and bone mineral density tended to be lower in the vegan group compared with the omnivore or lactovegetarian groups. Care must be given to ensuring an adequate intake of vitamin D especially in winter months in northern latitudes. The Institute of Medicine has released recommendations for intake of several nutrients related to bone health (63).

Besides vitamin D, various other dietary factors also influence calcium status. Numerous studies have demonstrated that increased intake of animal protein results in increased urinary calcium excretion. This relationship is not seen when plant protein is consumed (64). In addition, the ratio of dietary calcium to protein is thought to be important (65). This ratio in milk and dairy products is very favorable to a positive calcium balance (65). The ratio of calcium to protein in the diet of LOVs is higher than in omnivores and even higher than in vegans.

A high intake of sodium also increases calcium excretion (66). Some evidence indicates that vegans consume less sodium than LOVs or omnivores. However, investigators suggested that the characteristically increased consumption by vegans of oxalate- and phytate-containing foods may offset the benefits of their lower intakes of protein and sodium (58).

Although lower rates of hip fracture have been reported in populations worldwide having calcium intakes much lower than those in the United States, where fracture rates are higher, other factors such as genetic and lifestyle factors may play important roles. An optimal level of calcium intake under different dietary and lifestyle conditions remains to be determined.

As with all nutrients, obtaining an adequate calcium intake depends on food choices. Persons consuming relatively large amounts of animal protein, even when dairy products are not excluded, may need to give special attention to calcium intake. Vegans also may need to give attention to obtaining an appropriate intake, especially during periods of growth. In general, few other foods provide as concentrated a calcium source as dairy products; however, calcium is relatively widely distributed among plant foods. The content of bioavailable calcium in various food sources has been calculated and may be useful in guiding food choices (58). The calcium in high-oxalate vegetables such as spinach, Swiss chard, and beet greens is largely unavailable; however, kale, broccoli, Chinese cabbage, and mustard and turnip greens provide substantial amounts of available calcium. Legumes and some nuts and seeds also contribute to the calcium intake of vegetarians. Unfortified soy beverages provide negligible amounts, whereas calcium-set tofu and fortified soy milks are rich sources of calcium.

Zinc

Meat, fish, and poultry provide 40 to 45% of the zinc in the US diet; dairy foods and grain products contribute a little less than 20% each. Nonetheless, zinc intake among vegetarians is reported to be similar to that of omnivores. However, the lower availability of zinc from plant foods may result in somewhat lower zinc status among vegetarians compared with nonvegetarians. A lower zinc intake was found among vegetarian children and adolescents, but growth was not affected; in fact, vegetarians were slightly taller than nonvegetarian controls (67). Further research is needed to determine the functional consequences of lower absorption of zinc and other trace elements from vegetarian diets, as consumed in Western countries (68). Figure 103.2 illustrates that despite similar intakes of zinc and other minerals by consumers of vegetarian and nonvegetarian diets, the absorption for zinc and iron is reduced with vegetarian diets. A study of adolescent female

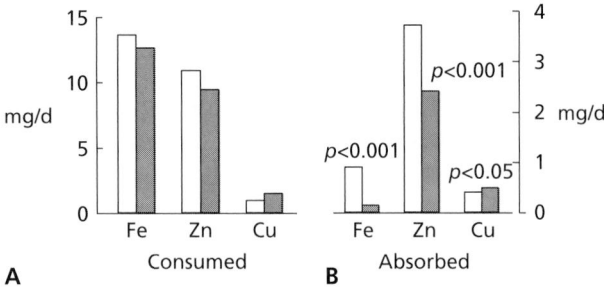

Figure 103.2. A and **B**. Contrast between the relative trace element content and the trace element bioavailability of experimental nonvegetarian *(open bars)* and vegetarian *(filled bars)* diets. (From Hunt JR. Am J Clin Nutr 2003;78[Suppl]:634S, with permission.)

vegetarians found no difference in dietary zinc intake by LOVs, semivegetarians, or omnivores (69). Further, the investigators found no differences in mean values for any indicator of zinc status, besides serum zinc, among the groups. Nonetheless, 24% of LOVs, 33% of semivegetarians, and 18% of omnivores had low serum zinc levels. An Australian study found that vegetarian women had significantly lower zinc intake than omnivores, but their serum zinc concentrations were not different (70). In men, the zinc intakes were similar between the groups, but the omnivores had significantly lower serum levels. Attention should be given to ensuring an adequate intake of foods that supply this nutrient.

Essential Fatty Acids

Vegetarian diets are typically low in α-linolenic acid (ALA, 18:3,n-3) and high in linoleic acid (LA, 18:2,n-6) (see Chapter 5 for fatty acids). This can inhibit the conversion of ALA to eicosapentanoic acid (22:5,n-3) and docosahexanoic acid (DHA, 22:6,n-3) (71), which are the precursors to important eicosanoids implicated in chronic disease prevention (see Chapter 5). If the intake of LA in the diet of vegetarians is high, their requirement for n-3 fatty acids may also be higher than that of omnivores (72). Sources rich in ALA such as flaxseed, walnuts, and soybean or canola oils should be included in the vegetarian diet, and the intake of oils rich in n-6 fatty acids should be decreased to optimize conversion to eicosapentanoic acid and DHA.

VEGETARIAN DIETS IN CHRONIC DISEASE PREVENTION

The association of vegetarian diets with lower risk of several chronic diseases is well documented. Various studies investigating these relationships have been reviewed (31, 73) and are the focus of two recent books (9, 74). The standardized mortality ratio for all-cause mortality is greatly reduced among vegetarians, who are known to consume more fruits, vegetables, and polyunsaturated fatty acids and less saturated fatty acids, cholesterol, and alcohol than

the general population (10, 11, 13, 14, 17, 73, 75). Vegetarians also smoke less, have a lower BMI, and may exercise more.

The specific health-promoting factors associated with a vegetarian lifestyle continue to be investigated, with particular attention currently focused on phytochemicals and the foods that contain them. These nonnutritive substances include a wide range of chemicals found in plant foods and are reviewed elsewhere (76, 77). These substances can alter various hormone actions and metabolic paths in beneficial ways. The advantages of fruits and vegetables are so well accepted that recommendations to include more of them in the diet are heard with increasing frequency. Some of the positive health effects of vegetarian diets may result from the increased intake of these foods.

Several major epidemiologic studies of vegetarians have focused on Seventh-Day Adventists, a conservative religious denomination. Adventists follow a broad range of dietary practices, from total vegetarianism to US American diets. Approximately half are vegetarians, and most are LOVs. Certain lifestyle characteristics, such as smoking and alcohol consumption, which can confound or modify the effects of other factors, are largely absent from this population. The Adventist Health Study has provided an opportunity to compare vegetarian and omnivorous dietary practices within a population with great similarity of other lifestyle factors. Overall mortality rates are lower among Adventists than in the general population. Although they die of similar diseases, they appear to develop these diseases at a later age (74).

Coronary Heart Disease

Lower risk of death from CHD among vegetarian populations is well established and not surprising, given their dietary and lifestyle characteristics resulting in lower body weight, lower blood pressure, and lower serum lipid levels (9, 11, 13, 14, 17, 74). An LOV vegetarian diet in an African-American population was also associated with a more favorable profile of blood lipid risk factors for premature CHD than the omnivorous diet (78). Multiple factors undoubtedly play roles in decreasing the risk seen among vegetarians.

An association between meat consumption and fatal ischemic heart disease was described in the Adventist Mortality Study, and data from the Adventist Health Study confirmed that relationship (79). Risk of fatal CHD was nearly twice as great in men who ate beef up to three times a week than in men who never ate any, and risk was more than twofold greater in men consuming beef three times a week or more. Meat eating did not change the risk of CHD for women.

The same analysis revealed other intriguing relationships. The risk of both nonfatal and fatal CHD was lower in those who consumed mainly whole wheat bread than in those who ate mainly white bread (79). Similarly, the risk of both nonfatal and fatal CHD was lower in those who ate nuts frequently than in those who ate nuts less than once a week. The protective effect of frequent consumption of nuts was found consistently among various subgroups including both vegetarians and nonvegetarians.

A carefully controlled dietary trial was subsequently conducted to investigate these relationships further (80). Moderate quantities of walnuts were incorporated into a National Cholesterol Education Program Step I isocaloric diet in place of fatty foods and visible oils, while maintaining fat at 30%. This diet resulted in a more favorable lipoprotein profile. The possible mechanisms mediating the beneficial effect of nuts have been reviewed (81).

To date, much of the research investigating the relationships between diet and CHD has focused on dietary factors related to modifying serum lipids. The rapid expansion since the mid-1990s of our understanding of various plant constituents has led to a rethinking of the relationship of diet with heart disease (82). Whereas great emphasis was placed on dietary fat, it is now suggested that other factors, such as a higher intake of antioxidants, may play important, if not decisive, roles. This is not to suggest that fat intake should be ignored, but rather that other factors should also receive attention (83).

Hypertension

Data from cross-sectional studies have shown that blood pressure and prevalence of hypertension are lower in vegetarians than in omnivores (74). This was also documented in African-Americans, a population with a well-recognized increased risk of hypertension (78). Confirmed hypertension occurred in significantly fewer vegetarians than semivegetarians and omnivores. Mean systolic blood pressure was significantly lower in black vegetarians than in black nonvegetarians but was higher than in white vegetarians or nonvegetarians, a finding suggesting that vegetarian dietary practices do not completely offset the risk of hypertension in the black population (78).

In contrast, the Health Food Shop Users cross-sectional study found no difference in blood pressure between vegetarians and omnivores (73). It was suggested that lifestyle factors other than avoidance of meat may be shared by vegetarians and other health-conscious persons and may affect blood pressure.

Randomized controlled trials introducing an LOV diet to meat eaters were reviewed (84). The review indicated that the reported blood pressure–lowering effect of vegetarian diets is between 5 and 10 mm Hg in systolic blood pressure and is independent of the effect of reducing body weight on lowering blood pressure.

The relationships between vegetarian diets and decreased risk of hypertension are complex because of the myriad dietary and lifestyle components that interact in this condition, as in other chronic diseases. None of the characteristics of the vegetarian diet alone—absence of meat, type of protein, a high ratio of polyunsaturated to saturated fat, or a high intake of fiber, potassium, or magnesium—has been identified as the active agent (85). The combined effect of several specific foods and/or nutrients may be responsible for the lower blood pressure seen in vegetarians.

Diabetes

Vegetarians may be at less risk of developing diabetes than omnivores. Among Adventist Health Study volunteers, vegetarians had lower rates of diabetes than omnivores. Nonvegetarian men, after adjusting for age and weight, were 1.8 times more likely to die of diabetes than vegetarian men. No difference, however, was seen among women (85). Furthermore, risk of death from diabetes ("diabetes" appearing on the death certificate) was greater with increasing meat consumption in men; that is, there was a dose-response relationship. In women, increased risk of death from diabetes was found only in those who consumed meat more than six times a week.

Various factors found among vegetarians have been suggested as protective for diabetes. Among these are lower body weight, lower serum cholesterol levels, high complex carbohydrate and fiber intakes, and lower fat and animal protein intakes. The benefits of high-carbohydrate, high-fiber diets in treating diabetes have been demonstrated (86).

Cancer

The German Vegetarian Study found that death from all cancers was reduced by 52% in vegetarian men and 26% in vegetarian women, compared with population expectations (87). More specifically, the standardized mortality rate for colon cancer was found to be 44 in men and 78 in women. Longer duration of vegetarian practices decreased the risk of cancer mortality.

The risk of death from cancer is considerably lower among Adventists as a whole than in an appropriate reference population (88). Lower risk would be expected for those sites associated with cigarette smoking or alcohol; however, the reduction in risk included nearly all major cancer sites, with a greater reduction for men than for women.

The relationships between dietary components and specific cancer sites were investigated in the Adventist population and recently reviewed (74). Multivariate analysis was used to control for factors other than the variable of interest. Frequent consumption of fruit (more than once daily versus less than three times weekly) was associated with a 75% reduction in risk of lung cancer, independent of past smoking status. The risk of stomach cancer was also greatly reduced in those who consumed fruit frequently. Raisins, dates, and other dried fruit provided significant protection against prostate cancer. Frequent consumption of tomatoes and dried beans also may protect against prostate cancer, whereas consumption of fish more than once a week may increase risk. No association with dietary factors, including animal fat, was found for breast cancer.

Striking protection against pancreatic cancer was afforded by frequent consumption of legumes; those consuming dried beans and peas more than twice a week had only one thirtieth the risk of those who consumed these foods rarely or not at all. An 80% reduction in risk of this cancer was associated with frequent consumption of raisins, dates, and other dried fruit.

Persons who ate beans more than twice a week had a 42% lower risk of developing colon cancer than those who ate beans less than once a week. A similar reduction was seen in those who consumed more fiber. In contrast, a somewhat greater risk was associated with eating meat, fish, or fowl several times each week. After adjusting for age, sex, and smoking history, frequent consumption of beef was associated with a more than twofold increase in risk of bladder cancer.

These results suggest that, with the exception of bladder and perhaps colon cancer, dietary factors other than the absence of meat are the protective agents in the reduced risk of cancer seen among vegetarians (74). Others reported an inverse relationship between milk intake and incidence of breast cancer (89). Thus, increasing attention is being focused on foods commonly consumed by vegetarians and the protective compounds they contain.

Osteoporosis

Studies of bone mineral status in vegetarians and omnivores have been reviewed (90). No differences were found in either cortical or trabecular bone. However, an earlier report suggested that postmenopausal vegetarian women are protected against bone loss and that their lower protein intake may be a major beneficial factor (90). A prospective study reported a small but significant increase in risk of forearm fracture for women who consumed more than 95 g/day of total protein, compared with those who consumed less than 68 g (91). A similar increase in risk was seen for animal protein, but no association was found with vegetable protein. Those who ate five or more servings per week of red meat had a higher risk of forearm fracture than those eating less than one serving a week.

Concern was expressed about the bone status of vegans (58). Recent reports have lent support to this concern, although to date few studies specifically of vegans have been conducted. Because leanness is also a risk factor for osteoporosis and because vegans are often leaner than the general population, it would be wise to give attention to their bone status. Investigators reported a higher risk of exceeding the lumbar spine fracture threshold and of being classified as osteopenic in vegan than in lactovegetarian postmenopausal Taiwanese women (92). Others reported significantly lower bone mass at several sites in Dutch adolescents who had followed a vegan macrobiotic diet in childhood (93). Children 3 to 13 years of age who avoided milk for a variety of reasons had smaller skeletons and lower bone mineral density, and they were at increased risk of prepubertal fractures (94, 95).

Bone density was compared with dietary intake in five counties in China, where calcium intakes differ widely (96). Bone density was approximately 20% higher from the fourth to well into the eighth decade of life in areas where more dairy products were consumed (calcium intake, 724 mg/day) compared with those where dairy products were not used (calcium intake, 230–359 mg/day). Protein intake in the former was 75 g/day versus 49 to 57 g/day in the latter counties. The lower protein intake reported in these Chinese persons did not confer protection against low bone density when calcium intake was very low.

Whereas it is recognized that animal products result in an acid response, it is less well recognized that grain products, including those from wheat and rice, also result in a net acid response (97). Investigators have suggested that vegetarians using relatively large amounts of these foods in the context of a diet low in calcium may be increasing their risk of less than optimal bone status, as seen in the macrobiotic vegan children and the Taiwanese women.

Many factors other than calcium affect bone status and risk of fractures. Nevertheless, a consistently low calcium intake combined with low vitamin D status and high fiber intake may place vegans at greater risk of low bone density. Earlier evidence suggested that the lower protein intake typical of vegans, especially protein from animal products, would be protective of bone status, because it may decrease the requirement for calcium. More recent evidence, however, suggests that a low intake of protein may be a risk factor for hip fracture in the elderly and that the potential negative effects of increased protein intake on metabolism are offset by an adequate intake of calcium (98, 99). In contrast to earlier studies, it was recently reported that low protein intake decreases calcium absorption (100). Investigators suggested that the hypercalciuria seen with high protein intake is a result of increased calcium absorption. The interactions of dietary protein and bone health have been reviewed (99). Other nutrients including vitamin D, potassium, and phosphorus can also influence the effects of protein on bone (101). Nonetheless, prospective studies and randomized trials are needed to answer the questions that still remain (102). The current understanding would suggest that it is important to consider the entire diet when planning for optimal bone health (103).

VEGETARIAN DIETS IN THE LIFE CYCLE

Risk of nutritional deficiencies is greatest during periods of growth, and adequate intake of all nutrients should especially be ensured at these times. The impact of vegetarian diets on various stages of the life cycle has been reviewed (9, 11).

Pregnancy and Lactation

LOV diets provide adequate nutritional support during pregnancy and lactation, but special attention is needed to obtain certain nutrients when a vegan or macrobiotic diet is followed. These nutrients include total energy, iron, vitamin B_{12}, calcium, vitamin D, and n-3 fatty acids. Vegetarian women are more likely to breast-feed their infants and to do so for a longer time than women in the general population. This necessitates continued attention to dietary intake. Guidelines for counseling pregnant vegetarians also have broader application to other groups (104).

The few reports of pregnant vegetarians suggest a possible increased risk of earlier labor and lower birth weight in those following a more limited diet, although no difference in incidence of pregnancy complications was reported (105). More concentrated energy sources may be necessary than are usually consumed on a vegan diet to ensure an appropriate pregnancy weight gain. Low serum ferritin levels are associated with an increased risk of prematurity and low birth weight, and therefore care should be taken to ensure an adequate intake of iron for all pregnant women.

Normally, enough vitamin B_{12} is deposited in the fetus to last for 6 to 12 months after birth, yet numerous cases of vitamin B_{12} deficiency have been reported in infants of vegan mothers, with the deficiency frequently developing before 6 months of age (106–108). The infants were totally breast-fed by vegan mothers who showed no clinical signs of deficiency, although later testing confirmed that they had low vitamin B_{12} status. Low maternal serum vitamin B_{12} levels were reflected in low vitamin B_{12} values in milk (109). Investigators have suggested that it is currently ingested vitamin B_{12} that is most available for placental transport and secretion in the breast milk (110). Thus, totally breast-fed infants born to vegan mothers may be at increased risk of vitamin B_{12} deficiency because of decreased vitamin B_{12} stores at birth coupled with low intakes of vitamin B_{12} from their mother's milk. In some cases, the deficiency has not been observed until the child is older (111, 112). Often, the child presents evidence of growth failure and developmental delays.

Certain features are characteristic of infants developing a vitamin B_{12} deficiency: increased fretfulness and apathy, decreased socialization and activity, and regression in motor control. The infants are typically very small for their age and show serious neurologic deficits. On testing, the vitamin B_{12} deficiency is apparent. The usefulness of magnetic resonance imaging in diagnosis and follow-up of patients with suspected diseases of myelination has been emphasized (107).

In most such cases, rapid improvement is noted after administration of vitamin B_{12}. Unfortunately, however, long-term neurologic deficits appear to occur in some cases (111, 113). A group of adolescents who had followed vegan macrobiotic diets to an average age of 6 years were found to have signs of impaired cognitive function even though they had consumed moderate amounts of animal products for a number of years (114, 115). An early deficiency of vitamin B_{12} may result in long-term impairment that can have an impact on daily living (115). Vegan women must understand the importance of consuming a reliable source of vitamin B_{12}, at least during pregnancy and lactation, and it must be included in the diets of infants and children.

Low vitamin D status and low calcium intake were found in lactating macrobiotic women (109). In view of the increased calcium needs in pregnancy and lactation, low vitamin D status and low calcium intake could result in bone demineralization. Adequate calcium and vitamin D must be ensured at these critical stages of the life cycle.

Essential fatty acids and their derivatives play important roles in fetal development, especially of the retina and central nervous system, and parturition (105). Although DHA, (22:6,n-3) is found in fishit is present in only small amounts in eggs and is absent from commonly consumed plant foods. In contrast to the low level of DHA, vegetarian diets contain high amounts of LA, 18:2,n-6. DHA can be synthesized in the body from ALA, 18:3,n-3; however, high levels of LA inhibit this process (see also Chapter 5). In comparison with omnivores, a lower proportion of DHA was found in the phospholipids present in plasma and umbilical cord artery blood, as well as in the milk, of vegan mothers (105). As expected, the erythrocyte lipids of their infants contained a lower proportion of DHA than those of infants breast-fed by omnivorous mothers or infants fed cow's milk formula. Investigators suggested that vegans should use soybean or canola oils, which have a lower ratio of AL to ALA, to facilitate the body's synthesis of DHA.

Infancy and Childhood

Concerns have been expressed regarding vegetarian diets for children whose vulnerability is considered greater than that of nonvegetarian children for nutrient deficiency, yet little evidence indicates that physical or intellectual growth has been harmed (10). The growth of Seventh-Day Adventist LOV children was found to be the same as that of omnivores, with no greater evidence of nutritional deficiencies (67). Although vegan children weighed less and were shorter than nonvegetarian controls, their growth was within normal ranges, and catchup occurred by about age 10 years (116). The lower growth early in life appeared related to the high bulk and low energy density of some vegetarian diets combined with the small stomach capacity of young children. Investigators reported significant catchup in height and in arm circumference-for-age, in boys and girls combined who had followed a macrobiotic diet in early childhood. However, both boys and girls were still significantly lower than reference values for height, and girls were lower than reference values for weight-for-height and for arm circumference-for-age (117). Multiple regression analysis showed that inclusion of moderate amounts of dairy products improved the growth of vegan children.

Inadequate weaning foods deficient in calories, vitamin D, calcium, iron, and vitamin B_{12} may be used by some vegan or macrobiotic parents, thus resulting in low growth and nutritional deficiencies. Similar diets continued into preschool years resulted in impaired growth, rickets, iron deficiency anemia, and vitamin B_{12} deficiency (118). Vegetarian food guides are available and can be helpful in planning diets for children and other age groups (119).

Adolescence

The few studies describing the nutritional status of vegetarian adolescents were reviewed, and suggestions were made for dietary management (120). Not everyone adopting a vegetarian diet understands the nutritional implications of excluding animal products, and care must be taken to ensure adequate intakes. This is especially important because intakes of some nutrients such as vitamin B_{12}, riboflavin, calcium, vitamin D, iron, selenium, and other trace elements are usually lower than the requirements in adolescent vegetarians (121).

Many young women opt to become vegetarians for reasons related to body image, body size, and weight (122). Thus, it is very common for girls and women who already have eating disorders such as anorexia nervosa, bulimia nervosa, and athletica nervosa (see Chapter 87) to disguise their disordered eating by adopting a vegetarian lifestyle (123).

Although some young girls choose vegetarianism as a way to restrict calories, a review of practices among adolescents show that well-planned vegetarian diets, when adopted for health reasons, can serve to sustain adequate physical growth (124). One study showed that preadolescent LOV girls were shorter than omnivores, but they were taller than omnivores later in adolescence (67). This finding suggests a delay in the pubertal growth spurt. They were also reported to experience a 6-month delay in onset of menarche. These findings appear to represent a delay in physical maturation that may be of benefit in adult life, particularly in relation to a lower risk of breast cancer that has been associated with later menarche (67). Investigators in Europe also reported that vegetarian children grow at least as well as omnivorous children, and both groups were close to the fiftieth percentiles for both height and weight (125).

Vegetarian diets may also be associated with menstrual cycle disturbances in young women. However, studies showed that age at menarche is similar in vegetarians and nonvegetarians (126), and the commonly reported delay in menarche for vegetarians did not take into account height, body weight, and socioeconomic status (127). Adolescent female vegetarians who experience weight changes or significant weight loss may experience missed cycles or amenorrhea, similar to omnivorous females under similar conditions (128). For weight-stable vegetarians with a normal BMI, however, no association with menstrual cycle disturbances was reported (124).

Compared with omnivores, LOV adolescents reported significantly greater intake of fruits, vegetables, and starchy foods and lower intake of dairy products, junk foods, and (as expected) meat (67). Thus, their dietary pattern more closely approximated current recommendations than that of the omnivorous controls. As noted previously, a larger proportion of LOVs and semivegetarians had low serum zinc levels than omnivores, although there was no difference in zinc intake (69). Similarly, more LOVs and semivegetarians than omnivores had low iron stores. They were, however, more likely to consume greater amounts of antioxidants and other presumably health-protective phytochemicals.

Adulthood and Elderly Persons

Adults may adopt vegetarian diets to lose weight, to decrease risk of chronic disease, or as part of a therapeutic regimen to control disease. As noted, vegetarians, and especially vegans, generally weigh less and have lower serum cholesterol levels and lower blood pressure. If no animal products are included in the diet, attention is warranted for those nutrients noted earlier as at risk. Low vitamin D levels were reported in some elderly vegetarians, as well as marginal iron and zinc status (11, 42, 129). Adequate vitamin D is particularly important in maintaining bone health in aging women, and care must be taken to ensure an adequate intake and/or exposure to sunshine.

Apart from the commonly reported association of bone density with low intakes of calcium, particularly in those consuming vegan diets, one study conducted on elderly vegetarians demonstrated that vegetarian diets that are rich in sodium but deficient in calcium predispose older vegetarians to hypertension (130). Therefore, calcium intake should be monitored in the elderly consuming a vegetarian diet.

Impaired absorption of vitamin B_{12} with advancing age, as seen in both vegetarians and omnivores, makes vitamin B_{12} deficiency increasingly common in vegetarians in this age group. Possibly, vegetarians, if they have reduced stores, may be at risk of an earlier manifestation of this deficiency. Furthermore, vitamin B_{12} deficiency in the elderly is rarely accompanied by anemia or megaloblastosis, and serum vitamin B_{12} levels in the elderly are often within the currently defined normal range (131). It was suggested that the cutoff for suspecting a vitamin B_{12} deficiency should be less than 258 pmol/L (<350 pg/mL), rather than less than 148 pmol/L (<200 pg/mL). Because a limited window of time exists for effective intervention in a vitamin B_{12} deficiency, particular attention must be directed to the status of this vitamin in elderly persons.

Women's Issues

At the time of menopause, some women choose to take hormone replacement therapy to reduce the severity of menopausal symptoms. However, because of the associated risk of hormone replacement therapy to breast cancer, plant phytoestrogens are being studied as an alternative therapy from which vegetarian women, as well as others, may reap great benefit. For instance, it has been observed that women in Japan, who consume more soy-containing foods than women in Western countries, experience less intense menopausal symptoms (132).

Breast cancer is another issue being debated with regard to vegetarian diets and reduced risk of disease. The American Cancer Society has indicated that women in populations eating a plant-based diet have a lower incidence of breast cancer than those consuming a Western-type diet. For example, mortality from breast cancer in the United States is five times greater than in China, four times greater than in Japan, and three times greater than in Mexico (133).

The biologic effects of soy protein, a common ingredient in vegetarian diets, were investigated in premenopausal women (134). The menstrual changes found in response to the inclusion of soy protein may be beneficial with respect to risk of breast cancer, and they may help to explain the lower risk of breast cancer in populations who consume significant amounts of soy. However, the isoflavones in soy may stimulate existing tumors in the breast, so women with current or previous breast cancer should be aware of this potential risk when they eat soy products (135). Other studies have shown that delayed onset of menarche, as has been observed in vegetarian adolescents, is associated with a reduced risk of breast cancer, presumably because of a lower plasma level and exposure to circulating estrogens.

A cohort of the Iowa Women's Health Study was evaluated for the potential role of heterocyclic amines and risk of breast cancer. A dose-response relationship was found between breast cancer risk and consumption of well-done meat (136). Other studies, however, did not demonstrate this relationship (137). Further studies on the relationship of consuming well-done red meat with breast cancer are therefore warranted.

The relationship between dietary fat intake and breast cancer has prompted numerous studies, some among vegetarians, many looking at various hormonal associations. However, most results to date are inconclusive. Although metaanalyses of various studies suggest that reducing the consumption of total fat to 20% energy or less may significantly reduce circulatory estradiol levels and breast cancer risk (138), no relationship between total fat intake and breast cancer risk has been demonstrated in various other studies.

VEGETARIAN DIETS IN CHRONIC DISEASE MANAGEMENT

Coronary Heart Disease

Numerous clinical trials have investigated diet and lifestyle changes in the treatment of CHD, with and without drug intervention. Regression of atherosclerosis has now been demonstrated in patients with advanced disease in multiple studies (139). Generally, the diets consumed were vegetarian or similar to vegetarian diets: low in fat, saturated fat, and cholesterol, and high in fiber. Other lifestyle factors were often incorporated in the treatment, such as exercise and stress management. As a result, any treatment effects of vegetarian-type diets are mixed with the effects derived from the other lifestyle factors. The benefits may best be ascribed to a "vegetarian lifestyle" than to a vegetarian diet alone.

For example, a very low-fat vegetarian diet has been used as part of comprehensive CHD treatment programs. Quantitative coronary angiography demonstrated regression of atherosclerosis in study subjects, compared with progression in controls, after 1 year and up to 12 years (140–142). Frequency, duration, and severity of symptoms, and clinical events were reduced in study subjects, whereas controls experienced progressive increases (relative risk, 2.47, for events in controls in the Lifestyle Heart Trial). A dose-response relationship was demonstrated with better outcomes in those with greater adherence to the treatment. However, very low-fat diets should be used with caution because some fats (i.e., those with n-6 and n-3 fatty acids) are essential in the human diet. Very low-fat vegetarian diets should include n-3 rich foods, such as flaxseed, and should emphasize monounsaturated fats such as those found in most nuts (see the earlier discussion of essential fatty acids and also Chapter 5). Just as vegetarian diets appear to provide a measure of primary prevention against CHD, they also contribute to secondary prevention and the reversal of CHD.

Hypertension

A vegetarian diet has been found helpful in managing hypertension (143). The DASH (Dietary Approaches to Stop Hypertension) diet is a combination diet that is rich in fruits, vegetables, and low-fat dairy products, including whole grains, fish, poultry, and nuts, and reduced in fats, red meats, sweets, and sugar-containing beverages. This food pattern is similar to a vegetarian diet and has been found to be comparable in lowering blood pressure in stage 1 isolated systolic hypertension (144, 145). The DASH diet also had favorable effects on serum lipids and on glycemic control, compared with the control diet.

Diabetes

A vegetarian diet may also be helpful in managing diabetes. Current recommendations for patients with diabetes include reducing the intake of total fat, saturated fat, and cholesterol, as well as increasing fiber. These changes may result in a food pattern similar to a vegetarian diet, especially if significant sources of plant proteins are included. Because patients with diabetes are prone to diabetic nephropathy, this change in protein source may be particularly appropriate. Evidence from patients with insulin-dependent diabetes suggests that isocaloric substitution of vegetable for animal protein results in beneficial effects on renal function (146).

Low-fat, high-fiber diets have effectively reduced serum glucose and cholesterol levels in patients with diabetes (86). In addition, such diets may help to control weight. Mean serum glucose and body weight were significantly reduced in patients with non–insulin-dependent diabetes mellitus who consumed a low-fat vegetarian diet without instituting other lifestyle changes (147). Thus, evidence indicates that vegetarian diets are not only compatible with therapeutic diabetic regimens but also may be beneficial in controlling the metabolic aberrations associated with diabetes. The Diabetes Care and Education Dietetic Practice Group of the American Dietetic Association has published a comprehensive resource for diabetes management in vegetarians (148).

Renal Disease

The importance of protein in the management of renal disease is recognized. Although a low protein intake is desirable, the use of vegetarian diets is often questioned because of their high phosphorus content relative to the quality and quantity of protein they contain. However, a review of the impact of vegetarian diets on renal disease provides evidence from both animal and human studies of potential benefits from such diets (149).

Plant proteins exert significantly different renal effects from animal proteins; the effects seem comparable to those achieved by reducing the total amount of dietary protein. In subtotally nephrectomized rats, soy protein, as compared with casein, resulted in less proteinuria, a lower glomerular filtration rate, milder renal histologic damage, and longer survival (150). In patients with diabetic nephropathy, a LOV diet that provided 1 g protein/kg/day reduced proteinuria while maintaining good nutritional status over 8 weeks (151). In addition, plant-based diets exert beneficial effects on the hyperlipidemias associated with renal disease, and soy-based diets reduce serum cholesterol independent of dietary fat (149). A carefully designed vegan diet was used successfully to manage mild chronic renal failure; this may be the diet of choice when a conventional low-protein diet is poorly tolerated (152).

Because plant foods provide more nonessential amino acids than do animal proteins, they generate more urea. Consequently, it may be more difficult to minimize uremic toxicity on a strictly plant-based diet in patients with severe chronic renal insufficiency (149). Fewer problems will be encountered on an LOV diet. In addition, a vegetarian diet may require an increase in phosphate binders in end-stage renal disease or in patients undergoing renal dialysis, and attention should be directed to using lower-potassium fruits, vegetables, and grains to compensate for the higher potassium content of some legumes, nuts, and seeds. Guidelines for planning a vegetarian diet for patients with renal disease are available (153).

Rheumatoid Arthritis

Claims are frequently made that special diets, including vegan or LOV diets, can alleviate the symptoms of rheumatoid arthritis. A review suggested that this claim is part of "the folklore of the disease" (154). Although some studies have been reported, most were poorly designed, did not include controls, and were not adequately blinded. Often, the subjects held a strong belief in the intervention. Clinically demonstrable improvements, rather than subjective responses, were not always used. Nonetheless, some patients may benefit from a vegetarian diet (155, 156).

DIETARY GUIDELINES FOR A HEALTHY VEGETARIAN LIFESTYLE

Dietary guidelines provide advice on the consumption of types of foods or food components related to public health. Therefore, they are intended to be population-based recommendations for health promotion and disease prevention (157) (see also Chapters 104 and 105). The following sections seek to highlight the vegetarian diet within the context of national diet recommendations, food guidance, and selection, as well as helpful suggestions for counseling current and prospective vegetarians, collectively and individually.

Dietary Recommendations

Vegetarian diets are quite consistent with both national and international dietary guidelines. For instance, a review of various studies showed consistently that vegetarians consumed less fat and cholesterol, and more polyunsaturated fat and dietary fiber, than nonvegetarians (155). Vegetarians throughout the life cycle consume substantially more vegetables, fruits, legumes, and nuts than nonvegetarians (19, 158–160), consistent with current dietary guidelines for disease prevention. Adolescent vegetarians were more likely to meet the Healthy People 2010 objectives than nonvegetarians, especially with respect to intakes of total fat and saturated fat, servings of fruits and vegetables, and consumption of fast food, fruit drinks, and regular sugared soda (161).

A prospective study of vegetarians found that the average nutrient intakes of all the subjects were close to the current US dietary reference intakes (22). In contrast, descriptive studies have demonstrated variable nutrient intakes among certain vegetarians, such as vegans, that do not comply with the average requirements for some essential nutrients (122). Although vegetarian diets can generally meet recommendations for essential nutrients, more restrictive vegetarian patterns may pose a challenge in this regard, unless carefully monitored and purposely balanced.

Food Guides

Food guides provide a framework for selecting the kinds and amounts of different types of foods, which can together provide nutritionally adequate diets (162). An example is the Loma Linda University Food Guide Pyramid (157), see Figure 103.3. Another example of a vegetarian food guide is the American Dietetic Association vegetarian food pyramids. It is important for vegetarians to make use of food guides that are specially designed for vegetarians. This ensures more appropriate balance in food selection based on the unique consumption patterns and typical energy intakes of vegetarians. Specific food guides developed for different types of vegetarians may also serve to provide food selection advice and improve overall diet quality.

Nutrition Counseling

A careful investigation of the dietary practices of persons who call themselves vegetarians is essential for the health professional to provide optimal counseling. General lifestyle practices that may affect health should be evaluated as well. The beliefs and attitudes that support these practices may affect a patient's willingness to follow suggestions. Those vegetarians adhering to more restrictive dietary practices, such as macrobiotics, may be less willing to seek or follow the advice of health care professionals. The attitude of the health professional will be perceived quickly, and a nonjudgmental approach is of utmost importance in establishing a productive relationship. Regardless of how persons identify themselves, so far as dietary practices are concerned, their actual dietary intake must be ascertained before an effective nutritional intervention can take place. Knowledge of why an individual follows particular dietary practices is also helpful in developing an appropriate approach to counseling. The differing reasons that persons adopt a vegetarian diet may affect their food choices and subsequently nutritional status. In addition, the rationale for a particular diet may be associated with other lifestyle

practices that can affect health. Thus, ascertaining these reasons and associated practices is an important aspect of a patient's history.

Throughout the life cycle of vegetarians, nutrition counseling can be very beneficial. Issues to be considered in counseling pregnant vegetarians are described earlier and are applicable to others as well (104). For infant feeding, clinicians should counsel their vegetarian clients about well-planned vegetarian diets and breast-feeding; those who are unable to breast-feed should be made aware of some appropriate soy-based formulas that are available. Vegetarian food guides with specific applications for vegetarian adolescents are available (119, 120). Foods that are sources of the nutrients most likely to be at risk are included in these guides. Bioavailable sources of calcium are also described (58). A vegetarian diet manual is available for use in various clinical conditions (163).

The basic principles for planning a vegetarian diet are the same as those for planning any other diet, with variety a key component. A diet restricted in either variety or amount can limit the intake of essential nutrients. Energy intake to maintain appropriate weight must be considered. Obtaining adequate calories may be a challenge on a vegan or macrobiotic diet, whereas avoiding excess calories may be equally challenging on an LOV diet that relies on full-fat dairy products (119). An emphasis on unrefined foods is appropriate in any diet. Many different ways exist to obtain the essential nutrients, and the health care provider should be aware of alternate sources for those nutrients commonly supplied by foods that are excluded from a given diet. The American Dietetic Association provides a very useful list of vegetarian food sources of nutrients (71). A registered dietitian can be very helpful in providing guidance, information, and counsel. An adaptable, creative, and sensitive approach will be most successful in providing dietary suggestions for persons whose dietary

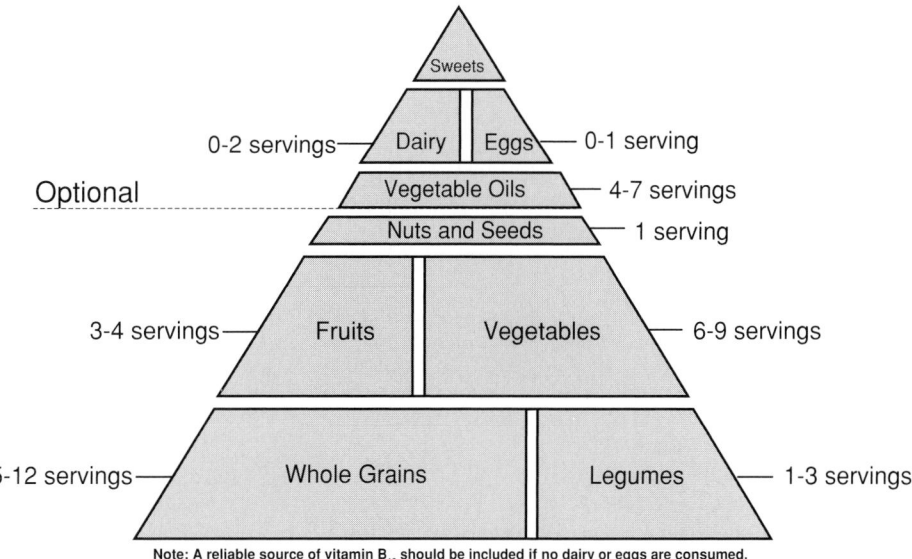

Figure 103.3. Loma Linda University Vegetarian Food Guide Pyramid. (Adapted from Sabaté J, ed. Vegetarian Nutrition. Boca Raton, FL: CRC Press, 2001:426.)

Note: A reliable source of vitamin B_{12} should be included if no dairy or eggs are consumed.

patterns and beliefs may differ from those of the health care provider.

Cultural sensitivity is another important aspect that clinicians need to consider when counseling current or prospective vegetarians. When persons who are practicing or contemplating a vegetarian lifestyle can include foods from their respective cultures and tastes, issues of compliance and long-term maintenance become less challenging. To accommodate persons wishing to adopt a vegetarian diet appropriately, nutrition counselors need to evaluate their clients' perceptions regarding the benefits and barriers to consuming a vegetarian diet. This will allow use of specially targeted strategies that could influence vegetarian nutrition knowledge, health beliefs, dietary behavior, and eventually public health (164, 165).

A reasonable approach to counseling a prospective vegetarian is to make sure that he or she (as well as family members) is involved in the planning process. This is beneficial for the following reasons: (a) it helps the counselor to understand the client's perspective and his or her family or other situations that could influence diet choice and patterns, (b) it engenders a trusting and interdependent relationship between the counselor and the client, and (c) it serves to motivate the client because the diet plans tend to be more individualized. An individualized vegetarian diet usually has the advantage of being more attainable and maintained on a long-term basis because such plans take into account factors such as food preferences, habits, family and lifestyle factors, social and environmental support, and barriers or benefits to compliance.

CONCLUSION

Current dietary recommendations call for increased consumption of plant foods in all diets. Evidence from populations consuming plant-based diets supports these recommendations. As one researcher said, "vegetables and fruits . . . are chemical powerhouses that produce dozens if not hundreds of unique and complex organic compounds, many of which are biologically active" (46). The potential health benefits, as well as issues of concern regarding vegetarian diets, have been described. The health professional has a responsibility to be informed regarding both, to encourage those dietary and lifestyle practices that promote health, and to provide alternatives to those that may be detrimental.

Acknowledgments

The generous reading of the manuscript and insightful suggestions of Patricia Dyett and John Kelly are gratefully acknowledged.

REFERENCES

1. Roe DA. J Nutr 1986;116:1355–63.
2. Whorton JC. Am J Clin Nutr 1994;59[Suppl]:103S–9S.
3. Murray Food Service Dir 1993;6:74.
4. Kushi LH, Cunningham JE, Hebert JR et al. Am Soc Nutr Sci 2001;[Suppl]:3056S–64S.
5. US Department of Agriculture and Health and Human Services. Nutrition and Your Health: Dietary Guidelines for Americans. 5th ed. Washington, DC: US Government Printing Office, 2000.
6. Krauss RM, Eckel RH, Howard B et al. Circulation 2000;102: 2296–311.
7. World Cancer Research Fund/American Institute for Cancer Research. Food, Nutrition and the Prevention of Cancer: A Global Perspective. Menasha, WI: Banta Book Group, 1997.
8. Stahler C. Vegetarian 1994;13:6–9.
9. Sabaté J, ed. Vegetarian Nutrition. Boca Raton, FL: CRC Press, 2001:1–551.
10. Messina VK, Burke KI. J Am Diet Assoc 1997;97:1317–21.
11. American Dietetic Association and Dietitians of Canada. J Am Diet Assoc 2003;103:748–65.
12. Dwyer JT. Annu Rev Nutr 1991;11:61–91.
13. Mutch PB, Johnston PK, eds. Am J Clin Nutr 1988;48 [Suppl]:707S–927S.
14. Johnston PK, ed. Am J Clin Nutr 1994;59[Suppl]:1099S–262S.
15. Johnston PK, Sabaté J, eds. Am J Clin Nutr 1999;70[Suppl]: 429S–634S.
16. Sabaté J, Rajaram S, eds. Am J Clin Nutr 2003;78[Suppl]: 601S–68S.
17. Messina M, Messina V. The Dietitian's Guide to Vegetarian Diets. Gaithersburg, MD: Aspen, 1996:1–511.
18. Sabaté J, Duk A, Lee CL. Am J Clin Nutr 1999;70[Suppl]: 601S–19S.
19. Haddad EH, Tanzman JS. Am J Clin Nutr 2003;78[Suppl]: 626S–32S.
20. Keinan-Boker L, Peters PH, Mulligan AA et al. Public Health Nutr 2002;5:1217–26.
21. Davey GK, Spencer EA, Appleby PN et al. Public Health Nutr 2003;6:259–69.
22. Spencer EA, Appleby PN, Davey GK et al. Int J Obes Relat Metab Disord 2003;6:728–34.
23. Haddad EH, Berk LS, Kettering JD et al. Am J Clin Nutr 1999; 70[Suppl]:586S–93S.
24. Rauma AL, Törrönen R, Hänninen O et al. Am J Clin Nutr 1995;62:1221–7.
25. Rauma AL, Mykkanen H. Nutrition 2000;16:111–9
26. Waldmann A. Koschizke JW, Leitzmann C et al. Eur J Clin Nutr 2003;57:947–55.
27. Robinson F, Hackett AF, Billington D et al. J Hum Nutr Diet 2002;5:323–9.
28. Appleby PN, Thorogood M, Mann JI et al. Int J Obes Relat Metab Disord 1998;22:454–60.
29. Kennedy ET, Bowman SA, Spence JT et al. J Am Diet Assoc 2001;4:411–20.
30. Sabaté J, Blix G. Vegetarian diets and obesity prevention. In Sabaté J, ed. Vegetarian Nutrition. Boca Raton, FL: CRC Press, 2001:91–108.
31. Dwyer JT. Am J Clin Nutr 1988;48:712–38.
32. Barr SI, Broughton TM. J Am Coll Nutr 2000;6:781–8.
33. Perry CL, Mcguire MT, Neumark–Sztainer D et al. J Adolesc Health 2001;6:406–16.
34. O'Conner MA, Touyz SW, Dunn SM et al. Med J Aust 1987; 147:540–2.
35. Janelle KC, Barr SI. J Am Diet Assoc 1995;95:180–6, 189.
36. Messina V, Mangels AR. J Am Diet Assoc 2001;101:661–69.
37. Young VR, Pellett PL. Am J Clin Nutr 1994;59[Suppl]: 1203S–12S.
38. Craig W. Am J Clin Nutr 1994;59[Suppl]:1233S–7S.
39. Nelson M, Bakaliou F, Trivedi A. Br J Nutr 1994;72:427–33.
40. Nathan I, Hackett AF, Kirby S. Br J Nutr 1996;75:533–44.

41. Thane CW, Bates CJ, Prentice A. Public Health Nutr 2003;6: 485–96.
42. Alexander D, Ball MJ, Mann J. Eur J Clin Nutr 1994;48: 538–46.
43. Hua NW, Stoohs RA, Facchini FS. Br J Nutr 2001;86:515–9.
44. Hunt JR. Am J Clin Nutr 2003;78[Suppl]:633S–9S.
45. Kandiah J. Plant Foods Hum Nutr 2002;57:197–204.
46. Koebnick C, Heins UA, Hoffmann I. et al. J Nutr 2001;131: 733–9.
47. Herbert V. Am J Clin Nutr 1994;59[Suppl]:1213S–22S.
48. Huang YC, Chang SJ, Chiu YT et al. Eur J Nutr 2003;42:84–90.
49. Obeid R, Geisel J, Schorr H. et al. Eur J Haematol 2002;69: 275–9.
50. Herrmann W, Schorr H, Obeid R et al. Am J Clin Nutr 2003;78: 131–6.
51. Refsum H, Yajnik CS, Gadkari M et al. Am J Clin Nutr 2001;74:233–41.
52. Herbert V. Am J Clin Nutr 1988;48:852–8.
53. Crane MG, Sample C, Patchett S et al. J Nutr Med 1994;4: 419–30.
54. Rauma AL, Törrönen R, Hänninen O et al. J Nutr 1995;125: 2511–5.
55. Specker BL, Miller D, Norman EJ et al. Am J Clin Nutr 1988; 47:89–92.
56. Dagnelie PC, van Staveren WA, van den Berg H. Am J Clin Nutr 1991;53:695–7.
57. Miller DR, Specker BL, Ho ML et al. Am J Clin Nutr 1991;53: 524–9.
58. Weaver CM, Plawecki KL. Am J Clin Nutr 1994;59[Suppl]: 1238S–41S.
59. Lamberg-Allardt C, Kärkkäinen M, Seppänen R et al. Am J Clin Nutr 1993;58:684–9.
60. Iq-bal SJ. J Hum Nutr Diet 1994;7:47–52.
61. Dagnelie PC, van Sraveren WA. Am J Clin Nutr 1994;59 [Suppl]:187S–96S.
62. Outila TA, Karkkainen MU, Seppanaen RH et al. J Am Diet Assoc 2000;100:434–41.
63. Food and Nutrition Board, Institute of Medicine. Dietary Reference Intakes: Calcium, Phosphorus, Magnesium, Vitamin D, and Fluoride. Washington, DC: National Academy Press, 1997.
64. Zemel MB. Am J Clin Nutr 1988;48:880–3.
65. Heaney RP. J Am Diet Assoc 1993;93:1259–60.
66. Evans CEL, Chughtai AY, Blumsohn A et al. Eur J Clin Nutr 1997;51:394–9.
67. Johnston PK, Haddad E, Sabaté J. Adolesc Med 1992;3: 417–37.
68. Hunt JR. Am J Clin Nutr 2003;78[Suppl]:633S–9S.
69. Donovon UM, Gibson RS. J Am Coll Nutr 1995;14:463–72.
70. Ball MJ, Ackland ML. Br J Nutr 2000;83:27–33.
71. ADA Reports. J Am Diet Assoc 2003;103:748–65.
72. Davis BC, Kris-Etherton PM. Am J Clin Nutr 2003;78[Suppl]: 640S–46S.
73. Thorogood M. Nutr Res Rev 1995;8:179–92.
74. Fraser, G. Diet, Life Expectancy, and Chronic Disease Studies of Seventh-Day Adventists and Other Vegetarians. New York: Oxford University Press, 2003:1–371.
75. Key TJ, Thorogood M, Appleby PN et al. BMJ 1996;313:775–9.
76. Steinmetz KA, Potter JD. Cancer Causes Control 1991;2: 427–42.
77. Knight D, Eden JA. Obstet Gynecol 1996;87:897–904.
78. Melby CL, Toohey ML, Cebrick J. Am J Clin Nutr 1994;59: 103–9.
79. Fraser GE, Sabaté J, Beeson WL et al. Arch Intern Med 1992;152:1416–24.
80. Sabaté J, Fraser GE, Burke K et al. N Engl J Med 1993;328: 603–7.
81. Sabaté J, Fraser GE. Curr Opin Lipidol 1994;5:11–6.
82. Fraser GE. Am J Clin Nutr 1994;59[Suppl]:117S–23S.
83. Hu FB, Willett WC. JAMA 2002;288:2569–78.
84. Beilin LJ. Am J Clin Nutr 1994;59[Suppl]:1130S–5S.
85. Snowdon DA, Phillips RL. Am J Public Health 1985;75:507–12.
86. Anderson JW, Zeigler JA, Deakins DA et al. Am J Clin Nutr 1991;54:936–43.
87. Frentzel-Beyme R, Chang-Claude J. Am J Clin Nutr 1994;59 [Suppl]:143S–52S.
88. Mills PK, Beeson WL, Phillips R et al. Am J Clin Nutr 1994; 59[Suppl]:136S–42S.
89. Knekt P, Järvinen R, Seppänen R et al. Br J Cancer 1996;73: 687–91.
90. Hunt IF. Adv Nutr Res 1994;9:245–55.
91. Feskanich D, Willett WC, Stampfer MJ et al. Am J Epidemiol 1996;143:472–9.
92. Chiu JF, Lan SJ, Yang CY et al. Calcif Tissue Int 1997;60:245–9.
93. Parsons TJ, van Dusseldorp M, van der Vliet M et al. J Bone Miner Res 1997;12:1486–94.
94. Black RE, Williams SM, Jones IE et al. Am J Clin Nutr 2002; 675–80.
95. Goulding A, Rockell JEP, Black RE et al. J Am Diet Assoc 2004;104:250–3.
96. Hu JF, Zhao XH, Jia JB et al. Am J Clin Nutr 1993;58:219–27.
97. Remer T, Manz F. J Am Diet Assoc 1995;95:791–7.
98. Munger RG, Cerhan JR, Chiu BC. Am J Clin Nutr 1999;69: 147–52.
99. Dawson-Hughes B. J Nutr 2003;133:852S–4S.
100. Kerstetter JE, O'Brien, Insogna KL. J Nutr 2003;133:855S–61S.
101. Spence LA, Weaver CM. J Nutr 2003;133:850S–1S.
102. Sellmeyer DE, Stone KL, Sebastian A et al. Am J Clin Nutr 2001;73:118–22.
103. Massey LK. J Nutr 2003;133:862S–5S.
104. Johnston PK. Am J Clin Nutr 1988;48:901–5.
105. Reddy S, Sanders TAB, Obeid O. Eur J Clin Nutr 1994;48: 358–68.
106. Michaud JL, Lemieux B, Ogier H et al. Eur J Pediatr 1992;151: 218–20.
107. Lovblad K, Ramelli G, Remonda L et al. Pediatr Radiol 1997; 27:155–8.
108. Grattan-Smith PJ, Wilcken B, Procopis PG et al. Mov Disorders 1997;12:39–46.
109. Specker BL. Am J Clin Nutr 1994;59[Suppl]:1182S–6S.
110. Higginbottom MC, Sweetman L, Nyhan WL. N Engl J Med 1978;299:317–23.
111. Centers for Disease Control and Prevention. MMWR Morb Mortal Wkly Rep 2003;52:61–4.
112. Rasmussen S, Fernhoff PM, Scanlon KS et al J Pediat 2001; 138:10–7.
113. Graham SM, Arvela OM, Wise G. J Pediatr 1992;121:710–4.
114. Van Dusseldorp M, Schneede J, Refsum H et al. Am J Clin Nutr 1999;69:664–71.
115. Louwman MWJ, Van Dusseldorp M, van de Vijver FJR et al. Am J Clin Nutr 2000;72:762–9.
116. Sanders TAB. Pediatr Clin North Am 1995;42:955–65.
117. Van Dusseldorp M, Arts IC, Bergsma JS et al. J Nutr 1996;126: 2977–83.
118. Dagnelie PC, van Staveren WA. Am J Clin Nutr 1994;59 [Suppl]:187S–96S.
119. Haddad EH. Top Clin Nutr 1995;10:7–16.
120. Johnston PK, Haddad EH. Vegetarian and other dietary practices. In: Richert VI, ed. Adolescent Nutrition: Assessment and

Management. New York: Chapman Hall, 1995;57–88, 637–45.

121. Larsson CL, Johansson GK. Am J Clin Nutr 2002;76:100–6.
122. Worsely A, Skrzypiec G. Appetite 1998;30:151.
123. Martins Y, Pliner P, O'Conner R. Appetite 1999;32:145.
124. Rajaram S, Dyett PA, Sabaté J. Nutrition and vegetarianism. In: Klimis-Zacas D, Wolinsky Ira, eds. Nutritional Concerns of Women. Boca Raton, FL: CRC Press, 2004:419–56.
125. Nathan I, Hackett AF, Kirby S. Eur J Clin Nutr 1997;51:20–5.
126. American Academy of Pediatrics, Committee on Nutrition. Nutritional aspects of vegetarian diets. In: Committee on Nutrition: Pediatric Nutrition Handbook. 3rd ed. Chicago: American Academy of Pediatrics, 1993:302.
127. Kissinger DG, Sanchez A. Nutr Res 1987;7:471.
128. Loucks AB, Heath EM. J Clin Endocrinol Metab 1994;78:910.
129. Brants HAM, Lowik RH, Westenbrink S et al. J Am Coll Nutr 1990;9:292–302.
130. Kwok TC, Chan TY, Woo J. Eur J Clin Nutr 2003;57:299–304.
131. Allen LH, Casterline J. Am J Clin Nutr 1994;60:12–4.
132. Somekawa Y, Chiguchi M, Ishibashi T et al. Obstet Gynecol 2001;97:109.
133. World Health Organization. World Health Statistics Annual 1996, Geneva: World Health Organization, 1997.
134. Cassidy A, Bingham S, Setchell KDR. Am J Clin Nutr 1994;60:333–40.
135. de Lomas ML. Ann Pharmacother 2001;35:1118.
136. Zheng W, Gustafson DR, Sinha R et al. J Natl Cancer Inst 1998;90:1724.
137. Ambrosone CB, Freudenheim JL, Sinha R et al. Int J Cancer 1998;75:825.
138. Wu AH, Oike MC, Stram DO. J Natl Cancer Inst 1999;91:529.
139. Superko HP, Krauss RM. Circulation 1994;90:1056–69.
140. Ornish D, Brown SE, Scherwitz LW et al. Lancet 1990;336:129–33.
141. Ornish D, Scherwitz LW, Billings JH et al. JAMA 1998;280:2001–7.
142. Esselstyn CB Jr. Prev Cardiol 2001;4:171–7.
143. Sacks FM, Svetkey LP, Vollmer W et al. N Engl J Med 2001;344:3–10.
144. Conlin PR, Chow D, Miller ER 3rd et al. Am J Hypertens 2000;13:949–55.
145. Moore TJ, Vollmer WM, Appel LJ et al. Hypertension 1999;34:472–7.
146. Kontessis P, Bossinakou I, Sarika L et al. Diabetes Care 1995;18:1233–40.
147. Nicholson AS, Sklar M, Barnard ND et al. Prev Med 1999;29:87–91.
148. Holzmeister LA, ed. On the Cutting Edge 1997;18:1–38.
149. Paggenkamper J. Top Clin Nutr 1995;10:22–6.
150. Fair DE, Ogborn MR, Weilar HA et a. J Nutr 2004;134:1504–7.
151. Teixeira SR, Tappenden KA, Carson L et al. J Nutr 2004;134:1874–80.
152. Barsotti G, Morelli E. Cupisti A. et al. Nephron 1996;74:390–4.
153. Paggenkamper J. J Renal Nutr 1995;5:234–8.
154. Darlington LG, Ramsey NW. Br J Rheumatol 1993;32:507–14.
155. Kjeldsen-Kragh J, Mellbye OJ, Haugen M et al. Scand J Rheumatol 1995;24:85–93.
156. Kjeldsen-Kragh J. Am J Clin Nutr 1999;70[Suppl]:594S–600S.
157. Haddad EH. Vegetarian diets and dietary guidelines for chronic disease prevention. In: Sabaté J. ed. Vegetarian Nutrition. Boca Raton, FL: CRC Press, 2001:371–410.
158. Bull NL, Barber SA. Hum Nutr Appl Nutr 1984;38A:288.
159. Donovan Um, Gibson R. J Adolesc Health 1996;18:292.
160. Haddad EH, Berk LS, Kettering JD et al. Am J Clin Nutr 1999;70[Suppl]:586S.
161. Perry CL, McGuire MT, Neumark-Sztainer D et al. Arch Pediatr Adolesc Med 2002;156:431–7.
162. Whitten C. Developing a vegetarian food guide. In: Sabaté J, ed. Vegetarian Nutrition. Boca Raton, FL: CRC Press, 2001:411–37.
163. Hodgkin G, Maloney S, eds. The Loma Linda University Diet Manual: A Handbook Supporting Vegetarian Nutrition. Loma Linda, CA: Seventh-Day Adventist Dietetic Association, 2003:1-1–1-16.
164. Lea E, Worsley A. Publ Health Nutr 2003;6:505–11.
165. Barr SI, Chapman GE. J Am Diet Assoc 2002;102:354–60.

SELECTED READINGS

ADA Reports. Position of the American Dietetic Association and Dietitians of Canada: Vegetarian diets. J Am Diet Assoc 2003;103:748–65.

Haddad EH. Vegetarian diets and dietary guidelines for chronic disease prevention. In: Sabaté J, ed. Vegetarian Nutrition. Boca Raton, FL: CRC Press, 2001:371–410.

Sabaté J, Rajaram S, eds. Am J Clin Nutr 2003;78[Suppl]:601S–68S.

104

DIETARY REFERENCE INTAKES: RATIONALE AND APPLICATIONS[1]

ALLISON A. YATES

HOW RECOMMENDED DIETARY ALLOWANCES
  AND RECOMMENDED NUTRIENT INTAKES
  BECAME DIETARY REFERENCE INTAKES 1655
    Origins of the Recommended Dietary
      Allowances 1655
    Melding of Nutrient Deficiency with Reduction
      of Risk Factors for Chronic Disease 1656
    Need for Additional Reference Values Beyond
      Recommended Dietary Allowances/
      Recommended Nutrient Intake 1656
    Current Uses of Recommended Intakes 1657
  DEVELOPMENT OF DIETARY REFERENCE INTAKES ...1658
    Categories of Dietary Reference Intakes 1658
    Model for Establishing Recommended Intakes ..1659
    Use of the Estimated Average Requirement 1662
    Use of the Adequate Intake 1665
    Establishing the Tolerable Upper Intake Level ...1665
    Nutrients Evaluated in the Dietary Reference
      Intake Process but without Tolerable Upper
      Intake Levels or Recommended Intakes 1667
    Energy and Physical Activity 1668
  NEW ASPECTS OF THE DIETARY
    REFERENCE INTAKES 1668
    Deficiency for What? 1668
    New Age Groups Selected 1668
    New Approaches to Infant Reference Values 1668
    Extrapolation when Data are Lacking 1669
    Evaluating the Role of Bioactive
      Food Components 1669
  INTERNATIONAL EFFORTS TO DEVELOP DIETARY
    REFERENCE INTAKES 1669
  CONCLUSION 1670

[1]**Abbreviations: AI,** adequate intake; **AMDR,** acceptable macronutrient distribution range; **BMI,** body mass index; **CV,** coefficient of variation; **DRI,** dietary reference intake; **EAR,** estimated average requirement; **EER,** estimated energy requirement; **FAO,** Food and Agricultural Organization; **FDA,** Food and Drug Administration; **LOAEL,** lowest observed adverse effect level; **NOAEL,** no observed adverse effect level; **RDA,** recommended dietary allowance (unless otherwise noted); **RNI,** recommended nutrient intake; **UF,** uncertainty factor; **UL,** tolerable upper intake level; **USDA,** US Department of Agriculture; **WHO,** World Health Organization.

HOW RECOMMENDED DIETARY ALLOWANCES AND RECOMMENDED NUTRIENT INTAKES BECAME DIETARY REFERENCE INTAKES

Quantitative reference values for nutrients used in food and nutrition planning have been available since the early 1900s, when recommended intakes for protein were included in early US Department of Agriculture (USDA) bulletins (1). Earlier dietary recommendations were generally given in the form of foods thought to prevent disease, such as scurvy (2). By the 1930s, quantitative nutrient recommendations were published by the British Medical Association (3), the USDA (4), the Canadian Council on Nutrition (5), and the League of Nations (6).

Origins of the Recommended Dietary Allowances

As the United States initiated preparations for war in 1940, major concerns were voiced regarding the nutritional status of military recruits in the United States, as well as concerns about preparedness in terms of health and fitness of the population (7). At that time, based on earlier USDA studies in the 1930s conducted by Hazel Stiebeling, it was estimated that at least one third of the US population was not properly nourished (7). Although the amount of food was adequate, given the clear evidence that nutrient deficiencies were present, the quality of the food was deemed inadequate.

The Consumer Protection Division of the National Defense Advisory Commission requested the National Research Council of the US National Academy of Sciences to convene a committee to develop national nutrition standards that would take into account the advances made in nutrition sciences over the previous decade and would advise the government on a national nutrition program (8). This committee, whose first meeting was held in November 1940, became the Food and Nutrition Board and proposed the first set of recommended dietary allowances (RDAs) in April 1941 (9). The extent of the concern for nutritional status of the population at that time was evident with the approval by the US Food and Drug Administration (FDA) of and the subsequent requirement for flour milling to enrich with thiamin, nicotinic acid, and iron (and subsequently riboflavin) (8).

The proposed RDAs covered the nutrients known at the time to be essential for human health (Table 104.1).

TABLE 104.1. CHANGES SINCE 1941 IN RECOMMENDED INTAKES FOR NUTRIENTS[a]

1941	1989	1997–2004
Protein	Protein	Protein
Calcium	Calcium	Calcium
Iron	Iron	Iron
Vitamin A	Vitamin A	Vitamin A
Thiamin	Thiamin	Thiamin
Vitamin C	Vitamin C	Vitamin C
Riboflavin	Riboflavin	Riboflavin
Nicotinic acid	Nicotinic acid	Nicotinic acid
Vitamin D	Vitamin D	Vitamin D
Calories	Energy	Energy[c]
	Vitamin K	Vitamin K
	Vitamin B_6	Vitamin B_6
	Folate	Folate
	Vitamin B_{12}	Vitamin B_{12}
	Vitamin E	Vitamin E
	Magnesium	Magnesium
	Phosphorus	Phosphorus
	Iodine	Iodine
	Selenium	Selenium
	Zinc	Zinc
	Chromium[b]	Chromium
	Copper[b]	Copper
	Fluoride[b]	Fluoride
	Pantothenic acid[b]	Pantothenic acid
	Biotin[b]	Biotin
	Manganese[b]	Manganese
	Molybdenum[b]	Molybdenum
	Potassium[d]	Potassium
		Sodium[c]
		Chloride[c]
		Total water[c]
		Choline
		Carbohydrate
		Total fiber
		Linoleic acid (n-6)[c]
		α-Linolenic Acid (n-3)[c]

[a] Unless otherwise noted, all recommended intakes are recommended dietary allowances.
[b] Estimated safe and adequate daily dietary intake.
[c] Adequate intake.
[d] Estimated minimum requirement.

Data on recommended dietary allowances from references 9 and 12, and date on dietary reference intakes from references 17, 19–21, 23, and 28.

By 1944, the RDAs (by that time, revised) were adopted by Canada and were used, to some extent, in Great Britain (10). Since 1941, the original RDAs have been revised nine times by the Food and Nutrition Board. In 1948, Canada released its own standards, which it continued to do through 1990, with the most recent update of the recommended nutrient intakes (RNIs) (11). The most recent revision of the RDAs, the tenth edition in 1989 (12), included recommended intakes for 27 nutrients in addition to energy (see Table 104.1), underscoring the growth in knowledge about the specific roles newly discovered nutrients played in preventing deficiency diseases. The 1989 RDAs and 1990 RNIs are given in Appendix Tables A-3-a and A-3-b.

Melding of Nutrient Deficiency with Reduction of Risk Factors for Chronic Disease

With this growth in knowledge over the last few decades, there has also been mounting evidence of the role essential nutrients and other important food components may play in maintaining health, decreasing risk of chronic disease, and thus potentially increasing longevity. Although at the beginning of the twentieth century, many deaths in the United States and Westernized countries were caused by acute illnesses and accidents, by the beginning of the twenty-first century, such deaths were much less frequent, with most now attributable to chronic diseases such as cancer and cardiovascular disease. The growing information on diet and disease relationships was reviewed and released in a report by the Food and Nutrition Board in 1989 (13) at the same time as the last edition of the RDAs, an indication that the two perspectives of how to approach the determination of dietary adequacy were coalescing—one from a deficiency viewpoint, and the other from a broader view of evaluating the role of diet and nutrition in causing or delaying chronic diseases.

Need for Additional Reference Values Beyond Recommended Dietary Allowances/Recommended Nutrient Intake

Two major changes in food composition and thus intake have evolved over the last few decades: the introduction into the marketplace and widespread use of dietary supplements and the voluntary fortification of foods with essential nutrients as well as potentially bioactive food components. The expectation that diet can ameliorate or delay the progression of chronic diseases, for which the symptoms may take years to develop, has fueled research to identify new roles for nutrients and ways to prevent the onset of disease. Because food is a common carrier for nutrients and bioactive food components, since the mid-1980s consumers have become increasingly convinced that through food or its component parts, health can be maintained and possibly improved. As a result, studies evaluating active components in food, whether considered essential nutrients or not yet proven to be required for maintenance of normal function, are now in the forefront of most research agendas set by public health groups to maintain and enhance the quality of life.

As consumer awareness has grown about the potential roles in health of specific nutrients or food components, to some extent as a result of the media's communicating benefit based on early stages of research, the demand for nutrients and food components in concentrated form in the marketplace has multiplied. As a result, concentrated sources of nutrients are now available and are easily attainable in the United States, at times replacing more traditional multivitamin/mineral supplements, some of which in the past provided nutrients frequently formulated at levels of 100% of the RDAs.

Consumer demand for enhanced dietary supplements has been accommodated by legislation in the United States (see Chapter 116) that requires the FDA to consider dietary supplements under much the same framework as they do traditional foods; thus, the FDA is to assume that dietary supplements are safe unless the agency can demonstrate an unreasonable risk of illness or injury when these supplements are consumed as directed on the label.

The RDA, defined as the ". . . levels of intake of essential nutrients considered, in the judgment of the Food and Nutrition Board on the basis of available scientific knowledge, to be adequate to meet the known nutritional needs of practically all healthy persons" (12), provide allowances for meeting known requirements. There has always been concern about consuming too much of a nutrient, because nutrients can cause toxicity if they are consumed in excess, just like other chemicals (see Chapter 38). In the past, however, little need existed for reference values for planning purposes to indicate how much was safe because nutrients were obtained from foods, and although occasional cases of toxicity resulted from ingestion of large amounts of single foodstuffs (e.g., cod liver oil), little concern was given to typical dietary variety.

By the 1980s, with the increasing availability of nutrient supplements, the need for reference intakes, in addition to RDAs, that would establish an amount that would not increase the risk of adverse consequences from overconsumption became evident for use in food and nutrition policy (Fig. 104.1).

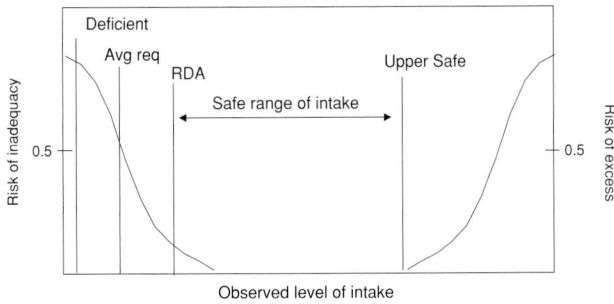

Figure 104.1. The concept of a safe range of intake was advanced in the writings of George Beaton and was subsequently discussed in reports on establishing nutrient requirements by a number of national and international organizations. As initially used by the Committee on Medical Aspects of Food Policy in the United Kingdom (15) in developing the first set of multiple reference intakes, the "safe range of intake" represents the range of intakes between what is the recommended intake that, as defined, should meet the needs of practically all healthy persons and the upper level at which there is no increased risk of adverse effects resulting from overconsumption. Included in this diagram are two additional reference values: the average requirement for a group of individuals and a deficiency level. The deficiency level is an intake level known to meet the needs of very few (in the population, and is defined as a level two standard deviations below the average requirement). Intakes at or below this level are assumed to be of great concern. RDA, recommended dietary allowance. (Adapted from Health and Welfare, Canada, 1983, in Food and Nutrition Board, Institute of Medicine. How Should the Recommended Dietary Allowances Be Revised? Washington, DC: National Academy Press, 1994:19, with permission.)

Although enrichment and fortification of the food supply have been components of public health policy in the United States since the 1930s, when the addition of iodine to salt to prevent goiter was instituted, addition of other nutrients and bioactive food components to foodstuffs has markedly increased since the mid-1980s. Federal guidelines developed in the 1970s regarding fortification of foods have been generally followed, but with the heightened interest in nutrients beyond their traditional role to prevent deficiency disease, the food industry has increasingly initiated voluntary fortification of their food products in response to the perceived needs of consumers and as a means to differentiate their product and thus encourage consumption. As more foods have been fortified, it has become possible for long-term overconsumption of some nutrients to lead to toxicity. Thus, the need to develop scientifically based determinations of reference values in addition to the RDAs became evident.

Current Uses of Recommended Intakes

Since their inception in 1941, the RDAs, being the only quantitative estimates available for nutrient needs, have been used in many different ways (Table 104.2) (14), such as the following: the basis for school lunch programs where only one meal is provided (e.g., the Child Nutrition Programs according to US federal statute are required to provide one third of the RDA in each school lunch); the basis for determination that adequate nutrition is provided so hospitals qualify for federal reimbursement for Medicare recipients; the yardstick when comparing adequacy of nutrient intakes of groups within the population (e.g., pregnant, low-income women) to determine whether dietary risk is present; and the basis for establishing safe levels of intake for free trade for dietary supplements or

TABLE 104.2. PAST USES OF RECOMMENDED DIETARY ALLOWANCES[a]

TYPICAL USERS

Federal and state agencies in nutrition programs and policies
Industry in formulating fortification guidelines
Nutrition researchers to evaluate requirements
State agencies in institutional feeding programs

EXAMPLES OF USES

Guide for procuring food supplies for groups of healthy persons
Basis for planning meals for groups, such as in correctional facilities
Reference point for evaluating the dietary intake of population subgroups, such as those who are low income
Component of food and nutrition education programs, such as the Food Guide Pyramid in the United States
Reference point for nutrition labeling of food and dietary supplements

[a] For a comprehensive list of uses of dietary reference standards, see the report on using the dietary reference intakes for dietary assessment (14) and for planning (25).

fortified foods (as proposed in 1997 in Codex Alimentarius deliberations).

Although much additional research has added to the ability to establish the requirement for a nutrient, it became evident to the Food and Nutrition Board and others involved in nutrition assessment and planning that one value, even if designated as applying to a specific age and life-stage group, was not always scientifically appropriate to use as the basis for all public health policy and programs as well as for client counseling (3). In Great Britain, multiple reference values were proposed in 1990 in an expansion of their RDAs (defined as recommended daily amounts) recognizing that ". . . incorporating the descriptive term 'recommended' has led many to believe it represents the minimum desirable intake for healthy life. In reality, for the great majority of the population, the RNI or RDA is substantially more than [an] individual needs" (15) (see Appendix Table A-4).

DEVELOPMENT OF DIETARY REFERENCE INTAKES

The dietary reference intakes (DRIs) represent a major expansion of past efforts to review nutrients and food components and to determine quantitative reference values (see Appendix A-2-a through A-2-g for specific values of DRIs for nutrients reviewed under the DRI process). The reports themselves (collectively a total of 11 as of this writing, with more than 4500 pages) provide significant detail about the rationale for selection of functional end points or criteria for adequacy and contain chapters on each nutrient reviewed and on the methods used to review the data, as well as general guidelines developed and continually revised as experience was gained with new nutrients. Thus, in this chapter, it is possible only to highlight some of the new or revised approaches taken.

In 1994, with the growing merging of diet and chronic disease relationships with nutrient recommendations, and with newer statistical evaluations of how best to estimate dietary inadequacy (16), the Food and Nutrition Board, after evaluating possible approaches to revamping the methodology used in the past, determined that an expanded approach to developing quantitative reference intakes was needed and proposed a framework that would encompass the following:

- The RDAs should incorporate concepts of risk reduction for chronic disease and developmental abnormalities for which sufficient data for efficacy and safety exist.
- Multiple reference points are needed instead of one number for each nutrient; thus, in addition to establishing recommended intakes and intakes for use in evaluating adequacy, estimates of upper limits of intakes should also be included.
- In addition to evaluating nutrients known to be essential to human life, other food components should also be reviewed using the same methodology.

- The process should be open and transparent, with adequate justification and rationale provided for the functional end points used to establish adequacy or adverse effects.

With these points as the conceptual base for developing new reference values, a joint effort was initiated in 1994 by the Food and Nutrition Board with Canadian and US scientists, sponsored by US federal agencies and Health Canada, and augmented by funding from private nonprofit organizations as well as a corporate donor fund. Given that more than just recommended intakes were to be established, a new term for the collective effort, DRIs, was adopted. Because some of the reference intakes proposed could not be considered "recommended" intakes (e.g., the tolerable upper intake level [UL]), the overall term "reference intake" was adopted.

A committee of national and international experts from both the United States and Canada was appointed to oversee the process (the Standing Committee on the Scientific Evaluation of Dietary Reference Intakes; see Fig. 104.2), along with two subcommittees: one appointed to apply the risk assessment model to nutrients, and the second to provide guidance on how to use the DRIs. Given the extensive analyses expected, groups of nutrients were reviewed by panels of experts with input from the subcommittees and the standing committee; six nutrient and two applications reports have been issued, in addition to short reports on the definition of dietary antioxidants, on defining dietary fiber, and on applying the risk assessment model to nutrients.

Using the procedures of the Institute of Medicine of the National Academies, committees of experts are formed and, while gathering data and information, hold open meetings to talk with others and hear from experts regarding specific topics; once the data are gathered, they are reviewed in closed deliberations, a report is drafted, and it is then reviewed anonymously by outside experts; the report is issued once it is approved for release as having met the statement of task which initiated the project.

Over the 11 years of developing the DRIs completed to date, more than 25 workshops and open meetings have been held, and 125 scientists have served as members and unpaid consultants of the DRI standing committee, subcommittees, and panels. In addition, as part of the procedures of the National Academies, more than 110 outside experts reviewed one or more of the reports before their release.

Categories of Dietary Reference Intakes

The categories of DRIs developed to date are given in Table 104.3. They include the following: the estimated average requirement (EAR) and its sibling for energy, the estimated energy requirement (EER); the RDA; the adequate intake (AI); the UL; and the acceptable macronutrient distribution range (AMDR). The Standing Committee

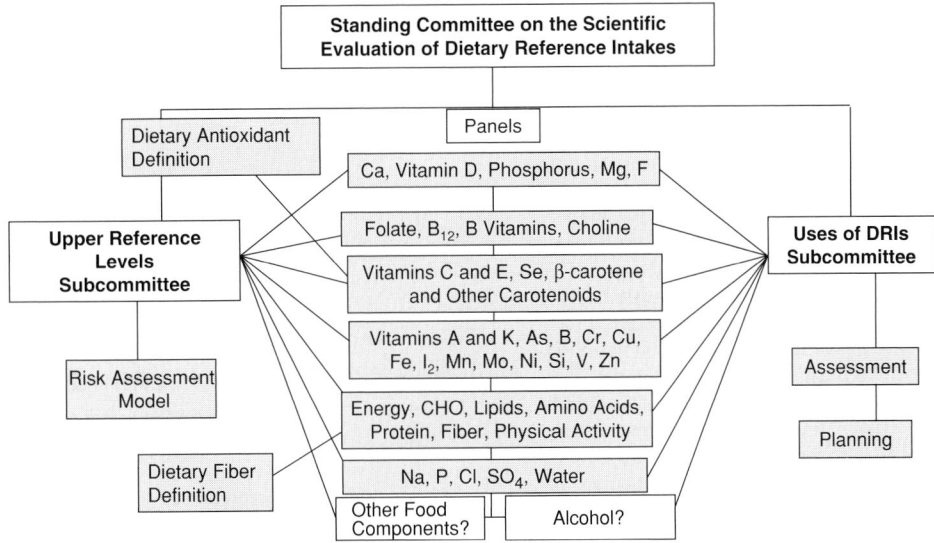

Figure 104.2. The organizational framework for the dietary reference intake (DRI) process of the Food and Nutrition Board (FNB), Institute of Medicine of the US National Academies. Initiated in 1994 with the publication of a white paper outlining this schema, the FNB Standing Committee on DRIs maintained oversight of the six panels and two subcommittees through 2004 with the completion of the report on electrolytes (28). *Shading* indicates reports issued and the order of the reports from panel deliberations as they were released between 1997 and 2004. A panel to review other food components as part of the DRI process was proposed as an original part of the DRI framework (3), but it has not yet been established. When the macronutrient panel was constituted, it was decided that a separate panel evaluating the role of alcohol in health and disease should be formed to consider this nutrient; this has yet to be established.

on DRIs initially planned to develop only three categories of DRIs for each nutrient for which the data were adequate: an EAR, an RDA, and a UL. However, with the first panel, it became apparent that for some nutrients, particularly those for which dose-response studies were not available, a surrogate RDA would have to be developed (17) (Fig. 104.3). This surrogate recommended intake, the AI, was not termed an RDA so all would realize that the data on which it was based were less conclusive than those of other nutrients with RDAs, and thus more judgment was involved in its determination. Its use is also different (Table 104.4).

Model for Establishing Recommended Intakes

Unlike past approaches to determining RDAs, a key feature of the DRI process is to evaluate explicitly all possible functional end points that could be used to determine adequacy and then to justify those used to establish a requirement. In evaluating the available evidence, attention is paid to observed intakes in healthy populations, epidemiologic observations, data from human balance studies, depletion-repletion studies, animal experiments, and biochemical indicators of adequacy, when functional outcomes, such as decreased rate of chronic disease, are not available. The model assumes a normal or at least symmetric distribution of requirements at varying levels of intake among similar individuals (Fig. 104.4). The EAR, as defined, is the best estimate of the requirement for a

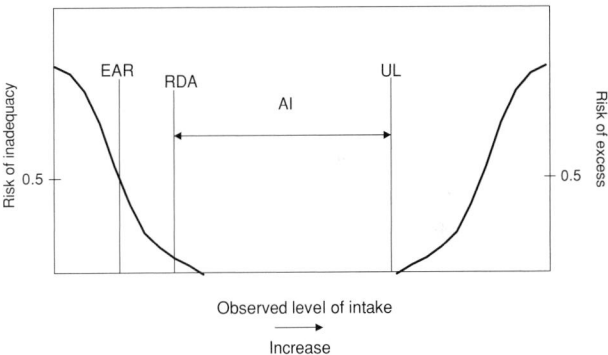

Figure 104.3. The dietary reference intake (DRI) model relating nutrient risk of inadequacy and excess includes four DRI categories. Unlike earlier concepts (as depicted in Figure 104.1), the DRI standing committee chose not to include a level of intake that was known to be deficient in almost all individuals, by realizing that the possibility of misuse of multiple values would increase with additional numbers and resulting from a lack of need for such a value in the United States and Canada. It was determined that with the estimated average requirement (EAR), it is possible to estimate the proportion of individuals whose diets are inadequate, and thus a lower value would not be needed. A new category was added, however, that of the adequate intake (AI). Note that the AI is not a range, but a specific level of intake that lies somewhere on the line indicated. Its relationship to an EAR and thus a recommended dietary allowance (RDA) is not known because it was not possible to determine an EAR from the data available. The AI is set at levels below the tolerable upper intake level (UL) and is likely greater than the RDA, if it were known. (From Food and Nutrition Board, Institute of Medicine. Dietary Reference Intakes for Calcium, Phosphorus, Magnesium, Vitamin D, and Fluoride. Washington, DC: National Academy Press, 1997, with permission.)

TABLE 104.3. CATEGORIES OF DIETARY REFERENCE INTAKES AND THEIR DEFINITIONS

DIETARY REFERENCE INTAKE	DEFINITION
AI (adequate intake)	The recommended average daily intake level based on observed or experimentally determined approximations or estimates of nutrient intake by a group (or groups) of apparently healthy people that are assumed to be adequate—used when an RDA cannot be determined.
EAR (estimated average requirement)	The average daily nutrient intake level estimated to meet the requirement of half the healthy individuals in a particular life stage and gender group[a]
RDA (recommended dietary allowance)	The average daily dietary nutrient intake level sufficient to meet the nutrient requirement of nearly all (97–98%) healthy individuals in a particular life stage and gender group
UL (tolerable upper intake level)	The highest average daily nutrient intake level that is likely to pose no risk of adverse health effects to almost all individuals in the general population; as intake increases above the UL, the potential risk of adverse effects may increase
AMDR (acceptable macronutrient distribution range)	The range of intakes for an energy yielding macronutrient associated with reduced risk of chronic disease while providing adequate intakes of essential nutrients; given as a percentage of energy intake

[a] In the case of energy, an estimated energy requirement (EER) is provided. The EER is defined as the average dietary energy intake that is predicted to maintain energy balance in a healthy adult of a defined age, gender, weight, height, and level of physical activity consistent with good health. In children and pregnant and lactating women, the EER is taken to include the needs associated with the deposition of tissues or the secretion of milk at rates consistent with good health.

Adapted from Food and Nutrition Board, Institute of Medicine. Dietary Reference Intakes for Energy, Carbohydrate, Fiber, Fat, Fatty Acids, Protein, and Amino Acids. Washington, DC: National Academy Press, 2002, with permission.

group of similar individuals. Although half of such persons will have their needs met at the EAR, half will not. The definition of the EAR implies a median, whereas the word "average" would indicate a mean. The decision to name this DRI "EAR" was made to follow precedent set by the United Kingdom (15), because if the distribution of requirements is symmetric, then the mean and median are the same (17). By definition, the EAR is increased by two standard deviations of the requirement to obtain the RDA, which should thus be a level of intake adequate to meet the needs of practically all (actually, 97.5%) of

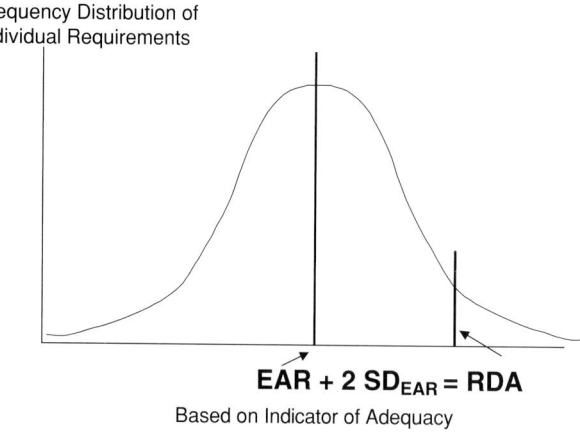

Frequency Distribution of Individual Requirements

EAR + 2 SD$_{EAR}$ = RDA

Based on Indicator of Adequacy

Increasing Intake

Figure 104.4. This graph depicts the theoretic model for establishing the estimated average requirement (EAR) and the recommended dietary allowance (RDA) from data on the nutrient requirements for a group of individuals of similar age, gender, and size. To establish an EAR in a population of similar individuals that is close to the mean requirement of the population, a normal or symmetric distribution of requirements is necessary. For the purposes of the dietary references intakes (DRIs), the RDA is defined as two standard deviations of requirements greater than the EAR, thus at a level of nutrient intake that will meet the needs of almost all (97.5%) of the individuals in the population. Of importance is the decision to base the requirements distribution on a specific indicator of adequacy or functional outcome. Different indicators or functional outcomes may result in different EARs, and thus RDAs.

individuals in the group. In the case of nutrients for which requirements are not symmetrically distributed, such as iron, it is necessary to use other statistical methods to establish both the EAR and RDA. See the iron chapter in the DRI report on micronutrients (20) for a discussion and estimation of the EAR and RDA for iron using modeling of the components the iron requirement.

Once the determination of which criterion or criteria of adequacy will be used for a given nutrient, then the data available indicating human response to varying levels of nutrient intake with that indicator are evaluated. In spite of the last century of research in human nutrition, dose-response data at varying levels of intake with large sample sizes have rarely been available for establishing nutrient requirements through the DRI process. In each case, the data used are documented, and the limitations are explained in the various DRI reports.

Adequate for What?

A key question in reviewing the available data has been which criterion of adequacy should be chosen. Depending on the criterion used, markedly different recommended intakes result. This is one reason that recommended intakes may be substantially different when comparing reference values from different organizations or countries. As an example, Figure 104.5 provides data analyzed by George Beaton for a group of women in the Netherlands

TABLE 104.4. USES OF THE VARIOUS CATEGORIES OF DIETARY REFERENCE INTAKES FOR HEALTHY INDIVIDUALS AND GROUPS

TYPE OF USE	FOR AN INDIVIDUAL[a]	FOR A GROUP[b]
Assessment	EAR: use to determine the probability that the usual intake of the individual is inadequate (if individual's usual intake is at the EAR, then there is a 50% probability that intake is inadequate) RDA: usual intake at or above this level has a low probability of inadequacy AI[c]: usual intake at or above this level has a low probability of inadequacy	EAR: use to estimate the prevalence of inadequate intakes within a group (the % of the group with intakes less than the EAR is the % whose intakes are inadequate) RDA: not used to assess intakes of groups AI[c]: for nutrients for which the AI is based on median intakes of a group of healthy individuals, a group intake at or above this level implies a low prevalence of inadequate intakes if the population intake and requirements distributions are similar
	UL: usual intake above this level may place an individual at risk of adverse effects from excessive nutrient intake AMDR: usual intake within the range given for each of the macronutrients with AMDRs minimizes the potential for diet-related chronic disease and allows for a diet that provides other essential nutrients	UL: use to estimate the percentage of the population at potential risk of adverse effects from excess nutrient intake AMDR: use to estimate the proportion of the population that falls outside the range to assess adherence to recommendations and determine concern level about adverse consequences
Planning	RDA: aim for this intake	EAR: use to plan an intake distribution with a low prevalence of inadequate intakes by planning so few individuals in the group consume less than the EAR
	AI[c]: aim for this intake	AI[c]: For nutrients for which the AI is based on median intakes of a group of healthy individuals, use to plan so the median intake of the group is at or above
	UL: use as a guide to limit intake; long-term intake of higher amounts may increase the potential risk of adverse effects AMDR: aim for maintaining intake between the range	UL: use to plan intake distributions with a low prevalence of intakes potentially at risk of adverse effects AMDR: use to plan intakes so the intakes of most of the group fall within the range; plan for the midpoint of the range initially and then evaluate

AI, adequate intake; AMDR, acceptable macronutrient distribution range; EAR, estimated average requirement; RDA, recommended dietary allowance; UL, tolerable upper intake level.

[a] Evaluation of true status requires clinical, biochemical, and anthropometric data.

[b] Requires statistically valid approximation of distribution of usual intakes.

[c] The AI is used as a guide for infants as it calculated based on the average intake from human milk for the midpoint of the age range. In the context of assessing groups, when the AI for a nutrient is not based on mean intakes of a healthy population, this assessment is made with less confidence.

Adapted from Food and Nutrition Board, Institute of Medicine. Dietary Reference Intakes for Energy, Carbohydrate, Fiber, Fat, Fatty Acids, Protein, and Amino Acids. Washington, DC: National Academy Press, 2002, with permission.

for whom data were available on dietary intake as well as biochemical measurements that could be used as criteria to establish AIs for iron. This figure demonstrates that at any given intake level (e.g., 8 mg/day of iron), if the cutoff for adequacy for hemoglobin is a less than 110 g/L, then the probability of being "inadequate" using this criterion will be 16% (16 times out of 100); if, instead, maintaining a normal level of iron-binding capacity is used, such as transferrin saturation, at this level of intake the probability of inadequacy is much higher, almost 60%. Moreover, if adequate storage in the form of ferritin were selected as the indicator or criterion of adequacy, there would be almost a 100% probability of inadequacy.

This example demonstrates how important it is to identify the criterion (and, at times, multiple criteria) chosen to establish adequacy of intakes. Depending on the public health goals and resources available, it may well be that,

for some situations, different criteria are appropriate to serve as the basis for food and nutrition policy.

Determination of the Coefficient of Variation of Requirements

The RDA for nutrients whose requirements are normally distributed thus depends on the EAR as well as on the spread of the distribution, because two standard deviations are added to determine the RDA; if the variation in requirements is small, the RDA will be close to the EAR; if it is broader, then it will be a larger amount. Although for nutrients with EARs, data may be sufficient to develop dose-response curves that allow for its calculation, in almost all cases errors in estimating the distribution of requirements were considered sizable enough to not attempt to estimate (14). If data on the variability of

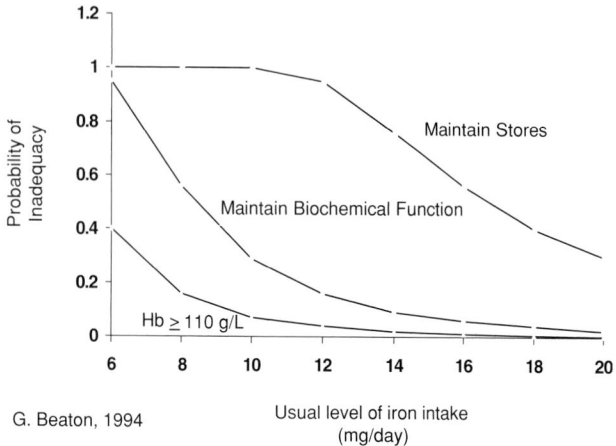

G. Beaton, 1994

Figure 104.5. The intake of a nutrient, in this example iron, and its relation to three different indicators of adequacy or functional outcomes in a group of similar individuals—menstruating women—is depicted in this graph. Although intake at a lower level, such as 8 mg, is adequate to prevent anemia when the cutoff for anemia is chosen as 110 g/L, to maintain normal iron-binding capacity (and thus biochemical function), a higher level of iron intake, 13 mg, is required; and to have storage iron, much higher levels of intake (>20 mg/day) are needed. This graph demonstrates the importance of explicitly identifying the criterion of adequacy used in establishing a requirement. (Courtesy of George Beaton.)

requirements for a nutrient are insufficient to calculate a standard deviation for the EAR, then the coefficient of variation (CV) for the EAR is assumed to be 10%.

The decision to use 10% as the default CV is based on the distribution of measured basal metabolism requirements of similar individuals (18), and on the distribution of protein requirements estimated to be 12.5% (18), both of which have been studied more extensively than other nutrients. For 6 of the 17 nutrients whose requirements were assumed to be normally distributed and that have EARs (vitamin A, copper, iodine, molybdenum, niacin, and carbohydrate), the CV applied differs from the default CV of 10%. In the case of copper, molybdenum, and niacin (19, 20), 15% was used, based on the variability in requirements in the few subjects observed; for vitamin A, 20% was used, based on the variability in the apparent half-life of vitamin A in liver stores (20); for iodine, 20% was applied, based on iodine turnover studies (20); and for carbohydrate, 15% was used, based on variability in brain glucose utilization (21).

Development of the Adequate Intake

When applying the theoretic model for some nutrients, data were inadequate or conflicting. In many cases, no dose-response data in humans were available to establish a level at which half of similar individuals would be adequate, based on the chosen criterion, and half would not be. For these nutrients, it was still necessary to provide a recommended intake for use as a goal for an individual person's intake, but to indicate that the reference value was not based on dose-

response information but on expert judgment and thus could not be used with the same degree of confidence. The AI was therefore established to fill this need.

As indicated in Table 104.1, certain nutrients have AIs rather than EARs and thus RDAs. In many cases, data indicated an intake level to which all individuals tested responded adequately, but intermediate levels of intake were not evaluated, a requirement to construct an EAR. In some cases, such as vitamin D, it was impossible to establish the amount synthesized or removed from stores in the few studies of adequacy available. In other cases, other nutrients may be able to fill the need, such as for methyl groups from folate and methionine in the case of choline, at different stages of life. Moreover, for others, such as manganese, the available data may provide only an indication that little evidence of deficiency exists in human diets as typically consumed. Because it is difficult to deplete individuals of a microelement such as manganese to observe the effects of deficiency, few data are available on how low an intake needs to be to produce deficiency signs in half of the individuals in a tested group. In these cases, the AI is based on intake data, usually the median estimated intakes, of individuals in a population relatively free of possible deficiency.

Not all AIs are based on median intakes, because some nutrients, such as fiber, are inadequate in the diets of many US residents and Canadians. Thus, using median intakes in the United States or Canada would not be scientifically appropriate. In these cases, the AI was derived from other data; in the case of fiber, the AI is based on a ratio of total dietary fiber to energy intake (14.5g/1000 kcal) from data indicating the level of decreased risk of cardiovascular disease (21) (see Chapter 4). In the case of calcium, another nutrient known to be lacking in many Western diets, the AI for adolescents is set at a level of desirable intake based on whole-body bone mineral accretion (17) (see Chapter 9).

Use of the Estimated Average Requirement

Although the EAR is the best estimate of the requirement for an individual for whom nothing else is known (by definition, it is no more than 50% more or less than a random individual needs), it will still underestimate the requirements of 50% of individuals. The RDA as defined is an amount that will meet the needs of almost all in a population subgroup. Thus, when planning a diet for an individual person, the RDA (and the AI for nutrients that have no RDA) is the correct reference intake value to use. However, when evaluating adequacy of intakes of groups, one of the most popular situations in which RDAs and RNIs have been applied in the past, the RDA is not the appropriate reference value, particularly when it is compared with the mean intake of a group.

The mean intake, although a useful descriptor, does not provide an understanding of the distribution of intakes of a group. Thus, with a broad distribution of intakes, such as one could have with a nutrient such as vitamin A, it is

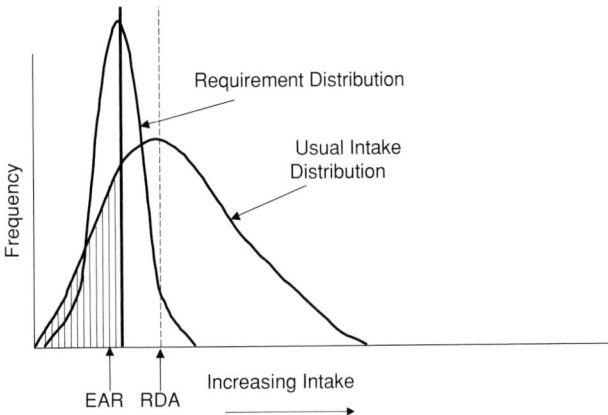

Figure 104.6. Of importance in assessing the adequacy of group intakes to determine the need for intervention or program planning is a tool to compare estimated intakes of nutrients. The estimated average requirement (EAR) serves this role. Using the EAR cut-point method (14, 25), the proportion of a population of similar individuals with intakes less than the EAR is equal to the portion of the population whose intakes are inadequate. In this graph, substantial portions of intakes of this population are below the EAR, whereas the recommended dietary allowance (RDA) and the mean usual intakes of the population are equal. This is one of the main reasons that the RDA should not be used to compare intakes; it does not adequately take into account the distribution of intakes in a group of individuals.

possible that some individual members of a group may have inadequate diets, whereas the mean of the group's intake is at or even above the RDA (Fig. 104.6).

To depict the relationship of the distribution of intakes of a group with their requirement more accurately, so the determination of the extent of inadequacy assessed more precisely, it is possible to use the EAR as the reference value to estimate inadequacy. Such use is statistically supported, given three caveats:

- The range of the variation in intake must be greater than the variation in requirements of the group.
- The variation of requirements must be symmetrically distributed.
- The usual intake of an individual is independent of that individual's requirement (e.g., this is not the case for energy).

If these assumptions are true, then it will be possible to estimate the percentage of individuals in a population whose intake is inadequate based on the criterion of adequacy chosen in establishing the EAR by using the EAR cut-point method (14, 22). The cut-point method works best when intakes are accurately measured and when the actual prevalence of inadequacy is neither very low nor very high. The striped area in Figure 104.6, representing the individuals in the group with intakes below the EAR, represents the prevalence of inadequacy in the group. Thus, in the example in Figure 104.6, although the RDA is approximately the same as the mean intake of the group, substantial proportions of the group's intakes are inade-

quate for the nutrient. The appropriate comparison therefore is with the percentage of intakes below the EAR.

Moreover, the cut-point method does not indicate whether a given individual is deficient; it is based on group information, and thus it can determine only the prevalence of inadequacy in the specific group. An example for data on vitamin C is given in Figure 104.7A. The percentage of nonsmokers with inadequate intakes (the proportion below the EAR: 21% for men and 10% for women) does not mean that this is the percentage of persons who would have clinical signs of scurvy. The criterion used in the establishing the EAR for vitamin C was the amount needed to maintain near-maximal neutrophil ascorbate concentration to handle oxidative stress (23).

Figure 104.7B shows similar data on vitamin C intakes from food and supplements of smokers from the same survey; the EAR was increased by 35 mg of vitamin C for smokers owing to the increased exposure to oxidative stress inducers (23). The data show that in these groups who smoke, there is a greater proportion with inadequate intakes: 52% for men and 30% for women, a finding indicating a decreased ability to handle oxidative stress.

When the Cut-Point Method Is Not Applicable

When the caveats or assumptions about symmetry (and thus normality) and variability in intakes being greater than variability in requirements are not met, the cut-point method to assess adequacy cannot be applied. A more labor-intensive approach can be used, however, called the probability approach (14). This was originally developed in an earlier Food and Nutrition Board report (16) for use in assessing population intakes. It compares each individual's usual intake for a nutrient with the distribution of requirements for that nutrient, obtains an individual probability of inadequacy, and then averages the individual probabilities across the group.

Using the probability approach, however, still requires that the estimated usual intake be independent of an individual's requirement and that the distribution of the requirements be known. The EAR cut-point method does not require that the distribution of the requirements be known, only that it is known to be less than the distribution of usual intakes. Usually, nutrient intakes vary much more than requirements, except in unusual situations in which individuals in the group consume the same food items and the same amounts on a daily basis, such as in an institutional setting where all foods provided are consumed.

Importance of Adjusting Intake Data When Assessing Intakes

Daily nutrient intake varies based on food choices and environmental conditions. Some nutrients are found in many foods in similar amounts (e.g., phosphorus), but some are isolated to specific foods or food groups, and thus intake from day-to-day can vary greatly depending on

A: Nonsmokers

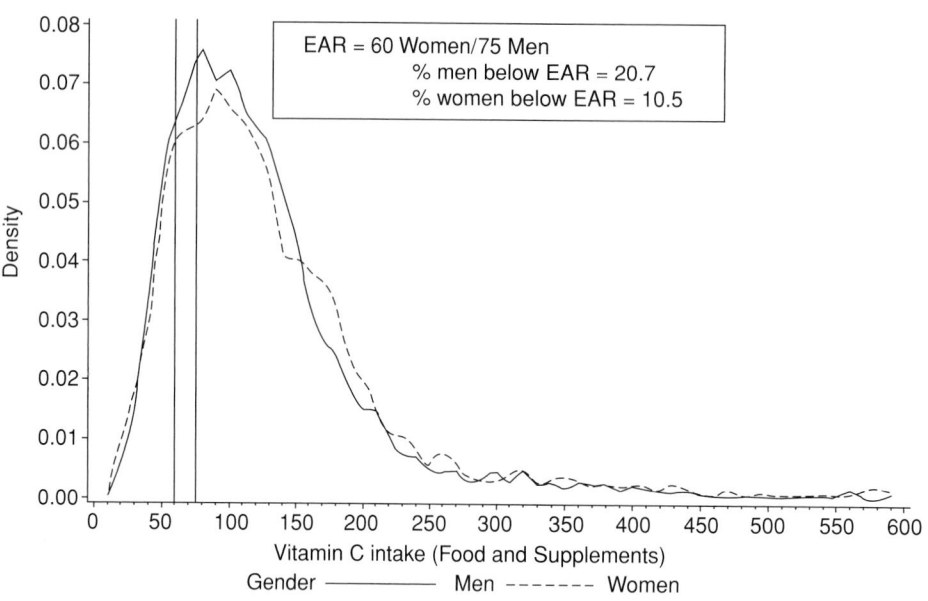

B: Smokers

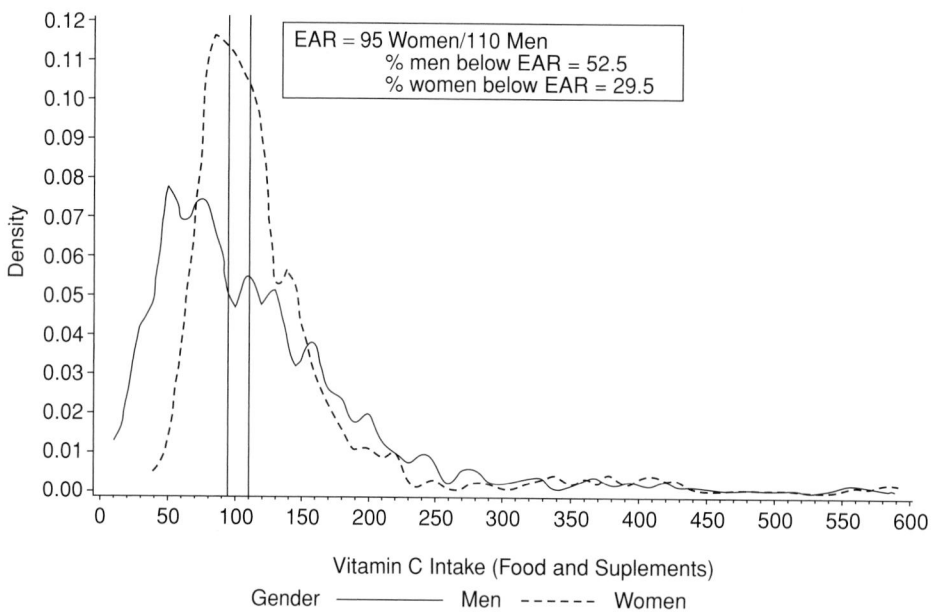

Figure 104.7. When the distribution of usual intakes of a nutrient is known, it is possible to estimate the prevalence of inadequacy for nutrients that have estimated average requirements (EARs). These data on vitamin C intake for smokers and nonsmokers are from the Third National Health and Nutrition Examination Survey (NHANES III), 1988 to 1994. The areas under the curves represent almost 100% of each population (the right tail of the distribution is not shown here). Data have been adjusted for within-person variability using the Iowa State University method (24). In **A**, the data for men and women who do not smoke, the prevalence of inadequate diets for vitamin C is almost 21% for men and more than 10% for women. Because the EAR is increased by 35 mg/day for smokers (**B**), the prevalence of inadequacy for women who smoke is almost 30%, and for men, about 52%. (Adapted from Food and Nutrition Board, Institute of Medicine. Dietary Reference Intakes for Vitamin C, Vitamin E, Selenium, and Carotenoids. Washington, DC: National Academy Press, 2003, with permission.)

what is consumed. For example, as described in the Institute of Medicine report on using DRIs to assess adequacy (14), the estimates of within-subject variation for adult women for nutrients in a 1994 to 1996 USDA dietary intake survey for some nutrients were high, such as for vitamin A (152%) and for vitamin B_{12} (294%), whereas for other nutrients, such as phosphorus, the estimate was 39%. This means that a 1-day food record obtained as a dietary recall cannot be considered as representing the usual intake of an individual for many nutrients.

TABLE 104.5. ZINC INTAKE PERCENTILES (mg/d), UNADJUSTED AND ADJUSTED FOR DAY-TO-DAY VARIANCE IN INTAKES[a]

	PERCENTILES						
	5th	10th	25th	50th	75th	95th	99th
Women 31–50 y							
Unadjusted	2.9	4.0	5.7	8.2	11.7	20.4	32.5
Adjusted	5.4`	6.1	7.3	9.1	11.1	14.9	18.5
Boys 14–18 y							
Unadjusted	4.9	6.1	8.4	12.8	19.1	32.8	47.0
Adjusted	8.4	9.6	11.7	14.3	17.5	24.0	30.3

[a] The estimated average requirement for women 31–50 y is 8 mg; for boys 14–18 y, 11 mg. The upper tolerable intake limit for women is 40 mg; for boys 14–18 y, 34 mg (20).

Data from ENVIRON Health Sciences analysis of 1994–96. Continuing Survey for Food Intakes by Individuals data, adjusted using the Iowa State University method (24).

To estimate intake as accurately as possible, nutrient intake data obtained from 1-day food records and used for assessment need to be adjusted to be more representative of usual intakes and thus more useful in assessing overall dietary adequacy of a given nutrient. The goal when adjusting intakes is to remove day-to-day variation in intakes for each individual to the extent possible, so almost all the resulting spread in the distribution of intakes is the result of interindividual variation in intakes. Adjustment methods are available to do so; an example of such an adjustment is provided in Table 104.5, using the Iowa State University method of adjustment on zinc intake data from a USDA survey (24). Without adjusting the data, the EAR cut-point method to assess adequacy would overestimate the percentage of the population group that was below their EAR, and a greater portion of the group would be determined to be inadequate with respect to zinc intake, thus producing a biased estimate of inadequacy. The adjustment acts to remove the day-to-day variation in individuals' intakes. The median intakes (fiftieth percentile) after adjustment are close to the nonadjustment median, compared with the distances between the adjusted and the nonadjusted data at the tails of the distribution. The tails have been brought in closer, thus decreasing the spread of the distribution (25).

Adjustment methods such as the Iowa State University method adjust intake distributions by having at least two independent recalls or dietary records for a subset of the group that is as representative as possible of the entire group. Independent recalls are those that are collected on nonconsecutive days. For more information on procedures to adjust intakes, see the DRI report on applications of the DRIs to dietary assessment (14), the earlier National Research Council report on nutrient adequacy (16), and Beaton's chapter on using reference values for individuals and populations (22). Suffice it that nutrient intake assessments using single-day food records are biased and are not necessarily representative of usual intakes.

Use of the Adequate Intake

The AI is a useful tool to plan diets (see Table 104.4), with the recognition that, although it is a recommended intake, it may be at or above the RDA (if known) for most nutrients. It is less useful in assessing adequacy of intakes of individuals or groups, because it does not have a specific relationship with requirements. The proportion of individuals in a population group whose intakes are above the AI can be estimated and assumed to be adequate, but it is not possible to use the AI as a cutoff similar to the EAR to determine the prevalence of inadequacy (14). One can determine only the prevalence of intakes below the AI, but not a make an assessment about adequacy. Thus, for assessment purposes, the AI is a less desirable the DRI. In many ways, it is similar to the RDAs of the past (12).

Establishing the Tolerable Upper Intake Level

Paralleling the need for quantitative estimates of how much of a nutrient is needed for adequacy is the need to determine at what point adverse effects are likely to result from overconsumption of a nutrient. In 1992, when the risk assessment model typically applied to chemical contaminants in the food supply was applied to nutrients (also "chemicals"), it resulted in an oral reference dose (RfD, an estimate of daily exposure levels likely to be without appreciable risk of deleterious effects) for zinc for children as determined by the US Environmental Protection Agency in 1992 lower than the recommended intake for children for zinc from the Food and Nutrition Board (26). This led both toxicologists and nutritionists to determine that the risk assessment model, which is based on determining the maximum amount unlikely to increase the risk of toxic effects, needed to be adapted for use with nutrients. Unlike chemicals and contaminants such as pesticides or food additives, a biologic need exists for specific nutrients in specific amounts.

Differences in outcome from risk assessments for nutrients versus contaminants resulted from the differences in the types of data available: (a) there is usually an absence of dose-response data in humans at high levels of nutrient intake; (b) few available human or animal *long-term* studies exist because those available typically determine toxicity of acute levels of ingestion; (c) few surveillance studies are available in which high intakes are estimated to establish a no observed adverse effect level (NOAEL) if dose-response data are lacking; (d) intakes in the few available studies are usually estimated based on supplement intake rather than total, thus not capturing intakes from foods, which may also be fortified; and (e) estimates of bioavailability may differ because of the nutrient source.

It was decided early on not to use the term "safe" when referring to upper levels because it could imply a utility in consuming levels of a nutrient beyond that needed to maintain health (the recommended intake). Thus, the term "tolerable" was chosen, to imply that the level of intake could be tolerated biologically.

Steps in Nutrient Risk Assessment

The steps in traditional toxicologic risk assessment were followed to establish ULs (27) (see Table 104.3). Risk is defined as the probability that an adverse effect will occur at some specified level of exposure. Risk assessment is a scientific exercise, which should not be influenced by value judgments.

- Hazard identification: The first step is not unlike the determination of the criterion or criteria to establish a requirement for a nutrient. For the DRI process, published literature regarding adverse effects resulting from ingestion on a long-term basis (usually over a few months to a few years) was reviewed by both experts in risk assessment on the DRI subcommittee on upper reference levels as well as experts in the nutrient under review on each nutrient panel. The review included evaluating causality, pharmacokinetic and metabolic data, mechanisms of toxic action, the quality and completeness of the database, and identification of distinct and highly sensitive subpopulations. Once documented, serious adverse effects were identified; the adverse effect appearing at the lowest level of intake was determined to be the critical data set for establishing the UL.
- Dose-response assessment: Using the data relating the critical adverse effect to intake, a NOAEL was identified (if possible), along with a lowest observed adverse effect level (LOAEL), and its relation to the critical end point was determined. In addition, an assessment of uncertainty was conducted: this includes evaluating the type, strength, and number of data used to establish the NOAEL and LOAEL, any data on variability in response, and the severity of the adverse effect.

  From this assessment, an uncertainty factor (UF) is derived. Depending on the clinical significance of observed adverse effects, the uncertainty factor will vary (Fig. 104.8). A UF for contaminants has typically been a factor of 100 or 1000 based on toxic levels seen in animals and then applied to humans; the UF for nutrients has characteristically been less than five when human data were available. The NOAEL (or, if one is not determinable, the LOAEL) is then divided by the UF to obtain the UL. The larger the UF, the lower the UL (see Fig. 104.8).
- Exposure assessment: To determine the extent of the potential risk of the adverse effect identified, nutrient intake data for the population are evaluated. For a few nutrients, based on differences in bioavailability or critical adverse effect, the UL pertains to intake from supplements and/or fortified foods. This is the case of the UL for magnesium, for which the adverse effect is diarrhea from the bolus amount present in the gut, and the

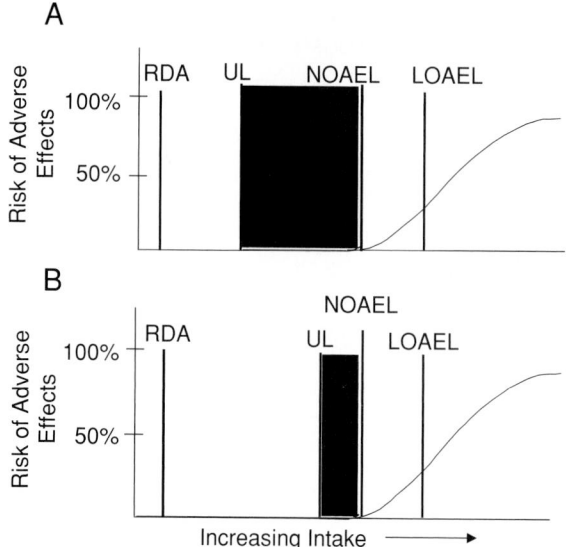

Figure 104.8. In applying the risk assessment model to determine the risk of adverse effects of excessive consumption of nutrients, it is necessary to determine the degree of uncertainty in the data used to establish the point at which no risk of adverse effects is predicted (in this figure, the NOAEL), or, if not available, the point at which the lowest level of adverse effects is apparent (the LOAEL). If significant uncertainty exists, then a larger uncertainty factor (UF) is applied (*gray area*, **A**), resulting in a lower tolerable upper intake level (UL). With less uncertainty (*gray area*, **B**), a higher UL is possible. To obtain the UL, the NOAEL (or LOAEL if no NOAEL is established) is divided by the UF. The UL represents an intake that is likely to result in no risk of adverse effects in sensitive individuals in the population. RDA, recommended dietary allowance. (Adapted from Food and Nutrition, Institute of Medicine. Dietary Reference Intakes for Water, Potassium, Sodium, Chloride, and Sulfate. Washington, DC: National Academy Press, 2004, with permission.)

UL applies to magnesium from supplements only. In the case of niacin and folate, the UL applies to intakes from fortified foods and supplements only.
- Risk characterization: Based on comparing the UL with intakes in specific subgroups of the population, it is possible to characterize the proportion of the population at possible risk of the critical adverse effect associated with the UL. Because the UL is established taking into account sensitive individuals in the population, it is not expected that all those whose usual or long-term intake exceeds the UL will demonstrate the adverse effect.

Limitations in Using Tolerable Upper Intake Levels

By definition, the UL is a level of intake at which there is expected to be no risk of adverse health effects for almost all individuals in the general population. As intake increases above the UL, the potential risk of adverse effects increases, but because of the lack of data, it is not possible to identify the slope of the risk curve (see Fig. 104.3). It can be assumed that intakes of a given nutrient by generally healthy people (and thus not under a health professional's care) at below the UL do not constitute risk.

In most cases, limited data were available because of the paucity of human studies. Studies conducted by investigators to evaluate potential health benefits of levels of intake above the UL and in which subjects are appropriately monitored for adverse effects will add to the body of knowledge and should not be curtailed. Likewise, use of higher levels of nutrients for specific purposes while under the supervision of a health care professional is not within the scope of the use of the UL. In the choice of the term tolerable, however, the DRI committees and panels pointed out quite strongly that there are no documented health benefits of intakes by the general population above the RDA or AI, and thus the ULs are not recommended intakes or desirable levels.

Application of the Model of Nutrient Risk Assessment to Macronutrients

As part of the DRI process, the risk assessment model has been applied to all nutrients reviewed, including macronutrients. Much of the evidence reviewed regarding intake of the energy-yielding nutrients fats and carbohydrates relates to their long-term effects on chronic disease.

The model was applied to food components such as cholesterol, *trans*-fatty acids, and saturated and total fat, but the dose-response data evaluated in the case of cholesterol, saturated fat, and *trans*-fatty acids indicated that a NOAEL did not exist (21) that as intakes decreased to zero, there continued to be demonstrable benefits in terms of decreased risk of cardiovascular disease. Thus, rather than providing a UL for a level at which there would be an expected and quantifiable risk, the recommendation is to decrease intake of these dietary fats as low as possible while consuming a nutritionally adequate diet.

In the case of added sugars, which were also evaluated, no UL was established because there was "no clear and consistent association between increased intake of added sugars and BMI" (21), although there was a trend toward dietary inadequacy with higher intakes of added sugars. Instead of providing a UL, the following statement was provided: "A maximal intake of 25% of energy from added sugars is suggested . . . . based on ensuring sufficient intakes of essential micronutrients that are for the most part [are] present in relatively low amounts in food and beverages that are major sources of added sugars in North American diets" (21).

These statement highlight one of the issues that must be considered when developing individual nutrient reference values: foods as consumed provide multiple nutrients and potentially bioactive food components, and eliminating a food that contains one nutrient to decrease the risk of disease, typically chronic disease, may potentially increase the risk of dietary inadequacy of other nutrients, just as consuming too much of one food can have adverse effects.

Nutrients Evaluated in the Dietary Reference Intake Process but without Tolerable Upper Intake Levels or Recommended Intakes

Not all the nutrients reviewed as part of the DRI process have ULs, and not all have AIs or RDAs. Two circumstances result in no UL: first, when data indicated no adverse consequences of consumption at high levels of intake on a long-term basis (e.g., vitamin B_{12}); second, when data on toxicity at short-term intakes were available, but no data on adverse effects likely to occur with long-term intakes (e.g., arsenic) could be found. Thus, it was decided to not provide ULs for those nutrients for which useful data were not available. The recommendation is made in the DRI reports that if there is no UL for a nutrient, then caution is warranted when consuming levels greater than those normally found in foods.

Tolerable Upper Intake Levels without Adequate Intakes/Recommended Dietary Allowances

For some nutrients (e.g., boron, nickel, and vanadium), data demonstrated their requirement in the diet of animals, with limited data on their beneficial role in human health, but the information was deemed inadequate to develop AIs or EARs. Because data indicated their potential toxicity, ULs exist for these elements. In the case of β-carotene, which was reviewed as part of the DRI process, no UL was established because of conflicting data when intakes at various levels were evaluated in long-term clinical trials (23).

Acceptable Macronutrient Distribution Ranges for Energy-Yielding Macronutrients

Nutrients such as fat, carbohydrate, and protein play multiple roles: they all serve as the source of energy, but specific types of each have independent roles in health. These independent roles are recognized by providing RDAs, AIs, or ULs, as in the case for specific indispensable amino acids or for dietary fiber. When functioning as energy sources, a specific amount of one type of energy source is not useful, because the total energy intake on a daily basis varies greatly depending on the individual, the environment, and energy expenditure. Research on risk factors correlated with chronic disease onset indicated that the *proportion* of each source is predictive of relative risk; modifying one results in a change in other energy sources if total energy intake is constant. Thus, for sources of energy related to chronic disease risk (for carbohydrate and fat: cardiovascular disease, obesity, and diabetes), AMDRs are expressed in the form of the percentage of energy consumed, primarily to give guidance to individual persons (see Table 104.4).

The lower level of the range can be considered the minimum amount needed, whereas the upper end of the range is the maximum amount. In assessing the diets of groups, the portion of the group with intakes outside the range can indicate concern about possible adverse consequences. In planning diets for groups, having the intakes of most of the group fall within the AMDR is the goal; initially, the mean of the range could be selected and then later evaluated to see whether the goal was attained (21).

In addition to protein, carbohydrate, and total fat, AMDRs were also established for two types of fatty acid: linoleic acid and α-linolenic acid (21). For these nutrients, the lower end of the range was the AI (to meet the needs for essential fatty acids), and the upper end of the range, in the case of linoleic acid, was set based on concerns about prooxidant effects of higher amounts, whereas for α-linolenic acid, it was set at the highest intakes from foods consumed by individual persons in the United States and Canada.

Energy and Physical Activity

Unlike past reference values for energy, the DRIs include estimates of energy requirements derived from energy expenditure studies using the doubly labeled water technique (21). Previous energy allowances were based on estimated time spent in various activities in addition to measured or predicted basal metabolic rates for different gender and life-stage groups at different levels of activity (12). Rather than developing an RDA (a level of energy intake that would be adequate for almost all the population), an EER is determined from regression equations derived from the doubly labeled water data based on gender, age, weight, height, and four levels of physical activity (sedentary, low active, active, very active) (21).

With the growing recognition of the importance of physical activity, the DRI process also reviewed the data and developed recommended levels of activity to both decrease risk of chronic disease and maintain body weight at less than body mass index (BMI) of 25. The recommended level of total activity is a greater than 1.6 physical activity level (the ratio of total energy expenditure to basal energy expenditure), and this is the equivalent of 60 minutes of moderate-intensity activity on a daily basis greater than sedentary levels (moderate activity is defined and is equivalent to walking at 3–4 miles/hour). This is the first time that a level of activity has been recommended as part of dietary recommendations; past energy allowances assumed a level of light to moderate activity (12).

NEW ASPECTS OF THE DIETARY REFERENCE INTAKES

Some features of the DRIs may represent new ways of approaching developing nutrient reference values. In each report, the methodology used in the review is described, and possible end points or criteria for adequacy and excess are delineated. It is useful to review some of the overarching approaches that are new within the DRI framework.

Deficiency for What?

The key question in establishing recommended intakes is this: What is the best indicator of a nutrient requirement? An important concept of each recommended intake is that there may be multiple criteria that could be used to establish a recommended intake, and that if a different criterion were chosen, it could well result in a different amount recommended. The amount of a vitamin to prevent a traditional deficiency may be much different from the amount of that vitamin to alter an indicator or biomarker known to be a risk factor for a specific chronic disease. Although the DRI process had an underlying requirement that each panel look at all possible end points, including those that could be biomarkers for chronic disease risk factor reduction, in many cases, the information was not adequate or sufficiently compelling to develop either an RDA or an AI based on such information. For some nutrients, in vitro or animal studies pointed to a relationship, but a lack of dose-response studies in humans prevented use of the relationship.

As a result, one of the major outcomes of the DRI process is that for each nutrient or food component reviewed, where there was an indication of a potential relationship, specific recommendations for further research are given. Recommended studies should provide the type of data needed to develop recommendations based on criteria or end points related to reduction of risk factors for chronic disease.

New Age Groups Selected

In initiating the DRI process, a key decision was that this was not to be a revision of the tenth edition of the RDAs or the RNIs; thus, all aspects were started from the beginning. The age groups used for recent RDAs (12) differed from those used for the RNIs (11), so a subgroup of the Standing DRI Committee contacted federal agencies and others in the United States and Canada to determine whether key age groups based on program planning and policies needed to be considered. In addition, new data on the onset of menarche as well as age at retirement indicated a need to revise groupings for these age periods. As a result, new age categories were established that took into account the age at which young children were entering institutional feeding settings (prekindergarten), as well as the age at which retirement appeared likely, potentially affecting energy requirements. For a discussion of these considerations, see Chapter 1 of the first DRI report issued (17).

New Approaches to Infant Reference Values

It was the experience of some of the experts on the DRI Standing Committee that, in the past, when the nutrient composition of human milk was compared to the RDAs for infants, human milk was cited as inadequate in a number of nutrients. To counter this false comparison, it was decided to provide AIs for infants based on nutrient content of human milk for all nutrients for which there was no evidence indicating that breast-fed infants should have supplementary amounts of a nutrient greater than those provided in human milk (17). The AIs for infants are thus based on the mean volume of intake midway through the first 6 months or the second 6 months of life. The concentration of the nutrient is calculated from human milk samples taken during the same period of infant feeding (birth–6 months or 7–12 months of age). During the second 6 months, estimates of the amount of a nutrient provided by consuming complementary foods are added to that obtained from human milk.

To assist infant formula manufacturers, if there are specific issues relative to bioavailability or source of a nutrient when provided in infant formula, then the information is discussed in a section on special considerations for that nutrient. Thus, for infants, most of the recommendations for the AI are less than previous RDA values (e.g., protein, vitamin D, thiamin, niacin, calcium, and zinc).

For two nutrients, iron and zinc, available data indicated that the nutrient content of human milk would not be adequate beyond 6 months of age (20). For these nutrients, EARs are established for infants 7 through 12 months of age; thus, the recommended intakes for these nutrients for this age group are RDAs.

Extrapolation When Data Are Lacking

Although much additional research has occurred related to human nutritional requirements, data were not usually available to determine nutrient requirements directly for each gender and life-stage group for all nutrients reviewed. Thus, available data were extrapolated to develop AMDRs, EARs, AIs, and ULs, and these extrapolation methodologies have been discussed comprehensively (19, 21). Nutrients required for energy metabolism were usually extrapolated on a metabolic body weight basis (B.Wt.$^{3/4}$). For nutrients involved in bone growth, extrapolation was based directly on body weight. For those nutrients distributed in the water space or other specific tissues, differences in the size of the tissues were used as the basis for extrapolation. Because of organ immaturity of infants and a concern about the ability to handle excess amounts, no ULs were established for infants, with the advice that infants should obtain nutrients from food (including human milk) or formula only.

Given that the data on adverse effects of overconsumption of nutrients were minimal in most cases, age and gender groups were frequently combined in establishing ULs; for some nutrients for which data were lacking for women, such as potassium (28), values obtained with men were applied to women. When adult values were based on available data, these values were usually extrapolated to children, elderly persons, or pregnant and lactating women, based on body size or based on differences in

route of ingestion, absorption, distribution, metabolism, or excretion. For vitamin E, boron, molybdenum, nickel, and vanadium, the ULs are based on animal studies, and thus the UF applied to each takes into account extrapolating animal data to humans.

Evaluating the Role of Bioactive Food Components

An increasingly important issue is how to approach establishing recommended intakes for bioactive food components. Initial plans of the DRI process (3) called for a panel to review other food components (see Fig. 104.2). This group of nutrients was held to the end of the initial reviews so more data would be available to evaluate the roles of these substances in health, and if any were determined to be sufficiently supported by available science, then quantitative recommendations and reference values would be developed.

Unlike most traditional nutrients, many of these substances are not stable; for example, the content of a compound such as catechin in grapeseed varies at least twofold depending on when the grapes are harvested, and processing produces significant changes as well. Polyphenolics such as catechins convert rapidly to epicatechins, which demonstrate significant differences in function in in vitro studies with platelet aggregation and antioxidant effects. If in vivo studies indicate a role in health for catechin, how is it to be evaluated? In addition, foods contain many polyphenolics, each having varying effects; how can they be evaluated collectively, labeled, and assayed for content if present?

These are questions that demonstrate the increased level of complexity in moving forward with the evaluation of bioactive components found in food and their role in health. Future emphasis on such evaluation will need to delineate how to establish the criterion of adequacy or excess to be used and how such substances can be effectively quantified to estimate intakes.

INTERNATIONAL EFFORTS TO DEVELOP DIETARY REFERENCE INTAKES

Initiated in the 1980s, the Committee on Medical Aspects of Food Policy of the United Kingdom was one of the first to develop multiple dietary reference values, publishing them in 1991 (15). As the DRI process was initiated, Canada joined the United States in developing the DRIs, and other countries were considering a similar framework. Following the release of the first DRI report on calcium and related nutrients in 1997 (17), the Health Council of the Netherlands released their first report on dietary reference values for calcium, vitamin D, and some of the B vitamins (29), which included EARs, RDAs, AIs, and ULs, using much the same definitions of these terms.

Subsequently, both China (30) and Japan (31) released DRIs for some nutrients, again providing the equivalent of

EAR, RDA, AI, and UL reference intakes, as did a joint effort of the nutrition societies in Austria, Germany, and Switzerland (32). Drafts are in final stages or out for comment in other countries: for example, nutritionists from ten countries in southeast Asia have joined together to develop DRIs for ten nutrients under the auspices of the International Life Sciences Institute of Southeast Asia (33). The Korean Nutrition Society is in the final stages of completing their DRIs (34), and Australia and New Zealand have combined efforts and released a draft document for comment, using similar reference categories (35).

In 2003, the Food Standards Agency's Expert Group on Vitamins and Minerals of the United Kingdom developed a risk assessment model to evaluate nutrients and recently issued their report on upper reference levels for nutrients for two categories of reference intakes, Safe Upper Levels and Guidance Levels (36). Similarly, the Scientific Committee on Food of the European Commission (now the Panel on Dietary Products, Nutrition, and Allergies of the European Food Safety Authority) issued guidelines in 2000 for the development of ULs for vitamins and minerals that were adopted in October 2000 and have been applied to a number of nutrients (37).

Internationally, the Food and Agricultural Organization (FAO) and the World Health Organization (WHO) jointly sponsored expert consultations on nutrient reference values for vitamins and minerals, energy, and protein (see Chapter 107). For vitamins and minerals, an FAO/WHO expert group developed the equivalent of RDAs, AIs, and ULs (38), with similar definitions of the reference values.

An international initiative organized by WHO/FAO to create a consensus on the scientific framework for risk assessment of nutrients (39) is under way in an effort to harmonize the various methods to evaluate data for ULs developed over the past decade by the organizations described earlier. An expert consultation will be held in 2005 to reach international agreement on the approach. Similarly, FAO/WHO is proposing an expert consultation (40) to develop new nutrient reference values to replace those last revised in 1988 (41).

CONCLUSIONS

A major aspect of the DRI process and of the work completed to date is the focus on incorporating the growing body of evidence of the role of nutrients and food components, beyond the prevention of known nutrient deficiency diseases in decreasing the risk of all noncommunicable diseases, to increase longevity and to improve the quality of life through diet-related benefits. The developing efforts over the last twenty years to incorporate concepts of risk factor reduction in quantifying nutrient requirements and recommendations will continue to increase. In looking at the factors that led to the development of DRIs in the United States and Canada, as well as ongoing activities globally, an agreed-on methodology of

how to incorporate such considerations on a scientific basis would be very useful.

No set of reference values can ever fully represent the state of the science because new data and research are continually updating and expanding the science base. Such new research leads inevitably to the need to review and possibly revise quantitative reference values. In addition, as the role of potentially bioactive food components in health becomes clear, either from beneficial or possibly adverse effects, they must be reviewed for inclusion in future evaluations. So the question is not should the DRIs be revised, but when and how?

Achieving consensus on the methods used to assess adequacy may result in altered EARs or AIs, and it is hoped that new data will provide enough levels of intake for whatever criterion is selected to be able to establish EARs for nutrients that at this point have AIs, thus allowing an enhanced ability to assess key nutrients at risk in a quantitative way. For example, since the first report on calcium and related nutrients was issued in 1997 (17), newer data indicate that the criteria for adequacy for vitamin D may need to be revised (42), incorporating as end points vitamin D function beyond that needed for adequate bone formation, to include noncalcemic functions related to downregulation of hyperproliferative cell growth, immune function, cardiovascular disease, or diabetes (see Chapter 20). The developing research base regarding knowledge of genetics, polymorphisms, and individual nutrient requirements (see Chapter 40) will play an increasingly important role in how quantitative human nutrient requirements and reference intakes are determined in the future.

Acknowledgments

The information contained in this chapter represents the combined efforts of more than 200 scientists in the United States and Canada over the last decade or more, and this work would not have been possible without the resources provided by the federal agencies, nonprofit foundations, and corporate sponsors identified in each of the DRI reports. The support of the Institute of Medicine and the chairs, members, consultants, and staff of the Food and Nutrition Board, all of whom worked on aspects of this project for at least a decade, have been critical to its development as it nears completion of this first phase. It is a tribute to all those involved, and especially to the late Vernon R. Young, first Chair of the DRI Committee, who, while questioning everything and wanting to have it right, moved the process forward by the grace of his wit, his intellect, and his quest for scientific validity.

REFERENCES

1. Atwater WA, Bryant MS. Bulletin No. 28. Washington, DC: US Department of Agriculture, 1902.
2. Lind, J. A Treatise of the Scurvy. London: A. Millar, 1753 (republished as Lind's Treatise on Scurvy. Edinburgh: University Press, 1953).
3. Food and Nutrition Board, Institute of Medicine. How Should the Recommended Dietary Allowances Be Revised? Washington, DC: National Academy Press, 1994:1–34.
4. Stiebeling HK. A dietary goal for agriculture. In: USDA: The Agricultural Situation. Washington, DC: US Department of Agriculture, 1937:18–20.

5. Canadian Council of Nutrition. Canadian Dietary Standards. Ottawa: Department of Pensions and National Health, 1938.

6. Technical Commission of the Health Committee, League of Nations. The Problem of Nutrition: Report on the Physiological Bases of Nutrition, vol 2. Geneva: League of Nations, 1936.

7. Dupont JL, Harper AE. Nutr Rev 2002;60:342–8.

8. Wilder RM. War Med 1941;1:143–7.

9. Committee on Food and Nutrition, National Research Council. Recommended Dietary Allowances. Washington, DC: National Research Council, 1941:1–13.

10. Roberts LJ. NY State J Med 1944;44:59–65.

11. Health and Welfare Canada. Nutrition Recommendations: The Report of the Scientific Review Committee. Ottawa: Canadian Government Publishing Centre, 1990:1–206.

12. Food and Nutrition Board, National Research Council. Recommended Dietary Allowances. 10th ed. Washington, DC: National Academy Press, 1989:1–285.

13. Food and Nutrition Board, National Research Council. Diet and Health: Implications for Reducing Chronic Disease Risk. Washington, DC: National Academy Press, 1989:1–749.

14. Food and Nutrition Board, Institute of Medicine. Dietary Reference Intakes: Applications in Dietary Assessment. Washington, DC: National Academy Press, 2000:1–288.

15. Committee on Medical Aspects of Food Policy. Dietary Reference Values for Food Energy and Nutrients for the United Kingdom: Report on Health and Social Subjects. no. 41. London: HMSO, 1991:1–210.

16. Food and Nutrition Board, National Research Council. Nutrient Adequacy: Assessment Using Food Consumption Surveys. Washington, DC: National Academy Press, 1986:1–146.

17. Food and Nutrition Board, Institute of Medicine. Dietary Reference Intakes for Calcium, Phosphorus, Magnesium, Vitamin D, and Fluoride. Washington, DC: National Academy Press, 1997:1–432.

18. Food and Agriculture Organization/World Health Organization/United Nations University. Energy and Protein Requirements. WHO Technical Report Series no. 724. Geneva: World Health Organization, 1985:1–207.

19. Food and Nutrition Board, Institute of Medicine. Dietary Reference Intakes for Thiamin, Riboflavin, Niacin, Vitamin B_6, Folate, Vitamin B_{12}, Pantothenic Acid, Biotin, and Choline. Washington, DC: National Academy Press, 2000:1–567.

20. Food and Nutrition Board, Institute of Medicine. Dietary Reference Intakes for Vitamin A, Vitamin K, Arsenic, Boron, Chromium, Copper, Iodine, Iron, Manganese, Molybdenum, Nickel, Silicon, Vanadium, and Zinc. Washington, DC: National Academy Press, 2001:1–773.

21. Food and Nutrition Board, Institute of Medicine. Dietary Reference Intakes for Energy, Carbohydrate, Fiber, Fat, Fatty Acids, Protein, and Amino Acids. Washington, DC: National Academy Press, 2002.

22. Beaton GH. Recommended dietary intakes: individuals and populations. In: Shils ME, Olson JA, Shike M, et al., eds. Modern Nutrition in Health and Disease. 9th ed. Baltimore: Williams & Wilkins, 1999:1705–25.

23. Food and Nutrition Board, Institute of Medicine. Dietary Reference Intakes for Vitamin C, Vitamin E, Selenium, and Carotenoids. Washington, DC: National Academy Press, 2003:1–507.

24. Nusser SM, Carriquiry AL, Dodd KW et al. J Am Stat Assoc 1996;91:1440–9.

25. Food and Nutrition Board, Institute of Medicine. Dietary Reference Intakes: Applications in Dietary Planning. Washington, DC: National Academy Press, 2003:1–237.

26. Smith JC Jr. Comparison of reference dose with recommended dietary allowances for zinc: methodologies and levels. In: Mertz W, Abernathy CO, Olin SS, eds. Risk Assessment of Essential Nutrients. Washington, DC: ILSI Press, 1994:127–43.

27. Food and Nutrition Board, Institute of Medicine. Dietary Reference Intakes: A Risk Assessment Model for Establishing Upper Intake Levels of Nutrients. Washington, DC: National Academy Press, 1998:1–77.

28. Food and Nutrition Board, Institute of Medicine. Dietary Reference Intakes for Water, Potassium, Sodium, Chloride, and Sulfate. Washington, DC: National Academy Press, 2004.

29. Health Council of the Netherlands. Dietary Reference Values: Calcium, Vitamin D, Thiamin, Riboflavin, Niacin, Pantothenic Acid, and Biotin. Publication no. 2000/12. The Hague: Health Council of the Netherlands, 2000.

30. Chinese Nutrition Society. Chinese Dietary Reference Intakes 2000 [trans.]. Beijing: China Light Industry Publishing House, 2000.

31. Japanese Health Nutrition Research Information Committee. Japanese Recommended Dietary Allowances: Dietary Reference Intakes [trans.]. 6th ed. Tokyo: Japanese Health Nutrition Research Information Committee, 1999:1–274.

32. Deutsche Gesellschaft für Ernährung (German Society of Nutrition), Österreichische Gesellschaft für Ernährung (Austrian Society of Nutrition), Schweizerische Gesellschaft für Ernährungsforschung (Swiss Society of Nutrition) et al. eds. Referenzwerte für die Nährstoffzefuhr (Recommended Values for Nutritional Intake). Frankfurt: Umschau Braus Verlag, 2000.

33. International Life Sciences Institute Southeast Asia annual report, 2004. Last accessed February 14, 2005, http://www.ilsi.org/file/AnnualRep11th.pdf.

34. Korean Nutrition Society. Proceedings [trans.] 2004;37:585-7.

35. Commonwealth Department of Health and Ageing, Australia, Ministry of Health, New Zealand. Nutrient Reference Values for Australia and New Zealand. Draft December 2004:1–312. Last accessed February 14, 2005: http://www.moh.govt.nz/moh.nsf/0/cc515a13536b3cb4cc256f6d000abde0?OpenDocument

36. Expert Group on Vitamins and Minerals. Safe Upper Levels for Vitamins And Minerals. London: Food Standards Agency, 2003:1–360.

37. European Commission. Guidelines of the Scientific Committee on Food for the Development of Tolerable Upper Intake Levels for Vitamins and Minerals. SCF/CS/NUTR/UPPLEV/11 Final. November 2000:1–11. Last accessed at http://europa.eu.int/comm/food/fs/sc/scf/out80a_en.pdf.

38. Food and Agriculture Organization/World Health Organization (FAO/WHO). Human Vitamin and Mineral Requirements. FAO/WHO Expert Consultation, Bangkok. Rome: Food and Agriculture Organization, 2001:1–290. Last accessed October 10, 2004: ftp://ftp.fao.org/es/esn/nutrition/Vitrni/pdf/TOTAL.pdf.

39. Food and Agriculture Organization/World Health Organization (FAO/WHO). Joint FAO/WHO Development of a Scientific Collaboration to Create a Framework for Risk Assessment of Nutrients and Related Substances: Background Paper and Request for Comment/Call for Information. Geneva: World Health Organization, October 2004:1–38. Last accessed November 24, 2004, http://www.who.int/ipcs.en.

40. Codex Committee on Nutrition and Foods for Special Dietary Uses. Report of the 26th session of the Codex Committee on Nutrition and Foods for Special Dietary Uses. Bonn: November 2004. Last accessed December 9, 2004, http://www.codexalimentarius.net/web/reports.jsp?lang=en.

41. Food and Agriculture Organization/World Health Organization (FAO/WHO)/Ministry of Trade and Industry, Finland. Recommended Nutrient Reference Values for Food Labelling Purposes. Report of a Joint FAO/WHO Expert Consultation on

Recommended Allowances of Nutrients for Food Labelling Purposes. Helsinki: September 12–16, 1988.

42. Holick MF. Am J Clin Nutr 2004;80[Suppl]:1678S–88S.

SELECTED READINGS

Beaton GH. Criteria of an adequate diet. In: Shils ME, Olson JA, Shike M, eds. Modern Nutrition in Health and Disease. 8th ed. Philadelphia: Lea & Febiger, 1994:1491–505.

Beaton GH. Recommended dietary intakes: Individuals and populations. In: Shils ME, Olson JA, Shike M et al., eds. Modern Nutrition in Health and Disease. 9th ed. Baltimore: Williams & Wilkins, 1999:1705–25.

Harper AE. Recommended dietary intakes: Current and future approaches. In: Shils ME, Olson JA, Shike M, eds. Modern Nutrition in Health and Disease. 8th ed. Philadelphia: Lea & Febiger, 1994:1475–90.

105 DIETARY GUIDELINES: NATIONAL PERSPECTIVES[1]

JOHANNA T. DWYER

GENERAL PRINCIPLES 1673
   Definition 1673
   Goals 1673
   Audiences 1674
   Assumptions 1674
   Approaches 1674
TYPES OF DIETARY GUIDELINES 1674
   Government-Sponsored Dietary Guidelines 1674
   Dietary Guidelines Issued by Other Groups 1674
CHARACTERISTICS OF EFFECTIVE DIETARY
   GUIDELINES 1674
DIETARY GUIDELINES DEVELOPMENT PROCESS 1675
   Information Needed to Formulate Guidelines . . .1675
   Developing the Scientific Rationale for
      Dietary Guidelines 1675
   Constructing and Modeling Food-Related
      Recommendations During Dietary
      Guideline Development 1677
COMMUNICATING AND IMPLEMENTING
   DIETARY GUIDELINES 1677
   Communicability 1677
   Actionability 1678
   Strategies for Implementation 1678
   Adoption and Use of Guidelines by Public
      and Private Groups 1678
   Procedures Used in Other Countries 1678
HISTORY OF DIETARY GUIDELINES: EXAMPLE
   OF THE UNITED STATES 1678
   Evolution of the *Dietary Guidelines*
      for Americans 1678
   1970s and 1980s: Dietary Goals for the
      United States and *Dietary Guidelines for*
      Americans: Emphasis on Balance and
      Moderation 1678
   1990s and Early 2000s: Convergence
      of Guidance 1679

Year 2000 Dietary Guidelines: Expanded
   Emphasis on Weight and Fitness 1679
Year 2005 Dietary Guidelines: Harmonization
   of Federal Guidance 1679
DIETARY GUIDELINES AND HEALTH OUTCOMES 1680
   Criteria 1680
   Available Evidence Not Definitive 1680
   Criticisms of the Dietary Guidelines 1680
   Clinical Trials of Dietary Guidelines? 1681
CONCLUSIONS 1681
   What Works Well 1681
   Needed Improvements 1681
   Challenges for the Future 1683
   Conclusion 1684

GENERAL PRINCIPLES

National dietary goals and guidelines are common in many countries today (1–5). This chapter focuses primarily on national dietary guidelines using examples from the United States. The observations have more general applicability because the processes used to formulate guidelines and issues involved are similar to those used in other countries.

Definition

Dietary guidelines are sets of advisory statements on diet for populations to promote overall nutritional well-being that relate to all diet-related conditions (6). This subset of dietary guidance has identifiable goals, assumptions, and approaches.

Goals

The immediate goal of dietary guidelines is to promote health by providing healthy consumers science-based advice on food choices and eating patterns. The ultimate goal is to optimize intakes of key nutrients and to change food-related behaviors in desirable directions from the health standpoint. These goals imply achieving adequacy with respect to the kinds and amounts of essential nutrients that are consumed, to avoid risks of dietary deficiency disease. In addition, they include lessening the risk of dietary excess and of diet-related chronic degenerative

[1]**Abbreviations: AMDR,** acceptable macronutrient distribution range for healthy adults; **ASCN,** American Society for Clinical Nutrition; **DRI,** dietary reference intake; **HEI,** Healthy Eating Index; **RFS,** recommended food score; **UL,** tolerable upper intake level; **USDA,** United States Department of Agriculture.

and noncommunicable diseases. The health goals are of prime importance in dietary guidelines; other reasons why people eat are not considered as explicitly, or with the same rigor.

Audiences

The primary purpose of dietary guidelines is to provide advice, nutrition information, and education to the general public, and not to guide experts. In practice, however, guidelines have dual purposes and target audiences. They also provide nutrition policy guidance to generalists for program planning efforts and guide health professionals in their work.

Assumptions

The eating recommendations in dietary guidelines should meet nutrition-related public health objectives. They must be authoritative, evidence based, and comprehensible (1). The advice is food based rather than nutrient based. Foods, rather than dietary supplements or modular sources of the energy providing macronutrients, are suggested to achieve most recommendations. The guidelines address total diet, particularly in Western countries in which dietary excess and imbalance as well as inadequacy may be a problem. Acceptable and affordable eating patterns are recommended. They are usually applicable to the generally healthy population, and not the ill.

Approaches

Dietary guidelines are qualitative statements, but they are often crafted to provide eating patterns that meet quantitative standards, such as the dietary reference intakes (DRIs) (7). Persons whose food choices are based on the guidelines should therefore have intakes of nutrients that fall within acceptable ranges.

TYPES OF DIETARY GUIDELINES

Government-Sponsored Dietary Guidelines

Eating is an intensely personal and often a private behavior, and therefore the rationale for government-sponsored guidance deserves examination. Government has a stake in providing advice and guidance to citizens about eating behavior. If authoritative dietary advice is widely disseminated and implemented, it may reduce risks of diet-related health problems, improve population health and productivity, and enhance the general welfare. Dietary guidelines may also help to shape government food and nutrition policy in more coherent and cost-effective directions. For these reasons, many governments have issued dietary guidelines (1, 8, 9). Government-sponsored dietary guidelines have limitations. Government money and staff are limited, and the process for developing official guidelines is slow and cumbersome Consensus must be achieved to develop clear and actionable recommendations. US law

requires that expert advisory committee nominations, deliberations, and meetings must all be public and preceded by public notice, to ensure transparency and stakeholder involvement, and this may be difficult.

Dietary Guidelines Issued by Other Groups

In most countries, dietary guidelines are also produced by other groups, including professional societies, disease-oriented voluntary associations, nonprofit groups, and individuals or companies (10). These nongovernment guidelines provide extensive and timely information on issues of special interest to particular target audiences, often in a consumer-friendly format. However, the presence of multiple and sometimes conflicting dietary guidelines may be confusing to the public. Some of these guidelines may be difficult to put into practice because they are do not take current food availability, food consumption patterns, or cost into account. In addition, the standards of evidence used in developing them vary. Consumers cannot distinguish which are well grounded in science and which are not.

CHARACTERISTICS OF EFFECTIVE DIETARY GUIDELINES

Effective dietary guidelines in all countries possess certain characteristics that set them apart from other forms of nutrition education (1, 3). Because government-sponsored dietary guidelines are official authoritative recommendations for healthy eating, they should be science based. They address the major diet-related nutrition problems in the population to which they are directed and attempt to mitigate them. They increase the probability of good health and of meeting nutrient needs. They focus on the totality of dietary intake, rather than only on a few specific foods or food groups. Moreover, because many some diet-related problems are caused by imbalances and excessive intakes, they address these issues as well.

Effective dietary guidelines are revised periodically to stay up to date, because science and nutritional problems change over time. Food choices suggested help individual persons to meet recommended eating patterns and are affordable and readily available.

Effective dietary guidelines are comprehensible to both the general public and to health professionals. These guidelines are disseminated and integrated with other nutritional guidance of a public health nature. Finally, if guidelines are to be integrated into food and nutrition policies, they are articulated and understood so policy makers in leadership positions who have the political will be able to implement them in other programs (8).

Dietary guidelines at present provide general principles, rather than highly specific guidance for specific subgroups. They are usually crafted to ensure that those who follow them meet quantitative dietary reference standards such as the DRIs.

Effective dietary guidelines link to and interconnect with other nutrition education efforts and authoritative guidance.

DIETARY GUIDELINES DEVELOPMENT PROCESS

The process of producing dietary guidelines begins with marshalling the scientific evidence and expert judgment to produce their scientific foundation for the recommendations.

Information Needed to Formulate Guidelines

Critical information needed includes data on current consumption of foods, including data on fortified foods and on nutrient-containing dietary supplements. Also needed are the current incidence, prevalence, and trends of diet-related public health problems. Data on links between diet or nutrients and disease and on whether dietary interventions are feasible are also useful (9).

Developing the Scientific Rationale for Dietary Guidelines

Judgment

Qualified experts in the areas under discussion must review and analyze the data and develop the scientific rationale for the recommendations. Even when systematic evidence-based reviews are used, the process is still somewhat subjective, although less so than when conclusions are reached by more arbitrary methods.

Expert Advisory Committee of Scientists

Scientific issues are best evaluated by scientific experts who are independent and free from bias. Advisory committees of such experts are useful in raising, addressing, and resolving scientific controversies that arise in formulating dietary guidelines. When the advisory committee is composed of members from outside of government, the danger of undue government pressure or excessive partisan political influence on the guideline formulation process is somewhat lessened.

A committee of unpaid, volunteer scientific experts is used in formulating the *Dietary Guidelines for Americans* (11). The experts are chosen from nominees after public announcement by the US Department of Agriculture (USDA) and the US Department of Health and Human Services, the two agencies that sponsor the report. In addition to scientific expertise, other factors must be considered, such as representation and balance in terms of race or ethnicity, gender, and geographic diversity, disciplinary expertise, and eminence. For the recommendations to be viewed as credible, the members of the expert committee must have open minds, must be unbiased, and must reveal and disclose potential conflicts of interest of a financial, ideologic, or institutional nature.

Methods for Reviewing the Scientific Evidence

Methods are needed to build the scientific case for the various dietary recommendations in dietary guidelines. Although scientists strive to review the literature completely and to base their conclusions on the best scientific evidence, it is now apparent that the methods used to review evidence in the literature may influence conclusions reached.

Until recently, the US dietary guidelines and perhaps many others were developed and revised using a consensus of expert opinion based on an expert review of reviews that was supplemented by newer studies. However, these processes are not always carried out in a systematic and comprehensive manner, and thus the conclusions reached may vary, even on the same question.

The 2005 dietary guidelines committee in the United States made the transition toward a more systematic, evidence-based approach (12). Structured, evidence-based reviews of the literature are formal methods for decision making about what types of literature and what data should be used in reviewing the evidence on associations among diet, health, and disease. The systems used for conducting these reviews vary, but all involve formulation of very specific questions about the problem or area of uncertainty being considered by experts in the field. Usually, the question has to do with a relationship between a dietary factor and some disease that is thought to be associated with it. The selection criteria that are used to survey studies and the analytic framework for evaluating them are also specified and applied. A comprehensive and systematic review of the literature using specific search terms and databases is then performed to find evidence on the topic. The literature identified is filtered and assessed in an objective manner for relevance to the question by examining abstracts of the studies or the full studies, if necessary. The evidence in each study is amassed and objectively assessed for its scientific quality. In general, more weight is paid to experimental studies such as randomized controlled trials, metaanalyses of several such trials, and quasiexperimental designs.

Observational studies such as cohort, case-control, cross-sectional, before-and-after studies and case series are given lesser weight because of the greater potential for confounding (13). One example of an evidence review is a monograph on assessing and treating overweight (14). Great emphasis is also placed on the definition of the interventions, the use of equal, reliable, and valid measures in the study, and assessment of each outcome separately in evaluating intervention studies. In addition, implementation of the design, avoidance of potential confounders, attrition, adjustment for intent to treat, and other possible influences are examined (15). All the available studies that meet the criteria are assessed, and metaanalyses are performed if appropriate. The conclusions, along with the strength of the supporting evidence, are then presented. Dietary guidelines can then be developed using this information (16, 17).

TABLE 105.1. DIETARY GUIDELINE IN VARIOUS EDITIONS OF THE DIETARY GUIDELINES FOR AMERICANS

1980	1985	1990	1995	2000	2005
Eat a variety of foods	→	→	→	Let the pyramid guide your food choices	Consume a variety of foods within and among the basic food groups while staying within energy needs
Maintain ideal weight	Maintain desirable weight	Maintain healthy weight	Balance the food you eat with physical activity to maintain or improve your weight	Aim for a healthy weight	Control calorie intake to manage body weight
				Be physically active each day	Be physically active each day
Avoid too much fat, saturated fat, and cholesterol	→	Choose a diet low in fat, saturated fat, and cholesterol	→	Choose a diet low in saturated fat and cholesterol and moderate in total fat	Choose fats wisely for good health
Eat foods with adequate starch and fiber	→				
Avoid too much sugar	→	Use sugars only in moderation	Choose a diet moderate in sugars	Choose beverages and foods to moderate your intake of sugars	Choose carbohydrates wisely for good health
		Choose a diet with plenty of vegetables, fruits, and grain products	Choose a diet with plenty of grains, vegetables, and fruits	Choose a variety of fruits and vegetables daily	Increase daily intake of fruits and vegetables, whole grains, and nonfat or low-fat milk and milk products
				Choose a variety of grains, including whole grains	Increase daily intake of fruits and vegetables, whole grains, and nonfat or low-fat milk and milk products
Avoid too much sodium	→	Use salt and sodium only in moderation	Choose a diet moderate in salt and sodium	Choose and prepare foods with less salt	Choose and prepare foods with little salt
If you drink alcohol, do so in moderation	→	→	→	→	If you drink alcohol, do so in moderation
				Keep foods safe to eat	Keep foods safe to eat

Table 105.1 shows that although both processes require expert judgment, the evidence provided and the review process are likely to be different and somewhat more comprehensive with systematic, evidence-based reviews than with less structured methods. For this reason, these reviews are being used more extensively in development of guidelines of all types.

Systematic, evidence-based reviews have rarely been used in reviewing the literature to formulate dietary guidelines, for several reasons. Very few nutritional data are available from randomized controlled clinical trials, especially when the question involves the effects of food or food patterns on health, rather than on more narrowly focused questions. When these data are available, the study groups may be so narrowly defined that the findings cannot be generalized to larger populations. Appropriate evidence is often unavailable, and therefore causal inference is limited. Consensus is currently lacking on the appropriate hierarchy and weighting for the quality and strength of evidence on questions about nutrition in the absence of randomized studies. Often, "hard" outcomes such as mortality or morbidity are unavailable, and so biomarkers or modifications of risk factors must be taken as the indicators of health effects, involving additional assumptions about the causal chain. The systematic review process was originally developed for assessing clinical evidence for the efficacy of interventions, such as drugs, on health. It may be less suitable for decision making involving dietary guidance.

The factors that must be weighed in providing advice on day-to-day eating decisions include not only health but food preferences, taste, cost, and other issues. In addition, government officials may not believe that the investment in structured reviews to answer questions relating to dietary advice more definitively is critical because downstream costs to government from inappropriate dietary advice are more difficult to reckon than are the costs of misjudging evidence for the efficiency of something such as a surgical procedure paid for by government funds. Finally, many nutrition scientists still lack familiarity with the systematic, evidence-based review process and often do not recognize its utility.

Staff

The voluntary nature of committee membership, the volume of new scientific information, and the limited time and money available for volunteers to meet together to formulate dietary guidelines place much of the burden of assembling relevant data and preparing it on the secretariat. In the United States, the secretariat consists of federal employees or consultants who are temporarily detailed and assigned to the task.

Public Comment

Public comment is helpful throughout the process. In the United States, mandatory public comment periods are built into the process to permit stakeholders to voice their opinions.

Role of Sponsoring Agencies in Adopting Advisory Committee Report and Issuing Guidelines

In the United States, the expert committee report and recommendations for the dietary guidelines are published separately. The USDA and the US Department of Health and Human Services, the two sponsoring cabinet level departments, retain the authority to accept, adapt, or reject the expert advisory committee's recommendations and to disseminate dietary guidelines. In fact, since 1980, committee recommendations have usually been followed by the agencies, with modifications restricted to slight changes in wording.

Constructing and Modeling Food-Related Recommendations During Dietary Guideline Development

The process of developing and testing food-based dietary guidelines is well described elsewhere and is summarized briefly here (4, 6, 9). Target foods or food patterns for public health nutrition programs are identified from an analysis of prevailing food and nutrient intakes. Major food sources of the nutrients of interest are then identified. Foods contributing substantially to population intakes because of their frequency of consumption are also noted. Foods or food patterns that are compatible with desirable nutrient intakes or that explain variations in nutrient intakes are identified. If data on food consumption are available at the level of the individual, key foods or food patterns fulfilling nutrient goals can be identified, and correlations between foods and nutrients in diets or the intakes of compliers and noncompliers with dietary guidelines can be assessed using factor analysis and discriminant function analysis. If nutrient-containing dietary supplement use is common, the contributions to total intakes must also be considered.

Once a tentative set of guidelines is developed, it is necessary to determine how well the proposed recommendations are likely to fit with current food availability and food consumption patterns. Modeling techniques help to estimate the likely effects of various possible recommendations on consumption. Successive approximations can be used to develop implementable recommendations that specify foods, portion sizes, and frequency of intake. Attainability, acceptability, and compatibility of the guidelines with existing dietary habits can be assessed by comparing recommended and actual consumption patterns.

COMMUNICATING AND IMPLEMENTING DIETARY GUIDELINES

Once the dietary guidelines have been determined, they must be communicated to the public (18).

Communicability

Dietary guidelines must be easy for consumers to understand, useful, realistic, practical, and flexible. Comprehensibility can be ensured by message testing before finalization of the messages. The recommendations and the foods or food groups that are mentioned must be stated in forms that are used by and are recognizable to the public. The foods suggested must be commonly used and available. To be flexible, information on how to adopt the dietary guidelines to individual eating habits and preferences is needed. Until recently in the United States, it was customary to have the scientific advisory committee craft the communications messages. Although this may have avoided an additional layer of review and interpretation and possible distortion, the committee members were not communication experts. The 2005 Dietary Guidelines for Americans committee provided specific recommendations for the content of the main dietary guidelines messages and supporting details, but they left the wording of the guidelines in consumer documents to communications experts. Detailed guidance on key messages, additional important information, and recommendations on means of achieving flexibility were provided in the 2005 report to ensure fidelity of translation of the science (12).

Actionability

Dietary recommendations are unlikely to be implemented if they stray too far from the realities of everyday life in terms of cost, current consumption patterns, food availability, and consumer preferences. Factors such as economics, food preferences, food habits, taste, fit with the existing food supply, and sustainability of the diet must also be considered in implementing dietary guidelines (19). These factors are equally, if not more, important in influencing dietary choice than is authoritative health advice.

Strategies for Implementation

Implementation requires political will and the expenditure of political capital by decision makers. Strategies to close gaps between guideline recommendations and current consumption include altering the types and amounts of foods consumed, stressing rich food sources of nutrients, using fortified food sources, and using dietary supplements for specific groups.

Adoption and Use of Guidelines by Public and Private Groups

Guidelines must also be understood and implemented in government policy. This includes other nutritional guidance, such as on food labels and graphics, and food programs. Voluntary coalitions of private and voluntary groups can help to disseminate these guidelines further.

Procedures Used in Other Countries

The examples in this chapter are drawn primarily from the evolution of the *Dietary Guidelines for Americans.* Canada has followed a somewhat different process in revising its dietary guidelines (20). Health Canada used two committees, a scientific committee and a communications and implementation committee. They deliberated and finally issued a more scientifically based document in 1977 entitled *Nutrition Recommendations for Canadians* and a set of guidelines targeted to the consumer entitled *Canada's Guidelines for Healthy Eating* in 1991. Australia, New Zealand, and the European countries have formulated dietary goals and guidelines using a variety of processes, and so has the World Health Organization (1, 9, 21, 22).

HISTORY OF DIETARY GUIDELINES: EXAMPLE OF THE UNITED STATES

Evolution of the Dietary Guidelines for Americans

Table 105.2 presents the recommendations in various editions of the *Dietary Guidelines for Americans* from 1980 until 2005 (12, 23–28). The early history of dietary guide-lines in the United States reveals that dietary recommendations reflect the nutrition-related problems of the era, the society's social context and physical environment, and the science of the times (29). Nutritionists' thinking about dietary guidance has evolved from an emphasis on deficiency, a foundation diet, getting enough to eat and enough of the essential nutrients to a gradual shift toward greater recognition of balance, variety, and moderation, and avoiding excess. Dietary advice has become increasingly complex over the past century, and so have the *Dietary Guidelines for Americans.* This document now includes not only goals of achieving nutrient adequacy but also goals relating to variety, moderation, balance, proportionality, and avoidance of excess to help consumers to make healthful food choices.

1970s and 1980s: Dietary Goals for the United States and *Dietary Guidelines for Americans:* Emphasis on Balance and Moderation

In the 1960s and 1970s, the associations between diet and certain chronic degenerative diseases became clearer. In 1977, the role of diet in chronic degenerative disease was examined in a series of oversight hearings by the US Senate Select Committee on Nutrition and Human Needs. The committee issued a staff report entitled *Dietary Goals for the United States* that provided national as well as individual targets for consumption. There was much discussion and dissent in Congress and in the nutritional community about the document's recommendations and its effects on production agriculture and the animal industry (8). To evaluate the evidence for the diet disease links, an expert group was assembled by the American Society for Clinical Nutrition (ASCN). It issued a set of recommendations that supported many, but not all, of those proposed in the Senate Select Committee report (30). In 1980, the USDA and the US Department of Health, Education and Welfare issued the first edition of the *Dietary Guidelines for Americans,* which reflected the ASCN guidelines (24). The ASCN guidelines, which gave qualitative goals, rather than the quantitative recommendations of the Senate Select Committee, were also incorporated into the first edition of *Healthy People,* recommendations from the National Academy of Sciences to the Department of Health, Education and Welfare on dietary and other objectives for promoting health and preventing disease in the United States (31).

Since the 1990s, professional organizations, voluntary groups, and government have been broadly supportive of the principles embodied in the *Dietary Guidelines for Americans,* and the process of formulating them has been marked with less bitterness. The authorizing legislation initially passed by Congress as part of the National Nutrition Monitoring and Related Research Act required the Secretaries of Agriculture and Health and Human Services jointly to publish a report entitled *Dietary Guidelines for Americans*

TABLE 105.2. TWO DIFFERENT DECISION-MAKING METHODS FOR GENERATING DIETARY GUIDELINES

	CONSENSUS OF EXPERT OPINION	EXPERT OPINION BASED ON STRUCTURED, SYSTEMATIC EVIDENCE-BASED REVIEW
Process	Recommendations are the opinions of the expert group as expressed in consensus and buttressed by appropriate citations in the scientific literature. Problems are identified by various processes, including expert opinion and public input, and by a relatively nonsystematic review of the literature. Expert opinion is used to obtain evidence and to produce the guidelines	Judgments of experts are based on evidence produced to respond to questions formally stated on the effectiveness of specific interventions using systematic reviews of the literature to answer questions using standardized methods and grading of the strength or weakness of the evidence.
Pros	It has historical precedent. Expert judgment can be used to a greater extent. Informal discussion is common. Many areas of nutrition have limited evidence, and so ultimately the verdict will rely heavily on judgment regardless of the process used. Costs are less. The process is more sensitive to public opinion and political climate.	It is considered "state of the art." It is transparent: systematically assembled evidence with explicit inclusion and exclusion criteria. Clear statements of what was considered relevant can be made. The strength of the evidence is stated and graded. New studies can be incorporated and evaluated in the body of the evidence. It may include formal processes to obtain consensus without a few powerful individuals' dominating the discussion.
Cons	Committee members have more personal influence on the process. Topics chosen to focus on and search of the literature may be limited. Opinions of experts are given more weight. Bias is possible because of incomplete knowledge of the literature and prior opinions of experts. Different experts include different types of searches even for the same topic.	It is expensive. It is time consuming, particularly early on in the process. Nonexperts often end up doing most of the work. Graders of the literature may not be expert and may operate mechanically in a manner that may miss important errors or findings. Literature searches may lag actual publications by many months or years. It is inherently conservative. The technique was originally designed for evaluating intervention studies, not nutritional questions. Results may be politically unsupportable.

(7 U.S.C.5341) every 5 years. Although that legislation has now expired, the reports continue to be issued (12, 24–28).

1990s and Early 2000s: Convergence of Guidance

Davis and Saltos provided a useful review of recommendations up until the 1990s (32). The USDA's Food Guide Pyramid and the first Healthy Eating Index (HEI), the tool for evaluating adherence to some of the guidelines, were also published during the 1990s (33).

Until 1995, only seven guidelines were included. In 2000, ten guidelines were provided, and they fell into three categories. In the 2005 version, there are nine guidelines and two major themes: consuming a variety of foods from the basic foods groups and controlling caloric intakes.

Year 2000 Dietary Guidelines: Expanded Emphasis on Weight and Fitness

Until the year 2000, the guidelines started with an emphasis on variety; after that, the first guideline emphasized aiming for fitness (aim for a healthy weight and be physically active each day). In the *Dietary Guidelines for Americans* published in 2000, after much debate over whether the USDA's Food Guide Pyramid should be mentioned, the pyramid concept was given a guideline of its own; the

"Eat a variety of foods" guideline of 1995 was changed to "Let the pyramid guide your food choices," to provide more specificity regarding meaning and to stress the guidelines goal of achieving variety among food groups. The guidelines also emphasized variety within food groups, endorsed the notion that plant foods were the foundation of the diet, stressed the necessity of proportionality in dietary choice, and added a food safety guideline (34–36).

Year 2005 Dietary Guidelines: Harmonization of Federal Guidance

Since the year 2000, the trend has been toward increasing fusion of the dietary guidelines with the newly reformulated DRIs for nutrients and the USDA's Food Guide Pyramid, which is currently being revised.

The emphasis on avoidance of overweight and sedentary lifestyles was maintained in the 2005 committee report. The major difference between the 2005 and 2000 and previous guidelines is that sugars were not explicitly mentioned in 2005, although a recommendation for limiting intakes of added sugars is provided under the topic listed as "Choose carbohydrates wisely," and also elsewhere when calorie intake levels are stressed.

The 2005 *Dietary Guidelines for Americans* required nearly 3 years for planning, implementation, and report production (11). The 2005 Dietary Guidelines Committee consisted of 13 members. The committee was unique in the challenges it faced, the systematic evidence-based review process it adopted, and the way in which its findings were communicated.

The major impetus for the 2005 revision was that dietary standards (the so-called DRIs) for all essential nutrients had been revised by the Food and Nutrition Board, Institute of Medicine, National Academy of Sciences (37–43) (see Chapter 104). A challenge to the committee was whether or how to incorporate concepts and quantitative targets such as tolerable upper intake levels (ULs) for several micronutrients and ranges of acceptable macronutrient distribution ranges for healthy adults (AMDRs), as well as guidance on energy needs and energy output in the presence of the country's obesity epidemic. Another challenge was to assess the effects of mandatory fortification of grains with folic acid and to incorporate the new science that had been published on clinical trials involving various nutrients since 2000.

The 2005 committee started its review "from scratch" (12). It set a new standard by incorporating more formal, systematic evidence-based reviews in the process of developing dietary guidance than in the past. Existing evidence reviews were used to document several key conclusions reached, and the committee conducted its own formal systematic evidence reviews for 34 major questions that arose during the course of its deliberations. The committee also used an evidence-based process for modeling food intakes and to develop some appreciation of the likely consumption outcomes of different scenarios. The original food modeling system, used to develop the USDA's Food Guide Pyramid, was updated to include current food consumption patterns and the most recent DRIs for nutrients (44).

Another innovation was that the 2005 guidelines committee report was solely a scientific report, rather than an amalgam of both a consumer document and a scientific justification. Communications experts were engaged to develop consumer versions of the guideline messages.

When translated into food, the 2005 guidelines give more emphasis to consumption of unsaturated fats and oils, whole grains, legumes, and dark green vegetables in dietary patterns.

DIETARY GUIDELINES AND HEALTH OUTCOMES

Criteria

The ultimate test of the success of dietary guidelines is that they improve dietary intakes. Long-term adherence to the guidelines should also improve health outcomes.

Available Evidence Not Definitive

Relatively little evidence is currently available on the extent to which the *Dietary Guidelines for Americans*

improve either dietary intakes or more general health outcomes. Few definitive studies and no clinical trials are available that have evaluated the diet or health outcomes of adhering to these dietary guidelines.

No perfect tool exists for assessing the eating patterns recommended by the *Dietary Guidelines for Americans.* Partial surrogate measures used to examine health outcomes include the recommended food score (RFS) (45), the HEI (33), the modified Dietary Guidelines Index (a modified version of the HEI to assess the Year 2000 Dietary Guidelines) (46), and the alternative HEI (47). The HEI is an index that assesses adherence to certain specific guidelines (fat, cholesterol saturated fat, sodium and variety) and to eating at least the minimum number of servings specified in the USDA's Food Guide Pyramid. It awards credits for meeting or exceeding the pyramid servings goals for variety, grains, vegetables, fruit, milk, and meat and for not exceeding the *Dietary Guidelines for Americans* for total fat, saturated fat, cholesterol, and sodium. US adults generally score about 64 out of a perfect HEI score of 100, a finding suggesting a great deal of room for improvement (33). Two studies assessed adherence to some of the guidelines as measured by a modified version of the HEI on both cardiovascular health and risk of all diet-related chronic degenerative disease as outcomes among a cohort of male health professionals. Cardiovascular disease risk was decreased, but other chronic disease was not decreased among those with higher scores on the modified HEI (48). Among a large cohort of female health professionals, only a weak relationship between such scores and cardiovascular disease was evident (49).

Kant and associates found associations with an RFS and health outcomes (45). In the National Health Interview surveys for 1987 to 1992, following recommended dietary behaviors was associated with decreases of 9% in female and 16% in male mortality rates (50).

Increasing scores on the modified HEI were associated with decreased total cancer incidence, and especially of colon cancer, in the Iowa Women's Health Study cohort (46). Adherence to the American Institute of Cancer Research's cancer prevention recommendations, which are similar in many respects to the *Dietary Guidelines for Americans,* was linked to decreases in morbidity and mortality in the same cohort (51). Another study used counts of daily servings of fruits, vegetables, and whole grains, an RFS, and the HEI to define diet quality and found that overall compliance with the *Dietary Guidelines for Americans* using these criteria protected against early age-related nuclear lens opacities in older women in the Nurses' Health Study cohort (52).

Criticisms of the Dietary Guidelines

Over the past decade, many alternative sets of dietary guidelines have been developed by persons who believed that the existing dietary guidelines fell short in one or more respects and that their versions were superior. However, to date, convincing differences in health outcomes have not been demonstrated.

One alternative sets of guidelines is based on the dietary patterns associated with lowest cardiovascular risk in large cohorts that have been followed prospectively (47). The problem is that the same cohorts were used for developing and testing the components that later became the new alternative guidelines. The alternative guidelines thus provide a self-fulfilling prophecy. Because of the problem of confounding that plagues cohort studies, additional tests are needed before alternative guidelines can be accepted. An independent test of such guidelines in other populations would be more convincing.

Today, data are lacking to decide which of the many competing dietary guidelines that have been issued in the United States is "best." Neither randomized trials nor other definitive tests of the effects of the *Dietary Guidelines for Americans* or for alternative recommendations are available. What can be said is that the differences among these guidelines are small. Compared with having no eating pattern at all, or food guides that focus only on achieving adequacy, any of these guidelines represent an improvement. Epidemiology has a role in developing dietary guidelines, but it is only one of many different types of relevant evidence (53–55). However, the current standard is an empiric test in a clinical trial, with the guidelines pitted against usual eating patterns or against each other.

Clinical Trials of Dietary Guidelines?

Observational studies have unavoidable problems of confounding, and therefore it is important to consider stronger research designs in the future. The health effects of the *Dietary Guidelines for Americans* could be examined experimentally in randomized clinical trials with intent-to-treat analyses using chronic disease biomarkers to determine whether those who followed the dietary guidelines had better diets, lesser risk factors, and better health than those who did not.

CONCLUSIONS

Those who wish to formulate dietary guidelines can learn much from the successes and failures of others since 1980. It is important to capitalize on successful strategies and to avoid those that have generated controversy and rancor.

What Works Well

During the 1970s, the process of formulating dietary goals and guidelines was marked by bitterness because it was viewed by the stakeholders as overly politicized. Ultimately, dietary guidelines are based on subjective decisions and not solely on science or logical processes. In the United States, after a stormy start in the 1970s, a process

for generating dietary guidelines evolved that seems to work well. The secret of success is to keep an appropriate balance between science and politics. The process of evaluating the science base and evidence for guidelines development has become institutionalized in the nutrition science establishment, rather than in congressional committees. In addition, the role of diet in chronic degenerative disease has become clearer, and a paradigm shift has occurred favoring the view that, in fact, such diet-disease relationships exist. Finally, nutrition scientists have become somewhat more sophisticated in giving advice to government (56).

The notion of authoritative nutritional guidance issued by government and endorsed by a panel of distinguished scientists is now well accepted. A rigorous process for declaring, reviewing, and disclosing conflicts of interest of scientific advisors is in place The public comment process and public deliberations are popular with stakeholders. The periodic and predictable review of the data every 5 years has become well accepted in most government circles. The practice of providing explicit documentation for the guideline recommendations and for further research is also expected and useful.

The dietary guidelines produce sound and durable nutritional guidance After 25 years, in spite of continual updating and much new science, the overall messages have remained remarkably constant, with only minor modifications.

Needed Improvements

Table 105.3 provides some suggestions for further strengthening the process of developing dietary guidelines in the future.

Goals

It is important to pay greater attention to the associations between adherence to the dietary guidelines and health outcomes. Outcome criteria for measuring adherence to the dietary guidelines need to be agreed on and measured (57). Adherence to the *Dietary Guidelines for Americans* should increase the likelihood of obtaining recommended intakes of nutrients and macronutrient intakes within acceptable macronutrient distribution ranges. For individuals, intakes should be at or above the recommended dietary allowances, below the ULs, and within the Food and Nutrition Board's newly established AMDRs for macronutrients. For groups, intake distributions should decrease the prevalence of intakes outside the ranges when the guidelines are followed. Adherence to the guidelines should also promote moderation, not only of salt, fat, and sugar, but also of alcoholic beverages and in intakes of foods that provide energy but few nutrients.

Adherence to the guidelines should also improve general health outcomes, including a physically active life and a body weight within healthy limits. Biomarkers for various

TABLE 105.3. RECOMMENDATIONS FOR FURTHER IMPROVING DIETARY GUIDELINES DEVELOPMENT

ISSUE AND RATIONALE	COMMENTS
Audience: If audience is both consumers and policy makers, ???	Policy needs must be addressed more explicitly in guidelines development, and more explicit policy statements need to be made.
Focus: The current focus is on maximizing population public health.	Adherence to dietary recommendations rarely succeeds by appeals to health alone. Broadening the focus to consider taste, food preferences, cost, equity, and sustainability issues may be helpful.
Budget: Adoption of an evidence-based review process for the dietary guidelines requires a large budget, especially in the first few years, when evidence bases on various questions must be developed.	Budgets and staff at the sponsoring agencies must be increased, or existing evidence-based practice centers or other expert groups must be enlisted to assist in the process. Once databases are established, maintenance should be less expensive.
Periodicity: Review and revisions every 5 years may be inappropriate and premature.	Most of the prior revisions in the dietary guidelines have been minor, suggesting that some of the revisions may not have been necessary. Some possible reasons for reviewing the dietary guidelines include changes in dietary reference intake standards or the food supply, need for harmonization with other guidelines, and evidence of ineffectiveness. Lengthening the intervals between reviews means loss of staff, budget, and continuity.
Process: Move from a consensus developed from expert opinion and informal review to formal processes for evaluating the evidence. Experts spend more time reviewing wording of public comments than discussing the science. Deliberations are public and reported verbatim, leading to posturing and making bargaining difficult.	Experts need to spent more time formulating evidence reviews, deliberating about them, examining past success/failure of implementation and adherence, and plans for future efforts.
Evidence: Evidence-based reviews are needed for many issues confronting the dietary guidelines committee suitable for population-based guidelines. More systematic reviews will permit more standardized and objective assessment of the evidence.	Better models must be developed for evidence-based reviews to generate dietary guidance for individuals within the population, including (a) models are needed for deciding what level of certainty is necessary for guidance in the absence of evidence from randomized clinical trials, (b) the hierarchy of evidence systems to evaluate individual research reports and systems on the strength of the evidence for dietary relationships, (c) science linking diet to chronic degenerative disease by specifying the strength of the evidence for each dietary guidelines statement.
	If evidence-based reviews are done of all the relevant questions confronting the dietary guidelines committee, they will exceed the goodwill and time of experts. The staff, time, and budgets of the federal agencies charged with carrying out these reviews are also likely to be exceeded.
	The means for developing and updating the evidence base in an ongoing fashion need to be put in place.
	Personnel and budgets must be greatly expanded if evidence-based reviews are to be employed more extensively in the future.
Politics: The dietary guidelines comprise a policy document developed by a combination of a political process and scientific deliberations. Acceptance or rejection for ultimate use is also a political process.	The guidelines process is inherently a hybrid model.
Product: The dietary guidelines are used by many different audiences, with differing wants and needs. The products need more tailoring for specific purposes.	Tailor specific products to specific audiences. The scientific justification for health professionals is appropriate as is. The consumer material needs additional review and revision by communications professionals. Policy and public health products have not yet been developed and should be.
Communication: Guidelines are meant to be communicated to consumers and policy makers. They are developed by a scientific expert panel with little expertise in either communication or policy.	A second tier of review by communications experts may be needed for consumer and policy applications; simply adding a member or members to the committee with the particular expertise may disrupt the process. Booklets for consumers may need to be developed and tested by communications professionals to ensure that intended messages are in fact communicated. Policy issues may be raised more explicitly in public comment periods and in charge to committee.
Implementation and application to population eating habits: In spite of widespread dissemination, there is little adherence to the dietary guidelines.	More research on means to bring about dietary behavior change in line with the dietary guidelines is needed.
	Specifically, studies are needed on the impact of dietary guidelines on populations by monitoring intakes, health behaviors, biomarkers of risk, and health outcomes.

TABLE 105.3. RECOMMENDATIONS FOR FURTHER IMPROVING DIETARY GUIDELINES DEVELOPMENT (continued)

ISSUE AND RATIONALE	COMMENTS
Application to individual eating habits: Dietary guidelines provide a description of healthful types of food choices but little tailored guidance for eating decisions by individuals.	Tailor guidelines to individuals.
Application to the food supply: Associations among the dietary guidelines recommendations, the food supply, and changes in the food supply are unclear.	Government and industry need to monitor and track these impacts better.
Research: Recommendations for further research provided by each dietary guidelines committee are rarely acted on before the next dietary guidelines committee begins, so evidence to answer many important questions is lacking.	Policy makers should implement dietary guidelines-related research.

chronic degenerative diseases should show changes in positive directions when the *Dietary Guidelines for Americans* are followed compared with a diet chosen haphazardly from what is available on the market. The public should be less likely to suffer from alcohol abuse and from "self-inflicted" food-borne illness owing to inappropriate food handling and storage.

Process

The establishment of a permanent secretariat within government would lessen the repeated work and confusion that result from disbanding and then restaffing dietary guidelines-related functions every 5 years. In addition, more attention needs to be paid to evidence-based reviews of the literature based on well-formulated questions and evaluation methods that are tailored to dietary studies. Because systematic evidence-based reviews are costly and labor intensive, additional resources are likely to be needed. A more systematic and formal means for considering and implementing the recommended research agendas developed by dietary guidelines committees would be helpful. The process of translating dietary guidelines into consumer-friendly advice with fidelity to the underlying scientific recommendations needs to be refined and formalized. More explicit attention needs to be paid to ensuring that eating according to the dietary guidelines is possible and reasonable from the economic standpoint and that it occurs (58). Partnerships among government, private, and voluntary groups for communicating the dietary guidelines need to be strengthened.

Communication

Over the past 25 years, dietary guidelines both in the United States and abroad have become more quantitative. Now they specify amounts, rather than simply the direction of consumption (e.g., eat less). This improvement makes the guidelines more actionable and measurable, but it also means that greater individualization in messages is needed. The appropriate balance between qualitative and quantitative statements needs to be given consideration. Appropriate levels of tailoring and individualization of the guidelines need attention. Guidelines or eating plans for those of different age, sex, and activity levels are biologically appropriate and useful. More tailoring of guidelines to those with different demographic characteristics, social or lifestyle habits, cultural beliefs, unique eating habits, and available food supplies may increase use of the guidelines, but such efforts will entail considerable market research and communication costs. Individualized, personalized guidelines designed for each individual's unique genetic endowment have also been suggested, but at present, the nutrigenomics sciences are not yet advanced enough to make this practical or valid (59).

Implementation

The cabinet-level departments of the federal government have many programs that may be affected by alterations in the *Dietary Guidelines for Americans*. Some programs are required by law to reflect these changes. In actuality, the extent to which programs and other guidance measures are linked to the dietary guidelines varies. More attention needs to be paid to harmonization among dietary guidelines, nutrient labels on foods and dietary supplements, and icons or graphics, such as the USDA's Food Guide Pyramid with respect to portion sizes and standards for nutrients. The potential for closer linkages exists, but a great deal remains to be done (60). Guidelines also should be linked to those of other countries

Challenges for the Future

Players

There has been agitation in some quarters for moving the dietary guideline development process from the two cabinet-level departments into the Institute of Medicine of the National Academy of Sciences, and this issue may be debated again in the next few years. No doubt, there are pros and cons to such a proposal. However, the National Academy of Sciences is not a government policy-making body that can impose its will on the executive departments of government. Such a development could distance the guidelines development process from the realities of health care delivery, food production, and consumption considerations. Although recommendations could be of scientific interest, they could fall short from the practical standpoint. The process would not necessarily be more transparent or accessible to stakeholders than it is currently. Moreover, the expertise of the secretariat within the relevant federal agencies would not be available.

Process

Standard setting always involves judgments, and good scientists disagree, particularly when the scientific evidence on an issue is not definitive, science is emerging, or the evidence is weak. For example, in the 2000 *Dietary Guidelines for Americans*, the sugars guideline was especially controversial (61, 62). Statements on the strength of the evidence would be particularly helpful with controversial guidelines.

Content

The call for age-specific guidelines continues, particularly for infants less than 2 years of age, adolescents, and elders more than 70 years of age (63, 64). Disease-specific guidelines are also popular as the distinctions among nutritional care, medical nutrition therapy, and population dietary guidelines are becoming blurred (17). Increasingly, dietary guidelines are being issued for those who are ill with specific diseases (65), and the trend is for dietetic practice guidelines to include dietary guidelines for patients (66). It will be a challenge to integrate all these recommendations into material useful for those at risk although not yet suffering from clinically evident disease.

Greater consideration is needed on the role of fortified foods and dietary supplements in guidelines development. Although food-based dietary guidelines are understandably focused on food, it is also true that dietary supplements are becoming increasingly common and contribute considerable amounts of some nutrients. Moreover, many foods are now fortified and have nutrient contributions beyond those of their basic commodities (67–70). At present, these realities are not taken into account in dietary guidelines modeling exercises. They need to be in the future, or more people could appear to have inadequate intakes of nutrients than would actually be the case.

There is a need to harmonize the proliferation of alternative dietary guidelines by voluntary and professional associations, each with slightly different emphases, to minimize consumer confusion. The existence of many different dietary guidelines directed toward the same groups may confuse the public.

Communication

Common types of dietary advice are likely to be appropriate for those with many chronic diseases, and thus there seems little point in having each organization issue its own guidelines (71).

Conclusion

The old adage that "all dietary problems are emotional, all solutions are technical, but all decisions are political" applies to dietary guidelines development. However, to improve nutritional guidance, scientists must continue to study nutritional problems and to generate the science needed to provide decision makers with the information needed to make wise decisions on dietary recommendations (56).

REFERENCES

1. Truswell AS. Dietary goals and guidelines: national and international perspectives. In: Shils ME, Olson JA, Shike M et al. Modern Nutrition in Health and Disease. 9th ed. Baltimore: Williams & Wilkins, 1999:1727–41.
2. Schneeman BO, Mendelson R. J Am Diet Assoc 2002;102:1498–500.
3. Dwyer J, Bermudez OI, Chwang LC et al. Dietary guidelines in three regions of the world. In: Berdanier CD, ed. Handbook of Nutrition and Food. Boca Raton, FL: CRC Press, 2002:353–71.
4. Sandstrom B. Public Health Nutr 2001;4:193–305.
5. Murphy SP. Nutrition guidelines to maintain health. In: Coulston AM, Rock CL, Monsen ER, eds. Nutrition in the Prevention and Treatment of Disease. San Diego: Academic Press, 2001:753–71.
6. Food and Agricultural Organization, World Health Organization. Food Based Dietary Guidelines. Rome: Food and Agricultural Organization, World Health Organization, 1995.
7. Dwyer J. Dietary reference intakes (DRI's): concepts and implementation. In: Johnson LR, ed. Encyclopedia of Gastroenterology. New York: Elsevier, 2004:613–23.
8. Dwyer J. Dietary recommendations and policy implications. In: Weininger J, Briggs GM, eds. Nuturition Update. New York: John Wiley, 1983:315–55.
9. Food and Agricultural Organization, World Health Organization. Preparation and Use of Food Based Dietary Guidelines. WHO Technical Report Series no. 880. Geneva: Food and Agriculture Organization, World Health Organization, 1998.
10. Dwyer JT. J Nutr 2001; 131:3074S–7S.
11. McMurray KY. J Am Diet Assoc 2003;103[Suppl 2]:10S–6S.
12. Dietary Guidelines Advisory Committee. Report of the Dietary Guidelines Advisory Committee on the Dietary Guidelines for Americans. Washington, DC: US Department of Health and Human Services, US Department of Agriculture, 2004.
13. National Health Service Centre for Reviews and Dissemination (CRD). CRD Report no. 4. Undertaking Systematic Reviews of Research on Effectiveness: CRD's Guidance for Those Carrying out or Commissioning Reviews. 2nd ed. York, UK: University of York, 2001.
14. National Heart, Lung and Blood Institute. Clinical Guidelines on the Identification, Evaluation, and Treatment of Overweight and Obesity in Adults: The Evidence Report. Publ. no. 98–4083. Bethesda, MD, National Institutes of Health, 1998.

15. Agency for Healthcare Research and Quality. Am J Prev Med 2001;20[Suppl]:21–34.

16. Cooper MJ, Zlotkin SH. J Am Diet Assoc 2003;103:28S–33S.

17. Myers E. J Am Diet Assoc 2003;103[Suppl 2]:34S–41S.

18. Committee on Dietary Guidelines Implementation, Thomas PR, ed. Improving America's Diet and Health: From Recommendations to Action. Washington, DC: National Academy Press, 1990.

19. Quandt SA. Social and cultural influences on food consumption and nutritional status. In: Shils ME, Olson JA, Shike M et al. Modern Nutrition in Health and Disease. 9th ed. Baltimore: Williams & Wilkins, 1999:1783–92.

20. Beaton GB. J Am Diet Assoc 2003;103:856–9.

21. Baghurst KI. J Am Diet Assoc 2003;103:7S–21S.

22. Joint WHO/FAO Expert Consultation on Diet, Nutrition and the Prevention of Chronic Disease. Diet, Nutrition and the Prevention of Chronic Diseases. Report of a Joint WHO/ FAO Expert Consultation Geneva Joint WHO FAO Expert Consultation on Diet, Nutrition and the Prevention of Chronic Disease Geneva: WHO, Technical Report Series no. 916–2002.

23. Hogbin M, Lyon J. Davis. Nutr Today 2003; 38:204–17.

24. US Department of Agriculture and US Department of Health and Human Services. Nutrition and Your Health: Dietary Guidelines for Americans. Home and Garden Bulletin no. 232. Washington, DC: US Government Printing Office, 1980.

25. US Department of Agriculture and US Department of Health and Human Services. Nutrition and Your Health: Dietary Guidelines for Americans. 2nd ed. Edition Home and Garden Bulletin no. 232. Washington, DC: US Government Printing Office, 1990.

26. US Department of Agriculture and US Department of Health and Human Services. Nutrition and Your Health: Dietary Guidelines for Americans. 3rd ed. Home and Garden Bulletin no. 232. Washington DC; US Government Printing Office, 1990.

27. US Department of Agriculture and US Department of Health and Human Services. Nutrition and Your Health: Dietary Guidelines for Americans. 4th ed. Home and Garden Bulletin no. 232. Washington, DC: US Government Printing Office, 1995.

28. US Department of Agriculture and US Department of Health and Human Services. Nutrition and Your Health: Dietary Guidelines for Americans. 5th ed. Home and Garden Bulletin no. 232. Washington, DC: US Government Printing Office, 2000.

29. Haughton B, Gussow JD, Dodds JM. J Nutr Ed 1987;19:169–75.

30. American Society for Clinical Nutrition. Am J Clin Nutr 1979;32[Suppl]:2610S–748S.

31. Public Health Service, US Department of Health, Education and Welfare. Healthy People: Surgeon General's Report on Health Promotion and Disease Prevention. PHS Publ. no. 70-55011. Washington, DC: US Department of Health, Education and Welfare, 1979.

32. Davis C, Saltos E. Dietary Recommendations and How They Have Changed Over Time. Washington, DC: US Department of Agriculture and Economic Research Service, 1995.

33. Kennedy ET, Ohls J, Carlson S et al. J Am Diet Assoc 1995;95:1003–9.

34. Keenan DP, Abusabha LR. J Am Diet Assoc 2001;101:631–4.

35. Schneeman BO. J Am Diet Assoc 2003;103[Suppl 2]:10S–6S.

36. Schneeman BO. J Am Diet Assoc 2001;101:742–3.

37. Food and Nutrition Board, Institute of Medicine. Dietary Reference Intakes for Energy, Carbohydrate, Fiber, Fat, Fatty Acids, Cholesterol, Protein, and Amino Acids. Part 1. Washington, DC: National Academy Press, 2002.

38. Food and Nutrition Board, Institute of Medicine. Dietary Reference Intakes for Energy, Carbohydrate, Fiber, Fat, Fatty Acids, Cholesterol, Protein, and Amino Acids. Part 2. Washington, DC: National Academy Press, 2002.

39. Food and Nutrition Board, Institute of Medicine. Dietary Reference Intakes for Water, Potassium, Sodium, Chloride and Sulfate. Washington, DC: National Academy Press, 2004.

40. Food and Nutrition Board, Institute of Medicine. Dietary Reference Intakes for Thiamin, Riboflavin, Niacin, Vitamin B_6, Folate, Vitamin B_{12}, Pantothenic Acid, Biotin, and Choline. Washington, DC: National Academy Press, 1998.

41. Food and Nutrition Board, Institute of Medicine. Dietary Reference Intakes for Vitamin A, Vitamin K, Arsenic, Boron, Chromium, Copper, Iodine, Iron, Manganese, Molybdenum, Nickel, Silicon, Vanadium, and Zinc. Washington, DC: National Academy Press, 2001.

42. Food and Nutrition Board, Institute of Medicine. Dietary Reference Intakes for Calcium, Phosphorus, Magnesium, Vitamin D, and Fluoride. Washington, DC: National Academy Press, 1997.

43. Food and Nutrition Board, Institute of Medicine. Dietary Reference Intakes for Vitamin C, Vitamin E, Selenium, and Carotenoids. Washington, DC: National Academy Press, 2000.

44. US Department of Agriculture. The Food Guide Pyramid. Home and Garden Bulletin no. 252. Washington, DC: US Government Printing Office, 1992.

45. Kant AK, Schatzkin A, Graubard BI et al. JAMA 2000;283:2109–15.

46. Harnack L, Nicodemus K, Jacobs DR et al. Am J Clin Nutr 2002;76:889–96.

47. McCullough M, Reskanich D, Stampfer MJ et al. Am J Clin Nutr 2002;76:1261–71.

48. McCullough ML, Feskanich D, Stampfer MJ et al. Am J Clin Nutr 2000;72:1214–22.

49. McCullough ML, Feskanich D, Rimm EB et al. Am J Clin Ntur 2000;732:1223–31.

50. Kant AK, Graubard BI, Schatzkin A. J Nutr 2004;134:1793–9.

51. Cerhan JR, Potter JD, Gilmore JM et al. Cancer Epidemiol Biomarkers Prev 2004;3:1114–20.

52. Moeller SM, Taylor A, Tucker KL et al. J Nutr 2004;134:1812–9.

53. Dietary Guidelines Advisory Committee. Report of the Dietary Guidelines Advisory Committee on the Dietary Guidelines for Americans. Beltsville, MD: US Department of Agriculture Agricultural Research Service, 2000.

54. Byers T. Am J Clin Nutr 1999;69[Suppl]:1304S–5S.

55. Truswell AS. Lancet 2001;357:1061–2.

56. Price DK. Government and Science: Their Dynamic Relation in American Democracy. New York: Oxford University Press, 1972.

57. Subcommittee on Interpretation and Uses of Dietary Reference Intakes and the Standing Committee on the Scientific Evaluation of Dietary Reference Intakes. Dietary Reference Intakes: Applications in Dietary Planning. Washington, DC: National Academy Press, 2003.

58. Guthrie JF, Smallwood DM. J Am Diet Assoc 2003;103:42S–9S.

59. Hoolihan LE. Nutr Today 2003;38:225–31.

60. Kennedy E. Dietary Guidelines, food guidance and dietary quality. In: Berdanier CD, ed. Handbook of Nutrition and Food. Boca Raton, FL: CRC Press, 2002:339–52.

61. Murphy SP, Johnson RK. Am J Clin Nutr 2003;78:827S–33S.

62. Frary CD, Johnson RK, Wang MQ. J Adolesc Health 2004;34:56–63.

63. McBean LD, Jarvis JK. Nutr Today 2003;38:218–24.

64. Life Sciences Research Office. Review and Assessment of the Scientific Basis for Dietary Guidelines for Children, Including Those of Less than Two Years of Age. Bethesda, MD: Life Sciences Research Office, American Society for Nutritional Sciences, 1999.

65. Neff LM. Nutr Clin Care 2003;6:51–61.

66. Hooper L, Griffiiths E, Abrahams B et al. J Hum Nutr Diet 2004;17:337–49.

67. Slexy U, Kersting M, Schultze-Pawlitscho V. Public Health Nutr 2003;6:697–702.

68. Stang J, Story MT, Harnack L et al. J Am Diet Assoc 2000; 100:905–10.

69. Sichert-Hellert W, Kerstling M, Alexy U et al. Eur J Clin Nutr 2000;54:81–6.

70. Sera-Majem L. Public Health Nutr 2001;4:101–7.

71. Eyre H, Kahn R, Robertson RM et al. Stroke 2004;35: 1999–2010.

SELECTED READINGS

Anderson GH, Blalock R, Harris S. J Am Diet Assoc 2003;103[Suppl 2]:3S–4S.

Dwyer J. Dietary recommendations and policy implications. In: Weininger J, Briggs GM, eds. Nutrition Update. New York: John Wiley, 1983:315–55.

Krebs-Smith S. J Nutr 2001;131:440S–535S.

Uauy Dagach R, Hertrampf E. Food based dietary recommendations: possibilities and limitations. In: Bowman BA, Russell RM, eds. Present Knowledge in Nutrition. 8th ed. Washington, DC: ILSI Press, 2001:636–49.

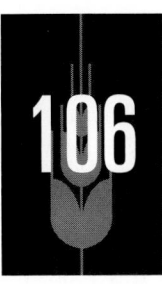

106 NUTRITION MONITORING IN THE UNITED STATES[1]

MARIE FANELLI KUCZMARSKI AND ROBERT J. KUCZMARSKI

HISTORICAL OVERVIEW 1688
NATIONAL NUTRITION MONITORING
    CORNERSTONE SURVEYS 1693
        Nationwide Food Consumption Survey 1693
        Continuing Survey of Food Intakes
            by Individuals 1694
        National Health and Nutrition
            Examination Survey 1695
        What We Eat in America: National Health
            and Nutrition Examination Survey 1696
OTHER NUTRITION MONITORING ACTIVITIES 1697
ACCOMPLISHMENTS AND LIMITATIONS OF THE
    NATIONAL NUTRITION MONITORING SYSTEM 1697
        Population Subgroup Coverage 1697
        Geographic Coverage .1698
CONCLUSION 1698

The nutrition monitoring program in the United States is regarded internationally for the quality, breadth, and detail of the nutrition and dietary data collected and has provided a benchmark for other countries for assessment of the health and nutritional status of their populations. A model national nutritional monitoring program has been described as one that possesses such features as a coordinated set of activities that responds to the diverse needs of its data users, provides data on a continuous basis, supports reliable inferences about all population groups and geographic areas,

[1]**Abbreviations: AMPM,** Automated Multiple Pass Method; **ASH,** Assistant Secretary for Health; **ARS,** Agricultural Research Service; **CDC,** Centers for Disease Control and Prevention; **CSFII,** Continuing Survey of Food Intake by Individuals; **DHHS,** United States Department of Health and Human Services; **DHKS,** Diet and Health Knowledge Survey; **IBNMRR,** Interagency Board for Nutrition Monitoring and Related Research; **JNMEC,** Joint Nutrition Monitoring Evaluation Committee; **LSRO,** Life Sciences Research Office; **NCHS,** National Center for Health Statistics; **NFCS,** Nationwide Food Consumption Survey; **NHANES,** National Health and Nutrition Examination Survey; **NHES,** National Health Examination Survey; **NNMRRA,** National Nutrition Monitoring and Related Research Act; **NNMRRP,** National Nutrition Monitoring and Related Research Program; **NNMS,** National Nutrition Monitoring System; **PedNSS;** Pediatric Nutrition Surveillance System; **PL,** public law; **PregNSS,** Pregnancy Nutrition Surveillance System; **USDA,** United States Department of Agriculture.

and assists state and local nutrition monitoring activities (1). The National Nutrition Monitoring and Related Research Program (NNMRRP) (Tables 106.1 and 106.2) in the United States is continually evolving. Despite its many accomplishments, it has known limitations with respect to these model features. For example, it does not completely describe the current dietary and nutritional status of selected subgroups of the US population, such as Native Americans residing on Indian reservations, Alaska Natives, persons without a place of residence (homeless persons), institutionalized persons, and persons with particular physiologic and nutritional characteristics. National nutritional surveys do provide data representative of the entire country and of major geographic regions, but not of states, counties, and cities.

Although various national surveys have been conducted since the 1930s, the US Congress and the executive branch of government did not mandate a comprehensive strategy for a coordinated program to strengthen existing national monitoring efforts until 1990. This strategy was designed to review and integrate the various federal surveys to provide timely, useful information that systematically addresses questions concerning the dietary and nutritional status of the US population. Thus, the National Nutrition Monitoring and Related Research Act (NNMRRA) of 1990, Public Law (PL) 101–445), was enacted to place the existing monitoring system, composed of interacting federal groups under an expanded program that includes related research. This program was designated to be guided by a specific 10-year plan under which action would be taken toward a goal of comprehensive national nutrition monitoring.

The NNMRRA defined nutrition monitoring as "the set of activities necessary to provide timely information about the role and status of factors that bear on the contribution that nutrition makes to the health of the people in the United States" (2). Nutrition monitoring is characterized by regular data collection, analysis and interpretation to provide a description of nutritional conditions in the population, and linkages with policy making and research. Monitoring provides a database for public policy decisions related to such issues as public health intervention programs, fortification, safety and labeling of the food supply, food assistance programs, and federally supported food service programs (3). It also assists in identifying

TABLE 106.1. GLOSSARY OF FEDERAL ACRONYMS

ARS: Agricultural Research Service
CDC: Centers for Disease Control and Prevention
CSFII: Continuing Survey of Food Intakes by Individuals
DHHS: Department of Health and Human Services
FASEB: Federation of American Societies for
    Experimental Biology
IBNMRR: Interagency Board for Nutrition Monitoring
    and Related Research
ICNM: Interagency Committee on Nutrition Monitoring
JNMEC: Joint Nutrition Monitoring Evaluation Committee
LSRO: Life Sciences Research Office (FASEB)
NFCS: Nationwide Food Consumption Survey
NHANES: National Health and Nutrition Examination Survey
NHES: National Health Examination Survey
NNMRA: National Nutrition Monitoring and Related
    Research Act
NNMRRP: National Nutrition Monitoring and Related
    Research Program
NNMS: National Nutrition Monitoring System
PedNSS: Pediatric Nutrition Surveillance System
PregNSS: Pregnancy Nutrition Surveillance System
USDA: United States Department of Agriculture
WIC: Women, Infants and Children

health and nutrition research priorities of public health significance such as food security and insecurity, thereby strengthening the research base for monitoring and policy making.

The five components of the US National Nutrition Monitoring System (NNMS) were specified in the 1987 Operational Plan as follows: (a) nutritional and health status measurements; (b) food consumption measurements; (c) food composition measurements and nutrient data banks; (d) dietary knowledge and attitude measurements; and (e) food supply and demand determinations (4). Although the titles of these components have been modified slightly in the 10-year plan for the NNMRRP, the content of these components remains essentially the same. See Table 106.2 for revised names.

This chapter provides a brief account of the historical development of the NNMS and the current NNMRRP (Table 106.3), describes the 2002 integration of the Continuing Survey of Food Intake by Individuals (CSFII) and the National Health and Nutrition Examination Survey (NHANES), and discusses the program's accomplishments and limitations. In the context of nutritional monitoring, *related health status* refers to health conditions that may be associated with nutritional variables, such as diabetes with obesity and osteoporosis with calcium. The terms *dietary status* and *nutritional status*, although often used interchangeably, have different connotations. Nutritional status encompasses anthropometric, biochemical, clinical, dietary, and sociodemographic factors. Dietary status is a more limited term that refers to intake of foods, beverages, both nonalcoholic and alcoholic, and nutrients, including supplements.

HISTORICAL OVERVIEW

In the late 1960s, concerns about the nutritional status of the US population emerged as reports about the existence of hunger and malnutrition were released (5). Between 1969 and 1977, the Senate Select Committee on Nutrition and Human Needs investigated not only the extent to which hunger existed in the United States but also how effective the federal government was in measuring this problem. Recognizing serious deficiencies in the federal nutrition monitoring efforts and identifying the need for a coordinated comprehensive NNMS, Congress sought to remedy the situation by legislative action.

The Food and Agriculture Act of 1977 (PL 95–113) required the secretaries of agriculture and health, education and welfare (currently health and human services) to:

> "formulate and submit to Congress . . . a proposal for a comprehensive nutritional status monitoring system, to include: 1) an assessment of a system consisting of periodic surveys and continuous monitoring to determine: the extent of risk of nutrition-related health problems in the United States; which population groups or areas of the country face greatest risk; and the likely causes of risk and changes in risk factors over time; 2) a surveillance system to identify remediable nutrition-related health risks to individuals or for local areas, in such a manner as to tie detection to direct intervention and treatment . . . ; and 3) program evaluations to determine the adequacy, efficiency, effectiveness and side effects of nutrition-related programs in reducing health risks to individuals and populations" (6).

The proposal for a comprehensive national nutritional monitoring system was submitted by the US Department of Health, Education and Welfare and the US Department of Agriculture (USDA) to Congress in 1978 (7). This proposal reviewed current federal, state, and local agency activities in the areas of nutritional and dietary status assessment, nutritional quality of foods, dietary practices and knowledge, and the impact of nutritional intervention programs. It acknowledged the deficiencies in existing nutritional and dietary assessment methods, recognized delays in data analysis and the publication of results, pointed out the inadequate coverage of certain target groups and geographic areas, and recognized the inadequate evaluation of nutrition intervention programs. Although the proposal contained a series of recommendations for improving and expanding the scope of federal nutrition monitoring activities, it lacked the following: a set of priorities, an assignment of tasks and a timetable for completion, a prospective plan, a reporting component to monitor progress of the NNMS, a timetable for publications, an assignment of responsibility for implementation, identification of costs, and identification of the relationship to the Joint Subcommittee on Human Nutrition Research (8).

At the request of the Committee on Science and Technology, a proposal was reviewed by the US General Accounting Office, which recommended that the departments develop an implementation plan for a national nutritional monitoring system to provide specific information on how and when the system could be implemented and on its

TABLE 106.2. PRINCIPAL NATIONAL NUTRITION MONITORING AND RELATED RESEARCH PROGRAM (NNMRRP) ACTIVITIES, SPONSORING FEDERAL AGENCIES, AND SURVEY DESIGNS

ACTIVITY	AGENCY	SURVEY DESIGN
Nutrition and related health measurements		
National Ambulatory Medical Care Survey	NCHS, CDC	Multistage, stratified, probability sample of licensed physicians in office-based patient care
NHANES	NCHS, CDC	Complex, multistage stratified, probability cluster sample of individuals in households
NHANES I Epidemiologic Follow-up Study	NCHS, CDC	Follow-up on NHANES I participants, aged 25–74 years in 1971–1975
Pediatric Nutrition Surveillance System	NCCDPHP, CDC	Convenience population of low-income children, 0–17 years of age, who participate in publicly funded health, nutrition, and food assistance programs
Pregnancy Nutrition Surveillance System	NCCDPHP, CDC	Convenience population of low-income, high-risk pregnant women who participate in publicly funded prenatal nutrition and food assistance programs
National Vital Registration System	NCHS, CDC	Vital registration system
What We Eat in America—NHANES	NCHS, CDC and BHNRC, ARS	Complex, multistage stratified, probability cluster sample of individuals in households
Food and nutrient consumption measurements		
CSFII	BHNRC, ARS	Multistage, stratified area probability sample of defined populations
Military Feeding Systems and Military Populations	USARIEM, MND	Varies with specific study
What We Eat in America—NHANES	NCHS, CDC and BHNRC, ARS	Complex, multistage stratified, probability cluster sample of individuals in households
Knowledge, attitudes, and behavior assessments		
Behavioral Risk Factor Surveillance System	NCCDPHP, CDC	Multistage, cluster telephone survey based on Waksberg method
Youth Risk Behavior Surveillance System	NCCDPHP, CDC	Representative sample of 9th–12th grade students and national household survey of a representative sample of persons 12–21 y of age
Diet-Health Knowledge Survey	BHNRC, ARS	Follow-up of CSFII meal planners using telephone interview
Health and Diet Survey	DMS, FDA	Telephone interviews with a national probability Waksberg sample selected by random digit dialing method
National Health Interview Survey	NCHS, CDC	Complex, multistage, stratified, probability cluster sample of households
Food composition and nutrient databases		
Food Label and Package Survey	CFSAN, FDA	Biennial probability survey of retail packaged foods using commercial market research data bases (A.C. Nielsen Scantrack)
National Nutrient Data Bank	BHNRC, ARS	NA
Nutrient Composition Laboratory	BHNRC, ARS	NA
Survey Nutrient Data Base	BHNRC, ARS	NA
Food supply determinations		
A.C. Nielsen Scantrack	ERS[a]	NA
Fisheries of the United States	DOC, NOAA/NMFS	NA
Total Diet Study	CFSAN, FDA	NA
United States Food and Nutrition Supply Series	CNPP	NA

ARS, Agricultural Research Service; BHNRC, Beltsville Human Nutrition Research Center; CDC, Centers for Disease Control and Prevention; CFSAN, Center for Food Safety and Applied Nutrition; CNPP, Center for Nutrition Policy and Promotion; CSFII, Continuing Survey of Food Intakes by Individuals; DMS, Division of Market Studies; DOC, Department of Commerce; ERS, Economic Research Service; FDA, Food and Drug Administration; MND, Military Nutrition Division; NA, not applicable; NCCDPHP, National Center for Chronic Disease Prevention and Health Promotion; NCHS, National Center for Health Statistics; NHANES, National Health and Nutrition Examination Survey; NMFS, National Marine Fisheries Service; NOAA, National Oceanic and Atmospheric Administration; USARIEM, United States Army Research Institute of Environmental Medicine.
[a] Primary sponsor.

cost. The US Department of Health and Human Services (DHHS) and USDA Joint Implementation Plan for a Comprehensive NNMS was submitted to Congress in 1981 (9). The plan made the assistant secretary of agriculture for food and consumer services, USDA, and the assistant secretary for health (ASH), DHHS, responsible for implementing compatible survey plans. It also identified and described the current efforts in nutrition monitoring conducted by the USDA and DHHS and proposed major goals and objectives for the NNMS. The two major objectives

TABLE 106.3. HISTORY OF NUTRITION MONITORING IN THE UNITED STATES FROM 1977 TO 2002

1977	Food and Agriculture Act (PL 95-113)
1978	Proposal to Congress for a comprehensive nutritional status monitoring system
1981	Joint implementation plan for a comprehensive national nutrition monitoring system
1986	First report to Congress: *Nutrition Monitoring in the United States: A Progress Report from the Joint Nutrition Monitoring Evaluation Committee*
1987	Operational Plan for the National Nutrition Monitoring System
1988	Interagency Committee on Nutrition Monitoring formed
1989	Second report to Congress: *Nutrition Monitoring in the United States: An Update Report on Nutrition Monitoring*
1990	National Nutrition Monitoring and Related Research Act (PL 101–445)
1991	Interagency Board for Nutrition Monitoring and Related Research formed; draft comprehensive plan published in the *Federal Register* on October 29
1992	National Nutrition Monitoring Advisory Council formed
1993	Comprehensive plan for the National Nutrition Monitoring and Related Research program signed by the president and transmitted to Congress
1993	First nutrition monitoring *Chartbook*
1995	Third report to Congress: *Third Report on Nutrition Monitoring in the United States*
1998	Memorandum of understanding to integrate the NHANES and CSFII signed by the NCHS, and ARS Expert Panel on Survey Integration formed
2000	Memorandum of understanding to implement the integrated dietary portion of a single, continuous survey was signed by NCHS and ARS
2002	Integrated survey, What We Eat in America—NHANES, fielded; workshop held on Future Directions for the Integrated Survey

ARS, Agricultural Research Service; CSFII, Continuing Survey of Food Intakes by Individuals; NCHS, National Center for Health Statistics; NHANES, National Health and Nutrition Examination Survey.

were (a) to achieve the best possible coordination of the NHANES and the Nationwide Food Consumption Survey (NFCS) and (b) to develop a reporting system to translate the findings from these two national surveys and other monitoring activities into periodic reports to Congress on the nutritional status of the US population. The plan described how to implement the first coordinated NHANES-NFCS survey in 1987. However, certain critical features were never fully addressed, and this deficiency inhibited achieving a comprehensive system (8).

In 1982 and 1983, the Subcommittee on Science, Research, and Technology and the Subcommittee on Department Operations, Research, and Foreign Agriculture jointly held hearings to review the system. They noted that coordination had improved but was still inadequate. The NNMS lacked a central focus, a provision for continuous monitoring, and a mechanism for evaluating food assistance programs.

In 1983, the Joint Nutrition Monitoring Evaluation Committee (JNMEC) was appointed. This federal advisory committee, jointly sponsored by the USDA and DHHS, was responsible for the first progress report to the Congress, as stipulated in the Joint Implementation Plan. The report, published in 1986, contained information on the nutritional status of the US population and made specific recommendations to improve the monitoring system (10). The JNMEC reported that the principal nutrition-related health problems experienced by the US population arose from overconsumption of fat, saturated fat, cholesterol, and sodium. Intakes of iron and vitamin C were low in certain population groups. In addition to reviewing available data, the Committee made 14 recommendations on how to improve nutrition monitoring efforts.

In 1987, the DHHS and the USDA published an operational plan for the NNMS, a revision of the 1981 Joint Implementation Plan (4). The operational plan described the goals of the operational phase, progress during the implementation phase (1981–1986), and proposed activities for the operational phase (1987–1996), including a calendar of events. The specific goals were to achieve a comprehensive system through coordination among NNMS components, thereby improving both information dissemination and exchange between data generators and users and Congress, as well as the research base for nutrition monitoring.

The operational plan did not stipulate a time for implementation of the comprehensive, coordinated system sought by the Congress. Given the lack of legislative mandate to establish such a system, it was unclear how this operational plan would be any more successful than the 1981 Joint Implementation Plan. In 1988, the Interagency Committee on Nutrition Monitoring was formed (11). The Committee was cochaired by the ASH, DHHS, and the assistant secretary of agriculture for food and consumer services, USDA. The purpose of this committee was to increase the effectiveness and productivity of federal nutrition monitoring efforts by improving planning, coordination, and communication among the agencies engaged in nutrition monitoring. The membership included representatives from DHHS Public Health Service agencies, USDA agencies, the Agency for International Development, the Bureau of Labor Statistics, the Census Bureau, the Department of Defense, and the Veterans Administration.

In 1989, the second progress report on nutrition monitoring, prepared by an ad hoc expert panel, was transmitted to the Congress. This report provided (a) an update to the 1986 report on the dietary and nutritional status of the United States population and (b) an in-depth analysis of the contributions of the NNMS to the assessment of iron nutriture and of dietary and nutritional factors related to cardiovascular disease (12). The expert panel concluded that the principal nutrition-related health problems experienced by the US population were related to overconsumption of selected nutrients, particularly food energy, fat, saturated fatty acids, cholesterol, sodium, and alcohol. Iron deficiency was cited as the most common single nutrient deficiency. The expert panel also offered several recommendations for improvements in the NNMS.

Between 1984 and 1990, several attempts were made to pass a legislative bill to establish a coordinated national nutrition monitoring and related research program (8, 13). This proposed legislation included developing a comprehensive plan to assess both the nutritional status and dietary intake of the US population as well as of the nutritional quality of the food supply. Provisions for conducting scientific research were also included. Finally, on October 22, 1990, the NNMRRA (PL 101–445) was signed into law (2).

The key monitoring provisions of this bill (Titles I and II) were as follows:

1. To establish an Interagency Board for Nutrition Monitoring and Related Research (IBNMRR), jointly chaired by an Assistant Secretary from the USDA and by an Assistant Secretary from the DHHS.
2. To establish a National Nutrition Monitoring Advisory Council of nine voting members who are not federal employees.
3. To develop and implement a 10-year comprehensive plan for a coordinated program designed to assess and report on a continuous basis the dietary and nutritional status of the US population, particularly infants and children, the aged, disadvantaged persons, minorities, and women; to develop and update nutrient data banks; to sponsor/conduct research to develop uniform indicators and methods for conducting and reporting nutrition monitoring activities; and to assist state and local government agencies in developing procedures and networks for nutrition monitoring and surveillance.
4. To publish at least once every 5 years or sooner a report to the Congress on the dietary, nutritional, and health-related status of the US population and the nutritional quality of food consumed in the United States.

In 1991, the IBNMRR was established through the expansion of the Interagency Committee on Nutrition Monitoring. About 20 agencies became members of the board (14). Board responsibilities included coordinating the scientific reports that describe the nutritional and health status of the US population, providing mechanisms for increased communication and collaboration among member agencies, and developing the annual budget report. The IBNMRR has not met since a joint meeting with the Interagency Committee on Human Nutrition Research in the late 1990s (15).

The National Nutrition Monitoring Advisory Council, composed of nine nonfederal members with expertise in the areas of public health, nutrition monitoring research, and food production and distribution, was established in 1992. The cochairpersons of the IBNMRR were ex officio nonvoting members of the Council. The Council was charged with providing scientific and technical advice on the development and implementation of the coordinated NNMRRP and advising the secretaries of the USDA and DHHS. The Council was also required to report to the secretaries annually on the effectiveness of the NNMRRP and to offer recommendations for enhancing the program's effectiveness. This Council identified six priorities for the NNMRRP: identifying ways to include high-risk subgroups of the population; integrating federal, state, and private data needs; determining the cost effectiveness of the NNMRRP; providing timely data dissemination; assessing nutrition monitoring research activities; and determining trends in NNMRRP data, especially those relating to measures of the food supply and to consumers' knowledge and attitudes towards nutrition and dietary guidance. The Council has not been active since 1996 (15).

The Ten-Year Comprehensive Plan for the NNMRRP described national nutrition monitoring activities for the period 1992 to 2002. A proposed plan was compiled by members of a DHHS-USDA working group and published on October 29, 1991 (16). After subsequent public comment and departmental revision periods, the plan was finalized. It was signed by the president and forwarded to Congress in January, 1993, and published in the *Federal Register* on June 11, 1993 (17). This plan was intended to be the guidance mechanism that provides direction to the federal and state agencies participating in the national nutritional monitoring program. It discussed a tentative course of action designed to address some of the recognized deficiencies in the NNMS.

The plan included three objectives at the national level and three at the state and local levels. The national objectives were to provide for a comprehensive NNMRRP through continuous and coordinated data collection, to improve the comparability and quality of data across the NNMRRP, and to improve the research base for nutrition monitoring. For each national objective, activities within the five components were delineated. The state and local objectives were to develop and strengthen state and local capacity for continuous and coordinated data collection that complements national nutrition surveys, to improve methodologies to enhance comparability of NNMRRP data across federal, state, and local levels, and to improve the quality of state and local nutrition monitoring data.

Chartbook I: Selected Findings from the National Nutrition Monitoring and Related Research Program was published in 1993. This resource highlighted dietary intake data from the Hispanic HANES and the 1989 and 1990 CSFII, changes in the food supply, progress in developing food composition methods, and selected dietary knowledge and attitudes of the US population (18). Chartbooks that display data with graphics and brief narratives were proposed intermediate to the scientific reports to Congress by DHHS and USDA. However, to date, no other chartbooks dedicated specifically to nutrition monitoring have been published.

In 1995, the third and last report on nutrition monitoring prepared by the Life Sciences Research Office (LSRO) and a group of expert consultants was transmitted to the president and Congress (19). This two-volume report provided an update to the 1989 report. Special emphasis was placed on the dietary and nutrition-related health status of the US population, and concerns for low-income and high-risk population subgroups were expressed. The expert consultants noted that a considerable gap existed between what US residents are eating and what they should eat and that some US residents do not get enough to eat. The increasing prevalence of overweight and the high proportion of the population with high serum cholesterol levels and hypertension were cause for public health concern. The expert consultants also provided recommendations for strengthening each component of the NNMRRP and indicated ways for overcoming its limitations.

Congressional appropriations and executive branch decisions about budget priorities have been the major determinants of the scope and number of nutrition monitoring and surveillance activities. Organizational changes in government contributed to a lowered visibility and support for nutrition monitoring. In 1987, The National Center for Health Statistics (NCHS) was moved from the Office of the ASH to the Centers for Disease Control and Prevention (CDC). This change meant that the NCHS director reported to the CDC director who reported to the ASH, rather than directly to the ASH, who had oversight for the NNMRRP and the Public Health Service. Consequently, the primary source of nutrition and health statistics for DHHS was removed from central oversight and support. In 1995, the USDA Human Nutrition Information Service was divided into two parts. Dietary survey functions moved to the Agricultural Research Service (ARS), and nutrition education was moved to the Center for Nutrition Policy and Promotion. This change meant that survey staff reported through a center director to an area director and then to the ARS Administrator and to a different under-secretary, the Under-Secretary for Research, Education, and Economics. Also in 1995, Public Health Service agencies were ordered to report directly to the Secretary of DHHS, and the ASH became an advisor to the secretary of the DHHS (15). The budgets of CDC and ARS did not expand during the 1990s to accommodate the costs of conducting the activities the agencies had pledged to undertake in the 10-year plan (15, 20). Thus, the USDA and the DHHS focused their efforts on improving survey methods and coordination to maximize efficiency given the limited funds available in government for nutrition monitoring.

In 1998, a memorandum of understanding to integrate the dietary data collection of the NHANES, sponsored by the NCHS of the DHHS, and the CSFII, sponsored by the ARS of the USDA, was signed (21). In the Conference Report (No. 106–948) accompanying the Agriculture, Rural Development, Food and Drug Administration, and Related Agency Appropriations Act (HR 4461) for fiscal year 2001, the conferees directed the USDA in consultation with DHHS to prepare and submit a report on the process of integrating NHANES and CSFII. The report was to include steps to accomplish goals set forth in the NNMRRA of 1990, to address the strengths and possible weakness of merging NHANES and CSFII, to identify funding needs, and to include recommendations for inclusion in reauthorization of the NNMRRA. The report, delivered to the Subcommittee on Agriculture, Rural Development, Food and Drug Administration, and Related Agency Appropriations in January, 2001, stated that both USDA and DHHS concluded that the advantages of merging the surveys significantly outweighed the potential disadvantages and that users of nutrition monitoring data would be convinced that the integration plan had considerable merit and would advance the goals of nutrition monitoring (22).

In 2001, the Council of the American Society for Nutritional Sciences formed a Working Group to review the status and future plans of the NNMRRP in terms of timeliness, budget, sampling and survey content, and evaluation of the impact of survey changes on the usefulness of the data for research and public policy. The Working Group was also charged to recommend research needed to strengthen the dietary measures in the integrated survey and to recommend approaches to ensure a comprehensive nutrition monitoring system that would meet the needs of program managers, researchers, and policy makers (23).

Because data from the NNMRRP are critical to the government, the Working Group recommended that Congress: (a) reauthorize an updated NNMRRA that addresses current public health priorities, data needs, and infrastructure requirements with adequate appropriations; (b) increase the appropriations for NHANES by a sufficient amount to allow a set of regularly collected nutrition indicators on an annual basis; (c) increase the appropriation for ARS by sufficient amount to provide for augmentation of the integrated design for dietary intake through the addition of 5000 sample persons; and (d) fund the grants program initially authorized under the NNMRRA. They also recommended that the DHHS and the USDA (a) establish a high level board to coordinate NNMRRP activities related to planning and budget and (b) continue to seek external advice about the design and conduct of the NNMRRP (23).

The Working Group believed that the integrated survey should improve the quality, timeliness, and usability of the survey data. An important research focus of the integrated survey is to establish relationships between dietary intake and health. To enhance estimates of usual food intake and support the analysis of the frequency of consumption of targeted foods and food habits of interest, the Working Group recommended that the current survey dietary collection of two 24-hour recalls be augmented by food frequency methods. They also recommended that additional information on an individual's knowledge related to diet and health be obtained. The Working Group also recognized the need for special research studies to develop methods to assess usual intake or biomarkers of usual dietary intake in surveys. It was clear from the statement of the American Society for

Nutritional Sciences Working Group that the nutrition monitoring program is underfunded and may be unable to meet future challenges (15, 23).

On January 22, 2002, another memorandum of understanding was signed by the ARS and NCHS to further the collaboration in data collection and implementation of the dietary portion of a single, continuous population-based national nutrition survey (21). The integrated survey, known as What We Eat In America—NHANES, was fielded in 2002. In June 2002, a workshop with representatives from federal agencies involved in research, surveillance, and policy, academia, and others involved with national nutrition data was held. Workshop objectives were to identify the strengths and limitations of the integrated survey and to recommend strategies to strengthen this survey and the NNMS. The three core themes addressed were the collection of food and dietary supplement intake, intake estimation, and food and supplement data and databases (21).

NATIONAL NUTRITION MONITORING CORNERSTONE SURVEYS

Between 1896, when the first food composition tables were published, and 2004, more than 100 federal nutrition surveys and surveillance activities have been conducted. A chronologic listing categorized by the measurement components has been published elsewhere (15, 24). Although many surveys and surveillance activities have been sponsored by a variety of agencies in the federal government,

three in particular, the NFCS, the CSFII, and the NHANES, were regarded as the cornerstones of national nutrition monitoring (Tables 106.4 and 106.5). In the early 1990s, the NFCS was discontinued. In 2002, the remaining periodic cornerstone NNMRRP surveys—CSFII and NHANES—were merged into a new continuous, integrated survey, What We Eat In America—NHANES. This survey is currently the primary source of nationally representative data on dietary intake of foods and beverages and on nutritional status.

Nationwide Food Consumption Survey

The involvement of the federal government in nutrition monitoring actually dates back to 1893, when the USDA received the first appropriation to conduct human nutrition research. The first national survey of household food consumption and dietary levels was conducted in 1936 to 1937 as part of the Consumer Purchases Study (25). Between 1942 and 1955, three nationwide studies on household food consumption (NFCS) were conducted by the Human Nutrition Information Service (26). These surveys collected information on household food use over 7 days and reflected food use from an economic perspective; that is, it included food used whether it is eaten, discarded, or fed to pets. The person primarily responsible for food preparation in a given household provided this information. Food distribution among members of the household was not taken into account. In the 1965 and subsequent NFCS (1977–1978, 1987–1988), data were

TABLE 106.4. NATIONAL FOOD SURVEYS CONDUCTED BY THE US DEPARTMENT OF AGRICULTURE FROM 1936 TO 1998

YEAR	SURVEY	TYPE OF DATA COLLECTED	DIETARY METHOD
1936–1937	Consumer Purchases Study	Household food use	7-d list recall, 7-d food inventory record
1942	Family Spending and Saving in Wartime	Household food use	7-d list recall
1948	Food Consumption of Urban Families	Household food use	7-d list recall
1955	Food Consumption of Households	Household food use	7-d list recall
1965–1966	Household Food Consumption Survey	Household food use and individual food intake	7-d list recall, 24-h dietary recall
1977–1978	NFCS	Household food use and individual food intake	7-d list recall 3 consecutive days: 24-h dietary recall plus 2-d diet records
1985–1986	CSFII	Individual food intake	Multiple 24-h dietary recalls over 1-y period
1987–1988	NFCS	Household food use and individual food intake	3 consecutive days: 24-h dietary recall plus 2-d diet records
1989–1991	CSFII	Individual food intake	24-h dietary recall plus 2-d diet records
1989–1991	DHKS	Dietary knowledge, behavior and attitudes	Telephone follow-up to CSFII
1994–1996	CSFII	Individual food intake	Two nonconsecutive 24-h dietary recalls, multiple-pass method.
1994–1996	DHKS	Dietary knowledge, behavior and attitudes	Telephone follow-up to CSFII
1998	CSFII	Individual food intake	Two nonconsecutive 24-h dietary recalls, multiple-pass method

CSFII, Continuing Survey of Food Intakes by Individuals; DHKS, Diet and Health Knowledge Survey; NFCS, Nationwide Food Consumption Survey.
Adapted from Dwyer J, Picciano MF, Raiten DJ et al. J Nutr 2003[Suppl];133:590S–600S, with permission.

TABLE 106.5. OVERVIEW OF THE NATIONAL HEALTH AND NUTRITION EXAMINATION SURVEYS

YEAR	SURVEY	TYPE OF DATA COLLECTED	DIETARY METHOD
1971–1974	NHANES I	Health and nutritional status of persons ages 1–74 y	24-h dietary recall, food frequency questionnaire
1976–1980	NHANES II	Health and nutritional status of persons ages 6 mo–74 y	24-h dietary recall, food frequency questionnaire
1982–1984	Hispanic HANES	Health and nutritional status of Mexican Americans, Cubans, and Puerto Ricans	24-h dietary recall, food frequency questionnaire
1988–1994	NHANES III	Health and nutritional status of persons ages ≥2 mo	24-h dietary recall, food frequency questionnaire, food security questions, vitamin/mineral supplement usage
1988–1994	Supplemental Survey of Older Americans	Health and nutritional status of persons aged 50+ y examined in NHANES III	Two 24-h recalls by telephone
1999–2001	Continuous NHANES	Health and nutritional status of persons all ages.	24-h dietary recall, targeted food frequency questions, food security questions, vitamin/mineral supplement usage
2002–2004	What We Eat in America—NHANES (Integrated Survey)	Health and nutritional status of persons all ages	Two nonconsecutive 24-h dietary recalls using Automated Multiple Pass Method, food security questions, vitamin/mineral supplement usage

NHANES, National Health and Nutrition Examination Survey.

obtained on dietary intakes and patterns of individuals, as well as on household food use (see Table 106.4).

The objectives of the NFCS were to describe current food consumption behavior, to identify changes in diet since the previous NFCS, and to assess the nutritional content of diets for their implications on policies relating to food production and marketing, food safety, food assistance, and nutrition education. Questions were also asked about the following: household characteristics; individual characteristics such as self-reported height, weight, and health status; participation in food assistance programs; and diet-related topics such as supplement use, alcohol consumption, use of salt at the table, and dieting (27).

The NFCS was designed to provide a multistage stratified area probability sample representative of the 48 conterminous states (26). The stratification plan took into account geographic location and degree of urbanization. In the 1987 to 1988 NFCS, households were drawn from nine geographic divisions and three urbanization classes as defined by the Bureau of the Census (27). This NFCS included two probability samples: one for the general population, the basic survey (households and individuals with all incomes), and one for the low-income survey (households with incomes consistent with eligibility for the Food Stamp Program).

The target sample for the basic 1987 to 1988 survey was about 6000 households and their approximately 15,000 individual members. The low-income survey targeted 2500 households and about 6000 individual members (28). The household response rate was 38% for the basic sample and 42% for the low-income sample (29). The individual response rate for the basic sample was 31% for individuals completing 1 day of intake and 25% for individuals who completed all 3 days of intake (28).

A survey is designed to represent the US population; if response rates are extremely low, it is questionable whether the data will provide an unbiased estimate of the dietary and nutritional status of the nation. USDA contracted with the LSRO of the Federation of American Societies for Experimental Biology to conduct an independent review of the impact of nonresponse on the estimates of food and nutrient intakes. The LSRO convened an Expert Panel of statisticians who noted that it was impossible to determine the extent to which nonresponse bias influenced the interpretation of the data. This panel consequently recommended that persons using the 1987 to 1988 NFCS data should exercise great caution and should recognize that the respondents may not be completely representative of subgroups when group comparisons are made. Comprehensive evaluations of the possible effects of nonresponse in the NFCS and of potential limitations in using the collected data have been published (28, 30).

Continuing Survey of Food Intakes by Individuals

The 1985 and 1986 CSFIIs constitute Series I. Series II began in 1989 and includes the 1990 and the 1991 CSFII. Series III began in 1994 and continued through 1996. This 3-year survey is popularly known as the "What We Eat in America Survey." The purpose of these surveys is to provide information on the dietary status of the US population and to monitor changes in dietary intakes. In addition, individuals identified as the main meal planners and preparers in the 1989 to 1991 CSFII were contacted to participate in the Diet and Health Knowledge Survey (DHKS), another NNMRRP activity sponsored by the USDA. The dietary data collected in the CSFII were then linked to an individual's nutrition knowledge and attitudes. The ARS conducted the 1998 CSFII as a supplement to the CSFII 1994 to 1996. The CSFII 1998 was responsive to the Food Quality Protection Act of 1996, which required the secretary of agriculture to provide the Environmental Protection Agency with information on food consumption patterns of a statistically valid sample of infants and children for estimating exposure to pesticide residues in the diets of children (31).

"Usual" intakes were assessed by a variety of dietary methods (see Table 106.4). The three-pass method for collecting dietary data was introduced in Series III of CSFII. This method was used to develop the USDA Automated Multiple Pass Method (AMPM), a computer-assisted interview based on five passes (32). The multiple-pass method is an approach that progressively records food and beverage intakes of individuals ranging from a general list of foods to specific characteristics of food items consumed.

The target population for Series I and II CSFII consisted of persons selected by sex and age residing in the 48 conterminous states in households with incomes at all levels (basic sample) and with incomes at or below 130% of poverty guidelines (low-income sample). The 1985 CSFII included men and women aged 19 to 50 years and children 1 to 5 years of age, whereas the 1986 CSFII included women 19 to 50 years of age and children 1 to 5 years of age (26). For the Series I CSFII, the basic sample included approximately 1300 households and their 2000 individual members. The 1985 low-income sample included about 1900 households and their 3400 individual members, whereas the 1986 low-income sample had about 1200 households and 2100 individual members. Individual response rates for women and children completing 1-day recalls were 71% for the basic sample and 65% for the low-income sample in 1985 and 66% for the basic sample and 75% for the low-income sample in 1986 (33).

The 1989, 1990, and 1991 CSFIIs were designed to obtain information on food intakes from all household members (men, women, and children of all ages). Like the 1985 and 1986 CSFIIs, these surveys had basic and low-income samples. Approximately 6700 households and their 15,000 individual members were included in the samples. Overall household response rate for the 1989 to 1991 CSFII was 67%. Individual response rates were 58% for those completing 1 day of dietary recall and 45% for those completing 3 days of dietary recall (19).

In the 1994 to 1996 CSFII, 20,126 individuals were selected as participants. Of these persons, 16,103 completed 1 day of intake (80% response rate) and 15,303 completed both days of intake (76% response rate) (31). Notable design changes from the first two series include a target population of noninstitutionalized persons in all 50 states, oversampling of the low-income population rather than a separate low-income survey, larger samples of young children and older adults, subsampling within households,

and the collection of 2 nonconsecutive days of food intake through in-person interviews rather than 3 consecutive days of food intake using a 1-day recall and a 2-day record (26). Using the same dietary collection methods, the 1998 CSFII collected data on 5559 children from birth through 9 years of age from all 50 states (31).

National Health and Nutrition Examination Survey

In 1967, the Senate Subcommittee on Employment, Manpower, and Poverty of the Committee on Labor and Public Welfare noted in a letter to President Lyndon Johnson that the conditions of malnutrition and widespread hunger had reached emergency proportions. In response to concerns regarding the existence of hunger and malnutrition and the lack of a monitoring system to determine the magnitude of the problem, Congress mandated, in Section 14 of the Partnership for Health Amendments of 1967, that the secretary of the Department of Health, Education and Welfare, in collaboration with other federal government and state officials, was to conduct a comprehensive survey to assess the incidence and location of serious hunger, malnutrition, and health problems. This action authorized the National Nutrition Survey, better known as the Ten State Nutrition Survey.

The Ten State Nutrition Survey, conducted from 1968 to 1970, was designed to select families randomly from the 1960 Bureau of Census enumeration districts, where the highest percentage of families had incomes below the Orshansky Poverty Index in the states of California, Kentucky, Louisiana, Massachusetts, Michigan, New York, South Carolina, Texas, Washington, and West Virginia. The sample population included middle- and upper-income persons who, because of changes in residential patterns subsequent to 1960, were living in selected enumeration districts. Nutritional status was assessed on the basis of dietary intakes and food patterns, dental examinations, and anthropometric and biochemical measurements. Information on nonnutritional factors that affect food intake (e.g., socioeconomic characteristics, health status, and income) was also gathered. The findings of the Ten State Survey indicated nutritional problems in selected age and sex groups (34).

While the Ten State Survey was still under way, in 1969, President Richard Nixon asked the secretary of the Department of Health, Education and Welfare to expand this survey to provide a description of the extent of hunger and malnutrition in the entire United States. In response, a Task Force on Nutritional Surveillance at the NCHS was formed and asked to plan and implement a survey that would provide an effective nutrition surveillance system. To minimize duplication with other surveys conducted by the NCHS and to permit nutritional variables to be correlated with other health status measurements already being collected in the National Health Examination Survey (NHES), a nutritional assessment component was added to the NHES to create the first NHANES: NHANES I.

Conducted between 1971 and 1974, NHANES I was the first health survey to assess dietary intake and other measures of nutritional status in a nationally representative sample of persons aged 1 to 74 years in the civilian, noninstitutionalized population in the United States (35, 36).

A major objective of the NHANES is the periodic assessment of the health and nutritional status of the United States population and the monitoring of changes in status over time. The second NHANES was conducted from 1976 to 1980 (37), and the third NHANES, from 1988 to 1994. The Hispanic HANES was conducted in the period 1982 to 1984 (38). This special survey included three Hispanic groups: Mexican-Americans residing in five southwestern states; Cubans in Dade County, Florida; and Puerto Ricans in the New York City metropolitan area.

Each of the cross-sectional NHANES surveys has used complex, stratified, multistage, probability, cluster sampling to select a representative sample of the civilian, noninstitutionalized population residing in households in the United States. Special oversampling techniques were used to ensure adequate representation of subgroups considered to be at high risk of malnutrition. NHANES II statistically selected a sample of 27,805 persons to represent the entire US population and selected subgroups. About 91% of those selected agreed to be interviewed, and 73% agreed to be interviewed and examined (33). In the full 6 years of data collection for the NHANES III, from 1988 to 1994, approximately 40,000 persons were selected, among whom 86% were interviewed and 78% were examined. The age range for the third NHANES has been expanded, beginning at 2 months, with no upper age limit (39).

In 1999, NHANES adopted a continuous data collection methodology to produce nationally representative data every year. This survey was designed to continue for approximately 6 years at 88 locations across the United States. Approximately 40,000 persons of all ages in households will be randomly selected to participate in the survey. Each 12-month cycle consists of about 7000 interviewed and 5000 examined persons. Respondents include whites as well as oversamples of African-Americans and Mexican-Americans to provide a representative sample by age, gender, and income level. Adolescents 12 to 19 years old, persons aged 60 years and older, and pregnant women are also oversampled (40).

Each single year and any combination of consecutive years of data collection comprise a nationally representative sample of the United States. Data release cycles of the continuous NHANES are described as NHANES 1999 to 2000, 2001 to 2002, and 2003 to 2004. For NHANES 1999 to 2000, 9965 persons were interviewed (82% response rate), and 9282 were examined (78% response rate). For NHANES 2001 to 2002, the interview sample size was 11,039, and the examined sample size was 10,477. Data can be analyzed for any 2-year cycle. However, it is strongly recommended that two or more 2-year cycles of continuous NHANES data be combined to provide estimates with greater statistical reliability (40).

The NHANES is unique in that it collects data on the health and nutritional status of the US population through interviews and direct physical examinations. Listings of the major parameters measured by sex and age for the 1999 to 2004 NHANES have been published elsewhere (41). The household interview data were collected by Computer Assisted Personal Interviewing and include demographic, socioeconomic, dietary, and health-related questions. A quantitative measure of intake of vitamins and minerals from supplements and a series of food security questions are also asked. Physical examinations include components such as anthropometric measurements, hematologic and biochemical assessments, and physical and dental examinations. The survey design, implementation strategies, and a compendium of all data collection instruments for the continuous NHANES are available electronically (42).

The NHANES is designed as a multipurpose survey. Some examples of the major uses of the data include the development of references such as growth charts (43), prevalence of overweight (44), evaluation and development of nutrition policy such as *Healthy People 2010* (45) and the *Dietary Guidelines for Americans* (46), and assessment of food fortification policies, such as folate status (47).

What We Eat in America: National Health and Nutrition Examination Survey

Launched in 2002, this continuous integrated survey interviews and examines a nationally representative sample of approximately 5000 persons per year. The main objective of the dietary component is to provide estimates of food and dietary supplement intakes that will guide dietary assessment, planning, research, and public health policy (48). The USDA's AMPM is used to collect two independent 24-hour dietary recalls. The AMPM is designed to engage the respondent more completely and provide more complete dietary recalls. Researchers at the Beltsville Human Nutrition Research Center of USDA have conducted extensive, biomarker-based validation studies of the AMPM to ensure its completeness and accuracy (49).

Dietary supplement intakes are estimated from a report of dietary supplement use over the past month. Because supplements can contribute a major and sometimes a larger proportion of micronutrient intakes than diet alone and may independently alter risk for developing selected chronic conditions, information on dietary supplements needs to be captured. The dietary supplement data collection methodology is still evolving, and the dietary supplement database needs to be more fully developed (50, 51).

A major advantage of integrating the CSFII and NHANES is that a single survey is less costly than maintaining two separate field operations to collect dietary recall data. Two days of dietary recall data are collected from each person so usual intakes can be estimated more reliably. Combining the assets of USDA and DHHS should also result in more timely release of data, which has been a past limitation of the NNMRRP. In addition, the dietary and nutritional data will be directly linked to the other health status data collected by NHANES on a continuous basis (22).

A major disadvantage of the integrated survey is the limited sample size. With the discontinuation of the CSFII, there was a yearly decrease of 5000 persons surveyed. With only 5000 persons examined each year, 2 years of data collection will be required before reliable analyses can occur. The DHKS, a telephone follow-up survey to a subsample of CSFII, was not included as a component of the integrated survey. Its discontinuation raised concerns because this survey was the only monitoring activity that linked understanding of diet and food choices to knowledge about nutrition (22). The return of a survey like the DHKS would provide data to better evaluate food assistance and nutrition education programs. ARS and NCHS are exploring approaches that could lead to a continuation of this survey in the future. Adequate funding and resources of two federal agencies are needed to carry out the integrated survey successfully. This change results in more pressure to ensure stability of funding for data collection and of research sufficient to enable the program to keep pace with the changing food supply, eating behaviors, and survey mechanisms.

OTHER NUTRITION MONITORING ACTIVITIES

In addition to the integrated survey, CSFII, and NHANES, several other survey and surveillance activities constitute the NNMRRP. The activities conducted on a regular basis and sponsoring federal agency are shown in Table 106.2. The periodicity of the activities varied. For example, food supply estimates were conducted annually, whereas the Food Label and Package Survey was done biennially. Many special surveys, such as the Women, Infants and Children Infant Feeding Study and the School Nutrition Dietary Assessment Study, were also conducted periodically as needs arose. A comprehensive compilation of NNMRRP activities with descriptions about survey design and objectives, sample sizes, and response rates is provided in the Directory of Federal and State Nutrition Monitoring Activities (39).

ACCOMPLISHMENTS AND LIMITATIONS OF THE NATIONAL NUTRITION MONITORING SYSTEM

The five components of the NNMRRP provide a considerable amount of valuable information that have advanced science and benefited the US population. The nutrition data collected in the NNMRRP are used by federal agencies, the private sector, and academia for a variety of purposes including the following: public policy, such as regulatory and nutrition programs; descriptive references such as biochemical indicators of nutrition status or dietary reference intakes; and research, such as health status, disease morbidity,

and mortality (15). Under the 10-year plan, the USDA and DHHS made significant progress in improving nutrition monitoring activities, specifically survey comparability, food composition data, federal state relations, and information dissemination and assessment of the effects of welfare reform on nutritional status and of food security of the population (52, 53).

Some of the major accomplishments linked to the 10-year plan include the development of the Federal and State Directory of Nutrition Monitoring Activities (39), the updating of the USDA food composition database (54), the development of a validated 18-item food security questionnaire for use at the national level and a six-item food security questionnaire for state and local use (55, 56), the use of improved anthropometric measures, the development of new child growth references (43), and the development of a dietary supplement database (50).

Historically, the common themes for NNMS improvement were as follows: more detailed information on racial, ethnic, and age groups; data that can support estimates for small geographic areas; improved timeliness and documentation of data; continuous or more frequent data collection; and increased dissemination of the data in general formats that facilitate access and analysis (57). Despite improvements of the latter three shortcomings, adequate coverage of high-risk population subgroups and estimates for small geographic areas are still limitations. These are discussed subsequently.

In the past, one of the major limitations of the NNMS was the inordinate delays that occurred in the processing and release of data from both the core and ancillary surveys. With improvements in technology, the use of computer-assisted dietary interviews, and of automation of selected data collection and processing systems, such as the dietary and physical examination components, the time required to disseminate data has been shortened. Data from the continuous NHANES are released in aggregate 2-year intervals to provide confidentially to respondents and improve analytic strength. The Internet and *Morbidity and Mortality Weekly Report* are used to distribute nutrition monitoring publications and survey data, and CD-ROMs are used to distribute survey data. The electronic transmission of data and information on key public health policy issues such as obesity trends and folate status have helped to meet the needs of public health administrators and nutrition policy makers.

Population Subgroup Coverage

The current What We Eat in America—NHANES and the earlier CSFII and NHANES provide data representative of the civilian, noninstitutionalized US population. Groups excluded from these surveys include active-duty military personnel residing on military installations and persons in institutions, such as long-term care hospitals, homes for the aged, convents, monasteries, and penal and mental institutions. Homeless people who do not have an address are excluded from all household surveys because lists of addresses within census tracts are used as the basic unit for sampling.

PL 101–445 mandated that the comprehensive plan include components to incorporate, in survey design, military and (where appropriate) institutionalized populations; to sample representative subsets of identifiable low-income populations such as Native Americans and the homeless; and to collect dietary and nutritional status measurements on preschool and school-age children, pregnant and lactating women, elderly persons, low-income populations, blacks, and Hispanics (2). However, no appropriations were granted to meet the cost of these activities.

As indicated in Table 106.2, a complex, multistaged, stratified probability method of sampling is used in national surveys. This method either limits or eliminates the sample size of some subgroups that may be at higher risk for nutritional problems. For example, selected subgroups, such as pregnant or lactating women and ethnic minority groups such as Asians and selected Hispanic subgroups, do not occur in the population in sufficient numbers to appear in the survey sample with adequate representation to make reliable detailed estimates of their nutritional and health status. To capture all population subgroups, other approaches such as special surveys or oversampling, a technique used to increase sample size, need to be implemented. For example, the What We Eat in America—NHANES oversamples African-Americans and Mexican-Americans, adolescents 12 to 19 years of age, and adults aged 60 years or older.

Geographic Coverage

Many users of NNMRRP data request that federal agencies provide information on defined geographic areas, such as cities, counties, and individual states. The design of federal surveys uses primary sampling units, consisting of a county or a contiguous group of small counties that are stratified by characteristics such as urbanization and income. However, confidentiality restrictions prohibit release of data with identification of limited geographic areas. Areas are selected randomly within regions to provide the most representative sample while minimizing operational costs. NHANES, CSFII, and the integrated survey are designed to provide a picture of the nation. Although regional data are available, representative state and local (city) data are not obtainable from these surveys.

The surveillance activities at the CDC effectively target high-risk populations in narrow geographic areas. These activities include the Pediatric Nutrition Surveillance System (PedNSS) and the Pregnancy Nutrition Surveillance System (PregNSS). The target populations for PedNSS and PregNSS consist of a convenience sample of low-income children and pregnant women, respectively, who participate in publicly funded health, nutrition, and food

assistance programs. Participation in the CDC system is voluntary. In 2002, 38 states, the District of Columbia, Puerto Rico, and six tribal governments participated in the PedNSS (58), and 33 states and five tribal governments participated in the PregNSS (59). The states involved in these two surveillance activities receive the data analysis results on a monthly, quarterly, or annual basis for use in program planning, management, and evaluation.

The comprehensive plan for the NNMRRP in PL 101–445 required the federal government to provide scientific and technical assistance, training, and consultation to state and local governments for the purposes of obtaining dietary and nutritional status data; of developing related databases; and of promoting the development of regional, state, and local data collection services so they may become an integral component of a national nutritional status network. A grants program to encourage and assist state and local governments in developing the capacity to conduct monitoring and surveillance of nutritional status, food consumption, and nutrition knowledge and to enhance nutrition services was also a provision of PL 101–445 (2). However, a recognized constraint of this legislation was that it had no statutory provision for additional funds to establish such programs.

CONCLUSION

Very little of the administrative infrastructure needed to maintain a fully coordinated system created by the NNMRRA remains in place. Nevertheless, the nutrition monitoring program in the United States is still considered the most comprehensive in the world. The NNMRRA has yet to be reauthorized. However, the activities mandated by the NNMRRA of 1990 can be carried out under other legislative authorities of USDA and DHHS without reauthorization. The NNMRRP requires not only support from the agencies that use the survey data for program planning, implementation, evaluation, and policy purposes but also advocacy from stakeholders and the research community. Taken together, the many national nutrition monitoring components provide an opportunity for the comprehensive and coordinated evaluation of the dietary status and the nutritional status of the US population as well as of selected population subgroups considered to be at high risk of developing nutrition-related health problems.

The NNMRRA (PL 101–445) was signed into law by the US Congress in 1990. Fifteen years after this act was passed, elements of the nutrition monitoring system remain. Some aspects of the monitoring system represent a long-time vision finally realized. For example, integration of the USDA national dietary intake survey into the DHHS NHANES may be considered a successful product resulting in cooperation, coordination, reduced duplication, and greater efficiency of combined resources. Although the What We Eat in America—NHANES and other elements of nutrition monitoring remain intact, failure to capitalize fully on nutrition monitoring legislation of the 1990s and carry it into the next decade has left the comprehensive NNMS in somewhat of a dormant state.

The What We Eat In America—NHANES remains the foundation of national nutrition monitoring in the United States. It allows documentation and monitoring of progress on prevalence and trends of existing nutrition related problems of public health concern, such as the current obesity epidemic (44). Obesity and related risk factors and comorbidities are influenced by dietary intake, physical fitness, body composition, and other factors. Emerging problems and solutions must continue to be monitored in the population. For example, related to the high-profile obesity epidemic in the United States, there are opportunities to monitor the impact of "natural experiments" that may occur on a national level. One contemporary example would be shifts that may have occurred in dietary macronutrient intakes associated with the various diets promoted by the popular media and supported by food industry changes and associated advertising. This incredible momentum of the low-carbohydrate, high-fat diet that may be widespread in the early 2000s should be monitored on the national level at which it could have a potentially positive impact on obesity and a potentially adverse future impact on other risk factors such as blood lipid levels and other diseases such as heart disease or cancer. Responses to environmental changes that may occur, such as the control of food and beverage vending machine availability and dietary choices or the impact of campaigns to promote fruit and vegetable consumption, should be monitored as well.

Translation of related research may inevitably result in changes not only to the food and beverage supply and dietary consumption practices, but also in the physical environment, physical activity, and other relevant behaviors. The comprehensive NNMRRP of the 1990s never realized its full potential in part because PL 101–445 was an example of authorization without appropriation, and this may represent a missed opportunity. Nevertheless, knowledge of the past can and should provide guidance to the future. The chronic disease nutrition-related health problems of today and the future likely will not be solved until more widespread food and beverage marketing changes occur. These changes may not come about in the absence of far reaching policy changes. All of this could be better informed by a reinvigorated coordinated national nutrition monitoring and related research program. In the United States, this could be achieved by an appropriate champion for the program from either the legislative or the executive branch, or ideally from both branches of the federal government.

REFERENCES

1. US General Accounting Office. Nutrition Monitoring: Establishing a Model Program. GAO/PEMD 95–19. Washington, DC: US General Accounting Office, 1995:1–88.
2. National Nutrition Monitoring and Related Research Act of 1990 (PL 101–445), Cong Rec 1990;136, Oct 22.
3. Forbes AL, Stephenson MG. J Am Diet Assoc 1984;84:1189–93.
4. US Departments of Health and Human Services and of Agriculture. Operational plan for the national nutrition monitoring system. Unpublished government report, 1987:1–47.
5. Ostenso GL. J Am Diet Assoc 1984;84:1181–5.
6. Food and Agriculture Act of 1977 (PL 95–113), Sec 1428. Cong Rec 1977;123, Sept 29.
7. US Departments of Health, Education and Welfare and of Agriculture. Proposal: A comprehensive nutritional status monitoring system. Unpublished US government report, 1978.
8. Porter D. A National Nutrition Monitoring System: Brief Background and Bill Review. CRS Report for Congress no. 88–199 SPR. Washington, DC: Congressional Research Service, 1988:1–50.
9. US Departments of Health and Human Services and of Agriculture. Joint implementation plan for a comprehensive national nutrition monitoring system. Unpublished government report, 1981:1–59.
10. US Departments of Health and Human Services and of Agriculture. Nutrition Monitoring in the United States: A Progress Report from the Joint Nutrition Monitoring Evaluation Committee. DHHS Pub. No. (PHS) 86–1255. Washington, DC: US Government Printing Office, 1986:1–356.
11. US Department of Health and Human Services, Interagency Committee on Nutrition Monitoring. Announcement of Committee Formation. 53 FR 26505 No. 134. Washington, DC: US Government Printing Office, 1988.
12. Life Sciences Research Office, Federation of American Societies for Experimental Biology. Nutrition Monitoring in the United States: An Update Report On Nutrition Monitoring. DHHS Pub. No. (PHS) 89–1255. Washington, DC: US Government Printing Office, 1989:1–158, 247 pp of appendices.
13. Nestle M. J Nutr Ed 1990;22:141–4.
14. Kuczmarski MF, Moshfegh A, Briefel R. J Am Diet Assoc 1994;94:753–60.
15. Woteki CE, Briefel RR, Klein JK et al. Nutrition Monitoring: A Statement from an American Society for Nutritional Sciences Working Group. 2002:1–44. Available at http://www.nutrition.org/cgi/data/132/12/3782/DC1/1. Last accessed June 2004.
16. US Departments of Health and Human Services and of Agriculture. Fed Reg 1991;56:55, 716–55, 767.
17. US Departments of Health and Human Services and of Agriculture. Fed Reg 1993;58:32, 752–32, 806.
18. Interagency Board for Nutrition Monitoring and Related Research. Nutrition monitoring in the United States. Chartbook 1: Selected findings from the National Nutrition and Related Research Program. Ervin B, Reed D, eds. DHHS Pub. No. (PHS) 93-1255-1. Hyattsville, MD: Public Health Service, 1993:1–136.
19. Life Sciences Research Office, Federation of American Societies for Experimental Biology. Third report on nutrition monitoring in the United States (Executive summary, 55 pp; vol 1, 365 pp; and vol 2, 354pp). Prepared for the Interagency Board for Nutrition Monitoring and Related Research. Washington, DC: US Government Printing Office, 1995.
20. Woteki CE. J Nutr 2003;133:582S–84S.
21. Dwyer J, Picciano MF, Raiten DJ. J Nutr 2003;133:576S–81S.
22. US Department of Agriculture. Integration of the National Health and Nutrition Examination Survey and the Continuing Survey of Food Intakes by Individuals. Unpublished government document, 2001:1–6.
23. Woteki CE, Briefel RR, Klein JK et al. J Nutr 2002;132:3782–3.
24. Briefel RR. Nutrition monitoring in the United States. In: Bowman BA, Russell RM, eds. Present Knowledge in Nutrition. 8th ed. Washington, DC: International Life Sciences Institute, 2001:617–35.

25. Stiebeling HK, Monroe D, Coons CM et al. Family Food Consumption and Dietary Levels: Five regions. Consumer Purchases Study. USDA misc. Pub. No. 405. Washington, DC: US Government Printing Office, 1941.

26. Dwyer J, Picciano MF, Raiten DJ et al. J Nutr 2003;133:590S–600S.

27. Hamma MY, Riddick HA. Fam Econ Rev 1988;2:24–7.

28. Life Sciences Research Office, Federation of American Societies for Experimental Biology. Impact of Nonresponse on Dietary Data from the 1987–88 Nationwide Food Consumption Survey. Bethesda, MD: Life Sciences Research Office, Federation of American Societies for Experimental Biology, 1991:1–39.

29. Interagency Board for Nutrition Monitoring and Related Research. Nutrition Monitoring in the United States: The Directory of Federal and State Nutrition Monitoring Activities. DHHS Pub. No. (PHS) 92-1255-1. Washington, DC: US Government Office, 1992:1–117.

30. US General Accounting Office: Nutrition monitoring: mismanagement of nutrition survey has resulted in questionable data. GAO/RCED 91–117. Gaithersburg, MD: US General Accounting Office, 1991.

31. Documentation Supplemental Children's Survey (CSFII 1998) to the 1994–96 Continuing Survey of Food Intakes by Individuals. Available at http://www.pop.psu.edu/data-archive/codebooks/csfii/doc.pdf. Last accessed June, 2004.

32. Raper N, Perloff B, Ingwersen et al. J Food Comp Anal 2004;17:545–55.

33. Interagency Committee on Nutrition Monitoring. Nutrition Monitoring in the United States: The Directory of Federal Nutrition Monitoring Activities. DHHS Pub. No. (PHS) 89-1255-1. Washington, DC: US Government Printing Office, 1989:1–64.

34. US Department of Health, Education and Welfare. Ten-State Nutrition Survey 1968–1970. DHEW Pub. No. (HSM) 72–8130-n-72-8133. Washington, DC: US Government Printing Office, 1972.

35. National Center for Health Statistics. Plan and Operation of the Health and Nutrition Examination Survey, United States, 1971–1973 (Part A: Development, Plan, and Operation). Vital and Health Statistics series 1, no. 10a. DHEW pub. no. (PHS) 79-1310. Washington, DC: US Government Printing Office, 1973:1–46.

36. National Center for Health Statistics. Plan and Operation of the Health and Nutrition Examination Survey, United States, 1971-1973 (Part B: Data Collection Forms of the Survey). Vital and Health Statistics series 1, no. 10b. DHEW Pub. No. (PHS) 79-1310. Washington, DC: US Government Printing Office, 1977:1–77.

37. National Center for Health Statistics. Plan and Operation of the Second National Health and Nutrition Examination Survey, 1976–80. Vital and Health Statistics series 1, no. 15. DHHS Pub. No. (PHS) 81–1317. Washington, DC: US Government Printing Office, 1981:1–144.

38. National Center for Health Statistics. Plan and Operation of the Hispanic Health and Nutrition Examination Survey, 1982–1984. Vital and Health Statistics series 1, no. 19. DHHS pub. no. (PHS) 85-1321. Washington, DC: US Government Printing Office, 1985:1–429.

39. Interagency Board for Nutrition Monitoring and Related Research. Bialostosky K, ed. Nutrition Monitoring in the United States: The Directory of Federal and State Nutrition Monitoring and Related Research Activities. Hyattsville, MD: National Center for Health Statistics. 2000, 267 pp. Available at http://www.cdc.gov/nchs/data/misc/direc-99.pdf

40. National Center for Health Statistics. NHANES Analytic Guidelines, June 2004. Available at http://www.cdc.gov/nchs/data/nhanes/nhanes_general_guidelines_june_04.pdf. Last accessed July, 2004.

41. US Department of Health and Human Services. National Health and Nutrition Examination Survey: 1999–2004. Survey Content 2003. Available at http://www.cdc.gov/nchs/data/nhanes/comp3.pdf. Last accessed June, 2004.

42. 2001–2002 National Health and Nutrition Examination Survey (NHANES) Survey Operations Manuals, Brochures, Consent Documents. Available at http://www.cdc.gov/nchs/about/major/nhanes/current_nhanes_01_02.htm. Last accessed July, 2004.

43. Kuczmarski RJ, Ogden CL, Guo SS et al. Vital Health Stat 2002;11:246.

44. Hedley AA, Ogden CL, Johnson CL et al. JAMA 2004;291:2847–50.

45. US Department of Health and Human Services. Healthy People 2010: Understanding and Improving Health. 2nd ed. Washington, DC: US Government Printing Office, 2000:1–76.

46. Wright JD, Kennedy-Stephenon J, Wang CY et al. MMWR Morb Mortal Wkly Rep 2004;53:80–2.

47. National Center for Health Statistics. MMWR Morb Mortal Wkly Rep 2000;49:962–5.

48. Murphy SP. J Nutr 2003;133[Suppl]:585S–89S.

49. Conway JM, Ingwersen LA, Moshfegh AJ. J Am Diet Assoc 2004;104:595–603.

50. Radimer KL. J Nutr 2003;133[Suppl]:2003S–7S.

51. Heimbach JT. J Nutr 2001;131[Suppl]:1335S–8S.

52. Anderson E, Steinfeldt LC, Ahuja JKC. J Food Comp Anal 2004;17:557–64.

53. Interagency Board for Nutrition Monitoring and Related Research, Survey Comparability Working Group. Improving Comparability in the National Nutrition Monitoring and Related Research Program: Population Descriptors. Hyattsville, MD: National Center for Health Statistics, 1992:1–135.

54. Dwyer J, Picciano MF, Raiten DJ et al. J Nutr 2003;133[Suppl]:624S–34S.

55. Guthrie JF, Nord M. J Am Diet Assoc 2002;102:904–6.

56. Hall B. Hunger Issue Brief. 2004; March:1–6. Available at http://www.centeronhunger.org/pdf/understanding.pdf. Last accessed June, 2004.

57. US General Accounting Office: Nutrition Monitoring: Data Serve Many Purposes; Users Recommend Improvements. GAO/PEMD 95–15. Washington, DC: US General Accounting Office, 1995:1–62.

58. Polhamus B, Dalenius K, Thompson D et al. Pediatric Nutrition Surveillance 2002 Report. Atlanta: Centers for Disease Control and Prevention, 2004:1–12. Available at http://www.cdc.gov/nccdphp/dnpa/pednss.htm. Last accessed August, 2004.

59. Centers for Disease Control and Prevention, personal communication. September 23, 2004.

SELECTED READINGS

National Nutrition Monitoring and Related Research Act of 1990 (PL 101–445). Congressional Record, October 20, 1990.

US Departments of Health and Human Services and of Agriculture. Ten-year comprehensive plan for the National Nutrition Monitoring and Related Research Program. Fed Reg 1993;58:32, 752–32, 806.

Supplement: Future Directions for What We Eat in America— NHANES: The integrated CSFII-NHANES. J Nutr 2003;133 [Suppl]:575S–635S.

107 FOOD-BASED DIETARY GUIDELINES FOR HEALTHIER POPULATIONS: INTERNATIONAL CONSIDERATIONS[1]

RICARDO UAUY, EVA HERTRAMPF, AND ALAN D. DANGOUR

EVOLUTION OF NUTRITIONAL RECOMMENDATIONS
FROM THE NATIONAL TO THE
INTERNATIONAL REALM 1701
BASIC CONSIDERATIONS IN DEFINING
NUTRITIONAL REQUIREMENTS AND
FOOD-BASED DIETARY GUIDELINES 1702
BASIC CONSIDERATIONS IN DEVELOPING
FOOD-BASED DIETARY GUIDELINES 1703
  Relevant Nutritional Problems 1703
  Nutrient Content of Foods and Bioavailability ...1704
  Nutritional Adequacy of Population
    Dietary Intakes 1704
  Access to Food and Nutritional Security 1707
  How to Accomplish Dietary Diversity
    in Practice 1707
MODIFICATION OF NUTRITIONAL QUALITY
OF PLANT AND ANIMAL FOODS 1707
STEPS IN THE DEVELOPMENT OF FOOD-BASED
DIETARY GUIDELINES 1708
VARIATIONS IN NATIONAL FOOD-BASED DIETARY
GUIDELINES 1710
EFFECT OF GENETIC VARIABILITY AND EPIGENETIC
FACTORS ON THE DEFINITION OF FOOD-BASED
DIETARY GUIDELINES: THE CASES OF CALCIUM
AND OF VITAMIN D 1710
GLOBAL FOOD-BASED DIETARY GUIDELINES:
ARE THEY POSSIBLE, DESIRABLE, AND
ACHIEVABLE? 1714

EVOLUTION OF NUTRITIONAL RECOMMENDATIONS FROM THE NATIONAL TO THE INTERNATIONAL REALM

The foods available to humans have varied over the course of evolution, depending on prevailing environmental conditions that affect climate, solar radiation, soil characteristics, and water resources. These conditions, fundamental for the development of agriculture in prehistoric times,

still play an important role in defining agriculture today. The human diet has similarly evolved from a predominantly hunter-gatherer or scavenger model to the present agriculture-based mode. Humans in preagricultural times depended on foraging plant foods such as seeds, fruits, and nuts as well as hunting small animals; if they inhabited the land-water interface, they were able to collect molluscs and algae and to catch fish (1). They were also likely to have been scavengers of meat that had been hunted by predators larger and stronger than humans. Agriculture evolved in very specific ecologic settings that facilitated the domestication and selection of the main food crops on which we currently rely. In these settings, wheat, corn, rice, and potatoes became the key food crops, supporting the expansion of human populations to the current levels of more than 6 billion persons (2).

Traditional dietary patterns have changed with time and have withstood the test of human evolution. Indeed, most naturally occurring dietary patterns meet or exceed the nutritional needs of populations, although this is not the case where social or economic conditions limit access to food (purchasing capacity) or where cultural practices restrict the choice of foods consumed. However, within the framework of our present understanding of food-health relationships, it seems likely that a large variety of foods can be combined in varying amounts to provide a healthy diet. Thus, it is difficult to determine a precise indispensable intake of individual foods that can, when combined with other foods, provide a nutritionally adequate diet under all conditions. The prevailing view is that a large set of food combinations is compatible with nutritional adequacy, but no given set of food can be extrapolated as absolutely required or sufficient across different ecologic settings. Recent trends in the globalization of food supply provide clear evidence that dietary patterns and even traditionally local foods can move across geographic niches.

The modern approach in defining nutritional adequacy of diets and dietary recommendations has progressed over the past 2 centuries in accordance with the scientific understanding of the biochemical and physiologic basis of human nutritional requirements in health and disease. The definition of essential nutrients and nutrient requirements has provided the scientific underpinnings for nutrient-based dietary recommendations. However, there are

---

[1]**Abbreviations: EAR,** estimated average requirement; **FAO,** Food and Agriculture Organization; **FBDGs,** food-based dietary guidelines; **RNI,** recommended nutrient intake; **SNP,** single-nucleotide polymorphism; **WHO,** World Health Organization.

obvious limitations to the reductionist nutrient-based approach, because people consume foods and not nutrients. Moreover, the effect of specific foods and of dietary patterns on health goes well beyond the combination of essential nutrients the food may contain. For example, if we neglect to integrate bioavailability or nutrient interactions in defining trace element recommendations, we will not be able to assess the true nutritional value of foods. In addition, factors unrelated to diet commonly play a key role on the health effect of diet; for example, parasitic infections, rather than iron deficiency, may be the cause of anaemia in many parts of the world (3). Similarly, if we continue to ignore or undervalue the key role of physical activity in achieving energy balance, dietary recommendations will fail to meet the goal of preventing obesity and other nutrition-related chronic diseases.

BASIC CONSIDERATIONS IN DEFINING NUTRITIONAL REQUIREMENTS AND FOOD-BASED DIETARY GUIDELINES

Since the early 1960s, expert committees have established nutrient-based recommendations for virtually every essential nutrient known to humankind (4–9). The quantitative definitions of nutrient needs and their expression as recommended nutrient intakes (RNIs) or dietary reference intakes have been important instruments of food and nutrition policy in many countries and have focused the attention of international bodies on necessary nutrient intakes. RNIs are customarily defined as the intake of energy and specific nutrients necessary to satisfy the requirements of a group of healthy individuals. This nutrient-based approach has served well to advance science but has not always fostered the establishment of nutritional and dietary priorities consistent with broad public health interests at national and international levels (10).

In contrast, food-based dietary guidelines (FBDGs) as instruments of policy are more closely linked to the diet-health relationships of relevance to the particular country or region of interest (11). FBDGs address health concerns related to dietary insufficiency, excess, or imbalance with a broader perspective, considering the totality of the effects of a given dietary pattern (12). A clear definition of nutritional requirements of the population has its role as a fundamental component of food and nutrition policy goals along with the priorities embodied in the FBDGs for improved nutrition, health, and well-being. In this setting, RNIs are used as a basic criteria to assess whether the proposed diet is sufficient to meet established nutrient recommendations. RNIs can also be used to support educational efforts in the implementation of dietary guidelines and to provide a basis for consumer information on the nutritional adequacy of specific foods.

The criteria used to estimate nutritional requirements have changed over time, as described in other chapters in this book (see Chapter 104). The main approaches used in establishing international recommendations are as follows:

1. The clinical approach is based on the need to correct or prevent nutrient-specific diseases associated with deficient intake. (Signs and symptoms of nutritional deficit and/or excess are provided in the nutrient-specific chapters of this book). This methodology is a highly specific but, for ethical reasons, clearly inappropriate method for establishing nutrient dose responses. However, information sporadically gathered from unintended outbreaks of deficit or excess can be used to define the levels of intake at which clinical signs or symptoms appear.

2. Functional indicators of nutritional sufficiency (molecular, cellular, biochemical, physiologic) can be used to assess nutritional normalcy and to define the limits for deficit and excess of specific nutrients. The approach is based on a defined set of biomarkers that are sensitive to changes in nutritional state and are specific in terms of identifying subclinical deficiency conditions. The use of balance data to define requirements should be avoided whenever possible because adaptation to intake may lead to equilibrium at a fairly wide range of intakes (9, 13, 14). In most cases, observed balance based on input-output measurements is greatly influenced by level of intake; that is, subjects adjust to high intakes by increasing output, and conversely they lower output when intake is low. The same applies to nutrient blood levels because these levels usually reflect levels of intake and absorption rather than functional state. The set of biomarkers that can be used to define requirements includes measures of nutrient stores, nutrient turnover, or critical tissue/organ pools.

3. The habitual consumption levels of "healthy" populations serve as a basis to establish a range of adequate intakes. In the absence of quantitative estimates based on the clinical or functional indicators of sufficiency, this criterion remains the first approximation to establishing requirements.

4. More recently, the concept of optimal nutrient intake has emerged and has influenced both scientists and the general public. The idea of optimal nutrient intake is based on the quest for improved functionality, be it in terms of muscle strength, immune function, or intellectual ability. The question "Optimal for what?" is usually answered by the suggestion that diet or specific nutrients can improve or enhance a given function, ameliorate the age-related decline in function, or decrease the burden of illness associated with loss of function. The goal is to add healthy life years and to prevent disability, in line with the use of disability-adjusted life years as a measure of health. However, the concept of optimal intake is too broad to be assessed quantitatively and is usually unsupported by appropriate population-based controlled studies. Thus, the preferred

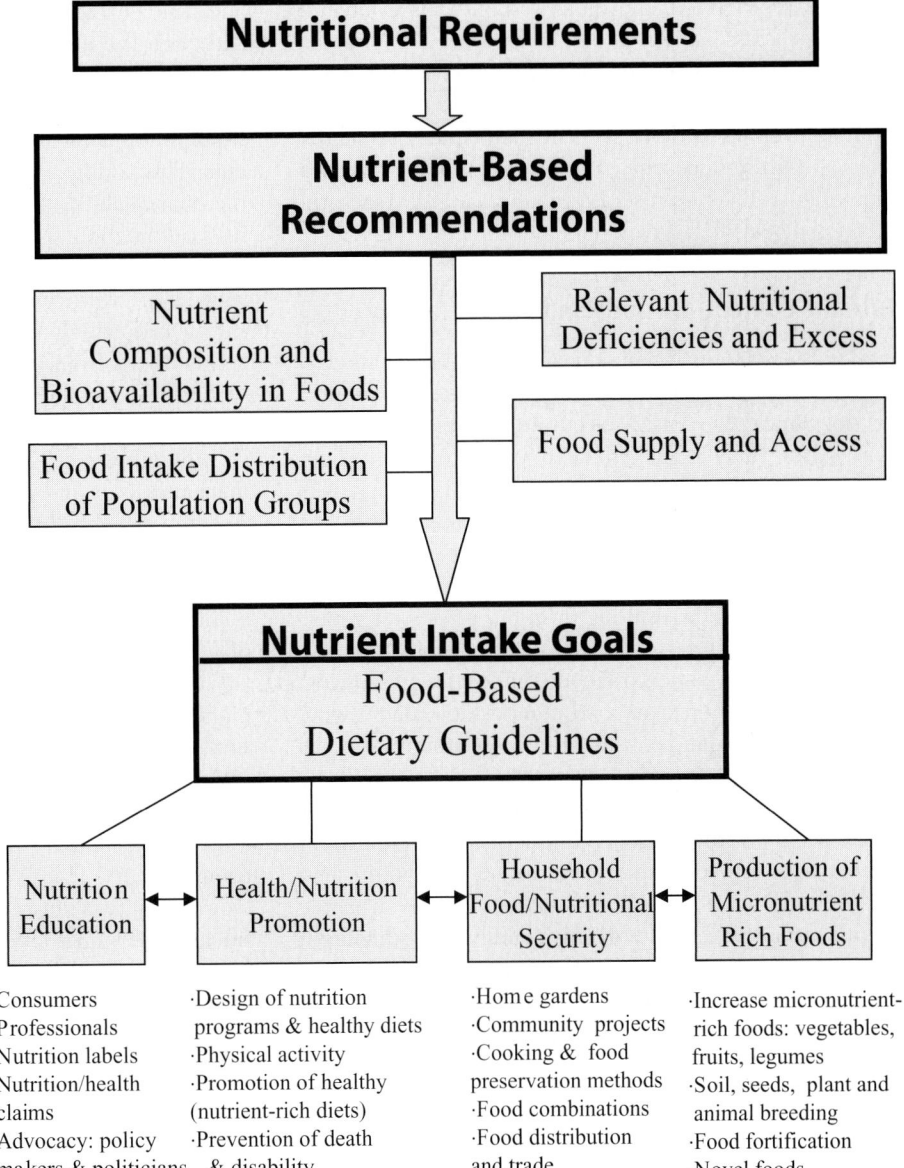

Figure 107.1. This schematic representation summarizes the process of defining food-based dietary guidelines (FBDGs), detailed descriptions of each step can be found in the text. The **bottom panel** presents the end uses of FBDGs and provides specific examples.

approach is to define clearly the goal that is of public health interest in relation to the intake of a specific nutrient or a given food (15). The selected goal should be directly related to a function of relevance to health or quality of life.

The quantified RNI estimates derived from these various approaches may differ for any given nutrient, although the implications of these differences in the establishment of FBDGs are usually minor (11, 12, 16). RNIs serve as the basis to establish nutrient intake goals that correspond to the desired target intakes that will achieve better health and nutrition for a given population within an ecologic setting. Their purpose is to promote overall health and/or to control specific nutritional disease induced by excess or deficit, as well as to reduce health risks considering the multifactorial nature of disease. Once nutrient intake

goals are defined, FBDGs can be established, by taking into account the customary dietary pattern, the foods available, and the factors that determine the consumption of foods and by indicating what aspects should be modified (Fig. 107.1). FBDGs consider the ecologic setting, socioeconomic and cultural factors, and the biologic and physical environments that affect the health and nutrition of a given population or community.

BASIC CONSIDERATIONS IN DEVELOPING FOOD-BASED DIETARY GUIDELINES

Relevant Nutritional Problems

The process of setting dietary guidelines is initiated by defining the significant diet-related public health problems in a given community (see Fig. 107.1). Once these problems are defined, the diet component is evaluated, including the assessment of dietary adequacy, by comparing available information on dietary intake with the RNIs. The purpose of nutrient intake goals in this situation is to promote overall health, to prevent specific nutritional disease, and to reduce the risk of diet-related diseases. Dietary guidelines represent a practical way to reach the nutritional goals for a given population.

Nutrient Content of Foods and Bioavailability

Accurate information on chemical composition of foods is needed to assess diets, to prevent and control micronutrient deficiencies, to ensure accurate information to consumers using nutrition labels, and to promote healthy diets. Unfortunately, food composition data for many regions of the world are insufficient or inadequate, thus limiting the assessment of dietary quality and the effectiveness of proposed interventions. The demand for data on nutrient composition of foods resulting from the process of generating FBDGs should serve to advocate for more complete and updated information on food composition worldwide. Stimulating an interest in food composition among government, industry, and consumer interest groups is crucial for this process.

The recognition of various situations in which deficiency occurs in the presence of adequate micronutrient content in the food supply has elicited great interest in determining the proportion of nutrients in food available for utilization by the body (bioavailability). We highlight here some aspects of particular relevance in defining optimal food combinations when establishing FBDGs.

Both food preparation and dietary practices need to be considered when attempting to attain vitamin A, vitamin C, folate, iron, and zinc dietary adequacy using food-based approaches. For example, it is important to recommend that vegetables rich in vitamin C, folate, and other water-soluble or heat-labile vitamins be cooked or steamed in small amounts of water over short periods of time. In the case of iron bioavailability, it is essential to reduce the intake of inhibitors of absorption and to increase the intake of enhancers in a given meal. Following this strategy, it is recommended to increase the intake of germinated seeds, fermented cereals and/or heat processed cereals, meats, and fruits or vegetables rich in vitamin C while avoiding the consumption of tea with meals. It should also be recommended to decrease the intake of high-fiber foods and high-polyphenol foods such as tea, coffee, chocolate, and herbal teas and to separate their intake from iron-rich meals (17).

In the case of zinc, flesh foods improve zinc absorption, whereas diets high in phytate, particularly diets based on unrefined cereals, inhibit zinc absorption. Zinc availability can be estimated according to the phytate/zinc (molar) ratio of the meal (18). Major cereal/tuber-based diets are clearly insufficient in vitamin A, vitamin C, folate, iron,

and zinc, in terms of both content and bioavailability. Although the inclusion of a few micronutrient-rich foods can be successfully used to achieve dietary adequacy, the optimal levels of folate, iron, and zinc commonly require a small amount of animal flesh as a source of micronutrients. This addition will improve nutrient density as well as the bioavailability of iron present in plant sources. A careful combination of plant foods, including legumes, fermented foods, sprouting seeds, and single-cell extracts such as brewer's yeast can also provide the required critical micronutrients for groups that opt to limit or exclude animal foods from their diet.

Figure 107.2 illustrates how food combinations serve to complement specific staple foods in providing a balance of specific nutrients. The figure presents information on key micronutrients and presents dietary adequacy in terms of recommended nutrient density. The figure demonstrates that rice alone, consumed in amounts that satisfy energy needs, is insufficient to meet micronutrient needs, but in combination with five or six small portions (around 50 g) of other foods, it can provide the necessary nutrient density to meet recommended nutrient densities. However, dietary diversification may remain insufficient to meet the nutritional needs of populations if the bioavailability of the micronutrients is poor. In this case, micronutrient fortification of centrally processed foods or at the household level may serve as an effective means to enhance micronutrient delivery. The effect of fortification on micronutrient bioavailability is illustrated in Figure 107.3, using iron fortification of wheat and maize as examples (19). The presence of inhibitors in the maize renders iron less bioavailable than in wheat, and this demands the use of iron compounds that can be better absorbed. At the same time, these compounds react with the food matrix and thereby limit the amount that can be used without affecting the sensory properties or the shelf-life of the food products made from the staple. Thus, both iron compound and compatibility of the food matrix are crucial in determining the amount of iron that can be included and effectively absorbed from the food (20).

Nutritional Adequacy of Population Dietary Intakes

A healthy diet can be attained in more than one way, given the variety of foods that can be combined. In practice, the set of food combinations compatible with nutritional adequacy is restricted by the level of food production that is sustainable in a given ecologic and population setting. In most countries, this restriction has been overcome because imported food can provide for a stable food supply independent of local food production. Of greater significance are the economic constraints that limit food supply at the household level, frequently the true underlying cause of nutritional deficiencies. The development of FBDGs recognizes this inherent variability and focuses on the food combinations that can best meet nutrient requirements,

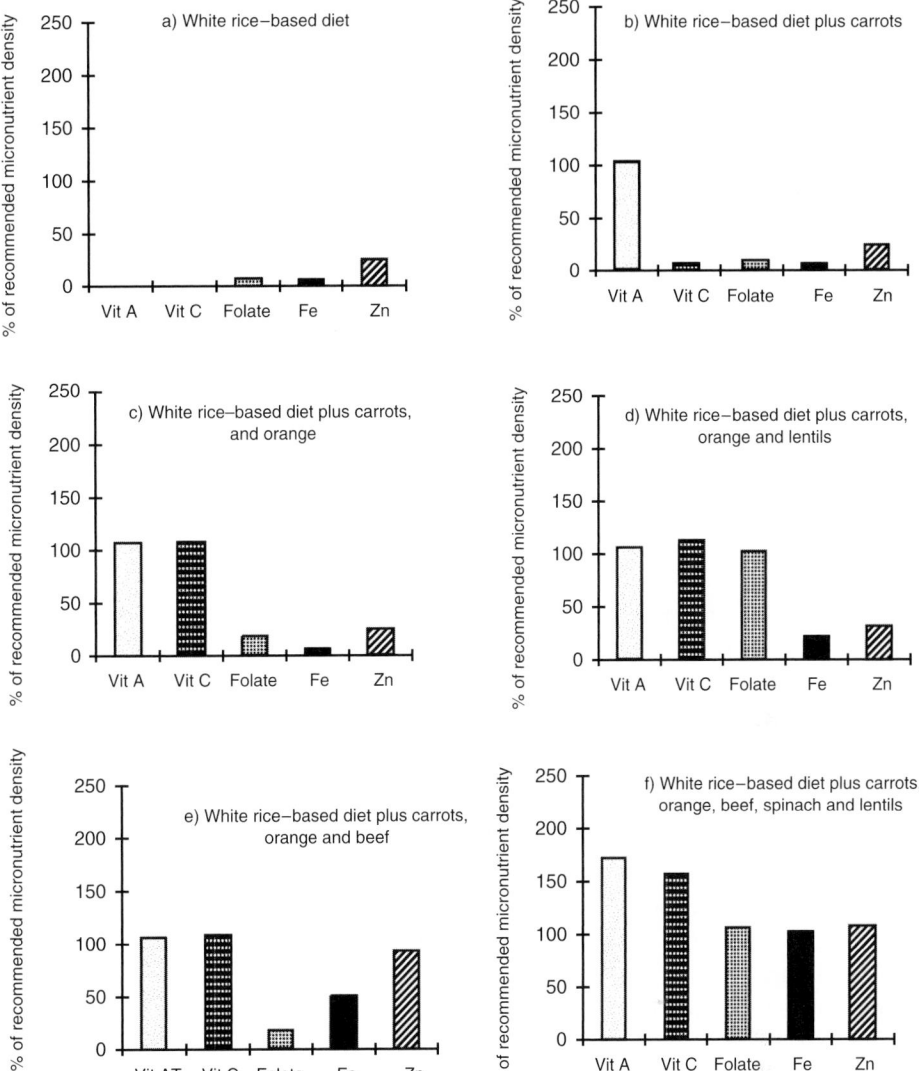

Figure 107.2. An example of food-based dietary diversification to meet micronutrient needs. A white rice–based diet has been enriched with small amounts of micronutrient-rich foods; vitamin A, vitamin C, folate, iron, and zinc adequacy is expressed as a percentage of recommended nutrient density values proposed in reference 11. Details of nutrient content and amount of food in the combinations can be found in reference 19.

rather than on how best to ensure that each specific nutrient is provided in adequate amounts (see Fig. 107.1).

The intake level that will meet specified criteria of nutritional adequacy, preventing risk of deficit or excess, is called the individual requirement. The criteria used to define individual requirements include a gradient of biologic effects related to the level of nutrient intake. This dose response is assumed to have a gaussian distribution if it has not been characterized; thus, a risk function of deficiency and excess can be derived.

The use of dietary recommendations in assessing the adequacy of nutrient intakes of populations requires good quantitative information of the distribution of usual nutrient intakes as well as knowledge of the distribution of requirements. The assessment of intake should include all sources of nutrient intake, that is, food, water, and supplements. Appropriate dietary and food composition data are essential to achieve a valid estimate of intakes. The day-to-day variation in individual intakes can be minimized by collecting intake data over several days. There are several statistical approaches to estimate the prevalence of inadequate intakes from the distribution of intakes and requirements. A simplified method is the estimated average requirement (EAR) cut-point approach, which defines the fraction of a population that consumes less than the EAR for a given nutrient. It assumes that variability of individual intakes is at least as large as the variability in requirements and that the distributions of intakes and requirements are independent of each other. The latter is commonly the case for vitamin and minerals but clearly it is not the case for energy intake. The EAR cut-point method requires a single population with a symmetric distribution around the mean. If these conditions are met, the prevalence of inadequate intakes corresponds to the proportion of intakes that fall below the EAR. It is clearly inappropriate to examine mean values of population intakes and take the proportion that fall below the RNI to define the population at risk of inadequacy. The relevant information is the proportion of intakes in a population group that is below the EAR (9, 21).

**% Fe absorption based on
fortificant and food matrix**

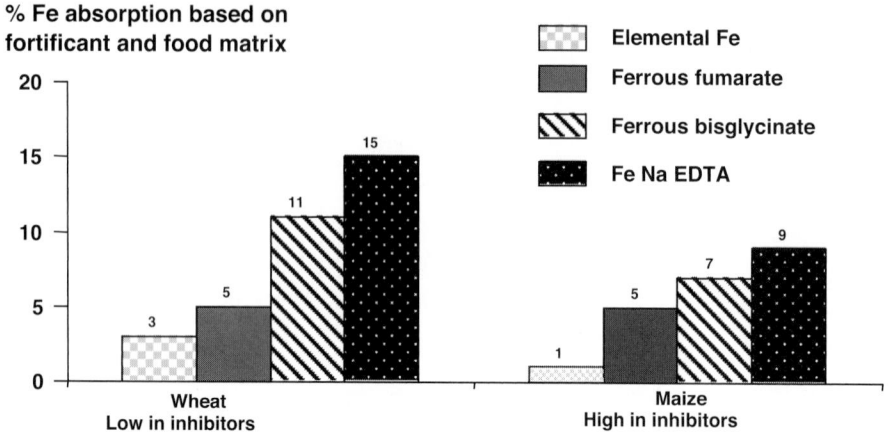

**Compatibility with food matrix
Max Fe load (mg/kg)**

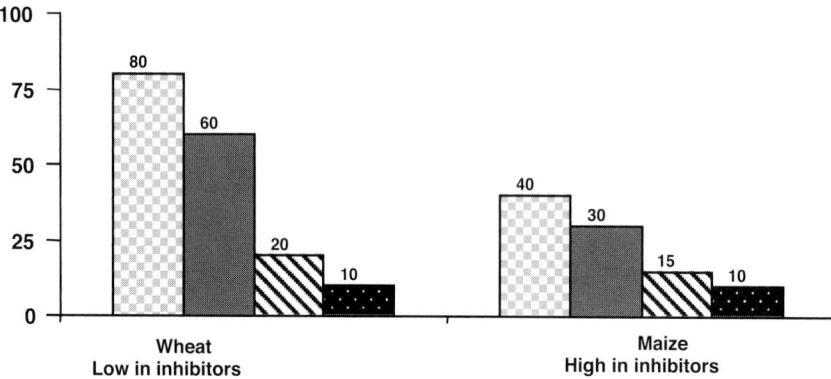

**Biologic impact
Fe absorbed mg per 100 g of product**

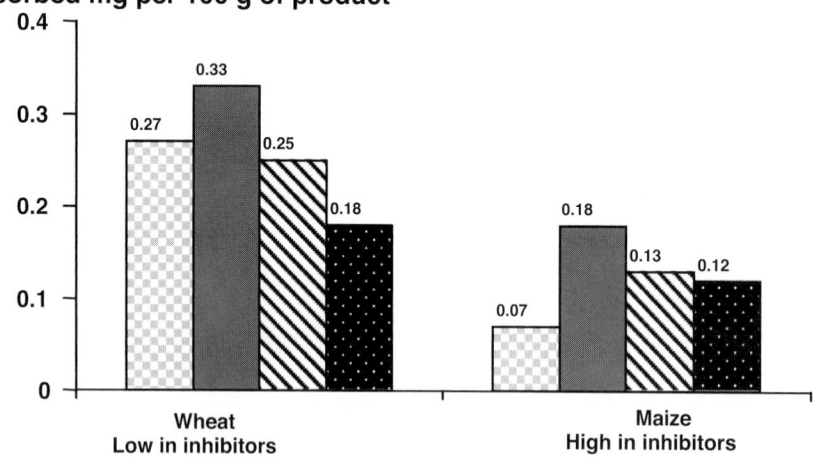

Figure 107.3. The biologic impact of iron fortification depends on the interaction of the iron fortificant and the food matrix, which determine the percentage of absorption, maximal iron load compatible with the food, and the resulting absorbed iron from the consumption of 100 g of the fortified food. Refined wheat flour represents a matrix with a low amount of inhibitors, whereas industrially produced maize dough for tortilla manufacturing is an example of a matrix with a high content of inhibitors [phytates, $Ca(OH)_2$]. The numbers on top of the bars correspond to respective value. Biologic impact is the product of percentage of absorbed iron and maximal iron load depending on the fortificant used and the food matrix; a small amount of iron derived from the matrix has been included in the final calculation. (Adapted from Uauy R, Hertrampf E, Reddy M. J Nutr 2002;132[Suppl]: 849S–52S.)

It is not absolutely necessary to define exact quantitative estimates of nutritional needs to assess the adequacy of FBDGs. Dietary quality can be assessed by comparing a given food combination with established recommendations. Because the household is the basic unit for food consumption under most settings, if there is enough food, individual members of the household can consume a diet within the recommended nutrient density values to

meet the need for specific nutrients. However, the problem of inappropriate intrahousehold food distribution escapes this analysis and should be considered, because children, women, and older people may not receive an equitable portion of foods with higher nutrient density (22). This possibility should be taken into account in establishing both general dietary guidelines and those specifically addressing the needs of vulnerable groups in the community. In addition, if the physiologic condition (i.e., pregnancy or rapid growth during infancy) does not increase energy needs in direct proportion to the increased requirements for specific nutrients, consumption of more of the same foods may not secure adequate protein, vitamin, or mineral intake to meet the recommended intakes for these situations. For these reasons, FBDGs usually exclude children less than 2 years of age and pregnant and lactating women. Specific guidelines for these groups have been established by some expert groups and international bodies.

Access to Food and Nutritional Security

Populations in developing countries often consume a monotonous diet out of need, rather than choice, because their access to different foods is often curtailed by economic factors. The percentage of increase in the consumption of a food item when income increases by 1% is called the elasticity of consumption of the given food item. Most staple foods such as rice, wheat, and corn have low income elasticity; that is, even if income increases greatly, the increase in the amount of staple foods eaten will be small. However, meat and animal food products have high income elasticity; that is, there is a large effect of income on consumption patterns. This can clearly be seen in that the amount of animal protein foods consumed by the wealthiest 20% of the world's population is four times larger than that consumed by the poorest 20%.

If access to food were not dependent on income but on need, the food available globally would be sufficient to meet the needs of humankind. A corollary to this conditional statement is that unless economic constraints in food consumption are overcome, dietary diversification will fail. The prevention of malnutrition of women and children through dietary means in economically deprived population groups will not work unless people have access to foods that are adequate in quantity and quality. This is part of the human-rights–based approach: the right to food (23). Food security cannot be determined based on the availability of food energy alone; nutritional security requires that all essential micronutrients are covered by the food supply. In the absence of major changes in income distribution in selected developing countries or major accelerations in economic growth in most of the developing world, other possible alternatives to achieve adequate dietary intake must be sought.

How to Accomplish Dietary Diversity in Practice

It is essential to work on strategies that promote and facilitate dietary diversification among the poor to achieve the complementation of cereal/tuber-based diets with micronutrient-rich foods. The following strategies have been used to promote dietary diversification within the implementation of food-based approaches (24).

Small-Scale Community Vegetable and Fruit Gardens

These projects should increase the production and consumption of micronutrient-rich foods at the community or household level. The success of such projects requires good knowledge and understanding of local conditions, as well as the involvement of women and overall community participation. These are key elements to support, achieve, and sustain the beneficial nutritional change at the household level. Conversely, land availability and water supply may be common constrains that often require local government intervention or support.

Household Production of Poultry, Fish, and Other Small Animals (Rabbits, Goats, Guinea Pigs)

These are excellent sources of highly bioavailable essential micronutrients, such as vitamin A, iron, and zinc. The production of animal foods at the local level may permit communities to access foods that otherwise would not be available because of their high costs. These types of projects also need some support to overcome the cost constraints of implementation and training of producers.

Implementation of Large-Scale Commercial Vegetable and Fruit Production

This initiative has the objective of providing micronutrient-rich foods at reasonable prices, through effective and competitive markets that lower consumer costs without reducing producers' prices.

Reduction of Postharvest Losses and Nutritional Value of Micronutrient-Rich Foods

Improvement of storage and food preservation facilities of fruits and vegetables significantly reduces postharvest losses. At the household level, the promotion of effective cooking methods (minimal cooking of vegetables) and practical ways of preserving foods (solar drying of seasonal micronutrient-rich foods, such as grapes, mangoes, peaches, and apricots), may significantly increase the access to bioavailable micronutrient-rich foods. At the commercial level, grading, packing, transport, and marketing practices can reduce losses and optimize income generation.

MODIFICATION OF NUTRITIONAL QUALITY OF PLANT AND ANIMAL FOODS

One possible alternative strategy for obtaining adequate nutrient intake, especially when food-based approaches are not feasible because of economic constraints, is the fortification of foods, especially dietary staples. Fortification refers to the addition of nutrients to a commonly eaten food. It can be single, with only one nutrient (fortificant) added, or multiple, to include two or more nutrients. Fortification should be seen as complementary to food-based strategies and not as a replacement to dietary diversification, and it can serve as a cost-effective measure to resolve micronutrient deficiencies until food-based approaches become feasible. Food-based approaches that require family incomes to reach a sufficient level to provide adequate high-quality, nutrient-dense foods can often take longer to implement but, once established, are generally sustainable. However, three essential conditions must be met in any fortification program: (a) the fortificant should be effective, bioavailable, acceptable, and affordable; (b) the selected food vehicle should be easily accessible and eaten in regular amounts by all sectors of society; and (c) detailed production instructions and monitoring procedures should be in place and enforced by law (17, 25).

The advent of new agricultural practices including improvement of soils and enhanced plant micronutrient content via classical plant breeding or genetic modification may also enhance the potential impact of food-based guidelines. These processes may provide new meaning to effective fortification for key micronutrients, because it may be possible to include bioavailable micronutrients into crops that are currently consumed as staples. Recent developments in genetic modification offer great promise in achieving micronutrient sufficiency from staple foods. For example, the introduction of rice varieties rich in iron-containing proteins and carotene may drastically change the way we approach prevention of micronutrient deficits (26, 27). The elimination of antinutritional factors that affect bioavailability of minerals either through traditional breeding or genetic modifications may also enhance the utilization of iron and zinc in regular plant foods.

The nutritional quality of animal foods can also be affected by production practices. For example, the type and quantity of fats present in monogastric animals may be determined by the feed provided; Thus, if chicken are free-range fed, they will have lower total fat and more n-3 fatty acids than if they are given a maize-based feed and constrained in their movements. Eggs can be enriched in long-chain n-3 fatty acids if animals are provided fish meal or flax seed in their feed. Pork fat can be improved in nutritional quality if animals are fed meals high in polyunsaturated fatty acids (e.g., soy oil) (28). Milk and meat from ruminants are more difficult to alter through diet because microbial fermentation in the rumen modifies ingested nutrients significantly. However, new techniques of microencapsulation do permit the delivery of nutrients beyond the rumen. Cattle living in constrained environments and given cereal-based diets have a higher total fat content than their pasture fed counterparts. Genetic modification also allows drastic changes in fatty acid composition of animal tissues; recently, the introduction of an n-3 desaturase gene from a worm, the nematode *Caenorhabditis elegans*, into mice produced a dramatic increase in docosahexaenoic acid content of milk and muscle from these mammals (29).

Novel methods such as these provide a way to enhance the nutritional quality of diets without having to modify consumption patterns drastically. These approaches may prove acceptable to food producers who are reluctant to change their traditional food productions systems and will allow consumers to maintain their customary diet and still achieve the desired nutrient intake goals.

STEPS IN THE DEVELOPMENT OF FOOD-BASED DIETARY GUIDELINES

FBDGs are an instrument and an expression of food and nutrition policy and should be based directly on diet and disease relationships of particular relevance to individual countries. Priorities in establishing dietary guidelines will thereby address the relevant public health concerns, whether they are related to dietary insufficiency or excess. In this context, meeting the nutritional needs of the population takes its place as one of the components of food and nutrition policy goals along with the priorities included in the FBDGs to improve health and nutrition for a given population. In addition, dietary guidelines serve to educate the public through the mass media and provide a practical guide in selecting foods by defining dietary adequacy. Advice for a healthy diet should provide both a quantitative and qualitative description of the diet to be understood by individuals, with information of both the size and number of servings per day. The Food and Agriculture Organization/World Health Organization (FAO/WHO) expert committee on Preparation and Use of Food Based Dietary Guidelines suggests following a systematic approach in developing FBDGs (11). This model, summarized in the following paragraphs, has been tested and used by various countries with necessary local adaptations to ensure better implementation.

The initial step is the establishment of a working group that includes all relevant stakeholders. Membership should be broad, representing private and government institutions, agricultural and food industry, communication and anthropology specialists, nutrition scientists, consumer organizations, and public health and medical nutritionists. There should be ample discussion of relevant nutrition problems of the region of interest based on up-to-date survey information, ideally representing different regions and population groups. Once identified, the dietary component of the public health nutritional problem should be defined. Dietary factors (nutrient excess, deficit, or imbalance) should be examined beyond mean population intakes, because overconsumption or underconsumption may occur in specific population groups. For example, there may be a shift in the overall population intake or a distinct subpopulation that does not consume the given nutrient. These problems should be addressed differently, in the first case increasing the nutrient intake for the complete population while in the latter case acting to increase the intake of the specific population subgroup of underconsumers. This may, however, represent a practical problem because in some cases it may be virtually impossible to identify such a subgroup, whereas in other situations, implementation strategies cannot be targeted to one particular group alone.

The working group should discuss and prioritize the set of major public nutrition problems that will be addressed by the FBDGs and explore the foods available to improve the nutritional problem. There may be a need to explore whether it is possible to change the pattern of agricultural production and food distribution. There may also be a need to modify food subsidies, apparent or hidden, or other government policies that affect food consumption. The economic constraints in implementing food-based approaches should be considered as well as the possible solutions. This will clearly be different for urban societies, which depend on an industrialized food supply, and self-sufficient farmers, who consume what they produce.

The working group should then define a set of FBDGs that will address the nutrient intake and food patterns that require modification while considering the relevant social, cultural, and economic factors. A statement discussed and approved by all working group members should support each guideline technically. This may include circulating the draft and receiving input from technical parties not present in the working group. All iterations necessary to bring about technical consensus should be explored. The final draft of this step, including the messages that will reach consumers, should then be pilot tested with consumer groups and modified to ensure understanding by the target group. The results of the pilot tests should be used in establishing the revised guidelines.

The final set of guidelines and supporting technical statements should then be released for ample critical public review by all relevant groups. The support of international technical experts and relevant United Nations agencies may be helpful at this stage. Recent experience suggests that the Internet can be used to enhance input from consumer groups. Subsequent to further modifications resulting from the public consultation process, the FBDGs will be ready for final approval, publication in various formats, and dissemination and implementation for general use. The lower portion of Figure 107.1 provides a summary of potential end users of the FBDGs.

The impact of FBDGs in modifying food intake patterns and the relevant public nutrition problems should be periodically assessed. Measures to enhance their applicability such as mass media and educational campaigns, incorporation into school curricula, and inclusion in other health promotion programs should be implemented. Based on periodic assessment, the guidelines should be reexamined and/or revised within a set period, normally every 5 to 10 years, to ensure that they remain current and scientifically valid.

Experience with FBDG over the past decade suggests that FBDGs offer a feasible, effective, and sustainable approach to promote healthy eating of the population in general and to address nutrition problems in vulnerable groups. These guidelines foster a practical, consumer-oriented approach to reach specific nutritional goals for a given population. A focus on foods and food groups helps in the development of clear, easy-to-understand, behavioral messages suitable for the target audience. FBDGs often go beyond the purview of "foods"; for example, they may promote a healthy weight, encourage physical activity, and provide advice about water and food safety. In this situation, they often act as part of a nation's plan of action to improve nutrition in a more general perspective.

Importantly, FBDGs must facilitate choices for consumers that are consistent with their preferences, food culture, and economic resources. Typically, such guidelines recommend a minimum number of servings from each of four to seven basic food groups. FBDGs also commonly suggest the need to limit intake of certain components of foods, such as saturated and *trans*-fatty acids, added sugars, and salt.

Food-based strategies also offer many benefits that go beyond the prevention and control of nutrient deficiencies (Table 107.1). For example, FBDGs:

- Help prevent and control both macronutrient and micronutrient deficiencies by addressing underlying causes.
- Support health promotion and preventive health.
- Should be cost-effective and sustainable.
- Can be adapted to different cultural and dietary traditions and to strategies that are feasible at the local level.
- Address multiple nutrition problems simultaneously.
- Minimize the risk of toxicity and adverse nutrient interactions because the amounts of nutrients consumed are within usual physiologic levels.

TABLE 107.1. KEY FACTORS IN DEVELOPING NATIONAL FOOD-BASED DIETARY GUIDELINES, ACCORDING TO THE JOINT FOOD AND AGRICULTURE ORGANIZATION/WORLD HEALTH ORGANIZATION CONSULTATION ON PREPARATION AND USE OF FOOD-BASED DIETARY GUIDELINES

Scientific evidence concerning diet-health relationships
Prevalence of diet-related public health problems
Food consumption patterns of the population
Nutritional requirements
Potential food supply
Composition of foods, including consideration of food preparation practices
Bioavailability of nutrients supplied by the mixed local diet
Sociocultural factors that relate to food choices and accessibility
Food costs

Data from Food and Agriculture Organization/World Health Organization (FAO/WHO). Preparation and Use of Food-Based Dietary Guidelines. Report of a joint FAO/WHO Expert Consultation, Nicosia, Cyprus. WHO/NUT/96.6. Geneva: World Health Organization, 1996.

- Support the role of breast-feeding and the special diet and care needs of infants and young children.
- Can foster the development of sustainable, environmentally sound food production systems.
- May serve to alert agricultural planners to the need to protect the micronutrient content of soils and crops.
- Build partnerships among governments, consumer groups, the food industry, and other organizations to achieve the shared goals of overcoming nutrition-related health problems.
- Empower people to become more self-reliant using local resources.
- May serve to support the addition of functional components found in specific foods (i.e., fiber).
- Provide opportunities for social interaction and enjoyment.

VARIATIONS IN NATIONAL FOOD-BASED DIETARY GUIDELINES

Many nations have developed FBDGs for their populations (Table 107.2). Dietary guidelines across countries tend to be similar in their purposes, development, and uses. They are intended for use by health professionals but also by members of the general population and thus are mostly worded in simple, concrete terms. The similarity among the guidelines of many nations is striking: they all place an emphasis on balance, moderation (especially with regard to fat, sugar, salt, and alcohol) and variety, and they all highlight the importance of consuming sufficient portions of fruits, vegetables, and grains. However, there are also several differences among guidelines, including the following:

- Total number of guidelines: They range from 5 to 15.
- Food groupings: The greatest variance is in the grouping of starchy foods.
- Difference in emphasis on particular foods, food groups, or nutrients: Examples include "Eat a piece of liver or meat at least once a week," "Consume animal foods in moderate amounts," and "Consume iron-rich foods."
- Specificity of recommendation: Examples include "Choose whole-grain and enriched products more often" and "Eat a variety of grains daily, especially whole grains."
- Substantial differences in the approach to the fat intake recommendation: Examples include "Keep fat consumption at 20% of energy intake" and "Do not abuse fats."
- Different approach to selection of types of fats: Examples include "One-third polyunsaturated, one-third monounsaturated, one-third saturated" and "Use soft, vegetable margarine or oil instead of hard margarine or butter."
- Guidelines also differ in their emphases on the following: limiting foods or ingredients such as sugar, salt, alcohol, food additives; actions necessary for weight

maintenance and the need for physical activity; chemical and microbiologic food safety; the positive and pleasurable aspects of food.

EFFECT OF GENETIC VARIABILITY AND EPIGENETIC FACTORS ON THE DEFINITION OF FOOD-BASED DIETARY GUIDELINES: THE CASES OF CALCIUM AND OF VITAMIN D

Two approaches have traditionally been employed to estimate average calcium requirement: the factorial method and the balance method (30). In the factorial method, the estimated physiologic requirements for calcium are summed, and estimated obligatory losses are then added to the total. Physiologic need for calcium varies at different life stages and includes the requirement for bone accretion during childhood and adolescence, skeletal maintenance requirements during adulthood, and the requirements to cover the costs of reproduction during both pregnancy and lactation. Obligatory or insensible losses include the amount lost on a daily basis from hair, skin, and nails and also the amount lost through feces and urine. Because calcium absorption can be modulated by the composition of the diet, habitual calcium intake, and physiologic state, the total requirement (physiologic need less obligatory losses) is then further adjusted to allow for average calcium bioavailability. In order that the requirement estimate covers 95% of the population, two standard deviations are then added to the estimate to obtain the RNI for the population.

The balance method for the estimation of calcium requirement relies on experimental data derived from carefully conducted balance studies, preferably over extended periods. In this method, study participants are fed diets containing varying levels of dietary calcium, and their calcium requirement is then usually determined by linear regression of calcium output on intake. The mean intake at which intake and output are equal (or balance is zero) can then be calculated. However, the process by which calcium is absorbed from the proximal small intestine depends on its concentration, with active transport being the main process at low calcium intakes, whereas at higher intakes most calcium is absorbed by diffusion. This results in a curvilinear relationship between intake and absorption, and thus simple linear regression models are not sufficient. Furthermore, zero balance is not appropriate for children, adolescents, and pregnant and lactating women, who require positive calcium balance. An alternative strategy, the intake at which the mean maximum positive balance occurs, has therefore been proposed (31). In this method, calcium balance is regressed on intake to determine the threshold intake above which there is no further increase in calcium retention.

A third method for setting calcium requirements has been proposed, namely, the setting of a dietary requirement

TABLE 107.2. COMPARISON OF DIETARY GUIDELINES AMONG COUNTRIES[a]

DIETARY GUIDELINE	COUNTRIES HAVING SIMILAR GUIDELINES	COUNTRIES MAKING DISTINCT VARIATIONS
Keep a healthy weight	Argentina (eat enough for adequate weight), Australia, Canada, China, Japan, Korea, Malaysia, Mexico, the Netherlands, New Zealand, Panama, Philippines, Singapore, Thailand, United Kingdom, United States, Venezuela	France: Weigh yourself every month
Engage in physical activity each day	Australia, Canada, China, France, Indonesia, Japan, Malaysia, Mexico, Philippines, South Africa, United States	Many combine weight and physical activity, mentioning balance
Use the pyramid as a guide for food choices	Variety: Argentina, Australia, Canada, Chile, China, Costa Rica, France, Germany, Guatemala, Hungary, Indonesia, Korea, Malaysia, Mexico (mentions Health Pyramid), New Zealand, Panama, Philippines, Singapore, South Africa, Sri Lanka, Thailand, United Kingdom, United States, Venezuela Five Steps to Healthy Eating: India	Japan (>30 different kinds of foods/d)
Eat a variety of grains daily (whole grains)	Argentina, Australia, Canada, Denmark, Germany, Guatemala (in all meals, including potatoes), Hungary (choose potatoes over rice), India, Malaysia, Mexico (preferably with legumes), Norway, Panama (includes roots), Singapore, South Africa (starchy foods), Thailand, United States	United Kingdom: Eat plenty of foods rich in starch and fiber
Consume a variety of fruits and vegetables	Argentina, Australia, Chile (increase your intake, mentions legumes), China, Denmark, France, Germany, Guatemala (green leafy, other vegetables, any fruit), Hungary (includes salads), India, Malaysia, Mexico, Norway, Panama (eating enough), Singapore, South Africa, Sri Lanka (leafy greens daily), Thailand, United States	Thailand: eat fiber-rich foods regularly Venezuela: eat the fiber that your body needs from daily consumption of vegetables
Be concerned with food safety	Argentina, China, Costa Rica (practice good hygiene), Indonesia, Philippines, Thailand, United States, Venezuela	
Select a diet low in saturated fat and cholesterol and moderate in total fat	Australia (but low-fat diets not suitable for children), Canada, Japan, the Netherlands, Mexico, New Zealand, Panama (total fat not mentioned), Singapore, South Africa, United States	Argentina: limit animal fat Chile: as above (prefer meats such as fish, turkey, or chicken), prefer vegetable oils China: as above, eat "light" diet Costa Rica, Thailand: moderate amounts of fat Denmark: only small quantities of butter, margarine and oil, choose low-fat dairy and meat products Germany, Hungary, United Kingdom: avoid too much fat India: fat eat least Malaysia: minimize fat in foods, choose prepared foods that are low in fat and cholesterol Norway: similar to Denmark Thailand: see Costa Rica Venezuela: consume moderate amounts of animal products; avoid excess animal fats
Moderate your intake of free sugars	Argentina, Australia, Chile, Costa Rica, Denmark, Germany, Hungary, India, Malaysia, Mexico, Panama, Singapore, Thailand, United Kingdom, United States	New Zealand (preprepared foods, drinks and snacks)

(continued)

TABLE 107.2. COMPARISON OF DIETARY GUIDELINES AMONG COUNTRIES[a] **(continued)**

DIETARY GUIDELINE	COUNTRIES HAVING SIMILAR GUIDELINES	COUNTRIES MAKING DISTINCT VARIATIONS
Limit salt intake	Argentina, Australia, Canada, Chile, China, Costa Rica, Denmark, Germany, Hungary, India, Japan, Korea, Malaysia, Mexico, the Netherlands, Panama, Singapore, South Africa, Thailand, United States, Venezuela	New Zealand (preprepared foods, drinks and snacks)
If you drink alcohol, do so in moderation	Argentina, Canada, China, France, Germany, Indonesia (avoid), Hungary (forbidden for pregnant women and children), Korea, Mexico, the Netherlands, New Zealand, Singapore, South Africa, United Kingdom, United States, Venezuela (alcohol not part of a healthy diet)	

[a] Most countries omit mention of cholesterol.

Data from Argentina, 1998; Australia, 1992; Canada, 1992; Chile, 1997; China, 1997; Costa Rica, 1997, Guatemala, 1998; Indonesia, 1995; Hungary, 1988; Japan, 1985; Korea, 1986; Malaysia, 1996; Mexico, 1993; the Netherlands, 1985; New Zealand, 1991; Panama, 1995; Philippines, 1990; Singapore, 1989; South Africa, 1998, preliminary; Sri Lanka, 1994; Thailand, 1991; United Kingdom, 1990; United States, 2000; Venezuela, 1990.

that maximizes function. In the case of calcium, optimal function refers specifically to minimizing the risk of osteoporosis and bone fracture. However, although it is potentially of great policy relevance, this approach has suffered from a difficulty in relating calcium status to long-term functional outcomes. More recently, calcium intake has been associated with a possible decreased risk of some components of the metabolic syndrome (obesity and hypertension [32]), and it is therefore possible that the critical function for calcium in the future may change from optimal bone mass to prevention of diet-related chronic disease.

The intake requirement for vitamin D is defined in a more pragmatic manner, by taking into account that vitamin D is a hormone, that it is synthesized in the skin, and that it has clearly defined deficiency states (unlike calcium). In general, recommended vitamin D intake is normally set as the level that, in the absence of sunlight, protects from the deficiency states of rickets or osteomalacia and results in a 25-hydroxyvitamin D level higher than that observed in disease states.

There is considerable variation in the requirement for calcium throughout the life course. Calcium needs are at their greatest during the period of growth in childhood and especially in adolescence (33). Requirements are also increased for women during pregnancy and lactation, and again after the menopause, which is accompanied by a dramatic and sustained rise in obligatory calcium loss (34). Aging also seems to be associated with decreased calcium absorption (35), although currently the evidence for an increased requirement in men is weak. Variation in the requirement for vitamin D within population groups appears to be largely a function of behavior, rather than physiologic need, because in general, reasonable exposure to sunlight will result in sufficient vitamin D levels throughout life. Older people are perhaps an exception to this rule because investigators have suggested that aging is

associated with a decreased ability for endogenous synthesis of vitamin D after exposure to sunlight (36).

Data used in the setting of calcium and vitamin D requirements come mostly, if not exclusively, from developed countries. Moreover, study populations are predominantly white postmenopausal women. Thus, data are potentially not truly representative of populations of different origins. Although this may not be a problem for some nutrients, it is proving to be a cause of concern for calcium and vitamin D. The main reason is a demonstrated difference among ethnic groups in markers of bone health such as the prevalence of osteoporosis; white subjects have considerably higher rates of osteoporosis or fracture than black subjects, even within the same country (37, 38). It has therefore been suggested that genetic differences among population groups may modulate bone density and thus fracture rates.

However, there is also sizeable variation in fracture rates within population groups, a finding supporting the suggestion that whereas genetics may prove important, lifestyle and dietary factors also play crucial roles in determining bone health (39, 40). The clear positive association between wealth and osteoporosis prevalence has led some researchers to state that osteoporosis is a disease of rich Western cultures (41). In addition, rather counterintuitively, a positive association also exists between the prevalence of fractures and dietary calcium intake, the so-called "calcium paradox."

To investigate this further, investigators demonstrated that significant positive relationships exist between mortality rate from falls (a surrogate marker for hip fracture rate) and calcium intake and also between mortality rate from falls and animal (but not plant) protein intake (42, 43). Calcium balance is clearly influenced by protein and sodium intake, and this led the most recent FAO/WHO expert group report to establish a higher calcium intake recommendation for populations consuming Western diets (high in protein and sodium). This recommendation concurs with the suggestion made earlier (41). However, Western populations also tend to live at higher latitudes, and a strongly significant positive relationship has also been demonstrated between mortality from falls and latitude (43). Latitude and the corresponding level of ultraviolet radiation affect vitamin D status, and vitamin D has long been known to promote calcium retention via the actions of 1,25(OH)$_2$ vitamin D on calcium absorption in the intestine and phosphorus reabsorption by the kidneys (44). These findings support a close link between calcium and vitamin D sufficiency and may also provide the solution to the calcium paradox.

Although most research has focused on the importance of calcium and vitamin D in bone health, emerging evidence also indicates that these nutrients play a role in other chronic diseases. For example, the findings of a recent large prospective study with a 16-year follow-up demonstrated that higher calcium intake is associated with a modest reduction in the risk of distal colon cancer (45). There appeared to be a threshold level above which no additional effect was seen, and the effect also seemed to be greater in women than in men. Given the known relationship between vitamin D status and calcium absorption, further analyses carried out taking into account vitamin D status demonstrated that the inverse relationship between calcium intake and distal colon cancer risk was greatest in those persons with higher vitamin D intake (45).

The intake of dietary calcium, specifically from dairy products, also seems to have an important impact on cardiovascular risk factors. Although the evidence is still limited, two prospective studies demonstrated a reduced risk of stroke subsequent to increased consumption of dairy products (46, 47). It has been hypothesized that hypertension and the associated conglomeration of disorders that arise in the metabolic syndrome are related to elevated intracellular calcium and depressed intracellular magnesium (48). The cellular concentrations of these two ions appear to be related to vasoconstriction, increased platelet aggregation, thrombosis, and insulin resistance, findings suggesting that increased dietary calcium intake may prove an important weapon in the prevention of the metabolic syndrome.

Considerable interest was aroused in the early 1990s by a report demonstrating an association between vitamin D receptor gene polymorphisms and bone turnover (49). Polymorphisms at four loci of the vitamin D receptor gene have been identified as being related to biologic variations in bone mass (50). Research aimed at determining the underlying mechanism behind this effect demonstrated that it is the regulatory effect of the vitamin D receptor gene on bone and mineral metabolism that leads to variation in bone mass. The vitamin D receptor alleles appear to have a differential action on intestinal calcium absorption and thereby affect the rate of accrual of bone mineral density and final peak bone mass (50).

This important effect has been demonstrated in both children and adults. For example, in a study on children aged 7 to 12 years, gene polymorphisms were found to be associated with both bone mineral density and rate of calcium absorption. The variation among genotypes in mean calcium absorption were considerable, with a maximum difference of more than 40%, resulting in an 8% change in bone mineral density (51). At the other end of the age spectrum, vitamin D receptor genotype has also been linked to calcium absorption in postmenopausal women, especially during periods of calcium restriction when calcium is mostly absorbed via active transport mechanisms (52). This important finding suggests that vitamin D receptor genotype may play a crucial role in determining bone health when calcium intake is low or marginal.

Vitamin D receptor polymorphisms also seem to affect the rate of age-related bone loss in older people, and this may influence a given person's likelihood of suffering from osteoporosis (53, 54). This field is complicated, however, and numerous conflicting results have also been reported (50). One reason for the lack of unanimity in findings may be the interaction between the various polymorphisms and other epigenetic factors such as habitual calcium intake, sun exposure, and degree of bone stress from weight-bearing physical activity.

Much recent research has focused on the role of isoflavones, derived from plants such as soy, in bone health. These compounds are structurally similar to mammalian estrogens and have thus been called phytoestrogens. This research gained prominence following the ecologic finding that Asiatic populations, who traditionally consume a diet high in isoflavones but low in calcium, had lower rates of hip fracture than white populations. A recent review of in vitro bone cell cultures, in vivo animal models, and human epidemiologic and dietary intervention studies concluded that the data were suggestive of a bone-sparing role of diets rich in phytoestrogens in the long term (55), although there was a need for more long-term studies. The results of one of the longest studies to date, a 12-month randomized controlled trial among approximately 200 postmenopausal women, were recently published and demonstrated that the loss of lumbar spine bone mineral content and of bone mineral density was significantly lower among those taking the isoflavone supplement rather than the placebo (56). Given the public health significance of osteoporosis, population-wide phytoestrogen supplementation, or dietary guidelines aimed at increasing isoflavone consumption perhaps in conjunction with increased calcium intake, may result, should further research support these current conclusions.

Current national-level recommendations and international consensus statements on dietary calcium and vitamin D intake requirements use traditional methods for estimating individual need, based exclusively on data collected in developed countries. However, it is now evident that apparent "need" varies tremendously both within and between populations. Clear interpopulation differences exist in markers of bone health that are contrary to those expected from calcium intake data, whereas within populations factors such as wealth, protein intake, isoflavone consumption, and degree of solar radiation significantly affect markers of calcium status. Based on the analysis of the complex interaction between calcium status and vitamin D status and the emerging information on the role of vitamin D receptor gene polymorphism in determining bone health, it is becoming progressively clear that it may not be possible or even desirable to give population-wide intake recommendations for calcium and vitamin D.

GLOBAL FOOD-BASED DIETARY GUIDELINES: ARE THEY POSSIBLE, DESIRABLE, AND ACHIEVABLE?

The possibility of defining one set of dietary guidelines is indeed attractive, considering the need for uniformity in the global village. Why should the optimal diet be different from one population to the next? Cultural and/or ethnic differences may result in the selection of population-specific foods to meet human nutritional needs but do not necessarily imply different dietary guidelines. The only justification for this would be a solid genetic basis for nutritional individuality. Indeed, present knowledge on genomics indicates that close to 30,000 genes encode the biologic basis of what makes us *Homo sapiens*, and around 3000 of these are key for most organic functions. Mutations in these 3000 genes occur infrequently (1 to 0.01 per 1000 births), but some will result in changed requirements to meet individual nutritional needs. In this manner, some humans are not able to metabolize phenylalanine and require a nearly phenylalanine-free diet, others cannot absorb zinc efficiently and thus require an intake several times the normal recommendation, and still others find the population average copper intake to be toxic, as in the case of Wilson disease. However, because these mutations are rare and occur similarly across different regions of the world, we need not establish specific recommendations for different populations (57–59).

More recently, we have begun to unravel the significance of changes in a given base pair of the DNA strand, so-called single-nucleotide polymorphisms (SNPs). These occur approximately once per 1000 base pairs, and although in most cases SNPs are silent, they can affect the expression of one or more genes and thus may have major consequences for nutrient metabolism. The concept of biochemical individuality coined by Garrod (60) acquires new meaning with the understanding of the intricate nature of gene expression and the interaction between genes and SNPs. At present, most agree close to 15 million distinct SNPs exist, and it these that make us truly unique.

At this stage, we are just beginning to discover the implications of genetic and epigenetic influences on nutritional needs of individuals and population groups. It remains to be seen whether biochemical or genomic

TABLE 107.3. HUMAN GENETIC POLYMORPHISMS THAT AFFECT RECOMMENDED NUTRIENT INTAKES

NUTRIENTS	GENE	POLYMORPHIC ALLELE	REFERENCE
Vitamins			
Folate	MTHFR	A222V	61
	CBS	844ins68	62
	GCPII	H475Y	63–65
Vitamin B$_{12}$	MTR	N919G	62
	MTRR	I22M	62
Vitamin D	VDR	Multiple	66
Minerals			
Iron	HFE	C282Y	67, 68
Copper	pATPase7–B	Multiple	69, 70
Zinc	SLC39A4	Several	71
Lipids			
	FABP–2	Multiple	72
	Apo B	Multiple	73, 74
	Apo C3	Multiple	75
	APO E	E2,E3,E4	76
Alcohol			
	ADH1B	ADH2°2	77–79
	ADH3	ADH3°1	80
	ALDH2	ALDH2°2	80
Carbohydrate			
Lactose	LD	Promoter	81

individuality leads to nutritional individuality, and if this is the case, we may to redefine the approach used to establish dietary recommendations. Table 107.3 summarizes gene polymorphisms that define specific nutritional needs based on current knowledge; this list will surely grow. For now, unless the genetic factor defines a special nutritional need that establishes a strong susceptibility for a given health disorder ,we do not consider genetics in defining nutritional recommendations. This may change as we increase our ability to detect these genetic conditions and do something about them, in terms of changing life-long exposure to given levels of nutrients.

Are global guidelines desirable? Undoubtedly, the answer must be "yes." However, universal guidelines present new problems and novel challenges. A single unified set of guidelines will fail to address cultural diversity and the complex social, economic, and political interactions between human and their food supply. Present user-needs of FBDGs have changed. It is no longer sufficient to prevent disease of mind and body; we now want to extend our healthy life years and minimize the loss of function associated with aging. The bottom panel of the scheme presented in Figure 107.1 serves to exemplify the different uses of dietary guidelines and also the expectations that may be associated with these different groups.

Are unified guidelines achievable? The answer to this is that for some guidelines this is certainly possible. However, as clearly demonstrated in the example of calcium and vitamin D, we cannot have a one-size-fits-all approach. Guidelines can most likely be harmonized following a unified approach to defining them, but there must be room to accommodate nutritional individuality. Global guidelines will fail unless they provide the necessary options for individuals and societies to select the foods they prefer and to combine them in the way that best suits their tastes and other sensory requirements. Most consumers will agree that food is far too important to be left solely in the hands of the experts.

REFERENCES

1. Eaton SB, Konner M. N Engl J Med 1985;312:283–9.
2. Mann C. Science 1997;277:1038–43.
3. Albonico M, Stoltzfus RJ, Savioli L et al. Int J Epidemiol 1998; 27:530–7.
4. Food and Agriculture Organization/World Health Organization (FAO/WHO). Calcium Requirements. Report of a joint FAO/WHO Expert Committee. WHO Technical Report Series no. 230. Geneva: World Health Organization, 1962.
5. Food and Agriculture Organization/World Health Organization (FAO/WHO). Requirements of Vitamin A, Thiamin, Riboflavin, and Niacin. Report of a joint FAO/WHO Expert Group. WHO Technical Report Series no. 362. Geneva: World Health Organization, 1967.
6. Food and Agriculture Organization/World Health Organization (FAO/WHO). Requirements of Ascorbic Acid, Vitamin D, Vitamin B_{12}, Folate, and Iron. Report of a joint FAO/WHO Expert Group. WHO Technical Report Series no. 452. Geneva: World Health Organization, 1970.
7. Food and Agriculture Organization/World Health Organization/ United Nations University (FAO/WHO/UNU). Energy and Protein Requirements. Report of a joint FAO/WHO/UNU Expert Consultation. WHO Technical Report Series no. 724. Geneva: World Health Organization, 1985.
8. World Health Organization (WHO). Diet, Nutrition, and the Prevention of Chronic Diseases. Report of a WHO Study Group, WHO Technical Report Series no. 797. Geneva: World Health Organization, 1990.
9. Food and Agriculture Organization/World Health Organization/International Atomic Energy Agency (WHO/FAO/IAEA). Trace Elements in Human Nutrition and Health. Geneva: World Health Organization, 1996.
10. Food and Agriculture Organization/World Health Organization (FAO/WHO). International Conference on Nutrition. World Declaration and Plan of Action for Nutrition. Rome: Food and Agriculture Organization and World Health Organization, 1992:1–50.
11. Food and Agriculture Organization/World Health Organization (FAO/WHO). Preparation and Use of Food-Based Dietary Guidelines. Report of a joint FAO/WHO Expert Consultation, Nicosia, Cyprus. WHO/NUT/96.6. Geneva: World Health Organization, 1996.
12. Uauy R, Hertrampf E. Food-based dietary recommendations: possibilities and limitations. In: Bowman B, Russell R, eds. Present Knowledge in Nutrition. 8th ed. Washington, DC: ILSI Press, 2001:636–49.
13. Hegsted DM, Linkswiler HM. J Nutr 1981;111:244–51.
14. Young VR. J Nutr 2002;132:621–9.
15. Koletzko B, Aggett PJ, Bindels JG et al. Br J Nutr 1998;80(Suppl 1):5S–45S.
16. US Departments of Agriculture and of Health and Human Services. Dietary Guidelines for Americans. 5th ed. Home and Garden Bulletin no. 232. Washington, DC: US Department of Agriculture, 2000:1–19.
17. Viteri FE. Prevention of iron deficiency. In: Prevention of Micronutrient Deficiencies. Tools for Policymakers and Public Health Workers. Washington, DC: National Academy Press, 1998:45–102.
18. Food and Agriculture Organization/World Health Organization/ International Atomic Energy Agency (WHO/FAO/IAEA). Zinc. In: Trace Elements in Human Nutrition and Health. Geneva: World Health Organization, 1996:72–104.
19. Oyarzun MT, Uauy R, Olivares S. Arch Latinoam Nutr 2001; 51:7–18.
20. Uauy R, Hertrampf E, Reddy M. J Nutr 2002;132[Suppl]: 849S–52S.
21. Food and Nutrition Board National Academy of Medicine. Dietary Reference Intakes: Applications in Dietary Assessment. Washington, DC: National Academy Press, 2001:1–306.
22. Messer E. Soc Sci Med 1997;44:1675–84.
23. Food and Agriculture Organization (FAO). Rome Declaration on World Food Security and World Food Summit Plan of Action. Rome: Food and Agriculture Organization, 1996.
24. Food and Agriculture Organization/International Life Sciences Institute (FAO/ILSI). Preventing Micronutrient Malnutrition: A Guide to Food-Based Approaches. Washington, DC: International Life Sciences Institute Press, 1997.
25. Lotfi M, Venkatesh-Mannar MG, Merx RJHM et al. Micronutrient Fortification of Foods: Current Practices, Research, and Opportunities. Micronutrient Initiative and International Agricultural Center, Ottawa, Canada 1996:1–108.
26. Guerinot ML. Science 2000;287:241–3.
27. Graham RD, Welch RM, Bouis HE. Adv Agron 2001;70:77–142.
28. Stewart JW, Kaplan ML, Beitz DC. Am J Clin Nutr 2001;74: 179–87.
29. Kang JX, Wang J, Wu L et al. Nature 2004;427:504.
30. Prentice A. Calcif Tissue Int 2002;70:83–8.
31. Matkovic V, Heaney RP. Am J Clin Nutr 1992;55:992–6.
32. McCarron DA. Am J Clin Nutr 1997;65[Suppl]:712S–6S.
33. Leitch I, Aitken FC. Nutr Abstr Rev Ser Hum Exp 1959;29: 393–411.
34. Nordin BEC, Need AG, Morris HA et al. Osteoporos Int 1999;9: 351–7.
35. Ebeling PR, Yergey AL, Vleira NE et al. Calcif Tissue Int 1994; 55:330–4.
36. Webb AR, Pilbeam C, Hanafin N et al. Am J Clin Nutr 1990;51: 1075–81.
37. Trotter M, Broman GE, Peterson RR. Am J Orthop 1960;42A: 50–8.
38. de Simone DP, Stevens J, Edwards J et al. J Bone Miner Res 1989;5:827–30.
39. Johnell A, Gullberg B, Allander E et al. Osteoporos Int 1992;2:298–302.
40. Xu L, Lu A, Zhao X et al. Am J Epidemiol 1996;144:901–7.
41. Hegsted DM. J Nutr 1986;116:2316–9.
42. Feskanich D, Willett WC, Stampfer MJ et al. Am J Epidemiol 1996;143:472–9.
43. Nordin BEC. Food Nutr Agric 1997;20:13–24.
44. Jones G, Strugnell SA, DeLuca HF. Physiol Rev 1998;78: 1193–231.
45. Wu K, Willett W, Fuchs C et al. J Natl Cancer Inst 2002;94: 437–46.
46. Abbott RD, Curb JD, Rodriguez BL et al. Stroke 1996;27:813–8.
47. Iso H, Stampfer MJ, Manson JE et al. Stroke 1999;30:1772–9.
48. Resnick L. Prog Cardiovasc Dis 1999;42:1–22.
49. Morrison NA, Yeoman R, Kelly PJ et al. Proc Natl Acad Sci USA 1992;89:6665–9.
50. Liu Y-Z, Liu Y-J, Recker RR et al. J Endocrinol 2003;177: 147–96.

51. Ames SK, Ellis KJ, Gunn SK et al. J Bone Miner Res 1999;14: 740–6.
52. Dawson-Hughes B, Harris SS, Finneran S. J Clin Endocrinol Metab 1995;80:3657–61.
53. Ferrari S, Rizzoli R, Chevalley T et al. Lancet 1985;345;423–4.
54. Brown MA, Haughton MA, Grant SF. J Bone Miner Res 2001; 16:758–64.
55. Setchell KRD, Lydeking-Olsen E. Am J Clin Nutr 2003;78 [Suppl]:593S–609S.
56. Atkinson C, Compston JE, Day NE et al. Am J Clin Nutr 2004; 79:326–33.
57. Risch NJ. Nature 2000;405:847–56.
58. Davey Smith G, Ebrahim S. Int J Epidemiol 2003;32:1–22.
59. Stover PJ. Physiol Genomics 2004;16:161–5.
60. Garrod A. Lancet 1902;2:1616–20.
61. Bailey LB. J Nutr 2003;33[Suppl]:3748S–53S.
62. Jacques PF, Bostom AG, Selhub J et al. Atherosclerosis 2003; 166:49–55.
63. Devlin AM, Ling EH, Peerson JM et al. Hum Mol Genet 2000; 9:2837–44.
64. Ordovas JM. Biochem Soc Trans 2002;30:68–73.
65. Afman LA, Trijbels FJ, Blom HJ. J Nutr 2003;133:75–7.
66. Uitterlinden AG, Fang Y, Bergink AP et al. Mol Cell Endocrinol 2002;197:15–21.
67. Griffiths W, Cox T. Hum Mol Genet 2000;9:2377–82.
68. Lee P, Gelbart T, West C et al. Blood Cells Mol Dis 2002;29: 471–87.
69. Bull PC, Thomas GR, Rommens JM et al. Nat Genet 1993;5: 327–37.
70. Hsi G, Cullen LM, Moira Glerum D et al. Genomics 2004;83: 473–81.
71. Dufner-Beattie J, Wang F, Kuo YM, Gitschier J et al J Biol Chem 2003 29;278:33474–81.
72. Weiss EP, Brown MD, Shuldiner AR et al. Physiol Genomics 2002;10:145–57.
73. Hbacek JA, Pistulkova H, Skodova Z et al. Ann Clin Biochem 2001;38:399–400.
74. Bentzen J, Jorgensen T, Fenger M. Clin Genet 2002;61:126–34.
75. Brown S, Ordovas JM, Campos H. Atherosclerosis 2003;170: 307–13.
76. Fullerton SM, Clark AG, Weiss KM, et al. Am J Hum Genet 2000;67:881–900.
77. Bosron WF, Li TK. Hepatology 1986;6:502–10.
78. Ferguson RA, Goldberg DM. Clin Chim Acta 1997;257:199–250.
79. McCarver DG. Drug Metab Dispos 2001;29:562–5.
80. Loew M, Boeing H, Sturmer T et al. Alcohol 2003;29:131–5.
81. Poulter M, Hollox E, Harvey CB, et al. Ann Hum Genet 2003;67:298–311.

108

THE NUTRITION TRANSITION: GLOBAL TRENDS IN DIET AND DISEASE[1]

BENJAMIN CABALLERO

GLOBAL TRENDS IN HEALTH AND DISEASE 1717
THE NUTRITION TRANSITION 1717
POPULATION TRENDS 1718
URBANIZATION 1718
DIETARY TRENDS 1719
PHYSICAL ACTIVITY 1720
POVERTY AND THE NUTRITION TRANSITION 1720
BIOLOGIC FACTORS: EARLY ORIGINS OF DISEASE . . .1721
POLICY IMPLICATIONS 1721

Diet has played a central role in the health and survival of the human population since the beginning of time. Over the past hundred years, however, dietary factors that modify disease risk have moved to the forefront, as the impact of infectious diseases was reduced by sanitation, antimicrobial therapy, and immunization. Closely linked to dietary practices, lifestyle is another critical element determining risk of disease. This chapter summarizes current global trends in these factors and their contribution to disease patterns, particularly in the developing world.

GLOBAL TRENDS IN HEALTH AND DISEASE

The past 30 years have witnessed a progressive decline in infant mortality in most areas of the world. Similar reductions in undernutrition and mortality occurred in the population of children younger than 5 years of age (1). Still, global health continues to be under the dark cloud of poverty: half the world population lives on less than $2 per day and about 20% on less than $1 per day, and poverty level continues to correlate strongly with several key risk factors, particularly underweight. At the onset of the new millennium, there were more than 170 million children suffering from undernutrition, and 3 million were dying every year of diseases aggravated by undernutrition (2). However, the persistent problem of undernutrition, primarily affecting infants and children, now coexists with the phenomenon of overnutrition, even within the same household (3, 4). About 1 billion adults are overweight, and more than 300 million are clinically obese (2). Overall, the disease burden

of the developing world, specifically that of countries in transition, is characterized by the emergence of noncommunicable, diet-related chronic diseases. More than 30% of mortality is related to only ten risk factors, among which overweight ranks fifth (2). Several other risk factors are also linked to diet and lifestyle, as shown in Table 108.1.

THE NUTRITION TRANSITION

The term *transition* has been used earlier to describe the epidemiologic transition (5), and it was applied by Popkin and others to describe trends associated with diet, food consumption, and chronic diseases that are occurring in the developing world (6, 7). This nutrition transition can be seen as part of the changes that shaped human health over the last half of the twentieth century, namely the demographic, economic, and technologic changes that many countries, but particularly developing countries, experienced over that period (8).

Although indices used to assess undernutrition are reasonably well established by consensus and use, there is less concurrence on how to assess overnutrition and its associated disease risk. Efforts to consolidate knowledge and to reach consensus on the global epidemic of obesity started only relatively recently (9). In adults, most of the bases supporting normative body mass index (BMI) cutoffs are founded on mortality risk of white populations from developing countries. However, the BMI-risk incremental slope is not identical for every population, and there is some consensus that BMI thresholds may need to be different for different countries and ethnic groups and perhaps even for predicting disease-specific risk. Furthermore, a given BMI level may be attained by very different weight-height combinations in developed and developing countries. In the latter, stunting during childhood results in a high proportion of relatively short adults, who can therefore attain any given BMI at a lower body weight than persons of normal height. Information on body fat amount and distribution becomes critical to interpret differences in BMI thresholds among stunted and nonstunted populations (10). It would be also desirable to develop standards based on indicators other than BMI, such as waist circumference. In children, the use of different growth curves in different populations complicates comparisons across countries or regions, although some statistical approaches to overcome this

---

[1] **Abbreviations: BMI,** body mass index; **GNP,** gross national product; **LDCs,** less-developed countries; **SES,** socioeconomic.

TABLE 108.1. TEN RISK FACTORS AND THEIR (%) CONTRIBUTION TO DISEASE BURDEN IN DEVELOPING COUNTRIES, EXPRESSED AS LOSS OF HEALTHY YEARS OF LIFE (DISABILITY-ADJUSTED LIFE YEARS)

COUNTRIES WITH HIGH MORTALITY	COUNTRIES WITH LOW MORTALITY
Underweight[a] (14.9)	Alcohol (6.2)
Unsafe sex (10.2)	Blood pressure (5.0)
Unsafe water, sanitation (5.5)	Tobacco (4.0)
Indoor smoke from fuels (3.6)	Underweight (3.1)
Zinc deficiency (3.2)	Overweight[a] (2.7)
Iron deficiency (3.1)	Cholesterol (2.1)
Vitamin A deficiency (3.0)	Low fruit and vegetable intake (1.9)
Blood pressure (2.5)	Indoor smoke from fuels (1.9)
Tobacco (2.0)	Iron deficiency (1.8)
Cholesterol (1.9)	Unsafe water, sanitation (1.8)

[a] Based on body mass index cutoffs of <19 (underweight) and >25 (overweight).

Data from World Health Organization. The World Health Report 2002. Geneva: World Health Organization, 2002.

limitation have been proposed (11). Finally, few developing countries have longitudinal national health surveys that can provide a precise evaluation of the impact of the nutrition transition on disease prevalence. More limited data sets are available for a number of countries, providing basic anthropometry and in some cases dietary intake data from food frequency or 24-hour-recall questionnaires. Food intake patterns can also be estimated, with well-recognized limitations, from country food balance sheets.

The nutrition transition has been driven by three major factors: population shifts, urbanization, and the globalization of food production and marketing. Technical advances in communications have played also an important role, by facilitating the rapid and extensive dissemination of cultural and lifestyle trends.

POPULATION TRENDS

For more than 2000 years, human population increased at a modest rate. In the mid-1800s, as mortality began to

decline in industrialized countries, growth rates rose progressively, but remained well below 1% until the 1920s. Highest growth rates were reached in the mid-1900s, but declined thereafter, as mortality continued to fall, with fertility rates following. By the end of the twentieth century, all but 16 countries had transitioned to lower fertility rates (12). This decline in population growth in the last half of the twentieth century is a key element in the modern nutrition transition. Declining fertility is associated with lower infant mortality and improved child survival, and lower mortality and increased life expectancy result in an increased number of persons who survive to ages when noncommunicable diseases are more prevalent. An important characteristic of this overall decrease in the rate of population growth is that it has affected primarily the younger generations, thus resulting in a relative increase in the older population. Growth projections for the next several decades predict a drastic increase in the population of persons more than 60 years of age (Fig 108.1). This aging of the world population will undoubtedly be associated with an increase in chronic, noncommunicable diseases.

URBANIZATION

Although at the end of the twentieth century the largest proportion of the world population was living in rural areas, it is anticipated that this trend will change dramatically over the next 15 years (13). As shown in Figure 108.2, the majority of people to be added to the world population in the next decade will reside in an urban rather than a rural environment.

Urban dwelling has several characteristics that greatly affect dietary intake and energy balance. First, the energy costs of basic survival activities (securing water, food, etc) are substantially lower. Second, labor energy demands are also reduced relative to typical rural work in the field. Similarly, food availability differs in quantity and composition, usually with an increase in total dietary energy and a higher proportion of fats and refined sugars (14). These factors combine to facilitate a positive energy balance and

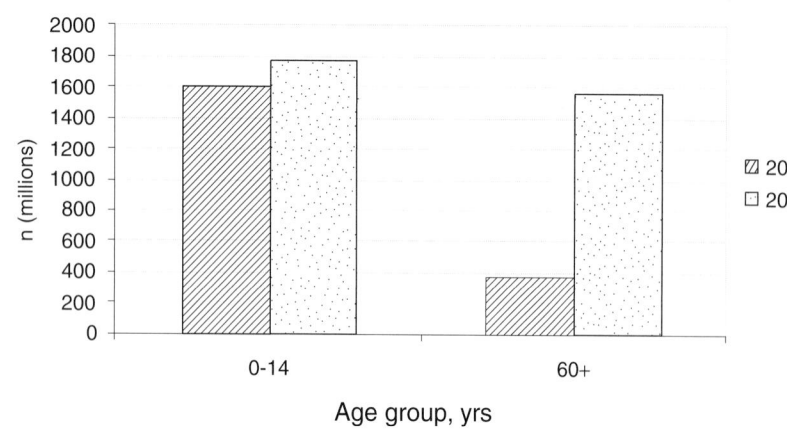

Figure 108.1. Contribution to the world population of two age groups, 0 to 14 years and 60+ years. The projections for the year 2050 show a sharp increase in the older group, whereas the younger group will show only minor increase. (Data from Zlotnik H. Demographic trends. In: Caballero B, Popkin BM, eds. The Nutrition Transition: Diet and Disease in the Developing World. London: Academic Press, 2002:71–108.)

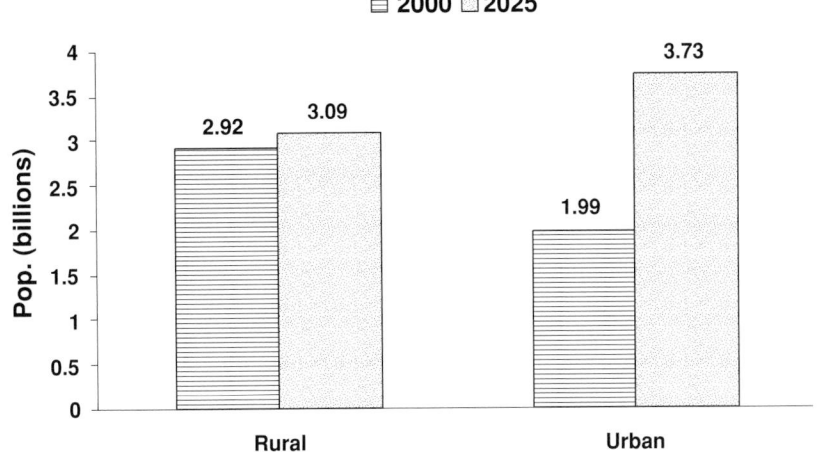

Figure 108.2. Distribution of the world population between rural and urban dwelling, in the year 2000 and projected to 2025. (Data from the United Nations Population Division. World Urbanization Prospects. New York: United Nations, 1988.)

consequent excess weight gain. Other factors characteristic of urban dwelling, such as television viewing, street violence, and the lack of open spaces, also facilitate an indoor, sedentary lifestyle and thus a further decline in energy expenditure.

Although it is usually linked to economic development, there is little evidence that urbanization, as it unfolds in developing countries, has helped improve the situation of those of lower socioeconomic status (SES). Using data from the World Bank, Haddad and associates reported an overall increase in urban poverty in less-developed countries (LDCs) in the last 20 years of the twentieth century (15). In 11 of the 14 countries examined, the prevalence of underweight children in urban areas also increased. Furthermore, some health indicators show a wider gap between the richest and the poorest in urban compared with rural populations (16, 17). Poverty may also have more negative consequences in urban than in rural areas. In the latter, families may be able to secure food by growing their own and may have developed social safety nets and survival strategies within their family and community. In the urban environment, conversely, families depend on their income to buy food and may have difficulty in replicating a support network in a culturally foreign environment, perhaps having left behind family members and friends. Food prices play an important role in food choices and food security in lower-income countries (18). When families need to spend 50% or more of their income in food, as is the case in many LDCs, food price becomes a powerful factor driving food choice. The diet pattern is thus strongly influenced by cost and is therefore highly susceptible to market conditions and sales strategies based on price manipulation.

DIETARY TRENDS

Over the past 20 to 30 years, major shifts in diet quantity and composition have occurred in the developing world. Per capita energy availability increased markedly over the past 30 years; in the developing world (excluding Sub-

Saharan Africa), this increase averaged around 600 kcal/day, and as much as 1000 kcal/day in China (19). Overall, LDCs have see n modest declines in consumption of cereals and pulses and an increase in animal food sources, whereas a low consumption of fruits and vegetables continues to be a concern. Figure 108.3 depicts trends in food sources in the developing world, including projections for the year 2030. Major contributors to the increase in total dietary energy intake are vegetable oils, particularly in lower-income LDCs. Table 108.2 shows recent changes in dietary fat availability in different regions of the world. The contribution of refined sugars and caloric sweeteners in general to the total energy intake of LDCs is less well documented. Unlike developed countries, where high-fructose corn syrup has largely replaced sucrose as a sweetener, sucrose is still the predominant

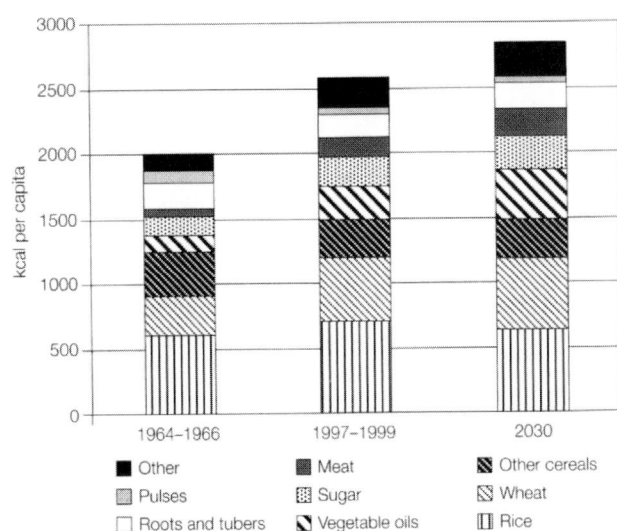

Figure 108.3. Dietary food sources accounting for total energy availability in developing countries, including projected changes to the year 2030. (Data from Food and Agriculture Organization. World Agriculture: Towards 2015/2030. Rome: Food and Agriculture Organization, 2002.)

TABLE 108.2. CHANGES IN THE WORLD SUPPLY OF DIETARY FAT, 1970–2000

	SUPPLY (g per capita/d)		
	1970	2000	CHANGE (%)
World	53	73	38
North Africa	44	64	45
Sub-Saharan Africa	41	45	9
North America	117	143	22
Latin America and Caribbean	54	79	46
China	24	79	229
East and Southeast Asia	28	52	86
South Asia	29	45	55
European Community	117	148	26
Eastern Europe	90	104	16
Near East	51	70	37
Oceania	102	113	11

Data from World Health Organization. Technical Report no. 916. Geneva: World Health Organization, 2003; and Food and Agriculture Organization. FAOSTAT. Rome: Food and Agriculture Organization, 2003.

caloric sweetener in LDCs. However, available projections indicate that fats will continue to be the main factor driving the increased dietary energy availability, with little if any increase in sugars (20).

The previous relationship between income and diet in poor countries led to the traditional concept that a low per capita gross national product (GNP) is associated with a diet that is low in fat and refined sugars and is plant based; this has been dramatically altered by global trends in food production and marketing. Using food balance data from developing countries, Drewnowski and others (3, 21, 22) have shown that current diets in intermediate-income countries have increasing proportions of calories derived from fat (primarily vegetable oils) and also from refined carbohydrates. A number of factors may explain these changes in diet composition. First, the increase in worldwide availability of relatively cheap vegetable oil (23, 24). Second, cultural perceptions of diet quality, influenced by commercial advertisement, have led to consumption of more products containing refined sugars. A quest for variety and convenience (i.e., prepared foods) have also been cited as important factors (22, 25). In a model to assess the impact of urbanization, Drewnowski and Popkin predicted a substantial increase in consumption of caloric sweeteners as urbanization increases (22). The contribution of fast food to these changes, although frequently mentioned, has not been clearly documented, but there is no doubt that over the past 10 years the number of fast food restaurants has increased dramatically in urban areas of the developing world.

PHYSICAL ACTIVITY

The energy demands of daily living are important contributors to total energy needs in rural populations. Securing food, water, and firewood consumes a significant portion

of daily caloric allowance, in addition to the energy spent at work. In the urban environment, the energy output needed for survival activities is sharply reduced, and the most common types of jobs are also lower in energy demands relative to rural work. As energy expenditure is reduced, persons find more and more difficult to match it with an equivalent reduction in dietary energy intake, particularly when energy-dense foods are widely available. The "Westernization" of lifestyle in LDCs has resulted in a continuing increase in sedentary, low-energy output activities, including television viewing and use of video games and computers. Economic growth tends to favor the service sector in many LDCs, fueled by outsourcing of jobs from developed countries by multinational corporations in search of lower labor costs (14). These jobs usually involve sedentary activities, thus further reducing total energy expenditure.

POVERTY AND THE NUTRITION TRANSITION

Until recently, it was generally considered that the highest risk of obesity and its comorbidities were in higher SES groups (26), and a linear correlation existed between per capita GNP and obesity prevalence. However, the nutrition transition has resulted in a more complex, less linear interrelationship among SES, GNP, and obesity. A recent analysis of data from 37 developing countries by Monteiro and associates (27) suggested that, although low-GNP countries (~$800/year) generally have a low prevalence of obesity, this prevalence increases rapidly in developing countries with an intermediate-level GNP (~$2,000/year). These authors demonstrated this shift by using data from two national surveys about 10 years apart in Brazil (Fig. 108.4). In the 1980s, the lower-SES population had more undernutrition and less obesity than the higher-SES group. Ten years later, the prevalence of both undernutrition and overnutrition was higher among the poor. Data

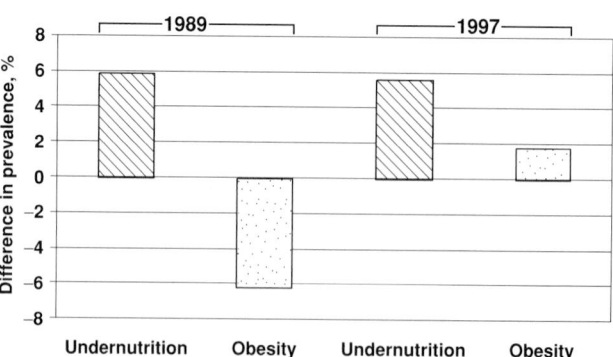

Figure 108.4. Relative contribution of undernutrition and overnutrition in low-socioeconomic status population of Brazil, in 1989 to 1997. The *bars* represent the difference in prevalences between the lower and upper quartiles of socioeconomic status in 1989 and 1997. The 1997 data show that the burden of overnutrition has also shifted to the poorer segment of the population. (Data from Monteiro CA, Conde WL, Popkin BM. Am J Public Health 2004;94:433–4.)

from China also suggested that income growth may have a negative effect on the diet of the urban poor (28). Although the causes of these shifts are complex, it is likely that in lower-income populations food availability is a limiting factor for energy intake, and frequent infections associated with a contaminated environment further increase energy requirements. As income increases, access to higher-fat, energy-dense foods may increase, allowing a higher total energy intake, which combined with lower energy output in physical activity would increase the risk of excess weight gain.

The increasing prevalence of obesity in intermediate-GNP countries results in the coexistence of undernutrition and overnutrition in the same population, even in the same family (4, 29, 30). By some estimates, as many as 60% of households in Southeast Asia may have at least one underweight and one obese member, frequently an underweight child-overweight mother pair (31). This "dual burden" poses a major challenge to the development of integrated prevention programs.

BIOLOGIC FACTORS: EARLY ORIGINS OF DISEASE

The relationship between nutritional status early in life and adult disease was brought to the forefront by a series of epidemiologic observations describing the association between low birth weight and diabetes, cardiovascular diseases, and respiratory disorders in adult life (32–34). Other studies extended these associations to include impaired growth during infancy and childhood, particularly when it is followed by a period of accelerated ("catch-up") growth (35, 36). Using medical records from Dutch populations who suffered severe nutritional deprivation during World War II, Susser and Stein (37) identified similar associations between fetal growth and subsequent risk of adult diseases. Overall, these data point to critical early periods of structural and functional differentiation, during which altered nutritional conditions may produce long-lasting effects (38, 39). The implications of this phenomenon for developing countries is significant because of their high prevalence of impaired fetal and postnatal growth, which would result in an additional risk burden for adult populations now facing the nutrition transition. Most of the initial evidence for the early origins hypothesis came from developed countries with predominantly white populations. A limited or biased availability of birth weight records is a limitation to performing similar studies in LDCs, but new evidence is emerging from well-designed studies in the Philippines (40), India (41), and other countries.

POLICY IMPLICATIONS

The evidence supporting the severe health impact of the nutrition transition in developing countries has been accumulating steadily for more than a decade. Today, a small number of chronic diseases associated with diet and lifestyle is responsible for well over half the world deaths. The magnitude of the problem and some possible interventions have been presented and discussed in a number of fora (42). There is ample consensus that three key modifiable risk factors are tobacco use, unhealthy diet, and physical inactivity. In the past 2 years, the international community, and particularly the World Health Organization, has defined a global operational framework for the implementation of tobacco control (43) and a strategy for diet, physical activity, and health (19). In addition, the enormous economic implications of chronic diseases for health care costs and productivity in developing countries are also becoming clear. Still, support and funding for a vigorous response to the problem have been limited so far, and only a few countries have included strategies to prevent noncommunicable diseases in their public health programs. Yach and associates pointed out that "one reason for this neglect has been the belief by governments and philanthropists that chronic diseases are afflictions of affluent populations who have led a life of sloth" (44) and added, "in reality, these diseases are now global problems that have been driven by profound changes in consumption patterns"

The difficulties in mounting such programs, however, cannot be minimized. The coexistence of undernutrition and overnutrition within households poses a major challenge to the development of focused, simple educational programs. Although in developed countries such programs can center on weight control, countries with a dual burden of malnutrition at both extremes will need to address the needs of undernourished children as well as those of overweight adults (45). However, several countries (e.g., Brazil, China) have begun to address specific risk factors, such as physical activity, thereby showing that it is possible to develop carefully targeted programs to reduce at least one or two of the key risk factors. It is also clear that fetal and early life undernutrition, important risk factors for adult diseases, can and should be addressed within the traditional health policy programs focused on maternal and child health. The possible protective effect of breast-feeding (46, 47) offers another opportunity to reduce the risk of obesity through those programs.

More difficult factors to address are the availability and cost of healthy foods. As noted earlier, because of the high impact of price elasticity on food choices in developing countries, eating patterns will be difficult to change without some form of market regulation and control, which may run counter to the "free market" principles demanded by many international lenders. However, an open global market, although potentially increasing variety, may not necessarily improve food quality as far as health is concerned.

Finally, although the main efforts should center on prevention, addressing the health care needs of those already suffering from chronic diseases is also imperative. Most persons with type 2 diabetes reside in LDCs, and India is the country with the largest number of diabetic patients in the world. As obesity continues to increase in the developing world, so will its comorbidities, unless specific interventions are put in place to break the links between excess adiposity and its complications.

REFERENCES

1. Caballero B, Maqbool A. International nutrition. In: Walker WA, Watkins JB, Duggan C, eds. Nutrition in Pediatrics. London: BC Decker, 2003:195–204.
2. World Health Organization. The World Health Report 2002. Geneva: World Health Organization, 2002.
3. Monteiro CA, Conde WL, Popkin BM. Am J Public Health 2004;94:433–4.
4. Doak CM, Adair LS, Bentley M et al. Int J Obes Relat Metab Disord 2005;29:129–36.
5. Omran AR. Milbank Mem Fund Q 1971;49:509–38.
6. Popkin BM. Nutr Rev 1994;52:285–98.
7. Caballero B, Popkin BM. The Nutrition Transition: Diet-Related Diseases in the Modern World. London: Academic Press, 2002.
8. Popkin BM. Public Health Nutr 1999;1:5–21.
9. World Health Organization. Obesity: Preventing and Managing the Global Epidemic. Geneva: World Health Organization, 1998.
10. Caballero B. J Nutr 2001;131:866S–70S.
11. Cole TJ, Bellizzi M, Flegal KM et al. BMJ 2000;320:1–6.
12. Zlotnik H. Demographic trends. In: Caballero B, Popkin BM, eds. The Nutrition Transition: Diet and Disease in the Developing World. London: Academic Press, 2002:71–108.
13. United Nations Population Division. World Urbanization Prospects. New York: United Nations, 1988.
14. Popkin BM. World Dev 1999;27:1905–16.
15. Haddad L, Ruel MT, Garrett JL. World Dev 1999;27:1891–904.
16. Menon P, Ruel M, Morris SS. http://www.ifpri.org/divs/fcnd/dp.htm. 2000.
17. Gwatkin DR, Guillot M, Heuveline P. Lancet 1999;354:586–9.
18. Regmi A, Deepak MS, Seale JL et al. Cross-Country Analysis of Food Consumption Patterns. Washington, DC: US Department of Agriculture/Economic Research Service, 2001:14–22.
19. World Health Organization/Food and Agriculture Organization. Diet, Nutrition and the Prevention of Chronic Diseases. Geneva: World Health Organization, 2003.
20. Food and Agriculture Organization. World Agriculture: Towards 2015/2030. Rome: Food and Agriculture Organization, 2002.
21. Popkin BM. Nutr Rev 2004;62:140S–3S.
22. Drewnowski A, Popkin BM. Nutr Rev 1997;55:31–43.
23. Popkin BM, Gordon-Larsen P. Int J Obes Relat Metab Disord 2004;28:2S–9S.
24. Smil V. Food production. In: Caballero B, Popkin BM, eds. The Nutrition Transition: Diet and Disease in the Developing World. London: Academic Press, 2002:25–50.
25. US Department of Agriculture/Economic Research Service. Changing Structure of Global Food Consumption and Trade. Washington, DC: US Department of Agriculture/Economic Research Service, 2001.
26. Sobal J, Stunkard AJ. Psychol Bull 1989;105:260–75.
27. Monteiro CA, Conde WL, Lu B et al. Int J Obes Relat Metab Disord 2004;28:1181–6.
28. Du S, Mroz TA, Zhai F et al. Soc Sci Med 2004;59:1505–15.
29. Doak CM, Adair LS, Monteiro C et al. J Nutr 2000;130:2965–71.
30. Garrett JL, Ruel MT. Stunted Child-Overweight Mother Pairs: An Emerging Policy Concern? Washington, DC: International Food Policy Research Institute, 2003; Discussion Paper no. 148.
31. Popkin BM, Horton SH, Kim S. Food Nutr Bull 2001;22:3–57.
32. Cheung YB, Low L, Osmond C et al. Hypertension 2000;36:795–800.
33. Eriksson JG, Forsen T, Tuomilehto J et al. Diabetes 1999;48:A72.
34. Forsen T, Eriksson J, Tuomilehto J et al. Ann Intern Med 2000;133:176–82.
35. Schroeder DG, Martorell R, Flores R. Am J Epidemiol 1999;149:177–85.
36. Martorell R, Stein AD, Schroeder DG. J Nutr 2001;131:874S–80S.
37. Susser M, Stein Z. Nutr Rev 1994;52:84–94.
38. Adair LS. Early nutrition conditions and later risk of disease. In: Caballero B, Popkin BM, eds. The Nutrition Transition: Diet and Disease in the Developing World. London: Academic Press, 2002:129–45.
39. McMillen IC, Adam CL, Muhlhausler BS. J Physiol (Lond) 2005 (in press).
40. Adair LS, Kuzawa CW, Borja J. Circulation 2001;104:1034–9.
41. Yajnik CS, Fall CH, Coyaji KJ et al. Int J Obes Relat Metab Disord 2003;27:173–80.
42. Bellagio Declaration. Nutrition and health transition in the developing world: the time to act. In: Caballero B, Popkin BM, eds. The Nutrition Transition: Diet and Disease in the Developing World. London: Academic Press, 2002:248–50.
43. World Health Organization. http://www.who.int/tobacco/framework/en/. 2005.
44. Yach D, Leeder SR, Bell J et al. Science 2005;307:317.
45. Caballero B N Engl J Med 2005; 352:1514-16.
46. von Kries R, Koletzko B, Sauerwald T et al. BMJ 1999;319: 147–50.
47. Dewey KG. J Hum Lancet 2003;19:9–18.

109 SPORTS NUTRITION[1]

MELVIN H. WILLIAMS

GENERAL DIETARY PRINCIPLES FOR ATHLETES 1723
DIETARY CARBOHYDRATE AND SPORTS
    PERFORMANCE 1724
        Dietary Supplements: Carbohydrate Metabolites .1725
DIETARY FAT AND SPORTS PERFORMANCE 1725
        Dietary Supplements: Fat Metabolites 1726
DIETARY PROTEIN AND SPORTS PERFORMANCE 1727
        Dietary Supplements: Protein, Amino Acids,
        and Metabolites....................1728
VITAMINS, VITAMINLIKE SUBSTANCES, AND SPORTS
    PERFORMANCE 1730
        Dietary Supplements: Vitamins and Vitaminlike
        Substances 1730
MINERALS AND SPORTS PERFORMANCE 1731
        Dietary Supplements: Minerals 1731
WATER/ELECTROLYTES AND SPORTS PERFORMANCE .1732
        Dietary Supplements: Water and Electrolytes ...1733
FOOD DRUGS AND SPORTS PERFORMANCE 1733
        Dietary Supplements: Food Drugs 1733
DIETARY SUPPLEMENTS AND SPORTS PERFORMANCE .1735
        Dietary Supplements: Miscellaneous Sport
        Supplements 1735
    SUMMARY AND CONCLUSIONS 1736

Sports are played worldwide by the young and old, male and female, and by amateurs and professionals, and successful sports performance may be the source of considerable fame and fortune. From a scientific perspective, sports performance by an athlete depends on human energy production, efficiency, and control, factors that are influenced primarily by genes and sports training. To be successful, athletes must be genetically endowed with the morphologic, psychologic, physiologic, and metabolic traits specific

[1]**Abbreviations: ACSM,** American College of Sports Medicine;
ADA, American Dietetic Association; **ATP,** adenosine triphosphate;
BCAA, branched-chain amino acid; **CLA,** conjugated linoleic acid;
CoQ$_{10}$, coenzyme Q$_{10}$, ubiquinone; **DC,** Dietitians of Canada;
FFA, free fatty acid; **fTRYP,** free tryptophan; **HGH,** human growth
hormone; **HMB,** β-hydroxy-β-methylbutyrate; **IOM-FNB,** Institute of
Medicine Food and Nutrition Board; **MCT,** medium-chain triglyceride;
PCr, creatine phosphate; **RDA,** recommended dietary allowance;
VO$_2$max, maximal oxygen uptake; **WADA,** World Anti-Doping Agency

to human energy characteristics vital to their sport. Such genetically endowed athletes must also receive proper physical and mental training to optimize energy utilization and prevent the premature development of fatigue. However, athletes may attempt to go beyond training and use substances and techniques, often referred to as ergogenics, in attempts to gain a competitive advantage. Doping, the use of prohibited techniques (blood doping, gene doping) and substances (amphetamines, anabolic steroids) has been curtailed in recent years through the efforts of the World Anti-Doping Agency (WADA), but various permitted nutritional ergogenic strategies and substances have been used since time immemorial.

Most Olympic training centers employ sports physiologists, psychologists, and biomechanists to help athletes increase their physical power, enhance their mental strength, and optimize their biomechanical ability. Depending on their specific sport, athletes train to optimize specific human energy performance attributes, such as aerobic power, anaerobic power, speed, strength, flexibility, reaction time, agility, balance, and coordination. Sports nutritionists advise athletes on various nutritional principles that may favorably influence human energy production, control, and efficiency. In general, sports nutrition involves the use of scientifically prudent dietary strategies and supplements during training or competition with the ultimate goal of maximizing sport performance. Given that all human energy processes are dependent on the nutrients in the foods we consume, every nutrient may be a potential ergogenic.

GENERAL DIETARY PRINCIPLES FOR ATHLETES

One of the key nutritional principles for the athlete is maintenance of an optimal body mass and composition. Excessive loss of body mass may impair sport performance and may also have significant health consequences. The female athlete triad, which includes disordered eating, amenorrhea, and osteoporosis, has been attributed to inadequate energy availability (1). Excess body mass, particularly fat, may impair performance in sports in which the body must move efficiently, such as distance running. Contrarily, excess body mass, particularly muscle, may enhance performance in sports dependent on absolute power production, such as putting the shot in track and field. Thus, achieving and maintaining an optimal body weight are important nutritional, and exercise, considerations for many athletes.

Another key nutritional principle for athletes is to prevent a nutrient deficiency that may impair performance. In general, the diet that is optimal for health is also optimal for sport performance. Sport nutritionists indicate that a diet rich in fruits, vegetables, whole grains, lean meats, and low-fat dairy products, stressing variety, balance, and moderation, will provide the nutrients needed by most athletes. In their joint position stand on nutrition and athletic performance, the American College of Sports Medicine (ACSM), American Dietetic Association (ADA), and Dietitians of Canada (DC) (2) noted that adequate energy intake derived from the macronutrients (carbohydrate, fat, and protein) and obtained from a wide variety of foods will provide adequate intake of the micronutrients (vitamins and minerals). Adequate intake of carbohydrate, essential fatty acids, protein, vitamins, minerals, and water is necessary to ensure optimal performance because a deficiency of any essential nutrient associated with human energy systems may impair performance. Thus, the ACSM, ADA, and DC (2) also noted that dietary supplements may be required by athletes who restrict energy intake, use severe weight-loss practices, or consume diets with low micronutrient density. Moreover, depending on the specific requirements of a given sport, nutritional intervention focusing on specific supplementation protocols may benefit some athletes.

In the United States, the Dietary Supplement Health and Education Act defined dietary supplements as something added to the diet, mainly vitamin, mineral, amino acid, herb or botanical, metabolite, constituent, extract, or a combination of any of these ingredients. Sports supplements are big business (3). Commodities include actual food products, including meals, and supplements specifically marketed to enhance sports performance.

Energy production during exercise is summarized in Chapter 47, and most nutritional ergogenics are theorized to enhance energy processes and delay the onset of fatigue, which may be defined as the inability to maintain energy production at the desired level. Nutrient supplementation could delay the onset of fatigue in various ways, such as providing energy substrate, enhancing energy-generating metabolic pathways, increasing oxygen transport, preventing catabolism of energy-generating cells, ameliorating psychologic functions, controlling body temperature, and facilitating loss of excess body fat. This chapter focuses mainly on the role of nutrient supplementation as a means to enhance sport performance.

DIETARY CARBOHYDRATE AND SPORTS PERFORMANCE

Carbohydrate oxidation increases progressively with increases in exercise intensity (4, 5), and carbohydrate is the primary dietary energy source for both high-intensity anaerobic (1–2 minutes) and aerobic (>3 minutes) exercise. Fatigue during anaerobic exercise is associated with adverse effects of muscle cell acidity caused by the rapid accumulation of lactic acid from anaerobic glycolysis, whereas fatigue during prolonged aerobic exercise may be associated with inadequate carbohydrate levels in the blood or muscles. Low blood glucose concentrations, or hypoglycemia, may impair central nervous system functions, inducing muscular weakness and fatigue. Depletion of muscle glycogen reduces energy production from aerobic glycolysis, a more efficient energy source than aerobic lipolysis. One proposed model suggests that, during exercise, energy is supplied in milliseconds via glycogenolysis, and one possible mechanism for muscle fatigue is that at low, but nonzero, glycogen concentrations, not enough glycogen is present to supply millisecond energy needs (6). Inadequate carbohydrate stores could also affect amino acid metabolism, inducing a decrease in serum branched-chain amino acids (BCAAs) and facilitating tryptophan uptake by the brain and formation of serotonin, which may induce fatigue. Thus, various carbohydrate supplementation strategies have been used in attempts to enhance aerobic endurance exercise performance. However, some investigators have suggested that carbohydrate supplementation may also be advisable for athletes involved in resistance, or strength, training (7).

Theoretically, carbohydrate supplementation may enhance sports performance if it helps to delay the onset of hypoglycemia, low serum BCAA levels, or muscle glycogen depletion, three metabolic responses associated with prolonged aerobic endurance exercise. In general, precompetition meals should contain a balanced macronutrient content, but the focus should be on carbohydrate because it is more readily digested and may help to bolster muscle glycogen stores. Numerous studies support the efficacy of carbohydrate supplementation during prolonged aerobic exercise tasks to improve performance (8–12). For example, marathoners ingesting carbohydrate compared with placebo beverages were able to run at a higher intensity during a competitive marathon, and yet the psychologic ratings of perceived exertion were similar in both groups of runners, a finding suggesting that carbohydrate may have permitted them to run at a faster rate with similar psychologic effort (13). Research also supports a beneficial role of carbohydrate for prolonged, intermittent high-intensity exercise tasks, such as multiple sprints in soccer (14). However, whether these ergogenic effects may be attributed to the effect of glucose on the central nervous system, either as a direct energy source for brain metabolism or through its effect on BCAA levels, or to its effect in the muscle as an energy source has not been determined. Moreover, fatigue may be delayed only temporarily because the amount of exogenous carbohydrate that may be consumed and oxidized during exercise is limited, approximately 1.0–1.7 g/minute (15).

Carbohydrate loading involves a very high-carbohydrate diet and exercise-tapering regimen several days before prolonged aerobic endurance competition and is designed to elevate endogenous muscle glycogen stores and to postpone fatigue. Based on earlier studies, one review (16) noted that carbohydrate loading could improve performance in which a set distance is covered as fast as possible by 2 to 3%, a finding supported by more recent research (17). However, Burke and others (18) found that a 3-day carbohydrate-loading regimen (9 g carbohydrate/kg), as compared with a moderate-carbohydrate diet (6 g carbohydrate/kg), did not enhance performance in a 100-km cycling trial, even though muscle glycogen content increased significantly. However, these investigators also provided carbohydrate during the exercise test and suggested that the availability of blood glucose during exercise may offset any detrimental effects on performance of lower preexercise muscle and liver glycogen concentrations. They also indicated that although the time to finish the 100-km ride (about 1.6 minutes faster with carbohydrate loading) was not statistically significant, such an effect, if real, could make a difference in the finishing order of top cyclists.

The ACSM, ADA, and DC (2) noted that, during times of high physical activity, energy and macronutrient needs, especially carbohydrate needs, must be met. Sports nutritionists have reported that the amount of carbohydrate recommended depends on the type of sport, level of fitness, body composition, and environmental conditions (19–21). Thus, the amount of carbohydrate needed by a person exercising to lose weight will be quite different from the amount needed by an athlete in training to run a marathon, particularly in the heat. In general, a daily intake of 5 to 7 g carbohydrate/kg body weight is recommended for the average athlete in training, whereas 7 to 10 g/kg is the recommended intake for endurance athletes. The recommended carbohydrate intake for endurance athletes would meet or exceed the upper level of the acceptable macronutrient distribution range of 45 to 65% of daily energy intake (22).

Increased carbohydrate intake would probably improve an athletes' training capacity, especially when rapid recovery between intense exercise bouts is required. Theoretically, this enhanced training would lead to improved performance in competition. Reviews of dietary strategies to promote glycogen synthesis after exercise indicated that supplementing at 30-minute intervals at a rate of 1.2 to 1.5 g carbohydrate/kg body mass/hour appears to maximize synthesis for 4 to 5 hours after exercise (23–25).

Dietary Supplements: Carbohydrate Metabolites

Several metabolites of carbohydrate have been theorized to possess ergogenic potential.

Pyruvate

Pyruvate, a three-carbon metabolite of glycolysis, is theorized to accelerate the Krebs cycle or to use glucose more efficiently. The limited research suggests that pyruvate supplementation is not ergogenic. For example, pyruvate supplementation (7 g/day for 1 week) failed to increase cycle time to exhaustion in well-trained male cyclists (26). However, earlier studies combining pyruvate with dihydroxyacetone, a metabolite in the citric acid cycle, reported an enhanced uptake of blood glucose by exercising muscle and an increase in ergometer endurance tasks in untrained male subjects (12). These findings are intriguing, but research is needed with trained subjects.

Ribose

Ribose is a five-carbon monosaccharide that comprises the sugar portion of adenosine triphosphate (ATP). Supplementation is theorized to increase ATP resynthesis and to promote faster recovery and exercise performance. However, studies reported that ribose supplementation had no effect on maximal resistance knee-extension exercise tests and ATP recovery (27) or on high-intensity exercise performance, as evaluated by repeat sprint cycling tests (28–30). The current data do not support an ergogenic effect of ribose supplementation.

DIETARY FAT AND SPORTS PERFORMANCE

Endogenous fat stores cannot produce energy anaerobically, but they can contribute significantly to energy production during aerobic endurance exercise. Adipose tissue free fatty acids (FFAs), muscle triglycerides, and dietary-derived fatty acids from plasma chylomicrons and very-low-density lipoproteins may provide FFAs as an energy source during exercise (31).

Exercise training can improve the ability to use fat as an energy source during exercise. A single bout of exercise, as well as exercise training, leads to an increased expression of genes in the skeletal muscle that increase the capacity for fat oxidation (32). Compared with untrained men, endurance-trained men use more fatty acids derived from both adipose tissue and muscle triglycerides as an energy source even during exercise intensity of 75 to 80% maximal oxygen uptake (VO$_2$max) (33). Several meticulous studies (4, 5) with well-trained male and female subjects exercising at 25, 65, and 85% of VO$_2$max revealed that the highest rate of fat oxidation was during exercise at 65% of VO$_2$max, but fat oxidation decreased significantly with greater exercise intensity as carbohydrate became the preferred fuel. The pattern of use of fat and carbohydrate during moderate- to high-intensity exercise is similar in trained men and women (5, 34). A high-fat diet may also induce rapid changes in genetic expression necessary for enhanced fatty acid transport and oxidation (35).

However, FFA oxidation generally is limited during exercise greater than 65% VO$_2$max and cannot meet energy demands of the muscle beyond 85% of VO$_2$max (36, 37). Various factors, such as inadequate transport of FFAs into the muscle cell and optimal muscle triglycerides lipase activity, may limit the ability to use fat as an energy source during high-intensity aerobic exercise (38, 39).

Theoretically, it may be advantageous for endurance athletes to optimize the utilization of fat as an energy source to spare enough liver and muscle glycogen for the later stages of an aerobic endurance contest. Jeukendrup (38) theorized that increased FFA availability would increase fat metabolism and decrease carbohydrate metabolism. In essence, the increased availability and oxidation of FFAs would generate more acetyl coenzyme A, which, in turn, would ultimately inhibit enzymes involved in carbohydrate breakdown. Such an effect could spare the use of muscle glycogen and enhance endurance performance.

Several sports nutritionists have challenged the dogma that endurance athletes need high-carbohydrate diets and suggest that endurance performance may benefit from high-fat diets, even diets that comprise more than 50% of the daily caloric intake (40). Proponents of the high-fat diet suggest that athletes can adapt to high-fat, low-carbohydrate diets and maintain physical endurance capacity, that high-fat diets can increase the muscle concentration of triglycerides, and that high-fat diets will increase use of fat as a fuel during exercise and decrease the use of carbohydrate, thus leading to enhanced endurance in prolonged aerobic exercise (40, 41).

The term *fat loading* has been used to describe both acute and chronic dietary techniques theorized to increase fat oxidation during exercise. Acute fat loading involves dietary strategies immediately before exercise, and several strategies have been used, including lipid infusion with heparin to increase serum FFAs. However, several studies employed practical protocols, such as consumption of high-fat meals (60–85% fat) several hours before testing or high-fat diets 1 to 2 days before testing. In general, research findings do not support an ergogenic effect of such dietary strategies, and such approaches may actually impair exercise performance in high-intensity tasks (12, 42).

Chronic fat loading has been studied with diets containing about 40 to 60% of daily caloric intake from fat and consumed for 5 to 14 days before testing, usually followed by 1 to 2 days of a high-carbohydrate diet. Several studies (43, 44) have reported significant improvements in endurance performance with such diets, but these studies may have experienced methodologic difficulties. However, one well-designed study using a chronic fat-loading protocol reported that endurance cyclists increased total fat oxidation, reduced carbohydrate oxidation, and significantly improved 20-km time trial performance by 1.4 minutes following 150 minutes of cycling at 70% VO_2max (45).

Contrarily, other well-controlled studies showed that chronic fat loading is not ergogenic. Although the percentage of dietary fat and the length of the protocol varied, studies showed no significant effect of chronic fat loading on 20-km road time performance in endurance-trained cyclists (46), an intense cycling time trial following cycling at 70% VO_2max for 2 hours (47, 48), a 1-hour cycling time trial following 4 hours at 65% VO_2max (49), a 50-km cycling trial (42), or 100-km cycling performance (50). However, although the results were not statistically significant, in several studies performance following the high-fat diet was better than the control diet. For example, in one study the investigators noted that although the main effects of the study were not significant, some evidence indicated enhanced ultraendurance cycling with a high-fat diet during training compared with a high-carbohydrate diet (50).

The results of several recent reviews are also equivocal. Several reviewers concluded that chronic high-fat diets may improve endurance capacity in cyclists and runners (51, 52). Conversely, other reviewers concluded such diets have no ergogenic effect (53–55). Some reviewers noted that ingestion of a high-fat diet by endurance-trained athletes results in substantially higher rates of fat oxidation and concomitant muscle glycogen sparing during submaximal exercise compared with an isoenergetic high-carbohydrate diet. Yet, despite marked changes in the patterns of fuel utilization that favor fat oxidation, this strategy does not provide clear benefits to the performance of prolonged endurance exercise (53). Other investigators noted that, overall, some evidence suggests that endurance performance, at best, can only be maintained after long-term adaptation to fat-rich diets when compared with carbohydrate-rich diets, and therefore long-term fat-rich diet usage cannot be recommended as a tool to improve endurance performance (54). This appears to be a balanced viewpoint.

The ACSM, ADA, and DC (2) noted that athletes need moderate amounts of dietary fat, about 20 to 25% of energy needs, to provide essential fatty acids and fat-soluble vitamins. An extremely low-fat diet (2% of energy) may reduce muscle triglycerides levels and total fat oxidation during exercise. In such a case, energy will be derived from carbohydrate and may lead to premature depletion, contributing to fatigue (56). However, excessive amounts of dietary fat may not be optimal. Although endurance athletes were able to maintain levels of high-intensity training while adapting to a high-fat diet over a 3-day period, the training sessions were associated with increased ratings of perceived exertion when compared with training with a high-carbohydrate diet (57). Three experts on fuel metabolism during exercise concluded that no evidence indicates that diets high in fat and restricted in carbohydrate enhance training (58).

Dietary Supplements: Fat Metabolites

Several different types of fats and fatty acids have been theorized to enhance sports performance.

ω-3 Fatty Acids

The production of specific eicosanoids from ω-3 fatty acid metabolism may stimulate human growth hormone (HGH) release (59), and several energy bars containing a blend of fish and vegetable oils with ω-3 fatty acids have been marketed for athletes. Several studies suggestive of an increased strength via an anabolic action of the ω-3 fatty acids were presented in a text on nutritional ergogenics, but some methodologic inconsistencies were found, and the studies have not appeared in peer-reviewed scientific journals (12). Currently, no support exists for an anabolic effect of ω-3 fatty acids.

Fish oil supplements have been shown to modulate the inflammatory response through alteration of the eicosanoid pathway, and they were theorized to prevent delayed-onset muscle soreness often associated with strenuous, repetitive eccentric muscle activity. However, no beneficial effects were reported following supplementation of 1.8 g of ω-3 fatty acids for 30 days (60).

Medium-Chain Triglycerides

Medium-chain triglycerides (MCTs) have been theorized to be ergogenic because of their more rapid absorption into the portal circulation, facilitated entrance into muscle cell mitochondria, and an oxidation rate comparable to that of exogenous carbohydrate. MCT supplementation, either alone or combined with carbohydrate, has been investigated as a means to enhance endurance exercise performance. Although earlier research revealed that MCT supplementation alone may actually impair endurance exercise performance, combining MCTs with carbohydrate is theorized to enhance endurance performance (12). However, more recent well-controlled studies with trained athletes using MCTs alone or combined with carbohydrate reported no significant ergogenic effect on muscle glycogen oxidation during 30 minutes cycling at 84% VO_2max (61), 100-km cycling time trial in eight endurance-trained male athletes (62), or an endurance treadmill test consisting of a 30-minute run at 85% VO_2max followed by a run to exhaustion at 75% VO_2max (63). MCT supplementation does not appear to be ergogenic, nor does a MCT-carbohydrate supplement provide any advantage over carbohydrate alone.

Conjugated Linoleic Acid

Conjugated linoleic acid (CLA) is a collective term for a group of isomers of linoleic acid, one of which is theorized to reduce lipid uptake by adipocytes. Because some animal research reported reduced body fat following CLA supplementation, dietary supplements have been marketed to humans, including athletes, for weight loss. However, although data are limited, more recent studies reported no significant effects of CLA supplementation on fatty acid metabolism or weight loss in healthy, weight-stable women (64) or on body mass and composition in experienced resistance-trained persons (65). Current research findings reveal no significant benefits of CLA supplementation to the physically active person.

DIETARY PROTEIN AND SPORTS PERFORMANCE

Dietary protein is of considerable importance to all athletes. Research indicates that adequate dietary protein is necessary to promote muscle tissue synthesis following exercise (12). Exercise also may use protein as an energy source during exercise. Sustained dynamic exercise stimulates amino acid oxidation, mainly of the BCAAs, and ammonia production in proportion to exercise intensity. If the exercise is intense enough, a net loss of muscle protein occurs as a result of decreased protein synthesis, increased catabolism, or both. Some of the amino acids are oxidized as fuel, and the rest provide substrates for gluconeogenesis (66). However, the energy contribution during exercise from protein is relatively minor (~5%) compared with carbohydrate and fat (67). Nevertheless, it is important to understand how dietary carbohydrate influences protein as an energy source during exercise. A low-carbohydrate diet leading to decreased muscle glycogen levels will lead to increased dependence on protein as an energy source. Exercise may also increase protein losses via proteinuria and sweat, although losses are relative minor (12).

Although factors regulating human muscle protein breakdown and synthesis are complex and interactive (68), both endurance and resistance training exercises increase skeletal muscle protein synthesis and breakdown in the postexercise recovery period (69), and such findings have stimulated research to determine protein requirements for physically active persons, a subject of continuing debate.

The Institute of Medicine Food and Nutrition Board (IOM-FNB), in their dietary reference intakes for protein (22), noted that little research had been conducted on the requirement for protein by persons engaged in strenuous physical activity. The IOM-FNB criticized the available studies and observed, for example, that although studies reported significant increases in amino acid oxidation during endurance exercise, the increased oxidation was measured around the time of the exercise itself and did not take into account the remaining part of the day. The IOM-FNB noted that the amount of protein oxidized, although significant, was small in comparison with the total daily amount of oxidation. Overall, the IOM-FNB concluded that in view of the lack of compelling evidence to the contrary, no additional dietary protein is suggested for healthy adults undertaking resistance or endurance exercise. Furthermore, Rennie (70) reported that muscle contractile activity enhances the anabolic response, so habitual training makes persons more efficient users of dietary protein, a finding suggesting that physically active people probably do not need to eat more protein and could likely manage perfectly adequately on less. Contrarily, based on available evidence, the ACSM, ADA, and DC (2), in their position stand on nutrition for athletes, concluded that protein requirements are higher in very active persons and suggested that resistance athletes need 1.6 to 1.7 g/kg body weight, whereas endurance athletes need approximately 1.2 to 1.4 g/kg.

Although these viewpoints are divergent, the available scientific data provide some support for several prudent recommendations regarding dietary protein intake for physically active persons, particularly for athletes who may be at risk of protein insufficiency, such as those in weight-control sports. First, all athletes should obtain at least the protein recommended dietary allowance (RDA) of approximately 0.8 to 1.0 g/kg body weight/day. Second, it may be prudent for athletes to consume more than the RDA, somewhat in the range recommended by the ACSM, ADA, and DC cited earlier. These recommendations approximate a 50 to 100% increase of the protein RDA, but they are well within the acceptable macronutrient distribution range of 10 to 35% of daily energy intake from protein. Third, these recommendations may be achieved from natural food sources in a healthy diet without the use of supplements. Fourth, eating strategies may also be an important consideration. Several investigators (24, 68, 70–72) reported that muscle protein synthesis appears to be very sensitive to increased availability of small amounts of essential amino acids in the blood, about 3.5 to 7.0 g of protein over an hour. However, although ingesting several doses of essential amino acids before exercise or during recovery will promote a net "anabolic" environment over 24 hours and may be a recommended protocol, it remains to be determined whether the acute effects of supplementation eventually lead to greater gains in muscle mass following habitual training (67). Overall, given these findings, consuming a small amount of protein and carbohydrate, such as a protein-carbohydrate energy drink, before or after exercise training, may be prudent behavior for many athletes (24, 73). Adequate carbohydrate is essential for muscle glycogen replenishment. Fifth, for endurance athletes, it is important to reinforce the viewpoint that carbohydrate is the main energy source. Besides its efficiency as a metabolic fuel during exercise, carbohydrate also provides a potent protein-sparing effect. Consuming sufficient carbohydrate will decrease reliance on protein during aerobic endurance exercise and will better maintain normal protein status in the body.

Dietary Supplements: Protein, Amino Acids, and Metabolites

Adequate protein intake is essential for all athletes. Protein continues to be a popular dietary supplement with athletes (74). Protein supplements have been recommended to athletes to enhance nitrogen retention and increase muscle mass, to prevent protein catabolism during prolonged exercise, to support an increased synthesis of hemoglobin, myoglobin, oxidative enzymes, and mitochondria during aerobic training, and to restore protein that may be lost in the sweat and urine during exercise. In general, however, research with protein supplements has shown no beneficial effects on strength, power, hypertrophy of muscle, or physiologic work capacity in athletes who obtain adequate dietary protein from natural food sources (12).

In recent years, specific types of protein compounds and amino acid supplements have been marketed to athletes and are among the most popular dietary supplements sold to athletes and physically active persons, particularly those involved in body building and strength training (74). Such commercial products have been studied for their ergogenic potential, including effects on strength and power as well as aerobic endurance performance.

Whey Protein and Colostrum

Whey and colostrum are two forms of protein that are theorized to be ergogenic. Whey protein isolates, extracted from the liquid whey produced during the manufacture of cheese or casein, are more than 90% protein and may contain other substances, including growth factors (75). Colostrum, or bovine colostrum, is the first milk secreted by cows and is a rich source of protein, carbohydrates, vitamins, minerals, and various biologically active components, also including growth factors (76). One theory of their ergogenicity is increased serum insulinlike growth factor, which could be anabolic, but research has not shown such increases following colostrum supplementation (77).

Whey supplementation has been shown to increase lean body mass and performance in some, but not all, strength tests more so than the placebo group (78), but other forms of protein may be just as effective because the placebo contained only carbohydrate. Colostrum supplementation did not enhance VO_2max (79) or performance in a 4-minute maximal rowing test (76), but it was shown to provide a small but significant improvement in a cycling time trial (79). Several studies (80, 81) evaluated the ergogenic effect of colostrum supplementation; these studies used whey protein as a placebo that could reveal whether colostrum supplementation produced any benefits beyond those attributed to whey protein alone. In general, the findings were negative, but a few were suggestive of some ergogenic effects. The current data should be regarded as preliminary, and additional research is merited.

Arginine

Arginine supplementation may be theorized to be ergogenic because it is a substrate for synthesis of nitric oxide, a potent endogenous vasodilator that may benefit blood flow and endurance capacity. Several studies involving patients with peripheral arterial disease or clinical symptoms of stable angina pectoris showed improved exercise capacity with arginine supplementation (82). However, research involving the independent effect of arginine supplementation on the aerobic endurance capacity of healthy athletes has not been uncovered (12).

Arginine, Ornithine, and Lysine

Arginine, ornithine, and lysine have been used in attempts to increase HGH production, the theory being to increase lean muscle mass and strength. However, a review of related studies revealed that well-controlled studies have not shown any increases in HGH release or increased muscle mass or strength (83).

Aspartates

Potassium and magnesium aspartates are salts of aspartic acid, an amino acid. They have been used as ergogenics, possibly by mitigating the accumulation of ammonia during exercise. The effect of aspartate supplementation on physical performance is equivocal, but about 50% of the available studies have indicated enhanced performance (12). Additional research is needed to study the potential ergogenicity and underlying mechanisms of these substances.

L-Tryptophan

L-Tryptophan is a precursor for serotonin, a brain neurotransmitter theorized to suppress pain. Free tryptophan (fTRYP) enters the brain cells to form serotonin. Thus, tryptophan supplementation has been used to increase serotonin production in attempts to increase tolerance to pain during intense exercise. However, well-controlled research indicates that L-tryptophan supplementation does not enhance high-intensity running or cycling performance (84) or aerobic endurance performance at 70 to 75% of VO$_2$max (85).

Branched-Chain Amino Acids

Some investigators believe that increased levels of serotonin may cause fatigue (86). During prolonged aerobic endurance exercise, muscle glycogen may become depleted, and the muscle may increase its reliance on BCAAs for fuel, thus decreasing the plasma BCAA:fTRYP ratio. Because BCAAs compete with fTRYP for entry into the brain, a low BCAA:fTRYP ratio would facilitate the entry of fTRYP to the brain and the formation of serotonin. Hypothetically, BCAA supplementation may delay central nervous system fatigue and enhance performance in prolonged aerobic endurance events by increasing the BCAA:fTRYP ratio and mitigating the formation of serotonin. The conclusions of several reviews are conflicting. One prominent investigator (87), although noting that more research is needed, indicated that ingestion of BCAAs reduces the perceived exertion and mental fatigue during prolonged exercise and improves cognitive performance after the exercise. She also suggested that, in some situations, BCAA ingestion may improve physical performance, such as during exercise in the heat or in actual competitive races when central fatigue may be more pronounced than in laboratory experiments. Other prominent investigators (88, 89) concluded that BCAA supplementation does not appear to affect fatigue or performance during prolonged exercise, and this appears to be the prevailing viewpoint, provided carbohydrate intake is sufficient.

Glutamine

Glutamine has been theorized as an anabolic substance, either by increasing HGH levels or by increasing muscle cell volume and stimulating protein synthesis. However, well-controlled studies (90, 91) did not show any ergogenic effects of glutamine supplementation on lean muscle mass or strength increase during training or on performance of multiple sets of resistance exercise to fatigue.

Glutamine is also an important fuel for some cells of the immune system; serum glutamine levels usually decrease following prolonged, strenuous exercise, and this decrease occurs concomitantly with transient immunodepression (92). Although earlier studies reported a lower incidence rate of infections in endurance athletes following glutamine supplementation (93), the current opinion is little support from controlled studies exists to recommend glutamine ingestion for enhanced immune function (89).

β-Hydroxy-β-Methylbutyrate

β-Hydroxy-β-methylbutyrate (HMB) is a byproduct of leucine metabolism in the human body and is currently marketed as calcium-HMB-monohydrate. Although the ergogenic mechanism is unknown, investigators have speculated that HMB may be incorporated into cell components or may influence cellular enzyme activity, in some way inhibiting the breakdown of muscle tissue during strenuous exercise and facilitating the response to training (94).

Some studies indicated that HMB supplementation (1.5–3.0 g/day) significantly increased lean tissue and strength in young untrained male subjects during the first 3 weeks of a resistance-training program (94), and similar findings were reported for older men and women undergoing resistance training (95). One study, using serum levels of several muscle enzymes as markers of muscle damage, suggested that prolonged HMB supplementation could help to prevent muscle damage following aerobic endurance exercise, such as in a 20-km run (96). Other investigators indicated that although some support exists for the claims that HMB supplementation may benefit young, untrained persons, the response of resistance-trained persons is less clear (97). Several well-designed studies have reported no significant effect of HMB supplementation on body composition, muscle strength, markers of muscle damage, muscle soreness, or muscle protein turnover in resistance-trained persons (98–101).

Currently, it would appear little evidence supports HMB supplementation as an ergogenic aid for strength- or endurance-trained persons.

VITAMINS, VITAMINLIKE SUBSTANCES, AND SPORTS PERFORMANCE

Most studies report that athletes consume high-calorie diets that contain the RDA of all nutrients, and they have few vitamin deficiencies (102). The prevailing viewpoint is that athletes will not need vitamin and mineral supplements if adequate energy to maintain body weight is consumed through a variety of foods (2, 103). However, individual athletes may be at risk, particularly those in weight-control sports, those who do not eat a well-balanced diet, and those who do not meet their energy needs (104). In such cases, vitamin supplements may be recommended to help prevent impaired exercise performance.

Dietary Supplements: Vitamins and Vitaminlike Substances

Vitamins are needed for numerous physiologic processes underlying sport performance, including coenzyme functions necessary for energy production from the macronutrients, formation of neurotransmitters and hormones, and prevention of oxidative damage associated with exercise. Studies have been conducted with virtually every individual vitamin to evaluate its ergogenic potential. In general, vitamin supplementation does not improve exercise performance in athletes with good nutritional status (12). Most research has focused on multivitamins, antioxidant supplements, and vitaminlike substances.

Multivitamins

The effect of multivitamins on exercise performance has been studied with various types of supplements, including B vitamin combinations and multivitamin-mineral preparations. Because many of the B vitamins are involved in the metabolism of carbohydrate, fat and protein, their ergogenic potential has been studied individually and in combination. Vitamins B_1, B_6, and B_{12} are believed to affect the formation of serotonin, an important neurotransmitter involved in relaxation. Research with large doses (60–200 times the RDA) of these vitamins showed increases in fine motor control and performance in pistol shooting (105), a sport activity in the pentathlon; this finding suggests that the beneficial effect was related to the role of these vitamins in promoting the development of neurotransmitters that induce relaxation. Additional research is merited. In general, however, although a deficiency of the B vitamins may impair both aerobic and anaerobic exercise performance, supplementation has not been shown to enhance performance in well-nourished persons (12).

The overall review of the literature supports the viewpoint that multivitamin-mineral supplements are unnecessary for athletes or other physically active persons who are on a well-balanced diet with adequate calories. Several well-controlled studies provided multivitamin-mineral supplements over prolonged periods (≤8 months) and reported no significant effects on both laboratory and sport-specific tests of physical performance (106, 107).

Antioxidants

Several antioxidant vitamins (β-carotene, vitamin C, vitamin E) have been studied individually or collectively in attempts to enhance exercise performance, to mitigate adverse effects of strenuous exercise on the immune system, or to reduce indices of muscle tissue damage following exercise.

Although vitamin C supplementation has been shown to improve physical performance in vitamin C–deficient subjects, research supports the general conclusion that vitamin C supplementation does not enhance physical performance in well-nourished persons (108). Vitamin E supplementation has also been studied as a means to enhance aerobic endurance capacity, possibly by maintaining integrity of the red blood cells and oxygen delivery. Vitamin E has been shown to enhance oxygen utilization during exercise at altitude (109), but it does not appear to be an effective ergogenic under sea level conditions (110). One review indicated that although vitamin E supplementation may increase tissue or serum vitamin E concentration, most evidence suggests no discernible effect on training or performance (111). Several reviews concluded that limited evidence suggests that dietary supplementation with antioxidants improves human performance, a finding indicating that these substances do not provide an ergogenic effect (112, 113).

Prolonged and intensive exertion, such as running ultramarathons, may impair the immune system and predispose to certain illnesses, such as upper respiratory tract infections. Large doses of vitamin C were claimed to strengthen the immune system and prevent upper respiratory tract infections, but more recent studies indicated that vitamin C supplementation and combined antioxidant vitamin supplementation are not effective countermeasures to exercise-induced immunosuppression (114, 115).

Preventing muscle tissue damage during strenuous exercise could be considered ergogenic, but principal investigators concluded that related research findings, mostly conducted with vitamin C, vitamin E, and β-carotene, did not provide clear evidence for the prophylactic effect of these substances on various types of muscle damage following exercise (116–118). Conversely, other reviewers concluded that dietary supplementation with antioxidant vitamins has favorable effects on lipid peroxidation and exercise-induced muscle damage, findings suggesting that antioxidant vitamin supplementation may be desirable for physically active persons under certain physiologic conditions by providing a larger protective margin

(119–122). Such conditions or situations could include regular heavy exercise, a suboptimal diet, or older athletes. In general, reviewers recommended a diet rich in antioxidant vitamins and minerals, but one group (123) recommended that athletes supplement with 100 to 200 mg of vitamin E daily to help prevent exercise-induced oxidative damage. However, all reviewers indicated that more research is needed to address this issue and to provide guidelines for recommendations to athletes, particularly because some beneficial physiologic processes during exercise may be mediated by oxidants and thus antioxidants may be counterproductive (122).

Coenzyme Q$_{10}$

Coenzyme Q$_{10}$ (CoQ$_{10}$), also known as ubiquinone, is a lipid with characteristics common to a vitamin. It is an antioxidant that may improve oxygen uptake in the mitochondria of the heart, and it has been used therapeutically for the treatment of cardiovascular disease (124). Theoretically, improved oxygen usage in the heart and skeletal muscles could improve aerobic endurance performance. However, studies showed that CoQ$_{10}$ supplementation to healthy, physically trained subjects did not influence lipid peroxidation, heart rate, VO$_2$max, anaerobic threshold, or cycling endurance performance (125–128). One study reported that CoQ$_{10}$ supplementation was associated with muscle tissue damage and actually impaired cycling performance compared with the placebo treatment (129).

Choline

Choline is involved in various metabolic roles in the human body, including the synthesis of acetylcholine. Significantly lower plasma choline levels were observed following a 42.2-km marathon, a finding suggestive as an etiologic factor in the development of fatigue because of the possibility of decreased acetylcholine production and resultant impaired muscular contractility (130). Choline supplementation was reported to accelerate synthesis and release of acetylcholine by neurons (131), but no data are available to support an ergogenic effect. Studies reported no beneficial effect of choline supplementation on various measures of endurance performance, such as cycling to exhaustion at 150 or 70% of VO$_2$max (132), marathon running time (133), or a run to exhaustion following a 4-hour treadmill exercise test carrying a total load of 34.1 kg (134).

MINERALS AND SPORTS PERFORMANCE

As with vitamins, athletes will not need mineral supplements if adequate energy to maintain body weight is consumed through a variety of foods (2). However, as noted previously, some athletes may not eat properly. Sports nutritionists have noted that calcium and iron are the two micronutrients most likely to be low in the diet, but supplements should be considered only if the diet cannot be

corrected (135). Young athletes should obtain adequate calcium during development of peak bone mass, and all female athletes should assess their dietary iron intake.

Dietary Supplements: Minerals

Minerals, functioning in our body as electrolytes or metalloenzymes, are involved in numerous metabolic processes important to sport performance, such as muscle contraction, enzyme activation, and oxygen transport. Various mineral supplements, mainly as mineral salts, have been used in attempts to enhance a variety of sports performances, including aerobic endurance, strength, and power.

Calcium

Most calcium in the body is used for bone formation, but calcium is also involved in numerous metabolic processes, including muscle contraction. Strenuous exercise has been shown to increase urinary calcium excretion, as much as 400 mg/day, and to reduce serum calcium levels (136, 137). Female athletes with disordered eating (anorexia athletica) are at high risk of premature osteoporosis (138). Calcium supplements may be recommended for some athletes, particularly those involved in strenuous exercise in weight-control sports, to optimize bone mass. However, there is a dearth of research regarding the effect of calcium supplementation on exercise performance (12).

Phosphates

Phosphates are found as components of various compounds in the body, including 2,3-diphosphoglycerate, which is essential for oxygen release from hemoglobin. An increased 2,3-diphosphoglycerate level is the prevalent theory underlying phosphate supplementation to endurance athletes. Although not all studies have shown ergogenic effects following phosphate supplementation, remarkably similar increases in VO$_2$max and aerobic endurance exercise performance were documented in four studies conducted between 1984 and 1990 (139–142). However, several confounding variables in previous research were identified in a 1994 review, with a recommendation for additional controlled study (143), but current research findings are still equivocal (12).

Magnesium

Magnesium is a component of more than 300 enzymes that play key roles in a variety of metabolic processes, such as muscle contraction, important to the athlete. One reviewer noted that although some evidence supports the hypothesis that magnesium may play a significant role in promoting strength and cardiorespiratory function in healthy persons and athletes, study designs limited the conclusions, and it is unclear whether these observations related to improvement of an impaired nutritional status or to a pharmacologic effect (144, 145). However, a meta-analysis of human supplementation studies indicated that the strength of the evidence favors those studies finding no effect of magnesium supplementation on any form of exercise performance, including aerobic, anaerobic-lactic acid, and strength activities (146).

Iron

Iron is one of the most critical minerals with implications for sports performance. Iron is a component of hemoglobin, myoglobin, cytochromes, and various enzymes in the muscle cells, all of which are involved in the transport and metabolism of oxygen for aerobic energy production. Female athletes may not obtain sufficient dietary iron, whereas strenuous exercise may increase body iron losses in a variety of ways, including hematuria and gastrointestinal losses (147–149). The prevalence of iron deficiency anemia is likely to be higher in athletic groups, especially in younger female athletes, than in healthy sedentary persons (150), and this condition impairs exercise performance (151).

The effects of iron supplementation on exercise performance depend on the iron status of the athlete. Iron supplementation to athletes with iron deficiency anemia should improve exercise performance. Iron supplementation to athletes with normal iron and hemoglobin status does not enhance performance, but athletes who train at altitude to produce erythropoietin and to optimize hemoglobin levels may benefit from iron supplementation (12). Whether iron supplementation improves performance in athletes who have iron deficiency without anemia, a condition of normal hemoglobin levels but reduced serum ferritin, is equivocal. One review noted that although iron supplementation can raise serum ferritin concentrations, increases in ferritin unaccompanied by increases in hemoglobin concentration have not been shown to improve endurance performance (152). However, several studies showed that iron supplementation may enhance the response to aerobic training in iron-depleted, nonanemic women (153, 154).

Zinc

Zinc is required for the activity of more than 300 enzymes, several involved in the major pathways of energy metabolism. Endurance athletes who adopt a diet rich in carbohydrate, but low in protein and fat, may decrease zinc intake; over time, this may lead to a zinc deficiency with loss of body weight, latent fatigue, and decreased endurance (155). Research regarding the ergogenicity of zinc supplementation to athletes is very limited, and the available research does not provide sufficient data to provide recommendations to athletes (144, 145).

Chromium

Chromium is an insulin cofactor, and its theorized ergogenic effect is based on the role of insulin to facilitate BCAA transport into the muscle. Chromium has been advertised for strength-type athletes to gain muscle and lose fat. Some early research data did suggest an increase in lean body mass and decreased body fat with chromium picolinate supplementation (156). However, this report was based on flawed studies. More contemporary research with better experimental design replicated these studies and showed that chromium picolinate supplementation does not increase lean muscle mass or decrease body fat and has no effect on muscular strength or intermittent, high-intensity, prolonged endurance performance in athletes or persons undergoing exercise training (157–163).

Boron, Vanadium, and Selenium

Boron has been marketed as an anabolic mineral, theoretically by increasing serum testosterone. However, this theory was based on research with elderly women and apparently has no application to healthy athletes. Research is limited, but it does not document an anabolic effect of boron supplementation (164). Vanadium has also been advertised for its anabolic potential, purportedly by enhancement of insulin activity. However, the limited data available do not support an anabolic effect of vanadium in young healthy persons (165). Selenium is essential for the functioning of various enzymes, including glutathione peroxidase involved in antioxidant activity. As with the vitamin antioxidants, the role of selenium supplementation is equivocal regarding its ability to prevent muscle tissue damage during intense exercise. However, several studies showed that selenium supplementation does not enhance VO_2max or aerobic and anaerobic running performance (12).

WATER/ELECTROLYTES AND SPORTS PERFORMANCE

Water is the milieu within which most nutrients in the body function, but for the athlete, one of its most important functions is to help optimize body water balance and body temperature regulation during exercise under warm environmental conditions. Excessive loss of body fluids via exercise-induced perspiration, which can range up to 3 L/hour, induces a state of hypohydration and affects numerous physiologic processes that may impair physical performance. Hypohydration decreases both intracellular and extracellular fluid volumes, particularly blood volume, with associated decreases in stroke volume, cardiac output, and endurance exercise performance (166, 167). Hypohydration may also induce an earlier onset of the anaerobic threshold and may adversely affect mental functioning (168, 169).

Sodium is involved in numerous metabolic functions, but of prime interest to the athlete is its role in maintenance of normal body fluid balance, particularly during very prolonged endurance events. Sodium is the main electrolyte in sweat, and over time, sodium deficits can lead to incomplete rehydration and muscle cramps. Potassium is also involved in numerous metabolic functions, but sweat losses of potassium are minor compared with losses of sodium and chloride, and hypokalemia is relatively rare (12).

Dietary Supplements: Water and Electrolytes

Fluid replacement is critical during prolonged exercise under warm environmental conditions, and it is one of the most thoroughly studied areas in sports nutrition. Electrolyte replacement is also an important consideration during very prolonged exercise.

Water

In brief, the key issue is prevention of hypohydration during an exercise session by hydrating well before the exercise task, drinking as much as is comfortable and practical during the session, and rehydrating adequately afterward in preparation for future exercise bouts (170). Hyperhydration before exercise may be helpful, but it has not been shown to be as effective as rehydration, which has been shown to decrease physiologic stress during exercise in the heat, as evidenced by a decreased heart rate response, lesser rise in the core temperature, and increased endurance performance (12). Athletes may hyperhydrate by consuming 500 to 1000 mL of fluid before exercise, rehydrate by consuming an amount of fluid about equivalent with the rate of sweat loss during exercise, and consuming about 120 to 150% of sweat losses after exercise to rehydrate rapidly (12, 171).

However, excessive intake of water before and during exercise may be potentially harmful. Hyponatremia (subnormal plasma sodium) may be caused from excessive sweat sodium losses or excessive water intake, but in athletes, the most likely cause is fluid overload (172, 173). Female athletes appear to be at increased risk. Hyponatremia may be mild, with symptoms such as bloating or mild nausea, or severe, with headache, vomiting, coma, and possible death from brain swelling and respiratory arrest (12, 174). Prevention is the key, and, as noted earlier, the current recommendation for rehydration during exercise is to consume amounts corresponding to fluid sweat losses during exercise.

Electrolytes

Sodium and chloride are the major electrolytes found in sweat, and potassium losses are much lower. Sodium intake is vital, and an increased beverage sodium chloride concentration (30–50 mmol/L; 1.7–2.9 g/L) may be beneficial during very prolonged exercise and during recovery (175–177). Athletes who sweat heavily are recommended to consume more salt in their daily diet. Potassium may be replaced through the daily diet, particularly one rich in fruits. Potassium supplements are not recommended because they may cause hyperkalemia and heart arrhythmias (178).

Sports Drinks

Sports drinks may be a very effective means to rehydrate during exercise. The major ingredient in sports drinks is water, but most also contain sodium chloride and carbohydrate. Research showed that although water rehydration may help to delay fatigue during endurance exercise, ingestion of water with carbohydrate was even more effective (179). Research also documented that sports drinks are one of the few nutritional food products that may enhance sport performance in exercise tasks in which performance may be impaired by dehydration and depleted endogenous carbohydrate reserves (8).

FOOD DRUGS AND SPORTS PERFORMANCE

Known as doping, pharmacologic ergogenic aids have been used to improve both physical and psychologic functions deemed important to sports performance. However, the use of most ergogenic drugs, such as amphetamines and anabolic steroids, is prohibited by WADA, which provides recommendations to the International Olympic Committee.

Dietary Supplements: Food Drugs

Some drugs are found naturally in foods, but they are also found in dietary supplements, sports drinks, and sports bars marketed to athletes. Two major food drugs are caffeine and ephedrine, which are used not only by elite athletes but also by people of all ages in attempts to improve athletic performance (180). Alcohol and sodium bicarbonate have also been studied as nutritional ergogenics.

Caffeine

Caffeine may affect metabolic processes important to sport performance either directly, as an adenosine receptor antagonist, or indirectly, through stimulation of the sympathetic nervous system. Originally, caffeine was theorized to enhance aerobic endurance performance through increased FFA oxidation and an associated sparing of muscle glycogen. However, current research does not support this hypothesis (181, 182), and it appears unlikely that increased fat oxidation with the associated glycogen sparing is the prime ergogenic mechanism underlying caffeine use as an ergogenic aid (183). Caffeine may affect exercise performance directly by increasing the force of muscle contraction (184) or via reduced psychologic perception of effort (185), but the mechanism underlying improved performance has not been determined.

Although not all studies have shown ergogenic effects of caffeine supplementation, several extensive reviews concluded that the available evidence supports moderate caffeine use (5 mg/kg) as an effective ergogenic aid. Although caffeine use does not appear to increase VO₂max, it does appear to enhance aerobic endurance performance (183,

186, 187). In one review, caffeine supplementation was calculated to improve 40-km cycling time trial performance by 55 to 84 seconds (188). Fewer studies with resistance exercise have been conducted, but the available literature suggests that caffeine could increase endurance in repeated muscle contractions (183). Caffeine use by athletes was restricted at one time, but it was removed from the WADA doping list in 2004.

Caffeine is found in some sports drinks. As a diuretic, it has been theorized to impair aerobic endurance performance. However, one review concluded that athletes will not incur detrimental fluid-electrolyte imbalances if they consume caffeinated beverages in moderation and eat a typical diet (189).

Ephedrine (Ephedra)

Like caffeine, ephedrine is a stimulant. *Ma Huang*, also known as Chinese ephedra, is an herbal preparation marketed for weight loss and increased energy. *Ma Huang* is herbal ephedrine and may be found in herbal teas and various dietary supplements. Several reviews concluded that research regarding the effect of ephedrine supplementation on sport performance is limited, but, in general, findings from reviews, including a meta-analysis, revealed no ergogenic effect on tests of aerobic endurance, strength, power, muscular endurance, reaction time, speed, or anaerobic capacity (190, 191). However, some research showed positive ergogenic effects of ephedrine alone and also an additive effect when it was combined with caffeine. Most of these studies involved physical performance tests of a military nature, such as a 10-km run while the subject was wearing a helmet and backpack weighing 11 kg (192–195). These studies used pharmaceutical grade ephedrine, not dietary supplements containing ephedra. No trial of ephedra and athletic performance has been reported (191).

Ephedrine use is prohibited by WADA. Moreover, ephedrine misuse may be associated with significant health risks in some persons, such as hypertension, heart palpitations and tachycardia, stroke, and death (196), and the sale of ephedra-containing dietary supplements was prohibited in 2004 by the US Food and Drug Administration.

Ethyl Alcohol (Ethanol)

Ethyl alcohol, a depressant, has been alleged to be ergogenic for aerobic endurance events, possibly by serving as an energy source, favorably affecting energy metabolism, or by modifying psychologic perceptions of fatigue. Its effects on exercise performance have been reviewed (12) and are summarized briefly. Although alcohol contains substantial energy, the available evidence suggests it is not used to any significant extent during exercise. Moreover, research also supports the finding that alcohol in small amounts does not beneficially affect VO$_2$max or other major physiologic variables associated with energy production during aerobic exercise. In general, alcohol does not significantly modify endogenous carbohydrate and fat utilization during exercise, but during prolonged exercise, some research indicates that alcohol may reduce gluconeogenesis by the liver and glucose uptake by the legs, effects that may impair endurance performance. Although most studies found that small amounts of alcohol do not enhance or impair aerobic endurance performance, some research indicated a significant decrease in aerobic endurance when alcohol is ingested before and during the exercise task. The available scientific data do not support an ergogenic role for alcohol in aerobic endurance exercise. Conversely, its use may be ergolytic. Nevertheless, alcohol use may reduce anxiety and associated side effects, such as hand tremor, and thus may benefit performance in some sports, such as archery and pistol shooting (12). Therefore, although WADA does not prohibit alcohol in most sports, its use is prohibited for a variety of sports in which anxiety reduction may enhance performance.

Sodium Bicarbonate and Citrate

Alkaline salts, such as sodium bicarbonate and sodium citrate, are described as antacids in the United States Pharmacopeia and have been studied as nutritional ergogenics. Sodium bicarbonate (0.3 g/kg) and sodium citrate (0.5 g/kg) supplementation may increase the alkaline reserve and may help to buffer lactic acid in the muscle cell. Ingestion of large amounts of these alkaline salts has high potential for gastrointestinal distress and may limit the use of this strategy by athletes in competition. However, a long-term loading protocol, or taking the same total amount of sodium bicarbonate spread over a 6-day period, may be just as effective and may not induce gastrointestinal distress (197). Alkaline salts are theorized to improve athletic performance in anaerobic-type events that depend primarily on anaerobic glycolysis. Research indicated that bicarbonate salt supplementation will increase the serum pH and may enhance performance in exercise tasks, particularly repetitive exercise tasks, that maximize energy production for 1 to 6 minutes. Not all studies showed ergogenic effects, but numerous laboratory and field studies supported a positive ergogenic effect of sodium bicarbonate supplementation. Several comprehensive reviews, including a meta-analysis reporting an effect size greater than 0.40 favoring sodium bicarbonate when compared with placebo conditions, or a mean performance improvement of 27%, concluded that sodium bicarbonate is an effective ergogenic (198, 199). Research conducted subsequent to these reviews provided mixed results, but, in general, about half of these more recent studies revealed beneficial effects of sodium bicarbonate or sodium citrate on exercise performance. Some beneficial effects have even been noted on prolonged aerobic endurance tasks, a finding that merits additional research (12, 200).

DIETARY SUPPLEMENTS AND SPORTS PERFORMANCE

As noted previously, sports supplements are big business. Consumers in the United States spend about $20 billion annually on dietary supplements, and sports supplements account for about 9% of sales; about 46% of physically active persons use supplements (3).

Dietary Supplements: Miscellaneous Sport Supplements

The effect on exercise performance of supplementation with vitamins, minerals, amino acids, and various metabolites was covered earlier, and this section briefly highlights the effects of other dietary supplements marketed to athletes.

Creatine

Creatine is a nitrogen-containing substance found naturally in small amounts in animal foods, particularly meat, but it may also be formed in the body from several amino acids. Oral creatine supplementation, usually as creatine monohydrate, particularly when consumed concomitantly with carbohydrate, was reported to increase muscle supplies of free creatine and creatine phosphate (PCr), a high-energy phosphagen (201). Performance enhancement was associated with enhanced ATP resynthesis from the increased PCr and a higher rate of PCr resynthesis from the free creatine (202, 203). Creatine is popular with athletes at all levels of competition, including middle and high school athletes (204).

Numerous studies and several major reviews, including a meta-analysis and a monograph, reported a significant ergogenic effect of creatine supplementation, particularly in repetitive, short-duration, high-intensity, short-recovery exercise tasks such as isotonic and isokinetic resistance tests, cycle ergometer sprint protocols, sprint running, and simulated match play in sports with intermittent sprinting (205–208). Creatine supplementation also consistently appears to increase body mass; short-term gains may be primarily water, but long-term gains associated with resistance training may be lean muscle mass (12), induced by increased myosin heavy-chain mRNA and protein expression (209). The prevailing opinion is that creatine supplementation is an effective ergogenic for strength and power athletes, but not for aerobic endurance athletes (210).

Carnitine

Carnitine, an amine, is derived from lysine and methionine. L-Carnitine is the active form that facilitates the transport of fatty acids into the mitochondria for oxidation, a function that theoretically could lead to a sparing of muscle glycogen during exercise. L-Carnitine also facilitates the oxidation of several amino acids and pyruvate, functions that could mitigate lactate production. However, research and detailed reviews of the available research did not support an ergogenic effect of L-carnitine supplementation on fuel utilization during exercise, maximal heart rate, anaerobic threshold, VO₂max, time to exhaustion in various anaerobic or aerobic exercise tasks, performance in either a marathon or a 20-km run, or body composition (211–214).

Inosine

Inosine is a nucleoside with a variety of potential ergogenic effects that could benefit either strength- or endurance-type athletes. No research is available relative to the effect of inosine supplementation on strength performance. Two studies did use the recommended supplementation protocol for endurance athletes and reported no beneficial effects on cardiovascular-respiratory or metabolic functions during submaximal or maximal exercise, nor was any effect noted on time to complete a simulated 4.83-km (3-mile) treadmill race. Both studies actually suggested that inosine could be ergolytic for certain athletic endeavors involving anaerobic glycolysis (215, 216).

Glycerol

Glycerol-induced hyperhydration, when compared with water hyperhydration alone, may result in greater fluid retention because the glycerol may help to maintain the osmolality of the blood, with better preservation of serum antidiuretic hormone levels. Such an effect could increase plasma volume and total body water, with potential beneficial effects for exercise performance and temperature regulation during exercise in the heat. Indeed, glycerol has been marketed in some sports drinks.

Not all studies showed positive effects of glycerol hyperhydration (217), but several showed that glycerol-induced hyperhydration increases body fluid retention and improves cardiovascular responses, temperature regulation, and cycling exercise performance under warm or hot environmental conditions (218–221). Reviews reached different conclusions regarding the ergogenic efficacy of glycerol supplementation. One review indicated that glycerol supplementation improves tolerance to exercise (222), others concluded that glycerol-induced hyperhydration appears to have no meaningful advantage during exercise-heat stress if euhydration is maintained (223, 224), whereas a third review suggested that additional research is needed to resolve the current equivocal findings (225). The third review appears most reasonable, particularly in sports in which the extra body mass needs to be moved, such as distance running (12).

Herbals and Botanicals

Herbal dietary supplements may be used to induce ergogenic effects in various ways. Some are theorized to enhance energy production, possibly by influencing metabolic pathways or enhancing physiologic factors important to exercise; increased mitochondrial oxidation, myocardial activity, capillarization, and hemoglobin concentration are some proposed mechanisms. Some of the most popular purported ergogenic herbals are theorized to modify favorably body composition, that is, to increase muscle mass and to decrease fat mass. Unfortunately, with a few exceptions, research investigating the ergogenic effects of herbal supplements is limited (226).

Ginseng. Ginsengs are preparations extracted from the roots of various genera of the plant family Araliaceae. Ginsengs contain a wide variety of chemical substances, the nature of which depends on the specific plant genus. Some of these substances, particularly glycosides, are theorized to be ergogenic, possibly by mitigating the stress of exercise. However, although the underlying mechanisms have not been determined, ginseng has been studied mainly as a means to enhance endurance performance.

Research findings relative to the effect of ginseng on endurance performance are equivocal. For example, one reviewer (227) indicated that controlled studies of Asian ginseng found improvement in exercise performance with use of standardized extracts, long duration of supplementation, large numbers of subjects, and elderly subjects. However, most studies reporting positive ergogenic effects were associated with improper research methodology (228). Several well-controlled studies reported no significant effect of *Panax ginseng, Eleutherococcus senticosus Maxim L* (regarded to be Siberian Ginseng), or a standardized ginseng extract on cardiovascular, metabolic, or psychologic responses to either submaximal or maximal exercise performance or on maximal performance capacity (229–232). Several reviews of well-designed studies concluded that compelling research evidence regarding the efficacy of ginseng use to improve physical performance in humans is absent (233, 234).

Hydroxycitrate. Hydroxycitrate, derived from a tropical fruit, has been hypothesized to modify citric acid cycle metabolism to promote fatty acid oxidation. However, the available evidence indicates that hydroxycitrate supplementation does not modify fat utilization during exercise in either sedentary persons or endurance-trained cyclists, much less confer an ergogenic effect (235, 236).

Prohormones. Several dietary supplements derived from plants are marketed as prohormones, such as dehydroepiandrosterone, androstenedione, and related substances, and they are theorized to function by stimulating testosterone production. Studies evaluated the effects of prohormone supplementation on serum testosterone levels, body composition, and exercise performance. Although high prohormone supplement doses (200–300 mg androstenedione) were shown to increase serum testosterone concentrations in some, but not all, studies, no associated ergogenic effects were noted on protein synthesis or metabolism, muscle mass or lean body mass, or muscle strength in men involved in resistance training (12, 237).

Other plant extracts, such as γ-oryzanol, *Tribulus terrestris,* and yohimbine, are also conjectured to elicit anabolic effects by stimulating the release of either testosterone or HGH. However, research is very limited and does not support an effect of γ-oryzanol supplementation on circulating concentrations of hormones (testosterone, HGH, insulin), vertical jump performance, or 1-RM muscular strength for the bench press and squat (238). *Tribulus terrestris* supplementation exerted no effect on body weight, body composition, maximal strength, or muscular endurance in resistance-trained male subjects involved in periodized resistance training (239), and no studies involving ergogenic effects of yohimbine were uncovered (12).

SUMMARY AND CONCLUSIONS

From time immemorial, athletes have used various nutritional strategies or dietary supplements to enhance their performance. Table 109.1 is based on current studies and reviews, and it indicates that although most dietary supplements have not been shown to enhance sport performance when added to a healthful, balanced diet, several dietary supplements may possess ergogenic properties. Others should not be used because they may possess health risks or are prohibited by WADA.

Athletes and clinicians should be aware that use of some dietary supplements may be associated with certain health risks and positive doping tests. For example, although creatine supplementation in recommended doses is generally regarded to pose no major adverse effects in healthy people, abnormal effects may occur when large amounts are consumed (206, 240). Excessive intake of many dietary supplements, even vitamins and minerals, may pose serious health risks. Athletes who may be tested for doping should also be aware that dietary supplements may contain prohibited substances. Some, such as ephedrine, may be listed in the Supplement Facts label, whereas others, such as anabolic steroids, may be added surreptitiously (12).

In summary, athletes benefit most from consumption of a balanced and varied healthful diet, but utilization of some dietary strategies and supplements may benefit athletes involved in certain types of athletic endeavors. Individuals may respond differently to various nutritional strategies or dietary supplements, so athletes and their advisors must be prepared to experiment, to optimize both training and performance (10).

TABLE 109.1 EFFICACY OF DIETARY STRATEGIES AND SUPPLEMENTS TO ENHANCE SPORTS PERFORMANCE IN WELL-TRAINED INDIVIDUALS

Perform as claimed
Caffeine
Carbohydrate
Creatine
Sodium bicarbonate
Sports drinks
Water

May perform as claimed but insufficient evidence
Aspartate salts
Carbohydrate/protein
Glycerol
Phosphate salts

Do not perform as claimed

Androstenedione	Dehydroepiandrosterone	Octacosanol
Antioxidant vitamins	Dimethylglycine	ω–3 Fatty acids
Arginine/ornithine	Fat loading	Ornithine
B vitamins	γ-Oryzanol	Pyruvate
Branched-chain amino acids	Ginseng	Ribose
Bee pollen	Glutamine	Selenium
Boron	Glycine	*Tribulus terrestris*
Calcium	Hydroxycitrate	Tryptophan
Carnitine	β-Hydroxy-β-methylbutyrate	Vanadium
Choline	Inosine	Vitamin A, D
Chromium	Iron	Vitamin C, E
Ciwujia	Lysine	Whey protein
Conjugated linoleic acid	Magnesium	Yohimbine
Colostrum	Medium-chain triglycerides	Zinc
Coenzyme Q10	Niacin	

Should not be used: dangerous or prohibited
Alcohol
Androstenedione/androstenediol
Dehydroepiandrosterone
Ephedrine

REFERENCES

1. Loucks AB. Exerc Sport Sci Rev 2003;31:141–8.
2. American College of Sports Medicine, American Dietetic Association, Dietitians of Canada. Med Sci Sports Exerc 2000;32:2130–45.
3. Dancho, CL, Manore MM. ACSM Health Fitness J 2001;5:7–12.
4. Romijn JA, Coyle EF, Sidossis LS et al. Am J Physiol 1993;265:E380–91.
5. Romijn, J, Coyle EF, Sidossis LS et al. J Appl Physiol 2000;88:1707–14.
6. Shulman R, Rothman D. Proc Nat Acad Sci 2001;98:457–61.
7. Haff GG, Lehmkuhl MJ, McCoy LB et al. J Strength Cond Res 2003;17:187–96.
8. Coombes J, Hamilton K. Sports Med 2000;29:181–209.
9. Hargreaves M. Carbohydrate replacement during exercise. In: Maughan R, ed. Nutrition in Sport. Oxford: Blackwell Science, 2000:112–18.
10. Lambert EV, Goedecke JH. Curr Sports Med Res 2003;2:194–201.
11. Peters EM. Curr Opin Clin Nutr Metab Care 2003;6:427–34.
12. Williams MH. Nutrition for Health, Fitness and Sport. Boston: McGraw-Hill, 2005.
13. Utter AC, Kang J, Robertson RJ. Med Sci Sports Exerc 2002;34:1779–84.
14. Welsh RS, Davis JM, Burke JR. Med Sci Sports Exerc 2002;34:723–31.
15. Jentjens RL, Achten J, Jeukendrup AE. Med Sci Sports Exerc 2004;36:1551–8.
16. Hawley J, Schabort EJ, Noakes TD et al. Sports Med 1997;24:73–81.
17. Walker JL, Heigenhauser GJ, Hultman E et al. J Appl Physiol 2000;88:2151–8.
18. Burke LM, Hawley JA, Schabort EJ et al. J Appl Physiol 2000;88:1284–90.
19. Burke LM, Cox GR, Cummings NK et al. Sports Med 2001;31:267–99.
20. Febbraio M. Sports Med 2001;31:47–59.
21. Manore, MM. ACSM Health Fitness J 2002;6:25–7.
22. Food and Nutrition Board, Institute of Medicine. Dietary Reference Intakes for Energy, Carbohydrates, Fiber, Fat, Protein and Amino Acids (Macronutrients). Washington, DC: National Academy Press, 2002.
23. Ivy JL. Can J Appl Physiol 2001;26:S236–45.
24. Ivy J, Portmans R. Nutrient Timing. North Bergen, NJ: Basic Health Publications, 2004.
25. Jentjens R, Jeukendrup AE. Sports Med 2003;33:117–44.

26. Morrison, MA, Spriet LL, Dyck DJ. J Appl Physiol 2000;89: 549–56.

27. Op 'T Eijnde B, Van Leemputte M, Brouns F et al. J Appl Physiol 2001;91:2275–81.

28. Berardi JM, Ziegenfuss TN. J Strength Cond Res 2003;17: 47–52.

29. Hellsten Y, Skadhauge L, Bangsbo J. Am J Physiol 2004;286: R182–8.

30. Kreider RB, Melton C, Greenwood M et al. Int J Sport Nutr Exerc Metab 2003;13:76–86.

31. Hawley JA. Med Sci Sports Exerc 2002;34:1475–6.

32. Tunstall RJ, Mehan KA, Wadley GD et al. Am J Physiol 2002;283:E66–72.

33. Coggan AR, Raguso CA, Gastaldelli A et al. Metabolism 2000; 49:122–8.

34. Roepstorff CH, Steffensen CH, Madsen M et al. Am J Physiol 2002;282:E435–47.

35. Cameron-Smith D, Burke, LM, Angus DJ et al. Am J Clin Nutr 2003;77;313–8.

36. Hawley JA. Med Sci Sports Exerc 2002;34:1475–6.

37. Van Loon LJ, Greenhaff PL, Constantin-Teodosiu D et al. J Physiol (Lond) 2001;536:295–304.

38. Jeukendrup AE. Ann NY Acad Sci 2002;967:217–35.

39. Spriet LL. Med Sci Sports Exerc 2002;34:1477–84.

40. Brown R, Cox C. Am J Med Sports 2001;3:75–86.

41. Stroud M. Proc Nutr Soc 1998;57:55–61.

42. Rowlands DS, Hopkins WG. Int J Sport Nutr Exerc Metab 2002;12:318–35.

43. Horvath PJ, Eagen CK, Fisher NM et al. J Am Coll Nutr 2000; 19:52–60.

44. Muoio DM, Leddy JJ, Horvath PJ et al. Med Sci Sports Exerc 1994;26:81–8.

45. Lambert EV, Goedecke JH, Syle C et al. Int J Sport Nutr Exerc Metab 2001;11:209–25.

46. Brown RC, Cox C. NZ J Sports Med 2000;28:55–9.

47. Burke LM, Angus DJ, Cox GR et al. J Appl Physiol 2000;89: 2413–21.

48. Burke LM, Hawley JA, Angus DJ et al. Med Sci Sports Exerc 2002;34:83–91.

49. Carey AL, Staudacher HM, Cummings NK. J Appl Physiol 2001;91:115–22.

50. Rowlands DS, Hopkins WG. Metabolism 2002;51:678–90.

51. Pendergast DR, Leddy JJ, Venkatraman JT. J Am Coll Nutr 2000;19:345–50.

52. Venkatraman, JT, Leddy J, Pendergast D. Med Sci Sports Exerc 2000;32:S389–95.

53. Burke LM, Hawley JA. Med Sci Sports Exerc 2002;34:1492–8.

54. Helge JW. Med Sci Sports Exerc 2002;34:1499–1504.

55. Kiens B. Can J Appl Physiol 2001;26:S56–63.

56. Coyle EF, Jeukendrup AE, Oseto MC et al. Am J Physiol 2001;280:E391–8.

57. Stepto NK, Carey AL, Staudacher HM et al. Med Sci Sports Exerc 2002;34:449–55.

58. Burke LM, Kiens B, Ivy JL. J Sports Sci 2004;22:15–30.

59. Bucci LR. Nutrients as Ergogenic Aids. Boca Raton, FL: CRC Press, 1993.

60. Lenn J, Uhl T, Mattacola C et al. Med Sci Sports Exerc 2002; 34:1605–13.

61. Horowitz JF, Mora-Rodriguez R, Byerley LO et al. J Appl Physiol 2000;88:219–25.

62. Angus DJ, Hargreaves M, Dancey J et al. J Appl Physiol 2000; 88:113–90.

63. Misell LM, Lagomarcino ND, Schuster V et al. J Sports Med Phys Fitness 2001;41:210–5.

64. Zambell KL, Horn WF, Keim NL. Lipids 2001;36:767–72.

65. Kreider RB, Ferreira MP, Greenwood M et al. J Strength Cond Res 2002;16:325–34.

66. Rennie MJ, Tipton KD. Annu Rev Nutr 2000;20:457–83.

67. Gibala MJ. Sports Sci Exchange 2002;15(4):1–4.

68. Wolfe RR. Can J Appl Physiol 2001;26:S220–7.

69. Fielding RA, Parkington J. Nutr Clin Care 2002;5:191–6.

70. Rennie MJ. Int J Sport Nutr Exerc Metab 2001;11:S170–76.

71. Levenhagen DK, Carr C, Carlson MG et al. Am J Physiol 2001;280:E982–93.

72. Wolfe RR. Am J Clin Nutr 2000;72:551S–7S.

73. Volek JS. Curr Sports Med Rep 2003;2:189–93.

74. Lawrence ME, Kirby DF. J Clin Gastroenterol 2002;35: 299–306.

75. Walzem RL, Dillard CJ, German JB. Crit Rev Food Sci Nutr 2002;42:353–75.

76. Brinkworth GD, Buckley JD, Bourdon PC et al. Int J Sport Nutr Exerc Metab 2002;12:349–63.

77. Kuipers H, van Breda E, Verlaan G et al. Nutrition 2002;18:566–7.

78. Burke DG, Chilibeck PD, Davidson KS et al. Int J Sport Nutr Exerc Metab 2001:11:349–64.

79. Coombes JS, Conacher M, Austen SK et al. Med Sci Sports Exerc 2002;34:1184–8.

80. Antonio J, Sanders MS, Van Gammeren D. Nutrition 2001;17: 243–7.

81. Hofman Z, Smeets R, Verlaan G et al. Int J Sport Nutr Exerc Metab 2002;12:461–69.

82. Cheng J, Baldwin SN, Baldwin SN. Ann Pharmacother 2001; 35:755–64.

83. Chromiak JA, Antonio J. Nutrition 2002;18:657–61.

84. Stensrud T, Ingjer F, Holm H et al. Int J Sports Med 1992;13:481–5.

85. van Hall G, Raaymakers JS, Saris WH et al. J Physiol (Lond) 1995;486:789–94.

86. Newsholme EA, Blomstrand E, Ekblom B. Br Med Bull 1992;48:477–95.

87. Blomstrand E. Amino Acids 2001;20:25–34.

88. Davis JM, Alderson NL, Welsh RS. Am J Clin Nutr 2000;72: 573S–8S.

89. Hargreaves MH, Snow R. Int J Sport Nutr Exerc Metab 2001; 11:133–45.

90. Antonio J, Sanders MS, Kalman D et al. J Strength Cond Res 2002;16:157–60.

91. Candow DG, Chilibeck PD, Burke DG et al. Eur J Appl Physiol 2001;86:142–9.

92. Castell L. Sports Med 2003;33:323–45.

93. Castell LM, Poortmans JR, Newsholme EA. Eur J Appl Physiol 1996;73:488–90.

94. Nissen S, Sharp R, Ray M et al. J Appl Physiol 1996;81: 2095–2104.

95. Vukovich MD, Stubbs NB, Bohlken RM. J Nutr 2001;131:2049–52.

96. Knitter AE, Panton L, Rathmacher JA et al. J Appl Physiol 2000;89:1340–4.

97. Slater GJ, Jenkins D. Sports Med 2000;30:105–16.

98. Kreider RB. Sports Med 1999;27:97–110.

99. Paddon-Jones D, Keech A, Jenkins D. Int J Sport Nutr Exerc Metab 2001;11:442–50.

100. Ransone J, Neighbors K, Lefavi R et al. J Strength Cond Res 2003;17:34–9.

101. Slater G, Jenkins D, Logan P et al. Int J Sport Nutr Exerc Metab 2001;11:384–96.

102. Armstrong L, Maresh C. Nutr Rev 1996;54:S148–58.

103. Manore MM. ACSM Health Fitness J 2001;5:33–5.

104. Benardot D, Clarkson P, Coleman E et al. Sports Sci Exchange Roundtable 2001;12(3):1–4.

105. Bonke D. Bibliotheca Nutritio et Dieta 1986;38:104–9.

106. Singh A, Moses DM, Deuster PA. Med Sci Sports Exerc 1992; 24:726–32.

107. Telford R, Catchpole EA, Deakin V et al. Int J Sport Nutr 1992; 2:135–53.

108. Gerster H. J Am Coll Nutr 1989;8:636–43.

109. Simon-Schnass I, Pabst H. Int J Vitamin Nutr Res 1988;58: 49–54.

110. Rokitzki L, Logemann E, Huber G et al. Int J Sport Nutr 1994;4:253–64.

111. Tiidus PM, Houston ME. Sports Med 1995;20:12–23.

112. Evans WJ. Am J Clin Nutr 2000;72:647S–52S.

113. Powers SK, Hamilton K. Clin Sports Med 1999;18:525–36.

114. Nieman DC. Can J Appl Physiol 2001;26:S45–55.

115. Nieman DC, Henson DA, McAnulty SR et al. J Appl Physiol 2002;92:1970–7.

116. Adams AK, Best TM. Physician Sportsmed 2002;30:37–44.

117. Goldfarb AH. Can J Appl Physiol 1999;24:249–66.

118. Sacheck JM, Blumberg, JB. Nutrition 2001;17:809–14.

119. Clarkson PM, Thompson HS. Am J Clin Nutr 2000;72: 637S–46S.

120. Evans WJ. Am J Clin Nutr 2000;72:647S–52S.

121. Ji LL. Ann NY Acad Sci 2002;959:82–92.

122. Sen CK Sports Med 2001;31:891–908.

123. Takanami Y, Iwane H, Kawai Y et al. Sports Med 2000;29:73–83.

124. Tran M, Mitchell TM, Kennedy DT et al. Pharmacotherapy 2001;21:797–86.

125. Bonetti A, Solito F, Carmosino G et al. J Sports Med Phys Fitness 2000;40:51–7.

126. Braun B, Clarkson PM, Freedson PS et al. Int J Sport Nutr 1991;1:353–65.

127. Laaksonen R, Fogelholm M, Himburg JJ et al. Eur J Appl Physiol 1995;72:95–100.

128. Snider IP, Bazzarre TL, Murdoch SD et al. Int J Sport Nutr 1992;2:272–86.

129. Malm C, Svensson M, Sjoberg B et al. Acta Physiol Scand 1996;157:511–12.

130. Conlay LA, Sabounjian LA, Wurtman RJ. Int J Sports Med 1992;13:S141–2.

131. Zeisel SH. Choline and phosphatidylcholine. In: Shils ME, Olson JA, Shike M et al, eds. Modern Nutrition in Health and Disease, 9th ed. Baltimore: Williams & Wilkins, 1999:513–23.

132. Spector SA, Jackman MR, Sabounjian LA et al. Med Sci Sports Exerc 1995;27:668–73.

133. Buchman AL, Awal M, Jenden D et al. J Am Coll Nutr 2000; 19:768–70.

134. Warber JP, Patton JF, Tharion WJ et al. Int J Sport Nutr Exerc Metab 2000;10:170–81.

135. Maughan RJ, Shirreffs SM, Bater-Jones ADG. Medicina Sportiva 2000; 4:E51–8.

136. Dressendorfer RH, Petersen SR, Lovshin SE et al. Int J Sport Nutr Exerc Metab 2002;12:63–72.

137. Klesges RC, Ward KD, Shelton ML et al. JAMA 1996;276: 226–30.

138. Gremion G, Rizzoli R, Slosman D et al. Med Sci Sports Exerc 2001;33:15–21.

139. Cade R, Conte M, Zauner C et al. Med Sci Sports Exerc 1984;16:263–8.

140. Kreider RB, Miller GW, Williams MH et al. Med Sci Sports Exerc 1990;22:250–6.

141. Kreider RB, Miller GW, Schenck D et al. Int J Sport Nutr 1992;2:20–47.

142. Stewart I, McNaughton L, Davies P et al. Res Q Exerc Sport 1990;61:80–4.

143. Tremblay MS, Galloway SD, Sexsmith JR. Can J Appl Physiol 1994;19:1–11.

144. Lukaski HC. Can J Appl Physiol 2001;26:S13–22.

145. Lukaski HC. Am J Clin Nutr 2000;72:585S–93S.

146. Newhouse IJ, Finstad EW. Clin J Sport Med 2000;10:195–200.

147. Shaskey DJ, Green GA. Sports Med 2000;29:27–38.

148. Horn S, Feller E. AMAA J 2003;16(1):5–6, 11.

149. Jones GR, Newhouse IJ, Jakobi JM et al. Can J Appl Physiol 2001;26:336–49.

150. Beard J, Tobin B. Am J Clin Nutr 2000;72:594S–597S.

151. Haas JD, Brownlie T. J Nutr 2001;131:676S–88S.

152. Garza D, Shrier I, Kohl HW et al. Clin Sports Med 1997;7: 46–53.

153. Hinton PS, Giordano C, Brownlie T et al. J Appl Physiol 2000; 88:1103–11.

154. Brownlie T, Utermohlen V, Hinton PS et al. Am J Clin Nutr 2002;75:734–42.

155. Micheletti A, Rosso R. Rifomo S. Sports Med 2001;31:577–82.

156. Evans GW. Int J Biosoc Med 1989;11:163–80.

157. Clancy SP, Clarkson PM, DeCheke ME et al. Int J Sport Nutr 1994;4:142–53.

158. Hallmark MA, Reynolds TH, DeSouza CA et al. Med Sci Sports Exerc 1996;28:139–44.

159. Pittler MH, Stevinson C, Ernst E. Int J Obes Relat Metab Disord 2003;27:522–9.

160. Trent LK, Thieding-Cancel D. J Sports Med Phys Fitness 1995; 35:273–80.

161. Walker LS, Bemben MG, Bemben DA et al. Med Sci Sports Exerc 1998;30:1730–37.

162. Davis JM, Welsh RS, Alerson NA. Int J Sport Nutr Exerc Metab 2000;10:476–85.

163. Livolsi JM, Adams GM, Laguna PL. J Strength Cond Res 2001;15:161–6.

164. Ferrando AA, Green NR. Int J Sport Nutr 1993;3:140–49.

165. Fawcett JP, Farquhar SJ, Walker RJ et al. Int J Sport Nutr 1996;6:382–90.

166. Cheuvront SN, Carter R, Sawka MN. Curr Sports Med Rep 2003;2:202–8.

167. Sawka MN, Montain SJ, Latzka WA. Comp Biochem Physiol A Mol Integr Physiol 2001;128:679–90.

168. Keneflick RW, Mahood NV, Mattern CO et al. J Strength Cond Res 2002;16:38–43.

169. Naghii MR. Nutr Health 2000;14:127–32.

170. Burke LM. Comp Biochem Physiol A Mol Integr Physiol 2001; 128:735–48.

171. Shirreffs SM, Maughan RJ. Exerc Sports Sci Rev 2000;28: 27–32.

172. Montain SJ, Sawka MN, Wenger CB. Exerc Sport Sci Rev 2001;29:113–7.

173. Speedy DB, Noakes TD, Schneider C. Emerg Med 2001;13:17–27.

174. Gardner JW. Mil Med 2002;167:432–4.

175. Rehrer NJ. Sports Med 2001;31:701–15.

176. Bergeron MF. Sports Sci Exchange 2000;13(3):1–4.

177. Twerenbold R, Knechtle B, Kakebeeke TH et al. Br J Sports Med 2003;37:300–3.

178. Parisi A, Alabiso A, Sacchetti M et al. J Sports Med Phys Fitness 2002;42:214–6.

179. Fritzsche RG, Switzer TW, Hodgkinson BJ et al. J Appl Physiol 2000;88:730–7.

180. Bouchard R, Weber AR, Geiger JD. Clin J Sport Med 2002;12:209–24.
181. Graham TE, Helge JW, MacLean et al. J Physiol (Lond) 2000;529:837–47.
182. Laurent D, Schneider KE, Prysaczyk WK et al. J Clin Endocrinol Metab 2000;85:2170–5.
183. Graham TE. Can J Appl Physiol 2001;26:S103–19.
184. Tarnopolsky M, Cupido C. J Appl Physiol 2000;89:1719–24.
185. Cole KJ, Costill DL, Starling RD et al. Int J Sport Nutr 1996;6:14–23.
186. Graham TE, Spriet LL. Sports Sci Exchange 1996;9(1):1–5.
187. Paluska SA. Curr Sports Med Rep 2003;2:213–9.
188. Jeukendrup AE, Martin J. Sports Med 2001;31:559–69.
189. Armstrong LE. Int J Sport Nutr Exerc Metab 2002;12:189–206.
190. Rawson ES, Clarkson PM. Ephedrine as an ergogenic aid. In: Bahrke MS, Yesalis CE eds. Performance-Enhancing Substances in Sport and Exercise. Champaign, IL: Human Kinetics, 2002:289–298.
191. Shekelle PG, Hardy ML, Morton SC et al. JAMA 2003;289:1537–45.
192. Bell DG, Jacobs I. Aviat Space Environ Med 1999;70:325–9.
193. Bell DG, McLellan TM, Sabiston CM. Med Sci Sports Exerc 2002;34:344–9.
194. Bell DG, Jacobs I, Ellerington K. Med Sci Sports Exerc 2001;33:1399–403.
195. Jacobs I, Pasternak H, Bell DG. Med Sci Sports Exerc 2003;35:987–94.
196. Haller CA, Benowitz NV. N Engl J Med 2000;343:1833–8.
197. McNaughton L, Thompson D. J Sports Med Phys Fitness 2001;41:456–62.
198. Matson LG, Tran ZV. Int J Sport Nutr 1993;3:2–28.
199. McNaughton LR. Bicarbonate and citrate. In: Maughan RJ, ed. Nutrition in Sport. Oxford: Blackwell Science, 2000:393–404.
200. Oopik V, Saaremets I, Medijainen L et al. Br J Sports Med 2003;37:485–9.
201. Preen D, Dawson B, Goodman C et al. Int J Sport Nutr Exerc Metab 2003;13:97–111.
202. Casey A, Greenhaff PL. Am J Clin Nutr 2000;72:607S–17S.
203. Yquel RJ, Arsac LM, Thiaudiere E et al. J Sports Sci 2002;20:427–37.
204. Metzl JD, Small E, Levine SR et al. Pediatrics 2001;108:421–5.
205. Kreider RB. Mol Cell Biochem 2003;244:89–94.
206. Terjung RJ, Clarkson P, Eichner ER et al. Med Sci Sports Exerc 2000;32:706–17.
207. Williams, MH, Kreider RB, Branch JD. Creatine: The Power Supplement. Champaign, IL: Human Kinetics, 1999.
208. Branch JD. Int J Sport Nutr Exerc Metab 2003;13:198–226.
209. Willoughby DS, Rosene J. Med Sci Sports Exerc 2001;33:1674–81.
210. van Loon LJ, Oosterlaar AM, Hartgens F et al. Clin Sci 2003;104:153–62.
211. Brass EP. Am J Clin Nutr 2000;72:618S–23S.
212. Heinonen OJ. Sports Med 1996;22:109–32.
213. Wagenmakers A. Med Sport Sci 1991;32:110–27.
214. Wachter S, Vogt M, Kreis R et al. Clin Chim Acta 2002;318:51–61.
215. Starling RD, Trappe TA, Short KR et al. Med Sci Sports Exerc 1996;28:1193–8.
216. Williams MH, Kreider RB, Hunter DW et al., Med Sci Sports Exerc 1990;22:517–22.
217. Magal M, Webster MJ, Sistrunk LE et al. Med Sci Sports Exerc 2003;35:150–6.
218. Anderson MJ, Cotter JD, Garnham AP et al. Int J Sport Nutr Exerc Metab 2001;11:315–33.
219. Scheett TP, Webster MJ, Wagoner KD. Int J Sport Nutr Exerc Metab 2001;11:63–71.
220. Lyons TP, Riedesel ML, Meuli LE et al. Med Sci Sports Exerc 1990;22:477–83.
221. Montner P, Stark DM, Riedesel ML et al. Int J Sports Med 1996;17:27–33.
222. Robergs RA, Griffen SE. Sports Med 1998;26:145–67.
223. Latzka WA, Sawka MN. Can J Appl Physiol 2000;25:536–45.
224. Lamb D, Shehata A. Sports Sci Exchange 1999;12(2):1–6.
225. Wagner DR. J Am Diet Assoc 1999;99:207–12.
226. Williams MH, Branch JD. Herbals as ergogenic aids. In: Bahrke MS, Yesalis CE, eds. Performance-Enhancing Substances in Sport and Exercise. Champaign, IL: Human Kinetics, 2002:209–25.
227. Bucci LR. Am J Clin Nutr 2000;72:624S–36S.
228. Bahrke MS, Morgan WP. Sports Med 1994;18:229–48.
229. Allen JD, McLung J, Nelson AG et al. J Am Coll Nutr 1998;17:462–6.
230. Dowling EA, Redondo DR, Branch JD et al. Med Sci Sports Exerc 1996;28:482–9.
231. Engels HJ, Kolokouri I, Cieslak TJ et al. J Strength Cond Res 2001;15:290–5.
232. Morris AC, Jacobs I, McLellan TM et al. Int J Sport Nutr 1996;6:263–71.
233. Bahrke MS, Morgan WP. Sports Med 2000;29:113–33.
234. Vogler BK, Pittler MH, Ernst E. J Clin Pharmacol 1999;55:567–75.
235. Kriketos AD, Thompson HR, Greene H et al. Int J Obes Relat Metab Disord 1999;23:867–73.
236. van Loon LJ, van Rooijen JJ, Niesen B et al. Am J Clin Nutr 2000;72:1445–50.
237. Earnest CP. Physician Sportsmed 2001;29:63–79.
238. Fry AC, Bonner E, Lewis DL et al. Int J Sport Nutr 1997;7:318–29.
239. Antonio J, Uelmen J, Rodriguez R et al. Int J Sport Nutr Exerc Metab 2000;10:208–215.
240. Poortmans JR, Francaux M. Sports Med 2000;30:155–70.

SELECTED READINGS

Antonio J, Stout JR, eds. Sports Supplements. Philadelphia: Lippincott Williams & Wilkins, 2001.

Bahrke MS, Yesalis CE, eds. Performance-Enhancing Substances in Sport and Exercise. Champaign, IL: Human Kinetics, 2002.

Dunford, M, ed. Sports Nutrition. Chicago: American Dietetic Association, 2005.

Maughan RJ, ed. Nutrition in Sport. Oxford: Blackwell Scientific, 2000.

Williams MH. Nutrition for Health, Fitness & Sport. Boston: McGraw-Hill, 2005.

110 SOCIAL AND CULTURAL INFLUENCES ON FOOD CONSUMPTION AND NUTRITIONAL STATUS[1]

SARA A. QUANDT

CONTRASTING NUTRITIONAL AND SOCIAL SCIENCES
    APPROACHES TO FOOD CONSUMPTION 1741
UNDERSTANDING WHY PEOPLE EAT WHAT
    THEY EAT: THEORETIC APPROACHES IN THE
    SOCIAL SCIENCES 1742
        Materialist Approaches to Food Consumption . . .1742
        Ideationist Approaches .1743
        Social Constructionist Approaches 1744
METHODS FOR STUDYING SOCIAL AND CULTURAL
    INFLUENCES ON FOOD CONSUMPTION 1746
IMPACT OF SOCIAL FACTORS ON NUTRITIONAL
    STATUS 1747
        Families and Food 1747
        Social Stratification and Nutritional Status 1747
        International Perspectives on Malnutrition 1748

The social sciences' approach to human nutrition complements that of the biologic and physical sciences. The latter approaches are used in other chapters of this book to describe the biologic mechanisms by which hunger and satiety are regulated in the organism, as well as the nutrient levels required for health and function. Despite a fair degree of uniformity among humans in these regulatory pathways and in nutrient needs, there is considerable variety in what humans eat and the extent to which they are successful in meeting their nutrient needs. It is on these latter issues that the social sciences focus.

This chapter describes social and cultural approaches to explaining why people eat what they eat. The goal is to show that understanding the social and cultural aspects of food consumption is critically important if nutrition scientists are to understand why groups of humans differ in nutritional status and how dietary change can be effected to correct problems of undernutrition and overnutrition. Attempts to change dietary habits cannot depend solely on nutrition education. Rather, they must recognize the way dietary habits are embedded in the social structure and culture of groups and must design interventions that are culturally appropriate.

This presentation begins with expanding the contrast between nutrition and social science approaches to food

consumption. It then gives an overview of the theoretic approaches used to study human dietary choices: materialist, ideationist, and social interactionist approaches. The data collection and analysis methods particular to such approaches are briefly summarized. The perspective then changes to an examination of the effects of social and cultural factors on food consumption and nutritional status. Whether social groups are defined at the level of family, social class, or world system, the patterning of these is evident in nutritional measures ranging from dietary quality to obesity to stature.

CONTRASTING NUTRITIONAL AND SOCIAL SCIENCES APPROACHES TO FOOD CONSUMPTION

Humans achieve and regulate their nutritional status by consuming foods, substances (vegetable, animal, mineral, or combination) that supply nutrients. Although food is composed of nutrients, cognizance of these nutrients and of their relationship to health and biologic functioning is neither necessary nor usual. What is—and what is not—food is defined socially and culturally. Thus, although some societies consider insects good to eat, others view them with disgust; some societies relegate maize to cattle feed, and others celebrate its harvest as a food for people. Nutrition science and the social sciences differ considerably in their approach to food consumption and the importance they attribute to contrasts such as these. The social science approach goes farther than food to focus on the patterning of foods into meals and on the meanings (both social and biologic) of such patterning (1–5).

The nutritional approach, which has been dominant in most research on food consumption, views food and eating in relation to the nutrient composition of foods and their instrumental roles in the physiologic functioning of the human body. Eating practices either promote development and function and should be encouraged or they impair these processes and should be discouraged. The nutrition perspective is functionally oriented, viewing food consumption as a means to an end. This perspective makes food habits and preferences secondary to the biologic activity of foods. The social and cultural factors surrounding food consumption become, thus, a barrier to

[1] **Abbreviation: GNP,** gross national product.

the objectives of nutrition, the consumption of a health-promoting diet.

Conceptually, the approach of social scientists (both anthropologists and sociologists of food) is quite different. Anthropologists and sociologists view food consumption as the "completion (most usually) of a culturally appropriate sequence of interpersonal cooking, feeding, and eating, involving social intercourse that leads towards culturally recognized consequences on bodily and mental life" (6). Thus, food consumption is a considerably more complex act than a nutritional/biologic perspective implies. Analytically removing food consumption from social and cultural contexts eliminates the nonbiologic qualities it embodies and transmits to the consumer.

Although the anthropologic and sociologic perspectives are not important to understanding the biology of nutrition, they are central to addressing questions that bear on the nutritional status and health of populations: How do food preferences and food habits arise? How do they become established in a society? How are they transmitted and changed? What roles do such diverse factors as gender and economics play in determining food consumption patterns? How do the symbolic aspects of food relate to consumption patterns? Why do variations in cultural or social factors correlate with variations in nutritional status such as obesity?

UNDERSTANDING WHY PEOPLE EAT WHAT THEY EAT: THEORETIC APPROACHES IN THE SOCIAL SCIENCES

As social and behavioral scientists have studied food consumption, it has become clear that many interconnected factors influence consumption. To help make sense of them, these factors have been organized into logically connected groups that constitute theoretic approaches. As in any science, the value of these theoretic approaches is in their power to generate predictions and hypotheses concerning food consumption in diverse circumstances, as well as to explain observations. For nutritionists, familiarity with some of the major theoretic approaches can be useful in understanding the causes of food consumption patterns they observe, as well as for predicting the outcome of interventions to change food behavior. Table 110.1 shows these approaches, as well as their key concepts.

Materialist Approaches to Food Consumption

Materialist approaches to food consumption are grounded in cultural ecology theory. Cultural ecology takes a systems approach to food consumption, modeling the interactions of the physical, cultural, and historical environments in producing food consumption patterns. Its focus on the physical environment leads some to classify it as geographic (7). Cultural ecology sets food consumption within the broader concept of foodways. These characterize populations and

TABLE 110.1. THEORETIC APPROACHES TO FOOD CONSUMPTION

NAME	APPROACH	KEY CONCEPTS
Materialism	Interactions of physical, cultural, social, and historical environments predict food consumption	Foodways
Ideationism	Food consumption reflects the way people conceptually organize the world and their social relations	Social Order Rules
Social constructionism	Food-related discourse produces subjective knowledge and self-understanding	Subjectivity Power

consist of all information surrounding the ways food is obtained, distributed, and processed, as well as consumed by a particular population (8, 9). Foodways are limited by the resources available within a specific environment. They can be considered adaptive to the extent that they promote health and functioning or maladaptive to the extent they prevent these outcomes. The history of maize consumption and deficiency disease provides illustration.

Katz and associates documented cross-cultural patterns in the techniques used to process maize for human consumption (10). They showed that dependence on maize as a primary staple occurs only when alkali processing techniques are used (e.g., soaking the kernels in lye or a wood ash solution before drying and grinding). Viewed biologically, this process alters the amino acid balance by enhancing the bioavailability of niacin. However, from a cultural standpoint, the importance for the consumer lies in the ability of the altered maize to be satisfactorily shaped into tortillas and other culturally preferred forms.

Katz and associates were able to find no examples of maize dependence without alkali processing. However, historians of medicine have identified significant health consequences of failure to carry out such processing under conditions where economic deprivation rendered foods other than maize unavailable. The pellagra epidemic in the southeastern United States in the early twentieth century is a case in point (11). Mill workers and tenant farmers who were forced by poverty to subsist on a diet of maize (made palatable by small amounts of salt pork and molasses) had high levels of pellagra, as a result of niacin deficiency. Goldberger's studies of pellagra made possible the ecologic analysis, situating the pellagra-inducing food consumption pattern in the economic context of cash cropping (cotton) in lieu of subsistence cropping (gardening) (12). The cultural ecology analysis of pellagra in the South links food consumption to the socioeconomic environment of social stratification and poverty.

Other food consumption patterns that have been analyzed from the perspective of cultural ecology include food taboos such as the Hindu proscription of beef consumption and the Jewish and Moslem of pork (13), as well as the prohibition of fish consumption in Africa (14).

Differing somewhat by drawing on world systems theory, but still squarely in the materialist domain, is Mintz's analysis of the remarkable increase in British sugar consumption in the eighteenth and nineteenth centuries (15). He linked the system of indentured servitude on the sugar plantations of the Caribbean to changes in work and income in England. Sugar consumption, he argued, increased, not so much because of a desire for sweets, but because of the working class's need for affordable calories.

Despite their utility in placing food consumption in context, materialist approaches have been criticized as overly functional explanations, relying too heavily on an attribution of rationality to human societies and better suited to post hoc explanation than prediction. Other theoretic perspectives focus far less on linking cultural practices to favorable biologic outcomes and center more on how societies think about food.

Ideationist Approaches

Rejecting functionalist or economic explanations for food consumption patterns, many anthropologists and sociologists have approached food consumption as a complex set of rules corresponding to the ways people organize their thinking about the world as a whole and reflecting the social interactions in which they engage. Such explanations avoid the pitfalls of teleologic thinking inherent in many materialist analyses, but their tendency to focus on aesthetic aspects of food or mundane details of eating sometimes leads nutritionists to overlook their importance.

Mary Douglas's studies of British meal patterns are classic structural analyses connecting the ordering of foods into daily, weekly, and annual cycles with ordering of social systems (16, 17). Based on observations carried out in British households of varying social class, Douglas declared meal consumption to be a ritual activity with rules regulating the order in which foods of different tastes, temperatures, and textures were permitted. Changes to the pattern (e.g., a single food for the evening meal rather than a central meat with starch and vegetable) created disharmony and unease for the participants, challenging their sense of order. From the most basic units of eating—tea and biscuits—Douglas showed how meals are used to symbolize and order social interactions. Principles of inclusion or exclusion and of hierarchy operated. Beverages were shared in British households with strangers and casual acquaintances, in contrast to meals, which were shared with family and close friends. Thus, to be invited into a home for a meal encoded a high degree of affiliation (literal or figurative kinship). To be offered only a drink excluded a guest from this circle and signified a social threshold over which the guest had not

crossed (16). By maintaining social boundaries, food consumption patterns helped to create and reinforce the social order (17). Similar analyses differentiating "proper meals" from snacks and other eating events were conducted more recently by Murcott (18) in South Wales and by Roos and I and our colleagues in the United States (19–21). We, too, found that meals are defined by where food is eaten and with whom it is eaten, in addition to by what is eaten.

Other ideationist analyses of food consumption patterns point to how the history of a people shapes present eating by providing organizing codes (22). Some show that the past is not so much a blueprint for present eating as a source of symbols or meanings that can be called on in a somewhat arbitrary way. One example of this is the use of African foods by contemporary African-Americans in the United States in the context of Kwanzaa to enhance the sense of African heritage and to reinforce their separateness from European-Americans. Few, if any, of the African dishes have been retained through time in the Americas. Rather, they have been researched and reintroduced for their symbolic value. Another example is the popularity of large "country" breakfasts in the United States. Although often consumed in relatively anonymous urban settings, they give the consumers a link to the agrarian past, with its connotations (accurate or not) of family, abundance, and a simpler, easier life. Roos and I and our colleagues studied older adults in the southeastern United States and noted the meanings attached to such meal patterns and the sense of loss often experienced as women living alone shift to a cold, uncooked breakfast (19, 20).

Even within meals, there are rules by which foods are combined or separated. A study by Drewnowski demonstrated the cognitive categories within which US adults think about common vegetables (23). Asking subjects to judge the similarity of pairs of vegetables as well as to rate the vegetables along attribute scales (e.g., weak to strong flavored, nutritious to nonnutritious), Drewnowski discovered that adults use the dimensions of calories, color, and convenience to think about vegetables. Vegetable preference is most closely linked to convenience, but compatibility of vegetables is associated with color contrast. Thus, vegetable combinations such as broccoli and cauliflower were more acceptable than broccoli and brussels sprouts.

The ideationist approaches to uncovering the grammar of food consumption patterns show that unwritten rules govern the seemingly mundane, everyday activity of eating. These rules vary from culture to culture, and indeed, they are often maintained by subgroups (e.g., ethnic groups) as a way of creating and reinforcing group identity. Social scientists studying food with ideationist approaches point to the implications for attempting dietary change (23). Although the substitution of a one type of food for another could create what more biologically oriented nutritionists would consider a better meal (e.g., replacing meat with fish or vegetables), such a change may be met with resistance because it violates the eater's sense of propriety (24), unless an effort is made to find cognitively acceptable substitutes.

Social Constructionist Approaches

Recently, the analysis of food consumption shifted to one that views preferences and choices as more fluid, marked by discontinuities and paradoxes. This "social constructionist" approach, like the ideationist approach, recognizes the importance of food as a domain in which individual persons define who they are in contrast to others. However, it focuses less on fixed patterns of food use and their reinforcement of social hierarchy and more on the way discourse, the patterning of language and behavior, around food produces meaning for individual consumers. Two concepts stand out in this approach. The first is subjectivity, the ways individual persons use experiences in their lives to understand themselves. This understanding is flexible, less rigid than "identity," depending on experiences with food and eating over time to create a subjective understanding of oneself. The second concept is power, a property that runs through food-related interactions between individuals and groups, creating subjective knowledge and self-understanding. Both these result, inter alia, in foods having relationships to gender, to age, and to life histories.

Gendered Foods

Contemporary Western society, as well as many non-Western societies, has a large body of assumptions about what foods are appropriate for men and what are appropriate for women (25). Women are expected to like sweets better than men and to use it to achieve certain ends, such as to make children behave (24). The concept of "light" foods is also used to describe women's foods, so salads, rather than potatoes and chicken, rather than red meat, should be consumed (24–27). Bourdieu highlights gender differences in preferences for fish among the working class in France (28). He notes that fish is considered women's food, because it has to be eaten in small mouthfuls, in the front of the mouth rather than the back and with considerable restraint to avoid bones. Such an eating style is antithetical to the understanding of a male body as powerful and large. Red meat and strong cheeses are considered more manly. By serving these to men and taking only small portions or eating fish or salads herself, women reinforce gender identities in the context of food. Such gender differences in foods are frequently and consistently reported by lay persons. Lupton for example surveyed residents of Great Britain and found a consistent association of "lighter" foods for women and "heavier" for men (24).

Roos and colleagues reported that within groups of men, differences in food preferences exist based on occupational class (29). Men in a blue collar occupation tended to favor meats, compared with those in a white collar occupation, who were more positive toward vegetables.

These findings suggest that the latter have less need to embrace higher-status foods to establish masculinity.

The notion of gendered foods is borne out in food consumption surveys (30). Women eat more fruit, more sweets, and less meat than men. Men also tend to eat larger quantities and frequently exaggerate their food consumption in surveys, whereas women underreport theirs.

Such patterns of gendered food ideology and consumption develop in the day-to-day interactions in which people engage. Meal times in Western households center on the serving of food, usually by women, in ways that meet expectations of men and children. DeVault, in her study of US families, documented the "invisible, caring work" of women, particularly wives and mothers, in catering to tastes, preferences, and schedules of family members (31). Hers and numerous other studies have shown that women often subordinated their own preferences to those of men (26, 32–34). Gittelsohn's detailed observations of intra-household food distribution patterns in Nepal extended the concept of gendered food interactions beyond Western cultures (35). He showed that at an early age, girls learn to eat only when served from the common pot, whereas boys learn to ask for more. As adults, these women eat last after the largest and choicest portions have gone to men and boys.

This pattern of social interactions over food, shaping female and male notions of relative power and status, is replicated across many cultures. Although studies tend to emphasize the normality and uniformity of such interactions, their linkage to gender relations is highlighted in the exceptions, domestic disputes. Several studies of divorced couples and of domestic violence noted the role played in precipitating problems by discontinuities between male and female behaviors and expectations related to food. In these studies, women not subordinating their own tastes to husbands' or not preparing foods as expected led to violence on the part of husbands (36, 37).

The social interactions surrounding food and the way that notions of gender are conveyed through them has been linked to the preponderance of eating disorders in women compared with men. Susan Bordo argued that Western culture demands self-control for all adults, but especially for women. Girls learn this through interactions concerning food and its relation to their body shape from an early age. Bordo contended that their bodies come to symbolize the arena in which control must be maintained, and women who are not thin embody a lack of self-control. By using self-starvation, women have a strategy for establishing control of the feminine emotions and appetites (38).

Age-Appropriate Foods

The domain of food is also used to differentiate age groups. Several studies have examined the interaction of parents and adolescents over food and the way adolescents use this interaction to declare their independence.

Although many dictums about feeding children have changed (e.g., forcing children to clean their plates is now recognized as creating the potential for overeating in adulthood), parents in Western societies are still expected to control their children's food intake. Through the discourse surrounding this control, children learn to define themselves within families and relative to adults (39, 40). Because eating is a domain used to reinforce relationships, it becomes one in which to redefine them. Hence, adolescents, particularly girls, resist parents by such acts as becoming vegetarian, skipping meals, and preparing their own food (24, 26, 41). Prättälä studied Finnish teenagers and found that they used "junk" food to differentiate themselves from adults (42). Although they knew well the nutritional benefits of the food served at family meals, they opted for "junk" food when with friends. This dual food preference was articulated in the contrast between parents and peers, and it served to help establish teens' subjective knowledge of themselves as leaving childhood. Roos studied preadolescents in the United States and found that they used age as the primary distinction around which to group food; "kid" food was always their stated preference, rather than "adult" food (43, 44).

Food and Life History

Social constructionist approaches have also been used to study the transmission of food habits from one generation to the next. Sharman studied dietary choices and allocation of resources in low-income African-American households, with special attention paid to the effects of federal food programs (45). After analyzing life histories from the women in these households, Sharman found that differences among women in the use of food derived in part from their experiences with it. In particular, she noted that the birth order of a woman—whether she was the oldest daughter or one of the youngest children of her mother—determined how much she was taught about food shopping, preparation, and meal formats. Eldest daughters knew more about these because they had been taught to assist their mothers, whereas younger children had not needed to know these things and came to adulthood with a different set of food-related knowledge, skills, and values. These formed the basis for food habits in households, but they were modified in the context of current activity patterns related to strategies for survival. For example, even women who preferred traditional cooked meals resorted to processed and quickly prepared foods when the demands of holding multiple low-wage jobs made the traditional meal impossible to prepare. Studies such as this demonstrate that even within the same family, there are differences in what ideas about food are transmitted. In addition, they show that dietary intake may not reflect nutrition knowledge or food preference, a finding of importance to nutrition educators.

Another study of the transmission of dietary practices through time focused on Italian-American communities (46–48). In this ethnic group, the interactions of social networks composed of adult sisters produced continuity of some food traditions, particularly for holiday or communally prepared meals. However, outside of this continuity, the experiences of members of individual households contributed to change in meal patterns consumed at everyday meals. A major factor determining dietary intake was the tradition of food exchange and regularly feeding persons besides household residents. In households monitored by the researchers, guests were present at meals or other food events from 30 to 50 times per month, and food exchanges between households occurred 16 to 29 times per month. For nutritionists, this study is important as one demonstrating how households overlap in determining the dietary intake and nutritional status of residents. Understanding the history of households, as well as ethnic-specific values related to reciprocity and obligations, helps to make sense of these food consumption patterns.

Ethnic Foods

Foods and cuisines are frequently categorized popularly or by nutritionists into "ethnic" or "regional" food patterns (e.g., Mexican food or Southern cuisine). Such labeling creates expectations of what foods will be eaten by members of a particular group or in a certain locale, expectations that are frequently not met as foodways change. Social scientists' current view of ethnicity as a process rather than a thing is useful in understanding why ethnic and regional foods are maintained and why they may change over time (49). Social scientists view self-ascribed membership in an ethnic group or in a regional population as a means by which persons establish an identity (50). This identity can be reinforced by any number of symbols or behaviors, from eating particular foods, to wearing characteristic clothing, to proclaiming one's allegiance to a particular sports team. As individual persons or groups choose to invest in a particular ethnic identity or reject it, they frequently do so through the symbols of food (51). For this reason, those studying the changes in foodways with immigration note that generational differences in food consumption patterns are not necessarily a continuum from native to US cuisine (52). Although members of the immigrant generation frequently try to maintain their foodways, the second generation rejects them in favor of newly available foods as they attempt to differentiate themselves from their parents. It is then, in third and subsequent generations, that there may be a conscious return to foods that provide identity with the original group or homeland. The content and context of such foods are often quite different from those of the immigrant generation, however. Substitutions are made based on available ingredients, ethnic foods may be consumed only on special occasions or as an accompaniment to foods of the dominant culture, or higher-status foods of the ethnic group may be substituted for those actually consumed by the immigrant generation.

Two factors complicate attempts to predict the food use of groups based on presumed ethnicity. The first is that ethnicity is frequently confounded by such variables as income, occupation, and education. It is thus impossible to know whether an ethnic group's consumption of a particular diet represents choices made to symbolize identity or simply limitations dictated by what is affordable to the group. Epidemiologists currently argue that one must exclude the possibility that health-related behaviors are not reflections of economic constraints before categorizing them as products of ethnicity (53). Those studying food use would do well to use similar caution.

The second factor complicating the prediction of food use based on ethnicity is that choosing so-called ethnic foods is a behavior readily open to anyone. In their analysis of eating in the United States, Root and de Rochemont argued that US eating reflects social relations (54). Ethnic foods (with the exception of perhaps German, Dutch, and British) have not melted into a single pot. Rather, they remain distinct and highly available. The consumption of foods from different ethnic groups (e.g., the spread of Vietnamese restaurants in the United States since the 1980s) symbolizes acceptance of the ethnic group, rather than membership in the group.

METHODS FOR STUDYING SOCIAL AND CULTURAL INFLUENCES ON FOOD CONSUMPTION

Methods used by social scientists to study food consumption differ substantially from those in which most nutritionists are trained (55). In those studies cited earlier, the two principal data collection methods used are open-ended interviewing and participant observation. Both these methods rely heavily on qualitative data, rather than on the quantitative data with which most nutritionists are familiar.

Open-ended interviewing is a technique designed to reveal how persons talk about a particular subject, the meaning they attach to it, and how they relate it to other aspects of their lives (56, 57). These are topics that, when approached directly, most people cannot articulate. Thus, the analysis and interpretation of the text a person produces in response to open-ended questioning become the sources of such insight. Open-ended interviewing can be conducted with one informant at a time or with groups. One-on-one interviewing is usually called "key-informant interviewing" because the informant has been chosen for being particularly knowledgeable about a specific domain of information. For example, a midwife with years of experience in a town, rather than a new mother, may be interviewed about infant feeding practices. When conducting key-informant interviews, it is possible to delve into how that person thinks about food without their responses being influenced by others. It is important to conduct several such interviews and to be aware of the type of sample

such persons comprise. In contrast to most quantitative research, which depends on a random or probability sample, most qualitative work uses an ethnographic sample. In such a sample, persons are chosen to provide breadth. Hence, the data produced are designed to give a better idea of the range of variation than of the central tendency (58, 59). For example, qualitative interviewing with an ethnographic sample can uncover the range of foods people classify as being for men versus women. A statistical sample would be necessary to then measure how these ideas about food are distributed in the population.

Group interviews are an increasingly popular alternative to key-informant interviewing for qualitative research. Group interviews about food consumption can be conducted with natural groups (e.g., neighbors or members of a class or club), expert groups (e.g., home economics extension agents for a group of counties), or focus groups (60). Focus groups are unacquainted persons who are brought together to participate in a facilitated discussion of a particular issue (61, 62). For example, the Best Start breast-feeding promotion intervention used focus groups of women to identify barriers to breast-feeding among low-income and minority group mothers (63, 64). Focus groups were also used to critique possible media messages for breast-feeding promotion. Group interviews, unlike key-informant interviews, have the potential for reactive effects as participants listen to others and shape their responses to topics introduced by the facilitator. For example, it may be more difficult for a participant to state a socially unacceptable opinion in a group than when alone. For this reason, it is important to conduct multiple group interviews with groups defined on theoretically relevant characteristics. In Best Start, separate groups were conducted with members of different ethnic groups, and mothers were interviewed separately from pregnant women because ethnicity and parity were expected to be linked to contrasting ideas about infant feeding. By doing this, it was possible to link different sets of ideas or beliefs with different groups, as well as to be assured that participants were not suppressing their opinions as a result of the presence of contrasting ideas from persons different from themselves.

Participant observation is a research method in which the researcher tries to fit into the group under study to interpret systematically the interviews conducted and observations made in such a role (65). In several of the studies described earlier (16, 46), researchers lived in homes of research subjects to observe and participate in meals.

Qualitative methods appear deceptively simple to those not trained in their use (66). However, they are extremely time-consuming and subject to established conventions of scientific rigor for their use within the social sciences that are analogous to the standards used in laboratory-based nutrition methods (67, 68). These include aspects of research design such as sampling, measurement, and analysis. Despite the lack of familiarity with these methods, their use by nutritionists in studies of food and nutrition either alone or in combination with other quantitative or nutritional methods (69, 70) can produce understanding of food consumption behaviors.

IMPACT OF SOCIAL FACTORS ON NUTRITIONAL STATUS

In addition to explaining the social and cultural patternings of food consumption, social science provides ways of examining the impact of social structures on nutritional status. Such an approach can help to identify points for intervention for both undernutrition and overnutrition.

Families and Food

The family is the basic social unit in which individual members are socialized into eating and that is organized to reflect larger societal patterns, such as age and gender roles. Some distinct patterns of nutritional status are attributable to variations in families (40). Several studies have examined the family environment's effect. Such indicators of family environment as levels of conflict and suppression of independence predict less adequate dietary intake among adult family members (71). For children, poor parenting skills, family conflict, and marital instability predict failure to thrive (72), as does a family environment with little physical contact and verbal interaction from mothers (73).

Other studies of families indicate that family size and birth order affect nutritional status. Their results support the "dilution model" of family resources (74). This model argues that greater numbers of children necessitate stretching resources (money, time, food), so the quality of the family's end product is lower. This end product can range from educational attainment of children to nutritional status. In general, children from large families are more likely to be stunted (short for age) than those from smaller families (75). The risk is particularly great for last-born children in large families (76). Such children have lower intakes of individual nutrients, and their diets are nutritionally inadequate overall compared with a reference standard (77) This pattern of poorer nutritional status of children in large families (78–80) or of high birth order (81–85), particularly in the context of poverty, has been documented in many populations, both Western and non-Western.

The effects of birth order sometimes differ when specific groups are examined, so it is the oldest child who is most at risk. Cecily Williams was the first to describe acute protein-energy malnutrition (86). She proposed the term "kwashiorkor," the name for the disease used by the Ga people of Ghana among whom she worked (87). Translated, kwashiorkor is literally the disease of the first born. Even without an understanding of the specific nutritional effects of abrupt weaning and transition to low nutrient-density gruels, the Ga recognized the adverse consequences for the weanling.

Because mothers and wives are responsible for feeding families in virtually all societies, it has been argued that women's participation in the labor force has a deleterious effect on nutritional status of family members. However, there is little support for this argument. In the United States, a comparison of diets of children of mothers employed outside the home with those not employed (88) found no evidence of either inadequate intake of nutrients or excessive intakes of fats. This lack of difference may be explained by other research that shows that working outside the home simply makes the production of family meals more difficult. Women simplify such meals (89), but they continue to produce them (32).

Research in developing countries that linked maternal employment and nutritional status demonstrated that children's nutritional status frequently improves as a result of their mothers' income-generating activities (90), particularly where women control the income. Women are more likely than men to direct extra cash income to feeding children, and in many cases it can smooth out the highs and lows of the agricultural cycles (91, 92). Hence, many interventions in developing countries that are aimed at improving child nutritional status take advantage of circumstances such as those in West Africa, where spousal incomes are customarily separated by introducing income-generating activities for women. However, maternal employment can sometimes impair child nutrition by diverting time from food preparation and child care activities (93, 94), so assessments of its impact depend on the situation.

Social Stratification and Nutritional Status

Whether measured by income, education, ethnic group, occupation, or composites of these, social stratification has a pronounced effect on nutrition-related health. Persons of higher social rank live longer and enjoy lower morbidity than do those of lower social rank. Sociologic analysis has shown that the effect of social rank on mortality is continuous, not just a difference between those of the highest and lowest ranks. Even within higher social classes, health and mortality differences parallel wealth and other measures (95, 96). These associations of social rank and health reflect the differences between groups in life course experience and are manifest in lifestyle differences.

In general, upper social classes have had greater access to high-quality diets, education, health care, and employment in higher-paying occupations that are not physically hazardous. These are associated with a lifestyle of more health-promoting behaviors, including more healthful diets, less smoking and other substance abuse, and lower rates of both chronic and infectious disease (97).

Class-related effects on nutritional status and dietary practices are evident in both historic and contemporary populations (98, 99). Persons of higher social class are taller. The secular trend in increasing stature correlates with social class, because stature increased earlier in upper than in lower classes. Today, diminished nutritional status can be linked to poverty.

The social class distribution of obesity, another measure of nutritional status, is marked in women in the United States and other developed countries. Women in lower-income groups, those with lower educational attainment, and those of minority status are on average the most obese (100). This finding is reinforced by preference for fatter body shape or greater acceptance of various body shapes among lower-class and minority women (101).

Conflicting explanations exist for the social stratification of nutritional status. Cultural explanations suggest that obesity has historically symbolized wealth and plenty. This view may continue among lower social classes, just as it predominates in many developing countries to the present (100, 102–104). In contrast, economic and social explanations point to the greater cost of a high-quality diet and the limits on opportunities for physical activity in poor neighborhoods (105, 106). One area of considerable interest is the apparent association of obesity with food insecurity and hunger. The issues surrounding this are complex (107). Drewnowksi and colleagues argued that the association of food insecurity and poverty with obesity reflects the high cost of a healthy and balanced diet. They suggested that the association of food insecurity and obesity is the result of far lower cost of energy-dense foods such as fats and sweets compared with food such as fruits and vegetables that are less dense (108, 109). Evidence suggests that class differences in dietary intake among adults may be decreasing. In a comparison of national food consumption surveys in the United States from 1965 to 1991, socioeconomic and racial differences in dietary quality decreased over time (103). However, this leveling of dietary quality may not be occurring in children, the most vulnerable age group, or it may not be sufficient to offset factors such as disease and stress that depress nutritional status (111).

International Perspectives on Malnutrition

Moving from national or population contexts to a worldwide perspective, social scientists have attempted to explain and to help alleviate overwhelming inequalities in nutritional status (112–113). One approach has been to note the association of numerous nutrition indicators (e.g., nutritional deficiency diseases, stunting, starvation, dietary quality) with a country's gross national product (GNP). The association of better nutritional status with higher GNP and greater evidence of malnutrition with lower GNP is clear (114, 115). Two contrasting perspectives have been taken to interpret this association. The first has predicted that increasing GNP will improve nutrition; the second has taken a historical approach to explore the interconnections of national economies and to predict the likelihood of ameliorating worldwide nutrition problems.

The idea that increasing GNP will lead to improvements in nutrition has produced a massive international economic development effort to raise the economic productivity of lower GNP countries (116, 117). Some early nutritional research challenged the utility of this approach. In a classic study of the transition from subsistence agricultural production to cash cropping, the latter was found to result in a decline in nutritional status as workers expended larger amounts of energy for lower nutrient intake (118). Likewise, a study in Mexico is exemplary of those that demonstrated that dietary shifts to a poor-quality diet accompanied participation in commercial agriculture (119). More recent studies suggest a more positive effect on nutrition, caused by greater available income being applied to family food purchases (120), thus resulting in improved nutritional status (121).

To explain these contradictory findings, other social scientists have been critical of the economic development approach to improving worldwide nutrition. They contend that such an approach may improve the GNP of countries. However, it results in similar gains for developed countries, thereby maintaining the same power relations and flow of resources from poor to rich countries. These investigators present a much less hopeful outlook for improving nutrition worldwide. This approach is referred to as a world systems perspective (122). Adherents argue that current inequalities between nations that lead to high levels of malnutrition in some countries with overnutrition in others reflect centuries-old patterns in which western Europe represented a core that economically exploited other peripheral countries with resources necessary for European lifestyles.

In recent years, countries at the periphery (those with the lowest GNP) have become dependent on imported foods from core countries (often surplus grain production) as they either exported their food or turned to industrial production of goods to be sold to core countries. Dependence on fluctuating supplies and prices, as well as the necessity of having cash to purchase food, has led to reduced food security and increased likelihood of hunger (123).

World systems theory suggests that nations at the periphery will have lower standards of living and greater nutrition problems. Data compiled from international sources (124, 125) bear this out. Ranking countries based on GNP and other aspects of development from periphery (e.g., Tanzania, Bangladesh, El Salvador) to semiperiphery (e.g., Egypt, Philippines, Mexico) to semicore (e.g., Brazil, Korea) to core (e.g., United States, Japan) results in a gradient in such measures as wasting, stunting, and prevalence of anemia in pregnant women (40). Both the economic development and world systems perspectives link nutritional status to such measures of national economic well-being as GNP. The latter, however, stresses the interdependence of economies and suggests that alleviating hunger and malnutrition around the world is far from simple.

Many of the concepts and findings presented in this chapter may seem, at first glance, self-evident. This is because all persons (including nutritionists) are members of families, communities, and societies, thus giving them ample opportunity to make observations related to the social and cultural aspects of food and nutrition. The social and behavioral sciences' value to modern nutrition lies in the rigorous methodology that these sciences can employ. This methodology, based usually on commonplace behaviors of observation and conversation, can be used critically to examine the content and distributions of ideas about food, as well as to investigate the relationship of nutritional status to social and cultural variation.

REFERENCES

1. Jerome NW, Kandel RF, Pelto GH, eds. Nutritional Anthropology. Pleasantville, NY: Redgrave, 1980:1–422.
2. Messer E. Annu Rev Anthropol 1984;13:204–49.
3. Quandt SA, Ritenbaugh C. Training Manual in Nutritional Anthropology. Special pub. no. 20. Washington, DC: American Anthropological Association, 1986:1–151.
4. Ritenbaugh C. J Nutr Educ 1982;13:12S–7S.
5. Mintz S. Annu Rev Anthropol 2002;31:99–119.
6. Khare R. Soc Sci Inform 1980;19:519–42.
7. Grivetti LE. Annu Rev Nutr 1981;1:47–68.
8. Harris M, Ross EB, eds. Food and Evolution: Toward a Theory of Human Food Habits. Philadelphia: Temple University Press, 1987:1–633.
9. Ritenbaugh C. Human foodways: A window on evolution. In: Bauwens EE, ed. The Anthropology of Health. St Louis: Mosby, 1978:111–20.
10. Katz SH, Hediger M, Valleroy L. Science 1974;184:765–73.
11. Etheridge EW. Pellagra: An unappreciated reminder of southern distinctiveness. In: Savitt TL, Young JH, eds. Disease and Distinctiveness in the American South. Knoxville, TN: University of Tennessee Press, 1988:100–19.
12. Goldberger J, Wheeler GA, Sydenstricker E. Public Health Rep 1920;35:2693–701.
13. Harris M. Cows, Pigs, Wars and Witches. New York: Vintage Books, 1974:1–276.
14. Simoons FJ. Ecol Food Nutr 1974;3:185–201.
15. Mintz S. Sweetness and Power: The Place of Sugar in Modern History. New York: Penguin, 1986.
16. Douglas M, Nicod M. New Soc 1974;30:744–7.
17. Douglas M. Daedalus 1972;101:61–81.
18. Murcott A. 'It's a pleasure to cook for him': Food, mealtimes and gender in some South Wales households. In: Gamarnikow E, Morgan D, Purvis J et al., eds. The Public and the Private. London: Heinemann, 1983:78–90.
19. Quandt SA, Vitolins MZ, DeWalt KM et al. J Appl Gerontol 1997;16:152–71.
20. Roos G, Quandt SA, DeWalt KM. Appetite 1993;21:295–8.
21. Quandt SA, McDonald J, Arcury TA et al. Gerontologist 2000; 40:86–96.
22. Barthes R. Toward a psychosociology of contemporary food consumption. In: Forster R, Ranum O, eds. Food and Drink in History: Selections from the Annales E-S-C. Baltimore: Johns Hopkins University Press, 1979:166–73.
23. Drewnowski A. J Am Coll Nutr 1996;15:147–53.
24. Lupton D. Food, the Body and the Self. London: Sage Publications, 1996:1–175.
25. Jensen KO, Holm L. Eur J Clin Nutr 1999;53:351–9.
26. Charles N, Kerr M. Women, Food and Families. Manchester, UK: Manchester University Press, 1988:1–244.
27. Visser M. Much Depends on Dinner: The Extraordinary History and Mythology, Allure and Obsessions, Perils and Taboos, of an Ordinary Meal. London: Penguin, 1986.
28. Bourdieu P. Distinction: A Social Science Critique of the Judgment of Taste. Cambridge, MA: Harvard University Press, 1984.
29. Roos G, Prättälä R, Koski K. Appetite 2001;37:47–56.
30. Patterson BH, Harlan LC, Block G et al. Nutr Cancer 1996;23: 105–19.
31. DeVault M. Feeding the Family: The Social Organization of Caring as Gendered Work. Chicago: University of Chicago Press, 1991:1–270.
32. Mennell S, Murcott A, van Otterloo AH. The Sociology of Food: Eating, Diet and Culture. London: Sage Publications, 1992:1–150.
33. McIntosh WA, Zey M. Food Foodways 1989;3:317–32.
34. Schafer RB, Bohlen JM. Home Econ Res J 1977;6:131–40.
35. Gittelsohn J. Soc Sci Med 1991;33:1141–54.
36. Burgoyle J, Charles D. You are what you eat: Food and family reconstitution. In: Murcott A, ed. The Sociology of Food and Eating. Aldershot, UK: Gower, 1983:152–63.
37. Ellis R. The way to a man's heart: Food in the violent home. In: Murcott A, ed. The Sociology of Food and Eating. Aldershot, UK: Gower, 1983:164–71.
38. Bordo S. Anorexia nervosa: Psychopathology as the crystallization of culture. In: Curt D and Heldke L, eds. Cooking, Eating, Thinking: Transformative Philosophies of Food. Bloomington, IN: Indiana University Press, 1992:28–55.
39. DeGarine I. Ecol Food Nutr 1972;1:143–63.
40. McIntosh WA. Sociologies of Food and Nutrition. New York: Plenum, 1996:1–314.
41. Brannen J, Dodd K, Oakley A et al. Young People, Health and Family Life. Buckingham, UK: Open University Press, 1994.
42. Prättälä R. Young people and food: Socio-cultural studies of food consumption patterns. Academic dissertation. Helsinki: University of Helsinki, 1989.
43. Roos G. Cultural Analysis of Children, Food and Gender in the United States. Ann Arbor, MI: University Microfilms, 1995.
44. Roos G. Ecol Food Nutr 2002;41:1–19.
45. Sharman A. From generation to generation: Resources, experience, and orientation in the dietary patterns of selected urban American households. In: Sharman A, Theophano J, Curtis K et al., eds. Diet and Domestic Life in Society. Philadelphia: Temple University Press, 1991;173–204.
46. Theophano J, Curtis K. Sisters, mothers, and daughters: Food exchange and reciprocity in an Italian-American Community. In: Sharman A, Theophano J, Curtis K et al., eds. Diet and Domestic Life in Society. Philadelphia: Temple University Press, 1991:147–72.
47. Theophano JS. It's Really Tomato Sauce but We Call It Gravy: A Study of Food and Women's Work among Italian-American Families. Ann Arbor, MI: University Microfilms, 1982.
48. Curtis K. I Can Never Go Anywhere Empty Handed: Food Exchange and Reciprocity in an Italian American Community. Ann Arbor, MI: University Microfilms, 1983.
49. Barth F. Ethnic Groups and Boundaries. Boston: Little, Brown, 1969.
50. Alba R. Ethnic Identity: The Transformation of White America. New Haven, CT: Yale University Press, 1990.
51. van den Berghe PL. Ethnic Racial Stud 1984;7:387–97.
52. Kalcik S. Ethnic foodways in America: Symbol and the performance of identity. In: Brown LK, Mussell K, eds., Ethnic and Regional Foodways in the United States. Knoxville, TN: University of Tennessee Press, 1985:37–65.

53. Kaufman JS, Cooper RS. Public Health Rep 1996;110:662–6.

54. Root W, de Rochemont R. Eating in America. Hopewell, NJ: Ecco Press, 1995:1–512.

55. Pelto GH, Pelto PJ, Messer E. Research Methods in Nutritional Anthropology. Food and Nutrition Bulletin Supplement 11. Tokyo: United Nations University, 1989.

56. Quandt SA, Arcury TA. Arthritis Care Res 1997;10:273–81.

57. Denzin NK, Lincoln TS, eds. Handbook of Qualitative Research. Thousand Oaks, CA: Sage Publications, 1994:1–643.

58. Werner O, Bernard HR. Cult Anthropol Methods 1994;6: 7–9.

59. Arcury TA, Quandt SA. Arthritis Care Res 1998;38:490–8.

60. Coreil J. Med Anthropol 1995;16:193–210.

61. Krueger RA. Focus Groups: A Practical Guide for Applied Research. Newbury Park, CA: Sage Publications, 1988:1–197.

62. Morgan DL, ed. Successful Focus Groups: Advancing the State of the Art. Newbury Park, CA: Sage Publications, 1993:1–271.

63. Bryant CA, Coreil J, D'Angelo SL et al. NAACOGS Clin Issues Perinat Women's Health Nurs 1992;3:723–30.

64. Coreil J, Bryant CA, Westover BJ et al. J Hum Lact 1991;11: 265–71.

65. Bernard HR. Handbook of Methods in Cultural Anthropology. Walnut Creek, CA: Altamira Press, 1998:1–816.

66. Gubrium JF. Gerontologist 1992;32:581–2.

67. Luborsky MR, Rubinstein RL. Res Aging 1995;17:89–113.

68. Creswell J. Qualitative Inquiry and Research Design. Thousand Oaks, CA: Sage Publications, 1998:1–402.

69. Steckler A, McLeroy KR, Goodman RM et al. Health Educ Q 1992;19:1–8.

70. Stange KC, Miller WL, Crabtree BF et al. J Gen Intern Med 1994;9:278–82.

71. Kintner M, Boss P, Johnson N. J Marriage Fam 1978;43: 633–41.

72. Chase P, Martin HP. N Engl J Med 1970;282:934–9.

73. Pollitt E, Leibel R. Biological and social correlates of failure to thrive. In: Greene LS, Johnston FE, eds. Social and Biological Predictors of Nutritional Status, Physical Growth and Neurological Development. New York: Academic Press, 1980: 173–200.

74. Blake J. Demography 1981;18:421–8.

75. Wray JD. Population pressure on families: Family size and child spacing. In: Study Committee of the Office of the Foreign Secretary, ed. Rapid Population Growth: Consequences and Policy Implications. Washington, DC: National Academy of Sciences, 1971:403–61.

76. Grant MW. Br J Prevent Soc Med 1964;18:35–9.

77. Kucera B, McIntosh WA. Ecol Food Nutr 1991;25:1–12.

78. Ighogboja SI. East Afr Med J 1992;69:566–71.

79. MacCorquodale DW, de Nova HR. Public Health Rep 1977;92:453–7.

80. Margo G, Lipschitz S, Joseph E et al. S Afr Med J 1976;50: 67–74.

81. Vella V, Tomkins A, Nviku J et al. J Trop Pediatr 1995;41: 89–98.

82. Reddaiah VP, Kapoor SK. Indian J Pediatr 1992;59:567–71.

83. Herold P, Sanjur D. Arch Latinoam Nutr 1986;36:599–624.

84. Hearst N. Int J Epidemiol 1985;14:575–81.

85. Grantham-McGregor SM, Desai P, Buchanan E. Trop Geogr Med 1977;29:165–71.

86. Williams CD. Arch Dis Child 1933;8:423–33.

87. Williams CD. Lancet 1935;2:1151–2.

88. Johnson RK, Smiciklas-Wright H, Croutier AC et al. Pediatrics 1992;90:245–9.

89. Kinsey J. Am J Agricult Econ 1983;65:10–9.

90. Wandel M, Holmboe-Otterson G. Food Nutr Bull 1992;14: 49–54.

91. Krieger J. Women, Men and Household Food in Cameroon. Ann Arbor, MI: University Microfilms, 1994.

92. Tripp R. J Trop Pediatr 1981;27:1407–16.

93. Popkin B, Florentino S. J Trop Pediatr 1976;22:1566.

94. Kumar S. The Role of the Household Economy in Child Nutrition at Low Incomes: A Case Study in Kerala. Cornell University Occasional Paper no. 95. Ithaca, NY: Cornell University Press, 1978.

95. Hertzman C, Frank J, Evans RG. Heterogeneities in health status and the determinants of population health. In: Evans RG, Barer ML, Marmor TR, eds. Why Are Some People Healthy and Others Not? Hawthorne, NY: Aldine de Gruyter 1994: 67–92.

96. Marmot MG. Social inequalities in mortality: The social environment. In: Wilkinson RG, ed. Class and Health: Research and Longitudinal Data. London: Tavistock, 1986:21–33.

97. Link BG, Phelan JC. Am J Public Health 1996;86:471–2.

98. Komlos J. On the significance of anthropometric history. In: Komlos J, ed. Stature, Living Standards and Economic Development. Chicago: University of Chicago Press, 1994:210–20.

99. Crooks DL. Yearbk Phys Anthropol 1995;38:57–86.

100. Sobal J, Stunkard AJ. Psychol Bull 1989;105:260–75.

101. Massara EB. Appetite 1980;1:291–8.

102. Brown PJ, Konner M. Ann NY Acad Sci 1987;499:29–46.

103. Ritenbaugh C. Cult Med Psychiatry 1982;6:347–61.

104. Bryant C. Soc Sci Med 1982;16:1757–65.

105. Morland K, Wing S, Diez Roux A. Am J Public Health 2002; 92:1761–7.

106. Molnar BE, Gortmaker SL, Bull FC et al. Am J Health Promot 2004;18:378–86.

107. Frongillo EA. J Nutr 2003;133:2225–31.

108. Drewnowksi A, Darmon N, Briend A. Am J Public Health 2004;94:1555–9.

109. Drewnowski A, Specter SE. Am J Clin Nutr 2004;79:6–16.

110. Popkin BM, Siega-Riz AM, Haines PS. N Engl J Med 1996; 335:716–20.

111. Miller JE, Korenman S. Am J Epidemiol 1994;140:233–43.

112. Berg A. The Nutrition Factor. Washington, DC: Brookings Institution, 1973.

113. Chambers R, Longhurst R, Pacey A, eds. Seasonal Dimensions of Rural Poverty. Totowa NJ: Allanheld-Osmun, 1981.

114. Périssé K, Sizaret F, François P. FAO Nutr Newslett 1969;7:2.

115. Timmer CP, Falcon WP, Pearson SR. Food Policy Analysis. Baltimore: Johns Hopkins University Press, 1983:1–301.

116. World Bank. The Assault on World Poverty: Problems in Rural Development, Education and Health. Baltimore: Johns Hopkins University Press, 1975.

117. Hoben A. Annu Rev Anthropol 1982;11:349–75.

118. Gross DR, Underwood BA. Am Anthropol 1971;72:725–40.

119. DeWalt KM. Nutritional Strategies and Agricultural Change in a Mexican Community. Ann Arbor, MI: UMI Research Press, 1983.

120. von Braun J. Production, employment, and income effects of commercialization of agriculture. In: von Braun J, Kennedy E, eds. Agricultural Commercialization, Economic Development, and Nutrition. Baltimore: Johns Hopkins University Press, 1994:37–64.

121. Pinstrup-Anderson P, Pelletier D, Alderman H, eds. Child Growth and Nutrition in Developing Countries: Priorities for action. Ithaca, NY: Cornell University Press, 1995.

122. Wallerstein I. The Modern World System: Capitalist Agriculture and the Origins of the European World Economy in the Sixteenth Century. New York: Academic Press, 1975.

123. Bernstein H, Crow B, Mackintosh M et al., eds. The Food Question: Profits vs. People. New York: Monthly Review Press, 1990.

124. World Bank. World Development Report 1993: Investing in Health. New York: Oxford University Press, 1993.

125. Levin HM, Pollitt E, Galloway R et al. Micronutrient deficiency disorders. In: Jamison DT, Mosley WH, Measham AR et al., eds. Disease Control Priorities in Developing Countries. New York: Oxford University Press, 1993:421–51.

SELECTED READINGS

Counihan C. The Anthropology of Food and Body: Gender, Meaning and Power. London: Routledge, 1999.

Counihan C, Van Esterik P. Food and Culture: A Reader. New York: Routledge, 1997.

Kiple KF, Ornelas KC, eds. The Cambridge World History of Food. New York: Cambridge University Press, 2000.

McIntosh WA. Sociologies of Food and Nutrition. New York: Plenum Press, 1996.

Mintz SW, Du Bois CM. The anthropology of food and eating. Annu Rev Anthropo 2002;31:99–119.

111 FADS, FRAUDS, AND QUACKERY[1]

STEPHEN BARRETT

VULNERABILITY TO QUACKERY 1752
MISLEADING CLAIMS 1752
   Claims for Foods 1753
   Promotion of Supplements 1754
   Advice from Retailers 1755
   Quality Control Problems 1756
DUBIOUS CREDENTIALS 1756
DUBIOUS DIAGNOSTIC TESTS 1757
QUESTIONABLE DIET PLANS 1757
QUESTIONABLE "DIET PILLS" 1758
DANGERS OF QUACKERY 1759
CONSUMER PROTECTION 1759

Food faddism can be defined as an unusual pattern of food behavior enthusiastically adopted by its adherents (1). It is commonly expressed by (a) beliefs that particular foods or food substances can cure diseases, (b) elimination of certain foods from the diet without adequate reason, and/or (c) emphasis on "natural" foods. Many aspects of food faddism become social movements that represent symbolic rebellions against authority, society–at large, or some imagined enemy.

Quackery can be defined as the promotion for profit of a medical scheme or remedy that is unproven or known to be false. This definition seeks to distinguish folk practices and neighborly advice from practices for financial gain. "Health fraud" has been defined in a similar way. However, because most people regard *fraud* as a deliberate attempt to deceive, the term *health fraud* is most appropriate when deliberate deception is involved.

Quack methods are sometimes referred to as "alternatives." Because ineffective methods are not true alternatives to effective ones, the terms *unscientific* or *dubious* are preferable. "Alternative" methods related to nutrition are discussed in Chapter 112.

---

[1]**Abbreviations: AIDS,** acquired immunodeficiency syndrome; **FASEB,** Federation of American Societies for Experimental Biology; **FDA,** Food and Drug Administration; **FTC,** Federal Trade Commission; **HDL,** high-density lipoprotein; **HIV,** human immunodeficiency virus; **LDL,** low-density lipoprotein; **PPA,** phenylpropanolamine; **RDA,** recommended dietary allowance; **USPSTF,** US Preventive Services Task Force.

Faddists and quacks urge everyone to distrust large food companies, government regulators, and scientific health professionals (2). This negative philosophy is essential because without it, there would be no reason to buy health–food industry products or consult "alternative" practitioners.

VULNERABILITY TO QUACKERY

Victims of quackery usually have one or more of the following characteristics:

1. *They are unsuspecting.* Many people believe that if something appears in print or in a broadcast, it must be true—or somehow it would not be allowed. People also tend to believe what others tell them about personal experience.
2. *They believe in magic.* Some people are easily taken in by the promise of an easy solution to their problem. Those who buy one fad diet book after another fall into this category.
3. *They are desperate.* Many people faced with a serious health problem that doctors cannot solve become desperate enough to try almost anything that arouses hope. Many victims of cancer, arthritis, multiple sclerosis, and acquired immunodeficiency syndrome (AIDS) are vulnerable in this regard.
4. *They are alienated.* Some people feel deeply antagonistic toward scientific medicine but are attracted to methods that are "natural" or otherwise unorthodox. They may also harbor extreme distrust of the medical profession, the food industry, drug companies, and government agencies.
5. *They are overconfident.* Despite P.T. Barnum's advice that one should "never try to beat a man at his own game," some strong-willed people believe they are better equipped than scientific researchers and other experts to tell whether a method works.

MISLEADING CLAIMS

Nutritional faddism and quackery are promoted with five basic fallacies:

1. *Our food supply is nutritionally inadequate because our soils are depleted and important nutrients are removed by food processing.* These claims encourage purchase of

"organic," "natural," and "health" foods. A typical example is this passage from a book by Earl Mindell (3), cofounder of the Great Earth chain of health food stores:

Much of our soil our food is grown in has been depleted of many vitamins and minerals, thanks to the overuse of fertilizers and chemicals. Then the food takes a long time to get to the supermarket.... The longer these foods are stored the more vitamins they lose. Many of the foods we eat have been heavily processed, meaning they have been crushed, heated, bleached, extracted, chemicalized and preserved.... Then we cook the food, destroying valuable enzymes and what's left of many vitamins. It's a wonder there's any nutrition at all left in our food by the time it gets to our tables!

2. *Vitamin and mineral deficiencies are common.* This claim is used to persuade people that everyone should take supplements. A typical example is this passage from *Prescription for Nutritional Healing* (4), a book that recommends supplements and/or herbs for more than 250 health problems:

The problem with most of us is that we do not get what we need from our modern diet. Even if you are not sick, you may not necessarily be healthy.... By understanding the principles of wholistic nutrition and knowing what nutrients we need, we can improve the state of our health, stave off disease, and maintain a harmonious balance in the way nature intended.

3. *Most health problems are the result of faulty diet and can be treated by "nutritional" methods.* These types of claims are used to market "food supplements," "health foods," and quack dietary methods.

4. *US residents are in danger of being poisoned by food additives and pesticide residues.* This claim, along with accusations that the food industry and government regulators are untrustworthy, is used to promote the sale of "organic" and "natural" foods.

5. *Personal experience is the best way to tell whether a health-related action is effective.* This claim encourages people to rely on testimonial evidence rather than scientific studies and prevailing medical beliefs.

Table 111.1 lists ways to spot nutrition quacks.

Claims for Foods

Many foods are promoted with slogans suggesting that they are safer, more nutritious, or have special therapeutic value. "Organically grown" foods are said to be grown without the use of "artificial" fertilizers or pesticides. The foods themselves are usually indistinguishable from "ordinary" foods but cost significantly more.

US Food and Drug Administration (FDA) market-basket studies indicate that pesticide residues are insignificant in the overall diet (5). Some studies have found that the pesticide content of "organically grown" and conventionally grown foods is similar (6). The largest such study measured the levels of more than 300 synthetic pesticides in about a thousand pounds of tomatoes, peaches, green bell peppers, and apples purchased in five cities. Traces were detected in 77% of conventional foods and 25% of

TABLE 111.1. THIRTY TIPS TO HELP SPOT VITAMIN PUSHERS AND FOOD QUACKS

1. When talking about nutrients, they tell only part of the relevant story.
2. They claim that most Americans are poorly nourished.
3. They recommend "nutrition insurance" for everyone.
4. They say that if you eat badly, you will be OK as long as you take supplements.
5. They say that most diseases are the result of faulty diet and can be treated with "nutritional" methods.
6. They allege that modern processing methods and storage remove all nutritive value from our food.
7. They claim that diet is a major factor in behavior.
8. They claim that fluoridation is dangerous.
9. They claim that soil depletion and the use of pesticides and "chemical" fertilizers result in food that is less safe and less nourishing.
10. They claim you are in danger of being "poisoned" by ordinary food additives and preservatives.
11. They charge that the recommended dietary allowances have been set too low.
12. They claim that under stress, and in certain diseases, your need for nutrients is increased.
13. They recommend "supplements" and "health foods" for everyone.
14. They say it is easy to lose weight.
15. They claim that sugar is a deadly poison.
16. They oppose pasteurization of milk and fluoridation of water.
17. They recommend a wide variety of substances similar to those found in your body.
18. They claim that "natural" vitamins are better than "synthetic" ones.
19. They suggest that a questionnaire can be used to indicate whether you need dietary supplements.
20. They promise quick, dramatic, miraculous results.
21. They routinely sell vitamins and other "dietary supplements" as part of their practice.
22. They use disclaimers couched in pseudomedical jargon.
23. They use anecdotes and testimonials to support their claims.
24. They offer phony "vitamins."
25. They display credentials not recognized by responsible scientists or educators.
26. They offer to determine your body's nutritional state with a single laboratory test.
27. They claim they are being persecuted by orthodox medicine and that their work is being suppressed because it is controversial.
28. They warn you not to trust your doctor.
29. They sue to intimidate their critics.
30. They encourage patients to lend political support to their treatment methods.

From Barrett S, Herbert V. The Vitamin Pushers: How the "Health Food" Industry Is Selling America a Bill of Goods. Amherst, NY: Prometheus Books, 1994.

organically labeled foods, but only one sample of each exceeded the federal limit (7). The amounts are small enough that the risk from pesticide residue is not worth worrying about and does not warrant paying higher prices.

Nutrients are absorbed by the plant in their inorganic chemical state regardless of whether the soil has been prepared with manure, compost, or manufactured fertilizer. Plants grow only if they receive enough nutrients, and their vitamin content is determined by their genes. Fertilizers can influence the mineral composition of plants, but these variations are rarely significant in the overall diet. A study encompassing 460 assessments of nine different fruits and vegetables done in the early 1990s found no significant difference in taste quality between "organic" and conventionally grown samples (8). Despite such facts, a 1990 federal law forced the US Department of Agriculture to establish standards for organic food "certification." The standards, which took effect in 2002, are embodied in a 26,000-word document that covers definitions, agricultural practices processing, and marketing claims.

The word "natural" is said by its proponents to designate foods that are minimally processed and contain no artificial additives or preservatives. This "no artificial additives or preservatives" is meant to imply that additives and preservatives (MES) pose a health risk. Actually, they help make our food supply safe, abundant, and palatable. Although one is occasionally found to pose a health hazard (e.g., sulfites), the vast majority appear safe, and the overall level in our food supply should not be a cause for concern or a reason to buy "natural" foods. The health food industry also circulates unfounded criticisms of food irradiation, milk pasteurization, and genetically engineered foods (9).

The term "health food" is commonly used to suggest that certain foods have special health-giving properties not found in "ordinary" foods. Some "health" foods are rich in various nutrients and can be a valuable part of a balanced diet. However, no food has any special health-promoting property beyond those of the nutrients it contains. FDA regulations permit food labels and packages to contain truthful and nonmisleading claims related to (a) calcium and osteoporosis, (b) sodium and high blood pressure, (c) dietary fats and heart disease, (d) dietary fats and cancer, (e) dietary fiber and cancer, (f) fiber and cardiovascular diseases, (g) oatmeal or oat bran and heart disease, (h) soy protein and heart disease, (i) folic acid and neural tube defects, and a few other relationships. The claims must be limited to the relationship between these conditions and a particular food component, rather than the specific product. The recommendation must also be consistent with a sound total diet (10, 11). Food advertising is primarily regulated by the Federal Trade Commission (FTC), which can apply similar criteria (12).

Promotion of Supplements

Although some dietary supplements are useful, US residents waste several billion dollars a year on products that are worthless or unnecessary. These products often are promoted with scare tactics and false promises. The most common sales pitch is "nutrition insurance," the idea that everyone needs vitamin and mineral supplements to be sure of getting enough. Some promoters falsely suggest

that it is difficult to balance one's diet, whereas others insist that our food supply is inadequate. The best strategy is to have an objective assessment of the quality of one's diet and to modify the diet or use supplementation for any remaining shortfall.

Another common ploy is the suggestion that supplementation is advisable to help deal with "stress." This idea was commercialized by distorting a 1952 National Academy of Sciences report (13). The report merely stated that people who are seriously ill or injured (some of whom have impaired appetite) might benefit from supplementation to prevent depletion of water-soluble vitamins, which have limited storage. However, in 1976, a major vitamin manufacturer began falsely advertising that "stress robs the body of vitamins" and that water-soluble vitamins must be replaced *daily* because the body cannot store them. Some manufacturers made no claims for their "stress" products but assumed that consumers would know their purpose. Several manufacturers falsely suggest that being active and elderly creates special needs that their products supposedly meet.

In the mid-1980s, the New York State attorney general secured consent agreements with two major "stress supplement" manufacturers to stop misrepresenting the need for their products. Since that time, the amount of direct advertising of "stress supplements" has greatly decreased. However, the Council for Responsible Nutrition, a trade organization that represents major supplement manufacturers and suppliers, has advertised that a busy lifestyle places US residents at nutritional risk. The advertisement included a narrowly worded "Vitamin Gap Test" suggesting that virtually everyone may have one or more "gaps." Council for Responsible Nutrition representatives maintain that virtually everyone needs supplements (14). In 1990, the FTC secured a consent agreement barring another large manufacturer from making unsubstantiated claims that any vitamin product is needed to replace nutrients lost as a result of athletic activities or "the stress of daily living." Such "stress" is not a true hypercatabolic state in which increased amounts of calories and nutrients are needed (see Chapters 89 and 91).

Many health food manufacturers market "ergogenic aids"—amino acid supplements falsely claimed to increase stamina, endurance, and muscle development. Some of these products are claimed to be "natural steroids" that release growth hormone (15). No scientific evidence indicates that these products actually release growth hormone, and this is fortunate, because if they did, acromegaly could result. David Lightsey, who coordinates the National Council Against Health Fraud's Task Force on Ergogenic Aids, has requested documentation from more than 80 companies that market "ergogenic aids." Fewer than half sent anything, and the rest submitted studies that were poorly designed or did not actually support product claims. Lightsey also checked statements that various teams were using certain products and found that management had neither endorsed the products nor encouraged their use (16).

The Federation of American Societies for Experimental Biology (FASEB) has criticized the widespread use of amino acids in supplements. Following extensive review, FASEB experts concluded the following: (a) single- or multiple-ingredient capsules, tablets, and liquid products are used primarily for pharmacologic purposes or enhancement of physiologic functions, rather than for nutritional purposes; (b) little scientific literature exists on most amino acids ingested for these purposes; (c) no scientific rationale has been presented to justify use of amino acid supplements by healthy persons; (d) safety levels for amino acid supplement use have not been established; and (e) a systematic approach to safety testing is needed (17).

In 2002, the Institute of Medicine's Food and Nutrition Board concluded the following: (a) there is no evidence that amino acids derived from usual or high intakes of protein from foodstuffs present any risk; (b) blood concentrations could be considerably higher when amino acids were consumed as supplements as opposed to a component of protein in food; (c) for some amino acids, studies in healthy persons indicated no evidence of adverse effects; and (d) for other amino acids, the data are insufficient to establish tolerable upper safe intakes (18). However, when there is a metabolic defect in the utilization of certain amino acids (see Chapter 58) or when renal insufficiency prevents excretion of normal metabolic products of an amino acid (see Chapter 36), there may be an undesirable effect.

Vitamin C, vitamin E, and ß-carotene are being vigorously promoted with claims that their antioxidant properties can help to prevent various diseases by blocking the harmful action of free radicals. Epidemiologic evidence indicates that diets containing significant amounts of fruits, vegetables, and grains are associated with a lower incidence of heart disease and certain cancers (19). However, it is not known which, if any, specific substances in the diet are responsible or whether taking doses of supplements higher than the recommended dietary allowance (RDA) will do more good than harm. Evidence exists, for example, that vitamin E can help to prevent atherosclerosis by interfering with oxidation of low-density lipoproteins (LDLs). However, vitamin E can also exert an anticoagulant effect. The issue can be settled scientifically by conducting long-term double-blind clinical studies that compare vitamin users and nonusers and measure death rates from all causes.

So far, clinical trials related to the prevention of cardiovascular disease and cancer have not been promising. The US Preventive Services Task Force (USPSTF) concluded the following:

The available evidence from randomized trials is either inadequate or conflicting, and the influence of confounding variables on observed outcomes in observational studies cannot be determined. As a result, the USPSTF could not determine the balance of benefits and harms of routine use of supplements of vitamins A, C or E; multivitamins with folic acid; or antioxidant combinations for the prevention of cancer or cardiovascular disease.

The USPSTF recommends against the use of beta-carotene supplements, either alone or in combination, for the prevention of cancer or cardiovascular disease (20).

In addition to marketing antioxidants, many companies are marketing products said to be concentrates of fruits and/or vegetables. Critics note, however, that it is not possible to condense large amounts of produce into a pill without losing fiber, nutrients, and many other phytochemicals (21). Although some products contain significant amounts of nutrients, these nutrients are readily obtainable at lower cost from foods.

Advice from Retailers

No special knowledge or training is required to become a salesperson at a health food store. Personnel in these stores typically obtain information by reading books and magazines that promote supplements and herbs for treatment of virtually all health problems. Retailers also obtain information from manufacturers and can attend seminars at trade shows sponsored by industry groups and trade magazines (14). Several large studies have demonstrated that the proprietors of these stores often give advice that is irrational, unsafe, and illegal:

- In 1983, investigators from the American Council on Science and Health made 105 inquiries at stores in New York, New Jersey, and Connecticut. Asked about eye symptoms characteristic of glaucoma, 17 of 24 store employees suggested a wide variety of products for a person not seen; none recognized that urgent medical care was needed. Asked over the telephone about sudden, unexplained 15-pound weight loss in 1 month's time, nine of 17 recommended products sold in their store; only seven suggested medical evaluation. Seven of ten stores carried "starch blockers" despite an FDA ban. Nine stores contacted made false claims of effectiveness for bee pollen, and ten stores did so for RNA (22).
- In 1989, volunteers of the Consumer Health Education Council telephoned 41 Houston-area health food stores and asked to speak with the person who provided nutritional advice. The callers explained that they had a brother with AIDS who was seeking an effective alternative against human immunodeficiency virus (HIV). The caller also explained that the brother's wife was still having sex with her husband and wanted to reduce or eliminate her risk of being infected. All 41 retailers offered products they said could benefit the brother's immune system, improve the woman's immunity, and protect her against harm from HIV. Thirty said they sold products that would cure AIDS. None recommended abstinence or using a condom (23).
- In 1993, posing as prospective customers, FDA agents visited local health food stores throughout the United

States. The investigators asked, "What do you sell to help high blood pressure?" "Do you have anything to help fight infection or help my immune system?" and/or "Do you have anything that works on cancer?" Of 129 requests for information, 120 resulted in recommendations of specific dietary supplements (24).

- In 1998, a researcher posing as the daughter of a patient with metastatic breast cancer inquired at 40 health food stores in Oahu, Hawaii. After products to assist in metastatic breast cancer care were mentioned and/or shown, if store personnel did not provide any further information, the researcher asked: (a) How does the product work? (b) Do you recommend any particular brand (if more than one brand available)? (c) Could I write down some prices? (d) How much of the product does my mother need to take per day? (e) Can the product(s) be taken together with the medication my mother is receiving from her physician? and (f) Is there anything else you can recommend? Personnel in 36 of the stores recommended one or more of 38 inappropriate products, the most common of which were shark cartilage (recommended by 17) and essiac (recommended by eight), and maitake mushrooms (recommended by seven) (25). Retailers who recommend products when customers describe symptoms violate state laws against the unlicensed practice of medicine or pharmacy, but they are rarely prosecuted.

About 100 companies market supplements through person-to-person (multilevel) sales. Virtually anyone can become a distributor by filling out a one-page application and buying a distributor kit for about $50. Most multilevel companies claim that their products can prevent or cure a wide range of diseases. A few companies merely suggest that people will feel better, look better, or have more energy if they use supplements.

Although pharmacists receive scientific training in nutrition, a study by *Consumer Reports* has cast considerable doubt on the ability of community pharmacists to give appropriate advice about supplements. When undercover investigators asked 30 pharmacists whether vitamins could relieve their nervousness or fatigue, 17 recommended vitamins, one recommended L-tryptophan, and only nine mentioned seeing a doctor (26).

Many supplement products are irrationally formulated. Several years ago, two dietitians examined the labels of vitamin products at five pharmacies, three groceries, and three health food stores in New Haven, Connecticut. Products were judged appropriate if they contained between 50 and 200% of the US RDA and no more than 100% of others for which estimated safe and adequate daily dietary intakes exist. Only 16 of 105 (15%) multivitamin-multimineral products met these criteria (27).

Few supplement products have any usefulness against disease, and most that do (e.g., niacin for cholesterol or triglyceride control and folic acid for lowering abnormal

blood levels of homocysteine) should not be taken without competent medical supervision.

Quality Control Problems

Although drugs are subject to rigorous quality control to ensure the nature, potency, and safety of ingredients, dietary supplements and herbs are not (28). The FDA has proposed adherence to good manufacturing practices but has not taken the necessary steps to require this standard.

ConsumerLab, which has tested hundreds of products since 1999, has reported that about 15% of the vitamins and minerals, 23% of the other supplements, and 38% of the herbals failed their evaluations. The most common reason for the failure was too little or none of the main ingredient. Other problems included the following: too much active ingredient; the wrong ingredient; dangerous or illegal ingredients; contamination with heavy metals, pesticides, or pathogens; "spiking" with unexpected ingredients; poor disintegration (which affects absorption); and misleading product information (29).

DUBIOUS CREDENTIALS

Since the early 1980s, many persons and groups have developed "credentials" intended to resemble those of established medical and nutritional organizations (14, 30). During this period, unaccredited correspondence schools and other organizations have issued a steady stream of "degrees" and other certificates intended to suggest that the recipient is a qualified expert in nutrition. The schools typically issue B.S., M.S., and/or Ph.D. "degrees" based on study of unscientific writings plus open-book tests that are scored quite liberally. The professional organizations typically grant immediate "professional memberships" and a fancy certificate for a modest fee. Household pets and nonexistent persons have achieved membership in several of these groups. Some organizations offer "certification" based on correspondence courses that invariably include unscientific teachings. The most significant of these is the C.N. (Certified Nutritionist) issued by the nonaccredited National Institute for Nutrition Education.

Such credentials have no legal or scientific standing but can be advertised or displayed in most states that do not regulate nutritionists. The American Dietetic Association is striving for increased regulation of nutritional practice and has gained passage of laws in 41 states.

In 1993, a 32-state survey sponsored by the National Council Against Health Fraud found that 286 (46%) of 618 "Yellow Page" listings under the heading "Nutritionists" were spurious, and 72 (12%) were suspicious. Listings were considered spurious if the advertiser used an invalid method of diagnosis, treatment, or nutritional assessment. Listings were rated suspicious if the practitioner did not comply with a request for information on credentials or methods used. Dubious nutrition practitioners were also found under the headings "Acupuncture," "Health and Diet Products,"

"Health, Fitness, and Nutrition Consultants," "Herbs," "Holistic Practitioners," "Weight Control Services," and "Wellness Programs." Many such listings were for chiropractors, homeopaths, naturopaths, holistic physicians, health food stores, and multilevel distributors for such companies as Herbalife International, Nu Skin International, Shaklee Corporation, and Sunrider International. The credentials used included C.C.N. (certified clinical nutritionist), C.N. (certified nutritionist), C.C.T. (certified colon therapist), C.M.T. (certified massage therapist), C.N.C. (certified nutrition consultant), H.M.D. (homeopathic medical doctor), L.Ac. (licensed acupuncturist), M.L.D. (manual lymph drainage), N.C. (nutrition counselor), N.D. (doctor of naturopathy), N.M.D. (doctor of nutrimedicine), and O.M.D. (oriental medical doctor). Of 24 persons identified as having a "Ph.D." in their ad, 17 had spurious credentials. Of 231 listings under the heading "Dietitians," 21 (9%) were spurious, including several from GNC stores (31). The best strategy to avoid entanglement with an unqualified nutritionist is to avoid *all* practitioners who sell supplements in their offices or espouse the statements listed in Table 111.1.

DUBIOUS DIAGNOSTIC TESTS

Unscientific practitioners use a variety of tests as a basis for prescribing supplements and/or making dietary recommendations. The most common such test is hair analysis, which is purported to detect "mineral imbalances" or the presence of "toxic minerals." The test is usually obtained by sending a small amount of hair from the nape of the neck to a commercial laboratory for analysis. The laboratory then issues a computerized report suggesting what supplements may be prescribed.

When 52 hair samples from two healthy teenagers were sent under assumed names to 13 commercial hair analysis laboratories, the reported levels of minerals varied considerably between identical samples sent to the same laboratory and from laboratory to laboratory. The laboratories also disagreed about what was "normal" or "usual" for many of the minerals. Literature from most of the laboratories suggested falsely that their reports were useful against a wide variety of diseases and supposed nutrient imbalances (32). A smaller study published in 2001 yielded similar findings (33). Properly performed, hair analysis has limited value as a research tool but little if any clinical application (34).

Supplement purveyors sometimes use "nutrient deficiency tests" to help them decide what their customers need. One type involves completion of a dietary history; another involves completion of a questionnaire about common symptoms that supposedly are signs of deficiency. The answers are then fed into a computer programmed to recommend supplements for everyone. Many such marketers claim that their supplements are individually customized.

Functional intracellular analysis (FIA), formerly called essential metabolics analysis (EMA), is performed by a laboratory that claims that most US residents have nutrient deficiencies and that "intracellular nutrient deficiencies" even occur in more than 40% of US residents who take multivitamins as "insurance." The test is performed by placing lymphocytes from the patient's blood into Petri dishes containing various concentrations of nutrients. A growth stimulant is added, and a few days later, technicians identify the dishes in which "greatest cell growth" takes place, which supposedly points to a deficiency. Properly performed, lymphocyte cultures have a legitimate role in testing for concentrations of certain nutrients, but they are not appropriate for general screening or for diagnosing nutrient deficiencies (14).

Some practitioners use data from legitimate laboratory tests but misrepresent their meaning. Chemistry profiles, which measure many different chemical characteristics of the blood, are a valuable screening test in scientific medical practice. However, dubious practitioners misuse the test by narrowing the normal ranges so healthy persons appear to have abnormalities, which are then used to recommend expensive supplements or special diets (14).

Some practitioners claim that food allergies may be responsible for virtually any symptom and can be treated with vitamin supplementation plus dietary restriction. To detect the alleged offenders, they assess the levels of various immune responses to foods. These levels, however, are not necessarily related to allergy and have nothing whatsoever to do with a person's need for supplements (35).

Although thousands of practitioners (mostly chiropractors) use the foregoing procedures, government regulatory agencies rarely attempt to stop them. Chapter 112 addresses this problem further.

QUESTIONABLE DIET PLANS

Many weight-reduction schemes are promoted to the public as a solution to obesity. Fad diet books typically have several things in common. They claim to offer a revolutionary new idea based on the author's personal experience. They suggest that certain nutrients, foods, or food combinations are either the key to weight reduction or the villains that prevent it. In addition, these books contain inaccurate biochemical information. Many fad diets are unbalanced and lack important nutrients.

Since the 1980s, many best-selling diet plans have emphasized proteins, some recommending "unlimited" amounts and others using small amounts. "Food-combining" schemes also have been popular. *Fit for Life*, which sold more than 3 million copies, claims that obesity caused accumulation of "toxic waste" from incomplete assimilation of foods eaten in the wrong combinations.

The most notorious high-protein (low-carbohydrate) plan has been the Atkins diet, which has four steps: a 2-week "induction" period, during which the goal is to reduce carbohydrate intake to less than 20 g/day; and three periods during which carbohydrate intake is progressively raised but kept below what Atkins calls "your critical carbohydrate level" for losing or maintaining weight (36). The dieter is permitted to eat unlimited amounts of noncarbohydrate foods "when hungry," but ketosis tends to suppress appetite. The plan calls for checking one's urine for ketone bodies to ensure that the desired level of ketosis is reached. Atkins also recommended large amounts of nutritional supplements.

A computer analysis of sample menus has found that the diet contained 59% fat and provided fewer servings of grains, vegetables, and fruits than recommended by the US dietary guidelines. The investigators also said that although the diet can produce short-term weight loss, long-term use is likely to increase the risk of both cardiovascular disease and cancer (37). A subsequent literature review found "insufficient evidence to make recommendations for or against the use of low-carbohydrate diets, particularly among participants older than age 50 years, for use longer than 90 days, or for diets of 20 g/d or less of carbohydrates." These reviewers noted that "weight loss while using low-carbohydrate diets was principally associated with decreased caloric intake and increased diet duration but not with reduced carbohydrate content" (38).

A controlled study of 63 people who were randomly assigned to either the Atkins diet or a conventional diet found that the Atkins group lost about 4% more weight for the first 6 months, but there was no significant difference between two groups at 1 year. The low-carbohydrate diet appeared to improve risk factors for heart disease, but the authors concluded that more research is needed on the safety and effectiveness of this regimen (39).

Low-carbohydrate diets are unsuitable for people with coronary artery disease, gout, or kidney disease. Before a low-carbohydrate diet is started, measurements should be made of the blood levels of creatinine (which reflects kidney function), uric acid (related to gout), and glucose (may detect diabetes, which can elevate triglyceride levels). Low-carbohydrate dieters should also monitor their blood lipid levels and stop the diet if their 3-month total or LDL cholesterol levels rise sharply. Among those whose cholesterol levels improve, the improvement is thought to be related to weight reduction, but no published study has examined the effect of the diet on the coronary arteries.

Because increasing the amount of carbohydrates in a diet can raise triglyceride levels and reduce high-density lipoprotein (HDL), a low-carbohydrate diet may be appropriate for obese persons with abnormally high triglyceride levels (40). As noted in Chapter 102, it is better to replace carbohydrate with monosaturated or polyunsaturated fat than with protein-fat containing foods, and the diet should contain fewer calories than expended. Future genetic research may be able to determine the diets that are best for persons with metabolic problems based on their genetic pattern.

The recent popularity of low-carbohydrate diets has encouraged food companies to market low-carbohydrate foods for people who want to "watch their carbs." Most of these foods are much higher in fat than the foods they are designed to replace. Thus, "low-carb" advertising is encouraging both dieters and nondieters to eat high-fat foods, which is exactly the opposite of what medical and nutrition authorities have been urging for decades.

QUESTIONABLE "DIET PILLS"

Questionable diet pills are marketed though retail outlets, direct mail solicitations, newspaper advertising, cable television infomercials, and the Internet. Typically, these pills are claimed to produce effortless, rapid, and permanent weight loss. Many are falsely claimed to block absorption of starch, fat, or calories, to flush fat out of the body, or to step up the body's "fat-burning system." Some contain a fiber (e.g., glucomannan or guar gum) that is claimed to curb appetite by absorbing water and swelling to fill the stomach. However, the amount of fiber is too small actually to fill the stomach, and even if it could, that would not necessarily curb a person's appetite. In 1990, guar gum was banned as a diet aid after the FDA received 17 reports of persons whose esophagus became blocked as a result of using tablets of "Cal-Ban 3000," a widely promoted guar gum product (41).

Spirulina, a dark-green powder or pill derived from algae, is said by its promoters to suppress appetite. However, no scientific evidence supports this claim.

Products containing *Gymnema sylvestre* are being touted as weight-control aids with claims that they block absorption of sugar. The leaves of this plant, when chewed, can prevent the taste sensation of sweetness. However, no evidence indicates that *Gymnema sylvestre* blocks absorption of sugar into the body.

Supplements containing chromium picolinate are promoted with unsubstantiated claims that this substance promotes fat loss and increases lean muscle mass. The FTC has stopped some companies from making such claims, but others have continued to do so.

A systematic review of scientific reports, including reviews and metaanalyses, has concluded that chitosan, chromium picolinate, *Garcinia cambogia*, glucomannan, guar gum, hydroxymethylbutyrate, plantago psyllium, pyruvate, yerba maté, and yohimbe have not been proven effective for reducing body weight. The reviewers stated: "None of the reviewed dietary supplements can be recommended for over-the-counter use" (42).

Products containing ma huang have been marketed as weight-loss aids even though they have not been proven safe or effective for this purpose. Ma huang is an herb that contains ephedrine, a nasal decongestant and nervous system stimulant. Ephedrine can raise blood pressure and therefore is hazardous to persons with high blood pressure. Deaths have been reported among users of stimulants containing ephedrine and caffeine. In April 2004, after concluding that ephedra poses an unreasonable risk of injury, the FDA banned its use as a dietary supplement ingredient.

The FDA is also planning to ban phenylpropanolamine (PPA), which has been used in weight-loss products as well as a nasal decongestant to relieve stuffy nose or sinus congestion. PPA can have a temporary effect on appetite, but no evidence indicates that it offers any long-term benefit for weight control, In 2001, the FDA announced that it plans to ban PPA in all drug products and asked manufacturers voluntarily to stop marketing them. The FDA warning was based on estimates that 200 to 500 strokes per year among persons 18 to 49 years old could be associated with PPA use. A study by scientists at Yale University in New Haven, Connecticut found an association between PPA use and hemorrhagic stroke in women (43). The study did not contain enough men to estimate the risk to men, but there is no reason to believe it is lower. The FDA's PPA information page provides comprehensive information (44).

DANGERS OF QUACKERY

Quackery's harm can be classified as economic, indirect, direct, psychologic, and societal (45). Individual economic damage can range from a few dollars a year for "nutrition insurance" to many thousands of dollars wasted on quack remedies for serious disease. Because everyone must eat, the potential market for nutritional quackery is immense. Indirect harm occurs when the use of an ineffective approach diverts someone from effective care. Direct harm occurs when a dubious method causes death (Fig. 111.1), serious injury, or unnecessary suffering. Psychologic harm arises when persons blame themselves for the failure of an ineffective remedy or when they mistaken conclude they have been helped and become more vulnerable to future deception. Quackery can also harm our democratic society when large numbers of people hold erroneous beliefs

about the nature of disease and the best way to deal with it. Limited resources can be wasted if funds are used to follow leads based on inadequate or faked data.

Between 1986 and 1990, the American Dietetic Association documented more than 500 cases of people harmed by inappropriate nutritional advice from bogus "nutritionists," health food store operators, and others. Privacy considerations, however, prevented the association from publishing a detailed analysis.

The tryptophan tragedy illustrates how inappropriate use of supplements can lead to disaster. In 1989, a form of L-tryptophan was implicated in an outbreak of eosinophilia-myalgia syndrome, a previously rare disorder characterized by severe muscle and joint pain, weakness, swelling of the arms and legs, fever, and rash. This amino acid had been promoted by the health food industry to treat insomnia, depression, premenstrual syndrome, and overweight, although it had not been proven safe and effective for these purposes. Within a year, more than 1500 cases were reported, with 27 deaths and many hospitalizations (46). When the outbreak's cause was identified, the FDA banned the sale of L-tryptophan products. The outbreak was traced to a Japanese bulk wholesaler that had used a new bacterial strain to produce the L-tryptophan sold to US manufacturers. Attorneys handling the resultant lawsuits state that more than 5000 users were injured, and total damages paid by the errant producer have exceeded $1 billion (47).

CONSUMER PROTECTION

Three federal agencies have responsibility for fighting quackery. The FDA has jurisdiction over the labeling of foods and drugs. Under federal law, any product "intended for use in the cure, mitigation, treatment or prevention of disease" is a drug. If a product is marketed with drug claims that lack FDA approval, the agency can issue a warning letter, initiate a seizure, obtain an injunction, and/or seek criminal penalties. The claim does not have to be on the product label itself. Any claim traceable to the manufacturer is considered part of the label. The FDA's enforcement ability was weakened by passage of the Dietary Supplement Health and Education Act of 1994 (see Chapter 116), which defines the term "dietary supplement" to include not only vitamins and minerals but also herbs, amino acids, and other substances intended "for use to supplement the diet by increasing total dietary intake." The law also shifted the burden of proof of product safety from manufacturers to the FDA and permits sellers to use third-party literature as sales aids. Since its passage, the consumer marketplace has been flooded with misleading claims, and even hormones, such as dehydroepiandrosterone (DHEA) and melatonin, are being hawked as supplements.

The FTC has jurisdiction over the advertising of nonprescription products that are marketed in interstate

---

In a study of 653 sick babies, every infant with colic had low blood potassium. "Improvement was dramatic," and the colic disappeared immediately, when physicians gave 500 to 1,000 milligrams of potassium chloride intravenously or 1,000 to 2,000 milligrams by mouth. These doctors found that most babies needed 3,000 milligrams of potassium chloride (⅔ teaspoon) before colic was corrected. They suggested that potassium be given to prevent colic, especially during diarrhea, when much of this nutrient is lost in the feces. Potassium is also lost when too much salt (sodium) is allowed a baby, and/or when pantothenic acid is so deficient that the adrenals become exhausted.

Figure 111.1. Fatal advice. In 1979, this passage from Adelle Davis' *Let's Have Healthy Children* persuaded the mother of 2-month-old Ryan Pitzer to administer potassium drops when he developed colic and became dehydrated. The potassium caused Ryan's heart to stop beating. Davis' advice was based on misrepresentation of a scientific study of infants hospitalized for severe gastroenteritis. The article had nothing do with colic and even warned that giving potassium to dehydrated infants could produce cardiac arrest. Ryan's parents sued Adelle Davis' estate, the book's publisher, and the manufacturer of the potassium drops and won out-of-court settlements totaling $160,000.

TABLE 111.2. WHERE TO COMPLAIN ABOUT NUTRITION-RELATED WRONGDOING

PROBLEM	AGENCIES TO CONTACT[a]
False advertising	Federal Trade Commission Bureau of Consumer Protection or regional office
	National Advertising Division, Council of Better Business Bureaus
Product marketed with false or misleading claims	Editor or manager of media outlet where ad appeared
	National or regional Food and Drug Administration office
	State attorney general
	State health department
	Local Better Business Bureau
	Congressional representatives
Bogus mail-order promotion	Chief Postal Inspector, US Postal Service
	Regional Postal Inspector
	State attorney general
Dubious telemarketing	State attorney general
	Federal Trade Commission Bureau of Consumer Protection or regional office
Improper treatment by licensed practitioner	Editor or station manager of media outlet where ad appeared
	Local or state professional society (if practitioner is a member)
	Local hospital (if practitioner is a staff member)
	State licensing board
	Quackwatch
Improper treatment by unlicensed person	Local district attorney
	State attorney general
	Quackwatch

[a]When more than one regulatory agency appears to have jurisdiction, contact each of them: Chief Postal Inspector, US Postal Service, Washington, DC 20260.
FDA, 5600 Fishers Lane, Rockville, MD 20857 or http://www.fda.gov/oc/buyonline/buyonlineform.htm
Federal Trade Commission Bureau of Consumer Protection, Washington, DC 20580 or https://rn.ftc.gov/pls/dod/wsolcq$.startup?Z_ORG_CODE=PU01
National Advertising Division, Council of Better Business Bureaus, 70 West 36th Street, New York, NY 10018.
Quackwatch, PO Box 1747, Allentown, PA 18105. Telephone: 610-437-1795.
For regional offices of federal agencies, consult the telephone directory under US Government. © 2004, Stephen Barrett, M.D.

commerce. It issues warnings, files complaints and negotiates settlements, going to court when necessary. It has a very powerful law but insufficient personnel to act against most violations it encounters. One notable FTC action was a 1994 consent agreement under which General Nutrition, Inc. paid $2.4 million dollars to settle charges that it had falsely advertised 41 products, most of which had been packaged by other manufacturers. The products included 15 alleged weight-control products, 18 alleged "ergogenic aids," five bogus hair-loss preventers, two alleged antifatigue products, and two purported disease-related products (14).

The US Postal Service has overlapping jurisdiction over products sold by mail. It has a strong law but has not pursued falsely advertised health products since the early 1990s.

Several state attorneys general have been active in combating quackery. However, their actions may not stop promoters from continuing their schemes out–of state. State and federal laws pertaining to quackery need strengthening (48).

The primary voluntary antiquackery forces in the United States are Quackwatch and the National Council Against Health Fraud, Inc. Both are nonprofit corporations. I operate Quackwatch with help from a network of consultants. It maintains 18 Web sites and publishes a free electronic newsletter. The National Council Against Health Fraud is a membership organization of health and nutrition professionals, educators, researchers, attorneys and other concerned citizens. Financed primarily by membership dues, it conducts research, maintains a Web site, publishes task force reports, serves as a clearinghouse, and helps victims of quackery to file lawsuits. Table 111.2 advises where to complain about nutrition-related wrongdoing.

REFERENCES

1. Schafer R, Yetley EA. J Am Diet Assoc 1975;66:129–33.
2. Barrett S, Jarvis WT, eds. The Health Robbers: A Close Look at Quackery in America. Amherst NY: Prometheus Books, 1993.
3. Mindell E. Dr. Earl Mindell's Live Longer and Feel Better with Vitamins and Minerals. New Canaan, CT: Keats Publishing, 1994.
4. Balch PA, Balch JF. Prescription for Nutritional Healing: A Practical A–Z Guide to Drug-Free Remedies Using Vitamins, Minerals, Herbs and Food Supplements. 3rd ed. New York: Avery (Putnam Group), 2000.
5. Food and Drug Administration Pesticide Program. Residues Monitoring 2001. Washington, DC: Food and Drug Administration, 2003.
6. Institute of Food Technologists Expert Panel on Food Safety and Nutrition. Food Technol 1990;44:123–30.
7. Consumer Rep 1998;63:12–8.
8. Basker D. Am J Alternative Agric 1992;7:129–36.
9. Whelan EM, Stare FJ. Panic in the Pantry. 2nd ed. Amherst, NY: Prometheus Books, 1992.
10. Fed Reg 1993;58:631–91, 2065–964.
11. Fed Reg 1996;61:296–337.
12. Federal Trade Commission. Enforcement Policy Statement on Food Advertising. Washington, DC: Federal Trade Commission, May 1994.
13. Pollack H, Halpern SL. Therapeutic Nutrition. Washington, DC: National Research Council, 1952.
14. Barrett S, Herbert V. The Vitamin Pushers: How the "Health Food" Industry Is Selling America a Bill of Goods. Amherst, NY: Prometheus Books, 1994.
15. Friedl KE. Performance-enhancing substances: Effects, risks, and appropriate alternatives. In: Baechle TR, ed. Essentials of Strength Training and Conditioning. Champaign, IL: Human Kinetics Press, 1994:188–209.
16. Lightsey D, Attaway JR. Natl Strength Conditioning J 1992;14:26–31.

17. Anderson SA, Raiten DJ, eds. Safety of Amino Acids Used as Ddietary Supplements. Bethesda, MD: Federation of American Societies for Experimental Biology, 1992.

18. Food and Nutrition Board, Institute of Medicine. Dietary Reference Intakes: Energy, Carbohydrate, Fiber, Fat, Fatty Acids, Cholesterol, Protein, and Amino Acids. Washington, DC: National Academy Press, 2002:78–109.

19. Jha P, Flather M, Lonn E et al. Ann Intern Med 1995;123:860–72.

20. Routine Vitamin Supplementation to Prevent Cancer and Cardiovascular Disease. US Preventive Services Task Force, New Topic, 2003. http://www.ahrq.gov/clinic/uspstf/uspsvita.htm

21. Consumer Rep Health 1995;7:133–5.

22. Stookey HE, Miller B, Meister K. ACSH News Views 1983;4:1, 8–9, 13–4.

23. Martin N. Nutr Forum 1990;7:16.

24. Food and Drug Administration. Unsubstantiated Claims and Documented Health Hazards in the Dietary Supplement Marketplace. Rockville, MD: Food and Drug Administration, 1993.

25. Gotay CC, Dumitriu D. Arch Fam Med 2000;9:692–8.

26. Consumer Rep 1986;51:170–75.

27. Bell LS, Fairchild M. J Am Diet Assoc 1987;87:341–3.

28. Rhodes RA. Update 2001;Nov/Dec:41.http://www.fdli.org/pubs/update/update/html

29. Cooperman T, Obermeyer W, Webb D, ConsumerLab.com's Guide to Buying Vitamins and Supplements: What's Really in the Bottle? White Plains, NY: ConsumerLab.com, 2003.

30. Raso J. Nutr Forum 1995;12:13–9.

31. Milner I. Nutr Forum 1995;11:19–22.

32. Barrett S. JAMA 1985;254:1041–5.

33. Seidel S, Kreutzer R, Smith D et al. Assessment of commercial laboratories performing hair mineral analysis. JAMA 2001; 285:67–72.

34. Hambidge KM. Am J Clin Nutr 1982;36:943–9.

35. Barrett S. http://www.quackwatch.org/01QuackeryRelatedTopics/Tests/allergytests.html, revised, June 14, 2003.

36. http://www.atkins.com. Accessed April 29, 2001.

37. Anderson JW, Konz EC, Jenkins DJ. J Am Coll Nutr 2000;19:578–90.

38. Bravata DM, Sanders L, Huang J et al. JAMA 2003;289: 1837–50.

39. Foster GD, Wyatt HR, Hill JO et al. N Engl J Med 2003;348:2082–90.

40. Jeppeson J, Chen YD, Zhou MY et al Am J Clin Nutr 1995;629:1201–5.

41. Barrett S. Nutr Today 1990;25:24–8.

42. Pittler MH, Ernst E. Am J Clin Nutr 2004:79:529–36.

43. Kernan WN, Viscoli CM, Brass LM et al. N Engl J Med 2000; 343:1826–32.

44. http://www.fda.gov/cder/drug/infopage/ppa/default.htm.

45. Jarvis W. How quackery harms. In Barrett S, Cassileth BR, eds. Dubious Cancer Treatment. Tampa: American Cancer Society, Florida Division, 1991:85–92.

46. Swygert LA, Maes EF, Sewell LE et al. JAMA 1990;264:1698–703.

47. Barrett S. Skeptical Inquirer 1995;19:6–9.

48. Barrett S. http://www.quackwatch.org/02ConsumerProtection/laws.html.

SELECTED READINGS

Barnes J, Anderson LA, Phillipson JD. Herbal Medicines: A Guide for Healthcare Professionals. London: Pharmaceutical Press, 2002.

Barrett S, Herbert V. The Vitamin Pushers: How the "Health Food" Industry Is Selling Americans a Bill of Goods. Amherst, NY: Prometheus Books, 1994.

Cooperman T, Obermeyer W, Webb D. ConsumerLab.com's Guide to Buying Vitamins and Supplements: What's Really in the Bottle? White Plains, NY: ConsumerLab.com, 2003.

About Herbs. http://www.mskcc.org/mskcc/html/11570.cfm.

Natural Medicines Comprehensive Database. http://www.naturaldatabase.com

Quackwatch. http://www.quackwatch.org.

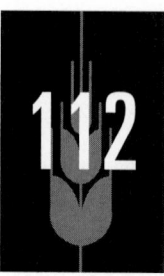

112 ALTERNATIVE NUTRITION THERAPIES[1]
STEPHEN BARRETT

UNSUBSTANTIATED CLAIMS .1763
"ALTERNATIVE" SYSTEMS 1763
    Chinese Medicine 1764
    Maharishi Ayur-Ved 1764
    Macrobiotics 1764
    Naturopathy 1765
    Natural Hygiene 1765
    Orthomolecular Therapy 1765
    Iridology 1766
    Metabolic Therapy 1766
    "Chiropractic Nutrition" 1766
    Colonic Irrigation 1767
    "Electrodiagnosis" 1767
    Herbs and Herbalism 1767
FAD DIAGNOSES 1768
    Hypoglycemia 1768
    "Environmental Illness" 1768
    "Yeast Infections" 1768
    "Leaky Gut Syndrome" 1769
    "Amalgam Toxicity" 1769
CHELATION THERAPY 1769
QUESTIONABLE CANCER THERAPIES 1769
    Laetrile 1770
    Gerson Method 1770
    Kelley/Gonzalez Metabolic Therapy 1770
    Shark Cartilage 1771
    Vitamin C 1771
POLITICAL CONSIDERATIONS 1771

The dictionary definition of the noun *alternative* is a choice between mutually exclusive possibilities. Until the late 1980s, in standard medical usage, it referred to choices among effective treatments. In some cases, they were equally effective (e.g., the use of radiation or surgery for

certain cancers); in others, the expected outcome differed, but there were reasonable tradeoffs between risks and benefits. During recent years, however, the word *alternative* has been applied to a multitude of unsubstantiated approaches that differ from standard medical ones.

To avoid confusion, alternative methods should be classified as genuine, experimental, or questionable. *Genuine* alternatives are comparable methods that have met science-based criteria for safety and effectiveness. Under the rules of science (and federal law), proponents who make health claims bear the burden of proof. It is their responsibility to conduct suitable studies and report them in sufficient detail to permit evaluation and confirmation by others. Methods can be evaluated by addressing four questions: (a) Has the method shown potential for benefit that clearly exceeds the potential for harm? (b) Have safety and efficacy been demonstrated by objective studies using adequate controls? (c) Have the methodology and results been published in peer-reviewed scientific journals? and (d) Have the results been replicated by others? Peer review is a process in which work is reviewed by others usually with equivalent or superior knowledge. The best scientific journals use experts for this purpose. Detailed standards for reporting and evaluating studies have been published (1).

Experimental alternatives are unproven but have a plausible rationale and are undergoing responsible investigation. The most noteworthy is the use of a 10% fat diet for treating coronary heart disease. *Questionable* alternatives are groundless because they lack a scientifically plausible rationale or have been disproved. The archetype is homeopathy, which claims that "remedies" so dilute that they contain no active ingredient can exert powerful therapeutic effects. When these three types of alternatives are lumped together, promoters of questionable methods can argue that because some have merit, the rest deserve equal consideration and respect. This chapter uses the word *alternative* in its "questionable" sense.

Another way to avoid confusion is sort methods into three groups: those that work, those that do not work, and those whose efficacy is uncertain. Most methods described as alternative fall into the second group. Arnold Relman, M.D., former editor of *The New England Journal of Medicine*, has expressed similar thoughts:

> There are not two kinds of medicine, one conventional and the other unconventional, that can be practiced jointly in a new kind of

[1]**Abbreviations: AK,** applied kinesiology; **B.E.S.T.,** bioenergetic synchronization technique; **DSHEA,** Dietary Supplement Health Education Act; **EDTA,** ethylenediaminetetraacetic acid; **FDA,** Food and Drug Administration; **NCCAM,** National Center for Complementary and Alternative Medicine; **NCI,** National Cancer Institute; **NIH,** National Institutes of Health; **OAM,** Office of Alternative Medicine; **TCM,** traditional Chinese medicine; **TM,** transcendental meditation.

"integrative medicine." Nor . . . are there two kinds of thinking, or two ways to find out which treatments work and which do not. In the best kind of medical practice, all proposed treatments must be tested objectively. In the end, there will only be treatments that pass that test and those that do not, those that are proven worthwhile and those that are not (2).

When someone feels better after using a product or procedure, it is natural to credit whatever was done. This can mislead, however, because most ailments resolve spontaneously, and those that persist can have symptoms that wax and wane. Even serious conditions can have sufficient month-to-month variation to enable spurious methods to gain large followings. In addition, taking action may temporarily relieve symptoms via the placebo effect. This effect is a beneficial change in a person's condition that occurs in response to some aspect of treatment but is not the result of the pharmacologic or physical aspects of the treatment. Belief in the treatment is not essential, but the placebo effect may be enhanced by such factors as faith, sympathetic attention, sensational claims, testimonials, and the use of scientific-looking charts, devices, and terminology. Another drawback of individual success stories is that they do not indicate how many failures may occur for each success. (In other words, no score is kept.) People unaware of these facts often give undeserved credit to alternative methods.

Practitioners of complementary and integrative medicine claim to synthesize the best of standard and "alternative" methods. However, no published data indicate the extent to which they actually use proven therapies or the extent to which they burden patients with medically useless methods. These practitioners typically claim credit for any improvement experienced by the patient and blame standard treatments for any negative effects. The result may undermine the patient's confidence in standard care, thereby reducing compliance or causing the patient to abandon it altogether (3).

Alternative nutrition therapies appeal to people who would like to take an active role in their treatment. These approaches are typically but falsely claimed to be safer and more effective than medically prescribed drugs. Government regulation of alternative products and practitioners is inadequate.

UNSUBSTANTIATED CLAIMS

When challenged about the lack of scientific evidence supporting what they espouse, alternative promoters may claim that (a) scientific reports (whose meaning they distort) back them up, (b) research is not necessary because they have seen with their own eyes that their methods are effective, (c) funds are not available for them to perform research, (d) the scientific establishment is unwilling to test their methods or look at their data, and (e) scientific journals are unwilling to consider their research because it poses a threat to the establishment. Each of these claims is incorrect. Preliminary research does not always require

TABLE 112.1. PLOYS USED BY "ALTERNATIVE" PROMOTERS

"Alternative" promoters offer solutions for virtually every health problem, including some they have invented. To those in pain, they promise relief. To the incurable, they offer hope. To gain a patient's allegiance, it is not necessary to persuade the patient that all the statements below are true. Just one may be enough.

"We really care about you!"
"We treat the whole patient."
"We attack the cause of disease."
"Out treatments have no side effects."
"We treat medicine's failures."
"Think positive!"
"Jump on the bandwagon."
"Our methods are time-tested."
"Backed by scientific studies"
"Take charge of your health!"
"Think for yourself."
"What have you got to lose?"
"If only you had come earlier."
"Science doesn't have all the answers."
"Don't be afraid to experiment."

funding but takes effort. The principal ingredients are careful clinical observations, detailed record-keeping, and long-term follow-up to "keep score." Proponents of alternative methods almost never do any of these things. Some even claim their concepts cannot be tested by scientific methods.

A study involving vitamin C illustrates why anecdotal evidence is not an appropriate substitute for carefully designed clinical trials. The study compared the effect of administering vitamin C supplements and placebo before and during colds. Although the experiment was supposed to be a double-blind study, half the subjects were able to guess which pill they were taking. When the results were tabulated with all subjects lumped together, the vitamin-treated group reported fewer colds per person over a 9-month period. Among the half who had not guessed which pill they had been taking, however, no difference in the incidence or severity of colds was found (4). This finding demonstrates how people who think they are doing something effective can report a favorable result even when none exists.

Each of the approaches described in this chapter has one or more of the following characteristics: (a) its rationale or underlying theory has no scientific basis, (b) it has not been demonstrated safe and/or effective by well-designed studies, (c) it is deceptively promoted (Table 112.1), or (d) its practitioners are not qualified to make appropriate medical diagnoses.

"ALTERNATIVE" SYSTEMS

Many alternative approaches involve nutrition-related issues. Proponents of these methods typically claim that (a) certain foods or nutrients have special ability to cure specific diseases, (b) certain foods are harmful and should be eliminated from the diet, and (c) "natural foods" are best. Most systems described in this section are also rooted in *vitalism*, the concept that bodily functions depend on a "vital force" that cannot be explained by the laws of physics and chemistry. Vitalistic proponents maintain that diseases should be treated by stimulating the body to heal itself rather than by "treating symptoms." Naturopaths, for example, claim that illness is caused by a disturbance of the body's natural healing force, which they can augment by "detoxification." Some vitalists assert that food can be "dead" or "living" and that "live" foods contain a dormant or primitive "life force" that humans can assimilate. None of these "energies" can be measured by scientific methods.

Chinese Medicine

Traditional Chinese medicine (TCM), also called Oriental medicine, is based on beliefs that the body's vital energy (*Chi* or *Qi*) circulates through 14 hypothetic channels called meridians, which have branches connected to bodily organs and functions (5). Illness and disease are attributed to imbalance or interruption of *Chi*. Acupuncture, herbs, and various other modalities are claimed to restore balance. A National Council Against Health Fraud task force has concluded the following: (a) acupuncture has not been proven effective for the treatment of any disease; (b) the greater the benefit claimed in a research report, the worse the experimental design; and (c) the best-designed experiments—those with the highest number of controls on variables—found no difference between acupuncture and control groups (6).

Many TCM practitioners are licensed acupuncturists. They are not permitted to prescribe drugs, but they are free to recommend dietary supplements and herbs. The diagnostic process they use may include questioning (medical history, lifestyle), observations (skin, tongue, color), listening (breath sounds), and pulse-taking. Medical science recognizes only one pulse, corresponding to the heartbeat, which can be felt in the wrist, neck, feet, and various other places throughout the body. TCM practitioners check six alleged pulses at each wrist and identify more than 25 alleged pulse qualities such as "sinking," "slippery," "soggy," "tight," and "wiry." TCM's "pulses" supposedly reflect the type of imbalance, the condition of each organ system, and the status of the patient's *Chi*. The herbs they prescribe are not regulated for safety, potency, or effectiveness. Although some cases of adverse effects from herbs have been reported (7), no systematic assessment of this problem has been published.

A study published in 2001 illustrates the nebulous nature of TCM practices. A 40-year-old woman with chronic back pain who visited seven acupuncturists during a 2-week period was diagnosed with "Qi stagnation" by six of them, "blood stagnation" by five , "kidney Qi deficiency" by two, "yin deficiency" by one, and "liver Qi deficiency" by one.

None of these alleged conditions can be quantified or verified by scientific means. The proposed treatments varied even more (8).

Maharishi Ayur-Ved

Proponents state that ayurvedic medicine originated in ancient times but was reconstituted in the early 1980s by the Maharishi Mahesh Yogi, who also popularized transcendental meditation (TM). Its origin is traced to four Sanskrit books called the *Vedas*—the most important scriptures of India, shaped sometime before 200 BCE. These books attributed most disease and bad luck to demons, devils, and the influence of stars and planets. Ayurveda's basic theory states that the body's functions are regulated by three "irreducible physiologic principles" called doshas, whose Sanskrit names are *vata*, *pitta*, and *kapha*. Like the Sun signs of astrology, these terms are used to designate body types as well as the traits that typify them. Like astrologic writings, ayurvedic writings contain long lists of supposed physical and mental characteristics of each constitutional type. Through various combinations of *vata*, *pitta*, and *kapha*, ten body types are possible. However, one's *doshas* (and therefore one's body type) can vary from hour to hour and season to season.

Ayurvedic proponents state that the symptoms of disease are always related to balance of the *doshas*, which can be determined by feeling the patient's wrist pulse or completing a questionnaire (9). Balance is supposedly achieved through "pacifying" diets, "purification" (to remove "impurities from faulty diet and behavioral patterns"), TM, and a long list of procedures and ayurvedic products, many of which are said to be formulated for specific body types. Some require the services of an ayurvedic practitioner. Although many of ayurvedic herbal products have been marketed with illegal claims, regulatory action by the US Food and Drug Administration (FDA) has been minimal.

Macrobiotics

Macrobiotics is a quasireligious system that advocates a semivegetarian diet. Macrobiotic diets have been promoted for maintaining general health and for preventing and treating cancer, acquired immunodeficiency syndrome, and other diseases. The optimal diet is said to balance "yin" and "yang" foods. It is composed of whole grains (50–60% of each meal), vegetables (25–30% of each meal), whole beans or soybean-based products (5–10% of daily food), nuts and seeds (small amounts as snacks), miso soup, herbal teas, and small amounts of white meat or seafood once or twice weekly (10). The yin/yang classification is not related to nutrient content but is based on the following: the food's color, pH, shape, size, taste, temperature, texture, water content, and weight; the region and season in which the food was grown; and how it is prepared and eaten. Some macrobiotic diets contain inadequate amounts of certain nutrients. Infants on macrobiotic diets have developed rickets and have had deficiencies of vitamin B_{12} and iron (11, 12).

Macrobiotics is promoted through books, local organizations, health food stores, unlicensed practitioners, and a few physicians. Practitioners typically base their recommendations on "pulse diagnosis" and other unscientific procedures related to Chinese medicine. These include "ancestral diagnosis," "astrologic diagnosis," "aura and vibrational diagnosis," "environmental diagnosis" (including consideration of "celestial influences" and tidal motions), and "spiritual diagnosis" (an evaluation of "atmospheric vibrational conditions" to identify spiritual influences, including "visions of the future") (13).

Today's leading proponent is Michio Kushi, founder and president of the Kushi Institute in Brookline, Massachusetts. Institute publications state that the macrobiotic way of life should include chewing food at least 50 times per mouthful (or until it becomes liquid), not wearing synthetic or woolen clothing next to the skin, avoiding long hot baths or showers, having large green plants in your house to enrich the oxygen content of the air, and singing a happy song every day (14). Kushi claims that cancer is largely the result of improper diet, thinking, and way of life and can be influenced by changing these factors. He recommends yin foods (e.g., tropical fruits) for cancers caused by excess yang, and yang foods (e.g., eggs and meat) for tumors that are predominantly yin (15). His books contain case histories of people whose cancers have supposedly disappeared after they adopted macrobiotic eating. However, the only reports of efficacy are testimonials by patients, many of whom also received standard medical treatment (16). The high-fiber diet can cause cancer patients to undergo serious weight loss (17).

Naturopathy

Naturopaths claim to remove the underlying causes of disease and to stimulate the body's natural healing processes (18). They maintain that diseases are the body's effort to purify itself and that cures result from increasing the patient's "vital force" by ridding the body of waste products and "toxins." However, they do not specify the chemical names of the "toxins," indicate how to measure them, or demonstrate that "detoxification" reduces the quantity in the body.

Although naturopaths say they emphasize prevention, they tend to oppose immunization. The doctor of naturopathy (N.D.) degree is available from four full-time naturopathy schools and a few correspondence schools. Naturopaths are licensed as independent practitioners in 13 states and may legally practice in a few others.

Most naturopaths believe that virtually all diseases are within the scope of their practice. Their methods include fasting, "natural food" diets, vitamins, herbs, tissue minerals, cell salts, manipulation, massage, exercise, colonic irrigation (see later), acupuncture, natural childbirth, minor

surgery, and applications of water, heat, cold, air, sunlight, and electricity. They may use radiation for diagnosis but not for treatment. "Detoxification" plays a prominent role. The most comprehensive naturopathic textbook recommends special diets, vitamins, minerals, and/or herbs for more than 70 health problems ranging from acne to acquired immunodeficiency syndrome (19). For many of these conditions, daily administration of ten or more products is recommended, some in dosages high enough to be toxic.

Natural Hygiene

Natural hygiene, an offshoot of naturopathy, is a philosophy of health and "natural living" that advocates a raw food diet of vegetables, fruits, and nuts. It also advocates periodic fasting and "food combining" (avoiding food combinations it considers detrimental) (20). Natural hygienists oppose immunization, fluoridation, and food irradiation and eschew most forms of medical treatment.

Orthomolecular Therapy

During the early 1950s, a few psychiatrists began adding massive doses of nutrients to the treatment of severe mental problems. The original substance used was niacin, and the therapy was termed *megavitamin therapy*. Since that time, the treatment regimen has been expanded to include other vitamins, minerals, hormones, and diets, any of which may be combined with mainstream drug therapy or electroconvulsive therapy.

Current proponents call this system *orthomolecular psychiatry*, a term meaning "the treatment of mental disease by providing an optimum molecular environment for the mind, especially substances normally present in the human body." Proponents claim that abnormal conditions are caused by molecular imbalances that can be corrected by administration of the "right" nutrient molecules at the right time. (*Ortho* is Greek for "right.") They also claim that their treatment is effective against many diseases. Their evaluations usually include laboratory tests that most physicians would consider questionable.

In 1973, an American Psychiatric Association task force report noted that megavitamin proponents used unconventional methods not only in treatment, but also in diagnosis. The report concluded that "the credibility of the megavitamin proponents is low" and "is further diminished by a consistent refusal over the past decade to perform controlled experiments and to report their new results in a scientifically acceptable fashion" (21). Additional claims that megavitamins and megaminerals are effective against psychosis, learning disorders, and mental retardation in children were debunked in reports by the nutrition committees of the American Academy of Pediatrics in 1976 and 1981 and by the Canadian Academy of Pediatrics in 1990, 2000, and 2004 (22). Both groups warned that there was no proven benefit in any of these conditions and that megadoses can have serious toxic effects. The 1976 report concluded that a "cult" had developed among followers of megavitamin therapy (23).

Iridology

Iridology is based on the notion that each area of the body is represented by a corresponding area in the iris of the eye (the colored area surrounding the pupil). Many of its practitioners are chiropractors or naturopaths, but it is also used by bogus nutritionists and by laypersons involved in multilevel marketing (24). Iridologists claim that states of health and disease can be diagnosed from the color, texture, and location of various pigment flecks in the eye. Iridology practitioners purport to diagnose "imbalances" and treat them with vitamins, minerals, herbs, and similar products. They may also claim that the eye markings can reveal a complete history of past illnesses as well as previous treatment. Two large objective trials involving prominent iridologists found that they could not distinguish between patients who had a disease (kidney or gallbladder disease) and those who were healthy. Nor did they agree with each other about who was ill (25, 26).

Metabolic Therapy

Proponents of "metabolic therapy" claim to diagnose abnormalities at the cellular level and correct them by normalizing the patient's metabolism. They regard cancer, arthritis, multiple sclerosis, and other "degenerative" diseases as the result of metabolic imbalance caused by a buildup of "toxic substances" in the body. They claim that scientific practitioners merely treat the symptoms of the disease, whereas they treat the cause by removing "toxins" and strengthening the immune system so the body can heal itself. The "toxins" are neither defined nor objectively measurable. "Metabolic" treatment regimens vary from practitioner to practitioner and may include a "natural food" diet, coffee enemas, vitamins, minerals, glandulars, enzymes, laetrile, and various other nostrums that are not legally marketable in the United States. The components of metabolic therapy vary from practitioner to practitioner. No controlled study has shown that any of its components has any value against cancer or any other chronic disease. However, many people find its concepts appealing because they do not seem far removed from scientific medicine's concerns with diet, lifestyle, and the relationship between emotions and bodily responses.

The most visible proponent of "metabolic therapy" was Harold Manner, Ph.D., a biology professor who announced in 1977 that he had cured cancer in mice with injections of laetrile, enzymes, and vitamin A. In fact, he had digested the tumors by injecting them with digestive enzymes, which cannot cure cancers that have metastasized. During the early 1980s, Manner left his teaching position and became affiliated with a clinic in Tijuana, Mexico. Although he claimed a high success rate in treating cancers, there is no evidence that he kept track of patients after they left his clinic (27). He died in 1988, but others continue to provide the same treatment.

"Chiropractic Nutrition"

Chiropractic is based on beliefs that most ailments are the result of spinal problems (28). Chiropractors can be divided into two main types: "straights" and "mixers." Straights tend to cling to the doctrine that most illness is caused by misaligned vertebrae ("subluxations") that can be corrected by "spinal adjustment." Mixers acknowledge that germs, hormones, and other factors play a role in disease, but they tend to regard mechanical disturbances of the nervous system as the underlying cause (through "lowered resistance"). In addition to spinal manipulation, mixers may use nutritional methods and various types of physiotherapy (heat, cold, traction, exercise, massage, and ultrasound). Chiropractors are licensed in all 50 states. They are not permitted to prescribe drugs or perform surgery, but most states permit them to prescribe dietary supplements, herbs, and homeopathic products.

Chiropractors who give nutritional advice typically recommend supplements that are unnecessary or are inappropriate for treating health problems. One such product is *Spine Align*, which, according to its manufacturer, can help repair, regenerate, correct, and normalize the spine. Its ingredients include "whole spinal column" (from cows), bone meal, silica, boron aminoate, copper gluconate, aromatic root beer, and potassium iodide. Many chiropractors espouse nutrition-related systems of diagnosis and treatment that lack scientific validity. The most noteworthy are applied kinesiology (AK), bioenergetic synchronization technique (B.E.S.T.), and contact reflex analysis.

AK is a pseudoscientific system of muscle testing and therapy based on assertions that specific muscle weaknesses are signs of disease in body organs. AK practitioners—most of whom are chiropractors—claim that nutritional deficiencies, allergies, and other adverse reactions to food substances can be detected by placing substances in the mouth or hand and testing muscle strength. "Good" substances supposedly make specific muscles stronger, whereas "bad" substances cause specific weaknesses. Treatment typically includes dietary modification, food supplements, acupressure, and spinal manipulation. Controlled studies of AK muscle-testing procedures have found no difference between results with test substances and those with placebos (29). Differences from one test to another may be the result of suggestibility, variations in the amount of force or leverage involved, and/or muscle fatigue.

B.E.S.T. practitioners claim that an imbalance in the patient's electromagnetic field causes unequal leg length, which the chiropractor can instantly correct by applying his or her own electromagnetic energy to proper points on the body. According to this notion, two fingers on each of the chiropractor's hands are North poles, two are South poles, and the thumbs are electromagnetically neutral. When imbalance is detected, the hands are held for a few seconds at "contact points" on the patient's body until "pulsation" is felt and the patient's legs test equally long. Proponents recommend that such testing be started early in infancy and continued at least monthly throughout life.

B.E.S.T.'s "nutritional" component is based on the notion that "patients can maintain life and vitality by consuming four times as much alkaline-forming as acid-forming foods." Proponents claim that saliva pH can reveal whether a person's symptoms are nutritionally or emotionally based and indicates whether the most effective method of care is nutritional supplementation and/or adjustive. For babies, a mixture of raw goat milk, carrot juice, and distilled water is said to be "an excellent replacement for infant formulas."

Contact reflex analysis resembles aspects of applied kinesiology and B.E.S.T. To diagnose a patient, the practitioner pulls on the patient's outstretched arm while placing a finger or hand on one of about 75 "reflex" points on the patient's body. If the patient's arm can be pulled downward, the disease corresponding to the reflex is said to be present. Large numbers of pills containing vitamins, minerals, dehydrated vegetables, plant enzymes, and/or freeze-dried animal organs are then prescribed to correct the alleged problems.

Many companies market supplements exclusively or primarily through chiropractic offices. Thousands of these products are intended for the treatment of disease, even though they are questionable and lack FDA approval for this use.

The percentage of chiropractors engaging in unscientific nutritional practices is unknown but appears to be substantial. A 1998 survey by the National Board of Chiropractic Examiners found that 90.4% of 3177 full-time practitioners who responded said they had used "nutritional counseling, therapy or supplements," and 43% said they had used AK within the previous 2 years (30). Chiropractors who prescribe supplements usually sell them to their patients for two to three times their wholesale cost. A typical regimen costs the patient several dollars per day. Chiropractic licensing authorities have not attempted to curtail inappropriate "chiropractic nutrition."

Colonic Irrigation

Some chiropractors and naturopaths advocate colonic irrigation as part of their treatment system. In this procedure, a rubber tube is passed into the rectum for a distance of up to 20 or 30 inches, and warm water is pumped in and out, a few pints at a time, typically using 20 or more gallons. Some practitioners add herbs, coffee, or other substances to the water. The procedure is said to "detoxify" the body. Its advocates claim that as a result of intestinal stasis, intestinal contents putrefy, and toxins are formed and absorbed, which causes chronic poisoning of the body.

This "autointoxication" theory was popular around 1900 but was abandoned by the scientific community during the 1930s. No such "toxins" have ever been identified, and careful observations have shown that persons in good health can vary greatly in bowel habits. Proponents may also suggest that fecal material collects on the lining of the intestine and causes trouble unless removed by laxatives, colonic irrigation, special diets, and/or various herbs or food supplements that "cleanse" the body. The falsity of this notion is obvious to doctors who perform intestinal surgery or peer within the large intestine with a diagnostic instrument. Fecal material does not adhere to the intestinal lining.

Colonic irrigation is not only therapeutically worthless but can cause fatal electrolyte imbalance. Cases of death from intestinal perforation and infection (from contaminated equipment) have also been reported (31).

"Electrodiagnosis"

Hundreds of alternative practitioners use devices purported to detect and treat "energy imbalances" said to signify organ dysfunctions, allergies, and other problems. This approach, called electrodiagnosis or electroacupuncture according to Voll (EAV), was initiated during the 1970s by a German physician who developed the first model of the device. Subsequent models include the *Vega, Dermatron, Accupath 1000,* and *Interro*. Proponents claim that these devices measure disturbances in the body's flow of "electromagnetic energy" along acupuncture meridians. Actually, they measure electrical resistance of the patient's skin when touched by a probe. One wire from the device goes to a brass cylinder covered by moist gauze, which the patient holds in one hand. A second wire is connected to a probe, which the operator touches to acupuncture points on the patient's other hand or foot. This completes a low-voltage circuit, and the device registers the flow of current. The information is then relayed to a gauge that provides a numeric readout. The size of the number actually depends on how hard the probe is pressed against the patient's skin (32). The treatment selected depends on the scope of the practitioner's practice and may include acupuncture, dietary change (to avoid supposed allergens), vitamin supplements, and/or homeopathic remedies.

Herbs and Herbalism

Herbs are used by folk healers, health food stores, herbalists, naturopaths, and other types of alternative practitioners. Some are prescribed at clinics devoted to the cure of specific diseases such as cancer. Some people also use herbs on their own initiative to maintain health, prevent specific diseases, and treat disease or ailments. Herbs may be obtained in various forms ranging from the plants themselves grown in gardens or harvested in the wild to processed herbal products such as pills. Herbal products have little or no nutritional value but are discussed in the chapter because federal law includes them it its definition of dietary supplements.

Many herbs contain hundreds or even thousands of chemicals that have not been completely cataloged. Some of these chemicals may turn out to be useful as therapeutic agents, but others could prove harmful. No legal standards exist for the processing, harvesting, or packaging of medicinal herbs, and the FDA does not require herbal products to adhere to any standards of identity or dosage. Many investigations have found products that did not have the amounts of ingredients listed on their label, and many products have been found to contain undeclared drugs and dangerous heavy metals.

Moreover, many herbal practitioners are nonphysicians who are not qualified to make appropriate diagnoses or to determine how herbal products compare to proven drugs. Thus, even if a substance is potentially useful, consumers cannot be certain what is in these products or how to use them. Adulteration, which can be accidental or deliberate, is another problem. In addition, the directions for use often fail to conform to research findings. A recent survey at 20 retail stores in and around Minneapolis found that only 43% of 880 products were labeled with the ingredients and dosage that had been used in published studies of the ingredients. The chosen herbs were echinacea, St. John's wort, ginkgo biloba, garlic, saw palmetto, ginseng, goldenseal, aloe, Siberian ginseng, and valerian. The actual ingredients were not measured, but the survey indicated that many formulations did not correspond to available research data (34).

To make a rational decision about an herbal product, it would be necessary to know what it contains, whether it is safe, how it interacts with drugs or other herbs, and whether it has been demonstrated to be as good or better than pharmaceutical products available for the same purpose. For most herbal ingredients, this information is incomplete or unavailable.

Even when a botanic product has some effectiveness, it may not be practical to use. Garlic, for example, has been demonstrated to lower cholesterol. However, prescription drugs are more potent for this purpose, and garlic has anticoagulant properties. No data are available to indicate the risk of combining garlic with other widely used products (vitamin E, ginkgo, fish oil, and aspirin) that can interfere with blood clotting.

FAD DIAGNOSES

Some practitioners misdiagnose large numbers of their patients with one or more conditions considered rare or even nonexistent by scientific practitioners. Some of these diagnoses are based on the patient's history (typically including fatigue and other common emotionally related symptoms), whereas others are based on inappropriate or misinterpreted laboratory tests.

Hypoglycemia

Many alternative practitioners diagnose "hypoglycemia" in large numbers of patients who report symptoms of nervousness or fatigue. The diagnosis of functional hypoglycemia should not be made unless a person on a balanced diet has symptoms 2 to 4 hours after eating, has a blood glucose level lower than 45 mg/100 mL whenever symptoms occur, and is immediately relieved of symptoms when the blood glucose level is raised. The glucose tolerance test is not reliable for evaluating most cases of suspected hypoglycemia (35). Low blood sugar levels without symptoms occur commonly in physiologically normal persons fed large amounts of sugar and are of no diagnostic significance.

"Environmental Illness"

"Clinical ecologists" claim that hypersensitivity to common foods and chemicals triggers dozens of symptoms that they label "environmental illness," or "multiple chemical sensitivity." They speculate that (a) although various substances alone may not cause trouble, low doses of different substances can add to or multiply each other's effects; (b) hypersensitivity develops when the total load of physical and psychologic stresses exceeds a person's tolerance; (c) hypersensitivities may be related to "immune system dysregulation" that can be difficult to diagnose and treat; (d) potential stressors include practically everything that modern humans encounter; and (e) the resultant symptoms can mimic almost any other condition (36). They base their diagnoses primarily on the results of "provocation" and "neutralization" tests, which are performed by having the patient report symptoms that occur within a specified period of time after suspected harmful substances are placed under the tongue or injected into the skin. If any symptoms occur, the test is considered positive, and lower concentrations are given until a dose is found that "neutralizes" the symptoms. Double-blind testing conducted by researchers at the University of California demonstrated that these procedures are not valid (37).

The American Academy of Allergy and Immunology, the nation's largest professional organization of allergists, has warned that "although the idea that the environment is responsible for a multitude of health problems is very appealing, to present such ideas as facts, conclusions, or even likely mechanisms without adequate support, is poor medical practice" (38). Chapter 95 describes the appropriate diagnosis of food allergies.

"Yeast Infections"

"Candidiasis hypersensitivity" is an alleged condition with multiple symptoms similar to those of "environmental illness." The American Academy of Allergy and Immunology regards this diagnosis as "speculative and unproven." Nevertheless, proponents claim that if a careful checkup does not reveal a cause for such symptoms, and a medical history includes antibiotic usage, a "yeast" problem is likely (39). The proposed treatment program includes food supplements, special diets, and treatment with antifungal drugs. In 1990, a double-blind trial found the antifungal drug nystatin was no better than a placebo for relieving systemic or psychologic symptoms attributed to "candidiasis hypersensitivity syndrome" (40).

"Leaky Gut Syndrome"

Proponents describe "leaky gut syndrome" (also called intestinal dysbiosis) as a condition in which the intestinal lining becomes irritated and porous so unwanted food particles, "toxins," bacteria, parasites, and *Candida* enter the bloodstream and result in a weakened immune system, digestive disorders, and eventually chronic and autoimmune disease. Treatment of this alleged condition can include dietary changes (e.g., not eating protein and starch at the same meal), "cleansing" with herbal products, "reestablishing good balance" of intestinal bacteria, and supplement concoctions claimed to strengthen and repair the intestinal lining.

"Amalgam Toxicity"

Alleged "amalgam toxicity" (also called "amalgam illness") is diagnosed by a few hundred dentists and physicians who claim that the mercury in amalgam fillings is toxic and causes a wide range of illnesses. They recommend replacing these fillings with other materials, which can cost thousands of dollars. Some recommend an elaborate program of supplements to minimize negative effects said to occur when the amalgam fillings are removed. The American Dental Association Council on Ethics, Bylaws, and Judicial Affairs considers the unnecessary removal of amalgam fillings "improper and unethical" (41). The leading antiamalgamist, a dentist, had his license revoked in 1996. The National Council Against Health Fraud has concluded that amalgam fillings are safe, that antiamalgam activities endanger public welfare, and that so-called "mercury-free dentistry" is substandard practice (42).

Many physicians accustomed to rendering the foregoing "fad diagnoses" have added chronic fatigue syndrome, Lyme disease, food allergies, and "parasites" to their list of overdiagnosed conditions.

CHELATION THERAPY

Chelation therapy is a series of intravenous infusions of disodium ethylenediaminetetraacetic acid (EDTA), vitamins, and various other substances. It is sometimes done by swallowing EDTA or other agents in pill form. Proponents claim that chelation is effective against coronary artery disease, peripheral vascular disease, Alzheimer disease, multiple sclerosis, amyotrophic lateral sclerosis, autism, and many other serious medical problems. However, (a) no

well-designed research has shown that chelation can help any of these conditions, (b) well-designed studies have yielded negative results (43), (c) further use for these conditions has no scientifically plausible rationale, and (d) using chelation instead of proven treatments (e.g., coronary bypass surgery) can have fatal consequences.

Many chelation therapists use hair analysis or other bogus laboratory tests to diagnose nonexistent "poisoning" with lead, mercury, or other heavy metals. Although chelation therapy can be used to treat actual heavy metal poisoning, genuine chelation therapy uses calcium EDTA and a much shorter timetable.

Some chelationists allege that childhood autism is caused by mercury toxicity and treatable with chelation. However, no scientific evidence indicates that autism has a toxic cause or is associated with abnormal levels of heavy metals. Some chelationists claim to treat "mercury poisoning" produced by amalgam dental fillings. However, the mercury in amalgam is chemically bound so significant amounts do not enter the body.

In 1998, the Federal Trade Commission secured a consent agreement barring the leading chelationist organization from falsely advertising that chelation therapy is effective against atherosclerosis or any other circulatory problem. The agreement is binding only on the group itself, not to its individual members. The National Council Against Health Fraud believes that chelation therapy is unethical and should be banned and that chelation therapy of autistic children should be considered child abuse (44).

QUESTIONABLE CANCER THERAPIES

The American Cancer Society describes alternative treatments as "unproven because they have not been scientifically tested, or they were tested and found to be ineffective" (45). These include corrosive agents, plant products, special diets and "dietary supplements," drugs, correction of "imbalances," biologic methods, devices, miscellaneous concoctions, and psychologic approaches. Many promoters combine methods to make themselves more marketable.

Promoters of questionable cancer treatment typically explain their approach in commonsense terms that appear to offer patients an active role: (a) cancer is a symptom, not a disease; (b) symptoms are caused by diet, stress, or environment; and (c) proper fitness, nutrition, and mental attitude allow biologic and mental defense against cancer. Nutrition-related methods are compatible with each of these "selling points" and therefore are highly marketable. They include fasting, megadoses of nutrients, consumption of raw foods, "detoxification," organ extracts, and various dietary regimens. The American Cancer Society advises that although dietary measures (e.g., eating more vegetables) may help to prevent certain cancers, no scientific evidence indicates that any dietary regimen is appropriate as a primary *treatment* for cancer (46).

Laetrile

Laetrile, which achieved great notoriety during the 1970s and early 1980s, is the trade name for a synthetic relative of amygdalin, a chemical in the kernels of apricot pits, apple seeds, bitter almonds, and some other stone fruits and nuts. Some promoters have called it "vitamin B_{17}" and falsely claimed that cancer is a vitamin deficiency disease that laetrile can cure. When subjected to enzymatic breakdown in the body, amygdalin forms glucose, benzaldehyde, and hydrogen cyanide. Some patients with cancer who were treated with laetrile have suffered nausea, vomiting, headache, and dizziness, and a few have died of cyanide poisoning (47).

Laetrile has been tested in at least 20 animal tumor models and found to have no benefit either alone or together with other substances. Studies of case reports of humans have also been uniformly negative, as has a clinical trial sponsored by the National Cancer Institute (NCI) (47–49).

In 1975, a patient sued in federal court to try to stop the FDA from interfering with the sale and distribution of laetrile. Early in the case, a sympathetic judge issued orders allowing patients with cancer to import a 6-month supply of laetrile for personal use if they could obtain a physician's affidavit that they were "terminal." A higher court partially upheld this ruling, but in 1979 the US Supreme Court ruled that it is not possible to be certain who is terminal and that even if it were possible, both terminally ill patients and the general public deserve protection from fraudulent cures. In 1987, after further appeals were denied, the judge who set up the affidavit system finally yielded to the higher courts and terminated it (50). Today, few sources of laetrile are available within the United States, but it still is used at Mexican clinics.

Gerson Method

Proponents of the Gerson diet claim that cancer can be cured only if toxins are eliminated from the body. They recommend "detoxification" with frequent coffee enemas and a low-sodium diet that includes more than a gallon a day of juices made from fruits, vegetables, and raw calf's liver. This method was developed by Max Gerson, a German-born physician who emigrated to the United States in 1936 and practiced in New York City until his death in 1959. Still available at a Mexican clinic, Gerson therapy is actively promoted by his daughter, Charlotte Gerson, through lectures, talk show appearances, and publications. Gerson protocols have included liver extract injections, ozone and coffee enemas, "live cell therapy," thyroid tablets, royal jelly capsules, linseed oil, castor oil enemas, clay packs, laetrile, and vaccines made from influenza virus and killed *Staphylococcus aureus* bacteria.

Charlotte Gerson claims that treatment at the clinic has produced high cure rates for many cancers. In 1986, however, a Gerson publicist admitted that patients were not monitored after they left the facility (51). Three naturopaths who visited the Gerson Clinic in 1983 were able to track 18 patients over a 5-year period (or until death) through annual letters or phone calls. At the 5-year mark, only one was still alive (but not cancer free); the rest had succumbed to their cancer (52).

A review of the Gerson rationale has concluded that (a) the "poisons" Gerson claimed were present in processed foods have never been identified, (b) frequent coffee enemas have never been shown to mobilize and remove poisons from the liver and intestines of patients with cancer, (c) there is no evidence that any such poisons are related to the onset of cancer, (d) there is no evidence that a healing inflammatory reaction exists that can seek out and kill cancer cells (53).

Kelley/Gonzalez Metabolic Therapy

In the 1960s, William Donald Kelley, D.D.S., developed a program for patients with cancer that involved dietary measures, vitamin and enzyme supplements, and computerized "metabolic typing." Kelley classified people as "sympathetic dominant," "parasympathetic dominant," or metabolically "balanced" and made dietary recommendations for each type. He claimed that his "Protein Metabolism Evaluation Index" could diagnose cancer before it was clinically apparent and that his "Kelley Malignancy Index" could detect "the presence or absence of cancer, the growth rate of the tumor, the location of the tumor mass, prognosis of the treatment, age of the tumor and the regulation of medication for treatment"(54).

In 1970, Kelley was convicted of practicing medicine without a license after witnesses testified that he had diagnosed lung cancer on the basis of blood from a patient's finger and prescribed dietary supplements, enzymes, and a diet as treatment. In 1976, following court appeals, his dental license was suspended for 5 years. However, he continued to promote his methods until the mid-1980s through his Dallas-based International Health Institute. Under the institute's umbrella, licensed professionals and "certified metabolic technicians" throughout the United States would administer a 3200-item questionnaire and send the answers to Dallas. The resultant computer printout provided a lengthy report on "metabolic status" plus detailed instructions covering foods, supplements (typically 100–200 pills per day), "detoxification" techniques, and lifestyle changes.

Treatment said to be similar is still provided today by Nicholas Gonzalez, M.D., of New York City, who claims to have analyzed Kelley's records and drafted a book about his findings. The manuscript was never published, but experts who evaluated its chapter on 50 cases found no evidence of benefit (55). Gonzalez says that he offers "10 basic diets with 90 variations" and typically prescribes coffee enemas and "up to 150 pills a day in 10 to 12 divided doses."

In 1997, a jury awarded $2.65 million in damages to a former Gonzalez patient. The woman had been diagnosed with an early stage of uterine cancer and underwent a hysterectomy. The woman testified that Gonzalez encouraged her to rely on his treatment instead of medically recommended radiation and chemotherapy. Later he claimed that her cancer was cured, even though it was progressing. It eventually damaged her spine and left her blind.

Shark Cartilage

Powdered shark cartilage is purported to contain a protein that inhibits the growth of new blood vessels needed for the spread of cancer. Although a modest effect has been observed in laboratory experiments, it has not been demonstrated that feeding shark cartilage to humans significantly inhibits blood vessel formation in patients with cancer. Even if direct applications were effective, oral administration would not work because the protein would be digested rather than absorbed intact into the body. Nevertheless, in 1993, CBS television's "60 Minutes" aired a program promoting the claims of biochemist entrepreneur I. William Lane, Ph.D., coauthor of *Sharks Don't Get Cancer*. The program highlighted a Cuban study of 29 patients with "terminal" cancer who received shark cartilage preparations. Narrator Mike Wallace filmed several of the patients doing exercises and reported that most of them felt better several weeks after the treatment had begun. The fact that "feeling better" does not indicate whether a cancer treatment is effective was not mentioned, nor was the fact that sharks do get cancer, even of their cartilage (56). NCI officials who reviewed the Cuban data called them "incomplete and unimpressive" (57). A subsequent study found shark cartilage ineffective against advanced cancer in adults with a life expectancy of at least 12 weeks (58).

Vitamin C

The claim that vitamin C is useful for treating cancer is largely attributable to Linus Pauling, Ph.D. During the mid-1970s, Pauling began claiming that high doses of vitamin C are effective in preventing and curing cancer. In 1976 and 1978, he and a Scottish physician, Ewan Cameron, reported that a group of 100 patients with terminal cancer who were treated with 10,000 mg of vitamin C daily had survived three to four times longer than historically matched patients who did not receive vitamin C supplements. However, Dr. William DeWys, Chief of Clinical investigations at the NCI, found that the patient groups were not comparable (59). The patient's receiving vitamin C were Cameron's, whereas the other patients were managed by other physicians. Cameron's patients were started on vitamin C when he labeled them "untreatable" by other methods, and their subsequent survival was compared with the survival of the "control" patients after they were labeled untreatable by their doctors. DeWys

found that Cameron's patients were labeled untreatable much earlier in the course of their disease, which meant that they entered the hospital before they were as sick as the other doctors' patients and would naturally be expected to live longer. Nevertheless, to test whether Pauling could be correct, the Mayo Clinic in Rochester, Minnesota conducted three double-blind studies involving a total of 367 patients with advanced cancer. All three studies found that patients given 10 g of vitamin C daily did no better than those given a placebo (60–62).

POLITICAL CONSIDERATIONS

The alternative movement is part of a general societal trend toward rejection of science as a method of determining truth. This movement embraces the postmodernist doctrine that science is not necessarily more valid than pseudoscience (63). In line with this philosophy, proponents of alternative approaches assert that scientific medicine (which they mislabel as allopathic, conventional, or traditional medicine) is but one of a vast array of health care options. Instead of subjecting their work to scientific standards, they would like to change the rules by which they are judged and regulated.

Research proposals normally are funded by competing on the basis of merit. A federal law passed in 1991 ordered the National Institutes of Health (NIH) to foster research into unconventional practices. The law was passed after proponents of questionable cancer treatments convinced several members of Congress that these treatments deserved more study than they had been receiving. To carry out the law's intent, the NIH established what became the Office of Alternative Medicine (OAM). In 1998, Congress upgraded the OAM into the NIH National Center for Complementary and Alternative Medicine (NCCAM), which now has an annual budget exceeding $110 million (64).

Proponents of alternative approaches trumpeted NIH's involvement as evidence that whatever they espouse is valid. Most press reports—even in medical publications—have contained little criticism and have featured the views of proponents and their satisfied clients. Few reporters make any effort to determine whether the alternative methods they mention are useful, promising, or nonsensical. To date, despite spending more than $200 million to fund studies, the OAM/NCCAM research program has not led to any recommendation that any method be adopted by mainstream medicine or abandoned by alternative proponents. Even if useful research eventuates, the benefit is unlikely to outweigh the publicity bonanza already given to worthless methods (65).

Additional publicity was generated by a 1993 *New England Journal of Medicine* report of a telephone survey concerning 16 types of "unconventional therapy." The authors concluded that 34% of the respondents had used at least one unconventional therapy during the previous year and that US residents made an estimated 425 million visits to providers of such therapy during 1990 (66). However, the methods these investigators selected included some that are medically appropriate, such as self-help groups, and some that are appropriate under proper circumstances (relaxation therapy, biofeedback, hypnosis, massage, and commercial weight-loss clinics). (67) Although the numbers of those using alternative methods were thus inflated, most commentators have accepted as gospel the idea that "One out of three Americans uses alternative therapies."

The most extensive survey (31,000 responses) of complementary and alternative medicine use among US residents age 18 years and older found that the most common practice is health-related prayer, used by 45.2%. When prayer was excluded, 36% of US adults used some form of complementary and alternative medicine during the previous months. About 18.9% reported using herbal products and other nonvitamin or nonmineral dietary supplements, 7.5% reported using chiropractic care, 2.8% reported using orthomolecular therapy, and 1.7% reported using homeopathy during the previous year. The percentages using ayurveda, naturopathy, and chelation therapy were between 0.0 and 0.2% (68).

Promoters of alternative approaches would like to weaken or overturn the laws that protect against methods that are ineffective or are promoted with misinformation. During the height of the laetrile controversy, 27 states legalized the manufacture and sale of laetrile within their borders. Within the past decade, a few states have passed "medical freedom of choice" bills. these prevent or make it difficult for their licensing boards to discipline practitioners who use an inappropriate treatment, as long as it does not directly threaten the life or health of the patient. A federal "Access to Medical Treatment Act" has been introduced to prevent the FDA from protecting the public against the sale and distribution of questionable drugs and devices. The 1976 Proxmire Amendment to the Food, Drug, and Cosmetic Act and the 1994 Dietary Supplement Health Education Act (DSHEA) prevent the FDA from regulating the dosage of vitamin, mineral, amino acid, and herbal products unless it can prove in court that a product is inherently unsafe. Although the American Medical Association Council on Scientific Affairs has urged that courses offered by medical schools on alternative medicine "present the scientific view of unconventional theories, treatments, and practice as well as the potential therapeutic utility, safety, and efficacy of these modalities" (69), pressure by proponents and the lure of grant money have led to the creation of courses, departments, and clinics that may promote unscientific methods (70).

Proponents claim that such laws increase individual freedom without increasing consumer risk. This is untrue. The basic principle of health-related consumer protection law is that products should not be marketed until demonstrated safe and effective by appropriate testing. Physi-

cians and drug companies wishing to test new products can obtain FDA permission by showing reasonable preliminary evidence of safety and potential usefulness. This policy is not oppressive; it simply requires that studies be carried out as outlined earlier in this chapter. "Medical freedom" laws facilitate the sale of worthless treatments and make it difficult to prevent unscientific practitioners from exploiting patients. The DSHEA permits the marketing of thousands of products that have no rational use.

REFERENCES

1. Standards of Reporting Trials Group. JAMA 1994;272:1926–31.
2. Relman AS. New Republic 1998;Dec 14.
3. Zwicky JF, Hafner AW, Barrett S et al. Reader's Guide to "Alternative" Health Methods. Chicago: American Medical Association, 1993.
4. Karlowski TR, Chalmers TC, Frenkel LD et al. JAMA 1975;246:2235–7.
5. Tai D. Acupuncture and Moxibustion. St Louis: CV Mosby, 1987.
6. National Council Against Health Fraud Task Force on Acupuncture. Clin J Pain 1991;7:162–6.
7. Okada F. Lancet 1996;348:5–6.
8. Kalauokalani D, Sherman KJ, Cherkin DC. South Med J 2001;94:486–92.
9. Lad V. Ayurveda: The Science of Self-Healing. Santa Fe, NM: Lotus Press, 1984.
10. Kushi M, Blauer B. The Macrobiotic Way. Wayne, NJ: Avery Publishing, 1985.
11. Dagnelie PC, van Staveren WA. Am J Clin Nutr 1989;50:818–24.
12. Anonymous. Am J Clin Nutr 1990;51:202–8.
13. Raso J. Nutr Forum 1990;7:17–21.
14. Anonymous. Macrobiotics: Standard Dietary and Way of Life Suggestions [flyer]. Brookline, MA: Kushi Institute, 1986.
15. Kushi M, Esko E. The Macrobiotic Approach to Cancer. Garden City Park, NY: Avery Publishing Group, 1991.
16. American Cancer Society. CA Cancer J Clin 1989;39:248–51.
17. Dwyer J. Nutr Forum 1990;7:9–11.
18. Pizzorno JE Jr. Let's Live 1988;56:64.
19. Pizzorno JE Jr, Murray MT, eds. A Textbook of Natural Medicine. 2nd ed. Philadelphia, WB Saunders, 1999.
20. Raso J. Nutr Forum 1990;7:33–6.
21. Lipton M, Ban TA, Kane FJ et al. Task Force Report on Megavitamin and Orthomolecular Therapy in Psychiatry. Washington, DC: American Psychiatric Association, 1973.
22. Nutrition Committee, Canadian Paediatric Society. Can Med Assoc J 1990;143:1009–13 [reaffirmed March 2004].
23. Committee on Nutrition, American Academy of Pediatrics. Pediatrics 1976;58:910–2.
24. Barrett S. http://www.quackwatch.org/01QuackeryRelatedTopics/iridology.html, revised July 23, 2001.
25. Simon A, Worthen DM, Mitas JA II. JAMA 1979;242:1385–7.
26. Knipschild P. BMJ 1988;297:1578–81.
27. South J. Nutr Forum 1988;5:61–7.
28. Homola S. Inside Chiropractic: A Patient's Guide. Amherst, NY: Prometheus Books, 1999.
29. Kenny JJ, Clemens R. J Am Diet Assoc 1988;88:698–704.
30. Christenson MG, ed. Job Analysis of Chiropractic: A Project Report, Survey Analysis, and Summary of the Practice of Chiropractic within the United States. Greeley, CO: National Board of Chiropractic Examiners, 2000.

31. Barrett S. http://www.quackwatch.org/01QuackeryRelatedTopics/gastro.html, revised December 7, 2003.

32. Barrett S. http://www.quackwatch.org/01QuackeryRelatedTopics/electro.html, revised April 26, 2004.

33. Barrett S. http://www.quackwatch.org/01QuackeryRelatedTopics/herbs.html, revised March 16, 2004.

34. Garrard J, Harms S, Eberly LE et al. Arch Intern Med 2003;163:2290–5.

35. Nelson RL. Mayo Clin Proc 1988;63:263–9.

36. Barrett S, Gots RE. Chemical Sensitivity. Amherst, NY: Prometheus Books, 1998.

37. Jewett DL, Fein G, Greenberg MH. N Engl J Med 1990;323:429–33.

38. American Academy of Allergy and Immunology. J Allergy Clin Immunol 1986;78:269–73.

39. Crook W. The Yeast Connection: A Medical Breakthrough. Jackson, TN: Professional Books, 1985.

40. Dismukes W. N Engl J Med 1990;323:1717–23.

41. Berry JH. J Am Dental Assoc 1987;115:679–85.

42. National Council Against Health Fraud. Position Paper on Amalgam Fillings. Peabody, MA: National Council Against Health Fraud, 2002.

43. Knudtson ML, Wyse DG, Galbraith PD et al. JAMA 2002;287:481–6.

44. National Council Against Health Fraud. Policy Statement on Chelation Therapy. Peabody, MA: National Council Against Health Fraud, 2002.

45. Bruss K, Salter MA, Galán E, eds. American Cancer Society's Guide to Complementary and Alternative Cancer Methods. Atlanta: American Cancer Society, 2000.

46. American Cancer Society. CA Cancer J Clin 1993;43:309–19.

47. Wilson B. http://www.quackwatch.org/01QuackeryRelatedTopics/Cancer/laetrile.html, revised Feb 17, 2004.

48. American Cancer Society. CA Cancer J Clin 1991;41:187–92.

49. Moertel C, Fleming TR, Rubin J et al. N Engl J Med 1982;306:201–6.

50. United States et al. v. Rutherford et al. Certiorari to the United States Court of Appeals for the Tenth Circuit. No. 78-605. Decided June 18, 1979.

51. Lowell J. Nutr Forum 1986;3:9–12.

52. Austin S, Dale EB, DeKadt S. J Naturopath Med 1994;5:74–6.

53. Green S. JAMA 1992;268:3224–7.

54. American Cancer Society. Kelley malignancy index and ecology therapy. In: Unproven Methods of Cancer Management. New York: Author, 1971.

55. US Congress, Office of Technology Assessment. Unconventional Cancer Treatments. OTA-H-405. Washington, DC: US Government Printing Office, 1990.

56. Barrett S, Herbert V. The Vitamin Pushers: How the "Health Food" Industry Is Selling America a Bill of Goods. Amherst, NY: Prometheus Books, 1994:370–5.

57. Mathews J. J Natl Cancer Inst 1993;85:1190–1.

58. Miller DR, Anderson GT, Stark JJ et al. J Clin Oncol 1998;16:3649–55.

59. DeWys WD. Your Patient and Cancer 1982;2:31–6.

60. Creagan ET, Moertel CG, O'Fallon JR et al. N Engl J Med 1979;301:687–90.

61. Anonymous. Proc Am Soc Clin Oncol 1983;2:92.

62. Moertel CG, Fleming TR, Creagan E et al. N Engl J Med 1985;312:137–41.

63. Sampson W. In: Gross PR, Levitt N, Lewis MW, eds. The Flight from Science and Reason. New York: New York Academy of Sciences, 1996:188–97.

64. Sampson WI. http://www.quackwatch.org/01QuackeryRelatedTopics/nccam.html, Accessed on Dec 10, 2002.

65. Barrett S. Nutr Forum 1993;10:1–5.

66. Eisenberg DM, Kessler RC, Foster C et al. N Engl J Med 1993;328:246–52.

67. Gorski T. http://Quackwatch.org/11Ind/eisenberg.html, Accessed on March 12, 2002.

68. Barnes PM, Powell-Griner E, McFann K et al. Advance Data Number 343, May 27, 2004.

69. Alternative Medicine: Report 12 of the AMA Council on Scientific Affairs (A-97), June 1997. http://www.ama-assn.org/ama/pub/article/2036-2523.html

70. Barrett S. http://www.quackwatch.org/01QuackeryRelatedTopics/peer.html, Accessed on June 14, 2004.

SELECTED READINGS

Barnes J, Anderson LA, Phillipson JD. Herbal Medicines: A Guide for Healthcare Professionals. 2nd ed. Chicago: Pharmaceutical Press, 2002.

Barrett S, Herbert V. The Vitamin Pushers: How the "Health Food" Industry Is Selling America a Bill of Goods. Amherst, NY: Prometheus Books, 1994.

Barrett S, Jarvis WT, eds. The Health Robbers: A Close Look at Quackery in America. Amherst, NY: Prometheus Books, 1993.

Barrett S, Jarvis WT, London WM et al. Consumer Health: A Guide to Intelligent Decisions. 6th ed. New York: McGraw-Hill, 2002.

Bruss K, Salter MA, Galán E, eds. American Cancer Society's Guide to Complementary and Alternative Cancer Methods. Atlanta: Author, 2000.

Quackwatch (http://www.quackwatch.org)

Zwicky JF, Hafner AW, Barrett S et al. Reader's Guide to "Alternative" Health Methods. Chicago: American Medical Association, 1993.

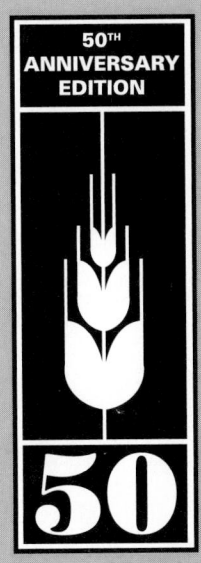

50TH ANNIVERSARY EDITION

50

PART VII

ADEQUACY, SAFETY, AND OVERSIGHT OF THE FOOD SUPPLY

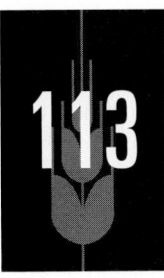

113 FOOD PROCESSING: NUTRITION, SAFETY, AND QUALITY[1]

JOHN W. FINLEY, DENISE M. DEMING, AND ROBERT E. SMITH

GENERAL PRINCIPLES 1777
   Historical Perspective .1777
   Why Food Processing .1777
CHEMISTRY IN FOOD PROCESSING 1778
   Control of Moisture .1778
   Lipid Oxidation 1778
   Browning 1779
THERMAL PROCESSING 1780
   Pasteurization 1781
   Canning 1782
   Baking 1782
   Extrusion 1783
   Breakfast Cereal Processing 1783
   Frying 1783
   Microwave 1784
IRRADIATION 1784
LOW-TEMPERATURE PROCESSING 1784
   Freezing 1784
   Dehydration 1784
   Concentration 1785
   Air Drying 1785
   Freeze Drying 1785
NEW APPROACHES IN PROCESSING 1785
   Ohmic Heating 1785
   High-Pressure Processing 1786
BIOTECHNOLOGY 1786
   Benefits 1786
   Consumer Concerns 1786
OVERVIEW OF NUTRIENT DAMAGE CAUSED BY
   PROCESSING 1787
SUMMARY 1787

GENERAL PRINCIPLES

Historical Perspective

Processing and preservation of foods can be traced to the earliest stages of civilization. The use of fire to "cook" food can be traced back to 8000 BCE. In northern climates,

[1]**Abbreviations: Aw,** water activity; **HPP,** high-pressure processing; **HTST,** high temperature, short time; **LTLT,** low temperature, long time; **OH,** ohmic heating; **UHT,** ultrahigh temperature.

ancient people used the cold environment and freezing temperatures to preserve their food. Fermentation was one of the earliest forms of preservation and food processing. For example, fermentation of grain to produce beer was reported in China as early as 2000 BCE. Preservation of milk was accomplished by combining fermentation and enzyme processing, resulting in what we know today as yogurt and cheese.

One of the most important advances in food preservation occurred in the eighteenth century, when Napoleon offered a reward for the development of a better means of food preservation to deliver an adequate supply of food for his army. Nicolas Appert demonstrated that when foods were adequately heated in sealed containers, spoilage was virtually eliminated. This was the birth of the canning industry. Fifty years later, Pasteur demonstrated that microorganisms were the major cause of food spoilage and that heat was the most effective means of preventing spoilage.

A safe food supply is the result of industry and government agencies working together to ensure appropriate handling, processing, packaging, distribution, and storage of foods. Although occasional breakdowns occur in the system, which sometimes necessitate the recall of foods, they are swiftly corrected. In fact, one of the reasons we hear about outbreaks of food-borne illness is that we have highly sophisticated means of tracing the sources of illness. Twenty-five years ago, it was difficult at best to track the source of food-borne illnesses beyond the immediate food consumed. Today, with data reporting systems and the tools of modern biotechnology, the Centers for Disease Control and Prevention can trace food illness outbreaks to single incidents in a processing plant. The result has greatly enhanced our ability to prevent food-borne illnesses.

Why Food Processing?

Food spoilage originates from three major causes: microbial, chemical, and enzymatic. Microbial contamination of food is impossible to eliminate because microorganisms originate in the soil, the water, and the air in the environment where the food is produced. However, control of endogenous microorganisms in food prevents spoilage, and because some of these organisms are pathogens, the safety of the food is also enhanced. The raw materials for foods come from living organisms, all of which contain multiple chemicals and enzymes.

Frequently, enzymes, which are essential for the life of the food organism, accelerate the postharvest loss of quality or spoilage of the food. For example, ethylene production by endogenous enzymes in tomatoes is important to the ripening process. After harvest, the production of ethylene in the tomatoes continues, and this can lead to overripening resulting in excessive softening of the fruit that renders it undesirable. One method to control postharvest ethylene production and to preserve the texture of tomatoes is to inactivate the enzymes by heat. Enzymatic activity can also be controlled through genetic engineering to extend the shelf life of the tomato and to enhance the thickness of resulting tomato paste.

Processing is also used to enhance the nutritive value of foods. For example, the carotenoids in fresh tomatoes are poorly absorbed; however, after thermal treatment, such as cooking or conversion to catsup, the carotenoids become more bioavailable. In raw corn, the vitamin niacin is not readily available, but the addition of calcium hydroxide (lime) during production of tortillas releases the niacin and increases the nutritive value of the corn.

Processing can also improve the flavor and texture of many food products and can provide convenience in preparation. The importance of quality as perceived by the consumer cannot be overemphasized. Antinutritional factors can be destroyed or eliminated by processing. For example, milling of grains into flour can be an effective way of removing mold and mold products associated with the bran layer.

Environmental factors such as pH, temperature, light, oxygen level, carbon dioxide level, and physical damage can significantly affect the shelf life of processed foods. Managing these factors can minimize spoilage and can increase nutrient retention.

CHEMISTRY IN FOOD PROCESSING

The essential elements of food processing are moisture control (increasing or decreasing water content and, more specifically, controlling the state and availability of water in the food) and thermal processing (heating or cooling).

Control of Moisture

One of the major roles of food processing in dry and intermediate-moisture foods is to control water. In reduced-moisture products, chemical and enzymatic reactions, as well as microbial growth, are influenced by water activity (Aw) of the product. For example, lipid oxidation is minimized at values of Aw between 0.3 and 0.4, whereas the browning reaction increases to a maximum at an Aw of approximately 0.7. Enzymatic activity and microbial growth tend to increase with Aw, as seen in Figure 113.1.

Aw in foods is controlled by the ratio of solutes and the moisture content of the food. Water in foods acts as a solvent and as plasticizer for macromolecules. The influence of solutes and Aw as it affects food quality and safety was reviewed in detail by Slade and Levine (1). The integrated understanding of water and glassy state dynamics focuses on the nonequilibrium nature of food products. The authors presented applicable information relevant to moisture management based on food polymer chemistry covering a broad range of food applications. Many of the applications described under drying, described later in this chapter, can be understood in greater detail through the application of food polymer chemistry.

Lipid Oxidation

Polyunsaturated fatty acids such as soy oil and fish oils are highly vulnerable to oxidation. Thus, a key concern in

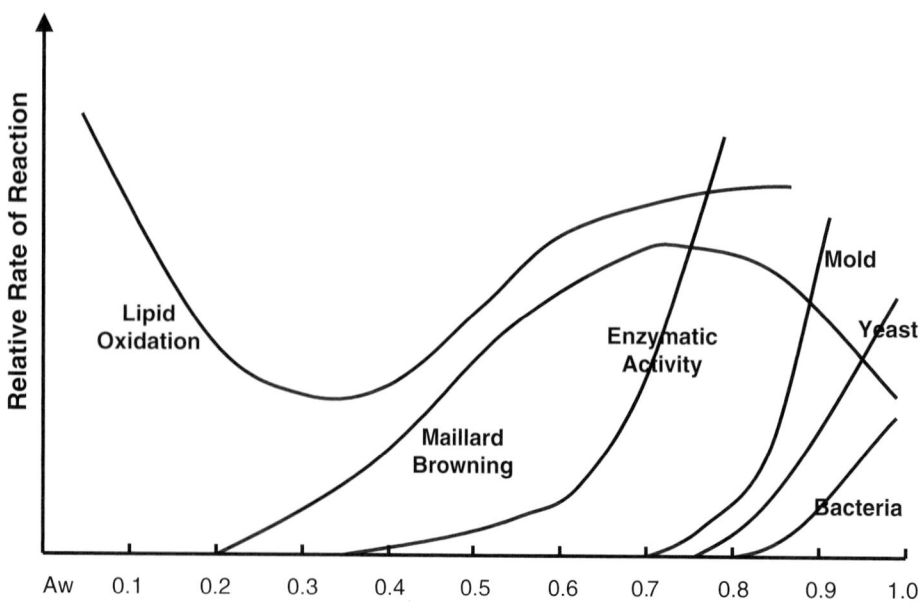

Figure 113.1. Influence of water activity on food chemistry and microbiology. (From Levine H, Slade L. Crit Rev Food Sci Nutr 1991;30:115–360, with permission.)

processing of foods containing highly unsaturated lipids is prevention of lipid oxidation. Fat-soluble vitamins, particularly vitamin E and the other tocopherol isomers, are important antioxidants that can provide protection against lipid oxidation in many food and oil systems.

The consequences of lipid oxidation are generally negative. The most obvious consequence is production of off-flavors in foods such as fishy notes in oils or grassy notes in vegetable oil products. However, mild oxidation during processing can contribute to positive flavors as in popcorn and fried foods. Oxidative stability can also be achieved by removal of metals such as iron and copper and ensuring that the oils do not contact metal surfaces and by protection from light and oxygen during processing, shipping, and storage.

Most foods are complex, heterogeneous systems in which the mobility of free radicals or oxygen permeation becomes the rate-controlling factor in lipid oxidation. Skibsted (2) used electron spin resonance/spin trapping to monitor these phenomena.

Many fat-containing systems are emulsions in which lipid oxidation is a major cause of quality deterioration in the food. The reaction mechanisms and factors that influence oxidation are different in emulsions from those in bulk lipids. McClements and Decker (3) reviewed the current understanding of the lipid oxidation mechanism in oil-in-water emulsions.

Muscle food quality is greatly affected by lipid oxidation and has been studied extensively for the effects on quality characteristics such as flavor, color, texture, nutritive value, and safety of the food. Lipid oxidation in muscle foods is initiated in the phospholipid-rich fraction in subcellular membranes that are high in polyunsaturated lipids. Oxidative damage to lipids may occur in the living animal because of an imbalance between the production of reactive oxygen species and the animal's antioxidant defense systems. Morrissey and colleagues (4) reviewed oxidation in muscle foods and the influence of vitamin E and other antioxidant micronutrients on lipid oxidation, color, water-holding capacity, and cholesterol oxidation in these foods.

ω-3 Polyunsaturated fatty acids are currently of great interest to the food and nutrition community because of their health benefits. Food products enriched in α-linolenic acid, eicosapentaenoic acid, and/or docosahexaenoic acid reduce some of the negative effects of linoleic acid, the major polyunsaturated fatty acid in our diet. Unfortunately, these fatty acids are extremely susceptible to lipid oxidation. As a result, the sensory and nutritional quality of foods enriched in ω-3 fatty acid can deteriorate quickly unless proper protection is afforded the products. The inherent instability and potential means of production have recently been reviewed (5).

Browning

The browning reaction was first described by Maillard in 1912 (6), when he reported the release of carbon dioxide

from the reaction of amino acids and sugars. Glucose and alanine react, first losing water, followed by the loss of carbon dioxide. Amadori (7) reported stable rearrangement products resulting from the reaction between amino acids and sugars. The Amadori rearrangement results in compounds that react further or degrade with continued heating, leading to the formation of colors and flavors associated with the browning reaction in foods.

In 1953, Hodge (8) clarified the understanding of the complex chemistry. Hodge's explanation described the Maillard reaction between glucose and an amino acid to yield an unstable glucosylamine that undergoes a reversible rearrangement, as described by Amadori, to yield an aminodeoxyketose. Glucose and fructose react in similar ways. These reactions can occur at room temperature during storage of foods, in vivo, and at high temperatures used in processing. Analogous reactions occur between proteins and reducing sugars both in foods and in vivo. The amino acids and sugars involved in the browning reaction lose their nutritional value. This is usually of minor consequence in the diet because the levels are relatively low. In fact, the Maillard browning reaction and associated reactions account for many of the positive attributes in cooked foods such as the aroma and flavor of cooked meat and baked products. Without the browning reaction, many products would not be as appealing. For example, a beef steak cooked to the same internal temperature in a microwave does not develop the reaction flavors that the same meat would achieve on the grill. The higher surface temperatures accelerate the development of flavors, aromas, and the brown color of foods.

Risk factors associated with the products of the Maillard reaction include loss of essential amino acids, particularly lysine, decrease in digestibility of glycosylated proteins, and production of antinutritional or toxic compounds (9). In highly processed or overcooked foods, concerns have been raised about potential carcinogenicity. One such Maillard reaction end product receiving much attention is acrylamide produced by the reaction of free asparagine and a carbonyl from a reducing sugar during the frying process (10, 11). The levels found in fried foods may reach up to 2500 ppb, although most foods are much lower than 50 ppb. Current data on acrylamide levels in foods is available through the Joint Institute for Food Safety and Applied Nutrition Web site (12). The significance of low levels of exposure of acrylamide is unknown at this time, but acrylamide is a neurotoxin and a purported animal carcinogen. However, a recent epidemiologic report failed to demonstrate any significant cancers related to dietary intake of acrylamide from food (13).

Strategies are emerging to prevent acrylamide formation in foods, including blanching (14), addition of divalent or trivalent metal ions (15), and enzymatically splitting the amide in asparagines (16). Any measures to reduce exposure to acrylamide in commercial foods, as well as those prepared by consumers in the home, must be assessed

TABLE 113.1. COMMON FOOD ANTINUTRIENTS AND ENZYMES REDUCED OR DESTROYED BY THERMAL PROCESSING

FOOD SOURCE	FACTOR	EFFECTS
Enzymes		
Cereal grains (higher moisture)	Amylase	Hydrolysis of starches
Whole grains	Proteases	Loss in dough strength
Milk	Lipase	Hydrolysis of fat, rancidity
Soy	Lipoxygenase	Lipid oxidation
Vegetables and fruit	Pectinase	Softening
Fish, shellfish, red cabbage	Thiaminase	Destruction of thiamin
Antinutrients		
Egg whites	Avidin	Biotin nonavailable
Soy beans	Lectins	Impaired nutrient absorption
Kidney beans	Hemagglutinins	Red blood cell aggregation
Turnips, beans, cabbage	Goitrogens	Limited iodine absorption
Chick peas	Lathyrogens	Disrupted collagen structure
Peas, beans, cereals	Amylase inhibitors	Slowed starch digestion
Potatoes, legumes, eggs	Trypsin inhibitors	Slowed protein digestion
Fish, shellfish, cabbage	Thiaminase	Destruction of thiamin

From Whitaker JR. Enzymes. In: Fennema O, ed. Food Chemistry. 3rd ed. New York: Marcel-Dekker, 1996:431–530, with permission.

thoroughly in terms of safety and quality. Two recent reviews (10, 17) summarized the current knowledge to date on acrylamide including analysis, levels in food, mechanisms of formation, and strategies of control.

THERMAL PROCESSING

In addition to killing pathogens and storage organisms, heat also causes multiple chemical changes in foods by inactivating enzymes. Some of these changes are highly beneficial and some are detrimental, especially when excessive heating occurs. An excellent example of the benefit of heating on food quality is the reduction of polyphenoloxidase activity in fruits, fruit juices, and vegetables. Typically, polyphenoloxidase oxidizes lower-molecular-weight phenolic compounds, thereby generating brown polymers in foods. Not only is this enzymatic browning aesthetically unpleasant, but also the oxidation of lower-molecular-weight phenolics represents a nutritional loss. More detail on the control of enzymes in food processing can be found in an extensive review by Ashie and colleagues (18). There is a growing body of evidence that phenolic compounds found in common fruits and vegetables act as antioxidants extending the shelf life of the products and also may act in vivo to scavenge reactive oxygen species, and some phenolic compounds have been shown to help delay or prevent chronic inflammatory diseases associated with aging (19).

Many foods contain enzymes in addition to polyphenoloxidase and antinutritional factors that are inactivated as a result of thermal processing. Fruits and vegetables are living organisms that have systems in place to protect the plant from invasion by microbes, insects, or other predators including humans. In many cases, we are eating the ungerminated seed. However, to preserve the food, we use thermal processing to arrest the reproductive mechanism

of the plant and to retain eating quality. Table 113.1 describes some representative antinutrients and enzymes that are reduced or eliminated by thermal processing, thereby resulting in enhanced quality, shelf life, or nutritive value (20).

Thermal processing of foods has advantages and disadvantages. Heat enhances the digestibility of proteins and complex carbohydrates. It also can enhance the quality of foods by destroying enzymes that damage flavor, color, or texture such as lipoxygenase and pectinases in fruits and vegetables. Nutrients such as vitamin B_6, folic acid, niacin, and carotenoids, in their native state, are often present in complexes limiting their bioavailability. Heat opens the complexes, and the nutrients became more available. Some foods also contain antinutritional factors, which are destroyed by heat.

Thermal processing comprises different methods of heat application including blanching, pasteurization, sterilization (e.g., canning), extrusion, microwaving, baking, and cooking in various forms. Table 113.2 summarizes some of the thermal processes applied to foods and their conditions, applications, advantages, and disadvantages (21).

Blanching is a heat treatment intended to inactivate enzymes, stabilizing the food product before further processing such as freezing, drying, or canning. Blanching is not intended to kill bacteria or sterilize the food. Blanching temperatures range from 75 to 95°C for 1 to 10 minutes using hot water, steam, microwave, or hot gas. Water blanching is used most often and affords the option of adding acid for pH control or other additives, which help to protect color or flavor retention in the product. Addition of acid enhances color retention, and minerals from the process water can improve the nutritive value of the final product.

Water-soluble vitamins and minerals tend to be lost during blanching, particularly water blanching. Vitamin C

TABLE 113.2. PARAMETERS AND BENEFITS OF THERMAL PROCESSING OPERATIONS

TREATMENT	TEMPERATURES	APPLICATIONS	ADVANTAGES	DISADVANTAGES
Blanching	75–95°C for 1–10 min	Fruits and vegetables for canning and freezing	Inhibition of damaging enzymes, air removal (canning)	Loss of water soluble vitamins and minerals
Pasteurization	LTLT: 63°C for 30 min HTST: 72°C for 10 s	Milk	Killing of pathogens, lipase; reduced spoilage organisms	Refrigeration required
UHT processing	135°C for <10 s	Milk, juices, puddings	Shelf stable, good flavor	Costly aseptic packaging
Canning	115–125°C for 10–120 min (303 can)	Fruits, vegetables, canned meats	Shelf stable	Nutrient losses, damaged texture
Baking	175–260°C for 4–30 min	Bread, cookies, sweet goods	Flavor development and preservation	Loss of vitamins from browning reaction
Frying	170->200°C	Potatoes, meat, fish	Flavor and texture development	Browning, thermal losses and high fat absorption
Extrusion	115–200°C for 10–90 s	Expanded snacks	Rapid processing, texture	High cost

HTST, high temperature, short time; LTLT, low temperature, long time; UHT, ultrahigh temperature.
From Nelson PE. Hortscience 1972;7:13–5, with permission.

losses from leaching into the water range from 10 to 50%, and thiamin losses range from 9 to 60% (22). Steam blanching retains more water-soluble vitamins because there is less leaching (23). Steam blanching can be used to process larger quantities of foods than microwave blanching (24).

Blanching of fruit greatly increased the radical-scavenging activity of the fruit juice, which is associated with higher recovery of anthocyanin pigments and total cinnamates (25). Table 113.3 summarizes blanching and drying conditions for a variety of fruits. It also shows fruits that do not require blanching before drying (26).

Pasteurization

The purpose of pasteurization is to eliminate pathogens, to reduce spoilage organisms, and to inactivate enzymes that can damage the quality of the product. In highly acidic

foods such as jellies and jams, pasteurization is sufficient to protect the product. Nutrient losses during pasteurization of acid products are minor because most nutrients are heat stable under acidic conditions (27).

Milk is a primary example of a pasteurized product. Milk is pasteurized under three different regimens:

1. Low temperature, long time (LTLT) (63°C for 30 minutes)
2. High temperature, short time (HTST) (72°C for 15 seconds)
3. Ultrahigh temperature (UHT) (135°C for <10 seconds)

The UHT process results in milk that is commercially sterile and does not require refrigeration. The higher the temperature is, the shorter the process time required to pasteurize the milk. The benefit of the HTST regimen is that there is equal or better killing of bacteria with considerably less nutrient loss. A 10°C change in process

TABLE 113.3. BLANCHING AND DRYING TIMES FOR SELECTED FRUITS

FRUIT	BLANCHING TIME		DRYING TIME	
	METHOD	MIN	METHOD	h
Apple	Steam	5	Sun	36–48
			Oven	8–12
Apricots	Steam	3–4	Sun	24–36
	Water	4–5	Oven	24–36
Figs	Not necessary		Sun	48–60
			Oven	12–20
Grapes, seedless	Not necessary		Sun	36–60
			Oven	12–20
Peaches	Steam	8	Sun	36–60
	Water	8	Oven	36–48
Pears	Steam	6	Sun	60
	Water	8	Oven	24–36

From Brady PL. Drying. In: Master Food Preserver Manual. Little Rock, AR: University of Arkansas Cooperative Extension Service, 1988, with permission.

temperature produces about a tenfold increase in bacterial kill. The same temperature increase doubles the rate of chemical reactions; thus, there is less chemical degradation of nutrients, as well as a significant benefit in killing microorganisms (28). Most milk in the United States is processed by the HTST process.

The UHT process is useful where refrigeration is not available. It is also used with specialty dairy products to obtain a longer shelf life. Pasteurization conditions for milk are targeted to eliminate the heat-stable pathogen *Coxiella burnetii*, the organism responsible for Q fever. Most vitamins in milk are stable to either LTLT or HTST conditions. The exclusion of oxygen during processing and storage helps to protect nutrients including folic acid, vitamin C, and vitamin B_{12}, which are vulnerable to oxidation. The UHT process is used to sterilize juices and other low-viscosity products such as ready-to-eat puddings. The flavor, texture, and nutritional quality of aseptically packaged materials is far superior to those of retorted products (28).

Canning

Canning, sometimes known as retorting, uses heat to sterilize food products commercially and thereby to extend their shelf life at ambient temperature. The retort process can also include glass or plastic jars, tray packs, and flexible pouches. The temperatures for sterilization vary depending on the food, but temperatures of the product typically exceed 80°C for extended times, depending on thermal conductivity of the product and the size and shape of the container.

The canning process destroys most pathogenic bacteria and spoilage organisms. The maximum allowable bacteria count is 1×10^{-12} per container. The residual bacteria are nonpathogenic organisms and spores that are extremely heat stable. The additional heat required to destroy these organisms would cause significant damage to the nutritive and organoleptic quality of the food (27).

Flame sterilization is an HTST process in which cans are rotated through gas burners. This process causes more convection in the container and therefore more rapid and even heating than other approaches. Products with high levels of particulates are amenable to such processing. Agitated retorts (gas fired or steam) result in more rapid and more even heating, which translates to less nutrient loss during the process (29).

The food industry is now using more retort pouches for food delivery. These pouches are heat-stable, flexible, heat-sealable, polymeric laminates capable of withstanding thermal processing temperatures. The polymeric laminates consist of layers of paper, polymers, and aluminum (30). Processing time can frequently be shorter because the pouches have a greater surface-to-volume ratio and the heat can penetrate to the center more rapidly. The result of less heat is lower potential for thermal damage of nutrients during processing and improved organoleptic quality.

Canning is widely used for juices, fruits, and vegetables. Vegetables are especially prone to extensive nutrient losses caused by long times at high temperatures required for sterilization. Several studies summarized by Prochaska and coworkers (31) demonstrated that the canning process adversely affects the nutrient content of most vegetables, especially peas and spinach and, to a lesser extent, tomatoes. When vegetables are canned, the water-soluble nutrients are distributed between the product and the water in the package. It has been reported that 30% of the thiamin is found in the liquid portion of canned vegetables (32). Minerals such as manganese, cobalt, and zinc migrate to the water surrounding spinach, tomatoes, and beans.

Several studies also demonstrated *trans-cis* isomerization of carotenoids in vegetables after canning. Significant increases in *cis* isomers of β-carotene of 30 to 50% were observed following canning of carrots and spinach (33, 34), the consequences of which may affect the vitamin A value of vegetables (35). However, thermal processing of lycopene-rich tomatoes and xanthophyll-rich vegetables resulted in relatively smaller increases in *cis*-lycopene (< 10%) (36, 37) and *cis*-xanthophylls (lutein, ~22%; zeaxanthin, ~17%), respectively (38).

Baking

Baking is one of the most popular forms of heat processing both commercially and in the home. Baking damages water-soluble vitamins, particularly thiamin and the basic amino acids, as a result of the browning reaction that takes place during the process. However, the same browning reaction produces many of the desirable flavors in baked products. The browning reaction is most intense in the outer layers (crust) of the baked product, where temperatures are the highest.

The temperatures reached in baking denature the cereal proteins and significantly enhance their digestibility. In fermented baked goods such as bread, the levels of some water-soluble vitamins are increased, but the increase is trivial in terms of the total diet. Similarly, it has been shown that action of the yeast releases some nutrients from complexes that exist in the raw grains (39).

Most vitamins are stable to the mildly acidic conditions of fermentation. In chemically leavened products such as cookies and crackers, the pH of the dough can become slightly alkaline, which results in losses of thiamin. Mild losses of riboflavin and niacin also occur in chemically leavened products. The niacin in grain is bound and consequently is poorly used by humans. However, the baking process appears to release the niacin, thus making it significantly more available. It is likely that this release of niacin is similar to the release of niacin in corn with alkaline treatment (40).

Most commercial baked goods in the United States are produced with fortified flour. The bread baking process does not appear to cause any significant damage to the availability of the fortified nutrients. However, yeast fermentation produces phytase, an enzyme that releases bound phytic acid, a strong chelating agent for minerals, particularly calcium and zinc. Chemical leavening has no effect on phytic acid (40).

Extrusion

Extrusion is a process in which foods are rapidly cooked under heat and pressure generated as the product progresses through an extruder barrel. Expansion occurs at the exit from the extruder. Extruders can also be used as chemical reactors to derivatize starch or other ingredients. Extrusion is a rapid and economical method to cook and simultaneously develop unique textures in food products. It is typically used in grain and soy-based products with applications in pet foods, expanded breakfast cereals, expanded or puffed snacks, textured vegetable proteins, meat analogs, and pasta.

Wide ranges of processing conditions are used in the extrusion of foods. Temperatures during extrusion processing range from 140 to 180°C with very high pressures at the outlet of the die (60–80 bar). The residence time is 15 seconds to 1 minute. The combination of high temperature and shear provides several benefits. Crisp snack extrusion starts with the ingredient (i.e., corn meal) at less than 18% moisture. In extrusion of products such as pasta and formed products, moistened flour (~30%) is forced through a dye to form the precise shape of the dye. Typical temperatures used for pasta extrusions are less than 60°C for 1 to 2 minutes. Ingredients for the formation of formed cereals may be precooked, whereas pasta doughs are uncooked.

The impact of extrusion on nutritional quality of products depends on the conditions. The cooking process in extrusion generally enhances digestibility of the starches and proteins and can be effective in removing antinutrients. Under more extreme conditions of extrusion, losses in lysine can take place (41). An additional advantage to extrusion is that the short exposure time of ingredients to high temperatures minimizes damage to vitamins.

Breakfast Cereal Processing

Ready-to-eat breakfast cereals are prepared in a variety of ways, resulting in products that are flaked, gun puffed, shredded, oven puffed, extruded, expanded, and clustered. The operations used to process cereals include blending, cooking, drying, tempering, flaking, toasting, extrusion, and gun puffing.

For cornflakes, field corn is dry milled to remove the bran and the germ. The remaining pieces, which represent one third to one half the original kernel, are combined with water, sugar, malt syrup, and salt. The mixture is then cooked in pressure vessels for 1 to 2 hours with steam at 15 to 18 psi. The grits are cooled and tempered and are then rolled at high pressure (≤40 tons) at temperatures of 43 to 46°C. The rolled flakes are then toasted for 90 seconds at temperatures from 274 to 329°C.

Wheat products typically start with whole soft wheat. The cooking process is similar to that for corn, although wheat cooks more rapidly than corn (30 minutes vs 1–2 hours). Flaking and toasting are similar to these processes in corn.

Gun puffing is usually done with whole rice or whole wheat. The grain is moistened and loaded into the pressure vessel, which is preheated to 200 to 260°C. The vessel is sealed and heated with gas flames until the internal pressure reaches 200 psi. When the pressure is achieved ,the gas is shut off, and the gun is fired by opening the lid on one end, releasing the grain, which expands with the sudden loss in pressure.

During shredding, wheat is cooked until the entire endosperm is translucent (30–35 minutes at boiling water temperatures). After cooking and cooling, the grain is held for about 24 hours. The wheat is then squeezed between two rollers, one of which is grooved. Multiple sets of rollers are used to lay down multiple layers of shreds. The shreds are then cut into biscuits and are baked at 200 to 315°C. Shredded wheat tends to be more susceptible to lipid oxidation than other ready-to-eat cereal products because the unsaturated fats are spread over the high surface area of the product.

Cereal grains are rich in B vitamins, iron, copper, and magnesium. Because of the heat treatments involved in production of breakfast cereals, labile vitamins such as thiamin are lost. These nutrients are generally replaced, and cereals are further supplemented with B vitamins, vitamin E, and minerals. Some ready-to-eat cereals provide 100% of the recommended dietary allowance for B vitamins and minerals (42).

Frying

Frying foods results in three major changes: (a) physical changes that result from water losses as steam and exchange of fat between the material being fried and the frying oil, (b) chemical interactions between the frying oil and the components in the food, and (c) changes in the food resulting from dehydration and high temperatures of frying (43). Fried foods are heated by direct contact with oil at temperatures ranging from 130° C to more than 200° C. The result is that the surface of the food reaches a much higher temperature than the internal portion, which rarely reaches 100°C.

Frying, like other forms of thermal processing, can result in a variety of chemical reactions, many of which lead to the fried flavors that consumers enjoy. In addition to changing flavor compounds in foods, the frying process also results in substantial oxidation of the frying oil. The rate of oxidation and polymerization of frying oils depends on temperature, time of use, and the chemical nature of the material being fried. Lipid oxidation results in reactive compounds that can interact with food components to affect nutritional quality. For example, aldehydes can react with lysine to render it unavailable. With increased lipid oxidation, there is also a greater likelihood that labile vitamins will be destroyed by reactive oxygen species.

Microwave

In microwave cooking, the energy from electromagnetic waves that are applied to the food induces vibration in any molecule that has a dipole moment. This vibration ultimately leads to the production of heat. Microwave processing is used in the food processing for a variety of products. Its greatest consumer impact is in home cooking. Industrially, microwave heating is used to temper meats for slicing. Frozen blocks of meat are brought to a uniform temperature just below freezing for cutting, slicing, or chopping. After cutting, the products are then reformed and refrozen.

The influence of microwave cooking on vitamin stability was reviewed by Gerster (44). In the review, it was concluded that when heat-sensitive vitamins such as vitamins C, B$_1$, and B$_2$ are used as markers, the retention or loss during blanching, cooking, and reheating of food in the microwave oven is comparable to the retention with conventional methods of heating. The same report suggested that thawing frozen food in a microwave resulted in somewhat higher nutrient retention than thawing in a refrigerator or at room temperature. The use of commercial microwave techniques to heat viscous fluids has been shown to be superior to conventional heating through a wall (heat exchanger or vessel) (45). When heating viscous liquids, Thorn and Yeow (46) reported greater thiamin retention at equivalent sporicidal levels.

IRRADIATION

Food irradiation is the process of exposing food to a controlled source of ionizing radiation for the purpose of reduction of microbial load, destruction of pathogens, extension of product shelf life, and/or disinfestations of produce (47). Irradiation has received approval for use in several food categories from the United States. The primary benefit of food irradiation is for safety. According to the Centers for Disease Control and Prevention (48), each year US residents suffer 76 million infections, 325,000 hospitalizations, and approximately 5000 deaths resulting from pathogen-contaminated foods. These events carry an estimated annual health care cost totaling $7 billion.

Ionizing radiation includes γ rays (from radioactive isotopes cobalt-60 or cesium-137), β rays generated by electron beam or "E-beam," and x-rays. The level of microbial reduction depends on the dose absorbed by the target food. γ Rays and x-rays are able to penetrate further into foods than β rays.

The need to eliminate bacterial pathogens from ready-to-eat food products by the use of irradiation must always be balanced with the maintenance of product quality. In general, macronutrient (protein, lipid, and carbohydrate) quality does not suffer as a result of irradiation, and minerals have been shown to remain stable. In most studies, vitamins have been shown to retain substantial levels of activity after irradiation. Vitamins A, C, and E are more sensitive, especially at higher levels of irradiation, and thiamin is most vulnerable. Irradiation has been shown to cause off-odors and flavors in milk, certain cheeses, eggs, and some fruits and vegetables; therefore, these products are not candidates for irradiation.

LOW-TEMPERATURE PROCESSING

Freezing

Freezing can significantly slow down microbial and chemical changes in food. Some chemical reactions can occur at freezer temperatures. This happens in foods such as fruit, vegetables, and meat that retain 2 to 5% of their total water content in the liquid phase. Freezing creates water crystals, which increase the solute concentration of this water and lower its freezing point, thereby enhancing the potential for chemical reactions. Additional problems occur because increased solute concentration causes movement of water by osmosis between food compartments. Ice crystal formation also ruptures the cell structure and causes components of the food to mix. Moreover, the complexity of these changes occurring in the food matrix makes it difficult to predict the effects on quality and shelf life of frozen foods.

When processed according to good manufacturing practices and consumed within their recommended storage lives, frozen foods often have a nutritional profile equivalent to that of their fresh counterparts (49). New processing developments can improve organoleptic properties, which may have significant effects on the nutritional value of frozen foods. Fletcher (49) described examples of potential new developments in freezing including less damaging blanching techniques, lower-temperature freezing, and the use of antifreeze proteins in foods systems (50, 51).

Dehydration

Several traditional and commercial processes are used to dehydrate foods. The effects of drying methods on nutrient stability are a function of temperature and time and vary greatly with the product being treated. For example, freeze drying results in the highest-quality products, with typical thiamin retention of 95%. Protein quality can be adversely affected by loss of available lysine as a result of the browning reaction. In the case of soy products, nutritional quality is improved as a result of the heat from drying, because the trypsin inhibitor activity is reduced.

Concentration

Liquid foods such as milk and juices are typically concentrated. Concentration methods range from heating under vacuum to membrane and freeze concentration. Thermal concentration under vacuum typically applies a vacuum of around 175 mm Hg, which allows water to be evaporated at 65°C. Freeze concentration is applied to foods that will not tolerate heating. Water is partially crystallized and is removed, thus enriching the juice. This method is typically applied to heat-sensitive liquid products to minimize nutrient losses.

Membrane processing is increasingly used for the removal and separation of desired fractions and well as for concentration. Membranes of various exclusion limits are applied to separate milk proteins, particularly whey. Whey proteins are fractionated, separating β-lactoglobulin, α-lactalbumin, and glycomacropeptide, and are now commercially available with minimal damage to functionality after drying.

Air Drying

Air-dried products are dehydrated under a constant stream of warm air until the moisture content is reduced. Herbs, spices, vegetables, and fruits are candidates for air drying. However, to maintain quality, these products must be prepared for drying as soon as possible after harvesting. Air-dried products are suitable for soups, dips and sauce mixes, bakery mixes, and canned foods.

During the first part of the drying process, the air temperature is relatively high, that is, 150 to 160°F (65–70°C), so moisture can evaporate quickly from the food. Because food loses heat during rapid evaporation, the air temperature can be high without increasing the temperature of the food. As soon as surface moisture is lost, however, the outside begins to feel dry, the rate of evaporation slows down, and the food becomes warm.

The air temperature must then be reduced to about 140°F (60°C). Toward the end of the drying process, the food can scorch easily, so careful monitoring is required at this stage. Each fruit and vegetable has a critical temperature, above which a scorched taste develops. The temperature should be high enough to evaporate moisture from the food, but not high enough to cook the food.

Rapid dehydration is desirable. The higher the temperature and the lower the humidity, the more rapid the rate of dehydration will be. The drying process can destroy some of the vitamins, especially A and C. Exposing fruit to sulfur dioxide before drying helps to retain vitamins A and C, but sulfur dioxide destroys thiamin.

Freeze Drying

Frozen food products are placed in a refrigerated vacuum system, and the ice in the product is sublimated into water vapor. The cell structure remains intact, and the products retain the color, shape, flavor, and nutritional value of the original ingredient better than other methods of drying. An advantage of freeze drying is that the finished product is easily rehydrated and is suitable for sauces, soups, noodle bowls, baby foods, and any other food product for which a high-quality, minimally processed ingredient is needed.

NEW APPROACHES IN PROCESSING

Ohmic Heating

Ohmic heating (OH) is a thermal process in which heat is internally generated by the passage of an alternating current through a material that serves as an electrical resistance (52). As an alternative to thermal methods, OH can ensure the benefits of safety and preservation of conventional heating while attenuating the thermal destruction of nutrients. More specifically, OH is a high-temperature, short-time method that can heat an 80% solids food product from room temperature to 129°C in approximately 90 seconds, and this method decreases the damaging effects of overprocessing at high temperatures.

The food industry's interest in OH stems from the development of aseptic processing of low-acid foods, particularly those that contain particulates and liquid. Conventional heating transfers heat from the liquid carrier to the particulates, so the time required to heat the interior of the particulate sufficiently results in overprocessing. However, overprocessing is avoidable in OH because both phases heat simultaneously, and under some conditions the particulates can heat faster than the liquid. This is called heating inversion and is not possible by traditional heating methods (53).

Sufficient heat is generated during OH to achieve pasteurization and sterilization temperatures in foods (54). In general, pasteurization involves heating high-acid foods (pH < 4.5) to 90 to 95°C for 30 to 90 seconds to inactivate vegetative bacteria, yeasts, molds, and lactobacilli. Because low-acids foods (pH > 4.5) can support the growth of *Clostridum botulinum*, they require heating to at least 121°C for a minimum of 3 minutes to achieve sterility. OH is an effective method to pasteurize milk and has been successful in producing high-quality viscous products and foods containing combinations of particulates such as meat, vegetables, pasta, or fruits, in a viscous medium (55).

Although OH is a unique thermal process with many potential uses, some major challenges currently hinder its full acceptance and commercialization. First, studies investigating the potential benefits of OH on nutrient retention in foods are limited, and more studies are needed to optimize critical process factors to achieve food safety and improve nutrient retention. Second, the commercialization of OH is limited by the lack of temperature monitoring techniques in continuous throughput systems and knowledge of critical processing factors affecting heating using OH.

High-Pressure Processing

One of the most successful new technologies for food preservation is high-pressure processing (HPP) to pasteurize foods nonthermally. HPP foods have been available in Japan since 1990 and in the United States and Europe since 1996. Many common foods are HPP processed including jams, fruit juices, acidic sauces and fruit used in yogurt (56), as well as dairy products, fish, and vacuum-packed meat products (57).

HPP involves the use of one or more pulses of high pressure applied isostatically to the food material; the pressure is applied equally throughout the material being processed (58). This method eliminates gradients in the food material, which are common in the application of heat and other processes. Pasteurization of vegetables or fruit is accomplished by applying a single pulse of pressure of 500 atmospheres (Mpa) at 20°C. Sterilization of vegetables is realized with two pulses of 1000 Mpa at 75°C. Some processes can go as high as 6000 Mpa. Because organoleptic properties of vegetables are changed when treated with pressure greater than 300 Mpa, the use of moderate pressures in combination with other treatment conditions appears to reduce populations of microorganisms while avoiding these undesirable changes (59).

In general, HPP can inactivate vegetative microorganisms, whereas bacterial spores appear to be more resistant to HPP. Environmental factors include pressure, time, temperature, and strain-to-strain differences. These factors make it more difficult accurately to predict that a specific HPP treatment, compared with a specific heat treatment, will inactivate microorganisms in a specific food material (58). However, several studies summarized by Knorr and coworkers (60, 61) indicate the possibility of reducing bacterial spores through a combination treatment of mild heat and HPP. Other combination techniques can also be effective in reducing spores. For example, the presence of bacteriocins can amplify the effect of HHP against *Bacillus coagulans* spores (62).

One of the important aspects of HPP is that food can be processed with minimal effect on color, flavor, taste, and texture and with little or no loss of vitamins (63). The minimal effects of HPP on nutrient stability are similar to the effects of freezing. For example, Farr reported that HPP treatment of nonpasteurized citrus juice resulted in a flavor profile similar to that of fresh-squeezed juice with no losses of vitamin C and a shelf life of up to 17 months (64). Few data are currently available on the effects of HPP on antinutrient stability.

HPP is also proving to be useful in optimizing the functional properties of food systems, especially in modifying the structure of animal or vegetable proteins. Galazaka and colleagues (65) discussed the potential effectiveness of HPP as a pretreatment tool to modify states of protein aggregation or gelation effectively, depending on the protein system, temperature treatment, solution conditions, and magnitude and duration of pressure application.

BIOTECHNOLOGY

Biotechnology has become an important and new aspect of food processing. In this context, we consider biotechnology as microbial, plant, and animal species altered by transfer of genes from another species. Microbial biotechnology has been used to enhance organisms for fermentation and particularly to produce enzymes for processing. New crops that resist certain pests, diseases, and herbicides are virtually the same as conventional crops. Stringent regulatory practices are in place to ensure that the approved crops are safe for animals and humans.

Benefits

Agricultural biotechnology has been widely adopted particularly in North America in soy and corn crops and in fruit trees. Soy that is modified to have herbicide resistance is of higher quality because it is lower in residual herbicides, and there is far less weed-seed contamination when the crop goes to the processor. Glyphosate-resistant soy is an excellent example of a transgenic crop. The products containing soy oil or protein from these crops are of higher quality with lower production costs. In addition, the technology facilitates low-till or no-till agriculture. Corn crops have been modified with resulting resistance against insects of the Lepidoptera order, the major pests against corn. Control of these insects significantly reduces insect damage and improves grain quality. Corn with fewer damaged kernels is less prone to mold infestation, thereby ensuring food and feed safety.

The Hawaiian papaya business has also benefited from insect resistance to the papaya ringspot virus through biotechnology. Collaborative efforts between Cornell University and the University of Hawaii resulted in the development of the new "rainbow papaya," which is no different from conventional fruit except that it is resistant to the virus (66).

The cheese industry has also been a major benefactor of biotechnology. Currently, 60% of all hard cheeses are produced using the enzyme chymosin. Chymosin replaces the need for rennet, normally prepared from calf stomach. Because it is produced by fermentation, it is much more cost effective and in many cases allows for the production of kosher cheese. The dairy production industry benefits from the inclusion of bovine somatotropin, which improves milk production by 10 to 15% (67).

Consumer Concerns

Although biotechnology offers many potential benefits, consumer concerns about the safety of biotechnology have reduced the momentum for development of new

TABLE 113.4. NUTRIENT LOSSES RESULTING FROM PROCESSING

NUTRIENT	HEAT	LEACHING	OXIDATION	ALKALI	ACID	LIGHT
			CAUSE OF NUTRIENT LOSS			
Ascorbic acid	X	X	X	X	X	X
Biotin				X		
Carotenoids	X		X		X	X
Cobalamin (B$_{12}$)			X	X		
Folic acid	X					X
Niacin		X				
Pantothenic acid	X			X	X	
Pyridoxine (B$_6$)				X		X
Riboflavin (B$_2$)	X		X	X		X
Thiamin (B$_1$)	X	X	X	X		X
Vitamin A	X		X			X
Vitamin D	X		X	X		X
Vitamin E			X			
Vitamin K				X	X	X
Minerals		X				
Flavonoids	X		X			X
Phenolics	X		X			X

From Harris RS. General discussion on stability of nutrients. In: Karmas E, Harris RS, eds. Nutritional Evaluation of Food Processing. 3rd ed. New York: Avi Publishing, 1988:3–5, with permission.

biotechnologic food products. Some of these concerns include antibiotic resistance, cross-pollination of crops, and introduction of allergens. The antibiotic resistance concern is based on whether or not antibiotic markers used in isolation of transformed plants can be transferred to bacteria in people or animals, thereby making medical antibiotics ineffective. Extensive global research concluded that transfer of the antibiotic resistance to bacteria is unlikely because several natural barriers inhibit their transfer, and the antibiotics used in transformed plants are not commonly used in the treatment of disease.

Outflow of genes from modified crops by pollination of weeds is another major consideration. Gene flow is a natural process that is promoted by insects and wind that results in exchange of DNA between crops and closely related weeds. In the United States, crops such as sorghum and sunflowers are more likely to cross-pollinate because they are grown in areas with high concentrations of weedy relatives. Such crops are much less likely to be candidates for transgene improvements.

Introduction of new food allergens into the food supply by modified crops is another major concern among consumers. Most food allergens (90%) come from a few sources: fish, peanuts, soy, milk, eggs, crustaceans, wheat, rice and tree nuts. An extensive protocol has been proposed to assess and screen new proteins to ensure that they are not likely allergens before their introduction into the food supply (68).

OVERVIEW OF NUTRIENT DAMAGE CAUSED BY PROCESSING

Food processing provides many benefits, but there are some costs in terms of damage or loss of nutrients. Vitamin and mineral losses during food handling, processing, storage, and delivery have several common causes. Heat is particularly destructive to nutrients, especially vitamins, but optimized combinations of temperature and time can minimize nutrient loss. In Table 113.4, some of the more common reasons for losses are summarized (69).

SUMMARY

Food processing is an integral part of our urbanized society. Processed foods provide us with choices of high-quality nutritious foods at reasonable prices. The modest chemical changes and losses in nutrients observed during food processing operations are generally outweighed by the benefits of enhanced food quality, safety, and preservation of foods and ingredients from farm to consumer.

REFERENCES

1. Levine H, Slade L. Crit Rev Food Sci Nutr 1991;30:115–360.
2. Skibsted LH. Czech J Food Sci 2000;18:5–7.
3. McClements DJ, Decker EA. J Food Sci 2000;65:1270–82.
4. Morrissey PA, Kerry JP, Galvin K. ACS Symp Series 2003;836:188–200.
5. Kamal-Eldin A, Yanishlieva NV, Eur J Lipid Sci Technol 2002;104:825–36.
6. Millard AC. C R Acad Sci 1912;154:66–8.
7. Amadori M. Atti R Accad Naz Linceri Mem Cl Sci Fis Mat Nat 1931;13:72.
8. Hodge JE. J Agric Food Chem 1953;1:928–43.
9. Friedman M. Annu Rev Nutr 1992;12:119–37.
10. Taeymans D, Wood J, Ashby P et al. Crit Rev Food Sci Nutr 2004;44:323–47.
11. Wedzicha B, Mottram DS. In: Abstracts of Papers, 227th ACS National Meeting, Anaheim, CA, March 28–April 1, 2004: AGFD–108.

12. Joint Institute for Food Safety and Applied Nutrition (JIFSAN). Acrylamide Infonet, http://acrylamide–food.org/data.

13. Erdreich LS, Friedman MA. Regul Toxicol Pharmac 2004;39:150–7.

14. Lindsay RC, Jang S. US Pat Appl Publ 2004;US 2004224066 A1 20041111:1–11.

15. Elder VA, Fulcher JG, Leung HK et al. US Pat Appl Publ 2004;Cont–in–part of US Series no. 247, 504:1–8.

16. Zyzak DV, Lin PYT, Sanders RA et al. US Pat Appl Publ 2004;US 2004101607 A1 20040527:1–21.

17. Stadler RH, Scholz G. Nutr Rev 2004;62:449–81.

18. Ashie IN, Simpson BK, Smith JP. Crit Rev Food Nutr 1996;36:1–30.

19. Finley JW. Food Technol 2004;58:42.

20. Whitaker JR. Enzymes. In: Fennema O, ed. Food Chemistry. 3rd ed. New York: Marcel Dekker, 1996:431–530.

21. Nelson PE. Hortscience 1972;7:13–5.

22. Fennema O. Effects of freeze preservation on nutrients. In: Karmas E, Harris RS, eds. Nutritional Evaluation of Food Processing. 3rd ed. New York: Avi Publishing, 1988:269–317.

23. Brewer MS, Klein BP, Rastogi BK et al. J Food Qual 1994;17:245–59.

24. Vaeth B, Rumm-Kreuter D, Demmel I. Ernaehrungs-Umschau 1990;37:472–8.

25. Rossi M, Giussani E, Morelli R et al. Food Res Int 2003;36:999–1005.

26. Brady PL. Drying. In: Master Food Preserver Manual. Little Rock, AR: University of Arkansas Cooperative Extension Service, 1988.

27. Lund D. Effects of heat processing on nutrients. In: Karmas E, Harris RS, eds. Nutritional Evaluation of Food Processing. 3rd ed. New York: Avi Publishing, 1988: 319–354.

28. IFT. Food Technol 1986;40:109–16.

29. Ryley J, Kajda P. Food Chem 1994;49:119–29.

30. Dietz JM, Erdman JW Jr. Nutr Today 1989;24:6–15.

31. Prochaska LJ, Nguyen XT, Donat N et al. Med Hypotheses 2000;54:254–62.

32. Borenstein B, Lachance PA. Effects of processing and preparation on the nutritive value of foods. In: Shils ME, Young VR, eds. Modern Nutrition in Health and Disease. 7th ed. Philadelphia: Lea & Febiger, 1988:672–84.

33. Chandler LA, Schwartz SJ. J Food Sci 1987;52:669–72.

34. Lessin WJ, Catigani GL, Schwartz SJ. J Agric Food Chem 1997;45:3728–32.

35. Deming DM, Baker DH, Erdman JW Jr. J Nutr 2002;132:2709–12.

36. Schierle J, Bretzel W, Buhler I et al. Food Chem 1997;59:459–65.

37. Nguyen ML, Schwartz SJ. Proc Soc Exp Biol Med 1998;218:101–5.

38. Updike AA, Schwartz SJ. J Agric Food Chem 2003;51: 6184–90.

39. Adams CE, Erdman JW Jr. Effects of home food preparation practices on nutrients. In: Karmas E, Harris RS, eds. Nutritional Evaluation of Food Processing. 3rd ed. New York: Avi Publishing, 1988:557–95.

40. Ranhotra GS, Bock MA. Effects of baking on nutrients. In: Karmas E, Harris RS, eds. Nutritional Evaluation of Food Processing. 3rd ed. New York: Avi Publishing, 1988:355–65.

41. Harper JM. Effects of extrusion processing on nutrients. In: Karmas E, Harris RS, eds. Nutritional Evaluation of Food Processing. 3rd ed. New York: Avi Publishing, 1988:365–92.

42. Nesheim RO, Lockhart HB. Cereal nutrition. In: Fast RB, Caldwell EF, eds. Breakfast Cereals and How They Are Made. St. Paul, MN: American Association of Cereal Chemists, 1993.

43. Pokorny J. Changes of nutrients at frying temperatures. In: Boskou D, Elmadfa, eds. Frying of Food. Lancaster, PA: Technomic Publishing, 1999:69–103.

44. Gerster H. Food Sci Nutr 1989;42:173–81.

45. Hernandez-Infante M, Sousa V, Monfalvo I et al. Plant Foods Hum Nutr 1998;52:199–208.

46. Thorn, M-L, Yeow YL. Proceedings of the 6th Conference of Asia Pacific Confederation of Chemical Engineers and the 21st Australias Chemical Engineering Conference, September 26-29,1993, Melbourne, Australia.

47. Smith JS, Pillai S. Food Technol 2004;58:48–55.

48. Centers for Disease Control and Prevention. MMWR Morb Mortal Wkly Rep 2004;53:338–43.

49. Fletcher JM. Freezing. In: Henry CJK, ed. Nutrition Handbook for Food Processors. Cambridge, UK: Woodhead Publishing, 2002:331–41.

50. Levine H, Slade L. Agric Food Chem 1989;1:315–96.

51. Griffith M, Ewart KV. Biotech Adv 1995;13:375–402.

52. Ruan R, Ye X, Chen P. Ohmic heating. In: Henry CJK, ed. Nutrition Handbook for Food Processors. Cambridge, UK: Woodhead Publishing, 2002.

53. Nott KP, Hall LD. Trends Food Sci Technol 1999;10:366–74.

54. Ranesh MN. Food preservation by heat treatment. In: Rahman RS, ed. Handbook of Food Preservation. New York: Marcel Dekker, 1999;95–172.

55. Zolati P, Swearingen P. Food Technol 1996;50:263–6.

56. Selman J. Food Sci Technol Today 1992;6:205–9.

57. Grant S, Patterson M, Ledward D. Chem Industry 2000;24:55–8.

58. Gould GW. Proc Nutr Soc 2001;60:463–74.

59. Arroyo G, Sanz PD, Prestamo G. J Appl Microbiol 1997;82:735–42.

60. Knorr D, Angerbach A. Trends Food Sci Technol 1998;9:185–11.

61. Knorr D, Ade-Omowaye BIO, Heinz V. Proc Nutr Soc 2002;61:311–8.

62. Roberts CM, Hoover DG. J Appl Bacteriol 1996;81:363–8.

63. Tewari G, Jayas DS, Holley RA. Sci Aliments 1999;19:619–61.

64. Farr D. Trends Food Sci Technol 1990;1:14–6.

65. Galazka VB, Dickinson E, Ledward DA. Curr Opin Colloid Interface Sci 2000;5:182–7.

66. Gonsalves D. Curr Top Microbiol Immunol 2002;266:73–83.

67. Bauman DE. Domestic Anim Endocrinol 1999;17;101–16.

68. Chassy BM. J Am Coll Nutr 2002;21[Suppl]:166S–73S.

69. Harris RS. General discussion on stability of nutrients. In: Karmas E, Harris RS, eds. Nutritional Evaluation of Food Processing. 3rd ed. New York: Avi Publishing, 1988:3–5.

SUGGESTED READINGS

Arnoldi A. Thermal processing and nutritional quality. In: Henry CJK, ed. Nutrition Handbook for Food Processors. Cambridge, UK: Woodhead Publishing, 2002.

Henry CJK, ed. Nutrition Handbook for Food Processors. Cambridge, UK: Woodhead Publishing, 2002.

Matser AM, Krebbers B, van den Berg RW et al. Advantages of high pressure sterilisation on quality of food products. Trends Food Sci Technol 2004;15:79–85.

US Department of Agriculture Eastern Regional Research Center. Irradiation of Ready–to–Eat Foods: 2003 Update. http://www.sciencedirect.com.

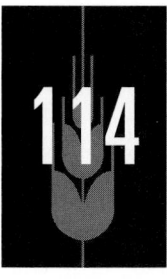

114 DESIGNING FUNCTIONAL FOODS[1]
WAYNE R. BIDLACK AND WEI WANG

THE FUNCTIONAL FOODS 1790
REGULATORY ISSUES 1791
    National Labeling Education Act 1791
    Dietary Supplement Health and Education Act ..1792
    Food and Drug Administration
        Modernization Act 1792
    Scientific Agreement Standards 1793
    Safety 1793
STATUS OF FUNCTIONAL FOODS AND
    THE UNITED STATES MARKET 1794
PHYSIOLOGICALLY ACTIVE COMPOUNDS 1795
    Isoprenoids 1795
    Phenolic 1801
    Animal-Derived Protein 1802
    Microbial 1803
DESIGNING FUNCTIONAL FOODS 1803
CONCLUSIONS 1805

Throughout evolution, each species, whether single cell or multicell, has sought a form of sustenance to provide nutrients for survival, growth, and reproduction. Human beings have selected a broader variety of foods of plant, animal, and microbial origin than most other species to provide the nutrients needed for existence (1–3). As a complex mixture of chemicals, food provides essential nutrients, requisite calories, and other physiologically active constituents needed for life and health. Yet very little is known about the physiologic effect of most substances found in foods.

The amount and composition of food consumed at various stages of life may impact the expression of certain diseases. Since 1980, epidemiologic studies have consistently

correlated diet as a factor in the etiology of the five leading causes of death in the United States: heart disease, certain types of cancer, stroke, non–insulin-dependent diabetes mellitus, and atherosclerosis (4, 5).

In the twentieth century alone, nutrition and food sciences have contributed to the enhanced development of an abundant, nutritious, and safe food supply supporting better health for people around the world. A new paradigm for optimal nutrition continues to evolve that would place emphasis on the positive aspects of diet, identifying components in addition to known nutrients that are physiologically active and that contribute to the prevention of disease onset. Understanding the mechanisms by which individual nutrients and nonnutrient constituents function physiologically should allow food scientists to truly design food products for a healthful diet. Thus, although genetic predisposition increases susceptible people's risk for some of these chronic diseases, especially with advancing age, optimal nutrition should enable people to achieve their maximum genetic potential and decrease their susceptibility to disease.

From the beginnings of recorded history, plant components (leaves, flowers, roots, and bark) have been identified and used in the treatment of specific diseases (6, 7). Even Hippocrates, the father of medicine, included food as a basic part of treatment to cure disease. Taken from many cultures, herbs and plants commonly used for treatment of specific disorders have been carefully identified. Modern analytic methods have identified more than 10,000 physiologically active constituents provided by the human diet, many of which have been developed into pharmaceutical agents.

Most epidemiologic evidence continues to correlate the positive effects of fruits, vegetables, and grains with lower incidence of cancer, coronary heart disease (CHD), and other diseases (5, 8). The most consistent finding was an inverse relationship between the risk for certain cancers and the consumption of fruits and vegetables, whole grains, fiber, and some types of fats (9). People who consume high amounts of fruits and vegetables have about one half the risk of developing cancer and a lower mortality rate from cancer (10–15). Fruits and vegetables are most effective against cancers involving epithelial cells, such as cancer of the lung, cervix, esophagus, stomach, colon, and pancreas, and for hormone-related cancers (16).

[1]Abbreviations: **ALF,** activation of lactoferrin; **bLF,** bovine lactoferrin; **CHD,** coronary heart disease; **CLA,** conjugated linoleic acid; **DSHEA,** Dietary Supplement Health and Education Act; **EC,** (-)-epicatechin; **ECG,** (-)-epicatechin-3-gallate; **EGC,** (-)-epigallocatechin; **EGCG,** (-)-epigallocatechin-3-gallate; **FDA,** Food and Drug Administration; **FDAMA,** Food and Drug Administration Modernization Act; **FOSHU,** Foods for Specified Health Use; **GM-CSF,** granulocyte-macrophage colony-stimulating factor; **GRAS,** generally recognized as safe; **LAB,** lactic acid bacteria; **LF,** lactoferrin; **NHP,** Natural Health Products; **NLEA,** National Labeling Education Act; **rhLF,** recombinant human lactoferrin.

The foods and herbs having the highest anticancer activity include garlic, soybeans, cabbage, ginger, licorice, and umbelliferous vegetables (carrots, celery, cilantro, parsley, and parsnips) (17). Modest effects are shown by onions, flax, citrus, tumeric, cruciferous vegetables (broccoli, Brussels sprouts, cabbage, and cauliflower), solanaceous vegetables (tomatoes and peppers), brown rice, and whole wheat.

Interestingly, the positive health correlations do not always agree solely with nutrient content. Nonnutrient constituents have been identified that contribute beneficial physiologic effects that may retard or prevent disease as well (17). Some of these include allyl sulfides in garlic and onions; phytates in grains and legumes; lignans in flaxseed and soybeans; isoflavones in soybeans; saponins in legumes; indoles and isothiocyanates in cruciferous vegetables; ellagic acid in grapes, strawberries, raspberries, and nuts; and a range of flavonoids, carotenoids, and terpenoids in various plant foods.

The new diet-health paradigm acknowledges the nutritious and healthful aspects of food, but goes beyond the role of food constituents providing essential nutrients for sustaining life and growth to one of preventing or delaying the premature onset of chronic disease later in life. Food and food products that combine these properties have been described by several different names, including designer foods, functional foods, or nutraceuticals. The promise of functional foods has emerged at a time when consumer interest in diet and health is at an all-time high (17, 18). The current nutraceutical market (19) includes vitamin, mineral, and herbal supplements ($6.4 billion); sports and herbal fortified beverages ($21.9 billion); diet and fiber aids ($0.8 billion); and meals, snacks, and meal replacements ($47.8 billion). Functional foods have already exceeded $20 billion and may double by the end of the decade. In the near term, foods will be enriched with new and unique physiologically active health components from unconventional sources.

THE FUNCTIONAL FOODS

The functional foods concept has unified the medical, nutritional, and food sciences. In general, functional foods are natural or formulated (designed) foods that will enhance physiologic performance or prevent or treat diseases (20). Since the early to mid-1990s, new technologies, such as biotechnology, genetic engineering, food processing, and product innovations, and mass production have enabled food scientists to design new healthful food products.

The functional food concept was first developed in Japan in the 1980s in response to increasing health care costs (21, 22). The Ministry of Health and Welfare in Japan initiated a regulatory system to approve certain foods with documented health benefits. These foods were identified as Foods for Specified Health Use (FOSHU).

By late 2001, more than 400 food products had been granted FOSHU status.

In the United States, functional food has no official legislative or regulatory definition. Functional foods include those items developed for health purposes as well as for physical performance. The Institute of Medicine (23) has defined functional foods as any modified food or food ingredient that may provide a health benefit beyond the traditional nutrients it contains.

Several related terms have been used to define different aspects of functional foods. Initially, the term designer foods was developed by the National Cancer Institute to describe foods that naturally contained or were enriched with nonnutritive, biologically active chemical components of plants (phytochemicals) that were potentially effective in reducing cancer risk (24). The term nutraceutical was used to identify "any substance considered a food or part of a food and provides medical or health benefits, including the prevention and treatment of disease" (25, 26). Nutraceuticals may range from isolated nutrients, dietary supplements, and diets to genetically engineered designer foods, herbal products, and processed products such as cereals, soups, and beverages. However, the term functional food may prove to be the best name for the category of foods containing physiologically active compounds that may provide a health benefit beyond basic nutrition.

In 1988, the orphan drugs amendment to the Federal Food, Drug, and Cosmetic Act provided medical foods with a legal definition: "a food which is formulated to be consumed or administered enterally under the supervision of a physician and which is intended for the specific dietary management of a disease or condition for which distinctive nutritional requirements based on recognized scientific principles, are established by medical evaluation." Medical foods differ from the general food supply because these foods frequently serve as the sole source of nutrition. Thus, medical foods are complex, formulated products designed to provide complete or supplemental nutritional support to individuals who are unable to ingest adequate amounts of food in a conventional form, or to provide specialized nutritional support to patients who have unique physiologic and nutritional needs associated with their conditions (27). Generally in their design and manufacture, medical foods require sophisticated and exacting science and technology comparable with that used in the manufacture of infant formulas and drugs; yet, medical foods are subject to much less scrutiny by the Food and Drug Administration (FDA) than virtually all other food categories. The 1990 National Labeling Education Act (NLEA) specifically exempted medical foods from the NLEA labeling provisions (28). There are no specific requirements for label information or substantiation of claims, formulations and compositional characteristics, manufacturing quality controls, or notification to the FDA of intent to market medical foods.

The relevance of any definition of functional foods will depend totally on an adequate description of these foods and substantiation of their health benefits (29). Traditional separation between food and medicine should be carefully defined to prevent creation of barriers that deter creation of functional foods that can provide health benefits to the general population.

REGULATORY ISSUES

During the 1990s, functional foods and nutraceuticals emerged as the dominant trend in the food industry in the United States and worldwide. The concept of foods that can provide health-enhancing and disease-preventing properties has been eagerly embraced by consumers, increasingly supported by scientific evidence provided by nutritional scientists, and legally endorsed by public policy and legislative mandates for food and supplement labeling (30). Marketing of products with health claims, reaching consumers with meaningful messages, and competitively positioning products in the functional food arena requires careful attention to regulatory issues and insight on how to communicate established product benefits to the consumer. Unfortunately, consumers are often more persuaded by association, emotion, and promises of well-being than by scientific statements and numerical documentation. Thus, accuracy in product labeling is essential and must be carefully regulated (31). The regulation of health claims for vegetables, fruits, and herbs, as with virtually all foods, is the responsibility of the FDA. Federal regulations control the language and detail of health benefits that may be conveyed on the product label, in the marketing literature, and in the product advertising.

A major dilemma is caused by the fact that functional foods exist at the interface between foods and drugs (32). In the past, compounds exerting this type of physiologic effect have been classified by the Federal Food, Drug, and Cosmetic Act of 1938 (33) as drugs, including all "articles intended for the diagnosis, cure, mitigation, treatment or prevention of disease." Thus, the legal categories displayed on a label referring to disease prevention or risk reduction has been limited to the following four categories (34):

- Ordinary food and nutrients. Health claims can be made on labels only when they are supported by the totality of publicly available scientific evidence, and then only after receiving regulatory approval from the FDA.
- Dietary supplements. Health claims based only on "evidence the statement is truthful and not misleading." The FDA must be notified of the statement, and the label must include a disclaimer stating that the agency has not evaluated the claim and that the product is not intended to diagnose, treat, cure, or prevent any disease.
- Medical foods. Health claims must be based on a somewhat higher standard (than for dietary supplements)

being backed by "sound scientific evidence." Medical foods do not require FDA approval for claims, although their packages must include disclaimers similar to those for dietary supplements.
- Drugs. Drug claims have the strictest standards, and must be proven safe and effective in FDA-approved and reviewed clinical trials.

Since 1973, FDA regulations have not allowed a food to be labeled representing that the food is adequate or effective in the prevention, cure, mitigation, or treatment of any disease or symptoms; if so stated, the product is deemed misbranded. These regulations have been amended to exempt FDA-approved health claims.

Three new labeling laws were created to regulate functional foods, nutraceuticals, and designer foods: the National Labeling Education Act of 1990 (NLEA) (35), the 1994 Dietary Supplement Health and Education Act (DSHEA)(36), and the 1997 FDA Modernization Act (FDAMA) (37). These changes have played an important role in the rapid development of functional food products (38).

National Labeling Education Act

The FDA, acting under congressional direction, wrote new regulations governing health claims on food labels. The first was the NLEA in 1990 (35), which was revised and became effective in 1993 (39). The basis for this change was an understanding that the food label serves as a primary nutrition education vehicle for the consumer. The NLEA carefully restricted what could be claimed on the label as well as what nutritional information must be disclosed.

The enactment of the NLEA established the health claim requirements for food labels. A health claim is a statement that expressly or by implication characterizes the relationship of any substance to a disease or health-related condition within the context of a total daily diet (39). The NLEA requires a prominent panel of nutrition facts, daily reference values, declaration of ingredients, nutrient content, and health claims.

Importantly, the NLEA requires that the evidence supporting a health or disease prevention claim submitted to the FDA must meet a standard of "significant scientific agreement". This must include agreement among experts in the field and be supported by publicly available evidence (40). Twelve health claims have been approved under these standards, involving the following: (a) calcium and osteoporosis; (b) dietary fat and cancer; (c) sodium and hypertension; (d) dietary saturated fat and cholesterol, and CHD; (e) fiber-containing grain products, fruits, and vegetables and cancer; (f) fruits, vegetables, and grain products containing fiber (soluble fiber) and risk of CHD; (g) fruits and vegetables and cancer; (h) folic acid and neural tube defects; (i) dietary noncariogenic carbohydrate sweeteners and dental caries; (j) soluble fiber from certain foods and risk of CHD; (k) soy protein and risk of CHD; and (l) stanols and sterols and risk of CHD (41).

A key factor needed to control health claims lies in the wording content of the claim, which should be consistent with the nature and scope of the scientific evidence. Four types of health claims have been identified: nutrient function claims, claims relating to dietary guidelines or a healthful diet, enhanced function claims, and reduction of disease risk claims. Considering that wording of nutrient function claims and dietary guidelines or a healthful diet are less complicated than are claims for enhanced function or reduction of disease, the authorization process should be handled accordingly.

Dietary Supplement Health and Education Act

The DSHEA (36) created structure/function claims for use on dietary supplements. These claims are limited to nutrients or dietary substances that have an established daily value, and they can only be made if a regulation is in place specifying criteria to meet the claim.

The description of a dietary supplement in the DSHEA (36) specifically includes (a) a product that is intended for ingestion in tablet, capsule, liquid, powder, soft gel, or gel cap, or if not in such form, is not represented as conventional food and is not represented for use as a sole item of a meal or of the diet, and is labeled as a dietary supplement; (b) a drug, antibiotic, or biologic, if the product had been marketed as a dietary supplement before such approval; (c) a food excluding the definition of food additive; (d) other than tobacco, intended to supplement the diet by increasing the total intake, that bears or contains one or more of the following dietary ingredients: a vitamin; a mineral; an herb or botanical; an amino acid; a dietary substance for use by people to supplement the diet by increasing the total dietary intake; or a concentrate, metabolite, constituent, extract, or any combination of these ingredients (42). The detailed description of supplements is not provided in any other regulatory policy worldwide. A definition of dietary supplement as broad as this allows for the addition of many ingredients with functional effects that span the food-drug spectrum in terms of use.

Under the DSHEA, dietary supplements are exempt from regulations as drugs and for the most part as food additives. Unfortunately, the DSHEA puts the burden of proof for safety of dietary supplements directly on the FDA and limits the agency's authority over their labeling.

With regard to functional foods, the DSHEA allows the use of structure/function claims and the dissemination of third-party literature. The FDA allows for two unqualified health claims. The first is an unqualified approval based on general science knowledge, and the second is an unqualified approval supported by an authoritative statement. However, both must state that the FDA has not evaluated the claim and that the dietary supplement is not intended to "diagnose, treat, cure, or prevent any disease."

Structure/function claims may describe how a dietary ingredient affects a structure or function in humans, or may describe general well-being from consumption of the ingredients. Although the FDA does not require preapproval, the manufacturer must submit a label notification to the FDA no later than 40 days after marketing the dietary supplement. The responsibility for accuracy and truthfulness remains with the manufacturer.

The DSHEA provides for statements of nutritional support, which can be applied to a wide variety of dietary ingredients (36). The following claims are allowed:

- To claim a benefit related to a classic nutrient-deficiency disease and disclose the prevalence of such a disease in the United States
- To describe the role of a nutrient or dietary ingredient intended to affect structure or function in humans
- To characterize the mechanism by which a nutrient or dietary ingredient acts to maintain such structure or function
- To describe the general well-being derived from the consumption of a nutrient or dietary ingredient

Dietary supplements have been drastically redefined by the DSHEA in terms of what they are and may contain. The use of such components in different food products and their suitability for claims in labeling depend on the application of the appropriate standards for safety of use and labeling criteria for a particular product category. In the general food supply, an inherent constituent of the food can be marketed unless it has been found to be "ordinarily injurious to health." As an intentional additive, a functional food component can be used to fortify a processed food, but it requires a stricter condition for "reasonable certainty of no harm" within the context of the total estimated exposure of the additive. According to the DSHEA, a dietary supplement is considered an unapproved food additive in terms of conventional food use because the supplement could be considered adulterated. A functional food component used in a supplement could be less safe than one that occurred naturally or that was intentionally added to a conventional food.

Food and Drug Administration Modernization Act

To streamline the authorization process, the FDAMA (37) was established. The FDA allows for a second type of unqualified health claim statement, the authoritative statement. The authoritative statement must be made by either a scientific body of the US government or the National Academy of Sciences regarding a nutrient and a condition or disease relationship. A food label can carry an authoritative statement with FDA approval (40). Three authoritative statements have been approved to date, involving choline, potassium, and risk of high blood pressure, and whole-grain foods and heart disease and certain cancers (41, 43). The FDAMA does not include dietary supplements in the provisions for health claims based on authoritative statements.

In July 2003, the FDA began allowing qualified health claims for foods in an effort to make it easier for food companies to make claims about the health benefits of their products, even if the science supporting these claims is not conclusive. This is a part of the initiative by the FDA to help consumers obtain accurate, up-to-date, and science-based information about the health consequences of these products. There are eight approved statements for qualified health claims and conditions for their use (41). They are rather long in an effort to be truthful and not misleading (43, 44).

Scientific Agreement Standards

By the end of 2000, the FDA had issued guidance to define its significant scientific agreement standard. The FDA concluded that the weight of the scientific evidence for these claims outweighed the evidence against the claims.

The language of the qualified health claim is dictated by a ranking of the levels A (significant, unqualified statement), B (scientific evidence supports the claim, but is not conclusive), C (some scientific evidence, but is limited and not conclusive), and D (very preliminary and limited scientific research and has little scientific evidence to support the claim). The rankings are based on an evaluation process rating the study design, study quality, and strength of the entire evidence. In addition, the FDA reviews the qualified health claim petitions using the following qualifications:

- The food is likely to have a significant impact on a serious or life-threatening illness.
- The strength of the evidence is considered.
- Consumer research has been provided to show the claim is not misleading.
- The substance of the claim has undergone FDA safety review.
- The substance has been adequately characterized so that the relevance of available studies can be evaluated.
- The disease is defined and evaluated in accordance with generally accepted criteria established by a recognized body of qualified experts.
- There is prior review of the evidence or the claim by a recognized body of qualified experts.

After an opportunity for public comment, the FDA will conduct a scientific review of the data either itself or by way of an appropriate third party. The review will be completed within 270 days of receipt of the petition, at which time the FDA will issue a letter to the petitioner setting the agency's determination as to whether to exercise enforcement discretion. A final rank based on the strength of the sum of evidence will be made from A to D.

Additional regulations may need to be created to clarify the product and label descriptions. The changes described in the DSHEA favor the development of functional food products in the form of dietary supplements. In the long term, the legislation may do little to stimulate scientific investigation into the potential role of functional food products in health promotion and disease prevention. However, consumer enthusiasm for products that truly provide health benefits will drive the development of supportive evidence that the claims are true and the products are truly efficacious. To date there has not been a systematic approach to the categorization of functional foods and their mechanisms of action in health promotion or disease prevention. Potential mechanisms are identified in Table 114.1, but the list may need to be revised further (45). New regulations may also be needed to ensure some kind of limited patent or copyright on a health claim for companies willing to make the research commitment to establish health efficacy.

Safety

Although significant evidence continues to accumulate showing that many phytochemicals may contribute to disease prevention and better health, very little effort is being made to test the long-term or possible toxic side effects of these agents. Addition of the phytochemicals, herbals, and other combinations of botanic components to food or taken as a dietary supplement has inherent risk simply because the number of consumers using the products are very high. In essence, the use of these products without

---

TABLE 114.1. CATEGORIZATION OF PHYSIOLOGICALLY ACTIVE FOOD COMPONENTS BY MECHANISM OF ACTION

Antioxidants, superoxide quencher, modifiers of oxidative damage and detoxification mechanisms related to oxidative stress; nitric oxide synthetase inducer, enhanced DNA repair, decreased DNA damage/modification

Antimutagens, anticarcinogens, and inducers of enzymes of xenobiotic phase II metabolism, inhibits tumor promotion; antimetastatic agents, inhibits cell proliferation, inhibits angiogenesis

Antimicrobial, antiviral bioactive substances

Enhancers of gastrointestinal function and colonic microflora, decreased risk for cancer and cardiovascular disease

Immunomodulators, stimulates immune function

Antiinflammatory agents

Neuroregulatory substances, improve psychologic condition, memory enhancement

Modulation of hormones relieves symptoms of menopause

Antihypertensives, control of blood pressure

Hypocholesterolemic agents, lowers serum cholesterol, reduces coronary heart disease

Diminishes allergenicity

Decreases platelet aggregation, reduces stroke

Stimulates bone repair, reduces osteoporosis

Inhibits macular degeneration

From Bidlack WR, Wang W. Designing functional foods. In: Shils ME, Olson JA, Shike M et al., eds. Modern Nutrition in Health and Disease. 9th ed. Baltimore: Williams & Wilkins, 1999:1823–34; and Ginnsman WH. Nutr Rev 1996;54:S33–7.

testing of dose controls or identification of possible contaminates has rapidly made their use a large uncontrolled human experiment. Although the majority of these materials have been consumed for thousands of years, there is little recorded history of actual outcomes of the consuming population.

Another aspect of self treatment with plant materials is efficacy and how treatment may affect other therapeutic regimens. Similar issues arose between drug-nutrient interactions 15 to 20 years ago, and package inserts now warn to avoid certain foods or the timing of ingestion that can diminish (or enhance) absorption of drugs and alter their efficacy. A similar case will be identified for specific phytochemicals, the form in which they are ingested, the foods they may interact with (affecting nutrient use), and the timing of consumption relative to drug therapy regimens.

The scientific development of functional foods and physiologically active ingredients is moving forward at a rapid pace, but cautious regulatory oversight must be provided to ensure safety. The General Accounting Office (46) has expressed concern, primarily noting a lack of regulations to guide companies on testing and presentation on product labels. Without such information, consumers incur a significant health risk unknown to them and that may be expressed by certain population subgroups. Companies need to be mindful of these safety issues to avoid liability issues.

Standard guidelines are needed for research evaluation and for label content and requirements, and a system is needed for recording and reporting health problems resulting from dietary intake of functional foods or supplements. The FDA has noted that the vast majority of these ingredients have not been cleared as generally recognized as safe (GRAS) or approved as food additives for most of the cases in which they were being used (47). Again, the company is placing itself at financial risk, while the consumer risks health consequences, and worse, a potentially beneficial nutraceutical/functional food could be eliminated from the marketplace because of a negative incident that may have been avoided with more development work. Thus, the use of plant materials and phytochemicals in functional foods to enhance the promotion of natural components for health may be premature. The consumer will respond best to products that show that they are safe and efficacious.

STATUS OF FUNCTIONAL FOODS AND THE UNITED STATES MARKET

In the United States and in other countries, regulations and/or recommendations for the use of functional foods continue to be developed. Nationally, the FDA enforces such regulations. Internationally, Codex (Codex Alimentarius Commission) is close to completing work on international guidelines for health claims, whereas a proposed

regulation on food claims recently went to the European Parliament in an attempt to standardize conditions across the European Union (48). To create more effective control of health claims, the United Kingdom created the Food Standards Agency, an independent national authority, to oversee their voluntary code of practice. The Canadian government created a new category called Natural Health Products (NHPs) to provide rapid access for the consumer to safe, efficacious, and high-quality products in an effort to establish stable regulations (49). The NHP regulations were established independent of food and drug regulations, yet are regulated as a subset of drugs to provide oversight and allow proper administration of NHPs. The regulatory concept of functional foods in Latin America is currently being discussed in several countries, including Brazil and Argentina. In China, functional food products are considered health foods. Recently, the Chinese government has announced its intention to improve the standards for these products, including restricting the use of curative claims. Functional foods were first commercialized in Japan as physiologically active foods in the 1980s, when a voluntary system was developed by the Ministry of Health and Welfare based on a list of approved foods and ingredients that assisted in the prevention or treatment of specific diseases that could merit the FOSHU label (22). With this exception, the definition of functional foods has yet to be legislatively defined in the United States or elsewhere in the world.

The functional foods market shows the extent of cultural differences between regions in the global marketplace. Products that appeal to Asian cultures may not appeal to Western consumers, and vice versa. Japanese products offer to improve intestinal health through the inclusion of oligosaccharides or active bacterial cultures, whereas the functional food market in the United States has emphasized products that relate to a reduction in the incidence of CHD or cancer. The functional food market is influenced by both personal and national health issues and consumer acceptability within each culture.

In the United States, the health product market was growing at 18 to 20%, with annual sales of $2.5 billion by 1988. At that time, projections were made that the functional food market would remain a high-growth business capable of reaching $9.0 billion by 1995 (50–52). In reality, the functional food market exceeded $20 billion by 2002, with a continuing 9% growth rate since 2001. This growth is more impressive when compared with the 3% and 3.5% growth rates seen for conventional foods and dietary supplements, respectively. Importantly, the sale of functional foods is now projected to reach more than $37 billion by 2007. A major growth category for functional foods is the snack foods and candies area, which is projected to increase to $11.5 billion by 2007 as well. As such, the health food products, natural and organic foods, dietary supplements, health foods, and functional foods market sales may exceed $75 billion and could reach $100 billion.

The increase in the market is credited to the availability of information, enabling consumer education and reasoned choices; to interest in personal control of individual and family health; to increasing costs of health care and pharmaceuticals; to labeling changes that allow informational health claims and a broader base of advertising; to acceptance by medical and health care professionals; and of course to the growth of the aging population, their health concerns, and their available disposable income. The specialty market may mature as the world functional food market grows and generates new products for import. The functional food market does not apppear to be a fad, it appears to be here for the long term.

PHYSIOLOGICALLY ACTIVE COMPOUNDS

There has been no evolutionary pressure on plants to cause development of food components that would protect humans from cancer and other diseases. Yet, diets rich in fruits and vegetables appear to do just that. Most likely these compounds developed as a part of the plants' own defense mechanisms against environmental insult and only fortuitously provide benefits to human beings. Similar positive effects are being identified for a few specific proteins isolated from animal sources as well.

The number of physiologically active food chemicals (plant, animal, and microbial) identified in the last 2 decades has increased dramatically because of greater emphasis on identifying the active component and its efficacy in laboratory animal, tissue culture, and human intervention models.

To provide a perspective on functional foods, a few of the more well-studied physiologically active compounds are listed in Table 114.2 (A, isoprenoids; B, phenolics; C, amino acid based; D, animal derived; E, fatty acids; and F, microbial) with identification of sources and biologic effects (45, 53–154). Identification of most nutraceutical and functional ingredients was initiated by epidemiologic surveys that correlated a positive health benefit with specific food groups, followed by narrowing the focus to determine the dietary intake of the individual foods. Researchers then examined the chemical constituents of these foods, isolating and identifying chemical structures and suggesting possible functions for these agents.

In an effort to show the complexity of these interactions, Figure 114.1 describes a model for chemically induced carcinogenesis and identifies the metabolic sites at which various classes of phytochemicals may provide protective effects (10, 155). In addition, these agents appear to be tissue-specific for the changes in tumor expression, as in the following examples. Agents in the carotenoid family expresses strong antioxidant activity but differ in their effects on the carcinogenic process. Lycopene, which is found in tomatoes, serves as a major singlet oxygen scavenger and appears to inhibit prostate cancer, whereas zeaxanthin, which provides the yellow color of corn, is a strong antioxidant as well but enhances immune function. Cruciferous vegetables are rich in isothiocyanates and indoles, which interact with liver enzymes involved in detoxification and excretion of potential carcinogens. These phytochemicals appear to inhibit cancer development specifically in the esophagus, colon, and lungs. Allyl sulfides, which occur in the allium family, also activate detoxification enzymes that break down carcinogens and their metabolites and enhance their excretion; importantly, they are inhibitors of cancer at different tissue sites located in the liver, lung, and breast. Berries and grapes contain ellagic acid, which reduces damage to DNA preventing cell transformation, especially in the esophagus. Capsaicin, which is found in spicy hot peppers, paprika, and chili powder, appears to block carcinogen binding to DNA and reduces tumors in the skin, mammary glands, colon, and forestomach. The metabolic pathways protecting the body are numerous and varied, efficiently clearing the daily low-dose exposures to dietary and environmental carcinogens, and are assisted by a variety of naturally occurring, physiologically active food components.

In many cases, animal experiments have been carried out to test the hypotheses of health benefits and mechanisms of action, whereas in others some human testing has been initiated. A decision on efficacy must look at the lowest dose needed for producing the effects, because higher doses increase the risk for toxicity. In addition, it becomes important to determine whether the same dose of the agent in the food has the same efficacy as the isolated compound. Very few physiologically active chemicals have been examined as thoroughly as needed.

It will be many years before we clearly understand the actual health benefits of these agents, either as natural ingredients, as food additives, or as dietary supplements. In many cases it may be determined that beneficial effects result from combinations of these chemicals provided by additive or synergistic effects. In all cases, the question of safety must be assured.

Only a few examples of basic and applied research are presented here to represent the exciting potential of some of these agents as future physiologically active agents that may be incorporated into functional foods. Each of the following examples has physiologic effects at levels found naturally in foods.

Isoprenoids

The major types of isoprenoids are identified in Table 114.2A. They include the carotenoids, limenoids (monoterpenes), saponins, tocopherols, and tocotrienols. Differing categories were initially identified for vitamin activities, as antioxidants, as inhibitors of cholesterol biosynthesis, but have now been found to inhibit carcinogenesis.

TABLE 114.2. PHYSIOLOGICALLY ACTIVE FOOD CHEMICALS THAT MAY PREVENT DISEASE

ACTIVE COMPOUNDS	FOOD SOURCE	POTENTIAL HEALTH BENEFIT	POSSIBLE MECHANISMS AND FUNCTIONS	REFERENCE
A. Isoprenoids				
Carotenoids lycopene carotene lutein/zeaxanthin	Tomatoes, carrots, yams, cantaloupe, spinach, sweet potatoes, citrus fruit, cantaloupe, apricots, mango, pumpkin, kale	Reduction of cancer and heart disease; reduction the risk of macular degeneration	Antioxidant activity; free radical scavenger; singlet oxygen scavenger; induction of cell-cell communication and growth control; inhibition of the proliferation of acute myeloblastic leukemia; modulation of mutagenesis, cell differentiation, and proliferation; differentiation and growth control of epithelial cells	53, 54, 55
Limonoids limonene	Citrus fruits	Chemoprevention of cancer	Inhibition of cell proliferation; Inhibition of isoprenylation of cell-growth-associated proteins; induction of phase II metabolizing enzymes, resulting in carcinogen detoxification	56, 57, 58
Saponins	Legumes, beans	Reduction of serum cholesterol; antimicrobial and anticarcinogenic activity	Binding bile acids, preventing cholesterol reabsorption, and increasing its excretion; inhibitory effect on certain cancer cells; stimulation of the immune system	59, 60, 61
Tocopherols Tocotrienols	Green leafy vegetables, nuts, grains, vegetable oil	Antioxidant; anticancer and hypocholesterolemic effects	Lowering free radicals; inhibition of lipid peroxidation; inhibition of proliferation of cancer cells; inhibition of HMG-CoA reductase (tocotrienols)	62, 63, 64
B. Phenolic compounds				
Coumarins	Vegetables, citrus fruits	Reduction in blood clotting; anticarcinogenic activity	Anticoagulants; inhibitors and inactivators of carcinogen and mutagen; scavengers of superoxide anion	65, 66, 67, 68
Tannins	Sorghum, hazelnuts, certain berries, grape seed (dry)	Cancer prevention; reduction of heart disease; antimicrobial	Antioxidant; inhibitors of superoxide radicals production and tumor promotion	69, 70, 71
Lignan	Oil seeds (flax, soy, rapeseed), whole-grain cereals (wheat, oats, rye), legumes, and various vegetables and fruit (particularly berries)	Reduction of heart disease Reduction of breast cancer risks	Inhibition of the production of oxygen free radicals by polymorphonuclear leukocytes in hypercholesterolemia; decrease in serum cholesterol, LDL-C, and lipid peroxidation product and increase in HDL-C and antioxidant reserve; inhibition of endogenous estrogens for premenopausal women	72, 73, 74, 75
Resveratrol	Grapes, red wine	Anticarcinogenic activity; cardiovascular protective effects	Antioxidant; antiproliferative effect; induction of growth inhibition and apoptosis; stimulation of eNOS expression and activity; phytoestrogen	76, 77, 78, 79, 80, 81
Flavonoids flavanones hesperetin naringenin	Citrus peel, citrus fruits	Reduction in the risk of coronary heart disease, osteoporosis, and cancer	Antioxidant; decrease in serum cholesterol by inhibiting HMG-CoA reductase and ACAT activities; reduction of HepG2 cell apoB secretion; hampering initial atherosclerotic events by blockage of induction of cell adhesion molecules to inhibit monocyte adhesion to stimulated endothelium; phytoestrogen; interacts with human sex hormone-binding globulin;	82, 83, 84, 85, 86, 87, 88, 89, 90, 91

TABLE 114.2. PHYSIOLOGICALLY ACTIVE FOOD CHEMICALS THAT MAY PREVENT DISEASE (continued)

ACTIVE COMPOUNDS	FOOD SOURCE	POTENTIAL HEALTH BENEFIT	POSSIBLE MECHANISMS AND FUNCTIONS	REFERENCE
			inhibition of bone loss in ovariectomized mice; suppression of cell proliferation	
flavonols quercetin myricetin kaempferol	Onions, grapes broccoli	Reduction in the risk of coronary heart disease and cancer; anti-inflammatory effect; inhibition of platelet activity.	Free radical scavengers; inhibition of inducible ICAM-1 expression; hampering initial atherosclerotic events involving endothelial CAM induction by interference with translocation and transactivation of NF-κB; inhibition of cyclooxygenase and phosphodiesterase enzymes; inhibition transcriptional activation of COX-2 and iNOS; increase in the nitric oxide release and decrease in the free radical and superoxide release in platelets	92, 93, 94, 95, 96
flavones apigenin luteolin	Parsley, celery, certain sweet peppers	Reduction in the risk of coronary heart disease and cancer; anti-inflammatory effect	Hampering initial atherosclerotic events involving endothelial CAM induction by interference with translocation and transactivation of NF-κB; inhibition of carcinogen-induced tumors in animals; inhibition of transcriptional activation of COX-2 and iNOS	93, 95, 96, 97
isoflavones genestein diazein	Soybeans, soy foods, legumes	Reduction in menopausal symptoms and osteoporosis; reduction of cancer and heart disease	Phytoestrogens (estrogenic and antiestrogenic activity); alleviation of the estrogen loss after menopause; maintenance of a positive calcium balance; inhibition of cell proliferation; inhibition of transcriptional activation of COX-2; decrease in cholesterol, low-density lipoprotein cholesterol, and TGs	95, 98, 99, 100, 101, 102, 103, 104
flavanols catechin epigallocatechin epigallocatechin gallate epicatechin gallate	Tea, red grapes, red wine	Reduction of cancer and heart disease	Inhibition of initiation, promotion, and progression of cancer; inhibition of carcinogen activation and binding of DNA-reactive species; antimetastatic agent; inhibitor of cell proliferation; antioxidant; reduction in free radical/oxidative damage; protection of red blood cell membrane from free radical–induced oxidation	105, 106, 107, 108, 109, 110, 111, 112
anthocyanins	Berries, cherries, red grapes	Reduction of the risk of coronary heart disease and cancer	Protects against oxidative stress; inhibits platelet aggregation; possesses vasoprotective properties; inhibits the growth of HL60 cells through the induction of apoptosis; reduces proliferation of human colon cancer cell lines	113, 114, 115, 116, 117, 118
C. Amino acid based				
Allyl S-compounds Diallyl disulfide Allicin	Garlic, onions, leeks, chives	Prevention of cancer; stimulation of immune function; free radical scavenger; reduction of serum cholesterol and serum TG	Inhibition of the proliferation of human tumor cells in culture; inhibition of the metabolic activation of the toxicant and carcinogen; inhibition of cholesterol biosynthesis	119, 120, 121, 122, 123
Isothiocyanates Sulforaphane	Cruciferous vegetables	Prevention of cancer	Mediation of chemopreventive activity by inhibition of cytochrome P450 involved in carcinogen activation and induction of phase II enzyme involved in carcinogen detoxification	124, 125, 126

(continued)

TABLE 114.2. PHYSIOLOGICALLY ACTIVE FOOD CHEMICALS THAT MAY PREVENT DISEASE (continued)

ACTIVE COMPOUNDS	FOOD SOURCE	POTENTIAL HEALTH BENEFIT	POSSIBLE MECHANISMS AND FUNCTIONS	REFERENCE
Indoles Indole-3-carbinol	Cruciferous vegetables	Prevention of cancer; reduction of chemical-induced tumors	Regulation of estrogen activity and metabolism and modulation of the estrogen receptor transcription activity; activation of a novel antiproliferative pathway; inhibits cytochrome P450 and induces GSH S-transferase	127, 128, 129
D. Animal-derived protein Lactoferrin	Milk	Stimulation of the immune system; antimicrobial agent; healing of gastrointestinal wounds	Stimulation of beneficial gut microflora; increase in the production and release of cytokines, which may affect the immune system; T-cell-dependent augmentation of natural killer cell activity; inhibition of the cell migration of certain gastrointestinal cell lines	130, 131, 132, 133
E. Fatty acids Conjugated linoleic acid	Dairy products, cheeses	Reduction of cancer, atherosclerosis, and obesity	Reduction of cell proliferation, alteration in the components of the cell cycle and induction of apoptosis; reduction of the LDL-to-HDL cholesterol ratio and total-to-HDL cholesterol ratio in rabbits; decrease in preadipocyte proliferation and differentiation into mature adipocytes; decrease in fatty acid and TG synthesis; increase in energy expenditure, lipolysis, and fatty acid oxidation	134, 135, 136, 137, 138, 139
Omega-3 fatty acids docosahexaenoic acid (DHA)/ eicosapentaenoic acid (EPA)	Salmon, tuna, other ocean fish, algae	Reduction in plasma triacylglycerol; reduction of heart disease; prevention of sudden cardiac death or fatal arrhythmias; antiinflammatory activity	Reduction in the total-to-HDL and LDL-to-HDL cholesterol ratios; increase in serum HDL cholesterol; reduction in endogenous production of TG-rich lipoproteins and increase in elimination of TG-rich lipoproteins; blockage of excessive sodium and calcium current in the heart; antithrombotic effect; decrease in monocyte and neutrophil chemotaxis; decreases in production of proinflammatory cytokines	140, 141, 142, 143, 144, 145
α-Linolenic acid	Green leafy vegetables, flaxseed, walnuts	Reduction of heart disease; prevention of sudden cardiac death or fatal arrhythmias	Decrease in serum LDL; blockage of excessive sodium and calcium current in the heart	145, 146, 147
F. Microbial compounds Prebiotics: nondigestible but fermentable oligosaccharides	Garlic, asparagus, chicory, barley, oatmeal	Intestinal fortification; stimulation of immune function; anticarcinogenic effects; hypolipidemia	Support growth of lactobacilli and bifidobacteria, which are found in the large intestine and are generally considered to be beneficial by stimulating the immune system and protecting body from infection; modulation of lipid metabolism	148, 149, 150, 151, 152, 153
Probiotics: living beneficial bacteria such as lactobacilli, bifidobacteria	Fermented dairy foods, such as yogurt, kefir	Enhancement of immune function; prevention of diarrhea; anticarcinogenic effects	Alter the intestinal microflora balance, inhibition the growth of harmful bacteria	150, 151, 154

ACAT, acyl-CoA: cholesterol acyltransferase; apoB, apoprotein B; CAM, cellular adhesion molecule; COX, cyclooxygenase; eNOS and iNOS, endothelial and inducible nitric oxide synthase; GSH, glutathione; HDL, high-density lipoprotein; HMG-CoA, 3-hydroxy-3-methyl-glutaryl-coenzyme A; ICAM, intercellular adhesion molecule; LDL, low-density lipoprotein; NF-κB, nuclear factor-κB; TG, triglyceride.

Modified from Bidlack WR, Wang W. Designing functional foods. In: Shils ME, Olson JA, Shike M et al., eds. Modern Nutrition in Health and Disease. 9th ed. Baltimore: Williams & Wilkins, 1999:1823–34.

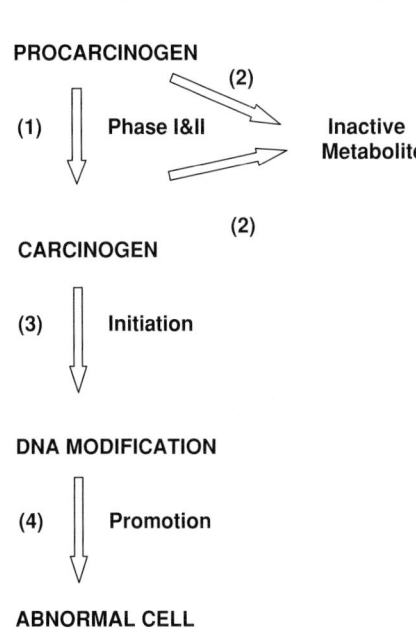

PROCARCINOGEN

(1) Phase I&II ⟶ (2) ⟶ **Inactive Metabolite**

(2)

CARCINOGEN

(3) Initiation

DNA MODIFICATION

(4) Promotion

ABNORMAL CELL

(5) Proliferation

TUMOR

1. Modification of carcinogen activation
   a. polyphenols
   b. alkyl sulfide
   c. isothiocyanates
   d. monoterpenes
   e. flavonoids

2. Modification of carcinogen detoxification
   a. alkyl cysteines
   b. isothiocyanates

3. Blocks initiation
   a. polyphenols
   b. indole
   c. sulfides
   d. flavonoids
   e. protease inhibitors

4. Blocks DNA reactive species
   a. carotenoids
   b. polyphenols
   c. flavonoids
   d. terpenes
   e. protease inhibitors
   f. sulfides
   g. indoles

5. Blocks cell proliferation
   a. monoterpenes
   b. vitamin A, precursors and metabolites

Figure 114.1. Anticancer activities of phytochemicals. (Data from Wattenberg LW. Chemoprevention of cancer by naturally occurring and synthetic compounds. In: Wattenberg LW, Lipkin M, Boone CW et al., eds. Cancer Chemoprevention. Boca Raton, FL: CRC Press, 1992:3–18; and Waladkhani AR, Clemens MR. Effect of dietary phytochemicals on cancer development. In: Watson RR, ed. Vegetables, Fruits, and Herbs in Health Promotion. Boca Raton, FL: CRC Press, 2001:3–18.)

Carotenoids

ß-Carotene has provided a model for the thorough research that is needed (156). The term carotenoids encompasses both carotene, which identifies the hydrocarbon forms, and the xanthophylls, which include carotenoid derivatives having one or more oxygen-containing functional groups (157). More than 600 distinct carotenoids and their glycosides have been identified. Most of the early research was focused only on ß-carotene, whereas many other carotenoids may have better health-supporting properties than those provided by ß-carotene. The success of ß-carotene research established the experimental models for studying other carotenoids and phytochemicals in general.

Important factors affecting carotenoid bioavailability include the release of the carotenoids from the physical food matrix in which they are ingested. Heating of food improves bioavailability, disassociating the protein-carotenoid complexes and enhancing dispersion of the crystalline carotenoid to form multilamellar lipid vesicles from lipid droplets resulting from bile salt and pancreatic lipase action. Nondigested lipids, such as sucrose polyesters, and some dietary fibers interfere with carotenoid absorption.

Movement of the carotenoid micelle into the mucosal cells of the duodenum appears to occur via passive diffusion, but may be species-specific (158). No intracellular binding proteins have been identified for the carotenoids, as have been reported for α-tocopherol, retinol, and cholecalciferol.

The transport of the carotenoids in plasma occurs exclusively within the lipoproteins. The distribution of ß-carotene, α-carotene, and lycopene in plasma lipoproteins is similar to the distribution of that for cholesterol. The dihydroxy carotenoids (lutein and zeaxanthin) are distributed 40 to 50% in the high-density lipoproteins, which is more similar to the pattern of distribution observed for α-tocopherol (159). Differential uptake and retention of different carotenoid species has been confirmed for several tissues. Characterization of the specificity of tissue distribution may contribute to further understanding of the physiologic role played by the carotenoids in influencing biologic processes.

The source of dietary carotenoid has an impact on transport from the intestine to the circulation. In one study, carotenoids were fed to 30 men over a 6-week period, and either of two supplementary doses of ß-carotene (30 and 12 mg) were compared with dietary intakes of carrots, broccoli, or tomato juice. The purified ß-carotene produced greater plasma response than did similar quantities of carotenoids provided from the food sources, suggesting a difference in bioavailability or interference by other dietary components (160).

Intestinal absorption, serum clearance, and interactions between ß-carotene and lutein have been evaluated in human subjects (161). Individual variances included ninefold differences for lutein and sixfold differences for ß-carotene. Comparison of individual doses versus combined doses indicated that ß-carotene significantly reduced lutein absorption by 40 to 45%, whereas lutein had mixed results on ß-carotene levels in the same patients (uniquely, half increased and half decreased). Thus, dietary intake is important but genetic regulation makes the major difference.

The role of ß-carotene and other carotenoids in relation to other isoprenoid antioxidants has been examined. Tocopherols, tocotrienols, ascorbic acid, and carotenoids react with free radicals, specifically peroxyl radicals, and with singlet oxygen. α-Tocopherol is the primary peroxyl radical scavenger in biologic lipid phases, such as membranes or low-density lipoproteins. Ascorbic acid is present in aqueous compartments, such as cytosol or plasma and other body fluids, and can reduce the tocopheroxyl radical. To regenerate these biologic agents, coupling occurs to nonradical reducing systems such as glutathione peroxidase. Carotenoids, such as ß-carotene, lycopene, and some oxycarotenoids, such as zeaxanthin and lutein, exert antioxidant function in lipid sites, quenching singlet oxygen and free radicals.

There is evidence for interactions with α-tocopherol and ascorbic acid. Using peroxidation of a microsomal membrane suspension as a model, ß-carotene was effective as an antioxidant at low oxygen tension (150 mm Hg PO_2); however, at higher oxygen tension (760 mm PO_2) ß-carotene became a prooxidant (162). Oxygen binds to the carotene radical to form peroxy radicals, which then become part of the propagation reaction stimulating lipid peroxidation. α-Tocopherol prevents the prooxidant effect of ß-carotene in a dose-dependent manner, either by decreasing the lipid free radicals or peroxyl radicals or the ß-carotene peroxyl radical directly.

Recent studies involving ß-carotene supplementation of smokers has indicated that there is no magic bullet. In reviewing these human experiments, Mayne (163) indicated that most had a negative effect on cancer expression in lung and possibly in cardiovascular disease. These studies suggested that other carotenoids in fruits and vegetables may be as or more important than ß-carotene. However, it may also have to do with the high dose of the ß-carotene supplement provided in these studies.

To date, dietary levels of the carotenoids have not been shown to cause adverse effects. Importantly, the role of other dietary phytochemicals cannot be ignored. Because diets rich in fruits and vegetables correlate highly with health benefits, any one phytochemical may not prove to be protective alone, but may well express protection in concert with other dietary components.

Monoterpenes

The monoterpenes, small ten-carbon isoprenoid units, are produced as secondary products of the mevalonic acid metabolic pathway in plants (56). This pathway initiates synthesis of the phytosterols, whereas in animals the mevalonic acid pathway leads to the formation of cholesterol and other sterols. Monoterpenes are found in the essential oil fraction of many fruits, herbs, and spices, as well as in barley oil, rice bran oil, olive and palm oil, and wine. Lesser amounts can be found in dairy products and eggs.

The isoprenoids were identified for their activity in reducing cholesterol biosynthesis in animals. However, more than 50 monoterpenes have been found to have substantial anticarcinogenic activity in a variety of cellular and animal models, inducing apoptosis; inducing phase II detoxification enzymes, glutathione-S-transferase and uridine diphosphoglucuronosyl transferase, essential for clearing carcinogen metabolites; and decreasing formation of DNA adducts. Not only do the monoterpenes inhibit carcinogenesis, but they also induce regression of mammary, liver, and pancreatic tumors in rats and express antitumor activity in various cell lines. Human studies have indicated that 0.5 mmol/day of isoprenoids will significantly lower serum cholesterol, whereas 20 times that amount is required to provide chemoprevention (with few side effects).

The two most researched monoterpenes, D-limonene and perillyl alcohol, are undergoing clinical trials for the treatment of advanced-stage cancers. Other important monoterpenes with antitumor effects are geraniol, menthol, and tocotrienol.

D-Limonene is found primarily in the essential oil fraction from orange peel and is often used as a flavor enhancer in drinks and foods. Dietary orange peel oil (1–5%) was found to inhibit the promotion and progression of chemically initiated mammary carcinogenesis in mice and subsequently to promote the regression of these tumors. Limonene has been found to decrease the incidence of many tumor types in animals, including lung adenomas and skin, liver, mammary, and stomach tumors (57). Currently, limonene is under investigation as a treatment for breast cancer in humans as an alternative to tamoxifen.

Perillyl alcohol is found in the essential oil fraction of mints, lavender, and cherries. It is the hydroxylated derivative of D-limonene and is five times more effective than limonene. By selectively inhibiting isoprenylation of small guanine nucleotide-binding proteins (G proteins) and by interacting with protein:prenyl transferases, perillyl alcohol has a significant role in cell growth.

Perillyl alcohol can also inhibit cell growth by regulating the synthesis of cholesterol, as well as inducing differentiation and increasing apoptosis activated by transforming growth factor β receptor as well as increased transforming growth factor β levels. Perillyl alcohol has been shown to inhibit colon and small intestine cancer and liver, pancreatic, mammary, and prostate cancer (58). Currently, the National Cancer Institute is carrying out phase I clinical trials for the use of perillyl alcohol for the treatment of advanced breast cancer in humans. There appears to be only slight renal and gastrointestinal toxicity associated with using this monoterpene up to 2 g/day.

Phenolic Compounds

Major types of phenolic compounds are identified in Table 114.2B. They include phenolic acids, flavonoids, tannins, coumarins, lignins, quinones, stilbenes, and curcuminoids. All exhibit strong antioxidant activity and may have beneficial chemopreventive activity (164).

Tannins

Tannins (tannic acid) are water-soluble polyphenols that are present in many plant foods. They have been reported to be responsible for decreases in feed intake, growth rate, feed efficiency, net metabolizable energy, and protein digestibility in experimental animals. Therefore, foods rich in tannins are considered to be of low nutritional value.

Incidences of certain cancers, such as esophageal cancer, have been reported to be related to consumption of tannin-rich foods such as betel nuts and herbal teas, suggesting that tannins may be carcinogenic. However, other reports indicated that the carcinogenic activity of tannins may be related to components associated with tannins rather than to the tannins themselves.

Interestingly, many reports indicated a negative association between tea consumption and incidences of cancers (70). Tea polyphenols, catechins, and many tannin components were suggested to be anticarcinogenic and may reduce the mutagenic activity of a number of mutagens. Because many carcinogens and/or mutagens are metabolized to free radical intermediates, which interact with cellular macromolecules, the anticarcinogenic and antimutagenic potentials of tannins may be related to their antioxidative property. The antimicrobial activities of tannins have been well documented, inhibiting growth of many fungi, yeasts, bacteria, and viruses. The antimicrobial properties seem to be associated with the hydrolysis of ester linkage between gallic acid and polyols initiated after ripening of many edible fruits. Tannins in these fruits thus serve as a natural defense mechanism against microbial infections.

Animal and human experiments indicate that tannins have other physiologic effects, such as to accelerate blood clotting, reduce blood pressure, decrease the serum lipid level, produce liver necrosis, and modulate immunoresponse. Thus, we must always be cognizant of the exposure dose and frequency.

Flavonols

Jasmine green tea is an excellent source of natural polyphenol antioxidants, specifically the catechins, including (-)-epicatechin (EC), (-)-epicatechin-3- gallate (ECG), (-)-epigallocatechin (EGC), and (-)-epigallocatechin-3-gallate (EGCG). The purified catechins showed a strong protection for red blood cell hemolysis in vitro induced chemically by an azo free radical initiator. Importantly, the effective dose for antioxidant activity occurred between 2.5 and 40 micromolar, and EGCG and ECG were most effective. However, only EGC and EC were found in the circulation after a gavage dose of jasmine tea, suggesting selective absorption, yet the tea still reduced red blood cell hemolysis (106).

The absorption, distribution, metabolism, and excretion of green tea catechins have been studied in animals and humans (165) and have been found in the systemic circulation after oral administration of green tea or green tea catechins in animals and humans. The unchanged catechins are in the low micrometer range, which is lower than the effective concentrations established in in vitro studies. However, more than 15 different metabolites have been identified after oral and intravenous administration, and the glucuronide, sulfate, and methylated catechin conjugates were determined to be present in the circulation at concentrations greater than those of the parent compound. The relationship of the catechin metabolites to biologic activity remains to be determined.

It has been consistently reported that there are large individual variations in the pharmacokinetics of green tea catechins and their metabolites reported in humans. High tissue levels of green tea catechins or derived metabolites are found in the gastrointestinal tract, kidney, and bladder. The tissue distribution pattern is related primarily to the site of metabolism (166).

The effects of green tea as a chemopreventive agent in multiple animal models are of great interest. Using either green tea infusion or isolated tea catechins, these polyphenolic compounds have proven to express a broad spectrum of anticarcinogenic activity. The effect of EGCG on leukemic blast cells from patients with acute myeloblastic leukemia indicated inhibition of proliferation. EGCG did not inhibit granulocyte-macrophage colony-stimulating factor (GM-CSF), but did block the stimulation of GM-CSF release by tumor necrosis factor-α or tetradecanoylphorbol acetate and blocked the modulation of c-kit, a receptor for stem cell factor on leukemic cells (107, 167).

Catechins are able to inhibit every stage of the carcinogenic process, including the development of tumors at different sites and in different organs, a wide array of enzymes involved in cell proliferation (such as protein kinase C, DNA polymerase, RNA polymerase, lipoxygenase, ornithine decarboxylase, cytochrome P450, and the induction of phase II enzymes), and a variety of indirect and direct chemical carcinogens and tumor promoters. Importantly, the results of animal experiments have consistently indicated that the effective concentrations of these phenolic compounds equal the levels found naturally in brewed tea (168).

Isoflavones

The soy isoflavones, genistein and daidzein, are representative phytoestrogens that function as chemopreventive agents against cancers, cardiovascular disease, and osteoporosis. However, in some of these experiments it has not been possible to separate the phytoestrogen effect from the effect of other components in the food. The isoflavonoids and lignins may play a significant inhibitory role in cancer development, particularly in the promotional phase of the disease, although recent studies suggest that genistein and/or daidzein may also participate in the initiation stage of carcinogenesis and induce cancers of the estrogen-sensitive reproductive organs in rodents (169, 170). Thus, at present no definite recommendations can be made regarding the dietary amounts needed for prevention of disease.

Phytoestrogens are present in the human diet in substantial amounts, especially in soybeans and soy foods (102). Three main classes of phytoestrogens exist—isoflavones, coumestans, and lignans. All are diphenolic compounds with structural similarities to natural estrogens and antiestrogens. The phytoestrogens have been shown to have many biologic effects in cell culture and in animals and humans. Phytoestrogens are estrogenic compounds found in plants that exert estrogenic effects on the central nervous system, induction of estrus, and stimulation of growth of the female genital tract in animals (98). Most of these effects are considered positive, although a few harmful effects have been reported.

Although the amount of phytoestrogen absorbed may be low relative to the dietary concentration, the level circulating in the blood may be 100 to 500 times that of naturally occurring estrogen and estradiol. Absorption is facilitated by hydrolysis of the sugar moiety on the phytoestrogen gastric hydrochloric acid and β-glucosidases in foods and by human gut bacterial β-glucosidases. When the diet is supplemented with soy products, the level of phytoestrogens can reach 1000 times the level of estradiol. Soy food processing appears to affect isoflavone bioavailability, and fermented tempeh appears to enhance absorption.

After absorption, isoflavones and lignans are conjugated with glucuronic acid and sulfate by hepatic phase II enzymes (uridine diphosphate-glucuronosyltransferase and sulfotransferase, respectively). These metabolic changes make the lipophilic compounds more water soluble and enhance their excretion. Urinary output indicated that the glucuronic acid derivatives were the primary excretory product.

Phytoestrogens can affect the menstrual cycle and the concentration of reproductive hormones in the blood of premenopausal women, but less so in postmenopausal women. Natural flavones, such as daidzein or coumestrol, inhibited the aromatase (placental) enzyme in vitro. Aromatase is the rate-limiting enzymatic step in estrogen synthesis in humans.

Genistein, the most abundant phytoestrogen, and coumestrol have been shown to enhance bone calcium retention in rats. They inhibit bone resorption and stimu-

late bone mineralization (101). Similar effects are noted after consuming soy protein products, which still contain the phytoestrogens. The protective effects are also observed in osteoporotic patients. The consumption of soy foods also includes a good source of dietary calcium to enhance the effect.

Genistein inhibits protein tyrosine kinase, an oncogene product that catalyzes tyrosine phosphorylation involved in tumor cell signal transduction and proliferation. Growth inhibition by genistein occurs in different human cancer cells, including melanoma cells and leukemia. Similarly, phytoestrogens inhibit endothelial cell proliferation in capillaries.

Genistein has also been shown to increase activities of antioxidant enzymes, such as superoxide dismutase, glutathione peroxidase and glutathione reductase, and liver cumene hydroperoxidase. These results suggest that genistein could work positively with other phytochemicals, having antioxidant activities, providing a broader cellular defense against free radical attack and oxidative damage.

Population studies and intervention trials have clearly shown a relationship between dietary phytosterol intake, as well as foods fortified with phytosterols, and a lowering of serum cholesterol levels in diverse population groups (171). In addition to increasing dietary fiber, soy protein foods and the incorporation of phytosterols into foods could have a major impact on the reduction of coronary artery disease risk of young adults.

Thus, most studies in humans, animals, and cell culture indicate that phytoestrogens play a role in prevention of menopausal symptoms, osteoporosis, cancer, and heart disease. Importantly, dietary supplementation with soy foods produces a similar response as noted for the isolated phytoestrogen supplement.

Animal-Derived Protein

Several animal proteins and lipids have been identified to support health properties and diminish the incidence of disease. Table 114.2D identifies lactoferrin (LF) as an example protein. Although not discussed in this section, Table 114.2E also indicates animal-derived fatty acids, such as conjugated linoleic acid (CLA) and ω-3 fatty acids.

Lactoferrin

An example of a physiologically active animal product is the milk protein, LF. Structurally similar to transferrin, it has been assumed to be an iron transport protein delivering maternal iron to the infant gut. LF binding sites have been identified on a variety of cells and tissues, but a high pI makes it difficult to characterize whether or not there are specific or nonspecific receptors. Several hypotheses for LF function have been made, including enhanced bioavailability of breast milk iron, an antimicrobial agent, and enhancement of immune response, including antibody production, complement activation, and natural killer cell function (172). The broad-spectrum antimicrobial properties of LF highlight the potential application of this protein as an enteral and parenteral antimicrobial factor, as well as a potential food additive (173). A patented process causes activation of LF (ALF) to provide many of the unique properties needed to be an effective antimicrobial agent, which enabled ALF to be approved by the FDA for meat applications (174).

The bacteriostatic effect of orally administered bovine LF (bLF) was evaluated on intestinal bacteria in the gut of mice fed bovine milk. Consumption of bovine milk increased the proliferation of Enterobacteriaceae, but with added bLF the proliferation was suppressed. Similar effects were noted when the gut was seeded with *Clostridium ramosum* as well as other species of *Clostridium*. Compared with other proteins, only bLF showed this effect. Interestingly, partial hydrolysis of bLF with pepsin, similar to digestive hydrolysis, did not alter the bacteriostatic effect—bLF still provided protection for infant animals from gastrointestinal infections (172).

Recombinant human LF (rhLF) has been produced and characterized. Addition of rhLF to infant formula will require further research, ensuring stability during processing and providing further evaluation of biologic activity through studies on large numbers of infants' intestinal microflora. Before implementing a new product with increased cost, the biologic effect must be confirmed and shown to be a clear benefit to the infant. Mature human milk contains 2 to 3 mg/mL of hLF, although most infant formulas currently contain no LF. bLF is naturally saturated only 20% with iron. At this level, benefits can be seen after 3 months of feeding, although not all studies indicate a need for LF supplementation.

Approval has been obtained to use ALF as a food additive. As a natural antimicrobial agent, it blocks microbial attachment to biosurfaces, such as the epithelial mucosa (adhesion is essential for colonization and replication); bacterial detachment occurs as ALF competes for the same attachment sites on the tissue; and the binding of ALF to the bacterial surface causes sequestration of iron and produces an antibacterial effect (174). In addition, ALF expresses broad-spectrum activity against both DNA and RNA viruses, blocking viral adhesion to eukaryotic cells. The recently approved application of ALF to beef carcasses to prevent *Escherichia coli* contamination included a patented application/spraying process to decrease microbial contamination. If not attached, there is no colonization or growth of *E. coli* and the risk for toxin production in ground meat is essentially eliminated.

Microbial

Lactic acid bacteria (LAB), such as lactobacilli and bifidobacteria, are among the predominant microorganisms in the gastrointestinal tract of humans and animals. Certain diseases, physiologic conditions, and aging could diminish LAB content and distribution resulting in gastrointestinal ailments. LAB prevents adherence of other organisms and decreases establishment and replication of several enteric mucosal pathogens using several antimicrobial mechanisms. LAB also releases various enzymes into the intestinal lumen, exerting synergistic effects on digestion and alleviating symptoms of intestinal malabsorption.

There are two mechanisms by which LAB can be enhanced to provide benefit to the gastrointestinal tract. Prebiotics, nondigestible oligosaccharides provided in food, pass unaltered through the stomach into the small intestine and reside in the large intestine, where they can be selectively metabolized and stimulate the growth and/or activity of one or more bacterial species residing in the colon (148). Thus, the number of indigenous probiotic bacteria would increase, providing a health benefit to the host. As a microbial dietary adjuvant, probiotic bacteria (bifidobacteria and some lactobacilli) beneficially affect the host physiology by modulating mucosal and systemic immunity as well as improving nutritional and microbial balance in the intestinal tract (154). In addition, probiotic-active substances include cellular complexes of LAB that have a great capacity to interact with the host mucosa and may beneficially modulate the immune system independent of LAB's viability.

Consumption of LAB-fermented dairy products may elicit antitumor and antimutagenic effects, which have been attributed to decreased activating enzymes and increased detoxification enzymes for carcinogens and mutagens, and decreased tumor promoting agents, leading to suppression of tumors. Specific cellular components in LAB strains induce strong adjuvant effects, including modulation of cell-mediated immune responses, activation of reticuloendothelial system, augmentation of cytokine pathways and regulation of interleukins, and tumor necrosis factor. In addition, the LAB enhances innate host defenses by production of natural antimicrobial substances. Oral administration of LAB is well tolerated and proven to be safe—use of fermented products has occurred over 5000 years and more importantly in 143 controlled human clinical trials (>700 subjects) studied between 1961 and 1998 (154). The future could incorporate greater acceptance of prebiotics and probiotics in prophylactic and therapeutic applications, thereby diminishing use of synthetic antimicrobial agents.

DESIGNING FUNCTIONAL FOODS

The new generation of functional foods represents an opportunity to apply food technology to enhance production of specific functional ingredients using gene transfer, genetic engineering, bioengineering, cell culture, and specialized breeding programs. Many of these processes have been used over the last decade in efforts to enhance the nutritional quality of the food supply, for example, breeding of meat animals to have lower body fat in an effort to control fat calories and cholesterol content per serving, and altering plant fatty acid content to achieve desired ratios of beneficial fatty acids in the extracted oil and to improve the nutritional quality of plant proteins. These efforts continue as a means of improving the diet without necessarily labeling them as functional foods. However, as the market grows these beneficial changes may become more marketable to the health-conscious consumer.

The examples of functional food products provided here are only representative of a larger effort to provide a healthful and safe diet. Some of the functional products identified here are already available in the marketplace, whereas others are being developed and some indicate opportunities for future project development. Designing of new delivery systems enables benefits from the use of each active functional food ingredient to be provided to a broader consumer population. A few current examples include:

- Soyfoods are a great example of a food source containing high-quality protein and naturally occurring phytoestrogens, such as isoflavones (Table 114.2B).
  - Tofu and other soy products are prepared using calcium coagulation of the protein, providing the food products with a ready source of calcium, high-quality protein, and phytoestrogens.
  - Flavoring of soy milk enhances consumption.
  - Textured soy protein can be formulated into a variety of new products, including meat substitutes.
  - Roasted soy nuts (soybeans) are a healthful snack food.
- Dairy products, including milk, cheese, yogurt, and protein (casein and whey) isolates
  - Partial hydrolysis of casein produces phosphopeptides, which enhance calcium absorption and may also yield other physiologic responses. These peptides have been added to other beverages as a natural product to enhance calcium absorption.
  - A nutraceutical milk has been developed, replacing fat with β-glucan + Oatrim (USDA) to lower cholesterol. (A similar fiber-based drink has been popular in Japan.)
  - Yogurt-based beverages can deliver live probiotic cultures (*Lactobacillus acidophilus* and *Bifidobacterium*).
  - Plant sterols can be added to milk and yogurt beverages to aid lowering of cholesterol.
  - Prebiotic oligosaccharides, such as inulin, cannot be digested, yet promote calcium absorption (an additional 18% above normal), and can be added to milk or yogurt.
  - LF, an iron-binding milk protein, has several unique properties, including antimicrobial functions (Table 114.2D). It has excellent potential to serve as a natural (GRAS) food additive, replacing other chemi-

cally derived agents, in sausages or canned meats or as a surface coating on carcasses (now USDA approved).
  - The dairy cow can be challenged with specific microorganisms, producing specific gamma globulins that can be isolated from the milk and used in therapeutic situations for calves (currently) and perhaps humans (in the future).
  - Modified natural cheese starter cultures to find a strain that will diminish cholesterol and reduce fat will produce a product that could be used in a variety of new functional food products.
- Blood recovered from slaughter houses has provided an opportunity to isolate several blood proteins for laboratory use, but also as a food ingredient (accepted in Europe, not the United States).
  - Albumin can be used as an egg white substitute.
  - The crude γ-globulin fraction can be fed to newborn animals to maintain their growth, serving as a natural antimicrobial agent.
  - Other blood components are isolated, purified, and developed into usable products.
- Dietary ω-3 fatty acids may reduce the risk of CHD (Table 114.2E). It can be obtained from ocean fish, although it comes from algae in their diet. A broader-based delivery system is sought to provide general access to ω-3 fatty acids as a food ingredient.
  - Designer oils containing eicosapentaenoic acid and docosahexanoic acid can be created and blended with other oils as ingredients to create specialty products, such as salad dressing, cooking oils, or margarine.
  - Growth incubators have been designed to promote the continuous production of the algae, allowing recovery and extraction of pure ω-3 fatty acids.
  - The algae can be incorporated into feed products for egg-laying poultry and for fish grown by aquaculture on fish farms.
  - Plant species are also being developed through breeding and biotechnology programs that will contain ω-3 fatty acids for use in an ever-increasing product category.
- Eggs are a nutritionally sound product delivered in a self-contained package. The contents can be nutritionally enhanced by altering the feed composition of the laying hens.
  - Addition of cholestyramine to the diet reduces the cholesterol content of eggs. Natural nutraceutical compounds may produce the same effect.
  - Chickens fed marigolds or dietary carotenoids incorporate greater ß-carotene levels into their egg yolks. Similar feeding of other phytochemicals could transform eggs into a functional food.
  - Chickens fed ω-3 fatty acids or algae incorporate the ω-3 fatty acids into the egg yolk, a rapidly growing consumer health product.

- Meat and dairy products contain bioactive fatty acids produced during stomach fermentation.
  - CLA is found in dairy products, meat, and certain plants. CLA appears to have health benefits against cancer, but also possibly in weight reduction (Table 114.2E).
- Cereal
  - Ready-to-eat breakfast cereals are one of the early functional foods, delivering the fiber and nutrient value in a palatable form.
  - Ready-to-eat breakfast cereal is coated with vitamins and some minerals, acting as a convenient nutrient delivery system, and should provide a delivery system for functional food ingredients.
- Margarines/spreads/cooking oils
  - Phytosterols, stanols, and sterols have esters that are GRAS-approved, food-grade ingredients, commercially available in margarine.
  - Phytosterols could be incorporated into other foods, such as chocolate candy, yogurt, and smoothies (health stores have added phytochemicals and herbs to smoothies for several years).
  - Esters of the phytosterols can be created using CLA, docosahexaenoic acid, or eicosapentaenoic acid to enhance the delivery of multiple phytochemicals in a single product. The esters are hydrolyzed during digestion, releasing the fatty acid ester.
  - Diglycerides can also be formed and incorporated into cooking oils, mayonnaise, spreads, salad dressings, and margarine. Diglycerides can reduce serum cholesterol as well.
  - Canola oil incorporated into butter can improve spreadability at lower temperatures.
  - Selection of plants to increase production of CLA esters would increase their availability in salad oils and many other functional foods.
- Orange juice
  - Calcium fortification of beverages, such as orange juice, and snack foods is not new but can contribute to bone repair and prevention of osteoporosis.
  - Nanodispersion of phytosterols, imbedded in a lecithin liposome, into orange juice enables more people to benefit from the cholesterol-lowering effects of the plant nutraceutical.
  - Other phytochemicals could be delivered by a similar mechanism.
- Chewing gum
  - Inclusion of zinc allows coating of the throat and possibly decreases colds.
  - Inclusion of cinnamic aldehyde was added to provide a cinnamon flavor, but was determined to act as an antimicrobial agent and to prevent bad breath.
  - Oligosaccharides were included (in Japan) as a prebiotic to promote beneficial bacteria in the gastrointestinal tract (Table 114.2F).

- Vitamins were included in a chewable form; other functional ingredients could be used as well.

To date, the average consumer has been willing to pay a higher price for health foods and nutritional and herbal supplement products. What price the consumer will consistently pay for these and future added-value products remains unknown. However, if the manufacturer can assure the consumer of an efficacious product that will provide an identifiable health benefit, they will spend more of their disposable income on "healthy" functional foods.

CONCLUSIONS

Given consumers' preference for more convenient and healthful foods, an improved knowledge of human nutritional and physiologic needs, and technological developments, the US food industry has been able to develop a wider variety of products. These include fortified foods, low-fat and low-calorie foods, functional foods (in which concentrations of one or more food constituents have been manipulated to enhance their contributions to a healthful diet), and most recently, foods produced by the emerging techniques of biotechnology (e.g., cereal grains with greater nutritional value). Taking a raw commodity such as wheat or soybeans and making it more nutritious, safer, more convenient, more acceptable, easier to prepare, or specific to the needs of special population groups adds immense value to the commodity.

It remains important to integrate a well-balanced diet, good lifestyle habits, environmental factors, and heredity. Without this connection, the designer-functional foods concept could be misinterpreted as offering some form of magic bullet. In the end, the consumer is responsible for maximizing his or her own health potential, and the food industry must deliver specific functional products that enable the consumer to optimize the individual genetic potential for long-term health and well-being.

REFERENCES

1. Bidlack WR. J Am Coll Nutr 1996;15:422–33.
2. National Research Council, Committee on Diet and Health. Diet and Health: Implications for Reducing Chronic Disease Risk. Washington, DC: National Academy of Science Press, 1989.
3. World Health Organization. Nutr Rev 1991;49:291–301.
4. US Public Health Service, Office of the Surgeon General. The Surgeon General's Report on Nutrition and Health. Publication No. 88–50210.Washington, DC: Department of Health and Human Services (Public Health Service), 1988.
5. Wise JA. Health benefits of fruits and vegetables: The protective role of phytonutrients. In: Watson RR, ed. Vegetables, Fruits and Herbs in Health Promotion. Boca Raton, FL: CRC Press, 2001:147–76.
6. Li TSC. Medicinal Plants: Culture, Utilization and Phytopharmacology. Lancaster, PA: Technomic Publishing, 2000.
7. McKenna DJ, Jones K, Hughes K et al. Botanical Medicines: The Desk Reference for Major Herbal Supplements. 2nd ed. New York: Haworth Herbal Press, 2002.

8. Verlangieri AJ, Kapeghian JC, el-Dean S et al. Med Hypotheses 1985;16:7–15.

9. American Institute for Cancer Research and the World Cancer Research Fund. Food, Nutrition and the Prevention of Cancer: A Global Perspective. Washington, DC: American Institute for Cancer Research, 1997:362–421.

10. Wattenberg LW. Chemoprevention of cancer by naturally occurring and synthetic compounds. In: Wattenberg LW, Lipkin M, Boone CW et al., eds. Cancer Chemoprevention. Boca Raton, FL: CRC Press, 1992:3–18.

11. Ziegler RG. Am J Clin Nutr 1991;53[Suppl]:251S–9S.

12. Steinmetz KA, Potter JD. Cancer Causes Control 1991;2: 325–57.

13. Steinmetz KA, Potter JD. Cancer Causes Control 1991;2: 427–42.

14. Patterson B, Block G, Rosenberger WF et al. Am J Public Health 1990;80:1443–9.

15. Block G, Patterson B, Subar A. Nutr Cancer 1992;18:1–29.

16. Greenwald P, Clifford CK, Milner JA. Eur J Cancer 2001; 166:948–65.

17. Goldberg G, ed. Plants: Diet and Health. The Report of a British Nutrition Foundation Task Force. Oxford: Blackwell Science, 2003.

18. Childs NM, Poryzees GH. J Consumer Market 1997;14: 433–47.

19. Finley JW. New opportunities to bring nutritionally superior food products to market. In: Shanidi I, Ho CT, eds. Phytochemicals and Phytopharmaceuticals. Champaign, IL: AOCS Press, 2000:22–31.

20. Wildman REC. Classifying nutraceuticals. In: Wildman REC, ed. Handbook of Nutraceutical and Functional Foods. Boca Raton, FL: CRC Press, 2001:13–31.

21. Arai S. Biosci Biotech Biochem 1996;60:9–15.

22. The FOSHU system is authorized by the Nutrition Improvement Law, Law No. 248, July 31, 1952, Amended by Law No. 101, May 24, 1995, and the Nutrition Improvement Law Enforcement Regulations, Ministerial Ordinance No. 41, July 1991, Amendment to Ministerial Ordinance No. 33, May 25, 1996.

23. Institute of Medicine, Committee on Opportunities in the Nutrition and Food Sciences. Thomas PR, Earl P, eds. Opportunities in the Nutrition and Food Sciences: Research Challenges and the Next Generation of Investigators. Washington, DC: National Academy Press, 1994:109.

24. Caragay AB. Food Technol 1992;46:65–8.

25. Anonymous. The Nutraceutical Initiative: A proposal for Economic and Regulatory Reform (White Paper). New York: Foundation for Innovation in Medicine, 1991.

26. DeFelice SL. Trends Food Sci Technol 1995;6:59–61.

27. Anonymous. Medical Food. Food Technol 1992;46:87–96.

28. Yetley EA, Moore RJ. Food Technol 1997;51:136.

29. Head RJ, Record IR, King RA. Nutr Rev 1996;54: S17–S20.

30. Childs NM. Marketing issues for functional foods and nutraceuticals. In: Wildman REC, ed. Handbook of Nutraceuticals and Functional Foods. Boca Raton, FL: CRC Press, 2001: 517–28.

31. Hyman PM. Legal developments in marketing foods with health claims in the United States. In: Watson RR, ed. Vegetables, Fruits and Herbs in Health Promotion. Boca Raton, FL: CRC Press, 2001:325–38.

32. Wrick KL. Cereal Foods World 1993;38:205–14.

33. Federal Food, Drug and Cosmetic Act of 1938. Pub L No. 75–717, 52 Stat 1040 (1938).

34. Neff J, Holman JR. Food Processing 1997;23:25–8.

35. Nutrition and Labeling Act of 1990. 21 U.S.C. § 343 (r)(3)(B)(i), implemented at 21 CFR101, 1990.

36. Dietary Supplement Health and Education Act of 1994. Pub L No. 103–417, 108 Stat 4325–35, 1994.

37. FDA Modernization Act of 1997. Pub L No. 105–114, 111 Stat 2296. Codified at 21 U.S.C. § 343(r)(3)(C) and (D), 1997.

38. Silverglade BA, Heller IR. Food Drug Law J 1997;52:313–21.

39. Food and Drug Administration. Fed Reg 1993;58:2478–536.

40. Deis RC. What's in a Claim? Labeling Functional Foods. Food Product Design FFA, 2003:15, 16, 19, 20, 22, 23.

41. Code of Federal Regulations Title 21, Food and Drugs, Part 101 (Food Labeling). Washington, DC: Food and Drug Administration, 2002.

42. Ginnsman WH. Nutr Rev 1996;54:S33–7.

43. Anonymous. Food Technol 2004;57:88–90.

44. Lucchina LA. Food Technol 2003;57:42–7.

45. Bidlack WR, Wang W. Designing functional foods. In: Shils ME, Olson JA, Shike M et al., eds. Modern Nutrition in Health and Disease. 9th ed. Baltimore: Williams & Wilkins, 1999: 1823–34.

46. Food Safety: Improvement Needed in Overseeing the Safety of Dietary Supplements and Functional Foods. Report RCED-00-156. Washington, DC: General Accounting Office, 2000.

47. Hasler C, Moag-Strahlberg A, Webb D et al. J Am Diet Assoc 2001;101:733–6.

48. Codex Alimentarius Commission. Proposed draft guidelines for use of health and nutrition claims. Codex Alimentarius. Rome, Italy, FAO/WHO, Alinorm 03/22, 2002.

49. Harwood M. Nutraceutical World 2004;March:42–5.

50. Hasler CM, ed. Regulation of Functional Foods and Nutraceuticals: A Global Perspective. Oxford: Blackwell, 2004.

51. Mongelsdorf ME, Bianchi A. Inc Magazine 1994:33.

52. Stibel GM, Devilbiss K. SPECTRUM Food Industry 1993; 30:1–12.

53. Stahl W, Sies H. Arch Biochem Biophys 1996;336:1–9.

54. Tyurin VA, Carta G, Tyurin YY et al. Lipids 1997;32:131–42.

55. Slattery ML, Benson J, Curtin K et al. Am J Clin Nutr 2000; 71:575–82.

56. Hohl RJ. Adv Exp Med Biol 1996;401:137–46.

57. Crowell PL, Siar Ayoubi A, Burke YD. Adv Exp Med Biol 1996;401:131–6.

58. Crowell P. J Nutr 1999;129:775S–8S.

59. Francis G, Kerem Z, Makkar HP et al. Br J Nutr 2002;88: 587–605.

60. Rao AV, Sung MK. J Nutr 1995;125:717S–24S.

61. Koratkar R, Rao AV. Nutr Cancer 1997;27:206–9.

62. Packer L, Weber SU, Rimbach G. J Nutr 2001;131:369S–73S.

63. Qureshi BA, Salser WA, Parmar R et al. J Nutr 2001;131: 2606–18.

64. Kling K, Yu W, Sanders BG. J Nutr 2001;131:161S–3S.

65. Booth SL, Charnley JM, Sadowski et al. Thromb Haemost 1997;77:504–09.

66. Hoult JR, Paya M. Gen Pharmacol 1996;27:713–22.

67. Cai Y, Baer-Dubowska W, Ashwood-Smith M et al. Carcinogenesis 1997;18:215–22.

68. Ednharder R, Tang X. Food Chem Toxicol 1997;35:357–72.

69. Santos-Buelga C, Scalbert A. J Sci Food Agric 2000;80: 1094–117.

70. Chung KT, Wong TY, Wei CI et al. Crit Rev Food Sci Nutr 1998;36:421–64.

71. Hagerman AE, Riedl KM, Jones GA et al. J Agric Food Chem 1998;46:1887–92.

72. Prasad K. Atherosclerosis 1997;132:69–76.

73. Prasad K. Circulation 1999;99:1355–62.

74. Potischman N. J Nutr 2003;133:875S–80.

75. McCann SE, Moysich KB, Freudenheim JL et al. J Nutr 2002; 132:3036–41.

76. Scarlatti F, Sala G, Somenzi G et al. FASEB J 2003;17: 2339–41.

77. Kuwajerwala N, Cifuentes E, Gautam S et al. Cancer Res 2002; 62:2488–92.

78. Estrov Z, Shishodia S, Faderl S et al. Blood 2003;102:987–95.

79. Ragione FD, Cucciolla V, Criniti V et al. J Biol Chem 2003;278: 23360–8.

80. Wallerath T, Deckert G, Ternes T et al. Circulation 2002; 106:1652–8.

81. Gehm BD, McAndrews JM, Chien PY et al. Natl Acad Sci USA 1997;94:14138–43.

82. van Acker FAA, Schouten O, Haenen GRMM et al. FEBS Lett 2000;473:145–8.

83. Bok SH, Lee SH, Park YB et al. J Nutr 1999;129:1182–5.

84. Borradaile NM, Carroll KK, Kurowska EM. Lipids 1999;34: 591–8.

85. Borradaile NM, de Dreu LE, Huff MW. Diabetes 2003;52: 2554–61.

86. Choi JS, Choi YJ, Park SH et al. J Nutr 2004;134:1013–9.

87. Dechaud H, Ravard C, Claustrat F et al. Steroids 1999;64: 328–34.

88. Hunter DS, Hodges LC, Vonier PM et al. Cancer Res 1999; 59:3090–9.

89. Chiba H, Uehara M, Wu J et al. J Nutr 2003;133:1892–7.

90. Tanaka T, Makita H, Kawabata K et al. Carcinogenesis 1997; 18:957–65.

91. Yang M, Tanaka T, Hirose Y et al. Int J Cancer 1997;73:719–24.

92. Kobuchi H, Roy S, Sen CK et al. Am J Physiol 1999;277: C403–11.

93. Choi JS, Choi YJ, Park SH et al. J Nutr 2004;134:1013–9.

94. Freedman JE, Parker C, Li L et al. Circulation 2001;103: 2792–8.

95. Liang YC, Huang YT, Tsai SH et al. Carcinogenesis 1999;20: 1945–52.

96. Liang YC, Tsai SH, Tsai DC et al. FEBS Lett 2001;496:12–8.

97. Huang YT, Kuo ML, Liu JY et al. Eur J Cancer 1996;32:146–51.

98. Kurzer MS, Xu X. Annu Rev Nutr 1997;17:353–81.

99. Peterson G, Barnes S. Cell Growth Differ 1996;7:1345–51.

100. Anderson JW, Johnstone BM. N Engl J Med 1995;333:276–82.

101. Ishimi Y, Miyaura C, Ohmura M et al. Endocrinology 1999;140: 1893–900.

102. Messina MJ. Am J Clin Nutr 1999;70:439S–50S.

103. Adams MR, Golden DB, Anthony MS et al. J Nutr 2002;132: 43–9.

104. Duncan AM, Phipps WR, Kurzer MS. Best Pract Res Clin Endocrinol Metabol 2003;17:253–71.

105. Dreosti IE. Nutr Rev 1996;54:S51–8.

106. Zhang A, Zhu QY, Luk YS et al. Life Sci 1997;61:383–94.

107. Asano Y, Okamura S, Ogo T et al. Life Sci 1997;60:135–42.

108. Lin JK, Lin YL, Liang YC et al. Modulating prooxidative mitotic signaling as action mechanisms of cancer chemopreventive agents including curcumin, epigallocatechin gallate, and other phytopolyphenols. In: Shamidi F, Ho CT, eds. Phytochemicals and Phytopharmaceuticals. Champaign, IL: AOCS Press, 2000:239–49.

109. Anderson RF, Fisher LJ, Hara Y et al. Carcinogenesis 2001; 22:1189–93.

110. Chung JY, Park JO, Phyu H et al. FASEB J 2001;15: 2022–4.

111. Zhang G, Miura Y, Yagasaki K. Nutr Cancer 2000;38:265–73.

112. Choi YJ, Kang JS, Park JHY et al. J Nutr 2003;133:985–91.

113. Prior RL. Am J Clin Nutr 2003;78:570S–8S.

114. Prior RL. Absorption and metabolism of anthocyanins: potential health effects. In: Meskin MS, Bidlack WR, Davies AJ et al., eds. Phytochemicals: Mechanisms of Action. Boca Raton, FL: CRC Press, 2004:1–19.

115. Camire ME. Bilberries and blueberries as functional foods and nutraceuticals. In: Mazza G, Qomah BD, eds. Herbs Botanicals and Teas. Lancaster, PA: Technomics Publishing, 2000:289–319.

116. Shanmuganayagam D, Beahm MR, Osman HE et al. J Nutr 2002;132:3592–8.

117. Katsube N, Iwashita K, Tsushida T et al. J Agric Food Chem 2003;51:68–75.

118. Kang SY, Seeram NP, Nair MG et al. Cancer Lett 2003;194: 13–9.

119. Sundaram SG, Milner JA. Biochim Biophys Acta 1996;1315: 15–20.

120. Hong JY, Wang ZY, Smith TJ et al. Carcinogenesis 1992;13: 901–4.

121. Gebhardt R, Bech H. Lipids 1996;31:1269–76.

122. Milner JA. Adv Exp Med Biol 2001;492:69–81.

123. Yeh YY, Liu L. J Nutr 2001;131:989S–93S.

124. Talalay P, Fahey JW. J Nutr 2001;131:3027S–33S.

125. Hecht SS. J Nutr 1999;129:768S–74S.

126. Hecht SS. Drug Metab Rev 2000;32:395–411.

127. Auborn KJ, Fan S, Rosen EM et al. J Nutr 2003;133:2470S–5S.

128. Firestone GL, Bjeldanes LF. J Nutr 2003;133:2448S–55S.

129. Xu M, Dashwood RH. Cancer Lett 1999;143:179–83.

130. Ganz T, Lehrer RI. Curr Opin Hematol 1997;4:53–8.

131. Shimizu K, Matsuzuwa H, Okada K et al. Arch Viral 1996;141: 1875–89.

132. Nakajima M, Shinoda I, Samejima Y et al. J Cell Physiol 1997; 170:101–5.

133. Lönnerdal B. Am J Clin Nutr 2003;77:1537S–43S.

134. Tanmahasamut P, Liu J, Hendry LB et al. J Nutr 2004;134: 674–680.

135. Belury MA. J Nutr 2002;132:2995–8.

136. Park Y, Albright K, Storkson J et al. Lipids 1999;34:243–8.

137. Evans M, Brown J, McIntosh M. J Nutr Biochem 2002;13: 508–16.

138. Nicolosi RJ, Rogers EJ, Kritchevsky D et al. Artery 1997;22: 266–77.

139. Pariza M, Park Y, Cook ME. Prog Lipid Res 2001;40:283–98.

140. Roche HM, Gibney MJ. Am J Clin Nutr 2000;71[Suppl]: 232S–7S.

141. Dwyer JH, Allayee H, Dwyer KM et al. N Engl J Med 2004; 350:29–37.

142. Calder PC. Lipids 2001;36:1007–24.

143. Kang JX, Leaf A. Am J Clin Nutr 2000;71[Suppl]:202S–7S.

144. Vanschoonbeek K, de Maat MPM, Heemskerk JWM. J Nutr 2003;133:657–60.

145. Leaf A, Kang JX, Xiao YF et al. Circulation 2003;107:2646–52.

146. Karvonen HM, Aro A, Tapola NS et al. Metabolism 2002;51: 1253–60.

147. Hu FB, Stampfer MJ, Manson JE et al. Am J Clin Nutr 1999; 69:890–7.

148. Gibson GR, Roberfroid MB. J Nutr 1995;125:1401–12.

149. Oku T. Nutr Rev 1996;54:S59–S66.

150. Gibson GR. Br J Nutr 1998;80[Suppl 2]:S209–S12.

151. Roberfroid MB. Am J Clin Nutr 2000;71:1682S–7S.

152. Taylor GRJ, Williams CM. Br J Nutr 1998;80[Suppl]:S225–30.

153. Delzenne NM, Kok NN. J Nutr 1999;129[Suppl]:S1467–70.

154. Naidu AS, Bidlack WR, Clemens RA. Crit Rev Food Sci Nutr 1999;38:13–126.

155. Waladkhani AR, Clemens MR. Effect of dietary phytochemicals on cancer development. In: Watson RR, ed. Vegetables,

Fruits, and Herbs in Health Promotion. Boca Raton, FL: CRC Press, 2001:3–18.

156. Omaye ST, Krinsky NI, Kagan VE et al. Fundam Appl Toxicol 1997;40:163–74.

157. Armstrong GA, Hearst JE. FASEB J 1996;10:228–37.

158. Parker RS. FASEB J 1996;10:542–51.

159. Goulinet S, Chapman MJ. Arterioscler Thromb Vasc Biol 1997;17:786–96.

160. Micozzi MS, Brown ED, Edwards BKK et al. Am J Clin Nutr 1992;55:1120–5.

161. Kostic D, White WS, Olson JA. Am J Clin Nutr 1995;62: 604–10.

162. Palozza P, Calviello G, Bartoli GM. Free Radical Biol Med 1995;19:887–92.

163. Mayne ST. FASEB J 1996;10:690–701.

164. Cai Y, Luo Q, Sun M et al. Life Sci 2004;74: 2157–84.

165. Cai Y, Chow H-HS. Pharmacokinetics and bioavailability of green tea catechins. In: Meskin MS, Bidlack WR, Davies AJ et al., eds. Phytochemicals: Mechanisms of Action. Boca Raton, FL: CRC Press, 2004:35–49.

166. Zhu M, Chen Y, Li RC. Planta Med 2000;66:444–7.

167. Liao S, Kao YH, Hiipakka RA Vitam Horm 2001;62:1–94.

168. Ho CT, Ferraro T, Chen Q et al. Phytochemicals in teas and rosemary and their cancer-preventive properties. In: Ho CT, Osawa T, Huang MT et al., eds. Food Phytochemicals for Cancer Prevention II. ACS Symposium Series. Washington, DC: American Chemical Society, 1992:2–19.

169. Adlercreutz H, Mazur W. Ann Med 1997;29:95–120.

170. Murata M, Midorikawa K, Koh M et al. Biochemistry 2004;43: 2569–77.

171. Lewis DS, Matvienko OA. Healthy foods phytosterol-fortified foods for primary prevention of coronary artery disease. In: Meskin MS, Bidlack WR, Davies AJ et al., eds. Phytochemicals: Mechanisms of Action. Boca Raton, FL: CRC Press, 2004; 121–43.

172. Hutchens TW, Lonnerdal B, eds. Lactoferrin: Interactions and Biological Functions. Totowa, NJ: Humana Press, 1997.

173. Naidu AS, Bidlack WR. Environ Nutr Interactions 1998; 2:35–50.

174. Naidu AS. Food Technol 2002;6:40–5.

115

FOOD ADDITIVES, CONTAMINANTS, AND NATURAL TOXICANTS AND THEIR RISK ASSESSMENT[1]

STEVE L. TAYLOR

FOOD ADDITIVES 1810
   Sorbitol and Hexitols .1811
   Sodium Nitrite 1811
   Sulfites 1812
   Tartrazine (Food, Drug, and Cosmetic
     Act Yellow No. 5) .1812
   Olestra 1812
   Saccharin 1812
NUTRITIONAL FOOD ADDITIVES 1812
   Niacin 1812
   Vitamin A 1813
   Infant Formula Misformulation 1813
UNSAFE FOOD ADDITIVES 1813
   Toxic Oil Syndrome 1813
FOOD CONTAMINANTS 1813
   Agricultural Chemicals 1814
   Chemicals Migrating from Packaging
     Materials and Containers 1816
   Industrial Chemicals 1816
   Natural Contaminants 1817
NATURAL TOXICANTS 1821
   Poisonous Animals 1821
   Poisonous Plants 1821
   Poisonous Mushrooms 1822
RISK ASSESSMENT 1823
   Basic Concepts of Risk Assessment 1824
   Risk Management 1824

Foods can be viewed as complex mixtures of chemicals. As noted throughout this book, many of those chemicals are nutrients needed to sustain life. However, many nonnutrients exist in foods also. Some of these nonnutrient components are toxic under certain circumstances of exposure, although fortunately under typical circumstances of exposure most are not. This chapter focuses on food additives,

food contaminants, and naturally occurring toxicants that can occur in foods. Food additives are intentionally added to foods, whereas food contaminants are either adventitious or unavoidable or both. Because food additives are carefully evaluated for safety before regulatory decisions are made regarding the approval of their addition to foods, food additives are generally not hazardous under normal circumstances of exposure. Food contaminants and naturally occurring toxicants are examples of chemical components that are more likely to be hazardous under certain circumstances of exposure. Certain nutrient components of food can also be potentially toxic under certain circumstances of exposure, and several of these situations serve as examples in this chapter. However, this occurs primarily when the nutrients are used as additives or supplements rather than as a consequence of the typical levels ingested with traditional dietary practices. In recent decades, the science of food toxicology has emerged as an approach toward understanding and assessing the risks posed by food additives, food contaminants, and naturally occurring toxicants.

Food toxicology could be defined as the science that establishes the basis for judgments about the safety of foodborne chemicals (1). The central axiom of toxicology as set forth by Paracelsus in the 1500s states: "Everything is poison. Only the dose makes a thing not a poison." Thus, all chemicals in foods, whether natural or synthetic, inherent, adventitious, or added, including nutrients, are potentially toxic. Most foodborne chemicals are not hazardous under typical circumstances of exposure. That is because the dose of each foodborne chemical ingested with traditional diets is insufficient to cause injury. Because all chemicals are toxic, the degree of risk posed by exposure to any specific foodborne chemical is determined by the dose, duration, and frequency of exposure (and especially in the case of allergies, the degree of sensitivity of the individual; see Chapter 95). The age-old wisdom about the benefits of eating moderate amounts of a varied diet protects most consumers from any harm. Unusual diets can sometimes result in toxic responses from chemicals that would normally be considered safe and desirable under more typical circumstances of exposure.

Acute adverse reactions to foods are defined as those adverse reactions occurring within hours to a few days after exposure to the particular foods and foodborne components

---

[1]**Abbreviations: ALA,** alimentary toxic aleukia; **BST,** bovine somatotropin; **Bt,** *Bacillus thuringiensis*; **DDT,** dichlorodiphenyltrichloroethane; **FD&C, Food, Drug,** and Cosmetic; **FDA,** United States Food and Drug Administration; **FEMA,** Flavor and Extract Manufacturers Association; **GRAS,** generally recognized as safe; **IGF-I,** insulinlike growth factor-I; **MSG,** monosodium glutamate; **PBBs,** polybrominated biphenyls; **PCBs,** polychlorinated biphenyls.

contained therein. Acute adverse reactions to foods can occur through many mechanisms, including infections (viral, bacterial, parasitic), various toxic responses or intoxications, and allergies and intolerances. Food allergies and intolerances are a major focus of Chapter 95 and are not discussed further in this chapter. Acute foodborne infections can be distinguished from intoxications by the onset time from the ingestion of the food to the development of symptoms. Infections typically develop 48 to 72 or more hours after ingestion of the offending food. Infections can be caused by pathogenic bacteria, viruses, parasites, or prions in the case of bovine spongiform encephalopathy; although all of these infectious agents are of considerable scientific interest because of their important roles in food safety, they are beyond the scope of this chapter. Acute foodborne intoxications usually result in the onset of symptoms within minutes to a few hours after the ingestion of the offending food. However, the diagnosis of foodborne intoxications can be more complicated because symptoms can ensue more slowly in situations in which exposure is more chronic. Foodborne infections are not discussed further in this chapter, but certainly can influence the nutritional status of affected persons.

Food intoxications encompass all food-associated illnesses that are caused by chemicals in food, although the chemical constituents of foods vary greatly in toxicity. All consumers are susceptible to most food intoxications. This chapter focuses on the various categories of chemical components that occur in foods (food additives, including nutrient additives; food contaminants, both man-made and naturally occurring; and nonnutrient components that can be classified as naturally occurring toxicants). In each case, illustrative examples will be discussed. The chapter concludes with a description of risk assessment approaches that are used to evaluate the comparative risks posed by individual food components.

FOOD ADDITIVES

Numerous chemical substances are knowingly added to foods to provide many different technical benefits, including not only flavorants and colorants but also acidulents, antimicrobial agents, sweeteners, and leavening agents; a list of the technical attributes provided by food additives is provided in Table 115.1. Nutrients are one category of food additives. Several thousand food additives exist, but many of these chemicals are used in rather small amounts. Food additives can be classified on the basis of their regulatory standing in the United States: (a) generally recognized as safe (GRAS) substances, (b) flavors and extracts, (c) direct additives, and (d) color additives.

In the United States, GRAS substances are those food ingredients that were in common use before the latest version of the Food, Drug, and Cosmetic (FD&C) Act that was enacted in 1958. The 1958 FD&C Act required United States Food and Drug Administration (FDA) approval of

TABLE 115.1. CATEGORIES OF FOOD ADDITIVES

Acidulents	Acetic acid
Anticaking agents	Magnesium silicate
Antimicrobial agents	Sodium benzoate
Antibrowning agents	Sodium bisulfite
Antioxidants	Butylated hydroxyanisole
Emulsifying agents	Lecithin
Nutrients	Ascorbic acid
Sequestrants	Citric acid
Stabilizers	Guar gum
Spices	Cinnamon
Oleoresins and extracts	Fennel oil
Flavorings	Ethyl butyrate
Enzymes	Glucose isomerase
Colorants, artificial	FD&C Yellow no. 5
Colorants, natural	Annatto
Sweeteners	Sucrose
Nonnutritive sweeteners	Aspartame

any newly developed food additives, but recognized the long history of safe use of many additives. More than 600 chemicals are on the FDA GRAS list, including such materials as sucrose, salt, butylated hydroxytoluene, and spices. Many nutrient ingredients are on the GRAS list also. Most of the common food ingredients on the GRAS list were in common use before 1958. From a legal standpoint, GRAS substances are not actually additives, but that distinction is seldom made by the consumer. Although GRAS substances were in common use before 1958, that does not necessarily imply that substantial toxicologic data exist for all of these substances. For example, the concern around sodium levels in the diet and hypertension ensued long after 1958, and salt and other sodium-containing ingredients such as monosodium glutamate (MSG) were placed on the GRAS list before this scientific information became available. Reviews of the safety of the GRAS substances have been conducted since 1958, and deficiencies in our information on their toxicity have been identified and corrected in some cases. Substances or certain uses of substances can be removed from the GRAS list if the FDA acquires evidence of some hazard to consumers.

Flavors and extracts represent a large percentage of the total number of food additives. The Flavor and Extract Manufacturers Association (FEMA) keeps a list of accepted flavors and extracts. FEMA is also responsible for evaluating the safety of the chemicals on the list. In essence, the FEMA list is a GRAS list for flavors and extracts. Over 1000 chemicals are on the FEMA list, although some of these chemicals and extracts are no longer used.

Direct food additives are the category for those new food additives that have been approved by the FDA since 1958. In reality, few approvals for new food additives have been granted in recent years. Extensive and costly safety data are required to gain FDA approval for a new food additive. Aspartame, a nonnutritive sweetener, is one of the most notable direct food additives in use in the United

States (and many other countries). Aspartame was approved as a nonnutritive sweetener for certain types of uses some years ago, and the consumption of this new additive has become substantial. More recently, Olestra, a noncaloric fat replacement, was approved for certain uses such as the deep-fat frying of chips. Although initially promising, Olestra usage has been somewhat limited. Aspartame and Olestra are examples of the types of substances for which potential usage levels are high enough to warrant the cost of acquiring the toxicologic information needed to gain food additive approval.

Color additives are regulated in a separate part of the FD&C Act. New artificial color additives must be approved by the FDA in much the same way that new food additives are approved. Some color additives have been banned since 1958 because of concerns about their possible chronic toxicity. A good example is FD&C Red no. 2, which is banned in the United States, although it is allowed in Canada and other countries. Conversely, FD&C Red no. 40 is allowed for use in the United States but banned in Canada.

The degree of hazard associated with the presence of additives in our foods is quite low for several reasons. First, the level of exposure to most food additives, especially flavoring ingredients, is rather low. Furthermore, the oral toxicity of food additives tends to be extremely low, especially with regard to acute toxicity. Some concerns have arisen about the chronic toxicity of a few of the many food additives, including saccharin, cyclamate, and others. Yet another reason for the low hazard associated with food additives is the established safety of many additives. Many food additives have been subjected to safety evaluations in laboratory animals. In these cases, the toxicity of these food additives is well known and exposure can be limited to levels far below any dose that would be hazardous. By contrast, the toxicity of naturally occurring chemicals in foods is often not known, and we cannot be certain that hazardous circumstances will not exist under certain conditions of exposure. Other food ingredients, particularly the GRAS substances, have long histories of safe use even if classic toxicologic evaluations in laboratory animals have not always been exhaustively performed.

The safety of some food additives is called into question. In some cases, the questions have revolved around evidence for weak carcinogenic activity in laboratory animals. Some additives, such as FD&C Red no. 2 and cyclamate, have been banned as a result of such evidence. Warning labels are required for saccharin. In addition to carcinogenicity, other concerns have arisen, such as the role of sugar in dental caries and abnormal behavioral reactions, the role of MSG in asthma, the role of aspartame in headaches and other behavior and neurologic reactions, and the role of Olestra in gastrointestinal complaints. The concerns range from acute toxicity, such as aspartame and headaches or MSG in asthma, to chronic toxicity, such as saccharin and bladder cancer or sugar in

dental caries. Although a detailed discussion of all of these issues is beyond the scope of this chapter, suffice it to say that many of these assertions have been questioned and remain to be validated.

A few illustrative examples will be discussed later. The examples include several food additives that have caused acute illness under certain conditions of exposure. These intoxications are usually the result of either excessive consumption of the additive or ingestion by an individual who has an abnormal degree of sensitivity to the additive. Misuse of food additives by consumers or food processors has also created hazardous situations on occasion. Saccharin is discussed briefly as an example of an additive for which chronic toxicity concerns exist. Many other examples could be cited for chronic toxicity concerns, including cyclamate and FD&C Red no. 2.

Sorbitol and Hexitols

Sorbitol and various other hexitols are commonly used alternative sweeteners. Dietetic food diarrhea associated with these polyol food additives is a good example of an intoxication resulting from the excessive consumption of a food additive. The hexitols and sorbitol are widely used sweeteners in dietetic foods. The hexitols and sorbitol are especially common in noncariogenic candies and chewing gum. Although these sugar alcohols are not as easily absorbed as sugar, they are equally as caloric as sugar, once absorbed. Because of their slow absorption, these sweeteners can cause an osmotic-type diarrhea if excessive amounts happen to be consumed. Several cases have been reported in which consumers were ingesting more than 20 g of these sweeteners per day (2, 3). The levels of hexitols and/or sorbitol used in foods varies, but in one case the ingestion of 12 pieces of hard candy over a short period provided 36 g of sorbitol and resulted in diarrhea (2).

Sodium Nitrite

Sodium nitrite has been used as an antimicrobial agent and color-fixing substance in processed meats for generations. When properly used, sodium nitrite presents little risk of acute intoxication because little free nitrite remains in the meat. Several foodborne intoxications have resulted from confusion about the identity of food ingredients, and at least one of these episodes involved sodium nitrite (2). Sodium nitrite is a white granular substance that can easily be confused with other salts, including sodium chloride, which is much less toxic. In the one incident, a small grocery store was repackaging additives such as sodium chloride, sodium nitrite, and MSG from bulk containers into home-use packets. Somehow, sodium nitrite was erroneously labeled as MSG. The mislabeled product was used in hazardous amounts by consumers, resulting in acute methemoglobinemia and at least one death (2).

Sulfites

Sulfites have been widely used as food additives for many years. Sulfites serve several important technologic functions, including as an antimicrobial agent, an inhibitor of enzymatic and nonenzymatic browning, a bleaching agent, and a dough conditioner. Several sulfites are approved as food ingredients, including sodium and potassium metabisulfite, sodium and potassium bisulfite, sodium sulfite, and sulfur dioxide. All these products yield sulfur dioxide at acidic pHs in food matrices. Sulfite-induced asthma is a good example of sensitivity to a food additive that afflicts only a small percentage of the population. Sulfite-induced asthma is discussed as one of the primary examples of a food intolerance reaction in Chapter 95.

Tartrazine (Food, Drug, and Cosmetic Act Yellow No. 5)

Tartrazine, also known as FD&C Yellow no. 5, is an approved artificial food color. This colorant has been widely used in foods and pharmaceuticals for many years. Tartrazine is another example of an additive, a color additive in this case, that is associated with adverse reactions in a sensitive subpopulation of consumers. Tartrazine has been implicated in the provocation of both asthma and chronic urticaria (hives) in some persons (4). However, unlike the situation with sulfite-induced asthma, the association of tartrazine in the provocation of asthma and chronic urticaria is controversial. Some studies have shown a cause-and-effect relationship, whereas other studies have not (5). Both asthma and chronic urticaria are chronic illnesses with symptoms that tend to flare up at unpredictable times. In some of the clinical trials of tartrazine, key pharmaceutical agents have been withdrawn from the human subjects before the tartrazine challenges. If the study is not designed carefully, the flare-up of the asthma or urticaria in such a trial could be because of either the administration of tartrazine or the withdrawal of the medication. The plethora of poorly designed clinical trials on tartrazine has led several groups to conclude that tartrazine may not actually provoke asthma or chronic urticaria (5, 6).

Olestra

Olestra received food additive approval more recently and can be used as a fat replacement. Because Olestra is poorly absorbed and is not metabolized, it does not provide the calories that would be obtained with fat in similar products. However, the use of Olestra has been associated with acute gastrointestinal complaints, including anal leakage (7). As with sulfites and tartrazine, only certain consumers seem to be affected. However, the prevalence and seriousness of such complaints is a matter of some controversy (7). Obviously, many consumers occasionally experience postprandial gastrointestinal maladies, which makes the association of such complaints with a particular ingredient rather challenging.

Saccharin

Saccharin was one of the first nonnutritive sweeteners approved for food use in the United States. High doses of saccharin have been shown to cause bladder cancer in laboratory animals (8). However, the extrapolation of these results to humans, who typically ingest much lower levels of the ingredient, has stimulated controversy. Thus, the carcinogenicity of saccharin to humans at typical levels of intake is uncertain at best, and saccharin remains on the market in the United States. Despite the uncertain relevance of the toxicologic data, warning labels remain on saccharin products indicating that saccharin is known to cause cancer in laboratory animals.

NUTRITIONAL FOOD ADDITIVES

Many food additives, including vitamins and minerals, serve nutritional functions. Although these functions are widely and appropriately viewed as beneficial, nutrients can occasionally be associated with adverse reactions. Because nutrients are chemicals and all chemicals are toxic at some dose, nutrients can exert toxic effects under some conditions of exposure. In fact, in the latest version of the Dietary Reference Intakes developed by the Institute of Medicine of the National Academy of Sciences, tolerable upper intake levels are provided for many of the common micronutrients (9). Although data on micronutrient toxicity are often scant, elevated levels of nutrients are clearly hazardous in some situations. For example, the intake of large amounts of vitamin A was hazardous to polar explorers consuming large amounts of polar bear liver (10). However, this would be one of the very few examples in which the ingestion of food (albeit an atypical food) was responsible for nutrient toxicity. More commonly, tolerable upper intake levels can only be exceeded by use of supplements or inappropriate addition of elevated levels when used as additives.

Niacin

As one example, excessive consumption of the B vitamin niacin can cause an acute onset of flushing, pruritus, rash, and burning or warmth in the skin, especially on the face and upper trunk (11), although gastrointestinal discomfort is also noted by some patients (12). Outbreaks have occurred from the excessive enrichment of flour used to make pumpernickel bagels (12) or corn meal (13). These episodes occurred as a result of inaccurate or inadequate labeling of food ingredient containers. The amount of niacin required to elicit such adverse reactions is at least 50 times the recommended dietary allowance (12, 13). The symptoms of niacin intoxication are acute, self-limited, and without sequelae.

Vitamin A

In addition to the example of polar bear liver noted earlier, the toxicity of vitamin A can also be illustrated by other more conventional, but also unwise, dietary choices. Vitamin A intoxication was reported in twin infants who were provided a diet consisting largely of pureed chicken livers, pureed carrots, milk, and vitamin supplements (2). Apparently, the mother of these infants initiated this diet because she did not trust commercial baby foods. After several weeks on this diet, the infants began to vomit and developed a skin rash. The symptoms disappeared when a more normal diet was instituted. The estimated intake of vitamin A and carotene was 44,000 IU/day, compared with the recommended dietary allowance of 1500 to 4500 IU/day for infants.

Infant Formula Misformulation

In 1980, a very serious outbreak occurred as the result of an error on the part of the processor (14). This manufacturer of soybean-based infant formula wished to market a version with a decreased sodium content despite a lack of evidence that such action would prevent the development of hypertension in the infants later in life. To achieve this marketing objective, the manufacturer removed the sodium chloride from the formula. Most infants receiving soybean formula survive on that formula as the sole source of nutrients. The removal of the sodium chloride resulted in a deficiency of chloride in the formula. The result was a condition known as metabolic alkalosis, characterized by lethargy, poor appetite, failure to gain weight, vomiting, and diarrhea. Several infants died as a result.

UNSAFE FOOD ADDITIVES

The preceding discussion centered on the use of ingredients that had been approved for addition to foods by some regulatory agency. Of course, the illegal and unscrupulous addition of chemicals that are not approved for addition to foods and that have not been tested for safety or that had a long history of safe use could be quite hazardous. Fortunately, few examples of such situations can be cited. The toxic oil syndrome that occurred in Spain several decades ago is the premier example.

Toxic Oil Syndrome

In the early 1980s, an epidemic occurred in Spain that was ultimately linked to the ingestion of unlabeled, illegally marketed cooking oils (15, 16). The dangers inherent with illicit food ingredients are emphasized by a total of 19,828 cases and 315 deaths recorded in this epidemic (17). The illicit cooking oil contained oils from both plant and animal sources. However, some of the oils were denatured and intended for industrial rather than food uses. The causative toxin in the oils remains unknown, although fatty acid anilides resulting from the denaturation process are suspected to be at least partially responsible (17, 18).

Multiple organ systems were involved in the clinical manifestations of this illness (17, 18). Initially, affected persons experienced fever, chills, headache, tachycardia, cough, chest pain, and pruritus. Physical examinations showed various skin exanthema, splenomegaly, and generalized adenopathy. Pulmonary infiltrates were noted in 84% of the affected persons, probably as the result of increased capillary permeability. The intermediate phase of the illness persisted from the second week after onset through the eighth week after ingestion. Gastrointestinal symptoms, primarily abdominal pain, nausea, and diarrhea, predominated during this intermediate phase. At this stage, clinical examination showed marked eosinophilia in 42% of patients, high immunoglobulin E levels, thrombocytopenia, abnormal coagulation patterns, and evidence of hepatic dysfunction with abnormal enzymes. Some persons became jaundiced, and many had hepatomegaly. The late phase of the illness, characterized initially by neuromuscular and joint involvement, developed in 23% of cases and began after 2 months of illness. Later, persons in this late phase of the illness developed vasculitis and a sclerodermalike syndrome. Affected persons complained of intense muscular pain, edema, and progressive muscular weakness. Muscular atrophy was apparent in some persons. Neurologic involvement included depressed deep tendon reflexes, anesthesia, and dysesthesia. Respiratory problems developed because of neuromuscular weakness and progressed to pulmonary hypertension and thromboembolic phenomena. The sclerodermalike symptoms included Raynaud phenomenon, sicca syndrome, dysphagia, and contractures caused by thickening collagen in the skin. Vascular lesions were noted in all organs, apparently resulting from endothelial proliferation and thrombosis. All patients in the late group had antinuclear antibody, and many had antibodies against smooth muscle and skeletal muscle (19). These pathologic and clinical features are consistent with an autoimmune mechanism for the illness. Because the precise causative agent and its mechanism have not been delineated, this serious epidemic may occur again if similar circumstances exist (17). In addition, because the causative agent has not been identified, it is unknown whether the toxin may be present in small amounts in other foods and thus may be producing or aggravating other clinical conditions (17).

FOOD CONTAMINANTS

Potentially hazardous chemicals may contaminate foods from various sources, including natural contaminants, agricultural chemicals, and industrial contaminants (Table 115.2). The natural contaminants can include mycotoxins from molds, phycotoxins from marine algae, and bacterial toxins. Other contaminants are man-made and have useful purposes, although not intended to occur in foods.

TABLE 115.2. CLASSIFICATION OF FOODBORNE CONTAMINANTS

Agricultural chemicals
  Insecticides
  Herbicides
  Fungicides
  Fertilizers
  Veterinary drugs and antibiotics
Chemicals migrating from packaging materials and containers
  Lead
  Tin
  Copper
  Zinc
Industrial chemicals
  Polychlorinated biphenyls
  Polybrominated biphenyls
  Mercury
Naturally occurring contaminants
  Bacterial toxins
    Staphylococcal enterotoxins
    Clostridium botulinum toxins
    Bacillus cereus toxins
    Bongkrek acid
    Tetrodotoxin (puffer fish poisoning)
  Mycotoxins
    Aflatoxins
    Fusarium toxins
    Penicillium toxins
  Algal toxins
    Ciguatera poisoning
    Paralytic shellfish poisoning
    Amnesic shellfish poisoning
    Diarrhetic shellfish poisoning
    Neurotoxic shellfish poisoning
  Insect-derived or mite-derived toxins

Agricultural Chemicals

Many different chemicals are used in modern agricultural practices. Residues of these agrichemicals can occur in raw and processed foods. Federal regulatory agencies evaluate the safety of such chemicals and regulate and monitor their use on plant food products and in food-producing animals (2). The major categories of agricultural chemicals include insecticides, herbicides, fungicides, fertilizers, and veterinary drugs, including antibiotics and hormones including bovine somatotropin (BST) and diethylstilbestrol.

Insecticides

Insecticides are applied to food crops to control insect pests. Insecticides fall into several major categories, including organochlorine compounds (dichlorodiphenyl-trichloroethane [DDT], chlordane, and others, many of which are now banned), organophosphate compounds (e.g., parathion and malathion), carbamate compounds (e.g., carbaryl and aldicarb), botanical compounds (e.g., nicotine and pyrethrum), and inorganic compounds (e.g., arsenicals).

Insecticide residues in foods are not particularly hazardous, especially on an acute basis, because of the exceedingly low residue levels of insecticides found in most foods. Certainly, large doses of insecticides can be toxic to humans. Some are neurotoxins, such as the organophosphates and carbamates, which are cholinesterase inhibitors and act by blocking synaptic nerve transmission. Insecticide residues in foods pose a low degree of hazard for several reasons: (a) the level of exposure is very low, (b) some insecticides are not very toxic to humans, (c) some insecticides decompose rapidly in the environment, and (d) many different insecticides are used, which limits the exposure to any one particular insecticide (1).

Acute food poisoning incidents attributable to the proper use of insecticides on foods are exceedingly rare. Most episodes of pesticide intoxications have resulted from the misuse of pesticides, including contamination of foods during storage and transport, the use of pesticides in food preparation because of their mistaken identity as common food ingredients such as sugar and salt, and their misuse in agricultural practice on crops for which they are not intended to be used (20).

Aldicarb poisoning is one of the best examples of acute food poisoning episodes associated with pesticides. In one noteworthy episode, an outbreak of aldicarb intoxication from watermelons occurred on the west coast in 1985 (21). The use of aldicarb on watermelons is illegal because excessive levels of aldicarb become concentrated in the edible portion of the melon. In this incident, several farmers used aldicarb illegally, resulting in consumer illnesses and the recall and destruction of thousands of watermelons. The outbreak involved a total of 1373 illness reports, with 78% classified as probable or possible aldicarb poisoning cases (21, 22). Thus, this episode is the largest known outbreak of pesticide poisoning in North America (21, 22). Aldicarb has also been involved in several other food poisoning outbreaks. These incidents were associated with ingestion of hydroponically grown cucumbers (22, 23). The symptoms of aldicarb intoxication include nausea, vomiting, diarrhea, and mild neurologic manifestations such as dizziness, headache, blurred vision, and loss of balance (21–23).

Chronic intoxications resulting from pesticide residues in foods have been a longstanding concern (24). For example, DDT is a known animal carcinogen. Because of these concerns for human health and additional concerns resulting from their potential for accumulation in the environment, many organochlorine pesticides have been banned or allowed only under very restricted use conditions. Despite the concerns, the evidence that the low residual amounts of insecticides on foods presents a carcinogenic risk to human consumers is not particularly strong.

Recently, several important crops, including corn and potatoes, have been genetically engineered for resistance to insects. These genetically engineered, insect-resistant crops contain a novel gene that produces a naturally occurring insecticidal protein toxin from *Bacillus thuringiensis* (Bt). Bt toxins have been used for decades in organic agriculture. The Bt proteins produced by the genetically engineered crops have been thoroughly examined and seem to be quite safe for human consumption (25).

Herbicides

Herbicides are applied to agricultural crops to control the growth of weeds. Classes of herbicides include chlorophenoxy compounds (e.g., 2,4-D), dinitrophenols (e.g., dinitroorthocresol), bipyridyl compounds (e.g., paraquat), substituted ureas (e.g., monuron), carbamates (e.g., propham), and triazines (e.g., simazine).

In most circumstances, herbicide residues in foods do not present any hazard to consumers. Food poisoning incidents have never resulted from the proper use of herbicides on food crops. The lack of hazard from herbicide residues is associated with the low level of exposure, their low degree of toxicity to humans and selective toxicity toward plants, and the use of many different herbicides, which limits exposure to any particular herbicide (2).

Most herbicides pose little hazard to humans simply because they are selectively toxic to plants. The bipyridyl compounds are an exception. The bipyridyl herbicides, including diquat and paraquat, are nonselective and are rather toxic to humans. These bipyridyl herbicides tend to exert their toxic effects on the lung (26). However, no food poisoning incidents have ever been attributed to inappropriate use of the bipyridyl compounds.

Fungicides

Fungicides are used to curtail the growth of molds on food crops. Important fungicide categories include captan, folpet, dithiocarbamates, pentachlorophenol, and the mercurial compounds. The hazards from foodborne fungicides are miniscule because exposure is quite low, most fungicides do not accumulate in the environment, and fungicides are typically not very toxic (2).

Several exceptions exist, including the mercurial compounds and hexachlorobenzene. Mercurial fungicides are often used to treat seed grains to prevent mold growth during storage. These seed grains are typically colored pink and are intended for planting rather than consumption. However, especially in times of famine, consumers are tempted to eat the seed grain. On several occasions, consumers have eaten these treated seed grains and developed mercury poisoning (20). Deaths have resulted in several severe episodes. More commonly, mild cases occur. Mild cases of mercury intoxication can be manifested in gastrointestinal symptoms such as abdominal cramps, nausea, vomiting, and diarrhea and dermal symptoms such as acrodynia and itching (20).

Hexachlorobenzene caused one of the most massive outbreaks of pesticide poisoning in recorded history. More than 3000 persons were affected in this incident in Turkey from 1955 through 1959 in which seed grain was consumed rather than planted (27). Hexachlorobenzene had been used to treat the seed grain. The symptoms were quite severe, with a 10% mortality rate, porphyria cutanea tarda, ulcerated skin lesions, alopecia, porphyrinuria, hepatomegaly, and thyroid enlargement (27).

Fertilizers

Fertilizers are typically combinations of nitrogen and phosphorus compounds. Nitrogen fertilizers are oxidized to nitrate and nitrite in the soil. Both nitrate and nitrite are hazardous to humans if these substances are ingested in large amounts (2). Infants are particularly susceptible to nitrate and nitrite intoxication (2). Fertilizers present little if any risk to consumers in most typical situations. However, some plants, such as spinach, can accumulate nitrate to hazardous levels if allowed to grow in overly fertilized fields (28). Because nitrite is more toxic than nitrate, the situation can be worsened if nitrate-reducing bacteria are allowed to proliferate on these foods.

Acute nitrite intoxications have occurred on occasion from the ingestion of spinach grown in overly fertilized fields (29). The problem results from consumption of nitrate-rich, unprocessed spinach in which conversion to nitrite has likely occurred because of bacterial action (28). As another example, improper storage of carrot juice has allowed the proliferation of nitrate-reducing bacteria resulting in the accumulation of hazardous levels of nitrite in the product (30). In low doses, the symptoms include flushing of the face and extremities, gastrointestinal discomfort, and headache; in larger doses, cyanosis, methemoglobinemia, nausea, vomiting, abdominal pain, collapse, and death can occur (28). The lethal dose of nitrite is estimated at about 1 g in adults (28).

Veterinary Drugs and Antibiotics

Food-producing animals can be treated with various veterinary drugs, especially antibiotics and hormones. If properly used, residues in foods are typically quite low. Acute food poisoning incidents have not occurred as a result of properly used veterinary drugs, including antibiotics and hormones (2). Concerns have arisen from the use of veterinary drugs. One of the best examples is penicillin. Penicillin is a common antibiotic used in animal as well as human health. Some consumers are allergic to penicillin primarily as a result of its use in human medicine. Questions exist regarding the potential for allergic reactions to penicillin residues resulting from its use in food-producing animals. However, the likelihood of allergic reactions to the very low levels of penicillin residues found in foods is quite remote (31).

Another example is BST. BST is a growth hormone specific for cows. BST has been approved to increase milk production in dairy cows. Concerns have arisen regarding the safety of the use of BST. However, the FDA has concluded that BST administration to dairy cows is safe because BST is biologically inactive in humans, recombinant BST is orally inactive and not absorbed, and native BST and recombinant BST are biologically indistinguishable (32). Some concerns have arisen regarding possible elevated levels of insulinlike growth factor-I (IGF-I) in milk from BST-treated cows. However, the FDA concludes that evidence for elevated milk levels of IGF-I in treated cows is weak and that whether absorption of biologically active IGF-I occurs in humans is not proven (32). So, although BST remains a safety issue in the minds of some consumers, the FDA asserts that milk from BST-treated cows poses no appreciable risk for consumers (32).

Chemicals Migrating from Packaging Materials and Containers

Foods are often packaged for convenience, shelf stability, and protection from microbial agents. These packages and containers also contain chemicals, and under certain circumstances, chemicals can migrate from the packaging material into the edible portion of the foods. Chemicals migrating from packaging materials into foods and beverages do not present a significant hazard. Various chemicals, including plastics monomers, plasticizers, stabilizers, printing inks, and others, do migrate at extremely low levels into foods. No known hazards exist resulting from any of the approved packaging materials used for food products.

Lead and tin are the main concerns associated with packaging materials. The storage of acidic foods in certain containers can result in the leaching of toxic heavy metals such as lead, tin, and zinc into the food. Contact of acidic beverages with copper can also release potentially hazardous levels of copper into the beverage. Cadmium and iron are also occasionally implicated in heavy metal intoxications associated with foods (33).

Lead

Environmental exposure to lead is a significant public health concern. However, exposure to lead via foods has always been a comparatively moderate contributor to overall environmental lead exposure. The migration of lead from lead-soldered cans was once a source of some concern. However, lead-soldered cans have been successfully phased out of use in the United States. Now, the main issue with lead contamination results from the occasional use of lead-based glazes on pottery or paint on glassware that may come in contact with acidic foods or beverages. Lead is a well-known toxicant that can affect the nervous system, the kidney, and bone.

Tin

Metal cans for food storage are typically constructed using tin plate. These cans have inner surfaces that are lined with a lacquer material when cans are used for acidic foods or beverages. The inappropriate use of unlacquered

cans for acidic food products such as tomato juice or fruit cocktail has resulted in cases of acute tin intoxication (34). Because tin is poorly absorbed, the primary symptoms are bloating, nausea, abdominal cramps, vomiting, diarrhea, and headache occurring 30 minutes to 2 hours after consumption of the acidic product (34).

Copper

One of the most common causes of acute copper poisoning, characterized primarily by nausea and vomiting, results from faulty check valves in soft drink vending machines (2). The check valves on soft drink vending machines prevent contact between the acidic, carbonated beverage and the copper tubing that delivers the water or ice in the machine. Several outbreaks of copper poisoning have resulted from such occurrences (35).

Zinc

The inappropriate storage of acidic foods or beverages in galvanized containers can result in acute zinc intoxication (33, 36). Episodes have involved fruit punch and tomato juice (33). Zinc is a potent emetic. The symptoms of zinc intoxication include irritation of the mouth, throat, and abdomen; nausea; vomiting; dizziness; and collapse (2).

Industrial Chemicals

Industrial and/or environmental pollutants have the potential to migrate into foods on occasion. In most circumstances, rather small and inconsequential (from a health perspective) residual amounts are found. On rare occasions, hazardous levels of such chemicals enter the food supply, often with devastating consequences from both a health and an economic perspective. A few prominent examples will illustrate the potential magnitude of this issue.

Polychlorinated Biphenyls and Polybrominated Biphenyls

Food contamination with polychlorinated biphenyls (PCBs) and polybrominated biphenyls (PBBs) has occurred on several occasions (2). PCBs and PBBs are quite persistent in the environment. These compounds are fat soluble, so they tend to accumulate in the fat depots of various organisms; concentrations often magnify upward along the food chain. PCBs and PBBs are considered to be toxic pollutants from industrial practices. PBBs are commonly used as fire retardants, and PCBs are frequently used in transformer fluid. PCBs and PBBs are not particularly worrisome as acute toxicants in foods. However, because they are lipid soluble, elimination from the body is slow and the chronic effects of exposure to these contaminants in foods are of concern. PBBs were involved in one of the most infamous industrial contamination incidents ever in the United States involving the accidental contamination of dairy feed in Michigan (37). This incident resulted in the destruction of many cows and their milk. Although the health consequences of this incident remain uncertain, the economic impact was considerable. PCBs were responsible for cases of human illness associated with contaminated rice bran oil in Japan in one of the most infamous international episodes of industrial contamination of foods (38). The PCBs leaked from a heat exchanger used to deodorize the oil. The resulting syndrome was called yusho (meaning "oil disease") by the Japanese. Yusho was characterized by chloracne, weakness, numbness of limbs, swelling of eyelids, discharges from the eyes, dark skin pigmentation, and liver damage (38, 39). Acute symptoms were evident at exposure doses as low as 0.5 g. The toxic effects were chronic in many of the victims, persisting for 8 years or more after exposure. Prolonged symptoms included chloracne, menstrual disturbances, fatigue, headache, fever, cough, digestive disturbances, and numbness of the extremities (38, 39). These symptoms were reproduced in a study on monkeys (40). Such incidents continue to occur periodically, although fortunately without the human toll experienced in the yusho episode. Leaking transformers have contributed to the contamination of feeds with PCBs, which led to the destruction of chickens, eggs, and egg-containing food products (2). Pollution of Lake Michigan with PCBs has reached sufficient levels in recent years that commercial fishing on Lake Michigan has ceased (2).

Mercury

Minamata disease, caused by mercury intoxication, is another classic example of food contamination by industrial pollutants. The episode occurred over a number of years and resulted from an industrial firm located on the shores of Minamata Bay in Japan that dumped mercury-containing wastes into the bay from 1953 until the early 1960s. In the bay, bacteria in the sediment converted the inorganic mercury into highly toxic methylmercury. Although elemental mercury is poorly absorbed from the gastrointestinal tract, organomercury compounds, including methylmercury, are much more efficiently absorbed and are thus more toxic as food contaminants. Fish in the bay became contaminated with the methylmercury, and consumers became ill from eating this fish. More than 1200 cases of mercury intoxication occurred among consumers of Minamata Bay fish (41). The symptoms included tremors and other neurotoxic effects and kidney failure.

Natural Contaminants

Contaminants can also enter the food supply through various natural means. Bacterial toxins, mycotoxins from molds, and phycotoxins from marine algae are relevant examples.

Bacterial Toxins

Pathogenic bacteria typically cause foodborne disease by the infectious route. The pathogenesis mechanism involves invasion of cells and tissues, multiplication, and symptom causation as a result of cellular injury, inflammation, and/or disturbance of key physiologic processes. Although infectious bacteria are properly viewed as contaminants of food, this chapter focuses on chemical contaminants. The infectious pathogens are living microorganisms and thus will not be considered further.

A few bacteria are toxigenic and produce exogenous toxins in foods before they are eaten. For these bacteria, the ingestion of the toxins initiates the disease process even if the bacteria are destroyed in processing or preparation. The best examples of bacterial intoxications are the staphylococcal enterotoxins and botulinal toxins.

The staphylococcal enterotoxins can be produced in foods by certain strains of *Staphylococcus aureus* (42). The *S. aureus* grows on foods under certain conditions such as temperatures between 10°C and 45°C and produces the enterotoxin during growth. When ingested, these protein enterotoxins cause nausea and vomiting with a rapid onset time of 1 to 6 hours. Staphylococcal food poisoning is one of the most common forms of foodborne disease, associated with about 16% of all confirmed bacterial foodborne disease outbreaks in the United States from 1973 to 1992 according to statistics compiled by the Centers for Disease Control and Prevention (42). Low microgram levels of the staphylococcal enterotoxins are sufficient to elicit symptoms (42). Nine distinct (but structurally related) enterotoxins have been identified as being produced by various strains of *S. aureus* (42). The enterotoxins are small proteins with molecular weights of 25,000 to 29,000 d. The enterotoxins bind to some as-yet-unidentified site in the small intestine and transmit a signal to the vomiting center in the brain. The enterotoxins are more stable to digestion than most proteins and are quite heat resistant. For this reason, staphylococcal food poisoning is often associated with foods that have been cooked after improper storage that allowed the proliferation of *S. aureus*.

The botulinal toxins are potent neurotoxins and can be produced in foods under anaerobic conditions by *Clostridium botulinum* (43). Toxin formation can occur in canned foods that have been improperly processed. The commercial canning process is predicated on the destruction of this organism and its spores so that the spores will not germinate, grow, and produce toxin on storage of the canned product. Seven toxin types have been identified as being produced by various strains of *C. botulinum*, although types A, B, and E are most commonly associated with foodborne illness (43). The botulinal toxins are proteins with a molecular mass of about 150 kDa (43). The neurotoxin inhibits the release of acetylcholine at the synapses and thus affects the peripheral nervous system. Botulinal toxins are among the most potent toxins known to humans. Clinical symptoms begin to develop 12 to 48 hours after exposure to the toxin, with weakness, dizziness, and mouth dryness occasionally accompanied by nausea and vomiting. Neurologic symptoms follow, including blurred vision, inability to swallow, aphasia, and weakness of the skeletal muscles. Symptoms can ultimately progress to respiratory paralysis and death. The vegetative cell of *C. botulinum* and the botulinal toxins are easily destroyed by heat. But the spores of *C. botulinum* are heat-resistant, will survive improper thermal processing, and will germinate and grow under suitable anaerobic conditions (43). Infant botulism is a related illness. In infant botulism, the spores enter the gastrointestinal system early in life before competitive microflora are in place to resist their germination and growth (43). The growth of *C. botulinum* ensues in the intestinal tract, where toxin production occurs and causes severe illness. Honey is one of the more frequent sources of the spores in the infant diet (43).

Several other examples exist of toxins produced by bacteria growing on foods. Histamine intoxication was discussed in Chapter 95 because it is an allergylike intoxication. Both diarrhetic and emetic syndromes can be caused by *Bacillus cereus*, another spore-forming microorganism that can occasionally provoke foodborne disease (44). Several other microbial toxins have only caused human illness in a few isolated circumstances.

Bongkrek food poisoning was once common in Indonesia but has never occurred in the United States (2). The symptoms of bongkrek food poisoning include hypoglycemia, severe spasms, convulsions, and death. Bongkrek is an Indonesian food composed of flat white cakes made from pressed coconut and fermented with the fungus *Rhizopus oryzae*. The cakes are wrapped in banana leaves during the fermentation. A toxin known as bongkrek acid is produced by *Pseudomonas cocovenenans*, a bacteria that can occasionally overgrow the fungus under some conditions. Bongkrek acid is a heat-stable unsaturated fatty acid (45). The bacterial overgrowth can be prevented by use of oxalis leaves rather than banana leaves. The oxalis leaves contribute to a rapid decrease in pH to about 5.5, which prevents the growth of *P. cocovenenans*. Bongkrek food poisoning has been largely eliminated even in Indonesia by the substitution of oxalis leaves for banana leaves.

Fermented corn flour poisoning was encountered in the People's Republic of China between 1961 and 1979 (2). A total of 327 cases with 101 deaths were reported during that period, associated with the ingestion of fermented corn flour. The disease had a short onset period and was characterized by abdominal discomfort, mild diarrhea, and vomiting. In severe cases, the disease progressed to jaundice, coma, delirium, oliguria, hematuria, rigidity of the extremities, urinary retention, toxic shock, and death. The bacterial toxin responsible for this illness is produced by *Flavobacterium farinofermentans*. This toxin was subsequently identified as bongkrek acid (46). Fermented corn flour poisoning can be prevented by properly controlling the fermentation of the corn flour, ensuring that the pH of the fermentation is sufficiently high. The fermented corn meal produced in the affected regions of China was made under conditions of neutral pH. Under alkaline conditions,

the growth of *F. farinofermentans* would be discouraged, and the toxin is unstable.

Tetrodotoxin or pufferfish poisoning could also probably be discussed in this section because it now seems as though the tetrodotoxins are produced by certain bacterial species. However, tetrodotoxin poisoning will be discussed with the algal toxins because it has traditionally fit with other seafood intoxications.

Mycotoxins

Mycotoxins are produced by a wide variety of molds that can grow on many different foods (47). The first recognition of mycotoxins emanated from the observation of domestic animals fed moldy animal feeds. Although their effects on humans are not clearly established, many of the mycotoxins are potentially hazardous to humans as well. Not all of the many mycotoxins are equivalently hazardous to humans.

From a historical perspective, ergotism was undeniably the first mycotoxin-associated illness recognized in humans (48). The mold responsible for ergotism is *Claviceps purpurea*, which infects the heads of rye and sometimes wheat, barley, and oats. The shriveled, purplish grain kernel contains the mycotoxin. The toxins involved in ergotism are known collectively as the ergot alkaloids, and ergotism can be manifested in two forms: gangrenous ergotism and convulsive ergotism. Gangrenous ergotism, also known as St. Anthony's fire, begins with a burning sensation in the feet and hands that is followed by a progressive restriction of blood flow to the hands and feet. This results in gangrene, which can lead to the loss of limbs. Convulsive ergotism is characterized by hallucinations leading to convulsive seizures and sometimes death. No outbreaks of ergotism have been recorded since the early 1950s.

Aspergillus molds are known to produce several types of mycotoxins, most notably the aflatoxins and ochratoxins (47). The aflatoxins are produced primarily by *A. flavus* and *A. parasiticus*, molds that often contaminate peanuts and corn. Several types of aflatoxins have been identified in legumes and cereals, including aflatoxins B and G. Dairy cows fed aflatoxin-contaminated grains or oilseeds are known to release a related form of aflatoxin, aflatoxin M, into their milk. The aflatoxins are potent carcinogens, especially affecting the liver (47). The role of aflatoxins in human carcinogenesis remains uncertain, but they are among the most potent animal carcinogens known. Ochratoxins are produced primarily by *A. ochraceus*, a mold that can contaminate cereals, peanuts, and tree nuts. Ochratoxin A is the most potent form. The ochratoxins affect the livers and kidneys of domestic animals, with the effects on the kidney being particularly damaging (47). The toxicity of ochratoxin to humans is unknown.

Fusarium molds produce numerous different mycotoxins, including the trichothecenes, fumonisins, and zearalenone (47). The trichothecenes are known human toxicants and are primarily contaminants of grains. Alimentary toxic aleukia

(ALA) was an illness described in the former Soviet Union owing to consumption of grains containing trichothecenes (48). ALA has four stages. The first stage begins with a burning sensation in the mouth and throat that proceeds down the esophagus to the stomach. This burning sensation is followed by diarrhea, nausea, and vomiting, occurring 1 to 3 days later and ceasing after about 9 days. The second stage occurs from about 2 weeks to 2 months after onset and involves bone marrow destruction, leukemia, agranulocytosis, anemia, and loss of platelets. At the end of this stage, small hemorrhages may occur on the skin. The third stage of ALA lasts from 5 to 20 days and involves total loss of bone marrow with necrotic angina, sepsis, total agranulocytosis, and moderate fever. The hemorrhages progress to become larger, and necrotic lesions appear on the skin. Bronchial pneumonia appears, along with abscesses and hemorrhages in the lungs. The fourth stage is death, with the mortality rate approaching 80% and dependent on the dose and frequency of exposure to the trichothecenes. Several trichothecene mycotoxins have been identified including T-2 toxin and deoxynivalenol, also known as vomitoxin (47). Although the involvement of particular trichothecene mycotoxins in ALA is uncertain because this illness occurred before any knowledge existed of these mycotoxins, T-2 toxin is thought to have been a primary causative agent (47).

Fumonisins are produced primarily by *F. verticillioides* and several other *Fusarium* species (47). These molds contaminate various grains and soybeans but are a particular problem with corn. The fumonisins have been implicated in equine leukoencephalomalacia, a fatal neurotoxic syndrome in horses, characterized by extensive necrosis of the white matter in the brain (47). The possible carcinogenicity of fumonisins remains an active area of scientific scrutiny. Although their effects on humans remain unknown, low-level contamination of grains with fumonisins seems to be fairly common.

Zearalenone is an estrogenic substance produced in grains by *F. graminearum* (48). It causes spontaneous abortions in pigs, but its effects on humans are unknown.

Penicillium molds produce many different mycotoxins, including ochratoxin, patulin, citrinin, cyclochlorotine, luteoskyrin, rugulosin, cyclopiazonic acid, citreoviridin, and penicillic acid (47). These mycotoxins cause various effects in domestic and laboratory animals, but their effects if any on humans are quite uncertain. Cyclochlorotine, luteoskyrin, and rugulosin are thought to perhaps be involved in yellow rice disease, another illness that like ALA occurred during World War II (47). Many other mycotoxins have been identified, although most of these others have received little scientific study.

Algal Toxins (Phycotoxins)

Marine algae are capable of producing certain potentially hazardous substances. These toxins are ingested by shellfish and fish, resulting in the development of potentially hazardous seafood. In some cases, the algal toxins are modified by the fish or shellfish, although that action does not necessarily detoxify them. In other cases, these algal toxins pass through the food chain from smaller organisms to larger ones; the largest ones are occasionally the most toxic. However, in all cases, the fish and shellfish are only toxic in circumstances in which they have the opportunity to feed on toxic marine algae. Several acute illnesses are associated with such seafood, including ciguatera poisoning, paralytic shellfish poisoning, neurotoxic shellfish poisoning, diarrhetic shellfish poisoning, amnesic shellfish poisoning, and tetrodotoxin poisoning (49).

Ciguatera Poisoning. Ciguatera poisoning results from the ingestion of fish that have fed on toxic dinoflagellate algae. Ciguatera poisoning is probably the most common cause of foodborne disease of chemical etiology on a worldwide basis. This foodborne illness is common throughout the Caribbean and much of the Pacific, but is now encountered around the world because of the improved distribution of fish (49–51). In the United States, the illness occurs most frequently in Florida, Hawaii, and the Virgin Islands (50–52). Fish that inhabit reef and shore areas in temperate regions, such as grouper, red snapper, barracuda, amberjack, kingfish, Spanish mackerel, mahi-mahi, sea bass, surgeon fish, and eels, are the most commonly implicated species, although many different fish species can be involved (52, 54). These fish acquire the toxic agent(s) by feeding on smaller fish that acquire the toxin from the poisonous planktonic algae (49, 55). Several species of dinoflagellate algae appear able to produce toxins of the type associated with ciguatera poisoning (30); *Gambierdiscus toxicus* is one of the most prominent (49, 51, 55).

Several toxins may be involved in ciguatera poisoning, but the major toxin is a lipid-soluble polyether compound with a molecular weight of 1112 known as ciguatoxin (54). Ciguatoxin has ionophoric properties (51, 54). Although the toxins accumulate in the liver and viscera of the fish, enough can enter the muscle tissues to result in ciguatera poisoning among humans ingesting these fish (56). The toxins are heat-stable and thus unaffected by processing or cooking practices (56).

The symptoms of ciguatera poisoning are somewhat variable. Perhaps this observation confirms the role of several different dinoflagellate algae and several different toxins in this syndrome (54). Gastrointestinal and neurologic manifestations are the predominant symptom (51, 54), although in some cases the gastrointestinal symptoms predominate, whereas in other cases the neurologic symptoms predominate (51). The gastrointestinal complaints include nausea, vomiting, diarrhea, and abdominal cramps. The neurologic symptoms include dysesthesia, paresthesia especially in the perioral region and extremities, pruritus, vertigo, muscle weakness, malaise, headache, and myalgia. A peculiar reversal of hot and cold sensations occurs in about 65% of all patients (51). In severe cases, the neurologic manifestations can progress to delirium, pruritus, dyspnea, prostration, brachycardia, and coma (51). Many patients recover within a few days or weeks. However, treatment can be difficult, and some deaths from cardiovascular collapse have been encountered (49, 56).

Paralytic Shellfish Poisoning. Paralytic shellfish poisoning occurs as the result of ingesting molluscan shellfish, such as clams, mussels, cockles, and scallops, that have become poisonous by feeding on toxic dinoflagellate algae (49). Although paralytic shellfish poisoning occurs worldwide, it is most commonly encountered along the Pacific and North Atlantic coasts of North America, the coastal areas of Japan, and the southern coast of Chile (49, 56). Toxic dinoflagellate algae belonging to *Alexandrium* spp. have been implicated in paralytic shellfish poisoning (49, 57). Because the blooms of the toxic dinoflagellates are quite sporadic, most shellfish will be hazardous only during the times of the blooms (56). In most shellfish species, the toxins are cleared from their systems within a few weeks after the end of the dinoflagellate bloom (58). However, a few species, such as the Alaskan butter clam, seem to retain the toxin for long periods (58). Neurotoxins known as saxitoxins are the causative agents involved in paralytic shellfish poisoning (49, 56, 59). Saxitoxins bind to and block the sodium channels in nerve membranes (49, 57). Processing and cooking have no effect on the toxicity of the heat-stable saxitoxins in the shellfish (58).

Because the saxitoxins can block nerve transmission, they are very potent neurotoxins. The symptoms of paralytic shellfish poisoning include a tingling sensation and numbness of the lips, tongue, and fingertips; followed by numbness in the legs, arms, and neck; ataxia; giddiness; staggering; drowsiness; incoherent speech progressing to aphasia; rash; fever; and respiratory and muscular paralysis (49, 57). Death from respiratory failure does occur with some frequency, usually within 2 to 12 hours, depending on the dose ingested (58). No antidotes are known, although the prognosis is good if the victim survives the first 24 hours of the illness (57, 58).

Amnesic Shellfish Poisoning. Amnesic shellfish poisoning was first recognized in 1987 as the result of an outbreak in Canada (60). This outbreak, involving ingestion of mussels from Prince Edward Island, was associated with more than 100 cases and at least four deaths (60, 61). A planktonic algae, *Nitzschia pungens*, which was blooming in an isolated area of Prince Edward Island at the time of the outbreak, was implicated as the source of the toxin (62). Domoic acid, a neuroexcitatory amino acid, was identified as the toxin (63). Amnesic shellfish poisoning is characterized by gastrointestinal symptoms and unusual neurologic abnormalities (60). The gastrointestinal symptoms include vomiting, abdominal cramps, and diarrhea usually occurring in the first 24 hours after onset of the illness. The neurologic symptoms, which had onset within 48 hours, were severe incapacitating headaches, confusion,

loss of short-term memory, and in a few cases, seizures and coma. Severely affected patients who did not die experienced prolonged neurologic sequelae including memory deficits and motor or sensorimotor neuronopathy or axonopathy (61).

Diarrhetic Shellfish Poisoning. Diarrhetic shellfish poisoning is associated with the ingestion of toxic clams, mussels, and scallops (49). In this case, the source of the toxin is a dinoflagellate algae of the genus *Dinophysis* (64). Most known outbreaks have occurred in Japan, Europe, and Chile (64). The symptoms of diarrhetic shellfish poisoning include severe diarrhea, nausea, vomiting, abdominal cramps, and chills that have an onset time within 30 minutes to a few hours after ingestion of contaminated shellfish (49). Spontaneous recovery typically occurs within 3 days (49). Several different toxins have been identified as produced by *Dinophysis* spp, including okadaic acid, pectenotoxins, and yessotoxin (49). Okadaic acid is a polyether compound (65), and it is the only one of these toxins that has been definitely proven to cause diarrheal symptoms (49).

Neurotoxic Shellfish Poisoning. Neurotoxic shellfish poisoning occurs in areas where so-called red tides have caused massive fish kills (49). Shellfish poisonings have been reported occasionally in association with these red tide episodes. Neurotoxic shellfish poisoning occurs primarily in the United States in coastal areas of Florida. The symptoms of neurotoxic shellfish poisoning are quite similar to those of ciguatera poisoning, which were described earlier. Symptoms begin within 30 minutes to a few hours and typically subside spontaneously within 2 days. Although the symptoms are similar to those of ciguatera, they are usually less severe. The algal species involved is thought to be *Gymnodinium breve*, which produces polyether brevetoxins that are structurally similar to certain ciguatoxins (49).

Tetrodotoxin or Pufferfish Poisoning. Tetrodotoxin poisoning is presented at this location in the chapter because it is a seafood-related illness that is perhaps best discussed in the context of ciguatera poisoning and paralytic shellfish poisoning. However, as mentioned earlier, the tetrodotoxins are likely bacterially produced, so this illness could have been described with the other bacterial contaminants. Pufferfish poisoning occurs primarily in Japan and China because those are the primary areas of the world where pufferfish are frequently consumed (66). More than 30 species of pufferfish are found worldwide, although most species are not considered to be toxic (58). The most hazardous pufferfish belong to the genus *Fugu*; these fish are considered in Japan and China to be delicacies (66). Pufferfish are also sometimes referred to as blowfish. The toxin in pufferfish is a potent neurotoxin called tetrodotoxin (49). For many years, the toxin was thought to be produced by the fish. More recently, new evidence suggests that marine bacteria may be the original source of the toxin (67). Tetrodotoxins are heat-stable and, like the saxitoxins, act by blocking the sodium channels in nerve cell membranes (49). The symptoms of tetrodotoxin poisoning usually begin with a tingling sensation of the fingers, toes, lips, and tongue, followed by nausea, vomiting, diarrhea, and epigastric pain (68). Twitching, tremors, ataxia, paralysis, and death often ensue (68). A fatality rate of about 60% occurs in untreated cases (58, 68). The tetrodotoxins accumulate in the liver, viscera, and roe of the pufferfish. Careful cleaning of the fish before ingestion of the edible muscle is required to safeguard against tetrodotoxin intoxication (57). Although tetrodotoxin was once thought to be a single chemical entity (58), it is now recognized that various bacteria belonging to species such as *Alteromonas*, *Vibrio*, and others can produce different but related forms of tetrodotoxin that vary in potency (49). Although tetrodotoxin poisoning is primarily associated with *Fugu* fishes, similar if not identical toxins occur in newts, frogs, marine snails, octopuses, crabs, starfishes, and other marine species (49).

Insect-Derived and Mite-Derived Toxins

Insect infestations occur frequently in the food supply and are considered by most consumers to be aesthetically undesirable. Although not generally appreciated, insects can produce chemicals, some of which are potentially hazardous, that remain in the foods even if the insects are removed. The common flour beetles, *Tribolium confusum* and *Tribolium castaneum*, produce o-benzoquinones (69). The o-benzoquinones are putative carcinogens based on experiments in laboratory animals, although their carcinogenicity for humans remains unknown (70). The o-benzoquinones are also mutagenic to the flour beetles themselves when insect contamination of the flour becomes high (70). No cases of human illness have been reported from the ingestion of foods contaminated with flour beetles.

However, several cases of human illness have been reported from the ingestion of foods contaminated with dust mites. Although dust mites are very common inhalant allergens, they can contaminate foods, sometimes in high numbers if food storage conditions are poor (71). Although cases appear to be rare, sufficient levels of dust mite allergens can be produced in the food to elicit allergic symptoms in susceptible consumers when the contaminated food is ingested. Because the dust mites are microscopic, the consumer would not be aware of the contamination.

NATURAL TOXICANTS

In addition to the naturally occurring contaminants, natural constituents of foods may be hazardous under some circumstances of exposure. Fungi, plants, and occasionally animals can contain hazardous levels of various naturally occurring toxicants. Of course, such fungi, plants, and animals should not be consumed as food, but are accidentally or intentionally consumed on occasion, resulting in foodborne illness. Beyond the poisonous species, many other plants and animals contain levels of naturally occurring toxicants that are probably not hazardous to humans ingesting typical amounts of these foods. However, the ingestion of abnormally large quantities of such foods and their naturally occurring toxicants is potentially hazardous. The naturally occurring toxicants in some plants are inactivated or removed during processing or preparation of foods before consumption, but the failure to adhere to such processing and preparation practices can result in foodborne illness.

Poisonous Animals

Acute intoxications occur with very few animal species, although several species of poisonous fish and other marine animals are known to exist (66, 72). Pufferfish is the most often cited example, although it now seems that the toxin in pufferfish may actually emanate from bacteria (67).

Furthermore, animal tissues and products are not generally hazardous if ingested in abnormally large quantities, at least not on acute basis. Of course, this statement does not take into account the nutritional concerns with cholesterol and saturated fats. Although overconsumption of cholesterol and saturated fat on a chronic basis may be considered potentially deleterious to health, these substances are not generally regarded as toxicants. In fact, animal tissues and products contain very few naturally occurring toxicants. The best example is vitamin A (2, 10). This example was discussed under the Food Additives section because vitamin A is also a food additive. Milk can occasionally contain hazardous substances, but these are typically contaminants that are secreted into the milk after the cow has eaten a poisonous plant (73). Ovomucoid, a protein in egg whites, is a trypsin inhibitor, but this activity is diminished by cooking (74). Molluscan shellfish may contain arsenic compounds, but typically at levels that are not considered to be especially hazardous (75). Additional examples are difficult to find.

Poisonous Plants

In contrast, a very large number of poisonous plants exist in nature (76). Classically, plants such as water hemlock and nightshade were used to poison one's enemies. Consumers purchasing foods from commercial sources usually avoid the ingestion of poisonous plants. However, intoxications occur each year among persons who have harvested their own foods in the wild (77). For example, an elderly couple died after preparing herbal tea from materials they had gathered in the forest surrounding their home. They mistook foxglove for comfrey; foxglove contains digitalis, a potent cardiotoxic substance (78). In another example, a team member in a desert survival course died after eating a salad prepared in part from jimsonweed (77). Jimsonweed contains tropane alkaloids, including atropine. Atropine has potent anticholinergic properties, and persons ingesting jimsonweed and other plants containing tropane alkaloids suffer neurotoxic effects. Although digitalis and atropine are both useful pharmaceutical agents, their ingestion from natural sources in uncontrolled doses can be fatal. Many more such examples could be cited.

Plant food products purchased from commercial sources rarely cause acute intoxications. However, occasional exceptions do exist. In one well-investigated episode, a commercial herbal tea sold to the Mexican American population in Arizona was contaminated with *Senecio longilobus*, a well-known poisonous plant (79). The herbal tea was called gordolobo yerba, and it was promoted as a cure for colic, viral infections, and nasal congestion in infants. The number of infants and others who ingested the hazardous tea is not known, but six infants died. This tea contained 1.5% of dry weight of pyrrolizidine alkaloids, and one of the deceased infants was estimated to have consumed 66 mg of the alkaloids over a 4-day period. *Senecio* plants contain a group of chemicals known as pyrrolizidine alkaloids that can cause both acute and chronic symptoms. Chronic low doses produce liver cancer and cirrhosis (58). The acute symptoms associated with the contaminated herbal tea included ascites, hepatomegaly, venoocclusive liver disease, abdominal pain, nausea, vomiting, headache, and diarrhea (79). The infants who died experienced liver failure.

Although the herbal tea episode involved acute intoxication, pyrrolizidine alkaloids can also cause chronic intoxications if ingested in smaller quantities over more extended periods of time (80). With such chronic low-level intake, the effects on the liver are cumulative, with irreversible liver damage occurring in small increments over months or even years. Eventually, cirrhosis and liver cancer are the principal manifestations of chronic intoxication with pyrrolizidine alkaloids. Several of the pyrrolizidine alkaloids are well-documented carcinogens in laboratory animals. The lifelong ingestion of herbal products containing low levels of potentially carcinogenic pyrrolizidine alkaloids presents unknown carcinogenic risks. For example, many herbal teas commonly contain lower levels of pyrrolizidine alkaloids that are not typically hazardous on an acute basis. Comfrey (*Symphytum officinale*) typically contains a total alkaloid level of 0.003 to 0.02%, including a pyrrolizidine alkaloid, symphytine, which is apparently insufficient to elicit acute illness. It is unknown whether chronic intake of comfrey tea would significantly increase the risk of development of liver cancer.

Thousands of alkaloids with varying degrees of toxicity are known to occur in plant tissues (80). Some, like the pyrrolizidine alkaloids in *Senecio*, are very hazardous, whereas others are much less hazardous. Some commonly consumed plant foods contain alkaloids at levels that are not considered to be acutely toxic at typical levels of consumption. Comfrey tea is one example.

In some cases, plant-derived foods contain naturally occurring toxicants at doses that are not acutely toxic at typical levels of consumption but that can be toxic when large quantities of the food are eaten. Examples include solanine and chaconine in potatoes, oxalates in spinach and rhubarb, furan compounds in mold-damaged sweet potatoes, and cyanogenic glycosides in lima beans, cassava, and many fruit pits (80). Because there are so many possible examples, the cyanogenic glycosides will serve as an illustrative example (58, 80). Cyanogenic glycosides can release cyanide from enzymatic action occurring during the storage and processing of the foods or on contact with stomach acid. Although wild varieties of lima beans can contain high and potentially hazardous levels of cyanogenic glycosides, the commercial varieties of lima beans contain minimal amounts of these cyanogenic glycosides, having a hydrogen cyanide yield of 10 mg/100 g of lima beans (wet weight). Because the lethal oral dose of cyanide for humans is 0.5 mg/kg, a 70-kg adult would have to ingest 35 mg of cyanide, an amount that would require the ingestion of at least 350 g of lima beans. Such levels of consumption are quite unlikely, and human illnesses from cyanide intoxication from ingestion of commercially harvested lima beans have not been reported. Wild varieties of lima beans contain much higher levels of the cyanogenic glycosides (up to 300 mg hydrogen cyanide/100 g). Other plant sources of cyanogenic glycosides also exist. In Africa and South America, cyanide intoxications have occurred from the consumption of cassava (58, 80). Cassava is sometimes ingested in large quantities in these areas because of a lack of other foods (58, 80). Acute cyanide intoxication has also occurred from the ingestion of fruit pits (58), including the grinding of pits with the fruit in food processors during the preparation of jams and wines. The symptoms of cyanide intoxication include a rapid onset of peripheral numbness and dizziness, mental confusion, stupor, cyanosis, twitching, convulsions, coma, and death (58).

In some cases, plant foods would be hazardous if eaten raw, but processing and preparation ensure the safety of these foods. In these situations, the toxic constituents of plants are inactivated or removed during processing and preparation. For example, raw soybeans contain trypsin inhibitors, lectins, amylase inhibitors, saponins, and various antivitamins (58). Fortunately, these toxicants are inactivated during the heating and fermentation processes used with soybeans. If these toxicants are not removed or inactivated, foodborne illness can occur. For example, raw kidney beans contain lectins that are typically inactivated during cooking. In the United Kingdom, immigrants who did not appreciate the importance of thorough cooking of kidney beans have ingested undercooked kidney beans, leading to the onset of nausea, vomiting, abdominal pain, and bloody diarrhea from the lectins (58).

Poisonous Mushrooms

Mushrooms are often poisonous, so the harvesting of mushrooms in the wild can be a hazardous practice. Incidents of mushroom poisoning occur each year in the United States (81). Poisonous mushrooms contain various naturally occurring toxicants that can be classified into groups I to VI (58, 82).

The group I toxins are the most hazardous. Group I toxins include amatoxin and phallotoxin. Amatoxin is characteristically produced by *Amanita phalloides*, the death cap mushroom. Acute amatoxin intoxication occurs in three stages. In the first stage, abdominal pain, nausea, vomiting, diarrhea, and hyperglycemia begin to develop 6 to 24 hours after ingestion of the mushrooms. A short period of remission then occurs. In the third and often fatal stage, severe liver and kidney dysfunction lead to hypoglycemia, convulsions, coma, and death. Death resulting from hypoglycemic shock occurs 4 to 7 days after the onset of symptoms.

The group II toxins are hydrazines. Gyromitrin, produced by *Gyromitra esculenta* or false morel mushrooms, is the best-known example. The symptoms elicited by ingestion of false morel mushrooms include a bloated feeling, nausea, vomiting, watery or bloody diarrhea, abdominal pain, muscle cramps, faintness, and ataxia occurring within 6 to 12 hours of ingestion.

Muscarine is the most characteristic of the group III toxins, which affect the autonomic nervous system. Muscarine occurs in fly agaric (*Amanita muscaria*), sometimes in association with the group I toxins. Symptoms include perspiration, salivation, lacrimation with blurred vision, abdominal cramps, watery diarrhea, constriction of the pupils, hypotension, and a slowed pulse occurring rapidly after the ingestion of the poisonous mushrooms.

Coprine is a group IV toxin that cause symptoms only when ingested with alcoholic beverages. Coprine is produced by *Coprinus atramentarius*. Symptoms include flushing of the neck and face, distension of the veins in the neck, swelling and tingling of the hands, metallic taste, tachycardia, and hypotension progressing to nausea and vomiting. Symptoms begin within 30 minutes of ingestion of the mushrooms but only if alcoholic beverages are also consumed simultaneously. Symptoms can persist for up to 5 days.

The group V and VI toxins are hallucinogenic, ostensibly exerting their actions on the central nervous system, causing hallucinations. The group V toxins include ibotenic acid and muscimol. The group V toxins cause dizziness, drowsiness followed by hyperkinetic activity, confusion, delirium, incoordination, staggering, muscular spasms, partial amnesia, a comalike sleep, and hallucinations beginning 30 minutes to 2 hours after ingestion. Fly agaric is a good source of the group V toxins.

The group VI toxins include psilocybin and psilocin. The symptoms of the group VI toxins include a pleasant or aggressive mood, anxiety, unmotivated laughter and hilarity, compulsive movements, muscle weakness, drowsiness, hallucinations, and sleep. Mexican mushrooms, *Psilocybe mexicana*, contain the group VI toxins. Symptoms usually begin within 30 to 60 minutes after ingestion of the mushrooms, and recovery is often spontaneous in 5 to 10 hours. When the dose of the group VI toxins is high, prolonged and severe sequelae, even death, can occur.

RISK ASSESSMENT

Clearly, foods contain a complex mixture of chemicals, including some that can certainly be hazards under various conditions of exposure. Obviously, consumers wish to avoid those chemicals that are serious acute hazards, such as the ones obtained from poisonous mushrooms or a known poisonous plant. Avoidance of these hazards seems reasonably easy, although species identification can require some expert judgment and knowledge if one is harvesting food in the wild. However, if one eats foods from the commercial marketplace, this potential hazard can largely be avoided. Commercial foods are evaluated for their safety to a greater or lesser extent. Most foods are considered safe based on a long history of safe use rather than on a formal toxicologic safety evaluation. However, worldwide regulatory agencies do generally prohibit the commercial sale and distribution of unsafe foods. As this chapter has shown, many examples exist of food components that are known to present hazards under some set of exposure conditions. Some of these components are naturally occurring constituents, whereas others are contaminants from various sources. Much of the knowledge of the toxicity of these particular components also comes from history—from health problems suffered by consumers that then lead to the identification of these particular hazardous chemicals. Most food components have never been thoroughly tested for toxicity, but there is no compelling reason to do so because of the history of the safe use of these foods. Toxicologic evaluation of whole foods is difficult and is not recommended because nutritional imbalances almost always create confounding problems. Toxicologic evaluation of every single chemical component of every food clearly would be an enormous task. However, scientists and regulatory agencies have assessed the risks associated with many of the foodborne chemicals that are known to have the potential to elicit human illness under some circumstances. Thorough risk assessments are required by regulatory agencies for substances such as food additives that will be intentionally added to foods. However, toxicologic evaluations are not required for naturally occurring toxicants. Thus, although toxicologic data often exist for naturally occurring toxicants, the data are often incomplete and have not been obtained in the structured manner that is followed for food additive risk assessments. However, sufficient data often exist for reasonable risk assessments. Risk assessments have been performed for many of the chemical components of foods that are known to have the potential to cause foodborne disease. Even nutrients have been subjected to risk assessments (9), because like all chemical constituents of foods, nutrients can produce adverse health consequences if intakes of any combination of food, water, dietary supplements, and pharmacologic agents are excessive.

Basic Concepts of Risk Assessment

Risk assessment is a scientific process intended to characterize the nature and likelihood of harm resulting from human exposure to agents in the environment. For foods, the focus is on the nature and likely harm associated with the ingestion of a particular chemical in the food supply or related materials (water, dietary supplements). Risk assessment is a process that uses all of the available scientific information on the risk and then applies uncertainty factors to arrive at recommendations regarding levels of exposure that are safe for most consumers. Risk management decisions can then be based on the knowledge of these acceptable levels of risk derived from risk assessment. For example, shellfish harvesting in an area could be banned if levels of a shellfish toxin (as discussed earlier) are identified in that area.

The US National Academy of Sciences developed an approach to risk assessment that has been applied to all sorts of environmental risks for many years (83). The risk assessment process requires that the available scientific information be organized in a rather specific way, but it does not require that the data be obtained by any specific scientific evaluation methods. Instead, all data that are available are reviewed by experts to determine whether they are germane to the risk assessment consideration and if they are reliable and were acquired by sound methodology.

The risk assessment approach developed by the National Academy of Sciences has four steps:

(a) Hazard identification involves the collection, organization, and examination of all information pertaining to the adverse effects of a given foodborne chemical. The nature of the adverse reaction will be described, and the level of evidence relating the particular chemical to that particular adverse reaction will be evaluated.

(b) Dose-response assessment determines the quantitative relationship between the oral dose of the foodborne chemical and the adverse effect in terms of incidence and severity. Experimental data from studies on laboratory animals are often used at this stage, but if sufficient information is available from actual human experiences, those data are extremely valuable as well. Obviously, detailed dose-response data are almost never available on humans because any experiments would be unethical.

(c) Exposure assessment examines the frequency, distribution, and level of intake of the foodborne chemical. Obviously, some naturally occurring constituents of certain foods are regularly encountered by every consumer of that food. Contaminants are more sporadic in terms of exposure. Exposure assessment is particularly critical in evaluation of chronic health hazards because an estimate of the level of intake over many years is a critical component of the risk assessment process. With an acute toxicant, one dose on one occasion may be sufficient to produce an adverse health effect, so the frequency of exposure can be a moot point—once is enough.

(d) Risk characterization involves taking the conclusions from these first three steps and then evaluating the risk. What is the likelihood that ingestion of a particular foodborne chemical at a particular dose (perhaps over some period of time) will result in an adverse health consequence? Scientific uncertainties are applied at this stage. In most circumstances, very fragmentary human data will be available because either the number of people exposed will have been small or the evaluation of the human episodes will be incomplete because of lack of adequate sampling, analytic methods, or other deficiencies. So, if human data are used, the risk assessor must apply some uncertainty factor to account for the possibility that some human subjects may be more susceptible than the ones for which data exist and to correct for possible data deficiencies. Even larger uncertainty factors are often applied when reliance is placed primarily on toxicologic data from studies on experimental animals. In these cases, an uncertainty factor must also be included to account for the extrapolation from experimental animals to humans. Therefore, the magnitude of the uncertainty factor applied to the available data in the risk characterization stage is dependent on the nature, volume, and quality of the toxicologic data.

Risk Management

Clearly, the management of the risk is intended to protect human health. The risk management process for foodborne chemicals is often not straightforward. Certainly, regulatory officials and others can be more cautious when the foodborne chemical is not an essential part of the diet. Therefore, the closing of a particular beach area to recreational shellfish harvesting, for example, can be done with ample precaution because no consequences beyond protection of human health arise from this activity. On the other hand, the establishment of upper reference intake levels for nutrients requires careful consideration (9) because nutrients are required in the diet; you want enough but not too much. With uncertainty factors, the window between optimal requirements for nutrients and upper reference intake levels can be quite narrow. In other examples, such as mycotoxins in grains, worldwide trade may be disrupted by overly cautious risk management decisions.

In all cases, special populations must be considered as well. Infants, elderly persons, those with particular chronic illnesses, and others may be at higher risk, but the goal would be protection of most consumers, including special groups.

Risk management decisions within worldwide regulatory agencies require careful judgment. Because of the weighing of factors differently in different regulatory jurisdictions, the same data can be evaluated in different countries but lead to differing regulatory decisions. Of course, if these decisions have trade implications, then serious arguments can ensue.

However, it should be emphasized that individual consumers often make critical risk management decisions as well. They often proceed without any evaluation of the available scientific information or any attempt at a risk assessment. For example, the decision to harvest wild mushrooms or herbs for herbal tea in the forest carries some risk depending on the individual's degree of expertise in species identification. Thus, many of the human experiences discussed in this chapter have resulted from decisions made by individual consumers without scientific evaluation rather than from decisions made through risk assessment by the commercial sector or worldwide regulatory agencies. Risk assessment and risk management are sound approaches, but frankly they are not always applied to the examples discussed in this chapter.

REFERENCES

1. Taylor SL. Food toxicology. In: Metcalfe DD, Sampson HA, Simon RA, eds. Food Allergy—Adverse Reactions to Foods and Food Additives. 3rd ed. Elmsford, NY: Blackwell Publishing, 2003:475–86.
2. Taylor SL. Chemical intoxications. In: Cliver DO, Riemann HP, eds. Foodborne Diseases. 2nd ed. San Diego: Academic Press, 2002:305–16.
3. Taylor SL, Byron B. J Food Prot 1984;47:249.
4. Lockey S. Ann Allergy 1959;17:719–25.
5. Bush RK, Taylor SL, Hefle SL. Adverse reactions to food and drug additives. In: Adkinson NF, Yunginger JW, Busse WW et al., eds. Middleton's Allergy Principles and Practice. 6th ed. St. Louis: Mosby, 2003:1645–63.
6. Stevenson DD. Tartrazine, azo, and non-azo dyes. In: Metcalfe DD, Sampson HA, Simon RA, eds. Food Allergy—Adverse Reactions to Foods and Food Additives. 3rd ed. Elmsford, NY: Blackwell Publishing, 2003:351–9.
7. Cheskin LJ, Miday R, Zorich N et al. JAMA 1998;279:150–2.
8. Munro IC. A case study: the safety evaluation of artificial sweeteners. In: Taylor SL, Scanlan RA, eds. Food Toxicology—A Perspective on the Relative Risks. New York: Marcel Dekker, 1989: 151–67.
9. Food and Nutrition Board, Institute of Medicine. Dietary Reference Intakes—A Risk Assessment Model for Establishing Upper Intake Levels for Nutrients. Washington, DC: National Academy Press, 1998:71.
10. DiPalma JR, Ritchie DM. Ann Rev Pharmacol Toxicol 1977;17: 133–48.
11. Press E, Yeager L. Am J Public Health 1962;52:1720–8.
12. Campana L, Redmond S, Nitzkin JL et al. JAMA 1983;250:160.
13. Burkhalter J, Shore M, Wollstadt L et al. MMWR Morb Mortal Wkly Rep 1981;30:11–2.
14. Linshaw MA, Harrison HL, Gruskin AB et al. J Pediatr 1980;96: 635–40.
15. Kilbourne EM, Rigau-Perez JG, Heath CW Jr et al. N Engl J Med 1983;309:1408–14.
16. de la Paz MP, Philen RM, Borda IA et al. Food Chem Toxicol 1996;34:251–7.
17. Condemi JJ. Unusual presentations. In: Chiaramonte LT, Schneider AT, Lifshitz F, eds. Food Allergy—A Practical Approach to Diagnosis and Management. New York: Marcel Dekker, 1988:231–54.
18. World Health Organization. Toxic oil syndrome—Current knowledge and future perspectives. Copenhagen: WHO Regional Publications, European Series No. 42, 1992.
19. Rodriguez M, Nogura AE, Del Villaras S et al. Arthritis Rheum 1982;25:1477–80.
20. Ferrer A, Cabral R. Food Addit Contam 1991;8:755–76.
21. Green MA, Heumann MA, Wehr HM et al. Am J Public Health 1987;77:1431–4.
22. Goldman LR, Beller M, Jackson RL. Arch Environ Health 1990; 45:141–7.
23. Goes EA, Savage EP, Gibbons G et al. Am J Epidemiol 1980; 111:254–60.
24. Concon JM, Food Toxicology, Part B, Contaminants and Additives. New York: Marcel Dekker, 1988:1371.
25. Sanders PR, Lee TC, Groth ME et al. Safety assessment of insect-protected corn. In: Thomas JA, ed. Biotechnology and Safety Assessment. 2nd ed. London: Taylor and Francis, 1998: 241–56.
26. Taylor SL, Nordlee JA, Kapels LM. Pediatr Allergy Immunol 1992;3:180–7.
27. Schmid R. N Engl J Med 1960;268:397–8.
28. Fassett DW. Nitrates and nitrites. In: Committee on Food Protection. Toxicants Occurring Naturally in Foods. 2nd ed. Washington, DC: National Academy of Sciences, 1973:7–25.
29. Spinios A. Munch Med Wochenschr 1964;106:1180–2.
30. Keating JP, Lell ME, Straus AW et al. N Engl J Med 1973;288: 825–6.
31. Dewdney JM, Edwards RG. J R Soc Med 1984;77:866–77.
32. Food and Drug Administration, Center for Veterinary Medicine. 1999. Report on the Food and Drug Administration's Review of the Safety of Recombinant Bovine Somatotropin. Available at: http://www.fda.gov/cvm/index/bst/RBRPTFNL.htm
33. Hughes JM, Horwitz MA, Merson MH et al. Am J Epidemiol 1977;105:233–44.
34. Barker WH Jr, Runte V. Am J Epidemiol 1972;96:219–26.
35. Hamel AJ, Drawbaugh R, McBean AM et al. MMWR Morbid Mortal Wkly Rep 1977;26:218.
36. Brown MA, Thom JV, Orth GL et al. Arch Environ Health 1964; 8:657–60.
37. Hecht A. FDA Consumer Dec 1976–Jan 1977:21–5.
38. Kuratsune M, Yoshimura T, Matsuzaka J et al. Environ Health Perspect 1972;1:119–28.
39. Higuchi K, ed. PCB Poisoning and Pollution. New York: Academic Press, 1976.
40. Allen JR, Norback DH. Science 1973;179:498–9.
41. Kurland LT, Faro SN, Siedler H. World Neurol 1960;1: 370–95.
42. Wong ACL, Bergdoll MS. Staphylococcal food poisoning. In: Cliver DO, Riemann HP, eds. Foodborne Diseases. 2nd ed. San Diego: Academic Press, 2002:231–48.
43. Parkinson NG, Ito K. Botulism. In: Cliver DO, Riemann HP, eds. Foodborne Diseases. 2nd ed. San Diego: Academic Press, 2002:249–59.
44. Griffiths MW, Schraft H. Bacillus cereus food poisoning. In: Cliver DO, Riemann HP, eds. Foodborne Diseases. 2nd ed. San Diego: Academic Press, 2002:261–70.

45. Van Veen AG. The Bongkrek toxins. In: Mateles RI, Wogan GN, eds. Biochemistry of Some Foodborne Microbial Toxins. Cambridge, MA: MIT Press, 1967:43–50.

46. Hu WJ, Zhang GS, Chu FS et al. Appl Environ Microbiol 1984;48:690–3.

47. Chu FS. Mycotoxins. In: Cliver DO, Riemann HP, eds. Foodborne Diseases. 2nd ed. San Diego: Academic Press, 2002:271–303.

48. Taylor SL. Naturally occurring toxicants in foods. In: Dulbecco R, ed. Encyclopedia of Human Biology. 2nd ed. San Diego: Academic Press, 1997:6:57–64.

49. Johnson EA, Schantz EJ. Seafood toxins. In: Cliver DO, Riemann HP, eds. Foodborne Diseases. 2nd ed. San Diego: Academic Press, 2002:211–30.

50. Bagnis R, Kuberski T, Laugier S. Am J Trop Med Hyg 1979;28:1067–73.

51. Russell FE, Egen NB. J Toxicol Toxin Rev 1991;10:37–62.

52. Lawrence DN, Enriquez MB, Lumish RM et al. JAMA 1980;244:254–8.

53. Morris JG Jr, Lewin P, Hargrett NT et al. Arch Intern Med 1982;142:1090–2.

54. Hokama Y, Miyahara JT. J Toxicol Toxin Rev 1986;5:25–53.

55. Bagnis R, Chanteau S, Chungue E et al. Toxicon 1980;18:199–208.

56. Taylor SL. Food Technology 1988;42:94–8.

57. Whittle K, Gallacher S. Br Med Bull 2000;56:236–53.

58. Taylor SL, Schantz EJ. Naturally occurring toxicants in foods. In: Cliver DO, ed. Foodborne Diseases. San Diego: Academic Press, 1990:67–84.

59. Shimizu Y. The chemistry of paralytic shellfish toxins. In: Tu AT, ed. Handbook of Natural Toxins, vol 3. Marine Toxins and Venoms. New York: Marcel Dekker, 1988:63–85.

60. Perl TM, Bedard L, Kosatsky T et al. N Engl J Med 1990;322:1775–80.

61. Teitelbaum JS, Zatorre RJ, Carpenter S et al. N Engl J Med 1990;322:1781–7.

62. Bates SS, Bird CJ, DeFreitas ASW et al. Can J Fish Aquatic Sci 1989;46:1203–15.

63. Wright JLC, Boyd RK, DeFreitas ASW et al. Can J Chem 1989;67:481–90.

64. Yasumoto T, Murata M, Oshima Y et al. Diarrhetic shellfish poisoning. In: Ragelis EP, ed. Seafood Toxins. Washington, DC: American Chemistry Society, 1984:207–16.

65. Yasumoto T, Murata M. Polyether toxins involved in seafood poisoning. In: Hall S, Stricharty G, eds. Marine Toxins—Origin, Structure and Molecular Pharmacology. Washington, DC: American Chemistry Society 1990:120–32.

66. Halstead BW. Fish toxins. In: Hui YH, Gorham JR, Murrell KD et al., eds. Foodborne Disease Handbook, vol 3. Diseases Caused by Hazardous Substances. New York: Marcel Dekker, 1994:463–96.

67. Yasumoto T, Yasumura D, Yotsu M et al. Agr Biol Chem 1986;50:793–5.

68. Mines D, Stahmer S, Shepherd SM. Emerg Med Clin North Am 1997;15:157–77.

69. Wirtz RA, Taylor SL, Semey HG. Comp Biochem Physiol 1978;61B:25–8.

70. Taylor SL, Hefle SL. Naturally occurring toxicants in foods. In: Cliver DO, Riemann HP, eds. Foodborne Diseases. 2nd ed. San Diego: Academic Press, 2002:193–210.

71. Sanchez-Borges M, Capriles-Hulett A, Fernandez-Caldes E et al. J Allergy Clin Immunol 1997;99:738–43.

72. Halstead BW. Other poisonous marine animals. In: Hui YH, Gorham JR, Murrell KD et al., eds. Foodborne Disease Handbook, vol 3. Diseases Caused by Hazardous Substances. New York: Marcel Dekker, 1994:497–528.

73. Beier RC, Nigg HN. Toxicology of naturally occurring chemicals in foods. In: Hui YH, Gorham JR, Murrell KD et al., eds. Foodborne Disease Handbook, vol 3. Diseases Caused by Hazardous Substances. New York: Marcel Dekker, 1994:1–186.

74. Doell BH, Ebden CJ, Smith CA. Qual Plant Foods Hum Nutr 1981;31:139–44.

75. Whanger PD. Factors affecting the metabolism of nonessential metals in foods. In: Hathcock JN, ed. Nutritional Toxicology, vol 1. New York: Academic Press, 1982:163–208.

76. Smith RA. Poisonous plants. In: Hui YH, Gorham JR, Murrell KD et al., eds. Foodborne Disease Handbook, vol 3. Diseases Caused by Hazardous Substances. New York: Marcel Dekker, 1994:187–226.

77. Huxtable RJ. Perspect Biol Med 1980;24:1–14.

78. Cooper L, Grunenfelder G, Blackmon J et al. MMWR Morbid Mortal Wkly Rep 1977;26:257–9.

79. Stillman AE, Huxtable R, Consroe P et al. Gastroenterology 1977;73:349–53.

80. Sinden SL, Deahl KL. Alkaloids. In: Hui YH, Gorham JR, Murrell KD et al, eds. Foodborne Disease Handbook, vol 3. Diseases Caused by Hazardous Substances. New York: Marcel Dekker, 1994:227–59.

81. Hughes JM, Horwitz MA, Merson MH et al. Am J Epidemiol 1977;105:233–44.

82. Spoerke DG Jr. Mushrooms: Epidemiology and medical management. In: Hui YH, Gorham JR, Murrell KD et al., eds. Foodborne Disease Handbook. vol 3. Diseases Caused by Hazardous Substances. New York: Marcel Dekker, 1994:433–62.

83. National Research Council. Risk Assessment in the Federal Government: Managing the Process. Washington, DC: National Academy Press, 1983.

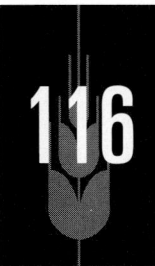

116 NUTRITION LABELING OF FOODS AND DIETARY SUPPLEMENTS[1]

KENNETH D. FISHER, ELIZABETH A. YETLEY, AND CHRISTINE L. TAYLOR

BASIS FOR NUTRITION LABELING 1827
    Misbranding 1827
    Right to Free Speech .1828
    Regulatory Categories 1828
    Procedures for Nutrition Labeling 1828
AMENDMENTS TO THE FOOD, DRUG,
    AND COSMETIC ACT OF 1938 1828
FIRST MAJOR COMPONENT OF NUTRITION
    LABELING: FACTS PANELS 1829
    Nutrition Facts Panel 1831
    Supplement Facts Panel 1832
    Meat and Poultry Labeling 1832
SECOND MAJOR COMPONENT OF NUTRITION
    LABELING: NUTRITION CLAIMS 1832
    Nutrient Content Claims 1833
    Health Claims 1834
OTHER LABELING STATEMENTS 1836
    Structure Function Claims 1836
    Product Quality and Warning Statements 1836
INTERNATIONAL NUTRITION LABELING 1836
FUTURE OF NUTRITION LABELING 1837

The chapter focuses on nutrition labeling in the United States as reflected in its evolution stemming from key amendments to the Food, Drug, and Cosmetic Act of 1938 (FD&C Act) (1), including the Nutrition Labeling and Education Act of 1990 (NLEA) (2) and the Dietary Supplement Health and Education Act of 1994 (DSHEA) (3). Certain recent court decisions that have affected nutrition labeling procedures are also identified.

Over the past 100 years, the history and evolution of nutrition labeling have reflected the dynamic interplay among changes in nutrition science, consumer concerns, and the interests of the food industry as well as court decisions and the role of government in fostering public health

and regulation of the food supply. This history and evolution of nutrition labeling of foods and dietary supplements have been addressed extensively in several reviews (4–8) and in previous editions of this textbook (9, 10). Major milestones in the development of nutrition labeling of foods and dietary supplements before 1999 were reviewed previously (4, 6). These reviews also discuss in detail the many public and private organizations that have and continue to play major roles in the development of nutrition labeling. This chapter focuses specifically on significant advances and changes in nutrition labeling of foods and dietary supplements since 1990.

BASIS FOR NUTRITION LABELING

The authoritative bases for nutrition labeling are often referred to as "anchors or drivers." They have been derived from several sources including continuing evolution of knowledge and scientific consensus on the role of nutrition in health and disease, congressional legislative mandates, development of regulation by the Food and Drug Administration (FDA), and judicial approval of FDA's implementation of these concepts into a comprehensive system for nutrition labeling of foods and dietary supplements.

Misbranding

The *legal authority* for nutrition labeling is derived from the misbranding provisions in the FD&C Act as amended (1). Nutrition labeling is based primarily on the fact that the food *label* and any accompanying *labeling* are legal documents subject to FDA regulation. Because the label and labeling are considered communication, or a form of "speech," between the food manufacturer and the food consumer, there is legal basis for the government to protect the consumer from misleading and inaccurate information on the label or in labeling. Consistent with this concept, the FD&C Act prohibits the interstate marketing of a misbranded food and subjects the food to enforcement action by FDA. A food is misbranded if, among other considerations, its labeling is *false or misleading*. The determination of false or misleading is based on both the truthfulness of any given label statement and the failure to reveal so-called *material facts* in light of the statement;

[1]**Abbreviations: DRI,** dietary reference intake; **DSHEA,** Dietary Supplement Health and Education Act of 1994; **DV,** daily value; **FDA,** Food and Drug Administration; **FDAMA,** FDA Modernization Act; **FD&C Act,** Food, Drug, and Cosmetic Act of 1938; **NAS,** National Academy of Sciences; **NLEA,** Nutrition Labeling and Education Act of 1990; **RDA,** recommended dietary allowance; **SSA,** significant scientific agreement; **USDA,** United States Department of Agriculture.

that is, labeling may be misleading not only because of what it states but also because of what it fails to state.

Failure to meet the standard of truthful and nonmisleading can be caused not only by *explicit* statements but also by *implied* statements, which are identified often through the combination of information from various parts of the label. In addition, considerations about the need for *material facts* form the rationale for requiring the declaration of the nutritional content on packaged foods; that is, in the absence of information about the nutritional content of foods, consumers are less able to select diets that maintain and promote health and reduce risks of disease.

Right to Free Speech

The First Amendment of the US Constitution protects against the prohibition of speech by individuals as well as speech reflecting commercial interests. These different types of speech have different legal precedents. In the case of commercial free speech, a government agency may restrict such speech when the prohibition is based on a substantial government interest such as protecting the consumer from false and misleading information. However, this "balancing act" between the manufacturer's right to commercial free speech and the government's interest in protecting the consumer is a challenging aspect of nutrition labeling in the marketplace, particularly in the area of health claims.

Regulatory Categories

Foods and drugs are defined as two separate *regulatory categories* on the basis of their *intended use,* and the regulatory requirements a manufacturer must follow to market products legally in either category vary (1). This distinction is particularly critical with respect to dietary supplements, which are regulated as foods, but are often used as preventive and therapeutic products by consumers.

The *regulatory category* "food" includes conventional foods, dietary supplements, infant formulas, and medical foods. Regulations governing each of these subcategories vary regarding how much and what type of FDA premarket notification and review are required, as well as regarding the final authorizations and provisions a manufacturer must meet. These include both similarities and differences in regard to nutrition labeling but also good manufacturing practices and reporting of adverse effects from use (standards for safety also vary among these food categories).

The *intended use* of a product is generally what the manufacturer indicates through explicit and implied claims and other information about the product. Food products in conventional food form are generally assumed to be consumed for their "taste, aroma, and nutritive value." Dietary supplements are intended to "supplement the dietary intake" of particular substances. A food or dietary supplement with label information suggesting that it is useful for the diagnosis, mitigation, treatment, or prevention of a disease would result in the product's being regulated as a drug.

Another type of information comprises the name and the representation of the product. Conventional foods must be identified on the principal display panel on a product label by their *common or usual name*. Dietary supplements must carry a *statement of identity* on the principal display panel that clearly identifies them as a dietary supplement or a specific type of supplement. Additionally, dietary supplements cannot represent themselves as conventional foods. The types of claims allowed on a "food" depend in part on its regulatory category.

Procedures for Nutrition Labeling

Implementation of nutrition labeling legislation by the FDA has occurred primarily through a multistep process termed *notice-and-comment rulemaking.* In this process, the FDA first proposes how it intends to regulate an issue, solicits public comment, and then finalizes the regulation based on public input to the proposal and further analysis. Both the proposed and final rules contain extensive preambles that describe the agency's rationale and the scientific evidence on which the agency has relied.

A major advantage of rulemaking in this manner is its fairness; that is, all interested stakeholders have an opportunity for input. In addition, any interested party can petition the FDA to create a new regulation or to amend an existing regulation. Once adopted and published, final rules carry the force and effect of law and are subject to enforcement. A major disadvantage of the *notice-and-comment rulemaking* process is the extensive time between development and publication of a proposed rule and revision and publication of a final rule or regulation. The FDA has in some cases published interim final regulations that allow the proposal to become effective while public comments are being collected and reviewed. Additionally, the FDA has issued *guidance documents* to assist stakeholders' in understanding the agency's reasoning and intent in the rulemaking. The FDA has issued several guidance documents since 1990 for a number of issues related to health claims (11–16).

AMENDMENTS TO THE FOOD, DRUG, AND COSMETIC ACT OF 1938

In the 50 years following passage of the FD&C Act, advances in nutritional science, governmental efforts to address public health issues, and increasing public interest in health and wellness focused national attention on the role of diet in health promotion and disease prevention. A major outcome of the 1960 White House Conference on Food, Nutrition, and Health was recognition in the public and private sectors of the need to improve nutrition labeling of foods (17).

Evolution of this effort led to Congressional enactment of the NLEA in 1990 (2). The NLEA amended the FD&C Act and specifically authorized the FDA to regulate nutrition labeling for food products. This landmark legislation, which built on, refined, and expanded many of the core components of nutrition labeling that had evolved since the early 1940s, made nutrition labeling mandatory for processed and packaged conventional foods and dietary supplements. It also expanded the emphasis of nutrition labeling to include macronutrients such as fats and enhanced FDA authority to set standards for serving sizes, define descriptors for nutrient content levels such as "high" and "low," and make provisions for specific disease risk reduction claims. The NLEA provided for voluntary nutrition labeling for fresh fruits and vegetables and seafood. The NLEA did not address advertising or labeling of restaurant foods.

The NLEA allowed the FDA the option of creating separate nutrition labeling regulations for dietary supplements. However, the agency concluded that both are foods, and as such both should be regulated by means of a consistent approach. Scientific issues related to using daily values (DVs) in place of recommended dietary allowances (RDAs) as well as concerns with regard to uniform nutrition labeling of foods and dietary supplements led to the passage of the Dietary Supplement Act (18). The Act did not change the NLEA provisions regarding nutrition labeling; it established a moratorium on implementation of NLEA provisions on labeling of dietary supplements for 1 year and use of new RDAs in regulations until late 1993.

The DSHEA was enacted by Congress in 1994 (3). The Act reiterated that dietary supplements are foods and that they could contain a broad range of ingredients including vitamins, minerals, botanicals, amino acids, and other substances intended to supplement the diet. The DSHEA also stated certain separate provisions for nutrition labeling of dietary supplements and specified modifications to the manner in which supplement labels were to declare nutrients and other dietary ingredients. Further, the DSHEA provided unique provisions for the use of so-called structure function claims.

In 1997, Congress passed the FDA Modernization Act (FDAMA) (19). Although it focused on regulation of drugs, the FDAMA included provisions for food and supplement health claims to be based on authoritative statements from certain scientific bodies. This process involved a notification to the FDA of intent to use an authoritative statement from a scientific body of the US government or the National Academy of Sciences (NAS) in lieu of an FDA review via the petition process. These consensus statements of recognized scientific bodies were advanced as an alternate to the approach of demonstrating significant scientific agreement (SSA) as implemented to meet the NLEA.

FIRST MAJOR COMPONENT OF NUTRITION LABELING: FACTS PANELS

On product labels, nutrition labeling includes two parts: (a) the Nutrition Facts Panel or the Supplement Facts Panel that includes information on nutrients per se and (b) nutrition claims.

The NLEA included several important provisions that initiated a critical and comprehensive effort to develop a system of nutrition labeling useful to the consumer. For example, the NLEA specifically stipulates that the nutrition information on the food label shall "be conveyed to the public in a manner which enables the public to readily observe and comprehend such information and to understand its relative significance within the context of the total daily diet" (2). The FDA concluded this requirement could be met through consideration of graphic design as well as the continued use of a reference intake value (20–22). The concept of reference intake values was originally developed as RDAs as the average daily nutrient intake level sufficient to meet the nutrient requirement of nearly all healthy individuals in a particular life stage and gender group (23). The FDA had used this concept in 1973 to develop a set of US RDAs that assisted consumers in interpreting voluntary nutrient declarations made on food labels. Research during the development of the NLEA label suggested that the best approach for assisting consumers was to list the quantitative amount of the reference intake value (as a percentage) present in a serving of the food; that is, the Facts Panel was to express nutrition information per serving of the food and as the percentage of the reference intake in that specified serving (Fig. 116.1). The original set of nutrient reference values (US RDAs) was modified and expanded during the implementation of the NLEA, and these values are now referred to as DVs. (24).

DVs are based on a standard serving size and thus provide consumers a way to determine readily whether a nutrient listing reflects a large or small amount of a "desirable" intake. In other words, a food that provides 20% or more of the DV in a single serving contains a "high" quantity of a nutrient, whereas a food with 2 to 5% of the DV is a low source. However, the benefit perceived by the consumer for a food high or low in a particular nutrient will vary depending on the nutrient; that is, foods high in saturated fat or sodium may be considered as undesirable, and in this case low-source foods should be sought, whereas the opposite may be true for nutrients such as calcium or fiber. Selecting foods with high or low levels of the nutrients of interest allows consumers to select their diets to meet public health goals. In this context, it is important to recognize that the DVs were established only as points of reference for nutrition labeling and should not be used to determine adequacy of the diet for individuals.

Currently, DVs for vitamins and minerals are generally based on the highest value for the age or gender groups

Nutrition Facts

Serving Size ¹/₁₂ package
(44g, about 1/4 cup dry mix)
Servings Per Container 12

Amount Per Serving	Mix	Baked
Calories	190	280
Calories from Fat	45	140

	% Daily Value**	
Total Fat 5g*	**8**%	**24**%
Saturated Fat 2g	**10**%	**13**%
Cholesterol 0mg	**0**%	**23**%
Sodium 300mg	**13**%	**13**%
Total Carbohydrate 34g	**11**%	**11**%
Dietary Fiber 0g	**0**%	**0**%
Sugars 18g		
Protein 2g		

Vitamin A	0%	0%
Vitamin C	0%	0%
Calcium	6%	8%
Iron	2%	4%

* Amount in Mix

** Percent Daily Values are based on a 2,000 calorie diet. Your daily values may be higher or lower depending on your calorie needs:

		Calories:	2,000	2,500
Total Fat	Less than		65g	80g
Sat Fat	Less than		20g	25g
Cholesterol	Less than		300mg	300mg
Sodium	Less than		2,400mg	2,400mg
Total Carbohydrate			300g	375g
Dietary Fiber			25g	30g

Calories per gram:
Fat 9 • Carbohydrate 4 • Protein 4

Figure 116.1. Nutrition Facts Panel.

listed among the RDAs provided for that nutrient (24). For those nutrients or substances to be listed on the label as required by the NLEA but for which there was there was no existing RDA, the FDA used the notice-and-comment rulemaking process to derive quantitative levels for a DV based on available consensus documents from the federal government and recognized scientific bodies (20–22).

When the development of a DV required a reference to caloric intake, a reference intake value of 2000 calories was used. The value was calculated on the basis of an average of the NAS recommended calorie (energy) allowance from the 1989 RDA table (25). The caloric reference

intake affects the manner in which nutrients are listed. For example, the consensus recommendation for saturated fat intake specified as 10% of calories. Thus, the DV of 20 g for saturated fat is based on a 2000-calorie diet.

The enactment of the Dietary Supplement Act in 1992 delayed the use of any new RDAs in the final regulations on nutrition labeling, even though the nutrition labeling provisions at that time were and still are based on data from the 1970s. Since that time, the NAS has published newer recommended intake values known collectively as dietary reference intakes (DRIs) (26). A recent study of the NAS provided recommendations on use of the DRIs to develop updated DVs (24). The study report suggested the use of the newer values as well as a population-adjusted average of the values, rather than the selection of the highest value. Moreover, the NAS expert panel recommended that the estimated average requirement (defined in detail in Appendix Section A-2-b-1 and discussed in Chapter 104) be used as the basis for the DVs in nutrition labeling. This approach was selected because a labeling reference value must, by nature, be population based and is not appropriately an expression of requirements for individuals. These recommendations should be included in any FDA notice-and-comment rulemaking concerning options for updating DVs.

Finally, appropriate nutrition labeling requires identification of serving sizes. The NLEA specified that serving sizes for foods were to be determined by the FDA and that they should specifically reflect the amount of food "customarily consumed and which is expressed in a common household measure that is appropriate to the food." Therefore, serving sizes were based on typical consumption among US consumers and were not recommendations for intake. The only possibility to meet this statutory directive at that time was to use the then-existing food consumption data from the late 1970s. These consumption data were used to establish the 139 serving sizes currently in use.

The specified serving sizes are important because they provide the basis on which the manufacturer determines the amount of nutrients listed within the Facts Panels, and therefore they affect all the quantitative declarations on the label. The larger or smaller the serving size is determines the greater or lesser quantity of the percentage of DV declaration. Moreover, serving sizes affect the manufacturer's ability to make nutritional claims about their products. This is because the criteria for claims are tied to the amount of the nutrient present per serving of food. The development of serving sizes was an extremely complicated task, but it proved to be a critical and useful component of nutrition labeling.

More comprehensive consumption data have been collected recently that reflect contemporary patterns of food consumption. There is an urgent need to use these data to update and revise the scientific basis for determination of serving sizes. Revision of serving sizes and subsequent modification of nutrition labeling would assist in consumer understanding of the importance of nutrient intakes in maintaining health, avoiding obesity, and further reduce risks of diseases.

Nutrition Facts Panel

An example of a Nutrition Facts Panel (Nutrition Panel) is shown in Figure 116.1. The entire label on any product has only a limited area for information. Therefore, the Nutrition Panel focuses on the "critical" nutrition information and so, in turn, includes those nutrients and food components considered of highest public health significance for the general population as well as nutrient content of the food per serving using a standardized format.

Nutrients Required to be Declared

When passed in November of 1990, the NLEA specified that consideration should be given to providing mandatory declarations for the following: total calories; calories from total fat; amount of total fat, saturated fat, cholesterol, sodium, total carbohydrates, complex carbohydrates, sugars, dietary fiber, total protein, and any vitamin, mineral, or other nutrients that would assist consumers in maintaining healthy dietary practices. These provisions of the NLEA were based on knowledge of and consensus on critical links between existing science and public health policy. However, in some cases, implementation of the congressional mandates was made difficult by the incomplete nature of available scientific knowledge and interpretations of available data. For example, the order in which the nutrients and food components would appear within the Nutrition Panel was a subject of extensive discussion. Because essentially all available dietary guidelines and consensus documents included recommendations to balance energy intake, maintain desirable body, avoid obesity, or reduce the prevalence of obesity, the FDA decided to highlight the most significant recommendations from these documents and guidelines to the general public by placing those food components at the top of the Nutrition Panel (22). Moreover, these reports suggest links between excessive body weight and the risk of certain chronic diseases, and obesity may exacerbate other disease conditions. Thus, the importance of calories to public health was marked by its being placed first at the very top of the panel.

As with calories, virtually all the consensus documents available at that time recommended that US residents reduce intakes of total fat as well as intakes of saturated fatty acids and cholesterol. In the early 1990s, a major public health focus was the use of diets containing no more than 30% of total calories from fat. Certain comments to the 1991 proposal focused on whether saturated fat should be defined as including all fatty acids containing no double bonds. Although some comments suggested that the amounts labeled should reflect only those

with "serum cholesterol–raising" effects, the FDA rejected the suggestion of including only those known to raise cholesterol and cited both available consensus reports and the legislation in making it mandatory. More recently, regulations were added in 2003 requiring the mandatory declaration of *trans* fat in this portion of the Nutrition Panel (27).

The same process of relying on scientific consensus documents in the notice-and-comment process was employed in identifying the scientific bases for inclusion of sodium, total carbohydrates, complex carbohydrates, sugars, dietary fibers, total protein, and vitamins and minerals. However, some nutrients presented special cases. For example, the NLEA identified sugars as a mandatory declaration to assist consumers in following dietary guidelines that recommended avoiding too much sugar. Because there was no consensus on quantitative intake for sugars, a DV could not be developed, and the declarations are listed as quantitative amounts. The scientific bases and documentation for these decisions were published in the preambles to the proposed and final rules (20, 21).

Similarly, label declarations for amounts of protein per serving were proposed because protein is a major component of the diet and is the source of essential amino acids. Thus, protein is declared as a quantitative amount (in grams) in the Nutrition Panel, but it is not required to be declared as a percentage of the DV. Further, label statements must indicate that the food is not a significant source of protein if and when the quality of the protein is below specified threshold levels.

Finally, limited space in the Nutrition Panel precluded the mandatory listing of all essential vitamins and minerals. Thus, the current mandatory declarations for vitamins and minerals list only those of which intakes present public health concerns, if they are present in a limited number of foods, or are important to chronic disease risk reduction. On the basis of these criteria, FDA proposed four mandatory declarations as a percentage of the DV for vitamin A, vitamin C, calcium, and iron.

Voluntary Declaration of Nutrient Requirements

The NLEA permitted voluntary nutrition information in addition to the mandatory declarations. Some, but not all, food labels have space to provide information about nutrients other than those deemed mandatory. Congress expected that this voluntary information would not interfere with the consumer's understanding of the required information. However, comments received during the rulemaking process confirmed that unlimited additional information on the nutrition label had the potential of being confusing or misleading. To address this matter, the FDA provided permission for certain voluntary nutrition information to be on the nutrition label. This included (a) vitamins and minerals that had an established RDA; (b) calories from saturated fat, polyunsaturated fat, monounsaturated fat;

(c) soluble and/or insoluble fiber; (d) sugar alcohols; (e) other carbohydrates; and (f) potassium. A format based on a linear array of vitamins and minerals voluntarily declared was provided to minimize label clutter.

Finally, although the nutrition labeling rules adopted to address the provisions of the NLEA attempted to be complete, they resulted in some complications that may be confusing to consumers. For example, to avoid misleading consumers, under certain conditions nutrients that would normally be declared on a voluntary basis are required to be declared; that is, if a voluntary nutrient is added to a food or if a claim is made about the nutrient on the label, the nutrient must be listed within the Nutrition Panel. For example, polyunsaturated fat content must be declared if monounsaturated fat is listed or if a cholesterol claim is made. Conversely, monounsaturated fat must be declared if polyunsaturated fat is listed or if a cholesterol claim is made. Additional information on analogous complex issues can be found in various FDA publications and in guidance documents.

Supplement Facts Panel

The DSHEA defined dietary supplements as a subcategory of foods and included special provisions for labeling of, and declarations on, dietary supplement products (3). The legislation stipulates that dietary supplements containing ingredients that do not have a DV are to be included within the Supplement Panel on such products. This is in contrast to the final regulation for conventional foods, which prohibits listing of substances lacking a DV in the Nutrition Panel. The DSHEA also requires that the information provided for vitamins and minerals, as well as other substances, include the quantity of each or for each within each proprietary blend. The listing of dietary ingredients may also include the source.

The Supplement Panel also differs in that it provides for the listing of ingredients that are not generally found in the classic vitamin-mineral supplement formulation. As shown in Figure 116.2, the Supplement Panel format is similar to that of the Nutrition Panel for conventional foods. In this way, it provides a similar and familiar format to help consumers with understanding the product label contents. Further, when an ingredient has no DV, it is placed in a section separated by a heavy line indicating that no DV has been established. Moreover, to address concerns that requiring declarations of the exact amounts of the ingredients in a blended product violated the manufacturer's free speech right to withhold the specific formulation of their product, the format provides for listing of the total amount of the proprietary blend and its ingredients without listing of quantitative amounts of each ingredient.

The authority to identify serving size provided by the NLEA was carried over to the DSHEA and has an important role of allowing consumers to compare products (see

Fig. 116.2A and B). However, the serving size issues for dietary supplements are quite different from conventional foods, for which serving size is the amount of the food customarily consumed based on national intake data. In the case of dietary supplements, no national intake data were available; thus, the amount customarily consumed is defined as the maximum amount recommended on the label by the manufacturer. Therefore, if a dietary supplement label indicates an intake of 3 teaspoons/day, for example, then the serving size for which the nutrition information is presented must be for 3 teaspoons (see Fig. 116.2C). Manufacturers are also allowed to list additional information that further defines the serving size, but such declarations are voluntary.

The DSHEA also requires that the term "dietary supplement" appear as part of the statement of identity of the product. This requirement is consistent with the requirement that the label of all packaged foods bear a statement of identity for the food. Statements of identity can be defined by the FDA in its regulations or can be the "common or usual name" of the product as determined by the wording or term commonly used in the marketplace. Although not directly relevant to nutrition labeling, the long regulatory history of clearly identifying all foods through statements of identity resulted in the final determination that the words "dietary supplement," or certain variations such as the actual name of the ingredient (e.g., vitamin C), should appear as part of the name on the label of the product. This requirement assists consumers in identifying a product as a dietary supplement, particularly when that may not be otherwise apparent.

Meat and Poultry Labeling

Although the NLEA applied only to FDA-regulated foods, meat and poultry products are regulated by the US Department of Agriculture (USDA). Companion nutrition labeling rules for meat and poultry products were implemented by the USDA at the same time that the FDA implemented the regulations in response to the NLEA (30, 31). The FDA and USDA have continued to coordinate their regulations related to nutrition labeling to maintain consistency even though responsibilities of the two agencies are governed by different laws.

SECOND MAJOR COMPONENT OF NUTRITION LABELING: NUTRITION CLAIMS

The NLEA provided for nutrient content and health label claims about the nutritional properties and benefits of food on a per serving basis. These claims are useful to consumers in selecting healthful foods and as an incentive to manufacturers to improve the nutritional profiles of their foods. Regulations for nutrition claims are applicable

Supplement Facts

Serving Size 1 Tablet

	Amount Per Serving	% Daily Value
Vitamin A (as retinyl acetate and 50% as beta-carotene)	5000 IU	100%
Vitamin C (as ascorbic acid)	60 mg	100%
Vitamin D (as cholecalciferol)	400 IU	100%
Vitamin E (as dl-alpha tocopheryl acetate)	30 IU	100%
Thiamin (as thiamin mononitrate)	1.5 mg	100%
Riboflavin	1.7 mg	100%
Niacin (as niacinamide)	20 mg	100%
Vitamin B$_6$ (as pyridoxine hydrochloride)	2.0 mg	100%
Folate (as folic acid)	400 mcg	100%
Vitamin B$_{12}$ (as cyanocobalamin)	6 mcg	100%
Biotin	30 mcg	10%
Pantothenic Acid (as calcium pantothenate)	10 mg	100%

Other ingredients: Gelatin, lactose, magnesium stearate, microcrystalline cellulose, FD&C Yellow No. 6, propylene glycol, propylparaben, and sodium benzoate.

A

Supplement Facts

Serving Size 1 Capsule

Amount Per Capsule		% Daily Value
Calories 20		
Calories from Fat 20		
Total Fat 2 g		3%*
Saturated Fat 0.5 g		3%*
Polyunsaturated Fat 1 g		†
Monounsaturated Fat 0.5 g		†
Vitamin A 4250 IU		85%
Vitamin D 425 IU		106%
Omega-3 fatty acids 0.5 g		†

* Percent Daily Values are based on a 2,000 calorie diet.
† Daily Value not established.

Ingredients: Cod liver oil, gelatin, water, and glycerin.

B

Supplement Facts

Serving Size 1 tsp (3 g) (makes 8 fl oz prepared)
Servings Per Container 24

	Amount Per Teaspoon	% Daily Value
Calories	10	
Total Carbohydrate	2 g	< 1%*
Sugars	2 g	†
Proprietary blend	0.7 g	
German Chamomile (flower)		†
Hyssop (leaves)		†

* Percent Daily Values are based on a 2,000 calorie diet.
† Daily Value not established.

C Other ingredients: Fructose, lactose, starch, and stearic acid.

Figure 116.2. A. Supplement Facts Panel for a multivitamin/mineral preparation. **B.** Supplement Facts Panel for a product containing ingredients with and without reference daily intake or daily reference values (DV) established. **C.** Dietary Supplement Panel for a proprietary blend of ingredients.

regardless of whether the claims are explicitly or implicitly stated.

Nutrient Content Claims

Nutrient content claims describe a nutrient level in a serving of a food, such as "low" in fat or "high" in calcium. The NLEA required that standard definitions for nutrient content claims (or "descriptors") be developed. Currently, nutrition labeling regulations permit 11 core content claims (i.e., free, low, lean, extra lean, high, good source, reduced, less, light, fewer, and more) as well as certain

synonyms. For example, "free" denotes an insignificant amount of the nutrient in the diet because absolute zero is analytically difficult to determine and to guarantee; similarly, at least 20% of the DV defines the term "high." Further information on these definitions can be found in materials on the FDA Web site and guidance documents (12). The rationale for the criteria and cutoff levels for nutrient content claims is described in the preamble to the proposed and final rules (28, 29).

The use of the defined descriptors for conventional foods was limited to nutrients for which a DV exists based on nutrient intake recommendations suggested by quantitative recommendations in the US dietary guidelines or by the NAS. Thus, a content claim that characterizes the level of conventional food ingredients, such as "high in garlic," is not permitted because no DVs exist for garlic.

Finally, label claims may describe organoleptic properties or suggest an added value as long as they are truthful and not misleading; however, such statements are not generally considered nutrient content claims. Nonetheless, such statements may be considered to be implied nutrient content claims and therefore subject to nutrient content regulations. For example, a claim such as "70% milk" could imply a claim about the level of calcium in the product.

At the time the 1993 nutrient content claim final rules were published, the term, "high potency" for use on dietary supplement labels was not defined. The FDA subsequently indicated that "high potency" could be claimed when a supplement contains 100% or more of the DV. At the same time, the FDA also provided for an antioxidant content claim allowing the use of "high," "good source," and "more" for supplement products containing vitamin C, vitamin E, and β-carotene (32).

Passage of the DHSEA in 1994 resulted in some differences between nutrient content claims for dietary supplements as compared with conventional foods; for example, the DSHEA provided for claims that characterize the percentage level of a dietary ingredient. In addition, the law permitted dietary supplement labels to bear claims for dietary ingredients for which no DV had been established. For instance, "95% glucosamine" is an allowable claim for dietary supplements but not for conventional foods. Quantitative amounts of the substance also must be included in the label claim. Other defined nutrient content claims such as "high" and "more" remain the same for both conventional foods and dietary supplements and are limited to those dietary ingredients that have DVs.

Health Claims

Despite accumulating scientific evidence that nutrients and related substances in food may increase or reduce the risk of certain chronic diseases, until passage of the NLEA in 1990, such claims were legally considered drug claims and were not allowed on foods. The NLEA amendments to the FD&C Act allow certain nutrition labeling claims, termed health claims, on food labels. The NLEA stated that health claims were to help consumers maintain healthy dietary practices and to protect them from unfounded health claims.

Health claims are limited to statements that explicitly or implicitly describe the role of dietary substances in reducing the risk of diseases. They cannot claim usefulness in the cure, treatment, mitigation, or prevention of a disease. Health claims differ from other types of food label claims and statements in that they require the presence of two components: a substance and a disease. Label statements that have only one of these components are not

health claims. Currently, nutrition labeling includes three types of health claims: (a) those authorized by provisions of the NLEA, (b) those meeting provisions of the FDAMA, and (c) those that are "qualified."

Health Claims Meeting the Significant Scientific Agreement Standard

The NLEA established that significant scientific agreement among experts qualified by training and experience to evaluate such relationships (SSA) is the basis for determining whether a health claim could be authorized. The SSA standard was based on the totality of available scientific evidence. SSA was seen as a high standard that would ensure consumer confidence because such claims, if well established, would be unlikely to be changed by new and evolving scientific evidence (13).

The SSA standard in the NLEA for conventional foods was not specified for dietary supplements. The NLEA left the decision as to a scientific substantiation standard for supplements to the discretion of the FDA. However, the agency found no scientific basis for different standard with dietary supplements and, in keeping with the concept of consistency, has applied the SSA standard to dietary supplements as well as to conventional foods since 1993. The Commission on Dietary Supplement labels reaffirmed this decision in 1997 (33).

The NLEA provided a petition process for the evaluation of additional substance-disease relationships. Since completion of NLEA-specified health claim evaluations in 1993, the FDA has authorized several petitioned claims meeting the SSA standard. As of late 2004, 12 health claims that meet the SSA substantiation have been authorized by the FDA (Table 116.1). The number of SSA-

---

TABLE 116.1. HEALTH CLAIMS BASED ON SIGNIFICANT SCIENTIFIC AGREEMENT (AS OF NOVEMBER 2004)[a]

Calcium and osteoporosis
Dietary lipids (fat) and cancer
Dietary saturated fat and cholesterol and risk of coronary heart disease
Dietary noncarcinogenic carbohydrate sweeteners and dental caries
Fiber-containing grain products, fruits, and vegetables and cancer
Folic acid and neural tube defects
Fruits and vegetables and cancer
Fruits, vegetables, and grain products that contain fiber, particularly soluble fiber, and risk of coronary heart disease
Sodium and hypertension
Soluble fiber from certain foods and risk of coronary heart disease
Soy protein and risk of coronary heart disease
Stanols/sterols and risks of coronary heart disease

[a] Information on specific health claims is contained in the Code of Federal Regulations 21 CFR 101.70 et seq. and at http://www.cfsan.fda .gov/~dmshclaims.html.

TABLE 116.2. NUTRIENT CONTENT AND HEALTH CLAIMS BASED ON AUTHORITATIVE STATEMENTS (AS OF NOVEMBER 2004)[a]

Nutrient content claims for choline-containing foods
Potassium and risk of high blood pressure and stroke
Whole-grain foods and risk of heart disease and certain cancers

[a] Information on specific health claims is contained in the Code of Federal Regulations 21 CFR 101.70 et seq. and at http://www.cfsan.fda .gov/~dmshclaims.html.

authorized claims may reflect the time, resources, and effort required to collate available pertinent data and to establish that the scientific evidence supporting a relationship between a substance and a disease is conclusive (34).

Concerned that the number of health claims authorized by the SSA substantiation process developed to implement the NLEA was limited, Congress included provisions in the FDAMA that provide an alternative approach for establishing SSA. Although validation of additional health claims was anticipated, only two claims were identified via this mechanism (Table 116.2). It is probable that the claims previously authorized under SSA criteria already reflected the diet and disease recommendations of authoritative bodies.

Qualified Health Claims

In 1993, when the final NLEA health claim decisions were made, supplement manufacturers were concerned that application of the SSA standard resulted in the denial of most supplement-related health claims. As a result, a series of legal challenges were initiated. These focused on whether the FDA could impose commercial speech bans to prevent truthful information on food product labels about a specified substance-disease relationship for which the available scientific evidence was insufficient to meet the SSA standard. This brought the issue of First Amendment rights of commercial free speech in direct conflict with NLEA requirements to prohibit health claims that did not meet the SSA standard.

Because of the impact of any court decisions on these First Amendment issues and their affect on the scope of nutrition claims, the FDA sought the advice of the NAS, using as case studies nutrient-disease relationships that had been evaluated at different points in time, to determine whether there were patterns of preliminary evidence that could reliably predict the future validity of a diet-health relationship (34). The NAS found no patterns of evidence that would predict clearly any change in the confidence of such relationships. Further, the report noted that confidence in nutrient-disease relationships may often change in unexpected directions.

Because federal courts historically have shown a preference for open disclosure over suppression of information in decisions related to First Amendment issues, courts hearing cases related to issue of free commercial speech have ruled that the FDA should consider the use of "disclaimer statements" on food labels for health claims that do not meet the SSA standard. The court rulings hold that disclaimer statements provide clarification for consumers as to the specific state of the science supporting the proposed claim. In other words, when the scientific evidence for health claims does not meet the SSA standard, the label statements for these claims were to be "qualified" by corrective disclaimers so as not to mislead consumers. For example, a qualifying disclaimer could state: "the evidence supporting the claim is not conclusive."

Consumer research to determine whether consumers can accurately discriminate among various levels of evidence for qualified claims and whether they can differentiate between qualified and SSA claims is expected to provide useful information for fully implementing a qualified health claims policy (35).

Based on the recommendations in the Institute of Medicine report and the decisions of the court, the FDA developed a grading system of evidence-based criteria by which the nature of the uncertainties in the evidence for qualified claims can be described. In 2003, the FDA issued this guidance, which is intended for use with qualified health claims when the levels of scientific evidence are less than those meeting the SSA standard http://www. cfsan.fda.gov/~dms/lab-qhc.html).

Using this guidance, the FDA currently handles petitions for qualified health claims on a case-by-case basis by means of a mechanism known as "enforcement discretion." Qualified health claims for which letters of enforcement discretion have been sent are noted in Table 116.3. Because these letters are not published in the *Federal Register,* interested persons are advised to check the

TABLE 116.3. QUALIFIED HEALTH CLAIMS (AS OF NOVEMBER 2004)[a]

Cancer risk
  Selenium and certain cancers
  Antioxidant vitamins and risk of certain cancers[b]
Cardiovascular disease
  Monounsaturated fatty acids from olive oil
  ω-3 fatty acids and coronary heart disease
  Walnuts and coronary heart disease
  Nuts and coronary heart disease
  B vitamins and vascular disease
  Folic acid, vitamin B_6, and vitamin B_{12} and vascular disease[c]
Cognitive function
  Phosphatidylserine and cognitive dysfunction and dementia
Neural tube defects
  Folic acid

[a] Information on specific health claims is contained in the Code of Federal Regulations 21 CFR 101.70 et seq. and at http://www.cfsan.fda .gov/~dmshclaims.html.
[b] Dietary supplements only.
[c] Qualified as follows: "0.8 mg folic acid in a dietary supplement is more effective in reducing the risk of neural tube defects than a lower amount in foods in common forms."

Center for Food Safety and Applied Nutrition Web site for not only decisions on qualified health claims, but also additions or changes to all authorized health claims.

OTHER LABELING STATEMENTS

Structure Function Claims

Historically, structure and function claims have been available for use on foods, dietary supplements, and drugs (16). Many persons often consider structure and function claims as "health claims," but they are not regulated as health claims in the context of nutrition labeling. These types of claims describe the effect of a substance on the structure or function of the body. In the case of conventional foods, these claims do not require FDA review or authorization, but the claim must be derived from the so-called nutritive value of the product. For dietary supplements, use of structure and function claims requires that manufacturers notify FDA of their intent to use the claim, but it does not require FDA review or authorization. Additionally, for dietary supplements, structure and function claims must be accompanied by a disclaimer that states that FDA has not reviewed or approved these claims. The DSHEA allowed dietary supplement structure and function claims to be based on nonnutritive as well as nutritive components of these products. Additional information on structure and function claims for foods and dietary supplements can be found in the Code of Federal Regulations, Chapter 21, Section 101.

Product Quality and Warning Statements

Product quality and warning statements may be required or voluntarily used on certain foods and dietary supplement, but they are not nutrition labeling. Some dietary supplement ingredients may be included in official compendia such as the US Pharmacopeia or the National Formulary. These compendia provide standards for quality, strength, purity, identity, chemical names, and packaging of the substance that may be recognized by the FDA. In these cases, manufacturers may voluntarily include label statements that indicate their product is in compliance with these standards. These "product quality statements" generally take the form of displaying the designation or logo of the sponsoring agency on the label (e.g., United States Pharmacopeia).

In addition, warning statements are a component of labeling regulations that address the "material facts" about the use of the product. The FDA may require mandatory label warnings for products that the agency has determined need additional information to allow consumers to more safely use the product. Such labeling is relatively commonplace on drugs, but for foods and dietary supplement labels, it has been unusual because such products are generally regarded as safe. Moreover, the existing warning statements have come into existence on a case-by-case basis. A commonly recognized warning statement is the label wording that persons with phenylketonuria should not consume foods or supplements that contain the amino acid phenylalanine.

INTERNATIONAL NUTRITION LABELING

The use of nutrition labeling in other countries is a relatively recent trend, and in some ways its development has mirrored the experience in the United States. However, differences in cultural perspectives on diet and health and differences in consumer's information needs have resulted in numerous approaches to nutrition labeling of foods. The labeling of dietary supplements has taken an even more diverse path, primarily because dietary supplements are regulated quite differently in that some countries and regions define supplements as a separate category from both foods and drugs, whereas others regard them as drugs.

Examples of recent regulatory programs that address nutrition labeling can be found in a number of countries and regions including Canada, Australia, and the European Union. Some programs are mandatory for all packaged foods, whereas others, such as the provisions within the European Union, are required under only certain conditions, such as when a nutrition claim is made about the food.

The United States as a nation led the way in conceptualizing and requiring a nutrition label on packaged foods, and its efforts most likely have served as a starting point for others. Although the US nutrition label may have been taken into account during the development of nutrition labels in other counties, each country has modified or added components germane to its interpretation of the science about diet and health, regulatory structure, or interface with stakeholders and consumers. These differences range from providing for only voluntary declarations for cholesterol within the European Union label, in contrast to the required declaration for the US label, to the use of 100-g portions as the basis for the label declarations within the European Union, in contrast to identified serving sizes in household measures within the United States (29).

The Codex Alimentarius is an international food standards program under the auspices of the Food and Agricultural Organization and the World Health Organization. Its goal is to facilitate international food trade and to guide the food industry while also protecting the consumer. The Codex Alimentarius has addressed nutrition labeling from the perspective of an international standard-setting body with the mission to both protect the consumer and facilitate trade (36). Early nutrition labeling efforts within Codex focused on guidelines for declarations related to concerns about nutrient deficiencies such as iron and certain vitamins. With the growing recognition of the importance of diet in the prevention of chronic disease, the Codex interest in expanding its guidelines to encompass a broader range of nutrients has become evident.

However, such internationally oriented efforts move slowly because of the need to attempt harmonization across a diverse set of interests. Further, because of the concern for international harmonization, Codex guidelines, by their nature, tend to be more generalized and less specific than are those derived from national public health legislation or regulations (36). The current Codex nutrition label guidelines advise that the nutrition label be required when a nutrition claim or representation is made on the label, at which point the declaration of a standard list of nutrients should be made. The premise is that the nutrition label requires the manufacturer to back up a claim by providing more information on the nutrient value of the product. The identified declarations are for energy, protein, available carbohydrate, and fat, as well as various provisions for additional declarations if claims are made about substances such as fatty acids. In the case of vitamins and minerals, 16 nutrient reference values have been specified for labeling purposes. Declarations for all nutrients are to be made both per 100-g portion and per serving.

FUTURE OF NUTRITION LABELING

Nutrition labeling is a work in progress and will continue to be influenced by the complex interactions of science, legislation, regulation, public policy, judicial decisions, and international trade policies. Its evolution also reflects ever-changing cultural aspects, consumer interests, and industry initiatives. Regardless of its level of development and use, nutrition labeling is a tool to assist citizens in selecting a nutritious diet and to motivate the food industry to improve the composition of marketed foods that will meet the health and nutritional needs of consumers. The extent to which nutrition labeling successfully meets these objectives is unknown. Achieving the full public health potential of nutrition labeling will require additional scientific research and possible modifications of laws, regulations, and public policies. Among the most critical needs are an improved understanding of consumer use of nutrition labeling for maintaining health, enhanced scientific knowledge of nutrient requirements and the relationship of dietary intakes to health outcomes, and a full understanding of the obstacles that impede industry improvements in food manufacturing and labeling that will best promote the healthfulness of marketed foods.

Several revisions to the current regulatory framework for nutrition labeling are of obvious high priority. For example, the current DVs and nutrients for which DVs are provided are derived primarily from RDAs that were established more than 30 years ago. The availability of the recently updated DRIs may provide a basis for updating the DVs used for nutrition labeling. The current amounts for reference serving sizes are also based on food consumption data that were collected several decades ago and need to reflect currently used serving sizes and types of food products. Consumer studies providing insights into consumer understanding of qualified health claims and other label information are needed to help inform the development of regulations. Potential modifications and expansions of substantiation criteria for nutrition claims and structure function claims will continue to be discussed by both US and international regulatory bodies. Additional rulemaking will likely be needed to sort out how best to resolve the competing requirements of commercial free speech versus prohibition of claims that do not meet SSA health claim standards.

Although scientific research can address the foregoing issues associated with meaningful nutrition information, public policy developed from science through legislation and regulation will influence whether existing nutrition labeling or any changes are contributing to health optimization and reduction of disease risks. If additional time, effort, and resources were available, public policy concerning nutrition labeling of foods and dietary supplements and the ability of the regulatory process to reflect new and important scientific findings in a timely manner would enhance the usefulness of nutrition labeling in this country and throughout the world.

REFERENCES

1. Federal Food, Drug, and Cosmetic Act. PL 75-717. 52 Stat.1040 (1938), as amended. 21 USC 201 et seq.
2. Nutrition Labeling and Education Act of 1990. PL101-535. November 8, 1990. 104 Stat. 2353, 21 USC.
3. Dietary Supplement Health and Education Act of 1994. PL103-417. October 25, 1994. Stat/4325-4335; 103rd Congress; 2nd sess.
4. US Department of Health and Human Services. The Surgeon General's Report on Nutrition and Health. Washington, DC: US Government Printing Office, 1988.
5. National Research Council, National Academy of Sciences. Diet and Health: Implications for Reducing Chronic Disease Risk. Report of the Committee on Diet and Health, Food and Nutrition Board. Washington, DC: National Academy Press, 1989.
6. Hutt PB. Annu Rev Nutr 1984;4:1–20.
7. Shapiro R, ed. Nutrition Labeling Handbook. New York: Marcel Dekker, 1995.
8. Pape SM, Kracov DA, Rubin PD. Dietary Supplements and Functional Foods: A Practical Guide to FDA Regulation. Tampa, FL: Thompson Publishing Group, 2001.
9. Forbes AL. National nutrition policy, food labeling, and health claims. In: Shils ME, Olson JA, Shike M, eds. Modern Nutrition in Health and Disease. 8th ed. Philadelphia: Lea & Febiger, 1994.
10. Forbes AL, McNamara SH. Food labeling, health claims, and dietary supplement legislation. In: Shils ME, Olson JA, Shike M et al., eds. Modern Nutrition in Health and Disease. 9th ed. Baltimore: Williams & Wilkins, 1999.
11. Labeling of Dietary Supplements. April 18, 2003, http://www.cfsan.fda.gov/~dms/ds-labl.html.
12. Nutrient Content Claims. September 7, 2004, http://www.cfsan.fda.gov/~dms/lab-nutr.html.
13. Health Claims that Meet Significant Scientific Aagreement (SSA). June 9, 2004, http://www.cfsan.fda.gov/~dms/lab-ssa.html.
14. FDA Moderization Act of 1997 (FDAMA) claims. June 9, 2004, http://www.cfsan.fda.gov/~dms/labfdama.html.

15. Qualified Health Claims. November 8, 2004. Available at: http://www.cfsan.fda.gov/~dms/lab-qhc.html.

16. Structure/Function Claims. June 9, 2004. Available at: http://www.cfsan.fda.gov/~dms/labstruc.html.

17. White House Conference on Food, Nutrition, and Health: Final Report. Washington, DC: US Government Printing Office, 1970.

18. Dietary Supplement Act of 1992 (Title II of the Prescription Drug User Fee Act of 1992). PL 102-571. October 29, 1992. 106 Stat.4499. 21 USC.

19. Food and Drug Administration Modernization Act of 1997. PL 105-115. Sections 303-304. 111 Stat. 2296. 21 USC.

20. Fed Reg 1990;55:29476–86.

21. Fed Reg 1991;56:60366–94.

22. Fed Reg 1993;58:2079–205.

23. Food and Nutrition Board, Commission on the Life Sciences, National Research Council. Recommended Dietary Allowances, 10th ed. Washington, DC: National Academy Press, 1968.

24. Food and Nutrition Board, Institute of Medicine. Dietary Reference Intakes: Guiding Principles for Nutrition Labeling and Fortification. Washington, DC: National Academy Press, 2003.

25. Food and Nutrition Board, Institute of Medicine. Nutrition Labeling: Issues and Directions for the 1990s. Washington, DC: National Academy Press, 1990.

26. Food and Nutrition Board, Institute of Medicine. Dietary Reference Intakes for Energy, Carbohydrate, Fiber, Fat, Fatty Acids, Cholesterol Protein, and Amino Acids (Macronutrients). Washington, DC: National Academy Press, 2002.

27. Fed Reg 2003;58:41433–506.

28. Fed Reg 1991;56:60421–77.

29. Fed Reg 1993;58:2302–426.

30. Fed Reg 1991;56:13564–74.

31. Fed Reg 1993;58:47624–8.

32. Fed Reg 1997;62:49868–81.

33. Report of the Commission on Dietary Supplements Labels to the President, Congress, and the Secretary of Health and Human Services. Washington, DC: US Government Printing Office, 1997.

34. Food and Nutrition Board, Institute of Medicine. Evolution of Evidence for Selected Nutrient and Disease Relationships. Washington, DC: National Academy Press, 2002.

35. FDA Task Force Report. Consumer Health Information for Better Nutrition Initiative. July 10, 2003. Available at: http://www.cfsan.fda.gov/~dms/nuttftoc.html.

36. Food and Agriculture Organization, World Health Organization. Codex Alimentarius Food Labelling Complete Texts. Rome: Food and Agriculture Organization, World Health Organization, 2001.

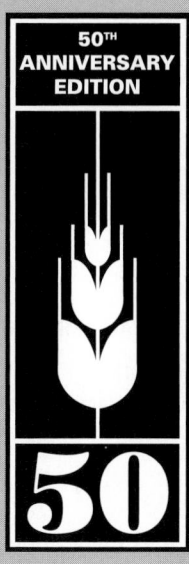

50TH
ANNIVERSARY
EDITION

PART VIII

APPENDICES

EDITORS:
ABBY S BLOCH
MAURICE E SHILS

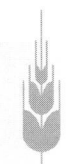

TABLE OF CONTENTS OF THE APPENDICES 10TH EDITION, MODERN NUTRITION IN HEALTH AND DISEASE

SECTION I. CONVERSION FACTORS, WEIGHTS AND MEASURES, AND METABOLIC WATER FORMATION / 1846

A-1 A-1-a. Conversion Factors between Traditional and SI Units / 1846
  A-1-b. Factors and Formulas Used in Interconverting Units of Vitamin A and Carotenoids / 1847
  A-1-c. Table of Atomic Weights: / 1848
    A-1-c-1. Alphabetic Order / 1848
    A-1-c-2. Order of Atomic Number / 1849
  A-1-d. Weights and Measures / 1850
  A-1-e. Water Formed in the Metabolism of Tissue and Caloric Sources / 1851

SECTION II. NATIONAL AND INTERNATIONAL RECOMMENDED DIETARY REFERENCE VALUES /1852

  Introduction to Section: Appendices Editors / 1852
A-2 United States and Canada: Dietary Reference Intakes (DRIs) 1997–2004 / 1852
  A-2-a. Introductory Comments: Appendices Editors / 1852
  A-2-b. Verbatim Excerpts from the Dietary Reference Intakes Texts / 1853
    A-2-b-1. Dietary Reference Intakes: Categories and Definitions / 1853
      A-2-b-1-a. Dietary Reference Intake Definitions / 1853
      A-2-b-1-b. Dietary Reference Intake Relations / 1853
    A-2-b-2. Comparison of Recommended Dietary Allowances and Adequate Intakes / 1854
    A-2-b-3. Tolerable Upper Level (UL) / 1855
    A-2-b-4. Using Dietary Reference Intakes to Assess Nutrient Intakes for Healthy Individuals and Groups / 1855
      A-2-b-4-a. Uses of Dietary Reference Intakes, Assessment and Planning Table / 1856
    A-2-b-5. Acceptable Macronutrient Distribution Ranges for Healthy Diets / 1856
    A-2-b-6. Cholesterol Summary / 1857
    A-2-b-7. Water, Potassium, Sodium, Chloride, and Sulfate / 1857
  A-2-c. Reference Height and Weights for Children and Adults in the United States / 1857
    A-2-c-1. Reference Heights and Weights (From NHANES III) / 1858
    A-2-c-2. New Reference Heights and Weights (IOM, 2002) / 1858
  A-2-d. Criteria and Dietary Reference Intakes by Life-Stage Group / 1859
      A-2-d-1-a. For Energy by Active Individuals / 1859
      A-2-d-1-b. Estimated Energy Requirements (EER) by Men and Women 30 Years of Age / 1860
    A-2-d-2. For Carbohydrate / 1861
    A-2-d-3. For Total Fiber / 1862
    A-2-d-4. For Total Fat / 1863
    A-2-d-5. For n-6 Polyunsaturated Fatty Acids (Linoleic Acid) / 1863
    A-2-d-6. For n-3 Polyunsaturated Fatty Acids (alpha-linolenic Acid) / 1864
    A-2-d-7. For Proteins / 1864
    A-2-d-8. For Total Water (Water, Food & Beverages) / 1865
    A-2-d-9. For Potassium / 1866
    A-2-d-10. For Sodium / 1867
    A-2-d-11. For Chloride / 1867
  A-2-e. Recommended Intakes for Individuals, Vitamins / 1868
  A-2-f. Tolerable Upper Limits (UL), Vitamins / 1869
  A-2-g. Recommended Intake for Individuals, Elements / 1870
  A-2-h. Tolerable Upper Limits (UL), Elements / 1871
A-3. United States, 1989 and Canada 1989-1990 / 1872
  Introductory Comments: Appendices Editors / 1872
  A-3-a. United States / 1872
    A-3-a-1. Recommended Dietary Allowances, United States Revised, 1989 / 1872
    A-3-a-2. Estimated Safe and Adequate Daily Dietary Intakes of Selected Vitamins and Minerals / 1873

A-3-b. Canada / 1873
 A-3-b-1. Summary of Examples of Recommended Nutrient Intake Based on Age and Body Weight Expressed as Daily Rates, Canada / 1873
 A-3-b-2. Summary of Examples of Recommended Nutrients Based on Energy Expressed as Daily Rates, Canada / 1874

A-4   United Kingdom: 1991 / 1874
  Dietary Reference Values / 1874
  A-4-a. Excepts from the Report / 1874
  A-4-b. Estimated Average Requirement for Energy / 1877
  A-4-c. Reference Nutrient Intakes for Protein / 1877
  A-4-d. Reference Nutrient Intakes for Vitamins / 1877
  A-4-e. Reference Nutrient Intakes for Minerals / 1878
  A-4-e-1. SI Units / 1878
  A-4-e-2. Traditional Units / 1879
  A-4-f. Safe Intakes / 1880
  A-4-g. Safe Upper Levels and Guidance Levels: Vitamins and Minerals—2003 / 1880

A-5   Japan: 1996 / 1881
  A-5-a. Dietary Allowances for Growth Period and Moderate Level of Physical Activity / 1881
  A-5-b. Dietary Allowances for Light Level of Physical Activity / 1882
  A-5-c. Dietary Allowances for Light Heavy Level of Physical Activity / 1883
  A-5-d. Dietary Allowances for Heavy Level of Physical Activity / 1883

A-6   Nutrient Reference Values for Australia and New Zealand including Recommended Dietary Intakes—2005 (Draft copy) / 1884
  A-6-a. Macronutrients Including Water / 1884
  A-6-b. B Vitamins / 1884
  A-6-c. Vitamins A, C, D, E, and K and Choline / 1885
  A-6-d. Minerals (EARs and RDIs) / 1885
  A-6-e. Minerals (EARs and RDIs Continued) / 1885
  A-6-f. Minerals (Adequate Intake) / 1886

A-7.   European Community Nutrient and Energy Intakes / 1886
  A-7-a   Recommendations and Nomenclature / 1886
  A-7-a-1. Multiple Values Proposed for Adults / 1887
  A-7-a-2. Nutrients with Acceptable Ranges of Intake / 1887
  A-7-a-3. Population Reference Intakes—Nutrients / 1888
  A-7-b. Tolerable Upper Intake Levels—2000 website / 1889
  A-7-c. Netherlands Health Council, Dietary Reference Values—2000 Reference / 1889
  A-7-d. German, Austrian, and Swiss Societies of Nutrition, Recommended Values for Nutritional Intakes—2000 Reference / 1889

A-8   International Dietary Recommendations / 1889
  A-8-a. World Health Organization Diet, Nutrition and the Prevention of Chronic Diseases—2003 (WHO/FAO) / 1889
  A-8-a-1. Intervening Throughout Life / 1889
  A-8-a-2. Ranges of Population Nutrient Intake Goals / 1889
  A-8-a-3. Summary of Strength of Evidence on Factors that Might Promote or Protect Against Weight Gain and Obesity / 1890
  A-8-a-4. Classification of Overweight in Adults According to BMI / 1890
  A-8-b. World Health Organization (WHO) / 1891
  A-8-b-1. Values for the Digestibility of Protein in Man / 1891
  A-8-b-2. Daily Average Energy Requirements and Safe Level of Protein Intake: / 1891
   A-8-b-2-a. Infants and Children Aged 3 Months to 10 Years / 1891
   A-8-b-2-b. Adolescents Ages 10 to 18 Years / 1891
   A-8-b-2-c. Adults / 1892
  A-8-b-3. Recommended Dietary Allowances of Vitamins and Minerals / 1892
  A-8-c. FAO/WHO Human Vitamin and Mineral Requirements—2001 / 1893

A-9   National Dietary Guidelines and Recommendations (United States) / 1893
  A-9-a. Dietary Guidelines for Americans, 2005 (Executive Summary) / 1893
  A-9-b. Management of High Blood Cholesterol and Related Risk Factors (NCEP) / 1896
  A-9-b-1. Cholesterol Levels and Coronary Heart Disease Risk / 1896
   A-9-b-1-a. ATP III Classification of LDL, Total, and HDL Cholesterol (mg/dL) / 1896
   A-9-b-1-b. Major Risk Factors (Exclusive of LDL Cholesterol) that Modify LDL Goals / 1896
  A-9-b-2. Role of Other Risk Factors in Risk Assessment / 1896
   A-9-b-2-a. Metabolic Syndrome / 1897
  A-9-b-3. Primary Prevention with LDL-Lowering Therapy / 1897
  A-9-b-4. Secondary Prevention with LDL-Lowering Therapy / 1897
  A-9-b-5. LDL-Lowering Therapy in Three Risk Categories / 1897

A-9-b-5-a. LDL Cholesterol Goals and Cutpoints for Therapeutic Lifestyle Changes (TLC) and Drug Therapy in Different Risk Categories / 1897

A-9-b-6. Therapeutic Lifestyle Changes in LDL-Lowering Therapy / 1897

A-9-b-6-a. Nutrient Composition of the TLC Diet / 1898

A-9-b-6-b. A Model of Steps in Therapeutic Lifestyle Changes (TLC) / 1898

A-9-b-7. Benefit Beyond LDL Lowering: The Metabolic Syndrome as a Secondary Target of Therapy / 1898

A-9-b-7-a. Clinical Identification of the Metabolic Syndrome / 1898

A-9-b-7-b. Management of Underlying Causes of the Metabolic Syndrome / 1899

A-9-b-8. Specific Treatment of Lipid and Nonlipid Risk Factors / 1899

A-9-b-8-a. ATP III Classification of Serum Triglycerides / 1899

A-9-b-9. Addendum—NCEP Report of 2004; Appendices Editors Comments / 1900

A-9-b-9-a. ATP III LDL-C Goals and Cutpoints for TLC and Drug Therapy in Different Risk Categories and Proposed Modifications Based on Recent Clinical Trial Evidence / 1900

A-9-b-9-b. Recommendations for Modifications to Footnote the ATP III Treatment Algorithm for LDL-C / 1900

SECTION III. ENERGY AND PROTEIN NEEDS AND ANTHROPOMETRIC DATA / 1901

A-10 Basal Metabolic Rate (BMR) and Resting Energy Expenditure (REE) Data / 1901

A-10-a. Nomogram for Estimation of Calorie Needs and Surface Area / 1901

A-10-b. Equation for Predicting Basal Metabolic Rate from Body Weight—FAO/WHO/UNU, 1985 / 1902

A-10-c. Examples of Predicted Basal Metabolic Rate (BMR) in Subjects of the Same Height but Different Weights, Predicted from Actual Weight and Median Acceptable Weight for Height—FAO/WHO/UNU, 1985 / 1902

A-10-d. Basal Metabolic Rates of Adolescent Boys and Grils—FAO/WHO/UNU, 1985 / 1903

A-10-e. BMR in Adult Men and Women in Relation to Height and Median Acceptable Weight for Height—FAO/WHO/UNU, 1985 / 1903

A-10-f. Equations for Prediction of Energy Expenditure—Germany, 2004 / 1903

A-10-f-1. Appendices Editors Comments / 1903

A-10-f-2. Measured REE, REE Adjusted for FFM, and REE Adjusted for FFM and FM in the Study Population / 1904

A-10-f-3. REE Plotted versus Body Weight or FFM in Various Age Groups / 1905

A-10-f-4. REE adjusted for FFM and adjusted for FFM and FM in Underweight, Normal Weight, Overweight, and Obese Women and Men / 1906

A-10-f-5. REE and Reference Intake Values Estimated by the Institute of Medicine or German, Austrian and Swiss Nutrition Societies (DACH) in Various Age and Weight Groups / 1907

A-11 Energy Expenditure and Requirements—WHO, 1985 / 1908

A-11-a. Derivation of Average Values of the Energy Cost of Three Grades of Physical Activity at Work for Women and Men / 1908

A-11-b. Average Daily Energy Requirement of Adults Whose Occupational Work is Classified as Light, Moderate, or Heavy, Expressed as a Multiple of BMR / 1909

A-11-c. Estimates of Energy Cost of Weight Gain / 1909

A-12 Frame Size, Elbow Breadth, and Height-Weight Tables / 1909

A-12-a. Frame Size and Elbow Breadth / 1909

A-12-a-1. Categories of Frame Size: Comments of A.R. Frisancho / 1909

A-12-a-2. Weight by Age and Percentiles for Adult Males of Small, Medium, and Large Frames / 1910

A-12-a-3. Weight by Age and Percentiles for Adult Females of Small, Medium, and Large Frames / 1911

A-12-b. Elbow Breadth by Percentiles of US Males and Females, 1–74 years—NHANES I and 11 Data Set / 1912

A-12-c. Changes in Weight and Height with Age / 1913

A-13 Body Mass Index Tables / 1914

A-13-a. Body Mass Index by Percentiles of US Males and Females, 1–74 years—NHANES I and 11 Data Set / 1914

A-13-b. Nomograph for Estimating Body Mass Index (Bray) / 1915

A-13-c. Body Mass Index Tables (NIH). / 1916

A-13-c-1. BMI Table 1. For Rapid calculation - to BMI of 35 / 1916

A-13-c-2. BMI Table 2. For Rapid calculation - to BMI of 54 / 1917

A-14 Physical Growth Standards: a-f: (NCHS-CDC) 2000

A-14-a. Weight-for-Length Percentiles / 1918

A-14-a-1. Girls: Birth to 36 months / 1918

A-14-a-2. Boys: Birth to 36 months / 1919

A-14-b. Length-for Age Percentiles / 1920

A-14-b-1. Girls: Birth to 36 months / 1920

A-14-b-2. Boys: Birth to 36 months / 1921

A-14-c. Weight-for-Age Percentiles / 1922

A-14-c-1. Girls: Birth to 36 months / 1922

　　　　　　　A-14-c-2.　Boys: Birth to 36 months / 1923
　　　　A-14-d.　Weight-for-Age Percentiles
　　　　　　　A-14-d-1.　Girls: 2 to 20 years / 1924
　　　　　　　A-14-d-2.　Boys: 2 to 20 years / 1925
　　　　A-14-e.　Stature-for-Age Percentiles / 1926
　　　　　　　A-14-e-1.　Girls: 2 to 20 years / 1926
　　　　　　　A-14-e-2.　Boys: 2 to 20 years / 1927
　　　　A-14-f.　Body Mass Index-for-Age Percentiles / 1928
　　　　　　　A-14-f-1.　Girls: 2 to 20 years / 1928
　　　　　　　A-14-f-2.　Boys: 2 to 20 years / 1929
　　　　A-14-g.　Velocity of Height Changes with Age: Tanner/Davies
　　　　　　　A-14-g-1.　Girls: 1 to 14 years / 1930
　　　　　　　A-14-g-2.　Boys: 1 to 14 years / 1931
A-15　Adult Weights and Heights / 1932
　　　　A-15-a.　Height (cm) by Age and Percentile for Males and Females, 1 to 74 Years / 1932
　　　　A-15-b.　Weight (kg) by Age and Percentiles for Males and Females, 1 to 74 Years / 1933
　　　　A-15-c.　Weight by Height in Percentiles for Males, 2 to 74 Years / 1934
　　　　A-15-d.　Weight by Height in Percentiles for Females, 2 to 74 Years / 1935
　　　　A-15-e.　Selected Anthropometric and Impedance Measures by Age and Sex, ages 12 to 79.9 years—NHANES III 2000 / 1936
　　　　　　　A-15-e-1.　For non-Hispanic Whites / 1936
　　　　　　　A-15-e-2.　For non-Hispanic Blacks / 1937
　　　　　　　A-15-e-3.　For Mexican-Americans / 1938
A-16　Anthropometric Data, 1990 / 1939
　　　　A-16-a.　Triceps Skinfold Thickness, by Percentiles for: / 1940
　　　　　　　A-16-a-1.　White Males and Females, 1 to 74 Years / 1940
　　　　　　　A-16-a-2.　Black Males and Females, 1 to 74 Years / 1941
　　　　A-16-b.　Subscapular Skinfold Thickness, by Percentiles for: / 1942
　　　　　　　A-16-b-1.　White Males and Females, 1 to 74 Years / 1942
　　　　　　　A-16-b-2.　Black Males and Females, 1 to 74 Years / 1943
　　　　A-16-c.　Upper Arm Circumference, by Percentiles for: / 1944
　　　　　　　A-16-c-1.　White Males and Females, 1 to 74 Years / 1944
　　　　　　　A-16-c-2.　Black Males and Females, 1 to 74 Years / 1945
　　　　A-16-d.　Upper Arm Muscle Area, by Percentile / 1946
　　　　　　　A-16-d-1.　Males, 18 to 74 Years / 1946
　　　　　　　A-16-d-2.　Females, 18 to 74 Years / 1946
　　　　A-16-e.　Summed Skinfolds (Triceps and Subscapular), by Percentile / 1947
　　　　　　　A-16-e-1.　Males, 18 to 74 Years / 1947
　　　　　　　A-16-e-2.　Females, 18 to 74 Years / 1947
　　　　A-16-f.　Percent Fat Weight by Percentiles for Males and Females, 18 to 74 Years / 1948
A-17　Body Fat Estimations From Skinfold Data / 1949
　　　　A-17-a.　Equivalent Fat Content, as a Percentage of Body Weight, for a Range of Values for the Sum of Four Skinfolds / 1949
　　　　A-17-b.　Percentage of Body Fat Estimation for Women from Age and Triceps, Suprailium, and Thigh Skinfolds / 1950
　　　　A-17-c.　Percentage of Body Fat Estimation for Men from Age and the Sum of Chest, Abdominal and Thigh Skinfolds / 1951
　　　　A-17-d.　Percentage of Body Weight of Adults Estimated from Sum of Tricep and Subscapular Skinfold Thicknesses, Males and Females / 1952
　　　　　　　A-17-d-1.　18–49 Years / 1952
　　　　　　　A-17-d-2.　50–74 Years / 1952
A-18　Growth and Anthropometric Data for Clinical Conditions / 1953
　　　　A-18 a.　Height and Weight Relations in Defining Obesity / 1953
　　　　　　　A-18-a-1.　Classification of Overweight and Obesity by BMI, Waist Circumference, and Associated Disease Risks / 1953
　　　　　　　A-18-a-2.　Selected BMI Units Categorized by Inches (cm) and Pounds (kg) / 1953
　　　　　　　A-18-a-3.　Age-Adjusted Prevalence of Overweight (BMI 25–29.9) and Obesity (BMI ≥30), Ages 20–74 Years 1960–94 / 1954
　　　　A-18 b.　Defining Obesity and Superobesity / 1955
　　　　　　　A-18-b-1.　85th and 95th Percentiles for BMI and TSF / 1955
　　　　　　　A-18 b-2.　5th to 95th Percentiles of Body Mass Index (in kg/m^2) / 1956
　　　　　　　A-18 b-3.　5th to 95th Percentiles of Triceps Skinfold Thickness (mm) / 1958
　　　　A-18 c.　Human Body Proportions for Assessing Amputees / 1960

A-18 d. Recommended Equations for Predicting Stature in Individuals Unable to Stand-Equations / 1961
A-18-e. Limb Lengths for Age of the Disabled Child / 1962
      A-18-e-1. Lower Leg—Girls: 3 to 16 Years / 1962
      A-18-e-2. Lower Leg—Boys: 3 to 18 Years / 1962
      A-18-e-3. Upper Arm—Girls: 3 to 16 Years / 1963
      A-18-e-4. Upper Arm—Boys: 3 to 18 Years / 1963

SECTION IV. NUTRIENTS, LIPIDS, AND ORGANIC COMPOUNDS IN BEVERAGES AND SELECTED FOODS / 1964

A-19 Beverages and Alcoholic Drinks—Calories and Selected Electrolytes / 1964
A-20 Dietary Fiber Content of Common Foods / 1965
A-21 Average Values for Triglycerides, Fatty Acids, and Cholesterol (Including ω-3 Fatty Acids) / 1968
    A-21-a. In Selected Foods and Oils / 1968
    A-21-b. In Marine Foods and Oils / 1975
    A-21-c. Names, Codes and Formulas of Various Fatty Acids / 1976
    A-21-d. Average Values for Total Fat, *Trans* Fatty Acids, and Total Saturated Fatty Acids Per Serving Portion / 1977
A-22 Protein and Minerals in Selected Common Foods / 1978
    A-22 a. Protein, Sodium, Potassium, Calcium, Phosphorus, and Magnesium / 1978
    A-22-b. Iron, Zinc, Copper, Selenium, and Manganese / 1981
A-23 Vitamins in Selected Common Foods / 1983
    A-23-a. Retinol Activity Equivalents (RAE), Vitamin D, α-Tocopherol (TOC), Vitamin C, Thiamin, Riboflavin, Niacin Equivalents, Vitamin B6, Vitamin B12, and Dietary Folate Equivalents (DFE) Content of Selected Foods per Serving Portion / 1984
    A-23-b. Vitamin K Content / 1987
    A-23-c. Retention of Nutrients in Cooked Vegetables / 1988
A-24 Organic Compounds of Interest in Selected Foods / 1989
    A-24-a. Caffeine / 1989
    A-24-b. Carnitine / 1990
    A-24-c. Choline / 1990
    A-24-d. Phenolic Phytochemicals / 1991
      A-24-d-1. Phenolic Phytochemical Content of Selected Foods / 1991
      A-24-d-2. Phenolic Phytochemical Content of Selected fruits / 1992
      A-24-d-3. Phenolic Phytochemical Content of Selected Beverages / 1992
      A-24-d-4. Phenolic Phytochemical Content of Selected Vegetables Foods / 1993

SECTION V. THERAPEUTIC DIETS / 1993

A-25 Medical Foods and Diets for Inherited Metabolic Diseases / 1994
    A-25-a. Formulation, Nutrient Composition, and Sources of Medical Foods for Selected Inborn Errors of Metabolism / 1995
    A-25-b. Average Nutrient Content of Serving List for Phenylalanine and/or Tyrosine and Protein-Restricted Diets / 1999
    A-25-c. Sample Diets Phenylketonuria (2 Weeks of Age): Weight 3.25 kg / 1999
    A-25-d. Recommended Phenylalanine, Tyrosine, Protein, Fat, Essential Fatty Acid, and Energy Intakes for Pregnant Women with Phenylketonuria / 2000
    A-25-e. Average Nutrient Content of Serving Lists for Methionine-Restricted Diets / 2001
    A-25-f. Sample Diets for Homocystinuria (2 wk Age): Weight 3.25 kg / 2001
    A-25-g. Average Nutrient Content of Equivalent Lists for Branched-Chain Amino Acid–Restricted Diets / 2002
    A-25-h. Sample Diets for Branched-Chain Ketoaciduria (2 wk of Age): Weight 3.25 kg / 2002
    A-25-i. Average Nutrient Content of Serving List for Isoleucine-, Methionine-, Threonine-, and Valine-Restricted Diets / 2003
    A-25-j. Sample Diets for Propionic Acidemia and Methylmalonic Acidemia / 2003
    A-25-k. Average Nutrient Content of Serving Lists for Lysine- and Tryptophan-Restricted Diets / 2004
    A-25-l. Sample Diets for Glutaric Acidemia Type I (2 wk of Age): Weight 3.25 kg / 2005
    A-25-m. Suppliers of Medications and Nutrition Supplements Required for Treatment of Urea Cycle Disorders / 2006
    A-25-n. Recommended Daily Nutrient Intakes (Ranges) for Infants and Children with Urea Cycle Disorders / 2006
    A-25-o. Sample Diet for A Urea Cycle Enzyme Defect (2 wk of Age): Weight 3.25 kg / 2006
    A-25-p. Galactose-Restricted Diet / 2007
A-26 Gluten Free Foods and Instructions / 2008
    A-26-a. Introduction / 2008
      A-26-a-1. Food Group Allowed or to be Avoided with Suggested Daily Intake / 2009
      A-26-a-2. Questionable Ingredients / 2010
      A-26-a-3 Additives that are Gluten-Free Safe / 2011
      A-26-a-4. Medications Allowed or to be Avoided / 2011
      A-26-a-5. Gluten-Free Pharmaceutical Excipients / 2012

A-26-b. Sources of Gluten-free Drug Information / 2012
A-26-c. Writing Effective Letters to Food Manufactureres / 2012
A-26-d. Appendices Editors' Comment / 2013
A-27 Lactose-Controlled Diets / 2013
A-27-a. Appendices Editors' Comment / 2013
A-28 Oxalate Content of Selected Foods / 2014
A-28-a. By Foods Groups / 2014
A-28-b. Foods to Use and Avoid / 2016
A-28-c. Oxalate Content of Foods per 100 grams and per Portion / 2017
A-28-d. Low-Oxalate Meal Suggestions / 2022
A-28-e. National Organizations / 2023

SECTION VI. WEBSITES OF INTEREST TO THE HEALTH PROFESSIONAL / 2024

A-29-a Agencies and Organizations—National and International / 2024
A-29-b Search Engines and Medical Journals / 2025
A-29-c Oncology Societies and Services / 2026
A-29-d Commercial Nutrition Product Websites / 2026

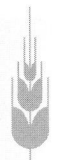

SECTION I CONVERSION FACTORS, WEIGHTS AND MEASURES, AND METABOLIC WATER FORMATION

Factors for converting nutrients expressed in metric or milliequivalent units into International System (SI) units.

1. Definitions
   a. Equivalent weight (EW) = atomic weight of element/ valence of ionic form. Example with magnesium: atomic wt = 24, valence = 2+; therefore EW = 12
   b. Quantity of an electrolyte in milliequivalents per liter (mEq/L) = mg of electrolyte/L/EW. Example: 48 mg of magnesium/L/12 = 4 mEq/L
   c. Quantity of an electrolyte in mg/dL = (mEq/L × EW)/10
   d. To convert mg/dL (= mg%) of an electrolyte to mEq/L: mg/dL × 10/EW = mEq/L
   e. 1 mol = 1 molecular or atomic weight of element or compound in grams (GMWt). In solutions this is usually expressed as moles per liter; i.e., 1 mol/L = 1 M; 1 mM

(mmol) = 1 mol × 10^{-3}, 1 μM (μmol) = 1 mol × 10^{-6}; 1 nM (nmol) = 1 mol × 10^{-9}

   f. (1) To convert mEq/L of an electrolyte or other ions in solution to mmol/L: mEq/L divided by valence = mmol/L; e.g., (a) 2 mEq/L of magnesium (Mg^{2+}) = 2/2 = 1 mmol/L; e.g., (b) 140 mEq Na^+/L = 140/1 = 140 mmol/L
      (2) To convert mg/dL to mmol/L: (mg/dL × 10/EW) divided by valence = mmol/L; e.g., 2 mg/dL of magnesium = (2 × 10/12) divided by 2 = 0.83 mmol/L
      (3) For organic substances: mmol/L = wt in mg/L/MW (in mg)

2. SI units for expressing clinical laboratory data
   These units are now widely used and are increasingly required for publication of scientific data in physical, biologic, and biomedical publication. Extensive SI conversion tables have been published together with an explanation of the rationale for their use and technical aspects of usage (1)

CONVERSION FACTORS FOR SELECTED COMPOUNDS OF NUTRITION INTEREST[a]

COMPONENT	(1) PRESENT UNIT	(2) CONVERSION FACTOR	(3) SI UNIT SYMBOL	(4) MASS CONVERSION FACTOR
Albumin (s)	g/dL	10	g/L	—
Aluminum (s)	μg/L	37.04	nmol/L	μg/27 = mol
Amino acids	(see ref. 3. p. 119 for individual amino acids)			
Amino acid nitrogen (p)	mg/dL	0.714	mmol/L	mg/14 = mmol
Ascorbic acid (p)	mg/dL	56.78	μmol/L	mg/176 = mmol
Calcium (s)	mg/dL	0.250	mmol/L	mg/40 = mmol
Calcium (s)	mEq/dL	0.500	mmol/L	mEq/2 = mmol
β-Carotene[b] (s)	μ/dL	0.0186	μmol/L	μg/536.85 μmol
Chloride (s)	mEq/L	1.00	mmol/L	mEq = mmol
Cholesterol (p)	mg/dL	0.0259	mmol/L	mg/386.6 = mmol
Cobalamin (B_{12})	pg/mL	0.738	pmol/L	pg/1355 = pmol
Copper (s)	μg/dL	0.157	μmol/L	μg/63.5 = μmol
Ethanol (p)	mg/dL	0.217	mmol/L	mg/46 = mmol
Folic acid	ng/mL	2.265	nmol/L	ng/441.4 = nmol
Glucose (p)	mg/dL	0.0555	mmol/L	mg/180.2 = mmol
Iron (s)	μg/dL	0.179	μmol/L	μg/55.9 = μmol
Phosphate (p) (as phosphorus)	mg/dL	0.323	mmol/L	mg/31 = mmol
Potassium (s)	mEq/L	1.000	mmol/L	mEq = mmol
Potassium	mg/dL	0.256	mmol/L	mg/39.1 = mmol
Magnesium (s)	mg/dL	0.411	mmol/L	mg/24.3 = mmol
Pyridoxal (B)	ng/mL	5.981	nmol/L	ng/167 = nmol
Retinol[b] (p,s)	μg/dL	0.0349	μmol/L	μg/286 = μmol
Riboflavfin (s)	μg/dL	26.57	nmol/L	μg/376 = nmol
Sodium (s)	mEq/L	1.00	mmol/L	mEq = mmol
Thiamin HCl (U)	μg/24 h	0.00298	μmol/d	μg/337 = μmol
α-Tocopherol (p)	mg/dL	23.22	μmol/L	μg/431 = μmol
Vitamin D_3	μg/dL	26.01	nmol/L	μg/384 = μmol
Calcidiol	ng/mL	2.498	nmol/L	ng/400 = nmol
Zinc (s)	μg/dL	0.153	μmol/L	μg/65.4 = μmol

[a] To convert metric or equivalent unit per unit volume (column 1) to SI units per liter (column 3), multiply by the conversion factor in column 2. p, plasma; s, serum; B, blood; U, urine.
[b] See Appendix Table A-1-b for detailed conversion figures for retinol and carotene.

References
1. Young DS. Ann Intern Med 1987;106:114. See also, Katz A, Ferraro M, Sluss PM et al. N Engl J Med 2004;351:1548–63.

3. Prefixes and symbols for decimal multiples and submultiples

FACTOR	PREFIX	SYMBOL	FACTOR	PREFIX	SYMBOL
10^9	giga	G	10^{-3}	milli	m
10^6	mega	M	10^{-6}	micro	μ
10^3	kilo	k	10^{-9}	nano	n
10^2	hecto	h	10^{-12}	pico	p
10^1	deca	da	10^{-15}	femto	f
10^{-1}	deci	d	10^{-18}	atto	a
10^{-2}	centi	c			

TABLE A-1-b. FACTORS AND FORMULAS USED IN INTERCONVERTING UNITS OF VITAMIN A AND CAROTENOIDS

Molecular mass:
  1 mol retinol = 286.44 g
  1 mol β-carotene = 536.88 g
  1 mol α-carotene = 536.88 g
  1 mol β-cryptoxanthin = 552.88 g
Units and conversion factors:
  1 μg retinol activity equivalent (RAE)[a]
  = 1 μg all-*trans* retinol
  = 2 μg all-*trans* β-carotene from supplements
  = 12 μg all-*trans* β-carotene from foods[b]
  = 24 μg other all-*trans* provitamin A carotenoids
  = 3.49 nmol all-*trans* retinol
  = 22.35 nmol all-*trans* β-carotene
  ~ 43.4 nmol other all-*trans* provitamin A carotenoids[c]
1 IU_a[d] (International Unit)
  = 0.3 μg all-*trans* retinol
  = 0.3 μg RAE
  = 0.6 μg β-carotene from supplements
  = 3.6 μg of β-carotene from fruits and vegetables
  = 7.2 μg of other all-*trans* provitamin A carotenoids
  = 1.05 nmol all-*trans* retinol
  = 1.12 nmol β-carotene from supplements
  = 6.7 nmol β-carotene from fruits and vegetables
  = 13 nmol of other all-*trans* provitamin A carotenoids

1 IU_c[e]
  = 0.05 μg RAE
  = 0.6 μg all-*trans* β-carotene from supplements
  = 3.6 μg of β-carotene from fruits and vegetables
  = 7.2 μg of other all-*trans* provitamin A carotenoids
Sample calculations (all-*trans* configurations of retinol and carotenoids are assumed):

1. 1 μg RAE = μg retinol + μg β-carotene in foods/12 + μg of provitamin A carotenoids/24
   A diet contains 500 μg retinol, 1800 μg β-carotene and 2400 μg of provitamin A carotenoids. Then:
     500 + 1800/12 + 2400/24 = 750 μg RAE
2. μg RAE = IU_a/3.33 + IU_c/20
   A diet contains 1667 IU_a of retinol and 3000 IU_c of β-carotene. Then:
     1667/3.33 + 3000/20 = 650 μg RAE
3. μg RAE = μg β-carotene/12 + μg other provitamin A carotenoids/24
   A serving of sweet potato contains 2400 μg of β-carotene and 480 μg of other provitamin A carotenoids. Then:
     2400/12 + 480/24 = 220 μg RAE
4. A supplement contains 5000 IU of vitamin A (half as β-carotene)[f]. Then:
     5000/3.33 = 1500 μg RAE

[a] The rationale for the unit RAE, Retinol Activity Equivalent, which replaces the previously defined RE (Retinol Equivalent) is discussed in "Dietary Reference Intakes for Vitamin A, Vitamin K, Arsenic, Boron, Chromium, Copper, Iodine, Iron, Manganese, Molybdenum, Nickel, Silicon, Vanadium, and Zinc," Institute of Medicine, 2001, and Chapter 19.
[b] β-carotene in foods refers to β-carotene in fruits and vegetables, not in supplements consumed with foods.
[c] This conversion is approximate because the molecular mass of different species of provitamin A carotenoids differs slightly from that of β-carotene, and from one another.
[d] IU_a, for retinol, and IU_c, for β-carotene, are now outdated terms that should be replaced, wherever possible, by RAE. The term IU and approximate conversion factors are included here for the purpose of converting IU values in older literature to current RAE equivalents. 1 μg retinol = 3.33 IU vitamin A activity from retinol (*WHO Expert Committee on Biological Standardization Eighteenth Report. Technical Report Series no. 329.* Geneva: WHO, 1966); 10 IU β-carotene = 3.33 retinol (WHO, 1966), where the value of 10 IU is based on 3.33 IU vitamin A activity × 3 (the relative vitamin activity of β-carotene in supplements versus in diets). To convert IU of β-carotene from foods to μg RAE, IU is divided by 20 (twice the previous value of 10).
[e] The equivalency of 1 IU_a = 1 IU_c is an assumption made in the United States Department of Agriculture's *Handbook* 8 (8.1–8.10). The equivalency of IU_c and μg RAE is based on the 2001 DRI conversion factors, footnote a.
[f] It is assumed that the portion of vitamin A from β-carotene has already been converted to an equivalent IU of vitamin A activity.
Prepared by A. Catharine Ross, (Ph.D).

TABLE A-1-c-1. ATOMIC WEIGHTS (ALPHABETIC ORDER)

ELEMENT	SYMBOL	ATOMIC NUMBER	ATOMIC WEIGHT	ELEMENT	SYMBOL	ATOMIC NUMBER	ATOMIC WEIGHT
Actinium	Ac	89	227.0277*	Mercury	Hg	80	200.59
Aluminum	Al	13	26.981538	Molybdenum	Mo	42	95.94
Americium	Am	95	243.0614*	Neodymium	Nd	60	144.24
Antimony	Sb	51	121.760	Neon	Ne	10	20.1797
Argon	Ar	18	39.948	Neptunium	Np	93	237.0482*
Arsenic	As	33	74.92160	Nickel	Ni	28	58.6934
Astatine	At	85	209.9871*	Niobium	Nb	41	92.90638
Barium	Ba	56	137.327	Nitrogen	N	7	14.0067
Berkelium	Bk	97	247.0703*	Nobelium	No	102	259.1010*
Beryllium	Be	4	9.012182	Osmium	Os	76	190.23
Bismuth	Bi	83	208.98038	Oxygen	O	8	15.9994
Bohrium	Bh	107	264.12*	Palladium	Pd	46	106.42
Boron	B	5	10.811	Phosphorus	P	15	30.973761
Bromine	Br	35	79.904	Platinum	Pt	78	195.078
Cadmium	Cd	48	112.411	Plutonium	Pu	94	244.0642*
Calcium	Ca	20	40.078	Polonium	Po	84	208.9824*
Californium	Cf	98	251.0796*	Potassium	K	19	39.0983
Carbon	C	6	12.0107	Praseodymium	Pr	59	140.90765
Cerium	Ce	58	140.116	Promethium	Pm	61	144.9127*
Cesium	Cs	55	132.90545	Protactinium	Pa	91	231.03588*
Chlorine	Cl	17	35.453	Radium	Ra	88	226.0254*
Chromium	Cr	24	51.9961	Radon	Rn	86	222.0176*
Cobalt	Co	27	58.933200	Rhenium	Re	75	186.207
Copper	Cu	29	63.546	Rhodium	Rh	45	102.90550
Curium	Cm	96	247.0704*	Rubidium	Rb	37	85.4678
Dubnium	Db	105	262.1141*	Ruthenium	Ru	44	101.07
Dysprosium	Dy	66	162.50	Rutherfordium	Rf	104	261.1088*
Einsteinium	Es	99	252.0830*	Samarium	Sm	62	150.36
Erbium	Er	68	167.259	Scandium	Sc	21	44.955910
Europium	Eu	63	151.964	Seaborgium	Sg	106	266.1219*
Fermium	Fm	100	257.0951*	Selenium	Se	34	78.96
Fluorine	F	9	18.9984032	Silicon	Si	14	28.0855
Francium	Fr	87	223.0197*	Silver	Ag	47	107.8682
Gadolinium	Gd	64	157.25	Sodium	Na	11	22.989770
Gallium	Ga	31	69.723	Strontium	Sr	38	87.62
Germanium	Ge	32	72.64	Sulfur	S	16	32.065
Gold	Au	79	196.96655	Tantalum	Ta	73	180.9479
Hafnium	Hf	72	178.49	Technetium	Tc	43	97.9072*
Helium	He	2	4.002602	Tellurium	Te	52	127.60
Holmium	Ho	67	164.93032	Terbium	Tb	65	158.92534
Hydrogen	H	1	1.00794	Thallium	Tl	81	204.3833
Indium	In	49	114.818	Thorium	Th	90	232.0381*
Iodine	I	53	126.90447	Thulium	Tm	69	168.93421
Iridium	Ir	77	192.217	Tin	Sn	50	118.710
Iron	Fe	26	55.845	Titanium	Ti	22	47.867
Krypton	Kr	36	83.80	Tungsten	W	74	183.84
Lanthanum	La	57	138.9055	Unununium	Uuu	111	272.1535*
Lawrencium	Lr	103	262.1097*	Uranium	U	92	238.02891
Lead	Pb	82	207.2	Vanadium	V	23	50.9415
Lithium	Li	3	6.941	Xenon	Xe	54	131.293
Lutetium	Lu	71	174.967	Ytterbium	Yb	70	173.04
Magnesium	Mg	12	24.3050	Yttrium	Y	39	88.90585
Manganese	Mn	25	54.938049	Zinc	Zn	30	65.39
Meitnerium	Mt	109	268.1388*	Zirconium	Zr	40	91.224
Mendelevium	Md	101	258.0984*				

Based on 1999 IUPAC Table of Standard Atomic Weights of the Elements.
* Relative atomic mass of the isotope of that element of longest known half-life.

TABLE A-1-c-2. ATOMIC WEIGHTS (ORDER OF ATOMIC NUMBER)

ATOMIC NUMBER	ELEMENT	SYMBOL	ATOMIC WEIGHT	ATOMIC NUMBER	ELEMENT	SYMBOL	ATOMIC WEIGHT
1	Hydrogen	H	1.00794	56	Barium	Ba	137.327
2	Helium	He	4.002602	57	Lanthanum	La	138.9055
3	Lithium	Li	6.941	58	Cerium	Ce	140.116
4	Beryllium	Be	9.012182	59	Praseodymium	Pr	140.90765
5	Boron	B	10.811	60	Neodymium	Nd	144.24
6	Carbon	C	12.0107	61	Promethium	Pm	144.9127*
7	Nitrogen	N	14.0067	62	Samarium	Sm	150.36
8	Oxygen	O	15.9994	63	Europium	Eu	151.964
9	Fluorine	F	18.9984032	64	Gadolinium	Gd	157.25
10	Neon	Ne	20.1797	65	Terbium	Tb	158.92534
11	Sodium	Na	22.989770	66	Dysprosium	Dy	162.50
12	Magnesium	Mg	24.3050	67	Holmium	Ho	164.93032
13	Aluminum	Al	26.981538	68	Erbium	Er	167.259
14	Silicon	Si	28.0855	69	Thulium	Tm	168.93421
15	Phosphorus	P	30.973761	70	Ytterbium	Yb	173.04
16	Sulfur	S	32.065	71	Lutetium	Lu	174.967
17	Chlorine	Cl	35.453	72	Hafnium	Hf	178.49
18	Argon	Ar	39.948	73	Tantalum	Ta	180.9479
19	Potassium	K	39.0983	74	Tungsten	W	183.84
20	Calcium	Ca	40.078	75	Rhenium	Re	186.207
21	Scandium	Sc	44.955910	76	Osmium	Os	190.23
22	Titanium	Ti	47.867	77	Iridium	Ir	192.217
23	Vanadium	V	50.9415	78	Platinum	Pt	195.078
24	Chromium	Cr	51.9961	79	Gold	Au	196.96655
25	Manganese	Mn	54.938049	80	Mercury	Hg	200.59
26	Iron	Fe	55.845	81	Thallium	Tl	204.3833
27	Cobalt	Co	58.933200	82	Lead	Pb	207.2
28	Nickel	Ni	58.6934	83	Bismuth	Bi	208.98038
29	Copper	Cu	63.546	84	Polonium	Po	208.9824*
30	Zinc	Zn	65.39	85	Astatine	At	209.9871*
31	Gallium	Ga	69.723	86	Radon	Rn	222.0176*
32	Germanium	Ge	72.64	87	Francium	Fr	223.0197*
33	Arsenic	As	74.92160	88	Radium	Ra	226.0254*
34	Selenium	Se	78.96	89	Actinium	Ac	227.0277*
35	Bromine	Br	79.904	90	Thorium	Th	232.0381*
36	Krypton	Kr	83.80	91	Protactinium	Pa	231.03588*
37	Rubidium	Rb	85.4678	92	Uranium	U	238.02891
38	Strontium	Sr	87.62	93	Neptunium	Np	237.0482*
39	Yttrium	Y	88.90585	94	Plutonium	Pu	244.0642*
40	Zirconium	Zr	91.224	95	Americium	Am	243.0614*
41	Niobium	Nb	92.90638	96	Curium	Cm	247.0704*
42	Molybdenum	Mo	95.94	97	Berkelium	Bk	247.0703*
43	Technetium	Tc	97.9072*	98	Californium	Cf	251.0796*
44	Ruthenium	Ru	101.07	99	Einsteinium	Es	252.0830*
45	Rhodium	Rh	102.90550	100	Fermium	Fm	257.0951*
46	Palladium	Pd	106.42	101	Mendelevium	Md	258.0984*
47	Silver	Ag	107.8682	102	Nobelium	No	259.1010*
48	Cadmium	Cd	112.411	103	Lawrencium	Lr	262.1097*
49	Indium	In	114.818	104	Rutherfordium	Rf	261.1088*
50	Tin	Sn	118.710	105	Dubnium	Db	262.1141*
51	Antimony	Sb	121.760	106	Seaborgium	Sg	266.1219*
52	Tellurium	Te	127.60	107	Bohrium	Bh	264.12*
53	Iodine	I	126.90447	109	Meitnerium	Mt	268.1388*
54	Xenon	Xe	131.293	111	Unununium	Uuu	272.1535*
55	Cesium	Cs	132.90545				

Based on 1999 IUPAC Table of Standard Atomic Weights of the Elements.
* Relative atomic mass of the isotope of that element of longest known half-life.

TABLE A-1-d. WEIGHTS AND MEASURES

VOLUMES:

APOTHECARIES' MEASURE	METRIC	HOUSEHOLD
1 fluid dram (fl dr)	4 milliliter (mL)	1 teaspoon (tsp)
2 fl dr	8 mL	1 dessert spoonful
½ fluid ounce (fl oz)	15 mL	1 tablespoon (Tbsp) (3 tsp)
1 fl oz	30 mL	2 Tbsp (⅛ cup)
1-½ fl oz	45 mL	1 jigger
2 fl oz	59 mL	4 Tbsp (¼ cup)
2-⅔ fl oz	80 mL	5-⅓ Tbsp (⅓ cup)
4 fl oz	118 mL	8 Tbsp (½ cup)
8 fl oz	237 mL	1 cup
16 fl oz	473 mL	1 pint (pt)
32 fl oz	947 mL	1 quart (qt)
128 fl oz	3785 mL	1 gallon (gal)
3.38 fl oz	1 deciliter (dL) (100 mL)	
2.11 pt	1 liter (L) (1,000 mL)	

WEIGHTS: AVOIRDUPOIS

	METRIC
	1 femtogram (fg) (10^{-15} g)
	1 picogram (pg) (10^{-12} g)
	1 nanogram (ng) (10^{-9} g)
	1 microgram (μg) (10^{-6} g)
1 grain (gr)	0.065 g (65 mg)
1 gram (0.035 oz)	15.432 gr
1 scruple (20 gr)	1.296 g
1 dram (dr) (= drachm) (27.3 gr)	1.77 g
1 oz (16 dr)	28.35 g
1 lb (16 oz)	453.59 g
1 ton (2000 lb)	0.91 metric tons
1.015 gr	1 milligram (mg) (10^{-3} g)
	1 centigram (cg) (10^{-2} g)
	1 decigram (dg) (10^{-1} g)
15.4 gr (0.035 oz)	1 gram (g)
2.2 lb	1 kilogram (kg) (10^3 g)

LENGTH/AREA:

	METRIC
1 angstrom (Å)	10 millimeter (mm)
¹⁄₂₅₀₀ inch (in)	1 micron (μ) (10^{-3} mm) = micrometer (μm)
0.039 in	1 mm
0.39 in	1 centimeter (cm)
1 in	2.54 cm
1 foot (ft) (12 in)	30.5 cm
39.4 in	1 meter (m)
1 yard (yd) (3 ft)	0.9 m
1 rod (5.5 yd)	4.95 m
1093.6 yd (0.62 mile)	1 kilometer (km)
1 mile (mi) (5280 ft)	1.61 km
1 acre (160 square rods)	0.4 hectare

TEMPERATURE CONVERSIONS:

F to C: 5/9 (F − 32)
C to F: (9.5 × C) + 32

ELECTROLYTE DATA:

ION		ATOMIC WT (1)	VALENCE (2)	EQUIVALENT Wt 1 ÷ 2
Bicarbonate	HCO_3^-	61.0	1	61.0
Calcium	Ca^{2+}	40.1	2	20.0
Chloride	Cl^-	35.5	1	35.5
Magnesium	Mg^{2+}	24.3	2	12.2
Phosphate	HPO_4^{2-}	96.0	2	48.0[b]
Potassium	K^+	39.1	1	39.1
Sodium	Na^+	23.0	1	23.0
Sulfate	SO_4^{2+}	96.1	2	48.0

TABLE A-1-e. WATER FORMED IN THE METABOLISM OF TISSUE AND CALORIC SOURCES

SOURCE	AMOUNT
Muscle	1 g yields 0.85 mL (0.1 mL from protein + 0.75 mL cellular water)
Mixed tissue	100 kcal yields 10 mL
Fat	1 g yields 1.0 mL
Protein	1 g yields 0.4 mL
Glucose	1 g yields 0.64 mL
Glucose • H_2O	1 g yields 0.60 mL
Mixed diet	100 kcal yields 20 mL

Example: High-glucose TPN solution

750 mL 10% amino acids	= 300 kcal yields 30 mL H_2O
1175 mL 50% glucose/water	= 2000 kcal yields 353 mL H_2O
143 mL 10% lipid	= 157 kcal yields 14 mL H_2O
Total: 2068 mL	= 2457 kcal yields 397 mL H_2O

Example: Glucose-lipid TPN solution

750 mL 10% amino acids	= 300 kcal yields 30 mL H_2O
750 mL 50% glucose/water	= 1275 kcal yields 225 mL H_2O
500 mL 20% lipid	= 1000 kcal yields 100 mL H_2O
Total: 2000 mL	= 2575 kcal yields 355 mL H_2O

Prepared by M. E. Shils.

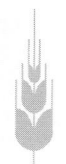
INTRODUCTION TO SECTION II

Chapter 103 of the ninth edition of *Modern Nutrition in Health and Disease* authored by George H. Beaton, Ph.D. is a comprehensive review of the historical development of nutritional standards and current controversial issues. It provides pertinent comments and recommendations concerning key national and international standards.

Key tables from the various national and international reports are included in this section. The reader is referred to the original reports for background statements and ancillary tables. Because the United Kingdom's Dietary Reference Values report is probably not easily available to readers in the United States, significant excerpts have been included in Table II-A-4a.

Some key text and important tables from the first six volumes of the new Food and Nutrition Board, Institute of Medicine Dietary Reference Intakes published between 1997 and 2004 are given in Tables A-2-c through A-2-h following subsections A-2-a and A-2-b. See also Dr. Allison Yates' Chapter 104. Earlier US and Canadian standards are reprinted for comparison with newer standards in A-3-a-1 to A-3-b-2.

We have been provided with a draft set of Nutrient Reference Values for Australia and New Zealand published for comment in December 2004 (Table A-6). We are aware that an updated and revised set of nutrient reference values have been published recently in Japan but were unable to obtain a translated set in English prior to publication. The ninth edition Japanese data have been reproduced (Table A-5.) As noted in A-7-b, A-7-c, and A-7-d revised European standards have been recently published.

Appendices Editors

A-2. UNITED STATES AND CANADA: DIETARY REFERENCE INTAKES: 1997–2004

A-2-a. Introductory Comments: Appendices Editors

This section has been changed appreciably from that of the previous edition by the addition of significant amounts of text, graphics, and tables from the six volumes of Dietary Reference Intakes (DRIs), published by the Institute of Medicine, Food and Nutrition Board between 1997 and 2004. The DRIs were developed through joint United States and Canadian efforts and are listed as values for both countries in subsection A-2. For those interested in comparing the changes in the DRIs from those of 1989 US Recommended Dietary Allowance (RDA) and 1990 Canadian recommendations, see subsection A-3.

Single-volume publications of *Recommended Dietary Allowances of the Food and Nutrition Board, National Academy of Sciences* were published between 1941 and 1989 and the periodic *Recommended Nutrient Intakes* (RNIs) that were published in Canada have been succeeded by a new series of cooperative publications titled *Dietary Reference Intakes*. In order of publication, they are listed as follows (but in the following text, the source reference is identified as IOM with the appropriate year):

Food and Nutrition Board, IOM. Institute of Medicine. Dietary Reference Intakes for Calcium, Phosphorus, Magnesium, Vitamin D, and Fluoride. Washington, DC: National Academy Press, 1997: pp 432.

Food and Nutrition Board, IOM. Dietary Reference Intakes for Thiamin, Riboflavin, Niacin, Vitamin B$_6$, Folate, Vitamin B$_{12}$, Pantothenic Acid, Biotin, and Choline. Washington, DC: National Academy Press, 1998: pp 564.

Food and Nutrition Board, IOM. Dietary Reference Intakes for Vitamin C, Vitamin E, Selenium, and Carotenoids. Washington, DC: National Academy Press, 2000b:506.

Food and Nutrition Board, IOM. Dietary Reference Intakes for Vitamin A, Vitamin K, Arsenic, Boron, Chromium, Copper, Iodine, Iron, Manganese, Molybdeum, Nickel, Silicon, Vanadium, and Zinc. Washington, DC: National Academy Press, 2001: pp 772.

Food and Nutrition Board, IOM. Dietary Reference Intakes for Energy, Carbohydrate, Fiber, Fat, Fatty Acids, Cholesterol, Protein, and Amino Acids. Washington, DC: National Academy Press, 2002.

Food and Nutrition Board, IOM. Dietary Reference Intakes for Water, Potassium, Sodium, Chloride, and Sulfate. Washington, DC: National Academy Press, 2004.

In addition to the Dietary Reference Intakes volumes, other volumes were published which relate to revision and application, such as the following:

Food and Nutrition Board, IOM. How Should the Recommended Dietary Allowances Be Revised? Washington, DC: National Academy Press, 1994. Dietary Reference Intakes: Applications in Dietary Assessment. Washington, DC: National Academy Press, 2000a.

Any of the IOM volumes can be ordered or read on line at http://www.nap.edu. Each of the nutrient volumes includes extensive review of the pertinent literature, nutrient needs, indications for estimating requirements, the biochemical, physiologic, and metabolic aspects of nutrients, in addition to the reference values of the various nutrients. IOM, 2002 also "provides guidance on appropriate macronutrient distribution thought to reduce risk of disease including chronic disease" by presenting "Acceptable Macronutrient Distribution Ranges" (AMDRs). This volume also summarizes research data related to disease with recommendations, such as for the levels of physical activity and energy expenditure estimated to maintain health and reduce risk of disease.

The overall project is a comprehensive effort involving large numbers of individuals active in nutrition-related sciences and medicine undertaken by the DRI Committee of the Food and Nutrition Board, IOM, National Academy of Science in collaboration with Health Canada.

The text is taken verbatim from the DRI volumes, including the definitions and use of the various forms of DRI defined so the data in the tables of specific nutrients are intelligible. All of the verbatim text and tabular and graphic material in subsections A-2-b through A-2-h are reprinted with permission from The National Academy of Sciences and The National Academies Press, Washington, D.C. Additional information on the DRIs is given in Chapter 104 by Dr. Allison Yates, formerly Director of the Food and Nutrition Board and Staff Study Director of the Standing Committee on the Scientific. Evaluation of the DRI's.

The Appendices Editors

A-2-b. Verbatim Excerpts from the Dietary Reference Intakes Texts

A-2-b-1. Dietary Reference Intakes: Categories

The reference values, collectively called the Dietary Reference Intakes (DRIs), include the Estimated Average Requirement (EAR), Recommended Dietary Allowance (RDA), Adequate Intake (AI), and Tolerable Upper Intake Level (UL) (Table A-2-b-1-a). Establishment of these reference values requires that a criterion be carefully chosen for each nutrient, and that the population for whom these values apply be carefully defined.

A requirement is defined as the lowest continuing intake level of a nutrient that, for a specific indicator of adequacy, will maintain a defined level of nutriture in an individual. The chosen criterion or indicator of nutritional adequacy upon which EARs and AIs are based is identified for each nutrient. The criterion may differ for individuals at different life stages. Particular attention is given throughout this report to the choice and justification of the criterion used to establish requirement values and the intake levels beyond which the potential for increased risk of adverse effects may occur.

The *Estimated Average Requirement* (EAR)[1] is the daily intake value that is estimated to meet the requirement, as defined by the specified indicator or criterion of adequacy, in half of the apparently healthy individuals in a life stage or gender group (see Figure A-2-b-1-b). (A normal or symmetrical distribution [median and mean are similar] is usually assumed for nutrient requirements).

TABLE A-2-b-1-a. DIETARY REFERENCE INTAKES DEFINITION

Recommended Dietary Allowance (RDA): the average daily dietary nutrient intake level sufficient to meet the nutrient requirement of nearly all (97–98%) healthy individuals in a particular life stage and gender group.

Adequate Intake (AI): the recommended average daily intake level based on observed or experimentally determined approximations or estimates of nutrient intake by a group (or groups) of apparently healthy people that are assumed to be adequate—used when an RDA cannot be determined.

Tolerable Upper Intake Level (UL): the highest average daily nutrient intake level that is likely to pose no risk of adverse health effects to almost all individuals in the general population. As intake increases above the UL, the potential risk of adverse effects may increase.

Estimated Average Requirement (EAR): the average daily nutrient intake level estimated to meet the requirement of half the healthy individuals in a particular life stage and gender group.[a]

---

[a] In the case of energy, an Estimated Energy Requirement (EER) is provided; it is the average dietary energy intake that is predicted to maintain energy balance in a healthy adult of a defined age, gender, weight, height, and level of physical activity, consistent with good health. In children and pregnant and lactating women, the EER is taken to include the needs associated with the deposition of tissues or the secretion of milk at rates consistent with good health.

This is equivalent to saying the randomly chosen individuals from the population would have a 50:50 chance of having their requirement met at this intake level. This use follows the precedent set by others that have used the term "Estimated Average Requirements" for reference values similarly derived but meant to be applied to population intakes (COMA, 1991). [(See Appendices Section A-4. Appendices Editors)].

The EAR's usefulness as a predictor of an individual's requirement depends on the appropriateness of the choice of the nutritional status indicator or criterion and the type and amount of data available.

The EAR serves three major functions: as the basis for the Recommended Dietary Allowance (RDA), as the primary reference point for assessing the adequacy of estimated nutrient intakes of groups (IOM, 2000a) and, together with estimates of the variance of intake, in planning for the intake of groups.

The *Recommended Dietary Allowance* (RDA) is an estimate of the minimum daily average dietary intake level that meets the nutrient requirements of nearly all (97–98%) healthy individuals in a particular life stage and gender group. The process for setting RDA depends on being able to set an EAR and estimating the variance of

---

[1] The definition of EAR implies a median as opposed to a mean, or average. The median and average would be the same if the distribution of requirements followed a symmetrical distribution and would diverge as a distribution became skewed

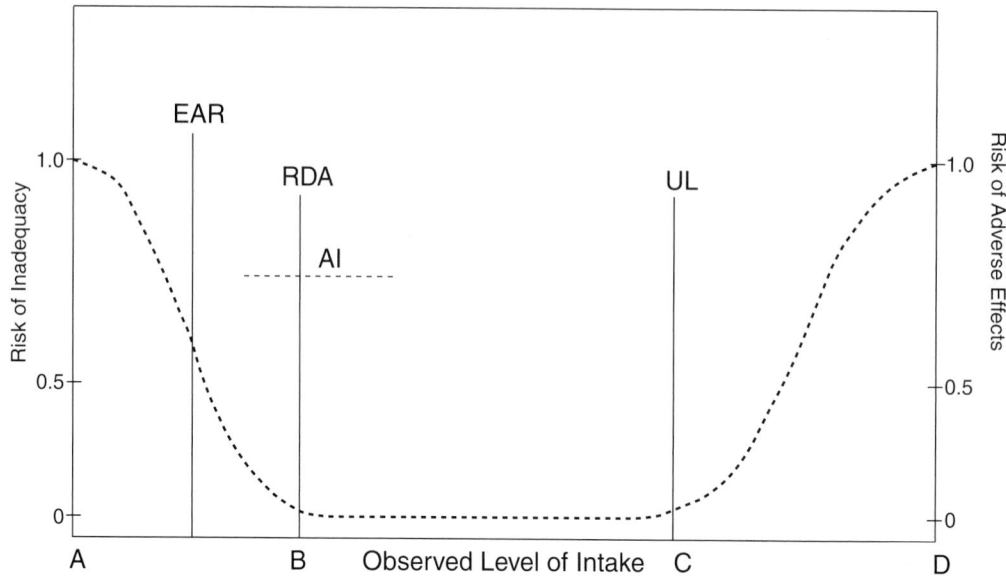

Figure A-2-b-1-b. Dietary Reference Intakes relations. This figure shows that the Estimated Average Requirement (EAR) is the intake at which the risk of inadequacy is estimated to be 0.5 (50%) to an individual. The Recommended Dietary Allowance (RDA) is the intake at which the risk of inadequacy would be very small—only 0.02 to 0.03 (2–3%). At intakes between the RDA and the Tolerable Upper Intake Level (UL), the risks of inadequacy and of excess are both estimated to be close to 0. At intakes above the UL, the potential risk of adverse effects may increase. A dashed line is used because the actual shape of the curve has not been determined experimentally.

the requirement itself. Note that if an EAR cannot be set due to limitations of the data available, no RDA will be set.

This approach differs somewhat from that used by the World Health Organization, Food and Agriculture Organization, and International Atomic Energy Agency (WHO/FAO/IAEA) Expert Consultation on *Trace Elements in Human Nutrition and Health* (WHO, 1996). That publication uses the term *basal requirement* to indicate the level of intake needed to prevent pathologically relevant and clinically detectable signs of a dietary inadequacy. The term *normative requirement* indicates the level of intake sufficient to maintain a desirable body store or reserve. In developing the RDA (and Adequate Intake [IA], see below) emphasis is placed instead on the reasons underlying the choice of the criterion of nutritional adequacy used to establish the requirement. It is not designated as basal or normative.

Adequate Intake. If sufficient scientific evidence is not available to calculate the EAR, a reference intake called an *Adequate Intake* (AI) is provided instead of an RDA. In the judgment of the Standing Committee on the Scientific Evaluation of Dietary Reference Intakes, the AI is expected to meet or exceed the amount needed to maintain a defined nutritional state or criterion of adequacy in essentially all members of a specific, apparently healthy, population. Examples of defined nutritional states include normal growth, maintenance of normal circulating nutrient values, or other aspects of nutritional well-being or general health.

For young infants for whom human milk is the recommended sole source of food for most nutrients for the first

4 to 6 months of life, the AI is based on the daily mean nutrient intake supplied by human milk for healthy, full-term infants who are exclusively fed human milk. The goal may be different for infants consuming infant formula for which the bioavailability of a nutrient may be different from that in human milk. For adults, the AI may be based on data from a single experiment, on estimated dietary intakes in apparently healthy population groups, or on a review of data from different approaches that, when considered alone, do not permit a reasonably confident estimate of an EAR.

A-2-b-2. Comparison of Recommended Dietary Allowances and Adequate Intakes

There is much less certainty about an AI value than about an RDA value. Because AIs depend on a greater degree of judgment than is applied in estimating an EAR and subsequently an RDA, an AI may deviate significantly from and be numerically higher than an RDA. For this reason, AIs must be used with greater care than is the case for RDAs. Also, an RDA is usually calculated from the EAR by using a formula that takes into account the expected variation in the requirement for the nutrient.

Both AI and RDA are used as a goal for individual intake. In general, the values are intended to cover the needs of nearly all apparently healthy persons in a life stage group. (For infants, the AI is the mean intake when infants in the age group are consuming human milk. Larger infants may have greater needs, which they meet by consuming more milk). The AI for a nutrient is expected to exceed the RDA for that nutrient, and thus it should cover the needs of more than 97 to 98% of individuals. The degree to which the AI exceeds the RDA is likely to differ among nutrients and population groups. As with RDAs, AIs for children and adolescents may be extrapolated from adult values if no other usable data are available.

For people who have diseases that increase specific nutrient requirements or who have other special health needs, the RDA and AI each may serve as the basis for adjusting individual recommendations. Qualified health professionals should adapt the recommended intake to cover higher or lower needs.

A-2-b-3. Tolerable Upper Intake Level (UL)

These are the highest level of daily nutrient intake that is likely to pose no risk of adverse health effects for almost all individuals in the specified life stage group (see Figure A-2-b-1-b). As intake increases above the UL, there is the potential for an increased risk of adverse effect. The term *tolerable* was chosen to avoid implying a possible beneficial effect. Instead, the term is intended to connote a level of intake that can, with high probability, be tolerated biologically. The UL is not intended to be a recommended level of intake, as there is no established benefit for healthy individuals if they consume a nutrient in amounts exceeding the recommended intake (the RDA or AI).

The UL is based on an evaluation conducted by using the methodology for risk assessment of nutrients. The need for setting ULs has arisen as a result of the increased fortification of foods with nutrients and the use of dietary supplements by more people and in larger doses. The UL applies to chronic daily use and is usually based on the total intake of a nutrient from food, water, and supplements if adverse effects have been associated with total intake. However, if adverse effects have been associated with intake from supplements or food fortificants only, the UL is based on nutrient intake from one or both of those sources only, rather than on total intake. As in the case of applying AIs, professionals should avoid very rigid application of ULs and first assess the characteristics of the individual or group of concern (e.g., source of nutrient, physiological state of the individual, length of sustained high intakes, etc.).

For some nutrients, data may not be sufficient for developing the UL. This indicates the need for caution in consuming amounts greater than the recommended intake; it does not mean that high intake poses no potential risk of adverse effects.

The safety of routine, long-term intake above the UL is not well documented. Although members of the general population should be advised not to routinely exceed the UL, intake above the UL may be appropriate for investigation within well-controlled clinical trials. Clinical trials of doses above the UL should not be discouraged as long as subjects participating in these trials have signed informed consent documents regarding possible toxicity and as long as these trials employ appropriate safe monitoring of trial subjects. (IOM, 2002:1-1-6).

There were insufficient data to set a UL for total fat, monounsaturated fatty acids, n-6 and n-3 polyunsaturated fatty acids, protein, or amino acids. While increased serum low density lipoprotein (LDL) cholesterol concentrations, and therefore risk of coronary heart disease, may increase at high intakes of saturated fatty acids, *trans* fatty acids, or cholesterol, a UL is not set for these fats because the level at which risk begins to increase is very low and cannot be achieved by usual diets and still have adequate intakes of all other required nutrients. It is thus recommended that saturated fatty acid, trans fatty acid, and cholesterol consumption be as low as possible while consuming a nutritionally adequate diet. Although there were insufficient data to set a UL for added sugars, a maximal intake level of 25 percent or less of energy is suggested to prevent the displacement of foods that are major sources of essential micronutrients (IOM, 2002:pS-4).

Dietary Fiber can have variable composition and therefore it is difficult to link a specific fiber with a particular adverse effect, especially when phytate is also often present. It is concluded that as part of an overall healthy diet Dietary Fiber will not produce significant deleterious effects in healthy individuals. Therefore, a Tolerable Upper Intake Level is not set for Fiber (IOM, 2002:p7–13).

A-2-b-4. Using Dietary Reference Intakes to Assess Nutrient Intakes of Groups

Suggested uses of Dietary Reference Intakes (DRIs) appear in Table A-2-b-4-a. The transition from using previously published Recommended Dietary Allowances (RDAs) and Reference Nutrient Intakes (RNIs) to using each of the DRIs appropriately will require time and effort by health professionals and others.

The Estimated Average Requirement (EAR) is the appropriate reference intake to use in assessing the nutrient intake of groups, whereas the RDA is not appropriate. When assessing nutrient intakes of a group it is important to consider the variation in intake in the same individuals from day to day, as well as underreporting. With these considerations, the prevalence of inadequacy for a given nutrient may be estimated by using national survey data and determining the percent of the population below the EAR.

Assuming a normal distribution of requirements, the percent of surveyed individuals whose intake is less than the EAR equals the percent of individuals whose diets are considered inadequate based on the criteria of inadequacy chosen to determine the requirement. For example, intake data from the Continuing Survey of Food Intakes by Individuals (1994–1996, 1998), which collected 24 hour diet recalls for 1 or 2 days, indicate that:

TABLE A-2-b-4-a. USES OF DIETARY REFERENCE INTAKES FOR HEALTHY INDIVIDUALS AND GROUPS

TYPE OF USE	FOR AN INDIVIDUAL[a]	FOR A GROUP[b]
Assessment	**EAR:** use to examine the probability that usual intake is inadequate. **EER**[d]**:** Use to examine the probability that usual energy intake is inadequate **RDA:** usual intake at or above this level has a low probability of inadequacy. **AI**[c]**:** usual intake at or above this level has a low probability of inadequacy. **UL:** usual intake above this level may place an individual at risk of adverse effects from excessive nutrient intake.	**EAR:** use to estimate the prevalence of inadequate intakes within a group. **EER:** use to estimate the prevalence of inadequate energy intakes within a group. **RDA:** do not use to assess intakes of groups. **AI**[c]**:** mean usual intake at or above this level implies a low prevalence of inadequate intakes. **UL:** use to estimate the percentage of the population at potential risk of adverse effects from excess nutrient intake.
Planning	**RDA:** aim for this intake. **AI**[c]**:** aim for this intake. **UL:** use as a guide to limit intake; chronic intake of higher amounts may increase the potential risk of adverse effects.	**EAR:** use to plan an intake distribution with a low prevalence of inadequate intakes. **EER:** use to plan an energy intake distribution with a low prevalence of inadequate intakes. **AI**[c]**:** use to plan mean intakes. **UL:** use to plan intake distributions with a low prevalence of intakes potentially at risk of adverse effects.

RDA = Recommended Dietary Allowance
EAR = Estimated Average Requirement
AI = Adequate Intake
UL = Tolerable Upper Level
[a] Evaluation of true status requires clinical, biochemical, and anthropometric data.
[b] Requires statistically valid approximation of distribution of usual intakes.
[c] For the nutrients in this report, AIs are set for infants for all nutrients, and for other age groups for fiber, n-6, and n-3 fatty acids. The AI may be used as a guide for infants as it reflects the average intake from human milk. Infants consuming formulas with the same nutrient composition as human milk are consuming an adequate amount after adjustments are made for differences in bioavailability. When the AI for a nutrient is not based on mean intakes of healthy populations, this assessment is made with less confidence.
[d] Estimated Energy Requirement (EER) may be used as the EAR for these applications

- Less than 5 percent of adults at that time consumed dietary carbohydrate at a level less than the EAR
- Less than 5 percent of children and adults consumed protein at levels less than the EAR
- Less than 5 percent of adults consumed *Dietary Fiber* at levels greater than the AI (IOM 2002:S-6-8)

A-2-b-5. Acceptable Macronutrient Distribution Ranges for Healthy Diets

Dietary Reference Intakes have been set for carbohydrate, *n*-6 and *n*-3 polyunsaturated fatty acids, protein and amino acids based on controlled studies in which the actual amount of nutrient provided or utilized is known or based on median intakes from national survey data (see Appendix Tables A-2-d-1 to A-2-d-7). A growing body of evidence has shown that macronutrients, particularly fats and carbohydrate, play a role in the risk of chronic diseases.

Although various guidelines have been established that suggest a maximal intake level of fat and fatty acids (e.g., American Heart Association [Krauss et al., 1996], *Dietary Guidelines for Americans* [USDA/HHS, 2000]), the scientific evidence suggests that individuals can consume moderate levels without risk of adverse health effects while increased risk may occur with the chronic consumption of

diets that are too low or too high in these macronutrients. Much of this evidence is based on clinical end points (e.g., risk of coronary heart disease [CHD], diabetes, cancer, and obesity), which are associations rather than distinct end points. Furthermore, because there may be factors other than diet that may contribute to chronic disease, it is not possible to determine a defined level of intake at which chronic disease may be presented or may develop.

Based on the evidence to suggest a role in chronic diseases, as well as information to ensure sufficient intakes of sufficient nutrients, Acceptable Macronutrient Distribution Ranges (AMDR) have been estimated for individuals. An AMDR is defined as a range of intakes for a particular energy source that is associated with reduced risk of chronic disease while providing adequate intakes of essential nutrients. The AMDR is expressed as a percentage of total energy intake because its requirement, in a classical sense, is *not* independent of other energy fuel sources or of the total energy requirement of the individual. Each must be expressed in relative terms to each other. A key feature of each AMDR is that it has a lower and upper boundary, some determined mainly by the lowest or highest value for the other judged to have an expected impact on health. If an individual consumes below or above this range, there is a potential for increasing the risk of chronic diseases shown to affect long term health, as well as increasing the risk of insufficient intakes of essential nutrients.

When fat intakes are low and carbohydrate intakes are high, intervention studies, with the support of epidemiological studies, demonstrate a reduction in plasma HDL, cholesterol concentration, an increase in the plasma total cholesterol: HDL cholesterol ratio, and an increase in plasma triglycerol concentration, all consistent with an increased risk of CHD. Conversely, interventional studies show that when fat intakes are high, many individuals gain additional weight. Weight gain on high-fat diets can be detrimental to individuals already susceptible to obesity and will worsen the metabolic consequences of obesity, particularly risk of CHD. Moreover, high-fat diets are usually accompanied by increased intakes of saturated fatty acids that can raise plasma LDL cholesterol concentrations and further heighten risk for CHD. Based on the apparent risk for CHD that may occur on both low- and high-fat diets, and the increased risk for CHD at higher carbohydrate intakes, an AMDR for fat and carbohydrate is estimated to be 20 to 35 and 45 to 65 percent of energy, respectively, for all adults. By consuming fat and carbohydrate within these ranges, the risk for CHD, as well as obesity and diabetes, may be kept to a minimum. Furthermore, these ranges allow for sufficient intakes of essential nutrients, while keeping the intake of saturated fat at moderate levels. To complement these ranges, the AMDR for protein is 10 to 35 percent of energy.

Based on usual median intakes of energy, it is estimated that a lower boundary level of 5 percent of energy will meet the Adequate Intake for linoleic acid. An upper boundary for linoleic acid is set at 10 percent of energy for three reasons: 1) individual dietary intakes of linoleic acid in the North American population rarely exceed 10 percent of energy, 2) epidemiological evidence for safety of intakes greater than 10 percent of energy are generally lacking, and 3) high intakes of linoleic acid create a pro-oxidant state that may predispose to several chronic diseases such as CHD and cancer. Therefore, an AMDR of 5 to 10 percent of energy is suggested for linoleic acid.

The AMDR for α-linolenic acid is set at 0.6 to 1.2 percent of energy. Up to 10 percent of this range can be consumed as eicosapentaenoic acid (EPA) and/or docosahexaenoic acid (DHA). The lower boundary of the range meets the Adequate Intake for α-linolenic acid. The upper boundary corresponds to the highest intakes from foods consumed by individuals in the United States and Canada. A growing body of literature suggests that diets higher in α-linolenic acid, EPA and DHA may afford some degree of protection against CHD. Because the physiological potency of EPA and DHA is much greater than that for α-linolenic acid, it is not possible to estimate one AMDR for all n-3 fatty acids.

A maximal intake of 25 percent of energy from added sugars is suggested. This maximal intake level is based on

ensuring sufficient intakes of essential micronutrients that are for the most part present in relatively low amounts in foods and beverages that are major source of added sugars in North American diets (IOM, 2002:S5–6).

A-2-b-6. Cholesterol Summary

Cholesterol plays an important role in steroid hormone and bile acid biosynthesis, and serves as an integral component of cell membranes. Given the capability of all tissues to synthesize sufficient amounts of cholesterol for their metabolic and structural needs, there is no evidence for a biologic requirement for dietary cholesterol. Therefore, neither an Adequate Intake nor Recommended Dietary Allowance was set for cholesterol.

There is much evidence to indicate a positive linear trend between cholesterol intake and low-density lipoprotein cholesterol concentration, and therefore increased risk of coronary heart disease (CHD). A Tolerable Upper Intake Level is not set for cholesterol because any incremental increase in cholesterol intake increases CHD risk. Because cholesterol is unavoidable in ordinary diets, eliminating cholesterol in the diet would require significant changes in patterns of dietary intake. Such significant adjustments may introduce undesirable effects (e.g., inadequate intakes of protein and certain micronutrients) and unknown and unquantifiable health risks. Nonetheless, it is possible to have a diet low in cholesterol while consuming a nutritionally adequate diet (IOM, 2002:9–1).

A-2-b-7. Water, Potassium, Sodium, Chloride, and Sulfate (IOM, 2004)

This volume provides a detailed review and summary of the biochemical and physiologic aspects of the controlling organ systems for absorption, utilization, and excretion of water and these ions, their body distribution, hormonal factors influencing them and their nutritional requirements in health and disease. Average intakes are given for all by lifestage groups (Appendix Tables A-2-d-8 thru A-2-d-11). Tolerable upper limits are also given for sodium and for chloride.

A-2-c. Reference Weights and Heights for Children and Adults in the United States

The reference weights and heights selected for children and adults are shown in Table A-2-c-1. These values were based on anthropometric data collected from 1988 to 1994 as part of the Third National Health and Nutrition Examination Survey (NHANES III) in the United States. When extrapolation to a different age group was conducted, these reference weights were used, except for iron, which used weights with known coefficients of variation that were required for factorial modeling. The median heights for the life stage and gender groups

TABLE A-2-c-1. REFERENCE HEIGHTS AND WEIGHTS FOR CHILDREN AND ADULTS IN THE UNITED STATES[a]

GENDER	AGE	MEDIAN BODY MASS INDEX (kg/m²)	REFERENCE HEIGHT, cm (in)	REFERENCE WEIGHT[b] kg (lb)
Male, female	2–6 mo	—	64 (25)	7 (16)
	7–11 mo	—	72 (28)	9 (20)
	1–3 y	—	91 (36)	13 (29)
	4–8 y	15.8	118 (46)	22 (48)
Male	9–13 y	18.5	147 (58)	40 (88)
	14–18 y	21.3	174 (68)	64 (142)
	19–30 y	24.4	176 (69)	76 (166)
Female	9–13 y	18.3	148 (58)	40 (88)
	14–18 y	21.3	163 (64)	57 (125)
	19–30 y	22.8	163 (64)	61 (133)

[a] Adapted from the Third National Health and Nutrition Examination Survey (NHANES III), 1988–1994.
[b] Calculated from body mass index and height for ages 4 through 8 years and older.

From Food and Nutrition Board, IOM. Dietary Reference Intakes for Vitamin A, Vitamin K, Arsenic, Boron, Chromium, Copper, Iodine, Iron, Manganese, Molybdeum, Nickel, Silicon, Vanadium, and Zinc. Washington, DC: National Academy Press, 2001:772.

through age 30 years were identified, and the median weights for these heights were based on reported median body mass index (BMI) for the same individuals. Because there is no evidence that weight should change as adults age if activity is maintained, the reference weights for adults ages 19 through 30 years were applied to all adult age groups. The reference weights chosen for this report were based on the most recent data set available from either country, with recognition that earlier surveys in Canada indicated shorter stature and lower weights during adolescence than did surveys in the United States. Reference weights are used primarily estimated when setting the Requirement or Tol-erable Upper Intake Level for children or when relating the nutrient needs of adults to body weight. This table was referenced in IOM 1997–2001b (IOM, 2001b:41).

Table A2-c-2 is based on new data on male and female body mass index and height for age data from the Centers for Disease Control and Prevention/National Center for Health Statistics Growth Charts. (IOM, 2002) (See Appendix Tables A-14-a to A-14-d). Ref. (Kuczmarski RJ, Ogden CL, Grummer-Strawn LM et al. CDC Growth Charts: United States Advance Data from Vital and Health Statistics. Hyattsville, MD:NCHS, 2002: 314:1–28.).

TABLE A-2-c-2. NEW REFERENCE HEIGHTS AND WEIGHTS FOR CHILDREN AND ADULTS IN THE UNITED STATES

SEX	AGE	PREVIOUS MEDIAN BODY MASS INDEX[a] (kg/m²)	NEW MEDIAN BODY MASS INDEX[b] (kg/m²)	NEW MEDIAN REFERENCE HEIGHT[b], cm (in)	NEW REFERENCE WEIGHT[c] kg (lb)
Male, female	2–6 mo	—	—	62 (24)	6 (13)
	7–12 mo	—	—	71 (28)	9 (20)
	1–3 y	—	—	86 (34)	12 (27)
	4–8 y	15.8	15.3	115 (45)	20 (44)
Male	9–13 y	18.5	17.2	144 (57)	36 (79)
	14–18 y	21.3	20.5	174 (68)	61 (134)
	19–30 y	24.4	22.5	177 (70)	70 (154)
Female	9–13 y	18.3	17.4	144 (57)	37 (81)
	14–18 y	21.3	20.4	163 (64)	54 (119)
	19–30 y	22.8	21.5	163 (64)	57 (126)

[a] Taken from male and female median Body Mass Index and height-for-age data from the Third National Health and Nutrition Examination Survey (NHANES III), 1988–1994; used in earlier DRI reports (IOM 1997, 1998, 2000a, 2000b, 2001).
[b] Taken from new data on male and female median body mass index and height-for-age data from the Centers for Disease Control and Prevention/National Center for Health Statistics Growth Charts (Kuczmarski et al., 2000).
[c] Calculated from CDC/NCHS Growth Charts (Kuczmarski et al., 2000); median body mass index and median height for ages 4 through 19 years.

From Food and Nutrition Board, IOM. Dietary Reference Intakes for Energy, Carbohydrate, Fiber, Fat, Fatty Acids, Cholesterol, Protein, and Amino Acids. Washington, DC: National Academy Press, 2002.

A-2-d. Criteria and Dietary Reference Intakes by Life-Stage Group

TABLE A-2-d-1-a. CRITERIA AND DIETARY REFERENCE INTAKE VALUES FOR ENERGY BY ACTIVE INDIVIDUALS BY LIFE-STAGE GROUP[a]

		ACTIVE PAL[b] EER (kcal/d)	
LIFE-STAGE GROUP	CRITERION	MALE	FEMALE
0 through 6 mo	Energy expenditure plus energy deposition	570	520 (3 mo)
7 through 12 mo	Energy expenditure plus energy deposition	743	676 (9 mo)
1 through 2 y	Energy expenditure plus energy deposition	1,046	992 (24 mo)
3 through 8 y	Energy expenditure plus energy deposition	1,742	1,642 (6 y)
9 through 13 y	Energy expenditure plus energy deposition	2,279	2,071 (11 y)
14 through 18 y	Energy expenditure plus energy deposition	3,152	2,368 (16 y)
>18 y	Energy expenditure	3,067[c]	2,403[c] (19 y)
Pregnancy			
14 through 18 y	Adolescent female EER plus change in TEE		
1st trimester	plus pregnancy energy deposition		2,368 (16 y)
2nd trimester			2,708 (16 y)
3rd trimester			2,820 (16 y)
19 through 50 y	Adult female EER plus change in TEE plus		
1st trimester	pregnancy energy deposition		2,403[c] (19 y)
2nd trimester			2,743[c] (19 y)
3rd trimester			2,855[c] (19 y)
Lactation			
14 through 18 y	Adolescent female EER plus milk energy		
1st 6 mo	output minus weight loss		2,698 (16 y)
2nd 6 mo			2,768 (16 y)
19 through 50 y	Adult female EER plus milk energy output		
1st 6 mo	minus weight loss		2,733[c] (19 y)
2nd 6 mo			2,803[c] (19 y)

[a] For healthy moderately active Americans and Canadians.

[b] PAL, physical activity level; EER, estimated energy requirement; TEE, total energy expenditure. The intake that meets the average energy expenditure of individuals at the reference height, weight, and age.

[c] Subtract 10 kcal/d for males and 7 kcal/d for females for each year of age above 19 y.

Addendum from text for A-2-d-1-a: The EER during pregnancy is derived from the sum of the TEE of the woman in the nonpregnant state plus median change in TEE of 8 kcal/wk plus the energy deposition during pregnancy of 180 kcal/d. Because TEE changes little and weight gain is minor during the first trimester, the additional energy is recommended during the second and third trimester only (IOM, 2002:5–62).

See Table A-2-d-1-b footnote for the physical activity coefficients for the various levels of physical activity (Appendices Editors).

From Food and Nutrition Board, IOM. Dietary Reference Intakes for Energy, Carbohydrate, Fiber, Fat, Fatty Acids, Cholesterol, Protein, and Amino Acids. Washington, DC: National Academy Press, 2002. This is Table S-1, p S-10, in this reference.

TABLE A-2-d-1-b. ESTIMATED ENERGY REQUIREMENTS (EER) FOR MEN AND WOMEN 30 YEARS OF AGE[a]

HT (m [in])	PAL[b]	WEIGHT FOR BMI OF 18.5 kg/m² (kg [lb])	WEIGHT FOR BMI OF 24.99 kg/m² (kg [lb])	EER, MEN (kcal/d) BMI OF 18.5 kg/m²	BMI OF 24.99 kg/m²	EER, WOMEN (kcal/d) BMI OF 18.5 kg/m²	BMI OF 24.99 kg/m²
1.45 (57)	Sedentary	38.9 (86)	52.5 (116)	1,777	1,994	1,564	1,691
	Low active			1,931	2,172	1,734	1,877
	Active			2,127	2,399	1,946	2,108
	Very active			2,450	2,771	2,201	2,386
1.50 (59)	Sedentary	41.6 (92)	56.2 (124)	1,848	2,080	1,625	1,762
	Low active			2,009	2,267	1,803	1,956
	Active			2,215	2,506	2,025	2,198
	Very active			2,554	2,898	2,291	2,489
1.55 (61)	Sedentary	44.4 (98)	60.0 (132)	1,919	2,167	1,688	1,834
	Low active			2,089	2,365	1,873	2,037
	Active			2,305	2,615	2,104	2,290
	Very active			2,660	3,027	2,382	2,593
1.60 (63)	Sedentary	47.4 (104)	64.0 (141)	1,993	2,257	1,752	1,907
	Low active			2,171	2,464	1,944	2,118
	Active			2,397	2,727	2,185	2,383
	Very active			2,769	3,160	2,474	2,699
1.65 (65)	Sedentary	50.4 (111)	68.0 (150)	2,068	2,349	1,816	1,982
	Low active			2,254	2,566	2,016	2,202
	Active			2,490	2,842	2,267	2,477
	Very active			2,880	3,296	2,567	2,807
1.70 (67)	Sedentary	53.5 (118)	72.2 (159)	2,144	2,442	1,881	2,057
	Low active			2,338	2,670	2,090	2,286
	Active			2,586	2,959	2,350	2,573
	Very active			2,992	3,434	2,662	2,917
1.75 (69)	Sedentary	56.7 (125)	76.5 (169)	2,222	2,538	1,948	2,134
	Low active			2,425	2,776	2,164	2,372
	Active			2,683	3,078	2,434	2,670
	Very active			3,108	3,576	2,758	3,028
1.80 (71)	Sedentary	59.9 (132)	81.0 (178)	2,301	2,635	2,015	2,211
	Low active			2,513	2,884	2,239	2,459
	Active			2,782	3,200	2,519	2,769
	Very active			3,225	3,720	2,855	3,141
1.85 (73)	Sedentary	63.3 (139)	85.5 (188)	2,382	2,735	2,083	2,290
	Low active			2,602	2,994	2,315	2,548
	Active			2,883	3,325	2,605	2,869
	Very active			3,344	3,867	2,954	3,255
1.90 (75)	Sedentary	66.8 (147)	90.2 (199)	2,464	2,836	2,151	2,371
	Low active			2,693	3,107	2,392	2,637
	Active			2,986	3,452	2,693	2,971
	Very active			3,466	4,018	3,053	3,371
1.95 (77)	Sedentary	70.3 (155)	95.0 (209)	2,547	2,940	2,221	2,452
	Low active			2,786	3,222	2,470	2,729
	Active			3,090	3,581	2,781	3,074
	Very active			3,590	4,171	3,154	3,489

[a] For each year below 30, add 7 kcal/day for women and 10 kcal/day for men. For each year above 30, subtract 7 kcal/day for women and 10 kcal/day for men.

[b] PAL = Physical activity level.

Where PA is the physical activity coefficient:

PA = 1.00 if PAL is estimated to be ≥ 1.0 < 1.4 (Sedentary)

PA = 1.12 if PAL is estimated to be ≥ 1.4 < 1.6 (Low Active)

PA = 1.27 if PAL is estimated to be ≥ 1.6 < 1.9 (Active)

PA = 1.45 if PAL is estimated to be ≥ 1.9 < 2.5 (Very Active)

Addendum from *text*:

Because of the direct impact of deviations from energy balance on body weight and of changes in body weight, body weight data represent critical indicators of the adequacy of energy intake. Energy requirements are defined as the amounts of energy that need to be consumed by individuals to sustain stable body weights in the range desired for good health (BMI from 18.5 up to 25 kg/m²) while maintaining lifestyles that include adequate levels of physical activity. Since any energy intakes above the Estimated Energy Requirement (EER) would be expected to result in weight gain and a likely increased risk of morbidity, the UL method is not applicable to energy. If weight gain was identified as the hazard, the lowest-observed-adverse-effect level (LOAEL) would be any intake above the EER for adults and the uncertainty factor would be one as there is no uncertainty in the fact that overconsumption of energy leads to weight gain. Thus, because of the adverse effects of excess weight gain, a UL for energy is not established, (Jony, 2002: 5–83).

From Food and Nutrition Board, IOM. Dietary Reference Intakes for Energy, Carbohydrate, Fiber, Fat, Fatty Acids, Cholesterol, Protein, and Amino Acids. Washington, DC: National Academy Press, 2002. This is Table 5-22 on p 5-58 in this reference.

TABLE A-2-d-2. CRITERIA AND DIETARY REFERENCE INTAKE VALUES FOR CARBOHYDRATE BY LIFE-STAGE GROUP

LIFE-STAGE GROUP	CRITERION	EAR (g/d)[a] MALE	EAR (g/d)[a] FEMALE	RDA (g/d)[b] MALE	RDA (g/d)[b] FEMALE	AI (g/d)[c]
0 through 6 mo	Average content of human milk					60
7 through 12 mo	Average intake from human milk plus complementary foods					95
1 through 3 y	Extrapolation from adult data	100	100	130	130	
4 through 8 y	Extrapolation from adult data	100	100	130	130	
9 through 13 y	Extrapolation from adult data	100	100	130	130	
14 through 18 y	Extrapolation from adult data	100	100	130	130	
>18 y	Brain glucose utilization	100	100	130	130	
Pregnancy						
14 through 18 y	Adolescent female EAR plus fetal brain glucose utilization		135		175	
19 through 50 y	Adult female EAR plus fetal brain glucose utilization		135		175	
Lactation						
14 through 18 y	Adolescent female EAR plus average human milk content of carbohydrate		160		210	
19 through 50 y	Adult female EAR plus average human milk content of carbohydrate		160		210	

[a] EAR, Estimated Average Requirement. The intake that meets the estimated nutrient needs of half of the individuals in a group.

[b] RDA, Recommended Dietary Allowance. The intake that meets the nutrient need of almost all (97–98%) of individuals in a group.

[c] AI, Adequate Intake. The observed average or experimentally determined intake by a defined population or subgroup that appears to sustain a defined nutritional status, such as growth rate, normal circulating nutrient values, or other functional indicators of health. The AI is used if sufficient scientific evidence is not available to derive an EAR. For healthy infants receiving human milk, the AI is the mean intake. **The AI is not equivalent to an RDA**.

From Food and Nutrition Board, IOM. Dietary Reference Intakes for Energy, Carbohydrate, Fiber, Fat, Fatty Acids, Cholesterol, Protein, and Amino Acids. Washington, DC: National Academy Press, 2002. This is Table S-2, p S-11, in this reference.

TABLE A-2-d-3. CRITERIA AND DIETARY REFERENCE INTAKE VALUES FOR *TOTAL FIBER* BY LIFE-STAGE GROUP

LIFE-STAGE GROUP	CRITERION	AI (g/d)[a]	
		MALE	FEMALE
0 through 6 mo		ND[b]	ND
7 through 12 mo		ND	ND
1 through 3 y	Intake level shown to provide the greatest protection against coronary heart disease (14 g/1,000 kcal) × median energy intake level (kcal/1,000 kcal/d)	19	19
4 through 8 y	Intake level shown to provide the greatest protection against coronary heart disease (14 g/1,000 kcal) × median energy intake level (kcal/1,000 kcal/d)	25	25
9 through 13 y	Intake level shown to provide the greatest protection against coronary heart disease (14 g/1,000 kcal) × median energy intake level (kcal/1,000 kcal/d)	31	26
14 through 18 y		38	36
19 through 30 y	Intake level shown to provide the greatest protection against coronary heart disease (14 g/1,000 kcal) × median energy intake level (kcal/1,000 kcal/d)	38	25
31 through 50 y	Intake level shown to provide the greatest protection against coronary heart disease (14 g/1,000 kcal) × median energy intake level (kcal/1,000 kcal/d)	38	25
51 through 70 y	Intake level shown to provide the greatest protection against coronary heart disease (14 g/1,000 kcal) × median energy intake level (kcal/1,000 kcal/d)	30	21
>70 y	Intake level shown to provide the greatest protection against coronary heart disease (14 g/1,000 kcal) × median energy intake level (kcal/1,000 kcal/d)	30	21
Pregnancy			
14 through 18 y	Intake level shown to provide the greatest protection against coronary heart disease (14 g/1,000 kcal) × median energy intake level (kcal/1,000 kcal/d)		28
19 through 50 y	Intake level shown to provide the greatest protection against coronary heart disease (14 g/1,000 kcal) × median energy intake level (kcal/1,000 kcal/d)		28
Lactation			
14 through 18 y	Intake level shown to provide the greatest protection against coronary heart disease (14 g/1,000 kcal) × median energy intake level (kcal/1,000 kcal/d)		29
19 through 50 y	Intake level shown to provide the greatest protection against coronary heart disease (14 g/1,000 kcal) × median energy intake level (kcal/1,000 kcal/d)		29

[a] AI, Adequate Intake. Based on 14 g/1,000 kcal of required energy.

[b] ND, not determined. The observed average or experimentally determined intake by a defined population or subgroup that appears to sustain a defined nutritional status, such as growth rate, normal circulating nutrient values, or other functional indicators of health. The AI is used if sufficient scientific evidence is not available to derive an Estimated Average Requirement (EAR). For healthy infants receiving human milk, the AI is the mean intake. **The AI is not equivalent to an RDA.**

From Food and Nutrition Board, IOM. Dietary Reference Intakes for Energy, Carbohydrate, Fiber, Fat, Fatty Acids, Cholesterol, Protein, and Amino Acids. Washington, DC: National Academy Press, 2002. This is Table S-3, p S-12, in this reference.

TABLE A-2-d-4. CRITERIA AND DIETARY REFERENCE INTAKE VALUES FOR TOTAL FAT BY LIFE-STAGE GROUP

LIFE-STAGE GROUP	CRITERION	AI (g/d)[a]	
		MALE	FEMALE
0 through 6 mo	Average consumption of total fat from human milk	31	31
7 through 12 mo	Average consumption of total fat from human milk and complementary foods	30	30
1 through 3 y		ND[b]	ND
4 through 8 y		ND	ND
9 through 13 y		ND	ND
14 through 18 y		ND	ND
>18 y		ND	ND
Pregnancy		ND	ND
14 through 18 y		ND	ND
19 through 50 y		ND	ND
Lactation		ND	ND
14 through 18 y		ND	ND
19 through 50 y		ND	ND

[a] AI, Adequate Intake.

[b] ND, not determined. The observed average or experimentally determined intake by a defined population or subgroup that appears to sustain a defined nutritional status, such as growth rate, normal circulating nutrient values, or other functional indicators of health. The AI is used if sufficient scientific evidence is not available to derive an Estimated Average Requirement (EAR). For healthy infants receiving human milk, the AI is the mean intake. **The AI is not equivalent to an RDA.**

From Food and Nutrition Board, IOM. Dietary Reference Intakes for Energy, Carbohydrate, Fiber, Fat, Fatty Acids, Cholesterol, Protein, and Amino Acids. Washington, DC: National Academy Press, 2002. This is Table S-4, p S-13, in this reference.

TABLE A-2-D-5. CRITERIA AND DIETARY REFERENCE INTAKE VALUES FOR *n*-6 POLYUNSATURATED FATTY ACIDS (LINOLEIC ACID) BY LIFE-STAGE GROUP

LIFE-STAGE GROUP	CRITERION	AI (g/d)[a]	
		MALE	FEMALE
0 through 6 mo	Average consumption of total *n*-6 fatty acids from human milk	4.4	4.4
7 through 12 mo	Average consumption of total *n*-6 fatty acids from human milk and complementary foods	4.6	4.6
1 through 3 y	Median intake of linoleic acid from CFSII[b]	7	7
4 through 8 y	Median intake of linoleic acid from CFSII	10	10
9 through 13 y	Median intake of linoleic acid from CFSII	12	10
14 through 18 y	Median intake of linoleic acid from CFSII	16	11
19 through 30 y	Median intake of linoleic acid from CFSII	17	12
31 through 50 y	Median intake of linoleic acid from CFSII	17	12
51 through 70 y	Median intake of linoleic acid from CFSII	14	11
>70 y	Median intake of linoleic acid from CFSII	14	11
Pregnancy			
14 through 18 y	Median intake of linoleic acid from CFSII		13
19 through 50 y	Median intake of linoleic acid from CFSII		13
Lactation			
14 through 18 y	Median intake of linoleic acid from CFSII		13
19 through 50 y	Median intake of linoleic acid from CFSII		13

[a] AI, Adequate Intake. The observed average or experimentally determined intake by a defined population or subgroup that appears to sustain a defined nutritional status, such as growth rate, normal circulating nutrient values, or other functional indicators of health. The AI is used if sufficient scientific evidence is not available to derive an Estimated Average Requirement (EAR). For healthy infants receiving human milk, the AI is the mean intake. **The AI is not equivalent to an RDA.**

[b] CSFII, Continuing Survey of Food Intake by Individuals.

From Food and Nutrition Board, IOM. Dietary Reference Intakes for Energy, Carbohydrate, Fiber, Fat, Fatty Acids, Cholesterol, Protein, and Amino Acids. Washington, DC: National Academy Press, 2002. This is Table S-5, p S-14, in this reference.

TABLE A-2-d-6. CRITERIA AND DIETARY REFERENCE INTAKE VALUES FOR *n*-3 POLYUNSATURATED FATTY ACIDS (α-LINOLENIC ACID) BY LIFE-STAGE GROUP

LIFE-STAGE GROUP	CRITERION	AI (g/d)[a]	
		MALE	FEMALE
0 through 6 mo	Average consumption of total *n*-3 fatty acids from human milk	0.5	0.5
7 through 12 mo	Average consumption of total *n*-3 fatty acids from human milk and complementary foods	0.5	0.5
1 through 3 y	Median intake of α-linolenic acid from CFSII[b]	0.7	0.7
4 through 8 y	Median intake of α-linolenic acid from CFSII	0.9	0.9
9 through 13 y	Median intake of α-linolenic acid from CFSII	1.2	1.0
14 through 18 y	Median intake of α-linolenic acid from CFSII	1.6	1.1
19 through 30 y	Median intake of α-linolenic acid from CFSII	1.6	1.1
31 through 50 y	Median intake of α-linolenic acid from CFSII	1.6	1.1
51 through 70 y	Median intake of α-linolenic acid from CFSII	1.6	1.1
>70 y		1.6	1.1
Pregnancy			
14 through 18 y	Median intake of α-linolenic acid from CFSII		1.4
19 through 50 y	Median intake of α-linolenic acid from CFSII		1.4
Lactation			
14 through 18 y	Median intake of α-linolenic acid from CFSII		1.3
19 through 50 y	Median intake of α-linolenic acid from CFSII		1.3

[a] AI, Adequate Intake. The observed average or experimentally determined intake by a defined population or subgroup that appears to sustain a defined nutritional status, such as growth rate, normal circulating nutrient values, or other functional indicators of health. The AI is used if sufficient scientific evidence is not available to derive an Estimated Average Requirement (EAR). For healthy infants receiving human milk, the AI is the mean intake. **The AI is not equivalent to an RDA.**
[b] CSFII, Continuing Survey of Food Intake by Individuals.

From Food and Nutrition Board, IOM. Dietary Reference Intakes for Energy, Carbohydrate, Fiber, Fat, Fatty Acids, Cholesterol, Protein, and Amino Acids. Washington, DC: National Academy Press, 2002. This is Table S-6, p S-15, in this reference.

TABLE A-2-d-7. CRITERIA AND DIETARY REFERENCE INTAKE VALUES FOR PROTEIN BY LIFE-STAGE GROUP

LIFE-STAGE GROUP	CRITERION	AI OR RDA FOR REFERENCE INDIVIDUAL (g/d)		EAR (g/kg/d)[a]		RDA (g/kg/d)[b]		AI
		MALES	FEMALES	MALES	FEMALES	MALES	FEMALES	(g/kg/d)[c]
0 through 6 mo	Average consumption of protein from human milk	9.1 (AI)	9.1 (AI)					1.52
7 through 12 mo	Nitrogen equilibrium + protein deposition	13.5	13.5	1.1	1.1	1.5	1.5	
1 through 3 y	Nitrogen equilibrium + protein deposition	13	13	0.88	0.88	1.10	1.10	
4 through 8 y	Nitrogen equilibrium + protein deposition	19	19	0.76	0.76	0.95	0.95	
9 through 13 y	Nitrogen equilibrium + protein deposition	34	34	0.76	0.76	0.95	0.95	
14 through 18 y	Nitrogen equilibrium + protein deposition	52	46	0.73	0.71	0.85	0.85	
>18 y	Nitrogen equilibrium	56	46	0.66	0.66	0.80	0.80	

[a] EAR, Estimated Average Requirement. The intake that meets the estimated nutrient needs of half of the individuals in a group.
[b] RDA, Recommended Dietary Allowance. The intake that meets the nutrient need of almost all (97–98%) of individuals in a group.
[c] AI, Adequate Intake. The observed average or experimentally determined intake by a defined population or subgroup that appears to sustain a defined nutritional status, such as growth rate, normal circulating nutrient values, or other functional indicators of health. The AI is used if sufficient scientific evidence is not available to derive an EAR. For healthy infants receiving human milk, the AI is the mean intake. **The AI is not equivalent to an RDA.**
[d] The EAR and RDA for pregnancy are only for the second half of pregnancy. For the first half of pregnancy the protein requirements are the same as those of the nonpregnant woman.
[e] In addition to the EAR and RDA of the nonlactating adolescent or woman.

From Food and Nutrition Board, IOM. Dietary Reference Intakes for Energy, Carbohydrate, Fiber, Fat, Fatty Acids, Cholesterol, Protein, and Amino Acids. Washington, DC: National Academy Press, 2002. This is Table S-7, p S-16, in this reference.

TABLE A-2-d-8. CRITERIA AND DIETARY REFERENCE INTAKE VALUES[a] FOR *TOTAL* WATER[b]

LIFE-STAGE GROUP	CRITERION	AI[c] (L/d) MALE		
		FROM FOODS	FROM BEVERAGES	*TOTAL* WATER
0 through 6 mo	Average consumption of water from human milk	0	0.7	0.7
			0.6	0.8
7 through 12 mo	Average consumption of water from human milk and complementary foods	0.2	0.9	1.3
			1.2	1.7
1 through 3 y	Median total water intake from NHANES III	0.4	1.8	2.4
4 through 8 y	Median total water intake from NHANES III	0.5	2.6	3.3
9 through 13 y	Median total water intake from NHANES III	0.6	3.0	3.7
14 through 18 y	Median total water intake from NHANES III	0.7		
>19 y	Median total water intake from NHANES III	0.7		
Pregnancy				
14 through 50 y	Median total water intake from NHANES III			
Lactation				
14 through 50 y	Median total water intake from NHANES III			

LIFE-STAGE GROUP	CRITERION	FEMALE		
		FROM FOODS	FROM BEVERAGES	*TOTAL* WATER
Pregnancy				
14 through 50 y	Median total water intake from NHANES III	0	0.7	0.7
Lactation		0.2	0.6	0.8
14 through 50 y	Median total water intake from NHANES III	0.4	0.9	1.3
		0.5	1.2	1.7
		0.5	1.6	2.1
		0.5	1.8	2.3
		0.5	2.2	2.7
		0.7	2.3	3.0
		0.7	3.1	3.8

[a] No UL established; however, maximal capacity to excrete excess water in individuals with normal kidney function approximately 0.7 L/hour.

[b] *Total* water represents drinking water, other beverages, and water from food.

[c] AI, Adequate Intake. The observed average or experimentally determined intake by a defined population or subgroup that appears to sustain a defined nutritional status, such as growth rate, normal circulating nutrient values, or other functional indicators of health. The AI is used if sufficient scientific evidence is not available to derive an EAR. **The AI is not equivalent to an RDA.**

From Food and Nutrition Board, IOM. Dietary Reference Intakes for Water, Potassium, Sodium, Chloride, and Sulfate. Washington, DC: National Academy Press, 2004. This is Table S-2, pp S-6 and 7, in this reference (reorganized).

TABLE A-2-d-9. CRITERIA AND DIETARY REFERENCE INTAKE VALUES[a] FOR POTASSIUM BY LIFE-STAGE GROUP

LIFE-STAGE GROUP	CRITERION	AI (g/day)[b]	
		MALE	FEMALE
0 through 6 mo	Average consumption of potassium from human milk	0.4	0.4
7 through 12 mo	Average consumption of potassium from human milk and complementary foods	0.7	0.7
1 through 3 y	Extrapolation of Adult AI based on energy intake	3.0	3.0
4 through 8 y	Extrapolation of Adult AI based on energy intake	3.8	3.8
9 through 13 y	Extrapolation of Adult AI based on energy intake	4.5	4.5
14 through 18 y	Extrapolation of Adult AI based on energy intake	4.7	4.7
>18 y	Intake level to lower blood pressure, reduce the extent of salt sensitivity, and to minimize the risk of kidney stones	4.7	4.7
Pregnancy			
14 through 50 y	Intake level to lower blood pressure, reduce the extent of salt sensitivity, and to minimize the risk of kidney stones		4.7
Lactation			
14 through 50 y	Intake level to lower blood pressure, reduce the extent of salt sensitivity, and to minimize the risk of kidney stones plus the amount of potassium in breast milk (0.4 g/d)		5.1

[a] No UL is established; however, caution is warranted given concerns about adverse effects when consuming excess amounts of potassium from potassium supplements while on drug therapy or in the presence of undiagnosed chronic disease.

[b] AI, Adequate Intake. The observed average or experimentally determined intake by a defined population or subgroup that appears to sustain a defined nutritional status, such as growth rate, normal circulating nutrient values, or other functional indicators of health. The AI is used if sufficient scientific evidence is not available to derive an EAR. **The AI is not equivalent to an RDA.**

From Food and Nutrition Board, IOM. Dietary Reference Intakes for Water, Potassium, Sodium, Chloride, and Sulfate. Washington, DC: National Academy Press, 2004. This is Table S-3, p S-8, in this reference.

TABLE A-2-d-10. CRITERIA AND DIETARY REFERENCE INTAKE VALUES FOR SODIUM

LIFE-STAGE GROUP	CRITERION FOR AI	AI[a] (g/d) MALE	FEMALE	UL[b] (g/d) MALE	FEMALE
0 through 6 mo	Average consumption of sodium from human milk	0.12	0.12	ND[c]	ND
7 through 12 mo	Average consumption of sodium from human milk and complementary foods	0.37	0.37	ND	ND
1 through 3 y	Extrapolation of Adult AI based on energy intake	1.0	1.0	1.5	1.5
4 through 8 y	Extrapolation of Adult AI based on energy intake	1.2	1.2	1.9	1.9
9 through 13 y	Extrapolation of Adult AI based on energy intake	1.5	1.5	2.2	2.2
14 through 18 y	Extrapolation of Adult AI based on energy intake	1.5	1.5	2.3	2.3
19 through 50 y	Intake level to cover possible daily losses, provide adequate intakes of other nutrients, and maintain normal function	1.5	1.5	2.3	2.3
51 through 70 y	Extrapolated from younger adults based on energy intake	1.3	1.3	2.3	2.3
>70 y	Extrapolated from younger adults based on energy	1.2	1.2	2.3	2.3
Pregnancy 14 through 50 y	Same as non-pregnant women		1.5		2.3
Lactation 14 through 50 y	Same as non-lactating women		1.5		2.3

[a] AI, Adequate Intake. The observed average or experimentally determined intake by a defined population or subgroup that appears to sustain a defined nutritional status, such as growth rate, normal circulating nutrient values, or other functional indicators of health. The AI is used if sufficient scientific evidence is not available to derive an EAR. **The AI is not equivalent to an RDA.**
[b] UL, Tolerable Upper Intake Level. Based on prevention of increased blood pressure.
[c] ND, Not determined. Intake should be from food or formula only.

From Food and Nutrition Board, IOM. Dietary Reference Intakes for Water, Potassium, Sodium, Chloride, and Sulfate. Washington, DC: National Academy Press, 2004. This is Table S-4, pp S-10 and 11, in this reference.

TABLE A-2-d-11. DIETARY REFERENCE INTAKE VALUES FOR CHLORIDE[*]

LIFE-STAGE GROUP	AI (g/d) MALE	FEMALE	TOLERABLE UPPER LIMIT (UL) (g/d)
0 through 6 mo		0.18	not set
7 through 12 mo		0.57	not set
1 through 3 y		1.5	2.3
4 through 8 y		1.9	2.9
9 through 13 y	2.3	2.3	3.4
14 through 18 y	2.3	2.3	3.6
19 through 30 y	2.3	2.3	3.6
31 through 50 y	2.3	2.3	3.6
51 through 70 y	2.0	2.0	3.6
>70 y	1.8	1.8	3.6
Pregnancy (14 through 50 y)		2.3	3.6
Lactation (14 through 50 y)		2.3	3.6

AI, Average Intake.
[*] Data taken from text in Chapter 6 of Food and Nutrition Board, IOM. Dietary Reference Intakes for Water, Potassium, Sodium, Chloride, and Sulfate. Washington, DC: National Academy Press, 2004.

TABLE A-2-e. RECOMMENDED INTAKES FOR INDIVIDUALS, VITAMINS, DIETARY REFERENCE INTAKES AND FOOD AND NUTRITION BOARD, INSTITUTE OF MEDICINE-NATIONAL ACADEMY OF SCIENCES

LIFE-STAGE GROUP	VITAMIN A (µg/d)[a]	VITAMIN C (mg/d)	VITAMIN D (µg/d)[b,c]	VITAMIN E (mg/d)[d]	VITAMIN K (µg/d)	THIAMIN (mg/d)	RIBOFLAVIN (mg/d)	NIACIN (mg/d)[e]	VITAMIN B6 (mg/d)	FOLATE (µg/d)[f]	VITAMIN B12 (µg/d)	PANTOTHENIC ACID (mg/d)	BIOTIN (µg/d)	CHOLINE (mg/d)[g]
Infants														
0–6 mo	400*	40*	5*	4*	2.0*	0.2*	0.3*	2*	0.1*	65*	0.4*	1.7*	5*	125*
7–12 mo	500*	50*	5*	5*	2.5*	0.3*	0.4*	4*	0.3*	80*	0.5*	1.8*	6*	150*
Children														
1–3 y	300	15	5*	6	30*	0.5	0.5	6	0.5	150	0.9	2*	8*	200*
4–8 y	400	25	5*	7	55*	0.6	0.6	8	0.6	200	1.2	3*	12*	250*
Males														
9–13 y	600	45	5*	11	60*	0.9	0.9	12	1.0	300	1.8	4*	20*	375*
14–18 y	900	75	5*	15	75*	1.2	1.3	16	1.3	400	2.4	5*	25*	550*
19–30 y	900	90	5*	15	120*	1.2	1.3	16	1.3	400	2.4	5*	30*	550*
31–50 y	900	90	5*	15	120*	1.2	1.3	16	1.3	400	2.4	5*	30*	550*
51–70 y	900	90	10*	15	120*	1.2	1.3	16	1.7	400	2.4[h]	5*	30*	550*
>70 y	900	90	15*	15	120*	1.2	1.3	16	1.7	400	2.4[h]	5*	30*	550*
Females														
9–13 y	600	45	5*	11	60*	0.9	0.9	12	1.0	300	1.8	4*	20*	375*
14–18 y	700	65	5*	15	75*	1.0	1.0	14	1.2	400[i]	2.4	5*	25*	400*
19–30 y	700	75	5*	15	90*	1.1	1.1	14	1.3	400[i]	2.4	5*	30*	425*
31–50 y	700	75	5*	15	90*	1.1	1.1	14	1.3	400[i]	2.4	5*	30*	425*
51–70 y	700	75	10*	15	90*	1.1	1.1	14	1.5	400	2.4[h]	5*	30*	425*
>70 y	700	75	15*	15	90*	1.1	1.1	14	1.5	400	2.4[h]	5*	30*	425*
Pregnancy														
≤18 y	750	80	5*	15	75*	1.4	1.4	18	1.9	600[i]	2.6	6*	30*	450*
19–30 y	770	85	5*	15	90*	1.4	1.4	18	1.9	600[i]	2.6	6*	30*	450*
31–50 y	770	85	5*	15	90*	1.4	1.4	18	1.9	600[i]	2.6	6*	30*	450*
Lactation														
≤18 y	1,200	115	5*	19	75*	1.4	1.6	17	2.0	500	2.8	7*	35*	550*
19–30 y	1,300	120	5*	19	90*	1.4	1.6	17	2.0	500	2.8	7*	35*	550*
31–50 y	1,300	120	5*	19	90*	1.4	1.6	17	2.0	500	2.8	7*	35*	550*

NOTE: This table (taken from the DRI reports, see www.nap.edu) presents Recommended Dietary Allowances (RDAs) in **bold type** and Adequate Intakes (AIs) in ordinary type followed by an asterisk (*). RDAs and AIs may both be used as goals for individual intake. RDAs are set to meet the needs of almost all (97–98%) individuals in a group. For healthy breastfed infants, the AI is the mean intake. The AI for other life-stage and gender groups is believed to cover needs of all individuals in the group, but lack of data or uncertainty in the data prevent being able to specify with confidence the percentage of individuals covered by this intake.

[a] As retinol activity equivalents (RAEs). 1 RAE = 1 µg retinol, 12 µg α-carotene, 24 µg α-carotene, or 24 µg β-cryptoxanthin. To calculate RAEs from REs of provitamin A carotenoids in foods, divide the REs by 2. For preformed vitamin A in foods or supplements and for provitamin A carotenoids in supplements, 1 RE = 1 RAE.

[b] As calciferol. 1 µg calciferol = 40 IU vitamin D.

[c] In the absence of adequate exposure to sunlight.

[d] As α-tocopherol. α-Tocopherol includes RRR-α-tocopherol, the only form of α-tocopherol that occurs naturally in foods, and the 2R-stereoisomeric forms of α-tocopherol (RRR-, RSR-, RRS-, and RSS-α-tocopherol) that occur in fortified foods and supplements. It does not include the 2S-stereoisomeric forms of α-tocopherol (SRR-, SSR-, SRS-, and SSS-α-tocopherol), also found in fortified foods and supplements.

[e] As niacin equivalents (NE). 1 mg of niacin = 60 mg of tryptophan; 0–6 months = preformed niacin (not NE).

[f] As dietary folate equivalents (DFE). 1 DFE = 1 µg food folate = 0.6 µg of folic acid from fortified food or as a supplement consumed with food = 0.5 µg of a supplement taken on an empty stomach.

[g] Although AIs have been set for choline, there are few data to assess whether a dietary supply of choline is needed at all stages of the life cycle, and it may be that the choline requirement can be met by endogenous synthesis at some of these stages.

[h] Because 10 to 30% of older people may malabsorb food-bound B12, it is advisable for those older than 50 years to meet their RDA mainly by consuming foods fortified with B12 or a supplement containing B12.

[i] In view of evidence linking folate intake with neural tube defects in the fetus, it is recommended that all women capable of becoming pregnant consume 400 µg from supplements or fortified foods in addition to intake of food folate from a varied diet.

TABLE A-2-f. TOLERABLE UPPER INTAKE LEVELS (UL^a), VITAMINS, DIETARY REFERENCE INTAKES (DRIs) AND FOOD AND NUTRITION BOARD, THE INSTITUTE OF MEDICINE, NATIONAL ACADEMY OF SCIENCES

LIFE-STAGE GROUP	VITAMIN A (μg/d)[b]	VITAMIN C (mg/d)	VITAMIN D (μg/d)	VITAMIN E (mg/d)[a,d]	VITAMIN K	THIAMIN	RIBOFLAVIN	NIACIN (mg/d)[d]	VITAMIN B$_6$ (mg/d)	FOLATE (μg/d)[d]	VITAMIN B$_{12}$	PANTOTHENIC ACID	BIOTIN	CHOLINE (g/d)	CAROTENOIDS[e]
Infants															
0–6 mo	600	ND[f]	25	ND	ND	ND	ND	ND	ND	ND	ND	ND	ND	ND	ND
7–12 mo	600	ND	25	ND	ND	ND	ND	ND	ND	ND	ND	ND	ND	ND	ND
Children															
1–3 y	600	400	50	200	ND	ND	ND	10	30	300	ND	ND	ND	1.0	ND
4–8 y	900	650	50	300	ND	ND	ND	15	40	400	ND	ND	ND	1.0	ND
Males, Females															
9–13 y	1,700	1,200	50	600	ND	ND	ND	20	60	600	ND	ND	ND	2.0	ND
14–18 y	2,800	1,800	50	800	ND	ND	ND	30	80	800	ND	ND	ND	3.0	ND
19–70 y	3,000	2,000	50	1,000	ND	ND	ND	35	100	1,000	ND	ND	ND	3.5	ND
>70 y	3,000	2,000	50	1,000	ND	ND	ND	35	100	1,000	ND	ND	ND	3.5	ND
Pregnancy															
≤18 y	2,800	1,800	50	800	ND	ND	ND	30	80	800	ND	ND	ND	3.0	ND
19–50 y	3,000	2,000	50	1,000	ND	ND	ND	35	100	1,000	ND	ND	ND	3.5	ND
Lactation															
≤18 y	2,800	1,800	50	800	ND	ND	ND	30	80	800	ND	ND	ND	3.0	ND
19–50 y	3,000	2,000	50	1,000	ND	ND	ND	35	100	1,000	ND	ND	ND	3.5	ND

[a] UL = The maximum level of daily nutrient intake that is likely to pose no risk of adverse effects. Unless otherwise specified, the UL represents total intake from food, water, and supplements. Due to lack of suitable data, ULs could not be established for vitamin K, thiamin, riboflavin, vitamin B$_{12}$, pantothenic acid, biotin, or carotenoids. In the absence of ULs, extra caution may be warranted in consuming levels above recommended intakes.

[b] As preformed vitamin A only.

[c] As α-tocopherol; applies to any form of supplemental α-tocopherol.

[d] The ULs for vitamin E, niacin, and folate apply to synthetic forms obtained from supplements, fortified foods, or a combination of the two.

[e] β-Carotene supplements are advised only to serve as a provitamin A source for individuals at risk of vitamin A deficiency.

[f] ND = Not determinable due to lack of data of adverse effects in this age group and concern with regard to lack of ability to handle excess amounts. Source of intake should be from food only to prevent high levels of intake.

From Dietary Reference Intakes for Calcium, Phosphorus, Magnesium, Vitamin D, and Fluoride (1997); Dietary Reference Intakes for Thiamin, Riboflavin, Niacin, Vitamin B$_6$, Folate, Vitamin B$_{12}$, Pantothenic Acid, Biotin, and Choline (1998); Dietary Reference Intakes for Vitamin C, Vitamin E, Selenium, and Carotenoids (2000); and Dietary Reference Intakes for Vitamin A, Vitamin K, Arsenic, Boron, Chromium, Copper, Iodine, Iron, Manganese, Molybdenum, Nickel, Silicon, Vanadium, and Zinc (2001). These reports may be accessed via www.nap.edu.

TABLE A-2-g. RECOMMENDED INTAKES FOR INDIVIDUALS, ELEMENTS, DIETARY REFERENCE INTAKES AND FOOD AND NUTRITION BOARD, THE INSTITUTE OF MEDICINE, NATIONAL ACADEMY OF SCIENCES

LIFE-STAGE GROUP	CALCIUM (mg/d)	CHROMIUM (µg/d)	COPPER (µg/d)	FLUORIDE (mg/d)	IODINE (µg/d)	IRON (mg/d)	MAGNESIUM (mg/d)	MANGANESE (mg/d)	MOLYBDENUM (µg/d)	PHOSPHORUS (mg/d)	SELENIUM (µg/d)	ZINC (mg/d)
Infants												
0–6 mo	210*	0.2*	200*	0.01*	110*	0.27*	30*	0.003*	2*	100*	15*	2*
7–12 mo	270*	5.5*	220*	0.5*	130*	11	75*	0.6*	3*	275*	20*	3
Children												
1–3 y	500*	11*	340	0.7*	90	7	80	1.2*	17	460	20	3
4–8 y	800*	15*	440	1*	90	10	130	1.5*	22	500	30	5
Males												
9–13 y	1,300*	25*	700	2*	120	8	240	1.9*	34	1,250	40	8
14–18 y	1,300*	35*	890	3*	150	11	410	2.2*	43	1,250	55	11
19–30 y	1,000*	35*	900	4*	150	8	400	2.3*	45	700	55	11
31–50 y	1,000*	35*	900	4*	150	8	420	2.3*	45	700	55	11
51–70 y	1,200*	30*	900	4*	150	8	420	2.3*	45	700	55	11
>70 y	1,200*	30*	900	4*	150	8	420	2.3*	45	700	55	11
Females												
9–13 y	1,300*	21*	700	2*	120	8	240	1.6*	34	1,250	40	8
14–18 y	1,300*	24*	890	3*	150	15	360	1.6*	43	1,250	55	9
19–30 y	1,000*	25*	900	3*	150	18	310	1.8*	45	700	55	8
31–50 y	1,000*	25*	900	3*	150	18	320	1.8*	45	700	55	8
51–70 y	1,200*	20*	900	3*	150	8	320	1.8*	45	700	55	8
>70 y	1,200*	20*	900	3*	150	8	320	1.8*	45	700	55	8
Pregnancy												
≤18 y	1,300*	29*	1,000	3*	220	27	400	2.0*	50	1,250	60	13
19–30 y	1,000*	30*	1,000	3*	220	27	350	2.0*	50	700	60	11
31–50 y	1,000*	30*	1,000	3*	220	27	360	2.0*	50	700	60	11
Lactation												
≤18 y	1,300*	44*	1,300	3*	290	10	360	2.6*	50	1,250	70	14
19–30 y	1,000*	45*	1,300	3*	290	9	310	2.6*	50	700	70	12
31–50 y	1,000*	45*	1,300	3*	290	9	320	2.6*	50	700	70	12

NOTE: This table presents Recommended Dietary Allowances (RDAs) in **bold type** and Adequate Intakes (AIs) in ordinary type followed by an asterisk (*). RDAs and AIs may both be used as goals for individual intake. RDAs are set to meet the needs of almost all (97 to 98 percent) individuals in a group. For healthy breastfed infants, the AI is the mean intake. The AI for other life stage and gender groups is believed to cover needs of all individuals in the group, but lack of data or uncertainty in the data prevent being able to specify with confidence the percentage of individuals covered by this intake.

From: Dietary Reference Intakes for Calcium, Phosphorus, Magnesium, Vitamin D, and Fluoride (1997); Dietary Reference Intakes for Thiamin, Riboflavin, Niacin, Vitamin B$_6$, Folate, Vitamin B$_{12}$, Pantothenic Acid, Biotin, and Choline (1998); Dietary Reference Intakes for Vitamin C, Vitamin E, Selenium, and Carotenoids (2000); and Dietary Reference Intakes for Vitamin A, Vitamin K, Arsenic, Boron, Chromium, Copper, Iodine, Iron, Manganese, Molybdenum, Nickel, Silicon, Vanadium, and Zinc (2001). These reports may be accessed via www.nap.edu.

TABLE A-2-h. TOLERABLE UPPER INTAKE LEVELS (UL^a), ELEMENTS, DIETARY REFERENCE INTAKES (DRIs) AND FOOD AND NUTRITION BOARD, THE INSTITUTE OF MEDICINE, NATIONAL ACADEMY OF SCIENCES

LIFE-STAGE GROUP	ARSENIC[b] (mg/d)	BORON (mg/d)	CALCIUM (g/d)	CHROMIUM	COPPER (µg/d)	FLUORIDE (mg/d)	IODINE (µg/d)	IRON (mg/d)	MAGNESIUM (mg/d)[c]	MANGANESE (mg/d)	MOLYBDENUM (µg/d)	NICKEL (mg/d)	PHOSPHORUS (g/d)	SELENIUM (µg/d)	SILICON[d]	VANADIUM (mg/d)[a]	ZINC (mg/d)
Infants																	
0–6 mo	ND[f]	ND	ND	ND	ND	0.7	ND	40	ND	ND	ND	ND	ND	45	ND	ND	4
7–12 mo	ND	ND	ND	ND	ND	0.9	ND	40	ND	ND	ND	ND	ND	60	ND	ND	5
Children																	
1–3 y	ND	3	2.5	ND	1,000	1.3	200	40	65	2	300	0.2	3	90	ND	ND	7
4–8 y	ND	6	2.5	ND	3,000	2.2	300	40	110	3	600	0.3	3	150	ND	ND	12
Males, Females																	
9–13 y	ND	11	2.5	ND	5,000	10	600	40	350	6	1,100	0.6	4	280	ND	ND	23
14–18 y	ND	17	2.5	ND	8,000	10	900	45	350	9	1,700	1.0	4	400	ND	ND	34
19–70 y	ND	20	2.5	ND	10,000	10	1,100	45	350	11	2,000	1.0	4	400	ND	1.8	40
>70 y	ND	20	2.5	ND	10,000	10	1,100	45	350	11	2,000	1.0	3	400	ND	1.8	40
Pregnancy																	
≤18 y	ND	17	2.5	ND	8,000	10	900	45	350	9	1,700	1.0	3.5	400	ND	ND	34
19–50 y	ND	20	2.5	ND	10,000	10	1,100	45	350	11	2,000	1.0	3.5	400	ND	ND	40
Lactation																	
≤18 y	ND	17	2.5	ND	8,000	10	900	45	350	9	1,700	1.0	4	400	ND	ND	34
19–50 y	ND	20	2.5	ND	10,000	10	1,100	45	350	11	2,000	1.0	4	400	ND	ND	40

[a] UL = The maximum level of daily nutrient intake that is likely to pose no risk of adverse effects. Unless otherwise specified, the UL represents total intake from food, water, and supplements. Due to lack of suitable data, ULs could not be established for arsenic, chromium, and silicon. In the absence of ULs, extra caution may be warranted in consuming levels above recommended intakes.

[b] Although the UL was not determined for arsenic, there is no justification for adding arsenic to food or supplements.

[c] The ULs for magnesium represent intake from a pharmacological agent only and do not include intake from food and water.

[d] Although silicon has not been shown to cause adverse effects in humans, there is no justification for adding silicon to supplements.

[e] Although vanadium in food has not been shown to cause adverse effects in humans, there is no justification for adding vanadium to food and vanadium supplements should be used with caution. The UL is based on adverse effects in laboratory animals and this data could be used to set a UL for adults but not children and adolescents.

[f] ND = Not determinable due to lack of data of adverse effects in this age group and concern with regard to lack of ability to handle excess amounts. Source of intake should be from food only to prevent high levels of intake.

From Dietary Reference Intakes for Calcium, Phosphorus, Magnesium, Vitamin D, and Fluoride (1997); Dietary Reference Intakes for Thiamin, Riboflavin, Niacin, Vitamin B₆, Folate, Vitamin B₁₂, Pantothenic Acid, Biotin, and Choline (1998); Dietary Reference Intakes for Vitamin C, Vitamin E, Selenium, and Carotenoids (2000); and Dietary Reference Intakes for Vitamin A. Vitamin K, Arsenic, Boron, Chromium, Cooper, Iodine, Iron, Manganese, Molybdenum, Nickel, Silicon, Vanadium, and Zinc (2001). These reports may be accessed via www.nap.edu.

A-3. UNITED STATES, 1989 AND CANADA, 1990

A-3-a. Introductory Comments: Appendices Editor

As noted in the text of II A-2-a, the 1989 RDA of the United States and the 1990 Recommended Nutrient Intakes of Canada have been revised and updated in a joint United States-Canada series of Dietary Reference Intakes in Section II A-2. What changes have occurred from the 1989–1990 data to those of the DRIs? Our review indicates that there are a number of differences, such as in the reference heights and weights, in the nutrients (micro and macro) that were included, in the categories of ages covered, in the nutrients levels classified as RDA, as well as in various increases or decreases in intake values and in major reviews of the impact of diseases on nutritional status and needs. Accordingly, we feel that inclusion of the two sets of data may be useful to those who having either a practical or intellectual interest in knowing the types and extent of changes from the "old" to the "new."

Appendices Editors

TABLE A-3-a-1. RECOMMENDED DIETARY ALLOWANCES,[a] REVISED 1989 (DESIGNED FOR THE MAINTENANCE OF GOOD NUTRITION OF PRACTICALLY ALL HEALTHY PEOPLE IN THE UNITED STATES)

CATEGORY	AGE (years) OR CONDITION	WEIGHT[b] (kg)	WEIGHT[b] (lb)	HEIGHT[b] (cm)	HEIGHT[b] (in)	PROTEIN (G)	VITAMIN A (μg RE)[c]	VITAMIN D (μgx)[d]	VITAMIN E (mg α-TE)[e]	VITAMIN K (μg)
Infants	0.0–0.5	6	13	60	24	13	375	7.5	3	5
	0.5–1.0	9	20	71	28	14	375	10	4	10
Children	1–3	13	29	90	35	16	400	10	6	15
	4–6	20	44	112	44	24	500	10	7	20
	7–10	28	62	132	52	28	700	10	7	30
Males	11–14	45	99	157	62	45	1000	10	10	45
	15–18	66	145	176	69	59	1000	10	10	65
	19–24	72	160	177	70	58	1000	10	10	70
	25–50	79	174	176	70	63	1000	5	10	80
	51+	77	170	173	68	63	1000	5	10	80
Females	11–14	46	101	157	62	46	800	10	8	45
	15–18	55	120	163	64	44	800	10	8	55
	19–24	58	128	164	65	46	800	10	8	60
	25–50	63	138	163	64	50	800	5	8	65
	51+	65	143	160	63	50	800	5	8	65
Pregnant						60	800	10	10	65
Lactating	1st 6 months					65	1300	10	12	65
	2nd 6 months					62	1200	10	11	65

CATEGORY	C (mg)	B$_1$ (mg)	RIBOFLAVIN (mg)	NIACIN (mg NE)[f]	B$_6$ (mg)	FOLATE (μg)	B$_{12}$ (μg)	Ca (mg)	Ph (mg)	Mg (mg)	Fe (mg)	Zn (mg)	I (μg)	Se (μg)
Infants	30	0.3	0.4	5	0.3	25	0.3	400	300	40	6	5	40	10
	35	0.4	0.5	6	0.6	35	0.5	600	500	60	10	5	50	15
Children	40	0.7	0.8	9	1.0	50	0.7	800	800	80	10	10	70	20
	45	0.9	1.1	12	1.1	75	1.0	800	800	120	10	10	90	20
	45	1.0	1.2	13	1.4	100	1.4	800	800	170	10	10	120	30
Males	50	1.3	1.5	17	1.7	150	2.0	1200	1200	270	12	15	150	40
	60	1.5	1.8	20	2.0	200	2.0	1200	1200	400	12	15	150	50
	60	1.5	1.7	19	2.0	200	2.0	1200	1200	350	10	15	150	70
	60	1.5	1.7	19	2.0	200	2.0	800	800	350	10	15	150	70
	60	1.2	1.4	15	2.0	200	2.0	800	800	350	10	15	150	70
Females	50	1.1	1.3	15	1.4	150	2.0	1200	1200	280	15	12	150	45
	60	1.1	1.3	15	1.5	180	2.0	1200	1200	300	15	12	150	50
	60	1.1	1.3	15	1.6	180	2.0	1200	1200	280	15	12	150	55
	60	1.1	1.3	15	1.6	180	2.0	800	800	280	15	12	150	55
	60	1.0	1.2	13	1.6	180	2.0	800	800	280	10	12	150	55
Pregnant	70	1.5	1.6	17	2.2	400	2.2	1200	1200	320	30	15	175	65
Lactating	95	1.6	1.8	20	2.1	280	2.6	1200	1200	355	15	19	200	75
	90	1.6	1.7	20	2.1	260	2.6	1200	1200	340	15	16	200	75

[a] The allowances, expressed as average daily intakes over time, are intended to provide for individual variations among most normal persons as they live in the United States under usual environmental stresses. Diets should be based on a variety of common foods in order to provide their nutrients for which human requirements have been less well defined. See text for detailed discussion of allowances and of nutrients not tabulated.

[b] Weights and heights of reference adults are actual medians for the U.S. population of the designated age, as reported by NHANES II. The median weights and heights of those under 19 years of age were taken from Hamill et al. (1979). The use of these figures does not imply that the height:weight ratios are ideal.

[c] Retinol equivalents. 1 retinol equivalent = 1 μg retinol or 6 μg β-carotene. See text for calculation of vitamin A activity of diets as retinol equivalents.

[d] As cholecalciferol. 10 μg cholecalciferol = 400 IU of vitamin D.

[e] α-Tocopherol equivalents. 1 mg d-α tocopherol = 1 α-TE. See text for variation in allowances and calculation of vitamin E activity of the diet as α-tocopherol equivalents.

[f] 1 NE (niacin equivalent) is equal to 1 mg of niacin or 60 mg of dietary tryptophan.

From Food and Nutrition Board, National Research Council. Recommended dietary allowances. 10th ed. Washington, DC: National Academy Press, 1989.

TABLE A-3-a-2. ESTIMATED SAFE AND ADEQUATE DAILY DIETARY INTAKES OF SELECTED VITAMINS AND MINERALS[a]

		VITAMINS	
CATEGORY	AGE (years)	BIOTIN (µg)	PANTOTHENIC ACID (mg)
Infants	0–0.5	10	2
	0.5–1	15	3
Children and adolescents	1–3	20	3
	4–6	25	3–4
	7–10	30	4–5
	11+	30–100	4–7
Adults		30–100	4–7

		TRACE ELEMENTS[b]				
CATEGORY	AGE (years)	COPPER (mg)	MANGANESE (mg)	FLUORIDE (mg)	CHROMIUM (µg)	MOLYBDENUM (µg)
Infants	0–0.5	0.4–0.6	0.3–0.6	0.1–0.5	10–40	15–30
	0.5–1	0.6–0.7	0.6–1.0	0.2–1.0	20–60	20–40
Children and adolescents	1–3	0.7–1.0	1.0–1.5	0.5–1.5	20–80	25–50
	4–6	1.0–1.5	1.5–2.0	1.0–2.5	30–120	30–75
	7–10	1.0–2.0	2.0–3.0	1.5–2.5	50–200	50–150
	11+	1.5–2.5	2.0–5.0	1.5–2.5	50–200	75–250
Adults		1.5–3.0	2.0–5.0	1.5–4.0	50–200	75–250

[a] Because there is less information on which to base allowances, these figures are not given in the main table of RDA and are provided here in the form of ranges of recommended intakes.

[b] Because the toxic levels for many trace elements may be only several times usual intakes, the upper levels for the trace elements given in this table should not be habitually exceeded.

From Food and Nutrition Board, National Research Council. Recommended dietary allowances. 10th ed. Washington, DC: National Academy Press, 1989:284.

TABLE A-3-b-1. SUMMARY OF EXAMPLES OF RECOMMENDED NUTRIENT INTAKE BASED ON AGE AND BODY WEIGHT EXPRESSED AS DAILY RATES, CANADA

AGE	SEX	WEIGHT (kg)	PROTEIN (g)	VIT. A (RE)[a]	VIT. D (µg)	VIT. E (mg)	VIT. C (mg)	FOLATE (µg)	VIT. B$_{12}$ (µg)	CALCIUM (mg)	PHOSPHORUS (mg)	MAGNESIUM (mg)	IRON (mg)	IODINE (µg)	ZINC (mg)
Months															
0–4	Both	6.0	12[b]	400	10	3	20	25	0.3	250[c]	150	20	0.3[d]	30	2[d]
5–12	Both	9.0	12	400	10	3	20	40	0.4	400	200	32	7	40	3
Years															
1	Both	11	13	400	10	3	20	40	0.5	500	300	40	6	55	4
2–3	Both	14	16	400	5	4	20	50	0.6	550	350	50	6	65	4
4–6	Both	18	19	500	5	5	25	70	0.8	600	400	65	8	85	5
7–9	M	25	26	700	2.5	7	25	90	1.0	700	500	100	8	110	7
	F	25	26	700	2.5	6	25	90	1.0	700	500	100	8	95	7
10–12	M	34	34	800	2.5	8	25	120	1.0	900	700	130	8	125	9
	F	36	36	800	2.5	7	25	130	1.0	1,100	800	135	8	110	9
13–15	M	50	49	900	2.5	9	30[e]	175	1.0	1,100	900	185	10	160	12
	F	48	46	800	2.5	7	30[e]	170	1.0	1,000	850	180	13	160	9
16–18	M	62	58	1,000	2.5	10	40[e]	220	1.0	900	1,000	230	10	160	12
	F	53	47	800	2.5	7	30[e]	190	1.0	700	850	200	12	160	9
19–24	M	71	61	1,000	2.5	10	40[e]	220	1.0	800	1,000	240	9	160	12
	F	58	50	800	2.5	7	30[e]	180	1.0	700	850	200	13	160	9
25–49	M	74	64	1,000	2.5	9	40[e]	230	1.0	800	1,000	250	9	160	12
	F	59	51	800	2.5	6	30[e]	185	1.0	700	850	200	13	160	9
50–74	M	73	63	1,000	5	7	40[e]	230	1.0	800	1,000	250	9	160	12
	F	63	54	800	5	6	30[e]	195	1.0	800	850	210	8	160	9
75+	M	69	59	1,000	5	6	40[e]	215	1.0	800	1000	230	9	160	12
	F	64	55	800	5	5	30[e]	200	1.0	800	850	210	8	160	9
Pregnancy (additional)															
1st trimester			5	0	2.5	2	0	200	0.2	500	200	15	0	25	6
2nd trimester			20	0	2.5	2	10	200	0.2	500	200	45	5	25	6
3rd trimester			24	0	2.5	2	10	200	0.2	500	200	45	10	25	6
Lactation (additional)			20	400	2.5	3	25	100	0.2	500	200	85	0	50	6

[a] Retinol equivalents.

[b] Protein is assumed to be from breast milk and must be adjusted for infant formula.

[c] Infant formula with high phosphorus should contain 375 mg calcium.

[d] Breast milk is assumed to be the source of the mineral.

[e] Smokers should increase vitamin C by 50%.

From Health and Welfare Canada, Nutrition recommendations. The report of the Scientific Review Committee, Ottawa: Supply and Services Canada, 1990. Reproduced with permission of the Minister of Public Works and Government Services Canada 1998.

TABLE A-3-b-2. SUMMARY OF EXAMPLES OF RECOMMENDED NUTRIENTS BASED ON ENERGY EXPRESSED AS DAILY RATES, CANADA

AGE	SEX	ENERGY (kcal)	THIAMIN (mg)	RIBOFLAVIN (mg)	NIACIN (ne[a])	n-3 PUFA[b] (g)	N-6 PUFA (g)
Months							
0–4	Both	600	0.3	0.3	4	0.5	3
5–12	Both	900	0.4	0.5	7	0.5	3
Years							
1	Both	1,100	0.5	0.6	8	0.6	4
2–3	Both	1,300	0.6	0.7	9	0.7	4
4–6	Both	1,800	0.7	0.9	13	1.0	6
7–9	M	2,200	0.9	1.1	16	1.2	7
	F	1,900	0.8	1.0	14	1.0	6
10–12	M	2,500	1.0	1.3	18	1.4	8
	F	2,200	0.9	1.1	16	1.2	7
13–15	M	2,800	1.1	1.4	20	1.5	9
	F	2,200	0.9	1.1	16	1.2	7
16–18	M	3,200	1.3	1.6	23	1.8	11
	F	2,100	0.8	1.1	15	1.2	7
19–24	M	3,000	1.2	1.5	22	1.6	10
	F	2,100	0.8	1.1	15	1.2	7
25–49	M	2,700	1.1	1.4	19	1.5	9
	F	1,900	0.8[c]	1.0[c]	14[c]	1.1[c]	7[c]
50–74	M	2,300	0.9	1.2	16	1.3	8
	F	1,800	0.8[c]	1.0[c]	14[c]	1.1[c]	7[c]
75+	M	2,000	0.8	1.0	14	1.1	7
	F[d]	1,700	0.8[c]	1.0[c]	14[c]	1.1[c]	7[c]
Pregnancy (additional)							
1st trimester		100	0.1	0.1	1	0.05	0.3
2nd trimester		300	0.1	0.3	2	0.16	0.9
3rd trimester		300	0.1	0.3	2	0.16	0.9
Lactation (additional)		450	0.2	0.4	3	0.25	1.5

[a] NE, Niacin equivalents.
[b] PUFA, Polyunsaturated fatty acids.
[c] Level below which intake should not fall.
[d] Assumes moderate (more than average) physical activity.

From Health and Welfare Canada. Nutrition recommendations. The report of the Scientific Review Committee. Ottawa: Supply and Services Canada, 1990. Reproduced with permission of the Minister of Public Works and Government Services Canada 1996.

A-4. DIETARY REFERENCE VALUES FOR FOOD ENERGY AND NUTRIENTS FOR THE UNITED KINGDOM (1)

Comments: To assist the reader in understanding the following tables taken from this Dietary Reference Values report, excerpts from its Introduction are given here. We make special note of the following:

1. The abbreviation RDA for nutrients differs from the RDA of the 10th RDA (1989) (Table II-A-23-a) and the recent Dietary Reference Intakes of the United States Food and Nutrition Board of the Institute of Medicine (Table II-A-2-b). The UK RDA refers to a group mean (see their paragraph 1.3 below).
2. The UK report defines three different sets of reference values as indicated in 1.3.8.
3. The figures in the various tables for individuals and groups are designated Dietary Reference Values (DRVs) rather than recommendations.

4. The values for protein, vitamins, and minerals given in the following tables are at the RNI level as defined in 1.3.8 below. These are statistically equivalent in derivation to the U.S. 1989 10th RDA and new U.S. dietary reference intakes. With the exception of the figures for energy (given as EAR), only the RNI values are included in these tables.

The Appendix Editors

A-4-a. Excerpts from the Report's Introduction (1)

1.3 Interpretation of the Terms of Reference
1.3.1 The definition of the Recommended Daily Amount (RDA) for a nutrient which was used in the previous Report of the Committee on Medical Aspects of Food Policy is "the average amount of the nutrient which should be provided per head in a group of people if the needs of practically all members of the group are to be met." This was

framed in an attempt to make it clear that the amounts referred to are averages for a group of people and not amounts which individuals must consume . . .

1.3.7 The Panel found no single criterion to define requirements for all nutrients. Some nutrients may have a variety of physiological effects at different levels of intake. Which of these effects should form the parameter of adequacy is therefore to some extent arbitrary. For each nutrient the particular parameter or parameters which were used to define adequacy are given in the text . . .

1.3.8 *Definition of Dietary Reference Values* Although information is usually inadequate to calculate the precise distribution of requirements in a group of individuals for a nutrient, it has been assumed to be normally distributed . . . This gives a notional mean requirement or Estimated Average Requirement (EAR) . . . The Panel has defined the Reference Nutrient Intake (RNI) as a point in the distribution, that is two notional standard deviations above the (EAR) . . . Intakes above this amount will almost certainly be adequate. At a point, two notional standard deviations (2 SD) below the mean, the Lower Reference Nutrient Intake (LNRI), represents the lowest intakes which will meet the needs of some individuals in the group. Intakes below this level are almost certainly inadequate for most individuals. For some nutrients the derivation of DRVs was not possible from these principles, and this is stated in the text. In particular, for those nutrients where no requirement could be defined (starches, sugars, fat and fatty acids), the DRVs are not derived on these principles, although analogous figures based on pragmatic judgements have been proposed (see original report).

1.3.9 At higher levels of consumption there may be evidence of undesirable effects. Guidance on such high levels of consumption is given in the text. The RNI . . . is the amount sufficient or more than sufficient to meet the nutritional needs of practically all healthy persons in a population, and therefore exceeds the requirements of most.

1.3.11 *Interpretation of Dietary Reference Values* For most nutrients the Panel found insufficient data to establish any of the DRVs with great confidence. There are inherent errors in some of the data, for instance in individuals' reports of their food intake, and the day-to-day variation in nutrient intakes also complicates interpretation. Even given complete accuracy of a dietary record, its relation to habitual intake remains uncertain, however long the recording period. The food composition tables normally used to determine nutrient intake from dietary records contain a number of assumptions and imperfections. Furthermore, there is uncertainty about the relevance of many biological markers, such as serum concentrations of a nutrient, as evidence of an individual's 'status' for that nutrient . . .

1.3.14 *Weights and standard age ranges* As requirements for most nutrients vary with both age and sex, the Panel has attempted to set DRVs for all such groups of the population. The Panel has sought new weight data for use in calculating DRVs for people of all ages in the United Kingdom . . . These weights are given in the table below for each of the standard age groups.

1.3.18 *Safe intakes* For some nutrients, which are known to have important functions in humans, the Panel found insufficient reliable data on human requirements and were unable to set any DRVs for these. However, they decided on grounds of prudence to set a safe intake, particularly for infants and children, and these are given in [Report] Table 1.6 [Appendix Table II-A-4-f]. The safe intake was judged to be a level or range of intake at which there is no risk of deficiency, and below a level where there is a risk of undesirable effects.

1.4 *Uses of Dietary Reference Values* These DRVs apply to groups of healthy people and are not necessarily appropriate for those with different needs arising from disease, such as infections, disorders of the gastro-intestinal tract or metabolic abnormalities. The DRVs for any one nutrient presuppose that requirements for energy and all other nutrients are met . . .

1.4.1 *For assessing diets of individuals*

1.4.1.1 The impression of most estimates both of individuals' nutrient intakes and of nutritional status, and thus of the estimation of the DRVs themselves, means that utmost caution should be used in

CHILDREN		MALES		FEMALES	
AGE	WEIGHT (kg)	AGE	WEIGHT (kg)	AGE	WEIGHT (kg)
0–3 mo (formula fed)	5.9	11–14 y	43.1	11–14 y	43.8
		15–18 y	64.5	15–18 y	55.5
4–6 mo	7.7	19–50 y	74.0	19–50 y	60.0
7–9 mo	8.9	50+ y	71.0	50+ y	62.0
10–12 mo	9.8				
1–3 y	12.6			Pregnancy	
4–6 y	17.8			Lactation: 0–4 mo	
7–10 y	28.3			4+ mo	

applying the figures to the interpretation (or assessment) of individual diets. Even with a perfect measure of an individuals's habitual intake of a nutrient (a difficult goal), the DRVs can give no more than a guide to the adequacy of diet for that individual.

1.4.1.2 If the habitual intake is below the LRNI it is likely that the individual will not be consuming sufficient of the nutrient to maintain the function selected by the Panel as an appropriate parameter of nutritional status for that nutrient, and further investigation, including biological measures, may be appropriate.

1.4.1.3 If the habitual intake is above the RNI, then it is extremely unlikely that the individual will not be consuming sufficient.

1.4.1.4 If the intake lies between the two, then the chances of the diet being inadequate (in respect of the chosen function parameter for any nutrient) fall as the intake approaches the RNI ... It is impossible to say with any certainty whether an individual's nutrient intake, if it lies between the LRNI and the RNI, is or is not adequate, without some biological measure in that individual.

1.4.2 *For assessing diets of groups of individuals*

1.4.2.1 When measures of individual diets are aggregated, one of the sources of imprecision is attenuated—that is intraindividual day to day variability. Assuming that the interindividual variability is random, then in a sufficiently large group, this source of imprecision is also diminished. Thus the group mean intake will more precisely represent the habitual group mean intake than any of the individual measures will represent individual intakes.

1.5 DRV for energy

1.5.1 ... RNIs for all nutrients, but not energy, can be set at the upper end of the range of requirements because an intake moderately in excess of requirements has no adverse effects, but reduces the risk of deficiency. For energy, however, this is not the case. Recommendations for energy have therefore always been set as the average of energy requirements for any population group. The Panel has therefore calculated EARs for energy, but not LRNIs or RNIs.

1.7 DRVs for protein ... The approach derived from estimates of basic nitrogen requirements with additions for specific situations such as growth and pregnancy, which was adopted by joint FAO/WHO/UNU Expert Consultation in 1985, has formed the basis of the Panel's deliberations and enabled calculations of DRVs including EARs shown in [Report] Table 1–3 [Appendix Table II-A-4-c].

REFERENCE

1. Report on Health and Social Subjects No. 41. Dietary Reference Values for Food Energy and Nutrients for the United Kingdom. Report of the Panel on Dietary Reference Values of the Committee on Medical Aspects of Food Policy. London: Her Majesty's Stationery Office, 1991.

TABLE A-4-b. ESTIMATED AVERAGE REQUIREMENTS (EARs) FOR ENERGY, UNITED KINGDOM[a]

AGE	EARs MJ/d (kcal/d) MALES	FEMALES
0–3 mo	2.28 (545)	2.16 (515)
4–6 mo	2.89 (690)	2.69 (645)
7–9 mo	3.44 (825)	3.20 (765)
10–12 mo	3.85 (920)	3.61 (865)
1–3 y	5.15 (1,230)	4.86 (1,165)
4–6 y	7.16 (1,715)	6.46 (1,545)
7–10 y	8.24 (1,970)	7.28 (1,740)
11–14 y	9.27 (2,220)	7.72 (1,845)
15–18 y	11.51 (2,755)	8.83 (2,110)
19–50 y	10.60 (2,550)	8.10 (1,940)
51–59 y	10.60 (2,550)	8.00 (1,900)
60–64 y	9.93 (2,380)	7.99 (1,900)
65–74 y	9.71 (2,330)	7.96 (1,900)
75+ y	8.77 (2,100)	7.61 (1,810)
Pregnancy		+0.80[b] (200)
Lactation		
1 mo		+1.90 (450)
2 mo		+2.20 (530)
3 mo		+2.40 (570)
4–6 mo (group 1)[c]		+2.00 (480)
4–6 mo (group 2)		+2.40 (570)
>6 mo (group 1)		+1.00 (240)
>6 mo (group 2)		+2.30 (550)

[a] See paragraph 1.5 in Table 11-A-4-a.
[b] Last trimester only.
[c] See original text for comments.
From Report on Health and Social Subjects: no. 41, Dietary reference values for food energy and nutrients for the United Kingdom. Report of the Panel on Dietary Reference Values of the Committee on Medical Aspects of Food Policy. London: Her Majesty's Stationery Office, 1991. This is the UK's Report Table 1.1.

TABLE A-4-c. REFERENCE NUTRIENT INTAKES FOR PROTEIN, UNITED KINGDOM[a]

AGE	REFERENCE NUTRIENT INTAKE[b] (g/d)
0–3 mo	12.5[c]
4–6 mo	12.7
7–9 mo	13.7
10–12 mo	14.9
1–3 y	14.5
4–6 y	19.7
7–10 y	28.3
Males	
11–14 y	42.1
15–18 y	55.2
19–50 y	55.5
50+ y	53.3
Females	
11–14 y	41.2
15–18 y	45.0
19–50 y	45.0
50+ y	46.5
Pregnancy[d]	+6
Lactation[d]	
0–4 mo	+11
4+ mo	+8

[a] See paragraph 1.7 in Table 11-A-4-a.
[b] These figures, based on egg and milk protein, assume complete digestibility.
[c] No values for infants 0–3 months are given by WHO. The RNI is calculated from the recommendations of Committee on Medical Aspects of Food Policy (COMA).
[d] To be added to adult requirement through all stages of pregnancy and lactation.
From Report on Health and Social Subjects: no. 41, Dietary reference values for food energy and nutrients for the United Kingdom. Report of the Panel on Dietary Reference Values of the Committee on Medical Aspects of Food Policy. London: Her Majesty's Stationery Office, 1991. This is the UK's Report Table 1.3.

TABLE A-4-d. REFERENCE NUTRIENT INTAKES FOR VITAMINS, UNITED KINGDOM[a]

AGE	THIAMIN (mg/d)	RIBOFLAVIN (mg/d)	NIACIN (NICOTINIC ACID EQUIVALENT) (mg/d)	VITAMIN B_6 (mg/d)[b]	VITAMIN B_{12} (μg/d)	FOLATE (μg/d)	VITAMIN C (mg/d)	VITAMIN A (μg/d)	VITAMIN D (μg/d)
0–3 mo	0.2	0.4	3	0.2	0.3	50	25	350	8.5
4–6 mo	0.2	0.4	3	0.2	0.3	50	25	350	8.5
7–9 mo	0.2	0.4	4	0.3	0.4	50	25	350	7
10–12 mo	0.3	0.4	5	0.4	0.4	50	25	350	7
1–3 y	0.5	0.6	8	0.7	0.5	70	30	400	7
4–6 y	0.7	0.8	11	0.9	0.8	100	30	400	—
7–10 y	0.7	1.0	12	1.0	1.0	150	30	500	—
Males									
11–14 y	0.9	1.2	15	1.2	1.2	200	35	600	—
15–18 y	1.1	1.3	18	1.5	1.5	200	40	700	—
19–50 y	1.0	1.3	17	1.4	1.5	200	40	700	—
50+ y	0.9	1.3	16	1.4	1.5	200	40	700	—[c]
Females									
11–14 y	0.7	1.1	12	1.0	1.2	200	35	600	—
15–18 y	0.8	1.1	14	1.2	1.5	200	40	600	—
19–50 y	0.8	1.1	13	1.2	1.5	200	40	600	—
50+ y	0.8	1.1	12	1.2	1.5	200	40	600	—[c]
Pregnancy	+0.1[d]	+0.3	—[e]	—[e]	—[e]	+100	+10[d]	+100	10
Lactation									
0–4 months	+0.2	+0.5	+2	—[e]	+0.5	+60	+30	+350	10
4+ months	+0.2	+0.5	+2	—[e]	+0.5	+60	+30	+350	10

[a] See paragraph 11-A-4-a for definition. [b] Based on protein providing 14.7% of EAR for energy. [c] After age 65 the RNI is 10 μg/day for men and women. [d] For last trimester only. [e] No increment. From Report on Health and Social Subjects: no. 41. Dietary reference values for food energy and nutrients for the United Kingdom. Report of the Panel on Dietary Reference Values of the Committee on Medical Aspects of Food Policy. London: Her Majesty's Stationery Office, 1991. This is the UK's Report Table 1–4.

TABLE A-4-e-1. REFERENCE NUTRIENT INTAKES FOR MINERALS (SI UNITS) UNITED KINGDOM[a]

AGE	CALCIUM (mmol/d)	PHOSPHORUS[b] (mmol/d)	MAGNESIUM (mmol/d)	SODIUM[c] (mmol/d)	POTASSIUM[d] (mmol/d)	CHLORIDE[e] (mmol/d)	IRON (µmol/d)	ZINC (µmol/d)	COPPER (µmol/d)	SELENIUM (µmol/d)	IODINE (µmol/d)
0–3 mo	13.1	13.1	2.2	9	20	9	30	60	5	0.1	0.4
4–6 mo	13.1	13.1	2.5	12	22	12	80	60	5	0.2	0.5
7–9 mo	13.1	13.1	3.2	14	18	14	140	75	5	0.1	0.5
10–12 mo	13.1	13.1	3.3	15	18	15	140	75	5	0.1	0.5
1–3 y	8.8	8.8	3.5	22	20	22	120	75	6	0.2	0.6
4–6 y	11.3	11.3	4.8	30	28	30	110	100	9	0.3	0.8
7–10 y	13.8	13.8	8.0	50	50	50	160	110	11	0.4	0.9
Males											
11–14 y	25.0	25.0	11.5	70	80	70	200	140	13	0.6	1.0
15–18 y	25.0	25.0	12.3	70	90	70	200	145	16	0.9	1.0
19–50 y	17.5	17.5	12.3	70	90	70	160	145	19	0.9	1.0
50+ y	17.5	17.5	12.3	70	90	70	160	145	19	0.9	1.0
Females											
11–14 y	20.0	20.0	11.5	70	80	70	260[f]	140	13	0.6	1.0
15–18 y	20.0	20.0	12.3	70	90	70	260[f]	110	16	0.8	1.1
19–50 y	17.5	17.5	10.9	70	90	70	260[f]	110	19	0.8	1.1
50+ y	17.5	17.5	10.9	70	90	70	160	110	19	0.8	1.1
Pregnancy	[c,f,e]	—[f]	—[f]	—[f]	—[f]	—[f]	*	*	*	*	*
Lactation											
0–4 mo	+14.3	+14.3	+2.1	*	*	*	*	+90	+5	+0.2	*
4+ mo	+14.3	+14.3	+2.1	*	*	*	*	+40	+5	+0.2	*

* No increment.

[a] See paragraph A-4-a for definition.

[b] Phosphorus RNI is set equal to calcium in molar terms.

[c] 1 mmol sodium = 23 mg.

[d] 1 mmol potassium = 39 mg.

[e] Corresponds to sodium 1 mmol = 35.5 mg.

[f] Insufficient for women with high menstrual losses where the most practical way of meeting iron requirements is to take iron supplements (see Table 28-2 in original report).

From Report on Health and Social Subjects: no. 41. Dietary reference values for food energy and nutrients for the United Kingdom. Report of the Panel on Dietary Reference Values of the Committee on Medical Aspects of Food Policy. London: Her Majesty's Stationery Office, 1991. This is the UK's Report Table 15.

TABLE A-4-e-2.   REFERENCE NUTRIENT INTAKES FOR MINERALS (TRADITIONAL UNITS), UNITED KINGDOM[a]

AGE	CALCIUM (mg/d)	PHOSPHORUS[b] (mg/d)	MAGNESIUM (mg/d)	SODIUM[c] (mg/d)	POTASSIUM[d] (mgl/d)	CHLORIDE[e] (mg/d)	IRON (mg/d)	ZINC (mg/d)	COPPER (mg/d)	SELENIUM (µg/d)	IODINE (µg/d)
0–3 mo	525	400	55	210	800	320	1.7	4.0	0.2	10	50
4–6 mo	525	400	60	280	850	400	4.3	4.0	0.3	13	60
7–9 mo	525	400	75	320	700	500	7.8	5.0	0.3	10	60
10–12 mo	525	400	80	350	700	500	7.8	5.0	0.3	10	60
1–3 y	350	270	85	500	800	800	6.9	5.0	0.4	15	70
4–6 y	450	350	120	700	1,100	1,100	6.1	6.5	0.6	20	100
7–10 y	550	450	200	1,200	2,000	1,800	8.7	7.0	0.7	30	110
Males											
11–14 y	1,000	775	280	1,600	3,100	2,500	11.3	9.0	0.8	45	130
15–18 y	1,000	775	300	1,600	3,500	2,500	11.3	9.5	1.0	70	140
19–50 y	700	550	300	1,600	3,500	2,500	8.7	9.5	1.2	75	140
50+ y	700	550	300	1,600	3,500	2,500	8.7	9.5	1.2	75	140
Females											
11–14 y	800	625	280	1,600	3,100	2,500	14.8[f]	9.0	0.8	45	130
15–18 y	800	625	300	1,600	3,500	2,500	14.8[f]	7.0	1.0	60	140
19–50 y	700	550	270	1,600	3,500	2,500	14.8[f]	7.0	1.2	60	140
50+ y	700	550	270	1,600	3,500	2,500	8.7	7.0	1.2	60	140
Pregnancy	—*	—*	—*	—*	—*	—*	—*	—*	—*	—*	—*
Lactation											
0–4 mo	+550	+440	+50	—*	—*	—*	*	+6.0	+0.3	+15	—*
4+ mo	+550	+440	+50	—*	—*	—*	*	+2.5	+0.3	+15	—*

* No increment.
[a] See paragraph II-A-4-a for definition.
[b] Phosphorus RNI is set equal to calcium in molar terms.
[c] 1 mmol sodium = 23 mg.
[d] 1 mmol potassium = 39 mg.
[e] Corresponds to sodium 1 mmol = 35.5 mg.
[f] Insufficient for women with high menstrual losses where the most practical way of meeting iron requirements is to take iron supplements (see Table 28.2 in original report).

From Report on Health and Social Subjects: no. 41. Dietary reference values for food energy and nutrients for the United Kingdom. Report of the Panel on Dietary Reference Values of the Committee on Medical Aspects of Food Policy. London: Her Majesty's Stationery Office, 1991. This is the UK's Report Table 1.5.

TABLE A-4-f. SAFE INTAKES, UNITED KINGDOM[a]

NUTRIENT	SAFE INTAKE[b]
Vitamins	
Pantothenic acid	
Adults	3–7 mg/d
Infants	1.7 mg/d
Biotin	10–200 μg/d
Vitamin E	
Men	Above 4 mg/d
Women	Above 3 mg/d
Infants	0.4 mg/g polyunsaturated fatty acids
Vitamin K	
Adults	1 μg/kg/d
Infants	10 μg/d
Minerals	
Manganese	
Adults	Above 1.4 mg (26 μmol)/d
Infants and children	Above 16 μg (0.3 μmol)/kg/d
Molybdenum	
Adults	50–400 μg/d
Infants, children, and adolescents	0.5–1.5 μg/kg/d
Chromium	
Adults	Above 25 μg (0.5 μmol)/d
Children and adolescents	0.1–1.0 μg (2–20 nmol)/kg/d
Fluoride	
Children over 6 years and adults	0.5 mg/kg/d (3 μmol/kg/d)
Children over 6 months	0.12 mg/kg/d (6 μmol/kg/d)
Infants under 6 months	0.22 mg/kg/d (12 μmol/kg/d)

[a] See paragraph II-A-4-a for definition.

[b] For some nutrients, which are known to have important functions in humans, the Panel found insufficient reliable data on human requirements and were unable to set any dietary reference values for these. However, they decided on grounds of prudence to set a safe intake, particularly for infants and children. The safe intake was judged to be a level or range of intake at which there is no risk of deficiency and below a level where there is risk of undesirable effects. They are not therefore intended as a "toxic level," and although exceeding these safe intakes would not necessarily result in undesirable effects, equally there is no evidence for any benefits. The Panel agreed that the safe range of intakes set for the nutrients need not be exceeded.

From Report on Health and Social Subjects: no. 41. Dietary reference values for food energy and nutrients for the United Kingdom. Report of the Panel on Dietary Reference Values of the Committee on Medical Aspects of Food Policy. London: Her Majesty's Stationery Office, 1991.) This is the UK's Report Table 1.6.

A-4-g. Safe Upper Levels for Vitamins and Minerals Expert Group on Vitamins and Minerals Food Standards Agency (UK). London, 2003[a].

---

[a] This and other selected references (Tables A-7-b, c & d) have been provided by Allison A. Yates, Ph.D., and are discussed with other national and international nutrient standards in her Chapter 104. This reference was not available to us at publication time. Appendices Editors

A-5. JAPAN

TABLE A-5-A. RECOMMENDED DIETARY ALLOWANCES FOR THE JAPANESE: DIETARY ALLOWANCES FOR GROWTH PERIOD AND MODERATE LEVEL (II) OF PHYSICAL ACTIVITY, JAPAN*

(AGE year)	REFERENCE HEIGHT (cm) MALE	FEMALE	REFERENCE BODY WEIGHT (kg) MALE	FEMALE	ENERGY (kcal) MALE	FEMALE	PROTEIN (g) MALE	FEMALE	FAT ENERGY RATIO (%)	CALCIUM (g) MALE	FEMALE	IRON (mg) MALE	FEMALE	VITAMIN A (IU) MALE	FEMALE	VITAMIN B$_1$ (mg) MALE	FEMALE	VITAMIN B$_2$ (mg) MALE	FEMALE	NIACIN (mg) MALE	FEMALE	VITAMIN C (mg)	VITAMIN D (IU)
0 month					120/kg		3.0/kg		45	0.5	0.5	6	6	1,300		0.2	0.2	0.3	0.3	4	4		400
2 month					110/kg		2.4/kg		45	0.5	0.5	6	6	1,300		0.3	0.3	0.4	0.4	6	6		
6 month					100/kg		2.8/kg		30–40	0.5	0.5	6	6	1,000		0.4	0.4	0.5	0.5	6	6		
1	80.2	79.1	10.57	10.07	960	920	30	30	25–30		0.5	7	7	1,000	1,000	0.4	0.4	0.5	0.5	6	6	40	100
2	89.6	88.4	12.85	12.36	1,200	1,150	35	35				7	7	1,000	1,000	0.5	0.5	0.7	0.6	8	8		
3	97.6	96.4	15.00	14.57	1,400	1,350	40	40				8	8	1,000	1,000	0.6	0.5	0.8	0.7	9	9		
4	104.7	103.6	17.12	16.74	1,550	1,500	45	45				8	8	1,000	1,000	0.6	0.6	0.9	0.8	10	10		
5	111.2	110.2	19.34	18.97	1,650	1,550	50	50				9	9	1,000	1,000	0.7	0.6	0.9	0.9	11	10		
6	117.2	116.2	21.70	21.25	1,700	1,600	55	50				9	9	1,200	1,200	0.7	0.7	0.9	0.9	11	11		
7	123.0	121.9	24.40	23.75	1,800	1,650	60	55				9	9	1,200	1,200	0.7	0.7	1.0	1.0	12	11		
8	128.6	127.5	27.42	26.60	1,900	1,750	65	60				10	10	1,200	1,200	0.8	0.7	1.0	1.0	13	12		
9	133.9	133.2	30.69	29.95	1,950	1,850	70	65				10	10	1,500	1,500	0.8	0.8	1.1	1.1	13	12		
10	139.2	139.7	34.34	34.23	2,050	1,950	75	70		0.6	0.6	10	10	1,500	1,500	0.8	0.8	1.1	1.2	14	13		
11	145.4	146.5	38.73	39.28	2,200	2,100	80	75		0.7		12	12	1,500	1,500	0.9	0.8	1.2	1.2	15	14		
12	153.0	151.6	44.31	43.92	2,350	2,250	85	75		0.8		12	12	1,500	1,500	0.9	0.9	1.3	1.3	16	15		
13	160.5	154.7	50.39	47.60	2,550	2,300	90	75		0.9	0.7	12	12	2,000	1,800	1.0	0.9	1.4	1.2	17	15		
14	166.0	156.5	55.69	50.38	2,650	2,300	90	75		0.9		12	12	2,000	1,800	1.1	0.9	1.5	1.2	17	15		
15	169.3	157.4	59.62	52.08	2,700	2,250	90	70		0.8		12	12	2,000	1,800	1.1	0.9	1.5	1.2	18	15		
16	171.0	158.0	61.93	52.92	2,750	2,200	80	65		0.8		12	12	2,000	1,800	1.1	0.9	1.5	1.1	18	15		
17	171.9	158.3	63.15	52.95	2,700	2,150	75	65		0.7		12	12	2,000	1,800	1.1	0.9	1.5	1.1	18	14		
18	172.3	158.5	63.53	52.53	2,700	2,100	75	60		0.7		12	12	2,000	1,800	1.0	0.8	1.4	1.1	18	14		
19	172.3	158.5	63.53	51.93	2,600	2,050	70	60				12	12	2,000	1,800	1.0	0.8	1.4	1.1	17	14		
20–29	171.3	158.1	64.69	51.31	2,550	2,000	70	60	20–25	0.6	0.6	10	12	2,000	1,800	1.0	0.8	1.4	1.1	17	13	50	
30–39	170.8	157.3	66.62	54.02	2,500	2,000	70	60				10	12	2,000	1,800	1.0	0.8	1.4	1.1	17	13		
40–49	168.8	155.9	66.19	55.49	2,400	1,950	70	60				10	12	2,000	1,800	1.0	0.8	1.3	1.1	16	13		
50–59	165.9	153.0	63.66	53.95	2,300	1,850	70	60				10	12	2,000	1,800	0.9	0.7	1.3	1.0	15	12		
60–64	163.4	150.6	61.12	51.28	2,100	1,750	70	60				10	10 (postmenopausal)	2,000	1,800	0.8	0.7	1.2	1.0	14	12		
65–69	162.1	149.1	59.28	49.53	2,100	1,700	70	60				10	10	2,000	1,800	0.8	0.7	1.2	1.0	14	12		
70–74	160.7	147.6	57.28	47.69	1,850	1,600	70	60				10	10	2,000	1,800	0.8	0.7	1.2	1.0	14	12		
75–79	159.3	146.1	55.30	45.83	1,800	1,500	65	55				10	10	2,000	1,800	0.8	0.7	1.2	1.0	14	12		
80–	157.3	143.9	52.85	43.67	1,650	1,400	65	55				10	10	2,000	1,800	0.8	0.7	1.2	1.0	14	12		

From Recommended Dietary Allowances for the Japanese, 5th rev. Supervised by Health and Nutrition Division, Ministry of Health and Welfare, 1996. With permission.

Notes to "Dietary allowances for the Japanese" (table)

1. The dietary allowances shown in Tables A-5-a–d are not to be applied to individuals without modification. Reference should be made to original report for application.

2. As for determination of the intensity of living activity, reference should be made to the "classification" for intensities of living activities as viewed from daily life (standards). Those falling under "I (light)" in the degree of intensity of living activities are recommended to expend calories equivalent to "II (moderate)" degree of intensity as listed in Table A-5-a by either changing the daily activities or engaging in additional physical activities.

3. The daily salt intake is recommended to be 10 g/day/person or less as previously.

4. Vitamin E (α-tocopherol equivalent) intake should preferably be 8 mg for adult males and 7 mg for adult females.

* The Japanese Ministry of Health, Labor and Welfare issued in 2005 new dietary reference allowances. These were not available in English at the time of book publication. Those interested in the published version of the new guidelines can obtain them from the following websites:

URL related to New guidelines

http://www.mhlw.go.jp/houdou/2004/11/h1122–2.html

http://www.mhlw.go.jp/houdou/2004/11/h1122–2a.html

http://www.mhlw.go.jp/houdou/2004/11/d1/h1122–2b.pdf

The last is the full version of guideline (PDF Files)

TABLE A-5-b. DIETARY ALLOWANCES FOR LIGHT LEVEL (I) OF PHYSICAL ACTIVITY

AGE (y)	ENERGY (kcal) MEN	ENERGY WOMEN	PROTEIN (g) MEN	PROTEIN WOMEN	FAT ENERGY RATIO (%)	CALCIUM (g) MEN	CALCIUM WOMEN	IRON (mg) MEN	IRON WOMEN	VITAMIN A (IU) MEN	VITAMIN A WOMEN	VITAMIN B₁ (mg) MEN	VITAMIN B₁ WOMEN	VITAMIN B₂ (mg) MEN	VITAMIN B₂ WOMEN	NIACIN (mg) MEN	NIACIN WOMEN	VITAMIN C (mg)	VITAMIN D (IU)
15	2,400	2,000	90	70	25–30	0.8	0.7	12	12	2,000	1,800	1.0	0.8	1.3	1.1	16	13	50	100
16	2,400	1,950	80	65		0.8		12	12	2,000	1,800	1.0	0.8	1.3	1.1	16	13		
17	2,600	1,900	75	65		0.7		12	12	2,000	1,800	1.0	0.8	1.3	1.0	16	13		
18	2,400	1,850	75	60		0.7		12	12	2,000	1,800	1.0	0.7	1.3	1.0	16	12		
19	2,350	1,850	70	60				12	12	2,000	1,800	0.9	0.7	1.3	1.0	16	12		
20–29	2,250	1,800	70	60	20–25	0.6	0.6	10	12	2,000	1,800	0.9	0.7	1.2	1.0	15	12		
30–39	2,200	1,750	70	60				10	12	2,000	1,800	0.9	0.7	1.2	1.0	15	12		
40–49	2,150	1,700	70	60				10	12	2,000	1,800	0.9	0.7	1.2	0.9	14	11		
50–59	2,050	1,650	70	60				10	12 (PMS)	2,000	1,800	0.8	0.7	1.1	0.9	14	11		
60–64	1,900	1,550	70	60				10	10	2,000	1,800	0.8	0.6	1.0	0.9	13	10		
65–69	1,800	1,500	70	60				10	10	2,000	1,800	0.7	0.6	1.0	0.9	12	10		
70–74	1,700	1,400	70	60				10	10	2,000	1,800	0.7	0.6	0.9	0.9	12	10		
75–79	1,600	1,350	65	55				10	10	2,000	1,800	0.7	0.6	0.9	0.9	12	10		
80	1,500	1,250	65	55				10	10	2,000	1,800	0.7	0.6	0.9	0.9	12	10		
Pregnancy 1–5 months	+150		+10		25–30		+0.3		+3		+0		+0.1		+0.1		+1	+10	+300
Additions 6–10 months	+350		+20				+0.3		+8		+200		+0.2		+0.2		+2	+10	+300
Lactation	+700		+20				+0.5		+8		+1400		+0.3		+0.4		+5	+40	+300

Note: Additions for pregnant and lactating women are shown for convenience. Their levels of physical activity should not be regarded uniformly as falling subject to the light level (1).
URL related to New guidelines

TABLE A-5-c. DIETARY ALLOWANCES FOR LIGHT-HEAVY LEVEL (III) OF PHYSICAL ACTIVITY

AGE (y)	ENERGY (kcal) MEN	WOMEN	PROTEIN (g) MEN	WOMEN	FAT ENERGY RATIO (%)	CALCIUM (g) MEN	WOMEN	IRON (mg) MEN	WOMEN	VITAMIN A (IU) MEN	WOMEN	VITAMIN B₁ (mg) MEN	WOMEN	VITAMIN B₂ (mg) MEN	WOMEN	NIACIN (mg) MEN	WOMEN	VITAMIN C (mg)	VITAMIN D (IU)
15	3,250	2,650	105	85		0.8		12	12	2,000	1,800	1.3	1.1	1.8	1.5	21	17		
16	3,250	2,600	95	80		0.8	0.7	12	12	2,000	1,800	1.3	1.0	1.8	1.4	21	17		
17	3,250	2,550	90	80		0.7		12	12	2,000	1,800	1.3	1.0	1.8	1.4	21	17		
18	3,200	2,500	90	75		0.7		12	12	2,000	1,800	1.3	1.0	1.8	1.4	21	17		
19	3,150	2,450	85	70	25–30			12	12	2,000	1,800	1.3	1.0	1.7	1.3	21	16	50	100
20–29	3,050	2,400	85	70				10	12 (PM♀)	2,000	1,800	1.2	1.0	1.7	1.3	20	16		
30–39	3,000	2,350	85	70		0.6	0.6	10	12	2,000	1,800	1.2	0.9	1.7	1.3	20	16		
40–49	2,900	2,300	85	70				10	12	2,000	1,800	1.1	0.9	1.6	1.3	19	15		
50–59	2,750	2,250	85	70				10	12	2,000	1,800	1.1	0.9	1.5	1.2	18	15		
60–64	2,500	2,050	80	70				10	10	2,000	1,800	1.0	0.8	1.4	1.1	17	14		
65–69	2,400	2,000	80	70				10	10	2,000	1,800	1.0	0.8	1.4	1.1	17	14		

TABLE A-5-d. DIETARY ALLOWANCES FOR HEAVY LEVEL (IV) OF PHYSICAL ACTIVITY

AGE (y)	ENERGY (kcal) MEN	WOMEN	PROTEIN (g) MEN	WOMEN	FAT ENERGY RATIO (%)	CALCIUM (g) MEN	WOMEN	IRON (mg) MEN	WOMEN	VITAMIN A (IU) MEN	WOMEN	VITAMIN B₁ (mg) MEN	WOMEN	VITAMIN B₂ (mg) MEN	WOMEN	NIACIN (mg) MEN	WOMEN	VITAMIN C (mg)	VITAMIN D (IU)
15	3,800	3,100	115	95		0.8		12	12	2,000	1,800	1.5	1.2	2.1	1.7	25	20		
16	3,800	3,050	115	95		0.8	0.7	12	12	2,000	1,800	1.5	1.2	2.1	1.7	25	20		
17	3,800	2,950	110	90		0.7		12	12	2,000	1,800	1.5	1.2	2.1	1.6	25	19		
18	3,750	2,950	110	90		0.7		12	12	2,000	1,800	1.5	1.2	2.1	1.6	25	19		
19	3,700	2,850	105	85	25–30			12	12	2,000	1,800	1.5	1.1	2.0	1.6	24	19	50	100
20–29	3,550	2,800	100	85				10	12 (PM♀)	2,000	1,800	1.4	1.1	2.0	1.5	23	18		
30–39	3,500	2,750	100	85		0.6	0.6	10	12	2,000	1,800	1.4	1.1	1.9	1.5	23	18		
40–49	3,400	2,700	100	85				10	12	2,000	1,800	1.4	1.1	1.9	1.5	22	18		
50–59	3,200	2,600	100	85				10	12	2,000	1,800	1.3	1.0	1.8	1.4	21	17		
60–64	2,900	2,350	95	80				10	10	2,000	1,800	1.2	1.0	1.6	1.3	19	16		
65–69	2,800	2,300	95	80				10	10	2,000	1,800	1.1	1.0	1.6	1.3	19	16		

A–6. NUTRIENT REFERENCE VALUES FOR AUSTRALIA AND NEW ZEALAND INCLUDING RECOMMENDED DIETARY INTAKES DRAFT: DECEMBER 2004

Appendices Editors Comment: These are draft tables from the joint Australian and New Zealand Nutrient Reference Values. The publication is produced under the aus-pices of the Commonwealth Department of Health (Australia), the Ministry of Health in New Zealand and is under the auspices of the National Health and Medical Research Council in Australia. Final tables available in 2005 may be found at the NHMRC website (http://www.nhmrc.gov.au). We express our appreciation for the opportunity to include them here.

TABLE A-6-a. NUTRIENT REFERENCE VALUES FOR AUSTRALIA AND NEW ZEALAND: MACRONUTRIENTS AND WATER

Age/gender group		Energy* Mj/day	Protein g/day			Dietary fats[†] Linoleic (n6) g/d		α –linolenic (n3) g/d		VLC n3 (DHA/EP A/DPA) mg/d		Carbohydrate g/d		Dietary Fibre g/day		Total Water[‡] (fluids) L/d	
		EER	AI	UIL		AI	UIL	AI	UIL	AI	UIL	AI	UIL	AI	UIL	AI	UIL
Infants **	0-6 mo.	1.8 - 2.7	10	BM		4.4	BM	0.5[†]	BM	-		60	BM	NP	NP	0.7 (0.7)	NP
	7-12 mo.	2.5 - 3.5	14	B/F		4.6	B/F	0.5[†]	B/F	-		95	B/F	NP	NP	0.8 (0.6)	NP
			EAR	RDI	UIL	AI	UIL	AI	UIL	AI	UIL			AI	UIL	AI	UIL
Children	1-3 years	3.2 - 5.5	12	14	NP	5	NP	0.5	NP	40	3000	NONE SET FOR OTHER AGES		12	NP	1.4 (1.0)	NP
	4-8 years	5.5 - 7.4	16	20	NP	8	NP	0.8	NP	55	3000			16	NP	1.6 (1.2)	NP
Boys	9-13 years	7.8 - 10.0	31	40	NP	10	NP	1.0	NP	70	3000			21	NP	2.2 (1.6)	NP
	14-18 years	10.6 - 12.5	49	65	NP	12	NP	1.2	NP	125	3000			23	NP	2.7 (1.9)	NP
Girls	9-13 years	7.3 - 8.9	24	35	NP	8	NP	0.8	NP	70	3000			17	NP	1.9 (1.4)	NP
	14-18 years	9.2 - 9.7	35	45	NP	8	NP	0.8	NP	85	3000			18	NP	2.2 (1.4)	NP
Men	19-30 years	10.3 - 13.5	52	64	NP	13	NP	1.3	NP	190	3000			25	NP	3.4 (2.6)	NP
	31-50 years	10.2 - 12.6	52	64	NP	13	NP	1.3	NP	190	3000			25	NP	3.4 (2.6)	NP
	51-70 years	10.2 - 12.6	52	64	NP	13	NP	1.3	NP	190	3000			25	NP	3.4 (2.6)	NP
	>70 years	8.3 - 10.8	52	64	NP	13	NP	1.3	NP	190	3000			25	NP	3.4 (2.6)	NP
Women	19-30 years	8.2 - 11.1	37	46	NP	8	NP	0.8	NP	90	3000			20	NP	2.8 (2.1)	NP
	31-50 years	8.4 - 10.0	37	46	NP	8	NP	0.8	NP	90	3000			20	NP	2.8 (2.1)	NP
	51-70 years	8.4 - 10.0	37	46	NP	8	NP	0.8	NP	90	3000			20	NP	2.8 (2.1)	NP
	>70 years	7.4 - 9.2	37	46	NP	8	NP	0.8	NP	90	3000			20	NP	2.8 (2.1)	NP
Pregnant	14-18 years	2nd trimest +1.4MJ	47 #	58 #	NP	10	NP	1.0	NP	110	3000			20	NP	2.4 (1.8)	NP
	19-30 years		49 #	60 #	NP	10	NP	1.0	NP	115	3000			22	NP	3.1 (2.3)	NP
	31-50 years	3rd trimest + 1.9MJ	49 #	60 #	NP	10	NP	1.0	NP	115	3000			22	NP	3.1 (2.3)	NP
Lactating	14-18 years		51	63	NP	12	NP	1.2	NP	140	3000			22	NP	3.5 (2.6)	NP
	19-30 years	+ 2.0-2.1MJ	54	67	NP	12	NP	1.2	NP	145	3000			24	NP	3.5 (2.6)	NP
	31-50 years		54	67	NP	12	NP	1.2	NP	145	3000			24	NP	3.5 (2.6)	NP

EAR—Estimated Average Requirement. RDI—Recommended Dietary Intake. AI—Adequate Intakes. UIL—Upper Intake Limit. * Energy needs are dependent on body size and activity. ** AI recommendations for Infants are based on amounts in breast milk. # In second and third trimesters only. [†] Recommendations for total n6 and total u3; total fat AI also set at 30–31 g/day for infants. [‡] Total water includes water from foods as well as fluids. BM—amount normally received from breast milk of healthy women. B/F—amount in breast milk and food. NP—Not Possible to set (may be insufficient evidence or no clear levels for adverse effects).

TABLE A-6-b. NUTRIENT REFERENCE VALUES FOR AUSTRALIA AND NEW ZEALAND: B VITAMINS

Age group/gender		Thiamine mg/day			Riboflavin mg/day			Niacin * mg/d niacin equivalents			Vitamin B6 mg/day			Vitamin B12 µg/day			Folate (folate equivs) mg/day			Panto-thenate mg/day		Biotin µg/day	
		AI	UIL		AI	UIL		AI	UIL		AI	UIL#		AI	UIL		AI	UIL#		AI	UIL	AI	UIL
Infants **	0-6 mo.	0.2	NP		0.3	BM		2	BM		0.1	BM		0.4	BM		65	BM		1.7	BM	5	BM
	7-12 mo.	0.3	NP		0.4	B/F		4	B/F		0.3	B/F		0.5	B/F		80	B/F		2.2	B/F	6	B/F
		EAR	RDI	UIL	EAR	RDI	UIL	EAR	RDI	UIL	EAR	RDI	UIL	EAR	RDI	UIL	EAR	RDI	UIL#	AI	UIL	AI	UIL
Children	1-3 yrs	0.4	0.5	NP	0.4	0.5	NP	5	6	10	0.4	0.5	30	0.7	0.9	NP	120	150	300	3.5	NP	8	NP
	4-8 yrs	0.5	0.6	NP	0.5	0.6	NP	6	8	15	0.5	0.6	40	1.0	1.2	NP	160	200	400	4	NP	12	NP
Boys	9-13 yrs	0.7	0.9	NP	0.8	0.9	NP	9	12	20	0.8	1.0	60	1.5	1.8	NP	250	300	600	5	NP	20	NP
	14-18 yrs	1.0	1.2	NP	1.1	1.3	NP	12	16	30	1.1	1.3	80	2.0	2.4	NP	330	400	800	6	NP	30	NP
Girls	9-13 yrs	0.7	0.9	NP	0.8	0.9	NP	9	12	20	0.8	1.0	60	1.5	1.8	NP	250	300	600	4	NP	20	NP
	14-18 yrs	0.9	1.0	NP	0.9	1.0	NP	11	14	30	1.0	1.2	80	2.0	2.4	NP	330	400	800	4	NP	25	NP
Men	19-30 yrs	1.0	1.2	NP	1.1	1.3	NP	12	16	35	1.1	1.3	100	2.0	2.4	NP	320	400	1000	6	NP	30	NP
	31-50 yrs	1.0	1.2	NP	1.1	1.3	NP	12	16	35	1.1	1.3	100	2.0	2.4	NP	320	400	1000	6	NP	30	NP
	51-70 yrs	1.0	1.2	NP	1.1	1.3	NP	12	16	35	1.4	1.7	100	2.0	2.4	NP	320	400	1000	6	NP	30	NP
	>70 yrs	1.0	1.2	NP	1.3	1.6	NP	12	16	35	1.4	1.7	100	2.0	2.4	NP	320	400	1000	6	NP	30	NP
Women	19-30 yrs	0.9	1.1	NP	0.9	1.1	NP	11	14	35	1.1	1.3	100	2.0	2.4	NP	320	400	1000	4	NP	25	NP
	31-50 yrs	0.9	1.1	NP	0.9	1.1	NP	11	14	35	1.1	1.3	100	2.0	2.4	NP	320	400	1000	4	NP	25	NP
	51-70 yrs	0.9	1.1	NP	0.9	1.1	NP	11	14	35	1.3	1.5	100	2.0	2.4	NP	320	400	1000	4	NP	25	NP
	>70 yrs	0.9	1.1	NP	1.1	1.3	NP	11	14	35	1.3	1.5	100	2.0	2.4	NP	320	400	1000	4	NP	25	NP
Pregnant	14-18 yrs	1.2	1.4	NP	1.2	1.4	NP	14	18	30	1.6	1.9	80	2.2	2.6	NP	520	600	800	5	NP	30	NP
	19-30 yrs	1.2	1.4	NP	1.2	1.4	NP	14	18	35	1.6	1.9	100	2.2	2.6	NP	520	600	1000	5	NP	30	NP
	31-50 yrs	1.2	1.4	NP	1.2	1.4	NP	14	18	35	1.6	1.9	100	2.2	2.6	NP	520	600	1000	5	NP	30	NP
Lactating	14-18 yrs	1.2	1.4	NP	1.3	1.6	NP	13	17	30	1.7	2.0	80	2.4	2.8	NP	450	500	800	6	NP	35	NP
	19-30 yrs	1.2	1.4	NP	1.3	1.6	NP	13	17	35	1.7	2.0	100	2.4	2.8	NP	450	500	1000	6	NP	35	NP
	31-50 yrs	1.2	1.4	NP	1.3	1.6	NP	13	17	35	1.7	2.0	100	2.4	2.8	NP	450	500	1000	6	NP	35	NP

EAR—Estimated Average Requirement. RDI—Recommended Dietary Intake. AI—Adequate Intakes. UIL—Upper Intake Limit. * UIL for nicotinic acid. For supplemental nicotinamide UIL is 1000 mg/day for men and 850 mg/day for nonpregnant women. Insufficient evidence for upper limits for nicotinamide in pregnancy and lactation or for children and adolescents. ** All infant AIs as based on estimates based on breast milk concentrations in healthy women and average volumes. # for Vit B6 UIL, set for pyridoxine. For folate UIL is for Intake from fortified foods and supplements as dietary folate equivalents. BM—amount normally received from breast milk for healthy women. B/F amount in breast milk and food. NP—to set (may be insufficient evidence or no clear level for adverse effects).

TABLE A-6-c. NUTRIENT REFERENCE VALUES FOR AUSTRALIA AND NEW ZEALAND: VITAMIN A, C, D, E AND K AND CHOLINE

Age group/gender		Vitamin A (retinol equivalents) µg/day			Vitamin C mg/day			Vitamin D µg/day		Vitamin E (α-tocopherol equivalents #) mg/day		Vitamin K µg/day		Choline mg/day	
		AI		UIL	AI		UIL*	AI	UIL	AI	UIL	AI	UIL	AI	UIL
Infants	0-6 mo.	250 (as retinol)		600	25		BM	5	BM	4	BM	2	BM	125	BM
	7-12 mo.	430		600	30		B/F	5	B/F	5	B/F	2.5	B/F	150	B/F
		EAR	RDI	UIL	EAR	RDI	UIL	AI	UIL	AI	UIL	AI	UIL	AI	UIL
Children	1-3 yrs	210	300	600	25	35	NP	5	NP	5	70	25	NP	200	1000
	4-8 yrs	275	400	900	25	35	NP	5	NP	6	100	35	NP	250	1000
Boys	9-13 yrs	445	600	1700	28	40	NP	5	NP	9	180	45	NP	375	1000
	14-18 yrs	630	900	2800	28	40	NP	5	NP	10	250	55	NP	550	3000
Girls	9-13 yrs	420	600	1700	28	40	NP	5	NP	8	180	45	NP	375	1000
	14-18 yrs	485	700	2800	28	40	NP	5	NP	8	250	55	NP	400	3000
Men	19-30 yrs	625	900	3000	30	45	NP	5	NP	10	300	70	NP	550	3500
	31-50 yrs	625	900	3000	30	45	NP	5	NP	10	300	70	NP	550	3500
	51-70 yrs	625	900	3000	30	45	NP	10	NP	10	300	70	NP	550	3500
	>70 yrs	625	900	3000	30	45	NP	15	NP	10	300	70	NP	550	3500
Women	19-30 yrs	500	700	3000	30	45	NP	5	NP	7	300	60	NP	475	3500
	31-50 yrs	500	700	3000	30	45	NP	5	NP	7	300	60	NP	475	3500
	51-70 yrs	500	700	3000	30	45	NP	10	NP	7	300	60	NP	475	3500
	>70 yrs	500	700	3000	30	45	NP	15	NP	7	300	60	NP	475	3500
Pregnant	14-18 yrs	530	700	2800	38	55	NP	5	NP	7	300	60	NP	420	3000
	19-30 yrs	550	800	3000	40	60	NP	5	NP	7	300	60	NP	450	3500
	31-50 yrs	550	800	3000	40	60	NP	5	NP	7	300	60	NP	450	3500
Lactating	14-18 yrs	780	1100	2800	58	80	NP	5	NP	12	300	60	NP	525	3000
	19-30 yrs	800	1110	3000	60	85	NP	5	NP	11	300	60	NP	550	3500
	31-50 yrs	800	1110	3000	60	85	NP	5	NP	11	300	60	NP	550	3500

EAR—Estimated Average Requirement. RDI—Recommended Dietary Intake. AI—Adequate Intakes. UIL—Upper Intake Limit. * Not possible to establish UIL for Vitamin C but 1000 mg/day would be a prudent limit. # One alpha-tocopherol equivalent is equal to 1 mg RRR alpha (or d-I) tocopherol; 2 mg beta tocopherol; 10 mg gamma tocopherol; 3 mg alpha decotrienol. The relevant figure for synthetic all-rac-alpha tocopherols (di-alpha tocopherol) is 14 mg.

TABLE A-6-d. NUTRIENT REFERENCE VALUES FOR AUSTRALIA AND NEW ZEALAND: MINERALS (EARs AND RDIs)

Age/gender group		Calcium* mg/day			Phosphorus mg/day			Zinc mg/day			Iron mg/day		
		AI		UIL	AI		UIL	AI		UIL	AI		UIL
Infants	0-6 mo.	210		BM	100		BM	2		4	0.27		20
	7-12 mo.	270		B/F	275		B/F	2.5	3.0	5	6.9	11.0	20
		EAR	RDI	UIL	EAR	RDI	UIL	EAR	RDI	UIL	EAR	RDI	UIL
Children	1-3 yrs	360	500	2500	380	460	3000	2.5	3	7	4.1	9	20
	4-8 yrs	520	700	2500	405	500	3000	3	4	12	4.1	10	40
Boys	9-13 yrs	800/1050	1000/1300	2500	1055	1250	4000	5.2	6	25	5.9	8	40
	14-18 yrs	1050	1300	2500	1055	1250	4000	10.5	13	35	7.7	11	45
Girls	9-13 yrs	800/1050	1000/1300	2500	1055	1250	4000	5.2	6	25	5.7	8	40
	14-18 yrs	1050	1300	2500	1055	1250	4000	5.9	7	35	7.9	15	45
Men	19-30 yrs	840	1000	2500	580	1000	4000	11.7	14	40	6	8	45
	31-50 yrs	840	1000	2500	580	1000	4000	11.7	14	40	6	8	45
	51-70 yrs	840	1000	2500	580	1000	4000	11.7	14	40	6	8	45
	>70 yrs	1100	1300	2500	580	1000	3000	11.7	14	40	6	8	45
Women	19-30 yrs	840	1000	2500	580	1000	4000	6.5	8	35	8	18	45
	31-50 yrs	840	1000	2500	580	1000	4000	6.5	8	35	8	18	45
	51-70 yrs	1100	1300	2500	580	1000	4000	6.5	8	35	5	8	45
	>70 yrs	1100	1300	2500	580	1000	3000	6.5	8	35	5	8	45
Pregnant	14-18 yrs	1050	1300	2500	1055	1250	3500	8.3	10	35	23	27	45
	19-30 yrs	840	1000	2500	580	1000	3500	8.9	11	40	22	27	45
	31-50 yrs	840	1000	2500	580	1000	3500	8.9	11	40	22	27	45
Lactating	14-18 yrs	1050	1300	2500	1055	1250	4000	9.1	11	35	7	10	45
	19-30 yrs	840	1000	2500	580	1000	4000	9.7	12	40	6.5	9	45
	31-50 yrs	840	1000	2500	580	1000	4000	9.7	12	40	6.5	9	45

TABLE A-6-e. NUTRIENT REFERENCE VALUES FOR AUSTRALIA AND NEW ZEALAND: MINERALS (EARs AND RDIs contd)

Age/gender group		Magnesium mg/day			Iodine µg/day			Selenium µg/day			Molybdenum µg/day		
		AI		UIL#	AI		UIL	AI		UIL	AI		UIL
Infants	0-6 mo.	30		BM	90		BM	12		45	2		BM
	7-12 mo.	75		B/F	110		B/F	15		60	3		B/F
		EAR	RDI	UIL	EAR	RDI	UIL	EAR	RDI	UIL	EAR	RDI	UIL
Children	1-3 yrs	65	80	65	65	90	200	20	25	90	13	17	300
	4-8 yrs	110	130	110	65	90	300	25	30	150	17	22	600
Boys	9-13 yrs	200	240	350	73	120	600	40	50	280	26	34	1100
	14-18 yrs	340	410	350	95	150	900	55	65	400	33	43	1700
Girls	9-13 yrs	200	240	350	73	120	600	40	50	280	26	34	1100
	14-18 yrs	300	360	350	95	150	900	55	65	400	33	43	1700
Men	19-30 yrs	330	400	350	100	150	1100	55	65	400	34	45	2000
	31-50 yrs	350	420	350	100	150	1100	55	65	400	34	45	2000
	51-70 yrs	350	420	350	100	150	1100	55	65	400	34	45	2000
	>70 yrs	350	420	350	100	150	1100	55	65	400	34	45	2000
Women	19-30 yrs	255	310	350	100	150	1100	45	55	400	34	45	2000
	31-50 yrs	265	320	350	100	150	1100	45	55	400	34	45	2000
	51-70 yrs	265	320	350	100	150	1100	45	55	400	34	45	2000
	>70 yrs	265	320	350	100	150	1100	45	55	400	34	45	2000
Pregnant	14-18 yrs	335	400	350	160	220	900	47	57	400	40	50	1700
	19-30 yrs	290	350	350	160	220	1100	47	57	400	40	50	2000
	31-50 yrs	300	360	350	160	220	1110	47	57	400	40	50	2000
Lactating	14-18 yrs	300	360	350	190	270	900	55	65	400	35	50	1700
	19-30 yrs	255	310	350	190	270	1100	55	65	400	36	50	2000
	31-50 yrs	265	320	350	190	270	1100	55	65	400	36	50	2000

TABLE A-6-f. NUTRIENT REFERENCE VALUES FOR AUSTRALIA AND NEW ZEALAND: MINERALS (ADEQUATE INTAKES)

Age/gender group		Copper mg/day		Chromium μg/day		Manganese mg/day		Fluoride mg/day		Sodium mg/day *		Potassium mg/day	
		AI	UIL	AI	UIL	AI	UIL	AI	UIL	AI	UIL	AI	UIL#
Infants	0-6 mo.	0.20	BM	0.2	NP	0.003	BM	0.01	0.7	120	700	400	NP
	7-12 mo.	0.22	B/F	5.5	NP	0.6	B/F	0.5	0.9	170	1000	700	NP
Children	1-3 yrs	0.7	1	11	NP	2.0	2	0.7	1.3	200-400	1400	3000	NP
	4-8 yrs	1.0	3	15	NP	2.5	3	1	2.2	300-600	1600	3700	NP
Boys	9-13 yrs	1.3	5	25	NP	3.0	6	2	10	400-800	1400	4400	NP
	14-18 yrs	1.5	8	35	NP	3.5	9	3	10	460-920	1600	4700	NP
Girls	9-13 yrs	1.1	5	21	NP	2.5	6	2	10	400-800	1600	4400	NP
	14-18 yrs	1.1	8	24	NP	3.0	9	3	10	460-920	1600	4700	NP
Men	19-30 yrs	1.7	10	35	NP	5.5	11	4	10	460-920	1600	4700	NP
	31-50 yrs	1.7	10	35	NP	5.5	11	4	10	460-920	1600	4700	NP
	51-70 yrs	1.7	1	35	NP	5.5	11	4	10	460-920	1600	4700	NP
	>70 yrs	1.7	10	35	NP	5.5	11	4	10	460-920	1600	4700	NP
Women	19-30 yrs	1.2	10	25	NP	5.0	11	3	10	460-920	1600	4700	NP
	31-50 yrs	1.2	10	25	NP	5.0	11	3	10	460-920	1600	4700	NP
	51-70 yrs	1.2	10	25	NP	5.0	11	3	10	460-920	1600	4700	NP
	>70 yrs	1.2	10	25	NP	5.0	11	3	10	460-920	1600	4700	NP
Pregnant	14-18 yrs	1.2	8	30	NP	5.0	9	3	10	460-920	1600	4700	NP
	19-30 yrs	1.3	10	30	NP	5.0	11	3	10	460-920	1600	4700	NP
	31-50 yrs	1.3	10	30	NP	5.0	11	3	10	460-920	1600	4700	NP
Lactating	14-18 yrs	1.4	8	45	NP	5.0	9	3	10	460-920	1600	4700	NP
	19-30 yrs	1.5	10	45	NP	5.0	11	3	10	460-920	1600	4700	NP
	31-50 yrs	1.5	10	45	NP	5.0	11	3	10	460-920	1600	4700	NP

A-7. EUROPEAN COMMUNITY NUTRIENT AND ENERGY INTAKES

A-7-a. Recommendations and Nomenclature: Excerpts from the Report (1)

. . . This Committee is attempting to give, as far as possible, three values to indicate the spread of needs.

. . . This Committee will call the intake that is enough for virtually all healthy people in a group the Population Reference Intake (PRI).

The Average Requirement (AR), the mean nutrient requirement of the group, according to the criterion chosen.

The Lowest Threshold Intake (LTI) is that which is 2 standard deviations below the mean. This is the intake below which, on the basis of our current knowledge, almost all individuals will be unlikely to maintain metabolic integrity according to the criterion chosen for each nutrient.

. . . In this report LTIs are often set on the prudent side, being not those intakes below which frank deficiency is almost certain, but rather those intakes below which there may be cause for concern for a substantial section of the population. Consequently, the PRI and LTI values are not always the means plus and minus two standard deviations.

For nutrients where the requirements are given in terms of energy intake, . . . the convention adopted in this report [gives] the PRIs and LTIs for average energy intakes.

The Committee has given only one value for increases during pregnancy or lactation; it considers it has inadequate information to give more with any confidence.

REFERENCE

1. Reports of the Scientific Committee for Food (31st Series: December 11, 1992). Published by the Commission of the European Communities. Luxembourg, 1993.

TABLE A-7-a-1. MULTIPLE VALUES PROPOSED FOR ADULTS (AMOUNTS PER DAY, UNLESS GIVEN IN OTHER TERMS. IF THAT FOR WOMEN IS DIFFERENT FROM THAT FOR MEN, IT IS GIVEN IN PARENTHESES)

NUTRIENT	AVERAGE REQUIREMENT	POPULATION REFERENCE INTAKE	LOWEST THRESHOLD INTAKES
Protein (g)	0.6/kg body wt	0.75/kg body wt	0.45/kg body wt
Vitamin A (μg)	500 (400[c])	700 (600)	300 (250)
Thiamin (μg)	72/MJ	100/MJ	50/MJ
Riboflavin (mg)	1.3 (1.1[c])	1.6 (1.3[c])	0.6
Niacin (mg niacin equivalents)	1.3/MJ	1.6/MJ	1.0/MJ
Vitamin B_6 (μg)	13/g protein	15/g protein	—
Folate (μg)	140	200	85
Vitamin B_{12} (μg)	1.0	1.4	0.6
Vitamin C (mg)	30	45	12
Vitamin E (mg α-tocopherol equivalents)		0.4/g PUFA[b]	4 (3[c])/day regardless of PUFA[b] intakes
n-6 PUFA[b] (as percentage of dietary energy)	1	2	0.5
n-3 PUFA[b] (as percentage of dietary energy)	0.2	0.5	0.1
Calcium (mg)	550	700	400
Phosphorus (mg)	400	550	300
Potassium (mg)	—	3100	1600
Iron (mg)	7 (10[d],6[c])	9 (16[d], 8[c])	5 (7[d], 4[c])
Zinc (mg)	7.5 (5.5[c])	9.5 (7[c])	5 (4)
Copper (mg)	0.8	1.1	0.6
Selenium (μg)	40	55	20
Iodine (μg)	100	130	70

[a] This is Table 37.1 in the original report.
[b] PUFA, polyunsaturated fatty acids.
[c] Postmenopausal women.
[d] PRI to cover 90% of women.

TABLE A-7-a-2. NUTRIENTS WITH ACCEPTABLE RANGES OF INTAKE

Pantothenic acid (mg)	3–12
Biotin (μg)	15–100
Vitamin D (μg)	0–10
Sodium (g)	0.575–3.5
Magnesium (mg)	150–500
Manganese (mg)	1–10

[a] This is Table 37.1 in the original report.

TABLE A-7-a-3. POPULATION REFERENCE INTAKES

AGE GROUP	PROTEIN (g/kg BODY wt/d)	N-6 PUFA[b] (% OF DIETARY ENERGY)	N-3 PUFA[b] (% OF DIETARY ENERGY)	VITAMIN A (µg/d)	THIAMIN (µg/MJ)	RIBOFLAVIN (mg/d)	NIACIN (mg/MJ)	VITAMIN B$_6$ (µg/g PROTEIN)	FOLATE (µg/d)	VITAMIN B$_{12}$ (µg/d)	VITAMIN C (mg/d)	CALCIUM (mg/d)	PHOSPHORUS (mg/d)	POTASSIUM (mg/d)	IRON (mg/d)	ZINC (mg/d)	COPPER (mg/d)	SELENIUM (µg/d)	IODINE (µg/d)
6–11 mo	1.6	4.5	0.5	350	100	0.4	1.6	15	50	0.5	20	400	300	800	6	4	0.3	8	50
1–3 y	1.1	3	0.5	400	100	0.8	1.6	15	100	0.7	25	400	300	800	4	4	0.4	10	70
4–6 y	1.0	2	0.5	400	100	1.0	1.6	15	130	0.9	25	450	350	1100	4	6	0.6	15	90
7–10 y	1.0	2	0.5	500	100	1.2	1.6	15	150	1.0	30	550	450	2000	6	7	0.7	25	100
Males																			
11–14 y	1.0	2	0.5	600	100	1.4	1.6	15	180	1.3	35	1000	775	3100	10	9	0.8	35	120
15–17 y	0.9	2	0.5	700	100	1.6	1.6	15	200	1.4	40	1000	775	3100	13	9	1.0	45	130
18+ y	0.75	2	0.5	700	100	1.6	1.6	15	200	1.4	45	700	550	3100	9	9.5	1.1	55	130
Females																			
11–14 y	0.95	2	0.5	600	100	1.2	1.6	15	180	1.3	35	800	625	3100	22[d] 18[e]	9	0.8	35	120
15–17 y	0.85	2	0.5	600	100	1.3	1.6	15	200	1.4	40	800	625	3100	21[d] 17[e]	7	1.0	45	130
18+ y	0.75	2	0.5	600	100	1.3	1.6	15	200[c]	1.4	45	700	550	3100	20[d] 16[e] 8[f]	7	1.1	55	130
Pregnancy	0.75 (+10 g/day)	2	0.5	700	100	1.6	1.6	15	400	1.6	55	700	550	3100	[g]	7	1.1	55	130
Lactation	0.75 (+16 g/day)	2	0.5	950	100	1.7	1.6 (+2 mg/day)	15	350	1.9	70	1200	950	3100	10	12	1.4	70	160

[a] Table 37.2 in the original report.
[b] Polyunsaturated fatty acids.
[c] Neural tube defects have been shown to be prevented in offspring by periconceptual ingestion of 400 µg folic acid per day in the form of supplements.
[d] To cover 95% of population.
[e] To cover 90% of population.
[f] Postmenopausal.
[g] Supplementation necessary.

A-7-b. Tolerable Upper Intake Levels for Vitamins and Minerals SCF/CS/NUTR/UPPLEV/1 Final. Nov 2000. http://europa.eu.int/comm/food/fs/sc/scf/out80a_eu.pdf. (Scientific Committee on Food of the European Commission)

This selected reference has been provided by Allison A. Yates, Ph.D., and is discussed with other national and international nutrient standards in her Chapter 104. Data are available from the website.

A-7-c. Netherlands Health Council Dietary Reference Values: Calcium, Vitamin D, Thiamin, Riboflavin, Niacin, Pantothenic Acid, and Biotin. Publ. no. 2000/12. The Hague.

This selected references has been provided by Allison A. Yates, Ph.D., and is discussed with other national and international nutrient standards in her Chapter 104. Data are available from the Hague.

A-7-d. German, Austria, and Swiss Societies of Nutritional Intake (Referenzwerte fur die Nahrstoffzefuhr) (Recommended values for nutritional intake) Umshau Frankfurt, 2000.

This selected reference has been provided by Allison A. Yates, Ph.D., and is discussed with other national and international nutrient standards in her Chapter 104. The data are available from the publisher in Frankfurt.

A-8. INTERNATIONAL DIETARY RECOMMENDATIONS

A-8-a. Diet, Nutrition and the Prevention of Chronic Diseases - WHO/FAO 2003*

A-8-a-1. **Intervening throughout life** (paragraph 4.5 in original document) There is a vast volume of scientific evidence highlighting the importance of applying a life-course approach to the prevention and control of chronic disease. The picture is, however, still not complete, and the evidence sometimes contradictory. From the available evidence, it is possible to state the following:

- Unhealthy diets, physical inactivity and smoking are confirmed risk behaviours for chronic diseases.
- The biological risk factors of hypertension, obesity and lipidaemia are firmly established as risk factors for coronary heart disease, stroke and diabetes.
- Nutrients and physical activity influence gene expression and may define susceptibility.
- The major biological and behavioural risk factors emerge and act in early life, and continue to have a negative impact throughout the life course.
- The major biological risk factors can continue to affect the health of the next generation.
- An adequate and appropriate postnatal nutritional environment is important.
- Globally, trends in the prevalence of many risk factors are upwards, especially those for obesity, physical inactivity and, in the developing world particularly, smoking.

- Selected interventions are effective but must extend beyond individual risk factors and continue throughout the life course.
- Some preventive interventions early in the life course offer lifelong benefits.
- Improving diets and increasing levels of physical activity in adults and older people will reduce chronic disease risks for death and disability.
- Secondary prevention through diet and physical activity is a complementary strategy in retarding the progression of existing chronic diseases and decreasing mortality and the disease burden from such diseases.

In Table A-8-a-2, attention is directed towards the energy-supplying macronutrients. This must not be taken to imply a lack of concern for the other nutrients. Rather, it is a recognition of the fact that previous reports issued by FAO and WHO have provided limited guidance on the meaning of a "balanced diet" described in terms of the proportions of the various energy sources, and that there is an apparent consensus on this aspect of diet in relation to effects on the chronic non-deficiency diseases. This report therefore complements these existing reports on

TABLE A-8-a-2. RANGES OF POPULATION NUTRIENT INTAKE GOALS

DIETARY FACTOR	GOAL (% OF TOTAL ENERGY, UNLESS OTHERWISE STATED)
Total fat	15–30%
Saturated fatty acids	<10%
Polyunsaturated fatty acids (PUFAs)	6–10%
n-6 Polyunsaturated fatty acids (PUFAs)	5–8%
n-3 Polyunsaturated fatty acids (PUFAs)	1–2%
Trans fatty acids	<1%
Monounsaturated fatty acids (MUFAs)	By difference[a]
Total carbohydrate	55–75%[b]
Free sugars[c]	<10%
Protein	10–15%[d]
Cholesterol	<300 mg/d
Sodium chloride (sodium)[e]	<5 g/d (<2 g/d)
Fruits and vegetables	≥400 g/d
Total dietary fibre	From foods[f]
Nonstarch polysaccharides (NSP)	From foods[f]

[a] This is calculated as: total fat—(saturated fatty acids + polyunsaturated fatty acids + *trans* fatty acids).
[b] The percentage of total energy available after taking into account that consumed as protein and fat, hence the wide range.
[c] The term "free sugars" refers to all monosaccharides and disaccharides added to foods by the manufacturer, cook or consumer, plus sugars naturally present in honey, syrups and fruit juices.
[d] The suggested range should be seen in the light of the Joint WHO/FAO/UNUExpert Consultation on Protein and Amino Acid Requirements in Human Nutrition, held in Geneva from 9 to 16 April 2002 (1).
[e] Salt should be iodized appropriately. The need to adjust salt iodization, depending on observed sodium intake and surveillance of iodine status of the population, should be recognized.
[f] See page 58, under "Non-starch polysaccharides" in original document. Table 6 in original documents

energy and nutrient requirements issued by FAO and WHO (1–4). In translating these goals into dietary guidelines, due consideration should be given to the process for setting up national dietary guidelines (4).

1. Protein and amino acid requirements in human nutrition. Report of a Joint WHO/FAO/UNU Expert Consultation. Geneva, World Health Organization, 2003 (in press).
2. Fats and oils in human nutrition. Report of a Joint FAO/WHO Expert Consultation. Rome, Food and Agriculture Organization

of the United Nations, 1994 (FAO Food and Nutrition Paper, No. 57).
3. Carbohydrates in human nutrition. Report of a Joint FAO/WHO Expert Consultation. Rome, Food and Agriculture Organization of the United Nations, 1998 (FAO Food and Nutrition Paper, No. 66).
4. Preparation and use of food-based dietary guidelines. Report of a Joint FAO/WHO Consultation. Geneva, World Health Organization, 1998 (WHO Technical Report Series, No. 880).

TABLE A-8-a-3. SUMMARY OF STRENGTH OF EVIDENCE ON FACTORS THAT MIGHT PROMOTE OR PROTECT AGAINST WEIGHT GAIN AND OBESITY[a]

EVIDENCE	DECREASED RISK	NO RELATIONSHIP	INCREASED RISK
Convincing	Regular physical activity High dietary intake of NSP (dietary fibre)[b]		Sedentary lifestyles High intake of energy-dense micronutrient-poor foods[c]
Probable	Home and school environments that support healthy food choices for children[d]		Heavy marketing of energy-dense foods[d] and fast-food outlets[d] High intake of sugars-sweetened soft drinks and fruit juices
	Breastfeeding		Adverse socioeconomic conditions[d] (in developed countries, especially for women)
Possible	Low glycaemic index Foods	Protein content of the diet	Large portion sizes High proportion of food prepared outside the home (developed countries) "Rigid restraint/periodic disinhibition" eating patterns
Insufficient	Increased eating Frequency		Alcohol

Table 7 in original document.

[a] Strength of evidence: the totality of the evidence was taken into account. The World Cancer Research Fund schema was taken as the starting point but was modified in the following manner: randomized controlled trials were given prominence as the highest ranking study design (randomized controlled trials were not a major source of cancer evidence); associated evidence and expert opinion was also taken into account in relation to environmental determinants (direct trials were usually not available).

[b] Specific amounts will depend on the analytical methodologies used to measure fibre.

[c] Energy-dense and micronutrient-poor foods tend to be processed foods that are high in fat and/or sugars. Low energy-dense (or energy-dilute) foods, such as fruit, legumes, vegetables and whole grain cereals, are high in dietary fibre and water.

[d] Associated evidence and expert opinion included.

TABLE A-8-a-4. CLASSIFICATION OF OVERWEIGHT IN ADULTS ACCORDING TO BMI[a]

CLASSIFICATION	BMI (kg/m2)	RISK OF COMORBIDITIES
Underweight	<18.5	Low (but risk of other clinical problems increased)
Normal range	18.5–24.9	Average
Overweight	>25.0	
Pre-obese	25.0–29.9	Increased
Obese class I	30.0–34.9	Moderate
Obese class II	35.0–39.9	Severe
Obese class III	>40.0	Very severe

Table 8 in original document.

[a] These BMI values are age-independent and the same for both sexes. However, BMI may not correspond to the same degree of fatness in different populations due, in part, to differences in body proportions. The table shows a simplistic relationship between BMI and the risk of comorbidity, which can be affected by a range of factors, including the nature and the risk of comorbidity, which can be affected by a range of factors, including the nature of the diet, ethnic group and activity level. The risks associated with increasing BMI are continuous and graded and begin at a BMI below 25. The interpretation of BMI gradings in relation to risk may differ for different populations.

Both BMI and a measure of fat distribution (waist circumference or waist : hip ratio (WHR)) are important in calculating the risk of obesity comorbidities.

Source: Obesity: preventing and managing the global epidemic. Report of a WHO Consultation. Geneva, World Health Organization, 2000 (WHO Technical Report Series, No. 894). Report of a Joint WHO/FAO Expert Consultation, WHO Technical Report Series 916, Geneva 2003

http://www.who.int/dietphysicalactivity/publications/trs916/en/gsfao_overall.pdf

A-8-b. World Health Organization, Nutrition Tables

TABLE A-8-b-1. VALUES FOR THE DIGESTIBILITY OF PROTEIN IN MAN[a]

PROTEIN SOURCE	TRUE DIGESTIBILITY (MEAN ± SD)	DIGESTIBILITY RELATIVE TO REFERENCE PROTEINS
Egg	97 ± 3	
Milk, cheese	95 ± 3 91	100
Meat, fish	94 ± 3	
Maize	85 ± 6	89
Rice, polished	88 ± 4	93
Wheat, whole	86 ± 5	90
Wheat, refined	96 ± 4	101
Oatmeal	86 ± 7	90
Millet	79	83
Peas, mature	88	93
Peanut butter	95	100
Soyflour	86 ± 7	90
Beans	78	82
Maize + beans	78	82
Maize + beans + milk	84	88
Indian rice diet	77	81
Indian rice diet + milk	87	92
Chinese mixed diet	96	98[b]
Brazilian mixed diet	78	82
Filipino mixed diet	88[c]	93
American mixed diet	96[c]	101
Indian rice + bean diet	78[c]	82

[a]See original reference for data sources.
[b]Relative to egg measured in the same study.
[c]Recalculated from apparent digestibility, using F_k = 12 mg N/kg (see original text).

From Energy and Protein requirements: report of a Joint FAO/WHO/UNU Expert Consultation. Technical report series no. 724, Geneva: World Health Organization, 1985:119.

TABLE A-8-b-2-a. ENERGY REQUIREMENTS AND SAFE LEVELS OF PROTEIN INTAKE (per day/per kg): INFANTS AND CHILDREN AGED 3 MONTHS TO 10 YEARS (SEXES COMBINED UP TO 5 YEARS)

AGE	MEDIAN WEIGHT (kg)	ENERGY REQUIREMENT ($kcal_{th}$/kg)	(kJ/kg)	SAFE LEVEL OF PROTEIN INTAKE (g/kg)[a]
Months				
3–6	7.0	100	418	1.85
6–9	8.5	95	397	1.65
9–12	9.5	100	418	1.50
Years				
1–2	11.0	105	439	1.20
2–3	13.5	100	418	1.15
3–5	16.5	95	397	1.10

		BOYS	GIRLS	BOYS	GIRLS	
5–7	20.5	90	85	377	356	1.00
7–10	27.0	78	67	326	280	1.00

[a] Minimum level considered safe.

From Diet, nutrition and the prevention of chronic diseases: report of a WHO Study Group. Technical report series no. 797. Geneva: World Health Organization, 1990:167–168.

TABLE A-8-b-2-b. ENERGY REQUIREMENTS AND SAFE LEVELS OF PROTEIN INTAKE (per day/per kg): ADOLESCENTS AGED 10 TO 18 YEARS

AGE YEARS	MEDIAN WEIGHT (kg)	ENERGY REQUIREMENT ($kcal_{th}$)	(kJ)	SAFE LEVEL OF PROTEIN INTAKE (g/kg)[a]
Boys				
10–12	34.5	2,200	9,200	1.00
12–14	44.0	2,400	10,000	1.00
14–16	55.5	2,650	11,100	0.95
16–18	64.0	2,850	11,900	0.90
Girls				
10–12	36.0	1,950	8,200	1.00
12–14	46.5	2,100	8,800	0.95
14–16	52.0	2,150	9,000	0.90
16–18	54.0	2,150	9,000	0.80

[a] Minimum level considered safe.

From Diet, nutrition and the prevention of chronic diseases: report of a WHO Study Group. Technical report series no. 797. Geneva: World Health Organization, 1990:167–168.

TABLE A-8-b-2-c. ADULTS[a]

WEIGHT (kg)	ENERGY REQUIREMENT						SAFE LEVEL OF PROTEIN INTAKE (g/d)[b]
	18–30 y		30–60 y		OVER 60 y		
	(kcal$_{th}$)	(kJ)	(kcal$_{th}$)	(kJ)	(kcal$_{th}$)	(kJ)	
Men							
50	2,300	9,700	2,350	9,700	1,850	7,700	37.5
55	2,400	10,100	2,450	10,100	1,950	8,300	41.0
60	2,550	10,600	2,500	10,400	2,100	8,600	45.0
65	2,700	11,300	2,600	10,900	2,200	9,100	49.0
70	2,800	11,700	2,700	11,200	2,300	9,600	52.5
75	2,900	12,300	2,800	11,800	2,400	10,000	56.0
80	3,050	12,900	2,900	12,000	2,500	10,400	60.0
Women							
40	1,700	7,200	1,900	7,900	1,650	6,800	30.0
45	1,850	7,700	1,950	8,300	1,700	7,100	34.0
50	1,950	8,200	2,050	8,500	1,800	7,500	37.5
55	2,100	8,600	2,100	8,800	1,900	7,900	41.0
60	2,200	9,200	2,200	9,000	1,950	8,200	45.0
65	2,300	9,800	2,250	9,400	2,050	8,500	49.0
70	2,450	10,300	2,300	9,600	2,150	8,900	52.5
75	2,550	10,800	2,400	10,000	2,200	9,300	56.0

[a] For a basal metabolic rate factor of 1.6.
[b] Minimum level considered safe.

From Diet, nutrition and the prevention of chronic diseases: report of a WHO Study Group. Technical report series no. 797. Geneva: World Health Organization, 1990:167–168.

TABLE A-8-b-3. RECOMMENDED DIETARY ALLOWANCES OF VITAMINS AND MINERALS

AGE	VITAMIN A[a,b] SAFE LEVEL (μg retinol/d)		FOLATE[b] (μg/d)		VITAMIN B$_{12}$[a] (μg/d)		VITAMIN C[c] (mg/d)		VITAMIN D[c] (μg/d)		IRON[a,d] ABSORBED (μg/kg/d)		ZINC[e] (mg/d)	
	M	F	M	F	M	F	M	F	M	F	M	F	M	F
Infants (mo)														
0–3	350		16		0.1		20		10		120		3.1	
4–6	350		24		0.1		20		10		120		3.1	
7–9	350		32		0.1		20		10		120		2.8	
10–12	350		32		0.1		20		10		120		2.8	
Children and adults (y)														
1–2	400		50		1.0		20		10		56		4.0	3.9
3–4	400		50		1.0		20		10		44		4.0	3.9
5–6	400		102		1.0		20		10		40		4.0	3.9
7–10	400		102		1.0		20		2.5		40		4.0	3.9
11–12	500		102		1.0		20		2.5		40		7.0	6.6
13–14	600		170		1.0		30		2.5		34	40	7.0	6.6
15–16	600	500	170		1.0		30		2.5		34	40	7.0	5.5
17–18	600	500	200	170	1.0		30		2.5		34	40	7.0	5.5
19+	600	500	200	170	1.0		30		2.5		18	43	5.5	5.5
Pregnant women	600		370 to 470		1.4		50		10				6.4 to 7.5	
Lactating women		850	270		1.3		50		10		24		13.7	
Postmenopausal women		500	170		1.0		30		2.5		18		5.5	

Note: A detailed exposition has been published by the WHO on trace elements and nutrition entitled "Trace elements in human nutrition and health." World Health Organization, Geneva, 343;1996.
[a] Adapted from reference 1.
[b] Minimum level considered safe.
[c] Adapted from reference 2; 2.5 μg of cholecalciferol is equivalent to 100 IU of vitamin D.
[d] The amount of absorbed iron is a variable proportion of the intake, depending on the type of diet.
[e] Adapted from reference 3.
[f] Requirements during pregnancy depend on the woman's iron status before pregnancy.

From Diet, nutrition and the prevention of chronic diseases; report of a WHO Study Group. Technical report series no. 797. Geneva: World Health Organization, 1990:169.

A-8-c. FAO/WHO Human Vitamin and Mineral Requirements. Rome: Food and Agriculture Organization, 2001:01–290; ftp://ftp.fao.org/es/esu/nutrition/vitrni/pdf/total. Data avilables from website.

This selected reference has been provided by Allison A. Yates, Ph.D., and is discussed with other national and international nutrient standards in her Chapter 104.

A-9. NATIONAL DIETARY GUIDELINES AND RECOMMENDATIONS

A-9-a. Dietary Guidelines for Americans, 2005 (Executive Summary)*

Appendices Editors Note: The introduction for the EXECUTIVE SUMMARY 2005 has been abbreviated but the statements given here are verbatim. The entire report may be found at http://www.health.gov/dietaryguidelines/dga2005/report/. The reader is directed to Chapter 105 by Dr. Johanna Dwyer for a review and history of the dietary guidelines.

The Dietary *Guidelines for Americans [Dietary Guidelines]* provides science-based advice to promote health and to reduce risk for major chronic diseases through diet and physical activity. The intent of the *Dietary Guidelines* is to summarize and synthesize knowledge regarding individual nutrients and food components into recommendations for a pattern of eating that can be adopted by the public. In this publication, Key Recommendations are grouped under nine interrelated focus areas. The recommendations are based on the preponderance of scientific evidence for lowering risk of chronic disease and promoting health. It is important to remember that these are integrated messages that should be implemented as a whole.

Taken together, they encourage most Americans to eat fewer calories, be more active, and make wiser food choices.

A basic premise of the *Dietary Guidelines* is that nutrient needs should be met primarily through consuming foods. Foods provide an array of nutrients and other compounds that may have beneficial effects on health. In certain cases, fortified foods and dietary supplements may be useful sources of one or more nutrients that otherwise might be consumed in less than recommended amounts. However, dietary supplements, while recommended in some cases, cannot replace a healthful diet.

Throughout most of this publication, examples use a 2,000-calorie level as a reference for consistency with the Nutrition Facts Panel. Although this level is used as a reference, recommended calorie intake will differ for individuals based on age, gender, and activity level. At each calorie level, individuals who eat nutrient-dense foods may be able to meet their recommended nutrient intake without consuming their full calorie allotment.

The recommendations in the *Dietary Guidelines* are for Americans over 2 years of age. It is important to incorporate the food preferences of different racial/ethnic groups, vegetarians, and other groups when planning diets and developing educational programs and materials. The *Dietary Guidelines* is intended primarily for use by policymakers, health care providers, nutritionists, and nutrition educators. The following is a listing of the *Dietary Guidelines* by chapter.

Adequate Nutrients Within Calorie Needs

Key Recommendations

- Consume a variety of nutrient-dense foods and beverages within and among the basic food groups while

---

* Dietary Guidelines for Americans 2005 complete report in addition to Secretary, DHHS and Secretary of Agriculture comments may be accessed from: http://www.healthierus.gov/dietaryguidelines/

Websites for the 2005 MyPyramid Graphic

Appendices Editors Note: The order of the following websites allows the health professional to move from the home page to sites that provide sequential programs for application of the graphic.

The USDA MyPyramid.gov home site: http://www.mypyramid.gov/index.html

The MyPyramid Web site provides information specifically for professionals, in addition to the content for consumers: http://www.mypyramid.gov/professionals/index.html

Anatomy of MyPyramid describes how the symbol can be used to teach MyPyramid's key concepts: http://www.mypyramid.gov/downloads/MyPyramid_Anatomy.pdf

MyPyramid Food Guidance System Educational Framework: Key concepts for educators: http://www.mypyramid.gov/downloads/MyPyramid_education_framework.pdf

MyPyramid Food Intake Patterns—The suggested amounts of food to consume from the basic food groups, subgroups, and oils to meet recommended nutrient intakes at 12 different calorie levels. http://www.mypyramid.gov/downloads/MyPyramid_Food_Intake_Patterns.pdf

MyPyramid Food Intake Pattern Calorie Levels—MyPyramid assigns individuals to a calorie level based on their sex, age, and activity level. http://www.mypyramid.gov/downloads/MyPyramid_Calorie_Levels.pdf

Sample Menus for a 2000 Calorie Food Pattern—Averaged over a week, this seven day menu provides all of the recommended amounts of nutrients and food from each food group. http://www.mypyramid.gov/downloads/sample_menu.pdf

Mini Poster of the Graphics: http://www.mypyramid.gov/downloads/MiniPoster.pdf

There are 12 food intake patterns that identify how much food an individual should eat for health. Below are the downloads available for consumers via MyPyramid. These can be viewed and printed by calorie level: http://www.mypyramid.gov/professionals/results_downld.html

choosing foods that limit the intake of saturated and *trans* fats, cholesterol, added sugars, salt, and alcohol.

- Meet recommended intakes within energy needs by adopting a balanced eating pattern, such as the USDA Food Guide or the DASH Eating Plan.

Key Recommendations for Specific Population Groups

- *People over age 50.* Consume vitamin B$_{12}$ in its crystalline form (i.e., fortified foods or supplements).
- *Women of childbearing age who may become pregnant.* Eat foods high in hemeiron and/or consume iron-rich plant foods or iron-fortified foods with an enhancer of iron absorption, such as vitamin C-rich foods.
- *Women of childbearing age who may become pregnant and those in the first trimester of pregnancy.* Consume adequate synthetic folic acid daily (from fortified foods or supplements) in addition to food forms of folate from a varied diet.
- *Older adults, people with dark skin, and people exposed to insufficient ultraviolet band radiation (i.e., sunlight).* Consume extra vitamin D from vitamin D–fortified foods and/or supplements.

Weight Management

Key Recommendations

- To maintain body weight in a healthy range, balance calories from foods and beverages with calories expended.
- To prevent gradual weight gain over time, make small decreases in food and beverage calories and increase physical activity.

Key Recommendations for Specific Population Groups

- *Those who need to lose weight.* Aim for a slow, steady weight loss by decreasing calorie intake while maintaining an adequate nutrient intake and increasing physical activity.
- *Overweight children.* Reduce the rate of body weight gain while allowing growth and development. Consult a healthcare provider before placing a child on a weight-reduction diet.
- *Pregnant women.* Ensure appropriate weight gain as specified by a healthcare provider.
- *Breastfeeding women.* Moderate weight reduction is safe and does not compromise weight gain of the nursing infant.
- *Overweight adults and overweight children with chronic diseases and/or on medication.* Consult a healthcare provider about weight loss strategies prior to starting a weight-reduction program to ensure appropriate management of other health conditions.

Physical Activity

Key Recommendations

- Engage in regular physical activity and reduce sedentary activities to promote health, psychological well-being, and a healthy body weight.
- To reduce the risk of chronic disease in adulthood: Engage in at least 30 minutes of moderate-intensity physical activity, above usual activity, at work or home on most days of the week.
  - For most people, greater health benefits can be obtained by engaging in physical activity of more vigorous intensity or longer duration.
  - To help manage body weight and prevent gradual, unhealthy body weight gain in adulthood: Engage in approximately 60 minutes of moderate- to vigorous-intensity activity on most days of the week while not exceeding caloric intake requirements.
  - To sustain weight loss in adulthood: Participate in at least 60 to 90 minutes of daily moderate-intensity physical activity while not exceeding caloric intake requirements. Some people may need to consult with a healthcare provider before participating in this level of activity.
- Achieve physical fitness by including cardiovascular conditioning, stretching exercises for flexibility, and resistance exercises or calisthenics for muscle strength and endurance.

Key Recommendations for Specific Population Groups

- *Children and adolescents.* Engage in at least 60 minutes of physical activity on most, preferably all, days of the week.
- *Pregnant women.* In the absence of medical or obstetric complications, incorporate 30 minutes or more of moderate-intensity physical activity on most, if not all, days of the week. Avoid activities with a high risk of falling or abdominal trauma.
- *Breastfeeding women.* Be aware that neither acute nor regular exercise adversely affects the mother's ability to successfully breastfeed.
- *Older adults.* Participate in regular physical activity to reduce functional declines associated with aging and to achieve the other benefits of physical activity identified for all adults.

Food Groups to Encourage

Key Recommendations

- Consume a sufficient amount of fruits and vegetables while staying within energy needs. Two cups of fruit and 2 1/2 cups of vegetables per day are recommended for a reference 2,000-calorie intake, with higher or lower amounts depending on the calorie level.

- Choose a variety of fruits and vegetables each day. In particular, select from all five vegetable subgroups (dark green, orange, legumes, starchy vegetables, and other vegetables) several times a week.
- Consume 3 or more ounce-equivalents of whole-grain products per day, with the rest of the recommended grains coming from enriched or whole-grain products. In general, at least half the grains should come from whole grains.
- Consume 3 cups per day of fat-free or low-fat milk or equivalent milk products.

Key Recommendations for Specific Population Groups

- *Children and adolescents.* Consume whole-grain products often; at least half the grains should be whole grains. Children 2 to 8 years should consume 2 cups per day of fat-free or low-fat milk or equivalent milk products. Children 9 years of age and older should consume 3 cups per day of fat-free or low-fat milk or equivalent milk products.

Fats

Key Recommendations

- Consume less than 10 percent of calories from saturated fatty acids and less than 300 mg/day of cholesterol, and keep *trans* fatty acid consumption as low as possible.
- Keep total fat intake between 20 to 35 percent of calories, with most fats coming from sources of polyunsaturated and monounsaturated fatty acids, such as fish, nuts, and vegetable oils.
- When selecting and preparing meat, poultry, dry beans, and milk or milk products, make choices that are lean, low-fat, or fat-free.
- Limit intake of fats and oils high in saturated and/or *trans* fatty acids, and choose products low in such fats and oils.

Key Recommendations for Specific Population Groups

- *Children and adolescents.* Keep total fat intake between 30 to 35 percent of calories for children 2 to 3 years of age and between 25 to 35 percent of calories for children and adolescents 4 to 18 years of age, with most fats coming from sources of polyunsaturated and monounsaturated fatty acids, such as fish, nuts, and vegetable oils.

Carbohydrates

Key Recommendations

- Choose fiber-rich fruits, vegetables, and whole grains often.
- Choose and prepare foods and beverages with little added sugars or caloric sweeteners, such as amounts

suggested by the USDA Food Guide and the DASH Eating Plan.
- Reduce the incidence of dental caries by practicing good oral hygiene and consuming sugar- and starch-containing foods and beverages less frequently.

Sodium and Potassium

Key Recommendations

- Consume less than 2,300 mg (approximately 1 tsp of salt) of sodium per day.
- Choose and prepare foods with little salt. At the same time, consume potassiumrich foods, such as fruits and vegetables.

Key Recommendations for Specific Population Groups

- *Individuals with hypertension, blacks, and middle-aged and older adults.* Aim to consume no more than 1,500 mg of sodium per day, and meet the potassium recommendation (4,700 mg/day) with food.

Alcoholic Beverages

Key Recommendations

- Those who choose to drink alcoholic beverages should do so sensibly and in moderation—defined as the consumption of up to one drink per day for women and up to two drinks per day for men.
- Alcoholic beverages should not be consumed by some individuals, including those who cannot restrict their alcohol intake, women of childbearing age who may become pregnant, pregnant and lactating women, children and adolescents, individuals taking medications that can interact with alcohol, and those with specific medical conditions.
- Alcoholic beverages should be avoided by individuals engaging in activities that require attention, skill, or coordination, such as driving or operating machinery.

Food Safety

Key Recommendations

- To avoid microbial foodborne illness:
  - Clean hands, food contact surfaces, and fruits and vegetables. Meat and poultry should not be washed or rinsed.
  - Separate raw, cooked, and ready-to-eat foods while shopping, preparing, or storing foods.
  - Cook foods to a safe temperature to kill microorganisms.
  - Chill (refrigerate) perishable food promptly and defrost foods properly.
  - Avoid raw (unpasteurized) milk or any products made from unpasteurized milk, raw or partially

cooked eggs or foods containing raw eggs, raw or undercooked meat and poultry, unpasteurized juices, and raw sprouts.

Key Recommendations for Specific Population Groups

- *Infants and young children, pregnant women, older adults, and those who are immunocompromised.* Do not eat or drink raw (unpasteurized) milk or any products made from unpasteurized milk, raw or partially cooked eggs or foods containing raw eggs, raw or undercooked meat and poultry, raw or undercooked fish or shellfish, unpasteurized juices, and raw sprouts.
- *Pregnant women, older adults, and those who are immunocompromised*: Only eat certain deli meats and frankfurters that have been reheated to steaming hot.

A-9-b. Management of High Blood Cholesterol and Related Risk Factors

A-9-b-1. Cholesterol Levels and Coronary Heart Disease Risk

The Third Report of the Expert Panel on Detection, Evaluation, and Treatment of High Blood Cholesterol in Adults (Adult Treatment Panel III, or ATP III) constitutes the National Cholesterol Education Program's (NCEP's) updated clinical guidelines for cholesterol testing and management (1).

While ATP III maintains attention to intensive treatment of patients with CHD, its major new feature is a focus on primary prevention in persons with multiple risk factors. Many of these persons have a relatively high risk for CHD and will benefit from more intensive LDL-lowering treatment than recommended in ATP II. ATP III continues to identify elevated LDL cholesterol as the primary target of cholesterol-lowering therapy. As a result, the primary goals of therapy and the cutpoints for initiating treatment are stated in terms of LDL.

The relationship between LDL cholesterol levels and CHD risk is continuous over a broad range of LDL levels from low to high. Therefore, ATP III adopts the classification of LDL cholesterol levels shown in Table A-9-b-1-a, which also shows the classification of total and HDL cholesterol levels.

Risk determinants in addition to LDL-cholesterol include the presence or absence of CHD, other clinical forms of atherosclerotic disease, and the major risk factors other than LDL (see Table A-9-b-1-b)

Diabetes counts as a CHD risk equivalent because it confers a high risk of new CHD within 10 years, in part because of its frequent association with multiple risk factors. Furthermore, because persons with diabetes who experience a myocardial infarction have an unusually high death rate either immediately or in the long term, a more intensive prevention strategy is warranted.

TABLE A-9-b-1-a. ATP III CLASSIFICATION OF LDL, TOTAL, AND HDL CHOLESTEROL (mg/dL)

LDL Cholesterol	
<100	Optimal
100–129	Near optimal/above optimal
130–159	Borderline high
160–189	High
≥190	Very high
Total Cholesterol	
<200	Desirable
200–239	Borderline high
≥240	High
HDL Cholesterol	
<40	Low
≥60	High

A-9-b-2. Role of Other Risk Factors in Risk Assessment

ATP III recognizes that risk for CHD is influenced by other factors not included among the major, independent risk factors (Table A-9-b-1-b). Among these are *life-habit risk factors and emerging risk factors*. The former include obesity, physical inactivity, and atherogenic diet; the latter consist of lipoprotein (a), homocysteine, prothrombotic and proinflammatory factors, impaired fasting glucose, and evidence of subclinical atherosclerotic disease. The *life-habit risk factors* are direct targets for clinical intervention, but are not used to set a lower LDL cholesterol goal of therapy. The *emerging risk factors* do not categorically modify LDL cholesterol goals; however, they appear to contribute to CHD risk to varying degrees and can have utility in selected persons to guide intensity of risk-reduction therapy.

A-9-b-2-a. Metabolic Syndrome. Many persons have a constellation of major risk factors, life-habit risk factors, and emerging risk factors that constitute a condition called the *metabolic syndrome*. Factors characteristic of the metabolic syndrome are abdominal obesity, atherogenic dyslipidemia (elevated triglyceride, small LDL particles, low HDL cholesterol), raised blood pressure, insulin resistance (with or without glucose intolerance), and prothrom-

TABLE A-9-b-1-b. MAJOR RISK FACTORS (EXCLUSIVE OF LDL CHOLESTEROL) THAT MODIFY LDL GOALS*

- Cigarette smoking
- Hypertension (BP □140/90 mmHg or on antihypertensive medication)
- Low HDL cholesterol (<40 mg/dL)[†]
- Family history of premature CHD (CHD in male first degree relative <55 years; CHD in female first degree relative <65 years)
- Age (men □45 years; women □55 years)*

* In ATP III, diabetes is regarded as a CHD risk equivalent.
† HDL cholesterol □60 mg/dL counts as a "negative" risk factor; its presence removes one risk factor from the total count.

botic and proinflammatory states. ATP III recognizes the metabolic syndrome as a secondary target of risk-reduction therapy, after the primary target—LDL cholesterol.

A-9-b-3. Primary Prevention With LDL-Lowering Therapy

Primary prevention of CHD offers the greatest opportunity for reducing the burden of CHD in the United States. The clinical approach to primary prevention is founded on the public health approach that calls for lifestyle changes, including: 1) reduced intakes of saturated fat and cholesterol, 2) increased physical activity, and 3) weight control, to lower population cholesterol levels and reduce CHD risk, but the clinical approach intensifies preventive strategies for higher risk persons. One aim of primary prevention is to reduce long-term risk (>10 years) as well as short-term risk (10 years). LDL goals in primary prevention depend on a person's absolute risk for CHD (i.e., the probability of having a CHD event in the short term or the long term)—the higher the risk, the lower the goal. Therapeutic lifestyle changes are the foundation of clinical primary prevention. Nonetheless, some persons at higher risk because of high or very high LDL cholesterol levels or because of multiple risk factors are candidates for LDL-lowering drugs. Recent primary prevention trials show that LDL-lowering drugs reduce risk for major coronary events and coronary death even in the short term.

A-9-b-4. Secondary Prevention With LDL-Lowering Therapy

Recent clinical trials demonstrate that LDL-lowering therapy reduces total mortality, coronary mortality, major coronary events, coronary artery procedures, and stroke in persons with established CHD. As shown in Table A-9-b-1-a, an LDL cholesterol level of <100 mg/dL is *optimal;* therefore, ATP III specifies an LDL cholesterol <100 mg/dL as the goal of therapy in secondary prevention.

A-9-b-5. LDL-Lowering Therapy in Three Risk Categories

The two major modalities of LDL-lowering therapy are *therapeutic lifestyle changes* (TLC) and *drug therapy.* The TLC Diet stresses reductions in saturated fat and cholesterol intakes. When the metabolic syndrome or its associated lipid risk factors (elevated triglyceride or low HDL cholesterol) are present, TLC also stresses weight reduction and increased physical activity. Table A-9-b-5-a defines LDL cholesterol goals and cutpoints for initiation of TLC and for drug consideration for persons with three categories of risk: CHD and CHD risk equivalents; multiple (2+) risk factors (10-year risk 10–20% and <10%); and 0–1 risk factor.

A-9-b-6. Therapeutic Lifestyle Changes in LDL-Lowering Therapy

ATP III recommends a multifaceted lifestyle approach to reduce risk for CHD. This approach is designated *therapeutic lifestyle changes (TLC).* Its essential features are:

- Reduced intakes of saturated fats (<7% of total calories) and cholesterol (<200 mg per day) (see Table A-9-b-6-1 for overall composition of the TLC Diet)
- Therapeutic options for enhancing LDL lowering such as plant stanols/sterols (2 g/day) and increased viscous (soluble) fiber (10–25 g/day)
- Weight reduction
- Increased physical activity

A model of steps in TLC is shown in Figure A-9-b-6-2. To initiate TLC, intakes of saturated fats and cholesterol are reduced first to lower LDL cholesterol. To improve overall health, ATP III's TLC Diet generally contains the recommendations embodied in the Dietary Guidelines for Americans 2000. One exception is that total fat is allowed to range from 25–35% of total calories provided saturated fats and *trans* fatty acids are kept low. A higher intake of total fat, mostly in the form of unsaturated fat, can help to reduce triglycerides and raise HDL cholesterol in persons with the metabolic syndrome.

TABLE A-9-b-5-a. LDL CHOLESTEROL GOALS AND CUTPOINTS FOR THERAPEUTIC LIFESTYLE CHANGES (TLC) AND DRUG THERAPY IN DIFFERENT RISK CATEGORIES.

RISK CATEGORY	LDL GOAL	LDL LEVEL AT WHICH TO INITIATE THERAPEUTIC LIFESTYLE CHANGES (TLC)	LDL LEVEL AT WHICH TO CONSIDER DRUG THERAPY
CHD or CHD Risk Equivalents (10-year risk >20%)	<100 mg/dL	≥100 mg/dL	≥130 mg/dL (100–129 mg/dL: drug optional* 10-year risk 10–20%:
2+ Risk Factors (10-year risk ≥20%)	<130 mg/dL	≥130 mg/dL	≥130 mg/dL 10-year risk <10%: ≥160 mg/dL
0–1 Risk Factor†	<160 mg/dL	≥160 mg/dL	≥190 mg/dL (160–189 mg/dL: LDL-lowering drug optional)

* Some authorities recommend use of LDL-lowering drugs in this category if an LDL cholesterol <100 mg/dL cannot be achieved by therapeutic lifestyle changes. Others prefer use of drugs that primarily modify triglycerides and HDL, e.g., nicotinic acid or fibrate. Clinical judgment also may call for deferring drug therapy in this subcategory.

† Almost all people with 0–1 risk factor have a 10-year risk <10%, thus 10-year risk assessment in people with 0–1 risk factor is not necessary.

After maximum reduction of LDL cholesterol with dietary therapy, emphasis shifts to management of the metabolic syndrome and associated lipid risk factors. The majority of persons with these latter abnormalities are overweight or obese and sedentary. Weight reduction therapy for overweight or obese patients will enhance LDL lowering and will provide other health benefits including modifying other lipid and nonlipid risk factors.

At all stages of dietary therapy, physicians are encouraged to refer patients to registered dietitians or other qualified nutritionists for *medical nutrition therapy*, which is the term for the nutritional intervention and guidance provided by a nutrition professional.

A-9-b-7. Benefit Beyond LDL Lowering: The Metabolic Syndrome as a Secondary Target of Therapy

Evidence is accumulating that risk for CHD can be reduced beyond LDL-lowering therapy by modification of other risk factors. One potential secondary target of therapy is the metabolic syndrome, which represents a constellation of lipid and nonlipid risk factors of metabolic origin. This syndrome is closely linked to a generalized metabolic disorder called *insulin resistance* in which the normal actions of insulin are impaired. Excess body fat (particularly abdominal obesity) and physical inactivity promote the development of insulin resistance, but some individuals also are genetically predisposed to insulin resistance.

The risk factors of the metabolic syndrome are highly concordant; in aggregate they enhance risk for CHD at any given LDL cholesterol level. For purposes of ATP III, the diagnosis of the metabolic syndrome is made when

TABLE A-9-b-6-a. NUTRIENT COMPOSITION OF THE TLC DIET

NUTRIENT	RECOMMENDED INTAKE
Saturated fat*	Less than 7% of total calories
Polyunsaturated fat	Up to 10% of total calories
Monounsaturated fat	Up to 20% of total calories
Total fat	25–35% of total calories
Carbohydrate†	50–60% of total calories
Fiber	20–30 g/day
Protein	Approximately 15% of total calories
Cholesterol	Less than 200 mg/day
Total calories (energy)‡	Balance energy intake and expenditure to maintain desirable body weight/prevent weight gain

* Trans fatty acids are another LDL-raising fat that should be kept at a low intake.
† Carbohydrate should be derived predominantly from foods rich in complex carbohydrates including grains, especially whole grains, fruits, and vegetables.
‡ Daily energy expenditure should include at least moderate physical activity (contributing approximately 200 Kcal per day).

three or more of the risk determinants shown in Table A-9-b-7-a are present. These determinants include a combination of categorical and borderline risk factors that can be readily measured in clinical practice.

Management of the metabolic syndrome has a two-fold objective: (1) to reduce underlying causes (i.e., obesity and physical inactivity), and (2) to treat associated nonlipid and lipid risk factors.

A-9-b-7-b. Management of Underlying causes of the Metabolic Syndrome. First-line therapies for all lipid and nonlipid risk factors associated with the metabolic syndrome are weight reduction and increased physical activity, which will effectively reduce all of these risk

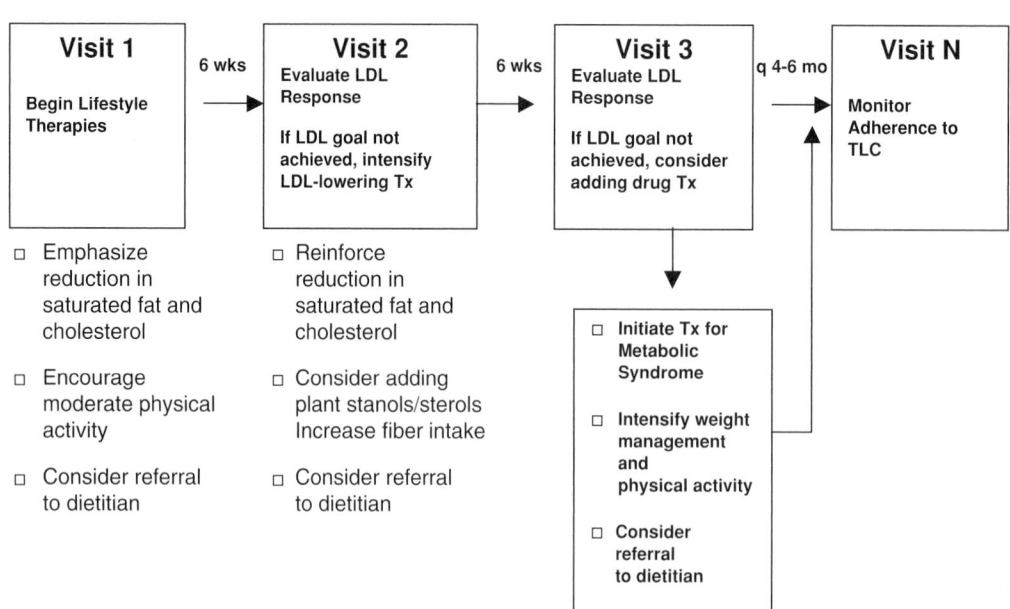

Figure A-9-b-6-b. A Model of Steps in Therapeutic Lifestyle Changes (TLC)

factors. Therefore, after appropriate control of LDL cholesterol, TLC should stress weight reduction and physical activity if the metabolic syndrome is present.

Weight control. In ATP III overweight and obesity are recognized as major, underlying risk factors for CHD and identified as direct targets of intervention. Weight reduction will enhance LDL lowering and reduce all of the risk factors of the metabolic syndrome. The recommended approaches for reducing overweight and obesity are contained in the clinical guidelines of the NHLBI Obesity Education Initiative.

Physical activity. Physical inactivity is likewise a major, underlying risk factor for CHD. It augments the lipid and nonlipid risk factors of the metabolic syndrome. It further may enhance risk by impairing cardiovascular fitness and coronary blood flow. Regular physical activity reduces very low density lipoprotein (VLDL) levels, raises HDL cholesterol, and in some persons, lowers LDL levels. It also can

lower blood pressure, reduce insulin resistance, and favorably influence cardiovascular function. Thus, ATP III recommends that regular physical activity become a routine component in management of high serum cholesterol.

A-9-b-8. Specific Treatment of Lipid and Nonlipid Risk Factors

Beyond the underlying risk factors, therapies directed against the lipid and nonlipid risk factors of the metabolic syndrome will reduce CHD risk. These include treatment of hypertension, use of aspirin in patients with CHD to reduce the prothrombotic state (guidelines for aspirin use in primary prevention have not been firmly established), and treatment of elevated triglycerides and low HDL cholesterol.

Elevated serum triglycerides. Recent meta-analyses of prospective studies indicate that elevated triglycerides are also an independent risk factor for CHD. Factors contributing to elevated (higher than normal) triglycerides in the general population include: obesity and overweight, physical inactivity, cigarette smoking, excess alcohol intake, high carbohydrate diets (>60% of energy intake), type 2 diabetes, chronic renal failure, nephrotic syndrome), certain drugs and genetic disorders.

A-9-b-8-a. ATP III Adopts the Following Classification of Serum Triglycerides:

- Normal triglycerides: <150 mg/dL
- Borderline-high triglycerides: 150–199 mg/dL
- High triglycerides: 200–499 mg/dL
- Very high triglycerides: ≥500 mg/dL

TABLE A-9-b-7-a. CLINICAL IDENTIFICATION OF THE METABOLIC SYNDROME

RISK FACTOR	DEFINING LEVEL
Abdominal Obesity*	Waist Circumference[†]
Men	>102 cm (>40 in)
Women	>88 cm (>35 in)
Triglycerides	≥150 mg/dL
HDL cholesterol	
Men	<40 mg/dL
Women	<50 mg/dL
Blood pressure	≥130/≥85 mmHg
Fasting glucose	≥110 mg/dL

*Overweight and obesity are associated with insulin resistance and the metabolic syndrome. However, the presence of abdominal obesity is more highly correlated with the metabolic risk factors than is an elevated body mass index (BMI). Therefore, the simple measure of waist circumference is recommended to identify the body weight component of the metabolic syndrome.

[†]Some male patients can develop multiple metabolic risk factors when the waist circumference is only marginally increased, e.g., 94–102 cm (37–39 in). Such patients may have a strong genetic contribution to insulin resistance. They should benefit from changes in life habits, similarly to men with categorical increases in waist circumference

1. Relevant text and tables taken from the National Cholesterol Education Program (NCEP) Expert Panel on Detection, Evaluation, and Treatment of High Blood Cholesterol in Adults (Adult Treatment Panel III). Third Report of the National Cholesterol Education Program (NCEP) Expert Panel on Detection, Evaluation, and Treatment of High Blood Cholesterol in Adults (Adult Treatment Panel III) final report. In JAMA. 2001;16:285:2486–97

A-9-b-9. Addendum- NCEP Report of 2004*

Appendices Editors Comment: Since the 2001 publication of the Executive Summary, the publication of five major clinical trials of statin therapy with clinical endpoints have been published. *This new report by NCEP committee reviews the results of these trials that led the committee to modify the ATP III treatment algorithm in terms of goals for* *various levels of risk.* These modifications are presented below in two tables: the first (*A-9-b-9-a*) states LDL-C goals and treatments and therapies at specific LDL levels; the second (*A-9-b-9-b*) is a statement of modifications in text form.

° Grundy SM, Cleeman JI, Merz NB, et al. for the Coordinating Committee of the National Cholesterol Education Committee. Circulation 2004;110:227–39.

TABLE A-9-b-9-a. ATP III LDL-C GOALS AND CUTPOINTS FOR TLC AND DRUG THERAPY IN DIFFERENT RISK CATEGORIES AND PROPOSED MODIFICATIONS BASED ON RECENT CLINICAL TRIAL EVIDENCE

RISK CATEGORY	LDL-C GOAL	INITIATE TLC	CONSIDER DRUG THERAPY**
High risk: CHD* or CHD risk equivalents[†] (10-year risk_20%)	<100 mg/dL (optional goal: <70 mg/dl)[≠]	≥100 mg/dL[#]	≥100 mg/dL[††] (<100 mg/dL: consider drug options)**
Moderately high risk: 2+ risk factors[‡] (10-year risk 10% to 20%)[§§]	<130 mg/dL[¶]	≥130 mg/dL[#]	≥130 mg/dL (100–129 mg/dL; consider drug options)[‡‡]
Moderate risk: 2_risk factors[‡] (10-year risk_10%)[§§]	<130 mg/dL	≥130 mg/dL	≥160 mg/dL
Lower risk: 0–1 risk factor[§]	<160 mg/dL	≥160 mg/dL	≥190 mg/dL (160–189 mg/dL: LDL-lowering drug optional)

* CHD includes history of myocardial infarction, unstable angina, stable angina, coronary artery procedures (angioplasty or bypass surgery), or evidence of clinically significant myocardial ischemia.

[†] CHD risk equivalents include clinical manifestations of noncoronary forms of atherosclerotic disease (peripheral arterial disease, abdominal aortic aneurysm, and carotid artery disease [transient ischemic attacks or stroke of carotid origin or >50% obstruction of a carotid artery]), diabetes, and 2+ risk factors with 10-year risk for hard CHD >20%.

[‡] Risk factors include cigarette smoking, hypertension (BP ≥140/90 mm Hg or on antihypertensive medication), low HDL cholesterol (<40 mg/dL), family history of premature CHD (CHD in male first-degree relative <55 years of age; CHD in female first-degree relative <65 years of age), and age (men ≥45 years; women ≥55 years).

[§§] Electronic 10-year risk calculators are available at www.nhlbi.nih.gov/guidelines/cholesterol.

[§] Almost all people with zero or 1 risk factor have a 10-year risk <10%, and 10-year risk assessment in people with zero or 1 risk factor is thus not necessary.

[≠] Very high risk favors the optional LDL-C goal of <70 mg/dL, and in patients with high triglycerides, non-HDL-C <100 mg/dL.

[¶] Optional LDL-C goal <100 mg/dL.

[#] Any person at high risk or moderately high risk who has lifestyle-related risk factors (eg, obesity, physical inactivity, elevated triglyceride, low HDL-C, or metabolic syndrome) is a candidate for therapeutic lifestyle changes to modify these risk factors regardless of LDL-C level.

** When LDL-lowering drug therapy is employed, it is advised that intensity of therapy be sufficient to achieve at least a 30% to 40% reduction in LDL-C levels.

[††] If baseline LDL-C is <100 mg/dL, institution of an LDL-lowering drug is a therapeutic option on the basis of available clinical trial results. If a high-risk person has high triglycerides or low HDL-C, combining a fibrate or nicotinic acid with an LDL-lowering drug can be considered.

[‡‡] For moderately high-risk persons, when LDL-C level is 100 to 129 mg/dL, at baseline or on lifestyle therapy, initiation of an LDL-lowering drug to achieve an LDL-C level <100 mg/dL is a therapeutic option on the basis of available clinical trial results.

TABLE A-9-b-9-b. RECOMMENDATIONS FOR MODIFICATIONS TO FOOTNOTE THE ATP III TREATMENT ALGORITHM FOR LDL-C

- Therapeutic lifestyle changes (TLC) remain an essential modality in clinical management. TLC has the potential to reduce cardiovascular risk through several mechanisms beyond LDL lowering.
- In high-risk persons, the recommended LDL-C goal is <100 mg/dL.
  - An LDL-C goal of <70 mg/dL is a therapeutic option on the basis of available clinical trial evidence, especially for patients at very high risk.
  - If LDL-C is ≥100 mg/dL, an LDL-lowering drug is indicated simultaneously with lifestyle changes.
  - If baseline LDL-C is <100 mg/dL, institution of an LDL-lowering drug to achieve an LDL-C level <70 mg/dL is a therapeutic option on the basis of available clinical trial evidence.
  - If a high-risk person has high triglycerides or low HDL-C, consideration can be given to combining a fibrate or nicotinic acid with an LDL-lowering drug. When triglycerides are ≥200 mg/dL, non-HDL-C is a secondary target of therapy, with a goal 30 mg/dL higher than the identified LDL-C goal.
- For moderately high-risk persons (2+ risk factors and 10-year risk 10% to 20%), the recommended LDL-C goal is <130 mg/dL; an LDL-C goal <100 mg/dL is a therapeutic option on the basis of available clinical trial evidence. When LDL-C level is 100 to 129 mg/dL, at baseline or on lifestyle therapy, initiation of an LDL-lowering drug to achieve an LDL-C level <100 mg/dL is a therapeutic option on the basis of available clinical trial evidence.
- Any person at high risk or moderately high risk who has lifestyle-related risk factors (eg, obesity, physical inactivity, elevated triglyceride, low HDL-C, or metabolic syndrome) is a candidate for TLC to modify these risk factors regardless of LDL-C level.
- When LDL-lowering drug therapy is employed in high-risk or moderately high-risk persons, it is advised that intensity of therapy be sufficient to achieve at least a 30% to 40% reduction in LDL-C levels.
- For people in lower-risk categories, recent clinical trials do not modify the goals and cutpoints of therapy.

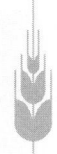

A-10. BASAL METABOLIC RATE (BMR) AND RESTING ENERGY EXPENDITURE (REE) DATA

TABLE A-10-a. NOMOGRAPH FOR ESTIMATION OF CALORIC NEEDS AND SURFACE AREA

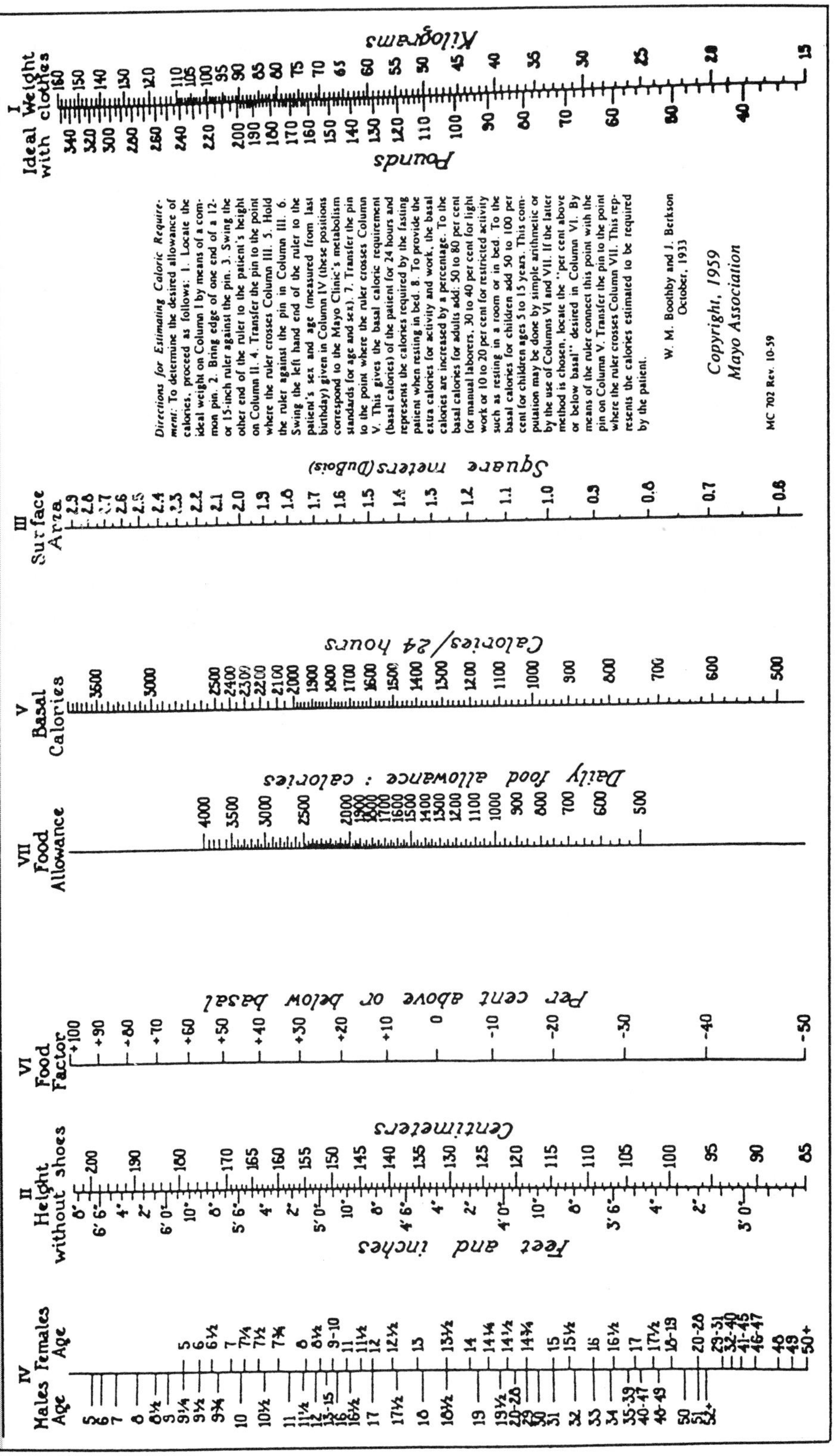

Directions for Estimating Caloric Requirement: To determine the desired allowance of calories, proceed as follows: 1. Locate the ideal weight on Column I by means of a common pin. 2. Bring edge of one end of a 12- or 15-inch ruler against the pin. 3. Swing the other end of the ruler to the patient's height on Column II. 4. Transfer the pin to the point where the ruler crosses Column III. 5. Hold the ruler against the left hand end of the ruler to the patient's sex and age (measured from last birthday) given in Column IV (these positions correspond to the Mayo Clinic's metabolism standards for age and sex). 7. Transfer the pin to the point where the ruler crosses Column V. This gives the basal caloric requirement (basal calories) of the patient for 24 hours and represents the calories required by the fasting patient when resting in bed. 8. To provide the extra calories for activity and work, the basal calories are increased by a percentage. To the basal calories for adults add: 50 to 80 per cent for manual laborers, 30 to 40 per cent for light work or 10 to 20 per cent for restricted activity such as resting in a room or in bed. To the basal calories for children add 50 to 100 per cent for children ages 5 to 15 years. This computation may be done by simple arithmetic or by the use of Columns VI and VII. If the latter method is chosen, locate the "per cent above or below basal" desired in Column VI. By means of the ruler connect this point with the pin on Column V. Transfer the pin to the point where the ruler crosses Column VII. This represents the calories estimated to be required by the patient.

W. M. Boothby and J. Berkson
October, 1933

Copyright, 1959
Mayo Association

MC 702 Rev. 10-59

I Ideal Weight with clothes — *Kilograms* / *Pounds*

III Surface Area — *Square meters (DuBois)*

V Basal Calories — *Calories/24 hours*

VII Food Allowance — *Daily food allowance : calories*

VI Food Factor — *Per cent above or below basal*

II Height without shoes — *Centimeters* / *Feet and inches*

IV Males Females Age

(From Pemberton, C.M., Gastineau, C.F.: Mayo Clinic Diet Manual. 5th Ed. Philadelphia, W.B. Saunders, 1981.)

TABLE A-10-b. EQUATIONS FOR PREDICTING BASAL METABOLIC RATE FROM BODY WEIGHT (W)[a]

AGE RANGE (y)	Kcal$_{th}$/d	CORRELATION COEFFICIENT	SD[b]	MJ/d	CORRELATION COEFFICIENT	SD
Males						
0–3	60.9 W − 54	0.97	53	0.255 W − 0.226	0.97	0.222
3–10	22.7 W + 495	0.86	62	0.0949 W + 2.07	0.86	0.259
10–18	17.5 W + 651	0.90	100	0.0732 W + 2.72	0.90	0.418
18–30	15.3 W + 679	0.65	151	0.0640 W + 2.84	0.65	0.632
30–60	11.6 W + 879	0.60	164	0.0485 W + 3.67	0.60	0.686
>60	13.5 W + 487	0.79	148	0.0565 W + 2.04	0.79	0.619
Females						
0–3	61.0 W − 51	0.97	61	0.255 W − 0.214	0.97	0.255
3–10	22.5 W + 499	0.85	63	0.0941 W + 2.09	0.85	0.264
10–18	12.2 W + 746	0.75	117	0.0510 W + 3.12	0.75	0.489
18–30	14.7 W + 496	0.72	121	0.0615 W + 2.08	0.72	0.506
30–60	8.7 W + 829	0.70	108	0.0364 W + 3.47	0.70	0.452
>60	10.5 W + 596	0.74	108	0.0439 W + 2.49	0.74	0.452

[a] Since the present report was compiled, the detabase for the equations contained in Schofield et al. Hum Nutr Clin Nutr 1985; 39(Suppl), has been slightly expanded. They therefore differ from the equations shown in this table, but the differences are negligible.
[b] Standard deviation of differences between actual BMR and predicted estimates.

From Energy and protein requirements: report of a Joint FAO/WHO/UNU Expert Consultation. Technical report series no. 724. Geneva: World Health Organization, 1985:71.

TABLE A-10-c. EXAMPLES OF PREDICTED BASAL METABOLIC RATE (BMR) IN SUBJECTS OF THE SAME HEIGHT BUT DIFFERENT WEIGHTS, PREDICTED FROM ACTUAL WEIGHT AND FROM MEDIAN ACCEPTABLE WEIGHT FOR HEIGHT

	MAN, AGE 40, HEIGHT 1.8 M			WOMAN, AGE 25, HEIGHT 1.5 M		
	POSITION IN RANGE[a]			POSITION IN RANGE[b]		
	UPPER	MEDIAN	LOWER	UPPER	MEDIAN	LOWER
BMI[b]	25	22	20	24	21	19
Wt (kg)	81.0	71.3	64.8	54.0	47.2	42.7
BMR[c] from actual wt						
kcal$_{th}$/d	1,820	1,710	1,630	1,290	1,190	1,120
MJ/day	7.61	7.15	6.82	5.39	4.98	4.68
BMR from median wt						
kcal$_{th}$/d	1,710	1,710	1,710	1,190	1,190	1,190
MJ/d	7.15	7.15	7.15	4.97	4.97	4.97

[a] Acceptable range of BMI (see Annex 2A in original reference).
[b] Body mass index = wt(kg)/ht²(m).
[c] Predicted from equations in Table A-10-b.

From Energy and protein requirements: report of a Joint FAO/WHO/UNU Expert Consultation, Technical report series no. 724. Geneva: World Health Organization, 1985:72.

TABLE A-10-d. BASAL METABOLIC RATES OF ADOLESCENT BOYS AND GIRLS

AGE (ys)	HEIGHT[a] (cm)	WEIGHT[b] (kg)	BMR[c] TOTAL (kcal_th/d)	(MJ/d)	BMR[c] per kg (kcal_th/d)	(MJ/d)
Boys
10–11	140	32.2	1,215	5.08	37.7	0.16
11–12	147	37.0	1,300	5.43	35.1	0.15
12–13	153	40.9	1,370	5.73	33.4	0.14
13–14	160	47.0	1,465	6.12	31.4	0.13
14–15	166	52.6	1,570	6.57	29.9	0.12
15–16	171	58.0	1,665	6.96	28.7	0.12
16–17	175	62.7	1,750	7.32	27.9	0.12
17–18	177	65.0	1,790	7.48	27.5	0.12
Girls
10–11	142	33.7	1,160	4.85	34.3	0.14
11–12	148	38.7	1,220	5.10	31.5	0.13
12–13	155	44.0	1,280	5.38	29.1	0.12
13–14	159	48.8	1,340	5.60	27.5	0.12
14–15	161	51.4	1,375	5.75	26.7	0.11
15–16	162	53.0	1,395	5.83	26.3	0.11
16–17	163	54.0	1,405	5.87	26.0	0.11
17–18	164	54.4	1,410	5.89	25.9	0.11

[a] Median height for age from NCHS standards.
[b] Median weight for height and age from Baldwin's standards (Annex 2(B) of original reference.)

From Energy and protein requirements: report of a Joint FAO/WHO/UNU Expert Consultation. Technical report series no. 724. Geneva: World Health Organization, 1985:72.

TABLE A-10-e. BASAL METABOLIC RATE IN ADULT MEN AND WOMEN IN RELATION TO HEIGHT AND MEDIAN ACCEPTABLE WEIGHT FOR HEIGHT[a] (VALUES GIVEN IN kcal_th WITH MJ IN PARENTHESES)

HEIGHT (m)	WEIGHTH[b] (kg)	18–30 y per kg per day	per day	30–60 y per kg per day	per day	>60 y per kg per day	per day
Men
1.5	49.5	29.0 (121)	1,440 (6.03)	29.4 (123)	1,450 (6.07)	23.3 (98)	1,150 (4.81)
1.6	56.5	27.4 (115)	1,540 (6.44)	27.2 (114)	1,530 (6.40)	22.2 (93)	1,250 (5.23)
1.7	63.5	26.0 (109)	1,650 (6.90)	25.4 (106)	1,620 (6.78)	21.2 (89)	1,350 (5.65)
1.8	71.5	24.8 (104)	1,770 (7.41)	23.9 (99)	1,710 (7.15)	20.3 (85)	1,450 (6.07)
1.9	79.5	23.9 (100)	1,890 (7.91)	22.7 (95)	1,800 (7.53)	19.6 (82)	1,560 (6.53)
2.0	88	23.0 (96)	2,030 (8.49)	21.6 (90)	1,900 (7.95)	19.0 (80)	1,670 (6.99)
Women
1.4	41	26.7 (112)	1,100 (4.60)	28.8 (120)	1,190 (4.98)	25.0 (105)	1,030 (4.31)
1.5	47	25.2 (105)	1,190 (4.98)	26.3 (110)	1,240 (5.19)	23.1 (97)	1,090 (4.56)
1.6	54	23.9 (100)	1,290 (5.40)	24.1 (101)	1,300 (5.44)	21.6 (90)	1,160 (4.85)
1.7	61	22.9 (96)	1,390 (5.82)	22.4 (94)	1,360 (5.69)	20.3 (85)	1,230 (5.15)
1.8	68	22.0 (92)	1,500 (6.28)	20.9 (87)	1,420 (5.94)	19.3 (81)	1,310 (5.48)

[a] BMR from equations in Table A-10-b rounded to 10 kcal_th.
[b] Weight taken as median acceptable weight for height: body mass index (wt/ht^2) = 22 in men, 21 in women.

From Energy and protein requirements: report of a Joint FAO/WHO/UNU Expert Consultation. Technical report series no. 724. Geneva: World Health Organization, 1985:72.

A-10-f. Equations for Prediction of Resting Energy Expenditure—Germany 2004

A-10-f-1 Appendices Editors Comments

This study by Müller and associates in Germany was conducted to establish resting energy expenditures (REE) in a modern affluent society and to compare the data with the most frequently used World Health Organization (WHO) equations of 1985 and others (1). This was a cross-sectional and retrospective analysis of data on REE and body composition obtained from 2528 subjects aged 5 to 91 years by seven different centers between 1985 and 2002).

Their data provide evidence that fat-free mass was a major determinant of the variance in REE of adults and that prediction was improved with the use of body mass index (BMI) group-specific prediction formulas particularly in seriously underweight subjects. Compared with the new data, WHO predictive equations systematically overestimated REE at low values and underestimated REE at high values.

1. Müller MJ, Bosy-Westphal A, Klaus S et al. World Health Organization equations have shortcomings for predicting resting energy expenditure in persons from a modern affluent population: generation of a new reference standard from a retrospective analysis of a German database of resting energy expenditure. Am J Clin Nutr 2004;80:1379–90.

TABLE A-10-f-2. MEASURED RESTING ENERGY EXPENDITURE (REE), REE ADJUSTED FOR FAT-FREE MASS (REE$_{adj1}$), AND REE ADJUSTED FOR FAT-FREE MASS AND FAT MASS (REE$_{adj2}$) IN THE STUDY POPULATION[1]

AGE (y)	REE		REE$_{adj1}$		REE$_{adj2}$	
	M	F	M	F	M	F
	MJ/d		*MJ/d*		*MJ/d*	
5–11	5.63 ± 0.99 [99]	5.35 ± 1.01[2] [89]	5.72 ± 0.58 [78]	5.54 ± 0.51 [68]	5.89 ± 0.57 [78]	5.70 ± 0.46[2] [68]
12–17	7.53 ± 1.21 [28]	6.18 ± 1.24[3] [27]	5.92 ± 0.88 [18]	5.03 ± 1.02[2] [16]	5.82 ± 1.02 [18]	5.17 ± 0.97 [16]
18–29	7.90 ± 1.66 [254]	5.77 ± 1.15[4] [398]	6.87 ± 1.22 [239]	6.42 ± 0.82[4] [362]	7.02 ± 1.19 [239]	6.55 ± 0.73[4] [362]
30–39	8.07 ± 1.72 [158]	6.33 ± 1.23[4] [145]	6.74 ± 1.11 [133]	6.60 ± 0.98 [125]	6.78 ± 1.08 [133]	6.53 ± 0.86[2] [125]
40–49	7.95 ± 1.61 [117]	6.46 ± 1.20[4] [182]	6.35 ± 0.84 [90]	6.55 ± 0.74[2] [152]	7.37 ± 0.81 [90]	6.42 ± 0.67 [152]
50–59	7.83 ± 1.20 [100]	6.26 ± 1.07[4] [213]	6.24 ± 1.06 [79]	6.38 ± 0.64[2] [181]	6.24 ± 0.90 [79]	6.27 ± 0.60 [181]
60–69	7.09 ± 1.21 [127]	5.78 ± 0.79[4] [258]	6.52 ± 1.00 [124]	6.53 ± 0.65 [242]	6.50 ± 0.92 [124]	6.41 ± 0.65 [242]
70–79	6.67 ± 0.77 [34]	5.38 ± 0.59[4] [88]	6.49 ± 0.82 [34]	6.57 ± 0.56 [88]	6.43 ± 0.75 [34]	6.50 ± 0.53 [88]
>80	6.04 ± 0.51 [8]	5.21 ± 0.54[4] [23]	6.22 ± 0.75 [8]	6.42 ± 0.60 [23]	6.26 ± 0.78 [8]	6.43 ± 0.57 [23]

[1] All values are $\bar{x}$ ± SD; *n* in brackets. Significant differences between age groups are not indicated. In two-factor repeated-measures ANOVA, the interaction term (sex × age) was significant for all 3 variables (ie, REE, REE$_{adj1}$, and REE$_{adj2}$).
[2–4] Significantly different from M (Mann-Whitney U test): [2]$P < 0.05$, [3]$P < 0.01$, [4]$P < 0.001$.

From 1. Müller MJ, Bosy-Westphal A, Klaus S et al. World Health Organization equations have shortcomings for predicting resting energy expenditure in persons from a modern affluent population: generation of a new reference standard from a retrospective analysis of a German database of resting energy expenditure. Am J Clin Nutr 2004;80:1379–90. Reproduced by permission of the *American Journal of Clinical Nutrition*, American Society for Clinical Nutrition.

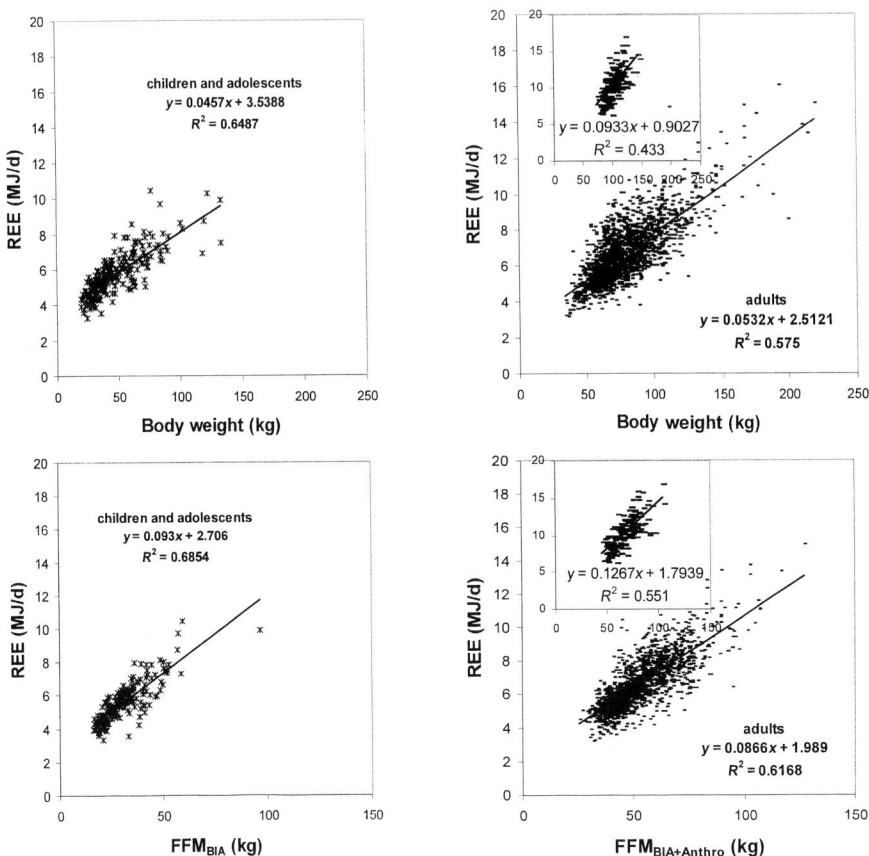

Figure A-10-f-3. Resting energy expenditure (REE) plotted against body weight or fat-free mass (FFM) in children and adolescents and in adults (total n = 2348). For the adults, data from 180 subjects whose REE was measured with a closed system are depicted in the insets. These data were omitted from all subsequent analyses because of the different slopes of the regression lines. Interaction terms between sex and weight and between sex and FFM were significant for adults but not for children and adolescents. FFM$_{BIA}$, FFM determined with the use of bioelectrical impedance analysis; FFM$_{BIA+Anthro}$, FFM determined with the use of bioelectrical impedance analysis or skinfold-thickness measurements.

From 1. Müller MJ, Bosy-Westphal A, Klaus S et al. World Health Organization equations have shortcomings for predicting resting energy expenditure in persons from a modern affluent population: generation of a new reference standard from a retrospective analysis of a German database of resting energy expenditure. Am J Clin Nutr 2004;80:1379–90. Reproduced by permission of the *American Journal of Clinical Nutrition*, American Society for Clinical Nutrition.

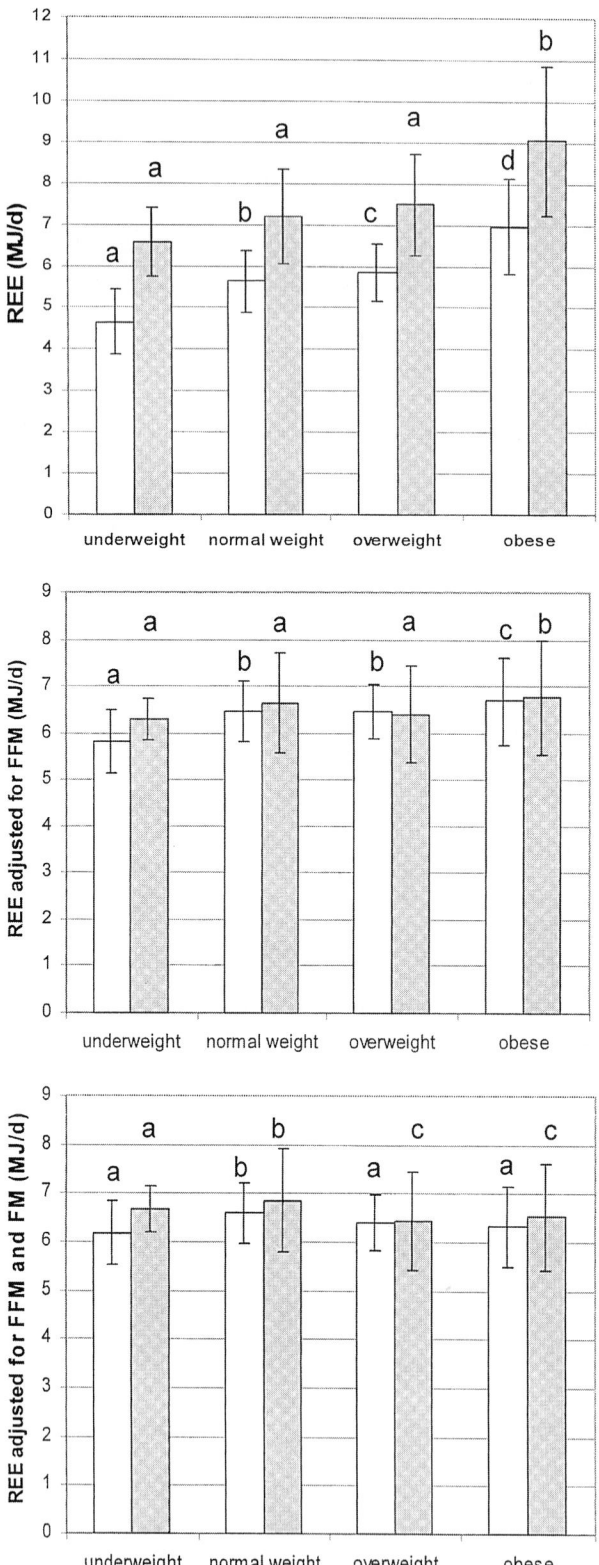

Figure A-10-f-4. Mean (±SD) resting energy expenditure (REE), REE adjusted for fat-free mass (FFM), and REE adjusted for FFM and fat mass (FM) in underweight (*n* = 98 F, 9 M), normal-weight (*n* = 551 F, 375 M), over-weight (*n* = 313 F, 220 M), and obese (*n* = 345 F, 194 M) women (□) and men (■). Bars with different letters are significantly different, *P* < 0.05 (ANOVA and Bonferroni post hoc test). Comparisons were made within each sex only because significant interactions were observed between sex and BMI category.

From 1. Müller MJ, Bosy-Westphal A, Klaus S et al. World Health Organization equations have shortcomings for predicting resting energy expenditure in persons from a modern affluent population: generation of a new reference standard from a retrospective analysis of a German database of resting energy expenditure. Am J Clin Nutr 2004;80:1379–90. Reproduced by permission of the *American Journal of Clinical Nutrition,* American Society for Clinical Nutrition.

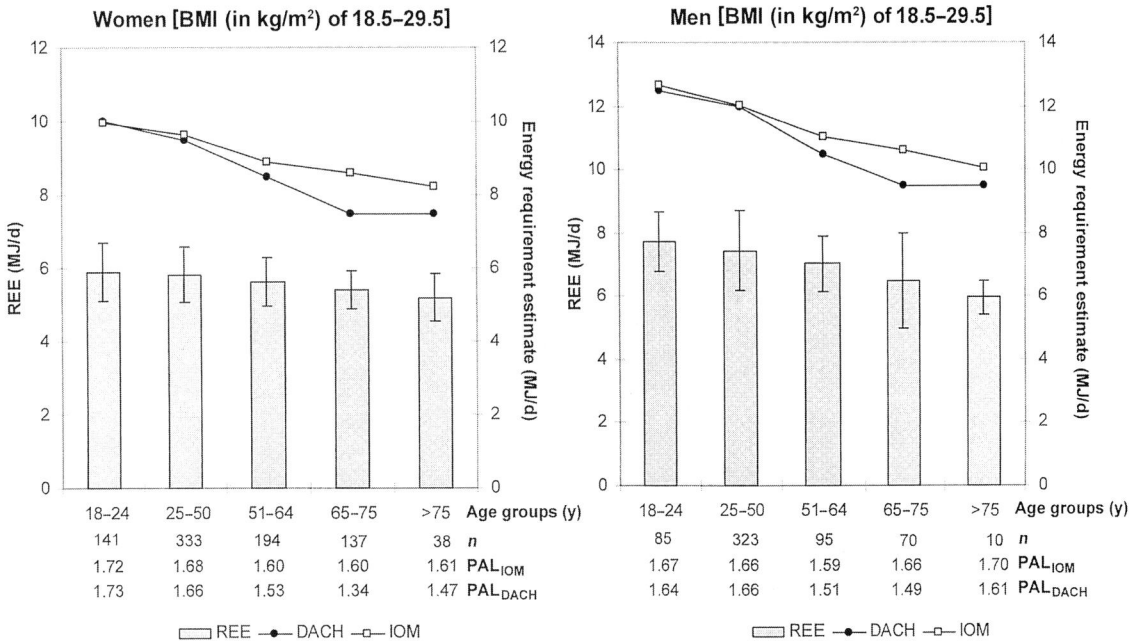

Figure A-10-f-5. Mean (±SD) measured resting energy expenditure (REE) and reference intake values for energy estimated by the Institute of Medicine (IOM) (40) or the German (D), Austrian (A), and Swiss (CH) societies for nutrition (DACH) (41) in 5 age groups of normal-weight and overweight women and men. Physical activity level (PALs) necessary to maintain body weight when following the recommendations from the IOM (PAL_{IOM}) or the DACH (PAL_{DACH}) were calculated as reference energy intake/REE.

From Müller MJ, Bosy-Westphal A, Klaus S et al. World Health Organization equations have shortcomings for predicting resting energy expenditure in persons from a modern affluent population: generation of a new reference standard from a retrospective analysis of a German database of resting energy expenditure. Am J Clin Nutr 2004;80:1379–90. Reproduced by permission of the *American Journal of Clinical Nutrition*, American Society for Clinical Nutrition.

A-11. ENERGY EXPENDITURE AND REQUIREMENTS. WORLD HEALTH ORGANIZATION—1985

TABLE A-11-a. DERIVATION OF AVERAGE VALUES OF THE ENERGY COST OF THREE GRADES OF PHYSICAL ACTIVITY AT WORK FOR WOMEN AND MEN[a]

	WOMEN[b]				MEN[c]			
	COST/MIN (kcal$_{th}$)	(kJ)	AVERAGE COST × BMR (gross)	(net)	COST/MIN (kcal$_{th}$)	(kJ)	AVERAGE COST × BMR (gross)	(net)
Light work								
75% of time sitting or standing	1.51	6.3			1.79	7.5		
25% of time standing and moving	1.70	7.1			2.51	10.5		
Average	1.56	6.5	1.7	0.7	1.99	8.3	1.7	0.7
Moderate work								
25% of time sitting or standing	1.51	6.3			1.79	7.5		
75% of time spent on specific occupational activity	2.20	9.2			3.61	15.1		
Average	2.03	8.5	2.2	1.2	3.16	13.2	2.7	1.7
Heavy work								
40% of time sitting or standing	1.51	6.3			1.79	7.5		
60% of time spent on specific occupational activity	3.21	13.4			6.22	26.0		
Average	2.54	10.6	2.8	1.8	4.45	18.6	3.8	2.8

[a] Times and energy costs of sitting, standing, moving around, and work tesks are composite values derived from published and unpublished data (Annex 5) in original reference.
[b] Based on young adult females (18–30 years). Wt 55 kg, BMR 0.90 kcal$_{th}$ (3.8 kJ)/min (Table A-10-b.)
[c] Based on young adult males (18–30 years). Wt 65 kg. BMR 1.16 kcal$_{th}$ (4.9 kJ)/min (Table A-10-b.)

From Energy and protein requirements: report of a Joint FAO/WHO/UNU Expert Consultation. Technical report series no. 724. Geneva: World Health Organization, 1985:76.

TABLE A-11-b. AVERAGE DAILY ENERGY REQUIREMENT OF ADULTS WHOSE OCCUPATIONAL WORK IS CLASSIFIED AS LIGHT, MODERATE, OR HEAVY, EXPRESSED AS A MULTIPLE OF BASAL METABOLIC RATE

	LIGHT	MODERATE	HEAVY
Men	1.55	1.78	2.10
Women	1.56	1.64	1.82

From Energy and protein requirements: report of a Joint FAO/WHO/UNU Expert Consultation. Technical report series no. 724. Geneva: World Health Organization, 1985:78.

TABLE A-11-c. ESTIMATES OF ENERGY COST OF WEIGHT GAIN[a]

	ENERGY COST	
SUBJECTS	(kcal$_{th}$/g)	(kJ/g)
Premature infants	4.9	20.5
Premature infants	5.7	23.8
Normal infants	5.6	23.4
Infants recovering from malnutrition	5.55	23.2
	4.6	19.2
	3.5	14.6
	4.4	18.4
	7.1	29.7
Adults recovering from anorexia nervosa	6.4	26.7
Adults, intentional overfeeding	8.2	34.3
Pregnancy Theoretic estimate[b]	6.4	26.7

[a] See original references for data sources.
[b] Calculated as 80,000 kcal$_{th}$ (335 mJ) stored for 12.5 kg of weight gain.

From Energy and protein requirements: report of a Joint FAO/WHO/UNU Expert Consultation. Technical report series no. 724. Geneva: World Health Organization, 1985:185.

A-12. FRAME SIZE, ELBOW BREADTH, AND HEIGHT-WEIGHT TABLES

. . . . three frame size categories, age- and sex-specific percentiles of Frame Index 2 were determined. Three categories of frame size were established—small, medium, and large—corresponding respectively to values below the 25th, from the 25th to the 75th, and above the 75th sex- and age-specific percentiles of Frame Index 2 [see original Table II.5 in Frisancho]. With these percentile cutoffs, 25%, 50%, and 75% of the sample of both males and females were classified as either small, medium, or large frame, respectively.

We decided to base the frame size classification on Frame Index 2 rather than on elbow breadth alone [because] weight increases until about the fifth decade in males and the sixth decade in females, while height starts declining by the fourth decade (see Table A-12-e) (1).

Weight not only varies with height and age but it is also influenced by factors such as body width, bone thickness, muscularity, and length of trunk relative to total height. . .

An appropriate evaluation of frame size requires a reliable measurement of elbow breadth . . . it should be measured accurately, not by simple manual touch as suggested by the Metropolitan Life Insurance Co., but with a broad faced calipers or other appropriate measuring devices. Otherwise estimations of desirable weight based on inappropriate frame size estimation may be unrealistic and subject to large errors.

A.R. Frisancho

REFERENCE

1. Frisancho AR. Anthropometric standards for the assessment of growth and nutritional status. Ann Arbor: University of Michigan Press, 1990.

A-12-a. Frame Size and Elbow Breadth

A-12-a-1. Categories of Frame Size: Excerpts from Comments of A. R. Frisancho (1)

The present classification is based upon a new index hereafter referred to as *Frame Index 2*, which is derived from measurements of *elbow breadth*, *height*, and *age*. The formula for calculating Frame Index 2 is:

$$\text{Frame Index 2} = [\text{elbow breadth (mm)/stature (cm)}] \times 100$$

TABLE A-12-a-2. MEANS, STANDARD DEVIATIONS, AND PERCENTILES OF WEIGHT (kg) BY AGE FOR ADULT MALES OF SMALL, MEDIUM, AND LARGE FRAMES

AGE (ys)	N	MEAN	SD	PERCENTILES								
				5	10	15	25	50	75	85	90	95
Males with small frames												
18.0–24.9	444	69.9	11.5	54.5	57.4	59.0	62.3	68.3	76.1	80.5	83.8	89.8
25.0–29.9	318	73.4	12.0	56.7	60.3	61.9	65.1	71.8	79.4	84.7	87.5	97.9
30.0–34.9	239	75.7	12.5	57.9	61.6	63.2	67.0	74.6	83.1	87.8	92.9	98.0
35.0–39.9	212	75.5	12.0	56.0	59.9	62.1	66.6	75.9	83.5	87.8	91.4	96.0
40.0–44.9	210	78.3	12.4	58.8	62.8	65.4	70.3	76.1	86.3	92.3	94.8	101.0
45.0–49.9	220	76.3	11.7	57.7	60.9	63.2	67.6	76.2	83.6	89.0	92.1	95.8
50.0–54.9	225	75.4	11.9	57.3	60.2	64.5	67.1	74.7	82.8	88.2	90.5	99.3
55.0–59.9	204	74.5	12.0	54.7	58.2	61.5	66.7	74.8	81.9	87.2	90.6	94.7
60.0–64.9	318	74.0	12.3	54.2	59.2	62.5	65.9	73.4	80.7	85.7	88.4	93.8
65.0–69.9	446	70.7	12.1	50.8	55.4	57.8	61.9	70.3	79.0	83.3	86.8	92.4
70.0–74.9	315	70.5	12.5	49.9	54.4	57.3	61.9	70.1	78.4	83.0	85.5	92.8
Males with medium frames												
18.0–24.9	877	74.0	12.7	57.5	60.6	62.3	65.3	71.5	80.3	86.0	91.6	99.6
25.0–29.9	627	77.0	13.2	58.5	61.8	64.5	68.4	75.9	84.1	88.3	92.4	100.4
30.0–34.9	473	78.5	12.9	59.8	63.0	65.9	69.5	77.8	85.8	91.1	93.8	98.8
35.0–39.9	419	80.5	12.8	58.7	64.8	68.4	72.9	80.4	87.4	91.5	95.9	102.5
40.0–44.9	414	80.1	12.4	60.8	64.2	67.9	71.9	79.3	88.1	92.4	96.8	102.6
45.0–49.9	436	80.7	13.0	60.3	65.1	67.1	71.9	79.8	88.7	93.3	96.7	101.3
50.0–54.9	441	79.0	13.7	58.4	62.5	65.8	70.0	78.3	86.3	91.7	96.6	103.1
55.0–59.9	404	78.8	12.7	59.9	64.5	66.7	70.5	77.9	85.3	91.1	95.4	102.2
60.0–64.9	629	76.7	11.9	58.3	61.5	64.5	68.7	76.3	84.4	88.4	91.6	97.8
65.0–69.9	886	75.0	12.2	56.1	59.5	62.5	66.9	74.5	82.9	86.9	90.8	97.2
70.0–74.9	627	73.6	12.2	54.3	58.3	61.1	65.5	72.6	81.0	86.1	89.8	93.9
Males with large frames												
18.0–24.9	433	77.5	15.4	58.2	61.3	62.6	67.4	74.7	85.0	91.2	95.0	104.9
25.0–29.9	310	84.3	17.4	61.2	66.0	68.4	72.6	82.2	91.6	99.8	102.8	115.2
30.0–34.9	233	86.5	16.6	65.5	68.4	70.2	75.2	85.4	94.0	101.6	106.7	116.7
35.0–39.9	206	85.0	15.0	59.6	67.4	71.8	75.4	84.1	93.1	98.9	104.1	113.3
40.0–44.9	205	85.8	16.4	63.7	67.7	68.8	74.3	84.9	94.5	100.3	107.4	113.3
45.0–49.9	215	85.5	16.5	62.7	67.0	69.4	74.0	84.0	94.0	101.3	105.9	119.2
50.0–54.9	216	84.7	14.7	64.4	66.9	68.8	73.3	83.1	94.3	101.7	103.6	108.4
55.0–59.9	199	85.7	15.7	64.5	67.1	70.3	74.8	84.5	93.5	100.5	103.5	121.1
60.0–64.9	313	82.1	14.6	61.5	66.6	69.3	73.1	80.7	89.4	94.5	98.9	107.7
65.0–69.9	440	79.5	13.8	57.0	61.5	64.9	70.4	78.9	87.8	93.0	96.3	104.0
70.0–74.9	310	77.1	13.8	55.3	59.9	63.6	67.9	76.7	84.1	90.5	95.8	101.4

From Frisancho AR. Anthropometric standards for the assessment of growth and nutritional status. Ann Arbor: University of Michigan Press, 1990, Table IV.22. With permission.

TABLE A-12-a-3. MEANS, STANDARD DEVIATIONS, AND PERCENTILES OF WEIGHT (kg) BY AGE FOR ADULT FEMALES OF SMALL, MEDIUM, AND LARGE FRAMES

AGE (ys)	N	MEAN	SD	PERCENTILES								
				5	10	15	25	50	75	85	90	95
Females with small frames												
18.0–24.9	652	56.2	8.7	44.0	46.1	48.0	50.3	55.1	60.9	64.4	66.9	71.5
25.0–29.9	487	56.9	9.5	44.1	47.3	48.6	50.9	55.6	61.1	64.5	67.6	72.6
30.0–34.9	413	59.1	10.0	45.7	48.2	50.0	52.7	57.6	63.4	68.1	71.8	77.7
35.0–39.9	369	61.1	11.4	45.8	48.2	50.8	53.4	59.5	66.7	71.9	76.0	79.5
40.0–44.9	353	60.6	9.4	48.1	50.3	51.8	54.5	59.1	66.1	70.0	73.6	80.3
45.0–49.9	244	61.4	11.1	46.3	47.8	50.8	53.6	60.3	67.3	71.4	75.1	80.8
50.0–54.9	257	61.3	10.8	46.3	49.1	51.7	54.5	60.3	66.9	71.0	73.1	78.4
55.0–59.9	224	61.3	11.1	47.3	49.5	52.2	54.7	59.9	65.3	70.2	73.6	81.5
60.0–64.9	351	61.9	11.0	46.4	48.9	50.6	54.2	60.9	68.5	71.7	74.0	82.2
65.0–69.9	491	61.1	10.7	44.9	48.4	50.7	53.6	60.2	67.4	71.7	74.0	79.3
70.0–74.9	369	60.6	12.1	42.6	45.9	48.5	51.6	60.2	67.0	72.3	75.4	81.0
Females with medium frames												
18.0–24.9	1,297	59.5	10.4	46.0	48.4	50.0	52.5	58.1	64.4	69.5	72.8	78.4
25.0–29.9	967	60.9	11.5	46.9	49.1	50.6	53.0	58.6	66.3	72.2	76.9	83.0
30.0–34.9	815	63.5	13.4	47.2	50.0	51.7	54.3	60.7	69.3	76.7	80.6	87.2
35.0–39.9	730	64.1	12.1	49.2	51.7	53.0	56.1	61.8	69.8	74.7	79.4	87.9
40.0–44.9	700	65.6	13.3	48.8	51.3	53.6	57.0	62.8	71.8	77.3	82.4	92.1
45.0–49.9	484	65.8	13.4	48.3	51.4	53.3	56.4	63.4	72.2	77.8	83.1	91.6
50.0–54.9	504	66.4	12.2	48.9	52.0	54.4	57.7	64.4	73.1	79.3	82.8	89.7
55.0–59.9	444	68.0	15.3	48.2	51.1	54.3	58.1	66.3	74.8	81.0	86.2	92.1
60.0–64.9	695	66.2	12.4	49.1	52.3	54.0	57.5	64.5	73.5	78.1	82.2	89.0
65.0–69.9	973	66.2	12.7	48.1	51.4	53.6	57.1	64.9	73.1	78.7	82.4	88.8
70.0–74.9	731	64.3	11.9	46.8	50.5	52.5	56.8	62.9	70.8	76.9	80.2	84.7
Females with large frames												
18.0–24.9	642	68.0	17.2	48.9	51.3	53.1	56.3	62.9	76.2	83.8	89.0	102.7
25.0–29.9	480	72.6	17.7	49.9	53.4	55.6	59.3	68.7	82.9	90.9	98.8	105.0
30.0–34.9	402	76.4	19.7	51.1	54.9	57.7	61.1	72.7	88.4	97.3	102.8	111.9
35.0–39.9	361	79.1	19.5	52.8	56.1	59.1	64.5	76.7	90.4	98.1	106.0	117.9
40.0–44.9	346	79.7	19.8	53.4	57.3	60.7	65.7	77.1	91.3	99.2	104.9	114.2
45.0–49.9	240	80.1	19.6	54.5	60.1	63.2	66.7	76.8	86.6	97.6	105.0	116.9
50.0–54.9	250	79.4	16.9	55.6	60.0	63.0	67.8	77.7	88.8	97.1	103.3	112.1
55.0–59.9	218	79.8	17.5	56.4	60.2	62.5	67.6	77.6	89.9	97.0	101.6	111.3
60.0–64.9	346	77.8	15.6	56.0	59.4	62.8	66.8	76.8	85.7	92.8	100.0	104.8
65.0–69.9	484	76.6	15.4	55.3	59.4	62.0	65.8	74.5	84.6	91.7	97.8	105.0
70.0–74.9	363	74.9	14.0	53.5	57.9	60.9	65.8	74.5	82.7	87.9	91.3	99.1

From Frisancho AR. Anthropometric standards for the assessment of growth and nutritional status. Ann Arbor: University of Michigan Press, 1990, Table IV.23. With permission.

TABLE A-12-b. MEANS, STANDARD DEVIATIONS, AND PERCENTILES OF ELBOW BREADTH (mm) BY AGE FOR MALES AND FEMALES 1 TO 74 YEARS

AGE (ys)	N	MEAN	SD	PERCENTILES								
				5	10	15	25	50	75	85	90	95
Males												
1.0–1.9	681	40.4	2.9	36.0	37.0	37.0	39.0	40.0	42.0	43.0	44.0	45.0
2.0–2.9	677	42.5	2.7	38.0	39.0	40.0	41.0	42.0	44.0	45.0	46.0	47.0
3.0–3.9	717	44.5	2.8	40.0	41.0	42.0	43.0	44.0	46.0	47.0	48.0	50.0
4.0–4.9	709	46.4	3.0	42.0	43.0	43.0	44.0	46.0	48.0	50.0	50.0	52.0
5.0–5.9	676	48.3	3.3	43.0	44.0	45.0	46.0	48.0	50.0	51.0	52.0	53.0
6.0–6.9	298	50.4	3.3	45.0	46.0	47.0	48.0	51.0	52.0	54.0	55.0	56.0
7.0–7.9	312	51.9	3.6	47.0	48.0	49.0	49.0	52.0	54.0	56.0	56.0	57.0
8.0–8.9	296	53.7	3.7	48.0	49.0	50.0	51.0	54.0	56.0	57.0	59.0	60.0
9.0–9.9	322	55.7	3.8	50.0	51.0	52.0	53.0	56.0	58.0	60.0	61.0	62.0
10.0–10.9	334	58.1	4.2	52.0	53.0	54.0	55.0	58.0	61.0	62.0	64.0	65.0
11.0–11.9	324	59.9	4.4	53.0	55.0	56.0	57.0	60.0	62.0	64.0	65.0	67.0
12.0–12.9	349	62.8	5.0	55.0	57.0	58.0	60.0	63.0	66.0	68.0	69.0	72.0
13.0–13.9	350	65.8	4.8	58.0	60.0	61.0	62.0	66.0	69.0	71.0	72.0	74.0
14.0–14.9	358	68.4	4.4	61.0	63.0	64.0	66.0	68.0	71.0	73.0	74.0	76.0
15.0–15.9	359	69.8	4.1	63.0	64.0	65.0	67.0	70.0	72.0	74.0	75.0	77.0
16.0–16.9	350	70.5	4.0	64.0	66.0	66.0	68.0	71.0	73.0	74.0	76.0	77.0
17.0–17.9	339	70.7	4.0	64.0	66.0	67.0	68.0	71.0	73.0	75.0	76.0	77.0
18.0–24.9	1,757	71.2	4.1	64.0	66.0	67.0	69.0	71.0	74.0	75.0	76.0	78.0
25.0–29.9	1,256	71.6	4.1	65.0	67.0	67.0	69.0	71.0	74.0	76.0	77.0	79.0
30.0–34.9	946	71.8	4.2	65.0	67.0	68.0	69.0	72.0	74.0	76.0	77.0	79.0
35.0–39.9	838	72.3	4.2	65.0	67.0	68.0	70.0	72.0	75.0	77.0	77.0	80.0
40.0–44.9	830	72.8	4.0	66.0	68.0	69.0	70.0	73.0	75.0	77.0	78.0	80.0
45.0–49.9	871	73.1	4.3	66.0	68.0	69.0	70.0	73.0	76.0	78.0	79.0	80.0
50.0–54.9	882	73.3	4.2	66.0	68.0	69.0	71.0	73.0	76.0	77.0	78.0	80.0
55.0–59.9	809	73.7	4.5	67.0	68.0	69.0	71.0	73.0	77.0	78.0	80.0	81.0
60.0–64.9	1,263	73.5	4.3	67.0	68.0	69.0	71.0	73.0	76.0	78.0	79.0	81.0
65.0–69.9	1,774	73.2	4.4	66.0	68.0	69.0	70.0	73.0	76.0	78.0	79.0	81.0
70.0–74.9	1,252	73.5	4.3	67.0	68.0	69.0	71.0	73.0	76.0	78.0	79.0	81.0
Females												
1.0–1.9	622	38.7	2.8	34.0	35.0	36.0	37.0	39.0	41.0	42.0	42.0	43.0
2.0–2.9	615	40.7	2.8	36.0	37.0	38.0	39.0	41.0	42.0	44.0	44.0	45.0
3.0–3.9	652	42.5	2.9	38.0	39.0	40.0	41.0	42.0	44.0	45.0	46.0	47.0
4.0–4.9	681	44.2	2.9	40.0	41.0	41.0	42.0	44.0	46.0	47.0	48.0	49.0
5.0–5.9	674	46.4	3.1	42.0	43.0	43.0	44.0	46.0	48.0	50.0	50.0	52.0
6.0–6.9	296	47.9	3.2	43.0	44.0	45.0	46.0	48.0	50.0	51.0	52.0	53.0
7.0–7.9	331	50.1	3.4	45.0	46.0	47.0	48.0	50.0	52.0	53.0	54.0	55.0
8.0–8.9	276	51.5	3.7	46.0	47.0	48.0	49.0	51.0	54.0	55.0	56.0	58.0
9.0–9.9	322	54.0	3.9	48.0	50.0	50.0	51.0	54.0	56.0	57.0	59.0	60.0
10.0–10.9	330	55.6	3.9	50.0	51.0	52.0	53.0	56.0	58.0	60.0	61.0	62.0
11.0–11.9	302	57.8	4.0	52.0	53.0	54.0	55.0	58.0	60.0	62.0	63.0	64.0
12.0–12.9	324	59.2	3.7	53.0	55.0	55.0	57.0	59.0	62.0	63.0	64.0	66.0
13.0–13.9	361	60.1	3.8	54.0	56.0	56.0	58.0	60.0	62.0	64.0	65.0	66.0
14.0–14.9	370	60.4	3.5	54.0	56.0	57.0	58.0	60.0	63.0	64.0	65.0	66.0
15.0–15.9	309	60.7	4.0	54.0	56.0	57.0	58.0	61.0	63.0	65.0	66.0	67.0
16.0–16.9	343	61.0	3.8	55.0	56.0	57.0	59.0	61.0	64.0	65.0	66.0	67.0
17.0–17.9	293	61.3	4.0	55.0	56.0	57.0	59.0	61.0	64.0	65.0	66.0	68.0
18.0–24.9	2,591	61.0	3.8	55.0	56.0	57.0	59.0	61.0	63.0	65.0	66.0	67.0
25.0–29.9	1,934	61.5	3.9	56.0	57.0	58.0	59.0	61.0	64.0	65.0	66.0	68.0
30.0–34.9	1,630	62.1	4.3	56.0	57.0	58.0	59.0	62.0	64.0	66.0	67.0	70.0
35.0–39.9	1,460	62.7	4.4	56.0	58.0	59.0	60.0	62.0	65.0	67.0	68.0	71.0
40.0–44.9	1,399	63.2	4.4	57.0	58.0	59.0	60.0	63.0	66.0	67.0	69.0	71.0
45.0–49.9	968	63.7	4.4	57.0	59.0	59.0	61.0	63.0	66.0	68.0	69.0	72.0
50.0–54.9	1,011	64.1	4.7	57.0	59.0	60.0	61.0	64.0	67.0	69.0	70.0	73.0
55.0–59.9	887	64.7	4.8	58.0	59.0	60.0	61.0	64.0	67.0	70.0	71.0	73.0
60.0–64.9	1,394	64.6	4.4	58.0	60.0	61.0	62.0	64.0	67.0	69.0	70.0	72.0
65.0–69.9	1,950	64.7	4.5	58.0	59.0	60.0	62.0	64.0	67.0	69.0	71.0	73.0
70.0–74.9	1,464	64.8	4.4	58.0	60.0	60.0	62.0	64.0	68.0	69.0	71.0	72.0

From Frisancho AR. Anthropometric standards for the assessment of growth and nutritional status. Ann Arbor: University of Michigan Press, 1990, Table IV.9. With permission.

TABLE A-12-c. CHANGES IN WEIGHT AND HEIGHT WITH AGE

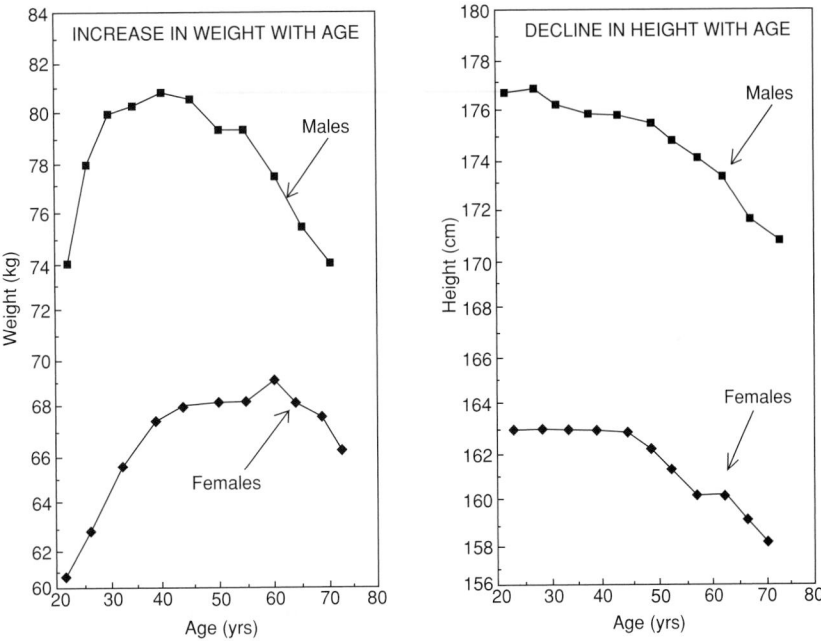

Relationship of weight and height to age among adults. Note that weight increases until about the fifth decade in males and sixth decade in females, while height begins to decline after the age of 40 years in both males and females. From Frisancho AR. Anthropometric standards for the assessment of growth and nutritional status. University of Michigan Press, Ann Arbor, 1990. Figure II.15.

A-13. BODY MASS INDEX TABLES

TABLE A-13-a. MEANS, STANDARD DEVIATIONS, AND PERCENTILES OF BODY MASS INDEX (w/s²) BY AGE FOR MALES AND FEMALES 1 TO 74 YEARS

AGE (ys)	N	MEAN	SD	PERCENTILES								
				5	10	15	25	50	75	85	90	95
Males												
1.0–1.9	366	17.3	2.4	15.2	15.6	15.9	16.4	17.1	18.0	18.6	19.0	19.6
2.0–2.9	664	16.2	1.3	14.3	14.6	15.0	15.4	16.2	17.1	17.5	17.8	18.4
3.0–3.9	716	16.0	1.4	14.2	14.6	14.8	15.1	15.8	16.6	17.1	17.5	18.2
4.0–4.9	709	15.7	1.3	13.9	14.2	14.5	14.9	15.6	16.4	16.8	17.2	17.8
5.0–5.9	675	15.6	1.5	13.8	14.1	14.3	14.7	15.5	16.3	16.8	17.2	18.1
6.0–6.9	298	15.8	1.9	13.7	14.1	14.3	14.8	15.3	16.4	17.2	18.0	19.3
7.0–7.9	312	16.0	1.8	13.7	14.1	14.3	14.9	15.6	16.7	17.5	18.2	19.5
8.0–8.9	296	16.3	2.2	13.8	14.3	14.6	15.0	15.9	17.1	18.0	19.1	20.1
9.0–9.9	322	16.9	2.4	14.1	14.6	14.8	15.3	16.3	17.7	19.0	19.9	21.8
10.0–10.9	334	17.7	2.8	14.6	15.0	15.3	15.8	17.1	18.7	19.8	21.2	23.4
11.0–11.9	324	18.4	3.6	14.7	15.1	15.7	16.2	17.4	19.8	21.5	22.5	25.3
12.0–12.9	349	18.9	3.5	15.2	15.7	16.1	16.7	17.9	20.2	21.7	23.7	25.8
13.0–13.9	348	19.5	3.5	15.6	16.4	16.6	17.2	18.7	20.7	22.2	24.0	25.9
14.0–14.9	359	20.3	3.3	16.5	17.0	17.5	18.1	19.5	21.6	23.1	24.2	26.4
15.0–15.9	359	20.8	3.1	16.8	17.5	18.0	19.0	20.4	22.0	23.4	24.1	26.6
16.0–16.9	349	21.9	3.3	18.0	18.5	19.0	19.6	21.3	23.0	24.8	25.9	27.3
17.0–17.9	338	21.8	3.5	17.8	18.4	18.9	19.5	21.1	23.4	24.9	26.1	28.3
18.0–24.9	1,755	23.6	3.8	18.8	19.6	20.1	21.0	23.0	25.5	27.2	28.5	31.0
25.0–29.9	1,255	24.9	4.3	19.5	20.4	21.1	21.9	24.3	27.0	28.5	30.0	32.8
30.0–34.9	947	25.7	4.2	19.9	21.0	21.9	23.0	25.1	27.8	29.3	30.5	32.9
35.0–39.9	839	25.9	4.0	19.7	21.0	21.9	23.3	25.6	28.0	29.5	30.6	32.8
40.0–44.9	829	26.2	4.0	20.4	21.5	22.2	23.4	26.0	28.5	29.9	31.0	32.5
45.0–49.9	871	26.3	4.2	20.1	21.5	22.4	23.5	26.0	28.6	30.1	31.2	33.4
50.0–54.9	882	26.1	4.2	19.9	21.1	22.0	23.3	25.9	28.2	30.1	31.3	33.3
55.0–59.9	807	26.2	4.3	19.8	21.3	22.1	23.5	26.1	28.5	30.2	31.6	33.6
60.0–64.9	1,261	28.8	3.8	20.1	21.3	22.0	23.4	25.6	28.0	29.4	30.4	32.4
65.0–69.9	1,773	25.5	4.0	19.1	20.5	21.4	22.7	25.5	27.8	29.6	30.7	32.3
70.0–74.9	1,257	25.3	4.0	19.0	20.3	21.4	22.6	25.1	27.7	29.3	30.5	32.3
Females												
1.0–1.9	333	16.7	1.5	14.4	14.9	15.2	15.7	16.7	17.6	18.2	18.6	19.3
2.0–2.9	610	16.0	1.5	14.1	14.4	14.7	15.1	15.9	16.8	17.3	17.8	18.4
3.0–3.9	651	15.7	1.4	13.6	14.1	14.4	14.7	15.5	16.4	17.0	17.5	18.0
4.0–4.9	678	15.5	1.4	13.6	13.9	14.2	14.6	15.3	16.2	16.7	17.2	18.0
5.0–5.9	673	15.5	1.7	13.3	13.7	14.0	14.5	15.2	16.3	16.9	17.5	18.6
6.0–6.9	296	15.5	1.7	13.5	13.7	13.9	14.3	15.2	16.2	17.0	17.5	18.7
7.0–7.9	331	15.9	1.9	13.7	14.1	14.2	14.7	15.4	16.8	17.5	18.3	19.6
8.0–8.9	276	16.5	2.7	13.8	14.1	14.4	14.9	15.8	17.4	18.7	19.8	21.7
9.0–9.9	322	17.3	3.1	14.0	14.6	14.8	15.3	16.5	18.1	19.8	21.5	23.3
10.0–10.9	330	17.7	3.1	14.0	14.5	15.0	15.6	16.9	18.9	20.7	22.0	24.1
11.0–11.9	303	18.9	3.8	14.8	15.3	15.6	16.3	18.1	20.3	21.8	23.4	26.2
12.0–12.9	324	19.6	3.7	15.0	15.6	16.2	17.0	18.9	21.2	23.1	24.6	27.0
13.0–13.9	361	20.4	4.1	15.4	16.3	16.7	17.7	19.4	22.2	23.8	25.2	28.6
14.0–14.9	370	21.1	3.9	16.5	17.1	17.7	18.4	20.3	22.8	24.7	26.2	28.9
15.0–15.9	309	21.1	3.8	17.0	17.5	18.0	18.8	20.3	22.4	24.1	25.6	28.7
16.0–16.9	343	22.1	4.0	17.7	18.3	18.7	19.3	21.1	23.5	25.7	26.8	30.1
17.0–17.9	293	22.5	4.7	17.1	17.9	18.7	19.6	21.4	24.0	26.2	27.5	32.1
18.0–24.9	2,592	22.9	4.6	17.7	18.4	19.0	19.9	21.8	24.5	26.5	28.6	32.1
25.0–29.9	1,935	23.7	5.2	18.0	18.8	19.2	20.1	22.3	25.6	28.4	30.8	34.3
30.0–34.9	1,633	24.8	5.9	18.5	19.4	19.9	20.8	23.1	27.2	30.4	33.0	36.6
35.0–39.9	1,461	25.3	5.8	18.7	19.5	20.2	21.3	23.8	28.0	31.0	33.1	36.9
40.0–44.9	1,399	25.7	5.9	18.8	19.8	20.5	21.5	24.2	28.3	31.6	33.7	36.6
45.0–49.9	969	26.0	6.2	19.0	20.1	20.8	21.9	24.5	28.6	31.4	33.4	37.1
50.0–54.9	1,012	26.3	5.5	19.2	20.3	21.0	22.4	25.2	29.2	32.1	33.8	36.5
55.0–59.9	887	26.9	6.1	19.2	20.5	21.3	22.8	25.7	30.1	32.7	34.7	38.2
60.0–64.9	1,392	26.7	5.5	19.3	20.7	21.4	22.9	25.8	29.7	32.1	33.8	36.6
65.0–69.9	1,952	26.8	5.5	19.5	20.7	21.7	23.0	26.0	29.6	32.0	33.8	36.6
70.0–74.9	1,467	26.6	5.3	19.3	20.5	21.5	23.0	26.0	29.5	31.7	33.1	35.8

From Frisancho AR. Anthropometric standards for the assessment of growth and nutritional status. Ann Arbor: University of Michigan Press, 1990. Table IV.5. With permission.

KNOW YOUR BODY MASS INDEX

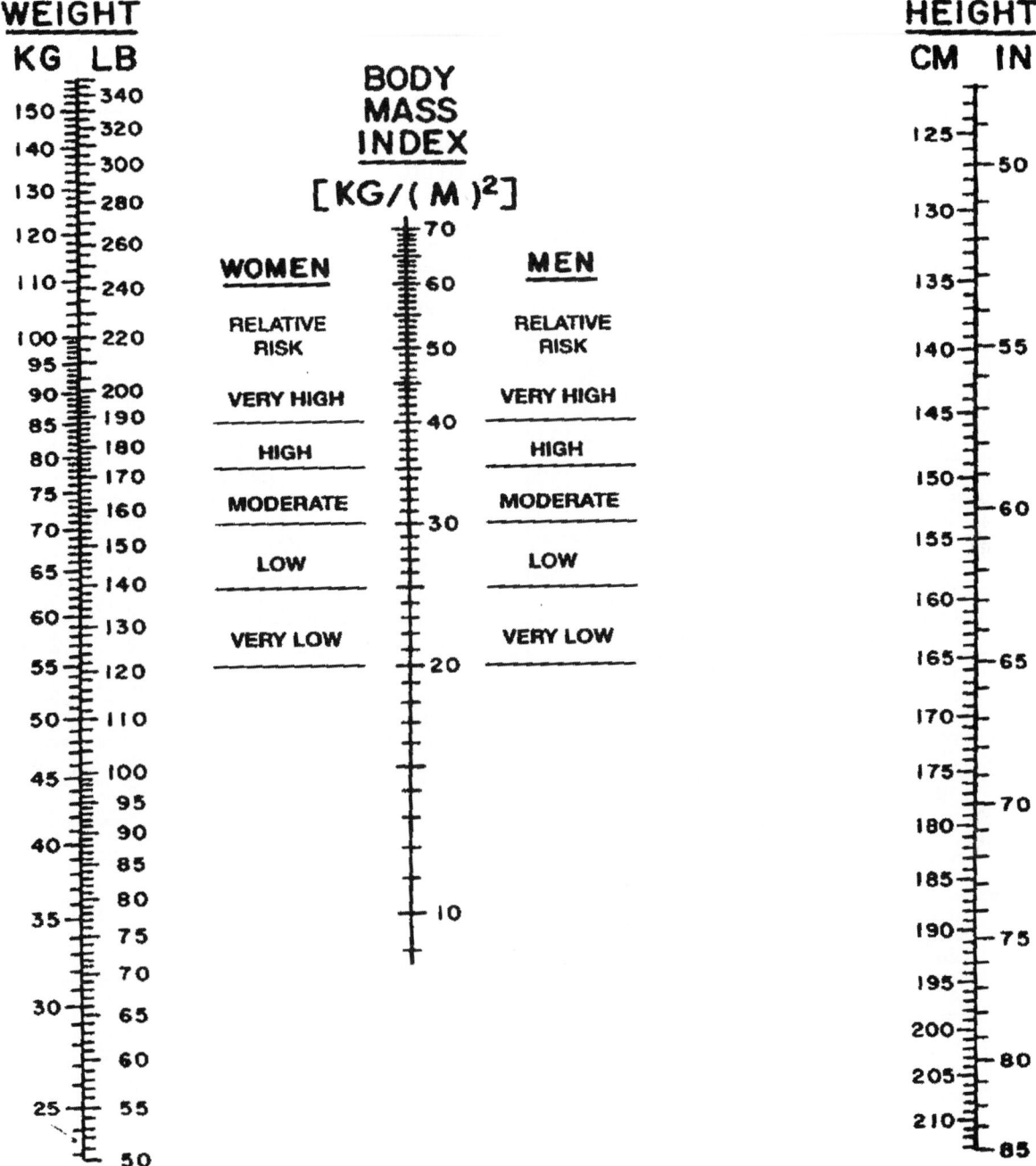

Figure A-13-b. Nomograph for determining body mass index and estimating relative risk.

Copyright 1978, George A. Bray, M. D.
Ref: Bray GA Am J Clin Nutr 1992;55(2 Suppl):488S-494S

A-13-c. BODY MASS INDEX TABLES (NIH), FOR RAPID CALCULATION

A-13-c-1. BODY MASS INDEX TABLE*

<u>**for BMI greater than 35, go to Table 2**</u>

To use the table, find the appropriate height in the left-hand column labeled Height. Move across to a given weight (in pounds). The number at the top of the column is the BMI at that height and weight. Pounds have been rounded off.

BMI	19	20	21	22	23	24	25	26	27	28	29	30	31	32	33	34	35
Height (inches)	Body Weight (pounds)																
58	91	96	100	105	110	115	119	124	129	134	138	143	148	153	158	162	167
59	94	99	104	109	114	119	124	128	133	138	143	148	153	158	163	168	173
60	97	102	107	112	118	123	128	133	138	143	148	153	158	163	168	174	179
61	100	106	111	116	122	127	132	137	143	148	153	158	164	169	174	180	185
62	104	109	115	120	126	131	136	142	147	153	158	164	169	175	180	186	191
63	107	113	118	124	130	135	141	146	152	158	163	169	175	180	186	191	197
64	110	116	122	128	134	140	145	151	157	163	169	174	180	186	192	197	204
65	114	120	126	132	138	144	150	156	162	168	174	180	186	192	198	204	210
66	118	124	130	136	142	148	155	161	167	173	179	186	192	198	204	210	216
67	121	127	134	140	146	153	159	166	172	178	185	191	198	204	211	217	223
68	125	131	138	144	151	158	164	171	177	184	190	197	203	210	216	223	230
69	128	135	142	149	155	162	169	176	182	189	196	203	209	216	223	230	236
70	132	139	146	153	160	167	174	181	188	195	202	209	216	222	229	236	243
71	136	143	150	157	165	172	179	186	193	200	208	215	222	229	236	243	250
72	140	147	154	162	169	177	184	191	199	206	213	221	228	235	242	250	258
73	144	151	159	166	174	182	189	197	204	212	219	227	235	242	250	257	265
74	148	155	163	171	179	186	194	202	210	218	225	233	241	249	256	264	272
75	152	160	168	176	184	192	200	208	216	224	232	240	248	256	264	272	279
76	156	164	172	180	189	197	205	213	221	230	238	246	254	263	271	279	287

* http://www.nhlbi.nih.gov/guidelines/obesity/bmi_tbl.htm

A-13-c-2. BODY MASS INDEX TABLE*

To use the table, find the appropriate height in the left-hand column labeled Height. Move across to a given weight. The number at the top of the column is the BMI at that height and weight. Pounds have been rounded off.

BMI	36	37	38	39	40	41	42	43	44	45	46	47	48	49	50	51	52	53	54
Height (inches)	Body Weight (pounds)																		
58	172	177	181	186	191	196	201	205	210	215	220	224	229	234	239	244	248	253	258
59	178	183	188	193	198	203	208	212	217	222	227	232	237	242	247	252	257	262	267
60	184	189	194	199	204	209	215	220	225	230	235	240	245	250	255	261	266	271	276
61	190	195	201	206	211	217	222	227	232	238	243	248	254	259	264	269	275	280	285
62	196	202	207	213	218	224	229	235	240	246	251	256	262	267	273	278	284	289	295
63	203	208	214	220	225	231	237	242	248	254	259	265	270	278	282	287	293	299	304
64	209	215	221	227	232	238	244	250	256	262	267	273	279	285	291	296	302	308	314
65	216	222	228	234	240	246	252	258	264	270	276	282	288	294	300	306	312	318	324
66	223	229	235	241	247	253	260	266	272	278	284	291	297	303	309	315	322	328	334
67	230	236	242	249	255	261	268	274	280	287	293	299	306	312	319	325	331	338	344
68	236	243	249	256	262	269	276	282	289	295	302	308	315	322	328	335	341	348	354
69	243	250	257	263	270	277	284	291	297	304	311	318	324	331	338	345	351	358	365
70	250	257	264	271	278	285	292	299	306	313	320	327	334	341	348	355	362	369	376
71	257	265	272	279	286	293	301	308	315	322	329	338	343	351	358	365	372	379	386
72	265	272	279	287	294	302	309	316	324	331	338	346	353	361	368	375	383	390	397
73	272	280	288	295	302	310	318	325	333	340	348	355	363	371	378	386	393	401	408
74	280	287	295	303	311	319	326	334	342	350	358	365	373	381	389	396	404	412	420
75	287	295	303	311	319	327	335	343	351	359	367	375	383	391	399	407	415	423	431
76	295	304	312	320	328	336	344	353	361	369	377	385	394	402	410	418	426	435	443

* http://www.nhlbi.nih.gov/guidelines/obesity/bmi_tbl2.htm

CDC Growth Charts: United States
Weight-for-Length Percentiles:
Girls, birth to 36 months

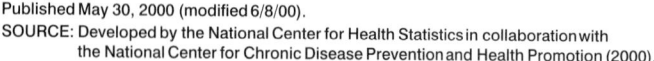

Length

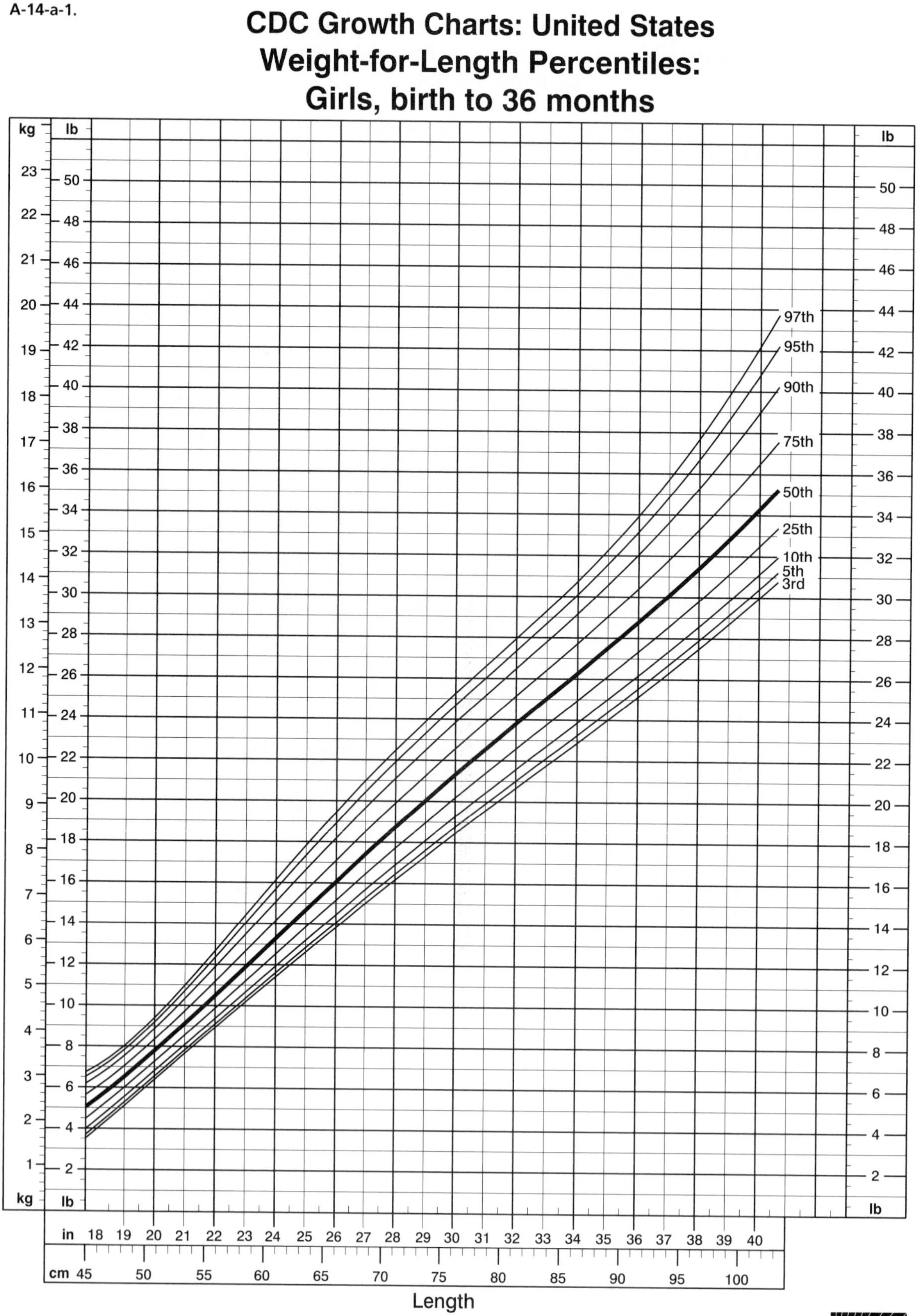

Published May 30, 2000 (modified 6/8/00).
SOURCE: Developed by the National Center for Health Statistics in collaboration with
the National Center for Chronic Disease Prevention and Health Promotion (2000).

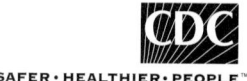

SAFER · HEALTHIER · PEOPLE™

A-14-a-2.

CDC Growth Charts: United States
Weight-for-Length Percentiles:
Boys, birth to 36 months

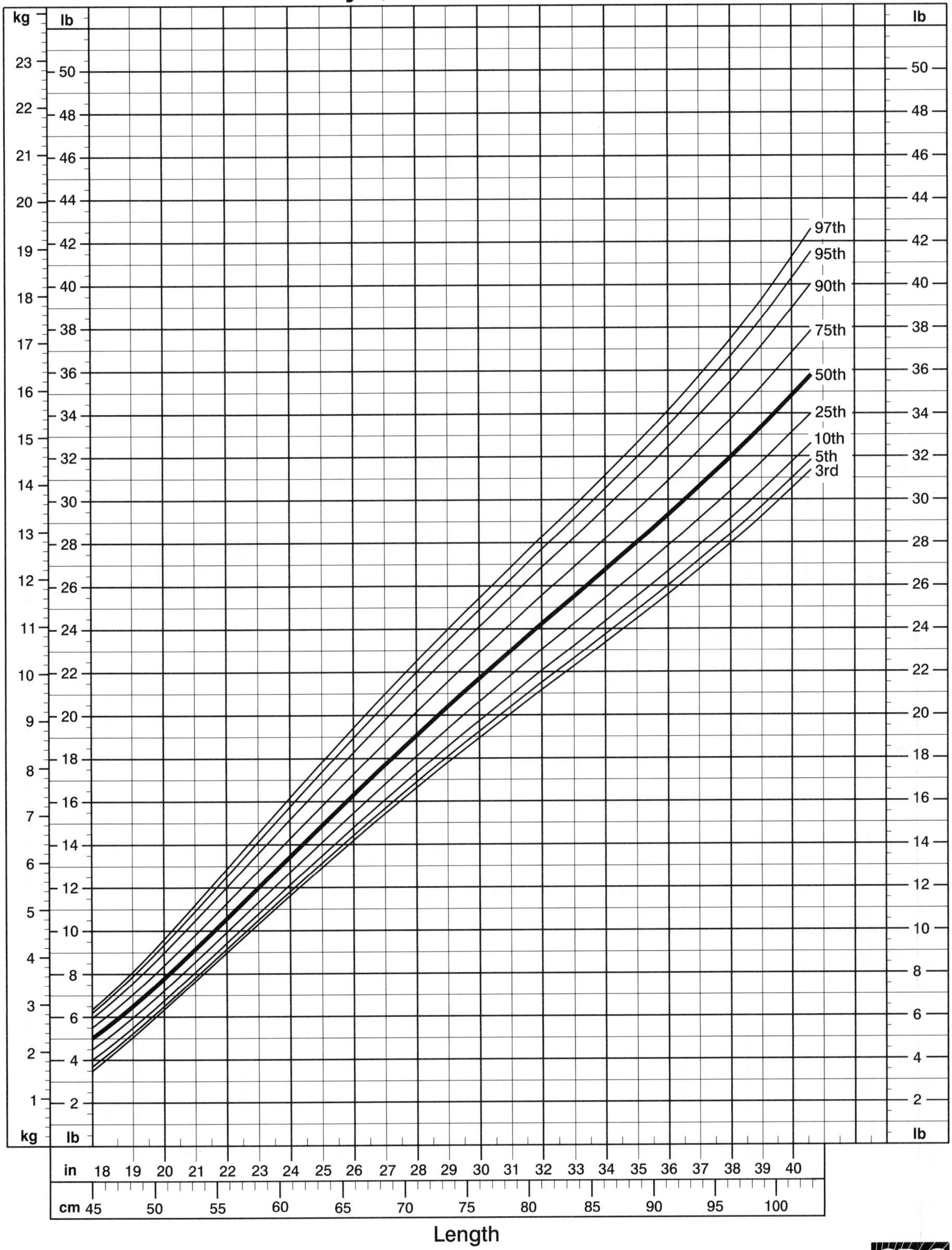

Length

Published May 30, 2000 (modified 6/8/00).
SOURCE: Developed by the National Center for Health Statistics in collaboration with
the National Center for Chronic Disease Prevention and Health Promotion (2000).

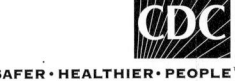

SAFER · HEALTHIER · PEOPLE™

A-14-b. Physical Growth—National Center for Health Statistics Percentiles, 2000

A-14-b-1.

CDC Growth Charts: United States
Length-for-Age Percentiles:
Girls, birth to 36 months

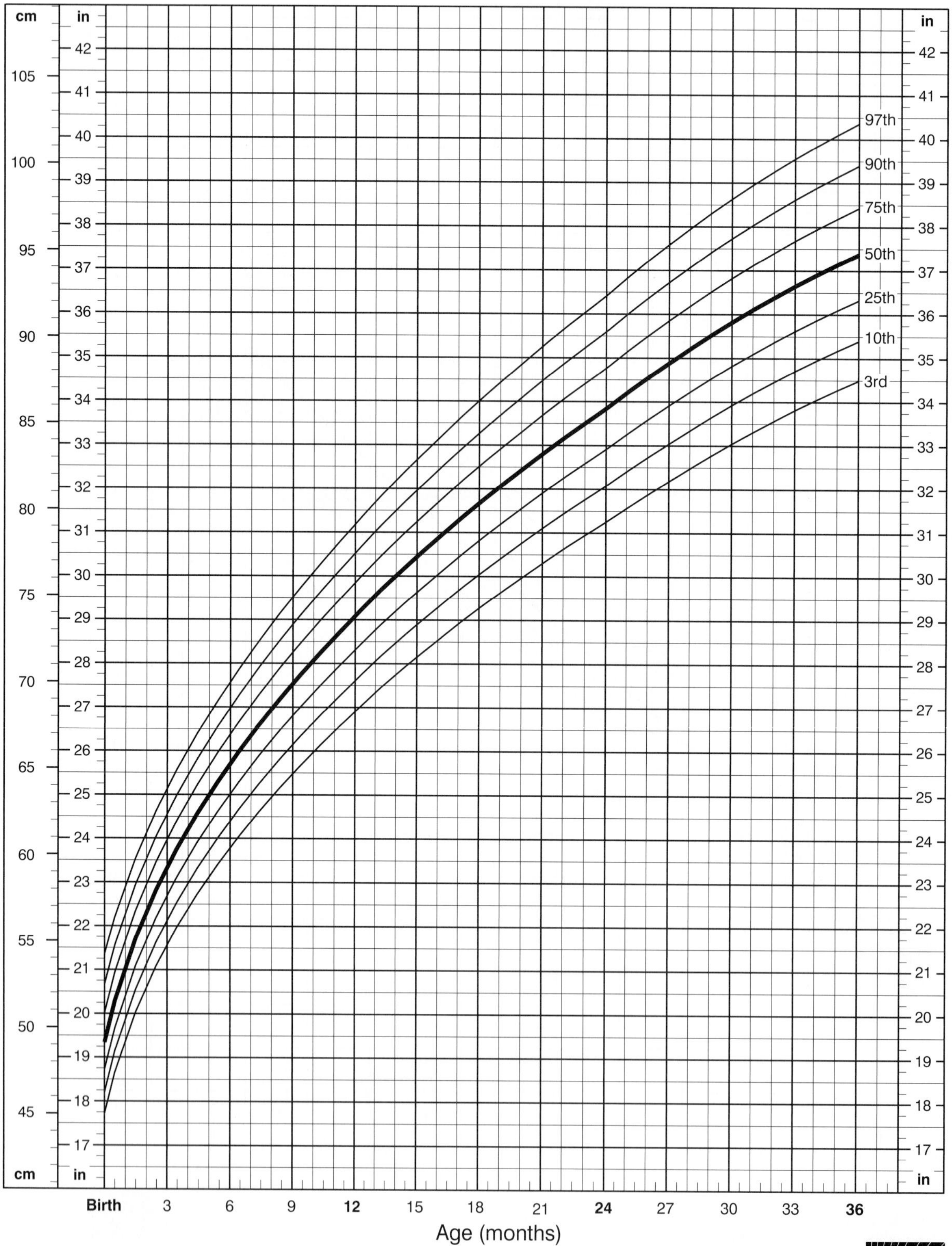

Age (months)

Published May 30, 2000.
SOURCE: Developed by the National Center for Health Statistics in collaboration with
   the National Center for Chronic Disease Prevention and Health Promotion (2000).

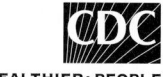

SAFER·HEALTHIER·PEOPLE™

A-14-b-2.

CDC Growth Charts: United States
Length-for-Age Percentiles:
Boys, birth to 36 months

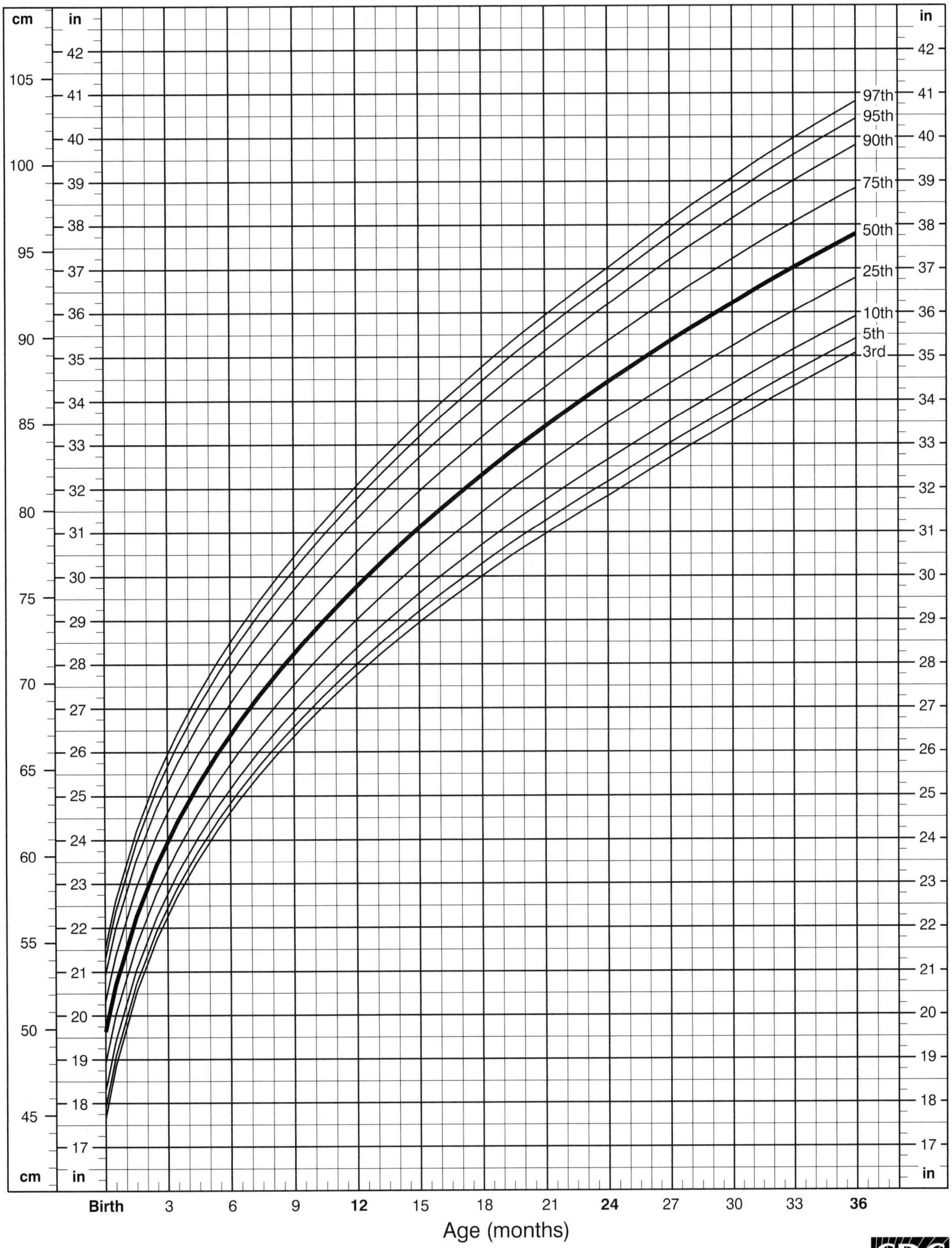

Published May 30, 2000.
SOURCE: Developed by the National Center for Health Statistics in collaboration with
the National Center for Chronic Disease Prevention and Health Promotion (2000).

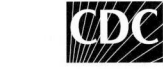

SAFER · HEALTHIER · PEOPLE™

A-14-c-1.

CDC Growth Charts: United States
Weight-for-Age Percentiles:
Girls, birth to 36 months

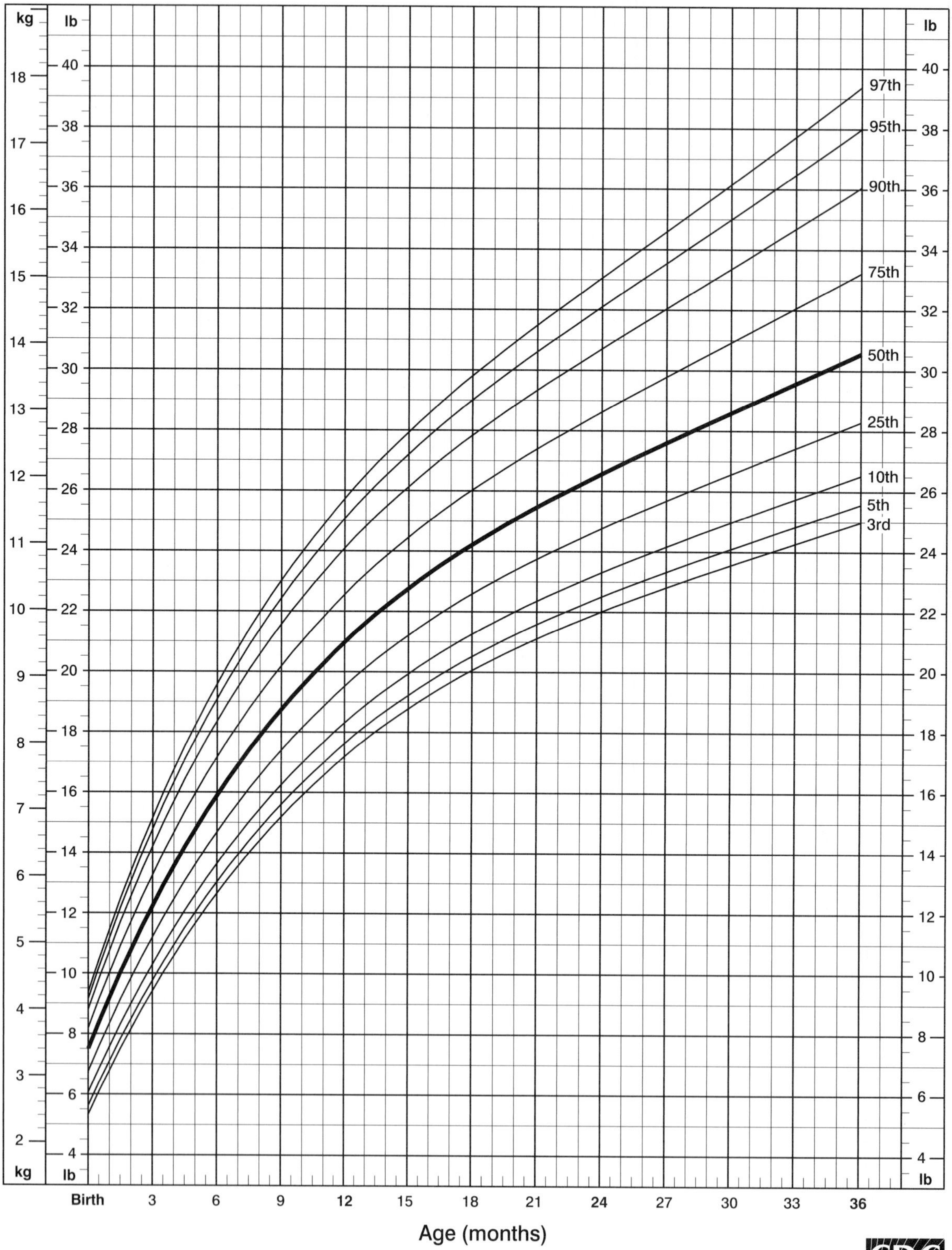

[Growth chart showing weight-for-age percentiles for girls from birth to 36 months, with percentile curves labeled 97th, 95th, 90th, 75th, 50th, 25th, 10th, 5th, and 3rd. The vertical axes show weight in kg (left inner, 2–18) and lb (4–40), and the horizontal axis shows Age (months) from Birth to 36.]

Age (months)

Published May 30, 2000.
SOURCE: Developed by the National Center for Health Statistics in collaboration with
the National Center for Chronic Disease Prevention and Health Promotion (2000).

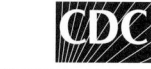

SAFER • HEALTHIER • PEOPLE™

A-14-c-2.

CDC Growth Charts: United States
Weight-for-Age Percentiles:
Boys, birth to 36 months

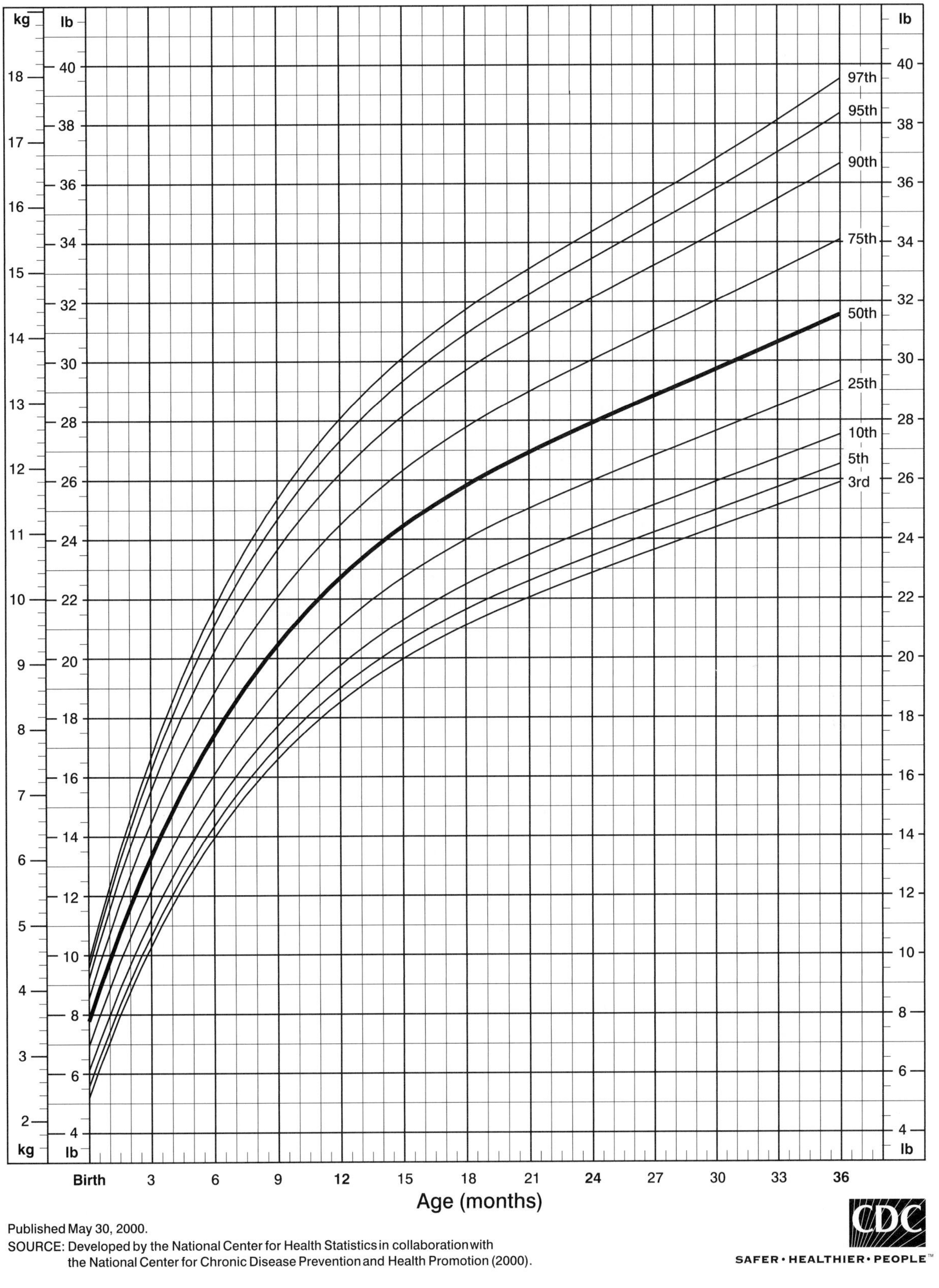

Age (months)

Published May 30, 2000.
SOURCE: Developed by the National Center for Health Statistics in collaboration with
the National Center for Chronic Disease Prevention and Health Promotion (2000).

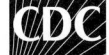

SAFER · HEALTHIER · PEOPLE™

A-14-d-1.

CDC Growth Charts: United States
Weight-for-Age Percentiles:
Girls, 2 to 20 years

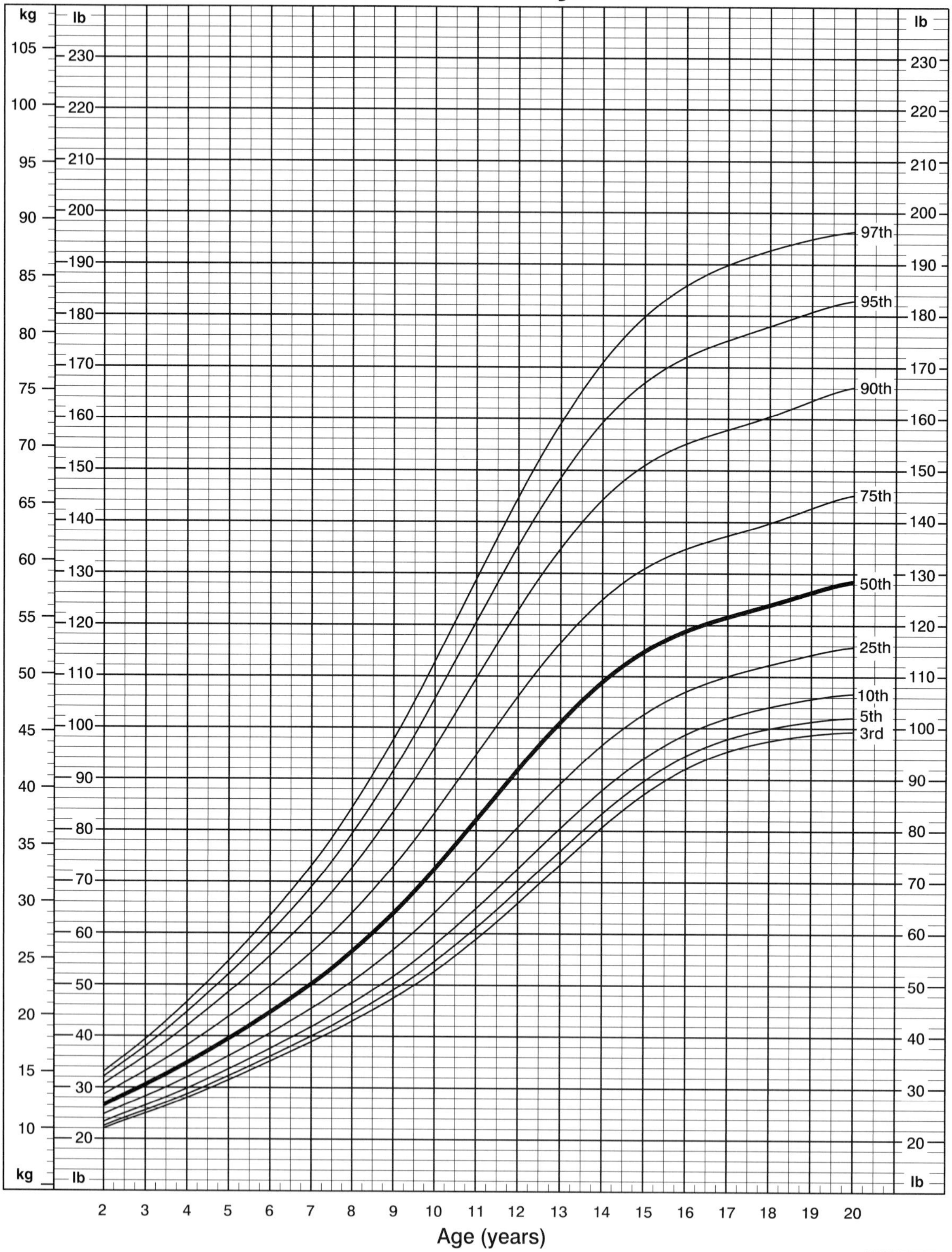

Age (years)

Published May 30, 2000.
SOURCE: Developed by the National Center for Health Statistics in collaboration with
the National Center for Chronic Disease Prevention and Health Promotion (2000).

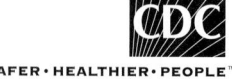

SAFER · HEALTHIER · PEOPLE™

A-14-d-2.

CDC Growth Charts: United States
Weight-for-Age Percentiles:
Boys, 2 to 20 years

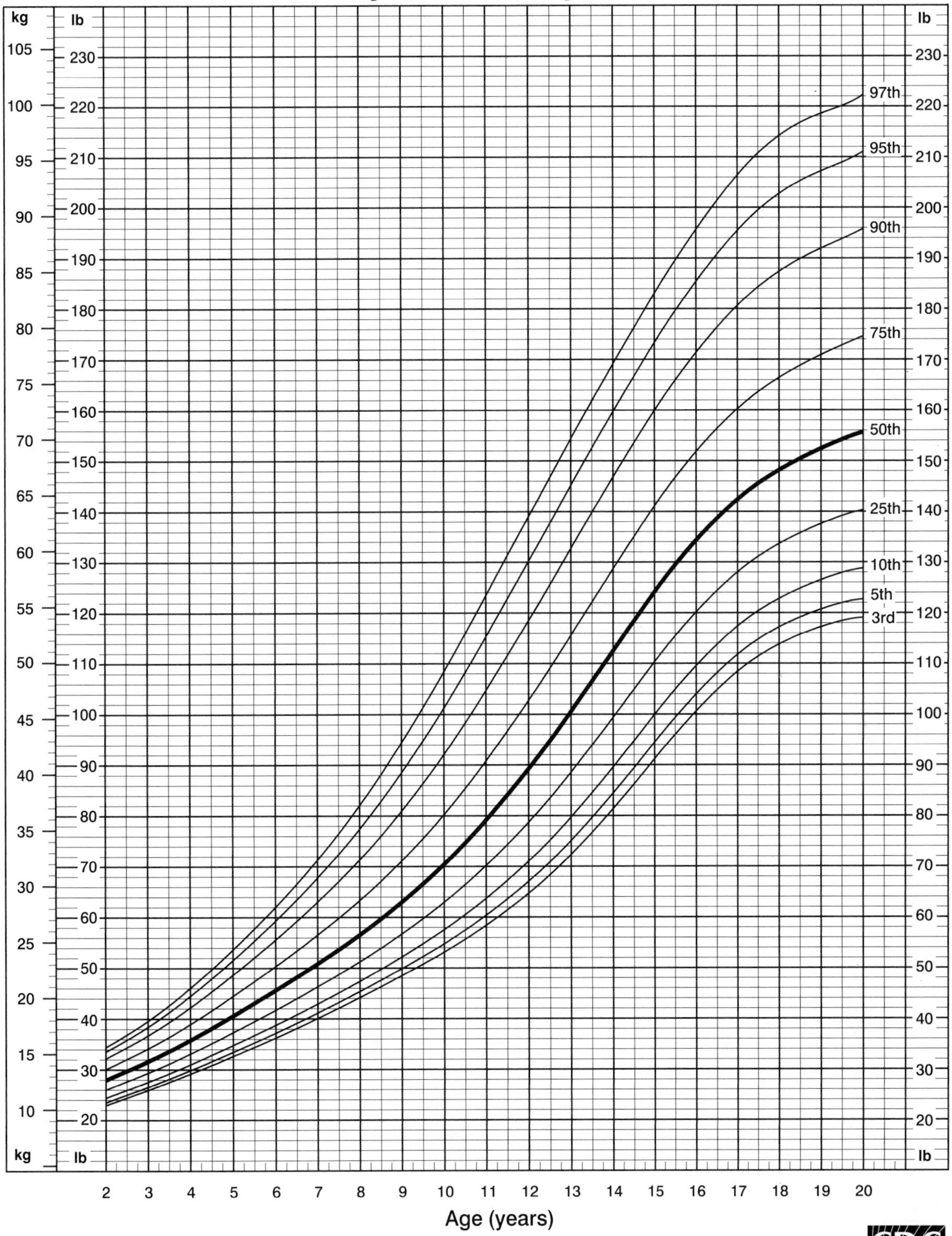

Age (years)

Published May 30, 2000.
SOURCE: Developed by the National Center for Health Statistics in collaboration with
the National Center for Chronic Disease Preventiona and Health Promotion (2000).

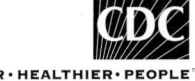

SAFER · HEALTHIER · PEOPLE™

A-14-C. Physical Growth—National Center for Health Statistics Percentiles, 2000

A-14-e-1.

CDC Growth Charts: United States
Stature-for-Age Percentiles
Girls, 2 to 20 years

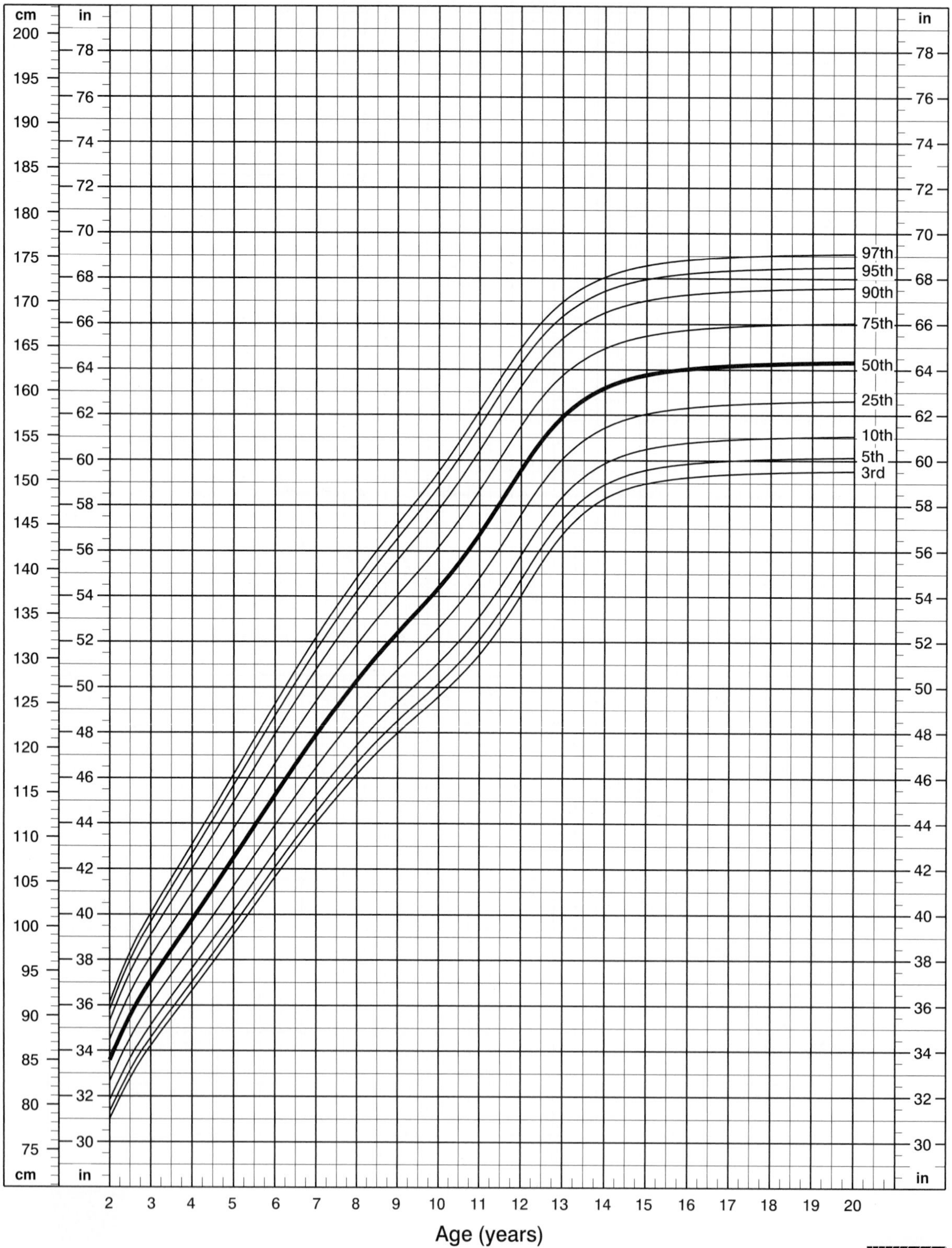

Age (years)

97th
95th
90th
75th
50th
25th
10th
5th
3rd

Published May 30, 2000.
SOURCE: Developed by the National Center for Health Statistics in collaboration with
the National Center for Chronic Disease Prevention and Health Promotion (2000).

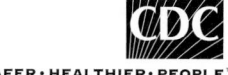

SAFER · HEALTHIER · PEOPLE™

A-14-e-2.

CDC Growth Charts: United States
Stature-for-Age Percentiles:
Boys, 2 to 20 years

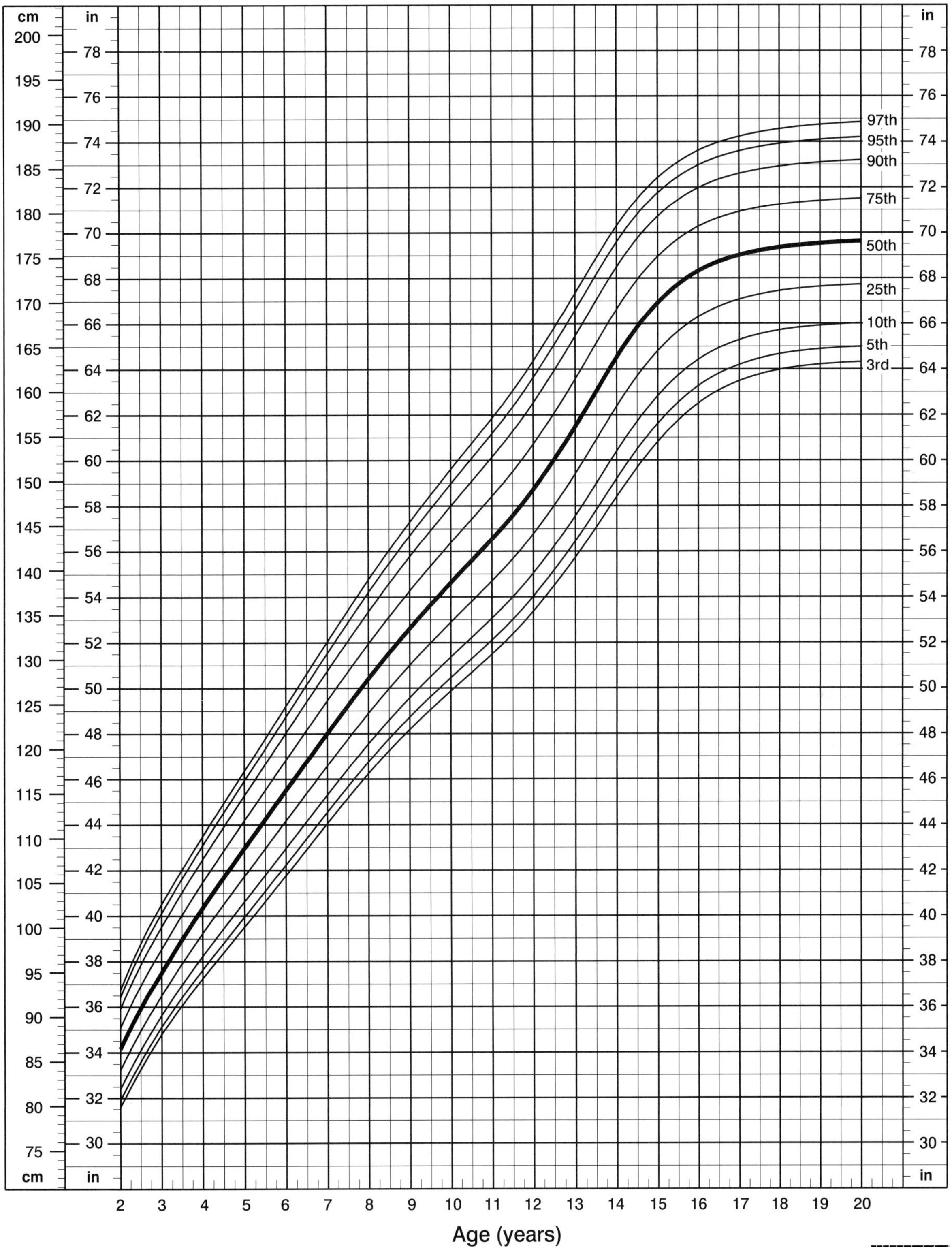

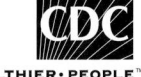

Published May 30, 2000.
SOURCE:Developed by the National Center for Health Statistics in collaboration with
the National Center for Chronic Disease Prevention and Health Promotion (2000).

SAFER · HEALTHIER · PEOPLE™

A-14-d. Physical Growth—National Center for Health Statistics Percentiles, 2000

A-14-f-1.

CDC Growth Charts: United States
Body mass index-for-Age Percentiles:
Girls, 2 to 20 years

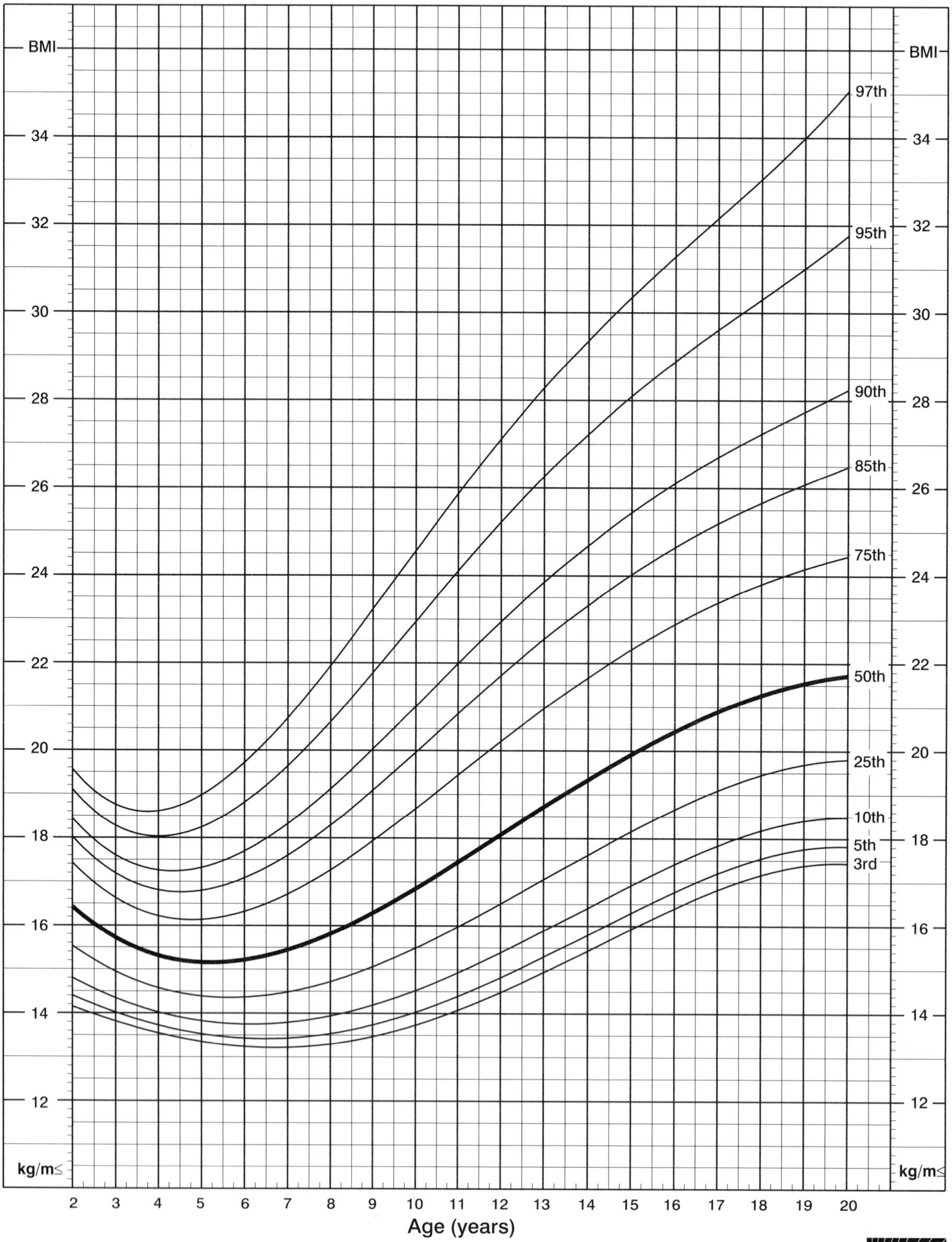

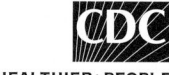

Published May 30, 2000.
SOURCE: Developed by the National Center for Health Statistics in collaboration with
the National Center for Chronic Disease Prevention and Health Promotion (2000).

SAFER ▪ HEALTHIER ▪ PEOPLE™

A-14-f-2.

CDC Growth Charts: United States
Body mass index-for-age percentiles:
Boys, 2 to 20 years

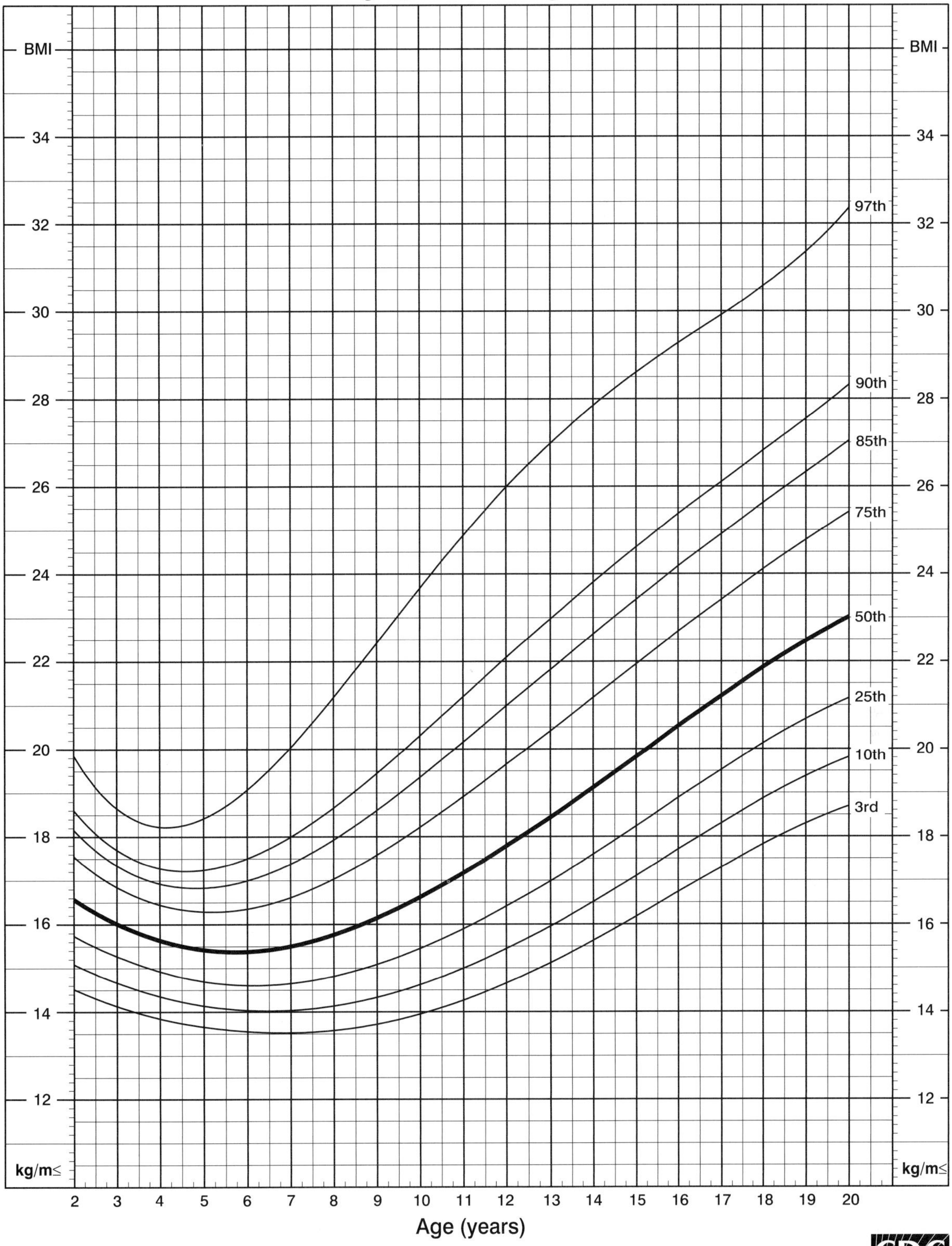

BMI

— 34

— 32

— 30

97th

— 28

90th

85th

— 26

75th

— 24

50th

— 22

25th

— 20

10th

3rd

— 18

— 16

— 14

— 12

kg/m≤

Age (years)

2 3 4 5 6 7 8 9 10 11 12 13 14 15 16 17 18 19 20

Published May 30, 2000.
SOURCE: Developed by the National Center for Health Statistics in collaboration with
the National Center for Chronic Disease Prevention and Health Promotion (2000).

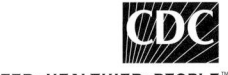

SAFER · HEALTHIER · PEOPLE™

A-14-e. Velocity of Height Changes with Age

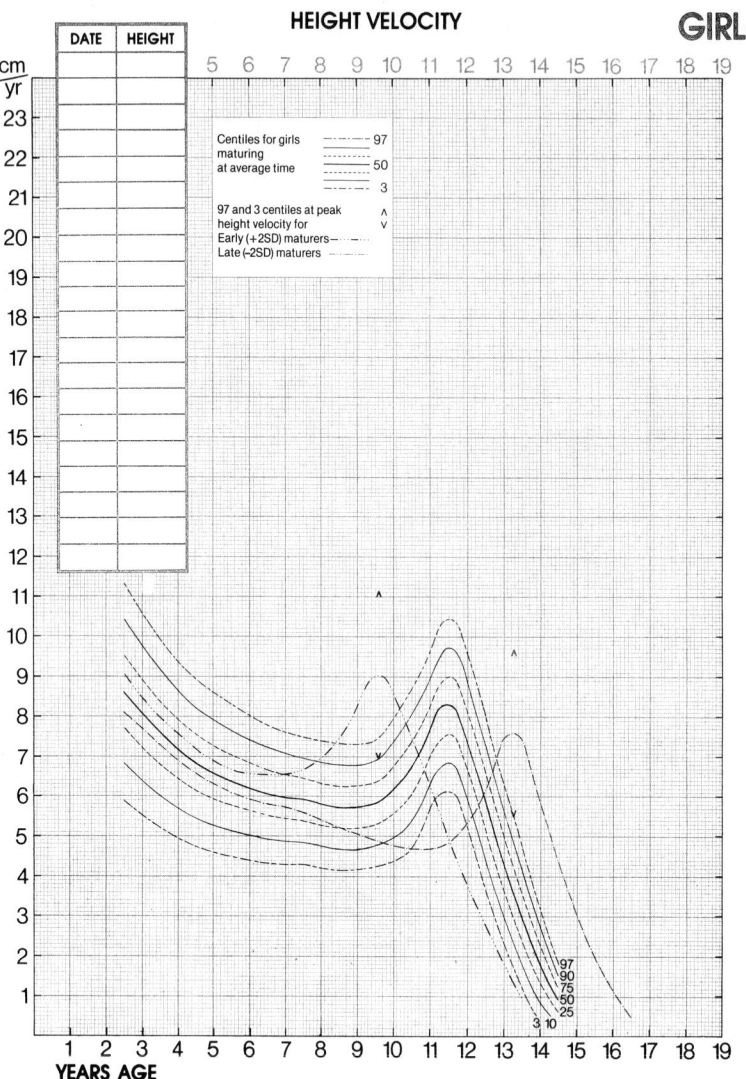

Figure A-14-e-1. Girls, 1 to 14 years.

From Tanner JM, Davies PSW. Journal of Pediatrics 1985:107.

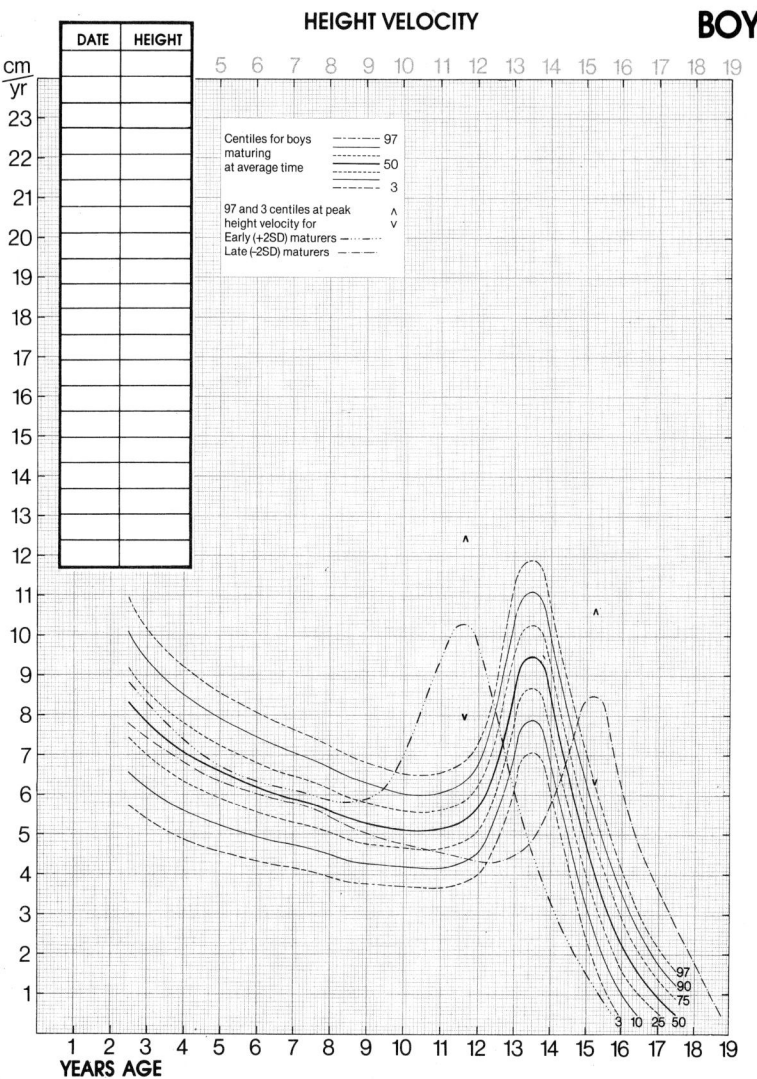

Figure A-14-e-2. Boys, 1 to 14 years.

From Tanner JM, Davies PSW. Journal of Pediatrics 1985:107.

A-15. ADULT WEIGHTS AND HEIGHTS

TABLE A-15-a. MEANS, STANDARD DEVIATIONS, AND PERCENTILES OF STATURE (cm) BY AGE FOR MALES AND FEMALES, 1 TO 74 YEARS

AGE (ys)	N	MEAN	SD	PERCENTILES 5	10	15	25	50	75	85	90	95
Males												
1.0–1.9	366	82.5	5.1	75.5	76.7	77.8	79.3	82.1	85.6	87.2	88.0	89.8
2.0–2.9	664	91.4	4.3	84.9	86.3	87.2	88.4	91.4	94.4	95.8	96.9	98.0
3.0–3.9	716	99.1	4.7	91.6	93.7	94.7	96.1	98.7	102.0	103.9	104.9	107.0
4.0–4.9	709	106.0	5.1	98.1	99.5	100.5	102.7	106.1	109.3	111.2	112.3	114.1
5.0–5.9	675	112.6	5.3	103.9	105.9	107.4	109.3	112.7	115.7	118.1	119.2	121.2
6.0–6.9	298	119.2	5.4	109.4	112.0	113.3	115.7	119.4	122.8	124.9	126.0	127.7
7.0–7.9	312	125.1	5.7	115.6	118.2	119.6	121.5	125.4	128.5	130.6	131.6	133.5
8.0–8.9	296	129.8	6.3	120.0	122.6	123.9	125.9	130.1	133.7	136.0	137.5	140.0
9.0–9.9	322	135.8	5.8	126.0	128.7	129.7	131.4	135.8	139.9	142.0	143.0	145.0
10.0–10.9	334	140.9	6.9	130.2	132.3	133.8	136.1	140.9	145.8	148.2	150.1	152.7
11.0–11.9	324	146.4	7.4	134.3	136.6	138.8	141.6	146.4	151.5	154.0	155.0	158.1
12.0–12.9	349	152.2	8.1	139.7	141.9	143.6	146.4	151.4	157.9	160.4	162.3	166.0
13.0–13.9	350	159.2	8.8	145.1	147.8	149.6	152.8	159.3	165.6	168.9	170.7	173.2
14.0–14.9	359	167.1	8.2	153.3	156.3	158.6	161.7	166.9	172.8	175.9	178.2	179.9
15.0–15.9	359	170.8	7.3	158.5	161.5	162.9	165.6	171.2	176.2	177.9	179.8	182.5
16.0–16.9	349	174.5	7.1	163.4	165.0	167.3	169.8	174.1	178.7	182.0	183.8	186.7
17.0–17.9	338	175.5	6.9	164.4	166.9	168.6	170.7	175.1	180.5	183.0	184.5	187.3
18.0–24.9	1,755	176.6	7.0	165.4	167.8	169.5	171.9	176.6	181.2	183.7	185.5	188.6
25.0–29.9	1,255	176.7	7.0	165.1	167.8	169.4	172.0	176.6	181.5	184.0	185.7	188.0
30.0–34.9	947	176.2	6.9	164.8	167.4	169.0	171.5	176.2	180.9	183.3	184.8	187.2
35.0–39.9	839	176.1	7.2	164.0	166.8	168.8	171.9	176.1	181.0	183.5	185.0	187.7
40.0–44.9	829	175.9	6.7	165.0	167.2	168.9	171.4	176.0	180.3	182.7	184.2	186.9
45.0–49.9	871	176.2	7.1	163.8	166.5	168.0	170.6	174.8	180.2	182.9	184.5	186.6
50.0–54.9	882	174.6	6.5	164.2	166.4	167.8	170.1	174.6	178.8	181.4	183.2	185.3
55.0–59.9	807	173.9	6.8	163.2	165.0	166.8	169.3	173.8	178.7	181.0	182.3	184.6
60.0–64.9	1,261	173.0	6.6	161.9	165.0	166.4	168.7	173.0	177.4	179.8	181.3	183.7
65.0–69.9	1,773	171.5	6.9	159.7	162.9	164.5	166.7	171.6	176.3	178.6	180.1	182.5
70.0–74.9	1,257	170.6	6.8	159.5	162.0	163.6	165.8	170.7	175.0	177.4	179.4	182.0
Females												
1.0–1.9	333	80.6	4.8	73.2	74.7	75.6	77.4	80.5	83.6	85.9	86.8	88.6
2.0–2.9	610	90.1	4.5	83.1	84.9	85.6	86.8	90.1	93.0	94.6	95.7	97.4
3.0–3.9	651	97.7	4.5	90.3	92.1	92.9	94.8	97.5	100.6	102.4	103.4	105.0
4.0–4.9	678	105.0	4.9	97.0	98.5	99.6	101.6	104.9	108.3	110.0	111.2	113.6
5.0–5.9	673	112.0	5.4	103.1	105.3	106.7	108.6	111.9	115.4	117.4	119.0	120.6
6.0–6.9	296	118.3	5.6	109.9	111.4	112.4	114.2	118.5	122.2	124.2	125.2	127.6
7.0–7.9	331	124.2	6.0	115.3	117.0	118.3	120.3	124.3	128.4	130.1	131.7	134.5
8.0–8.9	276	129.8	6.0	120.1	122.1	123.7	125.5	129.7	133.5	135.6	137.8	140.1
9.0–9.9	322	135.7	7.2	125.7	127.5	128.4	130.5	135.6	140.4	142.5	143.9	147.2
10.0–10.9	330	141.5	7.4	129.5	132.2	133.9	136.3	141.6	146.0	148.3	150.9	154.4
11.0–11.9	303	148.1	8.2	134.7	138.1	139.8	142.3	148.4	153.4	156.1	158.0	162.1
12.0–12.9	324	154.6	7.2	148.0	145.2	147.0	149.6	154.6	159.3	162.5	164.0	165.5
13.0–13.9	361	158.8	6.2	149.1	151.1	152.8	155.1	158.8	162.8	164.8	165.7	168.3
14.0–14.9	370	160.9	6.2	151.0	153.0	154.5	156.8	160.8	164.9	167.0	168.8	171.7
15.0–15.9	309	163.2	6.5	152.8	155.2	157.1	158.8	162.7	167.2	169.7	172.0	175.4
16.0–16.9	343	162.2	6.6	151.4	153.6	155.5	157.7	162.3	166.4	169.1	171.6	173.2
17.0–17.9	293	162.7	6.0	153.2	155.5	156.9	159.2	162.3	166.4	168.7	169.9	172.8
18.0–24.9	2,592	163.0	6.5	152.3	154.8	156.4	158.8	163.1	167.1	169.6	171.0	173.6
25.0–29.9	1,935	162.9	6.3	152.6	155.2	156.6	158.6	162.8	167.1	169.5	170.9	173.3
30.0–34.9	1,633	162.6	6.2	152.9	155.2	156.4	158.4	162.4	166.8	169.2	171.2	173.1
35.0–39.9	1,461	162.8	6.5	152.0	155.0	156.4	158.6	162.7	167.0	169.4	171.0	173.5
40.0–44.9	1,399	162.6	6.4	151.6	154.3	156.2	158.1	162.7	166.7	168.8	170.5	173.2
45.0–49.9	969	162.0	6.3	151.7	154.0	155.4	157.9	162.0	166.3	168.4	169.9	172.2
50.0–54.9	1,012	161.2	6.0	151.3	153.8	155.3	156.9	161.1	165.1	167.3	169.2	171.0
55.0–59.9	887	160.3	6.2	149.8	152.7	154.1	156.7	160.3	164.4	166.6	167.8	170.1
60.0–64.9	1,392	159.6	6.4	149.2	151.4	153.0	155.6	160.0	163.7	166.1	167.3	169.8
65.0–69.9	1,952	158.6	6.1	148.5	150.7	152.4	154.8	158.8	162.6	164.8	166.2	168.1
70.0–74.9	1,467	157.6	6.1	147.2	150.0	151.7	153.7	157.4	161.5	163.8	165.5	167.5

From Frisancho AR. Anthropometric standards for the assessment of growth and nutritional status. Ann Arbor: University of Michigan Press, 1990, Table IV. 1. With permission.

TABLE A-15-b. MEANS, STANDARD DEVIATIONS, AND PERCENTILES OF WEIGHT (kg) BY AGE FOR MALES AND FEMALES, 1 TO 74 YEARS

| AGE (ys) | N | MEAN | SD | PERCENTILES | | | | | | | | |
				5	10	15	25	50	75	85	90	95
Males												
1.0–1.9	681	11.8	1.7	9.6	10.0	10.3	10.7	11.6	12.6	13.1	13.7	14.4
2.0–2.9	677	13.6	1.7	11.1	11.6	11.9	12.5	13.6	14.6	15.2	15.8	16.6
3.0–3.9	717	15.7	2.1	12.8	13.4	13.8	14.4	15.5	16.8	17.5	18.1	19.4
4.0–4.9	709	17.7	2.4	14.1	15.0	15.4	16.1	17.5	19.0	20.0	20.6	21.5
5.0–5.9	676	19.9	3.0	16.0	16.7	17.1	17.8	19.6	21.4	22.4	23.5	25.4
6.0–6.9	298	22.6	3.7	17.5	18.8	19.4	20.2	21.9	24.0	26.0	27.7	30.0
7.0–7.9	312	25.1	4.2	19.0	20.4	21.2	22.2	24.7	27.2	28.7	29.9	33.1
8.0–8.9	296	27.7	5.2	21.5	22.7	23.5	24.5	26.8	29.7	31.8	33.6	37.3
9.0–9.9	322	31.3	6.3	23.6	24.7	25.7	27.1	30.3	33.6	37.1	40.3	43.2
10.0–10.9	334	35.4	7.8	26.2	27.7	28.5	30.2	33.8	38.6	42.1	45.6	53.1
11.0–11.9	324	39.8	10.0	28.3	30.0	31.5	33.4	37.6	43.3	48.6	52.3	58.6
12.0–12.9	349	44.2	11.1	30.8	32.8	34.4	36.6	42.2	49.0	53.9	59.0	66.9
13.0–13.9	348	49.8	11.6	34.6	37.1	38.7	41.6	48.5	56.1	60.3	65.2	69.6
14.0–14.9	359	56.9	11.9	41.3	44.0	45.9	49.2	55.3	63.0	66.4	70.1	76.9
15.0–15.9	359	61.0	11.2	44.7	48.6	50.8	54.2	60.0	66.2	70.4	74.4	81.3
16.0–16.9	349	66.8	11.9	51.7	54.2	55.7	59.0	64.8	72.9	77.8	81.6	89.0
17.0–17.9	339	67.5	12.2	51.1	54.1	56.5	59.3	65.7	72.5	78.0	83.3	91.4
18.0–24.9	1,758	73.9	13.4	56.4	59.8	61.6	64.8	71.4	80.5	86.3	91.5	99.9
25.0–29.9	1,256	77.9	14.6	58.7	61.8	64.5	68.1	76.0	84.8	90.6	95.1	103.4
30.0–34.9	948	79.8	14.4	59.8	63.3	66.3	69.8	78.4	87.4	93.4	96.8	103.0
35.0–39.9	840	80.3	13.6	58.4	62.9	66.6	72.2	79.8	87.8	92.4	96.7	102.8
40.0–44.9	830	81.0	13.8	60.7	64.3	67.9	71.9	79.6	89.4	94.3	98.8	104.8
45.0–49.9	871	80.8	14.0	60.0	64.0	66.8	71.4	79.7	89.2	94.0	97.2	103.6
50.0–54.9	882	79.5	13.9	58.7	93.3	66.2	70.0	78.0	87.4	93.3	99.3	103.6
55.0–59.9	808	79.4	13.9	58.2	63.0	66.4	70.2	78.5	86.8	92.9	97.1	103.5
60.0–64.9	1,263	77.3	13.1	57.9	61.8	64.5	68.8	76.8	84.9	89.3	92.5	100.0
65.0–69.9	1,774	75.0	13.0	55.1	58.5	61.5	66.4	74.5	83.2	88.0	91.8	97.2
70.0–74.9	1,257	73.7	12.9	53.9	57.5	60.4	65.2	73.0	81.3	86.3	90.4	95.9
Females												
1.0–1.9	622	10.9	1.4	8.7	9.2	9.5	9.9	10.8	11.8	12.4	12.8	13.4
2.0–2.9	615	13.0	1.6	10.8	11.2	11.6	12.0	12.8	13.9	14.6	15.1	15.9
3.0–3.9	653	15.0	2.1	11.8	12.6	13.0	13.6	14.7	16.2	17.1	17.6	18.6
4.0–4.9	682	17.1	2.4	13.7	14.3	14.7	15.5	16.8	18.4	19.4	20.1	21.3
5.0–5.9	674	19.5	3.2	15.3	16.2	16.8	17.3	19.0	21.0	22.4	23.6	25.3
6.0–6.9	296	21.8	3.6	17.0	17.7	18.6	19.4	21.3	23.7	24.8	26.5	28.9
7.0–7.9	331	24.7	4.5	19.2	19.8	20.6	21.9	23.8	26.5	28.7	29.9	32.7
8.0–8.9	276	28.1	6.3	20.9	21.9	22.6	24.0	26.9	30.4	33.3	35.1	39.9
9.0–9.9	322	32.0	7.5	23.7	24.8	25.6	26.8	30.7	34.7	38.9	41.7	46.5
10.0–10.9	330	35.7	8.4	25.6	27.0	27.9	29.6	33.9	39.2	44.1	46.5	52.4
11.0–11.9	303	41.8	11.0	29.1	30.5	31.6	34.3	39.8	46.3	52.8	56.9	61.9
12.0–12.9	324	47.1	10.7	32.5	34.3	36.3	39.1	45.9	53.0	58.5	61.2	66.7
13.0–13.9	361	51.5	11.7	37.2	39.3	40.6	44.3	49.6	55.7	61.6	66.8	76.2
14.0–14.9	370	54.7	11.2	40.3	42.9	44.8	47.3	52.7	60.0	64.9	69.5	75.6
15.0–15.9	309	56.4	11.6	43.4	45.3	46.6	48.6	54.2	60.3	65.2	69.5	79.4
16.0–16.9	343	58.2	11.7	43.4	46.1	47.5	50.8	55.7	62.8	68.9	73.1	80.8
17.0–17.9	293	59.7	13.3	43.2	46.4	49.2	51.9	57.4	63.3	69.4	74.7	86.0
18.0–24.9	2,592	60.8	12.8	45.6	48.4	50.0	52.6	58.3	65.4	71.5	76.1	84.3
25.0–29.9	1,935	62.8	14.2	46.6	49.0	50.7	53.4	59.4	68.4	76.1	81.6	90.8
30.0–34.9	1,633	65.6	16.1	47.5	50.1	52.0	54.9	61.5	72.2	80.5	86.5	97.9
35.0–39.9	1,461	67.1	15.8	48.6	51.7	53.1	56.4	63.3	73.7	82.0	88.1	98.2
40.0–44.9	1,399	67.8	16.1	49.2	51.8	54.0	57.0	64.0	75.1	83.3	89.8	99.1
45.0–49.9	969	68.2	16.3	47.8	51.4	53.5	57.1	64.9	75.9	83.0	87.4	98.4
50.0–54.9	1,012	68.3	14.8	48.8	51.9	54.4	58.1	65.8	75.8	83.1	88.4	97.1
55.0–59.9	888	69.2	16.3	48.6	52.2	54.5	58.2	66.3	77.2	85.2	89.4	98.5
60.0–64.9	1,393	68.0	14.2	48.5	51.7	54.1	58.1	66.0	75.8	82.1	86.0	94.1
65.0–69.9	1,954	67.5	14.2	47.8	51.4	53.9	57.7	65.7	74.8	80.8	86.1	93.9
70.0–74.9	1,468	66.0	13.6	46.5	50.1	52.4	57.0	64.5	74.4	79.7	83.3	88.8

From Frisancho AR. Anthropometric standards for the assessment of growth and nutritional status. Ann Arbor: University of Michigan Press, 1990, Table IV.2. With permission.

TABLE A-15-c. MEANS, STANDARD DEVIATIONS, AND PERCENTILES OF WEIGHT (kg) BY HEIGHT (cm) FOR MALES, 2 TO 74 YEARS

HEIGHT (cm)	N	MEAN	SD	PERCENTILES								
				5	10	15	25	50	75	85	90	95
Boys: 2 to 11 years												
84–86	75	12.1	1.1	10.7	10.9	11.1	11.3	11.9	12.8	13.1	13.5	14.3
87–89	170	12.8	1.1	11.2	11.4	11.7	12.0	12.7	13.4	13.8	14.2	14.6
90–92	207	13.5	1.0	11.9	12.1	12.5	12.8	13.6	14.2	14.6	14.9	15.2
93–95	278	14.4	1.2	12.7	13.0	13.4	13.6	14.3	15.1	15.5	15.8	16.3
96–98	310	15.0	1.3	13.3	13.6	13.8	14.2	15.0	15.6	16.1	16.4	17.0
99–101	300	16.0	1.3	13.9	14.4	14.7	15.1	15.9	16.7	17.2	17.6	18.3
102–104	290	16.9	1.4	15.1	15.4	15.6	15.9	16.8	17.7	18.0	18.5	19.3
105–107	291	17.6	1.6	15.4	15.9	16.2	16.6	17.5	18.4	19.0	19.4	19.8
108–110	298	18.7	1.7	16.7	17.0	17.1	17.6	18.5	19.6	20.1	20.5	21.3
111–113	274	20.0	2.2	17.0	17.8	18.1	18.7	19.6	21.0	21.7	22.4	23.4
114–116	223	20.9	2.2	18.6	19.0	19.2	19.6	20.5	21.7	22.3	22.7	23.6
117–119	199	21.9	2.3	19.0	19.6	20.2	20.5	21.5	23.0	23.8	24.3	26.0
120–122	177	23.3	2.4	19.8	20.8	21.2	21.9	23.1	24.5	25.4	26.0	27.3
123–125	174	25.0	2.8	21.5	22.0	22.7	23.4	24.5	26.2	27.0	28.2	30.0
126–128	185	26.5	3.8	22.6	23.1	23.8	24.3	25.9	27.8	29.4	30.6	32.0
129–131	174	27.6	3.1	23.5	24.4	24.7	25.6	27.3	28.9	30.0	31.0	32.9
132–134	180	29.3	3.5	25.1	25.7	25.8	26.8	28.5	31.0	33.0	34.4	35.4
135–137	175	31.4	4.6	26.2	27.1	27.6	28.5	30.4	33.0	34.9	37.4	41.5
138–140	150	33.5	4.7	28.2	28.9	29.4	30.5	32.3	35.1	37.8	39.9	42.0
141–143	153	36.1	5.0	30.4	31.3	31.8	33.0	34.9	38.2	40.5	43.3	45.4
144–146	114	38.9	6.6	31.6	32.7	33.1	35.1	37.6	41.2	43.9	46.3	50.7
147–149	87	40.9	6.8	33.6	34.3	35.3	35.9	39.2	43.8	47.3	51.5	56.7
Boys: 12 to 17 years												
144–146	59	38.1	5.5	31.1	32.4	33.6	34.6	36.5	40.3	42.1	46.1	53.0
147–149	77	40.9	7.1	33.6	34.0	34.7	36.5	38.3	43.8	47.4	49.4	59.8
150–152	103	43.4	6.6	36.3	37.2	38.0	38.7	41.4	46.5	51.5	54.7	56.7
153–155	106	45.9	7.9	36.5	38.1	39.1	40.6	43.7	49.7	51.9	55.2	60.9
156–158	113	48.5	9.2	39.9	40.7	41.3	42.5	45.8	50.0	57.9	62.0	67.3
159–161	146	51.1	9.2	40.8	42.9	43.9	45.6	48.6	53.6	60.9	65.4	68.4
162–164	177	54.8	8.9	44.7	45.9	46.9	49.1	53.2	58.4	61.8	64.3	69.1
165–167	197	57.3	9.2	47.1	48.8	49.9	51.3	55.3	61.0	64.8	68.6	73.3
168–170	235	61.4	10.4	49.2	51.4	52.4	55.0	59.9	65.5	69.6	72.5	79.1
171–173	233	62.8	8.8	51.4	53.4	54.8	56.9	61.3	66.1	71.2	73.7	78.2
174–176	202	66.7	10.9	52.3	55.7	57.4	60.0	64.8	71.2	75.5	81.4	89.9
177–179	166	68.8	12.0	55.8	58.7	59.6	61.6	66.3	72.3	75.5	79.6	88.0
180–182	103	71.8	9.7	60.2	60.9	62.1	64.0	70.1	79.5	82.2	85.2	88.7
183–185	64	73.5	9.1	62.4	63.6	65.4	67.8	72.1	77.3	79.4	89.9	91.1
Males: 18 to 74 years												
153–155	56	64.6	13.0	48.6	51.3	54.5	57.1	62.0	66.8	76.8	80.6	83.5
156–158	140	65.5	11.2	48.3	51.4	54.0	57.4	64.9	72.0	77.3	79.3	86.0
159–161	292	66.2	10.8	49.1	53.8	56.4	59.2	66.0	71.2	76.9	80.2	84.3
162–164	643	68.0	10.5	52.2	55.2	57.0	60.4	67.3	74.5	79.1	81.6	86.9
165–167	1,147	70.8	11.6	53.0	56.6	59.6	62.7	70.3	77.6	82.3	85.2	90.1
168–170	1,582	73.5	12.0	55.9	58.6	61.3	65.9	72.7	80.2	84.5	87.9	93.4
171–173	2,047	76.1	12.5	58.2	61.3	63.6	67.6	75.1	83.2	88.1	92.0	97.8
174–176	2,053	78.3	12.7	60.0	63.8	66.1	69.5	77.3	84.9	90.1	93.8	99.7
177–179	1,750	80.3	12.8	61.9	65.1	67.5	71.4	79.4	87.3	92.6	96.5	102.6
180–182	1,252	82.6	13.6	63.4	67.3	69.6	72.9	81.4	90.1	95.0	99.4	105.7
183–185	833	85.2	13.9	65.1	69.2	71.5	75.3	83.3	93.4	99.1	103.2	110.4
186–188	398	88.0	13.3	68.9	72.3	74.8	79.4	86.6	95.1	100.4	103.5	109.8
189–191	161	92.0	16.0	71.3	75.3	77.8	80.7	89.9	99.4	105.0	110.8	123.7
191–194	66	95.9	15.8	71.8	78.6	80.2	84.8	94.2	105.2	109.1	111.8	123.8

From Frisancho AR. Anthropometric standards for the assessment of growth and nutritional status. Ann Arbor: University of Michigan Press, 1990, Table IV.3. With permission.

TABLE A-15-d. MEANS, STANDARD DEVIATIONS, AND PERCENTILES OF WEIGHT (kg) BY HEIGHT (cm) FOR FEMALES, 2 TO 74 YEARS

HEIGHT (cm)	N	MEAN	SD	PERCENTILES								
				5	10	15	25	50	75	85	90	95
Girls: 2 to 10 years												
81–83	36	11.2	.8	10.1	10.2	10.3	10.4	11.0	11.7	12.1	12.6	12.6
84–86	118	11.9	.9	10.5	10.8	11.0	11.3	12.0	12.5	12.7	13.0	13.6
87–89	156	12.5	1.2	11.0	11.3	11.6	11.8	12.4	13.0	13.6	13.8	14.6
90–92	229	13.2	1.2	11.6	11.8	12.0	12.3	13.0	13.8	14.3	14.6	15.2
93–95	259	13.9	1.2	12.0	12.6	12.8	13.1	13.8	14.6	15.1	15.5	16.1
96–98	275	15.0	1.3	13.1	13.5	13.7	14.1	14.9	15.6	16.3	16.7	17.2
99–101	272	15.8	1.6	13.8	14.1	14.3	14.6	15.5	16.6	17.2	17.6	18.4
102–104	278	16.6	2.0	14.2	14.6	15.0	15.5	16.4	17.3	18.0	18.5	19.4
105–107	270	17.6	1.6	15.3	15.8	16.1	16.6	17.3	18.4	19.2	19.4	20.1
108–110	275	18.3	1.6	15.9	16.6	16.8	17.2	18.1	19.2	20.0	20.4	21.1
111–113	251	19.4	1.9	16.6	17.1	17.3	17.9	19.4	20.4	21.2	21.8	22.8
114–116	215	20.7	2.5	17.5	18.3	18.6	19.0	20.2	21.8	22.9	23.9	25.7
117–119	191	21.9	2.6	19.0	19.4	19.5	20.2	21.4	23.0	24.0	24.8	26.6
120–122	181	23.1	2.5	20.1	20.4	20.9	21.5	22.6	24.0	25.3	26.2	27.7
123–125	162	24.5	2.5	21.2	21.8	22.3	22.8	24.0	25.9	26.5	27.2	29.0
126–128	172	26.2	3.1	22.6	23.0	23.4	23.9	25.6	27.7	29.4	30.0	31.5
129–131	157	28.0	3.8	23.6	24.3	24.8	25.6	27.3	29.4	31.1	33.4	36.6
132–134	148	30.3	4.4	25.1	25.8	26.2	27.0	29.4	32.3	34.5	37.2	39.9
135–137	135	32.1	5.4	25.6	27.2	27.7	28.3	30.8	33.9	35.8	41.6	44.1
138–140	124	34.6	7.3	27.6	28.8	29.1	30.6	32.5	35.5	40.9	43.5	47.5
141–143	97	36.0	6.3	28.8	29.8	30.7	32.2	34.8	37.9	41.3	45.6	49.9
144–146	65	39.2	7.0	31.0	31.9	32.9	34.5	37.6	42.9	45.3	48.4	51.8
147–149	45	40.0	7.3	30.7	32.3	34.0	35.0	38.3	44.2	48.0	50.8	54.8
Girls: 11 to 17 years												
141–143	54	37.1	7.8	28.9	29.8	31.1	32.2	34.9	38.6	42.4	45.7	59.5
144–146	67	38.5	6.8	30.4	30.8	31.6	32.9	38.4	41.4	44.1	46.5	52.4
147–149	127	43.4	10.0	32.7	34.3	35.4	37.0	40.7	46.7	51.3	56.4	61.2
150–152	180	45.8	9.1	34.7	36.3	37.4	39.5	44.1	49.9	54.3	56.1	61.9
153–155	235	48.8	8.9	38.0	39.5	40.6	43.1	46.7	53.6	56.5	60.0	66.3
156–158	352	52.3	10.4	39.7	41.7	43.1	45.1	49.9	57.5	62.5	66.0	72.3
159–161	372	55.1	11.0	42.2	44.3	46.0	48.3	52.8	59.2	62.9	68.4	77.6
162–164	344	56.6	9.9	44.9	46.6	47.5	50.2	54.4	60.6	65.3	68.6	73.8
165–167	243	60.0	12.5	46.3	48.8	50.1	52.8	57.6	62.7	69.4	74.7	84.7
168–170	124	61.2	10.8	48.9	49.2	51.1	53.5	59.0	65.7	73.4	75.1	82.4
171–173	74	67.5	15.0	53.0	54.3	54.9	57.7	62.1	72.3	80.1	89.1	104.2
Females: 18 to 74 years												
141–143	64	55.9	10.2	39.2	41.3	43.9	49.0	56.5	63.3	64.9	67.7	76.6
144–146	178	57.1	14.2	38.7	42.0	44.3	48.1	54.3	64.4	71.3	74.6	82.0
147–149	430	59.4	13.2	41.5	44.6	46.8	50.1	56.9	66.9	71.9	76.1	84.8
150–152	928	61.1	13.2	43.1	46.5	48.1	51.5	59.0	68.3	74.3	78.4	86.2
153–155	1,685	63.0	13.7	45.3	47.5	49.8	53.2	60.7	70.2	77.3	81.6	88.6
156–158	2,670	63.8	14.6	46.6	49.1	50.8	53.5	60.7	70.9	77.1	82.3	90.0
159–161	3,041	65.3	14.5	47.7	50.2	52.0	55.2	62.3	72.6	79.4	84.6	92.9
162–164	2,849	66.9	14.6	49.4	51.5	53.4	56.6	63.5	74.2	81.4	86.0	94.9
165–167	2,327	68.2	15.3	50.3	52.8	54.9	57.8	64.5	74.7	82.4	88.6	98.2
168–170	1,327	69.5	15.1	52.5	54.7	56.5	59.2	65.4	76.1	83.5	90.1	99.4
171–173	685	71.8	15.8	54.1	55.9	57.9	60.5	67.6	78.9	86.1	93.9	105.0
174–176	334	72.9	17.3	56.1	57.9	59.6	62.3	68.4	77.6	85.7	93.1	106.9
177–179	97	75.3	16.5	57.6	59.9	60.7	64.4	71.2	81.8	89.6	102.1	112.8

From Frisancho AR. Anthropometric standards for the assessment of growth and nutritional status. Ann Arbor: University of Michigan Press, 1990, Table IV, 4. With permission.

A-15-e. Selected Anthropometric and Impedance Measures by Age and Sex, Ages 12 to 79.9 Years–NHANES III, 2000

TABLE 15-e-1. SELECTED ANTHROPOMETRIC AND IMPEDANCE MEASURES ACCORDING TO AGE AND SEX FOR NON-HISPANIC WHITES: NHANES III

AGE (ys)	ANTHROPOMETRIC MEASURE	NON-HISPANIC WHITE MALES				NON-HISPANIC WHITE FEMALES			
		N	MEAN	STANDARD DEVIATION	STANDARD ERROR	N	MEAN	STANDARD DEVIATION	STANDARD ERROR
12–13.9	Weight (kg)	88	51.7	12.3	1.5	101	52.1	13.3	1.6
	Stature (cm)		159.6	8.4	0.9		157.8	8.2	1.0
	BMI (kg/m^2)		20.1	3.5	0.4		20.9	4.7	0.6
	TBW (l)		31.3	6.3	0.8		28.5	4.2	0.6
	FFM (kg)		41.8	8.2	1.0		38.1	5.6	0.7
	TBF (kg)		10.0	6.0	0.7		14.0	8.7	1.0
14–15.9	Weight (kg)	82	68.3	20.5	2.5	120	57.8	10.5	1.2
	Stature (cm)		172.2	7.6	0.8		162.6	6.0	0.7
	BMI (kg/m^2)		23.0	6.3	0.8		21.9	3.8	0.4
	TBW (l)		40.6	7.0	0.9		29.9	3.7	0.5
	FFM (kg)		54.3	9.6	1.2		40.4	4.8	0.6
	TBF (kg)		14.0	12.2	1.6		17.4	6.9	0.8
16–17.9	Weight (kg)	96	70.9	13.8	1.6	104	61.1	14.5	1.7
	Stature (cm)		177.0	7.9	0.8		164.5	6.6	0.8
	BMI (kg/m^2)		22.6	4.0	0.5		22.5	4.9	0.6
	TBW (l)		43.1	6.2	0.8		30.7	4.0	0.5
	FFM (kg)		57.8	8.4	1.0		41.6	5.5	0.7
	TBF (kg)		13.1	7.5	0.9		19.5	10.1	1.2
18–19.9	Weight (kg)	76	73.1	15.0	1.9	90	63.7	15.0	1.9
	Stature (cm)		176.9	6.7	0.8		164.9	5.8	0.7
	BMI (kg/m^2)		23.3	4.2	0.6		23.4	5.5	0.7
	TBW (l)		43.2	5.8	0.8		31.9	4.2	0.6
	FFM (kg)		58.0	8.0	1.1		43.1	5.6	0.8
	TBF (kg)		15.1	8.5	1.1		20.6	10.3	1.3
20–29.9	Weight (kg)	384	79.2	16.6	0.9	426	63.2	14.3	0.8
	Stature (cm)		177.5	6.7	0.3		163.6	6.7	0.4
	BMI (kg/m^2)		25.1	4.9	0.3		23.6	5.1	0.3
	TBW (l)		45.5	6.9	0.4		31.8	4.5	0.3
	FFM (kg)		61.3	9.5	0.6		42.8	5.9	0.4
	TBF (kg)		17.9	8.7	0.5		20.5	9.6	0.6
30–39.9	Weight (kg)	436	84.0	17.1	0.9	543	69.1	18.0	0.9
	Stature (cm)		177.8	6.8	0.3		164.6	6.3	0.3
	BMI (kg/m^2)		26.5	4.6	0.3		25.5	6.5	0.3
	TBW (l)		47.2	7.6	0.4		33.5	5.1	0.3
	FFM (kg)		63.6	10.5	0.6		45.0	6.9	0.4
	TBF (kg)		20.4	8.5	0.5		24.1	12.3	0.6
40–49.9	Weight (kg)	410	86.0	17.0	0.9	454	70.7	16.8	1.0
	Stature (cm)		177.3	6.7	0.3		163.4	6.1	0.3
	BMI (kg/m^2)		27.3	4.9	0.3		26.6	6.5	0.4
	TBW (l)		48.0	7.8	0.5		33.3	5.2	0.3
	FFM (kg)		64.6	10.6	0.6		44.8	6.9	0.4
	TBF (kg)		21.3	8.5	0.5		25.9	10.9	0.6
50–59.9	Weight (kg)	396	86.9	15.0	0.8	454	73.9	17.4	1.0
	Stature (cm)		176.7	6.2	0.3		162.4	6.0	0.3
	BMI (kg/m^2)		27.8	4.6	0.3		28.0	6.4	0.4
	TBW (l)		47.9	6.5	0.4		33.8	5.1	0.3
	FFM (kg)		64.6	8.8	0.5		45.4	6.7	0.4
	TBF (kg)		22.3	8.3	0.5		28.6	11.6	0.7
60–69.9	Weight (kg)	465	84.9	14.7	0.8	447	70.3	15.1	0.9
	Stature (cm)		175.3	6.3	0.3		160.8	6.1	0.4
	BMI (kg/m^2)		27.6	4.2	0.2		27.2	5.6	0.3
	TBW (l)		46.2	6.6	0.4		32.5	4.8	0.3
	FFM (kg)		62.3	8.9	0.5		43.6	6.3	0.4
	TBF (kg)		22.7	7.7	0.4		26.7	9.9	0.6
70–79.9	Weight (kg)	447	79.3	13.3	0.7	538	67.1	14.5	0.8
	Stature (cm)		172.4	6.7	0.3		158.3	6.8	0.4

TABLE 15-e-1. SELECTED ANTHROPOMETRIC AND IMPEDANCE MEASURES ACCORDING TO AGE AND SEX FOR NON-HISPANIC WHITES: NHANES III (continued)

AGE (ys)	ANTHROPOMETRIC MEASURE	NON-HISPANIC WHITE MALES				NON-HISPANIC WHITE FEMALES			
		N	MEAN	STANDARD DEVIATION	STANDARD ERROR	N	MEAN	STANDARD DEVIATION	STANDARD ERROR
	BMI (kg/m²)		26.7	4.0	0.2		26.7	5.3	0.3
	TBW (l)		44.0	6.4	0.4		31.6	4.9	0.3
	FFW (kg)		59.1	8.6	0.5		42.3	6.5	0.4
	TBF (kg)		20.3	6.8	0.4		24.8	9.3	0.5

Adapted from Chumlea WC, Guo SS, Kuczmarski RJ et al. Body composition estimates from NHANES III bioelectrical impedance data. Int J Obes Relat Metab Disord 2002;26:1596–609. Provided by Drs Heymsfield and Baumgastner and refered to in their Chapter 49.

TABLE 15-e-2. SELECTED ANTHROPOMETRIC AND IMPEDANCE MEASURES ACCORDING TO AGE AND SEX FOR NON-HISPANIC BLACKS: NHANES III.

AGE (ys)	ANTHROPOMETRIC MEASURE	NON-HISPANIC BLACK MALES				NON-HISPANIC BLACK FEMALES			
		N	MEAN	STANDARD DEVIATION	STANDARD ERROR	N	MEAN	STANDARD DEVIATION	STANDARD ERROR
12–13.9	Weight (kg)	124	52.1	16.7	1.5	156	55.1	13.3	1.2
	Stature (cm)		157.9	10.1	1.0		159.6	7.3	0.7
	BMI (kg/m²)		20.7	5.2	0.5		21.5	4.4	0.4
	TBW (l)		30.7	7.0	0.7		29.3	4.1	0.4
	FFM (kg)		40.9	9.3	0.9		39.3	5.5	0.5
	TBF (kg)		11.2	9.1	0.9		15.8	8.7	0.8
14–15.9	Weight (kg)	131	64.4	15.4	1.4	102	62.0	16.3	1.8
	Stature (cm)		171.5	7.7	0.8		163.1	7.1	0.8
	BMI (kg/m²)		21.8	4.7	0.4		23.2	5.3	0.6
	TBW (l)		38.9	6.7	0.7		30.9	5.3	0.7
	FFM (kg)		52.2	9.0	0.9		41.8	7.0	0.9
	TBF (kg)		12.2	8.4	0.9		20.2	10.1	1.1
16–17.9	Weight (kg)	126	68.7	14.5	1.3	126	64.0	15.8	1.6
	Stature (cm)		173.8	7.2	0.7		163.9	7.0	0.7
	BMI (kg/m²)		22.7	4.1	0.4		23.8	5.7	0.6
	TBW (l)		41.2	6.6	0.7		31.0	4.2	0.5
	FFM (kg)		55.3	8.9	0.9		42.0	5.6	0.6
	TBF (kg)		13.4	7.3	0.8		22.0	11.4	1.1
18–19.9	Weight (kg)	118	74.7	16.4	1.5	110	65.8	18.6	2.0
	Stature (cm)		176.6	7.2	0.7		163.6	6.3	0.7
	BMI (kg/m²)		23.8	4.4	0.4		24.6	6.7	0.8
	TBW (l)		44.1	7.5	0.8		31.4	5.5	0.7
	FFM (kg)		59.2	10.2	1.0		42.6	7.1	0.8
	TBF (kg)		15.5	7.9	0.8		23.2	12.6	1.3
20–29.9	Weight (kg)	462	82.9	20.5	1.0	510	70.4	16.7	0.8
	Stature (cm)		177.1	7.4	0.4		163.7	6.1	0.3
	BMI (kg/m²)		26.3	5.8	0.3		26.2	6.0	0.3
	TBW (l)		46.1	8.0	0.4		32.8	4.9	0.3
	FFM (kg)		62.2	11.1	0.6		44.3	6.5	0.4
	TBF (kg)		20.7	11.4	0.6		26.0	11.3	0.6
30–39.9	Weight (kg)	454	82.9	17.9	0.9	569	76.7	20.2	1.0
	Stature (cm)		177.2	6.6	0.3		163.7	6.7	0.3
	BMI (kg/m²)		26.4	5.4	0.3		28.6	7.4	0.4
	TBW (l)		46.5	7.7	0.4		34.4	5.8	0.3
	FFM (kg)		62.6	10.5	0.5		46.4	7.8	0.4
	TBF (kg)		20.3	9.5	0.5		30.4	13.5	0.6
40–49.9	Weight (kg)	339	83.6	17.2	1.0	395	81.5	21.1	1.2
	Stature (cm)		176.5	7.3	0.4		164.2	6.1	0.4
	BMI (kg/m²)		26.8	4.8	0.3		30.2	7.4	0.4
	TBW (l)		46.1	7.5	0.5		35.8	6.0	0.4
	FFM (kg)		62.2	10.3	0.6		48.2	7.9	0.5
	TBF (kg)		21.4	8.7	0.6		33.3	14.1	0.8

(continued)

TABLE 15-E-2. SELECTED ANTHROPOMETRIC AND IMPEDANCE MEASURES ACCORDING TO AGE AND SEX FOR NON-HISPANIC BLACKS: NHANES III (continued)

AGE (ys)	ANTHROPOMETRIC MEASURE	NON-HISPANIC BLACK MALES				NON-HISPANIC BLACK FEMALES			
		N	MEAN	STANDARD DEVIATION	STANDARD ERROR	N	MEAN	STANDARD DEVIATION	STANDARD ERROR
50–59.9	Weight (kg)	191	83.7	19.4	1.4	231	80.7	19.4	1.5
	Stature (cm)		175.2	6.6	0.5		162.5	5.8	0.5
	BMI (kg/m^2)		27.2	5.7	0.4		30.6	7.1	0.6
	TBW (l)		45.9	8.5	0.7		35.2	5.8	0.5
	FFM (kg)		61.9	11.5	0.9		47.3	7.6	0.6
	TBF (kg)		21.8	9.7	0.8		33.4	12.9	1.0
			25.1	6.7	0.7		40.0	7.5	0.6
60–69.9	Weight (kg)	258	80.9	16.2	1.0	258	77.6	18.3	1.3
	Stature (cm)		173.6	6.6	0.5		161.1	6.3	0.5
	BMI (kg/m^2)		26.8	4.9	0.3		29.9	7.0	0.5
	TBW (l)		44.7	7.7	0.5		34.0	5.6	0.4
	FFM (kg)		60.1	10.3	0.7		45.7	7.3	0.6
	TBF (kg)		20.7	7.7	0.7		31.9	12.1	0.8
70–79.9	Weight (kg)	145	77.0	15.5	1.3	149	74.0	16.5	1.5
	Stature (cm)		171.6	7.1	0.7		159.4	5.7	0.6
	BMI (kg/m^2)		26.2	4.8	0.4		29.1	6.3	0.6
	TBW (l)		43.2	7.4	0.7		33.4	5.3	0.6
	FFM (kg)		58.0	10.0	0.9		44.7	6.8	0.7
	TBF (kg)		19.3	7.7	0.7		29.3	10.8	1.0

Adapted from Chumlea WC, Guo SS, Kuczmarski RJ et al. Body composition estimates from NHANES III bioelectrical impedance data. Int J Obes Relat Metab Disord 2002;26:1596–609.

Provided by Drs. Heymsfield and Baumgastner and refered to in their Chapter 49.

TABLE 15-e-3. SELECTED ANTHROPOMETRIC AND IMPEDANCE MEASURES ACCORDING TO AGE AND SEX FOR MEXICAN-AMERICANS: NHANES III

AGE (ys)	ANTHROPOMETRIC MEASURE	MEXICAN-AMERICAN MALES				MEXICAN-AMERICAN FEMALES			
		N	MEAN	STANDARD DEVIATION	STANDARD ERROR	N	MEAN	STANDARD DEVIATION	STANDARD ERROR
12–13.9	Weight (kg)	132	52.7	14.1	1.5	139	53.3	12.3	1.2
	Stature (cm)		156.0	9.2	0.9		155.4	6.5	0.7
	BMI (kg/m^2)		21.4	4.6	0.5		21.9	4.5	0.5
	TBW (l)		30.2	6.2	0.7		27.9	4.2	0.5
	FFM (kg)		40.3	8.2	0.9		37.3	5.3	0.6
	TBF (kg)		12.3	7.5	0.8		16.0	7.6	0.8
14–15.9	Weight (kg)	108	62.5	16.6	1.9	113	56.2	10.7	1.2
	Stature (cm)		167.2	8.5	0.9		157.7	6.0	0.7
	BMI (kg/m^2)		22.2	5.1	0.6		22.5	3.7	0.4
	TBW (l)		37.2	6.9	0.9		28.1	3.7	0.4
	FFM (kg)		49.8	9.3	1.2		37.8	4.8	0.6
	TBF (kg)		12.6	8.9	1.1		18.4	6.9	0.8
16–17.9	Weight (kg)	126	67.9	12.2	1.3	112	62.2	15.5	1.7
	Stature (cm)		170.5	6.7	0.7		159.3	5.8	0.7
	BMI (kg/m^2)		23.3	3.7	0.4		24.5	5.7	0.7
	TBW (l)		39.6	5.5	0.6		30.2	4.5	0.6
	FFM (kg)		53.0	7.5	0.9		40.5	6.0	0.7
	TBF (kg)		14.9	6.1	0.7		21.6	10.3	1.2
18–19.9	Weight (kg)	109	72.8	13.9	1.6	90	59.6	13.1	1.6
	Stature (cm)		171.9	6.3	0.7		157.7	5.7	0.7
	BMI (kg/m^2)		24.6	4.4	0.5		23.9	4.9	0.6
	TBW (l)		41.5	5.9	0.7		28.9	3.7	0.5
	FFM (kg)		55.7	8.0	1.0		38.8	4.9	0.7
	TBF (kg)		17.1	7.2	0.9		20.7	8.9	1.1
20–29.9	Weight (kg)	631	73.9	13.9	0.7	509	64.8	14.5	0.8
	Stature (cm)		170.0	6.4	0.3		157.6	6.2	0.3
	BMI (kg/m^2)		25.6	4.2	0.2		26.1	5.5	0.3
	TBW (l)		41.6	6.1	0.3		30.5	4.3	0.2

TABLE 15-e-3. SELECTED ANTHROPOMETRIC AND IMPEDANCE MEASURES ACCORDING TO AGE AND SEX FOR MEXICAN-AMERICANS: NHANES III (continued)

AGE (ys)	ANTHROPOMETRIC MEASURE	MEXICAN-AMERICAN MALES				MEXICAN-AMERICAN FEMALES			
		N	MEAN	STANDARD DEVIATION	STANDARD ERROR	N	MEAN	STANDARD DEVIATION	STANDARD ERROR
	FFM (kg)		55.7	8.3	0.4		40.8	5.6	0.3
	TBF (kg)		18.3	7.3	0.4		24.1	9.8	0.5
30–39.9	Weight (kg)	443	78.4	14.2	0.8	451	70.6	17.1	1.0
	Stature (cm)		170.6	7.0	0.4		156.9	6.3	0.4
	BMI (kg/m²)		26.9	4.3	0.2		28.6	6.4	0.4
	TBW (l)		43.4	6.5	0.4		32.2	4.8	0.3
	FFM (kg)		58.1	8.9	0.5		42.8	6.4	0.4
	TBF (kg)		20.3	7.1	0.4		27.8	11.5	0.6
40–49.9	Weight (kg)	361	82.0	14.5	0.9	334	73.4	13.9	0.9
	Stature (cm)		169.7	6.3	0.4		157.2	5.4	0.4
	BMI (kg/m²)		28.4	4.4	0.3		29.7	5.6	0.4
	TBW (l)		44.7	6.6	0.5		32.6	4.3	0.3
	FFM (kg)		59.8	8.9	0.6		43.5	5.5	0.4
	TBF (kg)		22.2	7.3	0.5		29.9	9.4	0.6
50–59.9	Weight (kg)	165	82.6	15.1	1.4	171	71.3	13.7	1.2
	Stature (cm)		169.3	6.0	0.5		155.7	5.4	0.5
	BMI (kg/m²)		28.7	4.5	0.4		29.5	5.5	0.5
	TBW (l)		45.0	7.1	0.7		32.1	4.4	0.4
	FFM (kg)		60.2	9.6	1.0		42.6	5.8	0.6
	TBF (kg)		22.4	7.1	0.7		28.7	9.0	0.8
			26.7	5.3	0.6		39.4	5.7	0.5
60–69.9	Weight (kg)	301	78.2	12.7	0.9	278	70.0	14.1	1.0
	Stature (cm)		168.3	6.0	0.4		154.3	5.9	0.4
	BMI (kg/m²)		27.6	4.0	0.3		29.5	5.9	0.4
	TBW (l)		42.6	5.9	0.4		31.6	4.6	0.4
	FFM (kg)		57.0	7.9	0.6		41.9	6.0	0.5
	TBF (kg)		21.2	6.7	0.5		28.1	9.3	0.7
70–79.9	Weight (kg)	118	72.3	12.5	1.4	101	65.0	13.0	1.5
	Stature (cm)		165.5	5.7	0.6		153.0	5.9	0.7
	BMI (kg/m²)		26.3	4.0	0.4		27.8	5.5	0.7
	TBW (l)		39.9	6.3	0.7		30.1	4.4	0.6
	FFM (kg)		53.1	8.3	1.0		39.8	5.6	0.7
	TBF (kg)		19.2	5.8	0.7		25.2	8.8	1.0

Adapted from Chumlea WC, Guo SS, Kuczmarski RJ et al. Body composition estimates from NHANES III bioelectrical impedance data. Int J Obes Relat Metab Disord. 2002;26:1596–609

Provided by Drs. Heymsfield and Baumgastner and refered to in their Chapter 49.

A-16. ANTHROPOMETRIC DATA, 1990

Anthropometric data are multiple and changing. Included here is basic material derived from Dr. Frisancho's publication *Anthropometric Standards for the Assessment of Growth and Nutritional Status*, Ann Arbor: University of Michigan Press, 1990. The interested reader is referred to this comprehensive publication for numerous other tables, graphs, and detailed text.

Appendices Editors

A-16-a. Triceps Skinfold Thickness, by Percentiles

TABLE A-16-a-1. TRICEPS SKINFOLD THICKNESS (mm) IN PERCENTILES BY AGE (years) FOR WHITE MALES AND FEMALES, 1 TO 74 YEARS

AGE (ys)	N	MEAN	SD	PERCENTILES									
				5	10	15	25	50	75	85	90	95
Males												
1.0–1.9	508	10.5	2.8	6.5	7.0	7.5	8.5	10.0	12.0	13.5	14.0	15.5
2.0–2.9	513	10.1	2.8	6.0	7.0	7.0	8.0	10.0	12.0	13.0	14.0	15.0
3.0–3.9	541	10.1	2.7	6.5	7.0	7.5	8.0	10.0	12.0	13.0	14.0	15.0
4.0–4.9	547	9.6	2.7	6.0	7.0	7.0	8.0	9.0	11.0	12.0	13.0	14.5
5.0–5.9	535	9.3	3.0	5.5	6.5	6.5	7.0	8.5	10.5	12.0	13.0	14.5
6.0–6.9	231	9.3	3.6	5.0	6.0	6.0	6.5	8.5	10.5	12.0	13.0	16.0
7.0–7.9	240	9.6	4.0	5.0	6.0	6.0	7.0	9.0	11.0	13.0	15.0	17.5
8.0–8.9	240	9.9	4.3	5.0	6.0	6.0	7.0	9.0	11.5	13.0	16.0	18.5
9.0–9.9	242	11.1	5.3	5.5	6.0	6.5	7.0	10.0	13.0	16.5	17.0	21.0
10.0–10.9	269	12.0	5.7	5.5	6.0	7.0	8.0	10.5	14.5	18.0	20.0	24.0
11.0–11.9	248	13.2	7.1	5.5	6.0	7.0	8.0	11.5	16.0	20.0	24.0	30.0
12.0–12.9	272	12.8	6.7	5.5	6.0	7.0	8.0	11.0	14.5	20.0	23.0	28.5
13.0–13.9	268	11.9	7.0	5.0	5.5	6.5	7.0	10.0	14.0	18.5	22.0	26.0
14.0–14.9	286	11.1	6.9	4.5	5.0	6.0	6.6	9.0	14.0	16.0	20.0	24.0
15.0–15.9	286	10.0	6.5	5.0	5.0	5.0	6.0	7.5	11.5	15.0	18.0	22.0
16.0–16.9	279	10.4	6.1	4.0	5.0	5.5	6.5	8.5	12.5	15.5	18.5	24.0
17.0–17.9	266	9.3	5.2	4.5	5.0	5.5	6.0	7.5	11.5	14.0	16.0	19.0
18.0–24.9	1,463	11.6	6.3	4.5	5.0	6.0	7.0	10.0	15.0	18.0	20.0	24.0
25.0–29.9	1,070	12.5	6.5	5.0	5.5	6.0	7.5	11.0	16.0	19.0	21.0	25.0
30.0–34.9	794	13.4	6.5	5.0	6.0	7.0	8.5	12.0	16.5	20.0	22.0	25.5
35.0–39.9	732	13.1	6.0	5.0	6.0	7.0	8.5	12.0	16.0	19.0	21.0	24.5
40.0–44.9	722	13.2	6.4	5.0	6.0	7.0	8.5	12.0	16.0	19.0	22.0	26.0
45.0–49.9	745	13.1	6.2	5.5	6.5	7.0	9.0	12.0	16.0	19.0	21.0	24.5
50.0–54.9	764	12.8	6.0	5.5	6.5	7.5	8.5	12.0	15.5	19.0	20.5	25.0
55.0–59.9	694	12.6	5.7	5.0	6.0	7.0	8.5	11.5	15.0	18.0	20.5	24.0
60.0–64.9	1,120	12.6	5.9	5.0	6.5	7.0	8.5	11.5	15.5	18.0	20.0	23.5
65.0–69.9	1,489	12.4	5.8	5.0	6.0	6.5	8.0	11.5	15.0	18.0	20.0	23.0
70.0–74.9	1,051	12.4	5.7	5.0	6.0	7.0	8.0	11.5	15.0	18.0	20.0	23.0
Females												
1.0–1.9	470	10.5	3.1	6.0	7.0	7.5	8.0	10.0	12.0	13.5	15.0	16.5
2.0–2.9	482	10.7	2.9	6.5	7.0	8.0	9.0	10.5	12.5	14.0	15.0	16.0
3.0–3.9	509	10.6	2.8	6.5	7.0	8.0	8.5	10.5	12.0	13.0	14.0	16.0
4.0–4.9	522	10.5	2.9	6.0	7.0	7.5	8.5	10.0	12.0	13.0	14.0	15.5
5.0–5.9	504	10.6	3.3	6.0	7.0	8.0	8.5	10.0	12.0	14.0	15.0	16.5
6.0–6.9	218	10.8	3.6	6.0	7.0	7.5	8.0	10.5	12.0	13.5	15.0	17.0
7.0–7.9	244	11.4	4.0	6.0	7.0	8.0	9.0	11.0	13.0	15.0	17.0	19.0
8.0–8.9	221	12.5	5.5	6.5	7.0	8.0	9.0	11.5	15.0	17.0	18.0	22.5
9.0–9.9	248	14.1	5.8	7.0	8.0	8.5	10.0	13.0	16.5	19.5	22.0	25.5
10.0–10.9	266	14.2	5.9	7.0	8.0	8.0	10.0	13.0	17.5	20.0	22.5	27.0
11.0–11.9	229	15.4	6.6	7.0	8.5	9.0	11.0	13.0	18.5	21.5	24.5	29.0
12.0–12.9	247	15.2	5.9	8.0	9.0	9.5	11.0	14.0	18.0	20.5	23.0	27.0
13.0–13.9	275	16.4	7.2	7.0	8.0	9.5	11.0	15.0	20.0	24.0	25.0	30.0
14.0–14.9	287	17.5	7.1	9.0	10.0	10.5	12.0	17.0	21.0	23.5	27.0	31.0
15.0–15.9	234	17.6	6.8	8.5	10.0	11.0	12.5	17.0	20.5	23.0	26.0	32.0
16.0–16.9	284	19.4	6.9	10.5	12.0	13.0	14.5	18.0	22.5	26.0	29.0	32.5
17.0–17.9	223	20.0	8.1	10.0	11.5	12.0	14.0	19.0	24.0	26.5	30.0	35.0
18.0–24.9	2,058	20.2	8.1	10.0	11.0	12.0	14.5	19.0	24.5	28.0	31.0	35.5
25.0–29.9	1,608	21.5	8.5	10.0	12.0	13.0	15.0	20.0	26.0	30.5	33.5	38.0
30.0–34.9	1,362	23.5	8.8	11.0	13.0	15.0	17.0	22.5	29.0	32.5	35.0	40.0
35.0–39.9	1,194	24.3	9.0	12.0	13.5	15.5	18.0	23.0	30.0	34.0	36.0	40.5
40.0–44.9	1,136	24.7	8.7	12.0	14.0	16.0	18.5	24.0	30.0	34.0	36.5	40.0
45.0–49.9	826	25.9	8.9	12.5	15.0	16.5	20.0	25.5	31.0	35.5	37.5	42.0
50.0–54.9	858	26.1	8.6	12.0	15.5	17.5	20.5	25.5	31.5	35.5	37.5	40.5
55.0–59.9	754	26.3	8.8	12.0	15.0	17.0	20.5	26.0	32.0	35.0	37.5	42.0
60.0–64.9	1,223	26.5	8.7	13.0	16.0	17.5	20.5	26.0	32.0	35.5	38.0	42.0
65.0–69.9	1,644	25.0	8.3	12.0	15.0	16.0	19.0	24.5	30.0	33.0	35.5	39.0
70.0–74.9	1,260	24.0	8.3	11.5	14.0	15.5	18.0	24.0	29.5	32.0	34.5	38.0

From Frisancho AR. Anthropometric standards for the assessment of growth and nutritional status. Ann Arbor: University of Michigan Press, 1990, Appendix B, Table 16. With permission.

TABLE A-16-a-2. MEANS, STANDARD DEVIATIONS, AND PERCENTILES OF TRICEPS SKINFOLD THICKNESS (mm) BY AGE (years) FOR BLACK MALES AND FEMALES, 1 TO 74 YEARS

AGE (ys)	N	MEAN	SD	PERCENTILES								
				5	10	15	25	50	75	85	90	95
Males												
1.0–1.9	157	10.2	3.0	6.0	7.0	7.0	8.0	10.0	12.0	12.5	13.5	15.0
2.0–2.9	142	9.6	3.1	5.0	6.0	6.5	7.0	10.0	11.0	13.0	14.0	15.0
3.0–3.9	151	9.0	2.6	6.0	6.0	6.5	7.0	9.0	10.5	12.0	12.0	13.5
4.0–4.9	150	8.2	2.4	5.0	5.5	6.0	7.0	7.5	9.5	11.0	11.0	12.0
5.0–5.9	122	7.5	3.0	4.5	5.0	5.0	5.5	7.0	8.5	10.0	11.0	13.0
6.0–6.9	60	7.4	4.1	4.0	4.0	5.0	5.0	6.5	8.0	9.5	10.0	13.0
7.0–7.9	67	7.1	3.6	4.0	4.0	5.0	5.0	6.0	8.0	9.0	11.0	13.0
8.0–8.9	49	7.8	3.9	4.0	4.0	5.0	6.0	7.0	8.0	10.0	11.5	15.0
9.0–9.9	74	7.6	3.5	3.5	4.0	5.0	6.0	6.5	9.0	10.5	12.0	17.0
10.0–10.9	60	9.5	5.5	5.0	5.0	5.5	6.0	7.5	11.0	13.0	16.5	20.0
11.0–11.9	71	9.8	6.0	4.0	5.0	5.0	6.0	8.0	11.0	15.0	18.0	25.0
12.0–12.9	71	10.0	6.9	4.0	4.0	4.5	6.0	8.0	11.0	17.0	18.0	24.0
13.0–13.9	74	8.0	4.2	3.0	4.0	5.0	5.0	6.5	9.0	11.5	14.0	19.0
14.0–14.9	68	7.6	3.9	3.5	4.0	4.5	5.0	7.0	8.5	10.0	12.5	17.0
15.0–15.9	64	9.3	6.9	4.5	5.0	5.0	6.0	6.7	9.0	12.0	18.0	28.0
16.0–16.9	66	8.0	5.1	4.0	4.0	4.5	5.5	6.5	9.0	11.0	12.0	17.0
17.0–17.9	62	7.8	5.1	4.0	4.0	4.5	5.0	6.5	8.5	10.0	12.0	20.0
18.0–24.9	253	9.6	7.0	3.0	4.0	4.5	5.0	7.0	12.0	15.0	18.5	23.5
25.0–29.9	160	10.3	7.7	3.5	4.0	4.3	5.0	8.0	12.0	17.0	21.0	24.0
30.0–34.9	120	11.8	7.4	3.5	4.0	5.0	6.0	11.0	15.5	18.5	20.0	23.5
35.0–39.9	83	11.7	7.7	4.0	4.5	5.0	7.0	10.0	15.0	17.0	19.0	24.0
40.0–44.9	89	11.7	7.1	4.0	5.0	6.0	6.0	10.0	14.2	17.0	20.5	25.5
45.0–49.9	112	11.8	7.5	3.0	4.5	5.5	6.0	10.0	15.0	18.0	21.0	30.0
50.0–54.9	105	11.2	6.4	3.5	4.0	5.0	6.0	10.0	15.0	16.0	19.0	25.5
55.0–59.9	104	11.2	7.2	3.0	4.0	5.0	5.5	10.0	14.0	19.0	22.0	28.0
60.0–64.9	126	11.8	7.0	4.0	5.0	5.5	7.0	10.0	16.0	20.0	22.0	24.5
65.0–69.9	254	10.7	6.8	4.0	4.5	5.0	6.0	9.0	13.0	15.0	19.0	25.0
70.0–74.9	186	9.8	5.3	4.0	4.5	5.0	6.0	9.0	12.0	15.0	16.0	19.0
Females												
1.0–1.9	134	10.2	2.9	6.0	6.0	7.0	8.0	10.0	12.0	13.0	14.0	15.0
2.0–2.9	119	9.8	2.7	6.0	6.5	7.0	8.0	10.0	11.0	12.0	13.0	16.0
3.0–3.9	127	9.4	3.2	5.5	6.0	7.0	7.0	9.0	11.0	12.0	13.0	15.0
4.0–4.9	147	9.4	3.2	5.0	6.0	6.5	7.0	9.0	11.0	12.0	13.5	16.0
5.0–5.9	163	9.6	4.0	5.0	5.5	6.5	7.0	8.5	11.5	13.0	15.0	18.0
6.0–6.9	72	9.1	3.9	4.5	5.5	6.0	7.0	8.0	10.0	12.0	12.0	18.5
7.0–7.9	81	10.0	4.4	5.0	6.0	6.5	7.5	9.0	12.0	13.0	15.0	18.0
8.0–8.9	54	10.4	4.5	5.0	6.0	7.0	7.0	9.0	12.0	15.0	17.5	19.0
9.0–9.9	71	11.1	5.7	5.5	6.0	6.5	7.0	10.0	13.0	17.0	20.0	21.0
10.0–10.9	61	13.0	7.0	5.5	6.5	7.5	8.0	10.0	17.5	19.5	22.0	24.5
11.0–11.9	67	13.6	7.7	5.0	6.5	7.5	8.0	11.5	17.5	22.0	23.0	30.0
12.0–12.9	71	14.7	7.6	6.0	7.0	7.0	9.0	12.5	19.0	25.0	26.0	31.0
13.0–13.9	82	16.3	8.1	6.0	8.0	8.5	10.5	15.5	20.5	24.0	25.0	34.0
14.0–14.9	79	15.5	7.7	6.5	8.0	9.0	10.5	13.5	19.0	24.0	27.0	32.0
15.0–15.9	73	16.1	8.8	6.0	8.0	9.0	10.0	14.0	20.0	23.0	27.5	40.0
16.0–16.9	54	18.9	7.5	8.0	11.0	11.5	12.0	18.5	24.0	26.0	31.0	33.0
17.0–17.9	66	15.9	6.9	7.0	9.0	9.0	12.0	14.0	20.0	24.0	27.0	28.0
18.0–24.9	473	19.3	8.9	8.0	9.0	10.5	12.5	17.0	25.0	30.0	32.0	36.0
25.0–29.9	275	22.8	10.2	8.5	10.5	12.0	15.0	22.0	29.0	32.2	35.0	40.5
30.0–34.9	236	25.0	11.0	8.0	10.0	13.0	16.0	24.0	32.0	35.5	40.0	45.0
35.0–39.9	235	26.6	10.7	10.0	12.0	15.0	18.0	26.0	33.5	37.0	40.8	46.0
40.0–44.9	231	26.8	10.0	11.0	14.0	15.5	20.0	27.0	35.0	37.0	40.5	42.0
45.0–49.9	125	27.1	11.7	10.0	12.0	14.0	19.0	26.0	34.0	40.0	42.0	50.0
50.0–54.9	135	29.5	10.9	10.0	13.5	16.5	22.0	30.5	37.5	41.0	42.5	46.0
55.0–59.9	119	28.7	12.0	8.5	13.0	15.0	20.0	28.0	37.5	41.0	43.0	50.0
60.0–64.9	152	27.7	10.1	12.0	15.0	17.0	21.0	27.0	34.5	39.5	40.5	46.0
65.0–69.9	282	25.6	9.6	10.0	13.0	15.5	18.5	25.5	31.0	35.0	38.0	44.0
70.0–74.9	196	24.3	9.3	10.0	13.0	15.0	17.0	24.0	30.0	33.0	37.0	40.5

From Frisancho AR. Anthropometric standards for the assessment of growth and nutritional status. Ann Arbor: University of Michigan Press, 1990, Appendix A, Table 16. With permission.

A-16-b. Subscapular Skinfold Thickness, by Percentiles

TABLE A-16-b-1. MEANS, STANDARD DEVIATIONS, AND PERCENTILES OF SUBSCAPULAR SKINFOLD THICKNESS (mm) BY AGE (years) FOR WHITE MALES AND FEMALES, 1 TO 74 YEARS

AGE (ys)	N	MEAN	SD	PERCENTILES								
				5	10	15	25	50	75	85	90	95
Males												
1.0–1.9	508	6.3	1.9	4.0	4.0	4.5	5.0	6.0	7.0	8.0	8.5	10.0
2.0–2.9	513	5.8	2.0	3.5	4.0	4.0	4.5	5.5	6.5	7.5	8.5	9.5
3.0–3.9	540	5.5	1.8	3.5	4.0	4.0	4.5	5.0	6.0	7.0	7.0	9.0
4.0–4.9	546	5.3	2.0	3.0	3.5	4.0	4.0	5.0	6.0	6.5	7.0	8.5
5.0–5.9	535	5.2	2.3	3.0	3.5	4.0	4.0	5.0	5.5	6.5	7.0	8.0
6.0–6.9	231	5.6	3.3	3.0	3.5	3.5	4.0	4.5	6.0	7.0	8.0	13.0
7.0–7.9	240	5.9	3.4	3.0	3.5	4.0	4.0	5.0	6.0	7.0	9.0	12.0
8.0–8.9	240	6.0	3.9	3.0	3.5	4.0	4.0	5.0	6.0	7.5	9.0	12.0
9.0–9.9	242	7.1	5.1	3.5	4.0	4.0	4.0	5.5	7.5	10.5	12.5	15.0
10.0–10.9	269	7.7	5.4	3.5	4.0	4.0	4.5	6.0	8.0	11.0	14.0	19.5
11.0–11.9	248	9.3	8.1	4.0	4.0	4.0	5.0	6.0	10.0	15.0	20.0	27.0
12.0–12.9	273	9.1	7.1	4.0	4.0	4.5	5.0	6.5	10.0	14.0	19.0	24.0
13.0–13.9	268	9.3	7.6	4.0	4.0	5.0	5.0	7.0	10.0	14.0	17.0	26.0
14.0–14.9	286	9.4	6.9	4.0	5.0	5.0	5.5	7.0	10.0	13.0	16.0	23.0
15.0–15.9	286	9.2	6.5	5.0	5.0	5.5	6.0	7.0	10.0	12.0	15.5	22.0
16.0–16.9	278	10.2	6.5	5.0	6.0	6.0	6.5	8.0	11.0	14.0	17.0	23.5
17.0–17.9	267	10.1	5.7	5.0	6.0	6.5	7.0	8.0	11.5	14.0	17.0	20.5
18.0–24.9	1,461	13.5	7.5	6.0	7.0	7.0	8.0	11.0	16.0	20.0	24.0	30.0
25.0–29.9	1,067	15.6	8.0	7.0	7.5	8.0	10.0	13.5	20.0	24.5	26.5	30.5
30.0–34.9	791	17.3	8.2	7.0	8.0	9.0	11.0	16.0	22.0	25.5	28.0	32.5
35.0–39.9	730	17.4	8.0	7.0	8.0	10.0	11.0	16.0	22.0	25.0	27.5	32.0
40.0–44.9	714	17.3	8.0	7.0	8.0	9.5	11.5	16.0	21.5	25.5	28.0	33.0
45.0–49.9	739	18.2	8.2	7.5	9.0	10.0	12.0	17.0	23.0	26.5	30.0	34.0
50.0–54.9	759	17.7	8.1	7.0	8.0	9.0	12.0	16.0	22.5	26.0	30.0	34.0
55.0–59.9	691	17.6	7.8	7.0	8.5	10.0	11.5	16.5	22.5	25.5	28.0	31.0
60.0–64.9	1,112	18.1	8.3	7.0	8.0	10.0	12.0	17.0	23.0	26.0	29.0	33.5
65.0–69.9	1,486	16.9	8.0	6.0	8.0	9.0	11.0	15.5	21.5	25.0	28.0	32.0
70.0–74.9	1,048	16.4	7.6	6.5	7.5	9.0	11.0	15.0	21.0	25.0	27.5	30.5
Females												
1.0–1.9	470	6.4	2.0	4.0	4.0	4.5	5.0	6.0	7.5	8.5	9.0	10.0
2.0–2.9	483	6.3	2.1	4.0	4.0	4.5	5.0	6.0	7.0	8.0	9.0	10.5
3.0–3.9	509	6.2	2.2	3.5	4.0	4.5	5.0	6.0	7.0	8.0	9.0	10.0
4.0–4.9	522	6.0	2.1	3.5	4.0	4.0	4.5	5.5	7.0	8.0	8.5	10.0
5.0–5.9	503	6.2	2.9	3.5	4.0	4.0	4.5	5.5	7.0	8.0	9.0	12.0
6.0–6.9	218	6.4	3.2	3.5	4.0	4.0	4.5	5.5	7.0	9.0	10.0	11.5
7.0–7.9	244	6.8	3.6	4.0	4.0	4.0	4.5	6.0	7.0	9.5	11.0	13.0
8.0–8.9	221	8.0	6.0	3.5	4.0	4.0	5.0	6.0	8.0	11.5	14.5	21.0
9.0–9.9	248	9.4	6.8	4.0	4.5	5.0	5.0	7.0	10.0	14.0	18.5	24.5
10.0–10.9	266	9.8	6.4	4.0	4.5	5.0	5.5	7.0	11.5	16.0	19.5	24.0
11.0–11.9	227	10.7	7.4	4.5	5.0	5.0	6.0	8.0	12.0	16.0	21.0	28.5
12.0–12.9	247	10.9	6.9	5.0	5.5	6.0	6.0	9.0	12.5	15.5	19.5	29.0
13.0–13.9	275	11.9	7.8	5.0	5.5	6.0	7.0	9.5	15.0	19.0	22.0	26.5
14.0–14.9	287	13.0	7.7	6.0	6.5	7.0	7.5	10.5	16.0	21.0	24.5	30.0
15.0–15.9	234	12.7	7.0	6.0	7.0	7.5	8.0	10.0	15.0	20.0	22.0	27.0
16.0–16.9	284	14.2	8.5	6.5	7.5	8.0	9.0	11.5	16.0	22.5	25.5	32.0
17.0–17.9	223	15.4	9.1	6.0	7.0	7.5	9.0	12.5	19.0	24.5	28.0	34.0
18.0–24.9	2,058	15.7	9.1	6.0	7.0	8.0	9.0	13.0	19.5	25.0	28.0	35.0
25.0–29.9	1,603	16.8	10.1	6.0	7.0	8.0	9.0	14.0	21.5	27.0	32.0	38.0
30.0–34.9	1,359	18.6	11.1	6.5	7.0	8.0	10.0	15.5	25.0	30.5	35.5	41.0
35.0–39.9	1,189	19.5	11.2	7.0	8.0	9.0	10.8	16.0	26.0	32.0	35.5	43.0
40.0–44.9	1,131	19.6	10.7	6.5	7.5	9.0	11.0	17.0	26.0	32.0	35.0	39.5
45.0–49.9	823	20.9	10.8	7.0	8.5	10.0	12.0	19.0	28.0	33.0	35.5	41.5
50.0–54.9	852	21.8	10.8	7.0	9.0	10.0	13.0	20.5	28.0	34.0	37.0	42.0
55.0–59.9	745	22.2	11.2	7.0	9.0	10.5	13.0	20.5	30.0	34.5	36.5	41.5
60.0–64.9	1,213	22.2	11.0	7.5	9.0	10.5	13.5	20.5	30.0	34.0	37.5	42.5
65.0–69.9	1,636	20.7	10.3	7.0	8.0	10.0	12.5	19.0	27.0	31.5	35.0	40.0
70.0–74.9	1,256	20.2	10.0	6.5	8.5	10.0	12.0	19.0	26.0	31.0	35.0	38.0

From Frisancho AR. Anthropometric standards for the assessment of growth and nutritional status. Ann Arbor: University of Michigan Press, 1990, Appendix B, Table 17. With permission.

TABLE A-16-b-2. MEANS, STANDARD DEVIATIONS, AND PERCENTILES OF SUBSCAPULAR SKINFOLD THICKNESS (mm) BY AGE (years) FOR BLACK MALES AND FEMALES, 1 TO 74 YEARS

AGE (ys)	N	MEAN	SD	PERCENTILES								
				5	10	15	25	50	75	85	90	95
Males												
1.0–1.9	157	6.6	2.0	4.0	4.0	4.5	5.0	6.0	8.0	8.5	9.0	10.5
2.0–2.9	142	6.1	2.1	4.0	4.0	4.5	5.0	6.0	7.0	8.0	9.0	10.0
3.0–3.9	151	5.4	1.7	3.5	4.0	4.0	4.5	5.0	6.0	6.5	7.0	8.5
4.0–4.9	151	5.0	1.4	3.0	3.5	4.0	4.0	5.0	5.5	6.0	6.5	7.5
5.0–5.9	122	5.0	2.2	3.0	3.0	3.5	4.0	4.5	5.0	6.0	7.0	8.0
6.0–6.9	60	5.1	3.5	3.0	3.0	3.0	4.0	4.0	5.0	5.5	6.5	11.0
7.0–7.9	67	5.2	3.0	3.0	3.5	3.5	4.0	4.5	5.0	6.0	7.0	10.0
8.0–8.9	49	5.7	3.0	3.5	3.5	4.0	4.0	5.0	6.0	7.5	9.0	11.0
9.0–9.9	74	5.6	3.6	3.0	3.5	3.7	4.0	5.0	6.0	7.0	8.0	11.0
10.0–10.9	60	7.3	5.7	4.0	4.0	4.0	4.5	5.0	7.0	8.0	12.0	19.0
11.0–11.9	71	7.6	5.9	4.0	4.0	4.5	5.0	5.5	7.0	10.5	14.5	21.0
12.0–12.9	71	8.3	7.3	4.0	4.0	4.0	4.5	5.5	7.0	16.0	18.0	22.0
13.0–13.9	74	6.9	3.8	3.0	4.5	5.0	5.0	6.0	8.0	8.5	9.5	17.0
14.0–14.9	68	7.4	4.6	4.0	4.5	5.0	5.0	6.0	8.0	8.0	11.0	16.0
15.0–15.9	65	10.4	8.4	5.0	5.0	6.0	6.5	8.0	10.0	14.5	17.0	24.0
16.0–16.9	66	9.6	4.7	5.5	6.5	7.0	7.0	8.0	10.0	13.0	14.5	17.5
17.0–17.9	63	9.5	4.9	5.0	6.0	6.0	6.5	8.0	10.5	12.0	14.0	16.0
18.0–24.9	253	12.7	7.9	6.0	6.5	7.0	8.0	10.0	15.0	18.5	22.5	29.0
25.0–29.9	159	14.5	9.4	6.5	7.0	7.5	8.0	11.0	17.0	24.0	28.0	38.0
30.0–34.9	120	17.4	9.9	6.0	8.0	9.0	10.0	15.0	22.0	25.0	30.0	36.0
35.0–39.9	88	19.0	10.1	7.0	8.0	10.0	11.0	17.0	24.0	26.5	33.0	35.5
40.0–44.9	87	17.2	9.4	6.5	7.5	8.5	10.0	15.0	22.0	25.0	30.0	35.0
45.0–49.9	111	17.9	10.7	5.0	6.5	7.0	9.0	16.0	25.0	29.0	31.5	35.0
50.0–54.9	103	17.4	10.1	6.0	7.0	7.5	9.0	15.0	25.0	28.0	30.0	36.0
55.0–59.9	103	17.7	10.0	5.0	6.5	7.0	9.5	15.0	24.0	27.0	30.5	35.0
60.0–64.9	126	18.0	9.6	6.0	7.5	8.0	10.5	16.0	24.0	27.0	30.5	39.5
65.0–69.9	253	16.3	9.6	5.0	6.0	7.0	9.0	14.0	21.0	25.5	30.0	37.5
70.0–74.9	185	15.8	9.2	6.0	6.0	7.0	8.0	13.5	21.0	26.0	30.5	35.0
Females												
1.0–1.9	134	6.6	1.9	4.0	5.0	5.0	5.0	6.5	8.0	8.5	9.0	10.0
2.0–2.9	119	6.4	2.9	4.0	4.0	4.5	5.0	6.0	7.0	8.5	9.5	12.0
3.0–3.9	127	5.7	2.2	3.0	4.0	4.0	4.5	5.0	6.5	7.0	7.5	9.0
4.0–4.9	147	6.0	2.7	3.5	4.0	4.0	4.5	5.0	7.0	8.0	9.0	11.0
5.0–5.9	163	6.0	3.1	3.5	4.0	4.0	4.0	5.0	6.5	8.0	10.0	12.0
6.0–6.9	72	6.1	4.1	3.0	4.0	4.0	4.0	5.0	6.5	7.0	7.5	12.0
7.0–7.9	81	6.4	2.9	3.5	4.0	4.0	5.0	5.5	7.0	8.0	10.0	12.0
8.0–8.9	54	7.1	4.7	4.0	4.0	4.0	4.5	5.0	7.0	11.5	14.0	16.0
9.0–9.9	71	7.9	5.5	4.0	4.0	4.5	5.0	6.0	8.0	10.0	13.5	24.0
10.0–10.9	61	9.5	6.8	4.0	4.5	5.0	5.5	6.5	11.0	16.0	17.0	23.6
11.0–11.9	67	10.8	8.4	5.0	5.0	5.0	6.0	8.0	12.0	15.0	20.0	30.5
12.0–12.9	71	13.4	10.1	5.0	5.5	5.5	6.5	9.0	16.0	26.5	30.0	36.0
13.0–13.9	82	13.5	7.6	5.5	6.5	7.0	8.0	12.0	16.5	20.0	25.0	28.4
14.0–14.9	79	13.1	8.1	6.0	6.0	6.0	7.5	10.0	17.0	19.5	27.0	33.5
15.0–15.9	72	13.8	9.1	6.0	7.0	7.5	8.0	10.0	16.5	20.0	26.5	35.0
16.0–16.9	54	17.1	10.0	7.0	8.0	9.0	10.5	14.0	20.0	27.0	33.0	40.5
17.0–17.9	66	14.9	7.9	6.5	7.0	8.0	9.0	12.0	20.0	24.0	27.0	30.0
18.0–24.9	472	17.9	10.2	6.5	7.5	8.0	10.0	15.0	24.0	29.0	32.0	38.0
25.0–29.9	272	21.6	11.3	7.0	8.5	10.0	12.0	20.5	28.0	34.5	37.0	41.5
30.0–34.9	235	25.2	13.1	7.0	9.0	11.0	14.5	25.0	34.5	40.0	43.0	49.0
35.0–39.9	233	26.1	11.9	7.0	9.5	12.0	16.5	27.5	34.0	38.0	40.6	45.0
40.0–44.9	227	27.2	12.3	8.0	11.0	13.0	18.0	27.5	35.0	40.0	44.0	48.0
45.0–49.9	122	27.8	12.9	9.5	11.0	12.5	17.0	28.0	37.0	41.0	44.0	50.0
50.0–54.9	131	30.7	12.5	10.0	13.5	16.0	22.0	30.5	38.0	43.1	47.8	52.5
55.0–59.9	118	28.8	13.1	7.0	9.0	13.0	21.0	28.0	37.0	44.0	47.5	54.5
60.0–64.9	149	28.0	12.0	8.5	12.0	14.0	20.0	28.0	35.5	39.0	44.0	50.0
65.0–69.9	277	25.1	11.5	7.5	9.5	11.0	16.0	25.0	32.0	37.0	40.4	45.5
70.0–74.9	197	22.9	10.5	7.5	9.9	11.0	14.0	22.0	31.0	35.0	37.0	40.0

From Frisancho AR. Anthropometric standards for the assessment of growth and nutritional status. Ann Arbor: University of Michigan Press, 1990, Appendix A, Table 17. With permission.

A-16-c. Upper Arm Circumference, by Percentiles

TABLE A-16-c-1. MEANS, STANDARD DEVIATIONS, AND PERCENTILES OF UPPER ARM CIRCUMFERENCE (cm) BY AGE (years) FOR WHITE MALES AND FEMALES, 1 TO 74 YEARS

AGE				PERCENTILES								
(y)	N	MEAN	SD	5	10	15	25	50	75	85	90	95
Males												
1.0–1.9	508	16.1	1.2	14.3	14.7	14.9	15.2	16.0	16.9	17.4	17.8	18.2
2.0–2.9	508	16.4	1.5	14.3	14.8	15.2	15.5	16.3	17.2	17.6	18.0	18.6
3.0–3.9	539	16.9	1.5	15.1	15.3	15.6	16.0	16.8	17.6	18.1	18.4	19.0
4.0–4.9	547	17.3	1.4	15.3	15.6	15.9	16.2	17.2	18.0	18.5	19.0	19.4
5.0–5.9	534	17.7	1.8	15.4	15.9	16.1	16.6	17.5	18.6	19.1	19.6	20.5
6.0–6.9	231	18.3	2.1	15.8	16.1	16.4	16.9	18.0	19.1	19.8	20.6	22.7
7.0–7.9	240	19.1	2.0	16.2	16.8	17.1	17.7	18.8	20.1	21.0	22.1	22.9
8.0–8.9	240	19.7	2.3	16.5	17.2	17.6	18.3	19.3	20.5	21.6	22.8	24.4
9.0–9.9	242	20.9	2.8	17.5	18.0	18.4	19.1	20.3	22.1	23.5	24.9	26.0
10.0–10.9	268	22.0	3.0	18.2	18.7	19.1	19.8	21.4	23.2	24.9	26.2	27.9
11.0–11.9	248	23.0	3.5	18.6	19.3	19.8	20.5	22.3	24.6	26.1	27.8	29.8
12.0–12.9	273	23.9	3.3	19.4	20.1	20.7	21.6	23.2	25.5	27.3	28.5	30.5
13.0–13.9	268	25.0	3.3	20.0	21.3	22.0	22.8	24.7	26.7	28.2	29.5	31.0
14.0–14.9	286	26.4	3.5	21.8	22.7	23.3	23.9	26.0	28.3	29.2	30.2	32.3
15.0–15.9	288	27.2	3.2	22.3	23.2	23.8	25.1	27.1	28.9	30.1	31.2	32.5
16.0–16.9	279	28.7	3.3	24.0	24.8	25.6	26.6	28.1	30.8	32.2	33.3	34.7
17.0–17.9	267	29.1	3.3	24.5	25.1	26.1	27.0	28.7	30.8	32.3	33.3	34.5
18.0–24.9	1,467	31.1	3.4	26.2	27.2	27.8	28.8	30.8	33.1	34.4	35.5	37.2
25.0–29.9	1,072	32.1	3.4	27.1	28.2	28.8	29.9	31.9	34.2	35.4	36.5	38.1
30.0–34.9	797	32.7	3.2	27.8	28.8	29.4	30.5	32.5	34.9	35.8	36.6	38.2
35.0–39.9	733	32.9	3.2	27.9	28.9	29.7	30.7	32.8	34.9	36.1	36.7	37.9
40.0–44.9	723	32.9	3.1	28.2	29.0	29.8	31.0	32.8	34.8	35.9	36.6	37.9
45.0–49.9	748	32.7	3.3	27.4	28.7	29.5	30.7	32.7	34.8	36.0	36.8	38.1
50.0–54.9	767	32.3	3.2	27.2	28.4	29.2	30.2	32.3	34.3	35.6	36.5	37.8
55.0–59.9	695	32.2	3.2	26.8	28.1	29.2	30.4	32.3	34.2	35.2	36.1	37.4
60.0–64.9	1,123	31.9	3.3	26.7	27.8	28.6	29.7	32.0	34.0	35.1	35.8	37.1
65.0–69.9	1,488	31.1	3.3	25.3	26.8	27.8	29.1	31.2	33.2	34.4	35.1	36.5
70.0–74.9	1,051	30.6	3.3	25.1	26.3	27.3	28.6	30.7	32.6	33.7	34.6	35.9
Females												
1.0–1.9	470	15.7	1.3	13.7	14.2	14.4	14.9	15.7	16.5	17.0	17.3	17.9
2.0–2.9	483	16.2	1.3	14.3	14.7	15.0	15.4	16.1	17.0	17.4	18.0	18.5
3.0–3.9	509	16.7	1.4	14.5	15.1	15.3	15.8	16.6	17.5	18.1	18.4	19.0
4.0–4.9	521	17.1	1.4	15.1	15.5	15.8	16.2	17.1	18.0	18.5	18.9	19.4
5.0–5.9	504	17.8	1.7	15.4	15.8	16.2	16.6	17.5	18.5	19.3	20.0	20.8
6.0–6.9	218	18.2	1.9	15.7	16.2	16.5	17.0	17.9	19.1	20.0	20.6	22.1
7.0–7.9	245	19.1	2.3	16.4	16.7	17.1	17.5	18.6	20.1	21.1	21.8	23.4
8.0–8.9	220	20.1	2.7	16.9	17.2	17.6	18.4	19.5	21.3	22.4	23.3	25.3
9.0–9.9	247	21.3	2.8	17.8	18.3	18.8	19.4	21.0	22.3	24.3	25.3	26.9
10.0–10.9	266	21.7	3.0	17.8	18.4	18.9	19.6	21.2	23.4	24.7	25.7	27.2
11.0–11.9	229	23.2	3.5	18.8	19.6	20.0	20.7	22.4	25.2	26.5	27.9	30.3
12.0–12.9	247	23.9	3.1	19.5	20.3	20.8	21.6	23.7	25.7	27.2	28.1	29.4
13.0–13.9	276	25.0	3.8	20.0	20.8	21.5	22.3	24.3	26.7	28.5	30.1	33.4
14.0–14.9	287	26.0	3.4	21.2	22.2	23.0	23.9	25.2	27.6	29.6	30.9	32.2
15.0–15.9	234	25.9	3.3	21.4	22.3	23.0	23.9	25.3	27.7	28.8	30.0	32.0
16.0–16.9	284	26.7	3.3	22.1	23.0	23.6	24.3	26.1	28.4	29.9	31.4	32.8
17.0–17.9	223	27.3	4.0	22.2	23.1	23.7	24.5	27.0	29.1	30.7	32.4	34.7
18.0–24.9	2,060	27.4	3.8	22.5	23.3	24.0	24.9	26.8	29.1	30.8	32.1	34.7
25.0–29.9	1,617	28.3	4.1	23.1	23.9	24.5	25.4	27.4	30.2	32.1	33.8	36.5
30.0–34.9	1,371	29.3	4.5	23.8	24.7	25.4	26.3	28.4	31.3	33.5	35.4	37.9
35.0–39.9	1,197	29.8	4.5	24.2	25.2	25.7	26.5	29.0	31.8	34.2	35.9	38.4
40.0–44.9	1,141	30.1	4.5	24.2	25.4	26.1	27.0	29.3	32.4	34.9	36.4	38.1
45.0–49.9	831	30.6	4.7	24.2	25.5	26.2	27.3	29.9	33.2	35.2	37.0	39.3
50.0–54.9	862	30.8	4.3	24.8	26.0	26.7	27.9	30.3	33.1	35.3	36.8	38.5
55.0–59.9	756	31.2	4.6	24.8	26.0	26.7	28.1	30.6	33.8	36.3	37.4	39.5
60.0–64.9	1,227	31.2	4.5	25.0	26.1	27.1	28.3	30.6	33.8	35.5	37.1	39.4
65.0–69.9	1,648	30.7	4.4	24.3	25.7	26.6	27.8	30.3	33.1	34.9	36.2	38.3
70.0–74.9	1,261	30.4	4.3	23.8	25.3	26.3	27.6	30.2	33.0	34.5	35.8	37.3

From Frisancho AR. Anthropometric standards for the assessment of growth and nutritional status. Ann Arbor: University of Michigan Press, 1990, Appendix B, Table 10. With permission.

TABLE A-16-c-2. MEANS, STANDARD DEVIATIONS, AND PERCENTILES OF UPPER ARM CIRCUMFERENCE (cm) BY AGE (years) FOR BLACK MALES AND FEMALES, 1 TO 74 YEARS

AGE (ys)	N	MEAN	SD	PERCENTILES 5	10	15	25	50	75	85	90	95
Males												
1.0–1.9	157	16.0	1.3	14.0	14.3	14.8	15.3	16.0	16.9	17.2	17.6	18.6
2.0–2.9	142	16.3	1.2	14.4	14.7	14.9	15.4	16.3	17.1	17.5	17.8	18.2
3.0–3.9	151	16.6	1.4	14.6	15.1	15.2	15.7	16.5	17.4	18.0	18.2	18.9
4.0–4.9	150	16.8	1.4	14.3	15.2	15.5	16.0	16.9	17.8	18.5	18.6	18.9
5.0–5.9	122	17.6	1.6	15.8	16.0	16.2	16.6	17.3	18.2	19.0	19.5	20.2
6.0–6.9	60	18.3	2.2	16.0	16.2	16.5	17.0	17.7	18.6	19.6	20.7	23.0
7.0–7.9	67	18.7	2.4	15.6	16.6	17.0	17.3	18.4	19.7	20.3	21.0	22.6
8.0–8.9	49	19.2	1.9	17.1	17.1	17.3	17.6	19.0	20.3	20.9	21.8	23.1
9.0–9.9	74	20.0	2.3	17.0	17.5	18.4	18.7	19.6	21.0	21.9	22.2	25.0
10.0–10.9	60	21.3	3.0	18.0	18.5	19.1	19.7	20.4	21.8	23.3	25.0	27.3
11.0–11.9	71	22.2	3.2	18.2	19.2	19.4	20.5	21.3	22.8	26.0	27.2	28.7
12.0–12.9	71	23.3	4.1	19.2	20.1	20.4	20.8	22.3	24.0	27.1	27.9	29.0
13.0–13.9	74	24.2	3.4	19.8	20.3	20.9	21.7	23.4	25.9	28.1	28.8	29.9
14.0–14.9	68	25.5	2.9	21.5	22.2	22.5	23.4	25.4	26.9	28.2	28.7	31.5
15.0–15.9	65	27.6	3.2	23.0	24.0	24.7	25.4	27.3	29.0	30.9	31.1	33.2
16.0–16.9	66	28.8	2.6	25.2	25.7	25.9	27.2	28.6	30.1	31.5	32.5	34.0
17.0–17.9	63	28.5	3.2	24.3	25.3	25.6	26.4	28.0	29.8	32.0	32.6	36.2
18.0–24.9	254	30.8	3.8	25.9	27.0	27.4	28.2	30.2	32.6	33.8	34.8	38.0
25.0–29.9	162	32.3	4.3	26.8	28.0	28.5	29.5	31.7	34.5	36.2	37.2	39.8
30.0–34.9	121	33.4	4.1	28.0	29.4	29.9	31.0	32.6	35.3	36.8	38.0	39.3
35.0–39.9	88	33.8	3.9	27.2	27.7	29.6	31.1	33.9	36.5	37.6	38.2	39.3
40.0–44.9	90	33.2	3.9	26.3	28.0	29.0	30.3	33.2	36.1	37.1	37.7	40.0
45.0–49.9	113	33.0	4.1	26.8	27.8	28.8	30.1	32.7	35.6	37.2	38.5	40.1
50.0–54.9	105	33.1	4.5	26.5	27.9	28.3	29.9	32.7	35.7	38.6	39.4	40.1
55.0–59.9	105	32.9	4.1	26.9	27.9	28.7	30.0	32.3	35.3	37.4	38.1	39.1
60.0–64.9	127	32.4	3.8	26.0	27.8	28.8	30.0	32.8	34.1	36.1	37.9	39.0
65.0–69.9	254	31.3	4.0	25.7	26.6	27.4	28.5	31.0	34.0	35.5	36.5	38.6
70.0–74.9	186	30.4	3.7	25.1	25.9	26.5	27.5	30.3	32.5	34.3	35.2	37.0
Females												
1.0–1.9	134	15.5	1.3	13.5	14.0	14.3	14.7	15.6	16.3	16.7	17.0	17.6
2.0–2.9	119	16.1	1.4	13.8	14.3	14.7	15.2	16.0	17.0	17.5	17.8	18.4
3.0–3.9	126	16.3	1.4	14.3	14.7	14.9	15.4	16.2	17.1	17.5	18.4	19.0
4.0–4.9	147	16.9	1.7	14.1	14.8	15.2	15.8	16.8	17.8	18.6	19.1	19.8
5.0–5.9	163	17.6	2.0	14.8	15.5	16.0	16.3	17.2	18.5	19.4	20.2	21.6
6.0–6.9	72	18.2	2.4	15.7	16.0	16.3	16.8	17.5	18.8	19.9	20.2	22.0
7.0–7.9	80	18.8	2.0	16.4	16.7	16.8	17.3	18.6	19.9	20.3	21.0	22.0
8.0–8.9	54	19.3	2.2	16.0	17.0	17.4	17.9	19.0	20.0	21.6	22.5	23.6
9.0–9.9	71	20.2	2.5	16.9	17.8	17.9	18.6	19.6	21.3	23.1	23.7	25.1
10.0–10.9	62	22.1	3.5	18.3	18.7	19.0	19.5	21.2	23.8	26.0	26.8	28.9
11.0–11.9	67	23.3	4.0	18.8	19.6	20.1	20.7	22.1	25.1	26.6	29.6	30.0
12.0–12.9	72	24.2	4.5	17.9	19.1	19.3	20.7	23.9	26.3	29.0	30.1	33.0
13.0–13.9	82	25.1	3.5	20.5	21.3	21.8	22.8	24.5	26.7	27.8	30.1	31.3
14.0–14.9	79	25.6	4.4	20.8	21.2	21.8	22.3	24.7	27.2	29.5	31.6	33.4
15.0–15.9	73	26.0	4.1	21.7	22.3	22.6	23.2	25.0	27.8	29.1	31.2	37.1
16.0–16.9	54	27.6	4.3	22.8	23.3	23.9	24.7	26.4	29.3	31.4	33.8	38.3
17.0–17.9	68	26.9	4.3	21.8	22.5	23.6	24.2	26.0	28.2	30.1	34.6	35.6
18.0–24.9	474	28.0	4.6	22.4	23.2	24.0	24.9	27.0	30.2	32.2	34.5	37.3
25.0–29.9	279	29.9	5.0	23.4	24.3	25.1	26.0	29.3	32.3	34.6	37.2	40.1
30.0–34.9	237	31.2	5.3	23.9	25.0	25.9	27.2	30.9	34.5	36.5	37.8	41.4
35.0–39.9	239	32.5	5.7	24.0	25.1	26.5	28.4	32.0	36.0	37.7	39.5	43.7
40.0–44.9	232	32.7	5.7	24.6	25.6	27.4	29.1	32.1	35.9	37.8	39.7	41.1
45.0–49.9	126	33.0	6.2	24.8	26.4	27.2	29.2	31.6	35.8	38.4	41.0	44.2
50.0–54.9	135	33.7	5.2	24.8	27.2	28.4	30.7	33.7	36.7	39.3	40.2	43.6
55.0–59.9	124	34.2	7.0	24.0	27.3	28.4	29.5	33.5	36.8	39.5	42.9	48.2
60.0–64.9	153	33.0	5.0	25.1	26.3	28.1	29.3	32.7	36.0	38.0	39.1	41.8
65.0–69.9	282	32.0	4.7	24.0	26.1	27.6	29.0	31.8	35.1	36.8	37.7	39.4
70.0–74.9	197	31.0	4.4	23.3	25.5	26.3	27.7	31.5	34.0	35.0	36.2	39.0

From Frisancho AR. Anthropometric standards for the assessment of growth and nutritional status. Ann Arbor: University of Michigan Press, 1990, Appendix A, Table 10. With permission.

A-16-d. Upper Arm Muscle Area, by Percentile

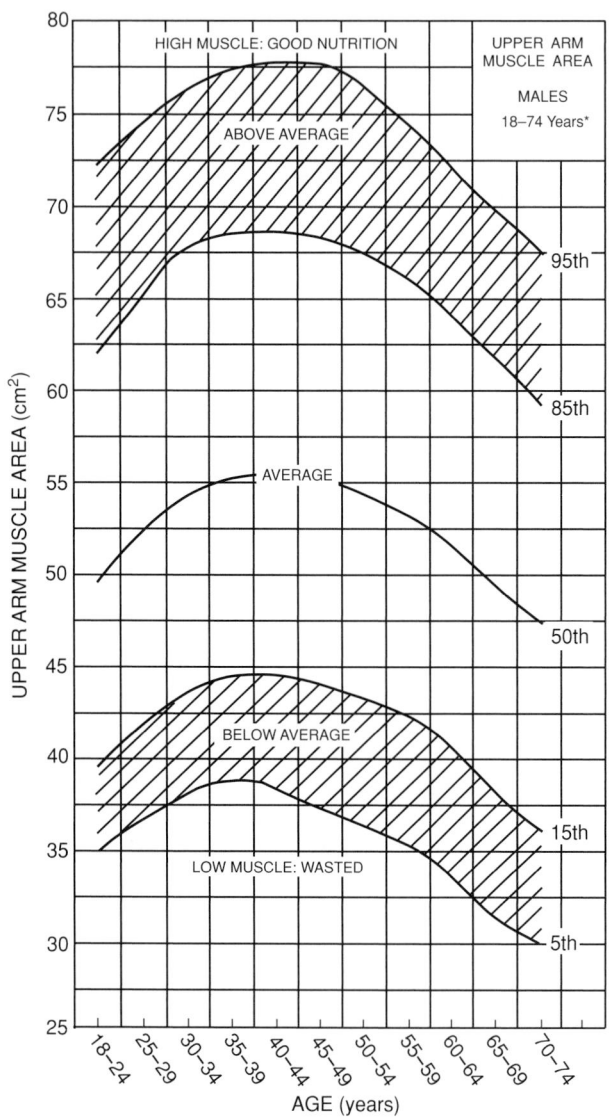

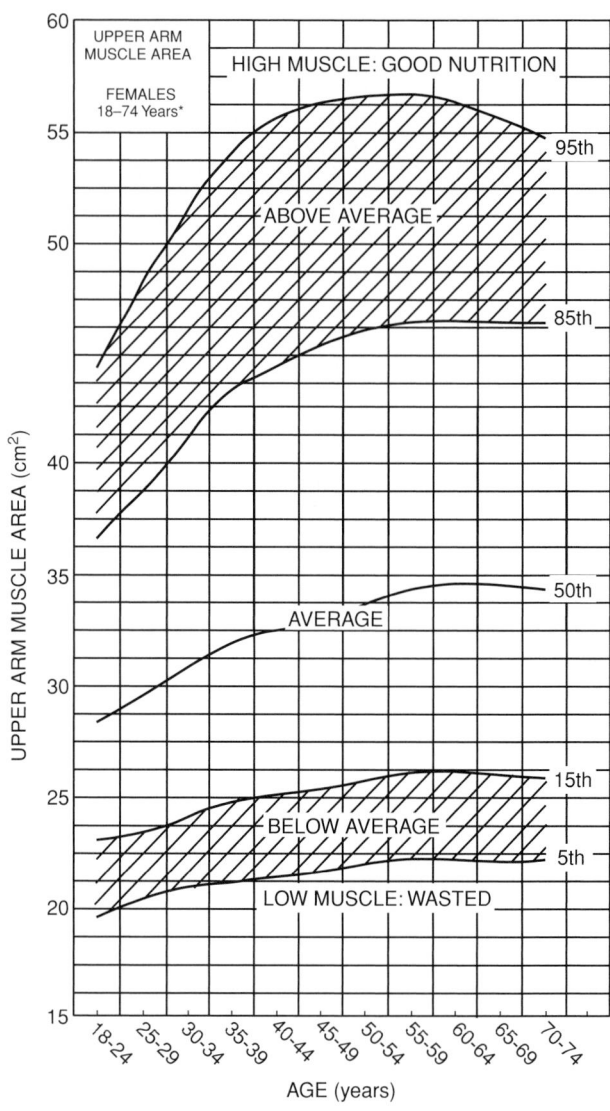

Figure A-16-d-1. Percentiles of Upper Arm Muscle Area (cm²) by Age for Males Ranging in Age from 18 to 74 Years.

Note: Values for males aged 18 years and older have been adjusted for bone area by subtracting 10.0 cm² from the calculated muscle area. From Frisancho AR. Anthropometric standards for the assessment of growth and nutritional status. Ann Arbor: University of Michigan Press, 1990. Figure IV.23.

Figure A-16-d-2. Percentiles of Upper Arm Muscle Area (cm²) by Age for Females Ranging in Age from 18 to 74 Years.

Note: Values for females aged 18 years and older have been adjusted for bone area by subtracting 6.5 cm² from the calculated muscle area. From Frisancho AR. Anthropometric standards for the assessment of growth and nutritional status. Ann Arbor: University of Michigan Press, 1990. Figure IV.26.

A-16-e. Summed Skinfolds (Triceps and Subscapular), by Percentile

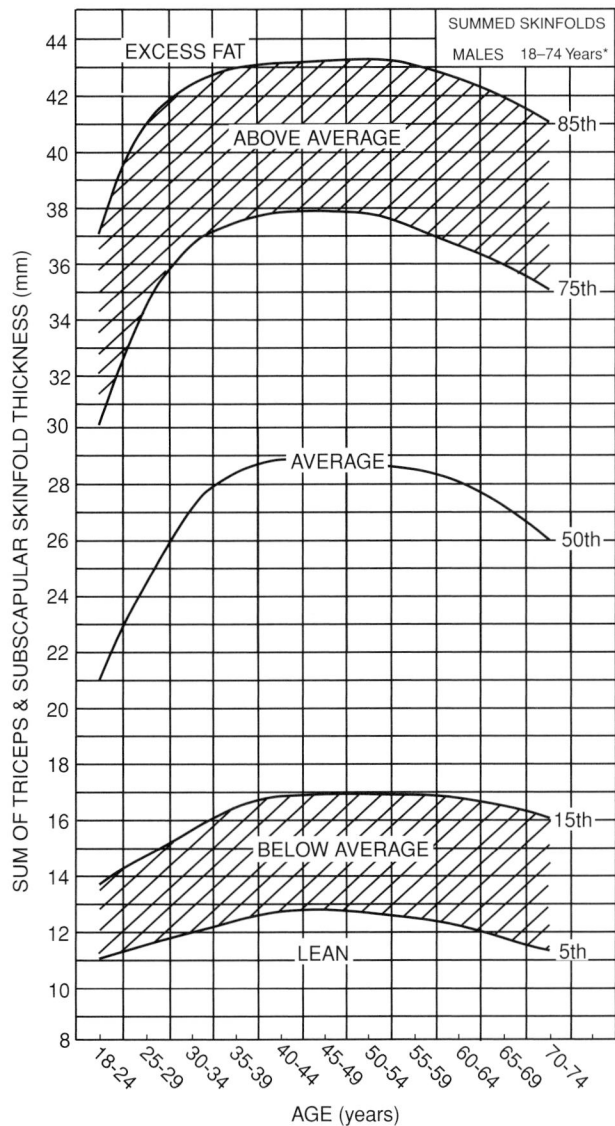

Figure A-16-e-1. Percentiles of Sum of Triceps and Subscapular Skinfold Thicknesses by Age for Males Ranging in Age from 18 to 74 Years

From Frisancho AR. Anthropometric standards for the assessment of growth and nutritional status. Ann Arbor: University of Michigan Press, 1990. Figure IV.39.

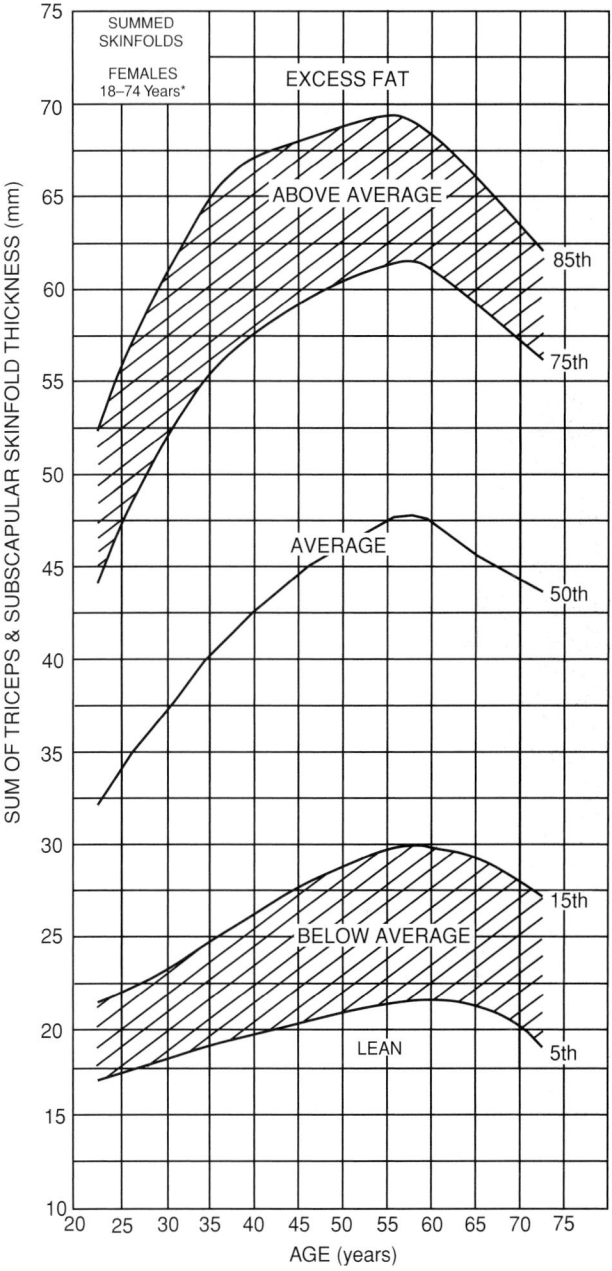

Figure A-16-e-2. Percentiles of Sum of Triceps and Subscapular Skinfold Thicknesses by Age for Females Ranging in Age from 18 to 74 Years

From Frisancho AR. Anthropometric standards for the assessment of growth and nutritional status. Ann Arbor: University of Michigan Press, 1990. Figure IV.42.

TABLE A-16-f. MEANS, STANDARD DEVIATIONS OF PERCENT FAT WEIGHT (%) IN PERCENTILES BY AGE FOR MALES AND FEMALES, 18 TO 74 YEARS

AGE (ys)	N	MEAN	SD	PERCENTILES 5	10	15	25	50	75	85	90	95
Males												
18.0–24.9	1,708	16.5	6.2	8.0	9.0	10.0	12.0	16.0	20.0	23.0	25.0	28.0
25.0–29.9	1,217	18.2	6.2	9.0	10.0	11.0	13.0	18.0	23.0	25.0	26.0	29.0
30.0–34.9	916	22.6	4.2	16.0	17.0	18.0	20.0	23.0	26.0	27.0	28.0	30.0
35.0–39.9	817	22.5	4.1	15.0	17.0	18.0	20.0	23.0	25.0	27.0	27.0	29.0
40.0–44.9	805	25.3	6.6	14.0	16.0	18.0	21.0	26.0	30.0	32.0	34.0	36.0
45.0–49.9	842	25.7	6.6	15.0	17.0	19.0	21.0	26.0	30.0	32.0	34.0	36.0
50.0–54.9	858	26.4	6.7	15.0	17.0	19.0	22.0	27.0	31.0	33.0	35.0	37.0
55.0–59.9	780	26.6	6.4	15.0	18.0	20.0	22.0	27.0	31.0	33.0	35.0	37.0
60.0–64.9	1,228	26.8	6.5	16.0	18.0	20.0	22.0	27.0	31.0	33.0	35.0	37.0
65.0–69.9	1,725	25.8	6.9	13.0	16.0	18.0	21.0	26.0	30.0	33.0	35.0	37.0
70.0–74.9	1,229	25.4	6.7	13.0	16.0	18.0	21.0	26.0	30.0	33.0	34.0	36.0
Females												
18.0–24.9	2,585	27.9	7.0	17.0	19.0	21.0	23.0	27.0	33.0	35.0	37.0	40.0
25.0–29.9	1,905	29.1	7.3	18.0	20.0	21.0	24.0	29.0	34.0	37.0	39.0	41.0
30.0–34.9	1,613	31.4	6.4	21.0	23.0	25.0	27.0	31.0	36.0	38.0	40.0	42.0
35.0–39.9	1,442	32.1	6.2	22.0	24.0	25.0	28.0	32.0	37.0	39.0	40.0	42.0
40.0–44.9	1,376	34.9	5.7	25.0	28.0	29.0	31.0	35.0	39.0	41.0	42.0	43.0
45.0–49.9	952	35.5	5.6	26.0	28.0	29.0	32.0	36.0	39.0	41.0	42.0	44.0
50.0–54.9	991	38.9	6.4	27.0	30.0	32.0	35.0	39.0	43.0	46.0	47.0	48.0
55.0–59.9	867	38.9	6.5	27.0	30.0	32.0	35.0	39.0	44.0	45.0	47.0	49.0
60.0–64.9	1,370	39.0	6.2	28.0	31.0	32.0	35.0	40.0	43.0	45.0	46.0	48.0
65.0–69.9	1,927	38.0	6.2	27.0	30.0	32.0	34.0	38.0	42.0	44.0	46.0	47.0
70.0–74.9	1,454	37.3	6.4	26.0	29.0	31.0	34.0	38.0	42.0	44.0	45.0	47.0

From Frisancho AR. Anthropometric standards for the assessment of growth and nutritional status. Ann Arbor: University of Michigan Press, 1990, Table IV, 19. With permission.

A-17. BODY FAT ESTIMATIONS FROM SKINFOLD DATA

Various investigators have developed equations for predicting the proportions of body fat by anthropometric measures of specific regions. Durnin and Womersley used four different skinfolds (Table A-17-a). Pollock, Schmidt, and Jackson have prepared tables based on three sites,

including thigh skinfolds (Tables A-17-b and A-17-c). Because some technicians have difficulty obtaining consistent results with thigh skinfold measurements, data also are available based on equations that do not use this skinfold.

See the discussion in Chapter 49 on the use of bioelectric impedance method for fat estimation; also see data in Appendix Tables 15-e.

Appendices Editors

TABLE A-17-a. EQUIVALENT FAT CONTENT, AS PERCENTAGE OF BODY WEIGHT, FOR A RANGE OF VALUES FOR THE SUM OF FOUR SKINFOLDS[a]

SKINFOLDS (mm)	MEN (age in years)				WOMEN (age in years)			
	17–29	30–39	40–49	50+	16–29	30–39	40–49	50+
15	4.8				10.5			
20	8.1	12.2	12.2	12.6	14.1	17.0	19.8	21.4
25	10.5	14.2	15.0	15.6	16.8	19.4	22.2	24.0
30	12.9	16.2	17.7	18.6	19.5	21.8	24.5	26.6
35	14.7	17.7	19.6	20.8	21.5	23.7	26.4	28.5
40	16.4	19.2	21.4	22.9	23.4	25.5	28.2	30.3
45	17.7	20.4	23.0	24.7	25.0	26.9	29.6	31.9
50	19.0	21.5	24.6	26.5	26.5	28.2	31.0	33.4
55	20.1	22.5	25.9	27.9	27.8	29.4	32.1	34.6
60	21.2	23.5	27.1	29.2	29.1	30.6	33.2	35.7
65	22.2	24.3	28.2	30.4	30.2	31.6	34.1	36.7
70	23.1	25.1	29.3	31.6	31.2	32.5	35.0	37.7
75	24.0	25.9	30.3	32.7	32.2	33.4	35.9	38.7
80	24.8	26.6	31.2	33.8	33.1	34.3	36.7	39.6
85	25.5	27.2	32.1	34.8	34.0	35.1	37.5	40.4
90	26.2	27.8	33.0	35.8	34.8	35.8	38.3	41.2
95	26.9	28.4	33.7	36.6	35.6	36.5	39.0	41.9
100	27.6	29.0	34.4	37.4	36.4	37.2	39.7	42.6
105	28.2	29.6	35.1	38.2	37.1	37.9	40.4	43.3
110	28.8	30.1	35.8	39.0	37.8	38.6	41.0	43.9
115	29.4	30.6	36.4	39.7	38.4	39.1	41.5	44.5
120	30.0	31.1	37.0	40.4	39.0	39.6	42.0	45.1
125	31.0	31.5	37.6	41.1	39.6	40.1	42.5	45.7
130	31.5	31.9	38.2	41.8	40.2	40.6	43.0	46.2
135	32.0	32.3	38.7	42.4	40.8	41.1	43.5	46.7
140	32.5	32.7	39.2	43.0	41.3	41.6	44.0	47.2
145	32.9	33.1	39.7	43.6	41.8	42.1	44.5	47.7
150	33.3	33.5	40.2	44.1	42.3	42.6	45.0	48.2
155	33.7	33.9	40.7	44.6	42.8	43.1	45.4	48.7
160	34.1	34.3	41.2	45.1	43.3	43.6	45.8	49.2
165	34.5	34.6	41.6	45.6	43.7	44.0	46.2	49.6
170	34.9	34.8	42.0	46.1	44.1	44.4	46.6	50.0
175	35.3					44.8	47.0	50.4
180	35.6					45.2	47.4	50.8
185	35.9					45.6	47.8	51.2
190						45.9	48.2	51.6
195						46.2	48.5	52.0
200						46.5	48.8	52.4
205							49.1	52.7
210							49.4	53.0

[a] Biceps, triceps, subscapular, and suprailiac of men and women of different ages.

From Dumin JVGA, Womersley J. Br J Nutr 1974;32:77–97, with permission.

TABLE A-17-b. PERCENTAGE OF BODY FAT ESTIMATION FOR WOMEN FROM AGE AND TRICEPS, SUPRALIUM, AND THIGH SKINFOLDS[a]

SUM OF SKINFOLDS (mm)	AGE TO THE LAST YEAR								
	UNDER 22	23 TO 27	28 TO 32	33 TO 37	38 TO 42	43 TO 47	48 TO 52	53 TO 57	OVER 58
23–25	9.7	9.9	10.2	10.4	10.7	10.9	11.2	11.4	11.7
26–28	11.0	11.2	11.5	11.7	12.0	12.3	12.5	12.7	13.0
29–31	12.3	12.5	12.8	13.0	13.3	13.5	13.8	14.0	14.3
32–34	13.6	13.8	14.0	14.3	14.5	14.8	15.0	15.3	15.5
35–37	14.8	15.0	15.3	15.5	15.8	16.0	16.3	16.5	16.8
38–40	16.0	16.3	16.5	16.7	17.0	17.2	17.5	17.7	18.0
41–43	17.2	17.4	17.7	17.9	18.2	18.4	18.7	18.9	19.2
44–46	18.3	18.6	18.8	19.1	19.3	19.6	19.8	20.1	20.3
47–49	19.5	19.7	20.0	20.2	20.5	20.7	21.0	21.2	21.5
50–52	20.6	20.8	21.1	21.3	21.6	21.8	22.1	22.3	22.6
53–55	21.7	21.9	22.1	22.4	22.6	22.9	23.1	23.4	23.6
56–58	22.7	23.0	23.2	23.4	23.7	23.9	24.2	24.4	24.7
59–61	23.7	24.0	24.2	24.5	24.7	25.0	25.2	25.5	25.7
62–64	24.7	25.0	25.2	25.5	25.7	26.0	26.7	26.4	26.7
65–67	25.7	25.9	26.2	26.4	26.7	26.9	27.2	27.4	27.7
68–70	26.6	26.9	27.1	27.4	27.6	27.9	28.1	28.4	28.6
71–73	27.5	27.8	28.0	28.3	28.5	28.8	28.0	29.3	29.5
74–76	28.4	28.7	28.9	29.2	29.4	29.7	29.9	30.2	30.4
77–79	29.3	29.5	29.8	30.0	30.3	30.5	30.8	31.0	31.3
80–82	30.1	30.4	30.6	30.9	31.1	31.4	31.6	31.9	32.1
83–85	30.9	31.2	31.4	31.7	31.9	32.2	32.4	32.7	32.9
86–88	31.7	32.0	32.2	32.5	32.7	32.9	33.2	33.4	33.7
89–91	32.5	32.7	33.0	33.2	33.5	33.7	33.9	34.2	34.4
92–94	33.2	33.4	33.7	33.9	34.2	34.4	34.7	34.9	35.2
95–97	33.9	34.1	34.4	34.6	34.9	35.1	35.4	35.6	35.9
98–100	34.6	34.8	35.1	35.3	35.5	35.8	36.0	36.3	36.5
101–103	35.3	35.4	35.7	35.9	36.2	36.4	36.7	36.9	37.2
104–106	35.8	36.1	36.3	36.6	36.8	37.1	37.3	37.5	37.8
107–109	36.4	36.7	36.9	37.1	37.4	37.6	37.9	38.1	38.4
110–112	37.0	37.2	37.5	37.7	38.0	38.2	38.5	38.7	38.9
113–115	37.5	37.8	38.0	38.2	38.5	38.7	39.0	39.2	39.5
116–118	38.0	38.3	38.5	38.8	39.0	39.3	39.5	39.7	40.0
119–121	38.5	38.7	39.0	39.2	39.5	39.7	40.0	40.2	40.5
122–124	39.0	39.2	39.4	39.7	39.9	40.2	40.4	40.7	40.9
125–127	39.4	39.6	39.9	40.1	40.4	40.6	40.9	41.1	41.4
128–130	39.8	40.0	40.3	40.5	40.8	41.0	41.3	41.5	41.8

[a] Percentage of fat calculated by the formula of Siri: percentage of fat = $(4.95/D_b - 4.5) \times 100$, where D_b = body density.

Reprinted with permission from Pollock ML, Schmidt DH, Jackson AS. Measurement of cardiorespiratory fitness and body composition in the clinical setting. Compr Ther 1980;6:12–27.

TABLE A-17-c. PERCENTAGE OF BODY FAT ESTIMATION FOR MEN FROM AGE AND THE SUM OF CHEST, ABDOMINAL, AND THIGH SKINFOLDS[a]

SUM OF SKINFOLDS (mm)	AGE TO THE LAST YEAR								
	UNDER 22	23 TO 27	28 TO 32	33 TO 37	38 TO 42	43 TO 47	48 TO 52	53 TO 57	OVER 58
23–25	9.7	9.9	10.2	10.4	10.7	10.9	11.2	11.4	11.7
26–28	11.0	11.2	11.5	11.7	12.0	12.3	12.5	12.7	13.0
29–31	12.3	12.5	12.8	13.0	13.3	13.5	13.8	14.0	14.3
32–34	13.6	13.8	14.0	14.3	14.5	14.8	15.0	15.3	15.5
35–37	14.8	15.0	15.3	15.5	15.8	16.0	16.3	16.5	16.8
38–40	16.0	16.3	16.5	16.7	17.0	17.2	17.5	17.7	18.0
41–43	17.2	17.4	17.7	17.9	18.2	18.4	18.7	18.9	19.2
44–46	18.3	18.6	18.8	19.1	19.3	19.6	19.8	20.1	20.3
47–49	19.5	19.7	20.0	20.2	20.5	20.7	21.0	21.2	21.5
50–52	20.6	20.8	21.1	21.3	21.6	21.8	22.1	22.3	22.6
53–55	21.7	21.9	22.1	22.4	22.6	22.9	23.1	23.4	23.6
56–58	22.7	23.0	23.2	23.4	23.7	23.9	24.2	24.4	24.7
59–61	23.7	24.0	24.2	24.5	24.7	25.0	25.2	25.5	25.7
62–64	24.7	25.0	25.2	25.5	25.7	26.0	26.7	26.4	26.7
65–67	25.7	25.9	26.2	26.4	26.7	26.9	27.2	27.4	27.7
68–70	26.6	26.9	27.1	27.4	27.6	27.9	28.1	28.4	28.6
71–73	27.5	27.8	28.0	28.3	28.5	28.8	29.0	29.3	29.5
74–76	28.4	28.7	28.9	29.2	29.4	29.7	29.9	30.2	30.4
77–79	29.3	29.5	29.8	30.0	30.3	30.5	30.8	31.0	31.3
80–82	30.1	30.4	30.6	30.9	31.1	31.4	31.6	31.9	32.1
83–85	30.9	31.2	31.4	31.7	31.9	32.2	32.4	32.7	32.9
86–88	31.7	32.0	32.2	32.5	32.7	32.9	33.2	33.4	33.7
89–91	32.5	32.7	33.0	33.2	33.5	33.7	33.9	34.2	34.4
92–94	33.2	33.4	33.7	33.9	34.2	34.4	34.7	34.9	35.2
95–97	33.9	34.1	34.4	34.6	34.9	35.1	35.4	35.6	35.9
98–100	34.6	34.8	35.1	35.3	35.5	35.8	36.0	36.3	36.5
101–103	35.3	35.4	35.7	35.9	36.2	36.4	36.7	36.9	37.2
104–106	35.8	36.1	36.3	36.6	36.8	37.1	37.3	37.5	37.8
107–109	36.4	36.7	36.9	37.1	37.4	37.6	37.9	38.1	38.4
110–112	37.0	37.2	37.5	37.7	38.0	38.2	38.5	38.7	38.9
113–115	37.5	37.8	38.0	38.2	38.5	38.7	39.0	39.2	39.5
116–118	38.0	38.3	38.5	38.8	39.0	39.3	39.5	39.7	40.0
119–121	38.5	38.7	39.0	39.2	39.5	39.7	40.0	40.2	40.5
122–124	39.0	39.2	39.4	39.7	39.9	40.2	40.4	40.7	40.9
125–127	39.4	39.6	39.9	40.1	40.4	40.6	40.9	41.1	41.4
128–130	39.8	40.0	40.3	40.5	40.8	41.0	41.3	41.5	41.8

[a] Percentage of fat calculated by the formula of Siri: percentage of fat = $(4.95/D_b - 4.5) \times 100$, where D_b = body density.

Reprinted with permission from Pollock ML, Schmidt DH, Jackson AS. Measurement of cardiorespiratory fitness and body composition in the clinical setting. Cornpr Ther. 1980;6:12–27.

TABLE A-17-d-1. MEAN PERCENTAGE BODY FAT WEIGHT BY SUM OF TRICEPS AND SUBSCAPULAR SKINFOLD THICKNESSES FOR ADULTS RANGING IN AGE FROM 18 TO 49 YEARS

MALES		FEMALES	
Summed Skinfold Thicknesses Range (mm)	Percentage Fat Weight (Mean ± SD)	Summed Skinfold Thicknesses Range (mm)	Percentage Fat Weight (Mean ± SD)
Age group: 18 to 24 years			
9 to 11	6.8 ± 1.0	8 to 17	15.5 ± 2.3
12 to 13	9.3 ± 0.7	18 to 21	19.8 ± 1.1
14 to 30	15.2 ± 3.1	22 to 44	27.0 ± 3.2
31 to 37	22.1 ± 0.8	45 to 52	34.1 ± 0.8
38 to 113	27.2 ± 3.0	53 to 130	39.5 ± 3.0
Age group: 25 to 29 years			
9 to 12	7.9 ± 1.2	9 to 17	15.3 ± 2.2
13 to 14	10.2 ± 0.4	18 to 22	20.1 ± 1.2
15 to 35	17.1 ± 3.3	23 to 48	28.1 ± 3.5
36 to 42	23.9 ± 0.7	49 to 58	35.9 ± 0.9
43 to 100	28.2 ± 2.6	59 to 116	40.9 ± 2.7
Age group: 30 to 34 years			
9 to 13	14.4 ± 1.1	9 to 18	18.4 ± 2.2
14 to 17	17.2 ± 0.9	19 to 24	23.3 ± 1.0
18 to 38	22.2 ± 2.1	25 to 55	30.6 ± 3.1
39 to 44	26.3 ± 0.5	56 to 64	37.2 ± 0.7
45 to 104	29.1 ± 1.7	65 to 117	41.3 ± 2.1
Age group: 35 to 39 years			
8 to 12	13.9 ± 1.1	8 to 19	19.5 ± 2.3
13 to 17	16.7 ± 0.9	20 to 25	23.8 ± 1.1
18 to 37	22.3 ± 2.0	26 to 57	31.4 ± 3.1
38 to 42	26.0 ± 0.4	58 to 66	37.7 ± 0.6
43 to 114	28.6 ± 1.8	67 to 112	41.3 ± 2.0
Age group: 40 to 44 years			
8 to 13	12.6 ± 1.6	8 to 20	22.9 ± 2.8
14 to 17	16.6 ± 1.1	21 to 27	27.8 ± 1.2
18 to 37	24.7 ± 3.1	28 to 58	34.5 ± 2.8
38 to 43	31.0 ± 0.8	59 to 67	40.2 ± 0.6
44 to 92	35.5 ± 2.7	68 to 115	43.2 ± 1.7
Age group: 45 to 49 years			
9 to 14	12.8 ± 2.0	8 to 21	23.4 ± 2.5
15 to 18	17.5 ± 1.1	22 to 27	27.8 ± 1.0
19 to 39	25.3 ± 3.3	28 to 59	35.0 ± 2.8
40 to 44	31.7 ± 0.6	60 to 69	40.5 ± 0.6
45 to 98	35.6 ± 2.7	70 to 117	43.6 ± 1.6

From Frisancho AR. Anthropometric standards for the assessment of growth and nutritional status. Ann Arbor: University of Michigan Press, 1990, Table IV. 20. With permission.

TABLE A-17-d-2. MEAN PERCENTAGE BODY FAT WEIGHT BY SUM OF TRICEPS AND SUBSCAPULAR SKINFOLD THICKNESSES FOR ADULTS RANGING IN AGE FROM 50 TO 74 YEARS

MALES		FEMALES	
Summed Skinfold Thicknesses Range (mm)	Percentage Fat Weight (Mean ± SD)	Summed Skinfold Thicknesses Range (mm)	Percentage Fat Weight (Mean ± SD)
Age group: 50 to 54 years			
8 to 13	12.9 ± 2.2	10 to 21	24.1 ± 3.1
14 to 17	17.5 ± 1.1	22 to 30	30.5 ± 1.5
18 to 37	25.7 ± 3.2	31 to 61	38.7 ± 3.0
38 to 43	32.3 ± 0.8	62 to 70	44.7 ± 0.7
44 to 94	36.8 ± 2.5	71 to 114	48.1 ± 1.8
Age group: 55 to 59 years			
9 to 13	13.2 ± 1.5	12 to 21	24.5 ± 2.2
14 to 18	18.5 ± 1.3	22 to 29	30.3 ± 1.4
19 to 37	26.2 ± 3.0	30 to 62	38.6 ± 3.2
38 to 43	32.3 ± 0.8	63 to 69	44.6 ± 0.5
44 to 86	36.4 ± 2.4	70 to 125	48.1 ± 2.2
Age group: 60 to 64 years			
9 to 14	14.1 ± 1.9	8 to 22	25.2 ± 2.7
15 to 18	18.6 ± 1.1	23 to 30	30.8 ± 1.3
19 to 37	26.1 ± 3.1	31 to 61	38.6 ± 3.0
38 to 43	32.2 ± 0.7	62 to 68	44.4 ± 0.5
44 to 94	36.9 ± 2.7	69 to 120	47.9 ± 1.9
Age group: 65 to 69 years			
8 to 12	12.0 ± 1.6	8 to 21	24.0 ± 2.9
13 to 16	16.6 ± 1.1	22 to 29	30.1 ± 1.4
17 to 36	25.2 ± 3.4	30 to 57	37.7 ± 2.8
37 to 42	31.9 ± 0.8	58 to 64	43.4 ± 0.5
43 to 102	36.4 ± 2.7	65 to 118	46.9 ± 2.1
Age group: 70 to 74 years			
9 to 12	12.0 ± 1.3	8 to 19	22.5 ± 2.9
13 to 16	16.6 ± 1.1	20 to 27	29.1 ± 1.4
17 to 35	24.7 ± 3.2	28 to 58	37.2 ± 3.1
36 to 41	31.3 ± 0.9	57 to 62	43.0 ± 0.6
42 to 90	35.8 ± 2.6	63 to 122	46.3 ± 2.0

From Frisancho, AR. Anthropometric standards for the assessment of growth and nutritional status. Ann Arbor, University of Michigan Press, 1990. Table IV. 21. With permission.

A-18. GROWTH AND ANTHROPOMETRIC DATA FOR CLINICAL CONDITIONS

A-18-a. Height and Weight Relations in Defining Obesity

TABLE A-18-a-1. CLASSIFICATION OF OVERWEIGHT AND OBESITY BY BMI, WAIST CIRCUMFERENCE, AND ASSOCIATED DISEASE RISKS

	BMI (kg/m^2)	OBESITY CLASS	DISEASE RISK[a] RELATIVE TO NORMAL WEIGHT AND WAIST CIRCUMFERENCE[b]	
			MEN ≤102 cm (≤40 in) WOMEN ≤88 cm (≤35 in)	>102 cm (>40 in) >88 cm (>35 in)
Underweight	<18.5		—	—
Normal	18.5–24.9		—	—
Overweight	25.0–29.9		Increased	High
Obesity	30.0–34.9	I	High	Very High
	35.0–39.9	II	Very High	Very High
Extreme Obesity	≥40	III	Extremely High	Extremely High

[a] Disease risk for type 2 diabetes, hypertension, and CVD.

[b] Increased waist circumference can also be a marker for increased risk, even in persons of normal weight.

From U.S. Department of Health and Human Services, National Institutes of Health, National Heart, Lung, and Blood Institute. Clinical guidelines on the identification, evaluation, and treatment of overweight and obesity in adults. The evidence report. Bethesda, MD; Preprint June 1998:228pp. This is Table ES-4 in the original report.

TABLE A-18-a-2. SELECTED BMI UNITS CATEGORIZED BY INCHES (cm) AND POUNDS (kg)

	BMI 25 kg/m^2	BMI 27 kg/m^2	BMI 30 kg/m^2
HEIGHT IN INCHES (cm)		BODY WEIGHT IN POUNDS (kg)	
58 (147.32)	119 (53.98)	129 (58.51)	143 (64.86)
59 (149.86)	124 (56.25)	133 (60.33)	148 (67.13)
60 (152.40)	128 (58.06)	138 (62.60)	153 (69.40)
61 (154.94)	132 (59.87)	143 (64.86)	158 (71.67)
62 (157.48)	136 (61.69)	147 (66.68)	164 (74.39)
63 (160.02)	141 (63.96)	152 (68.95)	169 (76.66)
64 (162.56)	145 (65.77)	157 (71.22)	174 (78.93)
65 (165.10)	150 (68.04)	162 (73.48)	180 (81.65)
66 (167.64)	155 (70.31)	187 (75.75)	186 (84.37)
67 (170.18)	159 (72.12)	172 (78.02)	191 (86.64)
68 (172.72)	164 (74.39)	177 (80.29)	197 (89.36)
69 (175.26)	169 (76.66)	182 (82.56)	203 (92.08)
70 (177.80)	174 (78.93)	188 (85.28)	207 (93.90)
71 (180.34)	179 (81.19)	193 (87.54)	215 (97.52)
72 (182.88)	184 (83.46)	199 (90.27)	221 (100.25)
73 (185.42)	189 (85.73)	204 (92.53)	227 (102.97)
74 (187.96)	194 (88.00)	210 (95.26)	233 (105.69)
75 (190.50)	200 (90.72)	216 (97.98)	240 (108.86)
76 (193.04)	205 (92.99)	221 (100.25)	246 (111.59)

Metric conversion formula = weight (kg)/height (m)^2 Non-metric conversion formula = [weight (pounds)/height (inches)^2] × 704.5

Example of BMI calculation:	Example of BMI calculation:
A person who weighs 78.93 kilograms and is 177 centimeters tall has a BMI of 25: weight (78.93 kg)/height (1.77 m)^2 = 25	A person who weighs 164 pounds and is 68 inches (or 5'8") tall has a BMI of 25: [weight (164 pounds)/height (68 inches)^2] × 704.5 = 25

From U.S. Department of Health and Human Services, National Institutes of Health, National Heart, Lung, and Blood Institute. Clinical guidelines on the identification, evaluation, and treatment of overweight and obesity in adults. The evidence report. Bethesda, MD; Preprint June 1998:228pp.

TABLE A-18-a-3. AGE-ADJUSTED PREVALENCE OF OVERWEIGHT (BMI 25–29.9) AND OBESITY (BMI ≥30), YEARS 20–74

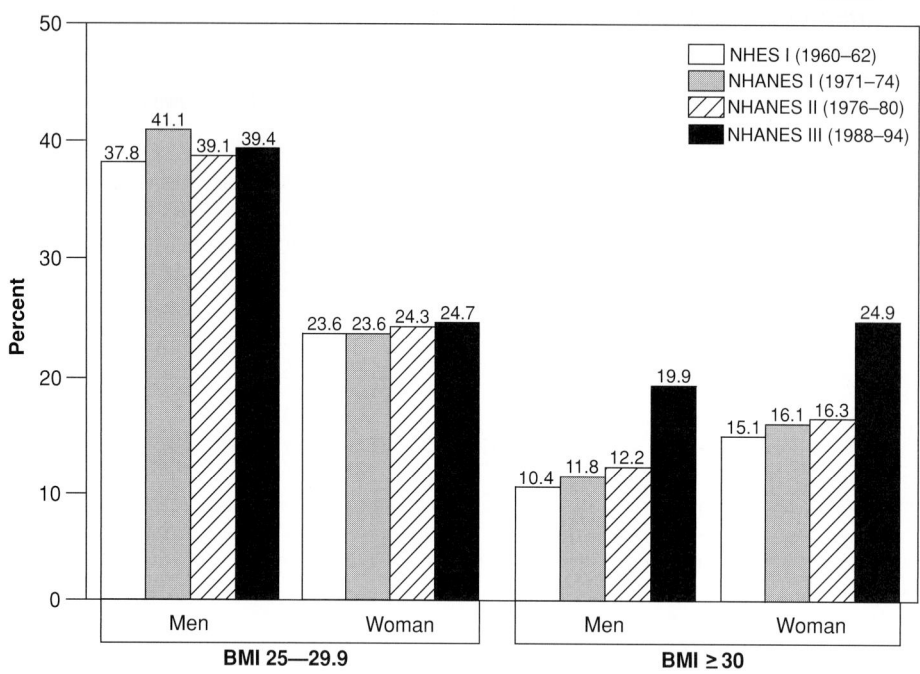

From Centers for Disease Control and Prevention. National Center for Health Statistics. United States 1960–94. This is Figure 1 in reference in Table A-18-a-1. above.

A-18-b. Defining Obesity and Superobesity

A-18-b-1. DEFINING OBESITY AND SUPEROBESITY USING 85TH AND 95TH PERCENTILES FOR BODY MASS INDEX AND TRICEPS SKINFOLD THICKNESS

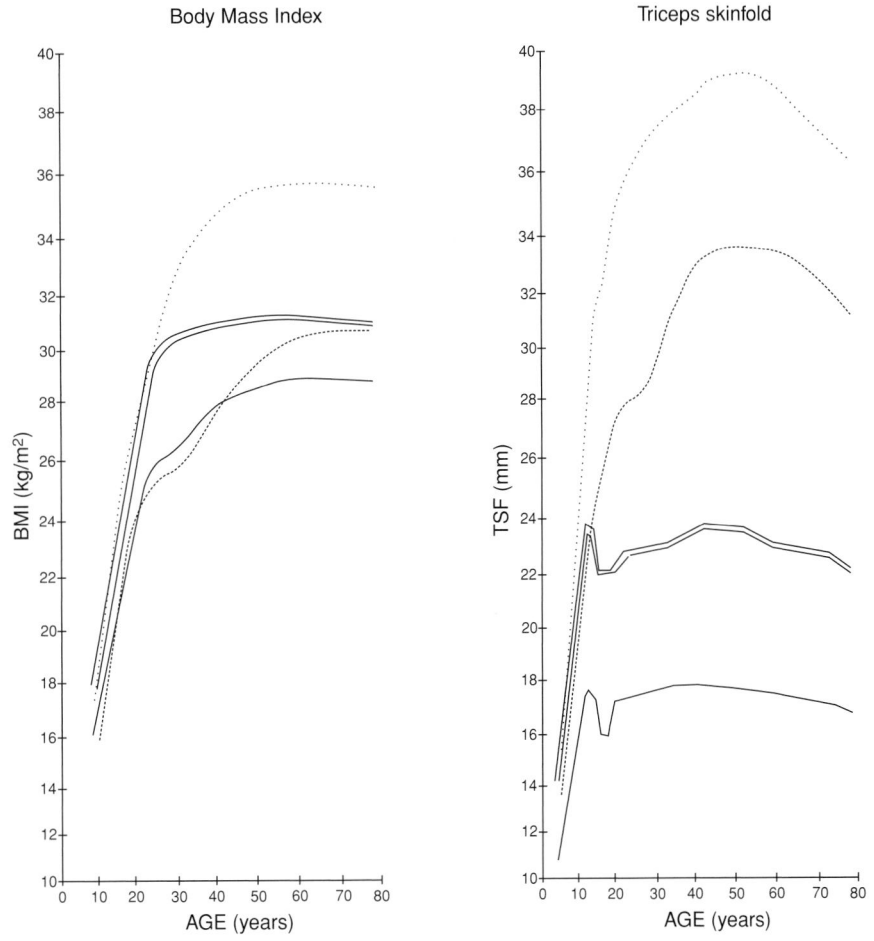

Smoothed 85th- and 95th-percentile body mass index (BMI) and triceps skinfold thickness (TSF) by age for males and females. ——— , 85th percentile for males; ········ , 85th percentile for females; ═══ , 95th percentile for males; ······· , 95th percentile for females. From Must A, Dallal GE, Dietz WH. Am J Clin Nutr 1991;53:839–846. These data were based on NHANES I data collected between 1971–1974 on 20,839 participants aged 6–74 years.

TABLE A-18-b-2. 5TH TO 95TH PERCENTILES OF BODY MASS INDEX (in kg/m²), AGES 6-74 YRS

AGE (y)	WHITES						BLACKS						POPULATION					
	n	5th	15th	50th	85th	95th	n	5th	15th	50th	85th	95th	n	5th	15th	50th	85th	95th
Males																		
6	117	12.93	13.46	14.62	16.52	17.75	47	12.68	13.66	14.49	16.83	18.58	165	12.86	13.43	14.54	16.64	18.02
7	122	13.30	13.88	15.15	17.31	18.98	40	13.11	14.03	14.98	17.29	19.56	164	13.24	13.85	15.07	17.37	19.18
8	117	13.67	14.31	15.70	18.10	20.22	30	13.54	14.41	15.49	17.76	20.51	149	13.63	14.28	15.62	18.11	20.33
9	121	14.04	14.75	16.24	18.88	21.45	55	13.98	14.81	16.00	18.26	21.45	177	14.03	14.71	16.17	18.85	21.47
10	146	14.42	15.19	16.79	19.67	22.66	29	14.41	15.21	16.53	18.78	22.41	177	14.42	15.15	16.72	19.60	22.60
11	122	14.81	15.64	17.35	20.47	23.87	44	14.86	15.62	17.06	19.32	23.42	169	14.83	15.59	17.28	20.35	23.73
12	153	15.21	16.11	17.93	21.28	25.01	50	15.36	16.06	17.61	19.85	24.39	204	15.24	16.06	17.87	21.12	24.89
13	134	15.69	16.65	18.57	22.12	26.06	42	15.89	16.64	18.28	20.62	25.26	177	15.73	16.62	18.53	21.93	25.93
14	131	16.16	17.22	19.25	22.97	27.02	42	16.43	17.22	18.94	21.54	26.13	173	16.18	17.20	19.22	22.77	26.93
15	128	16.57	17.79	19.94	23.82	27.86	43	16.97	17.79	19.56	22.50	27.05	175	16.59	17.76	19.92	23.63	27.76
16	131	17.00	18.35	20.63	24.63	28.69	40	17.51	18.37	20.19	23.45	27.95	172	17.01	18.32	20.63	24.45	28.53
17	133	17.29	18.72	21.13	25.44	29.50	33	17.86	18.77	20.70	24.41	28.89	167	17.31	18.68	21.12	25.28	29.32
18	91	17.50	18.95	21.46	26.08	29.89	28	18.05	19.03	21.09	25.06	29.35	120	17.54	18.89	21.45	25.92	30.02
19	108	17.77	19.25	21.88	26.53	29.98	24	18.32	19.35	21.51	25.38	29.62	137	17.80	19.20	21.86	26.36	30.66
20–24	423	18.62	20.26	23.09	27.02	31.43	82	18.43	19.84	22.59	25.76	32.00	514	18.66	20.21	23.07	26.87	31.26
25–29	582	19.10	21.02	24.17	28.15	31.89	81	18.48	20.26	23.87	27.81	32.68	671	19.11	20.98	24.19	28.08	31.72
30–34	390	19.45	21.58	24.90	28.76	32.04	63	18.44	20.75	24.49	29.34	32.95	466	19.52	21.51	24.90	28.75	31.99
35–39	394	19.44	21.82	25.29	29.17	32.12	49	18.58	20.90	24.47	29.99	33.09	451	19.55	21.71	25.25	29.18	32.23
40–44	412	19.44	21.87	25.54	29.34	32.21	58	18.67	20.91	24.66	30.61	33.27	474	19.52	21.75	25.49	29.37	32.41
45–49	466	19.39	21.84	25.61	29.36	32.15	81	18.73	20.90	24.70	30.83	33.45	532	19.45	21.72	25.55	29.39	32.40
50–54	452	19.31	21.78	25.60	29.29	32.04	75	18.82	20.87	24.61	30.62	33.52	531	19.35	21.66	25.54	29.31	32.27
55–59	406	19.23	21.70	25.58	29.23	31.95	57	18.92	20.81	24.47	30.40	33.59	468	19.25	21.58	25.51	29.24	32.18
60–64	327	19.14	21.60	25.54	29.17	31.87	46	19.02	20.75	24.32	30.16	33.67	378	19.15	21.49	25.47	19.17	32.08
65–69	888	19.06	21.50	25.49	29.10	31.78	184	19.12	20.67	24.15	29.90	33.77	1,084	19.05	21.39	25.41	29.08	31.98
70–74	616	18.98	21.39	25.41	29.01	31.69	129	19.21	20.60	23.97	29.60	33.86	752	18.94	21.29	25.33	28.99	31.87

	WHITES						BLACKS						POPULATION					
AGE (y)	n	5th	15th	50th	85th	95th	n	5th	15th	50th	85th	95th	n	5th	15th	50th	85th	95th
Females																		
6	118	12.81	13.37	14.33	16.14	17.59	42	12.52	13.40	13.83	16.24	16.06	161	12.83	13.37	14.31	16.17	17.49
7	126	13.18	13.82	15.00	17.16	18.99	47	12.88	13.79	14.55	17.36	17.95	174	13.17	13.79	14.98	17.17	18.93
8	118	13.57	14.27	15.68	18.19	20.39	35	13.25	14.17	15.26	18.49	19.84	153	13.51	14.22	15.66	18.18	20.36
9	125	13.96	14.72	16.35	19.21	21.78	47	13.63	14.57	15.98	19.64	21.71	173	13.87	14.66	16.33	19.19	21.78
10	152	14.36	15.18	17.02	20.23	23.15	41	14.02	14.96	16.69	20.79	23.57	194	14.23	15.09	17.00	20.19	23.20
11	117	14.76	15.64	17.69	21.24	24.48	43	14.41	15.36	17.39	21.96	25.44	163	14.60	15.53	17.67	21.18	24.59
12	129	15.17	16.11	18.36	22.25	25.53	47	14.83	15.77	18.11	23.15	27.27	177	14.98	15.98	18.35	22.17	25.95
13	151	15.59	16.55	18.91	23.13	26.46	47	15.33	16.23	18.78	24.41	28.90	199	15.36	16.43	18.95	23.08	27.07
14	141	15.89	16.89	19.29	23.87	27.31	49	15.77	16.66	19.24	25.46	30.29	192	15.67	16.79	19.32	23.88	27.97
15	117	16.21	17.23	19.69	24.28	27.89	47	16.20	17.07	19.67	26.04	31.40	164	16.01	17.16	19.69	24.29	28.51
16	142	16.55	17.59	20.11	24.68	28.45	30	16.65	17.48	20.11	26.68	32.51	173	16.37	17.54	20.09	24.74	29.10
17	114	16.76	17.84	20.39	25.07	28.95	44	16.92	17.81	20.45	27.38	33.38	159	16.59	17.81	20.36	25.23	29.72
18	109	16.87	18.01	20.58	25.34	29.23	29	17.04	18.06	20.78	27.92	33.18	140	16.71	17.99	20.57	25.56	30.22
19	104	17.00	18.20	20.80	25.58	29.37	37	17.20	18.35	21.11	28.40	33.27	142	16.87	18.20	20.80	25.85	30.72
20–24	956	17.47	18.61	21.38	25.78	31.25	261	17.26	18.97	22.38	28.81	35.19	1,244	17.38	18.64	21.46	26.14	31.20
25–29	1,093	17.90	19.05	21.94	27.16	32.79	191	17.64	19.70	23.88	31.03	36.82	1,307	17.84	19.09	22.10	27.68	33.16
30–34	900	18.21	19.48	22.47	28.38	34.07	180	18.23	20.41	25.06	32.28	37.79	1,092	18.23	19.54	22.69	28.87	34.58
35–39	815	18.48	19.84	22.99	29.25	34.77	185	18.66	21.00	25.87	32.98	38.45	1,017	18.51	19.91	23.25	29.54	35.35
40–44	799	18.61	20.13	23.48	29.90	35.04	183	18.76	21.60	26.61	34.06	39.12	999	18.65	20.20	23.74	30.11	35.85
45–49	519	18.67	20.40	23.91	30.38	35.09	79	18.66	21.97	27.07	34.75	39.26	603	18.71	20.45	24.17	30.56	36.02
50–54	529	18.76	20.62	24.30	30.66	35.09	83	18.52	22.19	27.32	35.11	39.35	615	18.79	20.66	24.54	30.79	35.95
55–59	416	18.84	20.83	24.69	30.93	35.08	74	18.38	22.40	27.52	35.50	39.49	492	18.88	20.86	24.92	31.00	35.88
60–64	394	18.92	21.04	25.08	31.20	35.04	68	18.21	22.60	27.71	35.92	39.64	463	18.96	21.06	25.29	31.21	35.80
65–69	958	18.99	21.25	25.46	31.46	34.98	194	18.01	22.79	27.87	36.32	39.77	1,157	19.03	21.25	25.66	31.40	35.70
70–74	711	19.06	21.45	25.84	31.70	34.91	134	17.78	22.93	28.00	36.67	39.88	848	19.09	21.44	26.01	31.58	35.58

From Must A, Dallal GE, Dietz WH. Am J Clin Nutr 1991; 54:773. Data source: NHANES I. With permission.

TABLE A-18-b-3. 5TH TO 95TH PERCENTILES OF TRICEPS SKINFOLD, THICKNESS, AGES 6–74 YRS

| | WHITES | | | | | | BLACKS | | | | | | POPULATION | | | | | |
| | | | | *mm* | | | | | | *mm* | | | | | | *mm* | | |
AGE (y)	n	5th	15th	50th	85th	95th	n	5th	15th	50th	85TH	95th	n	5th	15th	50th	85th	95th
Males																		
6	117	5.26	6.09	8.74	11.63	14.47	47	4.01	4.86	6.85	9.35	12.86	165	5.04	6.19	8.36	11.10	14.12
7	122	5.28	6.12	8.94	12.78	15.95	40	4.01	4.88	6.85	10.09	14.11	164	5.01	6.14	8.59	12.38	15.61
8	117	5.28	6.15	9.12	13.95	17.51	30	4.00	4.88	6.84	10.76	15.35	149	4.96	6.08	8.79	13.66	17.18
9	121	5.27	6.17	9.27	15.10	19.11	55	3.99	4.88	6.83	11.37	16.50	177	4.91	6.02	8.96	14.93	18.81
10	146	5.24	6.18	9.40	16.29	20.96	29	3.98	4.88	6.81	11.52	17.79	177	4.84	5.95	9.10	16.02	20.68
11	122	5.20	6.20	9.51	17.32	22.53	44	3.97	4.89	6.81	11.31	18.68	169	4.78	5.88	9.23	16.87	22.20
12	153	5.15	6.23	9.59	17.79	23.53	50	3.97	4.91	6.80	10.79	18.74	204	4.69	5.79	9.35	17.26	23.25
13	134	5.01	6.21	9.42	17.63	23.87	42	3.94	4.88	6.72	10.23	18.67	177	4.56	5.65	9.17	17.12	23.71
14	131	4.91	6.15	9.26	16.88	23.42	42	3.86	4.84	6.66	9.92	18.58	173	4.47	5.60	8.93	16.35	23.46
15	128	4.81	6.10	9.12	16.11	22.42	43	3.81	4.80	6.62	9.96	18.99	175	4.40	5.59	8.70	15.75	22.34
16	131	4.69	6.05	8.95	15.81	22.05	40	3.76	4.77	6.58	10.30	20.18	172	4.33	5.55	8.45	15.75	21.53
17	133	4.61	6.02	8.92	15.95	21.99	33	3.69	4.72	6.63	10.73	21.12	167	4.29	5.58	8.38	15.95	21.51
18	91	4.53	6.01	9.02	16.69	22.28	28	3.60	4.64	6.79	11.34	21.95	120	4.25	5.63	8.53	16.59	21.83
19	108	4.48	6.00	9.09	17.53	22.65	24	3.52	4.57	6.92	11.95	22.88	137	4.22	5.69	8.63	17.33	22.12
20–24	423	4.67	6.00	9.90	18.11	23.00	82	3.55	4.38	6.95	12.29	22.90	514	4.21	5.97	9.70	17.84	22.53
25–29	582	4.80	6.30	10.72	18.28	23.47	81	3.55	4.55	7.79	12.22	20.17	671	4.23	6.35	10.68	18.21	23.53
30–34	389	4.88	6.53	11.23	18.27	23.30	63	3.72	4.71	8.55	14.28	21.70	465	4.39	6.60	11.11	18.24	23.49
35–39	394	4.99	6.69	11.38	18.20	23.08	49	3.83	4.76	8.86	15.34	22.38	451	4.56	6.76	11.25	18.14	23.19
40–44	412	5.06	6.87	11.42	18.13	23.55	59	3.79	4.77	9.04	15.57	21.96	474	4.69	6.86	11.29	18.03	23.27
45–49	446	5.07	6.98	11.36	17.88	23.44	81	3.82	4.76	9.08	15.99	22.06	532	4.75	6.85	11.21	17.79	23.18
50–54	452	5.07	7.01	11.29	17.55	23.26	75	3.88	4.76	9.07	16.17	22.24	531	4.77	6.83	11.09	17.50	23.01
55–59	406	5.07	7.04	11.20	17.25	22.99	57	3.94	4.76	9.05	15.70	22.04	467	4.78	6.81	10.96	17.26	22.78
60–64	328	5.06	7.07	11.11	16.99	22.40	46	3.98	4.74	8.99	15.17	21.73	378	4.79	6.79	10.82	17.04	22.21
65–69	888	5.06	7.09	11.01	16.71	21.79	184	4.03	4.73	8.92	14.67	21.40	1084	4.78	6.76	10.68	16.81	21.59
70–74	615	5.05	7.10	10.91	16.48	21.23	129	4.07	4.72	8.85	14.04	20.92	751	4.76	6.72	10.54	16.61	20.96

AGE (y)	WHITES						BLACKS						POPULATION					
	n	5th	15th	50th	85th	95th	n	5th	15th	50th	85TH	95th	n	5th	15th	50th	85th	95th
				mm						mm						mm		
Females																		
6	118	5.65	6.96	10.19	13.48	15.47	42	4.90	6.10	7.99	13.71	14.94	161	6.00	6.76	10.01	13.44	15.57
7	126	6.06	7.42	10.89	14.93	18.08	47	5.09	6.33	8.60	15.27	17.20	174	6.24	7.17	10.68	14.94	17.89
8	118	6.52	7.86	11.60	16.35	20.60	35	5.29	6.57	9.22	16.82	19.41	153	6.47	7.58	11.36	16.41	20.18
9	125	6.94	8.31	12.31	17.74	23.07	47	5.51	6.83	9.85	18.40	21.65	173	6.71	8.01	12.05	17.85	22.47
10	152	7.37	8.77	13.02	18.84	24.84	41	5.73	7.09	10.47	19.63	23.76	194	6.95	8.44	12.74	19.01	24.38
11	117	7.80	9.23	13.74	19.82	26.23	43	5.96	7.36	11.08	20.72	25.84	163	7.20	8.87	13.43	20.13	26.15
12	129	8.17	9.68	14.44	20.97	27.73	47	6.21	7.62	11.68	21.58	27.53	177	7.45	9.31	14.13	21.25	27.98
13	151	8.49	10.19	15.14	22.00	29.08	47	6.50	8.05	12.22	21.86	29.17	199	7.78	9.84	14.87	22.25	29.51
14	141	8.78	10.76	15.77	22.99	30.22	49	6.81	8.53	12.56	21.71	30.48	192	8.15	10.37	15.47	23.27	30.86
15	117	9.06	11.29	16.39	24.08	31.48	47	7.11	8.94	12.95	21.77	30.54	164	8.46	10.85	16.03	24.32	32.22
16	142	9.34	11.83	17.03	24.85	32.35	30	7.41	9.35	13.36	22.06	30.07	173	8.78	11.34	16.62	25.12	33.22
17	114	9.55	12.18	17.45	25.48	32.95	44	7.67	9.70	13.75	23.03	30.46	159	9.03	11.66	17.02	25.80	33.83
18	109	9.66	12.29	17.67	26.22	33.51	29	7.87	10.03	14.19	24.94	31.42	140	9.21	11.79	17.24	26.51	34.26
19	104	9.79	12.46	17.95	26.95	34.07	37	8.08	10.37	14.59	26.92	32.32	142	9.41	11.97	17.50	27.23	34.74
20–24	956	10.29	12.86	19.02	27.52	34.45	261	8.20	11.20	17.59	28.48	33.54	1244	9.91	12.54	18.75	27.80	35.01
25–29	1,090	10.77	13.73	20.18	29.34	36.09	190	8.65	12.25	20.31	31.25	38.39	1307	10.44	13.45	20.02	29.58	36.43
30–34	897	11.23	14.47	21.18	30.72	37.41	180	9.05	13.36	22.26	33.41	40.44	1089	11.00	14.30	21.25	31.03	37.70
35–39	815	11.50	15.19	22.17	31.59	38.35	185	9.62	14.19	23.71	34.04	41.44	1017	11.36	15.08	22.35	32.00	38.55
40–44	799	11.56	15.66	22.74	31.98	38.81	183	9.89	14.55	24.90	34.92	42.00	999	11.46	15.53	23.02	32.69	39.16
45–49	519	11.56	15.92	23.04	32.25	38.94	79	9.96	14.65	25.28	35.52	42.42	603	11.47	15.78	23.41	33.11	39.43
50–54	528	11.53	16.04	23.22	32.34	38.68	83	10.00	14.68	25.51	35.23	42.75	615	11.43	15.92	23.65	33.21	39.12
55–59	416	11.49	16.15	23.40	32.23	38.10	73	10.03	14.69	25.78	34.77	42.40	491	11.38	16.05	23.89	32.98	38.51
60–64	393	11.44	16.23	23.56	31.74	37.14	68	10.02	14.67	26.05	33.68	41.27	462	11.31	16.16	24.10	32.30	37.44
65–69	959	11.38	16.29	23.70	31.21	36.13	194	9.97	14.60	26.30	32.47	40.22	1157	11.23	16.24	24.28	31.59	36.31
70–74	711	11.32	16.33	23.80	30.65	35.09	134	9.88	14.50	26.51	31.12	39.03	848	11.13	16.30	24.42	30.83	35.12

From Must A, Dallal GE, Dietz WH, Am J Clin Nutr 1991;53:839–46. Data source: NHANES I, With permission.

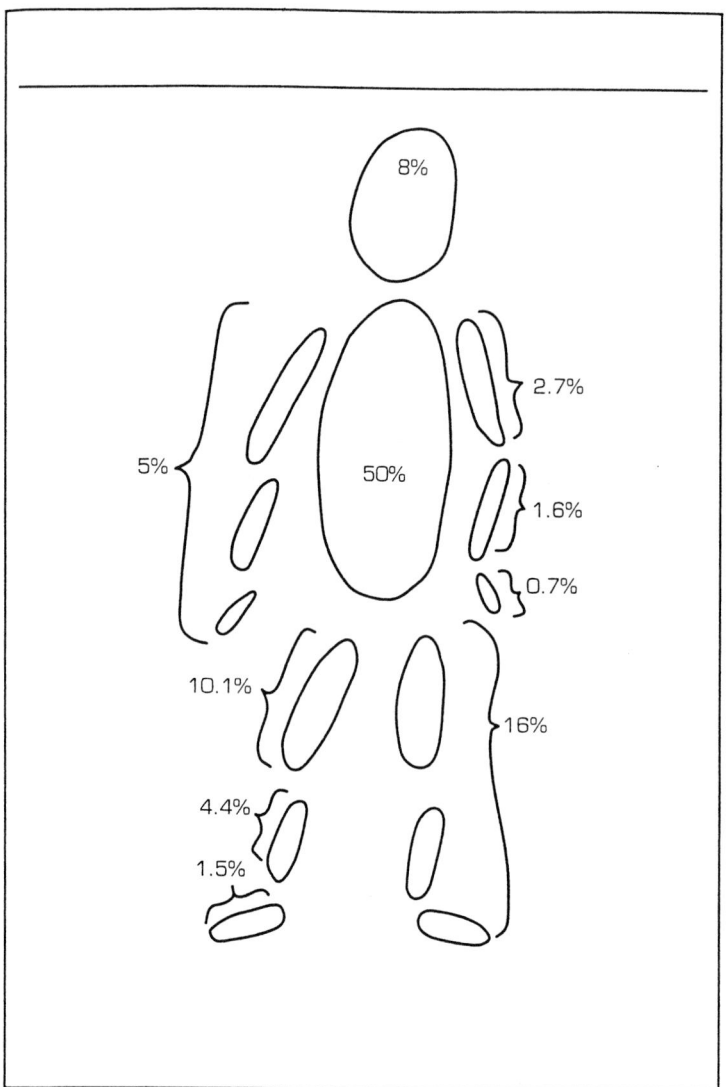

Figure A-18-c. Human Body Proportions for Assessing Amputees.

Ratio of segment weight to body weight based on 1955 data of Dempster and the 1969 data of Clauser et al (N = 21). From Osterkamp LK. J Am Dietetic Assn 1995;95:215–218. Current perspective on assessment of human body proportions of relevance to amputees.

TABLE A-18-d. RECOMMENDED EQUATIONS FOR PREDICTING STATURE IN INDIVIDUALS UNABLE TO STAND

GROUP	AGE GROUP	EQUATION[a]
White men	18–60	Stature = 1.88 (knee height) + 71.85
	17–67	Stature = 2.31 (knee height) + 51.1
	60–80	Stature = 2.08 (knee height) + 59.01
	17–67	Stature = 2.30 (knee height) − 0.063 (age) + 54.9
	17–67	Stature = 0.762 (arm span) + 40.7
Black men	18–60	Stature = 1.79 (knee height) + 73.42
	60–80	Stature = 1.37 (knee height) + 95.79
White women	18–60	Stature = 1.87 (knee height) − 0.06 (age) + 70.25
	22–71	Stature = 1.84 (knee height) + 70.2
	22–71	Stature = 1.91 (knee height) − 0.098 (age) + 71.3
	60–80	Stature = 1.91 (knee height) − 0.17 (age) + 75.00
	22–71	Stature = 0.693 (arm span) + 50.3
Black women	18–60	Stature = 1.86 (knee height) − 0.06 (age) + 68.10
	60–80	Stature = 1.96 (knee height) + 58.72
White boys	6–18	Stature = 2.22 (knee height) + 40.54
Black boys	6–18	Stature = 2.18 (knee height) + 39.60
Chinese boys	4–16	Stature = 1.75 (lower segment) + 26.56
	4–16	Stature = 0.92 (arm span) + 10.84
White girls	6–18	Stature = 2.15 (knee height) + 43.21
Black girls	6–18	Stature = 2.02 (knee height) + 46.59
Chinese girls	4–16	Stature = 1.81 (lower segment) + 22.75
	4–16	Stature = 0.93 (arm span) + 10.34

[a]Arm span, knee height, and stature are in cm; lower segment (subischial leg length) in cm = standing height minus sitting height; and age in years.

From Chapter 56 in 9th edition, Modern Nutrition in Health and Disease; see text for references, use, and source. With permission.

A-18-e. Limb Lengths for Age of the Disabled Child

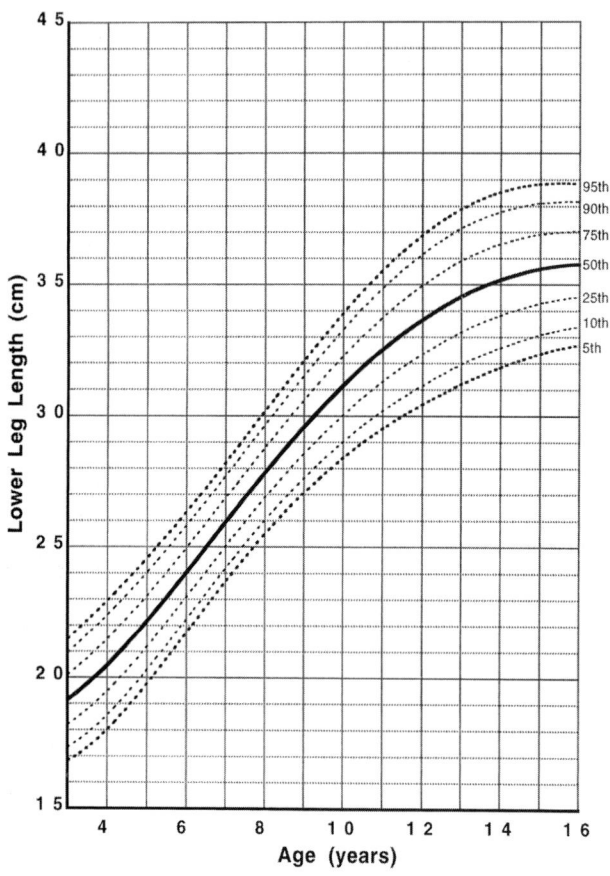

Figure A-18-e-1. Lower Leg Length: Girls 3-16 years.

Published in: Stallings VA, Zemel BS. Nutritional assessment of the disabled child. In: Sullivan PB, Rosenbloom L, eds. Feeding the disabled Child. London: Cambridge University Press 1996:62–76.

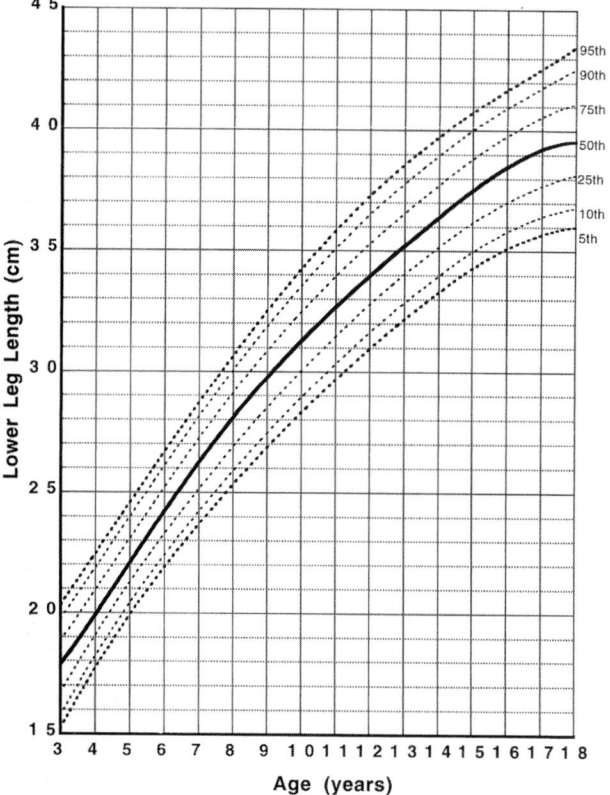

Figure A-18-e-2. Lower Leg Length: Boys 3-18 years.

Published in: Stallings VA, Zemel BS. Nutritional assessment of the disabled child. In: Sullivan PB, Rosenbloom L, eds. Feeding the disabled Child. London: Cambridge University Press 1996:62–76.

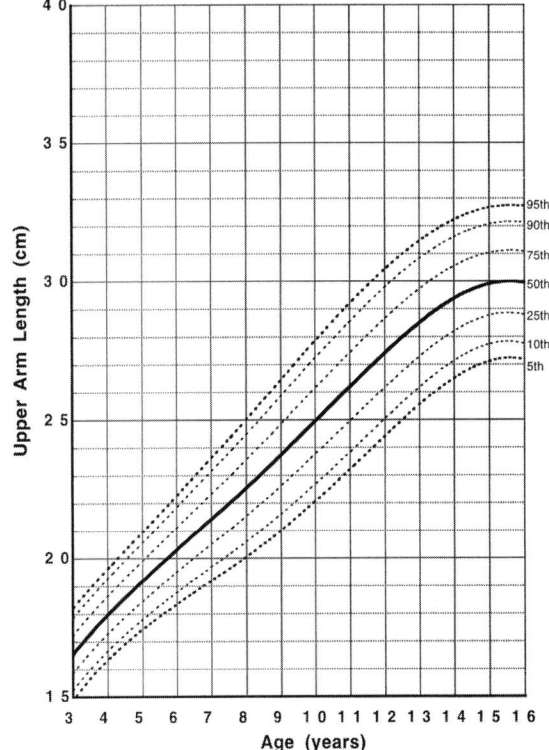

Figure A-18-e-3. Upper Arm Length: Girls 3-16 years.
Published in: Stallings VA, Zemel BS. Nutritional assessment of the disabled child. In: Sullivan PB, Rosenbloom L, eds. Feeding the disabled Child. London: Cambridge University Press 1996:62–76.

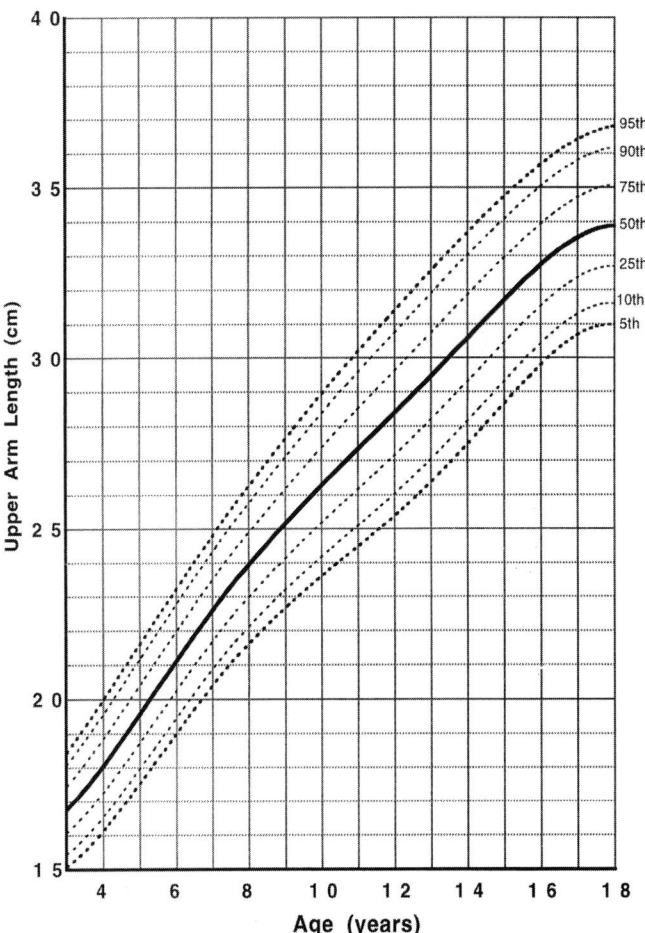

Figure A-18-e-4. Upper Arm Length: Boys 3-18 years.
Published in: Stallings VA, Zemel BS. Nutritional assessment of the disabled child. In: Sullivan PB, Rosenbloom L, eds. Feeding the disabled Child. London: Cambridge University Press 1996:62–76.

NUTRIENTS, LIPIDS, AND ORGANIC COMPOUNDS IN BEVERAGES AND SELECTED FOODS

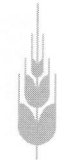

TABLE A-19. BEVERAGES AND ALCOHOLIC DRINKS: CALORIES AND SELECTED ELECTROLYTES (PER 100 mL)

BEVERAGE	CALORIES	SODIUM (mg)	SODIUM (mEq)	POTASSIUM (mg)	POTASSIUM (mEq)	PHOSPHORUS (mg)
Coffee, brewed, regular	2.0	2.0	0.1	54.0	1.4	1.0
Tea, brewed	1.0	3.0	0.1	37.0	1.0	1.0
Tea, herbal	1.0	1.0	<0.1	9.0	0.2	0.0
Cola, regular	43.0	4.0	0.2	1.0	<0.1	13.0
Cola, diet	1.0	5.0	0.2	6.0	0.2	11.0
Soda, fruit flavored, regular	50.0	12.0	0.5	2.0	0.1	1.0
Soda, lemon-lime, regular	42.0	11.0	0.5	1.0	<0.1	0.0
Root beer, regular	43.0	14.0	0.6	1.0	<0.1	0.0
Club soda, regular	0.0	21.0	0.9	2.0	0.1	0.0
Tonic water, regular	41.0	11.0	0.5	1.0	<0.1	0.0
Ginger ale, regular	41.0	11.0	0.5	1.0	<0.1	0.0
Soda, Dr. Pepper, regular	43.0	4.0	0.2	1.0	<0.1	12.0
Soda, Dr. Pepper, diet	1.0	5.0	0.2	6.0	0.2	11.0
Apple juice	49.0	3.0	0.1	125.0	3.2	7.0
Apricot nectar	59.0	3.0	0.1	121.0	3.1	10.0
Cranberry juice cocktail	61.0	2.0	0.1	19.0	0.5	2.0
Grape juice, canned	65.0	3.0	0.1	141.0	3.6	12.0
Grapefruit juice, unsweetened	41.0	1.0	<0.1	169.0	4.3	16.0
Orange juice, unsweetened	48.0	2.0	0.1	202.0	5.2	17.0
Peach nectar	61.0	1.0	<0.1	62.0	1.6	4.0
Pear nectar	62.0	1.0	<0.1	36.0	1.0	3.0
Pineapple juice, unsweetened	59.0	1.0	<0.1	142.0	3.6	8.0
Prune juice, unsweetened	77.0	4.0	0.2	299.0	7.7	27.0
Tomato juice, w/ salt	17.0	371.0	16.0	226.0	5.8	20.0
Tomato juice, w/o salt	17.0	10.0	0.4	226.0	5.8	20.0
Fruit punch	49.0	23.0	1.0	26.0	0.7	1.0
Beer, regular	41.0	5.0	0.2	25.0	0.6	12.0
Beer, light	28.0	3.0	0.1	18.0	0.2	12.0
Gin, rum, vodka, whiskey	217.0	1.0	<0.1	2.0	0.1	4.0
Wine, red	72.0	5.0	0.2	112.0	2.9	14.0
Wine, rose	71.0	5.0	0.2	99.0	2.5	15.0
Wine, white	68.0	5.0	0.2	80.0	2.1	14.0
Dessert wine, dry	126.0	9.0	0.4	92.0	2.4	9.0
Dessert wine, sweet	153.0	9.0	0.4	92.0	2.4	9.0

Note: Alcoholic beverages are customarily served in special glassware, the size of which tends to standardize the alcoholic content.

cordial glass = 20 mL	sherry glass = 60 mL	champagne glass = 150 mL
brandy glass = 30 mL	cocktail glass = 90 mL	tumbler = 240–360 mL
jigger = 60 mL	burgundy glass = 120 mL	mixing glass = 360 mL

Data from the Nutrition Data System for Research (NDS-R) version 5.0_35, 2004, with permission. Table complied and prepared by the Nutrition Coordinating Center, University of Minnesota, Minneapolis, MN.

TABLE A-20. DIETARY FIBER CONTENT OF COMMON FOODS

FOOD ITEM	SERVING SIZE	TOTAL FIBER PER SERVING (g)	SOLUBLE FIBER PER SERVING (g)	INSOLUBLE FIBER PER SERVING (g)
Cereals				
All Bran	⅓ cup	8.6	1.4	7.2
Benefit	¾ cup	5.0	2.8	2.2
Cheerios	1¼ cups	2.5	1.2	1.3
Corn flakes	1 cup	0.5	0.1	0.4
Cream of wheat, regular, uncooked	2½ tbsp	1.1	0.4	0.7
Fiber One	½ cup	11.9	0.8	11.1
40% Bran Flakes	⅔ cup	4.3	0.4	3.9
Grapenuts	¼ cup	2.8	0.8	2.0
Grits, corn, quick, uncooked	3 tbsp	0.6	0.1	0.5
Heartwise	1 cup	5.7	2.9	2.8
Nutri-Grain wheat	⅔ cup	2.7	0.7	2.0
Oat bran, cooked	¾ cup	4.0	2.2	1.8
Oat bran flakes	½ cup	2.1	0.8	0.3
Oat flakes	⅔ cup	2.1	1.0	1.1
Oatmeal, uncooked	⅓ cup	2.7	1.4	1.3
Product 19	1 cup	1.2	0.3	0.9
Puffed Rice	1 cup	0.2	0.1	0.1
Puffed Wheat	1 cup	1.0	0.5	0.5
Quaker Oat Squares	½ cup	2.2	0.8	1.4
Raisin Bran	¾ cup	5.3	0.9	4.4
Rice Krispies	1 cup	0.3	0.1	0.2
Shredded Wheat	⅔ cup	3.5	0.5	3.0
Shredded Wheat and Bran	⅔ cup	2.5	0.6	1.9
Special K	1 cup	0.9	0.2	0.7
Total, whole wheat	1 cup	2.6	0.6	2.0
Wheat flakes	¾ cup	2.3	0.4	1.9
Wheaties	⅔ cup	2.3	0.7	1.6
Grains				
Cornmeal	2½ tbsp	0.4	0.1	0.3
Flour, oat	2½ tbsp	1.8	1.0	0.8
rye	2½ tbsp	2.6	0.8	1.8
white	2½ tbsp	0.6	0.3	0.3
whole wheat	2½ tbsp	2.1	0.3	1.8
Macaroni, white, cooked	½ cup	0.7	0.4	0.3
whole wheat, cooked	½ cup	2.1	0.4	1.7
Noodles, egg, cooked	½ cup	1.4	0.4	1.0
spinach, cooked	½ cup	1.1	0.5	0.6
Popcorn, popped	3 cups	2.0	0.1	1.9
Rice, white, cooked	⅓ cup	0.5	trace	0.5
wild, cooked	⅓ cup	0.4	0.1	0.3

TABLE A-20. DIETARY FIBER CONTENT OF COMMON FOODS

FOOD ITEM	SERVING SIZE	TOTAL FIBER PER SERVING (g)	SOLUBLE FIBER PER SERVING (g)	INSOLUBLE FIBER PER SERVING (g)
Spaghetti, white, cooked	½ cup	0.9	0.4	0.5
whole wheat, cooked	½ cup	2.7	0.6	2.1
Wheat bran	½ cup	12.3	1.0	11.3
Wheat germ	3 tbsp	3.9	0.7	3.2
Breads and Crackers				
Bagel, plain	½	0.7	0.3	0.4
Biscuit, baked	1	0.5	0.3	0.2
Bread, bran	1 slice	1.5	0.2	1.3
cornbread	1–2-in cube	1.4	0.3	1.1
cracked wheat	1 slice	1.9	0.3	1.6
French	1 slice	0.9	0.3	0.6
mixed grain	1 slice	1.9	0.3	1.6
oatmeal	½ slice	1.2	0.3	0.9
pita, white	½ pocket	0.5	0.2	0.3
pumpernickel	1 slice	2.7	1.2	1.5
raisin	1 slice	1.2	0.3	0.9
rye	1 slice	1.8	0.8	1.0
sourdough	1 slice	0.8	0.3	0.5
white	1 slice	0.6	0.3	0.3
whole wheat	1 slice	1.5	0.3	1.2
Bread sticks	2	0.6	0.2	0.4
Bun, hamburger	½	0.7	0.2	0.5
Crackers, matzo	1	1.0	0.5	0.5
saltine	6	0.5	0.3	0.2
saltine, wheat	5	0.5	0.2	0.3
snack, whole wheat	4	2.0	0.3	1.7
wheat	5	0.6	0.2	0.4
English muffin	½	0.8	0.2	0.6
Melba toast, wheat	5 slices	1.8	0.4	1.4
Pretzels, hard	¾ oz	0.8	0.2	0.6
Roll, brown-and-serve	1 roll	0.8	0.3	0.5
Taco shell	2	1.4	0.2	1.2
Tortilla, corn	1	1.4	0.2	1.2
Tortilla, flour	1	0.7	0.3	0.4
Waffle, toasted	1	0.7	0.3	0.4
Fruits				
Apple, red, fresh w/skin	1 sml	2.8	1.0	1.8
Applesauce, canned, unswt	½ cup	2.0	0.7	1.3
Apricots, canned, drained	4 halves	1.2	0.5	0.7
dried	7 halves	2.0	1.1	0.9
fresh w/skin	4	3.5	1.8	1.7
Avocado, fresh, flesh only	⅛	1.2	0.5	0.7
Banana, fresh	½ sml	1.1	0.3	0.8
Blueberries, fresh	¾ cup	1.4	0.3	1.1

(continued)

TABLE A-20. DIETARY FIBER CONTENT OF COMMON FOODS

FOOD ITEM	SERVING SIZE	TOTAL FIBER PER SERVING (g)	SOLUBLE FIBER PER SERVING (g)	INSOLUBLE FIBER PER SERVING (g)
Cherries, black, fresh	12 lrg	1.3	0.6	0.7
Cherries, red, canned	½ cup	1.8	0.9	0.9
Currants, dried	2 tbsp	0.4	0.2	0.2
Dates, dried	2½ med	0.9	0.3	0.6
Figs, dried	1½	2.3	1.1	1.2
Fruit cocktail, canned	½ cup	2.0	0.7	1.3
Grapefruit, fresh	½ med	1.6	1.1	0.5
Grapes, red, fresh w/skin	15 sml	0.4	0.2	0.2
Grapes, white, fresh w/skin	15 sml	0.6	0.3	0.3
Kiwifruit, fresh flesh only	1 lrg	1.7	0.7	1.0
Mango, fresh, flesh only	½ sml	2.9	1.7	1.2
Melon, cantaloupe	1 cup cubed	1.1	0.3	0.8
honeydew	1 cup cubed	0.9	0.3	0.6
watermelon	1¼ cups cubed	0.6	0.4	0.2
Nectarine, fresh	1 sml	1.8	0.8	1.0
Orange, fresh, flesh only	1 sml	2.9	1.8	1.1
Peaches, canned, unswt	½ cup	2.0	0.7	1.3
fresh, w/skin	1 med	2.0	1.0	1.0
Pear, canned	½ cup	3.7	0.7	3.0
fresh, w skin	½ lrg or 1 sml	2.9	1.1	1.8
Pineapple, canned	⅓ cup	1.4	0.2	1.2
fresh	¾ cup	1.4	0.1	1.3
Plum, red, fresh	2 med	2.4	1.1	1.3
Prunes, dried	3 med	1.7	1.0	0.7
stewed, unswt, drained	¼ cup	1.6	0.9	0.7
Raisins, dried	2 tbsp	0.4	0.2	0.2
Raspberries, fresh	1 cup	3.3	0.9	2.4
Strawberries, fresh	1¼ cups	2.8	1.1	1.7

Vegetables

FOOD ITEM	SERVING SIZE	TOTAL	SOLUBLE	INSOLUBLE
Asparagus, cooked	½ cup	1.8	1.7	1.1
Bean sprouts, fresh	1 cup	1.6	0.6	1.0
Beets, flesh only, cooked	½ cup	1.8	0.8	1.0
Broccoli, cooked	½ cup	2.4	1.2	1.2
Brussel sprouts, cooked	½ cup	3.8	2.0	1.8
Cabbage, fresh	1 cup	1.5	0.6	0.9
red, cooked	½ cup	2.6	1.1	1.5

TABLE A-20. DIETARY FIBER CONTENT OF COMMON FOODS

FOOD ITEM	SERVING SIZE	TOTAL FIBER PER SERVING (g)	SOLUBLE FIBER PER SERVING (g)	INSOLUBLE FIBER PER SERVING (g)
Carrots, canned	½ cup	1.5	0.7	0.8
fresh	1 7½-in long	2.3	1.1	1.2
sliced, cooked	½ cup	2.0	1.1	0.9
Cauliflower, cooked	½ cup	1.0	0.4	0.6
Celery, fresh	1 cup chopped	1.7	0.7	1.0
Corn, whole kernel, canned	½ cup	1.6	0.2	1.4
Cucumber, fresh	1 cup	0.5	0.2	0.3
Green beans, canned	½ cup	2.0	0.5	1.5
French style, cooked	½ cup	2.8	1.1	1.7
Kale, chopped, frozen	½ cup	2.5	0.7	1.8
Lettuce iceberg	1 cup	0.5	0.1	0.4
Mushrooms, fresh	1 cup pieces	0.8	0.1	0.7
Okra, frozen, cooked	½ cup	4.1	1.0	3.1
Olives, canned	10 sml	1.0	0.1	0.9
Onion, cooked	½ cup chopped	2.0	1.1	0.9
fresh	½ cup chopped	1.7	0.9	0.8
Peas, green, canned	½ cup	3.2	0.4	2.8
green, frozen, cooked	½ cup	4.3	1.3	3.0
Pepper, green, fresh	1 cup chopped	1.7	0.7	1.0
Potato, sweet, canned	⅓ cup	0.8	0.3	0.5
sweet, flesh only, cooked	⅓ cup	2.7	1.2	1.5
Pumpkin, fresh, cooked	1 cup	1.2	0.4	0.8
Snow peas, fresh, cooked	½ cup	1.4	0.6	0.8
Spinach, cooked	½ cup	1.6	0.5	1.1
Squash, yellow, crookneck, frozen	½ cup	0.7	0.3	0.4
Tomato, canned	½ cup	1.3	0.5	0.8
fresh	1 med	1.0	0.1	0.9
sauce	⅓ cup	1.1	0.5	0.6
Turnip, cooked	½ cup	4.8	1.7	3.1
V-8 Juice	½ cup	0.7	0.2	0.5
Zucchini, sliced, cooked	½ cup	1.2	0.5	0.7

Legumes

FOOD ITEM	SERVING SIZE	TOTAL	SOLUBLE	INSOLUBLE
Black beans, cooked	½ cup	6.1	2.4	3.7
Black-eyed peas, canned	½ cup	4.7	0.5	4.2
Broad beans, no pods, cooked	½ cup	5.1	1.0	4.1
Butter beans, dried, cooked	½ cup	6.9	2.7	4.2

(continued)

TABLE A-20. DIETARY FIBER CONTENT OF COMMON FOODS

FOOD ITEM	SERVING SIZE	TOTAL FIBER PER SERVING (g)	SOLUBLE FIBER PER SERVING (g)	INSOLUBLE FIBER PER SERVING (g)
Chick peas, dried, cooked	½ cup	4.3	1.3	3.0
Garbanzo beans, canned	⅓ cup	2.8	0.3	2.5
Kidney beans, dk red, dried, cooked	½ cup	6.9	2.8	4.1
lt red, canned	½ cup	7.9	2.0	5.9
Lentils, dried, cooked	½ cup	5.2	0.6	4.6
Lima beans, canned	½ cup	4.3	1.1	3.2
Mung beans, dried, cooked	½ cup	3.3	0.7	2.6
Navy beans, dried, cooked	½ cup	6.5	2.2	4.3
Pinto beans, canned	½ cup	6.1	1.4	4.7
dried, cooked	½ cup	5.9	1.9	4.0
Split peas, dried, cooked	½ cup	3.1	1.1	2.0
White beans, Great Northern, canned	½ cup	7.2	2.2	5.0
Great Northern, dried, cooked	½ cup	5.0	1.4	3.6
Nuts and Seeds				
Almonds	6 whole	0.6	0.1	0.5
Brazil nuts	1 tbsp	0.5	0.1	0.4
Coconut, dried	1½ tbsp	1.5	0.1	1.4
fresh	2 tbsp	1.1	0.1	1.0
Hazlenuts (filberts)	1 tbsp	0.5	0.2	0.3
Peanut butter, smooth	1 tbsp	1.0	0.3	0.7
Peanuts, roasted	10 lrg	0.6	0.2	0.4
Sesame seeds	1 tbsp	0.8	0.2	0.6
Sunflower seeds	1 tbsp	0.5	0.2	0.3
Walnuts	2 whole	0.3	0.1	0.2

From the Manual of Clinical Dietetics. 5th ed. Chicago: American Dietetic Association, 1996; 847–51, with permission.

Adapted from Anderson JW. Plant Fiber in Foods. 2nd ed. HCF Nutrition Research Foundation Inc., PO Box 22124, Lexington, KY 40522, 1990.

Data from

Anderson JW, Bridges SR. Dietary fiber content of selected foods. Am J Clin Nutr 1988;47:440–447.

Food items analyzed by Anderson JW, Bridges SR, Siesel AE, 1989–1990.

Englyst HN, Bingham SA, Runswick SA, et al. Dietary fibre (non-starch polysaccharides) in fruit, vegetables, and nuts. J Hum Nutr Diet 1988;1:247–286.

Englyst HN, Bingham SA, Runswick SA, et al. Dietary fibre (non-starch polysaccharides) in cereal products. J Hum Nutr Diet 1989;2:257–276.

Ranhotra GS, Gelroth JA, Astroth K. Total and soluble fiber in selected bakery and other cereal products. Cereal Chem 1990;67:499–501.

Note: For additional information on fiber in foods, please see Marlett JA, Cheung T-F. Database and quick methods of assessing typical dietary fiber intakes using data for 228 commonly consumed foods. J Am Diet Assoc 1997; 97;1139–1148. and Marlett JA, Slavin JL. Position of the American Dietetic Association: health implications of dietary fiber. J Am Diet Assoc 1997; 97:1157–1159.

A-21. AVERAGE VALUES FOR TRIGLYCERIDES, FATTY ACIDS, AND CHOLESTEROL (INCLUDING ω-3 FATTY ACIDS)

TABLE A-21-a. AVERAGE VALUES FOR TRIGLYCERIDES, FATTY ACIDS, FATTY ACIDS (FA) (INCLUDING ω 3-FA), AND CHOLESTEROL IN SELECTED FOODS AND OILS (PER 100-g EDIBLE PORTION)[a]

FOOD NAME	FAT (g)	SFA (g)	MFA (g)	PFA (g)	M18:1 (g)	P18:2 (g)	P18:3 (g)	P:S	CHOL (mg)	S14:0 (g)	S16:0 (g)	S18:0 (g)	P20:5 (g)	P22:5 (g)	P22:6 (g)
Meats															
Liver, calf, cooked	6.90	2.56	1.49	1.09	1.28	0.61	0.08	0.43	561.00	0.00	1.40	1.16	0.00	0.00	0.00
Liver, pork, cooked	4.40	1.41	0.63	1.05	0.56	0.42	0.04	0.74	355.00	0.02	0.53	0.84	0.00	0.04	0.03
Kidney, beef, cooked	3.44	1.09	0.74	0.74	0.61	0.40	0.01	0.68	387.00	0.06	0.47	0.51	0.00	0.00	0.00
Kidney, pork, cooked	4.70	1.51	1.55	0.38	1.40	0.25	0.01	0.25	480.00	0.05	0.85	0.60	0.00	0.00	0.00
Brains, beef, cooked	12.53	2.92	2.50	1.44	2.00	0.03	0.00	0.49	2054.00	0.06	1.51	1.27	0.00	0.30	0.67
Brains, pork, cooked	9.51	2.15	1.72	1.47	1.10	0.09	0.12	0.68	2552.00	0.04	1.06	1.03	0.00	0.22	0.46
Beef, roast, chuck, trimmed, cooked	14.92	5.63	6.59	0.57	5.85	0.39	0.14	0.10	80.00	0.44	3.58	1.54	0.00	0.00	0.00
Beef, roast, chuck, untrimmed, cooked	25.98	10.52	11.16	0.90	10.04	0.61	0.27	0.09	84.00	0.85	6.45	3.07	0.00	0.00	0.00
Beef, steak, sirloin, trimmed, cooked	4.90	1.68	1.90	0.22	1.75	0.17	0.02	0.13	84.00	0.11	1.02	0.54	0.00	0.00	0.00
Beef, steak, sirloin, untrimmed, cooked	14.92	5.63	6.59	0.57	5.85	0.39	0.14	0.10	80.00	0.44	3.58	1.54	0.00	0.00	0.00
Beef, steak, tenderloin, T-bone, ribeye, trimmed, cooked	9.40	3.59	3.78	0.31	3.47	0.24	0.02	0.09	76.00	0.27	2.14	1.17	0.00	0.00	0.00
Beef, steak, tenderloin, T-bone, ribeye, untrimmed, cooked	19.76	7.82	8.31	0.71	7.49	0.48	0.19	0.09	79.00	0.63	4.79	2.31	0.00	0.00	0.00
Beef, roast, prime rib, trimmed, cooked	14.92	5.63	6.59	0.57	5.85	0.39	0.14	0.10	80.00	0.44	3.58	1.54	0.00	0.00	0.00
Beef, roast, prime rib, untrimmed, cooked	29.77	12.01	12.75	1.04	11.45	0.69	0.32	0.09	85.00	0.97	7.35	3.52	0.00	0.00	0.00
Lamb, chops, trimmed, cooked	13.31	4.76	5.83	0.87	5.40	0.71	0.08	0.18	88.00	0.42	2.56	1.64	0.00	0.00	0.00
Lamb, chop, untrimmed, cooked	29.82	12.77	12.52	2.17	11.33	1.63	0.46	0.17	97.00	1.19	6.45	4.08	0.00	0.00	0.00
Lamb, roast, leg, trimmed, cooked	9.17	3.28	4.02	0.60	3.72	0.49	0.05	0.18	92.00	0.29	1.76	1.13	0.00	0.00	0.00
Lamb, roast, leg, untrimmed, cooked	13.31	4.76	5.83	0.87	5.40	0.71	0.08	0.18	88.00	0.42	2.56	1.64	0.00	0.00	0.00
Pork, fresh, chop or roast, trimmed, cooked	10.13	3.54	4.49	0.85	4.02	0.73	0.02	0.24	83.00	0.12	2.20	1.12	0.00	0.00	0.00
Pork, fresh, chop or roast, untrimmed, cooked	15.15	5.35	6.68	1.30	6.00	1.12	0.03	0.24	81.00	0.18	3.32	1.70	0.00	0.00	0.00

FOOD NAME	FAT (g)	SFA (g)	MFA (g)	PFA (g)	M18:1 (g)	P18:2 (g)	P18:3 (g)	P:S	CHOL (mg)	S14:0 (g)	S16:0 (g)	S18:0 (g)	P20:5 (g)	P22:5 (g)	P22:6 (g)
Veal, cutlets or chop, trimmed, cooked	5.81	2.31	2.16	0.43	1.87	0.32	0.04	0.19	109.00	0.21	1.23	0.77	0.00	0.00	0.00
Veal, cutlets or chop, untrimmed, cooked	10.45	4.51	4.08	0.68	3.49	0.52	0.07	0.15	102.00	0.45	2.36	1.48	0.00	0.00	0.00
Chicken, light meat - unknown part, skin removed, cooked	4.51	1.27	1.54	0.98	1.30	0.74	0.04	0.77	85.00	0.04	0.87	0.32	0.01	0.02	0.03
Chicken, light meat - unknown part, with skin, cooked	9.97	2.80	3.92	2.12	3.23	1.83	0.08	0.76	74.00	0.08	2.07	0.56	0.01	0.02	0.03
Chicken, dark meat - unknown part, skin removed, cooked	10.50	3.28	3.04	2.91	2.48	2.43	0.12	0.89	82.00	0.07	1.90	0.89	0.00	0.04	0.06
Chicken, dark meat - unknown part, with skin, cooked	15.78	4.37	6.19	3.49	5.11	3.04	0.14	0.80	91.00	0.12	3.19	0.90	0.02	0.03	0.05
Duck, domestic, light meat, skin removed, cooked	1.18	0.38	0.21	0.31	0.17	0.21	0.01	0.82	86.00	0.01	0.17	0.12	0.00	0.01	0.01
Duck, domestic, light meat, with skin, cooked	9.97	2.80	3.92	2.12	3.23	1.83	0.08	0.76	74.00	0.08	2.07	0.56	0.01	0.02	0.03
Duck, domestic, dark meat, skin removed, cooked	4.31	1.45	0.98	1.29	0.81	1.05	0.04	0.89	112.00	0.03	0.76	0.43	0.00	0.02	0.03
Duck, domestic, dark meat, with skin, cooked	10.50	3.28	3.04	2.91	2.48	2.43	0.12	0.89	82.00	0.07	1.90	0.89	0.00	0.04	0.06
Ground beef, 5% fat (95% lean meat), cooked	6.55	2.85	2.74	0.35	2.45	0.25	0.05	0.12	76.00	0.15	1.52	1.05	0.00	0.00	0.00
Ground beef, 15% fat (85% lean meat), cooked	14.36	5.65	6.29	0.41	5.49	0.33	0.05	0.07	91.00	0.42	3.17	1.81	0.00	0.00	0.00
Ground beef, 25% fat (75% lean meat), cooked	18.21	7.01	8.04	0.43	7.00	0.36	0.04	0.06	89.00	0.56	3.98	2.17	0.00	0.00	0.00
Bologna, beef, regular	28.50	12.07	13.80	1.09	12.16	0.85	0.24	0.09	58.00	0.87	6.64	4.05	0.00	0.00	0.00
Frankfurter, all beef (Kosher), regular	29.57	11.69	14.31	1.18	12.43	1.01	0.18	0.10	53.00	0.87	6.48	3.56	0.00	0.00	0.00
Frankfurter, chicken	17.70	5.89	5.58	5.00	5.30	4.64	0.36	0.85	107.00	0.30	3.62	1.83	0.00	0.00	0.00
Frankfurter, regular, combination of meats	28.56	10.82	12.31	2.45	11.01	2.08	0.26	0.23	56.32	0.62	6.79	3.18	0.00	0.00	0.01
Ham, cured, trimmed	9.02	3.12	4.44	1.41	4.00	1.17	0.24	0.45	59.00	0.15	1.86	1.05	0.00	0.00	0.00
Ham, cured, untrimmed	15.20	5.04	7.07	1.78	6.61	1.62	0.16	0.35	62.00	0.16	3.19	1.65	0.00	0.00	0.00

(continued)

TABLE A-21-a. AVERAGE VALUES FOR TRIGLYCERIDES, FATTY ACIDS (FA) (INCLUDING ω 3-FA), AND CHOLESTEROL IN SELECTED FOODS AND OILS (PER 100g EDIBLE PORTION)ᵃ (continued)

FOOD NAME	FAT (g)	SFA (g)	MFA (g)	PFA (g)	M18:1 (g)	P18:2 (g)	P18:3 (g)	P:S	CHOL (mg)	S14:0 (g)	S16:0 (g)	S18:0 (g)	P20:5 (g)	P22:5 (g)	P22:6 (g)
Salami, hard or dry, beef and pork	34.39	12.20	17.10	3.21	15.40	2.87	0.33	0.26	79.00	0.51	7.60	4.00	0.00	0.00	0.00
Bacon, regular cut, cooked	49.24	17.42	23.69	5.81	21.96	4.89	0.79	0.33	85.00	0.62	10.98	5.67	0.00	0.00	0.00
Fish															
Cod, cooked	1.53	0.36	0.28	0.65	0.15	0.01	0.02	1.78	68.00	0.06	0.23	0.06	0.24	0.05	0.26
Trout, brook, cooked	4.86	1.43	1.38	0.92	0.20	0.09	0.00	0.64	63.00	0.06	0.29	0.10	0.18	0.09	0.15
Trout, rainbow, cooked	6.32	1.80	2.14	1.81	1.10	0.11	0.12	1.00	73.00	0.20	1.16	0.44	0.29	0.10	0.95
Trout, speckled, cooked	1.53	0.36	0.28	0.65	0.15	0.01	0.02	1.78	68.00	0.06	0.23	0.06	0.24	0.05	0.26
Trout, lake, cooked	8.47	1.47	4.17	1.92	1.85	0.22	0.20	1.30	74.00	0.24	1.05	0.19	0.26	0.24	0.68
Salmon, sockeye, cooked	10.97	1.92	5.29	2.41	1.34	0.11	0.06	1.26	87.00	0.26	1.01	0.16	0.53	0.13	0.70
Herring, smoked/kippered, canned and drained	12.37	2.79	5.11	2.92	2.07	0.18	0.14	1.05	82.00	0.76	1.85	0.15	0.97	0.08	1.18
Salmon, canned, drained, with salt	6.05	1.54	1.81	2.05	1.07	0.06	0.06	1.33	55.00	0.05	1.35	0.14	0.85	0.05	0.81
Sardines, canned in oil, drained	11.45	1.53	3.87	5.15	2.15	3.54	0.50	3.37	142.00	0.19	0.99	0.34	0.47	0.00	0.51
Tuna, canned, oil pack, regular, drained	8.21	1.53	2.95	2.89	2.84	2.68	0.07	1.88	18.00	0.03	1.42	0.09	0.03	0.00	0.10
Tuna, canned, water pack, regular, drained, not rinsed	0.82	0.23	0.16	0.34	0.09	0.01	0.00	1.44	30.00	0.02	0.16	0.06	0.05	0.01	0.22
Clams and mussels, cooked from fresh or frozen	1.95	0.19	0.17	0.55	0.07	0.03	0.01	2.94	67.00	0.03	0.12	0.04	0.14	0.10	0.15
Crab, hard-shell, Alaskan King, cooked	1.77	0.23	0.28	0.68	0.15	0.03	0.02	2.98	100.00	0.02	0.14	0.06	0.24	0.05	0.23
Lobster, cooked	0.59	0.11	0.16	0.09	0.10	0.01	0.00	0.85	72.00	0.01	0.08	0.02	0.05	0.00	0.03
Oyster, Pacific, cooked	4.60	1.02	0.78	1.79	0.38	0.06	0.06	1.75	100.00	0.16	0.71	0.14	0.88	0.04	0.50
Scallops, cooked	1.40	0.15	0.07	0.48	0.03	0.01	0.00	3.29	53.00	0.02	0.10	0.02	0.17	0.03	0.20
Shrimp, cooked	1.08	0.29	0.20	0.44	0.11	0.02	0.01	1.52	195.00	0.02	0.14	0.10	0.17	0.02	0.14
Caviar	17.90	4.78	4.63	7.41	3.17	0.08	0.02	1.55	588.00	0.21	3.56	0.29	2.74	0.23	3.80
Eggs/Dairy															
Eggs, whole, cooked	10.61	3.27	4.08	1.41	3.73	1.19	0.04	0.43	424.00	0.04	2.35	0.83	0.01	0.00	0.04
Eggs, yolk only, cooked	30.87	9.55	11.74	4.20	10.70	3.54	0.10	0.44	1281.00	0.10	6.86	2.42	0.01	0.00	0.11
Eggs, white only, cooked	0.00	0.00	0.00	0.00	0.00	0.00	0.00	0.00	0.00	0.00	0.00	0.00	0.00	0.00	0.00

FOOD NAME	FAT (g)	SFA (g)	MFA (g)	PFA (g)	M18:1 (g)	P18:2 (g)	P18:3 (g)	P:S	CHOL (mg)	S14:0 (g)	S16:0 (g)	S18:0 (g)	P20:5 (g)	P22:5 (g)	P22:6 (g)
Cream substitute, liquid, regular	7.13	1.65	4.32	1.17	4.32	1.14	0.03	0.71	0.00	0.03	0.86	0.75	0.00	0.00	0.00
Cream substitute, liquid, reduced fat or light	3.50	0.90	2.03	0.42	2.03	0.40	0.02	0.47	0.00	0.02	0.46	0.42	0.00	0.00	0.00
Cream substitute, powder, regular	35.48	32.53	0.97	0.01	0.97	0.00	0.01	0.00	0.00	5.99	3.75	6.34	0.00	0.00	0.00
Cream substitute, powder, reduced fat or light	15.70	3.80	11.50	0.20	11.50	0.20	0.00	0.05	0.00	0.00	1.12	2.69	0.00	0.00	0.00
Cream, half and half, 10–12% fat	11.50	7.16	3.32	0.43	2.89	0.26	0.17	0.06	37.00	1.16	3.03	1.39	0.00	0.00	0.00
Cream, light/coffee cream, 20% fat	19.31	12.02	5.58	0.72	4.86	0.44	0.28	0.06	66.00	1.94	5.08	2.34	0.00	0.00	0.00
Milk, buttermilk, 1% fat	0.88	0.55	0.25	0.03	0.22	0.02	0.01	0.06	4.00	0.09	0.23	0.11	0.00	0.00	0.00
Milk, skim	0.18	0.12	0.05	0.01	0.04	0.01	0.00	0.06	2.00	0.02	0.05	0.02	0.00	0.00	0.00
Milk, 1% fat	1.06	0.66	0.31	0.04	0.27	0.02	0.02	0.06	4.00	0.11	0.28	0.13	0.00	0.00	0.00
Milk, 2% fat	1.97	0.96	0.84	0.07	0.39	0.04	0.01	0.07	8.00	0.13	0.43	0.19	0.00	0.00	0.00
Milk, whole, 3.5 to 4% fat	3.34	2.08	0.97	0.12	0.84	0.08	0.05	0.06	14.00	0.34	0.88	0.41	0.00	0.00	0.00
American cheese, processed	31.25	19.69	8.95	0.99	7.51	0.61	0.38	0.05	94.00	3.21	9.10	3.80	0.00	0.00	0.00
American cheese, processed, reduced fat	14.10	8.85	4.13	0.41	3.47	0.27	0.15	0.05	53.00	1.45	3.93	1.61	0.00	0.00	0.00
Brie cheese	27.68	17.41	8.01	0.83	6.56	0.51	0.31	0.05	100.00	3.07	8.25	2.88	0.00	0.00	0.00
Cheddar cheese, natural	33.14	21.09	9.39	0.94	7.91	0.58	0.37	0.04	105.00	3.33	9.80	4.01	0.00	0.00	0.00
Cheddar cheese, reduced fat	7.00	4.34	2.08	0.22	1.85	0.16	0.07	0.05	21.00	0.89	1.98	0.87	0.00	0.00	0.00
Cottage cheese, regular or creamed, 4% fat	4.51	2.85	1.29	0.14	1.06	0.10	0.04	0.05	15.00	0.47	1.36	0.52	0.00	0.00	0.00
Cottage cheese, lowfat, 2% fat	1.93	1.22	0.55	0.06	0.45	0.04	0.02	0.05	8.00	0.20	0.58	0.22	0.00	0.00	0.00
Cottage cheese, 1% fat	1.02	0.65	0.29	0.03	0.24	0.02	0.01	0.05	4.00	0.11	0.31	0.12	0.00	0.00	0.00
Cream cheese, Neufchatel	23.43	14.80	6.77	0.65	5.66	0.45	0.20	0.04	76.00	2.35	6.88	2.99	0.00	0.00	0.00
Cream cheese, regular	34.87	21.97	9.84	1.27	8.38	0.77	0.49	0.06	110.00	3.60	10.54	4.05	0.00	0.00	0.00
Monterey Jack cheese, natural	30.28	19.07	8.75	0.90	7.37	0.64	0.26	0.05	89.00	3.61	7.76	3.42	0.00	0.00	0.00
Mozzarella cheese, part skim milk	20.03	12.67	5.73	0.63	5.15	0.45	0.18	0.05	54.00	2.12	6.45	2.57	0.00	0.00	0.00
Parmesan cheese, dry	30.02	19.07	8.73	0.66	7.74	0.32	0.35	0.03	79.00	3.38	8.10	2.68	0.00	0.00	0.00

(continued)

TABLE A-21-a. AVERAGE VALUES FOR TRIGLYCERIDES, FATTY ACIDS (FA) (INCLUDING ω 3-FA), AND CHOLESTEROL IN SELECTED FOODS AND OILS (PER 100g EDIBLE PORTION)[a] (continued)

FOOD NAME	FAT (g)	SFA (g)	MFA (g)	PFA (g)	M18:1 (g)	P18:2 (g)	P18:3 (g)	P:S	CHOL (mg)	S14:0 (g)	S16:0 (g)	S18:0 (g)	P20:5 (g)	P22:5 (g)	P22:6 (g)
Swiss cheese, natural	27.45	17.78	7.27	0.97	6.02	0.62	0.35	0.05	92.00	3.06	7.79	3.25	0.00	0.00	0.00
Swiss cheese, reduced fat	5.10	3.30	1.35	0.18	1.12	0.12	0.07	0.05	35.00	0.57	1.45	0.60	0.00	0.00	0.00
Sour cream, regular	19.31	12.02	5.58	0.72	4.86	0.44	0.28	0.06	66.00	1.94	5.08	2.34	0.00	0.00	0.00
Sour cream, reduced fat	12.00	7.47	3.47	0.45	3.02	0.27	0.18	0.06	39.00	1.21	3.16	1.45	0.00	0.00	0.00
Sour cream, lowfat	6.45	4.02	1.86	0.24	1.62	0.15	0.09	0.06	32.26	0.65	1.70	0.78	0.00	0.00	0.00
Yogurt, frozen, fruit or vanilla, whole milk 3–4% fat	3.60	2.33	0.99	0.10	0.82	0.07	0.03	0.04	13.00	0.38	0.99	0.36	0.00	0.00	0.00
Yogurt, frozen, fruit or vanilla, lowfat, 1–2% fat	1.89	1.20	0.53	0.06	0.45	0.04	0.02	0.05	7.41	0.20	0.51	0.20	0.00	0.00	0.00
Yogurt, plain, lowfat, 1–2% fat	1.55	1.00	0.43	0.04	0.35	0.03	0.01	0.04	6.00	0.16	0.42	0.15	0.00	0.00	0.00
Yogurt, fruit, nonfat, <1% fat	0.20	0.12	0.05	0.02	0.04	0.01	0.01	0.13	2.00	0.02	0.06	0.02	0.00	0.00	0.00
Yogurt, fruit, whole milk, 3–4% fat	3.24	1.98	0.91	0.13	0.80	0.10	0.05	0.07	9.74	0.32	0.84	0.37	0.00	0.00	0.00
Ice cream, regular, 11% fat, except chocolate	11.00	6.79	2.97	0.45	2.76	0.27	0.17	0.07	44.00	1.13	3.06	1.32	0.00	0.00	0.00
Ice cream, light, 7% fat, except chocolate	7.48	4.69	1.91	0.30	1.79	0.19	0.12	0.06	34.50	0.77	2.09	0.91	0.00	0.00	0.00
Ice cream, light, 4% fat, except chocolate	3.96	2.59	0.86	0.16	0.82	0.10	0.06	0.06	25.00	0.42	1.12	0.51	0.00	0.00	0.00
Sherbet, plain, regular	2.00	1.16	0.53	0.08	0.49	0.05	0.03	0.07	6.00	0.20	0.51	0.23	0.00	0.00	0.00
Fats/Oils															
Oil, canola	100.00	7.10	58.90	29.60	56.10	20.30	9.30	4.17	0.00	0.00	4.00	1.80	0.00	0.00	0.00
Oil, corn	100.00	12.70	24.20	58.70	24.20	58.00	0.70	4.62	0.00	0.00	10.90	1.80	0.00	0.00	0.00
Oil, sunflower	100.00	10.30	19.50	65.70	19.50	65.70	0.00	6.38	0.00	0.00	5.90	4.50	0.00	0.00	0.00
Oil, cottonseed	100.00	25.90	17.80	51.90	17.00	51.50	0.20	2.00	0.00	0.80	22.70	2.30	0.00	0.00	0.00
Oil, safflower	100.00	6.20	14.36	74.62	14.36	74.62	0.00	12.03	0.00	0.00	4.29	1.92	0.00	0.00	0.00
Oil, sesame	100.00	14.20	39.70	41.70	39.30	41.30	0.30	2.94	0.00	0.00	8.90	4.80	0.00	0.00	0.00
Oil, soybean (partially hydrogenated)	100.00	14.90	43.00	37.60	42.50	34.90	2.60	2.52	0.00	0.10	9.80	5.00	0.00	0.00	0.00
Oil, olive	100.00	13.45	73.90	10.00	72.29	9.21	0.79	0.74	0.00	0.00	10.93	1.98	0.00	0.00	0.00
Oil, peanut	100.00	16.90	46.20	32.00	44.80	32.00	0.00	1.89	0.00	0.10	9.50	2.20	0.00	0.00	0.00
Oil, coconut	100.00	86.50	5.80	1.80	5.80	1.80	0.00	0.02	0.00	16.80	8.20	2.80	0.00	0.00	0.00
Oil, palm	100.00	49.30	37.00	9.30	36.60	9.10	0.20	0.19	0.00	1.00	43.50	4.30	0.00	0.00	0.00

FOOD NAME	FAT (g)	SFA (g)	MFA (g)	PFA (g)	M18:1 (g)	P18:2 (g)	P18:3 (g)	P:S	CHOL (mg)	S14:0 (g)	S16:0 (g)	S18:0 (g)	P20:5 (g)	P22:5 (g)	P22:6 (g)
Oil, palm kernel	100.00	81.50	11.40	1.60	11.40	1.60	0.00	0.02	0.00	16.40	8.10	2.80	0.00	0.00	0.00
Shortening, vegetable	100.00	25.00	44.50	26.10	44.50	24.50	1.60	1.04	0.00	0.40	14.10	10.60	0.00	0.00	0.00
Margarine, regular, stick, salted, soybean oil	80.50	16.70	39.30	20.90	39.10	19.40	1.50	1.25	0.00	0.20	9.60	6.90	0.00	0.00	0.00
Margarine, spread, soybean oil	52.00	7.23	26.66	15.82	26.66	13.33	2.49	2.19	0.00	0.00	5.14	2.04	0.00	0.00	0.00
Margarine, diet, soybean oil	38.80	6.81	17.59	12.95	17.59	12.51	0.43	1.90	0.00	0.05	4.16	2.27	0.00	0.00	0.00
Lard	100.00	39.20	45.10	11.20	41.20	10.20	1.00	0.29	95.00	1.30	23.80	13.50	0.00	0.00	0.00
Butter, regular, salted	81.11	40.84	33.35	2.87	15.87	1.72	0.25	0.07	215.00	5.91	17.25	7.95	0.00	0.00	0.00
Oil, medium chain triglyceride	100.00	94.50	0.00	0.00	0.00	0.00	0.00	0.00	0.00	0.00	0.00	0.00	0.00	0.00	0.00
Mayonnaise, regular, commercial	79.40	11.80	22.70	41.30	22.50	37.10	4.20	3.50	59.00	0.10	8.50	3.10	0.00	0.00	0.00
Mayonnaise, low fat	33.09	5.21	8.07	17.95	8.02	16.04	1.92	3.45	35.00	0.03	3.48	1.39	0.00	0.00	0.00
Mayonnaise type dressing, regular	48.90	7.23	11.57	27.74	11.29	24.42	3.25	3.84	43.00	0.05	5.17	1.91	0.00	0.00	0.00
Mayonnaise type dressing, low fat	19.20	3.30	4.50	10.60	4.50	9.00	1.60	3.21	24.00	0.00	2.40	0.90	0.00	0.00	0.00
Salad dressing, French, regular	31.30	4.51	7.28	18.10	7.13	15.95	2.12	4.02	0.00	0.03	3.22	1.19	0.00	0.00	0.00
Salad dressing, Italian, regular	41.90	3.09	24.59	12.33	23.41	8.47	3.86	3.99	16.14	0.01	1.76	0.78	0.00	0.00	0.00
Salad dressing, ranch, regular	51.39	8.02	11.39	28.33	10.99	25.27	3.04	3.53	33.00	0.05	5.32	2.25	0.00	0.00	0.00
Salad dressing, 1000 island, regular	33.23	5.86	7.90	17.96	7.67	15.80	2.12	3.07	18.20	0.27	3.80	1.38	0.00	0.00	0.00
Salad dressing, French, reduced calorie	13.00	1.87	3.03	7.53	2.96	6.63	0.88	4.02	0.00	0.01	1.34	0.49	0.00	0.00	0.00
Salad dressing, Italian, reduced calorie	20.00	3.06	4.66	11.58	4.56	10.20	1.36	3.79	0.00	0.02	2.06	0.76	0.00	0.00	0.00
Salad dressing, ranch, reduced calorie	17.30	1.33	5.42	4.33	5.29	3.68	0.66	3.26	21.00	0.02	0.84	0.37	0.00	0.00	0.00
Salad dressing, 1000 island, reduced calorie	13.00	1.87	3.03	7.53	2.96	6.63	0.88	4.02	0.00	0.01	1.34	0.49	0.00	0.00	0.00
Miscellaneous															
Almonds, roasted, salted	55.17	4.21	34.79	13.52	34.58	13.52	0.00	3.21	0.00	0.00	3.30	0.91	0.00	0.00	0.00
Cashews, roasted, salted	47.77	8.48	25.92	8.55	25.62	8.48	0.07	1.01	0.00	0.02	4.27	3.51	0.00	0.00	0.00

(continued)

TABLE A-21-a. AVERAGE VALUES FOR TRIGLYCERIDES, FATTY ACIDS (FA) (INCLUDING ω 3-FA), AND CHOLESTEROL IN SELECTED FOODS AND OILS (PER 100g EDIBLE PORTION)[a] (continued)

FOOD NAME	FAT (g)	SFA (g)	MFA (g)	PFA (g)	M18:1 (g)	P18:2 (g)	P18:3 (g)	P:S	CHOL (mg)	S14:0 (g)	S16:0 (g)	S18:0 (g)	P20:5 (g)	P22:5 (g)	P22:6 (g)
Peanuts, roasted, salted	49.30	6.84	24.46	15.58	23.79	15.58	0.00	2.28	0.00	0.03	5.16	1.10	0.00	0.00	0.00
Walnuts	65.21	6.13	8.93	47.17	8.80	38.09	9.08	7.70	0.00	0.00	4.40	1.66	0.00	0.00	0.00
Peanut butter, regular, creamy or chunky	51.03	10.34	24.28	13.79	23.84	13.71	0.08	1.33	0.00	0.22	5.71	2.69	0.00	0.00	0.00
Olives, black	10.68	1.42	7.89	0.91	7.77	0.85	0.06	0.64	0.00	0.00	1.18	0.24	0.00	0.00	0.00
Candy bar or chips, dark chocolate, sweet or semi-sweet	30.00	17.75	9.97	0.97	9.89	0.91	0.06	0.05	0.00	0.15	7.72	9.47	0.00	0.00	0.00
Avocado	15.32	2.44	9.61	1.96	8.97	1.84	0.11	0.80	0.00	0.00	2.40	0.03	0.00	0.00	0.00
Coconut, fresh	33.49	29.70	1.43	0.37	1.43	0.37	0.00	0.01	0.00	5.87	2.84	1.73	0.00	0.00	0.00
Soybeans, cooked from dried	8.97	1.30	1.98	5.06	1.96	4.47	0.60	3.90	0.00	0.03	0.95	0.32	0.00	0.00	0.00
Peas, black-eyed, cooked from dried	0.53	0.14	0.04	0.23	0.04	0.14	0.08	1.63	0.00	0.00	0.11	0.02	0.00	0.00	0.00
Split peas, yellow or green, cooked from dried	0.39	0.05	0.08	0.17	0.08	0.14	0.03	3.06	0.00	0.00	0.04	0.01	0.00	0.00	0.00

[a] SFA, saturated fatty acid; MFA, monounsaturated fatty acid; PFA, polyunsaturated fatty acid; M18:1, oleic acid; P18:2, linoleic acid; 18:3, linolenic acid; S14:0, myristic acid; S16:0, palmitic acid; S18:0, stearic acid; P20:5, omega-3 (eicosapentaenoic acid); P22:5, omega-3 (docosapentaenoic acid); P22:6, omega-3 (docosahexaenoic acid).

Data from the Nutrition Data System for Research (NDS-R) version 5.0_35, 2004, with permission. Table compiled and prepared by the Nutrition Coordinating Center, University of Minnesota, Minneapolis, MN.

TABLE A-21-b. AVERAGE VALUES FOR TRIGLYCERIDES, FATTY ACIDS (FA) (INCLUDING ω-3 FATTY ACIDS[a], AND CHOLESTEROL OF MARINE FOODS AND OILS

FISH (100 g)	FAT (g)	CHOL (mg)	SFA (g)	MFA (g)	PFA (g)	M18:1 (g)	P18:2 (g)	P18:3 (g)	P20:5 (g)	P22:5 (g)	P22:6 (g)
Anchovy, European, raw	4.84	60.00	1.28	1.18	1.64	0.62	0.10	0.00	0.54	0.03	0.91
Bass, striped, raw	2.33	80.00	0.51	0.66	0.78	0.45	0.02	0.02	0.17	0.00	0.58
Bluefish, raw	4.24	59.00	0.92	1.79	1.06	0.68	0.06	0.00	0.25	0.06	0.52
Burbot, raw	0.81	60.00	0.16	0.13	0.30	0.10	0.01	—[b]	0.07	0.03	0.10
Carp, raw	5.60	66.00	1.08	2.33	1.43	1.15	0.52	0.27	0.24	0.08	0.11
Catfish, wild, raw	2.82	58.00	0.72	0.84	0.86	0.59	0.10	0.07	0.13	0.10	0.23
Catfish, farmed, raw	7.59	47.00	1.77	3.59	1.57	3.17	0.88	0.10	0.07	0.09	0.21
Cod, Atlantic, raw	0.67	43.00	0.13	0.09	0.23	0.06	trace[c]	trace[c]	0.06	0.01	0.12
Eel, all varieties, raw	11.66	126.00	2.36	7.19	0.95	2.77	0.20	0.43	0.08	0.07	0.06
Flounder, unspecified, raw	1.19	48.00	0.28	0.23	0.33	0.12	0.01	0.01	0.09	0.05	0.11
Haddock, raw	0.72	57.00	0.13	0.12	0.24	0.07	0.01	trace[c]	0.06	0.02	0.13
Halibut, raw	2.29	32.00	0.32	0.75	0.73	0.36	0.03	0.06	0.07	0.09	0.29
Herring, Atlantic, raw	9.04	60.00	2.04	3.74	2.13	1.52	0.13	0.10	0.71	0.06	0.86
Mackerel, Atlantic, raw	13.89	70.00	3.26	5.46	3.35	2.28	0.22	0.16	0.90	0.21	1.40
Mussel, blue, raw	2.24	28.00	0.42	0.51	0.61	0.20	0.02	0.02	0.19	0.02	0.25
Octopus, raw	1.04	48.00	0.23	0.16	0.24	0.06	0.01	0.00	0.08	0.01	0.08
Oyster, Eastern, wild, raw	2.46	53.00	0.77	0.31	0.97	0.12	0.06	0.05	0.27	0.06	0.29
Oyster, Eastern, farmed, raw	1.55	25.00	0.44	0.15	0.59	0.07	0.03	0.04	0.19	—[b]	0.20
Perch, all varieties, raw	0.92	90.00	0.18	0.15	0.37	0.07	0.01	0.01	0.08	0.03	0.17
Pike, walleye, raw	1.22	86.00	0.25	0.29	0.45	0.20	0.03	0.01	0.09	0.04	0.22
Pollock, Atlantic, raw	0.98	71.00	0.14	0.11	0.48	0.07	0.01	0.00	0.07	0.02	0.35
Sablefish, raw	15.30	49.00	3.20	8.06	2.04	4.07	0.16	0.10	0.68	0.17	0.72
Salmon, Chinook, raw	10.43	50.00	3.10	4.40	2.80	2.96	0.12	0.09	1.01	0.30	0.94
Salmon, coho, wild, raw	5.93	45.00	1.26	2.13	1.99	1.20	0.21	0.16	0.43	0.23	0.66
Salmon, coho, farmed, raw	7.67	51.00	1.82	3.33	1.86	1.72	0.35	0.08	0.38	—[b]	0.82
Sea bass, all varieties, raw	2.00	41.00	0.51	0.42	0.74	0.29	0.02	0.00	0.16	0.08	0.43
Smelt, rainbow, raw	2.42	70.00	0.45	0.64	0.88	0.41	0.04	0.05	0.28	0.02	0.42
Squid, all varieties, raw	1.38	233.00	0.36	0.11	0.52	0.05	trace[c]	trace[c]	0.15	trace[c]	0.34
Red snapper, all varieties, raw	1.34	37.00	0.28	0.25	0.46	0.16	0.02	trace[c]	0.05	0.06	0.26
Sole, raw	1.19	48.00	0.28	0.23	0.33	0.12	0.01	0.01	0.09	0.05	0.11
Sturgeon, all varieties, raw	4.04	60.00	0.92	1.94	0.69	1.43	0.07	0.10	0.19	0.04	0.09
Swordfish, raw	4.01	39.00	1.10	1.54	0.92	1.09	0.03	0.19	0.11	0.00	0.53
Trout, rainbow, wild, raw	3.46	59.00	0.72	1.13	1.24	0.61	0.24	0.12	0.17	0.11	0.42
Trout, rainbow, farmed, raw	5.40	59.00	1.55	1.54	1.80	1.06	0.71	0.06	0.26	0.00	0.67
Tuna, bluefin, fresh, raw	4.90	38.00	1.26	1.60	1.43	0.92	0.05	0.00	0.28	0.12	0.89
Whitefish, all varieties, raw	5.86	60.00	0.91	2.00	2.15	1.35	0.27	0.18	0.32	0.16	0.94
Cod liver oil	100.00	570.00	22.61	46.71	22.54	20.65	0.94	0.94	6.90	0.94	10.97
Herring oil	100.00	766.00	21.29	56.56	15.60	11.96	1.15	0.76	6.27	0.62	4.21
Menhaden oil	100.00	521.00	30.43	26.69	34.20	14.53	2.15	1.49	13.17	4.92	8.56
Salmon oil	100.00	485.00	19.87	29.04	40.32	16.98	1.54	1.06	13.02	2.99	18.23

[a] CHOL, cholesterol; SFA, saturated fatty acid; MFA, monounsaturated fatty acid; PFA, polyunsaturated fatty acid; M18:1, oleic acid; P18:2, linoleic acid; P18:3, linolenic acid; P20:5, eicosapentaenoic acid (EPA); P22:5, docosapentaenoic acid (DPA); P22:6 docosahexaenoic acid (DHA). The omega-3 fatty acids are P20:5, P22:5, and P22:6.

[b] Denotes lack of reliable data for nutrient.

[c] Trace is ≤0.005 g/100 g food.

Data from U.S. Department of Agriculture, Agricultural Research Service. 2004. USDA National Nutrient Database for Standard Reference, Release 17. Compiled by the Nutrition Coordinating Center, University of Minnesota, Minneapolis, MN, 2004.

TABLE A-21-c. NAMES, CODES, AND FORMULAS OF VARIOUS FATTY ACIDS

COMMON NAME	GENEVA NOMENCLATURE	CODE	FORMULA[a]
Short-chain saturated fatty acids			
butyric acid	butanoic acid	C4:0	$CH_3(CH_2)_2COOH$
Medium-chain saturated fatty acids			
caproic acid	hexanoic acid	C6:0	$CH_3(CH_2)_4COOH$
caprylic acid	octanoic acid	C8:0	$CH_3(CH_2)_6COOH$
caprio acid	decanoic acid	C10:0	$CH_3(CH_2)_8COOH$
lauric acid	dodecanoic acid	C12:0	$CH_3(CH_2)_{10}COOH$
Long-chain fatty acids			
myristic acid	tetradecanoic acid	C14:0	$CH_3(CH_2)_{12}COOH$
palmitic acid	hexadecanoic acid	C16:0	$CH_3(CH_2)_{14}COOH$
stearic acid	octadecanoic acid	C18:0	$CH_3(CH_2)_{16}COOH$
palmitoleic acid	9-hexadecaenoic acid	C16:1, n-7 *cis*	$CH_3(CH_2)_5CH=©CH(CH_2)_7COOH$
oleic acid	9-octadecaenoic acid	C18:1, n-9 *cis*	$CH_3(CH_2)_7CH=©CH(CH_2)_7COOH$
elaidic acid	9-octadecaenoic acid	C18:1, n-9 *trans*	$CH_3(CH_2)_7CH=©CH(CH_2)_7COOH$
linoleic acid	9, 12-octadecadienoic acid	C18:2, n-6, 9 all *cis*	$CH_3(CH_2)_4CH=©CHCH_2CH=©CH(CH_2)_7COOH$
α-linolenic acid	9, 12, 15-octadecatrienoic acid	C18:3, n-3, 6, 9 all *cis*	$CH_3CH_2CH=©CHCH_2CH=©CHCH_2CH=©CH(CH_2)_7COOH$
γ-linolenic acid	6, 9, 12-octadecatrienoic acid	C18:3, n-6, 9, 12 all *cis*	$CH_3(CH_2)_4CH=©CHCH_2CH=©CHCH_2CH=©CH(CH_2)_4COOH$
columbinic acid	5, 9, 12-octatrienoic acid	C18: n-6, cis, 9 cis, 13 *trans*	$CH_3(CH_2)_4CH=©CHCH_2CH=©CHCH_2CH_2CH=tCH(CH_2)_3COOH$
Very long chain fatty acids			
arachidic acid	eicosanoic acid	C20:0	$CH_3(CH_2)_{18}COOH$
behenic acid	docosanoic acid	C22:0	$CH_3(CH_2)_{20}COOH$
eicosenoic acid	11-eicosenoic acid	C20:1, n-9 *cis*	$CH_3(CH_2)_7CH=©CH(CH_2)_9COOH$
erucic acid	13-docosaenoic acid	C22:1, n-9 *cis*	$CH_3(CH_2)_7CH=©CH(CH_2)_{11}COOH$
brassidic acid	13-docosaenoic acid	C22:1, n-9 *trans*	$CH_3(CH_2)_7CH=tCH(CH_2)_{11}COOH$
cetoleic acid	11-docosaenoic acid	C22:1, n-11 *cis*	$CH_3(CH_2)_9CH=©CH(CH_2)_9COOH$
nervonic acid	15-tetracosaenoic acid	C24:1, n-9 *cis*	$CH_3(CH_2)_7CH=©CH(CH_2)_{13}COOH$
"Mead" acid	5, 8, 11-eicosatrienoic acid	C20:3, n-9, 12, 15 all *cis*	$CH_3(CH_2)_7CH=©CHCH_2CH=©CHCH_2CH=©CH(CH_2)_3COOH$
dihomo-γ-linolenic acid	8, 11, 14-eicosatrienoic acid	C20:3, n-6, 9, 12 all *cis*	$CH_3(CH_2)_4CH=©CHCH_2CH=©CHCH_2CH=©CH(CH_2)_6COOH$
arachidonic acid	5, 8, 11, 14-eicosatetraenoic acid	C20:4, n-6, 9, 12, 15 all *cis*	$CH_3(CH_2)_4CH=©CHCH_2CH=©CHCH_2CH=©CHCH_2CH=©CH(CH_2)_3COOH$
timnodonic acid	5, 8, 11, 14, 17-eicosapentaenoic acid	C20:5, n-3, 6, 9, 12, 15 all cis	$CH_3(CH_2CH=©CH)_5(CH_2)_3COOH$
clupanodonic acid	7, 10, 13, 16, 19-docosapentaenoic acid	C22:5, n-3, 6, 9, 12, 15 all *cis*	$CH_3(CH_2CH=©CH)_5(CH_2)_5COOH$
docosahexaeonic acid	4, 7, 10, 13, 16, 19-docosahexaenoic acid	C22:6, n-3, 6, 9, 12, 15, 18 all cis	$CH_3(CH_2CH=©CH)_6(CH_2)_2COOH$

[a] t, trans; ©, cis.

TABLE A-21-d. AVERAGE VALUES FOR TOTAL FAT, TOTAL TRANS FATTY ACIDS, AND TOTAL SATURATED FATTY ACIDS PER SERVING PORTION

FOOD NAME	SERVING PORTION	TOTAL FAT (g)	TFA (g)	SFA (g)
Animal products				
Ground beef, 25% fat (75% lean meat), cooked	1.0 oz	5.16	0.37	1.99
Chicken, dark meat, skin eaten, cooked	1.0 oz	4.47	0.10	1.24
Chicken, light meat, skin eaten, cooked	1.0 oz	2.83	0.06	0.79
Frankfurters, regular (combination of meats)	1.0 each - 10 per lb	12.85	0.32	4.87
Milk, whole	1.0 cup	8.15	0.24	5.07
Yogurt, lowfat (1–2% fat)	6.0 oz	1.84	0.05	1.19
Cheddar cheese, natural	1.0 oz	9.40	0.22	5.98
American cheese, processed	1.0 oz	8.86	0.22	5.58
Bread, Cookies, Crackers				
Bread, white	1.0 slice	0.90	0.16	0.13
Bread, whole wheat	1.0 slice	1.19	0.21	0.26
Italian bread	1.0 slice	0.70	0.14	0.17
Roll, dinner, white	1.0 medium	2.63	0.15	0.63
Roll, dinner, whole wheat	1.0 medium	1.51	0.27	0.33
Roll, hamburger or hot dog	1.0 medium	2.19	0.30	0.52
Taco shell	1 each - 5" diameter	3.01	0.90	0.43
Tortilla, flour, commercial type	1 each - 8" Diameter	3.05	0.48	0.75
Bagel, plain	1.0 medium	0.91	0.00	0.13
Muffin, plain, from commercial mix	1.0 medium	5.53	1.14	1.39
English muffin, white	1.0 each	1.03	0.00	0.15
Crackers, graham, plain	1.0 rectangle (2 squares)	1.31	0.38	0.32
Crackers, saltines	1.0 each	0.43	0.11	0.10
Crackers, whole wheat	1.0 each	0.56	0.17	0.16
Cake, prepared from mix, pudding type - added oil	1.0 cube (3" L × 3" W × 1.5" H)	10.05	0.42	2.04
Cookies sugar, bakery	1.0 each - 3" diameter	4.23	1.21	1.05
Cookies, chocolate chip, bakery	1.0 each - 2 1/4" diameter	4.22	0.63	1.52
Cookies, chocolate sandwich, commercial	1.0 medium	2.13	0.57	0.59
Doughnut, commercial cake	1.0 medium	10.79	2.44	2.47
Doughnut, commercial yeast	1.0 medium	13.67	2.60	3.26
Fats				
Butter, regular	1.0 tsp	3.84	0.23	1.93
Margarine, regular, stick, soybean oil	1.0 tsp	3.80	1.22	0.79
Margarine, spread, 75% fat, soybean oil	1.0 tsp	3.58	0.36	0.61
Margarine, liquid, regular	1.0 tsp	3.81	0.55	0.62
Shortening, vegetable, soybean/cottonseed	1.0 tsp	4.27	0.73	1.07
Oil, corn	1.0 tsp	4.54	0.01	0.58
Oil, olive	1.0 tsp	4.50	0.01	0.61
Mayonnaise, real, regular, commercial	1.0 tsp	3.64	0.00	054

Data from the Nutrition Data System for Research (NDS-R) version 5.0_35, 2004, with permission. Table compiled and prepared by the Nutrition Coordinating Center, University of Minnesota, Minneapolis, MN.

A-22. PROTEIN AND MINERALS IN SELECTED COMMON FOODS

TABLE A-22-a. PROTEIN, SODIUM, POTASSIUM, CALCIUM, PHOSPHORUS, AND MAGNESIUM CONTENT OF SELECTED COMMON FOODS PER SERVING PORTION

FOOD NAME	SERVING PORTION	PRO (g)	Na (mg)	K (mg)	Ca (mg)	P (mg)	Mg (mg)
Dairy products							
Eggs, whole, hard boiled	1.0 large	6.29	62.00	63.00	25.00	86.00	5.00
Cheese, cottage, uncreamed	1.0 oz	4.90	3.69	9.07	9.07	29.48	1.13
Cream, coffee/table, light (20% fat)	1.0 tbsp	0.41	6.00	18.30	14.40	12.00	1.35
Cream, sour, cultured	1.0 tbsp	0.39	5.75	17.54	13.80	11.50	1.29
Cream, sour, lowfat	1.0 tbsp	1.00	15.04	35.00	20.00	20.00	5.36
Cream, sour, nonfat/fat free	1.0 tbsp	0.47	21.15	19.35	18.75	14.25	1.50
Milk, buttermilk, fluid	1.0 cup	8.11	257.25	369.95	284.20	218.05	26.95
Milk, whole, 3.5–4% fat, fluid	1.0 cup	8.03	119.56	370.88	290.36	226.92	31.72
Milk, nonfat/skim, fluid	1.0 cup	8.35	127.40	406.70	301.35	247.45	26.95
Fats							
Butter, regular	1.0 tsp	0.04	25.49	1.14	1.14	1.14	0.09
Oil, corn	1.0 tsp	0.00	0.00	0.00	0.00	0.00	0.02
Oil, olive	1.0 tsp	0.00	0.14	0.05	0.05	0.00	0.00
Shortening, veg, soybean/cottonseed	1.0 tsp	0.00	0.00	0.00	0.00	0.00	0.00
Margarine, regular, stick, unsalted	1.0 tsp	0.04	1.32	1.80	1.28	0.95	0.09
Mayonnaise, real, commercial	1.0 tsp	0.05	26.03	1.56	0.83	1.28	0.05
Cereals							
Bran Flakes, Kellogg's	0.75 cup	2.90	207.35	171.10	15.37	156.60	40.60
Corn Flakes, Kellogg's	1.0 cup	1.96	203.00	25.20	1.96	14.00	3.08
Cream of Rice, cooked	1.0 cup	2.90	7.50	65.78	15.78	59.80	12.95
Cream of Wheat, instant	1.0 cup	3.50	292.62	38.01	104.91	33.99	13.60
Farina, enriched, cooked	1.0 cup	3.37	91.07	42.90	105.92	93.06	13.85
Oatmeal, cooked	1.0 cup	6.05	5.39	132.27	23.53	179.13	57.87
Wheat, puffed, plain	1.25 cup	2.44	0.75	54.60	3.60	49.65	19.95
Wheat, shredded, biscuit	1.0 item	2.39	1.61	97.75	10.12	84.18	27.14
Rice Krisples, Kellogg's	1.25 cup	2.05	318.78	43.89	5.28	45.87	13.20
Breads, cookies, crackers							
Bread, white, soft	1.0 slice	2.05	134.50	29.75	27.00	23.50	6.00
Bread, whole-wheat, soft	1.0 slice	2.75	149.40	71.44	20.41	64.92	24.38
Crackers, graham, plain	1 rectangle (2 squares)	0.51	78.06	23.85	3.46	5.71	4.16
Crackers, whole-wheat, low sodium	1.0 item	0.35	8.81	5.27	0.60	4.75	1.22
Crackers, saltines	1.0 item	0.27	34.32	6.38	5.32	6.99	1.61
Muffin, English, plain	0.5 item	2.19	132.24	37.34	49.59	37.91	5.99
Bread, Italian, enriched	1.0 slice	1.76	116.80	22.00	15.60	20.60	5.40
Rolls, hard, enriched	0.5 medium	2.48	136.00	27.00	23.75	25.00	6.75
Roll, hamburger/hotdog	1.0 medium	3.66	240.80	60.63	59.77	37.84	8.60
Cookies, vanilla wafer	5.0 medium	1.25	93.28	26.75	3.07	16.73	7.07
Meat/Fish							
Beef, roast, arm, trimmed, cooked	1.0 oz	8.11	19.28	112.26	2.27	61.80	7.65
Beef, roast, arm, untrimmed, cooked	1.0 oz	7.25	17.86	98.94	2.55	55.00	6.52
Ground beef, 5% fat (95% lean meat), cooked	1.0 oz	7.45	18.43	98.66	1.98	58.40	6.24
Ground beef, 15% fat (85% lean meat), cooked	1.0 oz	7.35	18.14	81.08	5.10	52.73	5.67
Ground beef, 25% fat (75% lean meat), cooked	1.0 oz	7.45	26.37	100.36	9.64	60.67	6.24
Beef, steak, sirloin, trimmed, cooked	1.0 oz	8.98	17.29	125.30	1.70	69.74	8.79
Beef, steak, sirloin, untrimmed, cooked	1.0 oz	7.54	17.86	101.49	1.70	62.37	7.09
Chicken/turkey, dark meat, no skin, cooked	1.0 oz	8.10	22.40	82.21	9.07	57.83	6.80
Chicken/turkey, light meat, no skin, cooked	1.0 oz	8.76	21.83	70.02	4.25	61.23	7.65
Lamb, all cuts, trimmed, cooked	1.0 oz	8.04	20.13	94.40	2.27	57.55	7.09
Lamb, all cuts, untrimmed, cooked	1.0 oz	7.42	22.96	89.30	5.95	55.28	6.52
Pork, roast/chop, fresh, trimmed, cooked	1.0 oz	8.17	14.17	102.91	1.70	62.94	6.80

TABLE A-22-a. PROTEIN, SODIUM, POTASSIUM, CALCIUM, PHOSPHORUS, AND MAGNESIUM CONTENT OF SELECTED COMMON FOODS PER SERVING PORTION (continued)

FOOD NAME	SERVING PORTION	PRO (g)	Na (mg)	K (mg)	Ca (mg)	P (mg)	Mg (mg)
Pork, roast/chop, fresh, untrimmed, cooked	1.0 oz	7.65	13.61	98.09	1.70	60.67	6.24
Veal, all cuts, lean/fat, cooked	1.0 oz	7.41	25.80	100.92	7.65	64.07	7.65
Bluefish, cooked	1.0 oz	6.69	18.71	157.06	3.69	76.83	10.77
Flatfish, cooked	1.0 oz	6.85	29.77	97.52	5.10	81.93	16.44
Cod, cooked	1.0 oz	6.85	29.77	97.52	5.10	81.93	16.44
Halibut, cooked	1.0 oz	6.85	29.77	97.52	5.10	81.93	16.44
Shrimp, cooked	1.0 oz	5.93	63.50	51.60	11.06	38.84	9.64
Tuna, can/oil, drained	1.0 oz	8.26	100.36	58.68	3.69	88.17	8.79
Tuna, can/water, low sodium	1.0 oz	7.23	57.55	67.19	3.12	46.21	7.65
Tuna, can/water, no salt	1.0 oz	7.23	14.17	67.19	3.12	46.21	7.65
Sweets							
Honey	1.0 tbsp	0.06	0.85	11.02	1.27	0.85	0.42
Ice cream, vanilla, light, 4% fat	0.5 cup	3.91	54.02	151.84	84.68	75.19	10.22
Ice cream, vanilla, regular, 11% fat	0.5 cup	2.52	57.60	143.28	92.16	75.60	10.08
Ice cream, vanilla, rich 16% fat	0.5 cup	3.75	65.27	167.99	125.19	112.35	11.77
Jam/ preserves, regular	1.0 tbsp	0.07	6.40	15.40	4.00	3.80	0.80
Sherbet, plain, regular	0.5 cup	0.81	34.04	71.04	39.96	29.60	5.92
Sugar, brown, packed	0.5 cup	0.00	42.90	380.60	93.50	24.20	31.90
Sugar, white granulated	1.0 tbsp	0.00	0.00	0.25	0.13	0.00	0.00
Juices							
Apple juice, can and bottle	6.0 fi oz	0.11	5.58	221.34	13.02	13.02	5.58
Apricot nectar, can	6.0 fi oz	0.70	5.65	214.61	13.18	16.94	9.41
Cranberry juice cocktail, bottle	6.0 fi oz	0.00	3.80	34.16	5.69	3.80	3.80
Grape juice, can and bottle	6.0 fi oz	1.06	5.69	250.47	17.08	20.87	18.98
Grapefruit, juice, can, unsweetened	6.0 fi oz	0.96	1.85	283.43	12.97	20.38	18.53
Lemon juice, can and bottle	1.0 tbsp	0.06	3.20	15.56	1.68	1.37	1.22
Orange juice, prep from frozen concentrate	6.0 fi oz	1.27	4.26	358.91	19.71	30.35	19.44
Pear nectar, can	6.0 fi oz	0.20	1.22	64.45	7.78	5.67	3.59
Pineapple juice, can	6.0 fi oz	0.60	1.88	251.25	31.88	15.00	24.38
Prune juice, can	6.0 fi oz	1.17	7.68	529.92	23.04	48.00	26.88
Tomato juice, can	6.0 fi oz	1.39	657.92	400.95	16.40	34.63	20.05
Tomato juice, can, low sodium	6.0 fi oz	1.39	18.23	400.95	16.40	34.63	20.05
Vegetables, Pasta, Rice							
Asparagus, can, spears	0.5 cup	2.59	347.27	208.12	19.36	52.03	12.10
Asparagus, cooked from frozen	0.5 cup	2.66	3.60	196.20	20.70	49.50	11.70
Beans, snap, green, can	0.5 cup	0.78	176.85	73.58	17.55	12.83	8.78
Beans, snap, green, boiled, drained	0.5 cup	0.93	5.63	78.75	30.63	19.38	15.00
Beans, snap, wax, boiled, drained	0.5 cup	0.93	5.63	78.75	30.63	19.38	15.00
Beets, can, whole	0.5 cup	0.74	158.11	120.62	12.23	13.86	13.86
Beets, boiled, drained	0.5 cup	1.37	62.76	248.58	13.04	30.97	18.75
Broccoli, boiled, drained	0.5 cup	1.50	5.34	68.87	16.01	23.77	6.31
Cabbage, green, boiled, drained	0.5 cup	0.77	6.00	72.75	23.25	11.25	6.00
Carrots, can, sliced, drained	0.5 cup	0.47	176.66	130.67	18.25	17.52	5.84
Carrots, boiled, drained	0.5 cup	0.85	51.48	177.06	24.18	23.40	10.14
Carrots, raw, whole	1.0 medium	0.63	21.35	197.03	16.47	26.84	9.15
Cauliflower, boiled, drained	0.5 cup	1.00	11.16	86.18	10.54	14.88	5.58
Celery, raw, stalk	1.0 medium	0.30	34.80	114.80	16.00	10.00	4.40
Corn, can, whole kernel, drained	0.5 cup	2.15	175.48	159.90	4.10	53.30	16.40
Corn, whole kernel, boiled, drained	0.5 cup	2.26	4.10	120.54	3.28	46.74	15.58
Cucumber, raw, sliced, with peel	0.5 cup	0.36	1.04	74.88	7.28	10.40	5.72
Green peas, can, drained	0.5 cup	3.76	214.20	147.05	17.00	56.95	14.45
Green peas, boiled, drained	0.5 cup	4.12	57.60	88.00	19.20	61.60	17.60
Potato, baked, with skin	1.0 medium	3.05	12.20	652.70	18.30	85.40	34.16
Potato, boiled, without skin	1.0 medium	2.09	6.10	400.16	9.76	48.80	24.40
Tomato, raw, red	1.0 medium	1.05	11.07	273.06	6.15	29.52	13.53
Tomato, red, can, stewed	0.5 cup	1.00	346.66	229.87	32.55	23.09	12.66

(continued)

TABLE A-22-a. PROTEIN, SODIUM, POTASSIUM, CALCIUM, PHOSPHORUS, AND MAGNESIUM CONTENT OF SELECTED COMMON FOODS PER SERVING PORTION (continued)

FOOD NAME	SERVING PORTION	PRO (g)	Na (mg)	K (mg)	Ca (mg)	P (mg)	Mg (mg)
Tomato, can, no salt added	0.5 cup	1.10	12.00	272.40	36.00	22.80	14.40
Noodles, egg, enriched, cooked	0.5 cup	3.80	5.60	22.40	9.60	55.20	15.20
Rice, white, enriched, parboiled, cooked	0.5 cup	2.35	0.88	30.62	8.75	37.63	10.50
Fruits							
Apple, raw, unpeeled	1.0 medium	0.26	0.00	158.70	9.66	9.66	6.90
Apple, raw, peeled	1.0 medium	0.19	0.00	144.64	5.12	8.96	3.84
Applesauce, can, unsweetened	0.5 cup	0.21	2.44	91.50	3.66	8.54	3.66
Apricot, can, light syrup	0.5 cup	0.75	4.64	198.82	10.97	15.60	8.86
Banana, ripe, raw, peeled	1.0 medium	1.22	1.18	467.28	7.08	23.60	34.22
Blueberries, raw	0.5 cup	0.49	4.35	64.53	4.35	7.25	3.63
Cherries, sweet, can, juice pack	0.5 cup	0.94	0.26	175.09	12.60	14.84	8.79
Grapefruit, raw, white	0.5 medium	0.88	0.00	189.44	15.36	10.24	11.52
Orange, raw	1.0 medium	1.23	0.00	237.11	52.40	18.34	13.10
Peach, raw	1.0 medium	0.69	0.00	193.06	4.90	11.76	6.86
Peach, can, light syrup	0.5 cup	0.56	6.06	118.88	3.28	13.32	6.28
Pear, raw, unpeeled	1.0 medium	0.65	0.00	207.50	18.26	18.26	9.96
Pineapple, can, juice pack	0.5 cup	0.52	1.25	151.89	17.43	7.47	17.43
Strawberries, raw, whole	0.5 cup	0.44	0.72	119.52	10.08	13.68	7.20

Data from the Nutrition Data System for Research (NDS-R) version 5.0_35, 2004, with permission. Table compiled and prepared by the Nutrition Coordinating Center, University of Minnesota, Minneapolis, MN.

TABLE A-22-b. IRON, ZINC, COPPER, SELENIUM, AND MANGANESE CONTENT OF SELECTED COMMON FOODS PER SERVING PORTION

FOOD NAME	SERVING PORTION	Fe (mg)	Zn (mg)	Cu (mg)	Se (μg)	Mn (mg)
Dairy products						
Eggs, whole, hard boiled	1.0 large	0.60	0.53	0.01	15.40	0.01
Cheese, cottage, uncreamed	1.0 oz	0.07	0.13	0.01	3.06	0.00
Cream, coffee/table, light (20% fat)	1.0 tbsp	0.01	0.04	0.00	0.09	0.00
Cream, sour, cultured	1.0 tbsp	0.01	0.04	0.00	0.09	0.00
Cream, sour, lowfat	1.0 tbsp	0.03	0.17	0.00	0.08	0.00
Cream, sour, nonfat/fat free	1.0 tbsp	0.00	0.08	0.00	0.80	0.00
Milk, buttermilk, fluid	1.0 cup	0.12	1.03	0.03	4.90	0.00
Milk, whole, 3.5–4% fat, fluid	1.0 cup	0.12	0.93	0.02	4.88	0.01
Milk, nonfat/skim, fluid	1.0 cup	0.10	0.98	0.02	5.15	0.00
Fats						
Butter, regular	1.0 tsp	0.00	0.00	0.00	0.05	0.00
Oil, corn	1.0 tsp	0.00	0.01	0.00	0.00	0.00
Oil, olive	1.0 tsp	0.03	0.00	0.00	0.00	0.00
Shortening, veg, soybean/cottonseed	1.0 tsp	0.00	0.00	0.00	0.00	0.00
Margarine, regular, stick, unsalted	1.0 tsp	0.00	0.01	0.00	0.00	0.00
Mayonnaise, real, commercial	1.0 tsp	0.02	0.01	0.00	0.08	0.00
Cereals						
Bran Flakes, Kellogg's	0.75 cup	8.12	3.77	0.15	3.05	1.22
Corn Flakes, Kellogg's	1.0 cup	8.40	0.08	0.02	1.43	0.07
Cream of Rice, cooked	1.0 cup	1.75	0.52	0.13	8.74	0.48
Cream of Wheat, instant	1.0 cup	9.44	0.32	0.09	6.60	0.29
Farina, enriched, cooked	1.0 cup	9.44	0.32	0.08	6.60	0.24
Oatmeal, cooked	1.0 cup	1.59	1.16	0.14	12.85	1.37
Wheat, puffed, plain	1.25 cup	0.66	0.46	0.09	18.46	0.30
Wheat, shredded, biscuit	1.0 item	0.72	0.63	0.07	1.36	0.84
Rice Krispies, Kellogg's	1.25 cup	1.82	0.46	0.07	5.08	0.35
Breads, cookies, crackers						
Bread, white, soft	1.0 slice	0.76	0.16	0.03	7.05	0.10
Bread, whole-wheat, soft	1.0 slice	0.94	0.55	0.08	10.38	0.66
Crackers, graham, plain	1 rectangle (2 squares)	0.29	0.04	0.01	1.92	0.05
Crackers, whole-wheat, low sodium	1.0 item	0.15	0.03	0.01	1.24	0.03
Crackers, saltines	1.0 item	0.11	0.05	0.01	0.98	0.04
Muffin, English, plain	0.5 item	0.71	0.20	0.04	5.73	0.10
Bread, Italian, enriched	1.0 slice	0.59	0.17	0.04	5.44	0.09
Rolls, hard, enriched	0.5 medium	0.82	0.24	0.04	9.78	0.12
Roll, hamburger/hotdog	1.0 medium	1.36	0.27	0.05	11.40	0.14
Cookies, vanilla wafer	5.0 medium	0.62	0.14	0.04	3.73	0.10
Meat/Fish						
Beef, roast, arm, trimmed, cooked	1.0 oz	0.70	1.48	0.03	6.46	0.00
Beef, roast, arm, untrimmed, cooked	1.0 oz	0.63	1.30	0.03	6.55	0.00
Ground beef, 5% fat (95% lean meat), cooked	1.0 oz	0.80	1.82	0.03	6.15	0.00
Ground beef, 15% fat (85% lean meat), cooked	1.0 oz	0.78	1.83	0.02	5.95	0.00
Ground beef, 25% fat (75% lean meat), cooked	1.0 oz	0.75	1.75	0.02	6.24	0.00
Beef, steak, sirloin, trimmed, cooked	1.0 oz	0.82	1.58	0.03	7.97	0.00
Beef, steak, sirloin, untrimmed, cooked	1.0 oz	0.82	1.20	0.03	7.40	0.00
Chicken/turkey, dark meat, no skin, cooked	1.0 oz	0.66	1.26	0.05	11.59	0.01
Chicken/turkey, light meat, no skin, cooked	1.0 oz	0.30	0.35	0.01	6.92	0.00
Lamb, all cuts, trimmed, cooked	1.0 oz	0.62	1.37	0.03	8.73	0.01
Lamb, all cuts, untrimmed, cooked	1.0 oz	0.50	1.27	0.04	7.63	0.01
Pork, roast/chop, fresh, trimmed, cooked	1.0 oz	0.28	0.80	0.00	12.25	0.00
Pork, roast/chop, fresh, untrimmed, cooked	1.0 oz	0.26	0.75	0.00	11.42	0.00

(continued)

TABLE A-22-b. IRON, ZINC, COPPER, SELENIUM, AND MANGANESE CONTENT OF SELECTED COMMON FOODS PER SERVING PORTION (continued)

FOOD NAME	SERVING PORTION	Fe (mg)	Zn (mg)	Cu (mg)	Se (μg)	Mn (mg)
Veal, all cuts, lean/fat, cooked	1.0 oz	0.33	1.22	0.04	3.20	0.01
Bluefish, cooked	1.0 oz	0.21	0.18	0.02	11.51	0.00
Flatfish, cooked	1.0 oz	0.10	0.18	0.01	16.50	0.01
Cod, cooked	1.0 oz	0.10	0.18	0.01	16.50	0.01
Halibut, cooked	1.0 oz	0.10	0.18	0.01	16.50	0.01
Shrimp, cooked	1.0 oz	0.88	0.44	0.05	11.23	0.01
Tuna, can/oil, drained	1.0 oz	0.39	0.26	0.02	21.55	0.00
Tuna, can/water, low sodium	1.0 oz	0.43	0.22	0.01	22.79	0.00
Tuna, can/water, no salt	1.0 oz	0.43	0.22	0.01	22.79	0.00
Sweets						
Honey	1.0 tbsp	0.09	0.05	0.01	0.17	0.02
Ice cream, vanilla, light, 4% fat	0.5 cup	0.06	0.53	0.01	1.46	0.00
Ice cream, vanilla, regular, 11% fat	0.5 cup	0.06	0.50	0.02	1.30	0.01
Ice cream, vanilla, rich 16% fat	0.5 cup	0.36	0.50	0.01	3.75	0.00
Jam/preserves, regular	1.0 tbsp	0.10	0.01	0.02	0.40	0.01
Sherbet, plain, regular	0.5 cup	0.10	0.36	0.02	0.96	0.01
Sugar, brown, packed	0.5 cup	2.10	0.20	0.33	1.32	0.35
Sugar, white granulated	1.0 tbsp	0.00	0.00	0.00	0.08	0.00
Juices						
Apple juice, can and bottle	6.0 fl oz	0.69	0.06	0.04	0.19	0.21
Apricot nectar, can	6.0 fl oz	0.72	0.17	0.14	0.00	0.06
Cranberry Juice cocktail, bottle	6.0 fl oz	0.28	0.13	0.03	0.00	0.37
Grape juice, can and bottle	6.0 fl oz	0.46	0.09	0.05	0.19	0.68
Grapefruit, juice, can, unsweetened	6.0 fl oz	0.37	0.17	0.07	0.19	0.04
Lemon Juice, can and bottle	1.0 tbsp	0.02	0.01	0.01	0.02	0.00
Orange juice, prep from frozen conc	6.0 fl oz	0.19	0.10	0.09	0.21	0.03
Pear nectar, can	6.0 fl oz	0.14	0.07	0.07	0.72	0.07
Pineapple juice, can	6.0 fl oz	0.49	0.21	0.17	0.19	1.86
Prune Juice, can	6.0 fl oz	2.27	0.40	0.13	1.15	0.29
Tomato juice, can	6.0 fl oz	1.06	0.26	0.18	0.91	0.14
Tomato juice, can, low sodium	6.0 fl oz	1.06	0.26	0.18	0.91	0.73
Vegetables, Pasta, Rice						
Asparagus, can, spears	0.5 cup	2.21	0.48	0.12	2.06	0.21
Asparagus, cooked from frozen	0.5 cup	0.58	0.50	0.15	1.53	0.17
Beans, snap, green, can	0.5 cup	0.61	0.20	0.03	0.27	0.14
Beans, snap, green, boiled, drained	0.5 cup	0.55	0.30	0.04	0.25	0.20
Beans, snap, wax, boiled, drained	0.5 cup	0.55	0.30	0.04	0.25	0.20
Beets, can, whole	0.5 cup	1.48	0.17	0.05	0.41	0.23
Beets, boiled, drained	0.5 cup	0.64	0.29	0.06	0.57	0.27
Broccoli, boiled, drained	0.5 cup	0.30	0.14	0.02	0.34	0.11
Cabbage, green, boiled, drained	0.5 cup	0.13	0.07	0.01	0.45	0.09
Carrots, can, sliced, drained	0.5 cup	0.47	0.19	0.08	0.29	0.33
Carrots, boiled, drained	0.5 cup	0.48	0.23	0.10	0.62	0.59
Carrots, raw, whole	1.0 medium	0.31	0.12	0.03	0.67	0.09
Cauliflower, boiled, drained	0.5 cup	0.25	0.08	0.01	0.37	0.09
Celery, raw, stalk	1.0 medium	0.16	0.05	0.01	0.36	0.04
Corn, can, whole kernel, drained	0.5 cup	0.71	0.32	0.05	0.57	0.14
Corn, whole kernel, boiled, drained	0.5 cup	0.29	0.33	0.03	0.57	0.10
Cucumber, raw, sliced, with peel	0.5 cup	0.14	0.10	0.02	0.00	0.04
Green peas, can, drained	0.5 cup	0.81	0.60	0.07	1.45	0.26
Green peas, boiled, drained	0.5 cup	1.22	0.54	0.08	0.80	0.22
Potato, baked, with skin	1.0 medium	1.32	0.44	0.14	0.49	0.27
Potato, boiled, without skin	1.0 medium	0.38	0.33	0.20	0.37	0.17
Tomato, raw, red	1.0 medium	0.55	0.11	0.09	0.49	0.13
Tomato, red, can, stewed	0.5 cup	0.52	0.18	0.10	0.74	0.14
Tomato, can, no salt added	0.5 cup	0.66	0.19	0.13	0.84	0.15
Noodles, egg, enriched, cooked	0.5 cup	1.27	0.50	0.07	17.36	0.21
Rice, white, enriched, parboiled, cooked	0.5 cup	1.05	0.43	0.06	6.56	0.41

TABLE A-22-b. IRON, ZINC, COPPER, SELENLUM, AND MANGANESE CONTENT OF SELECTED COMMON FOODS PER SERVING PORTION (continued)

FOOD NAME	SERVING PORTION	Fe (mg)	Zn (mg)	Cu (mg)	Se (μg)	Mn (mg)
Fruits						
Apple, raw, unpeeled	1.0 medium	0.25	0.06	0.06	0.41	0.06
Apple, raw, peeled	1.0 medium	0.09	0.05	0.04	0.38	0.03
Applesauce, can, unsweetened	0.5 cup	0.15	0.04	0.03	0.37	0.09
Apricot, can, light syrup	0.5 cup	0.39	0.14	0.10	0.13	0.07
Banana, ripe, raw, peeled	1.0 medium	0.37	0.19	0.12	1.30	0.18
Blueberries, raw	0.5 cup	0.12	0.08	0.04	0.44	0.20
Cherries, sweet, can, juice pack	0.5 cup	0.31	0.05	0.07	0.49	0.07
Grapefruit, raw, white	0.5 medium	0.08	0.09	0.06	1.79	0.02
Orange, raw	1.0 medium	0.13	0.09	0.06	0.66	0.03
Peach, raw	1.0 medium	0.11	0.14	0.07	0.39	0.05
Peach, can, light syrup	0.5 cup	0.36	0.11	0.07	0.38	0.06
Pear, raw, unpeeled	1.0 medium	0.42	0.20	0.19	1.66	0.13
Pineapple, can, juice pack	0.5 cup	0.35	0.12	0.11	0.50	1.40
Strawberries, raw, whole	0.5 cup	0.27	0.09	0.04	0.50	0.21

Data from the Nutrition Data System for Research (NDS-R) version 5.0_35, 2004, with permission. Table compiled and prepared by the Nutrition Coordinating Center, University of Minnesota, Minneapolis, MN.

A-23. VITAMINS IN SELECTED COMMON FOODS

TABLE A-23-a. RETINOL ACTIVITY EQUIVALENTS (RAE), VITAMIN D, α-TOCOPHEROL (TOC), VITAMIN C, THIAMIN, RIBOFLAVIN, NIACIN EQUIVALENTS, VITAMIN B6, VITAMIN B12, AND DIETARY FOLATE EQUIVALENTS (DFE) CONTENT OF SELECTED FOODS PER SERVING PORTION

FOOD NAME	SERVING PORTION	VIT. A RAE (μg)	D (μg)	VIT. E TOTAL α-TOC (mg)	C (mg)	THIAMIN (mg)	RIBO (mg)	NIACIN EQUIV (mg)	B-6 (mg)	B-12 (μg)	DFE (μg)
Dairy products											
Eggs, whole, hard boiled	1.0 large	84.00	0.64	0.51	0.00	0.03	0.26	1.36	0.06	0.56	22.00
Cheese, cottage, uncreamed	1.0 oz	2.29	0.00	0.03	0.00	0.01	0.04	0.87	0.02	0.24	4.25
Cream, coffee/table, light (20% fat)	1.0 tbsp	27.00	0.10	0.02	0.12	0.00	0.02	0.18	0.00	0.03	0.30
Cream, sour, cultured	1.0 tbsp	25.88	0.10	0.02	0.12	0.00	0.02	0.18	0.00	0.03	0.29
Cream, sour, lowfat	1.0 tbsp	29.02	0.04	0.01	0.08	0.02	0.03	0.36	0.02	0.08	1.01
Cream, sour, nonfat/fat free	1.0 tbsp	10.91	0.00	0.00	0.00	0.01	0.02	0.18	0.00	0.05	1.65
Milk, buttermilk, fluid	1.0 cup	18.38	0.02	0.15	2.45	0.08	0.38	1.64	0.08	0.54	12.25
Milk, whole, 3.5–4% fat,	1.0 cup	84.59	2.44	0.24	2.20	0.09	0.40	2.03	0.10	0.88	12.20
Milk, nonfat/skim, fluid	1.0 cup	149.45	2.45	0.10	2.45	0.09	0.34	2.22	0.10	0.93	12.25
Fats											
Butter, regular	1.0 tsp	40.25	0.07	0.07	0.00	0.00	0.00	0.00	0.00	0.01	0.14
Oil, corn	1.0 tsp	0.00	0.00	0.65	0.00	0.00	0.00	0.00	0.00	0.00	0.00
Oil, olive	1.0 tsp	0.32	0.00	0.54	0.00	0.00	0.00	0.00	0.00	0.00	0.00
Shortening, veg, soybean/cottonseed	1.0 tsp	0.00	0.00	0.34	0.00	0.00	0.00	0.00	0.00	0.00	0.00
Margarine, regular, stick, unsalted	1.0 tsp	40.65	0.00	0.70	0.00	0.00	0.00	0.00	0.00	0.00	0.05
Mayonnaise, real, commercial	1.0 tsp	3.77	0.01	0.07	0.00	0.00	0.00	0.00	0.03	0.01	0.37
Cereals											
Bran Flakes, Kellogg's	0.75 cup	187.44	1.00	3.69	15.66	0.38	0.44	5.66	2.03	6.00	672.80
Corn Flakes, Kellogg's	1.0 cup	138.46	1.06	0.03	6.16	0.36	0.43	5.18	0.50	1.51	169.96
Cream of Rice, cooked	1.0 cup	0.00	0.00	0.01	0.00	0.19	0.06	3.26	0.09	0.00	13.34
Cream of Wheat, instant	1.0 cup	0.00	0.00	0.04	0.00	0.17	0.07	2.22	0.03	0.00	60.03
Farina, enriched, cooked	1.0 cup	0.00	0.00	0.04	0.00	0.17	0.07	2.22	0.03	0.00	39.66
Oatmeal, cooked	1.0 cup	0.06	0.00	0.22	0.00	0.28	0.05	1.62	0.05	0.00	12.09
Wheat, puffed, plain	1.25 cup	0.05	0.00	0.16	0.00	0.09	0.06	1.29	0.02	0.06	30.90
Wheat, shredded, biscuit	1.0 item	0.08	0.00	0.08	0.00	0.06	0.03	1.78	0.09	0.00	9.89
Rice Krispies, Kellogg's	1.25 cup	153.12	1.02	0.04	6.37	0.38	0.46	5.38	0.50	1.49	175.89
Breads, cookies, crackers											
Bread, white, soft	1.0 slice	0.00	0.00	0.08	0.00	0.12	0.09	1.32	0.02	0.01	34.42
Bread, whole-wheat, soft	1.0 slice	0.05	0.00	0.22	0.00	0.10	0.06	1.76	0.05	0.00	14.18
Crackers, graham, plain	1 rectangle (2 squares)	0.00	0.00	0.10	0.00	0.04	0.03	0.47	0.01	0.00	10.00
Crackers, whole-wheat, low sodium	1.0 item	0.00	0.00	0.04	0.00	0.02	0.02	0.20	0.00	0.00	6.35
Crackers, saltines	1.0 item	0.02	0.00	0.05	0.00	0.02	0.01	0.14	0.00	0.01	3.86
Muffin, English, plain	0.5 item	0.00	0.14	0.03	0.00	0.13	0.08	1.61	0.01	0.01	38.76
Bread, Italian, enriched	1.0 slice	0.00	0.00	0.04	0.00	0.09	0.06	1.21	0.01	0.00	60.80
Rolls, hard, enriched	0.5 medium	0.00	0.00	0.08	0.00	0.12	0.08	1.58	0.01	0.00	37.75
Roll, hamburger/hotdog	1.0 medium	0.00	0.00	0.66	0.04	0.21	0.13	2.36	0.02	0.03	61.32
Cookies, vanilla wafer	5.0 medium	0.04	0.04	0.23	0.00	0.08	0.06	0.96	0.01	0.00	21.39
Meat/Fish											
Beef, roast, arm, trimmed, cooked	1.0 oz	1.23	0.17	0.04	0.00	0.03	0.06	2.34	0.12	0.57	2.27
Beef, roast, arm, untrimmed, cooked	1.0 oz	1.46	0.17	0.01	0.00	0.02	0.05	2.16	0.10	0.55	1.98

FOOD NAME	SERVING PORTION	VIT. A RAE (µg)	D (µg)	VIT. E TOTAL α-TOC (mg)	C (mg)	THIAMIN (mg)	RIBO (mg)	NIACIN EQUIV (mg)	B-6 (mg)	B-12 (µg)	DFE (µg)
Ground beef, 5% fat (95% lean meat), cooked	1.0 oz	1.18	0.13	0.10	0.00	0.01	0.05	2.35	0.12	0.70	1.98
Ground beef, 15% fat (85% lean meat), cooked	1.0 oz	1.46	0.12	0.12	0.00	0.01	0.05	2.07	0.10	0.71	1.70
Ground beef, 25% fat (75% lean meat), cooked	1.0 oz	1.61	0.11	0.14	0.00	0.01	0.05	2.02	0.12	0.83	3.40
Beef, steak, sirloin, trimmed, cooked	1.0 oz	1.18	0.20	0.04	0.00	0.03	0.08	2.71	0.16	0.70	3.40
Beef, steak, sirloin, untrimmed, cooked	1.0 oz	1.37	0.20	0.11	0.00	0.02	0.07	2.40	0.10	0.73	3.12
Chicken/turkey, dark meat, no skin, cooked	1.0 oz	5.10	0.09	0.18	0.00	0.02	0.07	2.53	0.10	0.10	2.55
Chicken/turkey, light meat, no skin, cooked	1.0 oz	2.55	0.06	0.08	0.00	0.02	0.03	5.19	0.17	0.10	1.13
Lamb, all cuts, trimmed, cooked	1.0 oz	0.00	0.17	0.05	0.00	0.03	0.09	3.28	0.05	0.73	5.95
Lamb, all cuts, untrimmed, cooked	1.0 oz	0.00	0.17	0.04	0.00	0.03	0.07	3.25	0.04	0.61	6.24
Pork, roast/chop, fresh, trimmed, cooked	1.0 oz	0.57	0.23	0.03	0.11	0.18	0.09	3.19	0.11	0.16	2.55
Pork, roast/chop, fresh, untrimmed, cooked	1.0 oz	0.57	0.28	0.05	0.11	0.17	0.08	3.10	0.10	0.16	2.27
Veal, all cuts, lean/fat	1.0 oz	0.00	0.43	0.14	0.00	0.02	0.09	3.67	0.09	0.45	4.82
Bluefish, cooked	1.0 oz	9.36	6.80	0.47	0.45	0.04	0.06	2.59	0.13	1.98	0.28
Flatfish, cooked	1.0 oz	3.12	0.54	0.54	0.00	0.02	0.03	1.95	0.07	0.71	2.55
Cod, cooked	1.0 oz	3.12	0.31	0.54	0.00	0.02	0.03	1.95	0.07	0.71	2.55
Halibut, cooked	1.0 oz	3.12	1.42	0.54	0.00	0.02	0.03	1.95	0.07	0.71	2.55
Shrimp, cooked	1.0 oz	19.82	1.01	0.14	0.62	0.01	0.01	2.06	0.04	0.42	1.13
Tuna, can/oil, drained	1.0 oz	6.52	1.67	0.34	0.00	0.01	0.03	5.02	0.03	0.62	1.42
Tuna, can/water, low sodium	1.0 oz	4.82	1.13	0.15	0.00	0.01	0.02	5.09	0.10	0.85	1.13
Tuna, can/water, no salt	1.0 oz	4.82	1.13	0.15	0.00	0.01	0.02	5.09	0.10	0.85	1.13
Sweets											
Honey	1.0 tbsp	0.00	0.00	0.00	0.11	0.00	0.01	0.03	0.01	0.00	0.42
Ice cream, vanilla, light, 4% fat	0.5 cup	100.98	0.03	0.07	0.15	0.03	0.12	0.90	0.02	0.23	3.65
Ice cream, vanilla, regular, 11% fat	0.5 cup	84.66	0.62	0.22	0.43	0.03	0.17	0.58	0.03	0.28	3.60
Ice cream, vanilla, rich 16% fat	0.5 cup	194.47	1.17	0.55	0.00	0.04	0.18	0.76	0.05	0.42	8.56
Jam/preserves, regular	1.0 tbsp	0.08	0.00	0.00	1.76	0.00	0.02	0.01	0.00	0.00	2.20
Sherbet, plain, regular	0.5 cup	7.28	0.02	0.02	4.29	0.02	0.07	0.23	0.02	0.09	5.18
Sugar, brown, packed	0.5 cup	0.00	0.00	0.00	0.00	0.01	0.01	0.09	0.03	0.00	1.10
Sugar, white granulated	1.0 tbsp	0.00	0.00	0.00	0.00	0.00	0.00	0.00	0.00	0.00	0.00
Juices											
Apple juice, can and bottle	6.0 fl oz	4.34	0.00	0.02	1.67	0.04	0.03	0.19	0.06	0.00	0.00
Apricot nectar, can	6.0 fl oz	105.89	0.00	0.08	1.13	0.02	0.03	0.49	0.04	0.00	1.88
Cranberry juice cocktail,	6.0 fl oz	1.11	0.00	0.00	45.01	0.02	0.02	0.07	0.04	0.00	0.00
Grape juice, can and bottle	6.0 fl oz	5.06	0.00	0.00	0.19	0.05	0.07	0.50	0.12	0.00	5.69
Grapefruit, juice, can, unsweetened	6.0 fl oz	3.09	0.00	0.07	54.09	0.08	0.04	0.43	0.04	0.00	18.53
Lemon juice, can and bottle	1.0 tbsp	0.11	0.00	0.01	3.78	0.01	0.00	0.03	0.01	0.00	1.53
Orange juice, prep from frozen concentrate	6.0 fl oz	8.56	0.00	0.17	73.43	0.15	0.03	0.38	0.08	0.00	82.54
Pear nectar, can	6.0 fl oz	1.29	0.00	0.25	2.06	0.01	0.03	0.05	0.01	0.00	3.61
Pineapple juice, can	6.0 fl oz	5.00	0.00	0.04	20.06	0.10	0.04	0.48	0.18	0.00	43.13

(continued)

TABLE A-23-a. (continued)

FOOD NAME	SERVING PORTION	VIT. A RAE (µg)	D (µg)	VIT. E TOTAL α-TOC (mg)	C (mg)	THIAMIN (mg)	RIBO (mg)	NIACIN EQUIV (mg)	B-6 (mg)	B-12 (µg)	DFE (µg)
Prune juice, can	6.0 fl oz	5.76	0.00	0.02	7.87	0.03	0.13	1.51	0.42	0.00	0.00
Tomato juice, can	6.0 fl oz	65.00	0.00	1.66	33.35	0.09	0.06	1.40	0.20	0.00	36.45
Tomato juice, can, low sodium	6.0 fl oz	65.00	0.00	1.65	33.35	0.09	0.06	1.40	0.20	0.00	36.45
Vegetables, Pasta Rice											
Asparagus, can, spears	0.5 cup	36.91	0.00	0.51	22.26	0.07	0.12	1.65	0.13	0.00	116.16
Asparagus, cooked from frozen	0.5 cup	40.20	0.00	1.09	21.96	0.06	0.09	1.43	0.02	0.00	121.50
Beans, snap, green, can	0.5 cup	24.92	0.00	0.09	3.24	0.01	0.04	0.31	0.02	0.00	21.60
Beans, snap, green, boiled, drained	0.5 cup	19.64	0.00	0.08	2.56	0.02	0.06	0.41	0.04	0.00	14.38
Beans, snap, wax, boiled, drained	0.5 cup	3.49	0.00	0.09	2.56	0.02	0.06	0.41	0.04	0.00	14.38
Beets, can, whole	0.5 cup	0.07	0.00	0.20	3.34	0.01	0.03	0.30	0.05	0.00	24.45
Beets, boiled, drained	0.5 cup	0.07	0.00	0.20	2.93	0.02	0.03	0.60	0.05	0.00	65.20
Broccoli, boiled, drained	0.5 cup	41.43	0.00	0.79	19.45	0.03	0.04	0.55	0.06	0.00	27.16
Cabbage, green, boiled, drained	0.5 cup	5.63	0.00	0.08	15.08	0.04	0.04	0.38	0.08	0.00	15.00
Carrots, can, sliced, drained	0.5 cup	456.92	0.00	0.31	1.97	0.01	0.02	0.57	0.08	0.00	6.57
Carrots, boiled, drained	0.5 cup	798.20	0.00	0.32	1.79	0.03	0.04	0.56	0.19	0.00	10.92
Carrots, raw, whole	1.0 medium	556.63	0.00	0.28	5.67	0.06	0.04	0.74	0.09	0.00	8.54
Cauliflower, boiled, drained	0.5 cup	0.21	0.00	0.02	19.41	0.02	0.03	0.36	0.05	0.00	25.42
Celery, raw, stalk	1.0 medium	5.00	0.00	0.14	2.80	0.02	0.02	0.13	0.03	0.00	11.20
Corn, can, whole kernel, drained	0.5 cup	3.14	0.00	0.11	6.97	0.03	0.06	1.15	0.04	0.00	40.18
Corn, whole kernel, boiled, drained	0.5 cup	7.24	0.00	0.04	2.54	0.07	0.06	1.57	0.11	0.00	25.42
Cucumber, raw, sliced, with peel	0.5cup	5.98	0.00	0.04	2.76	0.01	0.01	0.11	0.02	0.00	6.76
Green peas, can, drained	0.5 cup	22.67	0.00	0.32	8.16	0.10	0.07	1.12	0.05	0.00	37.40
Green peas, boiled, drained	0.5 cup	22.73	0.00	0.01	7.92	0.23	0.08	1.68	0.09	0.00	47.20
Potato, baked, with skin	1.0 medium	0.41	0.00	0.05	11.71	0.08	0.06	2.55	0.38	0.00	34.16
Potato, boiled, without skin	1.0 medium	0.41	0.00	0.06	9.03	0.12	0.02	2.10	0.33	0.00	10.98
Tomato, raw, red	1.0 medium	46.02	0.00	0.42	23.49	0.07	0.06	0.94	0.10	0.00	18.45
Tomato, red, can, stewed	0.5 cup	14.07	0.00	0.30	14.95	0.05	0.03	0.84	0.11	0.00	10.79
Tomato, can, no salt added	0.5 cup	18.60	0.00	0.43	17.04	0.05	0.04	1.05	0.11	0.00	9.60
Noodles, egg, enriched, cooked	0.5 cup	3.40	0.02	0.03	0.00	0.15	0.07	2.02	0.03	0.07	83.12
Rice, white, enriched, parboiled, cooked	0.5 cup	0.00	0.00	0.04	0.00	0.14	0.01	1.79	0.08	0.00	84.44
Fruits											
Apple, raw, unpeeled	1.0 medium	5.87	0.00	0.44	7.87	0.02	0.02	0.11	0.07	0.00	4.14
Apple, raw, peeled	1.0 medium	3.84	0.00	0.10	5.12	0.02	0.01	0.12	0.06	0.00	0.00
Applesauce, can, unsweetened	0.5 cup	2.75	0.00	0.01	1.46	0.02	0.03	0.23	0.03	0.00	1.22
Apricot, can, light syrup	0.5 cup	93.04	0.00	0.76	4.05	0.03	0.03	0.65	0.07	0.00	2.53
Banana, ripe, raw, peeled	1.0 medium	2.36	0.00	0.32	10.74	0.05	0.12	0.81	0.68	0.00	22.42
Blueberries, raw	0.5 cup	2.18	0.00	0.64	9.43	0.03	0.04	0.26	0.03	0.00	4.35
Cherries, sweet, can, juice pack	0.5 cup	2.34	0.00	0.10	5.47	0.04	0.05	0.48	0.03	0.00	3.13
Grapefruit, raw, white	0.5 medium	2.13	0.00	0.31	2.62	0.05	0.03	0.51	0.06	0.00	12.80
Orange, raw	1.0 medium	13.10	0.00	0.31	69.69	0.11	0.05	0.54	0.08	0.00	39.30
Peach, raw	1.0 medium	8.98	0.00	0.67	6.47	0.02	0.04	0.97	0.02	0.00	2.94
Peach, can, light syrup	0.5 cup	25.70	0.00	0.61	3.56	0.01	0.03	0.73	0.02	0.00	3.77
Pear, raw, unpeeled	1.0	4.15	0.00	0.80	6.64	0.03	0.07	0.17	0.03	0.00	11.62
Pineapple, can, juice pack	0.5 cup	2.39	0.00	0.01	11.83	0.12	0.02	0.52	0.09	0.00	6.23
Strawberries, raw, whole	0.5 cup	0.72	0.00	0.09	40.82	0.01	0.05	0.34	0.04	0.00	12.96

Data from the Nutrition Data System for Research (NDS-R) version 5.0_35, 2004, with permission. Table compeiled and prepared by the Nutrition Coordinating Center, University of Minnesota, Minneapolis, MN.

TABLE A-23-b. VITAMIN K (PHYLLOQUINONE) IN SELECTED FOODS TO INDICATE HIGH, MEDIUM, AND LOW SOURCES

FOOD NAME	SERVING PORTION	VITAMIN K (PHYLLOQUINONE) (μg)
Kale, cooked	1 cup	1062
Spinach, cooked	1 cup	888
Collards, cooked	1 cup	836
Beet greens, cooked	1 cup	697
Turnip greens, cooked	1 cup	529
Mustard greens, cooked	1 cup	419
Broccoli, cooked	1 cup	220
Brussels sprouts, cooked	1 cup	219
Collards, raw	1 cup	184
Noodles, egg, spinach, cooked	1 cup	162
Spinach, raw	1 cup	145
Asparagus, cooked	1 cup	144
Sauerkraut	1 cup	135
Endive, raw	1 cup	116
Lettuce, green leaf	1 cup	97
Broccoli, raw	1 cup	89
Cabbage, cooked	1 cup	73
Rhubarb, cooked	1 cup	71
Plums, dried (prunes), stewed	1 cup	65
Okra, cooked	1 cup	64
Lettuce, romaine	1 cup	57
Cabbage, raw	1 cup	42
Pumpkin, canned	1 cup	39
Peas, green, cooked	1 cup	38
Tuna, canned, oil pack, regular, drained	3 oz	37
Avocado, raw	1 medium	37
Celery, raw	1 cup	35
Sauce, pasta, spaghettl/marinara, ready-to-serve	1 cup	35
Green onions, raw (includes top and bulb)	1 medium	31
Kiwi fruit, raw	1 medium	31
Tomato paste	1 cup	30
Blueberries, fresh	1 cup	28
Plums, dried (prunes), uncooked	5 prunes	25
Artichokes, (globe or french), cooked	1 cup	25
Grapes, fresh	1 cup	23
Carrots, cooked	1 cup	21
Cucumber, with peel, raw	1 cup	17
Cauliflower, cooked from fresh	1 cup	17
Oil, canola	1 tbsp	17
Lettuce, iceberg	1 cup	13
Margarine, regular, tub, 80% fat	1 tbsp	13
Carrots, raw	1 carrot	10
Tomato, raw	1 medium	10
Oil, olive, salad or cooking	1 tbsp	8
Pears, raw	1 pear	8
Salad dressing, mayonnaise, soybean oil	1 tbsp	6
Tomatoes, stewed	1 cup	6
Raisins	1 cup	5
Oil, soybean, salad or cooking, hydrogenated	1 tbsp	3
Apple, fresh, with skin	1 medium	3
Liver, beef	3 oz	3
Cheddar cheese, natural	1 oz	1
Egg yolk only, cooked	1 large	<1
Peanut butter, regular, with salt	1 tbsp	<1

Data from U.S. Department of Agriculture, Agricultural Research Service. 2004. USDA National Nutrient Database for Standard Reference, Release 17. Compiled by the Nutrition Coordinating Center, University of Minnesota, Minneapolis, MN, 2004.

TABLE A-23-c. RETENTION OF NUTRIENTS IN COOKED VEGETABLES[a]

	ASCORBIC ACID (%)	THIAMIN (%)	RIBOFLAVIN (%)	NIACIN (%)	PANTOTHENIC ACID[b] (%)	VITAMIN B$_6$ (%)	FOLATE[c] (%)	VITAMIN A (%)
Potatoes								
Prepared from raw								
Baked in skin	80	85	95	95	90	95	90	—[d]
Boiled in skin	75	80	95	95	90	95	90	—
Boiled without skin	75	80	95	95	90	95	75	—
Fried	80	80	95	95	90	95	75	—
Hashed-brown[e]	25	40	85	80	—	—	65	—
Mashed	75	80	95	95	90	95	75	—
Scalloped and au gratin	80	80	95	95	90	95	75	—
Prepared from frozen								
French fried, heated	50	75	95	95	90	95	75	—
Baked, stuffed, heated	80	85	95	95	90	95	80	—
Hashed-brown	80	80	95	95	90	95	80	—
Sweet Potatoes								
Prepared from raw								
Baked in skin	80	85	95	95	90	95	90	90
Boiled in skin	75	80	95	95	90	95	90	85
Prepared from frozen								
Baked	80	80	95	95	90	95	80	90
Boiled	75	80	95	95	90	95	80	85
Tomatoes								
(prepared from raw, baked, boiled, or stewed)	95	95	95	95	95	95	70	95
Other vegetables (cooked in small or moderate amount of water until tender)								
Prepared from raw, drained								
Greens, dark and leafy[f]	60	85	95	90	95	90	65	95
Roots, bulbs, other vegetables of high starch and/or sugar content[g]	70	85	95	95	90	95	70	90
Other[h]	80	85	95	90	90	90	70	90
Prepared from frozen, drained								
Greens, dark and leafy[f]	60	90	95	90	95	90	55	95
Roots, bulbs, other vegetables of high starch and/or sugar content[g]	70	90	95	95	90	95	70	90
Other[h]	80	90	95	90	90	90	70	90

[a] % True retention = $\dfrac{\text{Nutrition content per g of cooked food} \times \text{g of food after cooking}}{\text{Nutrition content per g of raw food} \times \text{g of food before cooking}} = 100$

[b] Because of limited data, values are based on nutrient retention data from other cooked plant products.

[c] Values are based on limited data.

[d] Dashes denote lack of reliable data.

[e] Potatoes were pared, boiled, and held overnight before hashed-browning.

[f] Vegetables such as beet greens, Chinese cabbage, collards, mustard greens, spinach, Swiss chard, turnip greens, and other wild greens.

[g] Vegetables such as beets, carrots, green peas, lima beans, onions, parsnips, rutabagas, salsify, turnips, summer and winter squash, and other immature seeds of the legume group.

[h] Vegetables such as asparagus, bean sprouts, broccoli, brussels sprouts, cabbage, cauliflower, eggplant, kohlrabi, okra, and sweet peppers.

From Composition of foods, raw, processed, prepared. 1990 Supplement, Washington, DC: U.S. Department of Agriculture. Human Nutrition Information Service, Agriculture Handbook no. 8.

A-24. ORGANIC COMPOUNDS OF INTEREST IN SELECTED FOODS

TABLE A-24-a. CAFFEINE CONTENT IN Mg OF SELECTED COMMON FOODS PER SERVING PORTION

FOOD NAME	SERVING PORTION	CAFFEINE (mg)
Candy, milk chocolate	1.0 oz	7.37
Candy, semi-sweet chocolate	1.0 oz	17.58
Candy, sweet chocolate	1.0 oz	18.71
Chocolate, unsweetened, baking type	1.0 oz	57.83
Chocolate beverage mix, prepared with milk	8.0 fl oz	6.19
Cocoa mix, prepared	6.0 fl oz	3.26
Cocoa powder, unsweetened	1.0 tbsp	12.36
Coffee, brewed, regular	6.0 fl oz	103.01
Coffee, brewed, espresso	6.0 fl oz	376.51
Coffee, instant, regular, prepared	6.0 fl oz	58.56
Coffee, instant, decaffeinated, prepared	6.0 fl oz	2.20
Coffee, instant, cappuccino flavor, prepared	6.0 fl oz	58.91
Coffee, Instant, French flavor, prepared	6.0 fl oz	62.45
Coffee, mocha, with flavored syrup	6.0 fl oz	35.70
Cola beverage, regular	12.0 fl oz	37.20
Cola beverage, diet	12.0 fl oz	49.73
Ice cream, chocolate	0.5 cup	2.16
Milk, chocolate	8.0 fl oz	5.00
Pudding, chocolate	0.5 cup	1.73
Tea, brewed	6.0 fl oz	35.52
Tea, instant, unsweetened, prepared	6.0 fl oz	22.85
Tea, instant, unsweetened, lemon flavored, prepared	6.0 fl oz	19.64
Toppings, chocolate, fudge-type	1.0 tbsp	1.33
Topping, chocolate, syrup	1.0 tbsp	2.73

Data compiled from U.S. Department of Agriculture, Agricultural Research Service. 2004. USDA National Nutrient Database for Standard. Reference, Release 17, and the Nutrition Nutrition Data System for Research (NDS-R) version 5.0_35, 2004, with permission. Table compiled and prepared by the Nutrition Coordinating Center, University of Minnesota, Minneapolis, MN.

TABLE A-24-b. CARNITINE CONTENT OF SELECTED FOODS

FOOD ITEM	CARNITINE CONTENT[a]	FOOD ITEM	CARNITINE CONTENT[a]
Meat products		*Fruits*	
Beef steak	592 ± 260 (4)	Bananas	0.0056
Ground beef	582 ± 32 (3)	Apples	0.0002
Pork	172 ± 32 (3)	Strawberries	ND
Canadian bacon	146 ± 52 (3)	Peaches	0.0060
Bacon	145 ± 24 (3)	Pineapple	0.0063
Fish (cod)	34.6 ± 11.7 (3)	Pears	0.0107
Chicken breast	24.3 ± 8.0 (3)		
Dairy products		*Grains*	
Whole milk	20.4	White bread	0.912
American cheese	23.2	Whole-wheat	
Ice cream	23.0	bread	2.26
Butter	3.07	Rice (cooked)	0.090
Cottage cheese	6.96	Macaroni	0.780
Vegetables		Corn Flakes	0.078
Broccoli (fresh)	0.0228	*Nondairy beverages*	
(cooked)	0.0111	Grapefruit juice	ND
Carrots (fresh)	0.0408	Orange juice	0.012
(cooked)	0.0393	Tamoto juice	0.030
Green beans		Coffee	0.009
(cooked)	0.0189	Cola	ND
Green peas		Grape juice	0.093
(cooked)	0.0369		
Asparagus (cooked)	1.21	*Miscellaneous*	
Beets (cooked)	0.0195	Eggs	0.075
Potato (baked)	0.0800	Peanut butter	0.516
Lettuce	0.0066		

[a] Units are μmol/100 g (solid foods) or μmol/100 mL (liquids). ND, not detectable. Values for meat products are mean ± SD (number of observations in parentheses) and are based on precooked weight. Values reported are for total (nonesterified plus esterified) carnitine.
With appreciation to CJ Rebouche

Adapted from Rebouche CJ, Engel AG. J Clin Invest 1984;73:857-67.

TABLE A-24-c. CHOLINE CONTENT OF SOME COMMON FOODS

FOOD	CONCENTRATION (μmol/kg)[a]		
	CHOLINE	PHOSPHATIDYLCHOLINE	SPHINGOMYELIN
Apple	27	280	15
Banana	240	37	20
Beef liver	5,831	43,500	1,850
Beef steak	75	6,030	506
Butter	42	1,760	460
Cauliflower	1,306	2,770	183
Corn oil	3	12	5
Coffee	90	34	23
Cucumber	218	76	27
Egg	42	52,000	2,250
Ginger ale	2	4	3
Grape juice	475	15	5
Iceberg lettuce	2,930	132	50
Margarine	30	450	15
Milk (bovine, whole)	150	148	82
Orange	200	490	24
Peanut butter	3,895	3,937	9
Peanuts	4,546	4,960	78
Potato	511	300	26
Tomato	430	52	32
Whole wheat bread	968	340	11

[a] Choline, phosphatidylcholine and sphingomyelin were measured using a gas chromatography/mass spectrometry assay in foods prepared in the form that they would normally be consumed.
Courtesy of SH Zeisel

Modified from Zeisel SH. Biological consequences of choline deficiency. In: Wurtman R. Wurtman J, eds. Choline metabolism and Brain Function. New York: Raven Press, 1990; 75-99.

A-24-d. Phenolic Phytochemicals

TABLE A-24-d-1. PHENOLIC PHYTOCHEMICAL CONTENT OF SELECTED FOODS[a]

CLASS AND SUBCLASS	PHYTOCHEMICALS	FOOD OR BEVERAGE	QUANTITY (mg)[b]	REFERENCE
Flavonoids				
Flavonols	Quercetin, kaempferol, myricetin	Olives	270–830	25
		Onion	347	8
		Kale	321	6
		Leaf lettuce	308	8
		Cranberry	249	26
		Cherry tomato	17–203	8
		Broccoli	102	6
		Apple	21–72	10
		Beans, green/yellow	49	9
		Turnip greens	48	6
		Endive	46	6
		Tea, green leaves	30–45 g/kg DW[c]	27
		Apple juice	6–52	28
		Tea, black beverage	20	6
Flavones	Apigenin, luteolin	Celery	130	6
		Olives	6–29	25
Flavanols	Catechin, epicatechin	Pear	70–420	29
		Red wine	274	30
		Tea, green leaves	128–226 g/kg DW	27
		White wine	35	30
		Apple	23–30	31
Isoflavones	Genistein, daidzein	Soybeans, mature, dry	888–2,407	12,13
		Soy nuts	1,437–2,363	3,13,32
		Textured vegetable protein	1,175–1,191	13
		Soy flour	1,036–1,778	12,13,32
		Tofu	280–499	3,12,13,32
		Miso	256–540	3,13,32
		Soybeans, mature, fresh	182–205	3,12
		Soy milk	105–251	3,32
		Tofu yogurt	151	13
		Soy hot dog	116	13
		Soy cheese	7–74	13,32
		Soy sauce	13–23	3,32
Phenolic acids				
Hydroxycinnamic acids	Caffeic, ferulic, chlorogenic, neochlorogenic acids	Blueberry	1,881–2,112	2
		Cherry, sweet	290–1,280	33
		Pear	44–1,270	29,34
		Apple	2–258	29
		Orange	21–182	35
		Potato, white	100–190	36
		Grapefruit	25–60	35
		Cherry juice	124	37
		Apple juice	9–114	37
		Coffee beans	56 g/kg DW	38
Hydroxybenzoic acids	Ellagic, gallic acids	Raspberry	19–102	39,40
		Strawberry	21–89	39,40
		Grape juice, black	79	37
		Grape juice, green	110	37
Tannins				
Condensed	Catechin, epicatechin polymers	Lentils	3,800	41
		Black-eyed peas	141–1,774	21
		Grape, dark	43–64	2
		Grape, light	39–53	2
		Red wine	2,567	30
		White wine	239	30
		Apple juice	8–87	42

[a] Quantities given are a total of all phytochemicals included in the subclass. Quantities are not given for individual phytochemicals. For meaningful comparisons, only recent (since 1985) studies in which phenolics are reported as a percentage of the fresh weight of the food are included.
[b] DW = dry weight.
From King A, Young G. Characteristics and occurrence of phenolic phytochemicals. J. Am Dietetic Assoc. 1999;99:213–18 with permission.

TABLE A-24-d-2. PHENOLIC PHYTOCHEMICAL CONTENT OF SELECTED FRUITS[a]

| FRUIT | FLAVONOIDS | | | | PHENOLIC ACIDS | | CONDENSED TANNINS | REFERENCE |
	FLAVONOLS	FLAVONES	FLAVANOLS	ISOFLAVONES	HYDROXYBENZOICS	HYDROXYCINNAMICS		
					mg^b			
Apple	21–72		23–30			2–258		10,29
Blueberry						1,881–2,112		2
Cherry, sweet						290–1,280		33
Cranberry	249							26
Grape, light							39–53	2
Grape dark							43–64	2
Grapefruit						25–160		35
Olives	270–830							25
Orange		6–29				21–182		35
Pear			70–420			44–1,270	630,1,110	29,34
Raspberry					59–142			40,41
Strawberry					21–80			40,41
Tomato, cherry	17–203							8

[a] Content listed only for the phenolic phytochemical levels of fruits with relatively high concentrations (>30 mg/kg) of a specific phytochemical. If no content is listed under a specific phytochemical, that fruit has been less than 30 mg/kg of that phytochemical or no recent (since 1985) studies were found that quantified that chemical in that fruit in milligrams per kilogram fresh weight.
[b] Milligrams per kilogram fruit.

From King A, Young G. J. Am Dietetic Assoc. 1999;99:213–18 with permission.

TABLE A-24-d-3. PHENOLIC PHYTOCHEMICAL CONTENT OF SELECTED BEVERAGES[a]

| BEVERAGE | FLAVONOIDS | | PHENOLIC ACIDS | | CONDENSED TANNINS | REFERENCE |
	FLAVONOLS	FLAVANOLS	HYDROXYBENZOICS	HYDROXYCINNAMICS		
			mg^b			
Apple juice	6–52			9–114	8–87	28,37
Cherry juice				124		37
Coffee beans				56 g/kg DW		38
Grape juice, black			79			37
Grape juice, green			110			37
Red wine		274	95		2,567	30
White wine		56			239	30
Tea, black, brewed	20					6
Tea, green leaves	30–45 g/kg DW[c]	128–226 g/kg DW				27

[a] Content listed only for the phenolic phytochemical levels of fruits with relatively high concentrations (>30 mg/L) of a specific phytochemical. If no content is listed under a specific phytochemical, that fruit has less than 30 mg/kg of that phytochemical or no recent (since 1985) studies were found that quantified that chemical in that fruit in milligrams per liter fresh weight.
[b] Milligrams per liter juice.
[b] DW=dry weight.

From King A, Young G. J. Am Dietetic Assoc. 1999;99:213–18 with permission.

TABLE A-24-d-4. PHENOLIC PHYTOCHEMICAL CONTENT OF SELECTED VEGETABLES/FOODS[a]

VEGETABLE/FOOD	FLAVONOLDS			PHENOLIC ACIDS		REFERENCE
	FLAVONOLS	FLAVONES	ISOFLAVONES	HYDROXYCINNAMICS	CONDENSED TANNINS	
			mg[b]			
Celery		130				6
Beans, green and yellow snap	49					9
Black-eyed peas					141–1,774	21
Broccoli	102					6
Endive	46					6
Kale	321					6
Leaf lettuce	308					8
Lentils					3,800	41
Onion	347					8
Potato, white flesh				100–190		36
Turnip greens	48					6
Soybeans, mature, dry			882–2,407			12,13
Soybeans, mature, fresh			182–205			3,12
Soy nuts			1,437–2,363			3,13,32
Soy flour			1,036–1,178			12,13,32
Textured vegetable protein			1,175–1,191			13
Tofu			280–499			3,12,13,32
Soy milk			105–251			3,32
Miso			256–540			3,13,32
Soy sauce			13–23			3,32
Soy hot dog			116			13
Soy cheese			7–74			13,32
Tofu yogurt			151			13
Tofu ice cream			31			13

[a] Content listed only for the phenolic phytochemical levels of vegetables with relatively high concentrations (>30 mg/kg) of a specific phytochemical. If no content is listed under a specific phytochemical, that vegetable has less than 30 mg/kg of that phytochemical or no recent (since 1985) studies were found that quantified that chemical in that vegetable in mg/kg fresh weight.

[b] Milligrams per kilogram vegetable or food.

From King A, Young G. J. Am Dietetic Assoc. 1999;99:213–18 with permission.

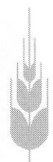

A-25. MEDICAL FOODS AND DIETS FOR INHERITED METABOLIC DISEASES

TABLE A-25-a. FORMULATION, NUTRIENT COMPOSITION, AND SOURCES OF MEDICAL FOODS FOR SELECTED INBORN ERRORS OF METABOLISM

DISORDER/MEDICAL FOODS	MODIFIED NUTRIENT(S) (mg/100 g)	PROTEIN EQUIVALENT (g/100 g)/SOURCE	FAT (g/100 g)/SOURCE	CARBOHYDRATE (g/100 g)/SOURCE	ENERGY (kcal/100 g)	MINERALS NOT ADDED
Aromatic Amino Acids *PKU and Hyperphenylalaninemia*						
Periflex[a]	PHE-0, TYR-1850, TRP-270, L-carnitine-20, taurine-520	20 L-Amino acids	17 Canola, hybrid safflower, fractionated coconut oils	40.5 Corn syrup solids	395[b] 411[c]	None
Phenex-1[d]	PHE-0, TYR-1500, TRP-170, L-carnitine-20, taurine-40	15 L-Amino acids	21.7 High-oleic safflower, coconut, soy oils	53 Corn syrup solids	480	None
Phenex-2[d]	PHE-0, TYR-3000, TRP-340, L-carnitine-40, taurine-50	30 L-Amino acids	14.0 High-oleic safflower, coconut, soy oils	35 Corn syrup solids	410	None
Phenex-2 Vanilla[d]	PHE-0, TYR-3000, TRP-340, L-carnitine-40, taurine-50	30 L-Amino acids	13.5 High-oleic safflower, coconut, soy oils	36 Corn syrup solids	410	None
XP Analog[a]	PHE-0, TYR-1370, TRP-300, L-carnitine-10, taurine-20	13 L-Amino acids	20.9 Peanut oil, refined lard, hydrogenated coconut oils	59 Corn syrup solids	475	None
XP Maxamaid[a]	PHE-0, TYR-2650, TRP-570; L-carnitine-20, taurine-140	25 L-Amino acids	<1.0 None added	62 Sucrose, hydrolyzed corn starch	350	None
XP Maxamum[a]	PHE-0, TYR-4030, TRP-890, L-carnitine-20, taurine added	39 L-Amino acids	<1.0 None added	45 Sucrose, hydrolyzed corn starch	340	None
Phenyl-Free-1[e]	PHE-0, TYR-1600, TRP-290; L-carnitine added, taurine-140	16.2 L-Amino acids	26 Palm olein, soy, coconut oils	51 Corn syrup solids, modified corn starch, sugar	500	Chromium Molybdenum
Phenyl-Free-2[e]	PHE-0, TYR-2200, TRP-290; L-carnitine, taurine added	22 L-Amino acids	8.6 Soy oil	60 Sugar, corn syrup solids, modified corn starch	410	None
Phenyl-Free 2HP[e]	PHE-0, TYR-4000, TRP-720; L-carnitine, taurine added	40 L-Amino acids	6.3 Soy oil	44 Sugar, corn syrup solids, modified corn starch	390	None
Tyrosinemia Types I, II, III						
Tyrex-1[d]	PHE-0, TYR-0; L-carnitine-20, taurine-40	15 L-Amino acids	21.7 High-oleic safflower, coconut, soy oils	53 Corn syrup solids	480	None
Tyrex-2[d]	PHE-0, TYR-0; L-carnitine-40, taurine-50	30 L-Amino acids	14.0 High-oleic safflower, coconut, soy oils	35 corn syrup solids	410	None
XPHE, TYR Analog[a]	PHE-0, TYR-0; L-carnitine-10, taurine-20	13 L-Amino acids	20.9 Peanut oil, refined lard,	59 Corn syrup solids	475	None

(continued)

DISORDER/MEDICAL FOODS	MODIFIED NUTRIENT(S) (mg/100 g)	PROTEIN EQUIVALENT (g/100 g)/SOURCE	FAT (g/100 g)/SOURCE	CARBOHYDRATE (g/100 g)/SOURCE	ENERGY (kcal/100 g)	MINERALS NOT ADDED
XPHE, TYR Maxamaid[a]	PHE-0, TYR-0; L-carnitine-20, taurine-140	25 L-Amino acids	hydrogenated coconut oils <1.0 None added	62 Sucrose, hydrolyzed corn starch	350	None
Tyros 2[e]	PHE-0, TYR-0; L-carnitine, taurine added	22 L-Amino acids	8.5 Soy oil	60 Corn syrup solids, modified corn starch, sugar	410	None
Homocystinuria–Pyridoxine Nonresponsive						
HCY Powder[e]	MET-0, CYS-810; L-carnitine, taurine added	22 L-Amino acids	8.5 Soy oil	61 Corn syrup solids, modified corn starch	410	None
Hominex-1[d]	MET-0, CYS-450; L-carnitine-20, taurine-40	15 L-Amino acids	21.7 High-oleic safflower, coconut, soy oils	53 Corn syrup solids	480	None
Hominex-2[d]	MET-0, CYS-900; L-carnitine-40, taurine-50	30 L-Amino acids	14.0 High-oleic safflower, coconut, soy oils	35 Corn syrup solids	410	None
XMET Analog[a]	MET-0, CYS-390; L-carnitine-10, taurine-20	13 L-Amino acids	20.9 Peanut oil, refined lard, hydrogenated coconut oils	59 Corn syrup solids	475	None
XMET Maxamaid[a]	MET-0, CYS-750; L-carnitine-20, taurine-140	25 L-Amino acids	<1.0 None added	62 Sucrose, hydrolyzed corn starch	350	None
XMET Maxamum[a]	MET-0, CYS-1180; L-carnitine-20, taurine-140	39 L-Amino acids	<1.0 None added	45 Sucrose, hydrolyzed corn starch	340	None
Organic Acids						
Maple Syrup Urine Disease						
Acerflex[a]	ILE-0, LEU-0, VAL-0; L-carnitine-20, taurine-140	20 L-Amino acids	17 Canola, hybrid safflower, fractionated coconut oils	40.5 Corn syrup solids	395	None
Ketonex-1[d]	ILE-0, LEU-0, VAL-0; L-carnitine-100, taurine-40	15 L-Amino acids	21.7 High-oleic safflower, coconut, soy oils	53 Corn syrup solids	480	None
Ketonex-2[d]	ILE-0, LEU-0, VAL-0; L-carnitine-200, taurine-50	30 L-Amino acids	14.0 High-oleic safflower, coconut, soy oils	35 Corn syrup solids	410	None
MSUD Analog[a]	ILE-0, LEU-0, VAL-0; L-carnitine-10, taurine 20	13 L-Amino acids	20.9 Peanut oil, refined lard, hydrogenated coconut oil	59 Corn syrup solids	475	None

Product		Protein source	Fat & source	Carbohydrate & source		Chromium Molybdenum
MSUD Diet Powder[e]	ILE-0, LEU-0, VAL-0; L-carnitine added, taurine-140	L-Amino acids	20 Corn oil	63 Corn syrup solids, modified corn starch	470	None
MSUD 2 Powder[e]	ILE-0, LEU-0, VAL-0; L-carnitine, taurine added	L-Amino acids	8.5 Soy oil	57 Corn syrup solids, modified corn starch	410	None
MSUD Maxamaid[a]	ILE-0, LEU-0, VAL-0; L-carnitine-10, taurine-140	L-Amino acids	<1.0 None added	62 Sucrose, hydrolyzed corn starch	350	None
MSUD Maxamum[a]	ILE-0, LEU-0, VAL-0; L-carnitine-20, taurine-140	L-Amino acids	<1.0 None added	45 Sucrose, hydrolyzed corn starch	340	None
Isovaleric Acidemia and Other Disorders of Leucine Catabolism						
I-Valex-1[d]	ILE-430, LEU-0, TRP-170, VAL-480; L-carnitine-900, GLY-1000, taurine-40	L-Amino acids	21.7 High-oleic safflower, coconut, soy oils	53 Corn syrup solids	480	None
I-Valex-2[d]	ILE-860, LEU-0, TRP-340, VAL-960; L-carnitine-1800, GLY-3020, taurine-50	L-Amino acids	14.0 High-oleic safflower, coconut, soy oils	35 Corn syrup solids	410	None
XLEU Analog[a]	ILE-400, LEU-0, TRP-260, VAL-450; L-carnitine-10, GLY-2500, taurine-20	L-Amino acids	20.9 Peanut oil, refined lard, hydrogenated coconut oils	59 Corn syrup solids	475	None
XLEU Maxamaid[a]	ILE-780, LEU-0, TRP-500, VAL-870; L-carnitine-20, GLY-3990, taurine-140	L-Amino acids	<1.0 None added	62 Sucrose, hydrolyzed corn starch	350	None
Propionic and Methylmalonic Acidemias						
Propimex-1[d]	ILE-120, MET-0, THR-100, VAL-0; L-carnitine-900, taurine-40	L-Amino acids	21.7 High-oleic safflower, coconut, soy oils	53 Corn syrup solids	480	None
Propimex-2[d]	ILE-240, MET-0, THR-200, VAL-0; L-carnitine-1800, taurine-50	L-Amino acids	13.0 High-oleic safflower, coconut, soy oils	35 Corn syrup solids	410	None
XMTVI Analog[a]	ILE-trace, MET-0, THR-0, VAL-0; L-carnitine added, taurine-20	L-Amino acids	20.9 Peanut oil, refined lard, hydrogenated coconut oils	59 Corn syrup solids	475	None
XMTVI Maxamaid[a]	ILE-trace, MET-0, THR-0, VAL-0; L-carnitine added, taurine-140	L-Amino acids	<1.0 None added	62 Sucrose, hydrolyzed corn starch	350	None
XMTVI Maxamum[a]	ILE-trace, MET-0, THR-0, VAL-0; L-carnitine added, taurine-140	L-Amino acids	<1.0 None added	45 Sucrose, hydrolyzed corn starch	340	None
Glutaric Acidemia Type I						
Glutarex-1[d]	LYS-0, TRP-0; L-carnitine-900, taurine-40	L-Amino acids	21.7 High-oleic safflower, coconut, soy oils	53 Corn syrup solids	480	None

(continued)

TABLE A-25-a. FORMULATION, NUTRIENT COMPOSITION, AND SOURCES OF MEDICAL FOODS FOR SELECTED INBORN ERRORS OF METABOLISM (continued)

DISORDER/MEDICAL FOODS	MODIFIED NUTRIENT(S) (mg/100 g)	PROTEIN EQUIVALENT (g/100 g)/SOURCE	FAT (g/100 g)/SOURCE	CARBOHYDRATE (g/100 g)/SOURCE	ENERGY (kcal/100 g)	MINERALS NOT ADDED
Glutarex-2[d]	LYS-0, TRP-0; L-carnitine-1800, taurine-50	30 L-Amino acids	13.0 High-oleic safflower, coconut, soy oils	35 Corn syrup solids	410	None
XLYS, TRY Analog[a]	LYS-0, TRP-0; L-carnitine, taurine-20	13 L-Amino acids	20.9 Peanut oil, refined lard, hydrogenated coconut oils	59 Corn syrup solids	475	None
XLYS, TRY Maxamaid[a]	LYS-0, TRP-0; L-carnitine added, taurine-140	25 L-Amino acids	<1.0 None added	62 Sucrose, hydrolyzed corn starch	350	None
XLYS, TRY Maxamum[a]	LYS-0, TRP-0; L-carnitine added, taurine-140	39 L-Amino acids	<1.0 None added	45 Sucrose, hydrolyzed corn starch	340	None
Urea Cycle Enzyme Defects						
Cyclinex-1[d]	Nonessential amino acids-0; L-carnitine-190, taurine-40	7.5 L-Amino acids	24.5 High-oleic safflower, coconut, soy oils	57 Corn syrup solids	510	None
Cyclinex-2[d]	Nonessential amino acids-0; L-carnitine-370, taurine-60	15 L-Amino acids	17.0 High-oleic safflower, coconut, soy oils	45 Corn syrup solids	440	None
WND 2	Nonessential amino acids-0; L-carnitine, taurine added	8.2 L-Amino acids	6.9 Soy oil	71 Corn syrup solids, modified tapioca starch	410	None
Pro-Phree[d]	Protein-0; L-carnitine-25, taurine-50	0	31.0 Palm, hydrogenated coconut, soy oils	60 Hydrolyzed cornstarch	520	None
PFD 2[e]	Protein-0; L-carnitine, taurine added	0	4.8 Soy oil	88 Corn syrup solids, sugar modified cornstarch	400	None
Protein-Free Diet Powder[e]	Protein-0; L-carnitine, taurine added	0	23.0 Corn oil	72 Corn syrup solids, modified tapioca starch	500	Chromium Molybdenum

[a] Scientific Hospital Supplies, North American Division, Gaithersburg, MD; 800-365-7354.
[b] Unflavored.
[c] Flavored.
[d] Ross Products Division, Abbott Laboratories, Columbus, OH; 800-551-5838.
[e] Mead Johnson Nutritional Division, Evansville, IN; 800-457-3550.

NOTE: values listed, although accurate at time of publication, are subject to change. The most current information may be obtained by referring to product labels. This table is referenced in the text of Chapter 58. It was prepared by Drs. Elsas and Acosta, the authors of that chapter.

TABLE A-25-b. AVERAGE NUTRIENT CONTENT OF SERVING LIST FOR PHENYLALANINE AND/OR TYROSINE AND PROTEIN-RESTRICTED DIETS

FOOD LIST	PHENYLALANINE (mg)	TYROSINE (mg)	PROTEIN (g)	CARBOHYDRATE (g)	FAT (g)	ENERGY (kcal)
Breads/cereals	30	20	0.6	7	0.0	30
Fats	5	4	0.1	0	5.0	60
Fruits	15	10	0.5	15	0.0	60
Vegetables	15	10	0.5	2	0.0	10
Free Foods A[a]	5	4	0.1	18	0.0	65
Free Foods B[a]	0	0	0	14	varies	55
Infant Formulas, Concentrate, 100 mL						
Enfamil with Iron[b]	116	134	3.0	13.9	7.6	135
Isomil Advance[c]	176	120	3.3	13.9	7.4	136
ProSobee[b]	198	138	4.0	13.5	7.2	135
Similac Advance[c] With Iron	118	116	2.8	14.6	7.3	136

[a] Very-low-protein pastas and breads not included.
[b] Mead Johnson Nutritionals Division, Evansville, IN; 800-457-3550.
[c] Ross Products Division, Abbott Laboratories, Columbus, OH; 800-551-5838.

This table is referenced in the text of Chapter 58. It was prepared by Drs. Elsas and Acosta, the authors of that chapter.

TABLE A-25-c. SAMPLE DIETS PHENYLKETONURIA (2 wk OF AGE): WEIGHT 3.25 kg

PRESCRIPTION	TOTAL	PER kg			
Phenylalanine, mg	179	55			
Tyrosine, mg	980	302			
Protein, g	9.8	3.0			
Energy, kcal	390	120			
Water, mL					

MEDICAL FOOD #1	AMOUNT	PHENYLALANINE (mg)	TYROSINE[a] (mg)	PROTEIN (g)	ENERGY (kcal)
Phenex-1	41 g	0	620	6.2	197
Similac Advance With Iron, Concentrate	126 mL	179	166	3.6	170
Table sugar	0.5 Tbsp	0	0	0.0	24
Water to make	600 mL				
Total		179	786	9.8	391

MEDICAL FOOD #2	AMOUNT	PHENYLALANINE (mg)	TYROSINE[a] (mg)	PROTEIN (g)	ENERGY (kcal)
Phenyl-Free 1	28 g	0	448	4.5	140
Enfamil With Iron, Concentrate	153 mL	179	206	4.6	206
Table sugar	1 Tbsp	0	0	0.0	48
Water to make	600 mL				
Total		179	654	9.1	394

MEDICAL FOOD #3	AMOUNT	PHENYLALANINE (mg)	TYROSINE[a] (mg)	PROTEIN (g)	ENERGY (kcal)
XP Analog	46 g	0	630	6.0	218
Similac Advance With Iron, Concentrate	128 mL	179	179	3.8	173
Water to make	600 mL				
Total		179	809	9.8	391

[a] Add L-tyrosine only if plasma tyrosine concentration is below the lower limit of the reference range. Reference range is 55–147 μmol/L.

This table is referenced in the text of Chapter 58. It was prepared by Drs. Elsas and Acosta, the authors of that chapter.

TABLE A-25-d. RECOMMENDED PHENYLALANINE, TYROSINE, PROTEIN, FAT, ESSENTIAL FATTY ACID, AND ENERGY INTAKES FOR PREGNANT WOMEN WITH PHENYLKETONURIA

TRIMESTER AND AGE	NUTRIENTS							
	PHENYLALANINE[a,b] (mg/d)	TYROSINE[b] (mg/d)	PROTEIN[c] (g/d)	FAT (g/d)	LINOLEIC ACID (g/d)	α-LINOLENIC ACID (g/d)	ENERGY[c] (kcal/d) MEAN	RANGE
Trimester 1 (0 < 14 wk gestation)								
15 < 19	200 < 820	≥7,600	≥76	36–132	13	1.4	2,500	1,600–3,400
19 < 24	180 < 800	≥7,400	≥74	47–124	13	1.4	2,500	2,100–3,200
≥24	180 < 800	≥7,400	≥74	47–132	13	1.4	2,500	2,100–3,400
Trimester 2 (14 < 27 wk gestation)								
15 < 19	200 < 1,000	≥7,600	≥76	36–132	13	1.4	2,500	1,600–3,400
19 < 24	180 < 1,000	≥7,400	≥74	47–124	13	1.4	2,500	2,100–3,200
≥24	180 < 1,000	≥7,400	≥74	47–132	13	1.4	2,500	2,100–3,400
Trimester 3 (27 < 41 wk gestation)								
15 < 19	330 < 1,200	≥7,600	≥76	36–132	13	1.4	2,500	1,600–3,400
19 < 24	310 < 1,200	≥7,400	≥74	47–124	13	1.4	2,500	2,100–3,200
≥24	310 < 1,200	≥7,400	≥74	47–132	13	1.4	2,500	2,100–3,400

[a] Recommended range of PHE intake covered about 80% of MPKUCS women studied. Initiate diet with the lowest amount recommended for trimester and age. Frequent monitoring of plasma PHE is essential to prevent deficiency or excess. Modify prescription based on frequent plasma PHE and TYR concentrations; intakes of PHE, TYR, protein and energy; and maternal weight gain. Recommended intake is from MPKUCS data (78).

[b] L-TYR is very insoluble in water. Consequently, any supplemental L-TYR should be mixed with fruit purees, mashed potatoes, or soup for ingestion. Recommended intake is from MPKUCS data (78).

[c] Modified from Dietary Reference Intakes (1). For some women, energy requirements may be greater than the upper limit of the range given, to obtain appropriate weight gain.

This table is referenced in the text of Chapter 58. It was prepared by Drs. Elsas and Acosta, the authors of that chapter.

TABLE A-25-e. AVERAGE NUTRIENT CONTENT OF SERVING LISTS FOR METHIONINE-RESTRICTED DIETS

FOOD LIST	METHIONINE (mg)	CYSTINE (mg)	PROTEIN (g)	FAT (g)	ENERGY (kcal)
Breads/cereals	20	20	1.2	0.0	55
Fats	2	0	0.1	2.0	50
Fruits	5	5	0.5	0.0	60
Vegetables	10	8	1.0	0.0	20
Free Foods A[a]	1	1	0.2	0.0	50
Free Foods B[a]	0	0	0.0	Varies	55
Infant Formulas, Concentrate, 100 mL					
Enfamil with Iron[b]	58	35	3.0	7.6	136
Isomil Advance[c]	84	36	3.3	7.4	136
ProSobee[b]	73	36	4.0	7.2	136
Similac Advance[c] With Iron	70	38	2.8	7.3	136

[a] Very low-protein pastas and breads not included.

[b] Mead Johnson Nutritionals Division, Evansville, IN; 800-457-3550.

[c] Ross Products Division, Abbott Laboratories, Columbus, OH; 800-551-5838.

This table is referenced in the text of Chapter 58. It was prepared by Drs. Elsas and Acosta, the authors of that chapter.

TABLE A-25-f. SAMPLE DIETS FOR HOMOCYSTINURIA (2 wk OF AGE): WEIGHT 3.25 kg

PRESCRIPTION	TOTAL	PER kg			
Methionine, mg	97	30			
Cystine, mg	975	300			
Protein, g	9.8	3.0			
Energy, kcal	390	120			
Water to make, mL	600				

MEDICAL FOOD #1	AMOUNT	METHIONINE (mg)	CYSTINE (mg)	PROTEIN (g)	ENERGY (kcal)
Hominex-1	39 g	0	176	5.8	187
Similac Advance With Iron, concentrate	138 mL	97	37	3.9	188
L-Cystine, 10 mg/mL	76 mL	0	760	0	0
Table sugar	4 g	0	0	0	15
Water to make	600 mL	0	0	0	0
Total		97	973	9.7	390

MEDICAL FOOD #2	AMOUNT	METHIONINE (mg)	CYSTINE (mg)	PROTEIN (g)	ENERGY (kcal)
XMET Analog	45 g	0	164	5.9	214
Similac Advance With Iron, concentrate	138 mL	97	37	3.9	188
L-Cystine, 10 mg/mL	79 mL	0	770	0	0
Water to make	595 mL				
Total		97	971	9.8	402

TABLE A-25-g. AVERAGE NUTRIENT CONTENT OF EQUIVALENT LISTS FOR BRANCHED-CHAIN AMINO ACID–RESTRICTED DIETS

FOOD LIST	ISOLEUCINE (mg)	LEUCINE (mg)	VALINE (mg)	PROTEIN (g)	FAT (g)	ENERGY (kcal)
Breads/cereals	18	35	25	0.5	0.0	30
Fats	7	10	7	0.1	8.0	70
Fruits	17	25	22	0.6	0.0	75
Vegetables	22	30	24	0.6	0.0	15
Free Foods A[a]	3	5	4	0.1	0.0	50
Free Foods B[a]	0	0	0	0.0	Varies	55
Infant Formulas, Concentrate, 100 mL						
Enfamil with Iron[b]	181	310	184	3.0	7.6	136
Isomil Advance[c]	148	270	152	3.3	7.4	136
ProSobee[b]	186	310	186	4.0	7.2	136
Similac Advance[c] With Iron	150	288	166	2.8	7.3	136

[a] Very-low-protein pastas and breads not included.
[b] Mead Johnson Nutritionals Division, Evansville, IN; 800-457-3550.
[c] Ross Products Division, Abbott Laboratories, Columbus, OH; 800-551-5838.

This table is referenced in the text of Chapter 58. It was prepared by Drs. Elsas and Acosta, the authors of that chapter.

TABLE A-25-h. SAMPLE DIETS FOR BRANCHED-CHAIN KETOACIDURIA (2 wk OF AGE): WEIGHT 3.25 kg

PRESCRIPTION	TOTAL	PER kg
Isoleucine, mg	163	50
Leucine, mg	229	70
Valine, mg	195	60
Protein, g	9.8	3.0
Energy, kcal	400	123
Water to make, mL	600	

MEDICAL FOOD #1	AMOUNT	ISOLEUCINE (mg)	LEUCINE (mg)	VALINE (mg)	PROTEIN (g)	ENERGY (kcal)
Ketonex-1	51 g	0	0	0	7.6	245
Similac Advance With Iron, concentrate	79 mL	118	228	131	2.2	107
Table sugar	13 g	0	0	0	0.0	50
Isoleucine, 10 mg/mL	4.6 mL	46	0	0	0.0	0
Valine, 10 mg/mL	6.4 mL	0	0	64	0.0	0
Water to make	600 mL	0	0	0	0.0	0
Total		164	228	195	9.8	402

MEDICAL FOOD #2	AMOUNT	ISOLEUCINE (mg)	LEUCINE (mg)	VALINE (mg)	PROTEIN (g)	ENERGY (kcal)
MSUD Analog	54 g	0	0	0	7.0	256
Isomil Advance, concentrate	84 mL	124	227	128	2.8	114
Polycose liquid	15 mL	0	0	0	0.0	30
Isoleucine, 10 mg/mL	3.4 mL	34	0	0	0.0	0
Valine, 10 mg/mL	6.6 mL	0	0	66	0.0	0
Water to make	600 mL	—	—	—	—	—
Total		158	227	194	9.8	400

MEDICAL FOOD #3	AMOUNT	ISOLEUCINE (mg)	LEUCINE (mg)	VALINE (mg)	PROTEIN (g)	ENERGY (kcal)
MSUD Diet Powder[a]	94 g	0	0	0	7.6	442
Enfamil With Iron, concentrate	73.3 mL	133	228	135	2.2	99
Isoleucine, 10 mg/mL	3 mL	30	0	0	0.0	0
Valine, 10 mg/mL	6 mL	0	0	60	0.0	0
Water to make	600 mL	—	—	—	—	—
Total		163	228	195	9.8	541*

[a] In order to supply adequate protein with MSUD Diet Powder, energy prescription must be exceeded.

This table is referenced in the text of Chapter 58. It was prepared by Drs. Elsas and Acosta, the authors of that chapter.

TABLE A-25-i. AVERAGE NUTRIENT CONTENT OF SERVING LIST FOR ISOLEUCINE-, METHIONINE-, THREONINE-, AND VALINE-RESTRICTED DIETS

FOOD LIST	ISOLEUCINE (mg)	METHIONINE (mg)	THREONINE (mg)	VALINE (mg)	PROTEIN (g)	FAT (g)	ENERGY (kcal)
Breads/cereals	25	10	25	35	0.70	0.0	30
Fats	5	2	5	5	0.10	5.0	30
Fruits	10	5	10	15	0.50	0.0	55
Vegetables	15	5	15	20	0.50	0.0	10
Free Food A[a]	4	2	4	5	0.10	Varies	65
Free Foods B[a]	0	0	0	0	0.00	Varies	55
Infant Formulas, Concentrate, 100 mL							
Isomil Advance[b]	148	84	128	152	3.82	7.4	136
Similac Advance[b] With Iron	150	70	154	166	2.80	7.3	136

[a] Very low-protein pastas and breads not included.
[b] Ross Products Division, Abbott Laboratories, Columbus, OH; 800-551-5838.

This table is referenced in the text of Chapter 58. It was prepared by Drs. Elsas and Acosta, the authors of that chapter.

TABLE A-25-j. SAMPLE DIETS FOR PROPIONIC ACIDEMIA AND METHYLMALONIC ACIDEMIA (2 wk OF AGE): WEIGHT 3.25 kg

PRESCRIPTION	TOTAL	PER kg
Isoleucine, mg	325	100
Methionine, mg	162	50
Threonine, mg	260	80
Valine, mg	276	85
L-Carnitine, mg	325	325
Protein, g	11.4	3.5
Energy, kcal	470	150

MEDICAL FOOD #1	AMOUNT	ISOLEUCINE (mg)	METHIONINE (mg)	THREONINE (mg)	VALINE (mg)	L-CARNITINE (mg)	PROTEIN (g)	ENERGY (kcal)
Propimex-1	34 g	41	0	34	0	366	5.1	163
Similac Advance With Iron, concentrate	166 mL	245	139	212	276	2	6.3	226
L-Isoleucine, 10 mg/mL	4 mL	40	—	—	—	—	—	—
L-Threonine, 10 mg/mL	2 mL	—	—	20	—	—	—	—
Polycose liquid	40 mL	—	—	—	—	—	—	80
Water to make	680 mL	—	—	—	—	—	—	—
Total		326	139	266	276	368	11.4	469

MEDICAL FOOD #2	AMOUNT	ISOLEUCINE (mg)	METHIONINE (mg)	THREONINE (mg)	VALINE (mg)	L-CARNITINE (mg)	PROTEIN (g)	ENERGY (kcal)
XMTVI Analog	39 g	—	—	—	—	4	5.1	185
Similac Advance With Iron, concentrate	166 mL	245	139	212	276	2	6.3	226
L-Isoleucine, 10 mg/mL	8 mL	80	—	—	—	—	—	—
L-Threonine, 10 mg/mL	5 mL	—	—	50	—	—	—	—
Polycose liquid	30 mL	—	—	—	—	—	—	60
L-Carnitine		—	—	—	—	319	—	—
Water to make	680 mL	—	—	—	—	—	—	—
Total		325	139	262	276	325	11.4	471

This table is referenced in the text of Chapter 58. It was prepared by Drs. Elsas and Acosta, the authors of that chapter.

TABLE A-25-k. AVERAGE NUTRIENT CONTENT OF SERVING LISTS FOR LYSINE- AND TRYPTOPHAN-RESTRICTED DIETS

FOOD LIST	LYSINE (mg)	TRYPTOPHAN (mg)	PROTEIN (g)	FAT (g)	ENERGY (kcal)
Breads/cereals	30	10	0.9	0.0	40
Fats	6	2	0.1	5.0	60
Fruits	20	5	0.6	0.0	45
Vegetables	20	5	0.5	0.0	15
Free Foods A[a]	5	1	0.1	0.0	55
Free Foods B[a]	0	0	0.0	Varies	60
Infant Formulas, Concentrate, 100 mL					
Isomil Advance[b]	200	42	3.3	7.4	136
Similac Advance[b] With Iron	226	44	2.8	7.3	136

[a] Very low-protein pastas and breads not included.
[b] Ross Products Division, Abbott Laboratories, Columbus, OH. 800 551-5838.

This table is referenced in the text of Chapter 58. It was prepared by Drs. Elsas and Acosta, the authors of that chapter.

TABLE A-25-I. SAMPLE DIETS FOR GLUTARIC ACIDEMIA TYPE I (2 wk OF AGE): WEIGHT 3.25 kg

PRESCRIPTION	TOTAL	PER kg
Lysine, mg	276	85
Tryptophan, mg	55	17
Protein, g	9.8	3.0
L-Carnitine, mg	325	100
Energy, kcal	390	128

MEDICAL FOOD #1	AMOUNT	LYSINE (mg)	TRYPTOPHAN (mg)	PROTEIN (g)	L-CARNITINE (mg)	ENERGY (kcal)
Glutarex-1	43 g	0	0	6.4	387	206
Similac Advance With Iron, concentrate	122 mL	276	54	3.4	2	166
Polycose Liquid	9 mL	0	0	0	0	18
Water to make	600 mL	—	—	—	—	—
Total		276	54	9.8	389	390

MEDICAL FOOD #2	AMOUNT	LYSINE (mg)	TRYPTOPHAN (mg)	PROTEIN (g)	L-CARNITINE (mg)	ENERGY (kcal)
XLYS, TRY Analog	49 g	0	0	6.4	5	233
Similac Advance With Iron, concentrate	122 mL	276	54	3.4	2	166
L-Carnitine		0	0	0	318	0
Water to make	600 mL	—	—	—	—	—
Total		276	54	9.8	325	399

This table is referenced in the text of Chapter 58. It was prepared by Drs. Elsas and Acosta, the authors of that chapter.

TABLE A-25-m. SUPPLIERS OF MEDICATIONS AND NUTRITION SUPPLEMENTS REQUIRED FOR TREATMENT OF UREA CYCLE DISORDERS

PRODUCT	SUPPLIER
Medications	
Sodium benzoate + sodium phenylacetate (Ammonul) (Intravenous) (IND)	Ucyclyd Pharma 8125 North Hayden Road Scottsdale, AZ 85258-2463 602-667-3914, 888-829-2593 (24 h)
Sodium phenylbutyrate powder and tablets (Buphenyl)	
Nutrition Supplements	
L-Arginine powder or capsules (free base)	Jo Mar Laboratories 251-B East Hacienda Avenue
L-Citrulline powder[a]	Campbell, CA 95008-6622 800-538-4545 FAX 408-374-5920
L-Arginine HCl[b] (R-Gene-10) (10% pyrogen-free solution)	Pharmacia & Upjohn 100 Route 206 North Peapack, NJ 07977 For emergencies, call 800 821-7000 (direct) Order from pharmaceutical distributor
L-Citrulline powder[a]	Seybridge Pharmacy 37 New Haven Road Seymour, CT 06483 203-888-0073: Peter Przybylski

[a]Amino acid powders have different densities. Consequently, they should be measured on a scale that reads in grams. A 1-week supply may be weighed and placed in a vial. The week's supply may then be mixed to a known volume in boiled water, capped, and stored in a refrigerator. The daily amount required may be measured in a disposable syringe or volumetric flask.

[b]Hyperchloremic acidosis may occur with high-dose L-arginine HCl. Consequently, plasma concentrations of chloride and bicarbonate should be monitored and bicarbonate administered if needed.

This table is referenced in the text of Chapter 58. It was prepared by Drs. Elsas and Acosta, the authors of that chapter.

TABLE A-25-n. RECOMMENDED DAILY NUTRIENT INTAKES (RANGES) FOR INFANTS AND CHILDREN WITH UREA CYCLE DISORDERS

	NUTRIENT		
AGE	L-ARGININE[a] (g/kg)	PROTEIN[b] (g/kg)	ENERGY[b,c] (kcal/kg)
Months			
0 < 1	500–100	2.2–1.5	155–120
1 < 2	500–100	2.0–1.5	150–115
2 < 3	500–100	1.9–1.3	145–110
3 < 4	400–100	1.5–1.2	140–105
4 < 5	400–100	1.4–1.0	135–100
5 < 6	400–100	1.3–1.0	130–95
6 < 7	400–100	1.2–0.9	125–90
7 < 8	300–100	1.1–0.8	120–85
8 < 9	300–100	1.1–0.8	115–80
9 < 10	300–100	1.0–0.8	110–80
10 < 11	300–100	1.0–0.8	105–80
11 < 12	300–100	1.0–0.8	105–80
Years			
1 < 2	300–100	1.3–0.8	110–105
2 < 3	300–100	1.2–0.8	105–100
3 < 4	300–100	1.1–0.8	100–95
4 < 7	300–100	1.0–0.7	95–85
7 < 11	300–100	1.0–0.7	85–65
11 < 19	300–100	1.0–0.6	60–40

[a]Not used with arginase deficiency.

[b]Based on fiftieth centile weight for age. Modify as needed to maintain normal linear growth and plasma NH_3 concentrations <50 μmol/L.

[c]Supply at least 1.5 mL fluid/kcal to infants, 1.0 mL/kcal to children.

This table is referenced in the text of Chapter 58. It was prepared by Drs. Elsas and Acosta, the authors of that chapter.

TABLE A-25-o. SAMPLE DIET FOR A UREA CYCLE ENZYME DEFECT (2 wk OF AGE): WEIGHT 3.25 kg

PRESCRIPTION	TOTAL	PER kg
L-Arginine,[a] mg	975	300
Protein, g	7.2	2.2
Energy, kcal	470	145
Water to make, mL	710	

MEDICAL FOOD #1	AMOUNT	L-ARGININE (mg)	PROTEIN (g)	ENERGY (kcal)
Cyclinex-1	69 g	0	5.2	352
Similac Advance With Iron, concentrate	71 mL	58	2.0	96
Polycose Liquid	11 mL	0	0	22
L-Arginine[a] (10 mg/mL)	92 mL	920	0	0
Water to make	710 mL	0	0	0
Total		978	7.2	470

[a]DO NOT use with arginase deficiency.

This table is referenced in the text of Chapter 58. It was prepared by Drs. Elsas and Acosta, the authors of that chapter.

TABLE A-25-p. GALACTOSE-RESTRICTED DIET

FOODS ALLOWED	FOODS EXCLUDED
Beverages	
Carbonated drinks; Isomil powder [a]; ProSobee Powder [b]; other formula powders made with soy protein isolate; fruit drinks free of apple, banana, orange, papaya, pear, pineapple, watermelon; tea	Beverages containing calcium caseinate or sodium caseinate; some cocoas and instant coffees (read labels); hot chocolate; imitation or filled milks; malted milk; milk — all untreated of any species and all products containing milk including buttermilk, whole, skim, dried, evaporated, or condensed; milk treated with lactobacillus acidophilus culture or lactase; Ovaltine; powdered soft drinks with lactose; soy milk containing carrageenan
Breads, Cereals, and Grains	
Breads, crackers, and rolls made without milk (contact bakeries in each geographic area for milkfree breads); Italian bread; some cooked and prepared cereals, soda crackers, and pasta (read labels); barley; buckwheat; oats; rye; rice; wheat	Prepared mixes such as biscuits, muffins, pancakes or waffles; some dry cereals (read labels carefully); instant Cream of Wheat; cereals, breads, crackers, French toast made with milk; zwieback containing milk
Cheeses/Other Milk Products None	All excluded
Desserts	
Water and fruit ices made with allowed fruit juices; gelatin; angel food cake; homemade cakes, pies, cookies made with allowed ingredients; puddings made with water; Isomil; ProSobee Powder; sorbets	Commercial cakes, cookies, and mixes; custard, ice cream, puddings, and sherbets made with milk; chocolate containing milk; Fig Newtons; pie crust made with butter or margarine that contains milk or soy flour
Eggs	
All	Omelets and soufflés containing milk,
Fats	
Margarines and salad dressings that do not contain milk or milk products, bacon, lard, nut butters, oils, shortening, some nondairy creamers (read label)	Margarines and dressings containing milk or milk products or soy, butter, cream, cream cheese, peanut butter with milk solid fillers, salad dressings containing lactose or milk products, nondairy creamers containing sodium or calcium caseinate, sour cream, whipping cream
Fruits [c, d]	
Canned, fresh, or frozen fruits that do not contain galactose and are not processed with lactose; apricot; avocado; cantaloupe; fruit cocktail; grapefruit; grapes, green; nectarines; peaches	Any canned or frozen fruits processed with lactose; apples; applesauce; banana; dates; figs; grapes, European; kiwi fruit; oranges; papayas; pears; persimmons, American; watermelon; juices containing excluded fruits
Legumes, Nuts, Seeds	
Peanut, peanut butter, nuts except hazelnuts	All legumes (dry beans and peas); hazelnuts; pumpkin, safflower, sesame, or sunflower seed kernel or flour
Meat, Fish, Poultry	
Plain beef, chicken, fish, ham, lamb, pork, veal, strained or junior meats that do not contain milk or milk products, kosher frankfurters	Creamed or breaded meat, fish, or fowl; sausage products such as cold cuts and wieners containing nonfat milk solids; brains; kidney; liver; pancreas; sweetbreads
Soups	
Clear consommés, cream soups, or soups made with nondairy creamers free of caseinate; vegetable soups made with allowed vegetables	Chowders, commercially prepared soups containing lactose, cream soups, vegetable soups made with excluded vegetables
Vegetables	
Canned, fresh, or frozen vegetables; artichokes; asparagus; bamboo shoots; bean sprouts, green; beets; cabbage; cauliflower; celery; chard; corn; cucumbers; eggplant; kale; lettuce; mushrooms, common; mustard greens; okra; parsley; parsnips; potatoes, white; radishes; rutabagas; spinach; turnips; squash, zucchini; all allowed vegetables not prepared with lactose	Any vegetable to which lactose, milk, or milk product is added during processing; breaded, buttered, or creamed vegetables; potatoes, instant; corn curls and frozen French fries if processed with lactose; bell peppers; broccoli; Brussels sprouts; carrots; onions; peas; pumpkin; sweet potatoes; tomatoes in any form; V-8 juice; yams
Miscellaneous	
Beet sugar; carob powder; corn syrup; gravy made with water (read label); honey, jelly, or marmalade; malt powder; molasses; olives; pickles; popcorn; monosodium glutamate, pure; seasonings and spices, pure; sugar candy, pure; sugar	Artificial sweeteners containing lactose, Bean-O, butterscotch, caramel, cocoa, chewing gum, dietetic preparations (read label), drugs such as estrogen or progestin, milk chocolate, monosodium glutamate extender, Neocalglucon, peppermint, spice blends if they contain lactose, toffee, vitamin and mineral preparations (read label)

[a] Ross Products Division, Abbott Laboratories, Columbus, OH 43215.
[b] Mead Johnson Nutritionals, Evansville, IN 47221.
[c] Reference 21.
[d] Matthews RH, Pehrsson R, Farhat-Sabet M. Sugar Content of Selected Foods: Individual and Total Sugars. USDA Home Economics Research Report no. 48. Washington, DC: US Government Printing Office, 1987.

This table is referenced in the text of Chapter 58. It was prepared by Drs. Elsas and Acosta, the authors of that chapter.

TABLE A-26. GLUTEN FREE FOODS AND INSTRUCTIONS

A-26-a. Introduction

The fraction of gluten protein in wheat that injures the intestine of susceptible persons is gliadin. The equivalent toxic protein fractions in barley, rye, and oats are prolamins. When all sources of gliadin and prolamin are removed from the diet, the intestine is able to regenerate, and normal function is usually restored.

Gliadin and prolamin may be either present in foods as a basic ingredient (i.e., listed as wheat, rye, oats, or barley) or added as a derivative when a food is processed or prepared. Thus, reading labels carefully is very important! A great deal of confusion occurs about the presence of gliadin- and prolamin-containing additives in foods. The following tables include lists of food groups, questionable ingredients, common additives that are safe as well as medications, and excipients.

Since flour and cereal products are quite often used in the preparation of foods, it is important to be aware of the methods of preparation used, as well as the foods themselves. This is especially true when dining out.

TABLE A-26-a-1. FOOD GROUPS WITH SUGGESTED DAILY INTAKE*

GRAINS — USE 6 TO 11 SERVINGS PER DAY

	FOODS ALLOWED	FOODS TO AVOID (IF SAFETY CANNOT BE ESTABLISHED)
BREADS	Specially prepared breads using only allowed flours: rice, potato, bean flours, nut flours, tapioca, corn, sorghum, buckwheat, millet, amaranth, quinoa, and tef are allowable; breads may be purchased ready-to-eat or as mixes to prepare at home	Those containing wheat, rye, oats, barley, triticale, kamut, graham, bulgar, couscous, or spelt flours. BEWARE: WHEAT-FREE does not always ensure gluten free! Breads made from "carob-soy flour" can contain 80% wheat flour!
CEREALS	Hot cereals: made from the allowable grains and seeds. Cold cereals: Special cereals made without malt or malt flavoring. Pastas made with appropriate flours	Those containing: wheat, rye, oats, barley, graham, wheat germ, malt or malt flavoring, bulgar, spelt, kamut, couscous
CRACKERS & SNACK FOODS	Rice wafers; rice crackers; plain corn and potato chips; rice cakes, pure corn tortillas; popcorn, caramel corn	Those with wheat, rye, oats, barley, or other questionable ingredients. READ LABELS CAREFULLY. Some coating mixes used on chips contain wheat flour! If the product shows 'brown rice syrup,' contact the manufacturer to check for "barley malt enzymes" used in processing.
SOUPS	Homemade broth and soup using allowed ingredients; a few canned soups; specialty dry soup mixes	Most canned soups and soup mixes; bouillon and bouillon cubes with hydrolyzed vegetable protein (HVP) or added ingredients not allowed
POTATO, RICE, PASTA AND OTHER STARCHES	White and sweet potatoes; yams; hominy; rice, wild rice; special pasta made from rice, soy, or corn; some Asian rice and bean thread noodles	Regular noodles; spaghetti or macaroni (semolina and Durham = wheat); most packaged or frozen rice or pasta side dishes

VEGETABLES—USE 3 TO 5 SERVINGS PER DAY

VEGETABLES	Use all plain, fresh, frozen, or canned; dried peas, beans, and lentils, some commercially prepared vegetables	Creamed vegetables, vegetables canned in sauce, some canned beans, commercially prepared vegetables and salads

FRUITS—USE 2 TO 4 SERVINGS PER DAY

FRUITS	All fresh, frozen, canned or most dried fruits; all 100% fruit juices; some canned pie fillings	Thickened or prepared fruits; some pie fillings

DAIRY—USE 2 TO 3 SERVINGS PER DAY

MILK	Fresh, dry evaporated or condensed milk; cream; sour cream; whipping cream; yogurt	Malted milk; some commercial chocolate drinks; some nondairy creamers
CHEESES Can be used for meat and milk groups.	All aged cheeses, such as cheddar, Swiss, Edam, and Parmesan; cottage cheese, cream cheese, pasteurized processed cheese	Any cheese product containing products to be avoided

PROTEIN—USE 2 TO 3 SERVINGS PER DAY

MEAT, FISH, POULTRY	All fresh meats, fish, other seafood, poultry; fish canned in oil, brine, or vegetable broth; some meat products, such as hot dogs and lunch meats	Prepared meats containing wheat, rye, or barley, such as: some sausages, hot dogs; bologna; luncheon meats; chili con carne; bread-containing products, such as Swiss steak, meat loaf and croquettes; tuna canned with hydrolyzed protein; turkey with hydrolyzed vegetable protein (HVP) injected as part of the basting solution. "imitation crab" containing wheat starch or other unacceptable filler; quick individually frozen (QIF) seafood.
EGGS	Plain or in cooking	Eggs in sauce made from wheat, rye, oats, or barley; usually wheat flour is used in white sauce

FATS AND SWEETS—USE SPARINGLY

FATS	Butter, margarine, vegetable oil, olive oil, hydrogenated butter, vegetable oil, nuts, peanuts, some salad dressings, mayonnaise	Some commercial salad dressings. Vinegars and distilled spirits do not contain protein and therefore are gluten free. All proteins, including gluten are too large to pass through the distillation process and are not found in the end product of distillation. Therefore distilled alcoholic spirits are safe, used in moderation. Malt vinegar may have a malt flavoring added after processing. Malt vinegar should be avoided.

(continued)

TABLE A-26-a-1. FOOD GROUPS WITH SUGGESTED DAILY INTAKE* (continued)

	FOODS ALLOWED	FOODS TO AVOID (IF SAFETY CANNOT BE ESTABLISHED)
DESSERTS	Cakes, cookies, quick breads, pastries, puddings made with allowed ingredients; cornstarch, tapioca and rice puddings; gelatin desserts, puddings; "expensive" ice cream with few, simple ingredients; sorbet, frozen yogurt, and sherbet	Commercial cakes, cookies, pies, etc., made with wheat, rye, barley, and spelt; products containing brown rice syrup made with barley malt enzyme
SWEETS	Jelly, jam, honey, brown and white sugar, molasses, most syrups, some candy, chocolate, pure cocoa, coconut, marshmallows	Some commercial candies; watch for malt/malt flavoring or "natural" flavoring; chocolate-coated nuts, which may be rolled in wheat flour; brown rice syrup made with barley malt enzyme
	BEVERAGES + MISCELLANEOUS	
BEVERAGES	Instant, ground coffee, and flavored coffee beans; instant tea; carbonated beverages; pure cocoa powder; wine and distilled spirits, such as rums, vodka, whiskey, etc.; some root beers	Grain beverages (such as Ovaltine), malted milk; ales; beer; some hard ciders; instant flavored coffees; some herbal teas with barley or barley malt added
MISC.	Spices (salt, pure pepper, cloves, ginger, nutmeg, cinnamon, allspice, etc.); herbs (oregano, rosemary, etc.); food coloring; flavoring extracts; yeast, baking soda, baking powder, cream of tartar, and dry mustard, vinegars, and olives; monosodium glutamate (MSG) made in the US	Some curry powders; some dry seasoning mixes; some gravy extracts; some meat sauces; most soy sauces; some chewing gum. Communion wafers/bread. Note: In Catholic communion, host crumbs are often added to the wine before it is served. A workable solution is to arrange to use a goblet of your own.

TABLE A-26-a-2. QUESTIONABLE INGREDIENTS

These questionable ingredients must be cleared with the manufacturer before they are eaten. A sample letter requesting information on questionable ingredients and packaging and processing ingredients is on the last page of this diet instruction.

	FOODS ALLOWED	FOODS TO AVOID (IF SAFETY CANNOT BE ESTABLISHED)
Dextrin		May be derived from wheat
"Hydrolyzed vegetable protein (HVP)" or "hydrolyzed protein," texturized vegetable protein (TVP), or vegetable protein	Those from soy, corn, or milk	Mixtures containing wheat, oats, and barley
"Flour" or "cereal products"	Rice flour, corn flour, cornmeal, potato flour amaranth, quinoa, tef, millet, buckwheat, and soy flour or any other allowed grains	Wheat, rye, barley, spelt, and other flours to be avoided
"Vegetable broth"	In the United States, must contain 2 or more of the following: beans, cabbage, carrots, celery, garlic, onions, parsley, peas, potatoes, green bell pepper, red bell pepper, spinach, or tomatoes; cannot contain any other ingredients. IT IS GLUTEN FREE.	
"Malt" or "malt flavoring"	Those from corn	Those derived from barley or barley malt syrup
"Brown rice syrup"	Rice only	Rice plus barley malt enzyme
"Starch"	In the United States, must be CORN STARCH (in food products only)	
"Modified starch" or "Modified food starch"	Arrowroot, corn, potato, tapioca, waxy maize, or maize	Wheat starch
"Vegetable gum"	Carob bean, locust bean, cellulose, guar, gum arabic, gum acacia, gum tragacanth, or xanthan gum.	Oat gum–rarely used due to cost.
"Soy sauce" or "Soy sauce solids"	Those which DO NOT contain wheat (SOY ONLY).	Those brewed from wheat and soy.
"Mono- and diglycerides"	Always gluten-free. When used in wet products, such as ice cream, there is no concern. In dry products, such as seasoning mixes, they must be 'dried' with a carrier. Those using a non-wheat-based carrier.	Those using wheat starch carrier in dry products. The problem is the carrier ingredients, not the mono and diglyceride

A-26-a-3. Additives That Are Gluten-Free Safe

(This list is not exhaustive)

Adipic acid
Annatto
Ascorbic acid
BHA
BHT
β-Carotene
Biotin
Calcium chloride
Calcium pantothenate
Calcium phosphate
Carboxymethylcellulose
Carrageenan
Citric acid
Corn sweetener
Corn syrup solids
Demineralized whey
Dextrimaltose
Dextrose
Dictyl sodium sulfosuccinate
Folic acid–folacin

Fructose
Fumaric acid
Gums: acacia, arabic, carob, bean,
    cellulose, guar, locust,
    tragacanth, and xanthan
Invert sugar
Lactic acid
Lactose
Lecithin
Magnesium hydroxide
Malic acid
Mannitol
Microcrystalline cellulose
Niacin–niacinamide
Polyglycerol
Polysorbate 60: 80
Potassium citrate
Potassium iodine
Propylene glycol monostearate
Propylgallate

Pyridoxine hydrochloride
Sodium ascorbate
Sodium acid pyrophosphate
Sodium benzoate
Sodium caseinate
Sodium citrate
Sodium hexametaphosphate
Sodium nitrate
Sodium silaco aluminate
Sorbitol
Sucrose
Sulfosuccinate
Tartaric acid
Thiamin hydrochloride
Tricalcium phosphate
Vanillin
Vitamins and minerals
Vitamin A (palmitate)

TABLE A-26-a-4. MEDICATIONS ALLOWED OR TO BE AVOIDED

Regulations for ingredients in medications are different than regulations for foods. Problem ingredients in medications are caused by inactive ingredients. **Only medications that come in direct contact with any part of the intestinal tract must be gluten-free.**
IV Drugs, Medicated Patches, Topical agents, and Inhalants do not contain ingredients with gluten.
Ask for the following statement to be put on all prescription drug orders "OR GLUTEN-FREE EQUIVALENT"

INGREDIENT	ALLOWED IF	AVOID IF SAFETY CANNOT BE ESTABLISHED)	NOTES
Starch	Made from corn, rice, tapioca or potato	Made from wheat	
Pregelatinized starch	From corn or tapioca starch	Wheat starch	Dextrin and maltose combined
Dextrimaltose		Processed by enzymatic action of barley malt on corn flour	
Flour, gluten, dusting powder		Unspecified source	
Malt, malt syrup			Derived from barley and used in production of other ingredients
Dextrin, dextrates, Cylcodextrins	From corn or potato starch	wheat	Derived from incomplete hydrolysis of starch
Maltodextrin	Derived from caramel color–in the United States; it is generally corn based	Wheat or oat maltodextrin	
Sodium starch glycolate (carboxymethyl starch)	From potato, corn, rice or tapioca starch	Made from wheat	
Caramel color		Derived from barley malt syrup or unidentified starch hydrolysates	Could also request "dyefree" drugs
Alcohol (distilled ethanol)			Distillation separates out pure ethanol from proteins in original starting matter

A-26-a-5. Gluten-Free Pharmaceutical Excipients

Acacia	Glucose	Propylene glycol
Alginic acid	Hydrogenated vegetable oil	Silicon dioxide
α Tocopherol	Hydroxypropyl cellulose	Simethicone
Ascorbic acid	Lactose	Sodium benzoate
Benzyl alcohol	Magnesium carbonate	Sodium lauryl sulfate
Calcium carbonate	Magnesium stearate	Sorbitol
Carboxymethylcellulose	Matitol	Stearic acid
Citric acid	Mannitol	Sucrose
Corn starch	Microcrystalline cellulose	Vanillin
Dextrose	Polydextrose	Xanthan gum
Docusate sodium	Povidone	Zinc stearate
Fructose		

* The material in Tables A-26-a through A-26-c have been provided through the kindness of The Gluten Intolerance Group with permission by Ms. Cynthia Kupper. Copyright © 2004 by the Gluten Intolerance Group ®
15110–10th Ave SW, Suite A, Seattle, WA 98166-1820
Phone: 206-246-6652   Fax: 206-246-6531
Email: info@gluten.net   Web site: www.gluten.net

A-26-b. Sources for Gluten-Free Drug Information

www.glutenfreedrugs.com (pharmacist controlled site)
www.stokesrx.com (some pharmacist assistance. Fee for service)
www.clanthompson.com (consumer controlled site. Updated frequently)

A-26-c. WRITING EFFECTIVE LETTERS TO FOOD MANUFACTURERS

It is important that you clarify questionable ingredients on food product labels and in medications before adding them to your gluten-free diet. Manufacturers are usually courteous and prompt when answering questions about their products. The accuracy of their reply often depends on what question is asked. The following letter format can be used as a sample when contacting a manufacturer. Remember to be very specific when asking questions.

Your address

Date

Dear Sir/Madam:

I am on a gluten-restricted diet for the treatment of celiac disease (dermatitis herpetiformis). I must avoid the 'gluten' protein found in wheat, rye, and barley, since they cause an immune response, which damages the lining of my intestine. I would like to be able to use your product (name product); however the ingredient listing does not provide adequate information for me to determine if it would be safe. Specifically, I need to know*

*Examples would be:
• What is the source of starch in your "food starch modified" ("food starch" or "modified food starch")?
• Are your "soy sauce solids" derived from wheat?
• What are the inactive ingredients used in the medication, including those used in the coatings and capsules?

Incidental ingredients, used in the packaging and processing, is another possible source of gluten contamination. I am relying on you to clarify if these substances contain gluten, since these incidental ingredients are not listed on the packaging.

Please send a copy of your response to:

The Gluten Intolerance Group of North America®
15110–10 Ave SW, Suite A
Seattle, WA 98166-1820

GIG® will be happy to share this information with their clients and health care professionals. If you have questions about these conditions and the dietary restrictions, please call our National Office at (206) 246-6652.

Thank you for your efforts on my behalf.

Sincerely,
Your Signature

A-26-d. Appendices Editors' Comment

The Gluten Intolerance Group that prepared these dietary suggestions and warnings has indicated that oats have the potential for contamination with gluten "although small quantities are safe" but recommend avoidance because of the danger of contamination. A letter to the editor of the New England Journal of Medicine with data provided by Tricia Thompson, M.S., R.D. was published recently in that journal. (1)

It contained several published references supporting the "safety of moderate amounts of uncontaminated oats." Nevertheless, Thompson obtained containers of rolled or steel-cut oats representing four different lots of three different commercial brands of oats sold in the United States and sent the unopened containers to an independent laboratory. The analytic procedure used employed a monoclonal antibody sensitive to the prolamins of wheat, barley, and rye, but insensitive to the prolamins of corn, rice, and oats. In this assessment, "oat samples were considered gluten-free if they contained 20 ppm or less of gluten in accordance with the current codes limit for naturally gluten-free foods." The results: "3 of the 12 oat samples contained gluten at levels of less the 20 ppm. The other 9 samples had gluten levels that ranged from 23 to 1807 ppm" (1).

Because all three brands had elevated gluten levels in at least two of the four samples with gluten as a contaminant from wheat, barley, or rye, it is apparent that there is a need for studies of other sources of oats and that the likelihood of gluten contaminated commercial oats must lead persons with celiac disease to view oats and oat-containing foods potentially as unsafe.

1. Thompson F. N Engl J Med 2004;351:2021–22.

A-27. LACTOSE-CONTROLLED DIETS

A-27-a. Appendices Editors' comment

In past editions, the Appendix table on lactose-controlled diets included text and tables of the lactose content of common foods and beverages, guidelines for food selection, and a sample menu. In this edition, we include a general statement about major and widespread changes resulting in the availability of milks of various fat content, ice cream, and cheeses that contain little or no lactose.

Some milk producers offer lactose- and fat-reduced milks of varying degrees, usually with a variety available in the same stores. Ultrapasteurized lactose-treated milks of the Lactaid brand are distributed by H.P. Hood, Inc (Lactaid phone number: 1-800-522-8243; www.lactaid.com). As noted in the ninth edition Appendix Table A-37, lactase-treated milk was available from McNeil CPC, 7050 Camp Hill Road, Fort Washington, PA 19034 and Dairy Ease products produced by Sterling Health, 90 Park Avenue, New York, NY 10016. Indicative of the demand is the action of at least one large supermarket company (Harris-Teeter of NC) in supplying lactose-free milk under its label.

At least one ice cream that a manufacturer prepares is "99% Lactose-Free Natural Vanilla" (Good Humor—Breyers Ice-Cream, P.O. Box 19007, Green Bay, WI 54307-9007; www.icecreamusa.com).

The Kraft Food Company (Kraft Food North America, Glen View, IL 60025, phone: 1-800-634-1984) in English and Spanish) and the Borden Co. state clearly (but in small print) on the label that specific cheeses "contain 0 g lactose per serving."

Undoubtedly, increasing numbers of milk-containing products that are very low in lactose are now available or will become so in the future as the demand increases. Such demand is best made directly to store managers and to food manufacturers.

Because one is never sure of the presence of lactose-containing ingredients unless clearly and specifically stated on product labels, lactose-intolerant persons should e-mail, write, or telephone food manufacturers whose products they need to question.

Lactose-intolerant persons are urged to read Chapter 74 because of its broad coverage; this includes the fact that there are disaccharidases in foods besides lactose; some persons are intolerant of one or more of them and should be aware of this possibility.

A-28. OXALATE CONTENT OF SELECTED FOODS

TABLE A-28-a. OXALATE CONTENT BY FOOD GROUP

FOODS	LITTLE OR NO OXLATE <2 mg OXALATE/SERVING EAT AS DESIRED	MODERATE-OXALATE CONTENT 2–10 mg OXALATE/SERVING LIMIT: TWO (½ CUP) SERVINGS/DAY OR TWO SERVINGS OF THE STATED SERVING SIZE	HIGH-OXALATE FOODS >10 mg OXALATE/SERVING AVOID COMPLETELY
Beverages/juices	Apple juice Beer, bottled Black coffee (brewed 5 min) Cranberry juice Diet Coke Grapefruit juice Lemonade or limeade Wine, red, rosé Pineapple juice Tap water (preferred for extra calcium) Orange soda (12 fl oz Minute Maid) Ginger ale (Schweppes) Root beer (Borg's and A&W) Aloe vera juice	Beer, Budweiser (12 fl oz) Coffee, any kind (8 oz serving) Cranberry juice (4 oz serving) Cocoa, Carnation dry Nescafe powder (1 tsp) Tomato juice (4 oz serving) Lipton tea (steeped 5 min)	Beer; Stout, Guiness, Draft, Lager, Tuborg, Pilsner Juices containing berries not allowed Ovaltine and other beverage mixes Tea, cocoa
Milk (2 or more cups)	Buttermilk Low-fat-milk Low-fat yogurt with allowed fruit Skim milk Whole milk	Yogurt plain, nonfat (1 cup)	
Meat group	Eggs Cheese, cheddar Lean lamb, beef, or pork Poultry Seafood	Sardines	Baked beans canned in tomato sauce Peanut butter Soybean curd (tofu)
Vegetables	Avocado Broccoli, boiled Brussels sprouts, boiled Cabbage, boiled Chive Potatoes, white, boiled Radishes Turnips, boiled Waterchestnuts	Asparagus Carrots, canned Cauliflower, boiled Corn, sweet white and yellow Cucumbers, peeled raw Onions, raw, boiled Green peas, boiled, canned Lettuce, iceberg, fresh Lima beans, cooked Parsnips Tomato, fresh, 1 small Mushrooms, fresh Escarole Kale, raw	Beans, boiled or raw: green, wax, dried Beets, boiled; tops, roots, and green Celery Chard, Swiss Collards Dandelion greens Eggplant, raw Leeks Mustard greens Okra Parsley, raw Peppers, green Pokeweed Potatoes, sweet Rutabagas Spinach Summer squash Watercress

Fruits	Avocado
	Banana
	Cherries, bing or sour
	Cranberries, canned
	Grapes, Thompson seedless
	Mangoes
	Melons: cantaloupe
	   casaba
	   honeydew
	   watermelon
	Nectarines
	Peaches, Hiley, canned
	Pineapple, canned, stewed
	Plums, green or Golden age
		Apple
		Apricots
		Black currants
		Cranberries, dried
		Grapefruit
		Orange
		Peaches, Alberta
		Pears, raw
		Plums, stewed
		Prunes, Italian
		Pineapple, Dole's
		Coconut
		Kiwi
			Berries
			Concord grapes
			Red currants
			Fruit cocktail
			Gooseberries
			Lemon peel
			Lime peel
			Orange peel
			Raspberries
			Rhubarb, canned, stewed
			Strawberries, canned
			Tangerine
			Plums, Damson

TABLE A-28-a. OXALATE CONTENT BY FOOD GROUP (continued)

FOODS	LITTLE OR NO OXLATE <2 mg OXALATE/SERVING EAT AS DESIRED	MODERATE-OXALATE CONTENT 2–10 mg OXALATE/SERVING LIMIT: TWO (½ CUP) SERVINGS/DAY OR TWO SERVINGS OF THE STATED SERVING SIZE	HIGH-OXALATE FOODS >10 mg OXALATE/SERVING AVOID COMPLETELY
Bread/starches	Pear, Bartlett, canned Orange juice fresh Papaya, Hawaiian Strawberries, fresh Cornflakes Macaroni, boiled Noodles, egg boiled Oatmeal, porridge Rice, boiled Wild rice, cooked Bread, white Barley, cooked	Cornbread Sponge cake Spaghetti, canned in tomato sauce Cornmeal, yellow, dry Cheerios (1 cup) Bagel (1 medium; 2 oz) Brown rice, cooked Garbanzo beans, canned Lentils, cooked Split peas, cooked Macaroni, cooked Spaghetti, cooked Corn tortilla (1 medium; 1.5 oz) English muffin (1 medium; 2 oz) Bread, whole wheat	Fruit cake Grits, white corn Soybean crackers Wheat germ Fig Newtons Graham crackers Popcorn (4 cups popped) Whole wheat flour
Fats and oils	Mayonnaise Salad dressing Vegetable oils Butter Margarine	Bacon	Nuts: Peanuts and pecans Sunflower seeds Mayonnaise (Heinz)

Miscellaneous	Jelly or preserves,
	  made with allowable fruits
	Lemon/lime juice, fresh
	Salt, pepper (1 tsp/day)
	Soups with allowed ingredients
	Sugar
	Honey (1 tbsp)
	Corn syrup (Karo)
	Unflavored gelatin (Knox), 1 pkt
	Maple syrup, pure
	Vanilla extract
	Oregano, dried (1 tsp)
	Apple cider vinegar (1 tsp.
	  Ralph's Supermarket)
	Nutmeg, dry (1 tsp)
	Cornstarch (1 tbsp)
		Vegetable soup
		Tomato soup
		Tofu (firm)
		Malt (1 tbsp)
		Basil, fresh (1 tbsp)
		Mustard, Dijon style (1 tbsp)
		Ginger, raw (1 tbsp sliced)
			Chocolate, plain
			Dry cocoa, plain
			Pepper (in excess of 1 tsp/day)
			Cinnamon, ground (1 tsp)

From Brzezinski E, Durning AM, Grasse B, Fusselman E, Ciaraldi T. Oxalate content of selected foods. The General Clinical Research Center, University of California, San Diego Medical Center. 1996:1–53. With permission.

TABLE A-28-b. FOODS TO USE AND AVOID

THESE CONTAIN SMALL AMOUNTS OF OXALATE 0–2 mg OXALATE PER SERVING (½ CUP)

VEGETABLES	FRUITS	BEVERAGES	MISCELLANEOUS
Broccoli	Avocado	Apple juice	Butter
Brussels sprouts	Banana	Barley water	Cheese, cheddar
Cabbage	Cherries	Beer, bottled	Chicken noodle soup
Cauliflower	Grapes, seedless	Cider	Cornflakes
Chives	Mangoes	Coca-Cola	Eggs
Cucumber	Melons	Grapefruit juice	Egg noodle (chow mein)
Lettuce	Peaches: canned	Lumonade	Fish (except sardines)
Mushrooms	Hiley	Lucozade, bottled	Jelly with allowed fruit
Onions	Stokes	Milk	Lemon Juice
Peas	Pineapple	Orange juice	Lime juice
Potato white	Plums:	Pepsi-Cola	Macaroni
Radishes	Golden Gage	Pineapple juice	Margarine
Rice	Green Gage	Sherry, dry	Meats
Turnips	Oxtail soup	Wine	Oatmeal, porridge
	Red plum jam		Poultry
	Sweets, boiled		

THESE ARE HIGH IN OXALATE >15 mg OXALATE PER SERVING (½ CUP)

Beans in tomato sauce	Berries;	Chocolate	Cocoa, dry
Beets	Black	Tuborg, Pilsner	Grits, white corn
Celery	Blue	Ovaltine (24 mg/8 oz)	Peanuts
Chard, Swiss	Green goose	Tea (132–181.2 mg/8 oz)	Pecans
Collards	Raspberries		Soybean crackers
Dandelion greens	Currants, red		Wheat germ
Eggplant	Grapes, concord		
Escarole	Lemon peel		
Leeks			
Okra			
Parsley			
Pepper, green			
Pokeweed			
Potato, sweet			
Rutabagas			
Spinach			
Squash, summer			

From Brzezinski E, Durning AM, Grasse B, Fusselman E, Ciaraldi T. Oxalate content of selected foods. The General Clinical Research Center, University of California, San Diego medical Center. 1996:1–53. With permission.

TABLE A-28-c. OXALATE CONTENT OF FOODS PER 100 GRAMS (~½ CUP) AND PER PORTION

FOOD	PORTION	mg/100 g	mg/PORTION
Cereals, grains, and cereal products			
Bagel, plain	1 medium; 55 g	12.37	6.804
Barley, cooked	1 cup: 156.25 g	3.46	5.404
Bread, white	1 slice; 25 g	4.9	1.225
Bread, whole wheat	1 slice;25 g	20.9	5.225
Cake, fruit	1 slice; 15 g	11.8	1.77
Cake, sponge	1 slice; 66 g	7.4	4.884
Cheerios	1 cup; 22.6 g	20.66	4.67
Corn tortilla	1 medium; 21.3 g	11.51	2.45
Cornflakes	1 cup; 22.7 g	2	0.454
Cornmeal, yellow	1 cup; dry; 138 g	6.25	8.624
Cornstarch	1 tbsp; 8 g	14.51	1.61
Crackers, soybean	1 ounce; 28.35 g	204	58.685
Egg noodle (chow mein)	1 cup; 45 g	1	0.45
English muffin, white	1 each; 58 g	10.22	5.93
Graham crackers (Keebler)	2 crackers; 14 g	12.41	1.74
Fig Newtons	1 each; 14.7 g	14.05	2.07
Garbanzo beans, canned	1 cup; 164 g	11.18	18.34
Grits, white corn	1 cup cooked; 242 g	41	99.22
Grits, white corn	1 cup dry; 156 g	41	63.96
Lentils, cooked	1 cup; 198 g	8.48	16.795
Macaroni, boiled	1 cup boil tender; 140 g	1	1.4
Macaroni, cooked soft	1 cup; 140 g	5.44	7.62
Oatmeal porridge	1 cup; 234 g	1	2.34
Popcorn, Orville Redenbacker, popped	single-serving bag; 4 cups = 50.39 g	33.29	16.777
Rice, brown, cooked	1 cup; 195 g	6.54	12.76
Rice, boiled	1 cup; 175 g	0	0
Spaghetti, boiled	1 cup boil tender; 140 g	1.5	2.1
Spaghetti, cooked soft	1 cup; 140 g	6.24	8.73
Spaghetti in tomato sauce	1 cup; 250 g	4	10
Split peas, cooked	1 cup; 196 g	4.83	9.48
Wheat germ	1 tbsp; 7.2 g	299	19.37
Wild rice, cooked	1 cup; 164 g	1.65	2.71
Whole wheat flour	1 cup; 120 g	25.03	30.031
Milk and milk products			
Butter	1 tbsp; 14 g	0	0
Cheddar cheese	1 ounce; 28.35 g	0	0
Margarine	1 tbsp; 14.1 g	0	0
Milk	1 cup; 244 g	0.15	0.366
Milk, whole	1 cup; 244 g	0.54	1.31
Yogurt, natural, nonfat plain	1 cup; 227 g	1	2.266
Meats, eggs and meat alternates			
Bacon, streaky, fried	1 strip; 6.3 g	3.3	0.21
Beef, canned, corned	3 oz; 85 g	0	0
Beef, topside roast	4 oz; 113.4 g	0	0
Chicken roast	4 oz; 113.4 g	0	0
Egg, boiled	1 medium; 50 g	0	0
Fish: haddock	4 oz; 113.4 g	0.2	0.23
plaice	4 oz; 113.4 g	0.3	0.34
sardines	4 oz; 113.4 g	4.8	5.42
Ham	4 oz; 113.4 g	1.6	1.81
Hamburger, grilled	4 oz; 113.4 g	0	0
Lamb, roast	4 oz; 113.4 g	trace	trace
Liver	4 oz; 113.4 g	7.1	8.02
Pork, roast	4 oz; 113.4 g	1.7	1.92
Tofu, raw firm	125 g	5.08	6.35
Vegetables			
Asparagus	1 cup; 180 g	5.2	9.36
Green beans, boiled	1 cup; 135 g	15	20.25
Beans in tomato sauce	1 cup	19	
Beetroot, boiled	1 cup; 170 g	675	1147.5
Beetroot, pickled	1 cup; 227 g	500	1135
Broccoli, boiled	1 cup; 155 g	trace	trace

(continued)

TABLE A-28-c. OXALATE CONTENT OF FOODS PER 100 GRAMS (~½ CUP) AND PER PORTION (continued)

FOOD	PORTION	mg/100g	mg/PORTION
Brussels sprouts, boiled	1 cup; 156 g	0	0
Cabbage, boiled	1 cup common; 70 g	0	0
Carrots, canned	1 cup; 146 g	4	5.84
Cauliflower, boiled	1 cup; 124 g	1	1.24
Celery	1 cup diced; 120 g	20	24
Chard, Swiss	1 cup raw; 36 g	645	232.2
Chard, Swiss	1 cup boiled; 175 g	645	1128.75
Chive	1 cup raw; 48 g	1.1	0.53
Collards	1 cup raw/boil; 128 g	74	94.72
Corn, yellow	1 cup; 165 g	5.2	8.58
Cucumber, raw	1 med whole; 301 g	1	3.01
Dandelion greens	1 cup raw; 55 g	24.6	13.53
Dandelion greens	1 cup boiled; 105 g	24.6	25.83
Eggplant	1 cup boiled; 96 g	18	17.28
Escarole	1 cup raw; 28 g	31	8.68
Kale	1 cup raw/boil; 130 g	13	16.9
Leek	1 cup raw/boil; 124 g	89	110.36
Lettuce	1 cup; 55 g	3	1.65
Lima beans	1 cup canned; 248 g	4.3	10.66
Mushrooms	1 cup raw/chopped; 70 g	2	1.4
Okra	1 cup boiled; 160 g	146	233.6
Onion, boiled	1 cup; 210 g	3	6.3
Parsley, raw	1 cup; 64 g	100	64
Parsnips	1 cup sliced/boil; 156 g	10	15.6
Peas, canned	1 cup; 170 g	1	1.7
Pepper, green	1 item; 74 g	16	11.84
Pokeweed	1 item; 136 g	476	
Potatoes, white boiled	1 item; 136 g	0	0
Potato, sweet	1 cup boil/mashed; 238 g	56	183.68
Radishes	1 each; 4.5 g	0.3	0.014
Rutabagas	1 cup boil; 170 g	19	32.3
Spinach, boiled	1 cup; 56 g	750	420
Spinach, frozen	1 cup frozen/boil; 205 g	600	1230
Squash, summer	1 cup sliced; 180 g	22	39.6
Tomato, raw	1 cup diced; 240 g	2	4.8
Turnips, boiled	1 cup; 156 g	1	1.56
Waterchestnut canned, whole slices	½ cup; 70 g	1.22	0.86
Watercress early, fine curled	1 cup raw; 34 g	10	3.4
Fruits			
Apple, raw	1 medium; 138 g	3	4.14
Apricot, w/o pit	1 each; 35.3 g	2.8	0.99
Avocado	1 California; 173 g	0	0
Avocado	1 Florida; 173 g	0	0
Banana, raw	1 medium peeled; 114 g	trace	trace
Berries: Black	1 cup; 144 g	18	25.92
blue	1 cup; 145 g	15	21.75
Berries: dew	1 cup; 144 g	14	20.16
Berries: green goose	1 cup; 150 g	88	132
raspberries, black	1 cup; 123 g	53	65.19
raspberries, red	1 cup; 123 g	15	18.45
Coconut fresh (flesh only)	45 g; 1.5 oz	2.14	0.96
Cranberries, dried	½ cup; 25 g	3.07	0.77
Cranberries, canned Ocean Spray	½ cup; 138 g	0.71	0.98
Cherries: bing	1 cup; 150 g	0	0
Cherries: sour	1 cup; 155 g	1.1	1.705
Currants: black	1 cup; 112 g	4.3	4.82
red	1 cup; 112 g	19	21.28
Fruit salad, canned	1 cup; 249 g	12	29.88
Grapes, red, fresh	1 cup; 92 g	0.52	0.475
Grapes: concord	1 cup; 160 g	25	40
Thompson seedless	1 cup; 160 g	0	0
Kiwi, fresh	1 medium; 76 g	2.6	1.97
Lemon, peel	1 tbsp; 6 g	83	4.98

TABLE A-28-c. OXALATE CONTENT OF FOODS PER 100 GRAMS (~½ CUP) AND PER PORTION (continued)

FOOD	PORTION	mg/100g	mg/PORTION
Lime, peel	1 Tbsp; 6 g	100	6
Melons: cantaloupe	1 cup; 160 g	0	0
casaba	1 cup; 170 g	0	0
honeydew	1 cup; 170 g	0	0
Mangoes	1 medium; 207 g	0	0
Mango, fresh	1 medium; 207 g	1.06	2.19
Nectarines	1 medium; 136 g	0	0
Orange, raw	1 medium; 131 g	4	5.24
Orange, Navel	1 medium; 140 g	2.18	3.06
Papaya, Hawaiian, fresh	1 medium; 304 g	1.99	6.065
Peaches: Alberta	1 medium; 87 g	5	4.35
canned	1 cup; 250 g	1.2	3
Hiley	1 medium; 87 g	0	0
stokes	1 medium; 87 g	1.2	1.044
Pears, Bartlett, canned	1 cup; 248 g	1.7	4.22
Pineapple, canned	1 cup; 252 g	1	2.52
Pineapple, Dole's (chunks, canned)	1/2 cup; 125 g	3.07	4.86
Plums: Damson	1 medium; 66 g	10	6.6
Golden Gage	1 medium; 66 g	1.1	0.73
Green Gage	1 medium; 66 g	0	0
Preserves: red plum, jam	1 tbsp: 20 g	0.5	0.1
strawberry, jam	1 tbsp; 20 g	9.4	1.88
Rhubarb: canned	1 cup; 240 g	600	1440
stewed, no sugar	1 cup; 242 g	860	2081.2
Strawberries, fresh	1 cup; 149 g	0.7	1.04
Strawberries, canned	1 cup; 254 g	15	38.1
Strawberries, raw	1 cup whole; 149 g	10	14.9
Watermelon	1 cup; 160 g	0	0
Nuts			
Peanuts, roasted	1 cup; 146 g	187	273
Pecans	1 cup; 110 g	202	222.2
Sunflower seeds, hulled, dry roasted, unsalted	1 oz; 28 g	18.9	5.29
Confectionery			
Chocolate, plain	1 oz; 28.35 g	117	33.17
Jelly with allowed fruit	1 tbsp; 20 g	0	0
Marmalade	1 tbsp; 20 g	10.8	2.16
Preserves: red plum jam	1 tbsp; 20 g	0.5	0.1
strawberry jam	1 tbsp; 20 g	9.4	1.88
Sweets, boiled (plain candies)	Hard candy 1 oz	0	
Beverages			
Barley water, bottled	1 cup; 237 g	0	0
Beer:	12 fl oz; 356 g		
bottled	12 fl oz	0	0
draft	12 fl oz	1	3.56
lager, draft, Tuborg, Pisner	12 fl oz	4	14.24
stout, Guiness draft	12 fl oz	2	7.12
Beer Budweiser	12 fl oz; 355 g	1.05	3.73
Cider	1 cup; 248 g	0	0
Coca-Cola	12 fl oz; 370 g	trace	trace
Coke	12 fl oz; 370 g	0.12	0.444
Coke, diet	12 fl oz; 354 g	0.1	0.35
Coffee (0.5 g Nescafe/100 mL)	1 tsp powder; 1.8 g	3.2	11.52
Coffee, black, brewed (brewed 4 min)	1 cup; 236 g	0.61	1.44
Coffee infusion:			
2 g per 100 mL infused 5 min		1	
4.4 g (1 tsp) per 100 mL infused 13 min		7.3	
Cocoa, Carnation Dry	1 pkt; 1 oz	7.69	2.184
Ginger Ale (Schweppes)	12 fl oz; 366 g	0.05	0.196
Lemon squash drink (lemonade)	12 fl oz; 349 g	1	3.49
Lucozade, bottled (soda)	12 fl oz; 350 g	0	0
Orange soda (Minute Maid)	12 fl oz; 372 g	0.24	0.91
Orange squash drink (orangeade)	12 fl oz; 372 g	2.5	9.3

(continued)

TABLE A-28-c. OXALATE CONTENT OF FOODS PER 100 GRAMS (~½ CUP) AND PER PORTION (continued)

FOOD	PORTION	mg/100g	mg/PORTION
Ovaltine drink, 2 g in 100 mL	1 tsp powder; 2.67 g	10	13.35
Pepsi Cola	12 fl oz; 370 g	trace	trace
Ribena concentrate (black currant drink)	12 fl oz; 360 g	2	7.2
Root beer (Borgs and A&W)	12 fl oz; 370 g	0.19	0.696
Sherry dry	1 cup; 240 g	trace	trace
Tea Indian:			
2-min infusion	1 cup; 237 g	55	130.35
4-min infusion	1 cup; 237 g	72	170.64
6-min infusion	1 cup; 237 g	78	184.86
Tea rosehip	1 cup; 237 g	4	9.48
Tea Lipton, steeped 5 min	1 cup; 237 g	3.74	8.86
Teas (steeped for 5 min w/o stirring, the tea bag then removed)			
Celestial Seasoning teas	1 cup; 250 mL		
Sleepytime	250 ml	0.99	
Peppermint	250 mL	1.71	
Wild Forest Blackberry	250 mL	0.9	
Mandarin Orange Spice	250 mL	0.9	
Cinnamon Apple Spice	250 mL	1.17	
R.C. Bigelow			
Cranberry Apple	250 mL	0.9	
Red Raspberry	250 mL	0.72	
I Love Lemon	250 mL	0.81	
Orange and Spice	250 mL	0.81	
Mint Medley	250 mL	1.71	
Sweet Dreams	250 mL	1.53	
Thomas J. Lipton			
Gentle Orange	250 mL	1.08	
Lemon Soother	250 mL	0.63	
Chamomile Flowers	250 mL	1.26	
Lyons Tetley Black Tea			
Tetley Tea (5-min steep)	250 mL	20.79	
Tetley Tea (1-min steep)	250 mL	10.8	
Tetley Tea (1-min steep with stirring)	250 mL	19.26	
Thomas J. Lipton			
Red Rose Classic Tea (5-min steep)	250 mL	11.97	
Red Rose Classic Tea (1-min steep)	250 mL	10.8	
Red Rose Classic Tea (1-min steep with stirring)	250 mL	15.75	
Green Tea R. Twining & Co.			
China Oolong Tea	250 mL	6.84	
Coffee			
Maxwell House (extra fine) coffee	250 mL	1.44	
Tomato juice	1 cup; 244 g	5	12.2
Wine:	1 cup; 236 g		
port	1 cup	trace	trace
rose	1 cup	1.5	3.54
white	1 cup	0	0
Fruit juices			
Aloe vera juice	1 cup; 250 g	0.83	2.07
Apple juice from concentrate	1 cup; 248 g	0.51	1.26
Apple juice	1 cup; 248 g	trace	trace
Cranberry juice	1 cup; 253 g	6.6	16.7
Cranberry juice from concentrate	1 cup; 252 g	0.31	0.78
Grapefruit juice	1 cup; 247 g	0	0
Orange juice	1 cup; 249 g	0.5	1.245
Pineapple juice	1 cup; 250 g	0	0
Miscellaneous			
Basil, fresh	1 tbsp; 2.5 g	115.6	2.89
Cinnamon, ground	1 tsp; 2 g	362.74	7.255
Cocoa, dry powder	1 cup; 86 g	623	535.78
Coffee, powder (Nescafe)	1 tsp; 1.8 g	33	11.52
Corn syrup, Karo	1 tbsp; 21 g	0.32	0.07

TABLE A-28-c. OXALATE CONTENT OF FOODS PER 100 GRAMS (~½ CUP) AND PER PORTION (continued)

FOOD	PORTION	mg/100g	mg/PORTION
Chicken noodle soup	1 cup; 241 g	1	2.41
Gelatin, unflavored Knox	1 pkt; 7 g	11.73	0.82
Ginger, raw	1 tbsp sliced; 6 g	115.03	6.902
Honey (clover)	1 tbsp; 21 g	1.51	0.32
Lemon Juice	1 cup; 244 g	1	2.44
Lime juice	1 cup; 246 g	0	0
Malt, powder	1 tbsp; 12.25 g	19.97	2.447
Maple syrup, pure	1 tbsp; 20 g	0.7	0.14
Mayonnaise, Heinz	1 tbsp; 14 g	11.98	1.677
Mustard, Dijon style	1 tbsp; 15 g	6.57	0.985
Nutmeg, dry	1 tsp; 2 g	63.76	1.275
Oregano, dried	1 tsp; 1.5 g	8.58	0.13
Ovaltine powder, canned	1 tsp; 2.67 g	10	13.35
Oxtail soup	1 cup; 376 g	1	3.76
Pepper	1 tsp; 2.1 g	419	8.8
Tomato soup	1 cup; 244 g	3	7.32
Vanilla extract, imitation	1 tsp; 5 g	0.42	0.021
Vegetable soup	1 cup; 241 g	5	12.05
Vinegar, apple cider Ralph's brand	1 tsp; 5 g	1.31	0.066

From Brzezinski E, Durning AM, Grasse B, Fusselman E, Ciaraldi T. Oxalate content of selected foods. The General Clinical Research Center, University of California, San Diego Medical Center. 1996:1–53. With permission.

Note: For references see original table, pp. 15–26.

TABLE A-28-d. LOW-OXALATE MEAL SUGGESTIONS

Select any one breakfast, lunch, dinner and snack/dessert combination from the meals/snack options below. Total oxalate will be less than 50 mg.

Oxalate values for meals rounded to nearest whole number.

Breakfast options	Oxalate (mg)

1. Banana Smoothie*
   1 standard slice white toast
   1 tsp margarine
   Bigelow Red Raspberry herbal tea
	15

2. 1 cup plain yogurt w/1 cup fresh strawberries
   Toasted plain medium bagel
   1 tsp margarine
   1 cup orange juice
	12

3. Two scrambled eggs (mixed with water)
   Three slices bacon, broiled or fried
   Whole English muffin with 1 tsp jelly
   1 cup cantaloupe chunks
   1 cup 1% or 2% lowfat milk
	8

4. 1 cup Cheerios
   1 cup 1% or 2% lowfat milk
   1 medium banana
   1 standard slice of white toast
   1 tsp margarine
	8

5. ½ fresh grapefruit
   1 poached egg
   1 standard slice white toast
   1 tsp margarine
   1 1/4 cup cornflakes
   1 cup 1% or 2% lowfat milk
	7

6. French Toast Bake* with 2 Tbsp
      maple syrup
   Fresh kiwi (1 medium) and ½ cup cantaloupe
   1 cup 1% or 2% lowfat milk
	12

7. 1 whole English muffin with ½ cup cottage
   cheese and tomato sliced (1/2 cup)
   1 cup orange juice
   1 cup 1% or 2% lowfat milk
	11

Lunch Options	Oxalate (mg)

1. California Chicken Sandwich*
   Picnic Potato Salad*
   1 cup Thompson seedless grapes
   12 fl oz Diet Coke
	9

2. Turkey burger: 3 oz ground turkey patty, grilled
                     1 white hamburger bun
                     1 Tbsp catsup
                     1 Tbsp mustard
   Sweet n Sour Cabbage*
   1 cup apple juice
	13

3. Cauliflower Curry*
   ½ cup steamed white rice
   1 medium fresh mango
   1 cup cranberry juice
   1 small white dinner roll
	11

4. 1 cup spaghetti in tomato sauce
   1 slice Italian bread with 1 tsp margarine
   Marinated Cucumbers*
   1 cup 1% or 2% lowfat milk
	13

5. Lettuce (1 cup) w/avocado slices (1/4 avocado)
   1 Tbsp mayonnaise style salad dressing
   1 cup beef noodle soup
   Roast turkey sandwich: 3 oz roast turkey,
                     1 Tbsp mayonnaise
                     2 slices white bread
	12

20 fresh bing cherries 1 cup 1% or 2% lowfat milk	

6. Chef's salad: 2 cups iceberg lettuce
                tomato wedges (½)
                hardboiled egg
                ½ cup water chestnuts,
                3 oz ham slices
                2 oz grated cheese
                ½ cup cucumber slices
                ½ medium carrot grated
   1 Tbsp mayonnaise-style salad dressing
   1 standard slice white bread
   1 tsp margarine
   1 cup honeydew melon
   12 oz diet soda
	12

7. Tuna salad sandwich: ½ cup tuna salad
      (made from tuna and mayonnaise),
      2 standard slices white bread
   Radishes (5 each) and 1 cup cucumber slices
   1 cup Thompson seedless grapes
   1 cup buttermilk
	11

Dinner Options	Oxalate (mg)

1. 1/2 roasted Cornish game hen
   California Wild Rice Salad*
   ½ cup green peas w/mushrooms
   1 small white dinner roll
   1 tsp margarine
   1 cup 1% or 2% lowfat milk
	11

2. Chicken Adobo*
   1 cup white rice boiled
   Salad: 1 cup iceberg lettuce
         ½ cucumber
         ½ carrot
         1 Tbsp mayonnaise-style salad dressing
   12 fl oz diet soda
   1 small plain white roll
   1 tsp margarine
	10

3. 4 oz poached salmon
   Angel Hair Saute*
   Watermelon Salad*
   1 cup sparkling water
	16

4. Sandra's Curry Chicken*
   1 cup steamed white rice
   ½ cup cooked carrots
   1 small white dinner roll
   1 tsp margarine
   1 cup apple juice
	13

5. 1 cup macaroni and cheese
   Tomato wedges (1 medium tomato)
   1 cup honeydew melon
   1 cup 1% or 2% lowfat milk
	6

6. Fish taco: 3 oz baked fish. 1/4 cup shredded
   iceberg lettuce, 1/2 medium tomato, avocado
   slices (1/4), 1 tsp lime juice, 2 small corn tortillas
   1 small corn on the cob
   1 tsp margarine
   12 fl oz diet soda
	11

7. 4 oz broiled steak
   1 medium baked potato
   ½ cup cooked cauliflower
   Small french roll
   2 tsp margarine
   8 fl oz lemonade without peel
	4

TABLE A-28-d. LOW-OXALATE MEAL SUGGESTIONS (continued)

Snack/Desserts	Oxalate (mg)		
		Graham crackers, 2 each	1.7
Watermelon Ice*	0	Sponge cake, 1 slice	4.9
Banana Ice Cream*	0	Fig Newtons, 2 each	4.2
Fruit Kabobs*	6	Popcorn, Orville Redenbacker popped, 2 cups	4.2

*Recipe in original document.
From Brzezinski E, Durning AM, Grasse B, Fusselman E, Claraldi T. Oxalate content of selected foods. The General Clinical Research Center, University of California, San Diego Medical Center. 1996:1–53. With permission. The 1998 edition has been updated to include several variations of some food choices and some new foods to further assist those attempting to follow a low-oxalate regimen.

A-28-e. National Organizations

National Kidney Foundation
30 East 33rd St. Suite 1100   (same)
New York, NY 10016
Phone: (800) 622-9010
          (212) 889-2210
Fax: (212) 689-9261

Oxalosis and Hyperoxaluria Foundation
201 East 19th Street, Suite 12E   (NEW)
New York, NY 10003
Phone: (212) 777-0470
Fax: (212) 777-0471
Toll Free: (800) OHF-8699
www.ohf.org

University of California San Diego Medical Center
General Clinical Research Center Nutrition Unit
200 West Arbor Drive
San Diego, CA 92103-8203
Phone: (619) 543-3580
Email: ebrzezinski@uscd.edu

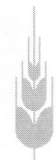

A-29-a. AGENCIES AND ORGANIZATIONS—NATIONAL AND INTERNATIONAL

Agency for Healthcare Research and Quality (AHRQ)	http://www.ahrq.gov
American Academy of Family Physicians	http://www.aafp.org
American Academy of Pediatrics	http://www.aap.org
American Diabetes Association	http://www.diabetes.org
American Dietetic Association	http://www.eatright.org
American Heart Association:	http://www.americanheart.org
American Obesity Association	http://www.obesity.org
American Medical Association	http://www.ama-assn.org
American Nurses Association	http://nursingworld.org
American Public Health Association	http://www.apha.org
American Society for Clinical Nutrition	http://www.faseb.org/ascn
American Society for Parenteral and Enteral Nutrition	http://www.clinnutr.org
Behavioral Counseling in Primary Care to Promote a Healthy Diet	http://www.ahrq.gov/clinic/uspstf/uspsdiet.htm
Centers for Disease Control and Prevention	http://www.cdc.gov/
Centers for Obesity Research and Education	http://www.uchsc.edu/core/
Codex Alimentarius (FAO/WHO)	http://www.codexalimentarius.net
Department of Agriculture Main Website	http://www.usda.gov/wps/portal/usdahome
Department of Agriculture, Agricultural Research Service:	http://www.ars.usda.gov/main/main.htm
Department of Agriculture, Economic Research Service:	http://www.ers.usda.gov/publications/foodreview/dec2002
Department of Health and Human Services:	http://www.os.dhhs.gov/2002
Department Health and Human Services-	http://www.healthfinder.gov
National Health Information Services:	http://www.cdc.gov
medical references, resources, fact sheets for	http://www.odphp.osophs.dhhs.gov
specific age groups, ethnicities and needs	
Department Health and Human Service- Aging	http://www.os.dhhs.gov/aging/index.shtml
Foods & Agriculture Organization of the United Nations	http://www.fao.org/
Food and Drug Administration	http://www.fda.gov
FDA's Center for Food Safety and Applied Nutrition	http://vm.cfsan.fda.gov/list.html
Food and Nutrition Board, IOM	http://www.nationalacademies.org/
Food Standards Australia New Zealand	http://www.foodstandards.gov.au/
Healthy Eating Index report	http://www.usda.gov/cnpp/healthyeating.html
Food and Agriculture Organization of the UN (FAO)	http://www.fao.org
Health Canada	http://www.hc-sg.ca
International Association for the Study of Obesity	http://www.iotf.org/
International Bibliographic Information on Dietary Supplements (IBIDS) database	http://dietary-supplements.info.nih.gov/Health_Information/IBIDS.aspx
International Food Information Council Foundation	http://ific.org
Institute of Medicine	http://www.iom.edu/
Medicare Official Website:	http://www.medicare.gov/
Medscape- integrated med information/edu	http://www.medscape.com/
National Center for Complementary and Alternative Medicine	http://nccam.nih.gov
National Institute of Child Health and Human Development	http://www.nichd.nih.gov
National Heart, Lung, and Blood Institute (NHLBI)	http://www.nhlbi.nih.gov/
NHLBI- Aim for a Healthy Weight	http://www.nhlbi.nih.gov/health/public/heart/obesity/lose_wt

NHLBI-
　information and resources on four key areas:
　cardiovascular health, asthma, sleep, and minority
　　populations:

http://hp2010.nhlbihin.net/

Natural Health Products Directorate, Canada

http://www.hc-sc.gc.ca/hpfb-dgpsa/
nhpd-dpsn/index.html

National Academies Press:

http://www.nap.edu/

The National Institute of Diabetes and Digestive and
　Kidney Diseases (NIDDK)

http://www.niddk.nih.gov/

NIDDK- Weight Control & Loss

http://www.niddk.nih.gov/health/nutrit/nutrit.html

National Institute of Environmental Health Sciences
　(NIEHS)

http://www.niehs.nih.gov

National Institutes of Health

http://www.nih.gov/

National Institutes of Mental Health (eating disorders)

http://www.nimh.nih.gov/publicat/eatingdisorders
.cfm

North American Association for the Study of Obesity

http://http://www.naaso.org

Nutrition and Aging information

http://www.fiu.edu/~nutreldr.

Nutrition Facts Panel on Food Labels

http://vm.cfsan.fda.gov/~dms/foodlab.html

Office of Dietary Supplements (ODS) at the NIH:
　　　OR

http://ods.od.nih.gov/
http://dietary-supplements.info.nih.gov/index.aspx

USDA's Food and Nutrition Information Center

http://www.nal.usda.gov/fnic

USDA's searchable nutrient database:

http://www.mal.usda.gov/fnic/foodcomp/search/

U.S. Government Official Web Portal

http://www.firstgov.gov

U.S. Government Nutrition Website

http://www.nutrition.gov/

World Health Organization

http://www.who.int

A-29-b. SEARCH ENGINES AND MEDICAL JOURNALS

Querying any search engine available on Internet for medical journals produces a huge array of options. For example, using Yahoo and selecting health as the topic, after typing in "medical journals" in the search box, categories of journals are displayed. Others sources for accessing on-line publications are listed below.

Google Scholar

http://scholar.google.com/

National Library of Medicine:

http://www.nlm.nih.gov

　Internet Grateful Med

http://igm.nlm.nih.gov

　MEDLINEplus

http://www.medlineplus.gov/

　MedlinePLUS News by date

http://www.nlm.nih.gov/medlineplus/
newsbydate.html

　NLM Gateway

http://gateway.nlm.nih.gov/gw/Cmd

　PubMed

http://www.ncbi.nlm.nih.gov/PubMed

American Journal of Clinical Nutrition

http://www.ajcn.org

Federation of American Societies for Experimental Biology

http://www.faseb.org

Annals of Internal Medicine

http://www.annals.org

Blood

http://www.bloodjournal.org

British Journal of Nutrition

http://www.cup.org/Journals/JNI.SCAT/nut/nut
.html

British Medical Journal

http://www.bmj.com/

Journal of the American Dietetic Association

http://www.eatright.org/

Journal of the American Medical Association

http://www.ama-assn.org/

Journal of Clinical Investigation

http://www.jci.org/

Journal of Clinical Oncology

http://www.jco.org

Journal of the National Cancer Institute

http://cancernet.nci.nih.gov/jnci/jncihome.html

Journal of Parenteral and Enteral Nutrition

http://www.clinnutr.org

Lancet

http://www.thelancet.com

McGill University list of e-journals

http://www.library.mcgill.ca/refshelf/ejournals.html

Nature Medicine

http://medicine.nature.com

New England Journal of Medicine   http://www.nejm.org
Proceedings of the National Academy of Sciences USA   http://www.pnas.org

A-29-c. ONCOLOGY SOCIETIES AND SERVICES

American Cancer Society: http://www.cancer.org/docroot/home/index.asp
Am Coll Surgeons Commission on Cancer: http://www.facs.org
American Institute of Cancer Research (AICR)   http://www.aicr.org
Cancer Information Service (CIS)   http://www.cis.nci.nih.gov
CancerNet   http://cancernet.gov
Cancer Research Institute (CRI)   http://www.cancerresearch.org
Memorial Sloan Kettering Cancer Center- About Herbs   http://www.mskcc.org/mskcc/html/11570.cfm
National Cancer Data Base (NCDB)   http://www.facs.org/dept/cancer/ncdb
National Cancer Institute (NCI)   http://www.cancer.gov
National Center for Complementary and Alternative Medicine   http://nccam.nih.gov
National Council Against Health Fraud   http://ncahf.org
Office of Cancer Complementary and Alternative Medicine   http://www3.cancer.gov/occam
OncoLink   http://www.oncolink.upenn.edu
Oncology Nursing Society   http://www.ons.org
OncoWeb (European School of Oncology)   http://www.oncoweb.com

A-29-d. COMMERCIAL NUTRITION PRODUCT WEBSITES

Abbott Laboratories   http://www.abbott.com/
Baxter International Incorporated   http://www.baxter.com/
B. Braun/McGraw   http://www.bbraunusa.com/
Bristol-Myers Squibb Company   http://www.bms.com/landing/data/index.html
Cambridge Nutraceutical   http://www.cambridgenutra.com/index.shtml
Mead Johnson Nutritionals   http://www.meadjohnson.com
Nestles Clinical Nutrition   http://www.nestleclinicalnutrition.com/
                                                                 home_content.html

Novartis Corporation (Sandoz)   http://www.novartis.com
Ross Products, a division of Abbott Laboratories   http://www.rosslabs.com
SHS North America   http://www.shsna.com/index1.htm

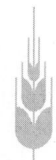

Page numbers followed by f indicate figures; page numbers followed by t indicate tables.

A

Abandonment, 1612
Abdominal adiposity
  elderly, 853
Abdominal fullness
  dietary fiber, 88–89
Abdominal pain
  with chronic pancreatitis, 1231
Abdominal Trauma Index (ATI), 1416
  sepsis risk, 1416t
Abetalipoproteinemia
  genetic defects, 405
  transfer protein deficiency, 1071–1072
  vitamin E deficiency, 397–399
Abortions
  with iodine deficiency, 305
Acarbose, 1062t
Acceptable macronutrient distribution range
    (AMDR), 1658–1659, 1660t, 1852
  for healthy diets, 1856–1857
Accutane, 366
ACD. See Acyl-coenzyme A dehydrogenase
    (ACD)
ACEI. See Angiotensin converting enzyme
    inhibitor (ACEI)
Aceruloplasminemia, 258t
  congenital, 260
Acesulfame potassium
  with diabetes mellitus, 1055t
Acetaminophen
  taurine interaction, 558
Acetazolamide
  for metabolic alkalosis, 184
Acetylcoenzyme A (CoA) carboxylase (ACC),
    499
Acid
  excretion, 178, 178f
  net production, 177–178, 178f
Acid base compensation
  predicting, 186t
Acid base diagnosis, 189–190
Acid base disorders, 176–186
  metabolic acidosis, 178–185
  metabolic alkalosis, 183–184
  respiratory acidosis, 184–185
  respiratory alkalosis, 185
  terminology, 176–177
Acidosis
  with chronic renal failure, 1499
  defined, 176–177
Acid secretion, 1182–1184
Acquired immunodeficiency syndrome (AIDS)
  chemical senses and diet, 703
  in infants and children, 996
  with malabsorption, 1149
Acrodermatitis enteropathica, 608
Action, 1611
  omitting to, 1611
Activity
  assessment of, 1031
  childhood obesity, 982–983
  programmed vs. lifestyle, 1035
Activity-related energy expenditure (AEE),
    720, 726

Acute diarrhea
  in infants and children, 992–994
Acute liver injury, 1236
Acute lung injury, 1467
Acute myocardial infarction
  with magnesium deficiency, 237
Acute pancreatitis, 1227–1228
  clinical assessment, 1227–1228
  clinical predictors or severity, 1228
  clinical presentation, 1227
  EN vs. TPN, 1229–1230
  glutamine for, 566
  imaging, 1228
  Ranson's criteria of severity, 1228t
  serum tests, 1228
  treatment, 1228–1230
Acute Physiology and Chronic Health
    Evaluation (APACHE-II), 1228
Acute promyelocytic leukemia (APL), 366
Acute renal failure
  amino acids, 1500–1502
  anabolic steroids, 1502–1503
  nutritional dialysis, 1502–1503
  nutritional therapy in, 1499–1505
  total parenteral nutrition, 1501t
Acute respiratory distress syndrome, 1467
Acute respiratory infection
  with malnutrition, 1405
Acyl-CoA oxidase
  deficiency, 969
Acyl-coenzyme A dehydrogenase (ACD),
    962–963
  defects, 965–966
Acyl-coenzyme A retinol acyltransferase
    (ARAT), 358
Adaptation
  diagnosis, 889–895
  disruption of, 889
  to starvation, 737–738, 738f
    characteristics, 739
    mechanisms, 741–742
Adaptive genes
  identification of, 634
Adaptive immunity, 674–675, 679–680
Additives
  gluten free safe, 2011
Adenine
  biosynthesis, 32–33
Adenosine diphosphate (ADP), 445f, 732
Adenosine triphosphate (ATP), 721, 732
  phosphorylation to oxidation yield, 137,
    138f
Adequate intake (AI), 797, 1658–1659, 1660t,
    1854
  comparison of, 1854–1855
  definition, 1853t
  development of, 1662
  use of, 1665
ADH. See Alcohol dehydrogenase (ADH)
Adiponectin, 640–642
Adipose tissue
  controlling meal size, 710–711
Adipose tissue hormones, 640–644
Adiposity rebound, 981

Adolescents, 818–827
  basal metabolic rate, 1903t
  calcium, 206
  caries free, 1157f
  magnesium deficiency treatment, 240
  manganese dietary reference intake values,
    327t
  nutritional requirements, 818–823
  nutrition effect on adult morbidity and
    mortality, 823–824
  obesity onset, 981
  riboflavin
    dietary reference intake value, 439t
  special nutritional problems, 823–827
  thiamin
    dietary sources, 427t
  vegetarian diets, 1648
  vitamin A requirements, 354t
  vitamin B6 recommended intakes, 457t
  vitamin D
    dietary reference intake values, 391t
  vitamin E dietary reference intakes,
    407t
  vitamin K, 423t
ADP. See Adenosine diphosphate (ADP)
Adulthood, 830–842
Advance care directives, 1618–1619
  inadequate, 1614
  lack of, 1614
Advanced dementia, 1618
Advance practice nurse
  roles of, 1603–1604
AEE. See Activity-related energy expenditure
    (AEE)
Aerobic fitness, 723–724
Aflatoxins, 1818
Africa
  selenium deficiency, 323
African dietary iron overload, 258t
African hemochromatosis, 260
Age-appropriate foods, 1744–1745
Aging
  anthropometry, 766–767
  chemosensory function, 701
  fitness, 724
  oral health, 1174
  photosynthesis
    previtamin D3, 380, 381f
  vitamin D absorption, 390
Agricultural biotechnology foods
  allergenicity of, 1520–1521
Agricultural chemicals, 1814–1815
Agricultural practices, 1708
AI. See Adequate intake (AI)
AIDS. See Acquired immunodeficiency
    syndrome (AIDS)
ALA. See Alimentary toxic aleukia (ALA)
Alanine, 25
  synthesis, 30–31, 1419f
Albendazole
  with fatty meal, 1542
Albumin, 288, 839t
  elderly, 853
  with malabsorption, 1146

Albumin (*Continued*)
  starvation, 740
  surgical complications, 1418f
Alcohol
  blood and urine studies, 1253f
  with chronic pancreatitis, 1231
  with diabetes mellitus, 1056
  with gout, 1328
  with hypercholesterolemia, 1085t
  inducing gastric emptying, 1181
  international dietary guidelines, 1712t
  osteoporosis, 1347
  osteosclerosis, 1321
  producing cobalamin malabsorption, 492
Alcohol abuse
  prevalence, 870–871
Alcohol dehydrogenase (ADH), 633
Alcoholic beverages
  calories, 1964t
  cancer, 1274
  Dietary Guidelines for Americans, 1895
  electrolytes, 1964t
  nutritional value of, 1246–1247
Alcoholic cardiomyopathy, 1255
Alcoholic cirrhosis
  iron overload, 261
Alcoholic hyperlipidemia, 1243
Alcoholic ketoacidosis, 1368
Alcoholic liver injury
  complications, 1240f
  sequential development, 1239f
Alcoholism, 1360
  angina pectoris, 1255
  bile salts, 1249
  with biotin deficiency, 503
  blood, 1255
  bone marrow, 1255
  electrolytes, 1252–1253
  with folic acid deficiency, 478
  heart, 1255
  liver, 1254
  minerals, 1252–1253
  nutritional status, 1247–1248
  nutritional therapy, 1255–1256
  pantothenic acid, 467
  protein intake, 1237
  salt retention, 1252
  stroke, 1254
  water retention, 1252
  zinc, 280
Alcohol metabolism, 633
Alcohol metabolizing isozymes, 633t
Aldehyde dehydrogenase (ALDH), 633
Aldehyde oxidase, 344
ALDH. *See* Aldehyde dehydrogenase
    (ALDH)
Aldicarb, 1814
Aldosterone, 164, 164
  with congestive heart failure, 1109
Aldosterone antagonists
  for hypokalemia, 165
Aldosterone blocking agent
  for congestive heart failure, 1111
Aldosterone deficiency, 166
Alendronate
  for osteoporosis, 1349
Alexandrium, 1820
Algal toxins (phycotoxins), 1819–1820
Alimentary toxic aleukia (ALA), 1818–1819
Alimentary tract, 1115–1141
Aliphatic amino acids, 22
Alkali
  food content, 177f
Alkalosis
  defined, 176–177

Allen, Frederick M., 1044
Allen Starvation Treatment, 1044
Allergenic foods
  residue detection, 1520
Allergens, 803
Allergy like intoxications, 1525–1527
All trans beta carotene
  structure, 353f
Alpha amino acids
  structural formulas, 23f
Alpha catecholamines, 168
Alpha-ketoglutarate dehydrogenase, 1368
Alpha ketoisocaproate
  leucine cellular transport, 40–41
Alpha linoleic acid. *See also* Polyunsaturated
    fatty acids (PUFA)
  DRI by life-stage group, 1864t
Alpha linolenic acid, 8, 1798t. *See also*
    Polyunsaturated fatty acids (PUFA)
  AMDR for, 1857
  phenylketonuria
    pregnancy, 2000t
Alpha melanocyte stimulating hormone
    (alpha-MSH), 712
Alpha tocopherol, 397, 1470
  adequacy of intake, 407
  assessment of, 407–408, 408t
  deficiency
    pathology, 406
  dietary fat, 399
  pathways, 401f
  preventing deficiency, 404t
  source, 406
  structure, 398f
  supplements, 408t
    controversy, 408
Alpha-Tocopherol Beta-Carotene (ATBC)
  group, 1470
  trial, 365, 1275
Alpha tocopherol transfer protein
  genetic defects, 404
Alstrom syndrome, 1021
Altermonas, 1821
Alternative movement
  political considerations, 1771–1772
Alternative promoters, 1763t
Alternative systems, 1763–1768
Aluminum
  bone, 1322–1323
  toxicity of, 1585
Alveolar minute ventilation
  defined, 1464t
Alzheimer disease, 1365–1366, 1618
  copper, 851
  glutamate, 32
AMA. *See* American Medical Association
    (AMA)
Amalgam toxicity, 1769
Amanita muscaria, 1823
Amanita phalloides, 1823
Amatoxin, 1823
Amblyopia
  deficiency, 1370
AMDR. *See* Acceptable macronutrient
    distribution range (AMDR)
American College of Cardiology
  Guidelines for Evaluation and
    Management of Heart Failure in
    Adults, 1108–1109
American Diabetes Association Exchange
    Lists, 1055t
American Heart Association
  Guidelines for Evaluation and
    Management of Heart Failure in
    Adults, 1108–1109

American Medical Association (AMA)
  statement of 1986, 1617
American Society for Parenteral and Enteral
    Nutrition (ASPEN), 1568
Amiloride
  for hypokalemia, 165
Amine oxidase, 287
Amino acid metabolism disorders
  infants and children
    daily requirements, 920t
Amino acids, 5–6, 21–56, 24t, 1728, 1755
  acute renal failure, 1500–1502, 1501t, 1505
  aliphatic, 22
  alpha
    structural formulas, 23f
  aromatic, 916–928
  branched chain, 1579
  commercially available mixtures, 998t
  concentrations, 26t
  defined, 22–25
  degradation, 27–28, 29t
  from dietary protein sources, 55
  dietary reference intakes in normal infants
    and children, 801t
  dispensable, 24, 24t
  distribution, 25–26
  egg protein, 25t
  energy contribution, 1579
  essential, 24t
    dietary reference intakes in normal
      infants and children, 801t
    for preterm infant formulas, 812t
  fluxes, 41, 41f
  incorporation into other compounds, 31–32
  indispensable, 24t
    vs. dispensable ratio, 54–55
  kinetics, 39–42
  liver protein, 25t
  molecular weights, 23
  muscle protein, 25t
  needs in disease, 55–56
  neutral, 22
  nonessential, 24, 24t
  optical activity, 23
  parenteral diet, 1428
  for preterm infant formulas, 812t
    1989 RDA *vs.* 2002 RDI, 819t
  recommended dietary allowances, 52t
  renal function, 1477
  requirements, 51–56, 54f
  splanchnic bed metabolism, 42
  sulfur, 22, 928–932
    biochemistry, 928
    measurement, 559
    RDA, 548
    structure, 546f
  synthesis, 27–28, 31t
  tracer methods, 36–37
  transport, 26–27, 27t
  vitamin B6, 454
    1989 *vs.* 2002 RDI, 831t
Aminoglycosides
  with Mg wasting, 233
Amino-nitrogen
  movement around glutamic acid, 28f
Aminorex
  adverse effects of, 1472
Aminothiols
  plasma, 547f
Amiodarone
  for congestive heart failure, 1112
Amitriptyline, 1360
Ammonia, 946–950
  biochemistry, 946
Amnesic shellfish poisoning, 1820

Amnestic deficit, 432
Amoxicillin
    gastrointestinal effects, 877t
Amphetamines, 1360
Amphotericin B
    with Mg wasting, 233
AMPM. *See* Automated Multiple Pass
        Method (AMPM)
Amputees
    human body proportions for, 1960f
Amylase, 1127–1128, 1136
    acute pancreatitis, 1228
Amylin
    affecting metabolism and food intake, 1046t
Amylopectin
    in starch, 66t
Amylose
    in starch, 66t
Amyotrophic lateral sclerosis
    glutamate, 32
    oxidative stress, 693
Anabolic steroids
    for acute renal failure, 1502–1503
    for cancer, 1301t
    for COPD, 1469
Anabolic support, 1394–1395
Anabolic therapy, 1394–1395
Anaphylactic shock
    with immunoglobulin E-mediated food
        allergy, 1514–1515
Ancient Greeks, 3
Anemia, 267
    blood count, 1437t
    with celiac disease, 1222–1223
    clinical consequences of, 1436–1437
    ferrous sulfate for, 5
    treatment of, 822
Anemia of chronic disease, 261
Angina pectoris
    with alcoholism, 1255
Angiotensin, 650–651
    with congestive heart failure, 1109
Angiotensin converting enzyme inhibitor (ACEI)
    chronic renal failure, 1479
    for congestive heart failure, 1111
Angiotensin II receptor blockers
    for congestive heart failure, 1111
Angiotensin receptor blockers (ARB)
    chronic renal failure, 1479
Animal-derived protein, 1802–1803
Animal feed
    determining fat content, 1708
Animal glue, 3
Anorexia
    cancer, 702
    elderly, 1532–1534, 1534–1535
Anorexia nervosa, 739, 825, 1353
Anovulation
    with iodine deficiency, 305
ANP. *See* Atrial natriuretic peptides (ANP)
Antacids
    copper interactions, 294
Anthocyanins, 583, 1797t
    absorption, 590
    biologic effects, 589–592, 591
    chemistry, 589–592
    gut metabolism, 590
    health effects, 585t
    metabolism, 590
    tissue metabolism, 590–591
    vascular permeability, 591
    vision, 591
Anthropometric equations
    predicting body density in female
        population, 761f

Anthropometric measure
    for Mexican-Americans, 1938t–1939t
    for non-Hispanic blacks, 1937t–1938t
    for non-Hispanic whites, 1936t–1937t
Anthropometry, 7540768
    aging, 766–767, 767t
    clinical applications of, 766
    error, 767–768, 767f
    measurements, 757, 757t
Antiarrhythmic agents
    for congestive heart failure, 1111–1112
Antibiotic-coated catheters, 1569
Anticoagulant agents
    for congestive heart failure, 1112
Anticonvulsants
    with folic acid deficiency, 479
Antidepressants, 1360
    associated with weight gain, 1021
    for cancer, 1301t, 1303
Antidiuretic hormone metabolism
    water, 188–189
Antidiuretic hormone release
    thirst, 167–169
Antiemetics
    for cancer, 1301t
Antiendomysial antibodies
    with celiac disease, 1223
Antienzymes
    in human milk, 790t
Antiepileptic drugs
    associated with weight gain, 1021
Antigliadin antibodies
    with celiac disease, 1223
Antigliadin immunoglobulin A antibodies
    celiac disease, 1221
Antihistamines
    for histamine poisoning, 1525–1526
Antiinflamatory agents
    cancer chemoprevention, 1285–1286
Antiinflammatory cytokines, 1392
Antioxidant network
    vitamin E, 398–399
Antioxidants, 692, 692
    arthritis, 1335–1336
    athletes, 1730
    sport nutrition, 1730–1731
Antipsychotic agents
    associated with weight gain, 1021
Antirachitic factor, 378
Antithiamin compounds, 427–428
APACHE-II. *See* Acute Physiology and
        Chronic Health Evaluation (APACHE-
        II)
Apigenin, 584, 1796t
APL. *See* Acute promyelocytic leukemia (APL)
Apnea of prematurity, 185
Apolipoprotein(s), 124
    A1 deficiency, 1072–1073, 1073t
    C-II deficiency, 1070
    C-III deficiency, 1088
    function, 125t
Apoproteins, 102–103
Apoptosis, 676–677
Apothecaries measure, 1850
Appendix, 1120
Appert, Nicolas, 1777
Appetite
    with cancer, 1295
Appetite questionnaire
    predicting weight loss in elderly, 1535t
Appetite stimulants
    for cancer, 1301–1302, 1301t
Applied kinesiology, 1766
Arachidonic acid, 92
    eicosanoid synthesis, 113f

Arachnia, 415
ARAT. *See* Acyl-coenzyme A retinol
        acyltransferase (ARAT)
ARB. *See* Angiotensin receptor blockers (ARB)
Arginine, 1579, 1728–1729, 1729
    cardiovascular system, 577–578
    chemical structure of, 572f
    clinical uses, 579t
    endocrine system, 578
    gastrointestinal tract, 578
    hematologic system, 578
    hypertension, 578
    immune system, 579
    metabolic pathway, 572f
    metabolism, 571–572
    Mg absorption, 229
    needs in disease, 56
    nitric oxide pathway, 572–575
    renal system, 579
    reproductive system, 579
    respiratory system, 576–577
    synthesis, 53
Arginine-nitric oxide synthase-cyclic
        guanosine monophosphate, 574f
Arginine paradox, 575
Aromatic amino acids, 916–928
    biochemistry, 916–925
    for inborn errors of metabolism,
        1995t–1996t
    metabolism of, 914f
Arrhythmias, 217
Arsenic, 339–340. *See also* Minerals
    absorption, 339–340
    analytic methods, 339
    bioavailability, 339–340
    chemistry, 339
    deficiency, 340
    dietary considerations, 340
    distribution, 340
    excretion, 340
    health effects, 340–341
    historical overview, 339
    mechanisms of action, 340
    metabolism, 340
    toxic effects, 340–341
    transport, 340
Arsenicism, 341
Arsine, 339
Arterial pressure, 1096f
Arteriovenous differences, 36
Arthritis
    antioxidants, 1335–1336
    nutritional aspects of, 1326–1327
        improving, 1326–1327
    oxidative stress, 693
Arthritis drug-nutrient interactions, 1327, 1327f
Artificial nutrition
    withdrawal of
        symptom management in, 1620t
Ascorbate recycling, 513
Ascorbic acid. *See* Vitamin C (ascorbic acid)
Aspartame, 1811
    with diabetes mellitus, 1055t
Aspartates, 1729
    synthesis, 30–31
ASPEN. *See* American Society for Parenteral
        and Enteral Nutrition (ASPEN)
Aspergillus, 1818
Aspirin
    vitamin E, 408
Aspirin-nutrient interactions, 1327f
Assessment, 751–754
Asthma, 1470
ATBC. *See* Alpha-Tocopherol Beta-Carotene
        (ATBC)

Atherogenesis
  phytosterols, 131–132
Atherogenic dyslipidemia, 1088–1092
  elevate apolipoprotein B, 1089
  etiology, 1089
  with hypertriglyceridemia, 1089–1090
  insulin resistance, 1091
  low-density lipoprotein cholesterol, 1091
  low high-density lipoprotein cholesterol,
    1090, 1091–1092
  small low-density lipoprotein, 1090, 1091
  treatment, 1090–1091
Atherosclerosis
  catechins, 588
  cholesterol, 124–127
  with diabetes mellitus, 1050
  lipid peroxidation, 106
Atherosclerotic cardiovascular disease
  lipoproteins, 1076–1077
  public health prevention of, 1077
Atherosclerotic vascular disease
  with magnesium deficiency, 238
Athletes
  antioxidants, 1730
  dietary principles, 1723–1724, 1723–1734
  dietary supplements
    arginine, 1728–1729
    aspartates, 1729
    beta-hydroxy-beta-methylbutyrate,
      1729–1730
    branched-chain amino acids, 1729
    glutamine, 1729
    L-tryptophan, 1729
    lysine, 1729
    ornithine, 1729
ATI. *See* Abdominal Trauma Index (ATI)
Atkins diet, 1757–1758
Atom % excess, 36
Atomic absorption spectrophotometry
  Mg, 231
Atomic model
  of body composition, 754
Atomic weights, 1848–1849
Atorvastatin
  for hypercholesterolemia, 1085t
ATP. *See* Adenosine triphosphate (ATP)
Atransferrinemia, 258t
  congenital, 260
Atrial natriuretic peptides (ANP), 651
At-risk surgical patient
  identification of, 1415–1416
Atropine, 1821–1822, 1822
Atwater, W.O., 13
Australia
  nutrient reference values, 1864t–1885t
Autoimmune thyroid disease
  with iodine excess, 306–307
Automated Multiple Pass Method (AMPM),
  1695
Autonomic nervous system
  branches of, 1124f
Autonomy, 1609
Autosomal dominant congenital cataracts,
  258t, 261
Autosomal recessive hypercholesterolemia,
  1069
Avoirdupois, 1850
Axokine
  for obesity, 1039
5-Aza-2'-deoxycytidine, 1285t

B
Bacillus cereus, 1818
Bacterial contamination
  with enteral feeding, 1564

Bacterial overgrowth syndrome, 1149
Bacterial toxins, 1817–1818
Bacteroides fragilis, 415
Baking, 1782–1783
Balance, 752–753
Balance method, 1323
  protein requirements, 49–50
Barber-Nejde Case, 1616
Bardet-Biedel syndrome, 1021
Bariatric surgery
  with diabetes mellitus, 1060
Barlow disease, 603
Basal energy expenditure (BEE), 1420–1421
Basal metabolic rate (BMR), 141–142, 1901t
  adolescent, 1903t
  equations for predicting from body weight,
    1902t
  estimating, 142t
  examples of predicted, 1902t
  during pregnancy, 773
Basal metabolism, 141–142
BCAA. *See* Branched chain amino acids
  (BCAA)
B cells, 671–672
  activation, 674–675
  adaptive immunity, 679
  receptor signaling, 675
  signaling, 674–675
  subsets, 672–673
Beaton, George, 1657f, 1660–1661
Beccari, Jacopo, 3
Beck Depression Inventory, 1030
Bedside gas exchange, 14–15
BEE. *See* Basal energy expenditure (BEE)
Beef consumption
  cultural ecology, 1743
Beef gelatin, 1519
Beer
  production of, 1777
Behavioral disorders
  affecting food intake, 1353–1360
Benedict, F.G., 13
Beriberi, 426, 430–431, 695
  cardiovascular, 599
  clinical manifestations of, 1368–1369
  infantile, 599
Beriberi heart failure, 1255
Beriberi neuropathy, 1369
Bernard, Claude, 12
BEST. *See* Bioenergetic synchronization
  technique (BEST)
Beta agonists
  Mg, 226
Beta blockers
  for congestive heart failure, 1111
Beta carotene
  alcoholism, 1249–1251
  antioxidant properties, 1755
  athletes, 1730
  cancer, 365
  intestinal metabolism, 358f
Beta Carotene and Retinol Efficacy Trial,
  365, 1467, 1470
Beta cryptoxanthin
  structure, 353f
Beta hydroxy beta methylbutyrate, 1729–1730
Beta hydroxy beta methylglutaryl
  coenzyme, 123
Betaine
  for homocystinuria, 930
  remethylation *vs.* transsulfuration, 552
Beta-oxidation enzymes, 962–964
  defects
    plasma carnitine levels in, 970t
    pregnancy-induced symptoms, 968

Beutler fluorescent test, 951–952
Beverages
  calories, 1964t
  electrolytes, 1964t
  gluten free foods, 2009t
  oxalate, 2014t, 2109t–2110t
  phenolic phytochemicals in, 1992t
Bexarotene, 1284t
BGP. *See* Bone gla-protein (BGP)
Bicarbonate
  carbon dioxide buffer system, 176
  maintaining high extracellular, 184t
Bile acids, 399
  conjugation
    taurine, 557
  malabsorption, 1149
  sequestrants
    for hypercholesterolemia, 1085
    with hypercholesterolemia, 1085t
Bile salts, 96–98, 1235–1236
  with alcoholism, 1249
  malabsorption of, 1145t
Biliary cirrhosis
  osteoporosis, 1322
Biliary fistulas
  with hypomagnesemia, 233
Biliary system
  function of, 1131
Billroth I procedure, 1186, 1186f
Billroth II procedure, 1186, 1186f
Binge eating disorder, 1022, 1031,
  1353–1354
Bioactive food components
  evaluating role of, 1669
Biochemical assessment
  elderly, 853–854
Bioenergetic synchronization technique
  (BEST), 1766
Bioimpedance analysis, 763–765
Biotechnology
  agricultural foods
    allergenicity of, 1520–1521
  benefits of, 1786
  consumer concerns, 1786–1787
Biotin, 498–505, 601
  absorption, 501–503
  adequate intake, 505t
  allowances, 505
  blood transport, 502
  carboxylases, 499–500
  central nervous system transport, 502
  chemistry, 499
  deficiency, 503–505, 601
    biochemical pathogens, 504–505
    brittle nails, 503
    clinical findings, 503–504
    diagnosis, 505
    etiology, 503
    laboratory findings, 504
  degradation, 499f
  dietary sources, 505
  in enteral feeding products, 1558t
  enzymes
    pathways, 500f
  historical background, 498
  intestinal absorption, 501
  intestinal uptake, 501
  liver uptake, 501–502
  measurement, 500–501
  metabolism, 499f, 500
  milk transport, 502–503
  placental transport, 502
  pregnancy, 777
  regulation, 498–499
  renal handling, 502

renal resorption, 501
requirements, 505
serum, 500t
structure, 498
toxicity, 505, 601
urine, 500t
Birth order, 1747
Bisphosphonates
for osteoporosis, 1349
Bitot spots, 370, 596
Black, Joseph, 11
Black foot disease, 341
Blacks
non-Hispanic
anthropometric measure, 1937t–1938t
Bladder cancer
fruits and vegetables, 1273
Blanching, 1780–1781, 1781t
Blaud, Pierre, 5
Bloch, Carl, 1401
Blood
iron, 5
Blood clotting factor V, 288
Blood clotting factor VIII, 288
Blood coagulation, 415
Blood glucose
metabolic regulation, 69–70
Blood mononuclear cells
Mg content, 232
Blood pressure
dietary fiber, 88
dietary salt, 155–156
metabolic syndrome, 1008–1009
potassium, 164
Blood triglycerides
dietary fiber, 88
Blood urea nitrogen (BUN), 839t–840t, 840
protein intake, 841
Blount disease, 984
BMD. *See* Bone mineral density (BMD)
BMI. *See* Body mass index (BMI)
BMR. *See* Basal metabolic rate (BMR)
BNP. *See* Brain natriuretic peptides (BNP)
Body circumferences, 760
Body composition, 751–768, 752f
aging, 767t
assessment of, 837
models of, 754–766
osteoporotic fractures, 1348
predicting from bioelectric impedance and
anthropometry, 764t
Body content
daily increments, 820t
Body density
predicting in females, 761f
Body fat
changes with age, 979–980
elderly, 854
Body fluids
composition of, 150–151
extracellular composition, 150
intracellular composition, 150–151
volume of, 150, 150t
Body fuel regulation, 1046–1048
Body mass
among athletes, 1723–1734
Body mass index (BMI), 979, 1013, 1014t, 1029
by age, 1914t
determining, 1915f
distribution of, 1079t
by inches and pounds, 1953t
mortality, 1015f, 1531
obesity, 765t
protein-energy malnutrition, 765t
rapid calculation tables, 1916f–1917f

rebound, 981
transition, 1717–1718
Body size, 1269–1270
Body weight, 757–758
interpretation of, 758
measurement of, 758
osteoporotic fractures, 1348
reference values, 765
Bombesin, 1123t
Bonaparte, Napoleon, 339
Bone
aluminum, 1322–1323
architecture, 1316–1317
ascorbic acid, 1321
calcium, 204
composition, 1314–1315
development, 1317
functions, 1318–1319
histomorphometry, 1324
homeostatic functions, 1319–1320
mechanical functions, 1318–1319
mineral, 1314
noncollagenous matrix proteins, 1315
nutritional deficiency, 838t
protein matrix, 1314–1315
remodeling, 1321
biochemical markers, 1325t
revision of, 1317–1318
structure, 1314–1315
Bone biology, 1314–1325
Bone cells
diagram of, 1317f
functions, 1315–1316
humoral factors acting on, 1316t
Bone gla-protein (BGP), 1315
Bone marrow
alcoholism, 1255
transplantation, 1306–1307
glutamine with, 567
for X-ALD, 973
Bone mass
change in, 1323–1324
feedback loop regulating, 1319f
Bone matrix
functions, 1315
Bone mineral density (BMD), 1321
adolescents, 821
assessment of, 1339–1340
direct measurement of, 1323–1324
nutritional determinants, 1342–1348
peak patterns, 1340–1341
vitamin A, 368
Bongkrek food poisoning, 1818
Boron, 339. *See also* Minerals
absorption, 342
analytic methods, 342
beneficial effects, 343
bioavailability, 342
chemistry, 341–342
dietary considerations, 343
distribution, 342
effects on periodontium, 1170t
excretion, 342
health effects, 343
historical overview, 341
mechanisms of action, 342–343
osteoporosis, 1347
sports nutrition, 1732
sports performance, 1732
tissue levels, 342t
toxicity, 343
transport, 342
Botanicals
athletes, 1736
sports nutrition, 1736

Botulinal toxins, 1817–1818
Bound galactose
enzymes degrading, 953
Bouvia Case, 1610
Bovine milk protein, 804
Bowel rest
with Crohn disease, 1215–1216
Boyle, Robert, 11
Brain
amino acids, 1363
lipids, 1363
Brain glucose transporter, 68
Brain natriuretic peptides (BNP), 651
Branched chain alpha ketoaciduria, 935–936
diagnosis, 936
equivalent lists, 937
nutrient requirements, 937
nutrition support, 937–939
screening, 936
stabilization, 935f
treatment, 936–937
Branched chain amino acids (BCAA), 22,
1579, 1729
medical food free of, 937
metabolism, 933f
restricted diets, 2002t
Branched chain ketoaciduria, 910
sample diets for, 2002t
Brazil
overnutrition, 1720f
undernutrition, 1720f
Breads
dietary fiber content of, 1965t
mineral content, 1981t
oxalate, 2015t
Breakfast
adolescents, 820
Breakfast cereal processing, 1783
Breast cancer
calcium, 1274
dairy products, 1273
dietary fat, 1628
dietary fiber, 88
genistein protective effects, 592
lactation impact on, 793–794
soy protective effects, 592
vitamin D, 1274
Breastfeeding, 803
childhood obesity, 982
with Crohn's disease, 1210
prevalence of, 785–786, 785f
psychologic advantages of, 803
Breath hydrogen test, 78, 1192–1193
Breathing
control of, 1462
Britain
selenium, 313
British meal patterns, 1743
Brittle nails
with biotin deficiency, 503
Brody-Kleiber relationship, 141
Brush border digestive enzymes, 1189
disaccharides, 1190t
starch, 1190t
Brush border membrane amino acid transport
systems, 1138t
Brush border membrane hydrolases, 1136
BS stimulated lipase, 98
Bulimia nervosa, 1353–1354
oral health, 1173–1174
BUN. *See* Blood urea nitrogen (BUN)
Bupropion
associated with weight gain, 1021
Bupropion SR
with diabetes mellitus, 1060

Burkitt lymphoma, 1260
Burning feet, 1370–1371
Butyrate
  dietary fiber, 86

C
Cachexia, 742, 1393–1394
  elderly, 1534
Cadmium
  poisoning, 1322
Caffeine
  calcium, 202
  food content, 1989t
  food drugs, 1733–1734
  osteoporosis, 1347
  sports nutrition, 1733–1734
Caffeine citrate, 185
Calbindin
  calcium, 195t
Calciferol. *See* Vitamin D (calciferol)
Calcitonin
  magnesium absorption, 229
  for osteoporosis, 1349
Calcitriol, 376, 1284t
  for chronic renal failure, 1498–1499
Calcium, 194–208, 604. *See also* Minerals
  absorption, 196–198, 197f, 198f
    physiologic factors affecting, 198–199,
      198t
  adolescents, 206, 821
  balance method for estimating
    requirements of, 1710
  bioavailability, 200–201
    sources of, 201t
  biologic roles, 194–195
  bone and teeth, 204, 1320
  bone mass, 1342–1343
  breast cancer, 1274
  cancer, 1274
  cell, 194–195
  cell proteins, 195t
  childhood, 206
  chronic renal failure, 1478–1479
  for chronic renal failure, 1495
  clinical disorders, 208–209
  colon cancer, 205, 1713
  deficiency, 204–205, 604
    tooth development, 1155t
  dietary reference intakes in normal infants
    and children, 801–802
  dietary sources, 200
  distribution in nature, 195
  effects on periodontium, 1170t
  elderly, 849–850
  endogenous fecal, 198–200
  in enteral feeding products, 1558t
  excretion, 198–200
  extracellular enzyme and protein cofactor,
    204
  factorial method for estimating
    requirements of, 1710
  food sources, 200–201
  fractures, 1343
  function method for estimating
    requirements of, 1712
  functions, 202–203
  homeostatic regulation, 195–196, 196f
  hypertension, 1713
  infants, 206
  intake adequacy, 207–208, 207f
  intestinal absorption, 227f
  intracellular messenger, 202–203, 203f
  intrauterine accretion rates during third
    trimester, 809t
  kidney stones, 205, 208

lactation, 207
  magnesium, 208
  malabsorption of, 1145t
  metabolism, 195–196, 198f
    in normal infants and children, 801–802
  nutrient nutrient interactions, 201–202
  osteoporosis, 205
  paracellular transport, 198
  parenteral diet, 1430
  parenteral nutrition, 1580
  peak bone mass, 206
  postmenopausal intake, 1343
  pregnancy, 207
  premenopausal intake, 1343
  1989 RDA *vs.* 2002 RDI, 819t
  requirements for, 205–206, 205t
    throughout life, 1712
  sports nutrition, 1731
  sports performance, 1731
  status assessment, 204
  sustained responses, 203–204
  toxicity, 208, 604
  transcellular transport, 198
  trigger proteins, 204
  urinary excretion, 200
  vegetarian diets, 1643
  1989 *vs.* 2002 RDI, 831t
Calcium balance, 1323
Calcium channel blocker (CCB)
  for congestive heart failure, 1111
  inducing gastric emptying, 1181
Calcium channels
  magnesium, 224
Calcium cystinate
  for homocystinuria, 930–931
Calcium-deficiency rickets, 604
Calcium paradox, 1712
Caldesmon
  calcium, 195t
Calmodulin
  calcium, 195t
Calneurin B
  calcium, 195t
Caloric intake
  with cancer, 1295
Calorie restriction, 743
Calories
  in alcoholic beverages, 1246
  defined, 136
  empty, 1629
  required to gain weight, 982t
Calorimetry
  historical development of, 4
  history of, 12–13, 14
  spreading to America, 13–14
Calretinin
  calcium, 195t
Calsequestrin
  calcium, 195t
cAMP. *See* Cyclic adenosine monophosphate
  (cAMP)
Cancellous bone, 1316
Cancer
  alcohol, 1274
  anabolic steroids, 1301t
  anorexia, 702
  antidepressants, 1301t, 1303
  carcinogenesis, 1281–1282
  carotenoids, 365
  catechins, 588
  chemical senses and diet, 702
  chemoprevention of, 1280–1288
    animal experiments, 1286–1287
    based on mechanism, 1282–1283
    clinical applications, 1288f

education, 1287–1288
    pharmacology of, 1283–1284, 1284t
    societal issues, 1287–1288
  depression, 1296
  diet relationship
    epidemiologic investigation, 1268–1269
    studies of, 1268t
  early lesions, 1282
  enteral feeding, 1298–1299
  gastrointestinal tract disturbances, 1296
  incidence of, 1291t
  lipid peroxidation, 106
  malnutrition with, 1291
    carbohydrate metabolism, 1292–1293
    energy expenditure, 1292
    etiology, 1292–1297
    lipid metabolism, 1293
    metabolic alterations, 1292
    metabolic alterations mediators,
      1293–1294
    protein metabolism, 1293
    significance of, 1291–1292
  mortality of, 1291t
  nutrition, 1297–1303
  nutritional support of, 1290–1308
  oxidative stress, 692–693
  pharmacotherapy, 1300–1303
  public health, 1267
  trends, 1290–1291
  vegetarian diets, 1645–1646
  vitamin B6, 458
Cancer prevention
  selenium, 318–319
Cancer therapies
  questionable, 1769–1771
Candida albicans
  parenteral nutrition, 1571
Candida aneurinolytica, 427
Candidate genes, 632–633, 634t
Candidiasis hypersensitivity, 1768–1769
Canning, 1782
Carbamazepine
  homocysteine interaction, 553
Carbohydrate-copper interactions, 294
Carbohydrate counting
  with diabetes mellitus, 1063
Carbohydrate intake, 1024
Carbohydrate intolerance, 77–78
Carbohydrate loading, 77, 1725
Carbohydrate metabolism
  cancer, 1292–1293
  hormonal regulation, 70–71
  prolonged fasting, 731–732
Carbohydrates, 62–80. *See also* Dietary
  carbohydrates
  absorption of, 1135–1137
  adolescents, 820
  in alcoholic beverages, 1246
  athletic performance, 77
  cancer, 1272
  cholesterol, 129
  chronic disease, 79–80
  for chronic renal failure, 1487t, 1494
  defined, 62–63
  dental caries, 1158–1161
  with diabetes mellitus, 1051–1052
  diagnostic tests, 78–79
  Dietary Guidelines for Americans, 1895
  DRI, 79
    by life-stage group, 1861t
  and elderly, 844t, 845–846
  energy, 137t
  energy substrate, 21
  enteral feeding, 1561
  in enteral feeding products, 1558t

vs. fat feeding
    short bowel syndrome, 1205–1206
in formulas, 805t
in formulas for term infants, 804t
heat equivalents, 137t
historical highlights, 62
in human milk, 788t, 789t, 790t
in hydrolyzed formulas and soy formulas,
    806t
in infant formulas, 806t
liver disorders, 1241–1242
liver regulation, 1236
in low birth weight infant formulas,
    813–814, 813t
low birth weight intake recommendations,
    810t, 811t
malabsorption of, 1145t
metabolites, 1725
for MHD or CPD, 1487t
for normal infants, 798
oxidants, 688
pregnancy, 775
1989 RDA *vs.* 2002 RDI, 819t
recommendations for term infant formulas,
    804t
tolerable upper intake for normal infants
    and children, 800t
UL
    for infants and children, 800t
    1989 *vs.* 2002 RDI, 831t
Carbon dioxide
    exercising, 720
    fatigue, 720
Carbon dioxide buffer system
    bicarbonate, 176
Carbon dioxide production, 139
    defined, 1464t
Carboxypeptidase A, 1137t
Carboxypeptidase B, 1137t
Carcinogenesis
    future directions, 1265
    molecular basis of, 1260–1265
    multistep model of, 1263
Cardiac beriberi (Shoshin), 1368–1369
Cardiac output
    defined, 1464t
    during pregnancy, 773
Cardiorespiratory fitness, 723–724
Cardiovascular beriberi, 599
Cardiovascular disease
    carotenoids, 365
Cardiovascular hormones, 650–651
Cardiovascular system
    arginine, 577–578
Caries. *See* Dental caries
Carnitine, 537–543
    absorption, 540–541
    analysis, 537–538
    athletes, 1735
    bioavailability, 540–541
    biochemical function, 538–539
    biosynthesis, 540
    chemistry, 537–538
    for chronic renal failure, 1493
    CoA, 538–539
    cycle defects, 964–968
    deficiency, 542
    dietary sources, 540–541
    drug actions, 542–543
    excretion, 541–542, 542f
    food content, 1990t
    historical development, 537
    homeostatic mechanisms, 540–541
    mitochondrial long-chain fatty acid
        oxidation, 538, 538f

nomenclature, 537–538
nutrient interactions, 542–543
proteins, 539–540
requirements, 543
sources, 540t
sports nutrition, 1735
status evaluation, 543
supplements
    for fatty acid metabolism defects, 972
synthesis, 31
transport, 541–542
Carnitine acetyltransferase (CAT), 537, 539
Carnitine acylcarnitine translocase, 539–540
Carnitine octanoyltransferase, 539
Carnitine palmitoyltransferase (CPT), 539,
    962
Carnitine palmitoyltransferase I (CPT I), 538
Carotenes, 1796t
    with malabsorption, 1146
    structure, 353f
Carotenoids, 9, 351–371, 360, 1470, 1796t,
    1799–1800
    antioxidant properties, 365–366
    bioavailability, 357–358
    interconverting factors and formulas, 1847
    intestinal absorption, 357
    structure, 353f
Carpenter syndrome, 1021
Carrel, Alexis, 655
Case controlled studies
    of diet effect on cancer, 1268t
Casein hydrolysate formula, 1518
CAT. *See* Carnitine acetyltransferase (CAT)
Catabolic stress
    failed adaptation, 740
Cataracts
    autosomal dominant congenital, 258t, 261
    oxidative stress, 693
CATCH. *See* Children's Activity Trial
    (CATCH)
Catechins, 587–588, 1797t, 1801
    absorption, 587–588
    biologic effect, 588
    dietary source, 587
    intake, 587
    metabolism, 587–588
Catecholamines, 649–650, 1389–1390
    fatty acids, 650
    lipolysis, 650
CAVH. *See* Continuous arteriovenous
    hemofiltration (CAVH)
CCB. *See* Calcium channel blocker (CCB)
CCK. *See* Cholecystokinin (CCK)
CDC growth charts
    body mass index-for-age percentiles,
        1928t–1929t
    length-for-age percentiles, 1920t, 1923t
    stature-for-age percentiles, 1924t, 1926t
    weight-for-age percentiles, 1921t–1922t,
        1925t, 1927t
    weight-for-length percentiles, 1918t–1919t
Celecoxib, 1284t
Celiac disease, 1148f, 1219–1224, 1521–1522
    anemia, 1222–1223
    associated diseases, 1222
    biochemistry, 1223
    clinical manifestations, 1221–1222
    dermatitis herpetiformis, 1222
    with folic acid deficiency, 478
    genetics, 1220
    hematology, 1222–1223
    historical background, 1219
    intestinal biopsy, 1223–1224
    investigations, 1222–1224
    malignancy with, 1222

pathogenesis, 1220–1221
pathology, 1219–1220
prevalence, 1219
radiology, 1223
treatment, 1224
treatment failure, 1224
Cell cycle, 1263–1265
    regulation, 1264f
Cells
    abnormal volume, 152–153
    in human milk, 790t
Cellular antioxidants, 689–692
Cellular function, 754
Cellular model
    of body composition, 755–756
Cellular retinoid binding protein (CRBP),
    351, 355–356
    hepatic metabolism, 359
Cellulose
    sources, 89
Central diabetes insipidus
    treatment, 171t
Central nervous system
    taurine, 557
Cephalic phase responses, 702t
Cereals
    dietary fiber content of, 1965t
    mineral content, 1978t, 1981t
    protein content, 1978t
    vitamins, 1984t
Cerebellar ataxia, 1370
Cerebral beriberi (Wernicke-Korsakoff
    Syndrome), 599
Ceruloplasmin (CP), 252t, 287–288, 608
CETP. *See* Cholesterol ester transfer protein
    (CETP)
Cheese
    dental caries, 1161
Cheese effect, 1547–1548
Chelation, 248, 1769
Chelators
    zinc, 273
Chemesthesis, 695–703, 697
Chemical senses, 695–703, 700–701
    food choice, 701–702
    nutrient utilization, 702
Chemosensory disorders, 698–699
    etiology, 699
    health implications, 699
    manifestations, 698–699
    prevalence, 699
    treatment, 699
Chemosensory function
    assessment, 697–698
    hedonics, 698
    identification, 697
    scaling, 697
    threshold sensitivity, 697
    time intensity, 698
Chemosensory systems, 696–697
CHF. *See* Congestive heart failure (CHF)
Chief cells, 1117
Child development, 868–869
Childhood obesity, 979–988
    activity, 982–983
    alternative therapy, 987–988
    behavioral environment, 982–983
    behavior modification, 987
    cardiovascular consequences, 984
    clinical assessment, 984–985
    clinical effects, 983–985
    consequences of, 983–984
    defined, 979–980
    dietary modification, 985–986
    education, 985

Childhood obesity (*Continued*)
  epidemiology, 980–983
  hepatic abnormalities, 984
  highly restrictive diets, 986
  history, 984–985
  increased activity, 986
  laboratory assessment, 985
  onset, 981
  orthopedic problems, 984
  outcome, 988
  pharmacotherapy, 987
  physical environment, 981–982
  physical examination, 985
  predicting syndrome X, 824
  prevalence, 980–981
  prevention, 988
  reduced inactivity, 986–987
  surgery, 987–988
  syndromes associated with, 983, 983t
  treatment, 985–988
Children, 1745
  acute diarrhea, 992–994
  biotin adequate intake, 505t
  calcium, 206
  with cancer
    malnutrition of, 1291
  caries free, 1157f
  cirrhosis, 297
  cobalamin dietary requirements, 489
  Crohn disease, 994–995
  dietary intake assessment, 877
  disabled
    limb lengths for age of, 1962f–1963f
  EER, 798
  EFAs, 118–119
  energy, 798–801
  energy requirements, 145–146
  epilepsy
    nutritional treatment of, 1378
  HIV, 996
  iodine, 303
  magnesium deficiency treatment, 240
  malnutrition, 1410f
  manganese dietary reference intake values,
    327t
  nutrient needs of, 797–802
  nutritional therapy, 996–997
  phosphorus, 211
  regional enteritis, 994–995
  riboflavin
    dietary reference intake value, 439t
  sulfur amino acids
    RDA, 548
  thiamin
    dietary sources, 427t
  with type 1 diabetes, 1056–1057
  with type 2 diabetes, 1057
  vegetarian diets, 1647–1648
  vitamin A requirements, 354t
  vitamin B6 recommended intakes, 457t
  vitamin D
    dietary reference intake values, 391t
  vitamin E dietary reference intakes, 407t
  vitamin K, 423t
Children's Activity Trial (CATCH), 824
Chile
  iodine excess, 309
China
  beer production, 1777
  obesity rates, 1026
  selenium, 313
  selenium deficiency, 323
  selenium toxicity, 322
Chinese medicine, 1764
Chiropractic nutrition, 1766–1767

Chlorhexidine, 1570
Chloride
  DRI by life-stage group, 1867t
  in enteral feeding products, 1558t
  intrauterine accretion rates during third
    trimester, 809t
  low birth weight intake recommendations,
    810t
  pregnancy, 777
  requirements for, 1857
Chlorpromazine, 1360
Chlorpropamide
  for polyuria, 170–171
Cholecalciferol, 8, 380f. *See also* Vitamin D
  (calciferol)
  cirrhosis, 1245
  and elderly, 846–847
  DRI, 844t
  with hypomagnesemia, 236
Cholecystokinin (CCK), 97–98, 1123t, 1231
  affecting metabolism and food intake,
    1046t
  secretion, 1130
Cholelithiasis
  short bowel syndrome, 1207
Cholestatic liver disease
  vitamin E deficiency, 397–399, 405
Cholesterol, 123–130, 1081
  after menopause, 1081
  atherosclerosis, 124–127
  ATP III classification of, 1896t
  carbohydrate, 129
  dietary fiber, 129–130
  Dietary Guidelines for Americans, 1896,
    1897t
  enriched low-density lipoproteins, 1082
  fat structure, 127
  food content, 1968t–1975t
  high total, 1067–1069, 1068t
  intracellular trafficking, 109–110
  linoleic acid, 127
  low
    genetic causes of, 1071–1072, 1072t
    triglycerides, 1071
  myristic acid, 127
  protein, 128–129
  raising fatty acids, 1080–1081
  requirements for, 1857
  structure of, 130f
  trans unsaturated fat, 127–128
Cholesterolemia
  phytosterols, 130–131
Cholesterol ester transfer protein (CETP),
  103
  deficiency, 1069, 1069t
Choline, 525–534, 603, 1731
  athletes, 1731
  carcinogenesis, 533
  deficiency, 533
    consequences, 531
  developing brain, 531–532
  dietary reference intake values, 526t
  dietary sources, 526
  in food, 527t, 528f
  food content, 1990t
  gene expression, 533
  intestinal absorption, 526–528
  liver injury, 1238–1239
  metabolism, 526–531, 529f
  with methotrexate, 530
  methyl group transfer, 528–530
  neuronal function, 532
  perinatal period, 528
  pregnancy, 777
  tissue distribution, 528

  transformation, 528
  uptake, 528
Choline kinase, 530
Choline phosphotransferase, 530
Chondroitin sulfate
  for osteoarthritis, 1330
Chromatin modifiers, 1285t
  cancer chemoprevention, 1286
Chromium, 332–336, 609. *See also* Minerals
  absorption, 334
  alcoholism, 1253
  bioavailability, 333
  biologic activity, 332
  chemistry, 332
  deficiency, 335, 609
    with diabetes mellitus, 1056
  diet, 332–334
  digestion, 334
  elderly, 851–852
  excretion, 334
  food source, 332–333
  functions, 334–335
  historical introduction, 332
  homeostatic regulation, 334
  intake adequacy, 333–334
  metabolism, 334
  nomenclature, 332
  nutrient-drug interrelationships, 333
  nutrient-nutrient interrelationships, 333
  parenteral nutrition, 1582t, 1583
  pregnancy, 778
  1989 RDA *vs.* 2002 RDI, 819t
  recommended intakes, 335–336
  requirements, 335–336
  sports nutrition, 1732
  sports performance, 1732
  status, 335
  storage, 334
  toxicity, 336, 609
  transport, 334
  1989 *vs.* 2002 RDI, 831t
Chronic disease
  cost, 1599
  management of, 1608–1609
  prevention of, 1608–1609
  team approach, 1598–1606
Chronic energy deficiency, 742–743
Chronic kidney disease (CKD), 1475
  National Kidney Foundation stages of,
    1476t
Chronic liver failure
  protein metabolism, 1237
Chronic liver injury, 1237
Chronic lung disease, 1467
Chronic metabolic acidosis, 165
Chronic obstructive pulmonary disease
  (COPD)
  anabolic steroids, 1469
  body mass index, 1468f
  malnutrition, 1468
  nutrient composition and administration,
    1469–1470
  nutritional supplementation, 1468–1469
Chronic pancreatitis, 1230–1233
  alcohol, 1231
  clinical presentation, 1231
  epidemiology, 1230
  etiology, 1230
  nutrition assessment, 1231–1232
  nutrition management, 1232
  pain management, 1233
  pathophysiology, 1230–1231
  patient monitoring, 1233
Chronic peritoneal dialysis (CPD), 1475
  recommended nutrient intake, 1487t

Chronic renal failure
  acidosis, 1499
  angiotensin converting enzyme inhibitor, 1479
  angiotensin receptor blockers, 1479
  calcitriol, 1498–1499
  dietary management of, 1486–1499
  dietary prescription, 1490
  experimental evidence of, 1478–1479
  human studies in, 1479–1481
  inflammation in, 1485
  metabolic consequences, 1482–1486
  nutritional consequences, 1482–1486
  recommended nutrient intake, 1487t
Chvostek and Trousseau sign
  with magnesium deficiency, 236
Chylomicron, 1135f
  atherosclerotic cardiovascular disease, 1077
  ethanol consumption, 1243
  half life, 358–359
  transport, 358–359
Chylomicronemia, 1087
Chymotrypsin, 1137t
Ciguatera poisoning, 1819–1820
Circulating (visceral) proteins
  assessment of, 837
Circulation
  discovery of, 11
Cirrhosis
  alcoholic
    iron overload, 261
  biliary
    osteoporosis, 1322
  children, 297
  diabetes, 1241
  malabsorption, 1237
  maldigestion, 1237
  protein intake, 1237
Cis-acting
  defined, 617t
Cisapride, 1182
Cisplatin
  carnitine interaction, 542
  with Mg wasting, 233
Citrate
  food drugs, 1734–1735
CKD. *See* Chronic kidney disease (CKD)
CLA. *See* Conjugated linoleic acid (CLA)
Claims
  health, 1834–1835
Cleft lip, 1156
Cleft palate, 1156
Clinical organic acidosis, 166
Clostridium barkeri, 312
Clostridium botulinum, 1817–1818
Clostridium thiaminolyticus, 427
Clozapine, 1360
  associated with weight gain, 1021
  for polyuria, 171
C-myc oncogene, 1260
CNAQ. *See* Mini-Council of Nutrition Appetite Questionnaire (CNAQ)
CoA. *See* Acetylcoenzyme A (CoA) carboxylase (ACC); Coenzyme A (CoA)
Cobalamin. *See* Vitamin B12 (cobalamin)
Cobalamin-folate interrelationship
  intracellular metabolism, 1447
Cocaine, 1360
  pregnancy, 779
Codex Alimentarius, 1836
Coenzyme A (CoA), 27–28, 463f
  cellular metabolism, 464
  metabolism, 464–465
  protein acetylation, 464

protein acylation, 464–465
  synthesis, 464
Coenzyme Q10, 1731
  athletes, 1731
Cognitive function, 1363
  micronutrient deficiencies, 1363–1364
Cohen syndrome, 1021
Cohort studies
  of diet effect on cancer, 1268t
Colchicine
  producing cobalamin malabsorption, 492
Colchicine-nutrient interactions, 1327f
Coley, William, 655
Colipase, 97
Collagen, 25
Colon
  epithelium, 1120
  structure of, 1119–1120
Colon cancer
  calcium, 205
  dietary fat, 1628
  dietary fiber, 88
  folate, 1274
  meat, 1272
  nutritional support of, 1306
  short bowel syndrome, 1202
Colonic irrigation, 1767
Color additives, 1811
Colorectal cancer
  calcium, 1274
  oncogenes, 1260
Colorectal tumorigenesis, 1263f
Colostrum, 1728
Columbinic acid, 115
Comfrey, 1822
Commercial nutrition product
  websites for, 2026
Communicability
  of dietary guidelines, 1677–1678
Communication systems, 1605
Community support, 1605
Complementary feeding, 806–807
Complex carbohydrates
  healthy diet, 1629
Compliance
  defined, 1464t
Conditioned aversions, 713
Conditioned orosensory control
  of meal size, 713
Conditioned orosensory negative feedback, 713
Cones, 362
Congenital aceruloplasminemia, 260
Congenital atransferrinemia, 260
Congenital heart disease, 992
Congestive heart failure (CHF), 1108–1113
  with alcoholism, 1255
  aldosterone, 1109
  aldosterone blocking agent, 1111
  angiotensin, 1109
  antiarrhythmic agents, 1111–1112
  anticoagulant agents, 1112
  clinical recognition, 1109–1110
  defined, 1108–1109
  epidemiology, 1109
  etiology, 1110
  medical therapy, 1111–1112
  nomenclature, 1108–1109
  nutritional deficiencies, 1112–1113
  nutritional management, 1112–1113
  nutritional support in, 1396
  obesity, 1113
  pathophysiology, 1109
  surgery, 1112
  treatment, 1110–1113

Conjugated fatty acids, 677–678
Conjugated linoleic acid (CLA), 127, 677–678, 1727, 1798t
  sports performance, 1727
Conjunctival xerosis, 370
Conroy case, 1616
Constipation
  with enteral feeding, 1564
Consumer awareness, 1656
Consumer protection, 1759–1760
Continuing Survey of Food Intake by Individuals (CSFII), 1688, 1694–1695
Continuing vegetative state, 1615
Continuous arteriovenous hemofiltration (CAVH), 1502
Contract reflex analysis, 1766–1767
Convenience foods
  Engels phenomenon, 866
Cooked vegetables
  nutrient retention in, 1988t
Cookies
  mineral content, 1981t
COPD. *See* Chronic obstructive pulmonary disease (COPD)
Copper, 286–297, 607–608. *See also* Minerals
  absorption, 291
  alcoholism, 1253
  Alzheimer disease, 851
  analysis, 289–290
  bioavailability, 291
  biochemical indices, 292
  biochemistry, 287–288
  bone and teeth, 1321
  cardiac function, 289
  central nervous system, 289
  chemistry, 286–287
  chemosensory function, 700
  cholesterol metabolism, 289
  connective tissue formation, 289
  deficiency, 295, 607, 1458–1459
  dietary consideration, 292–293
  dietary intake, 293–294
  dietary reference intake values, 293t
  dietary requirements, 292–293
  disease, 296–297
  effects on periodontium, 1170t
  elderly, 851
  in enteral feeding products, 1558t
  excretion, 291
  functional tests, 292
  genetic defects in metabolism, 297
  genetic regulation, 290–291
  historical highlights, 286
  homeostatic mechanisms, 291–292
  immune function, 289
  interactions, 294
  iron metabolism, 289
  melanin pigment formation, 289
  metabolism, 290–291, 290f
  migrating from containers, 1816
  molybdenum, 344
  osteoporosis, 1347
  parenteral nutrition, 296, 1582–1583, 1582t
  pregnancy, 778
  1989 RDA *vs.* 2002 RDI, 819t
  source, 293
  status evaluation, 292
  storage, 291
  stress, 296–297
  toxicity, 295–296, 608
  transfer, 291
  transport, 291
  1989 *vs.* 2002 RDI, 831t
Copper-binding proteins, 288

Copper-containing enzymes, 287–288
Copper-containing proteins, 287t
Coprine, 1823
Coprinus atramentarius, 1823
Cori cycle, 70
Cornea, 363
Corn flour poisoning, 1818
Cornstarch supplements
   for fatty acid metabolism defects, 972
Coronary heart disease
   dietary fiber, 87–88
   dietary index, 1633t
   vegetarian diets, 1644–1645, 1649
Cortical bone, 1317
Corticosteroids
   adverse effects of, 1472
Corticosteroids-nutrient interactions, 1327f
Corticotropin-releasing factor (CRF)
   mediating altered metabolism in cancer,
      1295
Cortisol, 645–646
   injury, 1390
Coumarins, 1796t
Courtois, Bernard, 300
Coxsackievirus B3
   selenium, 317
CP. *See* Ceruloplasmin (CP)
CPD. *See* Chronic peritoneal dialysis (CPD)
CPT. *See* Carnitine palmitoyltransferase
   (CPT)
Crackers
   dietary fiber content of, 1965t
   mineral content, 1978t
   protein content, 1978t
   vitamins, 1984t
Craniofacial development, 1155–1157
CRBP. *See* Cellular retinoid binding protein
   (CRBP)
C-reactive protein
   elderly, 853–854
Creatine
   athletes, 1735
   incorporation, 32
   sports nutrition, 1735
   synthesis, 32f
Creatinine, 839t
   synthesis, 32f
Credentials
   dubious, 1756–1757
Cretinism, 606
   endemic, 1364–1365
      historical highlights, 301
      with iodine deficiency, 304
CRF. *See* Corticotropin-releasing factor
   (CRF)
Critical care
   glutamine with, 566
Critical illness
   acute respiratory failure, 1465–1466
   metabolic requirements, 1465–1466
Croatia
   optimal iodine nutrition programs, 309
Crohn disease
   age disease duration, 1216
   breastfeeding, 1210
   enteral nutrition in, 1215–1216
      mechanism of action, 1216
      remission maintenance, 1216
   evidence-based therapeutic actions, 1215
   growth impairment, 1212, 1212t, 1213t
   in infants and children, 994–995
   long term nutritional support, 1216–1217
Crohn Disease Activity Index Score, 1594
Crop failure
   boron, 341

Cruzan case, 1613, 1617
CSFII. *See* Continuing Survey of Food Intake
   by Individuals (CSFII)
Cuban epidemic neuropathy, 1366–1367,
   1366t
Culture
   patient decision making, 1614
Curcumin, 1284t
Cushing syndrome, 1021
Cut-point method, 1663, 1705
14C-xylose breath test, 1149
Cyanidin, 590
Cyanocobalamin
   vs. hydroxocobalamin, 493t
Cyclic adenosine diphosphate, 445f
Cyclic adenosine monophosphate (cAMP), 224
   magnesium, 226
Cyclic compounds, 593
Cyclosporine
   with Mg wasting, 233
Cyproheptadine
   for cancer, 1301t, 1302
Cysteine, 22
   cellular form, 546
   chemistry, 546
   deficiency
      etiology, 557–558
   essential functions, 556–557
   estimated average requirement, 548
   excretion, 550
   glutathione synthesis, 556
   historical introduction, 545
   measurement, 559
   metabolism, 550–554, 554–556, 554f
      pathways, 554–555
   methionine sparing effect
      remethylation *vs.* transsulfuration, 552
   nomenclature, 546
   oxidation, 555–556
   plasma, 547f
   plasma level, 546–547
   protein synthesis, 556
   recommended intake, 547–548
   source, 547t
   toxicity, 559
   transport, 549
Cysteinesulfinate, 555
Cysteinylglycine
   plasma, 547f
Cystic fibrosis, 991–992, 1471
   vitamin E deficiency, 405
Cystine, 8
Cystinosis, 550
Cystinuria, 549
Cytidylyltransferase, 530
Cytochrome c oxidase, 288
Cytochrome P
   dietary factors modifying, 1547t
Cytokine, 655–665, 672t, 1391–1392
   adipose tissue, 640
   brain, 664
   cancer, 665
   carbohydrates, 663
   characteristics, 656–661
   circulating, 662f
   feedback regulation, 664f
   fever, 662–663
   history, 655–656
   human dynamics, 661–662
   hypermetabolic response, 1391t
   immunologic responses, 657f
   induced malnutrition, 742
   with infection, 1402–1403
   inhibitors
      for cancer, 1301t, 1302–1303

   integrated responses, 661–664
   iron, 662–663
   language, 659
   lipids, 663
   mediating metabolic response, 1420
   modulated behavior, 663
   neuroendocrine regulation, 663–664
   proteins, 663
   receptor binding, 659f
   receptor interactions, 657–659
   receptor structure, 658f
   reproductive tract, 664
   rheumatoid arthritis, 665
   septic shock, 665
   signal transduction, 657–659
   soluble receptors, 659–660, 660f
   systems, 660–661
   treatment with, 664
Cytosine
   biosynthesis, 32–33

D

Dacron cuff, 1569
Daidzein
   antagonizing tamoxifen, 592
Daily nutrient intakes
   adjusting, 1663–1775
Daily reference intakes
   for infants, 799t
Daily values (DV), 1829
Dairy products
   breast cancer, 1273
   cancer, 1272–1273
   gluten free foods, 2008t
   mineral content, 1978t, 1981t
   protein content, 1978t
   vitamins, 1984t
DARP. *See* Dissimilatory arsenate-reducing
   prokaryotes (DARP)
DASH. *See* Dietary Approaches to Stop
   Hypertension (DASH)
Data extrapolation, 1669
Dcytb. *See* Duodenal cytochrome b (Dcytb)
Dead-space ventilation
   defined, 1464t
Deafness
   with iodine deficiency, 305
Decision making
   family centered model, 1614
   patient autonomy model, 1614
Defensins, 1140
Deficiency amblyopia, 1370
Dehydration, 1784–1785
   elderly, 1534
   with enteral feeding, 1564
   infantile, 17–19
   types of, 158–159, 159f
Dehydroepiandrosterone (DHEA), 1759
Delayed hypersensitivity reactions, 1521
Deltanoids, 1285
Demeclocycline
   for hyponatremia, 175
Dementia, 1618
Demonstration and evaluation projects, 1605
Dendritic cells, 678–679
Dental caries, 1157–1163
   carbohydrates, 1158–1161
   early childhood, 1163
   factors affecting, 1161–1162
   interacting factors, 1159f
   permanent and primary dentition, 1158f
   sugar, 79
   water fluoridation, 1166f
Dental fluorosis, 1165–1166
Dental medicine, 1152–1175

Dentition
  development of, 1154t
Dentures, 1174
  alveolar process, 1169–1171
Deoxyadenosylcobalamin, 483
Depression
  with cancer, 1296
  with obesity, 1030
Dermatitis herpetiformis
  with celiac disease, 1222
Desaturase
  essential fatty acids, 108f
Descriptive studies
  of diet effect on cancer, 1268t
Desmopressin
  for polyuria, 170
Developing countries
  dietary foods sources, 1719f
Dextrose
  compatibility, 1591t
  Mg, 226
DHEA. *See* Dehydroepiandrosterone
  (DHEA)
DHKS. *See* Diet and Health Knowledge
  Survey (DHKS)
Diabetes
  oral health, 1174–1175
  vegetarian diets, 1645, 1649–1650
Diabetes Control and Complication Trial,
  1050
Diabetes gastroparesis, 1181–1182
Diabetes mellitus, 637, 1043–1064
  acesulfame potassium, 1055t
  alcohol, 1056
  bariatric surgery, 1060
  birth defects, 773
  chemical senses and diet, 703
  classification, 1044–1045, 1044t
  complications, 1048–1050
  diagnosis, 1045–1046, 1045t
  in elderly, 1536
  enteral feeding, 1559–1560
  epidemiology, 1045
  gestational, 781, 1044, 1058
    diagnosis, 1046t
  GLUT, 70–71
  historical overview, 1043–1044
  instructional meal plans, 1063–1064
  magnesium deficiency, 234
  metabolic derangements, 1048
  with nonalcoholic fatty liver disease,
    1244–1245
  nutritional assessment and education, 1063
  nutritional plan, 1051–1056, 1051t
  nutritional recommendations for, 1044t
  nutritional therapy, 1050–1051, 1050t
  nutrition and pharmacotherapy, 1061–1063
  pantothenic acid, 467
  physical activity, 1061
  types of, 1536t
  vitamin B6, 458–459
  weight management, 1059–1061
  zinc, 280
Diabetes Prevention Program, 1029, 1037
Diabetic foods, 1055–1056
Diabetic ketoacidosis (DKA), 1048–1049
Diagnostic tests
  dubious, 1757
Dialysis
  with biotin deficiency, 503
  chemical senses and diet, 703
  inflammation in, 1485
Diamine oxidase, 287
Diaphragm
  anatomy of, 1462–1463

Diarrhea
  with celiac disease, 1221
  with hypomagnesemia, 233
  infantile, 17–19
    early studies of, 17–18
  in infants and children, 992–994
  with malnutrition, 1404–1405
  mortality, 18
  protein-energy malnutrition, 904
  short bowel syndrome, 1204
Diarrhea epidemic, 18
Diarrhetic shellfish poisoning, 1820
Diazein, 1797t
Dicke, W.R., 1219
Dicumarol, 420
  structure, 420f
Diet
  childhood obesity, 982
  composition, 1024
  economics of, 1025
  global trends in, 1717–1722
Diet and Health Knowledge Survey (DHKS),
  1694
Dietary absorption
  short bowel syndrome, 1206f
Dietary adequacy
  standards for assessment, 843–844
Dietary Approaches to Stop Hypertension
  (DASH), 1102–1103, 1376
Dietary assessment
  elderly, 853, 853t
Dietary carbohydrates, 63–64, 65t
  sports performance, 1724–1725
  and sports performance, 1724–1725
Dietary cholesterol, 1081
  with hypercholesterolemia, 1085t
Dietary cysteine
  transport, 549
Dietary diversity, 1707
Dietary fats, 1024
  breast cancer, 1628
  calcium, 202
  cancer risk, 1628
  coronary heart disease incidence, 1627
  digestion of, 97t
  healthy diet, 1627
  hepatic triglycerides, 1243f
  with hypercholesterolemia, 1082–1083
  sport performance, 1725–1727
  type 2 diabetes risk, 1628
  word supply changes in, 1720t
Dietary fiber, 65–66, 83–89
  analytic determination of, 85–86
  blood pressure, 88
  blood triglycerides, 88
  breast cancer, 88
  butyrate, 86
  cancer prevention, 88, 1273–1274
  chemical nature of, 85–86
  cholesterol, 129–130
  defined, 84–85
  dietary reference intake value, 89
  effects on gastrointestinal physiology and
    energy, 86–87
  energy, 87
  food content, 1965t–1967t
  gastrointestinal distress, 88–89
  health benefits, 84–85
  with hypercholesterolemia, 1085t
  Mg, 228
  mineral bioavailability, 89
  overconsumption of, 88–89
  source of, 84
  sources, 89
  1989 *vs.* 2002 RDI, 831t

Dietary guidelines, 1632–1635, 1632t
  actionability, 1678
  adoption and use of, 1678
  approaches, 1674
  assumptions, 1674
  audiences, 1674
  characteristics of, 1674–1675
  clinical trials of, 1681
  communicating and implementing,
    1677–1678
  communication, 1683, 1684
  content, 1684
  criticisms of, 1680–1681
  defined, 1673
  development process, 1675
  evolution from national to international
    realm, 1701–1702
  expert advisory committee of scientists,
    1675
  future challenges, 1683–1684
  generation of, 1679t
  goals, 1673–1674
  government-sponsored, 1674
  and health outcomes, 1680–1681
  implementation strategies, 1678, 1683
  individualized, 1626–1627
  information needed for formulation,
    1675
  international comparison, 1711t–1712t
  national perspectives, 1673–1684
  needed improvements, 1681–1683
  players, 1683–1684
  procedures for use in other countries, 1678
  process, 1683, 1684
  public comment, 1677
  recommendation construction, 1677
  recommendations for improving
    development, 1682t–1683t
  scientific evidence review, 1675–1676
  scientific rationale development,
    1675–1676
  sponsoring agencies, 1677
  staff, 1677
  types of, 1674
  US history, 1678–1680
    balance and moderation, 1678–1679
    evolution of, 1678
    federal guidance harmonization, 1679
    guidance convergence, 1679
    weight and fitness, 1679
  in various editions, 1676t
Dietary Guidelines for Americans, 808
  2005, 1983–1996
Dietary Guidelines Index, 1680
Dietary indices
  validation of, 1634–1635
Dietary intake
  adolescents, 819
Dietary iron
  excess, 268
  intake, 262–263
Dietary lipids
  absorption, 98–99
  digestion and absorption, 96–99
Dietary methionine
  transport, 549
Dietary minerals
  sports nutrition, 1731–1732
Dietary phosphate
  Mg, 228
Dietary phospholipids
  liver, 1243–1244
Dietary protein
  sports performance, 1727–1730
  and sports performance, 1727–1728

Dietary reference intakes (DRI), 797, 830, 843–844, 1660f
  age groups, 1668
  assessing group nutrient intakes, 1855–1856, 1855t
  categories of, 1658–1659, 1660t
  definition, 1853t
  development of, 1658–1668
  elderly, 844t
  for healthy, 1661t
  international development of, 1669–1670
  model, 1659f
  new aspects, 1668–1669
  optimizing health, 830
  organizational framework for, 1659f
  rationale and application, 1655–1670
  recommended changes since 1941, 1656t
  relations, 1854f
  toxicity, 830
  US and Canada
    1997-2004, 1852–1875
  value
    dietary fiber, 89
  without tolerable upper intake levels, 1667
Dietary Reference Values for Food Energy and Nutrients for the United Kingdom, 1874–1876
Dietary salt
  blood pressure, 155–156
  with hypercholesterolemia, 1085t
Dietary sodium
  calcium, 202
Dietary status, 1688
Dietary Supplement Health Education Act (DSHEA), 1772, 1792
Dietary supplements
  arginine, 1728–1729
  athletes, 1728–1730
  carbohydrate metabolites, 1725
  colostrum, 1728
  defined, 1724
  electrolytes, 1733
  fat metabolites, 1726
  food drugs, 1733–1735
  food interactions, 1549, 1549t
  minerals, 1731–1732
  sports drinks, 1733
  sports performance, 1735–1736
  utilization, 1549t
  vitamins, 1730–1731
  water, 1733
  whey protein, 1728
Dietary trends, 1719–1720
Diet essentials
  nutritional classification of, 7–8
Diethylenetriamine pentaacetate
  chelating zinc, 280
Dietitians
  increased educational and practice opportunities, 1604–1605
  as Medicare/Medicaid providers, 1604
  roles of, 1604
Diet pills
  questionable, 1758–1759
Diet plans
  questionable, 1757–1758
Diets
  2000-kcal, 1064t
Differential mRNA display, 622
Digestion, 1182–1184
Digitalis, 1822
Digitalis glycosides
  for congestive heart failure, 1111
Digitalis intoxication, 166

Digoxin
  with enteral feeding, 1565
1,25-dihydroxyvitamin D, 386–387
  assays, 387–388
  cancer prevention, 387
Dinophysis, 1820
Direct amino acid oxidation method, 51
Directives
  problems in adherence to, 1600
Disabled children
  limb lengths for age of, 1962f–1963f
Disaccharidase depletions, 1179–1188
Disaccharides
  deficiency, 1150
  structure, 64f
Disease
  early origins of, 1721
  global trends in, 1717
  metabolic response to, 1381–1382
Dispensable amino acids, 24, 24t
  synthesis, 30–31, 30f
Dissimilatory arsenate-reducing prokaryotes (DARP), 340
Diuretics
  for congestive heart failure, 1111
Divalent metal transporter 1 (DMT1), 251, 252t
DKA. *See* Diabetic ketoacidosis (DKA)
D-lactic acidosis
  short bowel syndrome, 1207
D-limonene, 1800
DLW. *See* Doubly labeled water method (DLW)
DMT1. *See* Divalent metal transporter 1 (DMT1)
DNA array
  analysis, 622–623
  defined, 617t
DNA methylation, 1262–1263
DNA sequence polymorphisms, 628
Docosahexaenoic acid, 1798t
  for arthritis, 1335
Donnan equilibrium, 150
Dopamine beta hydroxylase, 288
Dopamines
  sweet taste, 709
Doping, 1723
Dorsolateral myelopathy
  in Cuban epidemic neuropathy, 1367
Doubly labeled water method (DLW), 15, 140–141
Douglas bag method, 140
Down syndrome, 1021
D-penicillamine-nutrient interactions, 1327f
DRI. *See* Dietary reference intakes (DRI)
Dronabinol, 1535
  for cancer, 1301t, 1302
Drug abuse
  poverty, 869–870
  pregnancy, 869–870
  prevalence, 870–871
Drug-nutrient interactions, 1539–1551
  altering physiologic functions, 1547
  classification of, 1540–1541
  clinical approach to, 1549–1550
  defined, 1540–1541
  diet, 1546
  enzymes, 1546
  ex vivo bioinactivations, 1541–1542
  factors contributing to, 1541f
  gastric acid secretion effect, 1543–1544
  gastrointestinal motility, 1543
  gastrointestinal tract binding and chelation interactions, 1545–1546

gastrointestinal tract enzymes, 1544–1545
  gastrointestinal tract transporter modulation, 1545
  genetics, 1546
  host factors, 1541
  incidence of, 1540, 1540t
  meal intake effect, 1542–1543
  mechanism, 1541–1547
  minimizing, 1542t
  presystemic clearance, 1544
DSHEA. *See* Dietary Supplement Health Education Act (DSHEA)
Dual energy x-ray absorptiometry (DXA), 1323–1324
DuBois, Eugene, 13
Dumas, Jean-Baptist, 12
Dumping syndrome, 1186–1187
Duodenal cytochrome b (Dcytb), 252t
Duodenitis
  with alcoholism, 1248
Duodenum
  anatomy of, 1118
  function of, 1129–1131
Durnin and Womersley formula, 760, 761f
DV. *See* Daily values (DV)
DXA. *See* Dual energy x-ray absorptiometry (DXA)
D-xylose, 1147
  with celiac disease, 1223
D-xylose test, 1146
Dye dilution method, 37, 37f
Dynorphins, 1123t
Dysbetalipoproteinemia, 1070–1071
Dysgeusia, 698–699
  hypothyroid, 700
Dyslipidemia
  with diabetes mellitus, 1058–1059
  drugs altering, 1074t
  metabolic syndrome, 1009–1010
Dysosmia, 698–699
Dysphagia, 878
  food property manipulation in, 878t
  symptoms of, 878t
Dyspnea
  with congestive heart failure, 1109
Dyssebacia, 599

E

EAR. *See* Estimated average requirement (EAR)
Early childhood caries, 1163
Eating
  assessment of, 1031
Eating disorder not otherwise specified (EDNOS), 1354
Eating disorders, 1353–1360
  adolescents, 825–826
  complications, 1356–1357
  developmental factors, 1355
  epidemiology, 1354
  etiology, 1354–1355
  evidence-based treatment, 1357–1358
  family, 1356
  genetics, 1354–1355
  inpatient treatment, 1358
  mass media, 1355
  medications, 1358
  nutritionists, 1358–1359
  outcomes, 1359
  outpatient treatment, 1357–1358
  peers, 1355–1356
  personality, 1355
  physical complications, 1356–1357
  prognosis, 1359

psychologic complications, 1356
   social and developmental complications, 1356
   sociocultural factors, 1355–1356
   treatment, 1357–1358
Ebeling, Albert, 655
Eclampsia
   with hypermagnesemia, 240–241
Edema
   with congestive heart failure, 1109
Edematous hypoalbuminemic malnutrition, 736–737
Edible oils, 1518
EDNOS. *See* Eating disorder not otherwise specified (EDNOS)
EER. *See* Estimated energy requirements (EER)
EFA. *See* Essential fatty acids (EFA)
EFAD. *See* Essential fatty acids deficiency (EFAD)
EGF. *See* Epidermal growth factor (EGF)
Egg protein
   amino acids, 25t
Eicosanoids, 665–668
   biosynthesis of, 112–114
   cyclooxygenase pathway, 666–667
   function, 112–114
   history, 665–666
   lipoxygenase pathway, 668
   syndrome, 666f
   synthesis of, 113f, 666
Eicosapentaenoic acid, 1798t
   for arthritis, 1335
   for cancer, 1301t
Elastase, 1137t
Elbow breadth, 1912t
   tables for, 1909
Elderly, 843–855, 1531–1537
   anthropometric assessment, 854
   current nutritional status, 843–853
   with diabetes mellitus, 1057
   glutamine, 568
   indicators of decline and mortality, 1531–1532
   metabolic diseases, 1536–1537
   minerals, 846–852
   nutritional assessment, 853–855
   nutritional factors increasing risk of poor health outcomes, 852–853
   nutritional needs, 843–853
   nutritional supplements, 852
   physiologic and metabolic factors altering nutrient needs, 846t
   vegetarian diets, 1648
   vitamin D, 389
   vitamins, 846–852
Electrodiagnosis, 1767
Electrogenic glucose-linked sodium transfer, 73
Electrolyte balance
   nonrenal control, 157
Electrolytes, 150, 896–898
   absorption of, 1132–1133, 1133f
   acute renal failure, 1501t
   daily reference intakes
      for infants, 799t
   dietary reference intakes in normal infants and children, 802–803
   extracellular fluids, 151t
   in formulas, 805t
      hydrolyzed and soy, 806t
      infant, 806t
      for term infants, 804t
   intracellular fluids, 151t

loss of, 157–159
   in low birth weight infant formulas, 813t, 814
   malabsorption of, 1145t
   in normal infants and children, 802
   parenteral diet, 1429–1430
   plasma, 150
   pregnancy, 776–777
   recommendations for term infant formulas, 804t
   sports nutrition, 1733
   sports performance, 1732–1733
   tolerable upper intake for normal infants and children, 800t
   UL
      for infants and children, 800t
      weights and measures, 1850
Electron transfer flavoprotein (ETF), 963
Elevated low-density lipoprotein cholesterol
   treatment algorithm for, 1086–1087, 1086t
Ellagic acid, 593
Ellison, Joseph, 1401
Elongase
   essential fatty acids (EFA), 108f
Emesis, 878
Empty calories, 1629
Enamel, 1153
Endemic cretinism, 1364–1365
   historical highlights, 301
   with iodine deficiency, 304
Endemic goiter
   historical highlights, 300–301
Endocrine glands
   arginine, 578
   hormones, 644–649
End-of-life issues, 1612
Endomorphins, 1123t
End stage renal disease
   osteoporosis, 1322
   vitamin B6, 459
Energy
   absorption
      short bowel syndrome, 1205f
   acute renal failure, 1501t, 1503–1504
   adolescents, 818–821
   balance, 138–139, 141f, 1269–1270
      components of, 1017–1018
      obese *vs.* nonobese, 1019
      short bowel syndrome, 1205
   body composition, 22t
   cancer, 1269
   for children
      tolerable upper intake, 800t
      UL, 800t
   chronic renal failure, 1487t, 1491–1492
   for CPD, 1487t
   density, 1024, 1033
   dietary fiber, 87
   dispersive x-rays
      Mg, 231
   DRI by life-stage group, 1859t
   EAR
      UK, 1877t
   endurance, 722f
   estimated requirements for, 1860t
   expenditure, 1017–1018, 1018t
      acquired immunodeficiency syndrome, 1383–1384
      cancer, 1292, 1382–1383
      environmental and behavioral influences, 1023–1024
      high-intensity exercise, 726–727
      injury and sepsis, 1382
      measurement of, 139–141
      organs, 45t

expenditure and requirements
      WHO, 1908t
   in formulas for term infants, 804t
   historical development of, 4
   homeostasis
      signals regulating, 80f
   in human milk, 789t
   imbalance
      consequences of, 1018–1019
   for infants, 798–801
      daily reference intakes, 799t
      tolerable upper intake, 800t
      UL, 800t
   intake, 1017–1018
      environmental and behavioral influences, 1024–1025
      measurement of, 139–141
   intake *vs.* output and stores, 752f
   low birth weight, 812
      infant formulas for, 813t
      intake recommendations, 810t, 811t
   malnutrition
      renal functions, 886–887
   metabolism, 10–15, 733–734
      adaptation to starvation, 741
   for MHD, 1487t
   needs, 136–147
      elderly, 844–845
   phenylketonuria
      pregnancy, 2000t
   physical activity, 1668
   1989 RDA *vs.* 2002 RDI, 819t
   recommended nutrients based on, 1874t
   requirements, 141–142, 1909t
      assessment of, 144–145
   stored in body, 1018
   stores
      body fuel regulation, 1046–1047
   substrates for, 21–22
   for term infant
      recommended formulas, 804t
   utilization, 137f
      1989 *vs.* 2002 RDI, 831t
   yielding macronutrients
      distribution ranges, 1667
Engel curves, 865, 865f
Enkephalins, 1123t
ENS. *See* Enteric nervous system (ENS)
Enteral feeding, 1554–1565
   amino acids, 1559
   for cancer, 1298–1299
   complications, 1563–1564
   contraindications, 1563
   controversial issues, 1563
   with cysteine deficiency, 558
   drugs, 1564–1565
   formulas, 1556–1557
      classification, 1556–1557
      composition, 1557–1558
      defined, 1556
   high-fat low carbohydrate, 1559
   history, 1554–1555
   hydration solutions, 1560
   immune modulating, 1559
   indications, 1562–1563
   infusion, 1563
   modular formulas, 1560
   nutrient absorption and utilization, 1560–1561
   nutrient content, 1558t
   pulmonary issues, 1466
   with taurine deficiency, 558
Enteric nervous system (ENS), 1116
   neurons in, 1124t

Enterochromaffin cells, 1117, 1129
Enteroclysis, 1147
Enterocyte brush border
    glycosidases, 65t
Enterocyte iron transport, 255f
Enterocytes, 1118
    iron metabolism, 255–256
Enteroendocrine cells, 1117, 1118–1119
Enteroglucagon, 1123t
Environment
    learning, 867–868
    nutrition, 867
Environmental illness, 1768
Enzymes
    antioxidants, 692
    chromosomal location, 917t–918t
    in human milk, 790t
Ephedrine (Ephedra), 1758
    food drugs, 1734
    sports nutrition, 1734
Epidermal growth factor (EGF), 652, 1123t
    magnesium, 226
Epigallocatechin, 1797t
Epigenetic
    defined, 617t
Epilepsy
    children
        nutritional treatment of, 1378
Epinephrine
    blood glucose, 72
    cardiovascular response to, 650
Epiphyses, 1316
Eplerenone
    for hypokalemia, 165
Ergosterol, 378
Erythroblasts
    iron metabolism, 256
Erythrocytes
    dysfunction, 218
    Mg content, 232
Erythrocyte transketolase
    activation assay, 430
Erythropoietin, 1476
    for anemia, 1484
Escherichia coli, 415
Esophageal cancer
    folate, 1274
    nutritional support of, 1304–1305
Esophagus, 1179
    anatomy of, 1116–1117
    dietary lipid digestion in, 96
    function of, 1128
Essential amino acids, 24t
    dietary reference intakes in normal infants
        and children, 801t
    for preterm infant formulas, 812t
Essential fatty acids (EFA), 92, 603–605
    childhood, 118–119
    deficiency, 603–604, 604
    desaturase, 108f
    with diabetes mellitus, 1053
    elongase, 108f
    functions of, 110–112
    infancy, 118–119
    nutrient interrelationships, 119
    pregnancy, 118
    requirements, 114–116, 114–120
    sports performance, 1727
    vegetarian diets, 1644
Essential fatty acids deficiency (EFAD),
    92–93
    high risk clinical situations, 119–120
    membrane phospholipids, 111
    symptoms, 115

Essential nutrients, 5t
Esterases, 399
Esterified retinol, 359
Estimated average requirement (EAR),
    1658–1659, 1660f, 1660t, 1663f,
    1853
    definition, 1853t
    for normal infants, 797
    use of, 1662–1663
Estimated energy requirements (EER),
    1658–1659
    adolescents, 819
    dietary reference, 145–146
    equations for, 146t
    in infants and children, 798
    for normal infants, 798–801
Estrogen, 648–649
    with choline deficiency, 531
    controlling meal size, 711
    for hypercholesterolemia, 1086
    for osteoporosis, 1349
ETF. *See* Electron transfer flavoprotein
    (ETF)
Ethacrynic acid
    with Mg wasting, 233
Ethanol
    food drugs, 1734
    sports nutrition, 1734
Ethanol, 716
    absorption, 1248–1249
    coronary protection, 1243
    digestion, 1248–1249
    effect on body weight gain, 1247f
    energy, 137t
    gastrointestinal tract, 1248–1249
    heat equivalents, 137t
    isocaloric substitution of carbohydrate,
        1246, 1246f
Ethanol abuse
    complications, 1242f
Ethanol consumption
    effects, 1240f
    hyperlipidemia, 1243
Ethanol metabolism
    dietary factors, 1253–1254
Ethics
    alternative approaches, 1610
Ethnic foods, 1745–1746
Ethyl alcohol
    food drugs, 1734
    sports nutrition, 1734
Etretinate, 366
Eubacterium, 415
Europe
    obesity rates, 1026
European Community
    nutrient and energy intakes, 1886–1889,
        1887t–1888t
Exchange Lists
    American Diabetes Association, 1055t
Exercise. *See also* Physical activity
    induced food allergy, 1515
    insulin, 649f
    lean tissue conservation, 739
    and long-term weight control, 1035
    osteosclerosis, 1321
    and short-term weight loss, 1035
    target for maintaining weight, 1035–1036
    training
        fat utilization, 1725
        resting energy expenditure, 727
        with weight loss, 727–728
Exocrine pancreatic insufficiency, 1297
Experimental alternatives, 1762

Expert opinion consensus
    for dietary guidelines generation, 1679t
Extracellular fluids
    electrolytes, 151t
    volume and osmolality regulation, 186–187
Extracellular volumes
    regulation of, 149–160, 154–157
Extracts, 1810
Extraordinary, 1612
Extrarenal acidosis
    genesis, 179f
Eye disease
    oxidative stress, 693
Eyes
    nutritional deficiency, 838t
Ezetimibe
    for hypercholesterolemia, 1085

F
FA. *See* Fatty acids (FA)
Factorial method
    protein requirements, 49
FAD. *See* Flavin adenine dinucleotide (FAD)
Fad diagnoses, 1768–1769
Failed adaptation, 739–740
Failure to thrive, 1171
Falls
    fractures, 1342
False morel mushrooms, 1823
Famciclovir
    food interactions, 1542
Familial defective Apolipoprotein B, 1068,
    1068t
Familial hypercholesterolemia, 1068–1069,
    1068t
Familial hypokalemia hypomagnesemia
    syndrome, 234
Familial isolated vitamin E (FIVE)
    with vitamin E deficiency, 404
Familial lecithin cholesterol acyltransferase
    deficiency, 1072
Familial lipoprotein lipase deficiency, 1070
Families
    childhood obesity, 982
    food, 1747
Family dissent
    decision making, 1617–1618
Fanconi syndrome, 179–180
Fast
    defined, 730
Fasting
    whole body adaptation, 46
Fasting chylomicronemia
    genetic causes of, 1070
Fasting hypoglycemia
    with acute liver injury, 1236
Fasting metabolism
    nutritional modification, 734–735
Fasting plasma glucose
    metabolic syndrome, 1007–1008, 1007f,
        1008f
Fasting plasma vitamin C, 515f
Fasting state
    body fuel regulation, 1047–1048
Fat(s). *See also* Dietary fats
    adolescents, 820
    breast cancer, 1269, 1270–1271
    calculation of, 761f
    chemistry, 93–95
    for chronic renal failure, 1487t
    colon cancer, 1271
    for CPD, 1487t
    daily reference intakes
        for infants, 799t

with diabetes mellitus, 1053
dietary considerations, 95–96
Dietary Guidelines for Americans, 1895
digestion, 1184
digestion of, 1134
distribution, 1013–1014
in elderly, 845, 1531–1532
    DRI, 844t
energy, 137t
energy substrate, 21
enteral feeding, 1561
in enteral feeding products, 1558t
in formulas, 805t
    for low birth weight infant, 813, 813t
    for term infant, 804t
    for term infants, 804t
gluten free foods, 2008t
heat equivalents, 137t
in hydrolyzed formulas and soy formulas,
    806t
in infant formulas, 806t
international dietary guidelines, 1711t
interpretation of, 758–760
intrauterine accretion rates during third
    trimester, 809t
liver regulation, 1236
loading, 1726
low birth weight intake recommendations,
    810t, 811t
lung cancer, 1471
malabsorption of, 1145t
measurement of, 758–760, 759
metabolism
    alterations in, 1419–1420
metabolites, 1726–1727
for MHD, 1487t
mineral content, 1978t, 1981t
for normal infants, 798
oxalate, 2015t
oxidation, 722
pantothenic acid, 465
phenylketonuria
    pregnancy, 2000t
pregnancy, 775
prostate cancer, 1271
protein content, 1978t
1989 RDA vs. 2002 RDI, 819t
reference values, 765
structure, 93–95
tolerable upper intake for normal infants
    and children, 800t
triglyceride fatty acid composition, 96t
UL
    for infants and children, 800t
vitamins, 1984t
weight, 1948t
Fat-free body mass
    calculation of, 761f
Fat free mass (FFM), 141, 142, 143, 736
Fat malabsorption syndrome
    vitamin E deficiency, 397–399, 405
Fat-soluble vitamins
    adolescents, 823
    alcoholism, 1249–1250
    cirrhosis, 1245
    in human milk, 789t
    pregnancy, 775
Fat substitutes
    with diabetes mellitus, 1053
Fatal advice, 1759f
Fatty acid metabolism
    defects, 964–969
        diagnosis, 969–971
            energy metabolism, 968

genetics, 971
            ketone bodies, 968
            riboflavin-responsive, 968
            treatment, 972–973
        sudden infant death, 971–972
Fatty acids (FA), 7, 92, 93–94, 677, 1578, 1798t
    biosynthesis of, 107–109
    codes, 94t, 1976t
    conjugated, 677–678
    food content, 1968t–1975t
    formulas, 94t, 1976t
    healthy diet, 1627
    in human milk, 789t
    names, 94t, 1976t
    oxidation
        lipids, 104–105
    requirements, 116–118
    transport hypothesis, 97f
    1989 vs. 2002 RDI, 831t
Fatty liver
    with alcohol consumption, 1242–1243
    with choline deficiency, 531
Favism, 1523–1524
FBDG. See Food-based dietary guidelines
    (FBDG)
FDA. See Food and Drug Administration
    (FDA)
FDAMA. See Food and Drug Administration
    Modernization Act (FDAMA)
Fear, 18
Federal acronyms
    glossary of, 1688t
Federal agencies, 1606
Federal Trade Commission (FTC), 1759
Fed state, 46, 731
    body fuel regulation, 1047
Feeding. See also Infant(s), feeding
    disorders, 876t
        anthropometry, 877–878
        assessment of, 877–879
        behavioral observations, 878–879
        classification of, 876–877
        diagnosis, 876–877
        history, 877
        medical conditions in, 876t
        medications causing, 877t
        physical examination, 877
        treatment, 879–880
    during later childhood, 808–809, 808t
    older infants, 804–807
    optimizing environment for, 876t
    toddlers, 807–808
    tubes, 1555–1556
Femur
    fractures
        osteoporosis, 1341–1342
Fenfluramine (Redux), 987
    adverse effects of, 1472
Fermentation
    dietary fiber, 86
Fermented corn flour poisoning, 1818
Ferritin, 252t
    elevated serum, 268
Ferrochelatase, 252t, 256
Ferroportin 1 (FPN1), 252t
Ferrous sulfate
    for anemia, 5
Ferroxidase II, 288
Ferroxidases, 287–288
Fertility
    lactation impact on, 794
Fertilizers, 1815
Fetal mortality
    iodine deficiency, 304

Fetus
    obesity onset, 981
FEV. See Forced expiratory volume in 1
    second (FEV$_1$)
FFA. See Free fatty acids (FFA)
FFM. See Fat free mass (FFM)
FGF. See Fibroblast growth factors (FGF)
Fiber. See also Dietary fiber
    for chronic renal failure, 1487t, 1494
    copper interactions, 294
    with diabetes mellitus, 1053–1054
    DRI in elderly, 844t
    elderly, 845–846
    enteral feeding, 1562
    in enteral feeding products, 1558t
    for MHD or CPD, 1487t
    1989 RDA vs. 2002 RDI, 819t
    zinc, 273
Fibroblast growth factors (FGF), 652
Fick, Adolf, 4, 720
Finland
    beta carotene, 365
    selenium, 313
Fish
    consumption
        cultural ecology, 1743
        gendered foods, 1744
    eye disease, 1072, 1073t
    household production of, 1707
    mineral content, 1978t, 1981t
    oil supplements
        sports performance, 1727
    protein content, 1978t–1979t
    vitamins, 1984t–1985t
Fitness
    defined, 721
    mortality, 724–725
FIVE. See Familial isolated vitamin E (FIVE)
Five-level model, 757
Flame atomic absorption spectrophotometry,
    328
    deficiency, 329
    toxicity, 329–330
Flame sterilization, 1782
Flatulence
    dietary fiber, 88–89
Flavanols, 1797t
Flavan-3-ols (catechins), 587–588
    absorption, 587–588
    biologic effect, 588
    dietary source, 587
    intake, 587
    metabolism, 587–588
Flavanones, 583, 1796t
    chemistry, 587
    dietary sources, 587
    health effects, 585t
    intakes, 587
Flavin adenine dinucleotide (FAD), 434, 963
Flavobacterium farinofermentans, 1818
Flavones, 583, 584
    health effects, 585t
Flavonoids, 582, 1796t
    analysis, 584
    classes of, 583–584
    health effects, 585t, 586t
    structure, 583f
Flavonols, 583, 1796t, 1801
    absorption, 586–587
    biologic effects, 587
    chemistry, 584–586
    dietary source, 584–586
    health effects, 585t
    intake, 584–586

Flavonols *(Continued)*
  metabolism, 586–587
  phenolic phytochemicals in, 1991t
Flavors, 1810
  fortification, 699
Fluids, 896–898
  absorption of, 1132–1133
  elderly, 846
  with gout, 1328
  loss of, 157–159
  in low birth weight infant formulas, 814
  malabsorption of, 1145t
  short bowel syndrome, 1204–1205
Fluid therapy, 159–160
Fluorescent indicators
  Mg, 231
Fluoride, 608–609. *See also* Minerals
  deficiency, 608
    tooth development, 1155t
  dental caries, 1163–1166
  dietary supplementation, 1165
  osteoporosis, 1347
  pregnancy, 778
  toxicity, 609, 1322
Fluorosis, 609
5-fluorouracil
  with malabsorption, 1297
Fluoxetine
  for eating disorders, 1358
Fluvastatin
  for hypercholesterolemia, 1085t
Fly agaric *(Amanita muscaria)*, 1823
Focus groups, 1746
Folate
  absorption, 1446–1447
  alcohol, 1455
  assay, 471–472
  cancer, 1274
  cellular uptake, 1446–1447
  deficiency, 1444–1445
    diagnosis, 1449–1550, 1449t
    megaloblastic sequelae, 1448t
    nutritional causes of, 1454
    pathogenesis of, 1454
    proliferating cells, 1447
    treatment, 1457
  elderly, 848
  in enteral feeding products, 1558t
  enterohepatic circulation, 1446–1447
  excretion, 1446–1447
  hematologic response to, 1457
  metabolism, 472f
  pathophysiology, 495t
  prophylaxis, 1453t
  retention, 1446–1447
  serum, 1450
  supplements, 1457–1458
  vegetarian diets, 1642
  1989 *vs.* 2002 RDI, 831t
Folate cobalamin interaction, 494–495
Folate-responsive neural tube defects,
    1455–1456
Foliate papillae, 696
Folic acid (pteroylmonoglutamic acid),
    470–480, 602
  absorption, 474
  alcoholism, 1249
  analytic methods, 471–473
  bioavailability, 474
  biochemical structure, 471f
  biochemistry, 470–471
  cobalamin interaction, 479
  deficiency, 475–479, 602, 1374–1375
    clinical features, 476

etiology, 478–479, 478t
    neurologic manifestations of, 1374–1375
    treatment, 479
  dietary considerations, 475
  dietary intake, 475t
  food fortification, 473–474
  historical background, 470
  homocysteine interaction, 479
  iron interaction, 479–480
  malabsorption of, 1145t
  metabolism, 474–475
  nutrition, 473–474
  oral cleft development, 1157t
  preconceptional health, 771–772
  supplements, 473–474
  toxicity, 602
  transport, 474
Folic acid deficiency
  alcoholism, 478
  with alcoholism, 1249
  anticonvulsants, 479
  with inflammatory bowel disease, 1213
Follow-up studies
  of diet effect on cancer, 1268t
Food
  additives, 1809–1825
    categories of, 1810t
  allergens, 1516
  allergy
    defined, 1512–1513
    exercise-induced, 1515
  avoidance, 1518–1520
  chemicals
    disease prevention, 1796t–1798t
  consumption
    ideationist approach, 1743–1744
    materialist approach, 1742–1743
    social and cultural influences on
        research, 1746–1747
    social constructionist approaches, 1744
    social sciences *vs.* nutritional approach
        to, 1741–1742
    theoretic approach, 1742–1746, 1742t
  contaminants, 1813–1814
    classification, 1814t
  cost
    food selection, 865–866
  culture
    food selection, 866
  drugs
    sports nutrition, 1733–1734, 1733–1735
  exchanges
    with diabetes mellitus, 1063–1064
  faddism, 1752
  groups
    Dietary Guidelines for Americans,
        1894–1895
    servings for energy intakes, 808t
  guidelines, 808t
  intake
    controls, 707–718
    regulation of, 1126–1127
    signals regulating, 80f
  intolerance
    defined, 1512–1513
  poisoning
    Bongkrek, 1818
  portions, 1024–1025
  preparation
    posture for, 1327f
  processing, 1777–1787
    air drying, 1785
    biotechnology, 1786–1787
    browning, 1779–1780

chemistry in, 1778–1780
    concentration, 1785
    effects on allergenicity, 1520
    extrusion, 1783
    freeze drying, 1785
    high-pressure, 1786
    historical perspective, 1777
    lipid oxidation, 1778–1779
    moisture control, 1778, 1778f
    new approaches to, 1785–1786
    nutrient damage, 1787, 1787t
    rationale, 1777–1778
  related injury, 1171
  restriction
    failed adaptation, 740
    physiologic responses to, 1619–1620
  safety
    Dietary Guidelines for Americans,
        1895–1896
    international dietary guidelines, 1711t
  spoilage, 1777–1778
  supplements
    promotion of, 1754–1755
  supply
    safety, 1777
  water restriction
    physiologic responses to, 1619–1620
Food(s)
  access to, 1707
  adverse reactions to
    classification of, 1513, 1513t
  antinutrients, 1780t
  bioavailability of, 1704
  cariogenic potential of, 1161
  claims for, 1753–1754
  components categorized by mechanism of
      action, 1793t
  and drugs, 716
  history of, 12–13
  irradiation, 1784
  life history, 1745
  low temperature processing, 1784–1785
  nutrient content of, 1704
  nutritional quality modification, 1707–1708
  potential energy contributions of, 136
  sensory properties, 695
  thermal processing, 1780–1784, 1781t
Food, Drug, and Cosmetic Act of 1938,
    1828–1829
Food and Drug Administration (FDA), 1759
Food and Drug Administration
    Modernization Act (FDAMA),
    1792–1793, 1829
Food and Drug Administration (FDA) Total
    Dietary Study, 227
Food-based dietary diversification, 1705f
Food-based dietary guidelines (FBDG), 1702
  calcium, 1710–1714
  defining, 1702–1703, 1703t
  developing, 1703–1707
  development of, 1708–1710, 1709t
  global, 1714–1715
  variations in national, 1710
  vitamin D, 1710–1714
Food-borne illness, 1777
Foods for Specified Health Use (FOSHU), 1790
Forced expiratory volume in 1 second (FEV_1)
  defined, 1464t
Forced vital capacity (FVC)
  defined, 1464t
Force generation, 723
Formula feeding, 803–804
Formulas. *See also* Infant(s), formulas
  composition of, 993t

nutrient content, 805t
nutrient content of, 805t
for term infants, 804t
FOSHU. *See* Foods for Specified Health Use (FOSHU)
14C-xylose breath test, 1149
Fourth International Study of Infarct Survival (ISIS-4), 237
FPN1. *See* Ferroportin 1 (FPN1)
Fractures
nutritional determinants, 1342–1348
Frame size, 1910t–1911t
tables for, 1909
Framingham Heart Study, 1330
Framingham Osteoarthritis Study, 1330
Frataxin, 252t
Free fatty acids (FFA)
exercise, 1725
in human milk, 790t
oxidation, 1725
transport of, 962
Free galactose
in diet, 953
Free speech
right to, 1828
Freezing, 1784
French botanists, 3
Friedreich ataxia, 258t, 261
Fructose
absorption, 74
with diabetes mellitus, 1055t
health impact, 79–80
liver utilization, 75f
metabolism, 74–76, 633
inborn errors, 75–76
transporter, 68
Fruits
adolescents, 820
cancer, 1273
dietary fiber content of, 1965t–1966t
drying times, 1781t
gluten free foods, 2008t
intake, 1024
international dietary guidelines, 1711t
lung cancer, 1470–1471
mineral content, 1983t
oxalate, 2014t, 2018t–2109t
phenolic phytochemicals in, 1992t
vitamins, 1986t
Frying, 1783–1784
FTC. *See* Federal Trade Commission (FTC)
Fumonisins, 1819
Functional assessment, 842
Functional fiber
defined, 85
Functional foods
designing, 1789–1805, 1803–1805
physiologically active compounds, 1795–1803
regulatory issues, 1791–1792
safety, 1793–1794
scientific agreement standards, 1793
US market, 1794–1795
Functional genomics
defined, 617t
Functional oral nutrition risk evaluation, 1168t
Fungicides, 1815
Fungiform papillae, 696
vitamin B, 700
Funk, Casimir, 6–7
Furosemide
with Mg wasting, 233

Fusarium, 1818, 1819
FVC. *See* Forced vital capacity (FVC)

G

Gait ataxia, 432
Galactose, 950–954
biochemistry, 950–951
cataracts, 74
in food and drugs, 953
metabolism, 74
restricted diet, 2007
transport, 74
Galactose metabolism
metabolic blocks, 950f
Galactosemia, 950–951, 1242
diagnosis, 952
diet termination, 954
formulas, 952–953
nutrient requirements, 952
nutrition support, 953–954
screening, 951–952
treatment, 952
Galactosyl transferase
with Mn, 326
Gallstones
with parenteral nutrition, 1589
GALT. *See* Gut-associated lymphoid tissue (GALT)
Gambierdiscus toxicus, 1819
Gamma-glutamylcysteine
plasma, 547f
Gamma tocopherol
health benefits, 408
structure, 398f
Garlic, 1768
Gas exchange
pioneers of, 11
Gastric accommodation, 1180
Gastric acid secretion, 1129–1130, 1130t
Gastric bypass, 1039–1040
Gastric cancer
nutritional support of, 1305
Gastric cells
secretory products, 1129f
Gastric emptying, 1128, 1181
alcohol, 1181
disorders of, 1181–1182
short bowel syndrome, 1201–1202
surgery, 1185–1186
Gastric fistula
sham feeding, 708f
Gastric gland, 1183f
Gastric hypersecretion
short bowel syndrome, 1204, 1207
Gastric inhibitory peptide (GIP)
affecting metabolism and food intake, 1046t
Gastric lipase, 1183
vs. pancreatic lipase, 1184
Gastric motility, 1179–1182
after meal, 1179–1182
during fasting, 1180–1181
Gastric secretion, 1182–1184
Gastric surgery, 1185–1186
Gastrin, 1123t, 1183, 1184
Gastrin cells, 1129
Gastritis
with alcoholism, 1248
Gastroesophageal disease
diet in, 1184–1185
Gastroesophageal reflux
oral health, 1173–1174
symptoms of, 879t
Gastroesophageal reflux disease (GERD)
diet in, 1184–1185

Gastrointestinal disorders
pediatric, 992
Gastrointestinal tract
arginine, 578
communication mediate responses, 1125f
enteric nervous system, 1121–1125
hormones, 1123t, 1125–1126
hypercatabolic state, 1393
immune system, 1140–1141
motility, 1121–1125
nutritional review of, 837t
during pregnancy, 773
structure of, 1115–1120
vasculature, 1120–1121
wall, 1116f
Gastrostomy, 1555–1556
Ga tribe, 881
GDM. *See* Gestational diabetes mellitus (GDM)
Gee, Samuel, 1219
Gemfibrozil, 1009
Gendered foods, 1744
Gene expression
nursing, 616f
nutritional regulation, 615–626, 618f
terminology, 617t
Gene knockout (null mutation) animals, 625
Gene polymorphism detection, 619
Generalized seizures
with magnesium deficiency, 236
Generally recognized as safe (GRAS), 1810
General surgical patients
nutritional screening, 1417–1418
Genes
adaptive
identification of, 634
nutrient regulation, 616
Genestein, 1797t
Genetics
defects, 8
disease management, 913–916
disorders
benefited by nutrition support, 910–913
nutrition treatment of, 911t–913t
drift, 629
modification, 1708
osteoporotic fractures, 1348
polymorphisms
affecting recommended nutrient intakes, 1714t
variation, 627–631
functional consequences of, 631–632
and gene expression, 631
nutrient metabolism and utilization, 632–633, 632t
origin of, 628–630
prevalence of, 627–628
and protein function, 631–632
Genistein, 1802
antagonizing tamoxifen, 592
Genomic organization and regulation, 615–616
Genomics
defined, 617t
Genotoxic xenobiotics, 628
GERD. *See* Gastroesophageal reflux disease (GERD)
Germany
REE prediction equations, 1903–1904
Gerson diet, 1770
Gestational diabetes mellitus (GDM), 781, 1044, 1058
diagnosis, 1046t
Gestational hypertension
with iodine deficiency, 305

GFR. *See* Glomerular filtration rate (GFR)
Ghrelin, 638, 1123t
  affecting metabolism and food intake, 1046t
  for cancer, 1301t
  elderly, 1533
Giardia lamblia
  with malabsorption, 1144, 1149
Ginseng
  athletes, 1736
  sports nutrition, 1736
GIP. *See* Gastric inhibitory peptide (GIP)
Gitelman syndrome, 234
Gliadin
  celiac disease, 1221
Glimepiride, 1062t
Glipizide, 1062t
Glomerular filtration rate (GFR), 1475,
    1490–1491
Glossitis
  with cobalamin deficiency, 490
Glossopharyngeal nerve, 696
GLP. *See* Glucagon like peptide (GLP)
GLP-1. *See* Glucagon like peptide-1 (GLP-1)
GLP-2. *See* Glucagon like peptide-2 (GLP-2)
Glucagon, 640
  affecting metabolism and food intake,
    1046t
  injury, 1390–1391
  magnesium absorption, 229
  secretion, 71–72
Glucagon like peptide (GLP), 1123t, 1203
Glucagon like peptide-1 (GLP-1), 637
  affecting metabolism and food intake,
    1046t
Glucagon like peptide-2 (GLP-2)
  short bowel syndrome, 1207
Glucerna, 1559
Glucoamylase, 1189, 1190t
Glucocorticoids
  blood glucose, 72
  medications
    osteoporotic fractures, 1348–1349
Gluconeogenesis
  vitamin B6, 455
Glucosamine
  for osteoarthritis, 1330
Glucose, 637
  alterations, 1420
  influence via insulin, 71t
  intolerance
    dietary fiber, 87
  liver utilization, 75f
  metabolism, 1572
    acquired immunodeficiency syndrome
      (AIDS), 1387
    cancer, 1386–1387
    injury and sepsis, 1386
  parenteral diet, 1428
  storage, 76–77
  tolerance
    cirrhosis, 1237
Glucose-dependent insulinotropic
    polypeptide. *See* Gastric inhibitory
    peptide (GIP)
Glucose-galactose malabsorption, 73
Glucose-6-phosphate dehydrogenase
    deficiency, 521
Glucose transporter (GLUT), 66–69, 1136
  family, 66t
  knockout mice, 69
  transgenic mice, 69
Glucose transporter 1 (GLUT 1), 67
  diagram, 67f
Glucose transporter 2 (GLUT 2), 68

Glucose transporter 3 (GLUT 3), 68
Glucose transporter 4 (GLUT 4), 68
  gene overexpression, 624f
Glucose transporter 5 (GLUT 5), 68
Glucosinolates, 593
Glucosuria
  Mg wasting, 233
GLUT. *See* Glucose transporter (GLUT)
Glutamate
  Alzheimer disease, 32
  amyotrophic lateral sclerosis, 32
  flux, 41
  neurodegenerative disease, 32
  synthesis, 30–31, 31
Glutamic acid, 1579–1580
Glutamine, 563–568, 1579–1580
  absorption, 563–564
  analytic methods, 563
  bioavailability, 563–564
  biochemistry, 563
  biosynthesis, 563
  chemical structure, 564f
  chemistry, 563
  with chemotherapy, 567
  deficiency, 564–565
  dietary requirements, 565
  digestion, 563–564
  enteral feeding, 1561
  excretion, 563–564
  flux, 41
  genetics, 563
  interorgan transport, 42
  metabolism, 564, 564f
  needs in disease, 56
  nutrient interaction, 568
  replacement therapy, 565–566
  safety, 568
  sports nutrition, 1729
  synthesis, 1419f
  therapeutic use, 566–567
  transport, 564
Glutamine supplementation
  with cancer, 1307
Glutamylcysteine
  plasma, 547f
Glutaric acidemia, 910
Glutaric acidemia type I, 945–946, 1997t
  sample diet for, 2005t
Glutathione
  plasma, 547f
  protein sulfhydryl redox cycle, 690–691
  structure, 690f
Glutathione peroxidase, 312
Gluten
  celiac disease, 1220, 1221
  dietary avoidance of, 1224
  mucosal changes, 1221
Gluten free drug information
  sources of, 2012
Gluten free foods, 1522, 2008–2103
  medications, 2011t
  questionable ingredients, 2010t
Gluten free pharmaceutical excipients, 2012
Glyburide, 1062t
Glycemic index, 78–79, 86
  diets based on, 1034
  of starchy foods, 1052t
Glycemic load, 78
Glycemic response
  with diabetes mellitus, 1051–1052
  dietary fiber, 87–88
Glycerol
  athletes, 1735
  sports nutrition, 1735

Glycerolipid
  synthesis, 1243
Glycine, 25, 30
  end-product approach, 37
  synthesis, 31
Glycogen, 1048
  breakdown, 76
  dietary manipulation of stores, 77
  formation, 76
  glucose storage, 76–77
  storage diseases, 76–77
  structure, 76f
Glycogenolysis
  vitamin B6, 455
Glycolysis, 721
Glycoproteins
  mediating altered metabolism in cancer,
    1293–1294
Goats
  household production of, 1707
Goblet cells, 1118–1119
Goiter, 606
  endemic
    historical highlights, 300–301
    iodine deficiency, 305
Goitrogens, 306
Gout
  alcohol, 1328
  defined, 1327
  dietary therapy, 1328–1329
  metabolic profile, 1328
Grains
  dietary fiber content of, 1965t
  gluten free foods, 2008t, 2009t
  international dietary guidelines, 1711t
Granulocytopenia
  with alcoholism, 1255
Grapefruit juice
  drug interaction, 587
  drugs with increased oral absorption, 1545t
  type IIA interactions, 1544
GRAS. *See* Generally recognized as safe
    (GRAS)
Grasbeck-Immerslund syndrome, 602
Graves disease
  with iodine excess, 306–307
Greater superficial petrosal nerve, 696
Green tea, 1801
Griseofulvin
  with fatty meal, 1542
Group interviews, 1746
Growth
  energy requirements, 144
  factors, 636–653
    adipose tissue, 640
  folate deficiency, 1454
  growth hormone effects on, 647f
  impairment
    nutrient deficiencies, 1213
    nutritional treatment of, 1214–1215
    pathophysiology, 1212–1213
  rates, 1269–1270
Growth hormone
  blood glucose, 72
  for cancer, 1301t
  composition of, 646–647
  for COPD, 1469
  deficiency, 1021
  short bowel syndrome, 1207
  for weight loss, 1535
Guanine
  biosynthesis, 32–33
Guinea pigs
  household production of, 1707

Gun puffing, 1783
Gustation, 696–697
Gut
    hormones
        affecting metabolism and food intake,
            1046t
    in host defense, 1424–1425
    as metabolic organ, 47–48
Gut-associated lymphoid tissue (GALT),
    1140, 1141f
Gymnodinium breve, 1820
Gynecologic cancer
    nutritional support of, 1306
Gyromitra esculenta, 1823
Gyromitrin, 1823

H
Haber-Weiss reaction, 686
Hair
    nutritional deficiency, 838t
Hallevorden-Spatz syndrome, 603, 1375
Haplotypes, 630
Haptocorrin, 488, 1127–1128
Harris-Benedict equation, 14, 1232, 1420–1421
Hartnup syndrome, 47, 448–449
Harvey, William, 11
Hashimoto disease
    with iodine excess, 306–307
HDL. *See* High density lipoproteins (HDL)
HDN. *See* Hemolytic disease of newborn
    (HDN)
Head and neck cancer
    nutritional support of, 1304
Health
    global trends in, 1717
Health Assessment Questionnaire, 1335
Health care
    costs
        difficulties meeting, 1600
    expenditures, 1599
    professionals
        conscience, 1612
        professional judgment, 1612
Health claims, 1834–1835, 1834t, 1835t
Health fraud, 1752
Health Professionals Follow-up Study, 1271
Healthy diet, 1625–1635
    alcohol, 1630
    calcium, 1630
    carbohydrates, 1628–1629
    dairy products, 1630
    formulating, 1627–1629
    fruits, 1629
    graphic representation of, 1633f
    indices representation of, 1633t
    processed meats, 1630
    protein, 1629
    quantity *vs.* quality, 1626
    salt, 1630
    validation, 1632–1635
    vegetables, 1629
    vitamin supplements, 1630–1631
Healthy eating index (HEI), 1633–1634,
    1633t, 1634t, 1680
Healthy foods
    availability of, 1721
    cost of, 1721
Healthy People 2010
    maternal and infant health, 772t
Healthy vegetarian lifestyle
    dietary guidelines for, 1650–1651
    dietary recommendations, 1650
    food guides, 1650–1651
    nutrition counseling, 1651–1652

Heart
    alcoholism, 1255
Heart disease
    congenital, 992
    dietary fiber, 87–88
    vitamin E, 408
Heart rate monitoring, 140–141
Heat
    history of, 12–13
HEI. *See* Healthy eating index (HEI)
Height
    changes with age, 1930f–1931f
    measurement of, 758
Height-weight
    age, 1913t
    tables for, 1909
Helicobacter pylori
    with iron deficiency, 268
    vitamin C, 520
Helsinki Heart Study, 1009
Hematologic diseases, 1436–1459
Hematologic system
    arginine, 578
Hematopoiesis, 670–671
Heme
    biosynthesis inhibition of, 915f
Heme biosynthesis
    vitamin B6, 455
Hemochromatosis, 260, 607
    juvenile, 258t
Hemolytic disease of newborn (HDN), 598
Hemorrhagic disease of newborn, 421
Hemosiderin, 252t
Hemostasis
    plasma proteins, 415–416
Hepatic alpha tocopherol transfer protein, 401
Hepatic coma, 1237
Hepatic dysfunction
    with cysteine deficiency, 558
    nutritional support in, 1396
    with parenteral nutrition, 1588–1589
    with taurine deficiency, 558
Hepatic encephalopathy, 1237
    amino acids, 1237–1238
    dietary treatment of, 1376–1377
    protein, 1237–1238
Hepatic gluconeogenesis, 731
Hepatic lipase, 1071
Hepatic lipase polymorphism, 1069, 1069t
Hepatic metabolism
    vitamin A, 359–362
Hepatolenticular degeneration, 297, 608
    copper, 1245
Hepcidin, 252t
Hephaestin, 252t
Herbalism, 1767–1768
Herbals, 1767–1768
    athletes, 1736
    sports nutrition, 1736
Herbicides, 1815
Hereditary
    nutrition, 867
Hereditary ataxias, 261
Hereditary fructose intolerance (HFI), 633
Hereditary hemochromatosis, 258–259
Hereditary (HLA-linked) hemochromatosis,
    258t
Hereditary sideroblastic anemia, 260
Hesperetin, 1796t
Hexachlorobenzene, 1815
Hexitols, 1811
Hexokinase, 1048
HFE protein
    mutations in, 259f

HFI. *See* Hereditary fructose intolerance
    (HFI)
hGH, human growth hormone (hGH)
High branched-chain amino acid formulas,
    1557–1558
High carbohydrate, high fiber exchange list,
    1054t
High density lipoprotein cholesterol
    genetic causes of, 1069t
High density lipoproteins (HDL), 103
    atherosclerotic cardiovascular disease, 1077
    ethanol consumption, 1243
    healthy diet, 1627
    tocopherols, 402
Highly selective vagotomy, 1186
High-pressure processing (HPP), 1786
High protein, low carbohydrate diet,
    1757–1758
High-risk patient, 837t
Hill, A.V., 721
Hippocrates, 507
Hippocratic tradition, 1609
Histamine, 1123t, 1183
Histamine poisoning, 1525–1527
    diagnosis of, 1525–1526
    preventive measures, 1527
    sources of, 1526
    symptoms of, 1525
    toxicology of, 1526
    treatment of, 1525–1526
Histidine, 52–53
HIV. *See* Human immunodeficiency virus
    (HIV)
HMB. *See* Hydroxy beta methylbutyrate
    (HMB)
HMG. *See* Hydroxy beta methylglutaryl
    (HMG)
Holotranscobalamin II, 485–486
Home enteral nutrition, 1564
    for cancer, 1299
Home parenteral nutrition, 1001–1002,
    1591–1593
    cost, 1593
Home total parenteral nutrition
    for cancer, 1300
Homocysteine, 30, 473, 848
    cellular form, 546
    chemistry, 546
    cobalamin, 485, 495
    dementia, 1375
    excretion, 550
    historical introduction, 545
    metabolism, 550–554
    needs in disease, 56
    nomenclature, 546
    plasma, 547f
    plasma level, 546–547
    stroke, 1375
    toxicity, 559
    transsulfuration, 551
Homocysteine methionine
    metabolism, 472f
Homocystinuria
    aromatic amino acids for, 1996t
    betaine, 930
    carrier state, 932
    diagnosis, 930
    dietary management, 554
    identification, 545
    metabolic bases, 553–554
    metabolic pathways, 929f
    nutrient requirements, 930–931
    nutrition support, 931–932
    reproductive performance, 932

Homocystinuria *(Continued)*
  sample diets for, 2001t
  screening, 929–930
  serving lists, 931
  treatment, 930
Homolog
  defined, 617t
Hooke, Robert, 11
Hookworm infection
  with malnutrition, 1405
Hormones, 636–653
  body fuel regulation, 1046
  for cancer, 1301, 1301t
  nutrient storage, 637t
Hospice, 1619
Hospitalists, 1600–1601
Host defenses
  malnutrition, 1465
Household production of small animals, 1707
HPP. *See* High-pressure processing (HPP)
Human dentition
  development of, 1154t
Human energy metabolism, 10–15
Human genetic polymorphisms
  affecting recommended nutrient intakes,
    1714t
Human genetic variation, 627–631
  origin of, 628–630
  prevalence of, 627–628
Human growth hormone (hGH)
  injury, 1431–1432
Human immunodeficiency virus
  infant, 996
Human immunodeficiency virus (HIV)
  with breastfeeding, 803
  chemical senses and diet, 703
  infant
    lactation impact on, 792
  in infants and children, 996
  lipodystrophy
    drugs altering, 1074t
  with malnutrition, 1405–1406
  oral infections, 1172
  SREBP, 1074
Human milk, 803
  bioactive components of, 790–791, 790t
  composition of, 786–787, 788t
    values of, 789t
  nutritional factors, 787–788
Human Nutrition Information Service, 1693
Humerus
  in tennis players *vs.* nonathletic controls,
    1319f
Hungry bone syndrome, 234
24-h urinary creatinine, 839t
24-h urinary urea nitrogen, 839t
Hyaluronan (hyaluronic acid), 150
  hydroxyl radicals, 688f
Hydration
  elderly, 846
  withdrawal of
    symptom management in, 1620t
Hydrazine sulfate
  for cancer, 1301t, 1302
Hydrogen peroxide, 686
Hydrolyzed formulas
  nutrient content, 806t
  nutrition, 806t
Hydroxy beta methylbutyrate (HMB),
    1729–1730
Hydroxy beta methylglutaryl (HMG)
  coenzyme, 123
Hydroxycitrate
  athletes, 1736
  sports nutrition, 1736

Hydroxyl radicals, 687f
Hydroxylysine, 25
3-hydroxy-3-methylglutaric aciduria, 941
  tandem mass spectrometry, 942t
3-hydroxy-3-methylglutaryl-coenzyme A
    reductase inhibitors
  for hypercholesterolemia, 1085
Hydroxyproline, 25
25-hydroxyvitamin D
  alternative metabolism, 384–385
  assays, 387
  to 1,25-dihydroxyvitamin D, 384
Hyperammonemia, 947
Hypercalcemia, 208, 604
  with diabetes mellitus, 1048–1049
  Mg wasting, 233
Hypercarotenosis, 596–599
Hypercatabolic response
  mediators of, 1389–1393
Hypercatabolic state, 1381–1396
  systemic and organ reactions, 1393–1394
Hypercholesterolemia, 1077–1088
  with aging, 1080
  alcohol, 1085t
  atorvastatin, 1085t
  dietary prevention of, 1078–1079
  drug therapy, 1084–1086
  etiology, 1077–1078
  lifestyle therapies, 1082–1083, 1085t
  maximal therapeutic lifestyle changes, 1084
  mild, 1079–1080
    genetic contribution to, 1079–1080
Hyperferritinemia, 258t, 261
Hyperglycemia, 1242
  carbohydrates, 1272
  with enteral feeding, 1564
  serum sodium, 152
Hyperhomocysteinemia
  metabolic bases, 553–554
  with vascular disease, 553
Hyperinsulinemia
  carbohydrates, 1272
Hyperkalemia, 166–167, 605
  clinical manifestations, 166–167
  with enteral feeding, 1564
  etiology, 166t
  treatment, 167, 167t
Hyperlipemia
  alcohol ingestion, 1243
  with childhood obesity, 984
Hyperlipidemia
  with alcohol consumption, 1242–1243
  alcoholic, 1243
Hypermagnesemia, 240–242, 606
  clinical presentations, 241–242
  with enteral feeding, 1564
  etiology, 240–241
  toxic effects, 241f
  treatment, 242
Hypermetabolic states
  physiologic characteristics of, 834, 834f
Hypernatremia, 175–176
  brain and muscle volume changes, 154f
  etiology, 175–176, 175t
  pathogenesis, 175–176
  treatment, 176
Hypernatremic dehydration, 18–19
  diet, 19
  epidemiology, 19
  insensible water loss, 18
  renal function, 18
Hyperosmolality
  signs, 153
Hyperparathyroidism
  elderly, 389

Hyperphagia
  genetics of, 715–716
Hyperphosphatemia, 220–221
  with enteral feeding, 1564
  treatment, 221
Hypertension
  alcohol, 1101
  arginine, 578
  calcium, 1099–2000
  carbohydrates, 1102
  chemical senses and diet, 703
  diet, 1102–1103
  gestational
    with iodine deficiency, 305
  insulin resistance, 1098–1099
  lipids, 1101–1102
  magnesium, 1100–1101
  with magnesium deficiency, 237–238
  obesity, 1098
  potassium, 1099
  prevention of, 1103
  protein, 1102
  public health implications, 1103–1105
  sodium chloride, 1095–1098
  treatment, 1103
  vegetarian diets, 1645, 1649
Hypertonic dehydration, 158
Hypertonic solution, 152
Hypertriglyceridemia
  carbohydrates, 1272
  with diabetes mellitus, 1059
  without chylomicrons
    genetic causes of, 1070–1071
Hyperuricemia, 1327–1328, 1478t
Hyperuricosuria, 521
Hypervitaminosis A, 596
Hypervitaminosis D, 597–598
Hypoalbuminemia
  starvation, 740
Hypoalbuminemic malnutrition, 833
Hypoalbuminemic stress syndrome, 833
Hypobetalipoproteinemia, 1072
  genetic defects, 405
Hypocalcemia, 604
  with hypomagnesemia, 235
Hypochromic anemia, 607
Hypogeusia, 608, 698–699, 700
  aging, 1174
  iron deficiency anemia, 700
Hypoglycemia, 1242, 1768
  with diabetes mellitus, 1048–1049
Hypokalemia, 164–166
  aldosterone antagonists, 165
  amiloride, 165
  clinical manifestations, 165
  etiology, 164t
  with hypomagnesemia, 236
  treatment, 165–166
Hypolactasia, 1190–1192
  etiology, 1192t
Hypomagnesemia, 234
  cardiac dysrhythmias, 236–237
  chronic latent, 237–239
  clinical presentation, 234–239
  diabetes mellitus, 234
  diagnosis, 232f
  etiology, 233t
  gastrointestinal disorders, 233
  laboratory animals, 234
  manifestations, 235t
  moderate to severe, 235–237
  neuromuscular manifestations, 236
  prevalence, 233–234
  renal disorders, 233–234
  treatment, 239–240

Hypometabolic states
  physiologic characteristics of, 834, 834f
Hyponatremia, 171–175
  brain and muscle volume changes, 153f
  diagnosis, 173
  differential diagnosis, 174f
  elderly, 846
  etiology, 171–173
  with normal effective osmolality, 171t
  pathogenesis, 171–173, 172f, 172t
  treatment, 173–175
Hypoosmolality
  signs, 152–153
Hypophosphatemia, 213–214, 604–605, 834–835
  effect of, 215–216
  erythrocyte dysfunction, 218
  etiology, 213t
  leukocyte dysfunction, 218–219
  metabolic acidosis, 219
  nervous system dysfunction, 219–220
  with phosphorus deficiency, 213t, 214–215
  platelet disorders, 219
  treatment, 220
  without phosphorus deficiency, 213–214, 213t
Hypophosphatemic cardiomyopathy, 217
Hyporeninemic hypoaldosteronism, 166, 187
Hyposmia, 698–699
Hypothalamic disorders
  causing obesity, 1021
Hypothyroidism, 304
  causing obesity, 1021
  iodine deficiency, 305
  with iodine excess, 306
Hypotonic dehydration, 158–159
Hypotonic solution, 152

I

IBNMRR. *See* Interagency Board for Nutrition Monitoring and Related Research (IBNMRR)
IBW. *See* Ideal body weight (IBW)
ICP. *See* Inductively coupled plasma (ICP)
IDD. *See* Iron deficiency disorder (IDD)
IDDM. *See* Insulin-dependent diabetes mellitus (IDDM)
Ideal body weight (IBW), 1465
Idiopathic intracranial hypertension
  nutritional treatment of, 1378
IDL. *See* Intermediate density lipoproteins (IDL)
IFN gamma. *See* Interferon gamma (IFN gamma)
Ifosfamide
  carnitine interaction, 542–543
IgA. *See* Immunoglobulin A (IgA) antibodies
IGF-1. *See* Insulin like growth factor-I (IGF-I)
IL1. *See* Interleukin 1 (IL1)
IL6. *See* Interleukin 6 (IL6)
Ileal resection
  short bowel syndrome, 1204
Ileum
  anatomy of, 1118
  short bowel syndrome, 1202
Imipramine, 1360
Immaturity
  with cysteine deficiency, 557–558
  with taurine deficiency, 557–558
Immune function
  vitamin B6, 455
Immune response
  effector mechanism, 661f
Immune system, 670, 1140–1141
  arginine, 579
  development of, 670–671

Immunity
  adaptive, 674–675, 679–680
  innate, 674–675, 677–678
Immunoblotting, 623–624
Immunocytochemistry, 624
Immunoglobulin A (IgA) antibodies
  celiac disease, 1221
Immunoglobulin E-mediated food allergy, 1512–1521, 1513f
  diagnosis of, 1517–1518
  minimal eliciting dose, 1519–1520
  persistence of, 1516
  prevalence of, 1516
  prevention of, 1516–1517
  sources of, 1515–1516
  symptoms of, 1514–1515, 1514t
  treatment of, 1518–1519
Immunohistochemistry, 624
Immunologic function
  glutamine effect on, 568
Inactivity
  childhood obesity, 983
Inborn errors of metabolism
  medical foods for, 1995t–1998t
  with neurologic manifestations, 1377t
Incomes
  leanness, 864f
Incompetent patient
  nutrition support of, 1614–1620
Incretins, 637–638
India
  optimal iodine nutrition programs, 309
Indian child cirrhosis, 608
Indicator amino acid oxidation method, 51–52
Indirect calorimetry, 1421
Indispensable amino acids, 24t
Indoles, 593, 1798t
Inductively coupled plasma (ICP)
  arsenic
    atomic emission spectrometry, 339
    mass spectrometry, 339
Industrial chemicals, 1816–1817
Infant(s)
  acute diarrhea, 992–994
  biotin adequate intake, 505t
  brain development
    lactation impact on, 791–792
  calcium, 206
  Crohn disease, 994–995
  daily reference intakes, 799t
  EER, 798
  EFAs, 118–119
  energy, 798–801
  energy requirements, 145–146
  feeding, 803–804
  formulas
    vs. bovine milk, 805–806
    misformulation of, 1813
  human immunodeficiency virus, 996
    lactation impact on, 792
  magnesium deficiency treatment, 240
  manganese dietary reference intake values, 327t
  morbidity
    lactation impact on, 793
  mortality
    iodine deficiency, 304
  normal
    daily reference intakes for, 799t
  nutrient needs of, 797–802
  nutritional therapy, 996–997
  obesity
    lactation impact on, 792
  older
    feeding, 804–807

  premature, 8
  reference values
    new approaches to, 1668–1669
  regional enteritis, 994–995
  riboflavin
    dietary reference intake value, 439t
  sulfur amino acids
    RDA, 548
  thiamin
    dietary sources, 427t
  vegetarian diets, 1647
  vitamin A requirements, 354t
  vitamin B6 recommended intakes, 457t
  vitamin D
    dietary reference intake values, 391t
  vitamin E dietary reference intakes, 407t
  vitamin K, 423t
Infantile beriberi, 599
Infantile dehydration, 17–19
Infantile diarrhea, 17–19
  early studies of, 17–18
Infantile scurvy (Barlow disease), 603
Infection, 1401–1410
  historical overview, 1401–1402
  zinc, 280
Inflammation
  anatomic localization of, 1215
Inflammatory bowel disease, 1209–1217
  absorption, 1211
  adjunctive nutritional therapy, 1214–1215
  diet, 1210
  digestion, 1211
  drug-nutrient interactions, 1211
  enteric losses, 1211
  fat absorption, 1210–1211
  with folic acid deficiency, 478
  glutamine for, 566
  growth impairment, 1212
  intensive nutritional support, 1214–1217
  intestinal effects, 1210–1211
  micronutrient deficiencies, 1213t
  nutritional assessment of, 1214t
  nutrition consequences, 1211–1213
  nutrition therapy for, 1213–1214
  pathogenesis, 1209–1210
  preoperative nutritional support, 1214
Information systems, 1605
Informed consent, 1610
Inheritance powder, 339
Inherited metabolic disease, 909–954
  beta-oxidation defects, 960–973
  genetic perspective, 909–910
INI. *See* Instant Nutritional Index (INI)
Injury
  anabolic agents, 1431–1432
  enteral diet, 1425–1426
  enteral feeding
    complications, 1427–1428
  enteral feeding access, 1426–1427
  enteral nutrition, 1424
  fat requirements, 1422
  glucose requirements, 1421
  metabolic response to, 1381–1382, 1382f, 1382t
  neuroendocrine consequences, 1383f
  nutritional support therapy monitoring, 1431
  parenteral diet, 1428–1429
  perioperative nutrition support, 1424
  physiologic response to, 1418–1419
  protein requirements, 1421–1422
  trace element requirements, 1423–1424
  vitamin requirements, 1422–1423
Injury Severity Score (ISS), 1416
Innate immunity, 674–675, 677–678

Inorganic elements
historical development of, 4–5
Inorganic sulfur
functions, 556
Inosine
athletes, 1735
sports nutrition, 1735
Inositol triphosphate (IP3), 224
Insecticides, 1814–1815
In silico
defined, 617t
In situ RNA hybridization, 618
Instant Nutritional Index (INI), 841
Institute of Medicine (IOM)
dietary reference intakes, 1852
Insulin
affecting metabolism and food intake,
1046t
for cancer, 1301t
fat storage, 639
glucose uptake, 638–639
GLUT, 70–71
injury, 1390
lipolysis, 639
magnesium, 226
absorption, 229
parenteral nutrition, 1571
protein storage, 639
resistance, 1005t
alcohol, 1241
dietary fiber, 87–88
dyslipidemia, 1074–1075
syndrome
in elderly, 1536
thrifty phenotype, 1074–1075
response
dietary fiber, 87
secretion, 637
metabolism, 71
timing of, 1062t
Insulin-dependent diabetes mellitus (IDDM),
1044
Insulin like growth factor-I (IGF-I), 651–652,
741–742, 1123t, 1212
elderly, 853
injury, 1432–1433
refeeding syndrome, 744
Insulin-responsive glucose transporter, 68
Insulin therapy
for diabetes mellitus, 1061–1062, 1061f
Integrated nutritional assessment scores,
841–842
Intellect
with iodine deficiency, 305
Intended use, 1828
Interagency Board for Nutrition Monitoring
and Related Research (IBNMRR), 1691
Interferon gamma (IFN gamma), 1391t
injury, 1392
mediating altered metabolism in cancer,
1294–1295
Interleukin
with congestive heart failure, 1109
Interleukin 1 (IL1), 1391–1392, 1391t
mediating altered metabolism in cancer,
1294
Interleukin 6 (IL6), 1391t
injury, 1392
mediating altered metabolism in cancer,
1294
Intermediate density lipoproteins (IDL)
lipid transport, 101
Intermediate metabolism
energetics of, 136–138

International dietary recommendations,
1889–1893, 1889t
International nutrition labeling, 1836–1837
Interstitial adipose tissue, 756
Interstitial retinoid-binding protein (IRBP),
356
Interventional studies
of diet effect on cancer, 1268t
Intestinal bacteria
biochemical reactions by, 1140t
Intestinal brush-border membrane hydrolase
activity, 1132t
Intestinal dysmotility
with cancer, 1296
Intestinal fistulas
with hypomagnesemia, 233
Intestinal folds, 1118f
Intestinal hormones and growth factors,
637–638
Intestinal microflora, 1139–1140, 1139t
Intestinal obstruction
with cancer, 1296
Intestinal resection
short bowel syndrome, 1202–1203
Intestines
dietary lipid digestion in, 96–98
propulsive reflexes, 1121f
transepithelial hexose transport, 72–73
Intracellular fluids
electrolytes, 151t
volume and osmolality regulation, 186–190
Intracellular volumes
regulation of, 149–160, 153
Intravenous dextrose preparations
osmolalities of, 1572t
Intravenous fluids
short bowel syndrome, 1204
Intravenous lipids
newer, 1577–1578
parenteral diet, 1428–1429
Intrinsic factor, 1184
Iodide (iodine), 300–310, 606. *See also*
Minerals
advocacy, 308
balance, 302
chemistry, 301
chemosensory function, 700
deficiency, 304–306, 606
abortions, 305
brain lesions pathogenesis, 1365
complications, 306
global, 309
neurologic deficits, 304–305
reproductive damage, 305
socioeconomic damage, 306
tooth development, 1155t
dietary sources, 304
distribution, 301
education, 308
in enteral feeding products, 1558t
excess, 303, 306–308
global, 309
global nutrition status, 309, 309t
historical highlights, 300–301
induced hyperthyroidism, 306
mean urinary, 303t
metabolism, 301–302
national nutrition programs, 308
nutrition assessment, 302–303
optimal nutrition, 309–310
parenteral nutrition, 1582
pregnancy, 778
properties, 301
recommended dietary intakes, 302t, 303–304

supplements, 307–308
thyroid hormones, 302
thyroid size, 303
toxicity, 606
urinary excretion, 302
Iodized oil, 308
Iodized salt, 307
Iodized water, 307–308
Iodothyronine deiodinases
selenium, 316
IOM. *See* Institute of Medicine (IOM)
Ion channels
magnesium, 224
Ionized serum magnesium, 232
Ion selective electrodes
ionized magnesium, 231
IP3. *See* Inositol triphosphate (IP3)
IRBP. *See* Interstitial retinoid-binding protein
(IRBP)
IRE. *See* Iron-responsive element (IRE)
Iridology, 1766
Iron, 248–268, 606–607. *See also* Minerals
absorption, 249–250, 1439–1440
adolescents, 821–822
alcoholism, 1252
assessment of, 266–267
average dietary intake, 263f
biochemistry, 248–249
as biologic resource, 248–249
blood, 5
calcium, 202
cell biology, 251–252
cellular uptake and storage, 251–252
chemosensory function, 700
chronic renal failure, 1497
cobalamin interaction, 495
copper interactions, 294
deficiency, 267–268, 606–607
adolescents, 1443
children, 1443
cognitive effects of, 1365–1366
conditions associated with, 268
cystic fibrosis, 1471
diagnosis, 1442
differential diagnosis, 1442–1443
infants, 1443
with inflammatory bowel disease, 1213
with PKU, 923
pregnancy, 1443
prevalence of, 1440–1442, 1441t
tooth development, 1155t
deficiency anemia, 865
after surgery, 1187
signs and symptoms of, 1441–1442
delivery, 250
dietary bioavailability, 263–264
measurement, 264
dietary reference intakes, 264–265
by life stage group, 1439t
dietary sources of, 1438–1439
effects on periodontium, 1170t
elderly, 850
elevated stores, 268
in enteral feeding products, 1558t
estimating requirements, 265–266, 265t
excess, 268
exogenous supply, 249–250
factorial modeling method, 265
flux, 250f
fortification, 1443–1444
biologic impact of, 1706f
gastrointestinal effects, 877t
generating free radicals, 249
hematologic disease, 1437–1438

historical background, 248
homeostasis, 252–253
with infection, 1409
intake, 262–263
kinetics, 249–250
loss, 251
malabsorption of, 1145t
manganese, 327
in medicine, 258–259
metabolism, 634
    clinical disorders affecting, 261–262
    genetic disorders affecting proteins,
        258–259, 258t
National Health and Nutrition Examination
    Survey III, 822t
nonheme bioavailability, 264f
normal distribution of, 1437t
in normal infants and children, 802
nutrition, 262–263
nutritional availability, 8–9
overload, 607
parenteral nutrition, 1581–1582
partitioning in body, 249
physiology, 249–250
potato density, 262t
preconceptional health, 772
pregnancy, 778–779
in protein, 249
proteins, 252t
public health, 1437–1438
1989 RDA *vs.* 2002 RDI, 819t
reclamation, 250–251
recommended dietary allowance, 264–265,
    264t, 1439t
regulation, 251
requirements for infants and children,
    1438t
reticuloendothelial system, 250
serum clinical chemistry values, 266t
sources of, 263t
sports nutrition, 1732
sports performance, 1732
storage depot, 251
tolerable upper levels of intake, 266
total dietary intake, 1440
toxicity, 607
vegetarian diets, 1641–1642
1989 *vs.* 2002 RDI, 831t
zinc interactions, 274
Iron deficiency disorder (IDD)
    cognitive function, 1364–1365
Iron regulatory protein (IRP), 252t, 254f
Iron-responsive element (IRE), 253
IRP. *See* Iron regulatory protein (IRP)
Isinglass, 1519
ISIS-4. *See* Fourth International Study of
    Infarct Survival (ISIS-4)
Isoflavones, 583, 591–592, 1797t, 1801–1802
    absorption, 591–592
    bone health, 1713
    dietary source, 591
    health effects, 586t
    intake, 591
    metabolism, 591–592
Isoleucine
    hepatic encephalopathy, 1238
    restricted diet, 2003t
Isomaltase, 1189, 1190t
Isoprenoids, 1795, 1796t, 1800
Isoprostanes, 106
Isothiocyanates, 593, 1797t
Isotonic dehydration, 158
Isotopes
    magnesium, 231

Isovaleric acidemia, 910, 939–941, 1997t
    diagnosis, 939–940
    nutrient requirements, 940
    nutrition support, 940–941
    screening, 939
    treatment, 940
ISS. *See* Injury Severity Score (ISS)

J

Jacob, François, 615
JAMA. *See* Journal of the American Medical
    Association (JAMA)
Japan
    functional foods, 1790
    iodine excess, 309
    iodine sources, 304
    obesity rates, 1026
    RDA
        for growth period and physical activity,
            1881t–1883t
    taurine, 548
Jejunal efflux
    short bowel syndrome, 1205f
Jejunal resection
    short bowel syndrome, 1204
Jejunostomy tubes, 1555–1556
Jejunum
    anatomy of, 1118
Jimsonweed, 1821
Joint Nutrition Monitoring Evaluation
    Committee (JNMEC), 1690
Joints
    nutritional deficiency, 838t
Joule
    defined, 136
Joule, James Prescott, 13
Journal of the American Medical Association
    (JAMA)
    end of life care series, 1618–1619
Journals
    websites for, 2025–2026
Juices
    fast
        defined, 730
    mineral content, 1979t, 1982t
    protein content, 1979t
    vitamins, 1985t
Justice, 1609
Juvenile hemochromatosis, 258t

K

Kaempferol, 1796t
Kashin-Beck disease, 318
Kayexalate, 167
Kefir
    lactose intolerance, 1195
Kelley/Gonzalez metabolic therapy, 1770–1771
Keshan disease, 312, 318, 323
Ketoacidosis, 180–181, 181f
    with alcohol consumption, 1242–1243
    alcoholic, 1368
Ketoaciduria
    branched chain, 910
        sample diets for, 2002t
3-ketoacyl-CoA thiolase
    deficiency, 967
Ketogenic diet, 1378
Ketoisocaproate (KIC)
    leucine cellular transport, 40–41
Ketonemia
    with diabetes mellitus, 1048–1049
Ketosis, 732–733
    with alcohol consumption, 1243
    biologic significance, 732–733

Key-informant interviewing, 1746
Khellin, 668
KIC. *See* Ketoisocaproate (KIC)
Kidney, 1475–1505
    disease, 1475
        National Kidney Foundation stages of,
            1476t
    failure
        nutritional support in, 1395–1396
    function of, 1475–1476
    malnutrition, 1476–1477
    during pregnancy, 773
    stones
        calcium, 205, 208
    transepithelial hexose transport, 72–73
Kleiber law, 14
Korsakoff psychosis, 431
Korsakoff syndrome, 1370
Krebs cycle, 27–28
K sparing diuretics
    for hypokalemia, 165
Kui, 1402
Kwashiorkor, 736–737, 833–834, 881,
    892–893, 894f, 1402, 1458, 1747
    diagnosis, 833t

L

LAB. *See* Lactic acid bacteria (LAB)
Laboratory studies, 835–841, 839t
Lactase, 1189, 1190t
    clinical assessment, 1192–1193
Lactase enzyme supplements, 1195–1196
Lactase nonpersistence (LNP), 1190–1192
    ethnicity, 1191t
Lactase-phlorizin hydrolase (LPH),
    1189–1196
    function, 1189–1190
    location, 1189–1190
Lactate, 721
Lactation, 784–795
    calcium, 207
    carbohydrate DRI, 1861t
    chloride DRI, 1867t
    elements
        DRI, 1870t
        UL, 1871t
    energy DRI, 1859t
    energy requirements, 144
    estimated energy requirements, 146–147
    folate deficiency, 1455
    future research, 795
    impact on breast cancer, 793–794
    impact on infant, 791–793
    impact on mother, 793–794
    iodine, 303
    iron dietary reference intakes, 1439t
    manganese, 326–327
    manganese dietary reference intake values,
        327t
    minerals
        recommended dietary allowances, 1872t
    n-3 polyunsaturated fatty acids (alpha-
        linoleic acid) DRI, 1864t
    n-6 polyunsaturated fatty acids (linoleic
        acid) DRI, 1863t
    phosphorus dietary reference intake values,
        212t
    potassium DRI, 1866t
    PUFA, 118
    riboflavin
        dietary reference intake value, 439t
    sodium DRI, 1867t
    sulfur amino acids
        RDA, 548

Lactation (*Continued*)
  thiamin
    dietary sources, 427t
    total fat DRI, 1863t
    total fiber DRI, 1862t
    total water DRI, 1865t
  vegetarian diets, 1647
  vitamin(s)
    DRI, 1868t
    recommended dietary allowances, 1872t
    UL, 1869t
  vitamin A, 354t, 367
  vitamin D DRI, 391t
  vitamin E DRI, 407t
Lactic acid bacteria (LAB), 1803
Lactic acidosis, 180
  etiology, 180t
  short bowel syndrome, 1207
Lactoferrin, 252t, 1798t, 1802–1803
Lactose
  calcium absorption, 201
  controlled diets, 2013
  deficiency
    serum glucose, 1248f
  hydrolyzed milk, 1195–1196
  intolerance, 78, 1193–1196, 1522–1523
    diet, 1193–1196, 1194t
    gastrointestinal transit effects,
      1194–1195
    gene therapy, 1196
  malabsorbed
    colonic adaptation to, 1196
  maldigestion, 1193
  metabolism, 633
  microbe-containing dairy foods, 1195
  source of, 1190t, 1519
  tolerance
    cocoa, 1195
Lactose-free bovine milk formula, 804
Lactovegetarian diet
  with rheumatoid arthritis, 1334
Laetrile, 1770
Laparoscopic adjustable gastric banding, 1040
Large intestines
  anatomy of, 1116f
  dietary fiber effects on, 86–87
  vitamin K, 415
L-arginine
  chemical structure of, 572f
Latent tetany
  with magnesium deficiency, 236
Later childhood
  feeding, 808–809
Latitude
  vitamin D3, 381–382, 382F
Lavoisier, Antoine Laurent, 12
Laxation
  dietary fiber, 86–87
LBW. *See* Low birth weight (LBW) infant
LCAT. *See* Lecithin cholesterol
    acyltransferase (LCAT)
LCD. *See* Low calorie diets (LCD)
LCFA. *See* Long chain fatty acids (LCFA)
LCHAD. *See* Long-chain 3-hydroxyacyl-CoA
    dehydrogenase (LCHAD)
LDC. *See* Less-developed countries (LDC)
LDL. *See* Low density lipoproteins (LDL)
Lead
  migrating from containers, 1816
  poisoning
    with iron deficiency, 268
Leaky gut syndrome, 1769
Lean tissue conservation
  energy balance, 738

protein intake, 738–739
  reference values, 765
Lean tissue loss
  protein energy deficiency, 737–738
Lean tissues, 762
LEARN, 1037
Learned food aversions (LFA)
  cancer, 702
  with cancer, 1296
Learning failure
  ecology of, 868
Lecithin, 1518
Lecithin cholesterol acyltransferase (LCAT)
  deficiency, 1072
Lecithin retinol acyltransferase (LRAT), 358
  hepatic metabolism, 359
Legumes
  dietary fiber content of, 1966t–1967t
Leicester Intravenous Magnesium
    Intervention Trial (LIMIT), 237
Leigh disease, 432, 599
Leiner disease
  with biotin deficiency, 503
Length, 1850
Length of stay
  hospitalists, 1601
Lennox-Gastaut syndrome, 1378
Leptin, 642–643, 711, 712, 741, 1039
  research, 716–717
Leptin-NPY, 1123t
LES. *See* Lower esophageal sphincter (LES)
Less-developed countries (LDC),
    1719–1720
Leucine, 25
  hepatic encephalopathy, 1238
  kinetics, 40f
  medical foods free of, 940
Leukocytes
  dysfunction, 218–219
Leukocytosis, 187
Leukotriene
  formation of, 112f
Levetiracetam
  food interactions, 1542
Levodopa
  food interactions, 1542
LFA. *See* Learned food aversions (LFA)
Liddle syndrome, 165
Liebig, Justus, 4, 12
Life extension, 743
Lignans, 593, 1796t
Likelihood of Malnutrition (LOM), 841
Limb fat area method, 759
LIMIT. *See* Leicester Intravenous
    Magnesium Intervention Trial (LIMIT)
Limonene, 1796t, 1800
Limonoids, 1796t
Lind, James, 507
Lingual lipase, 1179
Linoleic acid, 115. *See also* Polyunsaturated
    fatty acids (PUFA)
  cholesterol, 127
  DRI by life-stage group, 1863t
  phenylketonuria
    pregnancy, 2000t
Lipase
  acute pancreatitis, 1228
Lipid(s)
  absorption of, 98–99, 1133–1135
    with alcohol consumption, 1242–1243
  biosynthesis of, 107–110
  chemistry, 93–95
  chronic renal failure, 1479, 1492–1493
  digestion and absorption, 96–99

emulsions
    altered pulmonary function, 1576–1577
    catheter occlusion, 1576
    comparison of products, 1574t
    complications, 1576–1577
    composition, 1574
    immunity, 1577
    metabolism, 1574–1575
    microbial growth, 1576
    nitrogen retention, 1575
    safety, 1576
    stability, 1576
    tolerance, 1575
    total nutrient admixture, 1575–1576
  endogenous transport system, 100f,
    101–102
  exogenous transport system, 100–101, 100f
  fatty acid oxidation, 104–105
  human milk, 788t
  in human milk, 789t
  intracellular movement of, 107–110
  with magnesium deficiency, 238
  metabolic syndrome, 1008t
  metabolism, 99–104, 634
    cancer, 1293, 1388
    human immunodeficiency virus (HIV),
      1388–1389
    injury and sepsis, 1387–1388
  oxidants, 689
  peroxidation, 689f
  peroxidative modification, 105–106
  as pharmacologic vehicles, 1578
  solubility, 99–100
  structure, 93–95
  transfer proteins, 102–103
  transport, 99–104
  vitamin B6, 455
Lipid mobilizing factor (LMF)
  mediating altered metabolism in cancer,
    1294
Lipin, 351
Lipiodol, 308
Lipofuscin, 397, 406
Lipoproteins
  characteristics, 124t
  chronic renal failure, 1479
  dietary factors influencing, 103–104
  lipase deficiency, 1087–1088
  metabolism, 102–103, 1067–1075
    drugs altering, 1074, 1074t
    genetic disorders, 1067–1073
    history, 1067
  physical chemical characteristics of, 100t
  synthesis
    genetic defects, 405
Lithium, 1360
  associated with weight gain, 1021
  for hyponatremia, 175
Liver, 1235–1236
  alcoholism, 1254
  disease
    chemical senses and diet, 703
    nutritional therapy, 1237–1238
  failure
    protein metabolism, 1237
  glucose transporter, 68
  injury, 1236, 1237
    alcoholic complications, 1240f
    dietary intake, 1237
    maldigestion, 1237
    metabolic changes, 1237
    nutritional consequences, 1236–1237
    sequential development, 1239f
  intermediary metabolism, 1236

iron storage, 251
as metabolic organ, 47–48
nutrition effect on, 1245–1246
transplantation
osteoporosis, 1322
LMF. *See* Lipid mobilizing factor (LMF)
LNP. *See* Lactase nonpersistence (LNP)
Locura manganica (Manganese madness), 329
LOM. *See* Likelihood of Malnutrition (LOM)
Long bone
architecture of, 1316f
regions of, 1316f
Long chain fatty acids (LCFA), 95–96
Long-chain 3-hydroxyacyl-CoA
dehydrogenase (LCHAD)
deficiency, 966
Long-chain triglyceride mixtures, 1577–1578
Lorenzo's oil, 973
Lovastatin
for hypercholesterolemia, 1085t
Low birth weight (LBW) infant, 780–781
carbohydrate requirements, 813–814
energy requirements, 812
fat requirements, 813
fluid and electrolyte requirements, 814
formula composition, 813t
formulas
composition of, 813t
human milk, 816
Life Sciences Research Office
recommendations for, 811, 811t
mineral requirements, 814–815
nutrient intake recommendations, 810t
nutrient needs of, 809–815
nutrient requirements delivery, 815–816
nutritional management, 997
goals, 809–812
protein requirements, 812–813
vitamin requirements, 815
Low calorie diets (LCD), 1032
Low carbohydrate, high protein diets,
1033–1034
Low density lipoproteins (LDL)
atherosclerotic cardiovascular disease,
1076–1077
cholesterol
with diabetes mellitus, 1059
dietary fiber, 87
with hypercholesterolemia, 1078
healthy diet, 1627
lipid transport, 101
lowering dietary options, 1083
overproduction of, 1081–1082
reduced clearance of, 1082
tocopherols, 402
Low energy density diets, 1033
Lower esophageal sphincter (LES), 1179
Low fat diets, 1033
for childhood obesity, 985–986
Low high density lipoprotein
cholesterol
genetic causes of, 1073t
genetic causes of, 1072–1073
Low molecular weight carbohydrates
as dietary fiber, 84
Low molecular weight ligands, 288–289
Low-oxalate meal suggestions, 2022–2023
Low-protein diets (LPD), 1475
Lp(a), 1073
genetic causes of, 1074t
LPD. *See* Low-protein diets (LPD)
LPH. *See* Lactase-phlorizin hydrolase (LPH)
LRAT. *See* Lecithin retinol acyltransferase
(LRAT)

L-tryptophan, 1729, 1759
Lumina
dysfunction tests, 1149–1150
Lungs
cancer, 1470
fruits and vegetables, 1273
disease, 1467
injury, 1467
parenchyma, 1463
transplantation, 1471–1472
Lusk, Graham, 13
Lutein
intestinal absorption, 357
structure, 353f
Luteolin, 1796t
Lycopene, 1796t
cancer, 365
intestinal absorption, 357
source, 366
structure, 353f
Lymphoma
with celiac disease, 1222
Lysine, 1729
hepatic encephalopathy, 1238
historical development of, 6
metabolism of, 934f
restricted diet, 2004t
vegetarian diets, 1641
Lysyl oxidase, 287

M
Macedonia
optimal iodine nutrition programs, 309
Macrobiotic diets, 1639
Macrobiotics, 1764
Macrocytic anemia
defined, 483t
Macrominerals
pregnancy, 778
Macronutrients
anabolic support, 1394
current intakes, 1078t
disease, 1270–1272
human milk, 787–788
needs
elderly, 844–846
nutrient risk assessment, 1667
Macrophages
innate immunity, 677–678
iron metabolism, 256–257, 257f
Macrosatellite repeat sequences, 628
MADD. *See* Multiple acyl-CoA
dehydrogenation disorder (MADD)
Magendie, François, 3, 12
MAGIC. *See* Magnesium in Coronaries
(MAGIC) trial
Magnesium, 223–240, 605–606. *See also*
Hypermagnesemia; Hypomagnesemia;
Minerals
absorption
hormonal influences, 229
regulation, 228
alcoholism, 1252, 1255
analytic procedures for, 231
bioavailability, 228
biochemistry, 223–224
biologic indicators, 231–232
body composition, 225
body homeostasis, 227–229, 227f
calcium, 208
cellular homeostasis, 225–226, 226f
for chronic renal failure, 1496
combined lab testing, 232–233
deficiency, 605–606, 1323

with diabetes mellitus, 1056
dietary intake, 227
assessment, 230–231
distribution in adult, 225t
effects on periodontium, 1170t
elderly, 850
in enteral feeding products, 1558t
enzyme interactions, 223–224
filtration, 228–229
hypertension, 1713
intestinal absorption, 227–228, 227f
intrauterine accretion rates during third
trimester, 809t
ion channels, 224
malabsorption of, 1145t
need assessment, 229–230
osteoporosis, 1347
overdose, 241
parenteral diet, 1430
parenteral nutrition, 1580–1581
physiology, 223–224
pregnancy, 778
1989 RDA *vs.* 2002 RDI, 819t
recommended daily intakes, 229–230, 230t
renal regulation, 228–229
replacement therapy, 1430t
requirements, 229–231
sports nutrition, 1731–1732
sports performance, 1731–1732
status assessment, 231–232
sweat losses, 229
toxicity, 606
tubular absorption, 228–229
1989 *vs.* 2002 RDI, 831t
Magnesium in Coronaries (MAGIC) trial, 237
Magnesium load/retention test, 232
Magnesium salts
absorbability, 228
MAGPIE trial, 238–239
Maharishi ayur-ved, 1764
Ma huang, 1758
Maillard reaction, 1779–1780
Maintenance hemodialysis (MHD), 1475,
1491
monitoring nutritional status, 1488f
recommended nutrient intake, 1487t
Maize
cultural ecology, 1742
Major depression, 1359
Malabsorption, 1144t
assessment of, 1143–1150
with cancer, 1295, 1296–1297
with chronic pancreatitis, 1231
diet history, 1144
family history, 1144
laboratory studies, 1144–1150, 1145t
medical history, 1143–1144
pathogenesis of, 1149f
physical examination, 1144
with protein-losing enteropathy, 1297
syndrome
with folic acid deficiency, 478
with hypomagnesemia, 233
Malaise
with celiac disease, 1222
Malaria
with malnutrition, 1404
Maldigestion
with cancer, 1295
Malnutrition
acidosis, 1476
with cancer, 1291
with child mortality, 1403f
children, 1410f

Malnutrition *(Continued)*
  vs. disease, 830–832
  ecology of, 868
  history of, 14
  inducing gastric emptying, 1181
  with infection, 1403–1408
  with inflammatory bowel disease,
    1211–1212, 1211t
  international perspectives, 1748–1749
  nocturia, 1476
  poverty, 861, 863f
  prevention of, 1409–1410
  urine volume, 1476
Maltase-glucoamylase, 1196–1197
Mammary glands
  diagram of, 787f
  milk secretion, 786
Manganese, 326–330, 609–610. *See also*
    Minerals
  absorption, 328
  alcoholism, 1253
  analytic methods, 328
  associated enzymes, 326
  biochemistry, 326
  chemistry, 326
  deficiency, 609–610
  dietary considerations, 326–327
  dietary reference intake values, 327t
  in enteral feeding products, 1558t
  excretion, 328
  history, 326
  nutrient-nutrient interactions, 327
  osteoporosis, 1347
  parenteral nutrition, 327, 1582t, 1583
  pregnancy, 779
  tolerable upper intake levels, 330
  toxicity, 610
  transport, 328
Manganese madness, 329
Maple syrup urine disease, 935–936
  diagnosis, 936
  equivalent lists, 937
  nutrient requirements, 937
  nutrition support, 937–939
  organic acids for, 1996t
  screening, 936
  stabilization, 935f
  treatment, 936–937
Marasmic kwashiorkor, 834, 881, 892, 894f
Marasmic protein-energy malnutrition,
    892f
Marasmus, 832–833, 891–892, 892f
  diagnosis, 833t
  vs. kwashiorkor, 833t
Marijuana, 1360
  inducing gastric emptying, 1181
  pregnancy, 779
Masked megaloblastosis, 1457
Maternal diets
  recommendations for, 779–780
Maternal plasma volume
  during pregnancy, 773
Matrix Gla protein (MGP), 416
Maximum oxygen uptake, 724t
Mayow, John, 11
MCC. *See* Methylcrotonyl CoA carboxylase
    (MCC)
McCollum, E.V., 6
MCFA. *See* Medium chain fatty acids
    (MCFA)
McLaren, Donald, 1402
MCT. *See* Medium-chain triglyceride (MCT)
MDRD. *See* Modification of Diet in Renal
    Disease (MDRD)

Meals
  controlling food intake, 707–708
  control of number, 714–715
  control of size, 708–714, 710f
  direct and indirect controls, 713–714, 714f
  integrated response to, 1126–1132
  pancreatic secretion after, 1131t
  replacement
    with diabetes mellitus, 1059–1060
  social interactions, 1743
  stimuli-evoked responses, 1127
Measles
  with malnutrition, 1403–1404
Meat
  cancer, 1272
  labeling, 1832
  mineral content, 1978t, 1981t
  oxalate, 2014t, 2017t
  protein content, 1978t
  vitamins, 1984t
Mechanogrowth factor
  skeletal muscle hormones, 644
Medical care
  adequacy of, 1599–1600
Medical ethics
  changing views about, 1609–1610
Medical foods
  free of phenylalanine and tyrosine, 927
Medical journals
  websites for, 2025–2026
Medical nutrition therapy (MNT)
  protocols, 1604
  reimbursement for, 1604
Medical schools
  changes in, 1605–1606
Medical treatment
  right to refuse, 1610
Medications
  avoided with foods to maximize absorption,
    1543t
  causing anorexia in elderly, 1533t
  chronic renal failure, 1479
  taken with foods to maximize absorption,
    1543t
Mediterranean diet, 365
Mediterranean Diet Score, 1633t
Medium chain fatty acids (MCFA), 95–96
Medium-chain triglyceride (MCT),
    1577–1578, 1727
  sports performance, 1727
Megalin, 361
Megaloblastic anemia, 602
  defined, 483t
  with folic acid deficiency, 476, 477f
Megavitamin therapy, 1765
Megestrol acetate, 1307
  for cancer, 1301t
Meissner plexus, 1116
Melanocortins
  mediating altered metabolism in cancer,
    1295
Melanocyte stimulating hormone (MSH), 712
Melatonin, 1759
  for cancer, 1301t
Membrane phospholipids
  EFAD, 111
Membranes
  magnesium structural modification, 224
Memory loss
  choline, 532
Men
  cancer deaths in, 1281t
Menadione
  structure, 413t

Menaquinone, 415
Menaquinone-4
  metabolic role, 420
  structure, 413t
Menaquinone-9
  structure, 413t
Menarche
  breast cancer, 1269
Mendel, Lafayette, 6
Menkes disease, 297
Menkes steely hair disease, 607
Mental retardation
  with PKU, 918
Mercury, 1817
MET. *See* Metabolic equivalents (MET)
Metabolic acidosis, 165, 178–185, 219
  anion gap, 182t
  diagnosis, 182
  with Mg wasting, 234
  net acid excretion, 178–179, 179t
  renal acidosis, 179–180
  serum anion gap, 181, 181f
  treatment, 182–183
Metabolic alkalosis, 183–184
  acetazolamide, 184
  etiology, 183–184
  pathogenesis, 183–184
  treatment, 184
Metabolic balance, 1323
Metabolic body size, 14
Metabolic bone disease
  with parenteral nutrition, 1589–1591
Metabolic disease
  failed adaptation, 740
Metabolic equivalents (MET), 725
Metabolic rate
  in elderly, 1532, 1532f
Metabolic syndrome, 1004–1011, 1897, 1898
  blood pressure, 1008–1009
  clinical identification of, 1899t
  components of, 1006–1010
  underlying causes of, 1899
Metabolic therapy, 1766
Metabolomics
  defined, 617t
Metallothionein, 288
Metformin, 1062t, 1091
Methionine, 8, 22, 30, 471, 689f
  estimated average requirement, 548
  excretion, 550
  historical introduction, 545
  liver injury, 1238–1239
  metabolism, 550–554, 551f
  recommended intake, 547–548
  remethylation, 550–551
  remethylation *vs.* transsulfuration, 551–552
  restricted diet, 2003t
  source, 547t
  transmethylation, 550
  transport, 549
  vegetarian diets, 1641
Methionine free medical foods, 931
Methionine-restricted diets
  nutrient content, 2001t
Methotrexate
  folate, 1336
  with folic acid deficiency, 478
  food interactions, 1542
  nutrients, 1331
    interactions, 1327f
  for rheumatoid arthritis, 1336t
Methylarginines, 574–575
  chemical structure, 575f
Methylcobalamin, 483

3-methylcrotonyl-CoA
  tandem mass spectrometry, 942t
Methylcrotonyl CoA carboxylase (MCC), 499
3-methylcrotonylglycinuria, 941
Methylenetetrahydrofolate reductase
  (MTHFR) gene, 1626
3-methylglutaconic aciduria, 941
  tandem mass spectrometry, 942t
3-methylglutaryl-CoA lyase
  tandem mass spectrometry, 943t
3-methylhistidine
  degradation, 43–44
Methylmalonic acid (MMA), 485, 910, 1997t
  sample diet for, 2003t
  tandem mass spectrometry, 943t
Methylmalonic acidemia, 945
  tandem mass spectrometry, 944t
Methylphenidate
  for cancer, 1303
Metoclopramide, 1182
Mexican-Americans
  anthropometric measure, 1938t–1939t
MGP. See Matrix Gla protein (MGP)
MHD. See Maintenance hemodialysis
  (MHD)
Micellar bile salts, 98
Microarray analysis, 622f
Microbial, 1803
Microbial colonization
  with parenteral nutrition, 1570
Microbodies. See Peroxisomes
Microcytic anemia, 601
Microcytic hypochromic anemia, 606
Micronutrient malnutrition, 834–835
Micronutrients
  adolescents, 820–823
  anabolic support, 1395
  with diabetes mellitus, 1056
  human milk, 788
  supplementation
    bone and teeth, 1321
    short bowel syndrome, 1206, 1206f
Microsatellite instability, 1261–1262
Microsatellite repeat sequences, 628
Microwave, 1784
Miglitol, 1062t
Migraine
  dietary treatment of, 1376
Migrating myoelectric complex, 1121
Mild hypercholesterolemia, 1079–1080
  genetic contribution to, 1079–1080
Miliaria crystallina dermatitis, 329
Milk, 803
  bioactive components of, 790–791, 790t
  composition of, 786–787, 788t
    values of, 789t
  nutritional factors, 787–788
  oxalate, 2017t
  with rheumatoid arthritis, 1333
  riboflavin secretion, 437
Milk nutrients, 200t
Minamata disease, 1817
Mineral deficiency
  failed adaptation, 740
Mineralocorticoid, 167
Minerals, 604–610. See also Trace minerals;
  specific mineral
  absorption of, 1138–1139
  acute renal failure, 1504
  alcoholism, 1252–1253
  for children, 801–802
    recommended daily allowances, 921t
    UL, 800t
  for chronic renal failure, 1487t

for CPD, 1487t
DRI, 799t, 1870t
estimated safe and adequate daily dietary
  intake, 1873t
food content, 1978t–1980t
in formulas, 805t
  for infant, 806t
  for low birth weight infants, 813t,
    814–815
  for term infants, 804t
in human milk, 788t, 789t
in hydrolyzed formulas, 806t
for infants, 801–802
  DRI, 799t
  recommended daily allowances, 921t
  UL, 800t
intake recommendations
  for low birth weight infants, 810t, 811t
for MHD, 1487t
parenteral intakes of, 999t
recommended dietary allowances, 1872t
  WHO, 1892t
recommended intake
  based on age and body weight, 1873t
reference nutrient intakes
  UK, 1878t, 1879t
safe intakes
  UK, 1880t
safe upper levels
  UK, 1880t
in soy formula, 806t
sports nutrition, 1731–1732
sports performance, 1731–1732
status assessment, 841
tolerable upper intake for normal infants
  and children, 800t
UL, 800t, 1871t
Mini-Council of Nutrition Appetite
  Questionnaire (CNAQ), 1535t
Minimally conscious state, 1618
Mini Nutritional Assessment (MNA), 854,
  1535t
Minocycline, 1570
Minute ventilation
  defined, 1464t
Misbranding, 1827
Misleading claims, 1752–1756
Mismatch repair genes, 1261–1262
Mitochondria, 960
Mitochondrial beta-oxidation
  defects
    diagnosis, 970t
Mitochondrial fatty acid oxidation
  enzymes in, 962t
Mitochondrial iron metabolism, 254–255
Mixed acid base disorders, 185–186
Mixed venous blood
  defined, 1464t
MMA. See Methylmalonic acid (MMA)
MNA. See Mini Nutritional Assessment (MNA)
MNT. See Medical nutrition therapy (MNT)
Moderate hypercholesterolemia, 1081–1082
Modification of Diet in Renal Disease
  (MDRD), 1480, 1481
  test, 370
Molecular model
  of body composition, 754–755
Mole % excess, 36
Mole fraction, 36
Mole ratio, 36
Molybdenum, 339, 343–345, 609. See also
  Minerals
  absorption, 344
  analytic methods, 344

beneficial effects, 345
bioavailability, 344
chemistry, 343–344
deficiency, 609
dietary considerations, 344–345
distribution, 344
excretion, 344
health effects, 345
historical overview, 343
mechanisms of action, 344
parenteral nutrition, 1582t, 1584
pregnancy, 779
recommended dietary allowances, 345t
toxicity, 345, 609
transport, 344
Molybdenum-copper interactions, 294
Mono-adenosine diphosphate
  ribosyltransferases, 447–448
Monoamine oxidase, 287
  inhibitors
    associated with weight gain, 1021
Monoclonal antibodies
  for cancer, 1301t, 1302
Monocytes
  innate immunity, 677–678
Monod, Jacques, 615
Monodeficiency syndrome
  with celiac disease, 1222
Monogenic
  defined, 617t
Monomeric formulas, 1557
Monosaccharides
  absorption of, 1137f
  structure, 64f
Monosaturated fats
  with diabetes mellitus, 1053
Monoterpenes, 1800
Monounsaturated fatty acids (MUFA),
  93–94
Mood disorders, 1359
Morris, William, 339
Motilin, 1123t
Mouth, 1179
  dietary lipid digestion in, 96
  function of, 1127–1128
MSH. See Melanocyte stimulating hormone
  (MSH)
MTHFR. See Methylenetetrahydrofolate
  reductase (MTHFR) gene
Mucosa
  dysfunction tests, 1146–1147
MUFA. See Monounsaturated fatty acids
  (MUFA)
Mulder, Gerrit, 4
Muller, Johannes, 12
Multilumen catheters, 1569
Multiple acyl-CoA dehydrogenation disorder
  (MADD)
  deficiency, 967
Multiple sclerosis, 1376
Multitrace element additives
  parenteral nutrition, 1584–1585
Multivitamins
  athletes, 1730
  parenteral
    for children, 1587t
    composition of, 1586t
    FDA recommendations, 1422t
  sport nutrition, 1730
Muscarine, 1823
Muscle fiber
  types, 723, 723t
Muscle fiber necrosis
  aging, 724

Muscle mass
  elderly, 854
Muscle metabolic economy, 728f
Muscle protein
  amino acids, 25t
Muscle proteolysis, 733
Muscularis propria, 1116
Myeloneuropathy
  in Cuban epidemic neuropathy, 1367
Myocardial infarction
  with magnesium deficiency, 237
Myocardial ischemia
  with alcoholism, 1255
Myopathy, 216
Myricetin, 1796t
Myristic acid, 1081
  cholesterol, 127

N
NAD. *See* Nicotinamide adenine dinucleotide
    (NAD)
NADPH. *See* Nicotinamide adenine
    dinucleotide phosphate (NADPH)
NAFL. *See* Nonalcoholic fatty liver (NAFL)
NAFLD. *See* Nonalcoholic fatty liver disease
    (NAFLD)
Nails
  nutritional deficiency, 838t
Nandrolone
  for weight loss, 1535
Napoleon
  food preservation, 1777
Naringenin, 1796t
NASH. *See* Nonalcoholic steatohepatitis
    (NASH)
Nasoenteral tubes, 1555
Nasogastric tubes, 1555
Nateglinide, 1062t
National Center for Complementary and
    Alternative Medicine (NCCAM),
    1771
National Cholesterol Education Program
  cholesterol-lowering diet, 1082t
National Council Against Health Fraud,
    1760
National Health and Nutrition Examination
    Survey (NHANES), 1688, 1690,
    1695–1696, 1696–1697
  overview of, 1694t
  retinol, 359
National Health and Nutrition Examination
    Survey III (NHANES III), 227
  adolescents, 819
  magnesium intakes, 230
  plasma carotenoids, 360
  vitamin K, 423
National Labeling Education Act (NLEA),
    1790, 1791–1792
National Nutrition Monitoring and Related
    Research Act (NNMRRA), 1687, 1692
National Nutrition Monitoring and Related
    Research Program (NNMRRP), 1687,
    1689t, 1691, 1692
  geographic coverage, 1698
National Nutrition Monitoring System
    (NNMS), 1688, 1693
  accomplishments of, 1697–1698
  limitations of, 1697–1698
Nationwide Food Consumption Survey
    (NFCS), 1690, 1693–1694, 1694
Natriuretic peptides, 651
Natural contaminants, 1817–1818
Natural foods
  with enteral feeding, 1557

Natural Health Products (NHP), 1794
Natural hygiene, 1765
Natural killer cells, 678
Natural toxicants, 1821–1822
Naturopathy, 1765
NCCAM. *See* National Center for
    Complementary and Alternative
    Medicine (NCCAM)
Near optimal low-density cholesterol levels,
    1078–1079
NEAT. *See* Non-exercise associated
    thermogenesis (NEAT)
Negative energy balance, 1019
Negative-feedback control
  of meal size, 709–710
Neonatal health
  public health objectives, 771
Nephrons
  distribution of, 154f
  Mg absorption, 229f
Nephrotic syndrome, 1491
  nutritional alterations in, 1482
Nervous system
  beriberi of, 599
  dysfunction, 219–220
N-6 essential fatty acids
  requirements, 114–116
Net protein balance, 38
Net protein gain, 38
Neural hormones, 649–650
Neural tube closure
  choline, 531
Neural tube defects (NTD), 781, 1156
  diet, 1629
  folate, 1374–1375
Neurocrine VIP, 1123t
Neuroendocrine response
  cytokines, 1392–1393
Neuroimmunoendocrine response, 1389
Neuropeptide Y, 712–713
  mediating altered metabolism in cancer, 1295
Neurotoxic shellfish poisoning, 1820
Neutral amino acids, 22
Neutralization tests, 1768
New York Heart Association (NYHA)
  CHF classification, 1108
New Zealand
  nutrient reference values, 1864t–1885t
  selenium, 313
N-3 fatty acids, 677, 1578
  requirements, 116–118
NFCS. *See* Nationwide Food Consumption
    Survey (NFCS)
NHANES. *See* National Health and Nutrition
    Examination Survey (NHANES)
NHP. *See* Natural Health Products (NHP)
Niacin, 7, 442–450, 600–601, 1812
  adenosine diphosphate ribose cyclases,
    446–447
  antihyperlipidemic effects, 449
  biochemical pathways, 447f
  chemical structure, 443f
  chemistry, 442
  deficiency, 448–449, 600–601, 1371
  DRI in elderly, 844t
  elderly, 848
  in enteral feeding products, 1558t
  formulations, 449–450
  functions, 446–448
  historical background, 442
  manifestations, 448–449
  metabolism, 445–446
  nicotinamide adenine dinucleotide
    consuming enzymes, 446

nomenclature, 442
nutrient status, 449
oxidant induced cell injury, 449
oxidation reduction reactions, 446
as pharmacologic agent, 449
pyridine nucleotide synthesis, 446
recommended dietary allowances, 444t
toxicity, 600–601
toxicology, 450
1989 *vs.* 2002 RDI, 831t
Nickel, 339, 345–346
  absorption, 345
  alcoholism, 1253
  analytic methods, 345
  beneficial effects, 346
  bioavailability, 345
  chemistry, 345
  dietary considerations, 346
  distribution, 345
  excretion, 345
  health effects, 346
  historical overview, 345
  mechanisms of action, 346
  toxicity, 346
  transport, 345
Nicotinamide
  biochemical pathways, 447f
  chemical structure, 443f
Nicotinamide adenine dinucleotide (NAD)
  structure, 444f
Nicotinamide adenine dinucleotide
    phosphate (NADPH), 301
Nicotinic acid
  for type V hyperlipoproteinemia, 1088
NIDDM. *See* Non-insulin-dependent
    diabetes mellitus (NIDDM)
Nigerian seasonal ataxia, 432
Night blindness, 363, 370, 1250
Night eating syndrome, 1022
Nitric oxide, 575f
  airway effects, 576
  biologic functions of, 574t
  cardiovascular system, 577–578
  endocrine system, 578
  formation, 573f, 687f
  gastrointestinal tract, 578
  hematologic system, 578
  hypertension, 578
  immune system, 579
  inflammation effects, 576
  renal system, 578
  reproductive system, 579
  respiratory system, 576–577, 577t
  synthase enzymes, 573t
  vascular effects, 576
Nitrogen
  balance, 33–36
    technique, 35, 35f
  feces, 35
  historical development of, 3–4
  in human milk, 788t, 789t
  species, 687–688
Nitzschia pungens, 1820
NLEA. *See* National Labeling Education Act
    (NLEA)
NNMRRA. *See* National Nutrition
    Monitoring and Related Research Act
    (NNMRRA)
NNMRRP. *See* National Nutrition
    Monitoring and Related Research
    Program (NNMRRP)
NNMS. *See* National Nutrition Monitoring
    System (NNMS)
Nonalcoholic fatty liver (NAFL), 1245

Nonalcoholic fatty liver disease (NAFLD), 1244–1245
Nonalcoholic steatohepatitis (NASH), 1245
Nonenzymatic glycosylation pathway, 1049f
Nonessential amino acids, 24, 24t
Non-exercise associated thermogenesis (NEAT), 1020
Non-Hispanic blacks
anthropometric measure, 1937t–1938t
Non-Hispanic whites
anthropometric measure, 1936t–1937t
Non-insulin-dependent diabetes mellitus (NIDDM), 1044
Nonphysician clinical professionals, 1601, 1602–1603
Nonprotein respiratory quotient (NPRQ), 140
carbohydrate and fat utilization, 139f, 140t
Nonselective newborn screening
criteria for, 910t
Nonsteroidal antiinflammatory medications (NSAID)
for chronic pancreatitis, 1233
gastrointestinal effects, 877t
nutrient interactions, 1327f
Nonvertebral fractures
bone mass, 1341f
Norandrolone propionate
for cancer, 1301t
Norepinephrine
cardiovascular response to, 650
protein synthesis, 650
Normal infants
daily reference intakes for, 799t
nutrient needs of, 797–802
tolerable upper intake nutrient levels, 800t
Northern analysis, 617–618
mRNAs, 619f
N-3 polyunsaturated fatty acids (alpha-linoleic acid)
DRI by life-stage group, 1864t
N-6 polyunsaturated fatty acids (linoleic acid)
DRI by life-stage group, 1863t
NPRQ. See Nonprotein respiratory quotient (NPRQ)
NSAID. See Nonsteroidal antiinflammatory medications (NSAID)
NTD. See Neural tube defects (NTD)
Nuclear magnetic resonance spectroscopy
Mg, 231
Nuclear receptor ligands, 1284t
in cancer chemoprevention, 1283–1285
Nuclear retinoid receptors, 356
Nucleic acids
Mg structural modification, 224
oxidants, 688
Nucleotides
in human milk, 790t
Null mutation animals, 625
Nurses' Health Study, 368, 1271, 1481
Nutraceuticals, 1790
Nutramigen, 1554
Nutrient(s)
absorption of, 1132–1139
early ideas about, 3
essential, 5t
evolution of knowledge about, 3–9
required to be declared, 1831
requirement indicators, 1668
Nutrient content claims, 1833–1834
Nutrient deficiency
among athletes, 1724
oral soft tissues, 1166–1167
with risk factor reduction, 1656

Nutrient infusate, 998–999
composition, 998t
Nutrient requirements
voluntary declaration of, 1831–1832
Nutrient risk assessment
steps in, 1666
Nutrients interaction
vitamin B6, 455
Nutrition
assimilation
gastrointestinal disorders affecting, 878t
claims, 1832–1833
drug interactions, 869–871
indices
elderly, 854–855
labeling, 1827–1837
future of, 1837
learning, 867–868
monitoring
historical overview, 1688–1693, 1690t
support
history of, 1415
transition, 1717–1722
policy implications, 1721–1722
Nutritional amblyopia, 1370
Nutritional assessment, 835–842
Nutritional availability, 8–9
Nutritional deficiencies
physical findings of, 838t
Nutritional examination, 835
Nutritional food additives, 1812–1813
Nutritional frailty, 852–853
Nutritional genomics, 615–626
defined, 617t
historical perspective, 615
Nutritional history, 835, 836t
Nutritional myeloneuropathy, 1366–1367
Nutritional needs
modification of, 8–9
Nutritional neuropathy, 1366–1367
Nutritional optic neuropathy, 1370
Nutritional requirements
age-related determinants, 844
defining, 1702–1703
genetic variation, 1626
Nutritional security, 1707
Nutritional status, 1688
social factors, 1747–1749
social stratification, 1747–1748
Nutritional support
competent patient, 1610–1614
as ethical issue, 1608–1609
timing and route, 1466–1467
Nutrition Facts Panel, 1829, 1830f, 1831
Nutritionist
roles of, 1604
Nutrition-related wrongdoing
complaints to, 1760t
Nutrition Risk Index, 841
Nuts
dietary fiber content of, 1967t
oxalate, 2109t
NYHA. See New York Heart Association (NYHA)
Nystagmus, 432

O
OAM. See Office of Alternative Medicine (OAM)
Oattrim
with diabetes mellitus, 1053
Obesity, 1013–1027. See also Childhood obesity
adolescents, 981

age, 1016
age adjusted prevalence, 1015f, 1954t
ancient metabolism in modern world, 1026
assessment of, 1029–1030
axokine, 1039
balanced-deficit diets, 1032
behavioral counseling, 1040
behavior therapy for, 1036–1038, 1037t
BMI, 1955t–1959t
body fluids, 150
breastfeeding, 982, 1025–1026
cancer, 1269–1270
changes in rates, 1015
chemical senses and diet, 703
children, 1016
chronic renal failure, 1492–1493
classification of, 1030t
comorbidities, 1030t
congenital causes of, 1021
depression, 1030
diabetes, 1599
dietary counseling, 1040
dietary fiber, 87
dietary intervention, 1031–1032
dietary variety, 1025
drug-related causes, 1021–1022, 1022t
early environmental factors, 1025–1026
eating disorders associated with, 1022–1023
economic consequences, 1027
elderly, 853
energy balance disorder, 1016–1019
energy expenditure, 1020–1021
energy intake, 1020
environmental and behavioral influences, 1023–1024
epidemic onset, 1026–1027
epidemiology, 1014–1016
family studies, 1019–1020
food cost and availability, 1025
gender, 1015–1016
genes, 1020–1021
genetics, 1019–1020
height and weight defining, 1953t
with hypercholesterolemia, 1078–1079, 1083–1084
with aging, 1080
lean tissue conservation, 739
low-calorie diets, 1032, 1032t
meal replacements, 1032–1033
medical disorders causing, 1021
neuroendocrine disorders causing, 1021
with nonalcoholic fatty liver disease, 1244–1245
parental, 1026
pharmacologic treatment of, 1038–1039
physical assessment of, 1029–1030
polygenic interactions, 1020
portion-controlled servings, 1032–1033
preconceptional health, 772
prenatal influences, 1025
prevalence, 1016t
psychosocial evaluation, 1030–1031
public health, 1026–1027
race, 1016
screening for, 980f
self-monitoring, 1037
single gene defects, 1020
skinfold, 1955t–1959t
societal issue, 1026
socioeconomic status, 1016
stimulus control, 1037
stroke, 1599

Obesity (*Continued*)
surgical treatment of, 1039–1040
treatment
selection of, 1031–1034, 1031t
visceral adipose tissue, 756
worldwide rates, 1026
Obstructive lung disease, 1467–1468
OC. *See* Osteocalcin (OC)
Occupations
gendered foods, 1744
Ocular retinoid metabolism
vitamin A, 362–363
Oculoorogenital syndrome, 600
Odd-chain fatty acids
biotin deficiency, 504
Office of Alternative Medicine (OAM), 1771
Ohmic heating, 1785–1786
Oil
iodized, 308
Olanzapine, 1360
Older infants
feeding, 804–807
Older people. *See* Elderly
Olestra, 1811, 1812
with diabetes mellitus, 1053
Olfaction, 697
Omega-3-fatty acids, 1798t
Omeprazole
producing cobalamin malabsorption, 492
Oncogenes, 1260–1261, 1261t
Oncology
websites for, 2026
One carbon metabolism, 633
One-carbon units
vitamin B6, 454–455
One-on-one interviewing, 1746
Open-ended interviewing, 1746
Ophthalmoplegia, 432
Opiates
inducing gastric emptying, 1181
Opioids
sweet taste, 709
Opsoclonic cerebellopathy, 432
Optic neuropathy
in Cuban epidemic neuropathy, 1367
Optimal low-density cholesterol levels,
1077–1078
Oral antidiabetes drug therapy
for diabetes mellitus, 1062–1063, 1062t
Oral cancer, 1172
aging, 1174
Oral cavity
nutrient excesses, 1167–1168
Oral dietary therapy
for cancer, 1297–1298
Oral health
aging, 1174
Oral infections
immune deficiency disease, 1172
Oral intake
short bowel syndrome, 1206f
Oral iron therapy, 262
Oral rehydration solution
short bowel syndrome, 1205f
vs. standard WHO solution, 897f
Oral soft tissues, 1166
Oral surgery, 1171–1172
Oral tissues
cellular and structural characteristics of,
1152–1155
development of, 1155–1157
Ordinary, 1612
Organ failure
nutritional support in, 1395–1396

Organic acidemias
tandem mass spectrometry, 942t–944t
Organic acidosis, 180–181
Organic acids, 932–946
biochemistry, 932–934
for inborn errors of metabolism, 1996t
Organic compounds
food content, 1989t–1993t
Oriental medicine, 1764
Oriyas, 1402
Orlistat
with diabetes mellitus, 1060
for obesity, 1038–1039
Ornithine, 1729
Ornithine transcarbamylase deficiency
expression of, 947
Ortholog
defined, 617t
Orthomolecular psychiatry, 1765
Orthomolecular therapy, 1765–1766
Orthostatic hypotension
dietary treatment of, 1376
Osborne, Thomas, 6
Osmolality, 149–160
specific gravity, 152
Osmoregulation
taurine, 557
Osmotic diuresis
polyuria, 169
Osteoarthritis, 1329–1330
defined, 1329
nutrient intakes, 1329
nutrient status, 1329
obesity, 1329–1330
Osteoblasts
functions, 1315–1316
Osteocalcin (OC), 416, 1315
Osteoclasts
functions, 1315–1316
Osteocytes
bone mechanical function, 1318
functions, 1315–1316
Osteogenesis imperfecta, 1322
Osteomalacia, 597, 1321–1322
after surgery, 1187
Osteopenia, 1321
Osteoporosis, 604, 1321, 1339–1350, 1340f
alcohol, 1347
alendronate, 1349
alveolar bone, 1169
bisphosphonates, 1349
boron, 1347
caffeine, 1347
calcitonin, 1349
calcium, 205
copper, 851
with copper deficiency, 607
cystic fibrosis, 1471
epidemiology, 1340–1341
fractures
epidemiology, 1341–1342
lactation impact on, 794
with magnesium deficiency, 239
prevention, 1349
soy effects, 592
treatment, 1349–1350
vegetarian diets, 1646
Osteosclerosis
alcohol, 1321
Ovarian cancer
lactation impact on, 793–794
nutritional support of, 1306
Overweight
age-adjusted prevalence of, 1954t

BMI, 1890t
classification of, 1030t
with hypercholesterolemia, 1078–1079
Oxalate
breads, 2015t
food content, 2014t–2023t
national organizations, 2023
Oxalic acid
calcium absorption, 201
Oxaloacetate, 27–28
Oxandrolone
injury, 1433
Oxidants
macromolecules, 688–689
Oxidation products
toxicity, 106f
Oxidative stress, 685–688, 686f
arthritis, 693
disease, 692–693
oxygen species, 685–687
Oxygen consumption, 139
defined, 1464t

P

PA. *See* Proanthocyanidins (PA)
Packaging containers
chemical migrating from, 1816
PAEE. *See* Physical activity energy
expenditure (PAEE)
Paget disease of bone, 1322
PAL. *See* Physical activity level (PAL)
Palliative care, 1307–1308, 1619
Palmitic acid, 1080–1081
PAM. *See* Peptidylglycine alpha amidating
monooxygenase (PAM)
Pancreas
function of, 1131–1132
Pancreatic cancer, 1233
nutritional support of, 1305–1306
Pancreatic disorders, 1227–1234
Pancreatic enzymatic replacement,
1232–1233
Pancreatic hormones, 638–640
affecting metabolism and food intake, 1046t
Pancreatic islets
controlling meal size, 710
Pancreatic lipase, 96–98, 97
Pancreatic polypeptide, 1123t
Pancreatic proteases, 1137t
Pancreatic pseudocysts
with pancreatitis, 1230
Pancreatitis, 1227–1228. *See also* Acute
pancreatitis; Chronic pancreatitis
chronic, 1230–1233
clinical assessment, 1227–1228
clinical predictors or severity, 1228
clinical presentation, 1227
complications, 1230
EN *vs.* TPN, 1229–1230
glutamine for, 566
with hypomagnesemia, 233
Paneth cells, 1118–1119
Pantothenic acid. *See* Vitamin B5
(pantothenic acid)
Paracrine, 1123t
Paralytic shellfish poisoning, 1820
Parathyroid hormone (PTH)
bone, 1319
bone resorption, 1316
for chronic renal failure, 1495–1496
dysfunction, 1322
with hypomagnesemia, 235–236
Mg absorption, 229
for osteoporosis, 1350

Paravalbumin
  calcium, 195t
Parent-child interactions, 879t
Parenteral lipid emulsions, 999–1001
Parenteral multivitamins
  composition of, 1586t
    for children, 1587t
  FDA recommendations, 1422t
Parenteral nutrition, 1567–1594
  amino acids, 1578–1581
  Candida albicans, 1571
  carbohydrates, 1572–1573
  components, 1571–1588
  delivery systems, 1570–1571
  drug compatibility, 1591, 1591t
  glucose ventilatory response8, 1574
  hyperglycemia, 1573–1574
  indications for, 1568–1569, 1568t
  in infants and children, 997–1002
  lipids, 1574–1578, 1574t
  minerals, 1580–1582
  nomenclature, 1568
  organ function complications, 1588–1591
  pulmonary issues, 1466–1467
  requirements, 1571–1588
  serum glucose, 1573–1574
  short bowel syndrome, 1206–1207
  trace elements, 1581–1582, 1582t
  venous access, 1569–1570
  vitamins, 1585–1587
  water, 1571–1572
Parietal cells, 1117, 1129, 1183
Parkinson disease, 1365–1366
Paroxysmal nocturnal dyspnea, 1109
PARP. *See* Poly(ADP-ribose) polymerase
    (PARP)
Partial lipoprotein lipase deficiency, 1070
Partial pressure of oxygen in arterial blood
  defined, 1464t
Pasta
  mineral content, 1979t, 1982t
  protein content, 1979t
Pasteurization, 1781–1782
Pathologic anorexia
  in elderly, 1533–1534, 1533t
Patient decision making
  consequences, 1614
Patient education
  traditional *vs.* self-management, 1603t
Patient health literacy, 1600
Patient-physician differences
  resolution of, 1612
Patient-physician interaction
  decision making, 1610–1611
Patient Self Determination Act of 1990,
    1613–1614, 1618
Patterson-Kelly (Plummer-Vinson) syndrome,
    607
PC. *See* Pyruvate carboxylase (PC)
PCC. *See* Propionyl CoA carboxylase (PCC)
PCR. *See* Polymerase chain reaction (PCR)
PDGF. *See* Platelet-derived growth factors
    (PDGF)
Peak bone mass
  calcium, 206
Pediatric feeding problems, 875–880
Pediatric Nutrition Surveillance System
    (PedNSS), 1698
Pediatric palliative care
  attitude changes in, 1619
PEG. *See* Percutaneous endoscopic
    gastrostomy (PEG)
Pellagra, 448, 1371
  cultural ecology, 1742

Penicillamine
  chelating zinc, 280
  copper interactions, 294
  nutrient interactions, 1327f
Penicillium, 1819
Pentamidine
  with Mg wasting, 233
Pentoxifylline
  for cancer, 1301t, 1302
Pepsinogen, 1184
Peptic ulcers
  diet in, 1185
  short bowel syndrome, 1207
Peptides, 712
Peptide YY, 1123t
  affecting metabolism and food intake,
    1046t
Peptidylglycine alpha amidating
    monooxygenase (PAM), 287
Percutaneous endoscopic gastrostomy (PEG),
    1555–1556
Perillyl alcohol, 1800
Periodontal disease, 1168–1169
Periodontitis
  aging, 1174
Periodontium
  nutrient effects on, 1170t
Peripherally inserted central catheters
    (PICC) lines, 1569
Peripheral neuropathy
  in Cuban epidemic neuropathy, 1367
Peripheral parenteral nutrition (PPN), 1567
  acute renal failure, 1504
Peristalsis, 1121, 1128
Peristaltic reflex, 1122f
Perleche, 600
Pernicious anemia, 482, 491–492, 601
  defined, 483t
Peroxisomal beta-oxidation
  defects
    diagnosis, 971t
    metabolites, 971t
    enzymes of, 962t
Peroxisomal biogenesis defects, 968–969
Peroxisome proliferator activated receptor(s)
    (PPAR), 111, 1074
Peroxisome proliferator activated receptor
    alpha (PPAR alpha), 641
Peroxisomes, 960, 963–964
  beta-oxidation of fatty acids in, 961f
Persistent vegetative state (PVS), 1615
Personal Responsibility and Work
    Opportunity Reconciliation Act
    (PRWORA), 862
Peru
  optimal iodine nutrition programs, 309
PGE. *See* Prostaglandin E (PGE)
Phantom smells, 699
Phantom taste, 699
Pharmacodynamics
  defined, 1540
Pharmacokinetics
  defined, 1540
Pharyngeal cancer, 1172
Pharynx, 1179
PHE. *See* Phenylalanine (PHE)
Phenelzine, 1360
Phenolic acids
  phenolic phytochemicals in, 1991t
Phenolic compounds, 583, 1796t,
    1801–1802
Phenolic phytochemicals
  food content, 1991t–1993t
Phenols, 593

Phenothiazines
  inducing gastric emptying, 1181
Phentermine, 987
  for obesity, 1039
Phenylalanine (PHE), 8, 910
  flux, 41
  phenylketonuria
    pregnancy, 2000t
  restricted diet, 1999t
Phenylalanine-free medical foods, 922
Phenylketonuria (PKU), 910, 916–925
  aromatic amino acids for, 1995t
  chronic care, 919
  diagnosis, 919
  diet discontinuation, 924
  management problems, 922–923
  maternal, 924–925, 925t
  molecular biology, 916–919
  nutrient requirements, 919–921
  nutrition support, 919, 923
  pregnancy, 773, 2000t
  sample diets, 1999t
  screening, 919
  treatment, 919, 923–924
Phenytoin
  with enteral feeding, 1565
Phosphates
  Mg, 228
  sports nutrition, 1731
  sports performance, 1731
Phosphatidylcholine, 532
  biosynthesis, 530–531
Phospholipase A2
  calcium, 195t
Phospholipid(s), 94
  absorption, 99
  digestion, 99
  liver, 1243–1244
Phospholipid methyltransferase
  alcoholism, 1244
Phosphorus, 211–221, 604–605. *See also*
    Minerals
  absorption, 212
  bone and teeth, 1320
  chemistry of, 211
  in children, 211, 802
  chronic renal failure, 1478–1479
  for chronic renal failure, 1494–1495
  deficiency, 605
    tooth development, 1155t
  dietary reference intake
    in normal infants and children, 802
    values, 212t
  dietary sources, 212
  in enteral feeding products, 1558t
  functions, 213
  intrauterine accretion rates
    during third trimester, 809t
  metabolism of, 212–213
  in normal infants, 802
  osteoporosis, 1344
  parenteral diet, 1430–1431
  parenteral nutrition, 1580–1581
  pregnancy, 778
  properties of, 211
  1989 RDA *vs.* 2002 RDI, 819t
  renal handling, 212
  replacement therapy, 1431t
  total body content, 212
  toxicity, 605
  1989 *vs.* 2002 RDI, 831t
Phosphorus balance, 1323
Phosphorus deficiency
  effect of, 215–216

Photobiology, 378–382
  history, 378
Photoisiomerization, 362
Photosynthesis
  previtamin D3, 378–381
Phycotoxins, 1819–1820
Phylloquinone. *See* Vitamin K (phylloquinone)
Physical activity, 143–144
  adolescents, 824–825
  amount required, 725–726
  benefits of, 1036
  Dietary Guidelines for Americans, 1894
  economics of, 1025
  examples of, 1084t
  with hypercholesterolemia, 1084, 1085t
  improved function, 727
  for insulin resistance, 1091
  international dietary guidelines, 1711t
  LDC, 1720
  mortality, 724–725
  osteoporotic fractures, 1348
  weight maintenance, 725
Physical activity energy expenditure (PAEE),
    1017, 1018, 1023–1024
Physical activity level (PAL), 143
  adolescents, 819
Physical examination
  with chronic pancreatitis, 1231
  nutritional risk factors, 1167t
Physician-patient relations
  changing, 1600–1601
  changing attitudes in, 1601–1605
  chronic care model, 1602
  collaborative care, 1602
  collaborative care *vs.* traditional care, 1602t
  patient self-management, 1602
Physicians' Health Study, 319, 1470
  beta carotene, 365
Physiologic anorexia
  in elderly, 1532–1534, 1533f
Phytate
  copper interactions, 294
  zinc, 273, 274t
Phytic acid
  calcium absorption, 201
Phytochemicals, 582–593, 1790
  anticancer activities, 1799f
Phytoestrogens, 1802
Phytosterolemia, 1073
  genetic causes of, 1074t
Phytosterols, 130–132
  cholesterolemia, 130–131
  serum levels and atherogenesis, 131–132
  toxicity studies, 131–132
Piaglitizone, 1062t, 1091
Pica, 1441
PICC. *See* Peripherally inserted central
    catheters (PICC) lines
Picky eaters
  improving mealtime behaviors, 879t
PINI. *See* Prognostic Inflammatory and
    Nutritional Index (PINI)
Pitressin tannate
  for polyuria, 170
Pitting edema
  with congestive heart failure, 1109–1110
Pivalic acid
  carnitine interaction, 542
PKU. *See* Phenylketonuria (PKU)
Plants, 582, 583
  breeding, 1708
  enhanced micronutrients, 1708
  stanols
    with hypercholesterolemia, 1085t

Plasma aldosterone, 164
Plasma antioxidants, 692
Plasma branched chain amino acids
    fasting, 733
Plasma carotenoids, 360
Plasma electrolytes, 150
Plasma lipoproteins
  dietary factors influencing, 103–104
Plasma osmolality, 151–152
Plasma renin, 164
Plasma retinol, 359–360
  transport protein, 360–362
    tissue uptake, 361
    transport kinetics, 361
Plasma selenium, 320, 320f
Plasma transthyretin, 360
Plasma urea nitrogen (PUN)
  glomerular filtration rate, 1482f
Plasma vitamin A
  vitamin A storage, 360
Plasma vitamin E
  kinetics, 401
Platelet-derived growth factors (PDGF), 652
Platelet disorders, 219
Plummer-Vinson syndrome, 607
PNI. *See* Prognostic Nutritional Index (PNI)
Poisonous animals, 1821
Poisonous mushrooms, 1822–1823
Poisonous plants, 1821–1822
Polyacrylamide electrophoresis
  proteins, 623–624
Polybrominated biphenyls, 1816–1817
Polychlorinated biphenyls, 1816–1817
Polycystic ovary syndrome, 1021
Polygenic
  defined, 617t
Polymerase chain reaction (PCR), 619, 620f
Polymeric formulas, 1557
Polymorphisms, 627–634
Polyol pathway, 1049f
Polyols
  with diabetes mellitus, 1055t
Poly(ADP-ribose) polymerase (PARP), 442, 448
Polyunsaturated fat
  adolescents, 820
  healthy diet, 1627
Polyunsaturated fatty acids (PUFA), 8, 115,
    1798t
  AMDR for, 1857
  cholesterol, 127
  with Crohn's disease, 1210
  DRI by life-stage group, 1863t, 1864t
  lactation, 118
  lipid peroxidation, 106
  phenylketonuria
    pregnancy, 2000t
  tissue membrane, 111
Polyunsaturated polyenylphosphatidylcholines
    (PPC)
  cirrhosis, 1244
Polyuria, 169–171
  diagnosis, 170f
  differential diagnosis, 169–170
    osmotic diuresis, 169
  treatment, 170–171
  water diuresis, 169, 169t
Polyvinyl chloride (PVC) bags, 1570–1571
Poor. *See* Poverty
Population dietary intakes
  nutritional adequacy of, 1704
Population trends, 1718
Pork consumption
  cultural ecology, 1743
Pork gelatin, 1519

Porphyria cutanea tarda, 262
Porpranolol
  for polyuria, 171
Positional cloning, 623
Positive bone remodeling, 1324
Positive energy balance, 1019
Positive-feedback control
  of meal size, 708–709, 709f
Postoperative patients
  glutamine with, 567–568
Potassium, 605
  blood pressure, 164
  chronic renal failure, 1497
  deficiency, 605
  Dietary Guidelines for Americans, 1895
  dietary sources of, 161
  DRI by life-stage group, 1866t
  in enteral feeding products, 1558t
  food content, 161f
  intrauterine accretion rates during third
      trimester, 809t
  magnesium absorption, 229
  metabolism, 160–167
    disorders, 187–188
  parenteral administration of, 18
  parenteral diet, 1429–1430
  pregnancy, 777–778
  recycling, 162–164, 163f
  renal excretion, 161–162
  requirements for, 1857
  secretion at cortical collecting duct, 162f
  toxicity, 605
  transcellular flux, 160–164, 160f
Potential renal solute load (PSRL), 18
Poultry
  household production of, 1707
  labeling, 1832
Poverty
  behavior, 866–867
  consequences, 862–863
  defined, 861–862
  ecology of, 868
  family size, 862t
  food insecurity, 864–865
  growth, 863–864
  interventions, 871–872
  learning, 866–867
  malnutrition, 865–866
  micronutrient status, 864
  nutritional status, 863–865
  and nutrition transition, 1720–1721
  overnutrition, 864
  public policy, 871–872
PPA. *See* Propionic acidemia (PPA)
PPAR. *See* Peroxisome proliferator activated
    receptor(s) (PPAR)
PPC. *See* Polyunsaturated
    polyenylphosphatidylcholines (PPC)
PPI. *See* Proton pump inhibitor (PPI)
PPN. *See* Peripheral parenteral nutrition
    (PPN)
Prader-Willi syndrome, 1021
Pravastatin
  for hypercholesterolemia, 1085t
Prealbumin (transthyretin)
  elderly, 853
Prebiotics, 1798t
Preconceptional health, 771–773
Preeclampsia, 781
  with hypermagnesemia, 240–241
  with magnesium deficiency, 238–239
Pregnancy, 771–782
  adolescents, 826–827
    maternal growth during, 826

alcohol, 779
biotin, 777
caffeine, 779
calcium, 207
carbohydrate, 775
    DRI, 1861t
cardiac output, 773
chloride, 777
    DRI, 1867t
with choline, 777
    deficiency, 531
chromium, 778
cocaine, 779
copper, 778
with diabetes mellitus, 1057–1058
dietary supplements, 779–780
drug abuse, 869–870
EFAs, 118
electrolytes, 776–777
elements
    DRI, 1870t
    UL, 1871t
energy
    DRI, 1859t
    requirements, 144, 146–147, 774
exercise, 780
fluoride, 778
folate deficiency, 1454–1455
gastrointestinal problems, 780
herbal supplements, 779–780
hypertension, 781
illicit drugs, 779
iodine, 303, 778
iron
    dietary reference intakes, 1439t
    requirements, 1438
kidneys, 773
last trimester
    intrauterine accretion rates of, 809t
macrominerals, 778
magnesium, 778
manganese, 779
    DRI, 327t
marijuana, 779
maternal physiologic changes during, 773
minerals
    recommended dietary allowances, 1872t
nutrient requirements, 774–778
pantothenic acid, 777
phosphorus, 778
    DRI, 212t
potassium, 777–778
    DRI, 1866t
public health objectives, 771
PUFA DRI, 1863t, 1864t
respiratory system, 773
riboflavin
    DRI, 439t
selenium, 779
smoking, 779
sodium, 777
    DRI, 1867t
sulfur amino acids
    RDA, 548
thiamin
    dietary sources, 427t
third trimester
    intrauterine accretion rates of nutrients,
        809t
total fat DRI, 1863t
total fiber DRI, 1862t
total water DRI, 1865t
trace minerals, 778–779
vegetarian diets, 1647

vitamin(s)
    DRI, 1868t
    RDA, 1872t
    UL, 1869t
vitamin A, 367
    requirements, 354t
vitamin B6, 777
vitamin B12, 777
vitamin C, 521–522
vitamin D
    DRI, 391t
vitamin E
    DRI, 407t
water, 776–777
water-soluble vitamins, 775–776
weight gain, 773–774, 774t
Pregnancy Nutrition Surveillance System
    (PregNSS), 1698
Premature infants, 8
Preoperative patients
    glutamine with, 567–568
Prescriptions
    problems in adherence to, 1600
President's Commission for the Study of
    Ethical Problems in Medicine and
    Biomedical and Behavioral Research,
    1611–1612
Pressure ulcer
    zinc, 851
Preterm infant formulas
    essential amino acid recommendations for,
        812t
PRGP. See Proline rich Gla proteins (PRGP)
Priestley, Joseph, 11
Primary biliary cirrhosis
    copper, 1245
Primary polydipsia, 169
Principalism, 1609
Prion protein, 288
Proanthocyanidins (PA), 583
    absorption, 589
    analysis, 584
    biologic effect, 589
    chemistry, 588–589
    dietary source, 588–589
    health effects, 585t
    intakes, 588–589
    metabolism, 589
Probiotics, 1798t
Product quality, 1836
Professional societies, 1606
Prognostic Inflammatory and Nutritional
    Index (PINI), 1417
Prognostic Nutritional Index (PNI), 1417
Programmed cell death, 676–677
Progressive hyperphagic obesity, 1022–1023
Prohormones
    athletes, 1736
    sports nutrition, 1736
Proinflammatory cytokine peptides, 1391
Proinflammatory cytokines
    mediating altered metabolism in cancer,
        1294
Prolamin peptides
    celiac disease, 1221
Proline, 25
Proline rich Gla proteins (PRGP), 416
Prolonged fasting, 731–733
Promoter analysis, 621–622
Propionibacterium, 415
Propionic acidemia (PPA), 910, 941–945,
    1997t
    sample diet for, 2003t
    tandem mass spectrometry, 943t

Propionyl CoA carboxylase (PCC), 499
Prosky method, 85
Prospective studies
    of diet effect on cancer, 1268t
Prostaglandin
    formation of, 112f, 114f
    in human milk, 790t
Prostaglandin E (PGE)
    feedback regulation, 662f
Prostanoids
    for asthma, 1470
Prostate cancer
    calcium, 1274
    dairy products, 1273
    dietary fat, 1628
    fruits and vegetables, 1273
    lycopene, 365
    meat, 1272
    soy effects, 592
    vitamin D, 1274
Protein, 21–56, 1728
    above and below requirement level,
        735–736
    absorption, 46–47, 47f
    acute renal failure, 1500–1502
    adolescents, 820
    array
        defined, 617t
    biologic assays, 53–54
    bound biotin
        digestion, 501
    calcified tissue, 416
    calcium, 202
    calorie malnutrition, 1323
        tooth development, 1155t
    cancer, 1272
    catabolic rate
        assessment of, 837–838
    and children, 800t, 801
    cholesterol, 128–129
    for chronic renal failure, 1478, 1487t
    for CPD, 1487t
    deficiency, 735–737
    degradation, 43–44
    with diabetes mellitus, 1052–1053
    digestion of, 1137–1138, 1184
    DRI
        in elderly, 844t
        for infants, 799t
        by life-stage group, 1864t
    dysmetabolism, 833
    effects on periodontium, 1170t
    efficiency ratio, 53
    elderly, 845, 853–854
    energy, 137t
        substrate, 21
    energy deficiency, 737–740
        hemodynamic alterations, 898–899
        hyperthermia, 899
        hypothermia, 899
        infection, 898
        nutritional status homeostasis, 899–903
        severe anemia, 899
        severe vitamin A deficiency, 899
    energy malnutrition, 881–906, 895f, 1458,
        1484–1485
        adaptive responses, 883–887
        anthropometric measurements, 890–891
        biochemical changes, 896t
        biologic factors, 882–883
        cardiovascular functions, 886–887
        chronic renal failure, 1484t
        classification of, 889–890, 889t
        diarrhea, 904

Protein (*Continued*)
  dietary treatment of, 900–902, 900t, 901t, 902t
  education, 906
  in elderly, 1532
  endocrine changes, 884–885
  energy mobilization, 883–884
  environmental factors, 883
  enzyme, 884f
  epidemiology, 882–883
  etiology, 882–883
  flag sign, 894f
  food availability, 905–906
  hematology, 885–886, 886f
  hormonal changes, 885t
  host age, 883
  infection, 906
  inflammation, 1485–1486
  nutritional rehabilitation, 903–904
  obesity, 752f
  oxygen transport, 885–886
  pathophysiology, 883–887
  poor prognosis, 896t
  prevention and control, 905–906
  prognosis, 895–896
  protein breakdown and synthesis, 884
  severity classification, 890t
  social and economic factors, 882
  treatment, 896–905
  energy metabolism, 832–833
  in enteral feeding, 1560–1561
    products, 1558t
  food content, 1978t–1980t
  in formulas, 805t
    hydrolyzed, 806t
    for infants, 806t
    for low birth weight infants, 813t
    for term infants, 804t
  free diet
    nitrogen losses, 35t
  fuel, 722
  gluten free foods, 2008t
  heat equivalents, 137t
  historical development of, 4
  in human milk, 788t, 789t, 790t
  hydrolysates, 1518
  and infants, 800t, 801
  intrauterine accretion rates during third trimester, 809t
  liver regulation, 1236
  low birth weight, 812–813
    intake recommendations, 810t
  malabsorption of, 1145t
  malnutrition
    with alcoholism, 1247
  metabolism, 733–734
    adaptation to starvation, 741–742
    AIDS, 1385–1386
    cancer, 1385
    injury and sepsis, 1384–1385
    intermediary metabolism changes, 1419
  metabolites, 1728
  for MHD, 1487t
  minimum requirement, 735
  needs in disease, 55–56
  osteoporosis, 1344–1346
  oxidants, 688
  pantothenic acid, 465
  phenylketonuria
    pregnancy, 2000t
  PKU, 922
  pregnancy, 774–775
  quality assessment, 53–54
  1989 RDA *vs.* 2002 RDI, 819t

recommended dietary allowances, 50–51
recommended intakes, 50t
reference nutrient intakes
  UK, 1877t
renal function, 1477
requirements, 49–51
restricted diet, 1999t
scoring systems, 54
source of, 21
in soy formulas, 806t
and sports performance, 1727–1730
sulfhydryls
  oxidative reactions, 691f
synthesis, 42–43
tolerable upper intake
  for normal infants and children, 800t
turnover, 34f, 38f, 738
  measurement, 33–44, 33t
vegetarian diets, 1641
1989 *vs.* 2002 RDI, 831t
Protein kinase C
  calcium, 195t
Proteolysis-inducing factor
  mediating altered metabolism in cancer, 1293–1294
Proteomics
  defined, 617t
Prothrombin, 415
Prothrombin time, 839t
Proton pump inhibitor (PPI)
  with acid secretion, 1183–1184
  for chronic pancreatitis, 1232–1233
Protooncogenes, 1260
Provitamin A carotenoids, 352–353
Provocation tests, 1768
Proximal gastric vagotomy, 1186
PRWORA. *See* Personal Responsibility and Work Opportunity Reconciliation Act (PRWORA)
Pseudohyperkalemia, 166
Pseudohyponatremia, 171, 171t
Pseudomonas cocovenenans, 1818
Pseudotumor cerebri
  with childhood obesity, 984
PSRL. *See* Potential renal solute load (PSRL)
Psychotropic medications, 1360
  gastrointestinal effects, 877t
Pteroylmonoglutamic acid. *See* Folic acid (pteroylmonoglutamic acid)
PTH. *See* Parathyroid hormone (PTH)
PUFA. *See* Polyunsaturated fatty acids (PUFA)
Pufferfish, 1821
Pufferfish poisoning, 1818, 1820–1821
Pulmonary hypertension, 1472
Pulmonary insufficiency
  enteral feeding, 1559
Pulmonary pathophysiology, 1464–1465
Pulmonary physiology, 1463–1464
PUN. *See* Plasma urea nitrogen (PUN)
Purine
  biosynthesis, 32–33
  food content, 1328
PVC. *See* Polyvinyl chloride (PVC) bags
PVS. *See* Persistent vegetative state (PVS)
Pyloric sphincter, 1117
Pylorus, 1180
Pyridoxal
  structure, 453f
Pyridoxamine
  structure, 453f
Pyridoxine. *See* Vitamin B6 (pyridoxine)
Pyrimidine
  biosynthesis, 32–33

Pyrrolizidine alkaloids, 1822
Pyruvate, 28, 722, 1725
Pyruvate carboxylase (PC), 499
  with manganese, 326
Pyruvate dehydrogenase, 1368

Q
Quackery, 1752
  dangers of, 1759
  spotting, 1753t
  vulnerability, 1752
Quackwatch, 1760
Qualified health claims, 1835–1836, 1835t
Quality control, 1756
Quality guidelines
  inadequate adherence to, 1599–1600
Quality of care, 1605
Quality of life
  home parenteral nutrition, 1592–1593
Quantitative real-time polymerase chain reaction (Q-PCR), 620–621, 620f, 621f
Quercetin, 1796t
  absorption, 586
  biologic effects, 587
  dietary intake, 584
  metabolism, 586
Quietapine, 1360
Quinlan case, 1615
Quinolones
  nutrient interactions, 1551t

R
RA. *See* Retinoic acid (RA)
Rabbits
  household production of, 1707
Radiation
  glutamine with, 567
Radiation therapy
  inducing gastric emptying, 1181
Radioiodine studies, 302
Radionuclide gastric emptying study, 1182
Radius
  fractures
    osteoporosis, 1341
  in tennis players *vs.* nonathletic controls, 1319f
RAE. *See* Retinol activity equivalent (RAE)
Rales
  with congestive heart failure, 1109
Raloxifene, 1284t
  for osteoporosis, 1349–1350
Rapliginide, 1062t
RAR. *See* Retinoic acid receptors (RAR)
RA receptor response elements (RARE), 356
Ras oncogene, 1260
RBP. *See* Retinol binding proteins (RBP)
RBR. *See* Retinoid binding receptors (RBR)
RDA. *See* Recommended dietary allowances (RDA)
RDH. *See* Retinol dehydrogenase (RDH)
RE. *See* Retinol equivalent (RE)
Receptive relaxation, 1180
Recombinant erythropoietin
  functional iron deficiency with, 1444
Recommended dietary allowances (RDA), 1660f, 1660t, 1829, 1853–1854
  coefficient of variation, 1661–1662
  comparison of, 1854–1855
  current uses of, 1657–1658
  definition, 1853t
  in infants and children, 798
  model for establishing, 1659–1662
  for normal infants, 798

origins of, 1655–1656
past uses of, 1657t
revised 1989, 1972t
1989 values *vs.* 2002, 819t
1989 *vs.* 2002, 831t
Recommended Dietary Allowances of the Food and Nutrition Board, 1852
Recommended dietary reference values, 1852–1900
Recommended food score (RFS), 1680
Recommended Nutrient Intakes, 1852
Recommended nutrient intakes (RNI), 1702
Rectal cancer
meat, 1272
nutritional support of, 1306
Rectum
anatomy of, 1120
Red blood cell folate, 472–473
Redux, 987
adverse effects of, 1472
REE. *See* Resting energy expenditure (REE)
Refeeding syndrome, 743–744, 1357
Reference heights, 1857–1858, 1858t
Reference values, 765–766
need for additional, 1656–1657
Reference weights, 1857–1858, 1858t
Refractory celiac disease, 1224
Refsum disease, 969
Regional enteritis
with hypomagnesemia, 233
in infants and children, 994–995
Regulatory categories, 1828
REH. *See* Retinyl ester hydrolases (REH)
Related health status, 1688
Religious views, 1612
Remodeling transient, 1324
Renal acidosis, 179–180
genesis, 179f
Renal disease
chemical senses and diet, 703
with diabetes mellitus, 1058
vegetarian diets, 1650
Renal failure. *See also* Acute renal failure; Chronic renal failure
angiotensin converting enzyme inhibitor, 1479
angiotensin receptor blockers, 1479
calcitriol, 1498–1499
chronic, 1479–1499
hypermagnesemia, 241
progression of, 1477–1482, 1478t
Renal stones
short bowel syndrome, 1207
Renal system
arginine, 578
Renal tubular acidosis (RTA), 179–180
Renin, 164, 1476
Reperfusion injury
oxidative stress, 693
Reproductive system
arginine, 579
Resistance training, 728
Resistant starch, 64–65
as dietary fiber, 84
Resistin, 643–644
Respiratory acidosis, 184–185, 185t
Respiratory alkalosis, 185, 185t
Respiratory infection
with malnutrition, 1405
Respiratory insufficiency, 217–218
nutritional support in, 1395
Respiratory muscles, 1465
structure of, 1462–1463

Respiratory physiology
abbreviations, 1464t
terms, 1464t
Respiratory quotient (RQ), 139
defined, 1464t
Respiratory system
arginine, 576–577
development of, 1465
function of, 1462–1463
during pregnancy, 773
structure of, 1462–1463
Response element
defined, 617t
Resting energy expenditure (REE), 731, 734, 1017, 1211, 1901t, 1904t, 1905f–1907f
acute pancreatitis, 1229
cancer, 1383f
protein energy deficiency, 737
refeeding syndrome, 744
Resting metabolic rate (RMR), 1020, 1023
Resveratrol, 1796t
Retailers, 1755–1756
Retinal, 357
Retinal dehydrogenase, 361
Retinal pigment epithelium (RPE), 356
Retinin
calcium, 195
Retinitis pigmentosa
with vitamin E deficiency, 404
Retinoblastoma gene product, 1265f
Retinoic acid (RA), 351
embryonic development, 363–364
plasma, 361
tissues, 361
Retinoic acid receptors (RAR), 355, 356
Retinoic X receptors (RXR), 355, 356
Retinoid(s)
cancer, 366–367
dermatology, 366
emphysema, 367
excretion, 362
intestinal metabolism, 358f
metabolism, 355f, 362f
structure, 352f
use of, 366–367
vitamin A deficiency, 366
Retinoid binding receptors (RBR)
vitamin A, 355
Retinoid induced birth defects, 368
Retinoid receptors, 351
Retinol. *See* Vitamin A (retinol)
Retinol activity equivalent (RAE), 353
Retinol binding proteins (RBP), 351, 355
hepatic metabolism, 359
vitamin A, 355
Retinol dehydrogenase (RDH), 361
Retinol equivalent (RE), 353
Retinyl ester hydrolases (REH), 357
Retorting, 1782
Reverse transcriptase polymerase chain reaction, 619–620
Rexinoids, 1285
RFS. *See* Recommended food score (RFS)
Rhabdomyolysis, 216–217
Rheumatic diseases
defined, 1326
oxidative stress, 693
Rheumatoid arthritis, 1330–1331
body composition, 1332
defined, 1330
diet therapy, 1332–1333
fasting, 1333–1334
food allergy, 1333, 1333t

nutrient intakes, 1331
nutritional status, 1330–1331, 1331–1332, 1331t
vegetarian diets, 1333–1334, 1650
vitamins, 1331
Rhizopus oryzae, 1818
Rhodopsin, 362
Riboflavin. *See* Vitamin B2 (riboflavin)
Ribose, 1725
Rice
mineral content, 1979t, 1982t
protein content, 1979t
Rickets, 5, 208, 377, 377f, 597, 1321–1322
Rifampin, 1570
Rimonabant
for obesity, 1039
Risk assessment, 1823–1824
model, 1666f
Risk factors
contribution to disease burden in developing countries, 1718t
Risk management, 1824–1825
RMR. *See* Resting metabolic rate (RMR)
RNA interference
defined, 617t
gene expression, 625–626
RNase protection assays, 618–619
RNI. *See* Recommended nutrient intakes (RNI)
Rods, 362
Root caries, 1161–1162
Rosiglitazone, 1062t, 1091, 1284t
Rosuvastatin
for hypercholesterolemia, 1085t
Roux-en-Y gastric bypass
with diabetes mellitus, 1060
Roxarsone, 339
RPE. *See* Retinal pigment epithelium (RPE)
R protein, 1127, 1184
RQ. *See* Respiratory quotient (RQ)
RTA. *See* Renal tubular acidosis (RTA)
Rubner, Max, 13
Russia
optimal iodine nutrition programs, 309
RXR. *See* Retinoic X receptors (RXR)

S
Saccharin, 1812
dental caries, 1160
with diabetes mellitus, 1055t
S-adenosylmethionine
liver injury, 1238–1241
remethylation *vs.* transsulfuration, 552
Safe range of intake, 1657f
Salicylate-nutrient interactions, 1327f
Saliva, 1179
dental caries, 1161
oral health, 1172–1173
Salivary amylase, 1179
Salivary glands, 1127–1128
Salt
blood pressure, 155–156
with hypercholesterolemia, 1085t
international dietary guidelines, 1712t
iodized, 307
Salt replacement, 159
Saponins, 593, 1796t
Sarcopenia
elderly, 1534
Satiety
dietary fiber, 87
Saturated fat
with hypercholesterolemia, 1085t
1989 *vs.* 2002 RDI, 831t

Saxitoxins, 1820
SCFA. *See* Short chain fatty acids (SCFA)
SCHAD. *See* Short-chain 3-hydroxyacyl-CoA
    dehydrogenase (SCHAD)
Scheele, Carl Wilhelm, 11–12
Schiavo case, 1617–1618
Schilling test, 1145, 1146t
Schizophrenia, 1359–1360
Schofield equations, 142, 142t
Scottish Heart Health Study, 156
Scurvy, 6–7, 520, 603
    history, 507–508
    prevention, 521
    treatment, 521
Search engines
    websites for, 2025–2026
Season
    vitamin D3, 381–382, 382F
Seborrheic dermatitis
    with biotin deficiency, 503
Second Leicester Intravenous Magnesium
    Intervention Trial, 237
Secretin, 1123t
SeHCAT. *See* Selenium-75 homocholic acid
    taurine (SeHCAT) test
SELECT trial, 1275
Selenium, 5, 312–323, 320, 320f, 609, 678,
    1364–1365. *See also* Minerals
    absorption, 315
    alcoholism, 1251–1252
    amino acids, 313f
    analytic evaluation, 319–320
    bioavailability, 314
    biochemical evaluation, 320
    biochemical functions, 316–317
    biologic activity, 317
    blood levels, 319–320
    Britain, 313
    cancer, 1275
    cancer prevention, 318–319
    chemical forms, 312–313
    deficiency, 317–318, 609
        Africa, 323
    dietary, 313–314
    dietary *vs.* tissue forms, 314f
    elderly, 852
    excretion, 316
    food sources, 313–314
    healthy diet, 1631
    high risk clinical situations, 323
    with iodine deficiency, 305
    metabolic pool, 315f
    metabolism, 314–316
    nutrient-nutrient interrelationships, 314
    nutrient status, 319–320
    parenteral nutrition, 1582t, 1583–1584
    pregnancy, 779
    protein incorporation, 315–316
    1989 RDA *vs.* 2002 RDI, 819t
    recommended intakes, 320–322, 322t
    sports nutrition, 1732
    sports performance, 1732
    toxicity, 322–323, 609
    transport, 315
    urine samples, 319–320
    1989 *vs.* 2002 RDI, 831t
Selenium-75 homocholic acid taurine
    (SeHCAT) test, 1149
Selenocysteine, 312, 313f, 314f
Selenomethionine, 313f, 314f
Selenophosphate, 313
Selenophosphate synthetase, 317
Selenoprotein
    measurements, 320
    synthesis, 315f

Selenoprotein P, 317
Selenoprotein W, 317
Selenosis, 322–323
Semistarvation, 762
Senecio longilobus, 1822
Sensorineural deafness
    in Cuban epidemic neuropathy, 1367
Serine, 25
    synthesis, 31
Serotonin reuptake inhibitors
    associated with weight gain, 1021
Serum albumin, 839t
    with malabsorption, 1146
    starvation, 740
Serum amylase
    acute pancreatitis, 1228
Serum anion gap, 181–182, 181f
Serum carotene
    with malabsorption, 1146
Serum creatinine, 839t
Serum lipase
    acute pancreatitis, 1228
Serum low-density lipoprotein cholesterol
    classification, 1077t
Serum sodium
    hyperglycemia, 152
Serum T3
    iodine, 303
Serum T4
    iodine, 303
Serum thyroglobulin
    iodine, 303
Serum thyroid stimulating hormone
    iodine, 302–303
Serum triglycerides
    classification of, 1899
Serum urea nitrogen
    ratio to serum creatine, 1489–1490
Severe chronic anemia, 262
Severe hypercholesterolemia, 1082
Severe malnutrition
    dietary management of, 899t
Severe protein-energy malnutrition, 891
SGA. *See* Subjective Global Assessment (SGA)
Shark cartilage, 1771
Shellfish poisoning
    amnesic, 1820
    diarrhetic, 1820
Short bowel syndrome, 1147f, 1201–1207
    bowel atrophy, 1203
    bowel rest, 1204
    carbohydrate *vs.* fat feeding, 1205–1206
    complications, 1207
    defined, 1201
    diarrhea, 1204
    etiology, 1201, 1202t
    in infants and children, 995–996
    intestinal adaptation, 1203–1204
        hormonal factors, 1203
    pathophysiologic considerations, 1201–1202
    pharmacologic approaches promoting
        absorption, 1207–1208
    treatment, 1204
Short chain fatty acids (SCFA), 95–96, 1578
    dietary fiber, 86
Short-chain 3-hydroxyacyl-CoA
    dehydrogenase (SCHAD)
    deficiency, 967
Short-chain peptides, 1579–1580
Shoshin, 1368–1369
Shunt hemochromatosis, 261–262
SIADH. *See* Syndrome of inappropriate ADH
    secretion (SIADH)
Sibutramine
    for obesity, 1038

SIDS. *See* Sudden infant death syndrome
    (SIDS)
Silicon, 339, 346–347. *See also* Minerals
    absorption, 346
    analytic methods, 346
    beneficial effects, 347
    bioavailability, 346
    chemistry, 346
    dietary considerations, 347
    distribution, 346
    excretion, 346
    health effects, 347
    historical overview, 346
    mechanisms of action, 346–347
    toxicity, 347
    transport, 346
Silver sulfadiazine, 1570
Simvastatin
    for hypercholesterolemia, 1085t
Single nucleotide polymorphism (SNP), 628
    defined, 617t
Single skinfold method, 759
Sir2-like protein deacetylase, 448
SIRS. *See* Systemic inflammatory response
    syndrome (SIRS)
Sitosterolemia, 131–132
SI units
    conversion factors with traditional units,
        1846–1847
Skeletal disorders
    nutritional correlates, 1321–1322
Skeletal muscles
    composition of, 756
    hormones, 644
    sarcopenia
        aging, 724
Skeleton
    nutrient effects on, 1323–1324
    nutrients important to, 1320–1321
Skin
    nutritional deficiency, 838t
    nutritional review of, 837t
Skinfolds, 1947f
    body fat estimates from, 1949–1952
    equivalent fat content, 1949t–1952t
Sleep apnea
    with childhood obesity, 984
Sleeping metabolic rate (SMR), 141
SlimFast
    with diabetes mellitus, 1060
Slow twitch muscle fibers, 723, 723t
Small bowel
    bacterial overgrowth, 1297
    biopsy, 1147–1148
    desmoplastic reaction of, 1144f
    disorders
        osteoporosis, 1322
    malignancies of, 1297
    normal biopsy, 1147f
    short bowel syndrome, 1202
    transplantation, 1593
Small intestines
    anatomy of, 1116f, 1118–1119
    dietary fiber effects on, 86
    epithelium, 1118–1119
        organization, 1119f
        renewal, 1119
Small-scale community vegetable and fruit
    gardens, 1707
Smell, 695–703
Smith, Edward, 4
Smoking
    cessation
        associated with weight gain, 1022
        with hypercholesterolemia, 1084, 1085t

chemosensory function, 701
with Crohn's disease, 1210
osteoporotic fractures, 1348
with ulcerative colitis, 1210
vitamin C
EAR, 1664f
SMR. *See* Sleeping metabolic rate (SMR)
SNP. *See* Single nucleotide polymorphism (SNP)
SOD. *See* Superoxide dismutase (SOD)
Sodium
calcium, 202
chronic renal failure, 1496–1497
Dietary Guidelines for Americans, 1895
DRI by life-stage group, 1867t
in enteral feeding products, 1558t
hyperglycemia, 152
intrauterine accretion rates during third trimester, 809t
low birth weight intake recommendations, 810t
osteoporosis, 1346–1347
parenteral diet, 1429
pregnancy, 777
reabsorption of, 155, 155f
requirements for, 1857
sports performance, 1732–1733
Sodium bicarbonate
food drugs, 1734–1735
sports nutrition, 1734–1735
Sodium chloride
food content, 157, 157f
genetics, 1097
physiologic mechanisms, 1097–1098
Sodium citrate
sports nutrition, 1734–1735
Sodium-glucose transporters, 72–73
Sodium nitrite, 1811
Sodium polystyrene sulfonate (Kayexalate), 167
Soft drinks
adolescents, 819
Solution hybridization, 618–619
Somatostatin, 1123t
analog, 653
short bowel syndrome, 1207
cells, 1129
Sorbitol, 1811
South Africa
optimal iodine nutrition programs, 309
Southeast Asia
obesity rates, 1026
Soy
and breast cancer, 592
with diabetes mellitus, 1052–1053
formulas
nutrient content, 806t
health benefits, 592
sauce, 1519
Specific gravity
osmolality, 152
SPF. *See* Supernatant protein factor (SPF)
Spine
fractures
osteoporosis, 1342
Spiritual views, 1612
Spironolactone
for hypokalemia, 165
Spirulina, 1758
Spontaneous carpal pedal spasm
with magnesium deficiency, 236
Sports drinks, 1733
Sports nutrition, 1723–1737
antioxidants, 1730–1731
caffeine, 1733–1734

dietary supplements, 1735–1736
food drugs, 1733–1734
minerals, 1731–1732
vitamins, 1730–1731
water/electrolytes, 1732–1733
SREBP. *See* Sterol regulatory element-binding proteins (SREBP)
St. John's wort
type IIA interaction, 1544–1545
Staphylococcal enterotoxins, 1817
Staphylococcus aureus, 1817
Starch, 63
breakdown, 63–64
composition, 66f
dental caries, 1161
digestion of, 1136f
source of, 1519
Starvation
adaptation, 737–738
defined, 730
metabolic consequences of, 730–744
right to, 1610
stage, 739
whole body adaptation, 46
Statins
for hypercholesterolemia, 1085, 1085t
Stature, 757–758
by age, 1932t
equations for predicting, 759t
predicting in individuals unable to stand, 1961t
Steady-state relations, 751–752
Steatohepatitis, 1244–1245
Steatorrhea, 1237
with alcoholism, 1249
with celiac disease, 1223
with chronic pancreatitis, 1231
evaluation of, 1150f
with hypomagnesemia, 233
Stereoisomers, 23
Steroids, 96–98
for chronic pancreatitis, 1233
in human milk, 790t
Sterol regulatory element-binding proteins (SREBP), 1074
Sterols, 94–95
absorption, 99
digestion, 99
molecular structure, 95t
structure of, 130f
Stomach
anatomy of, 1116f, 1117
dietary fiber effects on, 86
function of, 1128–1129
phasic contractions, 1180
regional organization of, 1117f
short bowel syndrome, 1201–1202
tonic contractions, 1180
Stomach cancer
fruits and vegetables, 1273
vitamin C, 1275
vitamin E, 1275
Stoplight Diet, 985
Stress
protein requirements, 1422t
Stroke
alcoholism, 1254
dietary treatment of, 1376
Stroke volume
defined, 1464t
Strontium
osteoporosis, 1347
Structure function claims, 1836
Subacute necrotizing encephalomyelopathy (Leigh disease), 432, 599

Subcutaneous adipose tissue, 756
Suberoylanilide hydroxamic acid, 1285t
Subjective Global Assessment (SGA), 841–842, 854
Subscapular skinfold thickness, 1942t–1943t
Substance P, 1123t
Substance use disorders, 1360
Substrate metabolism, 1572–1573
Substrates
interorgan flow, 45f
Sucralose
with diabetes mellitus, 1055t
Sucrase, 1189, 1190t
Sucrase-isomaltase, 1196–1197
Sudden infant death syndrome (SIDS)
with biotin deficiency, 503
Sugar consumption
cultural ecology, 1743
Sugars, 66, 1024
and amphetamine, 716
dental caries, 79, 1160
international dietary guidelines, 1711t
Sugar tolerance tests, 78
Sulfasalazine
with folic acid deficiency, 479
Sulfasalazine-nutrient interactions, 1327f
Sulfate
requirements for, 1857
Sulfite-induced asthma, 1524–1525
Sulfite oxidase, 344
Sulfites, 1812
Sulforaphane, 1797t
Sulfur
food content, 177f
Sulfur amino acids, 22, 928–932
biochemistry, 928
homocystinuria, 928–929
measurement, 559
RDA, 548
structure, 546f
Sunscreens
vitamin D3, 381
Supernatant protein factor (SPF), 401
Super obesity
BMI, 1955t–1959t
skinfold, 1955t–1959t
Superoxide anion, 686
Superoxide dismutase (SOD), 288
with Mn, 326
Supplemental parenteral nutrition
acute renal failure, 1505
Supplement Facts Panel, 1829, 1832, 1833f
Supplements. *See also* Dietary supplements
fish oil
sports performance, 1727
Support programs
need for additional, 1605–1606
Suramin
for cancer, 1301t, 1302
Surgery
nutritional requirements, 1420–1424
physiologic response to, 1418–1419
Surgical patient
at-risk
identification of, 1415–1416
Survival
fasting, 735
starvation, 740–741
Sweeteners
with diabetes mellitus, 1054–1055
Sweets
gluten free foods, 2008t
mineral content, 1979t, 1982t
protein content, 1979t
vitamins, 1985t

Symphytum officinale, 1822
Syndrome of inappropriate ADH secretion
    (SIADH), 160, 172
Syndrome X, 1005, 1005t
Systematic evidence-based review
    for dietary guidelines generation, 1679t
Systemic inflammatory response syndrome
    (SIRS), 214, 1227
Systemic nutrition deficiencies
    skeletal manifestations of, 1323
Systems
    nutritional review of, 837t
Systems biology
    defined, 617t

T

Tacrolimus
    with Mg wasting, 233
Tangier disease, 1073, 1073t
Tannins, 1796t, 1801
    phenolic phytochemicals in, 1991t
TAP. *See* Tocopherol associated protein (TAP)
Tartrazine, 1812
Taste, 695–703, 696–697
    with cancer, 1295
Taste buds, 696
Taurine, 1579
    antioxidant effect, 557
    cellular form, 546
    chemistry, 546
    deficiency
        etiology, 557–558
    excretion, 550
    functions, 557
    historical introduction, 545–546
    measurement, 559
    nomenclature, 546
    plasma level, 546–547
    recommended intake, 548–549
    source, 548t
    synthesis, 31, 555–556
    toxicity, 559
Taurine chloramine, 557
TBAR. *See* Thiobarbituric acid reactive
        substances (TBAR)
TBW. *See* Total body water (TBW)
TCA cycle, 27–28
T cells, 673–674
    adaptive immunity, 679
    development, 673f
    signaling, 675–676
TCM. *See* Traditional Chinese medicine
        (TCM)
Tea
    flavonoids, 588
TEE. *See* Total energy expenditures (TEE)
Teeth, 1153f
    ascorbic acid, 1321
    calcium, 204
TEF. *See* Thermic effect of food (TEF)
Temperature
    conversions, 1850
Ten State Nutrition Survey, 1695
Terminally ill
    palliative care of, 1619–1620
Terminal respiratory units, 1463
Term infant formulas
    recommendations for, 804t
Term infants
    formulas, 804t
Testosterone, 647–648
    elderly, 1533
    sports nutrition, 1736
    for weight loss, 1535

Tetracycline-nutrient interactions, 1327f
Tetrahydrofolate (THF), 471
Tetrodotoxin, 1818
Tetrodotoxin poisoning, 1820–1821
TfR. *See* Transferrin receptors (TfR)
TGF. *See* Transforming growth factor alpha
        (TGF alpha)
TGRLP. *See* Triglyceride-rich lipoproteins
        (TGRLP)
Thailand
    optimal iodine nutrition programs, 309
Thalidomide
    for cancer, 1301t, 1302
T helper mediated B cell response, 675
Theophylline
    homocysteine interaction, 553
Therapeutic diets, 1994–2023
Therapeutic Lifestyle Changes (TLC), 1492
    ATP III goals, 1900t
    nutrient composition of, 1898t
    stages of, 1898f
Thermic effect of food (TEF), 143, 1017,
        1018, 1023
Thermochemical calorie
    defined, 136
Thermogenesis, 143
THF. *See* Tetrahydrofolate (THF)
Thiamin. *See* Vitamin B1 (thiamin)
Thiaminases, 427–428
Thiamin diphosphate dependent enzymes,
        431–432
Thiobarbituric acid reactive substances
        (TBAR), 106
Thiocyanate, 306
Thiocyanate toxicity, 1364
Thioredoxin reductases
    selenium, 316–317
Thioridazine, 1360
Thirst
    antidiuretic hormone release, 167–169
THOP II. *See* Trials of Hypertension
        Prevention Phase II (TOHP II)
Threonine
    metabolism, 933f
    restricted diet, 2003t
Thrombocytopenia
    with alcoholism, 1255
Thrombocytosis, 187
Thromboxane
    formation of, 112f
Thyroglobulin, 301
    iodine, 303
Thyroid cancer
    with iodine excess, 307
Thyroid hormones, 644–645
    blood glucose, 72
    iodine, 302
Thyroid stimulating hormone (TSH), 301
    iodine, 302–303
Thyroperoxidase (TPO), 301
Thyrotropin releasing hormone (TRH), 301
TIBC. *See* Total iron-binding capacity (TIBC)
Tibet
    selenium deficiency, 323
Tidal volume
    defined, 1464t
Time of day
    vitamin D3, 381–382, 382F
Tin
    migrating from containers, 1816
Tissue-system, 756
TLC. *See* Therapeutic Lifestyle Changes (TLC)
TMG. *See* Transmembrane Gla protein (TMG)
TML. *See* Trimethyllysine (TML)

TNF. *See* Tumor necrosis factor alpha (TNF
        alpha)
Tobacco
    inducing gastric emptying, 1181
Tobacco abuse
    prevalence, 870–871
Tobacco-alcohol amblyopia, 1370
Tocopherol. *See* Vitamin E (tocopherol)
Tocopherol associated protein (TAP), 401
Tocopherol transfer protein (TTP), 401
Tocotrienols, 1796t
Toddlers
    diet self-selection, 807
    eating habits, 807–808
    feeding, 807–808
    reduced food intake, 807
    self-feeding, 807
    self-selection diet, 807
Tolerable upper intake level, 1660t, 1855
    definition, 1853t
    establishing, 1665–1666
    for infants and children, 798, 800t
    limitations to, 1666–1667
    without AI/RDA, 1667
TONE. *See* Trial of Non-Pharmacologic
        Intervention in the Elderly (TONE)
Tongue, 696
Tooth bud, 1153
Tooth development
    nutrient deficiencies, 1155t
Topiramate
    for eating disorders, 1358
Total body energy, 752
Total body fat, 759
    vs. BMI, 752f
Total-body phosphate depletion, 605
Total body water (TBW), 150
Total caloric requirements
    estimating, 1420–1421
Total energy expenditures (TEE), 138, 845,
        1017, 1017f
    for normal infants, 798–801
Total fast
    defined, 730
Total fat
    DRI by life-stage group, 1863t
    1989 *vs.* 2002 RDI, 831t
Total fiber
    defined, 85
    DRI by life-stage group, 1862t
Total heat output
    calculation of, 140
Total iron-binding capacity (TIBC), 839t
Total lymphocyte count, 840t, 841
Total nutrient admixture system
    advantages and disadvantages of, 1576t
Total parenteral nutrition (TPN)
    acute renal failure, 1501t
    for cancer, 1299–1300, 1300
    with cysteine deficiency, 558
    metabolic complications, 1000t
    monitoring schedule, 1001t
    with taurine deficiency, 558
    weaning infants from, 1001
    withholding in cancer, 1308
Total retinol, 359
Total serum magnesium, 231–232
Total water
    DRI by life-stage group, 1865t
Toxic oil syndrome, 1813
TPN. *See* Total parenteral nutrition (TPN)
TPO. *See* Thyroperoxidase (TPO)
Trabecular bone, 1316, 1318f
Trace element combination products, 1584t

Trace elements
  acute renal failure, 1501t
  chronic renal failure, 1497–1498
  enteral feeding, 1561–1562
Trace minerals
  cirrhosis, 1245
  dietary reference intakes in normal infants
    and children, 802
  human milk, 788t
  in normal infants and children, 802
  osteoporosis, 1347–1348
  pregnancy, 778–779
Tracheobronchial tree, 1463
Traditional Chinese medicine (TCM), 1764
Traditional units
  conversion factors with SI units,
    1846–1847
Trans-acting factor
  defined, 617t
Transcobalamin I, 488
Transcobalamin II, 488
Transcriptome
  defined, 617t
Transcuprein, 288
Transepithelial hexose transport, 72–73
Trans fatty acids
  healthy diet, 1627–1628
  with hypercholesterolemia, 1083
Transfer protein deficiency
  abetalipoproteinemia, 1071–1072
Transferrin, 252t
Transferrin iron pool, 250
Transferrin receptor cycle, 253f
Transferrin receptors (TfR), 251, 252t
Transforming growth factor alpha (TGF
    alpha), 652
Transfusional hemochromatosis, 262
Transgenic animals, 624–625
Transketolase, 1368
Transmembrane Gla protein (TMG), 416
Transposable elements, 630–631
Transsulfuration
  redox and hormonal regulation, 552
Transthyretin
  elderly, 853
Transthyretin (TTR), 355, 360
  hepatic metabolism, 359
  vitamin A, 355
Tranylcypromine, 1360
Trauma patients, 1415–1416
Treatment
  denial as medically futile, 1612–1613
  refusal of, 1612
Trehalase, 1189, 1190t, 1197–1198
TRH. See Thyrotropin releasing hormone
  (TRH)
Trial of Hypertension Prevention, 1103
Trial of Non-Pharmacologic Intervention in
  the Elderly (TONE), 1103
Trials of Hypertension Prevention Phase II
  (TOHP II), 156
Triamterene
  for hypokalemia, 165
Tribolium castaneum, 1821
Tribolium confusum, 1821
Tribulus terrestris
  sports nutrition, 1736
Triceps skinfold thickness, 1940t–1941t
Tricyclic antidepressants
  associated with weight gain, 1021
  inducing gastric emptying, 1181
Triene:tetraene ratio, 115
Trigger proteins
  calcium, 204

Triglyceride-rich lipoproteins (TGRLP)
  atherosclerotic cardiovascular disease,
    1076–1077
  vitamin E, 400
Triglycerides, 93–94
  classification of, 1899
  food content, 1968t–1975t
  as fuel, 1018
  high, 1069–1070, 1070t
  low
    genetic causes of, 1072t
    low birth weight intake recommendations,
      811t
  without fasting chylomicronemia
    genetic causes of, 1071t
Trimethyllysine (TML), 31
Trophic agents
  parenteral nutrition, 1593–1594
Tropical amblyopia, 1370
Tropical sprue
  with folic acid deficiency, 478
Troponin C
  calcium, 195t
Truncal vagotomy, 1186
Trypsin, 1137t
Tryptophan, 7–8, 1729, 1759
  dietary considerations, 443–444
  historical development of, 5–6
  metabolic conversion, 443f
  metabolism of, 934f
  restricted diet, 2004t
  serotonin synthesis, 32
TSH. See Thyroid stimulating hormone
  (TSH)
TTP. See Tocopherol transfer protein (TTP)
TTR. See Transthyretin (TTR)
Tube feeding
  withdrawal of, 1616–1617
Tuberculosis
  with malnutrition, 1407–1408
Tumor necrosis factor alpha (TNF alpha),
    1391, 1391t
  with congestive heart failure, 1109
  mediating altered metabolism in cancer,
    1294
Tumors
  nutrition support effect on growth, 1303
Tumor suppressor genes, 1261, 1262t
Tungsten
  molybdenum, 344–345
Twenty-four-hour tracer balance method, 52
24-h urinary creatinine, 839t
24-h urinary urea nitrogen, 839t
25-hydroxyvitamin D
  alternative metabolism, 384–385
  assays, 387
  to 1,25-dihydroxyvitamin D, 384
Type 2 diabetes
  chromium, 852
Type 1 hyperlipoproteinemia, 1087–1088
Type III hyperlipoproteinemia, 1070–1071
Type II muscle fibers, 723, 723t
Type I muscle fibers, 723, 723t
Type V hyperlipoproteinemia, 1088
Tyramine
  drug-nutrient interactions, 1547–1548
  drugs interacting with, 1548t
  foods containing, 1548t
Tyrosinase, 288
Tyrosine, 8
  catecholamine synthesis, 32
  phenylketonuria
    pregnancy, 2000t
    restricted diet, 1999t

syndrome, 41
synthesis, 31
Tyrosinemia, 925–928, 925t
  aromatic amino acids for, 1995t–1996t
  diagnosis, 926
  nutrient requirements, 927
  nutrition support, 927–928
  serving lists, 927
  treatment, 926–927

U
Ubiquitin-proteosome proteolytic system
  (UPPS), 1394
Ubiquitous multitissue hormones and growth
  factors, 651–653
UCED. See Urea cycle enzyme defects
  (UCED)
UCP. See Uncoupling proteins (UCP)
Ulcerative colitis
  with hypomagnesemia, 233
Ultrasound
  with parenteral nutrition, 1570
Ultratrace elements, 339
Uncoupling proteins (UCP), 741
Undernutrition, 875, 1608
  learning failure, 867
Unesterified retinol, 359
United Kingdom
  obesity rates, 1026
  reference nutrient intakes, 1877t–1880t
United States Department of Agriculture
  national food surveys, 1693t
  Total Diet Study, 313
United States Department of Agriculture
  (USDA) Continuing Survey of Food
  Intakes by Individuals, 227
United States Food and Drug Administration
  Total Dietary Study, 227
United States Postal Service, 1760
Unsafe food additives, 1813
Unsubstantiated claims, 1763
Upper arm circumference
  by age, 1944t–1945t, 1946f
Upper gastrointestinal tract
  anatomy of, 1180f
UPPS. See Ubiquitin-proteosome proteolytic
  system (UPPS)
Uppsala Method of Theander, 85
Uracil
  biosynthesis, 32–33
Urbanization, 1718–1719
Urea cycle
  amino acid nitrogen disposal, 29f
  disorders
    recommended daily nutrient intakes,
      2006t
    sample diet for, 2006t
    treatment, 2006t
  inborn errors in, 946f
Urea cycle enzyme defects (UCED), 910,
  946–947, 1998t
  diagnosis, 948
  differential diagnosis, 948f
  serving lists, 950
  treatment, 948–950
Urea nitrogen
  ratio to serum creatine, 1489–1490
Uremia, 1483
Uremic acidosis, 179–180
Uric acid
  ethanol, 1253
Urinary creatinine, 839t
Urinary nitrogen
  excretion, 34f

Urinary urea nitrogen, 837–839, 839t
Urine
  magnesium excretion, 232
  nitrogen containing species, 35f
USDA. *See* United States Department of
    Agriculture (USDA) Continuing Survey
    of Food Intakes by Individuals

V
Vagotomy
  with antrectomy, 1186
Vagus nerve, 696
VA-HIT. *See* Veterans Affairs HDL
    Intervention Trial (VA-HIT)
Valine, 25
  hepatic encephalopathy, 1238
  restricted diet, 2003t
Valproate, 1360
Valproic acid
  carnitine interaction, 542
Valvulae conniventes, 1219
Vanadium, 339, 347–348. *See also* Minerals
  absorption, 347
  analytic methods, 347
  beneficial effects, 348
  bioavailability, 347
  chemistry, 347
  with diabetes mellitus, 1056
  dietary considerations, 348
  distribution, 347
  excretion, 347
  health effects, 348
  historical overview, 347
  mechanisms of action, 348
  sports nutrition, 1732
  sports performance, 1732
  toxicity, 348
  transport, 347
Vascular damage
  vitamin B6, 458–459
Vascular endothelial growth factors (VEGF),
  652
Vasopressin
  Mg absorption, 229
Vasopressin antagonists
  for hyponatremia, 175
Vegan diet
  with rheumatoid arthritis, 1335
Vegetables
  adolescents, 820
  cancer, 1273
  cooked
    nutrient retention in, 1988t
  dietary fiber content of, 1966t
  gluten free foods, 2008t
  intake, 1024
  international dietary guidelines, 1711t
  lung cancer, 1470–1471
  mineral content, 1979t, 1982t
  nutrient retention in, 1988t
  oxalate, 2014t, 2016t, 2017t–2018t
  phenolic phytochemicals in, 1993t
  protein content, 1979t
Vegetables intake, 1024
Vegetarian(s)
  BMI, 1640f
  dietary intake, 1639–1641
  energy intake, 1640
  nutritional status, 1639–1640
  weight, 1640
Vegetarian diets, 1638–1652
  biomedical literature, 1639t
  chronic disease management, 1649–1650
  chronic disease prevention, 1644–1645

defined, 1638–1639
diabetes, 1645, 1649–1650
historical context, 1638
life cycle, 1646
nutrient status, 1641–1642
trace elements, 1644f
trends in, 1639
weight loss, 1640–1641
Vegetarian food guide pyramid, 1651f
Vegetative state, 1615
VEGF. *See* Vascular endothelial growth
  factors (VEGF)
Venezuela
  selenium toxicity, 322
Ventilatory drive, 1465
Ventilatory requirements
  substrate supplementation, 1466
Verapamil
  food interactions, 1542
Vertical banded gastroplasty, 1040
Very low calorie diets (VLCD), 1032, 1034
  atherosclerotic cardiovascular disease,
    1077
  ethanol consumption, 1243
Very low density lipoproteins (VLDL)
  alpha tocopherol secretion, 400–401
  lipid transport, 101
  tocopherols, 402
Veterans Affairs HDL Intervention Trial
  (VA-HIT), 1009
Veterinary antibiotics, 1815–1816
Veterinary drugs, 1815–1816
Vibrio, 1821
Viral autoimmune disease
  oxidative stress, 693
Viral insertions, 628
Visceral adipose, 756
Visceral adiposity, 725
Visceral organs
  semistarvation, 756
Visceral proteins
  assessment of, 837
Vision
  vitamin A, 362–363
Visual cycle, 363
Visual system
  taurine, 557
Vitalism, 10
Vitamin(s), 595–606. *See also* Fat-soluble
    vitamins; Multivitamins
  absorption of, 1139
  acute renal failure, 1501t, 1504
  adolescents, 823
  for chronic renal failure, 1487t, 1498–1499
  for CPD, 1487t
  deficiency
    in elderly, 1536–1537, 1536t, 1537t
  discovery of, 6–7
  DRI, 1868t
    for infants, 799t
    in normal infants and children, 802
  enteral feeding, 1561–1562
  estimated safe and adequate daily dietary
    intake, 1873t
  food content, 1984t–1986t
  in formulas, 805t
  in formulas for term infants, 804t
  in hydrolyzed formulas and soy formulas,
    806t
  in infant formulas, 806t
  infants and children
    recommended daily allowances, 921t
  in low birth weight infant formulas, 813t,
    815

low birth weight intake recommendations,
  810t, 811t
for MHD, 1487t
nomenclature, 7
in normal infants and children, 802
parenteral intakes of, 999t
1989 RDA *vs.* 2002 RDI, 819t
recommendations for term infant formulas,
  804t
recommended dietary allowances, 1872t
  WHO, 1892t
recommended nutrient intake
  based on age and body weight, 1873t
reference nutrient intakes
  UK, 1877t
safe intakes
  UK, 1880t
safe upper levels
  UK, 1880t
sport nutrition, 1730–1731
sports performance, 1730–1731
status assessment, 841
structure, 379f
tolerable upper intake
  for normal infants and children, 800t
UL, 1869t
  for infants and children, 800t
Vitamin A (retinol), 6–7, 8, 351–371,
    359–360, 595–606, 678, 1470, 1813
  absorption, 356–362
  alcoholism, 1249–1250, 1250f, 1255
  analysis, 353
  assessment, 369–371, 369t
  biochemical indicators, 369–370
  birth defects, 368
  bone mineral loss, 368–369
  cellular differentiation, 363–364
  chemistry, 352–353
  chemosensory function, 700
  cirrhosis, 1245
  deficiency, 367, 595–596
    with iodine deficiency, 306
    neurologic disorders, 1367–1368
    tooth development, 1155t
  dietary assessment, 370
  effects on periodontium, 1170t
  and elderly, 846
  DRI, 844t
  embryonic development, 363–364
  in enteral feeding products, 1558t
  esterification, 358–359
  estimated average requirements, 354t
  eye signs, 370
  functions, 362–367
  hepatic metabolism, 359–362
  historical overview, 351–352
  immunity, 364–365
  with infection, 1408, 1408t
  interconverting factors and formulas, 1847
  intestinal metabolism, 356–360
  intoxication, 1367–1368
  liver, 370
  liver abnormalities, 368
  malabsorption of, 1145t
  osteoporosis, 1346
  physiologic processing, 355–362
  processing, 356f
  properties, 352–353
  public health assessment tools, 370–371
  recommended dietary allowances, 354,
    354t
  storage, 360
  supplements, 1401
  terminology, 352–353

toxicity, 367–371, 596
transport protein, 360–362
units, 353–354
upper level, 369
vitamin A storage, 360
in vivo kinetics, 360
1989 *vs.* 2002 RDI, 831t
Vitamin B, 7
chemosensory function, 700
effects on periodontium, 1170t
Vitamin B1 (thiamin), 426–432, 599–600
absorption, 428
alcoholism, 1255
beriberi, 1368
biochemistry, 426
cellular energy failure, 429
chemistry, 426
clinical response to, 432
deficiency, 429, 599
clinical manifestations of, 1368–1369
parenteral nutrition, 1587–1588
defined, 430–432
dietary sources, 426–427, 427t
DRI in elderly, 844t
elderly, 848
in enteral feeding products, 1558t
enzyme cofactor, 428–429
enzymes, 428f
excretion, 428
historical landmarks, 426
HPLC, 430
measurement, 430–432
neuronal cell death, 429–430
neuronal membranes, 429
oxidative stress, 429–430
sources, 427t
structure, 427f
toxicity, 599–600
turnover rates, 428t
1989 *vs.* 2002 RDI, 831t
Vitamin B2 (riboflavin), 434–439, 435f,
599–600
absorption, 436
assay, 435–436
biochemistry, 434–435
catabolism, 438
chemistry, 434–435
deficiency, 438, 599, 1371, 1458
dietary considerations, 439
dietary reference intake value, 439t
digestion, 436
and elderly, 848
DRI, 844t
in enteral feeding products, 1558t
erythrocyte assays, 436
excess, 438
excretion, 437–438
history, 434
metabolic interconversions, 437
metabolism, 436–437
natural flavins, 434
secretion, 437–438
sources, 848
toxicity, 600
transport, 436–437
urine excretion, 435–436
1989 *vs.* 2002 RDI, 831t
Vitamin B5 (pantothenic acid), 462–467,
602–603, 1375
absorption, 462–464
alcoholism, 467
analytic methods, 465
bioavailability, 464
biochemical assessment, 466–467

biochemistry, 462
blood concentration, 466
cellular metabolism, 464
chemistry, 462
clinical benefits, 467
deficiency, 467, 603
dietary components, 465
dietary intake, 466
dietary requirements, 465–466
digestion, 462–464
in enteral feeding products, 1558t
excretion, 462–464
genetic mutations, 467
historical highlights, 462
metabolism, 464–465
overconsumption, 467
physiologic aspects, 462–464
pregnancy, 777
protein acetylation, 464
protein acylation, 464–465
recommended intake, 466, 466t
source, 465t
synthesis, 464
urinary excretion, 466
Vitamin B6 (pyridoxine), 7, 452–459, 601,
1458
absorption, 453
aging, 458–459
amino acids, 454
assessment, 456t
bioavailability, 453–454
chemistry, 452–453
deficiency, 601, 1371–1372, 1458
drug interactions, 459
elderly, 849
in enteral feeding products, 1558t
functions, 454–455
historical overview, 452
for homocystinuria, 930
intoxication, 1372
metabolism, 453f, 454
nomenclature, 452–453
nutritional status, 456–457
pharmacologic therapy, 459
pregnancy, 777
recommended intakes, 457t
requirements, 457
source, 456
structure, 453f
toxicity, 459, 601
transport, 454
1989 *vs.* 2002 RDI, 831t
Vitamin B12 (cobalamin), 482–495, 601–602
absorption, 486–487, 486t, 487f, 1372,
1445–1446, 1451
alcoholism, 1249
analytic methods, 484–486
bioavailability, 486
biochemistry, 483–484
cellular, 485
cellular metabolism, 488
with chronic pancreatitis, 1231
deficiency, 489–494, 601–602, 1146t,
1372–1373, 1444–1445
diagnosis, 493, 1449–1550, 1449t, 1451
etiology, 491–492, 491t
hematologic features, 489
with inflammatory bowel disease, 1213
megaloblastic sequelae, 1448t
metabolic disorders, 492
neurologic features, 489–490, 1447–1448
neurologic manifestations, 1373–1374,
1373f
proliferating cells, 1447

signs and symptoms of, 1448–1449
subclinical, 490–491
treatment, 493–494, 493t, 1457
dietary causes
etiology, 491
dietary requirements, 488–489
elderly, 849, 1631
in enteral feeding products, 1558t
excretion, 488
hematologic response to, 1457
historical background, 482–483
interactions, 494–495
malabsorption of, 492, 1145, 1145t
metabolism, 472f, 488
pathophysiology, 495t
pregnancy, 777
primary dietary deficiency, 602
prophylaxis, 1453t
serum, 484–485, 485t, 1450
structure of, 483f
supplements, 1457–1458
terminology, 483t
transport, 488
vegetarian diets, 1642–1643
1989 *vs.* 2002 RDI, 831t
Vitamin C (ascorbic acid), 9, 507–522, 603,
1771
accumulation, 513–514
adverse effects, 521
alcoholism, 1249
as antioxidant, 510–511
antioxidant properties, 1755
for asthma, 1470
athletes, 1730
bioavailability, 517t
biochemistry, 509–512
blood adverse effects, 521
bone and teeth, 1321
cancer, 1274–1275
chemical properties, 508–509
content in human tissues, 513t
copper interactions, 294
deficiency, 520–521, 603, 1458
tooth development, 1155t, 1156
degradation, 508–509
dietary reference intakes, 521–522, 522t
DRI in elderly, 844t
EAR, 1664f
effects on periodontium, 1170t
elderly, 847–848
electron donor, 509–510
in enteral feeding products, 1558t
enzymatic functions, 510
excretion, 518
food sources, 514–516, 516t
formation, 508–509
functional consequences, 518–520
functions, 511t
gastrointestinal tract adverse effects, 521
gastrointestinal tract effects, 520
genetics, 520
history, 507–508
human tissue content, 513t
intake, 514–516
intestinal absorption, 516–517
intracellular concentration, 517f
kidney adverse effects, 521
measurement, 512
metabolism, 508f
nonenzymatic functions, 510–511
outcome studies, 518–519
oxidation reduction, 508–509
pantothenic acid, 465
pharmacokinetics, 514–518

Vitamin C (ascorbic acid) (*Continued*)
  pharmacologic doses, 520
  physiology, 512–514
  plasma concentration, 514
  pregnancy, 521–522
  as prooxidant, 511
  reductive functions, 510–511
  renal reabsorption, 518
  supplements, 1763
  tight control, 514–516
  tissue distribution, 512–514, 517
  transport, 513–514
  upper limit, 522
  urinary excretion, 519f
  utilization, 517–518
  in vivo functions, 514
  1989 *vs.* 2002 RDI, 831t
Vitamin D (calciferol), 8, 597–598, 678
  absorption
    aging, 390
  age-related bone loss, 1713
  alcoholism, 1251
  assays, 387–389
  biologic functions, 385–387
  bone and teeth, 1320–1321
  breast cancer, 1274
  calcium metabolism, 385–386
  cancer, 1274
  for chronic renal failure, 1495
  cirrhosis, 1245
  cutaneous production, 383f
  deficiency, 597
    with inflammatory bowel disease, 1213
    neurologic manifestations, 1376
    tooth development, 1155t, 1156
  deficiency epidemic, 388–389
  DRI, 391t
    in elderly, 844t
    in normal infants and children, 802
  effects on periodontium, 1170t
  elderly, 846–847
  in enteral feeding products, 1558t
  healthy diet, 1630–1631
  to 25-hydroxyvitamin D, 383–385
  with hypomagnesemia, 236
  intake requirement for, 1712
  intestinal absorption, 382–383
  intoxication, 392
  malabsorption of, 1145t
  metabolism, 383–385
    regulation of, 385
  in normal infants and children, 802
  osteoarthritis, 1330
  osteoporosis, 1343–1344
  phosphorus metabolism, 385–386
  physiologic actions, 392f
  recommended dietary allowance, 390–391
  resistant rickets, 1322
  serum, 383f
  sunlight, 389
  supplements, 390–392
  toxicity, 597–598
  vegetarian diets, 1643
  1989 *vs.* 2002 RDI, 831t
Vitamin D1, 376–393
Vitamin D₃
  serum, 381f
  supplements
    randomized trials of, 1345t
Vitamin E (tocopherol), 9, 396–408, 598–599, 678, 1796t
  absorption, 400f
    chylomicron, 400
  alcoholism, 1251–1252

antioxidant activity, 398–399
antioxidant properties, 1755
athletes, 1730
bile, 399–400
cancer, 1274–1275
chemistry, 397–399
chemosensory function, 700
cirrhosis, 1245
cystic fibrosis, 1471
deficiency, 598, 1458
  abetalipoproteinemia, 397–399
  etiology, 404–405
  neurologic manifestations, 1375–1376
  with selenium deficiency, 317
digestion, 399–400
distribution to tissues, 402–403
DRI, 406–409, 407t
  in elderly, 844t
effects on periodontium, 1170t
and elderly, 847
in enteral feeding products, 1558t
estimated average requirement, 406–407
excretion, 403
health benefits, 408
healthy diet, 1631
hepatic metabolism, 403
historical highlights, 397
interactions, 398–399
intestinal absorption, 399–400
kinetics, 401
lipid peroxidation, 106
liver disease, 1245f
malabsorption of, 1145t
membrane peroxidation, 691–692
metabolism, 403
nomenclature, 397–399
oxidation, 691f
oxidation products, 403
pancreatic secretions, 399–400
plasma transport, 400–401
requirements, 406
storage sites, 403
structure, 397–399, 398f
structure-function relationships, 399
total parenteral nutrition, 405
toxicity, 598
units, 398
1989 *vs.* 2002 RDI, 831t
Vitamin F
  effects on periodontium, 1170t
Vitamin K (phylloquinone), 412–424, 598–599
  absorption, 414–415
  adequate intake, 423t
  alcoholism, 1251
  analysis, 413–415
  bioavailability, 413–415
  biochemical role, 417–420
  bone and teeth, 1321
  cirrhosis, 1245
  deficiency, 420–422, 598–599
  dependent carboxylase, 417–418
  dependent clotting factors, 416f
  dependent gamma glutamyl carboxylase, 418f
  dependent proteins, 415–417
    source, 417
  dietary requirements, 423
  and elderly, 844t, 847
  in enteral feeding products, 1558t
  epoxide reductase, 419–420
  estimated average requirement, 423
  excretion, 414–415
  food content, 413–415, 1987t
  malabsorption of, 1145t

metabolism, 414–415
nomenclature, 413
osteoporosis, 1346
recommended dietary allowance, 423
reference values, 423
skeletal health, 422–423
source, 413–414, 413t
sources, 413–415
structure, 413, 413t
tissue calcification, 423
tissue metabolism, 419f
toxicity, 599
transport, 414–415
utilization, 413–415
1989 *vs.* 2002 RDI, 831t
Vitamin K deficiency bleeding (VKDB), 421
Vitamin X, 7
VKDB. *See* Vitamin K deficiency bleeding (VKDB)
VLCD. *See* Very low calorie diets (VLCD)
VLDL. *See* Very low density lipoproteins (VLDL)
Volumes, 1850
Von Gierke disease, 1242
Von Helmholtz, Hermann, 13
Von Jauregg, Julius Wagner, 655
Von Voit, Carl, 13

W
WADA. *See* World Anti-Doping Agency (WADA)
Waist circumference, 1013–1014, 1014t
  metabolic syndrome, 1006–1007
Warfarin, 420, 421
  for congestive heart failure, 1112
  food interactions, 1548–1549
  structure, 420f
Warning statements, 1836
Wasting syndrome, 1484–1485
Water
  absorption of, 1132, 1133f
  antidiuretic hormone metabolism, 188–189
  basal requirements, 159
  chronic renal failure, 1496–1497
  for chronic renal failure, 1487t
  for CPD, 1487t
  daily requirements, 159–160
  diuresis
    polyuria, 169, 169t
  DRI
    for infants, 799t
    in normal infants and children, 802–803
  fluoridation, 1164, 1164f
    dental caries, 1166f
  formed in metabolism of tissue and caloric sources, 1851
  intrauterine accretion rates during third trimester, 809t
  iodized, 307–308
  low birth weight intake recommendations, 810t
  for MHD, 1487t
  nonrenal control, 157
  in normal infants and children, 802
  pregnancy, 776–777
  replacement, 159
  requirements for, 1857
  soluble vitamins
    adolescents, 823
    alcoholism, 1249
    cirrhosis, 1245
    human milk, 788t, 789t
    pregnancy, 775–776
  sports nutrition, 1733